MW00862210

CIVETTA, TAYLOR, & KIRBY'S

Critical Care

FIFTH EDITION

Civetta, Taylor, & Kirby's

Critical Care

FIFTH EDITION

EDITED BY

A. Joseph Layon, MD, FACP
Co-Chairperson, Department of Pulmonary and Critical Care Medicine
System Director, Division of Critical Care Medicine
The Geisinger Health System
Danville, Pennsylvania
Professor of Medicine and Anesthesiology
The Geisinger Commonealth School of Medicine
Scranton, Pennsylvania

Andrea Gabrielli, MD, MBA, FCCM
Professor, Anesthesiology and Critical Care Medicine
University of Pennsylvania Perelman School of Medicine
Division Chief, Critical Care Medicine
Co-Director, Trauma ICU
Medical Director, PENN E-LERT® Telemedicine Program
Philadelphia, Pennsylvania

Mihae Yu, MD, FACS
Professor of Surgery
Vice-Chair of Education
University of Hawaii Department of Surgery
Program Director, Surgical Critical Care Fellowship
Director of Surgical Intensive Care
The Queen's Medical Center
Honolulu, Hawaii

Kenneth E. Wood, DO, FACP, FCCP, FCCM
Professor of Medicine-Program in Trauma
University of Maryland School of Medicine
Adjunct Professor, Institute for Systems Research
A James Clark School of Engineering
University of Maryland, College Park
University of Maryland Medical System
Director, University of Maryland Critical Care Network
Associate Chief Medical Officer
University of Maryland Medical Center
Chief Clinical Officer
Attending Staff, R Adams Cowley Shock Trauma Center
Baltimore, Maryland

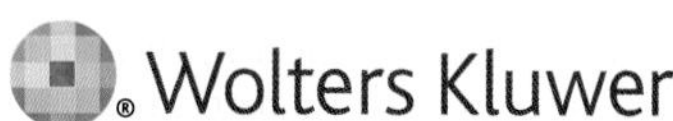

Philadelphia • Baltimore • New York • London
Buenos Aires • Hong Kong • Sydney • Tokyo

Acquisitions Editor: Keith Donnellan
Editorial Coordinator: David Murphy
Marketing Manager: Rachel Mante Leung
Senior Production Project Manager: Alicia Jackson
Design Coordinator: Elaine Kasmer
Manufacturing Coordinator: Beth Welsh
Prepress Vendor: Aptara, Inc.

5th edition

9 8 7 6 5 4 3 2 1

Printed in China

Library of Congress Cataloging-in-Publication Data

Names: Layon, A. Joseph, editor. | Gabrielli, Andrea, editor. | Yu, Mihae, editor. | Wood, Kenneth E., editor.
Title: Civetta, Taylor & Kirby's critical care / edited by A. Joseph Layon, Andrea Gabrielli, Mihae Yu, Kenneth E. Wood.
Other titles: Civetta, Taylor and Kirby's critical care | Critical care
Description: Fifth edition. | Philadelphia : Wolters Kluwer, [2018] | Includes bibliographical references and index.
Identifiers: LCCN 2017033400 | ISBN 9781469889849
Subjects: | MESH: Critical Care | Intensive Care Units
Classification: LCC RC86.7 | NLM WX 218 | DDC 616.02/8–dc23 LC record available at https://lccn.loc.gov/2017033400

This work is provided "as is," and the publisher disclaims any and all warranties, express or implied, including any warranties as to accuracy, comprehensiveness, or currency of the content of this work.

This work is no substitute for individual patient assessment based upon healthcare professionals' examination of each patient and consideration of, among other things, age, weight, gender, current or prior medical conditions, medication history, laboratory data and other factors unique to the patient. The publisher does not provide medical advice or guidance and this work is merely a reference tool. Healthcare professionals, and not the publisher, are solely responsible for the use of this work including all medical judgments and for any resulting diagnosis and treatments.

Given continuous, rapid advances in medical science and health information, independent professional verification of medical diagnoses, indications, appropriate pharmaceutical selections and dosages, and treatment options should be made and healthcare professionals should consult a variety of sources. When prescribing medication, healthcare professionals are advised to consult the product information sheet (the manufacturer's package insert) accompanying each drug to verify, among other things, conditions of use, warnings and side effects and identify any changes in dosage schedule or contraindications, particularly if the medication to be administered is new, infrequently used or has a narrow therapeutic range. To the maximum extent permitted under applicable law, no responsibility is assumed by the publisher for any injury and/or damage to persons or property, as a matter of products liability, negligence law or otherwise, or from any reference to or use by any person of this work.

LWW.com

CCS0917

To my children Maria, Nicolas, and Daniel—
who have taught me humility.
To my best friend and partner Susana E. Picado—
who taught me to be better.
To my green-eyed kid sister Serena M. Layon, 1953–2008—
suffering and dignity are reconcilable.
To those who struggle for justice and peace—no surrender.
To those on the path to becoming, rejecting the box of
conformity, we are fellow travelers.

—A. Joseph Layon

To the memory of my parents, Pietro and Giuliana
for showing me the right path in life.
To my brother Marco, the real smart guy of the family.
To my wife Elizabeth, little Rachelle, and soon to be with us
Vera for bringing endless joy to my life
To my students, friends, and colleagues worldwide
for being my drive to learn
To our patients: my inspiration for compassionate care.

—Andrea Gabrielli

To my Dad, General Jae Hung Yu and the Seventh Division
for their sacrifices and changing history for the better.
To my Mom, Esang Yoon who was the wind beneath
our wings.
To Dr. Thomas J. Whelan Jr. who continues to mentor me in
the practice of Surgery and Code of conduct.
To Joe and Judy Civetta who sparked my continuing love for
Critical Care and being the guiding light for all Peepsters.
And to my daughter Pearl (&CD)
who has the Master Key to All…

—Mihae Yu

Dedicated to the patients that we have the privilege
to serve; the interns, residents, fellows and advanced
practitioners we have the responsibility to teach; the nurses,
pharmacists, and therapists with whom we collaborate;
the authors who gave of their time to contribute and
my wife for her support and tolerance of yet another academic
project…..may this book serve as a resource to educate,
facilitate interdisciplinary collaboration and help fulfill
our mission of improving patient care.

—Kenneth E. Wood

Contributing Authors

Steven G. Achinger, MD, FASN
Department of Nephrology
Watson Clinic, LLP
Lakeland, Florida

Mustafa Ahmed, MD
Assistant Professor
Division of Cardiovascular Medicine
University of Florida
Gainesville, Florida

Kathleen M. Akgün, MD, MS
Assistant Professor
Department of Internal Medicine
VA-Connecticut, West Haven and Yale University School of Medicine
New Haven, Connecticut

Layth Al-Jashaami, MD
Clinical Assistant Professor
College of Medicine
University of Arizona
Phoenix, Arizona

Mayar Al Mohajer, MD
Associate Professor
Department of Medicine
University of Arizona
Tucson, Arizona

Rashid Alobaidi, MD
Faculty of Medicine and Dentistry
Department of Pediatrics and Critical Care Medicine
Department of Pediatrics
University of Alberta
Edmonton, Alberta, Canada

Kawther F. Alquadan, MD
Fellow in Nephrology
Division of Nephrology, Hypertension, and Transplantation
University of Florida
Gainesville, Florida

Adrian Alvarez, MD
Professor of Anesthesia
Hospital Italiano de Buenos Aires
Buenos Aires, Argentina

Marcelo Britto Passos Amato, MD, PhD
Associate Professor
Pulmonary Division
Heart Institute (Incor)
Hospital das Clínicas FMUSP
University of São Paulo
São Paulo, Brazil

Oya M. Andacoglu, MD
Abdominal Transplant Surgery Fellow
MedStar Georgetown Transplant Institute
Washington, DC

Sarah B. Anderson, MD
Maternal Fetal Medicine Fellow
University of Alabama at Birmingham
Birmingham, Alabama

Djillali Annane, MD, PhD
Professor in Critical Care Medicine
Dean of the Health Science Center
University of Versailles-Paris Saclay
Vélizy-Villacoublay, France
Head of the General ICU
Raymond Poincare Hospital (AP-HP)
Garches, France
Director of Lab Inflammation and Infection
Montigny-Le-Bretonneux, France

Massimo Antonelli, MD
Chair
Department of Anesthesiology and Intensive Care Medicine
Catholic University of Rome
A. Gemelli University Hospital
Rome, Italy

Juan M. Aranda, Jr., MD, FACC
Professor of Medicine
Division of Cardiovascular Medicine
University of Florida
Gainesville, Florida

Lennox K. Archibald, MD, PhD, FRCP (Lond), FRCP (Glasg), DTM&H
Hospital Epidemiologist
Attending Physician
Infectious Diseases Section
North Florida/South Georgia Veterans Health
Gainesville, Florida

Ganesh Asaithambi, MD
Vascular Neurologist
John Nasseff Neuroscience Institute
United Hospital
Allina Health
St. Paul, Minnesota

Andrew Davis Assaf
Internal Medicine Resident Physician Texas Health Presbyterian Hospital
Dallas, Texas

Juan Carlos Ayus, MD, FACP, FASN
Renal Consultants of Houston
Houston, Texas

Mariona Badia, MD, PhD
ICU Hospital Universitario Arnau de Vilanova
Lleida, Spain

Sanam Baghshomali, MD
Department of Neurology
Division of Neurocritical Care
University of Pennsylvania
Philadelphia, Pennsylvania

Sean M. Bagshaw, MD
Division of Critical Care Medicine
Faculty of Medicine and Dentistry
University of Alberta
Edmonton, Alberta, Canada

Claudia L. Barthold, MD
Department of Emergency Medicine
University of Nebraksa Medical Center
Omaha, Nebraska

Robert H. Bartlett, MD
Professor Emeritus of Surgery
University of Michigan
Ann Arbor, Michigan

Ribal Bassil, MD
Department of Neurology
University of Massachusetts Medical School
Boston, Massachusetts

Maher A. Baz, MD
Professor of Clinical Medicine
Division of Cardiothoracic Surgery
University of Kentucky
Lexington, Kentucky

Stacy G. Beal, MD
Medical Director
Microbiology, Core Laboratories, and Point of Care Testing
Department of Pathology, Immunology, and Laboratory Medicine
University of Florida College of Medicine
Gainesville, Florida

Erol V. Belli, MD
Thoracic Resident
Division of Thoracic and Cardiovascular Surgery
University of Florida
Gainesville, Florida

Giuseppe Bello, MD
Department of Anesthesia and Intensive Care
Agostino Gemelli Hospital
Università Cattolica del Sacro Cuore
Rome, Italy

Rinaldo Bellomo, MD, FRACP, FCICM
Professor of Intensive Care
School of Medicine
The University of Melbourne
Melbourne, Victoria, Australia

Jeffrey A. Bennett, MD
Clinical Associate Professor
Department of Radiology
The University of Florida
Gainesville, Florida

Pouya J. Benyamini, MD
General Surgery Residency Program
Department of Surgery
University of Hawaii
Honolulu, Hawaii

Eugene V. Beresin, MD, MA
Senior Educator in Child and Adolescent Psychiatry
Executive Director
The Clay Center for Young Healthy Minds
Massachusetts General Hospital
Professor of Psychiatry
Harvard Medical School
Boston, Massachusetts

Luca M. Bigatello, MD
Department of Anesthesia, Critical Care, and Pain Medicine
St. Elizabeth's Medical Center
Professor of Anesthesiology
Tufts University School of Medicine
Boston, Massachusetts

Paul B. Blanch, BA, RRT
Equipment Specialist with Respiratory Care Services (Retired)
Assistant in Anesthesia (Retired)
Shands Hospital and University of Florida College of Medicine
Gainesville, Florida

James C. Blankenship, MD, MHCM
Director, Cardiology and Cardiac Cath Labs
Geisinger Medical Center
Danville, Pennsylvania

Thomas P. Bleck, MD, MCCM
Professor of Neurological Sciences, Neurosurgery, Anesthesiology, and Medicine
Rush Medical College
Chicago, Illinois

Adrien Bougle, MD
Département d'Anesthésie, Réanimation
Institut de Cardiologie
Hôpital Universitaire La Pitié-Salpêtrière
Assistance Publique
Hôpitaux de Paris
Paris, France

Scott Allan Brown, MBA, BSN, RN, CIC
Director, Infection Control
University of Florida Health Shands Hospital
Gainesville, Florida

Eileen M. Bulger, MD
Professor of Surgery
University of Washington
Harborview Medical Center
Seattle, Washington

Frederick M. Burkle, Jr., MD, MPH, DTM, FAAP, FACEP
Senior Fellow and Scientist
Harvard Humanitarian Initiative Harvard University
Cambridge, Massachusetts
Senior International Public Policy Scholar
Woodrow Wilson International Center for Scholars
Washington, District of Columbia

Clay Cothren Burlew, MD, FACS
Director
Surgical Intensive Care Unit
Program Director
SCC and TACS Fellowships
Department of Surgery
Denver Health Medical Center
Professor of Surgery
University of Colorado School of Medicine
Denver, Colorado

Jennifer Bushwitz, PharmD
Clinical Pharmacy Specialist
Medical Intensive Care
Barnes-Jewish Hospital
St. Louis, Missouri

Patricia Marie Byers, MD, FACS
Professor of Surgery
Division of Trauma and Acute Care Surgery
Surgical Critical Care
Chief, Surgical Nutrition and Metabolic Surgery
The DeWitt Daughtry Family Department of Surgery
Miami, Florida

William G. Cance, MD
Professor of Oncology
Roswell Park Cancer Institute
Professor of Surgery
State University of New York at Buffalo
Buffalo, New York

Lawrence J. Caruso, MD
Associate Professor of Anesthesiology and Surgery
University of Florida College of Medicine
Gainesville, Florida

Juan C. Cendan, MD, FACS
Professor of Surgery
Chairman, Department of Medical Education
University of Central Florida College of Medicine
Orlando, Florida

Cherylee W. J. Chang, MD, FACP, FCCM
Medical Director
Neuroscience Institute/Neurocritical Care
Director
Stroke Center
Associate Clinical Professor of Medicine and Surgery
John A. Burns School of Medicine
University of Hawaii, The Queen's Medical Center
Honolulu, Hawaii

Kenneth K. Chen, MD
Assistant Professor of Medicine and Obstetrics and Gynecology
The Warren Alpert Medical School of Brown University
Providence, Rhode Island

Rex T. Chung, MD
Director
Surgical Simulation Laboratory
Cedars-Sinai Medical Center
Los Angeles, California

Cornelius J. Clancy, MD
Associate Professor of Medicine
Department of Medicine
University of Pittsburgh
Pittsburgh, Pennsylvania

Michael Coburn, MD
Professor and Chairman
Scott Department of Urology
Baylor College of Medicine
Houston, Texas

Vittoria Comellini, MD
Respiratory Disease Specialist
Alma Mater University
Department of Clinical, Integrated, and Experimental Medicine (DIMES)
Respiratory and Critical Care Unit
S. Orsola-Malpighi Hospital
Bologna, Italy

Jamie B. Conti, MD, FACC
Professor and Chief
Division of Cardiovascular Medicine
Department of Medicine
University of Florida
Gainesville, Florida

Mark S. Cooper, BMBCh, PhD, FRCP, FRACP
Professor of Medicine
Department of Endocrinology
Concord Repatriation General Hospital
Sydney, Australia

Eduardo Leite Vieira Costa, MD, PhD
Staff Physician
Cardiopulmonary Department
Pulmonary Division
Heart Institute (Incor)
University of São Paulo and Research and Education Institute
Hospital Sírio-Libanês (E.L.V.C.)
São Paulo, Brazil

Douglas B. Coursin, MD
Professor of Anesthesiology and Medicine
University of Wisconsin School of Medicine and Public Health
Madison, Wisconsin

Claudia Crimi, MD, PhD
Respiratory Intensive Care Unit
Azienda Ospedaliera per l'Emergenza Cannizzaro
Catania, Italy

Ettore Crimi, MD
Assistant Professor
Department of Anesthesia
University of Central Florida
Ocala Regional Medical Center
Ocala, Florida

Michael W. Cripps, MD, FACS
Department of Surgery
Division of Burn/Trauma/Critical Care
University of Texas Southwestern Medical Center at Dallas
Dallas, Texas

Kristina Crothers, MD
Professor of Medicine
Department of Medicine
Division of Pulmonary and Critical Care
University of Washington
Harborview Medical Center
Seattle, Washington

Gohar H. Dar, MD
Staff Intensivist
Cardiothoracic Anesthesia and Critical Care Medicine
Heart and Vascular Institute
Cleveland Clinic
Cleveland, Ohio

Rabih O. Darouiche, MD
VA Distinguished Service Professor
Departments of Medicine, Surgery, and Physical Medicine and Rehabilitation
Michael E. DeBakey Veterans Administration Medical Center
Baylor College of Medicine
Houston, Texas

Elizabeth Lee Daugherty, MD, MPH
Vice Chair for Clinical Affairs
Department of Medicine
Assistant Professor of Medicine
Division of Pulmonary and Critical Care Medicine
Department of Medicine
Johns Hopkins University School of Medicine
Baltimore, Maryland

Kimberly A. Davis, MD, MBA, FACS, FCCM
Professor of Surgery
Vice Chairman of Clinical Affairs
Chief of the Section of General Surgery, Trauma, and Surgical Critical Care
Yale School of Medicine
Trauma Medical Director
Surgical Director Quality and Performance Improvement
Yale New Haven Hospital
New Haven, Connecticut

Gennaro De Pascale
Professor
Department of Intensive Care and Anesthesiology
Catholic University of the Sacred Heart
Agostino Gemelli Hospital
Rome, Italy

Angela M. DeAntonio, MD, FCCP
Pulmonologist
Geisinger Health System
Wilkes-Barre, Pennsylvania

Chirag S. Desai, MD
Associate Professor of Surgery
Department of Surgery
University of North Carolina
Chapel Hill, North Carolina

Jack A. DiPalma, MD
Professor and Director
Division of Gastroenterology
University of South Alabama College of Medicine
Mobile, Alabama

Ericka Domalakes, MD
Clinical Instructor, MFM Fellow
Obstetrics and Gynecology
University of Kansas
Kansas City, Kansas

Karen Doucette, MD, MSc (Epi), FRCPC
Associate Professor and Director
Division of Infectious Diseases
Education Lead, Transplant Infectious Diseases Fellowship
Department of Medicine
University of Alberta
Edmonton, Alberta, Canada

Colin L. Doyle, MD
Fellow
Department of Surgery
University of Hawaii
Honolulu, Hawaii

Joep M. Droogh, MD, PhD
Intensivist
Medical Coordinator
Mobile Intensive Care Unit
Department of Critical Care
University Medical Center Groningen
Groningen, The Netherlands

Gary Duclos, MD
Service d'Anesthésie et de Réanimation
Hôpital Nord
Assistance Publique Hôpitaux de Marseille
Aix Marseille Université
Marseille, France

Quan-Yang Duh, MD
Professor and Chief
Section of Endocrine Surgery
University of California
San Francisco, California

Herbert L. DuPont, MD
Professor and Director
Center for Infectious Diseases
University of Texas School of Public Health
Mary W. Kelsey Distinguished Chair
University of Texas McGovern School of Medicine
Clinical Professor
Baylor College of Medicine
President
Kelsey Research Foundation
Houston, Texas

Pierre Durieux, MD, MPH
Associate Professor
Department of Medical Informatics and Public Health
Hôpital Européen Georges-Pompidou
Descartes University
Paris, France

Rodney K. Edwards, MD, MS
Professor and Chief
Section of Maternal-Fetal Medicine
Department of Obstetrics and Gynecology
University of Oklahoma Health Sciences Center
Oklahoma City, Oklahoma

A. Ahsan Ejaz, MD
Professor of Medicine
Division of Nephrology, Hypertension, and Transplantation
University of Florida
Gainesville, Florida

Elamin M. Elamin, MD, MSc, FACP, FCCP
Professor of Medicine
University of South Florida
Assistant Chief, Pulmonary
Critical Care and Sleep Medicine Section
James A. Haley Veterans Hospital
Tampa, Florida

Alyaa El Hazami, MD
Consultant Intensivist
Critical Care Department
King Faisal Specialist Hospital and Research Centre
Riyadh, Saudi Arabia

E. Wesley Ely, MD, MPH
Professor of Medicine
Associate Director of Research GRECC
Vanderbilt University Medical Center
Nashville, Tennessee

Timothy S. Eng, MD
Assistant Professor of Anesthesiology
University of Virginia Health System
Charlottesville, Virginia

Lisa M. Esolen, MD
Assistant Chief Quality Officer
Medical Director, Infection Control
Medical Director, Occupational Health
Geisinger Health System
Danville, Pennsylvania

Timothy C. Fabian, MD, FACS
Harwell Wilson Alumni Professor
Department of Surgery
University of Tennessee Health Science Center
Memphis, Tennessee

Samir M. Fakhry, MD, FACS
Charles F. Crews Professor
Chief
General Surgery
Department of Surgery
Medical University of South Carolina
Physician Leader
Surgical Acute and Critical Care Service Line
Charleston, South Carolina

Javairiah Fatima, MD
Assistant Professor of Surgery
Department of Vascular and Endovascular Surgery
University of Florida
Gainesville, Florida

Robert J. Feezor, MD, FACS
Associate Professor of Surgery
University of Florida
Gainesville, Florida

Joseph Feldschuh, MD
Teaching Attendant
New York University Medical School
New York, New York

Niall D. Ferguson, MD, FRCPC, MSc
Interdepartmental Division of Critical Care Medicine
University of Toronto
Toronto, Canada

Sebastian Fernandez-Bussy, MD
Assistant Professor of Medicine
Director, Interventional Pulmonology
Clinica Alemana-Universidad del Desarrollo
Santiago, Chile

Henry E. Fessler, MD
Professor of Medicine
Pulmonary and Critical Care Medicine
Johns Hopkins University School of Medicine
Baltimore, Maryland

J. Emanuel Finet, MD
Assistant Professor of Clinical Medicine
Department of Medicine
Krannert Institute of Cardiology
Indiana University
Indianapolis, Indiana

Jay A. Fishman, MD
Director
Transplant Infectious Disease and Compromised Host Program
Massachusetts General Hospital
Professor of Medicine
Harvard Medical School
Boston, Massachusetts

Sarah W. Flores, MD, MPH
Gastroenterologist
VA Northern California Health Care System
Mather, California

Timothy C. Flynn, MD, FACS
Professor of Surgery and Senior Associate Dean
University of Florida College of Medicine
Gainesville, Florida

Cory Franklin, MD
Director Emeritus
Medical Intensive Care Unit
Cook County Hospital
Chicago, Illinois

Michael A. Frölich, MD, MS
Professor
Department of Anesthesiology
The University of Alabama at Birmingham
Birmingham, Alabama

W. Craig Fugate
Administrator
Federal Emergency Management Agency 2009–2017
Washington, District of Columbia

Andrea Gabrielli, MD, MBA, FCCM
Professor, Anesthesiology and Critical Care Medicine
University of Pennsylvania Perelman School of Medicine
Division Chief, Critical Care Medicine
Co-Director, Trauma ICU
Medical Director, PENN E-LERT® Telemedicine Program
Philadelphia, Pennsylvania

Elizabeth Mahanna Gabrielli, MD
T32 Postdoctoral Research Fellow
Clinical Associate
Divisions of Critical Care Medicine, Neurocritical Care and Neuroanesthesia
Department of Anesthesiology and Critical Care Medicine
University of Pennsylvania Perelman School of Medicine
Philadelphia, Pennsylvania

Adam Gaffney, MD
Attending Physician
Division of Pulmonary and Critical Care Medicine
Cambridge Health Alliance
Cambridge, Massachusetts

Robert Peter Gale, MD, PhD
Haematology Research Centre
Department of Medicine
Division of Experimental Medicine
Imperial College London
London, United Kingdom

Rose B. Ganim, MD, FCCP, FACS
Thoracic Surgeon
Departments of Thoracic Surgery and General Surgery
Baystate Health
Springfield, Massachusetts

Joseph A. Garcia, MD
Department of Emergency Medicine
Henry Ford Hospital
Detroit, Michigan

Cynthia Wilson Garvan, PhD
College of Nursing
University of Florida
Gainesville, Florida

Achille Gaspardone, MD
Director
Division of Cardiology
Sant'Eugenio Hospital
Rome, Italy

Juan B. Ochoa Gautier, MD, FACS, FCCM
Associate Physician
Department of Critical Care Medicine
Geisinger Medical Center
Danville, Pennsylvania
Chief Medical Officer
Nestle Health Science USA
Florham Park, New Jersey

James A. Geiling, MD, MPH
Chief, Medical Service
VA Medical Center
White River Junction, Vermont
Professor of Medicine
Geisel School of Medicine at Dartmouth
Hanover, New Hampshire

David S. Gloss II, MD, MPH, TM
Section of Neurology
Charleston Area Medical Center
Charleston, West Virginia

Andreas Goetzenich, MD, PhD
Department of Thoracic and Cardiovascular Surgery
University Hospital RWTH
Aachen, Germany

Shankar Gopinath, MD, FAANS
Chief of Neurosurgery
Ben Taub Hospital
Baylor College of Medicine
Houston, Texas

Mollie Gowan, PharmD, BCPS, BCCCP
Clinical Specialist
Medical Intensive Care
Barnes-Jewish Hospital
S. Louis, Missouri

Michael C. Grant, MD
Assistant Professor
Department of Anesthesiology and Critical Care Medicine
The Johns Hopkins Medical Institutions
Baltimore, Maryland

Dietrich Gravenstein, MD
Chair, Division of Anesthesiology
Geisinger Health System
Danville, Pennsylvania

David M. Greer, MD, MA, FCCM, FAHA, FNCS, FAAN, FANA
Professor and Vice Chairman of Neurology
Department of Neurology
Yale School of Medicine
New Haven, Connecticut

Jeffrey Groeger, MD
Chief
Urgent Care Service
Memorial Sloan Kettering Cancer Center
Professor of Medicine
Weill Cornell Medical College
New York, New York

Angelika C. Gruessner, PhD
Professor
Department of Surgery
SUNY Upstate Medical University
Syracuse, New York

Rainer W. Gruessner, MD, FACS
Professor of Surgery
Chief of Transplantation
SUNY Upstate Medical University
Syracuse, New York

Cyrus Adel Hadadi, MD
Fellow in Cardiovascular Disease
Department of Cardiology
Geisinger Medical Center
Danville, Pennsylvania

Jonathan W. Haft, MD
Associate Professor
Department of Cardiac Surgery
University of Michigan Health System
Ann Arbor, Michigan

Ghady Haidar, MD
Clinical Assistant Professor of Medicine
Department of Medicine
Division of Infectious Diseases
University of Pittsburgh Medical Center
Pittsburgh, Pennsylvania

David J. Hall, MD
Resident
Department of Surgery
University of Florida
Gainesville, Florida

Laura Hammel, MD
Assistant Professor of Anesthesiology and Critical Care
University of Wisconsin Hospitals and Clinics
Madison, Wisconsin

Erica J. Hardy, MD, MMSc
Assistant Professor of Medicine (Clinical)
Divisions of Infectious Disease and Obstetric Medicine
The Warren Alpert Medical School of Brown University
Department of Medicine
Women & Infants Hospital
Providence, Rhode Island

Nicole P. Harlan, MD
Department of Medicine
Duke University Medical Center
Durham, North Carolina

Neil S. Harris, MBChB, MD
Clinical Associate Professor
Department of Pathology, Immunology, and Laboratory Medicine
University of Florida College of Medicine
Gainesville, Florida

Scott Alexander Harvey, MD, MS
Department of Surgery
University of Hawaii, Manoa
The Queen's Medical Center
Honolulu, Hawaii

Zubair A. Hashmi, MD
Director of Fellowship Program
Cardiothoracic Transplant Surgery and MCS
Indiana University Health
Indianapolis, Indiana

Michael S. Hayashi, MD, FACS
Trauma Medical Director
The Queen's Medical Center
Assistant Clinical Professor
The University of Hawaii
Honolulu, Hawaii

Stephen O. Heard, MD
Professor of Anesthesiology and Surgery
UMass Memorial Medical Center
University of Massachusetts Medical School
Worcester, Massachusetts

Bryce A. Heese, MD, MA
Associate Professor
Pediatrics
Medical Genetics
Children's Mercy Hospital
Kansas City, Kansas

Alan W. Hemming, MD, MSc, FACS, FRCSC
Professor and Chief
Transplantation Hepatobiliary Surgery
Department of Surgery
University of California Health System
San Diego, California

Phillip K. Henderson, DO
Assistant Professor of Medicine
College of Medicine
University of South Alabama
Mobile, Alabama

Santiago Herrero, MD, FCCP
Gijón General Hospital (Hospital of Cabuenes)
Principality of Asturian Health System (SESPA)
University of Oviedo, Government Principality of Asturias
Gijón, Asturias (Spain)

Dean R. Hess, PhD, RRT
Respiratory Care
Massachusetts General Hospital
Associate Professor of Anesthesia
Harvard Medical School
Boston, Massachusetts

Zoltan G. Hevesi, MD
Professor of Anesthesiology
University of Wisconsin
Madison, Wisconsin

Thomas L. Higgins, MD, MBA, MCCM
Chief Medical Officer and Interim President/CEO
Baystate Franklin Medical Center
Greenfield, Massachusetts
Professor of Medicine, Surgery, and Anesthesiology
Tufts University School of Medicine
Boston, Massachusetts

Gary M. Hochheiser, MD, FCCP
Chief
Division of Thoracic Surgery
Baystate Medical Center
Springfield, Massachusetts

Brian L. Hoh, MD, FACS, FAHA, FAANS
James and Newton Eblen Professor and Associate Chair of Neurosurgery
Chief
Division of Cerebrovascular Surgery
University of Florida
Gainesville, Florida

M. Barbara Honnebier†, MD, PhD
Pediatric and Adult Plastic and Reconstructive Surgery
Cranio-Maxillo-Facial Surgery
The Queens' Medical Center and Kapiolani
Medical Center for Women and Children
Honolulu, Hawaii

Srikanth Hosur, MD
Chief Medical Officer
The Geisinger Community Medical Center
Associate, Department of Critical Care Medicine
Scranton, Pennsylvania

David B. Hoyt, MD, FACS
Executive Director
American College of Surgeons
Chicago, Illinois

Laurence Huang, MD
Professor of Medicine
University of California San Francisco
Chief, HIV/AIDS Chest Clinic
Department of Medicine
Division of Pulmonary and Critical Care Medicine and HIV/AIDS Division
San Francisco General Hospital
San Francisco, California

Thomas S. Huber, MD, PhD
Professor and Chief
Division of Vascular Surgery
University of Florida College of Medicine
Gainesville, Florida

Maureen B. Huhmann, DCN, RD, CSO
Adjunct Faculty
Department of Nutrition Sciences
Rutgers University
Newark, New Jersey

David Inouye, MD, PhD
Assistant Professor of Surgery
John A. Burns School of Medicine University of Hawaii
Associate Medical Director
Surgical Critical Care
The Queen's Medical Center
Honolulu, Hawaii

†Deceased

Steven R. Insler, DO
Staff Physician
Department of Cardiothoracic Anesthesia and Critical Care Medicine
The Cleveland Clinic Foundation
Cleveland, Ohio

Nicole M. Iovine, MD, PhD
Hospital Epidemiologist
Department of Medicine
Division of Infectious Diseases and Global Medicine
University of Florida
Gainesville, Florida

James C. Jackson, PsyD
Research Associate Professor
Department of Medicine
Vanderbilt University School of Medicine
Nashville, Tennessee

Michael A. Jantz, MD
Associate Professor of Medicine
Division of Pulmonary, Critical Care, and Sleep Medicine
University of Florida
Gainesville, Florida

Edgar J. Jimenez, MD, FCCM
Vice President
Critical Care Medicine
Baylor Scott and White Health
Temple, Texas
Clinical Professor of Medicine
Texas A&M University
College Station, Texas

F. Elizabeth Jimenez, APRN, MSN, FNP-BC, CCRN
Assistant Professor
College of Nursing
University of Mary Hardin-Baylor
Belton, Texas

Aaron M. Joffe, DO, FCCM
Associate Professor
Department of Anesthesiology and Pain Medicine
Harborview Medical Center
University of Washington
Seattle, Washington

Firas Kaddouh, MD
Resident
Department of Neurology
University of Massachusetts Medical School
Worcester, Massachusetts

Atul Kalanuria, MD, FACP
Assistant Professor
Neurology, Neurosurgery, Anesthesia, and Critical Care
The Hospital of the University of Pennsylvania
Perelman School of Medicine
Philadelphia, Pennsylvania

Gautam Subbaiah Kalyatanda, MBBS, MD
Assistant Professor
Division of Infectious Disease and Global Medicine
University of Florida
Gainesville, Florida

Raja Kandaswamy, MD
Transplant Institute
MedStar Georgetown University Hospital
Washington, District of Columbia

Constantine Karvellas, MD, SM, FRCPC
Department of Critical Care Medicine
University of Alberta
Edmonton, Alberta, Canada

Paraskevi A. Katsaounou, MD
Assistant Professor of Pulmonary Medicine
Medical School University of Athens
Evangelismos Hospital
Athens, Greece

Jeffrey P. Keck, Jr., MD
Department of Anesthesia
SouthEast Health
Cape Girardeau, Missouri

Katherine Kemberling
Department of Critical Care Medicine
The Geisinger Medical Center
Danville, PA

Shravan Kethireddy, MD, FACP
Associate Physician
Department of Critical Care and Infectious Disease
Geisinger Medical Center
Danville, Pennsylvania

Khalid M. Khan, MBChB, MRCP
Associate Professor
MedStar Georgetown University Hospital
Washington, District of Columbia

Orlando C. Kirton, MD, FACS, MCCM, FCCP, MBA
Surgeon-in-Chief
Chairman of Surgery
Abington-Jefferson Health
Professor of Surgery
Sidney Kimmel Medical College of Thomas Jefferson University
Abington, Pennsylvania

Craig S. Kitchens, MD, MACP
Professor Emeritus
Department of Medicine
University of Florida
Gainesville, Florida

Charles T. Klodell Jr., MD
Medical Director, The Heart & Vascular Center
North Florida Regional Healthcare
Gainesville, Florida

Adam Klotz, MD
Associate Attending Physician
Memorial Sloan Kettering Cancer Center
Assistant Professor of Clinical Medicine
Weill Cornell Medical College
New York, New York

Marin H. Kollef, MD
Professor of Medicine
Division of Pulmonary and Critical Care Medicine
Washington University School of Medicine
St. Louis, Missouri

Karen A. Korzick, MD, MA, FCCP, FACP
Program Director
Critical Care Medicine
Vice Chair
Vice-Chair, Committee on Bioethics
Geisinger Medical Center
Danville, Pennsylvania

Anand Kumar, MD
Professor of Medicine, Medical Microbiology, and Pharmacology
Sections of Critical Care Medicine and Infectious Disease
University of Manitoba
Winnipeg, Manitoba, Canada

Emmanuel Kyereme-Tuah, MBChB, MD
Critical Care Medicine Fellow
Geisinger Medical Center
Danville, Pennsylvania

Franco Laghi, MD
Professor of Medicine
Department of Pulmonary and Critical Care Medicine
Stritch School of Medicine
Loyola University of Chicago
Maywood, Illinois
Staff Physician
Pulmonary and Critical Care Medicine
Edward Hines, Jr. VA Hospital
Hines, Illinois

Asad Latif, MD, MPH
Assistant Professor
Department of Anesthesiology and Critical Care Medicine
Johns Hopkins University School of Medicine
Baltimore, Maryland

A. Joseph Layon, MD, FACP
Co-Chairperson, Department of Pulmonary and Critical Care Medicine
System Director, Division of Critical Care Medicine
The Geisinger Health System
Danville, Pennsylvania
Professor of Medicine and Anesthesiology
The Geisinger Commonealth School of Medicine
Scranton, Pennsylvania

Daniel R. Layon
Resident in Orothopaedic Surgery
Virginia Commonwealth University
Richmond, Virginia

Gene T. Lee, MD
Assistant Professor
Department of Obstetrics and Gynecology
University of Kansas Medical Center
Kansas City, Kansas

Marc Leone, MD, PhD
Service d'Anesthesie et de Reanimation
CHU Nord
Chemin des Bourrely, France

Olivier Y. Leroy, MD
Intensive Care Unit
Centre Hospitalier Chatiliez
Tourcoing, Nord, France

Stephanie N. Lueckel, MD, MPH, FACS
Assistant Professor
Department of Surgery
Division of Trauma and Critical Care
Rhode Island Hospital
The Warren Alpert Warren Medical School of Brown University
Providence, Rhode Island

William R. Lynch, MD
Section of Thoracic Surgery
Department of Surgery
University of Michigan Medical Center
Ann Arbor, Michigan

Francisco Igor B. Macedo, MD
Department of Surgery
Providence Hospital and Medical Centers
Southfield, Michigan
Michigan State University
East Lansing, Michigan

John W. Mah, MD, FACS
Associate Professor
Department of Surgery
University of Connecticut School of Medicine
Farmington, Connecticut
Associate Director
Surgical Intensive Care
Hartford Hospital
Hartford, Connecticut

Sonal Mahajan, DO
Department of Internal Medicine
University of Chicago (Northshore)
Evanston, Illinois

Michael E. Mahla, MD
Professor of Anesthesiology
Chief, Division of Neuroanesthesia
Sidney Kimmel Medical College
Philadelphia, Pennsylvania

Elizabeth Manias, RN, BPharm, MPharm, MNStud, PhD, DLF-ACN, MPS, MSHPA
Professor
MMR Accredited Pharmacist
Certified Geriatric Pharmacist
Research Professor
Centre for Quality and Patient Safety Research
School of Nursing and Midwifery
Deakin University
Adjunct Professorial Fellow
Department of Medicine
Royal Melbourne Hospital
The University of Melbourne
Honorary Professor
Melbourne School of Health Sciences
The University of Melbourne
Melbourne, Australia

Edward M. Manno, MD, FNCS, FANA, FAHA, FCCM
Professor of Neurology and Neurosurgery
Vice Chair of Clinical Affairs
Department of Neurology
Northwestern University
Chicago, Illinois

Daniel R. Margulies, MD, FACS
Professor of Surgery
Director
Trauma and Acute Care Surgery
Department of Surgery
Cedars-Sinai Medical Center
Los Angeles, California

Paul E. Marik, MD, FCCM, FCCP
Professor of Medicine
Chief of Pulmonary and Critical Care Medicine
Department of Medicine
Eastern Virginia Medical School
Norfolk, Virginia

Claude Martin, MD
Professor of Anesthesia and Intensive Care Medicine
Nord University Hospital, ICU and Trauma Center
Marseille School of Medicine
Marseille, France

Mali Mathru, MD, FCCP
Professor
Department of Anesthesiology and Perioperative Medicine
University of Alabama at Birmingham
Birmingham, Alabama

Andrew Matragrano, MD
Associate
Department of Thoracic and Critical Care Medicine
Director
Pulmonary Function Laboratory
Geisinger Medical Center
Danville, Pennsylvania

Raimis Matulionis, MD
St. Elizabeth Medical Center
CAP Anesthesia
Department of Anesthesiology, Pain, and Critical Care Medicine
Boston, Massachusetts

Paul B. McBeth, MD, MASc, FRCSC
Clinical Assistant Professor of Surgery and Critical Care Medicine
University of Calgary
Calgary, Alberta, Canada

Matthew S. McKillop, MD, FACC, FHRS
Assistant Professor of Medicine
Department of Medicine
Division of Cardiovascular Medicine
North Florida/South Georgia VA Medical Center
University of Florida
Gainesville, Florida

Hiren J. Mehta, MD
Assistant Professor of Medicine
Division of Pulmonary, Critical Care, and Sleep Medicine
University of Florida
Gainesville, Florida

Niharika Mehta, MD
Assistant Professor of Medicine
Department of Medicine
Division of Obstetric Medicine
The Warren Alpert Medical School of Brown University
Providence, Rhode Island

Yatin B. Mehta, MD
Director
Adult Intensive Care Units
Geisinger Medical Center
Danville, Pennsylvania
Clinical Assistant Professor of Medicine
Temple University School of Medicine
Philadelphia, Pennsylvania

Kristin L. Mekeel, MD, FACS
Professor of Surgery
Division of Transplant and Hepatobiliary Surgery
University of California San Diego
San Diego, California

Guy Meyer, MD
Clinical Professor
Division of Respiratory and Critical Care Medicine
Hopital Européen Georges Pompidou
Assistance Publique Hopitaux de Paris
Paris, France

Erik H. Middlebrooks, MD
Assistant Professor of Neuroradiology
Director, K. Scott & E.R. Andrew Advanced Neuroimaging Lab
Department of Radiology
University of Florida
Gainesville, Florida

William M. Miles, MD
Professor of Medicine
University of Florida
Gainesville, Florida

Srilakshmi Mitta, MD
Assistant Professor of Medicine
Department of Medicine
Division of Obstetric Medicine
The Warren Alpert Medical School of Brown University
Providence, Rhode Island

Toshiki Mizobe, MD, PhD
Department of Anesthesiology
Kyoto Prefectural University of Medicine
Kyoto, Japan

Taro Mizutani, MD, PhD
Professor and Chairman
Department of Emergency and Critical Care Medicine
Faculty of Medicine
University of Tsukuba
Tsukuba, Ibaraki, Japan

Jerome H. Modell, MD, DSc(Hon)
Department of Anesthesiology
University of Florida College of Medicine
Gainesville, Florida

Tan-Lucien H. Mohammed, MD, FCCP
Associate Professor and Chief
Thoracic Imaging
Department of Radiology
University of Florida College of Medicine
Gainesville, Florida

Richard E. Moon, MD
Professor of Anesthesiology and Medicine
Duke University Medical Center
Durham, North Carolina

Ernest E. Moore, MD
Vice Chairman for Research Department of Surgery
University of Colorado
Editor, Journal of Trauma
Denver, Colorado

Frederick A. Moore, MD
Professor of Surgery
Head of Acute Care Surgery
Department of Surgery
University of Florida
Gainesville, Florida

Jan S. Moreb, MD
Professor of Medicine
Clinical Director, Hematologic Malignancies
Stem Cell Transplantation Program
Division of Hematology/Oncology
University of Florida
Gainesville, Florida

Thomas C. Mort
Assistant Clinical Professor
University of Connecticut School of Medicine
Subspecialty Chief
Critical Care Anesthesia
Hartford Hospital
Hartford, Connecticut

David W. Mozingo, MD, FACS
Professor of Surgery and Anesthesiology
Director
UF Health Shands Burn Center
Department of Surgery
University of Florida College of Medicine
Gainesville, Florida

Susanne Muehlschlegel, MD, MPH, FNCS, FCCM
Associate Professor of Neurology (Neurocritical Care)
Anesthesia/Critical Care and Surgery
University of Massachusetts Medical School
Worcester, Massachusetts

Michael J. Murray, MD, PhD
Department of Critical Care Medicine
Geisinger Medical Center
Danville, Pennsylvania

Ece A. Mutlu, MD, MBA, MSCR
Associate Professor of Medicine
Director, Clinical Research
Director, IBD Program
Rush University
Department of Internal Medicine
Division of Digestive Diseases and Nutrition
Section of Gastroenterology
Chicago, Illinois

Gökhan M. Mutlu, MD
Professor and Chief
Section of Pulmonary and Critical Care Medicine
The University of Chicago
Chicago, Illinois

Bhiken I. Naik, MBBCh
Assistant Professor of Anesthesiology and Neurosurgery
University of Virginia
Charlottesville, Virginia

Stefano Nava
Professor
Respiratory and Critical Care
Sant'Orsola-Malpighi Hospital
Alma Mater Studiorum
Department of Specialistic Diagnostic and Experimental Medicine (DIMES)
University of Bologna
Bologna, Italy

Minh Ly Nguyen, MD
Assistant Professor of Medicine
Department of Internal Medicine
Division on Infectious Diseases
Emory University School of Medicine
Atlanta, Georgia

M. Hong Nguyen, MD
Professor of Medicine and Clinical and Translational Science Institute
University of Pittsburgh
Pittsburgh, Pennsylvania

Bright I. Nwaru, PhD
Research Fellow
Asthma UK Centre for Applied Research
Centre for Medical Informatics
Usher Institute of Population Health Sciences and Informatics
University of Edinburgh
Edinburgh, United Kingdom

Jennifer A. Oakes, MD, FACEP
Associate Professor
Emergency Medicine and Medical Toxicology
Albany Medical College
Albany, New York

Uchenna R. Ofoma, MD, MS
Associate in Critical Care Medicine
Department of Critical Care Medicine
Geisinger Medical Center
Danville, Pennsylvania

Ronny Otero, MD
Assistant Professor
Emergency Medicine
University of Michigan
Ann Arbor, Michigan

Nimisha K. Parekh, MD, MPH, FACG, AGAF
Associate Clinical Professor
Director, Inflammatory Bowel Disease Program
Fellowship Program Director
University of California, Irvine
Irvine, California

Marcelo Park, MD, PhD
Intensive Care Unit, Emergency Department
Hospital das Clínicas
University of São Paulo
São Paulo, Brazil

Robert I. Parker, MD
Professor of Pediatrics
Chief, Pediatric Hematology/Oncology
Stony Brook University School of Medicine
Stony Brook, New York

Rohit P. Patel, MD
Director, Critical Care Ultrasound
Center for Intensive Care
Departments of Emergency Medicine, Anesthesiology, and Surgery
University of Florida Health
Gainesville, Florida

Karolina Paziana, MD
Department of Emergency Medicine
Johns Hopkins University
Baltimore, Maryland

V. Ram Peddi, MD
Transplant Nephrologist
Director, Kidney Transplant Research
Department of Transplantation
California Pacific Medical Center
San Francisco, California

Kevin Y. Pei, MD
Assistant Professor of Surgery
Department of Surgery
Yale School of Medicine
New Haven, Connecticut

Carl W. Peters, MD
Clinical Associate Professor of Anesthesiology
Division of Critical Care Medicine
University of Florida College of Medicine
Gainesville, Florida

Keith R. Peters, MD
Associate Professor of Radiology
Divisions of Neuroradiology and Interventional Neuroradiology
University of Florida College of Medicine
Gainesville, Florida

Michael R. Pinsky, MD, CM
Department of Critical Care Medicine
University of Pittsburgh Medical Center
Pittsburgh, Pennsylvania

Massimiliano Pirrone, MD
Dipartimento di Fisiopatologia Medico-Chirurgica e dei Trapianti
Università degli Studi di Milano
Milan, Italy

Lara Pisani, MD
Department of Clinical Integrated and Experimental Medicine (DIMES)
Alma Mater University
Respiratory and Critical Care Unit
Sant'Orsola-Malpighi Hospital
Bologna, Italy

Louis R. Pizano, MD, MBA, FACS
Professor of Surgery
University of Miami/Miller School of Medicine
Director
Surgical Critical Care and Trauma Surgery Fellowship Program
Jackson Memorial Hospital
Miami, Florida

S. Mark Poler, MD
Vice Chair, Anesthesiology
Geisinger Health System
Danville, Pennsylvania

Andrew N. Pollak, MD
The James Lawrence Kernan Professor and Chairman
Department of Orthopaedics
University of Maryland School of Medicine
Chief of Orthopaedics
University of Maryland Medical System
Baltimore, Maryland

David T. Porembka, DO, MCCM
Professor of Surgery
Avera Medical Center and Stanford University
Sioux Falls, South Dakota

Raymond O. Powrie, MD, FRCP
Chief of Medicine
Women and Infants Hospital of Rhode Island
Professor of Medicine and Obstetrics and Gynecology
The Warren Alpert School of Medicine of Brown University
Chief Medical Quality Officer
Care New England Healthcare System
Providence, Rhode Island

Peter J. Pronovost, MD, PhD, FCCM
Professor
Departments of Anesthesiology and Critical Care Medicine, Surgery, and Health Policy and Management
The Johns Hopkins University School of Medicine
Director
Armstrong Institute for Patient Safety and Quality
Sr. Vice President for Patient Safety and Quality
Johns Hopkins Medicine
Baltimore, Maryland

Issam I. Raad, MD, FACP, FIDSA, FSHEA
G. P. Bodey, Sr. Distinguished Professor and Chairman
Department of Infectious Diseases
Infection Control and Employee Health
The University of Texas MD Anderson Cancer Center
Houston, Texas

Alejandro A. Rabinstein, MD
Professor of Neurology
Mayo Clinic
Rochester, Minnesota

Dejan Radovanovic, MD
School of Respiratory Diseases
University of Milan
Milan, Italy

Amin Rahemtulla, MD
Consultant Haematologist
The Clementine Churchill Hospital
Sudbury Hill
Harrow, United Kingdom

Swarna Rajagopalan, MD
Neurocritical Care Fellow
University of Pennsylvania
Philadelphia, Pennsylvania

Judi Anne B. Ramiscal, MD
University of Hawaii Surgical Residency Program
Honolulu, Hawaii

G. Duemani Reddy, MD, PhD
Neurosurgeon
Department of Neurosurgery
Baylor College of Medicine
Houston, Texas

Andrew J. Redmann, MD
Department of Otolaryngology—Head and Neck Surgery
University of Cincinnati College of Medicine
Cincinnati, Ohio

Mary Jane Reed, MD, FACS, FCCM, FCCP
Associate in Critical Care Medicine and Surgery
Departments of Critical Care Medicine and General Surgery
Geisinger Medical Center
Danville, Pennsylvania
Clinical Assistant Professor of Medicine and Surgery
Temple Medical School
Philadelphia, Pennsylvania

Konrad Reinhart, MD, PhD
Department of Emergency Medicine and Surgery
Henry Ford Hospital
Wayne State University
Detroit, Michigan

Zaccaria Ricci, MD
Medical Doctor
Pediatric Cardiac Intensive Care Unit
Department of Cardiology and Cardiac Surgery
Bambino Gesù Children's Hospital
IRCCS
Rome, Italy

Winston T. Richards, MD
Department of Surgery
University of Florida
Gainesville, Florida

Emanuel P. Rivers, MD, MPH
Vice Chairman and Research Director
Department of Emergency Medicine
Attending Staff
Emergency Medicine and Surgical Critical Care
Henry Ford Hospital
Clinical Professor
Wayne State University
Detroit, Michigan

Claudia Robertson, MD
Professor of Neurosurgery
Baylor College of Medicine
Houston, Texas

Steven A. Robicsek, MD, PhD
Associate Professor of Anesthesiology and Neuroscience
University of Florida
Gainesville, Florida

Stefano Romagnoli, MD
Department of Health Science at University of Florence
Department of Anesthesia and Critical Care
Azienda Ospedaliero-Universitaria Careggi
Florence, Italy

Claudio Ronco, MD
Director
Department of Nephrology, Dialysis, and Transplantation
International Renal Research Institute of Vicenza (IRRIV)
San Bortolo Hospital
Vicenza, Italy

Martin D. Rosenthal, MD
Department of Surgery
University of Florida
Gainesville, Florida

Daniel T. Ruan, MD
Associate Surgeon
Department of Surgery
Harvard Medical School
Brigham and Women's Hospital
Boston, Massachusetts

Vivek Sabharwal, MD
Chairman
Department of Neurocritical Care
Ochsner Medical Center
New Orleans, Louisiana

Palash Samanta, MD
Fellow
Division of Infectious Diseases
Department of Internal Medicine
University of Pittsburgh Medical Center
Pittsburgh, Pennsylvania

Steven Sandoval, MD
Assistant Professor of Surgery
Medical Director, Burn Center
Stony Brook University Hospital
Stony Brook, New York

Thomas M. Scalea, MD
Physician in Chief
R. Adams Cowley Shock Trauma Center
Baltimore, Maryland

Denise Schain, MD, FACP
Clinical Associate Professor
Division of Infectious Diseases and Global Medicine
University of Florida College of Medicine
Gainesville, Florida

Carsten M. Schmalfuss, MD
Chief, Section of Cardiology
North Florida/South Georgia Veterans Health
Assistant Professor
Division of Cardiovascular Medicine and Department of Radiology
University of Florida
Gainesville, Florida

Eran Segal, MD
Director
Department of Anesthesia, Intensive Care and Pain Medicine
Assuta Medical Centers
Tel Aviv, Israel

Allen M. Seiden, MD
Professor
Department of Otolaryngology-Head and Neck Surgery
University of Cincinnati College of Medicine
Cincinnati, Ohio

Steven A. Seifert, MD, FAACT, FACMT
Professor
Department of Emergency Medicine
UNM Health Sciences Center
Medical Director
New Mexico Poison Center
University of New Mexico School of Medicine
Albuquerque, New Mexico

Donald R. Sessions
Special Operations Chief
Gainesville Fire Rescue
Emergency Manager, City of Gainesville
Gainesville, Florida

Daniel I. Sessler, MD
Michael Cudahy Professor and Chair
Department of Outcomes Research
Anesthesiology Institute
Cleveland Clinic
Cleveland, Ohio

Christoph N. Seubert, MD, PhD, DABNM
Professor of Anesthesiology and Neurosurgery
Chief, Division of Neuroanesthesia
Department of Anesthesiology
University of Florida
Gainesville, Florida

Carla M. Sevin, MD
Director
The ICU Recovery Center at Vanderbilt
Assistant Professor of Medicine
Division of Allergy, Pulmonary, and Critical Care Medicine
Vanderbilt University Medical Center
Nashville, Tennessee

Gregory A. Sgueglia, MD, PhD
Division of Cardiology
Sant'Eugenio Hospital
Rome, Italy

David M. Shade, JD
Associate Scientist
Departments of Epidemiology and Medicine
The Johns Hopkins University
Baltimore, Maryland

Stephen D. Shafran, MD, FRCPC, FACP, FIDSA
Professor
Division of Infectious Diseases
Department of Medicine
University of Alberta
Edmonton, Canada

Hameeda Shaikh, MD
Division of Pulmonary and Critical Care Medicine
Edward Hines, Jr. Veterans Affairs Hospital
Hines, Illinois

Marc J. Shapiro, MD, FACS, FCCM
Professor of Surgery and Anesthesiology
Department of Surgery
SUNY Stony Brook
Stony Brook, New York

Aziz Sheikh, OBE, MD, MSc
Professor
Asthma UK Centre for Applied Research
Centre for Medical Informatics
Usher Institute of Population Health Sciences and Informatics
The University of Edinburgh
Edinburgh, United Kingdom

Michiko Shimada, MD, PhD
Assistant Professor of Medicine
Division of Cardiology, Respiratory Medicine, and Nephrology
Hirosaki University Graduate School of Medicine
Hirosaki, Japan

Takeru Shimizu, MD, PhD
Assistant Professor
Department of Anesthesiology
Tsukuba University Hospital/Mito Kyodo General Hospital
Mito, Ibaraki, Japan

Yehuda Shoenfeld, MD, FRCP, MaACR
Zabludowicz Center for Autoimmune Diseases
Sheba Medical Center
Tel HaShomer, Israel
Incumbent of the Laura Schwarz-Kipp Chair for Research of Autoimmune Diseases
Tel Aviv University
Tel Aviv, Israel

Ora Shovman, MD
Zabludowicz Center for Autoimmune Diseases
Chaim Sheba Medical Center
Tel HaShomer, Israel

Avner Sidi, MD
Professor
Department of Anesthesiology
University of Florida College of Medicine
Gainesville, Florida

Ioanna Sigala, MD, PhD
Consultant Respiratory Physician-Intensivist
Department of Critical Care and Pulmonary Services
University of Athens Medical School
Evangelismos Hospital
Athens, Greece

Marc A. Simon, MD
Associate Professor of Medicine, Bioengineering, and Clinical Translational Science
Department of Medicine and Vascular Medicine Institute
University of Pittsburgh
UPMC Heart and Vascular Institute
Pittsburgh, Pennsylvania

Jennifer A. Sipos, MD
Associate Professor of Medicine
Director, Benign Thyroid Program
Division of Endocrinology and Metabolism
Wexner Medical Center at The Ohio State University College of Medicine
Columbus, Ohio

Christopher Lee Sistrom, MD, MPH, PhD
Department of Radiology
University of Florida College of Medicine
Gainesville, Florida

Andrew M. Skinner, MD
Chief Resident
Department of Medicine
University of Chicago (Northshore)
Evanston, Illinois

Robert N. Sladen, MBChB, FCCM
Allen Hymen Professor Emeritus of Critical Care
Anesthesiology at Columbia University Medical Center
College of Physicians & Surgeons of Columbia University
New York, New York

Angela A. Slampak-Cindric, PharmD, BCPS
Clinical Pharmacist, Adult Intensive Care
Director, PGY1 Pharmacy Residency Program
Geisinger Medical Center
Danville, Pennsylvania

Matthew S. Slater, MD
Professor, Department of Surgery
Head, Adult Cardiac Surgery Section
Director of Quality, Knight Cardiovascular Institute
Director, Multidisciplinary Heart Valve Program
Oregon Health and Sciences University
Portland, Oregon

Danny Sleeman, MD
Professor of Surgery
The DeWitt Daughtry Family Department of Surgery
Jackson Memorial Hospital
University of Miami School of Medicine
Miami, Florida

Wendy I. Sligl, MD, MSc, FRCPC
Associate Professor
Critical Care Medicine and Infectious Diseases
Adjunct Appointment, School of Public Health
University of Alberta
Edmonton, Canada

Marije Smit-Droogh, MD
Surgeon-Intensivist
Department of Critical Care
University Medical Center Groningen
University of Groningen
Groningen, The Netherlands

Howard K. Song, MD, PhD
Professor and Chief
Division of Cardiothoracic Surgery
Oregon Health and Science University
Portland, Oregon

Kelley A. Sookraj, MD
Trauma Surgical Critical Care Fellow
Department of Surgery
Ryder Trauma Center
Jackson Memorial Hospital
Miami, Florida

Chakrapol Sriaroon, MD
Senior Pulmonary and Critical Care Fellow
University of South Florida
Tampa, Florida

Petr Starostik, MD
Associate Professor
Director, Molecular Pathology
Department of Pathology, Immunology, and Laboratory Medicine
College of Medicine, University of Florida
Gainsville, Florida

Deborah M. Stein, MD, MPH, FACS
R. Adams Cowley Professor in Shock and Trauma
University of Maryland School of Medicine
Chief of Trauma
R. Adams Cowley Shock Trauma Center
University of Maryland Medical Center
Baltimore, Maryland

Andrew Stolbach, MD, MPH
Emergency Physician
Department of Emergency Medicine
Johns Hopkins University
Baltimore, Maryland

Christian Stoppe, MD
Department of Intensive Care Medicine
University Hospital RWTH
Aachen, Germany

R. Todd Stravitz, MD
Professor of Medicine
Medical Director of Liver Transplantation
Hume-Lee Transplant Center
Virginia Commonwealth University
Richmond, Virginia

Arturo Suarez, MD, D. ASA, D. ASE, FCCM
Assistant Professor of Anesthesiology
Department of Anesthesiology
Duke University
Durham, North Carolina

Kathirvel Subramaniam, MD
Associate Professor of Anesthesiology
University of Pittsburgh
Pittsburgh Pennsylvania

Michael Suk, MD, JD, MPH, FACS
Chairman and Service Line Director
Department of Orthopaedics
The Geisinger Health System
Danville, Pennsylvania

David E. R. Sutherland, MD, PhD
Department of Surgery
University of Minnesota
Minneapolis, Minnesota

Sankar Swaminathan, MD
Division of Infectious Diseases
Department of Medicine
University of Utah School of Medicine
Salt Lake City, Utah

Anita Szady, MD
University of Florida Health
Cardiology—Shands Hospital
Gainsville, Florida

Danny M. Takanishi, Jr., MD, FACS
Professor of Surgery
Associate General Surgery Residency Program Director
John A. Burns School of Medicine
University of Hawaii
Honolulu, Hawaii

S. Rob Todd, MD, FACS, FCCM
Associate Professor of Surgery
Michael E. DeBakey Department of Surgery
Baylor College of Medicine
Chief, General Surgery and Trauma
Ben Taub Hospital
Houston, Texas

Gaurav Trikha, MD
Fellow
Division of Hematology/Oncology
University of Florida
Gainesville, Florida

Jose Javier Trujillano, MD, PhD
ICU Hospital Universitario Arnau de Vilanova
Lleida, Spain

Krista L. Turner, MD
Trauma Medical Director
The Medical Center of Aurora
Aurora, Colorado

Kimi R. Ueda, PharmD, BCPS, FAST
Transplant Pharmacist
Barry S. Levin, M.D. Department of Transplantation
California Pacific Medical Center
San Francisco, California

Aditya Uppalapati, MD, MS, FCCP
Assistant Professor
Critical Care Medicine
Weill Cornell Medicine
Houston Methodist Hospital
Houston, Texas

Luis E. Urrutia, MD
Co-Director, Cardiothoracic and Vascular Intensive Care Unit
Departments of Critical Care Medicine and Cardiovascular Diseases
Geisinger Medical Center
Danville, Pennsylvania

Craigan T. Usher, MD
Clinical Associate Professor
Department of Psychiatry
Oregon Health and Science University
Portland, Oregon

Joseph Varon, MD, FACP, FCCP, FCCM, FRSM
Chief of Critical Care Services
Foundation Surgical Hospital of Houston
Past Chief of Staff
Professor, Department of Acute and Continuing Care
The University of Texas Health Science Center at Houston
Clinical Professor of Medicine
The University of Texas Medical Branch at Galveston
Professor of Medicine and Surgery, UDEM, UNE, UABC, UAT, Anahuac, UACH, USON, UPAEP
President
Dorrington Medical Associates, PA
Houston, Texas

Theodoros Vassilakopoulos, MD, PhD
Professor, Pulmonary and Critical Care Medicine
National and Kapodistrian University of Athens, Medical School
Pulmonary and Respiratory Insufficiency Unit
Critical Care Department
Evangelismos Hospital
Athens, Greece

Gloria Vazquez-Grande, MD
Critical Care Research Fellow
Section of Critical Care Medicine
Department of Medicine
University of Manitoba
Winnipeg, Canada

Alfredo Vazquez-Sandoval, MD
Assistant Professor of Medicine
Pulmonary/Critical Care and Allergy Medicine Division
Baylor Scott & White Healthcare
Texas A&M University Health Sciences Center
Houston, Texas

George C. Velmahos, MD, PhD, MSEd
John F. Burke Professor of Surgery
Harvard Medical School
Chief
Division of Trauma, Emergency Surgery, and Surgical Critical Care
Massachusetts General Hospital
Boston, Massachusetts

Nupur Verma, MD
Assistant Professor
Abdominal and Cardiac Imaging
Director of Abdominal CT
Director of Critical Care Imaging
Department of Radiology
University of Florida College of Medicine
Gainesville, Florida

Juan Vilaro, MD
Assistant Professor
Division of Cardiovascular Medicine
University of Florida
Gainesville, Florida

David B. Waisel, MD
Department of Anesthesiology, Perioperative and Pain Medicine
Boston Children's Hospital
Associate Professor of Anesthesia
Harvard Medical School
Boston, Massachusetts

Howard Waitzkin, MD, PhD
Distinguished Professor Emeritus, Sociology
University of New Mexico
Albuquerque, New Mexico
Adjunct Professor, Internal Medicine
University of Illinois
Rockford, Illinois

Hsiu-Po Wang, MD
Associate Professor of Internal Medicine
College of Medicine
National Taiwan University
Chief, Endoscopy Division
Chief, Department of Internal Medicine
National Taiwan University Hospital, Yun-Lin Branch
Taipei, Taiwan

Elizabeth Wenqian Wang, MD
Fellow
Department of Infectious Diseases
The Baylor University School of Medicine
Houston, Texas

Michael F. Waters, MD, PhD
Associate Professor
Departments of Neurology, Neuroscience, and Biomedical Engineering
University of Florida College of Medicine
Gainesville, Florida

Kenneth Waxman, MD
Director of Trauma and Surgical Education
Department of Surgical Education
Santa Barbara Cottage Hospital
Santa Barbara, California

Amanda Wehler, DO
Transfusion Medicine Director
Laboratory Medicine
Geisinger Health System
Danville, Pennsylvania

Carl P. Weiner, MD, MBA
K.E. Krantz Professor and Chair
Department of Obstetrics and Gynecology
University of Kansas School of Medicine
Kansas City, Kansas

Michaela A. West, MD, PhD
Emeritus Professor Surgery
University of California San Francisco
San Francisco, California

Peggy White, MD
Assistant Professor
Department of Anesthesiology
University of Florida College of Medicine
Gainesville, Florida

Eelco F. M. Wijdicks, MD, PhD
Division of Critical Care Neurology
Mayo Clinic
Rochester, Minnesota

William E. Winter, MD, FCAP, DABCC, FACB
Professor
Departments of Pathology, Immunology and Laboratory Medicine, Pediatrics, and Molecular Genetics and Microbiology
University of Florida
Gainesville, Florida

Linda L. Wong, MD
Professor and Associate Chairman
Department of Surgery
John A. Burns School of Medicine
Director
Liver Transplant Program
Queens Medical Center
Honolulu, Hawaii

Kenneth E. Wood, DO, FACP, FCCP, FCCM
Professor of Medicine-Program in Trauma
University of Maryland School of Medicine
Adjunct Professor, Institute for Systems Research
A James Clark School of Engineering
University of Maryland, College Park
University of Maryland Medical System
Director, University of Maryland Critical Care Network
Associate Chief Medical Officer
University of Maryland Medical Center
Chief Clinical Officer
Attending Staff, R Adams Cowley Shock Trauma Center
Baltimore, Maryland

Haviv Yadid Yael, MD
Head of General Intensive Care Unit
Sheba Medical Center
Ramat Gan, Israel

Jean-Pierre Yared, MD
Department of Cardiothoracic Anesthesia
Department of Outcomes Research
Director, Critical Care Medicine
Heart and Vascular Institute
Cleveland Clinic
Cleveland, Ohio

Dante D. Yeh, MD
Assistant Professor of Surgery
Department of Surgery
Division of Trauma, Emergency Surgery, and Surgical Critical Care
Massachusetts General Hospital
Boston, Massachusetts

Mihae Yu, MD, FACS
Professor of Surgery
Vice-Chair of Education
University of Hawaii Department of Surgery
Program Director, Surgical Critical Care Fellowship
Director of Surgical Intensive Care
The Queen's Medical Center
Honolulu, Hawaii

Joseph Zachariah, DO
Department of Neurointensive Care
Spectrum Health Hospital
Grand Rapids, Michigan

Katherine L. Zaleski, MD
Clinical Fellow
Department of Anesthesiology, Perioperative, and Pain Medicine
Boston Children's Hospital
Boston, Massachusetts

Arno L. Zaritsky, MD, FAAP, FCCM
Professor of Pediatrics
Eastern Virginia Medical School
Children's Hospital of The King's Daughters
Norfolk, Virginia

Jan G. Zijlstra, MD, PhD
Department of Critical Care
University Medical Center Groningen University of Groningen
Groningen, The Netherlands

Janice L. Zimmerman, MD
Head
Critical Care Division
Houston Methodist Hospital
Professor of Clinical Medicine
Weill Cornell Medicine
Houston, Texas

Andreas G. Zori, MD
Fellow
Division of Gastroenterology
Department of Medicine
University of Florida
Gainesville, Florida

Roberto T. Zori, MD
Professor and Chief
Division of Clinical Genetics and Metabolism
Department of Pediatrics
University of Florida
Gainesville, Florida

Preface

A preface is the remarks made before speaking or writing, from the Latin *prae*, in front of or before, and *fari*, to speak. It precedes or heralds whatever is coming—in this case, a book with 157 print and electronic chapters. As such, it is our last chance to tell the readers the story behind this work. Indeed, it is a story. For just as every lecture is a story told in a unique manner, every book, including ours is simply a story. In this case, a story of some of the most severely ill people in our world; of how we care for and think about them; of how we organize our care; of how we organize ourselves. This, in sum, is the textbook you have in your hands, on your computer screen.

This book began its life as an idea that was gestated and shared between three titans of Critical Care Medicine, Joe Civetta, Rob Taylor, and Bob Kirby. Joe died recently, and Bob is unwell. We four editors took the mantle from these men, vowing to make their textbook—now ours—the standard in our field. Without the work and dedication of these three men, there would be no 5th edition.

We have endeavored to make this textbook as useful and reader friendly as possible. Of course the science is as up-to-date as any text allows and the contributors are all experts in their fields. More than this, however, we sought to make the book completely portable by publishing it—in its entirety—online. The print version contains our best sense of the material needed immediately for the clinician caring for the critically ill patient. Further, we have shortened the book, decreasing the number of chapters from 178 to 157, decreasing to some extent the size of the printed version without compromising the clinical and basic science.

We continue to utilize the section organization, beginning with the social aspects of medicine, followed by monitoring and organ system pathobiology, and finally with specific disease states/syndromes. We have added new chapters. Most especially those dealing with what happens ***after*** the patient, the critically ill human for whom we care, leaves the ICU. This has, we think, received too little emphasis in the past.

Our colleagues at Wolters Kluwer and the production services group, Aptara kept us on time (more or less), on our toes, and provided us the encouragement needed as we headed into the last 5 miles of our marathon. Our colleagues and families have put up with us—quite an achievement and, for this, we thank them.

As with all the previous editions, we attempted to ensure that this book has an international flavor, and represents Critical Care Medicine today. As such, it is not an American book, but a text written by colleagues from throughout the world that deals with common issues, whether one practices in America, Asia, Europe, Antarctica, Africa, or Oceania.

Lastly, of course—as is often said and remains true—success has a thousand parents, failure only one. Whatever mistakes of omission or commission are found herein are ours and ours alone. We four editors share a friendship, have given each other guidance and moral support, and will share any failures and successes of our travail.

A. Joseph Layon
(ajlayon@geisinger.edu)
Danville, Pennsylvania

Andrea Gabrielli
(andrea.gabrielli@uphs.upenn.edu)
Philadelphia, Pennsylvania

Mihae Yu
(mihaey@hawaii.edu)
Honolulu, Hawaii

Kenneth E. Wood
(Kenneth.Wood@umm.edu)
Baltimore, Maryland

Video List

Chapter 25

Video 1 Parasternal long-axis view. Normal function with view through parasternal long axis of chest.

Video 2 Parasternal short-axis view. Normal function with view through parasternal short axis of chest at papillary muscle level.

Video 3 Apical view. Normal function of apical view of chest.

Video 4 Subcostal view. Normal size and function of ventricles in subcostal view.

Video 5 Left ventricular function. **A** and **B**: Systolic function hyperdynamic short and long axis. **C** and **D**: Systolic function poor short and long axis.

Video 6 Right ventricular failure. D sign showing possible elevated right-sided pressures or low left ventricular pressures. This can also occur in patients with obstructive lung disease.

Video 7 Pericardial effusion in parasternal long axis (**A**) and parasternal short axis (**B**).

Video 8 Lung sliding with A lines seen on both sides of chest indicated a normal aeration pattern, without pulmonary edema.

Video 9 Lung B lines. This pattern seen in both sides of the chest in multiple areas indicates pulmonary edema pattern.

Contents

CIVETTA, TAYLOR, & KIRBY'S

Critical Care

FIFTH EDITION

CHAPTER 1

Policy, Politics, and the Intensive Care Unit

ADAM GAFFNEY and HOWARD WAITZKIN

INTRODUCTION

The intensive care unit (ICU), located at the jagged interface between advanced biomedical technology and strained human biology, is sometimes perceived as an isolated silo within the larger health care universe. For some, this particular clinical setting may seem insulated from broader sociopolitical concerns facing the United States or the world. Practitioners or researchers in the field, it might be thought, could restrict their gaze to derangements in physiology, to the particularities of critical care pharmacology, to the evolving defenses of nosocomial microbes, and so on.

However, as we aim to demonstrate in this chapter, the many political and economic forces at play in society are very much at work in the ICU. Issues of health inequalities, of lack of insurance, of underinsurance, of the appropriate allocation of resources, and of social justice are as relevant to the practice of critical care medicine (CCM) as they are to any other medical specialty. Indeed, particularly in light of growing critical care expenditures, predicted future growth in ICU demand, and the unique ethical issues faced in the ICU, health policy considerations should be considered a primary concern to both practitioners and investigators in the field.

The ICU, in short, is very much an interlocking unit within the larger political economy of health care. An understanding of recent developments in health care reform in the United States—namely the enactment and ongoing implementation of the Affordable Care Act (ACA)—is therefore very relevant to those in the field. Therefore, this chapter takes the following approach. First, we provide a brief overview of the history of health care reform efforts in the United States to contextualize our present situation. Next, we detail the ramifications of the ACA, and how it does and does not affect the problems of uninsurance, underinsurance, long-term care, and costs, with a focus on CCM. We then very briefly address how nations outside the United States contend with these issues. Subsequently, we detail some unique ICU-specific policy considerations, including issues of regionalization, workforce, capital allocation, and cost control. Finally, after having outlined the problems of the US health care system both in and outside the ICU, we present a case for a national health program (NHP), which, in our opinion, will most adequately address these various problems.

A VERY BRIEF HISTORY OF HEALTH CARE REFORM IN THE UNITED STATES

In 2013, the journalist Steven Brill presented a shocking and widely discussed account of individuals who were brought to financial ruin as a result of encounters with the medical system (1). In this work, he tells the story of one man who is diagnosed with stage IV lung cancer and is given less than a year to live. As Brill describes, a single admission to the hospital—including time in an ICU—generates a massive bill. The family is underinsured—their policy has a limit—and so the man's widow is left under a mountain of debt in the wake of his death, with a trail of hospital bill collectors in hot pursuit. Such a tragic scenario would be impossible in many countries of the world that have systems of universal health care. However, despite passage of the ACA, some patients admitted to the ICU may still be exposed, to some extent, to the high costs of care. How has this situation come about?

A number of books have traced the rise and fall of health care reform efforts in the United States (2–7). These histories rely on varying sources, underscore different themes, and arrive at inconsistent conclusions, but together they provide a framework for understanding why, in the 21st century, the United States lacks a system of universal health care. At several key junctures, the country turned away from health care reform; in each instance, both "winners" and "losers" would draw on the lessons of the experience, for better or for worse, during subsequent battles.

The first pivotal junction occurred during the Progressive Era of the late 1910s, when reformers sought to pass state-level systems of "compulsory health insurance," mainly intended for industrial workers. The campaign met fierce opposition from the American Medical Association, insurers, and industrial corporations. Derided by its adversaries as a pro-German, pro-Bolshevik conspiracy, the health insurance movement did not survive World War I (8,9).

A next pivot occurred during the Great Depression. Despite the growth of the welfare state and the potent political mobilization during that era, Franklin Roosevelt ultimately deferred on a system of social health insurance as part of the New Deal, partially due to fear of provoking the resistance of key interest groups in health care, i.e., physicians (10).

The postwar era again saw a powerful push for a national health insurance scheme, which the administration of Harry Truman supported. However, a well-funded public relations campaign and the anti-communism associated with McCarthyism spelled doom to these broader legislative proposals for national health insurance (3,11). Simultaneous to the decline of national health insurance was the rise of the private health insurance industry. Health insurance companies received tax protection during World War II, and following the war health insurance became subject to collective bargaining (4). However, although collective bargaining won private insurance coverage for many families during these decades, many more were left behind, including the unemployed, the poor, and the elderly. The passage of Medicare and Medicaid in 1965 ameliorated these injustices, but represented an inadequate replacement for a universal system. Whereas Medicare was meant, at least to some extent, as a universal system for the elderly (12), Medicaid functioned as a "poor people's program," associated with inequities in access and quality.

During the 1970s, the Democratic Party turned away from national health insurance. By the end of the decade, for instance, Jimmy Carter was embracing a program more limited than that of Richard Nixon (6). However, following the social austerity and cutbacks of the Reagan years, a window of opportunity seemed to again open with the election of Bill Clinton in 1992. Yet, facing opposition from health care interests as well as critics across the political spectrum, the Clinton Health Plan also failed (3).

Another push for health care reform coincided with the election of 2008. However, as more than one observer has commented, Democrats, including Barack Obama, had by that time more or less abandoned the goal of a comprehensive NHP guaranteeing universal access to care (6,13). As a result, though the 2010 ACA increases access to health care for many, it will not accomplish the goal of universal health care.

THE US HEALTH CARE SYSTEM, THE AFFORDABLE CARE ACT, AND CRITICAL CARE MEDICINE

An appreciation of the core provisions of the ACA is important for practitioners and researchers in the field of CCM. Here, we review four specific shortcomings of the US health care system (lack of insurance, underinsurance, long-term care, and high costs) with a focus on the ICU, and analyze what the ACA does and does not do to address them.

Lack of Insurance, Insurance Disparities, and the ICU

As the result of the history recounted above, lack of insurance has remained one of the gravest deficiencies of the US health care system. More recently, however, the system has been further strained by a decade of falling rates of employer-sponsored health insurance (14). Furthermore, lack of insurance in America has always been characterized by stark racial disparities, with substantially higher rates among both Hispanics and blacks than among whites (14).

The negative health consequences of being uninsured on both access to care and outcomes have been well documented. For instance, in one large study using data from the NHANES database, among those with chronic illness, lack of insurance was associated with a significantly increased likelihood of having had no health visits in the previous year, having no "standard site of care" when ill, or identifying the ED as that "standard site" (15). Another study found that even after controlling for socioeconomic status, race, and various behavioral and health factors, the uninsured had a significantly increased risk of mortality (HR = 1.40; 95% CI = 1.06, 1.84) (16). The investigators used census data from 2005 to calculate that such an increased mortality rate translated into an estimated additional 35,327 deaths annually (16).

However, does insurance status affect the care of the critically ill in particular? In the past, uninsured patients might be "dumped"—rejected or transferred to other hospitals—by hospitals uninterested in assuming the financial liability for their care (17). Even critically ill patients have been "dumped" despite the obvious risk to health that such unnecessary transfers entailed (17). In part to address this issue, Congress passed the Emergency Medical Treatment and Active Labor Act (EMTALA) in 1986, which granted patients legal protection from being "dumped" by hospitals because of an inability to pay. More specifically, under the act, hospitals have to screen and stabilize patients with emergent conditions regardless of their means (18,19).

Given the emergent presentation of many critical conditions, it might therefore be assumed that insurance status would today be irrelevant for those experiencing a critical illness. However, there is accumulating evidence that insurance status may affect both processes of care and outcomes in the case of the critically ill. To illustrate this, let us consider the hypothetical but unremarkable case of an uninsured individual who develops a potentially emergent symptom—say acute dyspnea—that is the result of pneumonia complicated by severe sepsis, and consider the ways in which insurance status might affect her outcome.

First, before proceeding to the issue of inequalities in care, we should note that there are racial (20) and insurance-related (21) inequalities in the very incidence of critical illness. In one study, for instance, among the nonelderly, being uninsured increased the risk of a sepsis-associated hospital admission (21). Thus, this patient's insurance status, itself related to socioeconomic status, may have been an important risk factor for the onset of sepsis. But let us put that aside and focus on potential disparities in care. First, this individual may be more likely to delay presentation to an emergency facility after the onset of her symptom. This plausible phenomenon is supported by one study which found that among those with an acute myocardial infarction, uninsured patients were significantly more likely to delay seeking emergency care (even after controlling for a multitude of clinical and social factors) (22). For many clinical conditions, such delays can affect the efficacy of treatment. In this study, for instance, those with an ST-elevation acute myocardial infarction and a 6-hour or greater delay had a lower likelihood of being treated with a percutaneous coronary intervention or thrombolysis (22). It is plausible that the phenomenon described in this paper would be applicable to other symptoms and conditions, and might apply to our hypothetical patient. It also seems plausible that delays in care can worsen outcomes in the critically ill. For instance, one recent study found that patients with pneumonia and severe sepsis (like our patient) had an improved outcome if the first dose of antibiotics was administered within the first 6 hours of care (23). There is also some evidence that the uninsured may have reduced access to intensive care services (24).

In any event, let us assume that our hypothetical patient calls an ambulance. Even at this point, insurance status may potentially affect processes of care. Despite EMTALA, for instance, some have described instances in which unstable patients, some uninsured, were inappropriately brought, diverted, or transferred to a safety net hospital even when other hospitals were closer (19). Putting this possibility aside, let us assume that the patient arrives promptly at an appropriate facility. Again, even at this stage insurance status may impact outcome. An American Thoracic Society systematic review, for instance, found evidence of insurance-related inequalities in care delivery and outcomes (21). For instance, based on four studies that adjusted for potential confounders, the critically ill uninsured had elevated hospital mortality (OR 1.16, 95% CI 1.1–1.33) (24). The causes for this are no doubt multifactorial, but there is evidence that insurance status may affect provided services. For instance, in one large analysis, after adjustment for potential confounders, the uninsured had lower odds of receiving five common critical care procedures (25). Some ICU procedures, particularly when routinely performed, have no clinical benefit, as the story of pulmonary artery catheterization has demonstrated; so, receiving fewer procedures may not, in fact, be a bad thing. However, if we consider these procedures to be more generally "a proxy for ICU service use," as these investigators argue, then these findings may reflect broader inequalities in the overall level of service provided (25). Such differences, in other words, speak to *de facto* persistent insurance-related inequalities in the ICU.

How does the ACA affect the issue of insurance-related health inequalities? The law seeks to decrease lack of insurance through a patchwork of programs and mandates, as opposed to providing a universal benefit as a right of citizenship or permanent residency. The provisions of the ACA have been summarized elsewhere (26), but the relevant provisions can be briefly stated here. First, it creates an "individual mandate" that the uninsured purchase qualifying private health insurance, or otherwise, pays a penalty. To facilitate this mandate, the law creates online "exchanges" where qualifying plans are sold, and also offers subsidies to help those with low income purchase these plans. Second, the law creates an "employer mandate," in which employers with greater than 50 employees are required to provide insurance or pay a fee. Third, the law expands Medicaid for those with incomes up to 138% of the federal poverty level. The federal government will pay for 100% of this expansion until 2016, after which this contribution will decrease to 90% by 2020 (26,27). As the result of a decision by the Supreme Court in 2012, however, states are no longer required to participate in the Medicaid expansion. A total of 29 states are moving ahead with the Medicaid Expansion as of early 2015 (28). Poor people in the other states are simply being left to their own devices.

Even putting aside the unpredicted problem with the Medicaid expansion, the provisions of the ACA will not eliminate lack of insurance. For some, the purchase of insurance may still be, or seem, too costly; undocumented immigrants will also be excluded. Indeed, as demonstrated in Figure 1.1, according to the estimates of the Congressional Budget Office, a total of 27 million people will remain uninsured over the next decade (29). Thus, though the uninsured will be significantly reduced

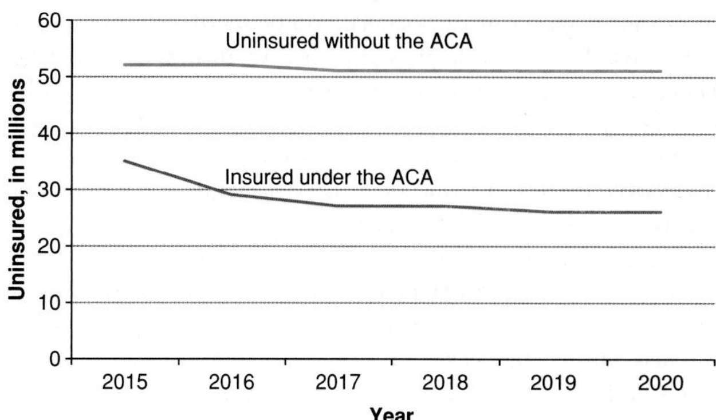

FIGURE 1.1 Estimated effects of the Affordable Care Act (ACA) on the uninsured. (Data from Congressional Budget Office. Insurance coverage provisions of the Affordable Care Act. CBO's March 2015 Baseline. Available at: https://www.cbo.gov/sites/default/files/cbofiles/attachments/43900-2015-03-ACAtables.pdf. Accessed May 2015.)

by the ACA, the problem will, by no means, be eliminated. Furthermore, inequalities between different types of insurance will endure. Many plans purchased on the ACA exchange, for instance, feature "narrow networks" that may limit access to care. Furthermore, though Medicaid currently functions as a crucial medical safety net for those with low income, inequalities in access to care have been described for participants in the program (30,31). Thus, in these two senses the ACA will not meet the endpoint of "universalism."

Underinsurance and the ICU

In another very important—and increasingly recognized—respect, the ACA will also not meet the standard of universal health care, and that is its failure to eliminate underinsurance. Though this is a problem no doubt predating the law, underinsurance is predicted to remain an important problem.

As long as there has been health insurance, there has been underinsurance. The concept, however, has been variably defined. For instance, in one study, individuals were defined as underinsured if they met one or more criteria for high financial exposure to health care costs (32). This included having out-of-pocket health care expenses 10% or more of income (or 5% for those with low income), or having out-of-pocket deductibles equal to or greater than 5% of income. Using these criteria, this study found that 20% of the nonelderly insured adult population—or 25 million people—were underinsured in 2007, which was up to 60% from 2003. The study further found that underinsurance affected both those with low income and those in the middle class. It found that the underinsured were more likely to avoid health care and to have increased likelihood of "financial stress" associated with health care, like putting health care costs on their credit card. In more recent years, underinsurance seems to have worsened. Indeed, a more recent study with similar methodology found that in 2014, 23% of nonelderly adults—or roughly 31 million people—were underinsured, which was approximately twice as many underinsured adults as 2003 (33).

One specific "cause" of underinsurance is health insurance plans that feature high levels of "cost sharing," or out-of-pocket money paid for health care at the time of use. The typical forms of cost sharing include co-payments (fixed fees for services or drugs), co-insurance (a percentage of the service or drug that is paid out of pocket), and deductibles (an amount that must be paid out-of-pocket before insurance coverage begins). In employer plans, the past decade has seen a substantial increase in such cost sharing. Over the last 9 years, the percentage of workers with single coverage with an annual deductible increased from 55% to 80%, while the amount of the average deductible approximately doubled (34).

Underinsurance and high out-of-pocket financial exposure more generally is problematic insofar as it deters individuals and families from seeking needed health care, and because it may unfairly burden the sick and those with low incomes (35,36). But is underinsurance a problem for CCM? To answer this question, we can first return to the issue of how financial barriers to care might result in avoidance or delay in seeking care, which may have important ramifications on critical care outcomes. Though one might think that those with potentially emergent symptoms would be insensitive to the costs of care, this does not appear to always be the case. Let us imagine, for instance, that the hypothetical patient we discussed in the previous section was insured, but had a high-deductible or emergency department co-payment. Might this affect her decision to seek care?

There is evidence that it might. One recent study compared a cohort of individuals who were transitioned to high-deductible health plans with a cohort that remained in a traditional HMO health plan (37). Among those of low socioeconomic status, the switch to the higher cost-sharing program was associated with reductions in "high-severity" Emergency Department visits, which included diagnoses like acute asthma exacerbations and head wounds. In other words, high cost sharing led some to avoid going to the emergency department, even when they needed it. Additionally, we earlier discussed how the uninsured with a myocardial infarction were more likely to experience delays in hospital presentation (22). This study additionally found that those who were insured but who had "financial concerns" were also more likely to experience delays in presentation. In other words, financial out-of-pocket exposure may result in delayed or foregone care, even in the case of emergencies.

Cost sharing may also adversely affect individuals with chronic pulmonary disease. High cost sharing discourages adherence to medication, including in those with chronic disease (38,39). One study found that when inhaler medications were subject to deductibles and co-insurance, the rate of emergency hospitalizations for COPD, asthma, and emphysema increased significantly (40).

Financial harm is another potential problem with underinsurance. The high costs of ICU care may impose severe financial strain for families at a particularly vulnerable time. A patient admitted to the ICU, for instance, might expect that the cost of the hospitalization would rapidly reach his or her increasingly high deductible.

Though the ACA provides some important protections (like outlawing caps on benefits, capping out-of-pocket costs, and preventing discrimination against those with pre-existing conditions), it does not eliminate the problem of underinsurance, for several reasons. First, it will do little to contain ongoing trends toward higher cost sharing in the employer insurance market. Furthermore, it may actually encourage this trend through the so-called Cadillac tax (41). The Cadillac tax was meant to address longstanding concerns that the tax exemption for employer-provided health insurance has encouraged the growth of overly generous plans. The tax, which was initially meant to go into effect in 2018 but has now been delayed, takes the form of a 40% excise tax—payable either by the insurer or the employer—on insurance plans that exceed a specified threshold (41). As a result, some employers have already moved to limit benefits in an attempt to evade hitting that threshold (41,42). Because the threshold is tied to overall inflation (and not to health care inflation, which is higher), one group has predicted that the number of those affected by the Cadillac tax will "grow rapidly over time," reaching 75.8% of all insurance plans for families by 2029 (43). Higher levels of cost sharing will be one way for insurers and employers to avoid paying this tax.

Second, the individual market insurance plans available through the ACA exchanges also incorporate substantial levels of cost sharing. The plans are divided into four metallic tiers—bronze, silver, gold, and platinum—that have actuarial values of 60%, 70%, 80%, and 90%, respectively. The out-of-pocket maximum for these plans can be as high as $13,200 for a family plan (though this depends on income), therefore requiring potentially high levels of cost sharing in the form of co-payments, co-insurance, and deductibles (44). For instance, in one recent survey, the average Bronze Plan had a medical deductible of $5,372 and a prescription drug deductible of $465 (44). Though there are cost-sharing subsidies for those making less than 250% of the federal poverty level, the burden of cost sharing may remain high for many middle-class families. Underinsurance will persevere; with financial barriers to care still in place, the United States will continue to lack a fully universal health care system.

Long-Term Care

The ordeal of surviving critical illness can, in some instances, leave patients profoundly disabled. Survivors of critical illness may be left with deficits in pulmonary function, neuromuscular strength, and cognitive capacity (45). They may face significant psychiatric sequelae including posttraumatic stress disorder, anxiety, and depression (45). Finally, they may have substantial, ongoing requirements for long-term care, whether in a facility or at home (45). Therefore, policy considerations around the question of long-term care should be central to practitioners and investigators in the intensive care field.

Simply stated, there is no "system" of long-term care in the United States. This reflects the historical development of long-term care in the United States, as recounted by Smith and Feng (46). In the 19th century, long-term care in the United States was provided in the tradition of the repressive English Poor Law (a centuries old system of relief for the poor), which essentially meant coupling public disgrace with the provision of benefits (so as to deter others from receiving such care) (46). In the early 20th century, however, long-term care recipients were progressively transferred to private boarding homes, which became the precursors for today's for-profit skilled nursing facilities (and which were sometimes part of publicly traded corporations) (46). The passage of Medicaid was another crucial pivot in this history. By providing a huge influx of resources for long-term care, the law resulted in a large increase in the number of nursing home beds, while simultaneously fostering the "medicalization and institutionalization" of long-term care (46).

Today, Medicaid remains the only real safety net for long-term care expenses for all but the very wealthy. According to one review, for instance, the cost for a nursing home for those paying out-of-pocket averages $75,000 a year (47). Those who are neither impoverished nor rich must, therefore, "spend down" their resources if they require long-term care services—until they reach a state of impoverishment—at which point Medicaid can be accessed. The ACA originally included a provision—the CLASS Act—which would have established a limited long-term care benefit. However, this would have been a voluntary program that provided only a limited set of benefits to a small section of the population (48). The benefits would have only partially reduced the costs of long-term care, and so would not have changed the fundamental dynamic of the "spend down" (48). Particularly as a result of its "voluntary" structure, the underlying finances were found to be profoundly flawed; given the impossibility of repairing the provision legislatively, the act was dropped altogether by the administration (49).

In contrast to the US experience, however, other nations have moved in the direction of providing long-term care as a universal benefit, including Germany (47,50–53), Japan (47,51), and the Netherlands (47). Despite the fact that these countries, unlike the United States, have a universal benefit for long-term care, they have public spending on long-term care that is only either slightly more (Japan) or slightly less (Germany) than the United States (51). These programs often also aim to provide long-term care services to patients in the setting of their home and community. Germany, for instance, encourages and financially supports care provision by family members (53).

To conclude, it is entirely true that the ACA may help many to avoid financial ruin because of an ICU admission. However, it may do little to help our patients who survive the ICU and go on to require long-term care. For those individuals, having to spend down the entirety of one's life savings to a state of pennilessness can perhaps fairly be compared with the stigma and scorn heaped on the unfortunate in the era of Poor Law–inspired long-term care.

Costs

The cost of health care is by no means a novel concern in the United States. Indeed, in 1927, a "Committee on the Cost of Medical Care" was formed to study this very problem (54). However, there can be no doubting that the problem of overall health care expenditure has reached a new state of urgency in more recent decades. From the comparative perspective, for instance, overall health care expenditures in the United States remain profoundly higher than other developed countries: in 2012, 16.9% of GDP was spent on health care in the United States, as compared to 11.6% in France, 10.9% in Canada, 11.3% in Germany, 10.3% in Japan, and 9.3% in the United Kingdom (55). These differences are particularly striking when we consider that these other nations spend less while covering the entirety of their populations.

However, it is true that the past 5 years has seen growth in US health care expenditures that is very low by historical standards (56). This slowdown in growth has been attributed in large part to the so-called Great Recession, though some provisions of the ACA have also been credited (56). In the long term, however, the ACA lacks potent cost-saving measures. Perhaps the ACA's greatest inadequacy in this regard is its failure to reduce our exceptionally wasteful spending on

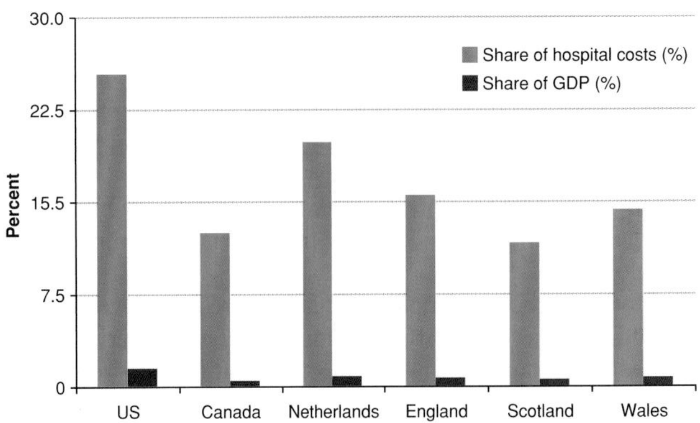

FIGURE 1.2 Total hospital administrative costs and spending, 2010. As per study authors, the numbers for Scotland and Wales are based on National Health Service hospitals only. Additionally, they note that the data for England, Scotland, and Wales are for April 1, 2010, to March 31, 2011. Data for France and Germany are not presented here given that data on these two specific metrics were not available for these two countries. The data for English share of GDP are inclusive of both NHS Trusts and Acute NHS Foundation Trusts. (Data from Himmelstein DU Jun M, Busse R, et al. A comparison of hospital administrative costs in eight nations: US costs exceed all others by far. *Health Aff (Millwood)* 2014;33:1586–1594.)

health care administration. Overall, data point to a rising proportion of health care dollars devoted to administrative costs, itself the result of our uniquely fragmented, multipayer health care system. For instance, from 1969 to 1999, the percentage of the US health care labor force devoted to administrative activities rose from 18.2% to 27.3% (57). By 1999, expenditures on health administration were $1,059 per capita in the United States, as opposed to the $307 per capita spent by Canada. Similarly, the proportion of total hospital costs spent on administrative activities increased from 23.5% in 2000 to 25.3% in 2011, even while they remained roughly stable in Canada (Fig. 1.2 gives greater detail on international comparisons) (58). Perhaps, more remarkable is the difference in administrative costs among nations: 1.43% of GDP goes to hospital administration in the United States, as compared to 0.41% and 0.51% in Canada and Scotland, respectively (58). Canada and Scotland both have single-payer systems with globally budgeted hospitals (in which hospitals receive a single payment to cover all operating expenses), allowing them to avoid not only the expense of interacting with multiple payers, but also eliminating patient-by-patient billing entirely (58). Nothing in the ACA will increase the administrative efficiency of the US health care system; doing so would require eliminating the problem of multiple payers and, like Canada and Scotland, globally budgeting hospitals.

The ACA does include a variety of other provisions that, it is hoped, will result in major savings. However, whatever their benefits and downsides may be, there is no strong evidence that many of these changes—for example, the expansion of the electronic medical record or the promotion of preventive medicine—will produce major cost savings (59,60).

As we will argue, an NHP could, conversely, facilitate substantial savings that could then be redirected to providing full coverage to both the uninsured and the underinsured, as well as the creation of new benefits (e.g., long-term care), without changing overall health care expenditures. Before we turn to the details of such a program, however, we will briefly discuss the health care system problems faced by other nations, and then explore some important policy issues specific to the ICU.

International Considerations

A comparative discussion of the health policy problems faced by other nations is well beyond the scope of this chapter. However, it does seem important to briefly emphasize that while the problems of the US health care system, as we have outlined, are to some extent unique to the country, they have important parallels, in both high- and low-income nations, throughout the globe.

However, before briefly discussing areas of overlap, we should first recognize the obvious divergence between the United States and other high-income nations with respect to health care: many industrialized nations have universal systems of health that are inclusive of either all or almost all of the population. A wide variety of explanations have been offered for why the United States failed to follow the developed world's lead in enacting a system of universal health care, and include such features of American political economy as the politics of race and the strength of powerful health care "stakeholders" (4). Navarro (61) emphasizes the importance of the labor movement (both through its unions and mass political parties) in the genesis of universalist national health programs in Europe. In any event, whether through the "Bismarck" model of health care reform (e.g., the social insurance model in Germany), the "Beveridge" model (e.g., the national health service in the United Kingdom), or some combination or variation thereof, systems of universal health care emerged in Europe and elsewhere in the industrialized world, mostly during the post–World War II period. To some extent, these developments represented a legal commitment to the notion of a right to health care that was proclaimed in such postwar documents as the constitution of the World Health Organization and the United Nations Universal Declaration of Human Rights.

At the same time, however, the universality of these systems has never been complete, and in some instances it has come under significant threat in recent years. For instance, though these systems have been very successful in facilitating universal access to care, they have not always eliminated the problem of underinsurance. Israel, for instance, has raised co-payments to such an extent that they now represent "a major bar to accessibility" to health care, especially for those with low incomes (62). In the Netherlands, meanwhile, concerns have been raised that health system privatization represents a turn away from universalism and a step toward tiered, inequitable access to health care (63). Similarly, some have argued that the 2012 Health and Social Care Act, passed by a Conservative-led government in the United Kingdom, is furthering the privatization of the English National Health Service and taking it away from its universalist foundations (64).

In the wake of the economic crisis of 2008, under the economic policy of austerity, the universality of the health care systems of many European nations has been the object of a more direct attack. Especially in the nations of Southern Europe (but also elsewhere, as in Ireland), the policy of health care austerity has meant reductions in insurance coverage, disrupted access to health care, and increases in co-payments (65). "The erosion of health coverage in a time of economic crisis across hard-hit countries is worrying both in terms of population health and for the future of the welfare state," as one observer puts it, also noting that "the universal nature of health systems has been consistently undermined, while demands for such publicly provided services are heightened" (65). Such changes have translated into a substantial rise in "unmet medical need" in nations like Greece (66). The onset of austerity policies has also been associated with increases in the suicide rate in Greece (67).

Low- and middle-income countries also face a range of challenges of their own. In particular, lack of access to quality health care remains a grave problem. The Indian health care system, for instance, is characterized by high out-of-pocket expenditures, regressive financing, low rates of insurance coverage, and deep inequalities in access along the lines of class, caste, and rural/urban geography (68). China, meanwhile, "turned its health system on its head" during the years of free-market reform in the 1980s: public funding for hospitals and rural health professionals evaporated as health care became increasingly an entrepreneurial endeavor (69). Out-of-pocket health care expenses became unaffordable for many, resulting in avoidance of health care (70,71). Recent reforms (69) may improve access for many Chinese, but comprehensive universal health care, without financial barriers to care, remains an aspiration in both nations.

In short, progress toward universal health care has proceeded very unevenly; even when it is achieved, it is by no means infallible. Moreover, the problems of being uninsured and underinsured, though particularly marked (among developed countries) in the United States, represent common weaknesses in the health systems of countries throughout the globe.

We now turn to health policy issues specific to the ICU.

POLICY CONSIDERATIONS IN THE ICU: COSTS, CAPITAL, DEMAND, SUPPLY

In 1952, Denmark was in the throes of a terrible epidemic of poliomyelitis. By late August, Blegdam Hospital had lost 27 patients to respiratory failure resulting from neuromuscular weakness (72). The hospital's chief physician, faced with the looming death of yet another patient—a 12-year-old girl—requested assistance from the anesthesiologist Björn Ibsen. Ibsen famously proceeded to recommend a tracheostomy and to carry out manual ventilation, thereby aborting her death (72,73). After this historic success, the protocol was soon repeated on all patients dying of respiratory failure from polio in the hospital (73). The life-saving capacity of this intervention was undeniable: the mortality rate fell from 87% to less than 40% (72).

To some extent, the "birth" of intensive care in Blegdam Hospital might be conceived as a sort of golden model of the potential beneficial effects of intensive care medicine. Patients were facing almost certain death from a condition that might be entirely reversible; with the temporary application of invasive, intensive medicine, lives were saved.

Juxtaposed to this inspiring story, however, is a more critical viewpoint that has emerged in the intervening decades. For instance, as one of us has previously studied, the rapid proliferation of critical care units in the United States was to a significant extent driven not by perceived needs and benefits, but by profit-driven corporate enterprises (74,75). Even putting that issue aside, it is increasingly recognized that the ICU might actually be harmful for some patients. To some extent, a glimpse of that reality may have already been apparent at the time of the 1952 polio epidemic. Bion and Bennet (76), for instance, have noted that even at the time, it was recognized that though "the new system of management produced many more survivors, it delayed death amongst patients destined not to survive". Some now see the ICU as representative of the worst of modern medicine: it is conceived as a highly invasive, enormously expensive site where dying is prolonged at the price of profound and unnecessary suffering. One can invoke the (sadly not unfamiliar) sight of a frail, elderly patient with advanced Alzheimer dementia, dying of multi-organ failure, chained to a respirator, invasive tubes, and central venous lines.

An essential goal of ICU policy is to steer the system away from the nonbeneficial interventions toward the beneficial. Achieving this goal is not always possible: Ibsen (76) could not, for instance, have predicted who was "destined not to survive"; he had to try and save all. But as CCM consumes increasingly large proportions of both health care and overall societal resources, it is clear that much more can and should be done to improve the rationale and appropriate use of these services.

Halpern et al. (77,78), for instance, have documented the rising resources devoted to intensive care medicine in two important papers. First, they noted that between 1985 and 2000, even though there was an 8.9% decrease in the number of hospitals and a 26.4% decrease in the number of hospitals beds, CCM beds actually *increased* by 26.2% (77). During this period, overall CCM costs rose to 190.4%, exceeding overall economic growth, resulting in about a half a percent of total GDP being devoted to critical care by 2000 (77). Between 2000 and 2005, similar trends continued: hospital beds continued to contract (though hospital days increased), while CCM beds continued to grow (78). The percentage of GDP devoted toward CCM rose to 0.66% (which did not account for physician costs that were privately billed) (78). "We surmise that in the current climate," the investigators noted, "the number and type of CCM beds will continue to increase without a 'plan,' simply as a response to increasing hospital admissions and days" (78). And in light of these trends, some have described an "impending critical care crisis," characterized by massive shortfalls in critical care physician staffing (79).

Are such trends problematic? We and others believe that they are. ICU care is one instance in which evidence points strongly to *supply-driven demand,* as convincingly argued by Gooch and Kahn (80). This situation is not necessarily driven by nefarious motives: we all want the best for our patients, and how could better observation and a greater intensity of nursing care be harmful, particularly when ample ICU beds are available? From the cost perspective, however, the phenomenon of supply-driven ICU demand is highly problematic, because it means that patients who will not benefit from ICU care may receive unnecessary care. The reality of supply-driven ICU demand was suggested by one cohort study (cited by Gooch and Kahn) conducted in Calgary, Alberta, involving patients whose clinical condition warranted activation of a rapid response system (81). In the multivariate analysis, if a rapid response was called when there were more empty beds, more patients were transferred to the ICU and fewer patients had a change in their goals of care from aggressive to "comfort" measures (81). Despite these differences, however, an absence of empty beds was not associated with greater hospital mortality (81). This finding suggests that having more beds available

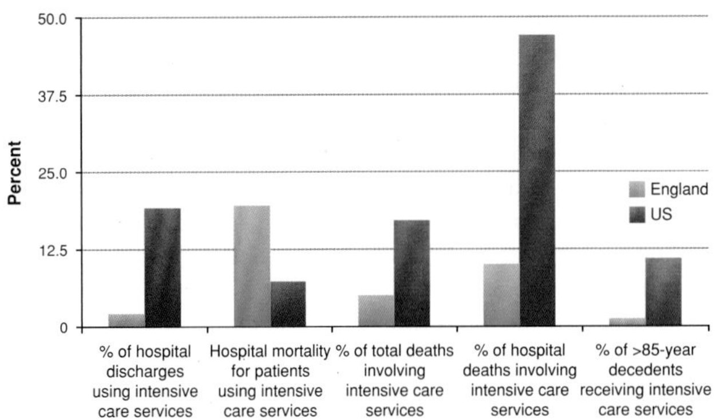

FIGURE 1.3 Use of the ICU at the end of life: US vs. England. US figures are based on data from seven states. Data from England is based on the 56% of ICU bed sample analyzed. (Data from Wunsch H, Linde-Zwirble WT, Harrison DA, et al. Use of intensive care services during terminal hospitalizations in England and the United States. *Am J Respir Crit Care Med* 2009;180:875–880.)

resulted both in greater use and greater intensity of care, without a corresponding improvement in overall outcomes.

Insights can also be gained from international comparisons. For instance, 2.2% of discharged patients received critical care services in English hospitals, as compared to 19.3% in the United States (Fig. 1.3) (82). ICU mortality is actually higher in England (suggesting sicker patients), but overall a much smaller proportion of *total deaths* involved critical care services in England (5.1%) as compared to the United States (17.2%) (82). Also, in England, only 1.3% of those aged over 85 died in an ICU, as compared to 11.0% in the United States (82). Another study (also cited by Gooch and Kahn), based on 102,346 admissions to ICUs in the United States and 70,439 in the United Kingdom, found that patients admitted to the ICU in the United States were older, less sick, less likely to die, and less likely to require mechanical ventilation (83), again suggesting the possibility that patients in the United States were less likely to need ICU services. From such studies, a complex picture emerges. On the one hand, patients in US ICUs are less sick overall, and are also less likely to die in the course of a single ICU stay, which is consistent with an overall increased use and supply of the ICU. On the other hand, in the United States (as compared to England), we are all more likely to be admitted to the ICU and to ultimately die there, even if we live to be older than 85.

Now the story is never so simple. For instance, it is also possible that NHS ICU spending and supply were too low during this period. After 2000, the English NHS pursued a major increase in the number of critical care beds, which was associated with a case mix–adjusted fall in hospital mortality thought consistent with a substantial improvement in outcomes (84). But in that case, a perceived inadequacy was met with a deliberate, planned expansion. In the case of the United States, there is simply no explicit effort to match ICU demand and supply, which results in significant and irrational regional differences in the availability of ICU infrastructure. For instance, within hospital referral regions, the number of ICU beds per 10,000 population ranges from 1.01 to 5.95 (85), a huge difference that is not explained by any obvious differences in need. There is also substantial variability in rates of ICU admission from hospital to hospital, a point emphasized by Gooch and Kahn (80). For instance, they cite a study involving Veterans Administration hospitals, in which—even after adjustment for important patient and hospital characteristics—rates of ICU admission ranged from 1.2% to 38.9% among hospitals for patients with "median predicted mortality" (86). Such variation in the availability of ICUs on the regional level and the utilization of ICUs on the hospital level speaks to two potential, intertwined problems: excess ICU capital and excessive ICU use (at least in certain regions or hospitals).

Against the indefinite expansion of supply, some have proposed other approaches. For instance, it has been argued that the regionalization of ICU services may help address the high costs and presumably lower efficiency of widely dispersed ICU capital. The model for such a reorganization comes, in part, from the experience with trauma care; some evidence points to an improvement in outcomes as a result of centering trauma care at certain hospitals (87). By restricting high-cost ICU infrastructure to particular regionalized centers, it has been proposed that the resulting efficiency gains and "economies of scale" might permit substantial savings and possibly improved outcomes (88). At the same time, as many have noted (88,89), there are several potential downsides to regionalization, foremost that it would involve moving patients away from their families and their communities at a crucial and trying time. Additionally, as has been recognized for some time (89), strong evidence that regionalization will reduce costs is still lacking.

From a broader perspective, however, we can perceive two overall narratives emerging. One is that we face a "crisis" in critical care, in which rising demand should be accommodated through aggressive efforts to further expand the critical care workforce (79). A second, which we favor, is a more skeptical perspective which maintains that the indefinite expansion of critical care services is neither sustainable nor necessarily beneficial. Kahn et al. (90), for instance, recently made this point in a perspective article titled the "Myth of the [Critical Care] Workforce Crisis". Instead of simply expanding ICU beds and training more ICU physicians, they contend that we should instead be looking to alternative solutions like regionalization. Indeed, they argue that states could legally regulate the growth in ICU beds, which would result in a lower ICU bed supply per capita over time.

We are sympathetic to the viewpoint of Kahn et al. (90). But we go further in contending that that an NHP is crucial to the goal of matching regional ICU demand and supply, and of regionalizing where appropriate and localizing where this is not the case. No doubt, more work needs to be done to better define the appropriate number of ICU beds per capita from the perspective of optimizing population health, and at present, there may be disagreements as to what this number should be. We also need more evidence with respect to where regionalization might improve outcomes and where it simply results in the estrangement of patients from families. More generally, we need to clarify who actually benefits from ICU care, and who would do equally well with less-invasive, less-intensive hospital care or palliative care. We likewise need to reduce inappropriate interventions that extend suffering without providing significant clinical benefit. However, we contend that an NHP will provide the critical organizational structure necessary to pursue these various goals. For instance, whatever the appropriate number of regional per capita ICU beds may be, without an NHP which explicitly allocates health care capital, it seems unlikely that such a goal will be met.

A NATIONAL HEALTH PROGRAM AND THE INTENSIVE CARE UNIT

As we saw earlier, the unique history of US health care politics has resulted in persistent deficiencies including lack of insurance, underinsurance, high costs, and an absence of key benefits even for the insured (i.e. long-term care). We subsequently told a related story: how the unplanned and disorganized growth of ICUs has led to a situation characterized by marked variation in the distribution of ICU infrastructure and the use of ICU services, as well as a lack of formal coordination on the regional level. In this final section, we describe how we would address these various deficiencies on the system-wide level, namely through the implementation of an NHP. The general framework for such a system (for the United States) has been outlined in three proposals (91,92,93). In the following outline of an NHP, we substantially rely on the detailed description of such a system as put forth in these documents.

The theoretical underpinning of an NHP is universalism. That is to say, unlike a patchwork system in which the poor partake in designated programs that provide certain benefits while those who are better off utilize separate private programs, the NHP would cover everyone. In this sense, the NHP would be more akin to Medicare than to Medicaid (though, as we will see, it would also address many of Medicare's inadequacies). The NHP would, simply put, function as a single-payer universal health insurance system, and would thereby entirely eliminate the problem of lack of insurance.

In terms of benefits, the NHP would provide the full spectrum of medical services. These services would include inpatient and outpatient medical care. However, they would also include mental health services, dental care, and palliative care, as well as prescription drugs. Importantly, it would cover these benefits without cost sharing; cost sharing, as previously discussed at length, deters patients from obtaining care and filling prescriptions, while also encouraging them to delay presentation to emergency rooms. With no financial liability at the time of care, underinsurance also would be eliminated. Additionally, some new benefits would be made available. Access to long-term care would become a universal benefit. As discussed, an emphasis on home and community solutions to those with long-term care needs—as opposed to institutionalization—would be an important aspect of this program.

We earlier discussed the enormous waste devoted to administrative overhead in the US health care system. In particular, we outlined how hospital administration has come to represent a huge cost in the United States. Hospital administrative expenses alone cost 1.43% of GDP in the United States (58), more than twice that of other developed countries and also more than twice that of total US critical care expenditures (78). Under an NHP, dramatic reductions in these expenditures can be expected. First, we already have evidence that Medicare (a public program) outperforms private insurance companies greatly with respect to administrative efficiency. For instance, the administrative overhead of traditional Medicare is estimated to be approximately 2.1% (94), whereas Medicare Advantage Plans run by private insurers have an overhead (including profits) closer to 13.6% (95). Second, providers, patients, and hospitals would no longer have to deal with a multiplicity of payers, greatly streamlining payment (and minimizing hassle for providers and patients alike). Third, hospitals would be allocated a "global budget," essentially a single sum of money that would cover all operating expenses for a given year. As a result, patient-level itemized billing could be discarded altogether.

An NHP could achieve additional savings through a number of measures. For instance, the system would, like other countries, negotiate directly with pharmaceutical companies over drug prices. One think tank has estimated that Medicare alone could save hundreds of billions of dollars over a decade through such negotiations (96). Another crucial aspect of an NHP is that it would facilitate a coherent system of health care capital planning. Until now, proliferation of medical resources and ICU beds has often been poorly planned and irrational. Insofar as the supply of health care drives demand—which as some have emphasized, clearly seems to be the case with ICU care (80)—such capital expenditures necessarily create new operating expenses. Thus, under an NHP, funding for new health care infrastructure would be independent from operating expenses, which will help to create a more sustainable and equitable distribution of health care capital. With respect to the ICU, an NHP would allow the country to make and meet regional goals for ICU beds per capita (whatever the precise goal may be). The NHP would help facilitate regionalization of specific ICU services, where appropriate. With global budgets in place, for instance, the financial incentives of having an ICU for individual hospitals will be attenuated. The focus could, therefore, be on meeting population needs in a coordinated fashion, not on the financial bottom line of particular institutions.

In sum, an NHP would provide health care for all as a right. By producing sufficient savings through reduced administrative spending and pharmaceutical expenditures, it could do so without an overall increase in health care expenditures. It would additionally be an important first step in the rational, regionalized, organized, and equitable distribution of ICU capital.

Key Points

- The Affordable Care Act expands access to health insurance, but does not resolve major problems in the US health care system including uninsurance, underinsurance, high costs, and administrative inefficiency.
- There is evidence that persistent insurance-related disparities may be detrimental to the health of those with acute and critical illness.
- The health care system still lacks adequate coverage for long-term care, which may be harmful to survivors of critical illness who are often left with significant disability.
- Overall spending on CCM is exceeding the rate of growth of the overall economy, necessitating that new ICU infrastructure is more rationally and explicitly planned.
- In the opinions of the authors, a single-payer NHP would best address the persistent deficiencies of the US health care system, both in and out of the ICU.

References

1. Brill S. Bitter pill: why medical bills are killing us. *Time*. February 20, 2013.
2. Funigiello PJ. *Chronic Politics: Health Care Security from FDR to George W. Bush*. Lawrence, KA: University Press of Kansas; 2005.
3. Gordon C. *Dead on Arrival: The Politics of Health Care in Twentieth-Century America*. Princeton, NJ: Princeton University Press; 2005.
4. Quadagno JS. *One Nation, Uninsured: Why the U.S. Has No National Health Insurance*. New York, NY: Oxford University Press; 2005.
5. Starr P. *The Social Transformation of American Medicine*. New York, NY: Basic Books; 1982.
6. Starr P. *Remedy and Reaction : The Peculiar American Struggle Over Health Care Reform*. Revised edition. New Haven, CT: Yale University Press; 2013.
7. Hoffman BR. *Health Care for Some: Rights and Rationing in the United States Since 1930*. Chicago, IL: University of Chicago Press; 2012.
8. Numbers RL. *Almost Persuaded: American Physicians and Compulsory Health Insurance, 1912–1920*. Baltimore, MD: Johns Hopkins University Press; 1978.
9. Hoffman B. *The Wages of Sickness*. Chapel Hill: The University of North Carolina Press; 2001.
10. Hirshfield DS. *The Lost Reform: The Campaign for Compulsory Health Insurance in the United States from 1932–1943*. Cambridge, MA: Harvard University Press; 1970.
11. Poen MM., Harry S. *Truman Versus the Medical Lobby: The Genesis of Medicare*. Columbia, MD: University of Missouri Press; 1979.
12. Navarro V. *The Politics of Health Policy: The US Reforms, 1980–1994*. Cambridge, MA: Blackwell; 1994.
13. Brill S. *America's Bitter Pill: Money, Politics, Backroom Deals, and the Fight to Fix Our Broken Healthcare System*. New York: Random House; 2015.
14. Kaiser Commission on Medicaid and the Uninsured. The uninsured: a prime – key facts about health insurance and the uninsured in America. Available at: http://kff.org/uninsured/report/the-uninsured-a-primer/. Accessed March 5, 2015.
15. Wilper AP, Woolhandler S, Lasser KE, et al. A national study of chronic disease prevalence and access to care in uninsured U.S. adults. *Ann Intern Med*. 2008;149:170–176.
16. Wilper AP, Woolhandler S, Lasser KE, et al. Health insurance and mortality in US adults. *Am J Public Health*. 2009;99:2289–2295.
17. Ansell DA, Schiff RL. Patient dumping: status, implications, and policy recommendations. *JAMA*. 1987;257:1500–1502.
18. Rosenbaum S. The enduring role of the emergency medical treatment and active labor act. *Health Aff (Millwood)*. 2013;32:2075–2081.
19. Rosenbaum S, Cartwright-Smith L, Hirsh J, Mehler PS. Case studies at Denver Health: 'patient dumping' in the emergency department despite EMTALA, the law that banned it. *Health Aff (Millwood)*. 2012;31: 1749–1756.
20. Soto GJ, Martin GS, Gong MN. Healthcare disparities in critical illness. *Crit Care Med*. 2013;41:2784–2793.
21. O'Brien JM Jr, Lu B, Ali NA, et al. Insurance type and sepsis-associated hospitalizations and sepsis-associated mortality among US adults: a retrospective cohort study. *Crit Care*. 2011;15:R130.
22. Smolderen KG, Spertus JA, Nallamothu BK, et al. Health care insurance, financial concerns in accessing care, and delays to hospital presentation in acute myocardial infarction. *JAMA*. 2010;303:1392–1400.
23. Menendez R, Torres A, Reyes S, et al. Initial management of pneumonia and sepsis: factors associated with improved outcome. *Eur Respir J*. 2012;39:156–162.
24. Fowler RA, Noyahr LA, Thornton JD, et al. An official American Thoracic Society systematic review: the association between health insurance status and access, care delivery, and outcomes for patients who are critically ill. *Am J Respir Crit Care Med*. 2010;181:1003–1011.
25. Lyon SM, Benson NM, Cooke CR, et al. The effect of insurance status on mortality and procedural use in critically ill patients. *Am J Respir Crit Care Med*. 2011;184:809–815.
26. Henry J, Kaiser Family Foundation. Summary of the Affordable Care Act. Available at: https://kaiserfamilyfoundation.files.wordpress.com/2011/04/8061-021.pdf. Accessed March 2, 2015.
27. Crowley RA, Golden W. Health policy basics: Medicaid expansion. *Ann Intern Med*. 2014;160:423–425.
28. Henry J, Kaiser Family Foundation. The ACA and Medicaid expansion. Available at: http://kff.org/report-section/the-aca-and-medicaid-expansion-waivers-issue-brief/. Accessed March 5, 2015.
29. Congressional Budget Office. Insurance coverage provisions of the Affordable Care Act—CBO's March 2015 Baseline. Available at: https://www.cbo.gov/sites/default/files/cbofiles/attachments/43900–2015–03-ACAtables.pdf. Accessed May 2015.

30. Bisgaier J, Rhodes KV. Auditing access to specialty care for children with public insurance. *N Engl J Med.* 2011;364:2324–2333.
31. Lyon SM, Douglas IS, Cooke CR. Medicaid expansion under the Affordable Care Act: implications for insurance-related disparities in pulmonary, critical care, and sleep. *Ann Am Thorac Soc.* 2014;11:661–667.
32. Schoen C, Collins SR, Kriss JL, Doty MM. How many are underinsured? Trends among U.S. adults, 2003 and 2007. *Health Aff (Millwood).* 2008;27:w298–309.
33. Collins SR, Rasmussen PW, Beutel S, Doty MM. The problem of underinsurance and how rising deductibles will make it worse: findings from the Commonwealth Fund Biennial Health Insurance Survey. *The Commonwealth Fund.* May 2015. Available at: http://www.commonwealthfund.org/publications/issue-briefs/2015/may/problem-of-underinsurance. Accessed January 13, 2016.
34. Henry J, Kaiser Family Foundation. 2014 Employer health benefits. Available at: http://kff.org/health-costs/report/2014-employer-health-benefits-survey/. Accessed March 3, 2015.
35. Lohr KN, Brook RH, Kamberg CJ, et al. Use of medical care in the Rand Health Insurance Experiment. Diagnosis- and service-specific analyses in a randomized controlled trial. *Med Care.* 1986;24:S1–S87.
36. Swartz K. Cost-sharing: effects on spending and outcomes. Robert Wood Johnson Foundation: the Synthesis Project 2010. Available at: http://www.rwjf.org/en/library/research/2011/12/cost-sharing–effects-on-spending-and-outcomes.html. Accessed January 13, 2016.
37. Wharam JF, Zhang F, Landon BE, et al. Low-socioeconomic-status enrollees in high-deductible plans reduced high-severity emergency care. *Health Aff (Millwood).* 2013;32:1398–1406.
38. Sinnott SJ, Buckley C, O'Riordan D, et al. The effect of co-payments for prescriptions on adherence to prescription medicines in publicly insured populations: a systematic review and meta-analysis. *PLoS One.* 2013;8:e64914.
39. Goldman DP, Joyce GF, Escarce JJ, et al. Pharmacy benefits and the use of drugs by the chronically ill. *JAMA.* 2004;291:2344–2350.
40. Dormuth CR, Maclure M, Glynn RJ, et al. Emergency hospital admissions after income-based deductibles and prescription copayments in older users of inhaled medications. *Clin Ther.* 2008;30(Part 1):1038–1050.
41. Health Policy Brief. Excise tax on 'Cadillac' plans. *Health Aff (Millwood).* 2013. Available at: www.healthaffairs.org/healthpolicybriefs/brief.php?brief_id=99. Accessed March 9, 2015.
42. Taylor K. Health care law raises pressure on public unions. *The New York Times.* August 4, 2013.
43. Herring B, Lentz LK. What can we expect from the "Cadillac tax" in 2018 and beyond? *Inquiry.* 2011;48:322–337.
44. Claxton G, Cox C, Rae M. *The Costs of Care with Marketplace Coverage.* Henry J Kaiser Family Foundation; 2015. Available at: http://kff.org/health-reform/issue-brief/the-cost-of-care-with-marketplace-coverage/. Accessed February 22, 2015.
45. Desai SV, Law TJ, Needham DM. Long-term complications of critical care. *Crit Care Med.* 2011;39:371–379.
46. Smith DB, Feng Z. The accumulated challenges of long-term care. *Health Aff (Millwood).* 2010;29:29–34.
47. Gleckman H. Long-term care financing reform: lessons from the U.S. and abroad. *The Commonwealth Fund.* February 2010. Available at: http://www.commonwealthfund.org/publications/fund-reports/2010/feb/long-term-care-financing-reform-lessons-from-the-us-and-abroad. Accessed January 13, 2016.
48. The Kaiser Commission on Medicaid and the Uninsured. Health care reform and the CLASS Act. Available at: http://kff.org/health-costs/issue-brief/health-care-reform-and-the-class-act/. Accessed March 17, 2015.
49. Gleckman H. Requiem for the CLASS Act. *Health Aff (Millwood).* 2011;30:2231–2234.
50. Cuellar AE, Wiener JM. Can social insurance for long-term care work? The experience of Germany. *Health Aff (Millwood).* 2000;19:8–25.
51. Campbell JC, Ikegami N, Gibson MJ. Lessons from public long-term care insurance in Germany and Japan. *Health Aff (Millwood).* 2010;29:87–95.
52. Geraedts M, Heller GV, Harrington CA. Germany's long-term-care insurance: putting a social insurance model into practice. *Milbank Q.* 2000; 78:375–401.
53. Harrington CA, Geraedts M, Heller GV. Germany's long-term care insurance model: lessons for the United States. *J Public Health Policy.* 2002; 23:44–65.
54. Committee on the Cost of Medical Care. *Medical Care for the American People: The Final Report of the Committee on the Costs of Medical Care, Adopted October 31, 1932.* New York, NY: Arno Press; 1972.
55. Organisation for Economic Co-Operation and Development. Health expenditure since 2000. Available at: http://stats.oecd.org/Index.aspx?DataSetCode = SHA. Accessed July 2, 2015.
56. Hartman M, Martin AB, Lassman D, Catlin A, The National Health Expenditure Accounts Team. National health spending in 2013: growth slows, remains in step with the overall economy. *Health Aff (Millwood).* 2015;34:150–160.
57. Woolhandler S, Campbell T, Himmelstein DU. Costs of health care administration in the United States and Canada. *N Engl J Med.* 2003;349:768–775.
58. Himmelstein DU, Jun M, Busse R, et al. A comparison of hospital administrative costs in eight nations: US costs exceed all others by far. *Health Aff (Millwood).* 2014;33:1586–1594.
59. Sidorov J. It ain't necessarily so: the electronic health record and the unlikely prospect of reducing health care costs. *Health Aff (Millwood).* 2006; 25:1079–1085.
60. Cohen JT, Neumann PJ, Weinstein MC. Does preventive care save money? Health economics and the presidential candidates. *N Engl J Med.* 2008;358:661–663.
61. Navarro V. Why Some countries have national health insurance, others have national health services, and the United States has neither. *Int J Health Serv.* 1989;19:383–404.
62. Gross AM. The right to health in Israel between solidarity and neoliberalism. In: Flood CM, Gross AM, eds. *The Right to Health at the Public/Private Divide: A Global Comparative Study.* New York, NY: Cambridge University Press; 2014.
63. Exter A. Health care access in the Netherlands: a true story. In: Flood CM, Gross AM, eds. *The Right to Health at the Public/Private Divide: A Global Comparative Study.* New York, NY: Cambridge University Press; 2014.
64. Davis J, Tallis R, eds. *NHS SOS.* London: Oneworld Publications; 2013.
65. Kentikelenis A. Bailouts, austerity and the erosion of health coverage in Southern Europe and Ireland. *Eur J Public Health.* 2015;25:365–366.
66. Reeves A, McKee M, Stuckler D. The attack on universal health coverage in Europe: recession, austerity and unmet needs. *Eur J Public Health.* 2015;25:364–365.
67. Branas CC, Kastanaki AE, Michalodimitrakis M, et al. The impact of economic austerity and prosperity events on suicide in Greece: a 30-year interrupted time-series analysis. *BMJ Open.* 2015;5(1):e005619.
68. Balarajan Y, Selvaraj S, Subramanian SV. Health care and equity in India. *Lancet.* 2011;377:505–515.
69. Blumenthal D, Hsiao W. Lessons from the East: China's rapidly evolving health care system. *N Engl J Med.* 2015;372:1281–1285.
70. Blumenthal D, Hsiao W. Privatization and its discontents: the evolving Chinese health care system. *N Engl J Med.* 2005;353:1165–1670.
71. Meng Q, Xu L, Zhang Y, et al. Trends in access to health services and financial protection in China between 2003 and 2011: a cross-sectional study. *Lancet.* 2012;379:805–814.
72. Hilberman M. The evolution of intensive care units. *Crit Care Med.* 1975; 3:159–165.
73. Reisner-Senelar L. The birth of intensive care medicine: Bjorn Ibsen's records. *.Intens Care Med.* 2011;37:1084–1086.
74. Waitzkin H. A Marxian interpretation of the growth and development of coronary care technology. *Am J Public Health.* 1979;69:1260–1268.
75. Waitzkin H. *Medicine and Public Health at the End of Empire.* Boulder, CO: Paradigm Publishers; 2011.
76. Bion JF, Bennett D. Epidemiology of intensive care medicine: supply versus demand. *Br Med Bull.* 1999;55:2–11.
77. Halpern NA, Pastores SM, Greenstein RJ. Critical care medicine in the United States 1985–2000: an analysis of bed numbers, use, and costs. *Crit Care Med.* 2004;32:1254–1259.
78. Halpern NA, Pastores SM. Critical care medicine in the United States 2000–2005: an analysis of bed numbers, occupancy rates, payer mix, and costs. *Crit Care Med.* 2010;38:65–71.
79. Kelley MA, Angus D, Chalfin DB, et al. The critical care crisis in the United States: a report from the profession. *Chest.* 2004;125:1514–1517.
80. Gooch RA, Kahn JM. ICU bed supply, utilization, and health care spending: An example of demand elasticity. *JAMA.* 2014;311:567–568.
81. Stelfox HT, Hemmelgarn BR, Bagshaw SM, et al. Intensive care unit bed availability and outcomes for hospitalized patients with sudden clinical deterioration. *Arch Intern Med.* 2012;172:467–474.
82. Wunsch H, Linde-Zwirble WT, Harrison DA, et al. Use of intensive care services during terminal hospitalizations in England and the United States. *Am J Respir Crit Care Med.* 2009;180:875–880.
83. Wunsch H, Angus DC, Harrison DA, et al. Comparison of medical admissions to intensive care units in the United States and United Kingdom. *Am J Respir Crit Care Med.* 2011;183:1666–1673.
84. Hutchings A, Durand MA, Grieve R, et al. Evaluation of modernisation of adult critical care services in England: time series and cost effectiveness analysis. *BMJ.* 2009;339:b4353.
85. Carr BG, Addyson DK, Kahn JM. Variation in critical care beds per capita in the United States: implications for pandemic and disaster planning. *JAMA.* 2010;303:1371–1372.

86. Chen LM, Render M, Sales A, et al. Intensive care unit admitting patterns in the veterans affairs health care system. *Arch Intern Med.* 2012;172: 1220–1226.
87. Kahn JM, Branas CC, Schwab CW, Asch DA. Regionalization of medical critical care: what can we learn from the trauma experience? *Crit Care Med.* 2008;36:3085–3088.
88. Nguyen YL, Kahn JM, Angus DC. Reorganizing adult critical care delivery: the role of regionalization, telemedicine, and community outreach. *Am J Respir Crit Care Med.* 2010;181:1164–1169.
89. Thompson DR, Clemmer TP, Applefeld JJ, et al. Regionalization of critical care medicine: task force report of the American College of Critical Care Medicine. *Crit Care Med.* 1994;22:1306–1313.
90. Kahn JM, Rubenfeld GD. The myth of the workforce crisis: why the United States does not need more intensivist physicians. *Am J Resp Crit Care Med.* 2014;191:128–134.
91. Woolhandler S, Himmelstein DU, Angell M, Young QD, Physicians' Working Group for Single-Payer National Health I. Proposal of the Physicians' Working Group for Single-Payer National Health Insurance. *JAMA.* 2003;290:798–805.
92. Himmelstein DU, Woolhandler S. A national health program for the United States: a physicians' proposal. *N Engl J Med.* 1989;320:102–108.
93. Gaffney A, Woolhandler S, Angell M, Himmelstein DU. Moving forward from the Affordable Care Act to a Single-Payer System. *Am J Public Health* 2016;106:987–988.
94. The Boards of Trustees of the Federal Hospital Insurance and Federal Supplementary Medical Insurance Trust Funds. 2014 annual report. Available at: http://www.cms.gov/Research-Statistics-Data-and-Systems/Statistics-Trends-and-Reports/ReportsTrustFunds/downloads/tr2014.pdf. Accessed March 19, 2015.
95. United States Government Accountability Office. Medicare advantage: 2011 profits similar to projections for most plans, but higher for plans with specific eligibility requirements. Available at: http://www.gao.gov/assets/660/659836.pdf. Accessed March 19, 2015.
96. Baker D. Reducing waste with an efficient medicare prescription drug benefit. Center for Economic and Policy Research, 2013.Available at: http://www.cepr.net/documents/publications/medicare-drug-2012–12.pdf. Accessed March 3, 2015.

CHAPTER 2

Life and Death in the ICU: Ethical Considerations

KATHERINE L. ZALESKI and DAVID B. WAISEL

"Death in the ICU is not always preventable and should neither be unduly hastened nor delayed." (1)

A BRIEF HISTORY OF END-OF-LIFE CARE

The modern history of end-of-life (EOL) care began with demands of patients to *refuse* treatments. In 1974, the American Medical Association asserted that "the purpose of cardiopulmonary resuscitation is the prevention of sudden unexpected death. Cardiopulmonary resuscitation is not indicated in cases of terminal irreversible illness where death is not unexpected" (2). Limiting resuscitation in patients with terminal illness was becoming acceptable.

In the 1976 case of Karen Ann Quinlan, the courts upheld the right to refuse potentially life-sustaining care when they permitted the ventilator to be disconnected from the supposed ventilator-dependent Quinlan (3). The *Quinlan* case was based on the general constitutional right to privacy. After mechanical ventilation was discontinued, Quinlan lived for nearly a decade, sustained by nasogastric feedings. The 1984 case of *Bartling* established the right for a competent person to refuse potentially life-sustaining care (4). For 6 months, Bartling, a competent adult patient with an incurable disease, received mechanical ventilation against his clear wishes, declaring, at one point, "While I have no wish to die, I find intolerable the living conditions forced upon me" (4). Similar in reasoning to *Quinlan,* the appellate court supported the right of a competent patient to refuse medical treatment based on the constitutional right to privacy.

The 1990 case of *Cruzan* brought about a crucial change in the right to refuse treatment (5). Several years before an incapacitating accident, Cruzan had expressed to a friend a desire not to live in a state of diminished capacity. Cruzan's surrogates wanted to withdraw treatment, but the Supreme Court of Missouri mandated continued care because Cruzan's informal statements did not meet Missouri's evidentiary standard of "clear and convincing evidence" of a patient's wish to terminate potentially life-sustaining care. The case was appealed to the United States Supreme Court, but unlike *Quinlan* and *Bartling,* the Supreme Court grounded the right of a competent patient to refuse treatment in the more powerful liberty interest of the Fourteenth Amendment, which states, "No State shall make or enforce any law which shall abridge the privileges or immunities of citizens of the United States; nor shall any State deprive any person of life, liberty or property . . . ." The decision upheld the rights of states to determine the standards for the level of certainty required, permitting Missouri to use the "clear and convincing evidence" standard, but also permitting other states to use different standards (5,6).

Intensive care unit (ICU) practices may also lead surrogates to demand care *for* their loved ones. Helga Wanglie, an 86-year-old patient in a persistent vegetative state who was receiving mechanical ventilation, is an archetypical case. The medical center believed that further therapy would be futile for Mrs. Wanglie and wanted to withdraw mechanical ventilation. When Mr. Wanglie refused the medical center request to stop mechanical ventilation, the medical center sought appointment of an independent guardian to supplant Mr. Wanglie as her guardian. In 1991, the Court declared that Mr. Wanglie was best able to be Mrs. Wanglie's surrogate (7,8); interestingly, a court ruled similarly in 2009 (9).

In the 1995 case of *Gilgun* (10), a jury supported a unilateral refusal of potentially life-sustaining care by the health care team. Catherine Gilgun had severe brain damage and was in a coma; the family refused any limitations on therapy. The Optimum Care Committee of the hospital agreed with the physicians that providing CPR was inadvisable. The legal division, believing the physicians were acting in the patient's best interest, approved the do-not-resuscitate order; following withdrawal of mechanical ventilatory support, she died.

Competent patients have a right to refuse potentially life-sustaining medical treatment (11). The modifier "potentially" is used before life-sustaining medical treatment to acknowledge that although clinicians may *believe* that a therapy is life sustaining, there is rarely certainty that the intervention *will* be life sustaining. For the incompetent patient, three hierarchical levels of judgment direct the decision-making process. The once competent patient's previously expressed preferences for EOL care should be followed as is best possible. When the patient's declared preferences are not known, *substituted judgment,* the surrogate's intimate knowledge of the patient's attitudes and beliefs, may be used to direct care. While these are two distinct categories, both levels require the surrogate to sufficiently know the patient to appropriately choose or interpret the patient's preferences. These standards put significant burdens on decision-makers who may have legitimate doubts about the appropriateness of their decisions. When a surrogate has to make decisions for a patient who has never been competent, such as a young child or a mentally disabled adult, substituted judgment is impossible, and the surrogate must rely on the *best interests standard.* The best interests standard requires the surrogate to make decisions based on the surrogate's view of what is best for the patient.

ADVANCE CARE PLANNING

Advance care planning permits patients to declare preferences for medical treatment if they become incapacitated. Respecting these preferences is how physicians honor the ethical principle of respect for autonomy, in which patients have the right to make substantially informed decisions about medical therapy and the resultant trajectory of their lives.

Advance care planning is designed to minimize the likelihood of undesired overtreatment and undertreatment of the patient. Three types of advance care planning are used: advance directive, durable power of attorney for health care decisions (DPAHC), and Physician Orders for Life-Sustaining Treatment (POLST). Although advance directives allow patients to declare the extent of desirable interventions, they are often unable to directly address the subtleties that characterize clinical situations. The difficulty of applying advance directives to clinical situations limits their effectiveness and leads some to prefer the greater flexibility provided by the DPAHC, in which the surrogate decision-maker can consider the specific details when making clinical decisions. DPAHCs permit patients to designate surrogate decision-makers—including nonfamily members—to make decisions for them, should they become unable to make such decisions for themselves. Surrogacy is not always effective, particularly for patients who do not make their preferences clearly known to the surrogate before losing their decision-making capacity. Surrogates may forget that they are merely a conduit to relay the preferences of the patient, and instead they feel responsible for the actions taken, thus limiting the wherewithal to make decisions that limit therapy.

Advance directives and DPAHCs are inadequately discussed, documented, disseminated, and followed. Interventions focusing on communication can increase the use of advance planning documents and may improve the quality of communication during the treatment process (12). In one study (13), a video improved the ability of patients and families to understand and use the terminology of CPR as compared to patients who were given the usual care of a standard pamphlet.

Over the past two decades, significant effort has been made to make advance care planning orders more portable and thus more actionable across health care settings. With these objectives in mind, the POLST Paradigm was started in Oregon in 1991 and has since spread nationally with the establishment of the National POLST Paradigm Task Force in 2004 (14). At present, all but six states have begun developing or have developed a POLST (also known as MOST, MOLST, POST, or TPOPP, among others, depending on region program). Although each state's program and documentation requirements differ, the paradigm aims to ensure that a patient's EOL care wishes are honored by promoting timely advance care planning discussions in the setting of a known condition and encouraging shared clinician–patient decision-making. The patient's wishes are recorded as a set of medical orders on a visible, portable, standardized form that will accompany the patient across different health care settings. POLST documents are meant to complement Advance Care Directives, and are intended for patients with an expected prognosis of one year or less.

The power of the POLST over advance directives is that POLST is rooted in using *physician orders*. Several small studies have demonstrated that care frequently matched the POLST instructions and that health care providers believe that the POLST facilitated EOL discussions and prevented unwanted resuscitation (15). Patients who have a POLST are more likely to die at home than those patients who only had an advance directive (16). POLST seems successful in transferring across settings, and that the preferences underlying a POLST are consistent with prior decisions and do not change over time (17).

Advance care planning should be used in conjunction with an ongoing alliance with surrogates. Successful conversations focus on advance care planning as an ongoing process and are designed to help guide decision-making. Discussion of practical questions permits intensivists to highlight the inherent uncertainties of prognostication in medicine and the value of speaking in likelihoods.

While competent patients may modify their previously declared preferences, demented patients who previously made an informed choice to limit certain therapy may express an interest in receiving that therapy (18). If a patient manifests evidence of decision-making capacity, such as being able to provide internally coherent reasoning, their wishes to receive therapy should be honored. However, the process of resolving this situation in a patient without decision-making capacity, and with almost no likelihood of *regaining* decision-making capacity, is more complex. It would be quite easy to simply provide therapy; however, that is unlikely to reflect their true desires if they had decision-making capacity. In this situation, it is better to choose therapy based on multiple sources, including significant others, documentation, and the best interests standard.

REQUESTS FOR TREATMENT BELIEVED TO BE INADVISABLE

A therapy is labeled physiologically futile when it cannot accomplish its intended physiological goal, for example, when mechanical ventilation cannot accomplish pulmonary gas exchange. But when referring to therapy that has a low likelihood of achieving the intended goal, it makes more sense to use the concept of *inadvisable care* rather than focus on the muddied concept of futile therapy (19).

A therapy may be considered inadvisable because of the burden to the patient, cost, or uncertain benefit. Policies to resolve differences of opinions about inadvisable care should be procedurally based. Good policies are public, reflect the moral values of the community, and include processes for identifying stakeholders, initiating and conducting the policy, starting an appeal process commencing appellate mechanisms, and determining relevant information. Discussions about inadvisable treatment should bear in mind qualitative and quantitative considerations. The qualitative aspects define the goals of the treatment, and the quantitative aspects define likelihood of achieving a defined result. When offering likelihoods of a result, clinicians should be clear whether the information used to form the estimation is from intuition, clinical experience, or rigorous scientific studies. Scoring systems useful for population-level predictions should be considered as contributory but not determinative for decision-making for individuals. Clinicians should keep in mind that the clinical value of a therapy changes over time, and that previously indicated therapies became outdated (20).

It is not surprising that patients and families ask for what clinicians may consider to be inadvisable care; media and lore spur false hopes. On a societal level, inadvisable care is expensive, with some estimating that 11% of ICU patients were receiving inadvisable care, meaning that in addition to the expense, ICU beds may not be available (21,22).

In 1999, the Texas State Legislature passed the Texas Advance Directives Act (TADA) (23). TADA allows attending physicians to refuse to honor a patient's advance directive or a treatment decision made by or on behalf of the patient if the physician deems the care to be futile ("futile" in this case means unlikely to accomplish a specific nonphysiologic goal, such as hospital discharge). In order for care to be withdrawn, TADA requires that the case be reviewed by an ethics or medical committee of which the physician is not a member, and that the patient or surrogate is given a 48-hour notice of and an invitation to the case review. The patient or surrogate must receive patient transfer policies and potential accepting physicians and facilities, TADA requires 10 days—from time of receipt of committee's findings—of continued care to allow for transfer in the event that care is deemed futile (23).

A survey of Texas Hospital Association member institutions demonstrated that only a minority of hospitals used TADA to review specific cases and that, among those that did, discontinuation of potentially life-sustaining therapy against the will of the patient or their representative occurred in few cases (24). Supporters of TADA believe that the statute allows the due process standard to be upheld while allowing for more timely resolution of EOL therapy disputes, presumably minimizing patient suffering (25,26). Opponents, however, question whether TADA is too effective in terminating care, and whether an ethics committee can truly appreciate and represent the breadth of cultural and socioeconomic backgrounds that inform the decisions of patients and their surrogates (27). Opponents argue that unilateral physician declarations are insufficiently respectful of patient autonomy and that negotiation nearly always resolves these problems, belying the need for unilateral action. Aside from Texas' statute, case law has generally supported physicians and hospitals unilaterally refusing to provide inadvisable treatment (20).

CARE OF THE DYING PATIENT

"End-of-life care seems too early until it is too late—too often." (28)

Management of pain, dyspnea, and other distressing physical and psychological symptoms needs to be integrated into the routine of intensive care. By aggressively providing medical, emotional, psychological, and spiritual care, the patient is able to focus on decision-making and related matters (Table 2.1). Poor-quality EOL care harms more than the patient; one-third of family members who had relatives die in the ICU had post-traumatic stress syndrome (29).

Good EOL care requires successful communication between families, nurses, other clinicians, and physicians. In one study, 10% of family members in the ICU believed they received contradictory information from clinicians, and more than half of family members did not know the roles for each clinician (30). Factors that improve communication among clinicians and family include minimizing hierarchy, implementing protocols for multidisciplinary communication, and using team training to improve communication skills and diminish the effects of differences in training (31). Studies indicate that assorted interventions improve communication, particularly when using a standardized approach to communicating with families (32,33), daily goal sheets and checklists (34,35), daily medical updates and additional support personal (36), and proactive EOL conferences (33). Some of the interventions decreased length of stay, mortality, and costs, and improved the response to bereavement. Given the variety of successes, it may be reasonable to suggest that simply having a reasonable protocol improves communication.

Patients and families prioritize effective and honest communication and shared decision-making, which enables patients and families to avoid undesirable therapy, prepare for the future, receive compassionate care, and have trust and confidence in the clinicians. Families are concerned about financial matters, and patients are concerned about an adequate environment for care and minimizing physical and emotional burdens on family members (37).

Race, socioeconomic status, and gender may affect receiving good EOL care. Difficulties associated as a member of a minority group include inadequate access to care secondary to finances, geography, and language differences; due to historical abuses, members of minority groups may mistrust the health care establishment. Mistrust may spur them to attempt every therapy and to forgo palliative care, even though these choices may not be in the best interests of the patient, because of the suspicion that clinicians are not making their recommendation in the patient's best interests.

The future of assessing EOL communication and decision-making may be the implementation of quality indicators. A Canadian panel of experts proposed 34 quality indicators within the four categories of Advance Care Planning, Goals of Care Discussion, Documentation, and Organizational/System Aspects (38). Table 2.2 lists 10 indicators that were rated "extremely important" by the panel.

Time-Limited Trials

While ethically equivalent, there is an emotional difference between withdrawing and withholding care. But trying and then withdrawing therapy is superior to withholding therapy, because a trial of therapy will let patients, families, and clinicians know whether the therapy could be applied with an acceptable benefit-to-burden ratio.

A time-limited trial is "an agreement between clinicians and a patient/family to use certain medical therapies over a defined period to see if the patient improves or deteriorates according to the agreed on clinical outcomes" (39). Time-limited trials may help advance the discussion when there is tension between shifting to full comfort measures and proceeding with potentially burdensome treatments.

Explicit goals, straightforward cases, and clear ownership of the process by a clinician or service improve the success of time-limited trials. Goals may either be broad, such as the ability to do certain activities by a specific time, such as following simple commands, or they may be narrow and based on data, such as ventilatory support or laboratory values. The decision about which type of goal to use is determined by the patient and family, the clinical issue, the clinician, and the habits of the unit.

Barriers to initiating time-limited trials include patients and surrogates not being ready or feeling pressured into doing a time-limited trial, clinicians disagreeing about whether to do a trial or the proposed timeline and goals of the trial, and when

TABLE 2.1 Quality End-of-Life Care

Honor Patient	Address Needs of Clinicians	Address Needs of the Family
• Have a system for continually evaluating and communicating EOL preferences. • Review therapies at specified intervals to assess whether they are legitimate and consistent with the patient's desires. • Treat iatrogenic events by outcome and not by etiology. • Consider whether care guidelines apply to the specific patient.	• Commit to a multidisciplinary practice that leads to respectful and productive collaboration and communication. • Provide ongoing education about palliative care and cultural beliefs. • Provide opportunities for bereavement, debriefing, and psychological support. • Provide time and space for professional conversations and personal reflections.	• Have a presentable senior team member inform family of bad news in private using nontechnical language. • Help families find meaning in the death of their loved one. • Accept, support, and comfort the family. • Assure family of patient comfort. • Enable family to be with and help the patient. • Clarify roles of clinicians to family.
• Reassess advance care planning continuously and by focusing on the patient. • Initiate EOL discussions early. • Withdraw ventilatory therapy in a manner that permits recognition of distress; aggressively treat discomfort with opioids and sedatives.	• Identify objectives. • Review medical facts and options for treatment. • Agree on a care plan and on criteria to define success or failure of a plan. • Understand and respect the narratives and perspectives of others. • Seek out perspectives on dying, dependence and loss of function. • Use multidisciplinary approach to keep family informed. • Provide sufficient time for questions.	• Perform EOL research. • Measure and assess EOL care. • Promote a change in attitude toward EOL care. • Maintain knowledge of EOL law. • Maintain knowledge of EOL guidelines and care.
Incorporate palliative care into intensive care	**Hold regular meetings with family and team to clarify intermediate and long-term goals**	**Work to improve EOL care**

→ Quality End-of-Life Care

TABLE 2.2 Top-Quality Indicators for Improving End-of-Life Communication and Decision-Making

Quality Indicator	Category
1. Since admission, a member of the health care team has talked to the patient and/or SDM about a poor prognosis or indicated in some way that the patient has a limited time left to live.	Goals of Care Discussion
2. Documentation of a Goals of Care is present in the medical record.	Documentation
3. The Goals of Care are present in the medical record is consistent with the patient's stated preferences.	Documentation
4a. Since admission, a member of the health care team has talked to the patient and/or SDM about the outcomes, benefits, and burdens (or risks) of life-sustaining medical treatments.[a]	Goals of Care Discussion
4b. Since admission, a member of the health care team has talked to the patient and/or substitute decision-maker about outcomes, benefits, and burdens of focusing on comfort care as the goal of the patient's treatment (e.g., palliative care or treating symptoms like pain without trying to cure or control their underlying illness).[a]	Goals of Care Discussion
6. Since the patient's admission, a member of the health care team has offered to arrange a time when the patient/SDM and/or their family can meet with the doctor to discuss the treatment options and plans.	Goals of Care Discussion
7. Before hospitalization, the patient discussed his/her preferences for using or not using life-sustaining treatments with their SDM.	Advance Care Planning
8. Before hospitalization, the doctor talked to the patient and/or a family member about a poor prognosis or indicated in some way that the patient has a limited time left to live.	Advance Care Planning
9. If the hospital uses a standardized folder or other strategy to locate ACP/Goals of Care documents in the medical record, these are present in the medical record.	Documentation
10. Since the patient's admission, a member of the health care team has asked if the patient or the SDM (if patient is incapable) had prior discussions or has written documents about the use of life-sustaining treatments.	Goals of Care Discussion

[a]Tied.
SDM, shared decision-maker.
From Sinuff T, Dodek P, You JJ, Barwich D, et al. Improving end-of-life communication and decision making: the development of a conceptual framework and quality indicators. *J Pain Symptom Manag.* 2015;49(6):1070–1080.

there is little evidence to drive decision-making (40). Rapid clinical course changes and mercurial decisions to abandon previously chosen timelines hinder successful time-limited trials. Concerns about changes in clinical courses affecting time-limited trials should be addressed at the beginning by clarifying expectations and potential outcomes.

Palliative Care

Palliative care is designed to improve the quality of life for patients and families by treating the symptoms and stress of a life-threatening illness. Table 2.3 lists the more extensive World Health Organization definition (41). The future of palliative care is centered on implementing systems of care, including ensuring that quality palliative care is available to all patients, and systems to evaluate outcomes (14,42). Defining and documenting quality measures such as adequate pain control as part of the electronic health record will provide global and individual assessments for institutions and clinicians.

Barriers to integrating palliative care and critical care include assuming that palliative care and critical care are mutually exclusive instead of complementary, confusing palliative care with hospice, and presuming palliative care hastens death. Clinician training in palliative care is inadequate, and clinicians and units are inadequately incentivized to provide quality palliative care, leaving them to prioritize higher profile concerns (43).

Palliative care and hospice have subtle but critical differences. Palliative care is for the patient with a serious illness, is not based on prognosis, can coexist with being in the ICU and receiving intensive care therapy, and does not require limitations on therapies, including resuscitation therapies. Hospice care is based on prognosis, usually has therapy limitations, particularly on resuscitation therapies, and is managed by the hospice team.

Palliative Sedation

Palliative sedation (also known as terminal sedation) is the administration of medications to decrease or obliterate consciousness to minimize or eradicate the patient's experience of distressing symptoms. Palliative sedation should be used only in extreme circumstances when all other interventions,

TABLE 2.3 World Health Organization Definition of Palliative Care

Palliative care is an approach that improves the quality of life of patients and their families facing the problem associated with life-threatening illness, through the prevention and relief of suffering by means of early identification and impeccable assessment and treatment of pain and other problems, physical, psychosocial, and spiritual.

Palliative care:

- Provides relief from pain and other distressing symptoms
- Affirms life and regards dying as a normal process
- Intends neither to hasten or postpone death
- Integrates the psychological and spiritual aspects of patient care
- Offers a support system to help patients live as actively as possible until death
- Offers a support system to help the family cope during the patient's illness and in their own bereavement
- Uses a team approach to address the needs of patients and their families, including bereavement counseling, if indicated
- Will enhance quality of life, and may also positively influence the course of illness
- Is applicable early in the course of illness, in conjunction with other therapies that are intended to prolong life, such as chemotherapy or radiation therapy, and includes those investigations needed to better understand and manage distressing clinical complications

From World Health Organization. WHO definition of palliative care. Available at: http://www.who.int/cancer/palliative/definition/en/. Accessed September 1, 2015.

TABLE 2.4 Common Criteria for Patient Eligibility for Physician-Assisted Suicide and Euthanasia

- The patient must clearly, voluntarily, and repeatedly request to die.
- The patient's judgment must not be distorted.
- The patient must have an incurable condition associated with severe, unrelenting, and intolerable suffering.
- The physician is obligated to ensure the request is not made out of inadequate comfort care.
- PAS should be done in context of a physician–patient relationship.
- Consultation with other experts should be made to review and verify the facts about prognosis and current comfort management.
- Document above and fulfill reporting requirements.

Data from Quill TE, Cassel CK, Meier DE. Care of the hopelessly ill. Proposed clinical criteria for physician-assisted suicide. *N Engl J Med.* 1992;327:1380–1384; Vincent JL. End-of-life practice in Belgium and the new euthanasia law. *Intens Care Med.* 2006;32:1908–1911.

such as multidisciplinary evaluation and the use of therapy not intended to affect consciousness, fail. It should be used only for symptoms that are present and the expected duration of symptoms. It should not be used in anticipation of distressing symptoms. Palliative sedation may be used temporarily, if other solutions for symptom management become available (43).

PHYSICIAN-ASSISTED SUICIDE AND EUTHANASIA

The term *physician-assisted suicide (PAS)* means that the physician makes a lethal dose of medicine available to the patient based on the patient's voluntary and competent request, but that the patient must perform the act of ingestion. While requiring the patient to perform the final act may protect against abuses, psychological pressure may defeat safeguards inherent in requiring the patient to self-ingest. The term *euthanasia* means that the physician administers the lethal medication directly on a patient's voluntary and competent request. Table 2.4 lists common criteria for patient eligibility for PAS and euthanasia. Similarly, *nonvoluntary* euthanasia means that the physician administers the medication but there has been no formal request by the patient. Nonvoluntary euthanasia has occurred in some European countries, and over the years the rate has been mostly stable. Arguments surrounding PAS and euthanasia center on the interpretations of the principles of respect for autonomy and beneficence, as well as the possible ramifications of legalization (Table 2.5).

In general, patients wished to hasten death when they worried about suffering and receiving a substandard quality of care in the future, when they were depressed, hopeless, and without adequate social support, and when they consider themselves a burden to others. PAS and euthanasia are legal in the Netherlands, Belgium, Luxembourg, and Canada (44), and is permitted in Switzerland (45); PAS is permitted in Oregon, Vermont (46), and Washington State (45,47).

In 1997, the State of Oregon in the United States legalized the Oregon Death with Dignity Act, which permitted terminally ill patients to receive prescriptions in lethal quantities for the purpose of self-administration. From 1998 through 2014, 859 patients took the medication out of 1,327 (65%) prescriptions written for patients (48). The most common diseases for patients choosing PAS were malignant neoplasms (78% of patients), amyotrophic lateral sclerosis (8.3% of patients), and chronic lower respiratory tract diseases (4.4% of patients). There has been a steady increase, albeit slow, of the number of prescriptions written and the number of deaths. In 1998, 23 patients received prescriptions, and 21 patients died from taking the prescriptions (48); in 2006, 65 patients

TABLE 2.5 Arguments for and Against Legalizing Physician-Assisted Suicide (PAS) and Euthanasia

Factor	For	Against
Autonomy Individuals have the right to make informed choices about their lives.	• Individuals should be permitted to decide whether the burdens of being alive outweigh the benefits.	• Requests for PAS or euthanasia are false expressions of autonomy because inadequate control of suffering—including pain, discomfort, loss of dignity, depression, the feeling of being a personal and financial burden, and "tiredness of life"—lead to poorly informed and forced choices.
Beneficence The obligation to do good for our patients.	• Doing good means physicians are obligated to help patients have a good death (as defined by the patient).	• Doing good means doing a better job of maintaining patients' comfort and dignity.
Nonmalfeasance The obligation to "do no harm."		• Physicians do not cause death.
Legalization	• Legal safeguards and public oversight (such as the yearly reporting by the Oregon Department of Human Services on the Death with Dignity Act) will prevent abuses.	• There will be concerns that clinicians may offer, feel pressure to offer, or be perceived to offer PAS/euthanasia for inappropriate reasons (e.g., race, gender, socioeconomic status). • Permitting PAS or euthanasia will discourage physicians from aggressively addressing the problems surrounding end-of-life care. • Permitting PAS or euthanasia will devalue the sanctity of life, thus further nudging society down the psychological slippery slope toward nonvoluntary euthanasia.

received prescriptions, and 35 patients died from taking the prescriptions (48); in 2014, 155 patients received prescriptions, and 105 people died from taking the prescriptions (48). The financial and educational status of patients did not seem to play a role in the request for PAD. Primary concerns of patients were loss of autonomy, inability to engage in enjoyable activities, and loss of dignity. Interestingly, losing control of bodily functions, the situation being hard on family, and inadequate pain control were cited less than half of the patients.

In 2013, in Washington State, 173 patients received prescriptions (47); of the 173 patients, 159 are dead, 119 patients ingested the medication, 26 patients died without ingesting the medication, and in 14 patients the ingestion status was unknown. Prescriptions in Washington State are also increasing in frequency, and the data for underlying illnesses are similar to Oregon's data.

DISTRIBUTIVE JUSTICE AND RATIONING IN THE ICU

Distributive justice refers to an equitable allocation of resources. Distributive justice can be viewed as a substantive request, such as determining a fundamental and inviolable level of health care for all members of a society; it can also be viewed as a process for achieving justice, using approaches including queuing and potential benefit to determine valid distribution. These approaches belie simplicity; consider the different interpretations of benefit, such as quality-adjusted life years, functional status, or the fair innings approach, which aims to level the playing field for characteristics such as gender that are not under control of the individual.

It is helpful to consider three taxonomic categories of rationing (49). The first is the limited availability due to external constraints, such as not giving a medication that is not on a formulary or diverting ambulances from an emergency department of an overfull hospital. This form of rationing is beyond the clinician's control.

A second category of rationing occurs from the following clinical guidelines. For example, local hospital policies may define pathways for evaluation of certain diseases, such as requiring a specific radiologic study before proceeding to a more costly study. Deviations from clinical guidelines should be based on patient characteristics and scientific literature, not on personal idiosyncrasies.

The third category of rationing is based on clinical judgment; it is used when there is ambiguity about how guidelines should be applied or when guidelines do not exist. Clinical judgment is imperfect; decisions about therapy are influenced by a patient's ethnicity, pre-illness employment status, the intensivist's interest in rationing, and the political power of clinical services.

Fair rationing policies have the decision-making process and rationale publically available, a framework for principled decision-making as a means for resolving disputes, and an appeal process (50). When considering rationing, one should recognize the difference between the statistical patient and the individual, or identifiable, patient. Clinical guidelines are developed in reference to the statistical patient. It is easier and more proper to discuss rationing using the statistical patient, such as whether society should spend dollars on preventive care, primary care, or tertiary care. When participating in those debates on a macro level, clinicians may wish to consider their obligation to their patient community as well as to society.

Clinical judgment refers to the known individual patient. When faced with an identifiable patient whose situation does not align precisely with guidelines or studies, it is improper for a clinician to determine and implement rationing based on distributive justice at the bedside (49).

Triaging is a special consideration of distributive justice. Utility principles encourage actions that maximize "the greatest good for the greatest number," and are at the heart of permitting unequal outcomes as long as overall health is maximized. For example, clinicians in the midst of a mass casualty will choose to provide discrete, rapid, and potentially life-sustaining care, such as chest tubes and endotracheal intubation, to many patients before devoting these resources to the treatment of a single resource-intensive head injury (51). Implicit in the utility principle is that like patients are treated similarly, without regard to other factors, such as socioeconomic status. The utility principle is suitable for a mass casualty situation in which all patients are equally unknown and no prior relationship with the patient has been established. It may, however, be less suitable for considering distribution of an absolute scarce resource, such as extracorporeal membrane oxygenation. In this case, many would suggest that the presence of a patient–physician relationship, current use of the resource, the appropriateness of the claim to the resource, and the idea that every person should have an equal chance to potentially life-sustaining resources should weigh heavily in these complicated balancing-act decisions.

Conscientious Objections

Conscientious objections can be defined as "as objections to providing or disclosing information about legal, professionally accepted, and otherwise available medical services based on a clinician's judgment that to do what is requested would be morally wrong"(52). These may include, for example, offering palliative sedation, or informing about the option of withdrawing nutrition and hydration. It is important to honor what would seem to be an inappropriate authority not to offer appropriate services, because there is value in enabling clinicians to maintain ethical integrity. On the other hand, permitting use of conscientious objections could harm vulnerable patients, burden other clinicians, and provide an out for those who wish not to honor professional commitments. The American Thoracic Society has made policy recommendations designed to protect clinicians' moral integrity and to protect patients' access to legitimate medical services (52). Institutions should develop policies and processes to manage and prospectively identify conscientious objections. Institutions should try to accommodate conscientious objections as long as there is no impediment to the patient's access to medical services or information, it will not create hardship for other clinicians, and the objection is not based on discrimination or other unjust reasons. A conscientious objection should not be considered a valid excuse to unilaterally forgo treatment of potentially inappropriate medical services; other mechanisms of resolution should be used in those cases.

HEALTH CARE ETHICS CONSULTATION IN THE ICU

Health care ethics consultation (HCEC) is defined as "a set of services provided by an individual or group in response to questions from patients, families, surrogates, health care providers, or other involved parties who seek to resolve uncertainty or conflict regarding value-laden concerns that emerge in health care" (53). The overriding goal of HCEC is to "improve the quality of health care through the identification, analysis, and resolution of ethical questions or concerns" (53). The process of HCEC is to gather relevant data, clarify relevant concepts and related normative issues, help identify a range of morally acceptable options within the context of the situation, and facilitate consensus among involved parties (54).

In larger adult hospitals, about half of all HCEC requests come from the ICU, and the most common categories relate to appropriate decision-making, goals of care, and EOL management. The most common topics were withdrawing or withholding treatment, patient wishes and respect for autonomy, and decision-making capacity (55,56). HCEC can help address treatment conflicts, reduce costs without diminishing quality, and limit inappropriate or unwanted interventions. In a randomized, prospective, cohort study in which addressing medical uncertainty or conflict were compared, patients in the intervention group, who received an ethics consultation, had a shorter length of ICU and hospital stays and significantly improved achievement of agreement of the goals of medical care (57). The frequency of HCEC will likely increase, given the aging population, continuing technological advances, the easy availability of information, and the increased participation of patients and families in determining care.

Key Points

- Treat patients and families with the grace and consideration you would want you and your family to be treated—that is, with respect for personal values, feelings, and preferences.
- Evaluate and implement continuing quality improvements in ICU communication and decision-making.
- POLST have the authority of physician's orders and are transferrable and actionable across clinical sites and states POLST is likely more effective in ensuring patient's wishes are followed than other forms of advance care planning.
- The concept of inadvisable care has replaced the concept of futility when considering whether to use a therapy with a low likelihood of success and a questionable benefit-to-burden ratio.
- Time-limited trials, trying a certain therapy over a defined period to see the benefits and burdens of therapy, is more ethically supportable than withholding therapy, because it gives an opportunity to see of a therapy provides an acceptable benefit-to-burden ration.
- Palliative care is designed to improve the quality of life for patients and families by treating the symptoms and stress of a life-threatening illness. It is complementary to critical care, is not based on prognosis, and requires no limitations on therapy.
- Palliative sedation, using sedation to depress consciousness to minimize the experience of distressing symptoms, only should be used as a last resort and to treat symptoms that are present.
- The process of HCEC is to gather data, interview stakeholders, clarify relevant concepts, identify morally acceptable options, and facilitate consensus among involved parties. HCEC may decrease ICU stay and improve agreement on goals of care.

References

1. Cook D, Rocker G, Giacomini M, et al. Understanding and changing attitudes toward withdrawal and withholding of life support in the intensive care unit. *Crit Care Med.* 2006;34(11 Suppl):S317–S323.
2. Standards for cardiopulmonary resuscitation (CPR) and emergency cardiac care (ECC). *JAMA.* 1974;227(Suppl):833–868.
3. *In the Matter of Karen Quinlan.* 70 N.J. 10,335 A.2d 647, cert. denied, 429 U.S. 922. 1976.
4. *Bartling v. Superior Court.* 163 Cal.App.3d 186 [209 Cal.Rptr. 220]. 1984.
5. Cruzan v. Director. Missouri Department of Health,110 S. Ct. 2841. 1990.
6. Bioethicists' statement on the U.S. Supreme Court's Cruzan decision. *N Engl J Med.* 1990;323:686–687.
7. *In re the Conservatorship of Helga M. Wanglie.* No. PX-91–283, District Probate Division, 4th Judicial District of the County of Hennepin, State of Minnesota. 1993.
8. Angell M. The case of Helga Wanglie: a new kind of "right to die" case. *N Engl J Med.* 1991;325:511–512.
9. *Betancourt v. Trinitas.* Superior Court of New Jersey, A-3849- 08T2. 1 A.3d 823 (N.J. Super. A.D. 2010). 2010.
10. *Gilgunn v. Massachusetts General Hospital.* Superior Court Civil Action No. 92–4820, Suffolk Co., MA.; verdict April 21. 1995.
11. Council on Ethical and Judicial Affairs, American Medical Association. Decisions near the end of life. *JAMA.* 1992;267:2229–2233.
12. Houben CH, Spruit MA, Groenen MT, et al. Efficacy of advance care planning: a systematic review and meta-analysis. *J Am Med Dir Assoc.* 2014; 15(7):477–489.
13. Wilson ME, Krupa A, Hinds RF, et al. A video to improve patient and surrogate understanding of cardiopulmonary resuscitation choices in the ICU: a randomized controlled trial. *Crit Care Med.* 2015;43(3):621–629.
14. Institute of Medicine. *Dying in America: Improving Quality and Honoring Individual Preferences Near the End of Life.* Washington, DC: The National Academies Press; 2015.
15. Fromme EK, Zive D, Schmidt TA, et al. Association between physician orders for life-sustaining treatment for scope of treatment and in-hospital death in Oregon. *J Am Geriatr Soc.* 2014;62(7):1246–1251.
16. Pedraza SL, Culp S, Falkenstine EC, Moss AH. POST forms more than advance directives associated with out-of-hospital death: insights from a state registry. *J Pain Symptom Manag.* 2015. doi: 10.1016/j.jpainsymman.2015.10.003
17. Hickman SE, Nelson CA, Smith-Howell E, Hammes BJ. Use of the physician orders for life-sustaining treatment program for patients being discharged from the hospital to the nursing facility. *J Palliat Med.* 2014;17(1):43–49.
18. Woien S. Conflicting preferences and advance directives. *Am J Bioeth.* 2007; 7(4):64–66.
19. Truong R, Devita M, Dagi F, et al. Consensus statement of the Society of Critical Care Medicine's Ethics Committee regarding futile and other possibly inadvisable treatments. *Crit Care Med.* 1997;25(5):887–891.
20. Swetz KM, Burkle CM, Berge KH, Lanier WL. Ten common questions (and their answers) on medical futility. *Mayo Clin Proc.* 2014;89(7):943–959.
21. Huynh TN, Kleerup EC, Wiley JF, et al. The frequency and cost of treatment perceived to be futile in critical care. *JAMA Intern Med.* 2013; 173(20):1887–1894.
22. Huynh TN, Kleerup EC, Raj PP, Wenger NS. The opportunity cost of futile treatment in the ICU. *Crit Care Med.* 2014;42(9):1977–1982.
23. Texas Health and Safety Code. Chapter 166. Advance Directives.
24. Smith ML, Gremillion G, Slomka J, Warneke CL. Texas hospitals' experience with the Texas Advance Directives Act. *Crit Care Med.* 2007; 35(5):1271–1276.

25. Fine RL. Point: the Texas advance directives act effectively and ethically resolves disputes about medical futility. *Chest.* 2009;136(4):963–967.
26. Jecker NS, Jecker NS. Futility and fairness: a defense of the Texas Advance Directive Law. *Am J Bioeth.* 2015;15(8):43–46.
27. Truog RD. Tackling medical futility in Texas. *N Engl J Med.* 2007; 357(1):1–3.
28. Nelson JE. Identifying and overcoming the barriers to high-quality palliative care in the intensive care unit. *Crit Care Med.* 2006;34(11 Suppl):S324–S331.
29. Azoulay E, Pochard F, Kentish-Barnes N, et al. Risk of post-traumatic stress symptoms in family members of intensive care unit patients. *Am J Respir Crit Care Med.* 2005;171(9):987–994.
30. Azoulay E, Pochard F, Chevret S, et al. Meeting the needs of intensive care unit patient families: a multicenter study. *Am J Respir Crit Care Med.* 2001; 163(1):135–139.
31. Schwarze ML, Bradley CT, Brasel KJ. Surgical "buy-in": the contractual relationship between surgeons and patients that influences decisions regarding life-supporting therapy. *Crit Care Med.* 2010;38(3):843–848.
32. Shaw DJ, Davidson JE, Smilde RI, et al. Multidisciplinary team training to enhance family communication in the ICU. *Crit Care Med.* 2014;42(2): 265–371.
33. Lautrette A, Darmon M, Megarbane B, et al. A communication strategy and brochure for relatives of patients dying in the ICU. *N Engl J Med.* 2007; 356(5):469–478.
34. Pronovost P, Berenholtz S, Dorman T, et al. Improving communication in the ICU using daily goals. *J Crit Care.* 2003;18(2):71–75.
35. Centofanti JE, Duan EH, Hoad NC, et al. Use of a daily goals checklist for morning ICU rounds: a mixed-methods study. *Crit Care Med.* 2014;1797–a803.
36. Ahrens T, Yancey V, Kollef M. Improving family communications at the end of life: implications for length of stay in the intensive care unit and resource use. *Am J Crit Care.* 2003;12(4):317–323.
37. Virdun C, Luckett T, Davidson PM, Phillips J. Dying in the hospital setting: a systematic review of quantitative studies identifying the elements of end-of-life care that patients and their families rank as being most important. *Palliat Med.* 2015;29:774–796.
38. Sinuff T, Dodek P, You JJ, Barwich D, et al. Improving end-of-life communication and decision making: the development of a conceptual framework and quality indicators. *J Pain Symptom Manag.* 2015;49(6):1070–1080.
39. Quill TE. Time-limited trials near the end of life. *JAMA.* 2011;306(13): 1483–1484.
40. Bruce CR, Liang C, Blumenthal-Barby JS, et al. Barriers and facilitators to initiating and completing time-limited trials in critical care. *Crit Care Med.* 2015;43(12):2535–2543.
41. World Health Organization. WHO Definition of palliative care. Available at: http://www.who.int/cancer/palliative/definition/en/. Accessed September 1, 2015.
42. Schenker Y, Arnold R. The next era of palliative care. *JAMA.* 2015; 314(15):1–2.
43. Aslakson R, Curtis JR, Nelson JE. The changing role of palliative care in the ICU. *Crit Care Med.* 2014;42(11):2418–2428.
44. *Carter v. Canada* (Attorney General), 2015 SCC 5 Title.
45. Steck N, Egger M, Maessen M, et al. Euthanasia and assisted suicide in selected European countries and US states: systematic literature review. *Med Care.* 2013;51(10):938–944.
46. Patient choice and control at end of life. Vermont Department of Health Web site. Available at: http://healthvermont.gov/family/end_of_life_care/patient_choice.aspx. Accessed November 3, 2015.
47. Washington State Department of Health. Washington State Department of Health 2013 Death with Dignity Act Report: Executive Summary. Available at: http://www.doh.wa.gov/portals/1/Documents/Pubs/422–109-DeathWithDignityAct2013.pdf. Accessed September 1, 2015.
48. Oregon Health Authority. *Oregon's Death with Dignity Act, 2014.* Salem, OR: Oregon Public Health Division.
49. Truog RD, Brock DW, Cook DJ, et al. Rationing in the intensive care unit. *Crit Care Med.* 2006;34(4):958–963.
50. Smith GP 2nd. Distributive justice and health care. *J Contemp Heal Law Policy.* 2002;18(2):421–430.
51. Moskop JC, Iserson K V. Triage in medicine, part II: Underlying values and principles. *Ann Emerg Med.* 2007;49(3):282–287.
52. Lewis-Newby M, Wicclair M, Pope T, et al. An official American Thoracic Society policy statement: managing conscientious objections in intensive care medicine. *Am J Respir Crit Care Med.* 2015;191(2):219–227.
53. Tarzian AJ, ASBH Core Competencies Update Task. Health care ethics consultation: an update on core competencies and emerging standards from the American Society for Bioethics and Humanities' Core Competencies Update Task Force. *Am J Bioeth.* 2013;13(2):3–13.
54. Aulisio MP, Arnold RM, Youngner SJ. Health care ethics consultation: nature, goals, and competencies: a position paper from the Society for Health and Human Values-Society for Bioethics Consultation Task Force on Standards for Bioethics Consultation. *Ann Intern Med.* 2000;133(1):59–69.
55. Wasson K, Anderson E, Hagstrom E, et al. What ethical issues really arise in practice at an academic medical center? A quantitative and qualitative analysis of clinical ethics consultations from 2008 to 2013. *HEC Forum.* September 30, 2015.
56. Moeller JR, Albanese TH, Garchar K, et al. Functions and outcomes of a clinical medical ethics committee: a review of 100 consults. *HEC Forum.* 2012;24(2):99–114.
57. Chen Y-Y, Chu T-S, Kao Y-H, et al. To evaluate the effectiveness of health care ethics consultation based on the goals of health care ethics consultation: a prospective cohort study with randomization. *BMC Med Ethics.* 2014;15(1):1.

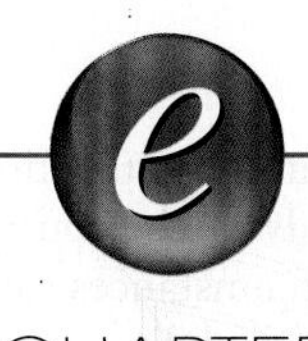

This chapter can be accessed in the accompanying eBook (see inside front cover for access instructions).

CHAPTER 3

Understanding Reactions of Patients and Families/Breaking Bad News to Patients

CRAIGAN T. USHER and EUGENE V. BERESIN

CHAPTER 4

Judicial Involvement in End-of-Life Decisions and Informed Consent

MICHAEL SUK, ANDREW M. SKINNER, SONAL MAHAJAN, and CORY FRANKLIN

END-OF-LIFE DECISIONS

Medical decision-making, as an extension of the physician–patient relationship, is grounded in ethical principles of autonomy and self-determination. From a legal perspective, it can be a matter of contractual obligation or civil duty. A basic assumption governing the shared responsibility is a "meeting of the minds" in the process of consultation and informed decision-making. Decisions made at the end of life, however, often lack clear direction and are fraught by mitigating medical and legal circumstances, leaving lingering doubt as to the final disposition of a patient's concern. It is in these areas that an often-reluctant judiciary has developed a growing body of case law guiding their role in the finality of life.

Foundational Principles

Informed Consent and the Right to Refuse Treatment

Informed consent is an ethical concept that all patients should understand and agree to the potential consequences of their care. It is typically the outcome of an open and deliberate conversation between medical provider and patient; once established, a treatment or procedure may ensue. Rooted in principles of autonomy and self-determination, the courts have long upheld that one's body may not be violated without proper approval.

A corollary to the right *to consent* to medical treatment is a patient's right *to not consent* (to refuse) medical treatment. In January 1908, Mary Schloendorff was admitted to New York Hospital to evaluate and treat a stomach disorder. During her stay at the hospital, she was diagnosed as having a fibroid tumor. The physician recommended surgery, which Schloendorff adamantly declined, although she did consent to an examination under ether anesthesia. During the procedure, the doctors performed surgery to remove the tumor. Afterwards, Schloendorff developed gangrene in the left arm, ultimately leading to the amputation of some fingers. Schloendorff blamed the surgery, and filed suit. Justice Benjamin Cardozo wrote the Court's opinion, in which he stated, "[e]very human being of adult years and sound mind has a right to determine what shall be done with his own body... [T]he doctrine of informed consent—a doctrine borne of the common-law right to be free from nonconsensual physical invasions—permits an individual to refuse medical treatment" (1).

Until recently, there were relatively few cases involving a patient's right to refuse care (2). However, technologic advances in medicine have made it possible to sustain life—or, alternatively stated, prolong dying—through artificial means (3). Generally speaking, it is the exercise of this "fundamental" right to refuse treatment that is at the center of most judicial intervention in treatment decisions. In particular, judicial intervention has been often sought out where there is disagreement between the desires of patients, surrogates, family, and/or providers regarding the terminal disposition of medical care.

Prolonging Life or Accelerating Death

The Case of Karen Ann Quinlan

In 1975, 22-year-old Karen Ann Quinlan went to a party at a friend's house and proceeded to consume a combination of diazepam and alcohol. Reportedly, she had been on a crash diet and had not eaten in the previous 2 days. Shortly afterwards she felt faint, and was quickly taken home and put to bed. When friends checked on her about 15 minutes later, they found she was not breathing. Paramedics were called and during the resuscitation, she regained a pulse but did not regain consciousness. Three days after admission, she was diagnosed as comatose and required a mechanical ventilator to assist her breathing; the coma was followed by a persistent vegetative state. At the time that the New Jersey Supreme Court considered the case, which was less than 1 year after her anoxic event, Quinlan had lost at least 40 pounds, and was in a permanent fetal-like position with her joints severely rigid and deformed (4).

Joseph and Julia Quinlan, believing that their daughter would not want to continue to live in this condition, requested the withdrawal of life support. Her physician refused, believing that the standard of care at that time prohibited withdrawal (5). After the physicians refused the request of her parents to disconnect Quinlan's ventilator, which they believed constituted extraordinary means of prolonging her life, her parents filed suit to force discontinuation from her ventilator. Complicating matters, hospital officials, too, faced threats of homicide charges if they complied with the parent's request.

The Quinlans filed a suit on September 12, 1975, to request that the extraordinary means prolonging Quinlan's life be terminated. The Quinlans' lawyer argued that Quinlan's right to make a private decision about her fate superseded the state's right to keep her alive, while Quinlan's court-appointed guardian argued that disconnecting her ventilator would be homicide. The suit was denied by New Jersey Superior Court Judge Robert Muir Jr. in November 1975, stating that Quinlan's doctors did not support removing her from the ventilator, that whether or not to do so was a medical, rather than a judicial, decision, and that doing so would violate New Jersey homicide statutes (4).

The Quinlans appealed the decision to the New Jersey Supreme Court. On March 31, 1976, the court granted their appeal, citing that the right to privacy was broad enough to encompass the Quinlans' request on Quinlan's behalf. The Court stated:

> [N]o external compelling interest of the State could compel Karen to endure the unendurable, only to vegetate a few measurable months with no realistic possibility of returning to any semblance of cognitive or sapient life. We perceive no thread of logic distinguishing between such a choice on Karen's part and a similar choice which, under the evidence in this case, could be made by a competent patient, terminally ill, riddled with cancer and suffering great pain; such a patient would not be resuscitated or put on a respirator [as testified by an expert neurologist in the case] and *a fortiori* would not be kept *against his will* on a respirator. (4)

Having found there was no compelling state interest to support interference with Karen's right to refuse life-prolonging treatment, the court addressed the contention that discontinuation of life-supporting treatment for Karen was inconsistent with the prevailing medical standards (6). Recognizing the uncertainty regarding potential civil and criminal liability for openly practicing the evolving medical standard of withholding or withdrawing such treatment, the Court carefully delineated a role for consultation with hospital ethics committees. And finally, with very little analysis, the court found that the termination of life support in circumstances such as Karen Quinlan's would not lead to criminal liability, concluding that while the state has the power to punish the taking of human life, that power does not extend to an individual's exercise of their privacy right to refuse medical treatment, and by extension, to a third party exercising that right for the patient.*

Quinlan's case continues to raise important questions related to moral theology, bioethics, euthanasia, legal guardianship, and civil rights. Her case has affected the practice of medicine and law around the world. A significant outcome of her case was the development of formal ethics committees in hospitals, nursing homes, and hospices.

The State Interest Test

Joseph Saikewicz, a 67-year-old man with the mental age of a 2½ years old, was a resident of the Belchertown State School in Belchertown, MA. In April 1976—1 month after the Quinlan decision—Saikewicz was diagnosed with acute myeloblastic monocytic leukemia. A *guardian ad litem* was appointed by the State to provide direction for Saikewicz's medical care. After reviewing the recommendation of Saikewicz's attending physicians which stated that the patient should not receive chemotherapy, the *guardian ad litem* recommended that Saikewicz go untreated, letting his disease run its natural course.

The *Saikewicz* court was presented with expert testimony indicating that acute myeloblastic monocytic leukemia was, at that time, incurable and inevitably fatal. Regardless, most capacitated patients chose to have chemotherapy, enduring its significantly unpleasant side effects even though the potential for remission was only 30% to 50% and, when it did occur, remission typically lasted for only 2 to 13 months. Thus, while chemotherapy was the normal medically indicated course of treatment, it could only provide the possibility of some uncertain and limited extension of life. Given Saikewicz's age and condition, the court was informed that left untreated, he would live for a matter of weeks or, at most, several months. Further, given his mental age, Saikewicz would not likely be able to comprehend the reasons to endure the treatment, nor appreciate its potential benefit and likely require restraint, which would cause him mental and physical anguish.

The court issued its order on July 9, 1976; Saikewicz died on September 4, due to bronchial pneumonia. On November 28, 1977, the *Saikewicz* court issued an opinion intended to provide comprehensive guidance in the review of cases related to the withholding of critical care in end-of-life situations, both for capacitated and incapacitated patients.

In its opinion, the *Saikewicz* court developed a four-pronged test to evaluate the "state's interest" and has been widely adopted by the courts in determining when an individual patient's ability to exercise her or his constitutional right to refuse treatment can be circumscribed:

(1) The preservation of life
(2) The protection of the interests of innocent third parties
(3) The prevention of suicide
(4) Maintaining the ethical integrity of the medical profession (7)

*When she was taken off the ventilator, Quinlan surprised many by continuing to breathe unaided, and was fed by artificial nutrition for 9 more years, until her death from respiratory failure in 1985.

Substituted Judgment

In addition to articulating the four state interests to be used in determining when a patient's fundamental right to refuse life-prolonging medical treatment may be denied, the *Saikewicz* court addresses the important question regarding the rights of an *incompetent* patient to forgo such treatment. The *Saikewicz* court believed that the "substituted judgment" standard would best preserve respect for the integrity and autonomy of the patient. In other words, the decision-maker's role would be to put himself/herself in Saikewicz's position and make the treatment decision the patient most likely would make were he competent. In this case, the court believed Saikewicz would have refused treatment.

"Clear and Convincing" Standard

In 1981, two cases involving the guardians of terminally ill, incapacitated patients objecting to the continued use of life-prolonging treatments further delineated the boundaries of "substituted judgment."

The first case was the 83-year-old Brother Joseph Fox; this patient suffered cardiac arrest and substantial brain damage; he was placed on a ventilator, and remained in a persistent vegetative state. Father Philip Eichner, a close friend, and leader of the Catholic order, acted as Fox's surrogate for medical decision-making. He reflected that in private conversations with Father Eichner, Fox had previously made it known that he would not have wanted to be maintained on a respirator in his present condition; the Court agreed.

In the second case, John Storar, a 52-year old man, profoundly mentally disabled since birth was diagnosed with terminal cancer of the bladder. With a prognosis for a very limited lifespan, palliative blood transfusions would be required frequently to maintain his daily activities; the Court refused to permit the withdrawal of treatment.

The key distinction between these cases according to the Court was the question of competence. The case of Brother Fox involved a man who was, at one time, competent for medical decision-making; this is as opposed to Storar who, at no time, had such capacity. The Court identified four key points that continue to provide us with guidance today:

(1) A patient's common-law right to determine the course of his own medical treatment is paramount to the doctor's obligation to provide needed medical care.
(2) Clear and convincing proof is required in cases where it is claimed that a person, now incompetent, left instructions to terminate life-sustaining procedures when there is no hope of recovery.
(3) An individual who was never competent at any time in his life is considered still a child and a parent may not deprive a child of life-saving treatment, however, well intentioned.
(4) Neither the common law nor the existing state statutes require persons to seek prior court approval in cases involving discontinuance of life-sustaining treatment for incompetent.

The Right to Die

The Case of Nancy Cruzan

On January 11, 1983, Nancy Cruzan lost control of her car and was thrown from the vehicle landing face down in a water-filled ditch. Paramedics found her with no vital signs, but they resuscitated her. After 3 weeks in a coma, she was diagnosed as being in a persistent vegetative state (8); surgeons inserted a feeding tube for her long-term care.

Rehabilitative efforts failed, and when it became apparent in 1988 that she had no medically reasonable chance of recovery, her parents—who were her court-appointed guardians—requested that the hospital terminates artificial nutrition and hydration measures. The hospital refused to do so without a court order, since the removal of the tube would cause Cruzan's death.

The Cruzans filed for, and received, a court order for the feeding tube to be removed. The trial court ruled that, constitutionally, there is a "fundamental natural right ... to refuse or direct the withholding or withdrawal of artificial death prolonging procedures when the person has no more cognitive brain function ... and there is no hope of further recovery" (9). The Court specifically noted that Nancy had effectively "directed" the withdrawal of life support by telling a friend earlier that year that if she were sick or injured, "she would not wish to continue her life unless she could live at least halfway normally" (9).

The State of Missouri appealed this decision. In a 4 to 3 decision, the Supreme Court of Missouri reversed the trial court's decision. It ruled that no one may refuse treatment for another person, absent an adequate living will "or the clear and convincing, inherently reliable evidence absent here" (10). The Cruzans appealed, and in 1989, the Supreme Court of the United States agreed to hear the case (11).

The legal question in this case was whether the State of Missouri had the right to require "clear and convincing evidence" in order for the Cruzans to remove their daughter from life support. Specifically, the Supreme Court considered whether Missouri was violating the Due Process Clause of the Fourteenth Amendment, which "protects individuals, conscious or unconscious, from such invasion by the state, without any particularized interest for that invasion" (12).

In a split 5 to 4 decision, the Court found in favor of the Missouri Department of Health. Upholding the Missouri Supreme Court's ruling, the United States Supreme Court ruled that nothing in the Constitution prevents the state of Missouri from requiring "clear and convincing evidence" before terminating life-supporting treatment (13).

The Court did rule that competent individuals have the right to refuse medical treatment under the Due Process Clause. However, with incompetent individuals, the Court upheld the state of Missouri's higher standard for evidence of what the person would want if they were able to make their own decisions. This higher evidentiary standard was constitutional, the Court ruled, because family members might not always make decisions that the incompetent person would have agreed with, and those decisions might lead to actions (like withdrawing life support) that would be irreversible (13). The Cruzan case:

(1) Recognized a "right to die" but carefully noted that this was not guaranteed by the Constitution
(2) Set out rules for what was required in order for a third party to refuse treatment on behalf of an incompetent person
(3) Established that, absent a living will or clear and convincing evidence of what the incompetent person would have wanted, the state's interests in preserving life outweigh the individual's rights to refuse treatment
(4) It left it to the states to determine their own right to die standards, rather than creating a uniform national standard (14)

Ongoing Challenges to the Right to Die

In February 1990, at the age of 27, Terri Schiavo suffered a cardiac arrest. She was resuscitated by paramedics, but never regained consciousness. Almost 9 years later, her husband, Michael Schiavo, petitioned the court to authorize removal of her feeding tube, arguing that Terri would not have wanted prolonged artificial life support without the prospect of recovery, and elected to remove her feeding tube. Schiavo's parents argued in favor of continuing artificial nutrition and hydration, and challenged Schiavo's medical diagnosis (15). The highly publicized and prolonged series of legal challenges presented by her parents, which ultimately involved state and federal politicians up to the level of President George W. Bush, caused a 7-year delay before Schiavo's feeding tube was ultimately removed.

In all, the *Schiavo* case involved 14 appeals and numerous motions, petitions, and hearings in the Florida courts; 5 suits in federal district court; extensive political intervention at the levels of the Florida state legislature, then-governor Jeb Bush, the US Congress, and President George W. Bush; and 4 denials of certiorari from the Supreme Court of the United States (16).

The *Schiavo* case did not change the landscape of legal authority surrounding the "right to die" as established by Quinlan and Cruzan. The courts recognized Schiavo as a permanently incapacitated patient and authorized her guardians to withdraw life-sustaining treatment—ventilator support and feeding tube—as compelled by "clear and convincing" evidence balanced against the four-pronged test of the State's interest. However, the prolonged nature of the case and its involvement of all three branches of government act as a testament to the ongoing controversy, emotion, and debate surrounding the withdrawal of life-sustaining treatment from a permanently incapacitated patient.

Conclusion

Decisions at the end of life have been made significantly more difficult with the advancement of technology that keeps physiologic functions intact in the absence of cognition. The cases reviewed here reflect the case of law authority that guides judicial involvement when conflict arises. Ultimately categorized as "right to die" cases, as illustrated by the *Schiavo* case, legal precedent does not eliminate controversy. What is clear, however, is that the individual power of medical decision-making to accept or refuse treatment is protected by the penumbra of the Due Process Clause of the Constitution of the United States. This individual right is balanced against the State's interest in the preservation of life and is more easily defended when one's wishes are made clear through legal instruments such as an advanced directive. In the case of incapacity, the courts struggle with their role in adjudicating these decisions and have established a standard of clear and convincing evidence to support the substituted judgment where incapacity exists.

INFORMED CONSENT

Informed consent is the process of providing patients with information about the risks, benefits, and potential alternatives to the care they are offered. Informed consent is an essential part of the therapeutic discussion and is central to the relationship created between patient and physician (17–20).

While the roots of the informed consent doctrine can be traced as far back as the Magna Carta, its practical basis was established in the early 20th century in the 1914 New York case *Schloendorff v. New York Hospital*, as noted above (1).

While *Schloendorff* is nearly synonymous with patient autonomy and informed consent today, at the time there was no specific mention of informed consent as an actual principle. The case did not address issues such as what amount or type of information is necessary for a patient to make appropriate care decisions, nor did it result in damage recovery.

The process of informed consent did not become an established part of American medical practice until the late 20th century. Two historical tragedies proved instrumental in the creation of the informed consent doctrine as we know it today. The first event was the Nuremberg Code (1946 to 1949), which was developed as a result of the notorious Nazi medical experiments at Dachau during World War II (21). This code provided that "voluntary consent of the human subject is absolutely essential" and "the person involved…should have sufficient knowledge and comprehension of the elements of the subject matter as to enable him to make an understanding and enlightened decision" (22).

The Tuskegee Syphilis Study (1932 to 1972), conducted under the direction of the United States government, marked the second event. The study resulted in the deliberate withholding of syphilis treatment from several hundred rural African-American males so that investigators could gain information regarding the serious complications of late-stage syphilis. When the facts surrounding this experiment finally became public, it raised the consciousness about the rights of patients and research subjects regarding what information doctors must disclose (23).

Unfortunately, a wide gap persists between the idealized elements of informed consent and current clinical practices. Too often, "informed consent" is simply another shopworn phrase of internal contradictions along the lines of "rush hour," "United Nations," or "reliable software." Simply put, when a harried medical student, nurse, or ward clerk hurries into a patient's room with a boilerplate form, the patient is expected to sign immediately; informed consent is thus often neither informed nor consent. A signed informed consent form is not the same as *getting* informed consent (24).

In this section, we discuss the current status of informed consent in the intensive care unit (ICU), stressing the principles of sharing information, making good faith attempts to understand patient values and decision-making processes, and finally, avoiding manipulation and coercion of the vulnerable ICU patient.

ETHICAL FOUNDATIONS OF INFORMED CONSENT

The ethical foundations of informed consent encompass the classic principles of autonomy, beneficence, and justice. These three virtues provide the moral framework for informed consent and present guidelines for appropriate clinical action (25).

Autonomy

Autonomy, from the Greek words for self (*auto*) and rule (*nomos*), refers to the capacity for self-governing and the patient's right to self-determination. This includes the right to select a course of medical therapy that best reflects individual values and preferences. A prerequisite of autonomy is that an individual maintains the right to hold certain beliefs and to exercise independent thought. From these principles arise the ability to choose a specific course of action, to act according to this preference, and to accept the consequences of that decision. This necessarily presumes an individual has access to relevant information and also possesses freedom from both internal and external constraints.

Practically speaking, before patients can reasonably form opinions regarding available therapeutic options, they must first appreciate the nature of their medical condition, recognize the range of possible interventions, and understand the possible risks, benefits, and consequences associated with each option. This is essentially the mental checklist the physician should perform when speaking with the patient. It is the physician's duty to ensure that the patient understands the medical diagnosis, the details of the proposed therapy, the available alternatives, and the consequences of refusal. Although the responsibility to provide this information lies with the physician, it is the patient who must ultimately integrate the facts and determine the most appropriate course of action.

Generally, autonomous action requires that individuals enter into the physician–patient relationship voluntarily and remain free to accept or refuse treatment without feeling coerced or intimidated; this is often not the case in the ICU. Patients frequently arrive in the ICU in a vulnerable condition, and are often admitted without their consent or knowledge; the additional stresses of critical illness leave them susceptible to fear, pain, or anxiety. With these factors in mind, the intensivist must maintain a balance between talking to the patient and making prompt therapeutic decisions. Given the emergent nature of developments in the ICU, it may be impractical to engage in extensive discussion about every procedure or therapy, but whenever possible, it is essential to provide patients with sufficient information to let them guide the overall course of their care. The balance between acting and letting the patient act characterizes the essence of informed consent in the ICU (26).

Beneficence

Beneficence—doing good—and its associated principle, nonmaleficence—not doing harm—embody the physician's obligation to provide benefit while refraining from committing harm. Beneficence requires the physician to treat illness, provide other appropriate care, and relieve pain; nonmaleficence compels the physician to avoid causing pain and refrain from committing unnecessary harm. It is unreasonable to expect physicians to completely avoid risk when treating patients, as many ICU therapies and interventions pose considerable risk to the patient and may also cause pain. The therapeutic relationship in the ICU represents a working relationship between physician and patient, balancing potential benefits against harms whenever possible. Physicians are not neutral observers and, as long as they avoid coercive techniques, it is certainly acceptable—and some would argue mandatory—for them to provide their professional recommendation based on their clinical experience (27).

Justice

The third principle, justice, is rarely a source of conflict between the individual physician and patient in matters of informed consent. Ideally, the rules of informed consent serve to motivate the social virtue of justice; when conflicts do occur, they relate more commonly to societal *versus* individual claims and, thus, do not involve the physician–patient relationship. An exception is organ transplantation, a situation in where the transplant surgeon's primary duty is directed to the proper allocation of organs rather than to a specific patient (28). Implicit in the relationship of justice to informed consent is the specific involvement of society's instrument of justice: the court.

LEGAL FOUNDATIONS OF INFORMED CONSENT

The development of legal opinions during the past century illustrates the evolution of the currently recommended standards of informed consent. The first use of the term *informed consent* was in 1957 by an unheralded attorney named Paul Gebhard, drawing on his experience in labor law negotiations (29). In *Salgo v. Leland Stanford Jr. University,* Gebhard used the term in a friend-of-the-court brief on behalf of the American College of Surgeons to refer to the requirement that physicians must disclose the relevant risks and benefits of a procedure to patients (30).

CURRENT ETHICAL MODELS OF THE PHYSICIAN–PATIENT RELATIONSHIP

Models of informed consent that propose strategies for presenting information to patients and discussing alternatives emanated from the paternalistic Hippocratic tradition. In the *physician-centered model*—alternatively known as the paternalist, parental, or priestly model—the physician is the authority figure and guardian (31). In prioritizing the principle of beneficence—doing good—the physician engages the patient in decision-making simply to provide relevant information and encourage acceptance of the proposed therapy. Historically, Hippocrates advocated "concealing most things from the patient while you are attending to him...." Similarly, in 1871, Oliver Wendell Holmes asserted, "Your patient has no more right to all the truth you know than he has to all the medicine in your saddlebags.... He should get only just so much as is good for him" (32).

In time, greater emphasis on patient self-determination emerged, along with a higher priority on patient autonomy. Consequently, the *informative model*—also known as the scientific, engineering, consumer, or independent choice model—emerged as an alternative patient-centered strategy. It minimized physician bias and value judgment, while acknowledging the physician as technician and source of information. This provided the patient with options regarding the range of medical choices, along with the risks and benefits of potential alternatives. In contrast to the physician-centered model, the informative model asserts the physician's duty to provide facts and medical knowledge without expressing bias toward any particular treatment strategy. Ultimately, only the patient determines which course of action best suits his/her values and goals.

By minimizing physician input, this departure from paternalism represented an attempt to achieve complete patient autonomy. Nevertheless, this remained an unsatisfactory strategy for achieving informed consent, as true informed consent requires an interactive process between physician and patient. In clinical practice, the physician–patient relationship is collaborative with both sides sharing responsibility for participation, with a common goal of enhanced understanding. Clearly, the physician must be more than a technical adviser; the ICU is where the physician's training, knowledge, and experience are most important in providing interpretive guidance about diagnosis and treatment. This means the patient may, on occasion, request and receive a great deal of information; other times, circumstances will dictate the physician as the primary decision-maker alone.

Two current models of shared decision-making propose mutual understanding through an interactive process. The first, the *interpretive model*, focuses on clarifying the patient's values and determining preferences regarding the goals of therapy. By serving as a counselor providing information and engaging the patient in a joint process to achieve understanding, the physician may help the patient recognize and express their preferences. A discussion of treatment options permits the patient to identify their own priorities and determine which option best realizes these values. Thus, physician guidance allows the patient to demonstrate autonomy and self-understanding.

The second model of shared decision-making, the *deliberative model*, requires the physician to provide clinical information and then elicit information from the patient regarding their understanding and goals. In representing an idealized interaction between physician and patient, the physician integrates medical information with the patient's values. In this model, the physician should express opinions and preferences regarding appropriate therapy. Patient autonomy is preserved through the patient's moral understanding and action.

These idealized models of the physician–patient relationship acknowledge that informed consent is a *process* of shared decision-making. Examining the values of both patient and physician contributes to decisions regarding treatment benefits or risks (33). The optimal model for the physician–patient relationship is one that achieves a level of interactive and shared decision-making, thereby prioritizing patient autonomy while still engaging the participation of a concerned physician (34).

CURRENT LEGAL STANDARDS OF INFORMED CONSENT

Considerable uncertainty and debate remain regarding the level of information a physician should reasonably provide for a patient to adequately appreciate the risks associated with any particular therapeutic intervention (35). The perpetual dilemma of informed consent in the ICU is that, in extreme situations of both benefit and risk, greater obligation lies on the physician to adhere strictly to the guiding principles of informed consent. At the same time, ICU patients, because of their weakened condition, may be less able to comprehend and make decisions. In any discussion of possible risks, a physician should routinely disclose to the patient the complications that would occur most commonly; a reasonable figure would be a complication with a probability of at least 1% to 5%. If the potential risk is particularly serious or potentially fatal, it seems obvious that even rare complications with less than a 1% probability should be mentioned (e.g., the vascular complications of routine central venous catheter placement). However, some might argue that the occasional one-in-a-million fatal complication is not the appropriate standard for disclosure (not to mention that some physicians may be unaware of such rare complications). Because opinions differ, no uniform legal standard exists that defines how much information is required to meet the standard of adequate disclosure (36). Consequently, three standards of disclosure have been developed and currently exist: the professional community standard, the reasonable patient standard, and the individual patient standard (37,38).

Standards of Disclosure

The Professional Community Standard

For decades, the professional community standard was the traditional standard for informed consent. According to this standard, a physician should provide the level of information that physicians in the community would communicate to patients in comparable situations. Courts would assess physician disclosure based on the standard practices of other physicians with similar training and experience, working under similar circumstances. Because of the imprecise definition of "professional community," the professional standard was used to justify a broad range of interpretation, albeit without solid grounding in clinical criteria. The "community" could range from very specific practice locations to a broad geographic region, or otherwise refer to a level of specialized training or experience. In some circumstances, even the opinions of a "respectable minority" of physicians would constitute an appropriate practice standard. As such, the expectation of what the physician should tell the patient was notoriously imprecise. It was difficult to define which specific surgical or procedure risks a physician should disclose to a patient. Furthermore, physicians often invoked the concept of "therapeutic privilege," which permitted them to withhold *all* information if they thought it would be harmful to the patient. This doctrine has fallen out of favor, both clinically and legally (25).

Critics cited not only the imprecision, but also the paternalistic nature of the professional community standard. According to this standard, the physician ultimately determined the threshold of risk that should be disclosed to the patient. The obvious problem with this model was that if the community standard did not include the disclosure of a potential complication or other information that a patient might reasonably want to know, the physician was not obligated to disclose it. For example, physicians might prescribe penicillin, and, while a potentially lethal anaphylactic reaction to the drug was possible, because it was rare, it would not necessarily merit mention as a complication. Although physicians could not be expected to divulge every possible complication of a procedure or adverse reaction to a drug, many still felt it unacceptable that the standard for providing information rested solely in the hands of the physician.

The Reasonable Patient Standard

In response to the paternalistic standard, and in concert with the trend toward greater emphasis on the patient's right to self-determination, American courts began recognizing an alternative reasonable patient standard to judge the adequacy of risk disclosure. Since it was unreasonable to expect a physician to disclose every potential risk associated with a particular treatment, the reasonable patient standard required the physician to disclose all information a reasonable person would need to make an informed decision. This new standard dictated that even rare complications should be explained to the patient if the consequences (death, severe injury) were such that a reasonable person would want to know them.

However, there are also problems with this model. For one, the physician must divine what a reasonable person would want to know. (Would a reasonable person want to know about anaphylactic responses to penicillin?) Second, the ICU, a setting where life and death decisions are commonplace, may not lend itself to the enforced neutrality of the reasonable person standard. The physician would be performing a grave disservice simply by reciting potential complications of endotracheal intubation to a patient in respiratory distress. Consequently, another standard was needed.

The Individual Patient Standard

In the ICU, the physician's input is critical to good decision-making, which is why the optimal model for physician–patient relationships is one of interactive and shared decision-making; the individual patient standard addresses this relationship. Based on interaction with the patient and understanding of their beliefs, the physician should disclose specific information, so the patient can reach a decision consistent with his or her principles. The distinction between the different standards is subtle but significant. Under the professional community standard, the physician asks, "What should I tell the patient?" Under the reasonable person standard, the physician asks, "What does a reasonable person want to know?" Under the individual person standard, the physician asks, "What does *this* patient want to know?" Obviously, the most idealized standard of disclosure, the individual person standard, is ultimately the most difficult to achieve. Courts may not require such an idealized standard in all cases, but when questions of informed consent arise, this is the standard courts are most likely to favor.

Adjustments of Standards

In discussing these legal standards, a note of caution is in order: These models represent guidelines for medical encounters where both parties—patient and physician—can interact. In the ICU, situations are constantly changing, life and death decisions are commonplace, and emergencies sometimes make the search for an ideal physician–patient relationship impractical. The long-term relationship between the patient and the primary physician does not apply; the intensivist is often meeting the patient for the first time under conditions of duress (39). For the patient, admission to the ICU is virtually always a stressful, and potentially overwhelming, situation where critical illness creates an unusual dependence and power imbalance. The patient may be unable to comprehend or express their wishes (see below, Competence and Decision-Making Capacity). Other times, when acute care is required, an autonomous patient may choose to relinquish medical decision-making at the physician's discretion (40).

When explaining the risks and benefits of any intervention, it is also important for physicians to use language patients can understand. This includes adequate translation non-English speaking patients and also making explanations as nontechnical as possible. Even in the best case, patients may have difficulty extracting important information from discussions with physicians. When physicians lapse into technical jargon, the anxious, frightened patient may have little or no opportunity to process what is being said. It is important that, when appropriate, physicians make use of translators, family members, and other intermediaries.

An extensive discussion regarding the risks and benefits of care are the desired standard, but in the ICU, sometimes less is more. In emergencies, the need to keep patients informed sometimes becomes a luxury that time and circumstance may not permit. Emergency circumstances, where a patient lacks decisional capacity and no proxy decision-maker is identifiable, do not realistically allow for voluntary consent. In truly emergent situations, if the patient lacks capacity, no proxy decision-maker is available, and the potentially life-saving intervention must be administered immediately, the "emergency exception" to informed consent permits the physician to intervene without obtaining formal informed consent. In these situations, the intensivist should document the emergent nature of the situation and the difficulty in obtaining informed consent.

COMPETENCE AND DECISION-MAKING CAPACITY

Hospitalized patients, especially those critically ill, often suffer from an impaired ability to comprehend, process, or analyze information. Under the influence of pain medication, sedation, or the physical and mental stresses of illness, even the healthiest ICU patient may not fully appreciate or be able to actively participate in health care decisions, as the emotional stresses of critical illness may temporarily compromise their decisional capacity (41). As one study noted, for very sick patients, the ability to perform simple cognitive tasks is impaired to the point an adult patient may temporarily function at the level of a 10-year-old (42). This presents unique challenges for critical care practitioners when discussing medically complex issues.

Definition of Terms: Competence Versus Capacity

Both "competence" and "capacity" refer to the patient's ability to make decisions. Although the terms are often used interchangeably, there is a distinction between their legal and medical definitions. Strictly speaking, *competence* refers to a legal determination, and does not refer specifically to the patient's ability to make appropriate health care decisions (43). A court decides whether or not a person is legally competent, and generally, when "competence" is used as a legal term, it refers to patients' ability or inability to conduct their personal affairs, but not necessarily to make health care decisions. It is unusual, but not unheard of, for petitioners to ask the court specifically to declare a patient incompetent to make medical

TABLE 4.1 The Five Elements Patients Must Understand to Determine Their Capacity

1. The diagnosis
2. The proposed therapy
3. The risks and benefits of the proposed therapy
4. The alternative options
5. The risks and benefits of refusal

From Franklin C, Rosenbloom B. Proposing a new standard to establish medical competence for the purpose of critical care intervention. *Crit Care Med.* 2000;28:3035–3038.

care decisions. More often than not, this legal determination regarding who decides care for a patient remains in limbo and is left to the patient's family and doctors.

If courts are not involved with a patient's ability to make decisions, health care providers commonly invoke the term "medical competence," but they are really referring to the patient's *capacity*. In contrast to legal competence, decision-making capacity is a clinical judgment, which specifically describes the patient's ability to make medical decisions. The physician's need to assess capacity arises when there is reason to question whether a patient can make decisions about care (44). When assessing the patient's capacity, i.e., what most observers refer to imprecisely as whether the patient is competent to consent to care, the examining physician must determine whether the patient understands the five basic elements of capacity (Table 4.1) (45). During an interview, if a patient demonstrates satisfactory understanding of these five facts, it can reasonably be inferred the patient possesses adequate decision-making capacity.

Informal Assessments

Informal assessments of a patient's cognitive abilities typically occur throughout physician–patient interactions. In the critically ill patient, mental status may fluctuate during the course of hospitalization or even during the course of the day. Unless presented with evidence to suspect otherwise, the treating physician should assume the default position that the patient remains capable of independent choice. If this ability is in question, the health care provider is obliged to demonstrate that the patient cannot make medical decisions. When the clinical situation suggests the patient is incapable of independent choice, a more formal evaluation may be initiated (46).

Physicians may be more likely to question the patient's mental capacity if the patient's choices appear unreasonable or contradict the physician's personal values. The patient who refuses a relatively low-risk, high-benefit intervention, or a terminally ill patient who insists on pursuing a painful intervention with little proven benefit, are both scenarios that may prompt a physician to question the patient's decision-making capacity. In these situations, the physician must first attempt to decipher whether the patient's seemingly illogical behavior is actually part of a rational thought process. A critically hemorrhaging patient who refuses a blood transfusion may be medically frustrating to care for, but this refusal becomes understandable once it is revealed the patient is a Jehovah's Witness. Similarly, the patient with end-stage metastatic cancer who has failed multiple rounds of chemotherapy may appear irrational for insisting on pursuing invasive experimental procedures. This seemingly irrational insistence may become more understandable in the context of an upcoming family event, anniversary, or graduation.

External and Emotional Factors

In the ICU, external factors, including sundowning, sedation, pain medication, or altered sleep patterns, may contribute to transient, reversible episodes of incapacity. Whenever possible, attempts should be made to minimize the impact of these influences and optimize the patient's cognitive status prior to making a capacity assessment. The patient's judgment is often compromised by emotional factors—anger, fear, denial, depression, or pain—this is especially true in both the ICU and in the emergency department. The common scenario of the 50-year-old executive with crushing substernal chest pain who denies he is having a heart attack and wants to sign out of the hospital is an example of how denial may compromise a patient's judgment.

Health care providers should recognize that the patient's decisions under those conditions may not be the same ones they would choose in a less stressful environment. The physician must attempt to ensure that external factors do not unduly influence the patient. True informed consent requires the patient's unhindered judgment; when that judgment appears to be unduly compromised, the physician should use appropriate measures such as family intervention, psychiatric consultation, or medication aimed at treating the specific problem. The frightened patient who refuses necessary medical care is often grateful if, after appropriate intervention, proper care is provided.

For particularly high-risk interventions or close-call scenarios, a second physician, generally someone with expertise in this area such as a psychiatrist or neurologist, may be consulted to evaluate the patient. In such cases, the physician should inform the consultant in advance about the situation so the consultant can conduct a focused interview and provide the necessary information.

Legal Interventions

In rare circumstances, questioning a patient's capacity means seeking a court determination of legal incompetence. In practice, resorting to court is rarely necessary. Rather than deferring to the court system, most states recognize the authority of a spouse, family member, or friend to make decisions in the best interest of the patient. However, when family members and health care providers cannot agree about the most appropriate course of action after attempts at resolution, a legal opinion may be the only option. Courts are generally reluctant to get involved in health care decisions, so this should generally be the last option.

SURROGATE DECISION-MAKING

Signing out of the Hospital Against Medical Advice

One of the most difficult situations for the ICU staff is the extremely uncooperative, combative patient. In most cases, these patients are reacting to fear, pain, illicit drug ingestion, or alcohol withdrawal. Usually, after appropriate sedation or analgesia, care can be rendered although occasionally a patient must be physically restrained. The indication for physical restraint is when patients present a risk to themselves or to others. In rare circumstances, despite the best efforts of the staff, a patient may refuse all treatments and demand to leave the hospital. The staff is then forced to reconcile the conflict between respecting the patient's rights and their duty to care for, and protect the patient from harm; there may be no easy resolution of this problem.

The right to leave the hospital against medical advice is the prerogative of the competent patient. If the patient meets the general test of medical competence as described in the five basic elements of capacity (see Table 4.1) (45), the patient must be permitted to leave the hospital, even if the staff disagrees with the decision or the decision seems irrational. However, all decisions by patients to leave against medical advice should be scrutinized by senior staff to ensure the patient truly is competent. Those decisions that appear irrational should be scrutinized with even more care. A classic example is the aforementioned 50-year-old male with an acute myocardial infarction, otherwise competent but who, in a fit of denial, demands to sign out of the hospital. All avenues should be used to get the patient to stay, including a detailed discussion of the situation and an appeal to family or friends who accompany the patient to the hospital. Ultimately, however, if the patient refuses to listen, because he is competent he must be permitted to leave. In such situations—very trying ones, indeed—health care providers must attempt to provide any appropriate care or workup before the patient leaves. Staff should avoid recriminations, and the patient should also be reassured he or she can return for care at any time.

Other situations are not so clear-cut. In many cases, the patient's competence is in question. Possible physiologic causes for the patient's condition, e.g., hypoxemia, electrolyte disturbances, sepsis, should be identified. If the patient cannot be deemed competent, staff may decide to institute treatment over the objection of the patient, which might even entail physical restraint. Failure to restrain when indicated carries a significant risk to both patient and health care providers. The classic counterpoint to the aforementioned myocardial infarction patient is the patient in a motor vehicle accident who appears intoxicated but wants to sign out of the hospital. If the physician suspects that the patient is intoxicated, based on clinical observation even before confirmation of blood alcohol concentration, the patient should not be allowed to leave until appropriate radiologic assessment of the head and neck have been performed.

Some health care providers are overly concerned with the liability they may incur by treating a patient against his or her wishes. When competence cannot be established with certainty, if the staff decides to restrain the patient, they may theoretically open themselves to charges of battery. Such an outcome, however, is extremely unlikely, and almost certainly less likely than the alternative of being charged with negligent discharge. The consequences of being responsible for the negligent death of unrestrained patients are far more serious than the responsibility for holding patients against their will for several hours. When the staff's actions are medically reasonable, they are acting in good faith, and they document their decision (see below, Documentation), the likelihood of successful litigation against them is remote.

Documentation

Every situation of implied consent, or a decision to leave the hospital against medical advice, requires *scrupulous* and *detailed* documentation. The information that should be included in the medical record is listed in Table 4.2. Specialty consultations with neurology or psychiatry are not mandatory but may be useful in assessing the patient and documenting the situation. In difficult cases, it may be necessary to involve a representative of the hospital's administration or legal counsel.

TABLE 4.2 Documentation of Patients Who Leave the Hospital Against Medical Advice

1. Description of the patient's condition
2. The basic questions used to assess the patient's competence
3. Risks, benefits, and alternatives of treatment
4. Urgency of the situation
5. Any attempts to contact family members or other potential surrogates (detail who, when, and what interaction occurred)

PATIENT COMPREHENSION OF CONSENT FORMS

There is no medical or legal consensus regarding which procedures require formal consent. As a general guideline, the greater the risk of the procedure, the greater need to discuss the risks and benefits more formally (34). This standard results in consent policies that vary significantly from hospital to hospital. One survey of informed consent practices found that while over 90% of hospitals surveyed required formal consent for gastrointestinal endoscopy, fiberoptic bronchoscopy, or medical research, fewer than 10% required consent for nasogastric intubation or bladder catheterization (47). Of note, requirements for consent varied between medical and surgical services, even within the same institution.

Achieving satisfactory informed consent may not always be possible, even when physicians explain the procedures to patients. In one study of patients who consented to moderately invasive bedside procedures (thoracentesis, paracentesis, bone marrow aspirate, or lumbar puncture), 90% of the patients surveyed reported the physician had explained the indication for the procedure, although only 70% could correctly recall the reason for the procedure. Although 86% of patients reported the physician had informed them of the risks of the procedure, only 57% could later name any of the risks (48). This raises the question of how effectively information is communicated to patients and how accurately patients understand and recall information presented to them.

To anticipate patients' needs and to simplify the consent process, many institutions use standardized consent forms that include essential information regarding particular procedures or interventions. The use of a standardized ICU admission consent package, describing and requesting consent for the most commonly performed procedures, can enhance the informed consent process (49). Standardized forms, however, do not necessarily guarantee clear communication. As a response to defensive medicine concerns, standardized consent forms may describe every possible adverse consequence instead of actually trying to inform the patient (50). Moreover, standardized lists of complications may fail to communicate the risks most relevant to any particular patient, especially in the ICU, where a patient's changing medical condition can present a dynamic series of risks and benefits. The risk of an iatrogenic pneumothorax from central venous catheter placement during mechanical ventilation carries different implications than the same complication when the catheter is simply placed for fluid replacement.

Despite these caveats, standardized consent forms for common procedures may be useful in initiating dialogue between patient and physician. Standardized consent forms may also be necessary for especially complex ICU surgical procedures such as organ transplantation or experimental surgery. In these situations, a detailed informational document provides patient and health care providers with a ready reference. The language of such forms should be reviewed periodically to ensure simplicity and reader-friendly, understandable language. Even when standardized forms are used, health care providers should enter a note in the patient's medical record detailing the conversation between the patient and physician.

RESEARCH CONSENT IN THE ICU

Like every specialty, critical care medicine has achieved progress through research involving the participation of volunteers (51). Critically ill patients represent a particularly vulnerable population, which raises concerns about their ability to give voluntary, autonomous consent to participate in clinical research (52). Ongoing critical care research recognizes a corresponding obligation to protect this vulnerable population. Requesting consent for voluntary participation in research differs fundamentally from discussing informed consent for therapeutic interventions. When discussing the risks, benefits, and alternatives of any therapeutic or diagnostic intervention, both the clinician and patient seek a course of action that would maximally benefit the patient. In contrast, the goal of research is to generate information that may benefit *future* patients but does not necessarily benefit the individual research participant (53). This creates a potential conflict of interest between researcher and patient, and thus, researchers must exercise particular caution in protecting patients' rights (54). Federal regulations, known as "the common rule," have been designed to protect this vulnerable population of research participants (55).

Patients participating in clinical research may misunderstand or overestimate the individual benefits of participation; alternatively, they may not fully recognize the potential risks (56). Although the possibility for personal benefit does exist, a patient might be randomized to a nontreatment arm of a trial or may alternatively receive experimental therapy with unexpected, hazardous side effects (54,57). Researchers are obligated to ensure that research participants recognize the additional risks and benefits of participation. Occasionally, this means a researcher may ask a research participant to accept a disproportionate share of risk with no prospect of additional individual gain. The precise limits of risk a vulnerable patient may be asked to accept have not been specifically defined (58).

The research consent process should clearly delineate the nature of the research and structure of the trial, specifically including details on any randomization process (59). In contrast to therapeutic interventions, informed consent for research represents a process that continues throughout the course of a clinical study. Consequently, routine updates for the patient may be necessary. Standardized consent forms may be helpful in communicating the relevant information, and the physician should ensure that information is clearly explained. During the study, clinical research consent forms may be used as reference documents. Because of concerns regarding literacy and language comprehension, the complexity of language should generally target comprehension for no higher than a sixth-grade reading level.

Since few patients are likely to have voiced their previous preferences regarding research participation, proxy decision-makers are left to infer the most appropriate actions in certain situations for patients without decision-making capacity. Emergency situations where patients cannot consent, and surrogates cannot be located, raise concerns about the ethics of conducting research in these cases. Although regulations have sought to protect potential research subjects, those regulations acknowledge that denying research participation to patients who cannot give consent may also deny them potentially beneficial therapy. A 1996 amendment to the Code of Federal Regulations for the Protection of Human Subjects permits emergency research with certain provisions if consent cannot be obtained (54,60). Clinical trials describe waivers of consent based on implied consent (61). Delayed consent is another mechanism that has been employed for clinical trials comparing two clinically acceptable therapies (62).

The Emancipated Minor Exception

Emancipated minors are children younger than 18 years of age (or whatever the age of majority is in the state of residence) who can decide their own medical care. The specific criteria for emancipated minors vary from state to state, but generally pertain to minors who are either married, pregnant, a parent, in the military, financially independent and living apart from their parents, or those who have been legally declared emancipated by the court. Pediatric critical care practitioners should be familiar with laws concerning the age of majority and emancipated minors in the state where they practice.

When the Parents or Surrogate and Health Care Team Disagree on the Care of a Critically Ill Child

This situation arises most commonly in end-of-life situations regarding the propriety and timing of providing care (63,64). These are obviously emotionally wrenching circumstances when health care professionals and parents or surrogates disagree. Health care providers may anticipate the termination of ventilator support in a severely brain-injured patient or a terminal cancer patient days, or even weeks, before parents or surrogates reach an understanding that this is the proper decision. Parents or surrogates may hold out unreasonable hope, however understandable, in the face of a child's impending death. Patience is usually the best approach, as time and reasoned discussion generally resolve these issues. This strategy requires the understanding that those involved may be at different stages of acceptance. Collegial communication eventually brings the concerned parties to an acceptable conclusion. It is imperative that critical care practitioners offer parents or surrogates sufficient opportunity to discuss their feelings and emotions. A distant, emotionally detached approach by the critical care provider is inappropriate and complicates the delivery of care.

When there is neither common ground nor hope of agreement between the critical care provider and parents or surrogates, the final resort is to resort to the courts. Practitioners should not undertake formal legal action lightly. Experience has shown that in most cases, attorneys, courts, and judges, rather than hearing such cases, prefer resolution outside the courtroom. Besides being expensive, the legal process requires time and energy, both physical and emotional, on the part of everyone involved. In this adversarial process between the critical care provider and parents or surrogates involving end-of-life decisions, medical professionals should keep in mind that, in some cases, courts have ruled against the medical team who originally instituted the proceedings (65). Whenever pediatric critical care practitioners consider going to court for resolution, they should consult the hospital's legal staff and ethics committee to explore other options and coordinate an optimal strategy for all parties involved. They should remember that the best interests of the pediatric patient are their paramount concern.

Key Points

- Rooted in principles of autonomy and self-determination, the courts have long upheld that one's body may not be violated without proper approval.
- A corollary to the right *to consent* to medical treatment is a patient's right *to not consent* (to refuse) medical treatment.
- The *Saikewicz* court developed a four-pronged test to evaluate the "state's interest" and has been widely adopted by the courts in determining when an individual patient's ability to exercise her or his constitutional right to refuse treatment can be circumscribed:
  - The preservation of life
  - The protection of the interests of innocent third parties
  - The prevention of suicide
  - Maintaining the ethical integrity of the medical profession
- In a patient who at no time had capacity, the Court identified four key points that continue to provide us with guidance today:
  - A patient's common-law right to determine the course of his own medical treatment is paramount to the doctor's obligation to provide needed medical care.
  - Clear and convincing proof is required in cases where it is claimed that a person, now incompetent, left instructions to terminate life-sustaining procedures when there is no hope of recovery.
  - An individual who was never competent at any time in his life is considered still a child and a parent may not deprive a child of life-saving treatment, however, well intentioned.
  - Neither the common law nor existing state statutes require persons to seek prior court approval in cases involving discontinuance of life-sustaining treatment for incompetent.
- In the Cruzan "right to die" case, the Court:
  - Recognized a "right to die" but carefully noted that this was not guaranteed by the Constitution
  - Set out rules for what was required in order for a third party to refuse treatment on behalf of an incompetent person
  - Established that, absent a living will or clear and convincing evidence of what the incompetent person would have wanted, the state's interests in preserving life outweigh the individual's rights to refuse treatment
  - Left it to the states to determine their own right to die standards, rather than creating a uniform national standard
- The roots of informed consent are to be found in the case of *Schloendorff v New York Hospital*, the Nuremberg Code, and the Tuskegee Syphilis Study.
- The ethical foundations of informed consent encompass the classic principles of autonomy, beneficence, and justice.
- The standards for informed consent vary.
  - Under the professional community standard, the physician asks, "What should I tell the patient?"
  - Under the reasonable person standard, the physician asks, "What does a reasonable person want to know?"
  - Under the individual person standard, the physician asks, "What does *this* patient want to know?"
- Emancipated minors are children younger than 18 years of age (or whatever the age of majority is in the state of residence) who can decide their own medical care. Specific criteria include minors who are married, pregnant, a parent, in the military, financially independent and living apart from their parents, or those who have been legally declared emancipated by the court.

References

1. Schloendorff V. *Society of New York Hospital.* 105 N.E. 92. (1914).
2. Karnezis, Patient's right to refuse treatment allegedly necessary to sustain life. 93 A.L.R.3d 67 (1979); and Cantor, A patient's decision to decline life-saving medical treatment: bodily integrity versus the preservation of life. *Rutgers L Rev.* 1973;26: 228, 229, and n.5.
3. In 1987, the Arizona Supreme Court wrote: "Not long ago the realms of life and death were delineated by a bright line. Now this line is blurred by wondrous advances in medical technology—advances that until recent years were only ideas conceivable by such science-fiction visionaries as Jules Verne and H.G. Wells. Medical technology has effectively created a twilight zone of suspended animation where death commences while life, in some form, continues." As the Arizona court notes, the rub is that "[s]ome patients, however, want no part of a life sustained only by medical technology. Instead, they prefer a plan of medical treatment that allows nature to take its course and permits them to die with dignity". *Rasmussen v. Fleming*, 154 Ariz. 207, 216 (1987).
4. In the Matter of Karen Quinlan. 355 A.2d 647, 655 (N.J. 1976).
5. In the Matter of Karen Quinlan. 355 A.2d 647, 655 (N.J. 1976). "It seemed to be the consensus not only of the treating physicians but also of the several qualified experts who testified in the case, that removal from the respirator would not conform to medical practices, standards and traditions."
6. In the Matter of Karen Quinlan. 355 A.2d 647, 667 (N.J. 1976).
7. Superintendent of Belchertown State School v. *Joseph Saikewicz.* (1977); 373 Mass. 728.
8. Cruzan's condition was described as "oblivious to her environment except for reflexive responses to sound and perhaps painful stimuli; …[having] a massive enlargement of the ventricles filling with cerebrospinal fluid in the area where the brain has degenerated and [her] cerebral cortical atrophy is irreversible, permanent, progressive and ongoing; …her highest cognitive brain function is exhibited by her grimacing perhaps in recognition of ordinarily painful stimuli, indicating the experience of pain and apparent response to sound; …her four extremities are contracted with irreversible muscular and tendon damage to all extremities." Cruzan v. Harmon. 760 S.W. 2d 408, 411 (Mo. 1989).

9. Cruzan v. Harmon. 760 S.W.2d 408, 434 (Mo. 1988).
10. Cruzan v. Harmon. 760 S.W.2d 408, 425 (Mo. 1988).
11. Gaudin AM. Cruzan v. Director. Missouri Department of Health: to die or not to die: that is the question: but who decides? *Louisiana Law Rev.* 1991;51(6):1308–1345.
12. The Due Process Clause of the Fourteenth Amendment states that no person shall be "deprived of life, liberty, or property without due process of law." Usually, "due process" refers to fair procedures. However, the Supreme Court has also used this part of the Fourteenth Amendment to establish rights that are not specifically listed in the Constitution, such as the right to privacy. Cruzan by Cruzan v. Director, Missouri Department of Health: Oral Argument—December 06, 1989 [Transcript]. The Oyez Project. IIT Chicago-Kent College of Law at Illinois Institute of Technology. December 6, 1989. Retrieved March 22, 2016.
13. Cruzan v. Director. Missouri Department of Health, 110 S. Ct. 2841 (1990).
14. Lewin T. Nancy Cruzan dies, outlived by a debate over the right to die. New York Times. 1990. Retrieved March 22, 2016.
15. Schiavo Timeline: Part 1. 1963 to 2003. University of Miami Ethics Programs.
16. Felos GJ. *Respondent Michael Schiavo's Opposition to Application for Injunction. Case No.: 04A-825.* Vol. 9. Blue Dolphin Publishing. 2005: Retrieved April 1, 2016.
17. Beauchamp T, Faden R. *A History and Theory of Informed Consent.* New York, NY: Oxford University Press; 1986.
18. Katz J. *The Silent World of Doctor and Patient.* Baltimore, MD: Johns Hopkins University Press; 2002.
19. Doyal L. Good clinical practice and informed consent are inseparable. *Heart.* 2002;87(2):103–105.
20. Nijhawan Lokesh P. Informed consent: issues and challenges. *J Adv Pharm Technol Res.* 2013; 3:134–140.
21. Meisel A. Legal and ethical myths about informed consent. *Arch Intern Med.* 1996;156:2521–2526.
22. *Trials of War Criminals before the Nuremberg Military Tribunals. Vols. I and II. The Medical Case.* Washington, DC: U.S. Government Printing Office; 1948.
23. Jones J. *Bad Blood.* New York, NY: The Free Press; 1981.
24. Feld AD. Informed consent: not just for procedures anymore. *Am J Gastroenterol.* 2004;99: 977–980.
25. Menikoff J. *Law and Bioethics.* Washington, DC: Georgetown University Press; 2001.
26. Cook D. Patient autonomy versus paternalism. *Crit Care Med.* 2001;29 (2 Suppl):N24–N25.
27. Quill TE, Brody H. Physician recommendations and patient autonomy: finding a balance between physician power and patient choice. *Ann Intern Med.* 1996;125:763–769.
28. Franklin C. Organ transplants: a doctor's dilemma. New York Times, 2000: A18.
29. *P.G. Gebhard, 69, Developer of the term 'informed consent' [obituary].* New York Times. August 26, 1997:A13.
30. Salgo V. Leland Stanford Jr. Univ. Bd. Of Trustees, 154 Cal App. 2d 560, 317 P.2d 170 (1957).
31. Emanuel EJ, Emanuel LL. Four models of the physician-patient relationship. *JAMA.* 1992;267:2221–2226.
32. Laine C. Patient-centered medicine: a professional evolution. *JAMA.* 1996; 275:152–156.
33. Brock DW. The ideal of shared decision making between physicians and patients. *Kennedy Inst Ethics J.* 1991;1:28–47.
34. Whitney SN, McGuire AL, McCullough LB. A typology of shared decision making, informed consent, and simple consent. *Ann Intern Med.* 2004; 140:54–59.
35. Bernat JL, Peterson LM. Patient-centered informed consent in surgical practice. *Arch Surg.* 2006;141:86–92.
36. Sprung CL. Informed consent in theory and practice: legal and medical perspectives on the informed consent doctrine and a proposed reconceptualization. *Crit Care Med.* 1989;17:1346–1354.
37. Karlawish JH. Shared decision making in critical care: a clinical reality and an ethical necessity. *Am J Crit Care.* 1996;5:391–396.
38. Piper A Jr. Truce on the battlefield: a proposal for a different approach to medical informed consent. *J Law Med Ethics.* 1994;22:301–313.
39. Schweickert W, Hall J. Informed consent in the intensive care unit: ensuring understanding in a complex environment. *Curr Opin Crit Care.* 2005; 11:624–628.
40. Lidz CW, Meisel A, Osterweis M, et al. Barriers to informed consent. *Ann Intern Med.* 1983;99:539–543.
41. Marzuk PM. The right kind of paternalism. *N Engl J Med.* 1985;313:1474.
42. Cassell EJ, Leon AC, Kaufman SG. Preliminary evidence of impaired thinking in sick patients. *Ann Intern Med.* 2001;134:1120–1123.
43. Berg JW, Appelbaum PS, Grisso T. Constructing competence: formulating standards of legal competence to make medical decisions. *Rutgers Law Rev.* 1996;48:345–371.
44. Brody H. Shared decision making and determining decision-making capacity. *Prim Care.* 2005;32:645–658.
45. Franklin C, Rosenbloom B. Proposing a new standard to establish medical competence for the purpose of critical care intervention. *Crit Care Med.* 2000;28:3035–3038.
46. Appelbaum PS, Grisso T. Assessing patients' capacities to consent to treatment. *N Engl J Med.* 1988;319:1635–1638.
47. Manthous CA, DeGirolamo A, Haddad C, et al. Informed consent for medical procedures: local and national practices. *Chest.* 2003;124: 1978–1984.
48. Sulmasy DP. Patients' perceptions of the quality of informed consent for common medical procedures. *J Clin Ethics.* 1994;5:189–194.
49. Davis N, Pohlman A, Gehlbach B, et al. Improving the process of informed consent in the critically ill. *JAMA.* 2003;289:1963–1968.
50. Hopper KD, TenHave TR, Tully DA, et al. The readability of currently used surgical/procedure consent forms in the United States. *Surgery.* 1998;123:496–503.
51. Drazen JM. Volunteers at risk. *N Engl J Med.* 2006;355:1060–1061.
52. Luce JM, Cook DJ, Martin TR, et al. American Thoracic Society. The ethical conduct of clinical research involving critically ill patients in the United States and Canada: principles and recommendations. *Am J Respir Crit Care Med.* 2004;170:1375–1384.
53. Silverman HJ, Luce JM, Lanken PN, et al. NHLBI Acute Respiratory Distress Syndrome Clinical Trials Network (ARDSNet). Recommendations for informed consent forms for critical care clinical trials. *Crit Care Med.* 2005;33:867–882.
54. Luce J. Is the concept of informed consent applicable to clinical research involving critically ill patients? *Crit Care Med.* 2003;31(3):153–160.
55. Karlawish JH. Research involving cognitively impaired adults. *N Engl J Med.* 2003;348:1389–1392.
56. Sacks CA, Warren CE. Foreseeable risks? Informed consent for studies within the standard of care. *N Engl J Med.* 2015;372(4):306–307.
57. Dunn LB. Enhancing informed consent for research and treatment. *Neuropsychopharmacology.* 2001;24:595–607.
58. Suntharalingam G. Cytokine storm in a phase 1 trial of the anti-CD28 monoclonal antibody TGN1412. *N Engl J Med.* 2006;355:1018–1028.
59. Weijer C. The ethical analysis of risk in intensive care unit research. *Crit Care.* 2004;8:85–86.
60. Bigatello LM, George E, Hurford WE. Ethical considerations for research in critically ill patients. *Crit Care Med.* 2003;31(3 Suppl):S178–S181.
61. Fisher M. Ethical issues in the intensive care unit. *Curr Opin Crit Care.* 2004;10:292–298.
62. Finfer S. A comparison of albumin and saline for fluid resuscitation in the intensive care unit. *N Engl J Med.* 2004;350:2247–2256.
63. Zawistowski CA. Ethical problems in pediatric critical care: consent. *Crit Care Med.* 2003;31(5 Suppl):S407–S410.
64. Cooke RW. Good practice in consent. *Semin Fetal Neonatal Med.* 2005;10:63–71.
65. Matter of Hofbrauer, 65 App. Div. 2d 108, 411 N.Y.S. 2d 416 (App. Div. 1978); 47 NY 2nd 648,419 NYS 2d 936, 393 NE 2d 1009 (1979).

CHAPTER
5

Collaborative Care: Physician and Nursing Interactions and the Foundation of a Successful Unit

ELIZABETH MANIAS

INTRODUCTION

This chapter examines collaborative care by considering meanings of collaborative care, the makeup of the critical care team, forms of communication, and team effort. Meanings associated with collaborative care are explored, with particular reference to benefits of collaborative care within the critical care context. The various interdisciplinary health professionals who make up the critical care team are described, including medical and nursing personnel, physician assistants, pharmacists, respiratory therapists, social workers, occupational therapists, physical therapists, and nutritionists. The forms of communication that take place in critical care settings are identified, including critical care rounds, clinical handovers, and admission and discharge practices. Also important is the team effort that needs to be employed for orientation of new team members, patient monitoring and observation, and communication with patients' families.

MEANINGS ASSOCIATED WITH COLLABORATION

Collaborative care involves communicating information, opinions, and feelings; sharing decision-making, tasks, and goals; negotiating power to enable equitable participation and mutual respect; and facilitating the uptake of effective treatment (1–3). Henneman et al. (4) described collaborative care as a joint venture with two or more health professionals working together to achieve a common goal. It is a cooperative endeavor in which individuals contribute willingly in planning and organizing patient care. Health professionals offer their expertise and share responsibility for final outcomes while other individuals acknowledge their involvement in the venture.

BENEFITS AND AIM OF CARE

The ultimate aim of collaborative care is to produce positive outcomes for patients. Positive outcomes of effective collaboration include a decline in nosocomial infections (5), improved patients' quality of life (6,7), lower mortality rates (8,9), reduced length of hospital or critical care stay (10,11), reduced cost of care (5,10), reduced unnecessary antibiotic use (12), reduced medication errors (13), and reduced adverse events such as oversedation and readmission to the intensive care unit (ICU) (5). Effective collaboration can have benefits for the health professional, the health care team, and the organization (14–16). For the health professional, benefits include feelings of self-worth, competence, and importance. For the health care team, collaboration can create opportunities for clarification of interactive roles and to enhance respect for, and collegiality between, individuals of various disciplines. For the organization, collaboration can promote productivity, retention, and satisfaction of employees (4,17).

HEALTH PROFESSIONALS WITHIN THE ICU

Various medical professionals have an input in patient care within the ICU, including the critical care medical director, ICU attending physicians, and ICU fellows and residents. Medical professionals from outside the ICU also play an important role and include consultants, surgical attendings (18,19), residents, and other ancillary personnel.

ICU Director

The ICU is overseen by a medical director with demonstrated competence in the provision of critical care services; this person is often responsible for the administrative organization of the ICU—Critical Care Medicine—physicians. The director manages the administrative aspects of the unit, including the development and implementation of policies and procedures, review of the appropriate use of critical care resources, and education of unit staff. Together with the nurse manager, the medical director assumes ultimate responsibility for the safety and appropriateness of services provided in the setting. Consequently, the medical director plays an important role in guiding patient care during unstable clinical situations that require careful titration of therapy, such as multi-organ failure and resuscitation procedures. This responsibility includes the need to communicate regularly with other health professionals and the family about patient goals of treatment. Usually, the medical director has final authority over admission and discharge practices of the unit.

Critical Care Medicine Attending Physicians

Critical care attending physicians, the specialists who staff the ICU, are primarily accountable for the day-to-day unit and patient management responsibilities. These individuals have expert knowledge in pathophysiology, physiology, pharmacology, and the technical aspects of monitors and invasive equipment, as well as competence in managing critically ill patients. Critical care attending physicians provide a leading role in dealing with the sensitivities associated with dying patients and their families. Also important are attributes related to the latest research and quality improvement activities, as well as facilitating education among health professionals in the unit. In the absence of the medical director, it is the critical care attending physicians who make decisions relating to the admissions and discharges of patients.

Critical Care Fellows

Fellows are required to undertake a specified period of the critical care experience, usually a 1-year fellowship in which they work at least 9 months in a critical care environment (e.g., a neurologic, trauma, surgical, cardiac, or medical intensive care unit), with the remaining 3 months involving either allocation to a clinical area (e.g., respiratory care or trauma service) or conducting research relevant to critical care. Fellows have comprehensive knowledge about the medical histories, surgical and diagnostic procedures, and laboratory data and medications relating to all patients in the ICU. Together with the critical care resident, they provide this information on ward-round presentations and in discussions with other health professionals, including consultants, surgeons, and nurses. Fellows review assessment charts of complicated patients with residents and they guide residents in managing patients with respect to issues such as setting mechanical ventilation parameters, providing hemodynamic support and invasive monitoring, prescribing antibiotics, and managing adverse events. Critical care attending physicians assist fellows in making appropriate patient care decisions and providing them with greater input at the beginning of their training compared to later in the training year, at which point fellows are expected to make more independent decisions.

Critical Care Residents

Residents are junior members of the medical staff who rotate through the ICU to learn fundamental principles of treating critically ill patients. They collaborate with critical care fellows in collecting patient assessment data and formulating a management plan. During their rotation in the ICU, they develop beginning-level competencies in treating patients with complex health care needs. Residents give patient presentations during ward rounds, where they are provided with feedback on their comprehension and understanding of patient assessment, management, and evaluation of care.

Critical Care Nurses

Critical care nurses provide comprehensive skilled care to critically ill patients by maintaining a continual presence at the bedside. Their extensive knowledge and expertise enable them to recognize changes in patients' clinical manifestations and implement strategies aimed at preventing worsening conditions and minimizing complications. They support patients and families by acting as their advocates and play an integral role in the decision-making process with the health care team. In the United States, critical care nurses may be certified through the American Association of Critical Care Nursing by undertaking specialized education and testing and are recognized as critical care registered nurses (CCRNs). In other countries such as Australia and the United Kingdom, critical care nurses may complete specialized postgraduate critical care qualifications at a university.

A nurse manager of the ICU provides clear lines of authority for critical care nurses and is accountable for the delivery of good-quality patient care from the nursing staff. This health professional must ensure that nursing practices address key standards of care. Aside from expertise in current advances in the field, the nurse manager also has experience with health information systems, risk management, and health care economics.

Advanced Practice Registered Nurses

Advanced practice registered nurses who work within the ICU include certified registered nurse anesthetists, clinical nurse specialists, and certified nurse practitioners. Certified registered nurse anesthetists, in conjunction with physician anesthesiologists, manage patients before, during, and following procedures that require anesthesia. They conduct patient assessment and prepare the patient for anesthesia by prescribing preprocedure medications, such as sedatives, antiemetics, and antihistamines. They also administer and maintain intravenous and gaseous anesthesia to ensure proper sedation and pain management, oversee patient recovery from anesthesia, and manage patients' immediate postoperative needs. Clinical nurse specialists conduct clinical education, consultation, research, and management. Certified nurse practitioners undertake direct patient care activities and research (20,21); their role in the care of ICU patients—partnered with and supervised by critical care medicine attendings—can be significant. Advanced practice registered nurses perform many of the interventions involved with conventional nursing practice. They also function autonomously and in collaboration with other health professionals in an effort to produce optimal patient outcomes. Compared to other critical care nurses, those in advanced practice roles require a greater depth and breadth of knowledge and a greater understanding in interpreting patient data and undertaking complex interventions. Advanced practice registered nurses are required to have completed additional postgraduate work, usually at master's level.

Physician Assistants

Physician assistants work under the supervision of a physician. They are trained to perform patient examination, to order and interpret clinical tests and imaging, to diagnose conditions, to order treatments, to develop management plans, to assist in clinical procedures, to perform minor surgical procedures, and to refer to medical specialists. Physician assistants complement and extend the critical care services provided by physicians. The role of physician assistant is very popular in the United States, and it is also practiced in other countries such as the United Kingdom, Canada, Australia, and Russia. The scope of practice for physician assistants generally varies between and within countries, and is largely directed by supervising physicians. Physician assistants and certified nurse practitioners—although somewhat differently trained—function interchangeably in the ICU.

CONSULTANTS OUTSIDE THE ICU

Consultants from services outside the ICU are specialists who provide important information about particular facets of patient management to the critical care team. To ensure time is used appropriately and constructively, the critical care team should discuss the issue of concern beforehand and provide a rational argument—and if possible a specific question to be answered—in seeking a consultant's opinion. It is usually the attending physician's role to write the consultant referral. Any suggestions provided by consultants should be discussed with the critical care team before treatment is implemented.

Surgical Attendings

Surgical attendings are surgeons who play an important role in managing surgical procedures required by critically ill patients. They interact with patients and their families about preoperative, intraoperative, and postoperative care, as well as long-term follow-up in terms of ensuring optimal recovery from surgery. Although surgical attendings conduct daily rounds in the ICU, specific aspects of patient management usually reside with the critical care team. In the context of the surgical team, surgical residents play much the same role as do critical care residents.

Pharmacists

Pharmacists are integral to patient care in a way that extends well beyond their traditional role of supplying and distributing medications. With the increasing sophistication of medications available, their role encompasses the education of physicians, nurses, and other health professionals in preparing, prescribing, administering, and monitoring medications for critical care patients. They have extensive knowledge about pharmacokinetics and pharmacodynamic principles associated with severe illness, poisoning and drug intoxication, sedation practices, pain relief, and antibiotic use.

Pharmacists also make up various medicinal preparations. For ICUs, these preparations commonly include total parenteral nutrition and the incorporation of cytotoxic agents, antibiotics, potassium, or opioids into intravenous fluids. These preparations are made up in laminar flow cabinets of hospital pharmacy departments under sterile conditions.

One of the most important tasks of pharmacists is to ensure medications are administered in a manner that promotes therapeutic efficacy and minimizes adverse outcomes. More specifically, they help physicians and nurses by coordinating the development, implementation, and evaluation of medication protocols or guidelines. For this reason, pharmacists attend ward rounds and team meetings to familiarize themselves with patients' medical conditions and how these affect medication therapy. The Society of Critical Care Medicine has released a position paper about the scope and practice of critical care pharmacy practice and service (22) and a pharmacy taskforce has produced an opinion paper on training and credentialing pharmacy services in critical care (23); critical care pharmacists are integral members of the ICU rounding team.

Respiratory Therapists

Respiratory therapists are involved with maintaining ventilation equipment and monitoring the airway management of critically ill patients. Airway management may include the provision of oxygen therapy, mechanical ventilation, and aerosol medication therapy. Respiratory therapists also titrate ventilation parameters to suit the breathing and hemodynamic patterns of patients, formulate weaning procedures, and provide patient and family education. Although respiratory therapists are well established in North America, they rarely exist in the United Kingdom, Europe, Australia, or Asia, where nurses are responsible for patients' respiratory equipment and clinical management of respiratory function in collaboration with physician consultation.

Social Workers

Social workers are integral members of the ICU team, providing a conduit to provide information about the ICU patient's management plans to family members. They possess specialized knowledge about health policies and services, social welfare systems, and community resources. With this knowledge to guide their practice, social workers are important advocates for critically ill patients and families. Examples of activities conducted by social workers include assisting in the adjudication of family–patient–health care team disagreements, leading team discussions in root cause analyses of adverse events, locating temporary accommodation for family members during patients' stay in hospital, and providing resources to help cover health care costs.

Occupational Therapists

Occupational therapists evaluate the impact of illness on the activities of critically ill patients at home, in work situations, and during recreational situations. They work synergistically with other health professionals to reduce patients' physical and psychological disabilities. Before patients are discharged, occupational therapists often visit the home environment to make comprehensive assessments of the current facilities and changes required to accommodate the patients' needs.

Physical Therapists

Physical therapists assess and treat critically ill patients with a temporary or permanent physical disability, with the aim of achieving the highest degree of recovery. Treatment modalities used by physical therapists include exercise, mobilization and manipulation, massage, splinting, the application of hot and cold compresses, suctioning of respiratory secretions, and electrical stimulation. Conditions treated include birth deformities, fractures, back strain, spinal injuries, strokes, and multiple sclerosis. Rehabilitation after surgery, such as open heart, orthopedic, and abdominal surgery, is another area of responsibility. An important and growing area for physical therapists is early mobilization of critically ill patients as a strategy for reducing muscle atrophy and improving muscle strength (24).

Nutritionists

The aim of nutritionists is to improve the nutritional health and promote recovery of the critical care patient. Nutritionists possess detailed knowledge of food principles that apply to health and disease states, the biochemical properties of food, the mechanisms underlying food absorption, metabolism, digestion and elimination, and the indications for nutritional support. They also have an in-depth understanding of the interactions of particular food products with medications commonly used in critical care.

Nutritionists play an important role in the decision to introduce parenteral or enteral feeding or other forms of nutrient supplementation for critically ill patients. Critically ill patients are susceptible to malnutrition as they undergo invasive procedures and diagnostic tests, and disease states may alter the digestive process of nutrients (25). In collaboration with physicians and nurses, nutritionists determine the precise requirements for energy, protein, vitamins, minerals, essential fatty acids, electrolytes, and water to be administered through parenteral or enteral feeding. Enteral feeds are usually made in a hospital diet kitchen, the process of which is supervised by nutritionists. Conversely, critical care pharmacists prepare parenteral nutrition solutions using sterile laminar flow environments.

FORMS OF COMMUNICATION

Health professionals interact with each other using different forms of communication, depending on the intended purpose. These forms of communication include critical care ward rounds, clinical handovers (hand-offs), and communication concerning admission and discharge of patients. Effective collaboration using these forms of communication is essential for the overall function of ICUs.

ICU Ward Rounds

ICU ward rounds are an important forum for health professionals to come together and discuss the daily goals of care. The goals of care serve various functions, which include recognizing patient problems, sharing information, initiating treatment, evaluating the effectiveness of changes in treatment, and increasing learning opportunities for the critical care staff (26). Ineffective patient care and decision-making can occur if the goals of care are not communicated clearly, leading to increased costs and the possibility of medical errors (27).

ICU rounds should be multidisciplinary and include various personnel in addition to the critical care physicians: the nurse unit manager, the specific nurse assigned to each patient, the pharmacist, the respiratory therapist, and others such as the social worker and nutritionist. Although some part of the ward round may be undertaken away from the bedside to prevent interruptions adversely affecting decision-making, the health care team must also be present at the bedside, since direct clinical assessment is integral to identifying problems. Such problems may include inappropriate mechanical ventilatory settings, patient agitation and confusion, an incorrectly positioned endotracheal tube, and pain as shown by abdominal guarding and inappropriate breathing.

Usually, the critical care fellow presents each patient with feedback provided by the critical care attending physician. In this manner, the ward round provides a formalized process of education and training for less-experienced medical personnel. It is also an opportunity for other health professionals to provide their feedback on various perspectives of the patients' care, including wound management, nutrition, and medication management. The critical care physician is then able to direct discussions and debates for planning patient care.

The ward round should be a structured process occurring at a designated time each day. Scheduled ward rounds allow health professionals to plan their attendance despite unexpected situations that can occur. Organizing the ward round as a haphazard process, where it is conducted at different times of day, may mean that certain health professionals will not be able to attend (28). A lack of representation at ward rounds by particular disciplines may adversely affect the range of opinions and possible therapies for patients. A well-organized ward round is more likely to become a creative space in which health professionals of different disciplines can contribute to developing strategic plans for patient care and to sharing openly their clinical activities with other individuals.

The patient presentation should be concise and clear without redundant and irrelevant information, such as unrelated details about the patients' past medical history or superfluous explanations of daily activities. There are several steps that should be followed to ensure the patient presentation functions smoothly (Table 5.1).

To improve the quality of care, a daily goals sheet can be used during ward rounds, with input from all health professionals. A daily goals sheet is a document that is completed during ward rounds and posted at the bedside of each patient. It summarizes the plan of prioritized activities for a patient

TABLE 5.1 Steps to Take for an Effective Ward Round

- Know who the patient is in terms of the patient's name, age, gender, and reason for admission to critical care.
- Summarize past medical treatments since admission in terms of when they happened, where they happened, and patient response. It may help to document information in the form of clear, concise points to which you can refer during the presentation. This process will enable you to update your colleagues quickly without having to look for information in voluminous medical histories.
- Assess current patient problems in an organized manner using a body systems approach.
- Discuss the plans for the day, including anticipated patient response.
- Ensure the patient's medical record and radiographs are readily available.
- Be sure that all medication orders and observation charts are readily accessible at the bedside.
- All key pathology investigation results should be available. The pathology laboratory may need to be contacted before the round commences to obtain all necessary results.
- Use the presentation as a time to seek information from members of the health care team to find out more about your patient's needs (e.g., social workers, physical therapists).
- Ensure the relevant health professionals know about changes made to treatment and the role played by the individual in this process.
- Determine if the patient's family members need to be contacted either during or following the ward round in relation to treatment decisions. Make arrangements to contact the family members for consultation or consent for procedures if needed.

TABLE 5.2 Sample Daily Goals Sheet

Name: ID No.:	Bed No.: Date:
Pathology tests and diagnostic procedures	Invasive lines, drains, catheters
Hemodynamic parameters	External specialist consultation
Medications (new prescriptions, changes to current medications)	Patient mobilization
Sedation, analgesia, muscle paralysis	Nutrition
Ventilation support	Family discussion, consent for procedures
Transfer to other units	Other
House staff team	

during the course of a day. Information recorded on the goals sheet depends on specific characteristics of the unit (Table 5.2). Since each sheet is a work-in-progress, it is usually discarded the day after use and not included in the patient's medical record. After introducing a daily goals sheet, past research has shown a significant reduction in the length of intensive care stay of patients from 6.4 to 4.3 days (27), as well as improved identification of new patient care issues and an individualized approach to patient management (29).

ICU Clinical Handover

The clinical handover is a verbal form of communication involving health professionals from one working shift communicating with those of the oncoming working shift. The purpose of the clinical handover is to enable effective transfer of responsibility and accountability from one health professional to another. While clinical handover has been shown to be a major source of communication failure and serious adverse events (30), health professionals rarely receive training in handover processes (31). Over recent years, standard operating procedures for clinical handover have been developed, which are tools (Table 5.3) or mnemonics that enable systematic communication of information with the ultimate goal of reducing communication failure and adverse events (32). A common clinical handover tool is the SBAR, which involves describing the patient's situation, background, assessment, and recommendation of care (33). Use of these tools helps to ensure important components of the patients' management and goals of care are addressed at clinical handover (34).

Another important aspect of clinical handover is attempting to involve patients and family wherever possible (35). Patient and family involvement in handover can assist in reducing communication breakdown and help to promote patient-centered care (36). Patients can participate in the conduct of clinical handover when they are nearing discharge from the ICU, which is a time they are likely to be conscious and alert.

Admission and Discharge Practices of ICUs

Consensus guidelines have been developed to provide general information about criteria and procedures for admission and discharge practices (37). These guidelines detail objective clinical parameters to assist health professionals in their decision-making about patient flow to and from the unit. Aside from consensus guidelines, organizational factors, which are closely linked to collaborative care, have been examined for associations between admission and discharge practices of critical care settings and patient mortality (38–40). Such organizational factors include open and closed systems and time of day.

TABLE 5.3 Steps to Ensure an Effective Clinical Handover

- Be on time for the clinical handover and come prepared with some form of communication device (e.g., tablet personal computer or paper and pen) to note down key aspects of the handover.
- Use a tool or mnemonic such as SBAR (situation, background, assessment, and recommendation) to facilitate a systematic approach to information conveyed.
- Take notes about changes in patient status and particular activities that need to be performed during the course of the shift.
- Ask questions of health professionals giving the clinical handover, especially if you are unfamiliar with or unclear about particular issues.
- Be respectful of the patients and families you are discussing. Avoid use of judgmental language, labeling or stereotyping patients, or making negative comments about them.
- Use correct terminology and professional language in describing patient diagnosis and treatment. Use only easily understood abbreviations that are typical of the critical care setting.
- Avoid repetition and irrelevant information.

OPEN AND CLOSED SYSTEMS

An organizational factor that has been examined in terms of admission and discharge practices is the open or closed system of care (19). In the *open system*, various health professionals are present in the unit, but physicians directing patient care have obligations at a site separate from the critical care setting, such as the operating room, or inpatient or outpatient areas. A physician with expertise in critical care may or may not be involved to assist with management of care in an open system arrangement. In a *closed system*, care is provided by a critical care–based team of physicians, nurses, pharmacists, respiratory therapists, and other health professionals (41).

In a cohort study, the medical records were examined of all consecutive high-risk surgical patients admitted to an ICU from 1996 to 1998 using an open format, and from 2003 to 2005 using a closed format (39). Mortality of patients was 25.7% in the open format group and 15.8% in the closed format group ($p = 0.01$). Mortality relating to a cardiopulmonary complication was higher in the open format group (12.2%) compared with the closed format group (8.3%; $P = 0.02$). Results suggest that a closed format was a more favorable environment than an open format in effort to minimize the effects of high-risk surgery.

TIME OF DAY

Another important organizational factor for admission and discharge practices is time of day, with specific attention to weekdays versus weekends and daytime versus nighttime. A cohort study of all 23,134 emergency admissions over a 3.5-year period showed that weekend critical care admissions were associated with an increased adjusted mortality compared with weekday admissions (odds ratio [OR] 1.20, 95% confidence interval [CI] 1.01–1.43) (42). The adjusted mortality was similar for admissions made after business hours compared with those made during business hours (OR 0.98, CI 0.85–1.13). On the other hand, the adjusted risk of death was higher after business hours as compared with during business hours (OR 6.89, CI 5.96–7.96). The time of discharge from the ICU was not associated with additional hospital mortality. In another study involving propensity score matching analysis of 2,891 consecutive patients, nighttime admission was associated with elevated risk of mortality (OR 1.73, CI 1.12–2.74, $P = 0.01$) (38). These findings provide evidence of the importance played by the organization of critical care services with respect to time of day.

FUNCTIONING AS A TEAM

The integral functioning of a critical care team goes beyond the interactions of health professionals. It also involves developing an understanding of unpredictable events that can lead to clinical crises. Providing support for new team members, monitoring and observing patients for changes in clinical outcomes, and facilitating the involvement of family members are crucial facets for the foundation of a successful collaborative unit.

New Team Members

Specialized health care requires a tailored form of orientation for health professionals entering the critical care setting. Experienced clinicians in critical care are faced with the challenge of how to deliver important information to new team members to facilitate effective learning. This challenge is compounded by difficulties associated with a shortage of appropriately trained nurses and physicians. Comprehensive preparation through orientation programs has been shown to be a vital component for retaining health professionals (43).

Orientation of newly employed health professionals to ICUs should be viewed as a shared responsibility among senior health professionals, educators, and new staff members. Sharing of responsibilities improves the effectiveness of the orientation process because it allows more efficient completion of activities relating to the orientation, promotes collegial relationships, and links knowledge with practice. Orientation should occur through a structured program with defined goals that are agreed on by all individuals concerned (44).

The new staff member needs to be matched with a primary mentor and a secondary mentor, based on their discipline backgrounds, past experiences, attitudes, and learning styles. This matching process should be a strategic rather than a random choice to stimulate critical thinking, encourage open communication, and stimulate further professional development. The designation of a mentor based on random choice often leads to the use of multiple mentors, leading to inconsistent and confusing messages being conveyed (45).

Learning opportunities should be structured using a combined learner-led, theoretical, and clinical program (43). Such a model facilitates the transfer of knowledge to the practice setting. Theoretical reference material provided to the new staff member should include information about unit policies and protocols, roles and responsibilities of various members of the health care team, and the pathophysiology, assessment, and treatment relating to common patient conditions observed in the unit.

Although new staff members are very likely to have a rich array of experiences, experienced mentors are also influenced by the critical care culture in which they are positioned. As a result, new staff members and experienced mentors could be accustomed to performing activities their own way, which may lead to conflict. New staff members may feel that their learning needs and past experiences are not adequately recognized while mentors may feel that their advice is being ignored. By identifying potential problems from the outset, the orientation process can be more individually adapted to the team member's specific needs, the focus of which is becoming part of the unit. Developing a sense of belonging can help to solidify collaboration between the new staff member and other health professionals.

Monitoring and Observation of Critically Ill Patients

Most patients in critical care require constant monitoring and observation, such as patients with multisystem organ failure, multiple trauma, and adult respiratory distress syndrome. The nurse:patient ratio in many parts of the world is generally 1:2 (18). However, in Australia, the nurse:patient ratio for carrying out nursing activities in ICUs is 1:1. As nurses maintain a constant presence at the bedside, they play a critical role in undertaking regular monitoring of patients, assist in the early diagnosis of impending problems, and recommend appropriate interventions to be administered.

Patients in critical care require clinical parameters to be measured hourly or more frequently if these parameters change quickly. Also important is the close observation of patients through physical methods of inspection, palpation, percussion, and auscultation. Comprehensive judgment should be used in interpreting the significance of information obtained to avoid the complacency that could occur with repetitious documentation of clinical parameters and observations.

Nurses' knowledge in conducting patient monitoring and observation is largely constructed by their ongoing experiences and education in the critical care context. On the other hand, medical residents and critical care fellows who work in critical care for a limited period have to rely on past experiences and knowledge as their major sources of information, which may not necessarily be compatible with the types of decisions required in critical care. As an illustration, in an ethnographic study on professional relationships (46), a critical care fellow with previous experience in anesthetics was confronted by a situation involving a patient who had gone to the operating room for a duodenal ulcer repair and returned to the critical care setting. Within an hour of the patient's return, the bedside nurse, who was a clinical nurse specialist, reported to the fellow that the patient was restless, cold, and not breathing well with the ventilator. Based on his past anesthetic experience, the fellow advised the nurse to extubate the patient. The nurse drew on her knowledge of similar patients in critical care and believed that the patient needed additional sedative and analgesic treatment rather than removal of the endotracheal tube. She presented the situation to the critical care attending who agreed with her view and requested that the patient receives further analgesic and sedative medications (5).

Critical care attending physicians are ultimately responsible for less-experienced medical personnel; however, these more-experienced physicians may be present in the unit only during discrete times of the day. Due to their lack of availability, critical care attending physicians may be able to address only a small portion of the educational needs of junior medical team members in explaining the significance of a patient's clinical parameters and observations. Instead, due to their constant presence in the environment, nurses provide a substantive component of the educational needs of critical care fellows and residents in interpreting data obtained from patient monitoring and observation.

Nurses and physicians collectively provide valuable knowledge in making decisions about information obtained from patient data. It is, therefore, important that any rigid role boundaries between them are broken down (9). Maintaining rigid role boundaries creates distrust and disrespect between nurses and physicians, thereby hindering future progression of informed decision making. In effect, nurses need to be accepted as the "eyes and ears" of all levels of the critical care medical team to extend their perceptual capabilities.

Communication with Family Members

The admission of a critically ill patient is a stressful time for families, especially in the current health care environment of advanced technology, greater sophistication of interventional treatment, and multiple health professionals providing care. This critical care event can adversely affect the functioning of family members and their ability to communicate and understand complex information (47). If miscommunication is allowed to occur, the likely outcomes are care fragmentation, family alienation, and the development of distrustful relationships between family members and health professionals, and among health professionals themselves. Such disagreements can result in poor-quality patient care. Collaboration among health professionals is required for the comprehensive support and involvement of family members. As nurses are continuously present at the bedside, they need to interact regularly with other health professionals involved in direct patient care to synthesize information in a way that can be easily communicated to family members (27).

In a descriptive study involving interviews with family members, and observations of interactions between family members and intensive care staff, Söderström et al. (47) found that initial impressions had a sustained effect on family members and influenced future interactions. Family members who understood explicit information and implicit messages were open in their interactions with staff, adjusted well to the critical care environment and were more accepting of the situation. In other words, a mutual understanding existed between these family members and critical care staff. Explicit information involved details about the rules and policies of the unit, the condition of the patient, and how to behave in front of the patient. There were also implicit messages inherent in the information. For example, the message "you can visit the patient freely" meant "as long as you do not disturb us in our work." In addition, the message "you can ask questions freely" was conveyed "as long as we find them relevant" (47). Unfortunately, some family members did not fully understand either the explicit information or the implicit messages, and consequently, they either became withdrawn and quiet, or more vocal in their communication by asking many questions. For these individuals, there was a mutual misunderstanding with staff. These family members did not adjust well to the environment and were either ignored or insulted by critical care staff.

It is important that nurses and physicians reflect on how they communicate with family members at initial meetings and in future interactions. Mutual understanding is more likely to occur if information is presented in a clear and unambiguous way. Family members need to have questions answered honestly, and they require regular communication about the patient's progress and prognosis, treatment received, and changes in patient condition (48). They need to be reassured that health professionals care about the patient and support family members in their coping strategies. Family members should be able to speak with the physician and bedside nurse daily, have flexible visiting hours, be able to assist with simple patient care if desired, and have a place where they can be alone.

SUMMARY

Underlying a health care system that is facing pressure to improve efficiency are critical care services, which are predicted to become more important as the population ages, as the boundaries within hospital areas and between health professionals become blurred, and as more specialized technology develops over time. Health professionals need to adapt their approach to collaborative care in a complex and ever-changing health care climate. By themselves, sophisticated technology and treatment are not sufficient to address the needs of patients and families—positive and conducive relationships are the critical drivers for improved care.

Key Points

- Collaborative care brings about positive outcomes for patients, their families, health professionals, the health care team, and the health care organization.
- The critical care setting is a complex organizational system comprising various health professionals who need to function as an interdependent team.
- The challenge is to understand how the roles and functions of health professionals fit with those of other professions, with the aim of developing solid working relationships.
- Health professionals need to interact with each other effectively using different forms of communication, including the ward round and clinical handover.
- The ward round needs to function as a structured process, occurring at a formally designated time every day.
- A daily goals sheet should be used during ward rounds, with input from nurses, physicians, and other health professionals to summarize the plan of prioritized activities for a patient during the course of a day.
- The clinical handover should be considered a time in which health professionals can develop strategic plans for patient care and share openly their clinical activities with each other.
- Organizational factors such as the presence of an open or closed unit and time of day can impact on collaborative

care. These factors can influence patient outcomes in relation to critical care admission and discharge.

- The integral functioning of a critical care team goes beyond the interactions of health professionals.
- Comprehensive preparation through orientation programs is a vital component for retaining newly employed health professionals in the ICU and bringing about collaborative care.
- Because of their constant presence, nurses provide a substantive component of the educational needs of critical care fellows and residents in interpreting data obtained from patient monitoring and observation.
- Collaboration among health professionals is required for the comprehensive support and involvement of family members of patients.

References

1. Leonard M, Graham S, Bonacum D. The human factor: the critical importance of effective teamwork and communication in providing safe care. *Qual Saf Health Care.* 2004;13:i85–i90.
2. Thomas E, Sexton J, Helmreich R. Translating teamwork behaviours from aviation to healthcare: development of behavioural markers for neonatal resuscitation. *Qual Saf Health Care.* 2004;13:i57–i64.
3. Zwarenstein M, Goldman J, Reeves S. Interprofessional collaboration: effects of practice-based interventions on professional practice and healthcare outcomes. *Cochrane Database Syst Rev.* 2009;(3):CD000072.
4. Henneman E, Lee J, Cohen J. Collaboration: a concept analysis. *J Adv Nurs.* 1995;21:103–109.
5. Jain M, Miller L, Belt D, et al. Decline in ICU adverse events, nosocomial infections and cost through a quality improvement initiative focusing on teamwork and culture change. *Qual Safety Health Care.* 2006;15:235–239.
6. Bekelman DB, Hooker S, Nowels CT, et al. Feasibility and acceptability of a collaborative care intervention to improve symptoms and quality of life in chronic heart failure: mixed methods pilot trial. *J Palliat Med.* 2014;17:145–151.
7. Khan B, Lasiter S, Boustani M. Critical care recovery center: an innovative collaborative care model for ICU survivors. *Am J Nurs.* 2015;115:24–31.
8. Wheelan SA, Burchill CN, Tilin F. The link between teamwork and patients' outcomes in intensive care units. *Am J Crit Care.* 2003;12:527–534.
9. Irwin RS, Flaherty HM, French CT, et al. Interdisciplinary collaboration the slogan that must be achieved for models of delivering critical care to be successful. *Chest.* 2012;142:1611–1619.
10. Curley C, McEachern JE, Speroff T. A firm trial of interdisciplinary rounds on the inpatient medical wards: an intervention designed using continuous quality improvement. *Med Care.* 1998;36(8 Suppl):AS4–AS12.
11. Schneiderman LJ, Gilmer T, Teetzel HD, et al. Effect of ethics consultations on nonbeneficial life-sustaining treatments in the intensive care setting: a randomized controlled trial. *JAMA.* 2003;290:1166–1172.
12. Rimawi RH, Mazer MA, Siraj DS, et al. Impact of regular collaboration between infectious diseases and critical care practitioners on antimicrobial utilization and patient outcome. *Crit Care Med.* 2013;41:2099–2107.
13. Manias E, Kinney S, Cranswick N, et al. Medication errors in hospitalised children. *J Paediatr Child Health.* 2014;50:71–77.
14. Boyle DK, Miller PA, Forbes-Thompson SA. Communication and end-of-life care in the intensive care unit: patient, family, and clinician outcomes. *Crit Care Nurs Q.* 2005;28:302–316.
15. Shirey MR. Authentic leaders creating healthy work environments for nursing practice. *Am J Crit Care.* 2006;15:256–267.
16. Vazirani S, Hays RD, Shapiro MF, et al. Effect of a multidisciplinary intervention on communication and collaboration among physicians and nurses. *Am J Crit Care.* 2005;14:71–77.
17. Costa DK, Barg FK, Asch DA, et al. Facilitators of an interprofessional approach to care in medical and mixed medical/surgical ICUs: a multicenter qualitative study. *Res Nurs Health.* 2014;37:326–335.
18. Brilli RJ, Spevetz A, Branson RD, et al. Critical care delivery in the intensive care unit: defining clinical roles and the best practice model. *Crit Care Med.* 2001;29:2007–2019.
19. Haupt MT, Bekes CE, Brilli RJ, et al. Guidelines on critical care services and personnel: recommendations based on a system of categorization of three levels of care. *Crit Care Med.* 2003;31:2677–2683.
20. Jackson A, Carberry M. The advance nurse practitioner in critical care: a workload evaluation. *Nurs Crit Care.* 2015;20:71–77.
21. Costa DK, Wallace DJ, Barnato AE, et al. Nurse practitioner/physician assistant staffing and critical care mortality. *Chest.* 2014;146:1566–1573.
22. Rudis MI, Brandl KM. Position paper on critical care pharmacy services. Society of Critical Care Medicine and American College of Clinical Pharmacy Task Force on critical care pharmacy services. *Crit Care Med.* 2000;28:3746–3750.
23. Dager W, Bolesta S, Brophy G, et al. An opinion paper outlining recommendations for training, credentialing, and documenting and justifying critical care pharmacy services. *Pharmacotherapeutics.* 2011;31:829–829.
24. Harris CL, Shahid S. Physical therapy–driven quality improvement to promote early mobility in the intensive care unit. *Proc Baylor Univ Med Center.* 2014;27:203-207.
25. Wischmeyer P. The evolution of nutrition in critical care: how much, how soon? *Crit Care.* 2013;17(Suppl 1):S7.
26. Ten Have ECM, Nap RE. Mutual agreement between providers in intensive care medicine on patient care after interdisciplinary rounds. *J Intensive Care Med* 2014;29:292–297.
27. Narasimhan M, Eisen LA, Mahoney CD, et al. Improving nurse-physician communication and satisfaction in the intensive care unit with a daily goals worksheet. *Am J Crit Care.* 2006;15:217–222.
28. Manias E, Aitken R, Dunning T. Graduate nurses' communication with health professionals when managing patients' medications. *J Clin Nurs.* 2005; 14:354–362.
29. Centofanti JE, Duan EH, Hoad NC, et al. Use of a daily goals checklist for morning ICU rounds: a mixed-methods study. *Crit Care Med.* 2014; 42:1797–1803.
30. Horwitz LI, Moin T, Krumholz HM, et al. Consequences of inadequate sign-out for patient care. *Arch Intern Med.* 2008;168:1755–1760.
31. Lane-Fall MB, Speck RM, Ibrahim SA, et al. Are attendings different? Intensivists explain their handoff ideals, perceptions, and practices. *Ann Am Thorac Soc.* 2014;11:360–366.
32. WHO Collaborating Centre for Patient Safety Solutions. Communication during patient handovers. *Patient Saf Solut.* 2007;1:1–4.
33. Haig K, Sutton S, Whittington J. SBAR: a shared mental model for improving communication between clinicians. *Jt Comm J Qual Patient Saf.* 2006; 32:167–175.
34. Ilan R, LeBaron CD, Christianson MK, et al. Handover patterns: an observational study of critical care physicians. *BMC Health Serv Res* 2012;12:11.
35. Manias E, Watson B. Guest editorial: Moving from rhetoric to reality: patient and family involvement in bedside handover. *Int J Nurs Stud.* 2014; 51:1539–1541.
36. Azoulay E, Chaize M, Kentish-Barnes N. Involvement of ICU families in decisions: fine-tuning the partnership. *Ann Intensive Care.* 2014;4:37.
37. Task Force of the American College of Critical Care Medicine, Society of Critical Care Medicine. Guidelines for intensive care unit admission, discharge, and triage. *Crit Care Med.* 1999;27:633–638.
38. Ju MJ, Tu GW, Han Y, et al. Effect of admission time on mortality in an intensive care unit in Mainland China: a propensity score matching analysis. *Crit Care.* 2013;17:R230.
39. van der Sluis FJ, Slagt C, Liebman B, et al. The impact of open versus closed format ICU admission practices on the outcome of high risk surgical patients: a cohort analysis. *BMC Surg.* 2011;11:18.
40. Orsini J, Butala A, Ahmad N, et al. Factors influencing triage decisions in patients referred for ICU admission. *J Clin Med Res.* 2013;5:343–349.
41. Park C, Chun H, Lee D, et al. Impact of a surgical intensivist on the clinical outcomes of patients admitted to a surgical intensive care unit. *Ann Surg Treat Res.* 2014;86:319–324.
42. Uusaro A, Kari A, Ruokonen E. The effects of ICU admission and discharge times on mortality in Finland. *Intensive Care Med.* 2003;29: 2144–2148.
43. Thomason TR. ICU nursing orientation and postorientation practices: a national survey. *Crit Care Nurs Q.* 2006;29:237–245.
44. Levett-Jones T, Bourgeois S. *The Clinical Placement.* 3rd ed. Marrickville: Elsevier; 2014.
45. Hardy R, Smith R. Enhancing staff development with a structured preceptor program. *J Nurs Care Qual.* 2001;15:9–17.
46. Manias E, Street A. The interplay of knowledge and decision making between nurses and doctors in critical care. *Int J Nurs Stud.* 2001;38:129–140.
47. Söderström IM, Saveman BI, Benzein E. Interactions between family members and staff in intensive care units—an observation and interview study. *Int J Nurs Stud.* 2006;43:707–716.
48. Al-Mutair AS, Plummer V, O'Brien A, et al. Family needs and involvement in the intensive care unit: a literature review. *J Clin Nurs.* 2013; 22:1805–1817.

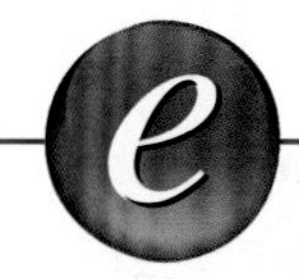

This chapter can be accessed in the accompanying eBook (see inside front cover for access instructions).

CHAPTER 6

Clinical Decision-Making

GUY MEYER and PIERRE DURIEUX

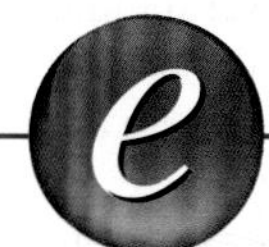

This chapter can be accessed in the accompanying eBook (see inside front cover for access instructions).

CHAPTER 7

How to Read a Medical Journal and Understand Basic Statistics

CHRISTOPHER LEE SISTROM and CYNTHIA WILSON GARVAN

CHAPTER 8

Quality Assurance, Safety, Outcomes, and External Compliance

ASAD LATIF, MICHAEL C. GRANT, and PETER J. PRONOVOST

INTRODUCTION

In response to the 1999 landmark report, *To Err is Human* (1), health care professionals have become increasingly attentive to improving the quality of care provided while mitigating any unintended harm. In the ensuing period, we have seen the evolution of global initiatives like the World Health Organization Patient Safety Programme, the strengthening of standards by international accreditation bodies like the Joint Commission, and even reimbursement becoming linked to quality with entities like the Centers for Medicare and Medicaid Service (CMS) progressively linking payments to health care outcomes rather than individual services. Yet, despite substantial progress made by the efforts of a wide variety of stakeholders to reduce harm in focused areas, quality gaps continue to rise in other areas, suggesting little comprehensive progress (2,3).

Quality gaps occur when clinicians fail to deliver care to qualifying patients commensurate with best practices or the available scientific evidence. These quality gaps result in less optimal care, and may lead to adverse events that cause direct patient harm. The individual concepts of health care quality and patient safety are naturally interwoven in this manner and, thus, can be considered almost interchangeable. High-quality care inherently leads to improved patient safety. Derived from the Institute of Medicine (IOM) (4), quality in health care is achieved when health services for patients result in the best possible outcome, no harm results from the care provided, and every aspect of care is consistent with current evidence-based knowledge given the patient's medical condition, comorbidities, and contraindications.

Although preventing quality gaps by providing care appropriate to the patient and condition appears a simple endeavor, proper adherence to these principles requires extensive review and improvement of existing health care delivery systems. The IOM considers health care quality a direct correlate of the level of improved health services and the desired health outcomes of individuals and populations (5). Therefore, quality improvement (QI) initiatives utilize systematic and continuous data-driven activities to exact measurable improvement in both the delivery of health care services and resultant patient outcomes. Given the direct link between health care delivery system quality and subsequent reduction in quality gaps, meaningful improvement in performance and quality often requires systematic change. In order to prevent quality gaps consistently, QI interventions adhere to basic principles that include evaluation of patient-centered outcomes through interpretation of measurable endpoints, multidisciplinary team-based collaboration, and evaluation of processes at the systems level, rather than at the individual provider level. By employing effective QI and forming predictable and reliable systems of care, organizations not only benefit directly, through improvements in health and process outcomes, but also indirectly, through heightened efficiency, more robust communication, more adaptive local culture, and potentially substantial cost savings.

No consensus exists regarding the best way to assess the current state of health care quality and patient safety (6–8). A recent panel of experts convened by the Agency for Health Care Research and Quality (AHRQ) reviewed the available literature (9), finding that most initiatives were based only on causal inferences to prove effectiveness. It is remarkable that health care still uses a limited range of approaches and models compared to the comprehensive intervention programs associated with other safety-focused industries. In this chapter, we will discuss the evaluation of compliance regarding quality in patient care, offer a framework for developing QI initiatives, discuss some implementation strategies, and examine several current tools and future directions for improving quality and safety in the intensive care unit (ICU) setting.

ASSESSING QUALITY OF PATIENT CARE

External Compliance Organizations

To Err Is Human served as a solemn reminder to all involved in the delivery of health care that further safeguards are critical for realizing much needed improvements in patient safety (1). An increased public awareness further fortified the impetus toward establishment of a systems-based approach and independent external evaluation to address this need through multiple mechanisms, at both local and national levels. The Joint Commission (JC), AHRQ, CMS, the Institute for Healthcare Improvement (IHI), VHA, Inc., and Leapfrog Group are just a few of the many organizations that have been focused on improving the quality of patient care over the years (10–18).

Evolution of External Performance Improvement Organizations

As a result of the 1999 IOM report, it was recommended to make the establishment of a center for patient safety a national priority. It further justified the development of mandatory and voluntary reporting systems as essential components in the evolution of a culture of safety and QI (1). In parallel, prior to that, the not-for-profit National Quality Forum was established at the behest of the President's Advisory Commission on Consumer Protection and Quality in the Health Care Industry (19). The mission of this entity was to lead national collaboration to promote the improvement of health and health care quality by establishing national consensus standards for measuring and publicly reporting on performance. In keeping with this, they helped formulate 30 novel standards directed at preventing adverse events and improving patient safety which were published in 2003, many of which were applicable to the ICU setting as well (20).

The JC has, as well, been an active contributor in the dissemination of improvements in patient safety and quality. Driven solely by health care professionals, JC was created to assist hospitals in improving quality of care and staff recruitment, and to offer accreditation of graduate medical education programs (12). Through the establishment of Medicare, and with the Social Security Amendments of 1965, any hospital accredited by JC was also eligible to participate in the Medicare Program. This was representative of the broader changes occurring in the health care sector, with the use of accreditation as an external QI evaluation mechanism. This introduced a governmental influence, which was soon followed by the public's use of accreditation as a proxy to evaluate the quality and safety of health care.

Today, other organizations and agencies are involved in the external evaluation of health care institutions. This list includes the National Committee for Quality Assurance, the American Medical Accreditation Program, the American Accreditation Health Care Commission/Utilization Review Accreditation Commission, and the Accreditation Association for Ambulatory Health Care; other agencies, such as the Foundation for Accountability, National Coalition on Health Care (NCHC), AHRQ, IHI, and Leapfrog Group also carry out unique roles in the assurance of safe, quality health care delivery (18). Each of these entities has differing missions and structures, making some better positioned to affect specialized environments like the ICU. However, most of the accrediting agencies share common tenets, similar to those established by JC at its inception as an accrediting body (8):

- Accreditation is a voluntary process.
- The evaluation of quality represents a cross-sectional analysis of the institution at the time of evaluation.
- The accreditation is based on previously defined standards and indicators of quality.
- The process of accreditation must occur periodically based on a fixed number of years.

The Joint Commission

The JC, previously known as the Joint Commission on Accreditation of Health Care Organizations (JCAHO), is the oldest accrediting body for health care worldwide and currently the largest hospital regulator in the United States. It has evolved significantly since it was first conceived as a standing committee of the American College of Surgeons in 1917, becoming an independent group in 1951 (12,15). This organization's role in the external accreditation process broadened in response to the dynamic changes that the health care environment experienced in the 1970s and 1980s. The escalating costs of health insurance threatened businesses in the globally competitive marketplace, resulting in the drive for cost containment and the eventual implementation of managed care and capitation payments. Concomitantly, rising costs of health insurance were continually passed on to employees, who were then responsible for copayments for health care services in addition to a rising proportion of employer-subsidized health insurance. In parallel, health care institutions were financially pressured to restructure and reorganize to meet the challenge of providing efficient, safe, and quality health care. Hence, this external accrediting agency took a national direction when, through the accreditation process, it began assisting the purchasers of health care services to make informed decisions regarding choice of health plans and providers. Finally, in response to public demand for representation in the development of policies and standards, JC added public members to its board and to its advisory committees in 1982 (12). This change was followed by the development of an Office of Quality Monitoring, which provides a mechanism to address public complaints pertaining to an institution's alleged noncompliance with standards, and discloses performance reports that detail the accreditation status of an institution and its performance in each of the standards on the JC website.

The accreditation process is still voluntary, as it was when this organization was first conceptualized in the early 1900s. It is noteworthy that approximately 50% of the JC standards have direct relevance to patient safety, and the remaining standards all have some indirect relationship (21–23). Therefore, the public, employers, insurers, and governmental agencies all tend to share the common belief that those institutions with accreditation provide a higher quality of professional care.

Institute for Health Care Improvement

The not-for-profit, Boston-based IHI was founded in 1991 as a by-product of the National Demonstration Project on Quality Improvement in Healthcare. Its website provides guidelines and tools for tracking both change in practice and outcomes (17). This organization has published a report in conjunction with the NCHC directly relevant to the ICU environment, entitled *Care in the ICU: Teaming Up to Improve Quality*. The basic premise is that improvements in ICU care that promote safety and quality are achievable now, based on evidence-based literature. IHI is a strong proponent for using care "bundles"—e.g., for patients on ventilators, or those with central lines – "rapid response teams," employing multidisciplinary rounds with daily goals assessment, and implementing the "intensivist-led model" of ICU care. They define a "bundle" as a "structured way of improving the processes of care and patient outcomes: a small, straightforward set of practices—generally three to five—that, when performed collectively and reliably, have been proven to improve patient outcomes" (17,24). The initiatives of the IHI are frequently closely aligned with JC, particularly in regards to their core measures.

The Leapfrog Group

This agency was founded in 2000, after a group of employers began the process of determining how best to approach the challenge of purchasing affordable, quality health care for their employees. Notably, this came on the heels of the IOM's report *To Err Is Human: Building a Safer Health System*, which recommended that large employers provide reinforcement for the provision of safe, quality health care through market pressure. The Leapfrog Group comprises a number of Fortune 500 corporations and spans a broad range of health care purchasers that represent more than 34 million individuals (10,15). CMS supports this group by propagating information-identifying facilities that achieve established standards. The Leapfrog Group proposes a tripartite approach to address the patient safety initiative, and estimated that it could save up to 58,300 lives and prevent more than 500,000 medication errors annually. The three recommendations included use of computerized physician order entry, increased evidence-based hospital referrals, and improved ICU physician staffing.

In common with proposals put forth by other organizations and agencies vested in patient safety and quality care in the ICU environment, the Leapfrog Group has conducted its own surveys to determine the degree to which institutions have been able to implement their recommendations. Significantly, some insurers have established incentives for health care facilities that integrate Leapfrog Group initiatives into their programs. The results have been promising, but not without its detractors from certain communities within the health care system. The American Hospital Association has questioned whether hospital should embrace standards promulgated by outside, or external, agencies, and challenged the costs needed to implement and sustain programs for computerized order entry and to employ qualified intensivists, who are already in short supply.

Evaluating Quality Improvement Initiatives

Though we are quick to compare current approaches and models of health care to other industrial surrogates, the nature of health care can differ significantly from other industries. It remains an unpredictable, dynamic environment with patient and provider behaviors that can be difficult to control. Health care does not enjoy a virtually fault-free operation as a starting point, which may preclude us from directly importing safety models from industries such as aviation and automobile manufacturing, which can easily pinpoint problems and have safe baselines. Health care's perspective also remains reactive, with an over-reliance on voluntary incident reporting and root cause analysis, rather than the more proactive approach of adjusting the process to prevent the adverse event from happening in the first place.

The greatest initial impediment to reforming health care quality and safety is the adoption of a universal framework to evaluate and monitor safety. Given the lack of rigorous appraisal of methodology and analysis employed by prior QI initiatives, the generalized research community has often labeled individual interventions as pseudo-science. The lack of rigor may be in part due to paucity of funding and research capacity, but also to a failure to develop pragmatic and scalable QI evaluation methods. Potentially novel and effective quality and safety initiatives garner less publicity than carefully controlled counterparts, leading to lost opportunity for advancement in the field. To begin to meet the lofty standards set by other areas of health research, we must set establish a framework for proper scientific discovery.

The ideal safety initiative would not only learn from past mistakes, but adapt to any unexpected present or future demands. Much like any formal research design, quality initiatives must:

- Review the theoretical basis for a proposed intervention and establish a hypothesis
- Employ valid and objective metrics
- Apply and describe consistent methodology and comprehensive process development, and
- Assess outcomes systematically

We will discuss these key elements to provide a simple framework that will help structure the approach to QI intervention (25).

Theoretical Basis

Most clinical research draws from extensive amounts of predefined molecular and physiologic data and principles that provide assumptions about how and why the single intervention should work even before it is demonstrated. Though one would expect similar standards to apply to improvement initiatives, this can prove most difficult given the wide-ranging diversity of foundational sciences including clinical medicine, human factors engineering, organizational psychology, and systems factors frameworks. As a result, a combination of qualitative and quantitative approaches is often needed to provide a meaningful understanding of safety and QI initiatives (26–28). For example, public attention attributed decreased central line–associated bloodstream infection (CLABSI) rates to the use of a checklist. However, the intervention also included and integrated a model for translating research evidence into practice with a comprehensive unit-based safety program (CUSP) to improve local safety and teamwork culture (29). Such a multifaceted approach was necessary to overcome local barriers, including social, emotional, cultural, and political ones, to affect a lasting change in provider behavior (30). Given that QI success can rarely (if ever) be attributed to a single intervention and is, rather, the result of a comprehensive multisystem endeavor, attempting to control for individual confounding and apply traditional research design would prove exceedingly challenging. Certainly, advancements can be made to current QI project design, but the answer may ultimately lie somewhere in between current less-exacting practice and excessive basic science standards.

Appropriate Measures

The challenge in monitoring patient safety stems from the fact that a patient can be harmed in innumerable ways, but only a limited number of measures exist for evaluating performance. The few publically reported performance measures that currently exist have done little to effectively evaluate safety (31). Even if organizations have scientifically sound measures in place, they often have an underdeveloped infrastructure for appropriately monitoring those endpoints. This problem is made all the more challenging as organizations are increasingly tasked with providing evidence that patients are safer. Ultimately, health care organizations are charged not only with establishing safety performance metrics, but also with creating information systems that recognize the dynamic nature of health care.

Good safety measures should have several qualities, such as importance, validity, and applicability to the local environment (32). Rather than conceptualize safety as a dichotomous variable—safe or unsafe—measures should be considered continuous—is it more safe than before? Ideally, measures should be quantifiable as rates or proportions to readily identify improvement in outcomes and processes, or they should be nonrate-based to enable evaluation of structure and context of care (33). Upon initial selection of a measure, its strategic importance should be assessed, both in the context of importance to the people responsible for improvement, and its importance given available effort, time, and resources. The measure should also maintain validity as upheld by existing supporting evidence, to ensure proper uptake and utilization. In that light, it must also be reliable and reproducible to minimize the potential for bias. Finally, any high-quality safety measure needs to be feasible and useful in its local environment to justify the commitment of potentially scarce resources. Data collection and analysis represents a significant organizational burden, and if any measure does not meet the standards of being an important, valid, and pragmatic way to guide improvement, efforts should be reconsidered. These qualities maintain the independent validity and objectivity of the individual measures, molding the overall initiative within the scientific methods framework instead of a less rigorous enterprise.

Detailing of Processes

Traditional clinical research relies on specific conserved methodology, but only limited guidance is available for successful implementation and evaluation of safety and QI initiatives in health care (34). This fact is underlined by management challenges that make it difficult to even report methods and results, such as the use of evolving multifaceted interventions and minimal dedicated data collection resources (35). Regardless, describing these practices in sufficient detail to allow replication should be a key requirement. The International Committee of Medical Journal Editors advises authors to "Describe statistical methods with enough detail to enable a knowledgeable reader with access to the original data to judge its appropriateness for the study and verify the reported results" (36). A recent review noted that several studies of prominent patient safety practices limited their descriptions to just a few sentences (9). While unique impediments to adequate reporting may exist in the QI infrastructure, several authors and guidelines have nonetheless recommended the practice (9,37,38).

Ironically, trials of complex multifaceted interventions, such as those used to improve safety and quality, would find detailing their processes of particular benefit. Given the evolving nature of most safety initiatives, detailing the encountered barriers and how they were addressed is of critical importance. The core intervention may be difficult to separate from the culture-based efforts to implement it, with the two often blending together over the course of the intervention. For example, the Keystone ICU project recognized the importance of leadership support and safety culture when is asked providers to change their practices to help reduce bloodstream infections, and therefore packaged them together as a safety practice (27,39).

Though some experts might believe that disentangling the co-interventions may not be meaningful, detailing then is crucial for any future replication and dissemination.

Assessment of Initiatives

Health care organizations are continuously adapting to address the dynamic nature of risks to patient safety. Dynamic systems theory suggests that all of the factors that influence safety and quality in the future cannot be completely defined today. Successful initiatives need to be able to incorporate multiple components, including anticipation of harm, sensitivity to local context and provider feedback, and the tracking of various outcomes.

Anticipation and Preparedness

In much the same way that clinical care delivery has preemptively adjusted treatment to satisfy predicted patient conditions, safety science is increasingly adopting a more proactive perspective as opposed to a reactive one. This approach relies on anticipation and foresight to predict potential problems. Unfortunately, as we have alluded to, there is usually no specific set of data that is explicitly relevant to anticipated harm. Instead, it remains a matter of fostering discussion and continually self-appraising, even in times of relative success and stability.

While the science of safety is ever evolving, some surrogate measures have proven promising. Hospitals that score higher on safety climate assessments are less likely to have patient safety events, a fact that serves to emphasize the importance of safety culture (40,41). What's more, programs like the Safer Clinical Systems curriculum run by the Health Foundation and Warwick Medical School have begun to develop the use of "safety cases," which provide an overall quantitative assessment of the likelihood that a variety of possible failures will occur based upon reported narratives of regular use. These cases stem from systematically examining processes of care to identify potential failures. Although these methods have not been widely adopted in health care, they provide reasonable starting points for further exploration of health care systems research.

Environmental Sensitivity and Feedback

Early identification of potential risk before a patient sustains direct harm is the hallmark of any well-constituted safety intervention program. To make this goal a reality, interventions must enable regular monitoring and response to appropriate information. The monitoring must also have sensitivity to variables within the local system and environment to allow researchers to develop, refine, and update interventions based on changes in the situation, including those outside normal operational activities (42). Examples of mechanisms that support sensitivity in health care organizations include safety walk-rounds, briefings and debriefings, operational rounds, the use of dedicated patient safety officers, and patient safety assessments (43,44).

Effective safety initiatives are tasked with identifying deviations from best practices and recognizing near-misses in an attempt to inform future operations. Health care organizations use a variety of formal and informal approaches to obtain information about safety in the context of care delivery. And while relevant information in this context can be gathered in a variety of ways, effective response is perhaps most important. The response must be prompt to mitigate the potential for growing patient risk, appropriate to the specific cultural environment, and discussed and integrated on multiple levels within the organization to obtain a comprehensive solution. Ultimately, the key is to ensure that the response to safety information engages frontline staff, because it will reassure them that their reports are being taken seriously.

Outcomes

Every clinical outcome relies on a formal assessment of associated outcomes. However, this assessment is often ignored when safety initiatives are evaluated, especially when the benefits are marginal, difficult to quantify, or may be outweighed by other effects (45,46). And though changes in the outcome of interest are often measured, tracking of the indirect consequences and costs is often ignored. It is important to note that certain practices, while not directly harmful, can undermine the original intent of the intervention and cause changes in practices or behaviors that lead to unintended consequences (47). An example is the regulation of resident work hours intended to decrease fatigue and thereby improve patient safety. This change was based on studies demonstrating decreased cognitive functioning in sleep-deprived individuals and the focused assessment of errors when physicians performed specific cognitive tasks in a simulated environment (47–49). When further analyzed, there were no definitive improvements in patient mortality, but there were some increases in complications (50–52). Another example is the use of computerized provider order entry systems. Even though these systems decrease medication errors, they might not reduce actual harm from adverse drug events (53). So it must be remembered that the outcome that we are measuring is often a surrogate marker, and changes in it do not necessarily affect the actual outcome of interest. Also, when operating within a complicated interwoven health care system, individual component changes can lead to unexpected collateral effects that need constant postintervention monitoring. These interactions can provide useful feedback to optimize system architecture and strengthen iterative processes.

Assessment of Contextual Factors

In much the same way, researchers evaluate the heterogeneity of treatment effects in clinical trials, one must appreciate the varied contextual factors to successfully implement a multifaceted safety intervention. Failure to adopt conceptually similar interventions in differing settings is likely associated with an inability to account for the influence of context (53,54). At least one published framework proposes the grouping of high-priority contexts into four domains (9): (a) structural characteristics of the organization; (b) leadership, culture, and teamwork; (c) patient safety tools and technologies; and (d) external factors.

Structural characteristics of organizations include geographic and demographic characteristics of hospital patrons and providers, organizational complexity, and financial status. These elements tend to be fixed and are unlikely to change. In contrast, local leadership, culture, and teamwork are all integrated concepts that can be altered appreciably with focused efforts (28). As previously reported, they can represent the backbone to the relative success or failure of safety initiatives, determining how an intervention is implemented and sustained. The use of specific tools for patient safety interventions can have a significant impact on deploying and managing culture-based components, and can be influenced relatively easily at the organizational level. These tools will be discussed in further detail later in this chapter. And finally, external factors consist of the overall environment in which the organization resides. While not under the direct influence of the organization, they often have a profound effect on patient safety and quality, often influencing crucial issues such as allocation of resources. Although the applications of the proposed high-priority contexts might vary based on the specifics of the initiative in question, evaluations should consider all of these contextual influences to be broadly applicable.

SPECIFIC IMPLEMENTATION METHODOLOGIES

After establishing the fundamental framework for a safety intervention program and considering the complexities of research design within the health care system format, successful QI requires a comprehensive strategy for implementation. It is imperative to use a systematic and multidisciplinary approach that involves relevant stakeholders in the pursuit of a common safety-based enterprise. In strategizing such an approach, it will help if a conceptual framework of safety issues and solutions is created to guide team efforts and ensure common points of dialogue. Some authors have described a consensus classification for patient safety practices in an effort to provide a common language for interpreting patient safety literature, whereas others have categorized patient safety efforts into general themes, which can be useful in focusing efforts to improve the culture of safety within a particular ICU (55,56). Here we provide examples of useful project frameworks for unit-based safety programs.

Translating Evidence into Practice (TRiP)

Although most available research funding has been devoted to understanding disease mechanisms and identifying therapy, little evidence describes how to effectively, efficiently, and safely deliver these therapies to patients. This omission only serves to further underline the ongoing issues with quality gap. Multiple methods seek to increase the reliable delivery of evidence-based therapies to patients. These methods include evidence-based medicine and clinical practice guidelines, professional education and development, assessment and accountability, patient-centered care, and quality management.

To better operationalize safety intervention "therapies," a four-step process has been developed and successfully used to translate research evidence into practice within the ICU (29,57). This model involves an interdisciplinary team taking ownership of the improvement project, is based on evidence and performance measurement, and encourages creation of a collaborative culture that is essential for sustaining results (Figure 8.1). The steps are described below:

1. *Summarize the evidence:* Rather than rely on the traditional practice of medicine wherein external consortiums provide impractical practice guidelines in the form of nonprioritized lists with ambiguous language, guidelines should be concisely summarized into individual key interventions based on the best evidence available. This practice serves to target interventions and aid in practical decision-making. For example, evidence supports the use of lung protective ventilation (LPV) for patients with acute respiratory distress syndrome, which can be concisely defined as providing a tidal volume <6 mL/kg of predicted body weight and a plateau pressure of <30 cm H_2O (58,59).
2. *Identify local barriers to practice compliance:* After establishing the key elements of the intervention, the next step is to identify and alleviate local barriers to effective implementation. Thus, researchers formally and systematically walk through the process, observe others performing key duties therein, and investigate the impediments to appropriate care. This exercise serves to reveal system defects or aspects of the process that prevent compliance with evidence-based practice. For example, intensivists may be aware of and agree with LPV use, but they may (a) find it difficult to know if they are actually compliant, or (b) fail to have access to elements vital to compliance. Although height is necessary in calculating predicted body weight, frequently it may be missing from the patient chart, resulting in unintentional noncompliance (60–67).
3. *Measure performance:* After choosing an intervention and developing specific practice behaviors, process measures (how frequently patients receive intended therapy) and outcome measures (how patient outcomes have improved) should be thoughtfully evaluated in the appropriate context. Each of these performance measures has its own relative strengths and weaknesses. Compliance with LPV strategy can vary considerably with each individual ventilator setting alteration during the course of a patient's ICU stay. Researchers must, therefore, structure the timing and frequency of measuring LPV compliance around certain clinical care parameters to ensure accuracy without becoming overly burdensome. Although potentially more burdensome, obtaining more frequent measures provides a better understanding of performance over the course of a patient's treatment course.
4. *Ensure all patients receive the therapy:* Ultimately, compliance of a unit or an organization with established practices requires similar adherence of QI teams with each element of the implementation model. Embedded into the final step of the TRiP model are the four E's of practice change:
   a. *Engage* clinicians, front-line staff, and organizational decision-makers alike by using local estimates of patient harm so that clinicians recognize the impact of noncompliance with evidence-based practices in their clinical area. For acute lung injury, this could be estimating the number of preventable deaths based on prevalence of LPV nonuse in such patients in an ICU.
   b. *Educate* involved parties to ensure that they know the evidence, agree with it, and understand the actions and resources needed to ensure compliance.
   c. *Execute* the intervention through a variety of individual tools (see below). This step should take the

Summarize the evidence
Identify interventions associated with improved outcomes
Select interventions with most benefit and least barriers to use
Convert the interventions to behaviors

Identify local barriers to implementation
Observe frontline staff performing the interventions
"Walk the process" to identify defects in implementation
Ask all stakeholders to share concerns and identify potential risks and benefits associated with implementation

Overall concepts
Place the problem within context of larger health care system
Use collaborative multidisciplinary teams both centrally and locally

Measure performance
Select measures (both processes and outcomes)
Develop and pilot feasibility of measures
Measure baseline performance

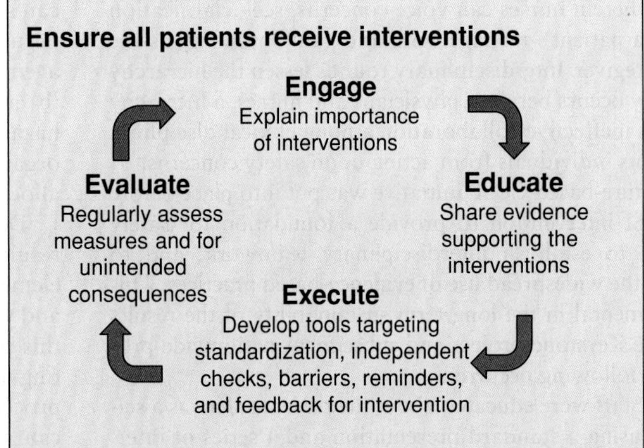
Ensure all patients receive interventions
Engage
Explain importance of interventions
Educate
Share evidence supporting the interventions
Execute
Develop tools targeting standardization, independent checks, barriers, reminders, and feedback for intervention
Evaluate
Regularly assess measures and for unintended consequences

FIGURE 8.1 A model for translating research evidence into practice. (Adapted from Pronovost PJ, et. al. Translating evidence into practice: a model for large-scale knowledge translation. *BMJ* 2008;337:963–965, with permission from BMJ Publishing Group Ltd.)

form of some standardized process intervention to ensure that all patients meeting certain criteria receive the intervention(s).

d. ***Evaluate*** the intervention with timely, accurate, appropriate, and consistent measures and serially report findings back to clinicians, staff, and leaders.

Comprehensive Unit-Based Safety Program

Although measuring harm and implementing effective therapies are important for patient safety, they are insufficient without teamwork and creation of a concomitant culture that embraces these directives (68). Repeated examples have shown that the pertinent elements of culture, such as failures in communication, lead to sentinel events in health care (69).

The CUSP is a comprehensive and longitudinal program designed to improve local culture and safety (70). Supported by a web-based project management tool, the CUSP has evolved significantly since its inception from an eight-step (70) to a five-step (71) program (Table 8.1). CUSP is designed to be adopted by individual work units or care areas, and to involve every individual who provides care within a given unit, from physicians to nurses, pharmacists, administrative clerks, and other support staff. The program also leverages support from senior leaders in the health care organization to provide financial, administrative, and other resource assistance.

TABLE 8.1 Comprehensive Unit-Based Safety Program

Pre-CUSP	Conduct a culture assessment as baseline to evaluate various domains (e.g., safety, teamwork, job satisfaction, unit- and hospital-level management). Should be repeated annually.
Step 1	Educate staff about the science of patient safety
Step 2	Engage frontline staff to identify locally relevant safety concerns. Provide mechanism for implementation and follow-up.
Step 3	Partner with senior executive. Set up monthly meetings to discuss safety issues and potential/existing initiatives
Step 4	Use defect investigation tool on regular basis (e.g., monthly or quarterly)
Step 5	Implement tool for improvement (e.g., teamwork, communication, culture).

The CUSP model, which was originally implemented in 2001 at two surgical ICUs at the Johns Hopkins Hospital, resulted in significant reductions in ICU length of stay, and medication errors, and even improvements in nursing turnover (72–74). This success was derived from emphasizing practical tools to investigate and learn from defects, improve teamwork and communication, and organize transitions of care within and between patient care areas. These elements empowered frontline staff with a strong baseline knowledge about the science of safety to recognize potential safety hazards and design interventions to eliminate them.

An intended byproduct of the CUSP initiative is gradual improvement in an individual unit's safety culture. Embedding patient quality and safety tasks into daily practice—for physicians, nurses, and staff alike—shifts workflow focus away from risk-provoking behavior and automatically prioritizes those same quality and safety tenets. The staff is provided a platform to share experiences with everyone in the unit, and the group is empowered to solve local problems in care delivery. For example, the creation of interdisciplinary rounds created a setting wherein nurses can voice concerns, seek clarification regarding a patient's management, and gain autonomy as the bedside caregiver. Interdisciplinary rounds lessen the hierarchy that usually occurs between physicians and nurses, a hierarchy that causes ineffective collaboration among clinical disciplines and prevents individuals from acting upon safety concerns.

The culture-based CUSP initiative was put into place before the CLABSI intervention to provide a foundation for safety awareness, to establish interdisciplinary teamwork, and to encourage the widespread use of evidence-based practices. This was instrumental in the long-term sustainability of the results (75). In the Keystone project and subsequent nationwide programs, the following occurred:

Step 1: Staff were educated about the patient safety as a science using a standard presentation and a series of interactive discussions.

Step 2: Staff were asked to identify how the next patient would be harmed on their unit, and what they would do to prevent this harm from occurring; a CUSP improvement team was formed to interpret the results and implement the work.

Step 3: Partnership with a senior hospital administrator was strongly encouraged. Their roles included reviewing the safety hazards identified by the unit staff with the improvement team, provide the institutional support and resources needed to implement appropriate risk reduction interventions, and hold staff accountable for mitigating hazards.

Step 4: Teams were trained to use a novel defect investigation tool, and asked to use it to address at least one defect each month.

Step 5: Teams were provided a variety of tools to improve communication and teamwork, and instructed to modify the tools to fit the local context and ensure ease of implementation.

Specific Tools for Quality Improvement

Briefings and Debriefings

Briefing and debriefing tools are designed to promote effective interdisciplinary communication and teamwork. A briefing is a structured review of the case at hand among all team members before any task is undertaken with the patient. A debriefing occurs after a procedure or situation in which the team reviews what worked well, what failed, and what can be done better in the future. Both have been used in the operating rooms (ORs), in hand-offs among the ICU nursing staff and intensivists, and between OR nursing and anesthesia coordinators (76–78).

A typical OR briefing will first introduce the relevant parties and establish anticipated roles of various team members. Next comes confirmation of the correct patient, site/side, and procedure, which coincides directly with the established JC "time-out" procedure, and assurance that all team members understand the important aspects of the intended procedure. A check of all necessary equipment (e.g., electrocautery) and medications (e.g., appropriate antibiotic) is then performed. Finally, to mitigate potential hazard, a concise discussion should take place regarding what plans are in place if procedure variables fall outside of intended practice parameters. A briefing will typically focus on a critical procedure, but it can also focus on unit management of a patient. Briefings may occur in an ICU setting, where attendings and nurse management meet to discuss (a) events that happened overnight, (b) admissions and discharges for the day, and (c) potential hazards that may occur during the day. This morning briefing organizes the ICU team, prioritizes the workflow for the unit, allocates resources, and mitigates potential hazards (78).

Debriefings occur after a formative event, regardless of the result. Often these are considered sessions for review of key elements of the procedure and discussion of relative merits and opportunities for improvement. Although constructive, this practice is often overlooked in the daily clinical care setting unless an unintended harm occurs or the consequence of a procedure is in question. Regular use of the debriefing strategy can serve not only to help establish root cause, but also to further educate providers for future similar patient encounters.

Learning from Defects

Most medical errors require the alignment of multiple failures within a system to occur. Reason's "Swiss cheese" model (Figure 8.2) illustrates how multiple failures, though insufficient by themselves to cause harm to the patient, can align to cause and adverse event in aggregate. The Learning from Defects tool is a less intensive version of a root cause analysis, allowing it to be implemented more frequently and with fewer resources to look at near-misses that would not necessarily trigger a hospital-level investigation. It provides a structured approach to help caregivers and administrators investigate a case and identify elements of a given system that contributed to the defect, while also providing a follow-up mechanism to ensure safety improvements are achieved. It does so by asking four basic questions: (a) what happened; (b) why did it happen; (c) how will you reduce the likelihood of this happening again; and (d) how will you know the risk has been reduced (79). Use of such a tool allows staff to investigate more incidents closer to the time of occurrence and to identify and mitigate a larger number of contributory factors. The learning-from-defects process can be implemented as part of the CUSP framework or as a key element in educational programs that focus on QI (80).

This form of retrospective identification, which shares overlap with key elements of debriefing, can be used to identify

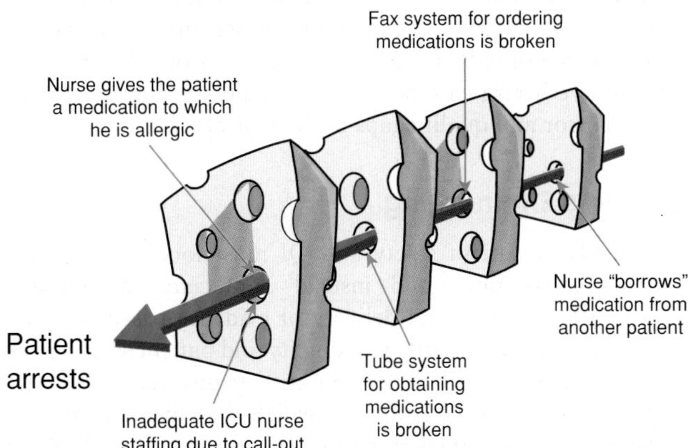
A Medication Error Story
Fax system for ordering medications is broken
Nurse gives the patient a medication to which he is allergic
Nurse "borrows" medication from another patient
Patient arrests
Tube system for obtaining medications is broken
Inadequate ICU nurse staffing due to call-out

FIGURE 8.2 The "Swiss cheese" model of a medical error. The events leading up to an adverse event involving a medication error are illustrated. The Swiss cheese model is a concept that originates from the work of James Reason, in which he proposes that the alignment of multiple system failures allows harm to reach a patient. His premise is that system failures occur often, but that health care professionals and other systems are built in to catch a failure (e.g., final safety check at the pharmacy to catch medication allergies). Couched in this way, it takes the alignment of several failures or defects to pass by and harm a patient. (Adapted from Reason J. Understanding adverse events: human factors. In: Vincent C, ed. *Clinical Risk Management*. London: BMJ Publications; 1995.)

medical errors and analyze contributing factors, thereby providing a learning opportunity, rather than just a way to recover from harm. The lessons will provide defense against recurrence of the same or similar harm and are essential to promoting a comprehensive culture of safety. The IOM has targeted incident reporting systems as a method to not only collect defect information, but also to investigate the causes, thereby improving safety (1,81). To make incident data useful, health care organizations can utilize a variety of formal (root cause analysis) or informal (Learning from Defects, case review) methods.

Checklists

As outlined, the care of any one patient may require any number of health care providers across multiple disciplines and levels of training. Hundreds of tasks, designed to implement dozens of therapies, may represent the balance of a single intensive care day. Given the natural limitations of human memory and attention, appreciation for and successful implementation of the associated choreography can prove nearly impossible.

These realities can lead to decreased compliance with proper protocols, increased error rates, and reduced efficiency (82,83). Using checklists to standardize processes ensures that all steps and activities are addressed, thereby reducing the risk of costly oversights or mistakes and improving outcomes. Checklists represent an organized list of essential elements or steps that need to be considered or performed for a given task. Lying somewhere between an informal cognitive aid and a protocol, checklists provide real-time guidance to users and serve as verification after task completion (84). Checklists are thus multifunctional as memory aids, evaluation frameworks, and tools to standardize and regulate processes. Ultimately, checklists facilitate care delivery by decreasing variability, and thus improving performance.

In large part, our understanding of checklist use in the workplace comes from industries outside of medicine. In aviation, checklists are now a mandatory part of routine operations and are highly regulated. They are used both in the course of normal practice and during emergency situations, providing a systematic approach to situation recovery. In product manufacturing, the smallest error during development can affect the quality of the final product, increase costs, and potentially harm the consumer. Checklists play a central role in ensuring that proper operating procedures are followed and quality standards are maintained. Quality assurance personnel use them routinely at multiple stages of the production process to evaluate whether required regulatory standards are being met. Checklists are an important component of standard operating procedures for manufacturing and distribution processes because they help to maintain product quality standards. A central theme among these exemplars is the reliance on precise execution to provide consistent quality and minimize error.

Although similar in enterprise, health care has been slow to adopt the use of checklists. Operationally, it can be challenging to standardize processes for the wide variability that exists between and even within patients. Nuanced patient comorbidities, individual physiology, and unforeseen events can continuously influence the approach to diagnosis, treatment, and even recovery, making the design and implementation of a standardized approach difficult. Socioculturally, health care providers, particularly physicians, are frequently resistant to standardized tools and approaches, viewing them as a restriction of their autonomy. Certainly, similar restraints have been overcome successfully in other industry, but universal adoption within health care will require a concerted effort focused on improving efficiency and outcome rather than catering to resistance.

Daily Goals Sheet

Since July 2001, the daily goals sheet has been used during multidisciplinary rounds in the ICUs at Johns Hopkins to improve communication (85). This tool is a one-page checklist that is completed every morning to document establishment of the care plan, set goals, and review potential safety risks for each patient. Posted at the bedside of the patient, the goals sheet is updated as needed based on the dynamic nature of patient care and used as an information sheet for all staff involved in the patient's care. This checklist can be modified for use on regular floor units and during OR sign-out.

The ICU version of a daily goals sheet can include the following questions:

- What needs to be done to move the patient closer to transfer or discharge?
- What is the patient's greatest safety risk?
- What are the plans for pain management, cardiovascular management, and respiratory management?
- Is it appropriate to evaluate the patient's rapid shallow breathing index?
- Is there any planned diuresis and nutritional support?
- Are any antibiotic levels needed?
- Can any lines, tubes, or drains be discontinued?
- Are any tests or procedures planned? Have consents and orders been completed?
- Consider key local safety initiatives, including family updates, or implementation of local protocols.

To evaluate the impact of the daily goals sheet, all care team members should answer two simple questions after rounding at each patient's bedside: (a) Do you understand the patient's goals for the day?; and, (b) Do you understand what work needs to be accomplished on this patient today? These questions were the impetus behind the development of this checklist. When asked initially, fewer than 10% of the residents and nurses time actually knew the care plan for the day. Traditional bedside rounds tended to focus as much or more on teaching staff about the disease than what work needed to occur to treat the patient. Approximately 4 weeks after Johns Hopkins implemented the daily goals sheet, 95% of the residents and nurses understood the goals for each patient (85). Moreover, length of stay in a surgical ICU at Johns Hopkins decreased from a mean of 2.2 days to just 1.1 days (85). Implementation of a daily goals sheet can also help improve communication and collaboration among nurses and physicians for individual patients, and lead to more effective coordination of daily care plans, and efficient movement of patients to ICU and even hospital discharge.

FUTURE DIRECTIONS

Simulation

Simulation is a powerful tool/technique that has been used in high-risk industries to improve safety and reduce errors (86,87). The potential benefits of simulation in health care include (88):

- Frequent training for emergencies (crisis resource management)
- Teamwork training (which is a weak link in the whole process of patient safety)
- Skills training and evaluation of competency before a trainee touches a patient
- Testing of new procedures and usability of new devices.

Health care takes place in a complex, high-stress environment that can affect human performance and patient outcomes. High-fidelity simulation allows us to not only examine human performance, but also analyze system-based problems. Although most medical simulation is still relatively new, it provides an opportunity to reorganize our "see one, do one, teach one" method of clinical training and better prepare trainees before they practice medicine. Education of health care staff is a vital part of any strategy to prevent errors. The benefits of simulation-based education include a pragmatic approach involving greater degree of interaction than traditional didactic sessions. It allows for the development of nontechnical skills along with assessment of technical skills. It facilitates real-time evaluation and feedback, assessment of practical and clinical judgment, as well as development of psychomotor and communication skills to optimize understanding of material and improve task execution (89–91).

Although a more thorough evaluation of the effect of simulation on patient safety might be necessary, just like in other industries, the face validity of this tool is likely to drive change and impact outcome. This impact will be especially apparent in the training domain, for both technical and nontechnical, or behavioral, skills (communication skills, leadership, task management, teamwork, situational awareness, and decision-making) (92,93). These behavioral skills are common contributors to critical events in health care (94). Simulation allows trainees to practice in an environment that is safe for the trainee and the patient. In addition, trainees are exposed to common, rare, and crisis situations, and can practice learned competencies and receive immediate feedback about their performance (95,96). A simulation-based approach has the potential to not only prevent similar errors from recurring, but to improve health care provider awareness to improve detection of error and quality gaps in the first place.

Systems Engineering

The fields of patient safety and QI must look beyond individual interventions and instead appreciate the ultimate goal—ensuring universal delivery of evidence-based therapies to eliminate harm. Health care quality and patient safety initiatives succeed only when collaborative teams account for the aspects specific to the system in which they live and operate. However, no individual system exists in a vacuum. While an individual checklist or learning-from-defects discussion may serve a function at the time of its use, it is a static tool that may become irrelevant over the dynamic course of a patient's care. The current siloed approach of targeting harms individually demonstrates a lack of understanding regarding when and where these synergies and discordances may be occurring, potentially leading to unintended, and sometimes harmful, consequences. Seemingly small personnel, resource, or architectural modifications can lead to domino effects at the individual and health system level given the interrelated nature of various systems. What's more, with the rapidly growing nature of health care technologies, providers are expected to deliver care that remains efficient and cost-conscious, yet robust enough to cover a range of disease and therapeutic complexities. Industries such as aerospace, defense, and information technologies have managed to thrive under similar conditions by integrating highly complex systems to function optimally without sacrificing principles of safety and quality. In them, harm is not perceived as being inevitable, but rather as a problem that can be overcome through a systems engineering approach (97).

Systems engineering is the practice of using core principles – termed systems methodology – to design systems architecture, language, and integration to satisfy a pre-determined goal. This approach contrasts with current health care strategy, wherein providers often address newly evolving problems by trying to retrofit current systems through "patches" or "work-arounds" because they are constrained by time and/or resources. By adopting systems engineering practices used ubiquitously in other surrogate industries, health care may more comprehensively alleviate systems defects by simply preventing them from occurring in the first place. All systems engineering initiatives follow a set of phases to either improve upon an existing system or develop a new system to solve a problem:

1. **System Concept Development:** To establish scope, the first phase in developing a new system is to define the problem, identify stakeholders and determine the goal. This step requires clear, concise language to adequately stage the overall initiative. *Example: Surgeons, intensivists, and administrators (stakeholders) believe nursing and provider workflow is significantly impeded in the ICU by redundant tasking (problem). They believe vital sign monitors should automatically input vital signs into the electronic medical record (EMR) and reduce time burden to bedside personnel (concise goal).*
2. **Requirements Analysis:** Individual stakeholders, with the aid of systems engineers, establish the necessary

requirements to successfully implement the system. They will make a rational appraisal of necessary financial, personnel, raw material and regulatory resources in order to provide a meaningful end product. *Example: Collaborators create a requirements list that includes raw elements (monitors, cables, hardware elements), personnel (programmers, engineers, software developers, construction), and so on to properly address the necessary systems architecture.*

3. **Functional Definition:** Define the system through a variety of diagrams geared toward simulating or prototyping the anticipated system. Here you establish the input, the intermediate steps and the final output product as well as all relevant components and interrelated subsystems. *Example: Numerous flow diagrams, object-oriented models, computer simulations, and even graphical user interfaces (GUIs) are prototyped to theoretically propose an optimal solution to the original problem.*
4. **Implementation:** Construct the system and properly integrate it among any pre-existing systems or subsystems in place. In the end, it should produce the expected output. *Example: All makes and models of individual existing monitors must work seamlessly in the new system, which must also be modified to current workflow (establish appropriate timing and ranges of vital signs).*
5. **Verification and Validation:** Over the life cycle of the new system, researchers must verify that the system meets the stated goals and validate the system under constraints of real-world operation. Predefined metrics are employed to ensure both endpoints. *Example: Intensivists review vital sign data to ensure accuracy, stakeholders observe workflow to comment on efficiency, and each provided feedback to systems architects to direct necessary modifications.*
6. **Iteration:** Through numerous cycles of the system, stakeholders may modify elements and improve upon them to optimize efficiency and integrate new goals. *Example: After vital signs are automatically input into the EMR, system checks may be set on subsequent cycles to notify providers if they fall outside of a preset range. This addition satisfies the original stated goal and improves upon the system through iteration.*

Application of such a systems engineering approach in health care has already begun in the ICUs in several settings. Project Emerge is an example of an active prototype developed at the Johns Hopkins Medical System and the University of California San Francisco to implement and track successful application of evidence-based practices to improve seven common harms in ICU patients. These include ICU-acquired delirium, venous thromboembolic events, CLABSI, ventilator-associated events, ICU-acquired weakness, provision of care inconsistent with patient goals, and loss of respect and dignity. Creating a model to address the chosen harms involved cataloging all the stakeholders, resources, and workflows associated with the evidence-based practices that contribute to the prevention of each harm. This detailed appraisal was necessary to gain insight regarding the interdependencies within the existing system. Based on this understanding, a generalizable, scalable framework was then developed, explicitly detailing the steps needed for harm reduction. A novel interface system was developed to allow providers to quickly visualize and assess successful application of known bundled elements of care to prevent the defined harms.

Similarly, researchers at the Mayo Clinic recognized issues surrounding burdensome interpretation of traditional electronic medical records; therefore, researchers created the Patient-centered Cloud-based Electronic System: Ambient Warning and Response Evaluation. This multicenter trial uses cloud-based technology to redesign the acute care interface system with built-in tools for prevention of provider error and practice surveillance.

Systems engineering principles can be applied within health care not only to establish new systems, but also to repair defects associated with existing ones. This practice has been successful across numerous industries with emphasis on safety amidst similarly complex infrastructure. Early returns in health care have been promising, and in an era of increasing emphasis on performance-based outcome, widespread utilization of systems methodology may be the link to engineering health care toward zero harm.

SUMMARY

Approaching QI and patient safety as a science is a relatively new concept and broad area of health care research that draws upon many disciplines. Many health care organizations have made concerted efforts to address the hazards that plague safety. Over the past several years, most of our efforts have been aimed at investigating causes and executing interventions to improve patient safety. Only now are researchers beginning to discuss how to evaluate these interventions and determine if patients are indeed safer. Evaluating our programs—and reliably answering whether patients are safer—will require valid measures and the ability to know whether we mitigated hazards, an area that is currently underdeveloped. Yet, the measurement model we describe in this chapter should move us in the right direction in developing new measures of safety.

To begin to improve patient safety and quality, we can implement collaborative projects that utilize proven models such as Translating Evidence into Practice (TRiP) and the Comprehensive Unit-based Safety Program (CUSP). Such initiatives foster a culture of safety where staff learns the interdependence between patient safety and quality, and why they are important, identify system failures in their workplace, and turn their efforts into safety and QI. Indeed, staff feels valued for their opinions and recognized when senior leaders listen. Once a more solid safety culture is established, interventions can be implemented more effectively through collaborative projects. The CUSP also provides feasible and reliable tools for collaboration to implement improvements in communication, teamwork, and adverse-event investigations. Collaborative projects are important because multiple sites that share the same goal can network to communicate successes and correct failures. The shared momentum increases sustainability.

Any QI program should provide a practical, goal-oriented toolset that will improve culture and lead to measurable improvements, using the principles described in this chapter as a guide. Additional research is necessary to identify other effective safety interventions. Links must be developed between the structural elements of health care delivery and patient safety outcomes. Given the evidence to date, it seems reasonable that all ICUs should be routinely assessing their culture of safety.

Although work is necessary at the organizational level, the question of whether our patients are safer and receiving the best quality of care possible can be meaningfully answered. Significant and very exciting improvements are beginning to be implemented throughout the United States and around the world. The critical care community must continue to develop the science of safety, but many of the foundations have clearly already been laid.

Key Points

- While providing care appropriate to the patient and their condition seems simple, doing so consistently requires proper adherence to QI principles including review and improvement of health delivery systems.
- Independent external evaluation and reporting systems are essential components in the evolution of a culture of safety and QI.
- Adoption of a common framework to evaluate and monitor safety is one of the greatest impediments to reforming health care quality and safety. The ideal initiative be designed to not only learn from past mistakes, but adapt to any unexpected present or future demands by being based on sound theory, using valid and objective metrics, application of a consistent methodology, and a systematic assessment of outcomes.
- A multidisciplinary approach involving all relevant stakeholders is necessary for successful QI initiatives. A conceptual framework of pertinent issues and solutions helps guide team efforts and ensure common point of dialogue. Examples of useful project frameworks include TRiP to operationalize safety intervention therapies, and CUSP to involve multiple levels of care providers in a work area while leveraging support from senior leaders.
- Using systems engineering to design system architecture, language, and integration with the existing health care environment to satisfy pre-determined QI and patient safety goals might help comprehensively alleviate systems defects by potentially preventing them from occurring in the first place.

REFERENCES

1. Institute of Medicine: Committee on Quality of Health Care in America. *To Err Is Human : Building a Safer Health System*. Washington, DC: National Academies Press; 1999:223.
2. Wachter RM. Patient safety at ten: Unmistakable progress, troubling gaps. *Health Aff (Millwood)*. 2010;29(1):165–173.
3. Downey JR, Hernandez-Boussard T, Banka G, Morton JM. Is patient safety improving? National trends in patient safety indicators: 1998–2007. *Health Serv Res*. 2012;47(1 Pt 2):414–430.
4. Institute of Medicine: Committee on Quality of Health Care in America. *Crossing the Quality Chasm: A New Health System for the 21st Century*. Washington, DC: National Academies Press; 2001.
5. Health Resources and Services Administration. *Quality Improvement*. Rockville, MD: U. S. Department of Health and Human Services Health Resources and Services Administration; 2011.
6. Auerbach AD, Landefeld CS, Shojania KG. The tension between needing to improve care and knowing how to do it. *N Engl J Med*. 2007; 357(6):608–613.
7. Shojania KG, Duncan BW, McDonald KM, Wachter RM. Safe but sound: patient safety meets evidence-based medicine. *JAMA*. 2002;288(4):508–513.
8. Leape LL, Berwick DM, Bates DW. What practices will most improve safety? Evidence-based medicine meets patient safety. *JAMA*. 2002;288(4):501–507.
9. Shekelle PG, Pronovost PJ, Wachter RM, et al. Advancing the science of patient safety. *Ann Intern Med*. 2011;154(10):693–696.
10. Simmons JC. Focusing on quality and change in intensive care units. *Qual Lett Healthcare Lead*. 2002;14(10):2–11, 1.
11. Centers for Medicare & Medicaid Services and The Joint Commission. Specifications manual for national hospital inpatient quality measures. http://www.jointcommission.org/specifications_manual_for_national_hospital_inpatient_quality_measures.aspx. Updated 2015.
12. Schyve PM. The evolution of external quality evaluation: Observations from the joint commission on accreditation of healthcare organizations. *Int J Qual Healthcare*. 2000;12(3):255–258.
13. Marinelli AM. Can regulation improve safety in critical care? *Crit Care Clin*. 2005;21(1):149–162.
14. Meyer GS, Battles J, Hart JC, Tang N. The US agency for healthcare research and quality's activities in patient safety research. *Int J Qual Health Care*. 2003;15(Suppl 1):i25–i30.
15. Angus DC, Black N. Improving care of the critically ill: institutional and health-care system approaches. *Lancet*. 2004;363(9417):1314–1320.
16. Gallesio AO, Ceraso D, Palizas F. Improving quality in the intensive care unit setting. *Crit Care Clin*. 2006;22(3):547–71.
17. *How to Improve*. http://www.ihi.org/resources/Pages/HowtoImprove/default.aspx.
18. Viswanathan HN, Salmon JW. Accrediting organizations and quality improvement. *Am J Manag Care*. 2000;6(10):1117–1130.
19. *National Quality Forum: About Us*. http://www.qualityforum.org/story/About_Us.aspx.
20. *30 Safe Practices for Better Health Care: Fact Sheet*. http://archive.ahrq.gov/research/findings/factsheets/errors-safety/30safe/30-safe-practices.html.
21. Saufl NM, Fieldus MH. Accreditation: A "voluntary" regulatory requirement. *J Perianesth Nurs*. 2003;18(3):152–159.
22. Catalano K, Fickenscher K. Complying with the 2008 national patient safety goals. *AORN J*. 2008;87(3):547–556.
23. *National Patient Safety Goals*. http://www.jointcommission.org/standards_information/npsgs.aspx. Updated 2015.
24. Stockwell DC, Slonim AD. Quality and safety in the intensive care unit. *J Intensive Care Med*. 2006;21(4):199–210.
25. Latif A, Holzmueller CG, Pronovost PJ. Evaluating safety initiatives in healthcare. *Curr Anesthesiol Rep*. 2014;4(2):100–106.
26. Bradley EH, Herrin J, Wang Y, et al. Strategies for reducing the door-to-balloon time in acute myocardial infarction. *N Engl J Med*. 2006; 355(22):2308–2320.
27. Pronovost P, Needham D, Berenholtz S, et al. An intervention to decrease catheter-related bloodstream infections in the ICU. *N Engl J Med*. 2006; 355(26):2725–2732.
28. Pronovost PJ, Berenholtz SM, Goeschel C, et al. Improving patient safety in intensive care units in Michigan. *J Crit Care*. 2008;23(2):207–221.
29. Pronovost PJ, Berenholtz SM, Needham DM. Translating evidence into practice: A model for large scale knowledge translation. *BMJ*. 2008;337:a1714.
30. Bosk CL, Dixon-Woods M, Goeschel CA, Pronovost PJ. Reality check for checklists. *Lancet*. 2009;374(9688):444–445.
31. Jha AK, Li Z, Orav EJ, Epstein AM. Care in U.S. hospitals–the hospital quality alliance program. *N Engl J Med*. 2005;353(3):265–274.
32. Pronovost PJ, Berenholtz SM, Needham DM. A framework for health care organizations to develop and evaluate a safety scorecard. *JAMA*. 2007;298(17):2063–2065.
33. Pronovost P, Holzmueller CG, Needham DM, et al. How will we know patients are safer? An organization-wide approach to measuring and improving safety. *Crit Care Med*. 2006;34(7):1988–1995.
34. The Commonwealth Fund Commission on a High Performance Health System. Why not the best? Results from the national scorecard on U.S. health system performance. 2008.
35. Davidoff F. Heterogeneity is not always noise: lessons from improvement. *JAMA*. 2009;302(23):2580–2586.
36. *Preparing for Submission*. http://www.icmje.org/recommendations/browse/manuscript-preparation/preparing-for-submission.html.
37. Glasziou P, Chalmers I, Altman DG, et al. Taking healthcare interventions from trial to practice. *BMJ*. 2010;341:c3852.
38. Davidoff F, Batalden P, Stevens D, Ogrinc G, Mooney S, SQUIRE Development Group. Publication guidelines for improvement studies in health care: evolution of the SQUIRE project. *Ann Intern Med*. 2008;149(9):670–676.
39. Pronovost PJ, Goeschel CA, Colantuoni E, et al. Sustaining reductions in catheter related bloodstream infections in Michigan intensive care units: observational study. *BMJ*. 2010;340:c309.
40. Hofmann D, Mark B. An investigation of the relationship between safety climate and medication errors as well as other nurse and patient outcomes. *Personnel Psychol*. 2006;59:847–869.
41. Singer SJ, Falwell A, Gaba DM, et al. Identifying organizational cultures that promote patient safety. *Health Care Manage Rev*. 2009;34(4):300–311.

42. Schulman PR. General attributes of safe organisations. *Qual Saf Health Care*. 2004;13 Suppl 2:ii39–ii44.
43. Frankel AS, Leonard MW, Denham CR. Fair and just culture, team behavior, and leadership engagement: the tools to achieve high reliability. *Health Serv Res*. 2006;41(4 Pt 2):1690–1709.
44. Vincent C, Burnett S, Carthey J. The measurement and monitoring of safety. 2013.
45. Stelfox HT, Bates DW, Redelmeier DA. Safety of patients isolated for infection control. *JAMA*. 2003;290(14):1899–1905.
46. Shojania KG, Jennings A, Mayhew A, Ramsay C, Eccles M, Grimshaw J. Effect of point-of-care computer reminders on physician behaviour: a systematic review. *CMAJ*. 2010;182(5):E216–E225.
47. Shojania S, Duncan B, McDonald K, Wachter R, Markowitz A, eds. *Making Health Care Safer. A Critical Analysis of Patient Safety Practices*. Rockville, MD: AHRQ Publication; 2001:E01–E058.
48. Pilcher JJ, Huffcutt AI. Effects of sleep deprivation on performance: a meta-analysis. *Sleep*. 1996;19(4):318–326.
49. Weinger MB, Ancoli-Israel S. Sleep deprivation and clinical performance. *JAMA*. 2002;287(8):955–957.
50. Laine C, Goldman L, Soukup JR, Hayes JG. The impact of a regulation restricting medical house staff working hours on the quality of patient care. *JAMA*. 1993;269(3):374–378.
51. Prasad M, Iwashyna TJ, Christie JD, et al. Effect of work-hours regulations on intensive care unit mortality in united states teaching hospitals. *Crit Care Med*. 2009;37(9):2564–2569.
52. Volpp KG, Rosen AK, Rosenbaum PR, et al. Mortality among hospitalized Medicare beneficiaries in the first 2 years following ACGME resident duty hour reform. *JAMA*. 2007;298(9):975–983.
53. Bates DW, Leape LL, Cullen DJ, et al. Effect of computerized physician order entry and a team intervention on prevention of serious medication errors. *JAMA*. 1998;280(15):1311–1316.
54. Koppel R, Metlay JP, Cohen A, et al. Role of computerized physician order entry systems in facilitating medication errors. *JAMA*. 2005; 293(10):1197–1203.
55. Dy SM, Taylor SL, Carr LH, et al. A framework for classifying patient safety practices: Results from an expert consensus process. *BMJ Qual Saf*. 2011; 20(7):618–624.
56. Pronovost PJ, Goeschel CA, Marsteller JA, et al. Framework for patient safety research and improvement. *Circulation*. 2009;119(2):330–337.
57. Pronovost PJ, Murphy DJ, Needham DM. The science of translating research into practice in intensive care. *Am J Respir Crit Care Med*. 2010; 182(12):1463–1464.
58. Fan E, Needham DM, Stewart TE. Ventilatory management of acute lung injury and acute respiratory distress syndrome. *JAMA*. 2005; 294(22):2889–2896.
59. Ventilation with lower tidal volumes as compared with traditional tidal volumes for acute lung injury and the acute respiratory distress syndrome. The acute respiratory distress syndrome network. *N Engl J Med*. 2000; 342(18):1301–1308.
60. Kalhan R, Mikkelsen M, Dedhiya P, et al. Underuse of lung protective ventilation: analysis of potential factors to explain physician behavior. *Crit Care Med*. 2006;34(2):300–306.
61. Young MP, Manning HL, Wilson DL, et al. Ventilation of patients with acute lung injury and acute respiratory distress syndrome: has new evidence changed clinical practice? *Crit Care Med*. 2004;32(6):1260–1265.
62. Rubenfeld GD, Cooper C, Carter G, Thompson BT, Hudson LD. Barriers to providing lung-protective ventilation to patients with acute lung injury. *Crit Care Med*. 2004;32(6):1289–1293.
63. Morris AH. Guideline adoption: a slow process. *Crit Care Med*. 2004; 32(6):1409–1410.
64. Schultz MJ, Wolthuis EK, Moeniralam HS, Levi M. Struggle for implementation of new strategies in intensive care medicine: anticoagulation, insulin, and lower tidal volumes. *J Crit Care*. 2005;20(3):199–204.
65. Akhtar SR, Weaver J, Pierson DJ, Rubenfeld GD. Practice variation in respiratory therapy documentation during mechanical ventilation. *Chest*. 2003;124(6):2275–2282.
66. Dennison CR, Mendez-Tellez PA, Wang W, Pronovost PJ, Needham DM. Barriers to low tidal volume ventilation in acute respiratory distress syndrome: survey development, validation, and results. *Crit Care Med*. 2007;35(12):2747–2754.
67. Umoh NJ, Fan E, Mendez-Tellez PA, et al. Patient and intensive care unit organizational factors associated with low tidal volume ventilation in acute lung injury. *Crit Care Med*. 2008;36(5):1463–1468.
68. Pronovost PJ, Nolan T, Zeger S, Miller M, Rubin H. How can clinicians measure safety and quality in acute care *Lancet*. 2004;363(9414):1061–1067.
69. Pronovost PJ, Weast B, Bishop K, et al. Senior executive adopt-a-work unit: a model for safety improvement. *Jt Comm J Qual Saf*. 2004;30(2):59–68.
70. Pronovost P, Weast B, Rosenstein B, et al. Implementing and validating a comprehensive unit-based safety program. *J Patient Saf*. 2005;1(1):33–40.
71. Pronovost PJ, King J, Holzmueller CG, et al. A web-based tool for the comprehensive unit-based safety program (CUSP). *Jt Comm J Qual Patient Saf*. 2006; 32(3):119–129.
72. Timmel J, Kent PS, Holzmueller CG, Paine L, Schulick RD, Pronovost PJ. Impact of the comprehensive unit-based safety program (CUSP) on safety culture in a surgical inpatient unit. *Jt Comm J Qual Patient Saf*. 2010; 36(6):252–260.
73. Pronovost P, Weast B, Schwarz M, et al. Medication reconciliation: a practical tool to reduce the risk of medication errors. *J Crit Care*. 2003; 18(4):201–205.
74. Pronovost PJ, Hobson DB, Earsing K. A practical tool to reduce medication errors during patient transfer from an intensive care unit. *J Clin Outcomes Manag*. 2004;11(1:26):29–33.
75. Pronovost PJ, Watson SR, Goeschel CA, et al. Sustaining reductions in central line-associated bloodstream infections in Michigan intensive care units: a 10-year analysis. *Am J Med Qual*. 2016;31(3):197–202.
76. Makary MA, Holzmueller CG, Sexton JB, et al. Operating room debriefings. *Jt Comm J Qual Patient Saf*. 2006;32(7):407–410, 357.
77. Makary MA, Holzmueller CG, Thompson D, et al. Operating room briefings: working on the same page. *Jt Comm J Qual Patient Saf*. 2006; 32(6):351–355.
78. Thompson D, Holzmueller C, Hunt D, Cafeo C, Sexton B, Pronovost P. A morning briefing: setting the stage for a clinically and operationally good day. *Jt Comm J Qual Patient Saf*. 2005;31(8):476–479.
79. Pronovost PJ, Holzmueller CG, Martinez E, et al. A practical tool to learn from defects in patient care. *Jt Comm J Qual Patient Saf*. 2006; 32(2):102–108.
80. Berenholtz SM, Hartsell TL, Pronovost PJ. Learning from defects to enhance morbidity and mortality conferences. *Am J Med Qual*. 2009;24(3):192–195.
81. Holzmueller CG, Pronovost PJ, Dickman F, et al. Creating the web-based intensive care unit safety reporting system. *J Am Med Inform Assoc*. 2005; 12(2):130–139.
82. Sexton JB, Thomas EJ, Helmreich RL. Error, stress, and teamwork in medicine and aviation: Cross sectional surveys. *BMJ*. 2000;320(7237):745–749.
83. Hockey GR, Sauer J. Cognitive fatigue and complex decision making under prolonged isolation and confinement. *Adv Space Biol Med*. 1996; 5:309–330.
84. Hales BM, Pronovost PJ. The checklist–a tool for error management and performance improvement. *J Crit Care*. 2006;21(3):231–235.
85. Pronovost P, Berenholtz S, Dorman T, et al. Improving communication in the ICU using daily goals. *J Crit Care*. 2003;18(2):71–75.
86. Fowlkes J, Dwyer D, Oser R, et al. Event-based approach to training. *Int J Aviation Psychology*. 1998;8:209–221.
87. Gaba D. Structural and organizational issues in patient safety: a comparison of health care to other high-hazard industries. *Calif Manage Rev*. 2000;43:83–102.
88. Cooper J. The role of simulation in patient safety. In: Dunn W, ed. *Simulators in Critical Care and Beyond*. Des Plaines, IL: Society of Critical Care Medicine; 2004:20–24.
89. Bird D, Zambuto A, O'Donnell C, et al. Adherence to ventilator-associated pneumonia bundle and incidence of ventilator-associated pneumonia in the surgical intensive care unit. *Arch Surg*. 2010;145(5):465–470.
90. Al-Tawfiq JA, Abed MS. Decreasing ventilator-associated pneumonia in adult intensive care units using the institute for healthcare improvement bundle. *Am J Infect Control*. 2010;38(7):552–556.
91. Chua C, Wisniewski T, Ramos A, et al. Multidisciplinary trauma intensive care unit checklist: impact on infection rates. *J Trauma Nurs*. 2010;17(3):163–166.
92. Fletcher G, Flin R, McGeorge P, et al. Anaesthetists' non-technical skills (ANTS): evaluation of a behavioural marker system. *Br J Anaesth*. 2003; 90(5):580–588.
93. Reader T, Flin R, Lauche K, Cuthbertson BH. Non-technical skills in the intensive care unit. *Br J Anaesth*. 2006;96(5):551–559.
94. Patey R, Flin R, Fletcher G, et al. Anaesthetists' nontechnical skills (ANTS). In: Hendricks K, ed. *Advances in Patient Safety: From Research to Implementation*. Washington, DC: Agency for Healthcare Research and Quality; 2005:325–326.
95. Grenvik A, Schaefer JJ III, DeVita MA, Rogers P. New aspects on critical care medicine training. *Curr Opin Crit Care*. 2004;10(4):233–237.
96. Salas E, Wilson KA, Burke CS, Priest HA. Using simulation-based training to improve patient safety: what does it take? *Jt Comm J Qual Patient Saf*. 2005;31(7):363–371.
97. Tropello SP, Ravitz AD, Romig M, Pronovost PJ, Sapirstein A. Enhancing the quality of care in the intensive care unit: a systems engineering approach. *Crit Care Clin*. 2013;29(1):113–124.

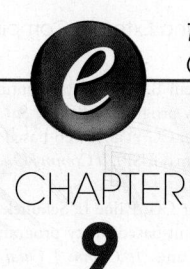

This chapter can be accessed in the accompanying eBook (see inside front cover for access instructions).

CHAPTER
9
The Virtual ICU and Telemedicine: Computers, Electronics, and Data Management

ERAN SEGAL

CHAPTER
10
Protecting the Health Care Practitioner

DENISE SCHAIN, SCOTT ALLAN BROWN, and NICOLE M. IOVINE

INTRODUCTION

Infection control is a key factor in protecting the health care worker (HCW) from infections that may be transmitted during patient care. This involves a complex interaction between patients, HCWs, and the hospital environment, and requires the use of specific measures to reduce the spread of infectious agents. In this chapter, we will review infection control guidelines as outlined by the Centers for Disease Control and Prevention (CDC), recommendations for vaccination in HCWs, and the application of these measures as they apply to common bacterial and viral agents in the health care setting.

HISTORICAL PERSPECTIVE

One of the pioneers of infection control was the Hungarian obstetrician Ignaz Semmelweis (1). While working on the obstetric wards at Allegemeines Krankenhaus in Vienna he became alarmed by the high rates of puerperal sepsis ("childbed fever"). He noted that the mortality rate on the delivery ward attended by midwives was much lower than the ward attended by physicians. Semmelweis postulated that women likely became ill when cared for by physicians who came directly to the obstetric ward after performing autopsies on women who had died of puerperal fever. However, autopsies were never performed by midwives. A colleague of Semmelweis, Jacob Kolletschka, died after he sustained a scalpel injury while performing an autopsy on a puerperal fever patient. His autopsy showed similar pathologic features to those patients. Semmelweis concluded that contact with infected autopsy tissue was the cause of puerperal fever when it was carried to the obstetrical patients on the physician ward. Semmelweis then implemented a simple measure asking the physicians to wash their hands with a chlorine solution after performing autopsies and prior to attending to obstetrical patients. Subsequent to this, the rates of puerperal fever decreased on the physician obstetric ward. To this day, hand hygiene is the central tenet for preventing the spread of infection. Further observations and advances have led to the modern era of infection control.

RECOMMENDED VACCINES FOR HCWS

A key component of protecting the HCW is vaccination. The Advisory Committee on Immunization Practices (ACIP) is a group of medical and public health experts that develops recommendations on how to use vaccines to control diseases in the United States. HCWs are at risk for exposure to serious, and sometimes deadly, diseases. The CDC and ACIP have published a list of recommended vaccines for HCWs (Table 10.1). These are general recommendations for HCWs who are not immunocompromised. If an HCW is pregnant or plans to become pregnant, all vaccine decisions should be discussed with her health care provider first. HCWs should not become

TABLE 10.1 CDC-Recommended Vaccines for Health Care Workers

Vaccine	Recommendations
Hepatitis B	HCWs lacking documented evidence of a 3-dose vaccine series and evidence of protective immunity defined as a HBsAg titer ≥10 mIU/mL should: • Receive the 3-dose vaccine series • Obtain a HBsAg titer 1–2 mo after the 3rd dose
Influenza	Annual vaccination with an inactivated (intramuscular) influenza vaccine
Measles, mumps, rubella (MMR)	[a]HCWs who have not had the MMR vaccine series, or those lacking serologic evidence of immunity also should receive 2 doses of MMR [b]MMR vaccine should not be administered to HCWs known to be pregnant or attempting to become pregnant or to immunocompromised HCWs
Varicella (chickenpox)	HCWs who have not had chickenpox, received the varicella vaccine, or lack serologic evidence of immunity should receive 2 doses of the varicella vaccine [b]Varicella vaccine should not be administered to HCWs known to be pregnant or attempting to become pregnant or to immunocompromised HCWs
Tetanus, diphtheria, pertussis (Tdap)	HCWs lacking documentation of prior Tdap vaccination should receive one dose of Tdap All HCWs should receive Td boosters every 10 yrs Pregnant HCWs should receive a dose of Tdap during each pregnancy
Meningococcal	HCWs who are routinely exposed to isolates of *N. meningitidis* should receive one dose

[a]Some health care institutions opt not to vaccinate HCWs born prior to 1957 based on the presumption of immunity from natural infection.
[b]HCWs should not become pregnant for at least 28 d after each dose of varicella vaccine, MMR vaccine, or any of the components of the MMR vaccine.
From Centers for Disease Control and Prevention. *Recommended Vaccines for Healthcare Workers.* Available at: http://www.cdc.gov/vaccines/adults/rec-vac/hcw.html.

pregnant for at least 28 days after each dose of varicella vaccine, MMR vaccine, or any of the components of the MMR vaccine. For specific recommendations, the full document is available on the CDC website (2).

PRECAUTIONS

In addition to vaccination, several types of precautions for use in patient care settings are critical to protecting the HCW. Making sense of them and knowing when to implement each can be confusing. The CDC has published guidelines outlining the recommended approach to infection control as well as the definition and application of the various precautions, including the specific personal protective equipment (PPE) to be used for each category. There are four types of precautions recommended in the CDC guidelines (3):

1. Standard (previously termed universal)
2. Contact
3. Droplet
4. Airborne

The CDC's 2007 Guideline for Isolation Precautions: Preventing Transmission of Infectious Agents in Healthcare Settings is available online (3). Appendix A of that document lists recommended precautions for an extensive list of diseases and conditions including links to updated information on emerging pathogens such as Ebola viral disease (EVD).

Standard Precautions

Standard precautions are those that are applied when the practitioner comes into contact with patients, regardless of the diagnosis. Standard precautions include hand hygiene before and after contact with every patient and between anatomic sites on the same patient. Based on the clinical task and setting, additional precautions may be required. When providing care or performing procedures during which the HCW may come into contact with blood and body fluids (including secretions and excretions, but excluding sweat), broken skin, and mucous membranes, use of PPE is required. This may include gloves, masks, eye protection, face shield, and/or gowns.

Other considerations include special handling of patient care equipment, including sharps and other instruments and correct disposal and cleaning of linen and other contaminated items. It is important to note that, while not all of these additional precautions apply in every circumstance, the standard precaution of hand hygiene is truly universal and must be done before and after every patient contact. Even in clinical situations where there has been no visual contamination with blood, body fluids, secretions, excretions, or contact with contaminated items, compliance with hand hygiene must be stressed. Hands must be cleaned immediately after gloves are removed if they were worn. In addition, hand hygiene should be performed whenever indicated to avoid transfer of microorganisms to other patients and the environment, such as after contact with intravenous tubing or a monitor even when there has been no direct patient contact. An alcohol-based hand sanitizer with at least 60% alcohol should be used for most routine care. Alcohol-based hand sanitizers have been shown to be more convenient, faster, and more efficient than hand washing (4,5), and many institutions have these available throughout patient care areas. However, alcohol-based regimens are not recommended in all situations. Hand washing with soap and water is recommended in situations where visible soiling on hands occurred or in environments where spores may be present such as when caring for patients with *Clostridium difficile*.

In order to decrease pathogens that can be transmitted on HCW clothing, there are now HCW clothing restrictions in Britain including the elimination of ties, except bow ties, and white coats with long sleeves. While these HCW clothing restriction proposals are not currently being practiced in the United States, some ICUs have instituted policies that HCWs wear only surgical scrubs while providing patient care and that white coats be removed prior to entering ICU rooms. At this time, these recommendations are not part of the CDC's standard precautions, but may become so in the future.

Gloves

Clean, nonsterile gloves are appropriate when contact with blood, body fluids, secretions, excretions, broken skin, mucous membranes, and items visibly contaminated by these fluids are expected. Gloves should be changed between tasks and procedures on the same patient if contact with material containing a high concentration of microorganisms occurs and between different anatomic sites on the same patient. Gloves should be removed immediately after use and hand hygiene performed before contact with the environment to avoid contamination of surfaces. Between contact with the next patient, hand hygiene must always be performed and new gloves donned if indicated; failure to do so is an infection control hazard (6). According to CDC guidelines, the use of gloves does not replace the need for hand hygiene. Gloves may have small, unapparent perforations or may be torn during use. Also, hands can become contaminated during removal of gloves (6) and clean gloves may be contaminated with dirty hands prior to donning making hand hygiene after glove removal critical.

Mask, Eye Protection, and Face Shield

The mucous membranes of the HCW, including those of the eyes, nose, and mouth, are at risk for exposure when performing procedures or patient care tasks that may generate aerosols or droplets. Bronchoscopy, open suctioning, and intubation are examples of aerosol-generating procedures (AGPs). Masks, goggles (eye protection), or face shields should be worn to protect the mucous membranes of the HCW.

Gowns

A clean, nonsterile gown that is fluid resistant or impermeable should be used during procedures and patient care activities when the clothing or skin of an HCW may be at risk for exposure or contamination. A gown should be worn if the patient is incontinent of urine or stool, has an ileostomy, colostomy, or wound drainage not covered, or contained by a dressing. Gowns should be removed immediately after patient contact and should not be worn outside of the patient's room. Hands may be contaminated during gown removal and hand hygiene should be performed prior to contact with the environment or other patients.

Patient Care Equipment and Linen

If patient care equipment is soiled with blood, body fluids, secretions, and excretions, the HCW should don appropriate PPE to prevent skin and mucous membrane exposures, contamination of HCW clothing, and transfer of microorganisms to other patients and the environment. Multi-use equipment should be appropriately cleaned or processed prior to being used for the care of another patient. Single-use items should be disposed of in the appropriate manner. Adequate procedures for the routine cleaning and disinfection of environmental surfaces, beds, bedrails, bedside equipment, and other high-touch surfaces should be established. Soiled linen should be handled and transported in a manner that prevents skin and mucous membrane exposure and contamination of HCW clothing (7).

Contact Precautions

Contact precautions are designed to reduce the risk of transmission of epidemiologically important microorganisms and certain infestations caused by lice or scabies. Transmission of these organisms or conditions may take place either by direct or indirect contact. Direct contact transmission from patient to staff includes physical transfer of microorganisms to the HCW from an infected or colonized patient. This usually takes place via skin-to-skin contact during patient care activities. Indirect transmission occurs when an HCW comes into contact with a contaminated intermediate object in the patient's environment, particularly high-touch surfaces such as monitors, medication pumps, bedrails, bedside tables, commodes, and sinks. Pathogenic organisms that can remain viable on the surfaces in the patient's environment for extended periods of time include methicillin-resistant *Staphylococcus aureus* (MRSA), vancomycin-resistant enterococcus (VRE), Gram-negative organisms such as *Pseudomonas* spp. and *Acinetobacter* spp., and *C. difficile* (6).

Contact precautions involve appropriate patient placement, hand hygiene, gloves, gowning, and precautions when transporting patients and when using patient care equipment. Patients should be placed in a private room if possible; however, the door to the room may be left open. When a private room is not available, the patient can be placed in a room with a patient who has colonization or active infection with the same microorganism but no other infection (cohorting). If a private room is not available and cohorting is not achievable, the epidemiology of the microorganism should be considered and the patient population taken into consideration when determining patient placement. An example of this would include the avoidance of placing an immunocompromised patient in the same room as a patient with a resistant organism.

Gloves and hand hygiene should be used as with standard precautions, and gowns should be used if there will be any contact with the patient, environmental surfaces, or items in a patient's room. However, unanticipated contact with the patient and/or the environment may occur. Therefore, many hospitals require a gown and gloves be worn upon entry to the room even if substantial contact with the patient or environment is not anticipated. Patient transport should be limited only to essential purposes, and if the patient is transferred out of the room, care should be taken to ensure minimal risk of transmission to other patients and environmental surfaces or equipment. Patient care equipment such as stethoscopes, thermometers, and intravenous pumps should be dedicated to a single patient (or cohort) to avoid sharing between patients, minimizing transfer of organisms.

Droplet Precautions

Droplet precautions aim to reduce the risk of spreading infectious agents when droplets formed by secretions are expelled from the respiratory tract during sneezing, coughing, talking, and open suctioning. Transmission in this manner occurs when infectious droplets greater than 5 μm in size come into contact with the mucous membranes (conjunctiva, nose, mouth) of an HCW. Droplet transmission requires close contact between the infected patient and the HCW, as droplets do not remain suspended in the air and generally travel only short distances, usually less than 3 feet. However, data from experimental studies with smallpox and experience during the severe adult respiratory syndrome (SARS) outbreak showed that droplets containing these viruses could reach persons up to 6 feet away. Because of this, the CDC suggests that masks and face protection be donned 6 to 10 feet from a source patient requiring droplet precautions. According to CDC recommendations, because droplets do not remain suspended in the air, special air handling and ventilation are not required to prevent droplet transmission, and the door to the patient's room may remain open (3).

Droplet precautions apply to any patient known or suspected to be infected with epidemiologically important pathogens that can be transmitted by infectious droplets, such as *Neisseria meningitidis*, influenza, *Bordetella pertussis*, rhinovirus, rubella, *Haemophilus influenzae* type B, adenovirus, *Mycoplasma pneumoniae*, and parvovirus B19. Patients should be placed in a private room or cohorted. Transport should be limited to essential purposes only. If transport becomes necessary, a surgical mask should be placed on the patient to minimize dispersal by droplets.

Hospitals should implement programs that encourage respiratory etiquette among patients, visitors, and HCWs. This includes covering sneezes and coughs with tissues which are then disposed of immediately, followed by hand hygiene. If tissues are not available sneezes or coughs should be covered by the upper arm or elbow and not directed into the hands. Visitors and patients may be asked to wear masks if they are experiencing upper respiratory symptoms (7). To prevent transmission to both patients and other HCWs, many hospitals require that HCWs with respiratory illnesses be medically evaluated prior to patient contact.

Airborne Precautions

Airborne precautions are designed to reduce the risk of transmission of respiratory infectious agents which are carried in airborne droplets less than or equal to 5 μm in size (droplet nuclei) or can attach to dust particles in the environment. Airborne transmission occurs by dissemination and inhalation of these droplet nuclei and dust particles which can be dispersed widely by air currents or may travel through ventilation systems. They may be inhaled by a susceptible host within the same room or by a patient several rooms or floors away from the source patient because a single ventilation system often serves multiple patient rooms. Therefore, special air handling and ventilation are required to prevent airborne transmission. Airborne precautions apply to patients known or suspected to be infected with epidemiologically important pathogens such as *Mycobacterium tuberculosis* (MTb), rubeola virus (measles), and varicella-zoster virus (VZV, chickenpox) (8). The patient should be placed in an airborne infection isolation (AII) room that has monitored negative air pressure in relation to the surrounding areas, 6 to 12 air exchanges per hour, and appropriate discharge of air outdoors or monitored high-efficiency filtration of room air before the air is recirculated to other areas in the hospital. The room door should be kept closed and the patient should remain in the room except for medically necessary tests. If a private AII room is not available, the patient should be cohorted with a patient infected with the same microorganism but with no other infection. Consultation with infection prevention and control professionals is advised before patient placement in the event no AII rooms are available (3).

An N95 or higher respirator must be worn to provide an adequate barrier to various airborne organisms including *M. tuberculosis* (9,10). Powered air-purifying respirators (PAPRs) may be used in these settings as well. PAPRs do not require fit testing and may be worn by HCWs with facial hair. Per CDC, HCWs with documented immunity to measles or chickenpox need not wear respiratory protection. However, hospital policies may dictate all HCWs wear respiratory protection regardless of immune status. Susceptible persons should not enter the room of patients known or suspected to have rubeola or VZV if immune caregivers are available. If susceptible persons must enter the room of a patient known or suspected to be infected with rubeola or VZV, they should wear an N95 respirator or PAPR.

Patient transport should be limited to the movement and transport of the patient from the room for essential purposes only. If transport or movement is necessary, minimize patient dispersal of droplet nuclei by placing a surgical mask on the patient. The patient is not required to wear an N95 respirator or PAPR during transport (3).

BLOOD-BORNE PATHOGENS

Handling of sharps (needles, scalpels, sutures and other sharp instruments or devices) during use, cleaning, or disposal should be done with extreme care to avoid percutaneous injury. Blood-borne pathogen training is mandatory for HCWs who have exposure to blood and body fluids per the Occupational Safety and Health Administration (OSHA) Blood-borne Pathogen Standard (11). Safe practices include never recapping any needle, avoiding manipulation of sharps using both hands, avoiding hand-off of a sharp from one HCW to another or using techniques that involve the point of a needle being directed toward any part of an HCW's body. Used needles should not be removed from disposable syringes by hand. Bending, breaking, or otherwise manipulating used needles should not be done. Used disposable syringes and needles, scalpel blades, and other sharp items should be placed in an appropriate puncture-resistant container which should be located as close as practical to the area in which the items are being used. Reusable sharps can be placed in a puncture-resistant container for transport to a reprocessing area. The Needlestick Safety and Prevention Act of 2000 directs employers to evaluate their medical devices on an ongoing basis and make efforts to convert as many devices as possible to safer products (11).

Human Immunodeficiency Virus

Human immunodeficiency virus (HIV) is the etiologic agent of acquired immunodeficiency syndrome (AIDS). Two species of HIV, HIV-1 and HIV-2, infect humans. HIV is transmitted primarily by exposure to blood and other body fluids from an HIV-infected patient. The three primary methods of transmission are via unprotected sexual intercourse, vertical transmission (mother to child), and contaminated needles (either occupational exposure or with the use of intravenous drugs of abuse). In the United States, blood products are screened for HIV, and transfusion-associated transmission essentially has been eliminated. Potentially infectious fluids include blood and blood-containing fluids; fluids from other sites such as semen, vaginal secretions, and cerebrospinal fluid (CSF); and, synovial, pleural, peritoneal, pericardial, and amniotic fluids.

After percutaneous or mucosal exposure, HIV replicates within dendritic cells and spreads via lymphatics to the bloodstream where CD4+ cells become infected. The delay in systemic spread leaves a "window of opportunity" for postexposure prophylaxis (PEP) using antiretroviral drugs. The most common HCW exposure is via percutaneous injury. Other types of exposures among HCWs include mucous membrane exposure, nonintact skin exposure, and bites. The average risk of HIV transmission to HCWs after a percutaneous injury is approximately 0.3% (12,13) and 0.09% after a mucous membrane exposure (14). Transmission of HIV via nonintact skin exposure has been documented (15); however, the risk for transmission via this route is much less than for mucous membrane exposures (16). The risk for transmission after exposure to fluids or tissues other than HIV-infected blood has not been quantified but is believed to be lower than for blood exposures.

Several factors may affect the risk of HIV transmission after an occupational exposure. Increased risk is associated with a larger quantity of blood from the source patient such as contained in a hollow bore needle, percutaneous injury that occurs during a procedure involving a needle placed directly into a vein or artery of the source patient, a deep tissue injury in the HCW and blood exposure from a patient with a high HIV viral load.

HIV Postexposure Management

Occupational exposures to HIV require urgent medical evaluation. The goal of postexposure management is to deliver HIV PEP to the HCW with a high-risk exposure within 2 hours. A number of occupational HIV PEP guidelines have been published (17,18). The initial step following an occupational exposure to blood and body fluids is prompt treatment of the exposure site including washing wounds and skin sites with soap and water and flushing mucous membranes with water. Squeezing the injured area to expel blood should not be done. The use of local antiseptics at the injury site is not contraindicated, although there is no evidence of efficacy.

The HCW should immediately report the exposure to facilitate rapid testing of the source patient for HIV, hepatitis B (HBV), and hepatitis C (HCV). PEP should be initiated for the HCW if indicated. The source patient should be tested for HIV immediately. FDA-approved rapid tests can produce HIV test results within 30 minutes, with sensitivities and specificities similar to those of first- and second-generation enzyme immunoassays (EIAs). Third-generation chemiluminescent immunoassays can detect HIV-specific antibodies 2 weeks sooner than conventional EIAs and generate test results in an hour or less. Fourth-generation combination p24 antigen—HIV antibody (Ag/Ab) tests produce both rapid and accurate results, and p24 antigen detection allows identification of most infections during the window period (the time period between HIV infection and the development of detectable HIV antibodies). Rapid determination of source patient HIV status provides essential information about the need to initiate and/or continue PEP. As per the U.S. Public Health Service Guidelines, regardless of which type of HIV testing is employed, all of the above tests are acceptable for determination of source patient HIV status (17). It is not necessary to investigate whether the source patient is in the window period unless acute antiretroviral syndrome is suspected (17). HIV RNA polymerase chain reaction (PCR) testing for routine screening of source patients is not recommended. As per the CDC, if the source patient is HIV negative, no further testing of the HCW is indicated. However, other guidelines recommend that if the source patient has been at risk for HIV exposure in the preceding 6 weeks, then an HIV RNA PCR should be performed on the source patient. Depending on the results, PEP is either continued or stopped (Figure 10.1) (18).

The severity of exposure is no longer used to determine the number of drugs to be offered in an HIV PEP regimen. A regimen of three or more antiretroviral drugs is now recommended for all occupational exposures to HIV. The drug regimen selected should have a favorable side-effect profile as well as a convenient dosing schedule to facilitate both adherence to the regimen and completion of the recommended 4-week course of PEP. As of 2015, the preferred HIV PEP regimen includes emtricitabine plus tenofovir with either raltegravir or dolutegravir. This once-a-day regimen is tolerable, potent, and conveniently administered, and it has been associated with minimal drug interactions (17). Expert consultation for HIV PEP is recommended for an exposure report delayed more than 72 hours, unknown source (needle in sharps disposal container or laundry), known or suspected pregnancy in the HCW, breastfeeding in the HCW, known or suspected resistance of the source HIV to antiretroviral agents, toxicity of the initial PEP regimen, or significant underlying illness in the HCW. HCWs should have follow-up within 72 hours of the occupational exposure regardless of whether they take PEP or not. If local expert consultation is not available, the National Clinicians' Post-Exposure Hotline (PEPline) can be consulted at 888-448-4911.

Hepatitis Viruses

Several hepatitis viruses have been described, including hepatitis A, B, C, D, E, and G. Hepatitis A and E are transmitted by the fecal/oral route, usually by contaminated food. They cause acute hepatitis that is generally self-limited and confers immunity to future infections. In a small percentage of cases, hepatitis E can develop into an acute severe liver disease that is often fatal, especially in pregnant women. Hepatitis D is caused by delta virus and can only replicate in the presence of HBV. By far, HBV and HCV pose the greatest threat to HCWs.

Hepatitis B

HBV is endemic in many parts of the world, causes both acute and chronic hepatitis, and is a major cause of hepatocellular carcinoma. The virus is transmitted through exposure to blood and body fluids. Routes of transmission include unprotected sexual contact, blood transfusions, use of contaminated needles and syringes, vertical transmission, and occupational exposure including needlesticks and mucous membrane exposure. As with many blood-borne viral pathogens, the risk of transmission from a blood and body fluid exposure is closely related to the volume of blood and the number of copies of virus present in the blood of the source patient. The percutaneous injury site should be washed with soap and water, and the mucous membrane flushed with water. Squeezing the injured area to expel blood should not be done.

Per the CDC guidelines, risk of transmission of HBV is also related to the HBV envelope antigen (HBeAg) status of the source patient. In patients who were both hepatitis B surface antigen (HBsAg) and HBeAg positive, the risk of developing clinical hepatitis from a needle injury was 22% to 31%. The risk of developing serologic evidence of infection was 36% to 62%. If the source patient was HBsAg positive with a negative HBeAg, the risk of developing clinical hepatitis from a needle injury was 1% to 6%, and the risk of developing serologic evidence of HBV infection was 23% to 37% (19). Blood exposure and percutaneous injuries are among the most efficient

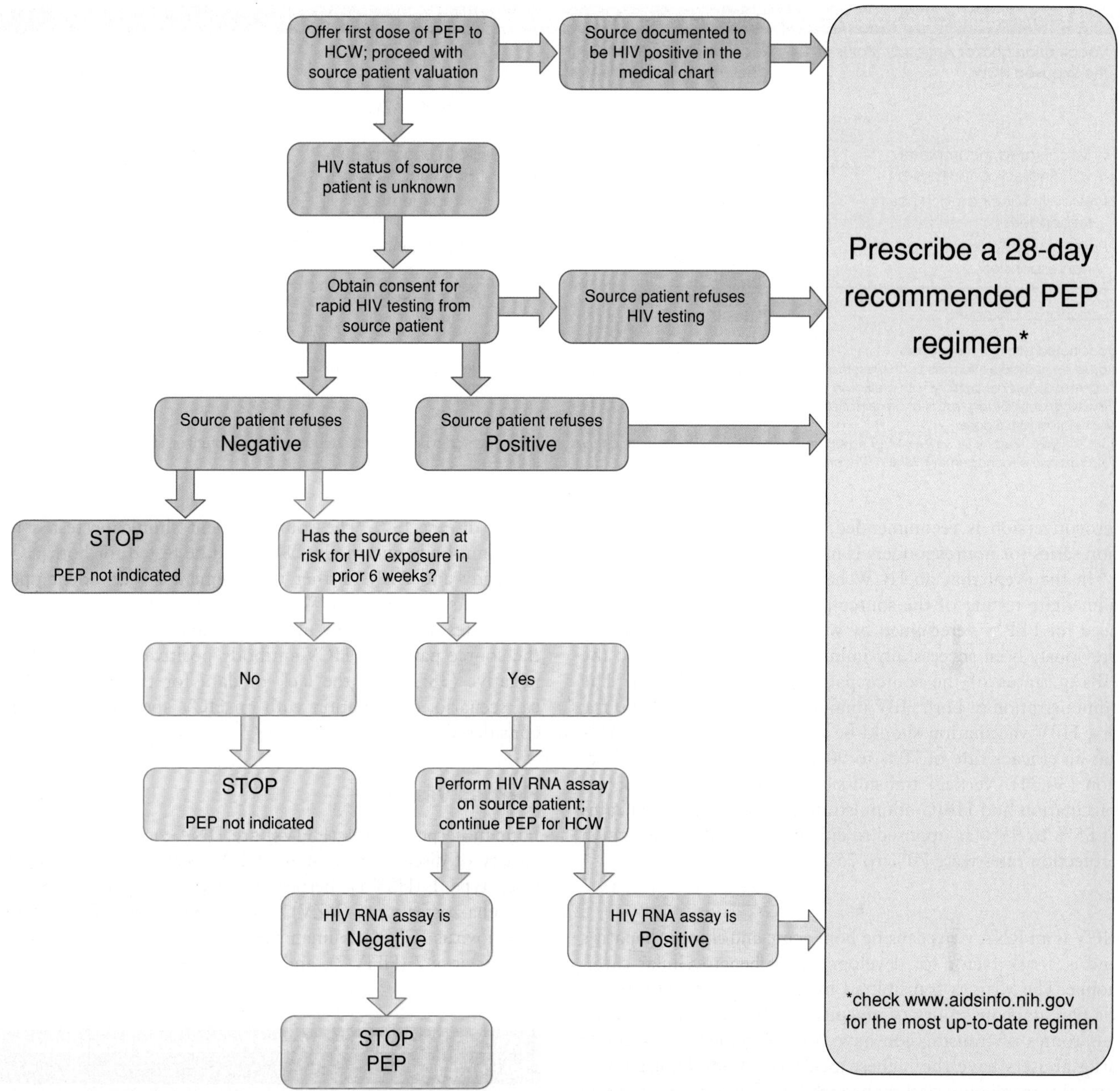

FIGURE 10.1 Health care worker HIV postexposure prophylaxis. The strategy for source patient evaluation and PEP recommended by the CDC is shown by the blue pathway. The orange pathway details additional steps recommended by other guidelines (18) when the source patient's rapid HIV test is negative. For both pathways, the choice of antiretrovirals for PEP (gray box) should be verified at www.aidsinfo.nih.gov, since the regimens change as new antiretrovirals become available.

modes of transmitting HBV since blood has the highest titers of HBV compared to other body fluids. HBsAg is also found in several other body fluids, including breast milk, CSF, stool, nasopharyngeal washings, saliva, semen, sweat, and synovial fluid (20). When investigations of outbreaks were performed, most infected HCWs could not recall a percutaneous injury but rather recalled caring for a patient who was HBsAg positive (21–24). HBV has been shown to survive in dried blood at room temperature for at least 1 week (25), and it is possible that contact with environmental surfaces is a potential risk for HBV transmission as has been shown in hemodialysis units (23,26–28).

The key factor in preventing HBV infection in the health care setting is vaccination. The OSHA Blood-borne Pathogen Standard requires employers to offer the HBV vaccine series to all employees who have exposure to blood-borne pathogens (11). The worker may opt out of the series but they can change their mind at any time and be given the vaccination series. HBV vaccination is part of the routine immunization schedule for infants and children in the United States; by the age of 18 months, children who are up to date on their vaccinations have been fully immunized for HBV. As with childhood vaccination, the protocol for adult immunization consists of three doses of the vaccine given intramuscularly in the deltoid muscle. For those whose HBV vaccination series is interrupted, there is no need to restart the series over again. Vaccination can resume based on where in the series the patient was at the time of the interruption. Follow-up testing to document

TABLE 10.2 Health Care Worker Postexposure Prophylaxis for Hepatitis B

Vaccination and/or Antibody Status of the Exposed HCW	Recommended Treatment When the Source Patient Is:		
	HBsAg POSITIVE	HBsAg NEGATIVE	Antibody status UNKNOWN or source not available for testing
Unvaccinated, incompletely vaccinated or nonimmune	HBIG ×1 and initiate or complete HBV vaccine series	Initiate or complete HBV vaccine series	Initiate or complete HBV vaccine series
Previously vaccinated,[a] known responder[b]	No treatment	No treatment	No treatment
Previously vaccinated,[c] known nonresponder[b]	HBIG ×2 separated by one month	No treatment	HBIG ×2 separated by one month
Previously vaccinated,[a] antibody response unknown[b]	HBIG ×1 and initiate revaccination	Initiate revaccination	HBIG ×1 and initiate revaccination

[a]Vaccinated with 3 or more doses.
[b]Based on available information on presentation. Responders are persons with previously documented adequate levels of serum antibody to HBsAg (≥10 mIU/mL); nonresponders are persons with previously documented inadequate response to vaccination (serum anti HBs <10 mIU/mL). Decision-making should not be delayed while awaiting anti-HBs test results at presentation.
[c]Vaccinated with 6 doses.
From Schillie S, Murphy TV, Sawyer M, Ly K, Hughes E, Jiles R, et al. CDC guidance for evaluating health-care personnel for hepatitis B virus protection and for administering postexposure management. *MMWR Recomm Rep.* 2013;62(RR-10):1–19.

seroconversion is recommended, and repeating the vaccination series for nonresponders is indicated.

In the event that an HCW has an occupational exposure immediate testing of the source patient should be done. The need for PEP is determined by whether or not the HCW has previously been successfully immunized against HBV and the HBsAg status of the source patient (Table 10.2) (29). The administration of both HBV immune globulin (HBIG) and the first HBV vaccination should be within 12 to 24 hours. This has an efficacy rate of 70% to 90% in preventing HBV infection (30,31). Vertical transmission studies using concurrent vaccination and HBIG administration report protection rates of 85% to 95% as opposed to either therapy alone for which protection rates were 70% to 75%.

HCV

HCV is an RNA virus causing both acute and chronic hepatitis and is a risk factor for development of hepatocellular carcinoma. The virus is transmitted by direct contact with blood via percutaneous injury or mucous membrane exposure. Various routes of transmission have been identified. Intravenous drug abusers have the highest incidence of developing HCV. Sexual transmission occurs through blood exposure, not body fluids such as semen or vaginal secretions. Vertical transmission is also possible, although this occurs infrequently. Mucous membrane or skin exposures, both intact and nonintact, rarely result in transmission of HCV. As with any percutaneous injury or mucous membrane exposure, washing the area with soap and water or flushing the mucous membrane site should be done immediately. Although data are limited on the survival of HCV in the environment, one study has suggested that HCV-RNA is resistant to drying at room temperature for at least 48 hours (32).

The average incidence of HCV seroconversion after percutaneous injury from an HCV-positive source is 1.8% (0% to 7%) (33,34). There is no vaccine for HCV, and antibodies which form after infection are not protective. Studies have shown no beneficial effect of immune globulin after an occupational exposure to HCV-infected blood, nor is there a recommendation for HCV PEP with the new HCV protease inhibitor agents (35,36). Postexposure management is aimed at the early detection of HCV infection and prevention of active disease (37). The source patient should be tested for HCV antibody and the HCW should be tested for both HCV antibody and ALT. Further management is dependent upon the results (Table 10.3). While it has been suggested that no further testing or follow-up is indicated for the HCW when the source patient is HCV-antibody positive and HCV RNA negative (38), given the lack of data for this specific clinical scenario, consultation with an HCV specialist should be considered.

Herpes Viruses

Human herpes viruses (HHVs) are DNA viruses that cause a variety of diseases in humans. HHVs include herpes simplex virus type 1 (HSV-1), herpes simplex virus type 2 (HSV-2), varicella-zoster virus (VZV), Epstein-Barr virus (EBV), cytomegalovirus (CMV), human herpes virus 6 (HHV-6), human herpes virus 7 (HHV-7), and human herpes virus 8 (HHV-8,

TABLE 10.3 Health Care Worker Postexposure Management for Hepatitis C

Clinical Scenario	Recommended Follow-up for the HCW
Source patient is HCV-antibody negative	No further testing or follow up
Source patient is unavailable or refuses testing	Follow up HCV antibody at 3 and 6 mo[a]
Source patient is HCV-antibody positive and HCV RNA negative[b]	No further testing or follow-up[b]
Source patient is positive for both HCV antibody and HCV RNA *and* Exposed worker is HCV-antibody negative	Consultation with an HCV specialist is recommended
Exposed worker tests positive for both HCV antibody and HCV RNA	Consultation with an HCV specialist is recommended

[a]HCV RNA should be measured in an exposed HCW if at any time the serum ALT becomes elevated to assess for acute HCV infection.
[b]Due to a lack of data for this clinical scenario, consultation with an HCV specialist should be considered.

also known as Kaposi sarcoma–associated virus). In the United States, the seroprevalence of HHVs varies. CMV seroprevalence has been documented to be 60% to 90% in the adult population. EBV and VZV seroprevalence is in the 80% to 95% range, while HSV-1 and HSV-2 antibodies are found in 50% to 70% and 30% to 50% of the adult population, respectively. Several HHVs cause similar clinical syndromes including vesicular skin lesions as well as organ involvement. After resolution of the primary infection, all members of the herpesvirus family establish and maintain latency and can reactivate to cause asymptomatic viremia or clinically significant infection.

HSV-1 and HSV-2 cause vesicles either in the oral or genital area. Standard precautions are indicated for HSV-1 and HSV-2 except in the case of severe infection when contact precautions are indicated. HSV-1 and HSV-2 can be transmitted to the HCW by direct contact with the lesions when standard precautions have not been followed. Primary infection with VZV causes chickenpox and VZV reactivation causes herpes zoster (shingles). VZV can be transmitted both by direct contact with the vesicles of chickenpox and shingles as well as via respiratory secretions during disseminated VZV infection. The recommended approach to patients with chickenpox includes both contact and airborne isolation. For patients with a localized shingles eruption, standard precautions should be used. Patients with disseminated herpes zoster infection should be placed on contact and airborne precautions. VZV-susceptible HCWs should not care for patients with VZV infections if immune HCWs are available (3).

One issue that arises in the clinical setting is the exposure of the nonimmune pregnant HCW to patients with CMV or VZV disease, as primary infection with either virus during pregnancy can be devastating to both mother and fetus. The transmission of CMV requires prolonged or recurrent close contact with any patient who is shedding the virus in body fluids and respiratory secretions. While there have been no conclusive recommendations regarding the precautions to be used by nonimmune pregnant HCWs with respect to patients with CMV, it would seem prudent to identify patients with active CMV infection so that these HCWs can be aware of the risk or be assigned to another patient. It must be recognized, however, that any patient can be shedding CMV without clinical signs or symptoms. This is the foundation for the CDC's strong recommendation of meticulous adherence to hand hygiene and standard precautions when providing care for any patient in any health care setting at any time as the best way to prevent CMV transmission. In patients with proven or suspected CMV pneumonitis, mask and eye protection may be a consideration in the nonimmune pregnant HCW.

A vaccine is available for VZV; it is a live, attenuated vaccine that is given in two doses spaced 4 to 8 weeks apart and is 70% to 90% effective in preventing infection and 95% effective in preventing severe disease up to 10 years after administration. For PEP, the VZV vaccine should be given to nonimmune exposed HCWs as soon as possible, but certainly within 120 hours. For nonimmune exposed HCWs for whom the VZV vaccine is contraindicated (immunocompromised or pregnant HCWs), provide VZV immune globulin (VZIG) within 96 hours. If VZIG is unavailable, intravenous immune globulin may be substituted. The vaccine is recommended for nonpregnant women of childbearing age, but not for pregnant women, with a further stipulation that women should not become pregnant for at least 1 month after each dose of the vaccine (39).

EMERGING PATHOGENS

Emerging pathogens are defined as agents of infectious diseases whose incidence is rising or threatens to rise in a defined time period and location. Such microorganisms may be entirely new, such as HIV; a known organism that has changed, such as pandemic influenza or the SARS coronavirus; or, a known organism that has spread to a new region, such as chikungunya virus in the U.S. Regardless of the pathogen, the type of PPE necessary to prevent the HCW from becoming infected with or transmitting the organism depends on two factors: (1) the organism's mode of transmission, and (2) the type of procedure(s) expected to be performed on the patient.

Ebola Viral Disease

Ebola is a filovirus, and the etiologic agent of EVD, first recognized during a 1976 outbreak in the Democratic Republic of Congo. More than 20 outbreaks have occurred since, mostly in central African countries. In 2014 to 2015, the largest recorded outbreak occurred in the west African nations of Sierra Leone, Guinea, and Liberia. As with prior outbreaks, many HCWs in the affected African nations contracted Ebola and died, a fact attributed to the difficulties in adhering to recommended infection control practices in a field hospital (40). However, transmission of Ebola to HCWs from an infected patient in an US hospital raised concern about appropriate PPE. Ebola is transmitted by contact with infected fluids or tissue with nonintact skin or mucous membranes, and by droplets that remained suspended in the air over short distances (<3 feet). By this logic, only contact and droplet precautions would be recommended (gown, gloves, surgical mask with eye protection). However, using this level of PPE, two HCWs in the United States contracted EVD (41). Given the complexity of medical care in acute care hospitals that includes AGPs such as intubation, and the inability to predict which patient will emergently need an AGP, the CDC recommends that HCWs wear an N95 respirator with eye protection or a PAPR in addition to gowns and gloves when caring for a suspected or confirmed EVD patient (40).

The CDC outlines a broad EVD preparedness plan that stresses early recognition as a key component of infection control and recommends four basic steps:

1. Initiate: Consider EVD when approaching a patient.
2. Identify: Assess the patient for EVD risk factors and evaluate for clinical signs and symptoms of EVD.
3. Isolate: If the assessment indicates the possibility of EVD, isolate the patient in a private room, limit staff contact, keep a log of persons who enter and leave the room, and don CDC-recommended PPE. An observer, ideally a trained observer, should be watching the PPE donning and doffing process to ensure that the HCW does not self-contaminate.
4. Inform: Alert hospital administration and the local or state health department.

Full details of the CDC's plan are available at www.cdc.gov/vhf/ebola/. The CDC also recommends that hospitals develop an EVD preparedness plan based on the Health Care Facility Preparedness Checklist for EVD (42).

Measles

Re-emerging pathogens are those that had been considered eradicated or controlled in the past but, nonetheless, show increasing incidence. An example of this type of pathogen that threatens HCWs is measles, that was declared eliminated in the United States in 2000 (43). However, due to declining vaccination rates in the United States and abroad, and due to the increased number of travelers from measles-endemic part of the world, outbreaks occur annually. Measles is of concern in the health care setting as it spreads via the airborne route and is one of the most infectious organisms known; >85% of nonimmune persons who share living space with a measles patient will contract measles (44). Patients with known or suspected measles should be placed in an AII room. Nonimmune HCWs should not enter the room of a known or suspected measles patient if immune care providers are available. If a nonimmune HCW becomes exposed to measles, vaccination within 72 hours is indicated or immune globulin within 6 days should be given as PEP (45). As a vaccine-preventable disease, the best means of protection for HCWs is to be immunized with two doses of the measles–mumps–rubella (MMR) vaccine (45) (Table 10.1). The MMR vaccine is contraindicated in pregnancy. Exposed nonimmune pregnant HCWs should be offered intramuscular immune globulin of 0.25 mL/kg (40 mg IgG/kg) (2).

Vector-Borne Diseases

Vector-borne diseases are transmitted to humans by rodents and arthropods, usually insects. Several viral illnesses have recently emerged or re-emerged in the United States. The chikungunya virus appeared for the first time in the western hemisphere in 2013 and is now endemic in the Caribbean. Dengue virus is endemic in the Caribbean and Central and South America but was eliminated from the continental United States. in 1946, except for sporadic cases along the southeastern border between Texas and Mexico. It re-emerged in Key West, Florida, between 2009 and 2010 (46). The mosquito vectors of chikungunya virus and dengue virus are found in the United States, and local transmission in the southeastern United States was documented (46,47). In 1993, hantavirus, carried by rodents, was identified in residents in the southwestern United States who suffering from a severe pulmonary syndrome later named hantavirus pulmonary syndrome (48). Despite the severity of the clinical syndromes caused by these viruses, they do not pose a risk to HCWs and standard precautions are recommended.

MULTIDRUG-RESISTANT ORGANISMS

Multidrug-resistant organisms (MDROs) are defined as microorganisms, predominantly bacteria, that are resistant to one or more classes of antimicrobial agents. Many are found in the community as well as hospital settings. Although the names of certain MDROs describe resistance to only one agent, such as MRSA or VRE, these pathogens are frequently resistant to additional antimicrobial agents. In 2013, for the first time, the CDC prioritized selected MDROs as "urgent", "serious" and "concerning" to reflect the danger they represent in the hospital setting (49). However, the risk to HCWs from MDROs has not been well defined. Therefore the careful adherence to standard and isolation precautions by HCWs affords the best means of protection.

Multidrug-Resistant Gram-Negative Bacteria

The bacteria of concern in this group include *Klebsiella pneumoniae, Escherichia coli, Acinetobacter baumanii, Pseudomonas aeruginosa, Salmonella*, and *Enterobacter* spp. Of particular concern are those Gram-negative bacteria (GNB) which have developed resistance to extended-spectrum beta lactam (ESBL) and carbapenem antibiotics (49). Some strains of these bacteria have acquired resistance to every antibiotic currently available in the United States, rendering the infections they cause untreatable. With the exception of *P. aeruginosa*, MDR GNB of clinical concern are primarily found in the gastrointestinal tract. Therefore, these patients should be placed on contact precautions. *P. aeruginosa* often infects the respiratory tract, and is a particular threat to cystic fibrosis (CF) patients (50). Although any patient with a resistant *P. aeruginosa* in a respiratory sample should be placed on droplet precautions, the 2013 Infection Prevention and Control Guideline for Cystic Fibrosis recommends that droplet and contact precautions be implemented when caring for all CF patients, regardless of respiratory tract culture results (51). *P. aeruginosa* also often infects wounds particularly in burn patients (52), and contact precautions are indicated for those patients. All these MDR GNB, however, can gain access to the blood stream, leading to high mortality. For example, the mortality rate for a bloodstream infection with a carbapenem-resistant *K. pneumoniae* is >50% (53). While adherence to indicated precautions will mitigate against colonization or infection with MDR GNB, the primary means by which HCWs can protect themselves is by 100% compliance with hand hygiene.

Methicillin-Resistant *Staphylococcus Aureus*

Serious MRSA infections declined in hospitals between 2005 and 2011, but still remain a major problem in both hospital and community settings (54). MRSA infections in the hospital are associated with both longer stays and higher costs (55,56). The U.S. National Healthcare Safety Network (NHSN) 2009–2010 reported that >50% of blood and urinary catheter associated infections caused by *S. aureus* were MRSA, as well as >40% of ventilator-associated pneumonia and surgical site infections (57). Methicillin resistance is mediated by the acquisition of a staphylococcal cassette chromosome (SCC) that harbors the *mecA* gene. Expression of the *mecA* gene leads to an altered penicillin-binding protein, PBP2a, which has a reduced affinity for β-lactam antibiotics.

Prevention of transmission is the most important step in controlling MRSA. Patients with MRSA infection in the hospital should be placed on contact precautions. However, hand hygiene remains a critical factor in preventing spread. HCWs must perform hand hygiene before and after any contact with a patient, even when gloves are worn as part of standard or contact precautions. Mask and eye protection are indicated if aerosols will be generated. Environmental surfaces have been implicated in the transmission of MRSA. In a meta-analysis of 127 investigations with 33,318 HCWs, 4.6% were found to be colonized or infected with MRSA. Poor infection control practices were implicated in both acquisition and transmission of MRSA by HCWs (58).

Vancomycin-Resistant Enterococcus

Enterococci are Gram-positive, facultative anaerobes that colonize the gastrointestinal tract. Two species in particular are associated with infection: *Enterococcus faecalis* and *Enterococcus faecium*. While many strains of enterococci remain susceptible to ampicillin, penicillin, and vancomycin, there has been an increase in the incidence of VRE. The NHSN reported that from 2009 to 2010, >80% of blood and urinary catheter associated infections and ventilator-associated pneumonia caused by *E. faecium* were resistant to vancomycin, as were >60% of surgical site infections (57). The rate of hospitalization with VRE doubled during the period 2003 to 2006 from 4.60 to 9.48 hospitalizations/100,000 population (59). VRE infections have been associated with adverse outcomes. The mortality rate from invasive VRE infections is significantly higher than infections with vancomycin-sensitive enterococci (60).

Risk factors for VRE colonization and infection include hospitalization longer than 72 hours, presence of significant underlying medical conditions (dialysis, cancer, transplant), previous antimicrobial treatment, care in the intensive care unit, and invasive devices (61). HCWs can become colonized in their gastrointestinal tracts, but the rate appears to be low and transmission to patients from this source has not been demonstrated. Transmission generally occurs from a colonized or infected patient to the hands of HCWs via direct contact with either the patient or contaminated environmental surfaces. VRE can survive from 30 minutes to 7 days on surfaces and equipment including stethoscopes (62). In general, the lack of proper hand hygiene appears to be the major factor in the spread of VRE from patient to HCW and back to other patients. Studies have shown a dramatic decrease in the incidence of VRE with the enforcement of proper hand hygiene, either with alcohol-based hand sanitizers or with routine hand washing (63). Proper environmental cleaning has been shown to also decrease the transmission of VRE (64). Patients who are known to be colonized or infected with VRE should be placed in contact isolation to prevent spread of the organism.

Clostridium Difficile

C. difficile is an anaerobic, spore-forming bacterium that causes pseudomembranous colitis, which manifests as diarrhea and can progress to toxic megacolon, sepsis, and death. An estimated 14,000 to 20,000 deaths/year are attributable to *C. difficile* infection (CDI) in the United States (65). CDI occurs when the enteric microbiota is altered by the use of antibiotics. Limiting the use and duration of antibiotics as well as choosing antibiotics with the narrowest appropriate spectrum is critically important to decreasing the risk CDI. The fluoroquinolones are one of the primary precipitating antibiotics, but cephalosporins, ampicillin, and clindamycin remain important predisposing antibiotics as well. However, every antibiotic has been associated with CDI. Suppression of gastric acid, advanced age, and severity of underlying illness are other factors associated with the increased risk (66). The organism produces two toxins, an enterotoxin (toxin A) and a cytotoxin (toxin B), which are responsible for diarrhea and colonic inflammation. Serologic testing using an enzyme-linked immunosorbent assay (ELISA) for detection of toxin A or B has a sensitivity of only 50% to 70% and is being supplanted by *C. difficile* toxin B gene PCR; the sensitivity of this PCR test is >95%.

Any patient with known or suspected CDI should be placed in contact precautions. While alcohol-based hand sanitizer may be used upon entering the room of a CDI patient, hand washing with soap and water must be performed upon exit because alcohol-based hand sanitizers do not kill *C. difficile* spores. The disease is spread from person to person via the fecal/oral route through ingestion of spores shed in the stool of infected patients. Such spores widely contaminate the infected patient's environment and can survive up to 70 days on surfaces and equipment. These spores can then be carried on the hands of HCWs who fail to practice proper hand hygiene and can be transmitted to other patients and areas of the hospital. Studies in which HCWs have been screened for *C. difficile* have reported carriage rates as high as 13%, whereas other studies did not detect HCW colonization. However, no studies have documented HCW *C. difficile* carriage to be associated with active CDI (67,68).

RESPIRATORY PATHOGENS

Mycobacterium Tuberculosis

MTb is the causative agent of tuberculosis. The disease is spread by aerosolized droplet nuclei from persons with active pulmonary infection when they cough, sneeze, speak, or spit. These droplet nuclei are 0.5 to 5 μm in diameter and remain suspended in the air. They can be dispersed widely by air currents or may travel through ventilation systems. About 40,000 droplet nuclei can be produced from a single sneeze and 3,000 from a single cough of an infected patient. The probability of transmission depends on several factors, including the quantity of droplet nuclei expelled, the effectiveness of ventilation, and the duration of exposure.

The most effective way to prevent transmission of MTb to the HCW is to identify patients at high risk of active MTb infection and place them in a negative pressure isolation room (AII) with airborne precautions until evaluation is complete. Patients at increased risk for exposure or infection with MTb include close contacts of persons with MTb, birth in or frequent prolonged visits to a high incidence country, residents and employees of high-risk congregate settings, and residence in medically underserved communities. Substance abuse is a specific comorbidity conferring increased risk of acquiring MTb (69). Since the mid-1990s, the majority of MTb cases in the United States have been diagnosed in emigrants from endemic areas.

Patients may have the classic presentation of pulmonary MTb with chronic symptoms including fever, night sweats, hemoptysis, fatigue, and weight loss. Immunocompromised individuals, including patients taking tumor necrosis factor alpha (TNFα) inhibitors, may have an atypical presentation with the acute onset of a fulminant pulmonary infection. Once placed in a negative pressure isolation room with airborne precautions, patients should have three expectorated or induced sputum specimens sent for acid-fast staining and culture for acid-fast bacilli (AFB). Patients with suspected MTb infection should not be removed from isolation until three adequate sputum specimens or specimens obtained by bronchoscopy or bronchoalveolar lavage have been obtained and are negative for AFB by smear (staining). AFB culture may take up to 6 weeks to grow on standard solid media and is, therefore, not used to decide on discontinuation of isolation. The growth of MTb using specific liquid culture media is significantly faster. The average time-to-growth detection with liquid culture is 10 to 14 days. Newer diagnostic techniques include nucleic acid amplification tests (NAAT) for MTb DNA can be used on both AFB-positive and AFB-negative body fluids. The positive predictive value of NAAT for TB is >95% in AFB smear-positive cases (70,71). The sensitivity for AFB NAAT in smear-negative cases is in the range of 50% to 80%, and it is not sufficiently sensitive to exclude the diagnosis of MTb in smear-negative cases (72).

Influenza Virus

Influenza viruses are RNA viruses which cause an acute febrile illness usually occurring during the winter months. However, influenza viruses circulate with low prevalence throughout the year and can cause infection at any time. The clinical manifestations include sudden onset of high fever, headache, myalgia, arthralgia, and cough. Transmission occurs via large droplets. Therefore, droplet precautions are used for patients who are admitted to the hospital with active or suspected influenza infection. While droplet precautions prevent spread, the mainstay of disease prevention is annual immunization. The Healthcare Infection Control Practices Advisory Committee (HICPAC) and ACIP recommend that all HCWs be vaccinated annually against influenza. The CDC recommends annual influenza vaccination for all persons aged 6 months and older with rare exceptions. Some hospitals have mandated annual influenza vaccination for all HCWs to prevent nosocomial transmission of influenza from HCWs to patients. For HCWs who opt out of influenza immunization, wearing a surgical mask may be required for all patient contacts during influenza season. There are two types of influenza vaccine. Because the live attenuated influenza vaccine results in replication of the virus in the respiratory epithelium with active viral shedding, the inactivated influenza vaccine is recommended for HCWs with direct patient contact.

Rapid influenza diagnostic test (RIDT) results are available in a little as 15 minutes. However, the sensitivity of RIDT ranges from 50% to 70%, and therefore, cannot exclude influenza infection if the result is negative, especially during periods when influenza disease prevalence is high. If the suspicion for influenza is high in a patient with a negative RIDT result, another respiratory specimen should be sent for influenza reverse transcriptase PCR (RT-PCR) testing if available. While awaiting test results, droplet precautions should be continued and antiviral treatment instituted. If RT-PCR testing is not available, the decision to treat is made on a clinical basis. Many hospitals will continue droplet precautions for any patient with an influenza-like illness to prevent transmission of other respiratory viruses (3).

Bordetella Pertussis

Pertussis, a respiratory illness commonly known as whooping cough, is a highly contagious disease caused by the bacterium *Bordetella pertussis*. Pertussis is spread by droplets created when infected person's cough or sneeze. Therefore, any patient with known or suspected pertussis should be placed in droplet isolation. Neither infection nor immunization produces lifelong immunity to pertussis as they do for diseases such as measles, indicating that previously immunized HCWs may not be fully protected against pertussis. In 2005, 2010, and 2012, substantial pertussis epidemics occurred. Cycles of pertussis occur and it is known that B. pertussis is continuing to circulate in a manner similar to that of the pre-vaccine era (73). Despite the possible limitations of pertussis immunization, the best way to protect against pertussis remains vaccination. PEP with a macrolide or trimethoprim–sulfamethoxazole is recommended for HCWs who have unprotected exposure to pertussis and are likely to expose a patient at risk for severe pertussis, including hospitalized neonates and pregnant women. Other HCWs can receive either PEP or be monitored daily for 21 days after pertussis exposure and treated at the onset of signs and symptoms suggestive of pertussis (2).

Neisseria Meningitidis

Neisseria meningitidis is the causative agent of meningococcal disease including meningitis and meningococcemia. The organism is transmitted by large droplets and patients with known or suspected meningococcal infection should be placed in droplet isolation. HCW who adhere to droplet precautions do not require antimicrobial chemoprophylaxis. PEP is only advised for HCWs who have had intensive, unprotected contact (not wearing a mask) with infected patients while performing mouth-to-mouth resuscitation, endotracheal intubation, endotracheal tube management, or close examination of the oropharynx. In HCWs who meet criteria for PEP, it is important to begin within less than 24 hours because secondary cases of *N. meningitidis* can occur rapidly after exposure. CDC recommendations for meningococcal PEP in adults, excluding pregnant and lactating women, include oral rifampin or oral ciprofloxacin. Rifampin may affect the reliability of oral contraceptives and female HCWs should be advised to use an alternative contraceptive method while taking rifampin. Pregnant or lactating women can receive a single intramuscular dose of ceftriaxone. Meningococcal vaccine has been used successfully to control community outbreaks but its use is not recommended for PEP in health care settings (74).

Respiratory Syncytial Virus

Respiratory syncytial virus (RSV) is a common respiratory virus that usually infects infants and children, resulting in a high rate of immunity in adults (75). RSV primarily causes a cold-like illness with or without fever but can also cause bronchitis, croup, and lower respiratory infections including bronchiolitis and pneumonia. It is spread by droplets and patients with known or suspected RSV infection should be placed in droplet isolation. However, nosocomial transmission appears to be exceedingly rare (76). The CDC recommends HCWs adhere to droplet precautions, and there is no PEP.

Coronaviruses

Coronaviruses (CoV) are common infectious agents that cause respiratory tract infection. First identified in the 1960s, there are now six coronaviruses known to infect humans including SARS-CoV (causing severe acute respiratory syndrome or SARS) and MERS-CoV (causing Middle East respiratory syndrome, or MERS). SARS-CoV was first recognized in China in November 2002, causing a worldwide outbreak between 2002 and 2003 with 8,098 probable cases and 774 deaths (77). Since 2004, there have been no reported cases of SARS-CoV infection.

MERS-CoV was first reported in Saudi Arabia in 2012 (78). This novel CoV causes a severe acute respiratory illness with a mortality rate of 30% to 40%. Diagnosis is made by RT-PCR, available in the United States through the CDC (79); no specific treatment is currently available. MERS-CoV, like other CoVs, is thought to spread by respiratory droplets, both large droplet and droplet nuclei, which are generated by infected persons through coughing and sneezing and by AGPs. However, the precise ways the virus spreads are not fully understood. Person-to-person spread of MERS-CoV, usually after close contact, such as caring for or living with an infected person, has been well documented. Infected patients have spread MERS-CoV to others in health care settings, such as hospitals, including to HCWs. These viruses may also transmitted by touching contaminated objects or surfaces then touching the mouth, nose, or eyes prior to performing hand hygiene. Patients with known or suspected SARS-CoV or MERS-CoV should be placed in an airborne isolation room with contact precautions. N95 or higher respiratory protection (PAPR) should be worn by HCWs and meticulous hand hygiene performed (80).

Key Points

- Hand hygiene is the most important intervention that can be performed to prevent illness in the health care practitioner.
- Standard precautions apply to contact with every patient.
- The CDC designates three levels of precautions in addition to standard precautions: airborne, droplet, and contact, and each delineates the PPE to be used by the health care practitioner.
- Additional precautions may be required based upon the nature of the task being performed and a patient's colonizing or infecting organism, symptoms, or other conditions.
- Certain vaccinations are recommended for all health care practitioners to prevent illness after exposures to infectious agents.
  - Exposed health care practitioners should under rapid evaluation and receive postexposure prophylaxis (if available) rapidly after a blood or body fluid exposure.

References

1. Wyklicky H, Skopec M. Ignaz Philipp Semmelweis, the prophet of bacteriology. *Infect Control.* 1983;4(5):367–370.
2. Immunization of health-care personnel: recommendations of the Advisory Committee on Immunization Practices (ACIP). *MMWR Recomm Rep.* 2011; 60(RR-7):1–45.
3. Siegel JD, Rhinehart E, Jackson M, Chiarello L. 2007 Guideline for isolation precautions: preventing transmission of infectious agents in healthcare settings. Available at: hppt://www.cdc.gov/ncidod/dhqp/pdf/isolation2007.pdf.
4. Boyce JM, Pittet D. Guideline for hand hygiene in health-care settings. Recommendations of the Healthcare Infection Control Practices Advisory Committee and the HICPAC/SHEA/APIC/IDSA Hand Hygiene Task Force. Society for Healthcare Epidemiology of America/Association for Professionals in Infection Control/Infectious Diseases Society of America. *MMWR Recomm Rep.* 2002;51(RR-16):1–45.
5. Widmer AF, Conzelmann M, Tomic M, et al. Introducing alcohol-based hand rub for hand hygiene: the critical need for training. *Infect Control Hosp Epidemiol.* 2007;28(1):50–54.
6. Garner JS. Guideline for isolation precautions in hospitals. Part I. Evolution of isolation practices, Hospital Infection Control Practices Advisory Committee. *Am J Infect Control.* 1996;24(1):24–31.
7. Centers for Disease Control and Prevention. Water, sanitation, and environmentally-related hygiene. Available at: http://www.cdc.gov/healthywater/hygiene/etiquette/coughing_sneezing.html.
8. Menkhaus NA, Lanphear B, Linnemann CC. Airborne transmission of varicella-zoster virus in hospitals. *Lancet.* 1990;336(8726):1315.
9. Fennelly KP. Personal respiratory protection against Mycobacterium tuberculosis. *Clin Chest Med.* 1997;18(1):1–17.
10. Li Y, Wong T, Chung J, et al. In vivo protective performance of N95 respirator and surgical facemask. *Am J Industrial Med.* 2006;49(12):1056–1065.
11. Bloodborne pathogens and needlestick prevention: occupational safety and health administration. Available at: https://www.osha.gov/SLTC/bloodbornepathogens/standards.html.
12. Bell DM. Occupational risk of human immunodeficiency virus infection in healthcare workers: an overview. *Am J Med.* 1997;102(5B):9–15.
13. Henderson DK, Fahey BJ, Willy M, et al. Risk for occupational transmission of human immunodeficiency virus type 1 (HIV-1) associated with clinical exposures: a prospective evaluation. *Ann Intern Med.* 1990; 113(10):740–746.
14. Ippolito G, Puro V, De Carli G. The risk of occupational human immunodeficiency virus infection in health care workers. Italian Multicenter Study. The Italian Study Group on Occupational Risk of HIV infection. *Ann Intern Med.* 1993;153(12):1451–1458.
15. Update: human immunodeficiency virus infections in health-care workers exposed to blood of infected patients. *MMWR Recomm Rep.* 1987; 36(19):285–289.
16. Fahey BJ, Koziol DE, Banks SM, Henderson DK. Frequency of nonparenteral occupational exposures to blood and body fluids before and after universal precautions training. *Am J Med.* 1991;90(2):145–153.
17. Kuhar DT, Henderson DK, Struble KA, et al. Updated US Public Health Service guidelines for the management of occupational exposures to human immunodeficiency virus and recommendations for postexposure prophylaxis. *Infect Control Hosp Epidemiol.* 2013;34(9):875–892.
18. New York State Department of Health. HIV prophylaxis following occupational exposure. Available at: http://www.hivguidelines.org/wp-content/uploads/2015/04/occPEP_Website-PDF_4-2-15.pdf.
19. Werner BG, Grady GF. Accidental hepatitis-B-surface-antigen-positive inoculations. Use of e antigen to estimate infectivity. *Ann Intern Med.* 1982; 97(3):367–369.
20. Bond WW, Petersen NJ, Favero MS. Viral hepatitis B: aspects of environmental control. *Health Lab Sci.* 1977;14(4):235–252.
21. Callender ME, White YS, Williams R. Hepatitis B virus infection in medical and health care personnel. *BMJ.* 1982;284(6312):324–326.
22. Chaudhuri AK, Follett EA. Hepatitis B virus infection in medical and health care personnel. *BMJ.* 1982;284(6326):1408.
23. Garibaldi RA, Hatch FE, Bisno AL, et al. Nonparenteral serum hepatitis: report of an outbreak. *JAMA.* 1972;220(7):963–966.
24. Rosenberg JL, Jones DP, Lipitz LR, Kirsner JB. Viral hepatitis: an occupational hazard to surgeons. *JAMA.* 1973;223(4):395–400.
25. Bond WW, Favero MS, Petersen NJ, et al. Survival of hepatitis B virus after drying and storage for one week. *Lancet.* 1981;1(8219):550–551.
26. Garibaldi RA, Forrest JN, Bryan JA, et al. Hemodialysis-associated hepatitis. *JAMA.* 1973;225(4):384–389.
27. Hennekens CH. Hemodialysis-associated hepatitis: an outbreak among hospital personnel. *JAMA.* 1973;225(4):407–408.
28. Snydman DR, Bryan JA, Macon EJ, Gregg MB. Hemodialysis-associated hepatitis: report of an epidemic with further evidence on mechanisms of transmission. *Am J Epidemiol.* 1976;104(5):563–570.
29. Schillie S, Murphy TV, Sawyer M, et al. CDC guidance for evaluating health-care personnel for hepatitis B virus protection and for administering postexposure management. *MMWR Recomm Rep.* 2013;62(RR-10):1–19.
30. Beasley RP, Hwang LY, Stevens CE, et al. Efficacy of hepatitis B immune globulin for prevention of perinatal transmission of the hepatitis B virus carrier state: final report of a randomized double-blind, placebo-controlled trial. *Hepatology.* 1983;3(2):135–141.
31. Weinbaum C, Lyerla R, Margolis HS; Centers for Disease Control and Prevention. Prevention and control of infections with hepatitis viruses in correctional settings. *MMWR Recomm Rep.* 2003;52(RR-1):1–36.
32. Piazza M, Borgia G, Picciotto L, et al. HCV-RNA survival as detected by PCR in the environment. *Boll Soc Ital Biol Sper.* 1994;70(5--6):167–170.
33. Antono SK, Raya RP, Irda Sari SY, et al. Occupational risk for human immunodeficiency virus, hepatitis B, and hepatitis C infection in health care workers in a teaching hospital in Indonesia. *Am J Infect Control.* 2010; 38(9):757–958.

34. Lanphear BP, Linnemann CC Jr, Cannon CG, et al. Hepatitis C virus infection in healthcare workers: risk of exposure and infection. *Infect Control Hosp Epidemiol*. 1994;15(12):745–750.
35. Henderson DK. Management of needlestick injuries: a house officer who has a needlestick. *JAMA*. 2012;307(1):75–84.
36. Larghi A, Zuin M, Crosignani A, et al. Outcome of an outbreak of acute hepatitis C among healthy volunteers participating in pharmacokinetics studies. *Hepatology*. 2002;36(4 Pt 1):993–1000.
37. Updated U.S. Public Health Service guidelines for the management of occupational exposures to HBV, HCV, and HIV and recommendations for postexposure prophylaxis. *MMWR Recomm Rep*. 2001;50(RR-11):1–52.
38. Corey KE, Servoss JC, Casson DR, et al. Pilot study of postexposure prophylaxis for hepatitis C virus in healthcare workers. *Infect Control Hosp Epidemiol*. 2009;30(10):1000–1005.
39. Enders G. Management of varicella-zoster contact and infection in pregnancy using a standardized varicella-zoster ELISA test. *Postgrad Med J*. 1985;61(Suppl 4):23–30.
40. Centers for Disease Control and Prevention. Ebola (ebola virus disease). Available at: http://www.cdc.gov/vhf/ebola/outbreaks/history/distribution-map.html.
41. Chevalier MS, Chung W, Smith J, et al. Ebola virus disease cluster in the United States–Dallas County, Texas, 2014. *MMWR Recomm Rep*. 2014; 63(46):1087–1088.
42. Centers for Disease Control and Prevention. Health care facility preparedness checklist for ebola virus disease (EVD). Available at: http://www.cdc.gov/vhf/ebola/pdf/healthcare-facility-checklist-for-ebola.pdf.
43. Katz SL, Hinman AR. Summary and conclusions: measles elimination meeting, 16-17 March 2000. *J Infect Dis*. 2004;189(Suppl 1):S43–S47.
44. Top FH. Measles in Detroit, 1935. I. Factors influencing the secondary attack rate among susceptibles at risk. *Am J Public Health*. 1938;28(8):935–943.
45. McLean HQ, Fiebelkorn AP, Temte JL, Wallace GS. Prevention of measles, rubella, congenital rubella syndrome, and mumps, 2013: summary recommendations of the Advisory Committee on Immunization Practices (ACIP). *MMWR Recomm Rep*. 2013;62(RR-04):1–34.
46. Locally acquired Dengue—Key West, Florida, 2009-2010. *MMWR Recomm Rep*. 2010;59(19):577–581.
47. Kendrick K, Stanek D, Blackmore C; Centers for Disease Prevention. Notes from the field: transmission of chikungunya virus in the continental United States–Florida, 2014. *MMWR Recomm Rep*. 2014;63(48):1137.
48. Duchin JS, Koster FT, Peters CJ, et al. Hantavirus pulmonary syndrome: a clinical description of 17 patients with a newly recognized disease. The Hantavirus Study Group. *N Engl J Med*. 1994;330(14):949–955.
49. Centers for Disease Control and Prevention. Antibiotic resistant threats in the United States, 2013:. Available at: http://www.cdc.gov/drugresistance/pdf/ar-threats-2013-508.pdf.
50. Lyczak JB, Cannon CL, Pier GB. Lung infections associated with cystic fibrosis. *Clin Microbiol Rev*. 2002;15(2):194–222.
51. Saiman L, Siegel JD, LiPuma JJ, et al. Infection prevention and control guideline for cystic fibrosis: 2013 update. *Infect Control Hosp Epidemiol*. 2014;35(Suppl 1):S1–S67.
52. Church D, Elsayed S, Reid O, et al. Burn wound infections. *Clin Microbiol Rev*. 2006;19(2):403–434.
53. Arnold RS, Thom KA, Sharma S, et al. Emergence of Klebsiella pneumoniae carbapenemase-producing bacteria. *South Med J*. 2011;104(1):40–45.
54. Centers for Disease Control and Prevention. Methicillin-resistant Staphylococcus aureus (MRSA) infections. Available at: http://www.cdc.gov/mrsa/healthcare/index.html.
55. Chaix C, Durand-Zaleski I, Alberti C, et al. Control of endemic methicillin-resistant Staphylococcus aureus: a cost--benefit analysis in an intensive care unit. *JAMA*. 1999;282(18):1745–1751.
56. Cosgrove SE, Qi Y, Kaye KS, et al. The impact of methicillin resistance in Staphylococcus aureus bacteremia on patient outcomes: mortality, length of stay, and hospital charges. *Infect Control Hosp Epidemiol*. 2005;26(2):166–174.
57. Sievert DM, Ricks P, Edwards JR, et al. Antimicrobial-resistant pathogens associated with healthcare-associated infections: summary of data reported to the National Healthcare Safety Network at the Centers for Disease Control and Prevention, 2009-2010. *Infect Control Hosp Epidemiol*. 2013;34(1):1–14.
58. Albrich WC, Harbarth S. Health-care workers: source, vector, or victim of MRSA? *Lancet Infect Dis*. 2008;8(5):289–301.
59. Ramsey AM, Zilberberg MD. Secular trends of hospitalization with vancomycin-resistant enterococcus infection in the United States, 2000–2006. *Infect Control Hosp Epidemiol*. 2009;30(2):184–186.
60. DiazGranados CA, Zimmer SM, Klein M, Jernigan JA. Comparison of mortality associated with vancomycin-resistant and vancomycin-susceptible enterococcal bloodstream infections: a meta-analysis. *Clin Infect Dis*. 2005;41(3):327–333.
61. Ostrowsky BE, Trick WE, Sohn AH, et al. Control of vancomycin-resistant enterococcus in health care facilities in a region. *N Engl J Med*. 2001; 344(19):1427–1433.
62. Cetinkaya Y, Falk P, Mayhall CG. Vancomycin-resistant enterococci. *Clin Microbiol Rev*. 2000;13(4):686–707.
63. Gordin FM, Schultz ME, Huber RA, Gill JA. Reduction in nosocomial transmission of drug-resistant bacteria after introduction of an alcohol-based handrub. *Infect Control Hosp Epidemiol*. 2005;26(7):650–653.
64. Hayden MK, Bonten MJ, Blom DW, et al. Reduction in acquisition of vancomycin-resistant enterococcus after enforcement of routine environmental cleaning measures. *Clin Infect Dis*. 2006;42(11):1552–1560.
65. Vital signs: preventing Clostridium difficile infections. *MMWR Recomm Rep*. 2012;61(9):157–162.
66. Dubberke ER, Carling P, Carrico R, et al. Strategies to prevent Clostridium difficile infections in acute care hospitals: 2014 update. *Infect Control Hosp Epidemiol*. 2014;35(Suppl 2):S48–S65.
67. van Nood E, van Dijk K, Hegeman Z, et al. Asymptomatic carriage of Clostridium difficile among HCWs: do we disregard the doctor? *Infect Control Hosp Epidemiol*. 2009;30(9):924–925.
68. Friedman ND, Pollard J, Stupart D, et al. Prevalence of Clostridium difficile colonization among healthcare workers. *BMC Infect Dis*. 2013;13:459.
69. Jensen PA, Lambert LA, Iademarco MF, Ridzon R. CDC Guidelines for preventing the transmission of Mycobacterium tuberculosis in health-care settings, 2005. *MMWR Recomm Rep*. 2005;54(RR-17):1–141.
70. Dinnes J, Deeks J, Kunst H, et al. A systematic review of rapid diagnostic tests for the detection of tuberculosis infection. *Health Technol Assessment*. 2007;11(3):1–196.
71. Update: Nucleic acid amplification tests for tuberculosis. *MMWR Recomm Rep*. 2000;49(26):593–594.
72. Lee HS, Park KU, Park JO, Chang HE, Song J, Choe G. Rapid, sensitive, and specific detection of Mycobacterium tuberculosis complex by real-time PCR on paraffin-embedded human tissues. *J Molec Dis*. 2011;13(4):390–394.
73. Cherry JD. Epidemic pertussis in 2012: the resurgence of a vaccine-preventable disease. *N Engl J Med*. 2012;367(9):785–787.
74. Cohn AC, MacNeil JR, Clark TA, et al. Prevention and control of meningococcal disease: recommendations of the Advisory Committee on Immunization Practices (ACIP). *MMWR Recomm Rep*. 2013;62(RR-2):1–28.
75. Eick AA, Faix DJ, Tobler SK, et al. Serosurvey of bacterial and viral respiratory pathogens among deployed U.S. service members. *Am J Prevent Med*. 2011;41(6):573–580.
76. Berger A, Obwegeser E, Aberle SW, et al. Nosocomial transmission of respiratory syncytial virus in neonatal intensive care and intermediate care units: a prospective epidemiologic study. *Pediatr Infect Dis J*. 2010;29(7):669–670.
77. Scales DC, Green K, Chan AK, et al. Illness in intensive-care staff after brief exposure to severe acute respiratory syndrome. *Emerg Infect Dis*. 2003; 9(10):1205–1210.
78. Rha B, Rudd J, Feikin D, et al. Update on the Epidemiology of Middle East Respiratory Syndrome Coronavirus (MERS-CoV) Infection and Guidance for the Public, Clinicians, and Public Health Authorities—January 2015. *MMWR*. 2015;64(3);61–62.
79. Schneider E, Chommanard C, Rudd J, et al. Evaluation of patients under investigation for MERS-CoV infection, United States, January 2013–October 2014. *Emerg Infect Dis*. 2015 Jul. doi: 10.3201/eid2107.141888.
80. Centers for Disease Control and Prevention. Middle East respiratory syndrome: information for healthcare professionals. Available at: http://www.cdc.gov/coronavirus/mers/hcp.html. Updated April 15, 2015. Accessed June 11, 2015.

CHAPTER
11

Transferring Critically Ill Patients

JOEP M. DROOGH, MARIJE SMIT-DROOGH, and JAN G. ZIJLSTRA

INTRODUCTION

Transfers of patients have occurred throughout the ages, and may be divided into three categories. *Primary transport* is the transfer of patients from injury site to first hospital contact. *Secondary transport* is the transport of patients from one hospital to another for continuing clinical care (interhospital transfer), and *intrahospital transport* is the transport between departments within the same hospital. This chapter will focus on interhospital and intrahospital transports.

Twenty years ago, approximately 11,000 patients per year required secondary transfers in the United Kingdom (1). Nowadays, nearly 1 in 20 intensive care unit (ICU) patients in the United States are transferred to another hospital (2,3). Moreover, and perhaps more worrisome, it is estimated that in the United States every year 4,000 mechanically ventilated patients who lost their lives might have been saved had they been transferred to a better qualified hospital (4). This illustrates that interhospital transfer of critically ill patients has played an important role for decades and is still of major importance today; it also speaks to the need—infrequently discussed—for the regionalization of critical care services.

The significance of transporting critically ill patients also applies to intrahospital transfers, as the availability of diagnostic tools, such as computerized tomography (CT), magnetic resonance imaging (MRI), angiography, and so forth, increases the need for transfer of the ICU patient through the hospital. While the goal during all such transfers is, and should be, to continue or improve the clinical care of the patient, the risks as well as the benefits of each transport event should be considered carefully prior to its initiation.

Transferring ICU patients, whether within or between hospitals, is a potentially challenging exercise and is, in our eyes, essentially a medical specialty with its own demands. As the same key factors apply both for intra- and interhospital transfers, we will not, further herein, discriminate between these two types of transfer, unless otherwise stated.

The Three Phases of Transport

Preparation begins with careful evaluation of the risks and benefits of the transport. The decision to move a patient should be made by the senior medical practitioner of the critical care team together with the physician accompanying the transport and the intensivist of the receiving facility (in case of a interhospital transport). The transport may be comprised of three phases: the preparatory phase, the transfer phase, and posttransport stabilization.

Preparatory Phase

This is generally the most significant stage as appropriate and detailed attention here minimizes problems in the other two phases.

- Stabilization of the patient before transport is an obvious goal, although other priorities may make this difficult to achieve. In general, all anticipated procedures should be performed before transport is considered *unless* this cannot be safely performed. Careful assessment of the patient's airway is critical, and adequate oxygenation and ventilation must be ensured. Patients who are combative, or who have decreased level of consciousness for whatever reason, are very carefully assessed for elective control of the airway *before* transport. The thinking that "...We will intubate once we get to the ICU..." may result in a patient with a compromised airway in the elevator. This is as true in patients with significant thermal injuries (especially inhalational injury), as it is in chest trauma, or respiratory distress. An apparently insignificant pneumothorax can progress rapidly—particularly with positive pressure ventilation—and tube thoracostomy should be considered. Once in place, chest tubes may be transported under water seal, and then, ideally, reattached to suction during any therapeutic or diagnostic procedure. If possible, vasoactive infusions are initiated in an attempt to obtain hemodynamic stability before any—and certainly before an elective—transport. Large-bore vascular access catheters should be in place, and volume resuscitation initiated in patients with shock, before transport is considered. When blood pressure cannot be stabilized, surgical exploration and control of bleeding must take precedence over any further diagnostic procedures.
- Communication and coordination are essential to the safe conduct of transport. When a patient is transferred to or from the critical care area, or between critical care areas, handoff information from physician to physician and nurse to nurse regarding the patient's condition, treatment, and management is mandatory. The reasons for the transport are adequately documented in the patient's chart and, critically, the patient handoff should be carried out in a flawless manner. Timing of arrival and procedures should be confirmed with personnel at the patient's destination, especially when CT, angiography, MRI, or nuclear medicine procedures are involved; mishaps are more likely when delays occur in these areas. Ideally, patient escort or security may arrange to clear the transport route and to have elevators standing by. A responsible physician from the ICU team should accompany the patient during transport.
- As resuscitative and scheduled medications, fluids, monitors, life-support equipment, airway supplies—including equipment for intubation and ventilation—and an oxygen supply, as well as adequate personnel need to be assembled, a checklist should be used to assist in preparation.

Transport Phase

During the transport phase, we attempt to maintain essentially the same level of care as the patient had in the critical care area. As such, we strive for the following:

- Monitor the patient and maintain stability
- Continue ongoing management

- Avoid iatrogenic mishaps
- Reduce the transport duration to a minimum

While transporting an ICU patient to and from ancillary locations, every attempt should be made to continue monitoring and care at the ICU level. Even monitoring modalities that are difficult to continue during the transport process may be re-initiated/continued when in a stationary location. By adhering to the principles of thorough preparation and minimizing time spent during the transport phase, we should decrease the potential for complications.

Posttransport Stabilization

When a patient returns to the ICU from a transport, no less attention should be paid to the posttransport stabilization phase than to the initial components of the process. Patients may continue to be at increased risk of secondary insults through the first 4 hours after return (5). Additional issues may have arisen during the transport/procedure, and therefore, handoff communication is essential. The primary team may not be aware of *all* of the problems that began in the OR/ED or during the transport, or important new findings may follow from a diagnostic procedure, thus a careful handoff is critical, and transport team members must review these issues with the critical care team, including the nurses, who are/will be caring for the patient. This communication is especially important for the trauma patients, who may have physicians from several disciplines involved in their care.

Monitoring

Perhaps more than any other patients, the critically ill demand that we individualize monitoring schemes, support systems, and the transport process. Guidelines have been set as the minimum acceptable standards:

- Continuous monitoring with periodic documentation of electrocardiogram and pulse oximetry
- Intermittent or continuous measurement and documentation of blood pressure, respiratory rate, and pulse rate
- Mechanically ventilated patients should have capnography to monitor ventilation. Airway pressure should be monitored and alarms set to indicate disconnects or excessively high airway pressures

SPECIAL CIRCUMSTANCES

Hemodynamically Unstable Patients

The importance of stabilization before transport cannot be overemphasized. Adequate large-bore venous access, resuscitation fluids, and blood products must be available throughout the transport. One person may need to be assigned the sole task of managing blood and fluid administration, especially if any significant amount of time is to be spent at an ancillary location. Patients with cardiovascular collapse may require multiple vasopressor and inotropic infusions, and these must be available during transport.

Neurotrauma Patients

Head injury is common in all age groups and remains a leading cause of morbidity and mortality in young adults. Once injured, the central nervous system is quite sensitive to secondary injury. Although the primary injury cannot be reversed, secondary injuries are prevented by optimal oxygenation (SpO_2 greater than 90%), eucapnia, systolic blood pressure no less than 90 mmHg, head of bed elevated at 30 to 45 degrees, and head in a neutral position. While these patients may require transport for diagnostic procedures not available in the ICU, transport may adversely impact intracranial pressure (ICP) or mean arterial pressure, resulting in compromised cerebral perfusion pressure and increasing risk of secondary ischemic injury.

Magnetic Resonance Imaging

The MRI can provide invaluable diagnostic information, but poses multiple management problems for the critically ill because of the effects of the magnetic field on monitoring and life-support equipment, physical isolation of the patient, and the frequently remote location of the scanner. If MRI is deemed necessary, careful planning is essential; with minor modification, most monitoring techniques are adaptable to the MRI suite. Because of patient isolation during the scan, particular attention should be paid to airway assessment.

Adverse Events

Irrespective of the type of transfer, there should always be an assessment of the benefit–risk ratio. Before the start of a transfer, one should always consider the risk of an adverse event occurring and, as noted above, plan the transport with care. A transfer should only take place if one can answer the following question in a positive manner: Does the indication for the transfer warrant the risk of an adverse event?

It is important to note that, depending on the definition of an adverse event, the incidence varies from 3% to as high as 75% (6,7). These events may be medical—most likely cardiovascular or respiratory in origin—or technical. The most common cardiovascular adverse events, with an incidence of up to 24%, are hypertension and hypotension, bradycardia and tachycardia, and dysrhythmias. Respiratory events are most often related to inadequate ventilation or desaturation, with an incidence as high as 15% (8–12).

Equipment failure or technical problems are common, occurring with an incidence of up to 36% (8,2–14). In fact, such misadventures may account for 46% of all incidents (15–17). The most common technical events are problems with the gas or electricity supply, defective equipment or, if transport is taking place outside of the institution, problems with the transport vehicle (13).

Prevention of Adverse Events

The impact of an adverse event during transfer may be more profound than in the ICU, because backup equipment and/or personnel may not be readily available. Efforts to minimize the incidence of adverse events, as well as to mitigate the effect of those events that do occur, are therefore of pivotal importance. Of note—and related to the detail above related to the Phases of Transport—with a skilled crew and teamwork, pretransport equipment checks, and careful examination of the patient, between 52% and 91% of adverse events may be prevented (11,16,18). This is most easily achieved by using a specialized transport team, specific transport training, and implementing preventive programs.

Mitigation of Adverse Events

Specialized Retrieval Teams Versus Standard Transportation

Ideally, the personnel accompanying a transported patient should comprise at least an experienced critical care physician and critical care nurse team. For intrahospital transports, both the patient's critical care nurse and physician often accompany the transport. There is evidence to suggest that, as with specialized interhospital transport teams, dedicated transport teams may do a better job with intrahospital transports, as well.

Studies comparing specialized with nonspecialized retrieval teams have shown lower adverse incident rates, decreased morbidity, and a reduction in acute physiologic abnormalities and mortality (11,12,19–23). Although, these data come primarily from retrospective cohort studies, there are other advantages of specialist transport teams as well:

- They are more familiar with transport-specific procedures and equipment (24).
- They do a better job in stabilizing the patient prior to the transfer (25).
- Front-end discontinuity is better addressed by an expert transport team. That is, there is less information loss, better treatment continuity, and less disruption of physiologic parameters during transfer (26,27).
- Nonspecialist teams have a higher incidence of dissatisfaction and stress (28).
- It is easier to maintain the expertise and training of a specialist team (24).

Transport Training

A small crew accompanying a critically ill patient during transport/transfer must not only be able to treat this patient with, at least, the same level of care as given at the referral ICU, but it must also be trained to deal with transport-specific problems. These problems include relative isolation, with little or no backup, inaccessibility of additional ICU equipment and treatment options, and working in a small moving compartment with significant noise (i.e., an ambulance, helicopter, or plane). Moreover, the crew must be able to deal with equipment failure, which means that technical knowledge of the equipment used is required. Therefore, the training of such a crew should focus on five items (29):

- *Preparation:* Thorough examination of the patient, review of laboratory results, EKG's, chest x-rays, and other results. In this way, one might be able to anticipate problems before they actually occur.
- *Teamwork:* Working with a small crew requires good communication skills; crew resource management training may be of value.
- *Equipment:* Equipment used is often different from the equipment used in the ICU because of its design for the transfer process. Additionally, there is the possibility of equipment failure. Hence, technical knowledge of the transport equipment is required.
- *Mobility:* Treating a patient while moving may be complicated. Consideration must be given as to what is possible while driving and what is not.
- *Safety:* Training for treating a patient while wearing a seat belt, communicating with the driver, and stowing unused equipment in a safe manner must all be simulated.

Although it has long been recognized that transfer teams should be trained before taking responsibility (13,30,31), training programs are not common in practice. In fact, only a few local training initiatives have been described (32,33), including one detailed crew resource management simulation training (29). This may lead to obvious problems alluded to above.

Implementing Preventive Programs

As an additional aid in preparation before transport/transfer, several pre-movement scoring cards and checklists have been developed (34–36). Just as the pre-flight checklists in aviation, the aim is to visualize potential transport/transfer risks so they can be acted upon before initiating the move. The scoring card developed by Berube for intrahospital transfers even showed a 20% reduction in adverse events when it was used (34). A checklist for intrahospital transports was published recently. This checklist covers all three phases of transport and can easily be adjusted for local use (Fig. 11.1) (37).

Equipment

The equipment used in the transport/transfer must comply with both ICU and transfer standards. As regards ICU standards, the equipment must meet ICU specifications, as one wants to maintain, minimally, the same level of care during a transport/transfer as while the patient is in the ICU. A standard equipment complement should be available for most critical care transports.

Suggestions for the kind of required equipment have been made (38–41). In general, an ICU monitor (for EKG, invasive/noninvasive pressures, capnography, and SpO_2 display), an ICU ventilator—preferably turbine driven and therefore independent of compressed air—a defibrillator, suction device, and airway management equipment, including a self-inflating resuscitation bag—to allow ventilation in the event of a malfunctioning ventilator—masks, oral airways, and a functioning laryngoscope with appropriate blades and endotracheal tubes, are mandatory. In certain cases, arterial and central venous lines and chest tubes are warranted. Basic resuscitation drugs such as epinephrine, atropine, and antidysrhythmic agents, as well as scheduled and anticipated medications (e.g., insulin, antibiotics, sedatives, and muscle relaxants) should also accompany the patient.

With regard to transfer standards, all electrical equipment should have prolonged battery life, and remaining charge should be properly displayed on the monitor. The equipment must be able to withstand vibration and shock, and thus be suitable for dealing with different transfer conditions—intrahospital as well as interhospital via ambulance, rotary-wing, or fixed-wing aircraft. The mounting of the equipment should follow national or international regulations. Preferably, all equipment are mounted on the transfer stretcher and, for safety, below the level of the patient. For intrahospital transports, a trolley or bed attachment to carry all equipment and drugs above is highly recommended.

Modes of Transport

The most common modes for interhospital transfers are by ground (ambulances) or air (fixed-wing or rotary-wing aircraft). In general, transfer by helicopters (rotary-wing aircraft) is considered for transfer distances greater than 80 km (50 miles) and fixed-wing aircrafts are used for distances greater than 240 km (150 miles). Although transfer by air may seem faster, one should bear in mind that mobilization times may be longer and transport by air often creates the need for additional transportation between landing site and hospital. These factors should be taken into consideration when deciding which mode of transport is going to be used. Furthermore, although transport by air might generate a reduction in transfer time, this has not been translated in a mortality reduction (42).

Apart from differences in transfer time, other issues must be considered when a transfer mode is to be chosen. These include risk, cost, mobilization time, influence of noise, vibrations and weather conditions, and the space required for patient care. Compared with air transport, ground transport has lower costs, more rapid mobilization times, lower risks—especially compared to rotary-wing transport—less noise and vibrations which could affect both patient and equipment, is less influenced by weather conditions and, in general, there is more space for patient care (again, especially compared to rotary-wing craft).

Organizational and Legal Aspects

The referral and the receiving team should make the assessment of the transfer risk–benefit ratio together, after which this should be discussed with the patient—if possible—and relatives. During transfer, the accompanying physician is responsible for both the patient's safety and treatment. This physician will have the best understanding of the risks of the transfer and will be the one to give the "go/no-go" decision for the transfer.

Since the transport/transfer is a continuation of the treatment, one is obliged to document all changes in the patient's physiology and in treatment; this record becomes part of the patient's medical record. During the formal handoff, the clinical situation before, during, and after transfer—as well

Patient label			
	Date	(dd/mm/yyyy)	
	Time of start transport	(hh/mm)	
	Time of arrival in ICU	(hh/mm)	
	Procedure		
	☐ CT-Scan	☐ MRI	☐ Angiography
	☐ Other		
	Purpose of transport		
	☐ Diagnostic	☐ Intervention	
	☐ Diagnostic and intervention		

Pre-transport

Equipment/materials	YES	NO	NA
Transport bag present			
Transport trolley fully charged			
Defibrillator present			
Manual resuscitation bag present			
Sufficient oxygen level			
Check length of i.v. tubes			
In case of MRI; extend length i.v. tubes			
Shut off necessary i.v. tubes			

Medication	YES	NO	NA
Sufficient intravenous medication			
Additional intravenous sedatives			
Additional intravenous inotropics			
Additional medication			
Additional infusion pump			
Additional intravenous fluids			
Stop enteral nutrition			
Stop enteral insulin			

In case of CT-Scan with contrast	YES	NO	NA
Intravenous cannula 18GA present			
Oral contrast administered			
If "YES":			
Renal protection according to protocol			

Monitor	YES	NO	NA
$EtCO_2$ monitoring present			
Check and set visual and audible alarm			

Transport ventilator	YES	NO	NA
Turn on the oxygen			
Put HME filter between ventilator and ET/TT			
Check and set visual and audible alarms			

ET/TT depth (cm)	

Administrative	YES	NO	NA
Register baseline vital signs overleaf			
Switch patient in PDMS to "Transport"			
Radiology department informed			
Fill in MRI safety questionnaire			

FIGURE 11.1 Example of an intrahospital transport checklist developed by Brunsveld-Reinders et al. (From Brunsveld-Reinders AH, Arbous MS, Kuiper SG, de Jonge E. A comprehensive method to develop a checklist to increase safety of intra-hospital transport of critically ill patients. *Crit Care.* 2015;19:214.)

During transport

At destination	YES	NO	NA
Plug in oxygen			
Plug in air			
Switch off oxygen & air on trolley			
Plug in transport trolley			
Check visibility on monitor during procedure			

Medication and fluids administered

Medication	Dosage	IV fluids	ml
Phenylephrine		Saline solution	
Midazolam		Voluven	
Propofol		Ringer's lactate	
....		....	
....		....	
....		....	

Vital signs	Pre-transport	20 min	40 min	60 min	Post-transport
Time	...../.....	...../.....	...../.....	...../.....	...../.....
HR/Rhythm					
BP					
MAP					
CVP					
PAP					
Vent mode					
FIO_2					
PEEP/PS					
RR					
Tidal volume					
Minute volume					
SpO_2					
$ETCO_2$					
GCS					
Pupil L/R					

**Only the clinical parameters that are also recorded in ICU*

During transport

Connecting patient	YES	NO	NA
Turn on humidifier			
Stop extra sedatives			
Start enternal nutrition			
Start enternal insulin			
Untangle i.v. tubes			
Switch patient in PDMS to "Back in ICU"			
Check level i.v. pump with PDMS			

Transport trolley	YES	NO	NA
Complement transport bag			
Change Oxygen tank if level < 50 bar			
Change HME filter			
Plug in transport trolley			
Report procedure in medical chart			
Change suction If used			
Report incidents			

Specify:

Physician: .... **Signature:** ....

Nurse: .... **Signature:** ....

FIGURE 11.1 *(Continued)*

as treatment given—should be extensively discussed. It is only after this formal handoff that the transfer has been completed.

For quality purposes, the transfer organization should keep record of all transfers.

Conclusion

Transporting critically ill patients is crucial to the public health system and will continue to be of vital importance in the future. Although every transport is a potential risk for our patient, it can be performed safely when circumstances are optimized. Transport teams with both experience in treating critically ill patients as well as insight into risks related to the actual transfer can provide such a safe transfer; this is as true with inter- as with intrahospital transports/transfers.

Key Points

- Interhospital transfer of critically ill patients should be carried out by specialized retrieval teams.
- All involved in transport should receive transfer training.
- Transfer training should focus on preparation, teamwork, equipment, mobility, and safety.
- Equipment used should meet both ICU and transfer standards.

ACKNOWLEDGMENT

The authors thank the previous edition's authors for their contributions.

References

1. Mackenzie PA, Smith EA, Wallace PGM. Transfer of adults between intensive care units in the United Kingdom: postal survey. *BMJ*. 1997;314:1455–1455.
2. Iwashyna TJ, Christie JD, Kahn JM, Asch DA. Uncharted paths: hospital networks in critical care. *Chest*. 2009;135:827–833.
3. Iwashyna TJ, Christie JD, Moody J, et al. The structure of critical care transfer networks. *Med Care*. 2009;47:787–793.
4. Kahn JM, Linde-Zwirble WT, Wunsch H, et al. Potential value of regionalized intensive care for mechanically ventilated medical patients. *Am J Respir Crit Care Med*. 2008;177:285–291.
5. Gentleman D, Jennett B. Audit of transfer of unconscious head-injured patients to a neurosurgical unit. *Lancet*. 1990;335:330–334.
6. Philpot C, Day S, Marcdante K, Gorelick M. Pediatric interhospital transport: diagnostic discordance and hospital mortality. *Pediatr Crit Care Med*. 2008;9:15–19.
7. Barry PW, Ralston C. Adverse events occurring during interhospital transfer of the critically ill. *Arch Dis Child*. 1994;71:8–11.
8. Gillman L, Leslie G, Williams T, et al. Adverse events experienced while transferring the critically ill patient from the emergency department to the intensive care unit. *Emerg Med J*. 2006;23:858–861.
9. Wallen E, Venkataraman ST, Grosso MJ, et al. Intrahospital transport of critically ill pediatric patients. *Crit Care Med*. 1995;23:1588–1595.
10. Rohan D, Dwyer R, Costello J, Phelan D. Audit of mobile intensive care ambulance service. *Ir Med J*. 2006;99:76–78.
11. Ligtenberg JJM, Arnold LG, Stienstra Y, et al. Quality of interhospital transport of critically ill patients: a prospective audit. *Crit Care*. 2005; 9:R446–R451.
12. Wiegersma JS, Droogh JM, Zijlstra JG, et al. Quality of interhospital transport of the critically ill: impact of a mobile intensive care unit with a specialized retrieval team. *Crit Care*. 2011;15:1122–1125.
13. Droogh JM, Smit M, Hut J, de Vos R, et al. Inter-hospital transport of critically ill patients; expect surprises. *Crit Care*. 2012;16:R26.
14. Hatherill M, Waggie Z, Reynolds L, Argent A. Transport of critically ill children in a resource-limited setting. *Intensive Care Med*. 2003;29:1547–1554.
15. Beckmann U, Gillies DM, Berenholtz SM, et al. Incidents relating to the intra-hospital transfer of critically ill patients. An analysis of the reports submitted to the Australian Incident Monitoring Study in Intensive Care. *Intensive Care Med*. 2004;30:1579–1585.
16. Flabouris A, Runciman WB, Levings B. Incidents during out-of-hospital patient transportation. *Anaesth Intensive Care*. 2006;34:228–236.
17. Papson JPN, Russell KL, Taylor DM. Unexpected events during the intrahospital transport of critically ill patients. *Acad Emerg Med*. 2007;14:574–577.
18. Henning R, McNamara V. Difficulties encountered in transport of the critically ill child. *Pediatr Emerg Care*. 2012;7:133–137.
19. Vos GD, Nissen AC, Nieman F, et al. Comparison of interhospital pediatric intensive care transport accompanied by a referring specialist or a specialist retrieval team. *Intensive Care Med*. 2004;30:302–308.
20. Edge WE, Kanter RK, Weigle CG, Walsh RF. Reduction of morbidity in interhospital transport by specialized pediatric staff. *Crit Care Med*. 1994; 22:1186–1191.
21. Macnab AJ. Optimal escort for interhospital transport of pediatric emergencies. *J Trauma: Injury, Infection, and Critical Care*. 1991;31:205–209.
22. Bellingan G, Olivier T, Batson S, Webb A. Comparison of a specialist retrieval team with current United Kingdom practice for the transport of critically ill patients. *Intensive Care Med*. 2000;26:740–744.
23. Ramnarayan P, Thiru K, Parslow RC, et al. Effect of specialist retrieval teams on outcomes in children admitted to paediatric intensive care units in England and Wales: a retrospective cohort study. *Lancet*. 2010;376:698–704.
24. Droogh JM, Smit M, Absalom AR, et al. Transferring the critically ill patient: are we there yet? *Crit Care*. 2015;19:749.
25. Britto J, Nadel S, Maconochie I, Levin M, Habibi P. Morbidity and severity of illness during interhospital transfer: impact of a specialised paediatric retrieval team. *BMJ*. 1995;311:836–839.
26. Wedel SK, Orr RA, Frakes MA, Conn AKT. Improving the incomplete infrastructure for interhospital patient transfer. *Crit Care Med*. 2013; 41:e21–e22.
27. Iwashyna TJ. The incomplete infrastructure for interhospital patient transfer. *Crit Care Med*. 2012;40:2470–2478.
28. Vos GD, Nieman FHM, Meurs AMB, et al. Problems in interhospital pediatric intensive care transport in the Netherlands: results from a survey of general pediatricians. *Intensive Care Med*. 2003;29:1555–1559.
29. Droogh JM, Kruger HL, Ligtenberg JJM, Zijlstra JG. Simulator-based crew resource management training for interhospital transfer of critically ill patients by a mobile ICU. *Jt Comm J Qual Patient Safe*. 2012;38:554–559.
30. Wallace PG, Ridley SA. ABC of intensive care. Transport of critically ill patients. *BMJ*. 1999;319:368–371.
31. Bion JF, Manji M. Transporting critically ill patients. *Intensive Care Med*. 1995;21:781–783.
32. Spencer C, Watkinson P, McCluskey A. Training and assessment of competency of trainees in the transfer of critically ill patients. *Anaesthesia*. 2004; 59:1248–1249.
33. Cosgrove JF, Kilner AJ, Batchelor AM, et al. Training and assessment of competency in the transfer of critically ill patients. *Anaesthesia*. 2005; 60:413–414.
34. Bérubé M, Bernard F, Marion H, et al. Impact of a preventive programme on the occurrence of incidents during the transport of critically ill patients. *Intensive Crit Care Nurs*. 2013;29:9–19.
35. Esmail R, Banack D, Cummings C, et al; Patient Safety and Adverse Events Team: Is your patient ready for transport? Developing an ICU patient transport decision scorecard. *Healthc Q*. 2006;9(Spec No.):80–86.
36. Jarden RJ, Quirke S. Improving safety and documentation in intrahospital transport: development of an intrahospital transport tool for critically ill patients. *Intensive & Crit Care Nurs*. 2010;26:101–107.
37. Brunsveld-Reinders AH, Arbous MS, Kuiper SG, de Jonge E. A comprehensive method to develop a checklist to increase safety of intra-hospital transport of critically ill patients. *Crit Care*. 2015;19:214.
38. Pearl RG, Mihm FG, Rosenthal MH. Care of the adult patient during transport. *Int Anesthesiol Clin*. 1987;25:43–75.
39. Warren J, Fromm RE, Orr RA, et al; American College of Critical Care Medicine. Guidelines for the inter- and intrahospital transport of critically ill patients. *Crit Care Med*. 2004;32:256–262.
40. Guidelines Committee of the American College of Critical Care Medicine; Society of Critical Care Medicine and American Association of Critical-Care Nurses Transfer Guidelines Task Force. Guidelines for the transfer of critically ill patients. *Crit Care Med*. 1993;6:931–937.
41. Vos GD, Buurman WA, van Waardenburg DA, et al. Interhospital paediatric intensive care transport: a novel transport unit based on a standard ambulance trolley. *Eur J Emerg Med*. 2003;10:195–199.
42. Borst GM, Davies SW, Waibel BH, et al. When birds can't fly. *J Trauma Acute Care Surg*. 2014;77:331–337.

CHAPTER 12

Post-ICU Syndrome and the Post-ICU Clinic

CARLA M. SEVIN and JAMES C. JACKSON

"Can we commit to the post-ICU phase of care in the same way we commit to intubations, pressors, antibiotics? We can."

Dr. Alison Clay, via Twitter

INTRODUCTION

With advances in critical care, deaths from critical illness have declined, resulting in an increasing survivorship every year. The victory is not, however, without cost. With this rise in survivorship has come a burgeoning awareness of the consequences of critical care, now known as the postintensive care syndrome (PICS). PICS has been defined as new or worsening dysfunction in one or more of the following domains after critical illness: cognitive, psychiatric, or physical (1). However, this must be acknowledged as a loose and changing definition of a yet incompletely understood syndrome representing the aftereffects of modern critical care. Recent iterations have acknowledged the adverse effects a critical illness may have on family members, expanding the definition to address the mental health of such family members, referred to as PICS-family (PICS-F). The effects of PICS and PICS-F are wide ranging, but can be grouped by functional domain.

POST-ICU SYNDROME

Physical Domain

Physical debility in survivors of critical illness is pervasive, severe, and often permanent (2,3). Even 5 years after a critical illness, a significant portion of ICU survivors remain impaired. While post-ICU pulmonary function may return to normal, symptoms of dyspnea persist and 6-minute walk distance (6MWD)—a measure of functional exercise capacity—rarely fully rebounds (3). In a group of young (mean age 45) acute respiratory distress syndrome (ARDS) survivors who required mechanical ventilation (MV), 6MWD did steadily improve over the first year after discharge from ICU, but never returned to age-predicted levels (3).

The effects of critical illness are even more pronounced in older patients. In a study of ICU patients older than 70 years, more than half experienced severe functional decline or early death after critical illness (4). MV, shock, and cognitive impairment were associated with increased risk of death and functional impairment at 30 days and 1 year after discharge from ICU. The majority of older ICU survivors require some level of enhanced care after discharge, either in a nursing or rehabilitation facility, or at home with services (5,6).

Substantial functional decline after critical illness is the norm rather than the exception (3,7–12). Survivors of severe sepsis often demonstrate a reduction in their ability to independently ambulate, bathe, use the toilet, dress, shop for and prepare complex meals, use the telephone, and effectively manage finances (10). In a large study of patients who had undergone more than 4 days of MV, only 15% returned directly home (8). In another study, 75% of patients who had survived 2 months after at least 2 days of MV displayed activities of daily living (ADL) impairment and dependency on caregivers (13). Two years after ICU discharge, 80% of ARDS survivors required care assistance, with resultant ill effects on their caregivers (14).

While acquired physical limitations appear to be a consequence of critical illness, the development of chronic or worsening morbidities that lead to rehospitalization is also a frequent outcome. An observational cohort study of survivors of severe sepsis and nonsepsis hospitalizations found that 67% of sepsis survivors were readmitted to the hospital in the year following discharge; 74% of their "alive days" were spent hospitalized or in postacute care facilities, and 65% of the cohort reported severe or complete functional dependency at 1 year (15). Readmission is common after an index hospitalization for sepsis, whether or not the patient was admitted to the ICU, though readmission is more likely if the patient spent time in the ICU. Other independent risk factors for readmission included severity of illness, hospital length of stay, medical comorbidities, and higher prehospitalization health care utilization (16).

Patients with weakness attributable to critical illness are diagnosed as having ICU-acquired weakness (ICUAW) (17). There is a subset of patients with ICUAW who have electrophysiologically documented axonal polyneuropathy (critical illness polyneuropathy, CIP) and another subset with documented myopathy (critical illness myopathy, CIM), which often co-occur and are termed critical illness neuromyopathy (CINM) (17). Approximately 50% of critically ill patients with sepsis, multiorgan failure, or prolonged MV have CINM, resulting in increased ICU and hospital stays and difficulties ambulating or breathing unassisted following discharge (17,18). These patients may experience neuromuscular abnormalities up to 5 years following discharge (19,20).

Additional serious physical sequelae of critical care include airway complications of prolonged MV (tracheal stenosis, vocal cord dysfunction), hypoxemic respiratory failure, vascular scarring and stenosis, anemia, chronic renal failure, peripheral gangrene with or without autoamputation, changes in taste and swallowing, malnutrition, usually with weight loss, and paresthesias. Disturbing to patients, but generally self-limited, are hair loss (telogen effluvium) (21) and nail changes (Beau's lines and onychomadesis) (Fig. 12.1) (22).

Cognitive Domain

Cognitive impairment after critical illness is a serious public health problem in its own right, one that is only now becoming

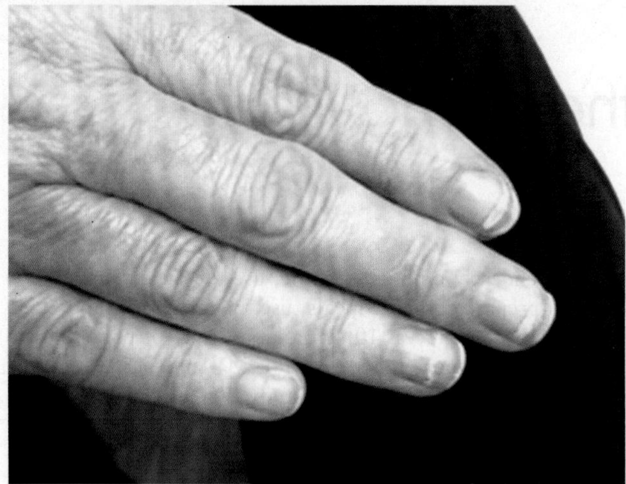

FIGURE 12.1 Onychomadesis after critical illness.

widely recognized. More than 25 prospective investigations, encompassing more than 3,000 patients, have assessed cognitive functioning after the ICU (23–29). Reports are consistent that cognitive impairment occurs in up to 60% of individuals, regardless of the reason for hospitalization (23,25,29). Nearly all survivors of ICU hospitalization are impaired at discharge (30) and these impairments tend to persist, although questions remain about trajectories of cognitive change over time (23). Although older age and pre-existing cognitive impairment increase susceptibility to cognitive disruptions within the context of critical illness and ICU hospitalization (25), even young and previously healthy individuals experience cognitive impairment after critical illness (31).

Cognitive problems in ICU survivors occur in areas of memory, attention, and executive functioning, all domains that have clear implications for daily functioning (32–36). The risk factors potentially associated with cognitive impairment after critical illness are many and include delirium, hypoxia, glucose and metabolic dysregulation, inflammation, and the effects of medications (e.g., sedatives and narcotics) (31). The extent to which each of these possible contributors affects cognitive outcomes is unclear; each is closely associated with the others and with ICU hospitalization more generally.

Much of the research pertaining to cognitive outcomes after critical illness has focused on delirium. Delirium is common during critical illness, though its prevalence has decreased in recent years (37–45). Contributors to the development of delirium are the subjects of intensive investigation and include genetic (e.g., APOE-4 allele), pathophysiologic (e.g., infection), medical (e.g., sedating medications), and environmental factors (e.g., chaotic ICU environment, dysregulation of sleep/wake cycle) (46–48). Cognitive vulnerability may also play a role (31). The exact mechanisms by which delirium confers a higher likelihood of cognitive dysfunction following critical illness have yet to be elucidated, though inflammation and neuronal death are each associated with delirium and may lead to untoward brain-related developments including brain atrophy (49).

A variety of mechanisms are believed to foster the development of cognitive impairment. A profound systemic inflammatory response is a common feature of critical illness (e.g., sepsis). The inflammatory response is characterized by production of proinflammatory cytokines (e.g., interleukin-6 [IL-6], IL-1, and tumor necrosis factor alpha [TNF-α] (50,51), which have been associated with Alzheimer's and vascular dementia, as well as cardiovascular disease (52,53). Inflammation may lead to a permanent shift in brain chemistry and likely is a major contributor to chronic brain dysfunction. Recent investigation using a mouse model of sepsis has revealed long-term neuroinflammation resulting in cognitive changes months after recovery from the acute illness (54).

Also common in critical illness is hypoxia, especially among patients with ARDS (55); hypoxia has been associated with significant memory decrements (56–58). Patients admitted to the ICU for critical illnesses are often geriatric; old age is a risk factor for pro-inflammatory responses, delirium, and cognitive decline (59–61). Pre-existing cognitive impairment, whether mild or severe, also appears to be a risk factor for cognitive impairment and accelerated decline following ICU hospitalization and critical illness (62). But younger patients are not spared, and the impact of cognitive impairment after critical illness is marked by profound decrements in functional status, independence, and employment in this population (63).

Psychiatric Domain

Critical illness is known to have significant impact on psychological outcomes of patients (64,65) and their families (66). Investigating psychological issues has been identified as a critical research priority by the Multisociety Strategic Planning Task Force for Critical Care Research (1). Psychological areas most frequently impacted include depression and posttraumatic stress disorder (PTSD).

Depression

Depression and depressive symptoms are common in the setting of critical illness and occur in nearly 30% of individuals (in contrast to 10% for any mood disorder in the general population) (67). Clinically significant depressive symptoms in patients after critical illness have been reported in over 30 studies (68). A recent analysis of ICU survivors showed that the risk of receiving a new prescription for a psychoactive medication in the 6 months after hospital discharge was 21 times greater than in the general population (69). Depression manifests in cognitive–affective symptoms but may result in somatic symptoms in ICU survivors in particular. These include fatigue and exhaustion, sleep disturbance, problems initiating physical activity, and preoccupation with health concerns (70). Depressive symptoms may increase the probability of developing recurrent critical illness, as individuals suffering from depression may make unwise and potentially harmful choices and engage in maladaptive health-related behaviors, such as smoking, sedentary lifestyle, alcohol consumption, malnutrition, and noncompliance with recommended preventive or treatment regimens. People with major depression die almost a decade earlier than their nondepressed counterparts from health conditions such as cardiovascular diseases, diabetes, and chronic obstructive pulmonary disease (COPD), likely due to early onset of maladaptive health behaviors (71,72). Health behavior change is a difficult process for many individuals, especially if those behaviors serve to momentarily enhance mood or reduce tension or fatigue (73). Conversely, a positive adaptive response to critical illness may be a renewed motivation to improve health behaviors. A subset of survivors of critical illness finds that their experiences, difficult as they

TABLE 12.1 **Patient Perspectives on Post-ICU Recovery: Clinical Vignettes**

Need for better post-ICU education and support	"It was/remains utterly baffling that my team . . . left me virtually to my own devices once I was released from their acute hospital, e.g. (1) almost totally passive with regard to physical therapy and (2) did not warn me/my family of potential subsequent issues (hallucinations, confusion, sense of helplessness, need for psychiatric consultation, etc.). To this day I doubt they know of the excruciating pain I experienced for nearly two months, the need to relearn to feed myself, stand, walk, etc." "My PCP, like all physicians, is overwhelmed. I don't think they get any feedback from the hospital about what went on." "I recently endured a long ICU stay and the delirium that was such an evil part of it. It is very important that those of us who have experienced this know that we are not alone and we are not crazy." "Even though I was hospitalized for pancreatitis, kidney failure, lung failure, blood clots, etc., the post-ICU experience was and is the worst part of my ongoing illness and sadly, no one even told us to expect it."
Cognitive impairment	"All should be right in my world but after my ICU stay I am a completely different person. I am slow, easily confused, look forward to nothing, scared of everything, not to mention the sleep issue – I am terrified to go to sleep because of the 'nightmares' I lived while in ICU (I have written over 50 of them down, some including sexual abuse, murder, being burned alive, etc.)." "My work suffers and I don't know how much longer I'll be able to go on with it (although I haven't admitted as much to my employer) and I tire incredibly easily . . . The past and present pain and uncertainty of my underlying physical conditions (pancreatitis, renal failure, etc.) are a comparative cakewalk compared to seeing severed heads in glass jars and being confused all the time. This is simply unsustainable." "I was lucky, about day 10 (in the ICU) I began to come out of it and everyone believed that I was normal with no problems but almost from my first day home I experienced depression, confabulation, short term memory problems, I would become lost in places that I was familiar with and I would find myself standing in a store staring at a shelf unaware how I got there or why I was there." "When I returned to work, the work I did before seemed foreign and unfamiliar." "I would tell my family and doctors that what I was experiencing was like having Alzheimer's and knowing it but nothing I said seem to being any aid so I figured there wasn't anything anyone could do. I became isolated and excluded from everyone, no one wanted to be around me." "I was unconscious, some 8 weeks (in the ICU), I had terrible nightmares, or so I thought . . . I have started to understand what really happened. This ordeal has completely changed my life. I can't work anymore, I can't handle any stress, I can't make decisions, my memory is terrible and I was only 39 when I went in for the surgery." "I also didn't finish my PhD behind this experience. I am different. I need help. I was once a very driven and smart person. Now I feel damaged and broken. My quality of life has really diminished. I am a mess, still."
Anxiety, depression, suicidal ideation	"Anyways, the ICU left me emotionally destitute. A part of me died in there. And I think he is dead forever. All of those experiences (even though they were not real) - were just too traumatic, too intense, and too real. I became incredibly despondent and checked out. I was dead inside. An emotional fuse burst." "I began to question my brain and my sanity. The emotions with the dreams all seemed connected to the emotions of the ICU delirium." "I really struggle with depression and anxiety. I can sleep for days at a time. I am irritable. I am paranoid. I no longer have any friends." "I spent 8 days in the ICU . . . and I am still tortured by the life changing experience that happened to me. I suffer from acute depression and anxiety, as well as changes in my personality and behavior. I am on medication, and know in my heart that without them I could not have any chance of a life." "I nearly ended my life a few times."
PTSD	"I suffer from ICU delirium and PTSD after being in a medically induced coma and in the ICU for months!! It's taking over my life I need answers and help!! My therapists don't understand it and I feel so alone, I hate my life now and just want to be me again."
Impact on family	"He doesn't know where he is . . . nothing hurts . . . we the family are hurting . . . because the body looks like my dad but he's not in it."

may be, are the gateway to significant growth and to a fundamental reordering of priorities. This "posttraumatic growth" occurs in up to a third of survivors of trauma and frequently results in increased gratitude, greater life satisfaction, and increased optimism and resilience (74,75).

Acute and Posttraumatic Stress

Acute distress symptoms are common during critical illness and are frequently followed by posttraumatic stress in the ICU recovery period (76,77). As many as one in two ICU survivors experience clinically significant symptoms of PTSD during the first year after ICU discharge, though recent investigations have suggested that the true prevalence of PTSD is between 10% and 20%. Still, this is nearly fourfold higher than the lifetime prevalence of posttraumatic stress symptoms in the general US population (76,78). PTSD may be driven by exposure to a variety of traumatic experiences, including the critical illness itself, the ICU environment, and delusional memories or delirious states (76,79). PTSD symptoms after critical illness often manifest in symptoms of avoidance, apprehension about discussing any signs or symptoms of a possible medical condition with providers, and reluctance to seek help. Patients may almost phobically avoid medical appointments, which can increase the likelihood of worsening symptoms (Table 12.1).

MANAGEMENT OF PICS AND THE POST-ICU CLINIC

Just as with ICU "bundles" or protocols for sepsis, ARDS, or diabetic ketoacidosis, protocols for ICU survivorship will be required in the future, and organizational change is key. The specific components of ICU follow-up have not been established, but stakeholders have created an agenda for what should be included for advancing research and practice in this realm (80). First, and critically important, is recognizing, preventing, and treating signs and symptoms of PICS. Second, we must identify and address needs and build institutional capacity to support survivors and families. Third, we must study and develop an understanding of barriers and facilitators to patient care across the spectrum of care environments.

Much of the work on long-term functional outcomes after critical illness has been epidemiologic and descriptive: what proportion of patients are discharged to home, what is their level of function, their perceived quality of life, how frequently are they readmitted, and how long do they survive? Important gaps remain in our knowledge about effective interventions to improve these outcomes through changes in practice as well as the optimal time points for intervention (i.e., during the episode of critical illness or later during the recovery period). Understanding such "phenotypes" of ICU survivors is a crucial next step (81).

Intensivists may be in the best position to understand the potential sequelae of the ICU experience, and should themselves be the ones caring for patients during the post-ICU recovery period. Doing so requires intensivists to have more knowledge, understanding, awareness, skills, and availability beyond the acute ICU stay. By some estimates, issues related to ICU survivorship are discussed during the index ICU episode only very rarely, and only 20% of hospitals have formal ways of communicating discharge follow-up planning to primary care providers (82). Even if intensivists are knowledgeable about survivorship, less than 5% of hospitals report having support groups for ICU survivors. Support groups could serve to identify the optimal time points for intervention while also providing needed care and support to patients, many of whom fall through the proverbial cracks following hospital discharge. And, while they are not yet widely recognized as valuable or effective, largely due to limited rigorous study to date, ICU follow-up clinics may be one important way to address the growing number of patients with PICS.

ICU follow-up clinics are not a new concept, but they have had some difficulty gaining traction in general practice. In the UK, about 30% of ICUs had a follow-up clinic program in 2006. Over half of those clinics were led by nurses, only 59% were funded by their affiliated hospital, and almost 90% of ICUs studied reported financial constraints (83). Another study of ICU follow-up clinics in the UK was unable to show a benefit in health-related quality of life (HRQoL) at 1 year among almost 300 patients participating in an ICU follow-up program (84). The lack of observed benefit may have been related to the fact that ICU follow-up clinics up to that time in the UK had developed in an *ad hoc* manner, were providing inconsistent service and staffing models, and were not uniformly available in hospitals across the country. All patients who required intensive care were eligible, raising the possibility that only a subset of patients would benefit from an aftercare program. The intervention consisted of a self-directed, manual-based recovery plan, introduced by a study nurse and formally reviewed in the clinic at 3 and 9 months. Although there was no difference in HRQoL or mortality between the groups, a third required medical specialist referral and another third needed referral for psychological services. The authors called for more work on the roles of early physical rehabilitation, delirium, cognitive dysfunction, and relatives in the ICU recovery process. An interdisciplinary team approach may improve outcomes through better coordination of care, but the optimal structure of such a team in a chaotic ICU environment with a variety of medical diagnoses and severity of illnesses is not yet clear (85).

TABLE 12.2 Wide-Ranging Implications of Postintensive Care Syndrome

Health care utilization
- Readmissions
- Emergency room visits
- Polypharmacy
- Primary care provider strain

Physical impairments
- Mortality
- Morbidity
  - Respiratory function
  - Endurance
  - Smoking
  - Nutrition
  - Drug effects

Cognitive effects
- Delirium
- Cognitive dysfunction
- Posttraumatic stress disorder
- Affective disorders

Socioeconomic factors
- Place of residence
- Driving
- Return to work
- Family and caregiver strain
- Financial stressors
- Quality of life

The wide array of affected functional domains has led to an emerging team-based approach to diagnosing and treating PICS. However, while awareness of post-ICU problems is becoming broader, evidence is lacking to guide diagnostic criteria and treatment options, and the absence of a defined team model has resulted in a patchwork of efforts around the United States and the world. Bookending the physical, cognitive, and psychiatric components of the syndrome are the wide-reaching systemic effects of this public health problem. These include, on the systems side, effects on health care utilization, and on the individual and family side, socioeconomic and quality-of-life factors (Table 12.2).

Clearly, this is a monumental collection of problems to be addressed in any one setting. And yet, by tailoring the post-ICU recovery approach to the individual patient, the intensivist may arrive at a high-yield, relatively low-resource intervention to minimize further morbidity and mortality.

Goals of an ICU Recovery Program

Screen for Known Complications

Although the long-term effects of critical illness are still being described, a number of common complications are known. Among the best studied of these is polypharmacy, most commonly, the unintentional and inappropriate continuation of medications started in the ICU setting (86). Common classes of inappropriately continued medications include antipsychotics, gastric acid suppressants, benzodiazepines, and inhaled bronchodilators and steroids. Without early intervention, inappropriate medication continuation often persists up to 1 year after hospital discharge, at the cost of millions of dollars and countless adverse drug events.

Conversely, previously appropriate medications may be stopped during critical illness and not restarted at hospital discharge (87). Due to rapidly changing clinical status, renal function, and hospital location or team, appropriate medications may be underdosed, overdosed, or lacking monitoring following hospital discharge. Careful medication reconciliation, pharmacy counseling, review of barriers to adherence, and implementation of medication compliance strategies are just a few ways a pharmacist can contribute to post-ICU recovery.

Pain is a common complaint after critical illness; unrelieved pain in the ICU increases the risk of chronic pain in the post-ICU period (88). Maladaptive hyperalgesia, whether induced by damage to peripheral or central nerve fibers, opioid administration or interruption, or inflammation, is further exacerbated in the post-ICU period by altered emotional and cognitive processing (89). Paresthesias are common; while therapeutic studies are lacking, neuropathic pain medications including gabapentin, capsaicin cream, SSRIs, and venlafaxine have been used (21).

Serious airway complications of prolonged MV, such as tracheal stenosis, are relatively rare, but can have potentially devastating effects. Thus, timely identification and subspecialty referral are key. Vocal cord dysfunction is more common, and often self-limiting. However, persistently symptomatic vocal cord pathology is best referred to otolaryngology, as targeted interventions and speech therapy can result in significant improvement.

Other subspecialty referrals common to the post-ICU period are wound care, plastic surgery, infectious diseases, and community mental health.

Above all, the systematic coordination of post-ICU care presents a unique opportunity for improvements in patient safety, recovery, and quality of life. Among the benefits of such coordinated (and potentially interdisciplinary) follow-up is the prevention of preventable readmissions, morbidity, and mortality.

Educate Patients and Families

In most cases, survivors of critical illness are unaware of the many difficulties they will potentially face as a consequence of their critical illness. Few lay people and relatively few professionals are familiar with literature that supports an association between sepsis, for example, and prolonged cognitive deficits, or with the voluminous evidence that links critical illness to the development of PTSD. Consequently, when new cognitive and mental health difficulties emerge or when old ones worsen, they have no particular context by which to understand them. In the absence of any understanding of the natural history or the "normal" clinical course of these conditions, patients often develop intense anxiety and are reluctant to talk about their fears with health care professionals. For these and many other reasons, proper education that both explains to patients what is happening, that is, describes what PICS is and normalizes it, helps set appropriate expectations, such as "these symptoms will probably persist for a time but will likely be better in 6 months to a year," and provides treatment recommendations—"consider focused cognitive rehabilitation with an occupational therapist or a rehabilitation psychologist for the treatment of attention deficits"—is a crucial part of post-ICU care.

Closely related to patient and family education is the education of outpatient medical providers, whether they are subspecialists, general practitioners, or mental health professionals (psychiatrists, psychologists, social workers). The disconnect between inpatient critical care providers and their outpatient counterparts has been well described; only infrequently do inpatient and outpatient physicians engage in professional "crosstalk." Accordingly, providers not involved in ICU care are rarely apprised of and sometimes not sensitive to the often profound debilities from which their patients now suffer. Primary care providers are extremely receptive to such information but without education, they are often as perplexed as survivors at the unusual constellation of symptoms they are seeing. Attempts to develop a primary care–based program to treat the sequelae of critical illness are underway, but have yet to be shown effective in improving outcomes (90). Post-ICU clinic personnel can play an invaluable role by bridging the gap between inpatient and outpatient providers. Outlining a summary of the ICU stay and current problems along with specific resources for the cognitive, mental health, and physical/functional decrements specific to PICS (sometimes referred to as a "health passport") may be a useful adjunct for patients, families, and medical teams.

Solidify Positive Change

Another issue central to ICU follow-up care involves solidifying changes that have already been made during critical illness. Whether active or passive, these changes can represent unique opportunities to improve health. For example, many patients arrive in the ICU with long histories of alcohol and nicotine use, patterns that predispose them to the development of critical illness (91,92). For such patients, a prolonged ICU hospitalization may represent the longest period of time they have been free of such substances in a lifetime. Similarly, many morbidly obese patients lose significant weight over the course of a critical illness—weight loss greater than 100 pounds is not unheard of—although this usually involves the loss of muscle as well as fat. In these instances, longstanding habits will rapidly re-emerge after patients return home unless active efforts are made to help make their new behaviors (e.g., smoking cessation) or conditions (e.g., decreased BMI) more permanent. ICU follow-up care providers can engage patients in smoking cessation programs, weight loss and nutrition programs, or alcohol treatment programs at the critical "teachable moment" between an ICU stay and the return to baseline function. These programs can be embedded in follow-up clinics—for example, smoking cessation programs can be delivered at little cost and require relatively little specialized expertise—or patients can be referred to appropriate specialists either at the hospital or in the community. An interdisciplinary team approach is especially well-suited to this type of health behavioral modification (Tables 12.3 and 12.4). While many of the impairments observed in the post-ICU period will improve over time, documenting them and explaining them to patients can serve as a powerful motivator in the pursuit of "best recovery."

Necessary and Desired Elements of an ICU Recovery Program

Little if any systematic study has been done of the crucial elements comprising ICU follow-up care. One of these is a dedicated ICU recovery center or clinic (Fig. 12.2), yet this is not the only method or model. Promising approaches that have

TABLE 12.3 Clinical Scenarios Highlighting Interdisciplinary Assessment and Intervention in an ICU Recovery Program

Scenario 1

Medication reconciliation and counseling find the patient to be taking a number of inappropriate medications, including omeprazole and quetiapine, which were prescribed in the ICU. The medications are stopped, decreasing the risk of *Clostridium difficile* colitis, QT prolongation, and excess somnolence, and freeing the patient from the financial burden of unnecessary medications.

Scenario 2

Medical evaluation reveals abnormal spirometry, low oxygen saturation, and a hoarse, airy voice. The patient is referred to voice clinic for airway evaluation and started on supplemental oxygen.

Scenario 3

A patient is seen for a cognitive assessment and displays severe but previously unrecognized cognitive impairment on screening tests of visuospatial and executive ability. He is advised not to drive and is referred for a formal driving evaluation.

Scenario 4

6MWD is severely decreased and the patient is having difficulty caring for her baby due to necrosis of the fingers and toes, a result of high-dose pressors in the ICU. Case management evaluation reveals the patient never received physical and occupational therapy prescribed at discharge because she did not have a PCP to receive the paperwork. CM arranges home therapy and assists the patient in finding an in-network PCP.

Scenario 5

At patient-centered consultation, review of spirometry shows early obstruction concerning for smoking-related lung disease. The patient reveals he stopped smoking in the ICU, but has been having cravings. After interdisciplinary review with psychology, pharmacy, and case management, a smoking cessation plan with behavioral and pharmacologic intervention is integrated into a Survivorship Care Plan.

TABLE 12.4 Institute of Medicine-Defined Key Elements of a Survivorship Program

Consensus elements

- Survivorship care plan
- Care coordination
- Health promotion
- Screening for "new" problems

High-need elements

- Late effects education
- Psychosocial assessment
- Psychosocial care
- Detailed medical assessment
- Education on survivorship

Strive elements

- Specialist referral
- Self-advocacy

a lower barrier to entry involve the use of telephone- or telehealth-related modalities to facilitate traditional interactions between patients and providers (93). Other potential models involve the use of peer guides or mentors or support groups. While peers have rarely been employed in post-ICU settings, they have proven to be highly effective in the management of patients with other chronic conditions such as diabetes, rheumatoid arthritis, and HIV/AIDS. These carefully selected individuals are matched by demographic and illness-related variables. As successful "navigators" of life after critical illness, they often have knowledge and insights about recovery that medical providers lack and can be particularly valuable in promoting effective recovery. Like peer mentoring programs, support groups have a long history of effectiveness with other groups but are in their infancy as applied to ICU survivors (94). They represent a relatively simple and cost-effective way to engage the needs of individuals after critical illness by using the considerable strengths and motivations of patients who are frequently highly motivated to help one another. Even more independent of the medical system are self-directed or manual-based recovery programs, such as those developed

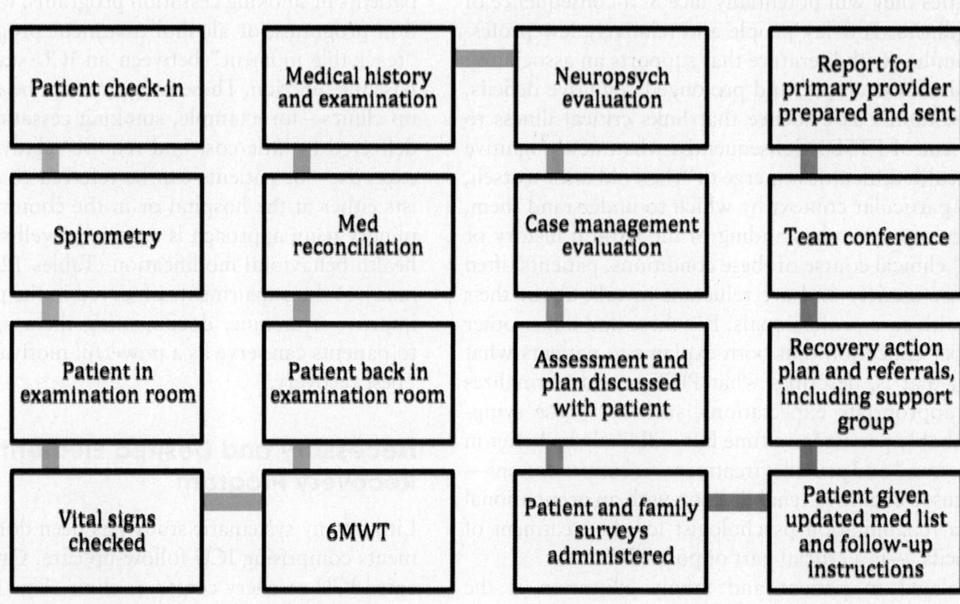

FIGURE 12.2 Sample ICU follow-up clinic flow.

in the United Kingdom (95). Several European studies have evaluated the potential benefits of keeping an intensive care diary, with promising effects on post-ICU anxiety, depression, quality of life, and PTSD in patients and families (96–102).

Barriers

Despite their promise, a number of barriers to the broad implementation of ICU follow-up care models exist, some easily dealt with and some difficult to surmount. Perhaps, chief among these barriers is the lack of insurance reimbursement for treatment that is viewed as highly experimental or lacking a significant evidence base. Closely related is the fact that few hospitals or hospital systems have the full complement of interdisciplinary resources needed to deliver comprehensive post-ICU care. Even when hospitals are prepared to offer services, patient and family buy-in may be lacking, as patients are often unaware of their limitations in the days and weeks after discharge, until they are placed in demanding situations that tax their newly depleted resources. Finally, due to the absence of research, it is unclear what the components of aftercare models should be. This uncertainty should invite humility but may also lead some individuals or organizations to hesitate to develop clinics due to very reasonable concerns about "getting things right."

As we have described throughout this chapter, ICU follow-up clinic models are innovative, potentially efficacious, and highly desired by both patients and providers alike. Still, they are not without controversy. Evidence for their effectiveness is lacking, but few studies have been done; similar models have been shown to be highly effective for other populations. There is clear evidence that this patient population is at risk for increased and potentially avoidable readmissions, as well as increased health care utilization overall (15,103,104). With the increase in survivors and the vacuum that currently represents post-ICU care, there is much interest despite little evidence for post-ICU clinics. Who might benefit from such clinics and for how long? There may be wisdom in targeting patients who are prone to respond to post-ICU care but as of now, we have no idea who they are. Identification of high-risk patients has been proposed by diagnosis (sepsis, ARDS), by physical functioning, by the presence of delirium, and others (MV, length of stay, severity of illness) (3,10,29,41,105,106); there is likely significant overlap among these. Questions also remain about the content of any interventions; for example, should they be generic in nature and mimic interventions done with other populations, or should they be tailored to the specific nuanced symptoms that exist in ICU survivors? What is the minimum effective intervention that can improve outcomes for ICU survivors? Though challenging, we must address the public health problem of survivorship created by the success of our field.

Key Points

- As advances in critical care have significantly improved mortality rates, concerns have begun to shift toward addressing the long-term outcomes of ICU survivors.
- PICS is an extremely common outcome among ICU survivors and it involves deficits in cognitive, physical, and psychiatric functioning.
- Mechanisms contributing to PICS are probably diverse. It is unlikely that a single common pathway drives the development of PICS.
- Little is known regarding how to optimally manage PICS as well as whether traditional approaches or tailored approaches are more effective.
- Post-ICU follow-up clinics may be a promising way to address the needs of those experiencing PICS. Such models have been broadly effective with other populations though rarely tried with ICU survivors.

References

1. Needham DM, Davidson J, Cohen H, et al. Improving long-term outcomes after discharge from intensive care unit: report from a stakeholders' conference. *Crit Care Med.* 2012;40(2):502–509.
2. Herridge MS. Building consensus on ICU-acquired weakness. *Intensive Care Med.* 2009;35(1):1–3.
3. Herridge MS, Tansey CM, Matte A, et al; Canadian Critical Care Trials Group. Functional disability 5 years after acute respiratory distress syndrome. *N Engl J Med.* 2011;364(14):1293–1304.
4. Ferrante LE, Pisani MA, Murphy TE, et al. Functional trajectories among older persons before and after critical illness. *JAMA Intern Med.* 2015;175(4):523–529.
5. Ely EW, Angus DC, Williams MD, et al. Drotrecogin alfa (activated) treatment of older patients with severe sepsis. *Clin Infect Dis.* 2003; 37(2):187–195.
6. Rady MY, Johnson DJ. Hospital discharge to care facility: a patient-centered outcome for the evaluation of intensive care for octogenarians. *Chest.* 2004;126(5):1583–1591.
7. Herridge MS, Cheung AM, Tansey CM, et al; Canadian Critical Care Trials Group. One-year outcomes in survivors of the acute respiratory distress syndrome. *N Engl J Med.* 2003;348(8):683–693.
8. Zilberberg MD, Luippold RS, Sulsky S, Shorr AF. Prolonged acute mechanical ventilation, hospital resource utilization, and mortality in the United States. *Crit Care Med.* 2008;36(3):724–730.
9. Herridge MS. Legacy of intensive care unit-acquired weakness. *Crit Care Med.* 2009;37(10 Suppl):S457–S461.
10. Iwashyna TJ, Ely EW, Smith DM, Langa KM. Long-term cognitive impairment and functional disability among survivors of severe sepsis. *JAMA.* 2010;304(16):1787–1794.
11. Barnato AE, Albert SM, Angus DC, et al. Disability among elderly survivors of mechanical ventilation. *Am J Respir Crit Care Med.* 2011; 183(8):1037–1042.
12. Wilcox ME, Brummel NE, Archer K, et al. Cognitive dysfunction in ICU patients: risk factors, predictors, and rehabilitation interventions. *Crit Care Med.* 2013;41(9 Suppl 1):S81–S98.
13. Im K, Belle SH, Schulz R, et al; QOL-MV Investigators. Prevalence and outcomes of caregiving after prolonged (> or = 48 hours) mechanical ventilation in the ICU. *Chest.* 2004;125(2):597–606.
14. Cameron JI, Herridge MS, Tansey CM, et al. Well-being in informal caregivers of survivors of acute respiratory distress syndrome. *Crit Care Med.* 2006;34(1):81–86.
15. Prescott HC, Langa KM, Liu V, et al. Increased 1-year healthcare use in survivors of severe sepsis. *Am J Respir Crit Care Med.* 2014;190(1):62–69.
16. Liu V, Lei X, Prescott HC, et al. Hospital readmission and healthcare utilization following sepsis in community settings. *J Hosp Med.* 2014; 9(8):502–507.
17. Stevens RD, Marshall SA, Cornblath DR, et al. A framework for diagnosing and classifying intensive care unit-acquired weakness. *Crit Care Med.* 2009;37(10 Suppl):S299–S308.
18. Latronico N, Shehu I, Seghelini E. Neuromuscular sequelae of critical illness. *Curr Opin Crit Care.* 2005;11(4):381–390.
19. Zifko UA. Long-term outcome of critical illness polyneuropathy. *Muscle Nerve Suppl.* 2000;9:S49–S52.
20. Fletcher SN, Kennedy DD, Ghosh IR, et al. Persistent neuromuscular and neurophysiologic abnormalities in long-term survivors of prolonged critical illness. *Crit Care Med.* 2003;31(4):1012–1016.
21. Volk B, Grassi F. Treatment of the post-ICU patient in an outpatient setting. *Am Fam Physician.* 2009;79(6):459–464.
22. Wester JP, van Eps RS, Stouthamer A, Girbes AR. Critical illness onychomadesis. *Intensive Care Med.* 2000;26(11):1698–1700.

23. Hopkins RO, Weaver LK, Collingridge D, et al. Two-year cognitive, emotional, and quality-of-life outcomes in acute respiratory distress syndrome. *Am J Respir Crit Care Med.* 2005;171(4):340–347.
24. Jackson JC, Hart RP, Gordon SM, et al. Six-month neuropsychological outcome of medical intensive care unit patients. *Crit Care Med.* 2003; 31(4):1226–1234.
25. Jones C, Griffiths RD, Slater T, et al. Significant cognitive dysfunction in non-delirious patients identified during and persisting following critical illness. *Intensive Care Med.* 2006;32(6):923–926.
26. Christie JD, DeMissie E, Gaughan C, et al. Validity of a brief telephone-administered battery to assess cognitive function in survivors of the adult respiratory distress syndrome (ARDS). *Am J Respir Crit Care Med.* 2004; 169:A781.
27. Sukantarat K, Burgess P, Williamson R, Brett S. Prolonged cognitive dysfunction in survivors of critical illness. *Anaesthesia.* 2005;60(9):847–853.
28. Rothenhausler HB, Ehrentraut S, Stoll C, et al. The relationship between cognitive performance and employment and health status in long-term survivors of the acute respiratory distress syndrome: results of an exploratory study. *Gen Hosp Psych.* 2001;23(2):90–96.
29. Girard TD, Jackson JC, Pandharipande PP, et al. Delirium as a predictor of long-term cognitive impairment in survivors of critical illness. *Crit Care Med.* 2010;38(7):1513–1520.
30. Santoro MJ, Girard TD, McCurley JL, et al. Cognitive impairment at discharge in intensive care unit survivors: data from the Awakening and Breathing Controlled (ABC) Trial. *Am J Respir Crit Care Med.* 2011; 183:A4119.
31. Pandharipande PP, Girard TD, Jackson JC, et al; BRAIN-ICU Study Investigators. Long-term cognitive impairment after critical illness. *N Engl J Med.* 2013;369(14):1306–1316.
32. Jefferson AL, Paul RH, Ozonoff A, Cohen RA. Evaluating elements of executive functioning as predictors of instrumental activities of daily living (IADLs). *Arch Clin Neuropsychol.* 2006;21(4):311–320.
33. Cahn-Weiner DA, Boyle PA, Malloy PF. Tests of executive function predict instrumental activities of daily living in community-dwelling older individuals. *Appl Neuropsychol.* 2002;9(3):187–191.
34. Royall DR, Chiodo LK, Polk MJ. Correlates of disability among elderly retirees with "subclinical" cognitive impairment. *J Gerontol A Biol Sci Med Sci.* 2000;55(9):M541–M546.
35. Burton CL, Strauss E, Hultsch DF, Hunter MA. Cognitive functioning and everyday problem solving in older adults. *Clin Neuropsychol.* 2006;20(3):432–452.
36. Insel K, Morrow D, Brewer B, Figueredo A. Executive function, working memory, and medication adherence among older adults. *J Gerontol B Psychol Sci Soc Sci.* 2006;61(2):P102–P107.
37. Ouimet S, Kavanagh BP, Gottfried SB, Skrobik Y. Incidence, risk factors and consequences of ICU delirium. *Intensive Care Med.* 2007;33(1):66–73.
38. Ely EW, Gautam S, Margolin R, et al. The impact of delirium in the intensive care unit on hospital length of stay. *Intensive Care Med.* 2001; 27(12):1892–1900.
39. Ely EW, Inouye SK, Bernard GR, et al. Delirium in mechanically ventilated patients: validity and reliability of the confusion assessment method for the intensive care unit (CAM-ICU). *JAMA.* 2001;286(21):2703–2710.
40. Ely EW, Margolin R, Francis J, et al. Evaluation of delirium in critically ill patients: validation of the Confusion Assessment Method for the Intensive Care Unit (CAM-ICU). *Crit Care Med.* 2001;29(7):1370–1379.
41. Ely EW, Shintani A, Truman B, et al. Delirium as a predictor of mortality in mechanically ventilated patients in the intensive care unit. *JAMA.* 2004; 291(14):1753–1762.
42. Dubois MJ, Bergeron N, Dumont M, et al. Delirium in an intensive care unit: a study of risk factors. *Intensive Care Med.* 2001;27(8):1297–1304.
43. Aldemir M, Ozen S, Kara IH, et al. Predisposing factors for delirium in the surgical intensive care unit. *Crit Care.* 2001;5(5):265–270.
44. Lin SM, Liu CY, Wang CH, et al. The impact of delirium on the survival of mechanically ventilated patients. *Crit Care Med.* 2004;32(11):2254–2259.
45. McNicoll L, Pisani MA, Zhang Y, et al. Delirium in the intensive care unit: occurrence and clinical course in older patients. *J Am Geriatr Soc.* 2003; 51(5):591–598.
46. Ely EW, Girard TD, Shintani AK, et al. Apolipoprotein E4 polymorphism as a genetic predisposition to delirium in critically ill patients. *Crit Care Med.* 2007;35(1):112–117.
47. Pandharipande P, Ely EW. Sedative and analgesic medications: risk factors for delirium and sleep disturbances in the critically ill. *Crit Care Clin.* 2006;22(2):313–327, vii.
48. Inouye SK, Charpentier PA. Precipitating factors for delirium in hospitalized elderly persons: predictive model and interrelationship with baseline vulnerability. *JAMA.* 1996;275(11):852–857.
49. Cunningham C. Systemic inflammation and delirium: important co-factors in the progression of dementia. *Biochem Soc Trans.* 2011;39(4):945–953.
50. Vitkovic L, Bockaert J, Jacque C. "Inflammatory" cytokines: neuromodulators in normal brain?*J Neurochem.* 2000;74(2):457–471.
51. Wilson CJ, Finch CE, Cohen HJ. Cytokines and cognition–the case for a head-to-toe inflammatory paradigm. *J Am Geriatr Soc.* 2002;50(12):2041–2056.
52. Heneka MT, O'Banion MK, Terwel D, Kummer MP. Neuroinflammatory processes in Alzheimer's disease. *J Neural Transm (Vienna).* 2010; 117(8):919–947.
53. Rubio-Perez JM, Morillas-Ruiz JM. A review: inflammatory process in Alzheimer's disease, role of cytokines. *ScientificWorldJournal.* 2012; 2012:756357.
54. Singer BH, Newstead MW, Zeng X, et al. Cecal ligation and puncture results in long-term central nervous system myeloid inflammation. *PLoS One.* 2016;11(2):e0149136.
55. Hopkins RO, Weaver LK, Pope D, et al. Neuropsychological sequelae and impaired health status in survivors of severe acute respiratory distress syndrome. *Am J Respir Crit Care Med.* 1999;160(1):50–56.
56. Wilson BA. Cognitive functioning of adult survivors of cerebral hypoxia. *Brain Inj.* 1996;10:863–874.
57. Stuss DT, Peterkin I, Guzman DA, et al. Chronic obstructive pulmonary disease: effects of hypoxia on neurological and neuropsychological measures. *J Clin Exp Neuropsychol.* 1997;19(4):515–524.
58. Kozora E, Filley CM, Julian LJ, Cullum CM. Cognitive functioning in patients with chronic obstructive pulmonary disease and mild hypoxemia compared with patients with mild Alzheimer disease and normal controls. *Neuropsychiatry Neuropsychol Behav Neurol.* 1999;12(3):178–183.
59. Bishop NA, Lu T, Yankner BA. Neural mechanisms of ageing and cognitive decline. *Nature.* 2010;464(7288):529–535.
60. Andrews-Hanna JR, Snyder AZ, Vincent JL, et al. Disruption of large-scale brain systems in advanced aging. *Neuron.* 2007;56(5):924–935.
61. Park DC, Reuter-Lorenz P. The adaptive brain: aging and neurocognitive scaffolding. *Annu Rev Psychol.* 2009;60:173–196.
62. Silbert BS, Scott DA, Evered LA, et al. Preexisting cognitive impairment in patients scheduled for elective coronary artery bypass graft surgery. *Anesth Analg.* 2007;104(5):1023–1028.
63. Norman BC, Jackson JC, Graves JA, et al. Employment outcomes after critical illness: an analysis of the bringing to light the risk factors and incidence of neuropsychological dysfunction in ICU survivors cohort. *Crit Care Med.* 2016[Epub ahead of print].
64. Bergbom-Engberg I, Haljamae H. Assessment of patients' experience of discomforts during respirator therapy. *Crit Care Med.* 1989;17(10): 1068–1072.
65. Huang M, Parker AM, Bienvenu OJ, et al; National Institutes of Health, National Heart, Lung, and Blood Institute Acute Respiratory Distress Syndrome Network. Psychiatric symptoms in acute respiratory distress syndrome survivors: a 1-year national multicenter study. *Crit Care Med.* 2016;44(5):954–965.
66. Cameron JI, Chu LM, Matte A, et al; RECOVER Program Investigators (Phase 1: towards RECOVER); Canadian Critical Care Trials Group. One-year outcomes in caregivers of critically ill patients. *N Engl J Med.* 2016;374(19):1831–1841.
67. Kessler RC, Chiu WT, Demler O, et al. Prevalence, severity, and comorbidity of 12-month DSM-IV disorders in the National Comorbidity Survey Replication. *Arch Gen Psychiatry.* 2005;62(6):617–627.
68. Davydow DS, Gifford JM, Desai SV, et al. Depression in general intensive care unit survivors: a systematic review. *Intensive Care Med.* 2009; 35(5):796–809.
69. Wunsch H, Christiansen CF, Johansen MB, et al. Psychiatric diagnoses and psychoactive medication use among nonsurgical critically ill patients receiving mechanical ventilation. *JAMA.* 2014;311(11):1133–1142.
70. Jackson JC, Pandharipande PP, Girard TD, et al; Bringing to light the Risk Factors And Incidence of Neuropsychological dysfunction in ICU survivors (BRAIN-ICU) study investigators. Depression, post-traumatic stress disorder, and functional disability in survivors of critical illness in the BRAIN-ICU study: a longitudinal cohort study. *Lancet Resp Med.* 2014;2(5):369–379.
71. Chang CK, Hayes RD, Broadbent M, et al. All-cause mortality among people with serious mental illness (SMI), substance use disorders, and depressive disorders in southeast London: a cohort study. *BMC Psychiatry.* 2010;10:77.
72. Katon WJ. Epidemiology and treatment of depression in patients with chronic medical illness. *Dialogues Clin Neurosci.* 2011;13(1):7–23.
73. Rozanski A. Integrating psychologic approaches into the behavioral management of cardiac patients. *Psychosom Med.* 2005;67 Suppl 1: S67–S73.

74. Seery MD, Holman EA, Silver RC. Whatever does not kill us: cumulative lifetime adversity, vulnerability, and resilience. *J Pers Soc Psychol.* 2010;99(6):1025–1041.
75. Zoellner T, Maercker A. Posttraumatic growth in clinical psychology: a critical review and introduction of a two component model. *Clin Psychol Rev.* 2006;26(5):626–653.
76. Davydow DS, Gifford JM, Desai SV, et al. Posttraumatic stress disorder in general intensive care unit survivors: a systematic review. *Gen Hosp Psychiatry.* 2008;30(5):421–434.
77. Parker AM, Sricharoenchai T, Raparla S, et al. Posttraumatic stress disorder in critical illness survivors: a meta-analysis. *Crit Care Med.* 2015;43(5):1121–1129.
78. Kessler RC, Wang PS. The descriptive epidemiology of commonly occurring mental disorders in the United States. *Annu Rev Public Health.* 2008; 29:115–129.
79. Jones C, Griffiths RD, Humphris G, Skirrow PM. Memory, delusions, and the development of acute posttraumatic stress disorder-related symptoms after intensive care. *Crit Care Med.* 2001;29(3):573–580.
80. Elliott D, Davidson JE, Harvey MA, et al. Exploring the scope of post-intensive care syndrome therapy and care: engagement of non-critical care providers and survivors in a second stakeholders meeting. *Crit Care Med.* 2014;42(12):2518–2526.
81. Iwashyna TJ. Trajectories of recovery and dysfunction after acute illness, with implications for clinical trial design. *Am J Respir Crit Care Med.* 2012; 186(4):302–304.
82. Govindan S, Iwashyna TJ, Watson SR, et al. Issues of survivorship are rarely addressed during intensive care unit stays: baseline results from a statewide quality improvement collaborative. *Ann Am Thorac Soc.* 2014;11(4):587–591.
83. Griffiths JA, Barber VS, Cuthbertson BH, Young JD. A national survey of intensive care follow-up clinics. *Anaesthesia.* 2006;61(10):950–955.
84. Cuthbertson BH, Rattray J, Campbell MK, et al; PRaCTICaL study group. The PRaCTICaL study of nurse led, intensive care follow-up programmes for improving long term outcomes from critical illness: a pragmatic randomised controlled trial. *BMJ.* 2009;339:b3723.
85. Kim MM, Barnato AE, Angus DC, et al. The effect of multidisciplinary care teams on intensive care unit mortality. *Arch Intern Med.* 2010;170(4):369–376.
86. Scales DC, Fischer HD, Li P, Bierman AS, et al. Unintentional continuation of medications intended for acute illness after hospital discharge: a population-based cohort study. *J Gen Intern Med.* 2015;31(2):196–202.
87. Bell CM, Brener SS, Gunraj N, et al. Association of ICU or hospital admission with unintentional discontinuation of medications for chronic diseases. *JAMA.* 2011;306(8):840–847.
88. Schelling G, Stoll C, Haller M, et al. Health-related quality of life and posttraumatic stress disorder in survivors of the acute respiratory distress syndrome. *Crit Care Med.* 1998;26(4):651–659.
89. Izard CE. Emotion theory and research: highlights, unanswered questions, and emerging issues. *Annu Rev Psychol.* 2009;60:1–25.
90. Schmidt K, Thiel P, Mueller F, et al; Smooth Study Group. Sepsis survivors monitoring and coordination in outpatient health care (SMOOTH): study protocol for a randomized controlled trial. *Trials.* 2014;15:283.
91. Clark BJ, Rubinsky AD, Ho PM, et al. Alcohol screening scores and the risk of intensive care unit admission and hospital readmission. *Subst Abus.* 2016:1–8.
92. Calfee CS, Matthay MA, Kangelaris KN, et al. Cigarette smoke exposure and the acute respiratory distress syndrome. *Crit Care Med.* 2015;43(9):1790–1797.
93. Cox CE, Porter LS, Hough CL, et al. Development and preliminary evaluation of a telephone-based coping skills training intervention for survivors of acute lung injury and their informal caregivers. *Intensive Care Med.* 2012; 38(8):1289–1297.
94. Mikkelsen ME, Jackson JC, Hopkins RO, et al. Peer support as a novel strategy to mitigate post-intensive care syndrome. *AACN Adv Crit Care.* 2016;27(2):221–229.
95. Jones C, Skirrow P, Griffiths RD, et al. Rehabilitation after critical illness: a randomized, controlled trial. *Crit Care Med.* 2003;31(10): 2456–2461.
96. Jones C, Backman C, Capuzzo M, et al; RACHEL group. Intensive care diaries reduce new onset post traumatic stress disorder following critical illness: a randomised, controlled trial. *Crit Care.* 2010;14(5):R168.
97. Jones C, Backman C, Griffiths RD. Intensive care diaries and relatives' symptoms of posttraumatic stress disorder after critical illness: a pilot study. *Am J Crit Care.* 2012;21(3):172–176.
98. Egerod I, Christensen D. A comparative study of ICU patient diaries vs. hospital charts. *Qual Health Res.* 2010;20(10):1446–1456.
99. Nydahl P, Knueck D, Egerod I. Extent and application of ICU diaries in Germany in 2014. *Nurs Crit Care.* 2015;20(3):155–162.
100. Garrouste-Orgeas M, Coquet I, Perier A, et al. Impact of an intensive care unit diary on psychological distress in patients and relatives*. *Crit Care Med.* 2012;40(7):2033–2040.
101. Knowles RE, Tarrier N. Evaluation of the effect of prospective patient diaries on emotional well-being in intensive care unit survivors: a randomized controlled trial. *Crit Care Med.* 2009;37(1):184–191.
102. Backman CG, Orwelius L, Sjoberg F, et al. Long-term effect of the ICU-diary concept on quality of life after critical illness. *Acta Anaesthesiol Scand.* 2010;54(6):736–743.
103. Lone NI, Gillies MA, Haddow C, et al. Five year mortality and hospital costs associated with surviving intensive care. *Am J Respir Crit Care Med.* 2016;194(2):198–208.[Epub ahead of print].
104. Unroe M, Kahn JM, Carson SS, et al. One-year trajectories of care and resource utilization for recipients of prolonged mechanical ventilation: a cohort study. *Ann Intern Med.* 2010;153(3):167–175.
105. Rydingsward JE, Horkan CM, Mogensen KM, et al. Functional status in ICU survivors and out of hospital outcomes: a cohort study. *Crit Care Med.* 2016;44(5):869–879.
106. Herridge MS, Chu LM, Matte A, et al; RECOVER Program Investigators (Phase 1: towards RECOVER) and the Canadian Critical Care Trials Group. The RECOVER program: disability risk groups and one year outcome after ≥ 7 days of mechanical ventilation. *Am J Respir Crit Care Med.* 2016[Epub ahead of print].

CHAPTER 13

Central Nervous System Physiology in Critical Illness

JOSEPH ZACHARIAH, ALEJANDRO A. RABINSTEIN, and EDWARD M. MANNO

INTRODUCTION

Critical care of acute neurologic states revolves around limiting or preventing secondary injury. A robust grasp of the physiology behind these secondary deteriorations is imperative in making appropriate treatment decisions. A rapidly growing body of literature keeps adding to our understanding of neurocritical care. In this chapter, we provide a foundation to conceptualize the basics of cerebrovascular physiology. Based upon these foundations, we will outline a rational approach to the treatment of both general and specific neurologic emergencies.

METABOLISM

The human brain represents only 2% of the total body mass, but accounts for approximately 20% of the cardiac output and oxygen consumption (1). The majority of cerebral oxygen consumption occurs at highly metabolically active grey matter structures. The relatively high metabolic activity of these cells is needed to sustain the electrical gradients of neurons required to transmit electrical signals, synthesize transmitters, and maintain the infrastructure of the cell (2).

The central nervous system utilizes intracellular stores of phosphocreatine and adenosine triphosphate (ATP) as its main energy source. These stores are constantly replenished through the aerobic oxidative phosphorylation of glucose at the inner membrane of the neuronal mitochondria. Glucose is the main substrate for brain metabolism, with specific glucose transferases in the capillary endothelium providing entry into the neuronal cytoplasm. The concept that the contribution of anaerobic metabolism to energy production in the brain is negligible, has been challenged by studies showing lactate being utilized by the mitochondrial tricarboxylic acid (TCA) cycle (3). Brain energy reserves are limited, thus electrical activity is inhibited within seconds, and cellular breakdown occurs within minutes, of lack of oxygen delivery to the neuron (4).

CEREBRAL BLOOD FLOW

Cerebral blood flow (CBF) is classically measured by the volume of blood in milliliters that supply 100 g of brain tissue per minute. The total average CBF is 50 to 55 mL/100 g/min. The CBF of grey matter is 70 to 75 mL/100 g/min, whereas white matter, which requires less blood flow, averages a CBF of 30 to 35 mL/100 g/min. CBF is lower than normal in areas of white matter hyperintensities, proportional to the intensity of signal changes (5). A spectrum of neuronal dysfunction arises once CBF decreases below 20 mL/100 g/min. Changes in electroencephalogram (EEG) or evoked potentials are noted with CBF of 16 to 18 mL/100 g/min; at 10 to 12 mL/100 g/min, ion pumps start to fail, resulting in cytotoxic edema. CBF under 10 mL/100 g/min produces frank ischemia with gross metabolic failure and membrane destabilization.

Measuring CBF

The study of modern cerebrovascular physiology began in the 1940s with Kety and Schmidt (6) describing a direct method for quantifying CBF based upon the Fick principle. The original Fick equation stated that oxygen uptake in the lung was equal to the product of cardiac output and the arteriovenous difference of oxygen (7). Kety (8) substituted nitrous oxide, an inert, nonmetabolizable, diffusible tracer, in place of oxygen. Thus, the accumulation of nitrous oxide in the brain was substituted for the absorption of oxygen in the lungs (9). This technique is still considered the gold standard for quantifying CBF, but it is invasive and limited to measuring only global CBF (10).

The development of external detection systems allowed for the use of radioactive tracers to measure regional CBF (rCBF); focal perfusion and washout of substances could thus be employed to determine flow into local regions of the brain. $Xenon^{133}$, a diffusible, gamma-emitting substance was used initially as an injection and later through inhalation. Perfusion and washout were calculated using a rotating gamma counter. Later, the application of computed tomographic techniques (Xenon CT) allowed for improved resolution of rCBF (11).

Single-photon emission computed tomography (SPECT) uses $technetium^{99}$ ligands to measure rCBF and is the most commonly used technique to measure CBF. $Technetium^{99}$ crosses the blood–brain barrier and is trapped within cells. The tracer accumulates in varying brain regions according to the rate of delivery—in turn determined by the local metabolic needs—and thus is a marker for rCBF; multidetector systems are used to provide images (12).

Positron emission tomography (PET) is similar to SPECT in that an external detector is used to measure an accumulated radioactive substance. The generation and use of positrons,

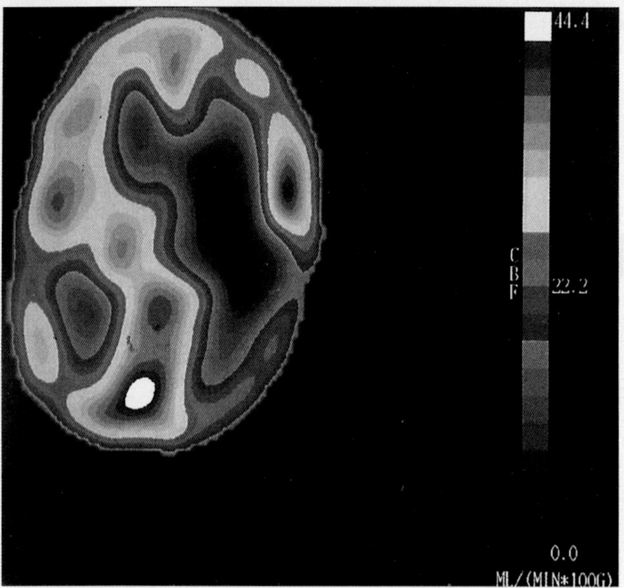

FIGURE 13.1 Positron emission tomography image of an intracerebral hemorrhage. Note central area of necrosis surrounded by area of decreased perfusion. (Courtesy of Michael Diringer, Washington University School of Medicine.)

TABLE 13.1 Normal Values for Cerebral Blood Flow and Metabolism

Cerebral blood flow (CBF)	50 mL/100 g/min
Systemic arterial oxygen content (CaO_2)	14–20 mL/100 mL
Jugular venous oxygen content ($CjvO_2$)	8–13 mL/100 mL
Jugular venous oxygen saturation ($SjvO_2$)	65%
Cerebral arterial–venous oxygen content difference ($(C(a\text{–}v)O_2 = CaO_2\text{–}CjvO_2)$)	6.3 mL/100 mL
Cerebral oxygen delivery ($CDO_2 = CBF \times CaO_2$)	10 mL/100 g/min
Cerebral metabolic rate of oxygen consumption $CMRO_2\text{–}CBF \times C(a\text{–}v)O_2$	3.5 mL/100 g/min

however, significantly improves resolution. A positron is an electron with a positive charge formed by the decay of radionuclides; it requires a cyclotron or linear accelerator for production. The collision of a positron with an electron produces two photons that are sent off at 180 degrees. The simultaneous detection of these photons allows for three-dimensional reconstruction of rCBF. In addition to measuring CBF, different radiolabeled ligands can be used to measure cerebral blood volume (CBV), glucose metabolism, or cerebral oxygen extraction. PET provides the highest quantifiable measure of rCBF and can be used for a variety of physiologic experiments (13). However, it is expensive, requires a cyclotron, and is, consequently, limited to a few academic centers (Fig. 13.1).

New techniques of bolus tracking in both magnetic resonance imaging (MRI) and computed tomography (CT) have allowed for acute assessments of cerebral perfusion. These techniques are known as CT perfusion and MR perfusion. In these techniques, a bolus of a contrast agent is detected either through changes in T_2 signal or Housenfield units. Estimations of CBF can be made by measuring the transit time required for these boluses to pass through cerebral tissue. These radiologic modalities are being used widely for the acute assessments of cerebral infarctions (14,15).

Regulation of CBF by Oxygen

Under normal conditions, CBF and regional distribution of oxygen are tightly coupled. Increases in cerebral metabolism lead to an increase in the delivery of oxygen and glucose to metabolically active tissue. The cerebral metabolic rate of oxygen consumption ($CMRO_2$) is the rate of oxygen utilization by cerebral tissue. It is calculated by the Fick method as the product of CBF and the cerebral oxygen arterial–venous difference of an inert nondiffusible substance. Direct and indirect methods exist to estimate both CBF and $CMRO_2$. Cerebral oxygen delivery (CDO_2) is the product of CBF and the oxygen-carrying capacity of hemoglobin. The normal mean capillary partial pressure of oxygen (PO_2) is approximately 65 mmHg, representing a difference between normal arterial PO_2 (PaO_2 = 90–95 mmHg) and venous PO_2 (PvO_2 = 35–40 mmHg). Normal values for standard measures of CBF, $CMRO_2$, and CDO_2 are listed in Table 13.1.

CDO_2 can also be affected by changes in the concentration of oxygen bound to hemoglobin. Hemoglobin has a high affinity for binding oxygen with greater than 90% of the hemoglobin binding sites for oxygen saturated at PaO_2 greater than 70 mmHg; increasing PaO_2 above this level, therefore, has little effect on oxygen delivery.

At PaO_2 below 50 mmHg, there is a rapid increase in CBF (Fig. 13.2). This is more significant in grey, as opposed to white, matter. There is a linear relationship between the arterial oxygen content and CBF in hypoxic states; however, the relationship between CBF and the PaO_2 is curvilinear (16). Vasoactive effects may be caused directly by oxygen or mediated though adenosine A_2 receptors (9). Several other mechanisms exist to maintain oxygen delivery to the brain. Cerebral hypoperfusion will lead to depolarization of medullary neurons controlling sympathetic output. This results in a compensatory increase in blood pressure and heart rate. Decreased cerebral perfusion leading to decreased arterial oxygen delivery to the cerebral capillary bed will lead to venodilation, lowering the postcapillary pressure and increasing flow across the capillary bed. Extraction of oxygen bound to hemoglobin is increased across

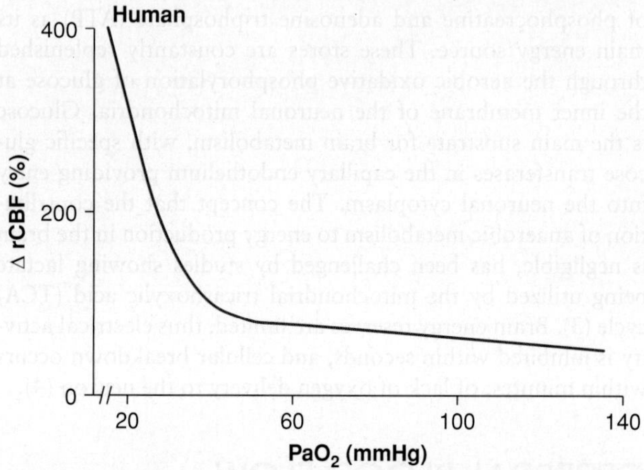

FIGURE 13.2 Alterations of regional cerebral blood flow (rCBF) to changes in arterial oxygen tension. Note oxygen tensions below approximately 50 mmHg lead to a sharp increase in rCBF. (From Golanov EV, Reisw DJ. Oxygen and cerebral blood flow. In: Welch KMA, Caplan LR, Reis DJ, et al., eds. *Primer on Cerebrovascular Disease*. San Diego, CA: Academic Press; 1997:58–60.)

the capillary bed as CBF continues to decrease. This increase in oxygen extraction can be detected by measuring oxygen concentration in jugular venous blood and comparing it to arterial oxygen content. Finally, increases in local hydrogen ion concentration will occur as ischemia develops, presumably due to lactate production from anaerobic metabolism. The resultant shift in the oxygen displacement curve of hemoglobin to the right will result in increased oxygen release from hemoglobin to the local cerebral tissue.

Regulation of CBF by CO_2

Changes in the partial pressure of carbon dioxide (PCO_2) have significant effects on CBF. One mmHg change in $PaCO_2$ can result in an approximately 2.5% to 4% change in CBF. This effect is more pronounced in the grey matter than in the white matter. The response curve of $PaCO_2$ is sigmoidal, with the CBF response flattening below 15 to 20 mmHg and above 100 mmHg. Vasodilation occurs at all vessel sizes, but is most pronounced on the smaller arterioles (9).

Changes in vessel diameter are mediated through alterations in cerebrospinal fluid hydrogen ion concentrations (CSF pH). The direct application of CO_2 or bicarbonate to pial arterioles does not affect vessel diameters. Since CO_2 is freely diffusible across the blood–brain barrier, changes in $PaCO_2$ will affect both CSF hydrogen ion and bicarbonate concentrations (17). The response of changes in hydrogen ion concentration is relatively short-lived, lasting only a few hours as the choroid plexus of the brain will compensate for changes in hydrogen ion concentration by adjusting the production of cerebrospinal fluid bicarbonate (18).

CEREBRAL AUTOREGULATION

Cerebral autoregulation refers to the capacity of CBF to remain constant despite changes in cerebral perfusion pressure (CPP). This intrinsic control allows for relative constant CBF over a wide range of CPP. The shape of the autoregulatory curve can be modified by a number of extrinsic factors: hypertension, hypocarbia, and increased sympathetic nerve activity will increase both the upper and lower ranges of autoregulation. Chronic hypotension, hypercarbia, and parasympathetic activity will lower the set points of autoregulation. The autoregulatory curve will shift upwards with advancing age. In the healthy, normotensive individual, CBF is relatively constant between CPP (or mean arterial pressure [MAP]) of 50 to 150 mmHg. Outside this range, CBF has a linear correlation with CPP, otherwise described as a pressure-passive phenomenon (Fig. 13.3) (18,19).

In most vascular beds, autoregulation occurs at the level of the arterioles. However, a significant proportion of vascular resistance in the cerebral circulation is modulated at the level of the cerebral arteries. In cats, dogs, and monkeys, approximately 40% of the cerebral vascular resistance is mediated by changes in the baseline pial artery diameter of vessels greater than 400 μm in diameter (19).

In response to hypotension, both cerebral arteries and arterioles will dilate to maintain constant CBF. Vessel dilation progresses from the largest vessels to the smallest in response to decreases in CPP (16). Cerebral arterioles will also continue to dilate below the lower limit of autoregulation (20). Further

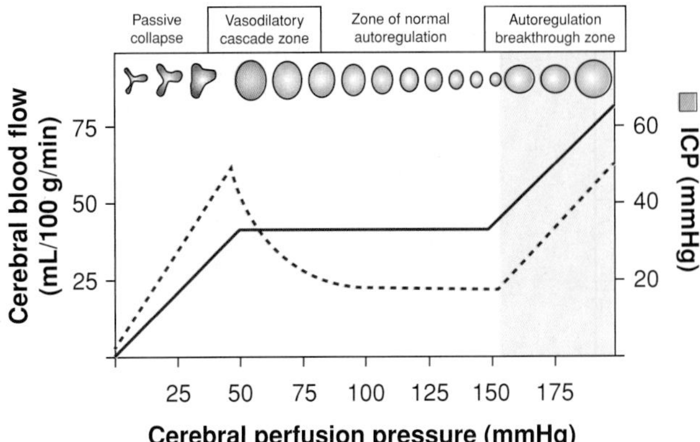

FIGURE 13.3 Cerebral autoregulatory curve with cerebral blood flow remaining constant between cerebral perfusion pressures (CPP) of 50 and 150 mmHg (*solid line*). Superimposed curve of cerebral blood volume (CBV) at variable CPP (*dotted line*). The top portion of the figure illustrates the cerebral arteriolar caliber. Note that at CPP below the level of cerebral autoregulation, arteries and arterioles begin to collapse (passive collapse). CBV decreases from a point of maximal dilation seen near the lower end of CA (vasodilatory cascade zone) to a constant blood volume (zone of normal autoregulation). Higher CPP leads to autoregulatory breakthrough and parallel increases in both CBF and CBV (autoregulatory breakthrough zone). ICP, intracranial pressure. (From Rose JC, Mayer SA. Optimizing blood pressure in neurological emergencies. *Neurocrit Care*. 2004;1:287–299.)

drops in pressure slow flow across the capillary bed and lead to an increase in the oxygen extraction coefficient from hemoglobin (21); continued hypotension progresses to ischemia. Oxygen deprivation leading to neuronal cell death proceeds through several distinctive steps. The high metabolic activity of neurons rapidly depletes oxygen-derived ATP and phosphocreatine stores, leading to failure of synaptic transmission. The EEG at this point becomes flat and consciousness is lost. Electrical failure occurs as CBF falls below 16 to 20 mL/100 g tissue/min and cerebral oxygen consumption falls below a third of its normal resting metabolism. Restoration of CBF after electrical failure, however, will lead to functional recovery of the cell. Further decreases in CBF to less than 10 mL/100 g/min will lead to energy failure needed to maintain the activity of the membrane sodium–potassium pump. As flow continues to decrease, membrane depolarizations occur and ionic gradients are lost as potassium effluxes out of the, and sodium and water enter, the cell, leading to the development of cytotoxic edema (Fig. 13.4).

In a similar fashion, cerebral pial arteries and arterioles will constrict as CPP (or MAP) increases. Maximal vasoconstriction occurs at CPP (MAP) of 160 to 170 mmHg. Above these pressures, passive dilation of the blood vessels occur with resultant autoregulatory failure, breakdown of blood–brain barrier, cerebral hyperperfusion, and development of vasogenic edema.

Several theories have been proposed to explain the mechanisms of cerebral autoregulation. These can be broadly categorized into myogenic, metabolic, and neurogenic (21).

The myogenic theory postulates that smooth muscle cells of the cerebral arteries and arterioles constrict or dilate in response to the transmural pressure that is generated across the vessel wall (22). This may be mediated by alterations in the position of the actin myosin filament in the vessel wall (23). Another theory is that changes in vessel wall shear stress induced by alterations in blood flow induce the release of

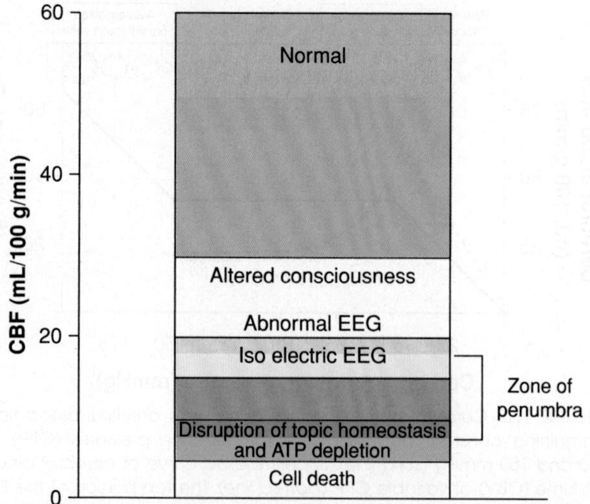

FIGURE 13.4 Blood flow thresholds for cerebral function and metabolism. As blood flow decreases, synaptic transmission and electrical activity ceases (electroencephalographic silence). Further decreases in flow lead to loss of ionic homeostasis and cell death. The ischemic penumbra describes brain tissue with blood flows below electrical failure but above membrane failure. CBF, cerebral blood flow; EEG, electroencephalogram; ATP, adenosine triphosphate. (From Veremakis CV, Lindner DH. Central nervous system injury: essential physiologic and therapeutic concerns. In: Civetta JM, Taylor RW, Kirby RR, eds. *Critical Care*. Philadelphia, PA: Lippincott–Raven Publishers; 1997:273–289.)

vasoactive substances from the vascular endothelium that subsequently leads to vessel wall constriction or dilation (24). The myogenic theory is supported by the rapidity by which cerebral autoregulation occurs. However, the myogenic theory by itself cannot account for all the regulation that occurs. In jugular venous hypertension, intravascular pressure is increased. This condition should lead to arterial vasoconstriction; however, vasodilation is most commonly found under these circumstances (25). It has, therefore, postulated that myogenic factors may play a significant role only when metabolic factors are not significant. Alternately myogenic factors may work synergistically with metabolic factors providing changes in vascular tone required to optimize the metabolic response (26).

The metabolic theory of pressure autoregulation postulates that the local changes in CBF found with changes in cerebral metabolic activity are mediated through the releases of local neurochemical substances from the nonvascular cells of the central nervous system (21). The tight coupling of flow to metabolism, and the timing of autoregulation support this postulated mechanism. Several substances have been implicated, including hydrogen ion, carbon dioxide, nitric oxide (NO), adenosine, potassium, and calcium (27). Experimental evidence exists in favor and against all of the postulated mediators (21,28–30); varying combinations have also been suggested. Most recently, changes in potassium levels mediated through alterations in calcitonin gene-related peptides have been suggested to be a mechanism of arteriolar dilation (31). Observations that changes in CPP alter the degree of endothelial oxygen tension suggest that this may be another important mechanism for autoregulation (32).

The direct role of neurogenic mechanisms on cerebral autoregulation is probably limited. The sympathetic and parasympathetic nervous systems play a role in modulating the cerebral autoregulatory curve, but direct neural control over small arteries or arterioles regulating focal changes in CBF does not occur. Other neurogenic mediators may be in a position to regulate vascular tone (33). The localization and central control of these nerves have so far proved elusive (21,34).

Measurement of Autoregulation

Severe TBI, infarcts, hemorrhagic strokes, and space-occupying lesions can result in impairment of cerebral autoregulation. As boundaries of autoregulation are exceeded, either hypoperfusion or hyperperfusion can occur, resulting in irreversible injury.

The index of autoregulation is calculated by a correlation coefficient between two factors within a time series. The coefficient ranges from −1 to +1 where a negative correlation is effective autoregulation and a positive correlation is impaired autoregulation. Several techniques utilized to calculate autoregulation indices include transcranial Doppler (TCD), intracranial pressure (ICP), partial pressure of brain oxygen ($PbtO_2$), and near-infrared spectroscopy (NIRS). Each of these techniques is surrogates of CBF and offer slightly different indices of autoregulation. Whether guiding therapy based on the status of autoregulation can improve functional outcomes in patients with critical brain injury remains to be elucidated.

ICP Waveform

The classical variations of ICP waveforms include pulse and respiratory components. The waves of ICP correlates with every pulse and represent large cerebral vessel pulsations. The pulse wave is made of three points: P1, P2, and P3. P1, otherwise known as the percussive wave, is produced by the direct transmission of the choroid plexus arterial pulsation; P2, also known as the tidal wave, represents brain compliance. In states of poor cerebral compliance, such as brain trauma, the P2 peak can be pathologically higher than the P1 peak. Closure of the aortic valve produces P3, the dicrotic wave which was previously thought to originate from the venous system. As ICP increases, all three components of the waveform increase in amplitude. However, as ICP continues to increase, P2 dominates and the waveform assumes a rounded appearance. Hypocapnia, on the other hand, will result in constriction of cerebral blood vessels and the amplitudes of all three P waves will be diminished.

ICP Dynamics

Normal ICP is usually between 5 and 8 mmHg, but can be as high as 15 mmHg in some circumstances. Beyond this, some degree of intracranial pathology should be suspected (35). Normal ICP fluctuates rhythmically approximately 3 to 5 mmHg. The sinusoidal pattern can be seen on an ICP pressure trace and was originally described by Traube and Hering (36). The origin of these waves is unknown, but may have to do with phasic constriction and dilation of the cerebral arterioles (37) or to changes in intrathoracic pressure during the phases of the respiratory cycle; as ICP increases, this variation is lost (38).

The ICP–volume curve demonstrates a relatively flat portion where increases in volume are accommodated with little change in pressure. At some inflection point, these processes are exhausted and small changes in volume lead to larger increases in ICP (Fig. 13.3). This pressure–volume curve may, therefore, represent the displacement of various fluids from the intracranial space.

The approximate contents of the intracranial cavity consist of brain parenchyma (75%), blood (20%), and CSF (5%). Most of the intracranial blood resides in the venous side of the circulation (35). According to the Monroe doctrine, the overall volume of the contents of the intracranial cavity must remain constant. Thus, any increase in the intracranial contents from venous engorgement, intracerebral hemorrhage, tumors, edema, etc. must be compensated by an equal displacement of fluids or tissue. The flat portion of the ICP–volume curve represents displacement of CSF into the more compliant spinal subarachnoid space. Progressive increases in volume lead to further displacement of venous and arterial blood. Finally, brain tissue is displaced and herniation occurs (Fig. 13.5) (39).

The ICP–volume curve can be affected by the speed and duration of changes that occur in the intracranial cavity. For instance, tumors can grow to large volumes before becoming problematic because the slow-growing process allows for a gradual increase in intracranial compliance. Conversely, an acute hemorrhage of the same size will not be tolerated.

Intracranial compliance can be determined by measuring the change in ICP to a given volume. A volume–pressure response (VPR) is estimated by measuring the ICP response to an infusion of sterile saline through an intraventricular catheter (40). Small changes in response to this increased volume suggest that the patient is on the flat portion of the volume–pressure curve. Increases in ICP greater than 4 mmHg in response to 1 mL of fluid would suggest that intracranial reserve is limited. A more widely used index to measure intracranial compliance has been the pressure–volume index (PVI); this index estimates the volume needed to increase ICP by a factor of 10 (41).

Spontaneous and sustained elevations in ICP were noted by Lundberg early in the history of study of cerebral hemodynamics (42). The origin of these "plateau waves" (or A waves) has been speculative until the 1980s when Rosner and colleagues observed that plateau waves were always preceded by drops in CPP. The decreases in CPP are largely a result of decreases in MAP, but could also be due to excess CSF volume, hypercarbia, or changes in vascular resistance induced by metabolic factors (43). Vasodilation in response to the drop in CPP would be responsible for the sustained rise in ICP (i.e., the generation of the plateau wave).

CPP Dynamics

CPP is defined as the pressure difference between MAP and mean jugular venous pressure. However, when ICP is greater than jugular venous pressure, ICP is substituted for jugular venous pressure. Thus, CPP is typically reported as (18):

CPP = MAP – ICP

In healthy controls, ICP is less than 5 mmHg and so CPP and MAP are nearly equal.

As previously noted, decreases in CPP will lead to an autoregulatory cerebral vasodilation increase in CBV. In the setting of altered intracranial compliance, ICP can increase with rising CBV. This increase in ICP in turn compromises CPP in a feedforward loop. The process is spontaneously reversed by an acute elevation of blood pressure—a phenomenon known as Cushing response. This sympathetic response probably occurs because of oligemia affecting the brainstem centers modulating sympathetic activity (44).

MECHANISMS OF BRAIN INJURY

Immediate Concerns

The most important features in managing acute neurologic injury are management of the airway, oxygenation, and circulation issues, careful and repeated monitoring of vital parameters, and neurologic status. Patients should be rapidly transported to a trauma center or stroke center for prompt

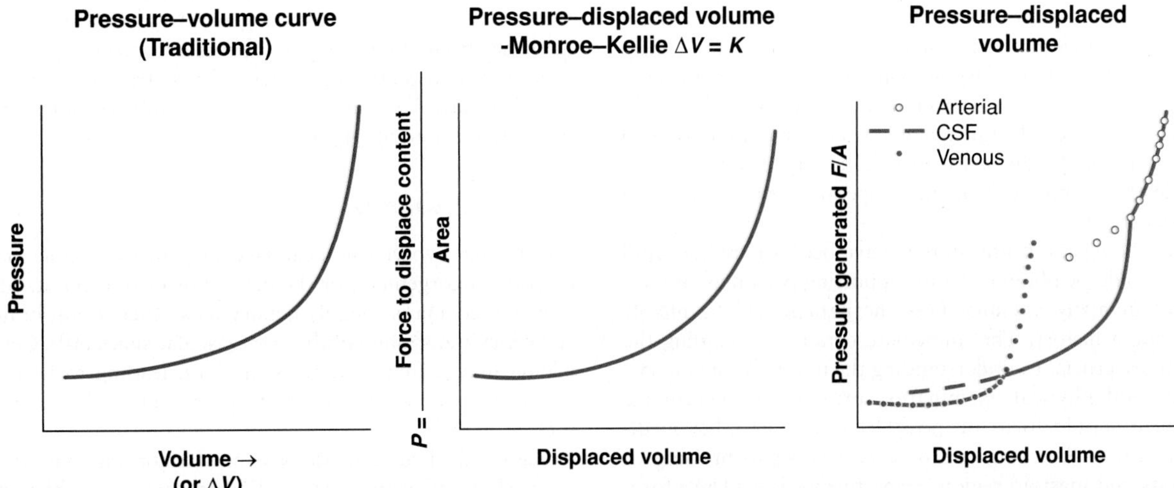

FIGURE 13.5 Three forms of the intracranial pressure volumes curves. The curve on the left represents the traditional teaching that compensatory mechanisms allow for small changes in pressure as intracranial volume increases. The middle section suggests that pressure may be better defined as the force per unit area needed to displace a certain volume of the intracranial contents. The last section suggests that the traditional pressure–volume curve actually represents superimposed displacement curves of varying substances in the cranial cavity. At low pressures (flat portion), cerebral spinal fluid is displaced downward into the compliant spinal subarachnoid space. As pressure increases, venous and arterial blood are displaced before brain parenchyma is displaced at very high pressures (cerebral herniation). CSF, cerebrospinal fluid. (From Rosner MJ. Pathophysiology and management of increased intracranial pressure. In: Andrews BT, ed. *Neurosurgical Intensive Care*. New York, NY: McGraw-Hill; 1993:57–112.)

head imaging with immediate medical or surgical management of expanding mass lesions (45).

The mechanisms of primary neurologic injury will vary depending upon the nature of the insult, but all will include, to some degree, the risk of secondary injury from cerebral hypoxia and ischemia. In head trauma, shearing injury develops due to different deceleration rates of grey and white matter. The resultant disruption of neurologic tracts is followed by a period of secondary ischemia. Prolonged seizure activity in status epilepticus (SE) leads to hippocampal ischemia, cell death and atrophy (46); a zone of ischemia surrounds all areas of cerebral infarction and cerebral hemorrhage (47).

The primary goal of acute neurologic management is to prevent secondary injury. This is attained by initiating measures to support CDO_2 and reduce cerebral metabolic demands. Hypoxemia ($SpO_2 < 90\%$), hypotension (generally systolic blood pressure < 90 mmHg), expanding mass lesions, persistent seizures, and intracranial hypertension all potentially worsen secondary injury by limiting CDO_2 and increasing cerebral metabolism. Immediate attention and correction of these problems can have a significant impact on both immediate and long-term outcome (45–47). A sense of urgency in the treating team is critical to provide early and aggressive resuscitative efforts (47).

The specific management of acute neurologic emergencies will vary according to the nature of the illness or injury; however, some general concepts can be applied to all neurologic emergencies. The basics of all life-support protocols focus on securing an adequate airway, restoring effective ventilation, and ensuring appropriate circulation. Loss of pharyngeal tone can lead to airway obstruction in patients with a depressed level of consciousness. Impairment of respiratory drive can occur after seizures, head trauma, anoxic injury, stroke, or metabolic disturbances. Decreases in cerebral perfusion are common after head or multisystem injury, shock, sepsis, or hemorrhage.

The acute management of neurologic injury must focus on the maintenance of CDO_2. To accomplish this goal, adequate oxygenation, respiration, and blood pressure must be assured. Airway control via endotracheal intubation (ETI) for the neurologic patient should be performed immediately in all patients with a Glasgow coma scale (GCS) sum score of ≤8. Supplemental oxygenation and, in patients with severe anemia, red blood cell transfusions—to a hemoglobin of 8 to 9 g/dL—should be given to provide adequate oxygenation. The role of glycemic control and temperature modulation will be discussed later.

Once the basics of life support have been secured, a rapid history should be obtained from supporting personnel or family since in many circumstances the patient will be unable to provide a history. The immediate details surrounding the incident are crucial to understanding the nature of the injury.

A general physical examination prior to the neurologic assessment should focus on possible trauma or other medical conditions. Raccoon eyes or a Battle's sign—bruising of the orbits and mastoid region, respectively—is evidence for a basilar skull fracture. In head trauma with a loss of consciousness, neck injury should be assumed and cervical stabilization should be used. A funduscopic examination may reveal papilledema or subhyaloid hemorrhages. Body or breath odors may suggest intoxication. New onset atrial fibrillation may be the only clue to the mechanism of a cerebral infarct. Subtle eye, finger, or limb movements may be the only signs of subclinical seizure activity.

A rapid neurologic assessment focusing on the level of consciousness, the cranial nerve examination, and any localizing features can be obtained within a few minutes. The GCS score is commonly used as a quantitative assessment of neurologic function (48). A new coma score, known as the FOUR score, has been developed and validated for application in the emergency room, medical intensive care unit, and the neurointensive care unit (Fig. 13.6) (49–52). The FOUR score has advantages over the GCS, especially in intubated patients as a third of the GCS score comprised of verbal responses. Moreover, the FOUR score identifies brainstem injury, locked-in syndrome, uncal herniation, and includes an assessment of the respiratory drive (49).

Emergent head imaging must be obtained as soon as the patient is considered hemodynamically stable to leave the emergency department or ICU. CT is the usual initial choice due to accessibility. A head CT without contrast is the best test to assess both for skull or bone fractures and for the presence of acute intracranial blood. Large intracerebral, epidural, or subdural hematomas may need emergent evacuation. New imaging techniques, such as CT perfusion and MRI perfusion–diffusion imaging, may be able to identify specific salvageable ischemic brain regions that are risk for infarction. Baseline laboratory studies to be assessed include serum glucose, electrolytes, complete blood count, prothrombin and activated partial prothrombin times, liver function tests, blood urea nitrogen, and creatinine levels.

The Brain Trauma Foundation guidelines recommends ICP monitoring for patients with severe head injury (defined as a GCS ≤ 8) and an abnormal CT scan. ICP monitoring is additionally recommended for severe head trauma and a normal CT scan if two or more of the following are present: abnormal motor posturing, age > 40 years, and systolic blood pressure < 90 mmHg (53). The practical value of other invasive monitoring modalities—such as local brain tissue oxygen monitoring—is less certain.

Specific treatment can be initiated once cardiopulmonary status has been stabilized and a general and neurologic assessment has been completed. Guidelines and protocols currently exist for prehospital management of head trauma, intravenous and intra-arterial lysis of cerebral thrombosis, intracerebral hemorrhage, and SE (45–47,54).

Cerebral Edema

Intracranial hypertension can be caused by expanding masses, cerebral engorgement, or the development of cerebral edema. Cerebral edema is roughly defined as an increase in brain tissue water and sodium of the extravascular space (10). Cerebral edema may compress brain structures, leading to herniation syndromes or reduce cerebral perfusion with subsequent infarction (55).

Cerebral edema can also be defined according to its location or mechanism of production. Edema can occur either inside the cells of the brain (intracellular) or outside the cells and the intravascular space in the interstitium (interstitial). While certain forms of cerebral edema may predominate, pure forms of either type of edema rarely exist. *Cytotoxic edema* is the term employed to describe the intracellular edema that develops after the loss of cell wall integrity (56). The terminology implies

Eye response

4 Eyelids open or opened, tracking, or blinking to command

3 Eyelids open but not tracking

2 Eyelids closed but open to loud voice

1 Eyelids closed but open to pain

0 Eyelids remain closed with pain

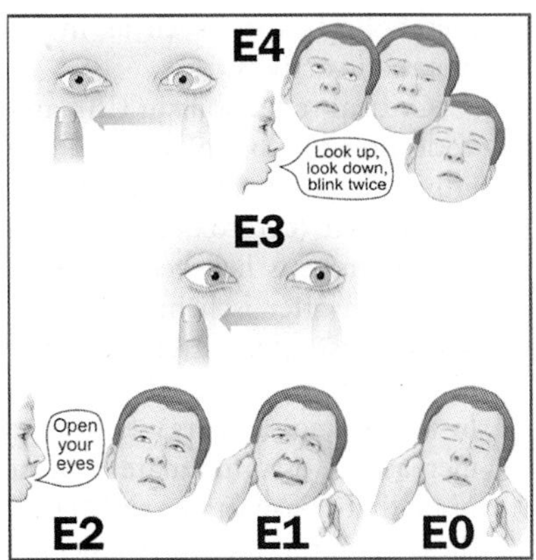

Eye response (E)
Grade the best possible response after at least three trials in an attempt to elicit the best level of alertness. A score of **E4** indicates at least three voluntary excursions. If eyes are closed, the examiner should open them and examine tracking of a finger or object. Tracking with the opening of 1 eyelid will suffice in cases of eyelid edema or facial trauma. If tracking is absent horizontally, examine vertical tracking. Alternatively, two blinks on command should be documented. This will recognize a locked-in syndrome (patient is fully aware). A score of **E3** indicates the absence of voluntary tracking with open eyes. A score of **E2** indicates eyelids opening to loud voice. A score of **E1** indicates eyelids open to pain stimulus. A score of **E0** indicates no eyelids opening to pain.

Motor response

4 Thumbs-up, fist, or peace sign to command

3 Localizing to pain

2 Flexion response to pain

1 Extensor posturing

0 No response to pain or generalized myoclonus status epilepticus

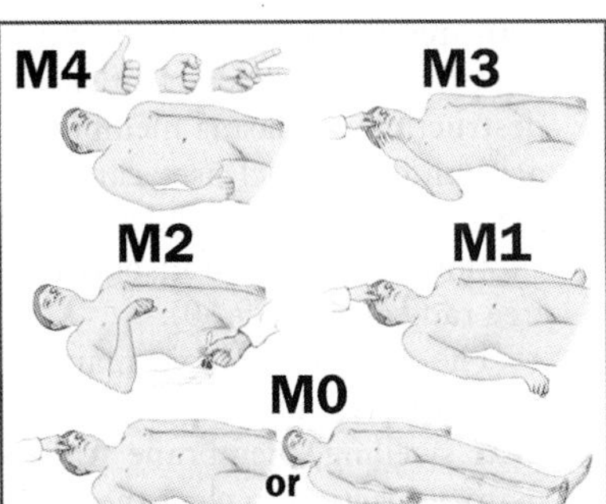

Motor response (M)
Grade the best possible response of the arms. A score of **M4** indicates that the patient demonstrated at least one of three hand positions (thumbs-up, fist, or peace sign) with either hand. A score of **M3** indicates that the patient touched the examiner's hand after a painful stimulus compressing the temporomandibular joint or supraorbital nerve (localization). A score of **M2** indicates any flexion movement of the upper limbs. A score of **M1** indicates extensor posturing. A score of **M0** indicates no motor response or myoclonus status epilepticus.

Brainstem reflexes

4 Pupil and corneal reflexes present

3 One pupil wide and fixed

2 Pupil *or* corneal reflexes absent

1 Pupil *and* corneal reflexes absent

0 Absent pupil, corneal, and cough reflex

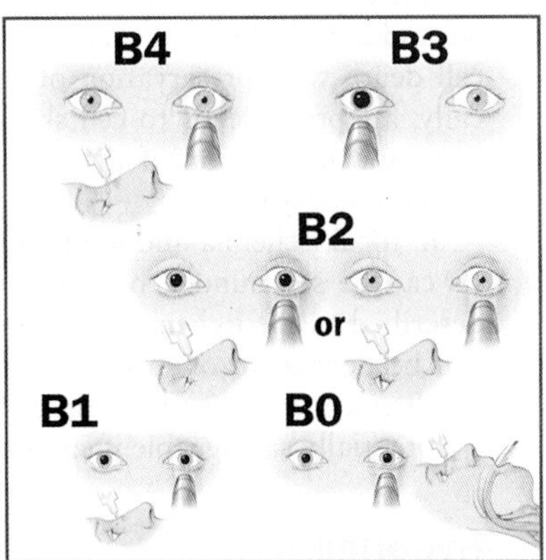

Brainstem reflexes (B)
Grade the best possible response. Examine pupillary and corneal reflexes. Preferably, corneal reflexes are tested by instilling two to three drops of sterile saline on the cornea from a distance of four to six inches (this minimizes corneal trauma from repeated examinations). Cotton swabs can also be used. The cough reflex to tracheal suctioning is tested only when both of these reflexes are absent. A score of **B4** indicates pupil and cornea reflexes are present. A score of **B3** indicates one pupil wide and fixed. A score of **B2** indicates either pupil or cornea reflexes are absent, **B1** indicates both pupil and cornea reflexes are absent, and a score of **B0** indicates pupil, cornea, and cough reflex (using tracheal suctioning) are absent.

Respiration

4 Not intubated, regular breathing pattern

3 Not intubated, Cheyne-Stokes breathing pattern

2 Not intubated, irregular breathing pattern

1 Breathes above ventilator rate

0 Breathes at ventilator rate or apnea

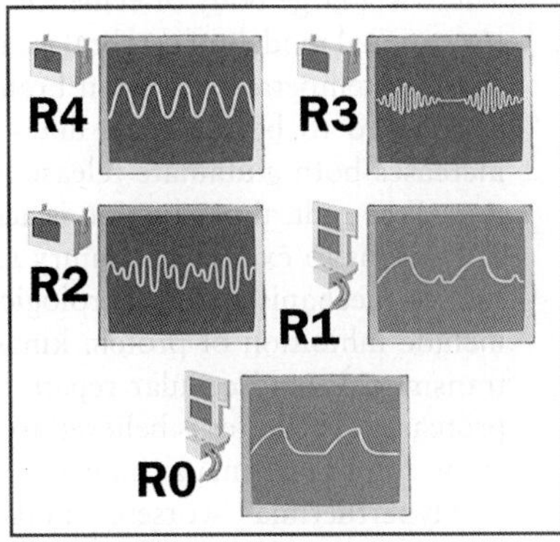

Respiration (R)
Determine spontaneous breathing pattern in a nonintubated patient and grade simply as regular **R4**, irregular **R2**, or Cheyne-Stokes **R3** breathing. In mechanically ventilated patients, assess the pressure waveform of spontaneous respiratory pattern or the patient triggering of the ventilator **R1**. The ventilator monitor displaying respiratory patterns is used to identify the patient-generated breaths on the ventilator. No adjustments are made to the ventilator while the patient is graded, but grading is done preferably with Pa_{CO_2} within normal limits. A standard apnea (oxygen-diffusion) test may be needed when patient breathes at ventilator rate **R0**.

FIGURE 13.6 Instructions for the assessment of the individual categories of the FOUR score. (From Wijdicks EFM, Bamlet WR, Maramattom BV, et al. Validation of a new coma scale: the FOUR score. *Ann Neurol*. 2005;58:585–593. © 2007. Mayo Foundation for Medical Education and Research.)

a toxic etiology but it is most often seen in cellular energy failure due to ischemia or hypoxia. *Vasogenic edema* represents an expansion of the interstitium due to disruption of the capillary blood–brain barrier, which allows extravasation of fluid from the intravascular space. Interstitial edema develops secondary to increases in the hydrostatic pressures of the ventricular system draining the CSF. Osmotic edema refers to the intracellular swelling that occurs due to rapid changes in brain sodium concentrations or due to osmotic dysequilibrium syndromes (10).

Hypoxic Ischemic Injury

Cerebral ischemia develops if cerebral oxygen utilization cannot meet metabolic demands. This can result from problems with CDO_2, increased metabolic demands, or impaired oxygen utilization. Decreases in CDO_2 can occur with decreases in CBF due to stroke, increased ICP, decreased cardiac output, or hypotension. Cerebral metabolic rate is increased with increased cerebral activity, seizures, or hyperthermia; blood loss or carbon monoxide poisoning can decrease oxygen-carrying capacity (57).

Cerebral ischemia can be categorized into focal and global causes. Focal ischemia occurs when there is severe or complete reduction of blood flow to one of the major arteries of the brain. Neurologic impairment develops in functional patterns attributable to the particular arterial distribution that is involved. This is caused most commonly by embolic or atherosclerotic large vessel occlusion. Global ischemia refers to severe reductions or cessation of blood flow to the entire brain. The most frequent cause is cardiac arrest, but can also be seen in any condition that leads to global cerebral hypoperfusion or hypoxia (2,57).

The various cellular components of the brain tissue exhibit selective vulnerability to ischemia. Neurons are most susceptible to cerebral ischemia followed by oligodendroglia, astrocytes, and endothelial cells. Specific neuronal populations also exhibit selective vulnerability to ischemia and hypoxia. The most susceptible neurons to anoxia are the CA_1 and CA_3 cell populations located in the medial hippocampus. These cells are the most widely connected and have the highest resting metabolic rate of all neurons. Similarly, highly metabolically active cells with high susceptibility to ischemia include the cerebellar Purkinje cells, cortical cell levels 3 and 5, and the medium-size neurons of the striatum (2,58).

Patterns of neuronal injury encountered with cerebral anoxia can be attributed to the selective ischemic vulnerability of varying cerebral cell types coupled with the different mechanisms by which ischemia or hypoxia can occur. Watershed or border-zone infarctions occur at the boundary between the perfusion territories of the large cerebral arteries. Cardiac, septic, and hemorrhagic shock are the most common etiologies for this pattern. Dysmyelination of the central white matter can develop in the setting of hypotension where hypoxia does not occur. Cerebral white matter is believed to be selectively vulnerable to this condition due to its decreased resting CBF compared to the more metabolically active grey matter (2).

Neuronal cell death is a product of both the severity and duration of ischemia. Thus, incomplete degrees of ischemia can be tolerated for longer periods of time. However, there is some critical threshold of ischemia which will ultimately lead to necrosis. The impact of ischemia can be modified by metabolic factors, such as hyperglycemia, temperature, and metabolic activity.

Critical reductions in CBF and cerebral oxygenation cause widespread failure of ionic pumps in cellular membranes, with efflux of potassium and influx of sodium and water causing cellular (cytotoxic) edema. Release of excessive amounts of glutamate is believed to mediate the process of excitatory cell death after ischemia. Normally glutamate, an excitatory neurotransmitter, is released into the synaptic cleft and rapidly cleared by energy-dependent cellular uptake mechanisms. In the setting of energy failure, extracellular glutamate levels increase. Most glutamate neurotoxicity is mediated through *N*-methyl-D-aspartate (NMDA) receptors. Stimulation of these receptors activates calcium channels that mediate calcium entry into the cell. Intracellular calcium subsequently activates a number of destructive enzymatic processes, including protease destruction of structural proteins, phospholipase destruction of plasma membranes with release of arachidonic acid and endonucleases capable of fragmenting DNA repair mechanisms. Mitochondrial uptake of calcium leads to interruption of electron transport and the development of oxygen free radicals (57,59,60).

The neuropathologic manifestations of cerebral ischemia are necrosis and apoptosis. Necrosis is characterized by cellular swelling, membrane wall lysis, and a resultant inflammatory reaction to clear the necrotic tissue; cells die in groups leaving large areas of necrotic tissue (61). Apoptosis is an organized and regulated form of cell death where intracellular and extracellular signals lead to a programmed process of cell death with preservation of the mitochondria. Pathologically, apoptosis leads to cell shrinkage, chromatin condensation, and dissolution of the cell membrane. Inflammation is not commonly seen.

In focal ischemia and infarction, a central region of necrosis can be surrounded by a potentially viable area of tissue described as the ischemic penumbra. The ischemic penumbra can be defined through CBF measures, electrophysiology, or biochemical and genetic methods. The penumbra is tissue that is potentially salvageable if circulation is restored.

Hyperthermia

There is a large body of evidence from experiments in laboratory animal models of cerebral ischemia showing that increases in brain temperature worsen brain injury (62); excitotoxicity is believed to be the most likely mechanism. Hyperthermia increases both glutamate release and extracellular concentration. Free radical production is accelerated and the sensitivity of neurons to excitotoxic injury is increased (63). Other postulated mechanisms for neurologic damage with hyperthermia include inhibition of protein kinases responsible for synaptic transmission and cellular repair, and the release of neuronal proteases. The latter is believed to be the mechanism for worsening cerebral edema at higher brain temperatures (64–67).

Hyperthermia worsens outcomes in ischemic stroke patients (68) with a 2.2-fold increase in morbidity and mortality for every 1-degree increase in temperature above 37.5°C (69). Similarly, these results have been extended to a neurologic intensive care unit population; hyperthermia in this population both worsened outcome and increased the length of stay (70).

Hyperglycemia

Hyperglycemia has been well documented to increase the infarct size and worsen outcome in ischemic stroke (71,72). More recent studies in patients treated with thrombolytics have supported these observations (73–76), although the negative effects of hyperglycemia may be limited to large vessel ischemia or occlusions (77). Hyperglycemia has also been associated with worse outcome in subarachnoid hemorrhage (SAH) (78); results in head trauma have been inconsistent (79,80).

Hyperglycemia in acute neurologic injury may be attributed to several different mechanisms. The most common proposed mechanism for the development of hyperglycemia is a hormonally induced stress response caused by the neurologic injury leading to an increase in catecholamine and cortisol release. Other proposed means by which hyperglycemia could occur in neurologic injury include uncovering of latent diabetes (72). Hyperglycemia may increase neurologic injury through a number of mechanisms. These include expansion of infarct size due to an associated reduction in perfusion (81), increases in cerebral metabolism (82) and cerebral edema (83), and potentiated calcium entry into neurons (84). The most widely supported mechanism of hyperglycemia-induced neuronal injury is through the production of free radicals causing oxidative stress and inflammation (85,86).

Insulin reduces ischemic brain damage in animal models of acute ischemia (87), perhaps through a direct neuroprotective role of insulin beyond the modulation of glucose levels (88). Insulin suppresses mediators of inflammation and coagulation, and increases endothelial NO release. The release of local NO could potentially lead to increased vasodilation and perfusion of the ischemic penumbra surrounding the core of infarcted tissue (89). A large (n = 1,400 subjects) multicenter insulin trial in ischemic stroke is currently underway, scheduled to complete in July 2018 (ClinicalTrials.gov Identifier: NCT01369069).

Hypoglycemia

Intensive glucose control comes at a cost of inadvertent hypoglycemia. An increase in mortality can be seen in even single episodes of severe hypoglycemia in ICU patients (90). Patients with glucose levels below 81 mg/dL (4.5 mMol/L) have been shown to have a higher mortality than patients with normal glucose levels (25.9% vs. 19.7%; OR, 1.42) (91). Factors such as CBF, and duration and degree of hypoglycemia can impact the degree of injury resulting from hypoglycemia. Neurotoxicity from hypoglycemia occurs as a result of oxygen free radical accumulation, activation of apoptotic pathways, and glutamate-mediated excitotoxicity (92). Studies with microdialysis and PET reveal increased glucose utilization in severe TBI patients (93) which would suggest against the need to maintain strict normoglycemia.

Blood Pressure

Hypertension is common after neurologic injury. The etiology is often multifactorial and may include underlying hypertension, catecholamine release to pain and stress, direct hypothalamic damage, or a physiologic response to volume depletion. In addition, cerebral autoregulation is disturbed to varying degrees after brain injury. Complete loss of autoregulation leads to CBF directly correlating with MAP. Disturbances in cerebral autoregulation can be global or focal, involving only areas adjacent to damaged brain.

The question whether the hypertension encountered during neurologic injury is pathologic or a normal compensatory and protective physiologic response has important therapeutic implications. In areas surrounding neurologic injury, the blood–brain barrier is often damaged. In these areas hypertension can lead to the development of cerebral edema by increasing the intravascular hydrostatic forces driving fluid into the interstitium of the brain. Brain area surrounding tumors, arteriovascular malformations, or local areas of trauma or infarction are particularly susceptible. Blood pressure management is often titrated to maintain systolic pressures between 110 and 140 mmHg after surgery to avoid the complications of postoperative edema and breakthrough hemorrhage. In severe carotid stenosis, the CPP to the affected cerebral hemisphere may be compromised leading to a shift of the cerebral autoregulatory curve downward. Postcarotid endarterectomy hypertension needs to be treated to avoid reperfusion injury (breakthrough hyperemia and hemorrhage). Reperfusion injury is also the main cause of hemorrhage after acute recanalization in ischemic stroke; thus, strict avoidance of severe hypertension is mandated in these patients.

Alternatively, over-aggressive management of hypertension after neurologic injury can be potentially deleterious. Brain areas with disturbed autoregulation may require a certain pressure to maintain adequate perfusion. An example of this is the development of plateau waves after head trauma produced by cerebral vasodilation in response to inadequate cerebral perfusion. Cerebral vasospasm after SAH is treated with induced hypertension. In selected small case series, induced hypertension has been used in the treatment of acute ischemic stroke (94). Optimal blood pressure should, therefore, to be titrated to the individual patient and disease process.

Cardiac Stunning

Cardiac stunning and neurogenic pulmonary edema can occur after acute neurologic catastrophes. This is most commonly seen after severe head trauma, SAH, SE, or intracerebral hemorrhage. The mechanism of cardiopulmonary damage is believed to occur through massive catecholamine release mediated by the sympathetic nervous system (95), the so-called Takotsubo cardiomyopathy (apical ballooning syndrome) (96). Studies on dogs revealed greater density of β-receptors in the apical myocardium as compared to the base (97); with a catecholamine surge, the adrenergic receptors become stunned resulting in apical ballooning.

Sympathetic innervation of the heart parallels the cardiac conduction system, which probably accounts for the noted electrocardiographic changes that can occur with severe neurologic injury. Deep T-wave inversions are usually reported as "cerebral T waves"; however, the spectrum of sympathetically induced electrocardiographic changes is broad and includes ST-elevations and depressions (102). Pathologically, cardiac contraction bands are seen surrounding the entry zone of the sympathetic endplates into the myocardium. These bands represent reperfusion injury from ischemic cardiac muscle.

The muscle dies in a hypercontracted state, which ultimately becomes calcified (98). Cardiac enzymes are elevated, but this finding does not necessarily implicate coronary artery disease. Clinically, myocardial contraction is impaired; cardiac output and ejection fractions are decreased; and pulmonary edema is common and may be cardiogenic, neurogenic, or both.

Serial echocardiography indicates that cardiac function usually improves over a course of 1 to 3 weeks. However, the diagnosis of catecholamine-induced cardiac stunning implies a more severe neurologic injury, complicates medical management, and usually portends a worse outcome (99).

Neurogenic Pulmonary Edema

In neurogenic pulmonary edema, sympathetic-mediated pulmonary venoconstriction is believed to create the excessive hydrostatic pressure necessary to develop pulmonary edema (100). The sympathetic nervous system also innervates contractile elements of the pulmonary endothelial cells; catecholamine-mediated contraction of these cells can lead to opening of the tight junctions of the capillaries, allowing protein to flux into the pulmonary parenchyma (101). The process is self-limited and positive pressure ventilation, often combined with induced diuresis, is typically adequate to improve oxygenation.

Sodium Metabolism and Homeostasis

Disturbances in sodium metabolism and homeostasis are found in a variety of neurologic diseases. Circulating levels of antidiuretic hormone (ADH) are elevated in a number of acute neurologic emergencies, secondary to a catecholamine-induced stress response. This raises the question of whether the hyponatremia encountered is truly resulting from inappropriate ADH release or just represents an appropriate but excessive response.

Hyponatremia can have significant implications for the management of the neurologic patient. Acute hyponatremia leads to the development of intracellular edema with expansion of the size of the neuronal cell body. Unlike other cells in our body, the neuron needs to maintain its cell size and integrity in order to transmit electrical signals. The cellular response of the neuron to intracellular edema is to extrude intracellular osmoles to reduce the intracellular osmolality and return the cell size to normal (102); thus, chronic hyponatremia can be tolerated well. However, cellular swelling in response to severe acute hyponatremia will lead to mental obtundation and seizures. Due to these considerations, intravenous hypotonic solutions should be avoided in the neurointensive care unit.

A self-limited, salt wasting nephropathy can develop after SAH. The process will lead to hyponatremia and volume depletion if not recognized and treated (103). The etiology of this process remains somewhat difficult to identify. In dogs and guinea pigs, the process is mediated through the renal sympathetic nerves; transection of these nerves will prevent salt wasting. This response is species-specific and not true for rats. The human mechanism is unclear (104). A variety of circulating hormones or substances have been proposed to initiate this response; the leading candidate is the B-isoform of atrial natriuretic peptide (ANP) which has been found in some series to be elevated prior to the development of hyponatremia and cerebral vasospasm (105).

Diabetes insipidus (DI) leading to hypernatremia is expected after pituitary surgery and is seen in any process that affects the hypothalamus or pituitary gland. Head trauma leading to a shearing injury of the pituitary stalk is a common cause for delayed DI. The diagnosis is made by the development of hypernatremia in the setting of a nondiuretic-induced hypotonic diuresis. This process must be differentiated from a postoperative diuresis; a normal postoperative diuresis will not spontaneously develop hypernatremia. Correction of the hypernatremia must be done slowly if hypernatremia has been maintained for more than a few hours (102). DI can rarely be seen in SAH patients as well; it is theorized that DI in this situation can be due to vasospasm of the vessels supplying the anterior hypothalamus.

General Therapeutic Considerations

Hypothermia. Hypothermia exerts neuroprotective effects in animal models through various mechanisms. However, its clinical application has been limited by disappointing results in randomized controlled clinical trials. At present, the only evidence-based indications for therapeutic hypothermia are postresuscitation coma—especially after witnessed out-of-hospital ventricular fibrillation arrest—and neonatal hypoxic encephalopathy.

Moderate hypothermia (33°C) was proven to be associated with improved neurologic outcomes in two randomized trials for global cerebral ischemia after cardiac arrest (106,107). Hypothermia must be induced early and maintained for 12 to 24 hours before proceeding to slow rewarming. Sedation and pharmacologic paralysis were instituted to prevent the hypermetabolism that occurs with shivering. A recent trial comparing hypothermia of 33°C versus 36°C demonstrated no difference in primary or secondary outcomes including mortality, functional outcomes in survivors, and adverse effects (108). While the target of temperature control can be debated, the intervention should be considered standard of care.

An initial trial hypothermia in severe TBI showed no difference in outcome between hypothermia and normothermia groups (109). A second trial (n = 232 patients) evaluating earlier induction of hypothermia was terminated because of futility (110); subgroup analysis showed a difference in favor of hypothermia among patients with surgically resectable hematoma (poor outcome 33% versus 69%; p = 0.02), but this was based on a very small number of patients. At this point hypothermia cannot be recommended as a routine treatment for severe TBI.

Hypothermia has been applied to patients with large ischemic stroke and patients with intracerebral hemorrhage (ICH) and associated brain edema in small case series with promising results (111,112). However, multicenter trials are necessary before hypothermia can be recommended for these indications.

Intubation

Medical complications are common after neurologic injury and they worsen outcome (99,113). Aspiration pneumonia is reported with depressed levels of consciousness, and early recognition and treatment are needed. ETI is required for neurologic patients that are unable to maintain airway patency or protect their airway from secretions. ETI portends a poor outcome for patients with ischemic and hemorrhagic strokes

(114). The timing of extubation in the neurologic patient is controversial since many patients remain intubated solely for airway protection. The usual practice is to keep patients intubated as long as they remain comatose; yet prolonged intubation in neurologic patients increases the rate of ventilator-acquired pneumonia, increases length of stay, and worsens outcomes. Early extubation based upon the patients' ability to control secretions is recommended (115). The value of early tracheostomy—by days 5 to 7 after intubation where there is no neurologic improvement—deserves further investigation.

SPECIFIC CONDITIONS AND TREATMENT OPTIONS

Head Trauma

Severe head trauma remains a significant source of morbidity and mortality in the United States accounting for approximately 50,000 deaths/year, and is the leading source of death for people less than 44 years of age (116). Historically, treatment has focused on the management of sustained intracranial hypertension, based largely on retrospective data obtained from the National Traumatic Coma data bank. Survival was greater than 80% in patients in whom the ICP was maintained <20 mmHg, compared to >90% mortality for patients that had uncontrollable sustained intracranial hypertension (117,118). Treatment, therefore, was designed to institute measures to decrease ICP. This could include diuresis, aggressive treatment of hypertension, keeping the patient relatively hypovolemic, and elevation of the head of bed.

The work by the Richmond group in the 1970s to 1980s largely changed the focus on treating head trauma from using measures designed to lower ICP to using measures designed to maintain adequate CPP. A recent study conducted in Bolivia and Ecuador compared ICP guided *versus* imaging and clinical examination guided therapy and found no significant difference in functional outcome or survival (119). The major criticism of this study is the questionable external validity in developed countries where pre- and posthospital care and resources, including rehabilitation, are plentiful. As per the Brain Trauma Foundation guidelines, ICP guided therapy in TBI is recommended for patients with GCS of 3 to 8 after resuscitation, abnormal CT scan of the head, and with two or more of the following at admission: age over 40, hypotension–systolic blood pressure <90 mmHg, and motor posturing (45).

Treatment thus shifted to include maintaining adequate blood volume and cerebral perfusion as well as treating sustained elevations in ICP. What constitutes an adequate CPP has been debatable and may vary under different conditions; however, the most recent Brain Trauma Foundation guidelines have recommended a CPP range of 50 to 70 mmHg (45).

Several studies have demonstrated an increase in mortality in TBI patients with brain tissue oxygen tension ($PbtO_2$) below 10 to 15 mmHg (120–122). More recently, brain tissue oxygen monitoring has been used in head trauma to guide therapy. Brain tissue oxygenation tension is measured by placement of a small flexible probe through a cranial bolt directly into the brain parenchyma. CBF and PET studies have reported good correlation with low oxygen tensions with low CBF measures and high oxygen extraction ratios (123,124).

A meta-analysis of trials comparing brain tissue oxygen guided therapy versus conventional ICP guided therapy concluded that $PbtO_2$ guided therapy significantly improved neurologic outcome (125). However, the historical controls had a very high mortality. For example, in a study of 53 patients, $PbtO_2$ guided therapy study was associated with decreased mortality compared to historical controls (mortality 25% vs. 44%, $p < 0.05$) (126); the average mortality rate across trauma centers was similar to the treatment arm rather than the historical control arm of this study. Another study with 139 patients had similar criticisms raised (127). In contrast, a study of 123 patients comparing $PbtO_2$ guided therapy to conventional ICP therapy showed not only no benefit in survival and outcome, but increased overall costs and ventilator-associated days in the treatment arm (128). Yet, these negative results could have been related to selection bias as the $PbtO_2$ monitors were placed at the discretion of the neurosurgeons and the treatment cohort had significantly worse neurologic presentation. The latest Brain Trauma Foundation guidelines from 2007 suggest consideration for the use of $PbtO_2$ monitoring with a level III evidence (45). The more recent Consensus Statement on Multimodality Brain Monitoring from the Neurocritical Care Society endorsed a stronger recommendation for the use of $PbtO_2$ monitoring in patients at risk of cerebral ischemia or hypoxia, such as those with severe TBI, but acknowledged that the quality of evidence to support this recommendation is low (129). The main limitation of $PbtO_2$ monitoring is that it only measures oxygenation in the close proximity of the catheter; location of the catheter should, therefore, be carefully individualized. Aiming for pericontusional tissue is often preferred because this is considered the area at highest risk for secondary injury (130).

A small study (n = 52 patients) evaluating 100% oxygen supplementation for 24 hours following TBI revealed statistically significant improvements in brain glucose, glutamate, lactate, lactate/glucose ratio, and lactate/pyruvate ratio. The ICP was also significantly decreased in patients receiving 100% oxygen. However, 3- and 6-month outcomes were not better than in controls (131). A Cochrane review of hyperbaric oxygen therapy for TBI identified 7 trials including 571 patients found a modest improvement in GCS associated with this treatment, but appropriately concluded that the therapy cannot be currently recommended because the trials were small and unblended, and, consequently, the estimates of benefit are not reliable (132).

Intracranial hypertension is treated through the removal of space-occupying lesions, decreasing cerebral edema or venous engorgement, or expanding the cranial vault. Expanding brain masses—tumors, subdural or epidural hematomas—need to be evacuated as soon as possible to avoid cerebral herniation and damage to important brain structures. Removal of CSF through an external ventricular drain is another means to reduce the intracranial volume. Placement of an external ventricular drain also allows for the direct measurement of ICP.

Hyperventilation is useful for the acute management of intracranial hypertension, as it rapidly decreases CBV through arteriolar vasoconstriction. Chronic hyperventilation is generally avoided due to concerns that prolonged vasoconstriction may worsen cerebral ischemia (133). The effect of hyperventilation on ICP is also self-limited, usually lasting only 3 to 6 hours. Thus, hyperventilation is optimally used for ICP control in the acute setting until some longer-acting strategy can be employed.

Osmotic agents are typically employed to lower ICP. Mannitol (20% solution) given in boluses of 0.25 to 1.0 g/kg lowers ICP through a number of mechanisms. The intravascular osmotic gradient created by mannitol can lead to extracellular fluid being drawn into the intravascular space and removed through an osmotic diuresis. Reductions in hemispheric brain water have been demonstrated in a rat stroke model after the administration of large boluses of mannitol. The effect, however, was small and delayed for several hours (134). More likely, mannitol exerts its effect on ICP by decreasing CBV. According to this theory, the osmotic gradient initiated by an infusion of mannitol causes an influx of extravascular water into the intravascular space. This leads to a decrease in blood viscosity due to a hemodilution of red blood cell mass and fibrinogen. The decrease in ICP can be explained through the use of the Hagen–Poiseuille equation. In this equation, flow is directly related to the fourth power of the radius of the cerebral vessel and inversely related to serum viscosity. If the flow remains constant and viscosity is reduced, then vessel diameter must decrease (39):

$$F = \frac{8dPr^4}{\pi nl}$$

where F is the flow; dP is the pressure gradient (CPP); r is the vessel diameter; n is the viscosity; and l is the vessel length. Then, assuming constant CBF and cerebral vessel reactivity, according to this equation, the radius of this vessel must decrease in response to both an increase in CPP and a decrease in viscosity (10). Rosner describes this as a passive vasoconstriction (39).

Hypertonic saline has been increasingly used in the treatment of brain trauma patients and it might be superior to mannitol for this indication (135). Hypertonic saline should also produce less risk of nephrotoxicity. Theoretically, its mechanism of action would be similar to that of mannitol, but hypertonic saline can increase cardiac output and indices less diuresis. Infusion of 30 to 60 mL of 23% sodium chloride is the most effective osmotic therapy to reverse severe surges in ICP and should be preferred in patients with signs of brain herniation (136).

An overall strategy for treating intracranial hypertension is to attempt to maintain the most optimal CPP and the lowest possible ICP. To attain this goal, other maneuvers may need to be used. Sedation and paralysis can be helpful to decrease ICP if chest wall compliance is high or if the patient is exhibiting respiratory dyssynchrony with the ventilator. Since the spinal venous plexus lacks valves, there is a theoretical concern that elevations in peak end expiratory pressures (PEEP) could be transmitted directly to the brain, thus increasing ICP. This is rarely problematic, but can occur if PEEP is maintained greater than 15 to 20 cm H_2O under conditions of increased pulmonary and decreased intracranial compliance (137).

Corticosteroids are useful in treating the vasogenic edema from tumors and meningitis. The use of glucocorticoids in head trauma, however, is not recommended as several randomized trials have found no therapeutic benefit (138–140).

Barbiturates are effective in lowering ICP by decreasing cerebral metabolism. Their use is generally reserved for cases of refractory intracranial hypertension. Dosing is often titrated to a burst suppression pattern monitored on the EEG. One randomized trial reported improved mortality (141) with barbiturate use. Barbiturate use in head trauma, however, remains debatable due to the limited quality of life of survivors (142). High-dose propofol (limited by the risk of propofol infusion syndrome) and hypothermia are alternative options for inducing metabolic suppression in patients with recalcitrant intracranial hypertension. Hemicraniectomy with duraplasty can be another alternative in very refractory cases (143). However, bifrontal craniectomy in patients with less severe intracranial hypertension cannot be recommended based on the negative results of the DECRA trial (144).

Seizure Control and Status Epilepticus

Seizures are common after neurologic injury and can worsen outcome by increasing metabolic demands beyond oxygen delivery capabilities. Anticonvulsant prophylaxis may be employed for patients with SAH, or intracerebral hemorrhages that abut or involve the cortical surface of the brain. Anticonvulsants are recommended during the first week after severe head trauma to prevent posttraumatic epilepsy (145). Immediate treatment of seizures should utilize generous dosing of benzodiazepines.

SE is a neurologic emergency associated with significant morbidity and mortality. Traditional definitions of SE that require 30 minutes of sustained seizure activity or nonarousal between sequential seizures have proved impractical to initiating timely treatment. A new operational definition advocates immediate treatment of all seizures that last >5 minutes (146). Protocols have been developed for the sequential application of anticonvulsants (146). Aggressive early initiation of treatment is important because SE becomes more difficult to control as seizures continue. Tachyphylaxis of antiepileptic medications is explained by receptor trafficking resulting in downregulation of GABA receptors and upregulation of NMDA receptors.

Tonic–clonic movements correlating with electrical seizure activity evolve through a progression of clinical stages until a form of electrical mechanical dissociation can occur. Over time, physical movements become progressively more subtle and can be manifested only by slight movements of the lips, fingers, or eyelids. It is important to note that nonconvulsive SE is often underrecognized. A common mistake is to assume seizures have resolved after loading with anticonvulsants and initiating pharmacologic paralysis. This underscores the importance of EEG monitoring to ensure seizures have been adequately treated. Attention to airway management and hemodynamics are important because many of the anticonvulsants will have respiratory and cardiovascular depressant effects.

Refractory SE is defined as SE that has not responded to the usual first- and second-line medications necessitating anesthetic infusions. Super refractory SE is a relatively new terminology to characterize an SE that continues despite 24 hours of anesthetic infusion. Propofol, midazolam, and thiopental or pentobarbital infusions under EEG monitoring are required for treatment. Propofol use has fallen into relative disfavor due to several case reports of deaths during infusions (147); it is not used in children with SE due to concerns over development of a propofol infusion syndrome (148).

Subarachnoid Hemorrhage

SAH from ruptured cerebral aneurysms has a high morbidity and mortality, with 15% of patients dying before reaching medical attention (149).

The care of patients with SAH can be divided into management before and after the ruptured aneurysm is secured. Management prior to aneurysmal treatment is designed to prevent rebleeding, which occurs in up to a quarter of patients with aneurysmal SAH (aSAH) and this risk is the highest within the first 2 days after aSAH. Neurosurgical repair or endovascular coil embolization of the aneurysm is, therefore, instituted as soon as possible.

Most patients will have acute elevations in blood pressure due to the significant pain stress and catecholamine surge that occurs after SAH. The management of blood pressure after SAH is controversial, but most neurosurgeons and neurointensivists will treat acute hypertension in patients with unsecured aneurysms. The rationale for treatment is based on the international cooperative aneurysmal trial (150) and a large Japanese observational study that noted a higher incidence of rebleeding in patients with sustained systolic elevations in blood pressure >160 mmHg (151). Blood pressure is preferentially treated with beta blockers which do not significantly affect CBF and can narrow the pulse pressure; hydralazine and ACE inhibitors have minimal effects on CBF. In general, nitroprusside is avoided due to concerns of cerebral venodilation and increases in ICP. Intravenous nicardipine is the drug of choice if intravenous titration of blood pressure is needed (149).

The use of antifibrinolytic agents (tranexamic acid, aminocaprioc acid) to prevent rebleeding is also controversial. Previously a mainstay of treatment, the use of antifibrinolytic agents was largely abandoned after studies revealed that the benefit from reduction in rebleeding was offset by increases in delayed ischemic complications when the drug was used for many days. However, a more recent randomized controlled trial showed rebleeding rates were significantly decreased without an increase in the rate of ischemic complications when tranexamic acid was started early and continued for no longer than 72 hours (152).

Acute hydrocephalus is common after SAH and requires prompt diversion of CSF through placement of an external ventricular drain or, alternatively, a lumbar drain when there is no obstruction to the CSF flow. Underrecognition of acute hydrocephalus is common and can be very detrimental to patients' outcomes. Similarly, premature discontinuation of CSF drainage is another common mistake with frequent deleterious consequences.

Once the aneurysm is secured, care focuses on the evaluation and treatment of cerebral vasospasm. Cerebral vasospasm is a pathologic narrowing of the basal cerebral arteries that occurs days after SAH. Pathologically, the cerebral vessels display intimal hyperplasia, collagen remodeling, and a diffuse cellular infiltrate (153). The process takes approximately 4 days to develop and resolves after approximately 2 weeks; it is initiated by some breakdown products of oxyhemoglobin found in the subarachnoid space. The likelihood of developing cerebral vasospasm is directly related to the amount of subarachnoid blood visualized on a 24-hour CT scan (154). Tobacco use and a high Hijdra sum score (>23) are predictive of developing vasospasm (155). The Hijdra sum score allocates 0 to 3 points based on the amount of blood noted in the 10 cisterns and fissures (156); intraventricular hemorrhage also contributes to the risk of vasospasm (157).

Cerebral vessel narrowing can be monitored by the use of TCD ultrasonography. Rising flow velocities often precede the development of neurologic deficits (153). Perfusion scans combined with noninvasive angiograms can be useful when it is unclear if the symptoms are caused by vasospasm. Conventional angiography is the gold standard for diagnosis of large-vessel vasospasm, but may fail to show any major abnormalities in symptomatic patients with vasospasm in more distal vessels.

Symptomatic vasospasm is treated with hemodynamic augmentation therapy, consisting of vasopressors and fluids to maintain isovolemia. Recalcitrant deficits may require interventional angioplasty or intra-arterial infusion of vasodilators—usually calcium channel blockers—to open the narrowed vessels.

Oral nimodipine, a calcium channel blocker, has been shown to improve functional outcomes in aSAH by reducing the risk of delayed ischemia; its routine use is recommended (158). Yet, it is important to make sure that its administration does not compromise the perfusion pressure as this effect will likely negate any benefits and might even increase the risk of infarction in patients with ongoing severe vasospasm.

Intracerebral Hemorrhage

ICH is bleeding that occurs directly into the brain parenchyma; it is classified as primary (or spontaneous) or secondary to underlying lesions. The most common etiology of ICH is hypertension, which weakens and ruptures the small perforating vessels of the basal cerebral arteries. Long-term anticoagulant use is becoming an increasing risk factor for ICH, especially in the elderly (159).

Clinically, ICH presents with severe headaches and focal neurologic deficits usually prompting immediate evaluation in an emergency room. Serial head CT studies have revealed that hematoma expansion occurs in approximate 40% of patients with ICH within the first 20 hours (160). A double-blinded randomized trial showed that the use of recombinant factor VII used within the first 4 hours of ictus decreased hematoma expansion, but did not result in improved functional outcomes and was associated with an increased risk of thromboembolic complications (161).

Acute hypertension is very common after ICH. Aggressive blood pressure control has been controversial because of theoretical concerns that it might cause ischemia around the hematoma. However, PET studies suggest that moderate control of hypertension is safe (162). Furthermore, a large randomized controlled trial comparing target systolic blood pressures of 140 versus 180 mmHg demonstrated a modest functional benefit in the intensive control arm (163). Another study addressing the question of rapid blood pressure control is currently ongoing and scheduled to be completed in July 2016 (ClinicalTrials.gov Identifier: NCT01176565).

A large randomized study evaluating surgical evacuation of supratentorial ICH did not report a benefit over medical management (164). Subgroup analysis did suggest a benefit to early evacuation of superficial hemorrhages. However, a follow-up study failed to show benefit even within this subgroup (165). Minimally invasive surgery with clot lysis using recombinant tissue plasminogen activator (tPA) has been shown to be safe (166). A phase III study is underway and scheduled to complete in September 2019 (ClinicalTrials.gov Identifier: NCT01827046). Corticosteroids have not shown any benefit in the treatment of ICH (167).

Ischemic Stroke

The use of thrombolytics has dramatically changed the management of acute ischemic stroke. The NINDS trial demonstrated improved 3-month outcomes in patients treated within 3 hours of onset with intravenous tPA (168); the treatment window has been expanded to 4.5 hours for select populations (169). Exclusion criteria for the extended window include the use of anticoagulants regardless of INR, age greater than 80, history of stroke, as well as diabetes and NIHSS > 25.

Several recent multicenter trials have shown that intra-arterial thrombectomy, in addition to intravenous alteplase, improves functional outcome in patients with severe acute ischemic stroke caused by a proximal intracranial vessel occlusion (170–172). This is in contrast to some previous endovascular studies which had failed to show benefit from intra-arterial interventions (173–175). The reason for the negative results of earlier studies is thought to be due to utilization of older generation clot retrieval devices and enrollment of patients without proven proximal intracranial vessel occlusion. Endovascular therapy should, therefore, be pursued in patients with disabling deficits from a large artery occlusion who fail to improve with intravenous thrombolysis—or have contraindications for its use—and do not already have a large established infarction on CT scan. For endovascular therapy to be effective, rapid intervention is essential.

Hypertension is common in the setting of an acute stroke and usually resolves within a few hours of ictus. Treatment to slowly decrease blood pressures, although in the current guidelines, has not shown to affect clinical outcome by recent studies (176–178). Hemorrhagic conversion of ischemic infarctions is increased with sustained systolic pressures over 180 mmHg and blood pressure must be below this limit prior to tPA administration (168). However, over-aggressive treatment of blood pressure is commonplace and can worsen the ischemic by compromising collateral flow.

Large hemispheric infarctions, defined as stokes involving over 50% of the middle cerebral artery (MCA) territory, are at risk for the subsequent development of cerebral edema and herniation (179). Close neurologic monitoring is required to identify any signs of deterioration. Treatments designed to lower ICP can be effective, but act as only a temporizing measure since cerebral tissue shifts and not increased ICP is most likely to be the source of neurologic deterioration (180). Hemicraniectomy has been proven effective in reducing mortality and improving functional outcomes in survivors among patients younger than 60 years when completed within 48 hours (181). Benefit is much more modest in older patients for whom decompressive hemicraniectomy can be lifesaving but may not prevent permanent severe disability (182).

SUMMARY

This chapter has attempted to provide an overview of cerebral vascular physiology and cerebral ischemia. A grasp of these principles is vital to understanding the nature of treatments designed to maintain adequate CBF and prevent secondary neurologic injury. Future treatments that focus on the details of critical care and maintaining tissue oxygenation show promise in improving outcome after neurologic injury.

Key Points

- A strong understanding of cerebral physiology is essential to construct a rational approach to the diagnosis and treatment of neurologic emergencies.
- Mechanisms of primary neurologic injury will vary depending upon the nature of the insult and these are often not modifiable. However, most critical neurologic and neurosurgical disease generate a risk secondary injury from cerebral hypoxia and ischemia, which can be ameliorated through optimal management.
- The primary goal of acute neurologic management is to prevent secondary injury.
- Hypoxemia, hypotension, expanding mass lesions, persistent seizures, and intracranial hypertension can all worsen secondary injury. Immediate attention and correction of these problems can have a significant impact on short- and long-term outcomes.
- Cerebral ischemia develops if cerebral oxygen utilization cannot meet the metabolic demand. This mismatch can result from problems with oxygen delivery, increased metabolic demands, or impaired oxygen utilization.
- Hemodynamic management should be adjusted to the specific neurologic diagnosis. Blood pressure goals are entirely different across different acute cerebral diseases and even vary depending on the timing from the acute injury.
- Cardiac stunning and neurogenic pulmonary edema can occur after acute neurologic catastrophes; they are most commonly seen after severe head trauma, SAH, SE, or intracerebral hemorrhage. Neurogenic cardiopulmonary damage is mediated by massive catecholamine release from the central sympathetic nervous system.
- There are multiple methods of invasive and noninvasive monitoring of cerebral function. All modalities have limitations and, consequently, it is best to apply them in combination and avoid interpreting their results in isolation.

References

1. Wieloch T. Molecular mechanisms of ischemic brain damage. In: Edvinsson L, Krause DN, eds. *Cerebral Blood Flow and Metabolism.* 2nd ed. Philadelphia, PA: Lippincott Williams & Wilkins; 2002:423–451.
2. Plum F, Pulsinelli WA. Cerebral metabolism and hypoxic-ischemic brain injury. In: Asbury AK, McKhann GM, McDonald WI, eds. *Diseases of the Nervous System: Clinical Neurobiology.* 2nd ed. Philadelphia, PA: W.B.Saunders; 1992:1002–1015.
3. Gallagher CN, Carpenter KL, Grice P, et al. The human brain utilizes lactate via the tricarboxylic acid cycle: a 13C-labelled microdialysis and high-resolution nuclear magnetic resonance study. *Brain.* 2009;132 (Pt 10):2839–2849.
4. Asbury AK, McKhann GM, McDonald WI. *Diseases of the Nervous System: Clinical Neurobiology.* 2nd ed. Philadelphia, PA: W.B. Saunders; 1992.
5. Brickman AM, Zahra A, Muraskin J, et al. Reduction in cerebral blood flow in areas appearing as white matter hyperintensities on magnetic resonance imaging. *Psychiatry Res.* 2009;172(2):117–120.
6. Kety SS, Schmidt CF. The determination of cerebral blood flow in man by the use of nitrous oxide in low concentrations. *Am J Physiol.* 1945; 143:53–66.
7. Fick A. Ueber die Messung des Blutquantums in den Herzventrikeln. *Sitz ber Physik-Med Ges Wurzburg.* 1870;2:16–28.
8. Marino P. Oxygen transport. In: Marino P, ed. *The ICU Book.* Philadelphia, PA: Lea and Febiger; 1991:14–24.
9. Ginsberg MD. Cerebral circulation: its regulation, pharmacology, and pathophysiology. In: Asbury AK, McKhann GM, McDonald WI, eds.

Diseases of the Nervous System. Clinical Neurobiology. Philadelphia, PA: W.B.Saunders; 1992:989.

10. Manno EM. When to use hyperventilation, mannitol, or corticosteroid to reduce increased intracranial pressure from cerebral edema. In: Rabinstein AA, Wijdicks EFM, eds. *Tough Calls in Acute Neurology.* Amsterdam: Elsevier; 2004:107–124.
11. Gur D, Good WF, Wolfson SK Jr, et al. In vivo mapping of local cerebral blood flow by xenon-enhanced computed tomography. *Science.* 1982; 215(4537):1267–1268.
12. Masdeu JC, Brass LM, Holman BL, et al. Brain single-photon emission computed tomography. *Neurology.* 1994;44(10):1970–1977.
13. Powers WJ, Raichle ME. Positron emission tomography and its application to the study of cerebrovascular disease in man. *Stroke.* 1985; 16(3):361–376.
14. Hunter GJ, Hamberg LM, Ponzo JA, et al. Assessment of cerebral perfusion and arterial anatomy in hyperacute stroke with three-dimensional functional CT: early clinical results. *AJNR Am J Neuroradiol.* 1998; 19(1):29–37.
15. Villringer A, Rosen BR, Belliveau JW, et al. Dynamic imaging with lanthanide chelates in normal brain: contrast due to magnetic susceptibility effects. *Magn Reson Med.* 1988;6(2):164–174.
16. Kontos HA, Wei EP, Navari RM, et al. Responses of cerebral arteries and arterioles to acute hypotension and hypertension. *Am J Physiol.* 1978; 234(4):H371–H383.
17. Traystman RJ. Regulation of cerebral blood flow by carbon dioxide. In: Welch KMA, Caplan LR, Reis DJ, et al., eds. *Primer on Cerebrovascular Disease.* San Diego, CA: Academic Press; 1997:55–58.
18. Ropper AH. Treatment of intracranial hypertension. In: Ropper AH, ed. *Neurological and Neurosurgical Intensive Care.* 3rd ed. New York, NY: Raven Press; 1993:29–52.
19. Shapiro HM, Stromberg DD, Lee DR, et al. Dynamic pressures in the pial arterial microcirculation. *Am J Physiol.* 1971;221(1):279–283.
20. Chillon JM BG. Autoregulation of cerebral blood flow. In: Welch KMA, Caplan LR, Reis DJ, et al, eds. *Primer on Cerebrovascular Disease.* San Diego, CA: Academic Press; 1997:51–54.
21. Chillon JM, Baumbach GL. Autoregulation: arterial and intracranial pressure. In: Edvinsson L, Krause DN, eds. *Cerebral Blood Flow and Metabolism.* 2nd ed. Philadelphia, PA: Lippincott Williams & Wilkins; 2002: 395–412.
22. Folkow B. Description of the myogenic hypothesis. *Circ Res.* 1964; 15(Suppl):279–287.
23. Bayliss WM. On the local reactions of the arterial wall to changes of internal pressure. *J Physiol.* 1902;28(3):220–231.
24. Rubanyi GM, Freay AD, Kauser K, et al. Mechanoreception by the endothelium: mediators and mechanisms of pressure- and flow-induced vascular responses. *Blood Vessels.* 1990;27(2–5):246–257.
25. Wei EP, Kontos HA. Responses of cerebral arterioles to increased venous pressure. *Am J Physiol.* 1982;243(3):H442–H447.
26. Osol G, Halpern W. Myogenic properties of cerebral blood vessels from normotensive and hypertensive rats. *Am J Physiol.* 1985;249(5 Pt 2): H914–H921.
27. Kuschinsky W, Wahl M. Local chemical and neurogenic regulation of cerebral vascular resistance. *Physiol Rev.* 1978;58(3):656–689.
28. Dirnagl U, Dreier J. Regulation of cerebral blood flow by ions. In: Welch KMA, Caplan LR, Reis DJ, et al., eds. *Primer on Cerebrovascular Disease.* San Diego, CA: Academic Press; 1997:75–77.
29. Magistretti PJ. Coupling of cerebral blood flow and metabolism. In: Welch KMA, Caplan LR, Reis DJ, et al., eds. *Primer on Cerebrovascular Disease.* San Diego, CA: Academic Press; 1997:70–75.
30. Winn RH. Adenosine and its receptors: influence on cerebral blood flow. In: Welch KMA, Caplan LR, Reis DJ, et al., eds. *Primer on Cerebrovascular Disease.* San Diego, CA: Academic Press; 1997:77–79.
31. Kitazano T, Heistad DD, Farachi FM. Role of ATP-sensitive potassium channels in CGRP-induced dilation of the basilar artery in vivo. *Am J Physiol Heart Circ Physiol.* 1993;265(2 pt 2):H581–H585.
32. Wei EP, Kontos HA. Increased venous pressure causes myogenic constriction of cerebral arterioles during local hyperoxia. *Circ Res.* 1984;55(2):249–252.
33. Edvinsson L. Neurogenic mechanisms in the cerebrovascular bed. Autonomic nerves, amine receptors and their effects on cerebral blood flow. *Acta Physiol Scand Suppl.* 1975;427:1–35.
34. Lou HC, Edvinsson L, MacKenzie ET. The concept of coupling blood flow to brain function: revision required? *Ann Neurol.* 1987;22(3):289–297.
35. Lindsey KW, Bone I, Callander R. *Neurology and Neurosurgery Illustrated.* 4th ed. Edinburgh: Churchill Livingstone; 2004:52.
36. Szidon JP, Cherniack NS, Fishman AP. Traube-Hering waves in the pulmonary circulation of the dog. *Science.* 1969;164(3875):75–76.
37. Newell DW, Aaslid R, Stooss R, et al. The relationship of blood flow velocity fluctuations to intracranial pressure B waves. *J Neurosurg.* 1992; 76(3):415–421.
38. Fan JY, Kirkness C, Vicini P, et al. An approach to determining intracranial pressure variability capable of predicting decreased intracranial adaptive capacity in patients with traumatic brain injury. *Biol Res Nurs.* 2010;11(4):317–324.
39. Rosner MJ. Pathophysiology and management of increased intracranial pressure. In: Andrews BT, ed. *Neurosurgical Intensive Care.* New York, NY: McGraw-Hill; 1993:57–112.
40. Miller JD, Garibi J, Pickard JD. Induced changes of cerebrospinal fluid volume. Effects during continuous monitoring of ventricular fluid pressure. *Arch Neurol.* 1973;28(4):265–269.
41. Marmarou A, Shulman K, Rosende RM. A nonlinear analysis of the cerebrospinal fluid system and intracranial pressure dynamics. *J Neurosurg.* 1978;48(3):332–344.
42. Lundberg N. Continuous recording and control of ventricular fluid pressure in neurosurgical practice. *Acta Psychiatr Scand Suppl.* 1960; 36(149):1–193.
43. Rosner MJ, Becker DP. Origin and evolution of plateau waves. Experimental observations and a theoretical model. *J Neurosurg.* 1984;60(2):312–324.
44. Schrader H, Lofgren J, Zwetnow NN. Regional cerebral blood flow and CSF pressures during the Cushing response induced by an infratentorial expanding mass. *Acta Neurol Scand.* 1985;72(3):273–282.
45. Brain Trauma Foundation; American Association of Neurological Surgeons; Congress of Neurological Surgeons. Guidelines for the management of severe traumatic brain injury. *J Neurotrauma.* 2007;24(Suppl 1): S1–S106.
46. Jauch EC, Saver JL, Adams HP Jr, et al. Guidelines for the early management of patients with acute ischemic stroke: a guideline for healthcare professionals from the American Heart Association/American Stroke Association. *Stroke.* 2013;44(3):870–947.
47. Morgenstern LB, Hemphill JC, Anderson C, et al. Guidelines for the management of spontaneous intracerebral hemorrhage: a guideline for healthcare professionals from the American Heart Association/American Stroke Association. *Stroke.* 2010;41(9):2108–2129.
48. Teasdale G, Jennett B. Assessment of coma and impaired consciousness. A practical scale. *Lancet.* 1974;2(7872):81–84.
49. Wijdicks EF, Bamlet WR, Maramattom BV, et al. Validation of a new coma scale: The FOUR score. *Ann Neurol.* 2005;58(4):585–593.
50. Eken C, Kartal M, Bacanli A, et al. Comparison of the full outline of unresponsiveness score coma scale and the Glasgow Coma Scale in an emergency setting population. *Eur J Emerg Med.* 2009;16(1):29–36.
51. Iyer VN, Mandrekar JN, Danielson RD, et al. Validity of the FOUR score coma scale in the medical intensive care unit. *Mayo Clin Proc.* 2009; 84(8):694–701.
52. Sadaka F, Patel D, Lakshmanan R. The FOUR score predicts outcome in patients after traumatic brain injury. *Neurocrit Care.* 2012;16(1):95–101.
53. Guidelines for the management of severe head injury. Brain Trauma Foundation, American Association of Neurological Surgeons, Joint Section on Neurotrauma and Critical Care. *J Neurotrauma.* 1996;13(11):641–734.
54. Brophy GM, Bell R, Claassen J, et al. Guidelines for the evaluation and management of status epilepticus. *Neurocrit Care.* 2012;17(1):3–23.
55. Rapoport SI. Brain edema and the blood-brain barrier. In: Welch KMA, Caplan LR, Reis DJ, et al., eds. *Primer on Cerebrovascular Disease.* San Diego, CA: Academic Press; 1997:25–28.
56. Klatzo I. Presidental address. Neuropathological aspects of brain edema. *J Neuropathol Exp Neurol.* 1967;26(1):1–14.
57. Bhardwaj A, Alkayed NJ, Kirsch JR, et al. Mechanisms of ischemic brain damage. *Curr Cardiol Rep.* 2003;5(2):160–167.
58. Auer RN Sutherland GR. Hypoxia and other related conditions. In: Graham DI, Lantos PL, eds. *Greenfields Neuropathology.* 7th ed. London: Arnold Publishers; 2002:233–280.
59. Astrup J, Symon L, Branston NM, et al. Cortical evoked potential and extracellular K+ and H+ at critical levels of brain ischemia. *Stroke.* 1977;8(1):51–57.
60. Choi DW. The excitotoxic concept. In: Welch KMA, Caplan LR, Reis DJ, et al, eds. *Primer on Cerebrovascular Disease.* San Diego, CA: Academic Press; 1997:187–190.
61. Kerr JF, Wyllie AH, Currie AR. Apoptosis: a basic biological phenomenon with wide-ranging implications in tissue kinetics. *Br J Cancer.* 1972; 26(4):239–257.
62. Ginsberg MD, Busto R. Combating hyperthermia in acute stroke: a significant clinical concern. *Stroke.* 1998;29(2):529–534.
63. Manno EM, Farmer JC. Acute brain injury: if hypothermia is good, then is hyperthermia bad? *Crit Care Med.* 2004;32(7):1611–1612.

64. Chen H, Chopp M, Welch KM. Effect of mild hyperthermia on the ischemic infarct volume after middle cerebral artery occlusion in the rat. *Neurology.* 1991;41(7):1133–1135.
65. Chen Q, Chopp M, Bodzin G, et al. Temperature modulation of cerebral depolarization during focal cerebral ischemia in rats: correlation with ischemic injury. *J Cereb Blood Flow Metab.* 1993;13(3):389–894.
66. Chopp M, Welch KM, Tidwell CD, et al. Effect of mild hyperthermia on recovery of metabolic function after global cerebral ischemia in cats. *Stroke.* 1988;19(12):1521–1525.
67. Morimoto T, Ginsberg MD, Dietrich WD, et al. Hyperthermia enhances spectrin breakdown in transient focal cerebral ischemia. *Brain Res.* 1997; 746(1–2):43–51.
68. Azzimondi G, Bassein L, Nonino F, et al. Fever in acute stroke worsens prognosis: a prospective study. *Stroke.* 1995;26(11):2040–2043.
69. Reith J, Jorgensen HS, Pedersen PM, et al. Body temperature in acute stroke: relation to stroke severity, infarct size, mortality, and outcome. *Lancet.* 1996;347(8999):422–425.
70. Diringer MN, Reaven NL, Funk SE, et al. Elevated body temperature independently contributes to increased length of stay in neurologic intensive care unit patients. *Crit Care Med.* 2004;32(7):1489–1495.
71. Capes SE, Hunt D, Malmberg K, et al. Stress hyperglycemia and prognosis of stroke in nondiabetic and diabetic patients: a systematic overview. *Stroke.* 2001;32(10):2426–2432.
72. Garg R, Chaudhuri A, Munschauer F, et al. Hyperglycemia, insulin, and acute ischemic stroke: a mechanistic justification for a trial of insulin infusion therapy. *Stroke.* 2006;37(1):267–273.
73. Alvarez-Sabin J, Molina CA, Montaner J, et al. Effects of admission hyperglycemia on stroke outcome in reperfused tissue plasminogen activator–treated patients. *Stroke.* 2003;34(5):1235–1241.
74. Baird TA, Parsons MW, Phan T, et al. Persistent poststroke hyperglycemia is independently associated with infarct expansion and worse clinical outcome. *Stroke.* 2003;34(9):2208–2214.
75. Leigh R, Zaidat OO, Suri MF, et al. Predictors of hyperacute clinical worsening in ischemic stroke patients receiving thrombolytic therapy. *Stroke.* 2004;35(8):1903–1907.
76. Williams LS, Rotich J, Qi R, et al. Effects of admission hyperglycemia on mortality and costs in acute ischemic stroke. *Neurology.* 2002;59(1): 67–71.
77. Bruno A, Biller J, Adams HP Jr, et al. Acute blood glucose level and outcome from ischemic stroke. Trial of ORG 10172 in Acute Stroke Treatment (TOAST) Investigators.*Neurology.* 1999;52(2):280–284.
78. Wartenberg KE, Mayer SA. Medical complications after subarachnoid hemorrhage: new strategies for prevention and management. *Curr Opin Crit Care.* 2006;12(2):78–84.
79. Cochran A, Scaife ER, Hansen KW, et al. Hyperglycemia and outcomes from pediatric traumatic brain injury. *J Trauma.* 2003;55(6):1035–1038.
80. Parish RA, Webb KS. Hyperglycemia is not a poor prognostic sign in head-injured children. *J Trauma.* 1988;28(4):517–519.
81. Duckrow RB, Beard DC, Brennan RW. Regional cerebral blood flow decreases during hyperglycemia. *Ann Neurol.* 1985;17(3):267–272.
82. Folbergrova J, Memezawa H, Smith ML, et al. Focal and perifocal changes in tissue energy state during middle cerebral artery occlusion in normo- and hyperglycemic rats. *J Cereb Blood Flow Metab.* 1992;12(1): 25–33.
83. Li PA, Shuaib A, Miyashita H, et al. Hyperglycemia enhances extracellular glutamate accumulation in rats subjected to forebrain ischemia. *Stroke.* 2000;31(1):183–192.
84. Berger L, Hakim AM. The association of hyperglycemia with cerebral edema in stroke. *Stroke.* 1986;17(5):865–871.
85. Dhindsa S, Tripathy D, Mohanty P, et al. Differential effects of glucose and alcohol on reactive oxygen species generation and intranuclear nuclear factor-kappa B in mononuclear cells. *Metabolism.* 2004;53(3):330–334.
86. Mohanty P, Hamouda W, Garg R, et al. Glucose challenge stimulates reactive oxygen species (ROS) generation by leucocytes. *J Clin Endocrinol Metab.* 2000;85(8):2970–2973.
87. Fukuoka S, Yeh H, Mandybur TI, et al. Effect of insulin on acute experimental cerebral ischemia in gerbils. *Stroke.* 1989;20(3):396–399.
88. Voll CL, Auer RN. Insulin attenuates ischemic brain damage independent of its hypoglycemic effect. *J Cereb Blood Flow Metab.* 1991; 11(6):1006–1014.
89. Aljada A, Saadeh R, Assian E, et al. Insulin inhibits the expression of intercellular adhesion molecule-1 by human aortic endothelial cells through stimulation of nitric oxide. *J Clin Endocrinol Metab.* 2000;85(7):2572–2575.
90. Krinsley JS, Grover A. Severe hypoglycemia in critically ill patients: risk factors and outcomes. *Crit Care Med.* 2007;35(10):2262–2267.
91. Egi M, Bellomo R, Stachowski E, French CJ, et al. Hypoglycemia and outcome in critically ill patients. *Mayo Clinic Proc.* 2010;85(3): 217–224.
92. Godoy DA, Di Napoli M, Rabinstein AA. Treating hyperglycemia in neurocritical patients: benefits and perils. *Neurocrit Care.* 2010;13(3): 425–438.
93. Bergsneider M, Hovda DA, Shalmon E, et al. Cerebral hyperglycolysis following severe traumatic brain injury in humans: a positron emission tomography study. *J Neurosurg.* 1997;86(2):241–251.
94. Rordorf G, Koroshetz WJ, Ezzeddine MA, et al. A pilot study of drug-induced hypertension for treatment of acute stroke. *Neurology.* 2001; 56(9):1210–1213.
95. Samuels MA. Cardiopulmonary aspects of acute neurologic diseases. In: Ropper AH, ed. *Neurological and Neurosurgical Intensive Care.* 3rd ed. New York, NY: Raven Press; 1993:103–119.
96. Connelly KA, MacIsaac AI, Jelinek VM. Stress, myocardial infarction, and the "tako-tsubo" phenomenon. *Heart.* 2004;90(9):e52.
97. Mori H, Ishikawa S, Kojima S, et al. Increased responsiveness of left ventricular apical myocardium to adrenergic stimuli. *Cardiovasc Res.* 1993;27(2):192–198.
98. Karch SB, Billingham ME. Myocardial contraction bands revisited. *Hum Pathol.* 1986;17(1):9–13.
99. Wartenberg KE, Schmidt JM, Claassen J, et al. Impact of medical complications on outcome after subarachnoid hemorrhage. *Crit Care Med.* 2006;34(3):617–623; quiz 624.
100. Smith WS, Matthay MA. Evidence for a hydrostatic mechanism in human neurogenic pulmonary edema. *Chest.* 1997;111(5):1326–1333.
101. Simon RP, Bayne LL. Pulmonary lymphatic flow alterations during intracranial hypertension in sheep. *Ann Neurol.* 1984;15(2):188–194.
102. Young GB, DeRubeis DA. Metabolic encephalopathies. In: Young GB, Ropper AH, Bolton CF, eds. *Coma and Impaired Consciousness. A Clinical Perspective.* New York, NY: McGraw-Hill; 1998:307–392.
103. Maroon JC, Nelson PB. Hypovolemia in patients with subarachnoid hemorrhage: therapeutic implications. *Neurosurgery.* 1979;4(3):223–226.
104. DiBona GF, Kopp UC. Neural control of renal function. *Physiol Rev.* 1997;77(1):75–197.
105. Sviri GE, Feinsod M, Soustiel JF. Brain natriuretic peptide and cerebral vasospasm in subarachnoid hemorrhage. Clinical and TCD correlations. *Stroke.* 2000;31(1):118–122.
106. Hypothermia after Cardiac Arrest Study Group. Mild therapeutic hypothermia to improve the neurologic outcome after cardiac arrest. *N Engl J Med.* 2002;346(8):549–556.
107. Bernard SA, Gray TW, Buist MD, et al. Treatment of comatose survivors of out-of-hospital cardiac arrest with induced hypothermia. *N Engl J Med.* 2002;346(8):557–563.
108. Nielsen N, Wetterslev J, Cronberg T, et al. Targeted temperature management at 33 degrees C versus 36 degrees C after cardiac arrest. *N Engl J Med.* 2013;369(23):2197–2206.
109. Clifton GL, Miller ER, Choi SC, et al. Lack of effect of induction of hypothermia after acute brain injury. *N Engl J Med.* 2001;344(8):556–563.
110. Clifton GL, Valadka A, Zygun D, et al. Very early hypothermia induction in patients with severe brain injury (the National Acute Brain Injury Study: Hypothermia II): a randomised trial. *Lancet Neurol.* 2011;10(2):131–139.
111. Staykov D, Wagner I, Volbers B, et al. Mild prolonged hypothermia for large intracerebral hemorrhage. *Neurocrit Care.* 2013;18(2):178–183.
112. Schwab S, Schwarz S, Spranger M, et al. Moderate hypothermia in the treatment of patients with severe middle cerebral artery infarction. *Stroke.* 1998;29(12):2461–2466.
113. Bae HJ, Yoon DS, Lee J, et al. In-hospital medical complications and long-term mortality after ischemic stroke. *Stroke.* 2005;36(11):2441–2445.
114. Gujjar AR, Deibert E, Manno EM, et al. Mechanical ventilation for ischemic stroke and intracerebral hemorrhage: indications, timing, and outcome. *Neurology.* 1998;51(2):447–451.
115. Coplin WM, Pierson DJ, Cooley KD, et al. Implications of extubation delay in brain-injured patients meeting standard weaning criteria. *Am J Respir Crit Care Med.* 2000;161(5):1530–1536.
116. Stone JL, Ghaly RF, Di Gianfilippo AD, et al. Acute head trauma management and pathophysiological principles. In: Stone JL, ed. *Head Injury and Its Complications.* Costa Mesa, CA: PMA Publishing; 1993:1–22.
117. Narayan RK, Kishore PR, Becker DP, et al. Intracranial pressure: to monitor or not to monitor? A review of our experience with severe head injury. *J Neurosurg.* 1982;56(5):650–659.
118. Veremakis C, Lindner DH. Central nervous system injury: essential physiologic and therapeutic concerns. In: Civetta JM, Taylor RW, Kirby RR, eds. *Critical Care.* 3rd ed. Philadelphia, PA: Lippincott-Raven; 1997: 273–289.

119. Chesnut RM, Temkin N, Carney N, et al. A trial of intracranial-pressure monitoring in traumatic brain injury. *N Engl J Med.* 2012;367(26): 2471–2481.
120. Bardt TF, Unterberg AW, Hartl R, et al. Monitoring of brain tissue PO2 in traumatic brain injury: effect of cerebral hypoxia on outcome. *Acta Neurochir Suppl.* 1998;71:153–156.
121. Valadka AB, Gopinath SP, Contant CF, et al. Relationship of brain tissue PO_2 to outcome after severe head injury. *Crit Care Med.* 1998; 26(9):1576–1581.
122. van den Brink WA, van Santbrink H, Steyerberg EW, et al. Brain oxygen tension in severe head injury. *Neurosurgery.* 2000;46(4):868–876.
123. Hemphill JC 3rd, Smith WS, Sonne DC, et al. Relationship between brain tissue oxygen tension and CT perfusion: feasibility and initial results. *AJNR Am J Neuroradiol.* 2005;26(5):1095–1100.
124. Johnston AJ, Steiner LA, Coles JP, et al. Effect of cerebral perfusion pressure augmentation on regional oxygenation and metabolism after head injury. *Crit Care Med.* 2005;33(1):189–195.
125. Nangunoori R, Maloney-Wilensky E, Stiefel M, Park S, et al. Brain tissue oxygen-based therapy and outcome after severe traumatic brain injury: a systematic literature review. *Neurocrit Care.* 2012;17(1):131–138.
126. Stiefel MF, Spiotta A, Gracias VH, et al. Reduced mortality rate in patients with severe traumatic brain injury treated with brain tissue oxygen monitoring. *J Neurosurg.* 2005;103(5):805–811.
127. Narotam PK, Morrison JF, Nathoo N. Brain tissue oxygen monitoring in traumatic brain injury and major trauma: outcome analysis of a brain tissue oxygen-directed therapy. *J Neurosurg.* 2009;111(4):672–682.
128. Martini RP, Deem S, Yanez ND, et al. Management guided by brain tissue oxygen monitoring and outcome following severe traumatic brain injury. *J Neurosurg.* 2009;111(4):644–649.
129. Le Roux P, Menon DK, Citerio G, et al. Consensus summary statement of the International Multidisciplinary Consensus Conference on Multimodality Monitoring in Neurocritical Care : a statement for healthcare professionals from the Neurocritical Care Society and the European Society of Intensive Care Medicine. *Intensive Care Med.* 2014;40(9):1189–1209.
130. Andrews PJ, Citerio G, Longhi L, et al. NICEM consensus on neurological monitoring in acute neurological disease. *Intensive Care Med.* 2008; 34(8):1362–1370.
131. Tolias CM, Reinert M, Seiler R, et al. Normobaric hyperoxia–induced improvement in cerebral metabolism and reduction in intracranial pressure in patients with severe head injury: a prospective historical cohort-matched study. *J Neurosurg.* 2004;101(3):435–444.
132. Bennett MH, Trytko B, Jonker B. Hyperbaric oxygen therapy for the adjunctive treatment of traumatic brain injury. *Cochrane Database Syst Rev.* 2012;12:CD004609.
133. Paczynski RP, He YY, Diringer MN, et al. Multiple-dose mannitol reduces brain water content in a rat model of cortical infarction. *Stroke.* 1997;28(7):1437–1443.
134. Shackford SR, Bourguignon PR, Wald SL, et al. Hypertonic saline resuscitation of patients with head injury: a prospective, randomized clinical trial. *J Trauma.* 1998;44(1):50–58.
135. Rickard AC, Smith JE, Newell P, et al. Salt or sugar for your injured brain? A meta-analysis of randomised controlled trials of mannitol versus hypertonic sodium solutions to manage raised intracranial pressure in traumatic brain injury. *Emerg Med J.* 2014;31(8):679–683.
136. Koenig MA, Bryan M, Lewin JL 3rd, et al. Reversal of transtentorial herniation with hypertonic saline. *Neurology.* 2008;70(13):1023–1029.
137. Dearden NM, Gibson JS, McDowall DG, et al. Effect of high-dose dexamethasone on outcome from severe head injury. *J Neurosurg.* 1986; 64(1):81–88.
138. Cooper PR, Moody S, Clark WK, et al. Dexamethasone and severe head injury: a prospective double-blind study. *J Neurosurg.* 1979;51(3):307–316.
139. Eisenberg HM, Frankowski RF, Contant CF, et al. High-dose barbiturate control of elevated intracranial pressure in patients with severe head injury. *J Neurosurg.* 1988;69(1):15–23.
140. Giannotta SL, Weiss MH, Apuzzo ML, et al. High dose glucocorticoids in the management of severe head injury. *Neurosurgery.* 1984;15(4):497–501.
141. Schalen W, Sonesson B, Messeter K, et al. Clinical outcome and cognitive impairment in patients with severe head injuries treated with barbiturate coma. *Acta Neurochir (Wien).* 1992;117(3–4):153–159.
142. Bullock MR, Chesnut R, Ghajar J, et al. Surgical management of traumatic parenchymal lesions. *Neurosurgery.* 2006;58(3 Suppl):S25–S46.
143. Temkin NR, Dikmen SS, Wilensky AJ, et al. A randomized, double-blind study of phenytoin for the prevention of post-traumatic seizures. *N Engl J Med.* 1990;323(8):497–502.
144. Cooper DJ, Rosenfeld JV, Murray L, et al. Decompressive craniectomy in diffuse traumatic brain injury. *N Engl J Med.* 2011;364(16):1493–1502.
145. Kumar MA, Urrutia VC, Thomas CE, et al. The syndrome of irreversible acidosis after prolonged propofol infusion. *Neurocrit Care.* 2005; 3(3):257–259.
146. Manno EM. New management strategies in the treatment of status epilepticus. *Mayo Clin Proc.* 2003;78(4):508–518.
147. Murdoch SD, Cohen AT. Propofol-infusion syndrome in children. *Lancet.* 1999;353(9169):2074–2075.
148. Manno EM. Subarachnoid hemorrhage. *Neurol Clin.* 2004;22(2):347–366.
149. Adams HP Jr, Kassell NF, Torner JC, et al. Early management of aneurysmal subarachnoid hemorrhage: a report of the Cooperative Aneurysm Study. *J Neurosurg.* 1981;54(2):141–145.
150. Ohkuma H, Tsurutani H, Suzuki S. Incidence and significance of early aneurysmal rebleeding before neurosurgical or neurological management. *Stroke.* 2001;32(5):1176–1180.
151. Hillman J, Fridriksson S, Nilsson O, et al. Immediate administration of tranexamic acid and reduced incidence of early rebleeding after aneurysmal subarachnoid hemorrhage: a prospective randomized study. *J Neurosurg.* 2002;97:771–778.
152. Manno EM, Gress DR, Schwamm LH, et al. Effects of induced hypertension on transcranial Doppler ultrasound velocities in patients after subarachnoid hemorrhage. *Stroke.* 1998;29(2):422–428.
153. Fisher CM, Kistler JP, Davis JM. Relation of cerebral vasospasm to subarachnoid hemorrhage visualized by computerized tomographic scanning. *Neurosurgery.* 1980;6(1):1–9.
154. Kistler JP, Crowell RM, Davis KR, et al. The relation of cerebral vasospasm to the extent and location of subarachnoid blood visualized by CT scan: a prospective study. *Neurology.* 1983;33(4):424–436.
155. Dupont SA, Wijdicks EF, Manno EM, et al. Prediction of angiographic vasospasm after aneurysmal subarachnoid hemorrhage: value of the Hijdra sum scoring system. *Neurocrit Care.* 2009;11(2):172–176.
156. Hijdra A, Brouwers PJ, Vermeulen M, et al. Grading the amount of blood on computed tomograms after subarachnoid hemorrhage. *Stroke.* 1990; 21(8):1156–1161.
157. Frontera JA, Claassen J, Schmidt JM, et al. Prediction of symptomatic vasospasm after subarachnoid hemorrhage: the modified fisher scale. *Neurosurgery.* 2006;59(1):21–27; discussion 7.
158. Connolly ES, Rabinstein AA, Carhuapoma JR, et al. Guidelines for the management of aneurysmal subarachnoid hemorrhage: a guideline for healthcare professionals from the American Heart Association/American Stroke Association. *Stroke.* 2012;43(6):1711–1137.
159. Brott T, Broderick J, Kothari R, et al. Early hemorrhage growth in patients with intracerebral hemorrhage. *Stroke.* 1997;28(1):1–5.
160. Mayer SA, Brun NC, Begtrup K, et al. Recombinant activated factor VII for acute intracerebral hemorrhage. *N Engl J Med.* 2005;352(8):777–785.
161. Mayer SA, Brun NC, Begtrup K, et al. Efficacy and safety of recombinant activated factor VII for acute intracerebral hemorrhage. *N Engl J Med.* 2008;358(20):2127–2137.
162. Mendelow AD, Gregson BA, Fernandes HM, et al. Early surgery versus initial conservative treatment in patients with spontaneous supratentorial intracerebral haematomas in the International Surgical Trial in Intracerebral Haemorrhage (STICH): a randomised trial. *Lancet.* 2005;365(9457):387–397.
163. Anderson CS, Heeley E, Huang Y, et al. Rapid blood-pressure lowering in patients with acute intracerebral hemorrhage. *N Engl J Med.* 2013;368(25):2355–2365.
164. Poungvarin N, Bhoopat W, Viriyavejakul A, et al. Effects of dexamethasone in primary supratentorial intracerebral hemorrhage. *N Engl J Med.* 1987;316(20):1229–1233.
165. Mendelow AD, Gregson BA, Rowan EN, et al. Early surgery versus initial conservative treatment in patients with spontaneous supratentorial lobar intracerebral haematomas (STICH II): a randomised trial. *Lancet.* 2013;382(9890):397–408.
166. Mould WA, Carhuapoma JR, Muschelli J, et al. Minimally invasive surgery plus recombinant tissue-type plasminogen activator for intracerebral hemorrhage evacuation decreases perihematomal edema. *Stroke.* 2013;44(3):627–634.
167. Gobin YP, Starkman S, Duckwiler GR, et al. MERCI 1: a phase 1 study of mechanical embolus removal in cerebral ischemia. *Stroke.* 2004;35(12): 2848–2854.
168. Tissue plasminogen activator for acute ischemic stroke. The National Institute of Neurological Disorders and Stroke rt-PA Stroke Study Group. *N Engl J Med.* 1995;333(24):1581–1587.
169. Hacke W, Kaste M, Bluhmki E, et al. Thrombolysis with alteplase 3 to 4.5 hours after acute ischemic stroke. *N Engl J Med.* 2008;359(13):1317–1329.
170. Campbell BC, Mitchell PJ, Kleinig TJ, et al. Endovascular therapy for ischemic stroke with perfusion-imaging selection. *N Engl J Med.* 2015; 372(11):1009–1018.

171. Goyal M, Demchuk AM, Menon BK, et al. Randomized assessment of rapid endovascular treatment of ischemic stroke. *N Engl J Med.* 2015; 372(11):1019–1030.
172. Berkhemer OA, Fransen PS, Beumer D, et al. A randomized trial of intra-arterial treatment for acute ischemic stroke. *N Engl J Med.* 2015; 372(1):11–20.
173. Broderick JP, Palesch YY, Demchuk AM, et al. Endovascular therapy after intravenous t-PA versus t-PA alone for stroke. *N Engl J Med.* 2013;368(10): 893–903.
174. Ciccone A, Valvassori L, Nichelatti M, et al. Endovascular treatment for acute ischemic stroke. *N Engl J Med.* 2013;368(10):904–913.
175. Kidwell CS, Jahan R, Gornbein J, et al. A trial of imaging selection and endovascular treatment for ischemic stroke. *N Engl J Med.* 2013; 368(10):914–923.
176. Potter J, Mistri A, Brodie F, et al. Controlling hypertension and hypotension immediately post stroke (CHHIPS): a randomised controlled trial. *Health Technol Assess.* 2009;13(9):1–73.
177. Robinson TG, Potter JF, Ford GA, et al. Effects of antihypertensive treatment after acute stroke in the Continue or Stop Post-Stroke Antihypertensives Collaborative Study (COSSACS): a prospective, randomised, open, blinded-endpoint trial. *Lancet Neurol.* 2010;9(8):767–75.
178. Sandset EC, Bath PM, Boysen G, et al. The angiotensin-receptor blocker candesartan for treatment of acute stroke (SCAST): a randomised, placebo-controlled, double-blind trial. *Lancet.* 2011;377(9767):741–750.
179. Frank JI. Large hemispheric infarction, deterioration, and intracranial pressure. *Neurology.* 1995;45(7):1286–1290.
180. Delashaw JB, Broaddus WC, Kassell NF, et al. Treatment of right hemispheric cerebral infarction by hemicraniectomy. *Stroke.* 1990;21(6):874–881.
181. Vahedi K, Hofmeijer J, Juettler E, et al. Early decompressive surgery in malignant infarction of the middle cerebral artery: a pooled analysis of three randomised controlled trials. *Lancet Neurol.* 2007;6(3):215–222.
182. Juttler E, Unterberg A, Woitzik J, et al. Hemicraniectomy in older patients with extensive middle-cerebral-artery stroke. *N Engl J Med.* 2014;370(12): 1091–1100.

CHAPTER

14

Lung Structure and Function

YATIN B. MEHTA and ANDREW MATRAGRANO

INTRODUCTION

Many aspects of cardiopulmonary life support are rooted in understanding the anatomy and physiology of the respiratory system. The purpose of this chapter is to review those aspects of normal structure and function of the lungs and chest wall that impact most directly on daily practice. Intentionally, we have only dipped tentatively into the physiology of pathologic conditions, as to attempt to do so would clearly exceed our page allocation and scope of this assignment. Nonetheless, we hope that this overview serves as a starting point by underlining the principles of undeniable clinical relevance.

ANATOMIC CONSIDERATIONS

Tracheobronchial Tree

A useful approach to understanding the tracheobronchial tree (Fig. 14.1) is that of Weibel (1), who numbered successive generations of air passages from the trachea to the alveolar sacs. In some sectors, there may be as few as eight generations, while in others, the air pathway may divide 23 times from the trachea (generation 0) to the alveoli (generation 23). It may be assumed that the number of passages in each generation is double that in the previous generation, and the number of passages in each generation is 2 raised to the power of the generation number. As a result there will be more than 8 million end branches called alveolar sacs.

The trachea has a mean diameter of 1.8 cm and a length of 11 cm. It is supported by U-shaped cartilage, which is joined posteriorly by smooth muscle bands. Despite the presence of cartilage, the posterior wall is deformable so that the trachea can be occluded by a pressure on the order of 50 to 70 cm H_2O. Within the chest, the trachea can be compressed by elevated intrathoracic pressure, as may occur during cough when the decreased diameter increases the efficiency of secretion removal. The tracheal mucosa is a columnar-ciliated epithelium containing mucous-secreting goblet cells. Cilia beat in a coordinated manner, creating an upward stream of mucus and foreign material; anesthetics render the cilial beat ineffective, and cilial movement of mucus and respiratory debris is also compromised by drying, which occurs in patients breathing dry gas through a tracheostomy.

The trachea bifurcates asymmetrically, with the right bronchus wider and better aligned with the long axis of the trachea; it is, thus, more likely, therefore, to receive aspirated material. Main, lobar, and segmental bronchi have firm cartilaginous support, which is horseshoe shaped; more distally, cartilage is arranged in irregular plates. Where cartilage is irregular and discontinuous, bronchial smooth muscle in helical bands forms a network (1,2). The bronchial epithelium is similar to that in the trachea, although the height of cells diminishes in more peripheral passages until it becomes cuboidal in bronchioles. Bronchi down to generation 4 are sufficiently regular to be individually named. By the third generation, total cross-sectional area of the respiratory tract is still minimal.

When bronchi in generations 1 through 4 are subjected to large changes in intrathoracic pressure, collapse occurs when intrathoracic pressure exceeds intraluminal pressure by about 50 cm H_2O. Collapse occurs in larger bronchi during a forced expiration since the greater part of the alveolar-to-mouth pressure difference is taken up in the segmental bronchi. Intraluminal pressure, particularly within larger bronchi, is well below intrathoracic pressure, particularly with emphysema. Collapse of larger bronchi limits peak expiratory flow in the normal subject (3).

Small bronchi extend through about seven generations, with diameter progressively falling from 3.5 to 1 mm. Since their number approximately doubles with each generation, the total cross-sectional area increases rapidly with each generation to a value at generation 11, which is about seven times the total cross-sectional area at the level of the lobar bronchi. Down to the level of true bronchi, air passages lie in close proximity to branches of the pulmonary artery in a sheath also containing pulmonary lymphatics. Distension of these lymphatics gives rise to classic cuffing seen with pulmonary edema. Small bronchi are not directly attached to pulmonary parenchyma and are not subject to direct traction. They rely on cartilage within their walls for patency and on transmural pressure, which is normally a positive gradient from the lumen to the intrathoracic space. Intraluminal pressure in small bronchi rapidly rises to more than 80% of alveolar pressure during forced expiration.

At the 11th generation, where diameter usually approximates 1 mm, cartilage disappears from the wall of airways, and structural rigidity ceases to be the factor maintaining patency. Beyond this level, air passages are embedded in pulmonary parenchyma, and traction from adjacent alveoli holds the air passages open. The caliber of the airways below the 11th generation is strongly influenced by lung volume, as forces holding the lumen open are greater at higher lung volumes. Airway closure may occur at reduced lung volumes.

In succeeding generations, the number of bronchioles increases more rapidly than caliber diminishes. The total cross-sectional area increases until, in terminal bronchioles, it is about 30 times the area at the level of the large bronchi. The flow resistance of the smaller air passages (<2 mm) approximates one-tenth of the total. Contraction of helical muscle bands wrinkles the cuboidal epithelium into longitudinal folds, which increases flow resistance and, in some cases, results in airway obstruction. Down to the terminal bronchiole level, air passages derive nutrition from bronchial circulation, and are influenced by systemic arterial blood gas levels; beyond this point, air passages rely on pulmonary circulation for nutrition (Table 14.1).

From the trachea to the smallest bronchioles, the functions of air passages are conduction and humidification. Beyond this

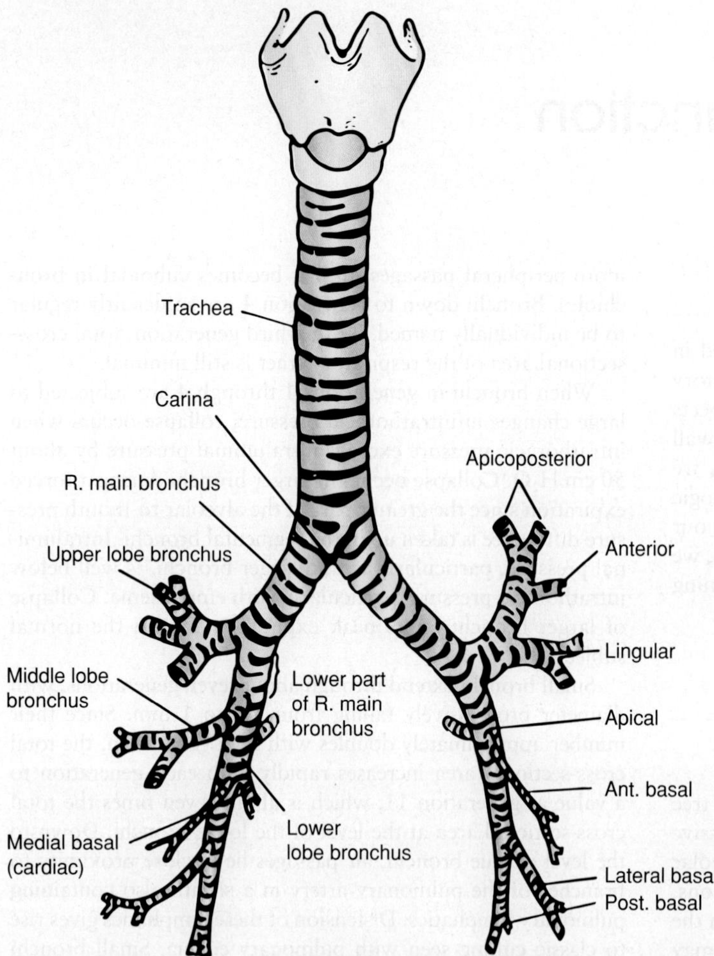

FIGURE 14.1 Named branches of the tracheobronchial tree, viewed from the front. (From Nunn JF. *Applied Respiratory Physiology.* 3rd ed. London: Butterworths; 1987, with permission.)

point there are acinar airways consisting of respiratory bronchioles, alveolar ducts and alveolar sacs where gas exchange occurs. At this point conduction transitions to convection and diffusion which is the main process in gas exchange. In the three generations of respiratory bronchioles, there is a gradual increase in the number of alveoli in the walls. The epithelium is cuboidal between the mouths of the mural alveoli in the earlier generations of respiratory bronchioles but becomes progressively flatter until it is entirely alveolar epithelium in the alveolar ducts. Like the conductive bronchioles, the respiratory bronchioles are embedded in the pulmonary parenchyma. The respiratory bronchioles have well-marked muscle layers, with bands looping over the opening alveolar ducts and the openings of mural alveoli. The total cross-sectional area at this level is in the order of hundreds of square centimeters.

The primary lobular terminal respiratory unit is the likely equivalent of the alveolus when considered from the standpoint of function. The primary lobule is defined as the zone supplied by a first-order respiratory lobule. There are approximately 130,000 primary lobules with a diameter of about 3.5 mm containing approximately 2,000 alveoli each.

Alveolar ducts (generations 20 to 22) arise from terminal respiratory bronchioles and differ from terminal respiratory bronchioles by having no walls other than the mouths of mural alveoli (approximately 20 in number); approximately half of alveoli arise from ducts. The last generation of air passages differs from the alveolar ducts solely in the fact that they are blind pouches. Approximately 17 alveoli arise from these alveolar sacs and account for half of the total number of alveoli. Because of this increase in cross-sectional area resistance decreases and airflow slows down thus facilitating gas exchange over a large surface area.

Alveoli

The total number of alveoli is approximately 300 million, but ranges from 200 to 600 million, corresponding to the height of the subject. The size of the alveoli is proportional to the lung volume; the alveoli are larger in the upper part of the lung due to higher negative pleural pressure, except at maximal inflation when the vertical size gradient disappears. The reduction in the size of alveoli and the corresponding reduction in the caliber of smaller airways in the dependent parts of the lung comprise the most important implications in gas exchange. During normal tidal breathing, most ventilator volume goes to lung bases. At functional residual capacity (FRC), the mean diameter is 0.2 mm (4).

Alveolar walls, which separate adjacent alveoli, consist of two layers of alveolar epithelium on a separate basement membrane enclosing the interstitial space. These layers contain pulmonary capillaries, elastin and collagen, nerve endings, and occasional neutrophils and macrophages. On one side of the interstitium, the capillary endothelium and alveolar epithelium are closely opposed, and the total thickness from gas to blood is usually less than 0.4 μm. This is the active side of the capillary, and gas exchange is more efficient at this

TABLE 14.1 Functional Anatomy of the Respiratory Tree

	Generation (Mean)	Number	Mean Diameter (mm)	Area Supplied	Cartilage	Muscle	Nutrition	Emplacement	Epithelium
Trachea	0	1	18	Both lungs	U-shaped	Links open end of cartilage			Columnar ciliated
Main bronchi	1	2	13	Individual lungs			From the bronchial circulation	Within connective tissue sheath alongside arterial vessels	
Lobar bronchi	2 ↓ 3	4 ↓ 8	7 ↓ 5	Lobes	Irregular shaped and helical plates	Helical bands			
Segmental bronchi	4	16	4	Segments					
Small bronchi	5 ↓ 11	32 ↓ 2,000	3 ↓ 1	Secondary lobules					
Bronchioles Terminal bronchioles	12 ↓ 16	4,000 ↓ 65,000	1 ↓ 0.5		Absent	Strong helical muscle bands		Embedded directly in the lung parenchyma	Cuboidal
Respiratory bronchioles	17 ↓ 19	130,000 ↓ 500,000	0.5	Primary lobules		Muscle bands between alveoli	From the pulmonary circulation		Cuboidal to flat between the alveoli
Alveolar ducts	20 ↓ 22	1,000,000 ↓ 4,000,000	0.3	Alveoli		Thin bands in alveolar septa		From the lung parenchyma	Alveolar epithelium
Alveolar sacs	23	8,000,000	0.3						

site. The opposite side of the capillary is usually more than 1 to 2 μm thick and contains collagen and elastin fibers in an expanded tissue space. Herein is situated the connective tissue framework, which maintains pulmonary geometry. Alveolar septa are generally flat due to the tension generated by elastic fibers and surface tension at the air–fluid interface. The surface tension of the alveolar lining fluid is modified in the presence of surfactant, which decreases surface tension at the air fluid interface. Both elastin fibers and the decrease in surface tension keep the alveoli open during the volume change of the respiratory cycles so that gas exchange can continue. Septa are perforated by fenestrations known as pores of Kohn, which provide collateral ventilation; this can be demonstrated between the air spaces supplied by large bronchi (2).

Alveolar Cellular Morphology

The alveoli are divided by septa lined by flattened, continuous epithelial cells covering the thin interstitium (5). This epithelium, in humans, consists primarily of two distinct cells—type I and type II—with occasional neuroendocrine cells. In addition, although not frequently a part of the alveolar wall, the alveolar macrophage is, in fact, normally present on the alveolar epithelial surface.

Type I Epithelium

The type I alveolar cell (squamous lining cell), although comprising only 8% of parenchymal lung cells and inconspicuous by light microscopy, covers approximately 95% of the alveolar surface area, and has a total volume twice that of the histologically more prominent type II cell. Its nucleus is small and flattened, covered by a thin rim of cytoplasm containing few organelles. The remainder of the cytoplasm is aligned in broad sheets measuring 0.3 to 0.4 μm in thickness and extending in all directions for 50 μm or more over the alveolar surface. Sheets of adjacent type I cells interdigitate, and individual plates may reach into neighboring alveoli by winding the septal tip or by extending through the alveolar pores. Localized gap junctions have been identified between adjacent type I cells and between type I and type II alveolar cells frequently in association with an occluding junction (6).

The cytoplasm of type I epithelium contains few organelles but numerous pinocytotic vesicles, which are thought to transport fluid or proteins across the air–blood barrier. Type I cells have shown the ability to take up intra-alveolar particulate material and, while this particle clearance may be small in comparison with alveolar macrophages and the mucociliary apparatus, movement of materials across type I epithelium may allow particles to be deposited in regional lymph nodes.

Type II Epithelium

The type II epithelial cell (granular pneumocyte) is cuboidal in shape and protrudes into the alveolar lumen, making it easily identified on light microscopy. These cells may occur in groups of two or three and are often located near corners where adjacent alveoli meet. The cytoplasm of type II epithelium is rich in organelles, including endoplasmic reticulum with ribosomes, Golgi complexes, mitochondria, and membrane-bound osmiophilic granules. There is evidence from ultrastructural, biochemical tissue culture, and immunologic studies that type II cells and their osmophilic granules supply alveolar surfactant. These granules appear to function in a storage capacity, although some aspects of surfactant synthesis may also occur. Release of granule contents into the alveolar lumen occurs by exocytosis.

A second major function of type II epithelium is repopulation of normal and damaged alveolar epithelium. The type I cell is thought to be incapable of replication. On the other hand, the type II population is mitotically active and repopulates the alveolar surface. In addition, cytoplasmic simplicity and the large surface area of type I cells make them susceptible to damage from a variety of stimuli. In such circumstances, type II cells proliferate and temporarily repopulate alveolar walls, providing epithelial integrity. In time, they transform into type I cells. This sequence has been demonstrated with pulmonary injury from a variety of agents including oxygen, nitrous oxide, and other chemicals. Microvilli cover the surface of type II cells, suggesting that these cells may function in resorption of fluid or other materials from the alveolar air space.

Alveolar Macrophage

Pulmonary macrophages can be divided into three groups based on anatomic locations: (a) airway macrophage situated within the lumen or beneath the epithelial lining of conducting airways; (b) interstitial macrophage found isolated or in relation to lymphoid tissue in the interstitial connective tissue space; and (c) alveolar macrophage located on the alveolar surface. The alveolar macrophage has been the most extensively studied due to its accessibility by bronchoalveolar lavage (7).

The alveolar macrophage ranges from 15 to 50 μm in diameter and is round in shape with a foamy granular cytoplasm; nuclei are eccentric and may be multiple within the cell. Ultrastructurally, macrophages show prominent cytoplasmic projections that appear as microvillus-like structures. The cytoplasm contains a well-developed Golgi apparatus, scattered mitochondria, endoplasmic reticulum, ribosomes, microtubules and microfilaments, and membrane-bound granules of varying appearance. These granules contain primary and secondary lysosomes.

Pulmonary alveolar macrophages differ from other macrophages by having aerobic energy production, increased mitochondria and mitochondrial enzymes, and more numerous and larger lysosomes. Alveolar macrophages are ultimately derived from bone marrow precursors, presumably by way of the peripheral blood monocyte. In addition, there is evidence for a population of alveolar interstitial macrophages capable of division and replenishment or augmentation of the alveolar macrophage population in the absence of a functioning bone marrow or in times of increased stress. The average lifespan of a pulmonary macrophage in the air space is estimated at 80 days. Various inhaled toxins, including cigarette smoke, have a negative effect on macrophage viability and activity.

The functions of the alveolar macrophage are numerous; they are the primary phagocytes of the innate immune system, clearing the air spaces of infectious, toxic, or allergic particles that have evaded the proximal mechanical defenses. Alveolar macrophages also function as regulators of innate alveolar defenses against respiratory infection by synthesizing wide array of cytokines (including ILs-1, 6 and TNF-α), chemokines (IL-8), and arachidonic metabolites. Using these cell-to-cell signals, alveolar macrophages initiate inflammatory responses and recruit activated neutrophils in to the alveolar spaces. Recent evidence suggests that the alveolar macrophages have equally important role in resolving inflammation within the airspace. As the inflammatory response resolves, neutrophils undergo programmed cell death, or apoptosis. During apoptosis, neutrophil surface membranes remain intact, containing potentially injurious cytoplasmic contents. If apoptotic neutrophils are not efficiently cleared, leak of intracellular proteases into the alveolus from devitalized neutrophils produce further tissue injury and perpetuate inflammation. Efficient clearance of apoptotic neutrophils not only reduced macrophage secretions of proinflammatory cytokines but also stimulates production of anti-inflammatory cytokines, such as transforming growth factor-β and IL-10 (8).

Pulmonary Vasculature

Pulmonary Arterial and Venous Circulation

The pulmonary circulation carries the same flow as the systemic circulation, but arterial pressure and vascular resistance are normally one-sixth as great (2). The media of the pulmonary arteries are half as thick as in the systemic arteries of the corresponding size. In larger vessels, the media consist mainly of elastic tissue, but in smaller vessels, they are mainly muscular, with a transition being in vessels of 1 mm in diameter. Pulmonary arteries lie close to corresponding air passages in connective tissue sheaths.

The transition to arterioles occurs at an internal diameter of 100 μm. These vessels differ radically from the systemic circulation, as they are virtually devoid of muscular tissue. There is a thin medium of elastic tissue separated from blood by the endothelium. There is little structural difference between the pulmonary arterioles and venules.

Pulmonary capillaries arise from larger vessels—the pulmonary arterioles—and form a dense network over the walls of the alveoli; the spaces between them are similar in size to the capillaries themselves. About 75% of the capillary bed is filled in the resting state, but the percentage is higher in the dependent parts of the lung. This gravity-dependent effect is the basis of the vertical gradient of ventilation/perfusion ratios. Inflation of alveoli reduces the cross-sectional area of the capillary bed and increases the resistance to blood flow. Pulmonary capillary blood is collected into venules, which are structurally similar to arterioles. Unlike pulmonary arteries, pulmonary veins run close to the septa, which separate segments of the lung.

Bronchial Circulation

At the level of terminal bronchioles, air passages and accompanying blood vessels receive nutrition from bronchial vessels, which arise from systemic circulation. Part of this bronchial circulation returns to the systemic venous beds but mingles with pulmonary venous drainage, contributing to shunt. It has been established that when pulmonary arterial pressure in animals is raised as by massive pulmonary emboli, pulmonary arterial blood is able to reach pulmonary veins without traversing the capillary bed. This physiologic arteriovenous communication may offer an explanation for abnormalities of gas exchange during anesthesia.

Pulmonary Lymphatics

There are no lymphatics visible in the interalveolar septa, but small lymph vessels commence at the junction between the alveolar and extra-alveolar spaces. A well-developed lymphatic system courses around the bronchi and pulmonary vessels, capable of containing up to 500 mL of lymph, and draining toward the hilum (9). Down to airway generation 11, lymphatics lie in a potential space around air passages and vessels, separating them from lung parenchyma. This space becomes distended with lymph and pulmonary edema and accounts for the characteristic "butterfly shadow" (also termed "bat-wing appearance") seen on a chest radiograph. In the hilum, lymphatic drainage passes through groups of tracheobronchial lymph nodes, where tributaries from superficial subpleural lymphatics contribute. Most of the lymph from the left lung enters the thoracic duct. Lymph from the right lung drains into the right lymphatic duct. Pulmonary lymphatics often cross the midline.

RESPIRATORY PHYSIOLOGY AND MECHANICAL VENTILATION

Positive pressure ventilation (PPV) as a life-sustaining measure first proved its merit during the polio epidemics of the 1950s. Since that time, the use of mechanical ventilatory (MV) support has been synonymous with the growth of critical care medicine. Early ventilation used neuromuscular blocking agents to provide control of patient respiratory efforts. Today, patient–ventilator interaction is critical, and there is a growing awareness of complications associated with neuromuscular blockade. Finally, there is increasing recognition that ventilators can induce various forms of lung injury, which has led to reappraisal of the goals of ventilatory support (10). While it seems that each manufacturer has introduced differing modes of MV, the fundamental principles of ventilatory management of critically ill patients remain unchanged.

PPV can be life saving in patients with hypoxemia or respiratory acidosis refractory to simpler measures. In patients with severe cardiopulmonary distress with excessive work of breathing, MV substitutes or supplements the action of respiratory muscles (11). In the setting of respiratory distress, respiratory muscles may account for as much as 40% of total oxygen consumption; in this circumstance, MV allows diversion of oxygen to other tissue beds that may be vulnerable. In addition, reversal of respiratory muscle fatigue, which may contribute to respiratory failure, depends on respiratory muscle rest. PPV can reverse or prevent atelectasis by allowing inspiration at a more favorable region of the pressure–volume curve describing pulmonary function. With improved gas exchange and relief from excessive respiratory muscle work, an opportunity is provided for the lungs and airways to heal. MV is not therapeutic in and of itself, and PPV may aggravate or initiate alveolar damage. These dangers of ventilator-induced lung injury have led to a reappraisal of the objectives of MV. Rather than seeking normal arterial blood gas values, it is often better to accept a degree of respiratory acidosis and possibly relative hypoxemia to avoid large tidal volumes and high inflation pressures.

MV may have hemodynamic effects as well. When applied to a passively breathing individual, PPV frequently lowers cardiac output (CO), primarily as a result of decreased venous return, especially when gas trapping occurs during passive inflation (12). In other circumstances, this form of ventilation may increase CO in the setting of impaired myocardial contractility because left ventricular afterload decreases with an increase in intrathoracic pressure. Alveolar distension compresses alveolar vessels, and the resulting increase in pulmonary vascular resistance and right ventricular afterload produces a leftward shift in the interventricular septum. Left ventricular compliance is decreased both by the bulging interventricular septum and increased juxtacardiac pressure from the distended lungs. There seems little doubt that adding MV or removing this support from critically ill patients can be a significant imposed stress.

MV strategies are clearly affected by underlying pulmonary disease. For example, in patients with acute respiratory failure, chronic obstructive pulmonary disease (COPD), asthma, or other conditions associated with a high residual volume, gas trapping develops in alveoli because patients have inadequate expiratory time available for exhalation before the next breath begins. Patients experiencing this "breath stacking" have a residual, peripheral positive end-expiratory pressure (PEEP). Also termed auto-PEEP, this retained peripheral gas makes triggering the ventilator more difficult, since the patient needs to generate a negative pressure equal in magnitude to the level of auto-PEEP in addition to the trigger threshold of the machine. This is one factor that may contribute to the patient's inability to trigger the ventilator despite the obvious respiratory effort. Auto-PEEP may be undetected because it is not registered routinely on the pressure manometer of the ventilator, although newer machines have software to detect auto-PEEP. In older machines, occluding the expiratory port of the circuit at the end of expiration in a relaxed patient causes pressure in the lungs and the ventilator circuit to equilibrate, and the level of auto-PEEP is displayed on the manometer (13).

LUNG MECHANICS

Respiratory Muscles

Air flows to and from the alveoli, driven by differences in pressure between the airway opening and the alveolus. During spontaneous breathing, mouth (atmospheric) pressure remains constant, while alveolar pressure fluctuates under the influence of changing pleural pressure and tissue recoil forces (14–16). The diaphragm powers inspiration both by displacing the abdominal contents caudally and by raising the lower ribs, expanding them outward by a bucket handle effect (17,18). This latter action is aided by the external intercostal muscles. Normal exhalation is passive. When faced with a large ventilatory requirement or with impeded gas flow due to airway obstruction or parenchymal restriction, the accessory muscles of respiration are recruited to aid inhalation. Forceful exhalation is assisted by the internal intercostal muscles. The phrenic nerves (C3–C5) innervate the diaphragm, while the spinal nerves (T2–L4) innervate the intercostal and abdominal muscles.

The primary disorders of respiratory muscle function are usefully considered as problems of the diaphragm or problems of the accessory respiratory muscles (18,19). When upright, patients with isolated paralysis of both hemidiaphragms can often sustain adequate ventilation by the coordinated use of the intercostal and abdominal muscles. First, the diaphragm is forced upward as the muscles contract to raise the abdominal pressure. The diaphragm then descends, aided by gravity, as muscle relaxation allows abdominal pressure to fall. This mechanism cannot work effectively in the supine position, a circumstance that explains why orthopnea is a prominent symptom of this disorder. Patients with spinal cord injury (quadriplegia) have the converse anatomic problem: The intact diaphragm provides adequate ventilation to meet the normal requirement, but paralysis of the expiratory musculature severely limits ventilatory reserve and coughing efficiency.

Pressure–Volume Relationships

The lung and its thoracic shell occupy identical volumes, except when air or fluid separates them (20–22). At any specified volume, the pressure acting to distend the lung is alveolar pressure minus pleural pressure, while the pressure across the chest wall is pleural pressure minus atmospheric pressure. The volume of the lung is determined uniquely by lung compliance (distensibility) and the pressure difference acting to distend it (transpulmonary pressure). Thus, static lung volume is the same whether the alveolar pressure is 0 and pleural pressure is –5, or if alveolar pressure is 25 and pleural pressure is 20. A similar relationship between the distending pressure, compliance, and volume also applies to the chest wall. When the chest wall muscles are relaxed at FRC, the tendency of the chest wall to spring outward balances the tendency of the lung to recoil to a smaller volume; movement away from this equilibrium point requires muscular effort (Fig. 14.2). Should

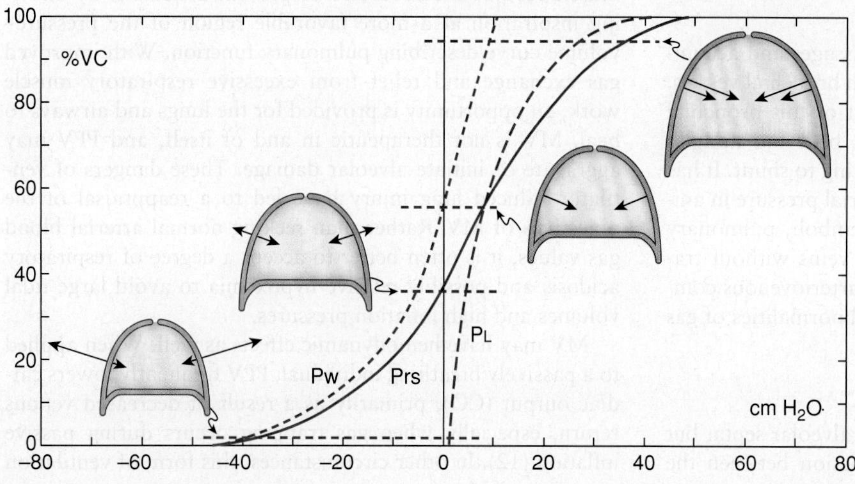

FIGURE 14.2 Static volume–pressure curves of the lung (P_L), chest wall (P_W), and total respiratory system (P_{rs}) during relaxation in the sitting posture. The static forces of the lung and the chest wall are pictured by the *arrows* in the side drawings. The dimensions of the *arrows* are not to scale; the volume corresponding to each drawing is indicated by the horizontal *broken lines.* (From Vassilakopoulos T, Zakynthinios S, Roussos C. Muscle function: basic concepts. In: Marini JJ, Slutsky AS, eds. *Physiological Basics of Ventilatory Support.* New York: Marcel Dekker; 1998:114, with permission.)

either the lung or the chest wall become less compliant (as in interstitial fibrosis or obesity), the pressure–volume curve shifts rightward and flattens, causing FRC to decrease (20). Conversely, an increased lung compliance (as in emphysema) allows a higher resting volume.

Pleural Pressure

The fraction of change in alveolar pressure sensed in the pleural space depends on the relative compliances of the lung (C_L) and chest wall (C_W). For a given change in alveolar pressure (ΔPa), the amount transmitted to the pleural space (ΔPpl) will be:

$$\Delta Ppl = \Delta Pa\ [C_L/(C_L + C_W)]$$

An inherently stiff chest wall would allow no volume change of the lung and complete transmission of a given increment in alveolar pressure to the pleural space. Conversely, an infinitely stiff lung would transmit none of it. Under normal circumstances, the lung and chest wall are almost equally compliant throughout the tidal range, so that approximately half of any change in alveolar pressure (as when PEEP is applied) is recorded in the pleural space. In clinical practice, average pleural pressure is estimated for clinical purposes as esophageal pressure (23).

Although clinicians speak fondly of pleural pressure as if it were a unique number, pleural pressure varies considerably throughout the chest because of hydrostatic gradients (which at FRC averages 0.37 cm H_2O/cm of vertical height). That translates in to higher pleural pressure (less negative) at lung bases due to weight of the lungs. At FRC, the average pleural pressure at midlung level is negative because the lungs are held open at greater than their relaxed volume. Pleural pressure surrounds the heart, the great vessels, and large airways, therefore affecting the vascular pressures measured at intrathoracic sites.

Effects of Changes in Lung Volume

Airway Resistance

Lung volume exerts a strong influence on airway resistance because resistance is inversely proportional to the fourth power of the radius of a conduit such as a bronchus. Pleural pressure surrounds the largest airways, while airways deeper within the lung are tethered open by the wall tension forces of the alveoli. Hence, as lung volume increases, the diameter of all airways increases, and resistance falls. Conversely, if a normal lung is held at a low resting lung volume, as in obesity, airway resistance will be high. In most restrictive diseases of lung tissue (e.g., interstitial fibrosis), the effects of heightened recoil on the airway diameter and driving force are usually more than sufficient to offset the effect of reduced volume, and flow rates are high relative to volume.

Pulmonary Vascular Resistance

Raising the lung volume has a different effect on the resistance of pulmonary vessels. Although the extra-alveolar vessels expand for reasons similar to those outlined for the airways, the capillaries are compressed as vascular pressures fall relative to alveolar pressure, and net pulmonary vascular resistance increases with each increment of lung volume above FRC (Fig. 14.3).

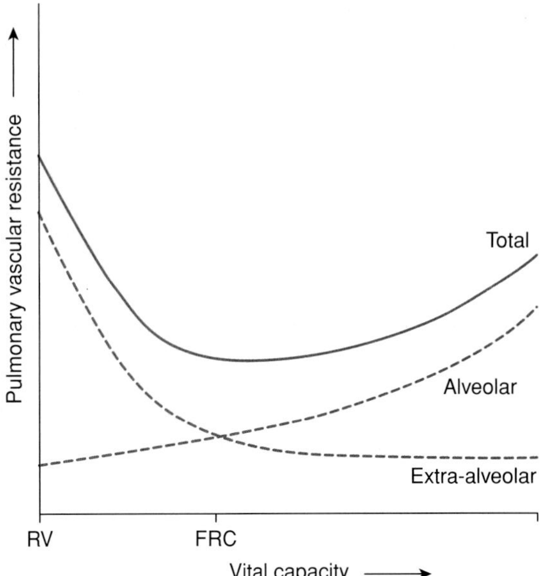

FIGURE 14.3 Schematic representation of the effects of changes in vital capacity on total pulmonary vascular resistance and the contributions to the total afforded by alveolar and extra-alveolar vessels. During inflation from residual volume (RV) to total lung capacity (TLC), resistance to blood flow through alveolar vessels increases, whereas resistance through extra-alveolar vessels decreases. Thus, changes in total pulmonary vascular resistance form a U-shaped curve during lung inflation. FRC, functional residual capacity. (From Murray JF. Circulation. In: *The Normal Lung: The Basis for Diagnosis and Treatment of Pulmonary Disease.* Philadelphia: WB Saunders; 1976:131, with permission.)

Muscular Force

The lung volume has an important effect on the maximal inspiratory and expiratory muscular forces that can be generated. The magnitude of these forces can be quantified by measuring the pressure recorded against the occluded airway. At total lung capacity (TLC), the lung and chest wall exert their highest recoil pressures. More importantly, the muscles of expiration are stretched maximally and are able to generate their highest contractile forces. If the occluded airway port is suddenly released, as during coughing, intraluminal airway pressure falls. The flexible posterior walls of the central airways invaginate, and the lumen narrows markedly to a slit. As gas accelerates to a high velocity through this narrow region, it shears mucus from the airway walls and delivers it to the oropharynx. To be maximally effective, a coughing effort must be forceful and start from a high lung volume. Gas flows should not be obstructed in small airways, and the glottis must be sealed to allow pressure within the airway to build. In critically ill patients, all of these conditions may be violated simultaneously. For intubated patients, a vital capacity greater than 20 mL/kg and a maximal expiratory pressure of 60 mmHg against an occluded airway at TLC are good predictors of an effective cough post extubation. The greatest negative end-inspiratory pressure can be generated at a residual volume where the muscle fibers of the diaphragm are stretched maximally to a position of favorable mechanical advantage. This encourages some patients to unintentionally misuse incentive spirometers that place emphasis on achieving a high flow rate rather than a high inhaled volume; they often exhale below FRC in order to take advantage of higher inspiratory muscle efficiency (and the relatively minor tendency of the chest wall to spring outward) at lower volumes.

Conversely, hyperinflation causes the diaphragm to work less effectively, adding to the sense of dyspnea experienced by patients with COPD (Fig. 14.3).

Position and Lung Volume

Position has an important influence on lung volume. In assuming a recumbent supine position, FRC falls approximately 25% to 30% (approximately 1,000 mL) in the adult, with most of the decrease occurring before the Fowler (30-degree) position (24). This reduction in lung volume occurs because the abdominal contents push the diaphragm upward. In either lateral recumbent position, the lung volume at FRC is only about 15% to 20% less than the upright sitting value because the nondependent (uppermost) lung maintains its sitting lung volume, or actually distends, partially offsetting the loss of volume from the lower lung. These observations have relevance for the nursing care of postoperative and critically ill patients.

Normal Pattern of Breathing

To provide fresh gas at 5 to 7 L/min to the lungs, the thoracic pump moves a stroke volume of 5 to 7 mL/kg at a frequency of 10 to 16 per minute. Once every 8 to 10 minutes, a sigh of two to four times the normal tidal volume occurs, which apparently serves to reverse the natural tendency for the individual alveoli to collapse when ventilated at a normal but monotonous volume. Breath-to-breath FRC changes continuously, at about a constant average value (25).

Dead Space

The bronchial, nasal, and pharyngeal passages do not participate in gas exchange. This anatomic dead space varies with airway caliber and lung volume, averaging roughly 2.2 mL/kg of lean body weight at FRC. Because approximately 50% of this dead space resides in the upper airways, orotracheal intubation and tracheostomy decrease anatomic dead space significantly (26). On the other hand, face masks and ventilator tubing unflushed by fresh gas can become an extension of the anatomic dead space, increasing the work of breathing. In addition to anatomic dead space, some volume of fresh gas (the alveolar dead space) reaches alveoli but does not participate in gas exchange because of inadequate perfusion. A portion of the increased ventilation requirement observed after a large pulmonary embolus results from this mechanism. Taken together, anatomic and alveolar dead space constitute the physiologic dead space—the volume of gas moved during each tidal breath that does not participate in gas exchange. The fraction of each tidal breath wasted in this fashion, the dead space volume-to-tidal volume (V_D/V_T) ratio, can be accurately approximated by the formula:

$$V_D/V_T = (PaCO_2 - PECO_2)/PaCO_2$$

where $PaCO_2$ and $PECO_2$ are the partial pressures of CO_2 in arterial blood and mixed expired gas, respectively. At a normal tidal volume, V_D/V_T increases with age; expressed as a percentage:

$$V_D/V_T = 24.6 + 0.17 \text{ (age in years)}$$

At very low tidal volumes, V_D/V_T rises to a high value because anatomic dead space does not decrease proportionately; nonetheless, even at tidal volumes theoretically below the anatomic dead space value, some alveolar gas exchange does occur. During exercise, the V_D/V_T may fall to 20% or less, owing both to large tidal breaths and better perfusion throughout the lung.

Flow Limitation

The rate of airflow depends on the pressure difference driving the flow and the resistance:

Flow = driving pressure/resistance

Flow rates during exhalation are volume dependent because the recoil pressure that drives gas flow, as well as the airway caliber, increases progressively with lung volume. Pressure generated by elastic recoil of the lung is greatest at high lung volumes. During unforced tidal breathing, the major site of airway resistance normally resides in the nasal passages, larynx, and uppermost tracheal airway. The average pleural pressure surrounding the airways varies from −2 cm H_2O to −10 cm H_2O, never reaching a positive value relative to the intraluminal pressure. As a result, there are no compressive pleural forces that tend to narrow the airway during passive exhalation. Forceful efforts to exhale raise the pleural pressure. Increased pleural pressure adds to the recoil pressure to boost alveolar pressure and thus potentially improves the driving pressure for gas flow. However, because pressure within the airway must decline progressively to zero as the airway opening is approached, positive pleural pressure also narrows the compressible intrathoracic airway at the equal pressure point and beyond. Above approximately two-thirds of maximal effort, each additional increment in pressure narrows the airway sufficiently to offset the increment in alveolar pressure. The maximal flow rate is then said to be effort-independent at that lung volume, and remains so at smaller lung volumes, so long as the forceful effort is sustained. According to classic teaching, the point within the airway where pleural pressure and intraluminal pressure are equal (the *equal pressure point*) determines where "critical narrowing" occurs (27). Normally, it resides in the trachea or main bronchi at high lung volumes and migrates toward the alveolus as forceful expiration proceeds. A less well-known theory of flow limitation is the *wave speed theory*. Although scientifically more defensible than the equal pressure point theory, it is less intuitive and less widely known. Both theories predict that once flow limitation occurs, flow rate is determined only by the recoil pressure of the lung and resistance of the airway segment upstream of the critical pressure point.

Reproducibility stemming from effort independence is the main reason why effort-independent, forced spirometry values (such as FEV_1) enjoy popularity as indices for evaluating airflow obstruction. Peak flow rate, which occurs before 25% of the vital capacity has been exhaled and all inspiratory flow rates are effort-dependent, is therefore less reproducible. There are some disadvantages in using maximal flow rates, however. Some patients with emphysema have such collapsible airways that flow rates demonstrate negative effort dependence (i.e., flow rates worsen with increasing effort).

Work of Breathing

Energy must be expended in moving gas to and from the alveoli, primarily against frictional and elastic forces (28–31). Under extreme ventilatory burdens, such exertion may contribute substantially to total oxygen consumption. The main portion of fractional resistance arises from collisions of gas molecules with the surfaces of the airway. Work done against friction depends strongly upon airway size, increasing rapidly as airway caliber narrows. For this reason, frictional work varies inversely with lung volume, which influences luminal diameter. When airways are narrowed by obstructive disease, a relatively small increase in resting lung volume can reduce the work dissipated against frictional forces substantially. During normal breathing, this increase in lung volume simultaneously imposes an additional elastic cost that partially offsets any frictional reduction.

The elastic forces that oppose inflation originate within the lung parenchyma and chest wall. The tendency for the thorax to recoil inward increases in nearly linear proportion to lung volume throughout the physiologic range. Diseases such as interstitial fibrosis and obesity may dramatically increase the effort required to distend the lung against recoil forces (20). When total work done against the combined frictional and elastic forces is plotted against lung volume, the minimum value normally occurs near FRC. Patients with airflow obstruction reduce their workload if they breathe at relatively high lung volumes, since frictional work may fall dramatically as lung volume increases. Dynamic hyperinflation contributes very substantially to the work of breathing (12,32). Conversely, patients with restrictive parenchymal disease may perform less total work at lower lung volumes as the reduction in elastic work more than compensates for the increase in frictional work. Under normal circumstances, FRC is set near the volume at which total work of breathing is minimized. In cases of advanced airflow obstruction, the end-expiratory lung volume may exceed the predicted FRC. Lung emptying is slowed and expiration is interrupted by the next inspiratory effort, before the patient has reached the static equilibrium volume. Positive alveolar pressure generated during this process is termed *dynamic hyperinflation,* and is quantified by stopping flow at end expiration. This allows auto-PEEP (intrinsic PEEP) to be approximated (12,33).

VENTILATION/PERFUSION RELATIONSHIPS

Distribution of Ventilation and Perfusion

Ventilation

Alveoli contiguous to the pleura are kept open by a positive distending pressure (Palv – Ppleural). At the same horizontal level, a net pressure—very nearly equal to pleural pressure—surrounds the alveoli deep within the lung parenchyma due to the phenomenon of interdependence, which links each alveolar wall to its immediate and distant neighbors. Although the alveolar distending pressures across a given horizontal slice of the lung are similar, the vertical gradient of pleural pressure—approximately 0.3 cm H_2O/vertical centimeter at FRC—causes a more negative pleural pressure at the apex of the upright lung than at the base (34,35). Consequently, the apical alveoli and airways are larger at FRC than their basal counterparts. However, as pleural pressure falls during inhalation, it does so unevenly; pressure falls most in the dependent regions closer to the diaphragm. This larger pressure swing, together with the fact that smaller alveoli are more compliant than larger ones, causes the bases to ventilate better than the apices. The same principles hold in the supine, prone, and lateral positions; uppermost lung regions are held open at higher volumes, but the dependent lung regions are better ventilated—a good rationale for periodically turning bedridden patients from side to side. These principles, which apply to spontaneous breathing, do not necessarily hold for patients receiving PPV in a passive mode.

Perfusion

The relationship of ventilation to dependency is fortunate, considering that the distribution of pulmonary blood flow follows a similar rule. Because of its low resistance, the normal pulmonary vascular bed is a low-pressure circuit, with resting pressures in the central arteries averaging approximately 25/10 mmHg (mean 15 mmHg). Pulmonary venous pressure is similar to that of the left atrium, oscillating between 3 and 10 mmHg with the cardiac cycle. Because the apices are positioned at least 10 cm above the hila in the upright position, many capillaries therein must "wink" open and closed at different phases of the breathing cycle during the tidal breathing cycle. Hydrostatic pressure adds to luminal pressure so that vessels in the dependent regions are relatively dilated and the driving pressure for flow is relatively high. Hence, perfusion improves markedly, proceeding from apex to base (36). This helps explain why emboli localize to the lower lobes and why collapse of the air spaces at the base can cause profound hypoxemia, while upper lobe atelectasis seldom does. Given the patient with unilateral parenchymal disease and a choice of placing the patient in either lateral position to improve gas exchange, the good lung should be placed dependent for two reasons: The good lung will receive a higher percentage of total ventilation and perfusion, and the bad lung will be subjected to higher distending pressures. One should be concerned, however, that mucus and other noxious liquids produced in the "bad" lung could flood the dependent "good" lung, unless precautions are taken. Although dependency causes both ventilation and perfusion per unit volume to increase, the effect on perfusion is more striking, and therefore the regional ventilation-to-perfusion ratio is highest at the apex and lowest at the base (35,36).

Regulation of Regional Perfusion

Blood flow through a lung region depends on the relationship between the alveolar pressure and pulmonary arterial and venous pressures. According to what is presently believed, if alveolar pressure exceeds arterial pressure, alveolar capillaries will pinch closed, and no blood will flow except through "corner" vessels that are subjected to different distending forces (37). If alveolar pressure is less than arterial pressure but exceeds venous pressure, flow through the region will be driven by the difference between arterial and alveolar (not venous) pressures. If venous pressure is higher than alveolar pressure, flow will be dependent on the arterial minus venous pressure difference, independent of alveolar pressure. Zones reflecting each of these conditions can be identified during tidal breathing (36,38–40). The influence of alveolar pressure on capillary patency is particularly important to consider when high levels of PEEP are applied to the airway. If alveolar pressure exceeds pulmonary venous pressure, balloon occlusion pulmonary (wedge) pressure will reflect alveolar—not pulmonary venous—pressure through at least a portion of the respiratory cycle.

Capillary Recruitment

Resistance has an inverse relation with flow, therefore, at a given lung volume, pulmonary vascular resistance falls as flow increases. Rising pulmonary arterial pressure recruits previously unperfused capillaries so that a fivefold increase in CO during exercise results in a smaller than twofold increase in mean pulmonary arterial pressure; the ventilation-to-perfusion match-up also becomes more uniform under these conditions. In a patient with a partially obliterated pulmonary vascular bed—for example, emphysema or interstitial fibrosis—no capillaries may remain to be recruited at rest. In this condition, even modest increments in CO or pulmonary vascular resistance cause pulmonary artery pressure to increase dramatically.

Active Vasoconstriction

Apart from the effect of capillary recruitment, pulmonary blood flow can be regionally controlled by active constriction of vascular smooth muscle. If vascular smooth muscle hypertrophy is due to chronic hypertension, the response to vasoconstricting stimuli may be exaggerated. Alveolar hypoxia exerts by far the most important influence on variations of local vascular tone (39). Normally, this property serves a useful purpose, diverting blood away from alveoli that are poorly ventilated. However, acting against a background of a restricted capillary bed, widespread hypoxic vasoconstriction may cause excessive pulmonary artery pressure and precipitate acute right ventricular failure, as in exacerbated COPD. Acidemia is a weaker stimulus to pulmonary artery vasoconstriction that adds to the effect of alveolar hypoxia.

Other stimuli can influence vasomotor tone. Hypertonic fluids, such as angiographic contrast media, can cause a striking vasoconstrictor response. This is believed to be a major mechanism causing sudden death in angiographic studies of patients with pulmonary hypertension (40). Vasoactive substances such as serotonin, histamine, and prostaglandin F_2-α released by clinical events such as pulmonary embolism produce notable vasoconstriction, while α-adrenergic vasopressors, such as norepinephrine, cause little response. Unfortunately, relatively few available drugs produce potent vasodilation. Prostacyclin (intravenous or aerosolized) and inhaled nitric oxide, however, are exceptions (41). Aminophylline, isoproterenol, and calcium channel blockers (e.g., nifedipine) also act as pulmonary vasodilators. In the outpatient setting, bosentan and sildenafil have an undeniable vasodilating effect, but over a longer term.

Regulation of Regional Ventilation

Ventilation to a given lung region depends not only on the stress (pressure difference) applied, but also on the regional compliance of that unit and the resistance to air entry (42,43). The product of resistance and compliance is known as the *time constant*, RC(τ), by analogy to electrical capacitors. A region with a low time constant (e.g., a stiff lung unit with open conducting airway) will fill and empty rapidly, and be relatively well ventilated for the amount of stress applied, compared to immediate neighbors having higher time constants. Healthy lungs depend upon contraction and relaxation of the bronchial smooth muscle to change the resistance and compliance of local units. Both β sympathetic and parasympathetic nerves innervate the bronchial smooth muscle. Vagal fibers are distributed throughout the tracheobronchial tree, while sympathetic fibers appear to concentrate in small airways. Under normal resting conditions, there is tonic vagal tone. Irritating stimuli, such as smoke, can trigger mild generalized bronchoconstriction, even among normal subjects, and localized bronchoconstriction occurs in an inflamed bronchus. Although found in some animal species, α receptors on bronchial smooth muscle are difficult to demonstrate in humans. Carbon dioxide bronchodilates while hypocarbia bronchoconstricts; diminished CO_2 delivery and resulting bronchoconstriction in conjunction with inflammatory mediators may partially explain the ventilation defects occasionally seen in the region of a pulmonary embolus. Hypoxemia and acidosis may also cause some degree of bronchoconstriction. Many circulating agents affect bronchial tone; epinephrine and other catecholamines that stimulate β_2 receptors bronchodilate, as do cholinergic blockers, certain prostaglandins, nitric oxide, and theophylline derivatives. Histamine, prostaglandin F_2-α, and perhaps α-adrenergic stimulators bronchoconstrict.

GAS EXCHANGE AND TRANSPORT

The Respiratory Quotient

The primary function of ventilation is to allow the exchange of CO_2 generated in body tissues for the O_2 available in the inspired gas mixture. In the adult of average size at rest, approximately 250 mL of oxygen are consumed by the tissues per minute, whereas 200 mL of CO_2 are generated—a respiratory quotient (CO_2/O_2 = RQ) of 0.8. Over a long period of time, the ratio of gases exchanged with the atmosphere, RER (respiratory exchange ratio measured in cardiopulmonary exercise from expired gas analysis), must equal the RQ. Transiently, however, this atmospheric exchange ratio may exceed or be less than RQ, as during hyper- or hypoventilation. Important increases in the CO_2 production relative to the oxygen consumption ratio can occur with the shift to a high-carbohydrate diet. Starvation and the development of certain metabolically stressful conditions (e.g., sepsis) reduce CO_2 generation.

Alveolar Gas Equation

Gases move between the blood and alveolar spaces by diffusing from areas of higher partial pressure to those with lower partial pressure (44). As fresh gas is inspired at local barometric pressure, it is warmed to body temperature and humidified before it reaches the carina. At saturation, the partial pressure exerted by water vapor at 37°C is 47 mmHg, independent of barometric pressure. Thus:

$$PiO_2 = FiO_2\ (P_B - 47)$$

where PiO_2 is the partial pressure of oxygen in the central airways, FiO_2 is the fraction of oxygen in the inspired gas mixture, and P_B is barometric pressure in millimeters of mercury. Barometric pressure falls with ascending altitude (45). Although 750 mmHg at sea level, P_B is 520 mmHg at 10,000 ft.

In the steady state, the partial pressure of oxygen at the alveolar level (P_AO_2) can be estimated from the simplified alveolar gas equation, which is based on the principle of conservation of mass:

$$P_AO_2 = PiO_2 - (PaCO_2)/RQ$$

$PaCO_2$, the partial pressures of CO_2 in arterial blood, and the alveolar PCO_2 of well-perfused units remain nearly equivalent, even in disease, so that $PaCO_2$ is usually measured and substituted. Transient episodes of hyperventilation and breath-holding can result in oxygen tensions that are considerably higher or lower than the values predicted.

Alveolar-Arterial Oxygen Tension Difference

The alveolar gas equation is worth remembering because the difference between calculated PAO_2 and measured PaO_2 (known variously as the A-a PO_2 difference, A-a DO_2, or the A-a gradient) provides a measure of the efficiency of gas exchange between the alveolus and the arterial blood. The normal A-a gradient increases with FiO_2 and with age. When supine, A-a DO_2 is approximately 10 mmHg for a healthy young person at sea level when breathing air and 100 mmHg while breathing 100% oxygen. Hyperventilation and hypoventilation do not noticeably affect it. The A-a DO_2 is a particularly useful index when monitoring patients who require supplemental oxygen.

Causes of Arterial Hypoxemia

Arterial oxygen content may fall due to one of six mechanisms: inhalation of a hypoxic gas mixture as in high altitude, hypoventilation, impaired diffusion of oxygen from alveolar space to pulmonary capillary, ventilation/perfusion mismatching, shunting of venous blood past alveolar capillaries, or admixture of abnormally desaturated systemic venous blood (34). A decrease in the barometric pressure, as at high altitude, will cause hypoxemia for obvious reasons. In the steady state and in accordance with the alveolar gas equation, hypoventilation will cause alveolar PO_2 (PAO_2) to fall as oxygen is consumed, but not replenished, at a sufficient rate. The impaired diffusion of oxygen can result in incomplete equilibration of alveolar and pulmonary capillary blood, but this appears to be of limited clinical importance except when the lung parenchyma is seriously abnormal, with decreased capillary surface area and a shorter blood transit time with increased CO, as seen in exercise. The increased distance for diffusion between the alveolus and erythrocyte, the decreased gradient for O_2 diffusion, and the shortened transit time of the red cell through the capillary all adversely influence diffusion (44). Under ordinary circumstances, however, none of these factors acting in isolation slows the equilibration sufficiently to prevent the saturation of end-capillary blood. Nonetheless, a combination of adverse influences may cause enough impairment of diffusion to contribute to hypoxemia (e.g., diffusion impairment probably contributes to the hypoxemia of a person with interstitial fibrosis during exercise).

Ventilation/Perfusion Mismatch

Regional mismatching of ventilation and perfusion is perhaps the most frequent cause of clinically important desaturation (e.g., COPD). *Regional* is the key word when the entire lung is considered. It is not the ratio of minute ventilation relative to total pulmonary blood flow that determines whether hypoxemia occurs, but rather whether ventilation and perfusion distribute appropriately (e.g., one lung could receive all ventilation and the other lung all perfusion, for an overall ventilation/perfusion [V/Q] ratio of 1.0). Units that are relatively poorly ventilated in relation to the perfusion they receive cause desaturation; high V/Q units contribute to alveolar and physiologic dead space, and hypoxemia. Unfortunately, overventilating some units to compensate for others that are underventilated may keep $PaCO_2$—but not PaO_2—at the proper level. Aliquots of blood exiting from different lung units mix gas *contents,* not partial pressures. For CO_2 content, which relates linearly to alveolar ventilation in the physiologic range, a unit with good ventilation can compensate for an underventilated unit. However, at normal barometric pressure, only a little more oxygen can be loaded onto blood with already saturated hemoglobin, no matter how high the oxygen tension in the overventilated units may rise. Hence, when equal amounts of blood from well and poorly ventilated units blend their contents, the result is blood with O_2 content halfway between them and a PaO_2 only slightly higher than that of the lower V/Q unit. Supplementing the FiO_2 will cause arterial hypoxemia to reverse impressively as the PAO_2 of even poorly ventilated units climbs high enough to achieve saturation. After breathing 100% oxygen for a sufficient period of time, only those units that are totally—or almost totally—unventilated will contribute to hypoxemia.

Shunt

Hypoventilation, impaired diffusion, and V/Q mismatching all respond to supplemental oxygen; however, hypoxemia caused by true shunt physiology is unresponsive to oxygen supplementation. Coronary veins draining directly in the left ventricle represents natural shunt that exist universally, but is seldom clinical significance. Units that are totally unventilated are unresponsive to oxygen therapy and contribute to intrapulmonary shunt. Shunt can also be intracardiac, as in cyanotic (right to left) congenital heart disease, or can result from the passage of blood between abnormal vascular communications within the lung, as occurs with pulmonary arteriovenous communications. If given oxygen for 15 minutes, the percentage of blood flow being shunted can be calculated from the formula:

$$Qs/Qt = [(CcO_2 - CaO_2)/(CcO_2 - CvO_2)] \times 100$$

where Qs denotes shunted blood flow, Qt denotes total blood flow, C denotes content, and c, a, and v denote end-capillary, arterial, and mixed venous, respectively (46). End-capillary PO_2 is assumed to equal PAO_2, which in turn is calculated from the simplified alveolar gas equation. Although it is best to measure mixed venous oxygen content directly, stable patients with presumed normal CO, hemoglobin, and oxygen consumption can reasonably be estimated to have a normal CvO_2, so long as arterial blood is near full saturation. For a patient breathing pure oxygen, a shunt fraction less than 25% can be estimated rapidly by dividing the A-a difference (670 – PaO_2) by 20, again with the proviso that the mixed venous oxygen content is normal. At lower inspired oxygen fractions, true shunt cannot be reliably estimated by an analysis of oxygen contents, but part of the CO perfusing unventilated alveoli, termed the venous admixture or physiologic shunt, can. Although V/Q mismatch, as well as true shunt, may contribute to a lower than normal PaO_2, any desaturation can be considered as if it originated from true shunt units. To calculate venous admixture, CcO_2 in the shunt formula is calculated from the ideal PAO_2 existing at that particular inspired oxygen fraction.

As the percentage of true shunt rises, supplemental oxygen becomes progressively less effective in raising PaO_2. When true shunt fraction is higher than 25%, little benefit accrues from raising the FiO_2 above 0.5. As a shunt increases, the P-to-F ratio becomes increasingly insensitive. These considerations have practical significance, because concentrations of oxygen higher than 0.5 markedly increase the risk of oxygen toxicity, but may have only marginal benefit in high shunt lungs (47). Hence, in patients with true shunt, FiO_2 can frequently be lowered out of the dangerous range without noticeably changing PaO_2. Conversely, at low shunt percentages, even small changes in shunt fraction or FiO_2 can cause major changes in PaO_2. If the venous admixture is due primarily to V/Q mismatching, the response to raising FiO_2 will depend on whether most admixture arises from units with nearly normal, moderately low, or very low V/Q ratios (48). If hypoxemia is caused by very low V/Q (but not shunt) units, little improvement may accrue until the FiO_2 approaches 1.0, at which point the PaO_2 rises abruptly.

Admixture of Abnormally Desaturated Venous Blood

Admixture of abnormally desaturated venous blood is a potentially important mechanism acting to lower PaO_2 in patients with impaired pulmonary gas exchange and reduced CO. The oxygen content of venous blood is determined by the interplay between oxygen consumption and oxygen delivery. O_2 consumption equals CO × [$CaO_2 - CvO_2$]. Oxygen delivery will be impaired if arterial content falls without a compensatory increase in tissue perfusion (e.g., anemia), or if tissue perfusion falls (e.g., shock). In the first instance, the peripheral tissues will strip the usual amount of oxygen from an already desaturated hemoglobin molecule, and the resulting venous O_2 content will drop, provided that O_2 consumption remains normal. In the second instance, venous content will fall as increased or normal amount of oxygen is removed from each unit volume of sluggishly passing blood.

If all returning venous blood goes to well-ventilated units, abnormally desaturated venous blood presents no problem, as blood exiting from the lung will be fully saturated. However, to the extent that venous admixture exists, reduced venous saturation translates into arterial desaturation. When lung parenchymal disease develops, patients with limited cardiac reserve are those at greatest jeopardy for serious desaturation by this mechanism. In such patients, there is a "positive feedback loop": arterial desaturation leads to venous desaturation, which adds to venous admixture and impairs arterial oxygenation further. Even with stable lung parenchymal disease, serious arterial desaturation can occur if CO falls disproportionately to oxygen consumption. Thus, in many intensive care patients, PaO_2 fluctuates considerably, independent of changes in the lungs.

GAS TRANSPORT AND STORAGE

Oxygen Carriage

In blood, hemoglobin binds the vast majority of oxygen, and plasma dissolves the remaining small fraction. The oxyhemoglobin dissociation relationship is curvilinear, with the knee of the curve at approximately 60 mmHg at normal pH (49). Acidosis, increased temperature, elevated $PaCO_2$, and increased erythrocyte 2,3-diphosphoglycerate (DPG) shift the curve rightward, mildly hampering loading at the alveolus but facilitating unloading of oxygen at the tissue level. At sea level, normal PaO_2 is age dependent, varying from approximately 100 mmHg at ages 20 to 80 mmHg at age 80. Because hemoglobin binding is 90% complete at a partial pressure of 60 mmHg and falls rapidly below that level, a PaO_2 of at least 60 mmHg and SaO_2 of at least 90% are commonly agreed to represent adequate oxygen loading, and are used as benchmark values for clinical purposes. Raising the PaO_2 10-fold raises the oxygen-carrying capacity a scant 12.5%. The volume of oxygen carried in 100 mL of blood can be calculated from the following formula:

$$CaO_2 = 1.39 \times [Hgb] \times \%saturation + 0.0034\ [PaO_2]$$

where Hgb is hemoglobin, expressed in grams per 100 mL of blood, and %saturation equals percentage of hemoglobin saturation. At normal rates of oxygen consumption and delivery, mixed venous blood has a PO_2 of 40 mmHg, a saturation of 75%, and an oxygen content of 15 mL oxygen per 100 mL of blood. The content difference between simultaneous arterial and mixed venous samples—the a-v O_2 content difference—averages 5 mL of oxygen per 100 mL of blood under normal circumstances. However, this difference widens when O_2 consumption is disproportionate to the rate of O_2 delivery to the tissues, as commonly occurs in states of low CO. Conversely, the difference will be narrow in sites of abnormally high blood flow, poor peripheral tissue oxygen utilization or if there are functional arteriovenous shunts in peripheral tissues.

CO_2 Carriage

Carbon dioxide is carried in the blood in three forms. The small proportion physically dissolved in plasma contributes little to CO_2 exchange between venous blood and the alveolus (about 10% of the total). CO_2 is also bound to blood proteins (mainly hemoglobin) more avidly by venous than by arterial blood. Approximately 30% of the CO_2 delivered to the alveolus is released from these "carbamino" compounds (50). Quantitatively, the majority of CO_2 carried in the blood takes the form of bicarbonate ion. With the help of erythrocyte carbonic anhydrase to speed its conversion to CO_2 as it reaches the alveolus, bicarbonate delivers approximately 60% of the total CO_2 offered for exchange.

Stores of O_2 and CO_2

Exclusive of the gas volume of the lungs, total body tissue stores of oxygen are small, scarcely more than 1 L. In addition, a considerable proportion of that stored volume is not available to the tissues without unacceptable reductions in PO_2 and the gradient for diffusion of oxygen at the tissue level. Following sudden cessation of the circulation, supplies are rapidly exhausted, and irreversible damage to certain vital organs occurs within minutes. The lungs act as a reservoir of approximately 500 mL of oxygen when breathing air; hence, PaO_2 falls more slowly during apnea than it does during circulatory arrest. It is for this reason that attempts to maintain adequate forward blood flow must not be interrupted during management of circulatory arrest. When filled with pure oxygen rather than air, the capacity of the lung reservoir is increased fivefold, and the duration of apnea before hypoxemia occurs is prolonged threefold or longer. Breathing oxygen does little to increase storage in blood and other body tissues, and PAO_2 falls precipitously upon returning to room air breathing. Thus, "preoxygenating" a patient before tracheal suctioning is ineffective if more than a few seconds elapse after oxygen is removed from the face, and is maximally effective when oxygen is continued up to the time that suction is applied. Similar considerations apply during endotracheal intubation; if the tube cannot be placed quickly and the patient continues to breathe spontaneously, the attempt to intubate should not be prolonged.

By comparison with oxygen stores, body stores of carbon dioxide are enormous—on the order of 100 times as great. As a result, it takes much longer for CO_2 to find a steady-state level after a step change in ventilation (51). Interestingly, $PaCO_2$ more rapidly achieves the steady-state value following a step *increase* in ventilation than following a step decrease. The $PaCO_2$ will have achieved its final value within 10 to 15 minutes after a ventilatory increase, although not for almost an hour or more following a decrease. These rules of thumb are helpful when deciding the time for arterial blood gas sampling during weaning efforts or when adjusting ventilator settings.

Consequences of Altered PaO_2, $PaCO_2$, and pH

Hypoxemia

Whether hypoxemia is tolerated well or poorly depends not only on the degree of desaturation, but also on compensatory mechanisms and the sensitivity of the vital organs to hypoxic stress. The major mechanisms of compensation are an increased CO to improve perfusion of vital tissues, due to capillary recruitment and changes in distribution of resistance, and increases in hemoglobin concentration. Other adaptations, such as improved downloading of oxygen by tissue acidosis and increased anaerobic metabolism, assume less importance until failure of the primary methods calls them into action, as occurs during circulatory arrest.

If a conscious individual without cardiac limitation or anemia is made mildly hypoxic over a short period of time, no important effect will be noted until PaO_2 falls below 50 to 60 mmHg. At that level malaise, light-headedness, mild nausea, vertigo, impaired judgment, and discoordination are the first symptoms, reflecting the extreme sensitivity of cerebral tissue to hypoxia (52). As minute ventilation increases, dyspnea develops, as seen at high altitude, and $PaCO_2$ levels fall unless mechanical problems, such as COPD, exist which can lead to hypercapnia. Marked confusion resembling alcohol intoxication appears as PaO_2 falls into the 35 to 50 mmHg range, especially in older individuals with ischemic cerebrovascular disease; heart rhythm disturbances also develop. Between 25 and 35 mmHg, renal blood flow decreases and urine output slows. Lactic acidosis appears at this level, even with normal cardiac function. The patient becomes lethargic or obtunded, and minute ventilation is maximal. At approximately 25 mmHg, the normal individual loses consciousness; and below that tension, minute ventilation falls due to depression of the respiratory drive center.

The sequence of events will be shifted to occur at progressively higher levels of PaO_2 if any of the major compensatory mechanisms for hypoxemia is defective. Even mild decreases in PaO_2 are poorly tolerated by an anemic patient with an impaired CO. In addition, critically ill patients may have impaired autonomic control of perfusion distribution due either to endogenous pathology (e.g., sepsis) or to vasopressor therapy.

Hyperoxia

At normal barometric pressure, venous and mean tissue oxygen tensions rise less than 10 mmHg above normal when pure oxygen is administered to healthy subjects; hence, nonpulmonary tissues are little altered. However, high concentrations of oxygen in the lung eventually replace nitrogen even in poorly ventilated regions, causing collapse of low V/Q units as oxygen is absorbed by venous blood faster than it is replenished. Diminished lung compliance results. More importantly, high oxygen tensions injure bronchial and parenchymal tissues. The toxic effects of oxygen are both time- and concentration-dependent (47). Several hours of pure oxygen breathing is sufficient to cause some sternal discomfort due to irritation of bronchial epithelium. Within 12 hours, histologic evidence of alveolar injury begins to develop. At high concentrations, parenchymal infiltration and fibrosis occur eventually, a process usually requiring days to weeks. However, many patients subjected to similar conditions undergo no detectable adverse changes. There is general agreement that very high oxygen concentrations are well tolerated for up to 48 hours. At concentrations of inspired oxygen less than 50%, clinically detectable oxygen toxicity is unusual; however long, such therapy is required.

Carbon Dioxide

Hypercapnia

The major waste product of oxidative metabolism, CO_2, is a relatively innocuous gas. Apart from its key role in regulation of ventilation, the clinically important effects of CO_2 relate to changes in cerebral blood flow, pH, and adrenergic tone. Hypercapnia dilates cerebral vessels and hypocapnia constricts them, a point of importance for patients with elevated intracranial pressure. Acute increases in CO_2 depress consciousness, probably a result of neuronal acidosis. Similar but slowly developing increases in CO_2 are well tolerated. Nonetheless, a higher $PaCO_2$ signifies alveolar hypoventilation, which causes a decrease in alveolar and arterial PO_2. With hypoxemia averted by supplemental oxygen, some outpatients with severe airflow obstruction continue to lead active lives despite higher than normal $PaCO_2$. The adrenergic stimulation that accompanies acute hypercapnia causes CO to rise and peripheral vascular resistance to increase. Diaphoresis and plethora are accompanying clinical signs. During acute respiratory acidosis, these effects may partially offset those of the hydrogen ion on cardiovascular function, allowing better tolerance of low pH than with metabolic acidosis of a similar degree. During acute respiratory acidosis, constriction of glomerular arterioles also occurs by adrenergic stimulation, sometimes producing oliguria. Muscular twitching, asterixis, and seizures may be observed at extreme levels of hypercapnia in patients made susceptible by electrolyte or neural disorders.

Hypocapnia

The major effects of acute hypocapnia relate to alkalosis and diminished cerebral blood flow. Abrupt lowering of $PaCO_2$ reduces cerebral blood flow and raises neuronal pH, causing altered cortical and peripheral nerve function. Sudden major reduction of $PaCO_2$ (e.g., shortly after initiating mechanical ventilation) can produce life-threatening seizures. Cardiac dysrhythmias are also an important consequence of abruptly lowering $PaCO_2$.

Hydrogen Ion Concentration

For mammalian cells to function optimally, hydrogen ion concentration must be rigidly controlled. The widest pH range that can be sustained for more than a few hours and is compatible with life is approximately 6.8 to 7.8 units. Although all organs malfunction to some extent during acidosis, cardiovascular function is perhaps the most impaired. Myocardial fibers contract less efficiently, systemic vessels react sluggishly to vasoconstrictive stimuli, vasomotor control deteriorates, blood pressure falls, dysrhythmias develop, and pulmonary hypertension is accentuated (53). As a result, defibrillation and cardiopulmonary resuscitation are especially difficult in an acidotic patient. In addition, acidosis profoundly affects neuronal performance, acts synergistically with alveolar hypoxia to cause pulmonary vasoconstriction, and blunts the action of adrenergic bronchodilators on the conducting airways. Each of these effects accelerates dramatically in severity as pH falls below 7.20; above this value, pH is not a major concern of itself, and should not prompt therapy aimed solely at pH correction. Indeed, the rightward shift of the oxyhemoglobin dissociation curve may improve tissue oxygen delivery if cardiovascular performance remains adequate. In this higher pH range, acutely developing acidosis is more alarming for what it signifies: Seriously compromised ventilatory, metabolic, or cardiovascular systems in need of urgent attention.

Alkalosis causes less apprehension among physicians than acidosis of a similar degree because the etiology is usually less life threatening. However, alkalosis is detrimental with regard to the release of oxygen to the tissues, shifting the oxyhemoglobin dissociation curve leftward. Raised pH does not exert the dangerously depressing influence on myocardium and blood vessels seen with a similar degree of acidosis. Furthermore, unless very abrupt and severe, the effects of raised pH on the brain are limited to confusion and encephalopathy. The major risk of extreme alkalosis appears to relate to cardiac dysrhythmias, which are caused in part by electrolyte shifts—decreased calcium, intracellular shift of potassium with intravascular hypokalemia—and diminished oxygen delivery.

To keep hydrogen ion concentration within narrow limits, its generation rate must equal the elimination rate. The hydrogen ion is generated in two ways: One by hydration of CO_2 from "volatile" acid (according to the reaction complex formula) and another by the production of fixed acid from the by-products of metabolism such as sulfates and phosphates (49,53). Ventilation eliminates the volatile acid load after reversal of the CO_2 hydration reaction in the lung capillaries, while the kidney excretes the bulk of the fixed acid load. Quantitatively, the lungs are much more important, as they eliminate a much greater acid load (53). If the excretion of CO_2 speeds or slows inappropriately, the result is respiratory derangement of the acid–base balance. If the excretion rate of fixed acid speeds or slows in relation to production, or if abnormal metabolic loads of acid or alkali develop that cannot be handled, metabolic acidosis or alkalosis occurs. A complete discussion of acid–base physiology is beyond the scope of this chapter.

Control of Ventilation

The respiratory center of the medulla modifies its own cyclic rhythm by integrating signals from many sources (54). These inputs, which may be of cortical, chemical, or reflex origin, cause changes in the timing frequency in the depth of tidal breathing. In general, each potential modifier of medullary activity is much more potent as a stimulus to increase breathing than as a depressant to retard the endogenous level of breathing set by the respiratory center. Efferent flow descends via the phrenic nerves to the diaphragm and via the spinal nerves to the intercostal and abdominal muscles. Control of output from the medullary respiratory center is an interactive process. For example, the precise effect of a given rise in $PaCO_2$ will depend on the levels of cortical arousal, PaO_2, and pH. The result of that neural output will depend on the ability of the ventilatory muscles to contract in a coordinated fashion and on the lungs to ventilate upon command.

Chemical Stimuli

Under normal resting conditions, cerebrospinal fluid (CSF) hydrogen ion concentration is the predominant influence over ventilation. As in the periphery, the ratio of bicarbonate concentration to PCO_2 determines pH. Unlike CO_2, which transports passively across the blood–brain barrier, the bicarbonate concentration of the CSF is maintained somewhat lower than in blood by an active process (the "brain kidney"). This mechanism is capable of making relatively rapid compensatory adjustments in bicarbonate so that CSF pH is restored almost completely to its normal resting value of 7.3 within 12 hours following a derangement (54,55). By comparison, the CO_2 crosses the juxtamedullary area quickly and passively. Thus, an abrupt rise in $PaCO_2$ precipitates CSF acidosis, prompting increased ventilation to restore pH balance. The potency of an increase in $PaCO_2$ wanes with time, as CSF bicarbonate rises to compensate. Conversely, the ventilatory compensation for sustained metabolic acidosis is maximized by carotid and aortic bodies in 12 or more hours following its onset, since initially peripheral pH receptors drive $PaCO_2$ to low levels and create CSF alkalosis, which temporarily limits the ventilatory increase.

$PaCO_2$ drives ventilation mainly through its effect on intracerebral hydrogen ion concentration. However, a rise in $PaCO_2$ also stimulates receptors at the carotid bifurcation, perhaps due to the peripheral pH receptors located there. The level of PaO_2 modifies the ventilatory response to CO_2, increasing it when hypoxemia occurs. Thus, when hypoxemia is relieved—as during treatment of the compensated COPD—$PaCO_2$ is expected to rise somewhat, even if the respiratory center is otherwise normally responsive to CO_2. The rise in CO_2 will be exaggerated if CO_2 sensitivity is reduced. Cortical depression, whether caused by sleep or sedative drugs, limits the response to CO_2, especially in patients with a previously blunted drive to breathe. Prolonged mechanical stress may also alter the sensitivity to chemical stimuli. Although the most common example of reduced CO_2 sensitivity occurs in chronic airflow obstruction, even normal individuals increase the CO_2 set point if made to breathe against resistance for an extended period of time. Teleologically, this occurs because total work of breathing lessens when $PaCO_2$ rises to make each tidal exchange more efficient.

PaO_2 is an important stimulus for ventilation only when the blood is significantly desaturated (54). Oxygen receptors located mainly in the carotid body send neural signals to the medulla. Extreme hypoxia depresses rather than stimulates ventilation by direct depression of the respiratory center. With advancing age, the ventilatory response to hypoxemia diminishes, perhaps a consequence of carotid artery sclerosis. Starvation and sedatives also attenuate the hypoxic ventilatory drive. Systemic acidosis is a very potent drive to ventilation, with its effect at least additive to that of hypoxemia when the two occur together, as they often do clinically. The receptors for peripheral blood pH are located in the carotid body.

Nonchemical Stimuli

Neural reflexes originating from receptors located within the lung or chest wall may drive ventilation. Thus, the hyperventilation that occurs during the early phases of asthma and pulmonary edema, as well as the chronic hyperventilation of interstitial fibrosis, may result from stimulation of normally quiescent receptors. Central neurogenic hyperventilation and Cheyne–Stokes breathing (on average, also a hyperventilatory pattern) usually result from intracerebral pathology and may be modified by neuromuscular input.

Clinical Disorders of Ventilatory Control

For therapeutic purposes, it is important when evaluating hypercapnia to distinguish patients with depressed drives ("won't" breathers) from those whose condition, such as COPD or neuromuscular disease, will not allow them to achieve normal alveolar ventilation ("can't" breathers). Many patients present with combined problems of drive and mechanics. For example, because advanced age and starvation may blunt ventilatory drives, an elderly patient with acutely elevated ventilation requirements and mechanical stress (e.g., pneumonia) often presents with a component of respiratory acidosis as well as hypoxemia. Clues to primary respiratory center dysfunction include no evidence of obstruction or neuromuscular disease, normal A-a DO_2, and the preserved ability to drive $PaCO_2$ considerably below normal with voluntary hyperventilation. Because a wide spectrum of response to PCO_2 and PaO_2 exist even among healthy normal subjects, it is not surprising that two otherwise indistinguishable patients with the same pulmonary pathology may set very different levels of alveolar ventilation.

Sleep routinely blunts the chemical drives to breathe (56–58). Many chronic disorders can depress the respiratory center function. Among these, hypothyroidism, narcotic overdose, and the obesity hypoventilation syndrome are perhaps the most reversible. The utility of respiratory center stimulants is limited. Stimulants are contraindicated for patients with problems confined to disordered mechanics, such as COPD, since dyspnea may worsen with little beneficial effect. Progesterone increases CO_2 drive in pregnant women and has been used therapeutically as a ventilatory stimulant for primary hypoventilation (59). Its maximal effect is delayed several days. Conversely, testosterone blunts CO_2 responsiveness (60). Newer drugs touted to selectively improve alertness (e.g., modafinil, atomoxetine) may prove useful when somnolence contributes to hypoventilation.

Key Points

- Understanding basic concepts in lung physiology are essential to achieve the goals of optimal oxygen delivery and aerobic cellular metabolism.
- The functions of the respiratory system include gas exchange, acid–base balance, phonation, pulmonary defense and metabolism, and the handling of bioactive materials.
- Ventilation and perfusion must be matched on the alveolar-capillary level for optimal gas exchange. Alveolar dead space and intrapulmonary shunt represent the two extremes of ventilation–perfusion ratios, infinite and zero, respectively.
- Tissue hypoxia can be a result of low alveolar P_{O2}, diffusion impairment, right-to-left shunts, or ventilation–perfusion mismatch (hypoxic hypoxia); decreased functional hemoglobin (anemic hypoxia); low blood flow (hypoperfusion hypoxia); or an inability of mitochondria to use oxygen (histotoxic hypoxia).
- Maintenance of adequate and safe alveolar-distending pressure, also referred as the *transpulmonary pressure* is essential during mechanical ventilation to avoid complications from under or over ventilation.

ACKNOWLEDGMENTS
We thank John J. Marini, David J. Dries, and John F. Perry, Jr. for their contribution to the last edition of this chapter.

References

1. Weibel ER. *Morphometry of the Human Lung*. Berlin: Springer; 1963.
2. Nunn JF. *Applied Respiratory Physiology*. 3rd ed. London: Butterworths; 1987.
3. Macklem PT, Wilson NJ. Measurement of intrabronchial pressure in man. *J Appl Physiol*. 1965;20:653–663.
4. Glazier JB, Hughes JM, Maloney JE, et al. Vertical gradient of alveolar size in lungs of dogs frozen intact. *J Appl Physiol*. 1967;23:694–705.
5. Fraser RG, Paré JA, Paré PD, et al. *Diagnosis of Diseases of the Chest*. 3rd ed. Philadelphia, PA: Saunders; 1988.
6. Crapo JD, Barry BE, Gehr P, et al. Cell number and cell characteristics of the normal human lung. *Am Rev Respir Dis*. 1982;126:332–337.
7. Hocking WG, Golde DW. The pulmonary-alveolar macrophage (two parts). *N Engl J Med*. 1979;301:580–587, 639–645.
8. Rubins J. Alveolar macrophages: wielding the double edge sword of inflammation. *Am J Resp Crit Care Med*. 2003;167:103–104.
9. Staub NC. J Pulmonary edema. *Physiol Rev*. 1974;54:678–811.
10. Dreyfuss D, Saumon G. Ventilator-induced lung injury: lessons from experimental studies. *Am J Respir Crit Care Med*. 1998;157:294–323.
11. Tobin MJ. Mechanical ventilation. *N Engl J Med*. 1994;330:1056–1061.
12. Pepe PE, Marini JJ. Occult positive end-expiratory pressure in mechanically ventilated patients with airflow obstruction: the auto-PEEP effect. *Am Rev Respir Dis*. 1982;126:166–170.

13. Chatburn RL, Primiano FP Jr. A new system for understanding modes of mechanical ventilation. *Respir Care*. 2001;46:604–621.
14. Loring SH. Mechanics of lungs and chest wall. In: Marini JJ, Slutsky AS, eds. *Physiological Basis of Ventilatory Support*. New York: Marcel Dekker; 1998:177–208.
15. Agostoni E, Mead J. Statics of the respiratory system. In: Fenn WO, Rahn H, eds. *Handbook of Physiology. Section 3: Respiration*. Vol. 1. Washington, DC: American Physiological Society; 1964:387–409.
16. Rodarte JH. Lung and chest wall mechanics: basic concepts. In: Scharf SM, Cassidy SS, eds. *Heart-Lung Interactions in Health and Disease*. New York: Marcel Dekker; 1989:221–242.
17. DeTroyer A, Loring SH. Actions of the respiratory muscles. In: Roussos C, Macklem PT, eds. *The Thorax*. 2nd ed. New York: Marcel Dekker Inc; 1994:535–563.
18. Vassilakopoulos T, Zakynthinos S, Roussos C. Muscle function: basic concepts. In: Marini JJ, Slutsky AS, eds. *Physiological Basis of Ventilatory Support*. New York: Marcel Dekker Inc.; 1998:103–152.
19. Roussos C, Macklem PT. The respiratory muscles. *N Engl J Med*. 1982; 307:786–797.
20. Sharp JT, Barrocas M, Chokroverty S. The cardiorespiratory effects of obesity. *Clin Chest Med*. 1980;1:103–118.
21. Otis AB, Fenn WO, Rahn H. Mechanics of breathing in man. *J Appl Physiol*. 1950;2:592–607.
22. Mead J. Mechanical properties of lungs. *Physiol Rev*. 1961;41:281–330.
23. Baydur A, Behrakis PK, Zin WA, et al. A simple method for assessing the validity of the esophageal balloon technique. *Am Rev Respir Dis*. 1982;126:788–791.
24. Marini JJ, Tyler ML, Hudson LD, et al. Influence of head-dependent positions on lung volume and oxygen saturation in chronic air-flow obstruction. *Am Rev Resp Dis*. 1984;129(1):101–105.
25. Tobin MJ. Breathing pattern analysis. *Intensive Care Med*. 1992;18:193–201.
26. Fowler WS. The respiratory dead space. *Am J Physiol*. 1948;154:405–416.
27. Hyatt RE. Expiratory flow limitation. *J Appl Physiol*. 1983;55(1 Pt 1):1–7.
28. Sassoon CSH, Mahutte CK. Work of breathing during mechanical ventilation. In: Marini JJ, Slutsky AS, eds. *Physiological Basis of Ventilatory Support*. New York: Marcel Dekker; 1998:261–310.
29. Tobin MJ. Respiratory monitoring in the intensive care unit. *Am Rev Respir Dis*. 1988;138:1625–1642.
30. Otis AB. The work of breathing. In: Fenn WO, Rahn H, eds. *Handbook of Physiolog., Section 3: Respiration*. Vol. 1. Washington, DC: American Physiology Society; 1964:463–476.
31. Aubier M, Viires N, Syllie G, et al. Respiratory muscle contribution to lactic acidosis in low cardiac output. *Am Rev Respir Dis*. 1982;126:648–652.
32. Kimball WR, Leith DE, Robins AG. Dynamic hyperinflation and ventilator dependence in chronic obstructive pulmonary diseases. *Am Rev Respir Dis*. 1982;126:991–995.
33. Hoffman RA, Ershowsky P, Krieger BP. Determination of auto-PEEP during spontaneous and controlled ventilation by monitoring changes in end-expiratory thoracic gas volume. *Chest*. 1989;96:613–616.
34. Otis AB, McKerrow CB, Bartlett RA, et al. Mechanical factors in distribution of pulmonary ventilation. *J Appl Physiol*. 1956;8:427–443.
35. Permutt S, Howell JB, Proctor DF, et al. Effect of lung inflation on static pressure-volume characteristics of pulmonary vessels. *J Appl Physiol*. 1961;16:64–70.
36. West JB, Dollery CT, Naimark A. Distribution of blood flow in isolated lung: Relation to vascular and alveolar pressures. *J Appl Physiol*. 1964;19:713–724.
37. Albert RK, Lakshminarayan S, Charan NB, et al. Extra-alveolar vessel contribution to hydrostatic pulmonary edema in in situ dog lungs. *J Appl Physiol*. 1983;54(4):1010–1017.
38. Riley RL, Cournand A. Analysis of factors affecting partial pressures of oxygen and carbon dioxide in gas and blood of lungs: theory. *J Appl Physiol*. 1951;4:77–101.
39. Peake MD, Harabin AL, Brennan NJ, et al. Steady-state vascular responses to graded hypoxia in isolated lungs of five species. *J Appl Physiol*. 1981; 51(5):1214–1219.
40. Peck WW, Slutsky RA, Hackney DB, et al. Effects of contrast media on pulmonary hemodynamics: comparison of ionic and nonionic agents. *Radiology*. 1983;149:371–374.
41. Sastry BK. Pharmacologic treatment for pulmonary arterial hypertension. *Curr Opin Cardiol*. 2006;21:561–568.
42. Mead J, Whittenberger JL. Physical properties of human lungs measured during spontaneous respiration. *J Appl Physiol*. 1953;5:779–796.
43. Grassino AE, Roussos C, Macklem PT. Static properties of the chest wall. In: Crystal RG, West JB, et al., eds. *The Lung: Scientific Foundations*. New York: Raven Press; 1991:855–867.
44. Forster RE. Diffusion of gases across the alveolar membrane. In: *Handbook of Physiology. Section 3*. Washington, DC: American Physiological Society; 1987.
45. West JB. The physiologic basis of high-altitude diseases. *Ann Int Med*. 2004;141:789–800.
46. Pontoppidan H, Geffin B, Lowenstein E. Acute respiratory failure in the adult. Parts 1–3. *N Engl J Med*. 1972;287:690–698, 743–752, 799–806.
47. Deneke SM, Fanburg BL. Normobaric oxygen toxicity of the lung. *N Engl J Med*. 1980;303:76–86.
48. Dantzker DR, Brook CJ, Dehart P, et al. Ventilation-perfusion distributions in the adult respiratory distress syndrome. *Am Rev Resp Dis*. 1979;120(5):1039–1052.
49. Corey HE. Stewart and beyond: new models of acid-base balance. *Kidney Int*. 2003;64(3):777–787.
50. Severinghaus JW. Simple, accurate equations for human blood O_2 dissociation components. *J Appl Physiol*. 1979;46:599–602.
51. Ivanov SD, Nunn JF. Influence of duration of hyperventilation on rise time of P-CO_2 after step reduction of ventilation. *Respir Physiol*. 1968; 5(2):243–249.
52. Kafer ER, Sugioka K. Respiratory and cardiovascular responses to hypoxemia and the effects of anesthesia. *Intl Anesthesiol Clin*. 1981;19: 85–122.
53. Kellum JA. Clinical review: reunification of acid-base physiology. *Crit Care*. 2005;9:500–507.
54. Younes M, Georgopoulos D. Control of breathing relevant to mechanical ventilation. In: Marini JJ, Slutsky AS, eds. *Physiological Basis of Ventilatory Support*. New York: Marcel Dekker; 1998:1–74.
55. Bisgard GE, Busch MA, Forster HV. Ventilatory acclimatization to hypoxia is not dependent on cerebral hypocapnic alkalosis. *J Appl Physiol*. 1986;60:1011–1015.
56. Weinhouse GL, Schwab RJ. Sleep in the critically ill patient. *Sleep*. 2006; 29:707–716.
57. Phillips B. Sleep, sleep loss, and breathing. *Southern Med J*. 1985;78: 1483–1486.
58. Skatrud JB, Dempsey JA. Interaction of sleep state and chemical stimuli in sustaining rhythmic ventilation. *J Appl Physiol*. 1983;55:813–822.
59. Sutton FD Jr, Zwillich CW, Creagh CE, et al. Progesterone for outpatient treatment of Pickwickian syndrome. *Ann Int Med*. 1975;83:476–479.
60. Matsumoto AM, Sandblom RE, Schoene RB, et al. Testosterone replacement in hypogonadal men: effects on obstructive sleep apnoea, respiratory drives, and sleep. *Clin Endocrinol*. 1985;22:713–721.

CHAPTER

15

Cardiovascular Physiology

LUIS E. URRUTIA, CYRUS ADEL HADADI, and JAMES C. BLANKENSHIP

"We are fearfully and wonderfully made..."
Psalm 139

INTRODUCTION

The function of the cardiovascular system is to circulate blood, essential for the maintenance of the internal environment of the human body. The cardiovascular system delivers oxygen-rich blood throughout the body by means of a synchronized intrinsic mechanical pump and electrical pacemaker, at an average of 60 to 100 heart beats per minute for a remarkable feat of over 2.5 billion beats in a lifetime. Despite advances in defining the underlying cellular and physiologic dynamics of the heart, it still remains a complex biomechanical pump that is not completely understood.

STRUCTURE OF THE HEART

Structure of Cardiac Myocytes

Cardiac myocytes are the main cell type of cardiac tissue (1). They have two important functions: to contract in response to an electrical stimulus, and to simultaneously transmit the electrical stimulus to neighboring cells.

Sarcomeres and mitochondria are the dominant components of cardiac myocytes (Fig. 15.1). These two structures are responsible for contraction and supply of energy, respectively. The cardiac sarcomere consists of actin filaments, built from actin monomers with associated troponin and tropomyosin; and myosin filaments. Cardiac myocytes are surrounded by the *sarcolemma*, a specialized plasma membrane that harbors the pumps responsible for ion exchange between the intracellular and the extracellular space. The sarcolemma forms a series of tubular invaginations, the *T tubules* or transverse tubules that increase the surface area of the cell and bring the extracellular environment into close proximity to intracellular structures. The *sarcoplasmic reticulum* (SR) is a network of tubes and cysts spreading throughout the cell. Together with the T tubules, the SR generates cyclic changes in the cellular calcium concentration.

Cardiac myocytes form a functional syncytium in which cells act in concert, both mechanically and electrically. This aspect requires sophisticated communication between cardiac myocytes at the intercalated discs, a specialized portion of the sarcolemma where individual cells make contact with each other and send processes deep into the neighboring cell. The heart contains three modifications of this prototypical ventricular cardiac myocyte: atrial cardiomyocytes located in the right and left atria, pacemaker cells located in the sinoatrial (SA) and atrioventricular (AV) nodes, and Purkinje cells located in the Tawara branches. Pacemaker cells have the ability to generate an action potential (AP), and Purkinje cells have the ability to transmit this AP with high speed. Both pacemaker and Purkinje cells are, in principle, myocytes, but with specialized electrical properties. On the other hand, atrial and ventricular myocytes have specialized mechanical properties, but they also have the ability to generate and propagate APs.

Electrical Cycle

The electrical cycle of the heart derives from the excitable nature of each cardiac myocyte. These are typical cells that are specialized in two major ways: to transmit electrical signals and to transduce that electrical signal into a mechanical function, contraction (Fig. 15.2).

Resting Membrane Potential

The resting membrane potential (E_m) is defined as the voltage difference across the cellular membrane—that is, between the inside and the outside of the cell. The cardiac myocyte is engulfed by the sarcolemma, a lipid bilayer with many voltage- and ligand-gated ion channels. The most significant elements of the sarcolemma that maintain the resting membrane potential and allow for electrical signals to be both generated and transmitted are the voltage-gated ion channels, the Na^+–Ca^{2+} exchanger and the Na^+-K^+-ATPase electrogenic pump. The resting membrane potential results from the open K^+ channels in the sarcolemma and the small "leak" of Na^+ through ion channels in the sarcolemma. The resting membrane potential is described by the Nernst equation, which takes into account the permeability of the sarcolemma and its ion gradients. The resting membrane potential is calculated to be approximately –85 mV for cardiac myocytes.

Action Potential

Within the SA node are pacemaker cells that have the important characteristics of *spontaneous diastolic depolarization.* The pacemaker cells undergo a gradual depolarization from their "resting" membrane potential of –65 mV to approximately –40 mV, which is the *threshold* at which an *AP* is initiated.

The pacemaking AP is a regenerative, all-or-none, event occurring when the membrane potential depolarizes to a level where a sufficient number of ion channels open, leading to an inward current that can begin a positive feedback loop (2). The predominant ion channels responsible for the AP in the SA node pacemaker cells are T- and L-type Ca^{2+} channels. The dependence on Ca^{2+} for the depolarizing current makes the SA and AV nodes particularly sensitive to pharmacologic manipulation with Ca^{2+} channel blockers. The configuration of the SA node AP is markedly different from that in the atrial and ventricular cardiac myocytes, where voltage-gated

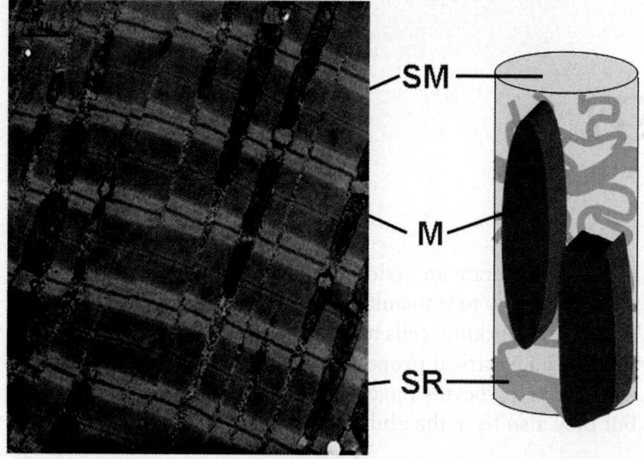

FIGURE 15.1 Internal structure of cardiomyocytes. The electron micrograph shows sarcomeres (SMs) and mitochondria (M), the dominant intracellular organelles. Sarcomeres form rods, which are surrounded by a web of sarcoplasmic reticulum (SR). Sarcomeres and mitochondria are oriented in parallel.

Na^+ channels predominate and provide the major fast inward current responsible for depolarization. Figure 15.3 provides examples of the APs from the SA node through the atria and the AV node down the bundle of His and Purkinje fibers into the ventricle. The rate of depolarization in the SA and AV nodes is considerably slower than in the rest of the heart. The reversal of the depolarization of the SA nodal pacemaker cells occurs at the peak of depolarization, with opening of delayed rectifier K^+ channels that provide the outward positive current to nullify the previous influx of positive ions, leading to repolarization of the cell. One of the most important ionic currents contributing to the automatic pacemaker ability of the SA node is the so-called "funny current," or I_f channel. The I_f channel is a mixed Na^+-K^+ inward current activated during diastolic depolarization, at approximately –40 mV, that is hyperpolarization activated and cyclical. It is named "funny current" due to its unusual properties of depolarization (3).

The AP in ventricular cardiac myocytes has a markedly different time course. As an AP passes from the conduction system to the ventricular cardiac myocytes, the voltage-gated Na^+ channels provide the positive inward current that depolarizes the ventricular myocyte. The entry of Na^+ is rapid, as can be seen from the fast upstroke of the AP, which has been named

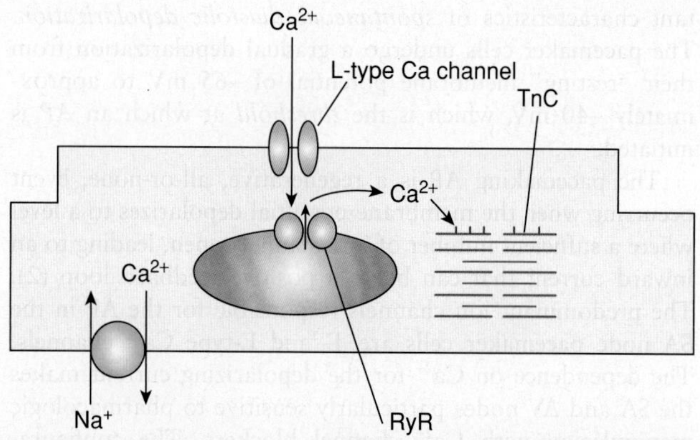

FIGURE 15.2 A schematic representing a cardiac myocyte demonstrating a few of the important Ca^{2+} regulatory sites. TnC represents troponin C and RyR represents the ryanodine receptor.

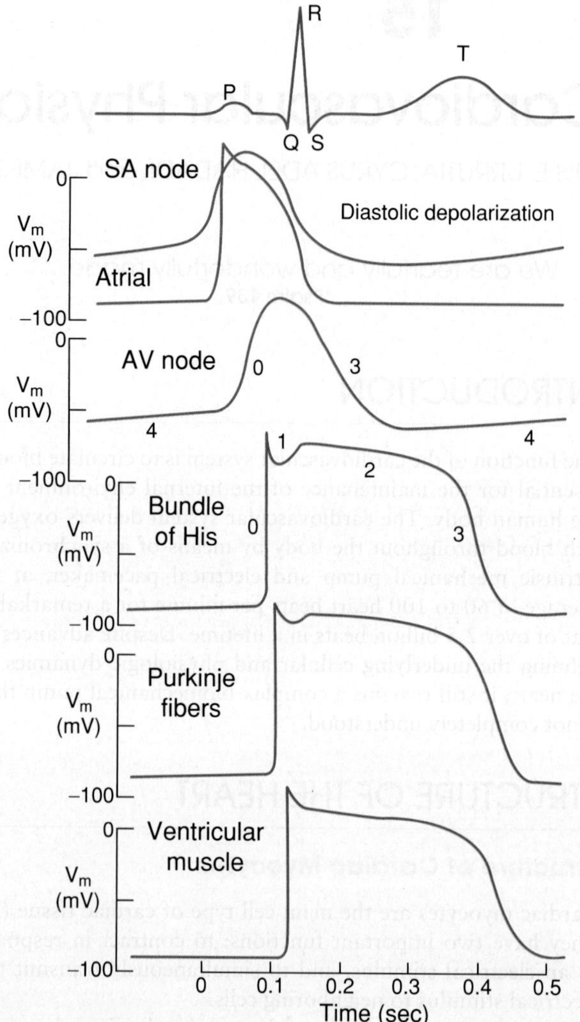

FIGURE 15.3 The surface electrocardiogram at the top of the figure and the action potential profiles throughout the heart and their temporal relationships to each other. SA, sinoatrial; AV, atrioventricular. (From Lynch C. Cellular electrophysiology of the heart. In: *Clinical Cardiac Electrophysiology: Perioperative Considerations*. Philadelphia, PA: JB Lippincott; 1994:1; with permission.)

phase 0, and is due in part to the kinetic characteristics of the voltage-gated Na^+ channel, which shows rapid activation and rapid inactivation (Fig. 15.4). The membrane potential moves toward the Nernst potential for Na^+, E_{Na^+}. *Phase 1* describes the notch in the AP that is seen at the initial reversal of the depolarization and is due to Na^+ channel inactivation and the transient outward flow of K^+ and inward flow of Cl^-. However, at this time, complete repolarization is delayed due to the opening of L-type voltage-gated Ca^{2+} channels, allowing the influx of Ca^+ and resulting in a plateau of the AP, known as *phase 2*. At the plateau, the membrane potential is held near 0 mV for about 100 milliseconds, which leads to the activation of an outward K^+ current. *Phase 3* describes the termination of the AP and the repolarization of the cell with the outflow of K^+ ions due to the opening of K^+ channels contributing to the delayed rectifier K^+ current. At *phase 4*, the cell has returned to its resting membrane potential, reestablishing its ion gradients with the activity of the Na^+-K^+-ATPase pump and the Na^+–Ca^{2+} exchanger. Ionic channels and currents that work in concert to accomplish the cardiac AP and its cyclical automaticity have

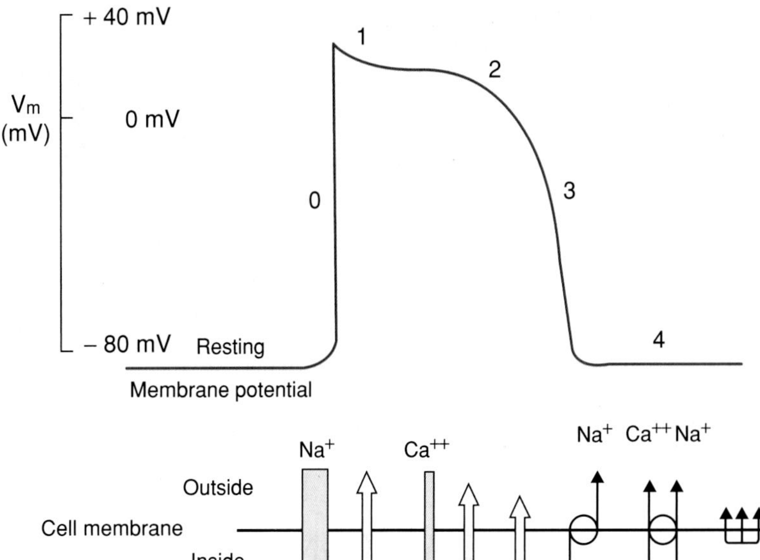

FIGURE 15.4 The ventricular cardiac myocyte action potential (AP). The numbers along the AP indicate the phases of the AP. The lower panel schematically represents the relative quantity and temporal relationship of the ionic movements involved in the AP.

highly complex organizational flows and structures that we are now beginning to understand. There are additional channels and mechanisms in the process of further investigation.

Given the importance of Na^+ and K^+ ion flow in the AP, any inborn or acquired defects in these channels may cause grave pathology. Over the past 20 years, multiple genes encoding for aberrant Na^+ and K^+ channels have been found to be responsible for inherited arrhythmias such as Brugada syndrome and long and short QT syndrome (4). These ion channel abnormalities, also known as cardiac channelopathies, can cause life-threatening arrhythmias such as ventricular tachycardia or fibrillation.

AUTONOMIC CONTROL OF THE CARDIAC ELECTRICAL ACTIVITY

The autonomic nervous system plays a major role in controlling the initiation of the heart beat and the rate of pacemaker firing. Both parasympathetic and sympathetic nervous inputs converge on the SA and AV nodal cells, exerting opposite influences on heart rate (5).

Parasympathetic Nervous System

The parasympathetic nervous system contributes nerve fibers from its cranial outflow through the cervical ganglia where preganglionic fibers course down to the cardiac plexus, and from there send postganglionic unmyelinated axons that impinge on the SA and AV nodal cells. The cardiac plexus is divided into a superficial and deep plexus; the superficial plexus is found at the base of the heart at the arch of the aorta, while the deep plexus is found on the anterior aspect of the trachea near its bifurcation. The parasympathetic fibers, carried by the vagus nerve, are cholinergic and release acetylcholine (ACh) when activated. ACh has three principal actions that result in the slowing of heart rate and a decrease in contractility: (a) activation of M2 muscarinic receptors in the SA and AV nodal cells, which (b) triggers a reduced spontaneous diastolic depolarization rate, which (c) reduces the slope of phase 0 of the AP, and thus results in a slower heart rate (5).

Sympathetic Nervous System

Sympathetic nervous input to the heart derives from preganglionic neurons in the upper four or five thoracic spinal segments. Axons pass to postganglionic neurons in thoracic and cervical ganglia. The cervical ganglia supply the superior, middle, and inferior cardiac nerves to the cardiac plexus, where they meet the thoracic cardiac nerves from the thoracic ganglia. Sympathetic nervous outflow then supplies the pacemaker cells in the SA and AV nodes, the conduction system, and both the atrial and ventricular myocytes. Norepinephrine, the major adrenergic synaptic mediator in the heart, activates specialized cardiac adrenergic receptors, the most important of which are the β_1, β_2 and α_1 receptors. Activation of β_1 and β_2 receptors leads to cardiac acceleration and increased contractility. Activation of the α_1 receptor also increases contractility. Table 15.1 illustrates the effects of adrenergic receptor activation.

TABLE 15.1 Main Effects of Receptor Activation of Adrenoreceptors

Receptor Class	Biologic Effect When Stimulated
α_1	Vasoconstriction, relaxation of GI smooth muscle, stimulation of salivary secretion
α_2	Inhibition of norepinephrine release from autonomic nerves, contraction of smooth muscle, platelet aggregation
β_1	Increased heart rate and contractility, GI smooth muscle relaxation
β_2	Bronchodilation, vasodilation, relaxation of visceral smooth muscle
β_3	Lipolysis

From Greenlee K, Militello MA. Cardiovascular medicine: essential pharmaceuticals. In: Griffin B, ed. *The Cleveland Clinic Cardiology Board Review*. 2nd ed. Philadelphia, PA: Lippincott Williams & Wilkins; 2013:882.

β-Adrenergic stimulation additionally leads to increased activation of I_f and accelerates diastolic depolarization, thus increasing the slope of phase 0 of the AP, so that a threshold is reached earlier. I_K activation and repolarization are thus faster, with the net result more frequent firing of the AP and a faster heart rate (5). Recent work has focused on the primacy of Ca^{2+} in regulating the pacemaker function of the SA node (6,7). When mechanoreceptors in the left and right atria sense increased venous return and resultant atrial stretch, an increase in sympathetic-mediated heart rate, known as the Bainbridge reflex, induces tachycardia in order to increase cardiac output (CO) and decrease intracardiac blood volume.

If both parasympathetic and sympathetic inputs to the heart are totally blocked, the heart rate actually *increases* due to the overriding parasympathetic inhibition seen in most individuals (5).

CONTRACTION–RELAXATION CYCLE

Initiating Events

The spontaneous and rhythmic electrical activity of the pacemaker cells must be transformed into regular and synchronized contraction and relaxation by the atrial and ventricular myocytes through a process described as excitation–contraction coupling. The electrical signal is uniformly passed through gap junctions from cardiac myocyte to cardiac myocyte, producing the AP. The unique characteristic of the AP essential for the initiation of the contractile process is the *plateau phase* (8). The plateau phase (Fig. 15.5) is due to the prolonged opening of the L-type Ca^{2+} channel, which provides an inward positive current of Ca^{2+}, thus maintaining the depolarization for a prolonged period. The entry of Ca^{2+} through the L-type channel initiates the sequence of events leading to contraction.

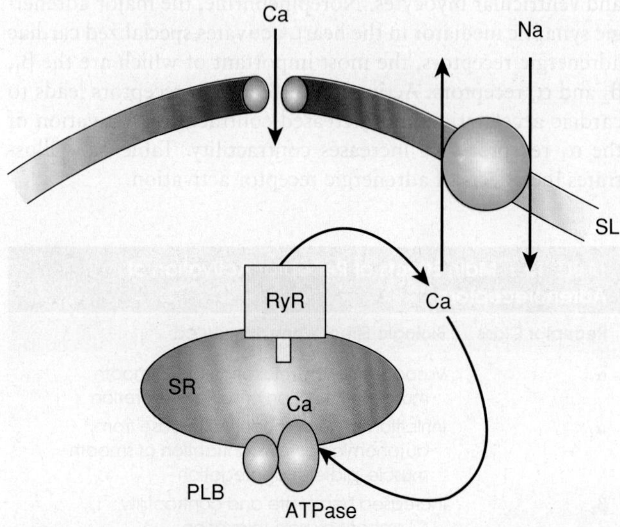

FIGURE 15.5 Proposed model of sarcoplasmic reticulum (SR) Ca^{2+} transport as a cardiac pacemaker. After a normal Ca^{2+} release, the SR Ca^{2+} uptake refills the SR with Ca^{2+} and triggers, via the ryanodine receptor, a local SR Ca^{2+} release, which triggers a Na^+–Ca^{2+} exchange current leading to the depolarization of the sinoatrial nodal cell. SL, sarcolemma; RyR, ryanodine receptor; SR, sarcoplasmic reticulum; PLB, phospholamban. (From Bers DM. The beat goes on. *Circ Res.* 2006;99:921; with permission.)

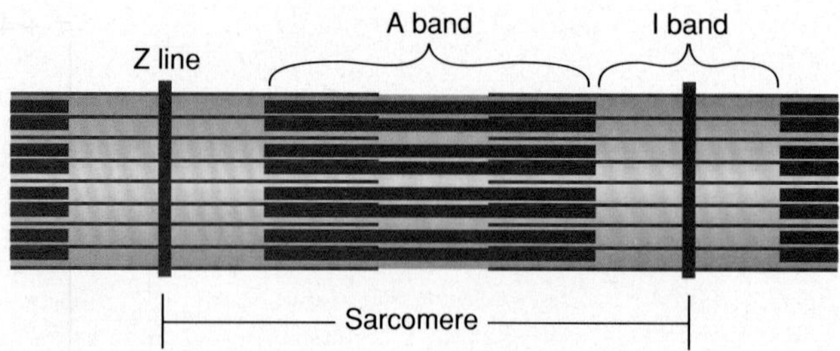

FIGURE 15.6 The sarcomere, the minimal unit of contraction in the cardiac myocyte. The A band demonstrates the overlap of thick and thin filaments. The I band represents the thin filaments anchored to the Z line.

Role of Calcium

The Ca^{2+} pump in the SR, known as the *SERCA* (sarcoendoplasmic reticulum calcium pump), transports Ca^{2+} from the cytosol back into the SR. Together with the Na^+–Ca^{2+} exchanger sarcolemmal protein, the SERCA sequesters Ca^{2+} in the SR in anticipation of the excitation–contraction–relaxation process.

Molecular Interactions

Ca^{2+} triggers the contractile process by interacting with the Ca^{2+}-binding protein, troponin C, which is an integral part of the sarcomere. The sarcomere is the smallest contractile unit and is defined from Z line to Z line (Fig. 15.6). The myofibrillar structure is made up of interacting filaments, termed thick and thin filaments. Thin filaments are polymers of actin monomers that are anchored to the Z line. The thick filament consists of myosin, a large protein made up of six subunits (Fig. 15.7). The thin filament consists of individual actin molecules that combine to form long polymer chains in a double helical array. Interposed along the actin double helix are complexes of tropomyosin (Tm) and troponin (Tn) (Fig. 15.8). Tropomyosin is a linear molecule that lies in the groove of the actin double helix. Tn is found at the amino terminal end of the Tm molecule. Tn consists of a complex of three protein components: TnT, TnI, and TnC. Each of these components has a unique function essential for contractility. TnT contains the binding site for tropomyosin and allows the Tn complex to be bound to Tm. TnI is an inhibitory subunit. TnC is a molecular switch that undergoes Ca^{2+}-mediated conformational change and activates the actin–myosin interaction (9,10).

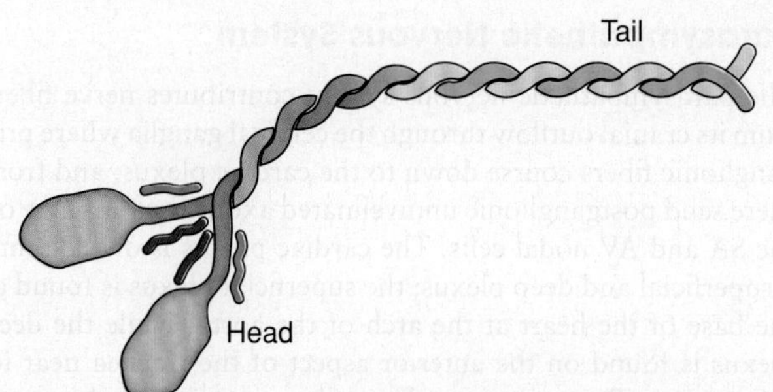

FIGURE 15.7 A schematic of the myosin molecule. A two-headed molecule with a flexible neck and an α-helical tail. The head contains a binding site for adenosine triphosphate. The head and neck have attached essential and regulatory light chains that are referred to in the text.

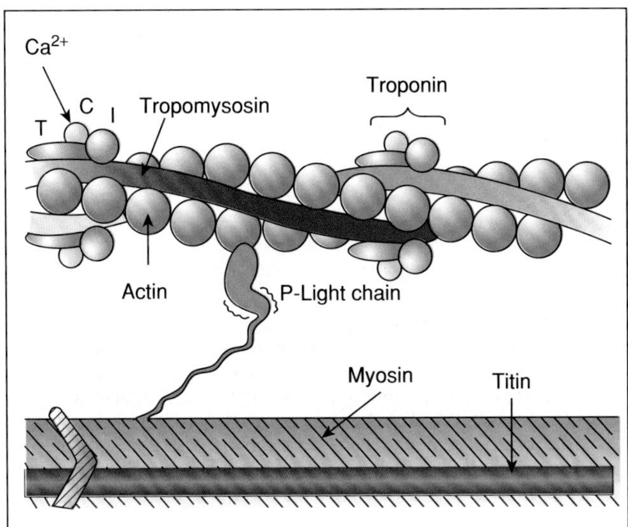

FIGURE 15.8 Schematic representation of protein interactions comprising the contractile apparatus in the cardiac myocyte. (From Ruegg JC. Cardiac contractility: how calcium activates the myofilaments. *Naturwissenschaften*. 1998;85:575; with permission.)

Cardiac Contraction Cycle

At the molecular level, contraction and force generation occur because of the interaction of the myosin head with actin (11). Two processes control contractility in the cardiac myocyte: the length of the sarcomere, and the intrinsic contractility of the contractile elements (12).

Positive peak *dP/dt*, the time differential of ventricular pressure, has been employed as a simple index of contractile function. While *dP/dt* is a simple concept, it is technically challenging to obtain, and is clearly dependent on preload, afterload, and heart rate. A further measure of contractility is the end-systolic pressure–volume relationship (ESPVR) (13). The ESPVR is derived from the pressure–volume loop, an illustration of ventricular volumes plotted against ventricular pressures over the events of a single cardiac cycle (Fig. 15.9). As can be seen in Figure 15.10, pressure volume loops may be generated at different ventricular volumes, and the slope of the line connecting the point of end systole on a family of loops gives a measure of contractility. However, even this measurement of contractility has been shown to yield inconsistent results (11).

Currently, one invasive measure of contractility that appears most consistent is the preload recruitable stroke work (PRSW) relationship. First proposed by Sarnoff and Berglund in 1954 (14), PRSW has been proven to have a linear relationship to the end-diastolic volume (EDV) (15). This index measures contractility despite changes in preload and afterload. The PRSW is obtained from the integrals of a family of pressure–volume loops, the measure of stroke work (SW), at varying EDVs (16–19) (Fig. 15.11).

In clinical practice, pressure–volume loops are not routinely performed due to their time-consuming nature, need for specialized catheters, and manipulation of the different loading conditions of the heart. With that *caveat*, pressure–volume loops provide a graphic representation of the active and passive properties of the heart as a pump. The shape and position of the pressure–volume loops have been of great value in characterizing the clinical picture. As shown in Figures 15.12 and 15.13, a particular pathologic state can be identified by the pressure–volume loop (20). The pressure–volume loop for patients with dilated cardiomyopathy and restrictive cardiomyopathy are markedly shifted to the right, while in hypertrophic cardiomyopathy, they are shifted to the left compared to normal individuals. Acute coronary ischemia also markedly alters the pressure–volume loops.

At the systemic level, the pressure–volume loop can be integrated over time by the eponymous Wiggers diagram of the cardiac cycle, as seen in Figure 15.14. The Wiggers diagram depicts the temporal relationship between cardiac flow and pressure changes, electrical activity, and auscultated heart sounds.

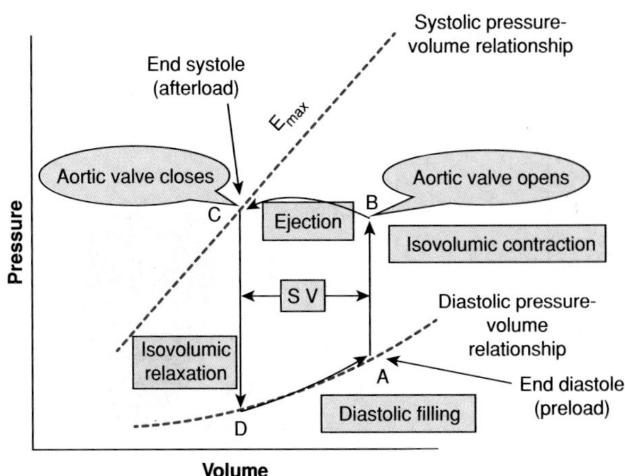

FIGURE 15.9 The pressure–volume loop. The *y* axis represents the pressure in the left ventricle, while the *x* axis represents the volume in the ventricle. Systole begins with the closure of the mitral valve and initiation of isovolumic contraction at time A. The aortic valve opens at time B for ventricular ejection. Systole occurs from time A to time C, aortic valve closure. Following time C, there is isovolumic relaxation and mitral valve opening at time D, followed by ventricular filling until time A. Diastole occurs from time C to time A. (From Lewis AM. Cardiovascular physiology: flow-volume loops. In: Griffin B, ed. *The Cleveland Clinic Cardiology Board Review.* 2nd ed. Philadelphia, PA: Lippincott Williams & Wilkins; 2013:37; with permission.)

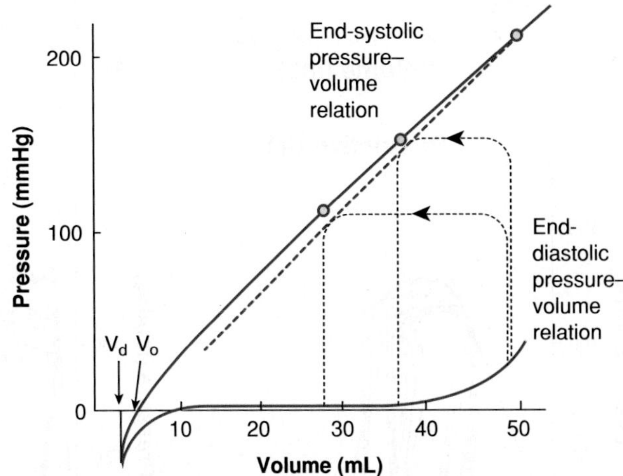

FIGURE 15.10 The pressure–volume loops in different ventricular volumes. The line connecting pressure–volume loops at end systole is a straight line called the end-systolic pressure–volume relationship. (From Sagawa K. The end-systolic pressure-volume relation of the ventricle: definition, modification, and clinical use. *Circulation.* 1981;63:1223; with permission.)

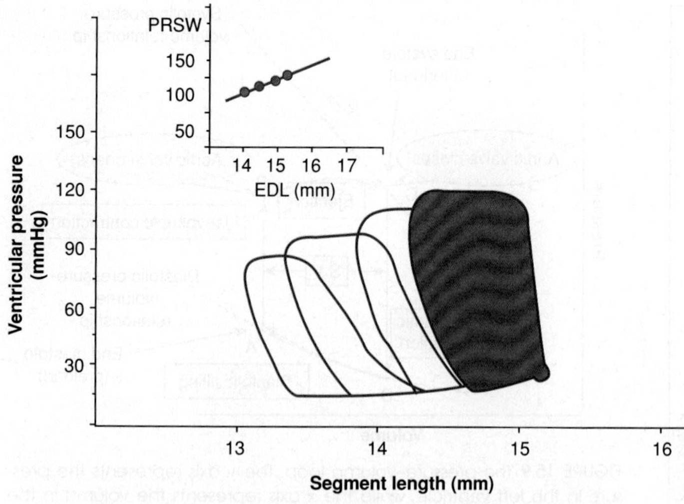

FIGURE 15.11 Pressure–segment length loop. In the inset, integrals of a family of pressure–segment length loops are plotted against end-diastolic segment length (EDL). The slope of this relationship, M_W, is a measure of contractility. (Adapted from Pagel PS, Kampine JP, Schmeling WT, et al. Comparison of end-systolic pressure-length relations and preload recruitable stroke work as indices of myocardial contractility in the conscious and anesthetized chronically instrumented dog. *Anesthesiology.* 1990;73:278.)

For the purposes of this text, we will focus on the left ventricle. At the beginning of ventricular systole, the electrical depolarization wavefront transmitted rapidly down the His-Purkinje fiber network, and represented by the R wave on the ECG, triggers the flood of incoming Ca^{2+} to the actin–myosin complex, excitation–contraction coupling, and the subsequent increase in myocardial contractility to peak dP/dt. Once the left ventricular pressure increases to greater than that of the left atrium (6 to 12 mmHg), within 20 milliseconds, the mitral valve closes and its acoustic reverberations create S1, the first heart sound. The movement of the valvular annulus back towards the atrium is represented by the *c wave* followed by the *x' descent* on the left atrial pressure waveform. On the pressure–volume loop, we observe *isovolumic contraction* as

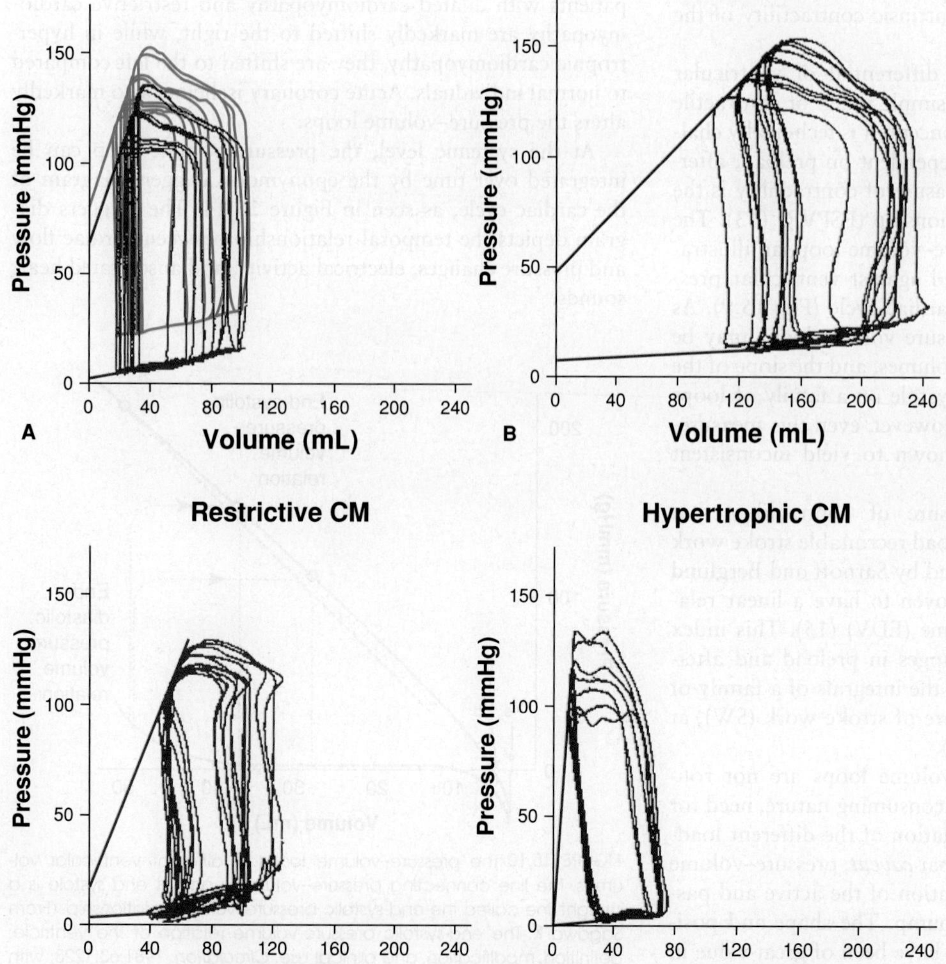

FIGURE 15.12 A comparison of pressure–volume loops of patients with distinct types of cardiomyopathy (CM) in comparison to a normal patient. (From Kass DA. Clinical ventricular pathophysiology: a pressure-volume view. In: Warltier D, ed. *Ventricular Function.* Baltimore, MD: Williams & Wilkins; 1995:131; with permission.)

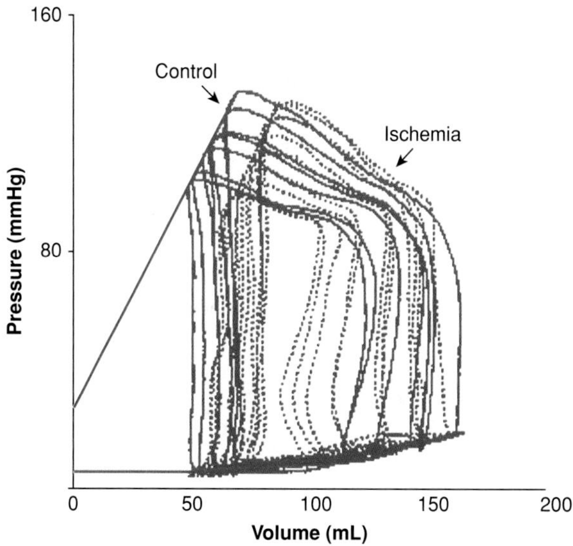

FIGURE 15.13 Pressure–volume loops from a patient prior to and during acute coronary occlusion. Note the marked shift to the right of the family of loops during the ischemic period. (From Kass DA. Clinical ventricular pathophysiology: a pressure-volume view. In: Warltier D, ed. *Ventricular Function*. Baltimore, MD: Williams & Wilkins; 1995:131; with permission.)

both the mitral and aortic valves are shut but actin–myosin complexes continue to be recruited and ventricular pressure increases; isovolumic contraction is the first phase of systole.

Once the left ventricular pressure surpasses the aortic pressure threshold, the aortic valve opens and *ejection* begins. Note on both the pressure–volume loop and the Wiggers diagram that during this phase there are two separate slopes: An initial steep slope representing *rapid ejection*, as blood quickly exits the ventricle into the aorta, and a second, shallower slope representing *delayed ejection* as the SR takes up available Ca^{2+}, decreasing its availability for actin–myosin cross-bridging.

At the end of delayed ejection, the ventricular pressure will have fallen well below the aortic pressure, and the aortic valve closes. The end of the delayed ejection phase represents the end of systole. Closure of the aortic valve creates the first component of S2, the second heart sound. On Wiggers diagram, the left ventricular *dicrotic notch* represents a transient increase in aortic pressure and on the pressure–volume loop, we observe *isovolumic relaxation* since both mitral and aortic valves are again closed. Isovolumic relaxation is the first phase of diastole. Complete ventricular repolarization at this time is represented by the T wave on the ECG.

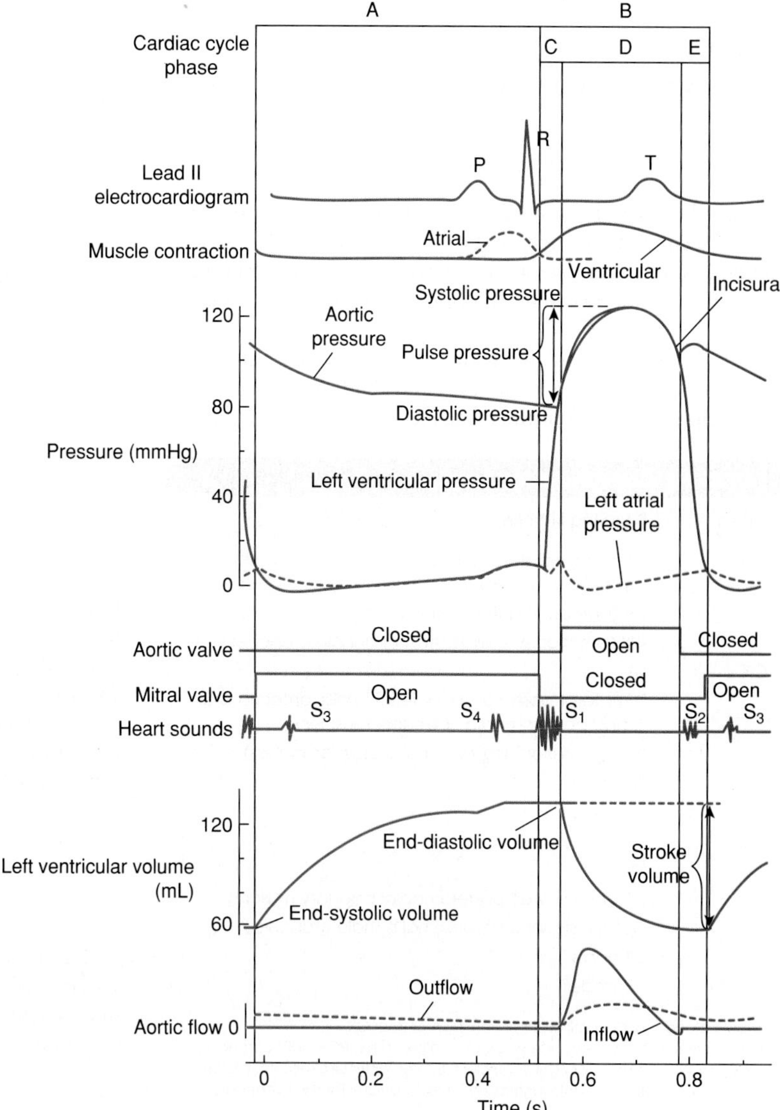

FIGURE 15.14 Modified Wiggers diagram illustrating the cardiac cycle. Cardiac cycle, left heart pump. Cardiac cycle phases: A, diastole; B, systole, which is divided into three periods; C, isovolumetric contraction; D, ejection; and E, isovolumetric relaxation. (From Mohrman DE, Heller JH. The heart pump. In: *Cardiovascular Physiology*. 8th ed. New York: McGraw-Hill Education; with permission.)

By comparing the end-systolic volume (ESV) to EDV on the pressure–volume loop, *stroke volume* of the ventricle and its derivative, the *ejection fraction* may be calculated. Average values for EDV, stroke volume, and ejection fraction are approximately 135 mL, 70 mL, and 50% to 55%, respectively.

As the ventricle relaxes and repolarizes, the left atrium has been filling with blood from the pulmonary veins. The corresponding increase in left atrial pressure is represented by the *v wave* on the left atrial pressure waveform. After complete ventricular relaxation, the pressure in the ventricle drops below the pressure in the left atrium, and the mitral valve opens. As the left atrial pressure drops, the v wave is followed by the *y descent*. *Rapid* or *early filling* subsequently occurs, contributing to approximately three-quarters of the ventricular filling. Atrial and ventricular pressures equalize during *diastasis*, with little net flow from one chamber to the other. Finally, the atrium undergoes its own depolarization and contraction, represented by the P wave on the ECG. Atrial systole, or the *atrial kick*, contributes the remaining one-quarter of the ventricular filling. On the left atrial pressure waveform, this is represented by the *a wave* followed by the *x descent*.

The electrical depolarization wavefront travels from the atrium down into the AV node and the His-Purkinje system, and the cycle restarts.

BLOOD FLOW AND BLOOD PRESSURE

Basic Hemodynamic Models

As stated above, the main purpose of the cardiovascular system is to circulate nutrient and oxygen-rich blood throughout the body and to remove its waste products for tissue homeostasis. The major vascular territories of the heart are noted in Table 15.2.

Any fluid that circulates within a closed system must conform to Newton's laws of motion and fluid dynamics. These laws help us understand the principles of flow hemodynamics

TABLE 15.2 Coronary Blood Supply

Artery	Supplied Structure
LAD	LV (anterior, lateral, and apical walls; anterolateral papillary muscle)
	RV (portion of anterior wall)
	IVS (anterior two-thirds, most of bundle branches)
CX	LA
	LV (lateral, posterior, and inferior[a] walls; anterolateral and posteromedial[a] papillary muscles)
	IVS[a] (posterior third, proximal bundle branches)
	SA node[a]
	AV node[a]
RCA	RA
	RV
	LV[a] (inferior wall, posteromedial papillary muscle)
	IVS[a] (posterior third, proximal bundle branches)
	SA node[a]
	AV node[a]

[a]Variable blood supply coming either from RCA or from CX.

LAD, left anterior descending artery; CX, circumflex artery; RCA, right coronary artery; LV, left ventricle; RV, right ventricle; IVS, interventricular septum; LA, left atrium; SA, sinoatrial; AV, atrioventricular; RA, right atrium; RV, right ventricle.

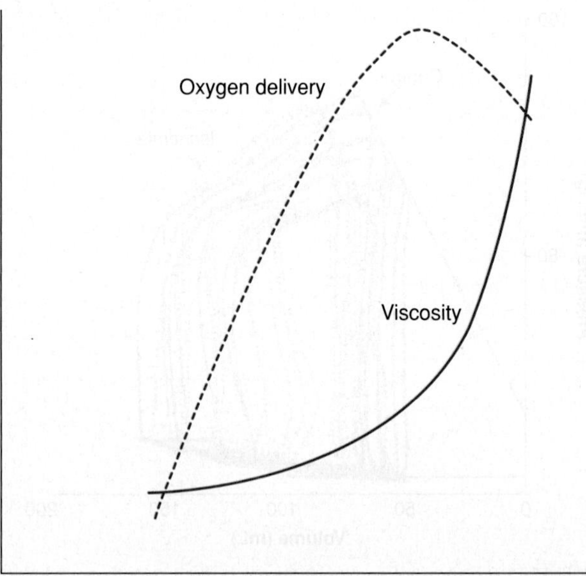

FIGURE 15.15 Effect of hematocrit on blood viscosity and oxygen delivery. Abnormally high hematocrits produce a sharp increase in viscosity, which raises vascular resistance to a point that oxygen delivery decreases. The decrease in oxygen delivery results from a decrease in cardiac output, which more than offsets the increase in oxygen-carrying capacity.

and can also be applied for our understanding of the cardiovascular system in both normal and abnormal conditions. Blood flow in the human body is in a constant state of flux, moving within areas that have different levels of resistance, pressure, and composition. For example, diseases such as anemia or polycythemia vera can change the hemoglobin content of blood, affecting its viscosity and thereby flow dynamics (Fig. 15.15).

Despite the fact that blood flow is not an ideal substrate for precise hemodynamic measurements, clinicians apply Newton's hemodynamic laws to approximate systemic conditions and obtain data pertinent to patient care given the variability of blood flow (pulsatility, viscosity, and composition) and the frequent need for invasive monitoring.

Cardiac Output

One of the primary parameters used in clinical medicine to describe blood flow is CO, which is the total volume of blood pumped by the ventricle per minute, expressed in L/min (22). CO can be measured *invasively* via the Fick equation, tracer dilution methods and contour analysis or *noninvasively* by estimation of flow or ventricular volumes using echocardiography, cardiac magnetic resonance (cMRI), Doppler ultrasound, and other tools.

The CO can be defined mathematically as the product of two factors, the heart rate and stroke volume:

$$CO = HR \times SV$$

Physiologic changes affecting either the heart rate or stroke volume will have a direct impact on systemic CO. Stroke volume is defined as the difference between EDV and ESV, that is, the volume of blood ejected by the ventricle in each heart beat.

$$SV = EDV - ESV$$

TABLE 15.3 Hemodynamic Variables

Variable	Normal Value
Mean arterial pressure	70–105 mmHg
Systolic blood pressure	90–140 mmHg
Diastolic blood pressure	60–90 mmHg
Central venous pressure	0–5 mmHg
Mean pulmonary artery pressure	10–20 mmHg
Systolic pulmonary pressure	15–25 mmHg
Diastolic pulmonary pressure	5–10 mmHg
Capillary wedge pressure	5–12 mmHg
Cardiac index (CI)	2.5–3.5 L/min/m^2
Stroke volume index (CI/heart rate)	36–48 mL/m^2
Systemic vascular resistance index	1,200–1,500 dyne-sec cm^{-5}/m^2
Pulmonary vascular resistance index	80–240 dyne-sec cm^{-5}/m^2

Stroke volume is determined by preload, cardiac contractility, and afterload conditions of the heart.

- Preload: The wall pressure caused by the volume of blood in the ventricle at end diastole, usually reported as a volume or pressure, the left ventricular end-diastolic pressure (LVEDP).
- Contractility: The force of cardiac muscle contraction. Ejection fraction is a surrogate indicator of contractility.
- Afterload: The load in systole against which the ventricle has to contract to successfully eject blood, usually reported as a pressure-flow product, the systemic vascular resistance (SVR). SVR is a correlate of left ventricular afterload in the absence of valvular heart disease.

CO increases with exercise and body size (21). In population studies with latent coronary artery disease (CAD), CO has been shown to decrease with age (22). More recently, echocardiography and radionuclide studies in populations without CAD have shown that CO is maintained by compensating for a slower heart rate by increasing left ventricular EDV (23).

In clinical practice, CO is normalized for body surface area given the wide range of patient sizes that can be encountered, which is then labeled the cardiac index (CI). The CI is obtained by dividing the CO over body surface area (Table 15.3). Figure 15.16 summarizes the major factors influencing cardiac output.

Fick Principle and Mixed Venous Oxygen Saturation

The Fick principle, described in the late 1800s by the German physiologist Adolph Fick, was the first method used to calculate cardiac output. The principle states that the total uptake of a substance by an organ or tissue is equal to the product of blood flow to the organ and the arterial-venous concentration difference, or gradient, of the substance. The arterial-venous gradient is the total amount of substance supplied to an organ minus the amount leaving the organ. This mathematical relationship can be rearranged to solve for blood flow.

$$\text{Cardiac output} = \frac{\text{O}_2 \text{ consumption (mL/min)}}{\text{AV O}_2 \text{ difference}}$$

$$\text{Cardiac output} = \frac{\text{O}_2 \text{ consumption (mL/min)}}{(\text{systemic arterial O}_2 \text{ sat} - \text{mixed venous O}_2 \text{ sat}) \times 1.36 \text{ Hb} \times 10}$$

Oxygen consumption at baseline can be measured by oxygen uptake through a metabolic hood. This process is cumbersome and time consuming as it requires a tight-fitting gas exchange mask. In most cardiac catheterization laboratories an *assumed* oxygen consumption of 125 mL/min/m^2 is used to facilitate calculations. Mixed venous oxygen saturation (MVO_2) is obtained by drawing a sample of blood from the distal port of a pulmonary artery catheter.

All invasive and noninvasive methods of CO measurement have limitations and pitfalls of which practitioners need to be aware. CO by the Fick Method can have significant error in the presence of intracardiac shunts or in nonsteady states (i.e., the critically ill). The *assumed* Fick equation estimates oxygen consumption based on patient weight instead of direct measurement, however this estimation can introduce significant error into the results. In a best case when using the *assumed* Fick equation, the error associated with measuring CO will be about 10% to 15%. Under less stringent conditions this variation can rise significantly (23). The Fick

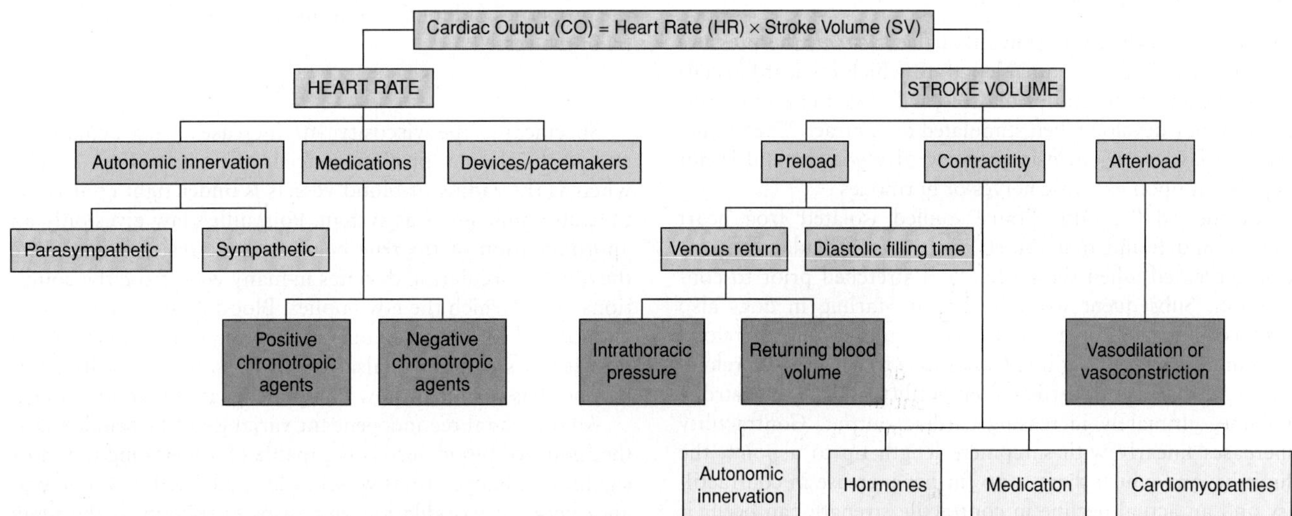

FIGURE 15.16 Major factors affecting cardiac output, divided by those primarily influencing the heart rate and those primarily influencing the stroke volume. (Valvular heart disease not included.)

method is the most accurate method for CO measurement in low CO states due to the large differences encountered in arterial and mixed venous oxygen saturations, thereby reducing errors in measurement of oxygen saturation (24,25). Other invasive methods to measure CO such as the *indicator dilution* or thermodilution method can have significant error in low CO states, arrhythmias, or severe tricuspid regurgitation. The indicator dilution method is most accurate in high output states.

Deoxygenated blood returning to the heart through the inferior and superior vena cava and coronary sinus will have different oxygen saturation levels due to the oxygen consumption ratios of tissues and organs. Inferior vena cava saturation is usually higher than superior vena cava saturation due to renal blood flow and lower oxygen extraction by the kidneys. Coronary sinus oxygen saturation is very low due to high myocardial oxygen extraction ratios but its systemic contribution is negligible due to its small volume. Normal pulmonary artery oxygen saturation (mixed venous O_2 saturation) is 70% to 75% as the normal tissue oxygen extraction is usually in the 25% to 30% range in humans.

In critical illness or in states of increased metabolic demand, tissue oxygen extraction increases throughout the body. In response, regulatory centers will attempt to maintain homeostasis by increasing oxygen delivery to tissue through an increase in cardiac output. MVO_2 can therefore be used as a surrogate marker for cardiac output, as it is decreased in low CO states such as congestive heart failure and can be severely decreased in cardiogenic shock. Isolated interpretation of MVO_2 should be done cautiously, as we know based on Fick's equation that MVO_2 can also be decreased in severe anemia and hypoxemia without a significant decrease in cardiac output.

Other applications of oxygen saturation in cardiovascular disease are in the diagnosis of intracardiac shunts. Measurement of oxygen saturations in various locations within the right heart chambers and vessels, termed an *oxygen saturation run*, can be diagnostic for clinically significant shunts such as ASD, VSD, and others (26). A significant increase or "step up" in oxygen saturation levels is noted in intracardiac shunts.

Frank–Starling Law

The Frank–Starling law states that the *preload*, the pressure associated with the maximal length to which myocardial cells are stretched at the end of diastole, will determine the active tension they develop when stimulated to contract. The Frank–Starling law is an intrinsic property of myocytes and is not dependent upon extrinsic nerves or hormones.

In the 1890s, Otto Frank studied isolated frog heart muscle and found that the strength of ventricular contraction increased when the muscle was stretched prior to contraction. Subsequent work by Ernest Starling in dogs also showed that increasing venous return and therefore preload also increased contractility. Conditions that increase preload cause an increase in cardiac contractility and thereby stroke volume, ultimately increasing cardiac output. Contractility increases linearly with sarcomere length up to a point, the limit beyond which there is no further increase in contractility and an actual decline in contractile strength can occur if further dilated.

Ohm's Law

Ohm's law of electron flow states that the current or flow between two points is proportional to the resistance between the two, so that the greater the resistance the lower the current or flow. Although in the strictest sense this law only holds true for a closed electrical circuit, it has been successfully applied to cardiovascular physiology.

$$I = \frac{V}{R}$$

$$\text{Flow}(Q) = \frac{\text{pressure gradient } (\Delta P)}{\text{resistance } (R)}$$

In order for blood flow to occur within the body, a pressure gradient must exist between two points. Blood will always flow from a high pressure region to a lower pressure region, such as from the left ventricle to aorta, aorta to cerebral circulation, or veins to right atrium. Flow is inversely proportional to vessel wall resistance.

Ohm's law is primarily used to calculate vascular resistance in patients in whom blood flow (by means of a pulmonary artery catheter) and blood pressure (by means of an arterial catheter) are measured simultaneously. In clinical practice, the SVR is calculated from the CO, the mean arterial blood pressure (MAP), and the central venous pressure (CVP):

$$\text{SVR} = (\text{MAP} - \text{CVP})/\text{CO}$$

Likewise, pulmonary vascular resistance (PVR) is calculated from the cardiac output, the mean pulmonary artery pressure (PAP_{mean}), and the pulmonary capillary wedge pressure (PCWP). The latter is measured after balloon occlusion of a branch of the pulmonary artery and is normally in equilibrium with left atrial pressure:

$$\text{PVR} = (\text{PAP}_{\text{mean}} - \text{PCWP})/\text{CO}$$

Poiseuille's Law

Resistance to blood flow is another important physiologic variable, one that constantly changes in response to external and internal factors. The resistance (R) to laminar flow through a rigid tube can be expressed by Poiseuille's law, which states that resistance depends on both the composition of blood and the properties of blood vessels, including length (L) and radius (r) of the vessel.

$$R = 8\eta\, L/\pi r^4$$

Specifically, the viscosity (η) increases with hematocrit and with plasma protein concentration (see Fig. 15.15), whereas the radius of blood vessels is under tight control by the autonomic nervous system. Poiseuille's law gives only an approximation of the true hemodynamic resistance because the human circulation deviates in many ways from the conditions under which the law applies. Blood vessels are not rigid and instead form branching and tapering elastic tubes; blood flow is not steady but pulsatile; flow is not necessarily laminar, but has turbulent flow components at certain locations.

Among the three independent variables of Poiseuille's law, the *radius* of blood vessels is capable of undergoing the most significant change. Total vessel radius, adjusted by a fine balance between vasodilation and vasoconstriction, is the *main regulator* of vascular resistance. SVR is the net result of the resistance generated by many vessels arranged both in series and in parallel.

Arterioles, in particular, are the main targets of the various regulatory mechanisms that lead to vasodilation or vasoconstriction. Because the resistances of the coronary, cerebral, and renal circulations are primarily controlled by local demand, the main factor that regulates total SVR is the net radius of arterioles in muscles, skin, and the gut.

Systemic arteries expand temporarily during systole, a mechanism that is used to store potential energy. Systemic veins and all pulmonary vessels expand and contract in order to accommodate changes in circulating blood volume. The degree to which vessels can expand is defined by their compliance (C):

$$C = \Delta V / \Delta P$$

where ΔV is the change in volume that corresponds to a certain change in transmural pressure, ΔP, the pressure difference between the inside and the outside of the vessel. The compliance is high in systemic veins and the pulmonary vasculature, which is why changes in blood volume will primarily affect the volume of these structures. In contrast, compliance is low in systemic arteries; as a result, their total volume is relatively stable, and they distend only minimally when the arterial pressure rises during systole. Compliance is inversely related to resistance; measurements have shown that SVR is normally about 10 times higher than the PVR (see Table 15.3).

In a steady state, blood flow is equal at any two cross sections in series along the circulation. Thus, the flow through the aorta equals the flow through all of the systemic capillaries. Although the aorta is the largest blood vessel, the combined cross-sectional area of the capillaries far exceeds the aortic cross section. As a result, the velocity of flow is much lower in the capillaries than in the aorta.

Laplace's Law

Laplace's law, first described in the 1700s, helps us understand the importance of vessel wall thickness as a compensatory mechanism of concentric *versus* eccentric ventricular wall hypertrophy in cardiomyopathies.

$$\text{Wall tension} = \text{pressure} \times \text{radius/wall thickness}$$

Laplace's law assumes that tension in the wall of a hollow cylinder is directly proportional to the cylinder's radius and the pressure across the wall caused by flow inside. Therefore, with luminal dilatation and increasing radius, wall tension will increase exponentially. For a similar level of blood pressure, large arteries that have an increased radius must have thicker walls when compared to smaller arteries so as to withstand the levels of wall tension. In an aortic aneurysm, in which the vascular wall is dilated, the process predisposes to an inescapable cycle where increases in wall tension potentiate further weakening of vessel walls, culminating in subsequent rupture.

In the left ventricle, conditions that typically increase ventricular afterload, such as hypertension or aortic stenosis, cause an increase in ventricular wall and cavity tension due to *pressure overload*. This pressure overload, over time, causes a pattern of *concentric* ventricular hypertrophy without an increase in ventricular radius. Dilated cardiomyopathies, however, typically cause a *volume overload* of the left ventricle with an increase in ventricular wall radius and tension. This increase in wall tension induces a compensatory increase in ventricular wall thickness of *eccentric* hypertrophy. This increase in muscle mass compensates for wall tension but also leads to an increase in oxygen consumption secondary to increased tissue requirements needed to generate the same blood pressure as in normal physiological states.

Generation of Blood Pressure

Although blood pressure is a poor indicator of CO and adequate tissue perfusion, it is still one of the two key measurements in cardiovascular hemodynamics alongside heart rate.

The pressure of the systemic circulation is produced by ejection of blood from the left ventricle. As a result of this ejection, blood is accelerated, and the elastic walls of the central blood vessels are slightly distended. This distension is crucial for normal circulatory function because it stores potential energy in vascular structures, resulting in a continuous flow of blood even after the actual ejection period is completed. Although the pressure during the ejection period (systolic blood pressure) is higher than the pressure after the ejection period (diastolic blood pressure), elastic recoil sustains the flow of blood at all times.

The difference between systolic and diastolic blood pressure is called pulse pressure. Pulse pressure is determined by the stroke volume and arterial compliance. A wide or increased pulse pressure can be seen in conditions that primarily increase systolic blood pressure or lower diastolic blood pressure. Conditions that increase systolic blood pressure do this by increasing stroke volume or decreasing arterial compliance (isolated systolic hypertension, old age with loss of arterial elastance and hyperkinetic states). Conditions that decrease diastolic blood pressure are severe aortic insufficiency, AV fistula, sepsis, and vasodilated states. A narrow pulse pressure is usually seen in conditions with low CO such as cardiogenic shock, cardiac tamponade, hemorrhage, or trauma. Although not well defined, normal values for pulse pressure are in the range of 30 to 40 mmHg.

An important indicator of the driving force of the circulation is the MAP. The MAP of one cardiac cycle is the area under the blood pressure curve ($\int P\,dt$) divided by the time of the cardiac cycle (Δt):

$$\text{MAP} = \int P\,dt / \Delta t$$

Determination of MAP by this equation requires invasive monitoring of a continuous blood pressure tracing. When blood pressure is measured by noninvasive techniques, MAP can be approximated from diastolic (DBP) and systolic (SBP) blood pressures by the following equation:

$$\text{MAP} = \frac{[(2 \times \text{DBP}) + \text{SBP}]}{3}$$

We also need to remember the noninvasive MAP formula is best applicable at lower heart rates approaching 60 beats per minute, as we are assuming a normal diastolic interval which is usually twice that of systole. When the heart rate increases, diastolic time decreases and the accuracy of the formula will decrease.

The MAP changes very little between the aorta and the small arteries. However, in arterioles and capillaries, a large pressure gradient exists, which eventually dissipates the mean pressure to a venous pressure value near zero. Despite the

TABLE 15.4 Distribution of Blood Volume

Element of Circulation	Blood Volume (%)
Systemic arteries	10–12
Systemic capillaries	4–5
Systemic veins	60–70
Pulmonary circulation	10–12
Heart	8–11

constant mean pressure in all small and large arteries, there are noticeable changes in systolic and diastolic blood pressures. The systolic blood pressure increases from proximal to distal arteries, whereas the diastolic blood pressure decreases in the same direction. This phenomenon, an observed increase in pulse pressure from central to distal vasculature, is caused by reflections of the pulse wave in the vascular tree.

Distribution of Blood Volume

The circulating blood volume in adults is 60 to 70 mL/kg for women and 70 to 80 mL/kg for men. In neonates, the blood volume is 80 to 90 mL/kg. More than half of the blood volume is present in the venous system, including venules, veins, and the cava (Table 15.4). As discussed above, the compliance of veins is about 10 times higher than that of systemic arteries. Thus, small changes in venous pressure are associated with large changes in venous volume, and the venous system serves as a reservoir to accommodate shifts in total blood volume.

Stroke volume and CO are highly sensitive to the degree of filling of the cardiac ventricles. Cardiac filling in turn depends on the central blood volume, which is defined as intrathoracic blood present in the heart, cava, pulmonary circulation, and intrathoracic arteries. The distribution of blood between the central (intrathoracic) compartment and the peripheral (extrathoracic) compartment can change with body position and with sympathetic tone. Redistribution of blood occurs mainly between compliant structures, such as the heart, the veins, and the pulmonary vasculature. The variable portion of the peripheral blood volume is located in the veins of the extremities and the abdominal cavity. In contrast, the blood volume in systemic arteries changes very little because of their low compliance. Changes in CVP can be used as an indicator of changes in central blood volume. Although this technique is widely employed in the practice of critical care, it is not very sensitive, and it is only accurate if a number of preconditions apply, such as normal cardiac function, normal intrathoracic pressures, and accurate positioning of the pressure transducer.

Just like the vascular resistance, blood volume and blood distribution are under endocrine and autonomic nervous control. Angiotensin II and aldosterone decrease renal excretion of sodium, which leads to an increase in total plasma volume. Atrial natriuretic peptide is released into the bloodstream when atria are stretched, causing increased renal sodium excretion, which therefore leads to a decrease in plasma volume. Erythropoietin is a hormone released by the kidneys that causes bone marrow to increase the production of red blood cells, which also increases total blood volume. The distribution of blood volume is sensitive to the sympathetic tone. High sympathetic outflow causes venoconstriction in addition to the constriction of arterioles. The main effect of venoconstriction is an increase of the central blood volume at the expense of the peripheral blood volume.

Key Points

- Blood flow in the human body is not a substrate that lends itself to precise or easy hemodynamic monitoring. In spite of this, clinicians can still apply Newton's laws of flow dynamics in order to obtain pertinent information and measurements that can be used clinically at bedside.
- Frank–Starling law states that cardiac *preload*, the pressure to which myocardial cells are stretched at the end of diastole, will influence cardiac contractility and therefore the stroke volume of the heart.
- Ohm's law states that blood flows from a high pressure area to a lower pressure area and that flow is inversely proportional to vessel wall resistance.
- Poiseuille's law states that vessel radius, vessel length, and blood viscosity determine resistance to blood flow within the vessel. Of these, vessel radius being the most significant.
- Laplace's law states that the larger the vessel radius the larger the wall tension required to withstand a given internal fluid pressure.

ACKNOWLEDGMENTS

We thank Drs. Michael Schlame and Thomas J. Blanck for their contributions to earlier editions of this chapter.

References

1. Rhoades RA, Tanner GA, eds. *Medical Physiology*. 2nd ed. Philadelphia, PA: Lippincott Williams & Wilkins; 2003.
2. Study R. The structure and function of neurons. In: Hemmings H, Hopkins P, eds. *Foundations of Anesthesia Basic and Clinical Sciences*. London: Mosby; 2000:179.
3. Boyett MR, Tellez JO, Dobrzynski H. The sinoatrial node: its complex structure and unique ion channel gene program. In: Zipes DP, Jalife J. *Cardiac Electrophysiology: From Cell to Bedside*. 5th ed. Philadelphia, PA: Saunders-Elsevier; 2009:131.
4. Tester DJ, Ackerman MJ. Single nucleotide polymorphisms and cardiac arrhythmias. In: Zipes DP, Jalife J. *Cardiac Electrophysiology: From Cell to Bedside*. 5th ed. Philadelphia, PA: Saunders-Elsevier; 2009:510.
5. Opie LH. *The Heart Physiology from Cell to Circulation*. 3rd ed. Philadelphia, PA: Lippincott-Raven; 1998.
6. Bogdanov KY, Maltsev VA, Vinogradova TM, et al. Membrane potential fluctuations resulting from submembrane Ca^{2+} releases in rabbit sinoatrial nodal cells impart an exponential phase to the late diastolic depolarization that controls their chronotropic state. *Circ Res*. 2006;99:979.
7. Bers DM. The beat goes on. *Circ Res*. 2006;99:921.
8. Barber MJ. Class I antiarrhythmic agents. In: Lynch C, ed. *Clinical Cardiac Electrophysiology: Perioperative Considerations*. Philadelphia, PA: JB Lippincott; 1994:85.
9. Bootman M, Higazi DR, Coombes S, et al. Calcium signaling during excitation-contraction coupling in mammalian atrial myocytes. *J Cell Sci*. 2006;119:3915.
10. Ruegg JC. Cardiac contractility: how calcium activates the myofilaments. *Naturwissenschaften*. 1998;85:575.
11. Blanck TJJ, Lee DL. Cardiac physiology. In: Miller RD, ed. *Anesthesia*. Vol. 1. Philadelphia, PA: Churchill Livingstone; 2000:619.
12. Katz AM, Lorell BH. Regulation of cardiac contraction and relaxation. *Circulation*. 2000;102(Suppl IV):69.
13. Sagawa K. The end-systolic pressure-volume relation of the ventricle: definition, modification, and clinical use. *Circulation*. 1981;63:1223.
14. Sarnoff SJ, Berglund EI. Starling's law of the heart studied by means of simultaneous right and left ventricular function curves in the dog. *Circulation*. 1954;9(5):706–718.
15. Glower DD, Spratt JA, Snow ND, et al. Linearity of the Frank-Starling relationship in the intact heart: the concept of pre-load recruitable stroke work. *Circulation*. 1985;71:994.

16. Pagel PS, Kampine JP, Schmeling WT, et al. Comparison of end-systolic pressure-length relations and preload recruitable stroke work as indices of myocardial contractility in the conscious and anesthetized chronically instrumented dog. *Anesthesiology*. 1990;73:278.
17. Lee W, Huang W, Yu W, et al. Estimation of preload recruitable stroke work relationship by a single-beat technique in humans. *Am J Physiol.* 2003;284:744.
18. Karunanithi MK, Feneley MP. Single-beat determination of preload recruitable stroke work relationship: derivation and evaluation in conscious dogs. *J Am Coll Cardiol.* 2000;35:502.
19. Baicu CF, Zile MR, Aurigemma GP, et al. Left ventricular systolic performance, function, and contractility in patients with diastolic heart failure. *Circulation.* 2005;111:2306.
20. Kass DA. Clinical ventricular pathophysiology: a pressure-volume view. In: Warltier D, ed. *Ventricular Function.* Baltimore, MD: Williams & Wilkins; 1995:131.
21. Costello FM, Stouffer GA. Cardiac output. In: Stouffer GA. *Cardiovascular Hemodynamics for the Clinician.* Madden: Blackwell Future; 2007:81.
22. Brandfonbrener M, Landowne M, Shock NW. Changes in cardiac output with age. *Circulation.* 1955;12:557–566.
23. Cheitlin MD. Cardiovascular physiology: changes with aging. *Am J Geriatr Cardiol.* 2003;12(1):9–14.
24. Kendrick AH, West J, Papouchado M, et al. Direct Fick cardiac ouput: are assumed values of oxygen consumption acceptable? *Eur Heart J.* 1988; 9:337–342.
25. Wolf A, Pollman MJ, Trindade PT, et al. Use of assumed versus measured oxygen consumption for the determination of cardiac output using the Fick principle. *Cath Cardiovasc Diagn.* 1998;43:372–380.
26. Costello FM, Stouffer GA. Detection, localization, and quantification of intracardiac shunts. In: Stouffer GA. *Cardiovascular Hemodynamics for the Clinician.* Madden: Blackwell Future; 2007:89.

CHAPTER

16

Renal Physiology and Its Systemic Impact

MICHIKO SHIMADA, KAWTHER F. ALQUADAN, and A. AHSAN EJAZ

INTRODUCTION

The primary function of the kidneys is to maintain volume, electrolyte, and acid–base homeostasis in the internal milieu. Rapid deterioration in kidney function or inability to maintain adequate urine output is termed acute kidney injury (AKI). After decades of conflicting definitions, current consensus defines AKI as an abrupt (within 48 hours) reduction in kidney function, defined as an absolute increase in serum creatinine above 0.3 mg/dL (>26.4 mmol/L), a percentage increase in serum creatinine above 50% (1.5-fold from baseline) in accordance with criteria established by the Acute Kidney Injury Network (AKIN) (1). Using this criterion, the incidence of AKI in adults in a district general hospital setting in the United Kingdom was reported to be 15,325 patients/million populations per year (2) and 39.3% in the critically ill patients in Finland (3). In a meta-analysis of 154 studies from North America, Northern Europe, and Eastern Asia, from high-income countries, and from nations that spent 5% or more of the gross domestic product on total health expenditure, the incidence of AKI among hospitalized patients was 21.6% in adults and 33.7% in children by AKIN criteria (4). AKI-associated hospital mortality is high (23.9%) (4), and worsens when renal replacement therapies are also required (5). AKI is also associated with increased length of intensive care unit (ICU) and hospital stay, increase in care on discharge, and an increase in hospital readmission within 30 days (2).

Knowledge of risk factors for AKI in the ICU can be helpful in the determination of clinical outcome and contribute to more defined risk assessment and management in this cohort (Table 16.1). This chapter briefly reviews pertinent renal physiology, the mechanisms and outcomes of ischemic AKI, the progression of chronic kidney disease and its impact on acute critical illness, and the principles of management of AKI. Specifics on the treatment of AKI and a detailed description of the various treatment modalities are to be found in later chapters of this textbook.

PHYSIOLOGY OF THE KIDNEY

General Anatomy

The ability of the kidney to maintain the equilibrium of the corporal fluids and electrolytes depends on three essential processes: (i) filtration of the circulating blood by the glomerulus to form an ultrafiltrate; (ii) reabsorption of specific solutes from the tubular fluid to the blood; and (iii) secretion from the peritubular capillary blood system to the tubular space. The functions of the kidney are dependent on the unique anatomic arrangement of its structures.

The afferent arteriole divides into several branches after entering the glomerular tuft and forms the capillary network present in the glomerulus (Fig. 16.1). The confluence of several capillaries forms the efferent arteriole which drains the blood from the glomerulus. During the ultrafiltration process, water and solutes pass through the endothelium, the glomerular basement membrane, and the slit-diaphragm between the podocytes. The determinant of the filtration of a substance is its size and charge. Substances with molecular radius of less than 2 nm are filtered freely, whereas the ionic charges of substances measuring between 2 and 4 nm determine the amount of their filtration; substances with molecular radius greater than 4 nm are not filtered.

The medullary region of the kidneys is characterized by low oxygen tension—10 to 15 mmHg—under normal conditions. The tubular segments located in this region—pars recta, or S3 segment of proximal tubule and medullary thick ascending limb—are characterized by active transport of Na^+, which is dependent on oxidative phosphorylation for energy. The high rates of oxygen consumption associated with the precarious blood flow in the medullary region are responsible for the vulnerability of this area to ischemia.

Glomerular Filtration Rate and Renal Plasma Flow

The glomerular filtration rate (GFR) and renal plasma flow (RPF) are rate measurements that help to characterize the status of renal function. The total rate at which fluid is filtered into all the glomeruli constitutes the *GFR*; normal GFR varies between 100 and 120 mL/min/1.73 m^2, depending on various factors including gender, age, and body weight. Changes in the GFR can result from changes in the glomerular permeability or capillary surface area or from changes in the net ultrafiltration. In a single glomerulus, the driving pressure for the glomerular filtration is determined by the difference of the gradient of the hydrostatic and oncotic pressures between the capillaries and the Bowman space.

The rate at which plasma flows through the kidney is called *RPF; renal blood flow* (RBF) is the volume of blood delivered to the kidney per unit time (1 to 1.2 L/min). RBF calculations are based on RPF and hematocrit:

$$\textit{Renal blood flow} = \textit{RPF} \,/\, 1 - \textit{hematocrit}$$

It is possible to measure the RPF using para-aminohippurate as a tracer in humans, with a normal value about 625 mL/min, but the test is not commonly used in clinical practice due to labor intensity and cost.

Autoregulatory Control of Renal Blood Flow

Despite the significant variations in mean arterial pressure (MAP), RBF and GFR remain constant, a phenomenon known as *autoregulation*. Autoregulation is affected via changes in diameter of the afferent arterioles in response to a combination of two mechanisms:

- *The myogenic reflex:* When the renal perfusion pressure increases, the afferent arteriole constricts automatically.

TABLE 16.1 Predictors of Acute Kidney Injury in the Intensive Care Unit

Risks	All patients OR N = 194[a]	Sepsis OR N = 2,442[b]	CV Surgery OR N = 43,642[c]	Trauma OR N = 153[d]
Demographics				
Age	0.93	1.1		2.82
Acute Clinical Setting				
High-risk surgery	1.51		1.98	
Sepsis	3.11			
High injury severity score				5.75–13.7
Emergency procedure			7.61	
Cardiopulmonary bypass			2.64	
Pre-existing Condition				
Chronic kidney disease	1.77	1.02	1.31–5.80[b]	
Cardiac failure	1.85		1.55	
Cancer	3.75		—	
Prior cardiac surgery			1.93	
COPD			1.26	
Hypertension (SBP >160 mmHg)			1.03–1.98[c]	
Peripheral vascular disease			1.51	
Clinical Findings				
Elevated A-a gradient	1.04			
Elevated serum bilirubin	3.6	9.7		
Hypotension				3.04
Hemoperitoneum				6.80
Long bone fractures				2.36
Morbid obesity	2.1		1.11	
APACHE II quartile	1.57			
Elevated CVP		1.5		

CV, cardiovascular; OR, odds ratio; COPD, chronic obstructive pulmonary disease; SBP, systolic blood pressure; CVP, central venous pressure.
[a]Chawla LS, Abell L, Mazhari R, et al. Identifying critically ill patients at high risk for developing acute kidney injury: a pilot study. *Kidney Int.* 2005;68:2274–2280.
[b]Yegenaga I, Hoste E, Van Biesen W, et al. Clinical characteristics of patients developing ARF due to sepsis/systemic inflammatory response. *Am J Kidney Dis.* 2004;43:817–824.
[c]Chertow GM, Lazarus JM, Christiansen CL, et al. Preoperative renal risk stratification. *Circulation.* 1997;95:878–884.
[d]Vivino G, Antonelli M, Moro ML, et al. Risk factors for acute kidney injury in trauma patients. *Intensive Care Med.* 1998;24:808–814.

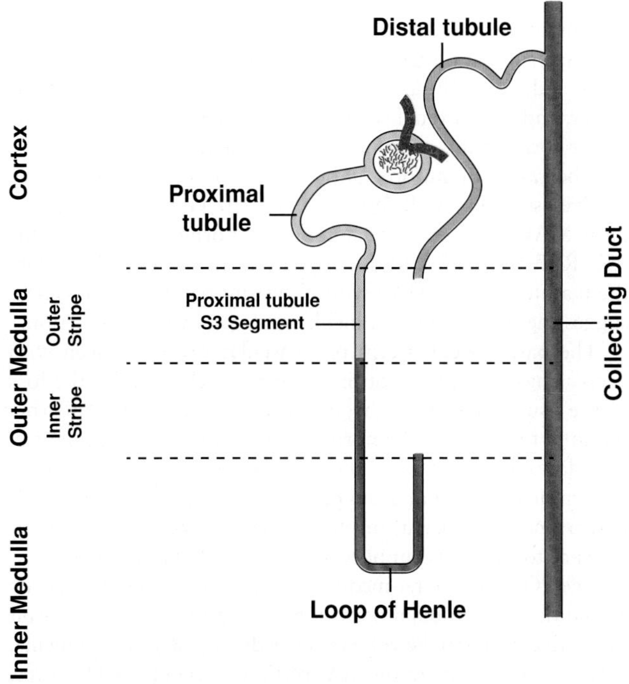

FIGURE 16.1 Nephron, the functional unit of the kidney.

- *Tubuloglomerular feedback:* Situations associated with an increased delivery of sodium chloride to the macula densa result in vasoconstrictive response of the afferent arteriole. The increased uptake of chloride ions by the macula densa cells leads to adenosine triphosphate (ATP) release into the surrounding extracellular space. ATP is then converted to adenosine, which binds to adenosine A_1 receptors causing afferent arteriolar vasoconstriction.

Basic Principles of Tubular Transport

The kidneys filter about 180 L of plasma per day, and all but 2 L are reabsorbed. This massive reabsorption is accomplished through several modifications of the glomerular ultrafiltrate, consisting of absorption and secretion of water and solutes before becoming the final urine. In general, three different tubular segments are involved in this process and can be recognized based on the differences in the function of their cells.

- The proximal tubule reabsorbs most of the filtered glucose, amino acids, low-molecular-weight proteins, and water (approximately 65%). Other solutes, such as sodium (Na^+), potassium (K^+), chloride (Cl^-), bicarbonate (HCO_3^-), phosphate (PO_4^-), and urea are also absorbed in this nephron segment. The terminal segment of the proximal tubule—the pars recta or S3—is responsible for the secretion of numerous drugs and toxins.

- The straight portion of the proximal tubule, the thin ascending and descending limbs, and the thick ascending limb constitute the region known as the loop of Henle. This region is responsible for the continuing reabsorption of the solutes that escaped the proximal tubules (sodium, potassium, chloride, calcium, magnesium ions). It is the major area responsible for the ability of the kidneys to concentrate or dilute the final urine. The principal luminal transporter expressed in the thick ascending limb is the sodium-potasium-2chloride cotransporter (NKCC2), which is the target of diuretics such as furosemide.
- The distal nephron is responsible for the final adjustments in the urine. Critical regulatory hormones such as vasopressin and aldosterone regulate the acid and potassium excretion and the urinary concentration at this segment. Thiazide diuretics act at the distal convoluted tubule through a thiazide-sensitive Na^+–Cl^-cotransporter on the apical membrane.

The Glomerulotubular Balance

The fact that the tubules tend to reabsorb a constant proportion of a glomerular filtrate rather than a constant amount is called *glomerular balance*. As an example, if the filtered load of Na^+ were increased by 10%, total Na^+ reabsorption in the tubules would also increase by 10%, keeping the final amount of Na^+ in the urine stable at 100 to 250 mEq/day. In the absence of this mechanism, even small changes in the GFR would cause major changes in the final amount excreted of any solute. The mechanisms responsible for this balance are not fully understood, but changes in the oncotic pressure in the peritubular capillaries and in the delivery of certain solutes (glucose and amino acids) to the proximal tubule are probably involved.

Control of Effective Circulating Volume via Integrated Mechanisms

Most volume-regulatory mechanisms in the kidney use the *effective circulating volume (ECV)*, or the degree of fullness of the vasculature, as the final target. Under normal conditions, the ECV varies in direct proportion to the extracellular fluid volume. As Na^+ is the most abundant extracellular solute, the kidney excretion or retention of Na^+ is a crucial step to control ECV. Osmoregulation is under the control of a single hormonal system, antidiuretic hormone (ADH), but volume regulation requires a complex set of redundant and overlapping mechanisms.

The kidneys are able to conserve water by excreting the solute load in concentrated urine in conditions of excess water loss. Similarly, in high water intake states, the urinary volume may increase to as high as 14 L/day, with an osmolality significantly lower than that of the plasma. Vasopressin or ADH regulates the water permeability in the distal nephron and is the principal hormone responsible for the determination of the urinary concentration and volume. Normally, the major stimulus to secretion of ADH is the plasma osmolality, but in situations of extracellular volume depletion, the set point to release ADH is shifted, and higher levels of this hormone are common even in hypotonic states.

The renin–angiotensin system plays a central role in the control of ECV. The afferent arteriolar cells that form part of the juxtaglomerular apparatus release renin in response to increased sympathetic nervous stimulation, reduced arterial blood pressure, or reduced delivery of sodium chloride (NaCl) to the macula densa region. Renin cleaves angiotensinogen into angiotensin I and is then converted to angiotensin II by the angiotensin-converting enzyme. Angiotensin plays important roles in the control of blood pressure and the effective circulatory fluid volume.

- Angiotensin II has the direct effect of increasing the sodium reabsorption in the proximal tubule (stimulation of Na^+/H^+ exchange).
- The aldosterone secreted by the adrenal glands in response to the angiotensin II stimulates sodium reabsorption in the distal nephron.
- Angiotensin II causes general arteriolar vasoconstriction, thereby increasing arterial pressure.

Increased renal sympathetic tone enhances renal salt reabsorption and often decreases RBF. In addition to its direct effects on renal function, increased sympathetic outflow promotes the activation of the renin–angiotensin system.

IMPACT OF ALTERED RENAL PHYSIOLOGY

Altered renal physiology can manifest as mild abnormalities in electrolyte and acid–base homeostasis or solute clearance to full-blown AKI that can progress to chronic kidney disease. The impacts of perturbed renal physiology and proposed pathogenesis are discussed.

Consequences of Aberrant Renal Blood Flow Autoregulation

RBF is dependent on systemic blood pressure and intrarenal vascular resistance. The autoregulatory mechanisms, through changes in vascular resistance, ensure that over a wide range of perfusion pressures RBF remains stable and glomerular filtration can be maintained. However, a substantial loss of renovascular response to neurohormonal stimuli follows ischemic AKI (6), related to increased renal vasoconstriction (7). Clinically this manifests as ischemic AKI, a syndrome that develops following a sudden transient drop in total or regional blood flow to the kidney resulting in tissue hypoxia, tubular and vascular injury, and loss of renal structure and function (Fig. 16.2). The severe form of this entity is known as acute tubular necrosis. An aberrant RBF autoregulation is also implicated in normotensive ischemic AKI. Whereas normal GFR is maintained until MAP falls below 50 mmHg, in normotensive ischemic AKI RBF and GFR can decrease by as much as 50% despite the maintenance of MAP within the autoregulatory range (8), suggesting the presence of heightened renal vasoconstriction.

The paradoxical rise in renovascular resistance seen with decreasing renal perfusion in ischemic AKI is due to the loss of the usual balance of vasoconstrictors and the vasodilators required to maintain the normal tone of the renal vasculature. The downstream consequence of aberrant responses to neurohormonal stimuli and the persistent vasoconstriction is that it worsens renal perfusion and impairs oxygen and nutrient delivery to the areas supplied by the postglomerular vessels.

The PO_2 in the outer medulla is about 10 to 15 mmHg; even a mild decrease in renal perfusion can lead to a hypoxic insult (oxidative stress) to the vulnerable medullary nephron segments. Tissue hypoxia can result in depletion of cellular ATP stores, increased intracellular calcium, and subsequent disruption of

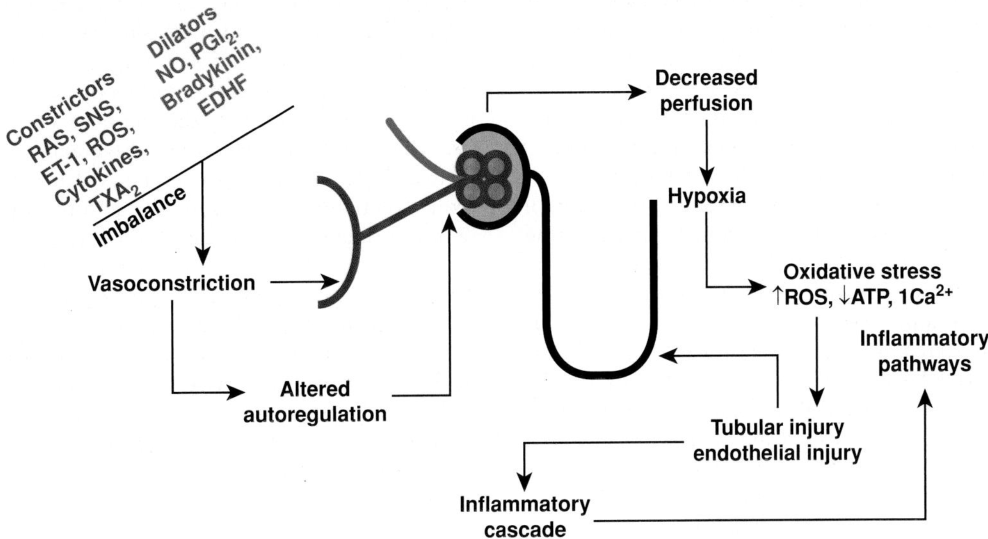

FIGURE 16.2 Schematic representation of the mechanisms of ischemic acute kidney injury. RAS, renin–angiotensin system; SNS, sympathetic nervous system; ET-1, endothelin-1; ROS, reactive oxygen species; TXA_2, thromboxane A_2; NO, nitric oxide; PGI_2, prostaglandin I_2; EDHF, endothelium-derived hyperpolarizing factor; ATP, adenosine triphosphate; Ca^{2+}, calcium.

actin cytoskeleton in the endothelial and vascular smooth muscle cells, with resultant hemodynamic impairment and tubular injury. Adenosine nucleotide metabolic products are not reused for the regeneration of ATP and are, instead, diverted through the degradatory pathways to generate xanthine and uric acid. Accumulation of adenosine and uric acid worsens vasoconstriction and renal perfusion via their effects on adenosine receptors and afferent arterioles, respectively. Cellular activation also leads to reactive oxygen species generation, phospholipase activation, and membrane lipid alterations (9).

Hypoxia, with subsequent reperfusion, leads to acute inflammatory changes. Inflammation is one of the major pathophysiologic pathways contributing to ischemic AKI. Ischemic injury to the vasa recta results in enhanced adherence of leukocytes to the vascular endothelial cells, sequestration of leukocytes, vascular congestion—that is, a no-flow phenomenon—cellular infiltration, production of inflammatory mediators, and generation of reactive oxygen species. Cytokines and chemokines, released from the injured cells, attract inflammatory cells to the site of injury and potentiate the inflammatory cascade. A similar inflammatory response is also seen in tubular cell injury, which is also capable of producing chemokines and inflammatory mediators. The inflammatory changes are most pronounced in the outer medullary stripe, the region that is most susceptible to hypoxic insult.

Numerous stress response mechanisms are rapidly activated in response to oxidative insults. Some of the pathways are preferentially linked to cell survival whereas others are proapoptotic; these pathways intersect and modulate each other's activities. Whether a particular insult leads to cell repair and survival—or death—depends on the nature and severity of the insult, the balance between the proapoptotic and antiapoptotic signals, and the basal state of the cells. Ongoing efforts to elucidate factors that play a role in microvascular endothelial injury and dysfunction, the role of immune system, the expression of adhesion molecules that facilitate leukocyte–endothelial interactions, the cytokine network, the cellular response to oxidative stress, and the gene activation patterns that regulate tissue injury and repair will result in a better understanding of the complex mechanisms involved in the pathogenesis of ischemic AKI.

Effect of Baseline Renal Function on New-Onset Acute Kidney Injury

RBF autoregulation is often impaired in the setting of chronic disease conditions such as hypertension, diabetes, and atherosclerosis. Additionally, endothelial dysfunction, chronic hypoxia, tubulointerstitial fibrosis, and vascular dropout may predispose the renal parenchyma to further damage. Consistent with these hypotheses, retrospective data suggests an increase in the risk of AKI from 1.95 to 40 times with increasing severity of renal dysfunction—for chronic kidney disease stage 3 through stage 5 patients compared to patients with estimated GFR in the stage 1 and 2 range (10). Nevertheless, the causal relationship between renal dysfunction and risk for AKI is uncertain despite assessments based on epidemiologic and outcome data that the two entities may be interconnected (11).

Effect on Fluid Balance

It is evident from the above discussion that acute deterioration in renal physiologic functions is synonymous with the entity of AKI in most clinical situations. A major complication of AKI is decrease in urine output and, hence, inability to maintain fluid balance. AKI complicates the implementation of fluid resuscitation strategies that are often utilized to optimize systemic hemodynamics in the critically ill patients. Fluid accumulation can contribute to tissue edema, impaired oxygenation and metabolite diffusion, disturbed cell–cell integrity, infections, delayed wound healing, and organ dysfunction. Indeed, positive fluid balance is a predictor of adverse outcomes in the critically ill patients (12–15). A 10% increase in body weight relative to baseline was reported to increase mortality and decrease the likelihood of renal recovery in critically ill patients (16). Fluid overload at dialysis initiation can double the adjusted odds ratio for death. In nondialyzed patients, less fluid accumulation at the peak of their serum creatinine was associated with better survival. Fluid balance can be particularly problematic in major surgery where a 3 to 6 kg increase in postoperative weight is not uncommon. It should be also noted that fluid overload may prevent or delay the diagnosis of AKI. Although dialysis is effective at volume removal, mortality has been shown to increase in relation to the proportion of dialysis days with fluid overload (16). An intriguing question is the causal relationship between fluid balance and AKI. Data from cardiac surgery suggests that positive fluid balance develops early in the intraoperative period (17) due to intravenous fluid bolus administered to treat hypotension (18). In pediatric surgery, fluid overload was associated with the development of AKI and more often preceded it than followed it (19). Moreover, the predictive power of positive fluid balance to diagnose AKI has been reported to be comparable to preoperative conventional (serum creatinine, GFR) and postoperative 24-hour novel biomarkers (urine neutrophil gelatinase–associated lipocalin, IL-18, and serum tumor necrosis factor-alpha [TNF-α] and monocyte chemoattractant factor-1) (15). Angiopoietin-2, a mediator of vascular permeability, was reported to positively correlate with fluid balance, pulmonary dysfunction, and death in sepsis patients (20). Despite these provocative data, the causative association between fluid balance and AKI has yet to be established.

Effect on Pulmonary Function

AKI negatively affects lung physiology significantly by altering the homeostasis of fluid balance, acid–base balance, and vascular tone (21). Most patients with acute respiratory failure receiving mechanical ventilation (MV) require some form of renal replacement therapy. Conversely, alterations in respiratory drive, mechanics, muscle function, and gas exchange are frequent consequences of uremia. The development of AKI predisposes patients to overall fluid overload, decreased plasma oncotic pressure, and leakage of fluid from pulmonary capillaries. The restrictive effects of pulmonary interstitial and alveolar edema, pleural effusion, and chest wall edema increase the work of spontaneous breathing and may contribute to the development of acute ventilatory failure. Additionally, the metabolic acidosis present in most instances of AKI increases the demand for ventilation through compensatory respiratory alkalosis, further disrupting the relationship between the patient's ventilatory needs and capabilities. Pulmonary edema and ventilation at low lung volumes can cause or worsen hypoxemia. Bidirectional kidney–lung cross-talk occurs in acute lung injury (ALI) and is deleterious for both organs. As previously mentioned, the renal medulla is sensitive to hypoxic injury and its presence results in activation of downstream inflammatory pathways and resultant AKI. Further, sympathetic overactivation, decreased cardiac output due to altered cardiopulmonary interaction, and release of proinflammatory mediators in ALI can affect renal vascular tone and renal cell viability (21).

AKI can necessitate several modifications in the management of MV. Higher airway pressure is required to maintain the same level of ventilation in the presence of pulmonary edema, pleural effusion, or total-body fluid overload. Airway mucosal edema can reduce effective airway diameter, predisposing to air trapping and intrinsic positive end-expiratory pressure, which can reduce venous return, further compromising cardiac function and increasing the risk of alveolar rupture. The management of ALI and acute respiratory distress syndrome (ARDS) using lung-protective ventilation strategies is made more difficult in the presence of metabolic acidosis, which increases ventilatory drive and worsens acidemia related to permissive hypercapnia. AKI has been reported to reduce ventilator-free days in cardiac surgery patients (22).

It is estimated that 8% to 10% of lung transplant patients who develop AKI require renal replacement therapy (23). Those with AKI following lung transplant surgery are noted to have reduced 5-year survival rates (30%) compared to patients without AKI (48.8%) (24). Patients with an episode of AKI are also at increased risk for chronic kidney disease and the risk appears to be similar irrespective of whether the patients had a complete or nonrecovery of the insult (25). AKI after lung transplantation is associated with longer duration of MV, increased hospital stay, and increased early mortality (26). As in other disease states, pre-existing renal disease also adversely affects clinical outcomes in this cohort. Those with pretransplant GFR less than 50 mL/min/1.73 m^2 have been shown to have a twofold increased risk for adverse outcomes compared to those with GFR above 50 mL/min/1.73 m^2 (27).

Effect on Neurobehavioral Function

Executive functions may be impaired in severe AKI due to accumulation of uremic toxins that impair cellular function. Although there is credible evidence for an association between functional and cognitive impairment and hyponatremia (28), the dose-response correlation of uremia with neurobehavioral changes in AKI are not available. This is confounded by the fact that although many solutes have been implicated, very few of them were actually investigated in clinical medicine for this purpose. Plasma concentrations of urea do not correlate with mental status changes (29), but several compounds including guanidine, uric acid, indoxyl sulfate, p-cresyl sulfate, IL-1-β, IL-6, TNF-α, and PTH appear to affect the cerebrorenal interaction (30). In dialysis patients, cognitive impairment is not uncommon and improves with dialysis therapy. In AKI, the effect of uremia, if any, is often complicated by concomitant metabolic derangements, medications, and underlying disease process. Although a trial and error approach to treatment is often utilized, causal relationship between them remains elusive in humans.

Effect on Drug Dosing

The pharmacokinetics of most drugs are altered in AKI; clearances of drugs are impaired, the half-lives are prolonged, or they accumulate in tissues and continue to exert their effects long after their administration. Some of the drugs are broken down into their metabolites with deleterious consequences; most of the drugs are not completely removable by dialysis due to their high protein binding. Many effective drug therapies cannot be used because of the risk of accumulation and toxicity; some drugs are removed by dialysis and require postdialysis supplementation. However, the varying clearances of the different continuous renal replacement therapies mandate the knowledge of the clearance of the particular modality used to effectively dose a particular drug. The minimum inhibitory concentration of antibiotics to treat severe infection may not be attained at their usual doses if the clearance of the drug is enhanced by renal replacement therapies and higher dosing regimens maybe required. Patients with acute or chronic kidney diseases, not on dialysis, also require careful consideration of drug dosing. The half-life of the drug, once-daily versus intermittent dosing regimens, bioavailability and volume of distribution between plasma and tissue compartments, acid–base dissociation constant of the drug, plasma protein binding, pharmacokinetics, and clearance are important considerations for drug dosing in these patients.

Implications of Altered Tubulointerstitial Function

Renal tubules are involved in electrolyte, acid–base, and fluid homeostasis and, therefore, alterations in their function may result in various disorders. Renal tubular dysfunction can be a consequence of medications, infections, crystalluria, rhabdomyolysis, acute and chronic inflammatory diseases, underlying diseases, and genetic causes. Alterations in tubular function in acute or chronic tubulointerstitial nephritis, for example, can be associated with imbalances of potassium, metabolic acidosis, and impaired urinary concentrating capacity. In critically ill patients, ischemia and non–ischemia-derived lactic acidosis can complicate chronic acidemia with resultant decrease in myocardial contractility, shift of oxyhemoglobin curve to the right, and interference of epinephrine binding to its receptor (31). An underlying renal tubular acidosis—for example, acquired or due to mutations in basolateral sodium bicarbonate cotransporter, NBCe1—may worsen after with treatment with ifosfamide or other medications that are toxic to the tubules. Nephrogenic diabetes insipidus is often due to acquired tubular structural damage, but may be complicated by mutations in the arginine vasopressin receptor 2 and vasopressin-sensitive water channel (aquaporin 2) gene that is associated with loss of water but normal conservation of sodium, potassium, chloride, and calcium. However, inactivating mutations in genes—SLC12A1, KCNJ1, CLCNKB, CLCNKA and CLCNKB in combination, or BSND—that encode the membrane proteins of the thick ascending limb of the loop of Henle have a complex polyuropolydipsic syndrome with loss of water, sodium, chloride, calcium, magnesium, and potassium, and treatment is difficult (32). Disturbances in sodium and potassium balance may also be due to loss—pseudohypoaldosteronism, Bartter and Gitelman syndromes—or gain of function gene mutations—Liddle syndrome (33). Careful attention to renal tubular functions is essential to avoid pitfalls in the critical care settings.

Effect of Acute Kidney Injury on the Progression to Chronic Kidney Disease

Several studies have advocated that AKI is a risk factor for progression to chronic kidney disease (CKD). In elderly patients, AKI without previous CKD, CKD without AKI, and AKI with CKD were associated with a 13-, 8.4-, and 41.2-fold increased risk for developing end-stage renal disease (ESRD) relative to those without kidney disease (34). Hematopoietic stem cell transplant patients who developed AKI within the first 100 days of stem cell transplant were reported to have an increased cumulative incidence of ESRD over time that reached 34% at 10 years (35). Additionally, dialysis requiring ARF was independently associated with a 28-fold increase in the risk of developing stage 4 or 5 CKD and more than a twofold increased risk of death (36). It however remains controversial whether an episode of AKI is itself responsible for the long-term poor prognosis rather than the progression of the underlying renal disease. Despite the notion of interconnectedness of the entities, the drivers of progression to CKD may include failed differentiation and atrophy during tubular regeneration and maybe independent of the processes that initiated them (37).

Clinical Outcomes Following Acute Kidney Injury

The outcome of AKI during a critical illness is of immense importance. The mean duration of inhospital AKI is 14 days. Most episodes resolve in the first month of evolution (38), and 11% of the patients require renal replacement therapy (39). However, the requirement for renal replacement therapy increases to over 70% when AKI is severe, that is, when associated with oliguria or severe azotemia (40,41). The usual ICU mortality approximates 5% without AKI, 23% with AKI, and over 60% with AKI requiring renal replacement therapy. Of the patients with AKI who expire, 78% do so within 2 weeks after the renal insult. The 90-day and 1-year survival of those who are discharged from the hospital are 64% and 50%, respectively (41). Interestingly, the ICU mortality of patients with ESRD is 11%, much lower than for AKI patients who do not need dialysis support (39). The increased mortality associated with the acute decline in renal function is not explained simply by loss of organ function. Recent data from a propensity-matched cohort study has shown that dialysis was associated with increased survival when initiated in patients with AKI who have a more elevated creatinine level (≥3.8 mg/dL) but was associated with increased mortality when initiated in patients with lower creatinine concentrations (42).

The recovery of renal function is influenced by many factors, including pre-existing chronic illness. In one review, only 41% of the patients were reported to be in good health 3 months before entry into the ICU (43); CKD has been reported in 30% of all patients admitted to the ICU (40,41,43). Most survivors of AKI recover renal function within 2 weeks, and 65% to 94% of them have independent renal function at discharge from the hospital (40,41,44). In 43.9 months of follow-up of patients from the Randomised Evaluation of Normal versus Augmented Levels of RRT (RENAL) study, patients with AKI had high long-term mortality (62% to 63%), but few required maintenance dialysis (5.1% to 5.8%) (5).

CHRONICALLY ALTERED RENAL PHYSIOLOGY

Chronic Kidney Disease

The injured kidney can repair itself and regain its structural and functional integrity quickly if the damage is mild. However with severe injury, parenchymal injury may lead to tissue fibrosis and progression to CKD. AKI increases the risk for ESRD; it has been postulated that the surviving renal tubular epithelial cells may have a role in fibrosis due to failure of differentiation and persistently high signaling activity that drives downstream events in the interstitium: inflammation, capillary rarefaction, and fibroblast proliferation (37).

Epidemiology of Chronic Kidney Disease

An increasingly elderly population with pre-existing renal dysfunction is treated in the ICU. The presence of CKD on admission to the ICU is associated with an increase in long-term mortality in survivors of AKI. Furthermore, recovery from AKI is often accompanied by residual renal dysfunction and the perils associated with CKD, which affects 10% of the US population (45).

In 2011, 113,136 patients in the United States started treatment for ESRD. The number of new cases of ESRD in people with diabetes or high blood pressure declined by about 2% in 2011 compared with 2010—the first decrease in more than 30 years; the projected ESRD incident count through 2020 is 150,722 patients, with a projected prevalent count of 784,613 (46). One reason for the discrepancy between the size of the CKD pool and the incidence of ESRD may be the premature cardiovascular death in many patients before progression to renal end stage. An independent, graded association was observed in a large, community based-population between reduced estimated GFR and the risk of death, cardiovascular events, and hospitalization (47). The 5-year mortality of patients with CKD stages 2, 3, and 4 are 19.5%, 24.3%, and 45.7%, respectively; 1.1%, 1.3%, and 19.9% progress to renal replacement therapy, respectively (48). The above data underscore the impact of pre-existing organ dysfunction on the prognosis of critically ill patients.

Chronic Kidney Disease as A Final Common Pathway

The U.S. National Kidney Foundation's Kidney Disease Outcomes Quality Initiative classification of CKD (Table 16.2) facilitates the development of appropriate management plans but does not provide information on the future risk of decline in renal function. Once renal damage reaches a certain threshold, the progression of renal damage is consistent, irreversible, and independent of initial insult. The characteristic histologic findings of tubular atrophy, interstitial fibrosis, and glomerulosclerosis in CKD of diverse causes suggest that multifactorial and complex interactions between numerous pathways of cellular damage by both cellular and humoral pathways contribute to their progression to a common final pathway. Brief overviews of the proposed mechanisms that are involved in the progression of CKD are provided in the following paragraphs.

TABLE 16.2 Definition and Classification of Chronic Kidney Disease (CKD)

DEFINITION

1. Kidney damage for ≥3 mo, as defined by structural or functional abnormalities of the kidney with or without decreased GFR, manifested by either:
   a. Pathologic abnormalities, or
   b. Markers of kidney damage, including abnormalities in the composition of the blood or urine, or abnormalities in imaging tests
2. GFR <60 mL/min/1.73 m^2 for 3 mo, with or without kidney damage

CLASSIFICATION

CKD stage	Description	GFR (mL/min/1.73 m^2)
I	Kidney damage with normal/increased GFR	≥90
II	Kidney damage with mild decreased GFR	60–89
III	Moderate decreased GFR	30–59
IV	Severe decreased GFR	15–29
V	Kidney failure	<15 (dialysis)

GFR, glomerular filtration rate.

The *hyperfiltration theory* emphasizes glomerular hemodynamic changes as the final common pathway in progressive CKD (49). Accordingly, renal injury from diverse causes results in hyperfunction of the remaining glomeruli. The sustained elevations in glomerular pressures and flows favor hyperfiltration and the loss of selectivity of the permeability of the glomerulus. The ensuing proteinuria causes tubular cell injury by "misdirected filtration"—the accumulation of glomerular filtrate outside of the Bowman space and into periglomerular space, creation of a cellular cover around the focus of misdirected filtration by interstitial fibroblasts, extension over the entire glomerulus leading to global sclerosis (50), luminal obstruction, and overwhelming the tubular mechanism by excessive uptake and degradation of filtered protein by the proximal tubule cells. The subsequent extravasation of the accumulated filtered plasma protein into the interstitium causes inflammatory reaction and tubulointerstitial fibrosis (51).

The *complement activation theory* maintains that the proteinuria-induced intraluminal activation of the terminal complement cascade, leading to the formation of C5b-9 membrane attack complex, is the principal mediator of chronic progressive interstitial damage and progressive renal failure in proteinuric renal disease, irrespective of primary glomerular injury. This is supported by the demonstration of increased urinary excretion of C5b-9 in nonimmunologic glomerular injury, correlation of tubulointerstitial deposition of the C5b-9 with interstitial myofibroblast accumulation and proteinuria, and the observation that, in experimental models, progressive interstitial injury was maintained only in hypocomplementemic animals.

The *chronic hypoxia theory* emphasizes chronic ischemic damage in the tubulointerstitium as a final common pathway in end-stage renal injury. The extent of tubulointerstitial damage is better correlated with impaired renal function than the degree of glomerular injury. The countercurrent arrangement of the descending postglomerular vessels and ascending vasa recta vessels, elevated vasa recta permeability to oxygen, and high metabolic requirement results in a graded fall in oxygen tension from the outer cortex to the inner medulla. In extensive tubulointerstitial injury, the loss and distortion of peritubular capillaries, increased transposition of extracellular matrix, vasoconstriction, glomerular damage, anemia, and oxidative stress impair oxygen supply to the corresponding regions. Hypoxia leads to apoptosis or epithelial–mesenchymal transdifferentiation and exacerbates fibrosis of the kidney and subsequent hypoxia, setting in motion the vicious cycle to ESRD (52).

The endothelium plays a crucial role in the maintenance of vascular tone and structure. Endothelium produces NO, a crucial mediator of vasodilation, inhibition of vasoconstrictor influences, antithrombosis, anti-inflammation, and antiproliferation. The generation of NO by nitric oxide synthase is inhibited by asymmetric dimethylarginine (ADMA). Elevated plasma ADMA levels are inversely related to GFR and significantly associated with progression of CKD (53,54). Elevated ADMA in CKD is not due to impaired urinary clearance, but to increased ADMA generation, synthesized by protein methyltransferase, and decreased degradation, mainly by dimethylarginine dimethylaminohydrolase. It is speculated that uremic oxidative stress is involved in the dysregulation of protein methyltransferase and dimethylarginine dimethylaminohydrolase (55).

Erythrocytes represent a major antioxidant component of blood. The generation of oxidants is amplified in anemia and also enhanced in CKD due to increased oxygen consumption by the remnant hyperfunctioning nephrons. Hypoxia of the tubular cells due to decreased delivery of oxygen may be the main link between interstitial fibrosis and tubular destruction. Hypoxia stimulates the production of extracellular matrix by tubular cells and renal interstitial fibroblasts and the release of profibrotic cytokines. Treatment with erythropoietin increases RBC mass, improves RBC survival by antiapoptotic effects, and decreases oxidative stress. Whether the correction of anemia can decrease the progression of CKD remains to be seen (56).

Renal microvasculature is maintained by the balance of angiogenic growth factors—alteration of which impairs capillary repair, causes loss of microvasculature, and leads to a decrease in GFR—and oxygen and nutrient supply to the tubules and interstitial cells. The progressive loss of the endothelium results in capillary collapse and development of glomerulosclerosis, impaired blood flow, and tubulointerstitial fibrosis. Increased expression of thrombospondin-1 and other antiangiogenic factors and decreased expression of vascular endothelial growth factor (VEGF) and other proangiogenic factors influence the renal microvasculature in progressive CKD. VEGF expression correlates with the severity of peritubular capillary loss and inversely correlates with the degree of tubulointerstitial inflammation; it is inhibited by macrophage-derived inflammatory cytokines (IL-10, IL-6, TNF-α) and angiotensin II, and modulated by NO—factors involved in the pathogenesis of renal injury (57).

TABLE 16.3 Impact of Chronic Kidney Disease on Other Organ Systems

Cardiovascular System
Blood pressure control
Inadequate sympathetic response due to autonomic dysfunction
Elevated frequency of cardiac tamponade leading to low blood pressure during dialysis
Coronary disease
High prevalence of severe coronary heart disease
Atypical presentation
False-positive elevations in creatine kinase and troponin T
Appropriate medical therapy is significantly underused
Dysrhythmias
High frequency caused by anatomic and biochemical abnormalities
Especially common during hemodialysis
Respiratory Failure
Pulmonary edema and/or pleural effusion
Restrictive effects of fluid retention contribute to the development of acute ventilatory failure
Metabolic acidosis
High demand for ventilation caused by acidosis makes the weaning a challenge
Auto-PEEP
Airway mucosal edema predisposes to air trapping and endogenous positive end-expiratory pressure
Central Nervous System
Uremic encephalopathy
Usually present when creatinine clearance level falls below 15 mL/min
Disequilibrium syndrome
Neurologic dysfunction caused by rapid correction of uremia

PEEP, positive end-expiratory pressure.

IMPACT OF CHRONIC KIDNEY DISEASE ON CRITICAL ILLNESS

CKD is associated with a decrease in structural and functional reserve. The renal capacity to autoregulate RBF; maintain normal systemic blood pressure; excrete solutes, fluids, electrolytes, and the daily acid load; and metabolize drugs is diminished (Table 16.3). The reduction in physiologic reserve influences drug dosing, treatment modality, and response to interventions in ICU patients. Here we briefly discuss a few issues relevant to the care of the critically ill patients.

Blood Pressure

Hypertension is a major cause of CKD. Hypertension in this population, especially with advanced kidney disease, is often driven by volume overload, sympathetic nervous system overactivity, elevated renin–angiotensin system, and decreased NO production from endothelial dysfunction. Even after initiation of dialysis and achieving dry weight optimal control of blood pressure requires time known as the lag phenomenon. Hypertension control may be complicated by the presence of autonomic dysfunction; this may result in supine hypertension and orthostatic hypotension complicating dialysis treatment of ICU patients who require removal of large quantities of fluid. Management requires excellent coordination of medication and dialysis modalities and prescription. Interestingly, significant downregulation of α- and β-adrenergic receptors can be present, plasma catecholamine levels are often elevated, and patients may be at increased risk of cardiac complications. Another vexing issue is chronic hypotension in dialysis patients. These patients are often poorly dialyzed due to difficulty in maintaining blood pressure on dialysis despite predialysis and intradialysis efforts to increase vascular tone and expand intravascular volume with medications, low dialysate temperatures, increased dialysate sodium and calcium concentrations, low ultrafiltration rates, and frequent administration of osmotic agents. This can be compounded by uremic pericardial effusion which can cause vasopressor-resistant hypotension that, if unrecognized, may have dire consequences for the patient, as the onset of cardiac tamponade can be rapid without premonitory signs.

Cardiac Dysrhythmias

Cardiac dysrhythmias are common in patients with chronic renal failure due to underlying left ventricular hypertrophy, calcific cardiomyopathy that involves the conducting tissues, a "disturbed" metabolic milieu, and chronic tissue hypoxia. An increased incidence of cardiac dysrhythmias is seen in patients with postoperative AKI that may be exacerbated with rapid fluctuations in hemodynamics and electrolyte concentrations in those requiring dialysis support. Atrial fibrillation is common in dialysis patients and its onset is more frequent on dialysis days. In case of hemodynamic instability, synchronized cardioversion is indicated for the treatment of atrial fibrillation. The adverse effects of antiarrhythmic medications are more common in reduced kidney function.

Chest Pain

The presence of renal dysfunction can influence the symptoms, manifestations, and progression of coronary syndromes. CKD affects outcome in patients with acute coronary syndrome and is an independent risk factor for the development of coronary artery disease and for more severe coronary heart disease; CKD is also associated with an adverse effect on prognosis from cardiovascular disease. Many dialysis patients with angina often have a fairly typical history of exercise-induced chest discomfort that is similar to those with normal renal function. However, silent myocardial ischemia is also common among patients with severe kidney disease. It has been speculated that the extremely poor prognosis among dialysis patients with an acute myocardial infarction may be due in part to a relatively increased number of atypical clinical presentations, resulting in both underdiagnosis and undertreatment. The presence of dyspnea alone due to an acute myocardial infarction in an individual scheduled to undergo a regular chronic dialysis procedure may be mistakenly attributed to volume overload. In addition, baseline abnormalities on the electrocardiogram, such as left ventricular hypertrophy, may mask characteristic changes with ischemia.

Disordered Consciousness

Uremic encephalopathy is an organic brain disorder that develops in patients with acute or chronic renal failure, usually when creatinine clearance falls, and remains, below 15 mL/min. Accumulation of toxins, increases in intracellular concentration of calcium in brain cells, and imbalances of neurotransmitter amino acids within the brain are thought to be responsible, although urea itself is not thought to be causative. Clinical manifestations vary with worsening uremia, but prompt identification and initiation of dialysis treatment can readily reverse the symptoms. Initiation of dialysis treatment can also lead to disordered consciousness, especially when advanced states of uremia are dialyzed for excessive lengths of time during their first treatment sessions—the *dialysis disequilibrium syndrome.*

GENERAL PRINCIPLES OF MANAGEMENT

Despite the remarkable progress achieved in understanding the pathophysiology of AKI, no specific pharmacologic agent has yet been approved for its treatment and prevention remains the principal element in its management.

The treatment of established AKI is based on the following principles:

- The preservation of RBF and optimal perfusion pressure favorably influences the deterioration of renal function.
- Correction of uremia, electrolyte, acid–base, endocrine, hematologic and nutritional disorders, and fluid imbalance can favorably affect outcome.
- The pharmacokinetics and clearance of drugs are altered in renal failure, and the appropriate dosage adjustment requires knowledge of the pharmacokinetic parameters of the drugs and clearance characteristics of the different renal replacement techniques.
- The treatment and complications of the primary conditions (e.g., sepsis) that causes AKI may determine the outcome of AKI.
- The appropriate integration of care provided by intensivists and organ specialists can favorably affect outcome.

In certain clinical situations, such as in cardiovascular surgery, ischemic AKI is strongly associated with occult renal ischemia—associated with poor cardiac performance, fixed atherosclerotic disease of the renal arteries and/or prolonged hypoxemia, and reduced renal functional reserve. Due to the silent nature of renal ischemia, prognostic stratification using reliable surrogates can guide clinical decision making (58–61). Recently, the use of atrial natriuretic peptides has been shown to improve dialysis-free survival in thoracic aortic aneurysm surgery patients with impaired renal function. However, the use of atrial peptides in AKI remains controversial—two major clinical trials have reported unfavorable outcomes whereas two smaller clinical trials have shown favorable outcomes.

The prevalence of AKI continues to rise; however, there are indications that the mortality of patients with this disorder may be declining. This decline in mortality is not due to the effects of newer drugs in the treatment, but rather, it is due to the increased cooperation between the intensivists and subspecialists, which has led to a concerted approach to treatment. This has resulted in increased awareness of disease states, early initiation and higher doses of dialysis treatments, maintenance of euglycemia, and other interventions that play important roles in reversing mortality.

Key Points

- Prevalence of AKI continues to increase.
- Mortality of AKI, despite improvements, remains high.
- Loss of autoregulation of RBF, vasoconstriction, and subsequent downstream effects potentiate the inflammatory cascade in AKI.
- Pre-existing organ dysfunction affects the prognosis of critically ill patients.
- Reduced kidney function as well as different renal replacement modalities influence drug dosing and response to interventions in the ICU.
- The treatment of AKI is based on the principle that the preservation of RBF and optimal perfusion pressure improves outcomes.
- AKI is a common finding in hospitalized patients.

References

1. Mehta RL, Kellum JA, Shah SV, et al; Acute Kidney Injury Network. Report of an initiative to improve outcomes in acute kidney injury. *Crit Care.* 2007; 11:R31.
2. Bedford M, Stevens PE, Wheeler TW, Farmer CK. What is the real impact of acute kidney injury?. *BMC Nephrol.* 2014;15:95.
3. Nisula S, Kaukonen KM, Vaara ST, et al; FINNAKI Study Group. Incidence, risk factors and 90-day mortality of patients with acute kidney injury in Finnish intensive care units: the FINNAKI study. *Intensive Care Med.* 2013;39:420–428.
4. Susantitaphong P, Cruz DN, Cerda J, et al; Acute Kidney Injury Advisory Group of the American Society of Nephrology. World incidence of AKI: a meta-analysis. *Clin J Am Soc Nephrol.* 2013;8:1482–1493.
5. Gallagher M, Cass A, Bellomo R, et al; POST-RENAL Study Investigators and the ANZICS Clinical Trials Group. Long-term survival and dialysis dependency following acute kidney injury in intensive care: extended follow-up of a randomized controlled trial. *PLoS Med.* 2014;11:e1001601.
6. Adams PL, Adams FF, Bell PD, Navar LG. Impaired renal blood flow autoregulation in ischemic acute kidney injury. *Kidney Int.* 1980;18:68–76.
7. Kelleher SP, Robinette JB, Conger JD. Sympathetic nervous system in the loss of autoregulation in acute kidney injury. *Am J Physiol.* 1984;246: F379–F386.
8. Abuelo JG. Normotensive ischemic acute kidney injury. *N Engl J Med.* 2007; 357:797–805.
9. Devarajan P. Update on mechanisms of ischemic acute kidney injury. *J Am Soc Nephrol.* 2006;17:1503–1520.
10. Hsu CY, Ordoñez JD, Chertow GM, et al. The risk of acute kidney injury in patients with chronic kidney disease. *Kidney Int.* 2008;74:101–107.
11. Chawla LS, Eggers PW, Star RA, Kimmel PL. Acute kidney injury and chronic kidney disease as interconnected syndromes. *N Engl J Med.* 2014;371: 58–66.
12. Alsous F, Khamiees M, DeGirolamo A, et al. Negative fluid balance predicts survival in patients with septic shock: a retrospective pilot study. *Chest.* 2000;117:1749–1754.
13. Wiedemann HP, Wheeler AP, Bernard GR, et al; National Heart, Lung, and Blood Institute Acute Respiratory Distress Syndrome (ARDS) Clinical Trials Network. Comparison of two fluid-management strategies in acute lung injury. *N Engl J Med.* 2006;354:2564–2575.
14. Dass B, Shimada M, Kambhampati G, et al. Fluid balance as an early indicator of acute kidney injury in CV surgery. *Clin Nephrol.* 2012;77:438–444.
15. Kambhampati G, Ejaz NI, Asmar A, et al. Fluid balance and conventional and novel biomarkers of acute kidney injury in cardiovascular surgery. *J Cardiovasc Surg (Torino).* 2013;54:639–646.
16. Bouchard J, Soroko SB, Chertow GM, et al; Program to Improve Care in Acute Renal Disease (PICARD) Study Group. Fluid accumulation, survival and recovery of kidney function in critically ill patients with acute kidney injury. *Kidney Int.* 2009;76:422–427.
17. Kambhampati G, Ross EA, Alsabbagh MM, et al. Perioperative fluid balance and acute kidney injury. *Clin Exp Nephrol.* 2012;16:730–738.
18. Parke RL, McGuinness SP, Gilder E, McCarthy LW. Intravenous fluid use after cardiac surgery: a multicentre, prospective, observational study. *Crit Care Resusc.* 2014;16:164–169.
19. Hassinger AB, Wald EL, Goodman DM. Early postoperative fluid overload precedes acute kidney injury and is associated with higher morbidity in pediatric cardiac surgery patients. *Pediatr Crit Care Med.* 2014;15:131–138.
20. van der Heijden M, Pickkers P, van NieuwAmerongenGP, et al. Circulating angiopoietin-2 levels in the course of septic shock: relation with fluid balance, pulmonary dysfunction and mortality. *Intensive Care Med.* 2009; 35:1567–1574.
21. Basu RK, Wheeler DS. Kidney-lung cross-talk and acute kidney injury. *Pediatr Nephrol.* 2013;28:2239–2248.
22. Horiguchi Y, Uchiyama A, Iguchi N, et al. Perioperative fluid balance affects staging of acute kidney injury in postsurgical patients: a retrospective case-control study. *J Intensive Care.* 2014;2:26–32.
23. Pham PT, Slavov C, Pham PC. Acute kidney injury after liver, heart, and lung transplants: dialysis modality, predictors of renal function recovery, and impact on survival. *Adv Chronic Kidney Dis.* 2009;16:256–267.
24. Xue J, Wang L, Chen CM, et al. Acute kidney injury influences mortality in lung transplantation. *Ren Fail.* 2014;36:541–545.
25. Wehbe E, Duncan AE, Dar G, et al. Recovery from AKI and short- and long-term outcomes after lung transplantation. *Clin J Am Soc Nephrol.* 2013;8:19–25.
26. Rocha PN, Rocha AT, Palmer SM, et al. Acute kidney injury after lung transplantation: incidence, predictors and impact on perioperative morbidity and mortality. *Am J Transplant.* 2005;5:1469–1476.
27. Osho AA, Castleberry AW, Snyder LD, et al. Assessment of different threshold preoperative glomerular filtration rates as markers of outcomes in lung transplantation. *Ann Thorac Surg.* 2014;98:283–289.
28. Shavit L, Mikeladze I, Torem C, Slotki I. Mild hyponatremia is associated with functional and cognitive decline in chronic hemodialysis patients. *Clin Nephrol.* 2014;82:313–319.
29. Meyers TW, Hostetter TH. Uremia. *N Engl J Med.* 2007;357:1316–1325.
30. Watanabe K, Watanabe T, Nakayama M. Cerebro-renal interactions: impact of uremic toxins on cognitive function. *Neurotoxicology.* 2014;44:184–193.
31. Sabatini S, Kurtzman NA. Bicarbonate therapy in severe metabolic acidosis. *J Am Soc Nephrol.* 2009;20:692–695.
32. Fujiwara TM, Bichet DG. Molecular biology of hereditary diabetes insipidus. *J Am Soc Nephrol.* 2005;16:2836–2846.
33. Bonny O, Rossier BC. Disturbances of Na/K balance: pseudohypoaldosteronism revisited. *J Am Soc Nephrol.* 2002;13:2399–2414.
34. Ishani A, Xue JL, Himmelfarb J, et al. Acute kidney injury increases risk of ESRD among elderly. *J Am Soc Nephrol.* 2009;20(1):223–228.
35. Shimoi T, Ando M, Munakata W, et al. The significant impact of acute kidney injury on CKD in patients who survived over 10 years after myeloablative allogeneic SCT. *Bone Marrow Transplant.* 2013;48:80–84.
36. Lo LJ, Go AS, Chertow GM, et al. Dialysis-requiring acute kidney injury increases the risk of progressive chronic kidney disease. *Kidney Int.* 2009; 76:893–899.
37. Venkatachalam MA, Griffin KA, Lan R, et al. Acute kidney injury: a springboard for progression in chronic kidney disease. *Am J Physiol Renal Physiol.* 2010;298:F1078–F1094.
38. Liano I, Liaño F, Pascual J; Madrid ARF Study Group. Epidemiology of acute kidney injury: a prospective, multicenter, community-based study. *Kidney Int.* 1996;50:811–818.
39. Clermont G, Acker CG, Angus DC, et al. Renal failure in the ICU: comparison of the impact of acute kidney injury and end-stage renal disease on ICU outcomes. *Kidney Int.* 2002;62:986–996.
40. Uchino S, Kellum JA, Bellomo R, et al. Beginning and ending supportive therapy for the Kidney (BEST Kidney) Investigators. Acute kidney injury in critically ill patients: a multinational, multicenter study. *JAMA.* 2005; 294:813–818.
41. Hegarty J, Middleton RJ, Krebs M, et al. Severe acute kidney injury in adults: place of care, incidence and outcomes. *QJM.* 2005;98:661–666.
42. Wilson FP, Yang W, Machado CA, et al. Dialysis versus nondialysis in patients with AKI: a propensity-matched cohort study. *Clin J Am Soc Nephrol.* 2014;9:673–681.
43. Silvester W, Bellomo R, Cole L. Epidemiology, management, and outcome of severe acute kidney injury of critical illness in Australia. *Crit Care Med.* 2001;29:1910–1915.
44. Bagshaw SM, Laupland KB, Doig CJ, et al. Prognosis for long-term survival and renal recovery in critically ill patients with severe acute kidney injury: a population-based study. *Crit Care.* 2005;9:R700–R709.
45. Radhakrishnan J, Remuzzi G, Saran R, et al. Taming the chronic kidney disease epidemic: a global view of surveillance efforts. *Kidney Int.* 2014; 86:246–250.
46. Gilbertson DT, Liu J, Xue JL, et al. Projecting the number of patients with end-stage renal disease in the United States to the year 2015. *J Am Soc Nephrol.* 2005;16:3736–3741.
47. Go AS, Chertow GM, Fan D, et al. Chronic kidney disease and the risks of death, cardiovascular events, and hospitalization. *N Engl J Med.* 2004; 351:1296–1305.
48. Keith DS, Nichols GA, Gullion CM, et al. Longitudinal follow-up and outcomes among a population with chronic kidney disease in a large managed care organization. *Arch Intern Med.* 2004;164:659–663.
49. Brenner BM, Meyer TW, Hostetter TH. Dietary protein intake and the progressive nature of kidney disease: the role of hemodynamically mediated glomerular injury in the pathogenesis of progressive glomerular sclerosis in aging, renal ablation, and intrinsic renal disease. *N Engl J Med.* 1982;307:652–659.
50. Kriz W, Elger M, Hosser H, et al. How does podocyte damage result in tubular damage? *Kidney Blood Press Res.* 1999;22:26–36.
51. Zandi-Nejad K, Eddy AA, Glassock RJ, et al. Why is proteinuria an ominous biomarker of progressive kidney disease? *Kidney Int.* 2004; 92:S76–S89.
52. Nangaku M. Chronic hypoxia and tubulointerstitial injury: a final common pathway to end-stage renal failure. *J Am Soc Nephrol.* 2006;17:17–25.
53. Fliser D, Kronenberg F, Kielstein JT, et al. Asymmetric dimethylarginine and progression of chronic kidney disease: the mild to moderate kidney disease study. *J Am Soc Nephrol.* 2005;16:2456–2461.
54. Ravani P, Tripepi G, Malberti F, et al. Asymmetrical dimethylarginine predicts progression to dialysis and death in patients with chronic kidney

disease: a competing risks modeling approach. *J Am Soc Nephrol.* 2005;16: 2449–2455.
55. Matsuguma K, Ueda S, Yamagishi S, et al. Molecular mechanism for elevation of asymmetric dimethylarginine and its role for hypertension in chronic kidney disease. *J Am Soc Nephrol.* 2006;17:2176–2183.
56. Rossert J, Fouqueray B, Boffa JJ. Anemia management and the delay of chronic renal failure progression. *J Am Soc Nephrol.* 2003;14:S173–S177.
57. Kang DH, Kanellis J, Hugo C, et al. Role of the microvascular endothelium in progressive renal disease. *J Am Soc Nephrol.* 2002;13:806–816.
58. Chertow GM, Lazarus JM, Christiansen CL, et al. Preoperative renal risk stratification. *Circulation.* 1997;95:878–884.
59. Chawla LS, Abell L, Mazhari R, et al. Identifying critically ill patients at high risk for developing acute kidney injury: a pilot study. *Kidney Int.* 2005; 68:2274–2280.
60. Yegenaga I, Hoste E, Van Biesen W, et al. Clinical characteristics of patients developing ARF due to sepsis/systemic inflammatory response. *Am J Kidney Dis.* 2004;43:817–824.
61. Vivino G, Antonelli M, Moro ML, et al. Risk factors for acute kidney injury in trauma patients. *Intensive Care Med.* 1998;24:808–814.

CHAPTER

17

Gastrointestinal Physiology

JUAN B. OCHOA GAUTIER, CARL W. PETERS, and MAUREEN B. HUHMANN

INTRODUCTION

The gastrointestinal (GI) tract is anatomically defined by the organs that comprise the tubular structure that extends from the mouth to the anus. In its simplest form, the GI tract serves the critical role in the ingestion, digestion (processing), and assimilation (absorption) of food. As such, in critical illness, the GI tract is the preferred route of delivery of nutrition (enteral nutrition [EN]) in critically ill patients.

Our understanding of the complexity and importance of the GI tract has grown dramatically with discovery of roles in addition to nutrition. The GI tract contains an active neuroendocrine system through which it interacts in a highly complex fashion with virtually all organs and systems in the body. Throughout the entire length of the GI tract is the site of the greatest concentrations of immune cells in the body, playing highly significant and complex roles in health and disease. Finally, there is the more recent appreciation of our symbiotic relationship with a healthy microbiome. Our gut is host to trillions of microorganisms, which—rather than passive bystanders—have essential roles in the defense against pathogens, in the processing and provision of vital nutrients, and in the fine tuning of immune responses.

The GI tract can be a source of critical illness. Multiple disorders, including critical illness, affect this organ and it can be, in itself, a source of life-threatening diseases; we discuss the most important of these below. Maintaining adequate GI function is, thus, paramount to the survival of the critically ill patient.

BASIC GASTROINTESTINAL ANATOMY, HISTOLOGY, AND PHYSIOLOGY

A Primer on Anatomy and Physiology

While GI tract is "simply" a tubular structure that extends from the mouth to the anus, in reality it is a highly complex system with multiple anatomically distinct organs. The *mouth* provides the initial entry of food into the GI tract. The main function of mouth is the mechanical breakdown of food into a manageable size that allow for the ingestion of food into the stomach and their mixing with GI secretions. The mouth, hypopharynx, pharynx, larynx, and the upper esophagus work in a complex and coordinated fashion to provide for the safe passage of food from the mouth into the esophagus, also known as swallowing.

The *esophagus* provides safe passage of food and saliva from the mouth and hypopharynx into the stomach. A critical function of the esophagus is to prevent the reflux of acid secretions from the stomach into the hypopharynx. The esophagus, like the mouth, is lined with a mucosal squamous epithelium.

During critical illness, swallowing can be severely affected by anatomic disruption (such as the placement of an endotracheal tube), neurologic illnesses, and medications. Alterations of swallowing is known as dysphagia and can lead to the aspiration of saliva (and the bacteria contained in the mouth), refluxed acid secretions from the stomach, and aspiration of ingested food into the airway; aspiration remains a significant cause of morbidity in the critically ill patient.

The *stomach* serves as a temporary repository of food, as well providing for the initial steps of digestion. Passage of chime—the mixture of food and GI secretions—into the duodenum is permitted by the *pylorus*.

The majority of nutrient absorption occurs in the small bowel, composed of the *duodenum, jejunum, and ileum*. The absorptive surface of the small bowel is significantly increased by villi (Fig. 17.1) (1).

The *colon* is composed of four portions, the ascending, transverse, descending, and the sigmoid colon. The colon is lined by a columnar epithelium with an abundance of goblet cells, cells that generate large amounts of mucous and are essential for the prevention of invasion of microorganisms in and through the intestinal wall. The last portions of the GI tract include the *rectum and anus* which provide sensitivity and continence to the presence of stool and flatus.

The mucosal lining of the entire GI tract is constantly renewed. In the small intestine and in the colon, mucosal cells arise from the crypts of Lieberkühn where pluripotent stem cell reside and can give rise to mature epithelial cells. The majority of the cells in the small bowel are mature enterocytes (absorptive cells). Goblet cells are cells that produce mucous and are particularly frequent in the colon. Paneth cells are long-lived cells localized in the small bowel with higher concentrations in the ileum. These cells play highly important antimicrobial roles through the secretion of antimicrobial peptides. Neuroendocrine cells, as their name implies, secrete a variety of hormones and interact with the autonomic nervous system. Tuft cells, relatively infrequent in number, play interesting roles in antigen "sampling" through guanine nucleotide–binding receptors (see below: The Immune System of the Gastrointestinal Tract) (2).

Gastrointestinal Functions

The GI tract provides four basic functions:

1. It serves to break down food, digest, and absorb nutrients (3).
2. A complex system of neuroendocrine functions that carefully regulates local and systemic metabolism in response to food, interacting with other organs and systems.
3. Starting from lymphoid tissues in the mouth and the hypopharynx, specialized immune cells and organs are distributed throughout the entire GI tract, providing us

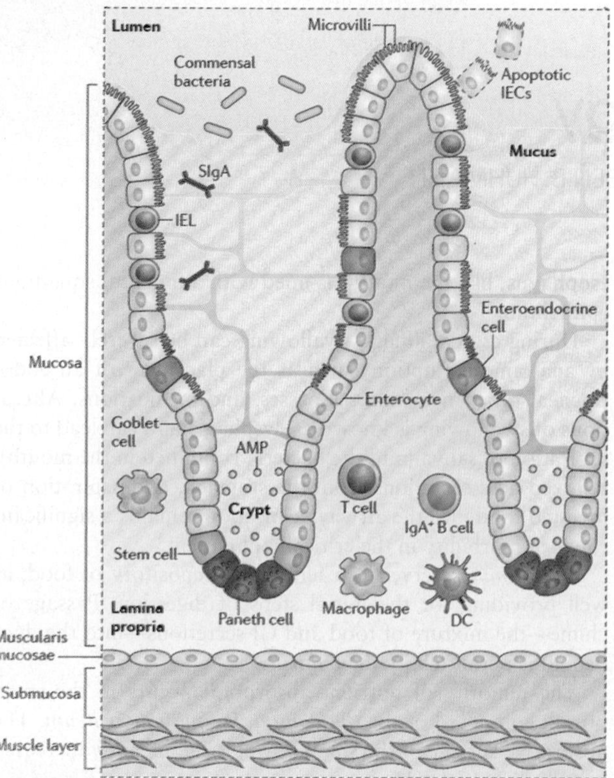

FIGURE 17.1 Schematic depiction of a villus. The villi are foldings of the intestinal epithelium that greatly increase the surface area in contact with the contents within the lumen. They are prominent in the small bowel, where completion of digestion and absorption of nutrients is paramount. Villi are absent in the colon. The cells facing the lumen are composed of a single layer of columnar epithelium consisting of different types of cells. At the base of the villus, stem cells are constantly dividing to produce enterocytes (the most abundant of all cells), goblet cells, neuroendocrine, and Paneth cells. Whereas enterocytes and goblet cells migrate toward the tip of the villus and are shed in just a few days, Paneth cells migrate toward the base (crypt). Goblet cells generate mucous and are most abundant in the colon. Paneth cells produce antimicrobial peptides (AMPs). The tuft cells (not depicted) constitute yet another cell type. Intraepithelial lymphocytes (IEL) can be found in between enterocytes. (From Mowat AM, Agace WW. Regional specialization within the intestinal immune system. *Nat Rev Immunol.* 2014;14(10):667–685. Reprinted by permission from Macmillan Publishers Ltd.)

protection from infection, while allowing (tolerating) the growth and proliferation of a healthy microbiome.

4. A healthy microbiome is essential for health, establishing a symbiotic relationship that permits the survival and growth of hundreds of bacterial species that live in the lumen but do not invade the walls of the GI tract.

Digestion and Absorption

The primary function of the GI tract is to process food, breaking it down mechanically and then, through digestion, convert it into the different substrates that are absorbed and subsequently serve all metabolic processes within the body. The mouth actively participates in the selection of the appropriate quantity and quality of food. Digestion also starts in the mouth with the secretion of amylase and initial breakdown of carbohydrates. In the stomach, the secretion of hydrochloric acid (HCl) by specialized parietal cells and pepsin by chief cells are essential for the initial digestion of protein into peptides. The acid environment also nearly sterilizes ingested food. Further digestion occurs in the duodenum where chyme mixes with bile and exocrine pancreatic secretions. The acid pH of chyme coming from the stomach is neutralized post pylorus by the secretion of bicarbonate. Completion of digestion occurs in the brush border of the small bowel mucosa. In addition, the secretion of fluid into the small bowel dilutes chyme to create an isotonic fluid.

Absorption of digested nutrients proceeds in the small bowel, starting proximally in the duodenum with the absorption of iron, proceeding with the absorption of amino acids, dipeptides, and tripeptides; lipids are broken down by lipases liberating mono- and diglycerides and essential fatty acids, which are surrounded by biliary salts to generate chylomicrons, which are absorbed in the distal ileum. Vitamin B_{12} is also absorbed in the ileum.

The volume of fluid secreted by the GI tract during digestion can be as high as 9 L; absorption of large amounts of this fluid is initiated in the small bowel. The ascending and transverse colon provide a large amount of absorption of fluid and electrolytes so that only a few 100 mL of water are evacuated in the stool.

Neuroendocrine Regulation

A normally functional GI tract has to be able to sense the amount and quality of the food, determine the rate of progression of the food bolus through the GI tract, communicate with other organs in the body to create the necessary metabolic and physiologic responses to a meal. To do this, highly specialized communication systems with distinct but overlapping functions had to be created.

The central and autonomic nervous systems interact with all anatomic and physiologic sites of the GI tract. For one, conscious issues of hunger and satiety, thirst and the desire for specific nutrients (water, sugar, lipids, salt, and others), which may appear as volitional and hedonistic brain functions, are a result of a careful interaction with the GI tract. Classic examples demonstrate an increase in salivation and release of gastric juices in response to a visual stimulus. Satiety is in part governed by hormones such as ghrelin and GLP1 providing another example for this interaction.

Mechanical progression of food and chyme is determined by peristaltic waves which, while promoting mixing of food and GI secretions, provide a measured aboral "wave" from the GI tract; peristalsis is governed by the autonomic nervous system.

The secretion of digestive enzymes is modulated by hormones secreted by specialized cells in the GI tract. In the stomach, gastrin produced by G cells increases the secretion of pepsin and HCl. In the pancreas, secretion of secretin increases the release of bicarbonate-rich pancreatic juice. Cholecystokinin increases the secretion of bile by the liver and contractility of the gallbladder.

Governing the communication between food, the GI tract, and the rest of the body are chemical messengers with different functions. Attempts to classify these messengers are difficult due to the constant growth and discovery of different substances and also to the overlapping functions of some of these. Nonetheless, a simple classification suggests the following categories:

1. Endocrine mediators (hormones). GI hormones are peptides released into the circulation generating local and

distant changes in tissue and organ physiology. Five GI hormones are recognized (although there are multiple unique peptides released from GI cells) and include:
   a. Gastrin
   b. Cholecystokinin
   c. Motilin
   d. Glucose-dependent insulinotropic peptide
   e. Ghrelin
2. Neurocrine messengers. These messengers, mediating communication between the nervous system and the GI tract, include acetylcholine, vasoactive intestinal polypeptide (VIP), substance P, nitric oxide (NO), cholecystokinin, 5-hydroxytryptamine, somatostatin, and calcitonin gene–related peptide.
3. Paracrine messengers mediate local communication between GI cells, and include molecules such as histamine, prostaglandins, somatostatin, and 5-hydroxytryptamine.
4. Immune/juxtacrine messengers, as the names implies, mediates communication between the immune system and the GI tract. Some examples are histamine, cytokines, reactive oxygen species, and adenosine (3).

The Immune System of the Gastrointestinal Tract

Diverse immune tissues are distributed across the entire GI tract where they play significant role in the prevention of invasion by microorganisms. Equally as important, proper immune function creates tolerance against antigenic stimuli that come from food and from symbiotic microorganisms, preventing autoimmune responses and self-injury. The immune system in the GI tract is modulated by nutrients such as vitamin A, by antigens of the microorganisms, and by bacterial products such as short-chain fatty acids.

Immune cells are not equally distributed across the GI tract with significant and dramatic variations in concentrations of cells from organ to organ. Thus, for example, the largest concentration of Th17 cells are located preferentially in the duodenum and jejunum. In contrast, the gut-associated lymphoid tissues (GALT) are preferentially distributed in the distal jejunum, ileum, and cecum. This suggests that there are highly different biologic roles in this distribution, which we are only beginning to delineate (1,3).

The GALT deserves special attention. In the distal small bowel, the GALT is organized in histologically distinct zones called Peyer patches. These contain numerous B-lymphocyte follicles which are flanked by smaller T-cell zones. The Peyer patches appear to be the main source of immunoglobulin A (IgA) in the small bowel. In addition, T lymphocytes are distributed across the intestine. Lymphocytes localized at the basement membrane between enterocytes and are called intraepithelial lymphocytes (IELs), and have a wide variety of regulatory and effector activities. Most frequently, IELs are T lymphocytes and are broadly divided into two categories: conventional (type A IELs) and unconventional (type B IELs).

Both helper T cells (CD4+) and cytotoxic T cells (CD8+) are observed in the lamina propria. Most of these T-cell subsets display a memory T phenotype possibly in response to the constant antigenic "sampling" that occurs at the level of the mucosa.

Of growing interest are the so-called innate lymphoid cells (ILCs) distributed across the small and large bowels, that play important and growing roles in the regulation of physiologic responses to antigenic stimuli and may also play pathologic roles during illness. There are three types of ILCs. Of these, the type 2 ILCs (ILC2) appear to play important roles in antigenic sampling. ILC2 cells proliferate in response to interleukin (IL)-25 which is in turn exclusively generated by tuft cells when activated by an antigenic stimulus. ILC2 cells play essential roles in generating type 2 humoral immune responses; ILC2 cells are also controlled by VIP.

Myeloid cells (macrophages and dendritic cells) are also distributed along the GI tract. Macrophages are the most abundant leukocytes in the intestinal lamina propria where they play essential homeostatic roles including phagocytosis, tissue repair, and healing. Intestinal dendritic cells are a distinct subset of dendritic cells as identified by their receptor signature (CD11c+, MHC class II+, CD64–, F4/80–, and expressing ZBTB46).

Disruption of immune responses are independent causative factors of illness. Such is the case of the inflammatory diseases such as celiac disease, Crohn disease, and ulcerative colitis.

The Gut Microbiome

Central to maintaining normal function of the GI tract is a healthy microbiome. While a microbiome exists all the way from the mouth to the anus, the duodenum and jejunum are nearly sterile. The microbial flora in the mouth and colon are distinct from each other and each one contains hundreds to over a thousand distinct bacterial and viral species and archaebacteria. Protozoa and helminths may also exist, although it is only recently that the role of these organisms in the maintenance of health for the overall microbiome has been recognized. Of all microbiomes the colonic microbiome has currently garnered the most interest.

Technologic advances using the tools of molecular biology have permitted a more complete and diverse mapping of the microbiome than otherwise could be afforded by attempting isolated cultures. In 2010, initiatives in the United States and in Europe created a complete mapping of the microbiome in distinct healthy individuals from different geographic, cultural, and genetic backgrounds. In these samples, over 750,000 distinct genes have been identified; thus, our microbiome contains multiple times more genes than our own cells (4).

Neither the type nor the proportion of bacteria is shared by all individuals. There is also an individual variation in the proportion of bacteria in a given individual in response to dietary changes, although there is a striking stability in bacterial species in a given individual across time.

A healthy microbiome exists in a symbiotic relation with its host that involves the creation of a "tolerant" immune response. The host provides food for bacteria, of which dietary fiber is particularly important. The host also provides for a healthy "temperature and oxygen-controlled" environment. In turn, the microbiome generates important nutrients such as short-chain fatty acids, and other micronutrients that feed the gut mucosa and can be absorbed and distributed systemically.

Disruption of the microbiome can occur as a result of multiple conditions. Acute and chronic alterations can occur as a result of diet. These alterations have been linked to obesity, cardiovascular diseases, and inflammatory bowel diseases such as Crohn disease. Acute disruption of the microbiome associated with antibiotic use causes GI intolerance in acute illness and diarrhea. *Clostridium difficile* colitis constitutes a classic illness associated with a disrupted microbiome, and is now being managed with interventions aimed at restoring microbial homeostasis.

SPECIFIC DISORDERS

Acute Pancreatitis

Acute pancreatitis, a disease process with a wide spectrum of clinical presentations and causes, can challenge any critical care physician. Only 10% to 15% of cases are severe enough to threaten patient survival, and these, therefore, likely involve the critical care physician. Gallstones and alcohol intake cause 85% of the cases of acute pancreatitis (5); the risk in heavy drinkers who also smoke heavily is increased fourfold. Other causes include hyperlipidemia, viral infections, and certain drugs such as propofol (6–8) (Table 17.1).

Of special importance to intensivists is the association between propofol, a medication commonly used for sedation of critically ill patients, and the presence of hypertriglyceridemia and acute pancreatitis. Devlin et al. (6) retrospectively studied 159 patients in the intensive care unit (ICU) with propofol sedation, finding that 29 (18%) patients developed hypertriglyceridemia and, among these 29 patients, three presented a clinical picture of acute pancreatitis. Their final recommendation was to monitor the serum triglycerides levels and pancreas enzymes after 48 hours on propofol.

The diagnosis of acute pancreatitis requires two of the following three criteria: (1) Abdominal pain consistent with acute pancreatitis; (2) pancreatic enzyme elevation to greater than three times the upper limit of normal; and (3) findings characteristic of acute pancreatitis on contrast-enhanced computed tomography (CT) of the abdomen (9). Thus, the usual initial workup for a patient with symptoms consistent with acute pancreatitis is to obtain serum amylase and lipase values and, generally, obtain an abdominal CT (see below). Severity of the disease may be defined using the guidance of the revised Atlanta criteria (Table 17.2). Note, however, that the degree of enzyme elevation at admission does not necessarily forecast eventual disease severity (10).

Acute pancreatitis due to pancreatic duct obstruction—as from a gallstone obstructing the duct—triggers the activation of endogenous pancreatic enzymes such as trypsin, causing autolysis and activation of the inflammatory response which may progress to organ failure (11). Alcohol-induced pancreatitis is more complex, inducing acinar cell dysfunction that leads to precipitation of secretions in the ducts, obstructing outflow (12).

TABLE 17.1 Classification System of Drug-Induced Acute Pancreatitis

Class Ia drugs: At least one case report with positive rechallenge, excluding all other causes, such as alcohol, hypertriglyceridemia, gallstones, and other drugs.

Class Ib drugs: At least one case report with positive rechallenge; however, other causes, such as alcohol, hypertriglyceridemia, gallstones, and other drugs were not ruled out.

Class II drugs: At least four cases in the literature; consistent latency (≥75% of cases).

Class III drugs: At least two cases in the literature; no consistent latency among cases; no rechallenge.

Class IV drugs: Drugs not fitting into the earlier described classes; single case report published in medical literature, without rechallenge.

From Badalov N, Baradarian R, Iswara K, et al. Drug-induced acute pancreatitis: an evidence-based review. *Clin Gastroenterol Hepatol.* 2007;5:648–661, with permission.

TABLE 17.2 Grades of Severity of Acute Pancreatitis

Mild acute pancreatitis
- No organ failure
- No local or systemic complications

Moderately severe acute pancreatitis
- Organ failure that results within 48 hrs (transient organ failure) and/or
- Local or systemic complications without persistent organ failure

Severe acute pancreatitis
- Persistent organ failure (>48 hrs)
  - Single organ failure
  - Multiple organ failure

From Banks PA, Bollen TL, Dervenis C, et al. Acute Pancreatitis Classification Working Group. Classification of acute pancreatitis—2012. Revision of the Atlanta classification and definitions by international consensus. *Gut.* 2013;62(1):102–111.

Bacterial seeding of necrotic pancreatic tissue can occur, most probably through bacterial translocation (BT) from the gut, and may lead to sepsis and delayed death (13); a severe aseptic inflammatory response to pancreatitis may be difficult to differentiate from a septic response due to bacterial contamination. Ideally, in all cases of severe acute pancreatitis, the extent of necrosis should be determined using the gold standard to make such determinations, contrast-enhanced CT. Furthermore, the CT can identify other life-threatening causes of SIRS and shock not uncommonly seen in such critically ill individuals, such as major bleeding and/or hollow viscus erosion/perforation.

After the first 2 to 4 weeks of the disorder it is often seen that initially sterile peripancreatic inflammatory fluid collections coalesce into structures known as *pseudocysts*, which often regress spontaneously, but may persist and become infected, warranting drainage. The patient may show a persistent inflammatory state, and can deteriorate with SIRS, sepsis, or septic shock. Although the presence of air bubbles in the pancreas on abdominal CT scan suggests infection, the gold standard to rule out this possibility is CT-guided needle aspiration of the necrotic pancreatic bed. Intervention, however, is not without hazard: "routine" drainage of pancreatic fluid collection often leads to infection in previous sterile collections (14), and thus the suspicion of infection must be convincing before intervention for drainage is undertaken. A variety of modalities of treatment exists to address infected fluid collections, ranging from percutaneous drainage to endoscopic procedures to minimally invasive or open necrosectomy. Studies of patients managed with percutaneous procedures have shown varying results (15). Transgastric drainage guided by endoscopic ultrasound is ideal in certain clinical situations (15), and may compare favorably with surgical intervention as experience develops (16). Surgical choices include the so-called VARD (video-assisted retroperitoneal debridement) technique with single or repeated procedures for removal of necrotic pancreatic tissue, or open complete necrosectomy with drain placement and continuous irrigation in the postoperative period (17). Clearly, with this variety of choices available for treatment, the decision for optimal treatment of a specific patient with acute pancreatitis must be individualized.

Clostridium difficile Colitis

The selective pressure of antibiotic use may lead to the disruption of normal fecal flora allowing the emergence of resistant organisms and causing disease. Best known of these organisms is *C. difficile*, which can cause diarrheal outbreaks in health care institutions. The emergence of a hypervirulent strain of *C. difficile* known as NAP1/B1/ribotype 027 which produces both toxins A and B—and is frequently fluoroquinolone-resistant—has been a problem of particular importance in ICUs in many countries. *C. difficile* colitis can be a lethal disease particularly if treatment is delayed or inadequate. There is an increased risk of developing severe *C. difficile* colitis in the chronically ill, the elderly, and immunosuppressed patients. Early identification and treatment are critical, and the presence of significant leukocytosis should trigger the possibility of such a diagnosis. The severity of disease ranges from asymptomatic carriage, through diarrhea that is mild in frequency and severity, up to a fulminant and rapidly progressive toxic state with profound leukocytosis, hypotension, hypoalbuminemia, and lactic acidosis; the latter condition warrants the most aggressive treatment regimen which often includes emergent surgery (18). Significant abdominal findings warrant radiologic investigation. An initial abdominal radiograph—a KUB (kidney, ureters, and bladder) study—may reveal significant small intestinal or colonic dilatation with pneumatosis in the colonic wall; abdominal CT scan is useful to assess colon integrity and to rule out other pathologies. Definitive diagnosis can be made using one of a variety of laboratory tests. However, the selected test should ***only*** be performed in individuals with diarrhea so as to avoid treatment of asymptomatic carriers (19). Combination testing designs including immunoassay for *C. difficile* glutamate dehydrogenase antigen followed by a rapid toxin A/B assay in screen-positive samples is a 92% accurate tactic with rapid turnaround (20). Polymerase chain reaction testing for *C. difficile* toxin genes is rapid with high sensitivity and specificity (21). It is important to remember that laboratory tests cannot distinguish between colonization and infection so it is important that diagnostic testing and treatment be made within the appropriate clinical context (22). The current mainstay of medical treatment includes the discontinuation of the inducing antibiotics, if possible (23) and the immediate initiation of oral vancomycin and/or metronidazole—the latter given either intravenously or orally. More serious disease warrants use of high-dose oral vancomycin, vancomycin retention enemas, and possibly fidaxomicin, although the expense of this new medication may limit its availability. The reader is referred to a recent review of treatment recommendations for more detail (24). Aggressive fluid resuscitation—guided by careful monitoring of the clinical condition and volume status—and timely surgical intervention, since this disease entity can progress rapidly to the point of need for surgery, are important to decrease mortality. Despite aggressive treatment of *C. difficile* infection (CDI), however, morbidity from this disease and a significant incidence of recurrence continue to be a problem. Adjunctive treatments such as dietary manipulations, the use of probiotics and toxin-binding agents, and restoration of the colonic flora through the use of fecal transplant are all treatments that are being investigated, although their exact roles are unclear (25). Fecal microbiota transplantation, the administration of fecal flora directly to the lumen of the colon or via a nasogastric (NG) or nasojejunal (NJ) tube to replete the eradicated normal gut bacterial flora, is sometimes used; it appears to have positive effects in recurrent CDI, although with low strength evidence (26). Effectiveness of administration via NG/NJ tube or rectally via colonoscope appears to be equal (27). Some promising findings that warrant further study have been seen in investigations of treatment of CDI with rifampin, rifaximin, nitazoxanide, tigecycline, monoclonal antibodies, and immunoglobulins (28).

Abdominal Compartment Syndrome

Increased intra-abdominal pressures (IAP) compromising blood flow to splanchnic organs have been described in an increased percentage of patients in the ICU. Elevated IAP can have a major negative impact on the functioning of all major body systems that are vital for life (29). Malbrain et al. from the European Community analyzed 265 consecutive patients in the ICU, measuring IAP via transduction of the urinary bladder; this work demonstrated that nonsurvivors tended to have higher IAP (30). Furthermore, patients with prior elevated IAP exhibited increased sepsis-related organ failure assessment (SOFA) scores. In an Argentinian study of 83 critically ill patients, 54% displayed intra-abdominal hypertension (IAH) (IAP_{mean} >12 mmHg) during ICU admission, with significantly higher ICU length of stay and hospital mortality (31). The 2013 consensus definitions from the World Society of Abdominal Compartment Syndrome are these: (1) Normal IAP is 5 to 7 mmHg in critically ill adults, as measured using 25 mL of distilled water instilled into the bladder; (2) IAH exists when the sustained or repeated IAP is greater than 12 mmHg; abdominal compartment syndrome (ACS) exists when the sustained IAP is greater than 20 mmHg and/or abdominal perfusion pressure ([mean arterial pressure] MAP–IAP) is less than 60 mmHg and associated with new organ dysfunction/failure (32). Severity is graded from one to four, based upon the IAP, with recommendations for management steps at each grade. A variety of risk factors for this condition exist. Management obviously involves reduction of the pathologically elevated IAP, most often by fluid removal, sedation and chemical paralysis, optimal patient positioning, decompression by NG drainage and, sometimes, by surgical decompression—decompressive laparotomy. Determining when abdominal decompression to improve splanchnic organ perfusion should be done remains controversial and is partially subjective (33). While this procedure can be life-saving, it is associated with considerable morbidity and mortality in both the short and long time frames.

Acute Mesenteric Ischemia

The splanchnic organs are perfused by three major arterial systems: those vessels radiating from the celiac axis (the left gastric, common hepatic, and splenic arteries) and perfusing the liver, stomach, and spleen; the superior mesenteric artery (SMA), supplying most of the small bowel and the right side of the colon; and the inferior mesenteric artery (IMA), supplying the left side of the colon, sigmoid, and superior portion of the rectum. Acute mesenteric ischemia may be caused by several conditions, such as classic arterial occlusion due to embolism (40% to 50% of cases), atherosclerosis, states of low cardiac output due to shock—including cardiogenic shock—mesenteric venous occlusion or, less frequently, arterial dissection, vasculitis, or nearby inflammatory conditions (34).

Manifestations of acute mesenteric ischemia may range from subtle findings of mild abdominal distention and/or mild pain to those of a devastating disease process of peritonitis, hypotension, circulatory collapse, and death. Reperfusion of the splanchnic organs with restoration of circulation to the affected organs may provoke a dramatic systemic inflammatory response (35). Difficulty in making a swift and accurate diagnosis, and in formulating and executing timely therapy, most often immediate surgical intervention, leads to staggering mortality: 60% to 80% (36).

Physical, laboratory, and radiologic findings in the patient with acute mesenteric ischemia can be difficult to analyze accurately. The presence of severe abdominal pain with few abdominal findings on physical examination in an individual (very often elderly) with risk factors is suggestive of mesenteric ischemia, and warrants immediate and aggressive investigation of this possibility. Patients with this condition—often sedated and mechanically ventilated ICU patients—making accurate abdominal examination quite difficult. Others may present with sudden overt peritoneal signs leading to pursuit of other acute abdominal conditions and delay in diagnosis. Laboratory investigation may reveal hemoconcentration and/or an otherwise unexplained metabolic acidosis or elevated lactate suggesting that progression to bowel injury has occurred. Occasionally, brisk lower GI tract bleeding or, more subtly, heme-positive stools may be discovered. Plain abdominal films are less specific, findings ranging from *normal* to the demonstration of ileus, portal vein air, air in the colonic wall, or free intraperitoneal air (Figs. 17.2 and 17.3). A contrast-enhanced abdominal CT scan is useful as it may identify the precise location of the compromised vessel (artery or vein) and the extent of visceral damage. Ominous signs such as air in the portal vein, the bowel wall, or free air in the peritoneal cavity may be seen. Bedside diagnostic laparotomy/laparoscopy is an option for patients too unstable to be moved for a radiologic study. Recently, treatment of acute mesenteric ischemia has evolved into a treatment strategy combining surgical and endovascular techniques. In suitable candidates, vascular occlusion of the SMA may be treated using catheters placed through the femoral or brachial artery to perform aspirative SMA embolectomy, SMA thrombolysis with recombinant tissue plasminogen activator (rtPA), or recanalization and stenting of the SMA. Such a procedure may be performed in combination with surgical intervention (37,38).

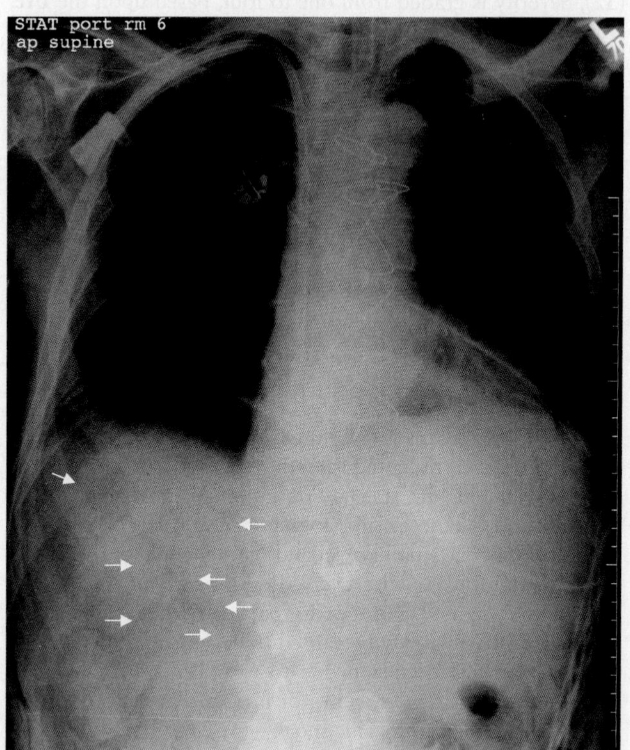

FIGURE 17.2 This abdominal plain film shows the presence of air inside the portal vein, a classic sign for mesenteric ischemia (*arrows*).

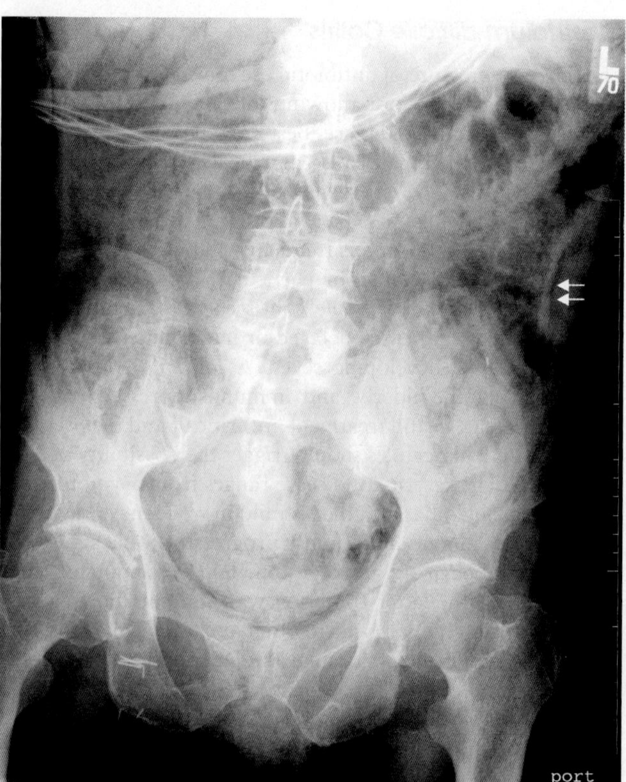

FIGURE 17.3 Note the colonic wall thickening and air bubbles in colonic wall—nonspecific signs for mesenteric ischemia (*arrows*).

Bacterial Translocation from the Gut

The GI tract performs a variety of critical physiologic functions. One among them is the maintenance of the physiologic gut mucosal barrier, which prevents the passage of bacteria—or bacterial products such as endotoxin—into the systemic circulation (39). It has been theorized that the failure of the GI tract to maintain its functional integrity during profound physiologic stress—as in major traumatic injuries or severe burns—may contribute to the phenomenon of multiorgan system failure (MOSF) (40); the exact nature of this morbid interaction, however, remains obscure (41).

It is recognized that, once the gut undergoes a predisposing condition, such as an ischemia–reperfusion insult, bacteria and endotoxins can traverse the intestinal barrier and seed distant organs such as mesenteric lymph nodes (MLNs), solid organs, and the bloodstream, a phenomenon termed *bacterial translocation*. Evidence from several studies has linked BT and the systemic inflammatory response with postoperative sepsis in up to 14% of cases (40,42–44), although BT may only be indicative of MOSF-associated pathologic gut permeability, rather than the cause of MOSF itself in this circumstance (45). Prevention of BT is essential, and is accomplished by careful maintenance of organ perfusion, judicious use of antibiotics, avoidance of excessive IV fluids, and the early institution of EN support (46) in preference to parenteral nutrition, although this assertion is controversial.

Extrahepatic Biliary Disease

Benign extrahepatic biliary disease (EBD) is a common reason for admission to the ICU, as it is often associated with sepsis and the inflammatory response. Epidemiologic data are startling: upward of 25 million Americans harbor gallstones, the consequences of which lead to the expenditure of more than $6 billion for medical and surgical treatment (47). The incidence of EBD increases with age, especially in women from all ethnic groups in the United States (48); it is particularly prevalent in native North Americans (49).

The most common form of EBD is "acute cholecystitis," resulting from cystic duct obstruction, causing increase in intraluminal pressure, venous congestion, and impairment of lymphatic drainage leading to inflammation and likely infection if unrelieved. The progression of acute inflammation of the gallbladder caused by cystic duct obstruction (50), to more serious conditions such as cholangitis—bacterial infection complicating biliary tract obstruction (51)—or emphysematous cholecystitis—infection with gas-forming anaerobic organisms (52)—with considerable morbidity and mortality may occur with delay in surgical consultation and in patients with chronic conditions such as diabetes mellitus or immunosuppression. The main cause of EBD is the presence of gallbladder calculi.

Cholecystitis in the absence of calculi ("acalculous cholecystitis," or ACC) may be observed in those with a variety of critical conditions requiring prolonged intensive care (sepsis, major trauma, substantial life-threatening burns), and who are kept without oral intake and/or are receiving total parenteral nutrition (TPN) (53). Usual findings are fever, hyperbilirubinemia, and right upper quadrant pain, although the only finding may be that of SIRS of obscure origin. Sepsis from acute ACC may be difficult to identify because studies such as ultrasound lose their accuracy in the critically ill (54–56). ACC carries the risk of considerable mortality (57).

The most appropriate initial study when EBD is suspected is *bedside ultrasound of the right upper quadrant,*which is rapid, noninvasive, and relatively accurate (58). Specific signs of inflammation are thickening of the gallbladder wall to greater than 3.5 mm, and/or pericholecystic fluid. Abdominal CT scan may also be helpful in demonstrating pericholecystic fluid and tissue inflammation; the obvious serious disadvantage of CT is the need to transport the patient outside the ICU. Major and minor ultrasound and CT criteria exist which, when combined with radionuclide testing—if movement to the nuclear radiology suite is advisable in a critically ill ICU patient—usually identifies AC or ACC if the intensivist recognizes often subtle findings and aggressively pursues diagnostic investigation. Of note is that nuclear cholescintigraphy has nearly perfect sensitivity in detection of acute cholecystitis (59), superior to ultrasound and CT, logistical difficulties notwithstanding.

The standard method of surgical treatment of acute cholecystitis is presently laparoscopic cholecystectomy (60). Alternatives to this approach, namely administration of antibiotics and analgesics, or nonsurgical but invasive procedures such as percutaneous transhepatic gallbladder drainage (PTGBD), percutaneous transhepatic gallbladder aspiration (PTGBA), endoscopic transpapillary gallbladder drainage and stenting (ETGBS), and endoscopic ultrasound-guided transmural gallbladder drainage (EUS-GBD) may be considered in the critically ill (61). The former two radiologic procedures provide long-term or transient, respectively, decompression and drainage of material from the enflamed gallbladder without the perils of general anesthesia, theoretically an attractive option to surgery in the critically ill. A Cochrane analysis was, however, unable to determine the role of percutaneous cholecystostomy compared to surgical treatment in the clinical management of high-risk surgical patients with acute cholecystitis (62). Procedures involving bile duct cannulation and placement of an intrabiliary pigtail drainage catheter or pigtail stent under endoscopic guidance show promising results nearly comparable to percutaneous procedures (63). A more recently developed procedure involves an endoscopically guided transgastric transmural needle followed by guidewire placement to the gallbladder and drainage tube or stent placement, offering the advantages of utility in the high-risk patient with perihepatic ascites and avoidance of the risks of percutaneous procedures in those with marginal coagulation function (64). As to the very critically ill patient with acute ACC, a study of 1,725 patients revealed improved outcomes with percutaneous drainage compared to surgical (laparoscopic or open) cholecystectomy (65).

Perforation of a Hollow Viscus

Perforation of a hollow viscus with resultant intra-abdominal sepsis is a common cause for ICU admission. As such, the intensivist will frequently manage these patients who present a picture of bacterial sepsis. Patients with colonic perforation may demonstrate varying degrees of septic shock, while those with perforated peptic ulcer disease most often present initially with chemical peritonitis and progress rapidly to bacterial peritonitis with time. Surgical management is obviously integral to such a patient's care, and thus coordination between the anesthesia, surgical, and critical care teams is of great importance.

The combination of an acute abdomen with rapid deterioration of the patient's condition should warrant investigation of the possibility of a perforated hollow viscus. In those abdominal infections caused by perforation of a hollow viscus, the accumulation of infectious material may reside within a confining space adjacent to the perforated organ, such as in the left lower quadrant in the case of a perforated diverticulum in the descending colon and eventually forming into an abscess cavity if not recognized, or more widespread as with a posterior perforating peptic ulcer (66). The emergent nature of the presentation will dictate the next step. Bedside plain abdomen films may demonstrate pneumoperitoneum (67); ultrasound may show, in experienced hands, pneumoperitoneum (68). CT scan may show very small volumes of free fluid and pneumoperitoneum, identify inflammatory changes of the duodenal wall and of surrounding organs (69), or small volumes of air and spillage from colonic perforation (70). Early source control—removal of inflammatory material—is integral to successful management of perforation-related peritonitis (71) sometimes employing a "damage control" surgical strategy in the sickest and most marginally compensated patients. Aggressive supportive and perioperative care is also crucial to optimize outcome, including proper selection of antimicrobial coverage (72).

The Abdomen as an "Unknown Source of Sepsis"

Evaluation of the abdomen as the source of sepsis in the ICU patient is difficult, and the stakes are quite high in that mortality from blood stream infection of abdominal origin is high (73). Clinical examination in a neurologically intact patient remains the gold standard used to rule out an acute surgical abdomen and the identification of the abdomen as a source of sepsis. This is not the case in many critically ill patients in whom neurologic impairment due to the primary disease, or resultant from sedation, abrogates good communication with the patient and a dependable clinical examination; indeed, performing a good clinical examination was not possible in 43% to 69% of patients in the ICU (74). Frequently, the elderly (75) or patients immunosuppressed by virtue of antirejection medication for organ transplant (76) may be unable to mount an inflammatory response such that peritoneal signs sufficient to facilitate immediate recognition are present; these patients may appear only to be "getting sick" despite gross peritoneal contamination. Particularly difficult are those who have had recent previous abdominal surgery and in whom an intra-abdominal septic complication could be a potential cause of critical illness.

How is one to open the "black box" of the abdomen and identify an occult source of sepsis? Several conditions—pancreatitis and mesenteric ischemia, for example—could develop during the ICU admission or may be the primary reason for presentation. The diagnostic approach in these patients is dictated by several factors including the severity of the critical illness, the availability of different diagnostic tools, and the availability of specialized consultants (Fig. 17.4). In patients with severe hemodynamic instability and/or marginal respiratory status, movement to radiologic suites or other diagnostic facilities may be quite difficult to accomplish safely. On the other hand, diagnostic procedures that require potentially risky (77) movement (from the standpoint of LOS but less likely mortality) from the ICU often change treatment, with a favorable risk–benefit ratio (78). Therefore, it is important for the critical care physician to identify the available tools that can assist him or her in the timely diagnosis and management of occult abdominal sepsis.

The use of radiologic tools such as plain abdominal films, CT scan, ultrasound, and nuclear medicine imaging require careful evaluation of the risks associated with the specific study versus the benefit from the information obtained. Safety of movement "to radiology" is a major consideration, as mentioned earlier; furthermore, intravenous radiocontrast material can produce serious toxicity such as acute kidney injury, as well as discomfort and pain. The information yielded by any of the studies may be poor or lead to misinterpretation, thereby increasing morbidity; thus, we discourage the use of diagnostic tests in a "fishing expedition" mode. The studies requested must be done to answer a *specific question or questions* and the results provided by the study should provide the answer. Nonetheless, CT has evolved with advances in practitioner experience and progress in engineering to be taking the lead in diagnosis with great accuracy of critical abdominal causes of sepsis and need for surgical or interventional radiologic intervention (79) even when prudent judgment mandates foregoing IV contrast (80).

Occasionally, the intensivist appeals to the surgeon to perform an exploratory laparotomy as a means to diagnose and treat intra-abdominal illness. Blind exploratory laparotomies, however, have yielded uniformly poor results, generally not identifying the source of infection, while significantly

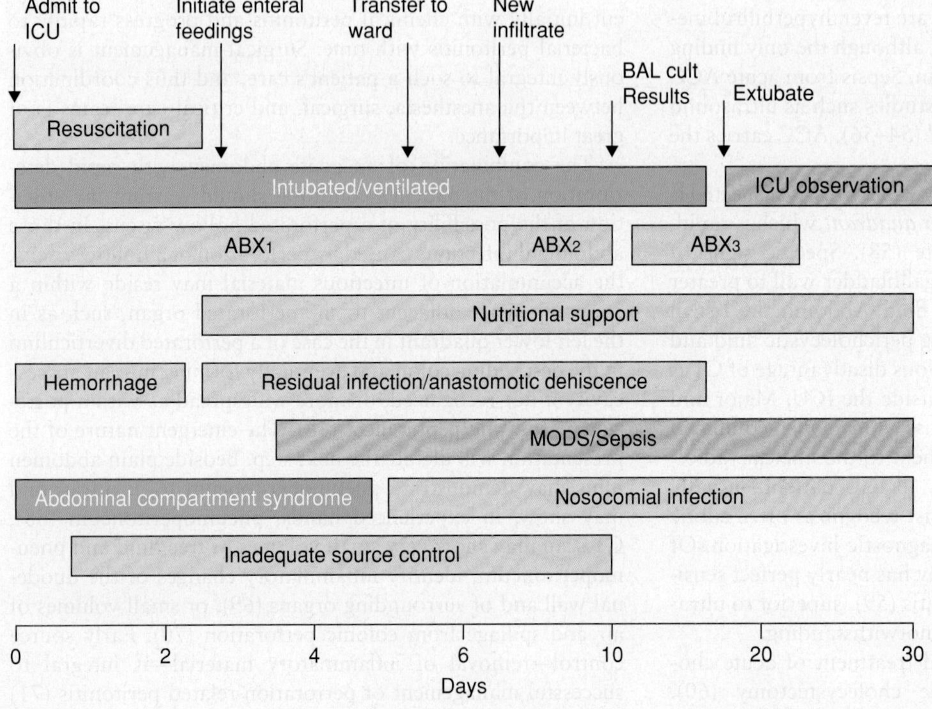

FIGURE 17.4 Scheme showing when, during the course of an intensive care unit admission, intra-abdominal problems are more likely to be seen, especially after abdominal or interventional procedures. ABX, antibiotics; BAL cult, bronchoalveolar lavage culture; ICU, intensive care unit; MODS, multiorgan dysfunction syndrome. (Adapted from Crandakk M, West MA. Evaluation of the abdomen in the critically ill patient: opening the black box. *Curr Opin Crit Care.* 2006;12:333–339, with permission.)

increasing morbidity or mortality (74). Other less aggressive modes of surgical diagnostic intervention exist, though less frequently used, including diagnostic peritoneal lavage (DPL), paracentesis (81), and bedside laparoscopy (82). Surgical intervention in critically septic patients is often managed in stages with multiple operations, with the intensivist supporting the patient through the sequential procedures (83).

GASTROINTESTINAL DYSMOTILITY AND INTOLERANCE

Normal GI motility permits a downstream (aboral) progression of secreted fluids and food through the GI tract. It also prevents bacterial overgrowth and provides the adequate contact of nutrients with the gut mucosa, thereby allowing digestion and absorption. Intolerance in enterally fed patients is documented at 30.5% to 33%, with higher levels of intolerance observed in critically ill patients (84,85). The definition of "intolerance" is somewhat subjective. In 2012 the Working Group on Abdominal Problems (WGAP) of the European Society of Intensive Care Medicine (ESICM) developed definitions for GI dysfunction (Table 17.3) (86). Loss of coordinated propulsive motor impulses may result in decreased digestion and absorption of food and liquids, GI intolerance, and the lack of passage of flatus or stool; this is called ileus. Ileus is therefore a functional intestinal obstruction in the absence of mechanical evidence of obstruction.

Ileus, in its worse clinical presentation, is a manifestation of organ (GI) dysfunction or failure. Ileus can result in ACS, severe electrolytic disturbances, and bacterial overgrowth. Furthermore, the presence of ileus precludes successful enteral nutritional interventions. For these reasons, adequate identification of ileus is an essential aspect of care of the critical care physician.

The diagnosis of ileus is often inaccurate and is based on significant preconceptions that are frequently erroneous. For example, it is often believed that surgical intervention on the GI tract results in ileus and that, postoperatively, this patient population should be kept without oral or enteral intake. Similar misconceptions are often observed with artificially established amounts of gastric residuals or NG outputs. Paradoxically, multiple patients are often kept without enteral intake, which only exacerbates GI dysfunction and provides an inadequate and/or inappropriate diagnosis of ileus.

Ileus must be carefully identified by radiographs and a thorough clinical assessment. Careful hydration and restoration of splanchnic blood flow through adequate resuscitation are essential. The judicious use of enteral nutritional support and avoiding prolonged time periods without enteral intake are essential to the prevention and treatment of ileus. Furthermore, the careful treatment of the cause of an ileus, such as sepsis, will often result in the spontaneous resolution of the GI process. Maintenance of fluid and electrolyte balance are also important.

ENTERAL NUTRITION

When to Feed?

Enteral nutrition (EN) has proven to be beneficial, and should be started as soon as possible in the ICU patient, as there are multiple studies demonstrating its benefits. For example, Moore et al. (87) found that starting early enteral nutrition (EEN) significantly decreased the risk of infections ($p < 0.05$). In contrast, the use of TPN (TPN)—particularly when selected instead of EEN—was associated with significant harm when performed by inexperienced personnel and/or if there was inadequate patient selection. In fact, a recent meta-analysis of 18 RCTs illustrated that EN was associated with decreases in infectious complications (p = 0.004) and ICU-LOS (p = 0.0003) when compared to parenteral nutrition (88).

The mechanisms that explain why EEN is superior to TPN are only partially understood. Routinely, patients on TPN achieve higher caloric goals than on EEN but, despite this practice, patients routinely do better in the absence of TPN. Thus, the benefits of EEN are not linked to the number of calories received by the patient. Starvation is associated with increased mucosal permeability along with increased expression of ICAM-1, favoring the migration of PMNs to the intestine wall

TABLE 17.3 European Society of Intensive Care Medicine (ESICM) Definitions for GI Dysfunction in the Critically Ill

AGI Grade	Definition	Manifestation
I	Increased risk of developing GI dysfunction or failure (a self-limiting condition)	Postoperative nausea and/or vomiting during the first days after abdominal surgery, postoperative absence of bowel sounds, diminished bowel motility in the early phase of shock
II	GI dysfunction (a condition that requires interventions)	Gastroparesis with high gastric residuals or reflux, paralysis of the lower GI tract, diarrhea, intra-abdominal hypertension (IAH) grade I (intra-abdominal pressure (IAP) 12–15 mmHg), visible blood in gastric content or stool. Feeding intolerance is present if at least 20 kcal/kg BW/day via enteral route cannot be reached within 72 hrs of feeding attempt
III	GI failure (GI function cannot be restored with interventions)	Despite treatment, feeding intolerance is persisting—high gastric residuals, persisting GI paralysis, occurrence or worsening of bowel dilatation, progression of IAH to grade II (IAP 15–20 mmHg), low abdominal perfusion pressure (APP) (below 60 mmHg). Feeding intolerance is present and possibly associated with persistence or worsening of MODS.
IV	Dramatically manifesting GI failure (a condition that is immediately life threatening)	Bowel ischemia with necrosis, GI bleeding leading to hemorrhagic shock, Ogilvie syndrome, abdominal compartment syndrome (ACS) requiring decompression

AGI, acute gastrointestinal injury.
From McClave SA, Taylor BE, Martindale RG, et al. Guidelines for the provision and assessment of nutrition support therapy in the adult critically ill patient: Society of Critical Care Medicine (SCCM) and American Society for Parenteral and Enteral Nutrition (A.S.P.E.N.). *JPEN J Parenter Enteral Nutr.* 2016;40(2):159–211.

compared with enteral-fed animals (89). Another interesting experiment showed that adding bombesin, an analogue of gastrin-releasing peptide, can recover the GALT in mice on TPN and, indeed, preserve the immune response to infections (90). Kudsk (91) reviewed the literature regarding EEN, finding fewer infections and better outcomes when such therapy was used. In addition, Andrad et al. (92) studied rats receiving either standard TPN or glutamine-enriched TPN. They found less BT in the group on glutamine-enriched TPN, suggesting that glutamine, an amino acid, improves the response to antigens and increases the IgA levels, as reported previously (93). Other authors have reported that EEN prevents GALT atrophy and the development of SIRS/MOD (94–96).

Monitoring Tolerance and Meeting Nutritional Goals

The typical critically ill patient receives less than 40% of their estimated needs (97); higher protein and calorie delivery in the ICU has been shown to significantly increase ventilator-free days (98). Achieving at least 80% of prescribed protein intake has been linked to improved survival (99). Appropriate prophylaxis for and management of feeding intolerance is an important component to meeting nutrition needs in critically ill patients (100,101). Feeding protocols can be effective in increasing the percentage of nutrition needs delivered (97).

SUMMARY

A healthy GI tract is essential for the survival of the patient with acute/critical illness. The GI tract can be a source of severe life-threatening acute illnesses that necessitate care in an ICU setting. On the other hand critical illness associated with hemodynamic instability, sepsis, and shock can cause significant alterations in GI function. An abnormal GI tract can worsen or perpetuate a persistent inflammatory–immunosuppressive response.

EN provides the healthiest and most appropriate form of nutrition in the critical care setting and should be used whenever possible. In addition to its roles in processing food, the GI tract plays other essential neuroendocrine and immunologic roles. Recently, increasing attention to the microbiome has been paid. A healthy microbiome can be severely disrupted during acute/critical illness. Restoring microbial homeostasis may prevent complications in the ICU and help in restoring health.

Key Points

- The classic role of processing and absorbing nutrients continues to be the main route by which patients are fed through their critical illness.
- There are important and specific roles for the different anatomic portions of the GI tract. Thus physiology of the GI can only be understood if we also understand the anatomy.
- The neuroendocrine system in the GI tract is of importance. Thus, the GI tract influences/affects the functions of distant organs/systems including the central nervous system.
- The GI tract is the single most important repository of immune tissues. The complexity is highlighted by the distribution and role of the cells of the immune system across the GI tract.
- There is an increasing awareness of the importance of the microbiome, distributed across the GI tract, in the maintenance of health and in the symbiotic relationship that exists with the host. A growing body of knowledge informs us to the importance of dysbiosis as a cause of disease and the impact of critical illness on microbiome balance.

References

1. Mowat AM, Agace WW. Regional specialization within the intestinal immune system. *Nat Rev Immunol.* 2014;14(10):667–685.
2. Gerbe F, Sidot E, Smyth DJ, et al Intestinal epithelial tuft cells initiate type 2 mucosal immunity to helminth parasites. *Nature.* 2016;529(7585):226–230.
3. Barret KE, ed. *Gastrointestinal Physiology.* 2nd ed. New York: McGraw-Hill Education/Medical; 2014.
4. Sandrini S, Aldriwesh M, Alruways M, Freestone P. Microbial endocrinology–host-bacteria communication within the gut microbiome. *J Endocrinol.* 2015;225(2):R21–R34.
5. Badalov N, Baradarian R, Iswara K, et al. Drug-induced acute pancreatitis: an evidence-based review. *Clin Gastroenterol Hepatol.* 2007;5:648–661.
6. Devlin JW, Lau AK, Tanios MA. Propofol-associated hypertriglyceridemia and pancreatitis in the intensive care unit: an analysis of frequency and risk factors. *Pharmacotherapy.* 2005;10:1348–1352.
7. Beger HG, Rau B, Mayer J, et al. Natural course of acute pancreatitis. *World J Surg.* 1997;21:130–135.
8. Yadav D, Lowenfels AB. The epidemiology of pancreatitis and pancreatic cancer. *Gastroenterology.* 2013;144(6):1252–1261.
9. Banks PA, Bollen TL, Dervenis C, et al. Acute Pancreatitis Classification Working Group. Classification of acute pancreatitis—2012. Revision of the Atlanta classification and definitions by international consensus. *Gut.* 2013;62(1):102–111.
10. Lankisch PG, Burchard-Reckert S, Lehnick D. Underestimation of acute pancreatitis: patients with only a small increase in amylase/lipase levels can also have or develop severe acute pancreatitis. *Gut.* 1999;44(4):542–544.
11. Lankisch PG, Apte M, Banks PA. Acute pancreatitis. *Lancet.* 2015;386(9988):85–96.
12. Apte MV, Pirola RC, Wilson JS. Mechanisms of alcoholic pancreatitis. *J Gastroenterol Hepatol.* 2010;25(12):1816–1826.
13. Capurso G, Zerboni G, Signoretti M, et al. Role of the gut barrier in acute pancreatitis. *J Clin Gastroenterol.* 2012;46 Suppl:S46–S51.
14. Kolvenbach H, Hirner A. Infected pancreatic necrosis possibly due to combined percutaneous aspiration, cystogastric pseudocyst drainage and injection of a sclerosant. *Endoscopy.* 1991;23(2):102–105.
15. Brun A, Agarwal N, Pitchumoni CS. Fluid collections in and around the pancreas in acute pancreatitis. *J Clin Gastroenterol.* 2011;45(7):614–625.
16. Bakker OJ, van Santvoort HC, van Brunschot S, et al. Dutch Pancreatitis Study Group. Endoscopic transgastric vs surgical necrosectomy for infected necrotizing pancreatitis: a randomized trial. *JAMA.* 2012;307(10):1053–1061.
17. Gooszen HG, Besselink MG, van Santvoort HC, Bollen TL. Surgical treatment of acute pancreatitis. *Langenbecks Arch Surg.* 2013;398(6):799–806.
18. Ofosu A. Clostridium difficile infection: A review of current and emerging therapies. *Ann Gastroenterol.* 2016;29(2):147–154.
19. Kufelnicka AM, Kirn TJ. Effective utilization of evolving methods for the laboratory diagnosis of Clostridium difficile infection. *Clin Infect Dis.* 2011;52(12):1451–1457.
20. Fenner L, Widmer AF, Goy G, et al. Rapid and reliable diagnostic algorithm for detection of Clostridium difficile. *J Clin Microbiol.* 2008;46(1):328–330.
21. Murad YM, Perez J, Nokhbeh R, et al. Impact of polymerase chain reaction testing on Clostridium difficile infection rates in an acute health care facility. *Am J Infect Control.* 2015;43(4):383–386.
22. Bagdasarian N, Rao K, Malani PN. Diagnosis and treatment of Clostridium difficile in adults: a systematic review. *JAMA.* 2015;313(4):398–408.

23. Goldstein EJ, Johnson S, Maziade PJ, et al. Pathway to prevention of nosocomial Clostridium difficile infection. *Clin Infect Dis*. 2015;60 Suppl 2: S148–158.
24. Surawicz CM, Brandt LJ, Binion DG, et al. Guidelines for diagnosis, treatment, and prevention of Clostridium difficile infections. *Am J Gastroenterol*. 2013;108(4):478–498.
25. Miller MA. Clinical management of Clostridium difficile–associated disease. *Clin Infect Dis*. 2007;45:S122–S128.
26. Drekonja D, Reich J, Gezahegn S, et al. Fecal microbiota transplantation for Clostridium difficile infection: a systematic review. *Ann Intern Med*. 2015;162(9):630–638.
27. Postigo R, Kim JH. Colonoscopic versus nasogastric fecal transplantation for the treatment of Clostridium difficile infection: a review and pooled analysis. *Infection*. 2012;40(6):643–648.
28. To KB, Napolitano LM. Clostridium difficile infection: update on diagnosis, epidemiology, and treatment strategies. *Surg Infect (Larchmt)*. 2014; 15(5):490–502.
29. Hecker A, Hecker B, Hecker M, et al. Acute abdominal compartment syndrome: current diagnostic and therapeutic options. *Langenbecks Arch Surg*. 2016;401(1):15–24.
30. Malbrain M, Chiumello D, Pelosi P, et al. Incidence and prognosis of intraabdominal hypertension in a mixed population of critically ill patients: a multiple-center epidemiological study. *Crit Care Med*. 2005; 33:315–322.
31. Vidal MG, Ruiz Weisser J, Gonzalez F, et al. Incidence and clinical effects of intra-abdominal hypertension in critically ill patients. *Crit Care Med*. 2008;36(6):1823–1831.
32. Kirkpatrick AW, Roberts DJ, De Waele J, et al; Pediatric Guidelines Sub-Committee for the World Society of the Abdominal Compartment Syndrome. Intra-abdominal hypertension and the abdominal compartment syndrome: updated consensus definitions and clinical practice guidelines from the World Society of the Abdominal Compartment Syndrome. *Intensive Care Med*. 2013;39(7):1190–1206.
33. De Waele JJ, Hoste EA, Malbrain ML. Decompressive laparotomy for abdominal compartment syndrome: a critical analysis. *Crit Care*. 2006; 10(2):R51.
34. Clair DG, Beach JM. Mesenteric ischemia. *N Engl J Med*. 2016;374(10): 959–968.
35. Vollmar B, Menger MD. Intestinal ischemia/reperfusion: microcirculatory pathology and functional consequences. *Langenbecks Arch Surg*. 2011; 396(1):13–29.
36. Oldenburg WA, Lau LL, Rodenberg TJ, et al. Acute mesenteric ischemia: a clinical review. *Arch Intern Med*. 2004;164(10):1054–1062.
37. Acosta S, Björck M. Modern treatment of acute mesenteric ischaemia. *Br J Surg*. 2014;101(1):e100–e108.
38. Acosta S. Mesenteric ischemia. *Curr Opin Crit Care*. 2015;21(2):171–178.
39. Gatt M, Reddy BS, MacFie J. Bacterial translocation in the critically ill–evidence and methods of prevention (Review). *Aliment Pharmacol Ther*. 2007;25(7):741–757.
40. Moore FA. The role of the gastrointestinal tract in postinjury multiple organ failure. *Am J Surg*. 1999;178(6):449–453.
41. Puleo F, Arvanitakis M, Van Gossum A, Preiser JC. Gut failure in the ICU. *Semin Respir Crit Care Med*. 2011;32(5):626–638.
42. Schmidt H, Martindale R. The gastrointestinal tract in critical illness. *Curr Opin Clin Nutr Metab Care*. 2001;4:547–551.
43. Achenson DWK. Microbial-gut interactions in health and disease. Mucosal immune responses. *Best Pract Res Clin Gastroenterol*. 2004;18:387–404.
44. MacFie J, Reddy BS, Gatt M, et al. Bacterial translocation studied in 927 patients over 13 years. *Br J Surg*. 2006;93:87–93.
45. Deitch EA. Gut-origin sepsis: evolution of a concept. *Surgeon*. 2012; 10(6):350–356.
46. Anastasilakis CD, Ioannidis O, Gkiomisi AI, Botsios D. Artificial nutrition and intestinal mucosal barrier functionality. *Digestion*. 2013; 88(3):193–208.
47. Stinton LM, Shaffer EA. Epidemiology of gallbladder disease: cholelithiasis and cancer. *Gut Liver*. 2012;6(2):172–187.
48. Everhart JE, Khare M, Hill M, Maurer KR. Prevalence and ethnic differences in gallbladder disease in the United States. *Gastroenterology*. 1999;117(3):632–639.
49. Everhart JE, Yeh F, Lee ET, et al. Prevalence of gallbladder disease in American Indian populations: findings from the Strong Heart Study. *Hepatology*. 2002;35(6):1507–1512.
50. Knab LM, Boller AM, Mahvi DM. Cholecystitis. *Surg Clin North Am*. 2014;94(2):455–470.
51. Lee JG. Diagnosis and management of acute cholangitis. *Nat Rev Gastroenterol Hepatol*. 2009;6(9):533–541.
52. Miyahara H, Shida D, Matsunaga H, et al. Emphysematous cholecystitis with massive gas in the abdominal cavity. *World J Gastroenterol*. 2013;19(4):604–606.
53. Huffman JL, Schenker S. Acute acalculous cholecystitis: a review. *Clin Gastroenterol Hepatol*. 2010;8(1):15–22.
54. Glenn F, Becker CG. Acute acalculous cholecystitis: an increasing entity. *Ann Surg*. 1982;195:131–136.
55. Boland G, Lee MJ, Mueller PR. Acute cholecystitis in the intensive care unit. *N Horiz*. 1993;1:246–260.
56. Ryu JK, Ryu KH, Kim KH. Clinical features of acute acalculous cholecystitis. *J Clin Gastroenterol*. 2003;36:166–169.
57. Laurila J, Laurila PA, Saarnio J, et al. Organ system dysfunction following open cholecystectomy for acute acalculous cholecystitis in critically ill patients. *Acta Anaesthesiol Scand*. 2006;50(2):173–179.
58. Yarmish GM, Smith MP, Rosen MP, et al. ACR appropriateness criteria right upper quadrant pain. *J Am Coll Radiol*. 2014;11(3):316–322.
59. Kiewiet JJ, Leeuwenburgh MM, Bipat S, et al. A systematic review and meta-analysis of diagnostic performance of imaging in acute cholecystitis. *Radiology*. 2012;264(3):708–720.
60. Yamashita Y, Takada T, Strasberg SM, et al. Tokyo Guideline Revision Committee. TG13 surgical management of acute cholecystitis. *J Hepatobiliary Pancreat Sci*. 2013;20(1):89–96.
61. Eachempati SR, Cocanour CS, Dultz LA, et al. Acute cholecystitis in the sick patient. *Curr Probl Surg*. 2014;51(11):441–466.
62. Gurusamy KS, Rossi M, Davidson BR. Percutaneous cholecystostomy for high-risk surgical patients with acute calculous cholecystitis. *Cochrane Database Syst Rev*. 2013;8:CD007088.
63. Itoi T, Coelho-Prabhu N, Baron TH. Endoscopic gallbladder drainage for management of acute cholecystitis. *Gastrointest Endosc*. 2010;71(6): 1038–1045.
64. Choi JH, Lee SS. Endoscopic ultrasonography-guided gallbladder drainage for acute cholecystitis: from evidence to practice. *Dig Endosc*. 2015;27(1):1–7.
65. Simorov A, Ranade A, Parcells J, et al. Emergent cholecystostomy is superior to open cholecystectomy in extremely ill patients with acalculous cholecystitis: a large multicenter outcome study. *Am J Surg*. 2013; 206(6):935–940.
66. Singh S, Khardori NM. Intra-abdominal and pelvic emergencies. *Med Clin North Am*. 2012;96(6):1171–1191.
67. Musson RE, Bickle I, Vijay RK. Gas patterns on plain abdominal radiographs: a pictorial review. *Postgrad Med J*. 2011;87(1026):274–287.
68. Nazerian P, Tozzetti C, Vanni S, et al. Accuracy of abdominal ultrasound for the diagnosis of pneumoperitoneum in patients with acute abdominal pain: a pilot study. *Crit Ultrasound J*. 2015;7(1):15.
69. Solomkin JS, Wittman DW, West MA, et al. Intraabdominal infections. In: Schwartz SI, Shires GT, Spencer FC, et al., eds. *Principles of Surgery*. 7th ed. New York: McGraw-Hill; 1999:1515–1550.
70. Zissin R, Hertz M, Osadchy A, et al. Abdominal CT findings in nontraumatic colorectal perforation. *Eur J Radiol*. 2008;65(1):125–132.
71. De Waele JJ. Early source control in sepsis. *Langenbecks Arch Surg*. 2010; 395(5):489–494.
72. Solomkin JS, Mazuski J. Intra-abdominal sepsis: newer interventional and antimicrobial therapies. *Infect Dis Clin North Am*. 2009;23(3): 593–608.
73. De Waele JJ, Hoste EA, Blot SI. Blood stream infections of abdominal origin in the intensive care unit: characteristics and determinants of death. *Surg Infect (Larchmt)*. 2008;9(2):171–177.
74. Crandall M, West MA. Evaluation of the abdomen in the critically ill patient: opening the black box. *Curr Opin Crit Care*. 2006;12:333–339.
75. Laurell H, Hansson LE, Gunnarsson U. Acute abdominal pain among elderly patients. *Gerontology*. 2006;52(6):339–344.
76. Spencer SP, Power N. The acute abdomen in the immune compromised host. *Cancer Imaging*. 2008;8:93–101.
77. Schwebel C, Clec'h C, Magne S, et al; OUTCOMEREA Study Group. Safety of intrahospital transport in ventilated critically ill patients: a multicenter cohort study. *Crit Care Med*. 2013;41(8):1919–1928.
78. Waydhas C. Intrahospital transport of critically ill patients. *Crit Care*. 1999;3:R83–R89.
79. Rubin GD. Computed tomography: revolutionizing the practice of medicine for 40 years. *Radiology*. 2014;273(2 Suppl):S45–S74.
80. Hill BC, Johnson SC, Owens EK, et al. CT scan for suspected acute abdominal process: impact of combinations of IV, oral, and rectal contrast. *World J Surg*. 2010;34(4):699–703.
81. Dever JB, Sheikh MY. Spontaneous bacterial peritonitis: bacteriology, diagnosis, treatment, risk factors and prevention. *Aliment Pharmacol Ther*. 2015;41(11):1116–1131.

82. Ceribelli C, Adami EA, Mattia S, Benini B. Bedside diagnostic laparoscopy for critically ill patients: a retrospective study of 62 patients. *Surg Endosc.* 2012;26(12):3612–3615.
83. Griggs C, Butler K. Damage control and the open abdomen–challenges for the nonsurgical intensivist. *J Intensive Care Med.* 2016;31(9):567–576.
84. Gungabissoon U, Hacquoil K, Bains C, et al. Prevalence, risk factors, clinical consequences, and treatment of enteral feed intolerance during critical illness. *JPEN J Parenter Enteral Nutr.* 2015;39(4):441–448.
85. Wang K, McIlroy K, Plank LD, et al. Prevalence, outcomes, and management of enteral tube feeding intolerance: a retrospective cohort study in a tertiary center. *JPEN J Parenter Enteral Nutr.* 2016 Feb 5 pii: 0148607115627142.
86. Reintam Blaser A, Malbrain ML, Starkopf J, et al. Gastrointestinal function in intensive care patients: terminology, definitions and management: recommendations of the ESICM Working Group on Abdominal Problems. *Intensive Care Med.* 2012;38(3):384–394.
87. Moore FA, Feliciano DV, Andrassy RJ, et al. Early enteral feeding, compared with parenteral, reduces postoperative septic complications: the results of a meta-analysis. *Ann Surg.* 1992;216:172–183.
88. Elke G, van Zanten AR, Lemieux M, et al. Enteral versus parenteral nutrition in critically ill patients: an updated systematic review and meta-analysis of randomized controlled trials. *Crit Care.* 2016;20(1):117.
89. Fukatsu K, Zarzaur BL, Johnson CD, et al. Enteral nutrition prevents remote organ injury and death after a gut ischemic insult. *Ann Surg.* 2001; 233:660–668.
90. DeWitt RC, Wu Y, Renegar KB, et al. Bombesin recovers gut-associated lymphoid tissue and preserves immunity to bacterial pneumonia in mice receiving total parenteral nutrition. *Ann Surg.* 2000;231:1–8.
91. Kudsk KA. Early enteral nutrition in surgical patients. *Nutrition.* 1998; 14:541–544.
92. Andrade M, Santos D, Fernandez S, et al. Prevention of bacterial translocation using glutamine: a new strategy of investigation. *Nutrition.* 2006; 22:419–424.
93. Sawai T, Goldstone N, Drongowski RA, et al. Effect of secretory immunoglobulin A on bacterial translocation in an enterocyte-lymphocyte coculture model. *Pediatr Surg Int.* 2001;17:275–279.
94. Avenell A. Glutamine in critical care: current evidence from systematic reviews. *Proc Nutr Soc.* 2006;65:236–241.
95. Wildhaber B, Yang H, Spencer A, et al. Lack of enteral nutrition: effects on the immune system. *J Surg Res.* 2005;123:8–16.
96. MacFie J. Enteral versus parenteral nutrition: the significance of bacterial translocation and gut-barrier function. *Nutrition.* 2000;16:606–611.
97. Heyland DK, Murch L, Cahill N, et al. Enhanced protein-energy provision via the enteral route feeding protocol in critically ill patients: results of a cluster randomized trial. *Crit Care Med.* 2013;41(12):2743–2753.
98. Elke G, Wang M, Weiler N, Day AG, Heyland DK. Close to recommended caloric and protein intake by enteral nutrition is associated with better clinical outcome of critically ill septic patients: secondary analysis of a large international nutrition database. *Crit Care.* 2014;18(1):R29.
99. Nicolo M, Heyland DK, Chittams J, et al. Clinical outcomes related to protein delivery in a critically ill population: a multicenter, multinational observation study. *JPEN J Parenter Enteral Nutr.* 2016;40(1):45–51.
100. Heyland DK, Cahill NE, Dhaliwal R, et al. Enhanced protein-energy provision via the enteral route in critically ill patients: a single center feasibility trial of the PEP uP protocol. *Crit Care.* 2010;14(2):R78.
101. McClave SA, Taylor BE, Martindale RG, et al. Guidelines for the provision and assessment of nutrition support therapy in the adult critically ill patient—Society of Critical Care Medicine (SCCM) and American Society for Parenteral and Enteral Nutrition (A.S.P.E.N.). *JPEN J Parenter Enteral Nutr.* 2016;40(2):159–211.

CHAPTER

18

Allergy and Immunology

JUAN B. OCHOA GAUTIER

INTRODUCTION

A vigilant immune system is necessary for the survival of all human beings, playing multiple and complex functions on a day-to-day basis. At the most basic level, our immune system is able to recognize self from foreign substances, organisms, or transplanted organs and tissues. The immune system also maintains basic vigilance over abnormal cell growth providing essential protection from tumors.

A central physiologic role of the immune system is the protection of the host from infection, a function that is essential for the survival of the critically ill patient. In addition, the immune system has the essential task, in concert with neurologic and endocrine systems, in coordinating a physiologic metabolic response, reprioritizing energy utilization, and protein anabolism and catabolism that leads to the reorganization of biologic functions necessary for the patient to survive an acute life-threatening illness. A normal immune response is vital for tissue remodeling and adequate wound healing. In essence, thus, an adequate immune response is central for the survival of all acutely ill and critically ill patients (1).

Universally, immune activation occurs in all illnesses. A physiologic immune response (also known as an inflammatory response) is conducive to survival of the patient, with the eventual resolution of the illness, adequate healing of wounds, and a restoration of normal metabolism. It is not surprising that there are instances where the immune responses are maladaptive, further aggravating the illness and even leading to the demise of the patient.

In the 1970s, it was recognized that excessive inflammatory responses (mostly of the innate immune system) in response to infections, burns, or injury, could set up severe metabolic and hemodynamic alterations associated with fever, hyperglycemia, metabolic acidosis, accumulation of lactate, hypotension, multiple organ failure and eventually death. In this model, it was predicted that the magnitude of the systemic inflammatory response was proportional to the severity of the infection or injury. Furthermore, it was thought that this early systemic inflammatory response (SIRS) would lead to a proportional compensatory anti-inflammatory response (CARS), which was proportional to the severity of the systemic inflammatory response characterized by dysfunction of adaptive immune responses, mainly observed T-lymphocyte dysfunction. T-lymphocyte dysfunction was, in turn, associated with increased susceptibility to infection by opportunistic organisms such as fungi. Accordingly, CARS could also have led to death from overwhelming infections (1,2) (Fig. 18.1).

Significant basic research, leading to multiple human observational studies, was based on understanding the sequential SIRS/CARS paradigm with an aim at identifying key triggers that led to early activation of the immune system. Clinical trials based on the premise of controlling excessive innate immune activation with the use of antibodies against cytokines such as tumor necrosis factor (TNF), or targeting toxins released by microorganisms such as endotoxin (lipopolysaccharide-LPS) uniformly failed to demonstrate a significant benefit in acutely ill/critically ill patients. Only one study utilizing activated protein C suggested a benefit, and then only in a subset of patients. However, even this failed to demonstrate a benefit in a phase IV postmarketing trial. Furthermore, in general, a focus on "enhancing" adaptive T-lymphocyte responses has also failed.

These humbling results demonstrate that the complexity of immune response is such that targeted intervention by blocking the action of a single cytokine is most probably going to fail to demonstrate clinical benefit. In this process, investigators have been forced to realize that the initial paradigm of the SIRS/CARS response, while extremely useful as a research tool, has significant flaws. Xiao et al. have demonstrated that both inflammatory and anti-inflammatory responses occur simultaneously which, in a patient that has a successful immune response, ultimately resolves. However, patients may have early severe immune dysfunction creating self-injury through uncontrolled innate immune responses–for example, excessive production of nitric oxide leading to vasodilation and hypotension—while having significant and simultaneous T-lymphocyte dysfunction. In addition, it is now recognized that "smoldering" and continued inflammation may persist for a long time leading—the so-called persistent inflammation–immunosuppression catabolism syndrome (PICS)— to prolonged illness with the ultimate demise of the patient after several months (3) (Fig. 18.2).

There is simply no "magic bullet" to normalize immune responses in the intensive care unit (ICU). A careful understanding of immune response, along with attention to detail at controlling the initial disease process and careful adherence to the prompt initiation of evidence-based therapy are all necessary as they remain the best mechanism to prevent and/or control on unregulated immune response.

STRUCTURAL AND FUNCTIONAL ORGANIZATION OF THE IMMUNE SYSTEM

Innate and Adaptive Immunity

The immune system is structurally and functionally divided into innate and adaptive immunity, which have evolved teleologically to provide sophisticated surveillance and coordinated responses (Table 18.1). Innate immunity—also called natural or native immunity—consists of cellular and biochemical defense mechanisms that are in place and are poised to respond rapidly to immune activation. There are several components of innate and primary immune responses including (a) physical and chemical barriers; (b) phagocytes (neutrophils, macrophages) and natural

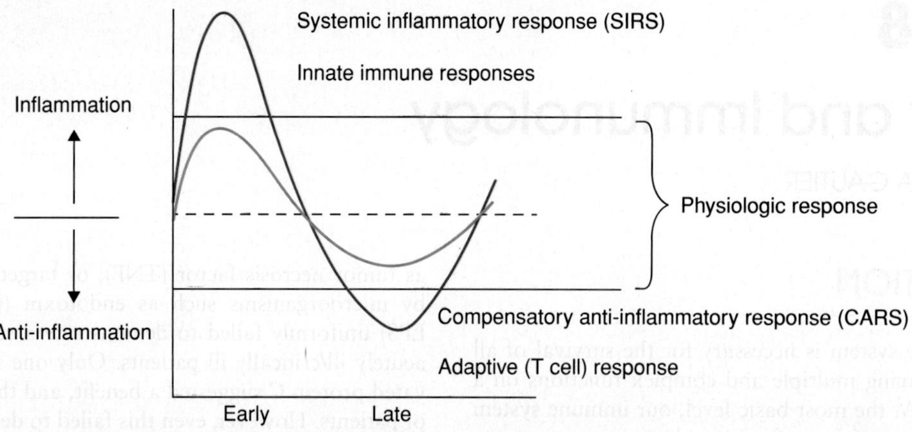

FIGURE 18.1 A historic paradigm was created to depict immune activation after injury or sepsis. It was thought that initial innate inflammatory response was followed by a compensatory anti-inflammatory adaptive immune response, which was proportional to the initial innate activation. Under physiologic circumstances, both the inflammatory and anti-inflammatory responses were self-contained (*blue line*). However, an excessive maladaptive inflammatory response would lead to self-injury, followed by increased susceptibility to infection from an equally maladaptive anti-inflammatory response (*red line*). This paradigm, dominant among investigators, led to the development of multiple clinical trials aimed at curtailing innate responses and/or enhancing adaptive immunity.

killer (NK) cells; (c) the complement system and acute-phase proteins; and (d) cytokines. Innate immune responses are nonspecific and, in acute illness, are typically activated by infections and may also be activated by tissue injury that can result from trauma, surgery, ischemia, and necrosis. Early recognition of invading organisms occurs through the recognition of pathogen-associated molecular patterns (PAMPs) by "microbial sensors" of which the best studied include the toll-like receptors (TLRs). Interestingly, TLRs also recognize molecules released from dead or dying tissues (alarmins and damage-associated molecular patterns). Thus, an immune response in response to infection shares common elements to that of immune responses induced after trauma or burns.

In contrast to innate immunity, the adaptive immune response is highly specific and is activated by exposure to infectious agents or molecules. The defining characteristics of adaptive immunity are exquisite specificity for distinct molecules and an ability to "memorize" and respond more vigorously to repeated exposure. Because of its specificity for a particular antigen, adaptive immunity is also referred to as antigen-specific immunity. Memory increases the rapidity, magnitude, and defensive capabilities with each successive exposure to a particular molecule.

Cellular Components of the Immune Response

Two cell families compose the cells of the immune response; myeloid cells and lymphocytes. Myeloid cells constitute

TABLE 18.1 Structural Division of Immune Responses

Innate immune responses
- First line of defense
- Nonspecific to the antigenic stimulus
  - Responds to both bacterial and tissue injury alike
- Provides cues to an adaptive immune response

Adaptive immune response
- Also called antigen-specific response
- Exquisite capacity to recognize foreign antigens
- Tolerance to self (antigens)
- Development of memory responses

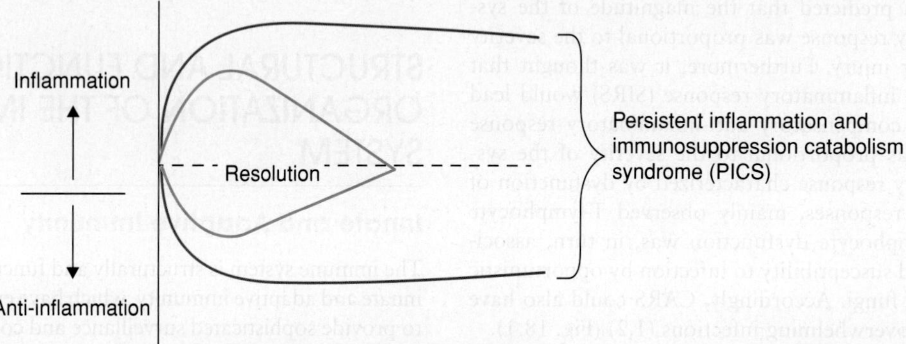

FIGURE 18.2 The possibility of studying the genomic response using new technologies has allowed a better understanding of the complexity of immune activation. A gargantuan effort performed by multiple centers studying the genomic response in different peripheral blood immune cells from both patients after injury and burns, as well as in normal volunteers receiving endotoxin. A virtual "genomic storm" was reported by Xiao and colleagues (2). Both innate inflammatory and adaptive anti-inflammatory responses occur simultaneously. Physiologic responses are self-contained and lead to resolution of illness (*blue lines*). On the other hand maladaptive responses lead to a persistent inflammatory and immunosuppressive syndrome that is also associated with severe muscle wasting and progression to malnutrition (*red lines*).

the most abundant nucleated hematopoietic cell lineage in humans. Classic ontogenic studies describe common myeloid progenitors (CMPs) eventually differentiate into three distinct mature cell lines: macrophages (derived from monocytes), dendritic cells (DCs), and granulocytes. Each of these cell lines play classic roles during immune activation directly functioning as effectors—such as in bacterial killing—while modifying immune and nonimmune physiologic functions.

Recently, an important group of mostly immature myeloid cell subpopulations have been identified playing key roles in immune responses in healthy individuals and during illness. These immature myeloid cells suppress lymphocyte function through two metabolic pathways involving the metabolism of arginine. Due to their suppressive functions, these cells are now called myeloid-derived suppressor cells (MDSCs). There are at least two subpopulations of MDSC, but it is possible there are more. MDSCs accumulate during pregnancy and appear to play an important role in preventing T-cell activation against the growing fetus. MDSCs also accumulate in certain cancers, during infection, and after physical injury (surgery or trauma) where they can cause severe immune suppression, worsening overall prognosis (4).

The main cells of adaptive immunity are lymphocytes; the two main subpopulations of which are designated B and T lymphocytes, which refer to the organs in which those cells are found to mature, bursa of Fabricius in birds (equivalent to bone marrow in mammals) and thymus, respectively. Lymphocyte responses are aided and modified in their provision of physiologic immunity by other cells, including myeloid cells (DCs, macrophages, monocytes, and others). Substances and molecules that induce specific immune responses, or are the targets of such responses, are termed antigens. There are two types of adaptive response: humoral immunity mediated by antibodies and B lymphocytes, and cell-mediated immunity, which involves T lymphocytes. The cardinal features of adaptive immune responses, besides specificity and memory, are diversity, which is the ability to respond to a large variety of antigens; specialization, considered as the optimal response for a particular antigen; self-limitation, allowing a regulated and finite immune response also known as immune homeostasis; and self-tolerance, a nonreactivity to self.

Both innate and adaptive immune responses can be divided into distinct phases: recognition of antigen, activation, and the effector phase of antigen elimination, followed by the return to homeostasis; and in the case of adaptive response, the maintenance of memory.

Lymphoid tissues are classified as generative or primary lymphoid organs, and as peripheral or secondary lymphoid organs. Primary lymphoid organs are bone marrow, where all lymphocytes arise and also where B lymphocytes mature, and the thymus, where T lymphocytes mature and reach a stage of functional competence. The peripheral lymphoid organs and tissues include lymph nodes, spleen, and the cutaneous and mucosal immune system. Specialized microenvironments within primary immune organs support immune cell growth and maturation, while secondary lymphoid organs are sites in which optimal adaptive immune responses are initiated and developed. Lymph nodes are sites of immune response to lymph-borne antigens, and the spleen is the major site of immune response to blood-borne antigens. Similarly, cutaneous and mucosal immune systems are specialized for the best response to potential antigens coming through skin and mucosal surfaces, respectively. Although some cells are permanently resident in one tissue, lymphocytes continuously "traffic" through the bloodstream and lymphatic system, from one peripheral (secondary) lymphoid tissue to another. Lymphocyte recirculation and migration to particular tissues are tightly regulated and mediated by adhesion molecules, chemokines, and their receptors, and depend on the cell maturation and activation stage.

The main cells of the immune system involved in the adaptive immune response are: antigen-specific lymphocytes, specialized antigen-presenting cells (APCs) that display antigens activate lymphocytes, and effector cells that function to eliminate antigens (microbes). Lymphocytes are exclusively capable of specifically recognizing and distinguishing different antigens; no other cell types are able to do so in our body. Lymphocytes consist of subsets that are different in their function, but are morphologically indistinguishable.

B lymphocytes are the only cells capable of producing antibodies. They recognize extracellular (soluble or cell surface) antigens and differentiate into antibody-secreting cells, thus functioning as the mediators of humoral immunity. T lymphocytes, the mediators of cellular immunity, consist of functionally distinct subpopulations. A growing complexity in the number of T-lymphocyte subpopulations is now recognized playing key distinct roles during health and disease. Attempts at understanding the role of T-lymphocyte subpopulations include identification of a functional state (naïve, memory, effector cells) and phenotypic differentiation based on the presence of specific receptors. Yet other mechanisms of differentiation of T-cell subsets are that of the production of specific cytokines and telomere length. There is a significant amount of controversy in the attempts to determine the biologic roles of T-lymphocyte subsets during health and disease. Furthermore, this area of knowledge is changing rapidly as new receptors, cytokines, and functional roles are identified. To complicate things further there are significant interspecies differences including different nomenclatures.

It has emerged that there is a significant overlap between the different T-cell subpopulations suggesting a continuum of differentiation. Nevertheless, it is important to understand the historically established subpopulations, how they are identified, and the biologic roles that these can play under different circumstances. The classic classification of T cells, divides them into helper T cells, cytolytic or cytotoxic T cells (CTLs), and regulatory T cells. NK cells are a third population of lymphocytes with receptors different from those of B and T cells and with major function involving innate immunity.

The use of monoclonal antibodies has allowed the identification of unique surface proteins, which are present only in a particular cell population. These surface proteins have thus been used as their characteristic identification marker(s). The standard nomenclature for these proteins is the CD (cluster of differentiation) numerical designation that currently consists of over 350 different molecules. The majority of characterized molecules, however, are present on more than one cell population, where their presence defines maturation stage or particular effector function. The classification of lymphocytes by CD antigen expression is now widely used in clinical medicine and experimental immunology. T lymphocytes express the CD3 receptor on the cell membranes. According to the CD classification, helper T cells are defined as CD3+ and CD4+; most CTLs are CD3+ and CD8+, while regulatory

T cells are a subgroup of helper cells with an additional low expression of the CD25 activation marker—the α-chain of the surface receptor for interleukin-2 (IL-2Rα)—and are defined as CD3+, CD4+, and CD25+. B cells are characterized with the expression of CD19, while NK cells express the CD56 molecule (1).

APCs are a cell population that are specialized to capture microbial and other antigens, process and present the antigens to lymphocytes, and provide signals that stimulate the proliferation and differentiation of lymphocytes. The major type of APC is the DC, which is found under the epithelia and in most organs, where it is poised to capture antigens and transport them to peripheral lymphoid organs. There are two major subtypes of DCs: myeloid and plasmacytoid. DCs are the most potent APCs capable of stimulating "naïve" T cells as they encounter antigens for the first time. Mature mononuclear phagocytes, tissue macrophages, also function as APCs in a T cell–mediated, adaptive immune response. Macrophages that have ingested microbes may activate "naïve" T cells while, in turn, effector T cells may stimulate the macrophages to more efficiently kill ingested pathogens. Follicular dendritic cells (FDCs) are cells present in the lymphoid tissue that trap antigens in the complex with antibodies or complement products and display those antigens for recognition by B lymphocytes.

After being stimulated by APCs, lymphocytes differentiate into effector cells. Differentiated effector helper T cells secrete cytokines (see below: Cytokines) and interact with and activate macrophages and B lymphocytes. Effector CTLs develop granules containing proteins that kill virus-infected and transformed host (tumor) cells; B cells differentiate into plasma cells that actively synthesize and secrete antibodies. Some antigen-stimulated B and T lymphocytes differentiate into memory cells whose function is to mediate rapid and enhanced responses to second and subsequent exposures to antigens.

Cytokines

These are proteins secreted by the cells of innate and adaptive immunity that mediate many of the functions of those cells. Cytokines are produced in response to microbes and other antigens, and different cytokines stimulate diverse responses of cells involved in immunity and inflammation. In the activation phase of the adaptive immune response, cytokines stimulate growth and differentiation of lymphocytes; in the effector phase, they modulate different cells for a variety of functions including proliferation, cytotoxicity or, alternatively, downregulation.

The number of cytokines, like T-lymphocyte subpopulations, has grown significantly. In some cases, the production of a specific cytokine is characteristic of particular T-lymphocyte subsets. Thus, for example, the production of interferon gamma (IFN-γ) is characteristically generated by NK and TH1 (helper T1) T cells upon activation. In contrast, the production of IL-4 is produced by TH2 (helper T2) cells. Cytokines exhibit multiple potent biologic activities including mediating innate immunity (IL-1, IL-6, and TNF-α); cytokines that control (either stimulate or modulate) adaptive immunity (IL-2, IL-4, IL-5, and IFN-γ); and those that stimulate hematopoiesis (IL-3, IL-7, and some growth factors) among others. Although different cells produce cytokines of innate and adaptive immunity, and those cytokines act on different target cells, this distinction is not absolute because cytokines produced during such reactions often have overlapping actions (1).

Antigen Recognition and Processing

Antigen recognition is the first phase of the adaptive immune response. Antibodies, major histocompatibility complex (MHC), and T-cell antigen receptors (TCRs) are the three classes of molecules used in adaptive immunity to recognize antigens. Antibodies produced in a membrane-attached form function as B-cell receptors for antigen recognition. The interaction of antigen with membrane antibodies initiates B-cell activation and, thus, constitutes the recognition phase of the humoral immune response. B-lymphocyte differentiation, upon activation, proceeds along two pathways: one that requires stimulation by helper T lymphocytes, the T cell–dependent pathway, or a second T cell–independent pathway. The antigens recognized by B cells may be in their native, nondegraded form and not require prior processing of the antigen by other immune system cells. In order to get help from T cells, however, B cells need to internalize the membrane antibody–antigen complex, degrade protein, and display it back on the cell surface membrane in complex with the class II MHC molecule. As explained below, T cells can recognize antigens only if they are processed and presented on the membrane surface of APCs in complex with the MHC molecules. Antibodies are also produced in a secreted form by activated B cells. In the effector phase of the humoral immune response, secreted antibody binds to antigens and triggers several effector mechanisms that eliminate the antigens. Although of the same antigen specificity, membrane-bound antibodies are involved in antigen recognition and B-cell activation, while secreted antibodies are responsible for triggering the effector phase of the humoral immune response and antigen clearance.

In contrast to B cells and their secreted antibodies that can recognize soluble as well as cell-associated antigens in their native form, T cells can only recognize antigens that are displayed on other cell surfaces and are degraded into fragments by the body's various APCs. The task of displaying (presenting) cell-associated antigens for recognition by T cells is performed by specialized proteins that are encoded by genes in a locus called the major histocompatibility complex. MHC molecules are integral components of the ligands that most T cells recognize, because the antigen receptors of T cells are actually specific for the complex of (foreign) peptide antigens and (self) MHC molecules.

MHC molecules are found on immune and nonimmune cells. There are two main types of MHC gene products: class I and class II MHC molecules, which sample different pools of protein antigens, cytosolic or intracellular antigens, and extracellular antigens that have been endocytosed, respectively. MHC class I molecules are present on virtually all nucleated cells where they display antigens to be recognized by CD8+ cytotoxic T lymphocytes. MHC class II molecules are found primarily on APCs and primarily activate CD4+ helper T cells. Once an antigen is engulfed by an APC, it is degraded to its peptide fragments. These antigen fragments are then integrated with the MHC molecule and transported to the cell membrane, where they are exposed to neighboring cells within a complex that includes either class I or class II MHC molecules. T lymphocytes subsequently recognize the MHC–antigen (MHC–Ag) complex and initiate antigenic response (1).

All T lymphocytes recognize an antigen by specific T-cell receptor (TCR) molecules expressed on their cell membrane. These TCR molecules function similarly to a lock and key with the MHC–Ag complex. Only a few T lymphocytes constituting one T-cell clone are specific for one particular antigen. In addition to T-cell receptor binding to the MHC–Ag complex, multiple membrane receptors are used in APC–T-cell interaction. Specificity of T-lymphocyte clones plays important physiologic functions. Specificity assures a graded T-cell response to infection, where upon activation, clonal expansion is sufficient to successfully eliminate the offending organism, cell, or foreign body. Typically, only one in a million T cells responds to a given antigenic stimulus.

Clonal expansion can, in fact, fail in some instances being now recognized as a major pathophysiologic mechanism in different illnesses. Toxic shock syndrome (TSS) is a severe and often fatal disease that may occur in response to an infection by *Staphylococcus aureus*, although it can also occur as a response to other organisms. TSS was famously described with the use of certain types of tampons (now off the market). In contrast to appropriately processed antigens that stimulate a limited number of T cells (one clone) bearing the same TCR (approximately one in a million circulating T cells), some bacterial proteins and toxins are able to stimulate T cells without first undergoing endocytosis and degradation. Those molecules, characterized as superantigens, can simultaneously stimulate T cells with different antigen specificity, and subsequently induce polyclonal activation with the extensive systemic release of cytokines. The stimulatory effect of superantigens is a consequence of direct binding to the class II MHC on APCs and the non–antigen-specific part of TCR on T cells, thus being able to activate 2% to 20% of all T cells. The massive T-cell activation results in the release of large amounts of inflammatory cytokines that induce T-cell anergy or death (apoptosis), which severely disturbs the ability of the immune system to respond appropriately to infection. As a consequence of the systemic effects of released cytokines, infected patients develop systemic effects including fever, endothelial damage, profound hypotension, disseminated intravascular coagulation, multiple organ failure, and death.

Clonal deletion and clonal inactivation are essential processes that eliminate some T-cell clones or prevent them from reacting to an antigenic stimulus. Some clones of T lymphocytes recognize self-antigens in local cells and tissues, and these need to be eliminated to avoid self-injury. Clonal deletion is a process that occurs under physiologic circumstances and is responsible for self-tolerance. However, clonal elimination may fail and is, indeed, what happens in some autoimmune diseases such as rheumatoid arthritis and possibly in inflammatory bowel disease (IBD) (1).

Immune Effector Functions

Antigen Clearance and Initial Immune Activation

Once the immune system recognizes an antigen, inflammation and clearance processes are initiated. Activation and the effector phase of the adaptive immune response are intended to eliminate antigen in the most appropriate and efficient way. For example, one set of components of the immune system is activated in response to the extracellular antigen (antibodies and helper T cells), while others are more effective in the elimination of the intracellular antigen (CTLs and NK cells). Regardless of the type of antigen, processes involved in the activation and effector phase of immune response induce changes in the surrounding tissue, defined as inflammation. The antigen clearance process is enhanced within inflamed tissues by increased vascular flow, altered vascular permeability, and the recruitment of immune cells. Those changes also produce four cardinal clinical signs of inflammation or ongoing immune response: warmness (*calor*), redness (*rubor*), swelling (*tumor*), and pain (*dolor*), often accompanied by malfunction of the involved organ (*functio laesa*).

Several physiologic mechanisms are involved in circulating inflammatory cell adhesion to vascular endothelium and subsequent traffic of immune cells from the circulation into tissues (diapedesis). The process of adhesion is governed by adhesion molecules such as L-selectin, LFA-1, and MAC-1 in immune cells and in endothelial cells (P-selectin, E-selectin, ICAM-1, and ICAM-2 molecules) after stimulation. Expression and function of these molecules is modulated by "early response" cytokines (TNF-α and IL-1) secreted by activated tissue macrophages and other APCs. Additionally, IL-8 production by endothelial cells and tissue fibroblasts is a major component of the chemotactic gradient facilitating neutrophil migration across the endothelial surface. Neutrophils are capable of direct recognition and phagocytosis of circulating antigens. After neutrophil phagocytosis, enzyme-laden lysosomes fuse with the antigen-containing phagosome, digesting and destroying the antigen. Neutrophils possess receptors for the Fc portion of immunoglobulins as well as receptors for complement components. Thus, opsonization or coating of antigens by immunoglobulins and complement markedly enhances phagocytic capability and antigen elimination (5).

The predominant mechanism for adequate reaction to, and rapid clearance of, extracellular antigen involves antibodies or immunoglobulins. Antibodies possess unique antigen specificity, thereby narrowing the inflammatory response to the specific antigenic target. Antibodies circulating in the bloodstream or interstitial fluid promptly recognize, and bind to, an antigen; but because antibodies do not directly perform any effector function, the elimination of antigen requires interaction of antibody with the components of innate immunity such as complement proteins or phagocytes and eosinophils. Antibody-mediated effector functions include neutralization of microbes or toxic microbial products, activation of the complement system, opsonization (coating) of antigens for enhanced phagocytosis, antibody-dependent cell-mediated cytotoxicity (ADCC), and immediate hypersensitivity in which antibodies trigger mast cell activation.

Antibodies

Antibodies are highly specific to a particular antigen. The molecular site at which the antibody recognizes an antigen is called an epitope. Specificity and effector functions of antibodies depend on their basic structure. An antibody molecule has a symmetric core structure composed of two identical light chains and two identical heavy chains. Both heavy chains and light chains consist of amino terminal variable (V) regions and carboxyl terminal constant (C) regions. While light- and heavy-chain amino terminal variable regions together participate in antigen recognition, only the constant regions of the heavy chains are involved in antibody effector functions.

Several different types of antibodies or immunoglobulins (Ig) exist and can be divided into distinct classes and subclasses on the basis of differences in the structure (heavy chain), tissue and biologic fluid distribution, functional capability, and timing of the immune response. In order from the highest to the lowest serum concentration, those classes of antibody molecules (also referred to as isotypes) are designated as IgG, IgA, IgM, IgD, and IgE.

Different classes of antibodies perform different effector functions. Among the most notable functions of immunoglobulins are opsonization and the capacity to activate complement. IgG, IgM, and IgA are also crucial for phagocytic cells to recognize an antigen (known as opsonization). Opsonization by IgG and IgM expedites the clearance of circulating antigens, whereas the secretion of IgA onto mucosal surfaces facilitates the clearance of invading organisms by mucosal surface macrophages and neutrophils. Because of its larger size, the function of IgM is confined primarily to the intravascular clearance of antigens, whereas IgG readily diffuses into the extravascular space. After being coupled with an antigen, antigen–antibody complexes—also termed immune complexes—are normally cleared by phagocytic and red blood cells. The clearance of immune complexes from the circulation is dependent on effective opsonization, binding of the immune complex–bound C3b fragment to CR1 on erythrocytes, and subsequent transport to the liver and spleen. IgD is primarily found on the surface of naïve B cells where it functions as the receptor for antigen recognition; a small amount of IgD is also secreted, generally along with IgM. The physiologic function for IgD appears that of activation of basophils. In contrast to other immunoglobulin classes, once secreted, IgE is present free in the serum for a very short time, since it binds rapidly to the specific receptor on basophils, eosinophils, and mast cells. Antigen activation of cell-bound IgE results in the immediate release of various mediators, including histamine, serotonin, and leukotrienes. Although IgE is commonly connected to the allergic reactions, the physiologic function of IgE seems to be an immediate response to antigen and the induction of vascular dilation, increased vascular permeability, and the recruitment of immune cells; another important immune function of IgE is to protect the host against parasites.

The complement system is capable of generating a broad series of inflammatory actions associated with antigen clearance. These actions include lysis of cells bearing antigen–antibody complexes, opsonization of antigens, chemotaxis of inflammatory cells, and generation of anaphylactic reactions. Complement activation may be accomplished by either the classic pathway, initiated by antigen–antibody complexes, or the alternate route initiated by antigenic protein aggregates, endotoxin, or insoluble compounds with certain surface characteristics. With sequential proteolysis of complement substrates, various complement fragments with neutrophil and eosinophil chemotactic properties, as well as vasodilatory effects, are generated that produce the previously mentioned cardinal signs of inflammation (6).

Cellular Involvement in Immune Response

The major cells involved in antigen clearance include APCs and lymphocytes, neutrophils, and various organ-specific structural cells or tissue macrophages. Although many antigens may be destroyed within mononuclear phagocytic cells by intracellular enzymes, some antigens may become sheltered within these cells. Elimination of these antigens requires additional activation from helper T cells, which predominates in the case of bacterial infection. In general, the helper population of T lymphocytes (CD4+) supports the function of mononuclear phagocytic cells and enhances antibody production by B lymphocytes, thus supporting the clearance of extracellular antigens. Activated T cells increase the secretion of cytokines that are crucial for regulation of the immune response.

On the basis of the pattern of cytokines secreted, CD4+ lymphocytes are subdivided into two major classes: Th1 or Th2. The cytokines secreted by the Th1 group of CD4+ cells, including IL-2 and IFN-γ, are potent stimulants of the cell-mediated immune response. Th2 CD4+ cells secrete cytokines such as IL-4 and IL-10 and IL-13 that stimulate humoral responses including the secretion of antibodies while exerting a regulatory role on cellular immune responses.

It is apparent that Th1 and Th2 responses are carefully orchestrated for successfully overcoming illness as could be seen in critically ill patients. A Th1 response is essential for the survival against infection, while a Th2 response prevents an excessive inflammatory response and sets the stage for healing of tissues. While understanding helper T cell responses as a dichotomous response is a significant oversimplification of immune response, it has served to understand how an imbalance between Th1 and Th2 can be a cause of illness. Thus, caution has to be exercised while interpreting the role of Th1 and Th2 cellular responses in complex processes such as seen in critically ill patients.

Increasing attention is being paid to the presence of different Th1 and Th2 subpopulations during health and disease. Predominance (also known as polarization) of Th1 responses appear to be a causative factor in continued unabated inflammation and self-injury in patients with Crohn disease; on the other hand a predominance of Th2 responses and the subsequent regulation of Th1 functions may worsen outcomes in patients with certain cancers, HIV, and tuberculosis (7).

The CD8+ population of T lymphocytes (CTLs) is essential for combating infection generating, for example, lysis of the infected cell such as is observed during viral infections. In a carefully orchestrated process, after exposure to processed antigen, and under the influence of the lymphokines IL-2 and IFN-γ, activated CD8+ cells proliferate, synthesize, and secrete membrane attack molecules, which result in lysis of the antigen-bearing cell. Besides the important role of the T lymphocyte in clearing microbial pathogens, CTLs are crucial for recognizing and eliminating self-transformed tumor cells. Tumor cells may express new antigens, which are presented on the cell surface within class I MHC molecules antigenic complexes. When functioning adequately, recognition of tumor cells arising in tissues is considered to be an essential and, in most cases, successful mechanism that of tumor surveillance and killing.

Similar to the cell lysis by CTLs, NK cells lyse neighboring cells by secreting membrane attack molecules (perforin and granzymes). Unlike the CTL response, the NK cell lysis of antigen-bearing cells does not seem to be antigen specific. Killer lymphocytes, the third major cytolytic cell population, are coated with surface receptors for antibodies. Killer lymphocytes may localize to antigen–antibody-coated cells, where they release their cytotoxic granules. Antibody recognition is crucial to this system, and killer lymphocyte function seems to be a component of antibody-dependent cytotoxicity.

NK cells and killer lymphocytes can be activated and made to proliferate in vitro under the influence of cytokines. These lymphokine-activated killer (LAK) cells may be reinfused into the body and have been investigated as cancer immunotherapy (8).

In addition to the primary immune APCs or professional APCs, structural cells, such as those of the endothelium, epithelium, and connective tissue, are also important to an effective immune response. Not only are these cells capable of secreting cytokines and inflammatory mediators, but after stimulation, they also express class II MHC molecules and may function in antigen presentation to T lymphocytes. Those cells, termed nonprofessional APCs, can play important physiologic roles. However, the activation of nonprofessional APCs by particular cytokines (IFN-γ) may underlie the organ dysfunction associated with chronic immune stimulation and inflammation (1).

Additional Factors and Mediators

Multiple additional inflammatory mediators from migrating leukocytes, such as proteases, oxygen radicals, leukotrienes, platelet-activating factors are released early on upon infection or after tissue injury, expanding the local inflammatory process. Conversely, several cytokines and soluble cytokine receptors are normally present to downregulate or limit the inflammatory response. Among these "anti-inflammatory" factors are IL-4, IL-10, IL-13, transforming growth factor (TGF)-β, other growth factors, and IL-1 receptor antagonist.

Myeloid-Derived Suppressor Cells and Arginine Metabolism

Increased numbers of myeloid cells are observed accumulating in the tumor and in lymphoid organs in patients with certain cancers. Similarly, myeloid cells accumulate rapidly in the spleen and in the circulation within hours of an injury or after surgery (9,10). These cells generally exhibit markers of immature myeloid cells and, given the appropriate growth stimuli, appear to exhibit the potential to differentiate in macrophages, granulocytes, or APCs. In cancer and after injury, immature myeloid cells are capable of suppressing T-lymphocyte function through two different enzymatic pathways that utilize arginine as a substrate; hence the name myeloid-derived suppressor cells (MDSCs). Nitric oxide synthase (iNOS) expression can be induced in myeloid cells through classic inflammatory stimuli including IL-1, TNF, and IFN-γ. Nitric oxide (NO) generated by iNOS can profoundly inhibit T-lymphocyte function. Conversely, anti-inflammatory stimuli such as IL-4, IL-13, and prostaglandin E_2 (PGE_2) induce arginase 1, which efficiently destroys arginine, an essential amino acid during T-lymphocyte activation. Arginine depletion inhibits T-lymphocyte function by acting on protein translation targeting the mammalian target of rapamycin (mTOR) and the general control nondepressible 2 (GCN2) serine/threonine-protein kinase (11).

Phenotypical and functional characteristics of arginine depletion have been described in T lymphocytes. Zhu et al. (4) first described these changes in cell cultures of T cells grown with limited arginine availability, demonstrating a decrease in the number of T-cell receptors on the cell membrane, an incapacity to proliferate, and a modest capacity to generate/utilize IL-2. It was later observed that expression of the ζ-chain, a peptide dimer whose concentrations significantly decrease in certain cancers and after trauma was exquisitely sensitive to arginine deprivation.

Immune suppression caused by MDSC through arginine depletion can be profound. Under physiologic circumstances, by accumulating in the placenta, arginine depletion may prevent fetal rejection. Under pathologic circumstances, MDSC may be part of an elaborate mechanism of tumor evasion, significantly worsening the prognosis of these patients. Loss of T-cell function (also known as anergy) is characteristically observed after trauma or after major surgery, and is associated with increased susceptibility to opportunistic infections such as *Candida albicans* and other fungal species (12).

Metabolic Effects of Immune Responses

Cytokines released into the systemic circulation as a consequence of either localized or systemic inflammation have been directly implicated in the pathophysiologic mechanisms of the organ dysfunction associated with major trauma, sepsis, and burns. If high plasma concentrations are achieved, IL-1, TNF-α, and IL-6 been shown to have profound effects on body metabolism and are capable of inducing hypotension, fever, and cachexia. Their functions have been implicated in the manifestations of septic shock, and their concentration correlates with mortality. In response to TNF-α, NO is produced by endothelial cells and, along with the other mediators, promotes smooth muscle relaxation and vasodilation.

HYPERSENSITIVITY REACTIONS INCLUDING ALLERGIES

Adaptive immunity serves the important function of host defense against microbial infections. However, the immune system is also capable of causing tissue injury and disease. Hypersensitivity reactions are a group of illnesses caused by immune responses leading to tissue injury and even death. Hypersensitivity is a term that arose from the clinical observations that an individual who has been exposed to an antigen instead of developing tolerance created a detectable clinical reaction becoming "sensitized" to subsequent encounters with the antigen. A common cause of hypersensitivity diseases is failure of self-tolerance, which, under physiologic conditions, ensures that the individual's immune system does not respond to his or her own antigens. Hypersensitivity diseases also result from uncontrolled or excessive responses against foreign antigens such as microbes and noninfectious environmental antigens (13).

Hypersensitivity diseases represent a clinically heterogeneous group of disorders that have been classified into four different types based on the nature of the abnormal immune response, the tissue injury caused, and the clinical manifestations that arise from these (Table 18.2).

Type I Hypersensitivity

Type I hypersensitivity reaction, also called immediate hypersensitivity, is the most prevalent type of hypersensitivity diseases and is characterized clinically as an allergic reaction. Type 1 hypersensitivity occurs when the patient has become "sensitized" to an otherwise innocuous antigen (also known

TABLE 18.2 Types of Hypersensitivity Responses

Type I
- Typically called as an "allergic" response
- Mediated by IgE
- Examples include asthma and allergic rhinitis

Type II
- Recruitment of inflammatory cells
- Tissues injury through activation of complement, recruitment of neutrophils and/or macrophages, and direct antibody effects against hormone receptors, clotting factors, or others.
- Examples include some vasculitis, glomerulonephritis, and myasthenia gravis

Type III
- Immune complex disease (antigen–antibody complex)
- Secondary damage through deposition of immune complexes in tissues
- Example includes serum sickness

Type IV
- Delayed-type hypersensitivity
- Examples include type I diabetes mellitus, rheumatoid arthritis, and inflammatory bowel disease

as allergen) to generate IgE antibodies, which are bound to mast cells, basophils, and eosinophils. Upon activation these cells degranulate, releasing a variety of mediators including histamine, leukotrienes, prostaglandins, and other substances. These mediators collectively cause increased vascular permeability, vasodilation, bronchial and visceral smooth muscle contraction, and local inflammation.

In clinical medicine, allergy is the most common disorder of the immune system, affecting up to 20% of all individuals in the United States. The most common clinical illnesses caused by type 1 hypersensitivity include allergic rhinitis (hay fever), bronchial asthma, atopic dermatitis (eczema), and food allergies.

A particularly concerning type I hypersensitivity is that which develops to certain medications such as antibiotics (penicillin). Severe, systemic allergic reactions can be life threatening, causing generalized edema, respiratory distress, hypotension among other manifestations and is called anaphylaxis. Anaphylactic reactions to medications can occur in hospitalized patients including those that arrived to the ICU.

Type II Hypersensitivity

Like type I, type II hypersensitivity is also mediated by antibodies other than IgE. Antibodies that react to an antigen can cause tissue injury by recruiting and activating inflammatory cells. Those antibodies are specific for antigens of particular cells or the extracellular matrix (generated in our own tissues). Antibodies against tissue antigens observed in type II hypersensitivity can cause disease by three main mechanisms.

1. Antibodies against antigens on circulating cells promote complement activation and cell lysis or phagocytosis. These antibodies are thought to be the cause of different illnesses including certain anemias, thrombocytopenia, and/or agranulocytosis.
2. Antibodies deposited in the tissue recruit neutrophils and macrophages, which in turn can release (through degranulation) their products and induce tissue injury. This is the case with blistering skin diseases, vasculitis, and some forms of glomerulonephritis.
3. Some antibodies to a hormone, hormone receptors, blood-clotting factors, growth factors, an enzyme, or a drug might cause disease or treatment failure by inactivating or activating vital biologic function of these molecules without inducing any inflammation and tissue damage. Diseases mediated by this mechanism include myasthenia gravis and hyperthyroidism.

Type III Hypersensitivity

Immune complex disease, or type III hypersensitivity, is caused by antibody–antigen complexes formed in tissues. In certain disease states, immune complexes may freely circulate or be deposited within tissues, stimulating inflammatory reactions throughout the body. Immune complexes easily activate and complement neutrophils that cause tissue injury. In contrast to the type II diseases, type III hypersensitivity diseases are often systemic, and include serum sickness and systemic lupus erythematosus (SLE) among others.

Serum sickness is characterized by the formation of circulating antigen–antibody complexes 7 to 10 days after injection of an antigenic protein into the body. With systemic deposition of the immune complexes, complement is activated and edema, rash, arthralgia, and fever result. Serum sickness can be observed after treatment with antithymocyte globulin (equine or rabbit origin) or snake antivenom (equine origin).

Type IV Hypersensitivity

Tissue injury may be due to T lymphocytes that activate the effector mechanisms of delayed-type hypersensitivity (DTH) or directly kill target cells. Such conditions are type IV hypersensitivity disorders. In those diseases, tissue injury results from the products of activated macrophages, such as hydrolytic enzymes, reactive O_2 species, NO, and proinflammatory cytokines. Many organ-specific autoimmune diseases are caused by hypersensitivity reactions induced by T cells, such as insulin-dependent diabetes mellitus, multiple sclerosis, rheumatoid arthritis, contact sensitivity, and IBDs.

IMMUNE DEFECTS AS A CAUSE OF CRITICAL ILLNESS

Life-threatening diseases can also occur when the immune system is incapable of mounting an immune response rendering the patient susceptible to recurrent and often unusual infections, increased susceptibility to tumors, and impaired wound healing. Immune defects can be congenital or acquired. Congenital diseases are not frequently observed in clinical practice; nevertheless, a short review of some of the common problems is discussed below to familiarize the critical care physician of their nature. In addition, due to the specialized nature of illnesses, suggested therapies are avoided in this chapter and the reader is encouraged to seek specialized information and early consultation with clinical immunologists.

Defective Complement Response

Defects of the complement system include deficiencies of individual complement component proteins, regulatory proteins, or complement receptors. Complement component deficiencies may be broadly grouped into early (C1–C4) or late-component (C5–C8) deficiencies. A predisposition to *Streptococcus pneumoniae* and *Haemophilus influenzae* infections are observed in patients deficient in early complement components. In contrast to patients with late-component deficiencies, patients with early-component deficiencies possess a uniquely higher incidence of autoimmune disease, especially SLE. In these patients, it has been suggested that the complement deficiency impairs effective clearance of circulating immune complexes, predisposing to autoimmune diseases. *Neisseria meningitidis* infections are recognized as sequelae of late-component deficiencies.

Complement Activation in Critical Illness

Complement activation is a central component to the innate immune response to injury. In addition, both the alternate and classic pathways of complement activation have been shown to be activated in septic shock. Like all immune functions, complement activation plays key physiologic roles. Nevertheless, a maladaptive complement response and also be observed. For example, an exaggerated immune response associated with complement activation has been observed in patients with H1N1 pneumonia (14). Complement depletion is observed in patients with septic shock and is associated with elevation of the dimer and coagulopathy. The correlation of complement depletion and other complement abnormalities with mortalities is however unclear (15).

Alterations in Immunoglobulin Production

Abnormalities of immunoglobulin production manifest most commonly as deficiencies, although the excessive production of immunoglobulins occasionally results in severe sequelae, as may occur in Waldenström macroglobulinemia. Infectious consequences result from most forms of immunoglobulin deficiency. The most common adult type of primary immunoglobulin deficiency is a selective deficiency of IgA. Although IgA deficiency has been associated with recurrent infections of the paranasal sinuses, pneumonia, and Giardiasis, many of these patients remain asymptomatic. The clinical consequences of hypogammaglobulinemia are more frequent in patients with the heterogeneous disorders that compose common variable hypogammaglobulinemia. Common variable hypogammaglobulinemia includes a group of disorders characterized by low or absent serum immunoglobulin levels and clinical manifestations that may be similar to IgA deficiency. Because the infections are usually recurrent and generally responsive to treatment, these patients may present in adulthood with bronchiectasis and lung destruction. Infections with encapsulated bacteria, such as *Haemophilus* and *Streptococcus*, are especially prevalent. The most frequently diagnosed immunoglobulin deficiency pattern in these patients is a decrease in all classes of immunoglobulins (16).

Among the many disorders associated with elevated serum concentrations of immunoglobulins, diseases associated with excessive IgM production are especially notable for acute clinical sequelae. Because of their size and structure, IgM globulins possess unique properties, including cold insolubility (cryoglobulins) and the potential to greatly increase blood viscosity. Excessive IgM production may result from as a response to mycoplasma and viral infections; alternatively, it can be a neoplastic-like B-lymphocyte response (Waldenström macroglobulinemia). The cold agglutinin response to infections rarely results in more than a mild hemolytic anemia, but the IgM levels associated with Waldenström macroglobulinemia may produce life-threatening consequences. Viscosity-related sequelae include confusion, coma, visual impairment, and congestive heart failure (17).

Illnesses Associated with Impaired Neutrophil Function

The most common abnormalities of phagocytic function are related to either an abnormal number or function of circulating neutrophils. The consequence of almost all neutrophil defects is infection, primarily bacterial and fungal, and, less commonly, viral. The incidence of infection among neutropenic patients correlates with the depression of the circulating neutrophil count and the duration of neutropenia. Neutropenia is graded based on absolute neutrophil count as mild (1,000 to 1,500 cells/μL), moderate (500 to 1,000 cells/μL), or severe (<500 cells/μL). The risk of infection increases proportionally as the circulating neutrophil count falls and is greater when the neutropenia persists over several days. Universally, patients with an absolute neutrophil count below 1,000 cells/μL have a substantially increased risk of infection over time, while serious infections are uncommon until more severe neutropenia develops with counts less than 500 cells/μL. With neutrophil counts below 100 cells/μL, the incidence of severe infection increases dramatically (1,18).

Acquired Defects in Immune Function

Acquired defects in lymphocyte- and macrophage-regulated immunity are the most common immunodeficiencies encountered in adults. Three major groups of disorders account for most of these disorders: acquired immunodeficiency syndrome (AIDS), lymphoid and hematologic malignancies, and iatrogenic immunosuppression. These diseases are associated with enhanced susceptibility to infections with common pathogens, as well as a unique predisposition to infections with opportunistic microorganisms.

As of 2015, some 37 million patients were living with AIDS, 1.2 million of these in the United States. HIV was identified as the cause of AIDS almost 35 years ago, spreading rapidly around the world. HIV targets CD4+ cells, eventually resulting in their depletion. Clinical manifestations of AIDS, mostly characterized by opportunistic infections and certain cancers (Kaposi sarcoma), are observed when CD4+ counts drop below 200 mm^3. Other immunologic abnormalities in patients with HIV include an accumulation of MDSCs, though their clinical significance is unknown. Severe pulmonary infections, frequently by organisms such as *Pneumocystis jirovecii, Listeria monocytogenes, Nocardia* sp., *Mycobacteria* sp., *Cryptococcus neoformans*, and cytomegalovirus are observed. Attempts to create a successful vaccine against HIV have failed so far. However, antiretroviral therapy has significantly prolonged the life of patients with HIV effectively preventing millions of deaths worldwide (19,20).

Iatrogenic Immune Suppression

A large number of medications affect immune function either as a side effect (e.g., chemotherapeutic agents) or as a targeted therapy. Chemotherapeutic agents used for the management of cancer patients may suppress the bone marrow decreasing lymphocytes and myeloid cells. Bone marrow suppression can generate a life-threatening susceptibility to infection and is also a limiting factor in aggressively treating patients with cancer (4).

Regulation of immune responses is particularly important in autoimmune diseases. With the greater knowledge of the immune system, it has become increasingly possible to provide highly targeted therapies in illnesses such as rheumatoid arthritis, lupus, IBD, and others with the use of so-called disease-modifying biologic agents. There are several major classes of biologic agents in this category, including antibodies against cytokine and depletion of B lymphocyte with anti-CD20 antibodies and the modulation of the B-cell receptor. Biologic modifiers are also used as a targeted therapy in transplanted patients to prevent organ rejection; these target T lymphocytes (21).

Corticosteroids

An essential response to sepsis and other acute injuries is that of the elevation of cortisol. There are multiple observations that suggest that inadequate elevations of cortisol response in critical illness can be maladaptive and are associated with poor outcomes. This is particularly important in sepsis.

Over 33 clinical trials have been performed to determine the clinical role of corticosteroids in sepsis. In addition to the endocrine role, corticosteroids also suppress immune function at multiple levels providing significant anti-inflammatory effects. A recent meta-analysis of the existing clinical trials as well as other levels of evidence suggest that careful use of corticosteroids in patients with septic shock is associated with a modest but significant decrease in mortality. Whether this beneficial effect is due to the endocrine role or the anti-inflammatory effect provided by corticosteroids (or both) is unclear.

Immunotherapy for Cancer Treatment

A central role of the immune system is to maintain vigilance to prevent the growth of malignancies. It is thus thought that failure of immune surveillance may be responsible for the clinical appearance of certain cancers. Immunotherapy involves the utilization of biologic response modifiers in an attempt to actively recruit the immune system to attack the tumor. Immunotherapy has gained a clear clinical role in certain tumors such melanomas and renal cell carcinomas and its role is expanding rapidly. Immunotherapeutic approaches can be classified as follows: cytokines (e.g., IL-12); cell-based therapies, which include vaccines and adoptive cell therapy; and immune checkpoint blockade, including PD-1 and CTLA-4 inhibitors. Immunotherapy may have significant side effects, including significant enhancement of inflammatory responses, such as is observed with the use of IL-2 (22).

IMMUNE RESPONSES IN CRITICAL ILLNESS

Immune activation plays a central role in the survival of all critically ill patients. Our understanding of immune responses has grown significantly in the past 15 years. From the early days of critical care, it was suggested that an abnormal immune response could cause systemic illness that affected multiple organs eventually leading to their failure. Significant progress at avoiding multiple organ systems failure (MOSF) has been made in critically ill patients with trauma or after surgery, and its incidence has decreased dramatically. No single intervention is responsible for this. Rather, the benefit has occurred with simple and clear attention to detail, early recognition of any issues, the avoidance of overly aggressive iatrogenic interventions, and a progressive knowledge of the organ physiology and adaptive responses.

Multiple organ failure continues to be observed in patients with sepsis. Sepsis has been recently redefined as a "life-threatening organ dysfunction caused by a dysregulated host response to infection." Septic shock is considered as a subset of patients with sepsis, which can be identified by persistent hypotension requiring vasopressor to maintain a MAP of at least 65 mmHg and are at substantially increased risk of mortality.

Multiple immunomodulatory agents, including cytokines, antibodies to cytokines, and soluble cytokine receptors, have been tested for the management of critical illnesses with particular interest in the management of septic shock. Whereas initial clinical trials suggested some efficacy of certain anti-endotoxin antibodies, studies in larger patient populations clearly demonstrated no benefit and perhaps a harmful effect; these results are not surprising, considering the complexity of the immune system regulatory mechanisms in critical illnesses.

A gargantuan effort in the past 15 years was done by multiple centers in an attempt to better understand the immune response in patients after trauma, burn victims, and in normal human beings receiving endotoxin. Using gene micro arrays and other technologies in isolated peripheral leukocytes, investigators demonstrated a "global reprioritization affecting over 80% of the cellular functions and pathways of the immune system" (2). They called these massive changes as a "genomic storm." Interestingly, there is a significant overlap and similarity between the genomic response of injury, burns, and volunteers receiving endotoxin. These findings demonstrate that innate immune responses are activated while simultaneously activating anti-inflammatory responses.

Based on these observations, investigators have begun understanding the determinants of maladaptive immune responses. As there is progressive success at managing early multiple organ failure, there are a growing number of patients who now survive the ICU. However, at least a number of these patients continue to have a subacute or chronic illness characterized by progressive loss of muscle mass, continued susceptibility to infections, pool wound healing, and eventual death. This persistent inflammation–immunosuppression catabolism syndrome appears to be our next challenge. Interestingly, the biggest determinants of poor outcomes in these patients are the continued T-cell dysfunction and the elevation in the expression of MDSCs expressing arginase. It remains to be seen whether interventions aimed at improving T-cell function and regulating MDSC activity will result in improved outcome (23).

SUMMARY

Appropriate immunologic responses are crucial to recovery from most critical illnesses. All aspects of immunity are tightly integrated, such that cell-mediated immune responses and humoral responses do not function as independently of each other, as was once thought. Similarly, almost all nonimmune cellular and organ functions, such as those responsible for hemodynamic stability and body metabolism, have been shown to be partially modulated by networking cytokine messages from the multiple immune system cells. The complex intercommunication among immune and nonimmune system cells manifests itself as many of the systemic symptoms commonly associated with acute illness, such as fever, hypotension, and protein depletion. Perturbation of the immune defense systems, whether on a congenital or acquired basis, complicates the recovery process and commonly prolongs otherwise curable illnesses.

A better understanding of the immune system has allowed or targeted interventions in autoimmune diseases. Conversely, immunotherapy involves the manipulation of the immune system at specific target levels to induce an immune response against cancer. Significant improvement in outcomes has been observed using both approaches. Significant side effects may also be present and may land the patient in the ICU. Because of the specialized nature of these new therapeutic approaches, it is strongly suggested that the intensivist consult clinical immunologists for help when these cases arise.

While targeted immune modulation has failed so far in the management of critically ill patients, progressive understanding of the pathophysiology of illnesses such as sepsis and injury allowed better control in the progression of these patients to the development of early multiple organ failure and death. Long-term survival of these patients is not possible. However, continued adaptive immune suppression associated with significant metabolic abnormalities in amino acid regulation and severe muscle loss (cachexia) occurs in the so-called persistent inflammatory immunosuppression cachexia syndrome. In the future, we expect to find immunotherapeutic approaches to overcome adaptive T-cell dysfunction and improve protein anabolism, resulting in long-lasting cure.

Key Points

- Activation of both inflammatory and anti-inflammatory responses occurrence is simultaneous during illness in all critically ill patients.
- A balanced/physiologic response leads to a self-limited immune response. A maladaptive/pathologic immune response can lead to organ failure and increased susceptibility to infection.
- The best mechanism to manage immune activation during critical illness is to control the illness for which the patient was admitted, paying attention to detail, following guidelines and protocols, and impeccable timing.
- Iatrogenic immune dysfunction can occur as a result of the treatment of several illnesses. Iatrogenic immune dysfunction may lead to increased susceptibility to opportunistic infections.
- Targeted therapy is now possible to generate immune suppression in illnesses such as autoimmune diseases. Immunotherapy using biologic response modifiers is now a useful tool for the treatment of certain cancers.

References

1. Paul WE. The immune system: introduction to immunology. In: *Fundamental Immunology*. 7th ed. Philadelphia, PA: Wolters Kluwer/Lippincot Williams & Wilkins; 2013.
2. Xiao W, Mindrinos MN, Seok J, et al. A genomic storm in critically injured humans. *J Exp Med*. 2011;208(13):2581–2590.
3. Vanzant EL, Lopez CM, Ozrazgat-Baslanti T, et al. Persistent inflammation, immunosuppression, and catabolism syndrome after severe blunt trauma. *J Trauma Acute Care Surg*. 2014;76(1):21–29.
4. Zhu X, Herrera G, Ochoa JB. Immunosuppression and infection after major surgery: a nutritional deficiency. *Crit Care Clin*. 2010;26(3):491–500.
5. Abbas KA, Lichtman HA. Innate immunity. In: Abbas KA, Lichtman HA, eds. *Cellular and Molecular Immunology*. 5th ed. Philadelphia, PA: Saunders; 2003.
6. Popovic P, Dubois D, Rabin SB. Immunoglobulin titers and immunoglobulin subtypes. In: Lotze MT, Thomson AW, eds. *Measuring Immunity*. San Diego, CA: Elsevier Academic Press; 2005:159.
7. Bretscher PA. On the mechanism determining the TH1/TH2 phenotype of an immune response, and its pertinence to strategies for the prevention, and treatment, of certain infectious diseases. *Scand J Immunol*. 2014;79(6):361–376.
8. Yamaguchi Y, Ohshita A, Kawabuchi Y, et al. Adoptive immunotherapy of cancer using activated autologous lymphocytes: current status and new strategies. *Hum Cell*. 2003;16(4):183–189.
9. Bryk JA, Popovic PJ, Zenati MS, et al. Nature of myeloid cells expressing arginase 1 in peripheral blood after trauma. *J Trauma*. 2010;68(4):843–852.
10. Makarenkova VP, Bansal V, Matta BM, et al. CD11b+/Gr-1+ myeloid suppressor cells cause T cell dysfunction after traumatic stress. *J Immunol*. 2006;176(4):2085–2094.
11. Talmadge JE, Gabrilovich DI. History of myeloid-derived suppressor cells. *Nat Rev Cancer*. 2013;13(10):739–752.
12. Ost M, Singh A, Peschel A, et al. Myeloid-derived suppressor cells in bacterial infections. *Front Cell Infect Microbiol*. 2016;6:37.
13. Janeway CA Jr, Travers P, Walport M, et al. Allergy and hypersensitivity. In: *Immunobiology: The Immune System in Health and Disease*. 5th ed. New York, NY: Garland Science; 2001.
14. Berdal JE, Mollnes TE, Wæhre T, et al. Excessive innate immune response and mutant D222G/N in severe A (H1N1) pandemic influenza. *J Infect*. 2011;63(4):308–316.
15. Ren J, Zhao Y, Yuan Y, et al. Complement depletion deteriorates clinical outcomes of severe abdominal sepsis: a conspirator of infection and coagulopathy in crime? *PLoS One*. 2012;7(10):e47095.
16. Pandit C, Hsu P, van Asperen P, Mehr S. Respiratory manifestations and management in children with common variable immunodeficiency. *Paediatr Respir Rev*. 2016;19:56–61.
17. Dimopoulos MA, Kastritis E, Ghobrial IM. Waldenstrom's macroglobulinemia: a clinical perspective in the era of novel therapeutics. *Ann. Oncol*. 2016;27(2):233–240.
18. Locke BA, Dasu T, Verbsky JW. Laboratory diagnosis of primary immunodeficiencies. *Clin Rev Allergy Immunol*. 2014;46(2):154–168.
19. Koff WC. A shot at AIDS. *Curr Opin Biotechnol*. 2016;42:147–151.
20. Act against AIDS. Centers for Disease Control and Prevention website. Available at: http://www.cdc.gov/actagainstaids/campaigns/hivtreatmentworks/index.html. Accessed October 9, 2016.
21. Suzuki S, Ishida T, Yoshikawa K, Ueda R. Current status of immunotherapy. *Jpn J Clin Oncol*. 2016;46(3):191–203.
22. Farkona S, Diamandis EP, Blasutig IM. Cancer immunotherapy: the beginning of the end of cancer?. *BMC Med*. 2016;14(1):73.
23. Gentile LF, Cuenca AG, Efron PA, et al. Persistent inflammation and immunosuppression: a common syndrome and new horizon for surgical intensive care. *J Trauma Acute Care Surg*. 2012;72(6):1491–1501.

CHAPTER 19

Invasive Pressure Monitoring: General Principles

DAVID M. SHADE, ELIZABETH LEE DAUGHERTY, and HENRY E. FESSLER

The sophistication of bedside intensive care unit (ICU) monitoring equipment and the precision of its displayed values may tempt clinicians to accept these data without question. However, critically ill patients place substantial demands on these measurement technologies. Although the technology is governed by rigorous industry standards, it is not foolproof. To ensure accuracy and recognize and correct sources of error, the practicing intensivist must be aware of key technical aspects of pressure transduction.

This chapter reviews the basic principles of vascular pressure measurement, including principles of wave transmission, transduction, signal processing, and recording. Clinical aspects of measuring vascular pressure, such as its indications and interpretation of findings, are covered in other chapters. The goal of this chapter is to equip the practicing clinician to select the appropriate measurement tool, optimize its performance, and recognize and correct its shortcomings.

WAVE TRANSMISSION

The technical demands for recording an accurate systemic or pulmonary arterial pressure are much more stringent than for venous pressures. In order to discern fine details within an arterial pressure signal, high fidelity is needed, but even a simple water manometer can measure a central venous pressure. Therefore, this chapter will focus on the measurement of arterial pressure. The engineering principles apply, however, in any setting in which high fidelity is essential.

Cardiac contraction generates a pressure wave that travels at wave speed, much faster than the propulsion of the stroke volume through the arteries. To be measured, this pressure wave must travel down the arterial tree and through a catheter, stopcocks, tubing, and a flush device, until finally terminating at the transducer. The pressure wave signal is invariably altered along the way. Signal modifications that are due to vascular characteristics often convey important clinical information. However, other signal modifications may be introduced by the external connecting tubing, catheters, and stopcocks. These changes can obscure important findings or mislead the clinician. These external connections are usually the weakest link between the patient and the bedside monitor, and every effort should be made to minimize the degradation of the signal occurring between the blood vessel and the transducer. Some familiarity with the vocabulary and physics of wave transmission is necessary to discuss how this goal can be achieved.

Natural Frequency

A measured pressure wave travels down the conducting tubing and deflects the transducer diaphragm, which rebounds and generates a reflected wave. When this reflected wave reaches the tip of the catheter, another reflected wave travels back toward the transducer. The oscillatory behavior of this system is determined by certain physical properties of its components (1–4). The *natural frequency* (f_n) of a system is the frequency at which a signal, such as a change in pressure, will oscillate in a uniform, frictionless tube. This frequency is measured in hertz (Hz), cycles per second. As will be seen, a higher f_n is desirable in a high-fidelity measuring device. Natural frequency decreases with increasing tube length, since at any given wave speed, a round trip in a longer tube simply takes more time. Natural frequency increases with wave speed, which in turn increases with tube radius and tube wall stiffness and decreases with the density of the conducting medium (5). Thus, short, wide, rigid tubing; a stiff transducer; and dense conducting media (e.g., saline rather than air) yield a higher f_n. For a fluid-filled catheter system:

$$f_n = \frac{1}{2\pi}\sqrt{\frac{\pi \bullet r^2 \bullet E}{\rho \bullet L}} \qquad [1]$$

where f_n is the natural frequency, r is the radius of the catheter, E is the elasticity (or stiffness) of the transducer and catheter walls, ρ is the density of the fluid (typically equal to 1), and L is the length of the catheter.

Damping

Pressure waves would reverberate forever in the absence of friction. However, friction is present in the pressure monitoring system due to the movement of the waves in the conducting tubing. Although there is no net flow in the system, minute amounts of the medium shift to and fro during wave transfer. The friction generated by the movement of the conducting medium decreases the amplitude of the reflected wave, or *damps* it. Stiffer transducer diaphragms and stiffer conducting tubing will result in less damping since smaller volumes are required to displace them. Damping is also influenced by the mass of the conducting medium since wave transmission requires acceleration and deceleration of that medium. Finally, tubing resistance, which impedes the minute amount of reciprocal flow needed for pressure wave transmission, causes dissipation of energy from the pressure wave and increases damping. The damping coefficient, zeta (ζ), is therefore calculated from the determinants of mass of the system, the tubing's length and radius, the density of the conducting medium, and the resistance of the system as calculated from Poiseuille's law:

$$\zeta = \frac{4\mu}{r^3}\sqrt{\frac{\rho L}{\pi E}} \qquad [2]$$

where E is the stiffness coefficient of the transducer and tubing ($\Delta P/\Delta V$), ρ is the density of conducting fluid, μ is the viscosity of conducting fluid, r is the tube radius, and L the tube length. Note that both natural frequency, f_n, and damping, ζ, are influenced by some of the same factors, but in opposite directions.

The undamped f_n of a pressure wave cannot be measured directly since friction and inertia cannot be eliminated in real systems, but it is instead possible to measure the wave's damped natural frequency, f_d. The f_d and ζ define the performance capacity of a catheter–tubing–transducer system, which must be adequate to accommodate the signal it is transducing (i.e., the pulse waveform) with the desired fidelity.

In an application of Fourier's theorem, the complex pulse wave may be considered to be composed of a group of simple sine waves of varied amplitude and frequency. Summed together, these simple sine waves represent the pulse wave, and with enough sine waves, the summation will reproduce the original pulse wave with great accuracy. The largest-amplitude sine wave component of the pulse wave has a frequency equal to the heart rate. The pulse wave is reproduced by summing this component and a series of *harmonics*, each with a smaller amplitude and a frequency that is some multiple of the primary frequency (second harmonic = 2 × primary frequency, etc.). Combining the first 6 to 10 harmonics results in a close representation of the actual pulse contour. Thus, a recording system must be able to capture a frequency at least 6 to 10 times the pulse rate with good fidelity to be able to faithfully record an arterial pressure tracing. A recording system that does not have good fidelity up to this frequency will appear smoother than the original waveform and may obscure important clinical information.

When the frequency of the harmonics that contribute meaningfully to the contour of the pulse wave approach the f_d of the recording system, considerable errors can occur. This effect is analogous to pushing a pendulum at its f_d, where a small, well-timed repetitive push can cause a large-amplitude oscillation. The effect of this phenomenon in a transducer system can be demonstrated using a test system like that illustrated in Figure 19.1. A pressure wave of a given amplitude is generated and simultaneously recorded by a high-fidelity reference transducer and by the tubing–transducer system being tested. As the range of pressure wave frequencies is varied, one can observe and compare the output recorded by both devices. The amplitude of the test transducer peaks at its damped natural frequency, when the input wave frequency is perfectly in phase with the reflected wave oscillating within the transducer system. Because adequate measurement demands that f_d exceeds the pulse rate by 6 to 10 times, to appropriately record pressure in a patient with a pulse of 120 (2 Hz; Hz = heart rate/60), f_d should exceed 12 to 20 Hz. Transducer–tubing systems commonly found in clinical use often meet this criterion by only a narrow margin (6).

In the same way that a pendulum pushed at its f_n in the absence of friction would spin continuously around its axis, a completely undamped transducer stimulated at its f_n would record a pressure of infinite amplitude. The relationship between the amplitudes of output and input signals is expressed in the *amplitude ratio*. When the amplitude ratio equals one, the transducer is reproducing the wave exactly. When it is greater than one, the transducer is amplifying the wave, and when it is less than one, the wave is being damped. Standard engineering equations can be used to calculate the amplitude ratio and the effects of different degrees of damping at varying frequencies, as is illustrated in Figure 19.2. In this figure, frequency ratios represent the relationship between the input frequency and the damped natural frequency of the system. When the frequency ratio equals one, the input wave is at exactly the transducer's natural frequency. In a system with little damping (low values of ζ), one sees a significant rise in the amplitude ratio when input frequencies approach f_d. When a system is "overdamped," the recorded system output drops significantly below the true amplitude at frequencies that are well below the natural frequency. *Critical damping* is the least amount of damping resulting in an amplitude ratio no greater than one and an output signal that is never amplified (7).

When choosing the ideal damping for a clinical transducer system, one targets the level of damping that extends the usable frequency range, the *bandwidth*, to the greatest degree. The most useful damping for a clinical transducer system is less than critical damping, or slight underdamping. Although the amplitude ratio is slightly greater than one near f_d (6,8), the amplification of the highest-frequency harmonics of a pulse wave does not generally result in clinically important errors and produces only small degrees of high-frequency "noise" on the resulting waveform.

There is an important relationship between the f_d and ζ necessary to accurately record a vascular pressure. If the f_d is well above 6 to 10 times the pulse, the system can accurately reproduce that wave over a wide range of zetas. High harmonics that will be distorted are of such minute amplitude

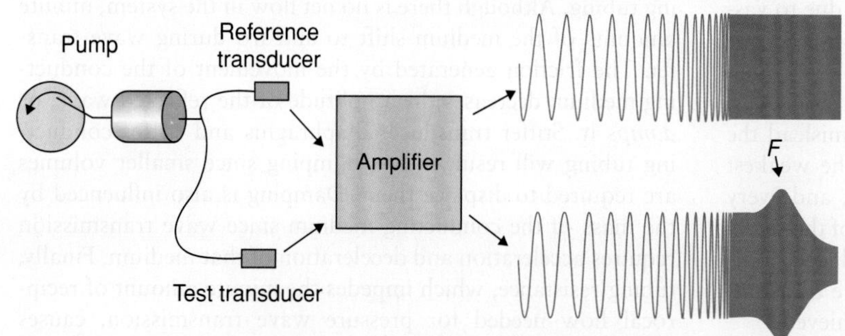

FIGURE 19.1 A device for bench testing the frequency response of pressure transducers and tubing. A pump generates a sinusoidal pressure through a range of frequencies. These are applied simultaneously to a high-fidelity reference transducer and the test transducer–tubing system. The output from the test transducer increases to a maximal amplitude at its natural frequency, designated *F*.

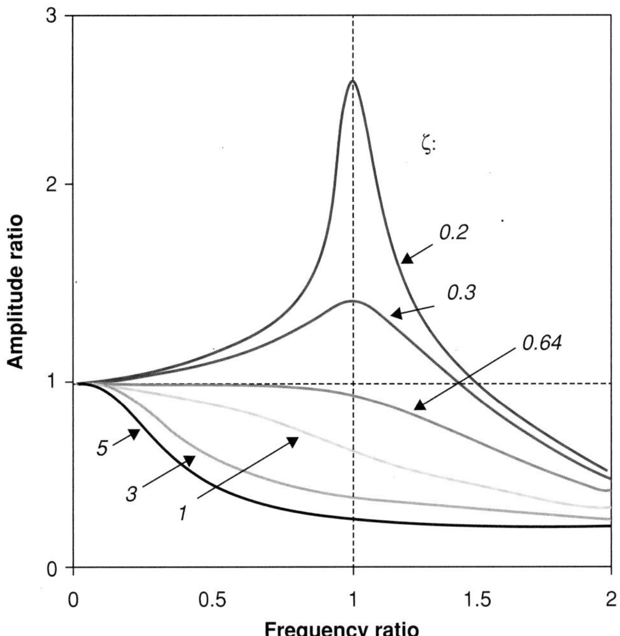

FIGURE 19.2 Effects of damping on transducer output. The frequency ratio is the ratio between the frequency at which the transducer is being stimulated and its natural frequency. The amplitude ratio is the ratio between the amplitudes of input to output signals. Different degrees of damping, zeta (ζ), are shown. With little damping, the output greatly amplifies the input over a wide range of frequencies and reaches maximum at the natural frequency. With extensive damping, the output amplitude falls at relatively low frequencies. At ζ of approximately 0.64, damping is critical (i.e., this is the lowest ζ where the amplitude ratio never exceeds one). However, this damping does not yield the broadest usable bandwidth. If one considers an amplitude ratio from 0.85 to 1.15 as reasonably accurate, then a ζ of 0.4 to 0.5 provides a greater bandwidth. This would mean that harmonics near the natural frequency would be amplified by up to 15%, and above the natural frequency they would be attenuated. However, if the natural frequency is high enough relative to the wave being studied, this will still yield acceptable accuracy.

that their amplification or attenuation will not distort the reproduced wave. Conversely, when f_d approaches frequencies that contribute meaningfully to the pulse wave, the values of ζ that allow for high-fidelity recording are more limited. Gardner (6) evaluated this relationship in a variety of commercially available transducers and found many of those systems to be barely adequate for pressure measurements in those critically ill patients with tachycardia and a hyperdynamic heart. Further, pulmonary artery waveforms have more high-frequency components than do systemic arterial waveforms. For this reason, careful selection of f_d and ζ are especially important in systems intended to measure pulmonary pressures, where any small errors may be clinically significant.

Standardized industry guidelines (9) ensure that the transducers themselves are appropriate for ICU use. Either the transducer's f_d or its usable bandwidth will be listed in the technical specifications. Bandwidths are generally described in terms of Hz either as "flat to X Hz," or "±15% to X Hz," indicating little distortion in the amplitude ratio up to the designated frequency. Guidelines require a frequency response range up to 200 Hz for typical external strain gage pressure transducers (9), and catheter tip micro-transducers may have a useable bandwidth up to 20,000 Hz (10,11).

TRANSDUCTION

Transducer Properties

For our purposes, transduction is the conversion of a pressure signal to an electrical one. Accurate conversion of signals requires several key system characteristics, including stability, linearity, adequate frequency response, lack of hysteresis, and freedom from noise.

Stability implies that the characteristics of the system remain constant over time. Both a system's gain and its baseline may be influenced by instability, or drift, resulting in errors. Baseline refers to the electrical signal corresponding to atmospheric pressure, and gain is the relationship between a change in pressure and a change in electrical signal. If the baseline of a system drifts from a pressure of 0 to 10 mmHg, the application of 100 mmHg would be recorded as 110 mmHg. In this case the applied pressure is measured accurately, but the starting point requires correction. If the gain has drifted, the starting point is correct, with a zero reading being equal to atmospheric pressure, but application of 100 mmHg would result in an incorrect electrical signal measuring 110 mmHg. A change in baseline is more easily detected and corrected, by rezeroing the transducer (exposing it to atmospheric pressure), than is instability in gain (generally requiring application of a known pressure).

Linearity indicates that electrical output remains linearly proportional to input throughout the range of measurement. Linear signals can be calibrated with few data points and linear amplifiers for such signals are relatively easy to design. With computer-based signal processing, linearity has become less important. Although most unprocessed output of pressure transducers is nonlinear, this problem may be corrected either through electronic or algorithmic processing or by setting the limits of a transducer's useable range to include only its most linear portion.

Frequency response describes a system's outputs in response to input signals of varying frequencies, usually in terms of *amplitude distortion* and *phase distortion*. Amplitude distortion refers to a change in the output amplitude ratio at different frequencies, as previously described. *Phase distortion* refers to the phase shift between input and output pressure waves that result from time lag. For example, the pulse displayed on the bedside display lags behind cardiac contraction by the momentary time it took for the pulse to travel down the arterial tree and external tubing. A constant phase shift is not problematic, as long as correction is made for this phenomenon when attempting to precisely synchronize events such as the electrocardiogram (ECG) and pulse. However, phase shift can be a significant problem in systems that cause different degrees of shift for inputs of varying frequency. Such a system would allow a different, frequency-dependent phase shift for the various components of a complex biologic wave and would produce a slurred output waveform.

Transducers should be free of *hysteresis*, in which the output signal varies with the system's recent history. That is, as it passes through the same pressure, a system with hysteresis will indicate a different value on the way down than on the way up. This characteristic would distort instantaneous recording of pulsatile signals.

Finally, a transducer should also introduce minimal *noise*, generally thought of as changes in the output signal introduced by environmental conditions. Both mechanical and electrical noise may influence vascular pressure measurement. Interference from patient movement, mechanical ventilation, fluorescent lighting, and nearby electronics should be minimized as much as possible. Transducer measurement systems may help to minimize noise through the use of electrical shielding.

Transducer Design

Several authors have reviewed the theory of transducer design (1,2,4,12,13). Manufacturers have addressed the four elements of transducer design we have discussed above in varied ways. The most commonly used design is known as a Wheatstone bridge. This design uses four strain sensors whose resistance changes when they are stretched or compressed. The bridge is designed such that all resistances are equal when no strain is applied to the transducer. When pressure is applied, two of the resistors are stretched and the others are compressed. The measured pressure is determined from the resulting imbalance of resistance between the pairs of resistors.

The strain sensors of most clinical transducers are etched from silicon (solid-state transducers). With this technology, transducers can be inexpensive enough to make them disposable after single use. This decreases processing costs and also limits their potential role in nosocomial infection. The transducers are durable and small, require minimal power and simple electronics, and are manufactured with a degree of uniformity that eliminates the need for tedious manual calibration of each transducer (14). Silicon's substantial changes in resistance with minimal changes in length give these strain gauges a high degree of sensitivity (15). This small requirement for volume displacement optimizes f_d and ζ. The Association for the Advancement of Medical Instrumentation and the American National Standards Institute have published manufacturing standards that dictate accuracy and safety characteristics for clinical transducers (9).

THE TUBING SYSTEM

Tubing

Although the fidelity of recorded pressures cannot exceed the capabilities of the transducer, performance is usually degraded below that optimal potential by other components between the transducer and the patient. Therefore, the most accurate waves can be recorded from microtransducer-tipped catheters that are inserted directly in a blood vessel without any tubing. For external transducers, every element added between the blood vessel and the transducer is a potential problem. The problems are minimized by designs that reduce ζ or increase f_d. Because damping is proportional to resistance, smaller intravascular catheters (16), clot, or kinking of the catheter will increase damping. Likewise, the mass of fluid in the catheter also increases damping, so catheter and tubing length should be minimized. Longer tubing systems have decreased f_d and reduce the usable bandwidth. Thus, if very long connecting tubes are used between the patient and transducer, more errors are likely than if the transducer is in close proximity to the blood vessel (17). Wave speed increases in stiffer tubes, so compliant tubing will also decrease f_d (12,16,18). Because air is compressible, bubbles increase the compliance of the system, both increasing damping and decreasing f_d. As an extreme illustration of this phenomenon, removing microscopic air bubbles by boiling the liquid used to fill the connecting tubing can double the f_d of a transducer system (8). Warmer room temperature can also alter f_d by softening tubing and expanding air bubbles (19). Finally, connections between tubing, tubing extenders, and transducers can also negatively affect the fidelity of the overall system.

Flush Systems

In the flush device, a mechanical resistor reduces high pressure in the flush bag to less than 1 mmHg at the transducer, while maintaining a continuous flow of solution to prevent clots (20,21). Depressing a lever or plunger bypasses the resistor, exposes the transducer to a square wave of pressure, and generates rapid flow into the patient. This can displace small clots or, as will be seen, can be used to test the intact recording system. Drip chambers should not be used in the tubing from the flush bag, or should be purged of air prior to use to eliminate risk of air embolization from turbulence during rapid flushes (21,22). Air dissolved under pressure in the flush bag can also form bubbles when decompressed in the tubing downstream from the flush device (19). These gradually collect and coalesce at stopcocks or connections and can impair the fidelity of recorded waveforms.

SIGNAL PROCESSING

Electronic Filtration and Analog-to-Digital Conversion

Transducer output may be electronically filtered to minimize noise, electrical interference, respiratory artifact, and other sources of error. Filtering can be applied either to the raw electrical signal with electronic circuits or after digital conversion with computer algorithms. Forms of filtration include low-pass filters, which attenuate high-frequency components; high-pass filters, which attenuate low-frequency components; and band-pass filters, which allow a specified range of frequencies to pass unaltered while attenuating frequencies surrounding above and below the specified band. Filters can vary in their cutoff frequencies, their extent of attenuation, and the sharpness of the transition from passage to blockage.

By first separating a pulse wave into systolic and diastolic portions, different filters may be applied to the regions to suit each component's anticipated characteristics. Although the manufacturer specifies a default set of filters, the clinician may select other options based on observation of the waveform. If the catheter–tubing–transducer combination has f_d that is sufficient for the measured waveform, a low-pass filter with a cutoff frequency just below f_d will attenuate excessive high-frequency noise without distorting the true waveform. Such selective filtering, like appropriate mechanical damping, extends the usable bandwidth.

Electrical transducer output is transmitted to a digital computer for further processing, analysis, recording, and display. The pressure waveform is transduced to a varying voltage signal which is then connected to a computer for conversion to a digital form.

The pressure waveform is processed further to calculate and display parameters such as systolic pressure, mean pressure, or pulmonary artery occlusion pressure, as numerical values. Vascular pressures change physiologically with the respiratory cycle. Vascular pressure measurements recorded within the thorax, such as pulmonary artery pressure, vary due to the changes in pleural pressure and respiration-induced changes in vascular filling. In vessels with low pressures, and particularly when pleural pressure changes are exaggerated due to disease or effort, the respiratory variation may confound clinical decisions. As a reflection of the state of cardiac filling, one is generally interested in the *transmural* pressure of intrathoracic vessels. However, the pressure on their surface is usually unmeasurable. Therefore, by convention, these vascular pressures are measured at end-expiration. Barring significant recruitment of expiratory muscles, pressure on the surface of vessels within the thorax is likely to be close to atmospheric pressure (regarded as zero) at end-expiration. For systemic arterial pressures, this rationale is less compelling. Mean arterial pressure, integrating pressures throughout the respiratory cycle, represents the average pressure driving arterial flow. Nevertheless, systolic and diastolic arterial pressures are also conventionally measured at end-expiration.

More advanced processing algorithms attempt to display digital values timed to end-expiration. Simply searching for the highest or lowest value within a time window (e.g., highest systolic value) is insufficient, because the phase difference between the respiratory cycle and the associated changes in vascular pressure differs when the patient is on positive pressure ventilation or breathing spontaneously. That is, inspiratory pleural pressure falls during spontaneous ventilation, rises during positive pressure ventilation, and changes biphasically during assisted ventilation. The highest systolic value will occur at end-expiration in the spontaneously breathing patient but not in patients on other modes.

For the measurement of pressures where accuracy is critical (such as the pulmonary artery wedge pressure), one should not rely on the displayed numerical pressure. End-expiration must be determined by inspecting the patient, and the simultaneous pressure measured directly from the waveform. An electronic cursor, placed manually or automatically and inspected for proper positioning, should be used to ensure end-expiratory values.

TROUBLESHOOTING

Simplicity and uniformity in transducer and catheter setup is key to minimizing opportunity for errors. Tubing should be stiff and designed for pressure monitoring, used with a minimum length and few stopcocks and connectors.

Zeroing

A common source of error is the zero reference level for pressure measurement. All pressures are measured relative to the horizontal plane at which the transducer is set to zero. When the transducer is connected to a fluid-filled catheter for the measurement of vascular pressure, any hydrostatic pressure imposed by the catheter will be sensed by the transducer. The recorded pressure will rise as the transducer is lowered, and vice versa. This continues to occur when the catheter is attached to a patient.

Most agree that vascular pressure should be referenced to the level of the heart; that is, the recording system should read zero pressure when the open end of a transduced fluid-filled tube is held at the horizontal plane of the heart. The optimal external anatomic landmark representing this plane remains a subject of debate. Many suggest the mid-axillary line (23,24), but others have recommended estimation of the uppermost boundary of the heart (25). For simplicity and uniformity, the mid-axillary line is best for general use. More complicated systems invite errors in practice, even if their perfect application could theoretically improve accuracy.

This anatomic reference level should be on the same horizontal plane, not of the transducer diaphragm, but of the port or stopcock that is opened to atmospheric pressure when the electronics are zeroed. The transducer itself could be in any convenient location. The amplifier will add or subtract the hydrostatic pressure of the fluid column between the zero point and the transducer. After zeroing, however, the height of the transducer relative to the zero level must remain fixed. For this reason, the zero reference level should be dictated by a unit-wide policy, and proper zero positioning should be confirmed prior to recording vascular pressure. If the transducer height moves, the zero reference level will change, resulting in erroneous readings. A parallel change in all the vascular pressures measured with the same transducer (e.g., central venous, pulmonary arterial, and wedge pressures), in a clinically stable patient, suggests a change in transducer level.

One simple way to provide consistency is to secure the transducer to the patient's arm near the heart and zero it using the port molded into the transducer body. This will allow fewer errors than attaching the transducer to an i.v. pole, in which case elevating the bed or sitting the patient up will change his or her horizontal relationship to the zero point. However, rezeroing to the cardiac level will be needed when patient orientation is changed (such as lateral decubitus or prone positions). Care must also be taken that the transducer has not rotated to a dependent position on the arm, or slipped to the elbow in a patient who is anything but completely flat.

Calibration

Modern disposable transducers are generally accurate to ±3% (26), are calibrated at the time of manufacture and do not require calibration in the field. Transducer accuracy can be compromised by mechanical trauma, overpressurization during assembly, or fluid entry on the ambient pressure side of the transducer diaphragm. Accuracy of a clinical transducer can be verified by calibration against a known pressure, such as with a mercury manometer.

Testing the Frequency Response

The catheter–tubing–transducer system allows simple bedside study. By using the flush device, one can apply a near square-wave pressure signal, and the features of the recorded output can be examined. When the flush device resistor is bypassed, a high-pressure signal is produced, which goes off-scale on the bedside monitor. When the lever is released, however, a square-wave low-pressure signal is generated, which falls within the range of the display. Proper functioning is indicated when this signal rapidly reverberates a few times and then decays back to the underlying vascular pressure.

If one records the effects of such a fast flush, those results may also be assessed quantitatively. The time between peaks of the oscillating signal is the round-trip travel time of the pressure wave to the catheter tip and back. It is equal to $1/f_d$. The decrease in amplitude of consecutive oscillations is from damping. ζ can be calculated from the amplitude ratio of consecutive oscillations A_1 and A_2 (1,6):

$$\zeta = -\ln \frac{\left(\frac{A_2}{A_1}\right)}{\sqrt{\pi^2 + \left[\ln\left(\frac{A_2}{A_1}\right)\right]^2}} \quad [3]$$

Using this equation, clinical engineers can evaluate their hospital's complete catheter–transducer subsystem. A related bench technique uses a "pop test," in which a balloon attached to a transducer and catheter system is popped with a needle to produce a "step" change in pressure. The Association for the Advancement of Medical Instrumentation publishes a comprehensive manual to guide the evaluation of pressure transducer systems by clinical engineering departments (19).

Overdamping Errors

Overdamping is a common problem that causes errors in the measurement of systolic and diastolic pressure. Overdamping is suggested during a bedside flush test by a gradual pressure decay or an undershoot and slow return to baseline without any oscillations (27). The effect of overdamping on the waveform is to first cause the wave to lose high-frequency details such as the dicrotic notch and a brisk systolic upstroke, or the a, v, and c waves of a venous pressure. With more damping, the wave will appear sinusoidal, reported systolic pressure will fall, and reported diastolic pressure will rise toward the mean arterial pressure. Even with extreme overdamping, the mean pressure remains accurate.

Numerous problems in the catheter–tubing–transducer subsystem can cause overdamping. These include air bubbles, blood clots, or fibrin within the catheter or tubing; catheter tips abutting a vessel wall; and kinks or partially closed stopcocks. Flushing or changing the tubing and obsessively purging air bubbles solves many overdamping problems. If the damped waveform is associated with kinking or thrombosis of the catheter, poor blood return, or sensitivity to minor catheter movement, it may need replacement.

Underdamping Errors

In tachycardic, hyperdynamic patients, excessive oscillation may be apparent in the pulse recording, especially at peak systole. This problem occurs when important harmonics of the pulse approach the transducer system's f_d. Underdamping causes systolic and diastolic pressure to be over- and underestimated, respectively. The excessive oscillations will also interfere with the algorithms used to calculate a digital display of systolic and diastolic pressure. Even manual estimation of these pressures from the bedside oscilloscope or printed record is inaccurate, since the pulse pressure is exaggerated.

The characteristics of the transducer system can be studied and optimized to reduce underdamping errors. During observation of a fast flush, oscillations that are widely spaced indicate a low f_d, which may poorly suit a patient whose pulse is dynamic with upper harmonics of high amplitude. Natural frequency is reduced by lengthy or compliant tubing or by bubbles. Removing unneeded tubing extensions and diligently clearing bubbles will bring the flush test oscillations closer together, and the waveform will show more detail with greater accuracy.

One would like to increase the damping of the system without decreasing its natural frequency. This effect can be achieved by reducing the amplifier high-pass filtration frequency just enough to eliminate the reverberations, as is outlined in most monitoring equipment user's manuals. Too much electronic damping will degrade the waveform just as would excess mechanical damping. Filtering should generally not be reduced below 12 Hz to avoid removing the higher-order harmonics contributing significantly to the systolic portion of the waveform. There are also mechanical devices that attach to a stopcock near the transducer and increase damping. These devices are designed to match the transducer impedance to that of the tubing, decreasing wave reflections without altering f_d (6,12).

Artifact that appears similar to underdamping can also occur when long, flexible catheters are vibrated by high-velocity blood flow, termed "catheter whip." This phenomenon should be suspected when long intravascular catheters are used in high-flow vessels of large diameter, such as long femoral or pulmonary artery catheters. Contributions of underdamping to the waveform appearance can be ruled out by inspecting the fast flush and optimizing the external tubing system. Artifact due to movement of the catheter tip is difficult to eliminate. In the pulmonary artery, stabilizing the catheter tip by inflating the balloon to measure a pulmonary artery occlusion pressure will remove the "whip." Measurement of mean pressures will also remain accurate.

FUTURE DIRECTIONS

Fifty years of engineering refinement have produced transducers that are many times more accurate than needed for most clinical decisions in critical care medicine. Basic knowledge of the physics of wave transmission and transduction and thoughtful bedside setup and inspection will minimize artifact. Further, simple, uniform protocols and education can reduce human errors. Once these steps are achieved, improved invasive vascular pressure measurement will not require greater accuracy in signal acquisition.

Instead, technical innovation is needed in data management. Enormous amounts of data are collected by bedside monitoring systems in the form of trend records. However, spurious values are recorded along with accurate ones. A nurse or doctor can easily recognize and discard such values (e.g., a pressure recorded while a stopcock is closed to draw blood, or while a patient is moving). However, it is a complex computational task to program this into a computer, and this field is in its infancy (28).

Another aspect of data management in need of innovation is alarms. Vascular pressure monitoring systems are only one of numerous sources of alarms in ICUs. Other sources include the ECG, oximetry, ventilators, infusion pumps, and virtually all mechanical devices at the patient's bedside. In a recent quality improvement review of alarm data from a 15-bed intermediate care unit in our hospital, an astounding 27,000 alarms were recorded in a 24-hour period. Furthermore, this number excluded equipment not monitored centrally (e.g., excluded were ventilators, infusion pumps, and bed alarms).

Over 90% of ICU alarms are either false alarms or of no clinical significance (29,30). These represent a major source of ambient noise and distract nurses from true alarms requiring intervention (28,31). Current alarm technology is simplistic. An alarm is triggered whenever a parameter falls above or below an acceptable range. On the other hand, clinically important trends do not trigger alarms until they fall outside of the range. Trend-based alarms (32) or use of artificial intelligence algorithms may someday improve the specificity of alarms (28).

SUMMARY

Invasive measurement of vascular pressure has become commonplace in the care and monitoring of the critically ill. However, decisions based on inaccurate or misleading information could prove costly. Simple, consistent setups that respect the physics of wave transmission will minimize errors. Critical evaluation of the quality of these data and recognition of the limitations of the technology will allow the clinician to optimize pressure recording fidelity.

Key Points

- *Natural frequency* is the frequency at which a wave oscillates in a tubing system.
- *Damping* is the attenuation of a wave due to friction.
- Natural frequency and damping characteristics set the performance limits of a system of a transducer and all its attached tubing and connectors.
- The pulse is a complex waveform whose accurate recording requires a system with adequate natural frequency and damping.
- Clinical pressure recording systems are optimized with proper setup, flushing, and zeroing.
- Use of the fast-flush device on a pressure transducer, and inspection of the resulting signal, can QC a measurement system and help diagnose potential sources of error.

ACKNOWLEDGEMENTS

The authors acknowledge the assistance of Stephanie Herrera and Kristen Kaiser in the preparation of this chapter.

References

1. Fry DL. Physiologic recording by modern instruments with particular reference to pressure recording. *Physiol Rev*. 1960;40:753–788.
2. van der Tweel LH. Some physical aspects of blood pressure, pulse wave, and blood pressure measurements. *Am Heart J*. 1957;53(1):4–17.
3. Kleinman B. Understanding natural frequency and damping and how they relate to the measurement of blood pressure. *J Clin Monit*. 1989; 5(2):137–147.
4. Hansen AT, Warburg E. The theory for elastic liquid-containing membrane manometers. *Acta Physiol Scand*. 1950;19:306–332.
5. Wilson TA, Hyatt RE, Rodarte JR. The mechanisms that limit expiratory flow. *Lung*. 1980;158(4):193–200.
6. Gardner RM. Direct blood pressure measurement–dynamic response requirements. *Anesthesiology*. 1981;54(3):227–236.
7. Fessler H, Shade D. Measurement of vascular pressure. In: Tobin MJ, ed. *Principles and Practice of Intensive Care Monitoring*. New York, NY: McGraw-Hill; 1997:91–106.
8. Shapiro GG, Krovetz LJ. Damped and undamped frequency responses of underdamped catheter manometer systems. *Am Heart J*. 1970;80(2): 226–236.
9. *Blood Pressure Transducers*. 2nd ed. Arlington, VA: Association for the Advancement of Medical Instrumentation; 1994.
10. Nichols WW, Walker WE. Experience with the Millar PC-350 catheter-tip pressure transducer. *Biomed Eng*. 1974;9(2):58–60.
11. Millar HD, Baker LE. A stable ultraminiature catheter-tip pressure transducer. *Med Biol Eng*. 1973;11(1):86–89.
12. Allan MW, Gray WM, Asbury AJ. Measurement of arterial pressure using catheter-transducer systems: improvement using the Accudynamic. *Br J Anaesth*. 1988;60(4):413–418.
13. Geddes LA. *The Direct and Indirect Measurement of Blood Pressure*. Chicago, IL: Year Book Medical Publishers; 1970.
14. Bailey RH, Bauer JH, Yanos J. Accuracy of disposable blood pressure transducers used in the critical care setting. *Crit Care Med*. 1995;23(1):187–192.
15. Geddes LA, Athens W, Aronson S. Measurement of the volume displacement of blood-pressure transducers. *Med Biol Eng Comput*. 1984;22(6):613–614.
16. Heimann PA, Murray WB. Construction and use of catheter-manometer systems. *J Clin Monit*. 1993;9(1):45–53.
17. Miller GS, Zbilut JP. Practical evaluation of catheter-transducer coupling systems for artifact. *Heart Lung*. 1983;12(2):156–161.
18. Hunziker P. Accuracy and dynamic response of disposable pressure transducer–tubing systems. *Can J Anaesth*. 1987;34(4):409–414.
19. *Evaluation of Clinical Systems for Invasive Blood Pressure Monitoring*. Arlington, VA: Association for the Advancement of Medical Instrumentation; 1992.
20. Gardner RM, Warner HR, Toronto AF, et al. Catheter-flush system for continuous monitoring of central arterial pulse waveform. *J Appl Physiol*. 1970;29(6):911–913.
21. Gardner RM, Bond EL, Clark JS. Safety and efficacy of continuous flush systems for arterial and pulmonary artery catheters. *Ann Thorac Surg*. 1977; 23(6):534–538.
22. Soule DT, Powner DJ. Air entrapment in pressure monitoring lines. *Crit Care Med*. 1984;12(6):520–522.
23. Pedersen A, Husby J. Venous pressure measurement. I. Choice of zero level. *Acta Med Scand*. 1951;141(3):185–194.
24. Yang SS. *From Cardiac Catheterization Data to Hemodynamic Parameters*. 3rd ed. Philadelphia, PA: Davis; 1988.
25. Courtois M, Fattal PG, Kovacs SJ Jr, et al. Anatomically and physiologically based reference level for measurement of intracardiac pressures. *Circulation*. 1995;92(7):1994–2000.
26. Gardner RM. Accuracy and reliability of disposable pressure transducers coupled with modern pressure monitors. *Crit Care Med*. 1996;24(5): 879–882.
27. Morris AH, Chapman RH, Gardner RM. Frequency of technical problems encountered in the measurement of pulmonary artery wedge pressure. *Crit Care Med*. 1984;12(3):164–170.
28. Imhoff M, Kuhls S. Alarm algorithms in critical care monitoring. *Anesth Analg*. 2006;102(5):1525–1537.
29. Tsien CL, Fackler JC. Poor prognosis for existing monitors in the intensive care unit. *Crit Care Med*. 1997;25(4):614–619.
30. Chambrin MC, Ravaux P, Calvelo-Aros D, et al. Multicentric study of monitoring alarms in the adult intensive care unit (ICU): a descriptive analysis. *Intens Care Med*. 1999;25(12):1360–1366.
31. Edworthy J, Hellier E. Alarms and human behaviour: implications for medical alarms. *Br J Anaesth*. 2006;97(1):12–17.
32. Schoenberg R, Sands DZ, Safran C. Making ICU alarms meaningful: a comparison of traditional vs. trend-based algorithms. *Proc AMIA Symp*. 1999;379–383.

CHAPTER

20

Noninvasive Cardiovascular Monitoring

UCHENNA R. OFOMA and LUIS E. URRUTIA

INTRODUCTION

Circulatory shock in the critically ill commonly occurs from trauma, hemorrhage, high-risk surgery, sepsis, anaphylaxis, burns, tension pneumothorax, and cardiac emergencies such as acute myocardial infarction (AMI) and pulmonary embolism (PE). Up to one-third of patients admitted to the intensive care unit (ICU) are in circulatory shock (1). Early recognition and aggressive therapy of shock by way of hemodynamic support are keys to successful resuscitation and mitigation of worsening organ dysfunction and failure in a broad spectrum of patient subgroups (2–6). Shock results from four potential but not exclusive pathophysiologic mechanisms (7,8): hypovolemia, cardiogenic factors, obstruction, or distributive factors. Identification of the main mechanism responsible for shock by clinical evaluation alone is difficult, especially in complex situations such as cardiac tamponade in a patient with trauma or septic shock in a patient with chronic heart failure (9). Furthermore, clinical assessment of cardiac output (CO) and intravascular volume status are very inaccurate (10). Hemodynamic measurements help with the determination of the type of shock, selecting appropriate therapeutic interventions, and evaluating the patient's response to therapy.

Hemodynamic monitoring and management has greatly improved during the past decade (11), with technologies evolving from very invasive to noninvasive (12,13), and a philosophical shift from more traditional static approaches to functional and dynamic approaches for monitoring (14). Traditional methods of hemodynamic monitoring—including blood pressure, pulse rate, central venous pressure (CVP), and arterial oxygen saturation—change minimally in early shock and are poor indicators of the adequacy of resuscitation (13,15). The measurements of stroke volume (SV) and CO are the fundamental aspects of current hemodynamic management and will be the focus of this chapter. Noninvasive continuous CO monitoring has potential clinical applications in the ICU, emergency department (ED), and operating room (OR) by way of establishing a diagnosis, risk stratification, and therapy guidance.

There are a variety of modalities that have been developed to provide for hemodynamic monitoring by invasive, minimally invasive, and noninvasive methods. CO measurement with a pulmonary artery catheter (PAC) using the bolus thermodilution method is the gold standard and reference method used to compare newer novel technologies (16,17). The PAC and other invasive methods are presented in detail elsewhere in this textbook. Minimally invasive methods include transesophageal Doppler and pulse contour analysis, with or without a dilution technique; noninvasive methods include CO_2 and inert gas rebreathing, transthoracic Doppler, thoracic bioimpedance cardiography, and bioreactance. Each of these methods has its own advantages and limitations; taken together they have the potential to create a robust multidimensional picture of patients' hemodynamic states and their responses to therapeutic interventions. When only one method is used, its limitations may obscure the real problem and limit clinical usefulness.

CO MONITORING BY ELECTRIC BIOIMPEDANCE

The technique of bioimpedance cardiography is based on the measurements of impedance (or resistance) to transmission of a small electrical current through the chest area (thoracic bioimpedance) or whole body (whole-body bioimpedance). Thoracic bioimpedance systems use pair of injecting and sensing electrodes applied at the base of the neck (thoracic inlet) and the costal margins (thoracic outlet), while whole-body systems use electrodes attached to limb extremities (17,18). Thoracic bioimpedance cardiography relies on the theory that the impedance of the thorax is dependent on the amount of fluid (blood and plasma) in the thoracic compartment; this represents conduits of low impedance, with higher impedance occurring in cardiac muscle, lungs, and fat. The varying amount of blood volume in the aorta during the cardiac cycle is thought related to the observed changes in impedance (19). The outer pairs of electrodes pass a small-amplitude (0.2–5.0 mA) alternating current at 40 to 100 kHz through the patient's thorax to produce an electrical field. The injected electrical signals travel predominantly down the aorta, which has lower electrical resistance than aerated lung. Each ventricular contraction propels the SV down the aorta, increasing aortic blood volume and aortic flow and lowering impedance. The impedance is sensed by the inner recording electrodes that capture the baseline impedance (Z_0) and the first derivative of the impedance waveform (dZ/dt) (20,21). Changes in aortic blood flow throughout the cardiac cycle are quantitatively related to changes in the electrical impedance. CO is computed based on mathematical equations under the assumption that thoracic impedance changes over time are proportional to the SV. Electrical velocimetry—a new bioimpedance method with a different algorithm for processing the impedance signal has demonstrated low accuracy and precision compared with pulmonary artery (22) and transthoracic (23) thermodilution techniques.

Numerous validation studies in diverse patient populations have been carried out to compare the performance of thoracic electrical bioimpedance with well-established reference methods. Data from very early studies showed inconsistent results when compared with the PAC thermodilution CO technique (24–27). Early meta-analyses reported mean percentage error of 37% (28) and poor agreement (29) between CO measurements obtained by thoracic cardiac impedance, a reference method. Improved newer-generation bioimpedance devices with upgraded computer technology and refined mathematical algorithms for CO calculation have also yielded contradictory results with regard to agreement with reference techniques and the ability to trend CO changes (30–35). A more recent meta-analysis of 13 validation studies of thoracic electrical bioimpedance reported an overall percentage error of 42.9% for thoracic bioimpedance measurements (36).

Thoracic electrical bioimpedance technology has several limitations. The clinical applicability of all thoracic electrical bioimpedance devices is highly dependent on electrode positioning, variations in patient age, gender, body size, and other physical factors like temperature and humidity that impact on electric conductivity between the electrodes and the skin (26,37,38). Its accuracy is further limited by electrical interference (e.g., from electrocautery), fluid in the thoracic compartment—pleural effusions, pericardial tamponade, pulmonary edema—changes in peripheral vascular resistance, cardiac dysrhythmias, and motion artefacts (39–42).

THORACIC BIOREACTANCE

Bioreactance devices were developed to overcome the limitations of bioimpedance devices by processing the impedance signals in a way that improves on the signal-to-noise ratio. In addition to changing resistance to blood flow (Z_0), changes in intrathoracic volume also produce changes in electrical capacitive and inductive properties that result in phase shifts of the received signal relative to the applied signal (17,43). Bioreactance represents the phase shift in voltage across the thorax; this almost exclusively depends on pulsatile flow. The bioreactance signal is therefore more closely related to aortic blood flow and less dependent on intra- and extravascular lung water (13,42). The only commercially available monitoring system assessing CO by bioreactance is the NICOM system (Cheetah Medical, Portland, OR).

Several studies have shown high correlation of CO measurements by bioreactance with that measured by thermodilution and pulse contour analysis (43–46). More recent studies have questioned the accuracy of the bioreactance cardiography. For example, a study of surgical patients treated for ovarian cancer showed that thoracic bioreactance did not reliably measure cardiac index (CI) compared with transpulmonary hemodilution (47).

Bioreactance cardiography can be performed in ventilated and nonventilated patients and can compute CO in patients with atrial and ventricular dysrhythmias (13). As with bioimpedance, electrical interference can alter bioreactance measurements.

ARTERIAL PULSE CONTOUR ANALYSIS AND PLETHYSMOGRAPHY

There are several devices being marketed for the noninvasive and continuous assessment of arterial blood pressure (ABP) and CO. The most commonly used are the CNAP, Finapres, and Clearsight systems. These devices function on two operating principles, the volume clamp method and pulse contour analysis.

In the first portion, the volume clamp method is used and a finger cuff is applied to the middle phalanx; the finger cuff is inflated and deflated so as to maintain a constant level of blood volume (48). The finger's arterial diameter is measured by sending infrared light through the tissue and measuring the absorption of light by the blood using a light detector integrated in the finger cuff. This photoplethysmographic signal controls the finger cuff pressure and the artery is kept at a constant diameter during the cardiac cycle. When the artery's diameter is constant, the cuff pressure must be equal to the intra-arterial pressure (42). From these measurements, the arterial waveform and pressures are calculated and used for pulse contour analysis. The brachial artery pressure is mathematically reconstructed from the finger cuff measurements and displayed on the monitor for continual display.

The pulse contour method then analyzes the systolic area under the arterial waveform curve—beginning of waveform to the dicrotic notch—for each beat. The arterial impedance is estimated from a three-element model to compute flow that has nonlinear pressure-dependent properties. The three determining elements are aortic impedance, Windkessel—or buffer—compliance, and peripheral resistance (49). The division of the systolic area by the impedance produces an estimate of the SV (50), and CO is derived.

This method has several drawbacks. Arterial impedance is an estimated parameter based on proprietary algorithms that are based on patient age, gender, height, and weight. The arterial waveform input can be degraded in patients with peripheral arterial disease, severe vasoconstriction, or edema of the extremities thereby yielding CO results that have limited accuracy (51–53). Additionally, studies have mostly been performed in cardiac surgery patients and have not been validated in the setting of valvular heart disease or significant tachydysrhythmias. Although the technology is promising, due to its noninvasive and continuous nature, the CO measurements do not meet the criteria for clinical interchangeability with the PAC, and further studies are needed to support its use in the critically ill shock patient (9).

RADIAL APPLANATION TONOMETRY

Applanation tonometry of the radial artery allows for continuous noninvasive monitoring of ABP without external calibration. Commonly used commercial devices are the T-Line System by Tensys Medical and SphygmoCor by AtCor Medical. The operating principle is the application of external pressure to the radial artery against a noncompressible surface (the radius). Once pressure is applied, the contact stress is transduced by a surface sensor into an electrical signal which provides continuous pulse recording of pressure with direct calibration over time. The degree of pressure that is needed to compress the vessel is in direct correlation to the instantaneous intraluminal pressure (54).

Tonometry studies in the critically ill have produced mixed results, with some studies citing a lack of reliability of systolic blood pressure (SBP) measurement (55), and wide agreement limits (56,57). Better correlation was shown with mean arterial pressure (MAP) and diastolic blood pressure (DBP). Additional draw backs are that systolic and diastolic blood pressures are derived from a scaled BP waveform through proprietary algorithms (T-system); that significant time is required before the initial reading is displayed when the system is initiated; and that readings are not available in the event of arm motion as the radial artery is being located by the device. Compared to the volume clamp method, this device does not appear to be as affected by arterial vasoconstriction and may yield CO measurements that have reasonable accuracy (58), but further studies are needed to support its use in the critically ill.

PULSE WAVE TRANSIT TIME

CO is estimated using the pulse oximeter waveform, arterial pressure, and electrocardiogram. The current commercial device on the market is esCCO by Nihon Kohden. The principle is that of an inverse correlation between pulse wave transit time and SV. So far, studies in the critically ill have not shown good correlation with transthoracic echocardiography (TTE) (59).

ECHOCARDIOGRAPHY

Since the early 1950s, when the first ultrasound (US) machine was used to examine the human heart, US has allowed us to "see" inside the human heart and gain a new understanding of its complex workings and physiology. As of today, cardiac US is the most advanced and cost-effective noninvasive hemodynamic monitor that we have at our disposal. There is no other device that can provide the wealth of information the echocardiogram (ECHO) does in a similar cost-effective manner, with real-time image assessment and without any known adverse side effects (60).

Given the appropriate acoustic windows, ECHO provides the intensivist with a complete hemodynamic assessment of the patient. Key hemodynamic and nonhemodynamic parameters such as left ventricular ejection fraction (LVEF), left ventricular end-diastolic volume (LVEDV), left ventricular end-systolic volume (LVESV), right ventricular function, pulmonary artery pressures, CO, and SV variation (SVV) can be obtained. Cardiac US has also been shown to alter the diagnosis and therapeutic management of patients in the ICU by 30% to 60% (61).

Over the last two decades, ECHO has replaced the need for invasive hemodynamic assessment (left and right heart catheterization) in valvular heart disease due to its accuracy, reliability, and noninvasive nature. Only in the setting of conflicting echocardiographic data do patients need to undergo additional hemodynamic testing. It is beyond the scope of this text to give an in-depth description of cardiac ultrasonography and its techniques. Below is a summary of key echocardiographic and hemodynamic parameters that are of importance for the critical care practitioner.

Left Ventricular Volumes and Ejection Fraction (LVEF)

The quantitation of left ventricular systolic function is critical to the proper evaluation of patients with cardiovascular disease (62). LVEF is a predictor of cardiovascular outcomes in the critically ill patient. The recommended method for quantification of left ventricular systolic function is the biplane method of discs (modified Simpson's rule) (63). The "eyeball" estimation of left ventricular systolic function is not recommended given the lack of reproducibility between readers and its subjective nature. The Simpson's technique requires the recording of an apical four-chamber view and an apical two-chamber view from which the endocardial borders are outlined in end-diastole and end-systole. Care must be taken to exclude the papillary muscles from endocardial border tracings and to locate the true apex of the ventricle. Failure to avoid these common mistakes will result in the underestimation of ventricular volumes (Fig. 20.1).

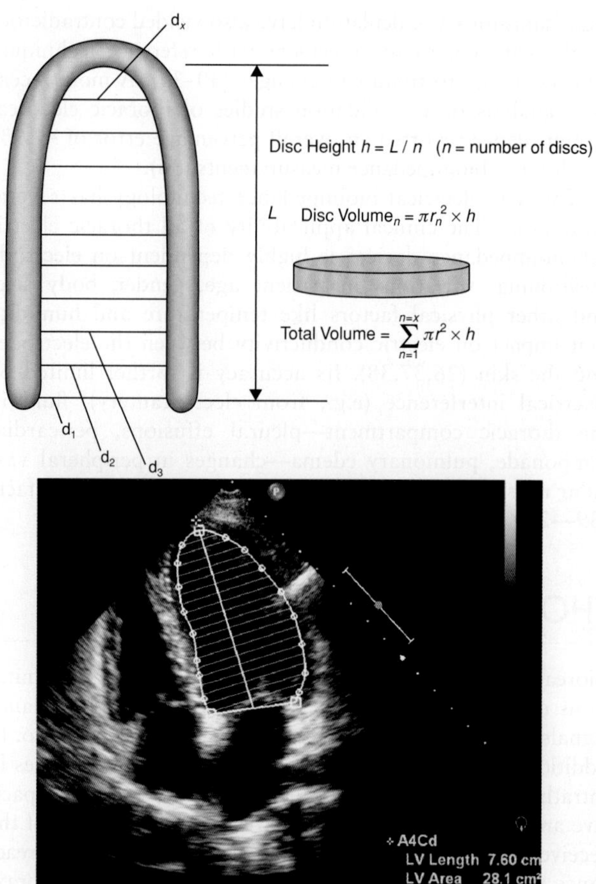

FIGURE 20.1 Schematic illustration of Simpson's rule of discs for calculating left ventricular volume. (From Armstrong WF, Ryan T. Evolution of systolic function of the left ventricle. In: *Feigenbaum's Echocardiography*. 7th ed. Philadelphia, PA: Lippincott Williams & Wilkins; 2010:127, with permission.)

$$\text{Ejection fraction (LVEF)} = \frac{\text{LVEDV} - \text{LVESV}}{\text{LVEDV}}$$

Ventricular volumes obtained by 2D-ECHO have usually yielded smaller volumes than those obtained by cardiac MRI or nuclear medicine studies. This is attributed to the difficulty in excluding trabeculae and the improper visualization of the true endocardial border. In the absence of significant mitral regurgitation, SV can be obtained by subtracting the LVESV from the LVEDV.

$$\text{SV} = \text{LVEDV} - \text{LVESV}$$

Linear measurements of left ventricular function, such as the Fractional shortening method, can be quite misleading when there are regional wall motion abnormalities present and, as such, is not recommended. LVEF is a marker of left ventricular contractility and is affected by conditions that alter the preload, afterload, and contractility of the heart. Severe valvular heart disease can affect these parameters and needs to be taken into consideration when interpreting LVEF.

Right Ventricular Systolic Function

ECHO evaluation of the right ventricular function is complex due to its unique crescent shape. Multiple studies have demonstrated the clinical utility of TAPSE, S' of the tricuspid annulus, and RIMP as surrogate measures of right ventricular ejection fraction (RVEF).

Tricuspid annular plane systolic excursion (TAPSE) is a one-dimensional measurement that represents longitudinal right ventricular function. It is measured by M-mode echocardiography with the cursor optimally aligned along the direction of the tricuspid lateral annulus obtained in the apical four-chamber view. TAPSE values less than 1.7 cm are highly suggestive of right ventricular systolic dysfunction (64). Tissue Doppler S' of the lateral tricuspid annulus has also been shown to correlate with measures of right ventricular systolic function. An S' velocity less than 9.5 cm/sec is indicative of RV systolic dysfunction (65).

CO and SV

CO is a key measurement in the management of the patient in shock. CO and SV can be obtained by a combination of Doppler and 2D US measurements. Pulse Doppler US allows us to measure intracardiac blood flow velocities; this is termed the velocity time integral or VTI. The VTI is the aggregate sum of blood flow velocities per heartbeat (SV) measured over time. By knowing the cross-sectional area through which blood flows through, we can then estimate blood volume (Figs. 20.2 and 20.3).

Stroke volume = cross-sectional area (CSA) × VTI Stroke volume = CSA (LVOT diameter squared × 0.785) × VTI LVOT

CO = stroke volume (SV) × heart rate (HR)

The preferred site for CSA measurement is the left ventricular outflow tract (LVOT) due to its minimal size variation during systole (66). CO measurements by the VTI method have been validated against invasive hemodynamic measurements with the PAC (67–70), and are reliable in the absence of valvular pathology.

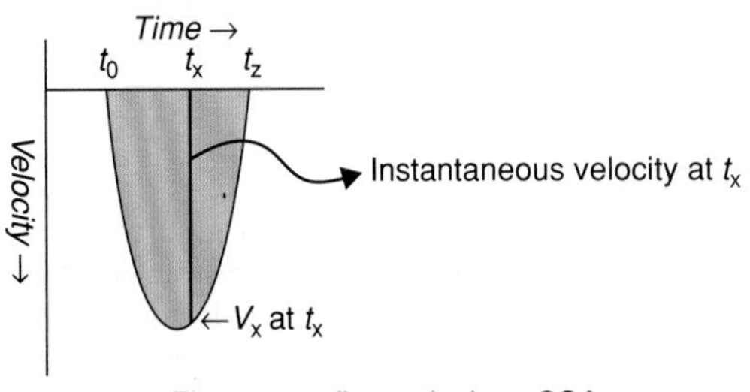

FIGURE 20.2 A schematic demonstrates the concept of flow quantification using the Doppler technique. (From Armstrong WF, Ryan T. Hemodynamics. In: *Feigenbaum's Echocardiography.* 7th ed. Philadelphia, PA: Lippincott Williams & Wilkins; 2010:219, with permission.)

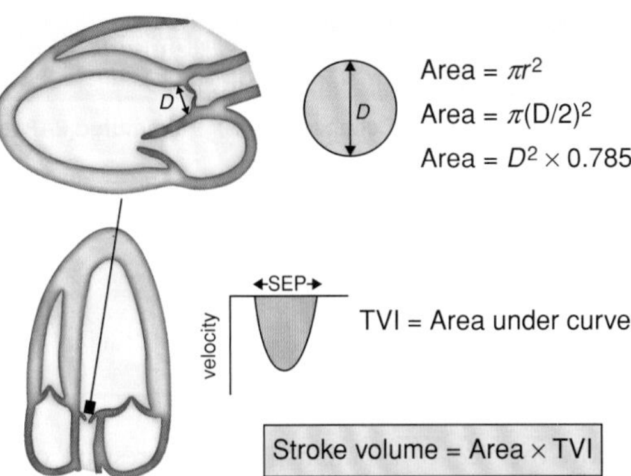

FIGURE 20.3 The method for quantifying stroke volume. (From Armstrong WF, Ryan T. Hemodynamics. In: *Feigenbaum's Echocardiography.* 7th ed. Philadelphia, PA: Lippincott Williams & Wilkins; 2010:219, with permission.)

Right Atrial Pressure/Central Venous Pressure

Right atrial pressure (RAP) or mean CVP can be estimated from the IVC diameter and its collapsibility on inspiration. Images are obtained of the intrahepatic portion of the inferior vena cava from the subcostal views. The combination of these two parameters (diameter and collapsibility) results in an accurate estimation of the mean RAP in patients who are not mechanically ventilated or who do not have elevated intra-abdominal pressures. In ventilated patients, an IVC diameter less than 1.2 cm appears to accurately identify patients with a RAP less than 10 mmHg. In this same group, if the IVC is small and collapsed it is suggestive of hypovolemia (64,65).

Another method to estimate RAP is through hepatic vein flow patterns obtained from the same subcostal views. Hepatic vein flow velocities have been validated in mechanically ventilated patients by a small number of patients (71) (Fig. 20.4 and Table 20.1).

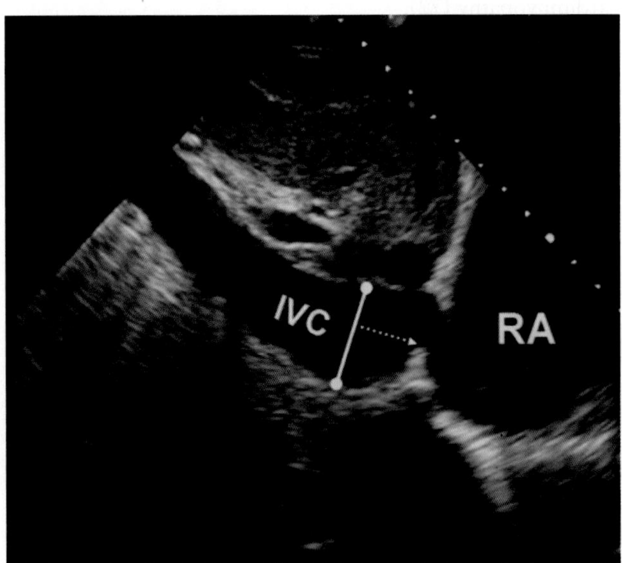

FIGURE 20.4 Inferior vena cava (IVC) view. Measurement of the IVC. The diameter (*solid line*) is measured perpendicular to the long axis of the IVC at end expiration, just proximal to the junction of the hepatic veins that lie approximately 0.5 to 3.0 cm proximal to the ostium of the right atrium (RA). (From Rudski LG, Lai WW, Afilalo J, et al. Guidelines for the echocardiographic assessment of the right heart in adults: a report of the American Society of Echocardiography. *J Am Soc Echocardiogr.* 2010;23:685–713, with permission.)

TABLE 20.1 Relationship Between IVC Diameter and Collapsibility with Estimated Right Atrial Pressure

IVC Diameter (cm)	IVC Collapsibility (%)	Estimated RAP (mmHg)
<2.1	>50	~3
<2.1	<50	~8
>2.1	>50	~8
>2.1	<50	~15

Systemic Vascular Resistance

If we know the SBP of a patient (by cuff pressure or arterial line), we can then calculate the MAP and obtain the estimated RAP and CO by cardiac US as already described above. We can then deduce systemic vascular resistance (SVR) by applying Ohm's law.

$$SVR = MAP - CVP/CO$$

Left Atrial Pressure

In the critically ill patient, left atrial pressure (LAP) measurements are not easily derived, nor should they be inherently trusted. Many factors need to be assessed and integrated clinically at the bedside. The parameter that best correlates with elevated LAP is E/e' ratio greater than 15 (<8 being normal). This ratio is obtained by pulse Doppler interrogation of the early mitral filling velocity (E) and then divided into the early diastolic mitral annular velocity (e') as obtained by tissue Doppler velocities. The ratio has been shown to accurately predict elevated filling pressures in the heart failure population. Factors that can cause significant variability are regional wall motion abnormalities affecting the basal myocardium, preload conditions, depressed systolic function, mitral annular calcification, tachyarrhythmia with E/A fusion, and hypertrophic cardiomyopathy (72).

Pulmonary Artery Systolic Pressure and Mean Pulmonary Artery Pressure

Pulmonary artery systolic pressure (SPAP) can be quantified by measuring the right ventricular pressure through the tricuspid regurgitation peak jet velocity. Because the RV systolic pressure (RVSP) and SPAP are—in the absence of pulmonary stenosis—similar; this approach provides a simple means of quantifying pulmonary artery pressures (71).

$$RVSP = 4 \times (\text{TR velocity})^2 + RAP$$

Mean pulmonary artery pressure (MPAP) can be obtained by pulsed Doppler interrogation of the RV outflow tract and obtaining the acceleration time (AT) of the pulmonic valve VTI. An AT less than 90 ms is suggestive of significant pulmonary hypertension (MPAP >25 mmHg). MPAP can also be deduced from the following formula:

$$MPAP = 70 - (0.45 \times AT)$$

Stroke Volume Variation and Fluid Responsiveness

Over the last decade there has been an increase in the number of studies emphasizing the importance of SVV and fluid responsiveness in the critically ill (15,60,73). ECHO can easily measure SV by pulse Doppler interrogation of the LVOT, the preferred site for this. By obtaining the VTI and SV measurements (described in the CO section, above) a fluid challenge is given and SV is remeasured. An increase in SV greater than 10% suggests volume responsiveness in the critically ill.

As with any technology, cardiac US has its own limitations and drawbacks. The first barrier is that of the human body and its acoustic windows. Air, a poor conductor of US waves, can impair and degrade image quality in those patients who have underlying lung disease or are mechanically ventilated. Further, acoustic windows may not be accessible due to postoperative pain, positional changes of the heart, drainage catheters, or skin dressings.

Another important barrier, which must be noted, is the learning curve and skill required in both the acquisition and interpretation of US images. This is a learned skill that requires dedicated training and will also be dependent on the power of the equipment used. Training requirements and expertise needed for analysis and interpretation of ECHO have been well delineated in professional society guidelines (74,75).

Finally, one of the biggest drawbacks of ECHO is its noncontinuous nature. Echocardiography provides a "snapshot in time" thereby limiting its ability to serve as a continuous monitoring tool in the critically ill patient.

SUMMARY

The future for hemodynamic monitoring is promising given new technologic advances on the horizon. The ideal hemodynamic monitor will be noninvasive, provide continuous display of key hemodynamic variables, be readily applicable with no significant learning curve, and help guide therapeutic interventions for improved outcomes. At this time the perfect hemodynamic monitor does not exist, either invasive or noninvasive. Our current monitors operate on different physiologic principles and assumptions of which critical care practitioners need to be thoroughly familiarized with. Additionally, most devices do not provide a complete hemodynamic picture but rather a partial one. Failure to understand the physiologic principles on which devices function will lead to misinterpretation and/or misdiagnosis in complex cardiovascular conditions. As of today, echocardiography is the most complete noninvasive hemodynamic monitor at our disposal but is limited by its noncontinuous monitoring capabilities and significant learning curve.

Key Points

- Continuous and noninvasive cardiac monitoring modalities are potentially innovative tools for the bedside assessment of hemodynamic parameters.
- The ideal hemodynamic monitor will be noninvasive, provide continuous display of key hemodynamic variables, be readily applicable with no significant learning curve, and help guide therapeutic interventions for improved outcomes.
- Currently there is no ideal hemodynamic monitor that is able to provide all hemodynamic variables in a reliable and continuous fashion.

- For many modalities, data regarding measurement performance in comparison with reference methods for CO assessment are conflicting.
- Each modality has its specific advantages and limitations regarding usefulness in the clinical setting.

ACKNOWLEDGMENT

The authors would like to thank William C. Shoemaker, Howard Belzberg, Charles C.J. Wo, George Hatzakis, and Demetrios Demetriades for their contributions to the earlier editions of the chapter.

References

1. Sakr Y, Reinhart K, Vincent JL, et al. Does dopamine administration in shock influence outcome? Results of the Sepsis Occurrence in Acutely Ill Patients (SOAP) Study. *Crit Care Med.* 2006;34(3):589–597.
2. Rivers E, Nguyen B, Havstad S, et al. Early goal-directed therapy in the treatment of severe sepsis and septic shock. *N Engl J Med.* 2001;345(19): 1368–1377.
3. Shapiro NI, Howell MD, Talmor D, et al. Implementation and outcomes of the Multiple Urgent Sepsis Therapies (MUST) protocol. *Crit Care Med.* 2006;34(4):1025–1032.
4. Lopes MR, Oliveira MA, Pereira VO, et al. Goal-directed fluid management based on pulse pressure variation monitoring during high-risk surgery: a pilot randomized controlled trial. *Crit Care.* 2007;11(5):R100.
5. Hamilton MA, Cecconi M, Rhodes A. A systematic review and meta-analysis on the use of preemptive hemodynamic intervention to improve postoperative outcomes in moderate and high-risk surgical patients. *Anesth Analges.* 2011;112(6):1392–1402.
6. Corredor C, Arulkumaran N, Ball J, et al. Hemodynamic optimization in severe trauma: a systematic review and meta-analysis. *Rev Brasil Terapia Intensiva.* 2014;26(4):397–406.
7. Weil MH, Shubin H. Proposed reclassification of shock states with special reference to distributive defects. *Adv Exper Med Biol.* 1971;23(0):13–23.
8. Vincent JL, De Backer D. Circulatory shock. *N Engl J Med.* 2013;369(18): 1726–1734.
9. Cecconi M, De Backer D, Antonelli M, et al. Consensus on circulatory shock and hemodynamic monitoring. Task force of the European Society of Intensive Care Medicine. *Intensive Care Med.* 2014;40(12):1795–1815.
10. Saugel B, Ringmaier S, Holzapfel K, et al. Physical examination, central venous pressure, and chest radiography for the prediction of transpulmonary thermodilution-derived hemodynamic parameters in critically ill patients: a prospective trial. *J Crit Care.* 2011;26(4):402–410.
11. Ramsingh D, Alexander B, Cannesson M. Clinical review: Does it matter which hemodynamic monitoring system is used?. *Crit Care.* 2013;17(2):208.
12. Alhashemi JA, Cecconi M, Hofer CK. Cardiac output monitoring: an integrative perspective. *Crit Care.* 2011;15(2):214.
13. Marik PE. Noninvasive cardiac output monitors: a state-of the-art review. *J Cardiothorac Vasc Anesth.* 2013;27(1):121–134.
14. Hadian M, Pinsky MR. Functional hemodynamic monitoring. *Curr Opin Crit Care.* 2007;13(3):318–323.
15. Marik PE, Cavallazzi R. Does the central venous pressure predict fluid responsiveness? An updated meta-analysis and a plea for some common sense. *Crit Care Med.* 2013;41(7):1774-1781.
16. Critchley LA, Lee A, Ho AM. A critical review of the ability of continuous cardiac output monitors to measure trends in cardiac output. *Anesth Analges.* 2010;111(5):1180–1192.
17. Jakovljevic DG, Trenell MI, MacGowan GA. Bioimpedance and bioreactance methods for monitoring cardiac output. *Best Pract Res Clin Anaesthesiol.* 2014;28(4):381–394.
18. Albert NM. Bioimpedance cardiography measurements of cardiac output and other cardiovascular parameters. *Crit Care Nurs Clin North Am.* 2006; 18(2):195–202, x.
19. Cotter G, Moshkovitz Y, Kaluski E, et al. Accurate, noninvasive continuous monitoring of cardiac output by whole-body electrical bioimpedance. *Chest.* 2004;125(4):1431–1440.
20. Shoemaker WC, Wo CC, Chan L, et al. Outcome prediction of emergency patients by noninvasive hemodynamic monitoring. *Chest.* 2001;120(2):528–537.
21. Charloux A, Lonsdorfer-Wolf E, Richard R, et al. A new impedance cardiograph device for the non-invasive evaluation of cardiac output at rest and during exercise: comparison with the "direct" Fick method. *Eur J Appl Physiol.* 2000;82(4):313–320.
22. Heringlake M, Handke U, Hanke T, et al. Lack of agreement between thermodilution and electrical velocimetry cardiac output measurements. *Intensive Care Med.* 2007;33(12):2168–2172.
23. Raue W, Swierzy M, Koplin G, Schwenk W. Comparison of electrical velocimetry and transthoracic thermodilution technique for cardiac output assessment in critically ill patients. *Euro J Anaesthesiol.* 2009;26(12): 1067–1071.
24. Appel PL, Kram HB, Mackabee J, et al. Comparison of measurements of cardiac output by bioimpedance and thermodilution in severely ill surgical patients. *Crit Care Med.* 1986;14(11):933–935.
25. Bowling LS, Sageman WS, O'Connor SM, et al. Lack of agreement between measurement of ejection fraction by impedance cardiography versus radionuclide ventriculography. *Crit Care Med.* 1993;21(10):1523–1527.
26. Marik PE, Pendelton JE, Smith R. A comparison of hemodynamic parameters derived from transthoracic electrical bioimpedance with those parameters obtained by thermodilution and ventricular angiography. *Crit Care Med.* 1997;25(9):1545–1550.
27. Shoemaker WC, Belzberg H, Wo CC, et al. Multicenter study of noninvasive monitoring systems as alternatives to invasive monitoring of acutely ill emergency patients. *Chest.* 1998;114(6):1643–1652.
28. Critchley LA, Critchley JA. A meta-analysis of studies using bias and precision statistics to compare cardiac output measurement techniques. *J Clin Monit Comput.* 1999;15(2):85–91.
29. Raaijmakers E, Faes TJ, Scholten RJ, et al. A meta-analysis of three decades of validating thoracic impedance cardiography. *Crit Care Med.* 1999;27(6):1203–1213.
30. Spiess BD, Patel MA, Soltow LO, Wright IH. Comparison of bioimpedance versus thermodilution cardiac output during cardiac surgery: evaluation of a second-generation bioimpedance device. *J Cardiothorac Vasc Anesth.* 2001;15(5):567–573.
31. Sageman WS, Riffenburgh RH, Spiess BD. Equivalence of bioimpedance and thermodilution in measuring cardiac index after cardiac surgery. *J Cardiothorac Vasc Anesth.* 2002;16(1):8–14.
32. Gujjar AR, Muralidhar K, Banakal S, et al. Noninvasive cardiac output by transthoracic electrical bioimpedance in post-cardiac surgery patients: comparison with thermodilution method. *J Clin Monit Comput.* 2008; 22(3):175–180.
33. Chakravarthy M, Rajeev S, Jawali V. Cardiac index value measurement by invasive, semi-invasive and non invasive techniques: a prospective study in postoperative off pump coronary artery bypass surgery patients. *J Clin Monit Comput.* 2009;23(3):175–180.
34. Simon R, Desebbe O, Henaine R, et al. [Comparison of ICG thoracic bioimpedance cardiac output monitoring system in patients undergoing cardiac surgery with pulmonary artery cardiac output measurements]. *Annal Franc Anesth Reanimation.* 2009;28(6):537–541.
35. Engoren M, Barbee D. Comparison of cardiac output determined by bioimpedance, thermodilution, and the Fick method. *Am J Crit Care.* 2005; 14(1):40–45.
36. Peyton PJ, Chong SW. Minimally invasive measurement of cardiac output during surgery and critical care: a meta-analysis of accuracy and precision. *Anesthesiology.* 2010;113(5):1220–1235.
37. Wang DJ, Gottlieb SS. Impedance cardiography: more questions than answers. *Curr Cardiol Rep.* 2006;8(3):180–186.
38. Sathyaprabha TN, Pradhan C, Rashmi G, et al. Noninvasive cardiac output measurement by transthoracic electrical bioimpedance: influence of age and gender. *J Clin Monit Comput.* 2008;22(6):401–408.
39. Critchley LA, Calcroft RM, Tan PY, et al. The effect of lung injury and excessive lung fluid, on impedance cardiac output measurements, in the critically ill. *Intensive Care Med.* 2000;26(6):679–685.
40. Critchley LA, Peng ZY, Fok BS, James AE. The effect of peripheral resistance on impedance cardiography measurements in the anesthetized dog. *Anesth Analg.* 2005;100(6):1708–1712.
41. Chamos C, Vele L, Hamilton M, Cecconi M. Less invasive methods of advanced hemodynamic monitoring: principles, devices, and their role in the perioperative hemodynamic optimization. *Periop Med.* 2013;2(1):19.
42. Saugel B, Cecconi M, Wagner JY, Reuter DA. Noninvasive continuous cardiac output monitoring in perioperative and intensive care medicine. *Br J Anaesth.* 2015;114(4):562–575.
43. Keren H, Burkhoff D, Squara P. Evaluation of a noninvasive continuous cardiac output monitoring system based on thoracic bioreactance. *Am J Physiol Heart Circ Physiol.* 2007;293:H583–H589.
44. Raval NY, Squara P, Cleman M, et al. Multicenter evaluation of noninvasive cardiac output measurement by bioreactance technique. *J Clin Monit Comput.* 2008;22(2):113–119.

45. Marque S, Cariou A, Chiche JD, Squara P. Comparison between Flotrac-Vigileo and bioreactance, a totally noninvasive method for cardiac output monitoring. *Crit Care*. 2009;13(3):R73.
46. Squara P, Denjean D, Estagnasie P, et al. Noninvasive cardiac output monitoring (NICOM): a clinical validation. *Intens Care Med*. 2007;33(7):1191–1194.
47. Kober D, Trepte C, Petzoldt M, et al. Cardiac index assessment using bioreactance in patients undergoing cytoreductive surgery in ovarian carcinoma. *J Clin Monit Comput*. 2013;27(6):621–627.
48. Thiele RH, Bartels K, Gan TJ. Cardiac output monitoring: a contemporary assessment and review. *Crit Care Med*. 2015;43(1):177–185.
49. Wesseling KH, Jansen JR, Settels JJ, Schreuder JJ. Computation of aortic flow from pressure in humans using a nonlinear, three-element model. *J Appl Physiol*. 1993;74(5):2566–2673.
50. Bubenek-Turconi SI, Craciun M, et al. Noninvasive continuous cardiac output by the Nexfin before and after preload-modifying maneuvers: a comparison with intermittent thermodilution cardiac output. *Anesth Analg*. 2013;117(2):366–372.
51. Fischer MO, Avram R, Carjaliu I, et al. Non-invasive continuous arterial pressure and cardiac index monitoring with Nexfin after cardiac surgery. *Br J Anaesth*. 2012;109(4):514–521.
52. Fischer MO, Coucoravas J, Truong J, et al. Assessment of changes in cardiac index and fluid responsiveness: a comparison of Nexfin and transpulmonary thermodilution. *Acta Anaesthesiol Scand*. 2013;57(6):704–712.
53. Hofhuizen C, Lansdorp B, van der Hoeven JG, et al. Validation of noninvasive pulse contour cardiac output using finger arterial pressure in cardiac surgery patients requiring fluid therapy. *J Crit Care*. 2014;29(1):161–165.
54. Drzewiecki GM, Melbin J, Noordergraaf A. Arterial tonometry: review and analysis. *J Biomechanics*. 1983;16(2):141–152.
55. Meidert AS, Huber W, Hapfelmeier A, et al. Evaluation of the radial artery applanation tonometry technology for continuous noninvasive blood pressure monitoring compared with central aortic blood pressure measurements in patients with multiple organ dysfunction syndrome. *J Crit Care*. 2013;28(6):908–912.
56. Saugel B, Fassio F, Hapfelmeier A, et al. The T-Line TL-200 system for continuous non-invasive blood pressure measurement in medical intensive care unit patients. *Intensive Care Med*. 2012;38(9):1471–1477.
57. Colquhoun DA, Forkin KT, Dunn LK, et al. Non-invasive, minute-to-minute estimates of systemic arterial pressure and pulse pressure variation using radial artery tonometry. *J Med Engin Technol*. 2013;37(3):197–202.
58. Wagner JY, Sarwari H, Schon G, et al. Radial artery applanation tonometry for continuous noninvasive cardiac output measurement: a comparison with intermittent pulmonary artery thermodilution in patients after cardiothoracic surgery. *Crit Care Med*. 2015;43(7):1423–1428.
59. Fischer MO, Balaire X, Le Mauff de Kergal C, et al. The diagnostic accuracy of estimated continuous cardiac output compared with transthoracic echocardiography. *Can J Anaesth*. 2014;61(1):19–26.
60. Barbier C, Loubieres Y, Schmit C, et al. Respiratory changes in inferior vena cava diameter are helpful in predicting fluid responsiveness in ventilated septic patients. *Intensive Care Med*. 2004;30(9):1740–1746.
61. Beaulieu Y. Bedside echocardiography in the assessment of the critically ill. *Crit Care Med*. 2007;35(5 Suppl):S235–S249.
62. Gaasch WH. Diagnosis and treatment of heart failure based on left ventricular systolic or diastolic dysfunction. *JAMA*. 1994;271(16):1276–1280.
63. Lang RM, Badano LP, Mor-Avi V, et al. Recommendations for cardiac chamber quantification by echocardiography in adults: an update from the American Society of Echocardiography and the European Association of Cardiovascular Imaging. *J Am Soc Echocardiol*. 2015;28(1):1–39.
64. Jue J, Chung W, Schiller NB. Does inferior vena cava size predict right atrial pressures in patients receiving mechanical ventilation? *J Am Soc Echocardiol*. 1992;5(6):613–619.
65. Rudski LG, Lai WW, Afilalo J, et al. Guidelines for the echocardiographic assessment of the right heart in adults: a report from the American Society of Echocardiography endorsed by the European Association of Echocardiography, a registered branch of the European Society of Cardiology, and the Canadian Society of Echocardiography. *J Am Soc Echocardiol*. 2010;23(7):685–713.
66. Quinones MA, Otto CM, Stoddard M, et al. Recommendations for quantification of Doppler echocardiography: a report from the Doppler Quantification Task Force of the Nomenclature and Standards Committee of the American Society of Echocardiography. *J Am Soc Echocardiol*. 2002;15(2):167–184.
67. Dubin J, Wallerson DC, Cody RJ, Devereux RB. Comparative accuracy of Doppler echocardiographic methods for clinical stroke volume determination. *Am Heart J*. 1990;120(1):116–123.
68. Huntsman LL, Stewart DK, Barnes SR, et al. Noninvasive Doppler determination of cardiac output in man: clinical validation. *Circulation*. 1983;67(3):593–602.
69. Lewis JF, Kuo LC, Nelson JG, et al. Pulsed Doppler echocardiographic determination of stroke volume and cardiac output: clinical validation of two new methods using the apical window. *Circulation*. 1984;70(3):425–431.
70. Temporelli PL, Scapellato F, Eleuteri E, et al. Doppler echocardiography in advanced systolic heart failure: a noninvasive alternative to Swan-Ganz catheter. *Circ Heart Fail*. 2010;3(3):387–394.
71. Nagueh SF, Kopelen HA, Zoghbi WA. Relation of mean right atrial pressure to echocardiographic and Doppler parameters of right atrial and right ventricular function. *Circulation*. 1996;93(6):1160–1169.
72. Ommen SR, Nishimura RA, Appleton CP, et al. Clinical utility of Doppler echocardiography and tissue Doppler imaging in the estimation of left ventricular filling pressures: a comparative simultaneous Doppler-catheterization study. *Circulation*. 2000;102(15):1788–1794.
73. Grocott MP, Dushianthan A, Hamilton MA, et al. Perioperative increase in global blood flow to explicit defined goals and outcomes after surgery: a Cochrane Systematic Review. *Br J Anaesth*. 2013;111(4):535–548.
74. Spencer KT, Kimura BJ, Korcarz CE, et al. Focused cardiac ultrasound: recommendations from the American Society of Echocardiography. *J Am Soc Echocardiol*. 2013;26(6):567–581.
75. Richard JC, Bayle F, Bourdin G, et al. Preload dependence indices to titrate volume expansion during septic shock: a randomized controlled trial. *Crit Care*. 2015;19:5.

CHAPTER
21

Hemodynamic Monitoring: Arterial and Pulmonary Artery Catheters

KEVIN Y. PEI and MIHAE YU

Since the introduction of the pulmonary artery catheter (PAC) in the 1970s, initial enthusiasm has been tempered by studies suggesting equivocal or potentially increased mortality when employed in the critically ill (1). Academic societies have convened expert panels to review the literature, poll society membership, and discuss important issues regarding PAC utilization; the usual conclusion calls for more rigorous, adequately powered, randomized, controlled trials (2). For many critical care practitioners, the benefits of PAC warrant its continued use in high-risk patients; interestingly, the PAC continues to be the gold standard by which noninvasive cardiac output (CO) monitoring is judged.

Inherent in the use of the PAC to improve outcomes is the assumption that flow-related variables such as cardiac output/cardiac index (CO/CI) and oxygen delivery (DO_2) are important for survival. Shoemaker et al. observed that survivors and nonsurvivors did not differ in traditional values of blood pressure (BP), heart rate (HR), urine output, and arterial oxygen tension (PaO_2). Contrary to conventional wisdom of the time, flow-related variables such as DO_2, oxygen consumption (VO_2), and CO were superior determinants of mortality (3,4). In addition, Bihari et al. (5) reported that as DO_2 was augmented in critically ill patients, VO_2 of the tissues increased suggesting, at least in part, that tissue consumption can become supply dependent. Mathematically, DO_2 and VO_2 are coupled because CO is on both sides of the equation; is this a true physiologic dependency? In a study using independent measurement of VO_2, Yu et al. (6) demonstrated that some but not all critically ill patients showed an increase in VO_2 as DO_2 improved. Titration of DO_2 until the VO_2 slope plateaus is an attractive but impractical theory as measurement of VO_2 is cumbersome. Perhaps an easier, and more clinically useful, end point of resuscitation is the mixed venous oxygen saturation (SvO_2)—a reflection of the balance between supply (DO_2) and demand (VO_2) (7).

The current body of literature regarding resuscitation to CI, DO_2, and SvO_2 goals (both for and against) is vast and beyond the scope of this chapter; nevertheless, these are important concepts and are summarized in the practice guidelines for PAC (2). Although global values of DO_2 are important, the exact threshold is unknown because they may not reflect oxygen transport at the cellular level. Until we have a tool to measure tissue-level oxygenation states (or one tissue bed that is a surrogate marker for the rest of the body), the amount of DO_2 necessary for tissue perfusion will remain controversial.

Over the decades, clinicians have progressed from treatment goals of BP, HR, and urine output to markers of anaerobic metabolism such as lactic acid and base deficit, and then to flow-related variables such as DO_2, VO_2, and SvO_2. While we have progressed in our goal-directed therapy, the whole concept has been called into question recently (8). Ideally, a user-friendly, noninvasive device could measure tissue oxygenation and the energy state of cells, thereby allowing clinicians to "titrate" DO_2 to meet tissue demands rather than aiming for a single global survival values of DO_2 and SvO_2 (3,4). Hemodynamic monitoring affords us the ability to treat the critically ill in a goal-oriented manner; we see these goals (BP, HR, urine output, DO_2, VO_2, and SvO_2) as complementary. While no existing technology is perfect in our pursuit to titrate resuscitation to cellular demands, we continue our quest to define superior end points of resuscitation and the modalities with which to improve cellular oxygen transport.

Once a standard of intensive care medicine, much controversy has befallen the PAC and its use in modern critical care. While literature on use of PAC is extensive and confusing, it is important for readers to critically evaluate the studies by asking the following questions.

1. Was the patient population appropriate to study design?
2. When was the PAC utilized during the course of illness and was there specific time-dependent goals? Timing of resuscitation is essential for successful outcome and studies stressing early resuscitative efforts (7,9–11) demonstrate better outcomes with DO_2 and SvO_2 goals than studies with no time specification (12,13). Given that early resuscitation potentially improves outcome, studies that demonstrate lack of benefit from PAC may be flawed if enrollment occurs within 48 hours of respiratory failure since resuscitation should be completed by 24 hours (14). Even among studies that call into question the utility of goal-directed therapy, early intervention itself seems to improve outcome (8).
3. What were the exclusion criteria? Studies excluding patients with acute cardiac or pulmonary problems would be deleting patients who would likely most benefit from PAC use. As an example, one study reporting no PAC advantage excluded patients who already had a PAC, chronic obstructive pulmonary disease (COPD), renal failure, acute myocardial infarct, and liver disease reported (14).
4. Patients with good cardiac function and reserve likely did not benefit from PAC use compared to high-risk patients. Their expected mortality would be lower and potentially "negate" benefits realized for the high-risk patients. Two studies that excluded patients with good cardiac function resulted in conflicting outcomes, most likely due to differences in treatment and timing of goal achievement (13,15).
5. What were the hemodynamic goals of the study: CI, DO_2, or SvO_2, or any one or combination of these? Our preference has been to use oxygen delivery indexed (DO_2I) rather than CI since the acceptable CI would vary with hemoglobin levels (16,17).

6. How was the treatment administered? Were fluids given to reach a certain pulmonary artery occlusion pressure (PAOP)? Is left ventricular stroke work index (LVSWI) an appropriate end point for fluid administration since a high BP would lead to an elevated LVSWI without an adequate preload (13)? How were fluids and blood given? Did large doses of inotropes (i.e., 200 μg/kg/min of dobutamine) possibly contribute to negative outcome (13)?
7. What percentage of study patients did not reach the goals? Was failure to reach goals due to inadequate effort by the treating team or due to the inherent inability of the patient's myocardium to respond to treatment? We demonstrated that in the initial phases of our prospective randomized trials, failure to reach DO_2I of 600 mL/min/m^2 or more occurred 46% of the time but decreased to 19% in the second part of the trial (15). High failure rates (>70%) to reach hemodynamic goals have been reported in some studies with negative outcome (13,18).

Differences in study design and treatment algorithm may contribute to different outcomes reported with PAC use. Nevertheless, our therapeutic armamentarium is limited, and as clinicians, there may still be benefit in continuing to optimize DO_2 with the aid of PAC—the ultimate goal is to satisfy the imbalance of supply and demand at the tissue level.

PEARLS

- Identify patients who may benefit from PAC insertion (Table 21.1).
- Insert the PAC early. The best treatment for MSOF is prevention. The majority of successful outcome studies suggest that timing is of the essence.
- Ensure proper readings. *No* information is better than *wrong* information leading to erroneous treatment. Studies have demonstrated an alarming degree of user error (18–20). A corollary is that infrequent use of PAC may lead to more error (both nursing and physician related).
- Have specific goals for the patient (i.e., DO_2, SvO_2). The goals may vary with disease process and clinical changes (17). For example, the preoperative patients may have a modest DO_2 goal (19) compared to shock patients (11,20). Older patients (>75 years of age) may have lower metabolic rates and need less DO_2 to meet tissue demands (6,15).
- Use of the PAC requires judgment. The "optimum" PAOP may vary compliance of the heart and degree of ventilator support. Similarly, a DO_2 goal is not fixed either.
- Individualize DO_2 to achieve normal values of traditional parameters (BP, HR, urine output), lactate levels, and SvO_2 levels. Additional monitoring of peripheral tissues is currently available such as gastrointestinal tonometry (21), transcutaneous pressure of O_2 ($PtcO_2$) and CO_2 ($PtcCO_2$) (22–24), and near-infrared spectroscopy (25). While orthogonal polarization spectral imaging of oral capillaries holds promise (26,27), further validation studies are needed.
- The PAC is a diagnostic tool that provides many parameters, but interpretation of the data is important. For example, central pressure may not give accurate information about the intravascular volume (28). Central and global values such as DO_2 and SvO_2 may not reflect adequate oxygenation state or cellular viability and function in all the tissue beds.

TABLE 21.1 Indications for Pulmonary Artery Catheter Insertion

Precautionary Reasons
For prevention of multisystem organ failure in high-risk patients (perforated viscus)
For preoperative assessment of high-risk patients with cardiac, pulmonary, and renal dysfunction
For management of high-risk patients postoperatively (major hemorrhage)
For patients with expected large fluid shifts: sepsis, bleeding, multiple trauma, burns, and cirrhosis
Treatment of Shock
Hypotension not relieved with fluid
Suspected cardiac event or cardiac compromise contributing to shock
Oliguria not responding to fluid
Patients with multiple organ dysfunction
For continuous SvO_2 monitoring
To Guide Treatment in Pulmonary Dysfunction
To differentiate cardiogenic causes of hypoxia from acute respiratory distress syndrome and guide fluid management
For monitoring cardiac output in patients requiring high-positive end-expiratory pressure (≥15 cm H_2O)
Treatment of Cardiac Dysfunction
Complicated myocardial infarction
Congestive heart failure with poor response to afterload reduction and diuretic therapy
Suspected tamponade or contusion from blunt chest injury
Pulmonary hypertension with myocardial dysfunction

INDICATIONS FOR PULMONARY ARTERY CATHETER INSERTION

Indications for PAC insertion (Table 21.1) have been broadly categorized to (a) precautionary measures in high-risk patients, (b) shock states, (c) pulmonary problems, and (d) cardiac dysfunction.

Preoperative intervention of high-risk surgical patients using PACs remains a controversial area and recommendations are vague in the American College of Cardiology/American Heart Association (ACC/AHA) guidelines (2,29). The key points are as follows: insert the PAC with enough time to achieve the hemodynamic goals (usually the day before), communicate with the anesthesiologist regarding the information obtained while in the intensive care unit (ICU), and monitor the patient in the ICU beyond 24 hours to allow for fluid shifts to occur.

The goals of preoperative invasive monitoring are to (a) optimize preload (plot the Starling curve, see below); (b) optimize CI and stroke volume index (SVI) by adjusting preload, afterload, and contractility (possibly by using inotropes); (c) maintain DO_2 to perfuse the rest of the body and prevent MSOF; (d) perfuse the coronaries by maintaining coronary perfusion pressure (CPP) and DO_2; (e) decrease myocardial work and myocardial oxygen consumption (MVO_2) by keeping systolic blood pressure (SBP) and HR normal; and (f) prevent myocardial infarct by avoiding significant changes (>15%) in HR and BP (19,30,31). Further details in utilization of PACs for treatment of high-risk patients, shock, and cardiopulmonary failure are covered in other chapters.

The PAC is inserted to obtain information beyond the physical examination. Clinical predictors of hemodynamic status in the critically ill patient, such as chest radiograph, jugulovenous distention, and urine output, are inaccurate (1,32). Physicians are correctly able to predict PAOP and CI only 30% to 70% of the time. The PAC provides the following information to guide therapy.

1. Central pressures in relationship to the right ventricle (RV) (i.e., central venous pressure [CVP] or right atrial [RA] pressure); central pressures in relationship to the left ventricle (i.e., PAOP to estimate left ventricular end-diastolic pressure [LVEDP])
2. Cardiac function measured as CO and presented as CI
3. SvO_2
4. Intrapulmonary shunt (*Qs*/*Qt*)

TABLE 21.2 Normal Hemodynamic Values

Hemodynamic Parameter	Normal Range
Systolic blood pressure	100–140 mmHg
Diastolic blood pressure	60–90 mmHg
Mean arterial pressure (MAP)	70–105 mmHg
Heart rate	60–100 beats/min
Right atrial (RA) or central venous pressure (CVP)	0–8 mmHg
Right ventricle systolic pressure	15–30 mmHg
Right ventricular diastolic pressure	0–8 mmHg
Pulmonary artery (PA) systolic pressure	15–30 mmHg
PA diastolic pressure	4–12 mmHg
Mean PA	9–16 mmHg
Pulmonary artery occlusion pressure (PAOP, wedge)	6–12 mmHg
Left atrial pressure (LAP)	6–12 mmHg
Cardiac output (L/min)	Varies with patient size
Cardiac index (L/min/m^2)	2.8–4.2 L/min/m^2
Right ventricular ejection fraction (RVEF)	40–60%
Right ventricular end-diastolic volume indexed (RVEDVI) to body surface area	60–100 mL/m^2
Hemoglobin	12–16 g/dL
Arterial oxygen tension (PaO_2)	70–100 mmHg
Arterial oxygen saturation	93–98%
Mixed venous oxygen tension (PvO_2)	36–42 mmHg
Mixed venous oxygen saturation (SvO_2)	70–75%

General Considerations

The technical aspects of PAC insertion are presented in "Vascular Cannulation." It is essential that the catheter be positioned and transduced properly, and a knowledgeable clinician must be able to reliably interpret the data (33–35). Physicians should understand the basic physical principles involved in catheterization, know the design of the catheter, and be able to recognize and remedy technical errors.

Although the modern PAC has features that were not available when it was introduced, the general principles of placement have not changed. If the PAC has fiberoptic bundles at the tip for continuous SvO_2 monitoring, external in vitro calibration is done prior to removing the catheter tip from the casing. The PAC is then flushed to assess the patency of its lumens and to fill the catheter with a noncompressible column of fluid capable of transmitting pressures. There is a distal port for monitoring the pulmonary artery pressures (PAPs) and a central port approximately 30 cm from the tip that will lie in the right atrium in the average, adult heart. For CO monitoring, a thermistor is located proximal to the tip to measure temperature changes (see Cardiac Output section). The catheter is placed through the protective sheath and the balloon is checked for integrity prior to insertion. The transducer is placed at the level of the patient's midaxillary line and zeroed to atmospheric pressure (phlebostatic point). If the transducer elevates above the patient level, the readings will be falsely low. Conversely, if the transducer falls below the patient level, the readings will be falsely high. This is typically noted in beds that are designed to rotate patients.

PRESSURE MEASUREMENTS

Normal hemodynamic values are presented in Table 21.2.

Pressure changes in the heart or vessels cause movement of the catheter, which is then converted to an electrical signal by a transducer. Electrical noise is filtered and the signal is amplified and displayed as a tracing on a bedside monitor. Before insertion, the function of the system is checked by shaking the catheter and seeing good waveforms on the monitor. If the waveform is dampened, the system should be flushed to rid the catheter and tubing of all air bubbles, and all connections should be tightened. After inserting the PAC 15 to 20 cm into the introducer sheath, the balloon is inflated and the catheter is gently advanced. The natural flow of blood from the vena cava through the heart and to the lungs guides the catheter to the pulmonary vasculature (36). While passing from the vena cava to a branch of the pulmonary artery, characteristic waveforms are displayed on the monitor (Fig. 21.1). Once the catheter is advanced to the "wedged" position (PAOP), the balloon is deflated and the catheter adjusted until 1.25 to 1.5 mL of inflation is needed to produce the PAOP tracing. The balloon should only be inflated long enough to record a measurement in order to avoid rupture of the artery or infarction of the downstream segment of lung. The balloon should always be deflated when withdrawing the catheter to avoid vascular and valvular injury. A chest radiograph is performed to assess for pneumothorax and may help to confirm proper position, the catheter should curve gently in the RV and sit in a larger branch of the pulmonary artery (Fig. 21.2). If there is not an obvious PAOP tracing, blood may be sampled from the distal port with the balloon inflated. The sample should have a higher PaO_2 and pH with a lower $PaCO_2$ than blood aspirated without occlusion (37). Proper placement is also indicated by the SvO_2 signal quality if using a fiberoptic catheter with continuous measurement. The quality of the signal may be altered by (1) fibrin clot at the tip of the catheter, (2) the tip situated against a vessel wall, (3) inserting the catheter too far, or (4) a hypovolemic with collapse of the vessel wall around the catheter tip. If the catheter is in too far, the PAOP tracing will continue to elevate and is called "overwedging" (Fig. 21.3). If this occurs, the balloon should be deflated and the catheter pulled back (≅1 cm) and the balloon inflated again

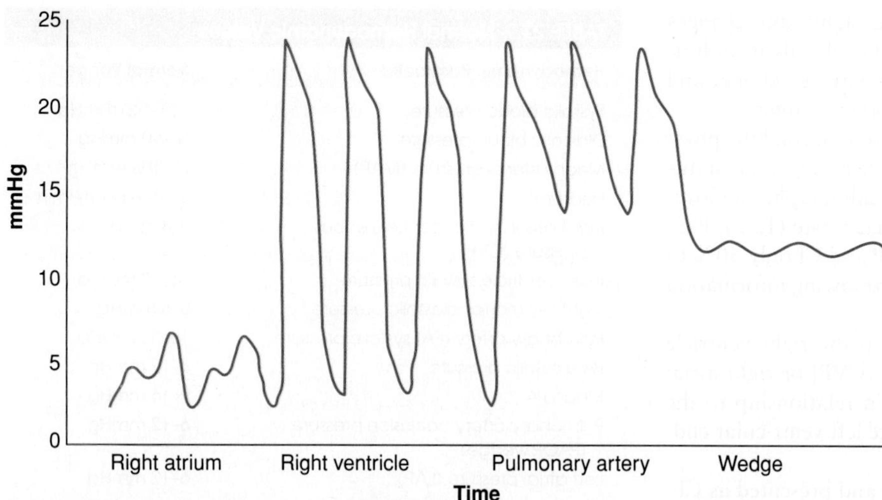

FIGURE 21.1 Waveforms seen during pulmonary artery catheter insertion.

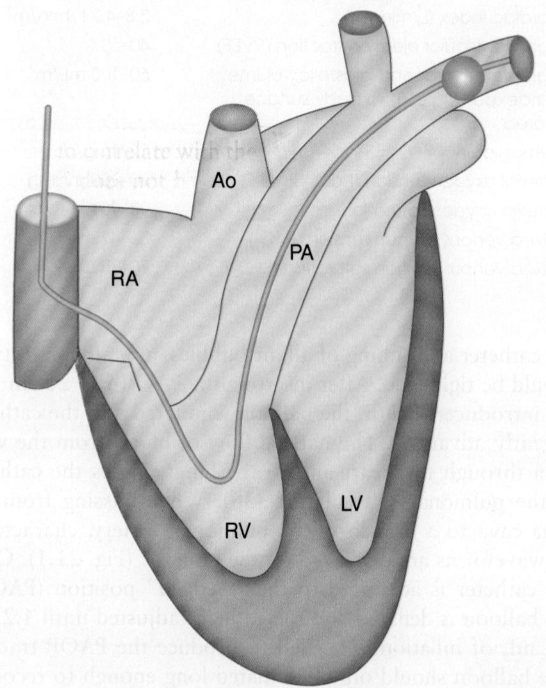

FIGURE 21.2 Proper position of the pulmonary artery catheter. RA, right atrium; RV, right ventricle; PA, pulmonary artery; LV, left ventricle; AO, aorta.

until a good tracing is seen with 1.25 to 1.5 mL of balloon inflation.

Because there is a tendency for materials to oscillate at their natural frequencies, the pressure signal may be distorted (38). This effect may be reduced by using noncompliant, short (<4 ft) tubing in the setup of the catheter and monitoring system. The loss of transmitted signal is referred to as damping, and catheters may be over- or underdamped. The degree of damping can be determined by a "fast-flush" device while demonstrating an optimal waveform (Fig. 21.4A). When the catheter is rapidly flushed, a square wave is produced, followed by a series of oscillations before the tracing returns to the baseline pressure reading (39). The appearance of the oscillations demonstrates the degree of damping. Underdamping, which occurs more frequently, is identified by several sharp oscillations and produces higher systolic pressure readings (Fig. 21.4B). Overdamping results in a rounded oscillation and results in lower readings, and may be due to clots, air bubbles, or kinking in the catheter (Fig. 21.4C). Another factor that may interfere with the signal is catheter whip, which results from contraction of the heart. The tracing will show high-frequency distortion and may be minimized by a high-frequency filter built into the transducer system (38).

Whether the patient is on mechanical ventilation (positive intrathoracic pressure at end inspiration) or spontaneously breathing (negative intrathoracic pressure at end inspiration),

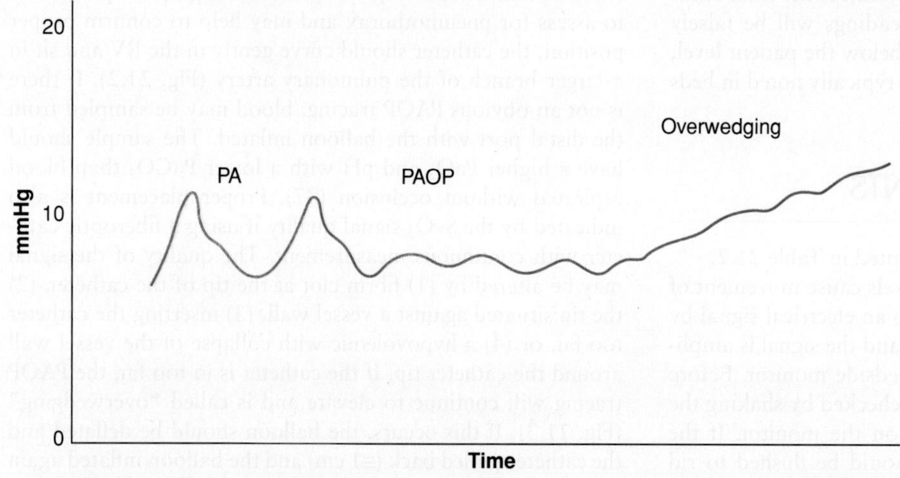

FIGURE 21.3 Overwedged tracing. PA, pulmonary artery; PAOP, pulmonary artery occlusion pressure.

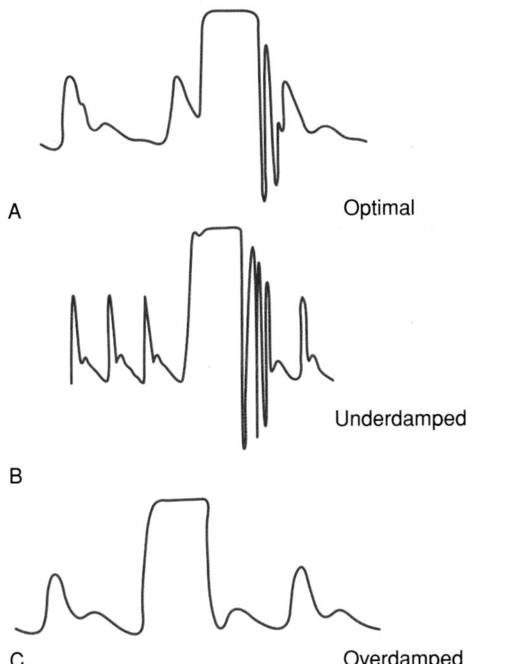

FIGURE 21.4 Checking transducer reliability by the "fast-flush square wave testing."

all pressure measurements should occur at end expiration when the intrathoracic pressure is closest to atmospheric pressure (Fig. 21.5). This point can be determined by watching the patient's respiratory movements or displaying the airway pressure tracing on the same monitor where the PAP is displayed. If respiratory variation is so pronounced that there is no flat end expiration, then it is best NOT to record a number (Fig. 21.6). In this situation, patients may need to be sedated, or if getting a PAOP is crucial, even paralyzed. Note that the approximation to atmospheric pressure is clearly affected by patients on extreme PEEP. It is ill advised to guess the PAOP; *no* information is better than *wrong* information.

The first characteristic waveform seen when inserting a PAC is the right atrium (RA) tracing (Fig. 21.7). The tracing can be seen while inserting the catheter or by transducing the right atrial pressure once the PAC is in position. There are two main positive pressure deflections, called the "a" and "v" waves. The "a" wave follows the P wave of the electrocardiogram (ECG) and is due to the pressure increase during atrial systole (Figs. 21.7 and 21.8). The "v" wave results from atrial filling against a closed tricuspid valve during ventricular systole. Between these two positive deflections is a small "c" wave due to tricuspid closure. Two negative deflections called the x and y descents occur when pressure in the atrium decreases. The x descent occurs during atrial relaxation. The y descent is

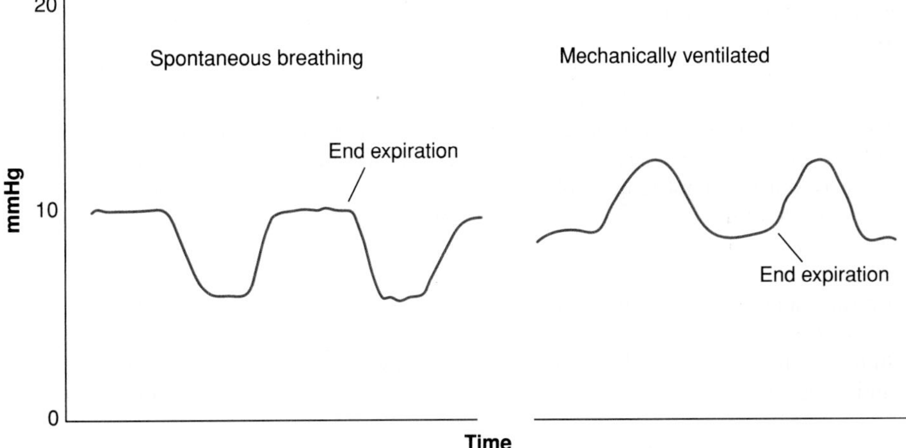

FIGURE 21.5 Reading of pulmonary artery occlusion pressure (PAOP) at end expiration. During spontaneous breaths, PAOP dips down during peak inspiration due to negative intrathoracic pressure. During mechanical ventilation, PAOP goes up during peak inspiration due to positive pressure ventilation and intrathoracic pressure. In both situations, PAOP should be read at end expiration.

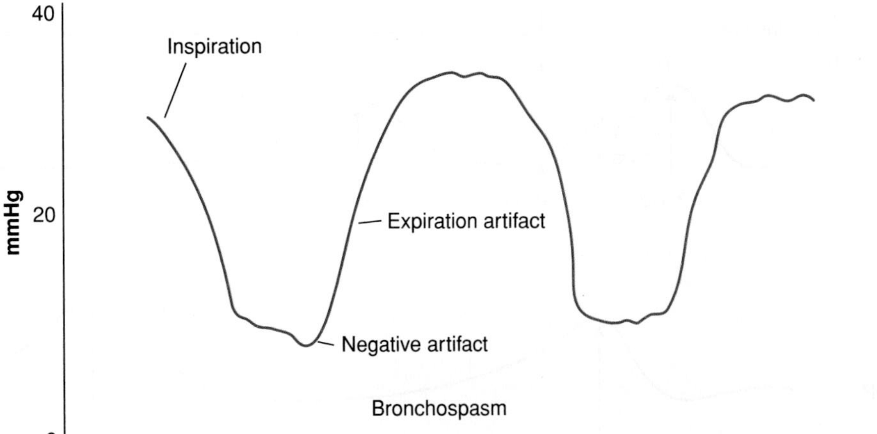

FIGURE 21.6 Excessive variation in pulmonary artery occlusion pressure with forced inspiratory and expiratory efforts precluding accurate measurement due to absence of a stable end-expiratory point.

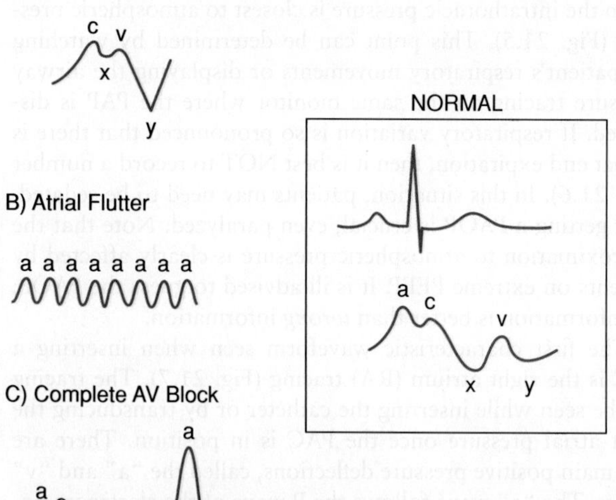

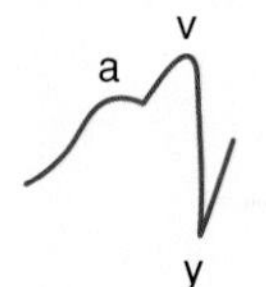

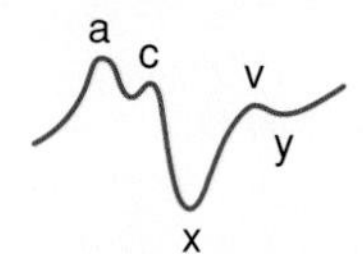

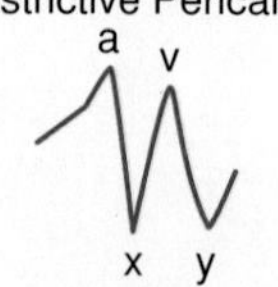

FIGURE 21.7 Pressure tracings from the right atrial port in normal and pathologic conditions (refer to text).

seen when the tricuspid valve opens and blood flows from the atrium to the ventricle.

The best estimate of CVP and PAOP is at end diastole when the atrium contracts. For CVP, where the "c" wave emerges from the "a" wave (also called the z-point) is the optimum reading point. If this point is not clear, read the pressure at the middle of the x descent. Certain patterns in the RA tracing may be seen in disease states (Fig. 21.7). For example,

- "a" waves may not be seen in patients with atrial fibrillation.
- Sawtoothed "a" waves will be present during atrial flutter.
- Large "a," or "cannon" waves occur during atrioventricular (AV) dissociation when the atrium contracts against a closed valve, or during complete heart block.
- A steep y descent is seen in tricuspid regurgitation and the x descent is not apparent.
- Both descents are prominent in RV infarction.
- Cardiac tamponade tends to cause loss of the y descent due to impairment of ventricular filling.
- In pericarditis, sharp a and v waves are followed by steep x and y descents.
- Large v waves are seen in mitral regurgitation, congestive heart failure, and ventricular septal defect due to the increase in atrial pressure.

Recognizing these patterns may suggest a diagnosis before a confirmatory echocardiogram is obtained.

The pressures observed in the right atrium range from 0 to 8 mmHg. Higher pressures may not necessarily mean fluid overload, but may reflect the volume of the right heart and the ability of the ventricle to eject that volume. There is little relationship between CVP and PAOP or left heart pressures in patients with valvular or coronary artery disease or when PAPs are elevated (40,41). Monitoring only the CVP can be misleading in patients with right heart failure, severe pulmonary disease, and most critically ill patients.

The next waveform seen is that of the RV (Fig. 21.1). The pressures here are higher with a wider difference between systolic and diastolic. If no RV waveform is seen after inserting the catheter 30 cm from the internal jugular or subclavian vein entry site, the catheter may be curling in the atrium or passing into the inferior vena cava. The catheter should be

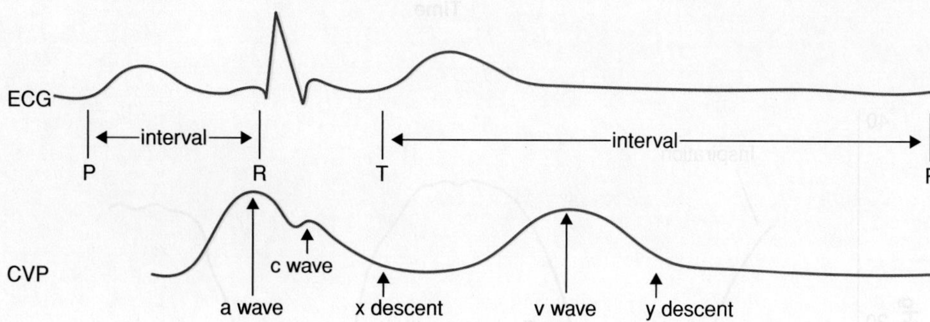

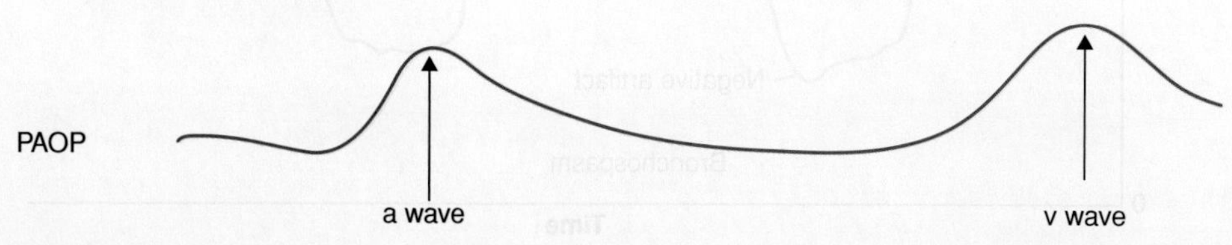

FIGURE 21.8 Reading of central venous pressure (CVP) and pulmonary artery occlusion pressure (PAOP) in relationship to the cardiac cycle (electrocardiogram).

expeditiously advanced through the ventricle both to avoid dysrhythmias and to keep the catheter from warming and softening. The RV systolic pressures generally range from 15 to 30 mmHg and diastolic pressures from 4 to 12 mmHg. In right heart failure, the RV diastolic pressures may be high enough that the waveform mimics the PA. Low RV pressures will be seen in hypovolemic shock and they will also be close to PA pressures. One concern at this point of insertion is causing a right bundle branch block (RBBB), or even complete heart block in patients with pre-existing left bundle branch block (LBBB) (42). However, the incidence of complete heart block appears to be no greater in patients with LBBB than without (43).

Once the catheter enters the pulmonary artery, the waveform shows an increase in diastolic pressure while the systolic pressure remains similar to the ventricle, sometimes referred to as the "step up" (Fig. 21.1). This transition may be difficult to discern when there is hypovolemia, tamponade, RV failure, or catheter whip. If there is no change in waveform after inserting the catheter 50 cm, it may be coiling in the ventricle and is at risk of knotting. A chest radiograph will discern the problem and fluoroscopy may be used to guide placement. Normal PA pressures range from 15 to 25 mmHg systolic over 8 to 15 mmHg diastolic. The beginning of diastole is marked by a dicrotic notch on the PA tracing, corresponding to the closure of the pulmonic valve (44). This incisura distinguishes the PA from the RV when RV diastolic pressures are elevated. As blood flows through the lungs to the left atrium, the PA pressure drops until it reaches a nadir at the end of diastole. Since the pulmonary circulation has low resistance, the diastolic pressure is able to decrease until it is just higher than PAOP. The highest PA systolic pressure occurs during the T wave of the corresponding ECG. The pulmonary circulation is very dynamic and is affected by acidosis, hypoxia, sepsis, and vasoactive drugs (38). An increase in CO may also paradoxically lower the PA pressures by a reflexive decrease in pulmonary vascular resistance (PVR) with fluid resuscitation and decreased sympathetic nervous system discharge (45).

The transition to the wedge position is noted by a drop in mean pressure from the PA. The PAOP usually ranges from 6 to 12 mmHg in normal states. PAOP most closely reflects LVEDP after atrial contraction and before ventricular contraction (Fig. 21.8). There are often no clear "a," "c," or "v" waves. The point 0.05 seconds after onset of QRS of the ECG is where the pressure best estimates LVEDP (46). When "v" waves are prominent such as in mitral insufficiency, the bottom of the "v" wave or the "a" wave may be used to measure the PAOP (Fig. 21.9). A prominent "v" wave may fool the novice into thinking that the catheter is not wedging. It is important to note the change in waveform from PA to v-wave tracing (although the two waves may look remarkably similar). One way of differentiation is that the "v" wave occurs later in the ECG cycle after the T wave while the PA wave occurs right after QRS (Fig. 21.9). There may be large "a" waves secondary to a decrease in left ventricle compliance (47); the point 0.05 seconds after initiation of QRS again best reflects LVEDP. Even though the measurements are correlated with the ECG and are done during end expiration, the PAOP may be exaggerated by respiratory muscle activity, especially during active or labored exhalation. Once the patient is adequately sedated, a short-acting paralyzing agent may be necessary to eliminate this effect (48) (Fig. 21.6).

Principles of Measuring Pulmonary Artery Occlusion Pressure

When the balloon is inflated, the blood flow in that segment of the pulmonary artery is occluded and the PAOP is measured. The pressure between the occluded pulmonary artery segment and the left atrium will equalize upon flow cessation (Fig. 21.10) which is analogous to closing off a pipe with pressures equalizing between the two ends (49). With the closed pipe analogy, there is a host of assumptions: PAOP ≅ PcP ≅ LAP ≅ LVEDP ≅ LVEDV, where PcP is pulmonary capillary pressure, LAP is left atrial pressure, and LVEDV is left ventricular end-diastolic volume. As long as there is no obstruction in this conduit, the relationship between PAOP and LVEDP may hold. The final assumption is equating pressure to volume by estimating LVEDV or "preload" with LVEDP. We will now assess the pitfalls with each of these assumptions.

1. PAOP ≅ PcP ≅ LAP. In the "closed pipe" analogy, the column of blood between the catheter tip and the left atrium should be patent and not narrowed by alveolar pressures. This occurs in the dependent areas of the lung, where the pressures from blood flow in the right atrium and pulmonary artery are greater than the alveolar pressure, or zone 3 in the West classification (50). In

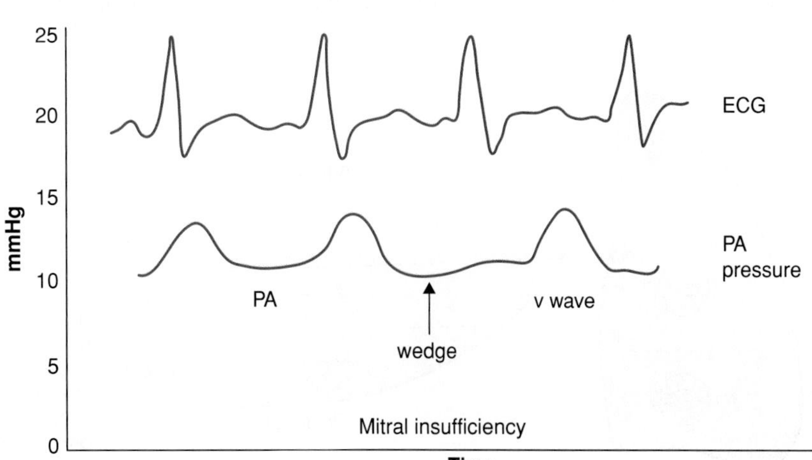

FIGURE 21.9 Regurgitant mitral valve generating a v wave seen during wedging. PA, pulmonary artery.

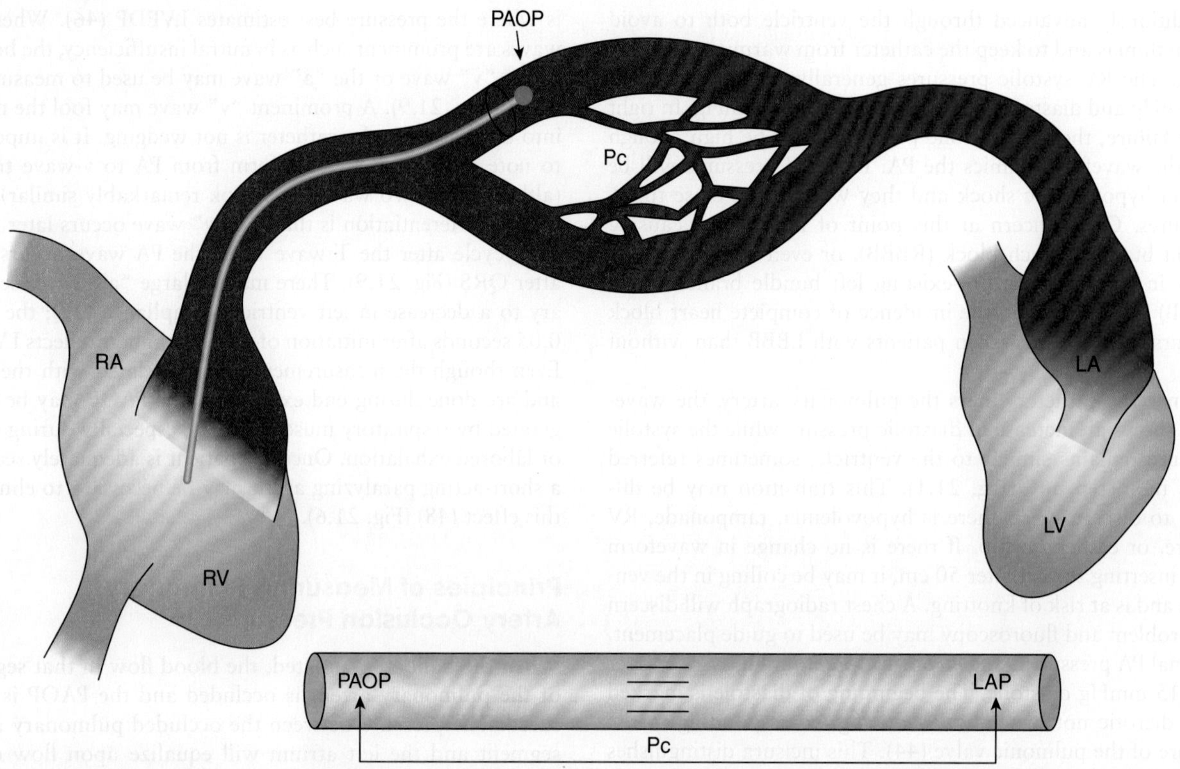

FIGURE 21.10 Closed pipe analogy: blocking of flow by the balloon with theoretical equalization of pressure in the conduit. RA, right atrium; RV, right ventricle; PAOP, pulmonary artery occlusion pressure; Pc, pulmonary capillary; LAP, left atrial pressure; LA, left atrium; LV, left ventricle.

other areas of the lung (zone 1 or 2), the pulmonary arteries may collapse from higher alveolar pressures and the wedge pressure may partially reflect alveolar pressure (Fig. 21.11). Because the PAC is directed by blood flow, it is more likely to pass into zone 3, where pulmonary arterial and venous pressures exceed alveolar pressures. This is especially true when the patient is supine, since there is greater volume of lung located in a dependent position (51). When pulmonary artery diastolic (PAD) pressure is lower than the PAOP, this implies incorrect positioning of the PAC (i.e., blood cannot flow in reverse direction), and may be due to transmission of alveolar pressures on the PAOP in non–zone 3 catheter position. Other factors that may cause errors in estimation of PAOP to LAP are pulmonary venous obstruction and respiratory variation as well as high ventilator support (PAOP reads higher than LAP).

The PAOP usually closely approximates the pulmonary capillary hydrostatic pressure (Pc). When there is an increase in PVR, the wedge pressure underestimates Pc. A difference of 2 to 3 mmHg between the PAOP and PAD pressure is a clue that there may be a discrepancy between PAOP and Pc (34). Hydrostatic pulmonary edema may therefore occur at lower wedge pressures. A method of calculating the Pc has been described by recording the rapid drop in pressure decline when the catheter balloon is inflated in the wedge position (52). The point where the rapid decline transitions to a more gradual slope before reaching the PAOP is the Pc (Fig. 21.12).

Increased intrathoracic pressure secondary to respiratory failure and the addition of PEEP in ventilated patients affects pulmonary vascular pressures. Up to about 15 cm H_2O, PAOP closely correlates with LAP (53). During higher PEEP states, the PAOP may not

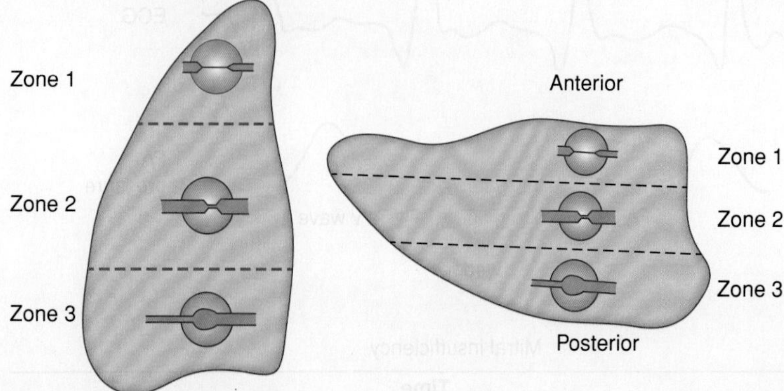

FIGURE 21.11 West lung zones. Zone 1: PAP < PalvP > PvP (there is no blood flow across the collapsed pulmonary capillary bed). Zone 2: PAP > PalvP > PvP (there is some flow since PAP is greater than PalvP). Zone 3: PAP > PalvP < PvP (pulmonary arteries are patent). PAP, pulmonary arterial pressure; PalvP, pulmonary alveolar pressure; PvP, pulmonary venous pressure.

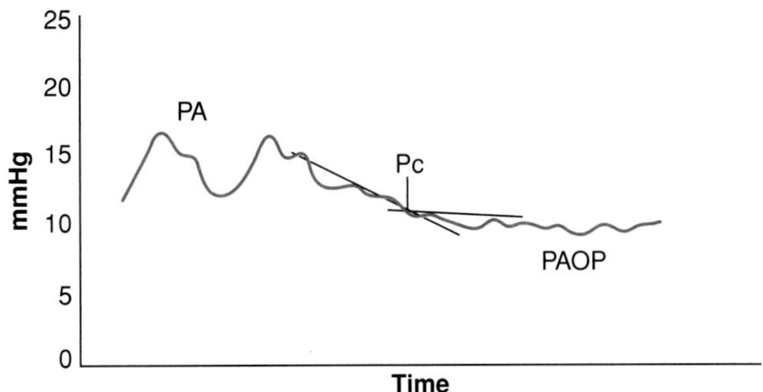

FIGURE 21.12 Estimation of pulmonary capillary pressure. PA, pulmonary artery pressure; Pc, pulmonary capillary pressure; PAOP, pulmonary artery occlusion pressure.

reflect the true filling pressure of the heart (i.e., pressure outside minus pressure inside the heart). Although the heart is seeing the high PEEP support at all times, on-PEEP PAOP is *not* giving the information that we need from the PAOP, which is the cardiac filling pressure. In general, 5 cm H_2O of PEEP is said to raise the measured PAOP by 1 mmHg, but a greater effect is seen in hypovolemic patients or when the catheter is not in West zone 3 (54). High PEEP may also turn zone 3 status to zone 2 or 1 by compressing the pulmonary artery and/or pulmonary vein. Another formula predicts that 50% of PEEP is transmitted to the pleural space (51). However, in noncompliant lungs, such as in the acute respiratory distress syndrome, the alveolar pressure is not effectively transmitted to the vasculature. Also, pulmonary disease is not homogeneous. In complicated cases, it is best to avoid formulas or assumptions. In order to more accurately correct for the effect of pressure transmitted during high PEEP ventilation, the intrapleural pressure may be measured directly with a catheter in the pleural space or distal esophagus and then subtracted from the PAOP. However, this is cumbersome and not often done.

Another method is to measure an "off-PEEP" wedge pressure by temporarily disconnecting the patient from the ventilator circuit and recording the nadir of the tracing (55). This nadir pressure better reflects LAP than the on-PEEP PAOP. The discontinuation should be brief (<1 second) so that a decrease in PaO_2 from derecruitment of alveoli does not occur (56). The brief off-PEEP state will not change physiologic conditions such as venous return and cardiac function. The procedure should be coordinated and done by trained personnel only when the PAOP is needed to make a clinical decision. The balloon is inflated first to ensure good position, then deflated. The FiO_2 may be increased temporarily for patient safety, the balloon reinflated, and at end expiration, the patient is disconnected from the ventilator for 1 second and then reconnected while the PAOP tracing is being recorded. The drop in PAOP upon ventilator disconnection is the off-PEEP PAOP (55). When done properly, it is extremely rare to cause hypoxia.

2. LAP ≅ LVEDP. LAP (and thus PAOP) will overestimate LVEDP if there is an obstruction between the left atrium and the left ventricle such as a myxoma or mitral stenosis. Mitral valve regurgitation also causes the PAOP to read higher than the true LVEDP because of the additional pressure of the retrograde flow of blood across the valve resulting in a large v wave (see Pressure Measurements Section). LAP (and thus PAOP) will underestimate LVEDP when severe aortic regurgitation causes premature closure of the mitral valve when the left ventricle is still filling. LAP (and PAOP) is higher when there is a left atrial kick in a failing heart and decreased ventricle compliance such as in ischemic states, left ventricular hypertrophy, and restrictive cardiomyopathies (57). This is especially true when LVEDP is greater than 25 mmHg.
3. LVEDP ≅ LVEDV. The pressure–volume relationship depends on the compliance of the ventricle and the transmural ventricular distending force. The compliance of the ventricles will change with ischemia, infarct, and hypertrophy. A stiff heart (myocardial hypertrophy) will need higher pressures to obtain the same amount of volume as a normal heart (Fig. 21.13). The transmural ventricular distending force (intracavitary pressure minus juxtacardiac pressure) will depend on the pressure inside and outside the heart. External forces elevating juxtacardiac pressures may be high ventilator support or pericardial tamponade, which may cause elevation of PAOP but may not reflect ventricular filling pressure.

Clinical Use of the Pulmonary Artery Occlusion Pressure

As long as the previously mentioned assumptions regarding the relationship between PAOP, LAP, and LVEDP have been evaluated, the PAOP may be used as an estimate of LAP with reasonable correlation (49,53). The optimum wedge pressure depends on the patient, but has been defined as the pressure where there is minimal increase in stroke volume or left ventricular stroke work. Although the normal PAOP values may be 10 to 14 mmHg (58,59), some patients require a high pressure to reach the optimum stroke volume (Fig. 21.14). Such optimization can be graphically illustrated using a Starling curve plotting SVI to PAOP (as an estimate of LVEDP). If vasoactive agents are started, the heart may now be on a different curve requiring new assessment of the optimum PAOP. The

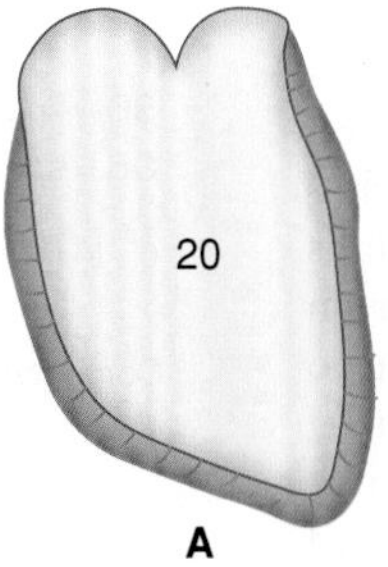

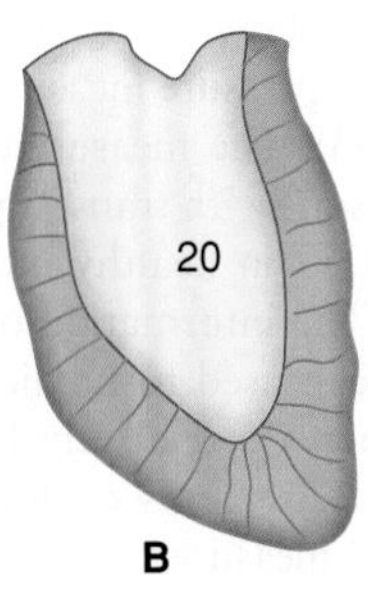

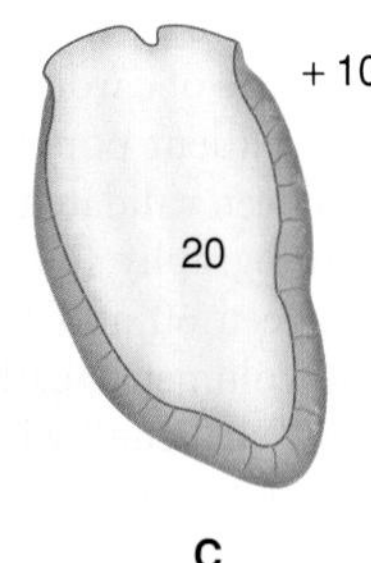

FIGURE 21.13 The same pulmonary artery occlusion pressure of 20 mmHg reflecting three different clinical conditions. **A:** Distended hypervolemic ventricle in a normal heart. **B:** Normal volume in a noncompliant heart (ventricular hypertrophy). **C:** Low volume in a normal ventricle with high juxtacardiac pressures such as high positive end-expiratory pressure.

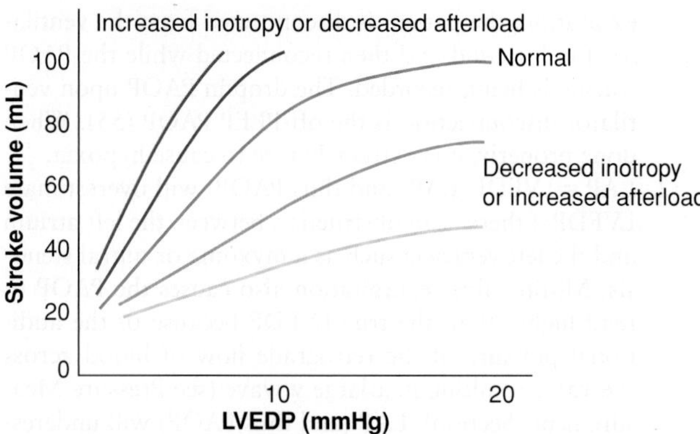

FIGURE 21.14 Frank–Starling curves (family of curves) showing the relationship between left ventricular end-diastolic pressure (LVEDP) and stroke volume (SV, mL/beat). Augmenting preload increases LVEDP with a concomitant increase in SV (up to a certain point). The effects of manipulating preload, afterload, and contractility and shifting to another curve can be seen.

optimum PAOP varies not only from patient to patient, but also temporally within the same patient as the clinical condition changes (such as vasoactive agents, myocardial compliance, and external forces around the heart). No set of values is broadly appropriate for all patients; in practice, each patient must be assessed *repeatedly,* further stressing the importance of judgment and expertise of the end user.

Elevated wedge pressures may help differentiate hydrostatic pulmonary edema from that caused by increased permeability. A PAOP of 24 mmHg or higher is associated with a tendency for hydrostatic edema (60). Lower wedge pressures may imply increase capillary permeability and traditionally, a PAOP of <18 mmHg has implied a pulmonary (or noncardiogenic) cause of lung edema. When there is an increase in PVR, the wedge pressure underestimates Pc and hydrostatic pulmonary edema may therefore occur at lower wedge pressures (see Fig. 21.12).

Volumetric PACs are designed with the ability to measure right ventricular ejection fraction (RVEF), from which the right ventricular end-diastolic volume indexed (RVEDVI) to body surface area (BSA) is calculated. Traditionally, the right heart function was deemed unimportant and thought to merely act as a conduit to funnel blood to the left ventricle. However, right heart dysfunction with septal deviation may impact LV compliance and contractility, and the function of RV is important when PAPs are elevated. The volumetric PACs have two additional electrodes that provide continuous measurement of the ECG and a thermistor with a rapid response. From beat-to-beat change in temperature, the ejection fraction (EF) is calculated. EF (%) = SVI/EDVI × 100, where SVI is stroke volume indexed and EDVI is end-diastolic volume indexed to BSA. CI/HR = EDVI − ESVI, where ESVI is end-systolic volume indexed to BSA (61). RVEDVI has been shown to be a more accurate measure of cardiac preload than pressure measurements in certain patient populations (62,63). The measurement of RVEF has been validated by comparisons with transesophageal echocardiography (64). The RVEDVI in healthy individuals falls between 60 and 100 mL/m^2. The information obtained from the volumetric catheter has been used to predict response to fluid challenge when the values are relatively low (<90 mL/m^2) (62). Much like other measurements of fluid responsiveness, the validity of the RVEF measurement is compromised by tachycardia (pulse >120 beats/min) and atrial fibrillation (irregular HR) (65).

CARDIAC OUTPUT

One's ability to meet increasing tissue oxygen demand by improving cardiac function is perhaps the single most important determinant in DO_2 and tissue perfusion. The evolution of CO measurement is fascinating in its simplicity and started with Adolf Fick, who in the 1870s proposed that uptake or release of a substance by an organ is the product of blood flow through that organ and the difference between arterial and venous values of that substance. The original "dye" was oxygen and the organ studied was the lung. Fick's equation stated: $CO = VO_2/(CaO_2 - CvO_2)$, where VO_2 is oxygen consumption, CaO_2 is arterial content of O_2, and CvO_2 is mixed venous content of O_2.

This principle is widely accepted as an accurate though invasive assessment of CO since a PAC must be placed to obtain accurate mixed venous oxygen content. Additionally, its practical use is limited by the cumbersome measurement of VO_2. Stewart (1897) and Hamilton (1932) utilized Fick's principles but used a known amount of dye injected into central circulation followed by serial peripheral arterial measurements of dye concentration (i.e., change in dye concentration over time), and calculated the flow. The area under the curve after plotting time (x axis) versus dye concentration (y axis) reflected the CO using the following equation: Cardiac output = Amount of dye injected/integral (dye concentration × function of time). The next revolutionary step in CO measurement was using temperature as the dye. Crystalloid solution (usually 10 mL, but 5 mL may be used in volume-restricted patients) is injected into the RA port at similar parts of the respiratory cycle (end expiration), within 4 seconds in a smooth manner (66). The thermistor near the tip of the PAC detects the change in temperature, and the change in blood temperature over time is proportional to the blood flow from the ventricle. Several measurements (three to five) should be taken and the average of the values (within 10% of each other) used. Principles of the modified Stewart–Hamilton equation calculate the CO (Fig. 21.15).

$$Q = \frac{VI\,(TB - TI) \times SI \times CI \times 60 \times CT \times K}{SB \times CB \quad \int_0^\infty \Delta TB\, dt}$$

Q = Cardiac Output
VI = volume of injectate
TI = injectate temperature
TB = blood temperature
CI = specific heat of the injectate (D5W = 0.965, saline = 0.997)
SI = specific gravity of the injectate (D5W = 1.018, saline = 1.005)
60 = seconds/minute
CT = correction factor (loss of thermal indicator due to time lost in injecting, catheter length, patient's temperature)

$$= \frac{TB - \text{mean temperature of the injectate delivered to the right atrium}}{TB - TI \text{ (preinjectate temperature)}}$$

SB = specific gravity of blood (1.045)
CB = specific heat of the blood (0.87)

$\int_0^\infty \Delta TB\, dt$ = integral of blood temperature change

$$\text{Computation constant (K)} = \frac{SI \times CI \times 60 \times CT \times VI}{SB \times CB} = \text{change with VI}$$

FIGURE 21.15 The modified Stewart–Hamilton equation for estimating cardiac output.

Although initial studies used iced solution as injectate, ambient temperature injectate is now the standard solution used with excellent reproducibility and correlation with its iced counterpart (67) and has less likelihood of reflexive bradycardia (68). It is important to note that iced injectate (0° to 5°C) is associated with higher reproducibility and the highest signal-to-noise ratio (69) and may be necessary in hypothermic patients. Falsely low CO will occur if an error in the system increases the change in temperature (which is in the denominator of the Stewart–Hamilton equation): the temperature probe reading the injectate is cooler than the actual injectate (or the solution is warmer than the temperature reading of the injectate), more than allotted "dye" amount is injected (>10 mL fluid), there is too rapid an injection, or the injection occurs during positive pressure ventilation. Falsely high CO may occur if the temperature probe measuring injectate reads warmer than the actual injectate (if the solution is cooler than the temperature reading of the injectate), less than the allotted amount of "dye" (<10 mL) is used, or the catheter has migrated distally with less change in temperature difference. Most institutions use temperature probes at the site of injection (RA port) so that variations in injectate temperature should not contribute to errors in CO measurements.

Another development in the evolution of measuring CO is the PAC with continuous cardiac output (CCO) monitoring (70,71). A heat element is embedded in the PAC to deliver small pulsations of heat, which is detected by a rapid-response thermistor placed distally to the heat source. The change in temperature detected is then used to calculate CO. Although intermittent bolus technology is still gold standard for measuring CO at the bedside, CCO values are reproducible and close to manual CO measurements, although discrepancies are observed at extremely low-flow states (70). Unlike the manual injection of crystalloid, the measurements are obtained at random parts of the respiratory cycle and are less subject to human error, which may account for some of the differences in the two techniques. It is important to note that the CCO value may not instantaneously reflect CO changes (e.g., while titrating inotropes), but the effect of treatment can be seen in seconds if using a continuous SvO_2 monitor. Due to the heat-generating wire coil in the distal end, these catheters must be removed before magnetic resonance imaging.

Starling Curves

Drs. Frank and Starling described the relationship between myocardial stretch and contractility. Myocardial stretch is an independent determinant of stroke work and the actin–myosin interaction has a linear correlation with the strength of systolic contraction up to a certain point. Given the heart's dynamic environment, a family of curves is more representative of the true preload-to-stroke volume relationship. Increasing afterload or decreasing contractility shifts the curve down and to the right (i.e., more stretch is necessary to produce a similar difference in stroke volume). One cannot stress enough the importance of reassessment after each therapy. For example, initiating afterload reduction may put the heart on a different Starling curve (to the left and up; see Fig. 21.14), but may decrease the preload. Unless more fluid is given to optimize the LVEDP (i.e., PAOP), the best stroke volume may not be achieved.

MIXED VENOUS OXYGEN SATURATION (SEE CHAPTER 24)

Specialized PACs with the ability to measure SvO_2 continuously using principles of reflection spectrophotometry are available (Fig. 21.16). Oxygen saturation is the ratio of hemoglobin bound to O_2 divided by total hemoglobin, and when measured at the tip of the PAC, reflects mixing of deoxygenated blood from superior and inferior vena cavae and coronary vessels. The SvO_2 value indicates the balance between DO_2 to the tissues and the amount consumed by the tissues before returning to the heart.

Rearranging the Fick's Equation

$$SvO_2(\%) = SaO_2 - \frac{VO_2}{CO\ (L/min) \times Hgb\ (g/dL) \times 1.36\ (mLO_2/g\ Hgb) \times 10}$$

Four factors determine the SvO_2 value: three parameters contributing to DO_2 (CO, hemoglobin, and SaO_2), and one parameter for O_2 consumption. Low SvO_2 suggests insufficient O_2 delivery or increased O_2 consumption. SvO_2 is also a harbinger of shock and may decrease before overt shock is apparent (15,16,23,72). SvO_2 has also regained popularity as an end goal of resuscitation with decreased mortality (7,73–75). Inadequate DO_2 can be the result of decreased CO, low hemoglobin, or low oxygen saturation. Increased consumption may occur due to activity, fever, hyperthyroid state, or repayment of oxygen debt. High SvO_2 suggests low cellular consumption such as in late sepsis, arteriovenous shunts (cirrhosis), or excessive inotrope use. Hypothermia, sedation, paralysis, anesthesia, hypothyroidism, and cyanide poisoning can also reduce VO_2. The catheter should also be checked to ensure that distal migration has not occurred leading to sampling of pulmonary capillary blood that is normally highly saturated (~100%). Inflating the balloon (wedging) should determine that the catheter is in too far if the PAOP tracing is seen with less than 1.25 mL of air.

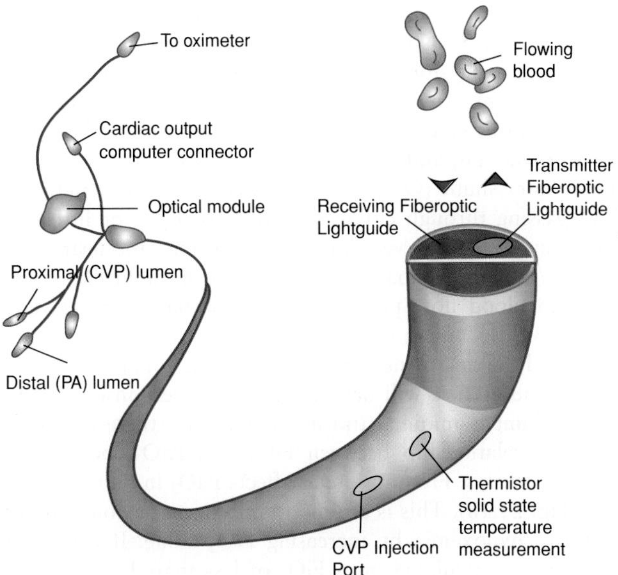

FIGURE 21.16 Fiberoptic catheter using principles of spectrophotometry.

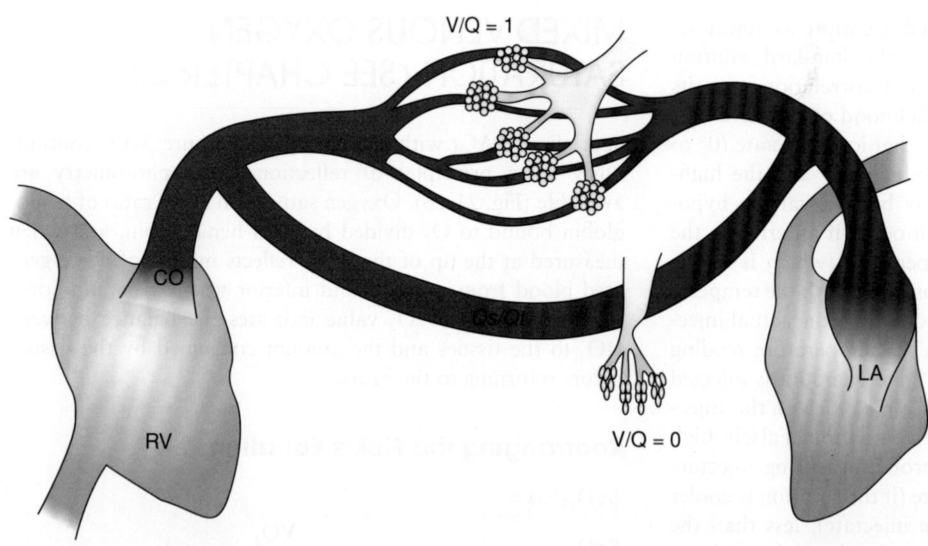

FIGURE 21.17 Intrapulmonary shunt (*Qs/Qt*) is the percentage of cardiac output (CO) not involved with gas exchange (goes through collapsed alveoli), with ventilation/perfusion V/Q = 0. LA, left atrium; RV, right ventricle.

Calibration by laboratory oximeter on a daily basis is important to check for drifting and whenever the values do not seem to correlate with the patient's clinical condition. Even if the PAC does not have continuous SvO_2 monitoring, SvO_2 can be checked by sending a blood sample from the distal PA port (by drawing slowly at the rate of 1 mL over 20 seconds to prevent sampling of pulmonary capillary blood) and sending it to the laboratory for oximeter analysis (direct saturation measurement and not arterial blood gas [ABG] analysis). If the PAC has continuous SvO_2 monitoring, a signal quality indicator is generated. If the signal intensity suggests poor quality, errors include (a) that PAC is in too far, (b) there are fibrin clots around the tip, (c) the catheter is touching the vessel wall, or (d) the patient may be hypovolemic. Repositioning the PAC or flushing the PA port may resolve this issue.

INTRAPULMONARY SHUNT (*Qs/Qt*)

Shunt refers to the portion (in %) of blood that flows (CO) from the right side of the heart to the left completely deoxygenated (Fig. 21.17). We will not discuss cardiac shunts in this chapter. Physiologic shunt = Anatomic shunt + Intrapulmonary shunt. Anatomic shunt refers to the direct drainage of the venous system to the left ventricle through the bronchial, thebesian, and pleural veins (~2%–5% of CO). Intrapulmonary shunt (*Qs/Qt*) is expressed as the percentage of CO passing through collapsed alveoli with no or little gas exchange so that the ventilation-to-perfusion ratio nears zero (i.e., V/Q = 0). Venoarterial admixture or shunt-like states refer to blood flow passing through partially open alveoli (i.e., V/Q <1). Acute or complete shunt will not respond to FiO_2 and the treatment is PEEP to open the collapsed alveoli. Venous admixture will demonstrate some response to FiO_2. If the shunt is minimal (normal condition), there is almost a linear relationship between FiO_2 and PaO_2, but as the shunt increases, FiO_2 no longer affects PaO_2 in a linear fashion (Fig. 21.18). This is an important concept as one cannot improve hypoxemia by increasing FiO_2 alone. If the shunt equation is calculated on a FiO_2 of less than 1.0, both the shunt and venous admixture will be captured in the equation. Intrapulmonary shunt (*Qs/Qt*) is calculated as ($CcO_2 - CaO_2$)/($CcO_2 - CvO_2$), where CcO_2 is the pulmonary capillary content of O_2, CaO_2 is the arterial content of O_2, and CvO_2 is the mixed venous content of O_2 (Table 21.3). Since pulmonary capillary blood cannot be sampled, the saturation is assumed to be 100%, which usually holds true when the FiO_2 is 1.0. It is important to understand the contribution of a low SvO_2 to PaO_2 if there is a moderate shunt (>20%). Any decrease in SvO_2 in a patient with more than 20% shunt will allow more deoxygenated blood to go into the arterial circulation, resulting in a lower PaO_2. This is called nonpulmonary cause of hypoxia. For example, if a patient with a 20% intrapulmonary shunt and a hemoglobin of 15 g/dL has an acute cardiac event, and the CO decreases from 5 to 3 L/min, the PaO_2 will decrease from approximately 80 to 65 mmHg (Fig. 21.19). If the same patient's hemoglobin is 10 g/dL, the PaO_2 will decrease from 70 to 55 mmHg. This demonstrates the importance of low SvO_2 contributing to lower PaO_2 (recall that hemoglobin affects the delivery portion of the SvO_2 equation). If the CO was not optimized prior to increasing PEEP, a potential further decrease in CO, SvO_2, and PaO_2 may have ensued. Another example: If a patient is agitated and the arterial saturation decreases, this may be due to increased VO_2 and low SvO_2 in a patient with a moderate intrapulmonary

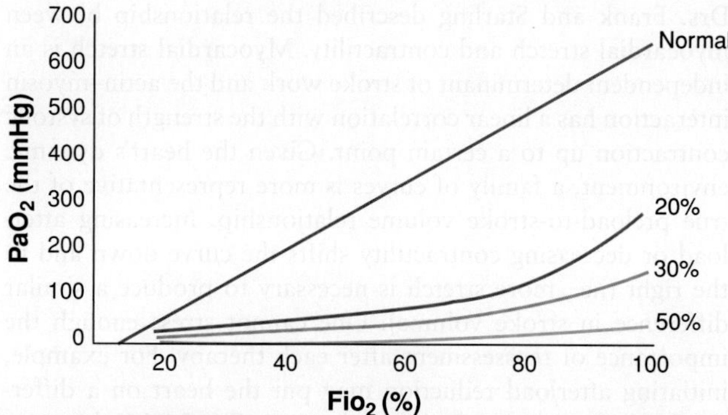

FIGURE 21.18 The effect of FiO_2 on PaO_2 depending on the degree of intrapulmonary shunts of 20%, 30%, and 50%. This is assuming that other parameters that affect SvO_2 such as cardiac output, hemoglobin, and oxygen consumption are remaining constant.

TABLE 21.3 Derived Calculations (All Indexed to Body Surface Area)

Parameter	Equation	Key	Normal	Units
Stroke volume indexed (SVI)	CI/HR or EDVI – ESVI	Amount of blood ejected with each contraction (per m^2)	30–65	mL/beat/m^2
Left ventricular stroke work index (LVSWI)	SVI × (MAP – PAOP) × 0.0136	External work for the left ventricle in 1 beat	43–61	g/m^2/beat
Right ventricular stroke work index (RVSWI)	SVI × (MPAP – CVP) × 0.0136	External work for the right ventricle in 1 beat	7–12	g/m^2/beat
Pulmonary vascular resistance indexed (PVRI)	$\frac{(MPAP - PAOP) \times 80}{CI}$	Resistance for right ventricle; 80 converts mmHg/min/L to dynes sec/cm^5	255–285	dynes sec/cm^5
Systemic vascular resistance (SVR)	$\frac{(MAP - CVP) \times 80}{CI}$	Resistance for left ventricle	1,970–2,390	dynes sec/cm^5/m^2
Arterial oxygen content of blood (CaO_2)	(Hgb × 1.36 mL O_2/gHgb × SaO_2) + (0.0031 × PaO_2)	Amount of oxygen in arterial blood, majority is carried by Hgb (1.36 mL of O_2/g of Hgb if blood is 100% saturated), very little is dissolved (0.0031 × PaO_2)	16–22	mL O_2/dL blood
Mixed venous oxygen content of blood (CvO_2)	(Hgb × 1.36 mL O_2/gHgb × SvO_2) + (0.0031 × PvO_2)	Amount of oxygen in mixed venous blood (sampled at the pulmonary artery)	12–17	mL O_2/dL blood
Arterial mixed venous oxygen content difference ($AVDO_2$)	$CaO_2 - CvO_2$	How much O_2 was consumed by the tissues before returning to the heart	3–5	mL O_2/dL blood
Delivery of oxygen indexed (DO_2I)	CaO_2 × CI × 10	Primary determinant of organ perfusion	500–600	mL O_2/min/m^2
Oxygen consumption indexed (VO_2I)	($CaO_2 - CvO_2$) × CI × 10	Oxygen consumed by the tissues	120–160	mL O_2/min/m^2
Intrapulmonary shunt (*Qs/Qt*)	($CcO_2 - CaO_2$)/($CcO_2 - CvO_2$) CcO_2 = (Hgb × 1.36 × 100% saturation) + (0.0031 × $PaAO_2$) $PaAO_2 = FiO_2$ × (760 mmHg – 47 mmHg) – ($PaCO_2$/ RQ)	% of CI that is not involved with gas exchange and goes to the arterial side deoxygenated; greater than 20% usually requires ventilator support. Since pulmonary capillary blood cannot be sampled, 100% saturation is assumed. 760 is atmospheric pressure at sea level; 47 is water vapor pressure.	3–5	% of cardiac output
Coronary perfusion pressure (CPP)	CPP = DBP – PAOP	The major determinant of flow in a fixed, diseased conduit is the pressure difference.	50–60	mmHg

CI, cardiac index (mL/min/m^2); HR, heart rate (beats/min); EDVI, end-diastolic volume index (mL/m^2); ESVI, end-systolic volume index (mL/m^2); MAP, mean arterial pressure; DBP, diastolic blood pressure (mmHg); PAOP, pulmonary artery occlusion pressure (mmHg); CVP, central venous pressure; Hgb, hemoglobin (g/dL); CcO_2, pulmonary capillary content of oxygen; PaO_2, partial pressure of oxygen in the alveoli; RQ, respiratory quotient VCO_2/VO_2 is 0.8 for a mixed fuel diet.

shunt, and not from an acute pulmonary event. Treatment is to decrease agitation and VO_2. There are times when severe cardiorespiratory compromise warrants titration of both CO and PEEP simultaneously in patients with life-threatening hypoxia. It is important to understand the interaction of one organ on the other and the relationship between PaO_2, hemoglobin, and CO (Fig. 21.19).

DERIVED VARIABLES

See Table 21.3 for the equations and normal values. Once flow and pressure variables have been obtained from the PAC, further hemodynamic calculations may be performed to ascertain a more complete clinical picture. Clinicians must understand the significance and pitfalls of these calculated values (most of which are automatically calculated by monitoring devices).

Stroke volume index (SVI): It is the quantity of blood ejected from the ventricle with each contraction (i.e., the difference between end-diastolic and end-systolic volumes). SVI accounts for the effect of the HR's contribution to CI, and is an important variable because one does not want to augment CI by causing tachycardia (Fig. 21.14). SVI varies with preload, afterload, and contractility. Preload is the theoretical stretch of ventricles at end diastole. According to Frank and Starling, the stretch of myocardium augments contractility to a certain point, and then CO is negatively affected by further increases (76). Afterload reflects the interplay between aortic compliance, peripheral vascular resistance, viscosity of blood, aortic impedance, and aortic wall resistance. Afterload is therefore the force that myocytes must overcome during each contraction and clearly more complex than an arbitrary division of the heart into left and right components. Contractility is the maximum velocity of myocardial fiber contraction; it is the myocytes' inherent ability, independent of preload. All these parameters are extremely dynamic and require frequent reassessment.

Left ventricular stroke work index (LVSWI): This estimates the work of the left ventricle in one beat. Work is the product of force and distance. Physiologically, this translates to the product of change in pressure and change in volume. Unfortunately,

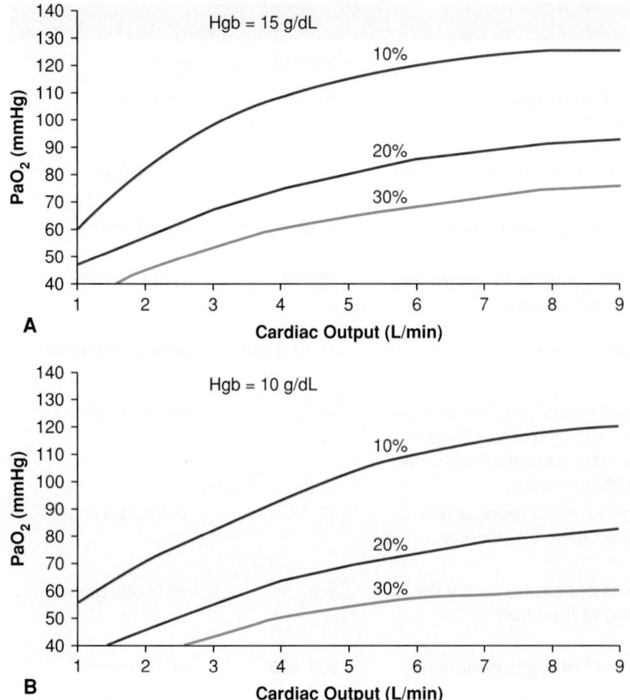

FIGURE 21.19 Relationship between PaO_2, cardiac output, and three different intrapulmonary shunt states (10%, 20%, and 30%) for patients with a hemoglobin of 15 g/dL **(A)** and 10 g/dL **(B)**. This graph demonstrates "nonpulmonary" causes for PaO_2 changes where a low cardiac output or low hemoglobin will impact PaO_2 depending on the degree of shunt.

current technology does not allow continuous measurements of both ventricular volumes at the bedside. Stroke work index is low in cardiogenic and hypovolemic shock, while it has been suggested that high LVSWI is associated with decreased mortality in trauma patients (77,78). It should be noted that not all work is alike since "good work" is associated with large volume change with little pressure, and "bad work" is associated with large pressure change with little volume movement (a reflection of compliance).

Right ventricular stroke work index (RVSWI): It is the right heart's ability to produce forward flow against the pulmonary circulation and estimates external work for the RV in one beat. The work generated by RV is markedly less than LV due to a relatively low pulmonary pressure system. In patients with pulmonary hypertension and consequent right heart failure, the RVSWI must compensate accordingly.

Pulmonary vascular resistance index (PVRI): It is the resistance for the RV. Resistance to blood flow is analogous to electrical circuit resistance defined by Ohm's Law. Resistance = Pressure/Flow. Physiologically, the pressure change between two vascular beds drives the flow (i.e., CI). PVRI reflects resistance in the pulmonary vasculature. Pulmonary hypertension exists when systolic PAP is greater than 35 mmHg or mean PAP is greater than 25 mmHg (79,80). In critically ill patients, the most common causes for elevated PAP are acute respiratory distress syndrome, acute LV dysfunction, and pulmonary embolism (79,81–85). Patients with comorbid conditions such as chronic pulmonary hypertension may suffer from interstitial lung disease, COPD, or liver or cardiac disease. The RV is exquisitely sensitive to increases in afterload and lacks the ability to overcome pulmonary hypertension with PAP greater than 40 mmHg (84). Subsequent decrease in CO is due to the combination of decreased RVSWI and decreased filling of the left ventricle as a result of interventricular septal deviation (86). Since CO is indexed to BSA, PVR should also be indexed and presented as PVRI.

Systemic vascular resistance index (SVRI): It is the resistance for the left ventricle. In the context of hyperdynamic states with high CI and decreased SVRI, the patient may be in distributive shock. Patients with low CI and high SVRI are in hypovolemic or cardiogenic shock. It is important to recognize that SVRI represents the interaction of vascular diameter and viscosity, neither variable is easily and reliably measured. SVRI is calculated; therefore error is introduced if any of its subcomponents carries inaccuracy. Since CO is indexed to BSA, SVR should also be indexed and presented as SVRI.

Arterial oxygen content of blood (CaO_2): It is the amount of oxygen carried in arterial blood. When evaluating delivery of oxygen, the CaO_2 is of critical importance. Each gram of hemoglobin carries 1.36 to 1.39 mL of oxygen if it is 100% saturated. Oxygen is poorly soluble in plasma and the dissolved oxygen contribution to arterial oxygen content is negligible. Therefore, saturation (SaO_2) plays a more important role than pressure of oxygen (PaO_2).

Mixed venous oxygen content of blood (CvO_2): It is the amount of oxygen carried in the mixed venous blood. Low mixed venous oxygen content has similar clinical implications as low SvO_2 and suggests decreased DO_2 or increased VO_2. Since the blood is sent for oximeter analysis for saturation value and not PvO_2, the PvO_2 value in the equation (Table 21.3) is usually substituted with the normal PvO_2 value of 40 mmHg since the amount dissolved is so small that a PvO_2 substitution of 0 to 70 mmHg will not make a difference in the calculation of CvO_2.

Delivery of oxygen indexed to BSA (DO_2I): It is the amount of oxygen delivered to the tissues by hemoglobin, arterial saturation, and flow (CI) (i.e., the product of CI and arterial oxygen content of blood). The survival benefit of titrating to a specific DO_2I value has been extensively studied as an end point of resuscitation with conflicting results. The controversy surrounding DO_2 augmentation is discussed in the beginning of this chapter (11,15,19,20,23,30,87–89).

Oxygen consumption indexed (VO_2I): There are two methods of assessing VO_2: Fick's principle and indirect calorimetry (90). Fick's principle states that the rate of diffusion of a known indicator (oxygen) is proportional to the product of concentration gradient and flow. Physiologically, this translates to the difference between arterial and mixed venous oxygen content multiplied by the CO. Consumption can also be assessed by indirect calorimetry and is typically 3.5 mL of oxygen/kg (91). Indirect calorimetry compares the difference between inspired and expired oxygen to carbon dioxide ratios. There is usually a discrepancy (either way) of up to 11% between Fick's principle and indirect calorimetry, partially explained by Fick's method not accounting for pulmonary VO_2 (92–95). Shoemaker first noted that a higher VO_2I of greater than 160 mL/min/m^2 was associated with survival (3,4). It may reflect cells' ability to increase metabolic rate and utilize oxygen during stressed states. The concept of "critical DO_2I" where VO_2 becomes delivery dependent has been described in certain disease states with values occurring at DO_2 of less than 450 mL oxygen/min/m^2 (96–98). Although the concept is attractive, it is difficult to use VO_2 as a therapeutic end point since VO_2 varies constantly depending on sedation, temperature, paralysis, loop diuretics, complete mechanical ventilation, vasoactive agents, and the progress of the underlying disease process (6,16).

Coronary perfusion pressure (CPP): In compliant vessels, flow to the coronary arteries can be augmented via coronary artery dilation. However, in patients with coronary artery disease with fixed vessels, flow depends on the pressure gradient between the two ends. Due to high LV pressures, coronaries feeding the LV fill during diastole, and maintenance of diastolic pressure is important. In patients undergoing preoperative optimization, nitroglycerin can be used to preferentially dilate healthy coronary vessels, thereby augmenting DO_2 to the myocytes. Generally CPP greater than 50 mmHg is desired, but there is individual variation.

SPECIAL COMMENT ON OBESITY AND DERIVED PARAMETERS

The validity of derived parameters indexed to BSA has been questioned in morbidly obese patients. Several studies have demonstrated that derived parameters indexed to BSA are appropriate and closely approximate indexing to body mass index. The large BSA in the obese patient may not affect these measurements (99–101).

COMPLICATIONS OF PULMONARY ARTERY INSERTION

PAC insertion is an invasive procedure and carries inherent risks (102–104). Complications related to central venous access are discussed in other chapters. The overall complication rate associated with PACs can be as high as 25%. The procedural risks are pneumothorax, hemothorax, and knotting of catheters. Multiple prospective and retrospective studies have reported the most common complications including infection, thrombosis, arrhythmias, new bundle branch blocks, and pulmonary artery rupture (105,106). Serious complications (PA rupture and cardiac perforation with tamponade) are infrequent, but they can be fatal if unrecognized. Although reports of PAC-related infection are up to 22%, consequential bacteremia is relatively rare (0.7%–2.2%) (107). Catheters inserted for greater than 3 days may be associated with more infectious and thrombotic complications (108,109). Arrhythmias were relatively common, occurring in up to 75% of insertions. However, clinically significant arrhythmias requiring treatment were rare; 3% developed new bundle branch blocks, but this complication was not associated with increased mortality (105,106). Pulmonary artery rupture is exceedingly rare with a reported incidence of 0.031% (110) but usually occurs in patients with pulmonary hypertension and can be fatal due to high pulmonary pressures. To prevent rupture, it is important to: 1) slowly inflate the balloon, 2) stop inflating when resistance is encountered, and 3) deflate when the waveform tracing demonstrates overwedging. Placement of PACs requires skilled operators who are trained to troubleshoot and recognize complications when they occur. As discussed earlier in this chapter, perhaps the most dangerous complication of PACs is the misinterpretation of information.

ARTERIAL LINES

Indications for invasive pressure monitoring are (a) hyperdynamic states including all forms of shock and (b) frequent blood sampling for blood gas analysis and laboratories. Other indications include monitoring of response to vasoactive agents and severe peripheral vascular disease precluding noninvasive BP monitoring. There are no true absolute contraindications.

Arterial cannulation is relatively safe with nonocclusive thrombosis and hematoma being the most common complications (111). Selection of anatomic site is an important consideration; percutaneous arterial catheters can be introduced in the radial, brachial, axillary, femoral, and dorsalis pedis arteries. Placement in brachial arteries is ill advised; it is an end artery and patients may develop ipsilateral hand ischemia in up to 40% of insertions (112,113). The radial artery remains the most popular placement site due to its ease of access and relatively low complication rates. A preprocedure Allen test assesses the patency of collateral arteries, but this test has poor correlation with distal flow and likelihood of hand ischemia (114,115).

Pressure Measurement

Continuous measures of SBP, diastolic blood pressure (DBP), and mean arterial pressure (MAP) are displayed with invasive arterial catheters. Four elements must be considered in direct pressure measurement: (a) energy content, (b) transformation of pressure pulse, (c) reflection of pressure wave, and (d) recording system. Each element can introduce error in invasive BP monitoring rendering the often large discrepancy between cuff and invasive pressures. The SBP is determined by the ventricular ejection velocity and volume and this pulse wave meets increasing impedance as the caliber of vessels decrease. Additionally, pulse amplification is proportional to distance from aorta; consequently, the radial artery pressure tends to be higher than aortic pressure.

Volume and velocity of left ventricular ejection, peripheral resistance, distensibility of arterial wall, and viscosity of blood determine the peak SBP. Usage of long tubing (≥4 feet) or microbubbles in the closed system can result in inaccurate measurements, specifically underdamping and falsely high SBP. Underdamping produces characteristic waveforms with sharp and overshooting upstroke and small, artifact pressure waves along the waveform. Overdamped tracings are caused by kinking, macrobubbles, or mechanical obstruction of tubing. Overdamped waveforms are characteristically diminished in their upstroke and exhibit loss of the dicrotic notch. The dynamic response of arterial monitoring circuits is assessed by a fast-flush square wave test (Fig. 21.4); a properly calibrated system produces one overdamped waveform followed by several oscillating overshoot waves (116).

Waveform analysis (Fig. 21.20) demonstrates the typical points associated with (a) systolic upstroke, (b) systolic peak, (c) systolic decline, (d) dicrotic notch, (e) diastolic runoff, and (f) end diastole. Examination of the arterial waveform provides useful information regarding a patient's clinical status. Left ventricular ejection produces the first, sharp upstroke at the beginning of aortic valve opening (Fig. 21.20, points 1 and 2). As the ventricular flow is dispersed peripherally, the waveform declines (point 3); this is also when the heart is in

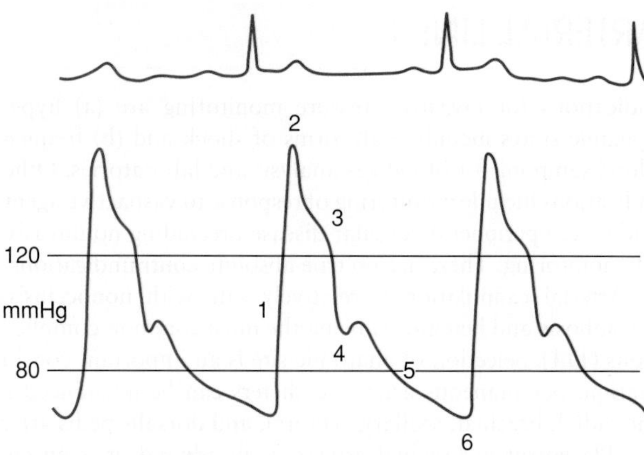

FIGURE 21.20 Arterial waveform analysis (see text for explanation of points 1–6).

isovolumetric relaxation and diastolic filling. Just prior to closure of the aortic valve and as a result of isovolumetric relaxation, there is a slight drop in pressure known as the incisura (at the aorta) or dicrotic notch (at the periphery) (point 4). Further decrease in the pressure waveform reflects the runoff to distal arterioles (points 5 and 6). More peripheral arteries exhibit narrower waveforms and higher systolic pressures and wider pulse pressures, although the MAP remains similar to central vessels. The etiology of varying pulse contours in the periphery is related to the elasticity, amplification, and distortion of smaller arteries (117). Various cardiac conditions produce characteristic arterial waveforms. In aortic stenosis, narrow waveform and loss of the dicrotic notch secondary to diseased valve are seen. Aortic regurgitation may exhibit widened pulse pressures and a sharp upstroke, sometimes accompanied by two peaks.

Systolic pressure variation (SPV): Variations in SBP and ventricular stroke volume are of greater magnitude in hypovolemic states (118). Theories on the etiology of this phenomenon relate to the characteristics unique to hypovolemia and include the following: (a) the superior vena cava is more easily collapsible, (b) there is an increased effect of transmural pressures in the right atrium, and (c) the preload and stroke volume relationship is on the steep portion of the Frank–Starling curve. Usually, a decrease in left ventricular stroke volume occurs with inspiration due to the positive pressure ventilation. Originally, Perel described SPV as two components (Fig. 21.21)—delta up (Δup) and delta down (Δdown)—while emphasizing the strong correlation between Δdown and hypovolemic states (119–121). Δup is the difference between maximum SBP and a reference SBP (usually at expiratory pause during mechanical ventilation). Δdown is similarly the difference between minimum SBP and reference SBP and represents a decrease in stroke volume during expiration. SPV greater than 10 mmHg indicates hypovolemia and suggests responsiveness to fluid challenge (122). SPV also has significant correlation with the left ventricular end-diastolic area by echocardiogram (123) and PAOP (124). Note that SPV, like stroke volume variation (SVV), may be sensitive to changes in volume status, but may not necessarily equate to actual intravascular blood volume.

Stroke volume variation (SVV): Arterial pressure variation during the respiratory cycle is a well-documented phenomenon (118). There exists normal fluctuations of arterial pressure during spontaneous respirations; however, pulsus paradoxus is observed when the ebb and flow of arterial pressures exceeds 10 mmHg. Reverse pulsus paradoxicus occurs in ventilated patients. Proprietary algorithms in new monitor devices analyze the pulse-to-pulse variation in a semicontinuous fashion with updates at 20-second intervals. SVV is not a measurement of absolute preload; rather, it is an assessment of response to fluid resuscitation (124–127). SVV greater than 9.5% to 15% is associated with fluid responsiveness. SVV is only approved for use in sedated, mechanically ventilated patients who are in sinus rhythm (rhythm must be regular or the variation may be due to irregular rate rather than volume status).

$$SVV = (SV\ maximum - SV\ minimum) /[(SV\ maximum + SV\ minimum)/2] \times 100$$

Available technology on the market: Several companies market continuous arterial catheter CO monitoring with several important distinctions. The main difference between the aforementioned technologies is that Lidco analyzes areas under a concentration curve, whereas FloTrac analyzes stroke volume based on pulse pressure variances. Each manufacturer has its own, largely proprietary algorithms. Over the years, manipulation of the algorithms attempted to mitigate errors introduced by various hyperdynamic states such as sepsis, no definitive outcome trial is available to guide the clinician in its use (128–130).

LidcoPlus (Lidco, Cambridge, UK): LidcoPlus combines the previously validated Lidco lithium indicator dilution calibration procedure with continuous pulse contour analysis for real-time CO assessment (131). A small amount of lithium chloride is injected in a vein and the concentration of arterial sampling over time produces a concentration-time curve. The area under this curve provides the CO by integral mathematics. The manufacturer recommends calibration every 8 hours. Studies have

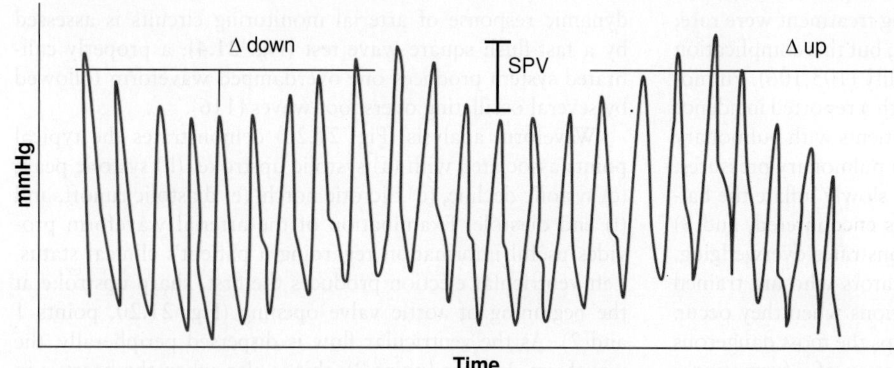

FIGURE 21.21 Systolic pressure variation (SPV).

shown that LidcoPlus provides similar CO results as traditional PACs over a wide range of hemodynamic states (132,133).

FloTrac (Edwards Lifesciences, Irvine, CA, USA): This features CCO and SVV without need for calibration utilizing an existing arterial catheter. Assumptions are made regarding the patient's vascular compliance given his or her age, weight, and height. Proprietary software analyzes waveform contours beat to beat and evaluates CO based on the concept that stroke volume is related to beat-to-beat pressure changes. The algorithm also takes into account the dynamic changes in vascular compliance by assessing the characteristic changes associated with alterations in vascular tone. Preliminary studies have demonstrated similar CO results compared to intermittent, bolus thermodilution techniques (134). Although the use of SVV has only been validated in heavily sedated patients without spontaneous respirations and in sinus rhythm, preliminary data confirm that SVV may be utilized in spontaneously breathing patients with quiet respirations.

The search for new, noninvasive, emerging technology continues. The literature on noninvasive hemodynamic monitoring devices is extensive; as of 2015, more than 1,500 articles attempt to compare various novel devices to address the complexities of hemodynamic monitoring. Devices encompassing bioimpedance, spectroscopy, pulse contour and wave analysis, and indwelling transesophageal echo all fail to address the clinical demand in a reliable manner and none has withstood the rigorous, randomized controlled clinical testing that demonstrates improved outcome (135). For now, the thermodilution technique is still gold standard.

SUMMARY

The value of any monitoring system is to impact outcomes. Although surrounded by controversy, there remains a group of patients who may benefit from invasive monitoring. It is imperative that technology is used by trained personnel who understand both the benefits and the limitations of the devices. Equally important is the concept of early resuscitation before the onset of multisystem organ failure. The next quantum leap in hemodynamic monitoring will allow us to optimize DO_2 to the tissue bed in a noninvasive platform. But until we can noninvasively and continuously monitor CO, cardiac preload, intravascular blood volume status, central SvO_2, and tissue oxygenation (see chapters 20, 22, 24, and 27), the PAC will likely continue to have a place in modern ICUs (136–138). To minimize the heterogeneity and often difficult to interpret data, future research should be focused on specific patient population, particularly in high-risk surgical patients (139,140).

Key Points

- Misinterpretation and inexperience in PAC likely contribute to lack of outcome benefit from its use.
- Clinicians should titrate flow variables during resuscitation to meet cellular level oxygen demand.
- The preload to stroke volume relationship governed by Frank–Starling's Law is a dynamic response to patient's clinical status.
- SVV has limited utility in patients who have spontaneous respiration and/or tachyarrhythmia.
- Until we can noninvasively and continuously monitor CO, cardiac preload, intravascular blood volume status, central SvO_2, and tissue oxygenation (see chapters 20, 22, 24, and 27), the PAC will likely continue to have a place in modern ICUs.

References

1. Connors AF. The effectiveness of right heart catheterization in the initial care of critically ill patients. SUPPORT Investigators. *JAMA*. 1996; 276:889–897.
2. Practice guidelines for pulmonary artery catheterization. *Anesthesiology*. 2003;99:988–1014.
3. Shoemaker WC, Elwyn DH, Levin H, et al. Use of nonparametric analysis of cardiorespiratory variables as early predictors of death and survival in postoperative patients. *J Surg Res*. 1974;17:301–314.
4. Shoemaker WC. Physiologic patterns in surviving and nonsurviving shock patients. *Arch Surg*. 1973;106:630.
5. Bihari D, Smithies M, Gimson A, et al. The effects of vasodilation with prostacyclin on oxygen delivery and uptake in critically ill patients. *N Engl J Med*. 1987;317:397–403.
6. Yu M, Burchell S, Takiguchi SA, et al. The relationship of oxygen consumption measured by indirect calorimetry to oxygen delivery in critically ill patients. *J Trauma*. 1996;41:41–50.
7. Rivers E, Nguyen B, Havstad S, et al. Early goal-directed therapy in the treatment of severe sepsis and septic shock. *N Engl J Med*. 2001;345: 1368–1377.
8. Mouncey PR, Osborn TM, Power GS, et al. Trial of early, goal-directed resuscitation for septic shock. *N Engl J Med*. 2015;372:1301–1311.
9. Moore FA, Haenel JB, Moore EE, et al. Incommensurate oxygen consumption in response to maximal oxygen availability predicts postinjury multiple organ failure. *J Trauma*. 1992;33:58–66.
10. Bishop MH, Shoemaker WC, Appel PL, et al. Relationship between supranormal circulatory values, time delays, and outcome in severely traumatized patients. *Crit Care Med*. 1993;21:56–63.
11. Fleming A. Prospective trial of supranormal values as goals of resuscitation in severe trauma. *Arch Surg*. 1992;127:1175.
12. Gattinoni L, Brazzi L, Pelosi P, et al. A trial of goal-oriented hemodynamic therapy in critically ill patients. *N Engl J Med*. 1995;333:1025–1032.
13. Hayes MA, Timmins AC, Yau E, et al. Elevation of systemic oxygen delivery in the treatment of critically ill patients. *N Engl J Med*. 1994;330: 1717–1722.
14. Wheeler AP, Bernard GR, Thompson BT, et al. Pulmonary-artery versus central venous catheter to guide treatment of acute lung injury. *N Engl J Med*. 2006;354:2213–2224.
15. Yu M, Burchell S, Hasaniya NW, et al. Relationship of mortality to increasing oxygen delivery in patients > or = 50 years of age: a prospective, randomized trial. *Crit Care Med*. 1998;26:1011–1019.
16. Yu M. Invasive and noninvasive oxygen consumption and hemodynamic monitoring in elderly surgical patients. *New Horiz*. 1996;4:443–452.
17. Yu M. Oxygen transport optimization. *New Horiz*. 1999;7:46.
18. Sandham JD, Hull RD, Brant RF, et al. A randomized, controlled trial of the use of pulmonary-artery catheters in high-risk surgical patients. *N Engl J Med*. 2003;348:5–14.
19. Berlauk JF, Abrams JH, Gilmour IJ, et al. Preoperative optimization of cardiovascular hemodynamics improves outcome in peripheral vascular surgery. *Ann Surg*. 1991;214:289–299.
20. Shoemaker WC. The efficacy of central venous and pulmonary artery catheters and therapy based upon them in reducing mortality and morbidity. *Arch Surg*. 1990;125:1332.
21. Gutierrez G, Palizas F, Doglio G, et al. Gastric intramucosal pH as a therapeutic index of tissue oxygenation in critically ill patients. *Lancet*. 1992;339:195–199.
22. Shoemaker WC, Bayard DS, Botnen A, et al. Mathematical program for outcome prediction and therapeutic support for trauma beginning within 1 hr of admission: A preliminary report. *Crit Care Med*. 2005;33:1499–1506.
23. Yu M, Chapital A, Ho HC, et al. A prospective randomized trial comparing oxygen delivery versus transcutaneous pressure of oxygen values as resuscitative goals. *Shock*. 2007;27:615–622.

24. Yu M, Morita SY, Daniel SR, et al. Transcutaneous pressure of oxygen. *Shock*. 2006;26:450–456.
25. Cohn SM, Nathens AB, Moore FA, et al. Tissue oxygen saturation predicts the development of organ dysfunction during traumatic shock resuscitation. *J Trauma*. 2007;62:44–55.
26. De Backer D, Creteur J, Preiser J-C, et al. Microvascular blood flow is altered in patients with sepsis. *Am J Respir Crit Care Med*. 2002;166: 98–104.
27. Boerma EC, Mathura KR, van der Voort PHJ, et al. Quantifying bedside-derived imaging of microcirculatory abnormalities in septic patients: a prospective validation study. *Crit Care*. 2005;9:R601.
28. Yamauchi H, Biuk-Aghai EN, Yu M, et al. Circulating blood volume measurements correlate poorly with pulmonary artery catheter measurements. *Hawaii Med J*. 2008;67:8–11.
29. Fleisher LA, Fleischmann KE, Auerbach AD, et al. 2014 ACC/AHA guideline on perioperative cardiovascular evaluation and management of patients undergoing noncardiac surgery: executive summary: a report of the American College of Cardiology/American Heart Association Task Force on Practice Guidelines. *Circulation*. 2014;130:2215–2245.
30. Boyd O, Grounds RM, Bennett ED. A randomized clinical trial of the effect of deliberate perioperative increase of oxygen delivery on mortality in high-risk surgical patients. *JAMA*. 1993;270:2699–2707.
31. Wilson RJ, Woods I. Cardiovascular optimization for high-risk surgery. *Curr Opin Crit Care*. 2001;7:195–199.
32. Eisenberg PR, Jaffe AS, Schuster DP. Clinical evaluation compared to pulmonary artery catheterization in the hemodynamic assessment of critically ill patients. *Crit Care Med*. 1984;12:549–553.
33. Iberti TJ, Daily EK, Leibowitz AB, et al. Assessment of critical care nurses' knowledge of the pulmonary artery catheter. *Crit Care Med*. 1994; 22:1674–1678.
34. Tuman KJ, Carroll GC, Ivankovich AD. Pitfalls in interpretation of pulmonary artery catheter data. *J Cardiothor Anesth*. 1989;3:625–641.
35. Connors AF Jr, McCaffree DR, Gray BA. Evaluation of right-heart catheterization in the critically ill patient without acute myocardial infarction. *N Engl J Med*. 1983;308:263–267.
36. Swan HJ, Ganz W, Forrester J, et al. Catheterization of the heart in man with use of a flow-directed balloon-tipped catheter. *N Engl J Med*. 1970; 283:447–451.
37. Morris AH, Chapman RH. Wedge pressure confirmation by aspiration of pulmonary capillary blood. *Crit Care Med*. 1985;13:756–759.
38. Sprung CL. The pulmonary artery catheter: methodology and clinical applications. *Crit Care Res Assoc*. 1993.
39. Daily EK, Schroeder JS. *Techniques in Bedside Hemodynamic Monitoring*. St. Louis: C. V. Mosby; 1981.
40. Sarin CL, Yalav E, Clement AJ, et al. The necessity for measurement of left atrial pressure after cardiac valve surgery. *Thorax*. 1970;25:185–189.
41. Civetta JM, Gabel JC. Flow directed-pulmonary artery catheterization in surgical patients: indications and modifications of technic. *Ann Surg*. 1972;176:753–756.
42. Thomson IR, Dalton BC, Lappas DG, et al. Right bundle-branch block and complete heart block caused by the Swan-Ganz catheter. *Anesthesiology*. 1979;51:359–362.
43. Shah KB, Rao TL, Laughlin S, et al. A review of pulmonary artery catheterization in 6,245 patients. *Anesthesiology*. 1984;61:271–275.
44. Sharkey SW. Beyond the wedge: clinical physiology and the Swan-Ganz catheter. *Am J Med*. 1987;83:111–122.
45. Zapol WM, Falke KJ. *Acute Respiratory Failure*. New York: Dekker; 1985.
46. Raper R, Sibbald WJ. Misled by the wedge? The Swan-Ganz catheter and left ventricular preload. *Chest*. 1986;89:427–434.
47. Fisher ML, De Felice CE, Parisi AF. Assessing left ventricular filling pressure with flow-directed (Swan-Ganz) catheters. Detection of sudden changes in patients with left ventricular dysfunction. *Chest*. 1975;68:542–547.
48. Schuster DP, Seeman MD. Temporary muscle paralysis for accurate measurement of pulmonary artery occlusion pressure. *Chest*. 1983;84:593–597.
49. Lappas D, Lell WA, Gabel JC, et al. Indirect measurement of left-atrial pressure in surgical patients–pulmonary-capillary wedge and pulmonary-artery diastolic pressures compared with left-atrial pressure. *Anesthesiology*. 1973;38:394–397.
50. West JB, Dollery CT, Naimark A. Distribution of blood flow in isolated lung; relation to vascular and alveolar pressures. *J Appl Physiol*. 1964;19:713–724.
51. O'Quin R, Marini JJ. Pulmonary artery occlusion pressure: clinical physiology, measurement, and interpretation. *Am Rev Respir Dis*. 1983;128: 319–326.
52. Cope DK, Allison RC, Parmentier JL, et al. Measurement of effective pulmonary capillary pressure using the pressure profile after pulmonary artery occlusion. *Crit Care Med*. 1986;14:16–22.
53. Lozman J. Correlation of pulmonary wedge and left atrial pressures. *Arch Surg*. 1974;109:270.
54. Sidebotham D. *Cardiothoracic Critical Care*. Philadelphia, PA: Butterworth-Heinemann; 2007.
55. Carter RS, Snyder JV, Pinsky MR. LV filling pressure during PEEP measured by nadir wedge pressure after airway disconnection. *Am J Physiol*. 1985;249:H770–H776.
56. De Campo T, Civetta JM. The effect of short-term discontinuation of high-level PEEP in patients with acute respiratory failure. *Crit Care Med*. 1979; 7:47–49.
57. Rahimtoola SH. Left ventricular end-diastolic and filling pressures in assessment of ventricular function. *Chest*. 1973;63:858.
58. Parker JO, Case RB. Normal left ventricular function. *Circulation*. 1979; 60:4–12.
59. Packman MI, Rackow EC. Optimum left heart filling pressure during fluid resuscitation of patients with hypovolemic and septic shock. *Crit Care Med*. 1983;11:165–169.
60. Guyton AC, Lindsey AW. Effect of elevated left atrial pressure and decreased plasma protein concentration on the development of pulmonary edema. *Circ Res*. 1959;7:649–657.
61. Zwissler B, Briegel J. Right ventricular catheter. *Curr Opin Crit Care*. 1998;4:177–183.
62. Diebel L, Wilson RF, Heins J, et al. End-diastolic volume versus pulmonary artery wedge pressure in evaluating cardiac preload in trauma patients. *J Trauma*. 1994;37:950–955.
63. Durham R, Neunaber K, Vogler G, et al. Right ventricular end-diastolic volume as a measure of preload. *J Trauma*. 1995;39:218–224.
64. Chang MC, Black CS, Meredith JW. Volumetric assessment of preload in trauma patients. *Shock*. 1996;6:326–329.
65. Bennett D, Boldt J, Brochard L, et al. Expert panel: The use of the pulmonary artery catheter. *Intensive Care Med*. 1991;17:I–VIII.
66. Conway J, Lund-Johansen P. Thermodilution method for measuring cardiac output. *Eur Heart J*. 1990;11:17–20.
67. Olsson B, Pool J, Vandermoten P, et al. Validity and reproducibility of determination of cardiac output by thermodilution in man. *Cardiology*. 1970;55:136–148.
68. Harris AP, Miller CF, Beattie C, et al. The slowing of sinus rhythm during thermodilution cardiac output determination and the effect of altering injectate temperature. *Anesthesiology*. 1985;63:540–541.
69. Elkayam U. Cardiac output by thermodilution technique: effect of injectate's volume and temperature on accuracy and reproducibility in the critically ill patient. *Chest*. 1983;84:418.
70. Tulzo Y, Belghith M, Seguin P, et al. Reproducibility of thermodilution cardiac output determination in critically ill patients: Comparison between bolus and continuous method. *J Clin Monitor Comput*. 1996;12: 379–385.
71. Seguin P, Colcanap O, Le Rouzo A, et al. Evaluation of a new semi-continuous cardiac output system in the intensive care unit. *Can J Anaesth*. 1998;45:578–583.
72. Burchell SA, Yu M, Takiguchi SA, et al. Evaluation of a continuous cardiac output and mixed venous oxygen saturation catheter in critically ill surgical patients. *Crit Care Med*. 1997;25:388–391.
73. Rivers E. The outcome of patients presenting to the emergency department with severe sepsis or septic shock. *Crit Care*. 2006;10:154.
74. Rivers EP, Nguyen HB, Huang DT, et al. Early goal-directed therapy. *Crit Care Med*. 2004;32:314–315.
75. Otero RM. Early goal-directed therapy in severe sepsis and septic shock revisited. *Chest*. 2006;130:1579.
76. Katz AM. Ernest Henry Starling, his predecessors, and the "law of the heart". *Circulation*. 2002;106:2986–2992.
77. Chang MC, Mondy JS, Meredith JW, et al. Redefining cardiovascular performance during resuscitation. *J Trauma*. 1998;45:470–478.
78. Martin RS, Norris PR, Kilgo PD, et al. Validation of stroke work and ventricular arterial coupling as markers of cardiovascular performance during resuscitation. *J Trauma* . 2006;60:930–935.
79. Barst RJ, McGoon M, Torbicki A, et al. Diagnosis and differential assessment of pulmonary arterial hypertension. *J Am Coll Cardiol*. 2004;43:S40–S47.
80. Chin KM, Kim NHS, Rubin LJ. The right ventricle in pulmonary hypertension. *Coron Artery Dis*. 2005;16:13–18.
81. Benza RL, Park MH, Keogh A, et al. Management of pulmonary arterial hypertension with a focus on combination therapies. *J Heart Lung Transplant*. 2007;26:437–446.
82. Girgis RE, Mathai SC. Pulmonary hypertension associated with chronic respiratory disease. *Clin Chest Med*. 2007;28:219–232.
83. O'Callaghan D, Gaine SP. Combination therapy and new types of agents for pulmonary arterial hypertension. *Clin Chest Med*. 2007;28:169–185.

84. Oudi.z RJ. Pulmonary hypertension associated with left-sided heart disease. *Clin Chest Med.* 2007;28:233–241.
85. Ryu JH, Krowka MJ, Swanson KL, et al. Pulmonary hypertension in patients with interstitial lung diseases. *Mayo Clin Proc.* 2007;82:342–350.
86. Zamanian RT, Haddad F, Doyle RL, et al. Management strategies for patients with pulmonary hypertension in the intensive care unit. *Crit Care Med.* 2007;35:2037–2050.
87. Fenwick E, Wilson J, Sculpher M, et al. Pre-operative optimisation employing dopexamine or adrenaline for patients undergoing major elective surgery: a cost-effectiveness analysis. *Intensive Care Med.* 2002;28:599–608.
88. Kern JW, Shoemaker WC. Meta-analysis of hemodynamic optimization in high-risk patients. *Crit Care Med.* 2002;30:1686–1692.
89. Yu M, Takanishi D, Myers SA, et al. Frequency of mortality and myocardial infarction during maximizing oxygen delivery. *Crit Care Med.* 1995; 23:1025–1032.
90. Hanique G, Dugernier T, Laterre PF, et al. Evaluation of oxygen uptake and delivery in critically ill patients: A statistical reappraisal. *Intensive Care Med.* 1994;20:19–26.
91. Severino Brandi L, Bertolini R, Calafà M. Indirect calorimetry in critically ill patients: clinical applications and practical advice. *Nutrition.* 1997; 13:349–358.
92. Peyton PJ, Robinson GJB. Measured pulmonary oxygen consumption: difference between systemic oxygen uptake measured by the reverse Fick method and indirect calorimetry in cardiac surgery. *Anaesthesia.* 2005; 60:146–150.
93. Bizouarn P, Blanloeil Y, Pinaud M. Comparison between oxygen consumption calculated by Fick's principle using a continuous thermodilution technique and measured by indirect calorimetry. *Br J Anaesth.* 1995;75:719–723.
94. Oudemans-van Straaten HM. Oxygen consumption after cardiopulmonary bypass—different measuring methods yield different results. *Intensive Care Med.* 1994;20:458–459.
95. Smithies M, Royston B, Makita K, et al. Comparison of oxygen consumption measurements. *Crit Care Med.* 1991;19:1401–1406.
96. Lorente JA, Renes E, GÓMez-Aguinaga MA, et al. Oxygen delivery-dependent oxygen consumption in acute respiratory failure. *Crit Care Med.* 1991;19:770–775.
97. Schumacker PT, Cain SM. The concept of a critical oxygen delivery. *Intensive Care Med.* 1987;13:223–229.
98. Appel PL. Relationship of oxygen consumption and oxygen delivery in surgical patients with ARDS. *Chest.* 1992;102:906.
99. Beutler S, Schmidt U, Michard F. Hemodynamic monitoring in obese patients: a big issue. *Crit Care Med.* 2004;32:1981.
100. Collis T, Devereux RB, Roman MJ, et al. Relations of stroke volume and cardiac output to body composition: the strong heart study. *Circulation.* 2001;103:820–825.
101. Stelfox HT, Ahmed SB, Ribeiro RA, et al. Hemodynamic monitoring in obese patients: the impact of body mass index on cardiac output and stroke volume. *Crit Care Med.* 2006;34:1243–1246.
102. Hadian M, Pinsky MR. Evidence-based review of the use of the pulmonary artery catheter: impact data and complications. *Crit Care.* 2006;10:S8.
103. Carrico CJ, Horovitz JH. Monitoring the critically ill surgical patient. *Adv Surg.* 1977;11:101–127.
104. McNally JB. Invasive monitoring with the Swan-Ganz catheter. *Ariz Med.* 1974;31:421–424.
105. Sprung CL, Elser B, Schein RMH, et al. Risk of right bundle-branch block and complete heart block during pulmonary artery catheterization. *Crit Care Med.* 1989;17:1–3.
106. Sprung CL, Pozen RG, Rozanski JJ, et al. Advanced ventricular arrhythmias during bedside pulmonary artery catheterization. *Am J Med.* 1982;72:203–208.
107. Payen D, Gayat E. Which general intensive care unit patients can benefit from placement of the pulmonary artery catheter? *Critical Care.* 2006; 10(Suppl 3):S7.
108. Sise MJ, Hollingsworth P, Brimm JE, et al. Complications of the flow-directed pulmonary-artery catheter. *Crit Care Med.* 1981;9:315–318.
109. Rosenwasser RH, Jallo JI, Getch CC, et al. Complications of Swan-Ganz catheterization for hemodynamic monitoring in patients with subarachnoid hemorrhage. *Neurosurgery.* 1995;37:872–876.
110. Kearney TJ. Pulmonary artery rupture associated with the Swan-Ganz catheter. *Chest.* 1995;108:1349.
111. Slogoff S, Keats AS, Arlund C. On the safety of radial artery cannulation. *Anesthesiology.* 1983;59:42–47.
112. Mortensen J. Clinical sequelae from arterial needle puncture, cannulation, and incision. *Circulation.* 1967;35:1118–1123.
113. Barnes RW. Complications of brachial artery catheterization: prospective evaluation with the Doppler ultrasonic velocity detector. *Chest.* 1974;66:363.
114. Barone JE, Madlinger RV. Should an Allen test be performed before radial artery cannulation? *J Trauma.* 2006;61:468–470.
115. Mangar D, Thrush DN, Connell GR, et al. Direct or modified Seldinger guide wire-directed technique for arterial catheter insertion. *Anesth Analg.* 1993;76:714–717.
116. Gardner RM. Direct blood pressure measurement: dynamic response requirements. *Anesthesiology.* 1981;54:227–236.
117. O'Rourke MF. Wave reflections and the arterial pulse. *Arch Intern Med.* 1984;144:366.
118. Michard F. Changes in arterial pressure during mechanical ventilation. *Anesthesiology.* 2005;103:419–428.
119. Perel A. Arterial pressure waveform analysis during hypovolemia. *Anesth Analg.* 1996;82:670–671.
120. Perel A. Assessing fluid responsiveness by the systolic pressure variation in mechanically ventilated patients. *Anesthesiology.* 1998;89:1309–1310.
121. Perel A. The value of delta Down during haemorrhage. *Br J Anaesth.* 1999; 83:967–968.
122. Rick JJ, Burke SS. Respirator paradox. *South Med J.* 1978;71:1376–1378.
123. Coriat P, Vrillon M, Perel A, et al. A comparison of systolic blood pressure variations and echocardiographic estimates of end-diastolic left ventricular size in patients after aortic surgery. *Anesth Analg.* 1994;78:46–53.
124. Preisman S. Predicting fluid responsiveness in patients undergoing cardiac surgery: functional haemodynamic parameters including the Respiratory Systolic Variation Test and static preload indicators. *Br J Anaesth.* 2005;95:746–755.
125. Berkenstadt H. Pulse pressure and stroke volume variations during severe haemorrhage in ventilated dogs. *Br J Anaesth.* 2005;94:721–726.
126. Berkenstadt H, Margalit N, Hadani M, et al. Stroke volume variation as a predictor of fluid responsiveness in patients undergoing brain surgery. *Anesth Analg.* 2001:984–989.
127. Michard F. Predicting fluid responsiveness in ICU patients. *Chest.* 2002; 121:2000.
128. Perner A, Faber T. Stroke volume variation does not predict fluid responsiveness in patients with septic shock on pressure support ventilation. *Acta Anaesthesiol Scand.* 2006;50:1068–1073.
129. Marik PE, Cavallazzi R, Vasu T, et al. Dynamic changes in arterial waveform derived variables and fluid responsiveness in mechanically ventilated patients: a systematic review of the literature. *Crit Care Med.* 2009;37:2642–2647.
130. Elstad M, Walloe L. Heart rate variability and stroke volume variability to detect central hypovolemia during spontaneous breathing and supported ventilation in young, healthy volunteers. *Physiol Meas.* 2015;36:671–681.
131. Linton R, Band D, O'Brien T, et al. Lithium dilution cardiac output measurement. *Crit Care Med.* 1997;25:1796–1800.
132. Kurita T, Morita K, Kato S, et al. Lithium dilution cardiac output measurements using a peripheral injection site comparison with central injection technique and thermodilution. *J Clin Monit Comput.* 1999;15:279–285.
133. Linton RA, Jonas MM, Tibby SM, et al. Cardiac output measured by lithium dilution and transpulmonary thermodilution in patients in a paediatric intensive care unit. *Intensive Care Med.* 2000;26:1507–1511.
134. McGee WT, Horswell JL, Calderon J, et al. Validation of a continuous, arterial pressure-based cardiac output measurement: a multicenter, prospective clinical trial. *Critical Care.* 2007;11:R105.
135. Thiele RH, Bartels K, Gan TJ. Cardiac output monitoring: a contemporary assessment and review. *Crit Care Med.* 2015;43:177–185.
136. Gidwani UK, Mohanty B, Chatterjee K. The pulmonary artery catheter: a critical reappraisal. *Cardiol Clin.* 2013;31:545–565, viii.
137. Reade MC, Angus DC. PAC-Man: game over for the pulmonary artery catheter? *Crit Care.* 2006;10:303.
138. Arora S, Singh PM, Goudra BG, et al. Changing trends of hemodynamic monitoring in ICU - from invasive to non-invasive methods: Are we there yet? *Int J Crit Illn Inj Sci.* 2014;4:168–177.
139. Balk E, Raman G, Chung M, et al. *AHRQ Technology Assessments: Evaluation of the Evidence on Benefits and Harms of Pulmonary Artery Catheter Use in Critical Care Settings.* Rockville,MD: Agency for Healthcare Research and Quality (US); 2008.
140. Leier CV. Invasive hemodynamic monitoring the aftermath of the ESCAPE trial. *Cardiol Clin.* 2007;25:565–571.

CHAPTER

22

Monitoring Tissue Perfusion and Oxygenation

DAVID INOUYE and KENNETH WAXMAN

Adequate tissue perfusion and oxygenation are necessary to maintain or restore homeostasis. When tissue oxygen delivery (DO_2) is inadequate to meet metabolic demands, shock ensues. Untreated, shock typically progresses to cellular dysfunction. The prompt recognition of and reversal from an early shock state may prevent the onset of cellular dysfunction. There is renewed interest in quantitative measurements of tissue perfusion in the context of shock detection and resuscitation. However the interpretation of these measurements in the many clinical conditions that manifest in shock are not well defined. This chapter outlines underlying principles of tissue perfusion and oxygenation and reviews some complexities of making clinically useful measurements with existing monitoring approaches.

There are multiple components of the circulation that contribute to cellular oxygenation, each of which is related to monitoring of tissue perfusion and oxygenation. Tissue perfusion is determined by cardiac output, the distribution of cardiac output to regional tissue beds, and the state of the microcirculation. Tissue oxygenation is determined by perfusion as well as by arterial oxygenation, nutritional blood flow, and cellular extraction of oxygen. This is a complex system, which is highly dynamic: Alteration of any component has physiologic impact upon other components (Fig. 22.1). Moreover, there is enormous heterogeneity within the circulation, both between organs and within organs. Hence tissue perfusion and oxygenation is never uniform between organs, nor even in particular tissue beds. Nonetheless, despite these complexities, there are several principles that allow useful monitoring to occur.

1. Peripheral perfusion and oxygenation monitors are not replacements for other commonly used monitors, but instead provide unique physiologic information.
2. A measured decrease in peripheral tissue perfusion may provide a significant and early warning of circulatory insufficiency.
3. In low-flow shock states (such as hemorrhagic or cardiogenic shock), there is a characteristic redistribution of regional blood flow, such that blood flow to the heart and brain is preserved, while peripheral blood flow is decreased. Blood flow to the skin decreases very early in this process; hence, monitoring skin perfusion is a very sensitive indicator of circulatory shock. Blood flow to other tissues such as the intestinal tract also decreases relatively early in shock, making the gut an alternative sensitive monitoring site. Unfortunately, in high-flow shock states (such as septic shock), the distribution of regional blood flow is less predictable, and interpretation of peripheral perfusion data becomes more complex.
4. A measured decrease in peripheral tissue oxygenation may be a significant warning of decreased tissue oxygenation or perfusion, hemoglobin concentration, arterial oxygenation, or increased cellular utilization of oxygen. Sorting out these alternative explanations for abnormal tissue oxygenation can lead to prompt diagnosis and treatment of the underlying problem.
5. Monitoring changes of tissue oxygenation in response to changes in cardiac output or arterial oxygen may provide meaningful clinical information. The use of these devices in response to physiologic challenges adds another dimension to their potential value.

MONITORING TECHNIQUES

Pulse Oximetry

Initially developed to measure oxygen saturation noninvasively, pulse oximetry technology now provides additional useful information in the care of critically ill patients. The incorporation of improved signal processing techniques and sensors has advanced pulse oximetry technology to obtain measurements of total blood hemoglobin, dyshemoglobin levels, and peripheral tissue perfusion. The ratio of the pulsatile to nonpulsatile components of the pulse oximetry waveform, frequently referred to as the perfusion index (PI), may provide a quantitative value of peripheral perfusion. Low values of PI are associated with increased severity of illness and decreased survival in patients with shock (1–4).

Pulse oximetry measurements of oxygen saturation in combination with tissue oxygen monitors can indicate whether low tissue oxygenation is due to arterial hypoxemia or to inadequate circulation. Similarly, oximetry measurements combined with oximetry-derived measurements of total blood hemoglobin and peripheral perfusion may provide an assessment of peripheral perfusion and oxygenation.

Transcutaneous Oxygen

In 1956 Clark developed a practical polarographic electrode to measure oxygen tension (5). Since then, the Clark electrode has become the standard for blood gas analysis. When the Clark electrode is placed into a heated probe, it can be used to measure transcutaneous oxygen. Heating the skin to 44°C or higher rapidly (over minutes) melts the lipoprotein barrier and allows diffusion of oxygen across the stratum corneum. Transcutaneous oxygen tension ($PtcO_2$) values may be site specific, sometimes with lower values in the extremities of patients with peripheral vascular disease. For critical care monitoring, most studies utilize the torso. Despite several confounding issues, transcutaneous oxygen monitoring provides useful physiologic data that are meaningfully related to tissue oxygenation.

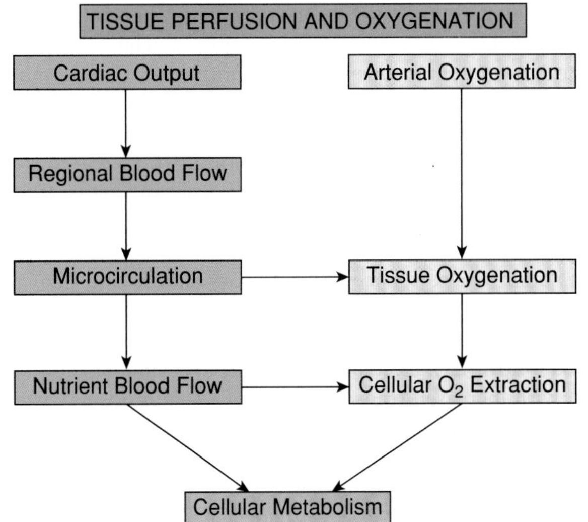

FIGURE 22.1 Tissue perfusion and oxygenation is determined by a complex interaction of systemic and regional blood flow and oxygenation, as well as by the state of the microcirculation and by cellular metabolism.

Experimental studies have shown that transcutaneous oxygen monitoring is sensitive to arterial oxygen tension (PaO_2) during normal cardiac output, but is more sensitive to perfusion in low-flow shock (6). In adult patients, $PtcO_2$ is approximately 80% of the PaO_2 during normal hemodynamic conditions. However, when blood flow is diminished, $PtcO_2$ also decreases. $PtcO_2$ is therefore related to both perfusion and oxygenation. When perfusion is normal, $PtcO_2$ varies with arterial oxygenation. When perfusion is inadequate, $PtcO_2$ varies with cardiac output. Hence, a normal $PtcO_2$ value indicates that both oxygenation and perfusion are relatively normal. A low $PtcO_2$ indicates that either oxygenation and/or cardiac output are inadequate. If arterial oxygenation is normal (as indicated by blood gases or pulse oximetry), low $PtcO_2$ indicates low-flow shock (7).

The relationship between $PtcO_2$ and PaO_2 can be quantitated, utilizing the $PtcO_2$ index, which is simply defined as $PtcO_2/PaO_2$. In a study that simultaneously measured cardiac index, $PtcO_2$, and PaO_2 in a large number of critically ill surgical patients, it was found that when cardiac output was relatively normal (cardiac index >2.2 L/min/m^2), the $PtcO_2$ index averaged 0.79 ± 0.12. In individual patients with these normal cardiac outputs, $PtcO_2$ varied linearly with PaO_2. When cardiac output decreased, however, the $PtcO_2$ index decreased as well. For patients with a cardiac index between 1.5 and 2.2 L/min/m^2, the $PtcO_2$ index averaged 0.48 ± 0.07. For patients with a cardiac index below 1.5 L/min/m^2, the $PtcO_2$ index was 0.12 ± 0.12 (7). These data confirm that when blood flow is relatively normal, $PtcO_2$ varies with arterial oxygenation. However, with low-flow shock, $PtcO_2$ becomes very sensitive to changes in cardiac output.

Clinical studies have demonstrated the usefulness of transcutaneous oxygen monitoring in detecting shock. When $PtcO_2$ monitors are placed during acute emergency resuscitation, low $PtcO_2$ values detect both hypoxemia and hemorrhagic shock. Moreover, the response of $PtcO_2$ during fluid infusion is a sensitive indicator of the efficacy of shock resuscitation (8,9).

Transcutaneous oxygen monitoring thus has benefit both as an early detector of shock and as a monitor to titrate resuscitation to a physiologic end point. It is noninvasive and inexpensive, and is therefore widely applicable for patients at risk, such as during emergency resuscitation of trauma and acute surgical emergencies, in the perioperative and postanesthesia period, and in the intensive care unit (ICU). However, while end points of successful resuscitation utilizing transcutaneous oxygen monitoring have been suggested, such values have not been validated in large prospective studies.

Tissue Oxygen Monitors

In addition to transcutaneous oxygen probes, alternative direct tissue oxygen monitoring techniques have been developed. An advantage of such tissue probes is that heating of the skin is not necessary. In addition, specific tissues can be monitored to provide organ-specific information. Probes may be placed into the subcutaneous tissue, which is very sensitive to low flow. They may also be placed into muscle, which is perhaps less sensitive to low flow, but more rapidly responsive to resuscitation. Probes may also be placed directly into organs. For example, specific probes are now available for placement in the brain to provide a measure of cerebral oxygenation.

Two techniques for direct tissue oxygen monitoring are available. Polarographic electrodes incorporated into needles have been most widely utilized. In addition, a technique utilizing the phenomenon of fluorescence quenching is available. Tissue oxygen probes contain a fluorescent compound that is O_2 sensitive, such that its fluorescent emission is diminished in direct proportion to the amount of O_2 present. Energy from the monitor is transmitted through fiberoptic elements to the florescent compound in the probe, resulting in the emission of light, which is then measured by sensors in the tissue probe. The intensity of the emitted light is inversely proportional to the tissue pO_2 (10).

Another method of tissue oxygen monitoring is transconjunctival. The conjunctiva of the eye does not have a stratum corneum, so oxygen is freely diffusible. Transconjunctival probes are placed against the eye, and allow continuous tissue oxygen monitoring without heating; the technology has been utilized both during anesthesia and shock (11).

Direct tissue oxygen monitoring devices offer alternatives to transcutaneous monitoring, with the potential advantages of more rapid initial readings, a variety of monitoring sites, and no heating necessary. However, there are little clinical data to determine the relative sensitivities and specificities of these various techniques.

Near-Infrared Spectroscopy

Near-infrared spectroscopy (NIRS) has been developed as a noninvasive measure of tissue oxygenation (12–15). NIRS measures the ratio of oxygenated hemoglobin to total hemoglobin (StO_2) in the microcirculation of the underlying muscle by measuring the absorption and reflectance of light. Using cutaneous probes placed upon the thenar eminence, values of 87% ± 6% have been measured in normal volunteers. Early clinical experience suggests that StO_2 values decrease during shock and increase with successful resuscitation. A recent multicenter trial in trauma patients suggested that a StO_2 value of 75% may be a therapeutic goal. This monitoring approach has potential value, as it provides convenient, continuous, noninvasive measurements. However, clinical data are limited. Tissue edema may be a confounding factor, as the distance between the probe and the underlying muscle affects measurements. Again, the sensitivity and specificity of this device compared to other tissue oxygen monitoring devices has not been studied. NIRS has been demonstrated to have a close relationship to base deficit in critically injured patients (15) as well as predicting development of organ failure in traumatic shock patients (16).

Gastric Tonometry

The mesenteric circulatory bed, particularly the gut mucosa, is prone to hypoperfusion and ischemia during shock. Tonometry has been developed as a technique to detect adequacy of gastrointestinal mucosal perfusion (17). The technique is based upon calculation of the gastrointestinal intramucosal pH (pHi). The basis of this measurement is that the gastrointestinal mucosal pCO_2 equilibrates with the gastric luminal pCO_2. Measurement of luminal pCO_2 was originally accomplished by placing a tube with an attached balloon into the stomach, allowing time for the CO_2 to diffuse; measuring pCO_2 in the balloon, assuming that luminal pCO_2 equals mucosal pCO_2; and then calculating pHi by the Henderson–Hasselbalch equation as follows:

$$\text{pHi} = 6.1 + \log(\text{HCO}_3^-) / (\text{pCO}_2) \times 0.031$$

Gastric pHi monitoring has recently been improved by utilizing gas tonometry without the need for balloons, utilizing capnography. This improvement decreases the lag time necessary for equilibration of carbon dioxide, and allows for more continuous measurements.

The potential usefulness of gastric tonometry has been suggested in clinical studies, in which pHi has been reported to reflect the severity of shock and to increase during successful resuscitation (17). However, the technique has not gained widespread acceptance, in part because the accuracy of the pHi measurement has been questioned. Utilization of arterial bicarbonate as an estimate of mucosal bicarbonate concentrations may be inaccurate. Measurements can also be altered by gastric acid secretion, because buffering of gastric acid by bicarbonate can produce CO_2 in the gastric lumen, which will confound the estimate of mucosal pCO_2. Enteral feeding may also affect pHi, although this effect is variable. To minimize these errors, it has been suggested that gastric feeding be withheld and antacid medication given prior to pHi monitoring. However, the variation and inaccuracies of gastric tonometry have limited its widespread application. Moreover, clear treatment end points have not been validated.

Several alternatives to gastric tonometry have been studied. Sublingual capnography is a less invasive technique, which shows promise as a sensitive indicator of tissue acidosis in shock models and in early clinical reports (18). This device was recalled in 2004 for infectious complications and may be reinstated in the future. Alternative luminal monitoring sites, such as the small intestine, rectum, and bladder, have also been proposed as monitoring sites for pHi monitoring (19).

Transcutaneous and End-Tidal Carbon Dioxide

Transcutaneous carbon dioxide may be measured using the Severinghaus carbon dioxide electrode. Because CO_2 is more diffusible than is O_2, heating of the probe is not necessary. In analogy with $PtcO_2$ monitoring, transcutaneous CO_2 parallels arterial values when cardiac output is relatively normal, although transcutaneous values are normally 10 to 30 mmHg higher than arterial. During low-flow shock, transcutaneous pCO_2 is increased, due to accumulation of carbon dioxide in the tissues due to inadequate perfusion (20). Increased transcutaneous pCO_2 may thus be utilized as an indicator of inadequate circulation, particularly if arterial pCO_2 is normal. In combination with low $PtcO_2$, increased transcutaneous pCO_2 gives additional evidence of circulatory shock. End-tidal CO_2 may also be utilized as a measure of perfusion; end-tidal CO_2 is decreased during low-flow states due to decreased pulmonary flow (21). Decreased end-tidal CO_2 values in combination with increased transcutaneous pCO_2 and normal arterial pCO_2 values are strong evidence of circulatory shock. This is an example of how combining noninvasive monitoring data can provide additional information.

TISSUE BLOOD FLOW

Measuring tissue blood flow can provide an indication of the adequacy of both cardiac output and regional blood flow. In critical illness, blood flow measurement has the particular potential to be combined with tissue oxygen monitoring to help determine if inadequate tissue oxygenation is due to perfusion deficits. Hence, a reliable tissue perfusion monitor has great appeal.

Many technologies have been developed to measure tissue perfusion. The best studied of these is laser Doppler. Laser Doppler utilizes analysis of scattering of light to determine quantitative blood flow in a small area around the probe (22). A variety of probes have been developed, which can be placed noninvasively onto the skin, or into tissues with needle probes. Laser Doppler measurements have been shown to be useful in detecting changes in blood flow under many experimental conditions. However, clinical utility has been limited due to the large variation in blood flow within tissues (23). Because of these variations, no normal values, no optimal values, and no therapeutic goal values for blood flow have been determined.

Numerous alternative approaches to monitoring tissue perfusion have also been developed. Measurement of local blood flow by thermal diffusion has been developed as an alternative to light scattering, and implantable probes using this technology are available. In addition, magnetic resonance imaging, positron emission tomography, and contrast-enhanced ultrasonography have been used to measure tissue perfusion, although these are not available as continuous monitoring devices. Videomicroscopy techniques such as fluorescence microangiography, orthogonal polarization spectral imaging, and sidestream dark field imaging can provide both visual imaging of the microcirculation and measurements of local blood flow (24–26). As with laser Doppler monitoring, validated clinical applications for these technologies have yet to be defined.

The Oxygen Challenge Test

An approach to utilize tissue oxygen monitoring in a more dynamic manner was proposed by Dr. Hunt's group in San Francisco (27,28). Endeavoring to assess adequacy of tissue

TABLE 22.1 Oxygen Challenge Test (29–31)

1. Select patients who have baseline arterial O_2 saturation over 90% on FiO_2 less than 0.6–0.8.
2. Obtain baseline transcutaneous (or tissue) pO_2 value.
3. Increase FiO_2 to 1.0.
4. After 5 min, repeat transcutaneous (or tissue) pO_2 measurement.
5. If transcutaneous (or tissue) pO_2 increases greater than 20–25 torr, patient can be assumed to have no flow-dependent oxygen consumption.
6. If transcutaneous (or tissue) pO_2 increases less than 20 torr, provide therapy to increase oxygen delivery until step 5 is met.

perfusion in postoperative patients, they measured subcutaneous pO_2 before and after patients breathed high-inspired O_2 concentrations. The expected response in well-perfused patients was a rapid increase in tissue pO_2. Many postoperative patients failed to demonstrate this response, which was, however, restored with intravenous fluid infusion. A physiologic explanation for the responses of tissue pO_2 to inspired O_2 is interesting. If there is no cellular O_2 deficit, then additional dissolved O_2 supplied after breathing O_2 is not required nor utilized by cells, and therefore results in increased tissue pO_2. However, if there is a cellular O_2 deficit (shock), then any additional dissolved O_2 would be rapidly utilized, and would thus not result in increased tissue pO_2. The tissue pO_2 response to inspired O_2 may then be a relatively rapid and minimally invasive method to detect cellular hypoxia. This approach, named the O_2 challenge test, was evaluated in trauma patients (29–31) (Table 22.1). The O_2 challenge test had 100% sensitivity and specificity in detecting flow-dependent O_2 consumption in invasively monitored patients in the ICU. It also appeared to be a very sensitive indicator of shock during acute resuscitation. This method, utilizing either transcutaneous or direct tissue O_2 monitors, has potential to detect which patients require fluid resuscitation, to provide a physiologic end point for resuscitation, and to detect the patients in whom initial resuscitation is inadequate and who therefore require additional monitoring and therapy. Using a noninvasive transcutaneous ($PtcO_2$) monitor, Yu et al. have studied the O_2 challenge test in patients in the ICU and have validated the sensitivity and specificity of the test in identifying patients in occult shock. In addition, their data have defined an increase in $PtcO_2$ of greater than 20 to 25 mmHg in response to a FiO_2 of 1.0 as a therapeutic end point (30,31). In a prospective randomized trial using the oxygen challenge test as an end point of resuscitation compared to the DO_2 variables from the pulmonary artery catheter, an improved survival was reported (31). Monitoring and treating the peripheral tissue oxygenation state does not exclude utilization of central hemodynamic parameters such as cardiac output and DO_2, but does allow manipulation of DO_2 to reach a specific goal of tissue perfusion rather than aiming for a general DO_2 value.

SUMMARY

Monitoring tissue perfusion and oxygenation provides important physiologic information. Increasing interest and use of noninvasive monitoring systems continue to demonstrate utility in the detection and treatment of shock. Great potential exists to develop these devices, which will provide sensitive and specific indications both of the severity of shock and end points for resuscitation. Such systems would provide a minimally invasive approach to improve the treatment of shock. To achieve acceptance and application of such systems will require quality clinical studies to determine and validate optimal treatment goals.

Key Points

- In addition to arterial oxygen saturation, pulse oximetry–derived measurements can provide noninvasive estimates of tissue perfusion and total hemoglobin. Low values of peripheral pulse index are associated with increased illness severity and mortality.
- A decreased transcutaneous oxygen value may be an early warning of decreased arterial oxygenation, decreased hemoglobin, or decreased cardiac output.
- The ratio of transcutaneous oxygen to arterial oxygen may be utilized as an end point of resuscitation, with a goal of 0.8.
- NIRS devices placed on the thenar eminence provide a measure of tissue oxygenation, with a normal value of 87% ± 6% saturation. Values less than 75% may indicate shock.
- Increased transcutaneous pCO_2 is an indicator of tissue acidosis.
- The presence of decreased end-tidal pCO_2 in the face of normal arterial pCO_2 is an indicator of low cardiac output.
- The response of transcutaneous or tissue oxygen monitors to an increased FiO_2 is an indication of the presence or absence of flow-dependent oxygen consumption. An increase in tissue oxygen of greater than 25 torr may be utilized as an end point of resuscitation.

References

1. Lima AP, Beelen P, Bakker J. Use of a peripheral perfusion index derived from the pulse oximetry signal as a noninvasive indicator of perfusion. *Crit Care Med.* 2002;30:1210–1213.
2. De Felice C, Latini G, Vacca P, Kopotic RJ. The pulse oximeter perfusion index as a predictor for high illness severity in neonates. *Eur J Pediatr.* 2002;161:561–562.
3. van Genderen ME, Lima A, Akkerhuis M, et al. Persistent peripheral and microcirculatory perfusion alterations after out-of-hospital cardiac arrest are associated with poor survival. *Crit Care Med.* 2012;40:2287–2294.
4. He H, Liu D, Long Y, Wang X. The peripheral perfusion index and transcutaneous oxygen challenge test are predictive of mortality in septic patients after resuscitation. *Critical Care.* 2013;17:R116.
5. Clark LC. Measurement of oxygen tension: a historical perspective. *Crit Care Med.* 1981;9:694–702.
6. Tremper KK, Waxman K, Shoemaker WC. Effects of hypoxia and shock on transcutaneous pO_2 values in dogs. *Crit Care Med.* 1979;7:526–531.
7. Tremper KK, Shoemaker WC. Transcutaneous oxygen monitoring of critically ill adults, with and without low flow shock. *Crit Care Med.* 1981;9:706–711.
8. Waxman K, Sadler R, Eisner M, et al. Transcutaneous oxygen monitoring of emergency department patients. *Am J Surg.* 1983;146:35–38.
9. Tatevossian RG, Wo CCJ, Velmahos GC, et al. Transcutaneous oxygen and CO_2 as early warning of tissue hypoxia and hemodynamic shock in critically ill emergency patients. *Crit Care Med.* 2000;28:2248–2253.
10. Shaw AD, Zheng L, Thomas Z, et al. Assessment of tissue oxygen tension: comparison of dynamic fluorescence quenching and polarographic electrode technique. *Crit Care.* 2002;6:76–80.
11. Abraham E, Smith M, Silver S. Conjunctival and transcutaneous monitoring during cardiopulmonary arrest and cardiopulmonary resuscitation. *Crit Care Med.* 1984;12:419–423.

12. Beilman GJ, Groehler KE, Lazaron V, et al. Near-infrared spectroscopy measurement of regional tissue oxyhemoglobin saturation during hemorrhagic shock. *Shock*. 1999;12:196–200.
13. Taylor JH, Mulier KE, Myers DE, et al. Use of near-infrared spectroscopy in early determination of irreversible hemorrhagic shock. *J Trauma*. 2005;58:1119–1125.
14. Crooks BA, Cohn SM, Bloch S. Can near-infrared spectroscopy identify the severity of shock in trauma patients. *J Trauma*. 2005;58:806–813.
15. Ikossi DG, Knudson MM, Morabito DJ, et al. Continuous muscle tissue oxygenation in critically injured patients: a prospective observational study. *J Trauma Injury Infect Crit Care*. 2006;61:780–790.
16. Cohn SM, Nathens AB, Moore FA, et al. Tissue oxygenation saturation predicts the development of organ dysfunction during traumatic shock resuscitation. *J Trauma*. 2007;62:44–55.
17. Guzman JA, Kruse JA. Continuous assessment of gastric intramucosal pCO_2 and pH in hemorrhagic shock using capnometric recirculating gas tonometry. *Crit Care Med*. 1997;25:533–537.
18. Creteur J. Gastric and sublingual capnometry. *Curr Opin Crit Care*. 2006; 12:272–277.
19. Walley KR, Friesen BP, Humer MF, et al. Small bowel tonometry is more accurate than gastric tonometry in detecting gut ischemia. *J Appl Physiol*. 1998;85:1770–1777.
20. Tremper KK, Waxman K. Transcutaneous monitoring of respiratory gases. In: Nochomovitz M, Cherniack NS, eds. *Non-Invasive Respiratory Monitoring*. New York: Churchill Livingstone; 1985:1–28.
21. Falk JL, Rackow EC, Weil MH. End-tidal carbon dioxide concentration during cardiopulmonary resuscitation. *N Engl J Med*. 1988;318:607–611.
22. Johnson JM, Taylor WF, Shepherd AP, et al. Laser-Doppler measurement of skin blood flow: comparison with plethysmography. *J Appl Physiol*. 1984;56:798–803.
23. Chang N, Goodson WH, Gottrup F, et al. Direct measurement of wound and tissue oxygen tension in postoperative patients. *Ann Surg*. 1983;197:470–478.
24. Waxman K, Formosa P, Soliman H. Laser Doppler velocimetry in critically ill patients. *Crit Care Med*. 1987;15:780–783.
25. Mcveigh ER. Emerging imaging techniques. *Circ Res*. 2006;14:879–886.
26. Eriksson S, Nilsson J, Sturesson C. Non-invasive imaging of microcirculation: a technology review. *Med Devices (Auckl)*. 2014;7:445–452.
27. Littooy F, Fuchs R, Hunt TK, Sheldon GF. Tissue oxygen as a real-time measure of oxygen transport. *J Surg Res*. 1976;20:321–325.
28. Jonsson K, Jensen AJ, Goodson WH, et al. Assessment of perfusion in postoperative patients using tissue oxygen measurements. *Br J Surg*. 1987;74: 263–267.
29. Waxman K, Annas C, Daughters K, et al. A method to determine the adequacy of resuscitation using tissue oxygen monitoring. *J Trauma*. 1994;36:852–858.
30. Yu M, Morita SY, Daniel SR, et al. Transcutaneous pressure of oxygen: a non-invasive and early detector of peripheral shock and outcome. *Shock*. 2006;26:450–456.
31. Yu M, Chapital A, Ho HC, et al. A prospective randomized trial comparing oxygen delivery versus transcutaneous pressure of oxygen values as resuscitative goals. *Shock*. 2007;27:615–622.

CHAPTER
23
Pulse Oximetry, Plethysmography, Capnography, and Respiratory Monitoring

S. MARK POLER

INTRODUCTION

Pulse oximetry and capnography are mainstays of physiologic monitoring, evaluating oxyhemoglobin saturation as a proxy for tissue availability of oxygen, and concentration of carbon dioxide being eliminated, respectively. Both technologies can provide additional information to the sophisticated clinician, as analysis of the shape and characteristics of continuous waveforms shows changing physiologic information. This large literature can only be superficially represented in the space of this general chapter. Ehrenfeld and Cannesson (1) have recently produced *Monitoring Technologies in Acute Care Environments*, an excellent resource for these and other monitoring technologies relevant to critical care.

Oxygen provides the essential metabolic oxidizer that must flow down a partial pressure gradient from alveolar gas to end-organ tissue. As the quantity of dissolved O_2 in blood is small relative to the quantity of the gas bound to hemoglobin, O_2 even at high partial pressures decreases rapidly to less than 100 torr as it diffuses from blood to tissue. This physiology must be kept in mind, even though not directly observed, for the oximetric assessment of hemoglobin in precapillary blood, this being where gas exchange with tissue occurs. In the reverse direction, the primary metabolic waste product, CO_2, must have a partial pressure gradient from tissue to exhaled gas in order to be eliminated at the rate of production; this is typically from a venous tension of about 46 torr to a normal of 40 torr in arterial blood (or equilibrated alveolar gas) (2).

Pulse oximetry is a ubiquitous *de facto* standard of care in ambulatory and inpatient facilities, emergency medical services (EMS), and low- and high-acuity patient care. Quickly and noninvasively obtaining oxygen saturation by pulse oximetry is often the first step in the decision-making process of caring for a patient. Continuous monitoring can detect acute or long-term deterioration of delivery of O_2 (DO_2) to tissue. It provides a measure of the essential supply of O_2 for oxidative metabolism, and can provide insight into pulmonary and cardiovascular function, metabolism, and dyshemoglobinemias. While conceptually convenient that the saturation of hemoglobin typically reaches 100% near a PaO_2 of 100 torr (2), this also exposes one of the principal shortcomings of pulse oximetry. Above about 100 torr, the increase of PaO_2 is not accompanied by a proportional increase in saturation. Below 100 torr, the nonlinearity of the sigmoid oxygen–hemoglobin binding relationship confounds easy conversion of saturation to the PaO_2 that provides the driving gradient for diffusion of O_2 into tissue and intracellular mitochondria. So, large changes in PaO_2 in blood do not have a simple relationship to hemoglobin saturation.

Until recently, tissue and mitochondrial PO_2 could not be easily assessed in clinical settings, except where tissue surfaces were accessible. These limitations are yielding to near-infrared spectroscopy (NIRS), new applications of pulse oximetry and, now, mitochondrial oximetry. Formerly tissue and mitochondrial PO_2 (PmO_2) tension could not be easily characterized because of technological limitations, though it was understood that at PmO_2 below 2 torr, oxidative metabolism is impaired, becoming anaerobic below 1 torr (3). More recently, methods including positron emission tomography (PET) and magnetic resonance imaging (MRI) have provided surveys of PO_2 in various tissues, and are largely consistent with the earlier data (4). These newer technologies are yielding new data dramatically changing the assessment of PO_2 sensitivity of oxidative metabolism in mitochondria at the end of the O_2 delivery pathway. Both O_2 tension and consumption can be characterized by O_2-dependent quenching of protoporphyrin fluorescence. This technique reports typical PmO_2 of 50–60 torr, and reveals metabolic adaptation below 70 torr (5). An endotoxin-induced model of sepsis in rats reports PmO_2 near 60 torr initially, decreasing to as low as 30 torr without fluid resuscitation (6).

Capnography assesses the elimination of CO_2, the principle end-product of oxidative metabolism (water not needing to be eliminated). While providing a snapshot of the steady elimination of CO_2 via the lungs, the shape of the capnogram can provide insight into the mechanics of ventilation, matching of cardiovascular and pulmonary function to metabolism. Attention to the ratio of partial pressures and content of O_2 and CO_2 in blood and exhaled gases contribute to evaluation of lung function or injury. Capnography and other monitors of respiratory function will be discussed in the second part of this chapter.

PULSE OXIMETRY

In 1864, Stokes (7) reported that the colored substance in blood carries oxygen. Hoppe-Seyler (8) subsequently crystallized and named hemoglobin, showing that the pattern of light absorption changed when shaken with air. Remarkably, in 1875, Paul Bert (9) recognized the cause of death for high-altitude balloonists to be low PaO_2, and during World War I hypoxia was recognized as cause of death for pilots flying to high altitudes, which became a much more compelling problem during World War II (10). Severinghaus (10) has written a fascinating historical review of oxygen and respiratory physiology, relating developments including pulse oximetry.

In 1937, Hertzman (11) described photoelectric plethysmography of fingers and toes to dynamically assess peripheral circulation. The device employed a beam from a headlight bulb through a finger or toe, then measured, by a shielded photoemissive photoelectric cell, employed in radios of that time. Measurement conditions were difficult, the photoelectric oscillations of variable blood content being amplified and recorded by a string galvanometer or oscillograph. Movement had to be minimized with a comfortable saddle or sling, and muscle relaxation was necessary. This method was also used through the nasal septum and results compared to digits.

In 1940, Squire (12) described a method to compute O_2 saturation employing red and infrared light passing through perfused and blanched tissue. Shortly thereafter, in 1941, Millikan and colleagues (13) coined the term *oximeter* and described a method for the continuous measurement of arterial saturation. A shell over the ear contained green and red light paths, absorption of green being proportional to total hemoglobin and red being proportional to oxygenated hemoglobin. Construction of a calibration curve allowed estimation of arterial O_2 saturation, having an accuracy of 5% in the top half of its range and 8% in the bottom half. In 1942, Goldie (14) reported another device continuously measuring oxygen saturation.

The winds of war accelerated development of oximetry during and after World War II. Prior instruments were required to be preset to known arterial saturation values, and could not be conveniently used in patients who had arterial hypoxia, nor could they be used for the actual determination of arterial O_2 saturation. Rather, these older devices could only be used for qualitative changes in saturation. Until the advent of semiconductors (transistors and LEDs), the goal of portable oximetry for high-altitude aviators was unattainable (10). As a result of these shortcomings, Wood and Geraci (15) improved on Millikan's design, incorporating a pressure capsule in a shell to blanch the pinna for calibration, developing a device that could continuously read the absolute value of arterial O_2 saturation from a pickup unit attached to the pinna of the human ear. This new design consisted of a photoelectric earpiece that allowed simultaneous measurement of the transmission of red and near-infrared light through either the normal heat-flushed ear or the bloodless ear. The difference distinguished the absorption by blood from other tissue, deriving percentage O_2 saturation; this device saw use only in clinical laboratories.

In 1963, Shaw developed an eight-wavelength ear oximeter; marketing it in 1970, it was expensive, large, and heavy, and had very limited sales (10). Subsequently in 1972, Aoyagi (16), in Japan, began work building on the theories and success of the Wood oximeter and employing the observations of Squire previously noted (10), creating a dye densitometry method in which two wavelengths of light were used; the ratio of the two optical densities was calculated to obtain a dye curve. This curve was expected to correspond to dye concentrations in blood. It was during this series of experiments that the importance of the pulsatile variations was first reported. After investigating the effect of this pulsatile component, using mathematical analysis of the Beer–Lambert law, it was concluded that calculating the ratio of two optical densities compensates for the pulsations; it was at this point that Aoyagi derived three main conclusions:

1. If the optical density of the pulsating portion is measured at two appropriate wavelengths and the ratio of the optical densities is obtained, the result must be equivalent to Wood's ratio.
2. With this method, arterial blood is selectively measured, and the venous blood does not affect the measurement. Therefore, the probe site is not restricted to the ear.
3. With this method, the reference for optical density calculation is set for each pulse. Therefore, an accidental shift of probe location introduces a short artifact and quick return to normal measurements.

By 1975, Aoyagi had developed a technique very similar to modern-day pulse oximeters. Two wavelengths of light, 630 and 900 nm, were chosen. From the transmitted light intensity data, the pulsation amplitude (AC) and the total intensity (DC) were obtained, and the ratio, AC/DC, was calculated. This ratio was obtained at both wavelengths of light to create a ratio of ratios that corresponded to SaO_2.

In 1980, Minolta (16) developed OXIMET using two optical fibers and precision optics. They adopted the finger as the probe site and proved that pulse oximetry was accurate. Nellcor introduced the N-100 in 1983, employing high-performance light-emitting diodes (LEDs), a sensitive and accurate photodiode, and a microcomputer. These technologic advances, development of monitoring standards in anesthesiology, and a coincident malpractice insurance crisis, led to the widespread clinical adoption of pulse oximeters in the 1980s, without benefit of a foundation in clinical effectiveness research. After such widespread adoption, it has been considered unethical to perform randomized control trials (RCT) necessary to document clinical effectiveness of the now ubiquitous technology.

As pulse oximeters have continued to improve, active research is being conducted in several key areas:

- Accuracy as it relates to optimum alarm-level setting
- A quick response time to desaturation, and auditory signal modulation to improve detection of change by clinicians (17,18)
- Ameliorating plethysmography and oximetry performance with poor tissue perfusion
- Eliminating motion artifact (16)
- Determination of hemoglobin concentrations noninvasively (see below)
- Photoplethysmographic assessment of cardiovascular volume status and cardiorespiratory balance
- Monitoring for respiratory depression during spontaneous breathing.

Theory

Oximetry is based on the Beer–Lambert law of optical wavelength-dependent absorption of light energy. Light intensity (*I*) decreases exponentially in proportion to a wavelength-dependent absorption coefficient (*a*), the concentration (*C*) of the absorbing substance, and the length (*L*) of the light pathway:

$$I = I_o e^{-aLC} \quad [1]$$

Rearranging the equation to employ the measured ratio of transmitted to incident light, we can define absorbance (*A*) as:

$$A = -\ln (I / I_o) = aLC \quad [2]$$

The absorption coefficient (*a*) is unique value for each wavelength and substance of interest. Oxygenated and reduced hemoglobins have different absorption coefficients across a spectrum of wavelengths, shown in Figure 23.1.

If we define C_o as the relative concentration of oxygenated hemoglobin (compared to the total amount of hemoglobin) and C_r as the relative concentration of reduced hemoglobin,

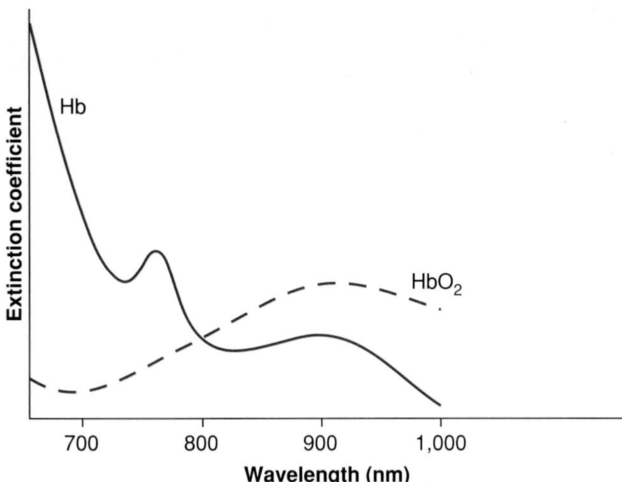

FIGURE 23.1 Absorption versus wavelength changes for oxygenated hemoglobin (HbO_2) and reduced hemoglobin (Hb).

we can then define the total absorbance of light at a given wavelength as:

$$A = \mathrm{WL}\,(a_o C_o + a_r C_r) \quad [3]$$

where W is the weight of hemoglobin per unit volume. Note that $C_o + C = 1.0$.

In Figure 23.1, it is seen that at a wavelength of 805 nm, the coefficient for oxygenated hemoglobin (a_o) and reduced hemoglobin (a_r) are the same, a unique instance enabling determination of total hemoglobin (oxygenated and reduced) in the light path. A measurement at this wavelength will give us a value for WL:

$$\mathrm{WL} = A_{805} \,/\, a_{805} \quad [4]$$

If we now measure at any other wavelength where a_r and a_o are not equal, we can exploit the ratio to eliminate WL and determine the relative concentration of oxygenated hemoglobin (C_o):

$$C_o = \frac{a_{805}}{a_o - a_r}\frac{A}{A_{805}} - \frac{a_r}{a_o - a_r} \quad [5]$$

All the absorption coefficients a are constants that depend on the physical media and wavelength. We can thus group those together and rewrite this equation as:

$$C_o = x\frac{A}{A_{805}} + y \quad [6]$$

This shows that we can measure the relative concentration of oxygenated hemoglobin by looking at the ratio of the absorbance (which we can measure) and adjusting with some known constants.

In a laboratory instrument we can have tight control of path length (a cuvette) and wavelength (a laser at 805 nm); these conditions are not possible for biologic or clinical application. For example, if we use a finger as our measurement compartment, Eq. [2] will generally hold, but we need to add the absorption of other finger tissues:

$$A_{\text{total}} = A_{\text{arterial}} + A_{\text{venous}} + A_{\text{other tissues}} \quad [7]$$

Since we are only interested in A_{arterial}, the other absorbance values need to be eliminated. This can be done by taking the time derivative of A_{total}. The volume of the tissue and venous components can be treated as constants since they do not vary nearly as much as arterial pulsations, so the time derivative of the venous and tissue components will be about zero. The pulsatile part of A_{total} is the arterial component with a nonzero time derivative. Hence the name "pulse" oximetry: It analyzes only the pulsatile portion of the absorbance.

When using a finger sensor, specific wavelengths are selected; LEDs emit light at specific wavelengths, 660 nm (red light) and 910 nm (infrared light), and have been employed for pulse oximetry. Other similar wavelengths can be chosen for particular designs (19). We can then define a ratio, R, as the ratio of the derivative of absorbances at two different wavelengths:

$$R = \frac{dA_1 \,/\, dt}{dA_2 \,/\, dt} \quad [8]$$

Applying similar logic as in the 805 nm case, we can derive an equation for C_o:

$$C_o = \frac{k_1 + k_2 R}{k_3 + k_4 R} \quad [9]$$

where constants k are a combination of the (oxygenated and reduced) absorption coefficients a at the two wavelengths. While these coefficients are only dependent on the physical optical properties of hemoglobin, in practice, the constants k in Eq. [9] are determined empirically by pulse oximeter manufacturers, and are generally unpublished. Simpler (19) and more exact (20) derivations are available.

PERFUSION INDEX

Perfusion index (PI), or peripheral flow index (PFI), is a simple ratio of the varying to the nonvarying absorbance in the infrared, since it is minimally affected by changes in oxyhemoglobin saturation affecting the red absorption. Conceptually, it is analogous to alternating (AC) and direct (DC) electrical currents, represented as a ratio (or as percentage, × 100):

$$\mathrm{PI} = (\mathrm{AC/DC})$$

PI changes with variation in peripheral perfusion. Relative change for an individual is useful, but variation between individuals can be considerable (19,21).

REASONS FOR ERRORS

Pulse oximetry fundamentally relies upon adequate perfusion of the vascular bed being monitored. Without a sufficient pulsatile signal, O_2 content cannot be adequately analyzed. Decreased perfusion may be caused by a variety of factors including hypotension, medications, ambient temperature, poor circulation, and so forth. Clinicians will often search multiple fingers, toes, and earlobes for a site that can provide a saturation value. Decreased perfusion, leading to the inability of the pulse oximeter to provide a saturation value, is very common. While central site probes may never be ubiquitous, their utility in patients with poor peripheral perfusion cannot be overstated. Since these central sites reflect carotid artery flow, they will rarely experience errors due to poor perfusion of the vascular bed. Sometimes even rotation of a pulse oximeter probe by 45 or 90 degrees on a digit can generate a usable signal that was otherwise inadequate.

Pulse oximeters are calibrated using saturation curves of healthy adult volunteers. They are, therefore, most accurate at high saturation levels and less so at low saturation levels (22,23). Unfortunately, from the clinical standpoint, low saturations pose the greatest dangers. Nonetheless, this is rarely of major consequence, as the clinical difference between a saturation of 83% and 80% is probably minimal. The utility of oximetry at low saturation is principally for rapid assessment of the direction of change with therapeutic interventions.

It is clinically important to be able to detect rapid hemoglobin desaturation with minimal delay. There is often, regrettably, a delay in numerical display of saturation due to the default moving average-calculated SpO_2 set by device manufacturers. However, many pulse oximeters annunciate a tone associated with saturation of each pulsation which audibly decreases even with small changes in saturation. That tone can be the clinician's earliest warning of deterioration of oxygenation (17,18). The delayed response time problem for pulse oximetry–detected desaturations can be partially overcome by reducing the user selectable averaging setting to the shortest duration, usually 2 seconds (24). However, because of an increased likelihood of false alarms and artifact, this is seldom done clinically. To overcome the problem of delayed response time, it is necessary to develop processing algorithms sensitive enough to detect changes quickly, while allowing for artifact rejection and avoiding false alarms, an area of active research.

Other sources of error have been explored by Trivedi and colleagues (25). The researchers looked at very common sources of error, including ambient light and motion artifact. Error rates with excess ambient light were as high as 63% for heart rate and 57% for saturation. For motion artifact, simulated with 2-Hz and 4-Hz tremors, all tested pulse oximeters showed clinically significant error rates in saturation with both movement artifact rates. Error rates were low in the 2-Hz motion for heart rate calculations; however, all devices failed at 4-Hz motion. Other investigators have also reported on the errors and false alarms associated with movement artifact (26–29). Additional sources of error include darkly pigmented skin (30,31), nail polish (32), thermal injuries to fingers and/or toes, and inaccessibility of the extremities. While unconventional, sometimes simply rotating application of a pulse oximeter probe on the axis of a finger or toe can improve signal and performance by changing the light path, though some report this maneuver is ineffective (32).

Another very common problem encountered is the lack of compatibility between probes and devices of the various manufacturers. van Oostrom and Melker (33) compared the accuracy of nonproprietary probes designed for use with a variety of pulse oximeters with that of their corresponding proprietary probes. A controlled signal was used on the Human Patient Simulator to simulate apnea. Statistical significance was not found in most of the comparisons, but in some instances the proprietary probes were closer to arterial oxygen than the nonproprietary probes. Thus, whether or not the manufacturer of the probe is the same as the manufacturer of the pulse oximeter may have importance. Table 23.1 summarizes the various reasons for errors (34).

TABLE 23.1 Reasons for Artifactual Measurement in Pulse Oximetry

Volume Artifacts	
Motion	Causes blood volume changes at the measurement site, resulting in difficulties calculating the saturation (35,36)
Low perfusion	Vasoconstriction, an inflated blood pressure cuff, etc., will cause the pulsatile portion of the plethysmogram to be small, causing difficulties calculating saturation (25)
Noise	
Light interference	Caused by other light sources, such as fluorescent lights, and other ambient light sources (25)
Electrical interference	Powerful radio-frequency signals can cause voltage fluctuations on the detector signal from the pulse oximeter probe (37)
Patient-related Interference	
Presence of carboxyhemoglobin and/or methemoglobin in blood	Will cause inaccurate calculation of saturation (38)
Dyes present in blood	Depending on the dye, inaccurate saturation calculation will result (39)
Skin pigmentation	Will cause a filtering of the light emitted by the pulse oximeter probe, and cause inaccurate saturation calculations (40)

As can be seen from Eq. [2], the intensity of light measured at the detector varies by path-length changes caused by the arterial pulsations. All other parameters in the equation are constant (at least within several minutes). Path-length changes are caused by volume changes at the sensor site, and for this reason, volume artifacts are a frequent problem. Other errors can be caused by light interference from sources outside of the measurement system or electrical interference, and will typically show up in the plethysmogram as additional waveform fluctuations. The effects of this noise are a distorted plethysmogram and can cause incorrect heart rates and saturations to be calculated. One last source of errors is the patient himself or herself, especially for smokers: Carboxyhemoglobin present in the blood can cause an inaccurate determination of saturation.

ALTERNATE-SITE PROBES

The standard location to measure pulse oximetry is the finger. Such probes are common and work well in many cases, but become unreliable with poor perfusion, vasoconstriction, and hypothermia. The *nasal septum* was explored as a possible monitoring site in 1937 (41). Groveman and colleagues (42) also explored the nasal septum, believing that it represents a constant picture of the internal carotid circulation and reflected cerebral flow. Cucchiara and Messick (43) showed that plethysmography from the nasal septum failed to estimate cerebral blood flow during carotid occlusion. In 1991, the nasal septum was explored during hypothermia (44). Fourteen patients were monitored every 20 minutes during major abdominal procedures. The nasal septum probe was superior to the finger probe in detecting a pulse during hypothermia. The authors concluded that monitoring at the nasal septum was more reliable than monitoring at the finger in hypothermic patients. They acknowledged several limitations, including use during nasal intubation, in patients with extremely small nostrils, or in the presence of a nasogastric tube.

Buccal probes have been evaluated as an alternative probe site. They were prepared by taping a malleable metal bar securely over the back of a disposable Nellcor finger probe and bending the metal bar and probe around the corner of a patient's mouth (45). It was determined that buccal SpO_2 was greater than finger SpO_2 and agreed more closely with SaO_2. The authors determined that buccal pulse oximetry is a viable alternative to the finger. Limitations included longer preparation time, difficult placement, and possible dislodgement during airway maneuvers.

Awad and colleagues (46) demonstrated that *the ear plethysmographic waveform* is relatively immune to vasoconstriction. They also determined that the photoplethysmographic width has a good correlation to cardiac output. They concluded that the ear is more suitable for monitoring hemodynamic changes than the finger.

Generally, any site that has an arterial bed and is thin enough to safely transmit red and infrared light through can be used for pulse oximetry. Several monitoring locations have become standard of care, including the fingers and toes. A flexible earlobe probe is also used quite frequently when the fingers and toes are inaccessible. Since finger probes work quite well for the majority of patients, it is unlikely that alternate-site probes will ever become ubiquitous. As the nasal septum, nares, cheek, and ear measure oxygenation from central sites, reflecting blood flow of the carotid arteries, their potential for measuring other physiologic parameters is only beginning to be explored.

Reflectance pulse oximetry has become available as an alternative, commonly applied to the forehead. It is less prone to motion artifact, may be less prone to errors due to poor perfusion from vasoconstriction of peripheral digits, and assesses a peripheral site derived from carotid perfusion (47). Nasal ala have also been employed as another site derived from carotid circulation (48).

OVERCOMING LIMITATIONS

Errors and interference on pulse oximetry can largely be eliminated or prevented. Volume/movement artifact can be reduced by ensuring that the measurement site is kept in place or moved slowly. Masimo (35) developed probes that use a third light source; with this additional measurement, it is possible to estimate nonarterial volume changes due to movement artifact. This allows for compensation for those artifacts and creates a more stable signal that is not as susceptible to motion artifact. Light interference can largely be eliminated by covering the measurement site through the use of a properly sized probe, or by external means such as towels or other covers. Patient-related artifacts can be reduced by fully understanding the patient's physiology, and by proper selection of the measurement site.

PHOTOPLETHYSMOGRAPHY

Photoplethysmography is the measurement of volume changes with light transmission. The photoplethysmograph (PPG) is displayed on most pulse oximeters; however, it is frequently ignored as oxygen saturation and pulse rate are the numbers of interest. There is an abundance of physiologic information that can potentially be extracted from this rarely used and noninvasively obtained signal.

Fundamentals

There are two main frequencies of variation in the value of light hitting the photodiode, and both are affected by absorption of the light by blood and various tissues. The low-frequency component (LFC)—DC or nonpulsatile component—represents the baseline amount of light hitting the detector. This value is affected by the total path traveled by the light; skin, bone, cartilage, adipose, blood, and so forth, all absorb light, and it is this relatively constant path that results in a baseline amount of light hitting the detector. This baseline amount fluctuates at a lower frequency than the heart rate. Since the biologic tissues in the path of the light are constant, with the exception of venous and arterial blood, the changes in the LFC correspond to changes in baseline blood volume in the path of the light. The majority of this baseline blood resides in the venous system.

The pulsatile cardiac component (PCC) corresponds to changes in the arterial blood volume with each heartbeat. The magnitude of change of the PCC with each heartbeat is related to stroke volume, and the area under the curve of each heartbeat is related to the volume of blood entering the vascular bed with each beat (49). The PCC is, therefore, a representation of flow into a vascular bed while the LFC is a representation of changes in venous volume (Figure 23.2A).

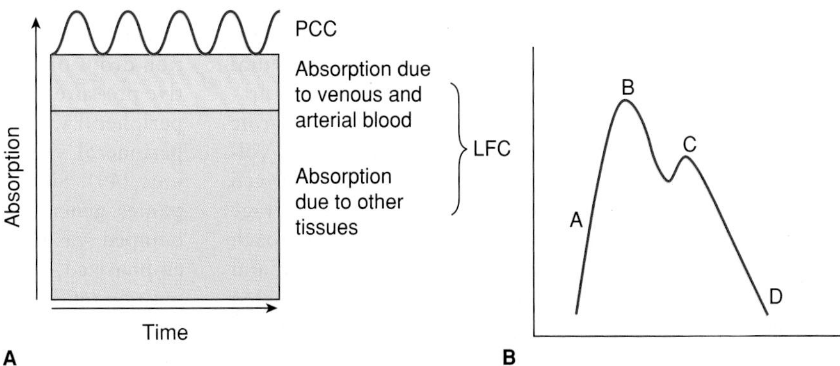

FIGURE 23.2 **A**: A graphic representation of the low-frequency component (LFC) and pulsatile cardiac component (PCC) from a typical finger probe. The PCC is typically less than 5% of the total signal acquired. **B**: A typical display of a processed pulse oximeter waveform. *A* represents the rate of maximum volume increase, *B* represents the point of maximum volume, *C* is the "dicrotic notch," and *D* is the minimal basal volume.

The typical pulse oximeter displays a processed waveform (Figure 23.2B). Since the raw data collected by the device corresponds to light hitting the photodiode, which is inversely related to blood volume, the waveform must be inverted to resemble an arterial pressure waveform. If the PPG was displayed as raw data and not inverted, point A would represent increasing light hitting the photodiode, corresponding to a decrease in blood volume, and point B would correspond to the point of maximum light hitting the photodiode, or the point of least blood in the vascular bed being monitored. Ideally, the plethysmograph would completely mimic the characteristics of an invasive arterial pressure tracing. Sometimes it comes very close. However, other factors influence the photoplethysmogram so that the waveform can be quite unlike an intra-arterial pressure. The steepness of the flow of the inflow phase A may be used as an indicator of ventricular contraction, and the amplitude of the phase may be used as an indicator of stroke volume (49). The vertical position of the dicrotic notch can be used as an indicator of vasomotor tone. Under most circumstances, the notch descends to the baseline during increasing vasodilation and climbs toward the apex with vasoconstriction (49). However, in many cases likely due to the variety of proprietary algorithms employed to process the PPG, unusual waveforms bearing little resemblance to the invasively measured arterial pressure waveform may be displayed by pulse oximeters, especially in conditions of poor peripheral perfusion (19,50,51).

Signal Processing

Prior to the advent of powerful personal computers, many researchers printed the PPG waveform and measured various parameters with a ruler; more recent efforts involve elaborate mathematical and signal processing models. Bhattacharya and colleagues (52) employed a novel concept aimed at detection of the dominant nonsinusoidal period and the extraction of the associated periodic component. This detection and extraction was performed with a moving window to accommodate the variations of the physiologic oscillations. They also characterized the system with a nonlinear dynamic system.

Most signal processing algorithms employed in pulse oximeters are proprietary and unpublished. The reasons and implications have been vigorously debated (51,53,54). Goldman and colleagues (35) from the Masimo Corporation published a detailed description of their signal extraction for error reduction. Masimo Signal Extraction Technology (SET) uses a new conceptual model of light absorption for pulse oximetry and employs discrete saturation transformed to isolate individual saturation components in the optical pathway. Johansson (55) processed the PPG signal using a 16th-order bandpass Bessel filter and a 5th-order bandpass Butterworth filter; a neural network analysis was then performed to determine respiratory rate. Nilsson and colleagues (56) employed three separate methods for the evaluation of the PPG (called the blood volume pulse) for changes caused by exercise. First, they derived a single parameter from the distribution found in the average histogram of the time-aligned beats. Their second approach analyzed the ratio observed between the first harmonic and higher harmonics in the signal. The third approach evaluated the dicrotic notch depth directly from the PPG waveform. Alian and Shelley further discussed the detrimental effects of excessive filtering and autogain on the utility and interpretation of the PPG, potential use of heart rate variability (HRV) as an index of autonomic nervous system activity, pulse transit time (PTT) as a correlate of arterial system rigidity, respiratory modulation as a guide to goal-directed fluid therapy, and artifacts due to venous engorgement from over-resuscitation or steep Trendelenburg positioning (19,50,51). Further significance of these findings will be elaborated below.

Uses of the Photoplethysmograph

The PPG is a noninvasively obtained window into many physiologic parameters. Since a pulse oximeter probe can be placed by those with minimal or no training and are found in virtually every aspect of medical care, there are many active research projects exploring the potential uses of the PPG (50,51).

Several researchers have attempted to construct mathematical relationships between the PPG and various indices of arterial mechanics. Kato and colleagues (57) measured the PPG from a finger pulse oximeter probe and pressure at the ipsilateral radial artery, simultaneously. The authors concluded that a four-element, two-compartment model can be applied to the PPG to determine peripheral vascular wall mechanics. Chowienczyk and colleagues (58) determined that PPG assessment may provide a useful method to examine vascular reactivity. Millasseau and colleagues, in 2002 (59), concluded that contour analysis of the digital volume pulse (DVP) provides a simple, reproducible, noninvasive measure of large artery stiffness, and, in 2003 (60), determined that indices of pressure wave reflection and large artery stiffness can be used as an index of vascular aging. Bortolotto and colleagues (61) concluded that the second derivative of the PPG and the pulse wave velocity can both be used to evaluate vascular aging in hypertensives.

Other researchers are exploring the use of the PPG for noninvasively determining respiratory rate. Changes in intrathoracic pressure during the respiratory cycle displace venous blood, affecting the LFC. These changes also affect cardiac return, changing the amplitude of the PCC. During spontaneous breathing, subatmospheric pressure during inspiration draws air and blood together into the lungs; blood is drawn from the vena cava into the right heart and pulmonary vascular bed; a minor decrease in peripheral venous pressure (PVP) ensues. Soon thereafter, the expiratory pressure normalizes the system. During positive pressure ventilation, the inspiration is driven by positive pressure, which raises intrathoracic pressure and reduces venous return to the right heart. Simultaneously, and very briefly, blood forced from the low-pressure pulmonary vascular bed increases return to the left heart as well as stroke volume (62). This is followed by a decrease in cardiac output as venous return into the central circulation drops off. The extent of the fluctuations caused by positive pressure ventilation depends on the state of filling of the peripheral vascular bed, the intrathoracic pressure changes, peripheral vasoconstrictor activity, and central blood volume (49). Since positive pressure ventilation often accompanies general anesthesia, which causes vasodilation and damped vasomotor response, respiratory fluctuations are emphasized. It was also discovered that early hypovolemia may be reflected in an exaggerated respiratory wave before other more classic signs of decreased urine output, tachycardia, or hypotension (49).

Nilsson and colleagues (63) extracted the cardiac- and respiratory-related components, applied a mathematic algorithm, and developed a new PPG device for monitoring heart rate and respiratory rate simultaneously; their study determined that the PPG has the potential for respiratory rate monitoring. Nilsson and colleagues (56) also hypothesized that the filling of peripheral veins is a major mechanism behind the LFC signal, and found that a correlation exists in the amplitudes of the LFC in the PPG and the respiratory variations in PVP ($p < 0.01$). Leonard and colleagues (64,65) concluded that baseline respiratory rate was easily identified from a pulse oximeter PPG using wavelet transforms. The study of Foo and Wilson (66) determined that the respiratory rate obtained from the PPG was significantly related to that estimated by a calibrated air pressure transducer during tidal breathing in the absence of motion artifact ($p < 0.05$). Nilsson and colleagues (56) concluded that respiration can be monitored by the PPG with high sensitivity and specificity regardless of anesthesia and ventilatory mode. Leonard and colleagues (67) continued their work by developing a fully automated algorithm for the determination of respiratory rate from the PPG.

Researchers have also been exploring the relationship between the PPG and volume status. Perel and colleagues (68) found that the difference between systolic pressure at end-expiration and the lowest value during the respiratory cycle (d-Down) correlated to the degree of hemorrhage. It also correlated with the cardiac output and the pulmonary capillary wedge pressure. Thus, the changes in systolic pressure with respiration, as demonstrated by arterial pressure waveforms (systolic pressure variation [SPV]) and its d-Down component, are accurate indicators of hypovolemia in ventilated dogs subjected to hemorrhage. Rooke and colleagues (69) also concluded that SPV and the d-Down appear to follow shifts in intravascular volume in relatively healthy, mechanically ventilated humans under isoflurane anesthesia. Building on this principle, Partridge (70) attempted to use pulse oximetry as a noninvasive method to assess intravascular volume status. The study showed that the PPG correlated with the systolic pressure variation ($r = 0.61$), which was previously shown to be a sensitive indicator of hypovolemia. Shamir and colleagues (71) investigated ventilation-induced changes in the PPG after removing and reinfusing 10% of the estimated blood volume in 12 anesthetized patients. The plethysmographic SPV was measured as the vertical distance between maximal and minimal peaks of waveforms during the ventilatory cycle and expressed as a percentage of the amplitude of the PPG signal during apnea. This was measured during five consecutive mechanical breaths before apnea and the mean value was obtained for analysis. The 10% loss of estimated blood volume resulted in increased heart rate without changes in mean arterial pressure. Both the PPG waveform changes and the SPV from the arterial blood pressure tracing increased significantly after blood withdrawal ($p < 0.01$). The changes in the PPG correlated with the changes in the SPV. After volume replacement, heart rate decreased while arterial pressure remained unchanged. There were no significant changes in the PPG waveform or the SPV with volume replacement. Fuehrlein and colleagues (72) investigated the use of PPG for volume status changes during blood donation and hemodialysis. They concluded that the PPG could be used to detect changes in volume status and vascular instability during hemodialysis and blood donation.

MULTIWAVELENGTH PULSE OXIMETRY

There is now an extensive literature concerning multiwavelength pulse oximetry, sometimes also called co-oximetry. Improvement of pulse oximetry performance, and new capabilities such as noninvasive estimation of concentrations of hemoglobin, carboxyhemoglobin, and methemoglobin are possible by using multiple wavelengths and new processing algorithms (73). Controlled studies in normal patients have reported generally good, but variable, correlations with laboratory determinations and trends in circulating hemoglobin concentrations, and responsiveness to blood and fluid administration (74). Because noninvasive results have not been reliably correlated with laboratory results, a debate continues concerning what is good enough or useful (54,75–77). The data have also demonstrated that there can be differences of 1 gm/dL in hemoglobin even between laboratory methods, as well as by oximetry (78). Correlation with laboratory values in low perfusion states, trauma resuscitation, and acute hemorrhage and circulatory changes have been less satisfactory than under more stable cardiovascular conditions (79). Assessment of hemoglobin concentration or trends in settings where laboratory determinations are not available or greatly delayed would have clear utility (80). The issues raised have contributed to the debate about which reference and transfusion triggers are appropriate, and how hemoglobin determinations could bias evidence or its application (53,81).

Rapid detection of high concentration of carboxyhemoglobin may be particularly significant for initial assessment of emergency patients. Detection of methemoglobins may be principally useful to avoid adverse effects of titratable drugs like nitroprusside (82).

A very interesting new development is Oxygen Reserve Index (ORI). ORI provides a graded, proportional change from 0 to 1 related to PaO_2 from about 98 to over 200 torr, above the 100% SpO_2 plateau with standard pulse oximetry (83). While this gradually increasing index is qualitatively proportional to changes in PaO_2, it gives an indication of change over a range of partial pressures where there was previously no indication of change PaO_2 after oxyhemoglobin reached full saturation, a useful feature for warning for impending desaturation or changes in lung function (84,85).

FUTURE DIRECTIONS OF OXIMETRY

While the foundational concepts of pulse oximetry are employed in many ways, innovation continues to provide improved performance and to break barriers and resolve limitations of previous generations of the technology. There is still room for improvement particularly at low saturations, for poor tissue perfusion, responsiveness to deterioration, alarm, and artifact management.

Clinically applicable assessment of mitochondrial oxidative state may probe previously inscrutable pathophysiology, for instance, in sepsis, hypoxia, and poor perfusion states (5).

Hemodynamic monitoring employing characteristics of PPG is beginning to realize objectives for cardiopulmonary optimization by noninvasive monitoring. Further investigation and pulse oximeter design optimization for PPG analysis will be needed (19).

Use of SpO_2 rather than directly measured SaO_2 in proportion to F_IO_2 as an index of severity of lung injury and risk stratification has the advantage of being noninvasive and easily trended, though not perfectly correlated (86–90).

NIRS assessment of various organs and particularly cerebral oxygenation is promising but not uncontroversial (91,92), having suffered from competing claims of manufacturers, lingering concerns about what is measured, and limited outcomes data (93,94). Use in evaluation of resuscitation from cardiac arrest is particularly intriguing (95). An unconventional approach to measuring jugular venous oxygenation is a promising method that may have utility for assessment of cerebral oxygen supply and demand matching (96).

CAPNOGRAPHY AND RESPIRATORY MONITORING

Capnometry refers to the measurement of carbon dioxide, regardless of the method used. Capnography describes the method of obtaining a capnogram, that is, a tracing of carbon dioxide concentration as a function of time or volume. A capnograph is the instrument used to generate a capnogram. Capnometry has become the minimal standard of practice for the American Society of Anesthesiologists since 1986—most recently amended in 2015—whenever a patient's airway is breached with an endotracheal tube, a laryngeal mask airway, or an esophageal tracheal airway (97). If CO_2 can be detected with each breath after placing the artificial airway, the clinician has the first and best—if not the only reliable—indication that the artificial airway is ventilating the patient's lungs rather than the esophagus and stomach. However, merely detecting carbon dioxide on one or two breaths is not sufficient. Persistence of capnograms with continuous ventilation is necessary, because there can be enough carbon dioxide insufflated in a stomach that even gas returned from a distended stomach can resemble a capnogram. With esophageal intubation, the concentration of carbon dioxide returned with each breath will decrease rapidly with dilution, and the waveform of the capnogram will not have the typical shape (see below). With impaired circulation, such as during CPR, capnograms will be diminished in amplitude, or may even be absent if the lungs are not perfused with blood. In this instance, an endotracheal tube should be evaluated for correct placement, but left in place even if there is no capnogram. Continuous capnograms should be expected with effective CPR that generates circulation of blood.

The delivery of CO_2 to gas exhaled from the lungs is the final step in a complex system. Cellular metabolism generates CO_2, which diffuses through local tissue and is absorbed by perfusing capillary blood. In blood, CO_2 is dissolved in plasma and buffered with proteins, principally hemoglobin. Venous blood flow delivers the CO_2 to the heart, which powers pulmonary perfusion, and delivers it to the lungs and, via ventilation, gathers it from the alveoli when a breath finally pushes it to the outside. Thus, the discovery of CO_2 after intubation of the patient's airway, while essential, is but the tip of the proverbial iceberg. In this section, we provide a clinician's overview of capnometry and its applications in the perioperative period and the intensive care unit.

HISTORY

Carbon dioxide and its measurement have enjoyed a colorful history (98–100). Jan Baptista van Helmont (1579–1644) recognized a spirit escaping from burning wood and called it gas sylvester (from Latin *silva* = wood and *silvester* = woody). The recognition that a gas could reside in something solid found expression in the term "fixed air" introduced by J. Black in 1755. He discovered the gas to be a constituent of carbonated alkali. Later, Antoine-Laurent de Lavoisier (1743–1794) showed the gas to be an oxide of carbon. What an extraordinary discovery: carbon (of coal and diamonds) connected with oxygen was a gas! John Tyndall (1820–1893) spoke of "perfectly colorless and invisible gases and vapors" such as carbonic acid (now called carbon dioxide) that could well absorb radiant energy. This insight enabled him to detect carbon dioxide in the exhaled gas. However, before capnography based on physical methods could gain a foothold in clinical practice, a chemical method described by John Scott Haldane (1860–1936) became the "gold standard." He caused a precisely measured volume of gas to be drawn into a closed system that made it possible to expose the gas to absorbents such as sodium or potassium hydroxide. These agents removed the carbon dioxide from the sample; the vanished volume was attributed to the absorbed CO_2. Refinements of this method were widely used, yet the methods were time consuming. Chemical methods, in general, destroy the gas to be measured and allow only snapshots of respiratory CO_2.

A number of methods exploited the physics of energy absorption. August Hermann Pfund (1879–1949), Professor of Optics in Baltimore, measured the effects of interposing more or less CO_2 between a heat source and a temperature sensor. Karl Friedrich Luft (1900–1999) employed infrared energy beamed through cells with and without CO_2, thus enabling the measurements of the energy absorbed by the gas in question. Later generations of this same principle gave rise to the currently most widely used infrared spectroscopic method of capnography.

Two other historical methods that were employed clinically for capnography, as well as other medical gas analyses, deserve mention. Both have been displaced by more economical—and less capable—infrared gas analyzers. One of the first methods used for clinical gas analysis, including capnography, was mass spectrometry, in which charged particles are separated by their mass when an ionized gas beam is passed through a magnetic field. The other was Raman scattering spectroscopy (101). Both of these spectrometers have other medical applications, including specialized gas analyses beyond needs for basic capnography. Gas mixtures add analytic considerations; nitrous oxide can interfere with PCO_2 measurement. Infrared gas analyzers cannot directly quantify nonpolar molecules, such as nitrogen and inert gases like helium and argon; together they represent the residual difference from atmospheric pressure after accounting for the reported gases and water vapor. Raman and mass spectrometry can directly quantitate mixtures even of nonpolar gases.

SITES OF MEASUREMENT

Capnography, herein examined, focuses on the detection and monitoring of CO_2 in the exhaled gases. There will always be small differences in PCO_2 between blood and different respired gas sampling sites. There must be at least a small difference in partial pressure of CO_2 to have a gradient for diffusion, even in health. With pathophysiology, increased gradients and mixing of gases from areas of lung with different ventilation–perfusion ratios will confound assumptions of uniform gradients. While direct measurement of alveolar CO_2 ($PACO_2$) is not clinically possible, the assumption that $PetCO_2$ will provide a valid proxy measurement is frequently not valid due to dilution of alveolar gas by admixture, either within the lung or the breathing apparatus before the measurement sampling point (102). This point is one of the most unappreciated errors for interpretation of capnograms and incorrect assertion of a-A gradient (103). Thus, capnograms from breath sampling sites without a closed connection to the trachea will be substantially diluted and distorted by the free diffusion of surrounding atmospheric air (100,104).

CO_2 can also be lost and consequently collected and measured from the skin (105), from the stomach (106), sublingually (107,108), and even the rectum (109), and other sites; these will not be discussed in this chapter.

STEADY OR UNSTEADY STATE

With modern methods, continuous readings of exhaled CO_2 tensions and volumes can be obtained. We speak of steady state when the partial pressure (tension, PCO_2) of carbon dioxide in different tissue and organ compartments and blood and alveolar gas have reached equilibrium, and when the input of CO_2 from metabolism equals the output of CO_2 via ventilation and, to a small extent, via skin, flatus, feces, and urine. A steady state can exist with high, normal, or low arterial, alveolar, or end-tidal CO_2 tension ($PaCO_2$, $PACO_2$, or $PetCO_2$); however, all too often, we do not have a steady state: Tissue depleted of CO_2 can absorb liters of the gas from blood until tissue PCO_2 and blood PCO_2 reach equilibrium; conversely, such tissue stores can contribute CO_2 to that generated by metabolism. For example, prolonged hyperventilation can exhaust tissue stores of carbon dioxide and bicarbonate. Under these conditions, the maintenance of a normal $PaCO_2$ requires less than normal ventilation because some of the metabolic CO_2 filters back into the tissues instead of being exhaled. Conversely, high tissue stores of CO_2 (e.g., after a cardiac and respiratory arrest) will call for greater than normal ventilation until steady state is once again reached. A depressed respiratory center (e.g., under the influence of an opiate) will lead to an imbalance of input and output as the tissues take up some of the CO_2 while the rest leaves the body in the exhaled gas. Once the tissues and blood reach equilibrium, steady state will once again supervene in the presence of elevated levels of $PaCO_2$, $PACO_2$, and $PetCO_2$. Renal compensation of metabolic acidosis or alkalosis, though much slower than respiratory changes, will also contribute to an unsteady state for many hours or days. The point is that capnograms can hide as much as they reveal, and thus the interpretation of capnograms calls for discerning clinicians.

CONVENTIONS OF MEASUREMENTS

Before describing the different methods of capnography, the conventions of reporting the tension or concentration of CO_2 present in the exhaled gas must be discussed. The tension of the gas can be reported in mmHg (torr), with normal end-tidal values between 35 and 45 mmHg, which translates into 4.67 and 6.0 kPa, respectively (1 kPa = 7.5 torr). The amount of CO_2 present in a gas sample can also be reported in percent or as a fraction of the volume of gas. Here caution needs to be exercised: 5.0% end-tidal PCO_2 (equal to the end-tidal fraction, Fet, 0.05) at a barometric pressure at sea level of 760 mmHg (101 kPa) would amount to 38 mmHg (5.05 kPa). However, many millions of people live in cities at altitude. Assume, for example, Mexico City with an ambient pressure of about 550 mmHg (73 kPa). Here, 5.0% end-tidal CO_2 would represent only 27.5 mmHg (3.65 kPa). The influence of the pressure exerted by water vapor (47 mmHg or 6.26 kPa at 37°C), which is not affected by barometric pressure but rises and falls as a function of temperature, also plays an important role at altitude (Table 23.2). As we wish to correlate alveolar gas tension with the tension of gases in blood (reported in mmHg or kPa), we prefer to report gaseous CO_2 not in percent, but as PCO_2 in mmHg or kPa.

METHODOLOGIES

Chemical

CO_2 goes into solution, combines with water to form carbonic acid, and establishes an equilibrium between dissolved CO_2 and bicarbonate. This reaction, which changes the pH, gives rise to chemical methods using pH indicators for the estimation of CO_2 concentration in moist gas, or colorimetric $etCO_2$ (Fig. 23.3).

Changes in temperature and the addition or removal of H^+ ions, in turn, affect the ratio of bicarbonate to carbonic acid, and dissolved CO_2, therefore, plays a crucial role in the acid-based equilibrium of blood, which is assessed by measuring pH and PCO_2 and calculating bicarbonate in blood. This is discussed in detail elsewhere in this book, as is the importance of buffers (primarily hemoglobin) and carbonic anhydrase, which accelerates the reaction:

$$CO_2 + H_2O \leftrightharpoons H_2CO_3 \leftrightharpoons HCO_3^- + H^+$$

TABLE 23.2 Carbon Dioxide and Barometric Pressure at 37°C

Barometric Pressure	End-Tidal PCO_2	End-Tidal Percent or Fraction of Volume	Alveolar Partial Pressure of Water Vapor	Alveolar Percent or Fraction of Water Vapor
Sea level at 760 mmHg	38 mmHg or 5.05 kPa	5.0% or Fet 0.05	47 mmHg or 6.26 kPa	6.2% or fe H_2O 0.06
Elevation[a] 550 mmHg	27.5 mmHg or 3.65 kPa	5.0% or Fet 0.05	47 mmHg or 6.26 kPa	8.5% or fe H_2O 0.08

[a]At altitude assuming hyperventilation to an end-tidal PCO_2 of 27.5 mmHg.

While hyperventilation can reduce the volume of carbon dioxide in the alveoli, it cannot reduce the tension of water vapor, which, as long as the temperature stays at 37°C, will remain at 47 mmHg. Some capnometers offer readings that assume dry or wet gas at 37°C.

f stands for fraction where 1 = 100% and 0.05 = 5%.

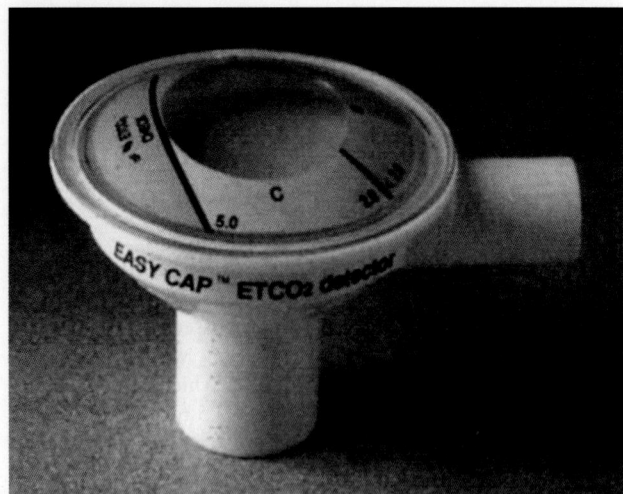

FIGURE 23.3 A device that detects CO_2 by chemically induced color change. (Courtesy of Nellcor, Inc.)

Sidestream and Mainstream (On-Airway) Capnography: Time-Based Methods

The gas to be analyzed has to be collected from the patient under conditions that prevent contamination of the gas with ambient air. Ideally, we would like to sample tracheal gas; that is rarely possible. A cuffed endotracheal tube with a port close to the mouth offers the next best opportunity to collect exhaled gas from the patient before it mixes with gas from the outside or the breathing circuit. First, we will take a look at the sidestream method.

Sidestream

On its way to the analyzer through a capillary, the gas cools (from body to room temperature) and the water vapor condenses, forming droplets. Two methods minimize the potential problem of having water obstruct the flow of gas or confound the spectroscopic analysis: Collecting capillaries made out of Nafion tubing enables the water vapor in the tube to diffuse through the tubing wall to equilibrate with the water vapor in air surrounding the tube. This leads to a reduction of water vapor burden in the capillary. The second, a more common method employs a water trap situated close to the analyzer.

Figure 23.4 shows a typical time-based capnogram obtained under ideal conditions. Here we plot the tension of carbon dioxide in the ordinate and time in the abscissa. Observe the angles α and β, both of which in a healthy individual approach 90 degrees. A respiratory pause at the end of exhalation will cause the plateau phase to become horizontal.

With the sidestream method, the costly analyzer can be kept out of the way; a thin, long aspirating capillary presents no encumbrance to the clinical team; and aspirated gas can be analyzed for CO_2 as well as other gases. Furthermore, gas can be aspirated from nasal prongs with minimal annoyance to a conscious patient. Commercial configurations are available that enable the simultaneous aspiration of gas from one nostril while delivering oxygen to the other nostril or to the mouth. However, in that application, contamination of the aspirated gas with room air or oxygen is possible, although several studies have shown clinically satisfactory results with these arrangements. At a minimum, such a system can provide evidence of ventilation and enable the recording of respiratory rates.

The sidestream method has two well-recognized drawbacks. The longer the capillary is, the longer the travel time for the gas from the patient to the analyzer. That causes the capnogram to be out of phase with simultaneously recorded flow or pressure tracings. The long travel also gives the leading edge of a gas a chance to mix with the gas it is replacing in the tubing, which produces slurring of the capnogram, particularly noticeable with rapid respiratory rates (Fig. 23.5).

Many sidestream capnometers aspirate up to 200 mL gas per minute into the analyzer. Premature newborns, with their small tidal volumes and high respiratory rates, will then develop capnograms that show false low end-tidal and false high inspiratory PCO_2 values. Two mechanisms contribute to these conditions: On the one hand, the tiny patient's tidal volume might be so low as to cause the capnograph to aspirate gas from the breathing tube, thus diluting the exhaled gas from the patient. On the other hand, the time constant of the capnograph may be too long to respond adequately to rapid breaths. Modern capnographs offer low rates of aspiration (30–200 mL/min) and short time constants (110).

Mainstream

Instead of aspirating a sample of respired gas with a sidestream system, it is possible to determine the concentration of carbon dioxide close to the patient's mouth in a "mainstream" or "on-airway" method (Fig. 23.6). The method eliminates two weaknesses of the sidestream system: Without a need to transport the gas through a capillary to the analyzer, mainstream capnograms show no slurring of the capnographic tracings. Of course, these advantages come with a (tolerable) cost: The carbon dioxide

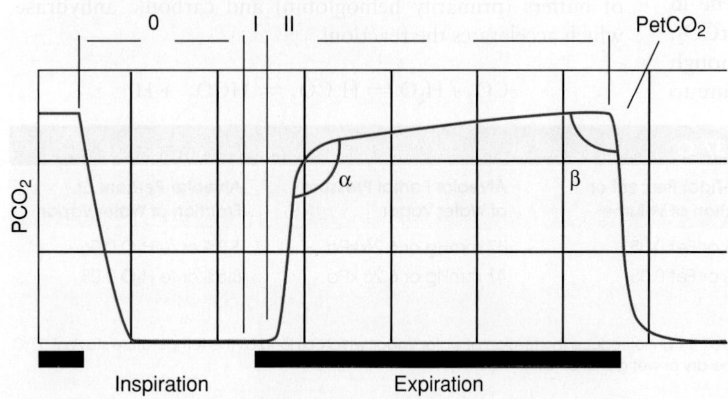

FIGURE 23.4 Capnogram showing exhaled PCO_2 versus time. Expiration shows phase I (dead space gas free of CO_2), phase II (rapid appearance of CO_2), and phase III (plateau). The α angle describes the transition from phase II to III and the β angle that from phase III to phase 0, the beginning of inspiration.

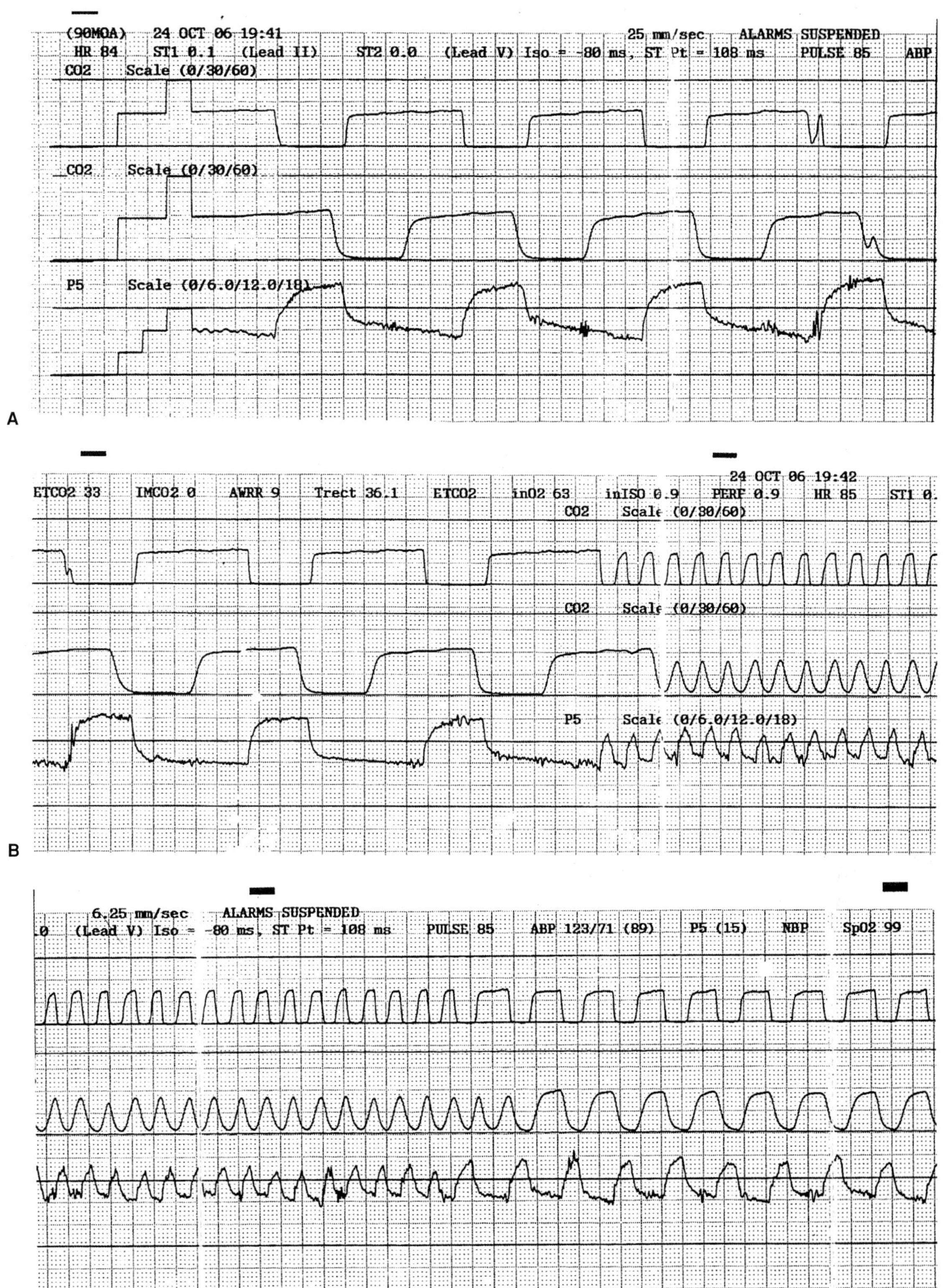

FIGURE 23.5 A: The top capnogram derives from an on-airway sampling location. The middle tracing is a capnogram from a sidestream device. Notice the on-airway waveform is a little more crisp than that from the sidestream device. The data were collected from a patient during mechanical ventilation. The increase in airway pressure is associated with the sudden disappearance of CO_2 and the drop in airway pressure signals exhalation. Travel time of gas in the capillary of the sidestream capnogram causes the on-airway curve to lag behind the pressure tracings. **B**: Increasing respiratory rate briefly to 60 breaths per minute eliminates the plateau in the sidestream-derived waveform with reduced end-tidal CO_2, while the on-airway device still shows a plateau. **C**: Dropping the rate to 30 breaths per minute results in the plateau reappearing in the on-airway device.

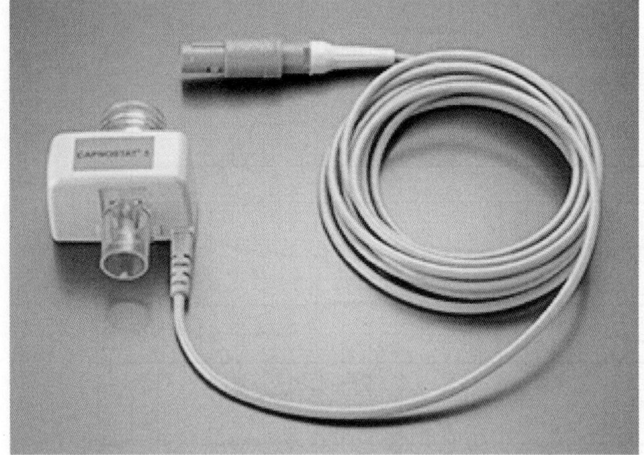

FIGURE 23.6 The Capnostat CO_2 sensor, a fully integrated gas measurement system, is shown assembled with an adult airway adapter. All of the signal acquisition and processing is performed within the sensor. This is accomplished by the use of microelectronics and digital signal processing. The capnogram along with calculated parameters such as end-tidal and inspired values are provided via a serial interface. (Courtesy of Respironics, Inc., Murrysville, PA.)

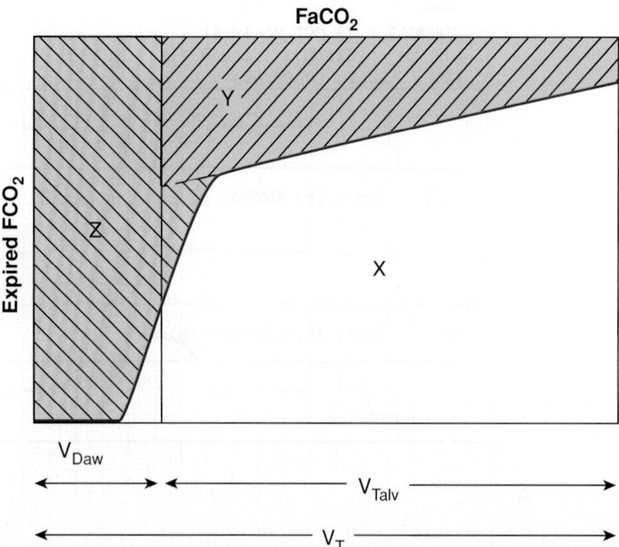

FIGURE 23.7 Schematic single-breath test. $FaCO_2$ represents the FCO_2 of a gas in equilibrium with arterial blood. Area X represents the volume of CO_2 in the breath. Area Y represents the alveolar dead space. The alveolar dead space fraction is given by Y/(X + Y). V_{Talv} is the alveolar tidal volume. The physiologic dead space fraction is represented by areas (Y + Z)/(X + Y + Z). Note that fractions are used, rather than partial pressures, in order that the areas may represent CO_2 volumes, actual or notional. Observe the top horizontal line of an invasively obtained $FaCO_2$. (Reproduced with permission from Fletcher R. In Gravenstein JS, Jaffe MB, Paulus DA, eds. *Capnography: Clinical Aspects.* Cambridge: Cambridge University Press; 2004:381.)

sensor must be brought close to the patient's mouth, which adds weight to the breathing circuit/endotracheal tube; in this position, the sensor is exposed to potential damage, and obtaining gas samples from a spontaneously breathing, nonintubated patient is more difficult than would be true from a sidestream system. Nevertheless, mainstream systems have been adapted for capnography even in nonintubated infants.

The mainstream, on-airway system avoids problems arising out of condensation of water vapor in the exhaled gas by heating of the sensor. At 37°C, water vapor will exert 47 mmHg, thus affecting—if not powerfully—the determination of PCO_2 in sidestream systems. Purists will, therefore, point out that mainstream capnography will give values more representative of alveolar gases than sidestream systems, a small advantage with no clinical significance.

Volume-Based Capnography

Instead of plotting the respired gas as a function of time, we can also plot it as a function of volume and concentration (111). This calls for a method to measure, breath by breath, the respired quantity of CO_2. Commonly, only the exhaled tidal volume is shown (Fig. 23.7).

Observe the following in Figure 23.7:

A: The tracing starts with the beginning of exhalation, which consists of dead space free of CO_2 (Phase I).

B: As the dead space is cleared, gas from the sequentially smaller and smaller airways, and finally alveoli, will be exhaled. A steeply rising concentration of carbon dioxide over volume reflects this phase (II). The phase ends in a distinctive knee and then transitions into a more or less horizontal phase (III).

C: The gently rising horizontal phase adds volume from distant lung segments.

D: The end-tidal value, normally about 40 mmHg, represents alveolar gas if lung function and tidal volume are normal.

E: The inspiratory limb of the breath is not recorded, as is the custom with volume-based capnograms.

The measurement of the exhaled volume presents challenges. Not only is the flow rate not uniform over the entire exhaled volume, but also the presence of water vapor, barometric pressure, composition of the exhaled gas (for example, in the presence of helium), configuration of the sensor, and response time of the flow meter can all affect the accuracy of the measurement (112).

Observe in Figure 23.7 the gap between the end-tidal value and the arterial CO_2 tension; thus, together with an arterial blood gas, the single-breath method enables the clinician to estimate the volume of CO_2 in the exhaled breath (*X*), the volume of the alveolar dead space (*Y*), and the volume of the anatomic dead space (*Z*). Fletcher (113) adopted an estimation of the "efficiency" of ventilation by drawing a horizontal line through the end-tidal concentration of CO_2 (Fig. 23.8). Ideal efficiency would be a square *X* region with *Y* approaching zero area.

Check of Capnograph

Before accepting the data provided by capnographs, check the technical details of the instruments, whether sidestream or mainstream and whether time or volume based. Calibration can be accomplished with a test gas, with references built into the instrument, and for mainstream systems with cells that mimic the presence of a known carbon dioxide concentration. When in doubt, the user can test his or her own exhaled gas. However, this will not test the linearity of the instrument.

For sidestream systems, check for a properly connected sampling system and patent tubing. When secretions or water droplets impede gas flow, the sidestream capnograph will report erroneous data. A break in the tubing or a loose connection can enable room air to dilute the sample. In a mainstream system, a leak between the sensor and patient can introduce artifacts. Gas other than the patient's exhaled gas can dilute the sample in all applications in which the sample is not taken

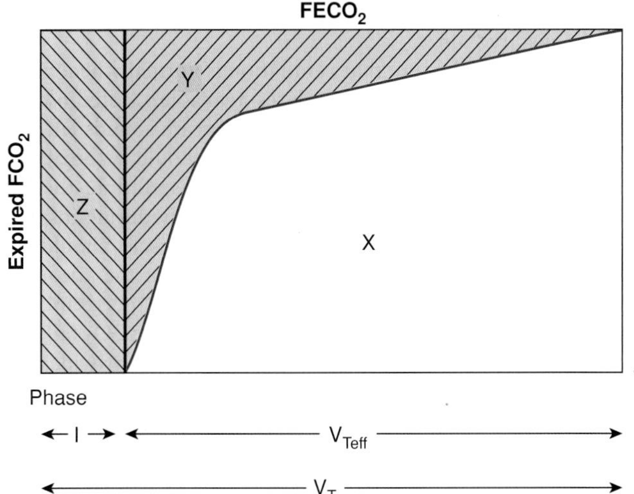

FIGURE 23.8 Definition of efficiency. The breath is divided into phase I, the ineffective part, and V_{Teff}, the effective part (which contains phases I and II). Efficiency is calculated from 100 times area X divided by areas (X + Y). In effect, efficiency is a noninvasive measure of ventilatory efficiency. (Reproduced with permission from Fletcher R. In Gravenstein JS, Jaffe MB, Paulus DA, eds. *Capnography: Clinical Aspects.* Cambridge: Cambridge University Press; 2004:382.)

from a port close to the endotracheal tube, as is true with aspiration of gas from nasal cannulae.

Pay attention to the patient's tidal volume. If the patient's tidal volume, whether spontaneous or not, is too small to deliver undiluted alveolar gas to the capnograph, the $PetCO_2$ will be falsely low; this concern arises particularly in premature newborns.

Respiratory rates affect the capability of the capnograph. Capnographs have limits to the rate of their response, usually expressed either as time needed for a 5% to 95% response or as time constant (Fig. 23.9). Consequently, with rapid respiratory rates, the instrument may not be able to reach a full response, and the end-exhaled values can present as falsely low and the inspired values falsely high.

Make sure the respired gas is free of gases that would confound the spectrographic analysis of CO_2, as can be true of nitrous oxide and helium. Many capnographs offer compensation for the presence of nitrous oxide. Helium causes the CO_2 concentrations to be read falsely low (114).

Cardiogenic Oscillations

Cardiogenic oscillations (Fig. 23.10) are a reminder that the lungs and heart share an enclosed space, causing gas to ebb and flow in the trachea as the cardiac volume changes with each beat in the enclosed chest. These oscillations can be seen with both sidestream and mainstream systems. The oscillations synchronous with the heart beat are thought to represent "the complex summation of transient alterations in the proportion of the total flow coming from different lung units and containing gases of different concentrations" (115).

INTERPRETATION

What is a Normal Capnogram?

A normal capnogram is a plot of CO_2 and time, which can be divided into inspiratory and expiratory segments, each one grouped in phases (see Fig. 23.4).

Inspiratory segment: The inspiratory phase, phase 0, is usually a flat line overlapping the zero (baseline) CO_2 concentration line, unless rebreathing is present. The latter part of the horizontal baseline is phase I of the expiratory segment. Phase 0 represents the dynamics of inspiration.

Expiratory segment: The expiratory segment, similar to a single-breath CO_2 curve, is divided into phases I, II, and III, and occasionally phase IV, which represents the terminal rise in CO_2 concentration.

Phase I: Phase I represents CO_2-free gas from the apparatus and anatomic dead space.

Phase II: Phase II consists of a rapid S-shaped upswing on the tracing due to mixing of dead space gas with alveolar gas.

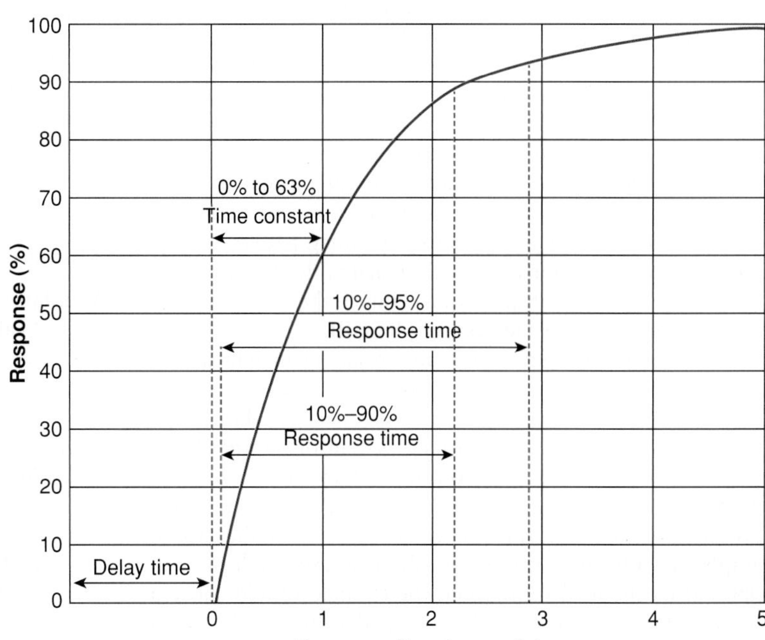

FIGURE 23.9 For sidestream sampling, total response time is equal to the delay or transit time in the sampling catheter plus the measurement rise time, which is expressed different ways. (Reproduced from Gravenstein JS, Paulus DA, Hayes TJ. *Capnography in Clinical Practice.* 2nd ed. Boston, MA: Butterworth-Heinemann; 1989.)

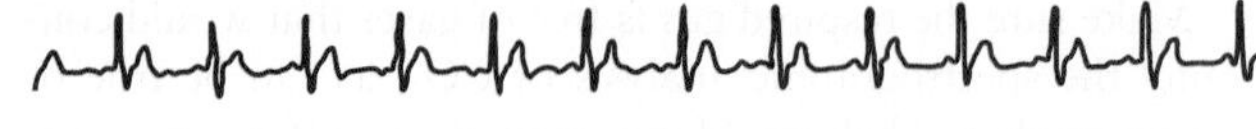

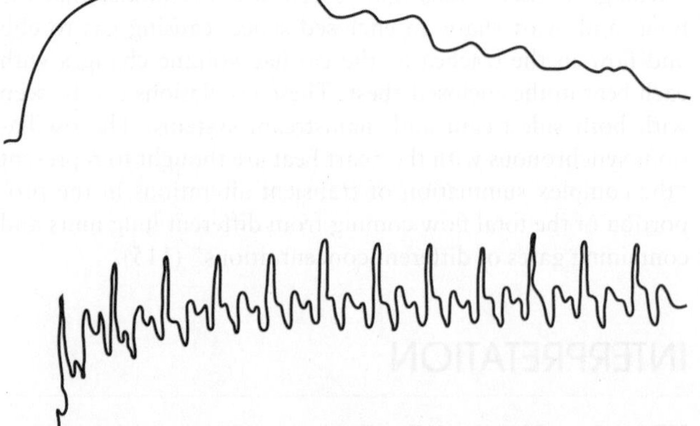

FIGURE 23.10 Simultaneous electrocardiogram and capnogram with cardiogenic oscillations and pneumotachygraph. Cardiogenic oscillations in this capnogram (**middle tracing**) were generated from a healthy volunteer who breathed into a mouthpiece, to which a pneumotachygraph (set at high sensitivity) and sidestream capnograph sampling connector were attached. An electrocardiogram (**top tracing**) was recorded simultaneously. Oscillations appeared on the capnogram only on the down-slope. The oscillation occurred at the same rate as the heartbeat, but 2 to 3 seconds after the pneumotachygraph because of the travel time of the gas in the sidestream capnograph. To generate a pneumotachygraph, the subject kept his glottis open after an exhalation was completed.

α Angle: The angle between phases II and III has been referred to as the α angle, and increases as the slope of phase III increases. Changes of the α angle correlate with sequential emptying of alveoli. In general, the more heterogeneous are functional units of the lung, and the wider one is the α angle.

Phase III: Phase III is the link between the α angle and the $PetCO_2$. Its slope increases with ventilation/perfusion (V/Q) mismatch, and it is determined by the gas-emptying sequence of the alveolar units. If the units empty synchronously, the CO_2 expired results in a smooth flat or slightly upsloping phase III. In patients with severe V/Q scatter and longer time constants, CO_2 emptying is sequential, resulting in a steeper rising slope of phase III. In general, the more severe the mismatch is, the steeper the slope. Factors such as changes in cardiac output, CO_2 production, airway resistance, breathing pattern (tachypnea), and low functional residual capacity (FRC) may further affect the V/Q status of the various units in the lung, and thus influence the height or the slope of phase III.

An incompetent expiratory valve resulting in rebreathing may affect the α angle and up-slope, the phase III of the capnograph—the ebb and flow of non-exhaled gas dilutes the $PetCO_2$, as in a "circle" breathing system of an anesthesia machine—a simultaneous recording of flow rate waveforms in both limbs can potentially differentiate this technical problem from an abnormal plateau of phase III of the capnograph. For a healthy, spontaneously breathing adult or with optimal mechanical ventilation, the α angle should show a smooth curve (see Fig. 23.4), end-tidal values of 35 to 45 mmHg, and a $PaCO_2$ (arterial) of only 3 to 4 mmHg higher than the end-tidal values. There would be no carbon dioxide in the inspired air.

How can we be sure that ventilation is normal when we do not have arterial blood gas analyses available? A stethoscope would be helpful in confirming normal breath sounds left and right. A spontaneously breathing patient should be breathing regularly, without a tracheal tug during inspiration; the left and right chest should rise equally and evenly during inspiration; and during expiration, the abdominal muscles should not contract. If clinical findings raise doubts about the adequacy of ventilation, even with a normal-appearing capnogram, the arterial blood gas should be analyzed. Should $PetCO_2$ fail reasonably to reflect $PaCO_2$, capnography can still provide useful trend data, but the clinician will now need to identify the reason for a larger than normal difference between $PetCO_2$ and $PaCO_2$.

The volume-based method provides a valuable opportunity to estimate the volume of CO_2 exhaled. Because no single breath equals the next, even with mechanical ventilation, several to many breaths need be sampled and averaged to arrive at a reasonable estimate. Volumetric capnography (plotting CO_2 concentration in relation to expired volume) has been used for real-time calculations of anatomic and physiologic dead space ventilation. Since anatomic dead space generally does not change rapidly, alterations of physiologic dead space measured in real time can indicate changes in the alveolar dead space component. While the information obtained from volumetric capnography could be theoretically useful to titrate ventilator parameters, its use is currently not widespread.

Normally, we expect 200 to 250 mL/min (about 2–3 mL/kg/min) of CO_2 to be produced by a resting, healthy, normothermic adult of average weight. Assuming steady state (ignoring small losses through skin, feces, and urine), the volume exhaled would represent the volume produced. Diet can change the respiratory quotient (RQ = carbon dioxide production/oxygen consumption), typically about 0.8.

What Are the Signs of an Abnormal Capnogram?

For a valid measurement of the tidal volume during mechanical ventilation, the exhaled rather than the inspired volume must be measured. Positive pressure during inspiration can cause gas to escape through a leak or around the endotracheal tube; such loss is less likely during passive expiration.

Equipment Related

Ventilator-Related Failures or Gas Leaks

1. **Leaks:** With mechanical ventilation, leaks in the breathing circuit are likely to spill gas during inspiration when the pressure in the system is high, and thus can lead to hypoventilation despite a properly calculated (but not measured) minute ventilation.
2. **Inspired CO_2:** In the absence of intentionally added CO_2, three mechanisms can lead to the appearance of inspired carbon dioxide:
   a. **Exhausted CO_2 absorber:** With a circle system, as used in anesthesia, an exhausted CO_2 absorber will cause rebreathing, evidenced by an increase of inspired CO_2, especially evident at low fresh gas flow.

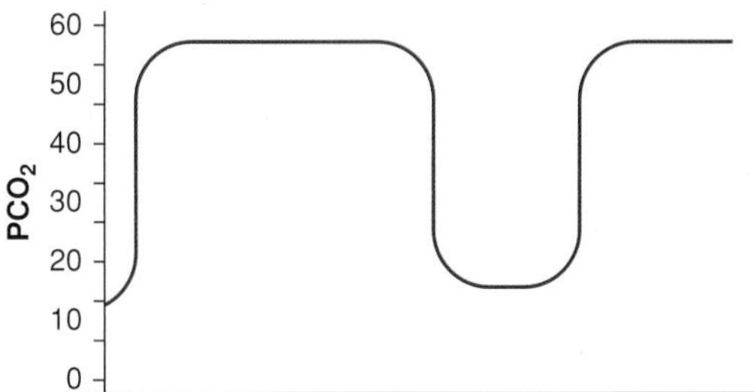

FIGURE 23.11 Incompetent expiratory valve leads to rebreathing of CO_2 in this time-based capnogram from a patient breathing from a circle system. Observe that the capnogram does not return to baseline during inspiration. Either an exhausted CO_2 absorber allows exhaled gas to return to the patient during inspiration or an expiratory valve stuck in the open position lets exhaled gas be admixed to the inspired gas during inspiration, indicating the presence of CO_2 in the inspired gas. High fresh gas flow can compensate for an exhausted CO_2 absorber but not for rebreathing through a faulty expiratory valve.

b. **Incompetent expiratory valve:** An incompetent expiratory valve will lead to rebreathing of the CO_2 deposited in the expiratory limb of the breathing circuit.

The two conditions described above, however, can be distinguished by simply raising the fresh gas flow to exceed minute ventilation: That will prevent rebreathing owing to an exhausted carbon dioxide absorber, but will not prevent rebreathing through a defective (stuck in the open position) expiratory valve. Whether an exhausted CO_2 absorber or a defective valve causes rebreathing of CO_2, the effect resembles the addition of dead space, which calls for an increase of minute ventilation lest CO_2 retention leads to rising $PACO_2$, $PaCO_2$, and $PetCO_2$ (Fig. 23.11).

c. **Incompetent inspiratory valve:** Malfunction of the inspiratory valve generates a typical capnogram (Fig. 23.12).

3. **Abnormal capnograms with normal production of CO_2**

Hyperventilation

Anxious people, and more often patients with central nervous system injuries, can hyperventilate to the point of inducing tetany; in healthy volunteers, a drop by 20 mmHg $PetCO_2$ induced tingling and tetany manifested by increased axonal excitability, presumably owing to reduced ionized calcium (116).

In the clinical setting, patients with an acute increase of intracranial pressure can be treated with transient hyperventilation in order to decrease cerebral blood flow known to fall with decreased $PaCO_2$. The capnogram will first briefly show increased and then decreased $PetCO_2$, eventually leading to reduced CO_2 tissue stores. However, be careful when observing an abnormally low $PetCO_2$; be sure that the low $PetCO_2$ is due to hyperventilation and not to other circumstances. For example, very low tidal volumes can show low $PetCO_2$ even though $PaCO_2$ is elevated due to CO_2 diffused into dead space (V_D). A mistaken diagnosis of hyperventilation and the decision to reduce minute ventilation would harm the patient.

Hypoventilation

Three clinical circumstances can lead to hypoventilation: drug- or disease-induced depression of the respiratory center, drug- or disease-induced muscle weakness, and airway obstruction. With the onset of hypoventilation, less CO_2 appears in the exhaled gas, CO_2 accumulates in the tissues, and venous PCO_2 rises. Eventually, the retained CO_2 levels reach a new equilibrium after renal compensation has reached its peak, a very low process taking days. There will be higher than normal levels of body stores of carbon dioxide, $PaCO_2$, $PACO_2$, and $PetCO_2$. Once a new steady state has been reached, and assuming unchanged metabolism, the amount of CO_2 exhaled per minute will be the same as before the perturbation; however, the end-expired values will be

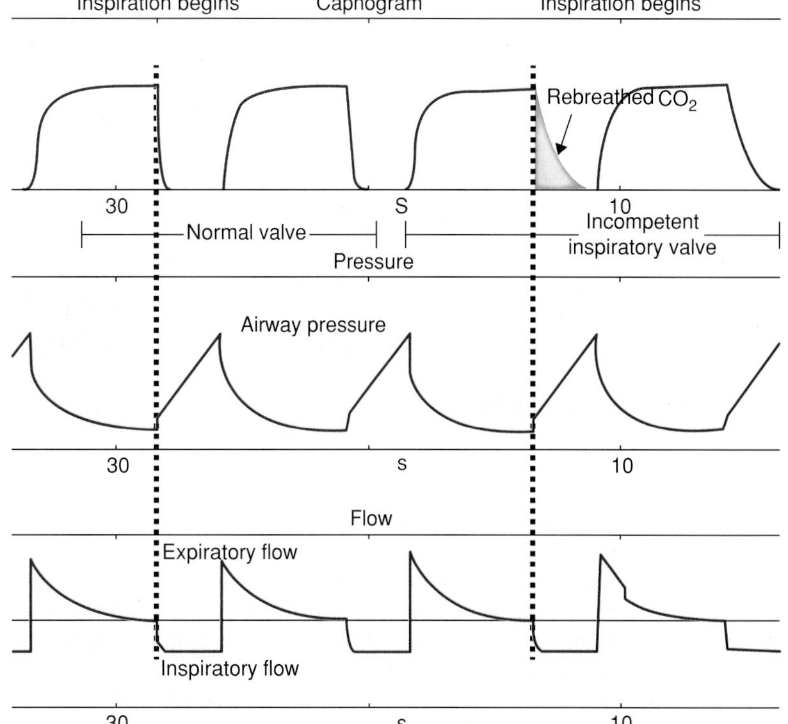

FIGURE 23.12 Illustration of the difference between normally functioning and incompetent inspiratory valves. Note that the CO_2 tracing in the normal capnogram rapidly drops to baseline at the start of inspiration (marked by increase in airway pressure (**center tracing**) and inspiratory flow (**bottom tracing**)). When the inspiratory valve is incompetent, exhaled CO_2 from the previous breath enters the inspiratory limb of the circle breathing system, and is rebreathed at the next breath. The presence of CO_2 in the inspiratory limb is evident from the widened capnogram (*shaded area*). (Generated with BreathSim software from Goldman JM, Ward DR, Daniel L. BreathSim, a mathematical model-based simulation of the anesthesia breathing circuit, may facilitate testing and evaluation of respiratory gas monitoring equipment. *Biomed Sci Instrum.* 1996;32:293–298.)

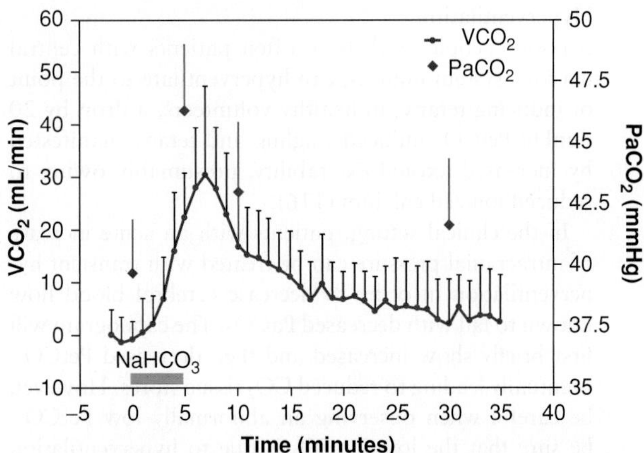

FIGURE 23.13 Time course of the changes in VCO_2 (ΔVCO_2) and $PaCO_2$ in 16 artificially ventilated critically ill patients during and after the infusion of 1.5 mmol/kg sodium bicarbonate over 5 minutes. (Reproduced with permission from Levraut J, Garcia P, Jiunti C, et al. The increase in CO_2 production induced by $NaHCO_3$ is affected by blood albumin and hemoglobin concentrations. *Intensive Care Med.* 2000;26:558.)

elevated. Instituting hyperventilation at this point will bring end-tidal values back toward "normal," at which point continued hyperventilation will result in respiratory alkalosis. In patients with elevated $PetCO_2$ on mechanical ventilation, clinicians should resist the temptation to increase minute ventilation without first going through a differential diagnosis of an elevated $PetCO_2$ lest they delay the treatment of an underlying process.

4. **Abnormal capnograms with increased production of CO_2**
Exogenous CO_2 Production
Bicarbonate infusion: Bicarbonate infused in the treatment of metabolic acidosis will dissociate under most clinical conditions (carbonic anhydrase being available) and directly liberate a nonmetabolic CO_2 load, about 1 L/50 mmol (Fig. 23.13).

Carbon dioxide insufflation: CO_2 insufflation during laparoscopic, thoracoscopic, vein harvest, and other operative procedures imposes extra respiratory excretion of many extra liters (at times >40 L in adults) of CO_2. Cardiac output and buffering capacity of blood will influence the rate of gas release. The blood carries much of the gas to the lungs, where increased ventilation is needed to maintain normal arterial gas values. Fortunately, after releasing the gas from the abdominal cavity, arterial blood gas values return toward normal over about an hour (117). Some surgeons like to flood the surgical field with CO_2. In case of venous aspiration of gas, the aspirate would be readily absorbed CO_2 rather than air containing close to 80% of poorly absorbed nitrogen (118).
Endogenous CO_2 Production
Shivering, as seen in patients with severe nervous system injuries or when emerging from anesthesia, can double the consumption of oxygen and thus the production of CO_2. Fever triggered by the liberation of pyrogens from infectious agents, toxins, or inflammation is the most common cause of increased CO_2 production.

Much rarer is malignant hyperthermia (MH), an autosomal dominant inherited disorder of skeletal muscle that sends CO_2 production into overdrive. In susceptible patients, halothane—and, to a lesser degree, other halogenated anesthetics—and succinylcholine can trigger the syndrome. A rising $PetCO_2$ provides the first warning many minutes before increasing blood or body temperature can be detected. The first impulse may be to increase ventilation, but unless there is other reason to suspect increased metabolic rate, MH should be considered. While the syndrome arises usually during anesthesia, it sometimes becomes manifest hours later, for instance, after arrival in the ICU. MH is often fatal condition if not detected promptly and vigorously with dantrolene, cooling, and fluids. Of course, in the treatment of MH, increasing minute ventilation becomes necessary, together with appropriate treatment of fever, hyperkalemia, and arrhythmias. If suspected, because of the immediately life-threatening nature of MH and a complex treatment regimen, assistance of an anesthesiologist or the Malignant Hyperthermia Association of the United States (www.mhaus.org) should be enlisted immediately.

Rarely, the neuroleptic malignant syndrome (NMS) is triggered by neuroleptic drugs such as prochlorperazine (Compazine), promethazine (Phenergan), clozapine (Clozaril), and risperidone (Risperdal). It is not the same syndrome as MH, but may have associated fever and increased metabolic rate. NMS has also been associated with nonneuroleptic agents that block central dopamine pathways (e.g., metoclopramide [Reglan], amoxapine [Asendin], and lithium) (119).

Severe cases of serotonin syndrome have also been reported to present with fever exceeding 41°C (120).

High metabolic activity with hyperthyroidism can become symptomatic after infection or trauma to the thyroid gland. Tachycardia, markedly increased O_2 consumption and CO_2 production, and raised body temperature characterize the syndrome. Muscle wasting in elderly hyperthyroid men can affect breathing and generate abnormal capnography.

5. **Abnormal capnograms with reduced production of CO_2**
If production of CO_2 is low, disproportionate ("normal") ventilation will represent hyperventilation. Numerous conditions can lead to a decrease of CO_2 production. Currently, the most common circumstance is iatrogenically decreased body temperature (e.g., as induced during cardiopulmonary bypass). Submersion in cold water, hypothyroidism, low muscle mass, and several mitochondrial diseases also decrease metabolism (121). Often the clinician will need to consider arterial blood gas values in order to correctly interpret normal and low $PetCO_2$.

CAPNOGRAPHY: CLINICAL APPLICATIONS

Obstructive Lung Diseases

Many patients with chronic obstructive pulmonary disease (COPD), including asthma, show typical capnographic features that include a slowly rising concentration of CO_2 in the expired tidal volume and alteration of the slopes of phase III; Figure 23.14 shows diagrammatically how impedance to air flow in sequential areas of the lungs contributes to uneven emptying of the lungs. Severe V/Q mismatch in patients with obstructive lung diseases will also cause CO_2 release, first from the high V/Q alveolar unit (low CO_2), and last from low V/Q alveolar units (high CO_2), contributing to the upsloping shape

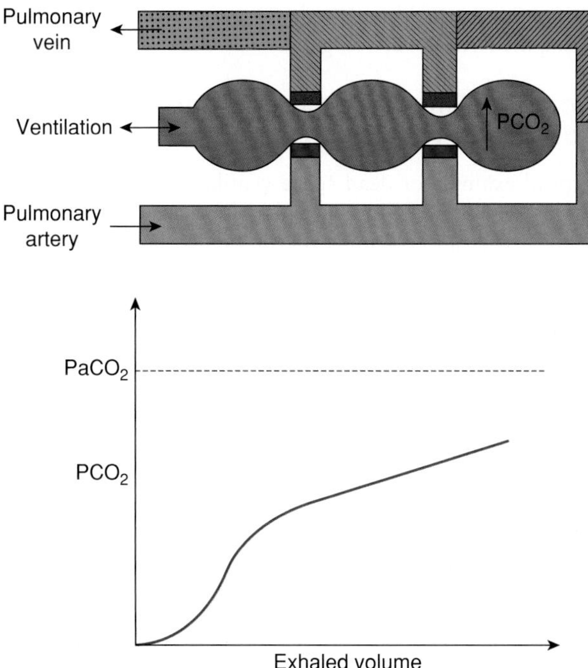

FIGURE 23.14 Diagram of ventilation/perfusion mismatch (i.e., chronic obstructive pulmonary disease) and the resulting volume-based capnogram. The diagram shows the narrowed air passages resulting in decreased ventilation of distal alveoli. (Reproduced with permission from Anderson JT. In Gravenstein JS, Jaffe MB, Paulus DA, eds. *Capnography: Clinical Aspects*. Cambridge: Cambridge University Press; 2004:192.)

of phase III (122). For these reasons, single values of $PetCO_2$ have proven unreliable as differential diagnosis indices in patients with obstructive disease compared to restrictive lung disease (123). When $PetCO_2$ differs from $PaCO_2$ because of V/Q mismatching, changes in the $PetCO_2$ may be seen with a corresponding increase, decrease, or no change in $PaCO_2$. In these cases, a direct measurement of dead space ventilation with volumetric capnography can be useful to predict the relationship between $PaCO_2$ and $PetCO_2$.

$PetCO_2$ during weaning from mechanical ventilation has been used with success to prevent dangerous, and frequently unrecognized, hypercapnia in patients with increased dead space ventilation (124). Unfortunately, in many cases, relevant hypercapnic episodes (increases of $PetCO_2$ of greater than 3 mmHg) can only be detected with a sensitivity of 82% and a specificity of 76%, making arterial sampling during weaning a frequent necessity. Despite these limitations, capnography may substantially reduce the number of arterial blood gas analyses necessary during weaning from mechanical ventilations (125). One can describe the degree of flattening by reporting an α angle as shown in Figure 23.15.

Ventilation/Perfusion Mismatch

In healthy individuals, the ventilation-to-perfusion ratio comes close to 1:1. Under the influence of gravity, the lower lungs are favored with perfusion over ventilation as compared to the upper lungs. Any pathologic condition that disturbs this balance can result in a mismatch. Under physiologic conditions, we expect the arterial CO_2 tension to be 3 to 5 mmHg higher than the end-tidal CO_2 tension. In general, neither end-tidal nor arterial CO_2 can exceed venous PCO_2. A conspiracy of ventilation–perfusion inequalities can raise or decrease arterial to alveolar PCO_2 differences depending on the patient's disease, position, ventilatory pattern and pulmonary perfusion pressure, and flow. Acute respiratory distress syndrome (ARDS) is an example of severe V/Q scatter. Low lung compliance and an increase in resistance imply longer time constants and sequential CO_2 emptying, resulting in a steeper rising slope of phase III of a time-based capnogram. Such a ventilatory disturbance in ARDS can be monitored with a real-time capnograph. However, when a significantly widened $PaCO_2$–$PetCO_2$ difference is observed, it is likely that coexisting significant dead space ventilation occurs. In these cases, direct measurement of dead space ventilation with volumetric capnography confirms the suspected diagnosis.

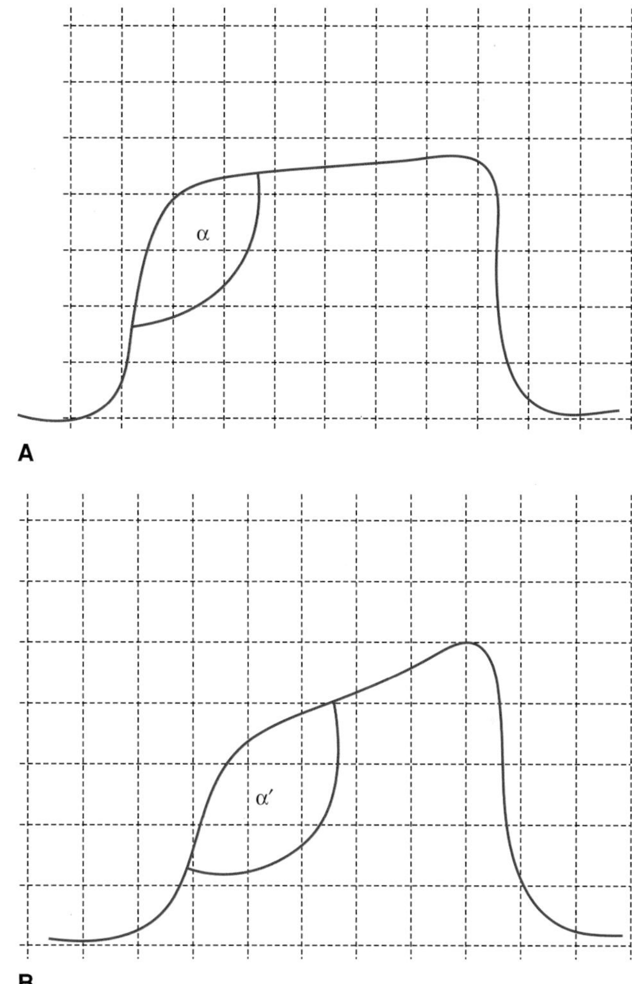

FIGURE 23.15 **A**: Normal capnogram showing α of 105 degrees. **B**: Capnogram during acute bronchospasm showing α of 140 degrees.

Recent reports in pediatric populations suggest that a dead space volume-to-tidal volume (V_D/V_T) ratio of 60% is a critical ratio for lack of reliability of $PetCO_2$ in patients with increased extravascular lung water (126). In this subset of patients with a particularly poor prognosis, a V_D/V_T ratio more than 65% identifies patients at risk for respiratory failure following extubation (126). This observation mirrors University of Florida experience in adult ARDS patients, whereas a V_D/V_T ratio more than 60% identifies patients with grave pulmonary dysfunction (127) and increased risk of death (128).

The $PaCO_2$–$PetCO_2$ difference in ARDS patients has recently found another interesting application. It has been

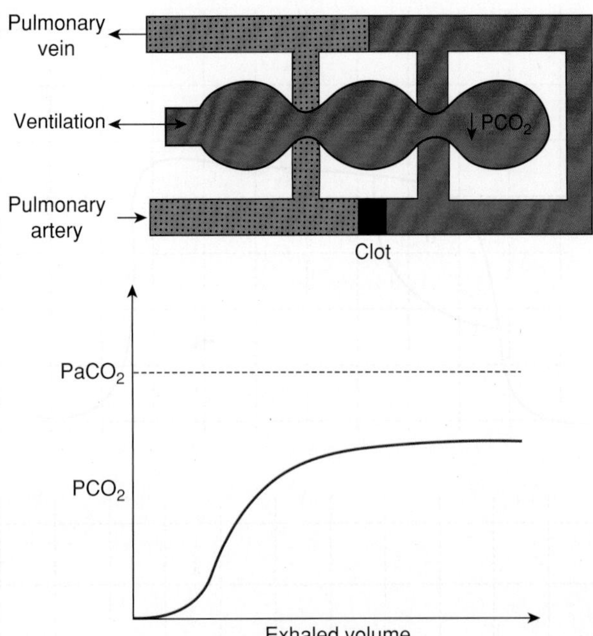

FIGURE 23.16 Diagram of ventilation/perfusion mismatch (i.e., chronic obstructive pulmonary disease) secondary to a clot (pulmonary embolus) on ventilated but not perfused alveoli and volume-based capnogram. (Reproduced with permission from Anderson JT. In Gravenstein JS, Jaffe MB, Paulus DA, eds. *Capnography: Clinical Aspects.* Cambridge: Cambridge University Press; 2004:192.)

theorized that the narrowing of this difference, while positive end-inspiratory pressure is applied, indicates the best possible recruitment of unstable alveoli without overdistension (129). In other words, calculating the V_D/V_T ratio in patients with a wide $PaCO_2$–$PetCO_2$ difference could be strategically useful to optimize positive end-expiratory pressure, thereby limiting promotion of excessive "West zone 1" in the lung.

Bronchial Intubation as an Example of a Shunt

With intubation of, usually, the right, mainstem bronchus, a classic example of a large shunt develops: one lung is perfused but not ventilated. About half of the cardiac output is shunted past the lung, and its desaturated blood is mixed with the saturated blood coming from the other lung. The mixing effect of the shunt is more pronounced for oxygen (46 mmHg PO_2 venous blood into 100 mmHg PO_2 arterial blood) than for CO_2 (46 mmHg PCO_2 venous blood into 40 mmHg PCO_2 arterial blood). The initial reduction of exhaled CO_2 results in a reduced $PetCO_2$ value until the system comes back into equilibrium. A partial and variable compensation for such a large shunt is caused by hypoxic pulmonary vasoconstriction, limiting the $PaCO_2$–$PetCO_2$ gap.

Pulmonary Embolism as an Example of Dead Space Ventilation

A typical example of dead space ventilation occurs when an embolus blocks perfusion such that lung tissue is ventilated but not perfused. Depending on the tidal volume of the nonperfused lung segment, the dead space being ventilated can substantially dilute the $PetCO_2$, leading to large differences between $PaCO_2$ and $PetCO_2$ (Fig. 23.16). In the same patient, the plateau of the CO_2 volume capnograph flattens (130). If the patient's respiratory drive is intact, alveolar hypoxia and increased alveolar dead space will result in increased minute ventilation with resultant low end-tidal PCO_2 values.

With ablation of this compensation, as in a patient who is chemically paralyzed, heavily sedated, or anesthetized, the $PaCO_2$ always increases from baseline, and the (a-ET)PCO_2 gap widens (131). The pulmonary artery angiogram, spiral chest computerized tomography, and scintillation V/Q lung scan remain the gold standards for diagnosing pulmonary embolism. Unfortunately, while capnography has the advantage of being noninvasive and practical at the bedside, it lacks specificity (132).

Low Cardiac Output State

Hemorrhagic shock represents the extreme of reduced pulmonary blood flow without, in this example, disturbance of lung function (Table 23.3). The reduced alveolar blood flow will prevent the matching of CO_2 elimination with systemic CO_2 production. As a result, $PetCO_2$ will decrease while the mixed venous PCO_2 will continue to increase (133). Positive pressure ventilation will enlarge the areas of the lungs receiving more ventilation than perfusion, which will exaggerate the impact of low perfusion pressure to the dependent areas of the lungs (134). However, if ventilation is maintained constant, the percent decrease in $PetCO_2$ directly correlated with the percent decrease in cardiac output ($r^2 = 0.82$) (135).

Cardiac Arrest

While capnography is well established as a tool to confirm correct endotracheal intubation (136–139), it has garnered growing interest in the interpretation of low blood flow states, primarily because of the difficulty in directly measuring low rates of blood flow, particularly during human cardiac arrest and resuscitation. It is much easier to measure end-tidal CO_2 as evidence of pulmonary blood flow than direct measurements of cardiac output.

With sudden cardiac standstill, the capnogram shows quickly vanishing CO_2 levels in the exhaled gas. Thus, continued ventilation will wash the CO_2 out of the unperfused

TABLE 23.3 Effect of Hemorrhagic Shock and Reduced Pulmonary Blood Flow on the Elimination of Carbon Dioxide

	Control → Shock Tissue	Control → Shock Venous	Control → Shock Arterial	Control → Shock $PetCO_2$
$PetCO_2$				38 → 15
PCO_2	50 → 120	45 → 96	40 → 25	
PO_2	45 → 10	40 → 15	97 → 300	
SO_2	65 → 15	70 → 20	99 → 99	

Modified from Ward KR. The basis for capnometric monitoring in shock. In: Gravenstein JS, Jaffe MB, Paulus DA, eds. *Capnography: Clinical Aspects.* Cambridge: Cambridge University Press; 2004:223–228.

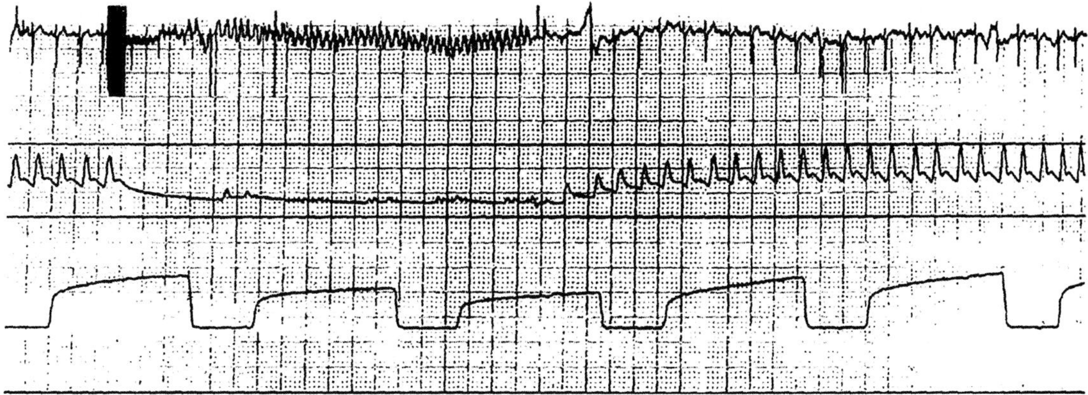

FIGURE 23.17 A patient undergoing the implantation of an automatic internal cardiac defibrillator was monitored with electrocardiogram (ECG; **top**), radial artery pressure (**middle**), and mainstream capnography (**bottom**). Induced ventricular fibrillation (*black area* in ECG) and defibrillation are apparent in the ECG tracing. Observe decay of arterial pressure. During absent pulmonary blood flow, the patient's lungs were ventilated and with two breaths the end-tidal PCO_2 fell from 35 mmHg before fibrillation to 22 mmHg.

lungs. After only a few breaths without alveolar perfusion, there will be very little CO_2 in exhaled breath (Fig. 23.17). Conversely, with re-establishment of circulation, the reappearance of capnograms provides welcome evidence of pulmonary perfusion. Amplitude of capnograms often improves dramatically with return of spontaneous circulation (ROSC) (140–142). Colorimetric changes of chemical indicators that detect exhaled CO_2 are not as reliable, do not distinguish gastric intubation well, deteriorate with even a small number of breaths, and are being displaced even for prehospital interventions (136,138,139,143,144).

During cardiac arrest, CO_2 will have accumulated in tissue and, because of acidosis development during shock and arrest, the addition of hydrogen ions will cause bicarbonate to be converted to CO_2. A number of recent studies have shown that $PetCO_2$ varies directly with cardiac output during cardiac arrest (145,146) and provides a useful indicator of the efficacy of resuscitation efforts. The relative effect of pharmacologic intervention during cardiopulmonary resuscitation (CPR) can also be assessed by the $PetCO_2$. For example, following the administration of epinephrine, the prior relationships of end-tidal CO_2 may be altered due to the changes in pulmonary and peripheral vascular resistance and preferential redirection of blood flow (147). In some instances, epinephrine may decrease pulmonary blood flow and end-tidal CO_2, while at the same time coronary perfusion pressure increases because of increased peripheral vascular resistance (148).

Investigators have used end-tidal CO_2 as a substitute for the measurement of blood flow in studies of CPR techniques (149,150). Because end-tidal CO_2 is directly related to cardiac output when minute ventilation is held constant, it is a useful tool for bedside real-time evaluation of effectiveness of chest compression. Unfortunately, if ventilation is not constant in any low state, including cardiac arrest, then end-tidal CO_2 levels are not helpful to assess cardiac output (142).

CAPNOGRAPHY STANDARDS IN THE INTENSIVE CARE UNIT

The American Association of Respiratory Care (AARC) strongly recommends the use of capnography in patients who are mechanically ventilated in the intensive care unit (ICU). However, when capnography is used as an indirect monitor of $PaCO_2$ in the critically ill patient, one has to consider limitations that can affect the accuracy of this technology, as listed below:

- The composition of the respiratory gas mixture may affect the capnogram, such as the use of high O_2 concentrations in critically ill patients (151).
- The breathing frequency may alter the slope of phase III and the $PetCO_2$ measured value (152).
- The presence of Freon, used as a propellant in metered-dose inhalers, can cause an transient increase of the $PetCO_2$ readings (153).
- Contamination of the monitor or sampling system by secretions or condensate, a sample tube of excessive length, a sampling rate that is too high, or obstruction of the sampling chamber can lead to distorted capnograms or erroneous measured concentrations.
- Use of filters can lead to falsely low $PetCO_2$ readings (154).
- Small tidal volume delivery, especially in neonates and pediatric patients, with low continuous flow rates that leak into the ventilator circuit, around the tracheal tube cuffs, or as a result of uncuffed tubes can result in a factitiously low $PetCO_2$ value (155).
- A low cardiac output state may result in an artificially low $PetCO_2$ value.
- In the presence of a carbonated beverage in the stomach, one may see several breaths with a factitiously elevated $PetCO_2$ value (156).
- Sampling exhaled breaths at any point in the breathing circuit where there is fresh gas flow (e.g., proximal to the dead space within the endotracheal tube) will produce dilution of the alveolar gas sample and distortion of the capnogram. Therefore, caution must apply to interpretation of the same $PetCO_2$ relative to PaO_2 as a true representation of the A-a gradient.

MONITORING FOR HYPOVENTILATION

Preventing patients from deteriorating to the point that intensive care is needed should be a major effort to improve the quality and safety of care for hospitalized patients. For patients who do not benefit from high nurse or physician to patient ratios in ICU settings, it is particularly important to provide suitable monitoring to prevent catastrophic outcomes (157). In many clinical circumstances, such as treatment of severe postoperative of nonsurgical pain with opioid analgesics, physiologic deterioration is often detectable for a period of time before severe and life-threatening deterioration (158). Periodic manual recording of SpO_2 is insufficient, and may be biased to higher values than are physiologically occurring for undisturbed patients, perhaps because of simple interaction and awakening of patients, or encouraging deep breaths (159). Failure-to-Rescue (FtR) includes a distressing proportion of preventable deaths, the end result of failure to detect deterioration and intervene while there is opportunity, before terminal events occur (157,160).

Given what has come before in this chapter, detection of hemoglobin desaturation as evidence of hypoventilation (161), and interruption of capnography or increasing $PetCO_2$ (162) would be expected signs of deterioration well before onset of catastrophic, life-threatening events (101,163). The characteristics of capnograms of nonintubated patient still provide useful information, though they frequently do not even approximate the normal characteristics of capnograms previously described (101,105). However, monitoring of pulse oximetry and capnography have not been as effective as hoped for prevention deaths during hospitalization. Their signals, alarm thresholds, and patterns of abnormality have not been integrated to become synergistic and more effective. Curry and Lynn (163) characterize three patterns of unexpected hospital death (PUHD), wherein conventional alarm settings for pulse oximetry or capnometry may produce alarm fatigue and may not avert FtR. The astute clinician should recognize patterns that might not evoke alarms. Type I, schematically represented in Figure 23.18, is characteristic of shock, microvascular circulatory failure of various causes. Type I progresses insidiously

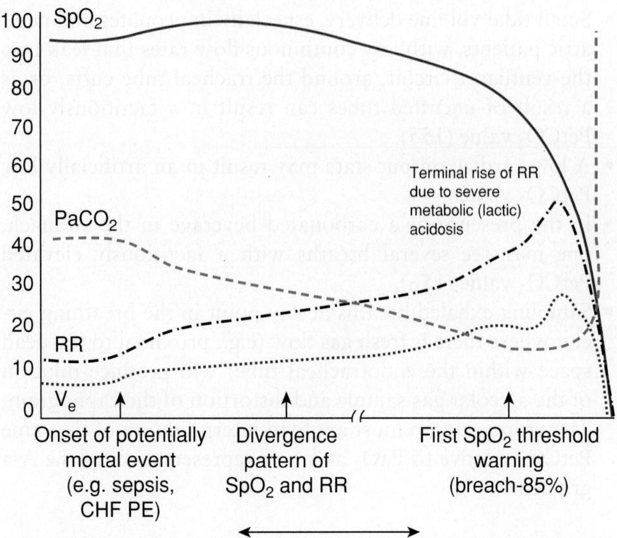

FIGURE 23.18 Type I pattern of unexpected hospital death. SpO_2, pulse oximetric oxyhemoglobin saturation; $PaCO_2$, arterial CO_2 concentration; V_e, minute ventilation; RR, respiratory rate. (Reproduced with permission from Curry JP, Lynn LA. Threshold monitoring, alarm fatigue, and the patterns of unexpected hospital death. *APSF Newslett.* 2011;26:33-35.) http://apsf.org/newsletters/pdf/fall_2011.pdf. Originally Published in Patterns of unexpected in-hospital deaths: a root cause analysis. Lynn LA, Curry JP. *Patient Saf Surg.* 2011 Feb 11;5(1):3.)

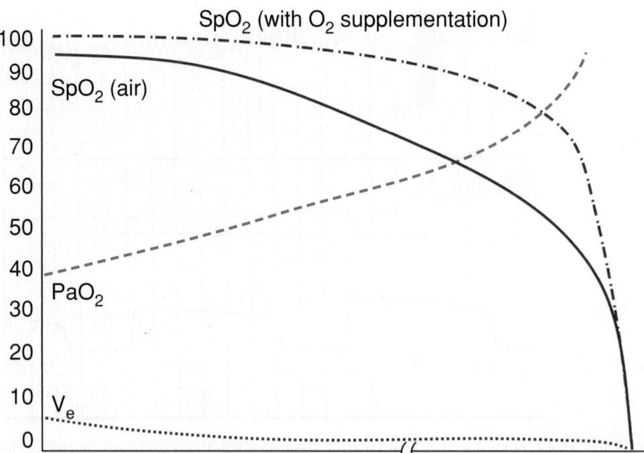

FIGURE 23.19 Type II pattern of unexpected hospital death. (Reproduced with permission from Curry JP, Lynn LA. Threshold monitoring, alarm fatigue, and the patterns of unexpected hospital death. *APSF Newslett.* 2011;26:33-35.) http://www.apsf.org/newsletters/pdf/fall_2011.pdf. Originally Published in Patterns of unexpected in-hospital deaths: a root cause analysis. Lynn LA, Curry JP. *Patient Saf Surg.* 2011 Feb 11;5(1):3.)

for extended periods before final precipitous decline in SpO_2, but often goes undetected because increasing hyperventilation, while below respiratory rate alarm thresholds, also maintains SpO_2 above alarm thresholds. Type II diagrammed in Figure 23.19 is perhaps most frequently due to opioid administration or other causes of hypoventilation, including changes in respiratory drive with aging and sleep (10). Increasing CO_2 contributes to narcosis, while supplemental oxygen can defer detection of hypoventilation by delaying recognition of respiratory deterioration as SpO_2 desaturation. Type III, illustrated in Figure 23.20, is due to airway obstruction and apnea. PCO_2 gradually increases contributing to narcosis, blunted respiratory response, eventually with SpO_2 decreasing below the "Lights out Saturation" where brain function ceases, and death follows without timely resuscitation.

Many patients do not tolerate oxygen masks, nasal cannulae, or sampling devices designed to improve capnography.

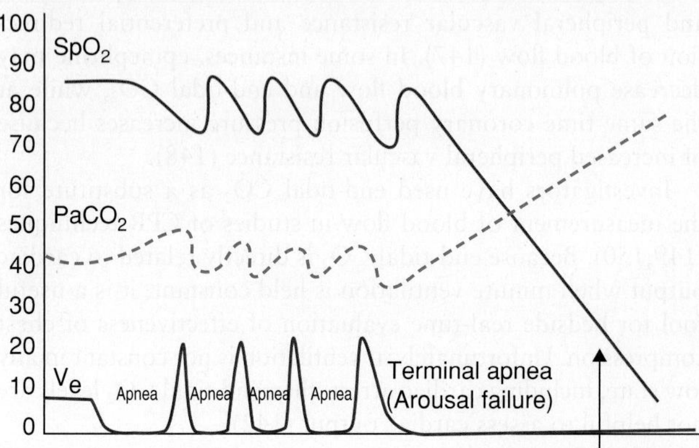

FIGURE 23.20 Type III pattern of unexpected hospital death. (Reproduced with permission from Curry JP, Lynn LA. Threshold monitoring, alarm fatigue, and the patterns of unexpected hospital death. *APSF Newslett.* 2011;26:33-35.) http://www.apsf.org/newsletters/pdf/fall_2011.pdf. Originally Published in Patterns of unexpected in-hospital deaths: a root cause analysis. Lynn LA, Curry JP. *Patient Saf Surg.* 2011 Feb 11;5(1):3.)

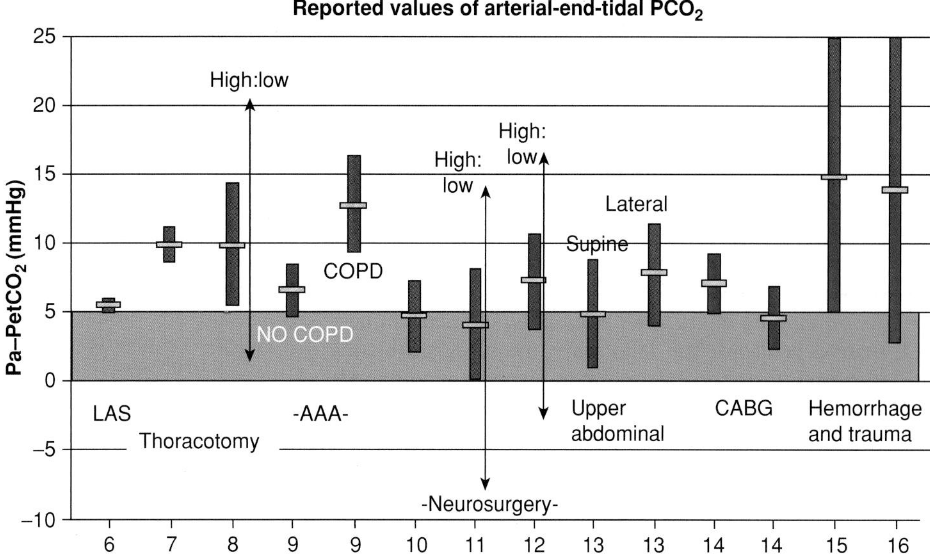

FIGURE 23.21 Intraoperative values of the arterial–end-tidal PCO_2 differences. The means ± standard deviation of the differences reported in 12 different articles are shown as vertical bars. The numbers on the horizontal axis are the references. The stippled area is the presumed "normal" value of 0 to 5 mmHg. The surgical procedure is identified. Note that surgical position, major diseases, and unstable cardiovascular status increase the difference. Note also the reported high and low values (*arrows*). COPD, chronic obstructive pulmonary disease; LAS, lower abdominal surgery; AAA, abdominal aortic aneurysmectomy; CABG, coronary artery bypass grafting. (Reproduced with permission from Wahba RWM, Tessler MJ. Misleading end-tidal CO_2 tensions: brief review. *Can J Anaesth.* 1996;43:862.)

For this reason, and to address the shortcomings of pulse oximetry and capnometry, alternative respiratory monitors are being developed. Devices to detect gas flow at the nostrils suffer the same intolerance as other devices positioned on the face. Acoustical devices to detect or characterize laryngotracheal gas flow have been developed (164,165), as have chest impedance monitors (166,167). Each has advantages, disadvantages, and differing ability to detect respiratory compromise. Any of them are superior to absence of monitoring for patients at increased risk, particularly to prevent some patients from needing intensive care (168). Further attention to human factors such as alarm tone characteristics may improve responsiveness of clinicians to deteriorating conditions (17). Wisdom to select and apply new and old monitoring technologies requires sophisticated understanding of the technologies themselves, underlying physiology and pathophysiology, and limitations in clinical application (169).

REVERSAL OF THE $PaCO_2$–$PetCO_2$ DIFFERENCE

A $PetCO_2$ higher than $PaCO_2$ or "reversed gradient" has been occasionally observed in pregnant and obese patients (170,171). The mechanisms for the reversals remain to be elucidated. However, this phenomenon has been appreciated only when phase III has a steep slope or when a terminal "step-up knee" of the waveform is present. As seen in Figure 23.21, a host of circumstances can be associated with large arterial to alveolar PCO_2 differences, rarely attributable to a single mechanism (171).

CONFIRMATION OF BRAIN DEATH

The diagnosis of brain death must meet many conditions, one of which is the unresponsiveness of the brainstem to rising CO_2 tensions in the absence of drug effects (172). In 2006, the Stroke Service of the Massachusetts General Hospital (173) presented a detailed description of apnea testing (most recently updated in 2011). Key features include, but are not limited to, criteria for body temperature and blood pressures, and call for an arterial pH of 7.35 to 7.45, preoxygenation, and a $PaCO_2$ of 35 to 45 mmHg for at least 20 minutes prior to discontinuation of mechanical ventilation. Higher PCO_2 thresholds may be appropriate if the patient was previously known to have chronically increased and compensated PCO_2. After discontinuation of ventilation, apnea is said to exist if $PaCO_2$ increases from 40 up to 60 mmHg, or a 20 mmHg or greater increase from the pretest baseline. Establishing normocapnia employing capnography prior to initiation of an apnea test can shorten the necessary time for evaluation and facilitate monitoring the course in increasing CO_2 (174).

CAPNOGRAPHY AND RESPIRATORY SUMMARY

The attention of physiologists and physicians has been recently focused on time and volume capnography to monitor the dynamics of CO_2 in critically ill patients as the result of respiratory and/or cardiovascular derangement. Therefore, capnographic features need to be interpreted in view of the clinician's knowledge of either factor. Despite its limitations, capnography can provide significant and clinically useful information, and may often allow life-saving diagnostic and therapeutic alterations. As capnographic technology improves and clinical experience of the intensivist accumulates, we anticipate more widespread use of this monitoring modality in the future.

Key Points

- The oxygen reserve index has extended the utility of pulse oximetry to reflect qualitatively changes in PaO_2 above the plateau of oxyhemoglobin saturation at about 100 torr, useful as a harbinger of deterioration or improvement in oxygenation not detectable by conventional pulse oximetry.

- Noninvasive measurement of hemoglobin concentration has utility, but has confounding factors do permit if to be a reliable alternative to laboratory measurements.
- New developments in measuring mitochondrial oxygen tension are changing concepts of oxidative metabolism in cells, and its sensitivity to pathophysiological states. Though not available for monitoring clinically, this raises hope of measuring oxygen utilization in tissue, rather than being limited to assessment of SaO_2 being delivered by blood.
- Assessing lung injury severity by pulse oximetry rather than dependence on laboratory measures of blood oxygenation is satisfactory, more expedient, noninvasive, and more amenable to trending change.
- Photoplethysmography complements EKG for evaluation of arrhythmias and their effect on cardiac output and evaluates interaction of respiration and cardiac filling, cardiac output and vascular elasticity in balance with peripheral perfusion (peripheral resistance).
- Advances in plethysmography improve targeted therapy for effective cardiovascular resuscitation, avoiding under- or overtreatment extremes.
- Incorporation of capnography in CPR protocols improves reliable determination of effective ventilation and resuscitative support of circulation.
- Widespread use of capnography and other monitors of respiratory function can provide early warning of respiratory deterioration before onset of catastrophic cardiopulmonary failures.
- Better integration of individual monitors into functional systems will be necessary to improve upon the insufficient performance of individual monitors with threshold alarms.

ACKNOWLEDGMENTS

The author thanks Johannes H. Van Oostrom, Brian Fuehrlein, Richard J. Melker, Michael B. Jaffe, David A. Paulus (deceased), and Joachim S. Gravenstein (deceased) for their contributions to the previous edition of this chapter.

References

1. Ehrenfeld JM, Cannesson M, eds. *Monitoring Technologies in Acute Care Environments*. New York, NY: Springer; 2014.
2. Collins J-A, Rudenski A, Gibson J, et al. Relating oxygen partial pressure, saturation and content: the haemoglobin–oxygen dissociation curve. *Breathe (Sheff)*. 2015;11:194–201
3. Nunn JF. *Applied Respiratory Physiology*. Boston, MA: Butterworths; 1977.
4. Carreau A, El Hafny-Rahbi B, Matejuk A, et al. Why is the partial oxygen pressure of human tissues a crucial parameter? Small molecules and hypoxia. *J Cell Mol Med*. 2011;15:1239–1253.
5. Mik EG. Measuring mitochondrial oxygen tension: from basic principles to application in humans. *Anesth Analg*. 2013;117:834–846.
6. Harms FA, Bodmer SI, Raat NJ, Mik EG. Non-invasive monitoring of mitochondrial oxygenation and respiration in critical illness using a novel technique. *Crit Care*. 2015;19:343.
7. Stokes G. On the reduction oxygenation of the colouring matter of the blood. *Philosoph Mag*. 1864;28:391.
8. Hoppe-Seyler F. Uber die chemischen und optischen Eigenschaffen des Blutfarbstoffs. *Arch Pathol Anat Physiol*. 1864;29:233–251.
9. Bert P. *La Pression Barométrique*. Paris: Masson;1878.
10. Severinghaus JW. High life: high altitude fatalities led to pulse oximetry. *J Appl Physiol*. 2016;120:236–243.
11. Hertzman A. Photoelectric plethysmography of the fingers and toes in man. *Proc Soc Exp Biol Med*. 1937;37:529.
12. Squire JR. Instrument for measuring quantity of blood and its degree of oxygenation in the web of the hand. *Clin Sci*. 1940;4:331–339.
13. Millikan G, Papenheimer J, Rawson A. Continuous measurement of oxygen saturation in man. *Am J Physiol*. 1941;133:390.
14. Goldie E. Device for continuous indication of oxygen saturation of circulating blood in man. *J Sci Instrument*. 1942;19:390.
15. Wood EH, Geraci JE. Photoelectric determination of arterial oxygen saturation in man. *J Lab Clin Med*. 1949;34:387–401.
16. Aoyagi T. Pulse oximetry: its invention, theory, and future. *J Anesth*. 2003; 17:259–266.
17. Paterson E, Sanderson PM, Paterson NA, et al. The effectiveness of pulse oximetry sonification enhanced with tremolo and brightness for distinguishing clinically important oxygen saturation ranges: a laboratory study. *Anaesthesia*. 2016;71:565–572.
18. Hinckfuss K, Sanderson P, Loeb RG, et al. Novel pulse oximetry sonifications for neonatal oxygen saturation monitoring: a laboratory study. *Hum Factors*. 2016;58:344–359.
19. Alian AA, Shelley KH. Photoplethysmography: analysis of the pulse oximetry waveform. In: Ehrenfeld JM, Cannesson M, eds. *Monitoring Technologies in Acute Care Environments*. New York, NY: Springer New York; 2014:165–178.
20. Zonios G, Shankar U, Iyer VK. Pulse oximetry theory and calibration for low saturations. *IEEE Trans Biomed Eng*. 2004;51:818–822.
21. Lima AP, Beelen P, Bakker J. Use of a peripheral perfusion index derived from the pulse oximetry signal as a noninvasive indicator of perfusion. *Crit Care Med*. 2002;30:1210–1213.
22. Severinghaus JW, Naifeh KH, Koh SO. Errors in 14 pulse oximeters during profound hypoxia. *J Clin Monit*. 1989;5:72–81.
23. Severinghaus JW, Naifeh KH. Accuracy of response of six pulse oximeters to profound hypoxia. *Anesthesiology*. 1987;67:551–558.
24. Grace RF. Pulse oximetry. Gold standard or false sense of security. *Med J Aust*. 1994;160:638–644.
25. Trivedi NS, Ghouri AF, Shah NK, et al. Effects of motion, ambient light, and hypoperfusion on pulse oximeter function. *J Clin Anesth*. 1997; 9:179–183.
26. Reich DL, Timcenko A, Bodian CA, et al. Predictors of pulse oximetry data failure. *Anesthesiology*. 1996;84:859–864.
27. Moller JT, Pedersen T, Rasmussen LS, et al. Randomized evaluation of pulse oximetry in. 20,802 patients. I. Design, demography, pulse oximetry failure rate, and overall complication rate. *Anesthesiology*. 1993;78:436–444.
28. Runciman WB, Webb RK, Barker L, Currie M. The Australian Incident Monitoring Study. The pulse oximeter: applications and limitations—an analysis of 2000 incident reports. *Anaesth Intensive Care*. 1993; 21:543–550.
29. Lawless ST. Crying wolf: false alarms in a pediatric intensive care unit. *Crit Care Med*. 1994;22:981–985.
30. Feiner JR, Severinghaus JW, Bickler PE. Dark skin decreases the accuracy of pulse oximeters at low oxygen saturation: the effects of oximeter probe type and gender. *Anesth Analg*. 2007;105:S18–S23.
31. Bickler PE, Feiner JR, Severinghaus JW. Effects of skin pigmentation on pulse oximeter accuracy at low saturation. *Anesthesiology*. 2005; 102:715–719.
32. Jubran A. Pulse oximetry. *Crit Care*. 2015;19:272–279.
33. van Oostrom JH, Melker RJ. Comparative testing of pulse oximeter probes. *Anesth Analg*. 2004;98:1354–1358.
34. van Oostrom JH, Mahla ME, Gravenstein D. The Stealth Station Image Guidance System may interfere with pulse oximetry. *Can J Anaesth*. 2005;52: 379–382.
35. Goldman JM, Petterson MT, Kopotic RJ, Barker SJ. Masimo signal extraction pulse oximetry. *J Clin Monit Comput*. 2000;16:475–483.
36. Jopling MW, Mannheimer PD, Bebout DE. Issues in the laboratory evaluation of pulse oximeter performance. *Anesth Analg*. 2002;94:S62–S68.
37. Block FE, Detko GJ. Minimizing interference and false alarms from electrocautery in the Nellcor N-100 pulse oximeter. *J Clin Monit*. 1986; 2:203–205.
38. Barker SJ, Tremper KK, Hyatt J. Effects of methemoglobinemia on pulse oximetry and mixed venous oximetry. *Anesthesiology*. 1989;70:112–117.
39. Vokach-Brodsky L, Jeffrey SS, Lemmens HJ, Brock-Utne JG. Isosulfan blue affects pulse oximetry. *Anesthesiology*. 2000;93:1002–1003.
40. Ralston AC, Webb RK, Runciman WB. Potential errors in pulse oximetry. I. Pulse oximeter evaluation. *Anaesthesia*. 1991;46:202–206.
41. Hertzman A. Photoelectric plethysmography of the nasal septum in man. *Proc Soc Exp Biol Med*. 1937;37:290–292.

42. Groveman J, Cohen DD, Dillon JB. Rhinoplethysmography: pulse monitoring at the nasal septum. *Anesth Analg*. 1966;45:63–68.
43. Cucchiara RF, Messick JM. The failure of nasal plethysmography to estimate cerebral blood flow during carotid occlusion. *Anesthesiology*. 1981;55:585–586.
44. Ezri T, Lurie S, Konichezky S, Soroker D. Pulse oximetry from the nasal septum. *J Clin Anesth*. 1991;3:447–450.
45. O'Leary RJ, Landon M, Benumof JL. Buccal pulse oximeter is more accurate than finger pulse oximeter in measuring oxygen saturation. *Anesth Analg*. 1992;75:495–498.
46. Awad AA, Stout RG, Ghobashy MA, et al. Analysis of the ear pulse oximeter waveform. *J Clin Monit Comput*. 2006;20:175–184.
47. Nesseler N, Frénel JV, Launey Y, et al. Pulse oximetry and high-dose vasopressors: a comparison between forehead reflectance and finger transmission sensors. *Intensive Care Med*. 2012;38:1718–1722.
48. Morey TE, Rice MJ, Vasilopoulos T, et al. Feasibility and accuracy of nasal alar pulse oximetry. *Br J Anaesth*. 2014;112:1109–1114.
49. Murray WB, Foster PA. The peripheral pulse wave: information overlooked. *J Clin Monit*. 1996;12:365–377.
50. Alian AA, Shelley KH. Respiratory Physiology and the impact of different modes of ventilation on the photoplethysmographic waveform. *Sensors (Basel)*. 2012;12:2236–2254.
51. Alian AA, Shelley KH. Photoplethysmography. *Best Pract Res Clin Anaesthesiol*. 2014;28:395–406.
52. Bhattacharya J, Kanjilal PP, Muralidhar V. Analysis and characterization of photo-plethysmographic signal. *IEEE Trans Biomed Eng*. 2001;48:5–11.
53. Shelley KH, Barker SJ. Disclosures: what is necessary and sufficient. *Anesth Analg*. 2016;122:307–308.
54. Cannesson M, Shafer SL. All boxes are black. *Anesth Analg*. 2016;122: 309–317.
55. Johansson A. Neural network for photoplethysmographic respiratory rate monitoring. *Med Biol Eng Comput*. 2003;41:242–248.
56. Nilsson L, Johansson A, Kalman S. Respiratory variations in the reflection mode photoplethysmographic signal: relationships to peripheral venous pressure. *Med Biol Eng Comput*. 2003;41:249–254.
57. Kato R, Sato J, Iuchi T, Higuchi Y. Quantitative determination of arterial wall mechanics with pulse oximetric finger plethysmography. *J Anesth*. 1999;13:197–204.
58. Chowienczyk PJ, Kelly RP, MacCallum H, et al. Photoplethysmographic assessment of pulse wave reflection: blunted response to endothelium-dependent beta2-adrenergic vasodilation in type II diabetes mellitus. *J Am Coll Cardiol*. 1999;34:2007–2014.
59. Millasseau SC, Kelly RP, Ritter JM, Chowienczyk PJ. Determination of age-related increases in large artery stiffness by digital pulse contour analysis. *Clin Sci (Lond)*. 2002;103:371–377.
60. Millasseau SC, Kelly RP, Ritter JM, Chowienczyk PJ. The vascular impact of aging and vasoactive drugs: comparison of two digital volume pulse measurements. *Am J Hypertens*. 2003;16:467–472.
61. Bortolotto LA, Blacher J, Kondo T, et al. Assessment of vascular aging and atherosclerosis in hypertensive subjects: second derivative of photoplethysmogram versus pulse wave velocity. *Am J Hypertens*. 2000;13:165–171.
62. Pinsky MR, Summer WR. Cardiac augmentation by phasic high intrathoracic pressure support in man. *Chest*. 1983;84:370–375.
63. Nilsson L, Johansson A, Kalman S. Monitoring of respiratory rate in postoperative care using a new photoplethysmographic technique. *J Clin Monit Comput*. 2000;16:309–315.
64. Leonard P, Beattie TF, Addison PS, Watson JN. Standard pulse oximeters can be used to monitor respiratory rate. *Emerg Med J*. 2003;20:524–525.
65. Leonard P, Grubb NR, Addison PS, et al. An algorithm for the detection of individual breaths from the pulse oximeter waveform. *J Clin Monit Comput*. 2004;18:309–312.
66. Foo JY, Wilson SJ. Estimation of breathing interval from the photoplethysmographic signals in children. *Physiol Meas*. 2005;26:1049–1058.
67. Leonard PA, Douglas JG, Grubb NR, et al. A fully automated algorithm for the determination of respiratory rate from the photoplethysmogram. *J Clin Monit Comput*. 2006;20:33–36.
68. Perel A, Pizov R, Cotev S. Systolic blood pressure variation is a sensitive indicator of hypovolemia in ventilated dogs subjected to graded hemorrhage. *Anesthesiology*. 1987;67:498–502.
69. Rooke GA, Schwid HA, Shapira Y. The effect of graded hemorrhage and intravascular volume replacement on systolic pressure variation in humans during mechanical and spontaneous ventilation. *Anesth Analg*. 1995;80:925–932.
70. Partridge BL. Use of pulse oximetry as a noninvasive indicator of intravascular volume status. *J Clin Monit*. 1987;3:263–268.
71. Shamir M, Eidelman LA, Floman Y, et al. Pulse oximetry plethysmographic waveform during changes in blood volume. *Br J Anaesth*. 1999; 82:178–181.
72. Fuehrlein B, Melker R, Ross EA. Alar photoplethysmography: a new methodology for monitoring fluid removal and carotid circulation during hemodialysis. *J Clin Monit Comput*. 2007;21:211–218.
73. Aoyagi T, Fuse M, Kobayashi N, et al. Multiwavelength pulse oximetry: theory for the future. *Anesth Analg*. 2007;105:S53–S58
74. Saito J, Kitayama M, Oishi M, et al. The accuracy of non-invasively continuous total hemoglobin measurement by pulse CO-oximetry undergoing acute normovolemic hemodilution and reinfusion of autologous blood. *J Anesth*. 2015;29:29–34.
75. Morey TE, Rice MJ, Gravenstein N. What is a reference standard? *Anesth Analg*. 2015;120:8–9.
76. Rice MJ, Gravenstein N, Morey TE. Noninvasive hemoglobin monitoring: how accurate is enough. *Anesth Analg*. 2013;117:902–907.
77. Hiscock R, Kumar D, Simmons SW. Systematic review and meta-analysis of method comparison studies of Masimo pulse co-oximeters (Radical-7™ or Pronto-7™) and HemoCue® absorption spectrometers (B-hemoglobin or 201+) with laboratory haemoglobin estimation. *Anaesth Intensive Care*. 2015;43:341–350.
78. Carabini LM, Navarre WJ, Ault ML, et al. A comparison of hemoglobin measured by co-oximetry and central laboratory during major spine fusion surgery. *Anesth Analg*. 2015;120:60–65.
79. Yang S, Hu PF, Anazodo A, et al. Trends of hemoglobin oximetry: do they help predict blood transfusion during trauma patient resuscitation. *Anesth Analg*. 2016;122:115–125.
80. Awada WN, Mohmoued MF, Radwan TM, et al. Continuous and noninvasive hemoglobin monitoring reduces red blood cell transfusion during neurosurgery: a prospective cohort study. *J Clin Monit Comput*. 2015;29:733–740.
81. Morey TE, Gravenstein N, Rice MJ. Let's think clinically instead of mathematically about device accuracy. *Anesth Analg*. 2011;113:89–91.
82. Shamir MY, Avramovich A, Smaka T. The current status of continuous noninvasive measurement of total, carboxy, and methemoglobin concentration. *Anesth Analg*. 2012;114:972–978.
83. Szmuk P, Steiner JW, Olomu PN, et al. Oxygen reserve index: a novel noninvasive measure of oxygen reserve—a pilot study. *Anesthesiology*. 2016;124:779–784.
84. Applegate RL, Dorotta IL, Wells B, et al. The relationship between oxygen reserve index and arterial partial pressure of oxygen during surgery. *Anesth Analg*. 2016 March 22 [Epub ahead of print].
85. Simpao AF, Gálvez JA. When seconds count, buy more time: the oxygen reserve index and its promising role in patient monitoring and safety. *Anesthesiology*. 2016;124(4):750–751.
86. Tripathi RS, Blum JM, Rosenberg AL, Tremper KK. Pulse oximetry saturation to fraction inspired oxygen ratio as a measure of hypoxia under general anesthesia and the influence of positive end-expiratory pressure. *J Crit Care*. 2010;25:542.e9–13.
87. Bilan N, Dastranji A, Ghalehgolab Behbahani A. Comparison of the SpO_2/FiO_2 ratio and the PaO_2/FiO_2 ratio in patients with acute lung injury or acute respiratory distress syndrome. *J Cardiovasc Thorac Res*. 2015;7:28–31.
88. Khemani RG, Thomas NJ, Venkatachalam V, et al. Comparison of SpO_2 to PaO_2 based markers of lung disease severity for children with acute lung injury. *Crit Care Med*. 2012;40:1309–1316.
89. Khemani RG, Rubin S, Belani S, et al. Pulse oximetry vs. PaO_2 metrics in mechanically ventilated children: Berlin definition of ARDS and mortality risk. *Intensive Care Med*. 2015;41:94–102.
90. Chen W, Janz DR, Shaver CM, et al. Clinical characteristics and outcomes are similar in ARDS diagnosed by oxygen saturation/FiO_2 ratio compared with PaO_2/FiO_2 ratio. *Chest*. 2015;148:1477–1483.
91. Hirsch JC, Charpie JR, Ohye RG, Gurney JG. Near infrared spectroscopy (NIRS) should not be standard of care for postoperative management. *Semin Thorac Cardiovasc Surg Pediatr Card Surg Annu*. 2010;13:51–54.
92. Tweddell JS, Ghanayem NS, Hoffman GM. Pro: NIRS is "standard of care" for postoperative management. *Semin Thorac Cardiovasc Surg Pediatr Card Surg Annu*. 2010;13:44–50.
93. Taillefer MC, Denault AY. Cerebral near-infrared spectroscopy in adult heart surgery: systematic review of its clinical efficacy. *Can J Anaesth*. 2005;52:79–87.
94. Wahr JA, Tremper KK, Samra S, Delpy DT. Near-infrared spectroscopy: theory and applications. *J Cardiothorac Vasc Anesth*. 1996;10:406–418.
95. Cournoyer A, Iseppon M, Chauny JM, et al. Near-infrared spectroscopy monitoring during cardiac arrest: a systematic review and meta-analysis. *Acad Emerg Med*. 2016.

96. Colquhoun DA, Tucker-Schwartz JM, Durieux ME, Thiele RH. Non-invasive estimation of jugular venous oxygen saturation: a comparison between near infrared spectroscopy and transcutaneous venous oximetry. *J Clin Monit Comput*. 2012;26:91–98.
97. Standards for basic anesthetic monitoring. American Society of Anesthesiologists website. https://www.asahq.org/~/media/Sites/ASAHQ/Files/Public/Resources/standards-guidelines/standards-for-basic-anesthetic-monitoring.pdf. Accessed April 4, 2016.
98. Jaffe MB. Brief history of time and volumetric capnography. In: Gravenstein JS, Jaffe MB, Paulus DA, eds. *Capnography: Clinical Aspects*. Cambridge: Cambridge University Press; 2004:341–354.
99. Jaffe MB. Time and Volumetric Capnography. In: Ehrenfeld JM, Cannesson M, eds. *Monitoring Technologies in Acute Care Environments*. New York, NY: Springer New York; 2014:179–191.
100. Kodali BS. Capnography outside the operating rooms. *Anesthesiology*. 2013;118(1):192.
101. Lawson D, Samanta S, Magee PT, Gregonis DE. Stability and long-term durability of Raman spectroscopy. *J Clin Monit*. 1993;9:241–251.
102. McSwain SD, Hamel DS, Smith PB, et al. End-tidal and arterial carbon dioxide measurements correlate across all levels of physiologic dead space. *Respir Care*. 2010;55:288–293.
103. Pekdemir M, Cinar O, Yilmaz S, et al. Disparity between mainstream and sidestream end-tidal carbon dioxide values and arterial carbon dioxide levels. *Respir Care*. 2013;58:1152–1156.
104. Kasuya Y, Akça O, Sessler DI, et al. Accuracy of postoperative end-tidal PCO_2 measurements with mainstream and sidestream capnography in non-obese patients and in obese patients with and without obstructive sleep apnea. *Anesthesiology*. 2009;111:609–615.
105. Rosner V, Hannhart B, Chabot F, Polu JM. Validity of transcutaneous oxygen/carbon dioxide pressure measurement in the monitoring of mechanical ventilation in stable chronic respiratory failure. *Eur Respir J*. 1999;13:1044–1047.
106. Groeneveld ABJ. Tonometry of partial carbon dioxide tension in gastric mucosa: use of saline, buffer solutions, gastric juice or air. *Crit Care*. 2000; 4:201–204.
107. Creteur J, De Backer D, Sakr Y, et al. Sublingual capnometry tracks microcirculatory changes in septic patients. *Intensive Care Med*. 2006; 32:516–523.
108. Maciel AT, Creteur J, Vincent J-L. Tissue capnometry: does the answer lie under the tongue. *Intensive Care Med*. 2004;30:2157–2165.
109. Weiss M, Schmitz A, Salgo B, Dullenkopf A. Rectal luminal $Pr(CO_2)$, measured by automated air tonometry, does not reflect gastric luminal $Pr(CO_2)$ in children. *J Anesth*. 2006;20:243–246.
110. Hagerty JJ, Kleinman ME, Zurakowski D, et al. Accuracy of a new low-flow sidestream capnography technology in newborns: a pilot study. *J Perinatol*. 2002;22:219–225.
111. Drummond GB, Fletcher R. Deadspace: invasive or not. *Br J Anaesth*. 2006;96:4–7.
112. Jaffe MB. Carbon dioxide measurement. In: Gravenstein JS, Jaffe MB, Paulus DA, eds. *Capnography: Clinical Aspects*. Cambridge: Cambridge University Press; 2004:399–412.
113. Fletcher R. Volumetric capnography: the early days. In: Gravenstein JS, Jaffe MB, Paulus DA, eds. *Capnography: Clinical Aspects*. Cambridge: Cambridge University Press; 2004:381–384.
114. Ball JAS, Grounds RM. Calibration of three capnographs for use with helium and oxygen gas mixtures. *Anaesthesia*. 2003;58:156–160.
115. Lauzon AM, Elliott AR, Paiva M, et al. Cardiogenic oscillation phase relationships during single-breath tests performed in microgravity. *J Appl Physiol*. 1998;84:661–668.
116. Macefield G, Burke D. Paraesthesiae and tetany induced by voluntary hyperventilation. Increased excitability of human cutaneous and motor axons. *Brain*. 1991;114:527–540.
117. Kazama T, Ikeda K, Kato T, Kikura M. Carbon dioxide output in laparoscopic cholecystectomy. *Br J Anaesth*. 1996;76:530–535.
118. O'Connor BR, Kussman BD, Park KW. Severe hypercarbia during cardiopulmonary bypass: a complication of CO_2 flooding of the surgical field. *Anesth Analg*. 1998;86:264–266.
119. Adnet P, Lestavel P, Krivosic Horber R. Neuroleptic malignant syndrome. *Br J Anaesth*. 2000;85:129–135.
120. Volpi-Abadie J, Kaye AM, Kaye AD. Serotonin syndrome. *Ochsner J*. 2013;13:533–540.
121. Morey TE. Carbon dioxide pathophysiology. In: Gravenstein JS, Jaffe MB, Paulus DA, eds. *Capnography: Clinical Aspects*. Cambridge: Cambridge University Press; 2004:257–268.
122. Strömberg NO, Gustafsson PM. Ventilation inhomogeneity assessed by nitrogen washout and ventilation-perfusion mismatch by capnography in stable and induced airway obstruction. *Pediatr Pulmonol*. 2000; 29:94–102.
123. Brown LH, Gough JE, Seim RH. Can quantitative capnometry differentiate between cardiac and obstructive causes of respiratory distress. *Chest*. 1998;113:323–326.
124. Saura P, Blanch L, Lucangelo U, et al. Use of capnography to detect hypercapnic episodes during weaning from mechanical ventilation. *Intensive Care Med*. 1996;22:374–381.
125. Niehoff J, DelGuercio C, LaMorte W, et al. Efficacy of pulse oximetry and capnometry in postoperative ventilatory weaning. *Crit Care Med*. 1988;16:701–705.
126. Hubble CL, Gentile MA, Tripp DS, et al. Deadspace to tidal volume ratio predicts successful extubation in infants and children. *Crit Care Med*. 2000;28:2034–2040.
127. Walsh BK, Crotwell DN, Restrepo RD. Capnography/capnometry during mechanical ventilation: 2011. *Respir Care*. 2011;56:503–509.
128. Nuckton TJ, Alonso JA, Kallet RH, et al. Pulmonary dead-space fraction as a risk factor for death in the acute respiratory distress syndrome. *N Engl J Med*. 2002;346:1281–1286.
129. Murray IP, Modell JH, Gallagher TJ, Banner MJ. Titration of PEEP by the arterial minus end-tidal carbon dioxide gradient. *Chest*. 1984;85: 100–104.
130. Schreiner M S, Leksell LG, Gobran SR, et al. Microemboli reduce phase III slopes of CO_2 and invert phase III slopes of infused SF6. *Respir Physiol*. 1993;91:137–154.
131. Nikodýmová L, Daum S, Stiksa J, Widimský J. Respiratory changes in thromboembolic disease. *Respiration*. 1968;25:51–66.
132. Patel MM, Rayburn DB, Browning JA, Kline JA. Neural network analysis of the volumetric capnogram to detect pulmonary embolism. *Chest*. 1999;116:1325–1332.
133. Weil MH, Bisera J, Trevino RP, Rackow EC. Cardiac output and end-tidal carbon dioxide. *Crit Care Med*. 1985;13:907–909.
134. Ward KR. The basis for capnometric monitoring in shock. In: Gravenstein JS, Jaffe MB, Paulus DA eds. *Capnography: Clinical Aspects*. Cambridge: Cambridge University Press; 2004:223–222.
135. Leigh MD, Jones JC, Motley HL. The expired carbon dioxide as a continuous guide of the pulmonary and circulatory systems during anesthesia and surgery. *J Thorac Cardiovasc Surg*. 1961;41:597–610.
136. Bhende MS, Thompson AE, Cook DR, Saville AL. Validity of a disposable end-tidal CO_2 detector in verifying endotracheal tube placement in infants and children. *Ann Emerg Med*. 1992;21:142–145.
137. Grmec S. Comparison of three different methods to confirm tracheal tube placement in emergency intubation. *Intensive Care Med*. 2002; 28:701–704.
138. Ornato JP, Shipley JB, Racht EM, et al. Multicenter study of a portable, hand-size, colorimetric end-tidal carbon dioxide detection device. *Ann Emerg Med*. 1992;21:518–523.
139. Vukmir RB, Heller MB, Stein KL. Confirmation of endotracheal tube placement: a miniaturized infrared qualitative CO_2 detector. *Ann Emerg Med*. 1991;20:726–729.
140. Hamrick JL, Hamrick JT, Lee JK, et al. Efficacy of chest compressions directed by end tidal CO_2 feedback in a pediatric resuscitation model of basic life support. *J Am Heart Assoc*. 2014;3(2):e000450.
141. Hartmann SM, Farris RW, Di Gennaro JL, Roberts JS. systematic review and meta-analysis of end-tidal carbon dioxide values associated with return of spontaneous circulation during cardiopulmonary resuscitation. *J Intensive Care Med*. 2015;30:426–435.
142. Kodali BS, Urman RD. Capnography during cardiopulmonary resuscitation: current evidence and future directions. *J Emerg Trauma Shock*. 2014;7:332–340.
143. Burns SM, Carpenter R, Blevins C, et al. Detection of inadvertent airway intubation during gastric tube insertion: capnography versus a colorimetric carbon dioxide detector. *Am J Crit Care*. 2006;15: 188–195.
144. Bhende MS, LaCovey DC. End-tidal carbon dioxide monitoring in the prehospital setting. *Prehosp Emerg Care*. 2001;5:208–213.
145. Kalenda Z. The capnogram as a guide to the efficacy of cardiac massage. *Resuscitation*. 1978;6:259–263.
146. Sanders AB, Atlas M, Ewy GA, et al. Expired PCO_2 as an index of coronary perfusion pressure. *Am J Emerg Med*. 1985;3:147–149.
147. Garnett AR, Ornato JP, Gonzalez ER, Johnson EB. End-tidal carbon dioxide monitoring during cardiopulmonary resuscitation. *JAMA*. 1987;257: 512–515.
148. Martin GB, Gentile NT, Paradis NA, et al. Effect of epinephrine on end-tidal carbon dioxide monitoring during CPR. *Ann Emerg Med*. 1990; 19:396–398.

149. Ornato JP, Levine RL, Young DS, et al. The effect of applied chest compression force on systemic arterial pressure and end-tidal carbon dioxide concentration during CPR in human beings. *Ann Emerg Med.* 1989;18:732–737.
150. Ornato JP, Gonzalez ER, Garnett AR, et al. Effect of cardiopulmonary resuscitation compression rate on end-tidal carbon dioxide concentration and arterial pressure in man. *Crit Care Med.* 1988;16:241–245.
151. Ammann EC, Galvin RD. Problems associated with the determination of carbon dioxide by infrared absorption. *J Appl Physiol.* 1968;25:333–335.
152. Graybeal JM, Russell GB. Relative agreement between Raman and mass spectrometry for measuring end-tidal carbon dioxide. *Respir Care.* 1994; 39:190–194.
153. Elliot WR, Raemer DB, Goldman DB, Philip JH. The effects of bronchodilator-inhaler aerosol propellants on respiratory gas monitors. *J Clin Monit.* 1991;7:175–180.
154. Hardman JG, Curran J, Mahajan RP. End-tidal carbon dioxide measurement and breathing system filters. *Anaesthesia.* 1997;52:646–648.
155. Branson RD. The measurement of energy expenditure: instrumentation, practical considerations, and clinical application. *Respir Care.* 1990;35: 640–656.
156. Li J. Capnography alone is imperfect for endotracheal tube placement confirmation during emergency intubation. *J Emerg Med.* 2001;20:223–229.
157. Taenzer AH, Pyke JB, McGrath SP. A review of current and emerging approaches to address failure-to-rescue. *Anesthesiology.* 2011;115:421–431.
158. Pyke J, Taenzer AH, Renaud CE, McGrath SP. Developing a continuous monitoring infrastructure for detection of inpatient deterioration. *Jt Comm J Qual Patient Saf.* 2012;38:428–431, 385.
159. Taenzer AH, Pyke J, Herrick MD, et al. A comparison of oxygen saturation data in inpatients with low oxygen saturation using automated continuous monitoring and intermittent manual data charting. *Anesth Analg.* 2014;118:326–331.
160. Weinger MB, Lee LA. No patient shall be harmed by opioid-induced respiratory depression. Proceedings of Essential Monitoring Strategies to Detect Clinically Significant Drug-Induced Respiratory Depression in the Postoperative Period conference. *APSF Newslett.* 2011;26:21,26–28.
161. Taenzer AH, Pyke JB, McGrath SP, Blike GT. Impact of pulse oximetry surveillance on rescue events and intensive care unit transfers: a before-and-after concurrence study. *Anesthesiology.* 2010;112:282–287.
162. Whitaker DK. Time for capnography—everywhere. *Anaesthesia.* 2011;66: 544–549.
163. Curry JP, Lynn LA. Threshold monitoring, alarm fatigue, and the patterns of unexpected hospital death. *APSF Newslett.* 2011;26:33–35. www.apsf.org/newsletters/pdf/fall_2011.pdf. Accessed October 1, 2016.
164. Jafarian K, Amineslami M, Hassani K, et al. A multi-channel acoustics monitor for perioperative respiratory monitoring: preliminary data. *J Clin Monit Comput.* 2016;30:107–118.
165. Atkins JH, Mandel JE. Performance of Masimo rainbow acoustic monitoring for tracking changing respiratory rates under laryngeal mask airway general anesthesia for surgical procedures in the operating room: a prospective observational study. *Anesth Analg.* 2014;119: 1307–1314.
166. Voscopoulos C, Brayanov J, Ladd D, et al. Special article: evaluation of a novel noninvasive respiration monitor providing continuous measurement of minute ventilation in ambulatory subjects in a variety of clinical scenarios. *Anesth Analg.* 2013;117:91–100.
167. Voscopoulos CJ, MacNabb CM, Brayanov J, et al. The evaluation of a non-invasive respiratory volume monitor in surgical patients undergoing elective surgery with general anesthesia. *J Clin Monit Comput.* 2015; 29:223–230.
168. Frasca D, Geraud L, Charriere JM, et al. Comparison of acoustic and impedance methods with mask capnometry to assess respiration rate in obese patients recovering from general anaesthesia. *Anaesthesia.* 2015; 70:26–31.
169. Cheifetz IM, Salyer J, Schmalisch G, Tobias JD. Classical respiratory monitoring. In: Rimensberger PC, ed. *Classical Respiratory Monitoring: Pediatric and Neonatal Mechanical Ventilation.* Berlin, Heidelberg: Springer Berlin Heidelberg; 2015:375–419.
170. Shankar KB, Moseley H, Kumar Y, Vemula V. Arterial to end tidal carbon dioxide tension difference during caesarean section anaesthesia. *Anaesthesia.* 1986;41:698–702.
171. Wahba RW, Tessler MJ. Misleading end-tidal CO_2 tensions. *Can J Anaesth.* 1996;43:862–866.
172. Scripko PD, Greer DM. An update on brain death criteria: a simple algorithm with complex questions. *Neurologist.* 2011;17:237–240.
173. Determination of brain death. Massachusetts General Hospital website. https://www2.massgeneral.org/stopstroke/protocolBrainDeath.aspx. Updated May 25, 2011. Accessed April 20, 2016.
174. Vivien B, Amour J, Nicolas-Robin A, et al. An evaluation of capnography monitoring during the apnoea test in brain-dead patients. *Eur J Anaesthesiol.* 2007;24:868–875.

CHAPTER

24

Venous Oximetry

COLIN L. DOYLE, MICHAEL S. HAYASHI, EMANUEL P. RIVERS, RONNY OTERO, JOSEPH A. GARCIA, KONRAD REINHART, ARTURO SUAREZ, and MIHAE YU

INTRODUCTION

During initial management of the critically ill patient, physiologic variables such as blood pressure (BP), heart rate (HR), urine output (UOP), cardiac filling pressures, and cardiac output (CO) are used to guide resuscitative efforts. Despite normalization of these variables, significant imbalances between systemic oxygen delivery ($\dot{D}O_2$) and demand result in decreases in central ($ScvO_2$) and mixed ($S\bar{v}O_2$) venous O_2 saturation levels and global tissue hypoxia (1–3). This global tissue hypoxia, if left untreated, leads to anaerobic metabolism, lactate production, and O_2 debt. The magnitude and duration of O_2 debt have been implicated in the development of the inflammatory response, multisystem organ failure (MSOF), and increased mortality (4–8). Early restoration of global tissue normoxia, aided by venous O_2 saturation monitoring has resulted in a reduction in inflammation, morbidity, mortality, and health care resource consumption (9,10). Herein we will review the physiologic principles and clinical utility of ($S\bar{v}O_2$) in the management of the critically ill patient.

MAJOR PROBLEMS

Patient Selection for Continuous Venous Oximetry

Continuous venous oximetry is likely most useful in patients at greatest risk of developing global tissue hypoxia. This includes patients with significant acute or chronic cardiopulmonary disease undergoing major surgical procedures and undergoing therapy that may interfere with their ability to increase O_2 delivery during times of stress. It is also useful in patients who require hemodynamic and ventilator support (11).

Goals of Venous Oximetry Monitoring

The goals of continuous venous oximetry vary depending on the initial condition of the patient. Venous oximetry can be used as an end point in early resuscitation, or as a monitoring device for high-risk patients at risk for developing global tissue hypoxia. The common goal is to ensure a balance between systemic O_2 delivery and demand. A stable and normal value for the $S\bar{v}O_2$ may indicate that further measurements are unnecessary. However, an abrupt decrease in $S\bar{v}O_2$ becomes a warning that investigation of oxygen delivery (comprised of CO, arterial oxygen saturation [SaO_2], and hemoglobin [Hgb] concentration), and systemic oxygen consumption $\dot{V}O_2$ is needed so that specific therapy may be directed toward the underlying disorder (Table 24.1) (12).

ESSENTIAL POINTS

1. A normal $S\bar{v}O_2$ range is 65% to 75% (0.65 to 0.75) and suggests that the O_2 supply is meeting the demands of the tissues, though some have suggested ranges 2% to 3% higher (13). Since $S\bar{v}O_2$ is a global value, a normal value does not guarantee the absence of ischemic tissues.
2. There are four determinants of $S\bar{v}O_2$: CO, Hgb concentration, CaO_2, and VO_2. In the critically ill patient, an abrupt change in $S\bar{v}O_2$ indicates that a change in O_2 transport–demand balance has occurred but does not identify which determinant has changed.
3. A decrease in $S\bar{v}O_2$ may be caused by a decrease in CO, Hgb concentration, or CaO_2, or an increase in $\dot{V}O_2$.
4. An increase in $S\bar{v}O_2$ is more difficult to interpret. It may indicate distal migration of the catheter which is easy to check by determining catheter position (see below). Patients may have a high CO, $\dot{V}O_2$, or CaO_2, especially during anesthesia or mechanical ventilation. If this is associated with persistent elevation of lactate levels, it is an ominous sign. In patients with cirrhosis, sepsis, and peripheral shunts, an abnormal distribution of peripheral blood flow may impair oxygen uptake so that $S\bar{v}O_2$ remains high. In cirrhosis, there is pathologic shunting between the arterial and venous systems in the liver causing a high CO and high $S\bar{v}O_2$. The septic state is accompanied by a peripheral O_2 deficit, which can be partially reversed by maintaining an above-normal CO and $\dot{D}O_2$ (14). Higher-than-normal $S\bar{v}O_2$ may be required in sepsis to overcome the defect in peripheral O_2 use. Patients with anatomic shunts such as ventricular septal defects and arterial–venous fistulas for hemodialysis also may have abnormal mixing of arterial and venous blood leading to higher venous O_2 saturations.
5. Pulse oximetry and mixed venous oximetry can be combined into a tool of continuous cardiac and pulmonary monitoring.
6. The difference between arterial and venous saturation (SaO_2–$S\bar{v}O_2$) is an estimation of arterial and venous O_2 content difference, and is inversely proportional to CO and directly proportional to O_2 consumption.
7. The ventilation/perfusion index ($\dot{V}/\dot{Q}$ I) gives an estimate of intrapulmonary shunt. Using saturation as an inference of O_2 content, respiratory dysfunction ($\dot{V}/\dot{Q}$ I) can be estimated from the equation $(1 - SaO_2)/(1 - S\bar{v}O_2)$.

ESSENTIAL TROUBLESHOOTING PROCEDURES

1. Continuous $S\bar{v}O_2$ measurements may drift and require daily calibration using laboratory co-oximetry.

TABLE 24.1 Normal Ranges, Units, and Derivation for Common Oxygen Transport Terms[a]

Parameter	Normal Range	Units	Derivation
PaO_2	(Varies with FiO_2)	mmHg	Measured
SaO_2	>0.92	(Fraction)	Measured
CaO_2	16–22	mL/dL	$(SaO_2 \times Hgb \times 1.38) + (PaO_2 \times 0.0031)$
$P\bar{v}O_2$	35–45	mmHg	Measured
$S\bar{v}O_2$	0.65–0.75	(Fraction)	Measured
$C\bar{v}O_2$	12–17	mL/dL	$(S\bar{v}O_2 \times Hgb \times 1.38) + (P\bar{v}O_2 \times 0.0031)$
$C(a - \bar{v})O_2$	3.5–5.5	mL/dL	$CaO_2 - C\bar{v}O_2$
$\dot{V}O_2$	180–280	mL/min	$C(a - \bar{v})O_2 \times CO \times 10$
$\dot{V}O_2$ indexed	120–160	mL/min/m^2	$C(a - \bar{v})O_2 \times CI \times 10$
$\dot{D}O_2$	700–1,400	mL/min	$CaO_2 \times CO \times 10$
$\dot{D}O_2$ indexed	500–600	mL/min/m^2	$CaO_2 \times CI \times 10$
OUC/O_2ER	0.23–0.32	(Fraction)	$\dot{V}O_2/\dot{D}O_2$

PaO_2, arterial oxygen tension; SaO_2, arterial oxygen saturation; CaO_2, arterial oxygen content; $P\bar{v}O_2$, mixed venous oxygen tension; $S\bar{v}O_2$, mixed venous oxygen saturation; $C\bar{v}O_2$, mixed venous oxygen content; $C(a - \bar{v})O_2$, arterial-venous oxygen content difference; $\dot{V}O_2$, oxygen consumption; $\dot{D}O_2$, oxygen delivery; OUC, oxygen utilization coefficient (extraction ratio); O_2ER, extraction ratio; FiO_2, fraction of inspired oxygen; Hgb, hemoglobin; CO, cardiac output.

[a]Normal ranges are approximate and may vary between laboratories.

2. Calibration should also be verified anytime the optical module is disconnected, or whenever the measurement is thought to be erroneous.
3. Distal migration of the pulmonary artery catheter (PAC) tip may cause a higher $S\bar{v}O_2$ reading due to proximity to pulmonary capillary blood, which is approximately 100% saturated. The catheter should be positioned in a large enough segment of the pulmonary artery to require no more than 1.25 mL of air in the balloon to occlude that segment.
4. Infusion of fluids or blood through the distal port of the catheter may alter the light signal and the reading.
5. Decreased light intensity signal or damping of the pulmonary artery (PA) tracing may indicate migration distally or fibrin around the optic bundles. If irrigation of the catheter does not correct the artifact, the catheter should be withdrawn and repositioned.
6. A change in $S\bar{v}O_2$ of greater than 10% in either direction requires investigation.

INITIAL THERAPY

1. If $S\bar{v}O_2$ is low in association with a low CO, optimization procedures with fluids or inotropic agents should occur immediately. When titrating inotropic infusions, *a lack of response* ($S\bar{v}O_2$ does not increase) suggests inadequate therapy. CO should be reassessed and treatment augmented.
2. In cases of respiratory dysfunction, arterial saturation (SaO_2) should respond to therapies such as increased fraction of inspired oxygen (FiO_2) and positive end-expiratory pressure (PEEP) within 8 to 10 minutes. If SaO_2 does not increase or if $S\bar{v}O_2$ decreases, either respiratory therapy has been ineffective or CO may be compromised.
3. After improvement in respiratory function, if the patient is receiving a high FiO_2, the FiO_2 may be decreased every 10 to 20 minutes if arterial and venous saturation remain stable. Increased difference in (SaO_2 – $S\bar{v}O_2$) usually correlates with a sudden decrease in CO.
4. A decrease in the arterial-venous oxygen concentration difference ($SaO_2 - S\bar{v}O_2$) in response to measure to alter CO indicates a successful intervention.

PHYSIOLOGY OF OXYGEN TRANSPORT

The process of O_2 transport includes loading O_2 into the red blood cells (hemoglobin) and delivering it to the tissue by the heart (CO), as well as utilization of the O_2 in the periphery and the return of deoxygenated blood to the right side of the heart. Several terms must be defined to understand the components of O_2 transport (absolute values should be indexed to body surface area):

- Oxygen delivery ($\dot{D}O_2$) is the volume of oxygen delivered (mL/min) from the left ventricle each minute:

$$\dot{D}O_2 = CO \times CaO_2 \times 10$$

Arterial content of oxygen (CaO_2) is the mL of O_2 in 100 mL of arterial blood:

$$CaO_2 = (Hgb \times 1.34 \text{ to } 1.39 \text{ mL } O_2/g \text{ of } Hgb \times SaO_2) + (0.0031 \times PaO_2)$$

Mixed venous content of oxygen ($C\bar{v}O_2$) is mL of O_2 in 100 mL of mixed venous blood:

$$C\bar{v}O_2 = (Hgb \times 1.34 \text{ to } 1.39 \text{ mL } O_2/g \text{ of } Hgb \times S\bar{v}O_2) + (0.0031 \times P\bar{v}O_2)$$

where $P\bar{v}O_2$ is the mixed pulmonary venous oxygen partial pressure.

- Oxygen demand is the cellular O_2 requirement to avoid anaerobic metabolism. Oxygen demand is the amount of O_2 required by the body tissues to function under conditions of aerobic metabolism. Because O_2 demand is determined at the tissue level, it is difficult to quantify clinically.
- Oxygen consumption ($\dot{V}O_2$) is the amount of O_2 consumed by the tissue, usually calculated by the Fick equation (Table 24.2):

$$\dot{V}O_2 = (CaO_2 - C\bar{v}O_2) \times CO \times 10$$

TABLE 24.2 Derivation of $S\bar{v}O_2$ from Fick Equation

1. $\dot{V}O_2 = C(a - \bar{v})O_2 \times CO \times 10$	Fick equation
2. $\dot{V}O_2/(CO \times 10) = C(a - \bar{v})O_2$	Divide by CO × 10
3. $\dot{V}O_2/(CO \times 10) = CaO_2 - C\bar{v}O_2$	Definition of $C(a - \bar{v})O_2$
4. $\dot{V}O_2/(CO \times 10) - CaO_2 = -C\bar{v}O_2$	Subtract CaO_2
5. $C\bar{v}O_2 = CaO_2 - (\dot{V}O_2/(CO \times 10))$	Multiply by −l.
6. $C\bar{v}O_2 = 1 - \dot{V}O_2/(CO \times 10 \times CaO_2)$	Divide by CaO_2
7. $C\bar{v}O_2/CaO_2 = 1 - \dot{V}O_2/\dot{D}O_2$	Definition of $\dot{D}O_2$
8. $S\bar{v}O_2 = 1 - \dot{V}O_2/\dot{D}O_2$	Definition of $S\bar{v}O_2$ if $SaO_2 = 1.0$

CO, cardiac output.

$\dot{V}O_2$ is a mechanism by which the body "protects" the O_2 demand created at the tissue level. Increased $\dot{V}O_2$ in early stages of shock is associated with increased survival. Oxygen consumption may increase by increasing CO, widening the arterial–venous O_2 content difference, or both. In the normal state, both CO and arterial–venous O_2 difference may increase by about threefold, providing a total increase of $\dot{V}O_2$ during times of stress to about ninefold above the resting state. Normally, $\dot{V}O_2$ and O_2 demands are equal; however, in times of great O_2 demand or times in which either CO or arterial–venous O_2 content difference cannot increase to meet the O_2 demand of the cells, demand may exceed $\dot{V}O_2$. When this occurs, an O_2 debt accumulates and anaerobic metabolism and lactic acidosis ensue (15).

- Oxygen uptake is the measured volume of O_2 removed from inspired gas each minute (using indirect calorimetry/metabolic gas monitor). Oxygen uptake differs slightly from $\dot{V}O_2$ in that the latter is a calculated value (from the Fick equation) and the former is the measured volume of O_2 taken up by the patient each minute. Oxygen uptake is measured by analyzing inspired and expired gas concentrations and inspired and expired volumes. Measurement of O_2 uptake may be useful for metabolic studies in assessing variations in $\dot{V}O_2$ as well as determining caloric needs.
- Oxygen utilization coefficient (OUC) or extraction ratio (O_2ER) is the fraction of delivered O_2 that is consumed:

$$\text{OUC or } O_2ER = \dot{V}O_2/\dot{D}O_2$$

- Therefore, the OUC defines the balance between O_2 supply (delivery) and demand (consumption) (Fig. 24.1).
- Oxygen transport is the process contributing to O_2 delivery and oxygen consumption.

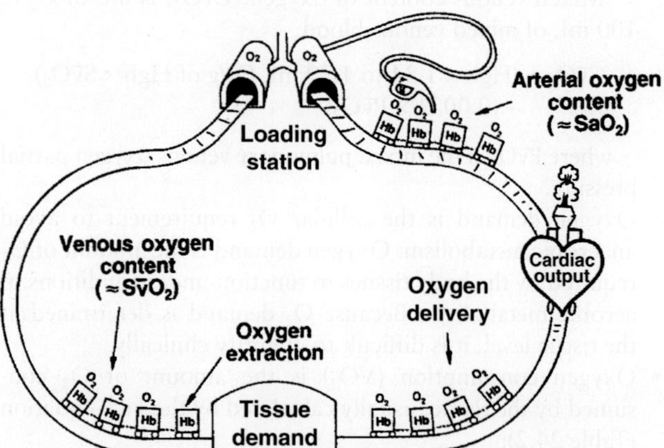

FIGURE 24.1 The physiology of oxygen transport and utilization.

ASSESSMENT OF OXYGEN TRANSPORT BALANCE

Oxygen transport balance may be assessed on several levels. First, examination of the patient may reveal signs of hypoperfusion, including altered mentation, cutaneous hypoperfusion, oliguria, tachycardia, and, when all compensatory systems have failed, hypotension. Unfortunately, these clinical signs are often late, nonspecific, and at times uninterruptible in critically ill patients. A more physiologic approach is to assess the determinants of O_2 transport balance individually by using the Fick equation. The arterial–venous O_2 content difference may be used to assess the relative balance between CO and $\dot{V}O_2$. An increase in the arterial–venous O_2 content difference indicates that either flow is decreased or consumption is increased.

When the Fick equation is solved for $S\bar{v}O_2$ (see Table 24.2), it becomes apparent that an inverse linear relation exists between $S\bar{v}O_2$ and O_2 utilization coefficients (11) if SaO_2 is maintained constant. $S\bar{v}O_2$ measured continuously is, therefore, an online indicator of the adequacy of the O_2 supply and of the demand in perfused tissues. The determinants of $S\bar{v}O_2$ are $\dot{V}O_2$, Hgb, CO, SaO_2, and, to a small degree, PaO_2. $S\bar{v}O_2$ represents the flow-weighted average of the venous O_2 saturations from all perfused tissues (Fig. 24.2).

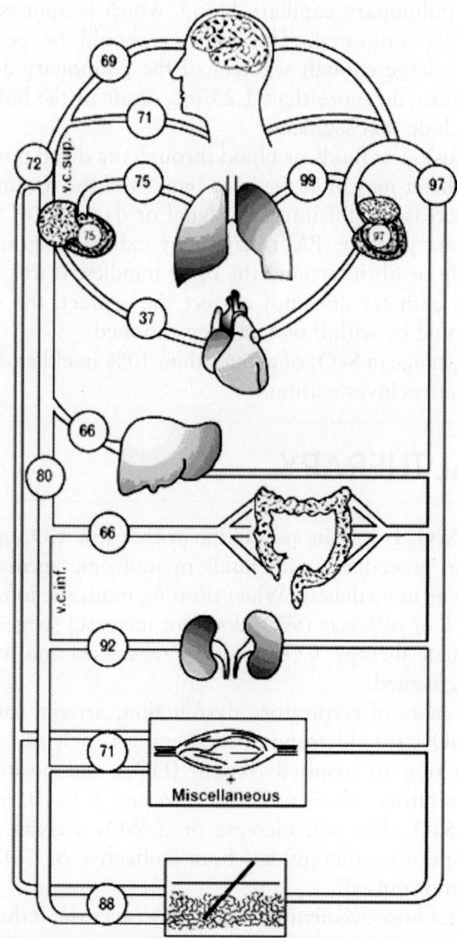

FIGURE 24.2 Venous oxygenation saturations of various organs. (From Reinhart K, Rudolph T, Bredle DL, et al. Comparison of central-venous to mixed-venous oxygen saturation during changes in oxygen supply/demand. *Chest*. 1989;95(6):1216–1221.)

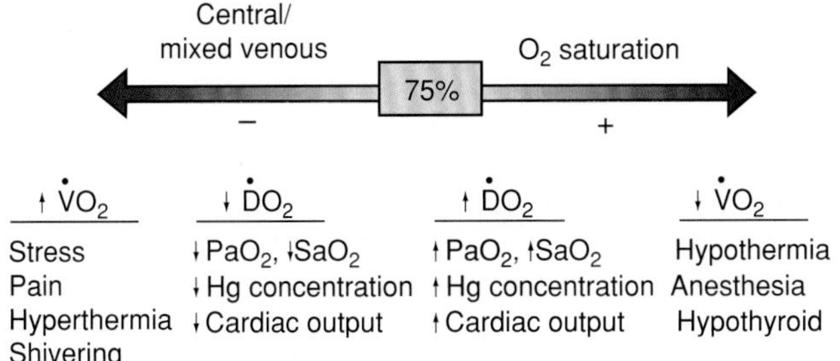

FIGURE 24.3 Variables that affect $S\bar{v}O_2$. (Adapted from Rivers EP, Ander DS, Powell D. Central venous oxygen saturation monitoring in the critically ill patient. *Curr Opin Crit Care.* 2001;7(3):204–211.)

Therefore, tissues that have high blood flow but relatively low O_2 extraction (kidney) will have a greater effect on $S\bar{v}O_2$ than will tissues with low blood flow, although the O_2 extraction of these tissues may be high (myocardium) (16,17).

The interpretation of $S\bar{v}O_2$ requires consistent and intact vasoregulation (5). When vasoregulation is altered—as in sepsis—O_2 uptake may be severely altered, causing a marked increase in $S\bar{v}O_2$. Septic patients can have a normal $S\bar{v}O_2$ while the hepatic venous saturation can be up to 15% lower (18,19). This reduced O_2 saturation was noted to arise from an increased regional metabolic rate rather than reduced perfusion. Flow-limited regional O_2 consumption may potentially exist despite the presence of a normal $S\bar{v}O_2$. Therefore, a normal $S\bar{v}O_2$ should not be considered as sole criteria to ensure optimal O_2 delivery in critically ill patients (Fig. 24.3) (20,21).

Although O_2 demand cannot be measured, the relative balance between consumption and demand is best indicated by the presence of excess lactate in the blood. Lactic acidosis implies that demand exceeds consumption, or O_2 supply dependency, and anaerobic metabolism is present (Fig. 24.4) (15,22,23). The relative balance between O_2 supply and demand can be assessed by the OUC (1). Calculation of this coefficient, however, requires the measurement of CO, Hgb, SaO_2, PaO_2, $S\bar{v}O_2$, and $P\bar{v}O_2$; the latter, a reflection of both PaO_2 and CO, is a better predictor of hyperlactatemia and death than either arterial PaO_2 or CO alone. A $P\bar{v}O_2$ below 28 mmHg is usually associated with hyperlactatemia and increased mortality (24). Blood lactate concentrations greater

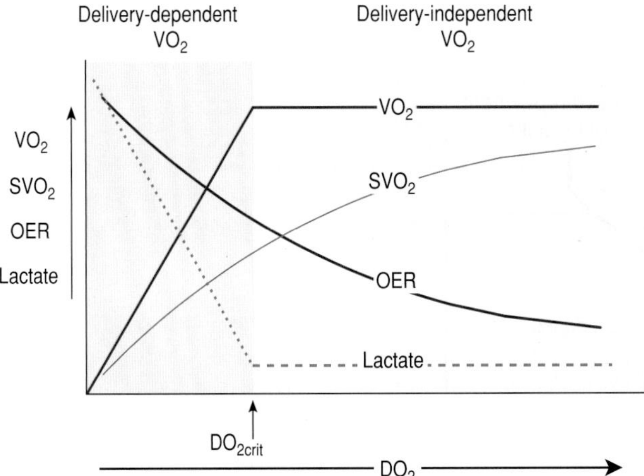

FIGURE 24.4 The relationship of oxygen transport variables and lactate levels.

than 4 mmol/L are unusual in normal and noncritically ill hospitalized patients and warrant concern. In hospitalized, non-ICU, nonhypotensive subjects, as well as in critically ill patients, a blood lactate concentration greater than 4 mmol/L portends a poor prognosis (25). Since serum lactate is a global measurement, a normal lactate is not a guarantee that all tissue beds are adequately perfused.

ARTERIAL VENOUS OXYGEN CONTENT DIFFERENCE

From the Fick principle, we learned that CO was equal to O_2 consumption divided by arterial venous O_2 content difference ($CaO_2 - CvO_2$). Even in the critically ill patient, it is unlikely that Hgb or total body O_2 consumption can change sufficiently minute to minute to affect the calculations. Therefore, $(Ca - \bar{v})O_2$ usually reflects changes in CO. In addition, immediate response to therapy—or lack thereof—can help tailor therapy more precisely and rapidly (26). Since the contribution of dissolved O_2 is minute ($0.0031 \times PaO_2$), and the factor (Hgb × 1.39 mL O_2/g Hgb) occurs in both sides of the equation, $(Ca - \bar{v})O_2$ can be estimated by subtracting the values of pulse oximetry and continuous mixed venous oximetry ($SaO_2 - S\bar{v}O_2$).

INTRAPULMONARY SHUNT

Although PaO_2 is affected by changes in respiratory function (intrapulmonary shunt), PaO_2 is also affected by changes in CO if there is a moderate intrapulmonary shunt (≥20%). For example, if 20% of CO is not involved with gas exchange—a shunt—and blood goes to the left side of the heart deoxygenated, any decrease in $S\bar{v}O_2$ will decrease PaO_2. Thus, although no change in pulmonary function has occurred, a decrease in CO—or even any factor that decreases venous O_2 content—lowers PaO_2 and increases the alveolar-to-arterial O_2 tension gradient (27). This nonpulmonary effect on PaO_2 is important to understand since treatment of intrapulmonary shunt is to increase PEEP, which would be disastrous if low CO was the cause for low PaO_2. The equation for intrapulmonary shunt is as follows:

$$\dot{Q}sp/\dot{Q}t = \frac{Cc - Ca}{Cc - C\bar{v}}$$

where $\dot{Q}sp/\dot{Q}t$ is physiologic shunt (% of cardiac output), Cc is capillary oxygen content, Ca is arterial oxygen content, and $C\bar{v}$ is venous oxygen content. We can simplify the shunt equation by ignoring the calculation of Hgb-carried oxygen by dropping (Hgb × 1.39) and substituting saturations of 100% for the pulmonary capillary saturation, pulse oximetry for arterial content, and mixed venous oximetry for venous content. The entire equation for pulmonary capillary content can be replaced by the term 1 (or 100% Hgb saturation). Because we have already substituted Sa for arterial content and $S\bar{v}$ for venous content, this estimation of physiologic shunt (the $(\dot{V}/\dot{Q}I)$) can be represented by Eq. [28]:

$$\dot{V}/\dot{Q}I = \frac{1 - SaO_2}{1 - S\bar{v}O_2}$$

For instance, if arterial saturation were 90% (or 0.9) and venous saturation were 60% (or 0.6), the Qs/Qt calculation would be

$$\frac{1-0.9}{1-0.6}=\frac{0.1}{0.4}=25\%$$

This estimation does not reflect the severity of respiratory failure as judged by the need to use, potentially, a higher FiO_2; thus, the equation needs to specify the patient's FiO_2 to be meaningful.

THE CONSEQUENCES OF TISSUE HYPOXIA

When compensatory mechanisms such as increased systemic O_2 extraction are exceeded, tissue hypoxia results with pathologic significance not only seen *in vitro* (4); low $S\bar{v}O_2$ is associated with the generation of inflammatory mediators and the impairment of mitochondrial O_2 use (29). The accumulation of global tissue hypoxia over time leads to O_2 deficits; the magnitude and duration of this O_2 debt has been associated with the generation of inflammatory biomarkers, morbidity, and mortality (Fig. 24.5) (8,29–33). Monitoring the $S\bar{v}O_2$, therefore, provides early and continuous data that may be acted upon immediately rather than waiting for laboratory results or markers of tissue hypoxia that signify an insult which has already occurred.

MONITORING OXYGEN TRANSPORT

Critically ill patients in the emergency department (ED), operating room (OR), and intensive care units (ICUs) may be grouped into three categories. *Category 1* consists of patients requiring intensive observation or monitoring. These patients may have major risk factors or may be admitted because of the nature of their illness or the nature of the therapy they are receiving. *Category 2* patients require intensive nursing care and often specialized technology and care facilities to direct therapy for major systemic illness. *Category 3* patients need continuous physician intervention for hemodynamic and other instabilities. Continuous venous oximetry may have clinical applications in each of these broad classes of patients. The three major objectives of monitoring critically ill patients are to ensure that the patient is stable, to provide an early warning system regarding untoward events, and to evaluate the efficiency and efficacy of interventions performed.

Category 1 patients undergoing hemodynamic and O_2 transport monitoring only because of underlying risk factors, who have a normal and stable $S\bar{v}O_2$, have an intact balance between O_2 supply and demand. Further assessment of CO and arterial and mixed venous blood gas analysis to reach that conclusion can be eliminated, and there is "safety in no (other) numbers." If the patient becomes unstable as manifested by a decreasing $S\bar{v}O_2$, the monitoring system will meet the second objective by providing an early warning of the imbalance in O_2 supply and demand. In this situation, although an alert has been given, the cause of the O_2 transport imbalance is not necessarily clear. The change in $S\bar{v}O_2$ is sensitive but not specific. In this clinical situation, it may be necessary to measure CO, SaO_2, and Hgb. When the cause of the imbalance is identified, specific therapy may be instituted to restore the O_2 supply–demand balance. While interventions are applied, the continuous assessment of supply–demand balance may be used to evaluate the efficacy of the intervention with instant feedback. Continuous CO methodology should supplement but not supplant mixed venous oximetry. This is particularly important in critical illness, defined as a nonsteady state, when changes in all elements of O_2 transport and use can be expected (33).

CONTINUOUS MIXED VENOUS MONITORING

$S\bar{v}O_2$ can be monitored continuously using infrared oximetry, based upon reflection spectrophotometry. Light is transmitted into the blood, and reflected off red blood cells and read by a photodetector in the receiving fiber-optic bundle (11). The amount of light reflected at different wavelengths varies depending on the concentration of oxyhemoglobin and hemoglobin (Fig. 24.6). The microprocessor uses the relative reflectances to calculate the oxyhemoglobin and total Hgb,

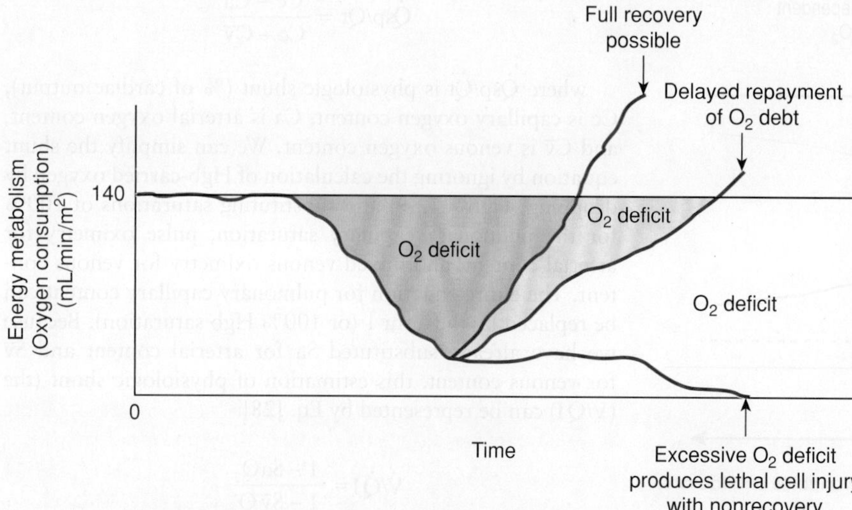

FIGURE 24.5 The concepts of oxygen debt (30–32).

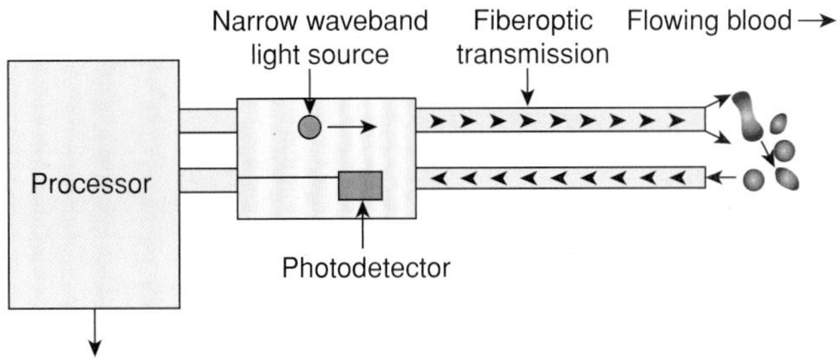

FIGURE 24.6 The technology of spectrophotometry. (Adapted from Rivers EP, Ander DS, Powell D. Central venous oxygen saturation monitoring in the critically ill patient. *Curr Opin Crit Care.* 2001;7(3):204–211.)

the fraction of which represents $S\bar{v}O_2$. The catheter used to measure venous O_2 saturation can be a pulmonary artery or a modified central venous catheter.

The continuous oximetry system must be calibrated before use by a co-oximetry measured sample (34). This may be done *in vitro* by positioning the catheter tip next to a target that reflects the transmitted light in such a manner that the microprocessor can be calibrated. After *in vitro* calibration, the O_2 saturation of the central venous system, right atrium, right ventricle, and PA can be measured while the catheter is being floated into the proper position. These measurements during the insertion of the catheter may be useful to rule out intracardiac left-to-right shunts.

Once the PAC—if this is the tool used—is in proper position, blood may be sampled through the distal port to calibrate or to verify the calibration of the system. The first *in vivo* calibration is usually done at 24-hours post-PAC insertion. A mixed venous sample is withdrawn and analyzed by laboratory co-oximetry. Blood drawn from the PA should be aspirated slowly (1 mL over 20 seconds) to prevent contamination by the highly oxygenated pulmonary capillary blood. The value obtained by the microprocessor at the time the blood sample is drawn is retained by the system. This may be compared against the value obtained from the laboratory sample, and, if a significant (>2%) difference exists, the instrument may be recalibrated to the laboratory co-oximeter value. The calibration should be verified at any time the optical module is disconnected from the catheter, whenever the measurement is suspected of being erroneous, and every 24 hours to ensure stability of the system.

Because it is crucial that red blood cells be flowing past the tip of the catheter, proper positioning in the PA is necessary. Distal migration of the PA catheter tip is a common source of error. When the catheter tip advances into the distal segments of the PA, a high or increased $S\bar{v}O_2$, a decreased light intensity signal, or damping of the PA tracing may become evident. If these signs are encountered, the distal lumen of the catheter should be irrigated with flush solution to remove fibrin on the catheter tip. If the pressure waveform is not restored to a proper PA tracing by irrigation, the catheter should be slowly withdrawn until the PA pressure tracing is restored. At this point, the PAC balloon may be slowly inflated until the pulmonary artery occlusion pressure (PAOP) tracing is observed. If this tracing is not produced by inflation of the balloon to maximum volume (1.5 mL), the catheter should be slowly advanced until an occlusion pressure tracing is observed. At that point, the balloon can be deflated again and then slowly reinflated until a PAOP tracing occurs. The volume required to restore this tracing should be at least 75% of the total capacity of the balloon. Using the maximum balloon volume to attain a PAOP tracing ensures that the catheter is in the proximal section of the PA and is, in fact, a physiologic confirmation of the catheter tip position.

Distal migration of the PAC may cause artifactually high O_2 saturation because highly saturated (approximately 100%) pulmonary capillary blood is sampled. The catheter tip may be lodged against a vessel wall or bifurcation, causing an alteration in the light intensity received by the fiber-optic bundles. A low-light intensity alarm must be corrected before the venous saturation measurement is considered reliable or before the system is recalibrated. Large fluctuations in the light intensity signal may indicate that the catheter tip is malpositioned but also may indicate a condition of intravascular volume deficit that allows compression or collapse of the pulmonary vasculature, especially during positive pressure ventilation (35).

CONTINUOUS CENTRAL VENOUS MONITORING

Early management of the critically ill patient is frequently performed outside the ICU. The time between the onset of critical illness and definitive ICU intervention may be prolonged and have outcome implications (36–38). Measurement of $S\bar{v}O_2$ requires placement of a PAC, which may not be feasible early in the resuscitation of adult, pediatric, and neonatal patients. However, central venous assess can be obtained in both ICU and non-ICU settings, making continuous $ScvO_2$ monitoring a convenient surrogate for $S\bar{v}O_2$.

Numerous animal and human models have examined the relationship between $S\bar{v}O_2$ and $ScvO_2$ obtained from the superior vena cava (SVC) and right atria (RA) (Fig. 24.7). SVC $ScvO_2$ is slightly lower and more accurately reflects $S\bar{v}O_2$ when patients are not in shock (39,40). The lower value of $ScvO_2$ in a nonstressed state can be explained by the low O_2 extraction of the kidneys which drain into the IVC and contribute to the $S\bar{v}O_2$ but not the $ScvO_2$ (41). RA $ScvO_2$ has a better correlation than SVC saturation and is not significantly different from $S\bar{v}O_2$ whether in shock or not (39). In patients in shock, a consistent reversal of this relationship occurs, with the $ScvO_2$ being greater than $S\bar{v}O_2$; this difference can range from 5% to 18% (39,40,42). Redistribution of blood flow away from the splenic, renal, and mesenteric bed toward the cerebral and coronary circulation, including more desaturated blood (<30%) from the coronary sinus contribute to this observation (39). Thus, $ScvO_2$ will consistently overestimate the true $S\bar{v}O_2$ under shock conditions. An interesting variation on this concept was recently demonstrated in liver transplant patients. A study of 30 patients undergoing liver transplant, in which samples from the RA and pulmonary artery were taken at several points during the procedure, found that the central venous and mixed venous O_2 saturation measurements were only concordant during the hepatectomy phase of the procedure and differed once the graft was in place. The proposed mechanism behind this finding is that increased $\dot{V}O_2$ of the

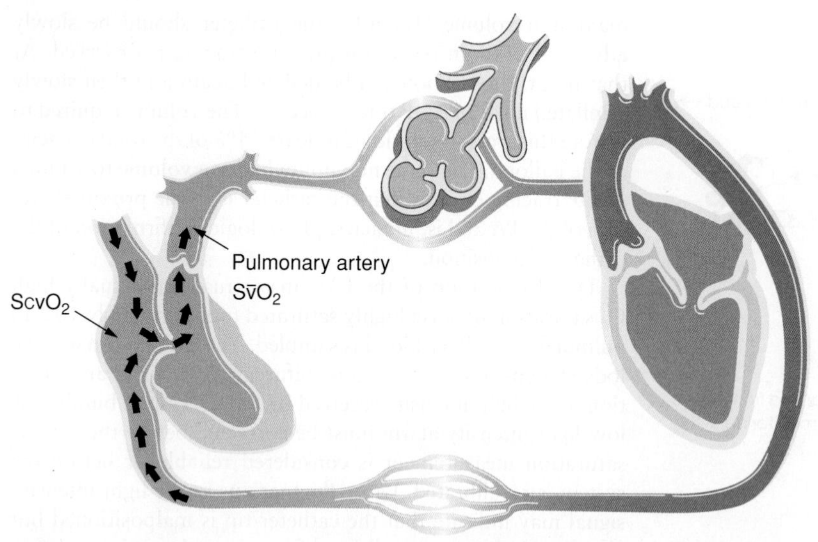

FIGURE 24.7 Central versus mixed venous oxygen saturation.

graft after reperfusion, causes the $S\bar{v}O_2$ to decrease relative to the $ScvO_2$, which is relatively unaffected by this change (43).

There has been considerable debate regarding whether $ScvO_2$ is a satisfactory substitute for $S\bar{v}O_2$, particularly in ranges above 65% (44–53). Although the absolute values of $ScvO_2$ and $S\bar{v}O_2$ differ, studies have shown close and consistent tracking of the two sites across a wide range of hemodynamic conditions (Figs. 24.8 and 24.9), thus making it clinically useful (46,54–66). The clinical utility or value of $S\bar{v}O_2/ScvO_2$ is in the lower ranges. The presence of a pathologically low $ScvO_2$ value—implying an even lower $S\bar{v}O_2$—is more clinically important than whether the values are equal. Goldman et al. (54) found that $ScvO_2$ below 60% showed evidence of heart failure or shock or a combination of the two. Hyperdynamic septic shock ICU patients seldom exhibit $S\bar{v}O_2$ levels <60% to 65%, which, if present and sustained, are associated with increased mortality (12,67). Studies examining the clinical utility of $ScvO_2$ early in the course of disease presentation routinely encounter values less than 50%, which are considered critical (3,68,69). At these values, venous saturations are actually 5% to 18% lower in the pulmonary artery (39,42) and 15% lower in the splanchnic bed (20). Thus, although

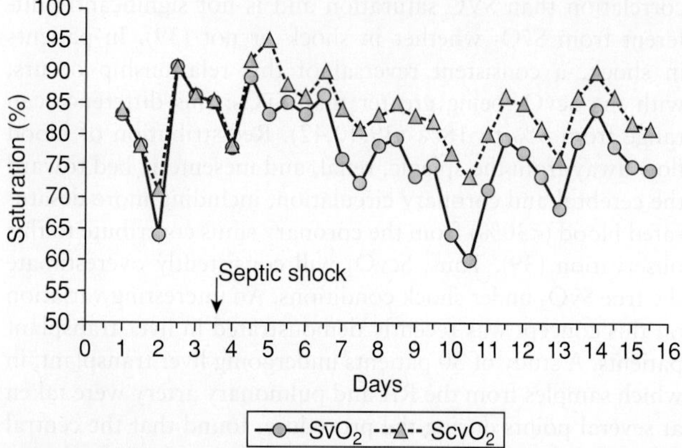

FIGURE 24.8 Central versus mixed venous oxygen saturation. (Adapted from Reinhart K, Rudolph T, Bredle DL, et al. Comparison of central-venous to mixed-venous oxygen saturation during changes in oxygen supply/demand. *Chest.* 1989;95(6):1216–1221.)

not numerically equivalent, these ranges of values have similar pathologic implications (54) and are associated with high mortality (24). Conversely, it has also been reported that patients with an $ScvO_2 > 90\%$ also had increased mortality (70); this can be explained by cellular injury resulting in lack of oxygen consumption.

The clinical utility of an end point of resuscitation is determined by whether it changes clinical practice and morbidity or mortality. Irrespective of whether the $ScvO_2$ equals $S\bar{v}O_2$, the presence of a low $ScvO_2$ in early sepsis portends increased mortality and correcting this value by a treatment algorithm (71) improves morbidity and mortality. The concept of the approximately 5% numeric difference between $S\bar{v}O_2$ and $ScvO_2$ (13) prompted the Surviving Sepsis Campaign to recommend reaching a $S\bar{v}O_2$ of 65% and/or $ScvO_2$ of 70% goal in the resuscitation portion of its severe sepsis and septic shock bundle (72,73). An $ScvO_2$ value of less than 70% has also been demonstrated to suggest a need for blood transfusion when accompanied by a hemoglobin of less than 10 g/dL and a central venous pressure (CVP) of 8 to 12 mmHg (13).

INTERPRETATION OF VENOUS OXYGEN SATURATION

The algorithm is presented in Figure 24.10. Mixed venous O_2 saturation values within the normal range (65% to 75%) indicate a normal balance between O_2 supply and demand, provided that vasoregulation is intact and a normal distribution of peripheral blood flow is present. Dysoxia usually develops when $S\bar{v}O_2$ decreases to 40% to 50%, though it may occur at higher values if oxygen extraction is impaired (13). Values of $S\bar{v}O_2$ greater than 75% indicate an excess of $\dot{D}O_2$ over $\dot{V}O_2$ and are most commonly associated with syndromes of vasoderegulation, such as cirrhosis and sepsis. High values also are seen in states of low $\dot{V}O_2$—hypothermia, muscular paralysis, sedation, coma, hypothyroidism, or a combination of these factors—hyperoxygenation, high CO, inability to consume O_2 and, rarely, cyanide toxicity.

Uncompensated changes in any of the four determinants of $S\bar{v}O_2$ may result in a decrease in the measured value, but in

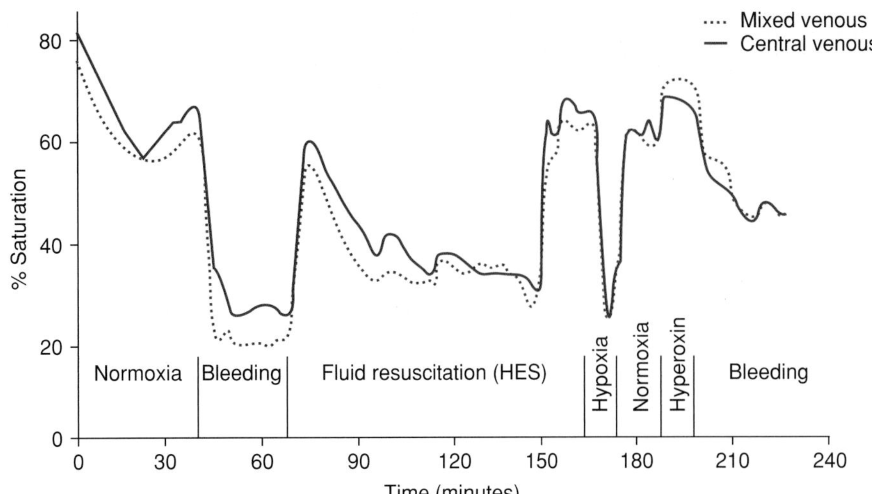

FIGURE 24.9 Central versus mixed venous oxygen saturation. HES, hydroxyethyl starch. (Adapted from Reinhart K, Rudolph T, Bredle DL, et al. Comparison of central-venous to mixed-venous oxygen saturation during changes in oxygen supply/demand. *Chest.* 1989;95(6):1216–1221.)

complex, critically ill patients, the correlation between changes in $S\bar{v}O_2$ and changes in any of the individual determining factors is low (74). In a study of the patients in a surgical ICU, no statistical correlation existed between changes in either PaO_2 or SaO_2 and $S\bar{v}O_2$. Although there was a statistically significant correlation between changes in $S\bar{v}O_2$ and CO and $\dot{D}O_2$, the coefficients of determination (r^2) were too low to allow prediction of CO, $\dot{V}O_2$, or $\dot{D}O_2$, from $S\bar{v}O_2$. Also, no statistical correlation existed between $S\bar{v}O_2$ and either arterial–venous O_2 content difference or calculated $\dot{V}O_2$. There was a significant inverse correlation between $S\bar{v}O_2$ and O_2 utilization coefficients, confirming the accuracy of the measurement and the reliability of $S\bar{v}O_2$ as an estimation of the O_2 utilization ratio—as long as SaO_2 is near 100%. The determinants of $S\bar{v}O_2$ are multifactorial, and, in critically ill patients, the degree of compensation for changes in one variable cannot be predicted (74). Patients with chronically impaired O_2 transport appear to tolerate very low $S\bar{v}O_2$ values better than acutely ill patients, presumably due to adaptive changes in the former group. Delayed lactate presentation may be seen in this group of patients (75,76).

It is useful, however, to appreciate the magnitude of change in $S\bar{v}O_2$ that would occur with an isolated change in any of the individual determinants. The relationship between the variables that contribute to $S\bar{v}O_2$ may not be linear (77). If no compensatory changes occur in $\dot{V}O_2$ or CO, Hgb must decrease by almost 50% (13 to 7.5 g/dL/L) before $S\bar{v}O_2$ decreases below the lower limit of the normal range (Table 24.3). The $S\bar{v}O_2$ changes would be even smaller because CO should increase in response to the acute anemia. However, if CO is fixed because of underlying cardiovascular disease, a decrease in Hgb will be reflected by a decrease in $S\bar{v}O_2$. Similarly, a small change in a patient with a low CO will have a greater effect on $S\bar{v}O_2$ than a larger change in a patient with a high CO (77).

The effect of arterial O_2 tension on $S\bar{v}O_2$ in the absence of other compensatory changes is demonstrated in Table 24.4. As long as SaO_2 is maintained in a relatively normal range, the direct effect on $S\bar{v}O_2$ is minimal. However, when there is sufficient arterial hypoxemia to produce arterial desaturation, the $S\bar{v}O_2$ falls in direct proportion to the change in SaO_2. Similarly, changes in CO (Table 24.5) and $\dot{V}O_2$ (Table 24.6) may

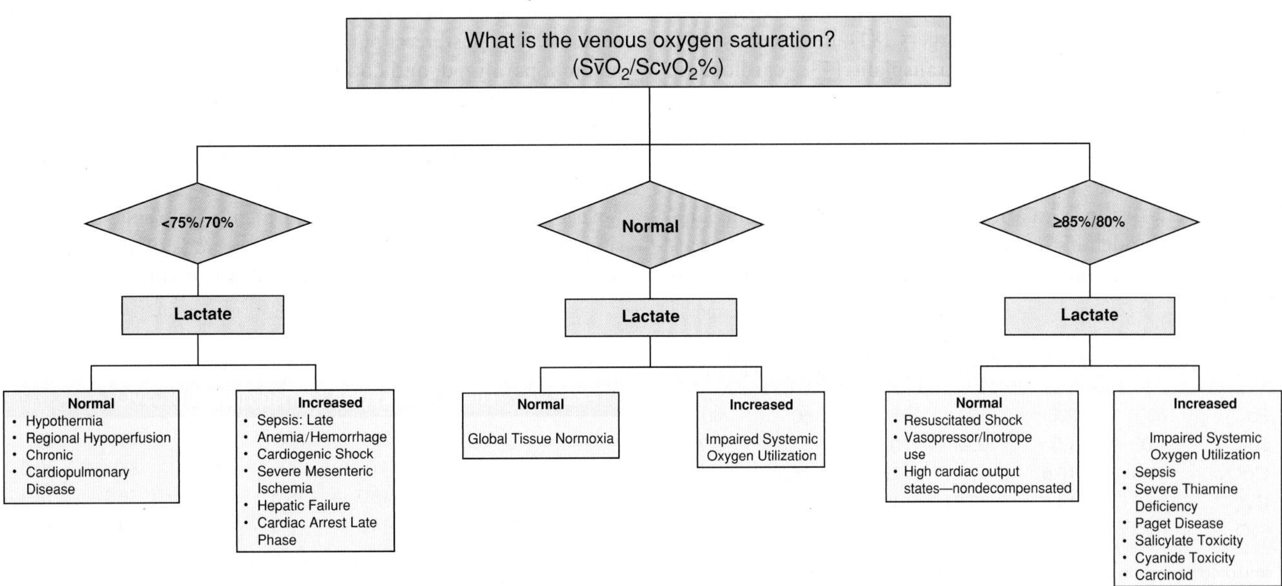

FIGURE 24.10 Diagnostic algorithm of $ScvO_2$/$S\bar{v}O_2$.

TABLE 24.3 Effect of Changes in Hemoglobin Concentration on $S\bar{v}O_2$

Hemoglobin	13	10	7.5	5
CaO_2	18.0	14.0	10.5	7.0
$C\bar{v}O_2$	14.0	10.0	6.5	3.0
$S\bar{v}O_2$	0.77	0.71	0.61	0.42

Calculated change in $S\bar{v}O_2$ caused by a change in hemoglobin (g/dL), assuming no compensatory changes in other determinants of $S\bar{v}O_2$; PaO_2 = 100 mmHg, SaO_2 = 0.98, $C(a - \bar{v})O_2$ = 4.0 mL/dL, and $\dot{V}O_2$ and cardiac output are not changed.

TABLE 24.5 Effect of Cardiac Output (CO) on $S\bar{v}O_2$

CO	10	7.5	5.0	4.0	3.0	2.0
$C(a-\bar{v})O_2$	2.5	3.3	5.0	6.3	8.3	12.5
CaO_2	18.3	18.3	18.3	18.3	18.3	18.3
$C\bar{v}O_2$	15.8	15.0	13.3	12.0	10.0	5.8
$S\bar{v}O_2$	0.87	0.83	0.73	0.66	0.55	0.31

Calculated effect of uncompensated changes in cardiac output (L/min) on $S\bar{v}O_2$, assuming hemoglobin = 13 g/dL, PaO_2 = 100 mmHg, SaO_2 = 0.98, and $\dot{V}O_2$ is fixed at 250 mL/min.

be shown to affect $S\bar{v}O_2$, although the magnitude of change in any of these individual parameters does not predict the magnitude of change in $S\bar{v}O_2$ because compensatory factors are usually involved. A decrease in $S\bar{v}O_2$ greater than 10% is likely to be clinically significant regardless of the initial value. A change from 70% to 60% may be associated with a large fractional change in CO if other factors did not change. On the other hand, a change from 60% to 50% is associated with a much smaller fractional change in CO but in the range of limited O_2 transport reserve and should raise more concern (Table 24.7).

When demand exceeds consumption, anaerobic metabolism must occur, and the eventual result is lactic acidosis. The lactate level, therefore, defines the balance between $\dot{V}O_2$ and O_2 demands. An elevated lactate implies either ongoing anaerobic metabolism (shock) or prior anaerobic metabolism and O_2 debt. A normal $S\bar{v}O_2$ implies the latter and a low $S\bar{v}O_2$, the former, in states of lactic acidosis, except in situations in which unloading cellular uptake or mitochondrial utilization are impaired.

CLINICAL USES OF MONITORING

$ScvO_2$ values have been used extensively in various clinical scenarios in critically ill patients. These include during and after cardiac arrest (CA) (78,79), in cardiac surgery patients (80), during and after cardiac failure (81), shock (82), acute myocardial infarction (54,84), general medical ICU conditions (85–87), postoperative cardiovascular procedures (87), trauma (88–90), vascular surgery (91,92), septic shock (9,12,67), hypovolemia (93,94), pediatric surgery (81), in neonates (95), lung transplantation (96), liver transplant (43), cardiogenic shock (97,98) and ECMO (99).

Cardiac Arrest

Management of the CA patient by advanced cardiac life support (ACLS) guidelines include physical examination (i.e., palpation of a pulse) and electrocardiographic monitoring. $ScvO_2$ monitoring during CA has been shown to be a diagnostic and therapeutic adjunct (100–102); CA patients routinely have $ScvO_2$ values of 5% to 20% during cardiopulmonary resuscitation (CPR). Failure to reach an $ScvO_2$ of at least 40% during the management of CA carries a 100% mortality even if the patient has an intermittent measurable blood pressure. These values are consistent with animal models ($S\bar{v}O_2$ < 43%) using cardiopulmonary bypass (103). $ScvO_2$ has also been used to confirm the presence or absence of sustainable cardiac activity during electromechanical dissociation (EMD) or a pulseless idioventricular rhythm where over 35% of these patients have been shown to have spontaneous cardiac activity (pseudo-EMD) (104). If the $ScvO_2$ is greater than 60% during CPR, return of spontaneous circulation (ROSC) is likely, and the pulse should be frequently rechecked if EMD was present. Between $ScvO_2$ values of 40% and 72%, there is a progressive increase in the rate of ROSC. When an $ScvO_2$ greater than 72% is obtained, ROSC has likely occurred. Continuous $ScvO_2$ monitoring also provides an objective measure to confirm the adequacy or inadequacy of CPR in providing $\dot{D}O_2$.

Postcardiac Arrest Care

In the immediate postresuscitation period, patients are frequently hemodynamically unstable and have a high frequency of rearrest. Blood pressure (1,101) may be rendered insensitive in the measurement of CO or DO_2 secondary to high systemic vascular resistance induced by catecholamine therapy. An abrupt or gradual decrease in $S\bar{v}O_2$, to less than 40% to 50%, indicates likelihood for rearrest. An $S\bar{v}O_2$ greater than 60% to 70% indicates hemodynamic stability. A study by Ameloot et al. (105) in postarrest patients who were intubated, placed in a coma, paralyzed, and cooled showed an optimal $S\bar{v}O_2$ range of 67% to 72%, with an odds ratio of 8.23 for mortality of patients outside of this range. A sustained extreme elevation of $S\bar{v}O_2$, greater than 80%, or venous hyperoxia, in the presence of a low $\dot{D}O_2$ and increased lactate levels carries a poor prognosis because it indicates an impairment of systemic O_2 utilization. This has been attributed to long periods of arrest and the use of large doses of vasopressors (106). If this derangement

TABLE 24.4 Effect of Variation in PaO_2 on $S\bar{v}O_2$

PaO_2	600	200	100	80	60	40
SaO_2	1.0	1.0	0.98	0.95	0.90	0.75
CaO_2	19.8	18.6	17.9	17.3	16.3	13.6
$C\bar{v}O_2$	15.9	14.6	13.9	13.3	12.3	9.6
$S\bar{v}O_2$	0.87	0.81	0.77	0.73	0.68	0.53

Calculated change in $S\bar{v}O_2$ caused by an uncompensated change in PaO_2 (mmHg), assuming hemoglobin = 13 g/dL, $C(a - \bar{v})O_2$ = 4.0 mL/dL, and $\dot{V}O_2$ and cardiac output are unchanged.

TABLE 24.6 Effect of Oxygen Consumption on $S\bar{v}O_2$

$\dot{V}O_2$	150	200	250	300	400	500
$C(a-\bar{v})O_2$	3.0	4.0	5.0	6.0	8.0	10.0
CaO_2	18.3	18.3	18.3	18.3	18.3	18.3
$C\bar{v}O_2$	15.3	14.3	13.3	12.3	10.3	8.3
$S\bar{v}O_2$	0.85	0.79	0.74	0.68	0.57	0.46

Effect of uncompensated changes in $\dot{V}O_2$ (mL/min) on $S\bar{v}O_2$, assuming hemoglobin = 13 g/dL, PaO_2 = 100 mmHg, SaO_2 = 0.98, and cardiac output is fixed at 5 L/min.

TABLE 24.7 Percentage of Error Resulting from Estimation of $P\bar{v}O_2$

	Measured Values of $S\bar{v}O_2$		
Factor	0.50	0.75	0.85
$C\bar{v}O_2$	1.2	0.8	0.7
$C(a-\bar{v})O_2$	1.2	2.6	4.8
$\dot{V}O_2$	1.2	2.6	4.8
$\dot{Q}sp/\dot{Q}t$	0.9	1.0	3.0

Theoretical maximum errors (%) in derived parameters if $P\bar{v}O_2$ is estimated at 20 and 50 mmHg for each saturation value measured. Maximum error is 4.8% only at the extreme of estimating $P\bar{v}O_2$, to be 20 mmHg when $S\bar{v}O_2$ is 0.85. The maximum error would be one-half of this amount if $P\bar{v}O_2$, is estimated to be 35 mmHg in all cases. These maximum predicted errors are not clinically significant.

is not corrected within the first 6 hours of the early postresuscitation period, the outcome is uniformly fatal (101). Venous hyperoxia can also be seen after acute myocardial infarction. Postexercise $S\bar{v}O_2$ overshoot and, hence, decreased systemic O_2 extraction during recovery represent a compensatory response of an enhanced peripheral vascular tone that maintains systemic arterial blood pressure in the setting of reduced CO by linking central and peripheral blood flow (107). As post-CA care now commonly incorporates hypothermia, it is also important to note that hypothermic therapy in post-CA patients has recently been shown to not affect the accuracy of the $S\bar{v}O_2$ measurement from the PAC. A study comparing 88 simultaneous values of $S\bar{v}O_2$ measured by PAC compared to blood gas samples drawn from the tip of the catheter in hypothermic postarrest patients showed no difference between the two modalities (105).

Traumatic and Hemorrhagic Shock

The standards of Advanced Trauma Life Support (ATLS) focus on normalization of vital signs (108). Studies have shown that vital signs are insensitive end points of resuscitation and outcome predictors in hemorrhage and trauma resuscitation (1,109). Scalea et al. (109) and Kowalenko and colleagues (110) have shown that patients presenting with trauma and hemorrhage required additional resuscitation or surgical procedures if the $ScvO_2$ remained less than 65%. Kremzar et al. (88) evaluated whether maintaining normal levels of $S\bar{v}O_2$ in patients with multiple injuries is more relevant to survival than maintaining above-normal levels of O_2 transport. For patients with multiple injuries, maintaining normal $S\bar{v}O_2$ values and increasing $\dot{D}O_2$ only if required are more relevant for survival than routine maintenance of above-normal O_2 transport values. In a series of 10 seriously injured patients requiring resuscitation and definitive operative control of hemorrhage, Karzarian and Del Guercio (89) found that improvement of the $S\bar{v}O_2$ was associated with improved survival. In this study, $S\bar{v}O_2$ was a valuable predictors of survival and was a helpful parameter to monitor during the resuscitative, operative, and immediate postoperative periods.

Acute and Chronic Heart Failure and Pulmonary Hypertension

Cardiogenic shock is characterized by decreased $\dot{D}O_2$, decreased $S\bar{v}O_2$, increased O_2ER, and evidence of tissue hypoxia—lactic acidosis and end-organ dysfunction—secondary to acute myocardial dysfunction (97,98). While $S\bar{v}O_2$ has been shown to have therapeutic and prognostic utility in patients with acute myocardial infarction (84,98,111,112), prospective outcome studies have not validated its clinical use in this patient population (113). Ander et al. (68) examined patients who presented with decompensated chronic severe heart failure (ejection fraction < 30%) who were stratified into normal and elevated lactate (>2 mmol/L) groups. There was a significant prevalence of "occult cardiogenic shock" ($ScvO_2$ 26.4% to 36.8%) in the presence of normal vital signs. Using a goal-oriented approach of preload, afterload, contractility, coronary perfusion, and heart rate optimization, these patients required additional therapy compared to their counterparts with normal lactate levels. $ScvO_2$ and brain natriuretic peptide (BNP) level predict hemodynamics associated with lower survival rates and may be useful as noninvasive markers of prognosis in epoprostenol-treated pulmonary arterial hypertension (PAH) patients (114).

Severe Sepsis and Septic Shock

$S\bar{v}O_2$ in sepsis is commonly referred to as an end point of low impact in clinical decisions because of the common perception that $S\bar{v}O_2$ is always increased in septic ICU patients. In septic shock the $S\bar{v}O_2$ is more difficult to interpret, as the O_2 demand may exceed $\dot{V}O_2$, meaning that $S\bar{v}O_2$ will not accurately reflect the relationship between $\dot{V}O_2$ and $\dot{D}O_2$ (116). Microcirculatory shunting is thought to explain the phenomenon of normal $S\bar{v}O_2$ in septic shock with multisystem organ failure from local tissue dysoxia (116). However, there are fundamental issues that render this modality clinically useful when applying it to the early stages of the supply-dependent phase of sepsis (global tissue hypoxia) where saturation is low in both animal (117,118) and human models of sepsis (111). During this phase, $S\bar{v}O_2$ is inversely correlated with lactate concentration ($r = -0.87$, $p < 0.001$). These data suggest that cellular O_2 utilization is largely maintained during rapidly fatal septic shock (119,120). These findings highlight the importance of early assessment and intervention. Identifying sudden episodes of supply dependency in septic ICU patients, that is, a sudden decrease in $S\bar{v}O_2$, has diagnostic and prognostic significance (10,12,67). Previous studies have examined $S\bar{v}O_2$-guided goal-directed therapy after ICU admission and have found no outcome benefit in general ICU patients (86). However, in a study evaluating early goal-directed therapy (EGDT) using multiple hemodynamic end points including $S\bar{v}O_2$ in the most proximal stages of hospital admission, patients presenting with severe sepsis and septic shock were randomized to 6 hours of EGDT or standard therapy before ICU admission. Both groups were resuscitated to a CVP higher than 8 mmHg and mean arterial pressure (MAP) over 65 mmHg; however, the treatment group was resuscitated to an $ScvO_2$ above 70% using additional therapies such as red cell transfusion, inotropes, and mechanical ventilation to reach this end point (Fig. 24.11). Over the initial 72 hours, there was a higher $ScvO_2$, lower lactate, lower base deficit, and higher pH in the EGDT versus the control group indicating more definitive resolution of global tissue hypoxia. Organ dysfunction, vasopressor use, duration of mechanical ventilation, and mortality were significantly reduced (9). This concept of EGDT has been reproduced in multiple studies and is one of the cornerstones of the resuscitation bundle recommended by the Surviving Sepsis Campaign (72). More recent studies have

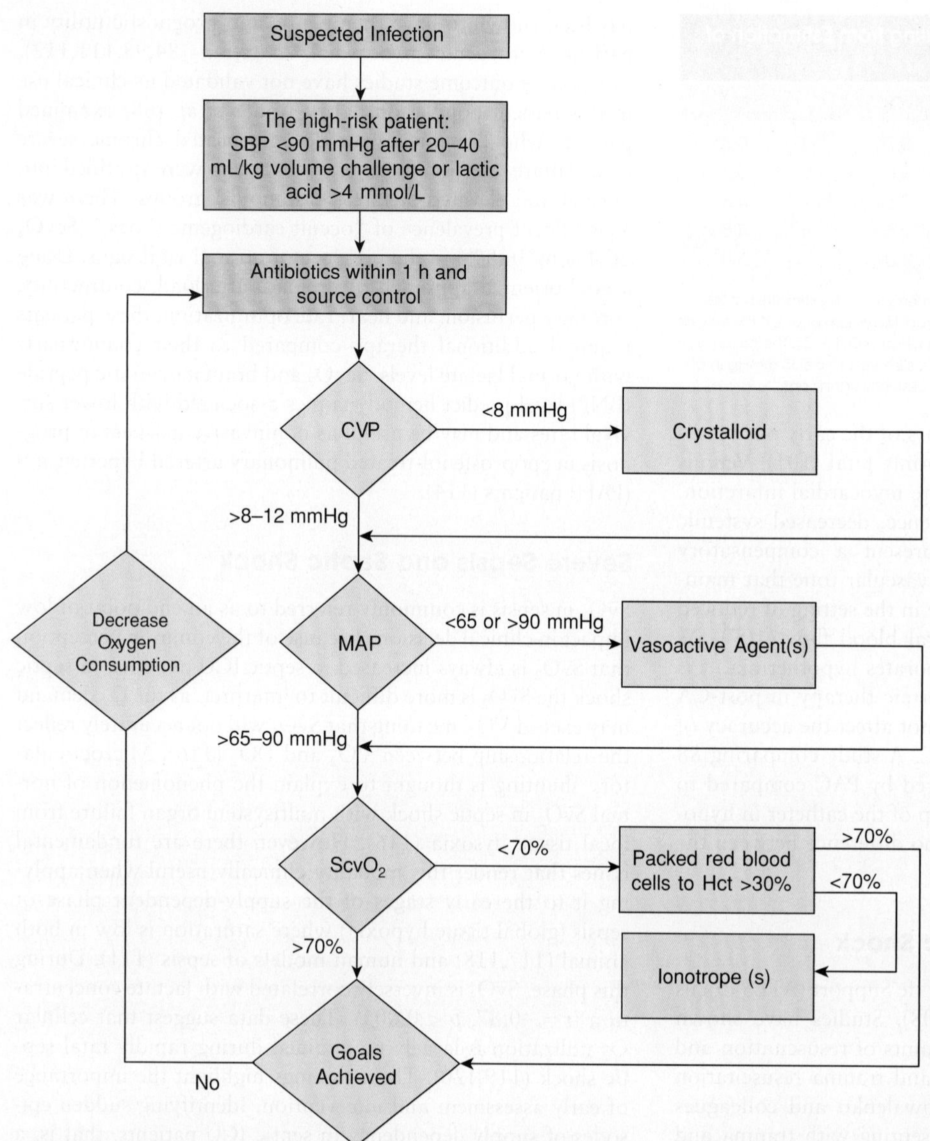

FIGURE 24.11 Early goal-directed therapy (EGDT) in severe sepsis and septic shock. CVP, central venous pressure; Hct, hematocrit; MAP, mean arterial pressure; SBP, systolic blood pressure; $ScvO_2$, central venous oxygen saturation. (Adapted from Rivers E, Nguyen B, Havstad S, et al. Early goal-directed therapy in the treatment of severe sepsis and septic shock. *N Engl J Med.* 2001;345(19):1368–1377.)

examined the relationship between $S\bar{v}O_2$ and fluid responsiveness, and have shown that baseline $S\bar{v}O_2$ in septic patients is a poor predictor of fluid responsiveness, measured as change in CI or change in SVI after a fluid challenge (116).

Pulmonary Embolus

Patients with massive pulmonary embolism (PE) and obstructive shock usually require hemodynamic stabilization, thrombolytics, and mechanical interventions. Krivec and colleagues (121) examined 10 consecutive patients hospitalized in the ICU with obstructive shock following massive PE in a prospective observational study. During hemodynamic optimization and infusion of thrombolytic therapy, heart rate, CVP, mean pulmonary artery pressure, and UOP remained unchanged, but the relative change of $S\bar{v}O_2$ at hour 1 was higher than the relative changes of all other studied variables ($p < 0.05$). Serum lactate on admission and at 12 hours correlated inversely with $S\bar{v}O_2$ ($r = -0.855$, $p < 0.001$). In obstructive shock after massive PE, $S\bar{v}O_2$ changes more rapidly than other standard hemodynamic variables.

Respiratory Failure

In 9 of 13 patients with hypoxemic respiratory failure requiring PEEP, there was a strong correlation ($r = 0.88$) between DO_2 and $S\bar{v}O_2$. Of the four patients not showing a good correlation, two had sepsis and two had nearly normal values of $S\bar{v}O_2$ and O_2 delivery at all levels of PEEP studied. Continuous measurement of $S\bar{v}O_2$ improves monitoring of patients, facilitates titration of respiratory therapies, detects abrupt changes in tissue O_2 consumption, and identifies levels of PEEP associated with greatest O_2 delivery (123).

Postoperative Thoracic and Cardiac Surgery Patients

Continuous $S\bar{v}O_2$ monitoring was examined in 19 patients as to its predictive value during the postoperative course after thoracotomy for a time period up to 60 hours. In all but 1 of the 10 patients with $S\bar{v}O_2$ less than 65% for at least 1 hour, complications occurred. A fall of $S\bar{v}O_2$ greater than 5% or a value below 60% predicted a period of hypotension in six patients. In two of them, this coincided with a period of ventricular dysrhythmias. In those with $S\bar{v}O_2$ above 65%, no postoperative complications such as arrhythmias, shock, respiratory dysfunction, or oliguria took place (82). Cardiac surgical patients are at risk of inadequate perioperative O_2 delivery caused by extracorporeal circulation and limited cardiovascular reserves (123,124). Four hundred and three elective cardiac surgical patients were enrolled in the study and randomly assigned to either the control or the protocol group. Goals of the protocol group were to maintain $S\bar{v}O_2$ over 70% and a lactate concentration of 2.0 mmol/L or less from ICU admission and up to 8 hours thereafter. The median hospital stay was shorter in the protocol group (6 vs. 7 days, $p < 0.05$), and patients were discharged faster from the hospital than those in the control group ($p < 0.05$). Discharge from the ICU was similar between groups ($p = 0.8$). Morbidity was less frequent at the time of hospital discharge in the protocol group (1.1% vs. 6.1%, $p < 0.01$) (125). Venous oximetry has also been shown to have clinical utility in weaning patients from ventricular assist devices (126,127).

There have been efforts to replace $S\bar{v}O_2$ with $ScvO_2$ in the cardiac surgery population, but these have shown that the two methods are not interchangeable. A study of 15 consecutive patients undergoing cardiopulmonary bypass for cardiac surgery using continuous fiber-optics to obtain 9,267 paired intraoperative and postoperative data points demonstrated that while concordance in the measurements and pattern of changes was seen in some patients, in others significant changes in $S\bar{v}O_2$ were not accompanied by changes in the $ScvO_2$ (128). These findings suggest that $ScvO_2$ is not a suitable replacement for $S\bar{v}O_2$ in cardiopulmonary bypass patients.

There may be utility to measuring $ScvO_2$ during cardiac surgery, however. Suehiro et al. (129) looked at 102 patients undergoing cardiac surgery with cardiopulmonary bypass and showed that the discrepancy between $S\bar{v}O_2$ and $ScvO_2$ intraoperatively was a better predictor of postoperative ICU stay and ventilator dependence than either marker alone, with a difference of 12% indicative of worse outcome. Similarly, a negative $ScvO_2 - S\bar{v}O_2$ gradient on postoperative day 1 in 156 cardiac surgery patients having undergone cardiopulmonary bypass had higher serum lactate levels, longer ischemia times, were older and considered higher operative risk. Patients with a negative gradient preoperatively also had lower SVI (41). The patient's cardiac function may have an impact on the relationship between $ScvO_2$ and $S\bar{v}O_2$, however. Gasparovic and colleagues (41) studied patients undergoing cardiac surgery with cardiopulmonary bypass, showing that $ScvO_2$ was strongly correlated with $S\bar{v}O_2$ in patients with a CI above 2 L/min/m^2 ($r^2 = 0.73$), but was weakly correlated in patients with a lower CI ($r^2 = 0.37$). Shahbazi et al. (130) demonstrated in 62 patients undergoing cardiac surgery with cardiopulmonary bypass that simultaneous measurements of $S\bar{v}O_2$ and lactic acid drawn from an arterial line did not correlate, stressing the importance of following $S\bar{v}O_2$ rather than relying of laboratory markers. Interestingly, this study did show a correlation between $S\bar{v}O_2$ and $ScvO_2$, though it used far fewer data points than the study by Lequeux and colleagues (128), mentioned above. The relationship between fluid responsiveness and $S\bar{v}O_2$ in cardiac or vascular surgery patients may differ from that of septic patients, described above. A recent study of patients undergoing cardiac and major vascular surgeries demonstrated a greater response in $S\bar{v}O_2$ among patients categorized as fluid responders based on increase in CI or SVI in response to a fluid bolus (131).

Vascular Surgery

In patients undergoing elective operations for aortic aneurysms ($n = 25$) and aortoiliac occlusive disease ($n = 6$), $S\bar{v}O_2$ was recorded throughout the operation. In all patients, unclamping the aorta resulted in a marked reduction of mean $S\bar{v}O_2$, with no change in the CO or SaO_2. The unclamping of tube grafts was associated with a significant reduction in arterial pH ($p < 0.01$) and in $S\bar{v}O_2$ ($p < 0.001$) when compared with unclamping of bifurcation grafts. Despite a longer clamp time, unclamping the second limb of a bifurcation graft resulted in a smaller decrease in $S\bar{v}O_2$ when compared with that observed after unclamping the first limb (12% vs. 6%, $p < 0.01$). The change in $S\bar{v}O_2$ after unclamping the second limb was only 2% in aortobifemoral grafts and 9% in aortobi-iliac grafts. Reperfusion via extensive pelvic and lumbar collaterals in patients with aortoiliac occlusive disease reduces the degree of $S\bar{v}O_2$ decrease after aortic unclamping. Monitoring the changes in $S\bar{v}O_2$ during different types of aortic reconstruction helps to define precisely the physiologic alterations that occur in the course of these operations (91,92).

Postoperative High-Risk Patients

$ScvO_2$ and other biochemical, physiologic, and demographic data were prospectively measured for 8 hours after major surgery. Data from 118 patients were analyzed; 123 morbid episodes occurred in 64 of these patients. The optimal $ScvO_2$ cutoff value for morbidity prediction was 64.4%. In the first hour after surgery, significant reductions in $ScvO_2$ were observed, but there were no significant changes in CI or DO_2I during the same period. Significant fluctuations in $S\bar{v}O_2$ occur in the immediate postoperative period and are not always associated with changes in DO_2, suggesting that O_2 consumption is also an important determinant of $ScvO_2$. Reductions in $ScvO_2$ are independently associated with postoperative complications (132–135).

Patients On ECMO

In patients being placed on extracorporeal membrane oxygenation (ECMO) devices, $S\bar{v}O_2$ has been shown to have prognostic importance. Preoperative $S\bar{v}O_2$ is predictive of the mortality of patients being placed on V–A ECMO, with 79.3% being the median $S\bar{v}O_2$ for survivors and 53.0% the median value for nonsurvivors in an observational study of 80 patients with cardiac failure, including adults and children (99). This finding is intriguing as the mean $S\bar{v}O_2$ of survivors exceeds the normal physiologic range; in this setting, it may prove useful in predicting who will benefit from such a resource-intense intervention.

Positioning Patients and Postural Changes

The effects of changes in positioning on $S\bar{v}O_2$ in critically ill patients with a low EF (≤30%) and the contribution of ($\dot{D}O_2$) and ($\dot{V}O_2$) variables to the variance in $S\bar{v}O_2$ were examined.

An experimental two-group repeated-measures design was used to study 42 critically ill patients with an EF of ≤30%. Patients were assigned randomly to one of two position sequences: supine, right lateral, left lateral; or supine, left lateral, right lateral. Data on $S\bar{v}O_2$ were collected at baseline, each minute after position change for 5 minutes, and at 15 and 25 minutes. A difference in $S\bar{v}O_2$ among the three positions across time was significantly different ($p < 0.0001$), with the greatest differences occurring within the first 4 minutes and in the left lateral position. $\dot{V}O_2$ accounted for a greater proportion of the variance in $S\bar{v}O_2$ with position change than did $\dot{D}O_2$ (136,137). Similar findings have been noted in $S\bar{v}O_2$ with orthostatic positioning and its superiority in reflecting central blood volume over CVP (93).

Neonates and Pediatric Patients

$S\bar{v}O_2$ has been shown to be clinically useful in pediatric patients (138). However, the challenges of PAC placement make monitoring of the shock state with $S\bar{v}O_2$ limited, making $ScvO_2$ a convenient surrogate (81,94). In an experimental model of neonatal sepsis, $S\bar{v}O_2$ significantly correlates with right atrial O_2 saturation ($r^2 = 0.88$). Animal studies suggest that $ScvO_2$ at the RA can be a sure, efficient, and easy alternative for the neonatal patient (139), particularly during therapeutic interventions such as mechanical ventilation and intravascular volume resuscitation (140); studies in patients have been less consistent. Simultaneous $ScvO_2$ and $S\bar{v}O_2$ values in children recovering from open heart surgery show $ScvO_2$ is consistently lower than $S\bar{v}O_2$. This difference may be secondary to residual intracardiac left-to-right shunting of blood or to altered distribution of systemic blood flow. The saturation difference between the two venous samples decreases during postoperative recovery, making a $ScvO_2$ blood sample an inadequate substitute for $S\bar{v}O_2$. Because $ScvO_2$ was frequently subnormal while $S\bar{v}O_2$ was in the normal range, monitoring of $S\bar{v}O_2$ could not be reliably used to rule out O_2 supply/demand imbalance during the early postoperative period in these patients (138,141). To overcome these clinical inconsistencies, a regression formula was derived:

$$S\bar{v}O_2 = 3 \times SVC + HIVC/4$$

where SVC is superior vena cava saturation and HIVC is high inferior vena cava saturation (64).

Validation of the clinical utility of $ScvO_2$ in children has the same challenges as in adults. A sepsis trial reported significant survival benefit when $ScvO_2$ was added to the pediatric model of septic shock. This study supports current recommendations by the American College of Critical Care Medicine for its use in neonatal and pediatric septic shock (Fig. 24.12) (142).

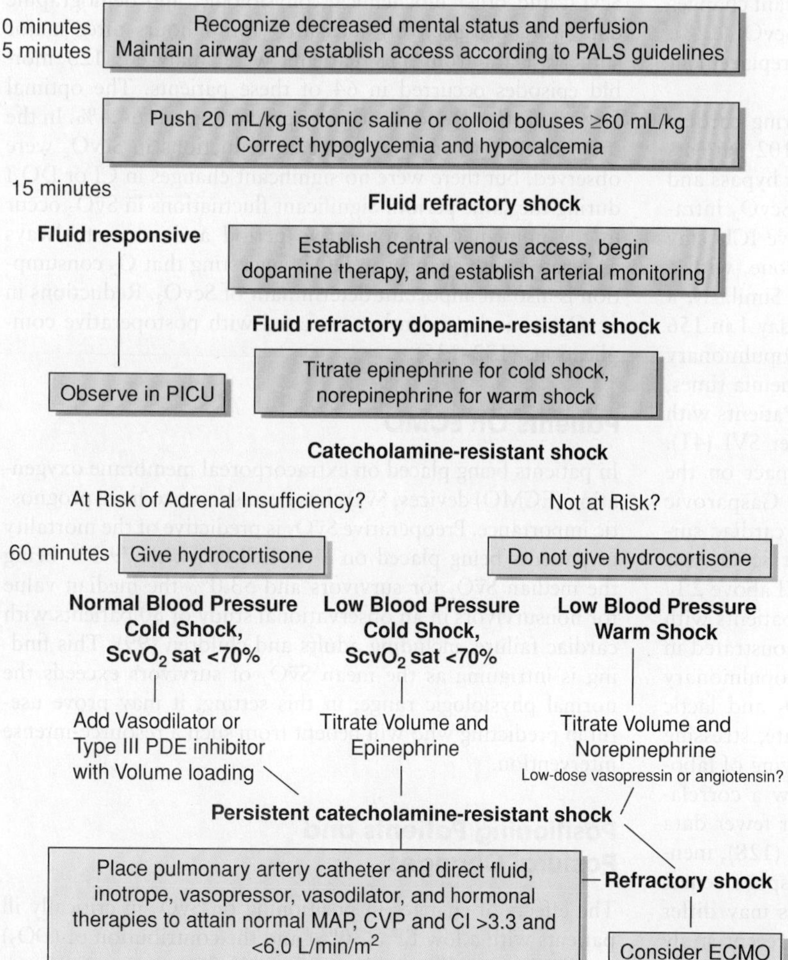

FIGURE 24.12 Pediatric advanced life support (PALS). CI, chlorine; CVP, central venous pressure; ECMO; extracorporeal membrane oxygenation; MAP, mean arterial pressure; PDE, phosphodiesterase; PICU, pediatric intensive care unit; $ScvO_2$, central venous oxygen saturation. (Adapted from Carcillo JA, Fields AI. Clinical practice parameters for hemodynamic support of pediatric and neonatal patients in septic shock. *Crit Care Med.* 2002;30(6):1365–1378.)

COST-EFFECTIVENESS

Economic analysis of the technology of venous oximetry is complex. Because of its variable use in many clinical situations, the direct association with one single variable to outcome and health care resource consumption is not a simple one. In quantitating the economic impact, one must assess prevention of additional resource use such as venous blood gases and nursing time, hemodynamic life-threatening events, and decreased health care resource consumption through improved morbidity and mortality. Significant reductions in the number of venous blood gas analyses, cardiac output measurement, and charges have been observed (123,143,144). Several studies have suggested that the increased cost of the fiber-optic catheter is not justifiable in terms of cost savings (145,146). However, in the treatment of sepsis and cardiothoracic patients, significant reductions in morbidity, mortality, and health care resource consumption have been observed with goal-directed algorithms using venous oximetry (125,147).

COMBINED VENOUS AND PULSE OXIMETRY

Pulse oximetry and continuous mixed venous oximetry can be combined into a useful tool if we understand the underlying physiology that allows certain inferences to be made as well as the limitations. The two devices together provide the capacity to evaluate simultaneous changes in the patient's cardiovascular and respiratory systems. Arterial oxygen tension and arterial oxygen saturation are related through the familiar oxyhemoglobin dissociation curve. SaO_2 values in the range of 70 to 95 reflect changes in PaO_2 and are useful in monitoring cardiorespiratory disease and directing therapy. Large changes in PaO_2 (80 to 600 mmHg) can occur with minimum changes in SaO_2. To maintain arterial oxygen delivery, we keep SaO_2 values between 90% and 95%. Below 90%, desaturation diminishes arterial oxygen content and oxygen delivery; above 95%, SaO_2 values no longer track PaO_2 values. At an Hgb value of 13 g/dL, fully saturated Hgb would carry 18.07 mL of oxygen. If arterial PO_2 was 100 mmHg, an additional 0.31 mL would be dissolved in plasma for a total oxygen content of 18.38 mL per 100 mL of blood. If PaO_2 fell to 75 mmHg and SaO_2 concomitantly dropped to 95%, Hgb-carried oxygen would be 18.07 times 0.95, or 17.17 mL. The dissolved oxygen would be 75 times 0.003, or 0.23, and total oxygen content would be 17.4 mL in 100 mL of blood. In the first example, total oxygen content was 18.38 mL. If the second oxygen content, 17.4 mL, is divided by 18.38 mL, the quotient is 0.95; thus, total oxygen content changed the same amount as did the arterial saturation. We can obtain the same information by comparing changes in SaO_2 alone without following either PaO_2 or calculating total oxygen content. The same is true for $S\bar{v}O_2$ and mixed venous oxygen content (28,148,150).

APPLICABILITY

There are many valuable bedside uses for simultaneous oximetry. For instance, if a patient's respiratory function has improved, high FiO_2 may be weaned quickly. We have found that changes can be made every 5 minutes. This contrasts to the usual clinical scenario using blood gases where after a change in FiO_2 (15-minute equilibration period), drawing of blood is done. If patients have severely depressed oxygenation, PEEP therapy can be augmented much more rapidly by monitoring $S\bar{v}O_2$. In the case of cardiovascular collapse associated with low $S\bar{v}O_2$, the response to blood and other fluid infusions as well as vasoactive drugs can be judged rapidly. If the intervention does not increase $S\bar{v}O_2$ quickly (within a few minutes), it probably has not been effective. Increased CO may result in increased oxygen consumption without a change in SaO_2 minus $S\bar{v}O_2$. This ability to judge the effectiveness of interventions quickly is certainly attractive and often gratifying to the clinician.

LIMITATIONS AND FUTURE QUESTIONS

In spite of studies questioning the value of $S\bar{v}O_2$ in ICU patients (101,141,146,150), there is considerable evidence that $ScvO_2$ may have a beneficial role in the early management of critically ill adults, children, and neonates (95,140). The ability to access this information earlier in the phases of critical illness is now a reality, and further studies are now in progress to confirm that early recognition and treatment of out-of-normal-range $ScvO_2$ values have significant outcome benefit.

CLINICAL EXAMPLES

Case 1

A 75-year-old male victim of a witnessed CA presents to the emergency department. After bystander CPR was performed, emergency medical services (EMS) initiates ACLS guidelines. He was found to be in ventricular fibrillation and was successfully defibrillated into normal sinus rhythm. He is admitted to the ICU.

Vital signs: Blood pressure (BP), 160/80; MAP, 106 mmHg; heart rate (HR), 130 beats per minute; respiratory rate (RR), 16 (bag/valve/mask); temperature, 36.4°C; SaO_2, 98% on 100% FiO_2; $ScvO_2$, 85%.

Arterial blood gas (ABG) (21%): pH, 7.20; $PaCO_2$, 31; PaO_2, 63; SaO_2, 93%; $NaHCO_3$, 18; base deficit, −5.

Complete blood count (CBC): White blood cells (WBC), 15.1; hemoglobin (Hb), 10.5; hematocrit (Hct), 31%; platelets (PLT), 400,000.

PA catheter: CI, 1.2/min/m^2; PAOP, 22 cm/H_2O; CVP, 26 cm/H_2O; systemic venous resistance (SVR), 5,600 dynes/s · cm^5.

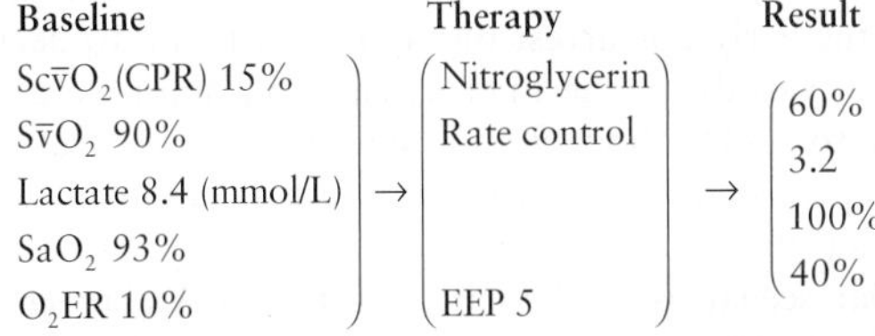

Baseline		Therapy		Result
$Sc\bar{v}O_2$(CPR) 15%		Nitroglycerin		60%
$S\bar{v}O_2$ 90%		Rate control		3.2
Lactate 8.4 (mmol/L)	→		→	100%
SaO_2 93%				40%
O_2ER 10%		EEP 5		

What's the Baseline?

This case (Fig. 24.13) illustrates several important elements. Namely, the interpretation of the $S\bar{v}O_2$ is limited without an

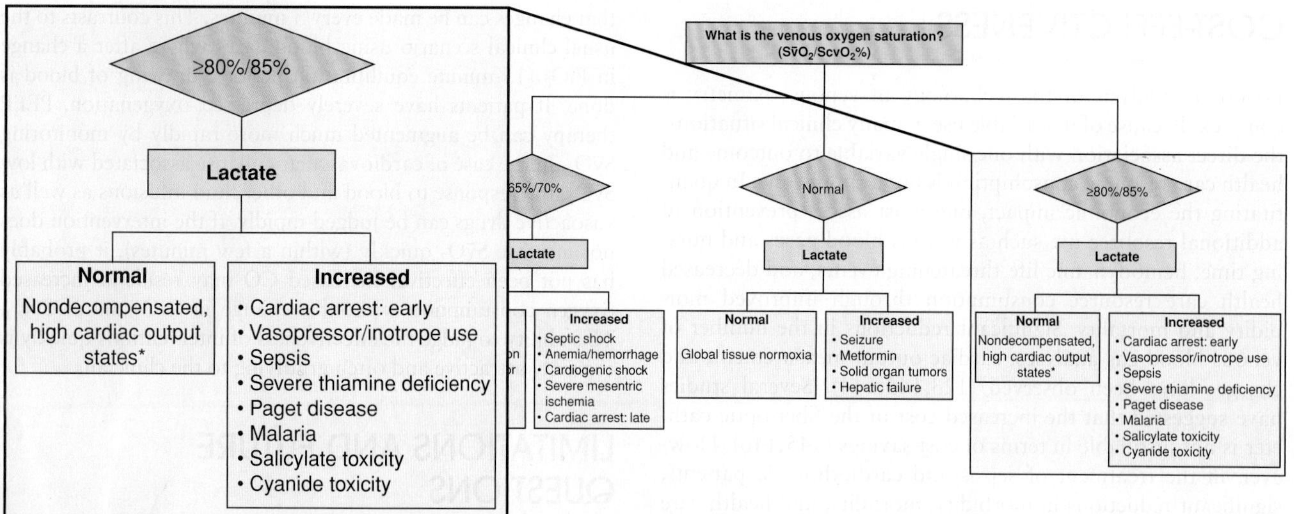

FIGURE 24.13 Baseline for Case 1.

ABG since a near-normal $S\bar{v}O_2$ value does not imply normal physiology. The oxygen extraction ratio (O_3ER) ($aO_2 - \bar{v}O_2$ difference/SaO_2) is only 10%. The value of $S\bar{v}O_2$ is also confounded by the presence of mild anemia. Hypoxemia and circulatory arrest with resultant hypoperfusion leads to anaerobic metabolism represented by the presence of lactic acidosis.

What's Happening?

The O_2ER is very low, and in the setting of CA, can possibly relate to the effects of vasopressors used during ACLS or the cytotoxic damage of global tissue hypoxia and reperfusion. This impairment of systemic O_2 utilization is manifest as mixed venous hyperoxia. Global tissue hypoxia ensues as a consequence of decreased perfusion and impaired tissue uptake resulting in lactic acidosis (79). It is notable that as treatment progresses with vasodilators, the O_2ER increases to 40% and lactate decreases.

What's the Interpretation?

The postresuscitative phase of CA is characterized by a complex array of hemodynamic perturbations (Fig. 24.14). O_2ER can be up to 90% during CA, and the failure to reach a $S\bar{v}O_2$ of 40% portends near 100% mortality (79). Once an ROSC is obtained, venous hyperoxia or an impaired O_2ER may be a temporary or permanent issue. The period immediately following multiple doses of vasopressors with ROSC is characterized by elevated circulating catecholamines and is termed the early postarrest phase. If efforts fail to decrease afterload, vasodilate the microcirculation, improve cardiac function to a $\dot{V}O_2$ above 90 mL/min/m^2 within 6 hours after CA and persistent lactic acidosis, death is imminent within 24 hours (79).

Similar scenarios to the early phase of CA characterized by an elevated $S\bar{v}O_2$ and lactic acidosis can also be seen with vasopressor-dependent shock, sepsis, severe thiamine deficiency, severe Paget disease, malaria, salicylate toxicity, and cyanide toxicity. The later post-ROSC phase demonstrating low $S\bar{v}O_2$ and persistent lactic acidosis is comparable to hepatic failure, sepsis, anemia/hemorrhage, cardiogenic shock, and severe mesenteric ischemia.

Case 2

A 66-year-old woman with a history of chronic obstructive lung disease (COPD) presents to the ED with a chief complaint of shortness of breath with fever for the past 4 days. She has had a cough productive of yellowish–greenish sputum and is tachypneic and in obvious respiratory distress.

Vital signs: BP, 140/80; HR, 118; RR, 24; temperature, 38.0°C; SpO_2, 88% on room air, 93% on 2 L/min O_2

ED course: The patient is noticeably more tachypneic and lethargic, so the patient is ultimately intubated for airway protection. Chest x-ray (CXR) study demonstrates a right lower lobe (RLL) infiltrate, consolidation, and airspace disease.

Hemodynamic monitoring in the ED: CVP, 16 cm/H_2O; $ScvO_2$, 44%; lactate, 1.9 mmol/L.

About 1 minute after intubation, $ScvO_2$ monitoring begins to rise; climbing to 58%. The patient is suctioned and copious thick sputum is removed. The patient's CVP improved to 8 cm

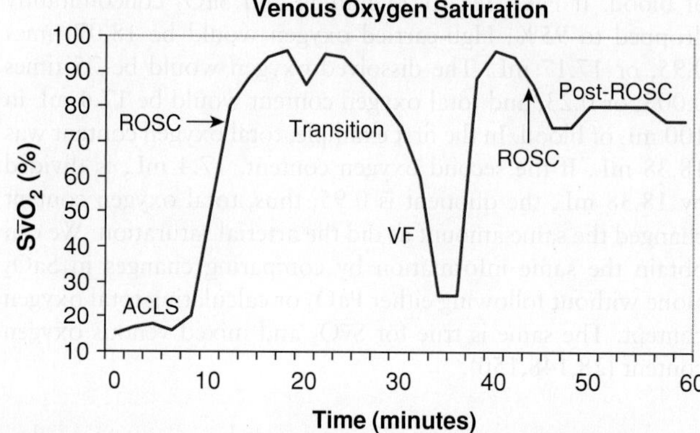

FIGURE 24.14 $S\bar{v}O_2$ response during resuscitation. ACLS, advanced cardiac life support; ROSC, return of spontaneous circulation; $S\bar{v}O_2$, mixed venous oxygen saturation; VF, ventricular fibrillation. (Adapted from Rivers EP, Martin GB, Smithline H, et al. The clinical implications of continuous central venous oxygen saturation during human CPR. *Ann Emerg Med.* 1992;21(9):1094–1101.)

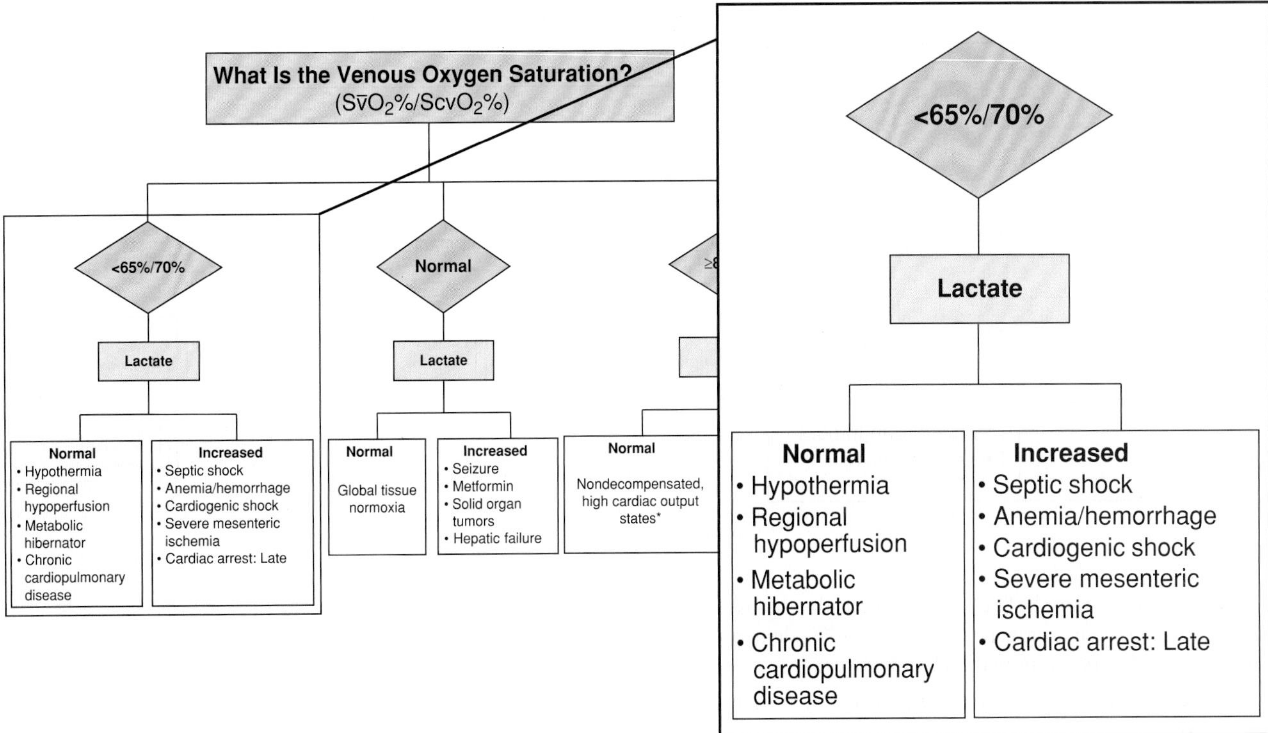

FIGURE 24.15 Baseline for Case 2.

H_2O after administration of a vasodilator. Repeat lactate reading increases 4.7 mmol/L.

Baseline		Therapy		Result
$Sc\bar{v}O_2$ 44%	→	Nitroglycerin	→	58%
Lactate 1.9 (mmol/L)		intubation		4.7
SaO_2 88%				100%
O_2ER 50%				40%

What's the Baseline?

This patient has hypoxia, respiratory distress, and relatively stable vital signs (Fig. 24.15). The fever and clinical complaint in the presence of three systemic inflammatory response syndrome (SIRS) criteria makes pneumonia a likely inciting condition. The patient also exhibits hyperlactatemia and central venous hypoxia (low $ScvO_2$).

What's Happening?

The patient has symptoms consistent with pneumonia and hypoxemia with an O_2ER of 50%. This increased O_2ER despite a normal blood pressure with an elevated CVP should alert the clinician of possible myocardial dysfunction.

What's the Interpretation?

The combination of three SIRS criteria and hyperlactatemia in the setting of infection heralds global hypoperfusion and organ dysfunction. The central venous hypoxemia reflects her O_2 delivery–dependent state. This illustrates the concept of cryptic septic shock. These patients are often clinically underrecognized due to the presence of seemingly normal vital signs in the face of tissue hypoxia. Interestingly, the presence of an elevated CVP would ordinarily imply normal or elevated intravascular volume, and in patients with a history of cardiac dysfunction, could lead the clinician to inappropriately administer a diuretic. In this case, a vasodilator was more appropriate therapy to improve CO by reduction of afterload. Patients with longstanding cardiopulmonary disease may have low venous saturation with normal lactate until they become delivery dependent. These have been characterized as metabolic hibernators (76).

The presence of SIRS criteria should prompt the clinician to consider obtaining a lactate level to stratify the severity of her condition. In certain patients who do not present initially with an elevated lactate, their history of concurrent medical conditions can create a state of ischemic preconditioning, also termed metabolic hibernation. This early recognition and treatment of the hypoperfused state was originally described by Rivers et al. where a protocolized approach to severe sepsis significantly improved morbidity and mortality. Similar hemodynamic conditions to this patient's *initial* presentation include hypothermia, a regional hypoperfused state, or congestive heart failure/cardiopulmonary disease.

Case 3

A 60-year-old male patient was brought to the ED from an assisted-living facility with a chief complaint of change in mental status. The patient has a past medical history significant for cerebral vascular accident (CVA), hypertension, schizophrenia, and diabetes. The patient was found slumped on a park bench.

Initially, the patient is nonverbal and presents with the following vital signs: BP, 110/40; HR, 120; RR, 24; temperature, 32°C; SaO_2, 96% on 2L O_2; Glasgow coma scale score, 11.

Physical examination: Patient receives 1-L bolus of isotonic crystalloid with mild increase in BP. The patient is taken to the monitored area of the ED because the nurse notices the patient

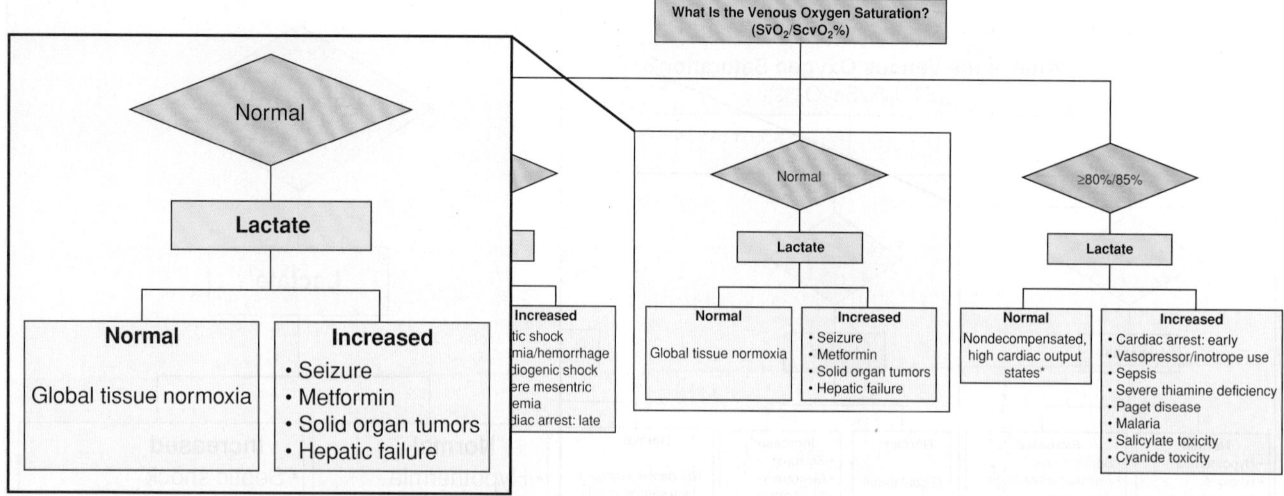

FIGURE 24.16 Baseline for Case 3.

is very slow to respond. The patient's bedside glucose is <50 mg/dL. The patient is given an amp of 50% dextrose. The patient's mental status immediately improves.

Labs: Na, 158; K, 5.2; Cl, 100; CO_2, 24; BUN, 90; creatinine, 1.8; glucose, 44; β-hydroxybutyrate, 8.0.

ABG: pH, 7.30; $PaCO_2$, 44; PaO_2, 100; SaO_2, 96%; HCO_3^-, 24; lactate, 2.0.

Hemodynamics: CVP, 1 cm H_2O, $ScvO_2$, 72%.

Hospital Course

Baseline	Therapy	Results
SaO_2: 96%	Fluids, thiamine, glucose	100%
$S\bar{v}O_2$ 72%		70%
O_2ER 25%		30%
Lactate 2.2% mmol/L		1.2 mmol/L

What's the Baseline?

This patient's mental status is altered, probably due to the combination of hypoglycemia and hypothermia (Fig. 24.16). His initial presentation and hemodynamic measurements indicate severe volume depletion. The patient is maintaining a normal blood pressure but has evidence of progressing hemodynamic instability. Given his history, toxicologic and metabolic derangements may be responsible for his hemodynamic embarrassment.

What's Happening?

The patient is exhibiting evidence of anion gap metabolic acidosis (which may be due to ketonemia [β-hydroxybutyrate] and mild lactic acidosis) as well as abnormal chemistry and blood gas data. His O_2ER is 25%, which is in the normal range. The patient is hypothermic, which may account for the central venous O_2 saturation in the normal range. His mental status may be accounted for by hypoglycemia.

What's the Interpretation?

The patient's extraction ratio may be slightly higher than expected but may be explained by a depressed metabolic rate associated with hypothermia. The near-normal lactate level on presentation may also be explained by a depressed metabolic rate despite the lack of substrate (glucose). The higher-than-expected O_2ER should be noted, and a search for disturbances of O_2 utilization should be considered. Entities that impair the tissues' ability to utilize O_2 consist of toxicologic and metabolic derangements including chronic thiamine deficiency, cyanide toxicity, and possibly severe acetaminophen toxicity.

Key Points

1. The mixed venous oxygen saturation may be represented as 1 – (systemic oxygen consumption/systemic oxygen delivery).
2. An imbalance between systemic oxygen delivery and consumption may result in either abnormally low values of mixed venous or central venous oxygen saturation when delivery is inadequate to meet demand, or abnormally high values when consumption decreases as a result of mitochondrial damage, altered vasoregulation, or with shunting. Both of these are associated with increased mortality.
3. Under normal conditions, central venous oxygen saturation will be higher than mixed venous oxygen saturation, but in a shock state, this relationship is consistently reversed. Regardless of which method is used, gross alterations in these values are ominous signs that require further investigation and/or intervention.
4. When oxygen demand is greater than consumption, a lactic acidosis will occur. This finding in combination with a low mixed venous oxygen saturation suggests a shock state, whereas if the saturation is normal, it implies a prior oxygen debt.
5. Because Hgb and oxygen consumption do not usually change rapidly, the difference between arterial oxygen content and venous oxygen content is usually indicative of a change in cardiac output.
6. Mixed venous oxygenation can be used to calculate the intrapulmonary shunt (1 – arterial saturation)/(1 – mixed venous saturation), which can be treated by increasing PEEP.

7. Specific nuances of mixed and central venous oxygen saturation monitoring in different patient populations exist and examples are highlighted in this chapter.
8. Using mixed venous oxygenation clinically requires knowledge of certain technical aspects of PACs which are reviewed in this chapter.

References

1. Wo CC, Shoemaker WC, Appel PL, et al. Unreliability of blood pressure and heart rate to evaluate cardiac output in emergency resuscitation and critical illness. *Crit Care Med.* 1993;21(2):218–223.
2. Cortez A, Zito J, Lucas CE, Gerrick SJ. Mechanism of inappropriate polyuria in septic patients. *Arch Surg.* 1977;112(4):471–476.
3. Rady MY, Rivers EP, Nowak RM. Resuscitation of the critically ill in the ED: responses of blood pressure, heart rate, shock index, central venous oxygen saturation, and lactate. *Am J Emerg Med.* 1996;14(2):218–225.
4. Karimova A, Pinsky DJ. The endothelial response to oxygen deprivation: biology and clinical implications. *Intensive Care Med.* 2001;27(1):19–31.
5. Beal AL, Cerra FB. Multiple organ failure syndrome in the 1990s: systemic inflammatory response and organ dysfunction. *JAMA* 1994;271(3):226–233.
6. Bihari D, Smithies M, Gimson A, et al. The effects of vasodilation with prostacyclin on oxygen delivery and uptake in critically ill patients. *N Engl J Med.* 1987;317(7):397–403.
7. Bakker J, Gris P, Coffernils M, et al. Serial blood lactate levels can predict the development of multiple organ failure following septic shock. *Am J Surg.* 1996;171(2):221–226.
8. Rivers EP, Kruse JA, Jacobsen G, et al. The influence of early hemodynamic optimization on biomarker patterns of severe sepsis and septic shock. *Crit Care Med.* 2007;35(9):2016–2024.
9. Rivers E, Nguyen B, Havstad S, et al. Early goal-directed therapy in the treatment of severe sepsis and septic shock. *N Engl J Med.* 2001;345(19):1368–1377.
10. Varpula M, Tallgren M, Saukkonen K, et al. Hemodynamic variables related to outcome in septic shock. *Intensive Care Med.* 2005;31:1066–1071.
11. Nelson LD. Continuous venous oximetry in surgical patients. *Ann Surg.* 1986;203(3):329–333.
12. Krafft P, Steltzer H, Hiesmayr M, et al. Mixed venous oxygen saturation in critically ill septic shock patients. The role of defined events. *Chest.* 1993;103(3):900–906.
13. Vallet B, Adamczyk S, Barreau O, Lebuffe G. Physiologic transfusion triggers. *Best Pract Res Clin Anaesthesiol.* 2007;21(2):173–181.
14. Wolf YG, Cotev S, Perel A, et al. Dependence of oxygen consumption on cardiac output in sepsis. *Crit Care Med.* 1987;15(3):198–203.
15. Kandel G, Aberman A. Mixed venous oxygen saturation. Its role in the assessment of the critically ill patient. *Arch Intern Med.* 1983;143(7):1400–1402.
16. Meier-Hellmann A, Hannemann L, Specht M, et al. Hepatic venous and mixed venous O_2 saturation during catecholamine therapy in patients with septic shock [in German]. *Anaesthesist.* 1993;42(1):29–33.
17. Reinhart K, Rudolph T, Bredle DL, et al. Comparison of central-venous to mixed-venous oxygen saturation during changes in oxygen supply/demand. *Chest.* 1989;95(6):1216–1221.
18. Takano H, Matsuda H, Kaneko M, et al. Hepatic venous oxygen saturation monitoring in patients with assisted circulation for severe cardiac failure. *Artif Organs.* 1991;15(3):248–252.
19. Ruokonen E, Takala J, Uusaro A. Effect of vasoactive treatment on the relationship between mixed venous and regional oxygen saturation. *Crit Care Med.* 1991;19(11):1365–1369.
20. Dahn MS, Lange MP, Jacobs LA. Central mixed and splanchnic venous oxygen saturation monitoring. *Intensive Care Med.* 1988;14(4):373–378.
21. Rivers EP, Ander DS, Powell D. Central venous oxygen saturation monitoring in the critically ill patient. *Curr Opin Crit Care.* 2001;7(3):204–211.
22. Bakker J, Vincent J-L. The oxygen supply dependency phenomenon is associated with increased blood lactate levels. *J Crit Care.* 1991;6:152–159.
23. Kruse JA, Haupt MT, Puri VK, et al. Lactate levels as predictors of the relationship between oxygen delivery and consumption in ARDS. *Chest.* 1990;98(4):959–962.
24. Kasnitz P, Druger GL, Yorra F, et al. Mixed venous oxygen tension and hyperlactatemia. Survival in severe cardiopulmonary disease. *JAMA.* 1976;236(6):570–574.
25. Aduen J, Bernstein WK, Khastgir T, et al. The use and clinical importance of a substrate-specific electrode for rapid determination of blood lactate concentrations. *JAMA.* 1994;272(21):1678–1685.
26. Wilson RF, Gibson D. The use of arterial–central venous oxygen differences to calculate cardiac output and oxygen consumption in critically ill surgical patients. *Surgery.* 1978;84(3):362–369.
27. Norwood SH, Civetta JM. Ventilatory support in patients with ARDS. *Surg Clin North Am.* 1985;65(4):895–916.
28. Rasanen J, Downs JB, Malec DJ, et al. Real-time continuous estimation of gas exchange by dual oximetry. *Intensive Care Med.* 1988;14(2):118–122.
29. Boulos M, Astiz ME, Barua RS, et al. Impaired mitochondrial function induced by serum from septic shock patients is attenuated by inhibition of nitric oxide synthase and poly(ADP-ribose) synthase. *Crit Care Med.* 2003;31(2):353–358.
30. Dunham CM, Siegel JH, Weireter L, et al. Oxygen debt and metabolic acidemia as quantitative predictors of mortality and the severity of the ischemic insult in hemorrhagic shock. *Crit Care Med.* 1991;19(2):231–243.
31. Rixen D, Siegel JH. Bench-to-bedside review: oxygen debt and its metabolic correlates as quantifiers of the severity of hemorrhagic and post-traumatic shock. *Crit Care.* 2005;9(5):441–453.
32. Siegel JH. The effect of associated injuries, blood loss, and oxygen debt on death and disability in blunt traumatic brain injury: the need for early physiologic predictors of severity. *J Neurotrauma.* 1995;12(4):579–590.
33. Snyder JV, Carroll GC. Tissue oxygenation: a physiologic approach to a clinical problem. *Curr Probl Surg.* 1982;19(11):650–719.
34. Nierman DM, Schechter CB. Mixed venous O_2 saturation: measured by co-oximetry versus calculated from PVO_2. *J Clin Monit.* 1994;10(1):39–44.
35. Nelson LD. Continuous monitoring of O_2 saturation. *Chest.* 1989;96(4):956–957.
36. Varon J, Fromm RE Jr, Levine RL. Emergency department procedures and length of stay for critically ill medical patients. *Ann Emerg Med.* 1994;23(3):546–549.
37. Lundberg JS, Perl TM, Wiblin T, et al. Septic shock: an analysis of outcomes for patients with onset on hospital wards versus intensive care units. *Crit Care Med.* 1998;26(6):1020–1024.
38. Lefrant JY, Muller L, Bruelle P, et al. Insertion time of the pulmonary artery catheter in critically ill patients. *Crit Care Med.* 2000;28(2):355–359.
39. Lee J, Wright F, Barber R, Stanley L. Central venous oxygen saturation in shock: a study in man. *Anesthesiology.* 1972;36(5):472–478.
40. Scheinman MM, Brown MA, Rapaport E. Critical assessment of use of central venous oxygen saturation as a mirror of mixed venous oxygen in severely ill cardiac patients. *Circulation.* 1969;40(2):165–172.
41. Gasparovic H, Gabelica R, Ostojic Z, et al. Diagnostic accuracy of central venous saturation in estimating mixed venous saturation is proportional to cardiac performance among cardiac surgical patients. *J Crit Care.* 2014;29(5):828–834.
42. Glamann DB, Lange RA, Hillis LD. Incidence and significance of a "step-down" in oxygen saturation from superior vena cava to pulmonary artery. *Am J Cardiol.* 1991;68(6):695–697.
43. Dahmani S, Paugam-Burtz C, Gauss T, et al. Comparison of central and mixed venous saturation during liver transplantation in cirrhotic patients: a pilot study. *Eur J Anaesthesiol.* 2010;27(8):714–719.
44. Edwards JD, Mayall RM. Importance of the sampling site for measurement of mixed venous oxygen saturation in shock. *Crit Care Med.* 1998;26(8):1356–1360.
45. Martin C, Auffray JP, Badetti C, et al. Monitoring of central venous oxygen saturation versus mixed venous oxygen saturation in critically ill patients. *Intensive Care Med.* 1992;18(2):101–104.
46. Faber T. Central venous versus mixed venous oxygen content. *Acta Anaesthesiol Scand Suppl.* 1995;107:33–36.
47. Dongre SS, McAslan TC, Shin B. Selection of the source of mixed venous blood samples in severely traumatized patients. *Anesth Analg.* 1977;56(4):527–532.
48. Rigg JD, Nightingale PN, Faragher EB. Influence of cardiac output on the correlation between mixed venous and central venous oxygen saturation. *Br J Anaesth.* 1993;71(3):459.
49. Varpula M, Karlsson S, Ruokonen E, Pettila V. Mixed venous oxygen saturation cannot be estimated by central venous oxygen saturation in septic shock. *Intensive Care Med.* 2006;32(9):1336–1343.
50. Chawla LS, Zia H, Gutierrez G, et al. Lack of equivalence between central and mixed venous oxygen saturation. *Chest.* 2004;126(6):1891–1896.

51. Martin GB, Carden DL, Nowak RM, et al. Central venous and mixed venous oxygen saturation: comparison during canine open-chest cardiopulmonary resuscitation. *Am J Emerg Med.* 1985;3(6):495–497.
52. Pieri M, Brandi LS, Bertolini R, et al. Comparison of bench central and mixed pulmonary venous oxygen saturation in critically ill postsurgical patients [in Italian]. *Minerva Anesthesiol.* 1995;61(7–8):285–291.
53. Turnaoglu S, Tugrul M, Camci E, et al. Clinical applicability of the substitution of mixed venous oxygen saturation with central venous oxygen saturation. *J Cardiothorac Vasc Anesth.* 2001;15(5):574–579.
54. Goldman RH, Klughaupt M, Metcalf T, et al. Measurement of central venous oxygen saturation in patients with myocardial infarction. *Circulation.* 1968;38(5):941–946.
55. Reinhart K, Rudolph T, Bredle DL, et al. Comparison of central-venous to mixed-venous oxygen saturation during changes in oxygen supply/demand. *Chest.* 1989;95(6):1216–1221.
56. Schou H, Perez de Sa V, Larsson A. Central and mixed venous blood oxygen correlate well during acute normovolemic hemodilution in anesthetized pigs. *Acta Anaesthesiol Scand.* 1998;42(2):172–177.
57. Cohendy R, Peries C, Lefrant JY, et al. Continuous monitoring of the central venous oxygen saturation in surgical patients: comparison to the monitoring of the mixed venous saturation. *Acta Anaesthesiol Scand.* 1996;40(8 Pt 1):956.
58. Berridge JC. Influence of cardiac output on the correlation between mixed venous and central venous oxygen saturation. *Br J Anaesth.* 1992;69(4): 409–410.
59. Scalea TM, Holman M, Fuortes M, et al. Central venous blood oxygen saturation: an early, accurate measurement of volume during hemorrhage. *J Trauma.* 1988;28(6):725–732.
60. Davies GG, Mendenhall J, Symreng T. Measurement of right atrial oxygen saturation by fiberoptic oximetry accurately reflects mixed venous oxygen saturation in swine. *J Clin Monit.* 1988;4(2):99–102.
61. Herrera A, Pajuelo A, Morano MJ, et al. Comparison of oxygen saturations in mixed venous and central blood during thoracic anesthesia with selective single-lung ventilation [in Spanish]. *Rev Esp Anestesiol Reanim.* 1993;40(6):349–353.
62. Wendt M, Hachenberg T, Albert A, et al. Mixed venous versus central venous oxygen saturation in intensive medicine. *Anasth Intensivther Notfallmed.* 1990;25(1):102–106.
63. Emerman CL, Pinchak AC, Hagen JF, et al. A comparison of venous blood gases during cardiac arrest. *Am J Emerg Med.* 1988;6(6):580–583.
64. Weber H, Grimm T, Albert J. The oxygen saturation of blood in the venae cavae, right-heart chambers, and pulmonary artery, comparison of formulae to estimate mixed venous blood in healthy infants and children [in German (author's transl)]. *Z Kardiol.* 1980;69(7):504–507.
65. Ladakis C, Myrianthefs P, Karabinis A, et al. Central venous and mixed venous oxygen saturation in critically ill patients. *Respiration.* 2001;68(3): 279–285.
66. Reinhart K, Kuhn HJ, Hartog C, Bredle DL. Continuous central venous and pulmonary artery oxygen saturation monitoring in the critically ill. *Intensive Care Med.* 2004;30(8):1572–1578.
67. Heiselman D, Jones J, Cannon L. Continuous monitoring of mixed venous oxygen saturation in septic shock. *J Clin Monit.* 1986;2(4):237–245.
68. Ander DS, Jaggi M, Rivers E, et al. Undetected cardiogenic shock in patients with congestive heart failure presenting to the emergency department. *Am J Cardiol.* 1998;82(7):888–891.
69. Rivers EP, Nguyen HB, Havstad S, et al. Early goal directed therapy in the treatment of severe sepsis and septic shock: an outcome evaluation [abstract]. *Chest.* 2000;118(4):87S.
70. Hartog C, Bloos F. Venous oxygen saturation. *Best Pract Res Clin Anaesthesiol.* 2014;28(4):419–428.
71. Task Force of the American College of Critical Care Medicine, Society of Critical Care Medicine. Practice parameters for hemodynamic support of sepsis in adult patients in sepsis. *Crit Care Med.* 1999;27(3):639–660.
72. Dellinger RP, Levy MM, Rhodes A, et al. Surviving Sepsis Campaign: international guidelines for management of severe sepsis and septic shock, 2012. *Crit Care Med.* 2013;41:580–637.
73. Rivers E. Mixed vs central venous oxygen saturation may be not numerically equal, but both are still clinically useful. *Chest.* 2006;129(3): 507–508.
74. Vaughn S, Puri VK. Cardiac output changes and continuous mixed venous oxygen saturation measurement in the critically ill. *Crit Care Med.* 1988;16(5):495–498.
75. Wiesemes R, Peters J. The role of mixed venous oxygen saturation in perioperative monitoring and therapy: a critical stock taking [in German]. *Anasthesiol Intensivmed Notfallmed Schmerzther.* 1993;28(5):269–278.
76. Rady M, Jafry S, Rivers E, et al. Characterization of systemic oxygen transport in end-stage chronic congestive heart failure. *Am Heart J.* 1994;128(4):774–781.
77. Squara P. Central venous oxygenation: when physiology explains apparent discrepancies. *Crit Care.* 2014;18(6):579.
78. Rivers EP, Martin GB, Smithline H, et al. The clinical implications of continuous central venous oxygen saturation during human CPR. *Ann Emerg Med.* 1992;21(9):1094–1101.
79. Rivers EP, Rady MY, Martin GB, et al. Venous hyperoxia after cardiac arrest: characterization of a defect in systemic oxygen utilization. *Chest.* 1992;102(6):1787–1793.
80. Waller JL, Kaplan JA, Bauman DI, Craver JM. Clinical evaluation of a new fiberoptic catheter oximeter during cardiac surgery. *Anesth Analg.* 1982;61(8):676–679.
81. de la Rocha AG, Edmonds JF, Williams WG, et al. Importance of mixed venous oxygen saturation in the care of critically ill patients. *Can J Surg.* 1978;21(3):227–229.
82. Krauss XH, Verdouw PD, Hughenholtz PG, et al. On-line monitoring of mixed venous oxygen saturation after cardiothoracic surgery. *Thorax.* 1975;30(6):636–643.
83. Muir AL, Kirby BJ, King AJ, et al. Mixed venous oxygen saturation in relation to cardiac output in myocardial infarction. *Br Med J.* 1970;4(730): 276–278.
84. Birman H, Haq A, Hew E, et al. Continuous monitoring of mixed venous oxygen saturation in hemodynamically unstable patients. *Chest.* 1984;86(5):753–756.
85. Gattinoni L, Brazzi L, Pelosi P, et al. A trial of goal-oriented hemodynamic therapy in critically ill patients. SvO_2 Collaborative Group. *N Engl J Med.* 1995;333(16):1025–1032.
86. Bracht H, Hanggi M, Jeker B, et al. Incidence of low central venous oxygen saturation during unplanned admissions in a multidisciplinary intensive care unit: an observational study. *Crit Care.* 2007;11(1):R2.
87. Polonen P, Ruokonen E, Hippelainen M, et al. A prospective, randomized study of goal-oriented hemodynamic therapy in cardiac surgical patients. *Anesth Analg.* 2000;90(5):1052–1059.
88. Kremzar B, Spec-Marn A, Kompan L, et al. Normal values of SvO_2 as therapeutic goal in patients with multiple injuries. *Intensive Care Med.* 1997;23(1):65–70.
89. Kazarian KK, Del Guercio LR. The use of mixed venous blood gas determinations in traumatic shock. *Ann Emerg Med.* 1980;9(4):179–182.
90. Rady MY. Patterns of oxygen transport in trauma and their relationship to outcome. *Am J Emerg Med.* 1994;12(1):107–112.
91. Powelson JA, Maini BS, Bishop RL, et al. Continuous monitoring of mixed venous oxygen saturation during aortic operations. *Crit Care Med.* 1992;20(3):332–336.
92. Norwood SH, Nelson LD. Continuous monitoring of mixed venous oxygen saturation during aortofemoral bypass grafting. *Am Surg.* 1986;52(2): 114–115.
93. Madsen P, Olesen HL, Klokker M, et al. Peripheral venous oxygen saturation during head-up tilt induced hypovolaemic shock in humans. *Scand J Clin Lab Invest.* 1993;53(4):411–416.
94. Madsen P, Iversen H, Secher NH. Central venous oxygen saturation during hypovolaemic shock in humans. *Scand J Clin Lab Invest.* 1993;53(1):67–72.
95. O'Connor TA, Hall RT. Mixed venous oxygenation in critically ill neonates. *Crit Care Med.* 1994;22(2):343–346.
96. Conacher ID, Paes ML. Mixed venous oxygen saturation during lung transplantation. *J Cardiothorac Vasc Anesth.* 1994;8(6):671–674.
97. Edwards JD. Oxygen transport in cardiogenic and septic shock. *Crit Care Med.* 1991;19(5):658–663.
98. Creamer JE, Edwards JD, Nightingale P. Hemodynamic and oxygen transport variables in cardiogenic shock secondary to acute myocardial infarction, and response to treatment. *Am J Cardiol.* 1990;65(20): 1297–1300.
99. Wagner K, Risnes I, Abdelnoor M, et al. Is it possible to predict outcome in cardiac ECMO? Analysis of preoperative risk factors. *Perfusion.* 2007;22(4):225–229.
100. Snyder AB, Salloum LJ, Barone JE, et al. Predicting short-term outcome of cardiopulmonary resuscitation using central venous oxygen tension measurements. *Crit Care Med.* 1991;19(1):111–113.
101. Rivers EP, Rady MY, Martin GB, et al. Venous hyperoxia after cardiac arrest: characterization of a defect in systemic oxygen utilization. *Chest.* 1992;102(6):1787–1793.
102. Nakazawa K, Hikawa Y, Saitoh Y, et al. Usefulness of central venous oxygen saturation monitoring during cardiopulmonary resuscitation: a comparative

case study with end-tidal carbon dioxide monitoring. *Intensive Care Med.* 1994;20(6):450–451.

103. Osawa H, Yoshii S, Abraham SJ, et al. Critical values of hematocrit and mixed venous oxygen saturation as parameters for a safe cardiopulmonary bypass. *Jpn J Thorac Cardiovasc Surg.* 2004;52(2):49–56.
104. Paradis NA, Martin GB, Goetting MG, et al. Aortic pressure during human cardiac arrest. Identification of pseudo-electromechanical dissociation. *Chest.* 1992;101(1):123–128.
105. Ameloot K, Meex I, Genbrugge C, et al. Accuracy of continuous thermodilution cardiac output monitoring by pulmonary artery catheter during therapeutic hypothermia in post-cardiac arrest patients. *Resuscitation.* 2014; 85(9):1263–1268.
106. Rivers EP, Wortsman J, Rady MY, et al. The effect of the total cumulative epinephrine dose administered during human CPR on hemodynamic, oxygen transport, and utilization variables in the postresuscitation period. *Chest.* 1994;106(5):1499–1507.
107. Sumimoto T, Sugiura T, Takeuchi M, et al. Overshoot in mixed venous oxygen saturation during recovery from supine bicycle exercise in patients with recent myocardial infarction. *Chest.* 1993;103(2):514–520.
108. Deakin CD, Low JL. Accuracy of the advanced trauma life support guidelines for predicting systolic blood pressure using carotid, femoral, and radial pulses: observational study. *BMJ.* 2000;321(7262):673–674.
109. Scalea TM, Hartnett RW, Duncan AO, et al. Central venous oxygen saturation: a useful clinical tool in trauma patients. *J Trauma.* 1990;30(12): 1539–1543.
110. Kowalenko T, Ander D, Hitchcock R, et al. Continuous central venous oxygen saturation monitoring during the resuscitation of suspected hemorrhagic shock [abstract]. *Acad Emerg Med.* 1994;1(2):A69.
111. Astiz ME, Rackow EC, Kaufman B, et al. Relationship of oxygen delivery and mixed venous oxygenation to lactic acidosis in patients with sepsis and acute myocardial infarction. *Crit Care Med.* 1988;16(7): 655–658.
112. Verdouw PD, Hagemeijer F, Dorp WG, et al. Short-term survival after acute myocardial infarction predicted by hemodynamic parameters. *Circulation.* 1975;52(3):413–419.
113. Kyff JV, Vaughn S, Yang SC, et al. Continuous monitoring of mixed venous oxygen saturation in patients with acute myocardial infarction. *Chest.* 1989;95(3):607–611.
114. Chin KM, Channick RN, Kim NH, et al. Central venous blood oxygen saturation monitoring in patients with chronic pulmonary arterial hypertension treated with continuous IV epoprostenol: correlation with measurements of hemodynamics and plasma brain natriuretic peptide levels. *Chest.* 2007;132(3):786–792.
115. Teboul JL, Hamzaoui O, Monnet X. SvO_2 to monitor resuscitation of septic patients: let's just understand the basic physiology. *Crit Care.* 2011;15(6):1005.
116. Velissaris D, Pierrakos C, Scolletta S, et al. High mixed venous oxygen saturation levels do not exclude fluid responsiveness in critically ill septic patients. *Crit Care.* 2011; 26;15(4):R177.
117. Griffel MI, Astiz ME, Rackow EC, et al. Effect of mechanical ventilation on systemic oxygen extraction and lactic acidosis during early septic shock in rats. *Crit Care Med.* 1990;18(1):72–76.
118. Hirschl RB, Heiss KF, Cilley RE, et al. Oxygen kinetics in experimental sepsis. *Surgery.* 1992;112(1):37–44.
119. Rackow EC, Astiz ME, Weil MH. Increases in oxygen extraction during rapidly fatal septic shock in rats. *J Lab Clin Med.* 1987;109(6): 660–664.
120. Astiz ME, Rackow EC, Weil MH. Oxygen delivery and utilization during rapidly fatal septic shock in rats. *Circ Shock.* 1986;20(4):281–290.
121. Krivec B, Voga G, Podbregar M. Monitoring mixed venous oxygen saturation in patients with obstructive shock after massive pulmonary embolism. *Wien Klin Wochenschr.* 2004;116(9–10):326–331.
122. Fahey PJ, Harris K, Vanderwarf C. Clinical experience with continuous monitoring of mixed venous oxygen saturation in respiratory failure. *Chest.* 1984;86(5):748–752.
123. Kirkeby-Garstad I, Sellevold OF, Stenseth R, et al. Marked mixed venous desaturation during early mobilization after aortic valve surgery. *Anesth Analg.* 2004;98(2):311–317.
124. Tweddell JS, Ghanayem NS, Mussatto KA, et al. Mixed venous oxygen saturation monitoring after stage 1 palliation for hypoplastic left heart syndrome. *Ann Thorac Surg.* 2007;84(4):1301–1310.
125. Polonen P, Ruokonen E, Hippelainen M, et al. A prospective, randomized study of goal-oriented hemodynamic therapy in cardiac surgical patients. *Anesth Analg.* 2000;90(5):1052–1059.
126. Termuhlen DF, Swartz MT, Pennington DG, et al. Predictors for weaning patients from ventricular assist devices. *ASAIO Trans.* 1988;34(2): 131–139.
127. Termuhlen DF, Swartz MT, Ruzevich SA, et al. Hemodynamic predictors for weaning patients from ventricular assist devices (VADs). *J Biomater Appl.* 1990;4(4):374–390.
128. Lequeux PY, Bouckaert Y, Sekkat H, et al. Continuous mixed venous and central venous oxygen saturation in cardiac surgery with cardiopulmonary bypass. *Eur J Anaesthesiol.* 2010;27(3):295–259.
129. Suehirö K, Tanaka K, Matsuura T, et al. Discrepancy between superior vena cava oxygen saturation and mixed venous oxygen saturation can predict postoperative complications in cardiac surgery patients. *J Cardiothorac Vasc Anesth.* 2014; 28(3):528–533.
130. Shahbazi S, Khademi S, Shafa M, et al. Serum lactate is not correlated with mixed or central venous oxygen saturation for detecting tissue hypo perfusion during coronary artery bypass graft surgery: a prospective observational study. *Int Cardiovasc Res J.* 2013;7(4):130–134.
131. Kuiper AN, Trof RJ, Groeneveld AB. Mixed venous O_2 saturation and fluid responsiveness after cardiac or major vascular surgery. *J Cardiothorac Surg.* 2013;8:189.
132. Pearse R, Dawson D, Fawcett J, et al. Changes in central venous saturation after major surgery, and association with outcome. *Crit Care.* 2005;9(6):R694–699.
133. Shoemaker WC, Thangathurai D, Wo CC, et al. Intraoperative evaluation of tissue perfusion in high-risk patients by invasive and noninvasive hemodynamic monitoring. *Crit Care Med.* 1999;27(10):2147–2152.
134. Bland RD, Shoemaker WC, Abraham E, et al. Hemodynamic and oxygen transport patterns in surviving and nonsurviving postoperative patients. *Crit Care Med.* 1985;13(2):85–90.
135. Donati A, Loggi S, Preiser JC, et al. Goal-directed intraoperative therapy reduces morbidity and length of hospital stay in high-risk surgical patients. *Chest.* 2007;132(6):1817–1824.
136. Gawlinski A, Dracup K. Effect of positioning on SvO_2 in the critically ill patient with a low ejection fraction. *Nurs Res.* 1998;47(5):293–299.
137. Lewis P, Nichols E, Mackey G, et al. The effect of turning and backrub on mixed venous oxygen saturation in critically ill patients. *Am J Crit Care.* 1997;6(2):132–140.
138. Schranz D, Schmitt S, Oelert H, et al. Continuous monitoring of mixed venous oxygen saturation in infants after cardiac surgery. *Intensive Care Med.* 1989;15(4):228–232.
139. Baquero Cano M, Sanchez Luna M, Elorza Fernandez MD, et al. Oxygen transport and consumption and oxygen saturation in the right atrium in an experimental model of neonatal septic shock [in Spanish]. *An Esp Pediatr.* 1996;44(2):149–156.
140. Hirschl RB, Palmer P, Heiss KF, et al. Evaluation of the right atrial venous oxygen saturation as a physiologic monitor in a neonatal model. *J Pediatr Surg.* 1993;28(7):901–905.
141. Rasanen J, Peltola K, Leijala M. Superior vena caval and mixed venous oxyhemoglobin saturations in children recovering from open heart surgery. *J Clin Monit.* 1992;8(1):44–49.
142. Carcillo JA, Fields AI. Clinical practice parameters for hemodynamic support of pediatric and neonatal patients in septic shock. *Crit Care Med.* 2002;30(6):1365–1378.
143. Orlando R III. Continuous mixed venous oximetry in critically ill surgical patients: 'high-tech' cost-effectiveness. *Arch Surg.* 1986;121(4):470–471.
144. Arnoldi D, Dechert R, Wise C. Use of continuous SvO_2 monitoring can decrease requirements for cardiac output determination in surgical ICU patients. *Crit Care Med.* 1995;23(1 Suppl):A22.
145. Pearson KS, Gomez MN, Moyers JR, et al. A cost/benefit analysis of randomized invasive monitoring for patients undergoing cardiac surgery. *Anesth Analg.* 1989;69(3):336–341.
146. Jastremski MS, Chelluri L, Beney KM, et al. Analysis of the effects of continuous on-line monitoring of mixed venous oxygen saturation on patient outcome and cost-effectiveness. *Crit Care Med.* 1989;17(2):148–153.
147. Huang DT, Angus DC, Dremsizov TT, et al. Cost-effectiveness of early goal-directed therapy in the treatment of severe sepsis and septic shock. *Crit Care.* 2003;7:S116.
148. Rasanen J, Downs JB, Hodges MR. Continuous monitoring of gas exchange and oxygen use with dual oximetry. *J Clin Anesth.* 1988;1(1):3–8.
149. Bongard FS, Leighton TA. Continuous dual oximetry in surgical critical care. Indications and limitations. *Ann Surg.* 1992;216(1):60–68.
150. Boutros AR, Lee C. Value of continuous monitoring of mixed venous blood oxygen saturation in the management of critically ill patients. *Crit Care Med.* 1986;14(2):132–134.

CHAPTER

25

Echocardiography

DAVID T. POREMBKA and ROHIT P. PATEL

INTRODUCTION

Echocardiography is a vital diagnostic modality for the intensivist. Echocardiography, both transthoracic (TTE) and transesophageal (TEE), has shown to improve diagnostic capability, obtain vital hemodynamic assessments, and allow repeated analysis of therapeutic outcomes after appropriate interventions (such as administration of fluids or start of inotropic agents) (1–8). Protocols have shown ultrasound examination can diagnose abnormalities and modify admitting diagnoses in 26% of patients, lead to changes in medical therapy in 18% of patients, and initiate invasive procedures in 22% of patients (1). As devices become more readily available at the bedside (e.g., handheld devices, hemodynamic TEE), examinations can become quicker and more repeatable for decision-making and guide response to therapies (2). Echocardiography lessens the potential for physician misdiagnosis, and because this mode is useful in indicating the most appropriate medical/surgical interventions, outcomes can be potentially improved (3–8). There is a trend toward performance of "limited" or "focused" ultrasound examinations by multiple subspecialist groups, which should be used to identify and treat focused findings such as pericardial tamponade, assess ventricular performance–systolic/diastolic function, assess marked right ventricular (RV) impairment, and volume responsiveness (9–12). Protocols generally emphasize performance by noncardiologists, time sensitive and performed serially, the examination investigates limited number of diagnoses, may encompass multiple anatomic areas, and does not replace a comprehensive echocardiogram examination (13–15). The purpose of these focused examinations is reducing time to life-saving interventions that may decrease morbidity and mortality and observe changes after clinical interventions (16). Despite the current trend to allow the intensivist to interpret basic echocardiography features, the importance of consulting with an expert in echocardiography in difficult cases cannot be overemphasized. By doing so, a bilateral dynamic interchange in learning, teaching, research, and clinical care can only improve and lead to better outcomes and a probable decrease in overall cost to health care and to the patient. Intensive care physicians should embrace echocardiography as an integral complement in the care of the critically ill patient (17,18). The use of ultrasound in critical care settings has been shown to be safe, accurate, repeatable, and provides data that may not be found with other routine methods of physical examination (19). Timely and accurate diagnoses are crucial in many situations (e.g., penetrating or blunt trauma-related cardiac structural damage or the presence of cardiac tamponade, aortic dissection/aneurysm, or traumatic injury, or shock not responding to conventional treatment).

The benefit of TEE compared to TTE includes better image capabilities in difficult to obtain imaging patients (patients with skin tapes, chest tubes, dressings, pneumothoraces, surgical wounds, severe obesity, body habitus, and emphysema), aortic pathology, cardiac valve anatomy and integrity, including endocarditis, and presence of thrombi in the atrial appendage. TEE can also be used as a guide in patients with atrial fibrillation undergoing electrical cardioversion. In a patient with shock, the clinician echocardiographers can quickly determine if there is inadequate ventricular systolic function or hypovolemia, and therapies can be implemented immediately and reassessed as frequently as needed (20–26). A relative contraindication in TEE is any known or suspected esophageal or gastric pathology, including recent esophageal or gastric surgery, undiagnosed gastrointestinal bleeding, esophageal varices in patients with portal hypertension (but TEE has been very useful during orthotopic liver transplantation), and suspected cervical spine injury. An uncooperative patient whose airway is not artificially secured is a relative contraindication unless adequate topical anesthesia is provided, or sedation even to the point of total control of the patient's airway with intubation. A penetrating esophageal injury, suspected or known by the mechanism of injury, remains an absolute contraindication to TEE. Critical care echocardiography is indicated in hypotension or hemodynamic instability of uncertain or suspected cardiac etiology (27–29).

TRAINING AND CERTIFICATION

Significant cognitive skills and knowledge are required when using TTE or TEE in the ICU (30–32). Echocardiography is an extension of the physical examination and encompasses data obtained from the use of invasive monitoring, handheld or portable TTE, and TEE. As described above, focused critical care echocardiography is preferred, and several guidelines are available in medical literature (33–35). Competence is different from certification, which is defined as the process by which competence is recognized by an external agency (33). As ultrasound grows in each specialty, there are more programs with competence-based training during residency or fellowship training (36). In fact, many medical schools are now incorporating ultrasound in the pre-clinical years in order to help students grasp anatomy through visualization of ultrasound, and as a result, this training should become easier for the individual throughout their graduate training years in all different specialties that are incorporating ultrasound into their curriculum (37,38). Appropriate level of training exists for varying specialties due to the varying limited diagnoses required to make accurate clinical decisions. Selective "training curriculum" is provided in specialties such as Emergency Medicine, Anesthesia, Surgery, and Critical Care Medicine (35,39–41). Comprehensive echocardiography requires substantial training to provide quality and avoid risks of misinterpretation. When focused cardiac ultrasound is employed,

TABLE 25.1 General Cognitive and Technical Echocardiography Knowledge

Indications and applications of TTE in critically ill patients
Indications and contraindications to the use of TEE
Knowledge of appropriate alternative diagnostic modalities
Ultrasound physics
Principles of M-mode echocardiography
Principles of 2D echocardiography
Principles of Doppler echocardiography and the Doppler examination
Color-flow imaging
Imaging techniques
Standard transducer positions
Standard cardiac views
Imaging platforms
"Knobology" of various platforms
Image acquisition and storage
Recognizing normal anatomy visualized by TTE and TEE
Recognizing common structural abnormalities
Ability to communicate the result of the examination to the patient and other physicians, and produce a written report

TTE, transthoracic echocardiography; TEE, transesophageal echocardiography.
Reproduced with permission from Mazraeshahi RM, Farmer JC, Porembka DT. A suggested curriculum in echocardiography for critical care physicians. *Crit Care Med.* 2007;35:S431–433.

formal training, mentoring, and proctored review of images are mandatory. Training should be combined with actual experience performing proctored focus cardiac examinations. Based on cardiology and cardiac anesthesiology experience, at least 50 supervised studies are required before one should function independently (Tables 25.1 to 25.4) (42,43).

SCANNING TECHNIQUES

The examination will be briefly presented. Adequate texts and atlases on this topic are numerous and can be easily accessed. With recent improvements in echocardiographic technologies, and two-dimensional and color-flow Doppler echocardiography, pulsed-wave Doppler echocardiography (PW), and

TABLE 25.2 Procedural Competency Assessment Based on Successful Interrogation of Cardiac Pathologic Conditions

Mitral valvular disease	20
Aortic valvular disease	20
Ventricular performance, RWMA or ischemic heart disease, volume assessment, and/or ventricular interactions	30
Aortic dissection and aneurysms	10
Aortic debris	10
Aortic trauma	30
Pericardial disease and pericardial tamponade	10
Endocarditis and complications	20
Identification of right-heart failure and pulmonary embolism	10
Intracardiac and extracardiac masses	10
Normal examinations	10
Esophageal intubations	10

RWMA, regional wall motion abnormality

Reproduced with permission from Mazraeshahi RM, Farmer JC, Porembka DT. A suggested curriculum in echocardiography for critical care physicians. *Crit Care Med.* 2007;35:S431–433.

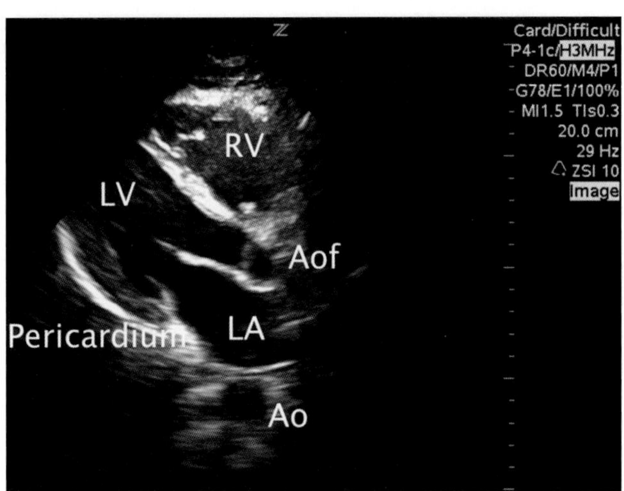

FIGURE 25.1 Parasternal long-axis view. Ao, descending aorta, Aof, aortic outflow tract; LA, left atrium; LV, left ventricle; RV, right ventricle. (See also Video 25-1.)

continuous-wave echocardiography (CW), excellent views can be obtained. For the surface examination, there are four major positions or approaches to the heart on the thorax. A discussion on the inferior vena cava (IVC) and aorta will also be made here as pathologies is illustrated later in the chapter.

Parasternal Long-Axis View

The transducer is placed in the left third, fourth, or fifth intercostal space, just lateral to the sternum. The probe marker should be directed toward the patient's right shoulder, which will place the left ventricular (LV) cavity on the left of the screen. Angulation, rotation, and fanning of the transducer can be made until the ideal parasternal long view is obtained. The ideal view includes bisection of the mitral valve and the aortic valve, and should include the LV chamber. The apex of the LV will not be in view. Depth should be adjusted to have the pericardium and descending aorta close to the bottom of the screen (Fig. 25.1).

Parasternal Short-Axis View

After obtaining ideal view of the parasternal long axis, the transducer is rotated 90 degrees clockwise. One can use the left hand to keep the transducer steady while rotating it clockwise in order to prevent movement of the actual location. Angling or fanning the probe from the right shoulder toward the right hip, one can go through the levels of investigation of the heart: pulmonary trunk, aortic valve, mitral valve, papillary muscle, and apex levels. The papillary muscle level is most frequently used for evaluation of systolic function and LV volume (Fig. 25.2).

Apical Four-Chamber View

With the patient positioned in as much left lateral decubitus as possible, the transducer should be placed at the apex of the heart, localized at the point of maximal impulse. The probe marker should be directed toward the 3-o'clock position. In older, obese, or abdominal surgery patients, the apex will be located laterally and superiorly, with the LV more horizontal

TABLE 25.3 Clinical Indication for the Use of Echocardiography in the ICU

Hypotension/Shock
1. Assessment of LV systolic function
 Global assessment of LV function
 Recognizing decreased LV function
 Defining overall contractility and ejection fraction
2. Assessment of RV function
 Recognizing signs of RV failure, including decreased RV systolic function, dilated RV, and dilated IVC
3. Global assessment of volume status including
 Recognizing hyperdynamic small LV
 Estimation of central venous pressure
 Measurement of IVC size and respiratory variation
4. Identification of pericardial effusion and tamponade
 Understanding tamponade physiology
 Recognizing signs of tamponade, including diastolic collapse of the RV free wall and RA wall

Hemodynamic Assessment
1. Measurement of cardiac output
 Understanding Doppler techniques for calibration of stroke volume
 Calculation of ejection fraction
 Calculation of stroke volume and cardiac output
2. Measurement of cardiac chambers size including
 LV size
 RV size
 LA size
 RA size
3. Estimating intracardiac pressures including
 RA pressure
 RV systolic pressure
 LA pressure
4. Evaluation of preload by
 Measurement of LV and RV end-diastolic area and volume
 Measurement of IVC size and respiratory variation
 Estimation of central venous pressure
5. Understanding echocardiographic signs of diastolic dysfunction
6. Global assessment of valvular function and integrity with Doppler

Myocardial Infarction Complications
1. Recognizing regional wall motion abnormalities
2. Recognizing rupture of free wall and septum
3. Recognizing acute mitral regurgitation
4. Identifying LV thrombus
5. Identifying pericardial effusion/tamponade
6. Recognizing echocardiographic signs of RV infarct

Postoperative (Cardiothoracic Surgery) Complications
1. Identifying LV and RV dysfunction
2. Identifying acute valvular dysfunction
3. Recognizing prosthetic valve dysfunction
4. Identifying pericardial effusion and tamponade

RV Dysfunction and Pulmonary Hypertension
1. Identifying echocardiographic signs of RV failure, RV dilation, and acute cor pulmonale
2. Measurement of central venous, RA, and RV systolic pressure

Valvular Dysfunction
1. Understanding the role of Doppler echocardiography in valvular dysfunction
2. Recognizing echocardiographic signs of aortic stenosis
3. Recognizing echocardiographic signs of aortic regurgitation
4. Recognizing echocardiographic signs of mitral regurgitation
5. Recognizing echocardiographic signs of tricuspid regurgitation

Pericardial Diseases
1. Identifying the presence of pericardial effusion and its location
2. Identifying echocardiographic signs of tamponade

Endocarditis
1. Identifying valvular vegetation or oscillating intracardiac mass
2. Recognizing valvular regurgitation
3. Recognizing prosthetic-valve dysfunction

Diseases of Aorta
1. Understanding the role of echocardiography in diagnosis of aortic dissection and aortic aneurysm
2. Measurement of aortic diameter in ascending aortic arch and abdominal aorta

Intracardiac Shunts
1. Understanding the role of contrast echocardiography with the use of agitated saline for finding intracardiac shunts

LV, left ventricle; RV, right ventricle; IVC, inferior vena cava; RA, right atrium; LA, left atrium.
Reproduced with permission from Mazraeshahi RM, Farmer JC, Porembka DT. A suggested curriculum in echocardiography for critical care physicians. *Crit Care Med.* 2007;35:S431–S433.

orientation. In the young, slender, or obstructive lung disease patients, the apex will be more medial and inferior, with the LV more vertical orientation. The depth also has to be increased from the parasternal view. The ideal view comprises the septum in the center of the screen and oriented vertically, with the mitral valve and tricuspid valve visualized together; RV maximal diameter is achieved through transducer rotation (Fig. 25.3).

TABLE 25.4 Summary of ACC/AHA Recommendations for Physicians in Echocardiography

Level of expertise	Duration (mo)	Number of studies performed	Cumulative number of studies interpreted	Annual studies to maintain competence
1	3	75	150	
2	6	150	300	300
3	12	300	750	500
Stress echo		100		100
TEE		50		25–50

Reproduced from Otto CM. *Textbook of Clinical Echocardiography*. 3rd ed. Philadelphia, PA: WB Saunders; 2004, with permission.
TEE, transesophageal echocardiography.

Subcostal (Subxiphoid) View

The transducer is placed below the xiphoid process, with the probe marker directed toward the 3-o'clock position (in cardiac presets on machine). A good amount of pressure must be placed downward with the probe almost flat on the skin (helpful to keep the palm of hand on the top portion of the probe to allow for direct contact of probe with skin). The image will be a four-chamber view, with the right side of the heart at the top of the screen, left heart at the bottom, and the apex on the right of the screen (Fig. 25.4).

Inferior Vena Cava

After proper visualization of subcostal view, with the image focused on the atrial–caval junction, the transducer

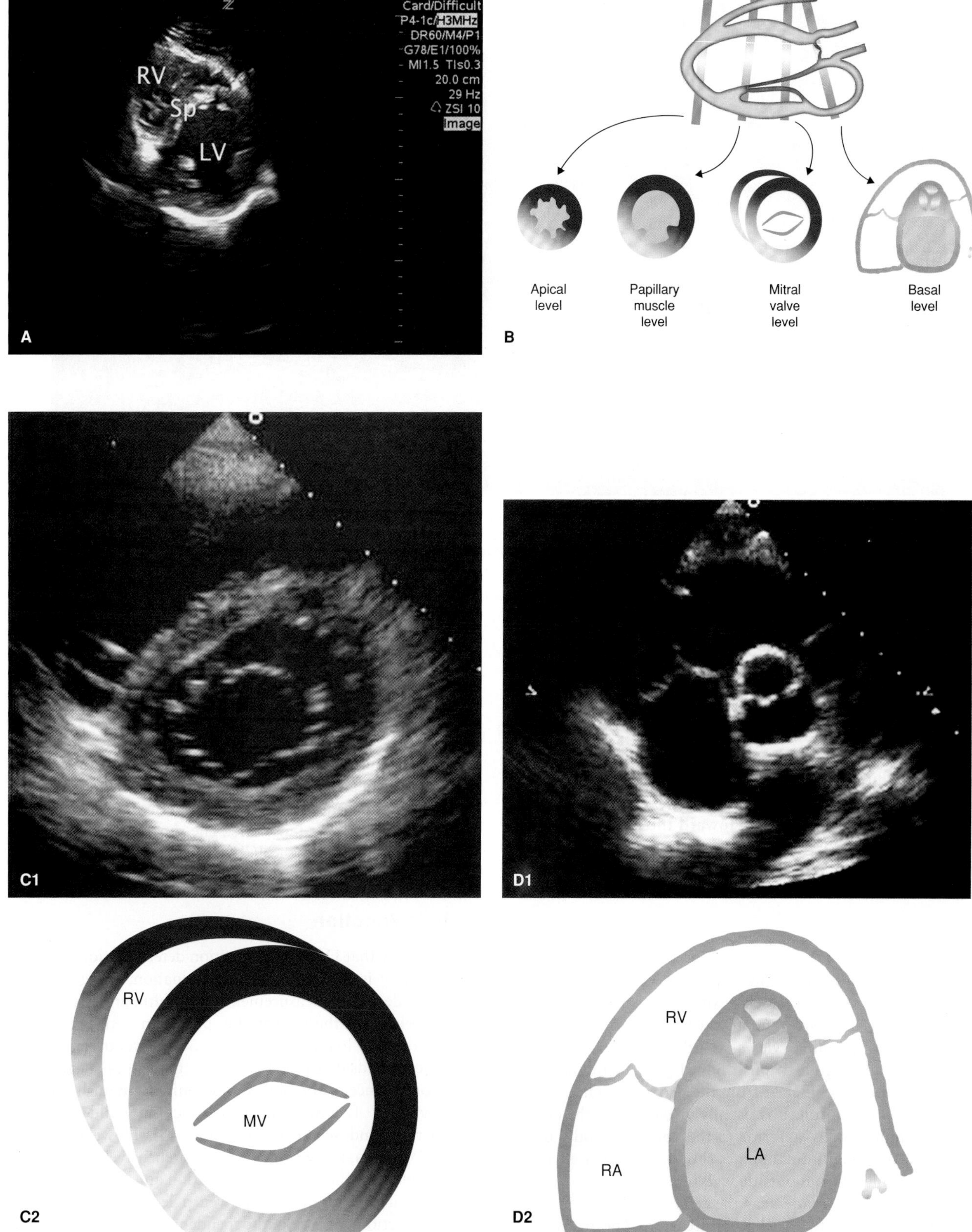

FIGURE 25.2 Parasternal short-axis view. **A**: Labeled view. LV, left ventricle, RV, right ventricle, Sp, interventricular septum. **B**: Schematic depiction of the various short-axis planes that can be derived from the parasternal long-axis view. Note that the planes are not exactly parallel but provide views of anatomy from apex to base. **C**: Short-axis view at the level of the mitral valve (MV) is demonstrated. **D**: Basal short-axis projection at the level of the aortic valve. (*continued*)

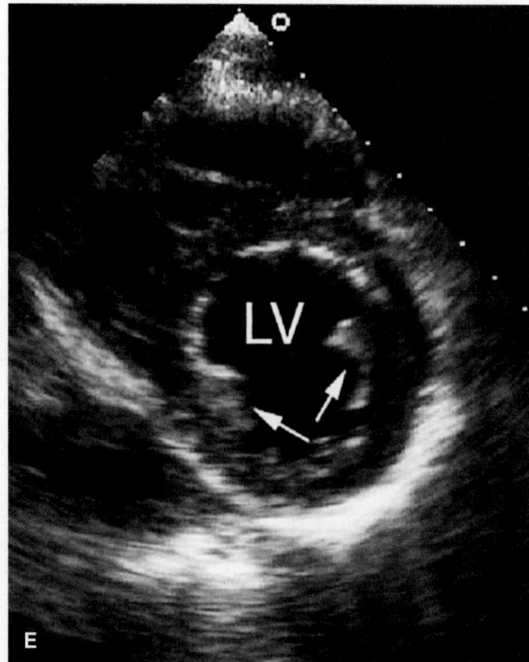

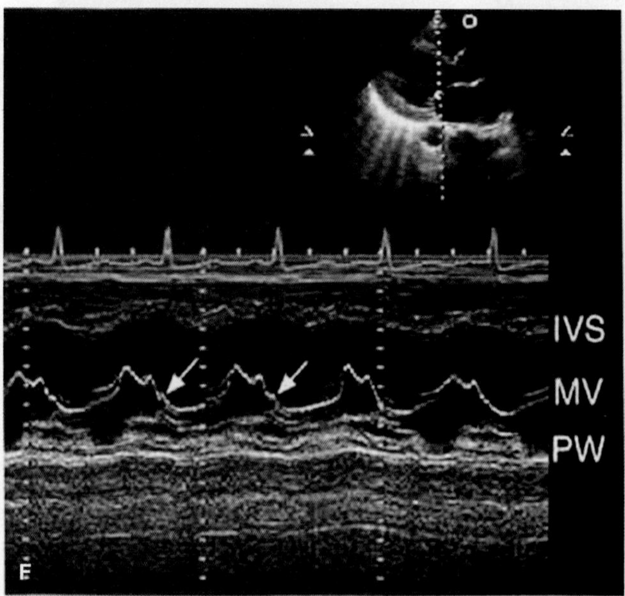

FIGURE 25.2 (*Continued*) **E**: A short-axis plane at the level of the papillary muscles (*arrows*) is shown. **F**: M-mode recording at the level of the mitral valve is shown. A B-bump is indicated by the *arrows*. IVS, interventricular septum; PW, posterior wall. (See also Video 25-2.) (**B–F**: From Feigenbaum H, Armstrong WF, Ryan T, eds. *Feigenbaum's Echocardiography*. 6th ed. Philadelphia, PA: Lippincott Williams & Wilkins; 2005, with permission.)

is rotated counter-clockwise and slightly angled with the marker oriented toward the 12-o'clock position. The IVC can be seen in longitudinal orientation. One must recognize the relationship between the aorta and the IVC, as they can be confused if not obtained in the manner described above. Pulsatility is seen more prominent in the aorta, although in some conditions the IVC can be seen as pulsating. The relationship can be confirmed by fanning the probe toward the left of the patient and back toward the right to identify both structures before evaluations are made. Visualization of the IVC draining into the RA is specific for identification (Fig. 25.5).

Aorta

The patient should be in the supine position. The probe marker is toward the 3-o'clock position for obtaining transverse views of the aorta and toward the 12-o'clock position for the longitudinal views. Gentle pressure is applied in the epigastric region to push bowel gas out of the way. The aorta should be imaged from the proximal celiac trunk to the distal bifurcation. It is usually visualized as the circular vessel immediately anterior to the vertebral body. Both transverse and longitudinal planes should be measured at its maximal diameter from outside wall to outside wall. A measurement should be made near the celiac trunk and another measurement distal to the iliac bifurcation. The transverse measurement is preferred due to "cylinder" effect and underestimation of aortic size in the longitudinal measurements. Abdominal aorta size greater than 3 cm and iliac arteries size greater than 1.5 cm are an indication of abnormal size (Fig. 25.6).

DIAGNOSIS AND TREATMENT

Ventricular Performance (Systolic and Diastolic Function)

Incidence of heart failure is considerable and rising, likely due to the increasing aging population. A better understanding of the evaluation and management of these patients has been acquired over the past few years. The reported incidences for systolic heart failure in the ICU are 61% and 68%, and for diastolic heart failure 16% to 39% (44–47).

Systolic Function

Experts agree that LV systolic function determination on echocardiography is multifactorial determination, using multiple views, modes, and measurements, and ultimately is a composite decision of the interpreting physician with perspective of the potential loading conditions on the ventricle (48). In critical care bedside evaluation, some guidelines suggest that basic competence of this skill should only distinguish between hyperdynamic function, normal function, mild–moderate dysfunction, and severe dysfunction (33). However, in the authors' opinion, knowledge of a comprehensive examination will complement the surface examination and appropriateness for further interrogation. The left ventricle function parameter, ejection fraction (EF), is load dependent (as well as fractional shortening, systolic time tissue velocity of the mitral annulus, and regional wall motion analysis [RWMA]) and is often used as an index of myocardial performance, and may be better in accuracy than pulmonary artery catheter–related parameters such as stroke volume, stroke volume index, and cardiac

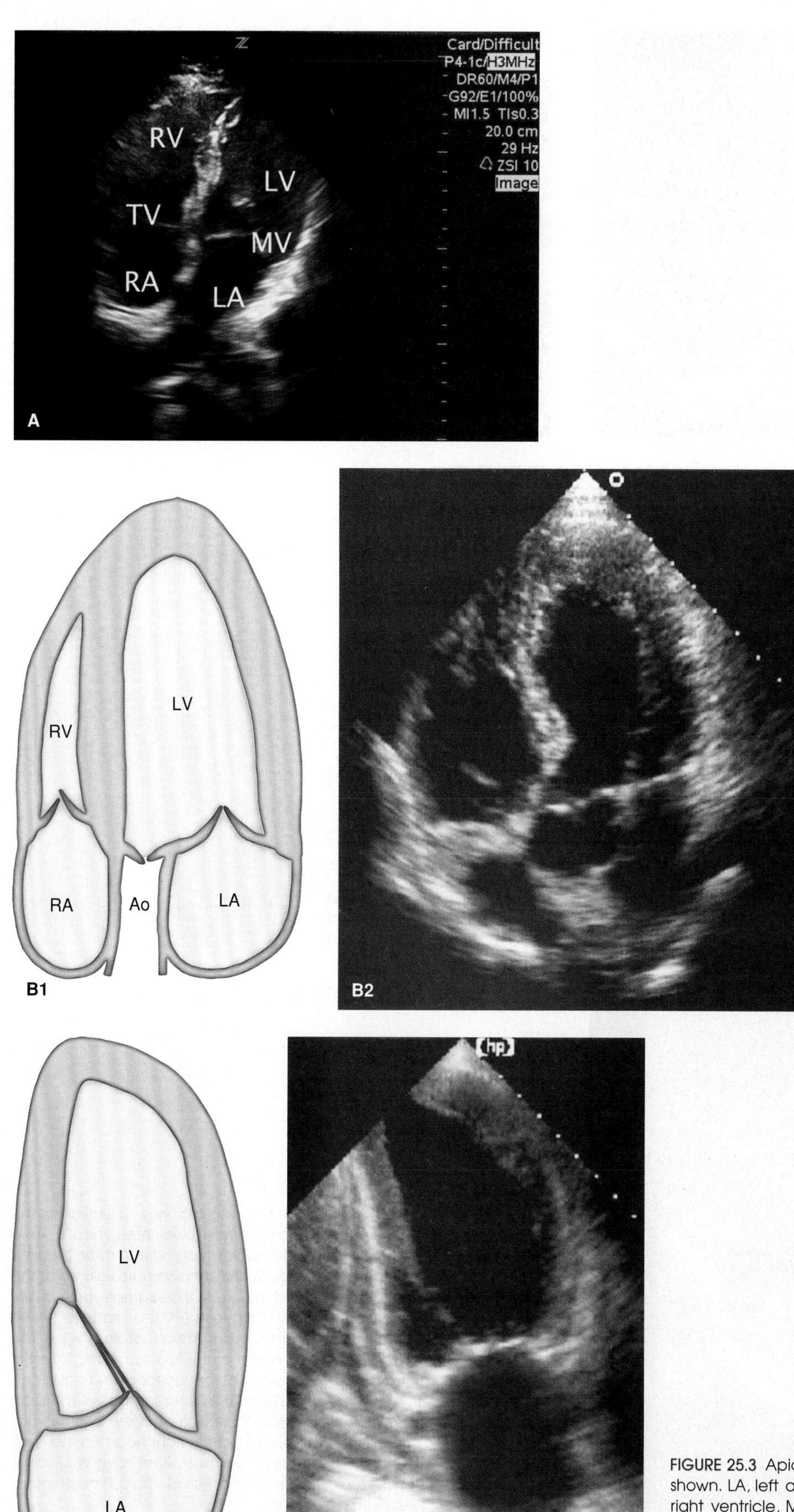

FIGURE 25.3 Apical view. **A**: The apical four-chamber view is shown. LA, left atrium; LV, left ventricle; RA, right atrium; RV, right ventricle, MV, mitral valve, TV, tricuspid valve. **B**: Starting from the four chamber, the transducer can be tilted to a shallower angle to produce a plane that includes the left ventricle outflow tract and proximal aorta (Ao). **C**: An apical two-chamber view is demonstrated. (*continued*)

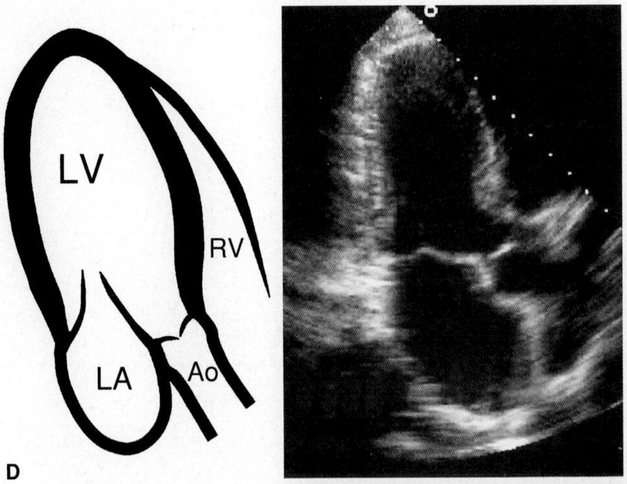

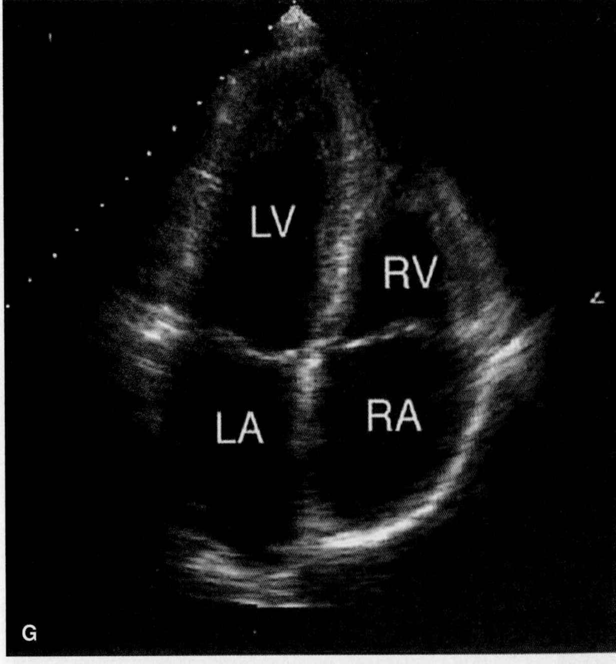

FIGURE 25.3 (*Continued*) **D**: The special long-axis view is similar to the parasternal long-axis view but is recorded from lower interspace. **E**: From the apical four-chamber view, pulsed Doppler imaging can often be used to record pulmonary venous flow by positioning the sample volume at the junction of the pulmonary vein and left atrium. In this example, pulmonary venous flow has three phases: a systolic phase (PV_s), a diastolic phase (PV_d), and a small wave of flow reversal during atrial systole (PV_a). **F**: The suprasternal notch also permits the aortic arch (AA) to be recorded in cross section. The plane allows visualization of the superior vena cava and demonstrates the right pulmonary artery (RPA) coursing below the arch and above the left atrium. **G**: The apical four-chamber view is sometimes recorded with this orientation that places just the right heart on the right. (See also Video 25-3.) (**B–G**: From Feigenbaum H, Armstrong WF, Ryan T, eds. *Feigenbaum's Echocardiography*. 6th ed. Philadelphia, PA: Lippincott Williams & Wilkins; 2005, with permission.)

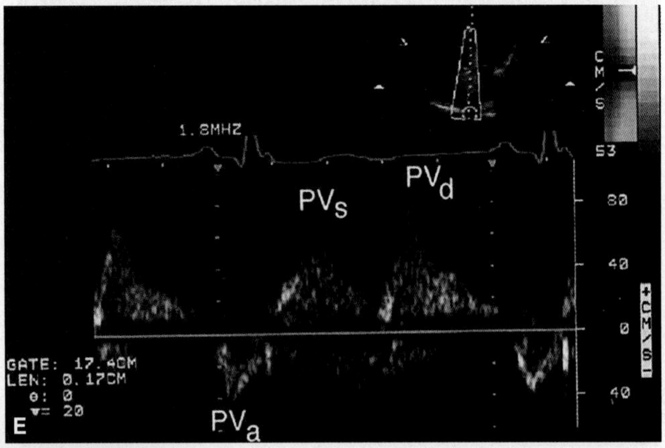

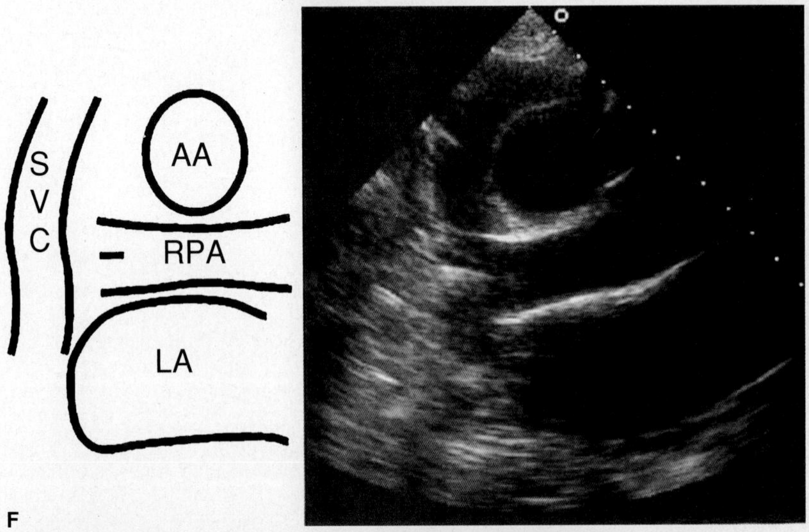

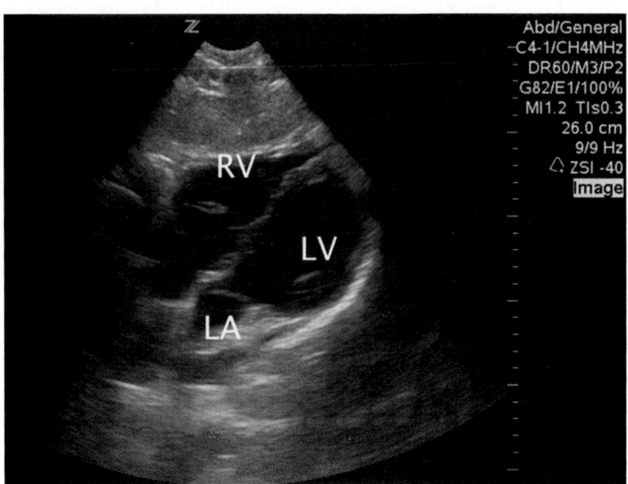

FIGURE 25.4 Subcostal view. Labeled view. LA, left atrium; LV, left ventricle; RA, right atrium; RV, right ventricle. (See also Video 25-4.)

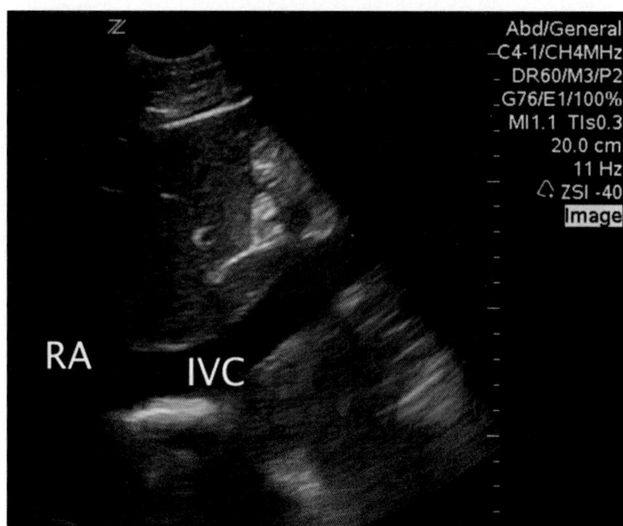

FIGURE 25.5 The inferior vena cava (IVC). RA, right atrium.

index (49). The strain and strain rate via echocardiography has been gaining favor as a useful parameter to evaluate load independently from indices of cardiac performance (50). The physician's capability to construct and interpret pressure/volume loops for the determination of contractility is a controversial issue, particularly in the setting of septic shock. How to intervene in the ventricular performance or optimization? What is preload? What are the goals of resuscitation and their end points? These are all reasonable questions, and show why echocardiography should be a part of the standard management of these critically ill patients and further investigations are needed to elucidate its efficacy and accuracy in the elusive patients (51–56). Even though left ventricular ejection fraction (LVEF) is a limited myocardial performance index, it is a strong predictor of clinical outcome in most cardiac abnormalities (57–59). Of interest, EF is more reliable as a general predictor of mortality, second only to age, than when used to quantify the extent of coronary artery disease or degree of perfusion defects (60,61). Surface approach echocardiography by the use of the modified Simpson rule is superior to estimating either intracardiac volume or LVEF (62,63). In fact, TEE in this situation underestimates volume by foreshortening the LV view with less incorporation of the apex. Volumetric measurements should be objectively quantified:

$$\text{LVEF} = (\text{LVEDV} - \text{LVESV})/\text{LVEDV}$$

where LVEDV refers to left ventricular end-diastolic volume and LVESV to left ventricular end-systolic volume. LVEF may also be calculated from LV dimensions measured with M-mode echocardiography at the mid-ventricular level (64,65). Three-dimensional echocardiography is currently the best practice technique for estimating volumes and EF with greater accuracy by minimizing the inherent problems of not being able to always obtain orthogonal foreshortened, short axis, and four-chamber views. Excellent comparative investigations with magnetic resonance imaging (MRI) and computed tomography (CT) with echocardiography reveal its accuracy as far as quantitative determinations (66,67).

The Doppler echocardiographic measure of systolic function is now a standard methodology in the interrogation of systolic function (68,69); acceleration (dV/dT) is easily measured by using spectral Doppler from the determination of peak

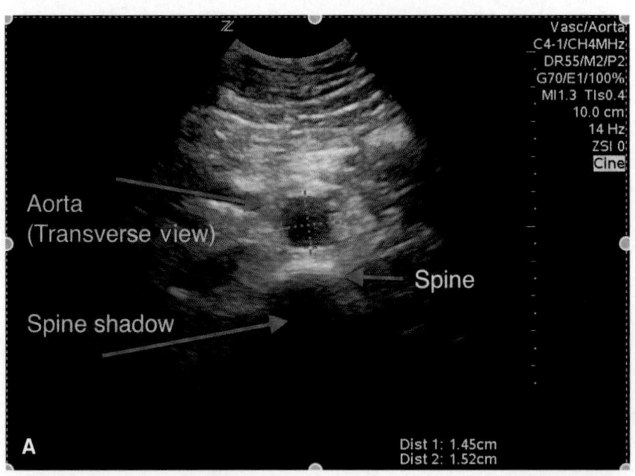

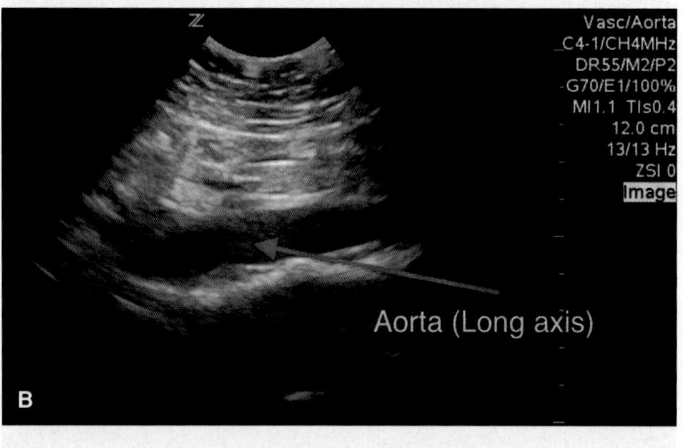

FIGURE 25.6 Aorta. A: Short-axis view, showing spine and spine shadow. B: Long-axis view, obtained by rotating the probe 90 degrees after acquiring the short-axis view.

outflow velocity and the time to achieve this determination. The first derivative of aortic velocity is the peak acceleration, and the slope from its onset to peak is the mean acceleration (70,71). Stroke volume is directly correlated with this velocity. By using the continuity equation, the determination of velocity of blood leaving a known chamber in relation to the cross-sectional area (CSA) of the orifice that the blood is flowing through, stroke volume can be calculated:

$$\text{Stroke volume} = \text{TVI} \times \text{CSA}$$

where TVI is the velocity–time integral on spectral Doppler (72). By multiplying by the heart rate, cardiac output is calculated. Diastolic volume and EF are determined using this same principle through the mitral valve:

$$\text{EF} = (\text{stroke volume/diastolic volume}) \times 100.$$

There are significant limitations to the methods described that include a rhythm other than sinus, and the accurate determination of the dimension of the orifice through which the blood flows is transverse (73).

Tissue Doppler imaging (TDI spectral analysis), by avoiding the limitations of the above techniques has gained acceptance (Fig. 25.7) (74).

TDI is also used in the evaluation of diastolic function and preload (75,76). Normal values of Doppler velocities (S) can be determined both in the pediatric and adult population (77,78). Ventricular length and afterload (a minor contributor) will affect this value (79,80); the lower the S-wave velocity, the more depressed the myocardial function will be, even at the point prior to the visualization of thickening of the left ventricle (81). In the context of existing diastolic function, the S-wave velocities will change in relation to worsening LV systolic function (82). A poor prognostic indicator of cardiac events in patients with heart failure is when the S velocities are greater than 5 cm/s (83). For example, TDI is a useful indicator that correlates with biopsies as well as regional segment abnormalities in heart transplant recipients who experience rejection, although difficulties do arise because of tethering (84–86).

Strain and strain rate analysis is becoming of greater use in echocardiography for evaluation of myocardial performance.

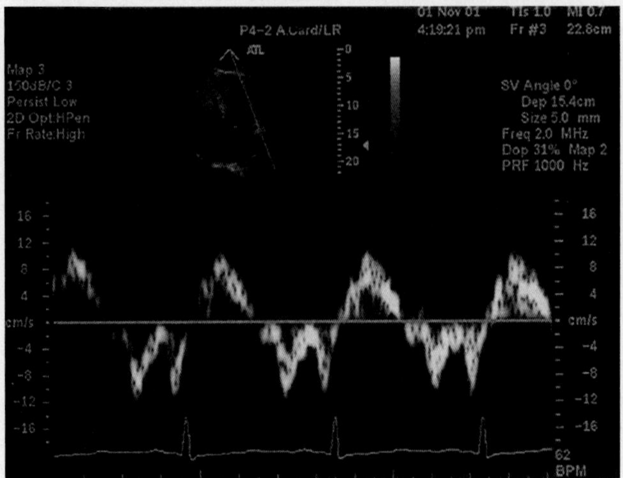

FIGURE 25.7 Normal spectral tissue Doppler. (From Dittoe N, Stulz D, Schwartz BP, et al. Quantitative left ventricular systolic function: from chamber to myocardium. *Crit Care Med.* 2007;35(8):S330–S339, with permission.)

In addition, TEE may not be readily available in the ICU (87). This technique measures the deformity of the LV segment during the cardiac cycle, with strain referring to relative change (%) and strain rate being the absolute of change (Fig. 25.8) (88).

Both strain and strain rate are being used in heart failure patients (resynchronization) for the early detection of myocardial ischemia and identification of viable myocardium (89–91). Technical limitations of this technique include a low signal-to-noise ratio, angle dependence, and a processing power that requires significant data storage and analysis (92). Nevertheless, it is independent of heart rate and afterload, although it is still influenced by preload due to the reliance on the initial diastolic dimension (93,94). Other potential advantages are the use of spectral tracking (which eliminates the angle effect), a feature that has been available only recently (95,96), and the backscatter/tissue characterization, which is similar to MRI in the evaluation of the myocardium (97–99).

Peak + dP/dT (typically recorded prior to opening of the aortic valve) is also commonly used, although some investigators believe it to be load independent in the presence of mitral regurgitation. It does have some prognostic importance (when less than 600 mmHg/s) in congestive heart failure (CHF) and valvular surgery (100,101). Other investigators believe that this index is influenced by preload and that stress-corrected, fiber-shortening velocity (V_{cf}) is a more viable index of CHF (102–104).

Lastly, the pseudonormalized Doppler total ejection isovolumic index (TEI) is a valid, load-independent measure of ventricular performance:

$$\text{Index} = (\text{ICT} + \text{IRT})/\text{ET}$$

where ICT is the isovolumetric time, ET is the ejection time, and IRT is the isovolumetric relaxation time (105,106). As ventricular function worsens (diastolic or systolic), this index increases (Fig. 25.9) (107).

Measuring systolic movement of the mitral annulus ring using M mode in the apical four-chamber view, mitral annulus postsystolic excursion (MAPSE) is another method of determining LVEF. Technical pitfalls are involved, due to the proper alignment of the M mode perpendicular to the annulus movement in order not to underestimate the systolic excursions. Intra- and interobserver variability is around 5% and is an independent predictor of 28-day mortality (108,109). MAPSE greater than 10 mm correlates with an EF greater than 55%, MAPSE less than 8 mm corresponds to a reduced EF, with 8 to 10 mm being and indeterminate zone regarding LV function.

Speckle tracking echocardiography (STE) is a novel and sensitive method for assessing myocardial deformation (strain). It can unmask dysfunction before it can be detected with conventional echocardiography. Unlike Doppler imaging, STE is an angle-independent process. It can be used in sepsis in the ICU, and can identify right ventricle and left ventricle dysfunction (110). STE may help identify higher-risk patients in the ICU and standardization of this technique is under current review (Fig. 25.10) (111).

Diastolic Function

Diastolic dysfunction is greatly underappreciated in the ICU (112,113). Research and clinical endeavors have emphasized systolic function. Since the addition of PW and CW Doppler

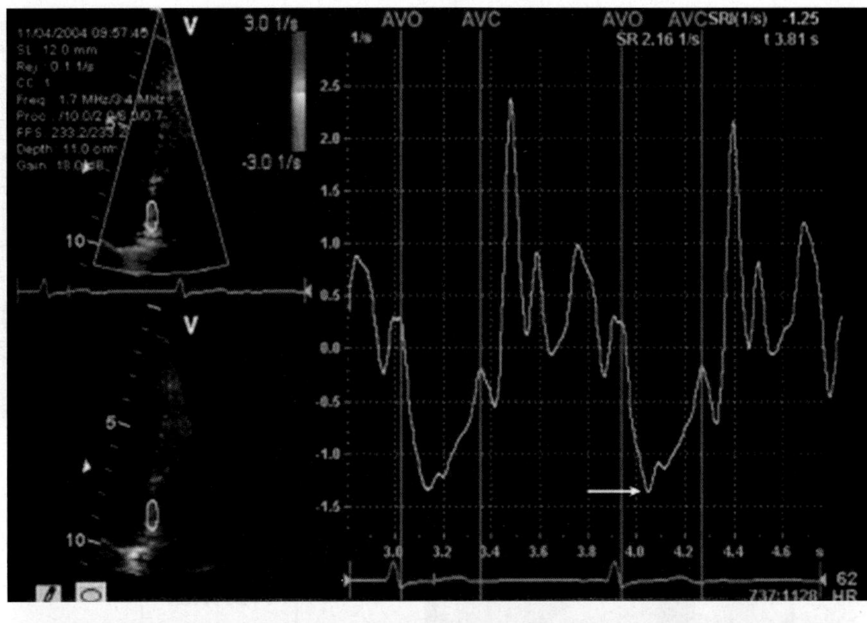

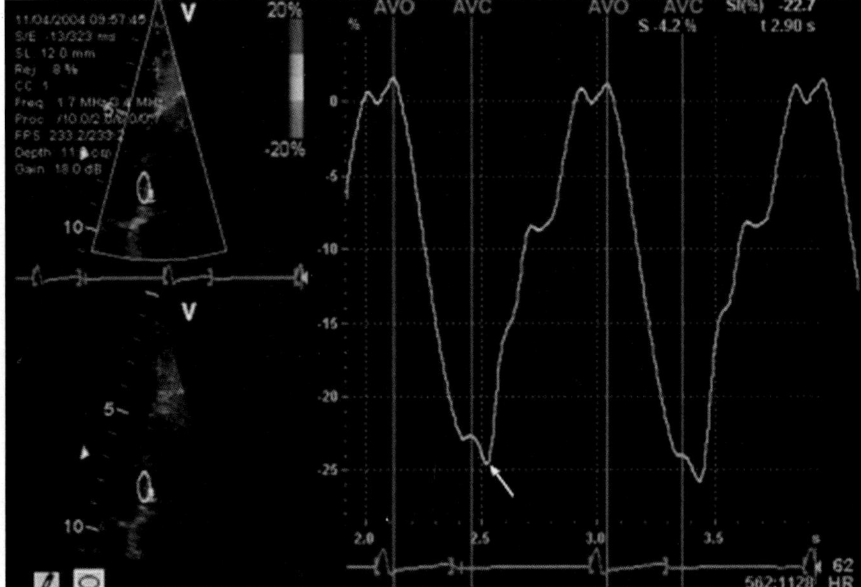

FIGURE 25.8 Recording of strain rate, which represents the rate of deformation; the peak negative strain rate (*arrow*) was $-1.3\ s^{-1}$. (From Oh JK, Seward JB, Tajik AJ. *The Echo Manual*. 3rd ed. Philadelphia, PA: Lippincott Williams & Wilkins; 2006, used with permission of Mayo Foundation for Medical Education and Research.)

echocardiography, the importance of diastolic dysfunction came to the forefront, especially when dealing with critically ill patients in whom clinical findings and hemodynamics can often be confusing and misleading. Diastolic dysfunction may be isolated but is usually associated with systolic dysfunction (112,114,115). Ventricular interactions may be a contributing influence in the presentation of echocardiographic findings.

Even though echocardiography provides a unique insight in LV dysfunction, there are significant difficulties with its use that must be appreciated (113). Diastole is associated with summation of the processes by which the heart loses its ability to generate force and shorten while returning to the precontractile state. Diastolic function is associated with relaxation and early ventricular filling or altered LV pressure/volume and stress–strain relationships. Many confounding factors interplay in early LV filling and compliance that, at times, may be diametrically opposed (Table 25.5) (116). Altered hemodynamics and loading conditions, as well as

TABLE 25.5 Factors Influencing the Left Ventricular End-Diastolic Pressure–Volume Relation (Chamber Stiffness)

Left ventricular physical properties
Left ventricular chamber volume and mass
Composition of the left ventricular wall
Viscosity, stress relaxation, creep
Factors intrinsic to the left ventricle
Myocardial relaxation
Coronary turgor
Factors extrinsic to the left ventricle
Pericardial restraint
Atrial contraction
Right ventricular interaction
Pleural and mediastinal pressure

Reproduced from Hoit BD. Left ventricular diastolic function. *Crit Care Med.* 2007;35:S340–S347, with permission.

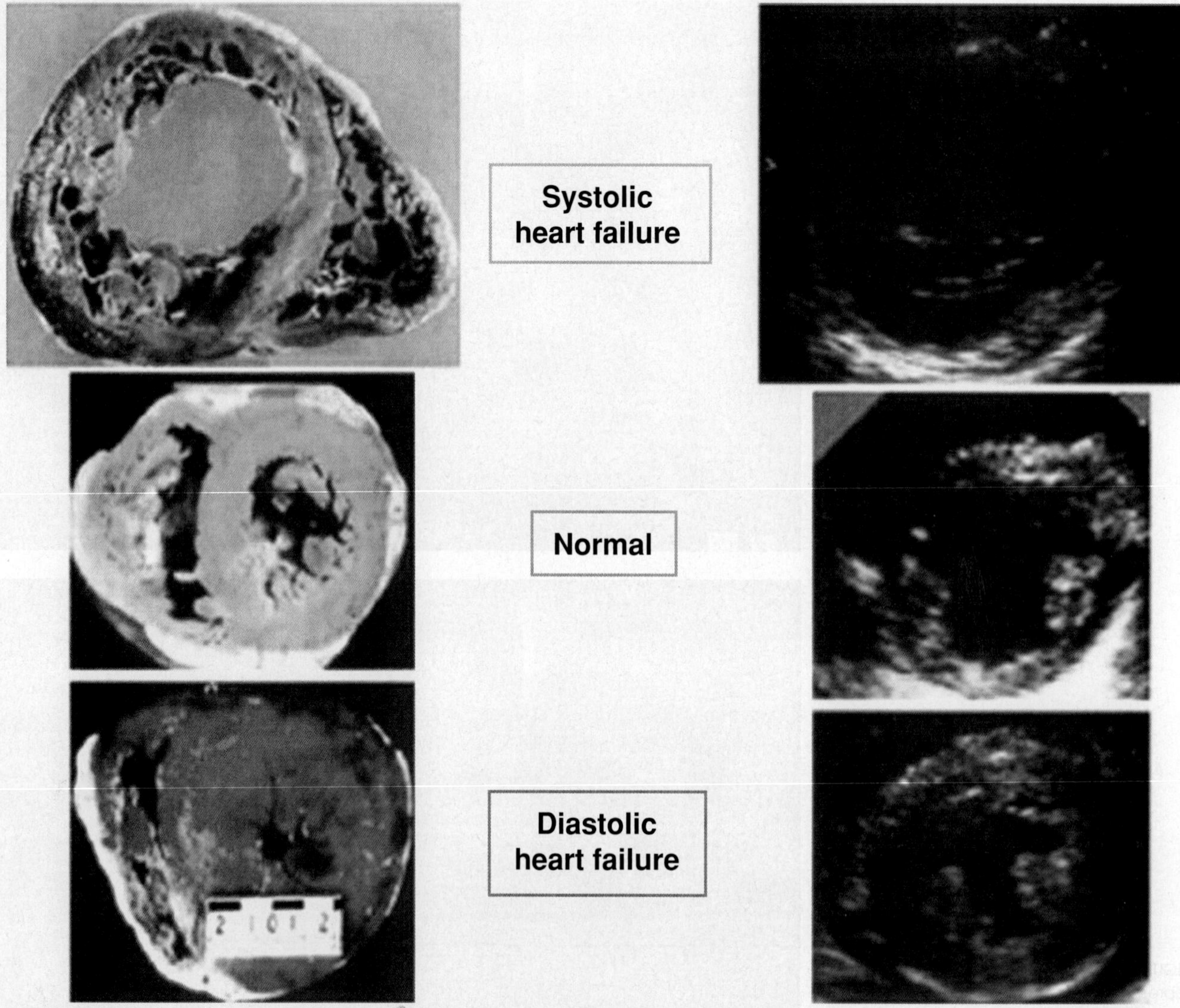

FIGURE 25.9 Ventricular remodeling in systolic and diastolic heart failure. **Left**: Autopsy examples. **Right**: Cross-sectional two-dimensional echocardiographic views of systolic and diastolic heart failures compared with normal are illustrated. In systolic heart failure, the left ventricular cavity is markedly dilated and wall thickness is not increased. In diastolic heart failure, the cavity size is normal or decreased and wall thickness is markedly increased. (Reprinted from Konstam MA. Systolic and diastolic dysfunction in heart failure? Time for a new paradigm. *J Card Fail.* 2003;9:1–3, with permission.)

tachycardia, are confounding issues in accurately determining the extent of LV diastolic dysfunction, particularly in patients who experience shock states—especially distributive events (sepsis, septic shock, systemic inflammatory response syndrome [SIRS], liver insufficiency); inflammatory mediators and cytokines affect all aspects of myocardial performance including atrial dysfunction and volume (116). Tachycardia can be an early deterrent in the accurate measurement of diastolic function (117).

Doppler indices can appreciate the complexities of LV relaxation. The rate of LV relaxation is estimated from the maximal rate of pressure decay ($-dP/dt_{max}$) and other indices (such as the relaxation half-time [RT]) (118). Tau (isovolumetric relaxation) reflects the aortic valve closure to mitral valve opening and appears to be a better index of relaxation because of the decreased load dependency (119).

Although the pressure/volume relationship of the left ventricle is more often emphasized, the pressure/volume relationship of the atria can also play an important role. Other extrinsic factors and myocardial ischemia may contribute to impairment of diastolic dysfunction. Despite the limitations discussed, echocardiography remains a viable tool for detecting the presence of diastolic dysfunction (112,113). Left atrium enlargement is the consequence of longstanding left atrium pressure and/or volume overload. Left atrium volume is sometimes called the HbA1c of study of diastolic dysfunction. Left atrium dilation is considered incompatible with preserved diastolic dysfunction. Quantification of left atrium volume according to body surface area (LA_{vol}/BSA) is as follows (120–122):

- LA_{vol}/BSA < 29 mL/m^2: normal
- LA_{vol}/BSA: 29–33 mL/m^2: mild
- LA_{vol}/BSA: 33–39 mL/m^2: moderate
- LA_{vol}/BSA > 39 mL/m^2: severe

The morphologic and functional differences between diastolic and systolic heart dysfunction are described in Table 25.6.

Diseases germane to the critically ill—such as metabolic derangements involving mitochondrial dysfunction as seen in

TABLE 25.6 Morphologic and Functional Changes in Diastolic vs. Systolic Heart Failure

Parameters	Diastolic Heart Failure	Systolic Heart Failure
Left ventricular cavity, size	Normal or decreased	Increased
Left ventricular mass	Increased	Increased
Mass/cavity	Increased	Normal or decreased
Wall thickness	Increased	Decreased
End-diastolic stress	Increased	Increased
End-systolic stress	Normal	Increased
End-diastolic volume	Normal	Increased
End-systolic volume	Normal or decreased	Increased
Ejection fraction	Normal	Decreased
Mechanical dyssynchrony	May be present	May be present
Left ventricular shape and geometry	Usually remains unchanged	Spherical

Reproduced from Chatterjee K, Massie B. Systolic and diastolic heart failure: differences and similarities. *J Card Fail.* 2007;13:569–576, with permission.

sepsis, SIRS, and liver insufficiency—or simply the postcardiac surgical patient status can affect the passive/active relaxation of the left ventricle (116,123–128). Comorbid conditions (hypertensive heart disease) and the presenting hemodynamic picture (the level of the atrial pressure and its rate of development) will also influence this relationship. Diastolic chamber stiffness is dependent on ventricular chamber characteristics (mass, volume) and myocardial stiffness, both load size- and chamber size–independent variables of passive chamber and myocardial properties (112,129,130).

The echocardiographic assessment is accomplished through several means: M-mode and two-dimensional echocardiography and Doppler techniques. LV diastolic pressure, diastolic function, and ventricular and atrial filling patterns are measured by flows through the pulmonary veins (left atrial [LA] filling) and annular velocities through the mitral valve orifice

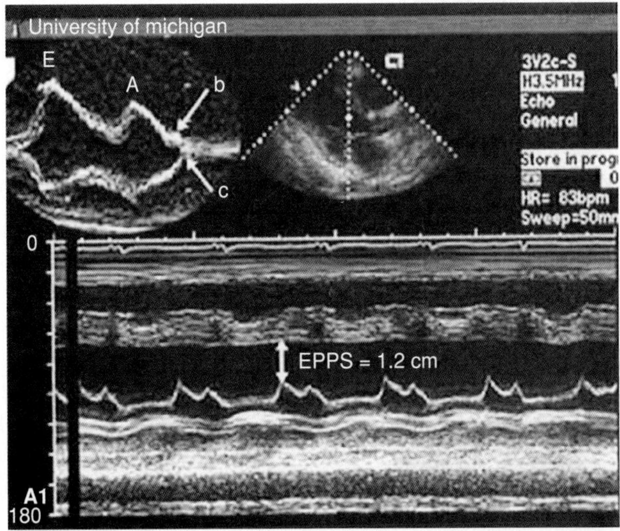

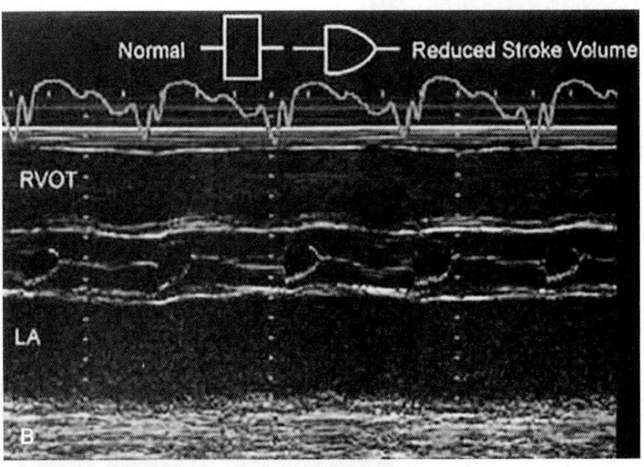

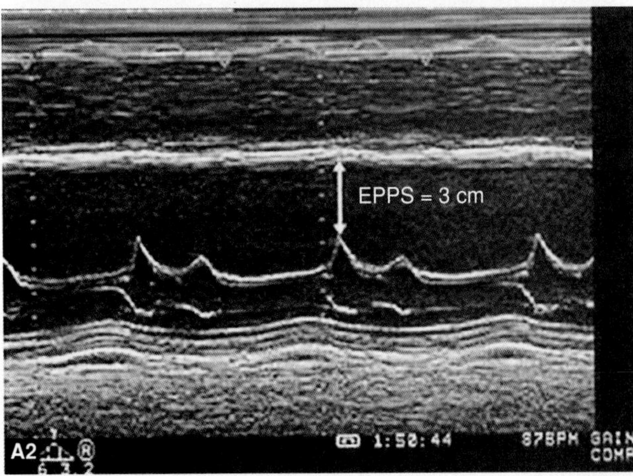

FIGURE 25.10 Left ventricular function. **A**: M-mode echocardiograms recorded in two patients with significant systolic dysfunction. **Top**: An E-point septal separation (EPSS) of 1.2 cm (normal M6 mm). **Bottom**: Recording in a patient with more significant left ventricular systolic dysfunction in which the EPSS is 3.0 cm. Also, note the interrupted closure of the mitral valve with a B bump (**top**), indicating an increase in the left ventricular end-diastolic pressure. **B**: M-mode echocardiogram recorded through the aortic valve in a patient with reduced cardiac function and decreased forward stroke volume. Note the rounded closure of the aortic valve, indicating decreasing forward flow at the end of systole. Normal and abnormal aortic valve opening patterns are noted in a schematic superimposed on the figure. (*continued*)

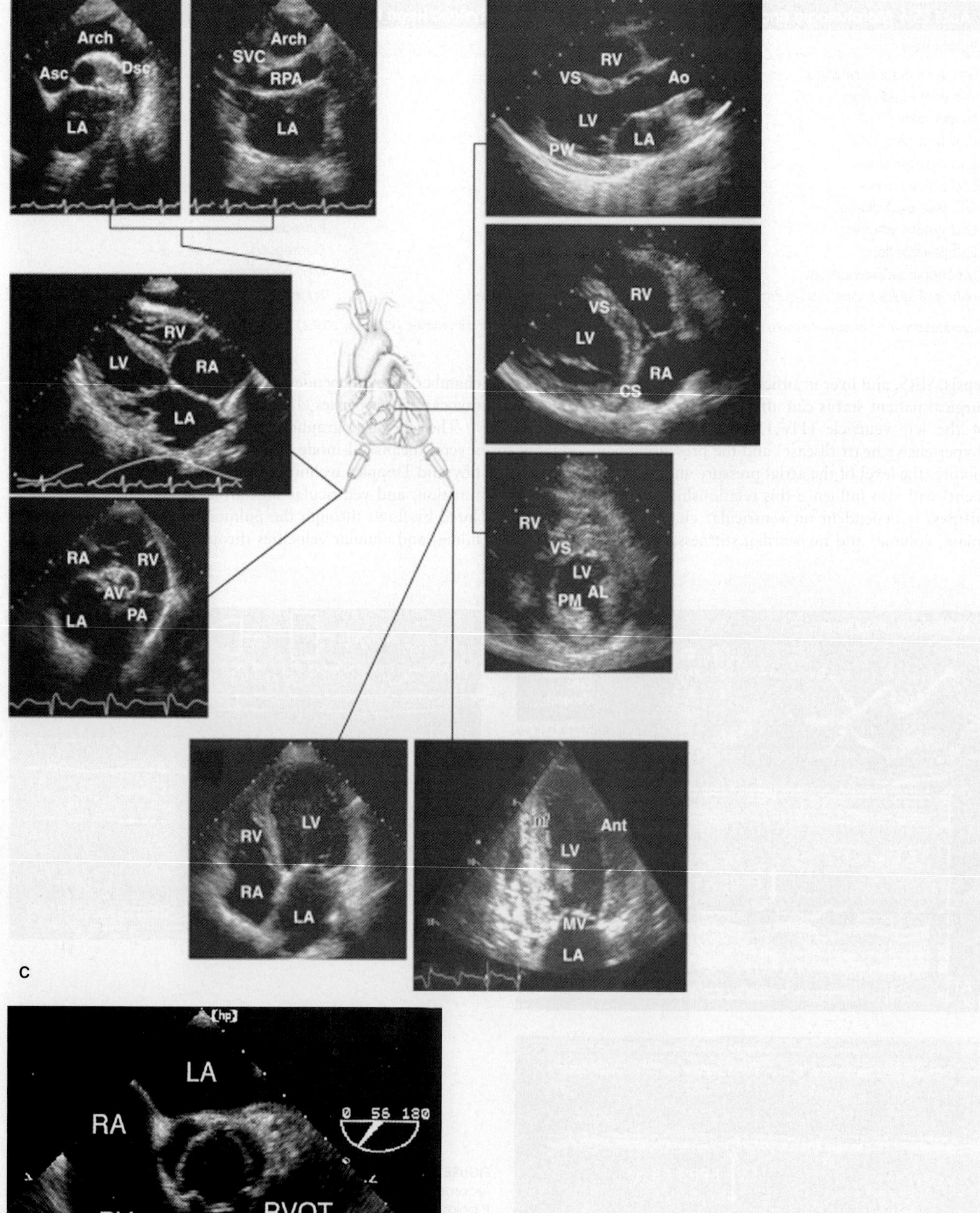

FIGURE 25.10 (*Continued*) C: Diagram of cardiac structures from standard tomographic planes: parasternal long-axis view (**left**), parasternal short-axis view (**upper right**), and apical four-chamber view (**lower right**). D: From the esophagus, the probe can be flexed to yield a basal short-axis projection. LA, left atrium; RA, right atrium; RV, right ventricle; RVOT, right ventricular outflow tract.

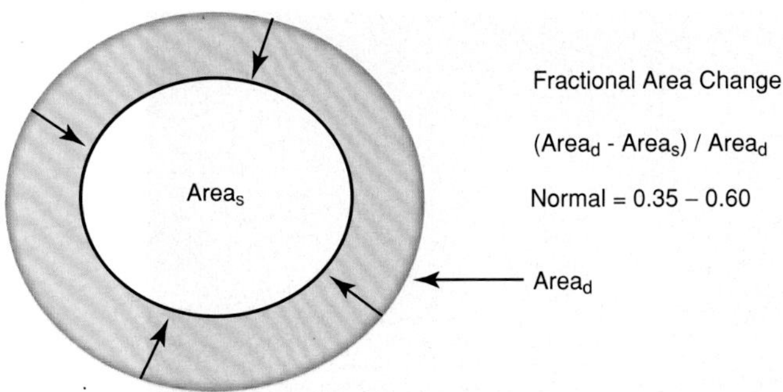

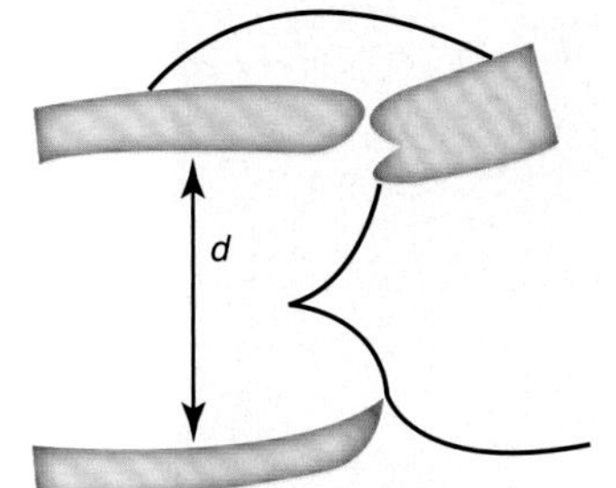

Area - Length volume determination

Area (A) = πr^2 or directly measured from a short axis view

Length = LV length from apical view

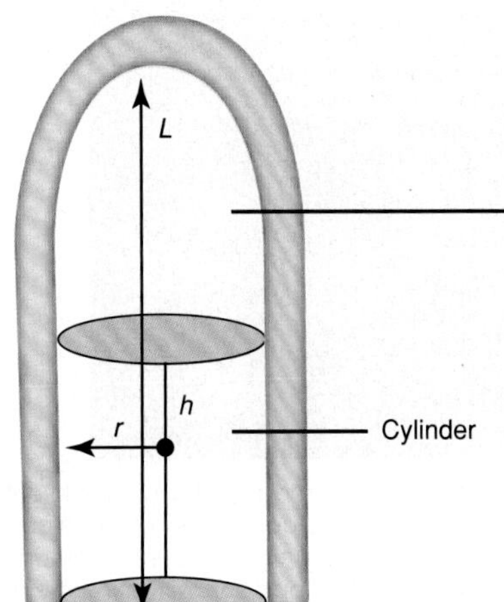

LV Volume = Volume$_{cone}$ + Volume$_{cylinder}$

$$V = A\,\frac{L}{2} + \frac{1}{3}\,A\,\frac{L}{2}$$

Cylinder Volume — Cone Volume

$$V = \frac{2}{3}AL$$

Alternately assuming a truncated ellipse

$$V = \frac{2}{6}AL$$

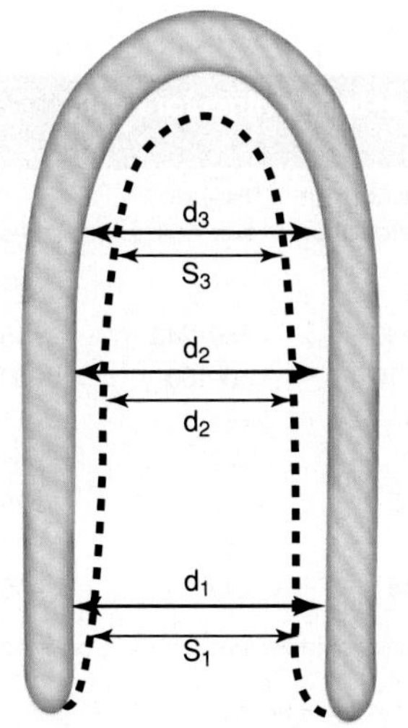

$$EF = K_{apex} + [(d_3^2 - S_3^2) + (d_2^2 - S_2^2) + (d_1^2 + S_1^2)]$$

K_{apex} = –5%, 0, +5%, +10% or + 15%

FIGURE 25.10 (*Continued*) **E**: Schematic representation of two-dimensionally derived measurements of left ventricular systolic function. **Top**: The methodology for determining fractional area change, which is defined by the formula in the figure. **Middle and bottom**: Using the geometric assumption that the left ventricular cavity represents a cylinder and cone configuration, the volume of each separate component can be calculated as noted. The overall left ventricular volume equals the sum of the two volumes. See text for further details. **F**: Schematic representation of a simplified method for determining the left ventricular ejection fraction from three separate minor-axis dimensions at the base, mid, and distal portions of the left ventricle in an apical view. The contribution of the apex is expressed as a constant (Kapex) ranging from –5% to +15%. (*continued*)

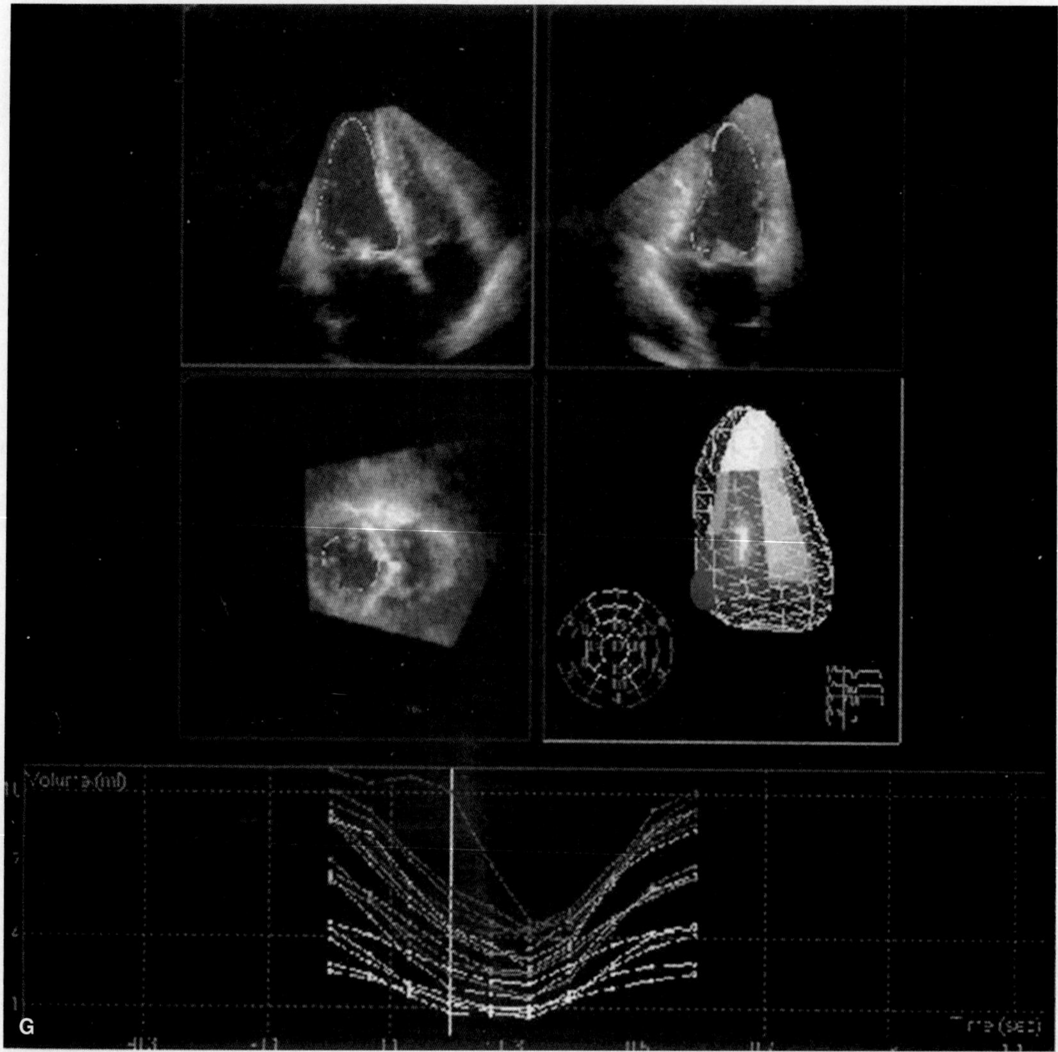

FIGURE 25.10 (*Continued*) G: The left ventricular volume cast (**lower right**) was created from 3D echocardiography imaging. Regional left ventricular volume changes are shown in the plot at the bottom. The color of each line corresponds to the segment of the same color in the left ventricular cast. (See also Video 25-5.) (**A,B,D–F**: From Feigenbaum H, Armstrong WF, Ryan T, eds. *Feigenbaum's Echocardiography*. 6th ed. Philadelphia, PA: Lippincott Williams & Wilkins; 2005, with permission. **G**: From Oh JK, Seward JB, Tajik AJ. *The Echo Manual*. 3rd ed. Philadelphia, PA: Lippincott Williams & Wilkins; 2006, used with permission of Mayo Foundation for Medical Education and Research.)

(LV filling) (112,131). By measuring these parameters, one can get a sense of prognosis and outcomes in patients with heart failure that can guide treatment (132). In addition, by using these Doppler techniques for measuring pulmonary artery pressures, the clinician can predict the extent of hospitalization and mortality (133). There are several patterns seen via PW Doppler through the mitral valve, which reflects the relationship between the LA and LV diastolic pressures. Normally, regarding the early/late filling pattern and ratio, E/A is greater than one. The deceleration time of E velocity (DT) and isovolumic relaxation time (IVRT) are other parameters obtained in the interrogation of this flow. Other patterns easily detected are restriction (E/A less than 2), pseudonormalization (E/A 1–1.5), and abnormal relaxation (E/A less than 1) (Table 25.7) (108). To clarify the second pattern, tissue Doppler index (TDI Ea [early annular] velocity) is measured through the mitral annulus. This technique measures high amplitude and low velocity of the myocardium (134). It appears that early diastolic annular velocity Ea is relatively load independent and should be completed in every patient (135). Ea will

TABLE 25.7 Classification of Left Ventricular Filling Patterns

	Normal	Abnormal Relaxation	Pseudo-normalization	Restriction
E/A ratio	1–1.5	<1	1–1.5	>2
DT, ms	160–240	≥240	160–240	≤150
IVRT, ms	60–100	≥110	60–100	<60
PV S/D ratio	~1[a]	>1	<1	<1
A_r duration	<A	>A	>A	>A
A_r vel, cm/s	<20	<35	>35	>25[b]
Ea, cm/s	>8	<8	<8	<8
V_p, cm/s	>45	<45	<45	<45

Reproduced from Hoit B. Left ventricular diastolic function. *Crit Care Med.* 2007;35:5340–5347, with permission.

[a]Young patients and athletes may have values of <1.

[b]If atrial contractile failure is present, the value will be <25 cm/s.

E/A, mitral E/A ratio; DT, decelerating time; IVRT, isovolumic relaxation time; PV S/D, pulmonary vein systolic and diastolic flow; A_r, atrial reversal flow of pulmonary vein; A, mitral A duration; vel, velocity; Ea, early mitral annular longitudinal tissue velocity; V_p, velocity of transmitral flow propagation.

decrease in the presence of elevated filling pressures associated with increases in early diastolic transmitral velocity. Of interest, the transmitral early diastolic velocity/tissue Doppler early diastolic annular velocity E/Ea correlates with pulmonary artery occlusion pressure and mean diastolic LV pressure over an extended range of EF (122,136–138).

Interrogation of the pulmonary venous patterns (PVF) is helpful in depicting diastolic dysfunction. Both modes of echocardiography (TTE and TEE) are useful, but invariably, TEE can only assess the flow characteristics usually in the left upper superior vein. The pattern seen is related to the suction effects of the LV and the LA. The systolic component represents LA filling during atrial relaxation (S1) and ventricular contraction (S2). The diastolic forward phase reflects the opening of the mitral valve. Atrial reversal flow represents retrograde flow during atrial contraction (less than 20 cm/s). The extent of reversal of atrial flow may also reflect elevated LA pressure with or without LV compliance changes (112).

Color M-mode Doppler is another method for identifying diastolic function abnormalities and is believed to be load independent (139). Thus, the propagation velocity (V_p) is inversely related to the time constant of LV relaxation (140). This method can be used with the *E* velocities and the IVRT to estimate pulmonary occlusion pressure (141). It is of interest that V_p may distinguish between restrictive and constrictive pericardial cardiomyopathies (139).

M-mode and two-dimensional echocardiography are underappreciated in diastolic function assessment. The timing and extent of LV thinning rate and wall motion as well as the duration of atrial contraction and early relaxation can provide useful data. Filling dynamics can be obtained by measuring, frame by frame, the LV volume with either apical four-chamber or short-axis views (142,143). Assessing ventricular volume and mass with M-mode echocardiography provides information of the ventricular pressure/volume relationship relating to operative chamber compliance. Also, a marker for duration and severity of diastolic dysfunction is LA volume (144).

TDI is an echocardiographic technique that directly measures myocardial velocities. Diastolic tissue Doppler velocities reflect myocardial relaxation and, in combination with conventional Doppler measurements, ratios (transmitral early diastolic velocity/mitral annular early diastolic velocity [E/Ea]). Ea is a relatively preload-independent measure of myocardial relaxation in patients with cardiac disease as compared to early transmitral velocity, and has been developed to noninvasively estimate LV filling pressure. Consequently, mitral E/Ea can help to establish the presence of clinical CHF in patients with dyspnea. However, E/Ea has a significant gray zone and is not well validated in a nonsinus rhythm and mitral valve disease. B-type natriuretic peptide (BNP) is a protein released by the ventricles in the presence of myocytic stretch and has been correlated to LV filling pressure and, independently, to other cardiac morphologic abnormalities. In addition, BNP is significantly affected by age, sex, renal function, and obesity. Given its correlation with multiple cardiac variables, BNP has high sensitivity, but low specificity, for the detection of elevated LV filling pressures. Taking into account the respective strengths and limitations of BNP and mitral E/Ea, algorithms combining them can be used to more accurately estimate LV filling pressures in patients presenting with dyspnea (145).

TABLE 25.8 Echocardiographic Left Ventricular Morphologic and Functional Characteristics in Primary Systolic and Diastolic Heart Failure Compared with Controls

	Controls	Systolic Heart Failure	Diastolic Heart Failure
LVEDV (mL)	102 + 12	192 + 10[a]	87 + 10
LVESV (mL)	46 + 11	137 + 9[a]	37 + 9
LVEF %	54 + 2	31 + 2[a]	60 + 2[b]
LV mass (g)	125 + 12	232 + 9[a]	160 + 9[b]
LV mass/volume	1.49 + 0.17	1.22 + 0.14	2.12 + 0.14[c]
NE pg/mL	169	287	306; $p = 0.007$
BNP pg/mL	3	28	56; $p = 0.02$

LVEDV, left ventricular end-diastolic volume; LVESV, left ventricular end-systolic volume; LVEF, left ventricular ejection fraction; LV, left ventricle; NE, norepinephrine; BNP, B-type natriuretic peptide.
[a]Systolic heart failure vs. controls, $p < 0.001$.
[b]Diastolic heart failure vs. controls, $p < 0.001$.
[c]Diastolic heart failure vs. controls, $p < 0.002$.
Reproduced with permission from Chatterjee K, Massie B. Systolic and diastolic heart failure: differences and similarities. *J Card Fail.* 2007;13:569–576.

In summary, systolic and diastolic dysfunction are two definitive entities or syndromes of heart failure. Even though the clinical symptoms and hemodynamic presentations may appear similar, the primary function and myocardial structural derangements are quite distinctive. There are marked advancements for treatment of systolic heart failure, but treatment for diastolic failure is still empiric. Echocardiography can serially follow and evaluate the treatment management of these patients (113), and in so doing, prognostic indicators can be detected (133,146). Therefore, the use of echocardiography in the syndromes of heart failure is crucial for enhancement of patient care and outcome. Even in sepsis, bedside evaluation of the ventricular function with echocardiography is a proven imaging tool (147). Left ventricular morphologic and functional characteristics in primary systolic and diastolic heart failure compared with controls are represented in Table 25.8.

Right Ventricular Assessment: Pulmonary Embolism and Right Ventricular Infarction

Findings of right heart failure in acute pulmonary embolism (PE) have higher mortality and morbidity (148). Chest CT or other modalities may not be feasible in certain critically ill patients (renal failure, unstable hypoxia, or hemodynamic instability). In these instances, a focused cardiac examination may help by ruling out other forms of shock, and may present with right heart strain and/or dilation. It has been suggested that echocardiography can be used to justify thrombolytics in certain patients who cannot get definitive diagnoses (149), but this suggestion has been questioned unless direct visualization of the proximal PE (150,151). TEE can diagnose large, central PEs with rare false positive results (152,153). This catastrophic cardiovascular event can either be underdiagnosed or overdiagnosed (154–159). A low cardiac output and RV failure post PE presages mortality because of the extent of distal obstruction. Early identification of these derangements, including the possible implementation of serial examinations, may assist in managing these critically ill patients by providing prognostic indicators, stratification for more intensive surveillance, and any necessary interventions (160). Even appropriate anticoagulation may not eliminate a PE. Several diagnostic tests are available, including a 64-cut chest CT, MRI, pulmonary angiography, and echocardiography (Fig. 25.11 and Table 25.9) (154).

The classic echocardiographic signs for a PE are the following:

- Dilation of the chamber and thinning of the right ventricle wall with global hypokinesis
- Pulmonic insufficiency
- Tricuspid insufficiency
- RA dilatation with decreased atrial function and abnormal atrial septal motion
- Septal flattening or paradoxical motion of the ventricular septum into the left ventricle
- Increased ratio of RV/LV dimensions
- Pulmonary artery hypertension
- Dilation of the pulmonary artery
- Identification of thrombi

If the patient's RV function is normal until the event, because of its innate inability to tolerate acute pressure overload, these echocardiographic events would occur acutely, and catastrophic events would result when 75% of the pulmonary vasculatures are obstructed. Earlier signs may manifest with as little as a 25% obstruction of the pulmonary vasculature (161). According to the International Cooperative Pulmonary Embolism registry, the presence of RV hypokinesis is associated with

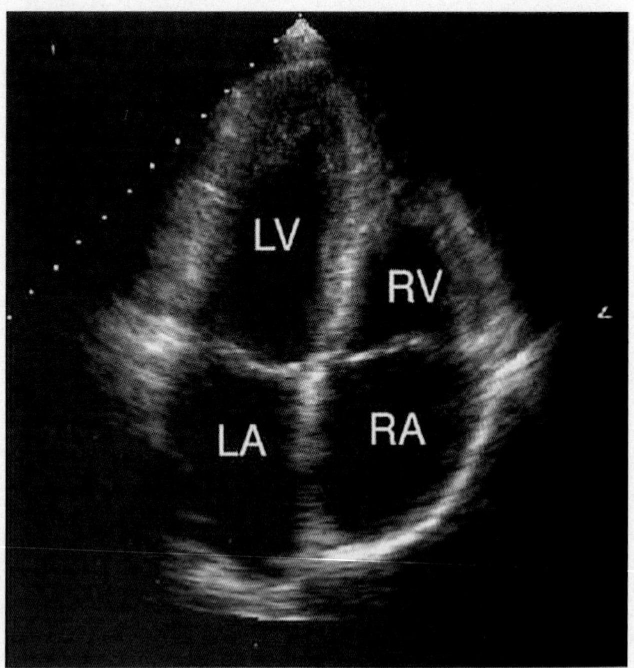

FIGURE 25.11 Enlarged right ventricle (RV) in parasternal short axis view. LV, left ventricle. (See also Video 25-6.)

TABLE 25.9 Imaging and Biomarker Findings Suggestive of Higher Risk in PE Patients

Source	Subjects, No.	Diagnostic Finding	Outcome	Sensitivity, % (95% CI)	Specificity, % (95% CI)	Positive Predictive Value, % (95% CI)	Negative Predictive Value, % (95% CI)
Echocardiography							
Ten Wolde et al., 2004 (161)	310	RV dysfunction	Hospital mortality		58†	5†	
Kucher et al., 2005 (162)	1,035	RV hypokinesis	30-day mortality	52.4 (43.7–61.0)	62.7 (59.5–65.8)	16.1 (12.8–19.9)	90.6 (88.1–92.7)
Contrast-enhanced CT							
Schoepf et al., 2004 (163)	454	RV/LV diameter >0.9	30-d mortality	78.2 (65.6–87.9)†	38.0 (33.3–43.0)†	15.6 (11.8–20.3)†	92.3 (87.0–95.5)†
van der Meer et al., 2005 (164)	120	RV/LV diameter >1.0	PE-related 90 day mortality	100†	45.1†	10.1 (2.9–17.4)	100 (94.3–100)
Troponin							
Pruszczyk et al., 2003 (165)	64	cTnT >0.01 ng/mL	Hospital mortality	100 (62.9–100)	57.0 (44.1–69.0)	25.8 (13.9–42.6)	98.5 (87.0–99.8)
Mehta et al., 2003 (166)	38	cTnI >0.04 ng/mL	Cardiogenic shock	85.7 (48.7–99.3)	61.3 (43.8–76.3)	33.3 (16.3–56.3)	95.0 (76.4–99.7)
Punukollu et al., 2005 (167)	33	cTnI >0.04 ng/mL	RV dysfunction	66.7 (43.7–83.7)	73.3 (48.0–89.1)	75.0 (50.5–89.8)	64.7 (41.3–82.7)
BNP							
Pruszczyk et al., 2003 (165)	79	NT-proBNP >600 pg/mL	Hospital mortality	100†	33†	22.7†	100†
Kucher et al., 2003 (168)	73	BNP >50 pg/mL	Combined end point*	95 (76–99)	60 (47–72)	48 (33–63)	97 (81–99)
Combined testing							
Binder et al., 2005 (169)	111	NT-proBNP >1,000 pg/mL and RV dysfunction	Combined end point†	61.1 (38.6–79.7)	79.6 (70.3–86.5)	36.7 (21.9–54.5)	91.4 (83.2–95.8)
Scridon et al., 2005 (170)	141	cTnI >0.1 ng/mL and RV/LV diameter > 0.9	30-d mortality	60.7 (42.4–76.4)	75.2 (66.5–82.3)	37.8 (25.1–52.4)	88.5 (80.6–93.2)

*Combined end point of death, cardiopulmonary resuscitation, mechanical ventilation, vasopressors, thrombolytics, catheter fragmentation, surgical embolectomy.
†Combined end point of cardiopulmonary resuscitation, mechanical ventilation, vasopressors, thrombolytics.
†Other values and CIs not reported.

increased mortality at 30 days even with a systolic systemic pressure greater than 90 mmHg (162).

If the patient exhibits pre-existing chronic pulmonary artery hypertension with RV hypertrophy, thrombosis of the right-sided circulation may be initially better tolerated. Eventually, RV failure will ensue and dominate the cardiovascular presentation (158,171). Morris-Thurgood and Frenneaux (172) describe RV and RA pressures with reversal of the transseptal diastolic pressure gradient when intravascular volume replacement is attempted to enhance diastolic ventricular interaction. In the situations where other diagnostic tests may fail, echocardiography is a useful diagnostic tool to determine RV afterload and associated hemodynamic findings significant for PE (154–158,162).

Tricuspid annular plane systolic excursion (TAPSE) is a measure of the distance of the systolic excursion of the RV annular segment along its longitudinal plane, obtained in the apical four-chamber view. TAPSE greater than 1.6 cm is considered indicative of normal RV function, less than 1.6 cm implies impaired RV function. One of the assumptions is that the displacement of the basal segment is representative of the entire RV. In a consensus document, it was summarized that the advantages include that it is simple, less dependent on optimal image quality, reproducible, and does not require sophisticated equipment or prolonged image analysis. It also commented disadvantages include that it is angle dependent, there are no large-scale validation studies, assumes a single segment represents the whole function, load dependent, and affected by LV dysfunction (173,174). In more recent reports, patients with TAPSE less than 1.6 cm had greater all-cause mortality at 30 days, and was also associated with most other markers of RV failure (RV end-diastolic diameter, RV/LV end-diastolic diameter, systolic pulmonary artery pressures) (174,175).

Right ventricular infarction and/or failure are one of the most difficult clinical entities to support. Diagnosis of isolated failure or biventricular failure alters the management of these complex patients. Inferior myocardial infarction is associated with RV infarction (35%) (176,177). The classic findings are tricuspid regurgitation, a dilated thinned RV, severe global hypokinesis, reduced descent of the base of the RV free wall (apical four-chamber view), and plethora of the IVC without any respiratory variations in its diameter. In diastole, there is flattening of the ventricular septum and occasional paradoxical motion and, at times, bulging of the septum into the LV, indicative of a right-sided pressure/volume overload situation. The RA may reveal right atrial hypertension with displacement of the interatrial septum (176–178). If there is coexisting patent foramen ovale (PFO) in the presence of RV and/or RA afterload, a right-to-left shunt is possible through the atrial septum, resulting in hypoxemia and thus complicating the clinical presentation. The identification of a PFO is greatly enhanced by choosing TEE over the surface approach (179).

Pericardial Disease and Tamponade

Echocardiography is an ideal technique to detect pericardial maladies such as pericardial effusions leading toward tamponade (acute vs. chronic), restrictive versus constrictive pericardial disease processes, and infiltrative processes, infective or not (congenital, neoplastic, metabolic, radiation-induced, iatrogenic, and traumatic) (180,181).

Pericardial effusions can readily be identified by either the surface or esophageal approach. In the parasternal long-axis view, the pericardial fluid is most frequently seen posterior to the left ventricle and atrium, and tapers anterior to the descending aorta. In larger effusions, it may be seen anterior to the right ventricle (Fig. 25.12). When the effusion is posterior and/or loculated (regional), the surface image may bypass its presence. Regional tamponade is not securely identified but may be juxtaposed to either ventricle and/or may involve the right atrium, vena cava, or pulmonary veins. The detection of a pericardial effusion ensures the diagnosis of a pericarditis. However, a patient with fibrinous acute pericarditis may often present with a normal echocardiogram. When fluid is detected, the clinician may proceed to drain it and determine if it is of an infectious cause (exudative), a complication of CHF (transudative), or traumatic in nature (hemorrhagic) (147).

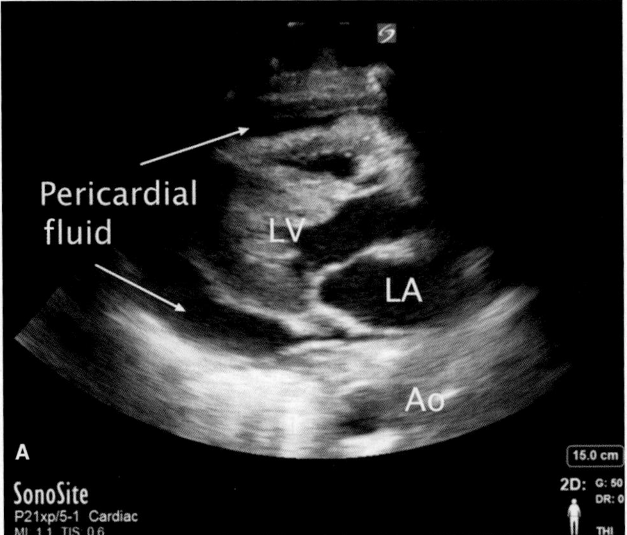

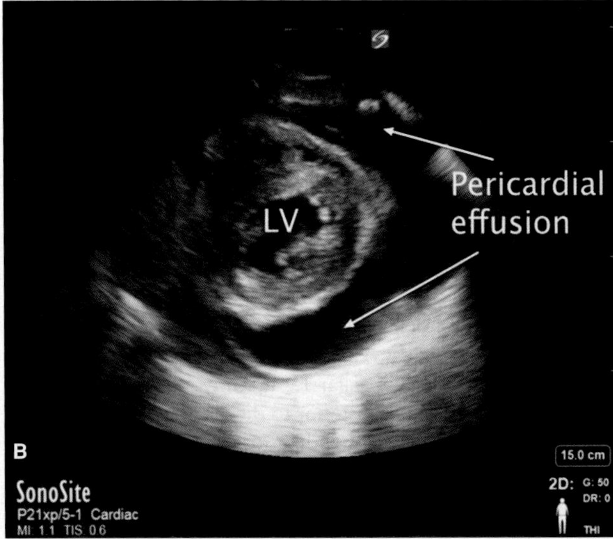

FIGURE 25.12 Pericardial effusion. **A:** Parasternal long axis showing pericardial effusion, seen tapering anterior to descending aorta (Ao). LV, left ventricle; RV, right ventricle; LA, left atrium. **B:** Parasternal short axis showing pericardial effusion. (See also Video 25-7.)

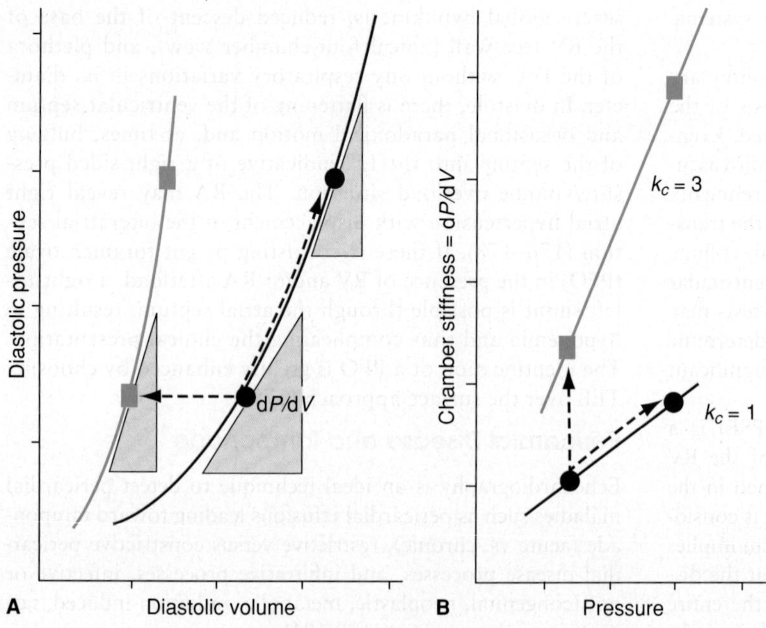

FIGURE 25.13 A: End-diastolic pressure–volume in two ventricles with differing passive diastolic properties. Chamber stiffness is d*P*/d*V* at any point on the end-diastolic pressure–volume relation. The stiffer chamber on the left has a steeper overall slope. B: Same data plotted as pressure versus chamber stiffness. Because of the exponential nature of the end-diastolic pressure–volume relation, the relation between chamber stiffness and pressure is a straight line whose slope is the chamber stiffness constant (k_c) that characterizes the overall slope of the end-diastolic pressure–volume relation. A similar relationship holds for stress and strain. (Reproduced from LeWinter MM, Osol G. Normal physiology of the cardiovascular system. In: *Hurst's the Heart*. 11th ed. New York, NY: McGraw-Hill; 2004:S342, with permission.)

In the syndrome of CHF (14%), myocardial infarction (15%), and valvular heart disease (21%), pericardial effusion is relatively common and may proceed to a tamponade syndrome (182,183). In cardiac surgical patients, the vast majority will have an effusion that presents usually on the second postoperative day and maximizes toward the 10th day (184). Fortunately, cardiac tamponade is unusual in these surgical patients, typically averaging 1% of the cases, with the exception of the cardiac transplanted patient in whom a higher frequency can result from repeated mediastinal procedures or rejection (185,186). Of interest, female gender, valvular intervention, and/or anticoagulants are predisposing factors (187).

An asymptomatic patient with chronic effusive pericarditis can present with a large effusion (188). Etiologic factors of this chronic process include uremia, neoplasm, tuberculosis (knobbed calcified pericardium), and connective tissue disorders (189). Typically, extensive effusion without any inflammatory disorders can be associated with a malignancy (188,190).

Echocardiography easily characterizes the relative contributions of cardiac enlargement or encroachment on the atrial/ventricular chambers and their ventricular and atrial performance, identifying underlying physiologic hemodynamic aberrations. Via M-mode echocardiography, one will see an echo-free space between the visceral and parietal pericardium dynamically throughout the cardiac cycle (Fig. 25.13).

If during systole there is a prominent separation, the fluid extent is deemed important. This modality is quite sensitive, as is two-dimensional echocardiography, which can detect small (less than 5 mm), moderate (5 to 10 mm), or large (greater than 10 mm) fluid amounts, as well as its global or regional involvement. As stated earlier, as the fluid volume increases, it will extend from the posterobasilar LV apically and then anteriorly, subsequently lateral and posterior to the LA (Fig. 25.14).

Drainage is performed for diagnostic purposes (e.g., infectious pathogens, cancer) or therapeutic reasons (hemodynamic compromise or pericardial tamponade) (187,191,192).

In regard to the end of this dynamic progression of fluid involvement, cardiac tamponade becomes a life-threatening event that must be correctly identified, diagnosed, and relieved in an expeditious fashion (193,194). Dynamic tamponade presentation depends on several physiologic considerations: the underlying ventricular performance; the rate of its development (increasing pericardial pressures in contrast to the intracardiac pressures with elevating venous pressures and decreasing to negative transmural pressures); the inherent intracardiac pressures, particularly of the ventricles; and the presenting intravascular volume or preload, especially in a hemorrhagic condition. If the patient has pre-existing RV afterload and/or pulmonary artery hypertension, the echocardiographic findings will be delayed because of the abnormal RV loading conditions. Normally, the diastolic collapse of the RV—depicted as abnormal posterior motion of the anterior RV wall during diastole—indicates that the pericardial pressure is exceeding the early diastolic RV pressure. In other words, the RV diastolic transmural pressure is negative (195). In contrast, if the patient's underlying LV systolic dysfunction is impaired, the

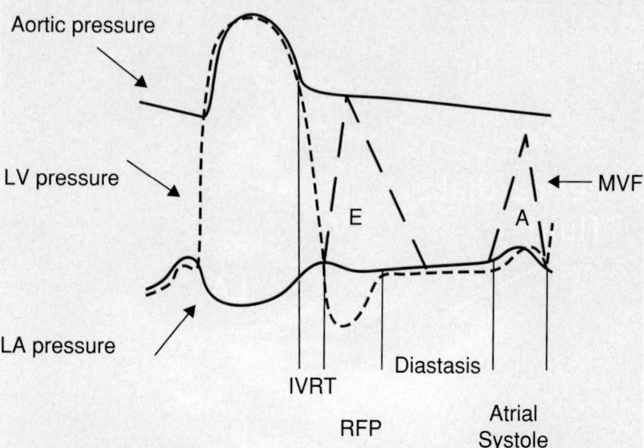

FIGURE 25.14 The four phases of diastole are schematically shown and include the isovolumic relaxation time (IVRT), which begins with aortic valve closure and extends to mitral valve opening, rapid early filling (RFP), diastasis, and atrial systole. Doppler E and A waves are superimposed. Note the points of left atrial–left ventricular (LA–LV) crossover and their relation to the mitral filling waves (MVF).

echocardiographic characteristics of tamponade will present earlier in the hemodynamic "fluid" progression with smaller volumes (196).

The echocardiographic indicators of pericardial tamponade include the following:

- Decrease in end-systolic and end-diastolic dimensions
- Relative increase in RV dimensions during spontaneous ventilation (inspiration) as compared to an increase in LV dimension
- RA diastolic collapse
- LV diastolic inversion
- Greater than 50% decrease in transmitral inflow
- Decrease in aortic flow velocities during inspiration

A large pericardial effusion (greater than 10 mm) may reveal a "swinging" heart throughout the cardiac cycle. In contrast, flow across the tricuspid valve and pulmonary flow velocities (PVFs) increase dramatically during inspiration, primarily in the systolic component of the PVF (197). Even though RV diastolic collapse is a sensitive indicator of tamponade, different loading conditions with varied ventricular performance will lower its specificity. RA diastolic volume is an even more sensitive (100%) marker for tamponade but, again, its specificity is not the best (198).

Of note, if the duration of RA diastolic collapse exceeds one-third of the cardiac cycle, the specificity increases (198). LA collapse is not usually detected (25%), but when it does exist, the specificity is markedly higher. LV diastolic collapse is much less common, probably due to the ventricular chamber properties (199–201). As in any dynamic hemodynamic setting, clinical conditions may vary, and pericardiocentesis is not necessary in every case of pericardial effusion. The absence of any chamber inversion has a high negative predictive value (92%), with the positive predictive value reaching 58%. Abnormal right-sided venous flows carry 82% and 88% positive and negative predictive values, respectively, for pericardial effusion (202).

If the pericardial fluid increases rapidly, the patient may initially have no prominent symptoms or may have only shortness of breath, with or without chest pain. Shortly thereafter, the patient will deteriorate to systolic hypotension, venous hypertension (distended jugular veins), and pulsus paradoxus. In the volume-depleted patient, these findings might not be initially present until rapid repletion of preload unmasks these characteristics (203).

Diastolic filling is also limited in constrictive pericarditis. Normal thickness of the pericardium does not preclude this diagnosis, which can be surgically confirmed in 28% of the cases of a negative series (204). The observed venous patterns of constrictive pericarditis from tamponade are characteristic. Because the ventricular chambers are fixed in volume by the pericardium, venous return is unimpeded during ejection, thereby ablating the normal venous surge during systole. Cardiac compression at end systole does not occur, so when the tricuspid valve opens the return of flow into the ventricle, it is of higher velocity, resulting in a biphasic venous return with a diastolic component faster than the systolic component (147). In contrast with tamponade, during inspiration in constrictive pericarditis, the decrease in intrathoracic pressure is not transmitted to the heart, and venous return does not fall (147,205). TEE measurement of the LV wall is markedly better than the surface approach (206,207).

The echocardiographic findings of this type of pericarditis include the flattening of the LV posterior wall, abnormal posterior septal motion in early diastole, rapid atrial filling, and the occasional premature opening of the pulmonic valve due to elevation of the RV pressure above the pulmonary artery pressure. Via the M-mode modality, there may be notching of the ventricular septum during early diastole or atrial systole secondary to a transient reversal of ventricular septal transmural pressure gradient (208). The above findings are not highly sensitive, yet a normal examination essentially excludes the diagnostic presence of constrictive pericarditis (209). Via two-dimensional echocardiography, the sonographer will detect dilation or lack of collapse of the hepatic veins and IVC, biatrial distention, and an abnormal contour between the LA and LV posterior walls. LV performance may be preserved unless there is a mixed pattern of restrictive–constrictive physiology (210,211). By applying Doppler techniques, the E velocities and E/A ratios on LV and RV inflow increase (due to the abnormal rapid early diastolic filling-restrictive pattern). In constrictive pericarditis, there is a prominent early diastolic velocity Ea when interrogated by tissue Doppler. The linear response to LA pressure increases, and the ratio of E/Ea is inverted (212).

When evaluating propagation velocity with color M-mode Doppler, the early diastolic transmitral flow is greater than 45 cm/s (212). These findings are counterintuitive to restrictive pathology and filling with reduced Ea (less than 8 cm/s) (213,214). A classic characteristic of constrictive pericarditis is when the mitral inflow velocity decreases up to 40% while flow through the tricuspid valve is greatly enhanced in the first cardiac cycle after inspiration. In concert, the respiratory variation in PVF is markedly influenced (215,216). When there is coexisting elevated LA pressure, this exaggerated transmitral inflow velocity may not be apparent (215,217). Even though there is an increased velocity in the PVF, especially during expiration, the ratio of S/D is reduced even further by affecting the diastolic component (218). Figure 25.15 describes in detail the comparisons and dissimilarities in the restrictive and constrictive pathologies (147).

Penetrating cardiac injury should be briefly presented here considering that it is a unique pathology with life-threatening lesions that are not always obvious by routine clinical examination (219). If the patient arrives at a definitive tertiary care setting alive, immediate control of the hemorrhage should be attempted, at times with an immediate thoracotomy in the emergency department or in the operating room (220,221). A bloody effusion may be contained in the pericardial space (if there is a contiguous pathway to the thorax) or extend externally, followed by profound shock and rapid death by exsanguination. The lesions have multiple configurations, ranging from a ventricular mural wound to small, irregular, and multiple lesions. In obvious cases, surface echocardiography may identify pericardial tamponade and/or large lesions (ventricular septal defect [VSD]). Following resuscitation, the clinician should further investigate the clinical picture via TEE, since small lesions—yet significant and potentially fatal—may be missed, including VSD, defects through valve leaflets, intracardiac thrombi, or regional tamponade (222,223). One of the largest studies to date on this topic is by Degiannis et al. (224). In a 32-month period, 117 patients with penetrating injuries of the mediastinum were evaluated retrospectively. A 17% mortality by stabbing was observed, whereas victims with gunshot wounds (GSW) revealed an expected higher mortality of 81% (194). Another series revealed a 7% occult injury,

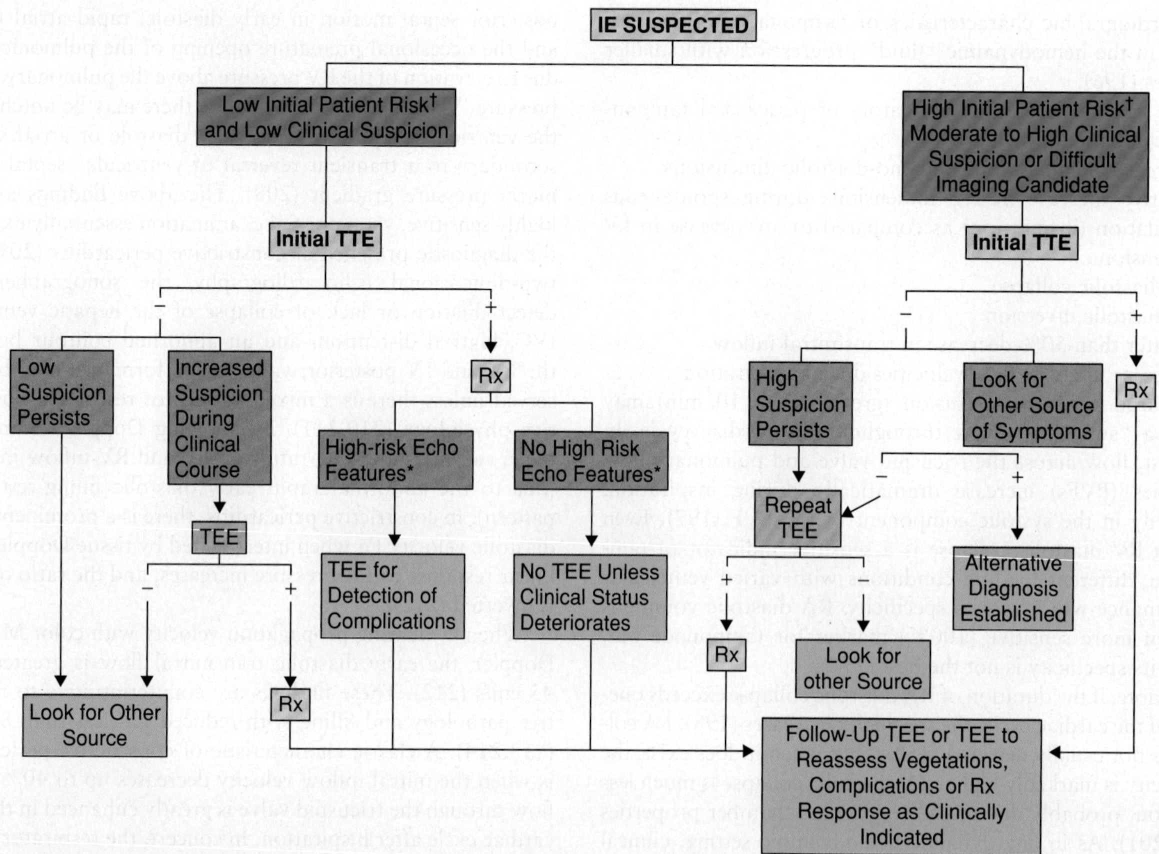

FIGURE 25.15 Approach to diagnostic use of echocardiography. IE, infective endocarditis; TTE, transthoracic echocardiography; TEE, transesophageal echocardiography. (Reproduced from Bayer AS, Bolger AF, Taubert KA, et al. Diagnosis and management of infective endocarditis and its complications. *Circulation*. 1998;98:2936–2948, with permission.)

with a similar mortality rate contrast between GSW and stab wounds (221). The clinician should always keep in mind that these patients are a complex challenge and that hemodynamic stability does not preclude an unexpected malady. Complacency should not occur (222,223).

Assessment of Myocardial Performance

Early focused echocardiography is recommended in circulatory and/or respiratory failure. It can improve early diagnostic accuracy from 50% (delayed performance after 15 minutes) versus 80% (performance immediate on presentation) (224). Although evaluation of the heart is mainstay, thoracic ultrasonography should include the evaluation of the pleura. The primary utility of thoracic ultrasound would be to exclude diagnoses like pericardial tamponade, severe ventricular systolic dysfunction, pulmonary fluid overload, and large pleural effusions.

In extrapolating the information reviewed in the sections of LV performance and pericardial disease, echocardiography is found to be an extremely useful diagnostic tool that can be used in a timely manner to delineate the cause of the shock state, whether hypovolemia, hyperdynamic derangements—type B metabolic lactic acidosis (sepsis, septic shock, liver failure, heavy metal poisoning)—and myocardial injury. An echocardiographic examination is easily performed, and the information obtained can avoid the placement of a PAC. The initial echocardiographic observation evaluates LV function and volume. In a hypovolemic condition, the ventricle exhibits systolic cavitary obliteration, with turbulence in the left ventricular outflow tract (LVOT) seen via color-flow Doppler. In extreme hypovolemia, the distal anterior leaflet of the anterior mitral valve in systole will cause obstruction to flow (225). This condition is amplified if relative hypovolemic states and tachycardia are observed in patients with hypertrophic obstructive cardiomyopathy (HOCM). Some of these echocardiographic indicators of a decreased preload state may be observed in patients who appear clinically normovolemic, regardless of baseline ventricular function (225).

Ventricular performance and ventricular interactions and loading conditions are quite complex in sepsis, SIRS, and septic shock. Echocardiography may clarify the effects of medical and/or pharmacologic interventions in these profoundly critically ill patients. However, often their physiologic effects are affected by the inherent (premorbid) chamber physical properties (pressure/volume characteristics) or fluid dynamics. A paradoxical response between survivors and nonsurvivors can be observed when a Frank–Starling curve is plotted against volume load in an animal model. The greater the end-systolic and end-diastolic volumes, the better the chance for survival (226). Furthermore, a paradoxical decrease in the slope of isovolumetric/pressure line (an index of contractility that is load independent) is associated with a decrease in cardiac compliance but increase in survival (227).

The effect of sepsis cardiomyopathy may result in a lower EF (which is load dependent) with high cardiac output, tachycardia, higher stroke volume, and elevated mixed venous saturation. As the patient deteriorates, hypotension occurs, impairment of cellular function follows, and the global ventricular volume response to resuscitation and fluid becomes ineffective (228–231). If there is no normalization of the above parameters within 48 to 72 hours, the chance for survival greatly diminishes. Persistent tachycardia is a marker of death. An apparent sympathovagal imbalance increases heart rate variability in the adult and pediatric patient populations. Atrial dysrhythmia and dysfunction are common in the clinical presentation and the progression of sepsis. TEE is obviously a valuable diagnostic tool for evaluating atrial function and volume by reviewing the LA appendage flow characteristics in concert with analysis of ventricular function and volume, ventricular interaction of dependency, transmitral inflow velocities, and pulmonary venous flow patterns (231,232).

In sepsis or SIRS, the right ventricle responds to fluid loading, but at some unknown end point, when the volume and pressure are exceedingly high, the compensatory response is no longer beneficial and mortality dramatically rises. A transitory increase of pulmonary artery pressure appears to be associated with increased mortality, but no serial investigations have been completed (233,234). In a clinical investigation by Poelaert et al. (235) based on transmitral inflow velocities and pulmonary venous flow patterns, patients with a decreased transmitral inflow velocity, abnormal pulmonary venous flow, and decrease in fractional area contraction are more likely to die as compared to two other subgroups. This pattern is particularly seen in older patients.

The hyperdynamic circulatory response of sepsis was earlier associated with a myocardial depressant factor (236) and presently is related to various mediators, cytokines, and humoral factors that are all related and intertwined (237). Interestingly, it is now known that there is a protective effect of early exposure to some of these mediators/cytokines that can induce the reversal of myocardial depression (228,230,238,239).

In summary, appreciating cardiac function in septic shock patients will assist in the determination of the pharmacologic interventions, fluid augmentation, and other modalities (240–242). It is intuitive reasoning that if the baseline cardiac junction is poor, the volume should be instilled judiciously and adjunct pharmacologic measures should be administered earlier and more aggressively. Echocardiography is a useful tool to initially identify and follow all hemodynamic variables. This diagnostic tool alone might suffice, but until further data are available, using it in conjunction with invasive monitoring is crucial (228,230,238,243).

Integration of Lung Ultrasound

Lung ultrasound has increasingly been incorporated into various components of critical care ultrasound evaluation of patients. In the well-known FAST (Focused Assessment with Sonography in Trauma), lung ultrasound is increasingly used to identify hemopneumothoraces with extended evaluation toward the lungs in the mid-axillary line. In evaluation of the cardiac function, it may be useful to evaluate the lungs to identify fluid overload states. Regardless of the function identified on cardiac evaluation, the finding of fluid overload during the lung examination suggests the patient may benefit from inotropic/vasopressor agents earlier in the course of the disease process (sepsis, multitrauma injury, cardiogenic shock). On the other hand, a patient with decreased cardiac function may benefit from judicious use of fluids if one can identify a lung examination that is not indicative of fluid overload state (e.g., CHF patients in septic shock). Several new studies over the past 10 years with growing terminologies with differences in evaluation, approach, nomenclature, and techniques of evaluation have led to international evidence-based recommendations for point-of-care lung ultrasound (244). Many times transportation of emergently ill patients is impossible and the ability to evaluate the lung at bedside can be very helpful in decision-making for the treatment plan. The "BLUE" protocol and "ICU Sound" protocol both found that diagnostic accuracy of lung ultrasound to differentiate dyspneic patients has increased greatly (1,245). The emergent question that must be answered when evaluating the hypotensive or critically ill patient is what is the fluid status of my patients (overload, depletion, euvolemic)? This can be answered by using ultrasound to evaluate the lung viscera/pleural interface and searching for "B" lines and "lung sliding." Lung sliding is the side-to-side movement of the pleural line with breathing. Lung sliding is the regular rhythmic movement synchronized with respiration that occurs between the parietal and visceral pleura that are in direct contact (without air between them). Lung sliding can be absent in pneumothorax, a mainstem intubation (on the left side), disease processes that affect the lung/chest wall interface such as pneumonia, acute respiratory distress syndrome (ARDS), and interstitial lung processes (inflammatory processes). The transducer is placed with the probe marker toward the patient's head and the operator should start the examination with the transducer on the sternum. The image obtained will be a shadow artifact from bony sternum. First, move toward the right anterior chest and then move laterally toward the posterior thorax. Multiple areas can be studied (Fig. 25.16). A more rapid two-region scan may be sufficient in some cases (anterior and mid-axillary chest positions in the supine patient). The view you should obtain here includes rib shadows, chest wall, and pleural interface. Lung sliding can be better appreciated by decreasing the ultrasound depth to maximize the lung/chest wall interface, approximately 1.5 cm below the rib shadow artifacts (Fig. 25.17). In a patient with no fluid overload state, "A lines" will be seen all throughout the lung fields. "A" lines are reverberation artifacts of the pleural line, hyperechoic, and horizontal (Fig. 25.18). "B" lines are vertical hyperechoic reverberation artifacts that arise from the pleural line and extend to the bottom of the ultrasound screen without fading. These lines can either be associated with lung

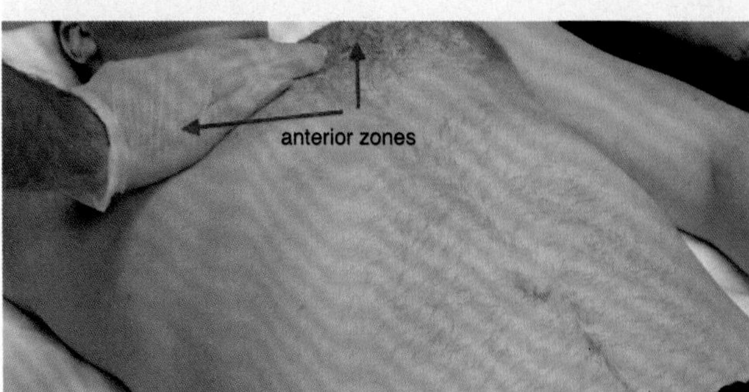

FIGURE 25.16 Anterior lung zones sites of evaluation: 1 to 2 cm lateral to the sternum and then in the upper/mid-axilla region.

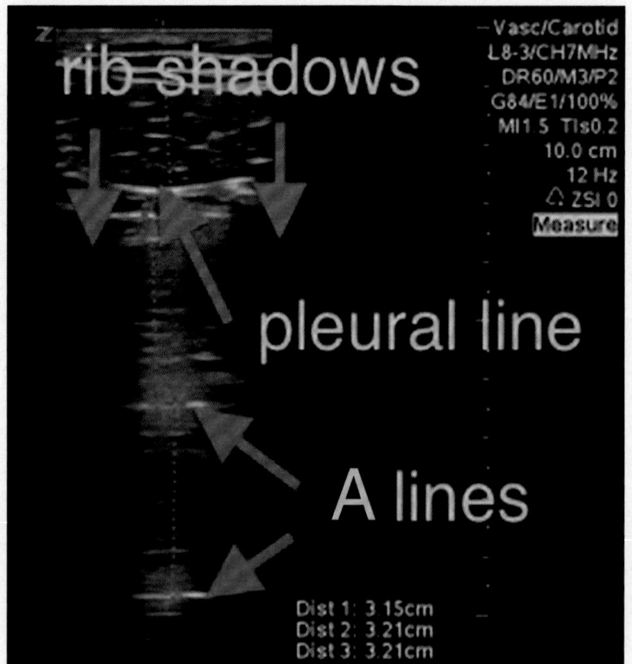

FIGURE 25.17 Pleural line and rib shadows seen with multiple hyperechoic horizontal lines artifacts of the pleural line.

sliding or not associated with lung sliding. B lines with lung sliding appear to move left and right on the screen similar to flashlights on the screen. B lines without lung sliding do not move with respiration. The anatomic and physical basis of B lines is not clear at this time, and could be related to alveolar wall thickening. Multiples of these lines are the sonographic sign of lung interstitial syndrome. A positive region is defined by the presence of more than three B lines in a longitudinal plane between the ribs, although it may be more important to perform serial examinations to see increase or decrease of these lines (Fig. 25.19). Focal B lines can be present in normal lung. In cardiogenic pulmonary edema, these B lines are

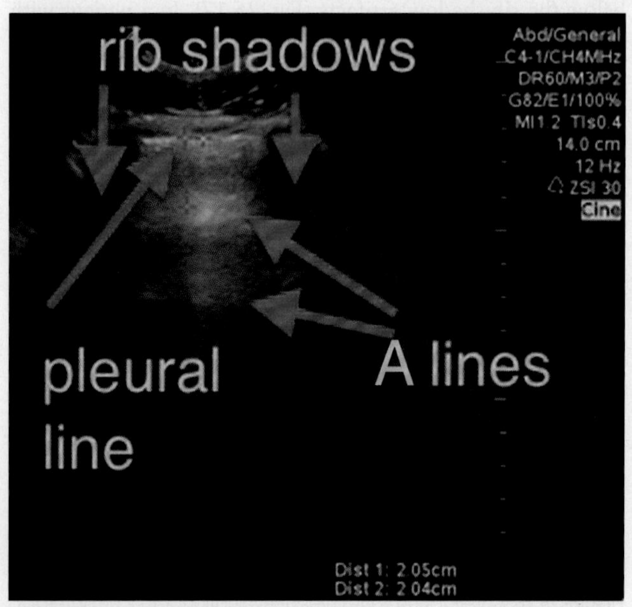

FIGURE 25.18 Lung A lines. (See also Video 25-8.)

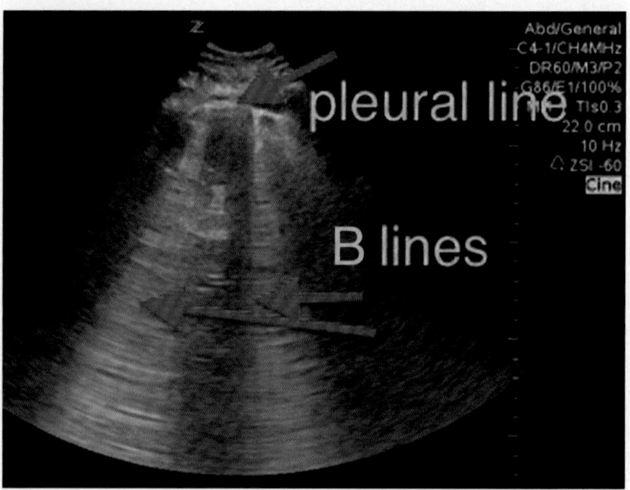

FIGURE 25.19 Lung B lines. (See also Video 25-9.)

associated with lung sliding, with homogenous distribution in anterior bilateral chest examination, and "spared" areas are not observed, and the pleural line is rarely involved (246). Pulmonary edema produces a transudate in this scenario, which is not supposed to generate inflammatory adherences (a factor that may affect lung sliding). In contrast, the findings in diffuse parenchymal lung disease include pleural line abnormalities (irregular, fragmented pleural line), subpleural abnormalities (small echo-poor areas), and nonhomogenous distribution of B lines. In ARDS, anterior subpleural consolidations, absence of lung sliding, "spared" areas of normal parenchyma, pleural line abnormalities (irregular fragmented pleural line), and nonhomogenous distribution of B lines can be found (247). Evaluation of B lines allows monitoring of response to therapy in cardiogenic pulmonary edema. Chest radiography can be used to diagnose pulmonary edema, but overall accuracy may be as low as 69% and findings of pulmonary edema can lag behind clinical changes (248,249). Many studies have now shown that lung ultrasound can be used to distinguish between cardiogenic and noncardiogenic causes of dyspnea (250,251). Also, B lines have been shown to correlate with more recognized methods of identifying pulmonary edema. Chest radiography (252), CT (253), pulmonary capillary wedge pressure, quantitative measurements of extravascular lung water, and natriuretic peptide levels have all been correlated to B lines using lung ultrasound (254,255). The presence of B lines has also been shown to be dynamic, disappearing in patients undergoing hemodialysis (256).

Inferior Vena Cava Assessment and Fluid Responsiveness

The IVC diameter and collapsibility can be measured just proximal to the entrance of the hepatic veins and can be used to determine volume status (Fig. 25.20). Positive pressure mechanical ventilation plays an important role in the accurate assessment of the IVC, and must be acknowledged when making volume status determinations. In spontaneously breathing patients, an IVC less than 2 cm and collapses greater than 50% is suggestive of a normal right atrium pressure. IVC diameter greater than 2 cm and collapses less than 50% suggests high right atrium pressures (173). In situations where they do not fit these descriptions, it

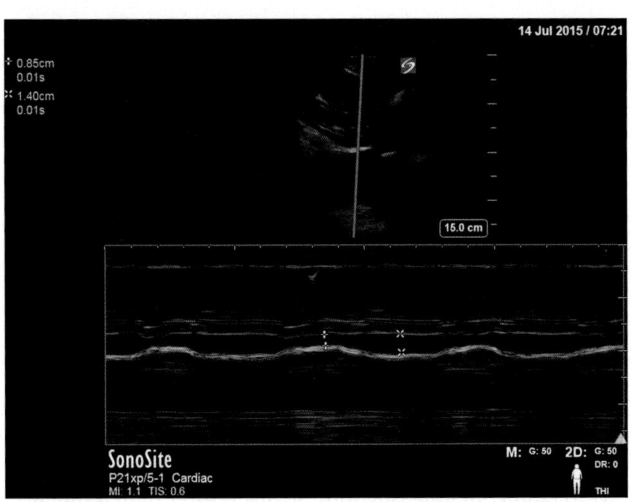

FIGURE 25.20 Inferior vena cava view with M mode showing collapsibility over a time period. (See also Videos 25-10 and 25-11.)

may be hard to make conclusions. It has an acceptable predictive value and reliability between operators (257,258). IVC collapsibility index is most studied for volume responsiveness, but other measures of subclavian, internal jugular, and femoral collapsibility have been suggested and are limited (259–261). The index is expressed as the difference between the value of the maximum and minimum diameters, divided by the maximum of the two values (Fig. 25.20). It was also shown that an i.v. bolus tends to produce an earlier response in the IVC, while the CVP response is more gradual (259).

However, in predicting fluid responsiveness as seen in an investigation 6 hours after cardiac surgery and in early hemorrhage, IVC collapsibility failed to be consistent (262,263). Variation of cardiac output and velocity time integral (an increase greater than 15%) after administration of 50 mL of crystalloid solution over 10 seconds can accurately predict fluid responsiveness (264). Echocardiographic assessment of changes in stroke volume due to passive leg elevation (at least 45 degrees) has shown to be useful to predict fluid responsiveness, but there has been no consensus value for change in stroke volume (265,266). Lastly, a controversial method to determine fluid responsiveness is measurement of the left ventricular end-diastolic area (LVEDA). LVEDA index (LVEDA/BSA) less than 5.5 cm/m^2 indicates significant hypovolemia. This measurement can be affected by LV hypertrophy, can be inaccurate if measured in area besides papillary muscle level, and requires too much technical skill (267).

Cardiopulmonary Resuscitation

Rationale for use in this setting is that nonarrhythmogenic cardiac arrest may be treatable, when due to tamponade, hypovolemic shock, or PE. Integration of focused echocardiography has been reviewed in many protocols, such as the FEEL protocol (268,269). It must be remembered that using ultrasound in cardiac arrest has not demonstrated to improve outcomes, and must be performed in a way not to cause interruptions in chest compressions. Subcostal views or modified apical views may be necessary. Newer technologies that allow visualization through transesophageal windows may be an optimal choice. Recently, large prospective studies are being performed to evaluate the information obtained and its prognostic capabilities (270). Other protocols have been created that combines lung and cardiac ultrasound mechanism and causes of cardiac arrest (271).

Trauma

Echocardiography is important in the evaluation of the trauma patient. It has been incorporated into the FAST examination (272). A clinician echocardiographer can rapidly diagnose and treat hemopericardium, which can be found in 11% of patients with penetrating truncal trauma and possible suggested improved outcome (273,274). A large amount of literature exists on FAST examination, but it is difficult to separate the cardiac component from abdominal and pleural ultrasound in terms of accuracy and utility (275).

The identification and pathogenesis of aortic trauma is better understood since TEE was added to the arsenal of the acute care physician. A vast number of these patients will succumb in the field due to extensive comorbid conditions, exsanguination, or tamponade. As expected, a significant number of patients (13% to 20%) will have been identified with this fatal injury (276), usually at postmortem; these deaths are second in frequency only to traumatic brain injury (TBI). A vast majority (75%) of blunt aortic injuries are due to motor vehicular crashes (276). If the patient arrives to the hospital trauma bay with vital signs, the presence of an aortic injury may be hidden or occult, considering that the physician is concentrating on other life-threatening conditions (e.g., TBI, intra-abdominal hemorrhage, pelvic injury, chest trauma, or pneumothoraces) (277). Of the patients who arrive to the hospital alive (33%), about a third of them will rapidly become hemodynamically unstable (278–281). Unless the clinician interrogates the aorta at the time of admission, this injury may be missed (282). Autopsy series reveal that the site of injury (acceleration–deceleration) is usually located near the aortic isthmus (54% to 65%), and multiple sites may be involved in extreme physical forces. In vertical acceleration–deceleration, the injury may occur at the root of the aortic valve (276,278,279,283). Aortography is not the gold standard, and the addition of TEE complements helical CT. If the patient is hemodynamically stable, high-definition (356-cut) CT may be the gold standard followed by TEE (Tables 25.10 and 25.11) (282). At present, if the patient is hemodynamically stable, CT angiography or a

TABLE 25.10 Transesophageal Echocardiography (TEE) and Angiography (Aortography or Contrast-enhanced Spiral Computed Tomography for Traumatic Aortic Imaging (TAI)

	Sensitivity, %	Specificity, %	NPV, %	PPV, %
Minor TAI (n = 7)				
TEE (n = 208)	100	100	100	100
Angiography (n = 206)	84	100	97	100
Major TAI (n = 33)				
TEE (n = 208)	97	100	99	100
Angiography (n = 206)	97	100	99	100
All TAI (n = 41)				
TEE (n = 208)	98	100	99	100
Angiography (n = 206)	83	100	96	100

NPV, negative predictive value; PPV, positive predictive value.
Reproduced with permission from Khalil A, Helmy T, Porembka DT. Aortic pathology: aortic trauma, debris, dissection, and aneurysm. *Crit Care Med.* 2007;35:S392–400.

TABLE 25.11 TEE and Helical Chest CT for the Identification of Traumatic Arterial Injuries in Severe Blunt Trauma

	Sensitivity (%)	Specificity (%)	NPV (%)	PPV (%)
Multiplane TEE	93	100	99	100
(*n* = 106)	(68–100)	(96–100)	(94–100)	(77–100)
Helical CT	73	100	95	100
(*n* = 99)	(45–92)	(96–100)	(89–99)	(71–100)

TEE, transesophageal echocardiography; CT, computed tomography; NPV, negative predictive value; PPV, positive predictive value.
Reproduced with permission from Vignon P. Hemodynamic assessment of critically ill patients using echocardiography Doppler. *Curr Opin Crit Care.* 2005;11:227–234.

64-cut chest CT should be performed initially, with TEE used to complement the diagnostic imaging modality (284). In these imaging schemes, most of the aorta is visualized. The benefit of TEE is its capability to visualize the aortic valve, the presence of aortic insufficiency, and the LV function and preload in real time, as well as identify pericardial effusions, especially when they are smaller, posterior, and loculated. These latter findings are typically not seen in the emergent FAST (focused assessment with sonography for trauma) examination commonly used in the trauma bay. Another benefit of TEE is color-flow Doppler identification of differential flow and/or turbulence as a sign of a potential injury (transection, subadventitial tear, intimal flap, intraluminal defect, or thrombus formation) (67,285–289). The detection of a periaortic hematoma or mediastinal hematoma may lead the physician to suspect an aortic injury (Table 25.12). The major disadvantages for echocardiography are reverberation artifacts, limited access to the superior ascending thoracic aorta, and the inability to adequately define the great vessels. However, in reviewing TEE investigations in aortic trauma, it is clear that the operator experience, training, and its availability are crucial to uniformly identifying or excluding aortic injury (290).

Aorta

Atherosclerotic Debris

Prior to the advent of enhanced diagnostic imaging techniques, clinicians routinely underappreciated the prevalence and importance of diseases affecting the aorta, particularly in patients following cardiac surgery and the general population in the critical care setting (282,291–301). Adverse events, such as a cryptogenic stroke, could previously not be explained until advancements were made for better resolution in head CT, MRI, carotid ultrasound with color-flow and Doppler capabilities, and TEE (300). Cardiac-originating embolism accounts for 15% to 30% of ischemic strokes in the general population. In the SPARC (Stroke Prevention Assessment of Risk in a Community) study, the incidence of detecting a plaque greater than 4 mm in the aorta of 588 randomly chosen patients (average age 66.9 years) was 43.7% (302). Of these, 29.9% presented lesions either in the arch or ascending portions of the thoracic aorta. The presence of a protruding debris or plaque described as greater than 4 mm approached 7.6% in the ascending aorta and 2.4% both in the arch and ascending portion are significant risk factors for complications (282,293,303). In another investigation, an atheromatous plaque greater than 4 mm was regarded as an independent risk factor for a central event (304). Because of the excellent acoustic window to the heart and thoracic aorta, TEE is considered to be one of the first diagnostic tools to evaluate the potential source for the embolic phenomenon (305–311). Although it remains insensitive to detecting smaller and irregular cardiac emboli and intra-aortic debris (312), it is a far superior diagnostic tool than TTE (313,314). TEE can easily identify the cause for a cerebral infarction, especially in the ascending aorta and its arch (315). Even if patients' underlying rhythm is sinus, patients with atherosclerotic plaques are at risk for stroke (316–318). Unfortunately, in the presence of pre-existing atrial fibrillation, the chance for such an embolic event greatly increases. If there is associated atherosclerotic debris, particularly protruding, pedunculated, and free-flowing debris, the issue of anticoagulation does not reduce the problem (319,320). In addition to atrial fibrillation, if there is concurrent presence of a PFO, the risks continue to rise (321). The existence of an atrial septal aneurysm increases the incidence for paradoxical embolism and stroke to 8.8% (322–324).

TABLE 25.12 Aortic Pathology: Computed Tomography for Trauma

Parameter	Hematoma Direct Signs	Periaortic Direct Signs	Direct Signs
No. patients	1,346	1,346	1,346
TN	671	1,258	1,299
FP	656	69	28
NPV, %	100	100	99.9
Sensitivity, %	100	100	95
Specificity, %	50	95	98
TAI	19	19	19
TP	19	19	18
PPV, %	3	22	39
FN	0	0	1

TN, true negative; FP, false positive; NPV, negative predictive value; TAI, traumatic aortic injury; TP, true positive; PPV, positive predictive value; FN, false negative.
Reproduced with permission from Khalil A, Helmy T, Porembka DT. Aortic pathology: aortic trauma, debris, dissection, and aneurysm. *Crit Care Med.* 2007;35:S392–400.

Thoracic Aortic Dissection

Thoracic aortic dissection is another potentially life-threatening event that can be detected by TEE. Besides TEE, other imaging techniques following the historical use of angiography, which continue to gain acceptance, are 64-slice chest CT and MRI (particularly for chronic evaluation), or a combination of the above (282,325–327). The incidence for aortic dissection approaches 4.5/1,000 and is ranked 13th in cause of death in Western societies (282,317–327). Common predisposing conditions are well known and have been documented in the IRAD (International Registry of Aortic Dissection) (e.g., hypertension 72%, atherosclerosis 31%, previous cardiac surgery 18%). In the population subgroup younger than 40 years of age, the predominant etiologic factors are Marfan syndrome, bicuspid aortic valve, or prior aortic surgery. Symptoms can range from chest pain and/or abdominal sharp constant tearing pain, back pain, syncope to the presence of tachycardia, hypotension, or hypertension (325). Diagnostic imaging needs to be urgently performed to assess the potential for immediate surgery, as well as to determine the preferred surgical approach. There are several classifications of dissections: type A or B, DeBakey, or Stanford. In patients with acute proximal aortic involvement, surgery is considered, as the mortality with this group is 20% by 24 hours and

30% by 48 hours (325). Most type B dissections (73%) have been managed medically with pharmacotherapy to lessen the shear forces and flow and distention of the aorta (325,328). The classic echocardiographic depiction for a dissection is a smaller true lumen, larger false lumen, and an intimal flap with a site. The presence of a thrombus in the false lumen reveals the propensity for a lower morbidity and mortality. These lesser untoward events are seen in patients when the flow is minimal or unidirectional versus bidirectional from the true to false lumens. At times, there may be several entry sites, and flow may not be limited to one area of the thoracic aorta. TEE visualizes the integrity or involvement of the aortic valve leaflets in type A dissections, and allows the evaluation of LV performance and RWMA and the detection of a pericardial effusion or tamponade.

A meta-analysis compared the accuracy of TEE, helical CT, and MRI for suspected thoracic aortic dissection results. In 1,139 patients (16 investigations), the pooled sensitivity varied between 98% and 100%, whereas the specificity ranged from 95% to 98%. There was a higher positive likelihood ratio comparison for MRI: mean 25.3 (11.1–57.1); for TEE, 14.1 (6.0–33.2); and helical CT, 13.9 (4.2–46.0). If patients' pretest probability was 5% (low risk), their likelihood of having a dissection approached 0.1% to 0.3%. In contrast, in high-risk patients with a 50% pretest probability, the presence of an aortic dissection ranged from 93% to 96% (329).

Aneurysms and Rupture

Thoracic aorta aneurysms may occur alone or in concert with an aortic dissection and typically are found in the elderly patient. This disease process is related to the presence of hypertension and atherosclerosis. Other population subsets for its occurrence are Marfan syndrome, bicuspid aortic valve (accelerated degeneration of the media), familial aortic aneurysmal disease, or annuloaortic ectasia. The ascending portion of the thoracic aorta can be noted via either echocardiographic modality, although TEE is the preferred choice. The aortic size is well characterized by gender and age. Once the dilatation reaches greater than 5 cm, there is an increased risk of rupture, and replacement is generally considered. After the size of the aorta expands past 6.0 cm, the risk for rupture and dissection reaches greater than 6.9% per year, with a mortality rate of 11.8% annually (330). TEE can assist in the decision process for root replacement or placement of a prosthetic device and reimplantation of the coronary arteries. In patients with bicuspid aortic pathology, there is greater than 50% of the patients will have root dilatation and aortic insufficiency (282,330,331).

The localized absence of the media in the aortic wall will result in possible rupture of the sinus of Valsalva. Usually, it will rupture into adjacent structures such as the cardiac chambers (RV or RA) or through the ventricular septum. TEE invariably will visualize the aneurysm (ventricular side of the aortic valve), particularly of the ventricular septum. The apical long and parasternal views may discriminate between this pathology and a membranous septum. In a nonruptured sinus of Valsalva aneurysm, echocardiography will visualize thinning of the wall that is larger than the other sinuses. The intensivist needs to be aware that this situation can be associated with endocarditis, syphilis, a potentially fatal rupture, a source of emboli, and fistulae communicating with ventricular chambers. In the latter case, a significant left-to-right shunting can be demonstrated by using color-flow Doppler echocardiography, with a continuous turbulent jet within the ruptured aneurysm into the receiving chamber (282,332–338). If the aneurysm communicates with the right atrium, the flow is continuous during systole and diastole. An increase in size of either the RA or RV will eventually occur (339–341).

Intramural Hematoma

A subpopulation of trauma patients will present with intramural hematoma (IMH), which arises from rupture of the vasa vasorum in the aortic medial wall layers, and is characterized by blood in the aortic wall in the absence of an intimal tear. IMH may be a precursor for the progression to a dissection. The associated prevalence is 10% to 30% of patients with a pre-existing dissection (342). Surgery is usually contemplated for type A dissection whereas intervention is warranted for a type B. The comparative mortality rates (medical vs. surgical), respectively, for types A and B are 36% versus 14% and 20% versus 14% (343).

Infective Endocarditis: Identification of Vegetations and Indications for Surgery

Infective endocarditis (IE) is a challenge to all disciplines, particularly for intensive care physicians who have to analyze how IE factors into the differential diagnosis of a fever of unknown origin. Recurrent positive blood cultures while the patient is on antibiotics may provide a clue to its existence, especially if the pathogens are Staphylococcus aureus, streptococci, and enterococci. However, there is an increasing incidence of culture-negative IE that includes such fastidious agents as Coxiella burnetii, Tropheryma whipplei, Legionella pneumophila, Bartonella spp., the HACEK group (Haemophilus spp., Actinomycetemcomitans, Cardiobacterium hominis, Eikenella corrodens, Kingella spp.), and fungi (including Candida, Histoplasma, and Aspergillus spp.) (344,345). The classic patient presentation with Janeway lesions, Osler nodes, Roth spots, and petechiae, and history of rheumatic heart disease is not seen in the developed world (346). However, in the industrial world, the risks are related to age, degenerated valvular disease, prosthetic valves, and the increasing incidence of nosocomial infections. Besides in HIV infection patients where it can be present in up to 90% of the cases, IE can be found increasingly in the younger population, with social trends such as body piercing and self-administered intravenous injection of recreational drugs, including HIV infection (40% to 90%; Tables 25.13 and 25.14) (344,345).

Perhaps more important than clinical findings, echocardiography is very useful for the identification of vegetations. Two fundamental predisposing factors are associated with the development of IE: cardiac endothelial injury and a microbiologic source. In endothelial injury, there is aberrant flow with a high-velocity jet directed onto the endothelial surface or increased shear stress through a narrow orifice. In the latter, there is a propensity for bacterial deposits downstream of the constriction via a Venturi effect. The detection of vibratory oscillations of vegetation or associated disruptive cardiac structures (torn leaflet, rupture of chordae tendineae) may indicate the presence of IE, as well as noting diastolic vibrations of the aortic valve or systolic vibrations of the mitral valve (M-mode echocardiography). Other characteristic findings involve structures that are in the path of a high-velocity jet as seen in valve regurgitation; these include motion of the valve that is chaotic and

TABLE 25.13 Definition of Infective Endocarditis (IE) According to the Modified Duke Criteria

Definite IE
Pathologic Criteria
Microorganisms demonstrated by culture or histologic examination of a vegetation, a vegetation that has embolized, or an intracardiac abscess specimen; or
Pathologic lesions; vegetation or intracardiac abscess confirmed by histologic examination showing active endocarditis
Clinical Criteria
2 major criteria; or
1 major criterion and 3 minor criteria; or
5 minor criteria
Possible IE
1 major criterion and 1 minor criterion; or
3 minor criteria
Rejected
Firm alternative diagnosis explaining evidence of IE; or
Resolution of IE syndrome with antibiotic therapy for <4 d; or
No pathologic evidence of IE at surgery or autopsy, with antibiotic therapy for <4 d; or
Does not meet criteria for possible IE as above

Reprinted with permission from Li JS, Sexton DJ, Mick N, et al. Proposed modifications to the Duke criteria for the diagnosis of infective endocarditis. *Clin Infect Dis.* 2000;30:633–638.

TABLE 25.14 Definition of Terms used in the Modified Duke Criteria for the Diagnosis of Infective Endocarditis (IE)

Major Criteria
Blood culture positive for IE
Typical microorganisms consistent with IE from 2 separate blood cultures:
Viridans streptococci, *Streptococcus bovis*, HACEK group, *Staphylococcus aureus;* or
Community-acquired enterococci in the absence of a primary focus; or
Microorganisms consistent with IE from persistently positive blood cultures defined as follows:
At least 2 positive cultures of blood samples drawn >12 h apart; or
All of 3 or a majority of 4 separate cultures of blood (with first and last sample drawn at least 1 h apart)
Single positive blood culture for *Coxiella burnetii* or antiphase IgG antibody titer >1:800
Evidence of endocardial involvement
Echocardiogram positive for IE (TEE recommended for patients with prosthetic valves, rated at least "possible IE" by clinical criteria, or complicated IE (paravalvular abscess); TTE as first test in other patients) defined as follows:
Oscillating intracardiac mass on valve or supporting structures, in the path of regurgitant jets, or on implanted material in the absence of an alternative anatomic explanation; or
Abscess; or
New partial dehiscence of prosthetic valve
New valvular regurgitation (worsening or changing or preexisting murmur not sufficient)
Minor Criteria
Predisposition, predisposing heart condition, or IDU
Fever, temperature >38°C
Vascular phenomena, major arterial emboli, septic pulmonary infarcts, mycotic aneurysm, intracranial hemorrhage, conjunctival hemorrhage, and Janeway lesions
Immunologic phenomena: glomerulonephritis, Osler nodes, Roth spots, and rheumatoid factor
Microbiologic evidence: positive blood culture but does not meet a major criterion as noted above[a] or serologic evidence of active infection with organism consistent with IE
Echocardiographic minor criteria eliminated

TEE, transesophageal echocardiography; TTE, transthoracic echocardiography; IDU, intravenous drug user.
[a]Excludes single positive cultures for coagulace-negative staphylococci and organisms that do not cause endocarditis.
Reprinted with permission from Li JS, Sexton DJ, Mick N, et al. Proposed modifications to the Duke criteria for the diagnosis of infective endocarditis. *Clin Infect Dis.* 2000;30:633–638.

independent; texture that is gray scale in relation to the myocardium; an amorphous shape; the presence of a fistula or abscess; and new onset of regurgitation for either native or prosthetic valves. There may be associated obstructions, perivalvular leaks, or dehiscence. With these findings, there are string-like mobile strands of vegetations or degenerative areas adjacent to the prosthetic device. In the mitral valve position, if there is a prosthetic device, TEE will easily identify these maladies. However, TTE is a better tool for visualizing the mechanical valve in the aortic position. Overall, TEE is a better diagnostic modality to visualize vegetations and associated complications. The sensitivities for TTE and TEE are 60% to 90% and 85% to 95%, respectively, while the specificities for both techniques (TTE and TEE) are far better: 90% to 98% (345,347–355). In the context of a negative TEE, the negative predictive value is only 90%; thus, maintaining good clinical judgment with clinical correlation is always a necessity (356–358). An algorithm proposed by Bayer et al. (359) can be used by the echocardiographer intensivist for this diagnostic dilemma (345,359). The most prominent indications for surgery are hemodynamic compromise or collapse from valve destruction, a persistent fever despite antibiotic treatment, and development of a fistula or abscess due to perivalvular spread of infection. Other indications are the presence of highly resistant organisms or aggressive pathogens, perioperative prosthetic valvular endocarditis, and large vegetations (greater than 10 mm). This latter indication is of particular concern given that the increasing size of the vegetation is associated with embolic events (344,355). A task force that includes input from the American Heart Association and the American College of Cardiology recently corroborated this last indication (360).

Myocardial Injury

In patients with acute myocardial infarction, echocardiography is a crucial tool in the diagnosis and exclusion of myocardial injury, especially in patients with chest pain and nondiagnostic electrocardiographic (ECG) findings. Other roles for echocardiography are evaluating the extent of myocardium at risk and involvement after reperfusion; evaluating viable myocardium; assessing patients with hemodynamic instability and related complications following infarction; and risk stratification.

Echocardiography is also commonly used for evaluating acute coronary syndromes (ACS) by measuring intraventricular dyssynchrony by tissue velocity and strain imaging (Fig. 25.21).

Resting and stress echocardiography are modalities for detecting ACS and complications of myocardial injury by prognostication using analysis of RWMA scoring, as well as assessing diastolic dysfunction and stress-induced alterations (361). All LV wall segments can be seen from the apical, parasternal, and occasionally subcostal views. The American Society of Echocardiography proposes a standard for this RWMA scoring by using either a 16- or 17-segment model

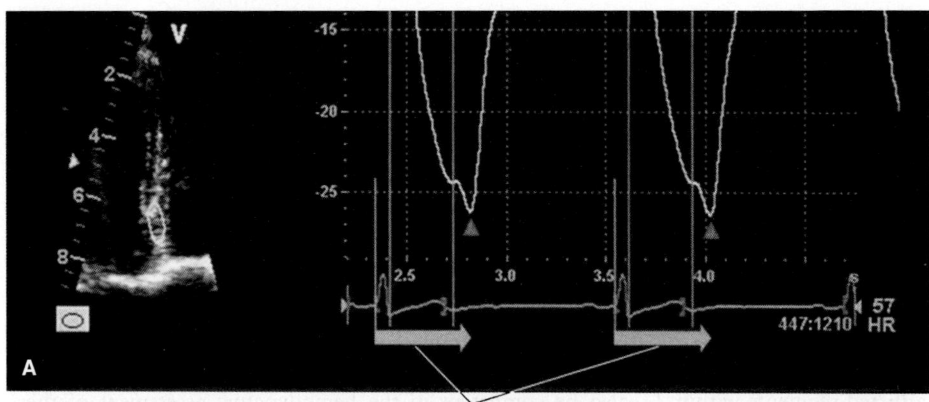

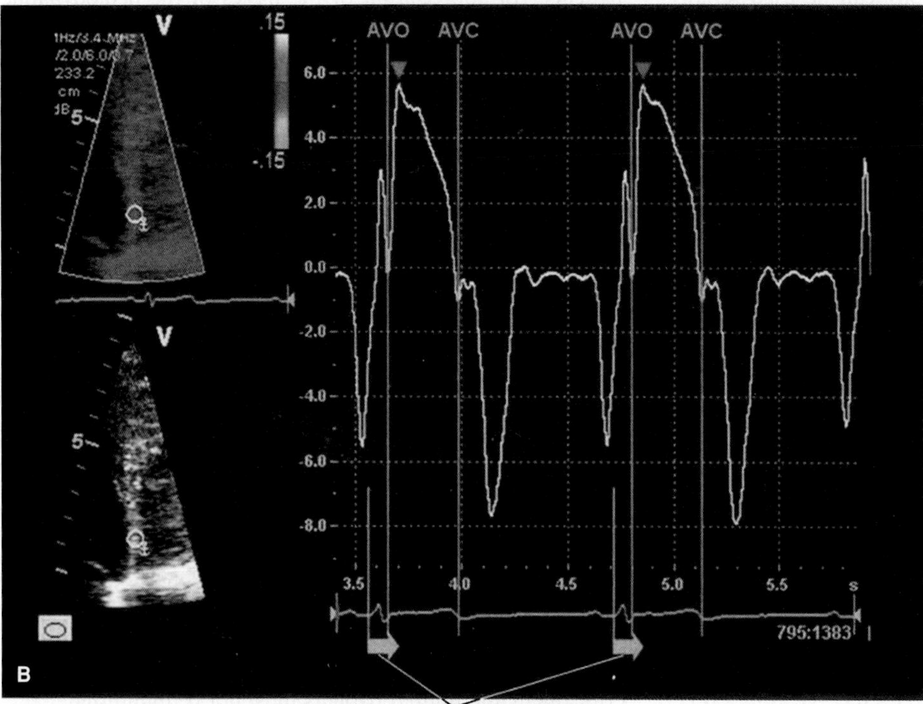

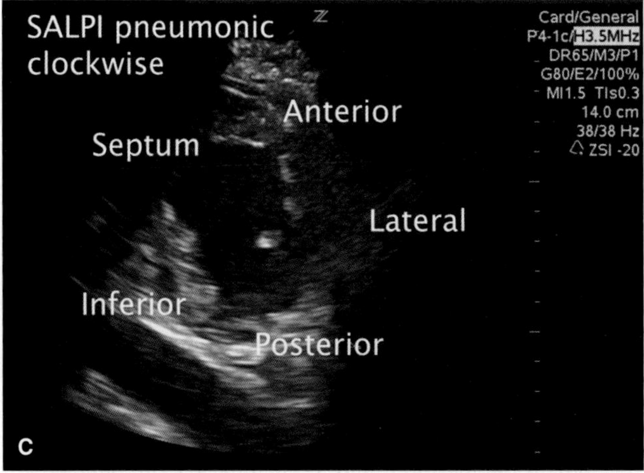

FIGURE 25.21 **A**,**B**: Measurement of intraventricular dyssynchrony by tissue velocity and strain imaging. **A**: Recording of strain from the basal segment of the ventricular septum from the apical four-chamber view. Time to peak systolic strain is measured from onset of QRS to the peak negative value including the postsystolic shortening. The timing of the peak negative strain is when shortening of the myocardium is maximum. **B**: Recording of tissue velocity from the basal segment of the ventricular septum. Peak systolic velocity is the positive wave during the ejection period. Time to peak tissue velocity is from onset of QRS to the positive peak velocity. The time interval is determined from 2 to 12 segments to measure intraventricular dyssynchrony. **C**: Wall motion abnormality image of LV in short axis showing segments using SALPI pneumonic, from septal position going clockwise. S, septum; A, anterior; L, lateral; P, posterior; I, inferior. (See also Video 25-12.) (**A**,**B**: from Oh JK, Seward JB, Tajik AJ. *The Echo Manual*. 3rd ed. Philadelphia, PA: Lippincott Williams & Wilkins; 2006, used with permission of Mayo Foundation for Medical Education and Research.)

(362). The benefit of observing RWMA is that the patient may be asymptomatic and hemodynamically may not exhibit any aberrations. However, not all RWMAs are related to myocardial ischemia, such as loading conditions applied to the heart, paced rhythms, and conduction delays. Typically, after reperfusion, there may be persistent RWMA representing a delayed return of normal function, which is described as a stunned myocardium. This physiology, as well as the existence of global transitory dysfunction such as hibernating myocardium, must be put into the clinical context of the patient's condition.

In patients with acute ST-elevation myocardial infarction (STEMI), the affected myocardium becomes an akinetic or dyskinetic segment. Following interventions (reperfusion), there is usually improvement in the afflicted segments within 24 to 48 hours, and echocardiography can be used serially to assess these patients for improvements or extension of the injury. Contrast echocardiography, low-dose dobutamine infusion, or strain imaging can also assess viability (363).

Complications

Numerous complications follow an acute myocardial infarction. Echocardiography is a mainstay in assessing these problems, which range from rupture of papillary muscle and VSDs to cardiopulmonary resuscitation (364).

Rupture

Acute free wall rupture also occurs less frequently in the postinterventional period (1.0%). About half of the ruptures will result in out-of-hospital sudden deaths. Following myocardial injury, the mortality of free wall rupture varies between 8% and 17%, with a significant number (40%) occurring within the first 24 hours and 85% after 1 week (176,365). Besides hemodynamic collapse or cardiac arrest, there may be severe bradycardia. Some patients may experience syncope, chest pain, or emesis. In these dire situations, echocardiography (TEE) is the diagnostic tool of choice. Pericardial effusions and/or cardiac tamponade may be found; keeping in mind that 25% of myocardial infarctions will have a pericardial effusion. Thrombus may exist, as well as the identification of flow via color-flow Doppler (366). Also, a pseudoaneurysm may form following a free rupture that is contained in a limited portion of the pericardial space, most frequently the posterior wall. A pseudoaneurysm is traditionally characterized by a small neck communication between the LV and the aneurysmal cavity (ratio less than 0.5). Color-flow Doppler may reveal flow, especially bidirectional (367).

Another cause for a new murmur is a ruptured papillary muscle (partial or complete) and mitral regurgitation (the extent of the murmur does not correlate with pathology). Extenuating circumstances for a new murmur may be LV regional or global remodeling, papillary muscle dysfunction with annular dilatation, or acute systolic anterior motion of the mitral valve. The latter cause is managed in a totally different way than with volume replacement, with primary intervention accomplished with beta-blockade and avoidance of vasodilators (368).

The most serious cause of new mitral regurgitation that must be acted on quickly is rupture of the posteromedial papillary segment. This acute problem may be even related to a small infarct corresponding to the circumflex or right coronary artery. The rupture may be complete or partial and is identified by color-flow Doppler imaging. After papillary muscle rupture and its discovery by TEE, surgery is imminent for mitral valve replacement, with or without coronary revascularization. In a series by Moursi et al. (369), in 65% of the patients with TEE, the head of the papillary muscle was observed in the LA. Another characteristic finding seen in these patients (90%) was some erratic motion in the body of the LV (176,369–371).

Hemodynamic and Valve Area Calculations

The intraoperative or perioperative physician expert in echocardiography must not only deal with the evaluation of ventricular function (global and regional), identification of aortic pathology, detection of masses, and visualization of normal abnormal pathology of native and prosthetic valves, but must also be competent in the hemodynamic assessment of these patients. An appreciation of the basics of the hemodynamic calculations sets the stage for the building blocks of accurate detection of flow hemodynamics and physiology that may affect the patient's clinical care (medical or surgical). The calculation of pressure gradient determination uses the Bernoulli equation. Additional valve area calculations use the continuity equation, pressure half-time and deceleration time, proximal isovelocity surface area (PISA), and effective regurgitant orifice. Similarly, the determination of valvular area is complex and based on several echocardiographic and Doppler principles evaluating the continuity equation pressure half-time method, deceleration time method, and planimetry. An extensive review of these topics is beyond the scope of this chapter but is available in all major textbooks on echocardiography (372,373).

CONTROVERSIES

Eventually, this field of critical care echocardiography should be encompassed in the training of the fellows in intensive care medicine. The implementation of training—basic skills versus full certification—is still being debated.

Having a remote echocardiographic team may be helpful in this short-term period, and the impact of echocardiography in critically ill and injured patients must not be minimized.

This imaging modality is crucial for timely medical and surgical interventions, and a subset of the total field of echocardiography should include intensive care medicine. In the meantime, collaborating with our cardiology colleagues is the key for better understanding of echocardiographic findings in the setting of a critical illness.

Key Points

- The critical care physician should have at the bedside the availability and expertise to correctly use echocardiography as a first-line diagnostic and monitoring tool as part of the basic physical examination.
- It is important to be familiar with assessment of volume and function of the ventricular chambers in multiple views to make final clinical decisions due to the varying patient population found in the intensive care units.
- The cardiac examination for evaluation of hemodynamics should benefit from the additional involvement of thoracic ultrasound evaluation for pulmonary edema through observation of sliding "A" versus "B" lines.

- The IVC size and collapsibility can be used but with caution noting recent use of diuretics or vasodilators as well as spontaneously breathing patient versus positive pressure.

REFERENCES

1. Manno E, Navarra M, Faccio L, et al. Deep impact of ultrasound in the intensive care unit: the ICU sound protocol. *Anesthesiology.* 2012;17: 801–809.
2. The hTEE approach. ImaCor website. Available at: http://imacorinc.com/htee/the-htee-approach.html.
3. Vignon P, Mentec H, Terre S, et al. Diagnostic accuracy and therapeutic impact of transthoracic and transesophageal echocardiography in mechanically ventilated patients in the ICU. *Chest.* 1994;106:1829–1834.
4. Bruch C, Comber M, Schmermund A, et al. Diagnostic usefulness and impact on management of transesophageal echocardiography in surgical intensive care units. *Am J Cardiol.* 2003;91:510–513.
5. Colreavy FB, Donovan K, Lee KY, et al. Transesophageal echocardiography in critically ill patients. *Crit Care Med.* 2002;30:989–996.
6. Wake PJ, Ali M, Carroll J, et al. Clinical and echocardiographic diagnoses disagree in patients with unexplained hemodynamic instability after cardiac surgery. *Can J Anaesth.* 2001;48:778–783.
7. Karski JM. Transesophageal echocardiography in the intensive care unit. *Semin Cardiothorac Vasc Anesth.* 2006;10:162–166.
8. Heidenreich PA, Stainback RF, Redberg RF, et al. Transesophageal echocardiography predicts mortality in critically ill patients with unexplained hypotension. *J Am Coll Cardiol.* 1995;26:152–158.
9. Mertens L, Seri I, Marek J, et al. Targeted neonatal echocardiography in the neonatal intensive care unit: practice guidelines and recommendations for training. Writing Group of the American Society of Echocardiography (ASE) in collaboration with the European Association of Echocardiography (EAE) and the Association for European Pediatric Cardiologists (AEPC). *J Am Soc Echocardiogr.* 2011;24(10):1057–1078.
10. Labovitz A, Bierig M, Goldstein SA, et al. Focused cardiac ultrasound in the emergent setting: a consensus statement of the American Society of Echocardiography and American College of Emergency Physicians. *J Am Soc Echocardiogr.* 2010;23:1225–1230.
11. Gunst M, Sperry J, Ghaemmaghami V, et al. Bedside echocardiographic assessment for trauma/ critical care: the BEAT exam. *J Am Coll Surg.* 2008;207(3):e1–e3.
12. Vieillard-Baron A, Slama M, Cholley B, et al. Echocardiography in the intensive care unit: from evolution to revolution? *Intensive Care Med.* 2008;34(2):243–249.
13. Jensen MB, SE, Larsen M, Schmidt MB. Transthoracic echocardiography for cardiopulmonary monitoring in intensive care. *Eur J Anaesthesiol.* 2004;21:700–707.
14. Pershad JMS, Plouman C, Rosson C, et al. Bedside limited echocardiography by the emergency physician is accurate during evaluation of the critically ill patient. *Pediatrics.* 2004;114:e667–e671.
15. Kimura B, Yogo N, O'Connell CW, et al. Cardiopulmonary limited ultrasound examination for "Quick-Look" bedside application. *Am J Cardiol.* 2011;108:586–590.
16. Manasia AR, Nagaraj HM, Kodali RB, et al. Feasibility and potential clinical utility of goal-directed transthoracic echocardiography performed by noncardiologist intensivists using a small hand-carried device (SonoHeart) in critically ill patients. *J Cardiothorac Vasc Anesth.* 2005;19:155–159.
17. Vieillard-Baron A, Slama M, Cholley B, et al. Echocardiography in the intensive care unit: from evolution to revolution? *Intensive Care Med.* 2008;34:243–249.
18. Price S, Nicol E, Gibson DG, et al. Echocardiography in the critically ill: current and potential roles. *Intensive Care Med.* 2006;32:48–59.
19. Lichtenstein D, Axler O. Intensive use of general ultrasound in the intensive care unit. Prospective study of 150 consecutive patients. *Intensive Care Med.* 1993;19:353–355.
20. Porembka DT. Importance of transesophageal echocardiography in the critically ill and injured patient. *Crit Care Med.* 2007;35:S414–430.
21. Nanda NC, Domanski MJ, eds. *Atlas of Transesophageal Echocardiography.* 2nd ed. Philadelphia, PA: Lippincott Williams & Wilkins; 2006.
22. Vannan MA, Lang RM, Rabowski H, et al., eds. *Atlas of Echocardiography.* Philadelphia, PA: Current Medicine; 2005.
23. Feigenbaum H, Popp RL, Wolfe SB, et al. Ultrasound measurements of the left ventricle: a correlative study with angiocardiography. *Arch Intern Med.* 1972;129:461–467.
24. Weyman AE. The year in echocardiography. *J Am Coll Cardiol.* 2006;47:856–863.
25. Mingo S, Benedicto A, Jimenez MC, et al. Dynamic left ventricular outflow tract obstruction secondary to catecholamine excess in a normal ventricle. *Int J Cardiol.* 2006;112:393–396.
26. Araujo AQ, Arteaga E, Ianni BM, et al. Relationship between outflow obstruction and left ventricular functional impairment in hypertrophic cardiomyopathy: a Doppler echocardiographic study. *Echocardiography.* 2006;23:734–740.
27. American College of Cardiology Foundation Appropriate Use Criteria Task Force; American Society of Echocardiography; American Heart Association, et al. ACCF/ASE/AHA/ASNC/HFSA/HRS/SCAI/SCCM/SCCT/SCMR 2011 Appropriate use criteria for echocardiography. A Report of the American College of Cardiology Foundation Appropriate Use Criteria Task Force, American Society of Echocardiography, American Heart Association, American Society of Nuclear Cardiology, Heart Failure Society of America, Heart Rhythm Society, Society for Cardiovascular Angiography and Interventions, Society of Critical Care Medicine, Society of Cardiovascular Computed Tomography, Society for Cardiovascular Magnetic Resonance American College of Chest Physicians. *J Am Soc Echocardiogr.* 2011;24:229–267.
28. Neskovic AN, Hagendorff A, Lancellotti P, et al. Emergency echocardiography: the European Association of Cardiovascular Imaging recommendations. *Eur Heart J Cardiovasc Imag.* 2013;14:1–11.
29. Neskovic AN, Edvardsen T, Galderisi M, et al. Focus cardiac ultrasound: the European Association of Cardiovascular Imaging viewpoint. *Eur Heart J Cardiovasc Imag.* 2014;15:956–960.
30. Mathew JP, Glas K, Troianos CA, et al. ASE/SCA recommendations and guidelines for continuous quality improvement in perioperative echocardiography. *Anesth Analg.* 2006;103:1416–1425.
31. Mathew JP, Glas K, Troianos CA, et al. American Society of Echocardiography/Society of Cardiovascular Anesthesiologists recommendations and guidelines for continuous quality improvement in perioperative echocardiography. *J Am Soc Echocardiogr.* 2006;19:1303–1313.
32. Quinones MA, Douglas PS, Foster E, et al. ACC/AHA clinical competence statement on echocardiography: a report of the American College of Cardiology/American Heart Association/American College of Physicians–American Society of Internal Medicine Task Force on clinical competence. *J Am Soc Echocardiogr.* 2003;16:379–402.
33. Mayo PH, Beaulieu Y, Doelken P, et al. American College of Chest Physicians/La Societe de Reanimation de Langue Francaise statement on competence in critical care ultrasonography. *Chest.* 2009;135;1050–1060.
34. Neri L, Storti E, Lichtenstein D. Toward an ultrasound curriculum for critical care medicine. *Crit Care Med.* 2007;35(5 Suppl):S290–S304.
35. Mazraeshahi RM, Farmer JC, Porembka DT. A suggested curriculum in echocardiography for critical care physicians. *Crit Care Med.* 2007; 35(8 Suppl):S431–S433.
36. Eisen LA, Leung S, Gallagher AE, Kvetan V. Barriers to ultrasound training in critical care medicine fellowships: a survey of program directors. *Crit Care Med.* 2010;38:1978–1983.
37. Rao S, van Holsbeeck L, Musial JL, et al. A pilot study of comprehensive ultrasound education at the Wayne State University School of Medicine: a pioneer year review. *J Ultrasound Med.* 2008;27:745–749.
38. DeCara JM, Kirkpatric NJ, Spencer KT, et al. Use of hand-carried ultrasound devices to augment the accuracy of medical student bedside cardiac diagnoses. *J Am Soc Echocardiogr.* 2005;18:257–263.
39. Douglas PS, Khandheria B, Stainback RF, et al. ACCF/ASE/ACEP/ASNC/SCAI/SCCT/SCMR 2007 appropriateness criteria for transthoracic and transesophageal echocardiography. *J Am Coll Cardiol.* 2007;50:187–204.
40. Mandavia DP, Hoffner RJ, Mahaney K, et al. Bedside echocardiography by emergency physicians. *Ann Emerg Med.* 2001;38:377–382.
41. Moore CL, Rose GA, Tayal VS, et al. Determination of left ventricular function by emergency physician echocardiography of hypotensive patients. *Acad Emerg Med.* 2002;9:186–193.
42. Quinones MA, Douglas PS, Foster E, et al. ACC/AHA clinical competence statement on echocardiography: a report of the American College of Cardiology/American Heart Association/ American College of Physicians–American Society of Internal Medicine Task Force on Clinical Competence. *J Am Coll Cardiol.* 2003;41(4):687–708.
43. Beaulieu Y. Specific skill set and goals of focused echocardiography for critical care clinicians. *Crit Care Med.* 2007;35:S144–S149.

44. Redfield MM, Jacobsen SJ, Burnett JC Jr, et al. Burden of systolic and diastolic ventricular dysfunction in the community: appreciating the scope of the heart failure epidemic. *JAMA*. 2003;289:194–202.
45. McMurray JJ, Pfeffer MA. Heart failure. *Lancet*. 2005;365:1877–1889.
46. Barker WH, Mullooly JP, Getchell W. Changing incidence and survival for heart failure in a well-defined older population, 1970–1974 and 1990–1994. *Circulation*. 2006;113:799–805.
47. Hogg K, Swedberg K, McMurray J. Heart failure with preserved left ventricular systolic function; epidemiology, clinical characteristics, and prognosis. *J Am Coll Cardiol*. 2004;43:317–327.
48. Perera P, Lobo V, Williams SR, Gharahbaghian L. Cardiac echocardiography. *Crit Care Clin*. 2014;30(1):47–92.
49. Pinsky MR, Vincent JL. Let us use the pulmonary artery catheter correctly and only when we need it. *Crit Care Med*. 2005;33:1119–1122.
50. Marwick TH. Measurement of strain and strain rate by echocardiography: ready for prime time? *J Am Coll Cardiol*. 2006;47:1313–1327.
51. Rivers EP, Kruse JA, Jacobsen G, et al. The influence of early hemodynamic optimization on biomarker patterns of severe sepsis and septic shock. *Crit Care Med*. 2007;35:2016–2024.
52. Huang DT, Clermont G, Dremsizov TT, et al. Implementation of early goal-directed therapy for severe sepsis and septic shock: a decision analysis. *Crit Care Med*. 2007;35:2090–2100.
53. Jones AE, Focht A, Horton JM, et al. Prospective external validation of the clinical effectiveness of an emergency department-based early goal-directed therapy protocol for severe sepsis and septic shock. *Chest*. 2007;132:425–432.
54. Nguyen HB, Smith D. Sepsis in the 21st century: recent definitions and therapeutic advances. *Am J Emerg Med*. 2007;25:564–571.
55. Roch A, Blayac D, Ramiara P, et al. Comparison of lung injury after normal or small volume optimized resuscitation in a model of hemorrhagic shock. *Intensive Care Med*. 2007;33:1645–1654.
56. Dellinger RP, Levy MM, Carlet JM, et al. Surviving sepsis campaign: international guidelines for management of severe sepsis and septic shock: 2008. *Intensive Care Med*. 2008;34(1):17–60.
57. Dittoe N, Stultz D, Schwartz BP, et al. Quantitative left ventricular systolic function: from chamber to myocardium. *Crit Care Med*. 2007;35:S330–S339.
58. Curtis JP, Sokol SI, Wang Y, et al. The association of left ventricular ejection fraction, mortality, and cause of death in stable outpatients with heart failure. *J Am Coll Cardiol*. 2003;42:736–742.
59. Wang TJ, Evans JC, Benjamin EJ, et al. Natural history of asymptomatic left ventricular systolic dysfunction in the community. *Circulation*. 2003;108:977–982.
60. Mock MB, Ringqvist I, Fisher LD, et al. Survival of medically treated patients in the coronary artery surgery study (CASS) registry. *Circulation*. 1982;66:562–568.
61. Sharir T, Germano G, Kavanagh PB, et al. Incremental prognostic value of post-stress left ventricular ejection fraction and volume by gated myocardial perfusion single photon emission computed tomography. *Circulation*. 1999;100:1035–1042.
62. Schiller NB, Shah PM, Crawford M, et al. Recommendations for quantitation of the left ventricle by two-dimensional echocardiography. American Society of Echocardiography Committee on Standards, Subcommittee on Quantitation of Two-Dimensional Echocardiograms. *J Am Soc Echocardiogr*. 1989;2:358–367.
63. Lang RM, Bierig M, Devereux RB, et al. Recommendations for chamber quantification: a report from the American Society of Echocardiography's Guidelines and Standards Committee and the Chamber Quantification Writing Group, developed in conjunction with the European Association of Echocardiography, a branch of the European Society of Cardiology. *J Am Soc Echocardiogr*. 2005;18:1440–1463.
64. Zamorano J, Cordeiro P, Sugeng L, et al. Real-time three-dimensional echocardiography for rheumatic mitral valve stenosis evaluation: an accurate and novel approach. *J Am Coll Cardiol*. 2004;43:2091–2096.
65. Teichholz LE, Kreulen T, Herman MV, et al. Problems in echocardiographic volume determinations: echocardiographic-angiographic correlations in the presence of absence of asynergy. *Am J Cardiol*. 1976;37:7–11.
66. Sugeng L, Mor-Avi V, Weinert L, et al. Quantitative assessment of left ventricular size and function: side-by-side comparison of real-time three-dimensional echocardiography and computed tomography with magnetic resonance reference. *Circulation*. 2006;114:654–661.
67. Feigenbaum H, Armstrong WF, Ryan T, et al. *Feigenbaum's Echocardiography*. 6th ed. Philadelphia, PA: Lippincott Williams & Wilkins; 2005.
68. Nishimura RA, Tajik AJ. Evaluation of diastolic filling of left ventricle in health and disease: Doppler echocardiography is the clinician's rosetta stone. *J Am Coll Cardiol*. 1997;30:8–18.
69. Oh JK, Hatle L, Tajik AJ, et al. Diastolic heart failure can be diagnosed by comprehensive two-dimensional and Doppler echocardiography. *J Am Coll Cardiol*. 2006;47:500–506.
70. Sabbah HN, Khaja F, Brymer JF, et al. Noninvasive evaluation of left ventricular performance based on peak aortic blood acceleration measured with a continuous-wave Doppler velocity meter. *Circulation*. 1986;74:323–329.
71. Bauer F, Jones M, Shiota T, et al. Left ventricular outflow tract mean systolic acceleration as a surrogate for the slope of the left ventricular end-systolic pressure-volume relationship. *J Am Coll Cardiol*. 2002;40:1320–1327.
72. Nishimura RA, Tajik AJ. Quantitative hemodynamics by Doppler echocardiography: a noninvasive alternative to cardiac catheterization. *Prog Cardiovasc Dis*. 1994;36:309–342.
73. Bouchard A, Blumlein S, Schiller NB, et al. Measurement of left ventricular stroke volume using continuous wave Doppler echocardiography of the ascending aorta and M-mode echocardiography of the aortic valve. *J Am Coll Cardiol*. 1987;9:75–83.
74. Vinereanu D, Khokhar A, Fraser AG. Reproducibility of pulsed wave tissue Doppler echocardiography. *J Am Soc Echocardiogr*. 1999;12:492–499.
75. Dokainish H, Zoghbi WA, Lakkis NM, et al. Optimal noninvasive assessment of left ventricular filling pressures: a comparison of tissue Doppler echocardiography and B-type natriuretic peptide in patients with pulmonary artery catheters. *Circulation*. 2004;109:2432–2439.
76. Hsiao SH, Huang WC, Sy CL, et al. Doppler tissue imaging and color M-mode flow propagation velocity: are they really preload independent? *J Am Soc Echocardiogr*. 2005;18:1277–1284.
77. Oki T, Tabata T, Mishiro Y, et al. Pulsed tissue Doppler imaging of left ventricular systolic and diastolic wall motion velocities to evaluate differences between long and short axes in healthy subjects. *J Am Soc Echocardiogr*. 1999;12:308–313.
78. Mori K, Hayabuchi Y, Kuroda Y, et al. Left ventricular wall motion velocities in healthy children measured by pulsed wave Doppler tissue echocardiography: normal values and relation to age and heart rate. *J Am Soc Echocardiogr*. 2000;13:1002–1011.
79. Pela G, Bruschi G, Montagna L, et al. Left and right ventricular adaptation assessed by Doppler tissue echocardiography in athletes. *J Am Soc Echocardiogr*. 2004;17:205–211.
80. Oki T, Fukuda K, Tabata T, et al. Effect of an acute increase in afterload on left ventricular regional wall motion velocity in healthy subjects. *J Am Soc Echocardiogr*. 1999;12:476–483.
81. Nagueh SF, Bachinski LL, Meyer D, et al. Tissue Doppler imaging consistently detects myocardial abnormalities in patients with hypertrophic cardiomyopathy and provides a novel means for an early diagnosis before and independently of hypertrophy. *Circulation*. 2001;104:128–130.
82. Yu CM, Lin H, Yang H, et al. Progression of systolic abnormalities in patients with "isolated" diastolic heart failure and diastolic dysfunction. *Circulation*. 2002;105:1195–1201.
83. Wang M, Yip GW, Wang AY, et al. Peak early diastolic mitral annulus velocity by tissue Doppler imaging adds independent and incremental prognostic value. *J Am Coll Cardiol*. 2003;41:820–826.
84. Mankad S, Murali S, Kormos RL, et al. Evaluation of the potential role of color-coded tissue Doppler echocardiography in the detection of allograft rejection in heart transplant recipients. *Am Heart J*. 1999;138:721–730.
85. Dandel M, Hummel M, Muller J, et al. Reliability of tissue Doppler wall motion monitoring after heart transplantation for replacement of invasive routine screenings by optimally timed cardiac biopsies and catheterizations. *Circulation*. 2001;104:I184–1191.
86. Shan K, Bick RJ, Poindexter BJ, et al. Relation of tissue Doppler derived myocardial velocities to myocardial structure and beta-adrenergic receptor density in humans. *J Am Coll Cardiol*. 2000;36:891–896.
87. Galderisi M, Cattaneo F, Mondillo S. Doppler echocardiography and myocardial dyssynchrony: a practical update of old and new ultrasound technologies. *Cardiovasc Ultrasound*. 2007;5:28.
88. Edvardsen T, Gerber BL, Garot J, et al. Quantitative assessment of intrinsic regional myocardial deformation by Doppler strain rate echocardiography in humans: validation against three-dimensional tagged magnetic resonance imaging. *Circulation*. 2002;106:50–56.
89. Hoffmann R, Altiok E, Nowak B, et al. Strain rate measurement by Doppler echocardiography allows improved assessment of myocardial viability in patients with depressed left ventricular function. *J Am Coll Cardiol*. 2002;39:443–449.
90. Voigt JU, Exner B, Schmiedehausen K, et al. Strain-rate imaging during dobutamine stress echocardiography provides objective evidence of inducible ischemia. *Circulation*. 2003;107:2120–2126.
91. Yu CM, Fung JW, Zhang Q, et al. Tissue Doppler imaging is superior to strain rate imaging and postsystolic shortening on the prediction of reverse

remodeling in both ischemic and nonischemic heart failure after cardiac resynchronization therapy. *Circulation.* 2004;110:66–73.
92. Gilman G, Khandheria BK, Hagen ME, et al. Strain rate and strain: a step-by-step approach to image and data acquisition. *J Am Soc Echocardiogr.* 2004;17:1011–1020.
93. Weidemann F, Jamal F, Kowalski M, et al. Can strain rate and strain quantify changes in regional systolic function during dobutamine infusion, B-blockade, and atrial pacing—implications for quantitative stress echocardiography. *J Am Soc Echocardiogr.* 2002;15:416–424.
94. Sutherland GR, Di Salvo G, Claus P, et al. Strain and strain rate imaging: a new clinical approach to quantifying regional myocardial function. *J Am Soc Echocardiogr.* 2004;17:788–802.
95. Teske AJ, De Boeck BW, Melman PG, et al. Echocardiographic quantification of myocardial function using tissue deformation imaging, a guide to image acquisition and analysis using tissue Doppler and speckle tracking. *Cardiovasc Ultrasound.* 2007;5:27.
96. Amundsen BH, Helle-Valle T, Edvardsen T, et al. Noninvasive myocardial strain measurement by speckle tracking echocardiography: validation against sonomicrometry and tagged magnetic resonance imaging. *J Am Coll Cardiol.* 2006;47:789–793.
97. Giglio V, Pasceri V, Messano L, et al. Ultrasound tissue characterization detects preclinical myocardial structural changes in children affected by Duchenne muscular dystrophy. *J Am Coll Cardiol.* 2003;42:309–316.
98. Dutka DP, Donnelly JE, Palka P, et al. Echocardiographic characterization of cardiomyopathy in Friedreich's ataxia with tissue Doppler echocardiographically derived myocardial velocity gradients. *Circulation.* 2000;102:1276–1282.
99. Sengupta PP, Krishnamoorthy VK, Korinek J, et al. Left ventricular form and function revisited: applied translational science to cardiovascular ultrasound imaging. *J Am Soc Echocardiogr.* 2007;20:539–551.
100. Kolias TJ, Aaronson KD, Armstrong WF. Doppler-derived dP/dt and -dP/dt predict survival in congestive heart failure. *J Am Coll Cardiol.* 2000;36:1594–1599.
101. Pai RG, Bansal RC, Shah PM. Doppler-derived rate of left ventricular pressure rise: its correlation with the postoperative left ventricular function in mitral regurgitation. *Circulation.* 1990;82:514–520.
102. Nixon JV, Murray RG, Leonard PD, et al. Effect of large variations in preload on left ventricular performance characteristics in normal subjects. *Circulation.* 1982;65:698–703.
103. Colan SD, Borow KM, Neumann A. Left ventricular end-systolic wall stress-velocity of fiber shortening relation: a load-independent index of myocardial contractility. *J Am Coll Cardiol.* 1984;4:715–724.
104. Carabello BA, Usher BW, Hendrix GH, et al. Predictors of outcome for aortic valve replacement in patients with aortic regurgitation and left ventricular dysfunction: a change in the measuring stick. *J Am Coll Cardiol.* 1987;10:991–997.
105. Yoshifuku S, Biro S, Ikeda Y, et al. Validation of TEI index in the estimation of cardiac function: an experimental study. *J Am Coll Cardiol.* 2002;39:372.
106. Tei C, Ling LH, Hodge DO, et al. New index of combined systolic and diastolic myocardial performance: a simple and reproducible measure of cardiac function–a study in normals and dilated cardiomyopathy. *J Cardiol.* 1995;26:357–366.
107. Miller D, Farah MG, Liner A, et al. The relation between quantitative right ventricular ejection fraction and indices of tricuspid annular motion and myocardial performance. *J Am Soc Echocardiogr.* 2004;17: 443–447.
108. Matos J, Kronzon I, Panagopoulos G, Perk G. Mitral annular plane systolic excursion as a surrogate for left ventricular ejection fraction. *J Am Soc Echocardiogr.* 2012;25:969–974.
109. Bergenzaun L, Ohlin H, Gudmundsson P, et al. Mitral annular plane systolic excursion (MAPSE) in shock: a valuable echocardiographic parameter in intensive care patients. *Cardiovasc Ultrasound.* 2013;1:6.
110. Orde SR, Pulido JN, Masaki M, et al. Outcome prediction in sepsis: speckle tracking echocardiography based assessment of myocardial function. *Crit Care.* 2014;18:R149.
111. Voigt JU, Pedrizzetti G, Lysyansky P, et al. Definitions for a common standard for 2D speckle tracking echocardiography: consensus document of the EACVI/ASE/Industry Task Force to standardize deformation imaging. *J Am Soc Echocardiogr.* 2015;28:183–193.
112. Hoit BD. Left ventricular diastolic function. *Crit Care Med.* 2007;35: S340–S347.
113. Chatterjee K, Massie B. Systolic and diastolic heart failure: differences and similarities. *J Card Fail.* 2007;13:569–576.
114. Kitzman DW, Gardin JM, Gottdiener JS, et al. Importance of heart failure with preserved systolic function in patients > or = 65 years of age. CHS research group. Cardiovascular health study. *Am J Cardiol.* 2001;87:413–419.
115. Vasan RS, Benjamin EJ, Levy D. Prevalence, clinical features and prognosis of diastolic heart failure: an epidemiologic perspective. *J Am Coll Cardiol.* 1995;26:1565–1574.
116. Merx MW, Weber C. Sepsis and the heart. *Circulation.* 2007;116:79–802.
117. Burns AT, Connelly KA, La Gerche A, et al. Effect of heart rate on tissue Doppler measures of diastolic function. *Echocardiography.* 2007;24: 697–701.
118. Mirsky I, Pasipoularides A. Clinical assessment of diastolic function. *Prog Cardiovasc Dis.* 1990;32:291–318.
119. Weiss JL, Frederiksen JW, Weisfeldt ML. Hemodynamic determinants of the time-course of fall in canine left ventricular pressure. *J Clin Invest.* 1976;58:751–760.
120. Oh JKS, Seward JB, Tajik AJ (Eds.). Assessment of diastolic function. In: *The Echo Manual.* Lippincott Williams & Wilkins; 2006.
121. Sohn DW, Chai IH, Lee DJ, et al. Assessment of mitral annulus velocity by Doppler tissue imaging in the evaluation of left ventricular diastolic function. *J Am Coll Cardiol.* 1997;30:474–480.
122. Nagueh SF, Middleton KJ, Kopelen HA, et al. Doppler tissue imaging: a noninvasive technique for evaluation of left ventricular relaxation and estimation of filling pressures. *J Am Coll Cardiol.* 1997;30:1527–1533.
123. Chopra M, Sharma AC. Distinct cardiodynamic and molecular characteristics during early and late stages of sepsis-induced myocardial dysfunction. *Life Sci.* 2007;81:306–316.
124. Rozenberg S, Besse S, Brisson H, et al. Endotoxin-induced myocardial dysfunction in senescent rats. *Crit Care.* 2006;10:R124.
125. Pirracchio R, Cholley B, De Hert S, et al. Diastolic heart failure in anaesthesia and critical care. *Br J Anaesth.* 2007;98:707–721.
126. Cinel I, Dellinger RP. Advances in pathogenesis and management of sepsis. *Curr Opin Infect Dis.* 2007;20:345–352.
127. Young JD. The heart and circulation in severe sepsis. *Br J Anaesth.* 2004;93:114–120.
128. Rudiger A, Singer M. Mechanisms of sepsis-induced cardiac dysfunction. *Crit Care Med.* 2007;35:1599–1608.
129. Burkhoff D, Mirsky I, Suga H. Assessment of systolic and diastolic ventricular properties via pressure-volume analysis: a guide for clinical, translational, and basic researchers. *Am J Physiol Heart Circ Physiol.* 2005;289:H501–H512.
130. Zile MR, Tomita M, Ishihara K, et al. Changes in diastolic function during development and correction of chronic LV volume overload produced by mitral regurgitation. *Circulation.* 1993;87:1378–1388.
131. Appleton CP, Firstenberg MS, Garcia MJ, et al. The echo-Doppler evaluation of left ventricular diastolic function: a current perspective. *Cardiol Clin.* 2000;18:513–546, ix.
132. Oh JK, Appleton CP, Hatle LK, et al. The noninvasive assessment of left ventricular diastolic function with two-dimensional and Doppler echocardiography. *J Am Soc Echocardiography.* 1997;10:246–270.
133. Ristow B, Ali S, Ren X, et al. Elevated pulmonary artery pressure by Doppler echocardiography predicts hospitalization for heart failure and mortality in ambulatory stable coronary artery disease: the Heart and Soul Study. *J Am Coll Cardiol.* 2007;49:43–49.
134. Garcia MJ, Rodriguez L, Ares M, et al. Myocardial wall velocity assessment by pulsed Doppler tissue imaging: characteristic findings in normal subjects. *Am Heart J.* 1996;132:648–656.
135. Miyatake K, Yamagishi M, Tanaka N, et al. New method for evaluating left ventricular wall motion by color-coded tissue Doppler imaging: in vitro and in vivo studies. *J Am Coll Cardiol.* 1995;25:717–724.
136. Dokainish H, Zoghbi WA, Lakkis NM, et al. Incremental predictive power of B-type natriuretic peptide and tissue Doppler echocardiography in prognoses of patients with congestive heart failure. *J Am Coll Cardiol.* 2005;45:1223–1226.
137. Ommen SR, Nishimura RA, Appleton CP, et al. Clinical utility of Doppler echocardiography and tissue Doppler imaging in the estimation of left ventricular filling pressures: a comparative simultaneous Doppler-catheterization study. *Circulation.* 2000;102:1788–1794.
138. Nagueh SF, Sun H, Kopelen HA, et al. Hemodynamic determinants of the mitral annulus diastolic velocities by tissue Doppler. *J Am Coll Cardiol.* 2001;37:278–285.
139. Takatsuji H, Mikami T, Urasawa K, et al. A new approach for evaluation of left ventricular diastolic function: spatial and temporal analysis of left ventricular filling flow propagation by color M-mode Doppler echocardiography. *J Am Coll Cardiol.* 1996;27:365–371.
140. Garcia MJ, Thomas JD, Klein AL. New Doppler echocardiographic applications for the study of diastolic function. *J Am Coll Cardiol.* 1998;32:865–875.

141. Gonzalez-Vilchez F, Ayuela J, Ares M, et al. Comparison of Doppler echocardiography, color M-mode Doppler, and Doppler tissue imaging for the estimation of pulmonary capillary wedge pressure. *J Am Soc Echocardiogr.* 2002;15:1245–1250.
142. Lawson WE, Brown EJ Jr, Swinford RD, et al. A new use for M-mode echocardiography in detecting left ventricular diastolic dysfunction in coronary artery disease. *Am J Cardiol.* 1986;58:210–213.
143. Hanrath P, Mathey DG, Siegert R, et al. Left ventricular relaxation and filling pattern in different forms of left ventricular hypertrophy: an echocardiographic study. *Am J Cardiol.* 1980;45:15–23.
144. Pritchett AM, Mahoney DW, Jacobsen SJ, et al. Diastolic dysfunction and left atrial volume: a population-based study. *J Am CollCardiol.* 2005;45:87–92.
145. Dokainish H. Combining tissue Doppler echocardiography and B-type natriuretic peptide in the evaluation of left ventricular filling pressures: review of the literature and clinical recommendations. *Can J Cardiol.* 2007;23:983–989.
146. Moller JE, Pellikka PA, Hillis GS, et al. Prognostic importance of diastolic function and filling pressure in patients with acute myocardial infarction. *Circulation.* 2006;114:438–444.
147. Vieillard-Baron A, Charron C, Chergui K, et al. Bedside echocardiographic evaluation of hemodynamics in sepsis: is a qualitative evaluation sufficient? *Intensive Care Med.* 2006;32:1547–1552.
148. Ribeiro A, Lindmarker P, Juhlin-Dannfelt A, et al. Echocardiography Doppler in pulmonary embolism: right ventricular dysfunction as a predictor of mortality rate. *Am Heart J.* 1997;34(3):479–487.
149. Torbicki A, Perrier A, Konstantinides S, et al.; ESC Committee for Practice Guidelines (CPG). Guidelines on the diagnosis and management of acute pulmonary embolism: the Task Force for the Diagnosis and Management of Acute Pulmonary Embolism of the European Society of Cardiology (ESC). *Eur Heart J.* 2008;29:2276–2315.
150. Miniati M, Monti S, Pratali L, et al. Value of transthoracic echocardiography in the diagnosis of pulmonary embolism: results of a prospective study in unselected patients. *Am J Med.* 2001;110(7):528–535.
151. Mansencal N, Vieillard-Baron A, Beauchet A, et al. Triage patients with suspected pulmonary embolism in the emergency department using a portable ultrasound device. *Echocardiography.* 2008;25(5):451–456.
152. Vieillard-Baron A, Qanadli SD, Antakly Y, et al. Transesophageal echocardiography for the diagnosis of pulmonary embolism with acute cor pulmonale: a comparison with radiological procedures. *Intensive Care Med.* 1998;24(5):429–433.
153. Pruszczyk P, Torbicki A, Kuch-Wocial A, et al. Diagnostic value of transoesophageal echocardiography in suspected haemodynamically significant pulmonary embolism. *Heart.* 2001;85(6):628–634.
154. Carlbom DJ, Davidson BL. Pulmonary embolism in the critically ill. *Chest.* 2007;132:313–324.
155. Kline JA, Hernandez-Nino J, Jones AE, et al. Prospective study of the clinical features and outcomes of emergency department patients with delayed diagnosis of pulmonary embolism. *Acad Emerg Med.* 2007;14:592–598.
156. Raisinghani A, Ben-Yehuda O. Echocardiography in chronic thromboembolic pulmonary hypertension. *Semin Thorac Cardiovasc Surg.* 2006;18:230–235.
157. Kucher N, Goldhaber SZ. Risk stratification of acute pulmonary embolism. *Semin Thromb Hemost.* 2006;32:838–847.
158. Cecconi M, Johnston E, Rhodes A. What role does the right side of the heart play in circulation? *Crit Care.* 2006;10(Suppl 3):S5.
159. Konstantinides SV. Acute pulmonary embolism revisited: thromboembolic venous disease. *Heart.* 2008;94:795–802.
160. Sanchez O, Trinquart L, Colobet I, et al. Prognostic value of right ventricular dysfunction in patients with haemodynamically stable pulmonary embolism: a systemic review. *Eur Heart J.* 2008;29:1569–1577.
161. ten Wolde M, Söhne M, Quak E, et al. Prognostic value of echocardiographically assessed right ventricular dysfunction in patients with pulmonary embolism. *Arch Intern Med.* 2004;164:1685–1689.
162. Kucher N, Rossi E, De Rosa M, et al. Prognostic role of echocardiography among patients with acute pulmonary embolism and a systolic arterial pressure of 90 mm Hg or higher. *Arch Intern Med.* 2005;165:1777–1781.
163. Schoepf UJ, Kucher N, Kipfmueller F, et al. Right ventricular enlargement on chest computed tomography: a predictor of early death in acute pulmonary embolism. *Circulation.* 2004;110:3276–3280.
164. van der Meer RW, Pattynama PM, van Strijen MJ, et al. Right ventricular dysfunction and pulmonary obstruction index at helical CT: prediction of clinical outcome during 3-month follow-up in patients with acute pulmonary embolism. *Radiology.* 2005;235:798–803.
165. Pruszczyk P, Bochowicz A, Torbicki A, et al. Cardiac troponin T monitoring identifies high-risk group of normotensive patients with acute pulmonary embolism. *Chest.* 2003;123:1947–1952.
166. Mehta NJ, Jani K, Khan IA. Clinical usefulness and prognostic value of elevated cardiac troponin I levels in acute pulmonary embolism. *Am Heart J.* 2003;145:821–825.
167. Punukollu G, Khan IA, Gowda RM, et al. Cardiac troponin I release in acute pulmonary embolism in relation to the duration of symptoms. *Int J Cardiol.* 2005;99:207–211.
168. Kucher N, Printzen G, Goldhaber SZ. Prognostic role of brain natriuretic peptide in acute pulmonary embolism. *Circulation.* 2003;107:2545–2547.
169. Binder L, Pieske B, Olschewski M, et al. N-terminal pro-brain natriuretic peptide or troponin testing followed by echocardiography for risk stratification of acute pulmonary embolism. *Circulation.* 2005;112:1573–1579.
170. Scridon T, Scridon C, Skali H, et al. Prognostic significance of troponin elevation and right ventricular enlargement in acute pulmonary embolism. *Am J Cardiol.* 2005;96:303–305.
171. Jardin F, Dubourg O, Gueret P, et al. Quantitative two-dimensional echocardiography in massive pulmonary embolism: emphasis on ventricular interdependence and leftward septal displacement. *J Am Coll Cardiol.* 1987;10:1201–1206.
172. Morris-Thurgood JA, Frenneaux MP. Diastolic ventricular interaction and ventricular diastolic filling. *Heart Fail Rev.* 2000;5:307–323.
173. Rudski LG, Lai WW, Afilalo J, et al. Guidelines for the echocardiographic assessment of the right heart in adults: a report from the American Society of Echocardiography endorsed by the European Association of Echocardiography, a registered branch of the European Society of Cardiology, and the Canadian Society of Echocardiography. *J Am Soc Echocardiogr.* 2010;23:685–713.
174. Kopecna D, Briongos S, Castillo H, et al. PROTECT investigators. Interobserver reliability of echocardiography for prognostication of normotensive patients with pulmonary embolism. *Cardiovasc Ultrasound.* 2014;12:29.
175. Lobo JL, Holley A, Tapson V, et al; PROTECT and RIETE investigators. Prognostic significance of tricuspid annular displacement in normotensive patients with acute symptomatic pulmonary embolism. *J Thromb Haemost.* 2014;12(7):1020–1027.
176. Wilansky S, Moreno CA, Lester SJ. Complications of myocardial infarction. *Crit Care Med.* 2007;35:S348–S354.
177. Kinch JW, Ryan TJ. Right ventricular infarction. *N Engl J Med.* 1994;330:1211–1217.
178. Goldberger JJ, Himelman RB, Wolfe CL, et al. Right ventricular infarction: recognition and assessment of its hemodynamic significance by two-dimensional echocardiography. *J Am Soc Echocardiogr.* 1991;4:140–146.
179. Manno BV, Bemis CE, Carver J, et al. Right ventricular infarction complicated by right to left shunt. *J Am Coll Cardiol.* 1983;1:554–557.
180. Porter TR, Shillcutt SK, Adams MS, et al. Guidelines for the use of echocardiography as a monitor for therapeutic intervention in adults: a report from the american society of echocardiography. *J Am Soc Echocardiogr.* 2015;28(1):40–56.
181. Lancellotti P, Price S, Edvardsen T, et al. The use of echocardiography in acute cardiovascular care: recommendations of the European Association of Cardiovascular Imaging and the Acute Cardiovascular Care Association. *Eur Heart J Acute Cardiovasc Care.* 2015;4:3–5.
182. Little WC, Freeman GL. Pericardial disease. *Circulation.* 2006;113:1622–1632.
183. Hoit BD. Pericardial disease and pericardial tamponade. *Crit Care Med.* 2007;35(Suppl):S355–S364.
184. Maisch B. Pericardial disease with a focus on etiology, pathogenesis, pathophysiology, new diagnostic imaging methods, and treatment. *Curr Opin Cardiol.* 1994;9:379–388.
185. Weitzman LB, Tinker WP, Kranzon I, et al. The incidence and natural history of pericardial effusion after cardiac surgery: an echocardiography study. *Circulation.* 1984;69:506–511.
186. Kuvin JT, Harati NA, Pandian NG, et al. Postoperative cardiac tamponade in the modern surgical era. *Ann Thorac Surg.* 2002;74:1148–1153.
187. Ciliberto GR, Anjos MC, Gronda E. Significance of pericardial effusions after heart transplantation. *Am J Cardiol.* 1995;76:297–300.
188. Tsang TS, Barnes ME, Hayes SN, et al. Clinical and echocardiographic characteristics of significant pericardial effusions following cardiothoracic surgery and outcomes of echo-guided pericardiocentesis for management: Mayo Clinic experience, 1979–1998. *Chest.* 1999;116:322–331.
189. Imazio M, Trinchero R. Triage and management of acute pericarditis. *Int J Cardiol.* 2007;118:286–294.
190. Slobodin G, Hussein A, Rozenbaum M, et al. The emergency room in systemic rheumatic diseases. *Emerg Med J.* 2006;23:667–671.

191. Kobayashi M, Okabayashi T, Okamoto K, et al. Clinicopathological study of cardiac tamponade due to pericardial metastasis originating from gastric cancer. *World J Gastroenterol*. 2005;11:6899–6904.
192. Taguchi R, Takasu J, Itani Y, et al. Pericardial fat accumulation in men at risk for coronary artery disease. *Atherosclerosis*. 2001;157:203–209.
193. Iacobellis G, Leonetti F. Epicardial adipose tissue and insulin resistance in obese subjects. *J Clin Endocrinol Metab*. 2005;90:6300–6302.
194. Seferovic PM, Ristic AD, Imazio M, et al. Management strategies in pericardial emergencies. *Herz*. 2006;31:891–900.
195. Degiannis E, Loogna P, Doll D, et al. Penetrating cardiac injuries: recent experience in South Africa. *World J Surg*. 2006;30:1258–1264.
196. Leimgrubber PP, Klopfenstein HS, Wann LS, et al. The hemodynamic derangement associated with right ventricular diastolic collapse in cardiac tamponade: an experimental echocardiographic study. *Circulation*. 1983;68:612–620.
197. Hoit BD, Gabel M, Fowler NO. Cardiac tamponade in left ventricular dysfunction. *Circulation*. 1990;82:1370–1376.
198. Hoit BD, Ramrakhyani K. Pulmonary venous flow in cardiac tamponade: influence of left ventricular dysfunction and the relation to pulsus paradoxus. *J Am Soc Echocardiogr*. 1991;4:559–570.
199. Gillam LD, Guyer DE, Gibson TC, et al. Hydrodynamic compression of the right atrium: a new echocardiographic sign of cardiac tamponade. *Circulation*. 1983;68:294–301.
200. Maisch B, Seferovic PM, Ristic AD, et al. Guidelines on the diagnosis and management of pericardial diseases executive summary: the Task Force on the Diagnosis and Management of Pericardial Diseases of the European Society of Cardiology. *Eur Heart J*. 2004;25:587–610.
201. Reydel B, Spodick DH. Frequency and significance of chamber collapses during cardiac tamponade. *Am Heart J*. 1990;119:1160–1163.
202. Fussman B, Schwinger ME, Charney R, et al. Isolated of left-sided heart chambers in cardiac tamponade: demonstration by two-dimensional echocardiography. *Am Heart J*. 1991;121:613–616.
203. Merce J, Sagrista-Sauleda J, Permanyer-Miralda G, et al. Correlation between clinical and Doppler echocardiography findings in patients with moderate and large pericardial effusions: implications for the diagnosis of cardiac tamponade. *Am Heart J*. 1999;138:759–764.
204. Roy CL, Minor MA, Brookhart MA, et al. Does this patient with a pericardial effusion have cardiac tamponade? *JAMA*. 2007;297:1810–1818.
205. Talreja DR, Edwards WD, Danielson GK, et al. Constrictive pericarditis in 26 patients with histiologically normal pericardial thickness. *Circulation*. 2003;108(15):1852–1857.
206. Pinamonti B, Zecchin M, Di Lenarda A, et al. Persistence of restrictive left ventricular filling pattern in dilated cardiomyopathy: an ominous prognostic sign. *J Am Coll Cardiol*. 1997;29:604–612.
207. Ling LH, Oh JK, Tei C, et al. Pericardial thickness measured with transesophageal echocardiography: feasibility and potential clinical usefulness. *J Am Coll Cardiol*. 1997;29:1317–1323.
208. Cheitlin MD, Armstrong WF, Aurigemma GP, et al. ACC/AHA/ASE 2003 guideline update for the clinical application of echocardiography: summary article. A report of the American College of Cardiology/American Heart Association Task Force on Practice Guidelines (ACC/AHA/ASE Committee for the Clinical Application of Echocardiography). *J Am Soc Echocardiogr*. 2003;16:1091–1110.
209. Tei C, Child JS, Tanaka H, et al. Atrial systolic notch on the interventricular septal echogram: an echocardiographic sign of constrictive pericarditis. *J Am Coll Cardiol*. 1983;1:907–912.
210. Engel PJ, Fowler NO, Tei CW, et al. M-mode echocardiography in constrictive pericarditis. *J Am Coll Cardiol*. 1985;6:471–474.
211. Hoit BD. Imaging the pericardium. *Cardiol Clin*. 1990;8:587–600.
212. D'Cruz IA, Dick A, Gross CM, et al. Abnormal left ventricular-left atrial posterior wall contour: a new dimensional echocardiographic sign in constrictive pericarditis. *Am Heart J*. 1989;118:218–132.
213. Ha JW, Oh JK, Ling LH, et al. Annulus paradoxus: transmitral flow velocity to mitral annular velocity ratio is inversely proportional to pulmonary capillary wedge pressure in patients with constrictive pericarditis. *Circulation*. 2001;104:976–978.
214. Oh JK, Hatle LK, Sinak LJ, et al. Characteristic Doppler echocardiographic pattern of mitral inflow velocity in severe aortic regurgitation. *J Am Coll Cardiol*. 1989;14:1712–1717.
215. Rajagopalan N, Garcia MJ, Rodriguez L, et al. Comparison of new Doppler echocardiographic methods to differentiate constrictive pericardial heart disease and restrictive cardiomyopathy. *Am J Cardiol*. 2001;87:86–94.
216. Pozzoli M, Traversi E, Cioffi G, et al. Loading manipulations improve the prognostic value of Doppler evaluation of mitral flow in patients with chronic heart failure. *Circulation*. 1997;95:1222–1230.
217. Sun JP, Abdalla IA, Yang XS, et al. Respiratory variation of mitral and pulmonary venous Doppler flow velocities in constrictive pericarditis before and after pericardiectomy. *J Am Soc Echocardiogr*. 2001;14:119–126.
218. Oh JK, Tajik AJ, Appleton CP, et al. Preload reduction to unmask the characteristic Doppler features of constrictive pericarditis. *Circulation*. 1997;95:796–799.
219. Troughton RW, Asher CR, Klein AL. Percarditis. *Lancet*. 2004;363: 717–727.
220. Krug EG, Mercy JA, Dahlberg LL, et al. The world report on violence and health. *Lancet*. 2002;360:1083–1088.
221. Gao JM, Gao YH, Wei GB, et al. Penetrating cardiac wounds: principles for surgical management. *World J Surg*. 2004;28:1025–1029.
222. Burack JH, Kandil E, Sawas A, et al. Triage and outcome of patients with mediastinal penetrating trauma. *Ann Thorac Surg*. 2007;83:377–382.
223. Asensio JA, Soto SN, Forno W, et al. Penetrating cardiac injuries: a complex challenge. *Injury*. 2001;32:533–543.
224. Jones AE, Tayal VS, Sullivan DM, et al. Randomized, controlled trial of immediate versus delayed goal-directed ultrasound to identify the cause of nontraumatic hypotension in emergency department patients. *Crit Care Med*. 2004;32(8):1703–1708.
225. Aboulhosn J, Child JS. Left ventricular outflow obstruction: subaortic stenosis, bicuspid aortic valve, supravalvar aortic stenosis, and coarctation of the aorta. *Circulation*. 2006;114:2412–2422.
226. Cesar S, Potocnik N, Stare V. Left ventricular end-diastolic pressure-volume relationship in septic rats with open thorax. *Comp Med*. 2003; 53:493–497.
227. Groban L, Dolinski SY. Transesophageal echocardiographic evaluation of diastolic function. *Chest*. 2005;128:3652–3663.
228. Azevedo LC, Janiszewski M, Soriano FG, et al. Redox mechanisms of vascular cell dysfunction in sepsis. *Endocr Metab Immune Disord Drug Targets*. 2006;6:159–164.
229. Bombardini T. Myocardial contractility in the echo lab: molecular, cellular and pathophysiological basis. *Cardiovasc Ultrasound*. 2005;3:27.
230. Assreuy J. Nitric oxide and cardiovascular dysfunction in sepsis. *Endocr Metab Immune Disord Drug Targets*. 2006;6:165–173.
231. Kumar A, Anel R, Bunnell E, et al. Pulmonary artery occlusion pressure and central venous pressure fail to predict ventricular filling volume, cardiac performance, or the response to volume infusion in normal subjects. *Crit Care Med*. 2004;32:691–699.
232. Donal E, Yamada H, Leclercq C, et al. The left atrial appendage, a small, blind-ended structure: a review of its echocardiographic evaluation and its clinical role. *Chest*. 2005;128:1853–1862.
233. Kortgen A, Niederprum P, Bauer M. Implementation of an evidence-based "standard operating procedure" and outcome in septic shock. *Crit Care Med*. 2006;34:943–949.
234. Krishnagopalan S, Kumar A, Parrillo JE, et al. Myocardial dysfunction in the patient with sepsis. *Curr Opin Crit Care*. 2002;8:376–388.
235. Poelaert JI, Trouerbach J, De Buyzere M, et al. Evaluation of transesophageal echocardiography as a diagnostic and therapeutic aid in a critical care setting. *Chest*. 1995;107:774–779.
236. Parrillo JE, Burch C, Shelhamer JH, et al. A circulating myocardial depressant substance in humans with septic shock: septic shock with a reduced ejection fraction have a circulating factor that depresses in vitro myocardial cell performance. *J Clin Invest*. 1985;76:1539–1553.
237. Fischer UM, Radhakrishnan RS, Uray KS, et al. Myocardial function after gut ischemia/reperfusion: does NF kappaB play a role? *J Surg Res*. 2009;152(2):264–270.
238. Barth E, Radermacher P, Thiemermann C, et al. Role of inducible nitric oxide synthase in the reduced responsiveness of the myocardium to catecholamines in a hyperdynamic, murine model of septic shock. *Crit Care Med*. 2006;34:307–313.
239. Martins PS, Brunialti MK, da Luz Fernandes M, et al. Bacterial recognition and induced cell activation in sepsis. *Endocr Metab Immune Disord Drug Targets*. 2006;6:183–191.
240. Pinsky MR, Teboul JL. Assessment of indices of preload and volume responsiveness. *Curr Opin Crit Care*. 2005;11:235–239.
241. Poeze M, Solberg BC, Greve JW, et al. Monitoring global volume-related hemodynamic or regional variables after initial resuscitation: what is a better predictor of outcome in critically ill septic patients? *Crit Care Med*. 2005;33:2494–2500.
242. Pinsky MR. Protocolized cardiovascular management based on ventricular-arterial coupling. In: Pinsky MR, Payen D, eds. *Functional Hemodynamic Monitoring*. New York: Springer-Verlag; 2005:381–394.
243. Axler O. Evaluation and management of shock. *Semin Respir Crit Care Med*. 2006;27:230–240.

244. Volpicelli G, Elbarbary M, Blaivas M, et al. International evidence-based recommendations for point-of-care lung ultrasound. *Intensive Care Med.* 2012;38(4):577–591.
245. Lichtenstein DA, Meziere GA. Relevance of lung ultrasound in the diagnosis of acute respiratory failure: The BLUE protocol. *Chest J.* 2008;134:117–125.
246. Reissig A, Copetti R. Lung ultrasound in community acquired pneumonia and in interstitial lung diseases. *Respiration.* 2014:87:179–189
247. Volpicelli G, Elbarbary M, Blaivas M, et al. International Liaison Committee on Lung Ultrasound for International Consensus Conference on Lung Ultrasound. International evidence-based recommendations for point-of-care lung ultrasound. *Intensive Care Med.* 2012;38:577–591.
248. Mueller-Lenke N, Rudez J, Staub D, et al. Use of chest radiography in the emergency diagnosis of acute congestive heart failure. *Heart.* 2006;92:695–696.
249. Gheorghiade M, Shin DD, Thomas TO, et al. Congestion is an important diagnostic and therapeutic target in heart failure. *Rev Cardiovasc Med.* 2006;7(Suppl 1):S12–S24.
250. Prosen G, Klemen P, Strnad M, Grmec S. Combination of lung ultrasound (a comet-tail sign) and N-terminal pro-brain natriuretic peptide in differentiating acute heart failure from emergency setting. *Crit Care.* 2011;15:R114.
251. Cibinel GA, Casoli G, Elia F, et al. Diagnostic accuracy and reproducibility of pleural and lung ultrasound in discriminating cardiogenic causes of acute dyspnea in the emergency department. *Intern Emerg Med.* 2011;7:65–70.
252. Jambrik Z, Monti S, Coppola V, et al. Usefulness of ultrasound lung comets as a nonradiologic sign of extravascular lung water. *Am J Cardiol.* 2004;93:1265–1270.
253. Lichtenstein D, Meziere G, Biderman P, et al. The comet-tail artifact: an ultrasound sign of alveolar-interstitial syndrome. *Am J Respir Crit Care Med.* 1997;156:1640–1646.
254. Agricola E, Bove T, Oppizzi M, et al. 'Ultrasound comet-tail images': a marker of pulmonary edema: a comparative study with wedge pressure and extravascular lung water. *Chest.* 2005;127:1690–1695.
255. Liteplo AS, Marill KA, Villen T, et al. Emergency thoracic ultrasound in the differentiation of the etiology of shortness of breath (ETUDES): sonographic B-lines and N-terminal pro-brain-type natriuretic peptide in diagnosing congestive heart failure. *Acad Emerg Med.* 2009;16:201–210.
256. Noble VE, Murray AF, Capp R, et al. Ultrasound assessment for extravascular lung water in patients undergoing hemodialysis. *Chest.* 2009;135:1433–1439.
257. Stawicki SP, Braslow BM, Panebianco NL, et al. Intensivist use of hand-carried ultrasonography to measure IVC collapsibility in estimating intravascular volume status: correlations with CVP. *J Am Coll Surg.* 2009;209:55–61.
258. Fields JM, Lee PA, Jenq KY, et al. The interrater reliability of inferior vena cava ultrasound by bedside clinician sonographers in emergency department patients. *Acad Emerg Med.* 2011;18:98–101.
259. Stawicki SP, Adkins EJ, Eiferman DS, et al. Prospective evaluation of intravascular volume status in critically ill patients: does inferior vena cava collapsibility correlate with central venous pressure? *J Trauma Acute Care Surg.* 2014;76(4):956–963.
260. Kent A, Patil P, Davila V, et al. Sonographic evaluation of intravascular volume status: can internal jugular or femoral vein collapsibility be used in the absence of IVC visualization? *Ann Thorac Med.* 2015;10(1):44–49.
261. Kent A, Bahner DP, Boulger CT, et al. Sonographic evaluation of intravascular volume status in the surgical intensive care unit: a prospective comparison of subclavian vein and inferior vena cava collapsibility index. *J Surg Res.* 2013;184(1):561–566.
262. Sobczyk D, Nycz K, Andruszkiewicz P. Bedside ultrasonographic measurement of the inferior vena cava fails to predict fluid responsiveness in the first 6 hours after cardiac surgery: a prospective case series observational study. *J Cardiothorac Vasc Anesth.* 2015;29:663–639.
263. Juhl-Olsen P, Vistisen ST, Christiansen LK, et al. Ultrasound of the inferior vena cava does not predict hemodynamic response to early hemorrhage. *J Emerg Med.* 2013;45:592–597.
264. Wu Y, Zhou S, Zhou Z, Liu B. A 10-second fluid challenge guided by transthoracic echocardiography can predict fluid responsiveness. *Crit Care (London).* 2014;18:R108.
265. Lu GP, Yan G, Chen Y, et al. The passive leg raise test to predict fluid responsiveness in children—preliminary observations. *Indian J Pediatr.* 2015;82:5–12.
266. Duus N, Shogilev DJ, Skibsted S et al. The reliability and validity of passive leg raise and fluid bolus to assess fluid responsiveness in spontaneously breathing emergency department patients. *J Crit Care.* 2015;30:e1–e5.
267. Cannesson M, Forget P. Fluid responsiveness monitoring in surgical and critically ill patients: clinical impact of goal directed therapy. *Anaesthesiology News.* 2010 September 1.
268. Breitkreutz R, Walcher F, Seeger FH. Focused echocardiographic evaluation in resuscitation management: concept of an advanced life support-conformed algorithm. *Crit Care Med.* 2007;35(5 Suppl):S150–S161.
269. Breitkreutz R, Uddin S, Steiger H, et al. Focused echocardiography entry level: new concept of a 1-day training course. *Minerva Anestesiol.* 2009;75:285–292
270. Nolan JP, Soar JZD, Biarent D, et al. REASON 1 trial: sonography in cardiac arrest. Available at: http://clinicaltrialsgov/ct2/show/NCT01446471.
271. Lichtenstein D, Malbrain ML. Critical care ultrasound in cardiac arrest: technological requirements for performing the SESAME-protocol—a holistic approach. *Anaesthesiol Intensive Ther.* 2015;47:471–481
272. Scalea TM, Rodriguez A, Chiu WC, et al. Focused Assessment with Sonography for Trauma (FAST): results from an international consensus conference. *J Trauma.* 1999;46(3):466–472.
273. Rozycki GS, Feliciano DV, Ochsner MG, et al. The role of ultrasound in patients with possible penetrating cardiac wounds: a prospective multicenter study. *J Trauma.* 1999;46(4):543–551.
274. Plummer D, Brunette D, Asinger R, et al. Emergency department echocardiography improves outcome in penetrating cardiac injury. *Ann Emerg Med.* 1992;21(6):709–712.
275. Melniker LA, Leibner E, McKenney MG, et al. Randomized controlled clinical trial of point-of-care, limited ultrasonography for trauma in the emergency department: the first sonography outcomes assessment program trial. *Ann Emerg Med.* 2006;48(3):227–235.
276. Feczko JD, Lynch L, Pless JE, et al. An autopsy case review of 142 nonpenetrating (blunt) injuries of the aorta. *J Trauma.* 1992;33:846–849.
277. Mattox KL, Wall MJ Jr. Historical review of blunt injury to the thoracic aorta. *Chest Surg Clin North Am.* 2000;10:167–182.
278. Dyer DS, Moore EE, Ilke DN, et al. Thoracic aortic injury: how predictive is mechanism and is chest computed tomography a reliable screening tool? A prospective study of 1,561 patients. *J Trauma.* 2000;48:73–682.
279. Karmy-Jones R, Carter YM, Nathens A, et al. Impact of presenting physiology and associated injuries on outcome following traumatic rupture of the thoracic aorta. *Am Surg.* 2001;67:61–66.
280. Chirillo F, Totis O, Cavarzerani A, et al. Usefulness of transthoracic and transoesophageal echocardiography in recognition and management of cardiovascular injuries after blunt chest trauma. *Heart.* 1996;75:301–306.
281. Minard G, Schurr MJ, Croce MA, et al. A prospective analysis of transesophageal echocardiography in the diagnosis of traumatic disruption of the aorta. *J Trauma.* 1996;40:225–230.
282. Khalil A, Helmy T, Porembka DT. Aortic pathology: aortic trauma, debris, dissection, and aneurysm. *Crit Care Med.* 2007;35:S392–S400.
283. Kodali S, Jamieson WR, Leia-Stephens M, et al. Traumatic rupture of the thoracic aorta. A 20-year review: 1969–1989. *Circulation.* 1991; 84(5 Suppl):III40–III46.
284. Rivas LA, Munera F, Fishman JE. Multidetector-row computerized tomography of aortic injury. *Semin Roentgenol.* 2006;41:226–236.
285. Braunwald E, Zipes DP, Libby P, et al., eds. *Braunwald's Heart Disease: A Textbook of Cardiovascular Medicine.* 7th ed. Philadelphia, PA: WB Saunders; 2004.
286. D'Cruz IA, ed. *Echocardiographic Anatomy: Understanding Normal and Abnormal Echocardiograms.* New York, NY: Mc-Graw-Hill/Appleton & Lange; 1995.
287. Porembka DT. Transesophageal echocardiography. *Crit Care Clin.* 1996; 12:875–918.
288. Fuster V, Alexander RW, O'Rourke RA, et al., eds. *Hurst's The Heart.* 11th ed. New York, NY: McGraw-Hill Professional; 2004.
289. Mathew J, Chakib A, eds. *Clinical Manual and Review of Transesophageal Echocardiography.* New York, NY: McGraw-Hill; 2005.
290. Cinnella G, Dambrosio M, Brienza N, et al. Transesophageal echocardiography for diagnosis of traumatic aortic injury: an appraisal of the evidence. *J Trauma.* 2004;57:1246–1255.
291. Bonomini F, Tengattini S, Fabiano A, et al. Atherosclerosis and oxidative stress. *Histol Histopathol.* 2008;23:381–390.
292. Mallika V, Goswami B, Rajappa M. Atherosclerosis pathophysiology and the role of novel risk factors: a clinicobiochemical perspective. *Angiology.* 2007;58:513–522.
293. Meissner I, Khandheria BK, Sheps SG, et al. Atherosclerosis of the aorta: risk factor, risk marker, or innocent bystander? A prospective population-based transesophageal echocardiography study. *J Am Coll Cardiol.* 2004;44:1018–1024.
294. Nzewi O, Slight RD, Zamvar V. Management of blunt thoracic aortic injury. *Eur J Vasc Endovasc Surg.* 2006;31:18–27.

295. Baguley CJ, Sibal AK, Alison PM. Repair of injuries to the thoracic aorta and great vessels: Auckland, New Zealand 1995–2004. *ANZ J Surg.* 2005;75:383–387.
296. Yu T, Zhu X, Tang L, et al. Review of CT angiography of aorta. *Radiol Clin North Am.* 2007;45:461–483.
297. Moustafa S, Mookadam F, Cooper L, et al. Sinus of valsalva aneurysms–47 years of a single center experience and systematic overview of published reports. *Am J Cardiol.* 2007;99:1159–1164.
298. Rustemli A, Bhatti TK, Wolff SD. Evaluating cardiac sources of embolic stroke with MRI. *Echocardiography.* 2007;24:301–308.
299. Sundt TM. Intramural hematoma and penetrating atherosclerotic ulcer of the aorta. *Ann Thorac Surg.* 2007;83:S835–S841.
300. Sharifkazemi MB, Aslani A, Zamirian M, et al. Significance of aortic atheroma in elderly patients with ischemic stroke: a hospital-based study and literature review. *Clin Neurol Neurosurg.* 2007;109:311–316.
301. Bossone E, Evangelista A, Isselbacher E, et al. Prognostic role of transesophageal echocardiography in acute type A aortic dissection. *Am Heart J.* 2007;153:1013–1020.
302. Meissner L, Whisnant JP, Khandheria BK, et al. Prevalence of potential risk factors for stroke assessed by transesophageal echocardiography and carotid ultrasonography: the SPARC study. Stroke Prevention Assessment of Risk in a Community. *Mayo Clin Proc.* 1989;64:862–869.
303. Cardiogenic brain embolism. The second report of the Cerebral Embolism Task Force. *Arch Neurol.* 1989;46:727–743.
304. Atherosclerotic disease of the aortic arch as a risk factor for recurrent ischemic stroke. The French Study of Aortic Plaques in Stroke Group. *N Engl J Med.* 1996;19:1216–1221.
305. Pearson AC, Labovitz AJ, Tatineni S, et al. Superiority of transesophageal echocardiography in detecting cardiac source of embolism in patients with cerebral ischemia of uncertain etiology. *J Am Coll Cardiol.* 1991;17:66–72.
306. Black IW, Hopkins AP, Lee LC, et al. Role of transoesophageal echocardiography in evaluation of cardiogenic embolism. *Br Heart J.* 1991; 66:302–307.
307. Pop G, Sutherland GR, Koudstaal PJ, et al. Transesophageal echocardiography in the detection of intracardiac embolic sources in patients with transient ischemic attacks. *Stroke.* 1990;21:560–565.
308. DeRook FA, Comess KA, Albers GW, et al. Transesophageal echocardiography in the evaluation of stroke. *Ann Intern Med.* 1992;117:922–932.
309. Vandenbogaerde J, De Bleecker J, Decoo D, et al. Transoesophageal echo-Doppler in patients suspected of a cardiac source of peripheral emboli. *Eur Heart J.* 1992;13:88–94.
310. Lee RJ, Bartzokis T, Yeoh TK, et al. Enhanced detection of intracardiac sources of cerebral emboli by transesophageal echocardiography. *Stroke.* 1991;22:734–739.
311. Albers GW, Comess KA, DeRook FA, et al. Transesophageal echocardiographic findings in stroke subtypes. *Stroke.* 1994;25:23–28.
312. Sansoy V, Abbott RD, Jayaweera AR, et al. Low yield of transthoracic echocardiography for cardiac source of embolism. *Am J Cardiol.* 1995;75:166–169.
313. Leung DY, Black IW, Cranney GB, et al. Prognostic implications of left atrial spontaneous echo contrast in nonvalvular atrial fibrillation. *J Am Coll Cardiol.* 1994;24:755–762.
314. Tunick PA, Rosenzweig BP, Katz ES, et al. High risk for vascular events in patients with protruding aortic atheromas: a prospective study. *J Am Coll Cardiol.* 1994;23:1085–1090.
315. Tunick PA, Kronzon I. Protruding atherosclerotic plaque in the aortic arch of patients with systemic embolization: a new finding seen by transesophageal echocardiography. *Am Heart J.* 1990;120:658–660.
316. Amarenco P, Cohen A, Tzourio C, et al. Atherosclerotic disease of the aortic arch and the risk of ischemic stroke. *N Engl J Med.* 1994;331:1474–1479.
317. Jones EF, Kalman JM, Calafiore P, et al. Proximal aortic atheroma: an independent risk factor for cerebral ischemia. *Stroke.* 1995;26:218–224.
318. Koren MJ, Bryant B, Hilton TC. Atherosclerotic disease of the aortic arch and the risk of ischemic stroke. *N Engl J Med.* 1995;332:1237.
319. Transesophageal echocardiographic correlates of thromboembolism in high-risk patients with nonvalvular atrial fibrillation The Stroke Prevention in Atrial Fibrillation Investigators Committee on Echocardiography. *Ann Intern Med.* 1998;128:639–647.
320. Black IW, Hopkins AP, Lee LC, et al. Left atrial spontaneous echo contrast: a clinical and echocardiographic analysis. *J Am Coll Cardiol.* 1991;18:398–404.
321. Zenker G, Erbel R, Kramer G, et al. Transesophageal two-dimensional echocardiography in young patients with cerebral ischemic events. *Stroke.* 1988;19:345–348.
322. Lechat P, Mas JL, Lascault G, et al. Prevalence of patent foramen ovale in patients with stroke. *N Engl J Med.* 1988;318:1148–1152.
323. Webster MW, Chancellor AM, Smith HJ, et al. Patent foramen ovale in young stroke patients. *Lancet.* 1988;2:11–12.
324. Gallet B, Malergue MC, Adams C, et al. Atrial septal aneurysm: a potential cause of systemic embolism-an echocardiographic study. *Br Heart J.* 1985;53:292–297.
325. Ince H, Nienaber CA. Diagnosis and management of patients with aortic dissection. *Heart.* 2007;93:266–270.
326. Haidary A, Bis K, Vrachiolitis T, et al. Enhancement performance of a 64-slice triple rule-out protocol vs 16-slice and 10-slice multidetector CT-angiography protocols for evaluation of aortic and pulmonary vasculature. *J Comput Assist Tomogr.* 2007;31:917–923.
327. Iezzi R, Cotroneo AR, Marano R, et al. Endovascular treatment of thoracic aortic diseases: follow-up and complications with multi-detector computed tomography angiography. *Eur J Radiol.* 2008;65(3):365–376.
328. Suzuki T, Mehta RH, Ince H, et al. Clinical profiles and outcomes of acute type B aortic dissection in the current era: lessons from the International Registry of Aortic Dissection (IRAD). *Circulation.* 2003;108(Suppl 1): II312–II317.
329. Shiga T, Wajima Z, Apfel CC, et al. Diagnostic accuracy of transesophageal echocardiography, helical computed tomography, and magnetic resonance imaging for suspected thoracic aortic dissection: systematic review and meta-analysis. *Arch Intern Med.* 2006;166:1350–1356.
330. Davies RR, Goldstein LJ, Coady MA, et al. Yearly rupture or dissection rates for thoracic aortic aneurysms: simple prediction based on size. *Ann Thorac Surg.* 2002;73:17–27; discussion 27–28.
331. Isselbacher EM. Thoracic and abdominal aortic aneurysms. *Circulation.* 2005;111:816–828.
332. Greiss I, Ugolini P, Joyal M, et al. Ruptured aneurysm of the left sinus of Valsalva discovered 41 years after a decelerational injury. *J Am Soc Echocardiogr.* 2004;17:906–909.
333. Vereckei A, Vandor L, Halasz J, et al. Infective endocarditis resulting in rupture of sinus of Valsalva with a rupture site communicating with both the right atrium and right ventricle. *J Am Soc Echocardiogr.* 2004;17:995–997.
334. Vincelj J, Starcevic B, Sokol I, et al. Rupture of a right sinus of Valsalva aneurysm into the right ventricle during vaginal delivery: a case report. *Echocardiography.* 2005;22:844–846.
335. Vural KM, Sener E, Tasdemir O, et al. Approach to sinus of Valsalva aneurysms: a review of 53 cases. *Eur J Cardiothorac Surg.* 2001;20:71–76.
336. Shah RP, Ding ZP, Ng AS, et al. A ten-year review of ruptured sinus of valsalva: clinico-pathological and echo-Doppler features. *Singapore Med J.* 2001;42:473–476.
337. Smith RL, Irimpen A, Helmcke FR, et al. Ruptured congenital sinus of Valsalva aneurysm. *Echocardiography.* 2005;22:625–628.
338. Banerjee S, Jagasia DH. Unruptured sinus of Valsalva aneurysm in an asymptomatic patient. *J Am Soc Echocardiogr.* 2002;15:668–670.
339. Ott DA. Aneurysm of the sinus of Valsalva. *Semin Thorac Cardiovasc Surg Pediatr Card Surg Annu.* 2006:165–176.
340. Patel ND, Williams JA, Barreiro CJ, et al. Valve-sparing aortic root replacement: early experience with the de paulis Valsalva graft in 51 patients. *Ann Thorac Surg.* 2006;82:548–553.
341. De Paulis R, Bassano C, Bertoldo F, et al. Aortic valve-sparing operations and aortic root replacement. *J Cardiovasc Med (Hagerstown).* 2007; 8:97–101.
342. Kamalakannan D, Rosman HS, Eagle KA. Acute aortic dissection. *Crit Care Clin.* 2007;23:779–800.
343. Maraj R, Rerkpattanapipat P, Jacobs LE, et al. Meta-analysis of 143 reported cases of aortic intramural hematoma. *Am J Cardiol.* 2000;86: 664–668.
344. Syed FF, Millar BC, Prendergast BD. Molecular technology in context: a current review of diagnosis and management of infective endocarditis. *Prog Cardiovasc Dis.* 2007;50:181–197.
345. Lester SJ, Wilansky S. Endocarditis and associated complications. *Crit Care Med.* 2007;35:S384–S391.
346. Silverman ME, Upshaw CB Jr. Extracardiac manifestations of infective endocarditis and their historical descriptions. *Am J Cardiol.* 2007;100: 1802–1807.
347. Erbel R, Rohmann S, Drexler M, et al. Improved diagnostic value of echocardiography in patients with infective endocarditis by transoesophageal approach. A prospective study. *Eur Heart J.* 1988;9:43–53.
348. Mugge A, Daniel WG, Frank G, et al. Echocardiography in infective endocarditis: reassessment of prognostic implications of vegetation size determined by the transthoracic and the transesophageal approach. *J Am Coll Cardiol.* 1989;14:631–638.
349. Shively BK, Gurule FT, Roldan CA, et al. Diagnostic value of transesophageal compared with transthoracic echocardiography in infective endocarditis. *J Am Coll Cardiol.* 1991;18:391–397.

350. Daniel WG, Mugge A, Grote J, et al. Comparison of transthoracic and transesophageal echocardiography for detection of abnormalities of prosthetic and bioprosthetic valves in the mitral and aortic positions. *Am J Cardiol.* 1993;71:210–215.
351. Pedersen WR, Walker M, Olson JD, et al. Value of transesophageal echocardiography as an adjunct to transthoracic echocardiography in evaluation of native and prosthetic valve endocarditis. *Chest.* 1991;100:351–356.
352. Reynolds HR, Jagen MA, Tunick PA, et al. Sensitivity of transthoracic versus transesophageal echocardiography for the detection of native valve vegetations in the modern era. *J Am Soc Echocardiogr.* 2003;16:67–70.
353. Alton ME, Pasierski TJ, Orsinelli DA, et al. Comparison of transthoracic and transesophageal echocardiography in evaluation of 47 Starr–Edwards prosthetic valves. *J Am Coll Cardiol.* 1992;20:1503–1511.
354. Zabalgoitia M, Herrera CJ, Chaudhry FA, et al. Improvement in the diagnosis of bioprosthetic valve dysfunction by transesophageal echocardiography. *J Heart Valve Dis.* 1993;2:595–603.
355. Jaffe WM, Morgan DE, Pearlman AS, et al. Infective endocarditis, 1983–1988: echocardiographic findings and factors influencing morbidity and mortality. *J Am Coll Cardiol.* 1990;15:1227–1233.
356. Dodds GA, Sexton DJ, Durack DT, et al. Negative predictive value of the Duke criteria for infective endocarditis. *Am J Cardiol.* 1996;77:403–407.
357. Lowry RW, Zoghbi WA, Baker WB, et al. Clinical impact of transesophageal echocardiography in the diagnosis and management of infective endocarditis. *Am J Cardiol.* 1994;73:1089–1091.
358. Vieira ML, Grinberg M, Pomerantzeff PM, et al. Repeated echocardiographic examinations of patients with suspected infective endocarditis. *Heart.* 2004;90:1020–1024.
359. Bayer AS, Bolger AF, Taubert KA, et al. Diagnosis and management of infective endocarditis and its complications. *Circulation.* 1998;98:2936–2948.
360. American College of Cardiology/American Heart Association Task Force on Practice Guidelines, Society of Cardiovascular Anesthesiologists, Society for Cardiovascular Angiography and Interventions, et al. ACC/AHA 2006 guidelines for the management of patients with valvular heart disease: a report of the American College of Cardiology/American Heart Association Task Force on Practice Guidelines (writing committee to revise the 1998 Guidelines for the Management of Patients with Valvular Heart Disease): developed in collaboration with the Society of Cardiovascular Anesthesiologists: endorsed by the Society for Cardiovascular Angiography and Interventions and the Society of Thoracic Surgeons. *Circulation.* 2006;114:e84–e231.
361. Armstrong WF, Zoghbi WA. Stress echocardiography: current methodology and clinical applications. *J Am Coll Cardiol.* 2005;45:1739–1747.
362. Cerqueira MD, Weissman NJ, Dilsizian V, et al. Standardized myocardial segmentation and nomenclature for tomographic imaging of the heart. A statement for healthcare professionals from the Cardiac Imaging Committee of the Council on Clinical Cardiology of the American Heart Association. *Int J Cardiovasc Imaging.* 2002;18:539–542.
363. Voigt JU, Lindenmeier G, Exner B, et al. Incidence and characteristics of segmental postsystolic longitudinal shortening in normal, acutely ischemic, and scarred myocardium. *J Am Soc Echocardiogr.* 2003;16:415–423.
364. Vignon P. Hemodynamic assessment of critically ill patients using echocardiography Doppler. *Curr Opin Crit Care.* 2005;11:227–234.
365. Raitt MH, Kraft CD, Gardner CJ, et al. Subacute ventricular free wall rupture complicating myocardial infarction. *Am Heart J.* 1993;126:946–955.
366. Mittle S, Makaryus AN, Mangion J. Role of contrast echocardiography in the assessment of myocardial rupture. *Echocardiography.* 2003;20:77–81.
367. Bunch TJ, Oh JK, Click RL. Subepicardial aneurysm of the left ventricle. *J Am Soc Echocardiogr.* 2003;16:1318–1321.
368. Bybee KA, Kara T, Prasad A, et al. Systematic review: transient left ventricular apical ballooning: a syndrome that mimics ST-segment elevation myocardial infarction. *Ann Intern Med.* 2004;141:858–865.
369. Moursi MH, Bhatnagar SK, Vilacosta I, et al. Transesophageal echocardiographic assessment of papillary muscle rupture. *Circulation.* 1996;94:1003–1009.
370. Birnbaum Y, Chamoun AJ, Conti VR, et al. Mitral regurgitation following acute myocardial infarction. *Coron Artery Dis.* 2002;13:337–344.
371. Hanlon JT, Conrad AK, Combs DT, et al. Echocardiographic recognition of partial papillary muscle rupture. *J Am Soc Echocardiogr.* 1993;6:101–103.
372. Otto CM. *Textbook of Clinical Echocardiography.* 3rd ed. Philadelphia, PA: WB Saunders; 2007.
373. Libby P, Braunwald E. *Braunwald's Heart Disease: A Textbook of Cardiovascular Medicine.* 8th ed. Philadelphia, PA: Elsevier Saunders; 2007.

CHAPTER

26

Temperature Monitoring

TOSHIKI MIZOBE and DANIEL I. SESSLER

INTRODUCTION

Well before the dawn of clinical thermometry, the temperature course of diseases such as malaria and enteric fever (typhoid and brucellosis) was well described in the *Corpus Hippocraticum* (circa 370–460 BC) (1). However, it was not until the 1590s when the astronomer Galileo invented the thermometer (which he termed "thermoscope") that humans could record temperature.

In 1612, Sanctorius of Justipolitanus at Padua first used thermometry to measure human body temperature. A major advance in temperature monitoring came in 1714 when Gabriel Fahrenheit invented the mercury thermometer (2); his scale, Fahrenheit, remains commonly used in England and the United States. However, another scale, Centigrade, invented by Anders Celsius in 1742, became popular in France and Germany. On the original Celsius scale, 0 degree was the temperature at which water boiled while 100 degrees was the temperature at which ice melted; Linnaeus reversed the scale in 1750.

Carl Reinhold Wunderlich developed the thermometer that was used clinically for over 130 years (3). It differed from previous ones in preserving the maximum temperature in any given session, presumably the one best representing core temperature. He published *Das Verhalten der Eigenwarme in Krankheiten* in 1868 in which he importantly suggested that fever is not a disease, but rather a sign of disease. His thermometers were 22.5 cm long and took 20 minutes to register.

Wunderlich and his colleagues determined axillary temperature four to six times daily on some 25,000 patients (representing several million observations), establishing the fever patterns for pregnancy, as well as various diseases, such as typhoid. He also established average normal body temperature as 98.6°F (37°C). He concluded "A physician who practiced medicine without employing the thermometer was like a blind man endeavoring to distinguish colors by feeling."

Clinical thermometry thereafter became a routine part of medical practice. By the 1860s, the axilla had been universally adopted as a convenient and reliable point of measurement. Only after use of alcohol and other germicidal agents became common in the late 1890s did sublingual placement replace the axilla as the most popular measurement site.

In 1875, Von Liebermeister first hypothesized that body temperature is regulated similarly in healthy and ill people, but that fever occurs in illness because the body's internal thermostat is set to a higher temperature. Edward Seguin and William Draper introduced thermometry and patient charting in New York City hospitals in the mid-1860s. Medical thermometry quickly spread from hospitals to general practitioners, and from there to nurses and the lay public. Mothers who could read a thermometer rendered invaluable service to their families in times of illness and provided important information for physicians. Seguin even concluded that thermometry was not only knowledge, but also represented social power.

TYPES OF CLINICAL THERMOMETERS

Electronic Contact

A thermistor is an electrical resistor in which resistance changes rapidly in response to temperature fluctuation. In general, resistance decreases exponentially with increasing temperature. A tiny amount of electrical power is required for measuring the resistance and for calibrating stored data in order to convert resistance data into temperature data. Thermocouples measure temperature by evaluating the tiny electrical potential (voltage) produced by the junction of two metals. Both thermistors and thermocouples are inexpensive, with a manufacturing cost as low as a few cents each, and are highly accurate. These thermometers are now by far the most commonly used.

Most products display the maximum temperature and provide an audible tone when the temperature increases slowly to 0.1°C in a preset time, generally in 8 seconds. Under-reading occurs occasionally, especially when measuring axillary temperature where the dry skin requires a longer time to achieve thermal equilibrium with the sensor. Some devices provide a predictive mode that tracks the changing resistance to estimate the final temperature. This results in a rapid temperature reading within several seconds, but somewhat compromises accuracy.

Infrared Thermometers

Optical infrared emission sensors can be used to measure surface temperature. Industrially, these devices are used to measure the temperature of objects that would be hard to otherwise measure, such as temperature of molten steel. However, they are also used medically to measure skin temperature. The magnitude and spectrum of the infrared energy emitted depend on the local temperature, efficiency of the surface for radiating electromagnetic radiation (emissivity), the filtering effect of any optical components, and the sensor temperature; the resulting signal is converted into a temperature.

International standards permit a lower accuracy (±0.2°C) in laboratory testing of clinical infrared thermometers than the corresponding standards of conventional contact thermometers (±0.1°C). Even larger errors are permitted when the ambient temperature is out-of-normal room temperature, about 18° to 26°C. Virtually instantaneous measurements are a major advantage of this type of device.

Zero-Heat-Flux Thermometers

The concept of zero-heat-flux thermometry dates to 1971 when Fox and Solman (4) proposed a method to monitor deep body temperature from the intact skin surface by creating a region of zero heat flow across the shell of the body from the core, thus exteriorizing deep body temperature. In practice, zero-heat-flux thermometers consist of a thermal insulator

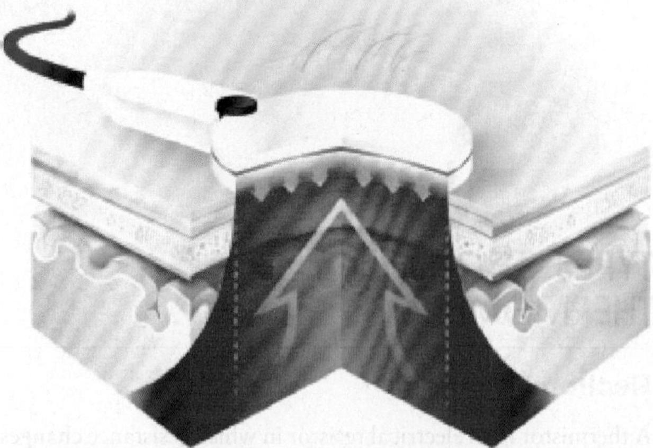

FIGURE 26.1 Zero-heat-flux cutaneous thermometer consists of a thermal insulator covered by an electric heater. The heater is servo-controlled to eliminate the heat flow through the insulator, at which point heater and skin temperatures are equal. Tissue temperature at the skin surface and just below the monitor must also be the same as subdermal temperature to avoid heat accumulation, which enables it to effectively measure tissue temperature approximately 1 to 2 cm below the skin surface. (From Eshraghi Y, Nasr V, Parra-Sanchez I, et al. An evaluation of a zero-heat-flux cutaneous thermometer in cardiac surgical patients. *Anesth Analg* 2014;119:543–549.)

attached to the skin which is covered by an electric heater that is servo-controlled to match temperature of the heater to temperature of the skin surface.

Because the Second Law of Thermodynamics specifies that heat can only flow down a temperature gradient, there can be no flow of heat across an insulating layer which has identical temperatures on the skin and ambient surfaces. The combination of the insulating layer and servo-controlled heater thus becomes a perfect insulator. Heat flowing from the core toward the skin surface thus cannot be dissipated through the monitor's insulating layer, and is reflected internally. After a suitable equilibration period, temperature of tissues 1 to 2 cm below the monitor resemble nearly equal temperature of deeper tissues (5). In appropriate body locations such as forehead and neck, temperature just below the skin surface is essentially core temperature (Fig. 26.1).

This device was originally manufactured in Japan with a heavy nondisposable probe that takes considerable time to reach thermal equilibrium (6). A new device is now available with a lightweight disposable probe that takes about 3 minutes to reach thermal equilibrium because of its low thermal mass (5). Forehead and neck zero-heat-flux thermometer measurements reflect core temperature in the pulmonary artery with a mean bias of −0.23° and −0.30°C, respectively. The average perioperative difference between forehead zero-heat-flux and pulmonary artery temperatures in elective cardiac surgery with CPB was −0.08° to −0.32°C, and 84% of measurements were within 0.5°C difference. It is likely that results are better in the target population of general surgical patients in whom temperature perturbations are lower and slower.

SITES OF TEMPERATURE MEASUREMENT

The core thermal compartment comprises well-perfused tissues whose temperature is uniform, and high, compared with the rest of the body. Core temperature is defined as the average temperature of the core compartment; it is not the highest temperature in the body, which may be found in the brain or liver. Core temperature can be evaluated in the pulmonary artery, distal esophagus, tympanic membrane with a contact probe, or nasopharynx with a probe inserted at least 10 cm.

The temperature equilibration rate between the blood and the organ measured is affected by various factors, such as the types of organ and the rate of temperature change. The average time lag between monitoring sites and the pulmonary artery (the gold standard) are reported as 5 minutes for the esophagus and forehead (zero-heat-flux measurement), 8 minutes for nasopharynx, 10 minutes for actual tympanic membrane, 15 minutes for rectum, and 20 minutes for bladder. Nasopharyngeal temperatures remain close to the brain temperature even during profound hypothermia, although the temperature gradients as large as 5°C have been observed between the brain and bladder and rectal temperatures (7).

The most common site of temperature measurement is probably under the tongue, at least in nonclinical environments. Unfortunately, hot and cold drinks, open-mouth versus close-mouth breathing, and tachypnea all affect oral temperature readings. However, nasogastric tubes do not interfere with oral temperature measurement (8–10). Carefully performed oral temperatures are remarkably accurate (11), while the accuracy of axillary temperature measurements is worse than at other sites, probably due to probe positioning (12). Axillary measurements are nonetheless usually suitable if care is taken to position the probe over the axillary artery and to keep the arm adducted.

Rectal temperature measurement is most accurate when the sensor is inserted more than 10 cm into the rectum; the rectal temperature correlates well with distal esophageal, bladder, and tympanic temperatures although, typically, it slightly exceeds the core value. However, this site responds slowly to rapid changes in body temperature (13). Consequently, rectal readings are often erroneous—sometimes by degrees—during heat stroke, malignant hyperthermia, and other situations where core temperature changes rapidly (14). It is thus a poor choice when, as usual, the purpose of monitoring is to detect rapid perturbations.

Tympanic membrane temperatures, obtained with a contact thermocouple or thermistor, are highly accurate core temperatures (15). By way of contrast, infrared aural canal "tympanic" temperatures do not actually evaluate the tympanic membrane and are far less accurate than actual tympanic membrane temperatures, thus possibly representing rather poorly the core temperature (16). Users must ensure that the aural canal is not obscured by cerumen and that the ear canal is straightened by manipulating the ear lobe so that the sensor can point directly at deeper sections of the canal which are nearer to core temperature (17). Even though infrared aural canal thermometers are often labeled as "tympanic," they do not actually "see" the tympanic membrane but extrapolate tympanic or core temperature from the skin temperature in the aural canal. Earphone-type infrared tympanic thermometer may work better than conventional infrared aural canal thermometers (18).

Distal esophageal temperature is an accurate core temperature monitoring site when patients are anesthetized or sedated, and the site is resistant to artifact (19). Probes are best situated in the lower third of the esophagus near the point of maximum heart sounds (about 45 cm from the nose in adults), but temperatures remain accurate over a broad range of insertion distances. Temperatures obtained from the proximal and mid-esophagus may be cooled by the ambient air because they are near the trachea and bronchi—although the artifact is generally small. Transesophageal echocardiography (TEE) may affect the esophageal temperature because heat is emitted by the probe. In intubated patients, the esophagus is usually the preferred temperature monitoring site since it provides true core temperature, measurements are easy to obtain using inexpensive probes, and the site is highly resistant to artifact.

Nasopharyngeal temperature monitoring is often used during general anesthesia or in adequately sedated patients. It is an excellent site and provides accurate and precise measurements of core temperature so long as probes are inserted at least 10 cm past the nares in adults. The nasopharynx is an excellent alternative to esophageal temperature and is sometimes preferable since access to the esophagus is restricted by laryngeal mask airways (20).

Urinary bladder temperature is measured by placing a probe in an indwelling urinary bladder catheter (IUBC). The measurement is affected by urinary flow during cardiopulmonary bypass and does not provide an accurate temperature measurement when urine flow is low (21). Under other circumstances, though, it is a reasonably accurate site.

Pulmonary artery temperature is measured by a sensor located at the distal end of the balloon-tipped, flow-directed pulmonary artery catheter. It is generally considered the single best core temperature measurement site, although obviously available in only a tiny fraction of patients. It is worth noting that brain temperature is slightly greater than pulmonary artery temperature, because core temperature at the pulmonary artery is the average value of the deep body structures. The gradient between core and brain temperatures tends to increase with fever and active cooling.

THERMOREGULATION

Precise control of core temperature is maintained by powerful thermoregulatory systems incorporating afferent inputs, central control, and efferent defenses. Efferent defenses can be broadly divided into autonomic responses (e.g., sweating and shivering) and behavioral responses (e.g., closing a window, putting on a sweater). Autonomic responses depend largely on core temperature and are mostly mediated by the anterior hypothalamus. In contrast, behavioral responses are roughly 50% determined by skin temperature and are controlled by the posterior hypothalamus (22).

Thermoregulation is maintained by feedforward and feedback pathways (23). Signals from cutaneous thermosensors that detect changes in environmental temperature are transmitted to the thermoregulatory center in the hypothalamus. The thermoregulatory center also receives signals from deep-tissue thermosensors which sense the body temperature. Effectors receiving efferent signals from the thermoregulatory center control thermoregulatory homeostasis. Recent studies suggest that the feedforward pathway may be more important than previously appreciated (Fig. 26.2).

Afferent Input

Dual detectors—cold sensors with myelinated A-δ fibers and warm sensors with unmyelinated C fibers—exist in the subcutaneous layer of the skin. The distribution density of cold sensors is several times greater than warm sensors. Skin temperature reflects a balance between body temperature and environmental conditions, thus serving as an "early warning" system for anticipated temperature changes to deeper tissues. Thermosensors are also located in brain areas such as the hypothalamus, midbrain, and spinal cord, and in deep thoracic and abdominal tissues. These deep sensors detect core body temperature.

TRP Channels as Putative Molecular Thermosensor

The transient receptor potential (TRP) channel superfamily in humans consists of 27 members that are subclassified into 6 subfamilies based on their sequence homology: TRPC (canonical), TRPV (vanilloid), TRPM (melastatin), TRPML (mucolipin), TRPP (polycystin), and TRPA (ankyrin). The TRP channel is a nonselective cation channel with six transmembrane domains, a pore-forming loop between the fifth and the sixth segments, and intracellular C-terminus and N-terminus (24).

Since finding the first temperature sensitive receptor, TRPV1 in 1997, 10 TRP channels (TRPV1, TRPV2, TRPV3, TRPV4,

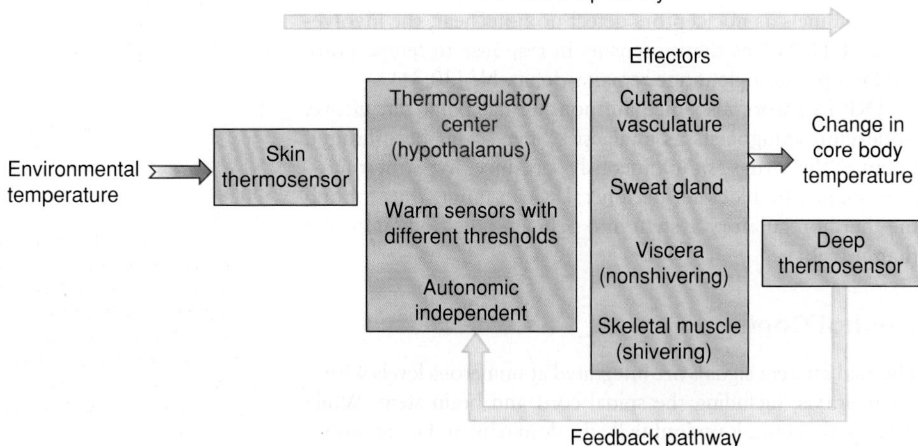

FIGURE 26.2 Thermoregulation. Signals from the cutaneous thermosensors detecting changes in environmental temperature are transmitted to the thermoregulatory center. The effectors receiving efferent signals control thermoregulatory homeostasis (feedforward). Also, the deep thermosensors detecting changes in body temperature transmit the afferent signals to the central controller (feedback).

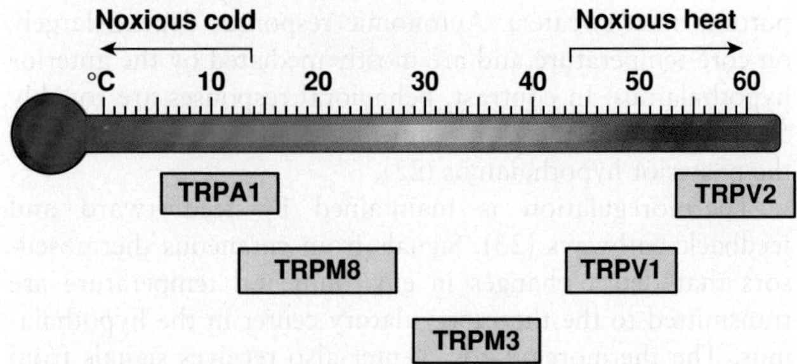

FIGURE 26.3 Temperature thresholds of five thermo-TRP channels on human sensory nerve. Although each thermo-TRP channel is activated within a narrow temperature range, these channels cumulatively cover a broad temperature range, from noxious cold (TRPA1 < 17°C) to noxious heat (TRPV2 > 52°C).

TRPM2, TRPM3, TRPM4, TRPM5, TRPM8, and TRPA1) have been reported to be highly temperature-sensitive. Furthermore, five of them—TRPV1, TRPV2, TRPM3, TRPM8, and TRPA1—are expressed on human sensory neurons (Fig. 26.3). Although each thermo-TRP channel is activated within a narrow temperature range; these channels cumulatively cover a broad temperature range, from noxious cold (TRPA1 < 17°C) to noxious heat (TRPV2 > 52°C). This feature strongly suggests that at least some thermo-TRP channels are the prime or sole molecular thermosensors responsible for the reception of peripheral temperature (25,26).

TRPV1 is expressed in A-δ and C fibers and is best characterized among TRP channels as the major receptor for capsaicin, one of the vanilloids, the spicy ingredient in hot chili peppers. As might be expected, TRPV1 antagonists cause hyperthermia as well as elevating the heat pain threshold in human patients (27).

In cultured neurons from TRPV1-deficient mice, no responses to heat (43° to 55°C) or capsaicin were observed, though heat responses at higher temperatures remained intact. Furthermore, these mice showed a longer latency to noxious heat, but normal latencies to pain stimuli (28). Subsequent studies revealed that TRP channels are polymodal nociception receptors that respond to various nociceptive stimuli such as membrane stretch, protons, and chemical ligands, as well as noxious heat. Hypothalamic TRPV1 channels are not activated at physiologically normal temperatures, as their response thresholds exceed 43°C (29).

Recent studies of TRP channels have indicated that additional TRP-independent mechanisms might play a major role in the transduction of physiologic thermal signals. Although TRP channels as nociceptors detect noxious heat, the involvement of TRPV1 as thermosensors in response to temperature within a physiologic range remains debatable (30,31).

TRP receptors also mediate nonthermal pain, but efforts to develop antagonists as analgesics have so far been limited because the drugs simultaneously produce hyperthermia—presumably, by blocking peripheral warm input, thus fooling the thermoregulatory system into believing the body is cooler than it truly is.

Central Control

Thermal afferent signals are integrated at numerous levels within the neuraxis, including the spinal cord and brain stem. While the hypothalamus is undoubtedly the dominant and most precise controller of body temperature, warm sensors are thought to mediate many of the stimulatory and inhibitory signals to effectors, as there are few cold sensors in the hypothalamus.

Core temperature varies with a daily circadian rhythm (32). Normal temperature is altered slightly by factors such as age (0.5°C lower in the elderly), time of day (1°C higher in the afternoon), time of menstrual cycle in women (higher near ovulation), and exercise (33). Nonetheless, core temperature is normally controlled to within a few tenths of a degree centigrade virtually irrespective of the environment (34). The thresholds triggering thermoregulatory defenses are uniformly about 0.3°C greater in women than in men, even during the follicular phase (34), and are an additional approximately 0.5°C greater during the luteal phase (35). However, men and women regulate core body temperature with comparable precision (Fig. 26.4).

Nonthermoregulatory cutaneous circulatory reflexes, including cardiopulmonary and arterial baroreceptor reflexes, modulate thermoregulatory vascular tone. Cardiopulmonary baroreceptor reflex controls peripheral vascular resistance in response to the change in blood volume through the central sympathetic nervous system and the renin–angiotensin pathway. The baroreceptor reflex is modified by the right atrial transmural pressure, which is the difference between central venous pressure and the intrathoracic pressure. Baroreflex loading, by increased right atrial pressure in patients placed in the leg-up position, results in an exaggeration of anesthesia-induced hypothermia because of attenuated peripheral vasoconstriction. In contrast, positive end-expiratory pressure (PEEP) ventilation decreases right atrial transmural pressure and, as a consequence, attenuates perioperative hypothermia (Fig. 26.5) (36,37).

Efferent Responses

The balance between heat production and heat loss determines body temperature; nonevaporative heat loss depends on the

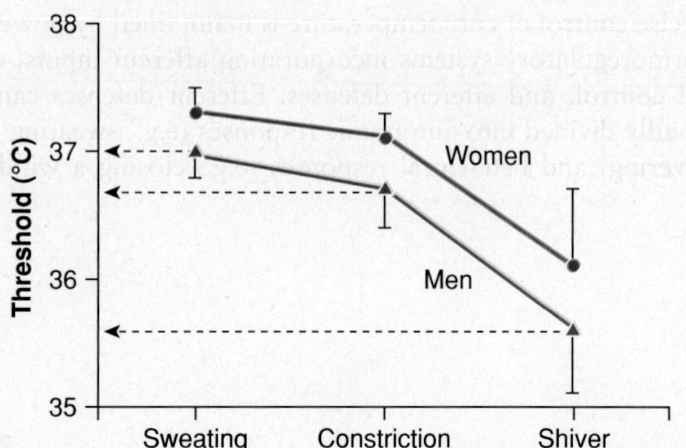

FIGURE 26.4 The thresholds (triggering core temperatures) for the three major autonomic thermoregulatory defenses: sweating, vasoconstriction, and shivering. Temperatures between the sweating and vasoconstriction threshold define the interthreshold range, temperatures not triggering autonomic responses. The thresholds are uniformly about 0.3°C greater during the follicular phase in women than in men, and are an additional ≈0.5°C greater during the luteal phase. However, men and women regulate core body temperature with comparable precision. Results are presented as means ±SD. (From Lopez M, Sessler DI, Walter K, et al. Rate and gender dependence of the sweating, vasoconstriction, and shivering thresholds in humans. *Anesthesiology* 1994;80:780–788.)

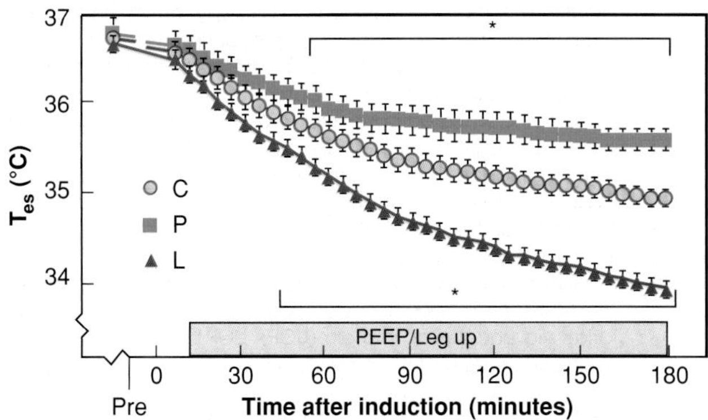

FIGURE 26.5 The esophageal temperature (T_{es}) after induction of anesthesia. Positive end-expiratory pressure (PEEP: 10 cm H_2O, P) or the leg-up position (L) was applied 10 minutes after induction of anesthesia. Baroreflex loading due to leg-up position exaggerates anesthesia-induced hypothermia because peripheral vasoconstriction is attenuated. Meanwhile, PEEP attenuated perioperative hypothermia because of stimulated vasoconstriction through baroreceptor unloading. Values are shown as mean ± SE. Significant difference compared with the control group (C). (From Nakajima Y, Mizobe T, Takamata A, Tanaka Y. Baroreflex modulation of peripheral vasoconstriction during progressive hypothermia in anesthetized humans. *Am J Physiol Regul Integr Comp Physiol* 2000;279:R1430–1436.)

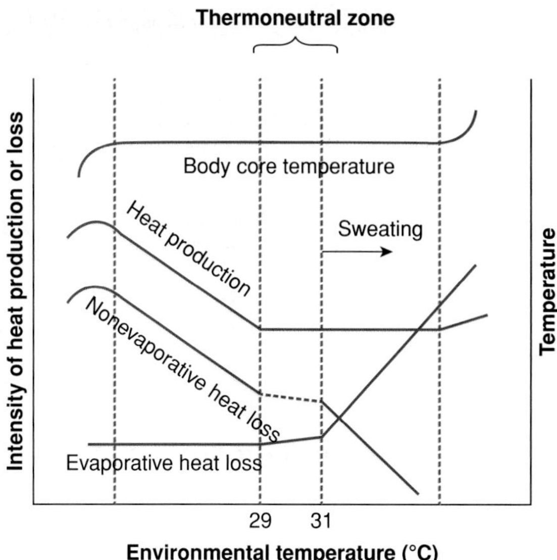

FIGURE 26.6 The thermoneutral zone is defined as the environmental temperature zone in which skin vascular tonus alone can maintain body temperature. The environmental temperature at which heat production increases, the lower critical temperature is 29°C; while the temperature at which evaporative heat loss starts, the upper critical temperature is 31°C.

difference between skin temperature and environmental temperature. Given that skin blood flow is a primary determinant of skin temperature—increased blood flow results in increased skin temperature—cutaneous vascular tone modulates heat loss. But when environmental temperature exceeds body temperature, evaporative heat loss—sweating—is the only way to lose heat.

Sweating is mediated by postganglionic cholinergic nerves that terminate on sweat follicles (38); these follicles apparently have no purpose other than thermoregulation. In this regard, they differ from most other thermoregulatory effectors that appear to have been co-opted by the thermoregulatory system but continue to play other important roles, such as vasomotion in blood pressure control and skeletal muscles in postural maintenance. Heat exposure can increase cutaneous water loss from trivial amounts to 500 mL/hr. Sweat loss in trained athletes can even exceed 1 L/hr. The process is remarkably effective, dissipating 0.58 kcal/g of evaporated sweat. In a dry, convective environment, sweating can thus dissipate enormous amounts of heat—perhaps up to 10 times the basal metabolic rate.

Cutaneous vasoconstriction is the first autonomic response to cold; metabolic heat is lost primarily via convection and radiation from the skin surface, and vasoconstriction reduces this loss. Active arteriovenous shunt vasoconstriction is adrenergically mediated. The shunts are vessels 100 μm in diameter and thus convey 10,000 times as much blood as a comparable length of 10-μm capillaries (laminar flow increases by the fourth power of radius) (39). Anatomically, they are restricted to the fingers, toes, nose, and nipples. Despite this restriction, shunt vasoconstriction is among the most commonly used and important thermoregulatory defenses. Roughly 10% of cardiac output (CO) traverses dilated arteriovenous shunts; consequently, shunt vasoconstriction increases mean arterial pressure by approximately 15 mmHg.

A major purpose of thermoregulatory vasoconstriction is to isolate core tissues from the environment and thus restrict peripheral-to-core heat transfer. The normal threshold (triggering core temperature) for vasoconstriction is approximately 36.5°C (34). Thermoregulatory vasoconstriction is more effective than might be imagined, but when environmental temperature is very low, heat production must increase if thermal homeostasis is to be maintained because maximal cutaneous vasoconstriction cannot compensate for the amount of heat loss. The *thermoneutral zone* can be defined as the range of environmental temperature over which cutaneous vasomotion alone can maintain body temperature (Fig. 26.6). The environmental temperature at which heat production increases, the lower critical temperature is about 19°C; while the temperature at which evaporative heat loss starts, the upper critical temperature is about 31°C.

In humans, shivering is the final autonomic response to be activated by cold exposure and is generally only observed when behavioral responses and vasoconstriction fail to maintain an adequate core temperature. The shivering threshold is approximately 35.5°C (34), which is about 1°C less than the vasoconstriction threshold. Shivering begins with the pectoralis muscles, but most shivering thermogenesis occurs in the extremities where the largest muscles are located. Typically, vigorous shivering doubles the metabolic rate (40,41), although greater increases can be sustained briefly (42,43).

An obvious consequence of shivering is the increased metabolic rate. This increase, which is analogous to exercise, provokes a substantial adrenergic response. For example, a reduction in core temperature of only 0.7°C increases norepinephrine (NE) concentration by 400% and oxygen consumption by 30%. When core temperature decreases to 1.3°C, NE concentration increases 700% and oxygen consumption doubles. As might be expected, shivering is associated with peripheral vasoconstriction and hypertension—although heart rate remains unchanged, as do plasma epinephrine and cortisol concentrations (44).

The interaction between thermal input, central control, and effector responses is shown in Figure 26.7, which also shows

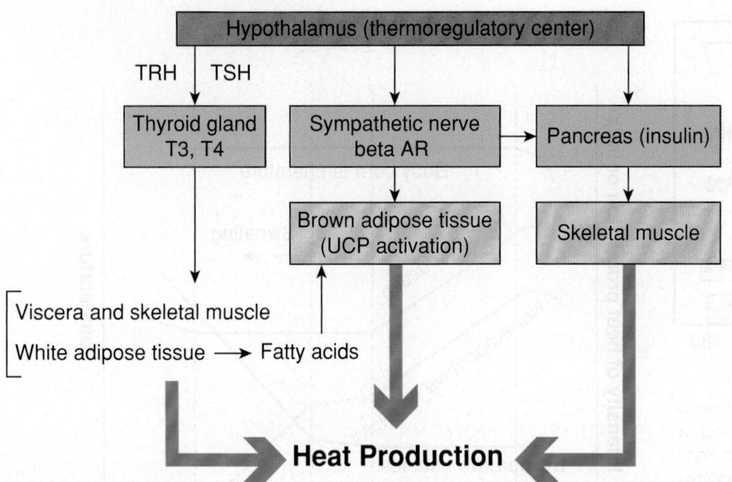

FIGURE 26.7 Thermoregulation and energy metabolism. In the sympathetic nervous system, norepinephrine (NE) is a primary neurotransmitter to activate beta-adrenergic receptor on the targeted organs (beta-2 receptors on the viscera, skeletal muscle and white adipose tissue (WAT); and beta-3 receptors on brown adipose tissue (BAT). The sympathetic nervous system also induces insulin secretion from pancreas which results in activated protein synthesis in skeletal muscles. Thyroid hormone stimulates oxidative phosphorylation and ATP synthesis in the mitochondria, which results in the activated energy metabolism in the targeted tissues. Also, thyroid hormone promotes thermogenesis by uncoupling oxidative phosphorylation via uncoupling protein (UCP). UCP1, expressed only in the mitochondria of BAT, facilitates the reflux of protons across the mitochondria down the proton gradient, bypasses ATP synthesis, and generates heat. Expression of UCP1 is required for BAT thermogenesis, and free fatty acids released from WAT serve as the main fuel for thermogenesis in BAT. Thermogenic capacity of BAT is reported about 344 W/kg whereas that of nonspecific tissue is about 4.1 W/kg.

the normal values for the major autonomic response thresholds. In the elderly, the vasoconstriction threshold is reduced (45). Similarly, the shivering threshold is significantly reduced in the elderly (46). Interestingly, abnormally reduced thresholds were not apparent in subjects less than 80 years of age, and even then in only a fraction of the population (Fig. 26.8).

The most powerful inhibitors of thermoregulation are general anesthetics. These drugs have been used to facilitate induction of hypothermia for cardiac surgery and during neurosurgery. In sufficient doses, especially when combined with neuromuscular blockers, anesthetics can essentially obliterate defenses against hypothermia.

Volatile anesthetics, such as desflurane and sevoflurane, have relatively little effect on sweating: even full anesthetic doses increase the sweating threshold by only about 0.5°C. In contrast, anesthetic gases markedly reduce the vasoconstriction and shivering thresholds. Interestingly, the threshold for each major cold defense is reduced synchronously, as if they are similarly controlled (Fig. 26.9) (47).

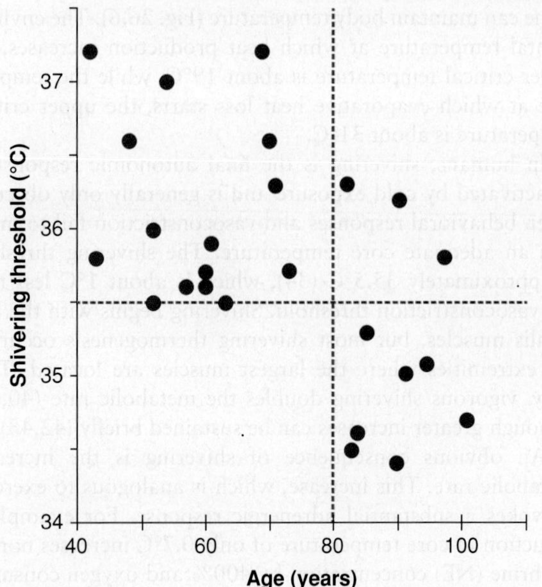

FIGURE 26.8 The effect of aging on the shivering threshold. Fifteen patients less than 80 years old (58 ± 10 year) (mean ± SD) shivered at 36.1 ± 0.6°C; in contrast, 10 patients aged 80 years or older (89 ± 7 year) shivered at a significantly lower mean temperature, 35.2 ± 0.8°C ($P < 0.001$). The shivering thresholds in 7 of the 10 patients 80 years or older was less than 35.5°C, whereas the threshold equaled or exceeded this value in all the younger patients. (From Vassilieff N, Rosencher N, Sessler DI, et al. The shivering threshold during spinal anesthesia is reduced in the elderly. *Anesthesiology* 1995;83:1162–1166.)

Neuromuscular blockers are not believed to have any effect on central control of thermoregulatory responses. But they obviously cause paralysis and thus prevent shivering. It is equally obvious though that muscle relaxants can only be given in the context of general anesthesia or substantial sedation and that paralyzed patients require mechanical ventilation. Muscle relaxants can be used as a treatment for shivering in intensive care units (48), but are not a substitute for adequate sedation and appropriate thermal management.

Thermogenesis and Energy Metabolism

All tissues generate heat which helps maintain body core temperature, especially the liver, brain, skeletal muscle, and brown adipose tissue (BAT). Most heat generation is simply a byproduct of organs doing their intended work. But to a modest extent, thermogenesis is regulated by the thermoregulatory center in the hypothalamus through both the sympathetic nervous and endocrine hypothalamic pituitary systems (Fig. 26.7). The two systems are known to regulate various metabolic processes in a synergistic and complementary fashion (49).

In the sympathetic nervous system, NE is the primary neurotransmitter to activate the beta-adrenergic receptor on target organs (beta-2 receptors on the viscera, skeletal muscle, and white adipose tissue (WAT); and beta-3 receptors on BAT). But the sympathetic nervous system also induces insulin secretion from pancreas which results in activated protein synthesis in skeletal muscles. Thyroid hormone, controlled primary by thyrotropin-releasing hormone (TRH) from the hypothalamus and secondary by thyroid-stimulating hormone (TSH) from the pituitary gland, binds with its intranuclear receptor in the target organs. Local activation of circulating serum thyroxine (T4) to the active form of triiodothyronine (T3), converted by the iodothyronine deiodinase type 2 (D2) with no change in the serum concentration of T3, is a main mechanism of thyroid hormone regulation.

D2, expressed in key thyroid-targeting tissue, is the primary enzyme responsible for the intracellular T3 regulation. Increased intracellular T3 stimulates oxidative phosphorylation and ATP

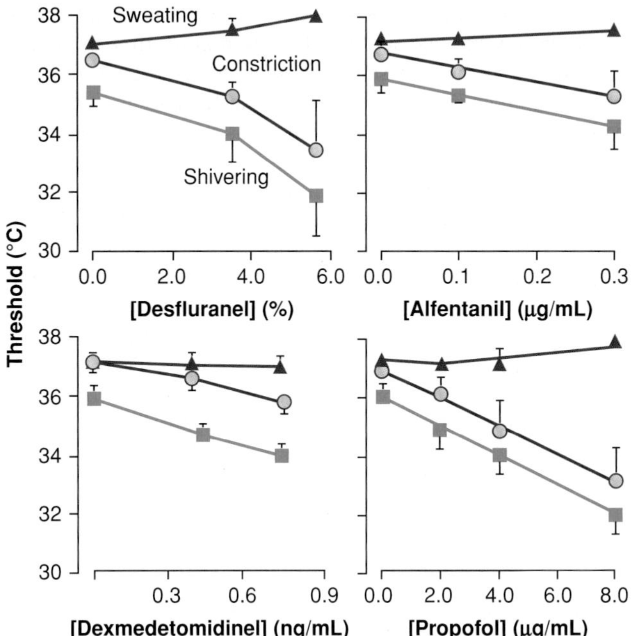

FIGURE 26.9 Concentration-dependent thermoregulatory inhibition by desflurane and isoflurane (halogenated volatile anesthetics), propofol (an intravenous anesthetic), and alfentanil (a μ-agonist opioid). General anesthetics are the most powerful known inhibitors of thermoregulatory control. The horizontal axis, in each case, spans a clinically relevant concentration range. The sweating (*triangles*), vasoconstriction (*circles*), and shivering (*squares*) thresholds are expressed in terms of core temperature at a designated mean skin temperature of 34°C. Anesthesia linearly, but slightly, increases the sweating threshold. In contrast, anesthesia produces substantial and comparable linear or non-linear decreases in the vasoconstriction and shivering thresholds. Typical anesthetic concentrations thus increase the interthreshold range (difference between the sweating and vasoconstriction thresholds) approximately 20-fold from its normal value near 0.2°C. Patients do not activate autonomic thermoregulatory defenses unless body temperature exceeds the interthreshold range; surgical patients are thus poikilothermic over a 3° to 5°C range of core temperatures. Isoflurane, 1%, and desflurane, 6%, have comparable anesthetic potency. Error bars smaller than the data markers have been deleted. (From Sessler DI. Perioperative hypothermia. *N Engl J Med* 1997;336:1730–1737. Copyright ©1997 Massachusetts Medical Society. Reprinted with permission from Massachusetts Medical Society.)

synthesis in the mitochondria which enhances energy metabolism. T3 also promotes thermogenesis by uncoupling oxidative phosphorylation via uncoupling protein (UCP). UCP1, expressed only in the mitochondria of BAT, facilitates the reflux of protons across mitochondria membranes; pumping protons back across the membrane is an ATP-requiring process that generates heat. Expression of UCP1 is required for BAT thermogenesis, which is synergistically regulated by both NE and T3. Unlike organs and other human tissues, heat production by BAT is entirely facultative.

Humans have both subcutaneous and visceral BAT. Recent studies using CT and PET imaging reveal substantial amounts of BAT in the subscapular, supraclavicular, and chest regions in adults (50), with younger and leaner subjects having more BAT. Also, cold exposure activates BAT within minutes, which is inhibited by beta-adrenergic antagonists. Persistent cold exposure affects BAT, resulting in increased expression of UCP1, increased mitochondria, and hyperplasia and hypertrophy via the sympathetic nervous system. In this process, free fatty acids released from WAT serve as the main fuel for thermogenesis in BAT. Thermogenic capacity of BAT is reported about 344 W/kg whereas that of nonspecific tissue is about 4.1 W/kg. Nonetheless, BAT contributes only small amounts to total metabolic heat production in adults and if it is clinically important, probably contributes more to long-term homeostasis (body weight stability) than protection against cold exposure.

TARGETED TEMPERATURE MANAGEMENT

Targeted temperature management (TTM), historically referred to as therapeutic hypothermia, is a clinical concept of therapeutic hypothermia followed by induced normothermia. However, it can also refer to fever prevention. While potentially applicable to most any tissue, clinical use has focused on the brain and heart (51).

Cardiac Arrest

Postcardiac arrest syndrome includes three characteristic phases of injury, largely identified in animal studies (Fig. 26.10). The first is the intra-arrest ischemic injury phase; it is due to absent

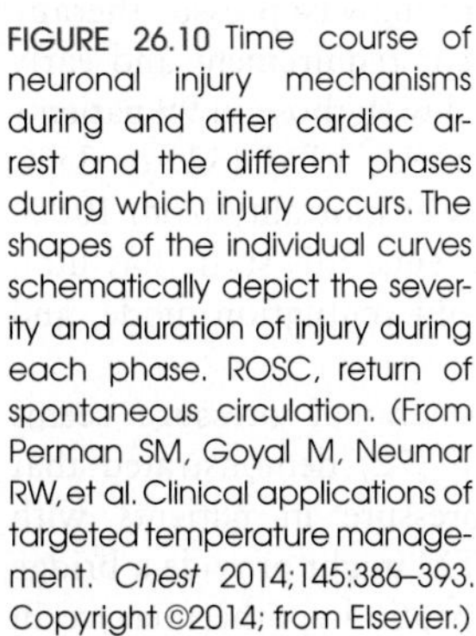

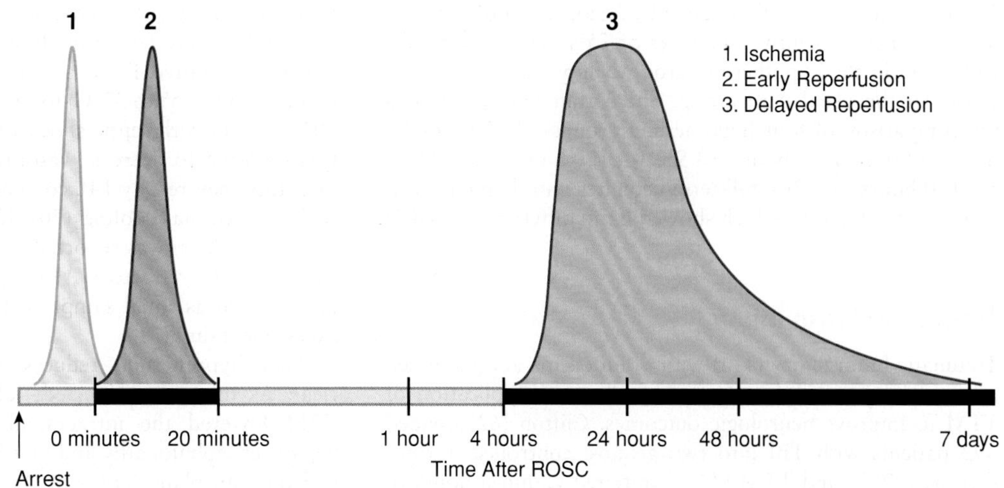

FIGURE 26.10 Time course of neuronal injury mechanisms during and after cardiac arrest and the different phases during which injury occurs. The shapes of the individual curves schematically depict the severity and duration of injury during each phase. ROSC, return of spontaneous circulation. (From Perman SM, Goyal M, Neumar RW, et al. Clinical applications of targeted temperature management. *Chest* 2014;145:386–393. Copyright ©2014; from Elsevier.)

blood flow, and results in energy failure, ischemic depolarization of cell membrane, release of excitatory amino acids, and cytosolic calcium overload. With return of spontaneous circulation, early reperfusion is associated with reactive oxygen generation and mitochondria calcium overload, which triggers apoptosis pathways. The delayed reperfusion phase is characterized by subsequent neuronal calcium overload, activation of pathologic proteases, and systemic inflammation. Each phase is regarded as a potential target of TTM with different therapeutic windows.

The first convincing human evidence for TTM was provided by two major clinical trials published in 2002 in patients who recovered spontaneous circulation after out-of-hospital cardiac arrest (CA). Forty-nine percent of patients randomized to TTM (33°C for 12 hours) were reported to have good neurologic outcomes at hospital discharge, compared with just 26% of patients with standard postarrest care (52). Furthermore, 55% of patients assigned to TTM (32° to 34°C for 24 hours) showed favorable neurologic outcomes 6 months after hospital discharge, compared with 39% patients of standard postarrest care (53). These two landmark studies were the basis for various guidelines that have defined the protocol framework of TTM as 32° to 34°C of target temperature with 12 to 24 hours duration (54,56).

Surprisingly, Nielsen et al. (57) reported in 2013 that hypothermia at a targeted temperature of 33°C did not show any benefits (overall mortality, or neurologic function at 180 days), as compared with a targeted temperature of 36° C in 950 comatose patients of out-of-hospital CA. This large trial included more patients than all previous randomized studies of TTM for CA and must thus be considered definitive. While no benefit was identified, no harm was apparent either at a targeted temperature of 33°C. The investigators suggest that controlling body temperature at 36°C, instead of allowing fever, may have been protective in the control group. Current evidence from large RCTs thus does not suggest that therapeutic hypothermia should be used routinely for out-of-hospital CA. But additional research is clearly necessary, and already in progress.

Neonatal Encephalopathy

In two randomized controlled trials of neonatal encephalopathy (239 and 325 infants, respectively) of TTM at 33.5°C for 72 hours, neither demonstrated reduced disability or death at 1.5 to 2 years (58,59). Subsequently, Azzopardi (60) reported improved neurocognitive outcomes of 75 survivors in middle childhood in the hypothermia group compared with 52 survivors in the usual care group. Shankaran (61) performed the comparison of four hypothermia groups—33.5°C for 72 hours, 32.0°C for 72 hours, 33.5°C for 120 hours, and 32.0°C for 120 hours—on 364 full-term neonates with hypoxic ischemic encephalopathy, which showed in no difference in NICU death.

Traumatic Brain Injury

Traumatic brain injury (TBI) with brain edema and increased intracranial pressure is associated with good application of TTM to improve neurologic outcomes. Clifton (62) divided 392 patients with TBI into two groups: controlled normothermia (37°C) and TTM (33°C) initiated within 6 hours of injury and maintained for 48 hours. There was no difference in Glasgow Outcome Score scale at 6 months after the injury between the groups. A subsequent randomized trial to investigate the efficacy of very early cooling for patients with TBI was stopped after a preliminary analysis showed no possibility of benefit (63).

A multicenter international trial assigned 225 children with severe TBI to either hypothermia therapy (32.5°C for 24 hours) initiated within 8 hours after injury, or to normothermia (37°C). At 6 months, 31% of the patients in the hypothermia group, as compared with 22% in the normothermia group, showed unfavorable outcomes ($p = 0.14$), such as severe disability and persistent vegetative state. There were 23 deaths (21%) in the hypothermia group and 14 deaths (12%) in the normothermia group ($p = 0.06$). Hypothermia therapy to pediatric TBI thus does not improve the neurologic outcomes or mortality (64).

Acute Myocardial Infarction

It is well established that hypothermia limits infarct size in animal models when initiated before or shortly after reperfusion (65,66). However, infarct sizes at 30 days were similar in 20 cooled and 21 normothermic patients (67). Furthermore, the Intravascular Cooling Adjunctive to Percutaneous Coronary Intervention (Part 1) (ICE-IT-1) showed no difference in door-to-balloon time or infarct size in patients randomized to TTM versus normothermia (68).

Aneurysm Surgery

To evaluate the effect of intraoperative cooling during open craniotomy in patients with subarachnoid hemorrhage (SAH), 1,001 patients were randomly assigned to intraoperative hypothermia (targeted core temperature of 33°C) and normothermia (targeted core temperature of 36.5°C). There were no differences in Glasgow Outcome Scores 90 days after surgery in the two groups. Nor were there differences in the duration of ICU stay, total length of hospitalization, or mortality. However, postoperative bacteremia was more common in patients assigned to hypothermia (5% vs. 3%) (69).

Other Potential Indications

Limited data suggest that hypothermia may prove beneficial for other indications. However, these applications of TTM remain largely speculative. For example, fever control to achieve normothermia (36.5° to 37°C) for 48 hours by external cooling in 101 patients with septic shock requiring vasopressor therapy was reported to decrease vasopressor requirement and early mortality (before Day 14), compared with those in 99 patients with no external cooling (70). In 1993, TTM (32° to 35°C for several days) was reported to lower mortality from 100% to 67% in 19 refractory ARDS patients; this study has limitations such as small sample size, old ventilation mode, and excess mortality (71).

That hypothermia reduces intracranial pressure seems clear. As might be expected, Jalan (72) demonstrated that TTM lowered the intracranial pressure in patients with hepatic encephalopathy and that TTM might provide a bridge to liver transplant. Trials of therapeutic hypothermia are in progress for stroke, sepsis, and various other conditions. A recent large trial, though, demonstrated worse long-term outcomes in patients with critical intracranial hypertension who were randomized to hypothermia—even though hypothermia reduced intracranial pressure.

Systemic Consequences of Hypothermia

Heart rate decreases during hypothermia because metabolic rate is reduced 6% per degree Centigrade. Bradycardia is mediated by a decrease in diastolic repolarization in the sinus node. Systemic vascular resistance increases, stroke volume remains normal, and CO decreases by 25% to 40% simply due to the reduction in heart rate; consequently, mean arterial blood pressure remains normal. A heart rate of 40 beats/min at 32°C is, therefore, perfectly normal and does not require treatment.

Mild hypothermia reportedly impairs left ventricular diastolic, but not systolic, function with decreased CO in anesthetized dogs (73). Trials of therapeutic hypothermia depends on prevention of hypovolemia, especially during induction of cooling, due to hypothermia-induced cold diuresis by increased venous return through increased systemic resistance as well as increased atrial natriuretic peptide and decreased reabsorption in the kidney. Hypovolemia is often accompanied by a rising plasma sodium concentration and consequent increase in osmolality.

The electrocardiogram of hypothermic patients often displays a notch on the downstroke of the QRS complex (Fig. 26.11), when core temperature reaches 33°C (74,75). However, cardiac dysrhythmias are rarely seen during therapeutic hypothermia, even in patients with myocardial ischemia (76). Profound hypothermia (<28°C), combined with electrolyte disorders, increases dysrhythmias such as atrial fibrillation, followed by ventricular tachycardia or ventricular fibrillation.

Overall, hypothermia has little effect on the respiratory system. Minute ventilation decreases during therapeutic hypothermia, but $PaCO_2$ remains normal because the metabolic rate decreases as well (77).

Circulating leukocyte concentrations decrease during hypothermia, and leukocytes become less effective (78). Impaired host defense may contribute to pneumonia risk, especially when therapeutic hypothermia exceeds 24 hours. Hypothermia inhibits the secretion of proinflammatory cytokines, impairs leukocyte migration, and reduces phagocytosis. Although infections are a common complication of therapeutic hypothermia, a systematic review and meta-analysis suggest that no increase in the overall risk of infection, such as pneumonia and sepsis (79). Nevertheless, fever is independently linked to adverse neurologic outcomes, increased hospital stay, and higher mortality in patients with neurologic injury (80). During hypothermia and controlled normothermia, blood is usually cultured daily because therapeutic hypothermia blunts symptoms of infection, including fever.

Prolonged hypothermia also decreases the number and function of platelets (<35°C) and delays clotting time (<33°C) (81). Even mild hypothermia increases blood loss and transfusion requirement in perioperative patients (82), but patients selected for TTM rarely have active bleeding. Perhaps consequently, no RCT has reported an increased risk of bleeding associated with therapeutic hypothermia. The bleeding risk in patients without active bleeding is thus considered low during therapeutic hypothermia (83,84).

During induction of therapeutic hypothermia, potassium shifts from the plasma into cells resulting in hypokalemia. However, caution should be used in correcting this condition because during rewarming potassium shifts back into the plasma which might lead to life-threatening hyperkalemia. Presumably, the risk of electrolyte disturbances is reduced by slow rewarming; phosphate concentration decreases similarly (85,86).

Urine output increases at induction of hypothermia as a result of decreased reabsorption in the ascending loop of Henle. It normalizes, however, when the patient reaches the target temperature (87). Volume status, potassium, and phosphate concentrations thus each require careful monitoring during therapeutic hypothermia. Hypomagnesemia is associated with poor neurologic outcome and increased mortality (88), and magnesium supplementation appears to improve neurologic outcome in SAH (89,90).

Although plasma lactate concentrations often increase to the maximum of 5 to 6 mMol/L in the induction phase of therapeutic hypothermia, probably due to vasoconstriction induced by hypothermia, these values remain stable in the maintenance phase. Among routine laboratory values,

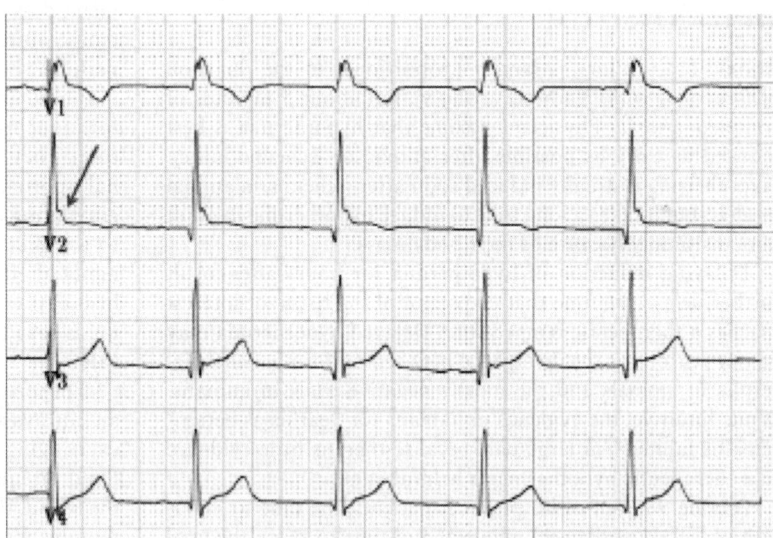

FIGURE 26.11 Electrocardiogram (EKG) changes during hypothermia treatment at a core temperature of 35.9°C. Note the slightly prolonged PR interval, slight widening of the QRS complex, increased QT interval, and Osborn wave (*arrow*). (From Polderman KH, Herold I. Therapeutic hypothermia and controlled normothermia in the intensive care unit: practical considerations, side effects, and cooling methods. *Crit Care Med* 2009;37:1101–1120. Copyright ©2009; with permission from Elsevier.)

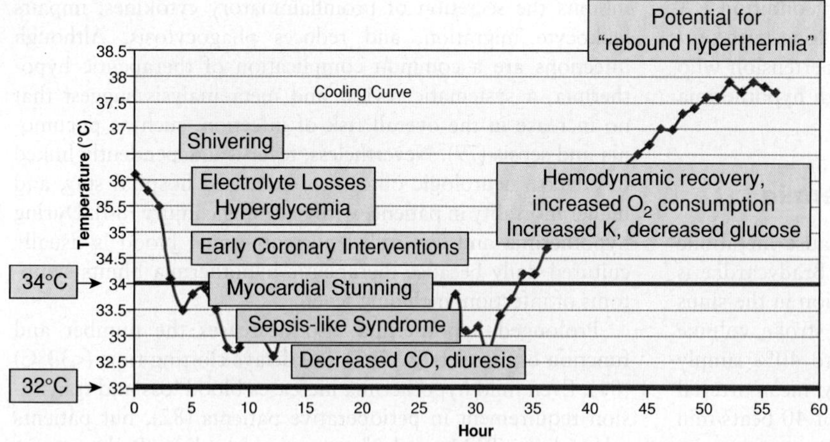

FIGURE 26.12 TTM-induced physiologic changes and resuscitation opportunities. Phase-specific physiologic findings have been observed during TTM. (From Perman SM, Goyal M, Neumar RW, et al. Clinical applications of targeted temperature management. *Chest* 2014;145:386–933. Copyright ©2014; with permission from Elsevier.)

mild increases in liver enzymes and serum amylase are often observed.

Severe hyperglycemia was thought to be associated with increased morbidity and mortality in critically ill patients (91,92). However, the most recent major study, NICE-SUGAR, currently concluded that a blood glucose target of 180 mg or less resulted in lower mortality than a target of 81 to 108 mg in critically ill patients (93). The optimal glucose concentration during therapeutic hypothermia remains unknown.

Mild hypothermia is associated with hyperglycemia, blood glucose variability, and increased insulin requirement. Enhanced glucose variability is a predictor of in-hospital mortality, independent of injury severity and mean blood glucose levels (94); whether controlling glucose improves outcomes remains to be determined.

The duration-of-action and plasma concentrations of most sedatives and analgesics, including neuromuscular blocking (NMB) agents, increase during hypothermia. The increase appears due to reduced activity of liver enzymes, reduced hepatic perfusion, and reduced biliary excretion of drugs (95,97). Typically, drug metabolism decreases by about a third at 34°C (98).

There are three clinical phases of TTM: induction phase, maintenance phase, and rewarming phase. Phase-specific adverse effects and physiologic changes are summarized in Figure 26.12 (51).

When to Start TTM

Anoxic brain injury is largely proportional to the duration of ischemia, with death occurring within about 5 minutes of complete anoxia. Physicians assume that hypothermia is best induced as early as possible after anoxic or ischemic injury. Hypothermia is usually induced soon after ischemia in animal models, but it takes a long time to induce hypothermia in adult humans simply because of their body mass.

Delaying induction of hypothermia for hours after insult further delays the time that elapses until the tissue-of-interest reaches a therapeutic temperature. Delayed hypothermia may be one reason for the divergence between uniformly beneficial results in animals and the mostly negative trials in humans. While intuitive, the evidence in humans for "earlier is better" remains limited—in large part because there is little evidence that therapeutic hypothermia is helpful at all.

Among 986 out-of-hospital CA patients, the time to initiation of TTM (median 90 minutes) and time to reach the goal temperature (<34°C, 260 minutes) was not associated with outcome (99). However, Mooney (100) reported that a 20% increase in the risk of death was observed for every hour of delay to initiation of TTM in 140 out-of-hospital CA patients. Using the International CA Registry (INTCAR) database (172 out-of-hospital CA patients), the odds of a poor neurologic outcome at transfer from ICU, as well as at hospital discharge and at postdischarge follow-up, increased with each 5-minute delay in initiating TTM (with a mean time of 94 minutes). Furthermore, the odds of a poor neurologic outcome at postdischarge follow-up increased for every 30-minute delay in time to target temperature (with a mean time of 309 minutes) (101). One trial specifically attempted to determine whether prehospital cooling improved outcomes after resuscitation after CA ($n = 1{,}364$). Prehospital cooling reduced core temperature at hospital arrival by 1.2°C and reduced the time to reach 34°C by about 1 hour, but it did not improve survival or neurologic status (102).

Cooling Methods

There is a general consensus that rapid infusion of 1 to 2 L of lactated Ringer solution at 4°C should be the initial cooling strategy in most patients. Each liter of fluid at 4°C reduces mean body temperature by 0.5°C in a 70-kg adult. However, the cooling is initially restricted to the core thermal compartment, thus producing about twice that much reduction in core temperature until heat redistributes between the core and peripheral thermal compartments (103).

There are various commercially available cooling devices for inducing hypothermia and maintaining targeted temperature. They can generally be divided into surface and internal approaches. Surface cooling is often accomplished with circulating cool water or cold packs (i.e., ice or gel), applied to the skin surface with various sorts of pads. Key determinants of efficacy are the amount of surface area covered and heat extraction efficiency of particular systems. Surface cooling is easy to initiate, relatively inexpensive, and presumably safe.

The principal alternative approach to surface cooling is an intravascular cooling system using central venous heat exchanging catheters through which cold fluid circulates. Fluid circulating through these catheters extracts heat from the blood, thus directly cooling the core. Endovascular cooling requires insertion of a relatively large central venous catheter

TABLE 26.1 The Characteristics of Cooling Methods

Phase of TTM	Parameter	Conventional	BR	CC	AS	CG
Induction	Noninvasive	O	O	O	O	X
	Cooling rate	X	O	X	O	O
	Mean °C/hr	0.32	1.33	0.18	1.04	1.46
Maintenance	Stability	X	X	X	X	O
	%	69.8	50.5	74.1	44.2	3.2
	Convenience of control	Cumbersome	Manual	Manual	Automatic	Automatic

Note: Stability is defined as the percentage of time the patient's temperature was 0.2°C below or above the targeted temperature.
Conventional, ice cold fluids and ice/cold packs; BR, water-circulating cooling system; CC, air-circulating cooling system; AS, gel-coated cooling system; CG, intravascular cooling system.
From Hoedemaekers CW, Ezzahti M, Gerritsen A, et al. Comparison of cooling methods to induce and maintain normothermia and hypothermia in intensive care unit patients: a prospective intervention study. *Crit Care* 2007;11:R91.

and is thus invasive and poses at least some risk. These systems also tend to be expensive. On the other hand, they directly cool the core and rapidly extract heat (104).

Hoedemaekers (105) compared the efficacy of several cooling devices for TTM (Table 26.1). The cooling rate was significantly higher with the water-circulating garments, gel-pads, and intravascular cooling systems than with the conventional cooling system or convective air cooling. After reaching the target temperature, core temperatures were out of range (±0.2°C), just 3.2% of the time with intravascular cooling which was far less than with any of the other cooling methods.

Intravascular cooling was compared with the water-circulating surface cooling in 167 CA patients (106). Time from CA to achieving 34°C was comparable with each device (270 minutes for intravascular vs. 273 minutes for gel-coated external cooling). Time from cooling initiation to a core temperature of 34°C was also similar, and there was no significant difference in survival with good neurologic function, either to hospital discharge or at follow-up after 6 to 12 months. There were significantly more episodes of continuous hyperglycemia in the external cooling group (70% vs. 48%), and significantly more hypomagnesemia in the intravascular cooling group (37% vs. 18%). The amount of shivering was similar in each group, probably because sufficient sedation was provided.

The same devices were also compared in the 80 other CA patients (107). There was no significant difference in neuron-specific enolase (a biomarker of brain injury) concentration at 72 hours, or clinical outcome between the two devices. The target temperature of 33°C was maintained more stable in the intravascular group (33.0° vs. 32.7°C). Bleeding complications were more frequent with the intravascular cooling system (44% vs. 18%).

Sedatives/Analgesics and Neuromuscular Blocking Agents

No current guidelines make specific recommendations for sedatives, analgesics, or muscle relaxants (54–56); whether sedation and blunting of thermoregulatory reflexes are necessary depends on the context. Patients recovering from CA or TBI are essentially poikilothermic and do not need drugs to facilitate cooling. In contrast, patients with stroke or acute myocardial infarction very much need pharmacologic intervention to prevent thermoregulatory vasoconstriction and shivering—and the hemodynamic consequences of each.

The best approach to inducing thermal tolerance appears to be a combination of buspirone and meperidine which reduces the shivering threshold to about 33.5°C with minimal impairment of ventilation (108). Dexmedetomidine also appears useful, and works even better in combination with meperidine (109–111). Meperidine is more effective than other opioids for control of shivering and is one of the only drugs that reduces the shivering threshold disproportionately to vasoconstriction (112,113).

A systematic review revealed that midazolam was most often used at doses between 5 mg and 0.3 mg/kg/hr in 39 of 68 ICUs, and that propofol was used in 13 ICUs at doses up to 6 mg/kg/hr. Fentanyl was used in 33 ICUs at doses between 0.5 and 10 μg/kg/hr, and 18 ICUs did not use any analgesics. NMB drugs, most often pancuronium, were routinely used to prevent shivering in 54 ICUs. Four ICUs used train-of-four monitoring of NMBs, and three ICUs used continuous monitoring of cerebral activity (114).

Bjelland (115) compared two protocols for sedation and analgesia during therapeutic hypothermia: midazolam and fentanyl versus propofol and remifentanil. Although time to target temperature was significantly shorter in patients administered propofol and remifentanil (13 vs. 37 hours), the propofol and remifentanil group required NE twice as often.

Rewarming

ERC Hypothermia After Cardiac Arrest Registry (ERC HACA-R) recommends a rewarming rate of 0.25° to 0.5°C/hr (116). In a retrospective cohort study of 128 patients, 6-month outcomes were similar with faster (>0.5°C/hr) and slower (< 0.5°C/hr) rewarming (117). Nonetheless, how best to rewarm patients remains essentially unknown and additional studies of the rewarming phase are very much required. In the meantime, the consensus among investigators and clinicians is that rewarming should be slow, generally over 12 or more hours.

Hyperthermia after discontinuation of active temperature management (i.e., postrewarming pyrexia defined as temperature > 38°C) was observed 69 of 167 patients (41%) who survived at least 24 hours after rewarming. Although postrewarming pyrexia was not associated with lower survival to discharge or worsened neurologic outcomes, higher maximal temperature (>38.7°C) was associated with worse neurologic outcomes—perhaps because patients with worse injuries were most likely to become febrile (118). Controlling shivering can be especially challenging in febrile patients.

FEVER

Hyperthermia is a generic term simply indicating a core body temperature exceeding normal values. In contrast, fever is a regulated increase in the core temperature targeted by the thermoregulatory system. Hyperthermia can result from a variety of causes and usually indicates a problem of sufficient severity that physician intervention is required. Fever is a special type of regulated hyperthermia that synchronously increases all thermoregulatory response thresholds. Fever thus represents an increase in the body's temperature set point. Fever is common among patients with neurologic injury and is associated with worse outcomes from stroke, although fever probably improves infectious outcomes (119,120).

Normal body temperature is neither set nor maintained by circulating factors. In contrast, fever results when endogenous pyrogens increase the thermoregulatory target temperature ("set point"). Identified endogenous pyrogens include IL-1, TNF, interferon alpha, and macrophage inflammatory protein-1 (121). Although it was initially believed that these factors acted directly on hypothalamic thermoregulatory centers, there is increasing evidence for a more complicated system involving vagal afferents. Most endogenous pyrogens have peripheral actions (e.g., immune system activation) in addition to their central generating capabilities (122,123).

Optimal treatment strategies for fever have yet to be established. Although active surface cooling of febrile patients makes intuitive sense, it is often either ineffective or counterproductive. This is principally because the febrile target set by the hypothalamus is in terms of *mean body* temperature, not core temperature. Weighted mean body temperature (for thermoregulatory purposes) is a linear combination of core and skin temperatures, with the skin contributing approximately 20% (124). Decreasing skin temperature 4°C will thus *increase* the target core temperature by about 1°C.

In intact patients, thermoregulatory defenses are more powerful than most types of surface cooling. The result is that active cooling fails to reduce core temperature, but does make patients highly uncomfortable, increases plasma catecholamine concentrations, augments metabolic rate, and provokes hypertension (Fig. 26.13) (125). However, in patients with impaired thermoregulatory defenses, surface cooling is an effective treatment for fever (126,127). The general strategy, then, is to distinguish active fever from passive hyperthermia. In the case of fever, treat the underlying fever trigger whenever possible because active cooling provokes considerable stress and usually is not especially effective. In the cases where hyperthermia appears passive or results from excessive heat production, simple cooling measures will usually be effective.

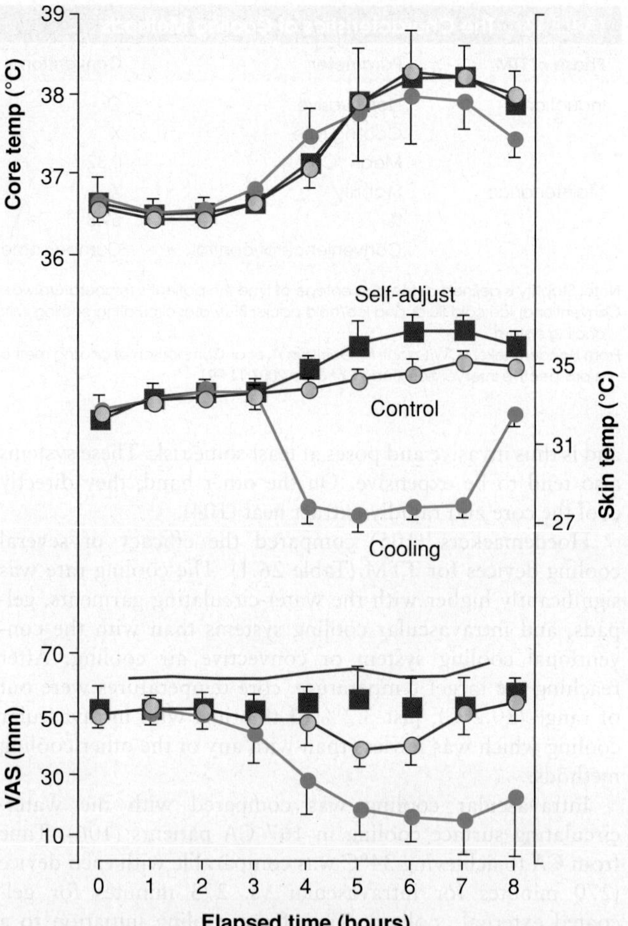

FIGURE 26.13 Change in core and skin temperature and thermal comfort after fever was induced by administration of interleukin-2, starting at elapsed time zero. The designated thermal management started after 3 elapsed hours and continued for 5 hours. This consisted of no treatment (control), self-adjustment per the subjects' comfort (self-adjust), and forced-air cooling (cooling). Thermal comfort is reported as millimeters on a visual analog scale (VAS), with 0 mm indicating the worst imaginable cold, 50 mm identifying thermoneutrality, and 100 mm being the worst imaginable heat. Active cooling made the subjects feel miserably cold, but did not reduce core temperature. Data are presented as means ± SDs. (From Lenhardt R, Negishi C, Sessler DI, et al. The effects of physical treatment on induced fever in humans. *Am J Med* 1999;106:550–555.)

Pharmacologic Cooling and Physical Cooling

Gozzoli (128) compared the effect of intravenous metamizol, intravenous propacetamol, and external cooling in febrile (>38.5°C) critically ill patients being mechanically ventilated. Although body temperature decreased significantly in all three groups, mean arterial pressure was the lowest with metamizol. Energy expenditure increased by 5% with external cooling, whereas it decreased by 7% and 8% with the metamizol and propacetamol groups.

Febrile patients with septic shock requiring vasopressors, mechanical ventilation, and sedation were allocated to external cooling ($n = 101$) to achieve normothermia (36.5° to 37°C) for 48 hours, or no external cooling ($n = 99$) (70). In the external cooling group, there were significantly more patients with a 50% vasopressor dose decrease within 12 hours of treatment (54% vs. 20%), but not at 48 hours (72% vs. 61%). Fourteen-day mortality was significantly lower in the external cooling group (19% vs. 34%), though with no significant difference in mortality rates of ICU discharge or hospital discharge between groups.

A meta-analysis of 5 randomized clinical trials in 399 patients admitted to ICU without neurologic injury was performed to investigate whether fever control (38.3° to 38.5°C)

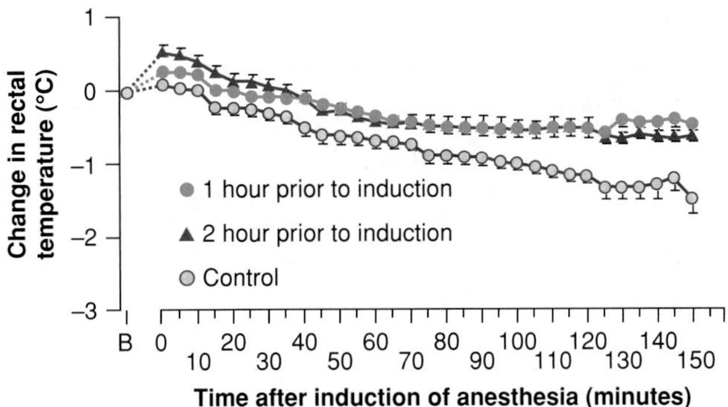

FIGURE 26.14 Changes in rectal temperature from baseline measurements throughout anesthesia in eight patients receiving amino acid infusion for 1 hour before and 1 hour of anesthesia, eight patients receiving amino acids for 2 hours before anesthesia, and eight patients receiving a nutrient-free saline solution for 1 hour before and 1 hour of anesthesia. Vertical bars, SEM of mean changes. (From Sellden E, Branstrom R, Brundin T. Preoperative infusion of amino acids prevent postoperative hypothermia. *Br J Anaesth* 1996;76:227–234; by permission of Oxford University Press.)

would affect mortality, compared with no control (40°). Although underpowered, no effect of fever treatment on mortality was found regardless of cooling methods (129).

Fever frequently occurs in critically ill patients, and various procedures are employed to cool patients, ranging from antipyretic medications (especially acetaminophen and NSAIDs) to surface cooling and intravascular cooling. Antipyretic treatments are administered routinely in these febrile patients both with and without infectious diseases. Despite the widespread use of acetaminophen in critical illness, prospective trials demonstrating the clinical benefit of acetaminophen are lacking (130,129). Overall, the effect of antipyretics on patient outcomes has been inconsistent and, consequently, there are no currently society-endorsed recommendations for antipyretics treatment on these critically ill patients (131,132). The impact of fever control on mortality of febrile critically ill patients thus remains unclear and further trials are needed—and in progress.

DIET-INDUCED THERMOGENESIS

The increase in energy expenditure after the ingestion of a meal or infusion of nutrients has been referred to as dietary-induced or nutrient-induced thermogenesis. Proteins or amino acids provoke a larger and longer response than carbohydrates or fats.

Intravenous infusion of 600 kJ (35 g) of amino acids increases energy expenditure in unanesthetized healthy volunteers by 20% and thus increases temperature of blood in the hepatic artery and vein by 0.3°C (133). Amino acid infusions increase resting core temperature by both increasing the thermoregulatory set point and increasing metabolic rate (134).

In patients having general anesthesia for lower abdominal surgery, continuous infusion of amino acids (240 kJ/hr) for 2 hours keeps core temperature about 0.3°C/hr higher than in patients not receiving the infusion (Fig. 26.14) (135). Furthermore, continuous infusion at a rate of 4 kJ/kg/hr for 2 hours before induction of spinal anesthesia prevents hypothermia (Fig. 26.15) (136). Perioperative amino acid infusion at a rate of 4 kJ/kg/hr for 4 hours improves esophageal temperature at the end of off-pump coronary artery bypass grafting by 0.6°C, and shortens the duration of mechanical ventilation, and ICU and hospital stays (137).

Fructose elicits the greatest thermogenesis among the various carbohydrates that have been tested. Oral intake of 75 g fructose in awake healthy volunteers increases arterial blood temperature by more than 0.2°C (138). Continuous infusion of fructose at a rate of 0.5 g/kg/hr for 4 hours in patients during general anesthesia for lower abdominal surgery increased their esophageal temperature at 3 hours after induction by 0.6°C. Fructose also increased the metabolic rate by approximately

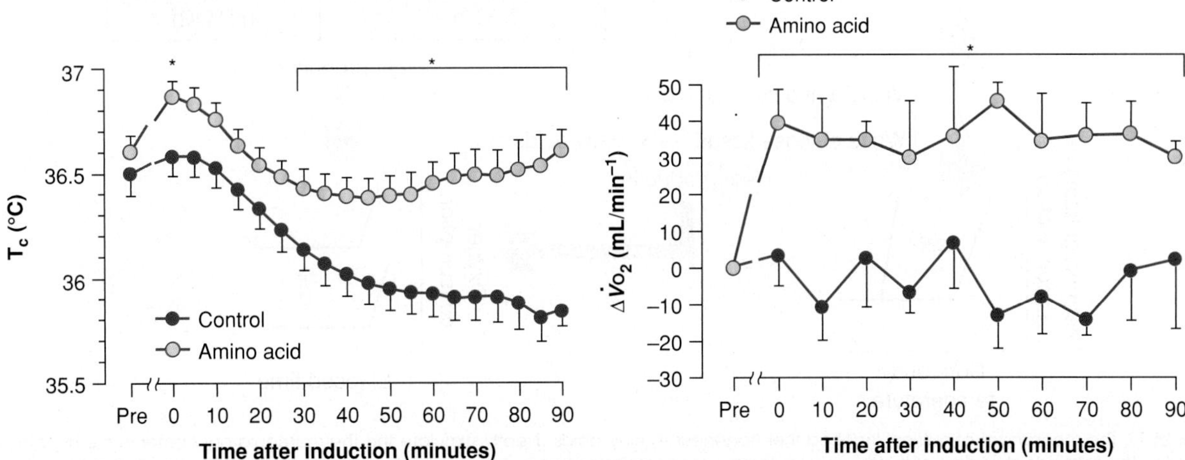

FIGURE 26.15 Change in tympanic-membrane core temperature (T_c) anesthesia. T_c values at 0 minute and after 30 minutes were significantly greater in the amino acid infusion group than the saline group. Data are presented as means ± SEMs. "Pre" indicates the period of pre-amino acid infusion. Asterisks (*) indicate statistically significant difference between the groups ($P < 0.05$). (From Kasai T, Nakajima Y, Matsukawa T, et al. Effect of preoperative amino acid infusion on thermoregulatory response during spinal anaesthesia. *Br J Anaesth* 2003;90:58–61; by permission of Oxford University Press.)

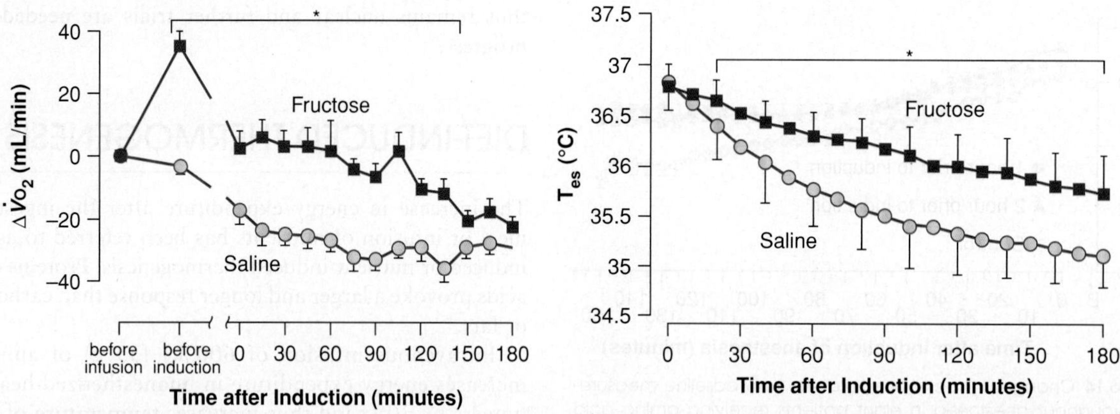

FIGURE 26.16 Core temperature measured at the distal esophagus (T_{es}) during surgery. Patients receiving the fructose infusion had significantly greater core temperatures than those receiving saline (*P = 0.001). Infusion was started 20 minutes after induction of anesthesia and continued until the end of the monitoring period (180 minutes after induction). Data are presented as mean ± SD for 10 patients in each group. (From Mizobe T, Nakajima Y, Ueno H, Sessler DI. Fructose administration increases intraoperative core temperature by augmenting both metabolic rate and the vasoconstriction threshold. *Anesthesiology* 2006;104:1124.)

20%, as well as increased the set point of thermoregulation (Fig. 26.16) (139).

Amino acid administration increases plasma insulin concentration, and increases phosphorylation of translation initiation components in protein synthesis. Infusion of amino acids thus increase oxygen consumption in anesthetized rats and help preserve core temperature. Interestingly, these changes were not observed in the somatostatin-treated rats (140,141). Recent evidence has identified a role for thyroid hormone (T3) in pancreatic islet development and insulin signaling. There is also central modulation and feedback by nutritional signals on TH pathway. The overall mechanism of nutrient-induced thermogenesis is shown in Figure 26.17 (142,143).

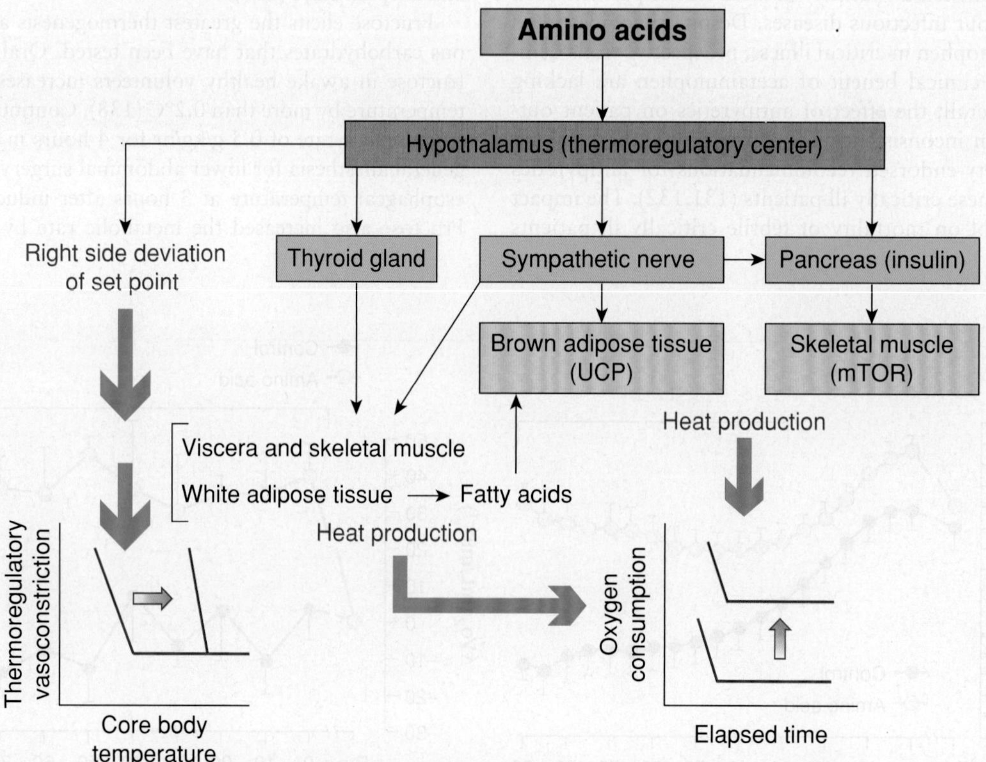

FIGURE 26.17 The mechanism of nutrient-induced thermogenesis. Amino acids directly stimulate the thermoregulatory center in the hypothalamus to develop the right side deviation of the thermoregulatory vasoconstriction threshold as well as to activate heat production through thyroid gland, sympathetic nervous system, and pancreas.

Key Points

- Reliable core temperature monitoring sites include the pulmonary artery, tympanic membrane (as measured with a contact thermocouple or thermistor), nasopharynx, and esophagus.
- Signals from cutaneous thermosensors are transmitted to the thermoregulatory center in the hypothalamus. TRP channels appear to be the most important thermosensors. Cutaneous vasoconstriction is the first autonomic response to cold. The normal threshold (triggering core temperature) for vasoconstriction is about 36.5°C. Shivering is the final autonomic response that is activated to cold and is generally only observed when behavioral responses and vasoconstriction fail to maintain an adequate core temperature. The shivering threshold is approximately 35.5°C, and vigorous shivering doubles the metabolic rate.
- Patients undergoing mild hypothermia exhibit decreased heart rate, increased systemic vascular resistance, normal mean blood pressure, and stroke volume. Minute ventilation decreases during therapeutic hypothermia, but $PaCO_2$ remains normal because of the decreased metabolic rate. The number of circulating leukocytes decreases. Prolonged hypothermia also decreases the number of circulating platelets and, more importantly, impairs their function. During induction of therapeutic hypothermia, potassium shifts from the plasma into cells resulting in hypokalemia. Conversely, during rewarming the shift of potassium back into the plasma. Urine output increases at induction of hypothermia. Gut motility decreases during hypothermia, which delays enteral feeding. Blood glucose concentrations increase in response to reduced insulin secretion.
- Current evidence does not strongly support therapeutic hypothermia for any indication in humans. But among potential indications, neonatal asphyxia is best documented. Hypothermia remains in common use for out-of-hospital CA, despite a large negative randomized trial. Despite the lack of high-quality supportive randomized data (and despite negative randomized data), TTM is also sometimes used for myocardial infarction, aneurysm surgery, sepsis, ARDS, hepatic encephalopathy, and pediatric TBI. Randomized trials of TTM are currently ongoing in adult TBI, ischemic stroke, sepsis, and pediatric CA.

References

1. Blumenthal I. Fever—concepts old and new. *J R Soc Med* 1997;90(7): 391–394.
2. Haller JS, Jr. Medical thermometry—a short history. *West J Med* 1985; 142(1):108–116.
3. Ring EF. The historical development of thermometry and thermal imaging in medicine. *J Med Eng Technol* 2006;30(4):192–198.
4. Fox RH, Solman AJ. A new technique for monitoring the deep body temperature in man from the intact skin surface *J Physiol* 1971;212 (Suppl):8P–10P.
5. Eshraghi Y, Nasr V, Parra-Sanchez I, et al. An evaluation of a zero-heat-flux cutaneous thermometer in cardiac surgical patients. *Anesth Analg* 2014; 119:543–549.
6. Harioka T, Matsukawa T, Ozaki M, et al. Deep-forehead temperature correlates well with blood temperature. *Can J Anesth* 2000;47:980–983.
7. Stone JG, Young WL, Smith CR, et al. Do standard monitoring sites reflect true brain temperature when profound hypothermia is rapidly induced and reversed? *Anesthesiology* 1995;82:344–351.
8. Erickson R. Thermometer placement for oral temperature measurement in febrile adults. *Int J Nurs Stud* 1976;13(4):199–208.
9. Heinz J. Validation of sublingual temperatures in patients with nasogastric tubes. *Heart Lung* 1985;14(2):128–130.
10. Tandberg D, Sklar D. Effect of tachypnea on the estimation of body temperature by an oral thermometer. *N Engl J Med* 1983;308(16):945–946.
11. Langham GE, Maheshwari A, Contrera K, et al. Noninvasive temperature monitoring in postanesthesia care units. *Anesthesiology* 2009;111:90–96.
12. Cork RC, Vaughan RW, Humphrey LS. Precision and accuracy of intraoperative temperature monitoring. *Anesth Analg* 1983;62(2):211–214.
13. Ramsey JG, Ralley FE, Whalley DG. Site of temperature monitoring and prediction of afterdrop after open heart surgery. *Can Anaesth Soc J* 1985; 32:607–615.
14. Iaizzo PA, Kehler CH, Zink RS, et al. Thermal response in acute porcine malignant hyperthermia. *Anesth Analg* 1996;82:803–809.
15. Benzinger M. Tympanic thermometry in surgery and anesthesia. *JAMA* 1969;209(8):1207–1211.
16. Imamura M, Matsukawa T, Ozaki M, et al. The accuracy and precision of four infrared aural canal thermometers during cardiac surgery. *Acta Anaesthesiol Scand* 1998;42:1222–1226.
17. Daanen HA. Infrared tympanic temperature and ear canal morphology. *J Med Eng Technol* 2006;30(4):224–234.
18. Kiya T, Yamakage M, Hayase T, et al. The usefulness of an earphone-type infrared tympanic thermometer for intraoperative core temperature monitoring. *Anesth Analg* 2007;105:1688–1692.
19. Crocker BD, Okumura F, McCuaig DI, et al. Temperature monitoring during general anaesthesia. *Br J Anaesth* 1980;52:1223–1229.
20. Lee J, Lim H, Son K, et al. Optimal nasopharyngeal temperature probe placement. *Anesth Analg* 2014;119:875–879.
21. Lilly JK, Boland JP, Zekan S. Urinary bladder temperature monitoring: a new index of body core temperature. *Crit Care Med* 1980;8:742–744.
22. Frank S, Raja SN, Bulcao C, et al. Relative contribution of core and cutaneous temperatures to thermal comfort, autonomic, and metabolic responses in humans. *J Appl Physiol* 1999;86:1588–1593.
23. Nakamura K. Central circuitries for body temperature regulation and fever. *Am J Physiol* 2011;301:R1207–R1228.
24. Vriens J, Nilius B, Voets T. Peripheral thermosensation in mammals. *Nat Rev Neurosci* 2014;15:573–589.
25. Caterina MJ, Schumacher MA, Tominaga M, et al. The capsaicin receptor: a heat-activated ion channel in the pain pathway. *Nature* 1997;389: 816–824.
26. Dhaka A, Uzzell V, Dubin AE, et al. TRPV1 is activated by both acidic and basic pH. *J Neurosci* 2008;29:153–158.
27. Gavva NR, Treanor JJ, Garami A, et al. Pharmacological blockade of the vanilloid receptor TRPV1 elicits marked hyperthermia in humans. *Pain* 2008;136:202–210.
28. Caterina MJ, Leffler A, Malmberg AB, et al. Impaired nociception and pain sensation in mice lacking the capsaicin receptor. *Science* 2000; 288:306–313.
29. McGaraughty S, Segreti JA, Fryer RM, et al. Antagonism of TRPV1 receptors indirectly modulates activity of thermoregulatory neurons in the medial preoptic area of rats. *Brain Res* 2009;1268:58–67.
30. Boulant JA. Counterpoint; heat-induced membrane depolarization of hypothalamic neurons; an unlikely mechanism of central thermosensitivity. *Am J Physiol Regul Integr Comp Physiol* 2006;290:R1481–R1484.
31. Romanovsky AA, Almeida MC, Garami A, et al. The transient receptor potential vanilloid-1 channel in thermoregulation: a thermosensor it is not. *Pharmacol Rev* 2009;61:228–261.
32. Mistlberger T, Rusak B. Mechanisms and models of the circadian time keeping system. In: Kryger MH, Dement WC, eds. *Principles and Practice of Sleep Medicine*. Philadelphia, PA: WB Saunders; 1989:141–152.
33. Crawford DC, Hicks B, Thompson MJ. Which thermometer? Factors influencing best choice for intermittent clinical temperature assessment. *J Med Eng Technol* 2006;30(4):199–211.
34. Lopez M, Sessler DI, Walter K, et al. Rate and gender dependence of the sweating, vasoconstriction, and shivering thresholds in humans. *Anesthesiology* 1994;80:780–788.
35. Stephenson LA, Kolka MA: Menstrual cycle phase and time of day alter reference signal controlling arm blood flow and sweating. *Am J Physiol* 1985;249:R186–R191.
36. Nakajima Y, Mizobe T, Takamata A, et al. Baroreflex modulation of peripheral vasoconstriction during progressive hypothermia in anesthetized humans. *Am J Physiol Regul Integr Comp Physiol* 2000;279(4):R1430–R1436.
37. Stauss HM. Baroreceptor reflex function. *Am J Physiol* 2002;283: R284–R286.

38. Brück K. Thermoregulation: control mechanisms and neural processes. In: Sinclair JC, ed. *Temperature Regulation and Energy Metabolism in the Newborn*. New York, NY: Grune & Stratton; 1978:157–185.
39. Hales JRS. Skin arteriovenous anastomoses, their control and role in thermoregulation. In: Johansen K, Burggren W, eds. *Cardiovascular Shunts: Phylogenetic, Ontogenetic and Clinical Aspects*. Copenhagen: Munksgaard; 1985:433–451.
40. Giesbrecht GG, Sessler DI, Mekjavic IB, et al. Treatment of immersion hypothermia by direct body-to-body contact. *J Appl Physiol* 1994;76: 2373–2379.
41. Horvath SM, Spurr GB, Hutt BK, et al. Metabolic cost of shivering. *J Appl Physiol* 1956;8:595–602.
42. Eyolfson DA, Tikuisis P, Xu X, et al. Measurement and prediction of peak shivering intensity in humans. *Eur J Appl Physiol* 2001;84:100–106.
43. Tikuisis P, Eyolfson DA, Xu X, et al. Shivering endurance and fatigue during cold water immersion in humans. *Eur J Appl Physiol* 2002;87:50–58.
44. Frank SM, Higgins MS, Fleisher LA, et al. Adrenergic, respiratory, and cardiovascular effects of core cooling in humans. *Am J Physiol* 1997; 272:R557–R562.
45. Khan F, Spence VA, Belch JJF. Cutaneous vascular responses and thermoregulation in relation to age. *Clin Sci* 1992;82:521–528.
46. Vassilieff N, Rosencher N, Sessler DI, et al. The shivering threshold during spinal anesthesia is reduced in the elderly. *Anesthesiology* 199;83: 1162–1166.
47. Sessler DI: Perioperative hypothermia. *N Engl J Med* 1997;336:1730–1737.
48. Fahey MR, Sessler DI, Cannon JE, et al. Atracurium, vecuronium, and pancuronium do not alter the minimum alveolar concentration of halothane in humans. *Anesthesiology* 1989;71:53–56.
49. Mullur R, Liu YY, Brent GA. Thyroid hormone regulation of metabolism. *Physiol Rev* 2014;94:355–382.
50. Lidell ME, Betz MJ, Enerback S. Brown adipose tissue and its therapeutic potential. *J Intern Med* 2014;276:364–377.
51. Perman SM, Goyal M, Neumar RW, et al. Clinical applications of targeted temperature management. *Chest* 2014;145:386–393.
52. Bernard SA, Gray TW, Buist MD, et al. Treatment of comatose survivors of out-of-hospital cardiac arrest with induced hypothermia. *N Engl J Med* 2002;346:557–563.
53. Hypothermia After Cardiac Arrest Study Group. Mild therapeutic hypothermia to improve the neurologic outcome after cardiac arrest. *N Engl J Med* 2002;346:549–556.
54. Advanced Life Support Chapter Collaborators. Part 8: advanced life support: 2010 international consensus on cardiopulmonary resuscitation and emergency cardiovascular care science with treatment recommendations. *Circulation* 2010;122:S345–S421.
55. American Heart Association. Part 9: post-cardiac arrest care. 2010 American Heart Association guidelines for cardiopulmonary resuscitation and emergency cardiovascular care. *Circulation* 2010;122:S768–S786.
56. Deakin CD, Nolan JP, Soar J, et al. European Resuscitation Council guidelines for resuscitation 2010 Section 4. Adult advanced life support. *Resuscitation* 2010;81:1305–1352.
57. Nielsen N, Wetterslev J, Cronberg T, et al. Targeted temperature management at 33°C versus 36°C after cardiac arrest. *N Engl J Med* 2013;369:2197–2206.
58. Shankaran S, Laptook AR, Ehrenkranz RA, et al. National Institute of Child Health and Human development Neonatal Research Network. Whole-body hypothermia for neonates with hypoxic-ischemic encephalopathy. *N Engl J Med* 2005;353:1574–1584.
59. Azzopardi D, Strohm B, Edwards AD, et al. TOBY Study Group. Moderate hypothermia to treat perinatal asphyxial encephalopathy. *N Engl J Med* 2009;361:1349–1358; *Erratum in N Engl J Med* 2010;362:1051–1052.
60. Azzopardi D, Strohm B, Marlow N, et al. Effects of hypothermia for perinatal asphyxia on childhood outcomes. *N Engl J Med* 2014;371:140–149.
61. Shankaran S, Laptook AR, Pappas A, et al. Effect of depth and duration of cooling on deaths in the NICU among neonates with hypoxic ischemic encephalopathy: a randomized clinical trial. *JAMA* 2014;312:2629–2639.
62. Clifton GL, Miller ER, Choi SC, et al. Lack of effect of induction of hypothermia after acute brain injury. *N Engl J Med* 2001;344:556–563.
63. Clifton GL, Valadka A, Zygun D, et al. Very early hypothermia induction in patients with severe brain injury (the National Acute Brain Injury Study: Hypothermia II): a randomized trial. *Lancet Neurol* 2011;10:131–139.
64. Hutchison JS, Ward RE, Lacroix J, et al. Hypothermia therapy after traumatic brain injury in children. *N Engl J Med* 2008;358:2447–2756.
65. Dae MW, Gao DW, Sessler DI, et al. Effect of endovascular cooling on myocardial temperature, infarct size, and cardiac output in human-sized pigs. *Am J Physiol Heart Circ Physiol* 2002;282:H1584–H1591.
66. Goetberg M, Olivecrona GK, Engblom H, et al. Rapid short-duration hypothermia with cold saline and endovascular cooling before reperfusion reduces microvascular obstruction and myocardial infarct size. *BMC Cardiovasc Disord* 2008;8:7.
67. Dixon SR, Whitbourn RJ, Dae MW, et al. Induction of mild systemic hypothermia with endovascular cooling during primary percutaneous coronary intervention for acute myocardial infarction. *J Am Coll Cardiol* 2002;40:1928–1934.
68. Grines CL. ICE-IT-1: intravascular cooling adjunctive to percutaneous coronary intervention (Part 1). A preliminary review of results TCT 2004. Available at: http://www.scribd.com/doc/40117148/ICE-IT-Presentation-TCT2004. Accessed October 23, 2012.
69. Todd MM, Hindman BJ, Clarke WR, et al. Mild intraoperative hypothermia during surgery for intracranial aneurysm. *N Engl J Med* 2005;352: 135–145.
70. Schortgen F, Clabault K, Katsahian S, et al. Fever control using external cooling in septic shock: a randomized controlled trial. *Am J Respir Crit Care Med* 2012;185:1088–1095.
71. Villar J, Slutsky AS. Effects of induced hypothermia in patients with septic adult respiratory distress syndrome. *Resuscitation* 1993;26:183–192.
72. Jalan R, O-Damink SW, Deutz NE, et al. Moderate hypothermia in patients with acute liver failure and uncontrolled intracranial hypertension. *Gastroenterology* 2004;127:1338–1346.
73. Fischer UM, Cox CS Jr, Laine GA, et al. Mild hypothermia impairs left ventricular diastolic but not systolic function. *J Invest Surg* 2005;18:291–296.
74. Osborn JJ. Experimental hypothermia: respiratory and blood pH changes in relation to cardiac function. *American Journal of Physiology* 1953;175: 389–398.
75. Polderman KH, Herold I. Therapeutic hypothermia and controlled normothermia in the intensive care unit: practical considerations, side effects, and cooling methods. *Crit Care Med* 2009;37:1101–1120.
76. Hypothermia After Cardiac Arrest Study Group. Mild therapeutic hypothermia to improve the neurologic outcome after cardiac arrest. *N Engl J Med* 2002;346(8):549–556.
77. Bernard SA, Buist M. Induced hypothermia in critical care medicine: a review. *Crit Care Med* 2003;31(7):2041–2051.
78. Bernard SA, Mac CJB, Buist M. Experience with prolonged induced hypothermia in severe head injury. *Crit Care (Lond)* 1999;3(6):167–172.
79. Geurts M, Macleod MR, Kollmar R, et al. Therapeutic hypothermia and the risk of infection: a systematic review and meta-analysis. *Crit Care Med* 2014;42:231–242.
80. Polderman KH. Induced hypothermia and fever control for prevention and treatment of neurological injuries. *Lancet* 2008;371:1955–1969.
81. Valeri CR, MacGregor H, Cassidy G, et al. Effects of temperature on bleeding time and clotting time in normal male and female volunteers. *Crit Care Med* 1995;23(4):698–704.
82. Rajagopalan S, Mascha E, Na J, et al. The effects of mild perioperative hypothermia on blood loss and transfusion requirement: a meta-analysis. *Anesthesiology* 2008;108: 71–77.
83. Michelson AD, MacGregor H, Barnard MR, et al. Hypothermia-induced reversible platelet dysfunction. *Thromb Haemost* 1994;71:633–640.
84. Watts DD, Trask A, Soeken K, et al. Hypothermic coagulopathy in trauma: effect of varying levels of hypothermia on enzyme speed, platelet function and fibrinolytic activity. *J Trauma* 1998;44:846–854.
85. Aibiki M, Kawaguchi S, Maekawa N. Reversible hypophosphatemia during moderate hypothermia therapy for brain-injured patients. *Crit Care Med* 2001;29(9):1726–1730.
86. Machida S, Ohta S, Itoh N, et al. [Changes in tissue distribution of potassium during simple hypothermia]. *Kyobu Geka* 1977;30(5):413–418.
87. Zeiner A, Sunder-Plassmann G, Sterz F, et al. The effect of mild therapeutic hypothermia on renal function after cardiopulmonary resuscitation in men. *Resuscitation* 2004;60(3):253–261.
88. Soliman HM, Mercan D, Lobo SS, et al. Development of ionized hypomagnesemia is associated with higher mortality rate. *Crit Care Med* 2003; 31:1082–1087.
89. Van den Bergh WM, Algra A, van Kooten F, et al. Magnesium sulfate in aneurysmal subarachnoid hemorrhage: a randomized controlled trial. *Stroke* 2005;36:1011–1015.
90. Temkin NR, Anderson GD, Winn HR, et al. Magnesium sulfate for neuroprotection after traumatic brain injury: a randomized controlled trial. *Lancet Neurol* 2007;6:29–38.
91. Van den Berghe G, Wilmer A, Hermans G, et al. Intensive insulin therapy in the medical ICU. *N Engl J Med* 2006;354:449–461.
92. Capes SE, Hunt D, Malmberg K, et al. Stress hyperglycemia and prognosis of stroke in non-diabetic and diabetic patients: a systematic overview. *Stroke* 2001;32:2426–2432.
93. The NICE-SUGAR Study Investigators. Intensive versus conventional glucose control in critically ill patients. *N Engl J Med* 2009;360:1283–1297.

94. Cueni-Villoz N, Devigili A, Delodder F, et al. Increased blood glucose variability during therapeutic hypothermia and outcome after cardiac arrest. *Crit Care Med* 2011;39:2225–2231.
95. Leslie K, Sessler DI, Bjorksten AR, et al. Mild hypothermia alters propofol pharmacokinetics and increases the duration of action of atracurium. *Anesth Analg* 1995;80:1007–1014.
96. Fukuoka N, Aibiki M, Tsukamoto T, et al. Biphasic concentration change during continuous midazolam administration in brain-injured patients undergoing therapeutic moderate hypothermia. *Resuscitation* 2004;60:225–230.
97. Caldwell JE, Heier T, Wright PMC, et al. Temperature-dependent pharmacokinetics and pharmacodynamics of vecuronium. *Anesthesiology* 2000; 92:84–93.
98. Tortorici MA, Kochanek PM, Poloyac SM. Effects of hypothermia on drug disposition, metabolism, and response: a focus of hypothermia-mediated alterations on the cytochrome P450 enzyme system. *Crit Care Med* 2007;35:2196–2204.
99. Nielsen N, Hovdenes J, Nilsson F, et al. Outcome, timing and adverse events in therapeutic hypothermia after out-of-hospital cardiac arrest. *Acta Anaesthesiol Scand* 2009;53:926–934.
100. Mooney MR, Unger BT, Boland LL, et al. Therapeutic hypothermia after out-of-hospital cardiac arrest. *Circulation* 2011;124:206–214.
101. Sendelbach S, Hearst MO, Johnson PJ, et al. Effects of variation in temperature management on cerebral performance category scores in patients who received therapeutic hypothermia post cardiac arrest. *Resuscitation* 2012;83:829–834.
102. Kim F, Nichol G, Maynard C, et al. Effect of prehospital induction of mild hypothermia on survival and neurological status among adults with cardiac arrest. *JAMA*2014;311:45–52.
103. Rajek A, Greif R, Sessler DI, et al. Core cooling by central-venous infusion of 4°C and 20°C fluid: Isolation of core and peripheral thermal compartments. *Anesthesiology* 2000;93:629–637.
104. Doufas AG, Akça O, Barry A, et al. Initial experience with a novel heat-exchanging catheter in neurosurgical patients. *Anesth Analg* 2002;95: 1752–1756.
105. Hoedemaekers CW, Ezzahti M, Gerritsen A, et al. Comparison of cooling methods to induce and maintain normothermia and hypothermia in intensive care unit patients: a prospective intervention study. *Crit Care* 2007;11:R91.
106. Tomte O, Draegni T, Mangschau A, et al. A comparison of intravascular and surface cooling techniques in comatose cardiac arrest survivors. *Crit Care Med* 2011;39:443–449.
107. Pittl U, Schratter A, Desch S, et al. Invasive versus non-invasive cooling after in- and out-of-hospital cardiac arrest: a randomized trial. *Clin Res Cardiol* 2013;102:607–614.
108. Mokhtarani M, Mahgob AN, Morioka N, et al. Buspirone and meperidine synergistically reduce the shivering threshold. *Anesth Analg* 2001;93: 1233–1239.
109. Doufas AG, Lin CM, Suleman MI, et al. Dexmedetomidine and meperidine additively reduce the shivering threshold in humans. *Stroke* 2003;34: 1218–1223.
110. Lenhardt R, Orhan-Sungur M, Komatsu R, et al. Suppression of shivering during hypothermia using a novel drug combination in healthy volunteers. *Anesthesiology* 2009;111:110–115.
111. Talke P, Tayefeh F, Sessler DI, et al. Dexmedetomidine does not alter the sweating threshold, but comparably and linearly reduces the vasoconstriction and shivering thresholds. *Anesthesiology* 1997;87:835–841.
112. Kurz A, Go JC, Sessler DI, et al. Alfentanil slightly increases the sweating threshold and markedly reduces the vasoconstriction and shivering thresholds. *Anesthesiology* 1995;83:293–299.
113. Kurz A, Ikeda T, Sessler DI, et al. Meperidine decreases the shivering threshold twice as much as the vasoconstriction threshold. *Anesthesiology* 1997;86:1046–1054.
114. Chamorro C, Borrallo JM, Romera MA, et al. Anesthesia and analgesia protocol during therapeutic hypothermia after cardiac arrest: a systematic review. *Anesth Analg* 2010;110:1328–1335.
115. Bjelland TW, Dale O, Kaisen K, et al. Propofol and remifentanil versus midazolam and fentanyl for sedation during therapeutic hypothermia after cardiac arrest: a randomized trial. *Intensive Care Med* 2012;38:959–967.
116. European Resuscitation Council After Cardiac Arrest Registry Study Group. Clinical application of mild therapeutic hypothermia after cardiac arrest. *Crit Car Med* 2007;35:1041–1047.
117. Bouwes A, Robillard LB, Binnekade JM, et al. The influence of rewarming after therapeutic hypothermia on outcome after cardiac arrest. *Resuscitation* 2012;83:996–1000.
118. Leary M, Grossestreuer AV, Iannacone S, et al. Pyrexia and neurologic outcomes after therapeutic hypothermia for cardiac arrest. *Resuscitation* 2013;84:1056–1061.
119. Kluger MJ. Is fever beneficial? *Yale J Biol Med* 1986;59:89–95.
120. Ginsberg MD, Busto R. Combating hyperthermia in acute stroke: a significant clinical concern. *Stroke* 1998;29(2):529–534.
121. Davatelis G, Wolpe SD, Sherry B, et al. Macrophage inflammatory protein-1: a prostaglandin-independent endogenous pyrogen. *Science* 1989;243(4894 Pt 1):1066–1068.
122. Blatteis CM. Role of the OVLT in the febrile response to circulating pyrogens. *Prog Brain Res* 1992;91:409–412.
123. Blatteis CM, Sehic E. Fever: how may circulating pyrogens signal the brain? *New in Physiological Sciences* 1997;12:1–9.
124. Cheng C, Matsukawa T, Sessler DI, et al. Increasing mean skin temperature linearly reduces the core-temperature thresholds for vasoconstriction and shivering in humans. *Anesthesiology* 1995;82:1160–1168.
125. Lenhardt R, Negishi C, Sessler DI, et al. The effects of physical treatment on induced fever in humans. *Am J Med* 1999;106:550–555.
126. Manthous CA, Hall JB, Olson D, et al. Effect of cooling on oxygen consumption in febrile critically ill patients. *Am J Resp Crit Care Med* 1995; 151:10–14.
127. Poblete B, Romand J-A, Pichard C, et al. Metabolic effects of i.v. propacetamol, metamizol or external cooling in critically ill febrile sedated patients. *Br J Anaesth* 1997;78:123–127.
128. Gozzoli V, Treggiari MM, Kleger GR, et al. Randomized trial of the effect of antipyresis by metamizol, propacetamol or external cooling on metabolism, hemodynamics and inflammatory response. *Intensive Care Med* 2004; 30:401–407.
129. Niven DJ, Stelfox HT, Laupland KB. Antipyretic therapy in febrile critically ill adults: a systematic review and meta-analysis. *J Crit Care* 2013; 28:303–310.
130. Jefferies S, Saxena M, Young P. Paracetamol in critical illness: a review. *Crit Care Resusc* 2012;14:74–80.
131. O'Grady NP, Barie PS, Bartlett JG, et al. Guidelines for evaluation of new fever in critically ill adult patients: 2008 update from the American College of Critical Care Medicine and the Infectious Diseases Society of America. *Crit Care Med* 2008;36:1330–1349.
132. Dellinger RP, Levy MM, Carlet JM, et al. Surviving Sepsis Campaign: International guidelines for management of severe sepsis and septic shock. *Crit Care Med* 2008;36:296-327; *Crit Care Med* 2008;36:1394–1396. Erratum.
133. Brundin T, Wahren J. Effects of i.v. amino acids on human splanchnic and whole body oxygen consumption, blood flow, and blood temperatures. *Am J Physiol* 1994;266(3 Pt 1):E396–E402.
134. Nakajima Y, Takamata A, Matsukawa T, et al. Effect of amino acid infusion on central thermoregulatory control in humans. *Anesthesiology* 2004; 100:634–639.
135. Sellden E, Branstrom R, Brundin T. Preoperative infusion of amino acids prevents postoperative hypothermia. *Br J Anaesth* 1996;76(2):227–234.
136. Kasai T, Nakajima Y, Matsukawa T, et al. Effect of preoperative amino acid infusion on thermoregulatory response during spinal anaesthesia. *Br J Anaesth* 2003;90(1):58–61.
137. Umenai T, Nakajima Y, Sessler DI, et al. Perioperative amino acid infusion improves recovery and shortens the duration of hospitalization after off-pump coronary artery bypass grafting. *Anesth Analg* 2006;103(6): 1386–1393.
138. Brundin T, Wahren J. Whole body and splanchnic oxygen consumption and blood flow after oral ingestion of fructose or glucose. *Am J Physiol* 1993;264(4 Pt 1):E504–E513.
139. Mizobe T, Nakajima Y, Ueno H, et al. Fructose administration increases intraoperative core temperature by augmenting both metabolic rate and the vasoconstriction threshold. *Anesthesiology* 2006;104(6):1124–1130.
140. Yamaoka I, Doi M, Nakayama M, et al. Intravenous administration of amino acids during anesthesia stimulates muscle protein synthesis and heat accumulation in the body. *Am J Physiol Endocrinol Metab* 2006; 290:E882–E888.
141. Yamaoka I, Doi M, Kawano Y, et al. Insulin mediates the linkage acceleration of muscle protein synthesis, thermogenesis, and heat storage by amino acids. *Biochem Biophys Res Com* 2009;386:252–256.
142. Szekely M. The vagus nerve in thermoregulation and energy metabolism. *Auton Neurosci* 2000;85:26–38.
143. Gobel G, Ember A, Petervali E, et al. Postalimentary hyperthermia: a role for gastrointestinal but not caloric signals. *J Therm Biol* 2001;26: 519–523.

CHAPTER

27

Blood Volume Measurement

JOSEPH FELDSCHUH

INTRODUCTION

Patients admitted to intensive care units are usually critically ill. They may be admitted with a variety of diagnoses such as sepsis, shock, cardiogenic shock, acute kidney failure, respiratory failure, and several other diagnoses. Regardless of how the patient is labeled with respect to the admitting diagnosis, it is very common for such critically ill patients to have major blood volume derangements. Such patients are often too ill to eat and may be fed only intravenously. Some of these patients are frequently intubated shortly after admission. Clinicians treating such patients are faced with major challenges in selecting the appropriate fluids and medications for treatment. It is not uncommon for patients with previously normal kidneys to develop acute kidney injury requiring temporary and sometimes permanent renal dialysis.

A common denominator is the clinical paradox of how to optimally treat patients who require external fluid support, selection of the correct fluid, and correction of electrolyte and blood protein abnormalities. Death rates vary between 20% and 45% in reported studies of septic and shock patients (1–4). Clinicians treating such patients use intravenous fluids such as normal saline, half-normal saline 5% dextrose and water, lactated Ringer's solution, packed red cells, fresh frozen plasma, 5% albumin solution, 25% albumin solution, as well a choice of intravenous electrolyte supplements such as potassium chloride.

Treatment decisions are based on the use of diagnostic tools such as chest x-rays, CAT scans, blood tests with particular emphasis on liver profiles, blood glucose levels, and serum lactate levels. Essential to the treatment goal is to enable a patient to survive restoration to normal of the blood volume (5). Clinicians recognize this problem and use many tests to estimate blood volume utilizing "surrogate" blood volume test rather than actual blood volume measurements. These surrogate tests include laboratory tests such as hemoglobin and hematocrits, which are frequently mistakenly used to estimate a person's blood volume. Hematocrit and hemoglobin are a reasonably accurate reflection of the patient's blood volume status only if the patient is in a healthy condition (6). In situations such as patients requiring admission to an intensive care unit, they are particularly likely to be misleading due to alterations caused by the underlying pathology as well as therapies which further cause blood volume derangements. An additional important factor is that achievement of a normal blood volume by itself, while a primary goal, must take into account the relationship between plasma volume and red cell volume. A patient with a normal blood volume with a red cell deficit of 55% and expanded plasma volume resulting in a total normal blood volume is very different from a patient with a normal blood volume, normal red cell volume, and normal plasma volume. Clinical maneuvers such as passive leg raising have been shown not to have a high correlation in response to fluid challenge (7,8).

Common confounding diseases, such as diabetes, renal disease, and sepsis, frequently result in hypoalbuminuria. Hypoalbuminuria is a major confounding factor in blood volume derangements and is a common cause of clinical errors in treating intensive care unit patients.

It is intuitively obvious that it is essential to provide effective circulation to all parts of the body. The kidneys are particularly susceptible to hypoperfusion. At rest, 25% of the blood volume is filtered by the kidney. Kidney function acts as the canary in the human organ profile. If the kidney fails, there is a markedly increased possibility of multiple-organ failure.

Multiple-organ failure is usually failure of therapy to restore effective circulation to the organs of the body. Multiple-organ system failure is often associated with derangements in blood volume which are difficult to recognize using surrogate measures which may lead to inappropriate therapy resulting in the death or severe morbidity of a surviving patient (1–3). The hematocrit and hemoglobin are often incorrect surrogates for blood volume measurement. Clinical maneuvers such as passive leg raising have been shown to have a poor correlation with actual blood volume. In most published studies involving this maneuver did not include actual blood volume measurements (7,8).

The goal of this chapter is to enable physicians to understand and recognize the various blood volume derangements that are commonly seen. A study by Yu et al. (5) showed that when blood volume measurement is used as part of goal-directed therapy in severely ill septic patients, there is an 8% death rate versus a 24% death rate when patients are treated without using blood volume measurements. In this series of patients, pulmonary artery catheterization as well as intensive therapy was used for all patients. The difference in results makes it clear, not surprisingly, that therapy based on accurate knowledge of the most fundamental underlying derangement in sepsis, namely blood compartment volumes, leads to markedly better survival rates.

Direct measurement of blood volume uses albumin I^{131} and is based on the indicator dilution principle (9). The concept is based on injecting a precise amount of albumin I^{131} into the circulation and obtaining timed samples at approximately 12, 18, 24, 30, and 36 minutes. Five-milliliter samples of the patient's blood are then separated into red cells and plasma, and the hematocrit is obtained on each timed sample. Albumin tagged with I^{131} behaves exactly as physiologic albumin (10). Albumin is a major carrier molecule for hundreds of substances within the human body. Albumin transudates across the capillary bed at approximately 0.05% to 0.25% per minute. At this rate, the albumin within the circulation turns over every 400 minutes (11).

In order to obtain an accurate blood volume measurement, it is essential that multiple samples be obtained to precisely measure the transudation rate so that a true "0" time blood volume measurement can be obtained. Standards are prepared in duplicate from a precisely matching injectate into a volumetric flask. The measured plasma volume can be accurately calculated from the ratio of the standard to the patient's blood volume. For example, if a standard manufactured from a 1,000-mL flask has 10,000 counts and the patient's plasma blood sample has 5,000 counts, the patient will have a plasma volume of 2,000 mL.

The technology for accurate measurement for blood volume has been known for more than 60 years. Blood volume measurements previously required 4 to 8 hours of technician time for preparation of standards, injectate, administration of tracer, collection of samples, individual measurements, and calculation of final results (9–15). Another impediment to accurate blood volume measurement was the need for an accurate norm for individual patients. In 1977, Feldschuh and Enson measured the blood volume in 160 healthy individuals who had a wide range of both heights as well as degrees of leanness and obesity (11,15). Their study demonstrated that blood volume was a curvilinear function rather than a linear function and that normal blood volume in healthy individuals varied from approximately 105 to 41 mL/kg in relation to the degree of leanness or obesity of the individual (16). The computation of individual norms from this data was time consuming. In June 1999, the FDA approved the Daxor BVA-100 Blood Volume Analyzer, which semi-automated blood volume measurement by providing a matching injectate and standards which could then be measured in a specialized semi-automated Geiger counter (10). The BVA-100 also computed the normal blood volume for each individual patient, eliminating another time-consuming step. The following information is provided by the BVA-100:

1. Total blood volume of the patient,
2. Red cell volume of the patient,
3. Plasma volume of the patient,
4. Normal values for the individual patients, i.e., total blood volume, total red cell volume, and total plasma volume of the patient.
5. Deviation from the predicted normal values in both milliliters and percentage,
6. Transudation rate of the albumin tracer. Normal rates of transudation are approximately 0.05% to 0.25% per minute. This information is particularly important in recognizing patients who have a capillary leak syndrome (5,11).
7. Normalized hematocrit. The instrument calculates the patient's adjusted or "normalized" hematocrit which is calculated from the measured blood volume compartments. The calculation reflects the difference between the predicted normal blood volume and the patient's measured blood volume (9). For example, patients who are hypovolemic, a common occurrence after surgery or acute hemorrhage will not have their hematocrit reflect the true extent of their blood volume depletion. The normalized hematocrit reflects the true nature of the patient's red blood volume status in another format which enables a clinician to more easily understand the blood volume derangements which are present. Patients who are hypovolemic will have a normalized hematocrit lower than the peripheral hematocrit and patients who are hypervolemic will have a normalized hematocrit which is higher than their peripheral hematocrit. The latter group may be considered to have a form of pseudo-anemia (17). These practices led to inaccurate blood volume measurements and when combined with inaccurate norms for individual patients, provided confusing results.

The development of an instrument which provides preliminary results in less than 30 minutes and highly accurate final results to ±2% in under an hour enables clinicians to analyze and treat blood volume compartment derangements which are at the core of treating sepsis on a timely basis (9). The injection kit is supplied with a collection kit which enables the entire injection and multiple-sample collection to be accomplished with a single venipuncture.

Clinicians have traditionally utilized hematocrit/hemoglobin measurements as a proxy for blood volume measurements despite the fact that it is well recognized that such measurements are only accurate if a patient is normovolemic. Critically ill patients who are frequently hypotensive and receive large quantities of fluids are particularly prone to be misdiagnosed using hematocrit/hemoglobin measurements. Patients who are hypervolemic will have their hematocrits depressed and may exhibit a pseudo-anemia while patients who are hypovolemic will have their hematocrits artificially elevated and have the severity of their anemia masked. Use of the normalized hematocrit helps to provide clarification for the clinician (5).

PHYSIOLOGY OF BLOOD VOLUME MAINTENANCE

The water in the body (total body water) is divided into two main compartments: the intracellular space (the water in the cells themselves) and the extracellular space. The extracellular space is further divided into the intravascular space and the interstitial space (the water between the cells and outside the vascular space). Although red blood cells are cellular, they are considered part of the vascular space.

Plasma and red blood cells account for more than 99% of the blood volume, while white cells and platelets account for less than 1%. Blood normally comprises approximately 7% of an average adult's body weight, but it can range anywhere from 4% to 10% depending on a person's gender and body composition. Women on average have an 8% lower blood volume and 18% lower red cell volume than men of identical height and weight. Leaner people tend to have a higher percentage of blood, while more obese people tend to have a lower percentage (11).

The most basic homeostatic mechanism in response to hemorrhage or sepsis is to restore a diminished normal blood volume to a normal blood volume. This process can be damaged by many confounding factors such as hypoalbuminemia, toxic damage to the capillaries resulting in a capillary leak syndrome, intravascular destruction of red cells, as well as other factors. Accurate correction of blood volume derangements is facilitated when clinicians can quantify the underlying derangements (5).

Plasma Volume Maintenance

The amount of plasma in the circulation adjusts constantly to maintain perfusion, temperature, and hemodynamics. A

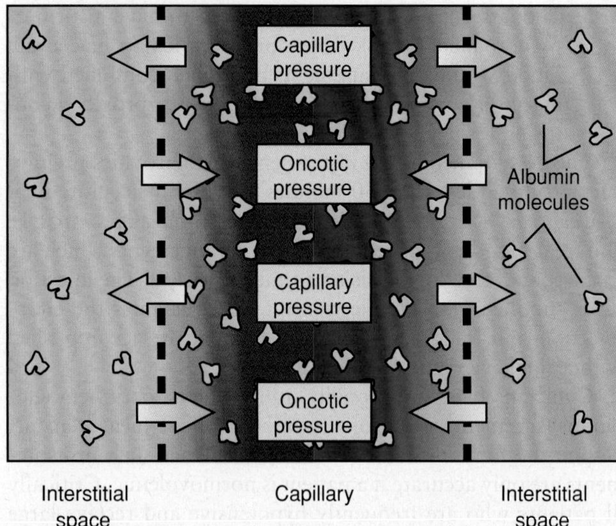

FIGURE 27.1 Dynamic equilibrium between hydrostatic (capillary) and oncotic pressures. Under normal conditions, there is a balance between the net hydrostatic pressure causing flux from the blood vessels into the interstitial space and the net oncotic pressure causing flux from the interstitial space into the blood vessels. The primary protein responsible for maintaining oncotic pressure is albumin, which occurs at a higher concentration in the blood vessels than in the interstitial space.

prime goal of plasma volume maintenance is to maintain a normal whole blood volume and to optimize perfusion to the organs and cells. The albumin and the kidneys play particularly important roles in plasma volume maintenance.

Albumin and Oncotic Pressure

The interstitial space functions in part as a reserve buffer of fluid, available as needed to provide additional fluid to the vascular space or accommodate excess fluid. Under normal circumstances, a constant flux of water across the capillary membranes between the vascular and interstitial spaces maintains a dynamic equilibrium. Hydrostatic pressure is higher in the vasculature than in the interstitial space, which causes water to flow out of the vascular space into the interstitial space. Counterbalancing this, the relatively higher concentration of albumin and other proteins in the vascular space results in a higher oncotic pressure, causing water to flow out of the interstitial space into the vascular space as described by Starling forces (Fig. 27.1). Albumin is the primary protein responsible for maintaining oncotic pressure (18). An adequate pool of albumin is needed to maintain the pressure gradient between the vascular and interstitial spaces, and a low enough capillary permeability is needed to keep albumin from transudating too quickly out of the circulation into the interstitial space. Normally, albumin transudates out of the plasma into the interstitial space at a rate of approximately 0.05% to 0.25% per minute (13). Albumin eventually returns to the circulation via the lymphatic system and re-enters the circulatory system via the thoracic duct. However, if too much albumin leaves the circulation too quickly, then the relative concentration of vascular albumin to interstitial albumin—and thus the oncotic pressure—decreases, causing a decrease in plasma volume. This can result in a capillary leak syndrome with a collapse of intravascular volume. Approximately 60% of the total body albumin is in the interstitial space (19).

The Kidneys and the Renin–Angiotensin–Aldosterone System

The kidneys are of particular importance in blood volume regulation. Under optimal circumstances, the kidneys' rate of excretion of sodium and water adjusts continually to maintain a normal whole blood volume.

When the kidneys receive decreased perfusion, the rennin–angiotensin– aldosterone (RAA) system is activated. The RAA system includes both rapid- and slow-response mechanisms. The rapid response, a rise in blood pressure caused by angiotensin-mediated vasoconstriction, occurs almost immediately. The slower response, an increase in plasma volume caused by the actions of aldosterone, can occur over the course of days. The kidneys' response is essentially primitive—they respond to changes in perfusion without being able to differentiate the cause. Thus, while the kidneys ideally function to regulate blood volume, sometimes their responses are maladaptive. For example, if an individual has a normal blood volume but has renal artery stenosis or heart failure, the RAA system is activated, vasoconstriction increases, and excess plasma volume is retained even if the individual has a normal or even expanded blood volume. In congestive heart failure patients, reduced cardiac output results in hypoperfusion of the kidneys and a maladaptive syndrome which results in increased retention of sodium and water resulting in an expanded plasma volume and blood volume (20,21).

The pituitary gland also plays a role in blood volume maintenance. It responds to increased concentration of solutes in plasma or decreased blood pressure by secreting antidiuretic hormone (ADH, also known as vasopressin), which stimulates water reabsorption in the kidneys, reducing urine output. Hyponatremia has been observed in intensive care units, particularly in septic patients. Like the kidneys, the pituitary gland responds to indicators of decreased volume without being able to differentiate the cause.

Red Blood Cell Volume Maintenance

Red cell volume is primarily maintained through a balance of production (erythropoiesis) and destruction (hemolysis). Red blood cells are created in the bone marrow and, at the end of their life span, hemolyzed in the spleen or the liver. In the presence of normal bone marrow function, the rate of red cell production is controlled by the hormone erythropoietin, which is produced by the kidney, with the rate of production affected by indicators of blood oxygenation. If red blood cells are lost (such as through hemorrhage), they can be replaced through the manufacture of new cells by the bone marrow. It can take days to months to replace lost red cells, depending on the amount lost and an individual's capacity for creating new red cells. A study of healthy males who donated two units of blood found that the subjects took a month to replace an average of 92% of the lost blood (22).

Difficulties in Estimating Blood Volume

Many of the measurements available in a clinical setting are indicators or proxy measurements for perfusion (local or systemic), vasomotor tone (local or systemic), or blood volume. These measurements may include:

- Blood pressure and heart rate
- Blood gases, including pH, base deficit, and lactic acid as estimates of perfusion

- Hematocrit and hemoglobin as surrogate tests for red cell volume
- Blood urea nitrogen (BUN)/creatinine as an estimate of kidney function
- Urine output as an estimate of kidney function and/or perfusion
- Invasive procedures such as pulmonary artery catheter (PAC) for determination of intravascular pressures
- Clinical maneuvers such as passive leg raising have been shown not to have a high correlation in response to fluid challenges (7,8)

None of these, however, is a direct measure of volume status. The physician in the critical care setting is faced with the difficult situation of administering or withholding fluids, blood, and blood components on the basis of these surrogate tests. In particular, hemoglobin and hematocrit are frequently inaccurate surrogate markers for blood volume. When using hematocrit or hemoglobin to estimate red cell volume, it is assumed that the whole blood volume remains normovolemic (euvolemic)—for example, that fluid replacement of lost red cells via plasma expansion is rapid but may not be complete. This is frequently not the case. Review articles on fluid management discuss a variety of complex factors to consider when estimating a patient's volume status (23,24), and clinical estimation is frequently inaccurate. Monitoring blood volume using clinical assessment and proxy measurements can be particularly misleading in the critical care setting, because compensatory responses to acute blood volume derangements occur at different rates. Changes in vasomotor tone may occur nearly instantaneously, while changes in plasma volume may occur over hours or days and may not completely compensate for lost red cells or albumin. Following acute blood loss, rapid changes in vasoconstriction, which can occur before any compensatory volume expansion takes place, may maintain a relatively normal peripheral blood pressure and hematocrit at the expense of organ perfusion. Administration of fluids, blood, or blood components can additionally complicate the diagnostic picture.

A 2003 study (25) compared clinical estimates of intravascular volume with estimates obtained by determining corrected left ventricular flow time from transesophageal Doppler imaging. Clinical estimates agreed with Doppler imaging results only 30% of the time. Therefore, it is clear that the Doppler imaging technique is not accurate for estimating blood volume.

It is a common intuitive assumption that achieving normovolemia facilitates effective perfusion and contributes to improved outcomes. Although no studies have explicitly evaluated clinical assessment against blood volume measurement in the critical care unit.

Additional recent studies have provided evidence that achieving normovolemia is a valid goal in a number of clinical settings. In a heart failure study performed at Columbia Presbyterian Hospital, among 43 nonedematous, hypervolemic patients had a 2-year mortality rate of 57%, while normovolemic and slightly hypovolemic patients had a 2-year mortality rate of 0%. The American College of Cardiology has previously recommended assessment of volume status as an important factor in the diagnosis and treatment of heart failure, but this was the first study to provide a clear association between measured blood volume and patient outcome with respect to treatment achieving normovolemia (20,21).

INTERPRETING BLOOD VOLUME MEASUREMENT RESULTS

Units of Measurement

In addition to absolute measurements, blood volume results for each compartment should be presented as the patient's deviation from his or her normal volume, both as a percent deviation and in milliliters. The percentage indicates the severity of the patient's blood volume, and the absolute quantity of the depletion can help guide treatment.

Relationship Between Whole Blood, Red Cell, and Plasma Volumes

When interpreting blood volume results, the whole blood volume should be considered first. Homeostatic mechanisms attempt to restore blood volume to normal even if it dilutes the remaining red cells (11). The relationship between the peripheral hematocrit and the normalized hematocrit will provide guidance for those not familiar with blood volume measurement results. Plasma volume results should be considered from the perspective of whether they are homeostatic or pathologic. For example, a patient with a diminished red cell volume should have an expanded compensatory or homeostatic expansion of the blood volume. Patients who have loss of red cells and hypoalbuminemia can be difficult to evaluate clinically unless a blood volume measurement, including red cell volume and plasma volume, is performed to elucidate the underlying derangement. Hypoalbminemia alters the normal ratio of one part plasma volume to three parts interstitial volume. Patients with severe hypoalbuminemia, therefore, will, out of necessity, require expanded interstitial volume, as manifested by peripheral edema, to achieve a normal blood volume.

The Rate of Transudation

Albumin I^{131} is an ideal tracer for measuring blood volume. Albumin normally transudates out of the circulation into the interstitial space at a rate of approximately 0.05% to 0.25% per minute (5,11). Obtaining a minimum of five-timed samples enables calculation of the transudation rate. Rates between 0.25% and 0.4% are suspicious for a capillary leak syndrome. Rates above 0.5% are strongly suggestive of a capillary leak syndrome. Capillary leak syndrome will result in hypoalbuminemia and hypovolemia. Sepsis and burn patients are classic examples of patients with these conditions. A major clinical error is to attempt to diurese patients who have hypoalbuminemia because they have evidence of peripheral edema, suggesting total body water. Such patients require an expanded interstitial volume to maintain a normal blood volume. Over diurising such patients to remove their peripheral edema will result in hypovolemia, hypoperfusion, and may result in renal failure or multiple-organ failure.

APPLICATIONS OF BLOOD VOLUME MEASUREMENT IN CRITICAL CARE

Undetected Hypovolemia

Early detection of hypovolemia is essential. By the time a patient becomes symptomatic, hypovolemia is often extreme, damage may have already occurred to critical organs (the gut and the kidneys are particularly susceptible), and deterioration may be rapid and unexpected (5).

In acute situations, the current primary measures used to track perfusion and evaluate fluid replacement requirements include pressure measurements (such as central venous pressure, intra-arterial or indirect auscultating blood pressure, and pulmonary artery catheter measurements) in conjunction with hematocrit/hemoglobin measurements. However, the body can respond to hypovolemia by initiating vasoconstrictive defense mechanisms, maintaining near-normal pressures even in the face of severe blood loss, and allowing the hypovolemia to remain undetected.

Hypovolemia is generally more dangerous and urgent than the same degree of hypervolemia, and sudden blood loss is more urgent than the same degree of chronic hypovolemia. A patient may tolerate a 40% increase in whole blood volume or an 80% increase in red cell volume for some time without suffering acute negative effects, but a 40% loss of blood or an 80% loss of red cells is an extreme medical emergency. A sudden loss of as little as 20% of the blood volume triggers an acute vasoconstrictive response, and a sudden 30% loss can lead to circulatory collapse. A rapid 40% to 45% loss is incompatible with life. Further, an already anemic or hypovolemic patient who experiences sudden blood loss will be less able to tolerate that loss than would a normovolemic or hypervolemic patient. Even after fluid resuscitation (whether after partially compensated shock or circulatory collapse), damage to the gut and kidneys may result in severe irreversible complications (26).

Undetected Hypervolemia

In the critical care unit, hypervolemia may be a result of comorbidities or iatrogenic causes such as excessive fluids. Chronic hypervolemia may develop slowly and is most frequently related to cardiac disease, particularly in heart failure. In contrast, acute hypervolemia is almost always iatrogenic. Particular attention must be paid to patients who are oliguric or in renal shutdown, as these patients cannot remove excess fluid through urine output. A major common clinical error is to equate evidence of fluid overload such as obvious edema as proof that the patient is hypervolemic. The patient may have paradoxical hypovolemia, particularly if the patient is also hypoalbuminemic. The patient may also have a capillary leak syndrome, which predisposes to hypovolemia. It is essential to avoid this mistake. An accurate blood volume measurement will quickly clarify the situation and save the lives of critically ill patients.

The hypervolemic patient is at risk for the development of pulmonary edema in response to increased pressure; hypoalbuminemia, which predisposes to pulmonary edema. Pulmonary hypertension as a maladaptive mechanism observed in chronic heart failure that may eventually lead to permanent pulmonary hypertension and worsening of heart failure.

Blood volume measurement can be used to accurately diagnose the presence and quantify the hypervolemia. Treatment can vary depending on the severity of the patient's hypervolemia and the patient's kidney function and may include fluid restriction, diuretic therapy, hemodialysis if the patient is in kidney failure, or ultrafiltration. It is important to remember that patients can usually tolerate moderate degrees of hypervolemia with minimal consequences as compared to the consequences of moderate hypovolemia (5).

The Bleeding Patient: When to Perform Blood Volume Measurement

If a patient has continuing massive bleeding such as, for example, greater than 100 mL/hr, blood volume measurement should be performed when the patient is semi-stabilized. Fluid pressures may be a helpful guide. In a patient who is bleeding at an estimated lower rate, for example, 60 mL/hr, a blood volume can be accurately performed and be quite useful. A patient losing 80 mL of blood per hour would lose 1920 mL of blood in a 24-hour period. This is a massive loss of blood. Since a blood volume measurement requires 40 minutes or less from the time of injection to completion of collection of five samples, such a patient would lose approximately 54 mL of blood. This would represent 1% to 3% of a patient's blood volume and lend a slight increase of inaccuracy to the measurement.

Each individual blood volume has a calculated degree of accuracy for that specific blood volume. If a measured blood volume had a measured accuracy of ±4% and a reported result of −30%, the result would still be very helpful in defining the patient as severely hypovolemic. It would also quantify the degree of the deficit.

Tracking Changes in Blood Volume and Performing Follow-Up Measurements

After an initial blood volume measurement, it is possible in a nonbleeding patient to track changes in blood volume with precise hematocrit measurements. If the patient's red cell volume remains stable, changes in the hematocrit reflect changes in blood volume as follows:

$$\text{Plasma volume} = \text{red cell volume} \times (1 - \text{hematocrit})/\text{hematocrit}$$

$$\text{Whole blood volume} = \text{red cell volume}/\text{hematocrit}$$

For example, consider a patient who is found to have a measured red cell volume of 2,000 mL, plasma volume of 4,000 mL, and hematocrit of 33%. This patient is diuresed, and the hematocrit rises to 40%. The new volume is equal to:

$$\text{Plasma volume} = 2{,}000 \text{ mL} \times (1 - 0.4)/0.4 = 3{,}000 \text{ mL}$$

$$\text{Whole blood volume} = 2{,}000/0.4 = 5{,}000 \text{ mL}$$

This relationship is particularly important to understand and can be used in analyzing changes in blood volume on patients undergoing renal dialysis. One study (27) demonstrated that in a nonbleeding patient undergoing acute volume changes, whether from dialysis or diuretics or ultra-filtration, it is possible to determine and quantify whether fluid being removed from the patient is primarily from the interstitial space or the intravascular space. This enables treatment choices to be made in direct response to blood volume compartment changes which are measured rather than rough estimates based on indirect surrogate measures.

If a nonbleeding patient receives a transfusion, the volume response may be roughly estimated based on the type of fluid transfused and its expected effect on the hematocrit; a follow-up blood volume measurement may be needed for precise quantification. If a patient is bleeding or otherwise experiences a change in red cell volume that cannot be reasonably estimated, blood volume changes cannot be tracked with precision via changes in hematocrit. A follow-up blood volume measurement should be performed 24 to 48 hours after treatment is initiated.

In general, changes in blood volume may correlate with changes in symptoms, hemodynamic measurements, or clinical status, but these relationships are not necessarily straightforward. In one study of acute decompensated heart failure patients (28) after 24 to 48 hours of treatment blood volume correlated better with some hemodynamic measurements than did brain natriuretic peptide (BNP) levels. However, no measurements correlated closely enough with blood volume results for any hemodynamic measurement to serve as a surrogate measure for volume status, or vice versa.

BLOOD VOLUME MEASUREMENTS IN COMMON CRITICAL CARE SITUATIONS

Shock

The presentation of symptoms in shock may not be straightforward and can complicate assessment of the patient's volume status, especially in situations where several factors contribute to shock. Blood volume measurement can be of major importance in understanding the underlying cascade of events that precipitate shock and determining appropriate treatment. In a patient with hypovolemia, even in conjunction with other contributing factors, appropriate transfusion and fluid replacement are needed before severe multiple-organ hypoperfusion and failure ensue.

For example, following a myocardial infarction, patients frequently become hypotensive. While cardiac damage usually plays a major, if not the predominant, role in the ensuing shock, blood volume derangements may play a significant additional role. A patient with a myocardial infarction (MI) may develop hypovolemia from severe vomiting, profuse sweating, or the use of anticoagulants. Sometimes blood loss secondary to gastrointestinal bleeding may trigger an MI. Because the blood loss may not be recognized as a precipitating factor in the MI, the patient may not be treated to restore volume. This may progress to renal or multiple-organ damage. Accurate assessment of the volume status and prompt treatment of volume derangements are important for all types of shock, even those that do not appear initially to be volume-related.

All patients who have shock from any cause should have a blood volume measurement to define the extent to which volume derangements, particularly hypovolemia, may be a causative factor. A patient who has a myocardial infarction may have hypovolemia either as a triggering factor or a secondary factor. It is essential to rapidly diagnose the patient and correct their hypovolemia with appropriate fluids. It has been demonstrated that clinical parameters, including information derived from PACs were not reliable in predicting blood volume in surgical intensive care patients (24).

Acidosis frequently develops from hypoperfusion and a shift to anaerobic metabolism, resulting in increased lactic acid production. Under these circumstances, the body's metabolic defense mechanisms, which are strongly geared to maintain a pH of 7.4, may be overcome. At a pH of 7.0 to 7.1, major deterioration of all functions including cardiac metabolism occurs. At a pH of 6.85 to 6.9, the body's metabolic systems are so diminished that death is imminent (29).

Acidosis may also develop from other underlying causes. For example, in diabetic acidosis, ketoacidosis develops from hyperglycemia. Hypovolemia may be a contributing factor, though, because the severely dehydrated patient may have localized ischemia.

Blood volume measurement may be helpful in elucidating the underlying cause of acidosis and determining optimal therapy. If the acidosis is caused by hypoperfusion related to diminished blood volume, aggressive and rapid therapy is needed before irreversible deterioration occurs. In situations such as diabetic acidosis, therapy should also be directed at correcting the underlying condition (such as hyperglycemia), correction of the electrolyte imbalance, and, most importantly, restoring the patient's blood volume derangement. There are a multitude of various combinations of red cell and plasma volume derangements which can only be defined and quantified by a blood volume measurement.

Hypoalbuminemia

Hypoalbuminemic patients, because of a shift in oncotic pressure, may be predisposed to edema formation in order to achieve a balance of hydrostatic and oncotic pressures that can maintain a normal blood volume. Rather than a normal ratio of 3:1 of extracellular to vascular volume, equilibrium between the two spaces may be reached at a ratio of 4:1 or 5:1. In such patients, the goal is to maintain a normal blood volume even if that means allowing an expanded extracellular volume. It is a common mistake to focus treatment on removal of obvious peripheral edema. Patients with hypoalbuminemia and/or capillary leak syndrome may require a larger volume of extracellular fluid in order to maintain a normal blood volume.

Therapeutic albumin is underutilized because of the inability to correctly quantify total body albumin. A common mistake is to misunderstand the size of the albumin pool and that it may take 12 to 24 hours for administered albumin to equilibrate in the albumin pool. Albumin has a half-life of 13 to 15 days (30). Approximately 60% of the body's albumin is in the interstitial space (25). A common misconception is to measure serum albumin concentrations 3 to 4 hours after administration of albumin and then measure albumin concentration 24 to 26 hours later and interpret the drop in albumin concentration as rapid metabolism of albumin instead of the prolonged equilibration period of albumin into the intravascular and interstitial pool. Hypoalbuminemia is a common problem seen in septic, diabetic, heart failure, renal and hepatic disease patients, which causes major blood volume derangements. These derangements can be quantified and appropriate therapy administered after blood volume measurement.

Hepatorenal Syndrome

In the hepatorenal syndrome, the liver and kidneys fail simultaneously. Frequently, this syndrome originates with liver damage that progresses to cirrhosis and portal hypertension, causing edema and ascites. If the patient is over diuresed to remove the edema, the patient becomes hypovolemic and the kidneys hypoperfused. If severe enough, this can lead to kidney failure, liver failure, and circulatory collapse.

Hepatorenal syndrome is essentially part of a cascade of circulatory decompensation that, if not corrected, usually results in multiple-organ failure and death. Quantifying the blood volume compartments of red cell volume and plasma volume is essential to detecting and correcting this situation. It is usually not possible to diurese a patient with liver damage to completely remove edema, because diuresis does not correct the underlying imbalance between intravascular and interstitial volume. A normal ratio of one part intravascular volume to three parts interstitial volume may now be altered so that the new ratio may be 1:5 or 1:6. After total body water reduction, the reduced fluid simply redistributes throughout the vascular and extravascular spaces in the same ratio. This situation is similar when using paracentesis to treat ascites. Because paracentesis only removes ascitic fluid and does not address the underlying fluid and pressure imbalance, the rapid removal of a large amount of ascetic fluid causes fluid to shift quickly from the vascular to the interstitial peritoneal space, resulting in hypovolemia, a drop in blood pressure, and collapse of the circulation.

Blood volume measurement can be performed on a patient with liver problems, edema, and/or ascites to determine what quantity of diuresis is possible without precipitating hypovolemia. A patient who is hypervolemic will be able to tolerate diuresis, and an edematous normovolemic patient should be diuresed only slowly and minimally, with careful follow-up. Some patients with edema and/or ascites may require a blood volume at the upper limit of normal in order to maintain adequate perfusion pressures. A patient who is hypovolemic should not undergo diuresis! Therapeutic use of albumin should be considered to help mobilize some of the acidic fluid and help maintain blood volume. Unfortunately, in late stages of the disease, the relief is relatively limited in time.

Diuretic Resistance

The term diuretic resistance is frequently used when patients do not respond to relatively large quantities of i.v. diuretics. To some extent the term may be a misnomer, because diuretic resistance may be a reflection of severe hypoperfusion. A patient in renal shutdown will obviously not respond to diuretics, and occasionally aggressive use of diuretics precipitates renal shutdown. To differentiate true diuretic resistance from hypoperfusion of the kidneys, blood volume measurement in conjunction with renal tests can be helpful. This differentiation is particularly important because aggressive use of diuretics in a patient with marginal perfusion to the kidneys caused by hypovolemia and hypotension may precipitate total renal shutdown. Hypoalbuminemia is a major confounding factor in treating patients with expanded total body water, as it predisposes to intravascular volume depletion.

A major common error is to equate the presence of obvious peripheral edema with evidence for intravascular volume expansion. This sometimes results in aggressive diuretic treatment in patients who have paradoxical hypovolemia that is further aggravated by the use of potent diuretics. Such patients are particularly susceptible to developing iatrogenic renal failure. Direct blood volume measurement can easily identify such patients and avoid inappropriate treatment that may lead to multiple-organ failure.

Cardiogenic and Noncardiogenic Pulmonary Edema

Cardiogenic pulmonary edema (caused by increased hydrostatic pressure in the alveoli), often secondary to hypervolemia, and noncardiogenic pulmonary edema (caused by damage to the membranes of the alveoli), also known as acute respiratory distress syndrome (ARDS), have different underlying causes and require different treatment approaches. The two conditions may present similar symptoms, and both are common in the critical care setting. When physical examination and noninvasive tests do not provide a definitive distinction, pulmonary capillary wedge pressure is often used to distinguish between the two, but results may be difficult to interpret in patients with pulmonary artery hypertension related to other conditions. Additionally, patients may have a combination of both conditions; increased hydrostatic pressure does not rule out damage to the alveoli. The relationship between blood volume and wedge pressures seems at best weak, with no correlation to central venous pressures (25).

Blood volume measurement, by detecting the presence or absence of hypervolemia, can be used in the differential diagnosis of cardiogenic and noncardiogenic pulmonary edema, especially in patients known to have pulmonary hypertension from other causes and in patients for whom invasive PAC is not desirable.

Hypervolemia is more likely to be present in a patient with cardiogenic pulmonary edema, while noncardiogenic pulmonary edema may develop in a patient with normovolemia or hypovolemia. However, because both conditions may coexist, hypervolemia does not rule out ARDS. These conditions must also be reviewed in the context of evaluating albumin, as hypoalbuminemia by itself will predispose to pulmonary edema. There have been documented cases of cardiac patients with pulmonary edema and hypoalbuminemia who are hypovolemic. Such patients need to be treated with 25% albumin and not treated with diuretics. The assumption that all patients with pulmonary edema and cardiac disease are hypervolemic may lead to inappropriate diuretic treatment.

Key Points

- While fluid resuscitation and blood volume management have long been mainstays in critical care, evaluation of blood volume has traditionally relied on assessment of the patient's clinical condition, which is often misleading, and surrogate measurements to estimate volume status, which are often inaccurate.
- Blood volume measurement has been traditionally difficult to estimate in critically ill patients, and the clinical utilization of rapid semi-automated radioisotopic blood volume measurement has shown to improve accuracy of that measurement.
- On the simplest level, blood volume measurement results can be used as an alternative guide to improve accuracy when estimating volume status.

References

1. Rivers E. Nguyen B. Havstad S, et al. Early goal-directed therapy in the treatment of severe sepsis and septic shock. *N Engl J Med*. 2001;345:1368–1377.
2. Tisherman SA. Barie P, Bokhari F, et al. Clinical practice guideline: end-points of resuscitation. *J Trauma*. 2004;57:898–912.
3. Jones AE, Brown MD, Trzeciak S, et al. The effect of a quantitative resuscitation strategy on mortality in patients with sepsis: a meta-analysis. *Crit Care Med*. 2008;36:2734–2739.
4. Murphy CV, Schramm GE, Doherty JA, et al. The importance of fluid management in acute lung injury secondary to septic shock. *Chest*. 2009;136:102–109.
5. Yu M, Pei K, Moran S, et al. A prospective randomized trial using blood volume analysis in addition to pulmonary artery catheter, compared with

pulmonary artery catheter alone, to guide shock resuscitation in critically ill surgical ill patients. *Shock*. 2011;35:220–228.

6. Marino P. Hemorrhage and hypovolemia. In: *The ICU Book*. 4th ed. Philadelphia, PA: Wolters Kluwer; 2014;195–215.
7. Mahjoub Y, Tuzeau J, Airapetian N, et al. The passive leg-raising maneuver cannot accurately predict fluid responsiveness in patients with intra-abdominal hypertension. *Crit Care Med*. 2010;36:1824–1829.
8. Cavallaro F, Sandroni C, Marano C, et al. Diagnostic accuracy of passive leg raising for prediction of fluid responsiveness in adults, systematic review and meta-analysis of clinical studies. *Intensive Care Med*. 2010;36:1475–1483.
9. Manzone TA, Dam HQ, Soltis D, et al. Blood volume analysis: a new technique and new clinical interest reinvigorate a classic study. *J Nucl Med Technol*. 2007;35(2):55–63.
10. Dworkin H, Premo M, Dees S. Comparison of red cell and whole blood volume as performed using both chromium-51 tagged red cells and iodine-125 tagged albumin and using I-131 tagged albumin and extrapolated red cell volume. *Am J Med Sci*. 2001;334(1):32.
11. Feldschuh J, Enson Y. Prediction of the normal blood volume. Relation of blood volume to body habitus. *Circulation*. 1977;56(4 Pt 1):605–612.
12. Smith HP. Blood volume studies II. Repeated determination of blood volume and short intervals by means of the dye method. *Am J Physiol*. 1920; 51:221.
13. Smith HP. The fate of an intravenously injected dye (brilliant vital red) with special reference to its use in blood volume determination. *Bull Johns Hopkins Hosp*. 1925;36:325.
14. Gergersen MI, Gibson JJ, Stead EA. Plasma volume determination with dyes, errors in colorimetry: use of the blue dye T-1824. *Am J Physiol (Proc)*. 1935;113:54–55.
15. Keys A, Brozek J, Henschel A, et al. *The Biology of Human Starvation*. Minneapolis, MN: University of Minnesota Press; 1950.
16. Feldschuh J, Katz S. The importance of correct norms in blood volume measurement. *Am J Med Sci*. 2007;334:41–46.
17. Takanishi DM, Yu M, Lurie D, et al. Peripheral blood hematocrit in critically ill surgical patients: an imprecise surrogate of true red cell volume. *Anesth Analg*. 2008;106:1808–1812.
18. Tullis JL. Albumin. 1. Background and use. 2. Guidelines for clinical use. *JAMA*. 1977;237:355–360, 460–463.
19. Mendez C, McClain C, Marsano L, et al. Albumin therapy in clinical practice. *Nutr Clin Pract*. 2005;20:314–320.
20. Androne AS, Katz SD, Lund L, et al. Hemodilution is common in patients with advanced heart failure. *Circulation*. 2003;107:226–229.
21. Mancini DM, Katz SD, Lang CC, et al. Effect of erythropoietin on exercise capacity in patients with moderate to severe chronic heart failure. *Circulation*. 2003;107:294–299.
22. Valeri CR, Ragno G, Srey R. Restoration of red blood cell volume following 2-unit red blood cell apheresis. *Vox Sang*. 2003;85:85–87.
23. Iregui MG, Prentice D, Sherman G, et al. Physicians' estimates of cardiac index and intravascular volume based on clinical assessment versus transesophageal Doppler measurements obtained by critical care nurses. *Am J Crit Care*. 2003;12:336–342.
24. Takanishi DM, Biuk-Aghai E, Yu M, et al. Availability of circulating blood volume alters fluid management in critically ill surgical patients. *Am J Surg*. 2009;197:232–237.
25. James KB, Troughton RW, Feldschuh J, et al. Blood volume and brain natriuretic peptide in congestive heart failure: a pilot study. *Am Heart J*. 2005;150:984.
26. Alrawi SJ, Miranda LS, Cunningham JN Jr, et al. Correlation of blood volume values and pulmonary artery catheter measurements. *Saudi Med J*. 2002;23:1367–1372.
27. Puri S, Park JK, Modersitzki F, Goldfarb DS.. Radioisotope blood volume measurement in hemodialysis patients. *Am J Kidney Dis*. 2014;18: 406–414.
28. Miller W, Mullan BP. Understanding the heterogeneity in volume overload and fluid distribution in decompensated heart failure is key to optimal volume management: role for blood volume quantitation. *JACC Heart Failure*. 2014;2:298–305.
29. Feldschuh J, Gambino R. Extreme central acidosis from Abbott epinephrine. *Am J Med*. 1983;74:30–32.
30. Vincent J-L, DeBacker D. Circulatory shock. *N Engl J Med*. 2013;369: 1726–1734.

CHAPTER

28

Neurologic Monitoring

STEVEN A. ROBICSEK, MICHAEL E. MAHLA, DIETRICH GRAVENSTEIN, and CHRISTOPH N. SEUBERT

Neurologic monitoring in the intensive care unit (ICU) is used either in a general sense as part of a system-based approach to assess one of the major bodily systems or with the specific intent to guide therapy and/or assess prognosis. Imaging studies of the central nervous system (CNS)—while not considered "monitoring" in the strict sense—play a central role in this assessment by establishing diagnoses and quantifying the extent of pathology. Important constraints for typical neuroradiologic imaging are presented in the first section below.

Many interventions in the ICU aimed at restoring or maintaining conditions that are favorable for recovery of the patient target the normal brain and, by extension, affect the results of neurologic monitoring. Therefore, an understanding of the parameters that affect the state of the brain is necessary as the context for interpreting the results of neurologic monitoring. These are presented in the second section, followed by a detailed discussion of available modalities for serial assessment or monitoring of the nervous system.

NEURORADIOLOGIC IMAGING

Routine imaging studies of the brain are important in the repeated assessment of a patient's neurologic status. Objective information, particularly about structural abnormalities, is essential to the clinical diagnosis. Computed tomography (CT) and magnetic resonance imaging (MRI) are the most commonly used studies. Continued or critically timed assessment may provide insight into the time course of an emerging or recovery from a pathologic process (1). Typical imaging workup for various clinical diagnoses in critical care medicine is presented in Table 28.1.

To maximize the utility of an imaging study, the requesting physician needs to be aware of the inherent strengths and weaknesses of the chosen imaging modality, as well as considerations such as morbid obesity, claustrophobia, the use of contrast agents, and metal implants (see www.mrisafety.com). Whereas the quality of CT images is simply degraded by patient movement, MRI images acquired in an uncooperative, moving patient may contain "spurious pathology" because of misregistration of anatomic structures. Contextual details of the clinical history should be provided to the interpreting radiologist so that the imaging protocol can be designed to optimize information. Finally, some thought should be given to the balance between the time spent obtaining the images and the risks to the patient from reduced, or delayed, care during imaging and transport. Given the rapid development in MRI modalities or in postacquisition processing, such a balance is frequently best achieved by consulting directly with the radiologist.

CT provides a map of the degree of radiographic absorption of intracranial structures. Generally, it is the test of choice for localizing blood and imaging bone. Newer, helical CT scanners make image acquisition a comparatively fast process. This allows the two- and three-dimensional reconstruction of arterial anatomy from images during the first pass of radiocontrast administration to obtain a CT arteriogram.

MRI provides a map of the response of hydrogen nuclei to external magnetic fields. It is more versatile than CT, provides better imaging of posterior fossa contents, and is considerably more time consuming. T1 weighting enhances the detection of lipids, methemoglobin (e.g., as the subacute residual of a hemorrhage), and concentrated protein (e.g., in a colloid cyst). A radiofrequency pulse prior to T1 image acquisition can suppress the enhancement of lipids ("fat suppression") and is an example of a protocol change that affects the resulting image. T2 weighting enhances the detection of unbound water such as in cerebrospinal fluid (CSF) (Fig. 28.1). A radiofrequency pulse prior to T2 image acquisition (fluid attenuation inversion recovery [FLAIR] imaging) can suppress the enhancement of CSF and improve the detection of edema. MRI can also be focused to detect moving elements such as in MR arteriography or venography or CSF flow studies. Axoplasmic motion of bulk water can be imaged with MRI to obtain a diffusion image (apparent diffusion coefficient [ADC] map). This axoplasmic motion stops shortly after brain ischemia; therefore, diffusion images provide the earliest radiographic evidence for the core zone of an ischemic stroke.

Contrast media distribute with the blood flow and can therefore accentuate areas of increased vascularity such as in inflamed tissue or areas of tumor-induced angioneogenesis. Contrast media also distribute into—and thereby highlight—brain structures that are missing a blood–brain barrier such as the pineal gland or pituitary stalk, or brain areas where the blood–brain barrier has been disrupted. Brain perfusion can be imaged following a bolus administration of contrast medium by both MRI and CT. The resulting map of the time to peak concentration of the contrast medium currently provides qualitative information on cerebral blood flow (CBF), although quantitative approaches are under development. Qualitative differences in CBF can be used to identify the ischemic penumbra of a stroke.

CEREBRAL METABOLISM

The cerebral metabolic rate for oxygen ($CMRO_2$) of the brain averages 3.0 to 3.8 mL O_2/min/100 g. Although only 2% of body weight, the human adult brain accounts for 15% to 20% of the resting oxygen consumption and about 25% to 30% of the glucose consumption of the body. To meet this high demand for oxygen and glucose, the brain requires a relatively high level of brain tissue perfusion (40 to 60 mL/min/100 g) of brain tissue. CBF is regulated by four primary factors: metabolic stimuli, chemical stimuli, perfusion pressure, and neural stimuli.

TABLE 28.1 Typical Imaging Procedures for Neurologic Diseases in Their Acute Phase

Neurologic Disease	Initial Imaging	Further Workup/Alternatives
Stroke	CT to rule out hemorrhage	Diffusion- and perfusion-weighted MRI to identify ischemic core and penumbra, respectively
Arteriovenous malformation	CT for hemorrhage	MR angiography or angiography as soon as possible
Intracerebral aneurysm	CT for subarachnoid hemorrhage	CT angiography or angiography to identify aneurysm; TCD for vasospasm
Brain tumor	MRI without and with contrast	
Traumatic brain injury	CT	MRI as indicated later
Multiple sclerosis	MRI without and with contrast	
Meningitis/encephalitis	CT without and with contrast	MRI without and with contrast after initial treatment
Intracranial abscess	CT without and with contrast	MRI without and with contrast even initially, if patient is stable
Granuloma	MRI without and with contrast	

CT, computed tomography; MRI, magnetic resonance imaging; TCD, transcranial Doppler ultrasonography.
Modified from Gilman S. Imaging the brain. First of two parts. *N Engl J Med.* 1998;338:812–820.

FLOW–METABOLISM COUPLING

In the normal brain, an increase in cerebral metabolism is rapidly matched by local increases in CBF. This is referred to as *regional flow–metabolism coupling* or *cerebral metabolic autoregulation* (2). CBF is thus linked to brain function and metabolism so that CBF varies in parallel with $CMRO_2$ (Fig. 28.2). Autoregulation and increased oxygen extraction are two compensatory responses to acute reductions in CBF (3–5). Oxygen extraction is able to vary within a narrow range. Misery perfusion occurs when oxygen extraction is increased as a response to increased $CMRO_2$, either when autoregulatory CBF compensation has been exceeded or uncoupling has occurred (6). As cerebral perfusion pressure (CPP) falls, CBF is maintained initially by resistance arteriole vasodilation (7). Severe ischemia results as CPP is further reduced; the capacity of CBF autoregulation and increased oxygen extraction is exhausted, and CBF falls as a function of pressure. Positron emission tomography (PET) studies indicate that this occurs with relatively preserved $CMRO_2$ in the penumbra of a focal ischemic area.

Several vasoactive metabolic mediators have been proposed for cerebral regulation, including hydrogen ion, potassium, CO_2, adenosine, glycolytic intermediates, phospholipid metabolites (2), and, more recently, nitric oxide (8). In humans, flow–metabolism coupling is evident during a variety of motor and cognitive tasks that can be mapped using CBF techniques (9).

The global relationship between CBF and $CMRO_2$ can be expressed by the Fick equation where $DajO_2$ is the arteriojugular difference in oxygen content:

$$CMRO_2 = DajO_2 \times CBF \quad \text{or} \quad DajO_2 = CMRO_2/CBF$$

In brain injury, during hypothermia, and under the influence of anesthetic agents, CBF and metabolism may become dissociated. In a series of 109 severe head injury patients, Bouma et al. reported that CBF measured within the first 6 hours after trauma was less than 18 mL/min/100 g (i.e., the threshold for cerebral ischemia) in one-third of the patients (10). Arterial vasospasm was an independent predictor of poor outcome (11). Secondary ischemic neurologic damage associated with systemic factors (e.g., hypotension or hypoxemia) and local factors (e.g., intracranial hypertension, hypoperfusion) worsened outcome. Disruption of normal homeostatic mechanisms such as pressure autoregulation (see below) may also aggravate cerebral ischemia. Mechanical hyperventilation used to reduce intracranial pressure (ICP) may be deleterious by decreasing CBF, and may thus also lead to ischemia (12).

Hypothermia

Cerebral protection by hypothermia is commonly attributed to cerebral metabolic suppression. The temperature coefficient (Q_{10}) is the factor by which $CMRO_2$ is decreased by a 10°C decrease in temperature. Between 37°C and 27°C, the temperature coefficient is 2.2, but between 27°C and 17°C—a temperature range during which electroencephalographic activity ceases—the temperature coefficient doubles to 4.5. Below 17°C, the Q_{10} returns to near 2.0 (Fig. 28.3). In the absence of electroencephalographic activity (e.g., during barbiturate coma), however, the Q_{10} remains near 2.0 over the entire temperature range. With moderate hypothermia (i.e., above 27°C), both CO_2 reactivity and autoregulation are intact while CBF and $CMRO_2$ remain coupled (13). Evidence suggests that there is a change in

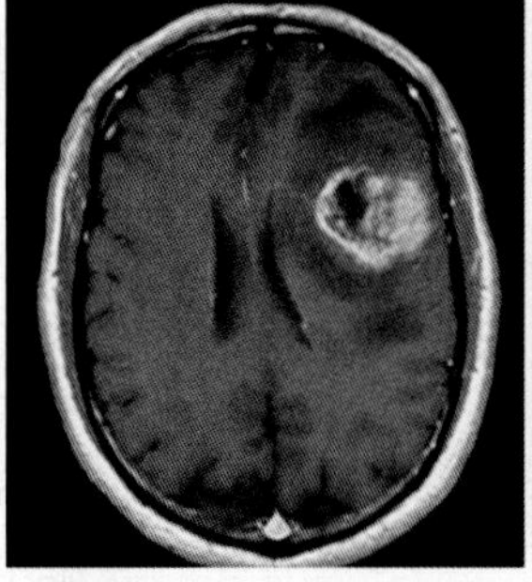

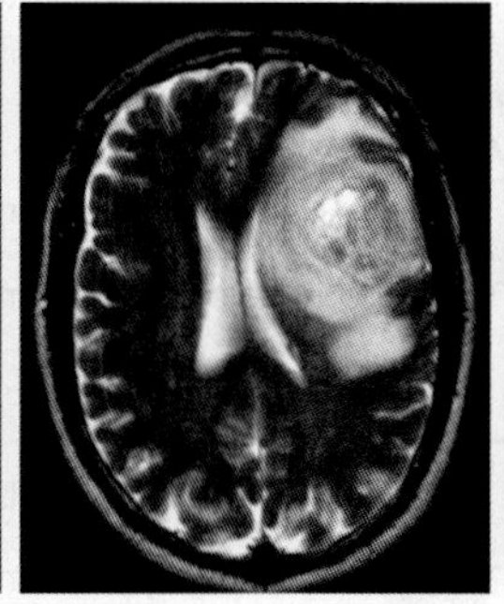

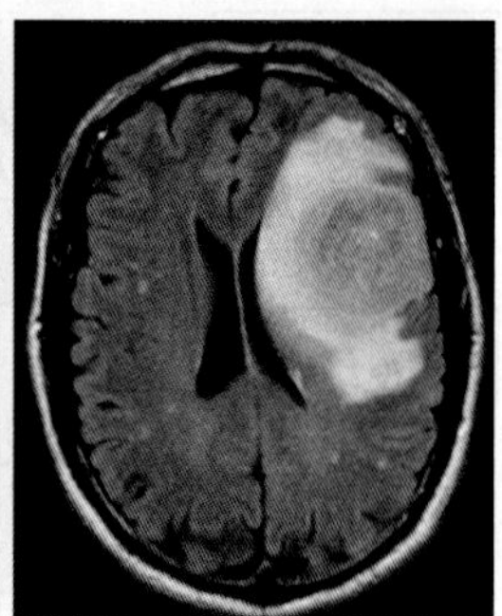

FIGURE 28.1. Magnetic resonance images from a patient with a glioblastoma multiforme. The axial, gadolinium-enhanced T1-weighted image demonstrates the enhancing tumor margin with its nonenhancing central necrosis. The axial, T2-weighted image shows water as a bright signal in perifocal edema and the central tumor necrosis, as well as in the cerebrospinal fluid, and the fluid attenuation inversion recovery image highlights only the edema around the tumor and suppresses the cerebrospinal fluid signal and the tumor necrosis. (Courtesy of Ilona Schmalfuss, MD.)

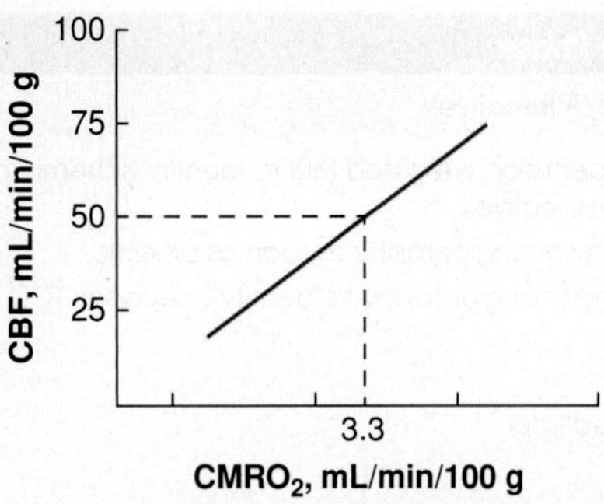

FIGURE 28.2. Flow–metabolism coupling in the central nervous system. As the metabolic needs of the brain, expressed as the cerebral metabolic requirement for oxygen ($CMRO_2$), increases, cerebral blood flow increases in parallel.

the coupling of blood flow and metabolism during deep cerebral hypothermia (below 25°C). Nonetheless, metabolic regulation remains a main determinant of CBF even during deep cerebral hypothermia (14).

Anesthetics

With the exception of ketamine, most intravenous and inhalational anesthetics depress cerebral metabolism (15,16), with consequent reductions in oxygen consumption ($CMRO_2$), CBF, and ICP with intact autoregulation (17). As $CMRO_2$ decreases, CBF is reduced proportionately because of flow–metabolism coupling. Flow–metabolism coupling usually remains intact after the administration of sodium thiopental and propofol (17), and cerebral oxygen saturation is expected to remain unaltered or improve. Etomidate, in contrast, can produce a rapid reduction in CBF accompanied by a slower reduction in $CMRO_2$ (18,19). This flow–metabolism coupled mismatch, resulting from a greater reduction in flow than demand, may induce significant, albeit transient, cerebral oxygen desaturation.

Propofol is believed to maintain cerebral autoregulation, and even high doses of this drug do not obtund autoregulation or carbon dioxide reactivity (20). The effect of propofol on flow–metabolism coupling is more controversial, with at least one study demonstrating intact coupling (21). Both increased and decreased cerebral oxygen extraction have been demonstrated with propofol, suggesting CBF–$CMRO_2$ uncoupling (22,23). Despite the fact that the retention of normal flow–metabolism coupling is thought to occur in only a proportion of head-injured patients, there is a paucity of data regarding the influence of propofol on flow–metabolism coupling after traumatic brain injury (TBI). It has been demonstrated that after TBI, flow–metabolism coupling remains intact during a step increase in propofol infusion rates (24), as is the case in noninjured patients (25).

Benzodiazepines and opiates appear to have limited intrinsic effects on CBF, $CMRO_2$, and CBF–$CMRO_2$ coupling (26,27). Because of their sedative properties, they cause a decrease in CBF and ICP that parallels the sedation-induced decrease in $CMRO_2$. As with all anesthetics, the decreased sympathetic tone caused by the sedation, on the other hand, risks a decrease in mean arterial pressure that may in fact diminish cerebral perfusion. Dexmedetomidine, an α_2-receptor agonist, is a recent and relatively expensive sedative. Similar to opiates and benzodiazepines, its effects on cerebral physiology appear to be caused by the sedation (28). Limited experience in traumatic brain-injured patients did not reveal any adverse effects (29).

Arterial Carbon Dioxide and Oxygen

Carbon dioxide is a potent cerebral vasodilator and thus a major determinant of CBF (Fig. 28.4) (30). At normotension, CBF increases almost linearly when the arterial partial pressure of carbon dioxide ($PaCO_2$) increases from 25 to 80 mmHg. Global CBF varies 2% to 4% for each millimeter of mercury change in $PaCO_2$ (31). The effects of $PaCO_2$ on cerebral circulation are regulated by a complex and interrelated system of mediators. The initial stimulus of CO_2-induced vasodilation is a decrease in brain extracellular pH (32), further mediated by nitric oxide, prostanoids, cyclic nucleotides, potassium channels, and a decrease in intracellular calcium concentration as a final common pathway.

Arteriolar tone has an important influence on how $PaCO_2$ affects CBF. Moderate hypotension impairs the response of the cerebral circulation to changes in $PaCO_2$, while severe hypotension abolishes it altogether (33). Similarly, $PaCO_2$ modifies pressure autoregulation, and from hypercapnia to hypocapnia, there is a widening of the autoregulation plateau (34). The response of cerebral vessels to CO_2 can be used therapeutically by instituting hyperventilation to decrease CBF, in turn

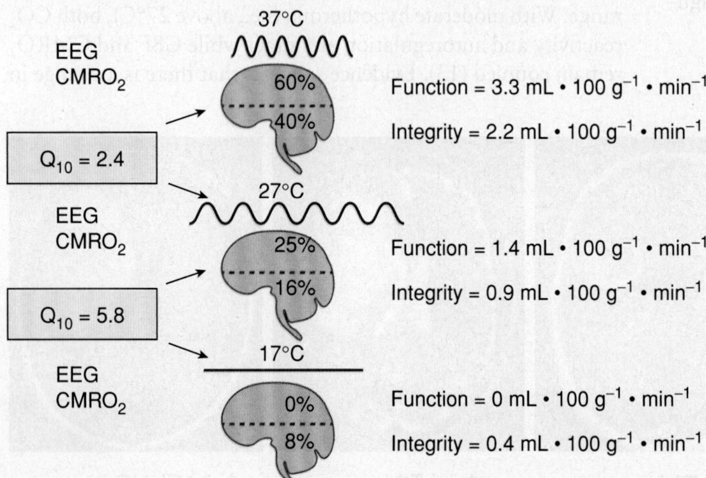

FIGURE 28.3. Theoretical interaction of temperature, brain function, metabolic requirements ($CMRO_2$), and calculated Q_{10} values. During temperature reduction from 37° to 27°C, function is maintained, and metabolism devoted to function and maintenance of integrity are presumed to be equally affected, with a slightly more than 50% reduction in $CMRO_2$ generating a Q_{10} value of 2.4. A further 10°C reduction in temperature to 17°C abolishes function, resulting in a step decrease in $CMRO_2$ such that the calculated Q_{10} value is 5.8. At this point, the total oxygen consumed by the brain is reduced to less than 8% of the normothermic value. (With permission from Black S, Michenfelder JD. Cerebral blood flow and metabolism. In: Cucchiara RF, Black S, Michenfelder JD, eds. *Clinical Neuroanesthesia*. 2nd ed. New York: Churchill Livingstone; 1998.)

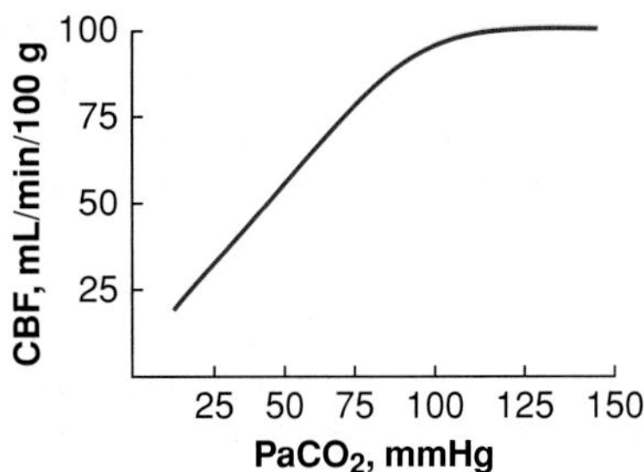

FIGURE 28.4. Effect of arterial CO_2 on cerebral blood flow.

reducing cerebral blood volume and ICP. Numerous studies on CO_2 reactivity have generally demonstrated that the response is preserved during intravenous or inhalation anesthesia (35). CO_2 reactivity has also been used to assess the adequacy of brain perfusion in patients with internal carotid artery stenosis or cerebrovascular disease. In severe head injury, intact CO_2 vasoreactivity is a good predictor of the effectiveness of hyperventilation or barbiturate therapy in controlling elevated ICP in individual patients (36). Furthermore, impaired cerebral CO_2 vasoreactivity is associated with a poor outcome in patients with severe head injury (37). On the other hand, hyperventilation has been found to increase oxygen extraction, cause misery perfusion, and thereby promote secondary brain injury (12).

Moderate changes in arterial PO_2 (PaO_2) do not significantly alter CBF. When PaO_2 falls below 50 mmHg, however, CBF increases so that cerebral oxygen delivery remains constant (30). Hypoxia acts directly on cerebral tissue to release lactic acid, adenosine, and prostaglandins, which contribute significantly to cerebral vasodilation. Hypoxia also acts directly on cerebrovascular smooth muscle to produce hyperpolarization and reduce calcium uptake, both mechanisms enhancing vasodilation.

Pressure Autoregulation

Pressure autoregulation refers to the ability of the brain to maintain total and regional CBF nearly constant despite large changes in systemic arterial blood pressure (Fig. 28.5), independent of flow–metabolism coupling (34). Autoregulation is generally expressed as the relationship between CBF and arterial blood pressure when cerebral venous and CSF pressures are low. It can be more precisely defined using the relationship between CBF and CPP that represents the difference between mean systemic arterial pressure and cerebral outflow pressure.

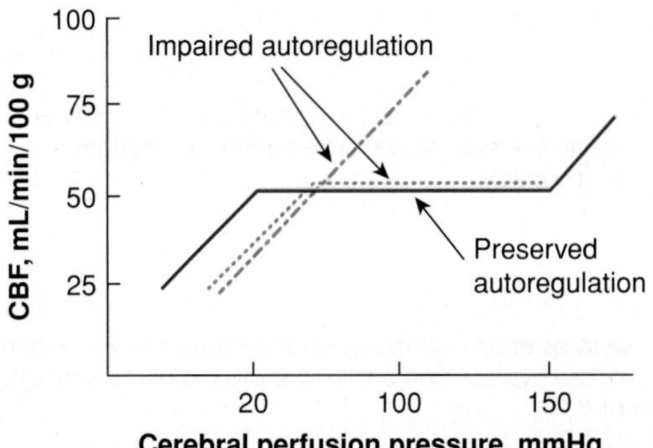

FIGURE 28.5. Preserved cerebral pressure autoregulation (*solid line*) keeps cerebral blood flow constant over a wide range of perfusion pressures. Impaired autoregulation (*dashed lines*) manifests as a shortened or even absent plateau of the autoregulation curve.

Because the cerebral venous system is compressible and may act as a "Starling resistor" or waterfall phenomenon (38), outflow resistance is governed by whichever pressure is higher—CSF pressure (ICP) or venous outflow pressure (jugular bulb pressure).

The cerebral vascular resistance (R) can be expressed as:

$$R = CPP/CBF = (8/\pi) \times h \times (l/r^4)$$

where $(8/\pi)$ is a constant for calculation, h = blood viscosity, l = length, and r = radius of the vessel. Importantly, the radius enters to the fourth power in the equation, making it the most efficient means of controlling vascular resistance.

In adults under normal conditions, CBF remains constant between a CPP of roughly 60 and 150 mmHg (34). The autoregulation curve is shifted to the right in hypertensive patients and to the left in neonates. At the lower limit of autoregulation, cerebral vasodilation is maximal, and below this level, CBF falls passively with CPP. Beyond the upper limit where vasoconstriction is maximal, the elevated intraluminal pressure may force the vessels to dilate, leading to an increase in CBF and damage to the blood–brain barrier (34,39). Metabolic mediators, such as adenosine, can also be involved in the low-pressure range of autoregulation (39).

Pressure autoregulation can be impaired in many pathologic conditions, including brain tumor, subarachnoid hemorrhage, stroke, or head injury. A loss of CBF regulatory capacity can be attributed to damage of the control system (e.g., cerebral vessels)—usually referred to as "paralysis" in the clinical literature (40)—or of the feedback mechanisms involved in the brain's hemodynamic control. Changes in the normal feedback mechanisms may include tissue acidosis, extracellular potassium increase, or alterations in cerebral neural pathways. Neurotransmitters can reach vasoactive levels in perivascular CSF as a result of synaptic overflow during neuronal activation or in pathologic conditions.

Neurogenic Regulation

A major difference between other systemic circulations and the cerebral circulation is the relative lack of humoral and autonomic control on normal cerebrovascular tone. Hence, a maximal stimulation of the sympathetic or parasympathetic nerves alters CBF only slightly (41). Furthermore, there is considerable evidence that indicates the existence of age-related differences in cerebral resistance vessels to neural stimuli. For example, both in vivo and in vitro, cerebrovascular constrictor responses to noradrenaline or electrical transmural stimuli are greater in fetal and neonatal animals than in adult animals. The mechanism for the age-related decrease is unclear, but could be the result of such factors as loss of number or affinity of α-adrenergic receptors with development. However, changes in cerebrovascular sensitivity to α-adrenergic stimuli may not occur with age in all species. Electrical or reflex activation of sympathetic nerves reduces CBF in adult rabbits. Sympathetic stimulation may protect the cerebral circulation from hyperemia associated with even modest elevations in arterial blood pressure.

Other Factors Regulating Cerebral Blood Flow

Although cardiac output hardly influences CBF in normal conditions, it may significantly influence flow to ischemic regions

(42,43). However, studies examining the possible relationship between changes in cardiac output and CBF have, for the most part, assessed the effect of drugs that increase cardiac output during either normotension or induced hypertension. Improving cerebral perfusion by volume loading is indirectly accomplished by improving blood rheology and directly accomplished by increasing systemic arterial pressure and preventing occult decreases in systemic pressure in hypovolemic patients.

Because blood viscosity is a major determinant of vascular resistance, CBF is inversely related with hematocrit (44). Nevertheless, a continuing controversy questions whether CBF is purely rheologic or a function of changes in oxygen delivery to the tissue (45). Bouma and Muizelaar have claimed that viscosity directly participates in cerebral hemodynamic autoregulation, termed *viscosity autoregulation* (39).

CEREBRAL FUNCTION

Clinical Examination

Cerebral function can be monitored with instrumentation or assessed clinically. As the discussion of individual monitoring modalities below shows, each monitor offers only a small window into the state of the CNS. Even in combination, current monitors have significant limitations in spatial and/or temporal resolution. A neurologic examination of an alert patient, on the other hand, can comprehensively assess the function of the CNS. Furthermore, it can be repeated as often as needed and requires neither expensive technical equipment nor specialized technologists.

In clinical practice, however, the neurologic examination has important limitations. First, the patient's clinical status or underlying disease may limit the amount of information obtainable by a clinical examination. Second, the results and, by extension, the utility of a neurologic examination may be constrained by therapeutic interventions that are frequently used in the ICU. For example, medications used for analgesia or sedation will alter the neurologic examination to varying degrees, making differentiation between drug effect and clinical deterioration very difficult. In an intubated patient who is treated with neuromuscular-blocking agents, the only evidence of recurrent generalized seizure activity may be increased ICP, while the postictal alteration of consciousness and the motor manifestations of the seizure go unnoticed. Finally, neurologic evaluations are performed intermittently and by examiners of variable skill, raising problems of reliability and reproducibility. Despite these limitations, the clinical examination forms the cornerstone of the neurologic assessment of ICU patients and typically directs further diagnostic or therapeutic interventions.

While a comprehensive discussion of a clinical neurologic examination is beyond the scope of this chapter, two aspects of the examination that are particularly pertinent to the ICU environment will be discussed in some detail. The first is the assessment of the level of consciousness, because of its ties to patient outcome for many different neurologic diseases. The second is the examination for assessing brain death, not only because it is a graded assessment of brainstem function, but also because it illustrates sources of error that may impact the results of the clinical neurologic examination in the ICU environment in general.

Level of Consciousness: Glasgow Coma Scale

The level of consciousness is typically assessed by the Glasgow coma scale (GCS). Numerical scores are assigned for best responses in the categories of eye opening, motor response, and verbal response (Table 28.2). The GCS was originally described more than 30 years ago for the continuous assessment of patients with TBI after the initial period of stabilization (46). Because its assessment is quick, objective, and relatively reliable (47), and because the resulting score is easily documented and communicated, the GCS has gained widespread use in emergency medicine and critical care patients. It has been incorporated into the Acute Physiology and Chronic Health Evaluation (APACHE) score (48) and the World Federation of Neurosurgical Societies (WFNS) grading of subarachnoid hemorrhage (49).

The level of consciousness is a reflection of the severity of many different disease states, and can be compromised not just by diseases of the CNS, but also at the extremes of a wide

TABLE 28.2 Glasgow Coma Scale

Category	Grading		Comments
Eye opening	Spontaneous	4	Swelling may interfere with testing.
	To voice	3	
	To pain	2	
	None	1	
Motor response	Follows commands	6	Avoid description of flexion as decorticate and extension as decerebrate because those terms denote an anatomic location of a lesion.
	Localizes pain	5	
	Withdraws to pain	4	
	Flexion to pain	3	
	Extension to pain	2	
	Flaccid	1	
Verbal response	Oriented	5	Impossible to assess in intubated patients. Some centers determine the response by inference and designate the final score with the subscript "T."
	Confused	4	
	Inappropriate	3	
	Incomprehensible	2	
	None	1	

The Glasgow coma score is the sum of the best attainable subscores in the categories of eye opening (E), motor (M), and verbal (V) responses. It ranges from 15 (E4 + M6 + V5) to 3 (E1 + M1 + V1).

variety of other organ dysfunctions common in critical care. Not surprisingly, therefore, the scores from a tool such as the GCS that assesses the level of consciousness may be associated with prognosis and outcome. For the GCS, an association of lower scores with worsened outcome has been shown for TBI (50), subarachnoid hemorrhage (51), brain abscess (52), survival after cardiac arrest (53,54), and septic encephalopathy (55). For example, in TBI, a GCS score greater than 7 suggests a 90% likelihood of an outcome of moderate disability or better, whereas a score less than 7 suggests an increased risk of death or persistent vegetative state that approaches 60% to 90% for a GCS score of 3 (50,56,57). New data suggest that, at least in children, early decompressive craniectomy significantly increases the likelihood of better outcome (only mild disability) (58). In aneurysmal subarachnoid hemorrhage, a GCS score less than 13 after initial treatment of increased ICP (i.e., WFNS grade 4 or 5) corresponds to a 60% to 90% chance of a poor functional outcome or death, whereas such outcomes only affect 14% of patients whose level of consciousness is unaffected (GCS 15, WFNS grade 1 or 2) (51).

Despite its widespread use and appeal, the GCS has several important limitations, even if applied correctly. One is the information loss inherent in reducing a graded assessment of three responses into a single number. The second is that mechanical problems such as swelling and endotracheal intubation may prevent proper assessment of eye opening and verbal response. In this setting, some clinicians assign the lowest component score, whereas others try to infer the "true" score from related neurologic findings, and still others add the subscript "T" to indicate an intubated patient. Third, sedatives and neuromuscular-blocking agents affect the GCS score upon repeated assessment. Finally, although the degree of brainstem involvement may reflect the severity of coma, the GCS provides limited information about brainstem function.

Determination of Brain Death

The determination of brain death for purposes of organ donation or withdrawal of life support is an area that has brought both the merits and the limitations of the neurologic examination into clear focus. Because the clinical determination of brain death requires a comprehensive and methodical assessment of the patient (59), its steps may serve as a guide to the neurologic examination of a comatose patient. An algorithm for the determination of brain death is shown in Figure 28.6. Given the gravity of the "therapeutic" consequences of the diagnosis of brain death, a prerequisite to its determination is a clinical picture, typically supported by imaging studies, that is consistent with the occurrence of brain death.

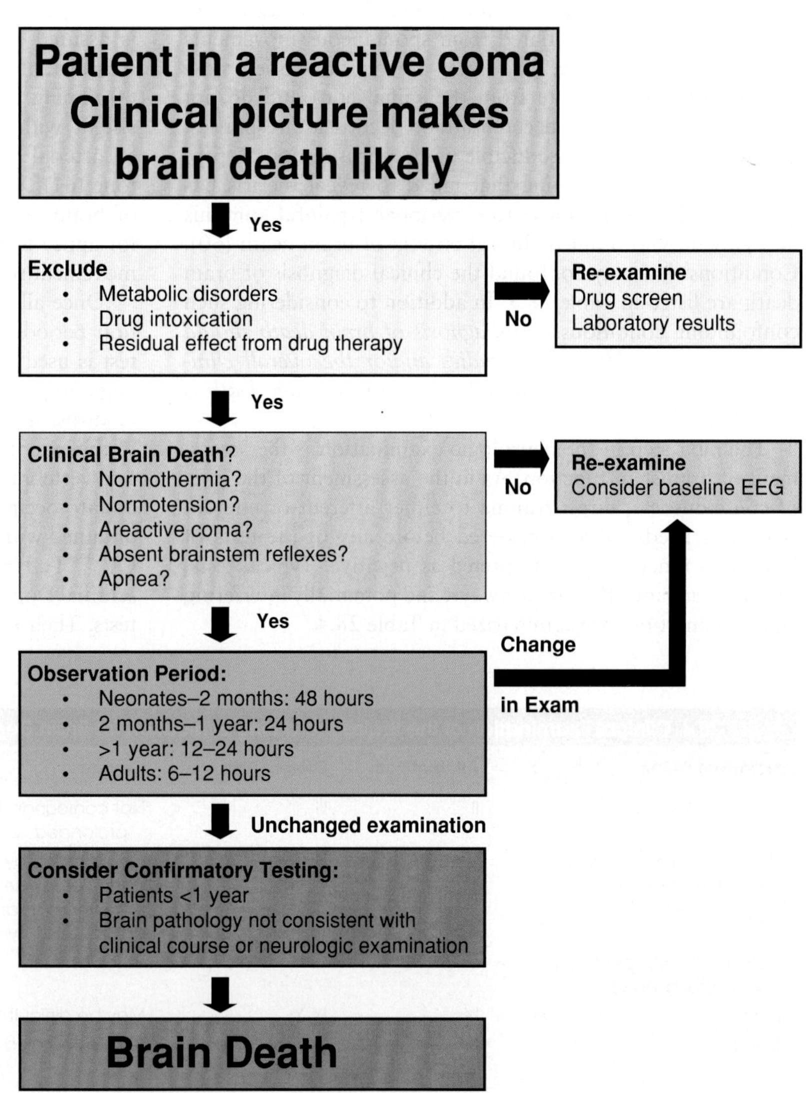

FIGURE 28.6. Evaluation of a patient in a coma.

TABLE 28.3 Neurologic States Resembling Brain Death

Disease State	Diagnostic Aids	Comments
Hypothermia	Core temperature <32°C Osborne waves on ECG[a] Drug screening	May cause CNS depression up to clinical brain death
Acute poisoning	Serum concentration measurements	In differentiating from brain death, consider antidote and/or document subtherapeutic drug concentration and/or wait for four elimination half-lives Direct CNS depressants may confound confirmatory testing of brain death because of $CMRO_2$–CBF coupling
Metabolic encephalopathy	Laboratory testing Intact lower brainstem function	Imaging studies should document structural CNS changes Imaging studies should document structural CNS changes
Akinetic mutism	Intact sleep–wake cycle	Imaging study shows frontal or mesencephalic brain lesion
Locked-in syndrome	Clinical course and imaging studies	Central locked-in syndrome: corticobulbar and corticospinal tracts are interrupted at the level of the base of the pons; vertical eye movements are intact Peripheral locked-in syndrome: Guillain–Barré syndrome, advanced amyotrophic lateral sclerosis, neuromuscular-blocking agents, organophosphate poisoning

[a]ECG, electrocardiogram; $CMRO_2$, cerebral metabolic requirement for oxygen; CBF, cerebral blood flow; CNS, central nervous system.

The first step in the neurologic examination for the determination of brain death is the determination of coma (i.e., lack of responsiveness to external stimuli due to unconsciousness as discussed above). Motor responses *elicited by the examination* need to be differentiated from spontaneous movements *during the examination.* The latter are typically brief, slow movements that originate from the spinal cord and do not become integrated into decerebrate or decorticate responses. Only rarely are they reproducible upon repeat testing. Reproducible partial eye opening that failed to reveal the iris has been described in response to a peripheral painful stimulus in a patient who fulfilled clinical criteria of brain death (60). Conditions that may confound the clinical diagnosis of brain death are listed in Table 28.3. In addition to considering such confounding conditions, the *diagnosis of brain death should be consistent with imaging studies and/or the overall clinical picture before the formal determination of brain death is considered.*

The next step in the neurologic examination is the assessment of brainstem function. As in the assessment of the level of consciousness, direct trauma to either afferent or efferent structures needs to be considered before any of the tests of brainstem function are interpreted as negative. Typical tests, their afferent and efferent pathways, and potentially interfering clinical conditions are summarized in Table 28.4.

To complete the diagnosis of brain death, an apnea test is performed to test the response to an acute decrease in the pH of CSF due to hypercarbia. Hypercarbia is induced by disconnecting mechanical ventilation while continued oxygenation is assured by both preoxygenation and apneic oxygenation. Absence of respiratory movements at an arterial PCO_2 of 60 mmHg or after an increase in PCO_2 of 20 mmHg is consistent with brain death. Apnea testing may be complicated by arterial hypotension due to loss of arterial and autonomic tone (61). While such hypotension corroborates the diagnosis of brain death, it makes the hemodynamic stability required for apnea testing difficult to attain. The apnea test may trigger movement responses, which reflect residual spinal activity (62).

Once all these criteria for brain death are met, an observation period followed by repeat assessment or a confirmatory test is used to reach a final diagnosis (see Fig. 28.6). Cerebral angiography is the gold standard among confirmatory tests. Contrast media is injected into the aortic arch and distributes to the external carotid circulation, whereas the internal carotid and vertebral arteries fill only to the level of the skull base and atlanto-occipital junction, respectively. Similar findings can be obtained with MR angiography or with single photon emission CT ^{99m}Tc-HMPAO. Electroencephalography (EEG) and transcranial Doppler (TCD) are also frequently used as confirmatory tests. Their role will be discussed in greater detail below.

TABLE 28.4 Clinical Examination of the Brainstem during Evaluation for Brain Death

Brainstem Reflex	Afferent Path	Efferent Path	Caveats
Pupillary light reaction	II	III	Not confounded by systemic drugs; absence may be caused by prolonged administration of neuromuscular-blocking agents
Ocular movements (oculocephalic reflex or caloric nystagmus)	VIII	III, VI	Confounded by damage from ototoxic drugs; cervical spine trauma may preclude testing of the oculocephalic reflex; voluntary ocular movements are sometimes the only finding that differentiates a "locked-in" syndrome from brain death
Corneal reflex/pressure on supraorbital nerve	V	VII	
Gag	IX	IX, X	May be difficult to assess in orotracheally intubated patient
Cough	X	X, cervical roots	Best tested by assessing the response to tracheal suctioning

Electrophysiologic Techniques

Neurophysiologic function testing has been used for more than 20 years as a diagnostic/prognostic tool in the ICU (63–66). Snapshots of function of different parts of the nervous system have been used to predict the most likely long-term function of the nervous system as a whole. This information helps the intensivist determine whether continued aggressive intensive care is appropriate given the patient's most likely long-term neurologic outcome. To a much lesser extent, neurophysiologic testing modalities have been used as continuous monitors of neurologic function in the patient who cannot be assessed neurologically, primarily because of the need for sedation (67–69). There are two main modalities of neurophysiologic function testing used in the intensive care unit: EEG and evoked potentials (EPs). For each modality, the theoretical basis for use and utility will be reviewed.

Electroencephalography

To understand how EEG can be used in the ICU, the clinician must first understand how scalp-recorded EEG is produced and what factors may affect the recordings. EEG activity is generated by neurons in the pyramidal layer of the cerebral cortex. The scalp-recorded EEG is produced by a summation of excitatory and inhibitory postsynaptic potentials (EPSPs and IPSPs), not actual cellular depolarization. EPSPs and IPSPs are produced by the spontaneous release of small packets of excitatory or inhibitory neurotransmitters from a nerve terminal that produce only very small changes in the postsynaptic membrane potential, insufficient to cause depolarization. As a result, the amplitude (voltage) of EEG electrical activity is much smaller than the electrocardiogram, ranging from less than 5 μV in the elderly to over 100 μV in the teenager. As a result, the EEG signal cannot be recorded remotely from the generator site, and practically speaking, EEG activity recorded from a single electrode only reflects cortical activity directly beneath the recording site. In addition, because the EEG signal is so small, poor electrode contact with the scalp may result in significant loss of signal.

Maintenance of ion fluxes associated with the production of the EEG is an energy-requiring process. Pharmacologic total suppression of the EEG will result in a 50% to 60% decrease in $CMRO_2$ (70,71). The decrease in oxygen requirement parallels the suppression of the EEG in cases of lesser suppression. An EEG that is merely slowed pharmacologically will be associated with a higher $CMRO_2$ than an EEG that is totally suppressed or flat.

The EEG is organized spatially and temporally, but patterns of organization are much more difficult for the clinician to recognize, primarily because few clinicians have significant experience with normal EEG patterns, pathologic EEG patterns, or drug-induced EEG patterns. EEG patterns are described primarily in terms of frequency (how fast voltage oscillations occur) and amplitude (size or voltage). Slower frequency ranges include δ (3 Hz or slower) and θ (3.5 to 7.5 Hz). These frequencies are not seen in the normal awake adult but are commonly seen in the naturally asleep adult or in the adult who is receiving therapeutic doses of sedative-hypnotic and/or analgesic drugs. Faster frequency ranges include α (8 to 13 Hz) and β (>13 Hz). Alpha frequencies (8 to 13 Hz) tend to be present on the posterior part of the head and are most prominent with the eyes closed. Alpha activity disappears with attention and concentration, replaced with faster β activity. Beta frequencies are commonly seen more toward the front of the head and are associated with increased "function" of a particular part of the brain. In the neurologically abnormal patient, θ and δ frequencies may be focal, associated with a specific loss of function, or more global, associated with generalized neurologic dysfunction. Generally, the more severe the neurologic damage/dysfunction, the slower the recorded EEG activity will be. For example, a patient with a receptive and expressive aphasia will likely demonstrate EEG slowing (θ and δ waves) over the dominant temporal lobe.

Sedative-hypnotic drugs produce a change in neurologic function that is likewise paralleled by EEG changes. The EEG changes associated with sedative-hypnotic drugs are predictable, related both to the drug used and the dosage of drug given. The vast majority of sedative-hypnotic drugs used in the ICU will produce identical, dose-related changes in the EEG. Table 28.5 shows EEG pattern changes associated with most drugs that would be used in the ICU environment. Dexmedetomidine sedation produces EEG patterns indicating that patients are more sedated than they actually are. Even a low-dose infusion produces a combination of slow delta oscillations with bursting 9- to 15-Hz spindles (72). Combinations of drugs, of course, will have different effects than when either drug is used alone. Specific data regarding the effect of combinations of drugs is limited and beyond the scope of this chapter. However, in general, both sedative and analgesic drugs will increase the primary effect of the drug being used in the higher dose as well as add effects of their own.

In summary, the scalp-recorded EEG reflects the function of closely underlying neuronal tissue. These functions may be altered by neurologic damage, pharmacologic means, normal changes in function associated with changes in alertness or sleep, or any combination of these factors. Thus, whether the EEG is used as a monitor or a diagnostic/prognostic tool, interpretation of data without a thorough knowledge of all factors that could influence recordings is not possible.

Diagnostic Electroencephalography in the Intensive Care Unit

Diagnostic EEG studies or EEG monitoring in the ICU is done primarily for one of three purposes: Brain death determination, monitoring for evidence of seizure activity or cerebral ischemia, and determination of drug effect for the purposes of titrating sedative and analgesic drugs or control of ICP.

Criteria for brain death vary from state to state, but in most states, a 16- to 32-channel isoelectric EEG on two consecutive recordings at least 24 hours apart can provide strong corroborating evidence for cessation of brain function (see Fig. 28.6). Because other factors affecting the EEG can produce an isoelectric EEG in the absence of brain death, the EEG cannot be used as the sole evaluation for brain death. Although it is likely that drug levels (see Table 28.5) will decline significantly over a 24-hour period, patients with massive drug overdose or impaired metabolic pathways may show an isoelectric EEG for much longer than 24 or 48 hours. In these cases, the neurologic examination may also not be useful because high drug levels may suppress even the most resistant reflex responses. Fortunately, other diagnostic testing methods, including other electrophysiologic and nonelectrophysiologic methods, may be helpful. EPs (see below), for example, are more resistant to drug effects than the EEG and can frequently be used to demonstrate brainstem and cortical function, even in the face

TABLE 28.5 Sedative-Hypnotic and Analgesic Drugs and the Electroencephalogram (EEG)

Drug and Dose	Effect on EEG Dominant Frequency	Effect on EEG Amplitude	Burst Suppression
Barbiturates			
Low dose	Fast frontal β activity	Slight ↑	Yes, with high doses
Moderate dose	Frontal α-frequency spindles	↑	
High dose	Diffuse δ → burst suppression → silence	↑↑↑ → 0	
Etomidate			
Low dose	Fast frontal β activity	↑	Yes, with high doses
Moderate dose	Frontal α-frequency spindles	↑	
High dose	Diffuse δ → burst suppression → silence	↑↑ → 0	
Propofol			
Low dose	Loss of α, ↑ frontal β	↑	Yes, with high doses
Moderate dose	Frontal δ, waxing/waning α	↑	
High dose	Diffuse δ → burst suppression → silence	↑↑ → 0	
Dexmedetomidine	Early appearance of high-amplitude δ frequency that increases with dose, Similar to opiates	↑	No
Ketamine			
Low dose	Loss of α, ↑ variability	↑↓	No
Moderate dose	Frontal rhythmic delta	↑	
High dose	Polymorphic δ, some β	↑↑ (β is low amplitude)	
Benzodiazepines			
Low dose	Loss of α, increased frontal β activity	↑	No
High dose	Frontally dominant δ and θ	↑	
Opiates			
Low dose	Loss of β, α slows	↔↑	No
Moderate dose	Diffuse θ, some δ	↑	
High dose	δ, often synchronized	↑↑	

δ, <3-Hz frequency; θ, 3.5–7.5-Hz frequency; α, 8–13-Hz frequency; β, >13-Hz frequency.

of an isoelectric EEG (73,74). In addition, an EEG recorded immediately after cardiac arrest may show an isoelectric pattern that subsequently recovers (75). Cortical EPs have also been demonstrated to be more reliable in assessing neurologic function immediately after an ischemic/anoxic insult (75). In summary, a scalp-recorded, 16- to 32-channel EEG is a helpful adjunct to the diagnosis of brain death, provided all other factors influencing the EEG are understood and controlled.

Continuous EEG monitoring in the ICU or, alternatively, sequential diagnostic EEG studies, have been described for detection of nonconvulsive seizure (NCS) activity (or seizure activity in the pharmacologically paralyzed patient) and for detection of cerebral ischemia (67–69,76–78). This type of monitoring requires multiple channels of information to obtain adequate monitoring coverage of the entire brain. A highly trained technologist observes the patient simultaneously with the EEG recording and operates the equipment and maintains recording electrodes during nursing care that will commonly dislodge them. The technologist also provides real-time neurophysiologic data to the clinicians caring for the patient. Processed EEG algorithms have been developed to facilitate detection of ischemia epileptiform and frank seizure activity during continuous EEG monitoring (79,80). Although the technology shows promise even in the hands of nonneurophysiologists (81), this technique has not yet evolved enough to eliminate the need for an on-site technologist with monitoring experience.

Continuous EEG monitoring in the ICU has demonstrated that NCSs are much more common than previously thought (77,78,82). NCSs have been reported following neurosurgical procedures, subarachnoid hemorrhage, CNS infection, head injury, and other conditions. In addition, there is evidence using neuron-specific enolase as a marker of neurologic injury that NCSs may produce neurologic damage and that seizure duration and time to diagnosis are significantly related to the extent of damage and long-term outcome. Without continuous EEG monitoring, NCSs cannot be detected, as they are not consistently and specifically associated with other findings such as hypertension and tachycardia (82).

The personnel and fiscal costs of continuous EEG monitoring have made it unfeasible except in the larger neurologic and neurosurgical ICUs, where many patients with conditions amenable to continuous monitoring require care (76). In addition, very little outcome data exist to demonstrate that such monitoring is overall cost effective. When considering real-time neurologic monitoring in the patient whose neurologic examination cannot be assessed, much work needs to be done to determine how continuous EEG monitoring will mesh with other neurologic monitoring modalities such as ICP, CBF, brain tissue pO_2 monitoring, TCD, and microdialysis monitoring. Theoretically and based on limited clinical data (76–81), there is much promise for continuous EEG monitoring when used as a part of a multimodality neurologic monitoring program.

Monitoring of Sedation by Processed Electroencephalogy

The use of the EEG to monitor the depth of sedation in patients in the ICU has been described extensively in the literature, and nearly all techniques utilize processed EEG rather than the unprocessed analog signal. Drug effect monitoring is generally accomplished using one or two channels of EEG information, generally recorded over the frontopolar region of the cerebral cortex. This location is chosen because application of surface recording electrodes is easy in this location (no hair) and most devices designed for this purpose have been validated using frontopolar recording locations. Usage of this smaller number of channels is based on the assumption that the drug effect will be similar in all areas of the brain. This assumption is generally valid except in the case of a patient with focal brain damage. In areas of damage, the drug effect will generally be greater than usual and must be interpreted in light of the abnormal baseline recording. None of the commercially available devices for monitoring drug effects on the EEG has been calibrated or validated appropriately for monitoring drug effects in the patient with the abnormal EEG, and relatively limited information is available on the use of EEG to monitor drug effects in neurologically damaged patients (83–86).

EEG drug effect monitoring is used most commonly for titrating sedative drugs, particularly in the pharmacologically paralyzed patient, but also for titration of barbiturate drugs or propofol used to control ICP (67–69,87,88). Devices used to monitor the drug effect utilize unprocessed, raw analog EEG in a fashion similar to ECG monitoring in the ICU or utilize one of three signal processing techniques: Power spectrum analysis, bispectral analysis (BIS), or EEG entropy analysis. Examples of commercial monitors include the BIS, the patient state index, SEDline, and entropy. Although the BIS monitor has been used and studied most widely among these monitors, the concepts discussed below should apply to other EEG-based monitors of sedation as well.

BIS (Aspect Medical Systems, Inc., Natick, MA) monitoring has been used in the intensive care setting to guide dosing of sedatives and reassure clinicians that paralyzed or agitated patients are amnestic but not excessively sedated (89). The BIS monitor processes EEG signals that are recorded from a self-adhesive electrode strip placed on the forehead. It calculates and displays a BIS value, a dimensionless number ranging from 0 to 100 that is derived from highly processed EEG data that includes EEG power, frequency, and bicoherence (90). Low BIS numbers indicate strong relationships among the EEG frequencies and reflect a condition consistent with a deep hypnotic state (Table 28.6). This relationship is valid despite the effects of age and infirmity on sensitivity to sedation (91,92).

Despite its obvious clinical utility, the aspects of imperfect performance of the BIS monitor are well known. For example, the BIS can decrease to numbers (20 to 50) consistent with deep general anesthesia during natural sleep without sedation

TABLE 28.6 Clinical Condition Expected with Bispectral Index Values

Value	Clinical Condition
100	Awake patient, amnesia unlikely
80	Sedated responsive patient, amnesia prominent unless significant event
70	Heavily sedated or unconscious patient, amnesia probable
60	General anesthesia, unresponsive to verbal stimuli
40	Deep hypnotic state
20	Burst suppression
0	Isoelectric electroencephalogram

(93). Moreover, although memory is less likely to form at lower BIS values, memory has been demonstrated even at a BIS in a range (40 to 60) associated with general anesthesia (94). Additionally, artifact from electromyographic, electrooculographic (95), or pacemaker generators (96) can produce significant but spurious BIS increases (from 50s to 80s), although the algorithm has been improved in the last decade to reduce the effects of such artifacts. This finding raises the possibility of overdosing nonrelaxed or paced patients when attempting to maintain a given BIS range. BIS values can also be driven higher by medications that are CNS stimulants, such as ketamine or methylphenidate (97). Dexmedetomidine, as discussed earlier, may produce EEG patterns that will result in lower BIS values at a comparable level of sedation (71,95). In such cases, the BIS may not reflect the level of hypnosis or sedation experienced by the patient. Therefore, when the sedative dosages required to achieve a desired BIS range exceed normal expectations, the possibility of an artifactual interference deserves consideration.

Perhaps the most significant issue with BIS or other monitors of cortical anesthetic drug effect are their inability to differentiate deep sedation from cerebral ischemia. Both conditions cause loss of higher frequency EEG waves (α and β slowing and δ and θ wave intrusion) and, in extreme states, both can produce burst suppression or isoelectric EEG patterns with a low BIS. When O_2 delivery decreases below a level sufficient to meet the $CMRO_2$, electrical function fails and BIS decreases. This may partly explain improved ICU outcomes when the BIS is maintained above 60 (98). Therefore, the determination that sedation is adequate based on having achieved a target BIS value should only be made when one is confident that cerebral perfusion is adequate.

Interpretation of BIS or, for that matter, any EEG-based monitor of sedation is best accomplished when the patient's pharmacologic support remains stable in the face of changing CPP or, conversely, the CPP remains adequate and stable during pharmacologic adjustments and BIS changes. As a corollary, the BIS can assist with guiding therapy when the adequacy of O_2 supply to the CNS is in question (99).

In summary, other than for drug effect monitoring, use of the EEG in the ICU remains relatively limited, primarily because of personnel costs and difficulty in maintaining stable technical conditions for monitoring multiple channels of information. As our understanding of underlying mechanisms for neurologic injury improves, we may be able to learn which monitoring modalities are most useful for a given clinical scenario and which can more specifically target EEG monitoring to a smaller area of the brain. In addition, as computing power continues to improve, signal processing technology will likewise improve, and EEG monitoring equipment that recognizes artifact and self-corrects technical problems may reduce the need for the continuous presence of highly trained personnel to operate the EEG in the ICU environment.

Peripheral Nerve Stimulation

The rate of recovery from neuromuscular-blocking agents depends upon the neuromuscular-blocking agent chosen, its dosing pattern (intermittent or continuous infusion), and numerous patient factors (e.g., pseudocholinesterase deficiency, hepatic or renal dysfunction, induced cytochrome P450 enzyme, organophosphate toxicity, among many others) (100). The suitability for extubation following prolonged neuromuscular blockade has traditionally relied upon functional strength testing, such as an ability to produce a negative inspiratory force or to sustain a head lift. Incomplete patient cooperation caused by sedation or confusion, among other reasons, can adversely affect these tests. Peripheral nerve stimulation (PNS), used for "muscle twitch" testing, or acceleromyography, complements such functional assessments by objectively revealing the condition of the neuromuscular junction, independent of patient participation.

Reliable interpretation of nerve stimulation requires uniform stimulation and placement parameters. Conventional PNS delivers current—adjustable up to 80 mA—in a train-of-four (TOF) series at 2 Hz as double-burst stimulation, as single shocks at 1.0 or 0.1 Hz, or by tetanic stimuli of 50 or 100 Hz. When tolerated, maximal current settings assure the best chance of delivering supra-threshold stimuli and activation of the greatest percentage of motor fibers despite changes of impedance or proximity, as can occur with electrode separation or desiccation, skin cooling, or peripheral edema. TOF and double-burst stimulation patterns do not require comparison to earlier responses for interpretation, and are therefore well suited for use in the ICU setting where recovery of neuromuscular function may take hours to days and may involve assessments by multiple providers.

Muscle twitch testing measures the force of muscle contractions in response to PNS. The ratio of the force between the last and first stimuli in a series (TOF or double-burst stimulation) best defines the percentage of acetylcholine receptors occupied by *nondepolarizing* neuromuscular-blocking agents in the neuromuscular junction, but is cumbersome to perform (101). Counting the loss of twitches in a TOF is a simpler method for assessing the level of block and has greater bedside utility (Table 28.7). In contrast, the TOF ratio does not change following the administration of a *depolarizing* neuromuscular-blocking agent such as succinylcholine. When depolarizing neuromuscular-blocking agents are used, the force of contraction diminishes equally across all stimuli and disappears altogether with sufficient dose. If an excessive depolarizing neuromuscular-blocking agent is administered, a prolonged phase II block emerges. TOF responses during a phase II block behave similarly to responses obtained following nondepolarizing neuromuscular-blocking agents.

The peripheral nerve stimulator is attached to a patient using two pre-gelled electrocardiogram electrodes, although needle electrodes can also be used. The electrodes should be placed closely (without the gels touching) to one another over a site where a nerve with motor function lies relatively superficial to the skin. Antegrade nerve conduction is improved if

TABLE 28.7 Percentage of Neuromuscular Junction Blockade with Nondepolarizing Neuromuscular-Blocking Agents and Corresponding Train-of-Four and Clinical Responses

Response	% Blockade
Train-of-four (0/4)	95
Train-of-four (1/4)	90
Train-of-four (2/4)	85
Train-of-four (3/4)	80
Train-of-four (4/4)	75
Sustained (≥5 sec) tetanus	50
Sustained (≥5 sec) head lift	25

the positive lead is applied to the proximal electrode. The current path between electrodes should not contain the muscle whose movement is being monitored. Separation of electrodes beyond several centimeters increases the probability that the PNS current may depolarize muscle directly, causing movement unrelated to conduction through the neuromuscular junction and thus, misinterpretation of the level of neuromuscular blockade.

Common sites for electrode placement are over the course of the ulnar nerve at the medial aspect of the wrist or over the ulnar groove at the elbow. Stimulation of the ulnar nerve activates the m. adductor pollicis and twitches the thumb. Placement of the electrodes anterior to the tragus will stimulate the facial nerve, which innervates the m. corrugator supercilii and furrows the eyebrow. Stimulation of the posterior tibial nerve posterior to the medial malleolus causes the m. flexor hallucis brevis and great toe to move.

Cold will weaken muscle strength even in the absence of neuromuscular-blocking agents, making PNS testing valuable in patients recovering from hypothermia (102). Patients who have had a stroke will experience an upregulation of acetylcholine receptor density on the muscle membrane as the affected muscles denervate. As a result, PNS on an affected limb will produce a TOF response that exceeds the response seen from the same site PNS on a normal limb. To avoid overdosing or prematurely extubating a patient based on TOF testing, PNS should be performed on sites unaffected by prior nerve injury.

PNS is particularly helpful for monitoring the level of relaxation achieved during the infusion of neuromuscular-blocking agents. PNS monitoring can help direct the rate of infusion and avoid excessive administration. Pharmacokinetic and pharmacodynamic models that illustrate the TOF response to PNS with succinylcholine and rocuronium neuromuscular-blocking infusions can be found at http://vam.anest.ufl.edu/simulations/simulationportfolio.php.

EVOKED POTENTIALS

The EEG is a recording of the spontaneous electrical activity of the cerebral cortex. In contrast, EPs are recordings of the electrical activity occurring within parts of the nervous system produced by activation of either sensory or motor systems. With the exception of motor-evoked responses recorded from muscle, EPs are much smaller than background EEG or muscle electrical activity, and the responses from repetitive stimuli must be averaged to be able to discern the responses from other background biologic signals and environmental noise. Auditory responses are very small (generally <0.5 μV) and require as many as 2,000 averaged responses to resolve the signal. Somatosensory responses are larger (0.5 to 10 μV) and require fewer responses to be visible. EPs are described in terms of latency (conduction time [milliseconds] from stimulus application to arrival at a generating site with onset or peak of response), amplitude (microvolts), and morphology (Fig. 28.7). Conceptually, amplitude is the more important parameter for ICU studies because voltage is related to the amount of functional neural tissue generating the response. With a nerve injury, however, signals will be conducted more slowly through the most damaged fibers. This situation spreads out the arrival times of conducted signals, desynchronizing the evoked response, decreasing its amplitude, and broadening its morphology.

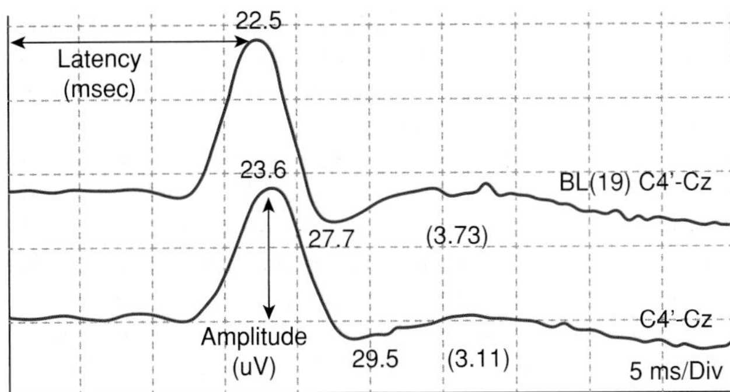

FIGURE 28.7. Latency is defined as the time from stimulus application to the onset or the peak of the response (peak latency shown here). Amplitude is the size (usually microvolts) of the evoked response.

In comparison with the EEG, EPs are much less susceptible to the effects of intravenous sedative-hypnotic drugs and are not significantly affected by intravenous analgesics (103). Auditory EP responses will not be altered significantly by any sedating or analgesic regimen used in the ICU today. Notably, based on known effects of opiates and sedatives on brainstem auditory-evoked potentials (BAEPs), patients admitted with opiate or sedative drug overdose and an isoelectric EEG will not show any significant abnormality of waves I through V related to the drug effect alone (73,74,103). Somatosensory evoked potentials (SEPs) are somewhat more susceptible to the effects of sedative drugs. Cortical SEPs do show significant increases in latency and decreases in amplitude with sedating medications (103), but generally, they will not be completely abolished even by enough sedative medication to render the EEG isoelectric (73,74,103). This is important to remember for the patient with drug overdose.

Table 28.8 is a summary of the different types of EPs that may be recorded or monitored in the ICU. The results of these tests are frequently used as prognostic indicators of intermediate and long-term neurologic function. Some large neurologic or neurosurgical ICUs are able to provide continuous real-time EP monitoring. Unlike EEG, which reveals only electrical function of the cortex, EPs reflect the function of nervous system tissue along the entire signal conduction pathway. The response to an electrical stimulus applied to a distal peripheral nerve is typically recorded as it is conducted centrally from the peripheral nerve, over the spinal cord (usually the cervical region), and over the cerebral cortex. Thus, the peripheral nervous system, spinal cord, brainstem, thalamus, internal capsule, and cerebral cortex are assessed with a single test. Generally, EPs are assumed to reflect the function of the surrounding neural tissue, whether cortical, subcortical, or spinal cord (Fig. 28.8). Where conduction times differ from normal or are observed to change helps to locate the stressed or damaged structure. Although it is possible to have unchanged EPs with very focal lesions in the brain or spinal cord causing profound neurologic deficit, this is uncommon. EPs usually reflect the function of the surrounding neural tissue and have been demonstrated as very effective at detecting a developing injury and in prognosticating the long-term effects of an existing neurologic injury. This section of the chapter will examine BAEPs, SEPs, and transcranial motor-evoked potentials (MEPs) and their use as diagnostic, prognostic, and monitoring tools in the ICU.

TABLE 28.8 Evoked Potentials (EPS) in the Intensive Care Unit

Type of EPs	Stimulus Type and Site	Recording Sites
Somatosensory	Electrical, peripheral nerve	Peripheral nerve, spinal cord, head
Brainstem auditory	Loud click, ear	Ear, head
Magnetic motor	Magnetic pulse, head	Spinal column, peripheral nerve, muscle
Electrical motor	Electrical, head	Spinal column, peripheral nerve, muscle

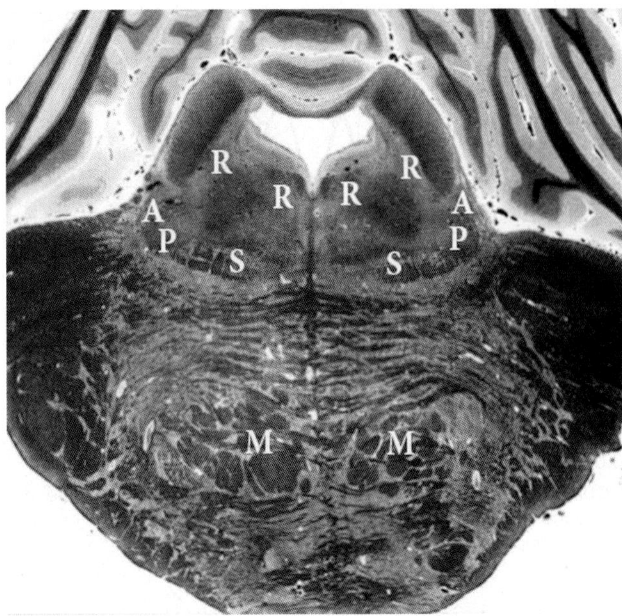

FIGURE 28.8. Section of the brainstem through the midpons. Note the relatively limited and separated territory of the brainstem actually monitored by evoked responses at this level. Function of the surrounding brainstem is assumed to be reflected by auditory and somatosensory function. Vital pathways and structures are near the auditory and somatosensory pathways. A, auditory pathway; P, pain pathway; S, somatosensory pathway; R, reticular formation; M, descending motor pathway.

BRAINSTEM AUDITORY-EVOKED POTENTIALS

The stimulus for the BAEP is a repetitive loud click applied via headphone or ear inserts. To interpret the information provided by BAEPs, the clinician must be aware of modes by which testing can fail. For example, cerumen in the ear canal may muffle the applied stimulus; trauma may anatomically disrupt the auditory apparatus (damage to the external auditory canal, tympanic membrane, middle ear apparatus; aminoglycoside antibiotics may damage the inner ear transduction system). Fortunately, the eighth nerve itself produces a recordable action potential (Fig. 28.9), and presence of this response confirms that the auditory stimulus has actually reached the nervous system. Confirmation of nervous system activation is an essential first step for all EPs and should precede any interpretation of waveforms. This step guards against equipment malfunction, technical issues, and incorrectly optimistic and

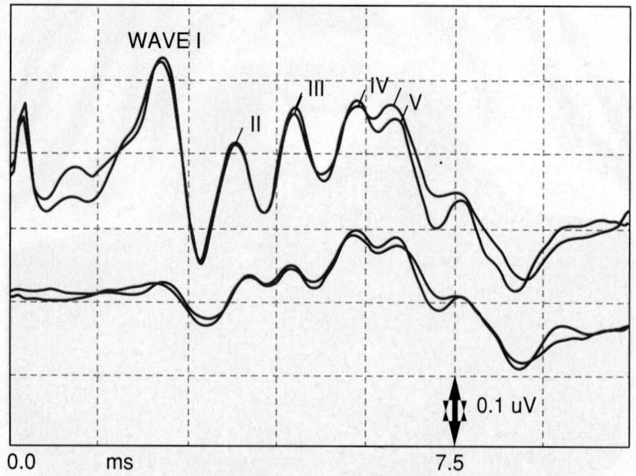

FIGURE 28.9. Normal brainstem auditory-evoked response. Note the presence of wave I, the eighth nerve action potential, which confirms that the auditory apparatus is being properly stimulated.

pessimistic interpretations. Without the presence of an eighth nerve action potential on the BAEP, no conclusions about the functioning of the more rostral auditory pathway can be made.

Figure 28.8 is a schematic representation of the auditory pathway in relationship to important brainstem and midbrain structures. The entire BAEP is generally completed within 10 milliseconds of the stimulus application. Because the auditory pathway has multiple synapses that produce recordable responses from the lower pons through the midbrain, if the recorded response demonstrates abnormalities at any level, significant neurologic impairment of the patient is likely because of the functional significance of nearby motor, sensory, autonomic, cranial nerve, and reticular activating system structures. Based on results from multiple studies, if the BAEP beyond the cochlear nerve action potential (wave I) is absent bilaterally, the CNS prognosis is grave with clinical and/or angiographic criteria often establishing brain death (63,66,104–106). Figure 28.10 shows BAEP and SEP recordings from three different patients who were comatose following trauma or surgery and were being evaluated for CNS function with EP recordings in the surgical ICU. Patient A had absent BAEPs beyond wave I and absent SEPs, and was determined to be brain dead within 24 hours of the EP studies. Patient B had a normal recording

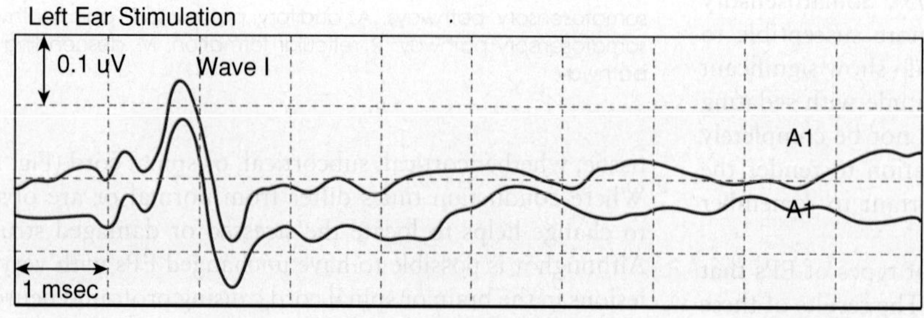

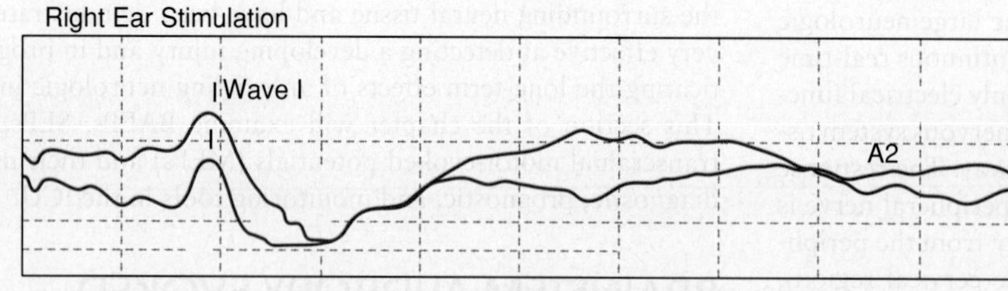

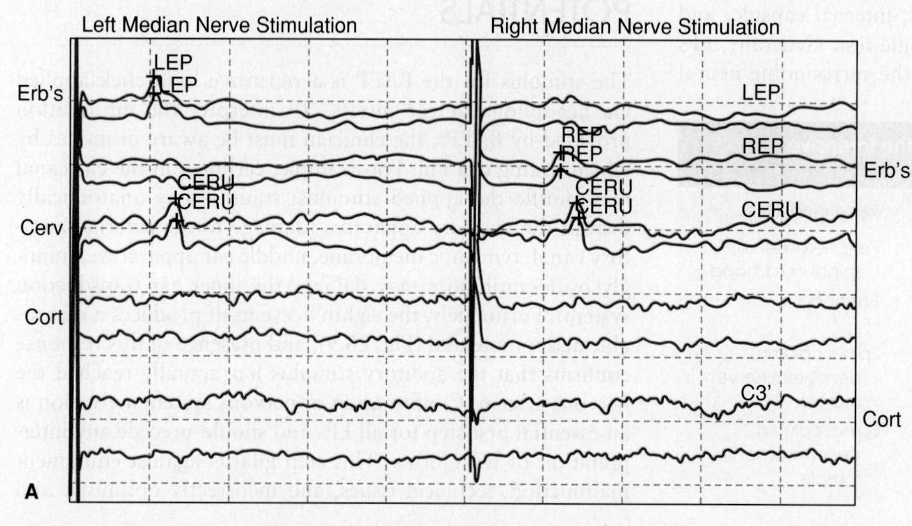

FIGURE 28.10. Neurophysiologic studies from three comatose patients. **A:** Brain-dead patient. This patient has no recordable evoked auditory response after wave I and no recordable somatosensory response after the cervical response. (*continued*)

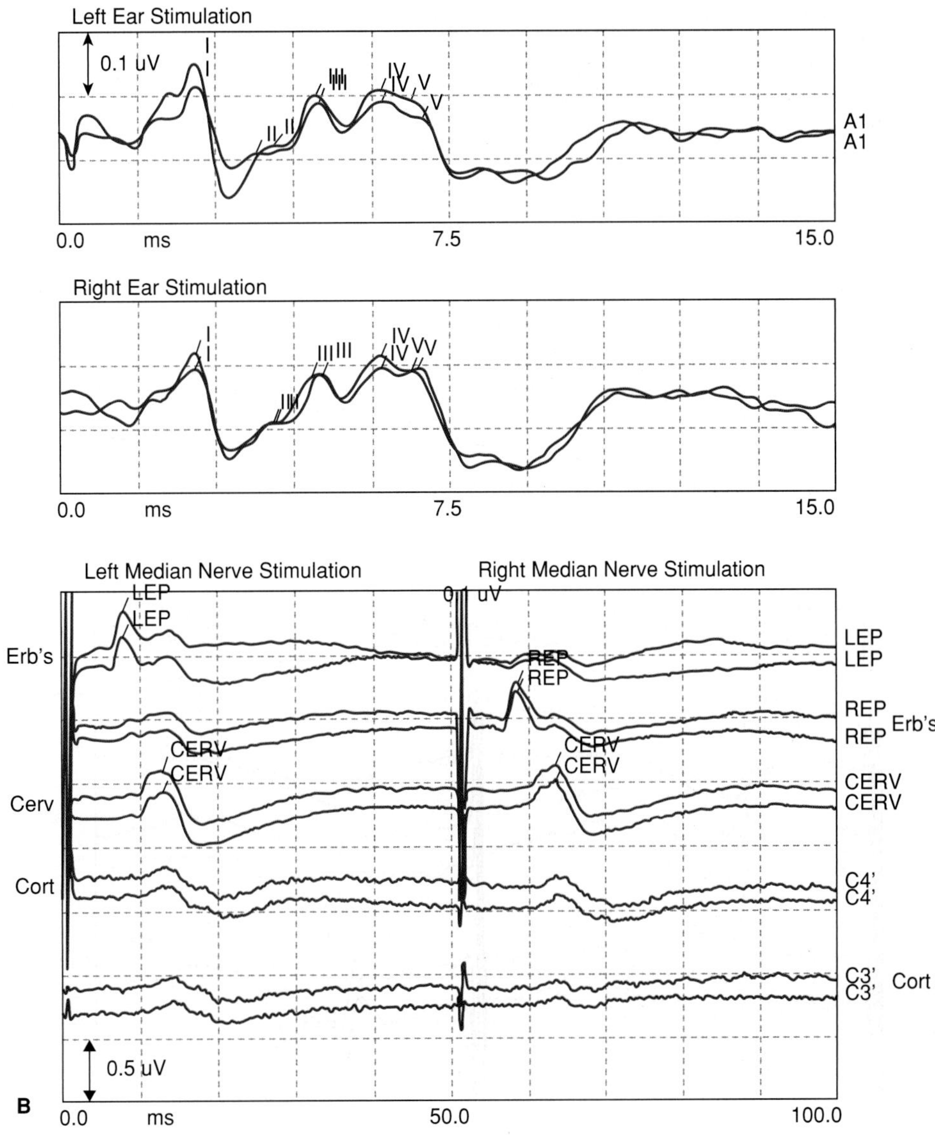

FIGURE 28.10. (*Continued*) **B:** Chronic vegetative state. This patient has an intact auditory-evoked response and no cortical somatosensory responses. (*continued*)

of waves I through V, but SEPs were absent. This patient had a prolonged hospital course and never recovered any higher neurologic function. Patient C had normal BAEPs and SEPs despite a severely impaired neurologic examination and difficult-to-control seizures at the time of the SEP study. Subsequent EP studies continued to show intact BAEPs and SEPs despite abnormal posturing and difficult-to-control seizures. This patient went on to recover independent neurologic function after many months of rehabilitation (107). These three patients exemplify the most common usage of EPs in the ICU, and their studies and outcome reflect what is documented in the literature. In summary, absent BAEPs beyond wave I indicate a high likelihood of a brain death outcome. Intact and normal BAEPs may indicate a good outcome, especially in the face of normal SEPs. If SEPs are absent bilaterally, the best likely outcome is a chronic vegetative state, even with normal BAEP waves I through V.

The auditory pathway continues rostrally, and responses may be recorded that are generated in the auditory cortex (middle-latency auditory-evoked responses). Limited clinical data suggest that presence of a normal middle-latency auditory response is a good a prognostic sign as the SEP in the comatose patient.

The stimulus for the SEP is repetitive electrical stimulation delivered to a peripheral nerve, most commonly the median nerve at the wrist or the posterior tibial nerve at the ankle, using surface electrodes or subdermal needle electrodes. The first response (a nerve action potential confirming pathway activation) is recorded proximally over the peripheral nerve or appropriate nerve plexus (Fig. 28.11). The next recorded response is generated in the lower brainstem and recorded with a surface electrode placed over the upper cervical spine. The primary initial cortical response at the rostral end of the somatosensory pathway is recorded over the cortex, contralateral to the side of stimulus application. Median nerve cortical SEPs usually occur 25 milliseconds from stimulus application or 50 milliseconds from stimulus application at the posterior tibial nerve. The normal SEP also contains responses that are later than the primary response. These responses, also generated by cortical neurons, are considered to be related to higher cognitive function. Most studies where SEPs are monitored or used for diagnosis and prognosis only analyze the initial primary cortical response occurring prior to 25 milliseconds. A few studies have also examined the prognostic significance of the later SEP or auditory responses (108,109), but the

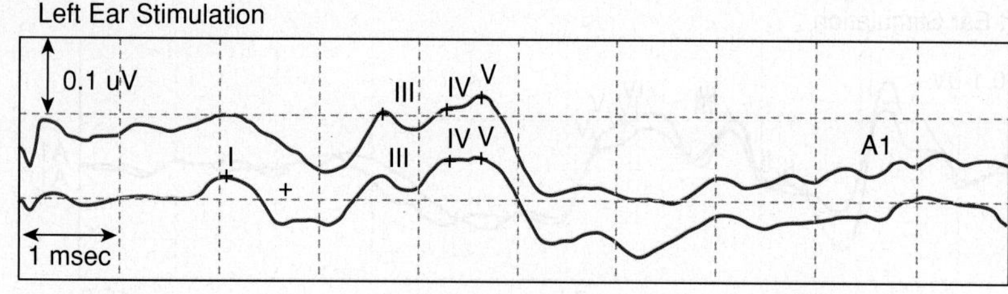

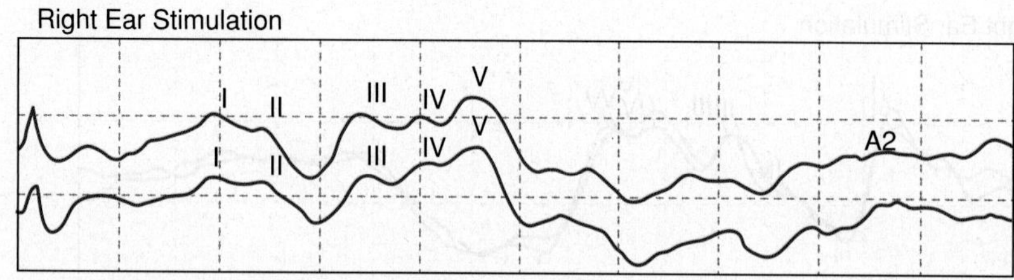

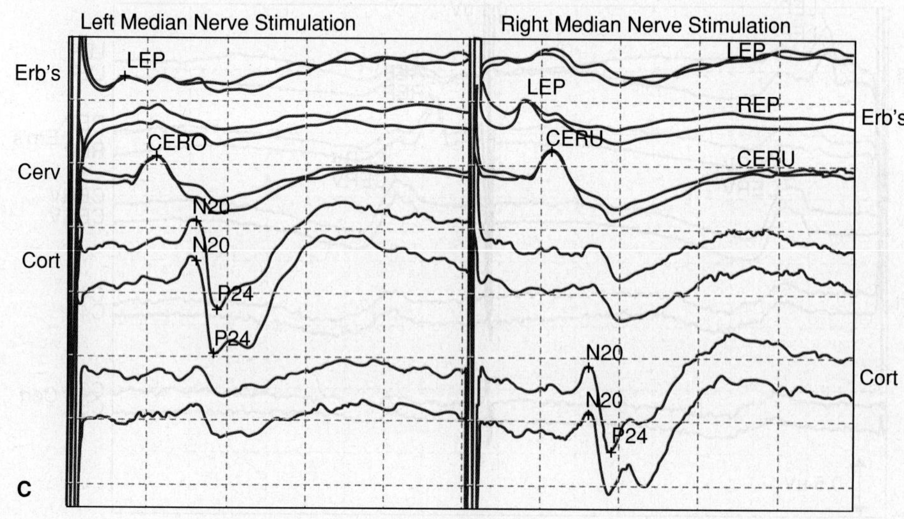

FIGURE 28.10. (*Continued*) **C:** Good outcome. This comatose patient has normal auditory- and somatosensory-evoked responses at all levels.

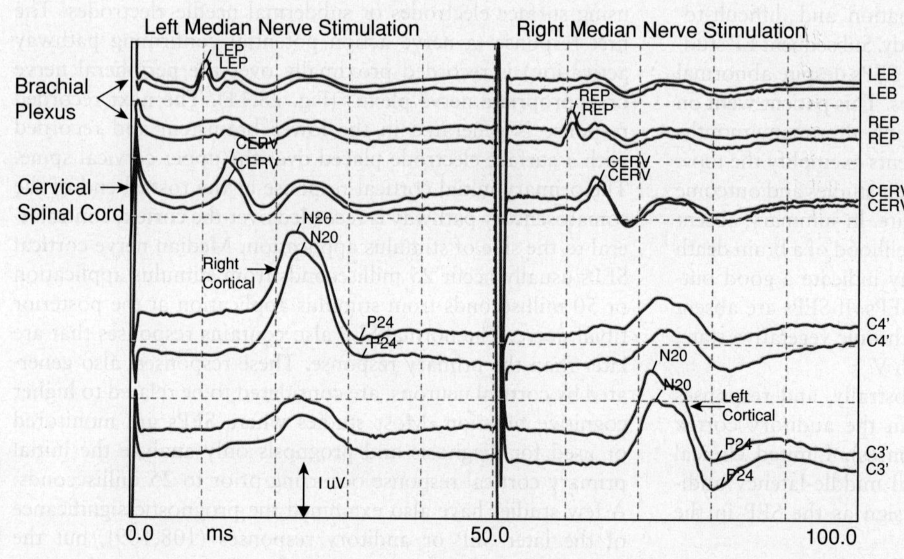

FIGURE 28.11. Normal median nerve somatosensory response. Reproducible responses at the brachial plexus and cervical levels confirm that a somatosensory stimulus is reaching the central nervous system. Without responses at both of these levels, conclusions about cortical functions cannot be made.

clinician should be aware that all of these later responses are highly influenced and easily abolished by any of the drugs used for sedation and analgesia in the ICU. In fact, later auditory responses have been used to gauge the depth of sedation in a fashion similar to the EEG bispectral index (109).

Figure 28.8 shows the somatosensory pathway schematically, together with the auditory pathway and nearby brainstem, midbrain, and cortical structures, in a single slice through the pons. As shown in the figure, the auditory and somatosensory pathways are separated far enough to include multiple important structures in the territory between them. The anatomic locations of the two separated pathways explain why neurologic outcome is usually better when both evoked response modalities show a normal response. The presence of cortical responses to a peripheral stimulus indicates that the involved subcortical nervous pathway is intact and that cortical neurons are still functional enough to be activated and produce a measurable electrical response, both of which are necessary for a good long-term neurologic outcome.

In summary, the presence of normal SEPs bilaterally, based on all available literature, is an excellent prognostic sign. The absence of any SEP cortical response is a poor prognostic indicator. The degree of bad outcome can be predicted by the BAEP. Intact and normal BAEPs with absent cortical SEPs predict a best outcome of a chronic vegetative state. Outcome may be worse, however, as BAEPs commonly deteriorate later with rostral-to-caudal CNS deterioration. Absent BAEP responses beyond wave I predict a high likelihood of brain death. Present but abnormal SEPs are associated with intermediate outcomes between good/high function and a chronic vegetative state (63,65,66,104–106,109–112).

The motor pathway may be tested by transcranial stimulation of the motor cortex. The cortex may be activated by a magnetic or electrical stimulus. A descending response may then be recorded over the spinal cord at multiple levels: The peripheral nerve and (most commonly) the muscle. Cortical stimulation, either electrical or magnetic, commonly activates the motor cortex governing the upper and lower extremities and produces a myogenic response that does not need to be averaged. The electrical stimulus intensity is quite high and is prohibitively painful in the awake subject. Thus, most of the limited work has been done using transcranial magnetic stimulation, which is much less painful and readily tolerated by the awake patient. What limited data are available indicate that results are mixed at best when using MEP testing as a prognostic indicator for long-term CNS outcome (113–116). Several carefully conducted studies also using SEPs indicate that SEPs are a much better prognostic indicator than MEPs (113,116). Much more work using MEPs needs to be done before any firm conclusions about their utility can be drawn.

CEREBRAL PERFUSION

This section of the chapter will examine methods that are available to monitor the adequacy of CBF. These monitors provide information that is complementary to the functional assessment discussed above, because function only becomes altered when CBF decreases by more than half.

The most common clinical measure aimed at ensuring adequate CBF is to maintain the CPP above the lower limit of cerebral autoregulation. Cerebral arterial circulation is normally autoregulated to maintain a constant CBF for a CPP between 70 and 150 mmHg. The accuracy of the CPP measurement should be confirmed in every patient. Because patients in the ICU are often positioned with their head elevated, calculating blood pressure goals that are corrected for the difference in vertical height between the external auditory meatus (as a landmark for the circle of Willis) and the blood pressure zero point (cuff, or arterial line zero point) are essential to defending the desired CPP. For every centimeter in vertical height between the two, the true blood pressure is approximately 0.75 mmHg lower in the head than displayed. Even in a semirecumbent adult, the height difference from the heart to the head can reach 27 cm, representing an arithmetic correction downward of 20 mmHg for blood pressure and CPP in the brain. Zero arterial transducers at the external auditory meatus or calculate the correction to achieve the target CPP.

Intracranial Pressure Monitoring and Waveform Interpretation

In cases of intracranial disease, the relevant pressure opposing adequate perfusion is the ICP. ICP reflects the dynamic interaction of tissues and fluids within a fixed volume, hard cranial shell of approximately 1,400 mL in an adult. Its contents can be divided into cerebral parenchyma, arterial and venous blood, and CSF components. The cerebral parenchyma accounts for 80% to 90% of the contents and includes intra- and extracellular fluid as well as cellular membranes. The volume of the blood together with the CSF makes up the remaining 10% to 20%. The Monroe–Kellie doctrine, as modified by Cushing at the turn of the 19th century, states that any increase in volume of one intracranial component occurs at the expense of another. Normal ICP in adults is 8 to 15 mmHg, and in babies, the pressure is 10 to 20 mmHg (less when measured through a lumbar puncture). Compensatory mechanisms stabilize ICP in response to slight changes in CBF, as well as CSF production and absorption. In the absence of effective compensatory mechanisms, an increase in the volume of any one of the components will lead to an exponential increase in pressure, as illustrated by the pressure–volume relationship (Fig. 28.12) described by Langfitt (117). Compensation may be achieved by any of the following: changes in the volume of CSF; the slight distention of the dura; changes in the intravascular volume, particularly in the venous channels; and compression or swelling of the brain. The rate of change in the volume of intracranial contents is important. For example, a rapid increase in volume produced by an epidural hematoma may overwhelm the compensatory mechanisms and produce a rapid increase in ICP, whereas a slowly growing brain tumor may produce a gradual displacement of structures within the cranial vault without a significant increase in ICP.

ICP is not static. Pressure fluctuations occur with cardiac systole due to distention of the intracranial arteriolar tree and respiration (i.e., ICP falling with each inspiration and rising with expiration). Straining or compression of neck veins can also cause a rise in pressure. A value in excess of 20 mmHg is almost always abnormal and should be treated. As the ICP increases, the cerebral venous pressure increases in parallel so as to remain 2 to 5 mmHg higher, or else the venous system would collapse. Because of this relationship, CPP can be satisfactorily estimated from mean arterial pressure at the external auditory meatus minus ICP.

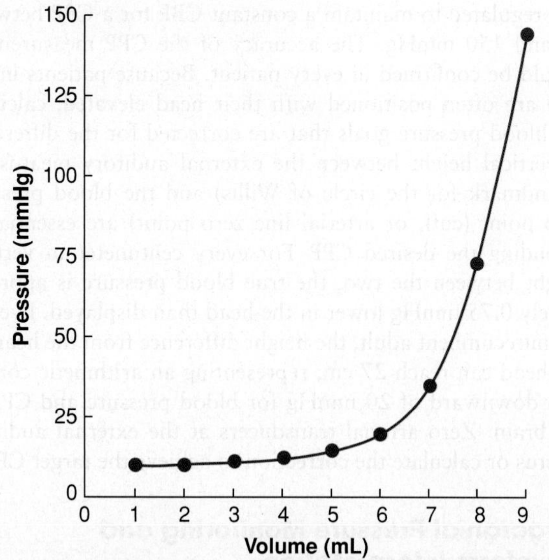

FIGURE 28.12. Pressure–volume relationship of the intracranial vault. Volume in milliliters (abscissa) of water added to a supratentorial extradural balloon in a monkey, 1 mL/hr. Pressure in millimeters of mercury (ordinate). (With permission from Langfitt TW. Increased intracranial pressure. *Clin Neurosurg.* 1969;16:43–71.)

Clinical deterioration in neurologic status is widely considered a sign of increased ICP. Bradycardia, increased pulse pressure, and pupillary dilation are accepted as signs of increased ICP.

The five methods most commonly used to monitor ICP are an intraventricular catheter, a subarachnoid or subdural bolt, a subdural catheteran intraparenchymal fiberoptic filament sensor, an extradural fiberoptic sensor. Each of these has its advantages and disadvantages. The intraventricular catheter is typically considered the gold standard. Its advantages include easy recalibration and a means to treat ICP elevations by removing CSF. However, it is the most invasive method and distorted intracranial pathology may necessitate several insertion attempts. The other devices are easier to place, but the accuracy of the recorded values may be more difficult to verify. All ICP monitors share a risk of infection of about 5%.

Patients who require ICP monitoring are generally considered to be those with a closed head injury and a GCS less than or equal to 8; in whom a CT scan shows significant brain distortion; with worsening neurologic status; in whom there is a need to sedate, paralyze, or operate in the context of an abnormal brain; with postoperative complications; and who are unconscious or in shock. The ICP data derived from such monitoring can serve as a useful therapeutic guide to clinical care.

The normal ICP waveform has three characteristic peaks (P1, P2, and P3) of decreasing height that correlate with the arterial pulse waveform (Fig. 28.13). The P1 (or percussion) wave originates from arterial systole and has a sharp peak and constant amplitude. The P2 (or tidal) wave is more variable and ends on the dicrotic notch. Elevation of the P2 component of the ICP waveform is thought to reflect decreased intracranial adaptive capacity and impaired autoregulation. However, sustained increases in ICP can occur without P2 elevation. The P3 (or dicrotic) wave follows the dicrotic notch and is venous in origin.

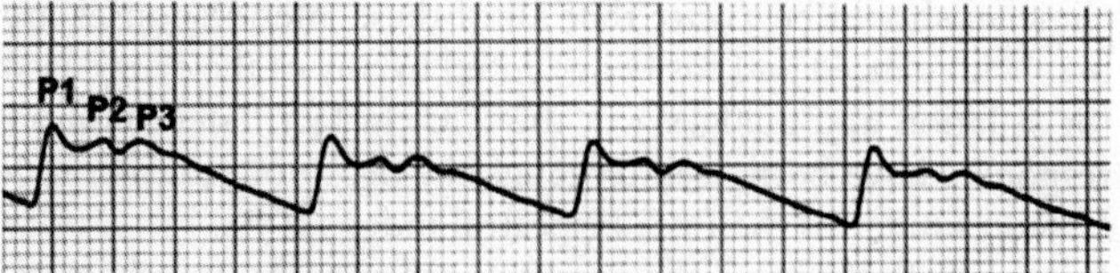

FIGURE 28.13. Intracranial pressure waveform showing the percussion wave (P1), tidal wave (P2), and dicrotic wave (P3). The timing of the peaks corresponds to the arterial pressure waveform. (Courtesy of Integra Neurosciences, Inc.)

When consecutive ICP waveforms are observed over time, three distinct patterns—first described by Lundberg in 1960 as A, B, and C waves—may be observed (118). A waves, now more commonly referred to as plateau waves, are pathologic (Fig. 28.14). There is a rapid rise in ICP up to 50 to 100 mmHg, followed by a variable period during which the ICP remains elevated ("plateau"), followed by a rapid fall to the baseline. These plateau waves typically last from 5 to 20 minutes. They are generally seen in patients with already elevated ICP. During a series of plateau waves, amplitude and duration may increase, leading to a "terminal" wave in which ICP may rise to levels that impede CBF. "Truncated" or atypical plateau waves that do not exceed 50 mmHg are early indicators of neurologic deterioration. B and C waves are smaller fluctuations in ICP thought to be related to respiration and autonomic fluctuations in blood pressure (Traube–Hering–Mayer waves), respectively. They are of little clinical significance.

Observing a normal CPP may be reassuring but must not be assumed to reflect normal CBF. Increased cerebrovascular resistance (e.g., because of carotid stenosis, cerebral vasospasm, or microcirculatory compromise) may cause ischemia despite normal CPP. Similarly, normal CPP may coexist with hyperemia in settings such as posttraumatic vasoparalysis, normal perfusion pressure breakthrough after resection of an arteriovenous malformation, or following carotid endarterectomy.

DIRECT CEREBRAL BLOOD FLOW MEASUREMENT

Several methods for determination of CBF exist (Table 28.9). They have the potential to provide insights into the pathophysiologic events in head injury or stroke, and help to direct therapeutic interventions.

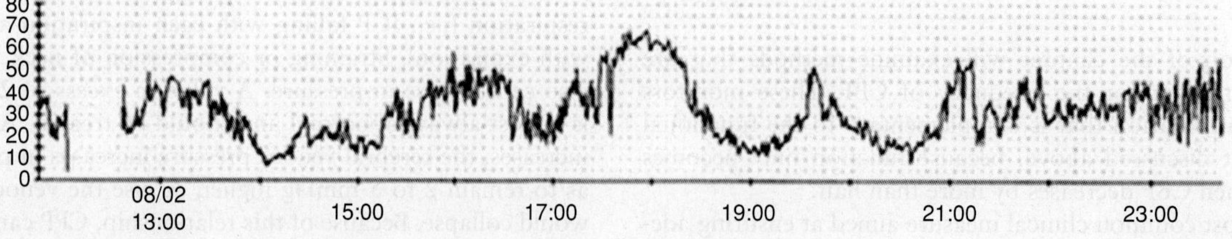

FIGURE 28.14. Lundberg plateau waves. The tracing of the intracranial pressure shows several pathologic increases of intracranial pressure, with plateaus lasting from 20 to 60 minutes. (Courtesy of Integra Neurosciences, Inc.)

TABLE 28.9 Techniques for Measuring Cerebral Blood Flow

Category	Technique	Resolution		Invasiveness	Cost
		Temporal	Spatial		
Bedside	Kety-Schmidt	15 min	Hemispheric	Jugular catheter	+
	^{133}Xenon wash-out	3–15 min	3–4 cm	Jugular catheter, radiation	+
	Arteriovenous difference in oxygen content, jugular venous oxygen saturation	<1 min	Global	Jugular catheter	+
	Double indicator dilution	3 min	Global	Jugular catheter, descending thoracic aortic catheter	+
	Near-infrared spectroscopy	<1 min	Local, bifrontal	No	+
	Thermal clearance probe	<1 min	Local, 1–2 cm	Exposed cortex	+
	Laser Doppler flow probe	<1 min	Local, 1–2 cm	Exposed cortex	+
Tomographic	Positron emission tomography	4–6 min/section	<1 cm	Radiation from positron emitter	+++++
	Stable Xenon computed tomography	4–6 min/section	<1 cm	Radiation from CT scan	+++
	Single photon emission tomography	4–6 min/section	<1 cm	Radiation from γ emitter	+++
	Magnetic resonance imaging	4–6 min/section	<1 cm	No	+++

Direct measurement of CBF is possible by determining the kinetics of wash-in or wash-out of an inert tracer compound in a variation of the method originally described by Kety and Schmidt (119). The most widely used measurement involves the administration of a radioactive isotope of ^{133}Xe per inhalation or intravenously, followed by measurement of the radioactivity wash-out, with γ detectors placed over specific areas of the brain. This method provides a spatial resolution of about 3 to 4 cm, depending on the number of detectors. In the normal brain, flow at different depths may be inferred from the early wash-out, which should reflect high-perfusion cortical gray matter and low-perfusion deeper white matter. An important disadvantage of the technique is its lack of sensitivity for focal areas of hypoperfusion, which are obscured by adjacent areas of adequate flow—a phenomenon described as "look-through."

Radiologic methods like SPECT, PET, Xenon-enhanced CT or perfusion CT, and MRI provide excellent spatial resolution, but are not available at the bedside. Some are used clinically as confirmatory tests in the determination of brain death. SPECT and magnetic resonance angiography, for example, show a "hollow skull phenomenon" and absent intracranial flow, respectively. Xenon-enhanced CT, and recently, perfusion CT scans have been used to obtain prognostic information and withhold unnecessarily aggressive therapy by assessing the severity of the decrease in CBF during stroke (120). Perfusion imaging allows the detection of a viable penumbra around areas of ischemia, which may be restored to normal function if the relative ischemia can be reversed.

Transcranial Doppler

An easy-to-apply, noninvasive bedside monitor that provides information on CBF is TCD ultrasound (121). The many applications of ultrasound imaging in the ICU setting have brought modern instrumentation to the ICU bedside, allowing TCD to be acquired based on color flow images of intracranial arteries against a backdrop of other intracranial structures as transcranial color-coded sonography (TCCS).

In TCD, ultrasound waves are used to measure the velocity of blood flow in the basal arteries of the brain and the extracranial portion of the internal carotid artery. These waves are transmitted through the relatively thin temporal bone, the orbit, or the foramen magnum (122). When they contact moving red blood cells, they are reflected at a changed frequency through the brain and skull back to a detector. The change in frequency as blood cells move toward or away from the ultrasound transmitter and detector is an example of the Doppler effect, and is related to velocity and direction of flow. Velocity increases during systole and decreases during diastole; blood in the center of the lumen moves faster than that near the vessel wall, producing a spectrum of flow velocities. This spectrum resembles the shape of the waveform produced by an intra-arterial pressure transducer (Fig. 28.15). The TCD probe emits ultrasound waves as short pulses. Because ultrasound travels through tissue at a constant velocity, assessment of flow at different distances from the transducer becomes possible by varying the time window during which the reflected ultrasound waves are received. Thus, each arterial segment at the base of the brain has a distinct signature in terms of depth of insonation and direction of flow. TCD measurements are most commonly (and easily) made in the middle cerebral and internal carotid arteries, but may also be measured in other vessels, including the anterior cerebral, anterior communicating, posterior cerebral, posterior communicating, and basilar arteries. In approximately 10% of patients, particularly elderly females, technically satisfactory recordings cannot be obtained because of increased skull thickness (122).

Although TCD allows the interrogation of all arteries that supply the brain, it cannot provide a simple assessment of global or hemispheric CBF. In the setting of acute stroke or traumatic arterial dissection, the mere patency of a vessel is an important question that has diagnostic, therapeutic, and prognostic implications (121–123). For example, the presence of blood flow indicates recanalization of a vessel and may be used to spare a patient the risks associated with thrombolytic therapy. Beyond the question of vessel patency, the link between TCD measurements and CBF is indirect and subject to one technical limitation and two principal assumptions inherent in the link. The technical limitation is that the accuracy with which the flow velocity can be determined depends on the

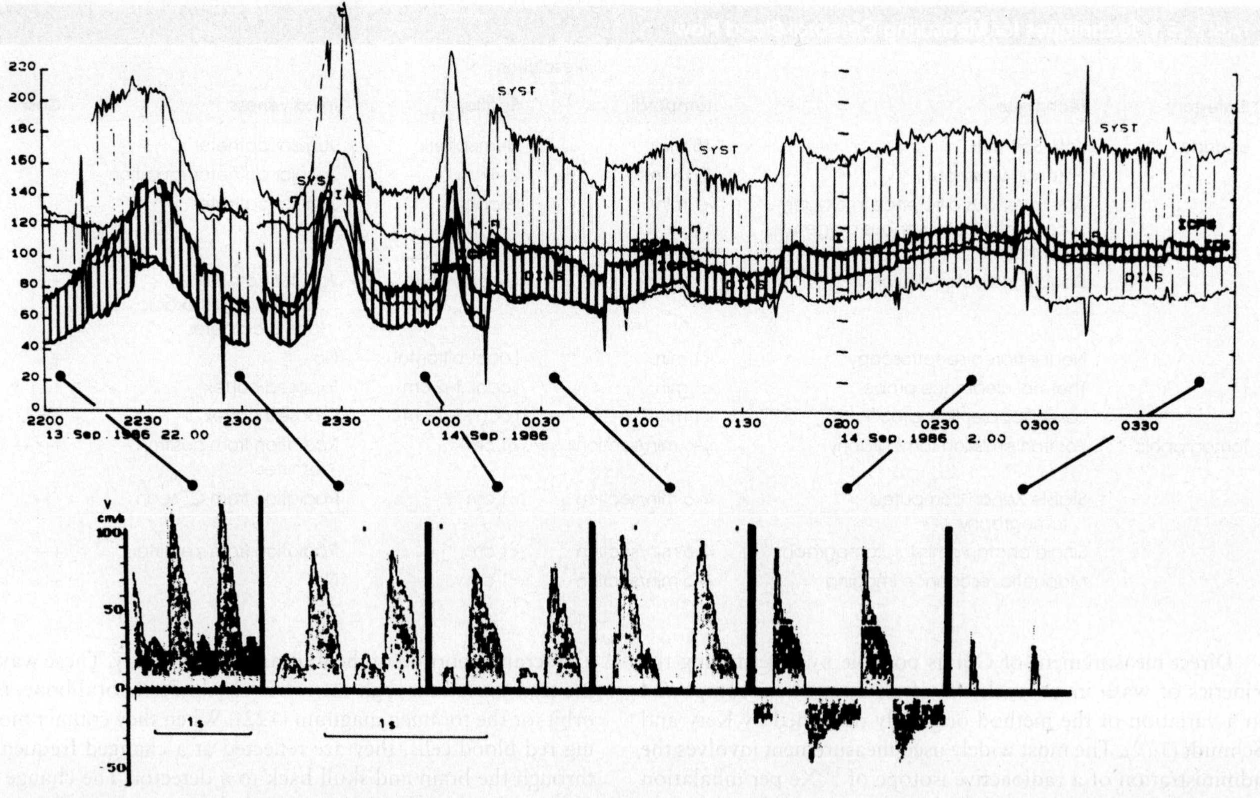

FIGURE 28.15. The flow velocity in intracerebral arteries shows a characteristic pattern of changes as intracranial pressure increases to the point of intracranial circulatory arrest and brain death. Initially, it resembles an arterial pressure waveform. (With permission from Hassler W, Steinmetz H, Gawlowski J. Transcranial Doppler ultrasonography in raised intracranial pressure and in intracranial circulatory arrest. *J Neurosurg*. 1988;68:745–751.)

angle of insonation. The variability of repeated measurements can be minimized by using a single examiner, provided a shift in brain structures caused by a mass lesion does not displace the artery. The two principal assumptions that have to be met for TCD-measured blood flow velocity to correspond to CBF are as follows:

1. Flow and flow velocity are directly related only if the diameter of the artery remains constant.
2. Second, the blood flow in the basal arteries of the brain must be directly related to cortical CBF.

These assumptions likely represent an oversimplification and have not been supported adequately by evidence. Specifically, radioactive Xenon-measured CBF does not correlate well with TCD-derived middle cerebral artery velocity during carotid endarterectomy or cardiopulmonary bypass (124–126). Likewise, normal variations in blood flow velocities are large (125).

Detection of Cerebral Vasospasm

TCD has been helpful in identifying vasospasm following aneurysmal subarachnoid hemorrhage and is typically used daily in these patients (127). As the diameter of the arterial lumen decreases with vasospasm, the velocity of blood flowing through the narrowed vessel must increase if flow is to be maintained. Using absolute flow velocity alone, detection and documentation of the severity and duration of vasospasm are possible, with a specificity that approaches 100% but with limited sensitivity. Flow velocities greater than 120 and 85 cm/sec identify patients at risk for angiographic vasospasm in middle cerebral and basilar artery territories, respectively (128). One important setting where absolute TCD flow velocity may underestimate the severity of vasospasm is that of increased ICP (129). Increases in ICP, however, lead to characteristic changes in the TCD waveform and increase the pulsatility index (see Fig. 28.15 and the following Section). Therapeutic dilation of stenotic arteries may not normalize TCD flow velocities immediately because of impaired autoregulation in the poststenotic vascular bed (130). Likewise, TCD cannot assess isolated distal vasospasm, which may account for as much as one-third of all cases of vasospasm (131).

Assessment of Intracranial Pressure and Confirmation of Brain Death

The TCD-generated waveform exhibits characteristic sequential changes as ICP increases (see Fig. 28.15) (132). As ICP increases, the systolic waveform becomes more peaked. As ICP nears diastolic blood pressure, diastolic flow diminishes and subsequently ceases. Once ICP exceeds diastolic blood pressure, TCD shows a pattern of to-and-fro movement of blood that indicates imminent intracranial circulatory arrest. This change in waveforms can be used to calculate a pulsatility index by relating the difference between peak systolic and end-diastolic velocity to the mean or to the systolic velocity. Such waveform analyses correlate well with ICP (133) but cannot replace ICP monitoring because autoregulation, vasospasm, or proximal arterial stenosis may alter the TCD signal independent of the ICP (121).

Clinical brain death demonstrates a characteristic blood flow velocity pattern (134,135). There is a short systolic inflow of blood, followed by an exit of blood (flow direction reverses) from the cranium during diastole. TCD is a validated confirmatory test in the diagnosis of brain death with a sensitivity that exceeds 90% and a specificity of 100% (136,137). Although TCD can ascertain the diagnosis in most patients at the bedside, a large craniotomy or an inadequate bone window may preclude the complete examination necessary to confirm brain death.

Jugular Venous Oxygen Saturation Monitoring

Jugular venous oxygen saturation ($SjvO_2$) monitoring has been touted as an indicator of cerebral oxygen homeostasis. Changes in $SjvO_2$ from the normal range (60% to 70%) provide indirect information on the state of $CMRO_2$, and because blood flow is normally linked to $CMRO_2$, indirect information on CBF as well. Approximately 50% to 70% of patients with severe head trauma (GCS $\leq$ 8) will have an episode of desaturation ($SjvO_2$ < 50%). Despite an ischemic threshold widely accepted to be $SjvO_2$ > 50% during the early hyperemic conditions following head injury, the clinical utility of $SjvO_2$ monitoring remains unsettled (138).

The complexity of catheter placement, robustness of data acquisition, sample collection, and results interpretation contribute to a limited utilization of $SjvO_2$ monitoring in victims of moderate to severe head injury (139). $SjvO_2$ is preferentially measured from the flow-dominant internal jugular vein (right 60%, left 25%, equal 15%) (140) to provide the best estimate of *whole* brain $CMRO_2$ conditions. Internal jugular vein size on ultrasound or CT provides a reasonable estimate of hemispheric dominance.

An increase in $SjvO_2$ indicates lowered $CMRO_2$ (less extraction) and/or increased or hyperemic CBF. A decrease in $SjvO_2$ (greater extraction) indicates increased $CMRO_2$, hypoxia/anemia, or oligemia. Observed changes in $SjvO_2$ might then help guide therapeutic interventions.

Abundant experience validates the association of jugular venous desaturation ($SjvO_2$ < 50%) with worsened neurologic outcome. Conversely, mortality in TBI was reduced 66% when monitoring and managing the cerebral extraction of oxygen with $SjvO_2$ in addition to CPP compared to management by CPP alone (141). $CMRO_2$ increased in patients with elevated ICP (ICP $\geq$ 20 mmHg) and normal to decreased cerebral extraction ("luxury perfusion") of oxygen with hyperventilation therapy. Elevated ICP associated with normal to increased cerebral extraction of oxygen was treated with mannitol, resulting in improved ICP and cerebral oxygenation.

Profound neurologic deterioration occurs with $SjvO_2$ desaturation to 30% or less (142). As cerebral circulatory arrest develops, the external carotid artery increasingly provides the blood sampled at the jugular bulb, and $SjvO_2$ then increases. In the clinical setting where brain death is expected, a ratio of mixed venous blood saturation to $SjvO_2$ less than 1 has been found to be highly sensitive (95%), specific (100%), and predictive (92%) for cerebral circulatory arrest (143).

The limitations of $SjvO_2$ monitoring may partly explain its decreasing use. Admixture of extracranial blood through collateral venous drainage into the superior sagittal, sigmoid, and cavernous sinuses or directly into the jugular bulb is believed to occur even when the catheter is correctly placed into the jugular bulb (144). When samples are drawn faster than 2 mL/min (145) or the catheter tip lies too far short of the jugular bulb, extracranial blood may further contaminate the specimen and spuriously elevate $SjvO_2$. Even a "clean" $SjvO_2$ sample does not distinguish between lateralizing differences in flow, metabolism, or brain injury. Thus, because $SjvO_2$ reflects a global average from a variety of brain regions, marked regional hypoperfusion may not be reflected by a change in $SjvO_2$ (146). Although $SjvO_2$ and brain tissue oxygen pressure ($PbtO_2$), a measure of regional ischemia, usually track in the same direction, maintaining $SjvO_2$ above conventional thresholds did not reliably protect against the occurrence of regional ischemic insults. Consequently, $SjvO_2$ cannot be used alone to direct hyperventilation or to alert clinicians to evolving hypocapnia-induced regional cerebral ischemia. It is now clear that "acceptable" hyperventilation may cause harm that remains clinically undetected by $SjvO_2$ (147).

$SjvO_2$ monitoring may be most useful as a trend monitor in patients with diffuse global brain injury and when it identifies saturations below the ischemic threshold. Normal range $SjvO_2$ can represent a "false-negative" measurement insofar as areas of regional ischemia may be present. Currently, the best technique for guiding therapy to a regional area of concern is with $PbtO_2$ monitoring.

Near-Infrared Spectroscopy

Near-infrared spectroscopy (NIRS) utilizes the minimal absorption and greater penetration of wavelengths in the infrared portion of the electromagnetic spectrum to evaluate changes in CBF and cerebral oxygenation. NIRS uses light with a wavelength between 700 and 1,300 nm to penetrate the scalp, skull, and brain (148) and offers the advantage of continuous, noninvasive monitoring of the cerebral cortex; it is typically done with one sensor each for the right and the left hemisphere of the brain. NIRS is currently best established for intraoperative use in cardiac surgery where neither confounding by intracranial pathology (edema, hematoma, or subarachnoid blood) nor strict differentiation between intracranial and extracranial contribution is of significant concern (149). In ideal circumstances, NIRS may be as sensitive in detecting progressive cerebral hypoxia as EEG (150), but spatial resolution is limited by the number of detectors. Further development in the technology will be required for NIRS to find a role in the ICU setting (128).

Brain Oxygen Monitoring

In contrast to most other techniques for evaluating brain oxygenation, tissue level monitoring offers both the advantage and disadvantage of robustly and continuously monitoring a very discrete region of tissue (151). Intraparenchymal direct oxygen partial pressure measurements ($PbrO_2$) are valuable in the management of cerebral perfusion and as well as with patients with TBI (152,153). They vary with CPP and can be used to define a physiologic lower limit of the CPP (154). The variability of $PbrO_2$ with cerebral perfusion can be used to define an oxygen reactivity index, which appears to reflect autoregulation. Diminished reactivity correlates with poorer outcome in subarachnoid hemorrhage and TBI (155,156).

In the 2007 Guidelines for the Management of Severe Head Injury (157), a brain tissue oxygenation threshold of less than 15 mmHg was adopted as a level III recommendation. Subthreshold levels of $PbrO_2$, particularly if severe or persistent, have been associated with increased morbidity and mortality in patients with severe brain injury. Van den Brink et al. studied

101 comatose, nonpenetrating head injury patients whose GCS score was greater than 8. Despite aggressive management of ICP and CPP, brain tissue hypoxia frequently occurred (158). The depth and duration of tissue hypoxia was associated with an unfavorable outcome and death at 6 months after injury. Such studies have recently been synthetized in a systematic review that confirmed the value of brain tissue oxygen monitoring (159). Research on optimal management strategies in the face of degreased $PbrO_2$ are still an active area of research (160,161). Giri et al. described that increases in inspiratory oxygen have little effect on $PbrO_2$ in normal tissue, whereas in the injured brain, $PbrO_2$ is increased as long as blood flow is present (162). Stiefel et al. reported in 2005 a management strategy in severe TBI that included $PbrO_2$ monitoring and therapy directed at maintaining brain oxygenation greater than 25 mmHg (163). Using this multimodal approach, they observed reduced patient mortality compared to CPP-directed therapy.

Cerebral Microdialysis

Microdialysis is a technique that can be combined with brain tissue oxygen monitoring within the same highly localized probe (164,165). Therefore, interpretation of the data will also be influenced by its location either in the penumbra of a lesion or in relatively normal brain. The intracerebral probe consists of a fluid path surrounded by a semipermeable membrane. This fluid path is perfused with a balanced salt solution that equilibrates with interstitial fluid from the brain. Therefore, the fluid returned from that fluid path contains substances from the brain in proportion to their local concentration, their specific membrane permeability, and the perfusate flow rate. Because the latter two do not change, the concentration of substances of interest can be followed over time. In the research context, this technique has been used to study topics as diverse as the role of excitotoxicity (166) or the proteomics of brain ischemia in stroke (167,168). The monitoring application closest to clinical utility, however, sets its sights considerably lower. It aims to determine the state of aerobic glucose utilization by following glucose concentrations directly or the ratio of metabolic intermediary products such as the pyruvate-to-lactate ratio. Ratiometric determinations of chemically similar molecules obviate the need to calibrate the probe based on the permeability of the substance(s) of interest. A decrease in the pyruvate-to-lactate ratio indicates an increase in anaerobic metabolism and/or mitochondrial dysfunction consistent with ischemia (166). Threshold values concerning for excessive substrate use of inadequate substrate delivery are a lactate/pyruvate ratio greater than 40 or a glucose concentration of less than 0.7 to 1 mmol/L (154). At this time, microdialysis is mostly used in conjunction with other monitors rather than as a stand-alone technique (128).

SUMMARY

Technologic advances in neurointensive care medicine have allowed for the successful treatment of severely injured patients. Early detection of the magnitude of the injury, damage control of coexisting diseases, prevention of secondary injury, and, ultimately, pharmacologic or surgical correction of neurodisorders are all primary objectives of the focused neurointensive care team. Effective neuromonitoring techniques are fundamental tools to achieve these goals. As the field of neurocritical care continues to emerge as a subspecialty dedicated to the treatment of critically ill patients with neurologic diseases, the neuromonitoring level of sophistication will increase in parallel, and so will our ability to monitor cerebral physiology and pathophysiology in real time.

Key Points

- Neuromonitoring requires an in-depth appreciation of neuroanatomy and neurophysiology.
- The foundation of monitoring is applied clinical evaluation.
- It is important to recognize the difference between systemic and cerebral circulation regulation to maintain neurologic integrity, autoregulation, and coupling of metabolism and oxygen delivery.
- Neuromonitoring has utility in determination of brain death, neurologic integrity, blood flow, and evaluation of blood flow.
- Continuous EEG may be used to evaluate seizure activity and depth of sedation.
- ICP monitoring provides dynamic information of compliance and pressure, which is useful following an intracranial insult.
- By providing complementary information about function, metabolism, and perfusion, multimodality monitoring may allow earlier identification of clinically important trends.
- Normal neurophysiologic monitoring signals are reassuring for current state and a patient's future recovery. Abnormal waveforms can be caused by a variety of benign or pathologic conditions and require investigation to interpret their significance.

References

1. Gilman S. Imaging the brain. First of two parts. *N Engl J Med.* 1998; 338:812–820.
2. Lou HC, Edvinsson L, MacKenzie ET. The concept of coupling blood flow to brain function: revision required? *Ann Neurol.* 1987;22:289–297.
3. Derdeyn CP, Videen TO, Yundt KD, et al. Variability of cerebral blood volume and oxygen extraction: stages of cerebral haemodynamic impairment revisited. *Brain.* 2002;125:595–607.
4. Kety SS, King BD, Horvath SM, et al. The effects of an acute reduction in blood pressure by means of differential spinal sympathetic block on the cerebral circulation of hypertensive patients. *J Clin Invest.* 1950;29:402–407.
5. Boysen G. Cerebral hemodynamics in carotid surgery. *Acta Neurol Scand Suppl.* 1973;52:3–86.
6. Derdeyn CP, Yundt KD, Videen TO, et al. Increased oxygen extraction fraction is associated with prior ischemic events in patients with carotid occlusion. *Stroke.* 1998;29:754–758.
7. Rapela CE, Green HD. Autoregulation of canine cerebral blood flow. *Circ Res.* 1964;15(Suppl):205–212.
8. Buchanan JE, Phillis JW. The role of nitric oxide in the regulation of cerebral blood flow. *Brain Res.* 1993;610:248–255.
9. Petersen SE, Fox PT, Snyder AZ, et al. Activation of extrastriate and frontal cortical areas by visual words and word-like stimuli. *Science.* 1990;249:1041–1044.
10. Bouma GJ, Muizelaar JP, Stringer WA, et al. Ultra-early evaluation of regional cerebral blood flow in severely head-injured patients using xenon-enhanced computerized tomography. *J Neurosurg.* 1992;77:360–368.
11. Lee JH, Martin NA, Alsina G, et al. Hemodynamically significant cerebral vasospasm and outcome after head injury: a prospective study. *J Neurosurg.* 1997;87:221–233.

12. Muizelaar JP, Marmarou A, Ward JD, et al. Adverse effects of prolonged hyperventilation in patients with severe head injury: a randomized clinical trial. *J Neurosurg*. 1991;75:731–739.
13. Michenfelder JD, Milde JH. The relationship among canine brain temperature, metabolism, and function during hypothermia. *Anesthesiology*. 1991;75:130–136.
14. Walter B, Bauer R, Kuhnen G, et al. Coupling of cerebral blood flow and oxygen metabolism in infant pigs during selective brain hypothermia. *J Cereb Blood Flow Metab*. 2000;20:1215–1224.
15. Stullken EH Jr, Milde JH, Michenfelder JD, et al. The nonlinear responses of cerebral metabolism to low concentrations of halothane, enflurane, isoflurane, and thiopental. *Anesthesiology*. 1977;46:28–34.
16. Alkire MT, Haier RJ, Barker SJ, et al. Cerebral metabolism during propofol anesthesia in humans studied with positron emission tomography. *Anesthesiology*. 1995;82:393–403.
17. Michenfelder J. *Anesthesia and the Brain*. New York, NY: Churchill Livingstone; 1988.
18. Milde LN, Milde JH, Michenfelder JD. Cerebral functional, metabolic, and hemodynamic effects of etomidate in dogs. *Anesthesiology*. 1985;63:371–377.
19. Edelman GJ, Hoffman WE, Charbel FT. Cerebral hypoxia after etomidate administration and temporary cerebral artery occlusion. *Anesth Analg*. 1997;85:821–825.
20. Matta BF, Lam AM, Strebel S, Mayberg TS. Cerebral pressure autoregulation and carbon dioxide reactivity during propofol-induced EEG suppression. *Br J Anaesth*. 1995;74:159–163.
21. Doyle PW, Matta BF. Burst suppression or isoelectric encephalogram for cerebral protection: evidence from metabolic suppression studies. *Br J Anaesth*. 1999;83:580–584.
22. Ederberg S, Westerlind A, Houltz E, et al. The effects of propofol on cerebral blood flow velocity and cerebral oxygen extraction during cardiopulmonary bypass. *Anesth Analg*. 1998;86:1201–1206.
23. Nandate K, Vuylsteke A, Ratsep I, et al. Effects of isoflurane, sevoflurane and propofol anaesthesia on jugular venous oxygen saturation in patients undergoing coronary artery bypass surgery. *Br J Anaesth*. 2000;84:631–633.
24. Johnston AJ, Steiner LA, Chatfield DA, et al. Effects of propofol on cerebral oxygenation and metabolism after head injury. *Br J Anaesth*. 2003;91:781–786.
25. Heath KJ, Gupta S, Matta BF. The effects of sevoflurane on cerebral hemodynamics during propofol anesthesia. *Anesth Analg*. 1997;85:1284–1287.
26. Citerio G, Cormio M. Sedation in neurointensive care: advances in understanding and practice. *Curr Opin Crit Care*. 2003;9:120–126.
27. Rhoney DH, Parker D Jr. Use of sedative and analgesic agents in neurotrauma patients: effects on cerebral physiology. *Neurol Res*. 2001;23:237–259.
28. Prielipp RC, Wall MH, Tobin JR, et al. Dexmedetomidine-induced sedation in volunteers decreases regional and global cerebral blood flow. *Anesth Analg*. 2002;95:1052–1059, table of contents.
29. Grille P, Biestro A, Farina G, Miraballes R. [Effects of dexmedetomidine on intracranial hemodynamics in severe head injured patients.] *Neurocirugia (Astur)*. 2005;16:411–418.
30. Kety SS, Schmidt CF. The effects of altered arterial tensions of carbon dioxide and oxygen on cerebral blood flow and cerebral oxygen consumption of normal young men. *J Clin Invest*. 1948;27:484–492.
31. Reivich M. Arterial pCO_2 and cerebral hemodynamics. *Am J Physiol*. 1964;206:25–35.
32. Brian JE Jr. Carbon dioxide and the cerebral circulation. *Anesthesiology*. 1998;88:1365–1386.
33. Harper AM. Autoregulation of cerebral blood flow: influence of the arterial blood pressure on the blood flow through the cerebral cortex. *J Neurol Neurosurg Psychiatry*. 1966;29:398–403.
34. Paulson OB, Strandgaard S, Edvinsson L. Cerebral autoregulation. *Cerebrovasc Brain Metab Rev*. 1990;2:161–192.
35. Eng C, Lam AM, Mayberg TS, et al. The influence of propofol with and without nitrous oxide on cerebral blood flow velocity and CO2 reactivity in humans. *Anesthesiology*. 1992;77:872–879.
36. Nordstrom CH, Messeter K, Sundbarg G, et al. Cerebral blood flow, vasoreactivity, and oxygen consumption during barbiturate therapy in severe traumatic brain lesions. *J Neurosurg*. 1988;68:424–431.
37. Berre J, Moraine JJ, Melot C. Cerebral CO_2 vasoreactivity evaluation with and without changes in intrathoracic pressure in comatose patients. *J Neurosurg Anesthesiol*. 1998;10:70–79.
38. Luce JM, Huseby JS, Kirk W, et al. A Starling resistor regulates cerebral venous outflow in dogs. *J Appl Physiol*. 1982;53:1496–1503.
39. Bouma GJ, Muizelaar JP. Cerebral blood flow, cerebral blood volume, and cerebrovascular reactivity after severe head injury. *J Neurotrauma*. 1992;9(Suppl 1):S333–348.
40. Langfitt TW, Weinstein JD, Kassell NF. Cerebral vasomotor paralysis produced by intracranial hypertension. *Neurology*. 1965;15:622–641.
41. Thiel A, Zickmann B, Stertmann WA, et al. Cerebrovascular carbon dioxide reactivity in carotid artery disease. Relation to intraoperative cerebral monitoring results in 100 carotid endarterectomies. *Anesthesiology*. 1995;82:655–661.
42. Tranmer BI, Keller TS, Kindt GW, et al. Loss of cerebral regulation during cardiac output variations in focal cerebral ischemia. *J Neurosurg*. 1992;77:253–259.
43. Todd MM, Weeks JB, Warner DS. The influence of intravascular volume expansion on cerebral blood flow and blood volume in normal rats. *Anesthesiology*. 1993;78:945–953.
44. Todd MM, Weeks JB, Warner DS. Cerebral blood flow, blood volume, and brain tissue hematocrit during isovolemic hemodilution with hetastarch in rats. *Am J Physiol*. 1992;263:H75–82.
45. Todd MM, Wu B, Maktabi M, et al. Cerebral blood flow and oxygen delivery during hypoxemia and hemodilution: role of arterial oxygen content. *Am J Physiol*. 1994;267:H2025–2031.
46. Teasdale G, Jennett B. Assessment of coma and impaired consciousness: a practical scale. *Lancet*. 1974;2:81–84.
47. Rowley G, Fielding K. Reliability and accuracy of the Glasgow Coma Scale with experienced and inexperienced users. *Lancet*. 1991;337:535–538.
48. Knaus WA, Draper EA, Wagner DP, et al. APACHE II: a severity of disease classification system. *Crit Care Med*. 1985;13:818–829.
49. Teasdale GM, Drake CG, Hunt W, et al. A universal subarachnoid hemorrhage scale: report of a committee of the World Federation of Neurosurgical Societies. *J Neurol Neurosurg Psychiatry*. 1988;51:1457.
50. Gennarelli TA, Champion HR, Copes WS, et al. Comparison of mortality, morbidity, and severity of 59,713 head injured patients with 114,447 patients with extracranial injuries. *J Trauma*. 1994;37:962–968.
51. Chiang VL, Claus EB, Awad IA. Toward more rational prediction of outcome in patients with high-grade subarachnoid hemorrhage. *Neurosurgery*. 2000;46:28–35.
52. Tseng JH, Tseng MY. Brain abscess in 142 patients: factors influencing outcome and mortality. *Surg Neurol*. 2006;65:557–562.
53. Edgren E, Hedstrand U, Kelsey S, et al. Assessment of neurological prognosis in comatose survivors of cardiac arrest. *BRCT I Study Group. Lancet*. 1994;343:1055–1059.
54. Niskanen M, Kari A, Nikki P, et al. Acute physiology and chronic health evaluation (APACHE II) and Glasgow coma scores as predictors of outcome from intensive care after cardiac arrest. *Crit Care Med*. 1991;19:1465–1473.
55. Eidelman LA, Putterman D, Putterman C, Sprung CL. The spectrum of septic encephalopathy. Definitions, etiologies, and mortalities. *JAMA*. 1996;275:470–473.
56. Kuhls DA, Malone DL, McCarter RJ, Napolitano LM. Predictors of mortality in adult trauma patients: the physiologic trauma score is equivalent to the Trauma and Injury Severity Score. *J Am Coll Surg*. 2002;194:695–704.
57. Massagli TL, Michaud LJ, Rivara FP. Association between injury indices and outcome after severe traumatic brain injury in children. *Arch Phys Med Rehabil*. 1996;77:125–132.
58. Mhanna MJ, Mallah WE, Verrees M, et al. Outcome of children with severe traumatic brain injury who are treated with decompressive craniectomy. *J Neurosurg Pediatr*. 2015:11–17.
59. Wijdicks EF. The diagnosis of brain death. *N Engl J Med*. 2001;344: 1215–1221.
60. Santamaria J, Orteu N, Iranzo A, Tolosa E. Eye opening in brain death. *J Neurol*. 1999;246:720–722.
61. Goudreau JL, Wijdicks EF, Emery SF. Complications during apnea testing in the determination of brain death: predisposing factors. *Neurology*. 2000;55:1045–1048.
62. Saposnik G, Bueri JA, Maurino J, et al. Spontaneous and reflex movements in brain death. *Neurology*. 2000;54:221–223.
63. Facco E, Munari M, Baratto F, et al. Multimodality evoked potentials (auditory, somatosensory and motor) in coma. *Neurophysiol Clin*. 1993;23: 237–258.
64. Fisher B, Peterson B, Hicks G. Use of brainstem auditory-evoked response testing to assess neurologic outcome following near drowning in children. *Crit Care Med*. 1992;20:578–585.
65. Pohlmann-Eden B, Dingethal K, Bender HJ, Koelfen W. How reliable is the predictive value of SEP (somatosensory evoked potentials) patterns in severe brain damage with special regard to the bilateral loss of cortical responses? *Intensive Care Med*. 1997;23:301–308.
66. Ruiz-Lopez MJ, Martinez de Azagra A, Serrano A, Casado-Flores J. Brain death and evoked potentials in pediatric patients. *Crit Care Med*. 1999;27:412–416.

67. Crippen D. Role of bedside electroencephalography in the adult intensive care unit during therapeutic neuromuscular blockade. *Crit Care.* 1997;1:15–24.
68. Freye E. Cerebral monitoring in the operating room and the intensive care unit—an introductory for the clinician and a guide for the novice wanting to open a window to the brain. Part II: sensory-evoked potentials (SSEP, AEP, VEP). *J Clin Monit Comput.* 2005;19:77–168.
69. Hirsch LJ. Continuous EEG monitoring in the intensive care unit: an overview. *J Clin Neurophysiol.* 2004;21:332–340.
70. Hall R, Murdoch J. Brain protection: physiological and pharmacological considerations. Part II: The pharmacology of brain protection. *Can J Anaesth.* 1990;37:762–777.
71. Steen PA, Newberg L, Milde JH, Michenfelder JD. Hypothermia and barbiturates: individual and combined effects on canine cerebral oxygen consumption. *Anesthesiology.* 1983;58:527–532.
72. Akeju O, Pavone KJ, Westove MB, et al. A comparison of propofol- and dexmedetomidine-induced electroencephalogram dynamics using spectral and coherence analysis. *Anesthesiology.* 2014;121:978–989.
73. Drummond JC, Todd MM, U HS. The effect of high dose sodium thiopental on brain stem auditory and median nerve somatosensory evoked responses in humans. *Anesthesiology.* 1985;63:249–254.
74. Sutton LN, Frewen T, Marsh R, Bruce DA The effects of deep barbiturate coma on multimodality evoked potentials. *J Neurosurg.* 1982;57:178–185.
75. Rothstein TL. Recovery from near death following cerebral anoxia: a case report demonstrating superiority of median somatosensory evoked potentials over EEG in predicting a favorable outcome after cardiopulmonary resuscitation. *Resuscitation.* 2004;60:335–341.
76. Kull LL, Emerson RG. Continuous EEG monitoring in the intensive care unit: technical and staffing considerations. *J Clin Neurophysiol.* 2005;22: 107–118.
77. Ronne-Engstrom E, Winkler T. Continuous EEG monitoring in patients with traumatic brain injury reveals a high incidence of epileptiform activity. *Acta Neurol Scand.* 2006;114:47–53.
78. Wartenberg KE, Mayer SA. Multimodal brain monitoring in the neurological intensive care unit: where does continuous EEG fit in? *J Clin Neurophysiol.* 2005;22:124–127.
79. Shi L, Agarwal R, Swamy MN. Model-based seizure detection method using statistically optimal filters. *Conf Proc IEEE Eng Med Biol Soc.* 2004; 1:45–48.
80. Subasi A. Selection of optimal AR spectral estimation method for EEG signals using Cramer-Rao bound. *Comput Biol Med.* 2007;37:183–194.
81. Diagnostic Accuracy of Electrographic Seizure Detection by Neurophysiologists and Non-Neurophysiologists in the Adult ICU Using a Panel of Quantitative EEG Trends. *J Clin Neuophysiol.* 2015;32: 324–30.
82. Abou Khaled KJ, Hirsch LJ. Advances in the management of seizures and status epilepticus in critically ill patients. *Crit Care Clin.* 2006;22:637–659.
83. Deogaonkar A, Gupta R, DeGeorgia M, et al. Bispectral Index monitoring correlates with sedation scales in brain-injured patients. *Crit Care Med.* 2004;32:2403–2406.
84. Fabregas N, Gambus PL, Valero R, et al. Can bispectral index monitoring predict recovery of consciousness in patients with severe brain injury? *Anesthesiology.* 2004;101:43–51.
85. Schnakers C, Majerus S, Laureys S. Bispectral analysis of electroencephalogram signals during recovery from coma: preliminary findings. *Neuropsychol Rehabil.* 2005;15:381–388.
86. Schneider G, Heglmeier S, Schneider J, et al. Patient State Index (PSI) measures depth of sedation in intensive care patients. *Intensive Care Med.* 2004;30:213–216.
87. Grindstaff RJ, Tobias JD. Applications of bispectral index monitoring in the pediatric intensive care unit. *J Intensive Care Med.* 2004;19:111–116.
88. Riker RR, Fraser GL, Wilkins ML. Comparing the bispectral index and suppression ratio with burst suppression of the electroencephalogram during pentobarbital infusions in adult intensive care patients. *Pharmacotherapy.* 2003;23:1087–1093.
89. Ozcan MS, Gravenstein D. The presence of working memory without explicit recall in a critically ill patient. *Anesth Analg.* 2004;98:469–470.
90. Rampil IJ. A primer for EEG signal processing in anesthesia. *Anesthesiology.* 1998;89:980–1002.
91. Ely EW, Truman B, Manzi DJ, et al. Consciousness monitoring in ventilated patients: bispectral EEG monitors arousal not delirium. *Intensive Care Med.* 2004;30:1537–1543.
92. Katoh T, Bito H, Sato S. Influence of age on hypnotic requirement, bispectral index, and 95% spectral edge frequency associated with sedation induced by sevoflurane. *Anesthesiology.* 2000;92:55–61.
93. Sleigh JW, Andrzejowski J, Steyn-Ross A, Steyn-Ross M. The bispectral index: a measure of depth of sleep? *Anesth Analg.* 1999;88:659–661.
94. Lubke GH, Kerssens C, Phaf H, Sebel PS. Dependence of explicit and implicit memory on hypnotic state in trauma patients. *Anesthesiology.* 1999;90:670–680.
95. Vivien B, Di Maria S, Ouattara A, et al. Overestimation of bispectral index in sedated intensive care unit patients revealed by administration of muscle relaxant. *Anesthesiology.* 2003;99:9–17.
96. Gallagher JD. Pacer-induced artifact in the bispectral index during cardiac surgery. *Anesthesiology.* 1999;90:636.
97. Johansen JW. Update on bispectral index monitoring. *Best Pract Res Clin Anaesthesiol.* 2006;20:81–99.
98. Chattopadhyay U, Mallik S, Ghosh S, et al. Comparison between propofol and dexmedetomidine on depth of anesthesia: a prospective randomized trial. *J Anaesthesiol Clin Pharmacol.* 2014;30:550–554.
99. Dunham CM, Ransom KJ, McAuley CE, et al. Severe brain injury ICU outcomes are associated with cranial-arterial pressure index and noninvasive bispectral index and transcranial oxygen saturation: a prospective, preliminary study. *Crit Care.* 2006;10:R159.
100. Chistyakov AV, Hafner H, Soustiel JF, et al. Dissociation of somatosensory and motor evoked potentials in non-comatose patients after head injury. *Clin Neurophysiol.* 1999;110:1080–1089.
101. Mazzini L, Pisano F, Zaccala M, et al. Somatosensory and motor evoked potentials at different stages of recovery from severe traumatic brain injury. *Arch Phys Med Rehabil.* 1999;80:33–39.
102. Moosavi SH, Ellaway PH, Catley M, et al. Corticospinal function in severe brain injury assessed using magnetic stimulation of the motor cortex in man. *J Neurol Sci.* 1999;164:179–186.
103. Banoub M, Tetzlaff JE, Schubert A. Pharmacologic and physiologic influences affecting sensory evoked potentials: implications for perioperative monitoring. *Anesthesiology.* 2003;99:716–737.
104. Goodwin SR, Friedman WA, Bellefleur M. Is it time to use evoked potentials to predict outcome in comatose children and adults? *Crit Care Med.* 1991;19:518–524.
105. Morgalla MH, Bauer J, Ritz R, Tatagiba M. [Coma. The prognostic value of evoked potentials in patients after traumatic brain injury]. *Anaesthesist.* 2006;55:760–768.
106. Nuwer MR. Electroencephalograms and evoked potentials. Monitoring cerebral function in the neurosurgical intensive care unit. *Neurosurg Clin N Am.* 1994;5:647–659.
107. Goodwin SR, Toney KA, Mahla ME. Sensory evoked potentials accurately predict recovery from prolonged coma caused by strangulation. *Crit Care Med.* 1993;21:631–633.
108. Lew HL, Dikmen S, Slimp J, et al. Use of somatosensory-evoked potentials and cognitive event-related potentials in predicting outcomes of patients with severe traumatic brain injury. *Am J Phys Med Rehabil.* 2003;82: 53–61; quiz 62-4, 80.
109. Lew HL, Poole JH, Castaneda A, et al. Prognostic value of evoked and event-related potentials in moderate to severe brain injury. *J Head Trauma Rehabil.* 2006;21:350–360.
110. Carter BG, Butt W. Review of the use of somatosensory evoked potentials in the prediction of outcome after severe brain injury. *Crit Care Med.* 2001;29:178–186.
111. Carter BG, Butt W. Are somatosensory evoked potentials the best predictor of outcome after severe brain injury? A systematic review. *Intensive Care Med.* 2005;31:765–775.
112. Fischer C, Luaute J. Evoked potentials for the prediction of vegetative state in the acute stage of coma. *Neuropsychol Rehabil.* 2005;15:372–380.
113. Zentner J, Ebner A. Prognostic value of somatosensory- and motor-evoked potentials in patients with a non-traumatic coma. *Eur Arch Psychiatry Neurol Sci.* 1988;237:184–187.
114. Dhand UK. Clinical approach to the weak patient in the intensive care unit. *Respir Care.* 2006;51:1024–1040.
115. Hemmerling TM, Le N. Brief review: neuromuscular monitoring: an update for the clinician. *Can J Anaesth.* 2007;54:58–72.
116. Heier T, Caldwell JE. Impact of hypothermia on the response to neuromuscular blocking drugs. *Anesthesiology.* 2006;104:1070–1080.
117. Langfitt TW. Increased intracranial pressure. *Clin Neurosurg.* 1969;16:43–71.
118. Steiner LA, Andrews PJ. Monitoring the injured brain: ICP and CBF. *Br J Anaesth.* 2006;97:26–38.
119. Kety SS, Schmidt CF. The nitrous oxide method for the quantitative determination of cerebral blood flow in man: theory, procedure, and normal values. *J Clin Invest.* 1948;27:476–493.
120. Drewer-Gutland F, Kemmling A, Ligges S, et al. CTP-based tissue outcome: promising tool to prove the beneficial effect of mechanical recanalization in acute ischemic stroke. *Rofo.* 2015;187:459–466.
121. White H, Venkatesh B. Applications of transcranial Doppler in the ICU: a review. *Intensive Care Med.* 2006;32:981–994.

122. Ringelstein EB, Biniek R, Weiller C, et al. Type and extent of hemispheric brain infarctions and clinical outcome in early and delayed middle cerebral artery recanalization. *Neurology*. 1992;42:289–298.
123. Manno EM. Transcranial Doppler ultrasonography in the neurocritical care unit. *Crit Care Clin*. 1997;13:79–104.
124. Halsey JH, McDowell HA, Gelmon S, Morawetz RB. Blood velocity in the middle cerebral artery and regional cerebral blood flow during carotid endarterectomy. *Stroke*. 1989;20:53–58.
125. Nuttall GA, Cook DJ, Fulgham JR, et al. The relationship between cerebral blood flow and transcranial Doppler blood flow velocity during hypothermic cardiopulmonary bypass in adults. *Anesth Analg*. 1996;82:1146–1151.
126. Weyland A, Stephan H, Kazmaier S, et al. Flow velocity measurements as an index of cerebral blood flow: validity of transcranial Doppler sonographic monitoring during cardiac surgery. *Anesthesiology*. 1994;81:1401–1410.
127. Sloan MA, Haley EC Jr, Kassell NF, et al. Sensitivity and specificity of transcranial Doppler ultrasonography in the diagnosis of vasospasm following subarachnoid hemorrhage. *Neurology*. 1989;39:1514–1518.
128. LeRoux P, Menon DK, Citerio G, et al. The international multidisciplinary consensus conference on multimodality monitoring in neurocritical care: a list of recommendations and additional conclusions: a statement for healthcare professionals from the Neurocritical Care Society and the European Society of Intensive Care Medicine. *Neurocrit Care*. 2014;21:S282–S296.
129. Klingelhofer J, Dander D, Holzgraefe M, et al. Cerebral vasospasm evaluated by transcranial Doppler ultrasonography at different intracranial pressures. *J Neurosurg*. 1991;75:752–758.
130. Giller CA, Purdy P, Giller A, et al. Elevated transcranial Doppler ultrasound velocities following therapeutic arterial dilation. *Stroke*. 1995;26:123–127.
131. Mizuno M, Nakajima S, Sampei T, et al. Serial transcranial Doppler flow velocity and cerebral blood flow measurements for evaluation of cerebral vasospasm after subarachnoid hemorrhage. *Neurol Med Chir (Tokyo)*. 1994;34:164–171.
132. Hassler W, Steinmetz H, Gawlowski J. Transcranial Doppler ultrasonography in raised intracranial pressure and in intracranial circulatory arrest. *J Neurosurg*. 1988;68:745–751.
133. Goraj B, Rifkinson-Mann S, Leslie DR, et al. Correlation of intracranial pressure and transcranial Doppler resistive index after head trauma. *AJNR Am J Neuroradiol*. 1994;15:1333–1339.
134. Newell DW, Grady MS, Sirotta P, Winn HR. Evaluation of brain death using transcranial Doppler. *Neurosurgery*. 1989;24:509–513.
135. Petty GW, Mohr JP, Pedley TA, et al. The role of transcranial Doppler in confirming brain death: sensitivity, specificity, and suggestions for performance and interpretation. *Neurology*. 1990;40:300–303.
136. Ducrocq X, Hassler W, Moritake K, et al. Consensus opinion on diagnosis of cerebral circulatory arrest using Doppler-sonography: task force group on cerebral death of the Neurosonology Research Group of the World Federation of Neurology. *J Neurol Sci*. 1998;159:145–150.
137. Hadani M, Bruk B, Ram Z, et al. Application of transcranial Doppler ultrasonography for the diagnosis of brain death. *Intensive Care Med*. 1999;25:822–828.
138. The Brain Trauma Foundation. The American Association of Neurological Surgeons. The Joint Section on Neurotrauma and Critical Care. Guidelines for cerebral perfusion pressure. *J Neurotrauma*. 2000;17:507–511.
139. Stocchetti N, Paparella A, Bridelli F, et al. Cerebral venous oxygen saturation studied with bilateral samples in the internal jugular veins. *Neurosurgery*. 1994;34:38–43; discussion 43–44.
140. Hatiboglu MT, Anil A. Structural variations in the jugular foramen of the human skull. *J Anat*. 1992;180(Pt 1):191–196.
141. Cruz J. The first decade of continuous monitoring of jugular bulb oxyhemoglobin saturation: management strategies and clinical outcome. *Crit Care Med*. 1998;26:344–351.
142. Gopinath SP, Valadka AB, Uzura M, Robertson CS. Comparison of jugular venous oxygen saturation and brain tissue PO_2 as monitors of cerebral ischemia after head injury. *Crit Care Med*. 1999;27:2337–2345.
143. Diaz-Reganon G, Minambres E, Holanda M, et al. Usefulness of venous oxygen saturation in the jugular bulb for the diagnosis of brain death: report of 118 patients. *Intensive Care Med*. 2002;28:1724–1728.
144. Shenkin GA, Harmel MH, Kety SS. Dynamic anatomy of the cerebral circulation. *Arch Neurol Psych*. 1948;60:12.
145. Matta BF, Lam AM. The rate of blood withdrawal affects the accuracy of jugular venous bulb. Oxygen saturation measurements. *Anesthesiology*. 1997;86:806–808.
146. Imberti R, Bellinzona G, Langer M. Cerebral tissue PO_2 and $SjvO_2$ changes during moderate hyperventilation in patients with severe traumatic brain injury. *J Neurosurg*. 2002;96:97–102.
147. Coles JP, Fryer TD, Coleman MR, et al. Hyperventilation following head injury: effect on ischemic burden and cerebral oxidative metabolism. *Crit Care Med*. 2007;35:568–578.
148. Kato T. Principle and technique of NIRS-Imaging for human brain FORCE: fast-oxygen response in capillary event. *Int Congress Series*. 2004;1270: 85–90.
149. Zauner A, Muizelaar JP. Measuring cerebral blood flow and metabolism. In: Reilly P, Bullock R, eds. *Head Injury*. London: Chapman & Hall; 1977:219–227.
150. Vernieri F, Tibuzzi F, Pasqualetti P, et al. Transcranial Doppler and near-infrared spectroscopy can evaluate the hemodynamic effect of carotid artery occlusion. *Stroke*. 2004;35:64–70.
151. Valadka AB, Furuya Y, Hlatky R, Robertson CS. Global and regional techniques for monitoring cerebral oxidative metabolism after severe traumatic brain injury. *Neurosurg Focus*. 2000;9:e3.
152. Manley GT, Hemphill JC, Morabito D, et al. Cerebral oxygenation during hemorrhagic shock: perils of hyperventilation and the therapeutic potential of hypoventilation. *J Trauma*. 2000;48:1025–1032; discussion 1032–1033.
153. Menzel M, Doppenberg EM, Zauner A, et al. Cerebral oxygenation in patients after severe head injury: monitoring and effects of arterial hyperoxia on cerebral blood flow, metabolism and intracranial pressure. *J Neurosurg Anesthesiol*. 1999;11:240–251.
154. Kirkman MA, Smith M. Intracranial pressure monitoring, cerebral perfusion pressure estimation, and ICP/CPP-guided therapy: a standard of care or optional extra after brain injury? *Br J Anesthesiol*. 2014;112:35–46.
155. Jaeger M, Schuhmann MU, Soehle M, et al. Continuous monitoring of cerebrovascular autoregulation after subarachnoid hemorrhage by brain tissue oxygen pressure reactivity and its relation to delayed cerebral infarction. *Stroke*. 2007;38:981–986.
156. Jaeger M, Schuhmann MU, Soehle M, Meixensberger J. Continuous assessment of cerebrovascular autoregulation after traumatic brain injury using brain tissue oxygen pressure reactivity. *Crit Care Med*. 2006;34: 1783–1788.
157. Bratton SL, Chestnut RM, Ghajar J, et al. Guidelines for the management of severe traumatic brain injury. X. Brain oxygen monitoring and thresholds. *J Neurotrauma*. 2007;24(Suppl 1):S65–S70.
158. van den Brink WA, van Santbrink H, Steyerberg EW, et al. Brain oxygen tension in severe head injury. *Neurosurgery*. 2000;46:868–876.
159. Nangunoori R, Maloney-Wilensky E, Stiefel M, et al. Brain tissue oxygen-based therapy and outcome after severe traumatic brain injury: a systematic literature review. *Neurocrit Care*. 2012;17:131–138.
160. Bardt TF, Unterberg AW, Hartl R, et al. Monitoring of brain tissue PO_2 in traumatic brain injury: effect of cerebral hypoxia on outcome. *Acta Neurochir Suppl*. 1998;71:153–156.
161. Valadka AB, Gopinath SP, Contant CF, et al. Relationship of brain tissue PO_2 to *outcome* after severe head injury. *Crit Care Med*. 1998; 26:1576–1581.
162. Giri BK, Krishnappa IK, Bryan RM Jr, et al. Regional cerebral blood flow after cortical impact injury complicated by a secondary insult in rats. *Stroke*. 2000;31:961–967.
163. Stiefel MF, Spiotta A, Gracias VH, et al. Reduced mortality rate in patients with severe traumatic brain injury treated with brain tissue oxygen monitoring. *J Neurosurg*. 2005;103:805–811.
164. Hillered L, Vespa PM, Hovda DA. Translational neurochemical research in acute human brain injury: the current status and potential future for cerebral microdialysis. *J Neurotrauma*. 2005;22:3–41.
165. Hillered L, Persson L, Nilsson P, et al. Continuous monitoring of cerebral metabolism in traumatic brain injury: a focus on cerebral microdialysis. *Curr Opin Crit Care*. 2006;12:112–118.
166. Zauner A, Bullock R. The role of excitatory amino acids in severe brain trauma: opportunities for therapy: a review. *J Neurotrauma*. 1995;12: 547–554.
167. Maurer MH, Berger C, Wolf M, et al. The proteome of human brain microdialysate. *Proteome Sci*. 2003;1:7.
168. Firlik AD, Rubin G, Yonas H, Wechsler LR. Relation between cerebral blood flow and neurologic deficit resolution in acute ischemic stroke. *Neurology*. 1998;51:177–182.

CHAPTER 29

Radiographic Imaging and Bedside Ultrasound

NUPUR VERMA and TAN-LUCIEN H. MOHAMMED

Imaging in the intensive care unit (ICU) plays an important and ever growing role in the diagnosis, management, and monitoring of critically ill patients. Portable technologies, such as radiography and ultrasound (US), are especially important in providing point of care imaging and guiding medical and surgical management. Image-guided procedures, with US, also assist in the care of these patients, allowing for confident placement of drainage catheters or stents, or guide sampling.

The portability of these modalities is especially appreciated in the ICU setting, where the patient is in need of continuous high level clinical monitoring and interventions, which often includes ventilator support. Imaging at the bedside allows the patient's clinical status to be further assessed while keeping them in the environment which best and most safely meets their medical needs.

RADIOGRAPHY

Portable chest radiographs are the most common radiologic examination performed in the ICU. Radiography of the ventilated patient is most often used to monitor cardiopulmonary status and position of catheters and tubes. Potential diagnoses which can be assessed include pulmonary edema, pneumonia, lobar collapse, and pneumothorax. Evaluation of the heart size, such as for sudden change in the setting of quick accumulating fluid with risk for tamponade, is also an advantage. Evaluation of support lines and devices may include evaluation for the placement of these devices, assessment of their function (e.g., effectiveness in draining pleural fluid), or to observe for change in their position compared to previous examinations. Current recommendations suggest performance of chest radiography for patient at admission or transfer, and when there is a clinical indication (1). Routine daily radiography of the ICU patient is not recommended without indication or change in status. However, given the critical nature of these patients and constant change in management, it is not uncommon for chest radiographs to be obtained frequently during the course of a patient's stay.

When compared to the alert, upright, outpatient examination, the portable anterior–posterior (AP) chest radiograph taken of the critically ill patient in the ICU has several limiting factors. These include technical factors such as lack of automatic exposure control which leads to less than optimal penetration, diminished distance from tube to the chest structures resulting in distorting enlargement, and lack of filters to reduce scatter (2). Additional patient factors such as poor inspiration, superimposition of structures, patient rotation and neck flexion, and overlying bedding and monitors often further limit the portable bedside radiograph. Familiarity with the appearance of these studies is important to avoid overdiagnosis and to effectively monitor for change with serial images.

Atelectasis

Areas of atelectasis or collapsed lung are not uncommon in the critically ill patient, especially those who are ventilated or have pleural effusions. Collapsed lung will be radiopaque (white) on radiography and is characterized by volume loss. The latter helps to differentiate it from pleural fluid or pneumonia which is space occupying. Radiographic patterns of lobar collapse are characteristic and include right upper lobe collapse, demonstrating the S-sign of Golden (Fig. 29.1). The most common etiology for atelectasis in the inpatient setting is mucus plugging or malpositioned endotracheal tube, the latter most often into the right mainstem bronchus (Fig. 29.2) (3). Complete atelectasis of a lobe due to aberrant positioning of the endotracheal tube or to a mucus plug in the right or left mainstem bronchus may lead to complete opacification of a lobe; the presence of mediastinal shift can assist in identifying volume loss and help differentiate it from complete thoracic opacification related to a large effusion (Fig. 29.3) (3).

Pleural Effusions

Pleural effusions are frequently seen in the setting of cardiogenic or noncardiogenic edema and can also relate to underlying pulmonary infection, volume resuscitation, or systemic illnesses or inflation. Effusions which are large but do not completely fill the chest will result in a gradient veil-like opacity, more opaque in the dependent chest in the supine patient, with blunting of the costophrenic angles (Fig. 29.4) (3). Additional signs include obscuration of the diaphragm border and lack of volume loss with contralateral mediastinal shift (see Fig. 29.3). Inclining the patient in their bed during radiography as much as 15 to 20 degrees or obtaining dependent positing of suspected hemithorax–decubitus chest radiographs—may aid in the diagnosis.

Alveolar Opacification

Infection is a particularly common cause of alveolar opacification in the intubated patient, with one in four patients having infection during an episode of respiratory failure (3). Infection or aspiration may result in a region of airspace opacification in the lung with air bronchograms (Fig. 29.5). The dependent positioning can suggest aspiration as the likely etiology in the high-risk patient, including those with altered mental status prior to intubation or had recent cerebrovascular accident. Diagnosing alveolar opacification as infection is, however, difficult due to the low specificity of its appearance (4). Multifocal alveolar opacification can also be seen in acute respiratory distress syndrome (ARDS), which manifests as less focal and more diffuse opacities in a ventilator dependent patient (Fig. 29.6) (4).

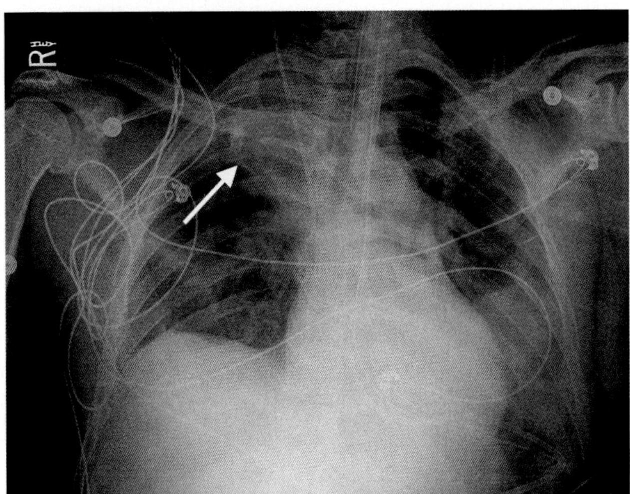

FIGURE 29.1 Patient with right upper lobe collapse and associated S-sign of Golden as demonstrated by the reverse S shape at the inferolateral border of the right upper lobe (*arrow*).

However, ARDS also can be difficult to differentiate from extensive infection or from volume overload, and the diagnosis is often facilitated by excluding failure related to volume overload or cardiac cause, and by decreased PaO_2/FiO_2 ratio (4). Potential etiologies include sepsis, inhalation of harmful substances such as chemical fumes, or pancreatitis.

Pulmonary Edema

Massive fluid resuscitation, burns, opiate overdose, cardiac or traumatic brain injury and a multitude of other etiologies can result in volume overload in the ICU patient. The most common pattern is a "batwing" appearance of perihilar airspace opacification, with bilateral pleural effusions (Fig. 29.7). Patients with cardiogenic pulmonary edema secondary to heart failure often have accompanying enlargement of the heart chambers or stigmata of recent or prior cardiac event or surgery. Diffuse bilateral parenchymal opacification may also be seen in alveolar edema (3). Cardiovascular status of the patient, clinical history, and volume status are helpful in differentiating edema from infection or ARDS.

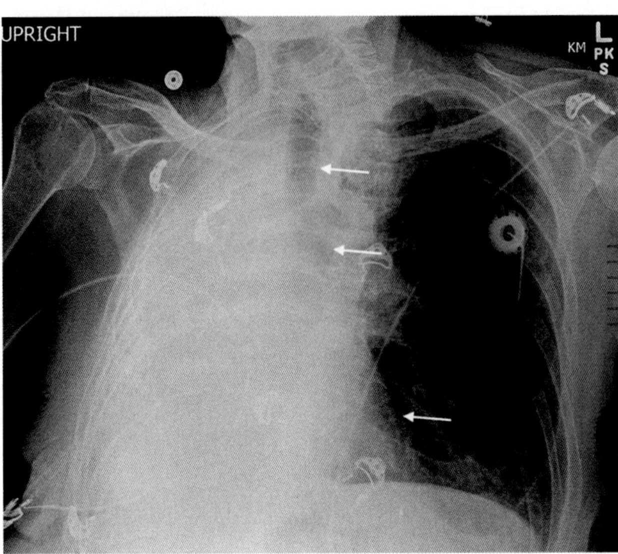

FIGURE 29.3 Patient with complete opacification of the right hemithorax. There is ipsilateral mediastinal shift as would be expected with atelectasis (*arrows*).

Pneumothorax

The critically ill patient is most often in the recumbent position, which can make the recognition of a pneumothorax

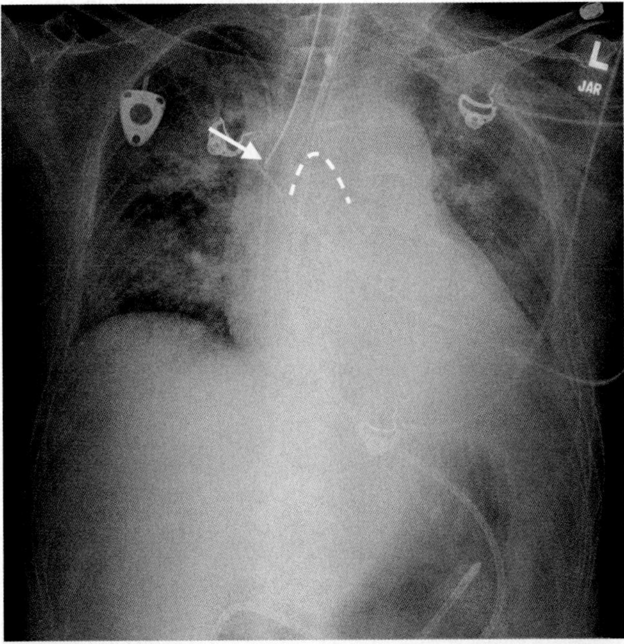

FIGURE 29.2 Placement of the endotracheal tube into the right mainstem bronchus (*arrow*), a not uncommon complication secondary to the more vertical orientation of the right main bronchus as compared to the left (carina; *dashed line*). There is associated atelectasis of the left lung and slight leftward cardiomediastinal shift.

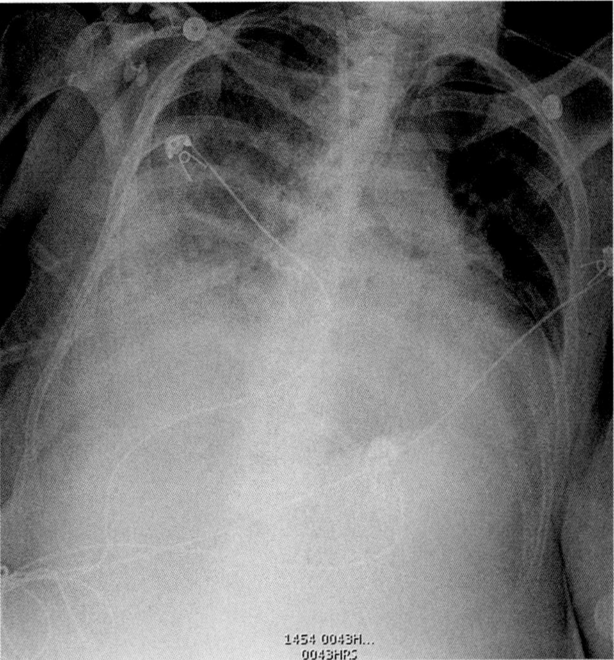

FIGURE 29.4 Right greater than left bilateral pleural effusions in a supine patient on portable anterior–posterior examination shows blunting of the costophrenic angles and obscuration of the hemidiaphragms.

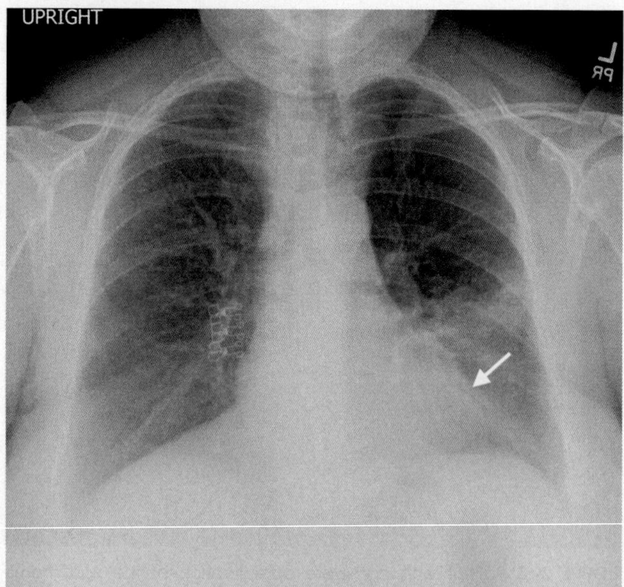

FIGURE 29.5 Airspace opacity with branching linear lucencies represents outlining of bronchi by surrounding alveolar consolidation and air bronchograms (*arrow*). Findings are concerning for lobar pneumonia in the right middle lobe.

difficult. A pneumothorax in the recumbent position may collect anteriorly, at the lung base, leading to the deep sulcus sign. The *deep sulcus sign* is the lucency at the lung base caused by air trapped in the most anterior portion of the pleural space in a recumbent patient (Fig. 29.8). Careful interrogation of a radiograph can also show the more easily recognized pleural reflection separate from the lateral thorax margin (Fig. 29.9). Pneumothorax in the ICU is often a complication of barotrauma, vascular access, or pleural drainage (5).

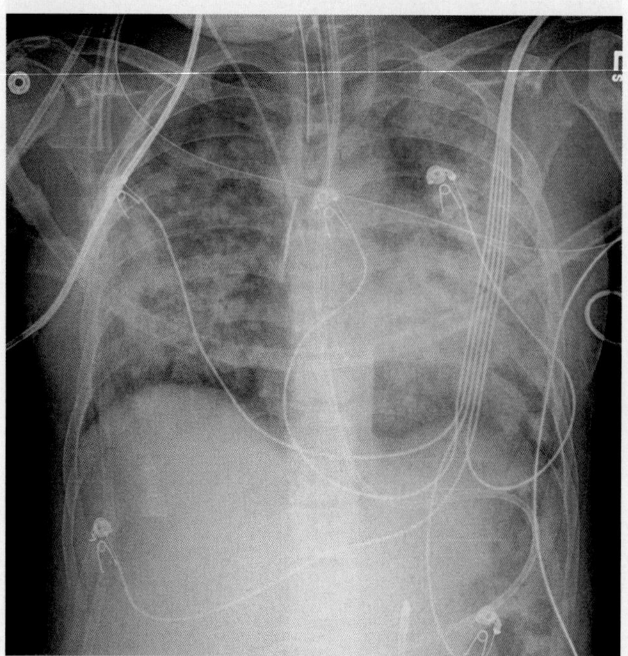

FIGURE 29.6 Intubated patient indicating respiratory failure. There are diffuse airspace opacities such as can be seen in the setting of adult respiratory distress syndrome.

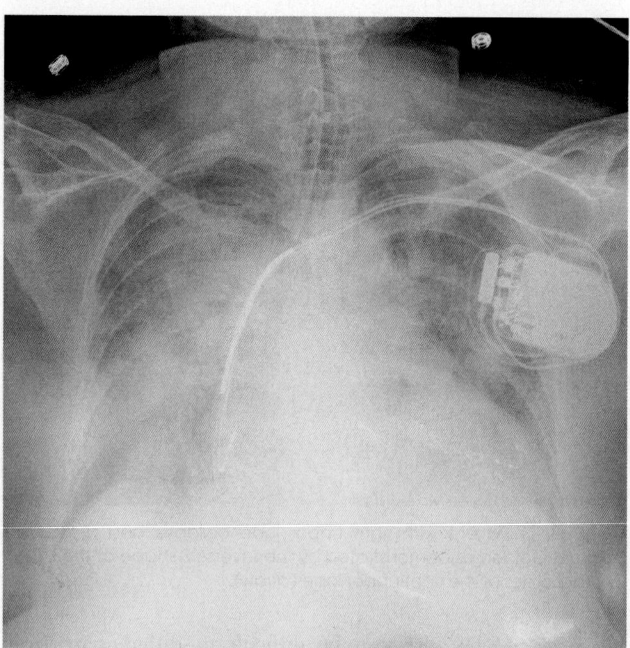

FIGURE 29.7 Batwing or perihilar opacities in a patient with cardiomegaly and bilateral pleural effusions; the latter is indicated by blunting of the costophrenic angles. This finding indicates pulmonary edema.

Support Lines and Tubes

The critical status of the ICU patient often requires the use of multiple support lines and tubes to monitor and administer therapy. Appropriate positioning after initial positioning should be performed with chest radiography to verify appropriate placement and to exclude complications such as atelectasis, pneumothorax, or hematoma.

Endotracheal Tube

The endotracheal tube (ET), is preferably located in the trachea 2 to 4 cm above the carina or projecting at the level of the clavicular heads (Fig. 29.10) (3,6). An ET that has been advanced too far caudally into the airway may enter one of the

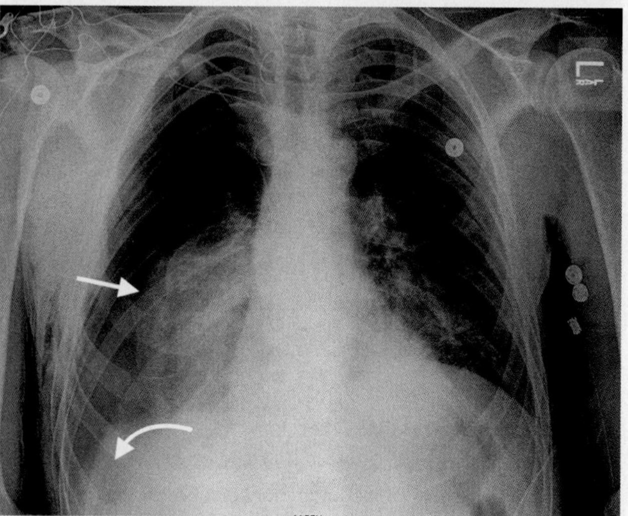

FIGURE 29.8 Chest radiograph demonstrates right basilar pneumothorax with deep sulcus sign (*curved arrow*). Note the large medially displayed right lower lung opacity caused by pneumonia (*straight arrow*).

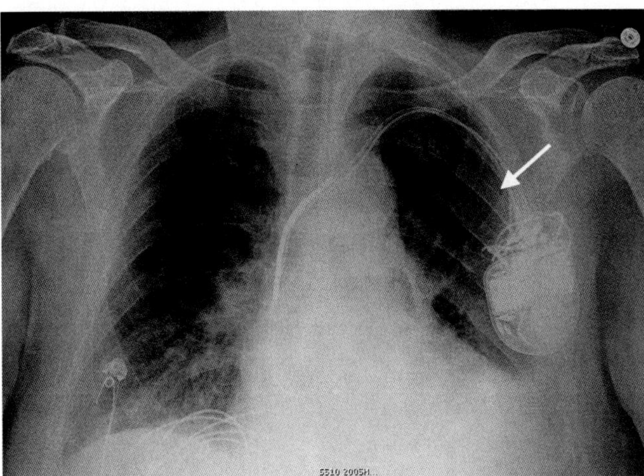

FIGURE 29.9 Subtle pneumothorax after left-sided thoracentesis (*arrow*). Note the thin radiodense pleural reflection.

two main bronchi and result in lobar collapse and atelectasis of the contralateral lobe (see Fig. 29.2).

Central Catheter Placement

Central venous catheters used for fluid, antibiotic administration, or parenteral nutrition can be placed into the subclavian or jugular veins with its tip most preferably projecting into the superior vena cava (SVC). Catheters that are advanced too far into the right heart or even into the inferior vena cava should be retracted, leaving the tip in the SVC. Some central venous access catheters, notably dialysis catheters, are designed to terminate in the right heart (7). The apex of the lung is in close proximity to the puncture site for a subclavian approach and thus is at risk for a pneumothorax. A peripherally inserted central catheter (PICC) is a long intravenous catheter usually advanced from a peripheral upper extremity vein with optimal positioning of its tip in the SVC (Fig. 29.11).

A pulmonary artery catheter (PAC) is usually placed via an introducer into the subclavian or jugular vein and advanced into either the right (most commonly) or left pulmonary artery to facilitate its use as a monitor of cardiac function. The PAC ideally should be positioned in the proximal right or left

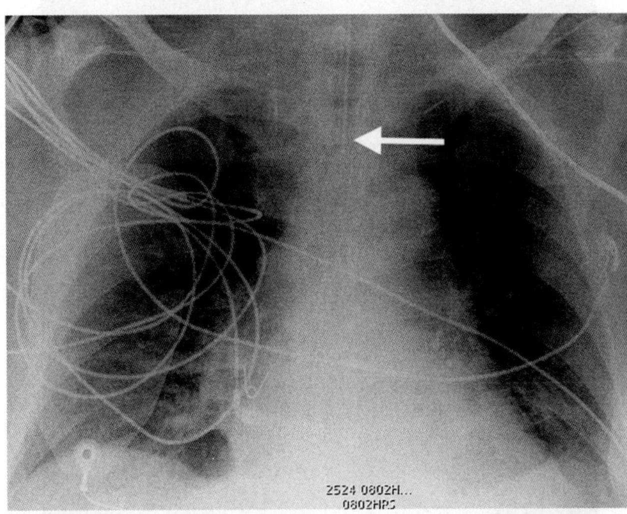

FIGURE 29.10 Satisfactory position of endotracheal tube, which terminates above the carina (*arrow*). This position is satisfactory for adequate ventilation to both lungs.

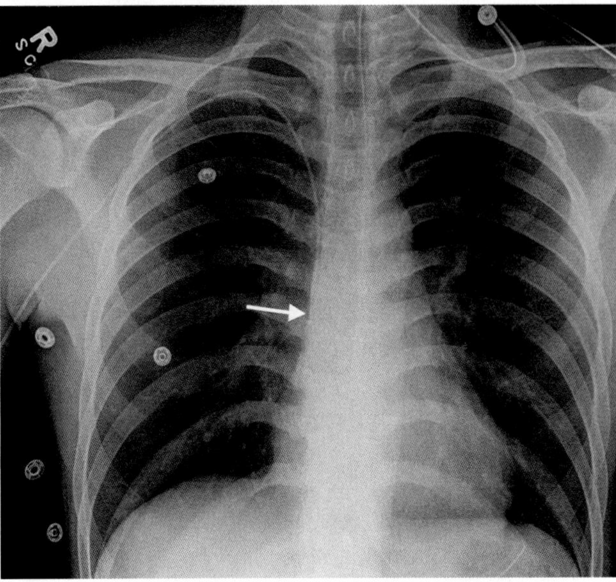

FIGURE 29.11 Right peripherally inserted central catheter terminates in the superior vena cava (*arrow*). Note the long course of the thin caliber catheter as it extends from the patient's right upper extremity centrally.

pulmonary artery (Fig. 29.12) (3). If the catheter is advanced too far distally, the balloon tip can cause pulmonary infarction. If placed too proximal, as in the right ventricle, the PAC could trigger dysrhythmias and result in potential inaccurate measurements (8).

Feeding Tube Placement

Feeding tube placement should always be subdiaphragmatic. The most optimal location is for the feeding tube's tip to extend into the proximal jejunum, as this best reduces the risk of reflux. If the position is ambiguous it can be confirmed by injection of a small amount of contrast and reimaging at bedside prior to use (Fig. 29.13). Nasogastric or orogastric (NG or OG)

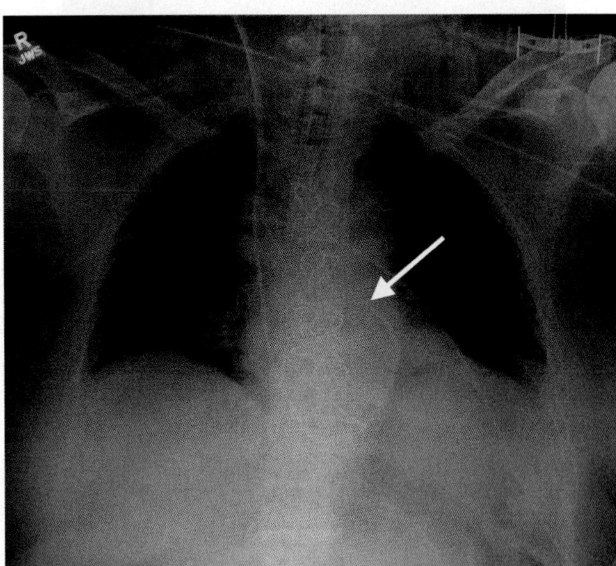

FIGURE 29.12 Pulmonary arterial catheter is present making a characteristic curve as it goes through the right atrium, right ventricle, pulmonary arterial outflow tract, and main pulmonary artery to terminate in the proximal right pulmonary artery (*arrow*).

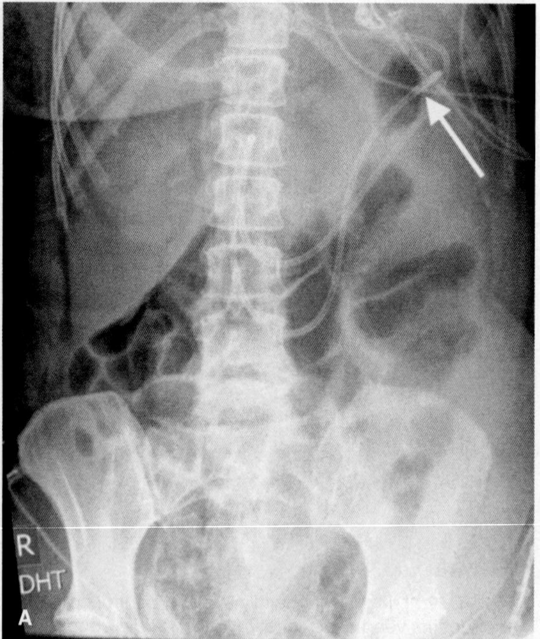

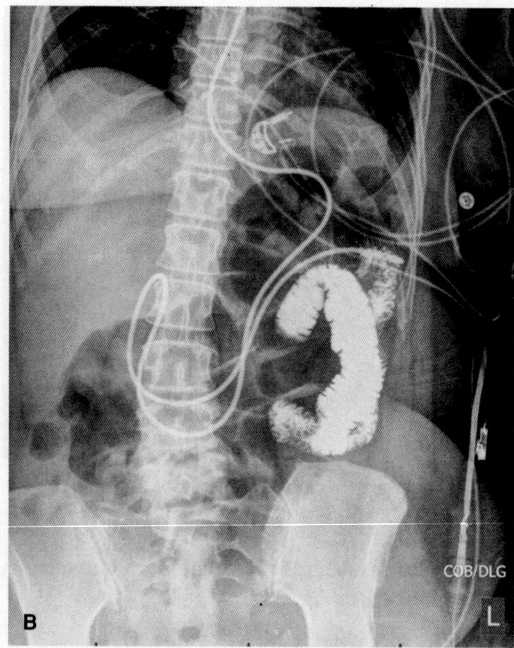

FIGURE 29.13 A: Feeding tube curved in the midabdomen, making it difficult to determine whether placement is postpyloric or curved on itself and terminating in the stomach (*arrow*). B: Subsequent bedside injection of a small volume of contrast shows feeding tube tip is in the small bowel, confirming postpyloric placement past the ligament of Treitz.

tubes are used for gastric decompression, administration of oral medications, and gastric pH monitoring. Most NG or OG tubes have a radiopaque stripe marking the length of the tube, with a side hole as a break in the marker. This side hole should be below the diaphragm to ensure that the tube resides in the stomach and thereby assists in decompression (Fig. 29.14) (3).

In patients with neurologic injuries, or in heavily medicated patients, the inability to protect their airway may lead to cannulation of the bronchus with the feeding tube, with the right lower lobe bronchus more often cannulated by the enteric tube because of its relatively straight course from the mouth (Fig. 29.15). Feeding tube malposition must be recognized to avoid the administering feeds into the lung (9).

Pneumoperitoneum

Portable radiography can allow the detection of free air in a patient suspected of having hollow visceral perforation. This may be seen in bowel ischemia, ulceration and perforation, or as an expected finding in the setting of recent surgery. In

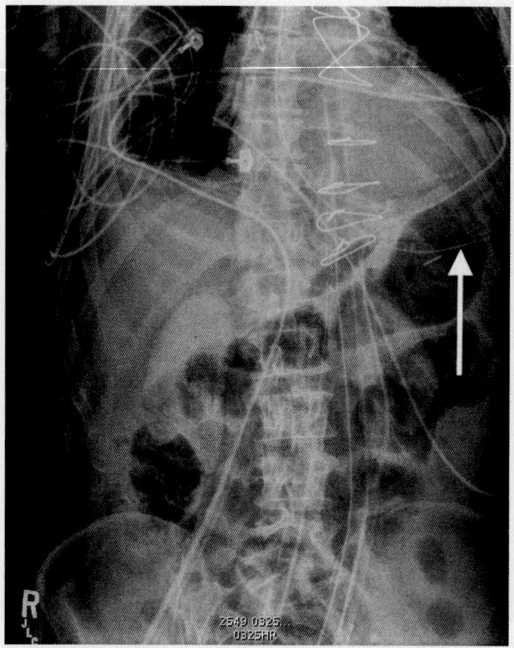

FIGURE 29.14 Nasogastric tube with side port and tip in the stomach (*arrow*). The number of drains and overlying electrodes make identification of the tube difficult in this critically ill patient.

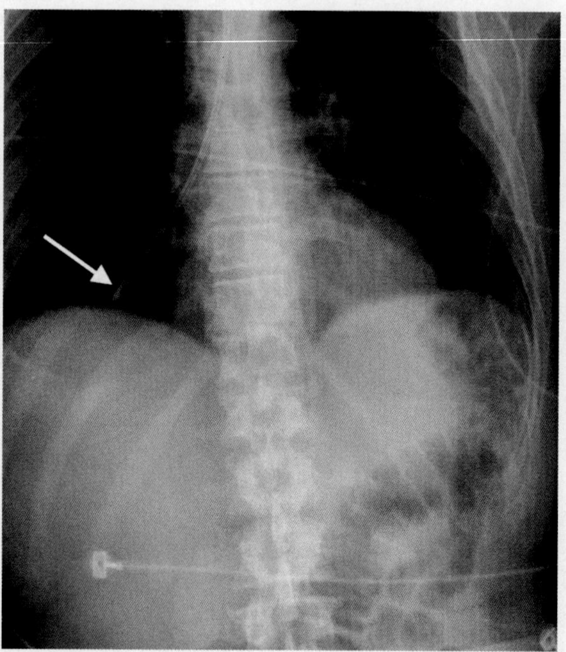

FIGURE 29.15 Feeding tube within the left mainstem bronchus (*arrow*). Inadvertent feeding of the patient will lead to infection (pneumonia).

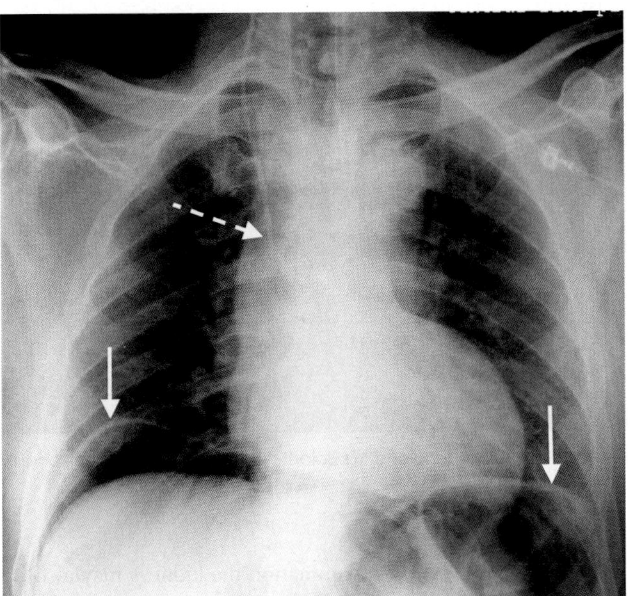

FIGURE 29.16 Pneumoperitoneum as seen by the radiolucency under the hemidiaphragm (*solid arrows*). This was identified on chest radiography and is often missed unless there is careful attention to interrogate the entire image. Right internal jugular catheter is in good position (*dashed arrow*).

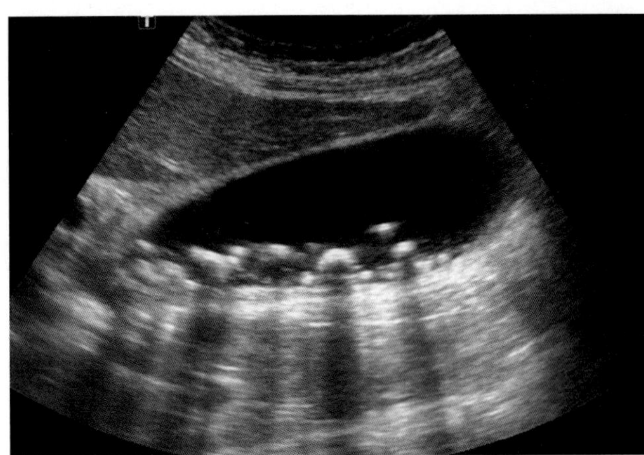

FIGURE 29.17 Multiple echogenic stones are present with stones in the gallbladder neck. There is no wall thickening or pericholecystic fluid to suggest acute cholecystitis in an ICU patient with fever.

the supine patient, a small volume of free air can be missed on radiography but a moderate to larger amount can be seen nondependently in the central abdomen or outlining bowel loops (10). Having the patient semiupright may be an option and can better show free air under the diaphragm (Fig. 29.16) (10). Other findings of the causative etiology, such as in bowel ischemia pneumatosis or portal vein gas, may also be seen.

ULTRASOUND IMAGING

US, because of its portability, lends itself to ease of use in the critically ill ICU patients. With its excellent soft tissue detail it is most commonly used to evaluate the liver, gallbladder, kidneys, bladder, and vasculature. Though, increasingly over the past two decades, it is playing a larger role in imaging of the chest. US can allow for diagnosis and follow-up for pneumothorax, pleural effusions, and also consolidation.

Cholecystitis

Acute cholecystitis in the ICU patient is not infrequent and often acalculous (11). US allows for portable imaging of these patients, with the sensitive US finding in acute cholecystitis being a distended, sludge or a stone-filled gallbladder with positive sonographic Murphy sign (Fig. 29.17); additional sonographic findings include wall thickening and pericholecystic fluid (Fig. 29.18A). Of note, the most sensitive examination finding of positive Murphy sign is often not able to be assessed in the ICU patients (11). In this case the consideration for diagnosis should be based on the additional findings and pretest probability. HIDA scan (Fig. 29.18B) may be used for further evaluation but requires moving the patient and is a lengthy examination, which may be problematic in the patient who needs close monitoring.

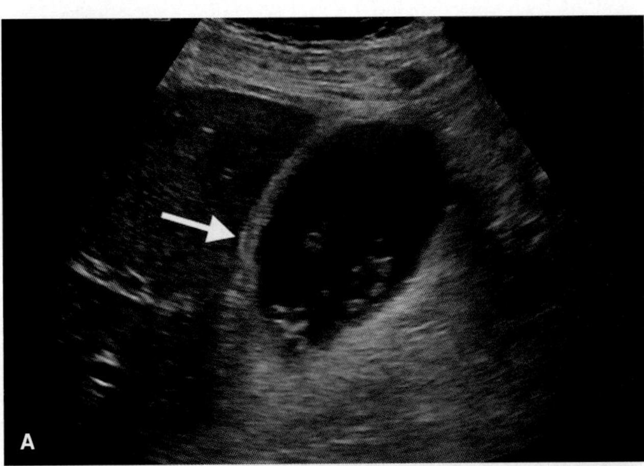

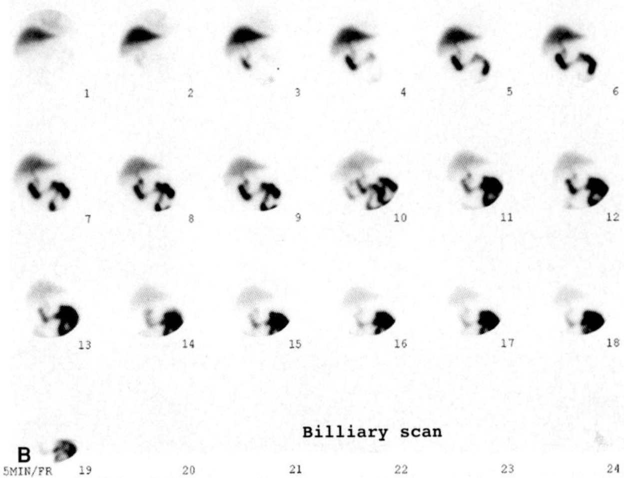

FIGURE 29.18 A: Multiple echogenic stones are present in the gallbladder with gallbladder wall thickening (*arrow*) in an ICU patient with hyperbilirubinemia and fever. Patient was subsequently diagnosed with acute cholecystitis. B: HIDA scan shows nonvisualization of the gallbladder which indicates obstruction of the cystic duct.

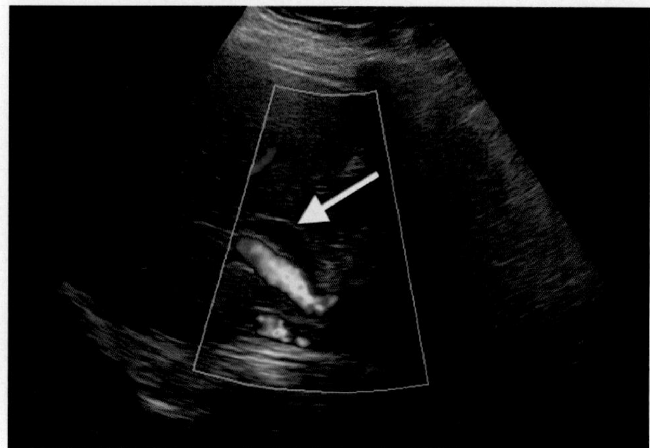

FIGURE 29.19 Ultrasound images shows dilated common bile duct (CBD; *arrow*) in a patient with distal CBD obstruction.

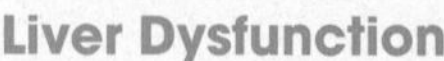

Liver Dysfunction

Liver dysfunction may be present in the ICU patient due to several factors, including shock, respiratory and metabolic disorders, chronic underlying liver disease or hepatitis, or therapy related (medication, transfusion, and total parenteral nutrition) (12). US may show increased hepatic echogenicity but predominately plays a role in excluding extrahepatic obstruction, from sludge or stones, as a cause for jaundice (Fig. 29.19).

Renal Failure or Obstruction

Renal failure may be due to any factor that increases patient's creatine, including medications, shock, or dehydration. This can be seen on sonography as increased echogenicity of the kidneys or increased corticomedullary differentiation (Fig. 29.20) (13).

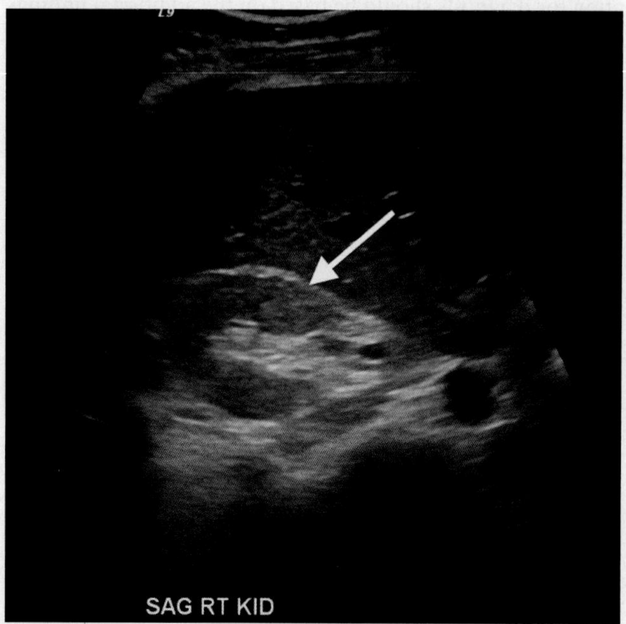

FIGURE 29.20 Ultrasound of a patient with declining renal function shows diffuse increased echogenicity of the kidney (*arrow*). This finding can be seen in acute renal failure. Comparison of renal echogenicity to the liver can be helpful in making this diagnosis.

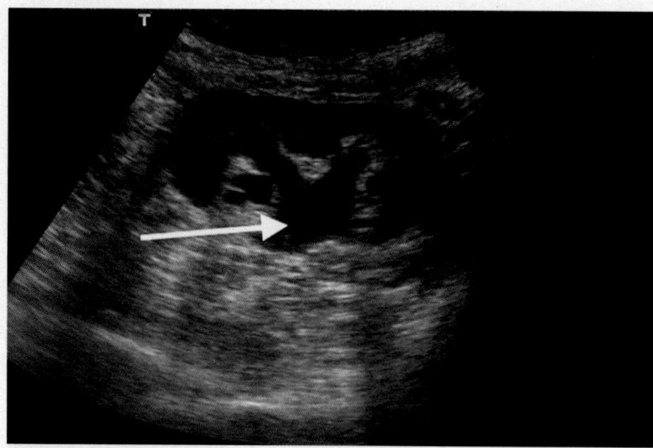

FIGURE 29.21 Ultrasound of a transplanted kidney shows hydronephrosis (*arrow*).

In infectious or systemic inflammation the kidneys may also be increased in size.

Renal obstruction may be due to clot or blood products or passage of a calculus (Fig. 29.21). It may also be due to intrinsic compression of the ureter from hematoma, nodes, or mass. Sonography can demonstrate hydronephrosis and its potential etiology, and also assist with placement of percutaneous drainage catheter. In the patient with decreased urine output, US of the bladder can confirm position of the Foley catheter and evaluate for debris or clot.

Pleural Effusions, Pericardial Effusions, and Ascites

US is well suited to image fluid, including fluid collections posttransplant or postoperatively, and free fluid in the chest or abdomen (14). The echogenicity of the fluid can help determine its complexity and US can also visualize septation or loculations that may make drainage difficult (Fig. 29.22). Pleural fluid and ascites can be drained with the aid of US guidance (14). This allows for a safer procedure while monitoring the amount of volume removed. Drainage catheters can also be placed for fluid or fluid collections with US assistance to help observe and document most optimal placement.

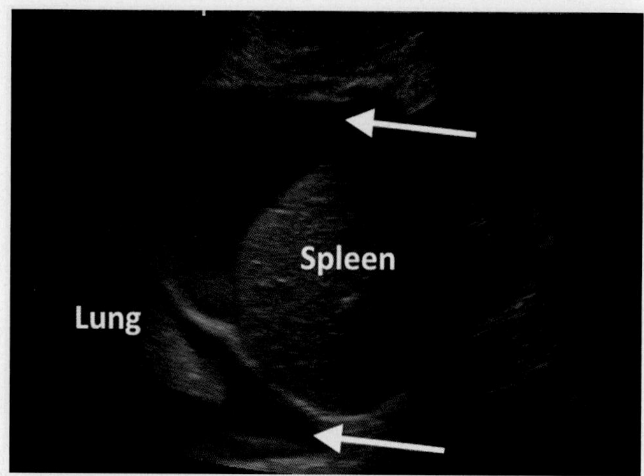

FIGURE 29.22 Ultrasound shows ascites surrounding the spleen as well as a left pleural effusion (*arrows*).

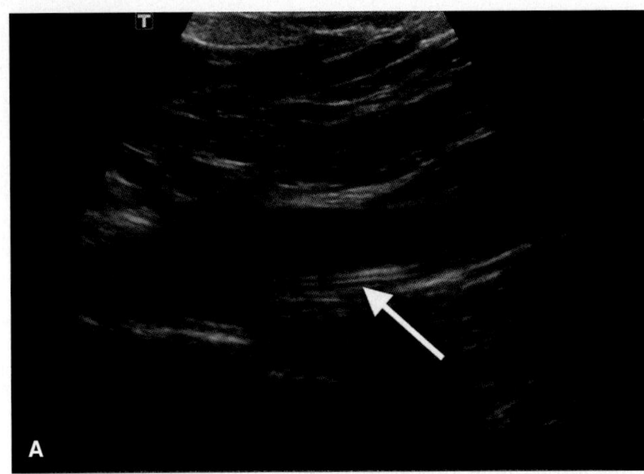

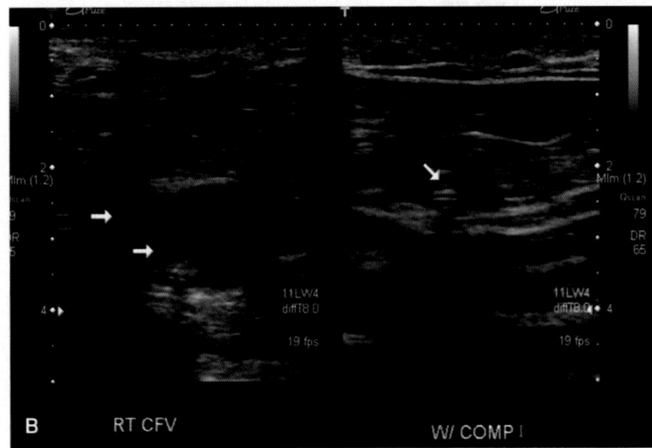

FIGURE 29.23 A: Deep venous thrombosis around a right femoral venous catheter is seen as echogenic clot (*arrow*). B: On compression image, there is incomplete compressibility of the vessel at the level of the nonocclusive thrombus (*arrows*).

Venous Thrombosis

Deep venous thrombosis (DVT) may be present in the ICU patient despite routine prophylaxis, given their multiple risk factors, along with the inciting nidus of indwelling catheters (15). Most DVTs are seen in the lower extremity and sonographic findings include visualization of echogenic thrombus in the vessel, incomplete venous compressibility, change in diameter of the vein, absent color Doppler flow, loss of spectral variability with Valsalva, or calf augmentation (Fig. 29.23) (16).

Key Points

- Imaging plays a key role in the management of the ICU patient and can help aid in diagnosis, guide management, and assist in performing procedures more proficiently and safely.
- Bedside radiography is the most common imaging for the ICU patient and should be used when there is admission or transfer, placement of a new support line or tube, or any change in clinical status of the patient.
- Ultrasonography allows for portable evaluation of the patient, while allowing them to remain on their ward. It can also be helpful in performing drainage procedures and placing drainage catheters.
- ICU patients are at increased risk for pulmonary infections, volume overload, hepatobiliary dysfunction, and DVT. Radiography and US at the bedside can assist in making these diagnoses.

References

1. Amorosa JK, Bramwit MP, Mohammed TL, et al. ACR appropriateness criteria routine chest radiographs in intensive care unit patients. *J Am Coll Radiol*. 2013;10:170–174.
2. Wandtke JC. Bedside chest radiography. *Radiology*. 1994;190:1–10.
3. Rubinowitz AN, Siegel MD, Tocino I. Thoracic imaging in the ICU. *Crit Care Clin*. 2007;23:539–573.
4. Winer-Muram HT, Rubin SA, Ellis JV, et al. Pneumonia and ARDS in patients receiving mechanical ventilation: diagnostic accuracy of chest radiography. *Radiology*. 1993;188:479–485.
5. Ding W, Shen Y, Yang J, et al. Diagnosis of pneumothorax by radiography and ultrasonography: a meta-analysis. *Chest J*. 2011;140:859–866.
6. Aronchick JM, Miller WT. Tubes and lines in the intensive care setting. *Semin Roentgenol*. 1987;32:102–116.
7. Vesely TM. Central venous catheter tip position: a continuing controversy. *J Vasc Interv Radiol*. 2003;14:527–534.
8. Elliott CG, Zimmerman GA, Clemmer TP. Complications of pulmonary artery catheterization in the care of critically ill patients: a prospective study. *Chest J*. 1979;76(6):647–652.
9. Kawati R, Rubertsson S. Malpositioning of fine bore feeding tube: a serious complication. *Acta Anaesthesiol Scand*. 2005;49:58–61.
10. Levine MS, Scheiner JD, Rubesin SE, et al. Diagnosis of pneumoperitoneum on supine abdominal radiographs. *AJR Am J Roentgenol*. 1991;156:731–735.
11. Molenat F, Boussuges A, Valantin V, Sainty JM. Gallbladder abnormalities in medical ICU patients: an ultrasonographic study. *Intensive Care Med*. 1996;22:356–358.
12. Hawker F. Liver dysfunction in critical illness. *Anaesth Intensive Care*. 1991;19:165–181.
13. Huntington DK, Hill SC, Hill MC. Sonographic manifestations of medical renal disease. *Semin Ultrasound CT MR*. 1991;12:290–307.
14. Goldberg BB, Goodman GA, Clearfield HR. Evaluation of ascites by ultrasound 1. *Radiology*. 1970;96:15–22.
15. Marik PE, Andrews L, Maini B. The incidence of deep venous thrombosis in ICU patients. *Chest J*. 1997;111:661–664.
16. Appelman PT, De Jong TE, Lampmann LE. Deep venous thrombosis of the leg: US findings. *Radiology*. 1987;163:743–746.

CHAPTER

30

Neuroimaging

JEFFREY A. BENNETT and ERIK H. MIDDLEBROOKS

INTRODUCTION

Appropriate care of the critically ill patient depends on rapid, accurate diagnosis. In critically ill patients, the frequent inability to obtain history or accurate physical assessment results in increasing dependence on neuroimaging. Modern computed tomography (CT) and magnetic resonance imaging (MRI) technology allow rapid assessment of the central nervous system (CNS) and can include or exclude life-threatening conditions with a high degree of confidence.

The availability of high-resolution imaging techniques allows CT and MRI images to be reformatted in any plane, enabling a more complete evaluation of fractures and soft tissue abnormalities. Contrast-enhanced CT angiograms provide accurate assessment of vascular abnormalities, and can frequently replace more invasive catheter-based cerebral angiograms. Three-dimensional images can be constructed from CT angiogram, which can be rotated to match what will be seen from a surgical approach. Anatomic imaging can also be supplemented with physiologic data obtained with CT, MRI, and nuclear medicine. This provides information about phenomena such as cerebral blood flow (CBF) and brain perfusion, cerebrospinal fluid (CSF) flow, or the rate and direction of diffusion of water in soft tissues. This type of data can clarify diagnoses such as brain infarction or abscesses, and can be used to investigate the effects of hydrocephalus, vasospasm, and brain herniation. The images also provide valuable prognostic information.

A wide range of pathophysiology exists in the CNS. The sensitivity and specificity of imaging for most CNS abnormalities is largely determined by selection of the most appropriate imaging parameters. Decisions such as choice of administered contrast agents, timing of the contrast administration, specific MRI sequences, and field-of-view can all have a major impact on the ability to detect an abnormality. If the imaging modality and protocol are not optimized for the clinical question, the likelihood of answering the clinical question will likely decrease.

The accurate interpretation of the images obtained then depends on a thorough knowledge of anatomy, normal anatomic variations, and pathophysiology. A basic knowledge of medical physics is also required to understand the imaging characteristics of both normal and abnormal tissues. Excellent communication between the radiologist and clinician is essential, as all radiologic studies must be interpreted in clinical context. It should be kept in mind that the hardest thing for the radiologist to do in real-time practice is to label a study as *normal* with great confidence. The consequences of incorrectly classifying a study as normal could obviously be very grave.

Excluding pathology with a high degree of confidence requires a great deal of training and is beyond the scope of this chapter; however, this section will serve as an introduction to the use of both standard and advanced imaging techniques as applied to the critically ill patient. The focus is on classic critical imaging findings of the brain and spine.

HERNIATION SYNDROMES

Many intracranial processes require immediate treatment to preserve brain function, and the urgency of any radiologic finding depends largely on the mass effect on normal neural tissue. This assessment must be made for all of the lesions subsequently described, and therefore is discussed first.

Pathophysiology

Intracranial pressure is determined by a delicate balance between neural tissue, intracranial blood volume, and CSF volume. Any space-occupying abnormality, such as a hematoma, tumor, or edema, adds volume to this confined space and increases pressure. Once the body's capacity to deal with this change in pressure is overcome, intracranial structures start to become displaced. Initially, sulci in the region of the abnormality become compressed. With increasing mass effect, brain herniation occurs. Brain herniation typically follows characteristic and predictable patterns, the most common of which are discussed in the following sections.

Diagnosis

Subfalcine Herniation

Subfalcine herniation refers to brain (typically the cingulate gyrus) being shifted across the midline underneath the falx cerebri (Fig. 30.1). Herniation below the falx cerebri tends to occur more anteriorly initially, as the falx cerebri is broader and more closely apposed to the corpus callosum when moving posteriorly.

Potential consequences of subfalcine herniation include compression of the anterior cerebral artery (ACA) or internal cerebral veins against the dura, which can result in brain infarction. Additionally, mass effect can cause compression of the ipsilateral lateral ventricle which can progress to obstruct the foramen of Monro. At this point, the contralateral lateral ventricle can become obstructed resulting in hydrocephalus. This is commonly referred to as "entrapment."

Transtentorial Herniation

Transtentorial herniation is the result of upward or downward displacement of brain structures through the incisura, which is an opening in the dura through which the brainstem passes. The plane of the incisura can be approximated on midline sagittal images by drawing a line from the dorsum sella to the junction of the vein of Galen and straight sinus (Fig. 30.2A). This line should normally bisect the interpeduncular fossa and tectum; the splenium of the corpus callosum should lie above this line.

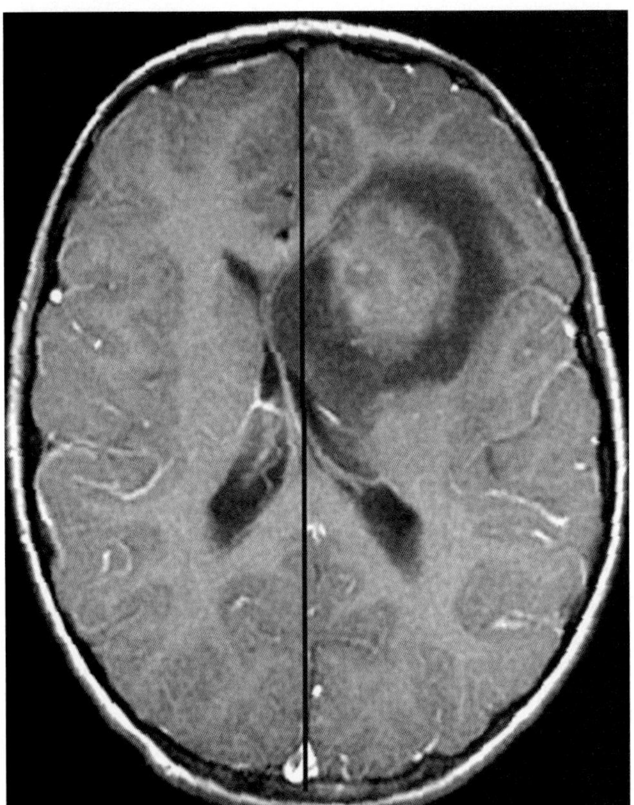

FIGURE 30.1 Postcontrast axial T1-weighted MRI. A large left frontal mass results in subfalcine herniation with shift of the ventricles and septum pellucidum to the right across midline (*black line*).

When there is downward transtentorial herniation from a supratentorial mass, the optic chiasm will be displaced toward the sella, the interpeduncular fossa will be compressed, the brainstem will appear buckled, and the splenium of the corpus callosum will lie below the plane of the incisura (Fig. 30.2B). There is resultant displacement of the midbrain and thalamus caudally.

When there is upward transtentorial herniation, usually from a cerebellar mass, the brainstem will be compressed against the clivus, the fourth ventricle will be compressed, and brainstem structures will become superiorly displaced with respect to the plane of the incisura.

On axial images, transtentorial herniation can be assessed by evaluating the circummesencephalic cisterns. With downward transtentorial herniation, the ambient cisterns and suprasellar cistern will become effaced (Fig. 30.3). When there is upward transtentorial herniation, the quadrigeminal plate cistern becomes effaced (Fig. 30.4).

Major complications of transtentorial herniation include vascular complications, hydrocephalus, and/or hemorrhage. Infarction in both the anterior and posterior circulation can occur from compression of major arteries against the dura. Hydrocephalus affecting the third and lateral ventricles can occur from obstruction of the aqueduct of Sylvius. A more portentous sign is the presence of midbrain and pontine hemorrhages referred to as *Duret hemorrhages*. These hemorrhages are typically the effect of reperfusion injury in vessels which were previously compressed and occluded by the mass effect.

Uncal Herniation

A specific subset of downward transtentorial herniation is herniation of the medial temporal lobe, specifically the uncus. This is usually the result of a medially directed vector from a middle cranial fossa lesion as opposed to the more downward-directed vector of traditional downward transtentorial herniation. Uncal herniation can be identified by displacement of the mesial portion of the temporal lobe, or the uncus, into the suprasellar cistern, causing effacement of the crural cistern.

As a result of its position medial to the uncus, the oculomotor nerve (cranial nerve III) may be compressed resulting in

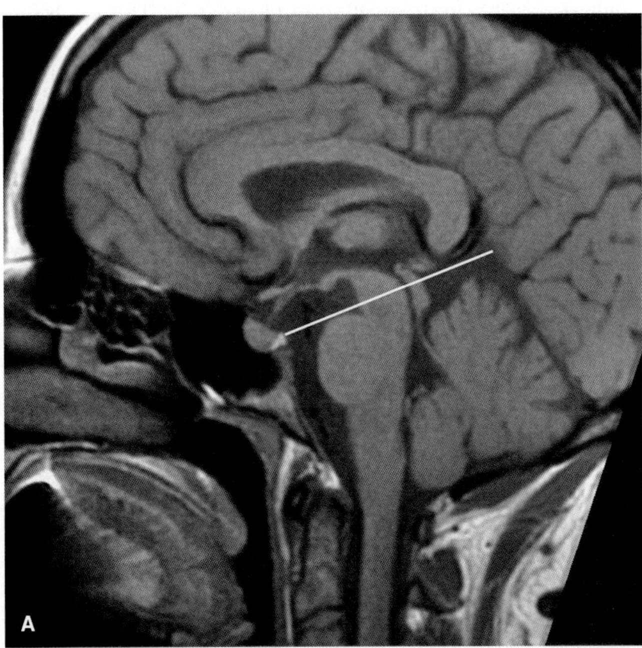

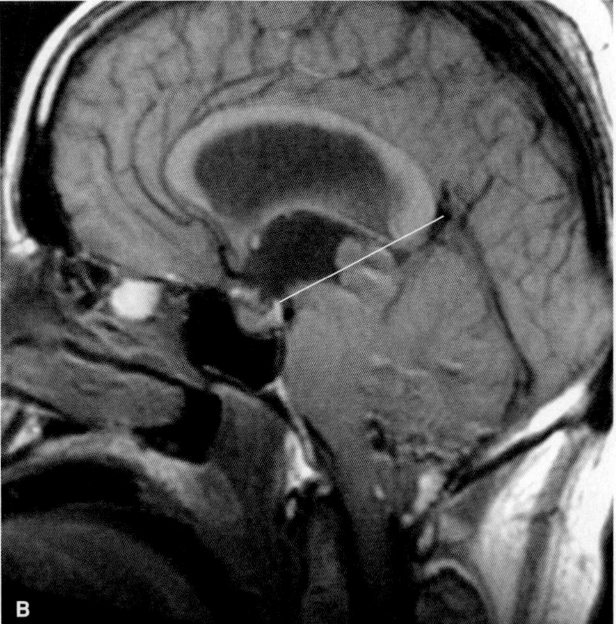

FIGURE 30.2 A: Normal midline sagittal T1-weighted MRI. The plane of the incisura (*white line*) runs from the posterior sella to the junction of the vein of Galen and the straight sinus. B: Sagittal T1-weighted MRI. A large tectal mass resulting in hydrocephalus and downward transtentorial herniation. Here, a line drawn along the plane of the incisura intersects the splenium of the corpus callosum and passes above the interpeduncular fossa.

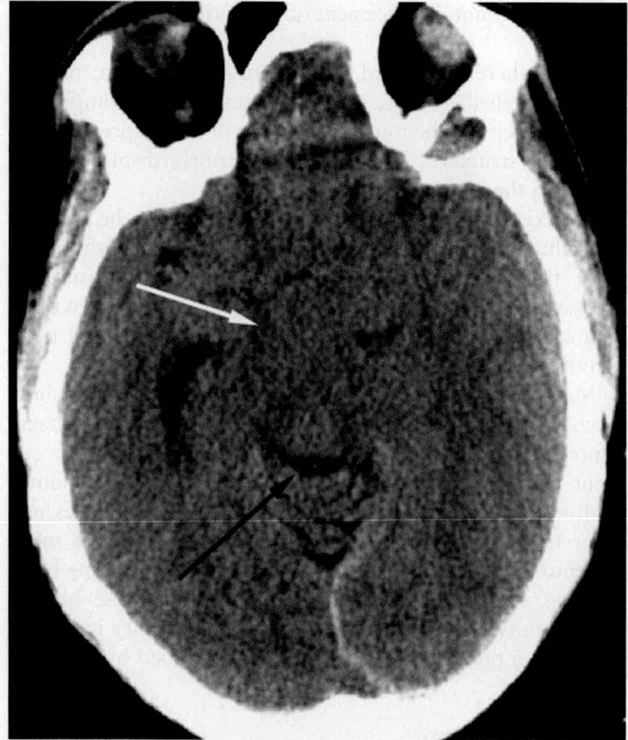

FIGURE 30.3 Axial CT image in a patient with supratentorial mass effect resulting in downward transtentorial herniation. There is effacement of the suprasellar and ambient cisterns (*white arrow*) with preservation of the quadrigeminal plate cistern (*black arrow*).

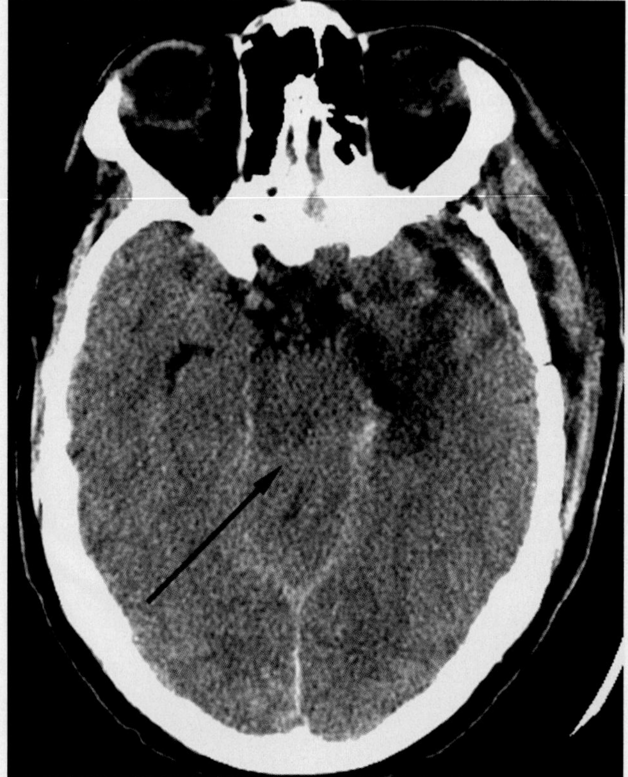

FIGURE 30.4 Axial CT image in a patient with posterior fossa mass effect resulting in upward transtentorial herniation. Notice the effacement of the quadrigeminal plate cistern (*arrow*).

a fixed and dilated ipsilateral pupil. Although less common, compression of the posterior cerebral artery (PCA) and/or anterior choroidal arteries can also occur. As the mass effect increases, the contralateral cerebral peduncle can be compressed against the tentorium cerebelli causing a hemiparesis on the side ipsilateral to the lesion leading to a false localization of the abnormality. The indentation of the tentorium on the cerebral peduncle has been classically termed *Kernohan notch* and can occasionally be visualized on imaging.

Tonsillar Herniation

Herniation of the cerebellar tonsils through the foramen magnum typically occurs as a result of a posterior fossa mass. By imaging, the cerebellar tonsils are displaced caudally through the foramen magnum. This can result in fourth ventricular outlet obstruction and hydrocephalus.

BRAIN EDEMA

Brain edema is a secondary effect of many pathologic conditions of the CNS. Recognition of brain edema is critical as it may often be the only sign of an underlying disease and can be the fatal endpoint of a variety of conditions due to the associated mass effect.

Pathophysiology

The two main types of brain edema are *vasogenic* and *cytotoxic*. *Cytotoxic edema* is related to cellular swelling, which typically occurs with cell damage such as infarction. *Vasogenic edema* occurs with leakage of fluid into the extracellular space, and is a common finding associated with many lesions including neoplasms and infection. A third type of brain swelling is less commonly discussed, but has critical implications. Loss of the brain's normal blood autoregulation, termed *dysautoregulation*, results in the rapid increase in intracerebral blood volume causing brain swelling and herniation. This syndrome is a frequent cause of death in head trauma.

The intracranial vascular compartment, unlike the brain itself, is compressible. Therefore, as there is increasing edema of any type within the confined space of the cranial vault, the intracranial pressure will also increase and have a detrimental effect on the vascular compartment. Normally, there is a reserve blood volume and autoregulation ensures continued adequate blood flow to the brain despite increased intracranial pressure. However, this only works up to a point. Brain death occurs once intracranial pressure exceeds the capacity for blood to flow to the brain.

Diagnosis

Cytotoxic edema is best detected with diffusion-weighted MRI. A distinguishing feature of cytotoxic edema is the involvement of gray matter resulting in loss of the normal gray–white differentiation. Identification of this characteristic is important as it limits the differential diagnosis. Cytotoxic edema localizing to the cortex is primarily related to vascular injury (i.e., arterial infarction), trauma, or infection. Infectious processes can result in cortical edema as a result of the infection itself (encephalitis) or from infection-related vasospasm causing secondary infarction. As opposed to cytotoxic edema,

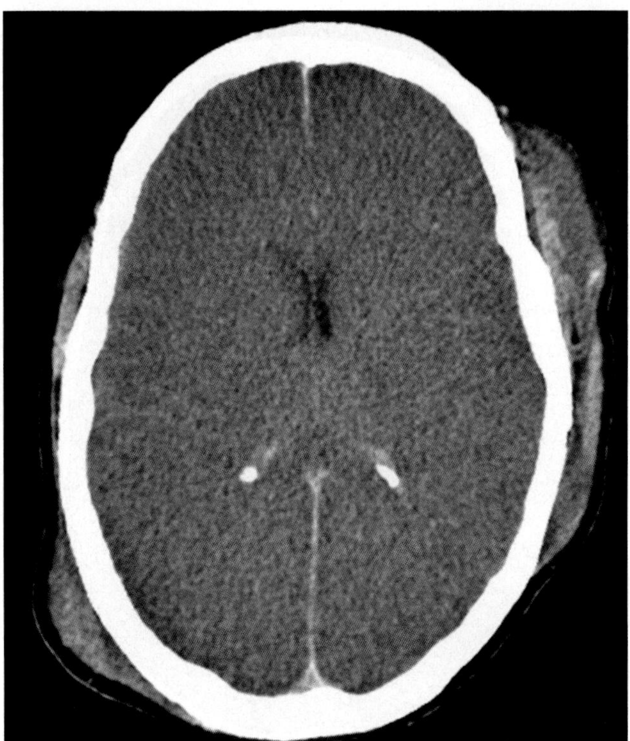

FIGURE 30.5 Axial noncontrast CT. There is diffuse brain edema with loss of normal gray–white differentiation, effacement of the sulci, and compression of the ventricles.

vasogenic edema typically affects white matter and spares the cortex leaving the gray–white differentiation intact. Unfortunately, the differential diagnosis remains broad in the setting of pure vasogenic edema as this is a common endpoint of the breakdown of the blood–brain barrier.

Brain dysautoregulation can be a difficult finding to appreciate on imaging. There is frequently no abnormal hypodensity, loss of gray–white junction, or other easily appreciable abnormality. The diffuse nature also means it is often symmetric in appearance making diagnosis all the more difficult. The secondary mass effect, including brain herniation or diffuse sulcal effacement, may be the only appreciable finding. The patients often have a profoundly abnormal Glasgow coma scale score despite the lack of readily apparent brain abnormality, such as hemorrhage.

All forms of brain edema typically result in secondary mass effect either in the region of edema or globally (Fig. 30.5). Once the increased intracranial pressure has resulted in sustained loss of blood flow, a nuclear medicine brain death study can be used to confirm the lack of intracranial blood flow; this study is often performed with Tc-99m diethylene triamine penta-acetate (DTPA) (Fig. 30.6). It is important to note that the brain death study will normalize within several days and therefore should be performed early when brain death is suspected.

INTRACRANIAL HEMORRHAGE

Early detection of acute intracranial hemorrhage can have a significant impact on patient outcomes. The hemorrhage itself can be a source of morbidity and mortality including localized brain damage, secondary mass effect, or hydrocephalus, to name a few. Additionally, identification of the source of hemorrhage may reveal a treatable cause which can decrease the incidence of subsequent hemorrhage.

Pathophysiology

Intracranial hemorrhage can result from a wide variety of causes, the majority of which are beyond the scope of this text. Some of the more common causes will be discussed here. As with all intracranial lesions, it is important to accurately localize hemorrhage on the imaging study, as this determines the most likely etiology and further workup and treatment. Moving from the outside in, this location can be extra-axial (i.e., epidural, subdural, or subarachnoid), intra-axial (i.e., involving the brain parenchyma itself), or intraventricular.

Diagnosis

Noncontrast CT is the study of choice in the evaluation of acute intracranial hemorrhage, as it is a rapid and accessible test, which produces high contrast between the high-attenuating (bright) clot and the low-attenuating (dark) CSF. MRI is also very sensitive for the detection of blood products, and the appearance of the blood on different sequences can be used to date the hemorrhage (1). Subarachnoid hemorrhage (SAH) is more commonly visualized on fluid-attenuated inversion recovery (FLAIR) images than conventional T1- and T2-weighted images since dilution of blood with CSF alters the normal evolution of blood products resulting in lack of the usual T1 and T2 signal characteristics. The FLAIR sequence is designed to suppress signal from the CSF so that it will appear dark; however, the presence of blood in the CSF results in incomplete suppression of CSF giving it a brighter appearance than normal (Fig. 30.7). However, this finding is not specific for hemorrhage

FIGURE 30.6 Tc-99m diethylene triamine penta-acetate brain death study. Projection images demonstrate no evidence of intracranial blood flow. There is increased activity over the nasal region (the "hot nose" sign commonly seen in brain death due to persistent external carotid arterial flow). Images from over the abdomen indicate perfusion of both kidneys, important information in a potential organ donor.

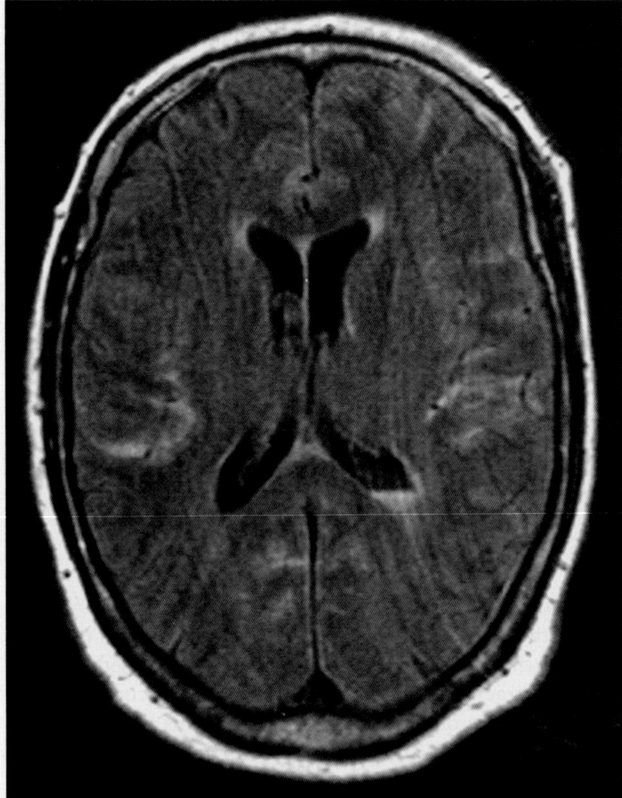

FIGURE 30.7 Axial fluid-attenuated inversion recovery (FLAIR) MRI. Subarachnoid blood is present as bright signal in the Sylvian fissures and sulci. A small amount of intraventricular hemorrhage is seen layering dependently in the left lateral ventricle.

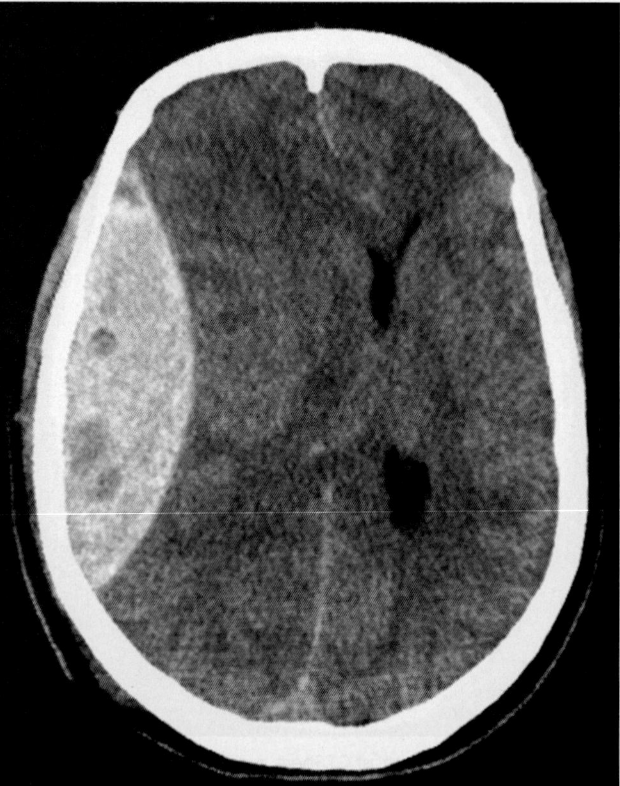

FIGURE 30.8 Axial noncontrast CT. Large right epidural hematoma with significant mass effect resulting in subfalcine herniation. Note the classic biconvex shape as the blood is confined by the frontoparietal suture anteriorly and the parietooccipital suture posteriorly. There was an associated parietal bone fracture (not visualized on this image).

and can also be seen from causes such as meningitis, neoplasm, propofol administration, or related simply to artifact. Susceptibility-weighted images (SWI) or gradient-recalled echo (GRE) sequences are also useful for the detection of blood products, as the hemoglobin affects the magnetic field in such a way as to decrease signal, the so-called susceptibility artifact. Thus, blood appears black on susceptibility images.

Epidural Hematoma

An epidural hematoma occurs in the potential space between the inner table of the calvaria and the dura. It usually results from a skull fracture lacerating a meningeal artery, although it can occur as a result of venous injury from trauma or surgery. The arterial pressure is sufficient to separate the bone from the dura except at the sutures where the dura is very tightly adherent. This results in the classic biconvex shape of the hemorrhage, which is confined by suture lines (Fig. 30.8). An epidural hematoma is a surgical emergency as it can continue to expand and result in considerable mass effect, brain herniation, and death.

Subdural Hematoma

A subdural hematoma is located between the dura mater and the arachnoid, and usually results from tearing of bridging veins that course from the cortex to the dura. It is differentiated from an epidural hematoma in that it crosses sutures and has a crescent shape (Fig. 30.9). The etiology can be trauma,

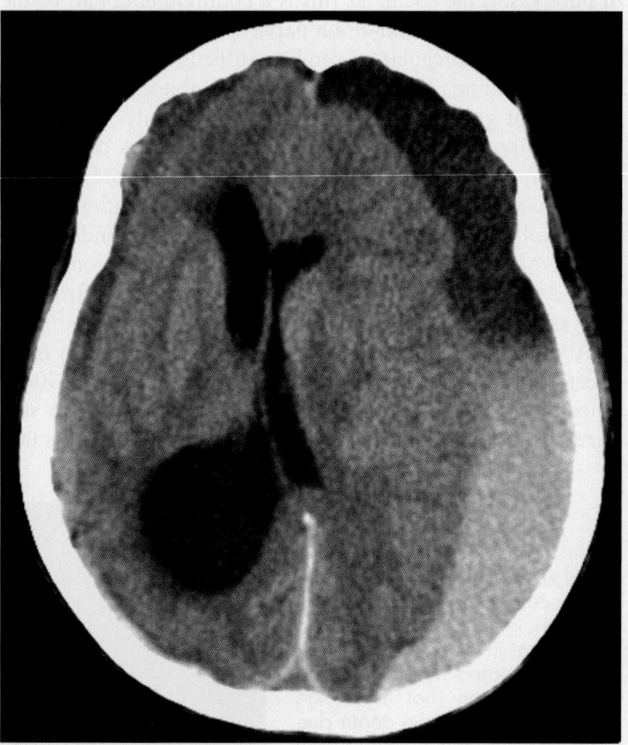

FIGURE 30.9 Axial noncontrast CT. Bilateral subdural hematomas, left greater than right. There is a fluid–fluid level on the left secondary to settling out of the blood products as the patient was in a prolonged supine position.

especially when there is rotational shear injury, but may also be secondary to a coagulopathy. Subdural hematomas are more common in elderly patients, where atrophy has resulted in a stretching of the bridging veins, predisposing them to injury.

Subarachnoid Hemorrhage

SAH is located between the arachnoid and pia mater, and therefore is detected on imaging studies as blood filling the sulci and basilar cisterns (Fig. 30.10). Although noncontrast CT is the imaging study of choice, small volume or subacute SAH may not be detectable with CT, and therefore a lumbar puncture to look for xanthochromia may still be warranted. Once an SAH has been diagnosed, an investigation of its cause is necessary. The leading cause is aneurysmal rupture. Arterial venous malformation (AVM) is a less common etiology. The most appropriate initial imaging study to search for a vascular abnormality is CT angiography (CTA) (Fig. 30.11). If an underlying etiology cannot be identified, a conventional angiogram is warranted. If this also is negative, the patient should be reimaged in 1 week to look for possible recanalization of a thrombosed aneurysm. In 10% of the cases no etiology will be identified.

Patients with SAH need to be monitored for vasospasm. This typically first appears around day 3, peaks at day 7, and then begins to subside becoming uncommon after day 14. Vasospasm is detected on CTA as constriction of vessels, often with compensatory physiologic dilatation of the more distal vessels. CT perfusion imaging can aid in determination of the physiologic significance of underlying vasospasm. If a patient with vasospasm has compensatory blood flow through collaterals maintaining their brain perfusion, they often can be followed or treated with modified triple-H therapy (euvolemia, hypertension [HTN] [mean arterial pressure 90 to 110 mmHg], and hemodilution). A patient with vasospasm and decreased perfusion may need endovascular intervention, which can be performed with an intra-arterial calcium channel blocker such as verapamil or by angioplasty (Fig. 30.12).

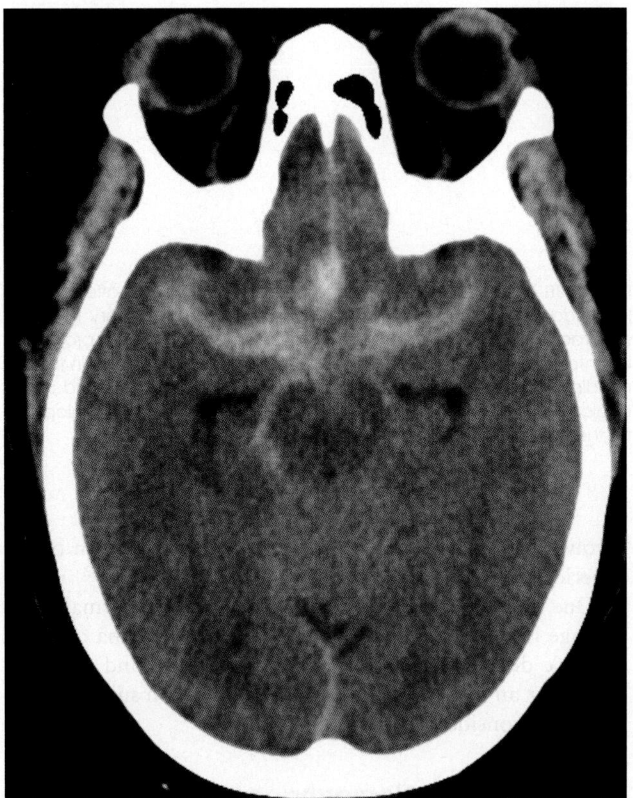

FIGURE 30.10 Axial noncontrast CT. Diffuse subarachnoid blood products fill the anterior interhemispheric fissure and the basilar cisterns. This patient was found to have a ruptured anterior communicating artery aneurysm.

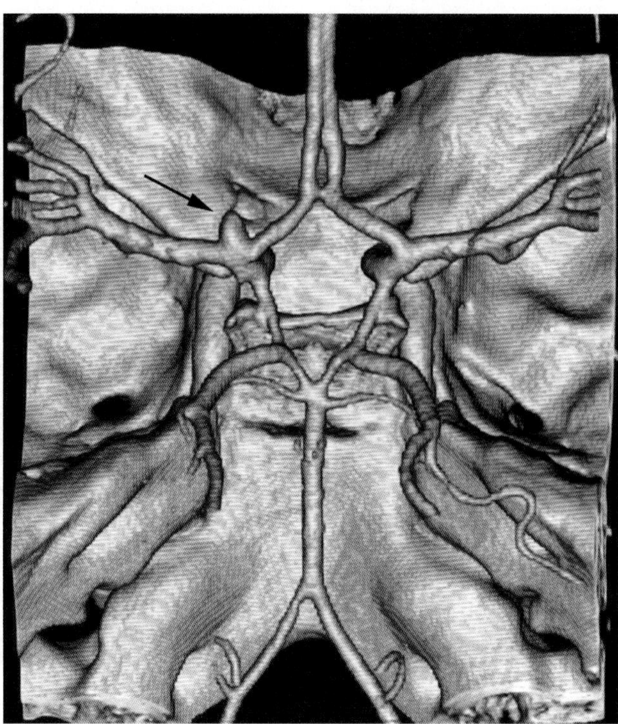

FIGURE 30.11 Volume surface–shaded rendering from a CT angiogram. There is a small aneurysm projecting anterosuperiorly at the origin of the middle cerebral artery on the right (*arrow*).

Intraparenchymal Hemorrhage

Intraparenchymal hemorrhage has many etiologies and can be divided into traumatic versus nontraumatic causes. Traumatic causes include blunt and penetrating injuries resulting in a contusion, or rotational forces resulting in shear injury and diffuse axonal injury (Fig. 30.13). Nontraumatic causes include HTN, amyloid angiopathy, hemorrhagic stroke, hemorrhagic tumor, coagulopathy, and venous obstruction. In the setting of nontraumatic injury, the underlying etiology may not be evident on CT or MRI and correlation with the clinical history is vital.

Parenchymal hemorrhage related to HTN usually occurs with an acute elevation of blood pressure in the background of chronic HTN. Chronic HTN produces small-vessel disease that leads to lipohyalinosis. This affects the penetrating arteries such as the lenticulostriates and thalamoperforators, and explains why hypertensive hemorrhage most commonly occurs in the basal ganglia and thalamus (Fig. 30.14).

Amyloid angiopathy is deposition of β-amyloid in the media and adventitia of small and midsized arteries of the leptomeninges and cortex. This leads to stenosis of the vessel lumen and weakening of the vessel wall, eventually resulting in the formation of microaneurysms. This predisposes patients to

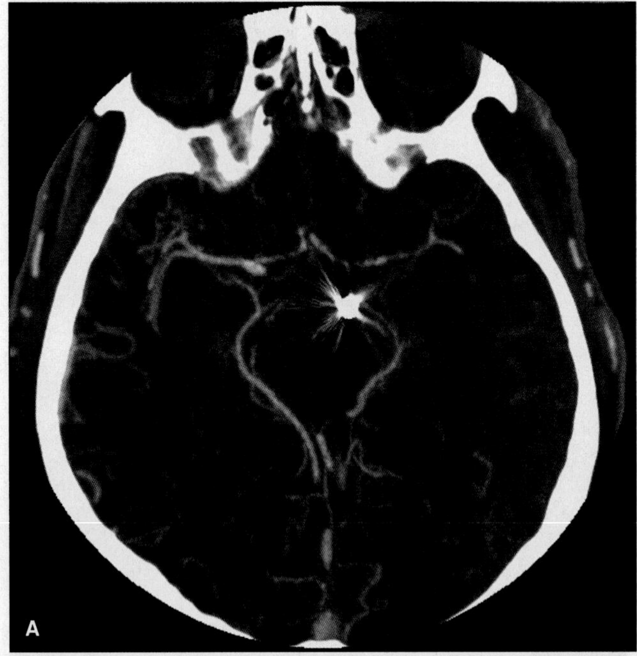

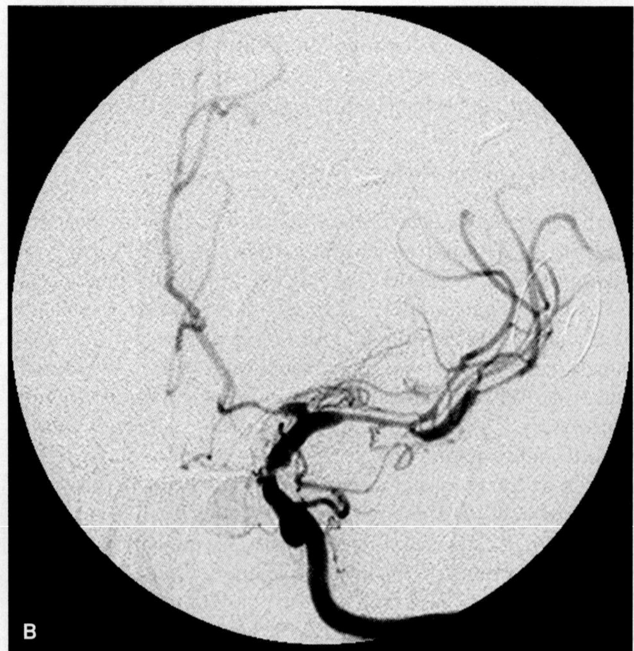

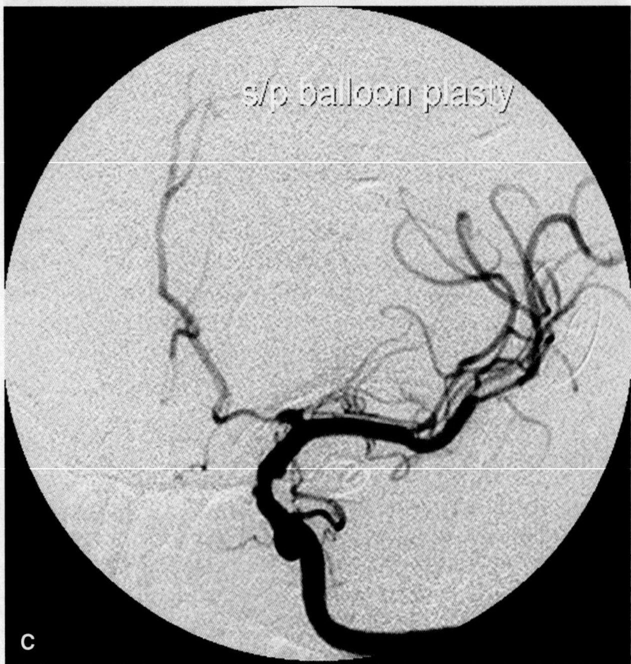

FIGURE 30.12 A: Axial CT angiography image. Vasospasm affecting the left middle cerebral artery and left posterior cerebral artery following subarachnoid hemorrhage and aneurysm coiling. B: Frontal projection left internal carotid artery angiogram also showing vasospasm in the left middle cerebral artery. C: Frontal projection left internal carotid artery angiogram showing normal size of the left MCA following angioplasty for the vasospasm.

intraparenchymal—typically lobar—hemorrhages, which can be large and multiple. The most common locations are the frontal and parietal lobes.

Another nontraumatic and often overlooked source of intraparenchymal hemorrhage is venous obstruction. This has many causes, including hypercoagulable states, pregnancy, infection, malignancy, and birth control pills. The location of hemorrhage is dependent on the vascular territory of the occluded vein, and does not correspond to a typical arterial territory. Vascular congestion follows venous obstruction, which eventually leads to cell death and venous infarction. This type of infarction tends to result in hemorrhage more frequently than arterial infarction. The hemorrhage may also involve both cerebral hemispheres if there is occlusion of the superior sagittal sinus.

One important subset of patients with parenchymal hemorrhage is young patients with no history of trauma or other systemic disease. Special care should be given, and a careful search for an underlying vascular malformation such as AVM should be considered.

Intraventricular Hemorrhage

In adults, intraventricular hemorrhage is usually secondary to extension from a parenchymal hemorrhage or reflux of SAH. Isolated intraventricular hemorrhage should raise the concern

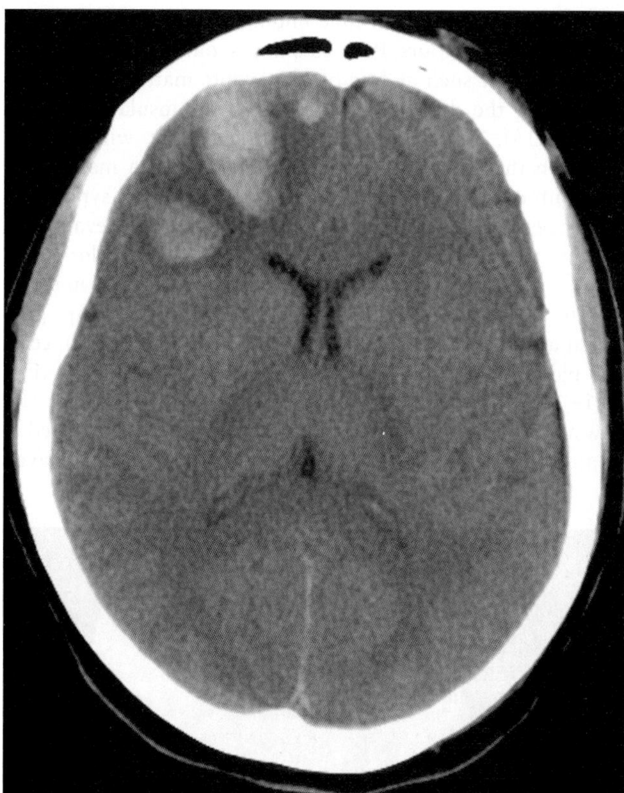

FIGURE 30.13 Axial noncontrast CT. Posttraumatic contusion (intraparenchymal hemorrhage) is present in the right frontal polar region with surrounding vasogenic edema.

for an AVM. In infants, germinal matrix hemorrhage occurs in premature newborns and frequently extends into the ventricular system. Intraventricular hemorrhage is important to recognize because it can commonly result in obstruction of normal CSF flow and therefore hydrocephalus may ensue.

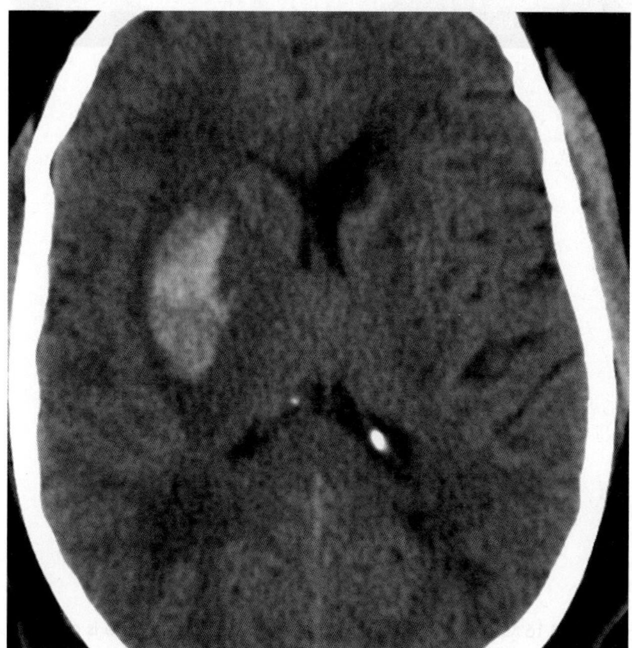

FIGURE 30.14 Axial noncontrast CT. Hypertensive-related hemorrhage into the right basal ganglia.

STROKE

Stroke is the clinical term used to describe a permanent nontraumatic brain injury with resulting neurologic deficit. It is important to remember that stroke is a clinical diagnosis with a wide variety of causes, although it is commonly used interchangeably with acute infarction. Rapid diagnosis of the cause of the clinical symptoms, particularly in the setting of infarction, is necessary as any delay decreases the likelihood of effective treatment and increases the incidence of complications.

Pathophysiology

Infarctions can be classified by their etiology as *ischemic,* secondary to hypoperfusion of an area of brain; *hemorrhagic,* from rupture of a vascular structure leading to bleeding into the brain; or secondary to a substrate deficiency such as hypoglycemia. More than 75% of strokes are due to ischemia.

Ischemic strokes can be thrombotic or embolic. In thrombotic strokes, clot forms locally on the wall of an artery leading to decreased blood supply. In an embolic stroke, a clot becomes dislodged from the heart or an extracranial vessel traveling to the brain and resulting in compromised blood supply. Both thrombotic and embolic strokes are secondary to blockage of arterial supply to an area of brain. However, in patients with a hypoperfusion state—hypotension, cardiac failure, dysrhythmia—decreased flow to the brain can result in damage to areas of brain with the least robust blood supply. This type of global hypoxic injury tends to occur first in the watershed areas of brain, for example, the ACA–middle cerebral artery (MCA) or

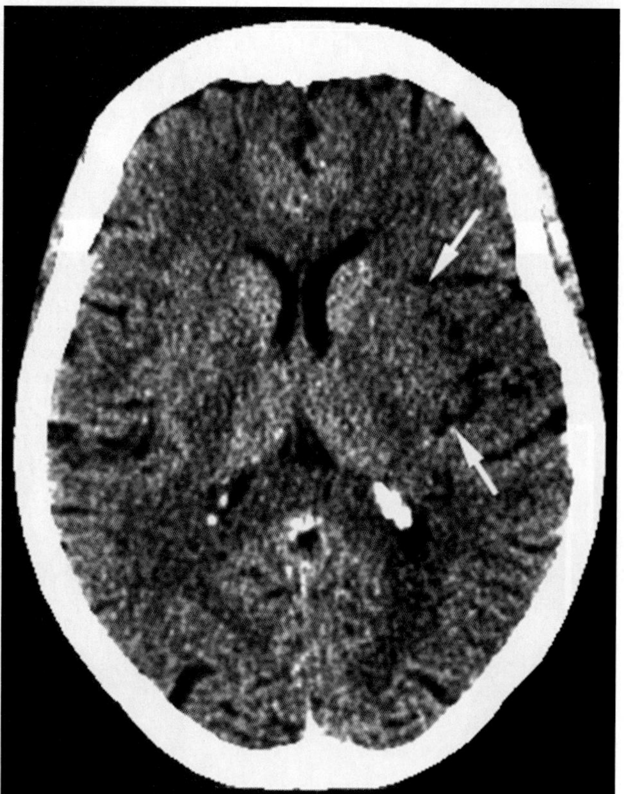

FIGURE 30.15 Axial noncontrast CT. Subtle loss of gray–white differentiation along the insular cortex on the left (*arrows*), the so-called insular ribbon sign.

the MCA–PCA watershed territories. Although far less common, stroke can also be the result of a venous occlusion. Predisposing factors include hypercoagulable states, pregnancy, meningitis, and sepsis. Blockage of venous outflow results in stasis of blood, which becomes deoxygenated, leading to subsequent neuronal death. Any venous structure can be involved, whether a cortical vein, a dural sinus, or the cavernous sinus. Venous infarcts should be considered in patients with ischemia affecting a nonarterial territory (2).

Diagnosis

Noncontrast CT should be obtained as the initial imaging modality in patients with new neurologic deficits suspected of having a stroke, as this imaging modality can rapidly identify patients with intracranial hemorrhage. Ischemic infarctions will often show no discernible findings on noncontrasted CT during the first 3 hours. Prior to 6 hours, only very subtle signs can be evident such as loss of gray–white matter distinction, haziness of the deep nuclei, or loss of the insular "ribbon" (Fig. 30.15). As time progresses, the patient will develop edema in the infarcted area, which can result in mass effect with shift of structures and potentially a herniation syndrome.

CT perfusion can often be rapidly obtained in evaluating patients for stroke (3,4). Perfusion CT produces color-coded maps of the brain at multiple levels showing differences in blood flow to areas of the brain. The most common color maps generated are time to peak (TTP), mean transit time (MTT), cerebral blood flow (CBF), and cerebral blood volume (CBV) (Fig. 30.16). MTT is the most sensitive measure to evaluate for any flow abnormality, but it is not specific. Flow will be prolonged in an area of ischemia or infarction, but also in areas with delayed

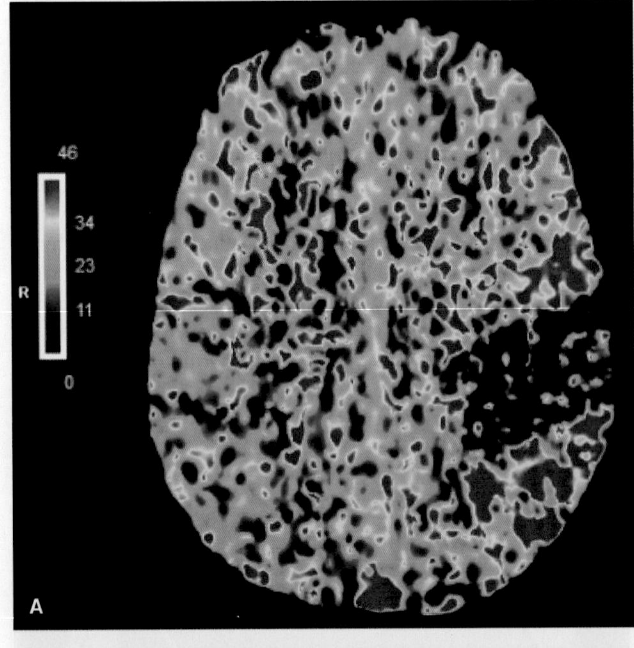

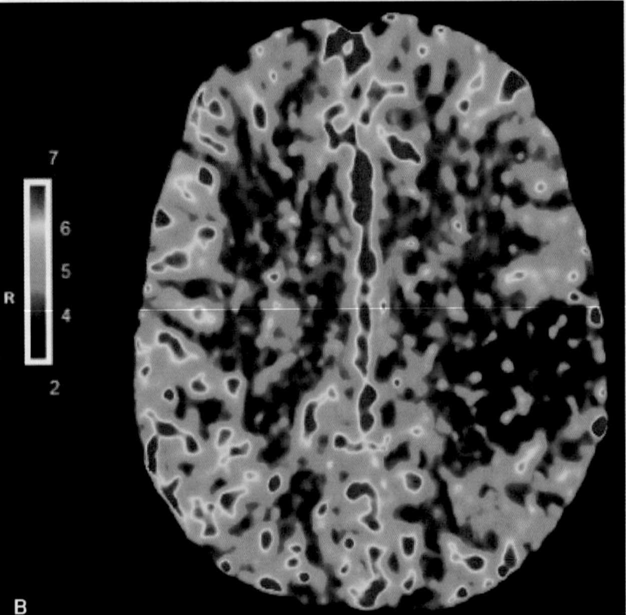

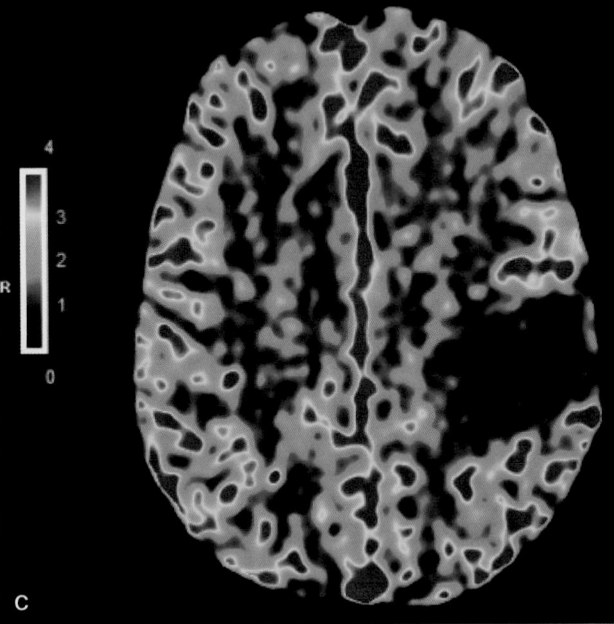

FIGURE 30.16 CT perfusion examination. A: Mean transit time is delayed to the left middle cerebral artery (MCA) territory. B: Cerebral blood flow is decreased in the left MCA territory. C: Cerebral blood volume is also decreased to the left MCA territory consistent with infarcted tissue.

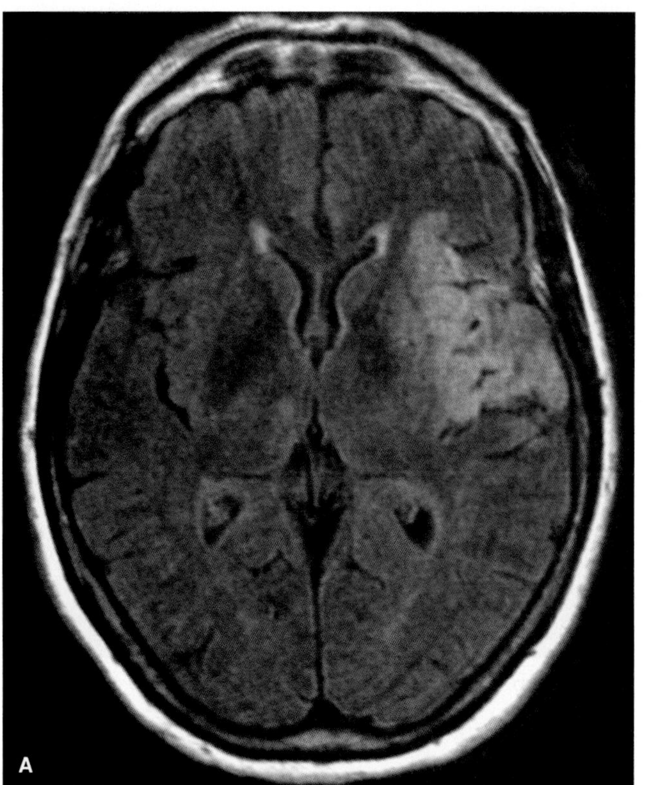

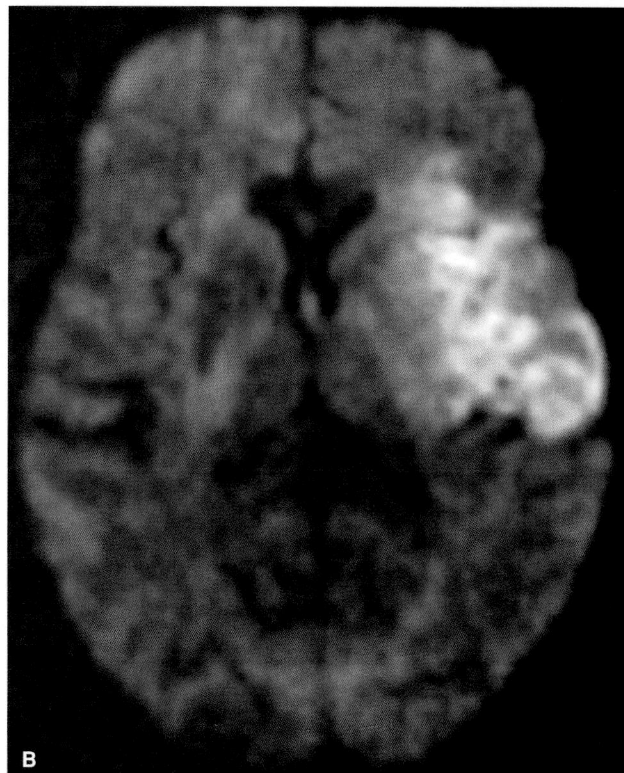

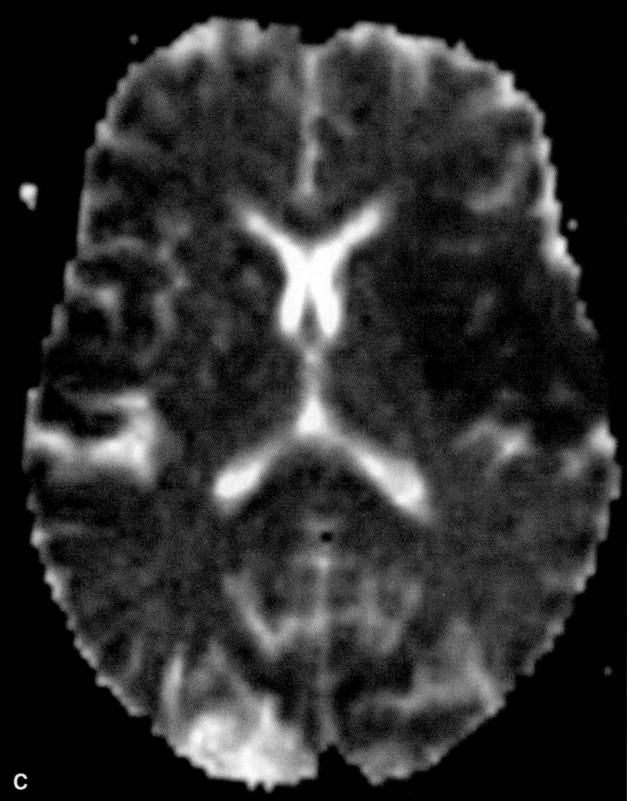

FIGURE 30.17 **A**: Axial FLAIR MRI. Cytotoxic edema is present as high signal in this patient with acute left middle cerebral artery (MCA) infarct. Axial diffusion-weighted MRI (**B**) and axial apparent diffusion coefficient (ADC) map (**C**) showing high signal on the diffusion image and low signal on the ADC map in the left MCA territory consistent with diffusion restriction and acute infarction.

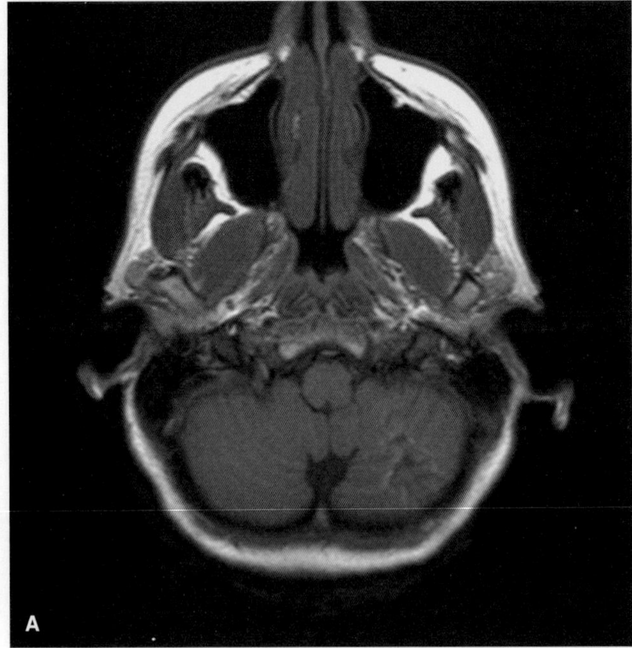

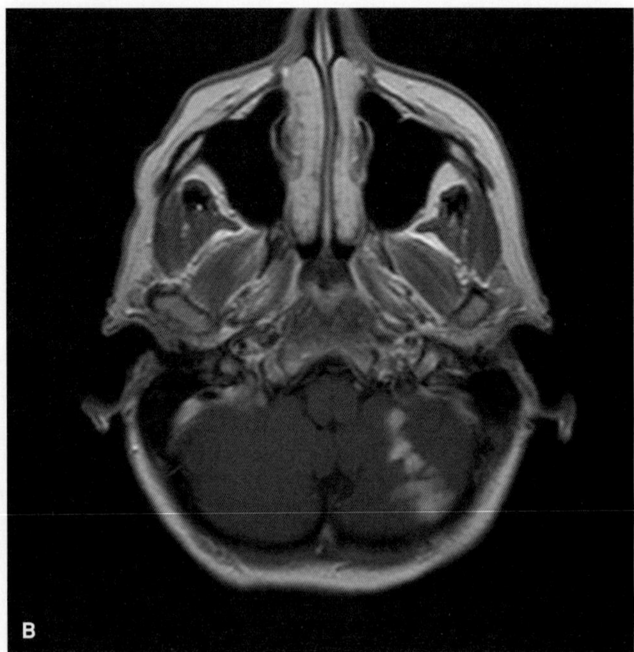

FIGURE 30.18 Precontrast (A) and postcontrast (B) axial T1-weighted MRI. Enhancing subacute infarct in the left posterior inferior cerebellar artery territory.

flow for any reason, such as regions distal to a vascular stenosis. Decreased CBF is present in areas of the brain either at risk for, or undergoing, infarct. CBV is the most specific indicator of an area undergoing infarction. An area of low CBF with normal to increased CBV represents an area of borderline ischemia which is currently compensated for by vasodilation. Once there is a decrease of both CBF and CBV, the tissue is undergoing infarction. Some limitations of perfusion CT include the need to administer intravenous contrast and long image acquisition times, requiring patients to hold completely still for 60 seconds. Similar perfusion information can be obtained with MRI perfusion, but CT with perfusion is often more rapidly accessible with fewer safety screening requirements than MRI.

MRI with diffusion-weighted imaging (DWI) is currently the gold standard for identifying acute cerebral infarction. DWI improves infarct detection to over 95% (Fig. 30.17A-C). DWI is positive in infarcted tissue within minutes. It is important to distinguish ischemia from infarction as those areas seen as having significant restriction of water movement on DWI are infarcted and not typically recoverable. Detection of ischemic, but not infarcted, tissue (penumbra) cannot be accurately determined on DWI alone and requires the application of perfusion imaging.

DWI identifies areas of decreased water motion in regions of infarction and displays them as bright areas (Fig. 30.17B). A few caveats are worth noting: first, restricted water diffusion is not specific to infarction and can be seen in other diseases such as infection or neoplasm; second DWI is unreliable in the presence of hemorrhage due to artifact from the magnetic effects of iron; finally, since DWI sequences are based on T2-weighted sequences, some areas with high T2 signals that are not secondary to restricted water diffusion can appear bright on diffusion imaging. Therefore, it is necessary to compare diffusion sequences with an apparent diffusion coefficient (ADC) map (Fig. 30.17C). Areas that are bright on diffusion and dark on ADC are true restricted diffusion.

Over time, the diffusion and ADC abnormalities will reverse as the stroke moves into a subacute phase. In evaluating for subacute stroke, contrast-enhanced T1-weighted MRI can show enhancement of a subacute infarct as soon as 2 to 3 days following the event. Contrast enhancement can persist for 8 to 10 weeks. The "2-2-2" rule is usually followed: The enhancement begins at 2 days, peaks at 2 weeks, and resolves by 2 months. Contrast enhancement is also seen with CT imaging of subacute stroke (Fig. 30.18).

INFECTION

CNS infections can progress rapidly, leading to stroke, hemorrhage, herniation, and death. Prompt recognition and initiation of therapy are therefore critical. Imaging can play an important role in evaluating for signs and complications of infection.

The discussion of CNS infection can take many different pathways, and may be divided into opportunistic and nonopportunistic infection, or specific pathogens can be studied individually. In the interest of simplicity, infection will be discussed anatomically.

Pathophysiology

Leptomeningitis, commonly referred to as meningitis, is an inflammatory infiltration of the pia and arachnoid meninges that can be caused by bacterial, viral, or fungal agents. Most commonly, the infection occurs via hematogenous dissemination. Pachymeningitis (involving the dura mater) is not a common manifestation of viral or bacterial infection, but can be seen with tuberculosis and fungal infections. Noninfectious etiologies such as sarcoid and carcinomatosis are more common causes of pachymeningeal disease and should also be considered. Infection can also spread to involve the ventricular lining (ventriculitis) or ependyma (ependymitis).

Focal pyogenic infections of brain parenchyma lead to cerebritis. Cerebritis is brain inflammation usually secondary to hematogenous dissemination of bacteria. Fungal and parasitic etiologies are also possible, but less common. The most common areas affected are the territories supplied by the MCA, specifically the frontal and parietal lobes.

Encephalitis is brain inflammation caused by a viral infection or a hypersensitivity reaction to a foreign protein. Sources include herpes simplex virus (HSV), mosquito-borne viruses, cytomegalovirus, and Epstein–Barr virus. Herpes encephalitis progresses rapidly and can result in death without prompt recognition and therapy. It is usually due to reactivation of latent HSV-1 virus in an immunocompetent patient, which ascends into the brain via the trigeminal and olfactory nerves.

Diagnosis

Imaging is insensitive for early meningitis and is often normal early in the course of infection (5). In fact, the most sensitive test for meningitis is a lumbar puncture, not an imaging examination. Imaging studies are more useful to evaluate for complications of meningitis. Noncontrast CT will often be relatively normal, but may show mild ventriculomegaly; contrast-enhanced CT can show enhancing material within sulci and cisterns. CTA can show evidence of vasculitis with multifocal areas of vessel irregularity.

MRI is a much more sensitive imaging modality for meningitis, but still is often normal in the earliest stages of infection. In leptomeningitis, FLAIR sequences can show high signal along the sulci from the proteinaceous material in the CSF (Fig. 30.19). Exudative material along the sulci will enhance in a serpiginous form on T1-weighted postcontrast images (Fig. 30.20). MRI is also useful to evaluate for complications of meningitis such as ventriculitis, abscess, and infarction. Infarcts are common complications of advanced meningitis. A vasculitis is caused by meningeal irritation, which potentially can progress to obstruction of arterial flow. Additionally, venous infarcts can be seen secondary to septic venous thrombosis (Fig. 30.21). Pachymeningitis, an infiltration of the dura, can be differentiated from leptomeningitis by its thick nodular enhancement pattern that closely approximates the calvaria and does not extend into the sulci.

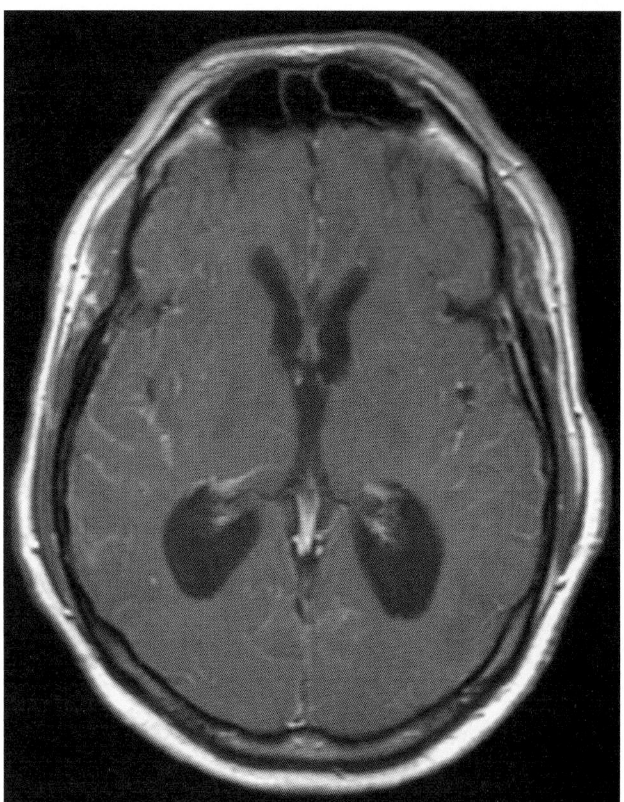

FIGURE 30.20 Postcontrast axial T1-weighted MRI. Leptomeningeal enhancement in the characteristic serpiginous pattern along the sulci in a patient with bacterial meningitis.

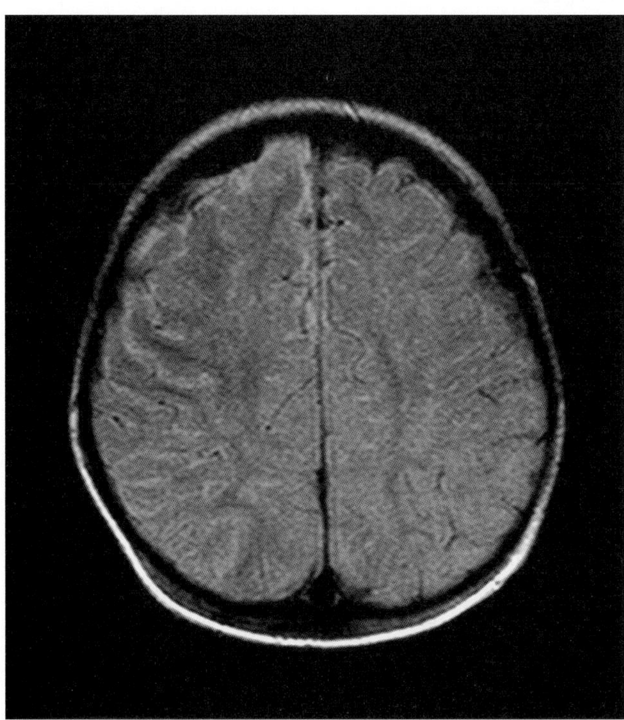

FIGURE 30.19 Axial fluid-attenuated inversion recovery (FLAIR) MRI. High signal in a serpiginous pattern along the sulci representing the high-protein inflammatory exudates in bacterial meningitis.

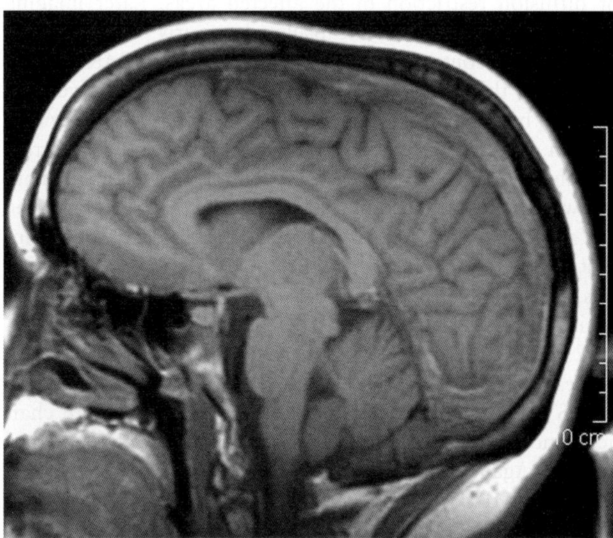

FIGURE 30.21 Sagittal T1-weighted MRI. High signal is seen within the superior sagittal sinus representing thrombus.

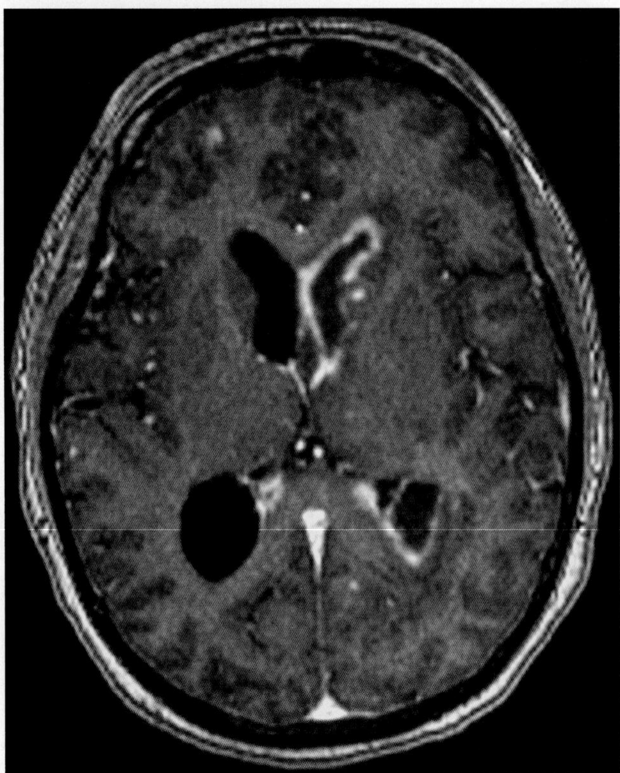

FIGURE 30.22 Postcontrast axial T1-weighted MRI. Enhancement is present along the ependymal lining of the left lateral ventricle consistent with ventriculitis.

Imaging exams are also frequently normal in the setting of ventriculitis and ependymitis. MRI is much more sensitive than CT and will demonstrate enhancement along the ventricular margins (Fig. 30.22). There will often be increased FLAIR signal surrounding the ventricles and the ventricles may appear enlarged. Keep in mind that this imaging appearance is not specific to infection; for example, lymphoma in an immunocompromised patient can have a similar appearance.

CT is also frequently normal in early cerebritis; however, MRI may demonstrate abnormal increased FLAIR signal or diffusion restriction in the affected areas. Later imaging features include an unencapsulated, poorly defined mass with patchy contrast enhancement on CT and MRI. If left untreated, this infectious, inflammatory mass will develop a capsule, become more organized, and eventually develop into a brain abscess. The capsule rim will enhance on postcontrast CT and MRI (Fig. 30.23A). FLAIR and T2-weighted imaging will often show prominent vasogenic edema surrounding the abscesses (Fig. 30.23B). Often, the capsule will be thinnest on the ventricular side, which may help in distinguishing this ring-enhancing lesion from a malignancy. Additionally, brain abscesses will show restricted diffusion centrally (Fig. 30.23C,D). The time course for the changes from cerebritis to abscess is approximately 2 weeks.

HSV encephalitis deserves special note due to more characteristic imaging findings and necessity of prompt antiviral therapy. Again, CT is insensitive to early features of this disease, but MRI will frequently show findings within 2 days of onset. Initially, edema is seen in the medial temporal lobe, insula, and inferior frontal lobe (Fig. 30.24). Occasionally this is unilateral, but more often asymmetric bilateral disease is present. Postcontrast imaging will show patchy vague enhancement in initial phases progressing to gyriform enhancement within 1 week. Hemorrhage is also a common finding.

An additional complication of CNS infection is development of an empyema. An empyema is a loculated collection of pus that can develop intracranially in either the subdural or epidural space. These are commonly referred to as subdural or epidural abscesses. These infections are considered a neurosurgical emergency and must be drained expediently. Most of these are supratentorial and present as an extra-axial collection. This fluid collection is often isodense to CSF on CT imaging, making MRI superior to CT in evaluating the extent and nature of this collection. On T1-weighted MRI, the fluid will be hyperintense to CSF because of proteinaceous material, pus, within it (Fig. 30.25). Often, prominent enhancement is present along the margins of the collection. Signal changes in adjacent brain parenchyma are also commonly seen secondary to cerebritis.

An empyema can develop as a complication of meningitis in younger patients. In older individuals, contiguous spread from a paranasal sinus or ear infection is the most common etiology. Occasionally, it can be difficult to determine if an epidural fluid collection is an abscess, effusion, or a hematoma, in which case follow-up CT examination may be useful. A key imaging feature is that subdural empyemas demonstrate restricted diffusion and a subdural effusion does not. An imaging pitfall is in differentiating a chronic subdural hematoma from a subdural empyema, as they may look similar. While empyema will have restricted diffusion on DWI, the magnetic effects of blood products in a subdural hematoma can result in the artifactual appearance of restricted diffusion.

SPINE

Injury to the spinal cord can be a source of significant morbidity and mortality and, too often, is irreversible. The spinal cord is protected by a bony spinal column and associated ligamentous structures; unstable injuries to the bony spinal column or ligaments predispose one to injury of the spinal cord. Recognition of these unstable injuries before spinal cord injury has occurred can help prevent significant morbidity or mortality.

Pathophysiology

The spine consists of both osseous and ligamentous components that transmit forces to allow movement while protecting the spinal cord and vertebral arteries. In terms of mechanical forces, the spine is divided into three columns.

- The anterior column includes the anterior longitudinal ligament and the anterior two-thirds of the vertebral body, disc, and annulus fibrosus.
- The middle column consists of the posterior third of the vertebral body, disc, posterior annulus, and the posterior longitudinal ligament.
- The facet joints, laminae, spinous processes, and interspinous ligaments comprise the posterior column. Interruption of at least two contiguous columns, including both osseous and ligamentous components, is generally considered unstable.

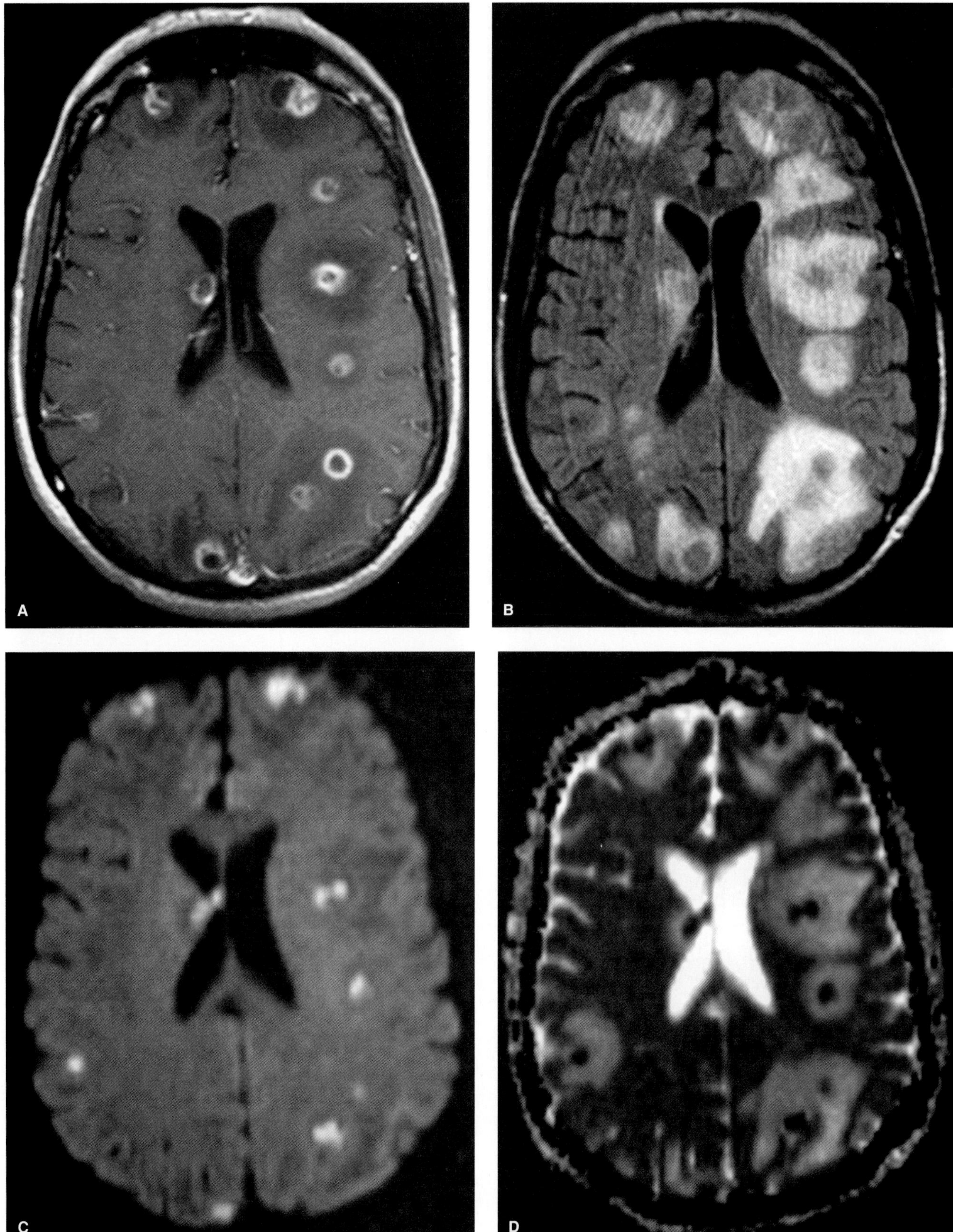

FIGURE 30.23 A: Postcontrast axial T1-weighted MRI: multiple rim-enhancing lesions. B: Axial fluid-attenuated inversion recovery (FLAIR) MRI. Prominent vasogenic edema surrounding the lesions. Axial diffusion (C) and axial apparent diffusion coefficient MRI (D) showing that the lesions demonstrate restricted diffusion, consistent with multiple brain abscesses. *Nocardia* was the causative agent in this patient.

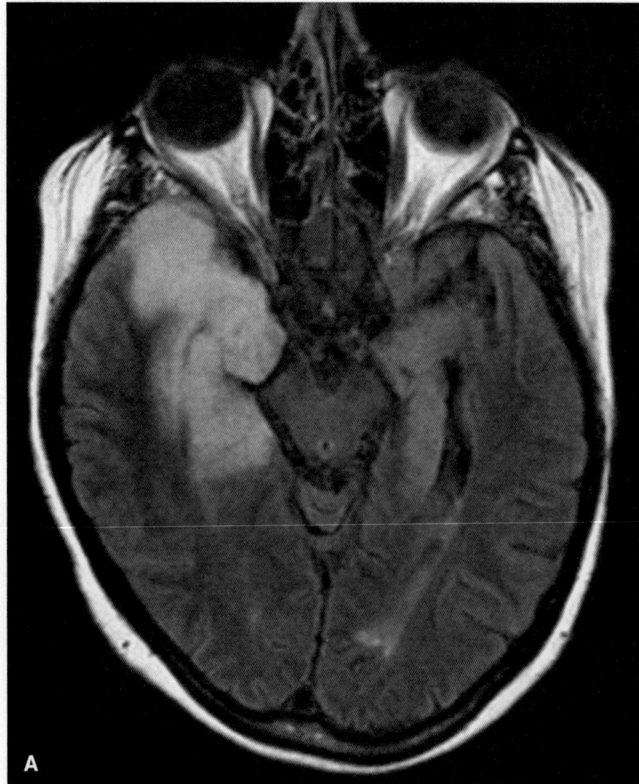

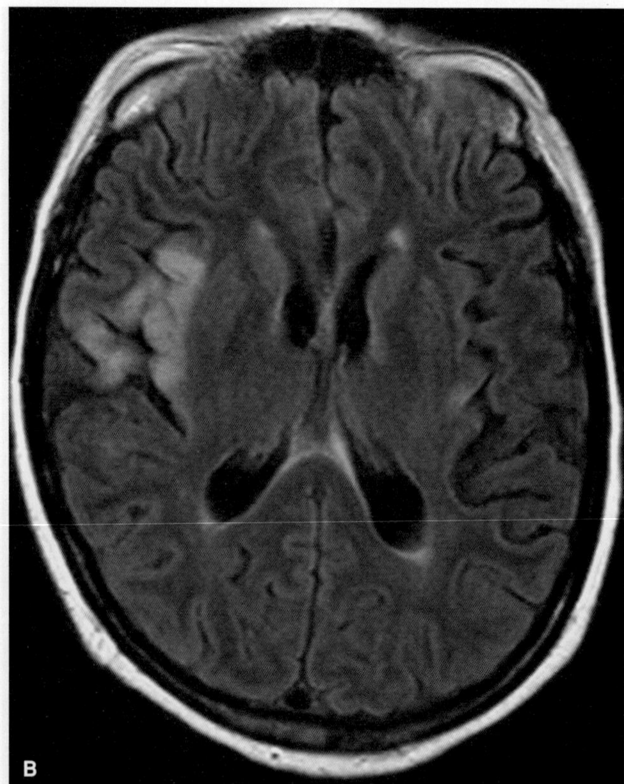

FIGURE 30.24 Axial FLAIR MRIs. Bilateral asymmetric edema is present in the temporal lobes (A) and insular cortex (B). This appearance should raise suspicion for herpes simplex virus encephalitis.

Diagnosis

Traditionally, radiographs were a primary means of assessing the spine for traumatic injury. CT has now largely replaced radiographs for assessing patients with a high risk of spinal column injury due to higher sensitivity and specificity. MRI has a much higher sensitivity and specificity for ligamentous or spinal cord injury; however, there is controversy surrounding the use of MRI in evaluating patients who have no evidence of fracture or misalignment on CT. There is currently no strong evidence that MRI, in the setting of completely normal CT, has any effect on patient outcomes; MRI is likely of little to no benefit unless the patient has unexplained focal neurologic symptoms suggesting underlying occult spinal cord injury.

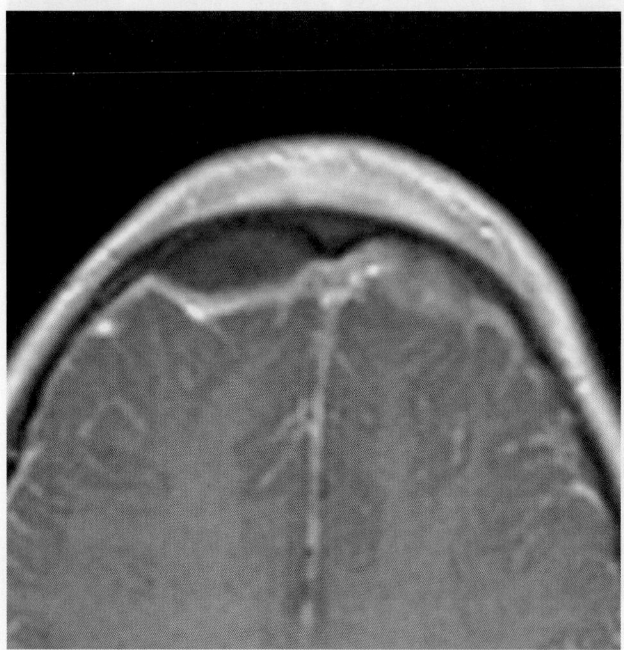

FIGURE 30.25 Axial postcontrast T1-weighted MRI. Extra-axial fluid collection adjacent to right frontal lobe with enhancement along the dural margin, consistent with a subdural empyema.

When evaluating any imaging study of the spine, the initial assessment must be made of appropriate alignment in both coronal and sagittal planes. Spinal alignment is assessed in the sagittal plane with the use of the anterior vertebral body line, posterior vertebral body line, spinolaminar line, and dorsal surface articular pillar lines (Fig. 30.26). The atlantoaxial and craniocervical relationship is evaluated with various measurements, including the basion–dens interval of 12 mm or less, the Power's ratio, and the atlantoaxial distance of less than 2 mm in an adult. Abnormal alignment, a widened facet joint, or widened intervertebral disc space raises suspicion for ligamentous injury, and should prompt additional imaging.

In the past, dynamic flexion and extension plain films were commonly used to assess for underlying ligamentous instability; however, recent studies have called into question their utility in the acute setting. In patients with acute spine injuries, a high percentage of flexion and extension radiographs will have insufficient flexion or extension effort to elicit a change in alignment due to natural protective reflexes. For this reason, flexion and extension radiographs have increasingly fallen out of favor. If there is high suspicion of underlying ligamentous injury, MRI with STIR (short tau inversion recovery) sequence is more sensitive for soft tissue injury. Increased signal within the ligaments on STIR images is consistent with ligamentous injury (Fig. 30.27).

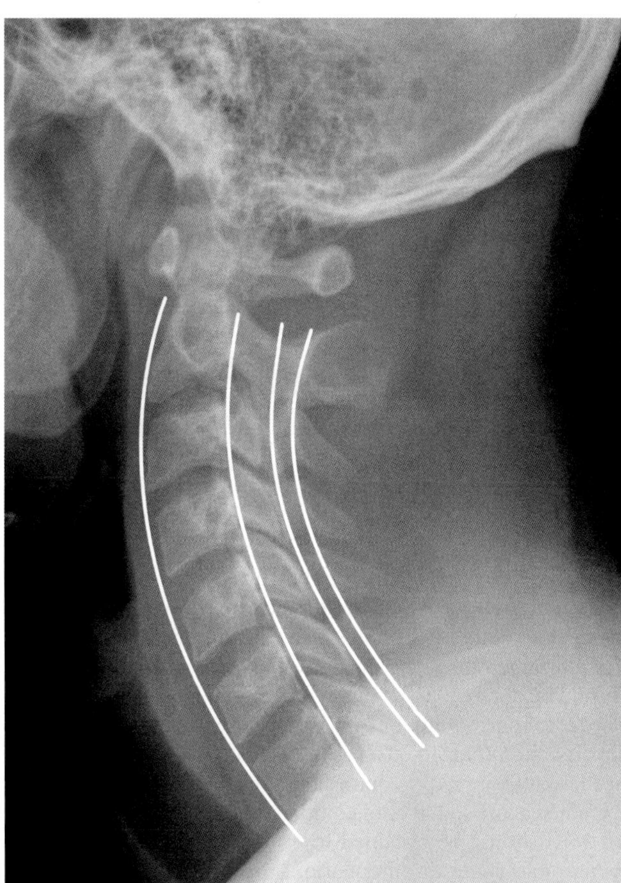

FIGURE 30.26 Normal lateral view of the cervical spine with normal smooth curvature of the anterior vertebral body line, posterior vertebral body line, dorsal surface articular pillar line, and spinal laminar line.

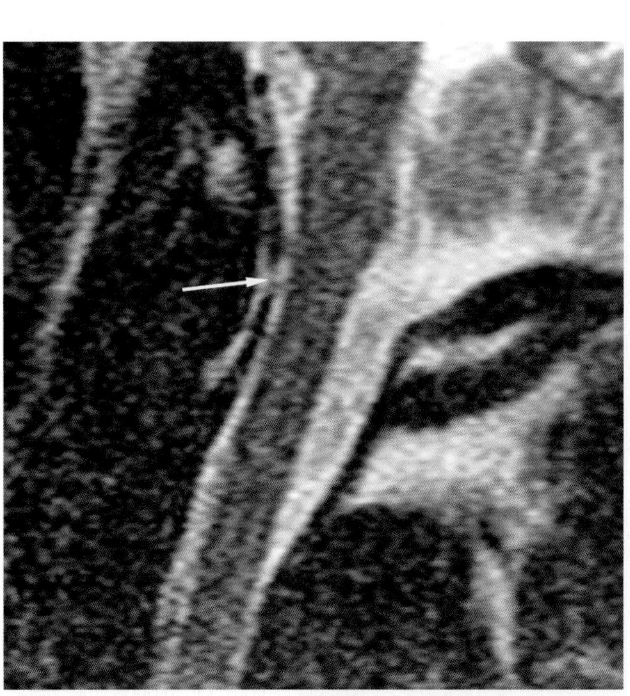

FIGURE 30.27 Sagittal short tau inversion recovery (STIR) MRI. Focal disruption of the posterior longitudinal ligament at the C2 level (*arrow*).

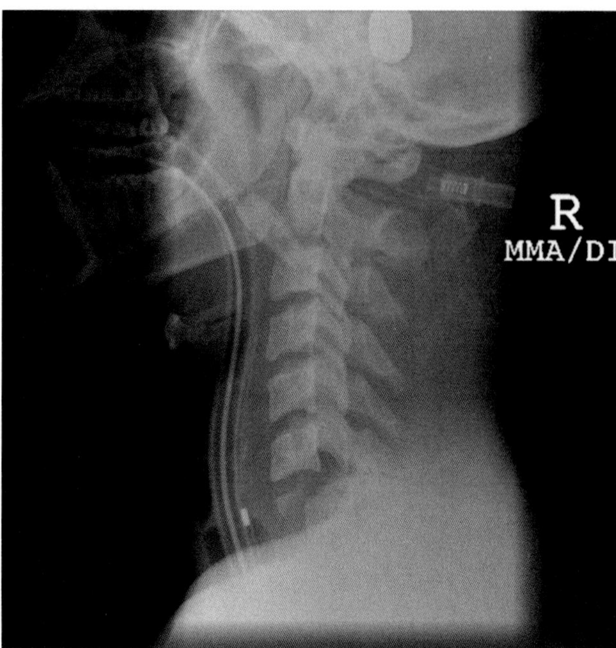

FIGURE 30.28 Lateral radiograph. Flexion teardrop fracture involving C7 with posterior subluxation of the C7 vertebral body. In this case, the teardrop was avulsed from the anterosuperior corner of the vertebral body, whereas an anteroinferior corner avulsion is more commonly seen.

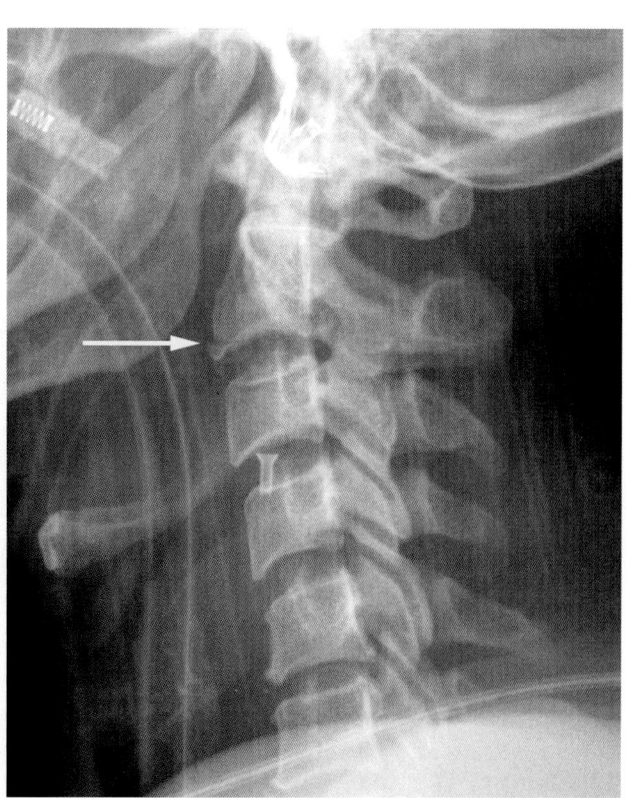

FIGURE 30.29 Lateral radiograph of the cervical spine. Extension teardrop fracture (*arrow*) with an avulsed bony fragment from the anteroinferior corner of C2.

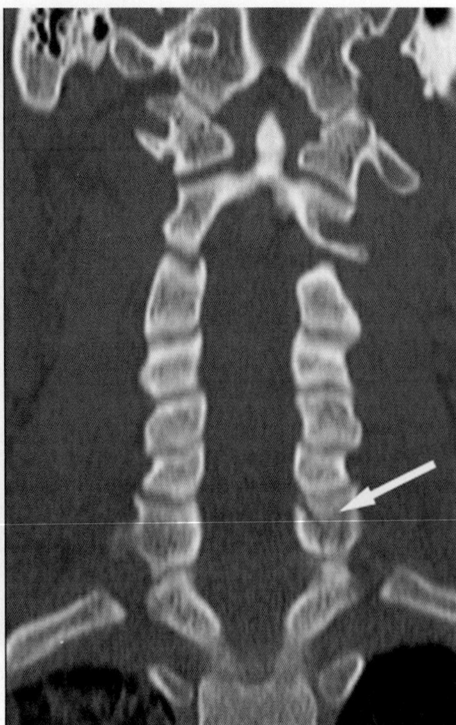

FIGURE 30.30 Coronal cervical spine CT reconstruction. Lateral flexion injury resulting in fracture of the left articular pillar of C7 (*arrow*).

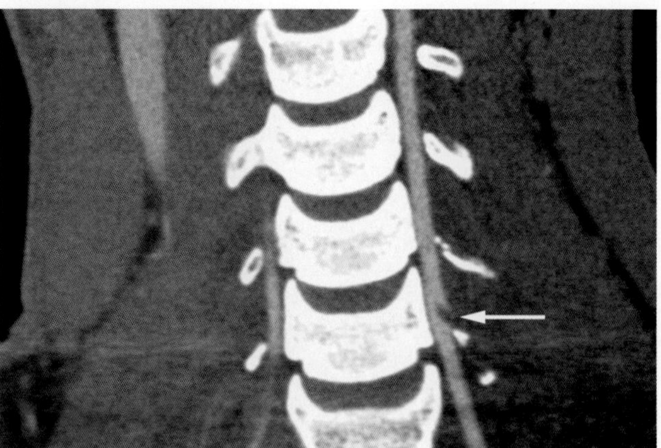

FIGURE 30.31 Coronal reformation of CT angiography. A focal defect is present in the left vertebral artery (*arrow*) immediately adjacent to transverse process fracture consistent with traumatic dissection.

Spine fractures are classified according to the mechanism of injury as axial load, hyperflexion, hyperextension, lateral flexion, or rotational injuries (Figs. 30.28–30.30). Variations of spine fractures are numerous and complex, the scope of which are beyond this text. For a comprehensive review of cervical spine trauma, refer to the suggested articles at the end of the chapter by Dreizin et al. (6) and Lustrin and colleagues (7). Often, the direction of forces involved in a spinal injury is complex, and variations and combinations of injury are seen. For example, dens fractures require a combination of flexion and extension as well as a shearing lateral force vector.

In addition to injury of the bony and ligamentous spinal column or spinal cord, vascular injury can also be associated with cervical spine trauma. The vertebral arteries arise from the subclavian arteries, usually entering the transverse foramen of the cervical vertebrae at C6. Should a fracture line cross the transverse foramen through which the vertebral artery runs, a CTA should be obtained to evaluate for traumatic injury. An intimal flap, focal narrowing, or even occlusion may be seen with vessel dissection (Fig. 30.31). Fractures that cross the carotid canal at the skull base may require similar evaluation with CTA.

When acute spinal cord compression symptoms are present, an MRI should be obtained to evaluate for a spinal epidural hematoma, acute disc herniation, or cord injury. Other than trauma, spinal epidural hematomas can be the result of anticoagulant therapy, vascular malformation, or systemic disease such as systemic lupus erythematosus. Even minor trauma can cause an epidural hematoma as the valveless venous plexus in the epidural space is prone to injury. MRI best demonstrates blood products in the epidural space (Fig. 30.32).

Spinal cord injury results in neurologic impairment. It can be caused by spinal cord compression from bony fragments, stretching injury, or impairment of the vascular supply—the anterior spinal artery in the overwhelming majority of cases. Symptoms are related to the level and severity of injury. MRI

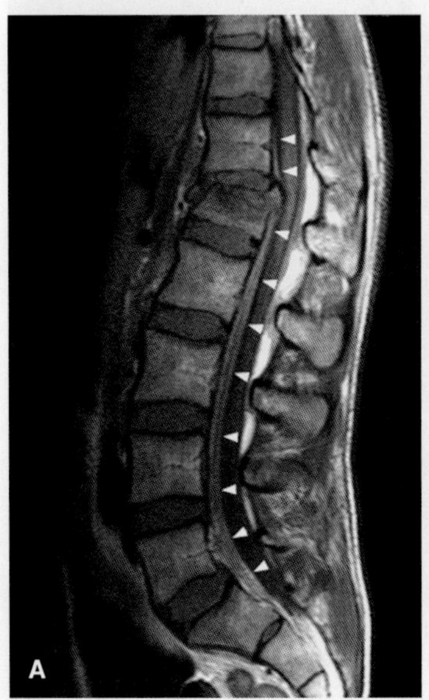

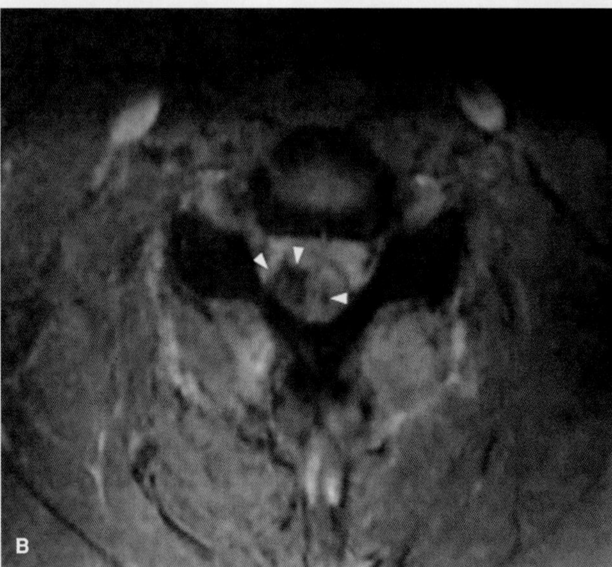

FIGURE 30.32 Sagittal (**A**) and axial (**B**) T1-weighted MRI of the lumbar spine in a patient with an L1 burst fracture. There is heterogeneous high signal intensity within the anterior epidural space extending from L1 through the upper sacrum representing epidural blood products (*arrowheads*).

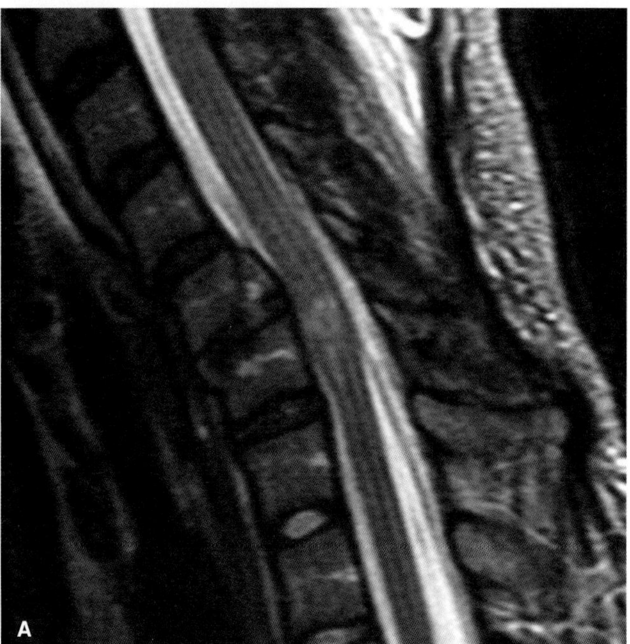

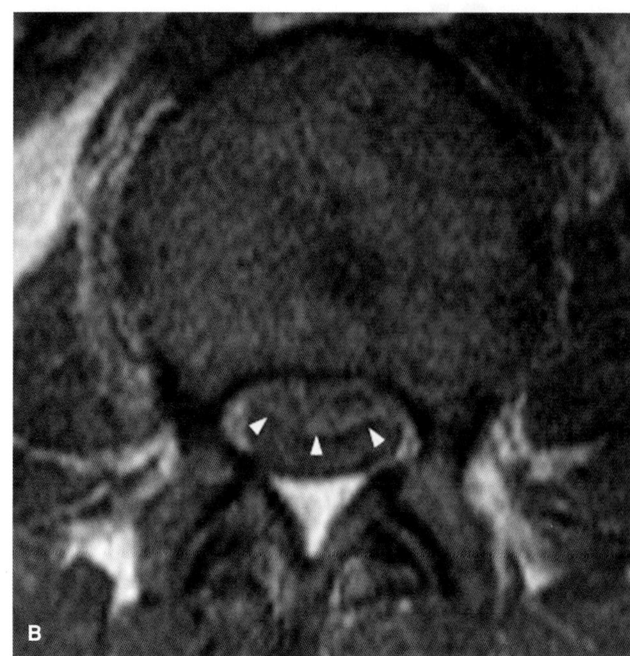

FIGURE 30.33 A: Sagittal T2-weighted MRI. A two-level fracture in the midcervical spine narrows the canal diameter and results in cord contusion manifested by high T2 signal in the cord. B: Axial gradient MRI. Areas of dark signal representing blood products are seen within the area of cord contusion (*arrowheads*).

is the imaging modality of choice in evaluating for cord and nerve root injury; increased T2 signal and enhancement are the hallmarks of injury (Fig. 30.33A). Cord contusions are often best visualized on gradient echo sequences, where the blood creates loss of signal and so appears black (Fig. 30.33B).

Key Points

- Neuroimaging may be a critical tool in the evaluation of the critically ill, particularly when their condition limits the ability to obtain accurate history and physical examination.
- Providing appropriate indications for the study is vital for the radiologist to determine the appropriate imaging parameters and sequences to be performed.
- Understanding the various patterns and locations of intracranial hemorrhage is often a valuable predictor in the acuity level, potential complications, and possible underlying etiology.
- In the acute stroke setting, imaging tools such as brain perfusion and noninvasive angiography can be valuable in determining the underlying etiology in order to appropriately triage patients for therapy.
- Although there is a wide variety of spinal fracture patterns, a basic pattern of image analysis with particular attention to alignment is the key tool in recognizing underlying spinal column injury.
- The use of flexion and extension radiographs to evaluate for underlying ligamentous injury in high-risk patients has generally fallen out of favor due to frequent inadequate flexion and extension effort by the patient and has been replaced by MRI.

References

1. Gomori JM, Grossman RI. Mechanisms responsible for the MR appearance and evolution of intracranial hemorrhage. *Radiographics*. 1988;8:427.
2. Leach JL, Fortuna RB, Jones BV, et al. Imaging of cerebral venous thrombosis: current techniques, spectrum of findings, and diagnostic pitfalls. *Radiographics*. 2006;26:S19–S41.
3. Lell MM, Anders K, Uder M, et al. New techniques in CT angiography. *Radiographics*. 2006;26:S45–S62.
4. Srinivasan A, Goyal M, Azri FA, et al. State-of-the-art imaging of acute stroke. *Radiographics*. 2006;26:S75–S95.
5. Offiah CE, Turnbull IW. The imaging appearances of intracranial CNS infections in adult HIV and AIDS patients. *Clin Radiol*. 2006;61(5):393–401.
6. Dreizin D, Letzing M, Sliker CW, et al. Multidetector CT of blunt cervical spine trauma in adults. *Radiographics*. 2014;34:1842–1865.
7. Lustrin ES, Karakas SP, Ortiz AO, et al. Pediatric cervical spine: normal anatomy, variants, and trauma. *Radiographics*. 2003;23:539.

CHAPTER

31

Point-of-Care Testing

WILLIAM E. WINTER, STACY G. BEAL, and NEIL S. HARRIS

INTRODUCTION

This chapter will focus on three aspects of laboratory testing in the intensive care unit (ICU) setting: choosing which point-of-care (POC) tests to offer, quality assurance (QA) in POC testing (POCT), and regulatory issues germane to POCT.

DEFINITION OF POINT-OF-CARE TESTING

POCT is the performance of laboratory tests in the immediate physical vicinity of the patient (1). A synonym for POCT is "near-patient testing." By definition, samples for POCT are not sent by courier or tube system to another geographically distant site.

POCT can be performed in the patient's home, business, or school; in a physician's office (e.g., a physician office laboratory [POL]); in a clinic; or near the patient's bedside in the hospital, emergency room, or operating room. POC tests can essentially be performed anywhere where trained personnel are present to provide patient care such as ICUs, operating rooms, ambulances, helicopters, ships, and airplanes. The most common POCT performed by patients is outpatient self-monitoring of blood glucose (SMBG) (2). In the outpatient setting, another commonly performed test—but far less common than SMBG—is self-testing for the prothrombin time-international normalized ratio (PT-INR) that is used to monitor and adjust warfarin doses in chronically anticoagulated patients (3).

Concerning inpatients, testing that is performed by medical technologists using central laboratory-type instruments near the patient's bedside can—geographically—qualify as POCT. However, such testing is outside the scope of this chapter, as such testing is really central laboratory testing in a noncentral laboratory location.

There are several strengths to POCT:

- Better sample stability between the time of sample drawing and analysis, often seconds in duration
- Shorter turnaround time (TAT); some results are available within a minute or less of sample acquisition
- Reduced sample volume requirements
- Immediate result availability to the respiratory therapist, nurse, or physician caring for the patient
- Opportunity for instantaneous notification of staff in cases of critical (e.g., "panic") values

CHOOSING WHICH TESTS TO RUN AT THE POINT OF CARE

POCT is most valuable when such test results immediately influence acute patient management (Tables 31.1 and 31.2) (1). An alternative way to provide rapid TATs is the placement of a satellite laboratory adjacent to the ICU or a tube system with direct sample delivery to a rapid response laboratory. Nevertheless, in resuscitations, it is difficult to argue against POCT being immediately adjacent to the patient.

If the test result will not immediately affect patient care, the higher cost of POCT compared with central laboratory testing is usually not justified. Also, POCT is usually not as accurate or precise as central laboratory testing, making central laboratory testing more advantageous in those regards. In addition, if a nurse or respiratory therapist is performing POCT, this takes time away from his or her direct patient care activities. Other experts argue that the time to perform POCT is no longer than the time it takes to draw and label a sample for transit to a central or satellite laboratory.

A list of tests appropriate for POCT in the ICU include arterial blood gas (ABG) analysis, sodium, potassium, ionized calcium, glucose, and lactate. In addition to pH, PaO_2, $PaCO_2$, and calculated bicarbonate and hemoglobin saturation—either estimated from the PaO_2 or measured directly via co-oximetry—ABG analysis provides a measurement of hemoglobin (g/dL) that can be of critical importance in postoperative patients or other patients who develop acute hypotension or manifest external evidence of bleeding, such as melena. If carbon monoxide poisoning or methemoglobinemia is present, dual-wavelength pulse oximetry will not reflect the true hemoglobin saturation. In such instances, hemoglobin saturation must be directly determined by co-oximetry or a multiwave pulse oximeter must be used. POCT for coagulation parameters is becoming increasingly important. Such tests include measurements of the PT-INR, the platelet count, thromboelastography (TEG), activated clotting time (ACT), plus a variety of more specialized tests such as the VerifyNow platelet function tests.

If cardiovascular intervention procedures are carried out in the ICU where heparin is administered in moderate to large doses, ACTs must be available within the unit to monitor heparin's effects. The ACT is monitored in such settings because such high doses of heparin will prolong the aPTT to infinity, as no clot forms. ACT is then monitored in place of the aPTT to determine when the arterial sheath can be removed. If an intravascular sheath is in place, the ACT is monitored to confirm that excessive anticoagulation is not present prior to sheath removal. The intensivist must be aware that while the term "ACT" is generic, ACT measurements performed on devices produced by different manufacturers are most often not equivalent. Thus, clotting time guidelines from one device are not necessarily transferable to another device, and such clotting guidelines must be determined for each manufacturer's ACT instrument.

While POC measurements of cardiac markers (troponin-I or troponin-T), markers of cardiac failure (B-type natriuretic peptide [BNP] or NT-proBNP [N-terminal-pro-B-type natriuretic peptide]), and emergency toxicology testing (ethanol, opiates,

TABLE 31.1 Point-of-Care Testing Recommendations for ICUs

Testing available at the point of care (POC), in a satellite laboratory adjacent to the ICU, or via rapid tube transport to a central laboratory
Arterial blood gases (includes hemoglobin concentration)
Lactate
Potassium (with or without sodium)
Glucose
Ionized calcium
Testing at a POC/satellite laboratory that is useful in special circumstances
Activated clotting time
Ionized magnesium
Examples of tests not justified at the POC or satellite laboratory
B-type natriuretic peptide/N-terminal-pro-B-type natriuretic peptide (BNP/NT-proBNP)
Cardiac markers
Endocrine testing
Iron studies (serum iron, total iron binding capacity, ferritin)
Lipid testing
Liver function testing
Prothrombin time, activated partial thromboplastin time
Renal function testing
Total magnesium
Toxicology testing

cocaine, PCP, and so forth) may be justified in the emergency room where patients require immediate triage (4), the performance of these tests at the POC in the ICU is not justified. The advantages of superior accuracy and reproducibility available through the central laboratory outweigh any TAT advantage of POCT. It is unlikely in the ICU that a cardiac marker result

TABLE 31.2 Examples of Laboratory Tests and the Decisions Based on their Results

Test	Possible Clinical Impacts
Arterial blood gases	Administration of oxygen or ventilator support
Lactate	If elevated: Need for more aggressive acute intervention with intravenous fluids, pressors, and/or improved ventilation
Na^+, K^+, Cl^-, total serum CO_2, Cr, blood urea nitrogen, serum and urine osmolality	Rates and type of fluid resuscitation or fluid restriction, need for fluid boluses, des-amino-d-arginine vasopressin (DDAVP) administration, fluid restriction for renal failure
Glucose	Attainment and maintenance of tight glycemic control
Ionized calcium	Need for intravenous calcium administration
Hemoglobin/ hematocrit	Assessment of need for transfusion of red blood cells
Platelet count	Assessment of need for platelet transfusions
Activated clotting time	Management of heparin anticoagulation and reversal of anticoagulation (e.g., protamine sulfate administration)
Prothrombin time, activated partial thromboplastic time, thrombin time, fibrinogen	Assessment of possible coagulopathy

TAT of less than 30 to 60 minutes will improve patient care. Likewise, there are no emergency decisions that need be made in the ICU or OR concerning renal function assessment, such as creatinine, blood urea nitrogen, and urinalysis, or liver function assessment, such as total protein, albumin, total and direct bilirubin, alanine aminotransferase (ALT), aspartate aminotransferase (AST), and alkaline phosphatase, that warrant routine POCT for these analytes in the ICU.

QUALITY ASSURANCE IN POINT-OF-CARE TESTING

Because many ICU decisions are based upon the results of laboratory analyses (Table 31.1), the intensivist must understand the strengths and the limitations of laboratory testing, whether performed in a central laboratory, in a satellite laboratory, or at the POC (1).

In order to provide quality results, an overview of QA concepts in laboratory testing follows. The *Clinical and Laboratory Standards Institute* (CLSI, previously named the National Committee for Clinical Laboratory Standards) defined QA as "the practice which encompasses all endeavors, procedures, formats and activities directed towards ensuring that a specified quality or product is achieved and maintained." QA programs encompass assessments of analytical quality control; monitoring of TATs, regulatory compliance, and success of proficiency testing; and supervision of personnel training and competency.

To provide quality results:

- Standard operating procedures (SOPs) must be developed and followed.
- Systems must be in place to recognize and solve random and systematic problems.
- Result reliability must be defined in terms of suitable precision and accuracy.

A QA program assesses all aspects of testing: preanalytical, analytical, and postanalytical events. Preanalytical issues concern proper patient identification and tube labeling, proper sample acquisition, appropriate transport to the central laboratory or to the POCT device (e.g., cooling of ABG samples), and timing of the test (e.g., proper timing for therapeutic drug monitoring). Analytical matters concern the instrument performance, and postanalytical issues concern proper result reporting (e.g., the correct result is reported on the correct patient).

Theoretically, the goal of laboratory testing is to produce timely and reliable (e.g., quality) measurements of analytes that assist in the diagnosis, management, and prevention of human diseases. "Analyte" is a generic term for any substance that is measured in any fluid; POC testing is most commonly carried out on blood or urine samples, and the source of blood can be arterial, capillary, or venous.

In the ICU setting, the sample of choice is usually whole blood drawn from an artery when measuring blood gases, or arterial or venous whole blood when, for example, measuring sodium, potassium, glucose, lactate, or ionized calcium. If patients are not in shock and display normal peripheral perfusion, a warmed finger or toe can be lanced to obtain a capillary whole-blood sample for glucose measurement. In the ICU setting, besides hematocrit and glucose measurements, there are no other common reasons to obtain capillary blood.

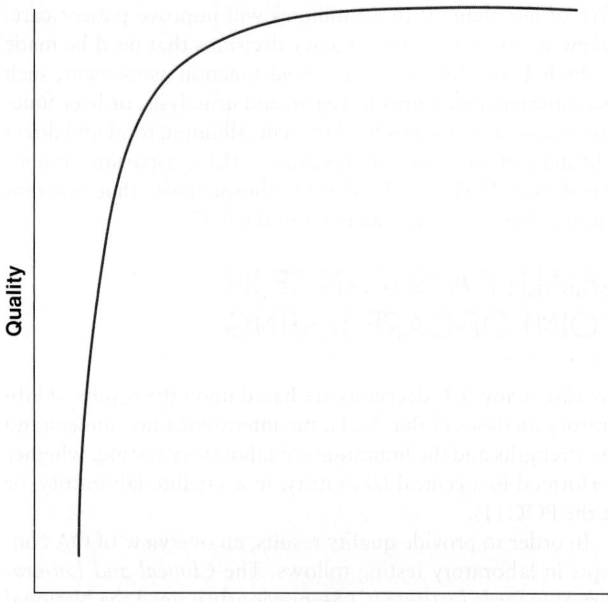

FIGURE 31.1 Relationship of quality to turnaround time (TAT).

The Value of Laboratory Test Results

The value of a test result can be conceptualized as the quality of the result divided by the TAT (Equation 1). This assumes that the laboratory data can be acted upon as soon as the data become available. Certainly, physiologic parameters that change the most rapidly attract and demand our attention, such as pH, $PaCO_2$, PaO_2, glucose, and potassium.

Quality results are accurate, and repeated measurements of the same sample demonstrate reproducibility (e.g., high precision; Equation 2). The central laboratory's ability to provide both quality results and a short TAT are often at odds with one another; more accurate and precise complex assays are usually more time consuming, and such tests may not be available on POCT devices. Figure 31.1 depicts a theoretical curve for the relationship of result quality (*y* axis) and TAT (*x* axis). If assay time is reduced below a certain limit, the quality of the assay will be reduced. On the other hand, significant delays in making critical clinical decisions can adversely affect patient outcome. We must also acknowledge that POC tests rarely, if ever, will be as accurate or precise as tests accomplished in the central laboratory.

Equation 1:

Value of a test ≈ quality of the result × turnaround time^{-1}

Note: Higher-quality results and lower turnaround times can provide higher-value tests.

Equation 2:

Quality of the result ≈ bias^{-1} × coefficient of variation^{-1}

Note: Reduced bias (e.g., higher accuracy) and reduced coefficients of variation (e.g., higher precision) improve the quality of the test result.

Desirable intrinsic characteristics of the assay for the diagnosis, management, or prediction of disease are a high sensitivity and specificity. In epidemiologic terms, *sensitivity* is the number of true positive results divided by the number of observations in a diseased population.

Sensitivity = true positives ÷ (true positives + false negatives)

Specificity is the number of true negative results divided by the number of observations undertaken in a nondiseased population.

Specificity = true negatives ÷ (true negatives + false positives)

In its broadest sense, TAT is the "vein to brain" time: The time it takes between sample acquisition (e.g., venipuncture: the *vein* time) to result recognition by the treating physician (i.e., the *brain* time). Usually TAT is defined as the duration of time between sample acquisition and result reporting. Unfortunately, the laboratory often has little control over factors that determine when a sample is delivered to the central laboratory after acquisition. Similarly, preanalytical problems frequently develop because the sample is not properly drawn, labeled, or preserved prior to delivery to the laboratory. To be of value, the correct sample must be drawn from the correct patient at the correct time in the correct volume and placed in the correct tube.

If the analysis produces the most accurate result possible, but the TAT is unacceptably long, the value of the result in patient management is significantly degraded. TAT is most important in the ICU setting when the test results are used to immediately alter the patient's care. Examples of such tests include ABG analysis for ventilated patients and glucose measurements in glycemic control protocols. There are many instances, however, where a TAT of several hours or more may be appropriate when the test is not used for immediate patient management (e.g., a karyotype result in a patient with suspected Down syndrome). Thus, the *required* TAT for any test result is *relative*. On the other hand, an instantaneous result that is not sufficiently accurate will not help—and may even hurt—the patient. It is wise to remember that bad data are worse than no data at all; physicians using bad data are misled.

Assay Performance: Precision

Precision is synonymous with reproducibility; for example, if aliquots of the original sample are retested, will the same result as the original result be observed (5)? Precision can be defined in terms of the assay's standard deviation (SD) and coefficient of variation (CV). When aliquots of a single sample are measured repeatedly, the histographic distribution of results will represent a bell-shaped curve. Other descriptions for such a distribution include a Gaussian distribution or parametric distribution.

The SD for an assay is the square root of the variance. The variance is calculated as follows: The difference between each individual value and the mean is squared, these values are summed, and the sum of the squares is then divided by the number of repeats minus one. Sixty-eight percentage of the repeats will fall within ±1 SD of the mean. Approximately 95% of the repeats will fall within ±2 SD of the mean, and approximately 99% of the repeats will fall within ±3 SD of the mean. This concept will be used in developing rules that will help us determine when an analysis and analyzer are or are not working properly.

CV is expressed as a percentage: The SD is divided by the mean multiplied by 100. While SDs have values with units—mg/dL for glucose or mmHg for pO_2—and are difficult to remember, CVs are unitless and allow easy comparisons among various analyses without needing to recall the specific SD or units. For example, electrolyte measurements using ion-selective electrodes usually display CVs of 1% to 2%. By way of comparison, analyses that use chemical reactions with spectrophotometric or electrical detection typically have CVs of 4% to 5%. As a consequence of their complex nature involving antigen–antibody interactions, immunoassays can show even greater variability, with CVs of 5% to 10%.

Precision can be further described as intra-assay or interassay reproducibility. Intra-assay precision is assessed when the same sample is run 10, 20, or more times in a single run. A "run" is the series of same analyses that are accomplished in a single day, shift, or other period of time during which the analyzer is believed to be analytically stable (e.g., does not require recalibration; many modern analyses are so stable that calibration may not be required for many days or longer). Intra-assay comparisons would not exceed 1 day.

Intra-assay precision is almost always superior to interassay precision; interassay precision is determined by measuring the same sample serially on different days (e.g., measuring the same sample once per day for 20 or more workdays in a row). For a typical chemical analysis, the intra-assay CV might be 5% and the interassay CV might be 7%. Clinicians do need to know the total imprecision—the combined intra-assay (e.g., same-day or same-shift reproducibility) and interassay (e.g., reproducibility over several days) imprecision—because some patients may be, for example, on ventilatory support for days or weeks with various degrees of pulmonary failure. While CVs (or SDs) cannot be added together to determine total imprecision, the intra-assay and interassay variances can be added together. The square root of the *total* variance then provides the SD, and the SD divided by the sample mean (multiplied by 100) provides the percentage CV.

Assay Performance: Accuracy

Accuracy is a measure of bias. *Bias* is the difference between the "real" (or "true") result and the measured result; bias can be positive or negative. A positive bias is present when the measured result exceeds the true result. A negative bias is found when the measured result is less than the true result. Bias must not be excessive; the bias that does exist must not lead to incorrect diagnosis, management, or disease prediction.

The true result of an assay may be difficult to define or determine. This is especially true when there is only one basic method available for the measurement of an analyte. For many measurements, the only method of analysis is the field method (i.e., the analytical procedure that is used in the central laboratories or at the POC). For example, pO_2 can only be measured using an oxygen-sensitive electrode. Reference methods, by definition, are more specific for the measurement of the analyte in question than the field method. Definitive methods are the best available methods of measurement with the highest specificity. Ideally, reference and definitive methods also have better precision than field methods. Because reference intervals (i.e., the "normal" ranges) are dependent on proper calibration, if there is a significant bias in calibration between the method used to establish the reference interval and the method in real-time use in the care of the patient, errors may be made in the interpretation of the result as to whether or not it falls within the reference interval, and to what degree the result may exceed or fall below the reference interval. On the other hand, relative change (i.e., the present result compared to a previous result) will not be affected by bias if instrument calibration is stable and the assay is precise. However, a lack of precision can have a major misleading effect on the interpretation of serial results. A lack of precision (i.e., imprecision) implies that larger absolute differences occur between serial measurements. With a highly precise assay, small serial differences are more likely to represent a true difference in the patient's condition. With a highly imprecise assay, larger serial differences are required to indicate a true difference in the patient's condition. To further complicate the consideration of a normal versus an abnormal result, we must consider biologic variation: The normal variation in a biologic measurement that can represent minute-to-minute or hour-to-hour fluctuations: Ultradian rhythms (e.g., luteinizing hormone [LH] or follicle-stimulating hormone [FSH] secretion); daily variations: Circadian rhythms (e.g., am vs. pm levels of cortisol); or variations greater than a day: Infradian rhythm (e.g., the menstrual period).

Analytical Sensitivity and Specificity

In analytical terms, sensitivity is the lowest concentration of an analyte that can reliably be measured. As measurements approach zero concentration of the analyte, the uncertainty of the measurement increases. At a certain point with a progressive decline in analyte concentration, the uncertainty of the measurement is so great that to report a lower number becomes meaningless. Analyzer manufacturers should define their lower limit of detection (LLD) to inform the user of the analyzer's expected analytical sensitivity. In addition, it is routine policy for laboratories to define their own LLD or, at a minimum, to confirm the manufacturer's stated LLD. In the ICU setting, LLD is most probably important in the measurement of glucose: "How low a glucose concentration can our POCT analyzer reliably report?" There are two forms of LLD. It is important to define which one the laboratory is using. One is the *Limit of Detection* (*LOD*) while the other is the *Limit of Quantitation* (*LOQ*). The LOD is the lowest concentration of an analyte that can reliably be distinguished from zero; the LOQ (also called the functional sensitivity) is the lowest concentration of an analyte that gives a reasonable precision, usually a CV of not more than 20%.

Analytical specificity is the certainty that the assay only measures the analyte of interest and does not measure other unintended substances in solution (e.g., "What is the assay's cross-reactivity to other analytes?"). Cross-reactivity is not usually an issue for POCT in ICUs based on the types of assays run in such situations. However, in the central laboratory, cross-reactivity can be a significant issue. For example, cardiac troponin-T or troponin-I measurements should not cross-react with skeletal muscle troponin-T or troponin-I. On the other hand, assay cross-reactivity is desirable if one wishes to test for a class of drugs (e.g., drug abuse testing for benzodiazepines, opiates, sympathomimetics, or barbiturates).

Quality Control Testing

For all inpatient testing, whether waived-regulated testing, moderate complexity testing, or high-complexity testing (see below), quality control must be assessed at least daily for all analytes measured on the device. For certain types of testing, such as radioimmunoassays or enzyme-linked immunosorbent assays (ELISAs), control testing may need to be performed with each run of patient samples.

To perform quality control testing, a sample of known concentration is measured with the device in question (5). This is the "control material" or, simply, the "control." The control material is usually available in a large volume and is prepared in many aliquots (e.g., >100) in a stable (e.g., frozen) form, so that the control material can be used over the course of many months to even longer than 1 year. If the control result for a run of samples falls within previously defined limits, the device and run are said to be "in control," and patient results can be reported. If the control result is outside defined limits, the device and run are said to be "out of control," meaning an analytical error has occurred and patient results cannot be reported. Another way to express an out-of-control run is to state that the run was "rejected" or "failed." Thus, before any patient results can be reported, the operator must ensure that the analyzer is functioning correctly. Clearly, the control material must be measured prior to the release of any patient results. For moderate- and high-complexity testing, at least two levels of control are usually assessed. For example, the mean value of one control can be near a clinical decision point, while the mean value of the other control value can be considerably above the clinical decision point.

If the assay is out of control, the operator must troubleshoot the problem. Possible causes of out-of-control runs include:

- Machine mechanical errors (e.g., pipetting too little or too much liquid)
- Outdated reagents
- Reagents that have lost potency due to heating or lack of refrigeration
- Degraded control materials
- Operator error (e.g., mislabeled or switched controls, as in reversing the low-level and high-level controls)
- Spectrophotometric error (e.g., bulb loss or degraded function)
- Detector error

Fortunately, most POCT devices, even if moderately complex, are self-contained, are fairly robust, and can be simply "fixed" by replacing the reagent cartridge. If nothing else, another POCT analyzer can be used.

James Westgard created a series of rules that can be used to determine if a run or device is in control or is out of control (5). These "Westgard rules," or their variations, are used essentially universally throughout the laboratory community. For each control material, the performance of the material is initially established by running this sample daily over the course of 20 to 30 days when the assay is otherwise known to be in control by using previously characterized control materials. From these data, the mean and the SD for the sample's measurement (e.g., the control material's "performance") on the device in question can be calculated.

Once the performance of the control material is known (i.e., its mean value and SD are established), this material can then be used to determine if subsequent runs are in control. If a single control value is 3 or fewer SDs away from the mean, the assay is in control and the results can be released. While, strictly speaking, being in control—a control result of +2 to +3 SDs above or −2 to −3 SDs below the mean—is a "warning," the operator should review previous control data and confirm that other instrument parameters are functioning normally.

TABLE 31.3 Westgard Quality Control Rules for a Single Level of Control

Rule Name	Rule Definition
1_{2s}	One control result is between 2 and 3 standard deviations (SDs) above or below the mean (warning only; all other rules are rejection rules)
1_{3s}	One control result greater than 3 SDs above or below the mean (random error)
2_{2s}	Two sequential control results between 2 and 3 SDs both above or both below the mean
2_{4s}	Two sequential control results with a total range of greater than 4 SDs (random error)
4_{1s}	Four sequential control results greater than 1 SD above or below the mean (systematic error)
10_m	Ten sequential control results above or below the mean (systematic error)

If the control result exceeds the mean value ±3 SDs, this is such an unlikely event (e.g., this should occur at random no more than in ~1% of all runs) as to suggest that the run is "out of control." A single out-of-control run represents the consequence of a random error. On the other hand, if in two sequential runs a control displays a warning result each time (on the same side of the mean), the second run is out of control. This is the 2_{2S} rule and demonstrates a probable systematic (i.e., nonrandom) error. The Westgard quality control errors are summarized in Table 31.3; systematic errors reflect recurrent errors such as short sampling and a degraded reagent, a constant interference, or loss of calibration.

For many POCT assays, the mechanics of the measuring device (e.g., electrodes) are designed into a single-use, disposable cartridge. In such cases, individual cartridges cannot be quality controlled, as measurement of a control material in the cartridge expends the cartridge. However, when such cartridges are manufactured using highly automated and monitored systems, the reproducibility of the manufacturing process can be so highly regulated that minimal variation exists among cartridges within a single manufacturing run, batch, or lot. While individual cartridges cannot be tested for quality control, the batch of cartridges can be assessed upon receipt by the health care institution by measuring a control material in one or more cartridges chosen at random from the batch received. Devices that use disposable cartridges can have their electronics or optics checked daily or more often via electronic quality control. In electronic quality control, a cartridge simulator is placed into the instrument to test if the instrument reports the proper result as defined for the simulator.

REGULATORY ISSUES IN POINT-OF-CARE TESTING

Laboratory testing, both at the POC and in satellite or central laboratories, is highly regulated by the Clinical Laboratory Improvement Amendments (CLIA) passed by the U.S. Congress in 1988. The shorthand term for the subsequent regulations is "CLIA 88" or, more simply, "CLIA." Laboratories that perform ex vivo tests on any human tissue or body fluid must be certified by the Secretary of Health and Human Services (HHS).

Analyses where a biologic sample is not intentionally removed from the body does not fall under CLIA regulations.

These types of analyses reflect *monitoring* and not *testing* according to CLIA. Examples of such analyses include measurement of the partial pressure of exhaled carbon dioxide, alcohol breathalyzers, exhalation of $^{13}CO_2$ after oral administration of ^{13}C-urea in search of *Helicobacter pylori* infection, transcutaneous bilirubinometers, pulse oximetry, and intermittent arterial sampling via indwelling cannula for blood gases when the blood is returned to the patient's body. Incidentally, workplace drug abuse testing does not fall under the CLIA regulations.

The CLIA laboratory certification program is operated by the Centers for Medicare and Medicaid Services (CMS), the Food and Drug Administration (FDA), and the Centers for Disease Control and Prevention (CDC). Specific information on CLIA can be found at http://www.fda.gov/medicaldevices/deviceregulationandguidance/ivdregulatoryassistance/ucm124105.htm (the FDA CLIA website that addresses complexity test categorizations and waivers); http://www.cms.hhs.gov/clia (the CMS CLIA website concerning program information, statistics, etc.); and http://wwwn.cdc.gov/clia/ (the CDC CLIA website regarding regulations).

Currently the FDA determines whether an in vitro diagnostic test (including the test system) is waived or nonwaived; nonwaived tests are further classified as moderate complexity or high complexity. Therefore, there are three major CLIA regulatory categories: waived testing, moderate-complexity testing, and high-complexity testing. The location of testing—POC versus satellite or central laboratory—does not define the complexity of the testing. Moderate-complexity testing can be performed immediately adjacent to the OR or ICU in a satellite laboratory, while, alternatively, a waived test (e.g., BNP) can be performed in a central laboratory.

The main differences between waived and nonwaived testing (from the regulatory perspective) are as follows.

- Method validation is needed for all nonwaived tests. For all FDA-approved nonwaived tests, the key principle is one of *verification*: verification of accuracy by comparing the results of the POC test with an assay for the same analyte either in the same laboratory or elsewhere, verification of precision (both within-run and run-to-run), and verification of the limit of detection (LOD) or limit of quantitation (LOQ) of the assay.
- All nonwaived tests require *proficiency testing* otherwise known as *external quality assurance (EQA)*. This is the means by which externally provided specimens are analyzed by the laboratory and the results are graded by an independent agency.
- Nonwaived tests, in some states, can only be performed by licensed personnel.

Waived Testing

Waived tests are defined as determinations that can be performed at any site by any operator following the manufacturer's recommendations. Theoretically, a waived test is a test that is so simple to perform that it is believed to carry little risk of error. CLIA describes waived tests as "simple procedures with little chance of negative outcomes if performed inaccurately." However in the real world, experience teaches us that even waived tests can be performed improperly and erroneous results from certain waived tests in various situations can undoubtedly lead to potentially serious or fatal adverse outcomes (e.g., underestimation or overestimation of the PT/INR in patients being treated with warfarin for anticoagulation).

A common misconception in the hospital setting is that waived POC tests can be plugged in, switched on, and used immediately by any and all operators, with perhaps an occasional glance at the instructions. There are however major differences in process between waived POC tests performed by the patient at home (e.g., SMBG, HbA_{1c} testing, pregnancy testing etc.) and waived POC tests run in the hospital setting.

Any waived hospital-based POC test will require that:

- The manufacturer's instructions need to be followed exactly as written.
- An SOP must be on file and readily available to all operators.
- Reagents need to be stored correctly.
- Controls need to be analyzed as recommended by the manufacturer.
- Results need to be documented in the electronic medical record.
- Documentation of operator competency needs to be performed.

Failure to comply with these requirements may shift the test category from a waived to a nonwaived high-complexity category; this is especially so if the manufacturer's instructions are not followed and the method is modified. High-complexity testing for practical purposes cannot be implemented in the POC setting.

Hospitals must develop procedures and policies that specify the circumstances in which waived test results are employed in patient management, services, and treatment. To achieve this, waived test results must be placed in the clinical record, along with the appropriate reference interval (i.e., the "normal range"). The need for confirmatory testing must be defined; for example, if the POCT blood glucose is less than 60 mg/dL or greater than 500 mg/dL, a blood sample is sent to the central laboratory for confirmation (note: the specific cutoffs depend upon the POCT analyzer). For inpatient waived testing to be performed properly, CLIA mandates that the staff executing the test must be identified, supervised, and qualified to perform the test. This requires adequate specific training and orientation to test performance and documentation of a satisfactory level of competence. This applies to all health care providers, including physicians. Competency must be demonstrated at the time of orientation training and yearly thereafter. Determination of competency must include at least two of the following four assessments.

- Performing a test on an unknown specimen
- Observation by a supervisor or qualified delegate
- Monitoring the user's quality control performance
- Written testing relevant to the waived test method

Other CLIA standards for inpatient waived testing include that written policies and procedures are readily available and kept up to date; quality control checks are defined and conducted on each procedure; and the quality control results are recorded and maintained for review.

Examples of waived tests are given in Table 31.4. Presently, there are at least 40 waived tests; the current list of waived tests and devices can be found at http://www.accessdata.fda.gov/scripts/cdrh/cfdocs/cfClia/testswaived.cfm.

TABLE 31.4 Examples of Waived Tests

B-type natriuretic peptide
Bladder tumor–associated antigen
Blood lead
Estrone 3-glucuronide
Fecal occult blood
Gastric occult blood, gastric pH
Hematocrit, spun
Hemoglobin (whole blood)
Hemoglobin A_{1c}
Ketones in blood
Lipids: Cholesterol, triglycerides, high-density lipoprotein cholesterol
Lithium
Nasal swab for influenza A/B
Platelet aggregation studies
Prothrombin time-international normalized ratio
Saliva fern test
Thyroid-stimulating hormone
Urine creatinine
Urine dipstick test strips (e.g., pH, specific gravity, protein, glucose, blood, ketones, urobilinogen, bilirubin, leukocytes, nitrites)
Urine human chorionic gonadotropin, luteinizing hormone (an LH ovulation test), follicle-stimulating hormone (FSH for menopause testing)
Urine microalbumin
Urine toxicology testing (e.g., cocaine, tetrahydrocannabinol (THC), amphetamines, methamphetamine, phencyclidine (PCP), barbiturates, tricyclic antidepressants, methylenedioxy-methamphetamine (MDMA), opiates, oxycodone, morphine, propoxyphene, etc.)
Various chemistry tests (e.g., total protein, total bilirubin, alanine aminotransferase, alkaline phosphatase, amylase, γ-glutamyl transpeptidase, blood urea nitrogen)
Various tests for infection (e.g., monospot, *Helicobacter pylori* antibodies, group A *Streptococcus*, vaginal aerobic/anaerobic organisms, adenovirus, respiratory syncytial virus)

Note: Approval of a test as being waived is device specific; listing a test in this table does not imply that all versions of the test are waived.

It is important to recognize that CLIA approval of a test as being waived is device specific: The test and the device are together approved as being waived for a specific analysis. For example, just because one manufacturer's test for blood glucose is waived does not mean that all single-use strip measurements of glucose by all manufacturers are waived.

A laboratory or health care unit performing only waived tests must obtain a certificate of waiver (COW). COW laboratories are required to follow manufacturers' test instructions, participate in the CLIA program, and pay applicable biennial certificate fees. This is relevant outside the formal boundaries of the hospital and ICU setting.

Moderate- and High-Complexity Testing

CLIA defines moderate-complexity tests as being more intricate than waived tests. Moderate-complexity testing is typically carried out on automated analyzers. Examples of such tests include blood counts and routine chemistries. High-complexity tests are still more complicated, usually involving nonautomated or complicated analyses requiring considerable technologist or laboratory professional judgment, such as cross-matching of blood, electrophoresis, or microbiology testing.

Seven categories are considered when classifying the complexity of a nonwaived test.

- Required operator knowledge
- Operator training and experience
- Preparation of reagents and materials
- Characteristics of the operational steps
- Calibration, quality control, and proficiency testing
- Test system troubleshooting and equipment maintenance
- Test result interpretation and judgment

For each category, the complexity of the test is scored: A score of 1 indicates the lowest level of complexity, and a score of 3 indicates the highest level. A score of 2 indicates complexity intermediate between 1 and 3. If the total score for the seven criteria is 12 or less, the test/device system is categorized as moderate complexity, whereas those test/device systems receiving scores above 12 are codified as high complexity.

Moderate- and high-complexity tests require quality control, proficiency testing, a QA program, and so forth. There are also specific and detailed requirements regarding personnel qualifications and, as an aside, the experienced laboratorian recognizes that their most important resource is a highly skilled staff. Excluding provider-performed microscopy (PPM), which is a subset of moderate-complexity testing, all nonwaived tests are generally the purview of the pathologist and the clinical laboratory, or supervised by the pathologist and the clinical laboratory. Similar to waived, but regulated, POC tests, all moderate-complexity tests performed at the POC are regulated and, at a minimum, require similar training, supervision, quality control, and proficiency testing as waived inpatient tests.

Many POC testing devices applicable to ICUs are of moderate complexity. Some POCT devices applicable to ICUs perform only blood gas measurements (pH, pO_2, pCO_2), while the option to perform co-oximetry may also be available. Other devices will measure Na^+, K^+, glucose, ionized Ca^{2+}, and/or lactate, in addition to blood gases. At least one device on the market has the capacity to measure cardiac markers and PT-INR in addition to the above parameters. Some devices can perform a wide battery of non–blood gas analyses and may not even be of moderate complexity (e.g., the Abaxis Piccolo POC Chemistry Analyzer [Abaxis North America, Union City, CA] performs 11 chemistry panels that are CLIA waived and regulated).While not attempting to provide an exhaustive list of all available blood gas analyzers, robust blood gas analyzers are available from a variety of manufacturers, including the following.

- Abbott Point of Care Inc., Princeton, NJ: iStat
- Siemens RAPIDPoint 500 Blood Gas System, Siemens Healthcare Diagnostics, Inc., Tarrytown, NY
- Accriva Diagnostics, San Diego, CA: Avoximeter 1000E Whole Blood Oximeter & Avoximeter 4000
- Nova Biomedical, Waltham, MA: Stat Profile pHOx Series
- Radiometer America Inc., Westlake, OH: ABL90 FLEX, ABL80 FLEX CO-OX and ABL80 FLEX

Some of these devices are completely mobile and hand-held (e.g., iStat), while other analyzers can be pole-mounted (Radiometer ABL80 and ABL90) or only require a small amount of bench space (e.g., they have a small "footprint").

There are important financial considerations in providing ICU POC testing. Which cost center is going to be responsible for financing the new equipment? Is the equipment going to be a capital purchase, a reagent rental, or an equipment lease? Will a service contract be needed (most likely "yes") and how much does this cost? Will the equipment require a laboratory information system (LIS) interface, and how much will that cost?

Intensivists should work closely with their hospital's clinical pathologists and POCT coordinators in determining what type of acute testing should be available in their ICU. With the emergence of improved glycemic control as a general principle of inpatient care, blood glucose testing must be available at the POC in ICUs. Such testing should be robust, accurate, and precise, and suffer from few, if any, critical interferences. These characteristics must also be sought in any POCT device that is brought into the ICU or OR. Likewise, the device must be FDA-approved approved for use in the care of critically ill patients.

The need for POCT for blood gas analysis and other tests depends on the ease of sample delivery to a satellite or central hospital laboratory and result TAT. In our satellite "STAT" laboratory located immediately outside the operating room complex and adjacent to many of the ICUs, 90% of blood gas results are reported in 10 minutes or less.

If blood gas analyses are performed in the ICU, unless personnel are added to the ICU staff, the work load is transferred, to some extent, to the ICU nursing or respiratory care staff from the laboratory staff. However, there may be time savings in the ICU if a sample does not need to be prepared for transit to the satellite or central laboratory, and it is this immediacy of the test result that *may* improve patient care. Nevertheless, it is very difficult to find evidence-based medicine studies that clearly demonstrate better patient outcomes that result from reduced laboratory TATs. Even if patient care is not markedly improved, reduced TATs may aid in transferring patients to the floor or home more quickly. Patients may be more rapidly weaned from ventilation, which may decrease the use of resources. After improving patient outcomes, the next most important outcome variable for most hospital administrators is the expense of care and the need to reduce those costs (6).

If the decision has been made to proceed with POCT in the ICU, the analyzer and the support system must be carefully chosen. Ideally, the POCT device should have the ability to easily interface with the LIS to enable laboratory data transfer, billing, quality control data management, and tracking of operator competency (7). The nursing staff or respiratory care staff who will perform the testing should have a voice in the analyzer choice. The device's reproducibility must be examined (i.e., the precision of the device) (5), and the device results should be correlated with those of the central laboratory in search of biases (i.e., the accuracy of the device) (5).

Just as important as the analyzer is the quality of the blood sample that will be used for testing. For example, blood for a glucose measurement that is drawn through a line through which glucose has been infused may give falsely elevated values unless a sufficient "blank" sample is drawn through the line—in other words, "clearing the line" beforehand. Recall that D5 has a glucose concentration of 5,000 mg/dL (50 times greater than normal) and D10 has a glucose concentration of 10,000 mg/dL (100 times greater than normal). Another example of such a preanalytical error is the exposure of blood to room air when blood gas testing is warranted. Blood samples exposed to room air can exhibit an increased pO_2, decreased pCO_2, and increased pH. When POCT devices that require cartridges are used, proper filling of the cartridge is essential to obtain a valid result. Wasting cartridges is expensive; in some systems, individual cartridges may cost several dollars, as opposed to pennies per test in a central laboratory.

Analytical interferences must be considered in the choice of ICU POCT instruments. An interference can bias a result. Examples of interferences affecting certain central laboratory tests include hyperlipidemia, hyperbilirubinemia, and hemolysis. At the POC, some blood glucose testing devices that use glucose dehydrogenase and the PQQ reagent (pyrroloquinolinequinone) display positive interferences when maltose is present in the patient's bloodstream. Maltose is used as a stabilizer in drugs such as intravenous immunoglobulin, and icodextrin that is used in dialysis is metabolized to maltose. This positive interference can lead to an overestimate of the blood glucose and subsequent overtreatment of "hyperglycemia," with severe or even fatal hypoglycemia as the consequence. Such devices have now been modified by the manufacturers to improve the analytical specificity and eliminate the maltose interference (Roche Accucheck Inform II). Glucose oxidase devices that use the patient's blood as a source of oxygen exhibit negative biases in the glucose measurement in cases of hypoxia or where the elevation is over approximately 5,000 ft. On the other hand, glucose oxidase devices that use ferrocene or ferricyanide display positive biases in blood glucose when the patient is hypoxic and negative biases when the patient is hyperoxic, such as a ventilated patient receiving supplemental oxygen.

Quality control for the POCT must be carried out and monitored as part of an overall QA program. All device operators will require initial training and competency testing. Cost per test must also be a consideration. POCT can be 10 or more times as expensive as central laboratory testing. In considering any POCT in the ICU, the pathologist and POCT coordinator must be involved in this process from the start, as this fosters a collegial relationship and best decision for the institution. In the end, the ultimate goal is to provide excellent patient care. New laboratory tests will continue to appear that will influence ICU care such as test panels for stroke and sepsis and improved cardiac risk panels. Prudent review of the medical literature and cooperation between the ICU staff and the laboratory staff will help determine where such testing is best carried out.

Key Points

- Every hospital and ICU is distinctive and has unique laboratory needs.
- The nursing staff, intensivists, POCT coordinators, and clinical pathologists should work together to define the appropriate testing mix for their institution.
- The take-home message for the intensivist and patient care staff is that POCT must be quality controlled to ensure a high reliability of test results.
- Intensivists and patient care staff must ensure that all regulatory rules are followed and enforced. This provides the best environment possible for the provision of accurate and precise laboratory test results.

References

1. Nichols JH. Point-of-care testing. In: Nichols JH, ed. *Point-of-Care Testing, Performance Improvement and Evidence-Based Outcomes*. New York: Marcel Dekker; 2003:1.
2. Winter WE. Point-of-care testing in the management of diabetes mellitus. In: Nichols JH, ed. *Point-of-Care Testing, Performance Improvement and Evidence-Based Outcomes*. New York: Marcel Dekker; 2003:235.
3. Nuttall GA, Santrach P. Hemoglobin and coagulation. In: Nichols JH, ed. *Point-of-Care Testing, Performance Improvement and Evidence-Based Outcomes*. New York: Marcel Dekker; 2003:353.
4. Christenson RH, Azzazy El-Badaway HME. Point-of-care testing for biochemical markers of acute coronary syndromes. In: Nichols JH, ed. *Point-of-Care Testing, Performance Improvement and Evidence-Based Outcomes*. New York: Marcel Dekker; 2003:379.
5. Westgard JO, Klee GG. Quality management. In: Burtis CA, Ashwood ER, Bruns DE, eds. *Tietz Textbook of Clinical Chemistry and Molecular Diagnostics*. St. Louis, MO: Elsevier Saunders; 2006:485.
6. Schallom L. Point of care testing in critical care. *Crit Care Nurs Clin North Am*. 1999;11:99.
7. Halpern NA. Point of care diagnostics and networks. *Crit Care Clin*. 2000; 16:623.

SECTION 4 **TECHNIQUES, PROCEDURES, AND TREATMENTS**

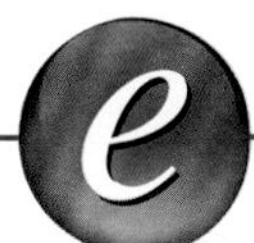

This chapter can be accessed in the accompanying eBook (see inside front cover for access instructions).

CHAPTER **32**

Clean and Aseptic Techniques at the Bedside

RABIH O. DAROUICHE and MAYAR AL MOHAJER

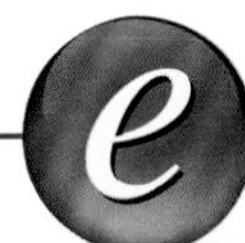

This chapter can be accessed in the accompanying eBook (see inside front cover for access instructions).

CHAPTER **33**

Vascular Cannulation

KELLEY A. SOOKRAJ and LOUIS R. PIZANO

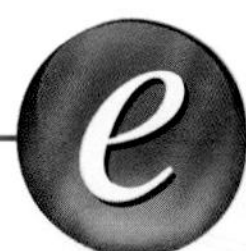

This chapter can be accessed in the accompanying eBook (see inside front cover for access instructions).

CHAPTER **34**

Temporary Cardiac Pacemakers

MATTHEW S. McKILLOP and JAMIE B. CONTI

This chapter can be accessed in the accompanying eBook (see inside front cover for access instructions).

CHAPTER 35

Important Intensive Care Procedures

DANIEL D. YEH and GEORGE C. VELMAHOS

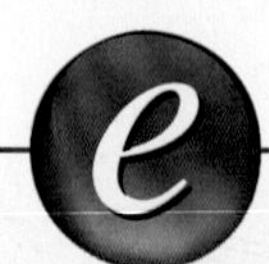

This chapter can be accessed in the accompanying eBook (see inside front cover for access instructions).

CHAPTER 36

Interventional Radiology

KEITH PETERS

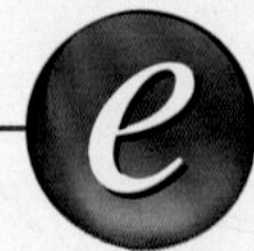

This chapter can be accessed in the accompanying eBook (see inside front cover for access instructions).

CHAPTER 37

Feeding Tube Placement

LAWRENCE CARUSO and DANIEL R. LAYON

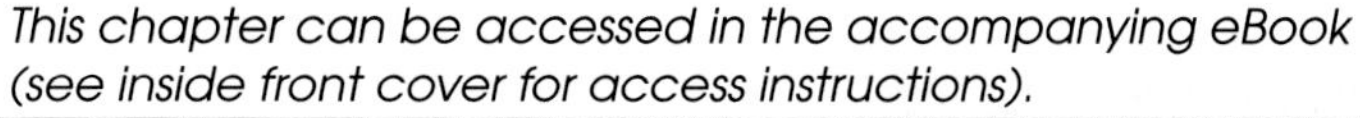

This chapter can be accessed in the accompanying eBook (see inside front cover for access instructions).

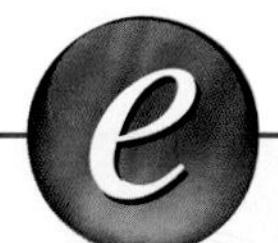

CHAPTER 38

Flexible Bronchoscopy

YATIN B. MEHTA and MICHAEL A. JANTZ

This chapter can be accessed in the accompanying eBook (see inside front cover for access instructions).

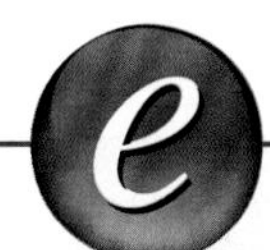

CHAPTER 39

Airway Management

TOM MORT and JEFF KECK

This chapter can be accessed in the accompanying eBook (see inside front cover for access instructions).

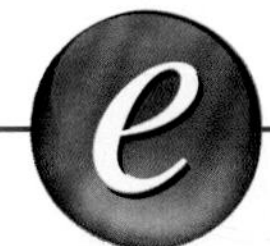

CHAPTER 40

Indications for and Management of Tracheostomy

JUDI ANNE B. RAMISCAL, MICHAEL HAYASHI and MIHAE YU

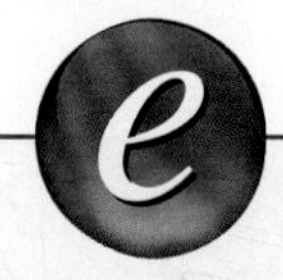

This chapter can be accessed in the accompanying eBook (see inside front cover for access instructions).

CHAPTER
41

Hyperbaric Oxygen Therapy

RICHARD MOON

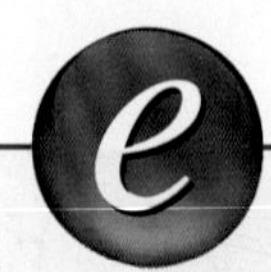

This chapter can be accessed in the accompanying eBook (see inside front cover for access instructions).

CHAPTER
42

Anesthesia

AVNER SIDI

CHAPTER 43

The Host Response to Injury and Critical Illness

CHRISTIAN STOPPE and ANDREAS GOETZENICH

INTRODUCTION

In 1794 John Hunter wrote: "There is a circumstance attending accidental injury which does not belong to disease—namely, that the injury has in all cases a tendency to produce both the disposition and the means of a cure." This first described the stress response, a biphasic physiologic response that, when uninterrupted by complications, has predictable characteristics and lasts 7 to 10 days. The early phase that occurs immediately following injury is characterized by a hyperinflammatory response with excessive release of mainly proinflammatory cytokines, chemokines, and reactive oxygen species. It lasts roughly for about 24 hours and is followed by a period of immune suppression that characteristically persists for about 5 to 7 days. The driving force for this second phase appears to lie with the need to mount an immune or inflammatory response to combat infection and facilitate repair of damaged tissues. Most markers for ongoing inflammation start to rapidly increase about 8 to 12 hours after the stimulus, and demonstrate peak levels on postinjury day 2, returning to baseline around day 7.

SURGERY, AN ELECTIVE TRAUMA

In the context of host response, there is little difference between accidental and surgical trauma. From a research perspective, the surgical intervention's projectable timeframe has enabled a better understanding of signaling pathways and mechanistic models. Simultaneously, strategies emerged to attenuate and modulate the overwhelming inflammatory response elicited by major surgery; many of these strategies failed to improve—or even worsened—clinical outcome. This suggests a "janiform" role of the physiologic stress reaction in the body's management of injury: While harmful if exaggerated, it is mandatory to induce regeneration and preservation strategies.

PATHOPHYSIOLOGY

David P. Cuthbertson was the first to study the host response to injury and in 1929 proposed a paradigm by which the body responded to injury: If the damage to the patient is not immediately fatal, there is a compensatory reaction in which vasoconstriction shunts blood away from the periphery and toward central organs, most notably the heart and brain; this promotes short-term survival. Hypothermia and oliguria are associated with a global decrease in oxygen consumption and energy expenditure; in an effort to expand plasma volume and avoid failed oxygen delivery, the body conserves salt and water by increasing aldosterone secretion (1). These effects are seen throughout the body in the first 24 hours after injury. Cuthbertson termed this sequence of events the "ebb" phase of traumatic shock. When death is not imminent, a second aspect of the response emerges, the key to which is an attempt to repair tissue damage, accomplished via the activity of white blood cells (WBCs). As part of the initial inflammatory response, the release of chemotactic mediators and involvement of the complement cascade trigger the migration of immune cells to the site of inflammation.

The immunologic defense capacity is determined by the functional interplay between the innate and the adaptive immune systems (2). The initial recognition of infectious agents or damage is carried out by the innate immune system; the sensing of pathogens is performed by specialized, sentinel immune cells, which are located in tissues with direct contact to the environment. The interaction between pathogen- and damage-associated molecular patterns (PAMPs/DAMPs) and their receptors results in induction of different signal transduction pathways and the transcription of various genes, which further results in an increased production of inflammatory and immunoregulatory cytokines (2).

As an important contributor to the innate immune system, inflammasomes—cytosolic protein complexes—assemble in response to DAMPs and PAMPs, resulting in the activation of caspase-1 and generation of the proinflammatory cytokines interleukin (IL)-1β and IL-18. The NLRP3 inflammasome is currently the most fully characterized and consists of NLRP3 (NACHT, LRR, and PYD domains-containing protein), ASC (apoptosis-associated speck-like protein containing a caspase recruitment domain), and caspase-1, which is its central effector protein. The inflammasome participates in both physiologic and pathologic inflammatory processes and contributes to several systemic diseases (3–5).

Inflammatory and immunoregulatory cytokines regulate the ensuing cellular and humoral immune response. Mouse strains with deletions in genes encoding cytokines or cytokine receptors show an increased susceptibility to infection (6). The uncontrolled increase of proinflammatory cytokines, in turn, frequently contributes to the development of organ dysfunctions and severe complications in patients with sepsis and septic shock. Cytokines act by binding cognate receptors expressed on target cells to activate signal transduction pathways, gene transcription, and the expression of downstream effector molecules. Additionally, release of chemotactic mediators triggers the migration of immune cells, and slowed circulation in the ebb phase allows WBCs to move toward the periphery and adhere to the endothelium. Neutrophils react first, with macrophages following. With restoration of the circulation, the process becomes active. It is characterized by phagocytosis and lysis of bacterial, viral, or fungal invaders, and removal of cellular debris. In addition, macrophages, lymphocytes, and antigen-presenting cells (APCs) secrete cytokines, which serve to further amplify the overall inflammatory response; to a great extent, these are growth factors such as vascular endothelial growth factor (VEGF) that facilitate repair of damaged tissue by stimulating angiogenesis and vasculogenesis.

The process of repair and recovery requires enormous amounts of energy, with a 2- to 20-fold increase in oxygen consumption and resting energy expenditure (REE). In sequence, body temperature rises, and oxygen consumption and carbon dioxide production increase (1,7). Monk et al. showed an increase in REE of up to 55% above predicted in trauma patients (8). Other studies demonstrated that survival is dependent partly on the ability to maintain hypermetabolism and adequate oxygen utilization (7,9–12). Because WBCs are, more or less, obligate glucose users, there is an associated increase in glucose requirements (13). After the first 24 hours, hepatic glycogen stores are depleted and a source of de novo glucose is required; this is generated by hepatic gluconeogenesis. However, adequate mobilization is not enough to ensure substrate delivery. Therefore, the response includes capillary dilatation to increase flow and improve delivery. Unfortunately, due to thrombosis in damaged tissue, most injured areas are avascular. To allow substrate delivery to these regions, capillary tight junctions separate allowing fluid and substrate to "leak" from the vasculature. Increased vascular permeability results in redistribution of extracellular fluid and plasma proteins to form edema and exudate (14). Glucose and other nutrients move down their concentration gradients across the extracellular matrix to areas of damage. Removal of waste requires an increase in renal blood flow and glomerular filtration to enable excretion of amino acid degradation products.

Early studies demonstrated that initiation of the flow phase is, in part, hormonally modulated. An initial, dramatic, release of endogenous catecholamines (15) is supplemented by alterations in the somatotropic system (growth hormone and insulin-like growth factor) such that anabolism is postponed and energy substrates are redirected to vital organs; both the thyroid and the gonadal axes are suppressed. Adrenocorticotropin hormone (ACTH) secretion is heightened by increased corticotropin-releasing hormone (CRH), arginine vasopressin (AVP), catecholamines, angiotensin II, serotonin, and some proinflammatory cytokines (IL-1, IL-2, IL-3, IL-6), tumor necrosis factor (TNF), macrophage migration inhibitory factor (MIF), and anti-inflammatory cytokines, including IL-10 and IL-1RA (16,17). ACTH stimulates the adrenal glands to produce glucocorticoids and mineralocorticoids; glucocorticoids and glucagon promote glucogenesis and glycogenolysis and induce peripheral insulin resistance, leading to increased glucose production (18), this, in turn, increases insulin secretion, producing an "insulin-resistant" state.

Hemorrhage and traumatized tissue further contribute to the excessive release of these mediators, which initiates the tissue repair by trafficking immune cells, such as macrophages to the injured tissue. In case of hemorrhage, the coagulation cascade is triggered by both the intrinsic and extrinsic pathways. This also serves to sustain and enhance immune cell migration and activation. In addition, fibroblasts at the edge of the wound divide, migrate toward the center, and produce collagen. New capillaries bud, and the neovascularization further supports the repair and tissue regenerating. Eventually the wound edges will fuse and consist of vascularized granulation tissue; this process is mediated by an increase in fibroblast growth factors, epidermal growth factor, platelet-derived growth factor, and VEGF (19,20).

This massive mobilization of defense mechanisms may also affect normal tissue. Therefore, one of the most important characteristics of the normal stress response is the balance between the inflammatory and the anti-inflammatory systems. This involves the proinflammatory cytokines TNF-α and MIF, which are released by the activated macrophages and various other cell types in response to infection, hypoxia, or harmful stimuli. TNF-α is capable of stimulating the medullary reticular formation and the hypothalamus in the brain; this activation of the hypothalamic–pituitary–adrenal axis ultimately causes increased anti-inflammatory activity. For example, glucocorticoids released as a result of this process limit the negative biologic consequences caused by inflammation (21). TNF-α also stimulates the dorsal vagal complex and alters the efferent vagal output; this is, in part, responsible for "sickness" behavior, such as anorexia and fever (22–24). More importantly, however, is neuromodulation of the immune response. The "inflammatory reflex" or the cholinergic anti-inflammatory pathway occurs when proinflammatory cytokines such as IL-1β and TNF-α stimulate the parasympathetic nervous system through receptors on the vagus nerve. The afferent input travels to the nucleus solitarius and is relayed to the dorsal motor nucleus, resulting in an increase in acetylcholine release at cholinergic nerve terminals in the areas of inflammation. Activated macrophages have acetylcholine receptors that, when stimulated, decrease the release of proinflammatory cytokines (25,26). Beside the release of anti-inflammatory markers, this balance of the systems is crucial in limiting the overall stress response.

Moore et al. (15) also observed changes in the size of body fluid compartments, an effect which ends 4 to 5 days after injury with a shift to anabolism. The vasculature contracts, fluid is removed from the extracellular space and either moves back into cells or is excreted by the kidneys, and the intracellular shift is accompanied by an influx of protein and electrolytes. While the physiologic "signal" that initiates this transition is still unknown, it is telling that the transition occurs at the completion of the first wave of angiogenesis. The generation of a new vascular highway obviates the need for nutrient concentration gradients, increased vascular permeability, as well as water and electrolyte conservation; with the latter no longer a priority, a brisk diuresis results. In addition, as the intracellular space expands, increases in intracellular anions and cations are required. As these must come from the vascular space, resolution of catabolism is accompanied by decreases in serum levels of potassium, magnesium, and phosphate ions and, therefore, diuresis and decreases in serum electrolytes are the hallmarks of resolution of the stress response.

The cellular immune response to normal inflammatory stimuli involves neutrophils, monocytes (macrophages), lymphocytes, and APCs. Neutrophils are recruited to areas of injury early in the process by chemoattractant molecules (chemokines) such as CXCL2, CXCL8, CXCL16, VEGF, MIF, which are released by endothelial cells, macrophages (most importantly), and fibroblasts (27,28). Their function is repair and regeneration, more precisely removal of cellular debris by phagocytosis through secretion of lytic molecules such as digestive enzymes and free radicals. While the influx of neutrophils is self-limited, the rest of the response, which starts within hours of neutrophil influx, may be more persistent. It consists of infiltration by macrophages, APCs, and lymphocytes. Macrophages are of key importance in innate immunity, a process that is nonspecific and involves natural barriers such as skin, natural killer (NK) cells, and chemicals in the blood that act immediately upon antigen introduction. Macrophages respond to stimulation with phagocytosis of foreign or damaged material and secretion of cytokines that stimulate inflammation and also function as growth factors. In addition, macrophages contribute to adaptive immunity by presenting antigens, a function that also is served by APCs. Depending on the local environment, macrophages undergo specific differentiation into M1 and M2 phenotypes. The M1 polarization corresponds with the classically activated macrophage and has an acute proinflammatory phenotype, whereas the alternative M2 polarization antagonizes the inflammatory response and are involved in the regulation of immunity, tissue repair, and wound healing (29).

Antigen-presenting cells, such as dendritic cells, capture antigens and transport them to lymph nodes, where they are presented to T cells, initiating cell-mediated immunity. Follicular dendritic cells have a similar function except that they present antigens to B cells and therefore initiate humoral immunity. Lymphocytes are the prime components of the adaptive immune response and have specific receptors for antigens. B cells produce antibodies and are mediators of humoral immunity; T cells recognize peptide fragments of protein antigens bound to APCs and are involved in cell-mediated immunity. T cells are further divided into CD4+ cells, which enhance or inhibit the immune response; CD8+ cells, which lyse other cells with intracellular pathogens; and NK cells, which do not express antigen receptors and contribute to innate immunity. Previous studies demonstrated that cytokines are centrally involved in regulation of adaptive immunity through control of T- and B-cell responses. The genetic deletion or immunoneutralization of specific cytokines was demonstrated to significantly reduce T-cell priming and memory responses, as well as cytokine production from T cells (30,31), and T cell–dependent antibody response. Activated T cells contribute to the auto/paracrine activation of IL-2, IL-2R, and IFN-γ production (32).

Adaptive immunity is antigen specific and can be divided into five phases. The first phase is presentation of the antigen to a B- or T cell by an APC. In the second phase, B- and T cells are activated, undergoing clonal expansion, differentiation, and antibody production. During the third or effector phase, antigens are eliminated. Decline is the fourth phase; the stimulus has been removed and there is apoptosis of immune cells and phagocytosis of cellular debris. This phase results in the surviving immune cells acquiring memory (33). As the process proceeds, there is a change in the phenotype of CD4+ T cells that is profoundly important. The early, protective phase of inflammation is characterized by an abundance of CD4+ T cells of the type 1 helper T-cell (T_h1) phenotype. This results in secretion of proinflammatory cytokines such as IL-2, TNF-α, and interferon-γ. The switch to reconstitution is accompanied by a predominance of type 2 helper T cells (T_h2), which secrete anti-inflammatory cytokines such as IL-4 and IL-10. In a normal stress response, immune function declines and the transition from T_h1 to T_h2 occurs by the fourth or fifth day; the switch from T_h1 to T_h2 may be hormonally mediated. It is known that cortisol and androgens, which are secreted in great quantities in catabolism, stimulate T_h2 cell production. Figure 43.1 and Table 43.1 provide an overview of the various contributors to the host response mechanisms after injury.

DIAGNOSIS

The stress response is considered to be adaptive and vital in order that an injury might be survived. However, many aspects of the process may become excessive or unbalanced; this converts an adaptive response into a pathologic one. Risk factors that predispose to the development of an abnormal response include inadequate or delayed resuscitation, persistent inflammatory or infectious sources, baseline organ dysfunction, age older than 65 years, immunosuppression, alcohol abuse, malnutrition, and invasive instrumentation (34).

This abnormal and pathologic response was termed systemic inflammatory response syndrome (SIRS). If SIRS is suspected to be from an infectious cause, then the condition is referred to as sepsis or the sepsis syndrome. Initially, the normal stress response, SIRS, and sepsis may mimic each other and clinically, there is often a subtle transition from one to the other.

The definitions of SIRS, sepsis, and severe sepsis were phrased in 1992 and 2001 by the Sepsis Consensus Conference and revised in part by the Surviving Sepsis Campaign guidelines in 2012. There is an open debate about the gold standard in measuring organ dysfunction and malperfusion (35) and consensus is currently sought via task forces and Delphi procedures.

While sepsis will be discussed in detail in a later chapter (see Chapter 46), the concomitant state of immune incompetence requires further discussion. Historically, sepsis has been viewed as a condition ruled by uncontrolled inflammation. However, an increasing number of studies indicate that sepsis is in fact a state of inflammatory failure (36–39), resulting from a dysbalance between pro- and anti-inflammatory mechanisms. More specifically, sepsis is associated with an alteration in the adaptive immune response (40). The early phase of sepsis resembles normal stress, in that there is a hormonal milieu that stimulates T_h2 responses and these responses are, indeed, observed; studies have shown that patients with sepsis have increased T_h2 cells and IL-10 and that these levels predict mortality (41,42). However, as sepsis progresses, there is a profound endocrinopathy and progressive energy (18). That is, chronic critical illness is associated with a loss of T-cell responsiveness on all levels (43); this may reflect enhanced lymphocyte apoptosis (44–46). Hotchkiss et al. also demonstrated that there were decreased levels of follicular dendritic cells, B cells, and CD4+ T cells at the time of death of septic patients, resulting in impaired antigen presentation, antibody

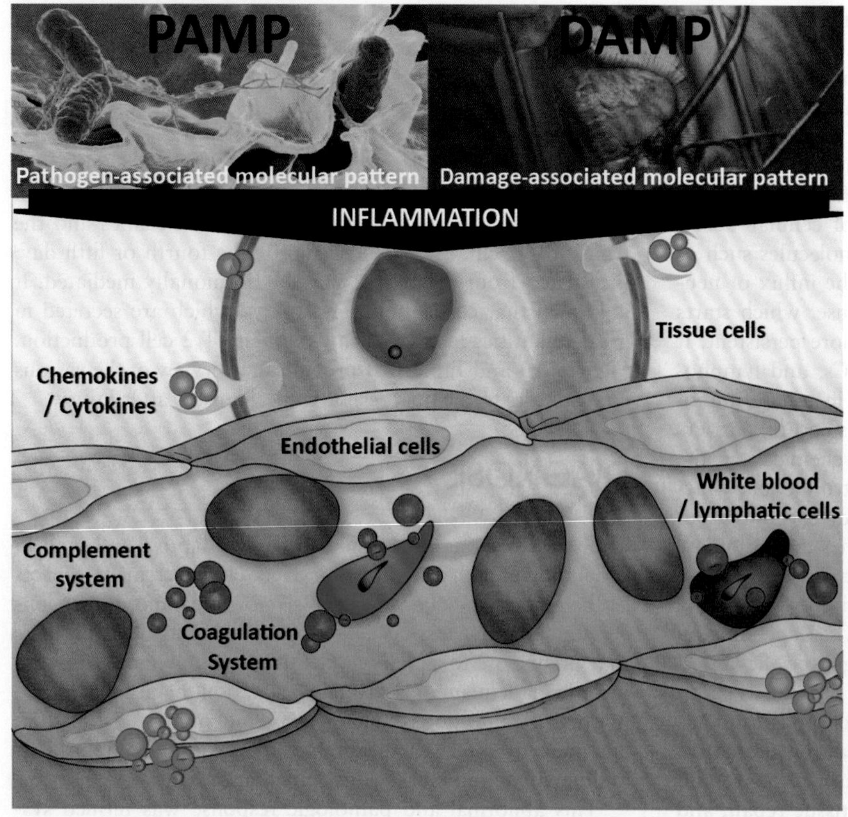

FIGURE 43.1 Contributors to the host response to injury. Occurrence and recognition of pathogen- or damage-associated molecular patterns initiate a broad and polyphonic response, triggering a range of immune-related and other cell types and inducing several complex protein pathways.

TABLE 43.1 Contributors to the Host Response to Injury[a]

Cellular Contributors
Organ-specific cells
- Cardiomyocytes
- Hepatocytes
- Others
Systemic cell types
- Adipose tissue
- Epithelial cells
- Endothelial cells
- Fibroblasts
Blood-Derived Contributors
Blood originated cells
- Neutrophils
- Macrophages/monocytes (M1, M2)
- Dendritic cells
- B cells, T cells (T_h1, T_h2), natural killer cells
- Thrombocytes
Complement system
- C3a, C5a, C5aR, C5b
Coagulation system
- Prothrombin, protein C
Chemokines/Cytokines
Proinflammatory
- Inflammasome (NLRP3/ASC/caspase-1)
- CXCL2, CXCL8, CXCL16,
- IL-1β, IL-2, IL-2R, IL-3, IL-6, IL-18, IFN-γ
- VEGF, MIF, TNF-α
Anti-inflammatory
- IL-4, IL-10, IL-1RA

[a]This list is by no means exhaustive but mentions, subjectively, the most important effectors in accordance with the chapter's text.

production, and B-cell and macrophage stimulation (44–46). The ultimate result of immunosuppression is the development of sequential infections, often invoking the decision to withdraw therapy.

One major contributor to the development of complications from inflammation is the presence of comorbidities. Chronic comorbid conditions are present in over 50% of patients with sepsis and are associated with increased mortality (47–49). This is of particular relevance as the concerned patient population is getting older and presenting with an increasing number of comorbid conditions. Diseases reported to increase the risk of the normal stress response developing into sepsis are diabetes mellitus (DM), human immunodeficiency virus (HIV), chronic liver disease, and cancer (47). Esper et al. conducted a retrospective analysis that reviewed patients with the diagnosis of sepsis in U.S. acute care hospitals within a 25-year follow-up, characterizing the type and source of infections and comorbid diseases. They found that men were more likely than women, and African Americans were more likely than Caucasians, to develop sepsis. Non-Caucasian patients who were septic were more likely to have concomitant DM, HIV, chronic renal failure, and alcohol abuse; Caucasians had higher incidences of cancer and chronic obstructive pulmonary disease (COPD). The presence of one comorbidity increased the risk of developing at least one-organ-system failure by 30%. Those with two comorbidities had a 39% chance, and those with three or more had a 45% chance of developing acute organ failure (50).

It is not difficult to imagine how baseline insufficiencies affect the stress response. For example, the ability to maintain a circulatory system capable of providing oxygen and nutrients to areas of injury is paramount to survival; in the setting of underlying coronary artery disease (CAD), this ability may be impaired. Kern et al. (51) found that patients with CAD have significantly decreased cardiac index and oxygen delivery and, not surprisingly, an increased oxygen extraction ratio during sepsis. They also showed that these patients had increased endothelial adhesion molecule expression, which may correlate with the severity of sepsis, shock, and organ failure and predict poor outcome (52,53). Chronic pulmonary disease, regardless of the etiology, increases the chance of intubation and the requirement for prolonged ventilatory support. Intubation places the patient at risk for ventilator-associated pneumonia, aspiration, and respiratory muscle atrophy, and is associated with a prolonged, cost-intense, treatment. A patient with chronic renal or liver failure is at risk for anemia, coagulopathy, and immunosuppression prior to being injured. With an impaired functional reserve in vital organs and responses, the stress response to injury has a high likelihood of progressing to a state of prolonged critical illness.

Beside these baseline characteristics, several relevant polymorphisms have been uncovered during the last decade, which are of importance for the development of innate immunity and susceptibility against associated complications (54). For example, the genotype of the proinflammatory cytokine TNF-α or MIF has been shown to affect susceptibility or clinical severity of different inflammatory or infectious diseases (55). In a large cohort of patients with pneumonia and at risk to develop septic shock, Yende et al. demonstrated that a high MIF expression genotype was associated with a significantly reduced mortality. These findings were unexpected, since an overwhelming inflammatory response was supposed to represent the most harmful stimulus within the pathophysiology of sepsis. Likewise, Calandra et al. reported the crucial role of MIF in macrophagic bactericidal properties. MIF-deficient macrophages exhibited an impaired killing of gram-negative bacteria that could be restored by an addition of recombinant MIF (56).

TREATMENT

Multiple clinical trials failed to show protective treatment-improved outcome in septic patients. The vast majority of trials focused on blocking the initial hyperinflammatory, cytokine-mediated phase of the disorder. Based on results from experimental studies where inhibition of TNF-α or IL1-β with neutralizing antibodies, soluble receptors, or receptor antagonists protected animals from the deleterious effects of high-grade bacteremia and endotoxemia, clinical trials aimed to confirm these findings in septic patients (57,58). Surprisingly, all studies failed to show any beneficial effects of pharmacologic antagonization of inflammatory mediators in sepsis (59). The underlying reasons remain speculative, but include the choice of heterogeneous patient cohorts. Furthermore, it is tempting to speculate that previous treatments were applied too late, when circulating levels of TNF-α and IL-1β had already returned to baseline values.

The last decade was shaped by substantial improvements in the treatment protocols emphasizing the necessity of early timing of treatment bundles, wherein anti-infectious therapies and restoration of adequate tissue perfusion were of particular relevance. Today, the majority of patients survive the initial hyperinflammatory phase, but are still exposed to severe complications during the protracted immunosuppressive phase (60). Deaths during this immunosuppressive phase result typically from failure to control the primary infection or the acquisition of secondary hospital-acquired infections (61). Therefore many attempts are under investigation, focusing on anticytokine and immunomodulatory therapies during this relevant period (61); additionally, emerging phase II clinical trials of immunotherapies have brought cautious optimism to the field, but need to be confirmed in large-scale multicenter trials (62–66). Further, there have been several experiments conducted with mice in septic or hemorrhagic shock showing increased mortality from immunosuppression after β-blockade (67,68). Adequate analgesia via epidural and intravenous use of agents such as opiates, α-blockers, and local anesthetics have been shown to both decrease inflammation and improve immune function (69–72).

Considering the prevention of both postoperative infection and excessive inflammation in cardiac surgery patients, recent evidence on corticosteroids provides conflicting evidence that attenuating the inflammatory response may result in clinical benefit. The dexamethasone for cardiac surgery trial randomized high-risk cardiac surgery patients to a single intraoperative dose of dexamethasone or placebo, but failed to demonstrate a benefit in treated patients (73). In the same vein, the Steroids In caRdiac Surgery (SIRS) Trial did not provide support for this hypothesis, stating that perioperative administration of pulse dose methylprednisolone did not reduce the risk of death at 30 days (74).

Trials of both medical devices and immune biologics aiming to eliminate the excessive inflammatory response are ongoing. Early results suggest complement inhibition to be a promising adjunctive therapy in infectious as well as noninfectious inflammatory disorders (75).

CONTROVERSIES

Given the multitude of failed clinical trials in septic patients, a better understanding of different immunologic phases seems mandatory to optimize the ongoing strategies of immune response modulation.

Recent experiences of failed studies on anti–toll-like receptor 4 (TLR-4), recombinant activated protein C, and anti–TNF-α therapies indicate that a higher precision is needed when trying to influence inflammatory pathophysiology (62–66). Furthermore, recent findings of a large clinical trial targeting oxidative stress in critically ill patients demonstrated no clinical benefit of antioxidant therapy and a trend toward increased mortality with glutamine administration (76). The reasons for the disappointing results are speculative; beside the question of dose and timing, adverse off-target effects may have contributed to their failure. Pertinent to possible off-target effects, it is important to remember that ROS are critical signaling molecules for cell homeostasis and adaptation to stress (e.g., hypoxia), processes that may be impaired with antioxidants. In addition, it has been recognized that ROS are critical signaling molecules essential for optimal function of innate and adaptive immunity. Both types of immunity are required to fight infection, a frequent contributor to morbidity and mortality in critically ill patients.

As many early-phase inflammatory cytokines operate concurrently and redundantly, identifying and targeting upstream triggers may generate therapies with broad downstream effects—yet not necessarily benefits. In the same way high precision surgery requires paramount knowledge of anatomy, immunomodulatory pharmacotherapy requires the same precision regarding signaling cascades and a detailed knowledge of consequences we are, perhaps, still lacking.

Key Points

- Injury is present in the form of elective surgery, trauma, infection, and other illnesses.
- The host response to injury is janiform. While harmful if exaggerated, it is mandatory to induce regeneration and preservation strategies.
- Balance is the hallmark of a physiologic host response. Pre-existing disease and persistent hypermetabolism offset this balance and pathologic conditions prevail.
- Both anti-inflammatory and proinflammatory strategies may offer therapeutic benefit restoring balance, yet so far most modulating therapies disappointed.

ACKNOWLEDGMENTS

The initial version of this chapter was written by Jamie Taylor and Clifford S. Deutschman, whom we thank.

References

1. Clowes GH Jr, O'Donnell TF, Blackburn GL, Maki TN. Energy metabolism and proteolysis in traumatized and septic man. *Surg Clin North Am.* 1976;56:1169–1184.
2. Janeway CA, Medzhitov R. Innate immune recognition. *Annu Rev Immunol.* 2002;20:197–216.
3. Guo H, Callaway JB, Ting JP. Inflammasomes: mechanism of action, role in disease, and therapeutics. *Nat Med.* 2015;21:677–687.
4. Drenth JP, van der Meer JW. The inflammasome: a linebacker of innate defense. *N Engl J Med.* 2006;355:730–732.
5. Mariathasan S, Monack DM. Inflammasome adaptors and sensors: intracellular regulators of infection and inflammation. *Nat Rev Immunol.* 2007;7:31–40.
6. Calandra T, Froidevaux C, Martin C, Roger T. Macrophage migration inhibitory factor and host innate immune defenses against bacterial sepsis. *J Infect Dis.* 2003;187(Suppl 2):S385–S390.
7. Cerra FB, Siegel JH, Border JR, et al. Correlations between metabolic and cardiopulmonary measurements in patients after trauma, general surgery, and sepsis. *J Trauma.* 1979;19:621–629.
8. Monk DN, Plank LD, Franch-Arcas G, et al. Sequential changes in the metabolic response in critically injured patients during the first 25 days after blunt trauma. *Ann Surg.* 1996;223:395–405.
9. Russell JA, Ronco JJ, Lockhat D, et al. Oxygen delivery and consumption and ventricular preload are greater in survivors than in nonsurvivors of the adult respiratory distress syndrome. *Am Rev Respir Dis.* 1990;141:659–665.
10. Shoemaker WC, Montgomery ES, Kaplan E, Elwyn DH. Physiologic patterns in surviving and nonsurviving shock patients: use of sequential cardiorespiratory variables in defining criteria for therapeutic goals and early warning of death. *Arch Surg.* 1973;106:630–636.
11. Hayes MA, Timmins AC, Yau EH, et al. Oxygen transport patterns in patients with sepsis syndrome or septic shock: influence of treatment and relationship to outcome. *Crit Care Med.* 1997;25:926–936.
12. Hayes MA, Yau EH, Timmins AC, et al. Response of critically ill patients to treatment aimed at achieving supranormal oxygen delivery and consumption: relationship to outcome. *Chest.* 1993;103:886–895.
13. Woolf N. *Pathology: Basic and Systemic.* London: WB Saunders; 1998.
14. Cuthbertson DP. Post-traumatic metabolism: a multidisciplinary challenge. *Surg Clin North Am.* 1978;58:1045–1054.
15. Moore FD, Olsen KH, McMurrey JD, Parker HV. *The Body Cell Mass and Its Supporting Environment.* Philadelphia, PA: Saunders; 1963.
16. Lenz A, Franklin GA, Cheadle WG. Systemic inflammation after trauma. *Injury.* 2007;38:1336–1345.
17. Rex S, Kraemer S, Grieb G, et al. The role of macrophage migration inhibitory factor in critical illness. *Mini Rev Med Chem.* 2014;14(14):1116–1124.
18. Van den Berghe G, de Zegher F, Bouillon R. Clinical review 95: acute and prolonged critical illness as different neuroendocrine paradigms. *J Clin Endocrinol Metab.* 1998;83:1827–1834.
19. Frank S, Hübner G, Breier G, et al. Regulation of vascular endothelial growth factor expression in cultured keratinocytes: implications for normal and impaired wound healing. *J Biol Chem.* 1995;270:12607–12613.
20. Werner S, Grose R. Regulation of wound healing by growth factors and cytokines. *Physiol Rev.* 2003;83:835–870.
21. Landry DW, Oliver JA. The pathogenesis of vasodilatory shock. *N Engl J Med.* 2001;345(8):588–595.
22. Goehler LE, Gaykema RP, Hansen MK, et al. Vagal immune-to-brain communication: a visceral chemosensory pathway. *Auton Neurosci.* 2000;85:49–59.
23. Hermann GE, Emch GS, Tovar CA, Rogers RC. c-Fos generation in the dorsal vagal complex after systemic endotoxin is not dependent on the vagus nerve. *Am J Physiol Regul Integr Comp Physiol.* 2001;280:R289–R299.
24. Emch GS, Hermann GE, Rogers RC. TNF-alpha activates solitary nucleus neurons responsive to gastric distension. *Am J Physiol Gastrointest Liver Physiol.* 2000;279:G582–G586.
25. Borovikova LV, Ivanova S, Zhang M, et al. Vagus nerve stimulation attenuates the systemic inflammatory response to endotoxin. *Nature.* 2000;405:458–462.
26. Bernik TR, Friedman SG, Ochani M, et al. Pharmacological stimulation of the cholinergic antiinflammatory pathway. *J Exp Med.* 2002;195:781–788.
27. Martin J, Duncan FJ, Keiser T, et al. Macrophage migration inhibitory factor (MIF) plays a critical role in pathogenesis of ultraviolet-B (UVB) – induced nonmelanoma skin cancer (NMSC). *FASEB J.* 2009;23:720–730.
28. Turner NA, Das A, O'Regan DJ, et al. Human cardiac fibroblasts express ICAM-1, E-selectin and CXC chemokines in response to proinflammatory cytokine stimulation. *Int J Biochem Cell Biol.* 2011;43:1450–1458.
29. Murray PJ, Wynn TA. Protective and pathogenic functions of macrophage subsets. *Nature Rev Immunol.* 2011;11:723–737.
30. Mizue Y, Ghani S, Leng L, et al. Role for macrophage migration inhibitory factor in asthma. *Proc Nat Acad Sci USA.* 2005;102:14410–14415.
31. Wang B, Huang X, Wolters PJ, et al. Cutting edge: deficiency of macrophage migration inhibitory factor impairs murine airway allergic responses. *J Immunol.* 2006;177:5779–5784.
32. Bacher M, Metz CN, Calandra T, et al. An essential regulatory role for macrophage migration inhibitory factor in T-cell activation. *Proc Nat Acad Sci USA.* 1996;93:7849–7854.
33. Abbas AK, Lichtman A, Pillai S. *Basic Immunology: Functions and Disorders of the Immune System.* Philadelphia, PA: Elsevier; 2014.
34. Orbach S, Weiss YG, Deutschman CS. The patient with sepsis or the systemic inflammatory response syndrome. In: Murray MJ, Coursin DB, Pearl RG, Prough DS, eds. *Critical Care Medicine: Perioperative Management.* Philadelphia, PA: Lippincott Williams & Wilkins; 2002:601–615.
35. Shankar-Hari M, Deutschman CS, Singer M. Do we need a new definition of sepsis? *Intensive Care Med.* 2015;41:909–911.
36. Lederer JA, Rodrick ML, Mannick JA. The effects of injury on the adaptive immune response. *Shock.* 1999;11:153–159.
37. Oberholzer A, Oberholzer C, Moldawer LL. Sepsis syndromes: understanding the role of innate and acquired immunity. *Shock.* 2001;16:83–96.
38. Ertel W, Kremer JP, Kenney J, et al. Downregulation of proinflammatory cytokine release in whole blood from septic patients. *Blood.* 1995;85:1341–1347.
39. Venet F, Bohé J, Debard AL, et al. Both percentage of γδ T lymphocytes and CD3 expression are reduced during septic shock. *Crit Care Med.* 2005;33:2836–2840.
40. Shelley O, Murphy T, Paterson H, et al. Interaction between the innate and adaptive immune systems is required to survive sepsis and control inflammation after injury. *Shock.* 2003;20:123–129.
41. Opal SM, DePalo VA. Anti-inflammatory cytokines. *Chest.* 2000;117:1162–1172.
42. Gogos CA, Drosou E, Bassaris HP, Skoutelis A. Pro- versus anti-inflammatory cytokine profile in patients with severe sepsis: a marker for prognosis and future therapeutic options. *J Infect Dis.* 2000;181:176–180.
43. Meakins JL, Pietsch JB, Bubenick O, et al. Delayed hypersensitivity: indicator of acquired failure of host defenses in sepsis and trauma. *Ann Surg.* 1977;186:241–250.
44. Hotchkiss RS, Swanson PE, Freeman BD, et al. Apoptotic cell death in patients with sepsis, shock, and multiple organ dysfunction. *Crit Care Med.* 1999;27:1230–1251.
45. Hotchkiss RS, Tinsley KW, Swanson PE. Depletion of dendritic cells, but not macrophages, in patients with sepsis. *J Immunol.* 2002;168:2493–2500.
46. Hotchkiss RS, Tinsley KW, Swanson PE, et al. Sepsis-induced apoptosis causes progressive profound depletion of B and CD4+ T lymphocytes in humans. *J Immunol.* 2001;166:6952–6963.

47. Angus DC, Linde-Zwirble WT, Lidicker J. Epidemiology of severe sepsis in the United States: analysis of incidence, outcome, and associated costs of care. *Crit Care Med.* 2001;29:1303–1310.
48. Alberti C, Brun-Buisson C, Burchardi H, et al. Epidemiology of sepsis and infection in ICU patients from an international multicentre cohort study. *Intensive Care Med.* 2002;28:108–121.
49. Martin GS, Mannino DM, Eaton S, Moss M. The epidemiology of sepsis in the United States from 1979 through 2000. *N Engl J Med.* 2003;348:1546–1554.
50. Esper AM, Moss M, Lewis CA, et al. The role of infection and comorbidity: factors that influence disparities in sepsis. *Crit Care Med.* 2006;34:2576–2582.
51. Kern H, Wittich R, Rohr U, et al. Increased endothelial injury in septic patients with coronary artery disease. *Chest.* 2001;119:874–883.
52. Sessler CN, Windsor AC, Schwartz M, et al. Circulating ICAM-1 is increased in septic shock. *Am J Respir Crit Care Med.* 2012;151:1420–1427.
53. Boldt J, Müller M, Kuhn D, et al. Circulating adhesion molecules in the critically ill: a comparison between trauma and sepsis patients. *Intensive Care Med.* 1996;22:122–128.
54. Lukaszewicz AC, Payen D. The future is predetermined in severe sepsis, so what are the implications? *Crit Care Med.* 2010;38(10 Suppl):S512–S517.
55. Teuffel O, Ethier MC, Beyene J, Sung L. Association between tumor necrosis factor-alpha promoter -308 A/G polymorphism and susceptibility to sepsis and sepsis mortality: a systematic review and meta-analysis. *Crit Care Med.* 2010;38:276–282.
56. Calandra T, Echtenacher B, Roy DL, et al. Protection from septic shock by neutralization of macrophage migration inhibitory factor. *Nat Med.* 2000;6:164–170.
57. Abraham E. Why immunomodulatory therapies have not worked in sepsis. *Intensive Care Med.* 1999;25:556–566.
58. Opal SM, Laterre PF, Francois B, et al; ACCESS Study Group. Effect of eritoran, an antagonist of MD2-TLR4, on mortality in patients with severe sepsis: the ACCESS randomized trial. *JAMA.* 2013;309:1154–1162.
59. Ranieri VM, Thompson BT, Barie PS, et al; PROWESS-SHOCK Study Group. Drotrecogin alfa (activated) in adults with septic shock. *N Engl J Med.* 2012;366:2055–2064.
60. Hotchkiss RS, Karl IE. The pathophysiology and treatment of sepsis. *N Engl J Med.* 2003;348:138–150.
61. Hotchkiss RS, Monneret G, Payen D. Sepsis-induced immunosuppression: from cellular dysfunctions to immunotherapy. *Nat Rev Immunol.* 2013;13:862–874.
62. Dolgin E. Trial failure prompts soul-searching for critical-care specialists. *Nat Med.* 2012;18:1000.
63. Opal SM, Fisher CJ Jr, Dhainaut JF, et al. Confirmatory interleukin-1 receptor antagonist trial in severe sepsis: a phase III, randomized, double-blind, placebo-controlled, multicenter trial. The Interleukin-1 Receptor Antagonist Sepsis Investigator Group. *Crit Care Med.* 1997;25:1115–1124.
64. Boomer JS, To K, Chang KC, et al. Immunosuppression in patients who die of sepsis and multiple organ failure. *JAMA.* 2011;306:2594–2605.
65. Hotchkiss RS, Coopersmith CM, McDunn JE, Ferguson TA. The sepsis seesaw: tilting toward immunosuppression. *Nat Med.* 2009;15:496–497.
66. Ward PA. Immunosuppression in sepsis. *JAMA.* 2011;306:2618–2619.
67. Schmitz D, Wilsenack K, Lendemanns S, et al. β-Adrenergic blockade during systemic inflammation: impact on cellular immune functions and survival in a murine model of sepsis. *Resuscitation.* 2007;72:286–294.
68. Oberbeck R, van Griensven M, Nickel E, et al. Influence of β-adrenoceptor antagonists on hemorrhage-induced cellular immune suppression. *Shock.* 2002;18:331–335.
69. Akural EI, Salomäki TE, Bloigu AH, et al. The effects of pre-emptive epidural sufentanil on human immune function. *Acta Anaesthesiol Scand.* 2004;48:750–755.
70. Wu CT, Jao SW, Borel CO, et al. The effect of epidural clonidine on perioperative cytokine response, postoperative pain, and bowel function in patients undergoing colorectal surgery. *Anesth Analg.* 2004;99:502–509.
71. Volk T, Schenk M, Voigt K, et al. Postoperative epidural anesthesia preserves lymphocyte, but not monocyte, immune function after major spine surgery. *Anesth Analg.* 2004;98:1086–1092.
72. Molina PE. Opioids and opiates: analgesia with cardiovascular, haemodynamic and immune implications in critical illness. *J Intern Med.* 2006;259:138–154.
73. Dieleman JM, Nierich AP, Rosseel PM, et al; Dexamethasone for Cardiac Surgery (DECS) Study Group. Intraoperative high-dose dexamethasone for cardiac surgery: a randomized controlled trial. *JAMA.* 2012;308:1761–1767.
74. Whitlock R, Teoh K, Vincent J, et al. Rationale and design of the steroids in cardiac surgery trial. *Am Heart J.* 2014;167:660–665.
75. Sun S, Zhao G, Liu C, et al. Treatment with anti-C5a antibody improves the outcome of H7N9 virus infection in African green monkeys. *Clin Infect Dis.* 2015;60:586–595.
76. Heyland D, Muscedere J, Wischmeyer PE, et al; Canadian Critical Care Trials Group. A randomized trial of glutamine and antioxidants in critically ill patients. *N Engl J Med.* 2013;368:1489–1497.

CHAPTER

44

Shock: General

S. ROB TODD, KRISTA L. TURNER, and FREDERICK A. MOORE

INTRODUCTION

Despite significant technologic advances and improved understanding of shock, it remains a diagnosis associated with significant morbidity and mortality. Hippocrates and Galen were the first to describe a "posttraumatic syndrome," then, in 1737, LeDran, a French surgeon, used the term *choc* to characterize a severe impact or jolt (1). However, it was not until 1867 that Edwin Morris popularized the term (2), defining shock as "a peculiar effect on the animal system, produced by violent injuries from any cause, or from violent mental emotions."

In the late 1800s, Fischer and Maphoter further delineated the pathophysiology of shock (3,4), with Fischer proposing a generalized "vasomotor paralysis" resulting in splanchnic blood pooling as the underlying mechanism, while Maphoter suggested that the clinical manifestations appreciated in shock were the result of the extravascular leakage of fluids. A variation of Fischer's theory was supported by Crile in 1899 (5).

In the early 1900s, Walter B. Cannon (6) proposed a toxin as the source of this altered capillary permeability and intravascular volume loss. Blalock (7) challenged this theory in 1930, charging that significant hemorrhage alone could account for insufficient cardiac output (CO) in shock states and that a circulating toxin was not needed. In the 1940s, Carl Wiggers (8) demonstrated that, following prolonged shock, irreversible circulatory failure could occur. At that time, hypotension was synonymous with shock, as blood pressure was the primary end point of resuscitation in shock. As such, volume resuscitation was the primary management strategy.

It was not until the turn of the 19th century that etiologies other than trauma were thought to cause shock; sepsis was first depicted as causing shock during the Spanish-American War (9). This was followed in 1906 with the description of anaphylactic shock. Subsequently, Tennant and Wiggers documented, in 1935, decreased myocardial contractility following coronary perfusion deprivation (10).

DEFINITION OF SHOCK

The definition of shock has historically been a moving target. Initially equated with hypotension (11,12), shock is now defined as an acute clinical syndrome resulting from cellular dysoxia, ultimately leading to organ dysfunction and failure (13). Cellular dysoxia or inadequate tissue perfusion is critical in diagnosing shock, as there are many other causes of organ dysfunction and failure that are not resultant from shock.

Note the emphasis on shock as a *syndrome,* as this constellation of signs and symptoms predictably follows a well-described series of pathophysiologic events (14). Its clinical presentation varies widely based on the underlying etiology, the degree of organ perfusion, and prior organ dysfunction.

CLASSIFICATION OF SHOCK

The incidence and prevalence of shock are poorly characterized for a multitude of reasons. First and foremost—even today—the definition of shock continues to lack consensus. As such, screening for shock tends to be inadequate, and thus it is underreported. Additionally, patients presumably die from shock in the prehospital setting. Taking these facts into account, one can readily appreciate why the reported incidence and mortality of shock varies widely.

Blalock's 1937 classification of shock (15) defined four categories: hematogenic or oligemic (hypovolemic), cardiogenic, neurogenic, and vasogenic. Subsequently, Weil and Shubin (16) characterized shock based on cardiovascular parameters. The categories included hypovolemic, cardiogenic, extracardiac obstructive, and distributive; Table 44.1 represents an adaptation of this system (17). It is important to appreciate that most shock states incorporate different components of each of the aforementioned shock categories.

Hypovolemic Shock

Hypovolemic shock represents a state of decreased intravascular volume. Inciting events include internal or external hemorrhage, significant fluid losses from the gastrointestinal tract (emesis, high-output fistulae, or diarrhea) or urinary tract (hyperosmolar states), and "third spacing" ("capillary leakage" into the interstitial tissues or the corporeal cavities) (see Table 44.1). Additional etiologies include malnutrition and large open wounds (burns and the open abdomen) (16,18).

The pathophysiology of shock is dependent upon its classification. Hypovolemic shock is characterized by a decrease in intravascular volume with resultant decreases in pulmonary capillary wedge pressure (PCWP) and CO (Table 44.2). There is a subsequent increased sympathetic drive in an attempt to increase peripheral vasculature tone, cardiac contractility, and heart rate. These, initially, beneficial measures ultimately turn detrimental, as their resultant hypermetabolic state predisposes tissues to localized hypoxia (14). Furthermore, the aforementioned increased peripheral vascular tone (systemic vascular resistance; SVR) may result in tissue ischemia via an inconsistent microcirculatory flow. In cases of severe hypovolemic shock, a significant inflammatory component coexists.

Cardiogenic Shock

Cardiogenic shock is defined as inadequate tissue perfusion due to primary ventricular failure. Its incidence has remained fairly stable, ranging from 6% to 8% (19–23). In the United States, it is the most common cause of mortality from coronary artery disease (CAD) (19). Despite medical advances, cardiogenic shock remains the number one cause of in-hospital

TABLE 44.1 Shock Classification

Hypovolemic

Hemorrhagic

- Trauma, gastrointestinal, retroperitoneal

Nonhemorrhagic

- Dehydration, emesis, diarrhea, fistulae, burns, polyuria, "third spacing," malnutrition, large open wounds

Cardiogenic

Myocardial

- Infarction, contusion, myocarditis, cardiomyopathies, pharmacologic

Mechanical

- Valvular failure, ventricular septal defect, ventricular wall defects

Dysrhythmias

Obstructive

Impairment of diastolic filling

- Intrathoracic obstructive tumors, tension pneumothorax, positive-pressure mechanical ventilation, constrictive pericarditis, pericardial tamponade

Impairment of systolic contraction

- Pulmonary embolism, acute pulmonary hypertension, air embolism, tumors, aortic dissection, aortic coarctation

Distributive

Septic, anaphylactic, neurogenic, pharmacologic, endocrinologic

mortality in patients experiencing a transmural myocardial infarction (MI), with rates ranging between 70% and 90% (21,24). Other causes include myocarditis, cardiomyopathies, valvular heart diseases, and dysrhythmias (Table 44.1).

The most common inciting event in cardiogenic shock is an acute MI. Historically, once 40% of the myocardium has been irreversibly damaged, cardiogenic shock may result. From a mechanical perspective, decreased cardiac contractility diminishes both stroke volume (SV) and CO (see Table 44.2). These lead to increased ventricular filling pressures, cardiac chamber dilatation, and ultimately univentricular or biventricular failure with resultant systemic hypotension; this further reduces myocardial perfusion and exacerbates ongoing ischemia. The end result is a vicious cycle with severe cardiovascular decompensation. Similar to hypovolemic shock, a significant systemic inflammatory response has been implicated in the pathophysiology of cardiogenic shock.

Obstructive Shock

In obstructive shock, external forces compress the thin-walled chambers of the heart, the great vessels, or any combination thereof. These forces impair either the diastolic filling or the systolic contraction of the heart (see Table 44.1). Large obstructive intrathoracic tumors, tension pneumothoraces, pericardial tamponade, and constrictive pericarditis limit ventricular filling, while pulmonary emboli (PE) and aortic dissection impede cardiac contractility.

The hemodynamic parameters witnessed in obstructive shock include increases in central venous pressure (CVP) and SVR, and decreases in CO and mixed venous oxygen saturation (SvO_2) (see Table 44.2). The PCWP and other hemodynamic indices are dependent on the obstructive cause. In pericardial tamponade, there is equalization of the right and left ventricular diastolic pressures, the CVP, and the PCWP (increased). However, following a massive PE, right ventricular failure leads to increased right heart pressures and a normal or decreased PCWP.

Distributive Shock

Distributive shock is characterized by a decrease in SVR. Septic shock is the most common form although, additionally, distributive shock includes the other oft-quoted classes of shock including anaphylactic, neurogenic, and adrenal shock (see Table 44.1). Physiologically, all forms of distributive shock exhibit a decreased SVR (see Table 44.2). Subsequently, these patients experience relative hypovolemia as evidenced by a decreased (or normal) CVP and PCWP. The CO is initially diminished; however, following appropriate volume loading, the CO increases.

CELLULAR ALTERATIONS

All forms of shock, especially hemorrhagic and septic, induce a host response that is characterized by local and systemic release of proinflammatory cytokines, arachidonic acid metabolites, and activation of complement factors, kinins, and

TABLE 44.2 Shock Hemodynamic Parameters

	CVP	PCWP	CO	SVR	$S\bar{v}O_2$
Hypovolemic	↓↓	↓↓	↓↓	↑	↓
Cardiogenic					
Left ventricular myocardial infarction	Nl or ↑	↑	↓↓	↑	↓
Right ventricular myocardial infarction	↑↑	Nl or ↑	↓↓	↑	↓
Obstructive					
Pericardial tamponade	↑↑	↑↑	↓ or ↓↓	↑	↓
Massive pulmonary embolism	↑↑	Nl or ↓	↓↓	↑	↓
Distributive					
Early	Nl or ↑	Nl	↓ or Nl or ↑	↑ or Nl or ↓	Nl or ↓
Early after fluid administration	Nl or ↑	Nl or ↑	↑	↓	↑ or Nl or ↓
Late	Nl	Nl	↓	↑	↑ or ↓

CVP, central venous pressure; PCWP, pulmonary capillary wedge pressure; CO, cardiac output; SVR, systemic vascular resistance; $S\bar{v}O_2$, mixed venous oxygen saturation; Nl, normal.

TABLE 44.3 Clinical Parameters of the Systemic Inflammatory Response Syndrome

1. Heart rate >90 beats/min
2. Respiratory rate >20 breaths/min, or $PaCO_2$ <32 mmHg
3. Temperature >38°C or <36°C
4. Leukocytes >12,000 cells/mm³ or <4,000 cells/mm³ or ≥10% juvenile neutrophil granulocytes

$PaCO_2$, arterial partial pressure of CO_2.

coagulation as well as hormonal mediators. Clinically, this is the systemic inflammatory response syndrome (SIRS). Paralleling this response is an anti-inflammatory response referred to as the compensatory anti-inflammatory response syndrome (sometimes abbreviated CARS). An imbalance between these responses appears to be responsible for increased susceptibility to infection and organ dysfunction (25–29).

Systemic Inflammatory Response Syndrome

In 1991, a consensus conference of the American College of Chest Physicians and the American Society of Critical Care Medicine defined SIRS as a generalized inflammatory response triggered by a variety of infectious and noninfectious events (30). They arbitrarily established clinical parameters through a consensus process; Table 44.3 summarizes the SIRS diagnostic criteria. At least two of the four criteria must be present to fulfill the diagnosis of SIRS. Note, this definition emphasizes the inflammatory process regardless of its etiology. Subsequent studies have validated these criteria as predictive of increased ICU mortality, and indicated that this risk increases concurrent with the number of criteria present. SIRS is characterized by the local and systemic production, and release, of multiple mediators, including proinflammatory cytokines, complement factors, proteins of the contact phase and coagulation system, acute phase proteins, neuroendocrine mediators, and an accumulation of immunocompetent cells at the local site of tissue damage (31).

Compensatory Anti-Inflammatory Response Syndrome

Shock stimulates not only the release of proinflammatory mediators, but also the parallel release of anti-inflammatory mediators (26). This compensatory anti-inflammatory response is present concurrently with SIRS (Fig. 44.1) (32). When these two opposing responses are appropriately balanced, the patient is able to effectively recover without incurring secondary injury from the autoimmune inflammatory response (25). However, overwhelming CARS appears responsible for post-shock immunosuppression, which leads to increased susceptibility to infections and sepsis (26,31,33). With time, SIRS ceases to exist and CARS is the predominant force.

Cytokine Response

Proinflammatory cytokines, tumor necrosis factor-α (TNF-α), and interleukin-1β (IL-1β) are key to the resultant inflammation (34,35). Secondary proinflammatory cytokines are released in a subacute fashion and include IL-2, IL-6, IL-8, platelet-activating factor (PAF), interferon-γ (IFN-γ), endothelin-1, leukotrienes, thromboxanes, prostaglandins, and the complement cascade (34,36).

IL-6 also acts as an immunoregulatory cytokine by stimulating the release of anti-inflammatory mediators such as IL-1 receptor antagonists and TNF receptors, which bind circulating proinflammatory cytokines (35). IL-6 also triggers the release of prostaglandin E_2 (PGE_2) from macrophages (35); PGE_2 is potentially the most potent endogenous immunosuppressant (35). Not only does it suppress T-cell and macrophage responsiveness, but it also induces the release of IL-10, a potent anti-inflammatory cytokine that deactivates monocytes (35). A listing of pro- and anti-inflammatory mediators may be found in Tables 44.4 and 44.5.

Cell-Mediated Response

Shock alters the ability of splenic, peritoneal, and alveolar macrophages to release IL-1, IL-6, and TNF-α, leading to decreased levels of these proinflammatory cytokines (35). Kupffer cells, however, have an enhanced capacity for production of proinflammatory cytokines. Cell-mediated immunity requires not only functional macrophage and T cells, but also intact macrophage–T-cell interaction (35). Following injury, human leukocyte antigen (HLA-DR) receptor expression is decreased, leading to a loss of antigen-presenting capacity and decreased TNF-α production. PGE_2, IL-10, and TGF-β all contribute to this "immunoparalysis" (25,35).

T-helper cells differentiate into either T_H1 or T_H2 lymphocytes; T_H1 cells promote the proinflammatory cascade through the release of IL-2, IFN-γ, and TNF-β, while T_H2 cells

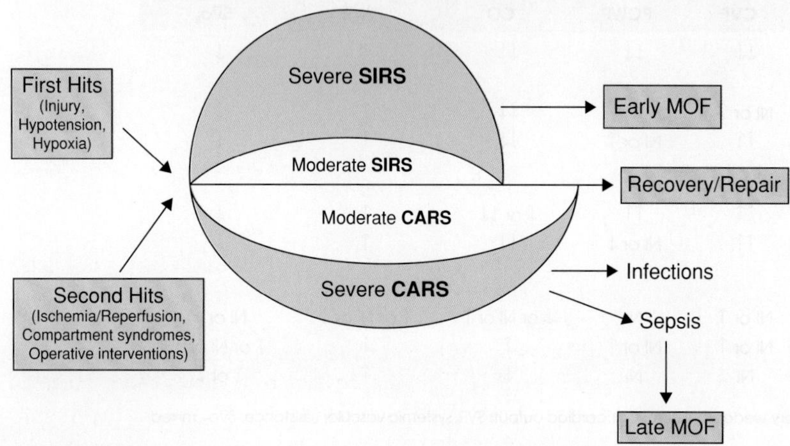

FIGURE 44.1 Postinjury multiple organ failure occurs as a result of a dysfunctional inflammatory response. SIRS, systemic inflammatory response syndrome; MOF, multiple organ failure; CARS, compensatory anti-inflammatory response syndrome.

TABLE 44.4 Proinflammatory Mediators

Mediator	Action
IL-1	IL-1 is pleiotropic. Locally, it stimulates cytokine and cytokine receptor production by T cells as well as stimulating B-cell proliferation. Systemically, IL-1 modulates endocrine responses and induces the acute phase response.
IL-6	IL-6 induces acute phase reactants in hepatocytes and plays an essential role in the final differentiation of B cells into Ig-secreting cells. Additionally, IL-6 has anti-inflammatory properties.
IL-8	IL-8 is one of the major mediators of the inflammatory response. It functions as a chemoattractant and is also a potent angiogenic factor.
IL-12	IL-12 regulates the differentiation of naive T cells into T_H1 cells. It stimulates the growth and function of T cells and alters the normal cycle of apoptotic cell death.
TNF-α	TNF-α is pleiotropic. TNF-α and IL-1 act alone or together to induce systemic inflammation as above. TNF-α is also chemotactic for neutrophils and monocytes, as well as increasing neutrophil activity.
MIF	MIF forms a crucial link between the immune and neuroendocrine systems. It acts systemically to enhance the secretion of IL-1 and TNF-α.

IL, interleukin; Ig, immunoglobulin; TNF, tumor necrosis factor; MIF, migration inhibitory factor.

TABLE 44.5 Anti-Inflammatory Mediators

Mediator	Action
IL-4	IL-4, IL-3, IL-5, IL-13, and CSF2 form a cytokine gene cluster on chromosome 5q, with this gene particularly close to IL-13.
IL-10	IL-10 has pleiotropic effects in immunoregulation and inflammation. It downregulates the expression of T_H1 cytokines, MHC class II antigens, and costimulatory molecules on macrophages. It also enhances B-cell survival, proliferation, and antibody production. In addition, it can block NF-κB activity, and is involved in the regulation of the JAK-STAT signaling pathway.
IL-11	IL-11 stimulates the T cell–dependent development of immunoglobulin-producing B cells. It is also found to support the proliferation of hematopoietic stem cells and megakaryocyte progenitor cells.
IL-13	IL-13 is involved in several stages of B-cell maturation and differentiation. It upregulates CD23 and MHC class II expression, and promotes IgE isotype switching of B cells. It downregulates macrophage activity, thereby inhibiting the production of proinflammatory cytokines and chemokines.
IFN-α	IFN-α enhances and modifies the immune response.
TGF-β	TGF-β regulates the proliferation and differentiation of cells, wound healing, and angiogenesis.
α-MSH	α-MSH modulates inflammation by way of three mechanisms: direct action on peripheral inflammatory cells; actions on brain inflammatory cells to modulate local reactions; and indirect activation of descending neural anti-inflammatory pathways that control peripheral tissue inflammation.

IL, interleukin; CSF, colony-stimulating factor; T_H, T helper; MHC, major histocompatibility complex; Ig, immunoglobulin; IFN, interferon; TGF, transforming growth factor; MSH, melanocyte stimulating hormone.

produce anti-inflammatory mediators (25,35). Monocytes/macrophages, through the release of IL-12, stimulate the differentiation of T-helper cells into T_H1 cells. Because IL-12 production is depressed following trauma, there is a shift toward T_H2, which has been associated with an adverse clinical outcome (25,35).

Adherence of the leukocyte to endothelial cells is mediated through the upregulation of adhesion molecules. Selectins such as leukocyte adhesion molecule-1 (LAM-1), endothelial leukocyte adhesion molecule-1 (ELAM-1), and P-selectin are responsible for polymorphonuclear leukocytes (PMNLs) "rolling" (25,37). Upregulation of integrins such as the CD11/18 complexes or intercellular adhesion molecule-1 (ICAM-1) is responsible for PMNL attachment to the endothelium (25). Migration, accumulation, and activation of the PMNLs are mediated by chemoattractants such as chemokines and complement anaphylotoxins (25). Colony-stimulating factors (CSFs) likewise stimulate monocyte- or granulocyto-poiesis and reduce apoptosis of PMNLs during SIRS. Neutrophil apoptosis is further reduced by other proinflammatory mediators, thus resulting in PMNL accumulation at the site of local tissue destruction (25).

Leukocyte Recruitment

Proinflammatory cytokines enhance PMNL recruitment, phagocytic activity, and the release of proteases and oxygen-free radicals by PMNLs. This recruitment of leukocytes represents a key element for host defense following trauma, although it allows for the development of secondary tissue damage (38–41). Recruitment involves a complex cascade of events culminating in transmigration of the leukocyte, whereby the cell exerts its effects (42). The first step is capture and tethering, mediated via constitutively expressed leukocyte selectin denoted L selectin; L selectin functions by identifying glycoprotein ligands on leukocytes and those upregulated on cytokine-activated endothelium (42). Following capture and tethering, endothelial E selectin and P selectin assist in leukocyte rolling or slowing (37,43–48). P selectin is found in the membranes of endothelial storage granules, termed Weibel–Palade bodies (45). Following granule secretion, P selectin binds to carbohydrates presented by P selectin glycoprotein ligand (PSGL-1) on the leukocytes (25). In contrast, E selectin is not stored, yet it is synthesized de novo in the presence of inflammatory cytokines (43,44). These selectins cause the leukocytes to roll along the activated endothelium, whereby secondary capturing of leukocytes occurs via homotypic interactions. The third step in leukocyte recruitment is firm adhesion, which is mediated by membrane-expressed β_1- and β_2-integrins (49–51). The integrins bind to ICAM, resulting in cell–cell interactions and ultimately signal transduction. This step is critical to the formation of stable shear-resistant adhesion, which stabilizes the leukocyte for transmigration (49–51).

Transmigration is the final step in leukocyte recruitment following the formation of bonds between the aforementioned integrins and immunoglobulin (Ig)-superfamily members (42). The arrested leukocytes cross the endothelial layer via bicellular and tricellular endothelial junctions in a process coined diapedesis (52). This is mediated by platelet endothelial cell adhesion molecules (PECAMs), proteins expressed on both the leukocytes and intercellular junctions of endothelial cells (42).

Proteases and Reactive Oxygen Species

Polymorphonuclear lymphocytes and macrophages are not only responsible for phagocytosis of microorganisms and cellular debris, but can also cause secondary tissue and organ damage through degranulation and release of extracellular proteases and formation of reactive oxygen species (ROS) or respiratory burst (25,39,40,41,53–55). Elastases and metalloproteinases, which degrade both structural and extracellular matrix proteins, are present in increased concentrations following trauma (25). Neutrophil elastases also induce the release of proinflammatory cytokines (25).

ROS are generated by membrane-associated nicotinamide adenine dinucleotide phosphate (NADPH)-oxidase, which is activated by proinflammatory cytokines, arachidonic acid metabolites, complement factors, and bacterial products (56,57). Superoxide anions are reduced in the Haber–Weiss reaction to hydrogen peroxide by superoxide dismutase located in the cytosol, mitochondria, and cell membrane (25). Hydrochloric acid is formed from H_2O_2 by myeloperoxidase, while the Fenton reaction transforms H_2O_2 into hydroxyl ions (25). These free ROS cause lipid peroxidation, cell membrane disintegration, and DNA damage of endothelial and parenchymal cells (58–60). Oxygen radicals also induce PMNLs to release proteases and collagenase as well as inactivating protease inhibitors (61).

Reactive nitrogen species cause additional tissue damage following trauma (62). Nitric oxide (NO), which induces vasodilation, is generated from L-arginine by inducible nitric oxide synthase (iNOS) in PMNLs or vascular muscle cells and by endothelial NOS (eNOS) in endothelial cells (62). iNOS is stimulated by cytokines and toxins, whereas eNOS is stimulated by mechanical shearing forces (62,63). Damage by reactive oxygen and nitrogen species leads to generalized edema and the capillary leak syndrome (62).

Complement, Kinins, and Coagulation

The complement cascade, kallikrein–kinin system, and coagulation cascade are intimately involved in the immune response to shock. They are activated through proinflammatory mediators, endogenous endotoxins, and tissue damage. The classic pathway of complement is normally activated by antigen–antibody complexes (Ig M or G) or activated coagulation factor XII (FXIIa), while the alternative pathway is activated by bacterial products such as lipopolysaccharide (64–66). Complement activation following trauma is most likely from the release of proteolytic enzymes, disruption of the endothelial lining, and tissue ischemia; the degree of complement activation correlates with the severity of injury. The cleavage of C3 and C5 by their respective convertases results in the formation of opsonins, anaphylotoxins, and the membrane attack complex (MAC) (64–66). The opsonins C3b and C4b enhance phagocytosis of cell debris and bacteria by means of opsonization (64,65). The anaphylotoxins C3a and C5a support inflammation via the recruitment and activation of phagocytic cells (i.e., monocytes, polymorphonuclear cells, and macrophages), enhancement of the hepatic acute phase reaction, and release of vasoactive mediators (i.e., histamine) (52,65). They also enhance the adhesion of leukocytes to endothelial cells, which results in increased vascular permeability and edema. C5a induces apoptosis and cell lysis through the interaction of its receptor and the MAC (52,65,66); additionally, C3a and C5a activate reparative mechanisms (65). C1 inhibitor inactivates C1s and C1r, thereby regulating the classic complement pathway. However, during inflammation, serum levels of C1 inhibitor are decreased via its degradation by PMNL elastases (65).

The plasma kallikrein–kinin system is a contact system of plasma proteases related to the complement and coagulation cascades. It consists of the plasma proteins FXII, prekallikrein, kininogen, and factor XI (FXI) (67). Activation of FXII and prekallikrein is via contact, when endothelial damage occurs and exposes the basement membrane (67). Factor XII activation forms factor XIIa (FXIIa), which initiates the complement cascade through the classic pathway, whereas prekallikrein activation forms kallikrein, which stimulates fibrinolysis through the conversion of plasminogen to plasmin or the activation of urokinase-like plasminogen activator (uPA) (67); tissue plasminogen activator (tPA) functions as a cofactor. Additionally, kallikrein supports the conversion of kininogen to bradykinin (67). The formation of bradykinin also occurs through the activation of the tissue kallikrein–kinin system, most likely through organ damage, as the tissue kallikrein–kinin system is found in many organs and tissues including the pancreas, kidney, intestine, and salivary glands. The kinins are potent vasodilators, increase vascular permeability and inhibit the function of platelets (67).

The intrinsic coagulation cascade is linked to the contact activation system via the formation of factor IXa (FIXa) from factor XIa (FXIa). Its formation leads to the consumption of FXII, prekallikrein, and FXI while plasma levels of enzyme–inhibitor complexes are increased (25). These include FXIIa-C1 inhibitor and kallikrein-C1 inhibitor. C1 inhibitor and α1-protease inhibitor are both inhibitors of the intrinsic coagulation pathway (68,69).

Although the intrinsic pathway provides a stimulus for activation of the coagulation cascade, the major activation following trauma is via the extrinsic pathway. Increased expression of tissue factor (TF) on endothelial cells and monocytes is induced by the proinflammatory cytokines TNF-α and IL-1β (69–71). The factor VII (FVII)–TF complex stimulates the formation of factor Xa (FXa) and ultimately thrombin (FIIa) (25). Thrombin-activated factor V (FV), factor VIII (FVIII), and FXI result in enhanced thrombin formation (25). Following cleavage of fibrinogen by thrombin, the fibrin monomers polymerize to form stable fibrin clots. The consumption of coagulation factors is controlled by the hepatocytic formation of antithrombin (AT) III (25). The thrombin–antithrombin complex inhibits thrombin, FIXa, FXa, FXIa, and FXIIa (72); other inhibitors include TF pathway inhibitor (TFPI) and activated protein C in combination with free protein S (72). Free protein S is decreased during inflammation due to its binding with the C4b-binding protein (68,72).

Disseminated intravascular coagulation (DIC) may occur following shock. After the initial phase, intra- and extravascular fibrin clots are observed. Hypoxia-induced cellular damage is the ultimate result of intravascular fibrin clots. Likewise, there is an increase in the interactions between endothelial cells and leukocytes (68–70,73). Clinically, coagulation factor consumption and platelet dysfunction are responsible for the diffuse hemorrhage (68,71). Consumption of coagulation factors is further enhanced via the proteolysis of fibrin clots to fibrin fragments (68,71). The consumption of coagulation factors is further enhanced through the proteolysis of fibrin clots to fibrin fragments by the protease plasmin (25,69,74).

Acute Phase Reaction

The acute phase reaction describes the early systemic response following shock and other insult states. During this phase, the biosynthetic profile of the liver is significantly altered. Under normal circumstances, the liver synthesizes a range of plasma proteins at steady-state concentrations. However, during the acute phase reaction, hepatocytes increase the synthesis of positive acute phase proteins (i.e., C-reactive protein [CRP], serum amyloid A [SAA], complement proteins, coagulation proteins, proteinase inhibitors, metal-binding proteins, and other proteins) essential to the inflammatory process at the expense of the negative acute phase proteins. The list of acute phase proteins, both positive and negative, is shown in Table 44.6 (75,76).

The acute phase response is initiated by hepatic Kupffer cells and the systemic release of proinflammatory cytokines IL-1, IL-6, IL-8, and TNF-α (77,78). The acute phase reaction typically lasts for 24 to 48 hours prior to its downregulation (35). IL-4, IL-10, glucocorticoids, and various other hormonal stimuli function to downregulate the proinflammatory mediators of the acute phase response (35); this modulation is critical. In instances of chronic or recurring inflammation, an aberrant acute phase response may result in exacerbated tissue damage (35).

The major acute phase proteins include CRP and SAA, the activities of which are both poorly understood (79,80). CRP was so named secondary to its ability to bind the C-polysaccharide of *Pneumococcus*. During inflammation CRP levels may increase by up to 1,000-fold over several hours depending on the insult and its severity (35). It acts as an opsonin for bacteria, parasites, and immune complexes; activates complement via the classic pathway; and binds chromatin (35). Binding chromatin may minimize autoimmune responses by disposing of nuclear antigens from sites of tissue debris (35). Clinically, CRP levels are relatively nonspecific and not predictive of posttraumatic complications. Despite this fact, serial measurements are helpful in trending a patient's clinical course (35).

SAA interacts with the third fraction of high-density lipoprotein (HDL3), thus becoming the dominant apolipoprotein during acute inflammation (81). This association enhances the binding of HDL3 to macrophages, which may engulf cholesterol and lipid debris. Excess cholesterol is then utilized in tissue repair or excreted (35). Additionally, SAA inhibits thrombin-induced platelet activation and the oxidative burst of neutrophils, potentially preventing oxidative tissue destruction (35).

TABLE 44.6 Acute Phase Proteins

Group	Individual Proteins
Positive acute phase proteins	
Major acute phase proteins	C-reactive protein, serum amyloid A
Complement proteins	C2, C3, C4, C5, C9, B, C1 inhibitor, C4-binding protein
Coagulation proteins	Fibrinogen, prothrombin, von Willebrand factor
Proteinase proteins	α_1-Antitrypsin, α_1-antichymotrypsin, α_2-antiplasmin, heparin cofactor II, plasminogen activator inhibitor I
Metal-binding proteins	Haptoglobin, hemopexin, ceruloplasmin, manganese superoxide dismutase
Other proteins	α_1-Acid glycoprotein, heme oxygenase, mannose-binding protein, leukocyte protein I, lipoprotein (a), lipopolysaccharide-binding protein
Negative acute phase proteins	Albumin, prealbumin, transferrin, apolipoprotein AI, apolipoprotein AII, α_2-Heremans–Schmid glycoprotein, inter-α-trypsin inhibitor, histidine-rich glycoprotein, protein C, protein S, antithrombin III, high-density lipoprotein

Positive acute phase proteins increase production during an acute phase response. Negative acute phase proteins are those that have decreased production during an acute phase response.

DIAGNOSIS OF SHOCK

Early diagnosis of shock affords the patient the best possible outcome. The patient in overt shock with hypotension and tachycardia is relatively easy to diagnose. However, more often than not, shock presents in more insidious forms, whereby underrecognition and delay in treatment can lead to a poor outcome. Moreover, the concurrent presence of mixed shock states can confuse the picture. Diagnosis of shock relies on both basic history and physical examination skills, as well as more advanced technology available to the clinician.

Numerous clues in a patient's history may help alert the physician to the possibility of impending shock. Large fluid losses via traumatic or gastrointestinal hemorrhage, third spacing from intra-abdominal surgery or pancreatitis, prolonged dehydration from vomiting or diarrhea, or insensible losses from burns may very easily tip the patient into hypovolemic shock. A history of infection, presence of indwelling catheters, or recent surgery may be implicated in septic shock. Neurogenic shock occurs almost exclusively after trauma, although limited forms are seen with spinal anesthesia. History of prolonged steroid use, particularly in the elderly, may indicate adrenal shock in the patient with hypotension postoperatively. Exposures to drugs, transfusions, or other allergens should be sought to rule out anaphylactic shock. Recent MI or cardiac intervention can lead to pump failure and cardiogenic shock. A detailed history is especially important for obstructive forms of shock, in which any intervention involving the chest can lead to either immediate or delayed compromise via cardiac tamponade or tension pneumothorax. Likewise, a history of deep venous thrombosis (DVT) or risk factors for thrombosis should alert the physician to the possibility of acute massive PE in the hypotensive patient.

Physical examination can provide more clues than just basic blood pressure measurements. As noted previously, hypotension alone is neither exclusive to shock nor absolute for a diagnosis, and therefore is only a small component of the physical examination. Certain findings may vary based on the type and timing of shock. The end result of any form of shock, however, is diminished end-organ perfusion. Therefore, any signs or symptoms of organ dysfunction should be considered as possible indicators of shock (Table 44.7). Often, the first sign of shock manifests as mental status changes, whether excitatory or somnolent in nature. The patient may appear diaphoretic and clammy in cardiogenic shock or warm and dry in early distributive shock. Heart rate may also be variable with

TABLE 44.7 Clinical Recognition of Shock

Organ System	Symptoms or Signs	Causes
CNS	Mental status changes	↓ Cerebral perfusion
Circulatory		
Cardiac	Tachycardia	Adrenergic stimulation, depressed contractility
	Other dysrhythmias	Coronary ischemia
	Hypotension	Depressed contractility secondary to ischemia or MDFs, right ventricular failure
	New murmurs	Valvular dysfunction, VSD
Systemic	Hypotension	↓ SVR, ↓ venous return
	↓ JVPs	Hypovolemia, ↓ venous return
	↑ JVPs	Right heart failure
	Disparate peripheral pulses	Aortic dissection
Respiratory	Tachypnea	Pulmonary edema, respiratory muscle fatigue, sepsis, acidosis
	Cyanosis	Hypoxemia
Renal	Oliguria	↓ Perfusion, afferent arteriolar vasoconstriction
Skin	Cool, clammy	Vasoconstriction, sympathetic stimulation
Other	Lactic acidosis	Anaerobic metabolism, hepatic dysfunction
	Fever	Infection

CNS, central nervous system; MDFs, myocardial depressant factors; VSD, ventricular septal defect; SVR, systemic vascular resistance; JVPs, jugular venous pulsations.

tachycardia compensating for diminished CO in the patient with intact sympathetic drive. Vasoplegic shock, such as neurogenic or adrenal (or in the β-blocked patient), may not have the compensatory increase in heart rate normally seen, and may itself provide a clue as to the type of shock. Tachypnea is almost universally seen, as the body tries to buffer the lactate produced in a state of tissue hypoxia. The kidneys provide a sensitive measure of adequate end-organ perfusion, as manifested by low urinary output. Cardiogenic shock has its own specific physical findings including increased venous jugular distension, acute pulmonary edema, and new murmurs or dysrhythmias.

Various modalities for evaluating shock may be used either alone or in combination. Pooling data from multiple sources, however, is often required to get an adequate picture of shock resuscitation. Basic laboratory studies such as lactate level, base deficit, hemoglobin (Hgb), creatinine, and cortisol may help provide evidence of or reason for shock. Likewise, a more advanced evaluation of shock may include echocardiogram, CVP monitoring, tissue oxygenation and capnography, or advanced methods of determining CO. Advantages and disadvantages of these more advanced modalities will be discussed later within the context of shock monitoring.

MANAGEMENT OF SHOCK

Optimal management of shock depends first and foremost on early recognition of the syndrome, determination of its etiology, and correction of the underlying source while supporting the patient hemodynamically. Rapidity and adequacy of shock resolution will help prevent secondary reperfusion injury and prolonged morbidity. Variables of shock resuscitation must be frequently reassessed and therapy adjusted accordingly.

The underlying goal of shock management is to improve tissue oxygen perfusion. This may be accomplished by manipulating one or multiple physiologic parameters involved in oxygen delivery (DO_2) and extraction. Forms of obstructive shock require the most prompt diagnosis, as continued mechanical impairment can be rapidly fatal. Adequate treatment of these etiologies can be just as rapid in the form of needle decompression for a tension pneumothorax or pericardiocentesis for cardiac tamponade. Management of distributive and hypovolemic forms of shock likewise involves source control early in the diagnosis. This may be in the form of hemorrhage control, removal of infected tissue (source control), or removal of an anaphylactic source. Once the inflammatory cascade has initiated, vasoactive medications are often used in addition to fluid provision to increase perfusion. Treatment of cardiogenic shock employs multimodality treatment including volume optimization, vasopressors, control of dysrhythmias, use of inotropes and the mechanical-assist devices, and early revascularization in primary myocardial ischemia (82).

Classically, all forms of shock are primarily treated with a combination of fluids and vasoactive agents. Deliberation is ongoing regarding the dosing and selection of these modalities for resuscitation, and will be examined here in greater detail.

Fluid Resuscitation

The initial treatment for all forms of shock is fluid administration. Provision of fluid helps restore perfusion and replace intravascular volume lost via hemorrhage, capillary leak, or redistribution. Intravenous fluid is readily available, inexpensive, easy to administer, and has low intrinsic morbidity. The etiology of shock and response to fluid will further dictate continued use of volume as primary therapy; however, all forms of shock potentially benefit from an initial fluid challenge (83). Deliberation should be given to the method of delivery, timing of administration, type of fluid, and volume of administration.

Route of Administration

The setting of shock dictates administration of fluid primarily via the intravenous route, which may be in the form of a peripheral or central venous catheter. Although the type of shock may guide the choice of catheter (i.e., an introducer catheter for a rapid infusion system or a triple lumen catheter for anticipated vasopressor therapy), the dictum of "two large-bore peripheral IVs" cannot be overstated (84). As per Poiseuille's Law, width and length of the catheter dictates flow; therefore, a long, narrow, peripherally inserted central catheter will be of little utility when infusing a large bolus of fluid quickly. In the severely volume-depleted patient with collapsed veins, obtaining percutaneous venous access can prove difficult; saphenous vein cut-downs or interosseous access, particularly in the trauma or pediatric patient, can provide means of fluid administration in these extreme situations.

Timing and Volume of Administration

For forms of hypovolemic shock in particular, the concept of early restoration of intravascular volume to prevent circulatory collapse has long been recognized. In the hemorrhagic patient, volume resuscitation combined with source control may limit or prevent a state of irreversible shock, or the "lethal triad" of hypothermia, coagulopathy, and acidosis (85,86). The importance of the timing of volume loading is also paramount in all forms of shock, particularly in sepsis (87). Amplification of the previously described immune response can potentially be avoided if perfusion is restored early in the pathophysiologic process (88). Often the resuscitation process begins in the prehospital phase, with ambulance personnel administering crystalloid *en route*. Standard fluid boluses in the patient with shock typically amounts to 20 to 30 mL/kg at a time.

Overly aggressive fluid resuscitation both early and late in the course can be harmful in some circumstances. The concept of hypotensive resuscitation in the patient in whom mechanical control of bleeding has not been achieved—whether in traumatic injury, aortic aneurysm rupture, or gastrointestinal bleed—advocates for limited early aggressive fluid administration. Measures to raise blood pressure, particularly with fluid administration, may be counterproductive in this setting. In the penetrating thoracic trauma patient, early administration of large volumes of crystalloid has been shown to increase bleeding and subsequent mortality. Pushing fluid and intravascular volume beyond the initial phases of ischemia may propagate reperfusion injury and can be detrimental to further recovery. Restrictive fluid therapies for resuscitation have emerged in an effort to reduce the cardiac, wound healing, and pulmonary complications associated with large crystalloid infusions. Once patients have been stabilized, a more restrictive strategy of fluid administration can prevent subsequent morbidity.

Continued fluid administration beyond an initial bolus relies more on the patient's pathology and response to treatment rather than on arbitrary numbers. Physical examination characteristics such as jugular venous distension, skin turgor, urine output, and basic vital signs may give clues to volume state, but are notoriously subject to interpretation. The examiner is often misled by the appearance of gross edema, insomuch as it has no bearing on effective extracellular fluid volume in the patient with capillary leak. New tools for approximating intravascular volume status are emerging to provide dynamic variables for the clinician to use when estimating appropriateness for further volume resuscitation. Measures such as stroke volume variation (SVV) and pulse pressure variation (PPV) can provide more accurate assessment of volume status and are replacing CVP and pulmonary artery pressures as primary tools in the ICU (89–92); these will be discussed further below.

Types of Fluid

Considerable debate abounds regarding the types of fluid to be administered for shock resuscitation. Often the determination to use crystalloid versus colloid depends on fluid availability, clinical scenario, and regional practice differences. The fact that there is so much debate over the preferred fluid type indicates the lack of conclusive evidence for the superiority of one fluid over another.

Crystalloids. Composed of varying amounts of electrolytes and sugar, crystalloids are inexpensive, require no special tubing or preparation, and pose little to no risk of adverse reaction. Crystalloids used in shock resuscitation are generally categorized as isotonic or hypertonic, describing the in vivo tonicity of the fluid. Typical isotonic crystalloids used are normal saline, lactated Ringer solution, or other commercially available combinations of electrolytes with sodium as the primary ion. Lacking protein components, the isotonic crystalloids readily distribute to the extracellular fluid compartment and will require larger volumes of infusion to maintain intravascular filling. Traditional philosophy dictates that a threefold volume of crystalloid to colloid is required for intravascular expansion; this ratio has recently been debated, however, and may actually be closer to a ratio of 1.5:1 when comparing crystalloid to 5% albumin (93).

Normal saline (0.9% saline solution) and lactated Ringer solution compromise the majority of isotonic crystalloid used for shock. Normal saline provides sodium with an equal amount of chloride for buffer; hypernatremia and hyperchloremic metabolic acidosis are therefore potential consequences of continued normal saline administration (94). Because of this, normal saline should be used for resuscitation typically only for head trauma patients, as hyponatremia can increase morbidity in this patient population.

While the tonicity is essentially the same, the electrolyte composition of lactated Ringer solution is physiologically closer to plasma, with inclusion of potassium and calcium, and reduction in chloride concentrations. Lactated Ringer is considered one of the "balanced" crystalloids as a different anion is used besides chloride to balance the cations in solution (95). A chloride restrictive strategy is associated with less acute kidney injury in the critical care setting, and therefore these types of balanced solutions are favorable.

Hypertonic Crystalloid. Combining the convenience of crystalloid with the tonicity of colloids, hypertonic saline (HTS) has emerged as an important tool in shock resuscitation. Hypertonicity of the sodium concentration promotes influx of fluid from the interstitial space. As such, HTS is advantageous for rapid, low-volume resuscitation for hypovolemic shock, particularly in situations where resources and space are limited, such as a combat setting. Hypertonic solutions also favorably impact immune modulatory function. Studies investigating hemorrhagic shock have found a decrease in neutrophil activation, and upregulation of anti-inflammatory cytokine production with use of HTS. Additional data suggest that HTS positively affects cardiac function in addition to volume expansion in septic shock (96,97).

While relatively safe compared to colloid infusion, the administration of high concentrations of sodium for volume resuscitation carries the concern for hypernatremia and hyperosmolarity. Compromise of renal function is likewise feared with high sodium and osmolar loads (98,99). Reports of hypokalemia, metabolic acidosis, and impaired platelet aggregation have also been documented with HTS use (100). Primary use of HTS is in the traumatic brain injury patient; small volumes should be used and electrolytes, creatinine, and serum osmolarity should be checked frequently to avoid the abovementioned complications.

Colloids. In reference to volume resuscitation, colloids generally consist of fluids that have a higher molecular weight based on composition consisting of protein or starches. These components increase the cost of colloids, make them susceptible to shortage, and mandate specialized tubing for delivery. The possibility of transfusion reaction is increased, as some of these compounds are derived from blood products. Likewise, allergic reactions can be noted with some of the synthetic formulations.

Conceptually, colloids more rapidly expand intravascular volume owing to their higher oncotic pressure. This effect may not necessarily persist beyond a few hours, especially in the critically ill patient in which capillary permeability is altered (101). In addition to more rapid volume expansion with less fluid infusion, this same increase in intravascular oncotic pressure has prompted the employment of colloids with the intent to reduce or prevent secondary edema; this effect has not been appreciated clinically, however. Studies reveal that edema formation is more dependent on fluid volume than on fluid type per se (102).

Albumin. First used for fluid resuscitation during World War II, albumin is a colloid derived from pooled human plasma and diluted with sodium. Preparations consist of 5% or 25% solution in quantities of 250 to 500 mL or 50 mL, respectively. As a blood product derivative, albumin is subject to disadvantages faced by other donated products—namely, periodic shortages, high acquisition costs, and refusal based on religious grounds. While transmission of viruses or other blood-borne diseases is theoretically a risk, only a few cases have been reported. Like any resuscitation fluid, patients are subject to sequelae of volume overload if infusion amounts are not monitored.

While indications for albumin use are broad, proven benefit to particular therapies is increasingly narrow. Numerous studies detailing poor prognosis with low serum albumin levels in critically ill patients prompted attempts to improve survival with intravenous supplementation (103–105). Compared with other colloid administration, albumin itself has no benefit in this patient population (106,107).

Albumin as a resuscitation fluid likewise has come under scrutiny. Previously, studies investigating albumin as a volume expander have been underpowered, prompting meta-analysis as the primary statistical measure of its worth. An initial Cochrane review comparing albumin to crystalloid examined 24 studies and found a 6% increase in absolute risk of death with albumin infusion (108). To confuse matters, subsequent meta-analysis of 55 studies showed no difference in mortality between albumin and crystalloid for resuscitation (109, 110). In 2004, the Saline versus Albumin Fluid Evaluation (SAFE) trial prospectively compared albumin to isotonic crystalloid for fluid resuscitation in a mixed ICU population (93); results showed no difference in morbidity or mortality overall with either fluid choice, although traumatic brain injury patients did show increased morbidity with albumin use. Subsequent multicenter studies demonstrated no difference in morbidity or mortality for albumin versus crystalloid in septic shock resuscitation.

Starches. Synthetic colloid polymers were developed for use in volume resuscitation in an attempt to retain the oncotic properties of albumin while decreasing cost and transfusion risk. Initial formulations of hydroxyethyl starch (HES) included high–molecular-weight moieties, accounting for an increased risk of coagulation and renal disturbances associated with their use (111–113). Lower–molecular-weight HES solutions were subsequently developed, with resultant fewer negative effects on bleeding, but concern for dose-dependent impaired renal function persisted (114).

While numerous studies have illustrated downregulation of proinflammatory cytokines with HES use, some of these results may be an effect of the efficiency of volume resuscitation, and not necessarily the fluid itself (115–117). Ongoing concerns about increase in renal failure and mortality in septic and mixed ICU populations prompted the U.S. Food and Drug Administration to add a warning regarding use of HES products in 2013. As such, HES use is not supported at this time.

Despite the theoretical advantage of colloids over crystalloids for shock resuscitation, there is no evidence from randomized controlled trials to demonstrate mortality difference. Studies demonstrating improved short-term gains with colloids use a heterogeneous population and/or fluid composition, making interpretation and application difficult. In larger studies, short-term physiologic gains made from colloid use do not translate in to longer-term improvement. As colloids are not associated with improvement in survival, and are considerably more expensive, it is hard to justify their use (118).

Special Fluid Considerations

Hemorrhagic Shock Resuscitation

Aggressive use of crystalloids during the Vietnam conflict resulted in improved mortality and reduction in renal failure, but also led to the emergence of acute lung injury and acute respiratory distress syndrome in the trauma population. Extensive use of crystalloids for trauma followed, with the popular concept of pushing fluids beyond supranormal resuscitation goals (119). Consequences of this large-volume approach are becoming more evident, with adverse cardiac, pulmonary, coagulation, and immunologic effects documented with massive crystalloid infusion (120).

With the recognition of the "blood lethal triad" of coagulopathy, acidosis, and hypothermia in the bleeding trauma patient, methods to physiologically break this cycle have come into play. Pushing crystalloids for shock resuscitation merely aggravates this pathway. Appropriate resuscitation in hemorrhagic shock includes measures such as damage control surgery and hemostatic resuscitation. The goals of damage control surgery are to stop ongoing hemorrhage and provide control of any visceral injury in a truncated manner such that the patient can return to the ICU for warming and resuscitation. Key to this approach is a massive transfusion strategy in which blood is provided in a balanced manner and in preference to crystalloid or other colloid during this time period. Since the patient bleeds whole blood, it makes physiologic sense to provide blood products in a manner that resembles that of whole blood. Major studies including PROMMTT and PROPPR have demonstrated survival benefits for hemorrhagic shock when providing platelets:FFP:RBC in as close to a 1:1:1 ratio as possible (121,122). The combination of early mechanical bleeding control with this hemostatic resuscitation is the current standard for hemorrhagic shock resuscitation.

Pharmacotherapy in Shock

Primary therapy for shock involves treating the cause and supplementation with fluids. When these modalities fail, vasopressors are typically employed as supplementation. Shock is not hypotension alone, however, and other agents can be used to compensate for the diminished tissue perfusion defined by this syndrome. Drugs used for shock will be examined here by the classifications of vasopressor, inotrope, and miscellaneous, although these categories may overlap to a degree.

Vasopressors

Vasopressors are generally given after an initial fluid bolus has failed or had marginal effect. Within the context of avoiding the consequences of excessive fluid administration, vasopressors may help limit volumes of fluid given; however, peripheral and end-organ vasoconstriction have their own adverse effects. Striking the balance between volume and vasopressors in the context of timing and type of shock is therefore a key component to resuscitation. With early recognition of shock, vasopressors can often be avoided by restoration of volume (123).

End-organ arterial autoregulation generally compensates for decreased MAP within a certain range; however, local vasoconstriction and vasodilatation may be unable to overcome extremes of perfusion. Administering catecholamine vasopressors may help improve MAP and therefore improve tissue perfusion by redistributing CO. The venous compartment also benefits from vasopressor therapy by decreasing compliance and therefore improving effective volume. Classifications of vasopressors consist of natural and synthetic versions of catecholamines (Table 44.8).

Norepinephrine. A naturally occurring vasopressor, norepinephrine is released by the postganglionic adrenergic nerves in response to stress. It has potent α-adrenergic effects, with less potent β_1-stimulation. The α-adrenergic effects lead to increased systolic and diastolic blood pressure, with the addition of increased venous return via decreasing venous capacitance; this subsequently leads to increased cardiac filling pressure. Effect on the coronary arterial flow is enhanced via the increase in diastolic blood pressure. The β-adrenergic effects lead to increased chronotropic function, although this is limited by the baroreflex of vasoconstriction, resulting in zero net change in heart rate. Enhanced inotrope stimulation and stroke volume are likewise negated by an increase in left ventricular afterload, leading to a limited increase in CO.

Historically, the exaggerated peripheral vasoconstrictive properties of the drug have promoted a level of distrust leading to the often quoted "leave 'em dead." These fears are largely unfounded at indicated dosing ranges, and use of the drug may actually enhance renal function (124). The drug is safe and easily titratable, and lacks the tachydysrhythmic properties of other frequently used agents for shock. Resurgence in the use of norepinephrine has occurred with the recognition of its beneficial properties, and is now recommended as the first-line vasopressor in the treatment of shock (125).

Epinephrine. Epinephrine is the major physiologic adrenergic hormone of the adrenal medulla and represents the maximum in catecholamine stimulation. The agent potently stimulates α_1-receptors with resultant marked venous and arterial vasoconstriction. These changes may lead to detrimental effects on regional blood flow, particularly on mesenteric and renal vascular beds. β-Effects lead to increased heart rate and inotropism. Due to counter effects of β_2-vasodilation, the diastolic blood pressure is only slightly affected, with a lesser degree of increase in MAP than seen with norepinephrine. Stimulation of β_2-receptors and blunting of mast cell response also makes epinephrine highly effective for anaphylaxis. Epinephrine has dose-dependent effects, with very low doses stimulating primarily β-receptors. This property makes epinephrine attractive as a primary inotrope; however, the range of that particular low dose

TABLE 44.8 Sympathomimetic Drugs

		Adrenergic Effects	Arrhythmogenic Potential			
Drug	**Usual IV dose**	**α**	**β**	**Dopa**		**Setting**
Dopamine	1–2 μg/kg/min[a]	1+	1+	3+	1+	Oliguria despite "normal" blood pressure
	2–10 μg/kg/min	2+	2+	3+	2+	Initial emergency treatment of hypotension (any cause)
	10–30 μg/kg/min	3+	2+	3+	3+	Alternative treatment for bradycardia
Dobutamine	2–30 μg/kg/min	1+	3+	0	2+	Cardiac shock Pulmonary edema with marginal blood pressure
Norepinephrine	0.01–0.1 μg/kg/min (0.5–80 μg/min)	3+	2+	0	2+	Initial emergency treatment of hypotension (any cause, especially sepsis)
Epinephrine	0.5–1 **mg**[b] (1:10,000) 0.01–0.3 μg/kg/min (1–200 μg/min)	1+	2+	0	3+	Cardiac arrest Severe hypotension and bradycardia
	0.3–0.5 **mg** SQ (1:1,000)[c]	2+	3+	0	3+	Anaphylaxis
Phenylephrine	0.1–1 μg/kg/min (20–200 μg/min)	3+	0	0	0	Distributive shock when no cardiac effect is desired
Isoproterenol	0.03–0.3 μg/kg/min (2–20 μg/min)	0	3+	0	3+	Refractory bradycardia
						Denervated hearts
Milrinone[d]	Load: 50 μg/kg over 10 min Then: 0.375–0.75 μg/kg/min	0	0	0	2+	Cardiogenic shock

Dopa, dopamine.
[a]Increases renal and splanchnic blood flow. No impact on AKI.
[b]Milligram doses are in bold to differentiate from micrograms.
[c]SQ: Subcutaneous dosing, may be repeated every 15–20 min.
[d]Phosphodiesterase inhibitors; require loading dose.

varies with each patient and titration may prove dangerous. Epinephrine is advocated as a secondary pressor for septic shock, and as the primary pressor for cardiac arrest resuscitation.

Dopamine. As the hormone precursor of norepinephrine and epinephrine, dopamine stimulates α-, β-, and dopaminergic receptors in a dose-dependent fashion. This results in mixed vasoconstrictive, inotropic, chronotropic, and vasodilatory effects.

Classically, "renal-dose" dopamine ranges from 0 to 5 μg/kg/min and results in vasodilation of renal and mesenteric vascular beds via dopamine receptors. Although this stimulation results in diuresis, the overall effect on renal function and need for renal replacement therapy is unchanged and may actually be worsened (126). Conversely, at high doses of 10 to 20 μg/kg/min, α-effects predominate, resulting in almost pure vasoconstriction. β-Receptor stimulation at middle doses of 5 to 10 μg/kg/min results in increased inotropic and chronotropic function leading to increased MAP similar to norepinephrine. However, without simultaneous activation of α-receptors at this dose, vasodilatation by dopamine receptors is unopposed and reflex tachycardia may predominate.

In the past, dopamine has been postulated as the first inotrope of choice in cardiogenic failure with hypotension (127). More recent recommendations, however, identify sympathetic inotropes such as dopamine as increasing mortality when used for primary left heart failure (128). Likewise, in septic shock, norepinephrine has a more reliable dosing profile and has demonstrated more beneficial outcomes compared to dopamine (129). Tachydysrhythmias are the predominant concern with dopamine, conversely making it potentially useful in shock with associated bradycardia.

Phenylephrine. Phenylephrine is a rapidly acting vasopressor with a short duration of action and pure α_1-receptor stimulation. As such, it increases MAP primarily by increasing SVR. Reflex bradycardia may develop; therefore, it is occasionally used for distributive shock in the face of tachydysrhythmias. This same unopposed increase in SVR also impairs CO in the patient with impaired pump function. The use of phenylephrine has since fallen out of favor, and is generally reserved for the pregnant patient with shock for whom other vasopressors may be detrimental or as rescue therapy in patients with a high CO and low SVR. Its rapid onset and short duration of action also makes it useful in the context of low intraoperative blood pressure due to vasodilatory inhaled anesthetics.

Inotropes

As a group, inotropic agents augment CO by increasing contractility. Sources of left ventricular failure are many, including exacerbation of congestive heart failure (CHF), acute infarction, or sepsis-related cardiomyopathy. The inflammatory state that accompanies some forms of cardiogenic shock may result in vasodilation instead of vasoconstriction, making particular inotropes less useful for restoration of tissue perfusion (130). As with other forms of pharmacotherapy for shock, inotropes should be used only in a short-term situation until underlying pathology can be corrected. Prolonged use can increase myocardial work and exacerbate ischemia.

Dobutamine. Dobutamine is a synthetic adrenergic agent derived from dopamine. Current formulation of the drug is as a racemic mixture, with the L-isomer stimulating α_1- and the D-isomer stimulating β_1- and β_2-receptors. This combined stimulation results in a net increase in inotropic and chronotropic parameters. In theory, vasodilatory (β_2) effects are limited, making dobutamine useful in increasing pump function without lowering blood pressure. In practice, some degree of vasodilation is encountered, resulting in decreased blood pressure and tachycardia acutely. With increase in CO, however, the BP generally corrects to normal. For this reason, adequate volume loading prior to initiation of dobutamine is emphasized. Likewise, the lack of increase in BP makes dobutamine a poor selection as monotherapy in primary cardiogenic shock. At higher doses, vasoconstriction may dominate leading to increased myocardial O_2 consumption (VO_2), so it should be used with caution in states where ischemia is present. Currently, dobutamine is the standard inotrope used in noncardiogenic shock (such as sepsis) when cardiac contractility is compromised (131).

Isoproterenol. With practically no α-adrenergic stimulation, isoproterenol functions as a pure β-agonist. β_1-Stimulation results in increased SV and heart rate, while β_2-stimulation induces vasodilatation. The net result is that of enhanced CO without the benefit of redistribution of blood flow. Increased myocardial VO_2 exacerbated by lack of coronary perfusion due to decreased diastolic pressures may lead to cardiac ischemia. Use of isoproterenol is generally limited to β-blocker overdose or in the atropine-resistant transplanted heart.

Phosphodiesterase Inhibitors. A novel agent in vasoactive treatment, milrinone is the most common synthetic phosphodiesterase III inhibitor. Reduction in this enzyme results in an increase in cyclic adenosine monophosphate (cAMP), a modulator of myocardial contractility. Additional increase in cAMP results in vasodilation, with the net effect of increasing CO and, at higher doses, tachycardia. This vasodilatory effect may decrease effective left ventricular preload, but may also benefit afterload reduction, reducing cardiac work. In the hypotensive patient, acute vasodilation may not be tolerated, thus, while not recommended in vasodilatory shock for this reason, milrinone may be used in specific situations for cardiogenic shock. These include advanced heart failure in patients awaiting heart transplant, in acute decompensation of CHF on standard medications, and in patients in cardiogenic shock with long-term β-blocker use (132). Amrinone is an additional agent in this class, but its use is limited by its side effect profile.

Levosimendan. Levosimendan is the singular drug in a new class of inotropic agents. Primary mechanism of action is by increasing the sensitivity of troponin C for calcium without enhancing influx of calcium itself. It also opens ATP-dependent potassium channels, leading to enhanced ventricular contractility without compromising diastolic function. This vasodilatory effect makes it particularly useful for myocardial protection. The drug is primarily used for acute and chronic heart failure; dosing is 0.05 to 0.2 μg/kg/min. It performs similarly to dobutamine for acute heart failure.

Vasopressin. Vasopressin is an attractive hormone for use in shock states not only for its vasoconstrictive properties but also for its antidiuretic effects. As a noncatecholamine vasopressor, it acts via V1 receptors to restore vascular tone. Catecholamine responsiveness may decrease over time during severe sepsis, possibly due to an increase in NO-induced vasodilatation. Likewise, studies of hemorrhagic and vasodilatory shock have demonstrated a relative deficiency of vasopressin. For this reason, vasopressin is often used at a low dose without titration, in the manner of hormone replacement. Potentiation of adrenergic agents makes vasopressin particularly useful in combination with norepinephrine, and has been recommended for the treatment of septic shock to reduce catecholamine administration (133). Although evidence from meta-analysis demonstrates decreased mortality with vasopressin administration versus norepinephrine in septic shock, a recent randomized control trial demonstrates no difference (134).

END POINTS OF RESUSCITATION

The primary goal in the management of shock is a return to normal tissue perfusion. If shock is recognized promptly, and timely, appropriate treatment strategies are implemented, reversal of its clinical signs may be appreciated. These include improvement in mental status, normalization of vital signs, and restoration of urine output. However, despite these findings, many patients remain in a state of occult hypoperfusion and ongoing tissue acidosis with resultant multiple organ failure and death (12,135). Consequently, better end points of resuscitation are needed to guide resuscitation efforts.

The holy grail of shock resuscitation in recent years has been that of achieving adequate end-organ DO_2. DO_2 is a function of cardiac index (CI), Hgb, and oxygen saturation (SaO_2), as seen in the Fick's equation. The use of DO_2 as a resuscitation end point has had varying results. In the 1970s, Shoemaker et al. (136) reviewed the physiologic patterns in surviving and nonsurviving shock patients, observing that survivors had significantly increased DO_2, VO_2, and CO values (DO_2 ≥600 mL/min/m^2, VO_2 ≥170 mL/min/m^2, and CI ≥4.5 L/min/m^2). In a subsequent prospective study, they documented decreased complications, lengths of stay, and hospital costs when employing these parameters as goals of resuscitation in high-risk surgical patients. Further work by Shoemaker's group and others have shown that utilization of this "supranormal resuscitation" strategy decreases morbidity and mortality in critically ill patients (137).

More recently, however, supranormal resuscitation has been associated with significant morbidity—ongoing tissue ischemia, abdominal compartment syndrome, coagulopathy, and CHF—and mortality. Velmahos et al. (138) documented improved survival in patients who achieved supranormal DO_2; however, they concluded that "this was not a function of the supranormal resuscitation, but rather the patient's own ability to achieve these parameters". As demonstrated here, the utilization of DO_2 and, more specifically, "supranormal resuscitation" in the management of shock has had varying degrees of success. Different strategies to monitor end-organ perfusion, as well as methods to assess volume responsiveness, are more commonly used.

Basic Hemodynamic Monitoring

Basic monitoring in patients with shock includes noninvasive vital sign measurements, cardiac rhythm, and urinary output and other clinical variables of end-organ perfusion. The hemodynamic profiles of shock are depicted in Table 44.2. It is these parameters that often guide the management of shock and, in that context, meticulous equipment calibration and documentation are essential (139,140). These measurements are subject to many potential artifacts as seen in Table 44.9 (14). Therefore, it is critical for the clinician to evaluate these variables in concert with the patient's clinical picture.

Invasive Hemodynamic Monitoring

Central venous catheters are commonly used in this patient population. As such, CVP measurements are readily available and were, in the past, often used as a rough guideline in the resuscitation of shock. It is increasingly recognized that there is actually very little correlation between intravascular volume status and CVP. As a consequence, utilization of CVP during shock resuscitation has fallen out of favor. Similarly, PACs can provide numerous additional hemodynamic parameters; however, it is not clear that the appropriate end point is the normalization of these values, nor is it clear how these end points should be achieved (141–144). Observational studies and meta-analysis have suggested that PACs may actually increase mortality, ICU length of stay, hospital costs, and resource utilization (145).

Blood and Serum Markers

Numerous laboratory values can provide some clues to degree and correction of shock. SvO_2 can be obtained from a PAC and provides an indication of the end result of DO_2 and VO_2; an approximation of this can also be obtained from a central venous catheter ($ScvO_2$), although the value will be higher. While both SvO_2 and $ScvO_2$ can be obtained continuously, and while initially considered essential to goal-directed resuscitation, both methods have fallen out of favor, both due to need for invasive monitoring, and due to equivalency of lactate clearance as a surrogate.

Base deficit is defined as the amount of base, in millimoles, required to increase 1 L of whole blood to the predicted pH based on the $PaCO_2$ (146). In shock states, the base deficit may serve as a surrogate marker for anaerobic metabolism and subsequent lactic acidosis if metabolic acidosis is the primary disorder and not a compensatory response (147). In this sense, it is superior to pH secondary to the many compensatory mechanisms in place to normalize pH (148). Base deficit has numerous confounders, so it should be used as a method to trend resuscitation and not as a stand-alone measure.

Serum lactate levels are used extensively in monitoring shock resuscitation. In patients suffering from noncardiogenic shock, Vincent et al. documented a correlation between initial serum lactate levels and patient outcomes (149). However, in shock resuscitation it is the lactate trend that is most predictive of mortality. Patients whose lactate levels normalized (serum levels <2 mmol/L) within 24 hours had less than 10% mortality, those who normalized between 24 and 48 hours had a 25% mortality, while those who did not normalize by 48 hours had over 80% mortality. Lactate measurement is now an integral part of the Surviving Sepsis Guidelines for monitoring resuscitation (125).

Esophageal Doppler

Esophageal Doppler measurement uses estimation of aortic velocity as a surrogate for CO. It also provides a reasonably accurate measure of SVV. Despite variable degrees of artifact with this method, it is well studied and provides the most accurate estimation of CO when compared to PAC measurements.

TABLE 44.9 Common Artifacts in Hemodynamic Measurements

Variable	Artifact	Causes	Comments/Corrective Action
Vascular pressures (including PCWP)	Preload overestimation	*Technical:*	
		Improper leveling of transducer	Avoid with rigid nursing protocols
		Improper calibration	
		Improper system frequency response	
		Respiratory:	
		Not recording pressures at end-expiration during mechanical ventilation	Avoid digital readouts Use analog tracings
		Active expiratory effort	Suspect with respiratory distress; consider neuromuscular blockade
		Positive end-expiratory pressure	Usually not significant with <10 cm H_2O PEEP
		Improper positioning of catheter tip	Suspect if tip in upper lobes on chest radiograph or PAD < PCWP
		Cardiac:	
		Mitral regurgitation	Read PCWP as post-A wave
		Mitral stenosis	Interpret with caution as preload estimate
		Acute changes in left ventricle compliance	Suspect in presence of myocardial ischemia
	Preload underestimation	*Technical:* as for overestimation	
		Respiratory:	
		Not recording pressures at end-expiration during spontaneous breathing	
Cardiac output	Inaccuracies	*Technical:*	
		Incorrect injectable volume; thermistor contact with vessel wall; incorrect computational constant	Inspect temperature curves; suspect if pulmonary artery waveform is damp-ened; follow rigid nursing protocol
		Cardiac:	
		Tricuspid regurgitation	Do not use in presence of significant tricuspid regurgitation
	Wide variation	*Technical:* as for inaccuracies	Delete measurements with >20% variation from the mean
		Respiratory:	
		Variable respiratory rate during mechanical ventilation	Average measurements throughout respiratory cycle
Mixed venous oxygen saturation	Inaccuracies	*Technical:*	
		Light reflecting against vessel wall, catheter kinking	Note computer error messages
		Presence of significant HgbCO	Measure HgbCO directly at least once
	Misinterpretation	Shifts in oxygen dissociation curve	Correlate with PvO_2 measurements
		Dependence on oxygen delivery	Correlate with oxygen delivery measurements
Extravascular lung water	Inaccuracies	Inaccurate measurement of cardiac output (as above)	Correlate cardiac output with regular thermodilution measurements
	Underestimation	Presence of significant areas of nonperfused lung	Measurements suspect in presence of significant regional disease (i.e., lobar pneumonia) or known vascular obstruction
Systemic vascular resistance	Inaccuracies	Inaccurate measurement of cardiac output (as above)	
		Inaccurate measurement of blood pressure	Measure directly (see above)

PCWP, pulmonary capillary wedge pressure; PEEP, positive end-expiratory pressure; PAD, pulmonary artery diastolic; HgbCO, carboxyhemoglobin; PvO_2, mixed venous oxygen partial pressure.

SVV is also extremely valuable from this method, with data supporting its use during perioperative resuscitation. Use is limited by discomfort to the patient and possible complications from insertion.

Near-Infrared Spectroscopy

Near-infrared spectroscopy (NIRS) is the measurement of the wavelength and intensity of the absorption of near-infrared light by a sample. In medicine, it uses chromophores such as Hgb to do so and allows for the measurement of tissue oxygenation, PO_2, PCO_2, and pH (150). Taylor et al. (151) documented a close correlation between tissue oxygenation measurements and hemodynamic parameters in a model of hemorrhagic shock. In this study, NIRS was also better able to differentiate "responder" from "nonresponder" animals in comparison to lactate levels or global DO_2. This technology is limited by cost and waveform interference.

Photoplethysmography

Similar to NIRS, photoplethysmography (PPG) uses measurement of intensity of light as it relates to a waveform produced peripherally. Essentially, PPG technology uses pulse oximeter data to calculate a variability index similar to PPV which is then used to predict fluid responsiveness. Although it does not correlate as well to intravascular measurements of PPV, it has the advantage of being noninvasive, less expensive, and easy to use.

Bioimpedance

Bioimpedance and bioreactance devices assess thoracic volume status based on noninvasive measurement of electrical current via Ohm's law. In theory, they can be used to roughly assess SV and, therefore, when multiplied times the heart rate, yield CO. Typically, they are most useful for measuring volume responsiveness. Although these are noninvasive and easy to use, they are limited by a large amount of artifact.

Arterial Waveform Analysis

Increasingly popular for assessing fluid responsiveness, arterial waveform analyzers estimate SV and CO. This can be done either with an arterial catheter or with both an arterial and venous catheter to improve accuracy in some devices. Measuring the variation in stroke volume during the respiratory cycle can estimate the SVV, which is a rough estimate of where the heart is on the Starling curve. These devices can be extremely useful when determining need for further fluid administration in patients who are mechanically ventilated. Use of SVV, instead of CVP, has favorable outcomes on perioperative patients in particular, as these individuals receive, in general, less fluid.

Key Points

- Shock is likely the most common life-threatening diagnosis made in the ICU.
- Despite technologic advances, it remains a significant source of morbidity and mortality.
- As the etiologies of shock are vast, the diagnosis of shock and its inciting source can be difficult to identify. Aggressive diagnostic testing is required to avoid irreversible cellular injury, multiple organ failure and, potentially, death.
- The primary goal in the management of shock is a return to normal tissue perfusion. This is attained via various volume resuscitation modalities, pharmacologic agents, and resuscitation strategies.
- Past and current research efforts continue in hopes of optimizing the diagnosis and management of shock with the ultimate goal of improving patient outcomes.

References

1. LeDran HF. *A Treatise, or Reflections Drawn from Practice on Gun-Shot Wounds*. London: England; 1737.
2. Morris EA. *A Practical Treatise on Shock after Operations and Injuries*. London: Hardwicke; 1867.
3. Fischer H. *Ueber den Shock. Samml Klin Vortr.* 1870:10.
4. Maphoter ED. Shock, its nature, duration, and mode of treatment. *BMJ.* 1879;2:1023.
5. Crile GW. *An Experimental Research into Surgical Shock*. Philadelphia, PA: JB Lippincott; 1899.
6. Cannon WB. *Traumatic Shock*. New York: D. Appleton and Company; 1923.
7. Blalock A. Experimental shock: the cause of the low blood pressure produced by muscle injury. *Arch Surg.* 1930;20:959–996.
8. Wiggers CJ. *The Physiology of Shock*. Cambridge, MA: Harvard University Press; 1950.
9. Report of the Surgeon General of the Army. 1900:318.
10. Tennant R, Wiggers CJ. The effect of coronary occlusion on myocardial contraction. *Am J Physiol.* 1935;211:351–361.
11. Wo CJ, Shoemaker WC, Appel PL, et al. Unreliability of blood pressure and heart rate to evaluate cardiac output in emergency resuscitation and critical illness. *Crit Care Med.* 1993;21:218–223.
12. Scalea TM, Maltz S, Yelon J, et al. Resuscitation of multiple trauma and head injury: role of crystalloid fluids and inotropes. *Crit Care Med.* 1994;22:1610–1615.
13. Mello PM, Sharma VK, Dellinger RP. Shock overview. *Semin Respir Crit Care Med.* 2004;25:619–628.
14. Jimenez EJ. Shock. In: Civetta JM, Taylor RW, Kirby RR, eds. *Critical Care*. 3rd ed. Philadelphia, PA: Lippincott–Raven Publishers; 1997:359.
15. Blalock A. Shock: further studies with particular reference to the effects of hemorrhage. *Arch Surg.* 1937;29:837–857.
16. Weil MH, Shubin H. Proposed reclassification of shock states with special reference to distributive effects. In: Hinshaw LB, Cox BG, eds. *The Fundamental Mechanisms of Shock*. New York: Plenum Press; 1972:13.
17. Kumar A, Parrillo JE. Shock: classification, pathophysiology, and approach to management. In: Parrillo JE, Dellinger RP, eds. *Critical Care Medicine*. 2nd ed. St. Louis, MO: Mosby, Inc.; 2002:371.
18. Warden GD. Burn shock resuscitation. *World J Surg.* 1992;16:16–23.
19. National Center for Health Statistics: Health, United States, 1986, DHHS Pub No (PHS) 87–1232, Washington, DC: US Government Printing Office; 1986.
20. Gruppo Italiano per lo Studio della Streptochinasi nell'Infarto Miocardico (GISSI). Effectiveness of intravenous thrombolytic treatment in acute myocardial infarction. *Lancet.* 1986;1:397–402.
21. Goldberg RJ, Gore JM, Alpert JS, et al. Cardiogenic shock after acute myocardial infarction: incidence and mortality from a community-wide perspective, 1975 to 1988. *N Engl J Med.* 1991;325:1117–1122.
22. Collaborative Group. Third International Study of Infarct Survival. ISIS-3 a randomised comparison of streptokinase vs tissue plasminogen activator vs anistreplase and of aspirin plus heparin vs aspirin alone among 41,299 cases of suspected acute myocardial infarction. *Lancet.* 1992;339:753–770.
23. The GUSTO Investigators. An international randomized trial comparing four thrombolytic strategies for acute myocardial infarction. *N Engl J Med.* 1993;329:673–682.
24. Hochman JS, Boland J, Sleeper LA, et al. Current spectrum of cardiogenic shock and effect of early revascularization on mortality: results of an international registry. SHOCK Registry Investigators. *Circulation.* 1995; 91:873–881.
25. Keel M, Trentz O. Pathophysiology of trauma. *Injury.* 2005;36:691–709.
26. Bone RC. Sir Isaac Newton, sepsis, SIRS, and CARS. *Crit Care Med.* 1996; 24:1125–1128.
27. Lyons A, Kelly JL, Rodrick ML, et al. Major injury induces increased production of interleukin-10 by cells of the immune system with a negative impact on resistance to infection. *Ann Surg.* 1997;226:450–458.
28. Malone DL, Kuhls D, Napolitano LM, et al. Back to basics: validation of the admission systemic inflammatory response syndrome score in predicting outcome in trauma. *J Trauma.* 2001;51:458–463.
29. Rangel-Frausto MS, Pittet D, Costigan M, et al. The natural history of the systemic inflammatory response syndrome (SIRS). A prospective study. *JAMA.* 1995;273:117–123.
30. American College of Chest Physicians/Society of Critical Care Medicine Consensus Conference: definitions for sepsis and organ failure and guidelines for the use of innovative therapies in sepsis. *Crit Care Med.* 1992;20:864–874.
31. Van Griensen M, Krettek C, Pape HC. Immune reactions after trauma. *Eur J Trauma.* 2003;29:181–192.
32. Neidhardt R, Keel M, Steckholzer U, et al. Relationship of interleukin-10 plasma levels to severity of injury and clinical outcome in injured patients. *J Trauma.* 1997;42:863–870.
33. Schroder O, Laun RA, Held B, et al. Association of interleukin-10 promoter polymorphism with the incidence of multiple organ dysfunction following major trauma: results of a prospective pilot study. *Shock.* 2004;21:306–310.
34. Dinarello CA. Proinflammatory cytokines. *Chest.* 2000;118:503–508.
35. Cook MC. Immunology of trauma. *Trauma.* 2001;3:79–88.
36. Giannoudis PV, Hildebrand F, Pape HC. Inflammatory serum markers in patients with multiple trauma. Can they predict outcome. *J Bone Joint Surg Br.* 2004;86:313–323.
37. Seekamp A, Jochum M, Ziegler M, et al. Cytokines and adhesion molecules in elective and accidental trauma-related ischemia/reperfusion. *J Trauma.* 1998;44:874–882.
38. Botha AJ, Moore FA, Moore EE, et al. Postinjury neutrophil priming and activation: an early vulnerable window. *Surgery.* 1995;118:358–364.

39. Cochrane CG. Immunologic tissue injury mediated by neutrophilic leukocytes. *Adv Immunol.* 1968;9:97–162.
40. Fujishima S, Aikawa N. Neutrophil-mediated tissue injury and its modulation. *Intensive Care Med.* 1995;21:277–285.
41. Smith JA. Neutrophils, host defense, and inflammation: a double-edged sword. *J Leuk Biol.* 1994;56:672–686.
42. Kubes P, Ward PA. Leukocyte recruitment and the acute inflammatory response. *Brain Pathol.* 2000;10:127–135.
43. Abbassi O, Kishimoto TK, McIntire LV, et al. E-selectin supports neutrophil rolling in vitro under conditions of flow. *J Clin Invest.* 1993; 92:2719–2730.
44. Bevilacqua MP, Pober JS, Mendrick DL, et al. Identification of an inducible endothelial-leukocyte adhesion molecule. *Proc Natl Acad Sci.* 1987; 84:9238–9242.
45. Geng J-G, Bevilacqua MP, Moore KL, et al. Rapid neutrophil adhesion to activated endothelium mediated by GMP-140. *Nature.* 1990;343:757–760.
46. Jones DA, Abbassi O, McIntire LV, et al. P-selectin mediates neutrophil rolling on histamine-stimulated endothelial cells. *Biophys J.* 1993; 65:1560–1569.
47. Kanwar S, Steeber DA, Tedder TF, et al. Overlapping roles for L-selectin and P-selectin in antigen-induced immune responses in the microvasculature. *J Immunol.* 1999;162:2709–2716.
48. Robinson SD, Frenette PS, Rayburn H, et al. Multiple, targeted deficiencies in selectins reveal a predominant role for P-selectin in leukocyte recruitment. *Proc Natl Acad Sci.* 1999;96:11452–11457.
49. Diamond MS, Springer TA. The dynamic regulation of integrin adhesiveness. *Curr Biol.* 1994;4:506–517.
50. Berlin C, Bargatze RF, Campbell JJ, et al. Alpha 4 integrins mediate lymphocyte attachment and rolling under physiologic flow. *Cell.* 1995; 80:413–422.
51. Hemler ME. VLA proteins in the integrin family: structures, functions, and their role on leukocytes. *Annu Rev Immunol.* 1990;8:365–400.
52. Schmidt OI, Infanger M, Heyde CE, et al. The role of neuroinflammation in traumatic brain injury. *Eur J Trauma.* 2004;30:135–149.
53. Goris RJ, te Boekhorst TP, Neytinck JK, et al. Multiple organ failure—generalized autodestructive inflammation? *Arch Surg.* 1985;120:1109–1115.
54. Martins PS, Kallas EG, Neto MC, et al. Upregulation of reactive oxygen species generation and phagocytosis, and increased apoptosis in human neutrophils during severe sepsis and septic shock. *Shock.* 2003;20:208–212.
55. Powell WC, Fingleton B, Wilson CL, et al. The metalloproteinase matrilysin proteolytically generates active soluble Fas ligand and potentiates epithelial cell apoptosis. *Curr Biol.* 1999;9:1441–1447.
56. Grote K, Flach I, Luchtefeld M, et al. Mechanical stretch enhances mRNA expression and proenzyme release of matrix metalloproteinase-2 (MMP-2) via NAD(P)H oxidase-derived reactive oxygen species. *Circ Res.* 2003;92: e80–e86.
57. Winterbourn CC, Buss IH, Chan TP, et al. Protein carbonyl measurements show evidence of early oxidative stress in critically ill patients. *Crit Care Med.* 2000;28:143–149.
58. Kazzaz JA, Xu J, Palaia TA, et al. Cellular oxygen toxicity. Oxidant injury without apoptosis. *J Biol Chem.* 1996;271:15182–15186.
59. Kretzschmar M, Pfeiffer L, Schmidt C, et al. Plasma levels of glutathione, alpha-tocopherol and lipid peroxides in polytraumatized patients; evidence for a stimulating effect of TNF alpha on glutathione synthesis. *Exp Toxicol Pathol.* 1998;50:477–483.
60. Shohami E, Beit-Yannai E, Horowitz M, et al. Oxidative stress in closed-head injury: brain antioxidant capacity as an indicator of functional outcome. *J Cereb Blood Flow Metab.* 1997;17:1007–1019.
61. Lewen A, Matz P, Chan PH. Free radical pathways in CNS injury. *J Neurotrauma.* 2000;17:871–890.
62. Laroux FS, Pavlick KP, Hines IN, et al. Role of nitric oxide in inflammation. *Acta Physiol Scand.* 2001;173:113–118.
63. Skidgel RA, Gao XP, Brovkovych V, et al. Nitric oxide stimulates macrophage inflammatory protein-2 expression in sepsis. *J Immunol.* 2002;169: 2093–2101.
64. Fosse E, Pillgram-Larsen J, Svennevig JL, et al. Complement activation in injured patients occurs immediately and is dependent on the severity of the trauma. *Injury.* 1998;29:509–514.
65. Mollnes TE, Fosse E. The complement system in trauma-related and ischemic tissue damage: a brief review. *Shock.* 1994;2:301–310.
66. Stahel PF, Morganti-Kossmann MC, Kossmann T. The role of the complement system in traumatic brain injury. *Brain Res Brain Res Rev.* 1998; 27:243–256.
67. Sugimoto K, Hirata M, Majima M, et al. Evidence for a role of kallikrein–kinin system in patients with shock after blunt trauma. *Am J Physiol.* 1998; 274:1556–1560.
68. Abraham E. Coagulation abnormalities in acute lung injury and sepsis. *Am J Respir Cell Mol Biol.* 2000;22:401–404.
69. Idell S. Coagulation, fibrinolysis, and fibrin deposition in acute lung injury. *Crit Care Med.* 2003;31:s213–s220.
70. Fan J, Kapus A, Li YH, et al. Priming for enhanced alveolar fibrin deposition after haemorrhagic shock: role of tumor necrosis factor. *Am J Respir Cell Mol Biol.* 2000;22:412–421.
71. Gando S, Kameue T, Matsuda N, et al. Combined activation of coagulation and inflammation has an important role in multiple organ dysfunction and poor outcome after severe trauma. *Thromb Haemost.* 2002;88:943–949.
72. Rigby AC, Grant MA. Protein S: a conduit between anticoagulation and inflammation. *Crit Care Med.* 2004;32:S336–S341.
73. Levi M, de Jonge E, van der Poll T. New treatment strategies for disseminated intravascular coagulation based on current understanding of the pathophysiology. *Ann Med.* 2004;36:41–49.
74. Lo EH, Wang X, Cuzner ML. Extracellular proteolysis in brain injury and inflammation: role for plasminogen activators and matrix metalloproteinases. *J Neurosci Res.* 2002;69:1–9.
75. Du Clos TW. Function of C-reactive protein. *Ann Med.* 2000;32:274–278.
76. Whicher JT, Evans SW. *Acute phase proteins. Hosp Update.* 1990:899.
77. Lennard AC. Interleukin-1 receptor antagonist. *Crit Rev Immunol.* 1995; 15:77–105.
78. Chikanza IC, Grossman AB. Neuroendocrine immune responses to inflammation: the concept of the neuroendocrine immune loop. *Bailliere's Clin Rheumatol.* 1996;10:199–225.
79. Emsley J, White HE, O'Hara BP, et al. Structure of pentameric human serum amyloid P component. *Nature.* 1994;367:338–345.
80. Gabay C, Kushner I. Acute-phase proteins and other systemic responses to inflammation. *N Engl J Med.* 1999;340:448–454.
81. Urieli-Shoval S, Linke RP, Matzner Y. Expression and function of serum amyloid A, a major acute-phase protein, in normal and disease states. *Curr Opin Hematol.* 2000;7:64–69.
82. Babaev A, Frederick PD, Pasta DJ, et al. Trends in management and outcomes of patients with acute myocardial infarction complicated by cardiogenic shock. *JAMA.* 2005;294:448–454.
83. Moore FA, McKinley BA, Moore EE, et al. Inflammation and the host response to injury, a large-scale collaborative project: patient-oriented research core—standard operating procedures for clinical care III. Guidelines for shock resuscitation. *J Trauma.* 2006;61:82–89.
84. American College of Surgeons. *Advanced Trauma Life Support for Doctors.* 7th ed. Chicago: American College of Surgeons; 2004.
85. Wiggers CJ. *Experimental Hemorrhagic Shock.* New York: Commonwealth Fund; 1950.
86. Bergstein JM, Slakey DP, Wallace JR, et al. Traumatic hypothermia is related to hypotension, not resuscitation. *Ann Emerg Med.* 1996;27:39–42.
87. Rivers E, Nguyen B, Havstad S, et al. Early goal-directed therapy in the treatment of severe sepsis and septic shock. *N Engl J Med.* 2001;345:1368–1377.
88. O'Neill PJ, Cobb LM, Ayala A, et al. Aggressive fluid resuscitation following intestinal ischemia-reperfusion in immature rats prevents metabolic derangements and down regulates interleukin-6 release. *Shock.* 1994;1:381–387.
89. Smith T, Grounds RM, Rhodes A. Central venous pressure: uses and limitations. In: Pinsky MR, Payen D, eds. *Functional Hemodynamic Monitoring. Update in Intensive Care and Emergency Medicine.* No. 42. New York: Springer-Verlag; 2005:99.
90. Marini JJ, Leatherman JW. Pulmonary artery occlusion pressure: measurement, significance, and clinical uses. In: Pinsky MR, Payen D, eds. *Functional Hemodynamic Monitoring. Update in Intensive Care and Emergency Medicine.* No. 42. New York: Springer-Verlag; 2005:111.
91. Singer M. Esophageal Doppler monitoring. In: Pinsky MR, Payen D, eds. *Functional Hemodynamic Monitoring. Update in Intensive Care and Emergency Medicine.* No. 42. New York: Springer-Verlag; 2005:193.
92. Vignon P. Hemodynamic assessment of critically ill patients using echocardiography Doppler. *Curr Opin Crit Care.* 2005;11:227–234.
93. Finfer S, Bellomo R, Boyce N. A comparison of albumin and saline for fluid resuscitation in the intensive care unit. *N Engl J Med.* 2004;350: 2247–2256.
94. Williams EL, Hildebrand KL, McCormick SA, et al. The effect of intravenous lactated Ringer's solution versus 0.9% sodium chloride solution on serum osmolality in human volunteers. *Anesth Analg.* 1999;88:999–1003.
95. Koustova E, Stanton K, Gushchin V, et al. Effects of lactated Ringer's solutions on human leukocytes. *J Trauma.* 2002;52:872–878.
96. Rhee P, Wang D, Ruff P, et al. Human neutrophil activation and increased adhesion by various resuscitation fluids. *Crit Care Med.* 2000;28:74–78.
97. Gushchin V, Stegalkina S, Alam HB, et al. Cytokine expression profiling in human leukocytes after exposure to hypertonic and isotonic fluids. *J Trauma.* 2002;52:867–871.

98. Khanna S, Davis D, Peterson B, et al. Use of hypertonic saline in the treatment of severe refractory posttraumatic intracranial hypertension in pediatric traumatic brain injury. *Crit Care Med.* 2000;28:1144–1151.
99. Huang PP, Stucky FS, Dimick AR, et al. Hypertonic sodium resuscitation is associated with renal failure and death. *Ann Surg.* 1995;221:543–554.
100. Kreimeier U, Messmer K. Small-volume resuscitation: from experimental evidence to clinical routine: advantages and disadvantages of hypertonic solutions. *Acta Anaesthesiol Scand.* 2002;46:625–638.
101. Fleck A, Hawker F, Wallace PI, et al. Increased vascular permeability: a major cause of hypoalbuminaemia in disease and injury. *Lancet.* 1985;1: 781–784.
102. Kohler JP, Rice CL, Zarins CK, et al. Does reduced colloid oncotic pressure increase pulmonary dysfunction in sepsis? *Crit Care Med.* 1981;9:90–93.
103. Blunt MC, Nicholson JP, Park GR. Serum albumin and colloid osmotic pressure in survivors and non-survivors of prolonged critical illness. *Anaesthesia.* 1998;53:755–761.
104. Golub R, Sorrento JJ Jr, Cantu RJ, et al. Efficacy of albumin supplementation in the surgical intensive care unit: a prospective, randomized study. *Crit Care Med.* 1994;22:613–619.
105. McCluskey A, Thomas AN, Bowles BJ, et al. The prognostic value of serial measurements of serum albumin in patients admitted to an intensive care unit. *Anaesthesia.* 1996;51:724–727.
106. Stockwell MA, Soni N, Riley B. Colloid solutions in the critically ill. A randomized comparison of albumin and polygeline. I. Outcome and duration of stay in the intensive care unit. *Anaesthesia.* 1992;47:3–6.
107. Boldt J, Hessen M, Mueller M, et al. The effects of albumin versus hydroxyethyl starch solution on cardiorespiratory and circulatory variables in critically ill patients. *Anesth Analg.* 1996;83:254–261.
108. Cochrane Injuries Group Albumin Reviewers. Human albumin administration in critically ill patients: systematic review of randomised controlled trials. *BMJ.* 1998;317:235–240.
109. Wilkes MM, Navickis RJ. Patient survival after human albumin administration: a meta-analysis of randomized, controlled trials. *Ann Intern Med.* 2001;135:149–164.
110. Alderson P, Bunn F, Li Wan Po A, et al. Human albumin solution for resuscitation and volume expansion in critically ill patients. *Cochrane Library.* 2006;3.
111. Treib J, Haass A, Pindur G. Coagulation disorders caused by hydroxyethyl starch. *Thromb Haemost.* 1997;78:974–983.
112. Cittanova ML, Leblanc I, Legendre C, et al. Effect of hydroxyethyl starch in brain-dead kidney donors on renal function in kidney-transplant recipients. *Lancet.* 1996;348:1620–1622.
113. Schortgen F, Lacherade JC, Bruneel F, et al. Effects of hydroxyethylstarch and gelatin on renal function in severe sepsis: a multicentre randomised study. *Lancet.* 2001;357:911–916.
114. Treib J, Haass A, Pindur G, et al. All medium starches are not the same: influence of the degree of hydroxyethyl substitution of hydroxyethyl starch on plasma volume, hemorrheologic conditions, and coagulation. *Transfusion.* 1996;36:450–455.
115. Schmand JF, Ayala A, Morrison MH, et al. Effects of hydroxyethyl starch after trauma-hemorrhagic shock: restoration of macrophage integrity and prevention of increased circulating IL-6 levels. *Crit Care Med.* 1995;23:806–814.
116. Handrigan MT, Burns AR, Donnachie EM, et al. Hydroxyethyl starch inhibits neutrophil adhesion and transendothelial migration. *Shock.* 2005; 24:434–439.
117. Dieterich HJ, Weissmuller T, Rosenberger P, et al. Effect of hydroxyethyl starch on vascular leak syndrome and neutrophil accumulation during hypoxia. *Crit Care Med.* 2006;34:1775–1782.
118. Perel P, Roberts I, Ker K. Colloids versus crystalloids for fluid resuscitation in critically ill patients. *Cochrane Database Syst Rev.* 2013:2:CD000567.
119. Shippy CR, Shoemaker WC. Hemodynamic and colloid osmotic pressure alterations in the surgical patient. *Crit Care Med.* 1983;11:191–195.
120. Cotton BA, Guy JS, Morris JA Jr, et al. The cellular, metabolic, and systemic consequences of aggressive fluid resuscitation strategies. *Shock.* 2006; 26:115–121.
121. Mouncey PR, Osborn TM, Power GS; ProMISe Trial Investigators. Trial of early, goal-directed resuscitation for septic shock. *N Engl J Med.* 2015; 372(14):1301–1311.
122. Holcomb JB, Tilley BC, Baraniuk S; PROPPR Study Group. Transfusion of plasma, platelets, and red blood cells in a 1:1:1 vs a 1:1:2 ratio and mortality in patients with severe trauma: the PROPPR randomized clinical trial. *JAMA.* 2015;313(5):471–482.
123. Mullner M, Urbanek B, Havel C, et al. Vasopressors for shock. *Cochrane Database Syst Rev.* 2004;3:CD003709.
124. Albanese J, Leone M, Garnier F, et al. Renal effects of norepinephrine in septic and nonseptic patients. *Chest.* 2004;126:534–539.
125. Dellinger RP, Levy MM, Rhodes A, et al. Surviving sepsis campaign: international guidelines for management of severe sepsis and septic shock: 2012. *Crit Care Med.* 2013;41(2):580–637.
126. Bellomo R, Chapman M, Finfer S, et al. Low-dose dopamine in patients with early renal dysfunction: a placebo-controlled randomised trial. Australian and New Zealand Intensive Care Society (ANZICS) Clinical Trials Group. *Lancet.* 2000;356:2139–2143.
127. Hollenberg SM, Kavinsky CJ, Parrillo JE. Cardiogenic shock. *Ann Intern Med.* 1999;131:47–59.
128. Sakr Y, Reinhart K, Vincent JL, et al. Does dopamine administration in shock influence outcome? Results of the Sepsis Occurrence in Acutely Ill Patients (SOAP) Study. *Crit Care Med.* 2006;34:589–597.
129. Martin C, Viviand X, Leone M, et al. Effect of norepinephrine on the outcome of septic shock. *Crit Care Med.* 2000;28:2758–2765.
130. Kohsaka S, Menon V, Lowe AM, et al. Systemic inflammatory response syndrome after acute myocardial infarction complicated by cardiogenic shock. *Arch Intern Med.* 2005;165:1643–1650.
131. Vallet B, Chopin C, Curtis SE, et al. Prognostic value of the dobutamine test in patients with sepsis syndrome and normal lactate values: a prospective, multicenter study. *Crit Care Med.* 1993;21:1868–1875.
132. Cuffe MS, Califf RM, Adams KF Jr, et al. Short-term intravenous milrinone for acute exacerbation of chronic heart failure: a randomized controlled trial. *JAMA.* 2002;287:1541–1547.
133. Landry DW, Oliver JA. The pathogenesis of vasodilatory shock. *N Engl J Med.* 2001;345:588–595.
134. Cooper DJ, Russell JA, Walley KR, et al. Vasopressin and septic shock trial (VASST): innovative features and performance. *Am J Respir Crit Care Med.* 2003;167:A838.
135. Abou-Khalil B, Scalea TM, Trooskin SZ, et al. Hemodynamic responses to shock in young trauma patients: need for invasive monitoring. *Crit Care Med.* 1994;22:633–639.
136. Shoemaker WC, Montgomery ES, Kaplan E, et al. Physiologic patterns in surviving and nonsurviving shock patients: use of sequential cardiorespiratory variables in defining criteria for therapeutic goals and early warning of death. *Arch Surg.* 1973;106:630–636.
137. Shoemaker WC, Appel PL, Kram HB, et al. Prospective trial of supranormal values of survivors as therapeutic goals in high risk surgical patients. *Chest.* 1988;94:1176–1186.
138. Velmahos GC, Demetriades D, Shoemaker WC, et al. Endpoints of resuscitation of critically injured patients: normal or supranormal? A prospective randomized trial. *Ann Surg.* 2000;232:409–418.
139. Eisenberg PR, Jaffe AS, Schuster DP. Clinical evaluation compared to pulmonary artery catheterization in the hemodynamic assessment of critically ill patients. *Crit Care Med.* 1984;12:549–553.
140. Connors AF Jr, McCafree DR, Gray BA. Evaluation of right heart catheterization in the critically ill patient without acute myocardial infarction. *N Engl J Med.* 1983;308:263–267.
141. Shoemaker WC, Bland RD, Appel PL. Therapy of critically ill postoperative patients based on outcome prediction and prospective clinical trials. *Surg Clin North Am.* 1985;65:811–833.
142. Bishop MH, Shoemaker WC, Appel PL, et al. Prospective, randomized trial of survivor values of cardiac index, oxygen delivery, and oxygen consumption as resuscitation endpoints in severe trauma. *J Trauma.* 1995;38:780–787.
143. Pinsky MR. Beyond global oxygen supply-demand relations: in search of measures of dysoxia. *Intensive Care Med.* 1994;20:1–3.
144. Shoemaker WC, Appel PL, Kram HB. Hemodynamic and oxygen transport responses in survivors and nonsurvivors of high-risk surgery. *Crit Care Med.* 1993;21:977–990.
145. Connors AF Jr, Speroff T, Dawson NV, et al. The effectiveness of right heart catheterization in the initial care of critically ill patients. SUPPORT Investigators. *JAMA.* 1996;276:889–897.
146. Thoren A, Elam M, Ricksten SE. Differential effects of dopamine, dopexamine, and dobutamine on jejunal mucosal perfusion early after cardiac surgery. *Crit Care Med.* 2000;28:2338–2343.
147. Balasubramanyan N, Havens PL, Hoffman GM. Unmeasured anions identified by the Fencl-Stewart method predict mortality better than base excess, anion gap, and lactate in patients in the pediatric intensive care unit. *Crit Care Med.* 1999;27:1577–1581.
148. Davis JW, Kaups KL, Parks SN. Base deficit is superior to pH in evaluating clearance of acidosis after traumatic shock. *J Trauma.* 1998;44:114–118.
149. Vincent J-L, Dufaye P, Berre J, et al. Serial lactate determinations during circulatory shock. *Crit Care Med.* 1983;11:449–451.
150. Horecker BL. The absorption spectra of hemoglobin and its derivatives in the visible and near infra-red regions. *J Biol Chem.* 1943;148:173–183.
151. Taylor JH, Mulier KE, Myers DE, et al. Use of near-infrared spectroscopy in early determination of irreversible hemorrhagic shock. *J Trauma.* 2005;58:1119–1125.

CHAPTER

45

Cardiogenic Shock

MARC A. SIMON and MICHAEL R. PINSKY

INTRODUCTION

Cardiogenic shock is characterized by primary myocardial dysfunction resulting in the inability of the heart to maintain an adequate cardiac output with subsequent compromising of metabolic requirements (Fig. 45.1). The clinical definition is a systolic blood pressure less than 90 mmHg or a blood pressure that has fallen to at least 30 mmHg less than the individual's baseline blood pressure in the presence of organ dysfunction and tissue hypoperfusion. The most common etiologies are myocardial infarction (MI) or cardiomyopathy with a superimposed hemodynamic stress. The exact incidence of cardiogenic shock is difficult to ascertain because of variability in diagnostic criteria and survival rates in the early phase of acute MI. The Multicenter Investigation of Limitation of Infarct Size trial (1) documented an incidence rate of cardiogenic shock in 7.5% of subjects who were admitted to the hospital after having an acute MI, a constant value from 1975 to 1997 (2). The Global Utilization of Streptokinase and Tissue Plasminogen Activator for Occluded Arteries (GUSTO-1) trial, GUSTO-III, and other thrombolytic trials have reported an incidences of 5% to 10% (3,4). Despite rapid advancement in pharmacologic thrombolytic therapy, mechanical revascularization techniques, and development of mechanical ventricular assist devices (VADs), cardiogenic shock remains a major clinical challenge with an associated high mortality. Historically, mortality rates were 81% as originally reported by Killip in 1967 (5). Early revascularization by angioplasty or surgery has been shown to reduce mortality from 63% to 50% at 6 months in the SHOCK trial (6). Improved survival in cardiogenic shock may be seen with an aggressive approach to diagnosis and management of the problem, with emphasis on early recognition and treatment of mechanical defects such as VSD, acute mitral insufficiency, and free wall rupture. Limitation of infarct size by minimizing the extent of infarcted tissue is the key component in all therapeutic strategies with the goal to maximize perfusion, limit irreversible cell death, and decrease potential for a secondary mechanical event.

PATHOPHYSIOLOGY

To understand the therapeutic approaches used to support left ventricular (LV) ejection and aid acutely decompensated hearts, it is important to understand the mechanisms underpinning LV systole. Systolic ventricular function is determined by preload, afterload, and contractility. Preload is the wall stress on the left ventricle prior to ejection. Operationally, we use LV end-diastolic volume to reflect this wall stress. Since measures of volumes can be difficult at the bedside, LV end-diastolic pressure, left atrial pressure, or pulmonary artery occlusion pressure (POAP) are often used as surrogates for LV end-diastolic volume. Afterload is the maximal LV wall stress during ejection. By LaPlace law, wall stress is proportional to the product of LV radius of curvature and transmural pressure. Under normal conditions maximal LV afterload occurs at the instant of aortic value opening. Contractility is a more difficult term to define and quantify. A reasonable definition is the amount of force capable of being produced by the contracting myocardium (7). On a cellular level, contractility is related to the integrity of the actin-myosin coupling, intracellular calcium (Ca^{2+}) flux rate and quantity. Functionally, one measures contractility by varying preload and afterload. Numerous measures have been attempted to quantify contractility with varying degrees of success depending upon the degree of true independence they have from preload or afterload. Measures of contractility include the maximal rate of isovolumic pressure development (dP/dt_{max}), the Frank–Starling law relating peak systolic activity (defined as either maximal developed pressure, volume ejected or the product of the two) directly to end-diastolic volume (8), and LV end-systolic pressure–volume relation (ESPVR) derived from pressure–volume loops. Systolic performance is the ability of the LV to empty. This is a function of end-systolic volume; a commonly used calculation is the LV ejection fraction (effective ejection fraction in the case of valvular regurgitation).

The most common etiology of cardiogenic shock is acute MI with a resultant loss of approximately 40% of functioning myocardium. Following MI, the final infarct size has been shown to correlate with the degree of LV dysfunction (9). Loss of myocardial function may occur in one massive MI or may result in a cumulative loss of pump function caused by serial smaller infarcts. Cardiogenic shock more commonly results from infarction of the left ventricle, although recent clarification of the potential role of the right ventricle in the precipitation of the shock state has been recognized. Additionally, acute mechanical complications of MI such as mitral insufficiency, free wall rupture, and acute VSD may result in cardiogenic shock during the periinfarct period, as does the late development of LV aneurysm (Table 45.1). Other causes of cardiogenic shock include end-stage or fulminant cardiomyopathy, myocarditis, acute chordal rupture causing valvular regurgitation, obstruction to LV ejection (severe aortic stenosis or hypertrophic cardiomyopathy) or LV filling (mitral stenosis or left atrial myxoma), or severe septic shock with myocardial depression.

Left Ventricular Acute Myocardial Infarction

Reduction in LV performance is one of the major complications of ischemic heart disease. Several classifications that attempt to standardize the clinical and hemodynamic presentation of MI have been proposed to aid in determining prognosis and the therapeutic approaches in patients with established cardiogenic shock or those who have the potential to progress to the shock state.

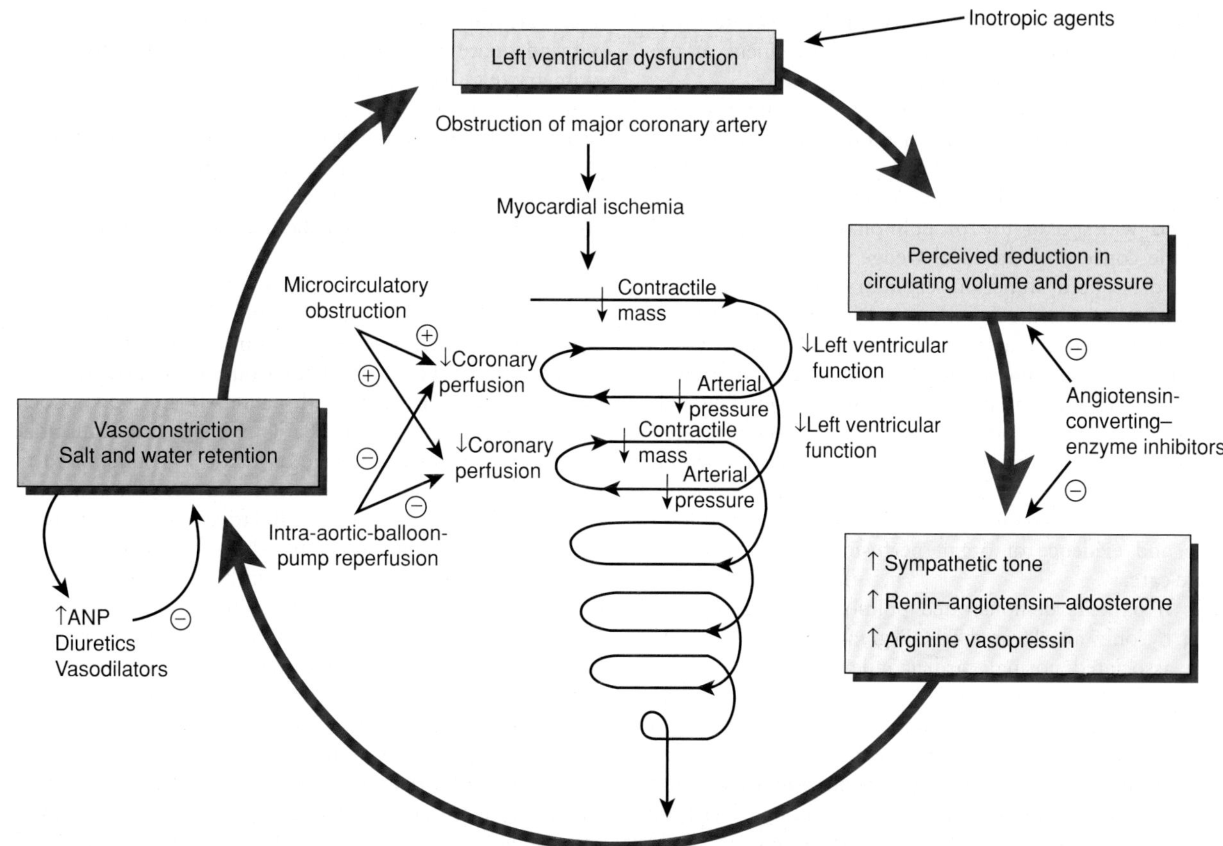

FIGURE 45.1 Neurohumoral and mechanical events that lead to death in patients with cardiogenic shock. ANP, atrial natriuretic peptide. (Used with permission from Francis GS. Neuroendocrine manifestations of congestive heart failure. *Am J Cardiol.* 1988;62(Suppl):9A–13A.)

The Killip classification on uses pure clinical bedside evaluation of the patient to establish prognostic indicators to predict the mortality associated with an acute MI using the physical findings of congestive heart failure (5).

- *Class I* patients developed no overt signs of congestive heart failure, and these individuals had a low in-hospital mortality rate. This subgroup represented approximately 40% to 50% of all patients who presented with an acute MI. The in-hospital fatality rate was approximately 6%.
- *Class II* patients demonstrated evidence of impaired ventricular function as manifest by persistent bibasilar rales and an audible third heart sound. This subset of patients accounted for approximately 30% to 40% of patients with acute MI. The in-hospital mortality rate of 17% was triple relative to Class I patients.
- Class *III* patients were characterized by the development of acute pulmonary edema, which was seen in approximately 10% to 15% of patients admitted to the hospital. A significant mortality rate of 38% was seen in this group treated conservatively before the thrombolytic era.
- *Class IV* patients had established cardiogenic shock with hypotension and signs of organ hypoperfusion. Cardiogenic shock occurred in 5% to 10% of infarct patients in this series but was associated with a high in-hospital mortality rate of 80%, which was a function of both severity of the underlying illness plus the limited availability of definitive treatment at the time this classification was proposed.

TABLE 45.1 Contributing Factors to the Development of Cardiogenic Shock in Myocardial Infarction

Loss of left ventricular function
Cumulative loss of myocardial tissue exceeding 40% of ventricular mass, particularly anterior infarcts
Myocardial infarction associated with bradyarrhythmias or tachyarrhythmias
Hypovolemia or hypervolemia
Right ventricular infarction
Mechanical defects
Papillary muscle dysfunction or rupture causing acute regurgitation
Ventricular septal defect
Ventricular pseudoaneurysm
Free wall rupture and/or cardiac tamponade

The group at Cedars Sinai Medical Center Los Angeles, also developed a clinical classification of heart failure associated with acute MI, which was subsequently refined by the availability of invasive hemodynamic monitoring using pulmonary artery catheters (PACs; Table 45.2) (10). The Cedars

TABLE 45.2 Hemodynamic Subsets and Mortality in Myocardial Infarction

Swan-Forrester Class	Cardiac Index (L/min/m²)	PAOP (mmHg)	Mortality Rate (%)
I	>2.2	<18	<3
II	>2.2	>18	9
III	<2.2	<18	23
IV	<2.2	>18	51

PAOP, pulmonary artery occlusion pressure.

Sinai classification also subdivided patients with acute myocardial into four subsets based on the measurement of the PAOP, cardiac index (CI), and clinical assessment.

Class I patients had no clinical evidence of pulmonary congestion or tissue hypoperfusion. Hemodynamic parameters measured in these subjects revealed the PAOP to be less than 18 mmHg and the CI to be in excess of 2.2 L/min/m^2. The advent and widespread use of pulmonary artery catheters clarified the concept of the ideal wedge that established the impact of diastolic dysfunction secondary to acute ischemia, with resultant impaired relaxation and elevated filling pressures being required to maintain adequate cardiac output.

Class I patients accounted for 25% of subjects admitted to the coronary care unit, and there was a low in-hospital mortality rate of 1%. Patients who on clinical grounds demonstrated no evidence of hypoperfusion or pulmonary congestion would not be expected to benefit from invasive cardiac monitoring. Frequent clinical reassessments; close attention paid to blood pressure and evidence of organ perfusion would represent adequate care.

Class II patients demonstrated pulmonary congestion as manifest by only an elevated PAOP greater than 18 mmHg with an associated normal cardiac index. Class II patients accounted for approximately 25% of patients admitted to the coronary care unit, but an 11% mortality rate was associated with this group. Mild pulmonary congestion is transiently seen in a significant percentage of patients admitted to the coronary care unit and has a multifactorial etiology. Diastolic dysfunction induced by ischemia with retrograde transmission of elevated filling pressures into the pulmonary venous circuit results in extravasation of fluid into the pulmonary bed when hydrostatic pressure exceeds oncotic pressure. Ischemic papillary muscle dysfunction with mild degrees of mitral insufficiency is also a potential cause of pulmonary congestion in this subgroup. Physical examination of these patients reveals mild to moderate rales and potentially an audible third heart sound associated with radiographic evidence of pulmonary venous hypertension. Dyspnea and orthopnea are the main symptoms superimposed on the clinical presentation of myocardial ischemia. Treatment in this group is centered on reduction of filling pressures to a level that relieves pulmonary venous congestion but does not result in an overzealous reduction of filling pressures below the ideal filling pressure as the reduced cardiac contractility will require some increased filling volume and pressure to maintain adequate stroke volume and perfusion pressure (Starling mechanism). Excessive diuresis should be assiduously avoided, especially in patients who were euvolemic before the onset of their infarct. Despite signs of pulmonary congestion, patients presenting with acute pulmonary congestion frequently are not intravascularly volume overloaded, and diuretic therapy may reduce filling pressures to a level that would impair cardiac output. It is often difficult to ascertain at the bedside which patients are actually euvolemic and which are hypervolemic. Afterload reduction therapy will benefit both groups of patients and may allow time to assess total effective circulating blood volume by indirect measures, such as the existence of hyponatremia, peripheral edema and S4 gallop. Inotropic agents should be considered in such a situation so that pulmonary congestion can be relieved by diuresis if afterload reduction is not immediately effective since the increased inotropic state mitigates against a reduction in cardiac output induced by any reduction in cardiac filling pressures. Oxygenation should be maintained with adequate arterial saturation that may be monitored by oximetry (e.g., SpO_2 >90%). Vasodilator therapies in the form of nitroglycerin or inotropic agents with vasodilating capacity such as dobutamine are effective to return the hemodynamic parameters to normal. The usefulness and risk–benefit ratio of invasive hemodynamic monitoring in this subgroup of patients are controversial, although these patients frequently may be managed on clinical grounds.

Class III patients are characterized predominantly by clinical evidence of hypoperfusion. Hemodynamic monitoring reveals a PAOP less than 18 mmHg and a CI of less than 2.2 L/min/m^2. The Class III subgroup accounted for approximately 15% of patients with acute MI and was associated with a 23% mortality rate. Patients in this subgroup may be extremely difficult to manage on clinical grounds, and treatment can be facilitated by invasive hemodynamic monitoring to establish the volume status. Relative hypovolemia is determined by measuring the PAOP, which falls below that of the ideal filling pressure as predicted in ischemic states. Excessive diuresis is extremely problematic in this group of patients and may further decrease cardiac output because of the preexistent relative hypovolemia. Class III patients require restoration of intravascular volume to increase filling pressures to a degree that ensures adequate cardiac output and organ perfusion.

Class IV patients demonstrated elevated PAOP in excess of 18 mmHg and a depressed CI of less than 2.2 L/min/m^2 and frequently manifested signs of cardiogenic shock with clinical evidence of organ hypoperfusion and dysfunction. This subgroup accounted for approximately 35% of patients with MI and was associated with an in-hospital mortality rate of approximately 50%. Class IV patients may have a mechanical defect such as acute mitral insufficiency, free wall rupture, or VSD underlying the acute MI; these are discussed separately. Oxygenation with the potential assisted ventilation in addition to inotropic and judicious use of vasodilator support is the recommended therapy in this subgroup.

Right Ventricular Infarction

Although isolated right ventricular (RV) infarction is rare, evidence of RV infarction and RV dysfunction is found in up to half of all infarcts and is clinically significant in nearly half of all inferior infarcts (11,12). The clinical diagnosis of RV infarction should be considered when elevated jugular venous pressure is accompanied by hypotension, while the lung fields are clear. But the diagnosis may be difficult to establish clinically unless hemodynamic measurements, special electrocardiographic leads, echocardiography, or nuclear imaging are performed (13). Right-sided precordial leads obtained by electrocardiography that demonstrates at least 1-mm ST elevation is approximately 70% sensitive in the diagnosis of RV infarction and confers a particularly poor prognosis (14). Echocardiography is an easily obtainable noninvasive study that demonstrates RV dilation and RV wall motion impairment. Radionuclide angiography currently is considered to be the most sensitive means to diagnose RV infarction, although more recent data suggest magnetic resonance imaging is comparable (15,16). A decrease in RV ejection fraction that is associated with wall motion abnormalities is more than 90% sensitive in the diagnosis of an RV infarction. Hemodynamic studies which are supportive of significant ischemic involvement of the right ventricle are manifested by increases in right atrial pressures plus demonstration of resistance to diastolic filling, as shown by blunting of the y-descent that follows tricuspid valve opening. A "square root" sign or "dip and plateau" pattern in the diastolic pressure curve is commonly demonstrated in RV infarctions but is not specific and may be associated with pericardial tamponade or restrictive cardiomyopathy (17).

The SHOCK trial registry reported on the clinical characteristics of patients presenting with isolated RV shock (18). Patients with RV shock compared to LV shock were younger, had a lower prevalence of previous MI (25.5% vs. 40.1%), a lower prevalence of anterior MI (11% vs. 59%), and a less multivessel disease (34.8% vs. 77.8%). As expected, the infarct-related vessel involved the right coronary artery more in RV shock (96% of cases) versus LV shock (27% of cases). These patients had a shorter median time between MI and the diagnosis of shock (2.9 vs. 6.2 hours) compared to patients with LV shock. Right atrial pressure was a highly significant distinguisher of right from LV shock (mean pressure 23.0 ± 9.9 vs. 14.2 ± 7.4 mmHg, $p = 0.0001$), while all other hemodynamic measures were similar. Interestingly, in-hospital mortality was not significantly different between RV and LV shock (53.1% vs. 60.8, respectively). Improvement in survival due to revascularization was similar between groups and multivariate analysis revealed that RV shock was not an independent predictor of lower in-hospital mortality (odds ratio 1.07, 95% confidence interval 0.54 to 2.13). This similarity in survival was despite patients with RV shock being younger, thus RV shock may carry a worse prognosis.

Cardiogenic shock in patients with RV infarction frequently represents a substantial loss of functioning myocardium and carries a poor prognosis. RV infarction accompanied by cardiogenic shock is frequently associated with a variety of conduction abnormalities, including a high-grade atrioventricular block or significant rhythm disturbances. The treatment of RV infarction complicated by cardiogenic shock centers around maintaining RV filling pressures and assurance of adequate volume. Hemodynamic measurements, including echocardiography, may facilitate the estimate of volume loading required. Nitrates, diuretics, and other predominantly vasodilating compounds should be avoided. Atrial fibrillation is frequently poorly tolerated by these patients and may require immediate electrical cardioversion. The use of digitalis in acute RV infarction, even in the presence of atrial fibrillation, is controversial. Adequate inotropic support with vasodilating inotropic agents such as dobutamine is used if cardiac output fails to optimize after adequate volume loading. Percutaneous revascularization should be considered as it has been shown to improve outcomes (19).

Mechanical Defects

A variety of mechanical defects may be associated with cardiogenic shock in the periinfarction stage (Table 45.3). MI resulting in cardiogenic shock from the appearance of mechanical defects such as acute mitral insufficiency, VSD, or free wall rupture represents a major complication and requires aggressive diagnostic and therapeutic interventions if the patient is expected to survive. Despite improvements in imaging techniques plus mechanical assist devices and emergency surgery, the mortality from these complications remains extremely high.

Acute Mitral Insufficiency

The mitral valve is a complicated apparatus and consists of the valvular annulus, leaflets, chorda tendineae, and papillary muscles plus potential functional alterations from involvement of the adjacent myocardium. Abnormalities affecting any of the components of the mitral valve may result in acute or chronic mitral insufficiency. The mitral valve annulus may be dilated and contribute to mitral insufficiency, although this complication is primarily associated with cardiomyopathies or connective tissue diseases such as Marfan syndrome rather than an acute MI. Calcification of the mitral valve annulus is common in the elderly and may alter coaptation of the mitral valve leaflets and result in mitral incompetence.

Acute mitral insufficiency caused by involvement of the valvular leaflets is associated with infective endocarditis from necrotizing organisms such as *Staphylococcus aureus* or *Enterococcus,* resulting in destruction of the valvular apparatus. Traumatic penetrating injuries that involve the valve itself are rare. Rupture of the chorda tendineae may also be seen in endocarditis or a variety of connective tissue diseases, including myxomatous degeneration or Marfan syndrome.

Chordal rupture that results in severe impairment of LV function depends on the number of involved structures and the rapidity with which the rupture occurs. Mitral insufficiency in the periinfarction state may result from involvement of the surrounding myocardium or papillary muscles. Papillary muscles located adjacent to the infarction zone may simply become dysfunctional because of alteration of synchrony of contraction related to ischemia or frank rupture from ischemic necrosis.

The degree of mitral insufficiency is a function of the degree of involvement and anatomic competence. The two papillary

TABLE 45.3 Complications of Myocardial Infarction

Characteristic	Ventricular Septal Rupture	Papillary Muscle Rupture	Papillary Muscle Dysfunction
Incidence	Unusual	Rare	Common
Murmur			
Type	Pansystolic	Early to pansystolic	Variable
Location	Left sternal border (95%)	Apex → axilla (50%)	Apex
Thrill	>50%	Rare	No
Clinical presentation	Left and right ventricular failure	Profound pulmonary edema	None to moderate LV failure
Catheterization	O_2 step-up in right ventricle	Large left atrial V wave	Mild to moderate elevation of left atrial pressure

Used with permission from Crawford MH, O'Rourke RA. The bedside diagnosis of the complications of myocardial infarction. In: Eliot RS ed. *Cardiac Emergencies.* Mount Kisco, NY: Futura; 1962.

muscles (posteromedial and anterolateral papillary muscles) have different ischemic vulnerabilities because of the blood supply from the coronary arteries. The anatomic vascular supply represents end arteries that are solely supplied by terminal portions of the coronaries, thus rendering the papillary muscles vulnerable to ischemic involvement during an acute MI. Papillary muscle dysfunction may result from intermittent ischemia during unstable angina or MI with involvement of the adjacent myocardium (20). Papillary muscle dysfunction is characterized by mild flow murmurs which may be grade I or grade II by auscultation. The anterolateral papillary muscle has a dual blood supply, which provides partial protection during ischemia. The diagonal branches of the left anterior descending and marginal branches from the circumflex supply blood to the anterolateral papillary muscle. The posteromedial papillary muscle is generally supplied solely from the posterior descending branch of the right coronary artery increasing its vulnerability to ischemic-related dysfunction.

Significant ischemia involving the papillary muscle that results in complete rupture with fulminant mitral insufficiency is generally fatal because of the marked volume load ejected retrograde into the left atria and pulmonary venous bed (21). However, if the major ischemia-related necrosis is distal and only involves rupture of the head of the papillary muscle, the resultant mitral insufficiency may be tolerated hemodynamically long enough to allow recognition, proper diagnosis, and surgical intervention. Mild ischemic involvement of the papillary muscle may be increased in hemodynamic significance in the presence of pre-existing LV dilation, which alters the ability of the mitral leaflets to coapt. Severe ischemia-related mitral insufficiency is more frequently a result of posteromedial papillary muscle necrosis resulting from inferior or posterior MIs although one-third of cases may result from anterior infarction (21,22). Less than half of cases present with electrocardiographic evidence of ST elevation or Q waves (22). RV papillary muscle rupture may occur but is uncommon. Involvement of papillary muscles in the right ventricle results in tricuspid insufficiency, which if severe may result in RV failure.

Papillary muscle rupture is a relatively uncommon complication and occurs in about 1% of patients having an acute ischemic event. The incidence has decreased in the thrombolytic era (23). After acute MI with cardiogenic shock, the incidence of acute severe mitral regurgitation is 6.9% (24). The peak incidence of papillary muscle rupture is within the first week with the majority occurring between days 3 and 5 after an acute MI. The diagnosis of papillary muscle rupture may be suspected on physical examination and has been facilitated with the advent of hemodynamic monitoring and echocardiography.

The physical examination in acute mitral insufficiency secondary to papillary muscle rupture differs from the findings associated with chronic valvular regurgitation. In the acute setting a palpable thrill is uncommon and the radiation of the murmur differs from chronic conditions. The systolic murmur is soft, decrescendo, generally ends before the second heart sound, and is best audible at the base of the heart as opposed to the apex with radiation to the neck or the top of the head.

Echocardiography and Doppler ultrasound has been a major advance in the diagnosis of acute mitral insufficiency and its clinical separation from other mechanical lesions associated with a new murmur (25). The left atrium and left ventricle are generally of normal size, and the ejection fraction is increased and frequently hyperdynamic. The mitral leaflet flails and may prolapse into the left atrium. Doppler ultrasound with color flow study determines the presence and severity of mitral insufficiency, presence of an intracardiac shunt and quantifies the degree of mitral regurgitation. Data from the SHOCK trial which randomized patients with cardiogenic shock within 36 hours of an acute MI demonstrated that the severity of mitral regurgitation quantified by Doppler echocardiography is an independent predictor of survival (26).

Pulmonary artery catheter placement with measurement of PAOP and cardiac output is useful in mitral insufficiency. The presence of a regurgitant wave in the PAOP tracing may be visible in acute mitral regurgitant lesion, especially when there is no evidence of a step-up in oxygen concentration in the right atria or right ventricle. Pulmonary artery catheterization is not necessary for diagnosis but the use of invasive monitoring allows optimization of cardiac output, filling pressures, and adjustment of inotropic, vasodilator and diuretic therapy on the basis of induced changes in pressures.

Ventricular Septal Defect

Rupture of the interventricular septum may present in a similar clinical manner as mitral insufficiency with the abrupt onset of congestive heart failure plus a new murmur, making the two conditions difficult to separate on clinical grounds. Rupture of the interventricular septum also occurs in the first week after the acute ischemic event with a peak incidence occurring between days 3 and 5. The prevalence rate of acute ventricular septal defects (VSDs) after an infarction is difficult to accurately determine but occurs within the range of 0.5% to 2.0% and is the cause of death in approximately 5% of all fatal MIs. Incidence of VSD as a cause of cardiogenic shock after acute MI in the SHOCK trial registry was 3.9% (24). Blood supply to the septum is supplied by septal perforating branches of the left anterior descending vessel and acute VSD is more common in anterior MIs. These patients frequently have multivessel disease and are older patients experiencing an initial MI (27).

The diagnosis of acute VSD may be inferred on clinical grounds but frequently requires more sophisticated evaluation to accurately diagnose and quantify the defect which is located in the muscular septum and may be multiple. The physical examination in acute VSD depends on the magnitude of the shunt, which is, in turn, a function of the size of the ventricular defect, RV compliance, pulmonary artery pressures, and the inotropic state. A significant VSD is associated with the characteristic findings of shock in addition to a new holosystolic murmur associated with a precordial thrill. A precordial thrill may be palpated in approximately 50% of patients with an acute VSD and is a function of the magnitude of pressure gradient between the two chambers.

The diagnosis of VSD and its separation from acute mitral insufficiency has been greatly facilitated by the advent of noninvasive and invasive diagnostic procedures. Two-dimensional echocardiography combined with Doppler flow study generally identifies a significant defect (28). Contrast echocardiography using microbubble techniques also may aid in the diagnosis of acute VSD and establish the presence of an intracardiac shunt. Pulmonary artery catheterization demonstrates the absence of a V wave in the PAOP tracing and an increase in oxygen saturation by about 10% in the right ventricle compared with the right atrium. The mortality rate for septal defects is significant, with approximately 25% of patients dying within the first 24 hours and a 50% mortality rate at 1 week. Less than 10% survive 1 year when treated solely with medical therapy (29). When occurring in the setting of cardiogenic shock, in-hospital mortality for MI patients with VSDs has been reported as high as 87% (24).

Free Wall Rupture and Tamponade

Free wall rupture is a major complication of MI and is difficult to diagnose premortem. The prevalence of this complication is unknown but may occur in up to 8% of all MIs with approximately one-third occurring in the first 24 hours after the onset of the ischemic event and the peak incidence between days 5 and 7 (30). The SHOCK trial registry reported a 1.4% incidence of free wall rupture as a cause of cardiogenic shock after acute MI (24). Rupture of the free wall is a major cause of mortality in acute ischemic events and is associated with large transmural infarcts with inadequate collateral circulation. This serious complication occurs more commonly in elderly hypertensive patients. Involvement of the left ventricle is the rule, although free wall rupture involving the right ventricle has been reported. Rupture of the free wall is frequently associated with the ventricular remodeling process in which a segmental infarction results in elevated LV and diastolic pressure with expansion of the infarcted area. Expansion involves thinning of the affected area with regional hypertrophy in the adjacent region surrounding the infarct. A disproportionate dilatation occurs in the infarcted area and the risk of free wall rupture is enhanced with high shearing forces and elevated pressures. Free wall rupture generally occurs in the border zone between the infarcted area and the normal surrounding myocardium. The advent of thrombolytic therapy has been postulated to potentially increase the risk of free wall rupture although not definitely confirmed. Thrombolytic therapy may actually minimize the extent of myocardial necrosis and decrease free wall rupture. The use of agents such as corticosteroids, previously used to blunt inflammatory response and infarct size, has been associated with increased risk of free wall rupture.

Cardiac rupture is a catastrophic event resulting in sudden cardiac death unless a pseudoaneurysm forms. Hemopericardium with cardiac tamponade is difficult to diagnose early enough to institute definitive therapy. Cardiac tamponade after acute MI also may be secondary to hemorrhagic pericarditis but massive hemopericardium is usually due to cardiac rupture with rapid development of electromechanical dissociation and death. The diagnosis of free wall rupture is difficult but should be suspected with sudden hypotension, elevated jugular venous pressures, muffled heart sounds, and a pulsus paradoxus. Echocardiography can document the presence of pericardial fluid and occasionally demonstrates the perforated free wall (31,32). The classic signs of tamponade are present on echocardiography and are caused by the rising intrapericardial pressure compressing the right atrium and right ventricle, resulting in equalization of pressures and RV diastolic collapse. Definitive therapy involves pericardiocentesis plus volume and pressure support with early surgical intervention being necessary for salvage. Untreated free wall rupture is universally fatal although isolated instances of successful aggressive intervention with surgical therapy have been reported (33).

Left Ventricular Aneurysm

LV aneurysm is a relatively common complication of MI and may occur in up to 15% of MI survivors (34). A true aneurysm has a wide base with the ventricular walls composed entirely of myocardium, compared with a pseudoaneurysm, which generally has a narrow base with the walls consisting of pericardium and thrombotic debris. True aneurysms have a relatively low risk of free wall rupture but are associated with increased mortality due to sudden death from ventricular arrhythmias, emboli from mural thrombus, and progressive loss of LV contractile function (35). Aneurysms may develop early in the postinfarction period and can be asymptomatic or present with significant deterioration of LV function. The presence of LV aneurysm may be inferred by persistent ST elevation in the absence of chest pain or enzyme leakage (36).

Echocardiography demonstrating dyskinesis is a valuable tool in diagnosing aneurysms as is LV angiography. LV angiography demonstrates paradoxic systolic distention during ventricular contraction. Successful treatment of the aneurysm may be achieved with resection of the involved myocardium, frequently in combination with saphenous vein or mammary artery bypass grafting because of the high associated prevalence of multivessel coronary artery disease. Surgical resection has been advocated in the presence of post-MI arrhythmias to eliminate the substrate for ventricular tachycardia, but electrophysiologic mapping techniques are necessary to demonstrate that the origin of the arrhythmia arises from the LV aneurysm.

DIAGNOSIS

The clinical manifestations of cardiogenic shock are a function of the underlying cause, and mechanical defects must be aggressively sought because the need for definitive therapy is differs markedly different by cause (Fig. 45.2). Clinical recognition of the shock syndrome frequently requires prompt and aggressive stabilization procedures to be instituted before the definitive diagnosis of the underlying cause. A history and physical examination should be obtained with special attention to mental status, jugular venous pulsations, quality and intensity of heart sounds, presence and localization of a murmur, and presence of oliguria. Diagnostic tests such as electrocardiogram, portable chest radiograph, arterial blood gases, and echocardiography frequently provide adequate clinical information to make a diagnosis and initiate stabilization therapy. A quarter of patients presenting with cardiogenic shock secondary to predominant LV dysfunction do not have evidence of pulmonary congestion (37).

TREATMENT

Percutaneous Revascularization

Prior to 1999, interventions for the management of cardiogenic shock complicating acute MI were not systematically studied. The landmark SHOCK trial demonstrated that a strategy of early revascularization by angioplasty or surgery reduced mortality from 63% to 50% at 6 months (6). This finding has resulted in a major paradigm shift in the management of cardiogenic shock. The first branch-point in the decision algorithm is whether or not shock is present in the setting

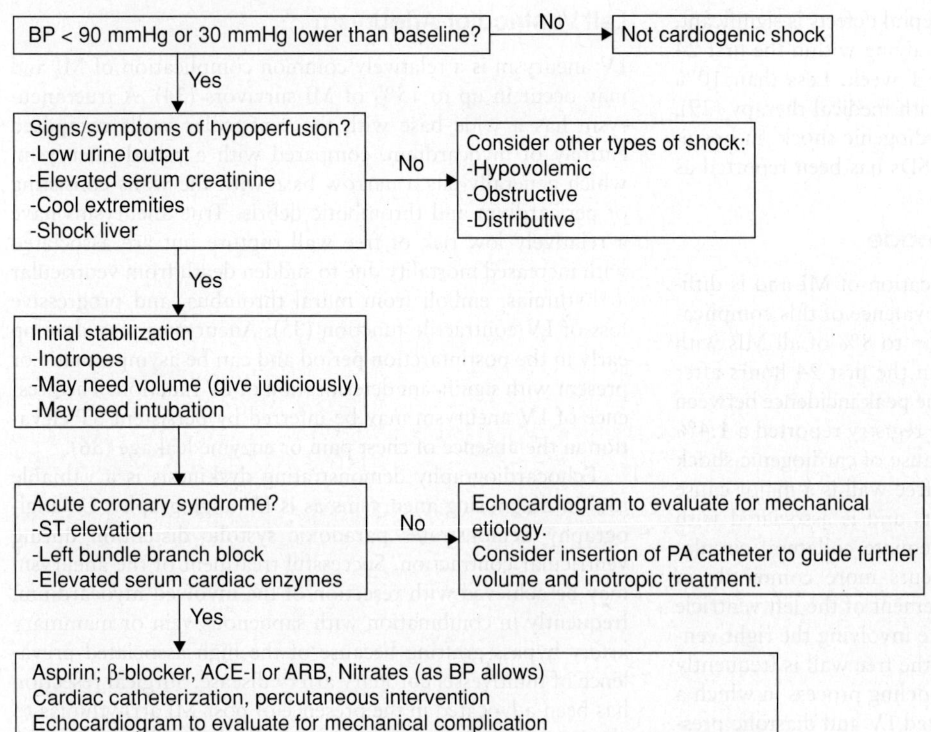

FIGURE 45.2 Management algorithm for cardiogenic shock. ACE-I, angiotensin converting enzyme inhibitor; ARB, angiotensin II receptor blocker.

of an acute MI. If shock is present, patients should undergo immediate coronary angiography with percutaneous intervention if feasible. Primary coronary artery stenting is now recommended for patients with ST elevation or left bundle branch block who develop shock and are suitable for revascularization, irrespective of time delay and need for transfer to a facility capable of coronary intervention (38,39). Thrombolytic therapy may be used if patient is not considered a candidate for percutaneous intervention (39,40).

The SHOCK trial studied patients with onset of shock within 36 hours of an MI and randomized the patients to immediate revascularization versus initial medical stabilization. Almost all patients required inotropes or vasopressors. Treatment in the revascularization group (64% of patients) was angioplasty or stenting (stents were not available at the beginning of the trial in 1993, but were actively used by the end of the trial in 1998) and coronary artery bypass graft surgery in 36%. In a subgroup analysis, survival was similar between percutaneous and surgically revascularized patients (55.6% vs. 57.4% at 30 days and 51.9% vs. 46.8% at 1 year, respectively) despite a higher incidence of diabetes and multivessel disease in those patients surgically revascularized (41).

Thrombolytic therapy was used in 49% of patients in the revascularization group and in 63% of the medical therapy group. There was no difference in survival at 30 days (53.3% in the revascularization group vs. 44.0% in the medical therapy group), likely a result of improved medical therapy. Age over 75 years was associated with significantly higher 30-day mortality. Follow-up reports have shown persistent benefit to early revascularization with survival rates of 47% versus 34% at 1 year, 33% versus 20% at 6 years (42,43). Of the patients surviving to hospital discharge (143/302), 6-year survival was 62% versus 44% (43).

An exciting aspect of the SHOCK trial was the registry that was created from patients screened for enrollment but not randomized, whose data were reported separately in a dedicated supplement to *J Am Coll Cardiol* in September 2000. This registry described 1,190 patients and is the largest prospectively collected database for cardiogenic shock (24). Etiology of shock from the registry was LV failure (78.5%), acute severe mitral regurgitation (6.9%), ventricular septal rupture (3.9%), isolated RV shock (2.8%), and tamponade from free wall rupture (1.4%). Electrocardiographic site of infarction was anterior (55%), inferior (46%), posterior (19%), lateral (32%), apical (11%), with multiple sites present in half of the cases. There was ST elevation, Q waves, or new left bundle branch block in 79% of cases. Systolic blood pressure averaged 88 mmHg with a mean heart rate of 96/min. Of the subset of patients with invasive hemodynamics measured, PAOP was 23 mmHg, CI was 2.08 L/min/m^2, and LV ejection fraction was 33%. In-hospital mortality averaged 60% and ranged from 55% for acute severe mitral regurgitation, isolated RV shock, and tamponade to 87% for ventricular septal rupture. Of the 717 patients who underwent coronary angiography, 15.5% had significant left main stenosis, 53.4% had three-vessel disease. Coronary artery disease severity also correlated with in-hospital mortality: no or single-vessel disease was associated with a 35% mortality rate as compared with three-vessel disease with a mortality rate of 50.8% (44).

Since the SHOCK trial, stenting has replaced angioplasty alone as the primary treatment for ischemic coronary artery disease because it carries a reduced incidence of restenosis. One recent case series has shown that stenting for cardiogenic shock decreased mortality compared to angioplasty alone (from 68% to 43%) (45). Primary coronary artery stenting is now recommended for patients with ST elevation or left bundle branch block who develop shock within 36 hours of acute MI and are suitable for revascularization that can be performed within 18 hours of shock onset (38). Thrombolytic therapy may be used if early revascularization is not available (40).

While drug-eluting stents which slowly elute a pharmacologic agent (currently either sirolimus or paclitaxel) are now widely used instead of bare metal stents due to their proven efficacy in reducing the incidence restenosis, to date they have not been studied in the setting of cardiogenic shock (46,47).

Pharmacologic Limitation of Infarct Size

Several pharmacologic interventions have been used during acute MI to minimize the extent of irreversible ischemic damage and decrease the likelihood of subsequent development of cardiogenic shock. Quantitative measurements of the extent of myocardial damage by electrocardiographic mapping and creatine kinase (CK) release are imprecise and frequently limit quantitative assessment of the potential therapeutic impact of pharmacologic interventions. Calcium channel blockers, beta-adrenergic receptor blockers (β-blockers), and nitrates have been the main agents that have undergone clinical analysis to minimize myocardial damage, whereas a variety of experimental or uncommonly used therapies have been evaluated in small-scale clinical trials. Nitrates are complex pharmacologic agents with arterial and venodilating activity in addition to other potential beneficial effects, such as alteration of prostacyclin metabolism. Nitrates when administered as topical, oral, or sublingual agents, are predominately venodilators with subsequent venous pooling, decreased venous return, and lowering of PAOP. Reduction in venous return and optimization of PAOP decreases LV volume and improves subendocardial perfusion, thus reducing wall stress with the potential for minimizing infarct extent. Nitrates also have effects on systemic vascular resistance and epicardial coronary arteries, with resultant reduction of impedance to LV ejection and increase in coronary blood flow.

Intravenously administered nitroglycerin has a more balanced arterial and venodilating effect. Clinical trials demonstrate that intravenous nitroglycerin administered at a level to decrease mean aortic pressure by 10% (48), results in a decrease in extension of MI, improves LV ejection fraction and survival (49). Intravenous nitrates minimize the magnitude of infarct size as monitored by CK, and alter infarct expansion with reduction in the subsequent remodeling process and progression to congestive heart failure. Intravenous nitrates are potent vasodilators and require careful blood pressure monitoring to prevent significant hypotension and paradoxical bradycardia. Nitrates may result in a beneficial redistribution of coronary flow to the subendocardium without the coronary steal syndrome, a major detriment of other potent intravenous vasodilators such as nitroprusside.

Calcium channel blockers are important agents in managing patients with classic and vasospastic angina. The calcium channel blocking agents decrease systemic vascular resistance, decrease oxygen demand and increase coronary flow, improving the balance between supply and demand. At pharmacologic doses, these agents also may have other potentially beneficial effects including antiplatelet activity.

Despite the documented beneficial effect of these agents in hypertension and angina, calcium channel blockers have not been proven to be beneficial in the treatment of MI and do not definitely limit infarct size. Studies using nifedipine have been unable to demonstrate benefit in patients with acute MI. Diltiazem has been advantageous in non–Q wave infarction in the Diltiazem Reinfarction Study (50). However, the Multicenter Diltiazem Postinfarction Trial was not able to document a benefit to the administration of diltiazem in the postinfarction state when compared with placebo (51). Subgroup analysis demonstrated a mortality benefit with diltiazem therapy when no pulmonary congestion was present. However, mortality was increased when diltiazem was administered to subjects whose infarction was complicated by pulmonary congestion implying that this agent should not be used in patients with cardiogenic shock. Studies performed in Denmark using intravenous verapamil followed by oral administration did not demonstrate a benefit. Later studies using only oral verapamil demonstrated a mortality reduction although these trials have not been reconfirmed (52). Currently, the evidence for using calcium channel blockers for the treatment of acute MI to limit infarct size and progression to cardiogenic shock is limited.

β-Adrenergic blocking agents have been used in treating hypertension, atrial fibrillation, and a variety of ischemic conditions. β-Blockers act predominantly by decreasing myocardial oxygen demand caused by the negative chronotropic and inotropic activities of these agents. β-Blockers may have several other potentially beneficial effects including antiplatelet activity, regression of LV hypertrophy, and reduction in sudden cardiac death. Clinical trials using β-blockade in acute MI have yielded conflicting results. The Goteborg trial administered metoprolol or placebo to subjects having an acute MI and demonstrated a significant reduction in mortality at 90 days in the group randomly assigned to β-blocker therapy (53). Early administration of metoprolol was associated with a reduction in estimated infarct size, which presumably has an effect on early and long-term survival. Despite the fact that β-blockers are not commonly used as antiarrhythmic agents, there was a documented decrease in sudden cardiac death in the β-blocker group, which has been shown to be secondary to an increase in ventricular fibrillatory threshold.

The Metoprolol in Acute Myocardial Infarction trial was able to demonstrate that the early administration of intravenous metoprolol followed by oral maintenance dose in acute MI was associated with a decrease in mortality in a high-risk subgroup of infarct patients (54). A subgroup study of the Goteborg Metoprolol trial found that early treatment with metoprolol in patients with suspected acute MI and signs of heart failure resulted in significantly reduced mortality at 3 months (10% vs. 19%) which persisted to 1 year (14% vs. 27%) compared to those who did not receive metoprolol (55). Propranolol, a noncardioselective β-blocker, has not uniformly been demonstrated to decrease mortality or limit infarct size when administered early in acute MI patients. However, the Beta-Blocker Heart Attack trial demonstrated reduced mortality when propranolol was administered after the acute phase of the infarction had subsided (56). Intravenous atenolol was studied in the First International Study of Infarct Survival trial and demonstrated a 15% reduction in the early mortality of infarct patients who were given oral atenolol after the intravenous loading doses (57). β-Blockers also have been combined with thrombolytic therapy to limit infarct size. The Thrombolysis in Myocardial Infarction trial (TIMI II-B) studied the impact of three 5-mg boluses of metoprolol administered at 5-minute intervals followed by oral metoprolol compared with thrombolysis plus oral metoprolol. The TIMI II-B trial demonstrated a decrease in nonfatal reinfarctions and recurrent ischemic episodes in the group who received immediate intravenous metoprolol followed by oral therapy compared with the delayed subgroup. More recently, the CAPRICORN (Carvedilol Post Infarct Survival Control in Left Ventricular Dysfunction) trial studied carvedilol (6.25 to 25 mg twice a day in addition to standard therapy of aspirin, angiotensin-converting enzyme [ACE] inhibition, and thrombolysis) versus placebo in a high-risk group of acute MI patients (n = 1,959) with LV ejection fraction of 40% or less. Patients were treated for a mean of 1.3 years. All-cause mortality was lower in the carvedilol group than in the placebo group (58). Patients who had echocardiography demonstrated significantly higher LV ejection fraction and decreased LV end-systolic volume in the carvedilol group at 6 months (59). Another post hoc analysis of CAPRICORN study found that carvedilol suppressed atrial arrhythmias (2.3% vs. 5.4%) as well as ventricular arrhythmias (0.9% vs. 3.9%) compared to the control group (60). The beneficial effect on ventricular remodeling, in addition to the antiarrhythmic effect may be one of the mechanisms by which carvedilol decreased mortality after acute MI in patients treated with ACE inhibitors. Use of β-blockers in acute MI, while now standard of care, must be undertaken with caution because of the potential of precipitating atrioventricular block, reactive airways disease, and hypotension (61).

ACE inhibitors have been administered orally and intravenously in clinical trials to halt progression to congestive heart failure in the SAVE (Survival and Ventricular Enlargement) and Consensus-II trials. The SAVE study used captopril in over 2,000 patients who had an acute anterior MI when enrolled during the period from 3 to 16 days after the acute myocardial event (62). All patients with ejection fractions below 40% were randomized to receive oral captopril or a placebo. Patients receiving captopril demonstrated less congestive heart failure, less recurrent MIs, less hospitalizations, and improved mortality over a 42-month period. The Consensus-II (Cooperative New Scandinavian Enalapril Survival Study) trial used intravenous enalapril in the early phase of infarction followed by oral enalapril but there was no mortality benefit when compared with placebo (63). A review of the major post-MI heart failure trials such as SAVE, AIRE (Acute Infarction Ramipril Efficacy), TRACE (Trandolapril Cardiac Evaluation) between 1992 and 1995, calculated that ACE inhibitors produced a relative risk reduction of 16% while β-blockade in addition to ACE inhibition in CAPRICORN trial demonstrated an additional relative risk reduction of 23% (64). Oral ACE inhibitors are attractive agents because of their effects on hemodynamics, microcirculation, and angiotensin-mediated vasoconstriction and should be administered especially in anterior infarcts with significant reductions in ejection fraction unless there are contraindications (hyperkalemia, known drug sensitivity).

Selective aldosterone blockade with eplerenone for patients with LV ejection fraction of 40% or less after acute MI has been studied in one large, placebo-controlled trial EPHESUS (Eplerenone Post-Acute Myocardial Infarction Heart Failure Efficacy and Survival Study). Eplerenone (in addition to treatment with β-blockers and ACE inhibitors) reduced all-cause mortality by 15%, cardiovascular mortality by 17%, heart failure hospitalizations by 23%, and sudden cardiac death by 21% (65). These outcomes were even more marked in the subgroup of patients with LV ejection fraction of 30% or less. In this group, all-cause mortality was reduced by 21%, cardiovascular mortality by 23%, sudden cardiac death by 33%, and heart failure mortality or hospitalization by 25% (66).

Angiotensin receptor blockade for LV ejection fraction of 40% or less after acute MI has been studied in the VALIANT (Valsartan in Acute Myocardial Infarction Trial) trial (67). This was a multicenter, double-blind, randomized, active-controlled, parallel-group study comparing the efficacy and safety of long-term treatment with valsartan, captopril, and their combination in high-risk patients after MI. This compared three treatment groups consisting of patients receiving standard therapy plus valsartan (n = 4,909), valsartan plus captopril (n = 4,885), or captopril alone (n = 4,909). Valsartan treatment alone resulted in similar outcomes as captopril treatment alone and thus these agents can be used interchangeably. The combination of valsartan plus captopril increased the rate of adverse events (hypotension and renal dysfunction more commonly with valsartan; cough, rash, and taste disturbance more commonly with captopril) with no change in survival.

Adjunctive antiplatelet therapy with the glycoprotein IIb/IIIa inhibitor abciximab during emergent coronary artery stenting for cardiogenic shock has been shown to reduce mortality from 43% to 33% in one case series (45). The glycoprotein IIb/IIIa inhibitor eptifibatide used for non–ST-elevation MI or unstable angina in the PURSUIT (Platelet Glycoprotein IIb/IIIa in Unstable Angina: Receptor Suppression in Using Integrilin Therapy Trial) reduced 30-day mortality in the subset of patients developing cardiogenic shock (68). Bivalirudin may be used as an antiplatelet agent for acute MI instead of a glycoprotein IIb/IIIa inhibitor, however it has had mixed results in cardiogenic shock and so is left to the operator's discretion (69,70). Clopidogrel in addition to aspirin is now standard of care after percutaneous coronary intervention and has been shown to decrease 1-year mortality in the setting of ST-elevation MI (71). However, clopidogrel significantly increases the risk of postoperative bleeding in patients requiring surgical intervention. More recent data from the ISAR-SHOCK registry suggest that prasugrel may be superior to clopidogrel in patients with acute MI complicated by cardiogenic shock (72).

Several agents have been used in small studies as adjunctive therapy in acute MI but have not reached widespread clinical use. Myocardial damage may be potentiated by the presence of reactive oxygen radicals and free radical scavengers such as superoxide dismutase or catalase may provide potential benefit. Free radical scavengers have been shown to be effective when administered before the onset of experimental infarcts and definitive clinical studies are currently ongoing.

Glucose insulin potassium infusions (polarizing solution) have been used for several years to reduce infarct size by altering free fatty acid metabolism (73). Polarizing solution consists of 300 g of glucose, 50 units of regular insulin, and 80 mMol of potassium in 1 L of water delivered at 1.5 mL/kg/hr. Ejection fraction and wall motion abnormalities have been noted to improve after administering this solution resulting in decreased mortality. Polarizing solution has not been studied extensively in double-blind, placebo-controlled trials and routine administration of this solution has not reached clinical acceptance.

Hyaluronidase may have anti-inflammatory activity and modulate the immune response postulated to play some role in the extent of infarct size. Hyaluronidase has been administered in small clinical studies and was associated with improved mortality and decreased development of Q waves implying myocardial salvage. There are no large-scale clinical trials available (74).

Thrombolysis

Thrombolysis induced by pharmacologic agents or direct angioplasty is an attractive treatment for reestablishing coronary perfusion to minimize the extent of MI and progression to cardiogenic shock. The open artery hypothesis postulates that clinical outcome is dependent on maintaining adequate coronary perfusion to minimize ischemic damage mediated by vascular occlusion secondary to an intravascular thrombus. Recent trials of coronary thrombolysis GISSI (Gruppo Italiano per lo Studio della Sopravvivenza nell'Infarto Miocardio), ISIS (International Study of Infarct Size), GUSTO (Global Utilization of Strategies to Open Occluded Coronary Arteries) demonstrate the prevalence of cardiogenic shock in approximately 2% to 3% of acute MIs on arrival to the hospital with an additional 3% to 4% subsequently developing cardiogenic shock with a combined total of 7% (3,75). Early progression to cardiogenic shock is characterized demographically by elderly patients, the presence of anterior infarctions, low ejection fractions, diabetes, and previous MIs. Despite the theoretic attractiveness of administering recombinant tissue plasminogen activators or streptokinase in patients with established or impending cardiogenic shock, the mortality associated with cardiogenic shock remains high despite thrombolytic therapy with survival rate being only 35% as reported in GISSI-I and GISSI-II trials (76). Prompt administration of thrombolytic agents within the first hour of acute MI may result in improved survival rates if reperfusion of the infarct-related artery can be sustained. Low coronary perfusion pressures in cardiogenic shock may play a potential role in the poor clinical outcome of these patients after thrombolytic therapy.

In vitro experimental infarct studies with reduced perfusion pressure have shown decreased diffusion of thrombolytic agents into clots with resultant impaired fibrinolysis (77). Enhanced pressure increases the rate of dissolution of an intravascular thrombus implying that in cardiogenic shock with systemic hypotension, a reduced transcoronary pressure gradient may decrease efficacy of thrombolytic agents. The metabolic abnormalities associated with cardiogenic shock including lactic acidosis also may alter the conversion of plasminogen to plasmin and limit the efficacy of these drugs in clot lysis. Failure from lytic agents to sustain vascular patency in patients with cardiogenic shock is an indication for early cardiac catheterization and direct angioplasty if no contraindications exist. Persistent hypotension, nonevolving ST elevation, continuing clinical evidence of myocardial ischemia, CK elevations, and clinical instability are potential indications for rescue coronary angioplasty which may result in increased survival (78). Rescue angioplasty has not been systematically studied in randomized controlled trials comparing it to thrombolytic therapy. If thrombolytic therapy does not result in establishment of coronary perfusion, angioplasty should be considered as a therapeutic option. The SHOCK trial reported 49% of patients in the revascularization group received thrombolytic therapy and the early intervention group had a survival benefit (see section above) (6). Additionally, the SHOCK trial reported a survival benefit due to thrombolytic therapy (in-hospital mortality of 54% vs. 64%) (40). Cardiogenic shock secondary to mechanical defects such as papillary muscle dysfunction also has been treated successfully with percutaneous transluminal coronary angioplasty (PTCA), resulting in improved mitral regurgitation with resolution of cardiogenic shock (79).

Thrombolytic agents should be administered to patients with acute MI who demonstrate evidence of the shock state if there are no contraindications in patients not considered candidates for percutaneous intervention (39). Failure of evidence of reperfusion is an indicator for rescue angioplasty.

Pharmacologic Agents

Inotropic Agents

The effectiveness of various inotropic agents in cardiogenic shock depends on the cause and underlying pathophysiologic mechanism of the shock state. With systemic hypotension, adequate perfusion of the coronary arteries must be maintained (Fig. 45.3).

Dopamine. Dopamine is an endogenous catecholamine with positive inotropic properties secondary to stimulation of α- and β-adrenergic receptors plus dopaminergic receptors, which have been divided into two subtypes: DA_1 and DA_2 (80,81). DA_1 receptors are postsynaptic and induce dilation of the coronary, renal, and mesenteric vasculature. DA_2 receptors are located in autonomic ganglia and in the postganglionic sympathetic nervous system. Stimulation of DA_2 receptors blocks the release of endogenous catecholamines from intraneuronal storage sites. The effect of dopamine on α- and β-activity is dose related. Low infusion dosages of dopamine (2 to 5 µg/kg/min) result in positive inotropic activity secondary to stimulation of the β_1-receptors. α-Receptor stimulation occurs at dosages above 10 µg/kg/min and results in a secondary increase in systemic vascular resistance caused by peripheral vasoconstriction. In addition to the inotropic effect, dopamine results in increased atrioventricular conduction from adrenergic stimulation. The effects of dopamine are thus dose dependent, and pharmacologic activity is a function of the amount of dopamine infused corrected for body weight. The individual response may be variable and unless the clinical situation warrants large pressor doses to maintain blood pressure, dopamine infusion should begin at a low rate (1 µg/kg/min) and gradually be increased to clinical responsiveness. Cardiogenic shock with low tissue perfusion accompanied by hypotension may be treated in a more aggressive manner with progressively increasing doses of dopamine at 5-minute intervals.

Low-dose dopamine infusion results in stimulation of DA_2 receptors and minimal or no changes in heart rate, cardiac output, or blood pressure. Stimulation of DA_2 receptors results in renal vasodilation and increases glomerular filtration rate, renal blood flow, and sodium excretion. Reduction in cardiac output in shock frequently results in shunting of blood away from the renal vasculature and induction of a prerenal state with elevated blood urea nitrogen-to-creatinine ratios and sodium retention. Dopamine reverses the redistribution of cardiac output, increases the amount of sodium presented to the loop of Henle, which allows increased efficacy of diuretics such as furosemide or bumetanide.

Medium dosing ranges of dopamine (5 to 10 µg/kg/min) result in an increase in cardiac output, which may also improve volume status by increasing renal blood flow. The

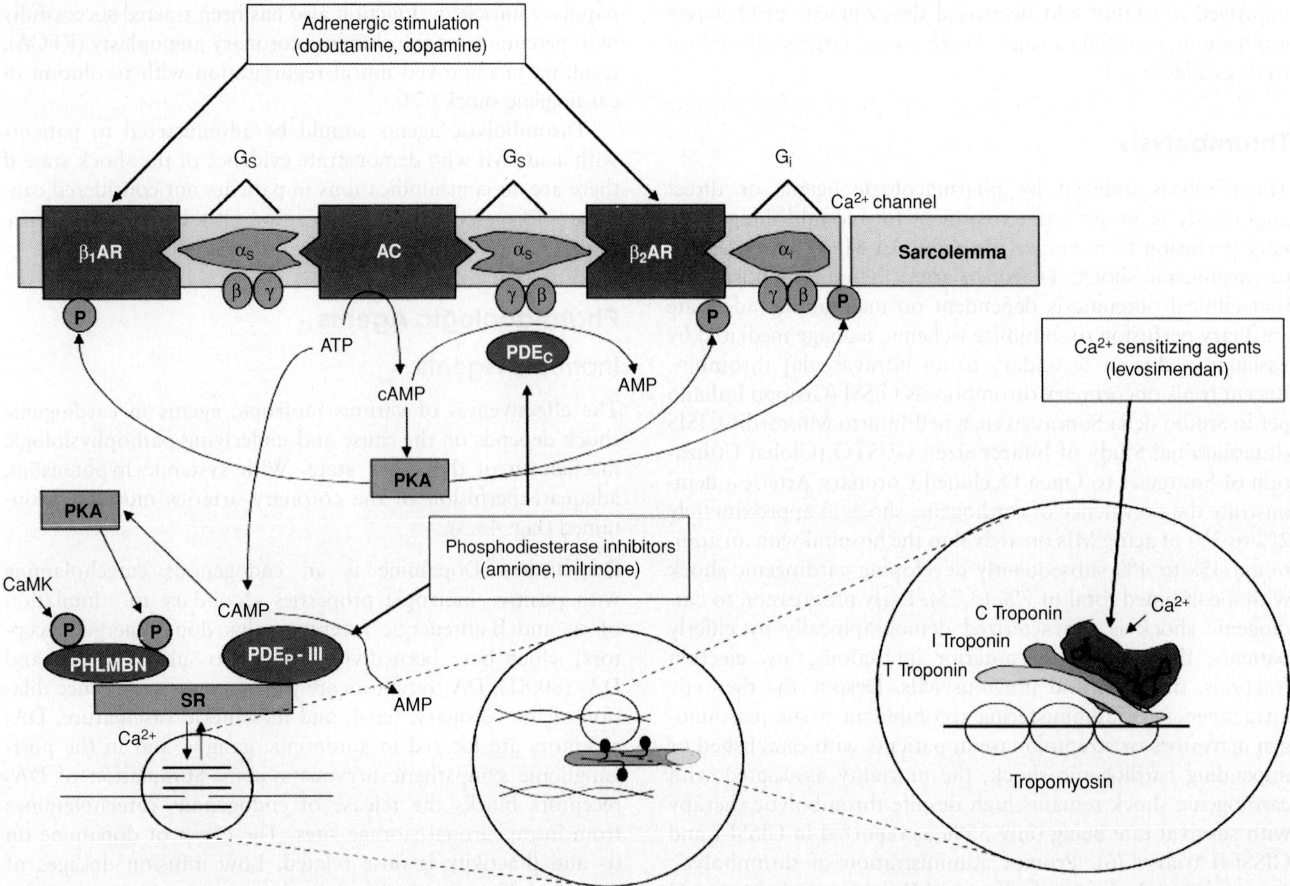

FIGURE 45.3 Mechanisms of action of inotropic drugs. β_1AR, β_1-adrenergic receptor; β_2AR, β_2-adrenergic receptor; AC, adenyl cyclase; AMP, adenosine monophosphate; ATP, adenosine triphosphate; Ca^{2+}, calcium; CaMK, calmodulin-activated kinase; cAMP, cyclic AMP; Gi, inhibitory G protein with α, β, and γ subunits; Gs, stimulatory G protein with α, β, and γ subunits; P, phosphorus; PDEc, cytosolic phosphodiesterases; PDEp – III, particulate, SR-associated PDE III; PHLMBN, phospholamban; PKA, cAMP-dependent protein kinase A; SR, sarcoplasmic reticulum. (Used with permission from Garcia Gonzalez MJ, Dominguez Rodriguez A. Pharmacologic treatment of heart failure due to ventricular dysfunction by myocardial stunning: potential role of levosimendan. *Am J Cardiovasc Drugs.* 2006;6:69–75.)

cardiac effects of dopamine in this dosing range are secondary to stimulation of the β_1-adrenergic receptors caused by a secondary release of norepinephrine. The effect of dopamine is indirect and depends on a pre-existent adequate storage level of endogenous catecholamines. Longstanding congestive heart failure is frequently associated with reduction in sympathetic receptors in the myocardium and the efficacy of dopamine may be limited if prolonged congestive heart failure was present before the shock syndrome. Dopamine infusion at this dose generally does not result in alterations of venous return secondary to venodilation, and right atrial and PAOP may not decrease. Dopamine may be combined with either direct vasodilating compounds or other inotropic agents such as dobutamine, which combine inotropism with vasodilation. Medium dosing range infusions of dopamine are generally safe and effective in maintaining blood pressure. Acid–base status and electrolyte levels should be optimized to avoid potential induction of arrhythmias with resultant malignant ventricular arrhythmias or marked sinus or supraventricular tachycardias, which would increase myocardial oxygen demand.

High-range dopamine infusions (>10 μg/kg/min) result in activation of α-adrenergic receptors and a secondary norepinephrine release with vasoconstriction and increased systemic vascular resistance. Patients in cardiogenic shock may need much higher doses of dopamine and ranges up to 50 μg/kg/min have been used. Strict attention to volume status and repeated examinations for signs of excessive vasoconstriction is necessary. A central venous line is used for higher dopamine doses due to tissue necrosis should the solution extravasate. Dopamine may interact with certain coadministered drugs. Tricyclic antidepressants may increase the pressor response of direct-acting sympathomimetics and decrease the sensitivity to indirect-acting sympathomimetics. Because dopamine has direct and indirect effects on the vasculature, this agent should be used with caution, especially with overdoses of the tricyclic drugs (82). Although not commonly used, the rauwolfia alkaloids may potentiate the pressor response of direct-acting sympathomimetics resulting in hypertension. Monoamine oxidase inhibitors may increase pressor response of dopamine (83). Dopamine is an endogenous catecholamine that is degraded by catechol-o-methyltransferase and is not effective when administered in oral doses.

Dobutamine. As opposed to dopamine, which is an endogenous catechol and immediate precursor of norepinephrine and epinephrine, dobutamine is a synthetic agent that stimulates predominantly β_1-adrenoreceptors (Table 45.4) (84). Dobutamine is a direct-acting agent unlike dopamine and does not require the presence or release of intramyocardial norepinephrine to modulate its effects. Mild activation of β_2- and

TABLE 45.4 Dobutamine

Adrenergic Receptor	Site	Action
β_1	Myocardium	Increase atrial and ventricular contractility
	Sinoatrial node	Increase heart rate
	Atrioventricular conduction system	Enhance atrioventricular conductions
β_2	Arterioles	Vasodilation
	Lungs	Bronchodilation
α	Peripheral arterioles	Vasoconstriction
DA_1	Postsynaptic	Dilation of coronary, renal, and mesenteric vasculature
DA_2	Autonomic ganglia and postganglionic sympathetic nervous system	Decreased release of endogenous catechols

α-receptors may be seen with this agent, but significantly less when compared with β_1-receptors. Administration of dobutamine results in a direct inotropic stimulation plus a secondary reflex vasodilation with reduction of systemic vascular resistance and an increase in cardiac output.

The pharmacologic mechanism of dobutamine is complicated because of its asymmetric structure and racemic mixture. The positive and negative isomers have been evaluated as to their relative activities in in vitro studies and it seems that the positive isomer is predominantly responsible for the activation of the β-receptors. The administration of dobutamine alters stimulation of β-receptors in a differential manner with an increased binding affinity for the predominantly cardiac β_1-adrenergic receptors with a direct inotropic effect. The inotropic effects of this agent are not coupled with an increased rate of arrhythmias when compared with epinephrine and norepinephrine and there seems to be less adverse electrophysiologic effects when compared with dopamine. Although a mild vasodilator, there are no major effects on arterial blood pressure due to an increase in cardiac output and stroke volume. The increase in cardiac output results in improved renal blood flow and enhanced ability to excrete sodium and water. Dobutamine is effective in cardiogenic shock, assuming that the underlying etiology is not caused by valvular or subvalvular stenosis and the pharmacologic infusion does not result in significant hypotension and this agent may be combined with dopamine to maintain blood pressure.

Norepinephrine. Norepinephrine is a powerful α-adrenergic agonist that results in significant peripheral vasoconstriction when administered within the usual dosage range of 2 to 8 μg/min. Norepinephrine is generally instituted in the treatment of cardiogenic shock after failure of volume correction and dopamine to maintain adequate cardiac output and blood pressure (80). Norepinephrine is a naturally occurring catecholamine that has both α- and β_1-adrenergic activity. Although generally associated with an increase in cardiac output, increases in systemic vascular resistance and mean aortic blood pressure may affect cardiac output adversely. The pressure work of the left ventricle and oxygen consumption are increased and blood may be shunted away from various organ beds because of volume redistribution secondary to catecholamine sensitivity. Oliguria and azotemia from impaired renal blood flow may be worsened secondary to the norepinephrine-mediated vasoconstriction if occult hypovolemia is coexistent. Norepinephrine has been associated with increased irritability of the ventricle with an increased electrical instability and potential adverse rhythm disorders. Clinical response will vary depending on the advantageous effects of increased perfusion pressure and cardiac output weighed against the detrimental effects of increased myocardial oxygen consumption and shunting from visceral organs.

Digitalis Preparations. The use of digitalis in general and cardiogenic shock specifically has been controversial because of theoretic objections involving the use of this agent and the lack of controlled clinical trials documenting a beneficial impact on mortality (84). Digitalis glycosides have complex mechanisms of action whose inotropic activity is modulated by increasing the availability of intracellular calcium secondary to inhibition of sodium–potassium ATPase. Inhibition of this ubiquitous enzyme, which is found not only in cardiac tissue but also in the central nervous system, gastrointestinal tract, and kidney, results in calcium influx by the activation of the sodium–calcium exchange mechanism. The level of free cytosolic calcium regulates the activity of tropomyosin with increased interactions between actin and myosin filaments and increased contractility. Alterations in contraction are caused by variations in levels of cytosolic calcium which can be moved in and out of the sarcoplasmic reticulum.

The increase in cardiac output after administration of digitalis is modest when compared with the more powerful intravenous inotropes such as dobutamine, dopamine, and norepinephrine. Digitalis increases the refractory period at the atrioventricular node and decreases conduction velocity resulting in a negative chronotropic effect in patients with atrial fibrillation. An advantage is that digitalis lacks the negative inotropic activity of other agents that have been used to slow the rate in atrial fibrillation, including β-blockers and calcium channel blockers such as diltiazem and verapamil (85). Digitalis increases vagal tone, decreases levels of norepinephrine in chronic heart failure possibly from decreased activity of the peripheral sympathetic nervous system, resets baroreceptor sensitivity, and may enhance natriuresis from increased cardiac output.

Digitalis withdrawal has been associated with worsening heart failure in a randomized, double-blind, placebo-controlled study of digitalis withdrawal in patients also treated with ACE inhibitors. However, the role of digitalis in cardiogenic shock is limited due to a modest increase in cardiac output although the autonomic effects of this agent with decreases in the heart rate in atrial fibrillation is clinically beneficial.

Isoproterenol. Isoproterenol has both β_1- and β_2-adrenergic properties with increased myocardial contractility, heart rate, and cardiac output without vasoconstriction. The powerful chronotropic and inotropic activities of this agent increase myocardial work and oxygen. Isoproterenol is infrequently used in heart failure or cardiogenic shock unless the shock state is associated with bradyarrhythmias that do not respond to other therapies or with acute valvular insufficiency if blood pressure and volume status are maintained. Isoproterenol thus has a limited role in the acute management of cardiogenic shock.

Phosphodiesterase Inhibitors. Amrinone and milrinone are bipyridine derivatives that inhibit cellular levels of phosphodiesterase (86). Inhibition of this key enzyme results in increased levels of cyclic AMP in cardiac muscle with resultant enhancement of protein phosphorylation by protein kinase with increased inotropic and chronotropic activities. The methylxanthines were known to nonspecifically inhibit phosphodiesterase activity and result in mild enhancement of the inotropic state. Both amrinone and milrinone have been shown in experimental and clinical studies to increase cardiac output in patients with severe congestive heart failure or cardiogenic shock (87).

Administering these agents results in reduction of central filling pressures and increases in stroke volume and cardiac output. The chronotropic effects of amrinone and milrinone are modest but a mild increase in heart rate may be observed. Large doses may result in severe peripheral vasodilation, hypotension, and tachycardia. The phosphodiesterase inhibitors have been studied in patients with pump failure after MIs and at a dose of 200 μg/kg/hr, has been shown to improve cardiac function. Comparison in clinical trials of amrinone to other vasodilating inotropes such as dobutamine documented a greater decrease in systemic and pulmonary venous pressures in the group that received amrinone (88). The vasodilating activity of the phosphodiesterase inhibitors while increasing cardiac output may result in significant hypotension, requiring concomitant administration of sympathomimetic amines with at least partial α-activity such as norepinephrine. The side effect profile of the phosphodiesterase inhibitors relates mainly to hematologic and gastrointestinal effects. Nausea, vomiting, and diarrhea occur in many patients. Thrombocytopenia is common with amrinone (approximately 15%), although the marked decreases in platelet counts to levels under 50,000 seems to be relatively rare and may require dose reduction. Milrinone is more potent on a milligram basis when compared with amrinone and also has effects on the inotropic state and ventricular relaxation. Incidence of thrombocytopenia seems less (<5%) than with amrinone. Enoximone is an imidazole derivative that also results in phosphodiesterase inhibition, increases levels of cyclic AMP and contractile force in isolated muscle preparations (89). Intravenous enoximone results in an increase in CI with a decrease in right-sided filling pressures with minimal impacts on systemic vascular resistance and heart rate. Enoximone is currently undergoing a variety of controlled trials, seems to have a relatively mild side effect profile and thrombocytopenia is uncommon with the use of this agent.

Glucagon. Glucagon is uncommonly used in cardiogenic shock but has a potential advantage in that it has a different mechanism of action from other sympathomimetic amines and does not require β-receptor stimulation to exert its inotropic effects (90,91). Glucagon is administered in a dosing range of 4 to 6 mg intravenously, which may be followed by a constant infusion of 4 to 12 mg/hr. Glucagon administration increases cardiac output by approximately 20%, which is associated with a decrease in peripheral vascular resistance with less myocardial oxygen demand when compared with norepinephrine. The indications for glucagon have not been delineated, although it seems justifiable to administer this agent to patients with cardiogenic shock who do not respond to conventional therapy or cannot tolerate other agents because of the development of significant arrhythmias or hematologic toxicity.

Levosimendan. Levosimendan is the first of a new class of inotropic agents called calcium sensitizers. Its mechanism of action involves increasing calcium sensitivity by binding to troponin C and stabilizing it in the calcium-induced conformation. This augments the effect of calcium binding to troponin C. Additionally, at high concentrations levosimendan inhibits phosphodiesterase 3, which also results in increased intracellular calcium concentration. These effects result in increased myocardial contraction associated with increased intracellular calcium transients (92). It improves myocardial contractility without increasing oxygen requirements and induces peripheral and coronary vasodilation with a potential antistunning, anti-ischemic effect (93). Given its vasodilatory properties, it is not primarily for cardiogenic shock but more for low-output heart failure. In addition to calcium sensitization, levosimendan also stimulates ATP-sensitive potassium ion channels that are suppressed by intracellular ATP and acts synergistically with nucleotide diphosphates. This mechanism may contribute to the vasodilator action and may protect cardiomyocytes against ischemic damage (94). A loading dose of 6 to 24 mg/kg over 10 minutes followed by an infusion of 0.1 mg/kg/min for 50 minutes, increased to 0.2 mg/kg/min for an additional 23 hours has been well tolerated (93). Initial clinical experience suggests that levosimendan causes dose-dependent increases in stroke volume and cardiac index, with minimum increase in heart rate (95). There are dose-dependent decreases in PAOP, right atrial, pulmonary arterial, and mean arterial pressures. The hemodynamic effects of levosimendan appear to be more pronounced than those seen with dobutamine (96) and are sustained up 24 hours after discontinuation of infusion due to an active metabolite (97). An initial clinical trial found no significant adverse events (95). Data from two published clinical trials indicate that levosimendan is associated with improved 6-month survival compared with dobutamine or placebo although the studies were not powered to look at this outcome (96,98,99). There are several other trials not yet published but presented at national meetings, which report a survival benefit of levosimendan compared with dobutamine or placebo. However, a 24-hour infusion of levosimendan had no effect on 6-month survival compared with dobutamine for patients with acutely decompensated heart failure in the SURVIVE trial reported at the American Heart Association Scientific Sessions in 2005 but not yet published (96). The European Society of Cardiology's 2005 guidelines on the diagnosis and treatment of acute heart failure include the use of levosimendan in patients with symptomatic low cardiac output secondary to systolic dysfunction without severe hypotension (100). This drug is not FDA approved, although it is available in some European countries.

Surgical Intervention

Surgical intervention in acute MI has been used to limit infarct size by direct revascularization or to correct the mechanical defects of an acute ischemic event such as VSDs, acute mitral insufficiency, free wall rupture, or LV aneurysm. Surgical intervention for revascularization in acute MI had been contraindicated on theoretic grounds because of the presumed high morbidity and mortality rates from cardiac catheterization and operative interventions during the unstable period of acute MI. A variety of clinical studies determined that coronary bypass surgery could be performed in an expeditious manner with low mortality. Bypass surgery has been used as primary therapy in acute MI with an overall operative rate of approximately 5% for transmural infarctions and a highly acceptable long-term mortality rate (101,102). Early revascularization (<6 hours) by direct PTCA, intravenous or intracoronary thrombolytic agents, or bypass surgery in selected patients represents the treatment of choice. Congestive heart failure that occurs in the post-MI state may be amenable to revascularization by surgical interventions although large-scale, controlled, randomized studies are lacking. However, several surgical series have reported on early and long-term survival of patients with an acute MI complicated by cardiogenic shock receiving coronary artery bypass surgery (101,103). Surgical intervention in cardiogenic shock is fraught with considerable clinical problems and requires the presence of surgically accessible and potentially viable myocardium. Surgical intervention has the advantage of reestablishing flow not only in the infarct-related artery but in vessels not involved in the acute ischemic process but significantly obstructed. Viability of the myocardium in the periinfarction state may be difficult to determine secondary to problems with the acute delineation of stunned, hibernating, or irreversibly damaged myocardium. Nitroglycerin or dobutamine enhancement of ejection fraction is an indirect method of determining viability but is time consuming in a period where early revascularization is of prime importance.

Indications for surgical intervention in cardiogenic shock have not been completely delineated but should be considered in patients who fail to respond to volume correction and inotropic therapy. Failure of conventional medical interventions for cardiogenic shock should result in consideration of intra-aortic balloon counterpulsation (IABP), a temporizing measure before revascularization. Historically, emergent coronary artery bypass surgery preceded by placement of intra-aortic balloon pump, has demonstrated improved survival rates in cardiogenic shock to approximately 75%. The SHOCK trial registry reported a 28% in-hospital mortality for the 290 patients undergoing coronary artery bypass surgery, which is comparable to other reported series (24,104). In a subgroup analysis of the SHOCK trial, survival was similar between percutaneous and surgically revascularized patients (55.6% vs. 57.4% at 30 days and 51.9% vs. 46.8%, respectively, at 1 year) despite a higher incidence of diabetes and multivessel disease in those patients surgically revascularized (41). Thus, surgical revascularization has an important role in patients with more extensive coronary artery disease.

Surgery for acute mitral insufficiency associated with cardiogenic shock in the postinfarction state is the only available definitive therapy. The impact of acute mitral insufficiency on LV performance may be underestimated by studying ejection fraction since the left ventricle ejects retrograde into the low compliance left atrial and pulmonary venous system. Medical therapy with inotropic support and systemic peripheral vasodilation improves regurgitant flow as calculated by the regurgitant fraction. Severe mitral insufficiency is associated with a variety of adverse pathophysiologic changes that result in a poor survival after surgical intervention, but the results are significantly better than medical treatment that results in essentially 100% mortality if marked mitral insufficiency is associated with cardiogenic shock.

Surgical intervention is generally required for acute VSDs, which occur in the muscular portion of the interventricular septum and may be multiple. Two anatomic types of acute VSDs have been described. A VSD resulting from occlusion of a posterior descending coronary artery that arises from the right coronary is associated with a defect located in the inferobasilar region of the septum. Anteroseptal MIs, which are associated with thrombotic occlusion of the left anterior descending, are associated with mid-apical to anterior defects in the septum. The physiologic impact of a left-to-right shunt is a function of the quantitative amount of involved myocardium plus associated LV dysfunction, pulmonary artery pressures, and RV compliance. A significant left-to-right shunt markedly decreases forward flow with poor peripheral perfusion and the clinical characteristics of cardiogenic shock. If the LV end-diastolic pressure is markedly elevated, left-to-right shunting will also occur during diastole and is associated with an extremely high 24-hour mortality rate of approximately 25% (29,103). Medical treatment alone is associated with a 20% survival beyond 60 days, and 1-year survival of less than 10%.

Surgical intervention in acute VSDs requires early and aggressive diagnostic and therapeutic interventions. Despite IABP and optimization with medical management, refinements in surgical technique have improved 1-year survival to 32% without coronary artery bypass. Evaluation of clinical trials that attempt to postpone therapy to improve the healing process have been questioned because this eliminates the most severely ill patients from definitive therapy and introduces a selection bias into the implications of therapy. Early surgical intervention with direct patch grafts plus coronary artery bypass may result in survival rates of up to 75%.

LV free wall rupture is a surgical disease even with a clotted hemopericardium tamponading further extravasation of blood into the pericardial space. The diagnosis of free wall rupture may be extraordinarily difficult on clinical grounds, and signs of pericardial tamponade should be actively sought. Pericardiocentesis with decompression of the pericardial space may be lifesaving in the short term but represents only a temporizing procedure. Cardiac rupture is essentially fatal but surgical intervention may be successful with direct over-sewing of the defect if recognized and managed in a timely fashion (30,105).

LV aneurysm as a cause of cardiogenic shock may require surgical intervention as a definitive therapy. The remodeling process, which begins after an acute ischemic event with regional thinning and expansion of the infarct zone, may result in progressive decrease in LV performance and cardiogenic shock. If the aneurysmal dilation of the left ventricle involves more than 20% of the LV mass, severe impairment of pumping ability ensues and potentially requires surgical intervention if poor response to medical management including intra-aortic balloon pumping. Surgical intervention for aneurysms should be optimized in timing with adequate healing and fibrosis.

Mechanical Circulatory Support

The intra-aortic balloon pump has been in clinical use for over 20 years to increase diastolic coronary arterial perfusion and to decrease LV afterload (106). The intra-aortic balloon pump is a temporizing measure that does not increase myocardial oxygen demand and results in reduction of ventricular diastolic volume and reduces pulmonary congestion with an increase in cardiac output. The intra-aortic balloon pump is the most widely used circulatory assist device in patients with cardiogenic shock because of the ease of insertion either percutaneously or surgically. Effective counterpulsation results in stabilization and potential reversal of the shock state with improvement in peripheral perfusion but does require an adequate systemic pressure and LV performance to maximize its use. Profoundly hypotensive patients respond poorly to intra-aortic counterpulsation and the IABP has limited efficacy.

Balloon pumping in selected patients allows optimization of blood pressure, cardiac output, and tissue perfusion in patients with cardiogenic shock while further diagnostic procedures are performed. Hemodynamic effects of IABP include the following (in percent change): Peak aortic systolic pressure (10% to 15%), diastolic intra-aortic pressure (70%), arterial end-diastolic pressure (10%), peak ventricular pressure (10%), LV end-diastolic pressure (10%), *dp/dt* (10%), systemic vascular resistance (no change), mean arterial pressure (no change), CI (10% to 15%), pulmonary capillary resistance (10% to 15%). Intra-aortic balloon pump may be used prophylactically in patients with mechanical defects such as acute mitral insufficiency or VSD to increase coronary perfusion, allow time for healing, and restore cardiac output toward normal. The impact of IABP on long-term survival is controversial and depends on the indications for insertion, hemodynamic status, and etiology of the cardiogenic shock. Patient selection is a key issue and early insertion of the intra-aortic balloon may result in increased clinical benefit rather than procrastination until overt low flow state has developed. The addition of IABP to thrombolytic therapy for acute MI complicated by cardiogenic shock has been studied in a randomized clinical trial. There was no overall mortality benefit but the subgroup of patients with Killip class III or IV benefitted with a 6-month mortality rate of 39% for combined therapy versus 80% for fibrinolysis alone (107). The SHOCK trial registry also reported a survival benefit with intra-aortic balloon pumping in addition to thrombolytic therapy (47% vs. 63% in-hospital mortality), but these results were heavily affected by higher revascularization rates in the group receiving intra-aortic balloon pump (68% vs. 20%) (40). More recently, the IAPP SHOCK trial reported no significant benefit in Acute Physiology and Chronic Health Evaluation (APACHE) II scores, CI or systemic inflammatory activation (108).

Patients who are not expected to significantly benefit from intra-aortic balloon pump are elderly patients, with severe peripheral vascular disease, and large MIs exceeding 40% of LV myocardium. The overall survival rate of patients with cardiogenic shock treated with the IABP is approximately 40%. For subjects who required balloon insertion for large MIs without a significant mechanical obstruction, the survival rate was only 27%. Complications may be documented in up to 30% of patients who undergo intra-aortic balloon pumping and relate mainly to local vascular problems, including surgical trauma, emboli, infection, and hemolysis.

Extracorporeal membrane oxygenation may also be considered for temporary mechanical support in cardiogenic shock. Results have been mixed, with no improvement on infarct size but some benefit in cardiac enzyme release, diastolic function, and coronary blood flow (109,110). Survival rates are generally low in these extremely ill patients, with 24% to 42% surviving to discharge from hospital (111,112).

Left ventricular assist devices ($LVAD_d$) function as prosthetic ventricles but require a sternotomy for insertion. Assist devices may be used to support LV performance, RV performance, or a combination, depending on the underlying condition. The indications for insertion of an LVAD have traditionally involved failure of medical and temporary mechanical support in the presence of the potentially salvageable myocardium and particularly as a bridge to cardiac transplantation. The Thoratec extracorporeal LVAD (Thoratec, Pleasanton, CA) has been used a bridge to cardiac transplantation. Insertion of the Thoratec device in patients with severe LV dysfunction allowed survival to transplant in approximately 75% of 29 patients (113). Outcomes continue to improve with advances in care and technology. The Heartmate II LVAD (Thoratec, Pleasanton, CA) and HeartWare (HeartWare Inc., Framingham, MA) have reported survival rates of 91% at 6 months and 84% to 85% at 1 year (114,115). Some LVADs are now approved for chronically ill patients too sick for cardiac transplantation as an alternative (destination therapy). The REMATCH (Randomized Evaluation of Mechanical Assistance in the Treatment of Congestive Heart Failure) trial was the first to demonstrate improved outcomes in chronically ill patients too sick for cardiac transplantation as an alternative (destination therapy) to routine medical care (116). The device used in REMATCH was the HeartMate XVE, which is no longer made, and the HeartMate II is now approved as destination therapy (117) and the HeartWare is completing.

There is retrospective data that early mechanical support as a bridge to transplantation, after acute MI complicated by cardiogenic shock improves survival compared with a strategy of early revascularization (118). The technology has now advanced to include several other continuous flow pumps that offer the potential advantage of greater mechanical longevity, thus making them truly a lifelong option. Complications include hemolysis, thromboembolism, and infection, which have been decreased with increasing experience.

There are several percutaneous continuous rotary flow VADs that do not require sternotomy and can be used, or are under evaluation, for temporary support. These include the TandemHeart (Cardiac Assist, Pittsburgh, PA), Impella (Abiomed, Danvers, MA) and the CircuLite Synergy (HeartWare Inc., Framingham, MA). The TandemHeart and Impella are currently FDA approved while the CircuLite is approved in Europe and in clinical trial in the United States. Use of these devices has increased substantially and has been associated with a decrease in mortality rates and hospital costs (119).

Controversies and Emerging Therapies

Ventricular Assist Devices to Promote Myocardial Recovery

Hemodynamic unloading and myocardial rest after VAD placement may lead to recovery of native cardiac function, allowing for removal of the device without cardiac transplantation (120,121). VAD support is also associated with decreases in neurohormonal activation, alterations in myocyte calcium handling, and improvement in the proinflammatory cytokine milieu (122,123). Histologic analysis of the explanted heart at the time of transplantation demonstrated decreased fibrosis and myocyte size after VAD placement (124–126). Despite these salutatory changes as a result of VAD support, the frequency of bridge to recovery (BTR) in chronically supported subjects remains low, in the range of 3% to 10% in various series (127–130).

Autologous Stem Cells

Stem cells offer the hope of biologically rebuilding damaged myocardium due to their ability to differentiate into cardiomyocytes. There has been a substantial amount of research into the biology of various stem cells and now several clinical trials have been reported, with mixed results. Most trials have looked at stem cells delivery percutaneously by intracoronary catheter after acute MI in numbers ranging from 30 to 100 patients. The BOOST (Bone Marrow Transfer to Enhance ST-elevation Infarct Regeneration) trial found 6% improvement in ejection fraction compared to control but no significant difference at 18 months (131,132). The ASTAMI (Autologous Stem Cell Transplantation in Acute MI) trial found no difference in ejection fraction at 4 and 6 months, respectively although Janssens et al. reported improved regional wall motion and decreased infarct size (133,134). TOPCARE-CHD (Transcoronary Transplant of Progenitor Cells after MI with Chronic Ischemic Heart Disease) trial found 2.9% improvement in ejection fraction at 3 months, while REPAIR-AMI (Intracoronary Administration of Bone Marrow-derived Progenitor Cells in Acute Myocardial Infarction) trial reported a 2.5% improvement in ejection fraction at 4 months (135,136). Multiple studies are currently underway including evaluating safety and efficacy of stem cells implanted during surgery for VAD installation as well as coronary artery bypass surgery with depressed ventricular function, and percutaneously for chronic angina. While this is a very promising therapy, considerable issues remain including the risk of generating an arrhythmic focus, the best cell type, the amount of local myocardial blood flow necessary, the best method to deliver the cells to the myocardium, and the number of cells necessary.

Clenbuterol

Clenbuterol is a β_2-adrenergic–receptor agonist that induces skeletal muscle hypertrophy and improves contraction. It also has been found to cause cardiomyocyte hypertrophy without apoptosis (137). In a recently reported single center study, 15 patients requiring LVAD support were treated with clenbuterol in addition to lisinopril, carvedilol, spironolactone, and losartan (138). There was sufficient myocardial recovery to explant the LVAD in 11 of 15, for whom 4-year survival was 89%, quality-of-life scores were almost normal, and mean LV ejection fraction was 64%. These patients all had heart failure due to nonischemic cardiomyopathy without histologic evidence of active myocarditis. These data remain unconfirmed in any larger trials.

Tissue Engineered Patches

Patches made from decellularized extracellular matrix may be another useful solution to biologic regeneration of myocardium. The patch retains biologically active substances such as growth factors providing paracrine as well as mechanical support for regrowth of cardiomyocytes. These devices are still in preclinical testing but have shown improvements in regional function in an MI model (139).

Key Points

- Clinical criteria used to establish the diagnosis of cardiogenic shock include absolute or relative hypotension, which is defined as a systolic blood pressure less than 90 mmHg or a blood pressure that has fallen to at least 30 mmHg less than the individual's baseline blood pressure. Cardiogenic shock thus may be a complication in patients with chronic hypertension who have an acute cardiac event that results in a decrease in blood pressure, but not to the 90 mmHg systolic level, if signs of organ dysfunction and tissue hypoperfusion exist.
- The exact incidence of cardiogenic shock is difficult to ascertain because of variability in diagnostic criteria and survival rates in the early phase of acute MI but seems to range from 5% to 10%.
- The mortality rate for cardiogenic shock in the setting of acute MI is exceedingly high despite significant improvements due to a strategy of early revascularization.
- Bedside clinical criteria that provide evidence of reduced organ perfusion include oliguria, confusion, peripheral cyanosis, and evidence of peripheral vasoconstriction.
- An accurate definition of cardiogenic shock also requires persistence of the shock state after correction of extracardiac conditions, such as hypovolemia or a variety of metabolic abnormalities including significant disturbances in acid–base metabolism, electrolyte abnormalities, or arrhythmias.
- The PAOP is frequently in excess of 18 mmHg, and the CI is usually less than 2.2 L/min/m^2.
- Cardiogenic shock in the setting of acute MI warrants pharmacologic intervention to limit infarct size and includes using heparin, aspirin, nitrates, β-blockers, calcium channel blockers, or a combination thereof. Primary coronary artery stenting is now recommended for patients with ST elevation or left bundle branch block who develop shock and are suitable for revascularization, irrespective of time delay and need for transfer to a facility capable of coronary intervention. Thrombolytic therapy may be used if patient is not considered a candidate for percutaneous intervention.
- Hemodynamic management includes optimization of preload and afterload and augmentation of contractility, when appropriate, with agents such as dobutamine, dopamine, norepinephrine, digitalis preparations, or phosphodiesterase inhibitors.
- Surgical intervention in MI has been used to limit infarct size by direct revascularization or correction of mechanical defects of an acute ischemic event such as VSDs, acute mitral insufficiency, free wall rupture, or LV aneurysm.
- Mechanical assist devices such as the IABP are used as temporizing measures to optimize blood pressure, cardiac output, and tissue perfusion in patients with cardiogenic shock while further diagnostic procedures and disease staging are performed. Newer percutaneous VADs providing 2 to 5 L/min blood flow are now available and are associated with improved outcomes.

ACKNOWLEDGMENT

This work supported in part by NIH grants HL103455 and TR000005.

References

1. Hands ME, Rutherford JD, Muller JE, et al. The in-hospital development of cardiogenic shock after myocardial infarction: incidence, predictors of occurrence, outcome and prognostic factors. The MILIS Study Group. *J Am Coll Cardiol.* 1989;14:40–46.
2. Goldberg RJ, Samad NA, Yarzebski J, et al. Temporal trends in cardiogenic shock complicating acute myocardial infarction. *N Engl J Med.* 1999;340:1162–1168.

3. Holmes DR Jr, Bates ER, Kleiman NS, et al.; the GUSTO-I Investigators. Contemporary reperfusion therapy for cardiogenic shock: the GUSTO-I trial experience. *J Am Coll Cardiol.* 1995;26:668–674.
4. Hasdai D, Holmes DR Jr, Topol EJ, et al. Frequency and clinical outcome of cardiogenic shock during acute myocardial infarction among patients receiving reteplase or alteplase: results from GUSTO-III. Global use of strategies to open occluded coronary arteries. *Eur Heart J.* 1999;20:128–135.
5. Killip T III, Kimball JT. Treatment of myocardial infarction in a coronary care unit: a two year experience with 250 patients. *Am J Cardiol.* 1967;20:457–464.
6. Hochman JS, Sleeper LA, Webb JG, et al.; SHOCK Investigators. Early revascularization in acute myocardial infarction complicated by cardiogenic shock: should we emergently revascularize occluded coronaries for cardiogenic shock. *N Engl J Med.* 1999;341:625–634.
7. Noble MI. Problems concerning the application of concepts of muscle mechanics to the determination of the contractile state of the heart. *Circulation.* 1972;45:252–255.
8. Sagawa K, Maughan WL, Suga H, Sunagawa K. *Cardiac Contraction and the Pressure-Volume Relationship.* New York: Oxford University Press; 1988.
9. Mathey D, Biefield W, Hanrath P, Effert S. Attempt to quantitate relation between cardiac function and infarct size in acute myocardial infarction. *Br Heart J.* 1974;36:271–279.
10. Forrester JS, Diamond G, Chatterjee K, Swan HJ. Medical therapy of acute myocardial infarction by application of hemodynamic subsets (first of two parts). *N Engl J Med.* 1976;295:1356–1362.
11. Andersen HR, Falk E, Nielsen D. Right ventricular infarction: frequency, size and topography in coronary heart disease: a prospective study comprising 107 consecutive autopsies from a coronary care unit. *J Am Coll Cardiol.* 1987;10:1223–1232.
12. Kinch JW, Ryan TJ. Right ventricular infarction. *N Engl J Med.* 1994;330:1211–1217.
13. Andersen HR, Nielsen D, Falk E. Right ventricular infarction: diagnostic value of ST elevation in lead III exceeding that of lead II during inferior/posterior infarction and comparison with right-chest leads V3R to V7R. *Am Heart J.* 1989;117:82–86.
14. Zehender M, Kasper W, Kauder E, et al. Right ventricular infarction as an independent predictor of prognosis after acute inferior myocardial infarction. *N Engl J Med.* 1993;328:981–988.
15. Dell'Italia LJ, Starling MR, Crawford MH, et al. Right ventricular infarction: identification by hemodynamic measurements before and after volume loading and correlation with noninvasive techniques. *J Am Coll Cardiol.* 1984;4:931–939.
16. Sato H, Murakami Y, Shimada T, et al. Detection of right ventricular infarction by gadolinium DTPA-enhanced magnetic resonance imaging. *Eur Heart J.* 1995;16:1195–1199.
17. Goldstein JA, Barzilai B, Rosamond TL, et al. Determinants of hemodynamic compromise with severe right ventricular infarction. *Circulation.* 1990;82:359–368.
18. Jacobs AK, Leopold JA, Bates E, et al. Cardiogenic shock caused by right ventricular infarction: a report from the SHOCK registry. *J Am Coll Cardiol.* 2003;41:1273–1279.
19. Bowers TR, O'Neill WW, Grines C, et al. Effect of reperfusion on biventricular function and survival after right ventricular infarction. *N Engl J Med.* 1998;338:933–940.
20. Tcheng JE, Jackman JD Jr, Nelson CL, et al. Outcome of patients sustaining acute ischemic mitral regurgitation during myocardial infarction. *Ann Intern Med.* 1992;117:18–24.
21. Sharma SK, Seckler J, Israel DH, et al. Clinical, angiographic and anatomic findings in acute severe ischemic mitral regurgitation. *Am J Cardiol.* 1992;70:277–280.
22. Thompson CR, Buller CE, Sleeper LA, et al. Cardiogenic shock due to acute severe mitral regurgitation complicating acute myocardial infarction: a report from the SHOCK trial registry. Should we use emergently revascularize occluded coronaries in cardiogenic shock? *J Am Coll Cardiol.* 2000;36:1104–1109.
23. Leor J, Feinberg MS, Vered Z, et al. Effect of thrombolytic therapy on the evolution of significant mitral regurgitation in patients with a first inferior myocardial infarction. *J Am Coll Cardiol.* 1993;21:1661–1666.
24. Hochman JS, Buller CE, Sleeper LA, et al. Cardiogenic shock complicating acute myocardial infarction—etiologies, management and outcome: a report from the SHOCK trial registry. Should we emergently revascularize occluded coronaries for cardiogenic shock? *J Am Coll Cardiol.* 2000;36:1063–1070.
25. Kisanuki A, Otsuji Y, Kuroiwa R, et al. Two-dimensional echocardiographic assessment of papillary muscle contractility in patients with prior myocardial infarction. *J Am Coll Cardiol.* 1993;21:932–938.
26. Picard MH, Davidoff R, Sleeper LA, et al. Echocardiographic predictors of survival and response to early revascularization in cardiogenic shock. *Circulation.* 2003;107:279–284.
27. Menon V, Webb JG, Hillis LD, et al. Outcome and profile of ventricular septal rupture with cardiogenic shock after myocardial infarction: a report from the SHOCK trial registry. Should we emergently revascularize occluded coronaries in cardiogenic shock? *J Am Coll Cardiol.* 2000;36:1110–1106.
28. Harrison MR, MacPhail B, Gurley JC, et al. Usefulness of color Doppler flow imaging to distinguish ventricular septal defect from acute mitral regurgitation complicating acute myocardial infarction. *Am J Cardiol.* 1989;64:697–701.
29. Gray RJ, Sethna D, Matloff JM. The role of cardiac surgery in acute myocardial infarction. I. With mechanical complications. *Am Heart J.* 1983;106:723–728.
30. Bates RJ, Beutler S, Resnekov L, Anagnostopoulos CE. Cardiac rupture: challenge in diagnosis and management. *Am J Cardiol.* 1977;40:429–437.
31. Assmann PE, Roelandt JR. Two-dimensional and Doppler echocardiography in acute myocardial infarction and its complications. *Ultrasound Med Biol.*1987;13:507–517.
32. Buda AJ. The role of echocardiography in the evaluation of mechanical complications of acute myocardial infarction. *Circulation.* 1991;84:I109–I121.
33. Pappas PJ, Cernaianu AC, Baldino WA, et al. Ventricular free-wall rupture after myocardial infarction: treatment and outcome. *Chest.* 1991;99:892–895.
34. Visser CA, Kan G, David GK, et al. Echocardiographic-cineangiographic correlation in detecting left ventricular aneurysm: a prospective study of 422 patients. *Am J Cardiol.* 1982;50:337–341.
35. Heras M, Sanz G, Betriu A, et al. Does left ventricular aneurysm influence survival after acute myocardial infarction? *Eur Heart J.* 1990;11:441–446.
36. Arvan S, Varat MA. Persistent ST-segment elevation and left ventricular wall abnormalities: a 2-dimensional echocardiographic study. *Am J Cardiol.* 1984;53:1542–1546.
37. Menon V, White H, LeJemtel T, et al. The clinical profile of patients with suspected cardiogenic shock due to predominant left ventricular failure: a report from the SHOCK trial registry. Should we emergently revascularize occluded coronaries in cardiogenic shock? *J Am Coll Cardiol.* 2000;36:1071–1076.
38. Levine GN, Bates ER, Blankenship JC, et al. 2011 ACCF/AHA/SCAI guideline for percutaneous coronary intervention: a report of the American College of Cardiology Foundation/American Heart Association Task Force on Practice Guidelines and the Society for Cardiovascular Angiography and Interventions. *J Am Coll Cardiol.* 2011;58:e44–e122.
39. O'Gara PT, Kushner FG, Ascheim DD, et al. 2013 ACCF/AHA guideline for the management of ST-elevation myocardial infarction: a report of the American College of Cardiology Foundation/American Heart Association Task Force on Practice Guidelines. *Circulation.* 2013;127:e362–e425.
40. Sanborn TA, Sleeper LA, Bates ER, et al. Impact of thrombolysis, intra-aortic balloon pump counterpulsation, and their combination in cardiogenic shock complicating acute myocardial infarction: a report from the SHOCK trial registry. Should we emergently revascularize occluded coronaries for cardiogenic shock? *J Am Coll Cardiol.* 2000;36:1123–1129.
41. White HD, Assmann SF, Sanborn TA, et al. Comparison of percutaneous coronary intervention and coronary artery bypass grafting after acute myocardial infarction complicated by cardiogenic shock: results from the Should We Emergently Revascularize Occluded Coronaries for Cardiogenic Shock (SHOCK) trial. *Circulation.* 2005;112:1992–2001.
42. Hochman JS, Sleeper LA, White HD, et al. One-year survival following early revascularization for cardiogenic shock. *JAMA.* 2001;285:190–192.
43. Hochman JS, Sleeper LA, Webb JG, et al. Early revascularization and long-term survival in cardiogenic shock complicating acute myocardial infarction. *JAMA.* 2006;295:2511–2515.
44. Wong SC, Sanborn T, Sleeper LA, et al. Angiographic findings and clinical correlates in patients with cardiogenic shock complicating acute myocardial infarction: a report from the SHOCK trial registry. Should we emergently revascularize occluded coronaries for cardiogenic shock? *J Am Coll Cardiol.* 2000;36:1077–1083.
45. Chan AW, Chew DP, Bhatt DL, et al. Long-term mortality benefit with the combination of stents and abciximab for cardiogenic shock complicating acute myocardial infarction. *Am J Cardiol.* 2002;89:132–136.
46. Moses JW, Leon MB, Popma JJ, et al. Sirolimus-eluting stents versus standard stents in patients with stenosis in a native coronary artery. *N Engl J Med.* 2003;349:1315–1323.

47. Stone GW, Ellis SG, Cox DA, et al. A polymer-based, paclitaxel-eluting stent in patients with coronary artery disease. *N Engl J Med.* 2004;350:221–231.
48. Flaherty JT, Becker LC, Bulkley BH, et al. A randomized prospective trial of intravenous nitroglycerin in patients with acute myocardial infarction. *Circulation.* 1983;68:576–88.
49. Jugdutt BI, Warnica JW. Intravenous nitroglycerin therapy to limit myocardial infarct size, expansion, and complications: effect of timing, dosage, and infarct location. *Circulation.* 1988;78:906–919.
50. Gibson RS, Boden WE, Theroux P, et al. Diltiazem and reinfarction in patients with non-Q-wave myocardial infarction: results of a double-blind, randomized, multicenter trial. *N Engl J Med.* 1986;315:423–429.
51. The Multicenter Diltiazem Postinfarction Trial Research Group. The effect of diltiazem on mortality and reinfarction after myocardial infarction. *N Engl J Med.* 1988;319:385–392.
52. Hansen JF; the Danish Study Group on Verapamil in Myocardial Infarction. Treatment with verapamil during and after an acute myocardial infarction: a review based on the Danish Verapamil Infarction Trials I and II. *J Cardiovasc Pharmacol.* 1991;18(Suppl 6):S20–S25.
53. Herlitz J, Hjalmarson A, Swedberg K, et al. The influence of early intervention in acute myocardial infarction on long-term mortality and morbidity as assessed in the Goteborg metoprolol trial. *Int J Cardiol.* 1986;10:291–301.
54. Hjalmarson A, Elmfeldt D, Herlitz J, et al. Effect on mortality of metoprolol in acute myocardial infarction: a double-blind randomised trial. *Lancet.* 1981;2:823–817.
55. Herlitz J, Waagstein F, Lindqvist J, et al. Effect of metoprolol on the prognosis for patients with suspected acute myocardial infarction and indirect signs of congestive heart failure (a subgroup analysis of the Goteborg Metoprolol Trial). *Am J Cardiol.* 1997;80:40J-4J.
56. Viscoli CM, Horwitz RI, Singer BH. Beta-blockers after myocardial infarction: influence of first-year clinical course on long-term effectiveness. *Ann Intern Med.* 1993;118:99–105.
57. Mechanisms for the early mortality reduction produced by beta-blockade started early in acute myocardial infarction: ISIS-1. ISIS-1 (First International Study of Infarct Survival) Collaborative Group. *Lancet.* 1988;1:921–923.
58. Dargie HJ. Effect of carvedilol on outcome after myocardial infarction in patients with left-ventricular dysfunction: the CAPRICORN randomised trial. *Lancet.* 2001;357:1385–1390.
59. Doughty RN, Whalley GA, Walsh HA, et al. Effects of carvedilol on left ventricular remodeling after acute myocardial infarction: the CAPRICORN Echo Substudy. *Circulation.* 2004;109:201–206.
60. McMurray J, Kober L, Robertson M, et al. Antiarrhythmic effect of carvedilol after acute myocardial infarction: results of the Carvedilol Post-Infarct Survival Control in Left Ventricular Dysfunction (CAPRICORN) trial. *J Am Coll Cardiol.* 2005;45:525–530.
61. Roberts R, Rogers WJ, Mueller HS, et al. Immediate versus deferred beta-blockade following thrombolytic therapy in patients with acute myocardial infarction: results of the Thrombolysis in Myocardial Infarction (TIMI) II-B Study. *Circulation.* 1991;83:422–437.
62. Pfeffer MA, Braunwald E, Moye LA, et al.; the SAVE Investigators. Effect of captopril on mortality and morbidity in patients with left ventricular dysfunction after myocardial infarction: results of the survival and ventricular enlargement trial. *N Engl J Med.* 1992;327:669–677.
63. Swedberg K, Held P, Kjekshus J, et al. Effects of the early administration of enalapril on mortality in patients with acute myocardial infarction: results of the Cooperative New Scandinavian Enalapril Survival Study II (CONSENSUS II). *N Engl J Med.* 1992;327:678–684.
64. McMurray J, Pfeffer MA. New therapeutic options in congestive heart failure: Part I. *Circulation.* 2002;105:2099–2106.
65. Pitt B, Remme W, Zannad F, et al. Eplerenone, a selective aldosterone blocker, in patients with left ventricular dysfunction after myocardial infarction. *N Engl J Med.* 2003;348:1309–1321.
66. Pitt B, Gheorghiade M, Zannad F, et al. Evaluation of eplerenone in the subgroup of EPHESUS patients with baseline left ventricular ejection fraction <or=30%. *Eur J Heart failure.* 2006;8:295–301.
67. Pfeffer MA, McMurray JJ, Velazquez EJ, et al. Valsartan, captopril, or both in myocardial infarction complicated by heart failure, left ventricular dysfunction, or both. *N Engl J Med.* 2003;349:1893–1906.
68. Hasdai D, Harrington RA, Hochman JS, et al. Platelet glycoprotein IIb/IIIa blockade and outcome of cardiogenic shock complicating acute coronary syndromes without persistent ST-segment elevation. *J Am Coll Cardiol.* 2000;36:685–692.
69. Bonello L, De Labriolle A, Roy P, et al. Bivalirudin with provisional glycoprotein IIb/IIIa inhibitors in patients undergoing primary angioplasty in the setting of cardiogenic shock. *Am J Cardiol.* 2008;102:287–291.
70. Pourdjabbar A, Hibbert B, Maze R, et al. bivalqirudin for primary percutaneous coronary interventions in patients with cardiogenic shock: outcome assessment in the capital STEMI registry. *Can J Cardiol.* 2014;30: S68.
71. Zeymer U, Gitt AK, Junger C, et al. Effect of clopidogrel on 1-year mortality in hospital survivors of acute ST-segment elevation myocardial infarction in clinical practice. *Eur Heart J.* 2006;27:2661–2666.
72. Orban M, Mayer K, Morath T, et al. Prasugrel vs clopidogrel in cardiogenic shock patients undergoing primary PCI for acute myocardial infarction: results of the ISAR-SHOCK registry. *Thromb Haem.* 2014;112:1190–1197.
73. Rackley CE, Russell RO Jr, Rogers WJ, et al. Glucose-insulin-potassium infusion in acute myocardial infarction: review of clinical experience. *Postgrad Med.* 1979;65:93–99.
74. Henderson A, Campbell RW, Julian DG. Effect of a highly purified hyaluronidase preparation (GL enzyme) on electrocardiographic changes in acute myocardial infarction. *Lancet.* 1982;1:874–876.
75. Grella RD, Becker RC. Cardiogenic shock complicating coronary artery disease: diagnosis, treatment, and management. *Curr Probl Cardiol.* 1994;19:693–742.
76. Gruppo Italiano per lo Studio della Streptochinasi nell'Infarto Miocardico (GISSI). Effectiveness of intravenous thrombolytic treatment in acute myocardial infarction. *Lancet.* 1986;1:397–402.
77. Cox RH. Mechanical aspects of large coronary arteries. In: Santamore WP, Bove AA, eds. *Coronary Artery Disease: Etiology, Hemodynamic Consequences, Drug Therapy and Clinical Implications.* Baltimore, MD: Urban and Schwartzenberg; 1982:19–38.
78. Stack RS, Califf RM, Hinohara T, et al. Survival and cardiac event rates in the first year after emergency coronary angioplasty for acute myocardial infarction. *J Am Coll Cardiol.* 1988;11:1141–1149.
79. Shawl FA, Forman MB, Punja S, Goldbaum TS. Emergent coronary angioplasty in the treatment of acute ischemic mitral regurgitation: long-term results in five cases. *J Am Coll Cardiol.* 1989;14:986–991.
80. Mueller H, Ayres SM, Giannelli S Jr, et al. Effect of isoproterenol,l-norepinephrine, and intraaortic counterpulsation on hemodynamics and myocardial metabolism in shock following acute myocardial infarction. *Circulation.* 1972;45:335–351.
81. Goldberg LI. Cardiovascular and renal actions of dopamine: potential clinical applications. *Pharmacol Rev.* 1972;24:1–29.
82. Teba L, Schiebel F, Dedhia HV, Lazzell VA. Beneficial effect of norepinephrine in the treatment of circulatory shock caused by tricyclic antidepressant overdose. *Am J Emerg Med.* 1988;6:566–568.
83. Horwitz D, Goldberg LI, Sjoerdsma A. Increased blood pressure responses to dopamine and norepinephrine produced by monoamine oxidase inhibitors in man. *J Lab Clin Med.* 1960;56:747–753.
84. Kelly RA, Smith TW. Digoxin in heart failure: implications of recent trials. *J Am Coll Cardiol.* 1993;22:107A–112A.
85. Sarter BH, Marchlinski FE. Redefining the role of digoxin in the treatment of atrial fibrillation. *Am J Cardiol.* 1992;69:71G–78G.
86. Honerjager P. Pharmacology of bipyridine phosphodiesterase III inhibitors. *Am Heart J.* 1991;121:1939–1944.
87. Benotti JR, Grossman W, Braunwald E, et al. Hemodynamic assessment of amrinone: a new inotropic agent. *N Engl J Med.* 1978;299:1373–1377.
88. Klein NA, Siskind SJ, Frishman WH, et al. Hemodynamic comparison of intravenous amrinone and dobutamine in patients with chronic congestive heart failure. *Am J Cardiol.* 1981;48:170–175.
89. Dage RC, Kariya T, Hsieh CP, et al. Pharmacology of enoximone. *Am J Cardiol.* 1987;60:10C–14C.
90. Goldstein RE, Skelton CL, Levey GS, et al. Effects of chronic heart failure on the capacity of glucagon to enhance contractility and adenyl cyclase activity of human papillary muscles. *Circulation.* 1971;44:638–648.
91. Scholz H. Inotropic drugs and their mechanisms of action. *J Am Coll Cardiol.* 1984;4:389–397.
92. Hasenfuss G, Pieske B, Castell M, et al. Influence of the novel inotropic agent levosimendan on isometric tension and calcium cycling in failing human myocardium. *Circulation.* 1998;98:2141–2147.
93. De Luca L, Colucci WS, Nieminen MS, et al. Evidence-based use of levosimendan in different clinical settings. *Eur Heart J.* 2006;27:1908–1920.
94. Yokoshiki H, Katsube Y, Sunagawa M, Sperelakis N. The novel calcium sensitizer levosimendan activates the ATP-sensitive K+ channel in rat ventricular cells. *J Pharmacaol Exp Ther.* 1997;283:375–383.
95. Slawsky MT, Colucci WS, Gottlieb SS, et al. Acute hemodynamic and clinical effects of levosimendan in patients with severe heart failure. *Circulation.* 2000;102:2222–2227.
96. Mebazaa A, Barraud D, Welschbillig S. Randomized clinical trials with levosimendan. *Am J Cardiol.* 2005;96:74G–79G.

97. Kivikko M, Lehtonen L, Colucci WS. Sustained hemodynamic effects of intravenous levosimendan. *Circulation.* 2003;107:81–86.
98. Moiseyev VS, Poder P, Andrejevs N, et al. Safety and efficacy of a novel calcium sensitizer, levosimendan, in patients with left ventricular failure due to an acute myocardial infarction: a randomized, placebo-controlled, double-blind study (RUSSLAN). *Eur Heart J.* 2002;23:1422–1432.
99. Follath F, Cleland JG, Just H, et al. Efficacy and safety of intravenous levosimendan compared with dobutamine in severe low-output heart failure (the LIDO study): a randomised double-blind trial. *Lancet.* 2002;360:196–202.
100. Nieminen MS, Bohm M, Cowie MR, et al.; the Task Force on Acute Heart Failure of the European Society of Cardiology. Executive summary of the guidelines on the diagnosis and treatment of acute heart failure: *Eur Heart J.* 2005;26:384–416.
101. DeWood MA, Heit J, Spores J, et al. Anterior transmural myocardial infarction: effects of surgical coronary reperfusion on global and regional left ventricular function. *J Am Coll Cardiol.* 1983;1:1223–1234.
102. DeWood MA, Notske RN, Berg R Jr, et al. Medical and surgical management of early Q wave myocardial infarction. I. Effects of surgical reperfusion on survival, recurrent myocardial infarction, sudden death and functional class at 10 or more years of follow-up. *J Am Coll Cardiol.* 1989;14:65–77.
103. Fox AC, Glassman E, Isom OW. Surgically remediable complications of myocardial infarction. *Prog Cardiovasc Dis.* 1979;21:461–484.
104. Bolooki H. Emergency cardiac procedures in patients in cardiogenic shock due to complications of coronary artery disease. *Circulation.* 1989;79:I137–I148.
105. Shapira I, Isakov A, Burke M, Almog C. Cardiac rupture in patients with acute myocardial infarction. *Chest.* 1987;92:219–223.
106. Cohn LH. The role of mechanical devices. *J Cardiac Surg.* 1990;5:278–281.
107. Ohman EM, Nanas J, Stomel RJ, et al. Thrombolysis and counterpulsation to improve survival in myocardial infarction complicated by hypotension and suspected cardiogenic shock or heart failure: results of the TACTICS trial. *J Thromb Thrombolysis.* 2005;19:33–39.
108. Prondzinsky R, Lemm H, Swyter M, et al. Intra-aortic balloon counterpulsation in patients with acute myocardial infarction complicated by cardiogenic shock: the prospective, randomized IABP SHOCK Trial for attenuation of multiorgan dysfunction syndrome. *Crit Care Med.* 2010;38:152–160.
109. Zhu GJ, Sun LN, Li XH, et al. Myocardial protection of early extracorporeal membrane oxygenation (ECMO) support for acute myocardial infarction with cardiogenic shock in pigs. *Heart Vessels.* 2015;30:669–674.
110. Brehm C, Schubert S, Carney E, et al. Left anterior descending coronary artery blood flow and left ventricular unloading during extracorporeal membrane oxygenation support in a swine model of acute cardiogenic shock. *Artif Organs.* 2015;39:171–176.
111. Doll N, Kiaii B, Borger M, et al. Five-year results of 219 consecutive patients treated with extracorporeal membrane oxygenation for refractory postoperative cardiogenic shock. *Ann Thorac Surg.* 2004;77:151–157.
112. Combes A, Leprince P, Luyt CE, et al. Outcomes and long-term quality-of-life of patients supported by extracorporeal membrane oxygenation for refractory cardiogenic shock. *Crit Care Med.* 2008;36:1404–1411.
113. Farrar DJ, Hill JD, Gray LA Jr, et al. Heterotopic prosthetic ventricles as a bridge to cardiac transplantatio: a multicenter study in 29 patients. *N Engl J Med.* 1988;318:333–340.
114. Starling RC, Naka Y, Boyle AJ, et al. Results of the post-U.S. Food and Drug Administration-approval study with a continuous flow left ventricular assist device as a bridge to heart transplantation: a prospective study using the INTERMACS (Interagency Registry for Mechanically Assisted Circulatory Support). *J Am Coll Cardiol.* 2011;57:1890–1898.
115. Slaughter MS, Pagani FD, McGee EC, et al. HeartWare ventricular assist system for bridge to transplant: combined results of the bridge to transplant and continued access protocol trial. *J Heart Lung Transplant.* 2013;32:675–683.
116. Rose EA, Gelijns AC, Moskowitz AJ, et al. Long-term use of a left ventricular assist device for end-stage heart failure. *N Engl J Med.* 2001;345:1435–1443.
117. Slaughter MS, Rogers JG, Milano CA, et al. Advanced heart failure treated with continuous-flow left ventricular assist device. *N Engl J Med.* 2009;361:2241–2251.
118. Tayara W, Starling RC, Yamani MH, et al. Improved survival after acute myocardial infarction complicated by cardiogenic shock with circulatory support and transplantation: comparing aggressive intervention with conservative treatment. *J Heart Lung Transplant.* 2006;25:504–509.
119. Stretch R, Sauer CM, Yuh DD, Bonde P. National trends in the utilization of short-term mechanical circulatory support: incidence, outcomes, and cost analysis. *J Am Coll Cardiol.* 2014;64:1407–1415.
120. Gorcsan J III, Severyn D, Murali S, Kormos RL. Non-invasive assessment of myocardial recovery on chronic left ventricular assist device: results associated with successful device removal. *J Heart Lung Transplant.* 2003;22:1304–1313.
121. Frazier OH, Delgado RM III, Scroggins N, et al. Mechanical bridging to improvement in severe acute "nonischemic, nonmyocarditis" heart failure. *Congest Heart Fail.* 2004;10:109–113.
122. James KB, McCarthy PM, Thomas JD, et al. Effect of the implantable left ventricular assist device on neuroendocrine activation in heart failure. *Circulation.* 1995;92:II191–II195.
123. Goldstein DJ, Moazami N, Seldomridge JA, et al. Circulatory resuscitation with left ventricular assist device support reduces interleukins 6 and 8 levels. *Ann Thorac Surg.* 1997;63:971–974.
124. Barbone A, Holmes JW, Heerdt PM, et al. Comparison of right and left ventricular responses to left ventricular assist device support in patients with severe heart failure: a primary role of mechanical unloading underlying reverse remodeling. *Circulation.* 2001;104:670–675.
125. Bruckner BA, Stetson SJ, Perez-Verdia A, et al. Regression of fibrosis and hypertrophy in failing myocardium following mechanical circulatory support. *J Heart Lung Transplant.* 2001;20:457–464.
126. Zafeiridis A, Jeevanandam V, Houser SR, Margulies KB. Regression of cellular hypertrophy after left ventricular assist device support. *Circulation.* 1998;98:656–662.
127. Farrar DJ, Holman WR, McBride LR, et al. Long-term follow-up of Thoratec ventricular assist device bridge-to-recovery patients successfully removed from support after recovery of ventricular function. *J Heart Lung Transplant.* 2002;21:516–521.
128. Mancini DM, Beniaminovitz A, Levin H, et al. Low incidence of myocardial recovery after left ventricular assist device implantation in patients with chronic heart failure. *Circulation.* 1998;98:2383–2389.
129. Hetzer R, Muller JH, Weng Y, et al. Bridging-to-recovery. *Ann Thorac Surg.* 2001;71:S109–113.
130. Simon MA, Kormos RL, Murali S, et al. Myocardial recovery using ventricular assist devices: prevalence, clinical characteristics, and outcomes. *Circulation.* 2005;112:I32–I36.
131. Wollert KC, Meyer GP, Lotz J, et al. Intracoronary autologous bone-marrow cell transfer after myocardial infarction: the BOOST randomised controlled clinical trial. *Lancet.* 2004;364:141–148.
132. Meyer GP, Wollert KC, Lotz J, et al. Intracoronary bone marrow cell transfer after myocardial infarction: eighteen months' follow-up data from the randomized, controlled BOOST (BOne marrOw transfer to enhance ST-elevation infarct regeneration) trial. *Circulation.* 2006;113:1287–1294.
133. Janssens S, Dubois C, Bogaert J, et al. Autologous bone marrow-derived stem-cell transfer in patients with ST-segment elevation myocardial infarction: double-blind, randomised controlled trial. *Lancet.* 2006;367:113–121.
134. Lunde K, Solheim S, Aakhus S, et al. Intracoronary injection of mononuclear bone marrow cells in acute myocardial infarction. *N Engl J Med.* 2006;355:1199–1209.
135. Assmus B, Honold J, Schachinger V, et al. Transcoronary transplantation of progenitor cells after myocardial infarction. *N Engl J Med.* 2006;355:1222–1232.
136. Schachinger V, Erbs S, Elsasser A, et al. Intracoronary bone marrow-derived progenitor cells in acute myocardial infarction. *N Engl J Med.* 2006;355:1210–1221.
137. Yacoub MH. A novel strategy to maximize the efficacy of left ventricular assist devices as a bridge to recovery. *Eur Heart J.* 2001;22:534–540.
138. Birks EJ, Tansley PD, Hardy J, et al. Left ventricular assist device and drug therapy for the reversal of heart failure. *N Engl J Med.* 2006;355:1873–1884.
139. Kochupura PV, Azeloglu EU, Kelly DJ, et al. Tissue-engineered myocardial patch derived from extracellular matrix provides regional mechanical function. *Circulation.* 2005;112:I144–I149.

CHAPTER

46

Sepsis and Septic Shock

GLORIA VAZQUEZ-GRANDE and ANAND KUMAR

INTRODUCTION

Septic shock (shock due to infection) and sepsis-associated multiple-organ failure are the dominant cause of death in intensive care units (ICUs) of the industrialized world. As many as 800,000 cases of sepsis are admitted every year to American hospitals—comparable to the incidence of first myocardial infarctions—with half of those developing septic shock (1). Historically, the mortality associated with sepsis and septic shock has approximated 50% to 75% (2–4). The major advance in the therapy of septic shock was the development of antibiotic therapy 50 years ago, resulting in a reduction in sepsis-associated mortality to the 30% to 50% range (2,3). The past 40 years has seen a gradual year-to-year increase in the incidence of sepsis (5), with resultant total deaths due to sepsis in the United States (US) increasing even though overall mortality has fallen from 27.8% to 17.9% during that period (5). The total death toll from sepsis is estimated to be comparable to that from myocardial infarction and far exceeds the impact of illnesses such as acquired immune deficiency syndrome (AIDS) or breast cancer (1,6).

The total number of cases continues to gradually increase due to a burgeoning population of patients with a chronic and high degree of susceptibility to infection—age, AIDS, organ failure, transplants, and other chronic illness—increased use of invasive medical devices, and increased use of cytotoxic agents for autoimmune disease, transplants and malignancy, all of which are at high risk for sepsis. Current estimates suggest a doubling of total US cases by 2050, despite a population increase of only 33% (1). Despite major advances in technology and constant refinement of our understanding of sepsis pathophysiology, numerous clinical trials have failed to produce any new drugs with consistent beneficial effects on this patient population. Nonetheless, the last 50 years have seen a gradual improvement in mortality, perhaps related to improvements in supportive care (5,7).

Definitions

Deriving from the verb *sepo* meaning "rot," the first introduction of the term *sepsis* occurs in the poems of Homer (circa eighth century bc) (8). Over the intervening 2,700 years, through Homer, Hippocrates, Aristotle, and Galen to current-day physicians, the term has continued to be used virtually unchanged in meaning. Hugo Schottmuller modernized the term with his 1914 definition "Septicemia is a state of microbial invasion from a portal of entry into the blood stream which causes signs of illness" (9). From the time of Schottmuller's definition of septicemia until recent years, terms such as septicemia, sepsis, toxemia, and bacteremia were all used interchangeably to indicate patients exhibiting systemic responses to infection.

A significant problem with the term "septicemia" (as defined by Schottmuller) is that most patients with a septic response cannot be documented to have bacteremia/fungemia and many with bacteremia/fungemia (e.g., endocarditis, catheter-related infection) do not exhibit overt sepsis. Recognizing that upcoming, large-scale clinical trials of novel sepsis therapies would require more consistent and precise definitions of the septic response, consensus definitions were developed in 1991 (10). These criteria were developed primarily as a tool to enhance the ability to perform clinical sepsis research; however, the terminology soon entered the clinical lexicon. These consensus definitions were revised in 2001 with an extended list of clinical and laboratory variables in order to accommodate the clinician's perspective (11) and a new revision of definitions is imminent. Current and previous definitions follow.

Infection

A microbial phenomenon characterized by an inflammatory response to the presence of microorganisms or the invasion of normally sterile host tissue by these organisms.

Bacteremia

The presence of viable bacteria in the blood: The presence of other organisms in the blood should be described in like manner—viremia, fungemia, etc. Bacteremia can either be transient, sustained, or intermittent.

Systemic Inflammatory Response Syndrome

The systemic inflammatory response to a variety of severe clinical insults, including but not limited to infection. A variety of other clinical insults including pancreatitis, ischemia, multiple trauma and tissue injury, hemorrhagic shock, immune-mediated organ injury, and exogenous administration of inflammatory mediators such as tumor necrosis factor (TNF) or other cytokines may lead to systemic inflammatory response syndrome (SIRS). Previous criteria for SIRS are enumerated in Table 46.1. The more recent revision to sepsis definitions removed these SIRS criteria while retaining the concept. However, some understanding of these criteria remains crucial for the intensivist/clinical researcher as most trials in the past 25 years have been predicated on patients having three or more of these criteria.

Sepsis

The systemic response to infection: This response is similar to SIRS, except that it must be thought to result from an infection. The previously accepted definition required at least two of the four SIRS criteria in the presence of documented or suspected infection. The recent revision of the criteria enumerates

TABLE 46.1 Definition of Systemic Inflammatory Response Syndrome (10)

Systemic inflammatory response syndrome (SIRS): The systemic inflammatory response to a wide variety of severe clinical insults manifests by two or more of the following conditions:

- Temperature >38° or <36°C
- Heart rate >90 beats/min
- Respiratory rate >20 breaths/minor $PaCO_2$ <32 mmHg
- White blood cell count >12,000/μL, <4000/μL, or 10% immature (band) forms

multiple potential diagnostic criteria for sepsis (Table 46.2) and no longer specifically requires the discarded elements of the SIRS criteria.

Severe Sepsis

Sepsis associated with organ dysfunction, perfusion abnormalities, or hypotension: Organ system dysfunction can be described by organ failure scoring systems (12,13).

TABLE 46.2 Revised Diagnostic Criteria for Sepsis (11)

Infection[a], documented or suspected, and some of the following[b,c]:

General variables
- Fever (core temperature > 38.3°C)
- Hypothermia (core temperature < 36°C)
- Heart rate > 90 min^{-1} or > 2 SD above the normal value for age
- Tachypnea
- Altered mental status
- Significant edema or positive fluid balance (> 20 mL/kg over 24 hr)
- Hyperglycemia (plasma glucose > 120 mg/dL or 7.7 mmol/L) in the absence of diabetes

Inflammatory variables
- Leukocytosis (WBW count > 12,000 μL^{-1})
- Leukopenia (WBC count < 4,000 μL^{-1})
- Normal WBC count with > 10% immature forms
- Plasma C-reactive protein > 2 SD above the normal value
- Plasma procalcitonin > 2 SD above the normal value

Hemodynamic variables
- Arterial hypotension[b] (SBP < 90 mmHg, MAP < 70, or an SBP decrease > 40 mm Hg in adults or < 2 SD below normal for age)
- SvO_2 > 70%
- Cardiac index > 3.5 L/min/m^2

Organ dysfunction variables
- Arterial hypoxemia (PaO_2/FiO_2 < 300)
- Acute oliguria (urine output < 0.5 mL/kg/hr or 45 nmol/L for at least 2 hr)
- Creatinine increase > 0.5 mg/dL
- Coagulation abnormalities (INR > 1.5 or aPTT > 60 s)
- Ileus (absent bowel sounds)
- Thrombocytopenia (platelet count < 100,000 cells/μL)
- Hyperbilirubinemia (plasma total bilirubin > 4 mg/dL or 70 mmol/L)

Tissue perfusion variables
- Hyperlactatemia (> 1 mmol/L)
- Decreased capillary refill or mottling

WBC, white blood cell; SBP, systolic blood pressure; MAP, mean arterial blood pressure; $S\bar{v}O_2$, mixed venous oxygen saturation; INR, international normalized ratio; aPTT, activated partial thromboplastin time.

[a]Infection defined as a pathologic process induced by a microorganism.

[b]SvO_2 sat > 70% is normal in children (normally, 75–80%), and CI 3.5–5.5 is normal in children; therefore, *neither* should be used as signs of sepsis in newborns or children;

[c]Diagnostic criteria for sepsis in the pediatric population are signs and symptoms of inflammation plus infection with hyper- or hypothermia (rectal temperature > 38.5 or < 35°C), tachycardia (may be absent in hypothermic patients), and at least one of the following indications of altered organ function: altered mental status, hypoxemia, increased serum lactate level, or bounding pulses.

Septic Shock

Sepsis with hypotension despite adequate fluid resuscitation, in conjunction with perfusion abnormalities: Standard abnormalities in an adult include mean arterial pressure (MAP) below 60 mmHg, systolic blood pressure (SBP) below 90 mmHg, or a drop in SBP greater than 40 mmHg from baseline.

Multi-Organ Dysfunction Syndrome

Presence of altered organ function in an acutely ill patient, such that homeostasis cannot be maintained without intervention: Primary multi-organ dysfunction syndrome (MODS) is the direct result of a well-defined insult in which organ dysfunction occurs early and can be directly attributable to the insult itself. Secondary MODS develops as a consequence of a host response and is identified within the context of SIRS.

The relationship of many of these conditions to each other is demonstrated in Figure 46.1. An understanding of sepsis definitions has become increasingly important since most clinical trials in the last two decades have utilized modified version of the 1991 sepsis definitions, usually requiring three rather than two SIRS criteria, in their entry criteria. The concept of a compensatory anti-inflammatory response (CARS) has also been introduced after the demonstration that traditional anti-inflammatory mediators were also elevated during sepsis (14). Over a decade after the second consensus conference, a consensus has emerged that further updating is required in order to incorporate advances in the understanding of sepsis pathophysiology and the fundamental role of the host response in producing self-harm (15). A simple example of the problem with current definitions is provided in one study that demonstrated that "the need for two or more SIRS criteria to define severe sepsis excluded one in eight otherwise similar patients with infection, organ failure, and substantial mortality and failed to define a transition point in the risk of death" (16).

EPIDEMIOLOGY

Although the sepsis syndromes—from sepsis to septic shock—have been a major burden on human health in both the developed and undeveloped world, epidemiologic information has been surprisingly rare. In North America, this has been caused by the earlier lack of consensus definitions of these syndromes and, more recently, the absence of syndrome-specific diagnostic codes for sepsis within the International Classification of Disease (ICD) coding system. In the last 20 years, the development of consensus definitions and application of computerized hospital and government administrative databases has allowed substantial insight into the problem.

According to the Centers for Disease Control and Prevention (CDC), sepsis rates doubled between 2000 and 2008 (17). Martin et al. (5) have estimated 660,000 annual cases of sepsis in the United States during 2000 (adjusted rate 240/100,000 population) using an analysis of ICD-9 codes associated with National Hospital Discharge Survey data. With the exception of a single major study with much higher values (1), estimates for severe sepsis from sites across North America and Europe have been fairly consistent at 50 to 80/100,000 population (18–22); these cases account for approximately 10% to 15% of all ICU admissions (19,20,22–24). Approximately 25% of

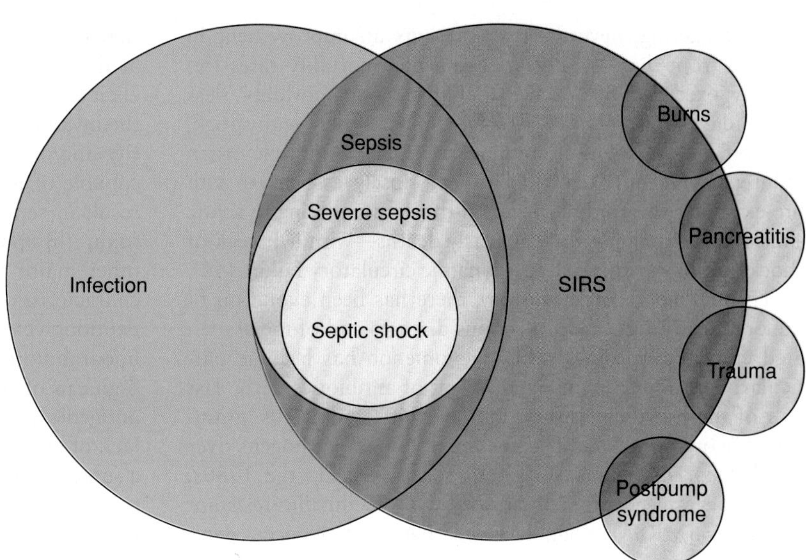

FIGURE 46.1 Venn diagram showing the relationship between infection and other sepsis-associated terms. The intersection of systemic inflammatory response syndrome and infection defines sepsis. Severe sepsis is a subset of sepsis defined by the presence of organ failure. Septic shock is a subset of severe sepsis in which the organ failure is cardiovascular (i.e., shock). Patients with certain inflammatory conditions (e.g., extensive burn injury pancreatitis, major trauma, postpump syndrome) may demonstrate a "septic" appearance without the presence of infection required for a diagnosis of sepsis. SIRS, systemic inflammatory response syndrome. (Adapted from Bone R, American College of Chest Physicians/Society of Critical Care Medicine Consensus Conference. Definitions for sepsis and organ failure and guidelines for the use of innovative therapies in sepsis. *Crit Care Med.* 1992;20:864–874.)

cases of sepsis (25) and 50% to 75% of cases of severe sepsis progress to septic shock (23). Septic shock represents between 5% and 8% of all ICU admissions (24,26). In the United States, the cost of sepsis and severe sepsis ranges from $22,000 to $60,000 per episode at a total cost of approximately $20 billion annually in 2011 (1,27,28); sepsis and related conditions represent the 11th leading cause of death in the United States in 2010 according to the CDC (29).

The incidence of sepsis increased approximately 9% per year between 1979 and 2001, with the greatest relative increase in fungal infections. In addition, since late 1980s, gram-positive pathogens have been numerically dominant over gram-negative organisms. However, coding rates for certain specific infections, including pneumonia, have dropped (30). Reasons for this increase include:

- An aging population with increased predisposition to illness
- An increased proportion of the subpopulation has conditions that predispose to systemic infection including chronic organ failure (e.g., cirrhosis, renal failure, cardiomyopathy, chronic obstructive pulmonary disease [COPD]) and other conditions (e.g., diabetes, cancer, HIV, etc.)
- Extensive utilization of invasive diagnostic and therapeutic modalities (indwelling catheters and devices), which lead to breakdown of native resistance to infection
- Widespread use of immunosuppressive chemotherapies for a wide range of diseases (asthma, inflammatory bowel disease, rheumatoid arthritis, systemic lupus erythematosus, and other autoimmune diseases, as well as transplants)
- Increased coding due to greater clinical awareness, which could be a confounder of the increased incidence of sepsis in the last decade (30).

Recently, reported trends detailing severe sepsis incidence and outcomes show important discrepancies. Gaieski et al. (31) showed a 3.5-fold variation in annual incidence of septic shock (from 300 to 1,031 cases/100,000) using the Nationwide Inpatient Sample US hospital population database with four different validated methods for identification of sepsis. These methods were also associated with a twofold difference in mortality (ranging from 14.7% to 29.9%), although all methods estimated a similar annual increased incidence of approximately 13% from 2004 to 2009. Other studies, comparing septic shock in different countries, show large discrepancies in incidence and mortality rates (e.g., Australia and New Zealand 22% mortality vs. Italy 61%) (38). This highlights the need for uniform and consistent method for definitions across national registries to facilitate assessment and outcome comparisons between hospitals across the world.

With respect to individual characteristics, age is a substantial risk factor for sepsis, severe sepsis, and septic shock (1,5,32). Patients over the age of 65 are approximately 13-fold more likely to develop sepsis compared to others (5). Similarly, septic shock is 18-fold more likely in those over 80 years of age compared to those in the 20- to 29-year-old age group (26). Given that the average age of the North American population is increasing and that the incidence of all the sepsis-related syndromes is markedly elevated in the elderly (26), the fact that the average age of patients with sepsis has climbed over the last few decades should be no surprise (1,5). The fact that septic shock is substantially a geriatric illness is reflected in the median age of 67 years (32). The persistent 60:40 male:female preponderance in sepsis, severe sepsis, and septic shock may have its origins in men's increased predisposition to smoking-associated cases of pneumonia and peptic ulcer disease or gastrointestinal malignancy–associated gastric and bowel perforation (1,5,20,23,25,26). Nonwhite ethnic groups are also at substantially increased risk, particularly blacks (5). However, low socioeconomic status is a substantial risk factor for septic shock, with a fourfold increased risk in the lowest quintile of income compared to any other quintile (26). In this context, it is unclear whether ethnicity may be relevant only as a marker of socioeconomic status. Comorbidities are common in patients with sepsis, as might be expected given an average age of 55 to 65 for sepsis and perhaps higher for septic shock (5,22,32–36). Diabetes, COPD, renal failure, congestive heart failure, and malignancy can each be found in 10% to 20% of patients with sepsis or septic shock. Approximately one-half of patients with severe sepsis have at least one major medical comorbidity (5); patients with septic shock have an even higher incidence (over 90%) of major comorbidities. Alcoholism and substance abuse substantially increases risk of sepsis and death from sepsis and septic shock (37).

As might be expected, mortality increases with the severity of the septic syndrome. Mortality for sepsis is below 15%, for severe sepsis 25% to 50%, and for septic shock over 50% (1,5,18–20,23–25,32,38). This mortality rate for septic shock, while staggering, nevertheless represents an improvement in survival from that of 35 years ago when mortality rates frequently exceeded 80% (39,40). Early septic mortality (less than 3 days) appears to be associated most closely with shock, with other deaths within the first week due to multiple organ failure; later deaths tend to be most closely associated with pre-existing comorbidities (41). Of those succumbing to septic shock, approximately 75% are early deaths—within 1 week of shock—primarily due to hyperdynamic circulatory failure (42).

Throughout recorded history, there has been evolution of the organisms that cause infectious diseases and of the associated clinical syndromes. This phenomenon has become particularly pronounced since the advent of antibiotics in the last half of the previous century. By the 1960s and 1970s, gram-negative organisms had become the dominant pathogens over *Staphylococcus aureus* and Streptococci. During the 1980s, resistant gram-positive organisms (i.e., methicillin-resistant *S. aureus* [MRSA], coagulase-negative staphylococci, penicillin-resistant *Streptococcus pneumoniae,* and enterococci) re-emerged as major pathogens. Gram-positive cocci account for approximately 40% to 50% of single isolates (excluding fungi) in sepsis and septic shock (23,32,38,43–45). In a recent study involving 14,000 ICU patients in 75 countries, gram-negative bacteria were isolated in 62% of patients with severe sepsis who had positive cultures, gram-positive bacteria in 47%, and fungi in 19% (46).

Most recently, yeast and other fungi have demonstrated a remarkable increase in contribution to sepsis (5% of total) and septic shock (8.2% of total) with an increase of about 10% per year (5,32,44,45). *Candida albicans* remain numerically dominant (about 60% of total fungal infections) but fluconazole-resistant yeasts are the most rapidly increasing species (47–49).

Other major concerns in recent years include the emergence of extended spectrum β-lactamase (ESBL; reliably sensitive only to carbapenems) (50) and carbapenemase-resistant (51) gram-negative bacilli, vancomycin-resistant enterococci (52), and an endemic strain of virulent MRSA in the community (53). In addition, concerns regarding sporadic cases of vancomycin-resistant *S. aureus* (VRSA) are growing (54).

In terms of the clinical infections associated with sepsis syndromes, lower respiratory tract infections dominate at 25% to 50% of the total in most studies (5,20,23,25,33,34,38,43,55). Intra-abdominal infections account for a disproportionate fraction of cases of severe sepsis (10% to 32%) relative to their contribution to ICU infections (5% to 7%) (44,56). Intra-abdominal infections may have an even greater role in septic shock where they accounted for 29% of cases of septic shock in a recent study (32). Conversely, the urinary system accounts for as much as 16% to 31% of ICU infections, but only 8% to 11% of cases of severe sepsis and septic shock (20,25,32,43,44,56). Positive blood cultures are found typically in only one-third of all cases of sepsis, and one-third are reported to have negative cultures from all sites (55,57).

PATHOGENESIS OF SEPSIS, SEVERE SEPSIS, AND SEPTIC SHOCK

Sepsis and septic shock or sepsis-associated multiple organ failure typically begin with a nidus of infection (e.g., pneumonia, peritonitis, urinary tract infection, abscess); within that nidus, the organism replicates. Eventually, the infection at the inciting focus releases sufficient microbial antigens to elicit a systemic inflammatory response designed to eliminate the invading microbes (Fig. 46.2). A large number of constitutive and/or inducible elements of invasive microorganisms are capable of inciting the systemic inflammatory responses that result in sepsis and septic shock (Table 46.3). Beyond endotoxin (lipopolysaccharide; LPS) of gram-negative bacteria, other major triggers of the systemic inflammatory response characteristic of sepsis include various exotoxins (all bacteria), peptidoglycans (streptococci), and teichoic acid (*S. aureus*); lipoarabinomannan of mycobacteria; and mannoproteins and β-glucan of fungi (58). Bacterial DNA may possess sufficient antigenic properties—based on unique CG repetitions and lack of deoxyribonucleic acid (DNA) methylation—to initiate a substantial inflammatory response independent of other bacterial elements (59,60,61); bacterial ribonucleic acid (RNA) may able to do the same (62). Recent investigations suggest a surprising commonality of signaling mechanisms in septic shock via toll-like receptors (TLRs) from a broad range of etiologic agents (60,63–66).

Despite the large number of potential elements of pathogenic microorganisms that can drive the septic response, endotoxin of gram-negative bacteria remains the prototype of such factors and the model for subsequent research. This antigen is thought to be central in initiation of the powerful host response during infection with these organisms (67). LPS and other antigens interact with immune cells—particularly macrophages—resulting in the induction of proinflammatory cytokines such as TNFα) and interleukin-1β (IL-1β) secreted by monocytes, macrophages and other cells (Fig. 46.2) (68). These cytokines initiate a complex signaling sequence involving release of secondary mediators—platelet-activating factor, leukotrienes, prostaglandins—monocytes and endothelial tissue factor expression, inducible nitric oxide synthetase (iNOS) induction, microvascular coagulation, cell-adhesion molecule upregulation and apoptosis (69–72). To maintain homeostasis, and likely as part of a feedback mechanism, several anti-inflammatory mediators are also released, including IL-10, transforming growth factor-β (TGFβ), and IL-1 receptor antagonist (IL-1ra). If homeostasis cannot be maintained, progressive and sequential dysfunction of various organ systems (i.e., MODS) may occur. If the inflammatory stimulus is particularly intense or if there is limited cardiovascular reserve, effects on the cardiovascular system as manifested by septic shock may dominate the clinical presentation.

MICROBIAL ANTIGEN SIGNALING

As the prototypical and best-studied microbial antigen, an understanding of signaling cascade of endotoxin is instructive. Endotoxin is an amphiphilic macromolecule located on the outer cell wall membrane of gram-negative bacteria. It is composed of lipid A, a diglucosamine-based acylated phospholipid, and a polysaccharide side chain (Fig. 46.3) (73,74). The polysaccharide chain is composed of a short, highly conserved, proximal section (core polysaccharide) and a highly variable, longer distal oligosaccharide side chain. The core polysaccharide and lipid A are sometimes referred to as the core glycolipid. The highly conserved lipid A moiety is the toxic element of endotoxin and can reproduce the manifestations of

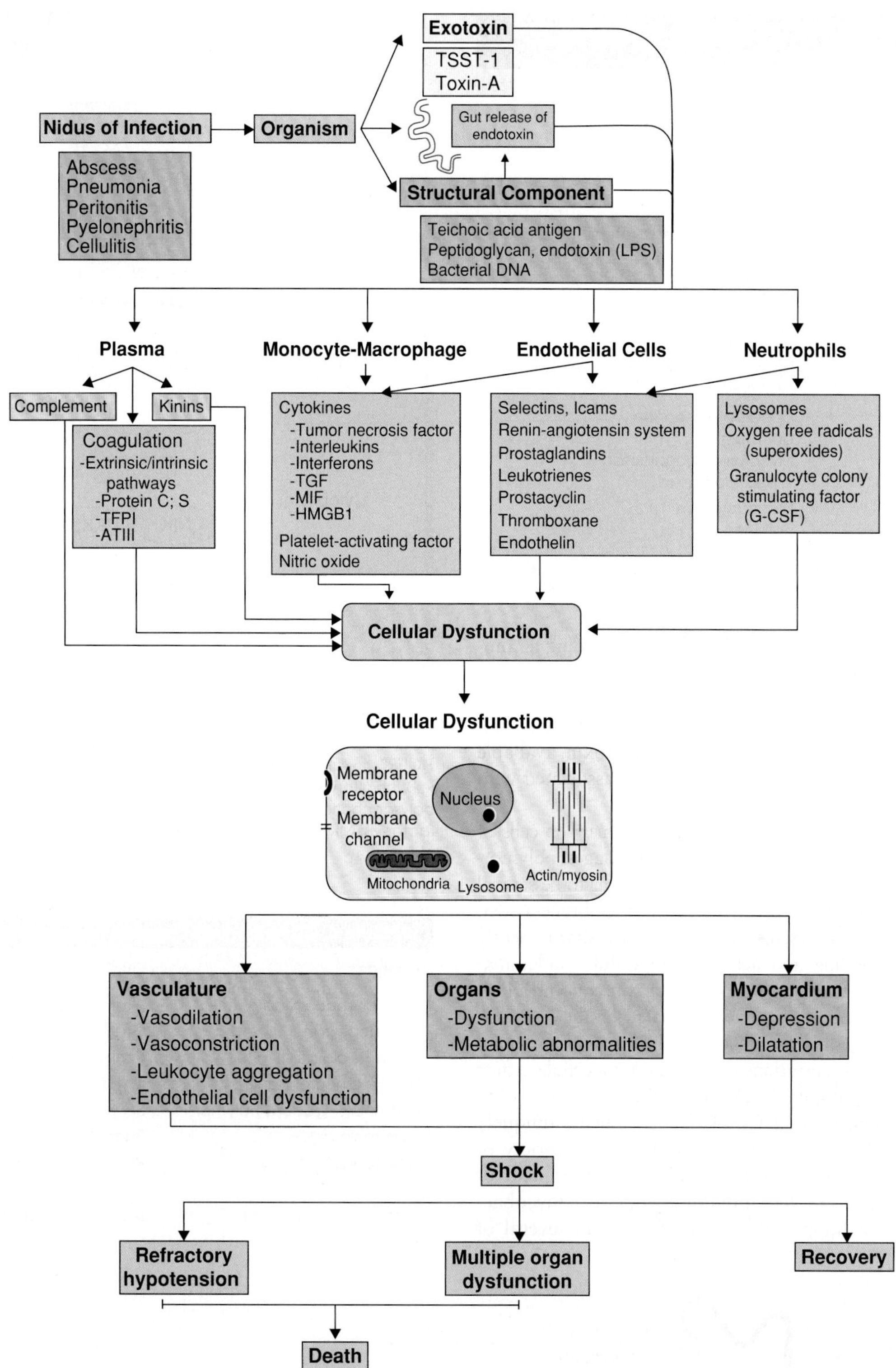

FIGURE 46.2 Pathogenesis of sepsis and septic shock. TSST-1, toxic shock syndrome toxin 1; Toxin A, *Pseudomonas* toxin A; LPS, lipopolysaccharide; TFPI, tissue factor pathway inhibitor; ATIII, antithrombin III; TGF, transforming growth factor; MIF, macrophage migration inhibitory factor; HMGB1, high mobility group box 1 protein. (Adapted from Parrillo JE. Pathogenic mechanisms of septic shock. *N Engl J Med.* 1993;328:1471–1477.)

endotoxic shock when administered alone (74–79). As a circulating form in the plasma, endotoxin exists in a multimeric, aggregate form.

Lipopolysaccharide binding protein (LBP) is an acute-phase reactant protein present in plasma (73,80,81). The levels increase with inflammatory stimulation. LBP catalyzes the transfer of endotoxin from serum aggregates to either serum lipoproteins such as high-density lipoprotein (HDL) leading to endotoxin neutralization or to CD14 receptors (either membrane-bound [mCD14] or soluble [sCD14]), the putative primary LPS receptor (Fig. 46.4). The degree to which endotoxin is shunted through either pathway appears to have a significant role in the

TABLE 46.3 Elements of Microorganisms Capable of Inducing Septic Response

Microorganism	Component
Gram-negative bacteria	Lipopolysaccharide Peptidoglycan Porins Lipoproteins Lipopeptides Lipid A associated proteins Pili Exotoxins DNA/RNA
Gram-positive bacteria	Exotoxins Peptidoglycan Lipoteichoic and teichoic acids DNA/RNA
Mycobacteria	Lipoarabinomannan Lipomannan Mycolyarabinogalactan–peptidoglycan
Fungi	Mannoproteins β-glucan

(Adapted from Heumann D, Glauser MP, Calandra T. Molecular basis of host-pathogen interaction in septic shock. *Curr Opin Microbiol.* 1998;1:49–55.)

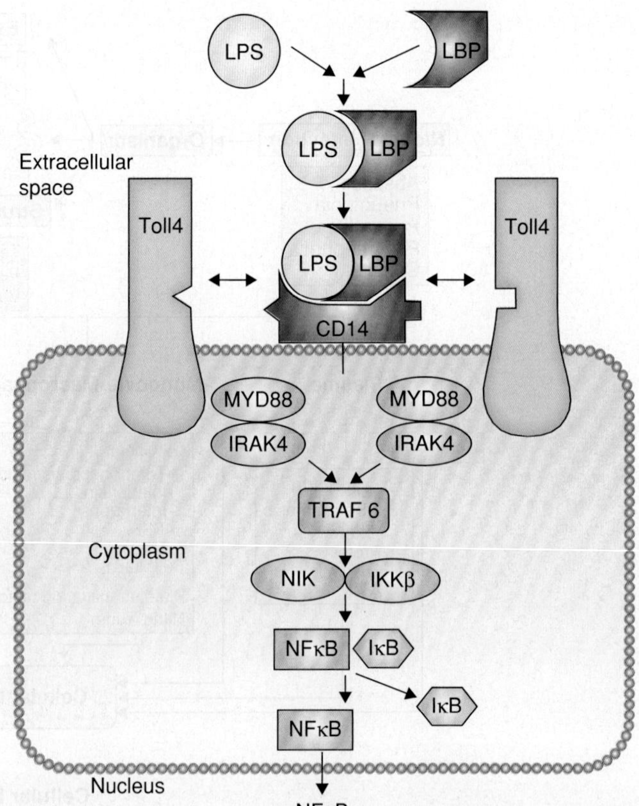

FIGURE 46.4 Endotoxin signaling pathway related to CD14 and TLR4. I-κB, inhibitory κB; IKK, I-κB kinase; IRAK, IL-1R-associated kinase; LPS, lipopolysaccharide, LBP, lipopolysaccharide-binding protein; NF-κB, nuclear factor-κB; NIK, nuclear factor κB-inducing kinase; TLR, toll-like receptor.

phenotypic physiologic response (58). LBP, by forming a complex with endotoxin monomers, appears to enhance the ability of endotoxin to bind CD14 and allows cellular activation at relatively low endotoxin concentrations (73,81). Although LBP appears to be a specific carrier molecule for endotoxin, available data suggests that other microorganism toxins associated with sepsis may use similar carrier proteins (82,83).

CD14, a glycoprotein receptor, is found primarily on cells of the myelomonocytic lineage (monocytes, macrophages, polymorphonuclear leukocytes) (84). Although there appear to be several other membrane-associated LPS receptors, membrane-associated CD14 (mCD14) represents the only receptor that is clearly involved in LPS binding and activation of cellular inflammatory responses. In contrast to the low endotoxin concentrations required to activate CD14—an effect mediated by the LBP–LPS interaction (85)—other receptors such as CD18 appear to require exceptionally high concentrations of LPS to elicit a cellular effect suggesting a lack of physiologic relevance (86).

Recent data suggests that CD14, far from being uniquely a receptor for LPS, may also bind ligands from a variety of pathogens including peptidoglycan and lipoteichoic acid of gram-positive bacteria, lipoarabinomannan of mycobacteria, and chitin of fungi (Table 46.4) (58,87). In several of

TABLE 46.4 CD14 Binding-capable Microbial Products

Ligands	Origin
Lipopolysaccharide	Gram-negative bacteria
Peptidoglycan	Gram-positive bacteria
Lipoteichoic acid	Gram-positive bacteria
Lipoarabinomannan	*Mycobacterium tuberculosis*
Rhamnose–glucose polymers	*Streptococcus* species
Polyuronic acids	Bacteria
Acylpolygalactoside	*Klebsiella pneumoniae*
Chitin	Yeast
Amphiphilic molecules	*Staphylococcus aureus*

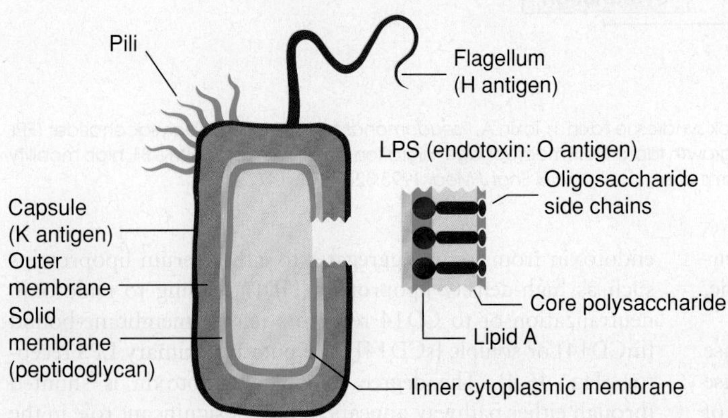

FIGURE 46.3 Endotoxin (lipopolysaccharide). Endotoxin is a component of the cell wall of gram-negative bacilli. (Adapted from Young LS, Martin WJ, Meyer RD, et al. Gram-negative rod bacteremia: microbiologic, immunologic, and therapeutic considerations. *Ann Intern Med.* 1977;86:456–471.)

these, binding is serum dependent suggesting the possibility of serum carrier/binding proteins similar to LBP (82). This convergence of receptor signaling mechanisms may explain why downstream intracellular signaling events (activation of NF-κB, MAP kinases, etc.) and cellular responses (cytotoxicity, cytokine generation, etc.) appear to be so highly conserved in sepsis due to different etiologic agents. Although elements of different microorganisms bind and activate CD14, limited data suggests that the precise binding sites vary.

Despite the importance of CD14, the receptor lacks the ability to initiate intracellular signaling on its own because of the lack of an intracytoplasmic signaling domain. CD14 signaling requires the involvement of the most recently discovered (and most central) element of microbial antigen–mediated signal transduction, the TLRs (64,88–91). The original toll receptor was initially described as an essential component of embryogenesis of Drosophila (92). In mammals, various TLRs have been shown to have a crucial role in the recognition of microbial antigens and initiation of the immune response. TLR4 and, to a lesser extent, TLR2 have been implicated in signaling associated with endotoxin (65,89,90,91,93). TLR4 appears to be co-expressed and forms a plasma membrane complex with mCD14; mCD14 appears to bind with the LPS–LBP complex to enable transfer to TLR-4 and an accessory protein MD-2 (94). The mCD14, acting as a receptor for other non-LPS microbial antigens, also appears to have a role in TLR2 signaling (95). The exact nature of the CD14–TLR interaction remains undetermined. However, interaction of CD14 and TLR4 stimulates downstream activity of the intracellular domain of TLR to generate NF–kB and other intracellular mediators that drive the response to LPS. Notably, the intracellular domain of the TLRs is shared in common with the IL-1 receptor. Several other TLR receptors are known to be involved in microbial antigen signaling from a variety of pathogens including gram-positive and gram-negative bacteria, fungi, mycobacteria, and viruses (Table 46.5).

Besides the TLR pathways, other important routes of microbial antigen signaling exist. In particular, some gram-positive organisms produce potent exotoxins that are implicated in the pathogenesis of toxic shock syndromes. These include the toxic shock syndrome toxin-1 associated with staphylococcal toxic shock and pyrogenic toxins predominantly associated with Group A streptococci. These exotoxins appear to be superantigens in that they are able to activate broad polyclonal groups of lymphocytes resulting in massive cytokine generation and toxic shock (96,97).

Cytokines

The concept of a SIRS has already been discussed in the context of sepsis. The notion of an innate anti-inflammatory response termed CARS during sepsis also exists (14). This model

TABLE 46.5 Toll-like Receptors and Their Ligands (515–517)

Receptor	Ligand	Origin
TLR1 (with TLR2)	Triacyl lipopeptides	Bacteria, mycobacteria
	Soluble factors	*Neisseria meningitidis*
TLR2 (with TLR1 or TLR6)	Lipoproteins, lipopeptides	Various pathogens
	Lipoteichoic acid	Gram-positive bacteria
	Peptidoglycan	Bacteria
	Lipoarabinomannan	Mycobacteria
	Phenol-soluble modulin, porins	*Staphylococcus epidermidis, Neisseria*
	Atypical LPS	*Leptospira interrogans, Porphyromonas gingivalis*
	Glycoinositolphospholipids, glycolipids	*Trypanozoma, Toxoplasma, Plasmodium*
	β-glucan, mannan	Fungi
	Core and NS3 proteins, dUTPase, glycoproteins	Hepatitis virus, Epstein-Barr virus, Cytomegalovirus
	HSP70	Host
TLR3	Double-stranded RNA	Viruses
TLR4	LPS	Gram-negative bacteria
	O-linked mannan	Fungi
	Taxol	Plants
	Fusion and envelope protein	Respiratory syncytial virus, mouse mammary tumor virus
	HSP60	*Chlamydia pneumoniae*
	HMGB1, HSP70, fibronectin, fibrinogen	Host
TLR5	Flagellin	Flagellated bacteria
TLR6 (with TLR2)	Diacyl lipopeptides, lipoteichoic acid, β-glucan	*Mycoplasma*, gram-positive bacteria, fungi
TLR7	Single-stranded RNA	Viruses, bacteria
	Imidazoquinoline, loxoribine, bropirimine	Synthetic compounds
TLR8	Single-stranded RNA	Viruses, bacteria
	Imidazoquinoline	Synthetic compounds
TLR9	CpG-containing DNA	Bacteria, viruses, fungi
	Homozoin	*Plasmodium falciparum*
TLR10 (±TLR1 or TLR2)	Lipopeptides (prediction)	
TLR11	Flagellin	Flagellated bacteria
TLR12	Profilin	Apicomplexan parasites
TLR13	23S RNA	Bacteria

LTA, lipotechoic acid; LPS, lipopolysaccharide; dsRNA, double-stranded RNA; ssRNA, single-stranded RNA.

suggests that a clinical insult such as infection or injury initiates a pro-inflammatory response that is countered by an endogenous anti-inflammatory reaction. The aggregate responses produce endogenous circulating mediators (e.g., cytokines, soluble receptors, adhesion molecules, growth factors, eicosanoids), which lead to systemic phenomenon such as septic shock or immunosuppression. Clinical manifestations and patient outcome are dependent on the balance between pro-inflammatory and anti-inflammatory elements. Predominance of the inflammatory response corresponds to SIRS and may lead to cardiovascular compromise, shock, and organ dysfunction. However, a predominance of anti-inflammatory mediators produces a state of immune paralysis associated with propensity to infection and inability to fight infection; both may ultimately lead to death. In patients with sepsis, duration of monocyte inactivation—a potential manifestation of CARS—correlates with mortality (98). If the counter-inflammatory response is able to balance the inflammatory stimuli—while the infecting microorganism is effectively cleared—homeostasis is achieved and clinical recovery will occur. In this model, sepsis has a dynamic nature based on the development and balance of the above-described responses (Fig. 46.5). This interplay is influenced by the nature of the inflammatory injury and the genetically determined variability of the host immune response (99,100).

Pro-inflammatory cytokines have multiple effects including the stimulation of production and release of other pro-inflammatory mediators. TNFα, IL-1β, and IL-6 are the best-known pro-inflammatory cytokines and have overlapping and synergistic effects in stimulating the inflammatory cascade. The next phase in the cytokine response to infection is the endogenous counter-inflammatory cascade in response to the systemic activity of pro-inflammatory cytokines. Cytokine inhibitors (e.g., IL-1ra, soluble TNF receptor) and anti-inflammatory cytokines (e.g., TGF-β, IL-4, IL-10, IL-13) are involved in this phase of the response. Other cytokines like HMGB1 may be involved even later in the syndrome. Thus, the cytokine network in sepsis involves pro-inflammatory cytokines, anti-inflammatory cytokines, and cytokine inhibitors (Table 46.6). It is the balance between these cytokines at different time points that determine clinical manifestations and outcome of sepsis.

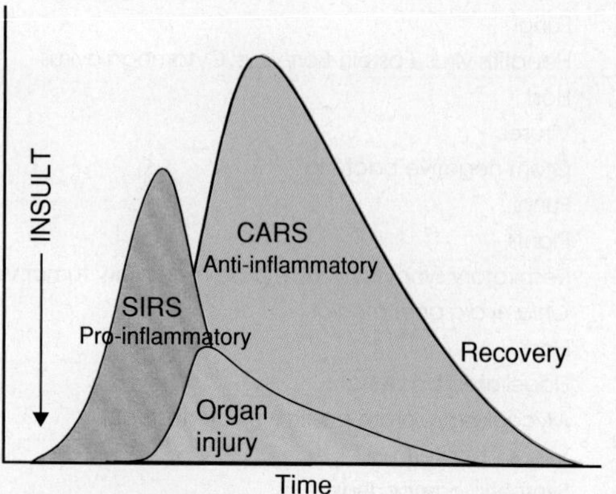

FIGURE 46.5 The dynamic cytokine inflammatory response. Sepsis is associated with an early transient dominance of proinflammatory cytokines corresponding to the systemic inflammatory response syndrome (SIRS) and the onset of organ damage. After this initial phase, the anti-inflammatory pathways of a compensatory anti-inflammatory response syndrome (CARS) become active with the development of a refractory state characterized by a decreased capacity of mononuclear cells to produce proinflammatory cytokines. Recovery occurs if homeostasis is reestablished. (Adapted from van der Poll T, van Deventer SJ. Cytokines and anticytokines in the pathogenesis of sepsis. *Infect Dis Clin North Am.* 1999;13:413–426.)

TABLE 46.6 Major Pro- and Anti-inflammatory Cytokines and Receptors in Sepsis

Pro-inflammatory Cytokines
Tumor necrosis factor-α (TNFα)
Interleukin-1β (IL-1β)
Interleukin-2 (IL-2)
Interleukin-6 (IL-6)
Interleukin-12 (IL-12)
Interferon-γ (IFN-γ)
Macrophage migration inhibitory factor (MIF)
High mobility group 1 protein (HMG-1)
Anti-inflammatory Cytokines
Transforming growth factor (TGF-β)
Interleukin-4 (IL-4)
Interleukin-6 (IL-6)
Interleukin-8 (IL-8)
Interleukin-9 (IL-9)
Interleukin-10 (IL-10)
Interleukin-11 (IL-11)
Interleukin-13 (IL-13)
Cytokine Inhibitors
Soluble TNF receptors
Type I
Type II
Interleukin-1 receptor antagonist (IL-1ra)

Nitric Oxide

Another important mediator, nitric oxide (NO), has a vital role in normal intracellular signal transduction (101). NO is synthesized by a family of enzymes called NO synthases (NOS) that incorporate nitrogen from one of the guanidine terminals of L-arginine with molecular oxygen to form NO and L-citrulline. Three distinct NOSs have been purified, cloned, and characterized: (a) neuronal NOS or nNOS, (b) inducible NOS or iNOS, and (c) endothelial NOS or eNOS, reflecting the cell types from which they were originally identified.

NO has several important roles in infection, sepsis, and septic shock. The iNOS gene is induced in immunoactivated cells; NO formed by these cells plays a role in host defense against bacterial, viral, and protozoan infections. Of particular importance in relation to septic shock, NO is the mediator through which endothelial cells normally cause relaxation of adjacent smooth muscle (101). Endothelial cells, through eNOS, produce picomolar quantities of NO in response to a number of vasodilatory stimuli such as shear stress, acetylcholine, and bradykinin. This NO diffuses to adjacent smooth muscle and activates guanylate cyclase to produce cyclic GMP (cGMP), which effects vascular relaxation. Activity of endothelial NOS is regulated and is calcium- and calmodulin-dependent.

During septic shock, an iNOS capable of producing nanomolar quantities of NO is generated in endothelium and vascular smooth muscle (101,102). Following generation, activity of this iNOS is unregulated and constant. NO-mediated generation of cGMP explains the profound loss of arterial vascular tone and venodilation seen in septic shock (102,103) and may, in part, explain irreversible vascular collapse seen late in

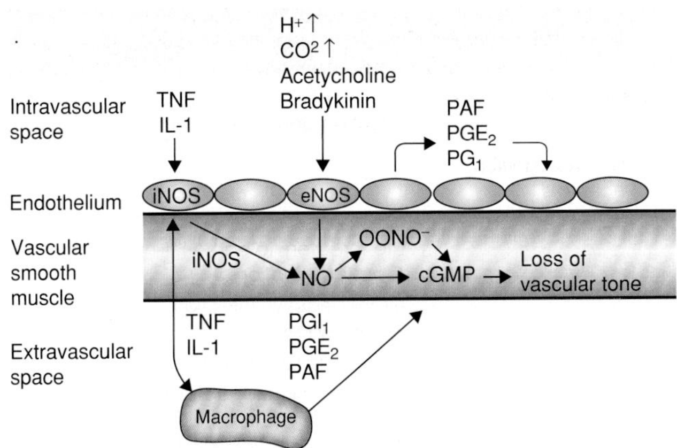

FIGURE 46.6 Physiologic and pathophysiologic vasodilatory factors relevant in sepsis and septic shock. IL-1, interleukin-1β; TNF, tumor necrosis factor-α; NO, nitric oxide; iNOS, inducible nitric oxide synthetase; eNOS, endothelial nitric oxide synthetase; $ONOO^-$, peroxynitrite; PAF, platelet activating factor; PGE_2, prostaglandin E_2; PGI_2, prostacyclin; cGMP, cyclic GMP. (Adapted from Bloos F, Thomas-Ruddel D, Ruddel H, et al. Impact of compliance with infection management guidelines on outcome in patients with severe sepsis: a prospective observational multi-center study. *Crit Care.* 2014;18(2):R42.)

hemorrhagic shock (104) (Fig. 46.6). A potential role for NO in inflammation-associated edema and third-spacing during shock has also been suggested (105). The *in vitro* myocardial depressant effects of TNFα, IL-1β, and serum from septic humans may be mediated by a similar NO and cGMP-dependent pathway (106,107). TNFα, IL-1β, and IFN-γ have been identified as key mediators of iNOS activation. An alternative pathway by which NO may play a role in the cardiovascular pathophysiology of shock and sepsis involves production of peroxynitrite (ONOO–), a highly reactive oxidant, from the interaction of superoxide (OH–) and nitric oxide (NO–) (108).

Hemostasis

The coagulation cascade represents a highly conserved antimicrobial defense mechanism common to even the most primitive complex organisms such as the Limulus horseshoe crab. The hemolymph of the horseshoe crab, one of the oldest complex organisms still in existence, clots rapidly in response to minute quantities of endotoxin or β-(1,3) glucan, a component of fungi. Pathogens are immobilized in the clot allowing subsequent elimination (109,110). Similarly, cells of the innate immune system of vertebrates are now recognized to generate thrombi as an antimicrobial defense, to immobilize pathogens in the thrombus matrices in order to mediate host protection (111,112). This commonality of purpose and function of the coagulation and inflammatory systems in elimination of invading microbes has persisted in evolution to present-day mammals including humans (113). These systems, in sharing common activation pathways, are inextricably linked.

While both these systems are normally highly adaptive in nature, excessive activity of the coagulation and inflammation pathways can result in vascular injury, aberrant tissue blood flow, tissue damage, and, ultimately, organ dysfunction. Clinical and laboratory investigations have established that, in conjunction with the cytokine cascade, the coagulation system has a key role in inflammatory states such as sepsis (Fig. 46.7) (114–116). A critical process in sepsis-induced coagulopathy is the activation of the extrinsic pathway (114).

During the normal hemostatic response, exposure of blood to nonvascular cell-bound tissue factor in the subendothelial layer initiates the extrinsic pathway through the binding of tissue factor to activated factor VII. The resulting enzyme complex, in turn, activates factor IX of the intrinsic pathway and factor X of the common pathway. With factor V as a cofactor, activated factor X cleaves prothrombin to form thrombin; thrombin then converts fibrinogen to fibrin, which results in clot formation (117).

In sepsis, however, the expression of tissue factor is either directly or indirectly induced by inflammatory cytokines. Overexpression of proinflammatory cytokines such as TNFα, IL-1β, and IL-8 are thought to upset the balance toward a procoagulant state (72,115,118). TNFα and IL-1β, for example, can induce expression of tissue factor in circulating monocytes and endothelial cells (115). The vascular endothelial injury resulting from inflammation can also further expose tissue factor in subendothelial tissue and perivascular cells. Endothelial injury

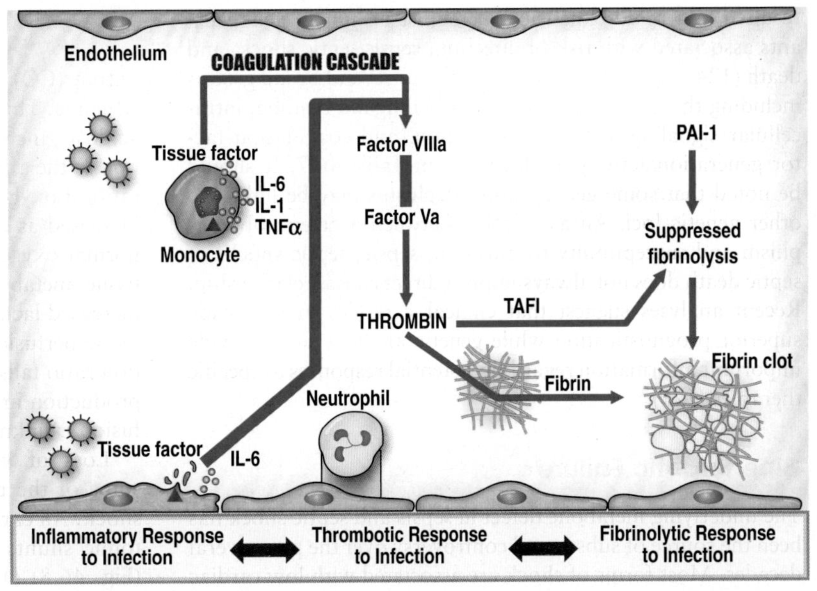

FIGURE 46.7 Cytokines induce the endothelial cell to shift from an antithrombotic to a prothrombotic phenotype. Expression of tissue factor by monocytes, and perhaps a subset of endothelial cells, initiates coagulation through the extrinsic system in patients with severe sepsis and septic shock. At the same time, fibrinolysis is inhibited through the release of thrombin activatable fibrinolysis inhibitor (TAFI) and plasminogen-activator inhibitor-1 (PAI-1). TNFα, tumor necrosis factor-α; IL-1, interleukin-1β; IL-6, interleukin-6. (Courtesy of the National Initiative on Sepsis.)

also inhibits the production and activity of anticoagulants such as proteins C and S, the heparin–antithrombin complex, and thrombomodulin. Loss of native anticoagulant function is indicated by decreased activity and circulating levels of protein C (119,120), antithrombin III (ATIII) (115,120), and tissue factor pathway inhibitor (TFPI) (121,122) in patients with severe sepsis and septic shock.

Current evidence suggests that the pathogenesis of sepsis is associated with (a) systemic activation of coagulation resulting in consumption of coagulant factors, (b) suppression of the anticoagulant system by the same proinflammatory mediators that activate coagulation, and (c) early activation followed by later suppression of fibrinolysis (see Fig. 46.7) (72,115). While the coagulation cascade is clearly activated in sepsis, the specific inciting events and the molecular linkages between inflammation and coagulation are being elucidated (72,115–117). Given observational studies demonstrating depletion of anticoagulant factors—decreased activity levels of protein C (72,116), ATIII (115,117), and TFPI (35)—in patients with severe sepsis and septic shock, such molecules may be useful as markers of the presence or severity of sepsis as well as potential therapeutic targets.

Host Genetic Factors

Although the characteristics of the pathogen have much to do with the occurrence of clinical infection and progression to sepsis and septic shock, a growing body of data suggests that genomic variations between patients are equally important. These genomic variations in microbial and cell signaling, innate immunity, coagulation, and inflammatory stress cytokine responses appear to explain individual variations in susceptibility to infection, sepsis/septic shock, and septic death. They likely explain why identical organisms cause fulminant disease with septic shock in some, but minimal clinical illness in others. The importance of inheritable elements in susceptibility and mortality risk of life-threatening infections is demonstrated by adopted twin studies demonstrating remarkable convergence in the causes of death (including sepsis/infection) of such individuals (123).

The advent of complete gene mapping via high-throughput analysis techniques (e.g., microarray gene chips, etc.) has resulted in a rapid expansion of the list of human gene variants associated with risk of infection, sepsis/septic shock, and death (124–128). These markers fall into several broad groups including those involved with microbial ligand binding, intracellular signaling, cytokine generation, and coagulation factor generation/activity as described in Table 46.7. It should be noted that some genetic polymorphisms may be linked to other genetic loci. An association between a given polymorphism and susceptibility to infection, sepsis, septic shock, or septic death does not always imply a direct causal relationship. Recent analyses suggest that clinical variables may provide superior prognostication while genetic analyses may provide important information regarding potential responses to specific therapies (129).

TABLE 46.7 Human Genetic Markers Associated with Risk of Infection and Sepsis/Septic Shock (125–128)

Gene Product Group/ Gene Product	Infection/Sepsis Association
Pattern Recognition Receptors	
TLR2	Tuberculosis Life-threatening bacterial infections *S. aureus* infections
TLR4	Gram-negative infection Septic shock
TLR5	*Legionella sp* infection
CD14	Septic shock and septic shock mortality Isolation of pathogenic bacteria in infection
Mannose-binding lectin	Bacterial infections Isolation of pathogenic bacteria in infection
Intracellular proteins	
IRAK4	Recurrent gram-positive infections
Cytokines	
TNFα	Sepsis, septic shock, septic mortality Meningococcal mortality
TNFβ	Sepsis and septic mortality
IL-6	Septic mortality
IL-10	Sepsis and septic mortality CAP severity and mortality Pneumococcal septic shock
IFNγ	Infection
MIF	Sepsis and sepsis-induced acute lung injury
IL-1Ra	Sepsis and septic mortality
Coagulation factors	
PAI-1	Meningococcal sepsis, septic shock, septic mortality, vascular complications Septic mortality
Protein C	Septic organ dysfunction and mortality
TAFI	Meningococcal and septic mortality
Fibrinogen-β	Septic mortality
Factor 5 (Leiden)	Septic mortality, pressor use, purpura fulminans

Bioenergetic Failure

The underlying metabolic defect in sepsis and septic shock has been the source of substantial controversy over the past several decades. Most forms of shock are associated with low cardiac output (CO) and tissue hypoperfusion leading to overt tissue ischemia. This results in anaerobic glycolysis with intracellular acidosis, increased lactate, and high-energy phosphate depletion in the affected tissues. Blood oxygen extraction ratio (the ratio of oxygen consumed divided by the oxygen delivered) is increased as tissues maximize oxygen extraction to maintain normal oxygen consumption. During septic shock, the same tissue metabolic phenomenon of intracellular acidosis and increased lactate production is noted. However, CO and total tissue perfusion is typically increased and the oxygen extraction ratio falls. The explanation for tissue acidosis and lactate production in septic shock in the presence of tissue hyperperfusion is unknown.

Loss of vascular autoregulatory control may explain some of the typical metabolic findings of sepsis and septic shock. An early theory postulated the existence of microanatomic shunts between the arterial and venous circulations (Fig. 46.8) (130). During sepsis, these shunts were said to

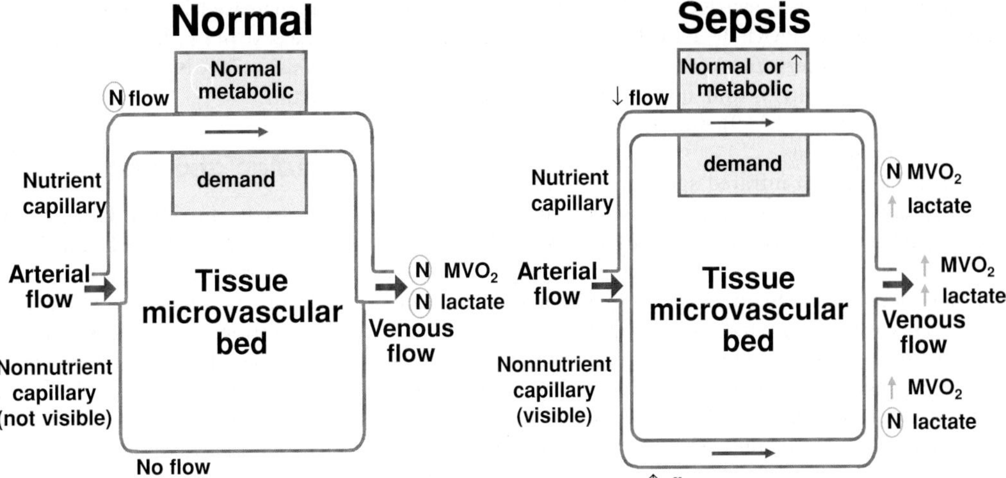

FIGURE 46.8 Microanatomic shunting in sepsis and septic shock. One explanation of the increased lactatic acidosis and mixed venous oxygen saturation (MVO_2) found in septic shock is the potential presence of opening of nonnutrient blood vessels between the arterial and venous vascular beds.

result in decreased systemic vascular resistance (SVR) and increased mixed venous oxygen saturation (MVO_2) (131). The resultant decrease in perfusion to tissue beds with normal or even increased metabolic demand could generate tissue ischemia and lactic acid. However, while microanatomic shunting has been noted in localized areas of inflammation, systemic evidence of this phenomenon in sepsis and septic shock is lacking (131–135). Another theory involving "functional" shunting due to defects of microcirculatory regulation in sepsis has also been proposed (Fig. 46.9) (136,137). Overperfusion of tissues with low metabolic requirements would result in increased MVO_2 and narrowing of the arteriovenous oxygen content difference. Relative vasoconstriction of vessels supplying more metabolically active tissues would result in tissue hypoxia and lactate production due to anaerobic metabolism. Observations that some capillary beds may be occluded by platelet microaggregates, leukocytes, fibrin deposits, and endothelial damage support this theory (132,136,138). Additional support comes from studies demonstrating evidence of supply-dependent oxygen consumption in sepsis (139–143). Updated versions of this theory suggest that sepsis is associated with a decrease in capillary density (resulting in an increased diffusion distance for oxygen) and the capillaries also suffer a dynamic process of intermittent perfusion resulting in heterogeneous microvascular blood flow. This leads to a variable oxygen extraction in the tissues, generating hypoxic zones even when the overall blood flow to the organ is preserved (144,145). Both of these theories of the metabolic defect of energy metabolism in sepsis and septic shock fall within the category of "stagnant" hypoxia as described by Barcroft in 1920 (146).

A third theory of the metabolic presentation of sepsis and septic shock suggests that circulating mediators cause an intracellular metabolic defect involving substrate utilization. This results in bioenergetic failure with high-energy phosphate (ATP and phosphocreatine) depletion and lactate production (147–149). Increased MVO_2 could then be explained by perfusion, which is maintained in excess of tissue oxygen utilization capability. This phenomenon has been termed "histotoxic" (146) or "cytopathic" (149) hypoxia. Potential mechanisms to explain this form of hypoxia include (a) structural damage to the mitochondrial membranes with proton leak across the inner membrane (150); (b) impairment/inactivation of the pyruvate dehydrogenase complex, decarboxylating pyruvate to acetyl-CoA (151); (c) inhibition of key enzymes by NO in the citric acid cycle, the Krebs cycle, and electron transport chain (152); (d) inhibition of enzyme complexes by peroxynitrite (153); (e) disturbances caused

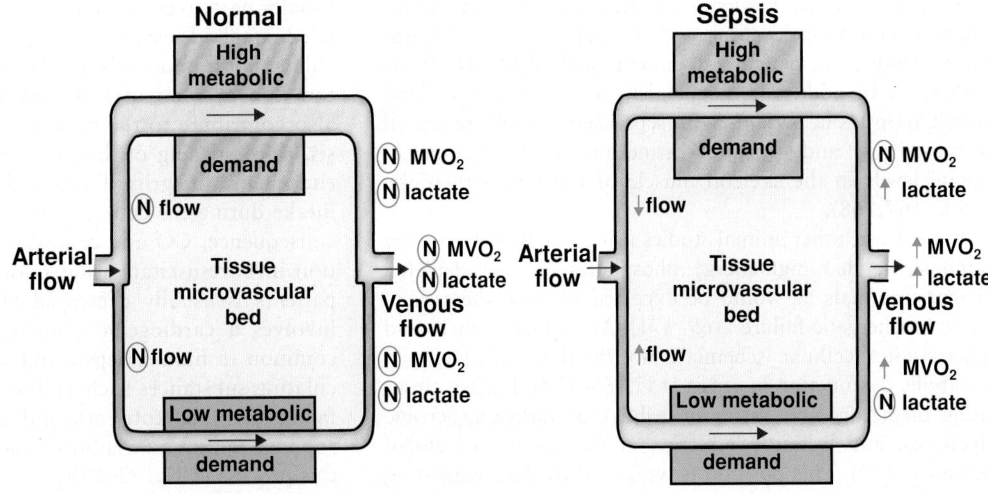

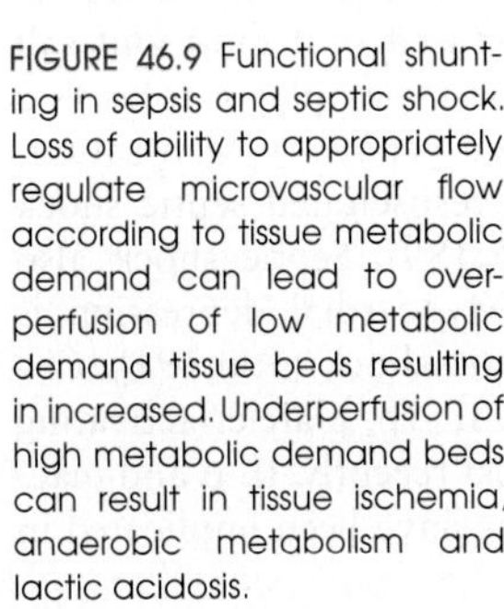
FIGURE 46.9 Functional shunting in sepsis and septic shock. Loss of ability to appropriately regulate microvascular flow according to tissue metabolic demand can lead to overperfusion of low metabolic demand tissue beds resulting in increased. Underperfusion of high metabolic demand beds can result in tissue ischemia, anaerobic metabolism and lactic acidosis.

by reactive oxygen species (ROS) (154); and (f) poly(ADP-ribose) polymerase (PARP-1) activation (155). Observations demonstrating preservation of tissue PO_2 (156), absence of tissue hypoxia (157), and impairment of mitochondrial function (149,152,158,159) during sepsis and septic shock support this possibility.

In particular, near-infrared spectroscopy (NIRS) has been used to examine the issue of mitochondrial function in a primate model of septic shock using live *Escherichia coli* infusion. NIRS demonstrated the presence of mitochondrial dysfunction in skeletal muscle in animals with experimentally induced sepsis. This was manifested by an impairment of oxidation of cytochrome aa3 with reperfusion after transient ischemia in septic animals compared to controls (159). Another primate study demonstrated early disturbance of mitochondrial redox state in skeletal muscle and brain during live *E. coli* bacteremia; of note, these changes occurred before the onset of overt hemodynamic alterations (160). In a limited, observational study, uncoupling of tissue oxyhemoglobin levels and mitochondrial oxygen consumption as indicated by cytochrome aa3 redox state (indicating mitochondrial oxidative stress) predicted the development of multiple-organ failure in patients with major trauma (161). These data particularly support the possibility of decreased ability of mitochondria to utilize oxygen as a potential cause of decreased tissue high-energy phosphate in sepsis.

All of these theories of septic bioenergetic metabolism would be expected to result in a deficit of tissue high-energy phosphates during septic shock. A series of studies using biochemical analysis of harvested tissues and nuclear magnetic resonance (NMR) spectroscopy of septic animals have suggested that high-energy phosphate reserves are decreased in animal models of septic or endotoxic shock (147,162,163). It can be argued that in many of these studies, animals were inadequately fluid resuscitated resulting in tissue hypoperfusion. However, animals in at least one study (147) were clearly adequately resuscitated (CO and tissue oxygen tension were maintained comparable to shams) and demonstrated similar evidence of high-energy phosphate depletion (skeletal muscle biopsy) along with an increase in lactate/pyruvate ratio during rat peritonitis induced by cecal ligation and perforation (147). In one of the few human studies of critically ill patients, most of whom were septic, the acetoacetate/β-hydroxybutyrate ratio (a marker of mitochondrial redox state) rose significantly in nonsurvivors compared to survivors (164). Evidence of increased acetoacetate/β-hydroxybutyrate ratio along with an increase in ATP degradation products in critically ill patients with sepsis also exists (165,166). In addition, independent studies using skeletal muscle biopsies in patients with sepsis/septic shock observed decreased ATP and phosphocreatine but variable changes in lactate levels in the skeletal muscle of patients with septic shock (167,168).

In contrast, other animal studies using NMR spectroscopy demonstrate that high-energy phosphates are not depleted in septic animals as would be expected in these theories of septic bioenergetic failure (169–171). According to these and other studies, cellular ischemia is not the dominant factor in metabolic dysfunction in sepsis (157,169–174). Rather, circulating mediators may result in cellular dysfunction, aerobic glycolysis, and lactate production in the absence of global ischemia (170). This position is weakened by data suggesting that increased lactate in septic shock is also associated with decreased pH (which would not be expected in aerobic glycolysis) (170). Nonetheless, ongoing controversy of this issue remains.

Cardiac and Vascular Responses

Prior to the introduction the balloon-tipped pulmonary artery catheter (PAC) and echocardiography to assess cardiovascular performance, much of our understanding of septic hemodynamics was based on clinical findings. Two distinct clinical presentations of septic shock were proposed: Warm shock characterized with high CO, warm dry skin, bounding pulses, and hypotension; and cold shock characterized with low CO, cold clammy skin, and diminished pulses (175). These two presentations were thought to represent a progressive continuum starting with "warm" shock (in the initial hemodynamically well-compensated phase) and progressing to "cold" shock (indicating decompensation) culminating in death. This notion was supported by studies showing a correlation between survival and a high cardiac index (CI) (175,176). A major problem with this interpretation was that all these studies used central venous pressure (CVP) as a reflection of left ventricular end-diastolic volume (LVEDV) and adequacy of fluid resuscitation. The central role of adequacy of intravascular volume status to CI and survival was suggested in a handful of studies of that time (177,178). Based on evidence collected over the past five decades, CVP is now accepted to be a poor measure of preload in critically ill patients, particularly those with sepsis and septic shock (179). Adequately resuscitated septic shock patients typically exhibit a persistent hyperdynamic state, high CO, and low SVR (180,181). In nonsurvivors, this hyperdynamic state usually persists until death (42,182).

More than any other form of shock, distributive and, particularly, septic shock, involves substantial elements of the hemodynamic characteristics of other shock categories. All forms of distributive shock involve decreased mean SVR. Before fluid resuscitation, distributive shock also involves a hypovolemic component with decreased CVP and pulmonary artery occlusion pressure. The primary cause of this relative hypovolemia is an increase of the vascular capacitance due to venodilation. This phenomena has been directly supported in animal models of sepsis (183–187) and is reinforced by the fact that clinical hypodynamic septic shock (low CO) can usually be converted to hyperdynamic shock (high CO) with adequate fluid resuscitation (42,175,188). Relaxation of vascular smooth muscle is attributed to a number of the mediators known to circulate during sepsis. These same mediators also contribute to the second cause of hypovolemia in sepsis, third spacing of fluid to the interstitium due to loss of endothelial integrity. Further, decreased oral fluid and salt intake during the course of the illness may play a role. As a consequence, CO and central/mixed venous oxygen saturation in unresuscitated and poorly resuscitated septic shock patients is usually decreased (188,189). Septic shock also involves a cardiogenic element. Myocardial depression is common in human sepsis and septic shock (190,191). Circulating substances such as TNFα, IL-1β, platelet activating factor (PAF), leukotrienes, and, most recently, IL-6 and macrophage migration inhibitory factor have been implicated in this process (107,192–199).

ORGAN SYSTEM DYSFUNCTION DUE TO SEPSIS AND SEPTIC SHOCK

Central Nervous System

Sepsis-associated encephalopathy (SAE) (Table 46.8) is the most common neurologic manifestation of sepsis and septic shock, occurring in 8% to 80% of patients with sepsis (200–203). The likely reason for the divergent frequencies of the syndrome in studies is the difficulty of separating out the condition in patients with superimposed hypotension, sedation, hypoxemia, acidosis, electrolyte disturbances, hypoglycemia or hyperglycemia, hypothermia or hyperthermia, or concurrent hepatic or renal failure or encephalopathy. SAE can be an early feature of infection particularly in the elderly and might appear before other systemic features of sepsis are obvious. It is primarily a clinical diagnosis of exclusion requiring the presence of altered mentation with an extracranial source of infection. While deficits can range from impairment of higher cognitive functions to delirium or coma, asterixis, myoclonus, and seizure activity are highly atypical (200,203). Electroencephalography (EEG) examination can provide supportive evidence although changes are nonspecific (204). The occurrence and severity of SAE (graded by EEG or Glasgow coma scale) appears to be associated with increased mortality (to as high as 70%) (200,205). Although no specific markers for SAE exist (206–208), changes in EEG (204) and somatosensory evoked potentials (SSEPs) (209) have been investigated as diagnostic tools for SAE. Imaging studies using magnetic resonance imaging (MRI) and computed tomography (CT) have demonstrated changes in SAE similar to those that are observed in other neurologic disorders such as stroke. The pathophysiology of SAE is, as yet, not completely understood; there is recent evidence suggesting it is driven by inflammatory mediators that, even in the absence of direct parenchymal infection, cause endothelial cell activation, microvascular dysfunction, changes in blood–brain barrier permeability, and alterations of amino acid and neurotransmitter levels (207,208,210,211).

TABLE 46.8 Organ System Dysfunction in Sepsis and Septic Shock

CNS
Septic encephalopathy
Critical illness polyneuropathy/myopathy
Heart
Tachycardia
Supraventricular tachycardia
Ventricular ectopy
Myocardial depression
Pulmonary
Acute respiratory failure
Adult respiratory distress syndrome
Kidney
Prerenal failure
Acute tubular necrosis
Gastrointestinal
Ileus
Erosive gastritis
Pancreatitis
Acalculous cholecystitis
Colonic submucosal hemorrhage
Transluminal translocation of bacteria/antigens
Liver
Intrahepatic cholestasis
Hematologic
Disseminated intravascular coagulation
Thrombocytopenia
Metabolic
Hyperglycemia
Glycogenolysis
Gluconeogenesis
Hypertriglyceridemia
Immune system
Neutrophil dysfunction
Cellular immune (T-cell/macrophage) depression
Humoral immune depression

Critical illness-associated neuromuscular syndromes (inclusive of critical illness polyneuropathy and myopathy) are the most common causes of neuromuscular problems in the ICU (212). The primary clinical manifestation of this condition is muscle weakness. Since many patients who are in the ICU with sepsis and septic shock require ventilatory support, the initial overt manifestation may be either respiratory failure or failure to wean from ventilation. Studies have suggested an incidence of between 35% to 50%, based on clinical criteria, and 40% to 80% based on EMG/nerve conduction studies (213–215). Although the disorder is commonly noted later in the recovery phase of sepsis and septic shock, EMG/nerve conduction data suggest that the onset is much earlier (concurrent or within days of the onset of septic shock) (216,217). The condition is a predominantly peripheral motor neuropathy in association with the presence of the systemic inflammatory response. Physical findings may include difficulty in weaning from mechanical ventilation (MV), symmetric paresis greater in the lower extremities, reduced deep tendon reflexes and ataxia (213); a distal sensory neuropathy is also common. Approximately 25% of patients who are awake after a week of MV have significant weakness that lasts at least a week (218). The condition is considered to be an element of, and is closely associated with, the occurrence of MODS.

Cardiac

The major clinically apparent manifestations of shock on the heart are due to sympathoadrenal stimulation. Heart rate is almost universally increased in the absence of disturbances of cardiac conduction; the degree of increase is predictive of outcome (42). In addition, catecholamine-driven supraventricular tachycardias and ventricular ectopy with ischemic electrocardiography (ECG) changes, particularly in patients predisposed to myocardial ischemia, may be found.

Like the brain, the blood supply to the heart is autoregulated, rendering it resistant to sympathetically driven vasoconstriction and shock-related hypoperfusion. Perfusion of the heart is unchanged or even increased during sepsis and septic shock (219,220). The occurrence of septic myocardial depression has been addressed; circulating myocardial depressant substances contribute to myocardial depression in sepsis and septic shock (221,222). This has been linked to decreased β-adrenoreceptor affinity and density (223–225) as well as potential defects of intracellular signal transduction involving NO, G proteins, cAMP, and cGMP (107,226–229).

Systolic function in sepsis and septic shock is characterized by reversible (7 to 10 days in survivors) biventricular dilatation and decreased ejection fraction (EF) (189,191,230,231). Despite this reduction in EF, CO is maintained at a higher than normal level, secondary to an increase in LVEDV. This phenomenon is most marked in survivors; nonsurvivors tend to maintain EF and EDV (182). In addition, these patients exhibit a flattening of the Frank–Starling relationship with significantly smaller increases in left ventricular stroke work index in response to similar LVEDV increments when compared to nonseptic critically ill controls (190). Sepsis is also characterized by a markedly reduced inotropic response to infusion of exogenous catecholamines (232). Compared to survivors, nonsurvivors demonstrate a flattened Starling response and blunted inotropic response to catecholamines (190,232).

Although septic myocardial depression is a transient phenomenon in survivors, myocardial cell injury as evidenced by increased troponin levels does occur (233,234). Serum troponin is elevated in almost half of patients with septic shock, without myocardial creatine kinase [CK-MB] elevation or ischemic EKG changes (235). A correlation between LV dysfunction and troponin I (TnI) positivity has been shown (234). Serum TnI correlated with left ventricular dysfunction and was an independent predictor of need for inotropic/vasopressor support, adverse outcomes, and mortality in septic shock patients (235). Whether the clinically inapparent myocardial cell injury that is the source of elevated troponin contributes to, or is a consequence of, septic shock is yet to be determined. Elevated levels of cardiac troponin, while a common marker of myocardial injury in the context of myocardial ischemia, does not specifically suggest myocardial infarction in other contexts.

Respiratory System

Early respiratory responses to sepsis include tachypnea and hyperventilation; gas exchange may be mildly abnormal. Later in the course of sepsis, patients may develop diffuse alveolar damage consistent with acute respiratory distress syndrome (ARDS). Infections account for about 50% of all cases of ARDS. These infections can involve local pneumonia or distant foci of infection associated with sepsis or septic shock. The risk of ARDS in association with sepsis increases with the severity of the syndrome: sepsis to septic shock (236). From 40% to 60% of patients with gram-negative septic shock develop ARDS; sepsis is the single condition most closely associated with progression to acute lung injury or ARDS with an incidence of 40% (237). Several comorbid factors increase the risk of ARDS, including chronic alcohol abuse, chronic lung disease, and severe acidemia (237). Most patients with septic ARDS also have other organ failure, i.e., MODS. Death is more commonly due to MODS or the underlying sepsis, rather than ARDS, although the impact of low tidal volume ventilation in ARDS studies suggest that the lung injury may still have a significant role, perhaps as a source of persistent inflammatory stimulation (237–239). The mortality of ARDS/MODS is approximately 40%, although some reports suggest that it may be falling (237,240). Failure to improve in the first week is associated with progression of the syndrome and poor prognosis, as are MODS, chronic liver disease, and age; interestingly, indices of oxygenation and ventilation are not predictive (237).

Kidney

Acute kidney injury (AKI) is a major complication of sepsis and septic shock, occurring with increasing frequency in relation to the severity of the syndrome, from 16% to 19% with sepsis to 51% with septic shock (38,236,241). Sepsis is the leading cause of acute tubular necrosis (ATN) in some ICU studies, accounting for 45% to 70% of all AKI (242). In adult and pediatric data in economically developed countries, sepsis accounts for 26% to 50% of all AKI compared with 7% to 10% of primary kidney disease–associated AKI (243–245). Sepsis-associated AKI is distinct from AKI without sepsis, driven by a number of characteristic pathophysiologic mechanisms, carrying a unique profile of timing—onset, duration—and being associated with different short- and long-term outcomes (246). Sepsis-associated AKI is associated with a worse outcome, both ICU and in-hospital mortality rates are significantly increased for patients with sepsis-associated AKI compared with patients with AKI without sepsis: ICU mortality rate 19.8% versus 13.4%; in-hospital mortality rate 29.7% versus 21.6% (243). Similarly, sepsis-associated kidney failure is associated with a substantially higher mortality risk (75%) than nonsepsis-associated failure (45%); within this group, septic shock mortality is higher (80%) than for those with severe sepsis (70%) (236,242). Compared with nonsepsis-associated acute kidney failure, patients with sepsis-related acute kidney failure are significantly older and sicker, require MV more often, and present later in the hospital course more frequently (242).

Gastrointestinal

The gut is relatively sensitive to circulatory failure due to the responsiveness of the splanchnic vasculature to vasoconstrictive stimulation by extrinsic factors. In addition, gut tissues may have increased sensitivity to proinflammatory cytokine-driven inflammatory injury. Typical clinical gut manifestations of hypoperfusion, sympathetic stimulation, and inflammatory injury associated with sepsis and septic shock include ileus, erosive gastritis, pancreatitis, acalculous cholecystitis, and colonic submucosal hemorrhage (247). In addition, enteric ischemia produced by circulatory shock and free radical injury with resuscitation may breach gut barrier integrity (248,249). Some theories propose that enteric bacteria and antigens (notably endotoxin) may translocate from the gut lumen to the systemic circulation during gut ischemia resulting in irreversible shock (250) and MODS (251).

Liver

Two major forms of organ injury can be seen in the liver with sepsis and septic shock (252,253). "Shock liver" (ischemic hepatitis) associated with massive ischemic necrosis and major elevations of transaminases, which can occur with septic shock, is atypical in the absence of extensive hepatocellular disease (254). When it does occur, it can contribute substantially to lactic acidosis since the liver accounts for the majority of clearance of serum lactate; hypoglycemia may also be seen. Centrilobular injury with mild increases of transaminases and lactate dehydrogenase is much more common. Transaminases usually peak within 1 to 3 days of the insult and resolve over 3 to 10 days. In both cases there are only mild increases in bilirubin and alkaline phosphatase early in the early phase. Despite the production of acute-phase reactants in early sepsis and septic shock, synthetic functions may be impaired with decreased generation of prealbumin, albumin, and hepatic coagulation factors (increased prothrombin time [PT]). After or independent of the occurrence of septic shock, evidence of biliary stasis with increased bilirubin and alkaline phosphatase may be present (253). Increases in transaminases are modest.

Hematologic

Sepsis and septic shock are associated with a range of hematologic disorders including overt disseminated intravascular coagulation (DIC), thrombocytopenia, and coagulopathy. Thrombocytopenia and coagulopathy are multifactorial in nature; bone marrow suppression, consumption, and medications can contribute to thrombocytopenia, while consumption and decreased liver production of coagulant factors as well as malnutrition—leading to depleted Vitamin K stores—contribute to coagulopathy. Nonetheless, whenever these findings are present, early DIC is possible.

Septic shock is the single most common cause of DIC, characterized by microangiopathic hemolysis, consumptive thrombocytopenia, consumptive coagulopathy, and microthrombi with tissue injury. Overt DIC occurs in one-quarter to one-half of cases of gram-negative sepsis (255,256). Although gram-positive sepsis has been thought to be less closely associated with DIC, the frequency of occurrence is quite similar (255,257). The occurrence of DIC in sepsis is associated with a doubling of projected mortality (255,256). DIC may also represent both a driver, and manifestation, of MODS. The deposition of microvascular thrombi can cause significant endothelial injury and inflammatory responses leading to ischemic and inflammatory tissue injury, the basis of MODS.

A prolonged PT and aPTT, hypofibrinogenemia, elevated level of fibrin-split products, and the presence of the D-dimer herald the onset of DIC. Since it is due to simultaneous systemic activation of coagulation and fibrinolysis cascades, it can be differentiated from the coagulopathy of liver failure by determination of endothelial cell–produced factor 8, which is normal or increased with hepatic dysfunction. The pathogenesis of this disorder is linked to activation of tissue factor on endothelial cells and macrophages, probably by pro-inflammatory cytokines induced by exogenous bacterial toxins (256,258).

Metabolic

Specific, predictable, and overlapping metabolic alterations occur in both sepsis and shock. Hyperglycemia is very common for two major reasons. Early in sepsis, when hemodynamic dyshomeostasis initiates compensatory responses, endogenous catecholamines are released as a consequence of enhanced sympathoadrenal stimulation. In addition, increased release of adrenocorticotropic hormone (ACTH), glucocorticoids, and glucagon, with concomitant decreased release of insulin results in glycogenolysis and gluconeogenesis (259,260). Increased epinephrine also results in skeletal muscle insulin resistance, sparing glucose for use by glucose-dependent organs such as the heart and brain (261). In addition, pro-inflammatory, stress-related cytokines such as TNFα, IL-1β, and IL-6 contribute to insulin resistance in peripheral tissues (262). Pharmacologic therapies of sepsis and shock including catecholamine vasopressors/inotropes, steroids, and total parenteral nutrition can add to these effects. It is notable that, despite insulin resistance, the increased metabolic demands of sepsis also result in increased overall glucose uptake and utilization (263).

With the evolution of sepsis to septic shock, metabolic responses progress. Late in shock, hypoglycemia may develop, possibly due to glycogen depletion or failure of hepatic glucose synthesis (264). Fatty acids are increased early in sepsis but fall later with hypoperfusion of adipose-containing peripheral tissue (263,265). Hypertriglyceridemia is often seen during shock as a consequence of catecholamine stimulation and reduced lipoprotein lipase expression induced by circulating TNFα (260,263,266). Increased catecholamines, glucocorticoids, and glucagon also increase protein catabolism resulting in a negative nitrogen balance (260,265).

Endocrine

Endocrine abnormalities are frequently underappreciated in sepsis and septic shock. Notable alterations in levels of pituitary, adrenal, thyroid, growth, and sex hormones are known to occur (262,267–273). In recent years, "relative" adrenal insufficiency in septic shock has received substantial attention; few septic patients exhibit overt adrenal insufficiency. Relative bradycardia and a nontoxic appearance in a patient with septic shock are suggestive of this possibility. These are often elderly patients who have survived an initial episode of septic shock and either fail to fully recover or suffer a relapse. However, a considerable body of literature suggests that a suboptimal cortisol response—within the normal range—to sepsis and septic shock can have deleterious effects including prolonged pressor dependence and increased mortality. Estimates of the frequency of adrenal insufficiency in septic shock vary wildly from 0% to 95% (274,275). In great part, this is due to the use of varying definitions based on baseline or cosyntropin-stimulated cortisol levels or changes in levels from baseline in response to cosyntropin. Common definitions in septic shock patients include random cortisol below 700 nmol/L (25 μg/dL), peak postcosyntropin level of 500 to 550 nmol/L (18 to 20 μg/dL), or post-cosyntropin change in cortisol of 200 to 250 nmol/L (7 to 9 μg/dL) (267,274,276,277). Interestingly, pituitary dysfunction may play a role in many patients with adrenal insufficiency, as 85% of critically ill patients have decreased levels of ACTH (278).

Abnormalities of thyroid hormones are also present in sepsis and septic shock, although the clinical significance is less certain. In humans, serum T4 and T3 levels fall shortly after the onset of severe clinical infection. Euthyroid sick syndrome is manifested by low serum levels of thyroid hormones in clinically euthyroid patients with severe nonthyroidal systemic illness; decreased T3 levels are most common. Patients with more severe or prolonged illness also have decreased T4 levels; serum reverse T3 (rT3) is increased. Patients are clinically euthyroid and do not have clinically significant thyroid-stimulating hormone (TSH) elevations.

Sepsis and septic shock are clearly associated with perturbations of a variety of hormones including insulin, TSH, thyroxin, ACTH, cortisol, growth hormone (279), and sex hormones; perturbations of hormones of the posterior pituitary should be expected. In addition to abnormal prolactin levels (280), sepsis and septic shock are accompanied by relative deficiencies of vasopressin/antidiuretic hormone (ADH) levels. Vasopressin, produced in the hypothalamus and stored in the posterior pituitary gland, is released in response to hyperosmolarity. Hypotension, as seen in shock states, is an even more powerful stimulus for release. Recent human studies have suggested a relative deficit of circulating vasopressin in patients with septic shock, relative to those with cardiogenic or hypovolemic shock. This deficiency may be related to depletion of neurohypophyseal stores in combination with NO-mediated inhibition of production (262,272). Clinically, vasopressin exerts powerful vasopressor effects in hypotensive patients, particularly those with septic shock. To some extent, this effect appears to be mediated through re-establishment of reduced sensitivity to catecholamine (281).

DIAGNOSIS OF SEPSIS

Ideally, each patient with evidence of sepsis would undergo a thorough evaluation at presentation prior to the initiation of therapy. In the context of sepsis and septic shock, circumstances are rarely ideal so an abbreviated initial assessment focusing in critical diagnostic and management planning elements is frequently necessary. To assure rapid initiation of effective therapy, a presumptive diagnosis of severe sepsis and septic shock is mandated; the criteria for this presumptive diagnosis should be highly inclusive and based primarily on clinical criteria.

The initial presumptive diagnosis of sepsis with organ dysfunction (severe sepsis) may be made in the presence of the following elements:

- Suspected infection based on a minimal clinical constellation of localizing—for example, dyspnea, cough, purulent sputum production, dysuria, pyuria, focal pain, local erythema, etc.—and systemic signs and/or symptoms of sepsis (Table 46.9).
- Clinical evidence of organ dysfunction—for example, hypotension with peripheral hypoperfusion, oliguria, hypoxemia, obtundation, etc.

Similarly, an initial diagnosis of septic shock is established in the presence of suspected infection with sustained hypotension absent a definitive alternate explanation.

The initial presumptive diagnosis of severe sepsis or septic shock is based on clinical criteria and does not require microbiologic, radiographic, or other laboratory evidence of specific infection or organ injury. Only a clinical suspicion of infection and organ failure is necessary. For the most part, available laboratory tests or imaging studies represent supportive, not diagnostic, elements. This clinical approach allows parallel, rapid initiation of empiric antimicrobials and supportive measures.

Although a suggestive clinical examination is sufficient for the presumptive diagnosis of severe sepsis and septic shock, more authoritative investigations (both laboratory and radiologic) are generally required for confirmation. For this reason, the definitive diagnosis of severe sepsis and septic shock involves a broader range of clinical and laboratory evidence of sepsis (Table 46.10) and organ dysfunction (arterial hypotension, lactic acidosis, or any organ dysfunction variables in Table 46.2). Establishment of a definitive diagnosis can help to more specifically target antimicrobial therapy and trigger specific therapies such as surgical source control.

TABLE 46.9 Clinical Symptoms/Signs for Presumptive Diagnosis of Severe Sepsis/Septic Shock

Fever or hypothermia
Chills, rigors
Tachycardia
Widened pulse pressure
Tachypnea or hyperpnea
Confusion, decreased level of consciousness or delirium
Decreased urine output
Hypotension

TABLE 46.10 Supportive/Confirmatory Findings for Severe Sepsis/Septic Shock

Leukocytosis, leukopenia, increased immature white blood cell forms, toxic granulation, Dohle bodies
Thrombocytopenia ± increased INR or prothrombin time
Increased D-dimer or fibrin split products
Increased serum bilirubin, AST/ALT, C-reactive protein
Serum pro-calcitonin elevation
Metabolic acidosis with anion gap
Serum lactate elevation
Respiratory alkalosis or acidosis
Mixed venous saturation > 70%
Diagnostic imaging findings
Positive microbiologic or pathologic samples for abnormal presence of microorganisms, leukocytes, or tissue necrosis

History

The initial history should focus on two major areas: The key symptoms with respect to diagnosis of sepsis and of the specific site of infection, and the key factors that would modify initial empiric therapies such as antimicrobials, fluid resuscitation and, possibly, vasopressors or inotropes. With respect to symptoms, constitutional complaints are entirely nonspecific. The classic pattern of fever, rigors, and chills is common, but far from universal. Fatigue, malaise, anxiety, or confusion may be observed, particularly in the elderly; yet occasionally, the elderly, the immunocompromised (nonspecific immune dysfunction due to chronic organ failure), and the immunosuppressed (specific immune defects) patient may present without such symptoms.

Fever is a common feature of infection and/or sepsis. Fever is caused by a direct effect of inflammatory mediators such as IL-1β on the hypothalamus. The fever response may be suppressed in septic shock and may be absent in the elderly, immunocompromised, or immunosuppressed; hypothermia in septic shock is associated with reduced CO and portends a poor prognosis (282). Septic encephalopathy, manifested by disorientation or confusion, is especially common in elderly individuals. Apprehension, anxiety, and agitation may all occur early in the course. With severe disease (i.e., septic shock) or progression of sepsis, overt encephalopathy with decreased level of consciousness and coma may occur. Hyperventilation with respiratory alkalosis can be seen even before the onset of metabolic acidosis as a consequence of cytokine-mediated stimulation of the respiratory center in the medulla. Localizing symptoms as described in Table 46.11 may be more helpful in determining the septic etiology of the constitutional manifestations of sepsis.

The key historical factors used to modify initial therapies include antimicrobial sensitivities/allergies, recent infections/antimicrobial use, locale of infection acquisition (i.e., nosocomial

TABLE 46.11 Localizing Clinical Symptoms and Signs in Severe Infections

	History	Physical Examination
CNS	Headache, neck stiffness, photophobia	Meningismus (neck stiffness), focal neurologic signs (weakness, paralysis, paresthesia)
Head and neck	Earache, sore throat, sinus pain, or swollen lymph glands	Inflamed or swollen tympanic membranes or ear canal, sinus tenderness, pharyngeal erythema and exudates, inspiratory stridor, and cervical lymphadenopathy
Pulmonary	Cough (especially if productive), pleuritic chest pain, and dyspnea	Dullness on percussion, bronchial breath sounds, and localized crackles
Cardiovascular	Palpitations, syncope	New regurgitant valvular murmur
Intra-abdominal	Abdominal pain, nausea, vomiting, diarrhea, purulent discharge	Abdominal distention, localized tenderness, guarding or rebound tenderness, and rectal tenderness or swelling
Pelvic/genitourinary	Pelvic or flank pain, vaginal or urethral discharge, and urinary frequency and urgency	Costovertebral angle tenderness, pelvic tenderness, pain on cervical motion, and adnexal tenderness
Skin/soft tissue/joint	Localized limb pain or tenderness, focal erythema, edema, and swollen joint	Focal erythema or purple discoloration (subcutaneous necrosis), edema, tenderness, crepitus in necrotizing infections (Clostridia and gram-negative infections), petechiae, purpura, erythema, ulceration, and bullous formation and joint effusion

Courtesy of Steve Mink and Satendra Sharma.

versus community), and major comorbidities. The existence of comorbidities—for example, HIV infection, chemotherapy, hematologic malignancy, neutropenia resulting in immunosuppression or chronic renal, heart, liver, or other organ failure, COPD, dementia, inflammatory bowel diseases, diabetes, or invasive catheters/devices—resulting in immunocompromise, mandate the use of extended spectrum antimicrobial therapy. Chronic renal, liver, or heart failure may also influence the choice and volume/dose of antimicrobials, resuscitation of fluids and vasopressors. Recent antimicrobial use and nosocomial or institutional acquisition of infection may also mandate consideration of extended spectrum antimicrobial therapy in order to adequately cover nosocomial pathogens.

Physical Examination

The physical examination focuses on ensuring patient stability and on rapid localization of the site of infection; it first ensures the airway is patent, breathing is satisfactory, and vital signs and peripheral perfusion are acceptable.

Tachypnea and tachycardia are almost universal. Normothermia and fever are consistent with sepsis, but hypothermia should be of concern due to the association with shock/hypoperfusion. All patients with sepsis should be observed for signs of hypoperfusion—mottling, pallor, diaphoresis, impaired capillary refill in nail beds. An acutely ill, flushed, and toxic appearance is common in the septic patient particularly early in the course. In the early stages of sepsis, CO is well maintained or even increased. Skin and extremities are warm; capillary refill is normal. As sepsis progresses, venodilation results in reduced CVP and venous return; hypovolemic manifestations—with hypotension, reduced stroke volume, and CO with signs of tissue hypoperfusion—then develop. As patients are aggressively fluid resuscitated, a hyperdynamic circulatory state, albeit with distributive shock, again dominates the clinical picture and will usually persist until recovery or death.

The most common sites of infection causing sepsis and septic shock are in order of frequency respiratory, abdominal, urinary, and soft tissue infections. Abdominal infections are more closely associated with septic shock, while urinary infections are more common in sepsis; intravascular catheters are a frequently overlooked source of infection and sepsis. A recent study suggested that central venous catheters might account for up to 3.7% of cases of septic shock (32). Similarly, cases of *Clostridium difficile*–related septic shock are often overlooked in the absence of overt toxic megacolon. Adding to the difficulty of managing the ICU patient with sepsis and/or septic shock, many patients have simultaneous infection at more than one site.

Laboratory Studies

Patients with sepsis require urgent laboratory testing to help make a firm diagnosis and to evaluate the severity of the illness. Sepsis and septic shock typically present with somewhat different though naturally overlapping laboratory parameters (Table 46.12). Laboratory tests usually start with a complete blood count (CBC); hemoglobin is often decreased, often due to the presence of chronic disease, but may be, occasionally, increased in patients with substantial interstitial third spacing and relative hypovolemia. The white cell count is increased in sepsis but may transiently normalize or even drop below normal range with progression to septic shock. Although this phenomenon has been linked to gram-negative septic shock, it can be seen in septic shock due to any pathogen; leukopenia in this setting has been linked to poor outcome. Toxic granulation and the presence of Dohle bodies are also seen more frequently with progression to more severe disease. Similarly, a marked left shift with increasing immature forms (bands) is more common in septic shock. Platelets often respond as an acute-phase reactant, with increases early in infection/sepsis; however, platelets fall with septic shock reaching a nadir around day 5 in survivors.

In contrast, the international normalized ratio (INR) may be mildly abnormal at the onset of sepsis (due to malnourishment) and is usually most abnormal at the onset of septic shock. Fibrinogen is an acute-phase reactant, usually elevated with the onset of infection/sepsis; however, levels will drop with septic shock especially if DIC intervenes. Fibrin split products and D-dimers are very sensitive markers of progression of sepsis and are almost universally elevated with septic shock.

TABLE 46.12 Key Laboratory Values in Infection/Sepsis versus Septic Shock

	Sepsis	Septic Shock
Hb	N or ↓ (chronic disease)	↑ (hemoconcentration)
WBC	↓ + left shift	↑, N or ↓
- marked left shift with metamyelocytes, toxic granulation and/ or Dohle bodies		
Platelets	N or ↑	N or ↓
PT/INR	N or ↑ (malnutrition)	↑↑
Fibrinogen	N or ↑	N or ↓
Fibrin split products/ D-dimer activity	↓	↓↓
Glucose	N or ↑	↑↑
Cr/BUN	N or ↑	↑↑
Bilirubin	N, late ↑	↑, late ↑↑
AST/ALT	N	↑-↑↑
Albumin	N or ↓ (malnutrition)	↓↓ (endothelial leakage/interstitial redistribution)
ABG	Respiratory alkalosis	Metabolic acidosis
HCO_3^-	N	↓
Lactate	N	↑-↑↑
C-reactive protein	↑	↑↑
Procalcitonin	↑	↑↑
Blood culture positivity	5% – 10%	30% – 40%

↑ increase, ↑↑ marked increase, ↓ decrease, ↓↓ marked decrease, N normal.
Hb hemoglobin, WBC white blood cell count, PT prothrombin time, INR international normalized ratio, Cr/BUN serum creatine and blood urea nitrogen, AST/ALT serum aspartate transaminase and alanine transaminase, ABG arterial blood gas, HCO_3^- serum bicarbonate concentration.

Serum creatinine and blood urea nitrogen (BUN) may actually be decreased due to increased renal blood flow in the early hyperdynamic phase of sepsis, but will increase with the onset of septic shock. An increase in serum creatinine denotes increased mortality risk even within a few hours of the onset of septic shock. Similarly, elevated serum lactate is closely correlated with increased mortality risk in septic shock.

Septic patients should have both site-specific and blood cultures obtained prior to initiation of antimicrobial therapy. In the case of septic shock, though, antimicrobial therapy should never be delayed in order to accommodate these cultures because of the antimicrobial delay-dependent increase in morality risk (32). Gram stain should be performed on all site samples. Although there are some data to suggest that Gram stain is not useful in the initial management of certain infections—nosocomial pneumonia, peritonitis due to bowel perforation—a good specimen, appropriately read, can provide invaluable information.

Imaging Studies

Although in most cases the clinical examination will localize the source of infection with a reasonable degree of confidence, basic radiographic imaging can be very useful in cases where an obvious site of infection is not apparent. Advanced imaging studies (CT, MRI, ultrasound) rarely yield information regarding localization of the infection that has not been provided by the clinical examination and basic imaging studies. However, these techniques may be highly useful when definitive or precise localization and/or delineation of extent of disease are required.

A chest radiograph should be obtained in most patients admitted to the hospital with sepsis. Elderly, immunocompromised, and immunosuppressed patients with occult sepsis will often be found to have a pulmonary source on radiographic examination. Supine and upright or lateral decubitus abdominal films are useful if bowel perforation is of concern. In the appropriate clinical context of crepitus, bullae, hemorrhage, or foul smelling exudate with intense local pain, evidence of gas in soft tissues on plain extremity radiographs is almost pathognomonic of necrotizing soft tissue infection with clostridia or facultatively anaerobic gram-negative bacilli.

CT scan with contrast is the preferred imaging modality to rule out intra-abdominal, intracranial, epidural, perinephric, and soft tissue abscesses, as well as retroperitoneal abscess or mediastinal infection. They can also be useful for localization of bowel wall injury and assessment of necrotizing soft tissue infections, although MRI is preferred for the latter.

Ultrasound is the initial imaging modality of choice for biliary sepsis and obstructive uropathy, although CT scan is also sensitive and specific. In recent years, the adoption of low-cost ultrasound imaging devices and the dissemination of expertise to emergency and critical care physicians has opened new avenues in the use of ultrasound techniques for the diagnosis and management of life-threatening infections, sepsis, and septic shock.

MANAGEMENT OF SEVERE SEPSIS AND SEPTIC SHOCK (THE SEPSIS SIXPACK)

To optimize outcome in sepsis with organ dysfunction (severe sepsis), the initiating triggers and downstream organ dysfunction must be addressed; this requires monitoring and therapeutic elements. With respect to the initiating triggers, antimicrobials and, where possible, surgical and nonsurgical source controls are mandated. Organ dysfunction is addressed through direct supportive measures. The most immediate of these, fluid and vasopressor/inotropic administration, support the circulatory system. However, MV and dialysis have also been shown to improve outcome in severe sepsis and septic shock.

Six major areas in the evaluation and treatment of severe sepsis can be identified. These include:

- Fluid resuscitation
- Antimicrobial therapy
- Invasive and noninvasive monitoring
- Vasopressors and inotropes
- Specific therapy
- Supportive therapy

Fluid Resuscitation

The development of shock in patients with sepsis involves disturbances of global and regional perfusion. Initially, ventricular filling pressures as reflected by CVP and pulmonary wedge pressure (PWP) are decreased; consequently, venous return falls, resulting in decreased CO. Although an increase in insensible losses and decreased fluid intake may contribute to this effect, NO-mediated venular dilatation and loss of endothelial barrier integrity—resulting in a drop in colloid oncotic pressure from loss of albumin into the interstitium—probably play a dominant role (283,284). A significant degree of hypovolemia is almost universal in early, untreated severe sepsis or septic shock. Available data suggest that initial isotonic fluid deficits can exceed 10 L (285).

Management of sepsis requires consideration of both global and regional perfusion defects making the establishment of goals for therapy more complex than for other forms of shock. Support of global perfusion takes initial precedence. Since hypovolemia is a major factor in the hypotension and hypoperfusion of early septic shock, foremost among the appropriate initial therapeutic considerations is infusion of intravascular fluids; resuscitation should be rapidly implemented by, first of all, placement of large-bore peripheral IV catheters. Fluid administration can improve global perfusion indices—blood pressure, CO, and MVO_2/central venous oxygen saturation ($ScvO_2$)—and may reveal the presence of regional perfusion disturbances and/or myocardial depression that might require therapy with vasopressors/inotropes.

The three issues to consider in optimizing fluid resuscitation are the type of fluid used, the rapidity of infusion, and the amount of fluid administered.

Initial resuscitation of septic patients should be aimed at rapid intravascular volume expansion. The view that intravascular fluid depletion plays a central role in the pathogenesis of early septic shock has been recognized since the mid-20th century. Several studies suggested that septic shock is associated with reduced total circulating blood volume (176,177). Since almost all untreated patients with severe sepsis or septic shock have a significant element of hypovolemia, a hypodynamic circulation with decreased CO is typical prior to fluid resuscitation. This hypovolemia is probably the basis of early observations that death in sepsis was associated with decreased CO. The patients in those studies were clearly inadequately resuscitated by current standards (176,177). Additional support for the central importance of functional hypovolemia in early septic shock comes from more recent demonstration that the venous oxygen saturation is decreased in early, preresuscitation septic shock, consistent with the findings in other forms of hypodynamic shock (188).

Aggressive fluid loading is the standard early therapy of septic shock and results in the generation of a hyperdynamic circulatory state in over 90% of patients (286). Rapid fluid resuscitation may reveal severe sepsis without shock in a significant subset of patients with apparent septic shock (285). Increased total blood volume has been associated with higher CO and with increased survival in human septic shock (177), and intravascular volume dependence of the hyperdynamic circulatory state in sepsis has been confirmed in animal models (185). Although the demonstration that resuscitation from hypovolemia improves outcome in traumatic shock dates back to the early work of Cannon in 1923 (287) and Cournand in 1943 (288), clear evidence that early aggressive fluid resuscitation improves outcome in septic shock is limited to a small series of pediatric septic shock (289). On the other hand, a major study of life-threatening infection with shock in children in an under-resourced setting found an increase in mortality with aggressive fluid resuscitation (290).

Initial fluid resuscitation should be titrated to specific clinical end points. Aggressive fluid loading in patients with septic shock can increase total blood volume, CO, DO_2, and VO_2, while reducing lactic acidosis (139). Older studies have suggested that increased blood volume associated with normalization of CO is associated with improved survival (176,177).

In the absence of early invasive or echocardiographic monitoring, clinical end points can be used for titration of fluid resuscitation. Since both initial heart rate and blood pressure have been shown to be associated with outcome in septic shock as well as hypovolemic shock (42,291–293), standard goals may include:

- Heart rate $\leq$ 100 beats/min
- SBP $\geq$ 90 mmHg
- MAP $\geq$ 60 to 65 mmHg
- Urine output $\geq$ 0.5 mL/kg/hr

It should be noted that these clinical parameters may underestimate initial resuscitative requirements in critically ill subjects including those with septic shock (294–296).

Mortality in both septic and other forms of shock has also been associated with increased arterial lactate and base deficit levels (297). Normalization of these parameters can be used to augment clinical end points for titration of fluid resuscitation (298). However, both parameters represent relatively late responses to cellular stress, and resolution may similarly lag the following implementation of effective resuscitation (299).

Initial fluid resuscitation should be achieved using isotonic crystalloid solutions. Effective fluid resuscitation can be delivered with either isotonic crystalloid (e.g., normal saline, Ringer lactate) or colloid solutions (e.g., human albumin); all of these solutions are equally effective if titrated to the same clinical end points. Given the difference in distribution of such compounds, it typically requires approximately fourfold more crystalloid to achieve the same hemodynamic effect as a given amount of colloid (300). Several animal and human studies have pointed out theoretical advantages to colloids in limiting interstitial fluid accumulation—which may benefit ARDS—in sepsis and septic shock (301–303). However, no clinical study has suggested improved clinical outcomes—morbidity or mortality—with colloid solutions (304,305). Although the severe sepsis subset of one recent randomized controlled trial (RCT) trended toward a more favorable outcome with albumin resuscitation (306), another (meta-analytic) study suggested an opposite trend toward increased mortality with albumin use (305,307). In a recent multicenter RCT, albumin and crystalloids versus crystalloids alone showed no difference in mortality (308).

By way of contrast, the use of hydroxyethyl starches in sepsis results in increased mortality, AKI, and a higher use of renal replacement therapy (309–311). These results motivated a warning from the U.S. Food and Drug Administration against the use of hydroxyethyl starches in critically ill adults (312). Fewer data are available addressing the effect of resuscitation using albumin or gelatin colloid solutions on the risk for AKI.

For these reasons, isotonic crystalloids are recommended as the initial resuscitative solution for severe sepsis and septic shock. The development of a hyperchloremic acidosis can be anticipated with the use of large volumes of 0.9% saline solution; use of lactated Ringer solution or another balanced salt solution (PlasmaLyte) may limit this effect. Hypertonic saline is not recommended in the routine resuscitation of septic shock.

Rapid volume expansion (500 mL of isotonic crystalloid every 10 to 30 minutes) should be continued until clinical and physiologic treatment targets are met. Vasopressor/inotropic support is required if fluid infusion alone fails to achieve physiologic response targets. Early aggressive resuscitation to achieve physiologically normal hemodynamic goals reduces subsequent morbidity and mortality in patients with septic shock. In a pediatric population with septic shock, rapid fluid resuscitation in the first hour of presentation to hospital improved survival (289). In an adult study, the effect of early goal-directed therapy (EGDT) to normal physiologic values in patients presenting to an emergency department with severe sepsis or septic shock was examined (313). All patients, both conventional and goal-directed therapy groups, were resuscitated in the emergency room for the first 6 hours to standard hemodynamic end points of CVP at least 8 mmHg, MAP at least 65 mm Hg, and urine output at least 0.5 mL/kg/hr. The experimental EGDT group, in addition, was managed using an experimental protocol to achieve both the standard goals and a central venous oxygen saturation ≥ 70%, as measured by an oximetric central venous catheter. During the 6 hours of their protocolized emergency room support, the experimental group received 1.5 L more fluid than the control group, and a substantially larger fraction of the patients in the experimental group achieved the physiologic resuscitative goals (99.2% vs. 86.1%); overall mortality was significantly lower in the EGDT group.

As of 2004, the Surviving Sepsis Campaign guidelines endorsed this form of EGDT (314). Since that time, three large international multicenter RCTs between 2014 and 2015, and a systematic review/meta-analysis have failed to show an improvement in survival with the use of EGDT compared to nonprotocolized usual care or protocol-guided care targeting clinical end points like MAP and end-organ perfusion (315–317). These data suggest a clear lack of improvement in outcomes using formal EGDT.

Antimicrobial Therapy and Source Control

Historically, critically ill patients with overwhelming infection have not been considered a unique subgroup comparable to neutropenic patients for purposes of selection of antimicrobial therapy. However, critically ill patients with severe sepsis and septic shock, like those with neutropenia, are characterized by distinct differences from the typical infected patient that impact on the optimal management strategy. These differences include:

- Marked alterations in antibiotic pharmacokinetics
- Increased frequency of hepatic and renal dysfunction
- High prevalence of unrecognized immune dysfunction
- Predisposition to infection with resistant organisms

Marked increase in frequency of adverse outcome if there is a failure of rapid initiation of effective antibiotic therapy. Critical management decisions in this patient group must often be made emergently in the absence of definitive data regarding the infecting organism and its sensitivity pattern, patient immune status and organ function. Since outcomes in severe sepsis and septic shock are strongly influenced by the rapidity of administration of an appropriate antimicrobial regimen at the first presentation, a particularly thoughtful and judicious approach to initial empiric antimicrobial therapy is required (318–320).

Empiric antibiotic regimens should approach 100% coverage of pathogens for the suspected source of infection. Initial administration of inappropriate antimicrobials increases morbidity in a wide range of infections; the occurrence of initiation of inappropriate antimicrobial therapy may occur as frequently as 17.1% in community-acquired and 34.3% in nosocomial bacteremia admitted to the ICU (320). Similarly, 18.8% and 28.4% of septic shock cases were initially treated with inadequate antimicrobial therapy in another large study (55). Retrospective studies have shown that the risk of death increases from 30% to 60% in ICU bacteremia (4,319) and 70% to 100% in gram-negative shock (4) when the initial empiric regimen fails to cover the inciting pathogen. More recent data suggest that the relative increase in survival of septic shock with inappropriate initial antimicrobial therapy is reduced approximately fivefold (range 2.5- to 10-fold in selected subgroups) to about 10% (55). These findings of sharply increased mortality risk with initial inadequate antimicrobial therapy apply to serious infections caused by gram-negative and gram-positive bacteria as well as *Candida* species (4,55,321–324).

As a consequence, empiric regimens should err on the side of overinclusiveness. The most common cause of initiation of inappropriate antimicrobial therapy is a failure of the clinician to appreciate the risk of infection with antibiotic-resistant organisms, either otherwise uncommon organisms with increased native resistance or antibiotic-resistant isolates of common organisms. Selection of an optimal antimicrobial regimen requires knowledge of the probable anatomic site of infection; the patient's immune status, risk factors and physical environment; and the local microbiologic flora and organism resistance patterns. Risk factors for infection with resistant organisms include prolonged hospital stay, prior hospitalization, and prior colonization or infection with multiresistant organisms.

Superior empiric coverage can be obtained through the use of a local antibiogram or infectious disease consultation (325). Although not routinely required, extended spectrum gram-negative regimens, vancomycin, and/or antifungal therapy may be appropriate in specific, high-risk cases with severe sepsis (Table 46.13). In addition, given that 90% to 95% of patients with septic shock have comorbidities or other factors

TABLE 46.13 Indication for Extended Empiric Antibiotic Therapy of Severe Sepsis/Septic Shock

↑ Gram-negative Coverage
Nosocomial infection
Neutropenic or immunosuppressed
Immunocompromised due to chronic organ failure (liver, renal, lung, heart, etc)
↑ Gram-positive Coverage (Vancomycin)
High level endemic MRSA (community or nosocomial)
Neutropenic patient
Intravascular catheter infection
Nosocomial pneumonia
Fungal/Yeast Coverage (Triazole, Echinocandin, Amphotericin B)
Positive relevant fungal cultures
Neutropenic fever or other immunosuppressed patient unresponsive to standard antibiotic therapy
Prolonged broad-spectrum antibiotic therapy
Consider empiric therapy if high-risk patient with severe shock

MRSA, methicillin-resistant *Staphylococcus aureus*.

that make them high risk for resistant organisms, it may be appropriate to initially treat all patients with septic shock using a combination of antimicrobials that result in a broadly expanded spectrum of coverage for the first few days. This approach should yield improved initial appropriateness of antimicrobial coverage and ensure that high-risk patients are not inappropriately categorized as low risk.

Intravenous administration of broad-spectrum antimicrobial should be initiated immediately (preferably less than 30 minutes) after the clinical diagnosis of septic shock. Appropriate intravenous empiric broad-spectrum therapy should be initiated as rapidly as possible in response to clinical suspicion of infection in the presence of hypotension, i.e., presumptive septic shock. While a differential diagnostic list is always appropriate, an assumption that hypotension is caused by anything other than sepsis in the setting of documented or suspected infection should be avoided in the absence of very strong data indicating a specific alternate etiology. Retrospective studies of human bacteremia, pneumonia, and meningitis with sepsis suggest that mortality in sepsis increases with delays in antimicrobial administration (318,324,326–328). One major retrospective analysis of septic shock has suggested that the delay to initial administration of effective antimicrobial therapy is the *single strongest predictor of survival* (32). Initiation of effective antimicrobial therapy within the first hour following the onset of septic shock–related hypotension was associated with 79.9% survival to hospital discharge. For every additional hour to effective antimicrobial initiation in the first 6 hours after the onset of hypotension, survival dropped an average of 7.6%. With effective antimicrobial initiation between the first and second hours after hypotension onset, survival had already dropped to 70.5%. With effective antimicrobial therapy delay to 5 to 6 hours after hypotension onset, survival was just 42.0%, and by 9 to 12 hours 25.4%. The adjusted odds ratio of death was already significantly increased by the second hour after hypotension onset and the ratio continued to climb with longer delays. Another recent study demonstrated similar reductions in mortality with delays to administration of appropriate antimicrobials with severe sepsis (329).

Substantial delays before initiation of effective therapy have been shown several studies of serious infections (318,328,330,331). In septic shock, the median time to delivery of effective antimicrobial therapy following initial onset of recurrent/persistent hypotension was 6 hours (32); studies have suggested improving time to antimicrobial therapy over the last decade (329,332,333).

A potential survival advantage may exist if a pathogenic organism can be isolated in severe infections including septic shock. Every effort should be made to obtain appropriate site-specific cultures in order to allow identification and susceptibility testing of the pathogenic organism; however, such efforts should not delay antimicrobial therapy.

Antimicrobial therapy should be initiated with dosing at the high end of the therapeutic range in all patients with life-threatening infection. Early appropriate antimicrobial therapy is the central element in management of septic shock. However, clearance of pathogens will not begin until therapeutic levels of the antimicrobials in the circulation are achieved. This is most easily achieved by initiating antibiotic therapy with high-end dosing regimens (334,335). In some cases, for example, colistin, loading doses may be useful (334,335). In addition, pharmacokinetic indices of efficacy such as time above the pathogen minimal inhibitory concentration (MIC) for β-lactams and peak concentration (Cp) or area under curve (AUC) divided by the pathogen MIC for fluoroquinolones and aminoglycosides is optimized with high-end dosing (336).

Early in sepsis, before the onset of hepatic or renal dysfunction, CO is increased in many patients. In association with increased free drug levels due to decreased albumin levels, drug clearance can be transiently increased via augmented renal clearance (337). As the illness progresses, ICU patients with sepsis or septic shock exhibit substantially increased volumes of distribution though clearance rates may decrease. Consequently, suboptimal dosing of antibiotics is common in these conditions (338–344). Such data are most well developed in reference to aminoglycosides, but also exists for fluoroquinolones, β-lactams, and carbapenems (338–345). Failure to achieve targets on initial dosing has been associated with clinical failure with aminoglycosides (346,347). Similarly, clinical success rate for treatment of serious infections tracks with higher peak blood levels of fluoroquinolones (nosocomial pneumonia and other serious infections) (334,348–350) and aminoglycosides (gram-negative nosocomial pneumonia and other serious infections) (334,351,352). Although there are extensive data in experimental animals and less serious human infections, data for optimization of outcomes in critically ill, infected patients using β-lactams is relatively limited (334,353,354). One retrospective study has shown improved survival in a more acutely ill subset patients with *Pseudomonas* bacteremia when treated with extended infusions rather than standard intermittent dosing of piperacillin/tazobactam (355). In another randomized study, superior clinical cure was noted with continuous infusion of several different kinds of β-lactams in patients with severe sepsis (356).

Achievement of optimal serum concentrations of aminoglycosides (peak antibiotic serum concentration to pathogen MIC ratio of 12 or higher) and longer periods of bactericidal β-lactam and carbapenem serum concentrations (minimum time above MIC in serum of 60% of dosing interval) are appropriate targets (348,357,358). This can most easily be attained with once-daily dosing of aminoglycosides (359). For β-lactams and related antibiotics, increased frequency of dosing, given identical total daily dose, is recommended. For example, piperacillin/tazobactam can be dosed at either 4.5 g every 8 hours or 3.375 g every 6 hours for serious infections; all things being equal, the latter would achieve a higher time above MIC and should be the preferred dosing option. A similar dosing approach should be used for other β-lactams in critically ill patients with life-threatening infections. Limited data suggest that continuous infusion of β-lactams and related drugs may be even more effective particularly for relatively resistant organisms (334,355,356,360–364).

Multidrug antimicrobial therapy is preferred for the initial empiric therapy of septic shock. Probable pathogens should be covered by at least two antimicrobials with different bactericidal mechanisms during initial therapy of septic shock, although monotherapy is sufficient for less severe forms of sepsis. Given that highly resistant organisms are increasingly endemic in the critical care environment, multidrug antimicrobial therapy will reduce the probability of failure to cover these organisms. In addition, most patients with septic shock, even those without specific pre-existing immune defects, exhibit significant deficits of neutrophil and monocyte function during the course of their illness (365–371). Further, malnutrition and organ dysfunction, for example, renal or hepatic failure, which are common in ICU patients, suppress cell-mediated immunity. Based on these data, septic shock patients likely have reduced ability to clear infection and may be best managed with multidrug therapy similar to that recommended for patients with neutropenic sepsis (372,373).

The only prospective, controlled study to specifically compare multiple versus single antimicrobial therapy in a broad range of severe sepsis or septic shock patients failed to show efficacy (374). Several meta-analyses have similarly failed to demonstrate a benefit of combination therapy in mortality in immunocompetent patients with sepsis (375,376). A meta-analysis in neutropenic sepsis suggested little incremental benefit of combination therapy in this setting (377). As a consequence, for most infectious diseases, physicians and other experts suggest that there is no advantage to multidrug therapy in serious infections including bacteremia (376,378).

Despite this, analyses of the sickest subset of patients with gram-negative bacteremia, with or without shock, have tended to suggest improved survival with the use of two or more antibiotics to which the causative organism is sensitive (379–382). Similarly, at least two retrospective and one prospective analyses of the most severe critically ill patients with bacteremic pneumococcal pneumonia suggested improvement in outcome if two or more effective agents were used (383–385). This occurred even as patients with pneumococcal bacteremia with a lower severity of illness demonstrated no such benefit (383). A secondary analysis of a prospective study of community-acquired pneumonia has shown benefit with multidrug therapy compared to monotherapy, but only in the subset of septic shock (386). In addition, a propensity matching study of a large cohort of adult septic shock has shown a survival advantage with combination therapy (387).

Based on the possibility that any benefit in survival with combination therapy may be restricted to only the most critically ill subset of patients, a stratified meta-analysis/meta-regression of 60 sepsis data-sets, derived from 48 individual studies (388), was performed. The power of the study was enhanced by splitting data from 12 studies into mutually exclusive groups of septic shock/critically ill and nonseptic shock/noncritically ill and by excluding studies where a structural bias would favor an equivalence outcome—for example, a highly potent β-lactam versus a less potent β-lactam and a second agent; studies of neutropenic sepsis were also excluded. Notably, it was required that the pathogen was known to be sensitive to both agents in the combination therapy group. Although the same absence of significant benefit of combination therapy overall was found, stratification of the data-sets by baseline (monotherapy) mortality risk showed a consistent substantial benefit in terms of clinical cure and survival with combination therapy in the most severely ill subset of patients.

Although highly suggestive, these retrospective analyses cannot be considered definitive. While waiting for appropriately designed RCTs, combination of empiric antibiotic therapy for several days with two drugs of different mechanisms of action is appropriate for patients in septic shock. Monotherapy is reasonable for patients who are not critically ill and/or at high risk of death.

Empiric antimicrobial therapy should be adjusted to a narrower regimen within 48 to 72 hours if a plausible pathogen is identified or if the patient stabilizes clinically (i.e., resolution of shock). While several retrospective studies have demonstrated that inappropriate therapy of bacteremic septic shock yields increased mortality (4,319,321–324), none have suggested that early narrowing of therapy is detrimental if the organism is identified or if the patient is responding well clinically. This approach will maximize appropriate antibiotic coverage of inciting pathogens in septic shock while minimizing selection pressure toward resistant organisms. Although it is tempting to continue a broad-spectrum regimen in the roughly 15% of improving patients who are culture negative for a potential pathogen, intensivists must recognize that a strategy of broad-spectrum initial antimicrobial therapy will only be sustainable if overuse of these agents can be avoided. Aggressive de-escalation of antimicrobial therapy within 48 to 72 hours after initiation is required.

Where possible, early source control should be implemented in patients with severe sepsis, septic shock, and other life-threatening infections. Source control is a critical issue in the management of infection associated with severe sepsis. Infections found in ICU patients frequently require source control for optimal management. The need for such source control may initially be overlooked in many common ICU infections—pneumonia-associated bacterial empyema, decubitus ulcers, *C. difficile* colitis. Causes of septic shock where source control may be required are noted in Table 46.14.

Source control may include removal of implanted or tunneled devices, open surgical or percutaneous drainage of infected fluids or abscesses, and surgical resection of infected tissues. In a broader sense, it is inclusive of elimination of inciting chemotherapies—antibiotics driving *C. difficile* colitis or chemotherapy causing gut injury. Efforts to identify infections requiring invasive forms of source control frequently require rapid (less than 2 hours) radiographic imaging (often CT scan) or, if clinical status and findings are supportive, direct and immediate surgical intervention without an imaging effort. With rare exceptions, surgical source control should follow aggressive resuscitative efforts in order to minimize intraoperative morbidity and mortality. In some cases—rapidly progressive necrotizing soft tissue infections, bowel infarction—optimal management mandates simultaneous aggressive resuscitation and surgical intervention. Subgroup analysis in at least one large prospective severe sepsis study has suggested that failure to implement adequate source control is associated with increased mortality (389). Earlier surgical intervention has been shown to have a significant impact on outcome in certain rapidly progressive infections such as

TABLE 46.14 Common Sources of Severe Sepsis/Septic Shock Requiring Urgent Source Control

Toxic megacolon or *C. difficile* colitis with shock
Ischemic bowel
Perforated viscus
Intra-abdominal abscess
Ascending cholangitis
Gangrenous cholecystitis
Necrotizing pancreatitis with infection
Bacterial empyema
Mediastinitis
Purulent tunnel infections
Purulent foreign body infections
Obstructive uropathy
Complicated pylonephritis/perinephric abscess
Necrotizing soft tissue infections (necrotizing fasciitis)
Clostridial myonecrosis

necrotizing fasciitis and abdominal sepsis (333,390–392). In a large retrospective study of septic shock, time from hypotension to implementation of source control was found to be highly correlated with outcome (393).

The necessity for, or efficacy of, source control efforts should be reassessed within 12 to 36 hours following admission and/or source control efforts based on clinical response.

Vasopressors and Inotropes

Following fluid resuscitation, patients with septic shock demonstrate persistent vasomotor dysfunction characterized by regional perfusion deficits with systemic hypotension despite normal or increased CO. Clinical manifestations may include lactic acidosis and ongoing progression of organ failure. Until recently, the only available approach to correction of regional perfusion defects was vasopressor therapy; vasopressors, however, do not represent a specific therapy for this problem. Their primary use is to increase systemic arterial pressure to a range that potentially sustains the ability of the vasculature to autoregulate flow on a tissue and organ level (394,395). In this way, vital organ perfusion can be supported—potentially at the expense of peripheral perfusion—until definitive therapy, infection source control, and antibiotics can be implemented.

The aim of vasopressor/inotropic therapy in septic shock is simply the optimization of critical organ and tissue perfusion. However, the specific global and/or regional perfusion goals required to achieve this result are complex and controversial. While specific targets can be suggested, therapy for each patient must be highly individualized and dynamic. Appropriate goals will change over time and should be re-evaluated on a continuing basis.

If hypotension or clinical evidence of tissue hypoperfusion persists after adequate fluid resuscitation of septic shock, vasopressor therapy is indicated, norepinephrine and dopamine are both effective as initial therapy. A target MAP of 65 mmHg is sufficient in most cases. Initiation of vasopressor support is dependent on the patient's clinical status following fluid resuscitation. If systemic hypotension in association with evidence of tissue/organ hypoperfusion—oliguria, obtundation, lactic acidosis—persists, vasopressor support is indicated. Selection of a vasopressor agent is based on an individualized assessment of the patient's needs. The patient's hemodynamic presentation, the anticipated cardiovascular effect of each vasoactive agent, based on the distribution of receptor activity, and the physician's experience and comfort with each drug should be considered. As a consequence of the variety of factors that may play a role in vasopressor selection, septic shock patients with a predominantly distributive hemodynamic pattern can be appropriately and effectively managed with one of several vasopressors including dopamine, norepinephrine, or phenylephrine.

Ideally, patients should have achieved the targeted intravascular volume status prior to initiation of vasopressors. Although vasopressors can be used to maintain blood pressure for brief periods while intravascular volume is repleted, the infusion of high-dose vasopressors to volume-depleted patients may substantially aggravate ischemic organ injury. In a recent retrospective, multicenter observational study, initiation of vasoactive agents within the first hour after shock onset, which occurred in association with decreased fluid resuscitation during that period, was associated with increased mortality (396). Another study from the same data-set has shown that delays in vasopressor initiation in septic shock on the order of several hours are not associated with increased mortality (397). Although selection of the target blood pressure is dependent on a variety of factors including the pre-existence of poorly controlled hypertension or renal dysfunction and the propensity to adverse toxicity, a goal of 65 mmHg appears to be adequate in most cases (398).

Studies suggesting norepinephrine is superior to dopamine are less than definitive (399–405). No controlled study has directly assessed norepinephrine and dopamine in terms of survival and few have compared the two agents with respect to markers of organ dysfunction. A single, large, multicenter RCT has shown that first-line use of dopamine is associated with more dysrhythmic events than norepinephrine but no difference in mortality in septic shock cases was noted (405). Studies assessing the effects of these agents on renal and splanchnic perfusion have been mixed with neither agent demonstrating conclusive superiority (400,401,404,406–412). Norepinephrine may have more powerful vasopressor activity than dopamine (413); its inotropic effects are mediated by direct activity on myocardial β-adrenoreceptors. Dopamine pressor effects are weaker than those of norepinephrine and inotropic effects are substantially indirect, through stimulation of release of myocardial catecholamine stores; excessive tachycardia may be more common with dopamine. In addition, dopamine may exert significant immunosuppressive effects through suppression of prolactin production from the hypothalamus (414). Phenylephrine, a relatively pure α-adrenergic agonist, has minimal or absent inotropic effects and tends to cause reflex bradycardia. For that reason, it can be very useful in the context of excessive tachycardia or concurrent tachyarrhythmias. However, phenylephrine consistently decreases CO and has an increased propensity to cause ischemic complications; it is not recommended as first-line vasopressor therapy. Despite potent inotropic and vasopressor activity, epinephrine is not commonly utilized as the initial pressor therapy in septic shock because it can generate profound tachycardia, tissue ischemia, and metabolic disturbances. However, one multicenter RCT has suggested similar outcomes in septic shock when epinephrine alone was compared with norepinephrine in combination with dobutamine (415).

Dobutamine is indicated for patients with low CI or other evidence of hypoperfusion following achievement of adequate BP. Milrinone can be used as an alternate agent if the response to dobutamine is suboptimal. In some cases of septic shock, clinical or laboratory evidence of hypoperfusion—oliguria, altered mentation, decreased mixed venous oxygen saturation, increased lactic acidosis—persists despite an adequate blood pressure. In this circumstance, the patient may require a higher blood pressure or assessment of CO, via PAC, echocardiography, or other method of CO evaluation, to determine the need for inotropic support. In the small proportion of septic shock patients who manifest overt myocardial depression following fluid resuscitation, dobutamine, or milrinone may be indicated. Dobutamine can increase CI in septic shock, although the inotropic response is frequently blunted relative to normal subjects (232,416). If catecholamine responsiveness is inadequate, low-dose milrinone may be effective since its inotropic activity is mediated through an alternate mechanism (417). When using either agent, patients must be adequately fluid resuscitated; severe hypotension can result if intravascular volume is deficient when either dobutamine or milrinone is initiated (232,417).

Although the aim of inotropic therapy in severe sepsis/septic shock is to improve CI and tissue perfusion, specific goals have been controversial; the currently recommended target is a CI within the normal range, approximately 2.5 to 4 L/min/m^2. The utility of MvO_2/$ScvO_2$ as global indices of tissue perfusion adequacy in severe sepsis and septic shock is also uncertain. Limited studies suggest that an MVO_2/$ScvO_2$ below the normal range (65% to 70%) may indicate inadequacy of resuscitation and/or total perfusion in early septic shock (188). If other hemodynamic targets have been achieved, an MvO_2 below 65% may represent an appropriate indication to increase DO_2 by starting inotropic agents. Recommendations to increase MvO_2 are based on mixed evidence; no benefit was noted in a randomized trial of goal-directed therapy using MvO_2 in critically ill patients after the onset of organ dysfunction (418,419). Although EGDT targeting a $ScvO_2$ of at least 70% was associated with improved outcome in one single-center RCT (313), large confirmatory trials have failed to replicate this finding (315–317).

Continuous infusion of vasopressin (0.01 to 0.04 U/min) exerts a strong pressor effect and may be beneficial in catecholamine-resistant septic shock following adequate volume resuscitation. Vasopressin levels in septic shock patients are known to be decreased (420). Studies have also demonstrated that i.v. infusion of vasopressin in patients with septic shock results in a profound pressor response (273,421,422), an effect that is absent with even larger amounts of vasopressin in normotensive patients (272). A randomized, controlled, double-blind trial of 4-hour infusion of norepinephrine and vasopressin in high-dose pressor-dependent shock has demonstrated significant improvement in urine output and creatinine clearance along with a concomitant reduction in conventional vasopressor requirements in the vasopressin group (422). Another RCT has demonstrated that while vasopressin can spare the need for high doses of sympathomimetic agents, outcome is not affected (423). A recent meta-analysis of nine RCTs has shown that vasopressin use in vasodilatory shock is safe, facilitates weaning of catecholamines, and may be associated with reduced mortality relative to norepinephrine alone (424). Because of the relatively prolonged pharmacologic effect of the drug, vasopressin should be utilized only after hemodynamic stabilization with standard agents (catecholamines) has been attempted.

At high dose, over 0.04 U/min, vasopressin may produce increased blood pressure, bradycardia, dysrhythmias—premature atrial contractions, heart block—severe peripheral vasoconstriction, decreased CO, myocardial ischemia, myocardial infarction, and cardiac arrest. In patients with vascular disease, even relatively modest doses can precipitate peripheral vascular insufficiency, mesenteric ischemia, or myocardial infarction. Given these potential side effects, the minimal amount of vasopressin required should be used to achieve desired blood pressure goals. In addition, since vasopressin appears to be a pure vasopressor in the context of vasodilatory shock, CO will usually fall.

Administration of "low"- or "renal"-dose dopamine (1 to 4 μg/kg/min) in order to maintain renal or mesenteric blood flow in sepsis and septic shock is not recommended. While concurrent infusion of "low"-dose dopamine during human septic shock does mitigate a decrease in renal perfusion that can occur as a consequence of norepinephrine infusion, the clinical benefit of this therapy is questionable (425,426). Low-dose dopamine infusions also cause a mild transient diuresis in the absence of other vasopressors in nonoliguric critically ill patients (427,428). However, "low"-dose dopamine does not prevent the development of renal dysfunction in these patients including those with sepsis and septic shock (429,430).

Invasive and Noninvasive Monitoring

Controversy exists regarding the most appropriate monitoring methods for determination of adequacy of resuscitation in patients with severe sepsis and septic shock. The range of monitoring that must be considered in each patient begins with observation by specially trained nursing personnel, through routine noninvasive devices—continuous electrocardiographic monitors, intermittent mechanical sphygmomanometry, end-tidal carbon dioxide sensors, percutaneous oximetry—to commonly used invasive, arterial, central venous, and pulmonary artery catheters, and nonroutine noninvasive—bedside echocardiography techniques. Before the advent of basic hemodynamic monitoring in the 1950s and early 1960s, clinical examination and manual sphygmomanometry were the only available methods for assessment of cardiovascular status. Clinical judgment correctly predicts the hemodynamic profile (including CO and central venous/PWPs) of critically ill patients only about half of the time (431,432).

CVP has been considered a useful measure of intravascular volume since the early studies of hypovolemic shock in young men following battlefield trauma (287,288). However, CVP may be much less reliable as a reflection of left ventricular preload in older patients with a variety of cardiopulmonary disorders as are typically found in a modern day ICU (179,433). While low filling pressures may reliably indicate hypovolemia in most patients, the presence of a normal or even elevated CVP can be misleading in patients in whom right ventricular afterload is elevated or right ventricular contractility impaired (434).

The pulmonary capillary wedge pressure (PCWP) obtained by using a PAC has been considered to reflect intravascular volume more reliably than CVP. In addition, the device allows thermodilution-based derivation of CO (431,432,435). Although the PAC had gained widespread acceptance, significant questions about its use have been raised; the last decade has seen a rapid decrease in its frequency of deployment. Several studies have questioned the relationship of PAC-derived, pressure-based, estimates of ventricular preload in specific groups of critically ill patients (433) and, more recently, even in normal subjects (436). In addition, the lack of randomized trials demonstrating benefit and the association of PAC with excess mortality in two observational cohorts have led to concerns regarding the clinical utility of and safety of PACs (437,438). Given these data, the monitoring need using a PAC remains only in a small subgroup of septic patients where there is significant diagnostic uncertainty and poor response to standard therapy. Intermittent echocardiography, although requiring somewhat more training, appears to provide equivalent or superior data to the intensivist (439,440).

Patients with established septic shock should have continuous monitoring of blood pressure, oxygen saturation, ECG, and urine output in a closed ICU staffed with full-time dedicated intensivists and critical care-trained nurses. Several studies have demonstrated reduced mortality with decreased length of stay and overall cost for a wide range of individual conditions are obtained when critically ill patients are cared for in closed ICU's staffed with full-time dedicated intensivists and nurses (441–445). Similar improvements in outcome of sepsis and septic shock have been documented with the use of dedicated intensivists in closed ICUs (446). Among the practice differences associated with the use of full-time intensivists is a greater use of invasive monitoring (444).

Patients requiring vasopressor agents for a prolonged period or at high dose should be strongly considered for insertion of an arterial pressure catheter for continuous blood pressure monitoring and to facilitate frequent measurements of arterial blood gases and chemistry. Accurate, continuous monitoring of blood pressure may be required for optimal assessment of severity of shock, response to fluid resuscitation, and titration of vasopressors and inotropes. However, intense peripheral vasoconstriction may occur during shock as a consequence of the vascular compensatory response to hypotension or due to administration of vasopressors. Clinical ausculatory and noninvasive mechanical methods can be highly inaccurate in this setting (447,448). Patients with sustained shock, particularly those requiring vasopressor support, should be assessed for placement of an intra-arterial catheter for continuous blood pressure monitoring. However, such catheters should be preferentially placed in peripheral sites in nonend arteries—radial, dorsalis pedis—and should be used with caution in patients at high risk for vascular disease.

Despite this, at least one retrospective analysis of vasopressor-dependent shock has suggested increased mortality in association with the use of arterial catheters, although confounding by illness severity is an obvious concern of such analyses (449).

If volume resuscitation requirements exceed 2 L, placement of central venous catheter for monitoring of CVP and for vasopressor/inotrope infusion should be considered. An initial target CVP of at least 8 mmHg is recommended. Alternately, intermittent echocardiographic monitoring may be implemented. Fluid deficits during septic shock in adults typically range from 5 to 10 L (285). In the absence of significant cardiopulmonary dysfunction, CVP should accurately assess intravascular volume status. However, cardiopulmonary dysfunction is not uncommon in patients with septic shock, either as an underlying predisposition to critical illness/sepsis or as a consequence of the injury, ARDS, myocardial depression. Low CVP remains indicative of hypovolemia; elevated or normal CVPs in this patient group may not necessarily indicate euvolemia. CVP monitoring should be entertained if substantial amounts of fluid resuscitation are required in order to ensure that overt hypovolemia is adequately addressed. The initial target CVP should be ≥8 mmHg with additional increases indicated by the effect of fluid boluses on CO. The overall goal is to provide adequate CO and tissue perfusion using the lowest necessary cardiac filling pressures.

Although not universally available, echocardiography has become a very important tool for the guidance for fluid therapy (450). Fluid responsiveness can be evaluated by respiratory variations in aortic flow velocity (variations greater than 20% in aortic velocity time integral [VTI]) (451) and respiratory variations in peak aortic flow (variations over 12% predict fluid responsiveness in patients with septic shock) (452). Respiratory variations in superior (453,454) and inferior (455,456) vena cava diameter can predict fluid responsiveness in mechanically ventilated patients.

Invasive monitoring using a PAC is not recommended for routine use in patients with severe sepsis or septic shock. At least one major, prospective, nonrandomized multicenter study has suggested increased length of stay, costs, and mortality in a cohort of risk-matched patients receiving a PAC in first 24 hours after ICU admission (457). A multicenter, randomized, controlled trial involving 676 subjects with shock (primarily septic), ARDS, or both demonstrated no difference in organ failure–free days, renal support needs, vasopressor requirements, MV, ICU/hospital length of stay or mortality (14- and 90-day) between subjects randomized to pulmonary artery catheterization and controls (458). A second smaller randomized trial of 200 patients (about 100 with sepsis) also demonstrated no mortality difference with or without the use of PAC (459). Other smaller studies including one randomized trial in high-risk operative patients failed to demonstrate excess mortality with PAC use (460,461). In contrast, one meta-analysis of RCTs demonstrated reduced mortality risk in surgical ICU patients treated with PAC, but no effect on mortality in medical or mixed ICU patients (462). On the basis of the total data available, routine use of PAC in patients with sepsis or other critical illness cannot be recommended.

Initiation of invasive cardiac monitoring using a PAC may be considered if there has been an inadequate response to fluid resuscitation, if there is clinical suspicion of intravascular fluid volume overload or if the patient has impaired cardiac function. While the maintenance of a blood pressure adequate for autoregulation of blood flow to vital organs and tissues is the first objective in the resuscitation of septic shock, support of global perfusion is also critical. Adequacy of global perfusion cannot always be reliably inferred from clinical examination or CVP/arterial pressure monitoring (431,435,463). Patients who respond poorly to fluid resuscitation or are at high risk for fluid resuscitation–related complications may benefit from a PAC. A substantial degree of variability in the relationship between PCWP and end-diastolic volumes makes it difficult to specify target PCWP goals that ensure adequate CI and tissue perfusion (436,464,465). In general, a PCWP titrated to at least 12 to 15 cm H_2O can optimize cardiac function (179). If hypotension persists, a higher PCWP may be beneficial as assessed by measuring the effect of additional fluids on CI. An elevated PCWP may risk the development or aggravation of ARDS (466,467). Specific groups that may require higher PCWP include those with congestive heart failure, left ventricular hypertrophy, restrictive or constrictive heart disease, or increased intrathoracic pressures including those on high levels of positive end-expiratory pressure (PEEP). The increasing penetration of echocardiography techniques into the ICU setting may obviate the need for PAC consideration in many situations.

Specific Therapy

As discussed, patients with severe sepsis and septic shock must first be treated using appropriate resuscitation, broad-spectrum antimicrobials, source control, and physiologic support of organ function in the ICU. Immunomodulatory therapy has only been evaluated in association with adequate treatment based on these four elements.

In the last few decades, the dominant hypotheses regarding the pathogenesis of septic shock and septic organ dysfunction had focused on inflammatory and coagulation mediators. Approximately 30 clinical trials have been performed evaluating both nonspecific inhibitors of inflammation such as nonsteroidal anti-inflammatory drugs and high-dose glucocorticoids, specific immunomodulatory agents such as monoclonal antibodies against TNFα and IL-1 receptor antagonist (468,469) and combined coagulation/inflammatory modulators such as drotrecogin-α (activated), TFPI, and antithrombin III (33–35,57). Despite an expenditure of over $1 billion, these studies have failed to demonstrate a consistent survival benefit.

Although large multicenter clinical trials of modulation of the coagulation cascade for treatment of sepsis with organ failure have been performed with several agents—for example, antithrombin III (34), TFPI (35)—only drotrecogin-α (activated) was initially shown to improve mortality (33); as a result, it was licensed in 2001. However, a subsequent large clinical trial in septic shock failed to confirm this benefit and the product was subsequently removed from the market. No novel immune/coagulation modulating experimental agent currently has regulatory approval.

Intravenous immune globulin (IVIG) should be considered for patients suffering from streptococcal toxic shock syndrome. The potential utility of polyclonal immune globulin preparations for severe sepsis and septic shock in general is uncertain at present. One meta-analysis has suggested that sepsis-related mortality is significantly reduced when IVIG is used in the management of such patients (470). A small RCT of trauma patients has also demonstrated a reduced incidence of septic complications including pneumonia and other infections, other than catheter-related infections, although ICU length of stay and mortality were not reduced (471). Evidence favoring the use of polyclonal immunoglobulin for defined invasive streptococcal infections including streptococcal septic shock is more definitive. A case-matching study has demonstrated improved 30-day survival in patients treated with intravenous polyclonal immune globulin while a RCT—aborted prematurely due to low enrollment—has shown decreased early sepsis-related organ failure with a trend toward improved survival (472). These results have been supported by other observational studies (473).

Immunosuppressive doses of corticosteroids are contraindicated in the management of sepsis and septic shock. In the past, high-dose steroids had been advocated for sepsis with organ failure in order to dampen inflammatory responses and minimize organ dysfunction (474). Several large multicenter RCTs have definitively demonstrated that administration of high-dose (15 to 30 mg/kg methylprednisolone equivalent) corticosteroids fail to improve outcome in adult septic shock (475–478). In some of these studies, mortality in specific subgroups appeared to be increased with steroid treatment (476).

Supportive Therapy

Although specific therapies for septic shock continue to be developed, general supportive care, in conjunction with antibiotics, remains the mainstay of care. Fluid and vasopressor/inotropic supports have been addressed earlier in this chapter. In addition, there has been an explosion of data in recent years regarding the efficacy of other elements of supportive care including ventilatory strategies, intensity of dialysis, endocrine support, and glycemic management. In other key areas, for example, nutritional support, definitive data are lacking. Nonetheless, it is likely that an aggressive approach to optimization of supportive care, in combination with anti-infective therapy and resuscitative efforts, can improve morbidity and mortality. For that reason, application of appropriate support modalities in a timely manner should be the standard of care of septic patients in all ICUs.

Intensive renal replacement therapy (daily intermittent dialysis or continuous renal replacement therapy) is indicated for severe sepsis or septic shock with renal failure. Indications for acute dialysis in the ICU population are not dissimilar to those for other patients but there is substantial uncertainty of the ideal approach. The indications include volume overload, electrolyte imbalance, acid–base disturbances, elevated BUN, uremic pericarditis, or uremic encephalopathy. The optimal timing for initiation is uncertain; while earlier initiation sounds intuitively attractive, available data is inconsistent on the issue (479). ICU patients, especially those with acute renal failure, may have altered hemodialysis kinetics such that standard intermittent dialysis may offer suboptimal urea clearance kinetics despite apparently equivalent doses. Compared to standard intermittent dialysis, daily hemodialysis has been shown to yield higher urea clearance and improved mortality in ICU patients with acute renal failure (480). Similarly, another study has demonstrated that higher urea clearance with continuous veno-venous hemodialysis yields reduced mortality (481). However, two subsequent large multicenter RCTs failed to demonstrate benefit including faster liberation from dialysis, reduced organ failure development, or decreased mortality with higher daily clearance rates (482,483). Patients in all these studies were critically ill but not exclusively septic. Given the ease of use, continuous renal replacement therapies will likely continue to the primary modality used in ICU despite the lack of a clear-cut outcome improvement.

Peritoneal dialysis is not appropriate since even high-frequency exchanges yield relatively low urea clearance kinetics. A study of infection-related acute renal failure that included cases of sepsis demonstrated increased mortality among those treated with peritoneal dialysis compared to those treated with hemodialysis (484).

Intensive insulin therapy maintaining blood glucose of 4.4 to 6.1 mmol/L (80 to 110 mg/dL) is harmful in critically ill ICU patients with severe sepsis. Hyperglycemia is a recognized risk factor for increased mortality in the critically ill independent of APACHE II score (485). One single-center, nonblinded RCT indicated that tight glycemic control in surgical ICU patients undergoing MV—mostly postcoronary artery bypass graft or other cardiovascular surgery—reduces the incidence of severe sepsis and decreases mortality primarily because of a decreased incidence of multiple organ failure with septic foci (486). This data is consistent with other clinical and experimental studies suggesting the presence of granulocyte dysfunction and increased risk of infection in postoperative surgical patients with persistent hyperglycemia (487). However, another single-center RCT by the same group failed to demonstrate similar improvements in critically ill medical patients (488). Subsequently, the Normoglycemia in Intensive Care Evaluation–Survival Using Glucose Algorithm Regulation (NICE-SUGAR) trial, an international multicenter prospective RCT, was performed to definitively test the hypothesis that intensive glucose control reduces mortality at 90 days. In this study, intensive glucose control increased mortality among adults, both surgical and nonsurgical, in the ICU: A blood glucose target of 180 mg/dL or lower resulted in lower mortality than did a target of 81 to 108 mg/dL (489). Patients with a primary diagnosis of sepsis accounted for between 20% and 25% of patients in the study. Meta-analyses, both including and excluding the NICE-SUGAR trial, have supported this finding (490,491).

Stress-dose steroids should not be routinely administered at presentation to patients with septic shock. Several previous large randomized, double-blind, multicenter trials have definitively demonstrated that administration of immunosuppressive (15 to 30 mg/kg methylprednisolone equivalent) corticosteroids fail to improve outcome in adult septic shock (475–478). However, some evidence had suggested low "stress-dose" corticosteroids may be beneficial. A "relative" adrenal insufficiency was proposed to exist in a substantial subset of patients with septic shock (276,492). Among other deleterious effects, adrenal insufficiency can result in impairment of catecholamine sensitivity (492–494). Administration of stress-dose steroids (150 to 300 mg hydrocortisone daily equivalent) to patients with septic shock can decrease pressor requirements while suppressing inflammatory markers (493,495,496). One RCT demonstrated that 7 days of therapy with hydrocortisone 50 mg IV every 6 hours and fludrocortisone 50 μg orally once daily generated a significant reduction in mortality in patients with relative adrenal insufficiency (497). Subgroup analysis showed that this improvement was restricted to those who fail to respond to ACTH challenge—about 75% of septic shock patients—with an increase in serum cortisol of at least 250 nmol/L (9 μg/dL). These data were taken to suggest that patients with pressor-dependent septic shock should undergo ACTH challenge on admission followed immediately by initiation of stress-dose steroid therapy. If the ACTH stimulation test was within normal limits, corticosteroids were discontinued. If the test results indicated "relative" adrenal insufficiency, hydrocortisone and fludrocortisone were often continued for 7 days or as otherwise clinically indicated.

The major uncertainty with regard to stress-dose steroid therapy had been the appropriate test and value of serum cortisol to indicate adrenal insufficiency. Various studies supported using random cortisol levels of between 275 and 950 nmol/L (10 to 35 μg/dL) during the acute stress or increments of cortisol of 250 nmol/L (9 μg/dL) within the first hour following ACTH stimulation (276,492,497). Although no definitive data existed as to which cutoff value was the best, many clinicians considered a random value of less than 400 nmol/L (15 μg/dL) to be sufficiently suggestive of relative adrenal insufficiency during the shock state to initiate and continue "stress"-dose therapy. Similarly, a value greater than 950 nmol/L (35 μg/dL) during shock has been thought to be sufficiently normal to discontinue stress-dose therapy without further assessment. Values between those two extremes were interpreted to be an indication for ACTH challenge with a response of less than 250 nmol/L (9 μg/dL) supporting the need for steroid therapy. Unfortunately, one major study challenged these accepted cutoffs in the critically ill by questioning the scientific validity of using total as opposed to free serum concentrations of serum cortisol in such patients (498).

Of greatest concern, a major, multicenter placebo-controlled double-blind RCT of septic shock has failed to confirm an improvement in survival regardless of ACTH responsiveness (499,500). The steroid group did exhibit a reduction in pressor days and total number of organ failures, due to faster resolution of cardiovascular failure, but also had a higher incidence of super-infections and associated sepsis/septic shock events (499,500). Confounding these results, the steroid regimen (hydrocortisone alone) differed from the regimen used in the previous positive study and also could be implemented as late as 72 hours following the onset of septic shock.

Based on these data, "stress"- or "low-dose" steroid therapy should not be considered part of the routine management of septic shock pending further definitive trials. Neither should assessment of ACTH response be routinely assessed. Corticosteroids may hold some utility to reduce the amount or hasten liberation from vasopressors.

Endotracheal intubation and MV should be considered early in the management of all patients with sepsis with organ failure. Airway intubation is indicated for all patients with impaired airway protection reflexes, for example, as a consequence of cerebral hypoperfusion or septic encephalopathy, refractory hypoxemia, respiratory acidosis, or respiratory distress associated with ongoing hypotension/hypoperfusion. Though not yet addressed by systematic studies, clinical experience suggests that respiratory arrest is a significant risk in such patients. These observations are consistent with observations of respiratory muscle compromise and respiratory failure in animal models of septic shock (506,507).

Low-volume (6 to 8 mL/kg ideal body weight), pressure-limited ventilation is indicated in patients with sepsis-associated ARDS. Animal and human studies have suggested that high levels of PEEP and large tidal volumes are associated with increased pulmonary generation of pro-inflammatory cytokines (501,502) and ventilation-induced lung injury (503). ARDS represent a manifestation of MODS which may occur in conjunction with severe sepsis and septic shock. Septic patients with bilateral persistent opacities in association with an acute and persistent defect of oxygenation (PaO_2/FiO_2 ratio of no more than 300, 200, and 100 for mild, moderate, and severe ARDS, respectively) and no clinical evidence of cardiogenic cause fits criteria for the new definition of this syndrome (504). A single large multicenter RCT has demonstrated that ventilation of critically ill patients with ARDS using a low tidal volume, 6 to 8 mL/kg ideal body weight, reduces all-cause absolute mortality by 10%—from 40% to 30%, a 25% relative risk reduction. Available evidence also suggests the use of low-volume, pressure-limited ventilation strategy during surgery also improves clinical outcomes in high-risk abdominal source septic patients (505). Patients with severe sepsis or septic shock who meet criteria for ARDS and potentially those at high risk for ARDS should be ventilated with a low-volume, pressure-limited strategy.

Enteral feeding should be implemented within 24 hours of admission to the ICU for most patients with sepsis and septic shock. parenteral feeding should only be utilized if enteral feeding is not possible despite best efforts. Meta-analyses suggest that early enteral feeding lowers risk of infection and improves survival compared to delayed feeding in the critically ill (508). These findings are consistent with animal studies demonstrating that enteral nutrition maintains gut mucosal integrity, decreases bacterial translocation, and limits the systemic inflammatory response to bacterial toxins (509). Diminished bowel sounds should not prevent a trial of enteral feeding. Few patients will fail to tolerate enteral feeding if a small bowel tube is utilized. Studies of parenteral feeding in the ICU have, in general, failed to demonstrate an improvement in mortality in critically ill patients (510). Other studies demonstrate the superiority of enteral over parenteral feeding in critically ill patients with respect to costs and complications including risk of infection (509,511). Despite these data, a recent large multicenter RCT comparing early parenteral and enteral feeding found no difference in infection risk or mortality (512). Pending additional confirmatory studies, however, enteral feeding should still be preferred.

A hemoglobin target of 7 g/dL is sufficient during the resuscitation of septic shock in patients not known to have an acute coronary syndrome. The Transfusion Requirements in Critical Care (TRICC) Trial, a randomized study of a conservative (7 g/dL target) versus liberal (9 g/dL target) transfusion strategy yielded similar survival in critically ill adult ICU patients (513). However, the applicability to septic shock has been uncertain given the results of the pivotal EGDT study by Rivers and colleagues (313) which suggested improved survival using a resuscitation protocol that included a hemoglobin target of 9 g/dL. This question has recently been answered in a large multicenter RCT which showed the absence of a difference in the frequency of occurrence of either ischemic events, other adverse events or deaths in adult septic shock patients—patients with acute coronary syndrome excluded—treated with a liberal or conservative transfusion target identical to those in the TRICC trial (514). This approach is supported by the recent studies which have failed to replicate the findings of the original Rivers trial (313,315–317). A conservative transfusion threshold of 7 g/dL is appropriate in the majority of adult patients with septic shock.

CONCLUSION

Severe sepsis and septic shock continue to be a major cause of mortality and morbidity among patients requiring ICU support. In recent years, both basic and clinical research in the field has accelerated substantially. This has led to the publication of an increasing number of studies with major implications regarding the appropriate management of patients with these conditions.

TABLE 46.15 Timeline of Implementation of Recommended Diagnostic and Therapeutic Interactions

Time	Resuscitation	Antimicrobials	Vasopressors/ Inotropes	Monitoring	Specific Therapy	Supportive Therapy
1st hr	-Initiation of crystalloid fluid resuscitation (500 mL every 10–15 min) titrating to HR < 100, MAP ≥ 65 mmHg and urine output ≥ 0.5 mL/hr	-Initiation of empiric, broad-spectrum, high dose antimicrobial therapy with 2 or more cidal drugs where possible		-Implement continuous monitoring of ECG, arterial saturation, blood pressure and UO		-Supplemental oxygen -Consider intubation and mechanical ventilation prior to overt respiratory distress
1–8 hrs	-Titrate fluid resuscitation to elimination of base deficit and normalization of serum lactate	-Initiate radiographic investigation for localization and delineation of infection -Implement source control if necessary	-Initiate vasopressor therapy if circulatory shock persists following adequate fluid resuscitation -Initiate Inotropes if CI or SVO2 are persistently decreased	-ICU transfer with full monitoring support -Arterial catheter assessment -If shock persists with >2 L crystalloid resuscitation, venous catheter assessment ± placement (goal CVP ≥8 mmHg)		
8–24 hr	-Dynamic evaluation of resuscitative goals (based on clinical and invasive monitoring end points)		-Consider vasopressin if shock refractory to first-line vasopressors persists	-If persistently pressor-dependent after 3–5 L crystalloid infusion, CVP ≥ 8 achieved, suspicion of intravascular volume depletion or limited cardiovascular reserve, echocardiogram or PAC placement (initial goal PWP 12–15 mmHg)—may be inserted earlier if clinically indicated	-Consider polyclonal immunoglobulin therapy for streptococcal toxic shock	-Initiate enteral feeding
>24 hr		-Narrow antimicrobial regimen depending on isolation of pathogenic organisms and/or clinical improvement -Reassess necessity for or efficacy of source control		-Consider PAC in vasopressor-dependent patients with progressive respiratory, renal or multiple organ dysfunction		-Intensive hemodialysis therapy for renal failure -Low-pressure, volume-limited ventilation for ARDS

Many of these new studies have refuted several different therapies that had previously been accepted including drotrecogin-α (activated), low-dose corticosteroids, tight glucose control, and EGDT (33,313,486,497). Nonetheless, outcome can most likely be improved by taking a systematic approach to therapy as described in Table 46.15. Studies focusing on antimicrobial and supportive elements of therapies clearly demonstrate that close attention to established treatments can have a substantial impact on survival in severe sepsis and septic shock.

Key Points

- The incidence of sepsis and septic shock continues to rise although the case fatality rate has fallen in recent years.
- Sepsis can be defined as the systemic response to severe infection. Sepsis causing organ failure is termed severe sepsis; when that organ failure is cardiovascular in nature with persistent hypotension and tissue hypoperfusion, septic shock exists.
- Increasing age and male gender are risk factors for the development of severe sepsis and septic shock.
- A multitude of organisms including bacteria and fungi can cause sepsis, severe sepsis, and septic shock.
- Microbial antigens, pro- and anti-inflammatory cytokines, coagulation factors, and intracellular mediators all play a role in the generation of the septic response.
- Nitric oxide appears to be a central mediator of cardiovascular collapse in septic shock.
- Genetic factors have been shown to be associated with infection and sepsis predisposition and outcome.
- In order to allow early initiation of appropriate therapy, the initial diagnosis of septic shock should be made on clinical grounds based on suspicion/documentation of infection, persistent hypotension, and the absence of an obvious alternate cause.
- The initial history should focus on two major areas: Key symptoms with respect to diagnosis of sepsis and of the specific site of infection, and key factors that would modify initial empiric therapies such as antimicrobials, fluid resuscitation, and, possibly, vasopressors or inotropes.
- The initial physical examination should focus on ensuring patient stability and on rapid localization of the site of infection.
- Management of sepsis requires consideration of both global and regional perfusion defects making the establishment of goals for therapy more complex than for other forms of shock.
- Initial resuscitation of septic patients should be aimed at rapid intravascular volume expansion to specific clinical end points using isotonic crystalloid solutions.
- If vasopressor therapy is indicated, norepinephrine and dopamine are both effective as initial therapy; a target MAP of 65 mmHg is sufficient in most patients.
- Early appropriate antimicrobial therapy and source control (where indicated) are key determinants of survival in septic shock.
- Invasive monitoring using a PAC is not recommended for routine use in patients with severe sepsis or septic shock.

References

1. Angus DC, Linde-Zwirble WT, Lidicker J, et al. Epidemiology of severe sepsis in the United States: analysis of incidence, outcome, and associated costs of care. *Crit Care Med.* 2001;29:1303–1310.
2. Finland M, Jones WF, Barnes MW. Occurence of serious bacterial infections since the introduction of antibacterial agents. *JAMA.* 1959;84:2188–2197.
3. Hemminki E, Paakkulainen A. Effect of antibiotics on mortality from infectious diseases in Sweden and Finland. *Am J Public Health* 1976;66:1180–1184.
4. Kreger BE, Craven DE, McCabe WR. Gram-negative bacteremia. IV. Reevaluation of clinical features and treatment in 612 patients. *Am J Med.* 1980;68(3):344–355.
5. Martin GS, Mannino DM, Eaton S, Moss M. The epidemiology of sepsis in the United States from 1979 through 2000. *N Engl J Med.* 2003;348(16):1546–1554.
6. Minino AM, Heron MP, Smith BL. Deaths: preliminary data for 2004. *Natl Vital Stat Rep (CDC).* 2006;54(19):1–52.
7. Friedman G, Silva E, Vincent JL. Has the mortality of septic shock changed with time. *Crit Care Med.* 1998;26(12):2078–2086.
8. Geroulanos S, Douka ET. Historical perspective of the word "sepsis". *Intensive Care Med.* 2006;32:2077.
9. Budelmann G, Budelmann G. [Hugo Schottmuller, 1867–1936. The problem of sepsis]. *Internist(Berl).* 1969;10(3):92–101.
10. Bone R, American College of Chest Physicians/Society of Critical Care Medicine Consensus Conference. Definitions for sepsis and organ failure and guidelines for the use of innovative therapies in sepsis. *Crit Care Med.* 1992;20:864–874.
11. Levy MM, Fink MP, Marshall JC, et al. 2001 SCCM/ES Intensive Care Med./ACCP/ATS/SIS International Sepsis Definitions Conference. *Crit Care Med.* 2003;31(4):1250–1256.
12. Marshall JC, Cook DJ, Christou NV, et al. Multiple organ dysfunction score: a reliable descriptor of a complex clinical outcome. *Crit Care Med.* 1995;23(10):1638–1652.
13. Ferreira FL, Bota DP, Bross A, et al. Serial evaluation of the SOFA score to predict outcome in critically ill patients. *JAMA.* 2001;286(14):1754–1758.
14. Bone RC, Bone RC. Immunologic dissonance: a continuing evolution in our understanding of the systemic inflammatory response syndrome (SIRS) and the multiple organ dysfunction syndrome (MODS). *Ann Intern Med.* 1996;125(8):680–687.
15. Czura CJ. "Merinoff symposium 2010: sepsis"—speaking with one voice. *Mol Med.* 2011;17:2.
16. Kaukonen KM, Bailey M, Pilcher D, et al. Systemic inflammatory response syndrome criteria in defining severe sepsis. *N Engl J Med.* 2015;372(17):1629–1638.
17. Hall MJ, National Center for Health Statistics C. Inpatient care for septicemia or sepsis: a challenge for patients and hospitals. NCHS Data Brief 2011. Available at: www.cdc.gov/nchs/data/databriefs/db62.pdf.
18. Padkin A, Goldfrad C, Brady AR, et al. Epidemiology of severe sepsis occurring in the first 24 hrs in intensive care units in England, Wales, and Northern Ireland. *Crit Care Med.* 2003;31(9):2332–2338.
19. Finfer SBR, Lipman J, French C, et al. Adult-population incidence of severe sepsis in Australian and New Zealand intensive care units. *Intensive Care Med.* 2004;30:589–596.
20. Brun-Buisson C, Meshaka P, Pinton P, Vallet B. EPISEPSIS: a reappraisal of the epidemiology and outcome of severe sepsis in French intensive care units. *Intensive Care Med.* 2004;30(4):580–588.
21. Sundararajan V, Macisaac CM, Presneill JJ, et al. Epidemiology of sepsis in Victoria, Australia. *Crit Care Med.* 2005;33(1):71–80.
22. Danai P, Martin GS. Epidemiology of sepsis: recent advances. *Curr Infect Dis Rep.* 2005;7:329–334.
23. Brun-Buisson C, Doyon F, Carlet J, et al. Incidence, risk factors, and outcome of severe sepsis and septic shock in adults: a multicenter prospective study in intensive care units. *JAMA.* 1995;274:968–974.
24. Annane D, Aegerter P, Jars-Guincestre MC, et al. Current epidemiology of septic shock: the CUB-Rea Network. *Am J Resp Crit Care Med.* 2003;168(2):165–172.
25. Sands KE, Bates DW, Lanken PN, et al. Epidemiology of sepsis syndrome in 8 academic medical centers. *JAMA.* 1997;278(3):234–240.
26. Pakhale S, Roberts D, Light B, et al. A geographically and temporally comprehensive analysis of septic shock: impact of age, sex and socioeconomic status. *Crit Care Med.* 2005;33(12):103.
27. Zhan C, Miller MR, Zhan C, Miller MR. Excess length of stay, charges, and mortality attributable to medical injuries during hospitalization. *JAMA.* 2003;290(14):1868–1874.
28. Torio CM, Andrews RM. National inpatient hospital costs: the most expensive conditions by payer, 2011. Healthcare Cost and Utilization

Statistical Brief #160, AHRQ 2013. Available at: www.hcup-us.ahrq.gov/reports/statbriefs/sb160.pdf.
29. Murphy SL, Xu J, Kochanek KD. Deaths: preliminary data for 2010. *National Vital Statistic Reports*. 2012;60(4):1–51. Available at: www.cdc.gov/nchs/data/nvsr/nvsr60/nvsr60_04.pdf.
30. Rhee C, Gohil S, Klompas M. Regulatory mandates for sepsis care—reasons for caution. *N Engl J Med*. 2014;370(18):1673–1676.
31. Gaieski DF, Edwards JM, Kallan MJ, Carr BG. Benchmarking the incidence and mortality of severe sepsis in the united states. *Crit Care Med*. 2013;41(5):1167–1174.
32. Kumar A, Roberts D, Wood KE, et al. Duration of hypotension before initiation of effective antimicrobial therapy is the critical determinant of survival in human septic shock. *Crit Care Med*. 2006;34(6):1589–1596.
33. Bernard GR, Vincent JL, Laterre PF, et al. Recombinant human Protein C Worldwide Evaluation in Severe Sepsis (PROWESS) study group: efficacy and safety of recombinant human activated protein C for severe sepsis. *N Engl J Med*. 2001;344(10):699–709.
34. Warren BL, Eid A, Singer P, et al. High-dose antithrombin III in severe sepsis: a randomized controlled trial. *JAMA*. 2001;286(15):1869–1878.
35. Abraham E, Reinhart K, Opal S, et al. Efficacy and safety of tifacogin (recombinant tissue factor pathway inhibitor) in severe sepsis: a randomized controlled trial. *JAMA*. 2003;290(2):238–247.
36. Abraham E, Laterre PF, Garg R, et al. Drotrecogin alfa (activated) for adults with severe sepsis and a low risk of death. *N Engl J Med*. 2005;353(13):1332–1341.
37. O'Brien JM Jr, Lu B, Ali NA, et al. Alcohol dependence is independently associated with sepsis, septic shock, and hospital mortality among adult intensive care unit patients. *Crit Care Med*. 2007;35(2):345–350.
38. Rangel-Frausto MS, Pittet D, et al. The natural history of the systemic inflammatory response syndrome (SIRS): a prospective study. *JAMA*. 1995;273(2):117–123.
39. Loeb HS, Cruz A, Teng CY, et al. Haemodynamic studies in shock associated with infection. *Br Heart J*. 1967;29(6):883–894.
40. Weil MH, Shubin H, Biddle M. Shock caused by gram-negative microorganisms. *Ann Intern Med*. 1964;60:384–400.
41. Kasal J, Jovanovic Z, Clermont G, et al. Comparison of Cox and Gray's survival models in severe sepsis. *Crit Care Med*. 2004;32(3):700–707.
42. Parker MM, Shelhamer JH, Natanson C, et al. Serial cardiovascular variables in survivors and nonsurvivors of human septic shock: heart rate as an early predictor of prognosis. *Crit Care Med*. 1987;15:923–929.
43. Alberti C, Brun-Buisson C, Burchardi H, et al. Epidemiology of sepsis and infection in ICU patients from an international multicentre cohort study. *Intensive Care Med*. 2002;28(2):108–121.
44. Richards MJ, Edwards JR, Culver DH, Gaynes RP. Nosocomial infections in medical intensive care units in the United States. *Crit Care Med*. 1999;27(5):887–892.
45. Wisplinghoff H, Bischoff T, Tallent SM, et al. Nosocomial bloodstream infections in US hospitals: analysis of 24,179 cases from a prospective nationwide surveillance study. *Clin Infect Dis*. 2004;39(3):309–317.
46. Vincent J, Rello J, Marshall J, et al. International study of the prevalence and outcomes of infection in intensive care units. *JAMA*. 2009;302(21):2323–2329.
47. Macphail GL, Taylor GD, Buchanan-Chell M, et al. Epidemiology, treatment and outcome of candidemia: a five-year review at three Canadian hospitals. *Mycoses*. 2002;45(5–6):141–145.
48. Berrouane YF, Herwaldt LA, Pfaller MA. Trends in antifungal use and epidemiology of nosocomial yeast infections in a university hospital. *J Clin Microbiol*. 1999;37(3):531–537.
49. Abi-Said D, Anaissie E, Uzun O, et al. The epidemiology of hematogenous candidiasis caused by different Candida species. *Clin Infect Dis*. 1997;24(6):1122–1128.
50. Giamarellou H, Giamarellou H. Multidrug resistance in gram-negative bacteria that produce extended-spectrum beta-lactamases (ESBLs). *Clin Microbiol Infect*. 2005;11(Suppl 4):1–16.
51. Doi Y, Paterson DL. Carbapenemase-producing Enterobacteriaceae. *Semin Resp Crit Care Med*. 2015;36(1):74–84.
52. Murray BE, Murray BE. Vancomycin-resistant enterococcal infections. *N Engl J Med*. 2000;342(10):710–721.
53. Miller LG, Perdreau-Remington F, Rieg G, et al. Necrotizing fasciitis caused by community-associated methicillin-resistant Staphylococcus aureus in Los Angeles. *N Engl J Med*. 2005;352(14):1445–1453.
54. From the Centers for Disease Control. Staphylococcus aureus resistant to vancomycin—United States, 2002. *JAMA*. 2002;288(7):824–825.
55. Kumar A, Ellis P, Arabi Y, et al. Initiation of inappropriate antimicrobial therapy results in a five-fold reduction of survival in human septic shock. *Chest*. 2009;136(5):1237–1248.
56. Vincent JL, Bihari DJ, Suter PM, et al. The prevalence of nosocomial infection in intensive care units in Europe: results of the European Prevalence of Infection in Intensive Care (EPIC) study. *JAMA*. 1995;274(8):639–644.
57. Ranieri VM, Thompson BT, Barie PS, et al. Drotrecogin alfa (activated) in adults with septic shock. *N Engl J Med*. 2012;366(22):2055–2064.
58. Heumann D, Glauser MP, Calandra T. Molecular basis of host-pathogen interaction in septic shock. *Curr Opin Microbiol*. 1998;1(1):49–55.
59. Hemmi H, Takeuchi O, Kawai T, et al. A toll-like receptor recognizes bacterial DNA. *Nature*. 2000;408(6813):740–745.
60. Bauer S, Kirschning CJ, Hacker H, et al. Human TLR9 confers responsiveness to bacterial DNA via species-specific CpG motif recognition. *Proc Natl Acad Sci USA*. 2001;98(16):9237–9242.
61. Sparwasser T, Miethke T, Lipford G, et al. Bacterial DNA causes septic shock. *Nature*. 1997;386(6623):336–337.
62. Alexopoulou L, Holt AC, Medzhitov R, Flavell RA. Recognition of double-stranded RNA and activation of NF-kappaB by toll-like receptor 3. *Nature*. 2001;413(6857):732–738.
63. Dziarski R, Wang Q, Miyake K, et al. MD-2 enables toll-like receptor 2 (TLR2)-mediated responses to lipopolysaccharide and enhances TLR2-mediated responses to gram-positive and gram-negative bacteria and their cell wall components. *J Immunol*. 2001;166(3):1938–1944.
64. Yang RB, Mark MR, Gray A, et al. toll-like receptor-2 mediates lipopolysaccharide-induced cellular signalling. *Nature*. 1998;395(6699):284–288.
65. Lien E, Sellati TJ, Yoshimura A, et al. Toll-like receptor 2 functions as a pattern recognition receptor for diverse bacterial products. *J Biol Chem*. 1999;274(47):33419–33425.
66. Schwandner R, Dziarski R, Wesche H, et al. Peptidoglycan- and lipoteichoic acid-induced cell activation is mediated by toll-like receptor 2. *J Biol Chem*. 1999;274(25):17406–17409.
67. Manocha S, Feinstein D, Kumar A, Kumar A. Novel therapies for sepsis: antiendotoxin therapies. *Exp Opin Invest Drugs*. 2002;11(12):1795–1812.
68. Martich GD, Boujoukos AJ, Suffredini AF. Response of man to endotoxin. *Immunobiology*. 1993;187(3–5):403–416.
69. Ing DJ, Zang J, Dzau VJ, et al. Modulation of cytokine-induced cardiac myocyte apoptosis by nitric oxide, Bak, and Bcl-x. *Circ Res*. 1999;84:21–33.
70. Albelda SM, Smith CW, Ward PA. Adhesion molecules and inflammatory injury. *FASEB J*. 1994;8:504–512.
71. Balligand JL, Ungureanu-Longrois D, Simmons WW, et al. Cytokine-inducible nitric oxide synthase (iNOS) expression in cardiac myocytes. *J Biol Chem*. 1994;269:27580–27588.
72. Esmon CT. Role of coagulation inhibitors in inflammation. *Thromb Haemost*. 2001;86(1):51–56.
73. Heumann D. CD14 and LBP in endotoxemia and infections caused by gram-negative bacteria. *J Endotoxin Res*. 2001;7(6):439–441.
74. Raetz CR, Ulevitch RJ, Wright SD, et al. Gram-negative endotoxin: an extraordinary lipid with profound effects on eukaryotic signal transduction. *FASEB J*. 1991;5(12):2652–2660.
75. Rietschel ET, Kirikae T, Schade FU, et al. Bacterial endotoxin: molecular relationships of structure to activity and function. *FASEB J*. 1994;8(2):217–225.
76. Hellman J, Warren HS. Antiendotoxin strategies. *Infect Dis Clin North Am*. 1999;13(2):371–386.
77. Kumar A, Zanotti S, Bunnell G, et al. Interleukin-10 blunts the human inflammatory response to lipopolysaccharide without affecting the cardiovascular response. *Crit Care Med*. 2005;33(2):331–340.
78. Kumar A, Bunnell E, Lynn M, et al. Experimental human endotoxemia is associated with depression of load-independent contractility indices: prevention by the lipid a analogue E5531. *Chest*. 2004;126(3):860–867.
79. Suffredini AF, Reda D, Banks SM, et al. Effects of recombinant dimeric TNF receptor on human inflammatory responses following intravenous endotoxin administration. *J Immunol*. 1995;155(10):5038–5045.
80. Le Roy D, Di Padova F, Tees R, et al. Monoclonal antibodies to murine lipopolysaccharide (LPS)-binding protein (LBP) protect mice from lethal endotoxemia by blocking either the binding of LPS to LBP or the presentation of LPS/LBP complexes to CD14. *J Immunol*. 1999;162(12):7454–7460.
81. Schumann RR, Leong SR, Flaggs GW, et al. Structure and function of lipopolysaccharide binding protein. *Science*. 1990;249(4975):1429–1431.
82. Heumann D, Barras C, Severin A, et al. Gram-positive cell walls stimulate synthesis of tumor necrosis factor alpha and interleukin-6 by human monocytes. *Infect Immun*. 1994;62(7):2715–2721.
83. Mattsson E, Rollof J, Verhoef J, et al. Serum-induced potentiation of tumor necrosis factor alpha production by human monocytes in response to staphylococcal peptidoglycan: involvement of different serum factors. *Infect Immun*. 1994;62(9):3837–3843.

84. Wright SD, Ramos RA, Tobias PS, et al. CD14, a receptor for complexes of lipopolysaccharide (LPS) and LPS binding protein. *Science.* 1990;249(4975):1431–1433.
85. Hailman E, Lichenstein HS, Wurfel MM, et al. Lipopolysaccharide (LPS)-binding protein accelerates the binding of LPS to CD14. *J Exp Med.* 1994;179(1):269–277.
86. Ingalls RR, Golenbock DT, Ingalls RR, Golenbock DT. CD11c/CD18, a transmembrane signaling receptor for lipopolysaccharide. *J Exp Med.* 1995;181(4):1473–1479.
87. Kusunoki T, Hailman E, Juan TS, et al. Molecules from Staphylococcus aureus that bind CD14 and stimulate innate immune responses. *J Exp Med.* 1995; 182(6):1673–1682.
88. Kirschning CJ, Wesche H, Merrill AT, Rothe M. Human toll-like receptor 2 confers responsiveness to bacterial lipopolysaccharide. *J Exp Med.* 1998;188(11):2091–2097.
89. Hoshino K, Takeuchi O, Kawai T, et al. Cutting edge: toll-like receptor 4 (TLR4)-deficient mice are hyporesponsive to lipopolysaccharide: evidence for TLR4 as the Lps gene product. *J Immunol.* 1999;162(7):3749–3752.
90. Takeuchi O, Hoshino K, Kawai T, et al. Differential roles of TLR2 and TLR4 in recognition of gram-negative and gram-positive bacterial cell wall components. *Immunity.* 1999;11(4):443–451.
91. Chow JC, Young DW, Golenbock DT, et al. Toll-like receptor-4 mediates lipopolysaccharide-induced signal transduction. *J Biol Chem.* 1999;274(16): 10689–10692.
92. Tauszig S, Jouanguy E, Hoffmann JA, Imler JL. Toll-related receptors and the control of antimicrobial peptide expression in Drosophila. *Proc Natl Acad Sci U S A.* 2000;97(19):10520–10525.
93. Lien E, Means TK, Heine H, et al. Toll-like receptor 4 imparts ligand-specific recognition of bacterial lipopolysaccharide. *J Clin Invest.* 2000;105(4): 497–504.
94. Muroi M, Ohnishi T, Tanamoto K, et al. MD-2, a novel accessory molecule, is involved in species-specific actions of Salmonella lipid A. *Infect Immun.* 2002;70(7):3546–3550.
95. Muroi M, Ohnishi T, Tanamoto K, et al. Regions of the mouse CD14 molecule required for toll-like receptor 2- and 4-mediated activation of NF-kappa B. *J Biol Chem.* 2002;277(44):42372–42379.
96. Muller-Alouf H, Alouf JE, Gerlach D, et al. Human pro- and anti-inflammatory cytokine patterns induced by Streptococcus pyogenes erythrogenic (pyrogenic) exotoxin A and C superantigens. *Infect Immun.* 1996; 64(4):1450–1453.
97. Cohen J, Cohen J. The immunopathogenesis of sepsis. *Nature.* 2002;420 (6917):885–891.
98. Docke WD, Randow F, Syrbe U, et al. Monocyte deactivation in septic patients: restoration by IFN-gamma treatment. *Nat Med.* 1997;3(6):678–681.
99. Mira JP, Cariou A, Grall F, et al. Association of TNF2, a TNF-alpha promoter polymorphism, with septic shock susceptibility and mortality: a multicenter study. *JAMA.* 1999;282(2):561–568.
100. Holmes CL, Russell JA, Walley KR. Genetic polymorphisms in sepsis and septic shock: role in prognosis and potential for therapy. *Chest.* 2003; 124(3):1103–1115.
101. Nathan C. Nitric oxide as a secretory product of mammalian cells. *FASEB J.* 1992;6:3051–3064.
102. Lorente JA, Landin L, Renes E, et al. Role of nitric oxide in the hemodynamic changes of sepsis. *Crit Care Med.* 1993;21(5):759–767.
103. Kilbourn RG, Gross SS, Jubran A, et al. N-methyl-L-arginine inhibits tumor necrosis factor-induced hypotension: implications for the involvement of nitric oxide. *Proc Natl Acad Sci U S A.* 1990;87:3629–3633.
104. Thiemermann C, Szabö C, Mitchell JA, Vane JR. Vascular hyporeactivity to vasoconstrictor agents and hemodynamic decompensation in hemorrhagic shock is mediated by nitric oxide. *Proc Natl Acad Sci.* 1993;90:267–271.
105. Kubes P. Nitric oxide modulates microvascular permeability. *Am J Physiol.* 1992;262(2):H611–H615.
106. Kumar A, Thota V, Dee L, et al. Tumor necrosis factor-alpha and interleukin-1 beta are responsible for depression of in vitro myocardial cell contractility induced by serum from humans with septic shock. *J Exp Med.* 1996;183(3):949–958.
107. Kumar A, Krieger A, Symeoneides S, et al. Myocardial dysfunction in septic shock. Part II: role of cytokines and nitric oxide. *J Cardiothorac Vasc Surg.* 2001;15(4):485–511.
108. Beckman JS, Beckman TW, Chen J, et al. Apparent hydroxyl radical production by peroxynitrite: implications for endothelial injury from nitric oxide and superoxide. *Proc Natl Acad Sci U S A.* 1990;87(4):1620–1624.
109. Muta T, Iwanaga S, Muta T, Iwanaga S. Clotting and immune defense in Limulidae. *Progr Mol Subcell Biol.* 1996;15:154–189.
110. Nachum R, Nachum R. Antimicrobial defense mechanisms in Limulus polyphemus. *Progr Clin Biol Res.* 1979;29:513–524.
111. Engelmann B, Massberg S. Thrombosis as an intravascular effector of innate immunity. *Nature Rev Immunol.* 2013;13(1):34–45.
112. Loof TG, Schmidt O, Herwald H, Theopold U. Coagulation systems of invertebrates and vertebrates and their roles in innate immunity: the same side of two coins? *J Innate Immun.* 2011;3(1):34–40.
113. McGilvray ID, Rotstein OD, McGilvray ID, Rotstein OD. Role of the coagulation system in the local and systemic inflammatory response. *World J Surg.* 1998;22(2):179–186.
114. Wheeler AP, Bernard GR. Treating patients with severe sepsis. *N Engl J Med.* 1999;340:207–214.
115. Gando S, Nanzaki S, Sasaki S. Activation of the extrinsic coagulation pathway in patients with severe sepsis and septic shock. *Crit Care Med.* 1998;26(12):2005–2009.
116. Mesters R, Helterbrand J, Utterback BG. Prognostic value of protein C concentrations in neutropenic patients at high risk of severe septic complications. *Crit Care Med.* 2000;28(7):2209–2216.
117. Rosenberg RD, Aird WC. Vascular-bed-specific hemostasis and hypercoagulable states. *N Engl J Med.* 1999;340(20):1555–1564.
118. van der Poll T, Bueller HR, tenCate H, et al. Activation of coagulation after administration of tumor necrosis factor to normal subjects. *N Engl J Med.* 1990;322(23):1622–1627.
119. Esmon NL, Esmon CT. Protein C and the endothelium. *Semin Thromb Hemostat.* 1988;14:210–215.
120. Mesters R, Mannucci PM, Coppola E. Factor VIIA and anti-thrombin III activity during severe sepsis and septic shock in neutropenic patients. *Blood.* 1996;88:881–886.
121. Abraham E. Tissue factor inhibition and clinical trial results of tissue factor pathway inhibitor in sepsis. *Crit Care Med.* 2000;28(9 Suppl):S31–S33.
122. Abraham E, Reinhart K, Svoboda P, et al. Assessment of the safety of recombinant tissue factor pathway inhibitor in patients with severe sepsis: a multicenter, randomized, placebo-controlled, single-blind, dose escalation study. *Crit Care Med.* 2001;29(11):2081–2089.
123. Sorensen TI, Nielsen GG, Andersen PK, et al. Genetic and environmental influences on premature death in adult adoptees. *N Engl J Med.* 1988;318(12): 727–732.
124. Namath A, Patterson AJ. Genetic polymorphisms in sepsis. *Crit Care Nurs Clin North Am.* 2011;23(1):181–202.
125. Arcaroli J, Fessler MB, Abraham E, et al. Genetic polymorphisms and sepsis. *Shock.* 2005;24(4):300–312.
126. Lin MT, Albertson TE, Lin MT, Albertson TE. Genomic polymorphisms in sepsis. *Crit Care Med.* 2004;32(2):569–579.
127. Texereau J, Pene F, Chiche JD, et al. Importance of hemostatic gene polymorphisms for susceptibility to and outcome of severe sepsis. *Crit Care Med.* 2004;32(5 Suppl):S313–S319.
128. Papathanassoglou ED, Giannakopoulou MD, Bozas E, et al. Genomic variations and susceptibility to sepsis. *AACN Adv Crit Care.* 2006;17(4):394–422.
129. Man M, Close S, Shaw A, et al. Beyond single-marker analyses: mining whole genome scans for insights into treatment responses in severe sepsis. *Pharmacogenom J.* 2013;13(3):218–226.
130. Udhoji VN, Weil MH. Hemodynamic and metabolic studies on shock associated with bacteremia. *Ann Intern Med.* 1965;62:966–978.
131. Cohn JD, Greenspan M, Goldstein CR, et al. Arteriovenous shunting in high cardiac output shock syndromes. *Surg Gynecol Obstet.* 1968;127: 282–288.
132. Thijs LG, Groenveld ABJ. Peripheral circulation in septic shock. *Appl Cardiopulm Pathophysiol.* 1988;2:203–214.
133. Wright CJ, Duff JH, McLean APH, MacLean LD. Regional capillary blood flow and oxygen uptake in severe sepsis. *Surg Gynecol Obstet.* 1971;132:637–644.
134. Finley RJ, Duff JH, Holliday RL, et al. Capillary muscle blood flow in human sepsis. *Surgery.* 1975;78:87–94.
135. Cronenwett JL, Lindenauer SM. Direct measurement of arteriovenous anastomic blood flow in the septic canine hindlimb. *Surgery.* 1979;85: 275–282.
136. Dantzker D. Oxygen delivery and utilization in sepsis. *Crit Care Clin.* 1989;5: 81–98.
137. Wolf YG, Cotev S, Perel A, Manny J. Dependence of oxygen consumption on cardiac output in sepsis. *Crit Care Med.* 1987;15:198–203.
138. Shoemaker WC, Chang P, Czer L, et al. Cardiorespiratory monitoring in postoperative patients. I. Prediction of outcome and severity of illness. *Crit Care Med.* 1979;7:237–242.
139. Haupt MT, Gilbert EM, Carlson RW. Fluid loading increases oxygen consumption in septic patients with lactic acidosis. *Am Rev Resp Dis.*1985;131:912–916.
140. Samsel RW, Nelson DP, Sanders WM, et al. Effect of endotoxin on systemic and skeletal muscle oxygen extraction. *J Appl Physiol.* 1988;65:1377–1382.

141. Vincent JL, Roman A, DeBacker D, et al. Oxygen uptake/supply dependency: effects of short-term dobutamine infusion. *Am Rev Resp Dis.* 1990;142:2–8.
142. Fenwick JC, Dodek PM, Ronco JJ, et al. Increased concentrations of plasma lactate predict pathological dependence of oxygen consumption on oxygen delivery in patients with adult respiratory distress syndrome. *J Crit Care.* 1990;5:81–87.
143. Gutierrez G, Pohil RJ. Oxygen consumption is linearly related to oxygen supply in critically ill patients. *J Crit Care.* 1986;1:45–53.
144. De Backer D, Orbegozo Cortes D, Donadello K, Vincent J-L. Pathophysiology of microcirculatory dysfunction and the pathogenesis of septic shock. *Virulence.* 2014;5(1):73–79.
145. Edul VSK, Enrico C, Laviolle B, et al. Quantitative assessment of the microcirculation in healthy volunteers and in patients with septic shock. *Critical care medicine* 2012;40(5):1443–1448.
146. Barcroft J. On anoxaemia. *Lancet.* 1920;2:485–492.
147. Astiz M, Rackow EC, Weil MH, Schumer W. Early impairment of oxidative metabolism and energy production in severe sepsis. *Circ Shock.* 1988;26:311–320.
148. Mizock B. Septic shock: a metabolic perspective. *Arch Intern Med.* 1984; 144:579–585.
149. Fink MP. Cytopathic hypoxia. Mitochondrial dysfunction as mechanism contributing to organ dysfunction in sepsis. *Crit Care Clin.* 2001;17(1): 219–237.
150. Crouser ED, Julian MW, Huff JE, et al. Abnormal permeability of inner and outer mitochondrial membranes contributes independently to mitochondrial dysfunction in the liver during acute endotoxemia. *Crit Care Med.* 2004;32(2):478–488.
151. Vary TC, Hazen S. Sepsis alters pyruvate dehydrogenase kinase activity in skeletal muscle. *Mol Cell Biochem.* 1999;198:113–118.
152. Brealey D, Brand M, Hargreaves I, et al. Association between mitochondrial dysfunction and severity and outcome of septic shock. *Lancet.* 2002;360(9328):219–223.
153. Radi R, Rodriguez M, Castro L, Telleri R. Inhibition of mitochondrial electron transport by peroxynitrite. *Arch Biochem Biophys.* 1994;308:89–95.
154. Galley HF. Oxidative stress and mitochondrial dysfunction in sepsis. *Br J Anaesth.* 2011;107(1):57–64.
155. Goldfarb RD, Marton A, Szabó É, et al. Protective effect of a novel, potent inhibitor of poly (adenosine 5 -diphosphate-ribose) synthetase in a porcine model of severe bacterial sepsis. *Crit Care Med.* 2002;30(5):974–980.
156. VanderMeer TJ, Wang H, Fink MP. Endotoxemia causes ileal mucosal acidosis in the absence of mucosal hypoxia in a normodynamic porcine model of septic shock. *Crit Care Med.* 1995;23(7):1217–1226.
157. Hotchkiss RS, Rust RS, Dence CS, et al. Evaluation of the role of cellular hypoxia in sepsis by the hypoxic marker [18F] fluoromisonidazole. *Am J Physiol.* 1991;261:R965–R972.
158. King CJ, Tytgat S, Delude RL, Fink MP. Ileal mucosal oxygen consumption is decreased in endotoxemic rats but is restored toward normal by treatment with aminoguanidine. *Crit Care Med.* 1999;27(11):2518–2524.
159. Simonson SG, Welty-Wolf K, Huang YT, et al. Altered mitochondrial redox responses in gram negative septic shock in primates. *Circ Shock.* 1994;43(1):34–43.
160. Griebel JA, Moore FA, Piantadosi CA. In-vivo responses of mitochondrial redox levels to Escherichia coli bacteremia in primates. *J Crit Care.* 1990;5:1–9.
161. Cairns CB, Moore FA, Haenel JB, et al. Evidence for early supply independent mitochondrial dysfunction in patients developing multiple organ failure after trauma. *J Trauma Injury Infect Crit Care.* 1997;42(3):532–536.
162. Mori E, Hasebe M, Kobayashi K, Iijima N. Alterations in metabolite levels in carbohydrate and energy metabolism of rat in hemorrhagic shock and sepsis. *Metabolism Clin Exp.* 1987;36:14–20.
163. Tanaka J, Sato T, Kamiyama Y, Jones RT, et al. Bacteremic shock: aspects of high-energy metabolism of rat liver following Escherichia coli injection. *J Surg Res.* 1982;33:49–57.
164. Yassen KA, Galley HF, Lee A, Webster NR. Mitochondrial redox state in the critically ill. *Br J Anaesth.* 1999;83(2):325–327.
165. Grum CM, Simon RH, Dantzker D, et al. Evidence for adenosine triphosphate degradation in critically ill patients. *Chest.* 1985;88:763–767.
166. Ozawa K, Aoyama H, Yasuda K, et al. Metabolic abnormalities associated with postoperative organ failure: a redox theory. *Arch Surg.* 1983;118(11): 1245–1251.
167. Bergstrom J, Bostrom H, Furst P, et al. Preliminary studies of energy-rich phosphagens in muscle from severely ill patients. *Crit Care Med.* 1976;4(4):197–204.
168. Liaw KY, Askanazi J, Michelson CB, et al. Effect of injury and sepsis on high-energy phosphates in muscle and red cells. *J Trauma Injury Infect Crit Care.* 1980;20(9):755–759.
169. Song SK, Hotchkiss RS, Karl IE, Ackerman JJ. Concurrent quantification of tissue metabolism and blood flow via 2H/31P NMR in vivo. III. Alterations of muscle blood flow and metabolism during sepsis. *Magn Reson Med.* 1992;25:67–77.
170. Hotchkiss RS, Karl IE. Reevaluation of the role of cellular hypoxia and bioenergetic failure in sepsis. *JAMA.* 1992;267:1503–1510.
171. Solomon MA, Correa R, Alexander HR, et al. Myocardial energy metabolism and morphology in a canine model of sepsis. *Am J Physiol.* 1994;266:H757–H768.
172. Hotchkiss RS, Song SK, Neil JJ, et al. Sepsis does not impair tricarboxylic acid cycle in the heart. *Am J Physiol.* 1991;260:C50–C57.
173. Chaudry IH, Wichterman KA, Baue AE. Effect of sepsis on tissue adenine nucleotide levels. *Surgery.* 1979;85:205–211.
174. Geller ER, Tankauskas S, Kirpatrick JR. Mitochondrial death in sepsis: a failed concept. *J Surg Res.* 1986;40:514–517.
175. MacLean LD, Mulligan WG, McLean APH, Duff JH. Patterns of septic shock in man: a detailed study of 56 patients. *Ann Surg.* 1967;166:543–562.
176. Nishijima H, Weil MH, Shubin H, Cavanilles J. Hemodynamic and metabolic studies on shock associated with gram-negative bacteremia. *Medicine (Balt).* 1973;52:287–294.
177. Weil MH, Nishijima H. Cardiac output in bacterial shock. *Am J Med.* 1978;64:920–922.
178. Blain CM, Anderson TO, Pietras RJ, Gunnar RM. Immediate hemodynamic effects of gram-negative vs gram-positive bacteremia in man. *Arch Intern Med.* 1970;126:260–265.
179. Packman MI, Rackow EC. Optimum left heart filling pressure during fluid resuscitation of patients with hypovolemic and septic shock. *Crit Care Med.* 1983;11:165–169.
180. Winslow EJ, Loeb HS, Rahimtoola SH, et al. Hemodynamic studies and results of therapy in 50 patients with bacteremic shock. *Am J Med.* 1973;54:421–432.
181. Krausz MM, Perel A, Eimerl D, Cotev S. Cardiopulmonary effects of volume loading in patients with septic shock. *Ann Surg.* 1977;185:429–434.
182. Parker MM, Suffredini AF, Natanson C, Ognibene FP, et al. Responses of left ventricular function in survivors and non-survivors of septic shock. *J Crit Care.* 1989;4:19–25.
183. Teule GJ, Van Lingen A, Verweij-van Vught MA, et al. Role of peripheral pooling in porcine Escherichia coli sepsis. *Circ Shock.* 1984;12:115–123.
184. Natanson C, Fink MP, Ballantyne HK, et al. Gram-negative bacteremia produces both severe systolic and diastolic cardiac dysfunction in a canine model that simulates human septic shock. *J Clin Invest.* 1986;78:259–270.
185. Carroll GC, Snyder JV. Hyperdynamic severe intravascular sepsis depends on fluid administration in cynomolgus monkey. *Am J Physiol.* 1982;243:131–141.
186. Teule GJ, Den Hollander W, Bronsveld W, et al. Effect of volume loading and dopamine on hemodynamics and red cell distribution in canine endotoxic shock. *Circ Shock.* 1983;10:41–50.
187. Magder S, Vanelli G. Circuit factors in the high cardiac output of sepsis. *J Crit Care.* 1996;11(4):155–166.
188. Donnino M, Nguyen HB, Rivers EP. A hemodynamic comparison of early and late phase severe sepsis and septic shock. *Chest.* 2002;122(4):5S.
189. Kumar A, Haery C, Parrillo JE. Myocardial dysfunction in septic shock. Part I. Clinical manifestation of cardiovascular dysfunction. *J Cardiothorac Vasc Anesth.* 2001;15(3):364–376.
190. Ognibene FP, Parker MM, Natanson C, et al. Depressed left ventricular performance. Response to volume infusion in patients with sepsis and septic shock. *Chest.* 1988;93:903–910.
191. Parker MM, Shelhamer JH, Bacharach SL, et al. Profound but reversible myocardial depression in patients with septic shock. *Ann Intern Med.* 1984;100:483–490.
192. Garner LB, Willis MS, Carlson DL, et al. Macrophage migration inhibitory factor is a cardiac-derived myocardial depressant factor. *Am J Physiol.* 2003;285(6):H2500–H2509.
193. Eichenholz PW, Eichacker PQ, Hoffman WD, et al. Tumor necrosis factor challenges in canines: patterns of cardiovascular dysfunction. *Am J Physiol.* 1992;263:H668–H675.
194. Vincent JL, Bakker J, Marecaux G, et al. Administration of anti-TNF antibody improves left ventricular function in septic shock patients: results of a pilot study. *Chest.* 1992;101:810–815.
195. Hosenpud JD, Campbell SM, Mendelson DJ. Interleukin-1-induced myocardial depression in an isolated beating heart preparation. *J Heart Transplant.* 1989;8:460–464.
196. Massey CV, Kohout TR, Gaa ST, et al. Molecular and cellular actions of platelet-activating factor in rat heart cells. *J Clin Invest.* 1991;88: 2106–2116.
197. Schutzer KM, Haglund U, Falk A. Cardiopulmonary dysfunction in a feline septic model: possible role of leukotrienes. *Circ Shock.* 1989;29:13–25.

198. Werdan K, Muller U, Reithmann C. "Negative inotropic cascades" in cardiomyocytes triggered by substances relevant to sepsis. In: Schlag G, Redl H, eds. *Pathophysiology of Shock, Sepsis and Organ Failure*. Berlin: Springer-Verlag; 1993:787–834.
199. Pathan N, Hemingway CA, Alizadeh AA, et al. Role of interleukin 6 in myocardial dysfunction of meningococcal septic shock. *Lancet.* 2004;363(9404):203–209.
200. Papadopoulos MC, Davies DC, Moss RF, et al. Pathophysiology of septic encephalopathy: a review. *Crit Care Med.* 2000;28(8):3019–3024.
201. Sprung CL, Peduzzi PN, Shatney CH, et al. Impact of encephalopathy on mortality in the sepsis syndrome. The Veterans Administration Systemic Sepsis Cooperative Study Group. *Crit Care Med.* 1990;18(8):801–806.
202. Pine RW, Wertz MJ, Lennard ES, et al. Determinants of organ malfunction or death in patients with intra-abdominal sepsis: a discriminant analysis. *Arch Surg.* 1983;118(2):242–249.
203. Young GB, Bolton CF, Austin TW, et al. The encephalopathy associated with septic illness. *Clin Invest Med.* 1990;13(6):297–304.
204. Young GB, Bolton CF, Archibald YM, et al. The electroencephalogram in sepsis-associated encephalopathy. *J Clin Neurophysiol.* 1992;9(1): 145–152.
205. Kollef MH, Sherman G. Acquired organ system derangements and hospital mortality: are all organ systems created equally? *Am J Crit Care.* 1999;8(3):180–188.
206. Piazza O, Russo E, Cotena S, et al. Elevated S100B levels do not correlate with the severity of encephalopathy during sepsis. *Br J Anaesth.* 2007;99(4):518–521.
207. Iacobone E, Bailly-Salin J, Polito A, et al. Sepsis-associated encephalopathy and its differential diagnosis. *Crit Care Med.* 2009;37(10 Suppl): S331–S336.
208. Siami S, Annane D, Sharshar T. The encephalopathy in sepsis. *Crit Care Clin.* 2008;24(1):67–82.
209. Zauner C, Gendo A, Kramer L, et al. Impaired subcortical and cortical sensory evoked potential pathways in septic patients. *Crit Care Med.* 2002;30(5):1136–1139.
210. Taccone FS, Castanares-Zapatero D, Peres-Bota D, et al. Cerebral autoregulation is influenced by carbon dioxide levels in patients with septic shock. *Neurocrit Care.* 2010;12(1):35–42.
211. Taccone FS, Su F, Pierrakos C, et al. Cerebral microcirculation is impaired during sepsis: an experimental study. *Crit Care.* 2010;14(4):R140.
212. De Jonghe B, Lacherade JC, Durand MC, et al. Critical illness neuromuscular syndromes. *Crit Care Clin.* 2006;22(4):805–818.
213. Leijten FS, Harinck-de Weerd JE, Poortvliet DC, et al. The role of polyneuropathy in motor convalescence after prolonged mechanical ventilation. *JAMA.* 1995;274(15):1221–1225.
214. Bercker S, Weber-Carstens S, Deja M, et al. Critical illness polyneuropathy and myopathy in patients with acute respiratory distress syndrome. *Crit Care Med.* 2005;33(4):711–715.
215. Lorin S, Sivak M, Nierman DM. Critical illness polyneuropathy: what to look for in at-risk patients. *J Crit Illness.* 1998;13(10):608–612.
216. Tennila A, Salmi T, Pettila V, et al. Early signs of critical illness polyneuropathy in ICU patients with systemic inflammatory response syndrome or sepsis. *Intensive Care Med.* 2000;26(9):1360–1363.
217. Tepper M, Rakic S, Haas JA, et al. Incidence and onset of critical illness polyneuropathy in patients with septic shock. *Netherlands J Med.* 2000;56(6):211–214.
218. De Jonghe B, Sharshar T, Lefaucheur JP, et al. Paresis acquired in the intensive care unit: a prospective multicenter study. *JAMA.* 2002;288(22):2859–2867.
219. Cunnion RE, Schaer GL, Parker MM, et al. The coronary circulation in human septic shock. *Circulation.* 1986;73:637–644.
220. Dhainaut JF, Huyghebaert MF, Monsallier JF, et al. Coronary hemodynamics and myocardial metabolism of lactate, free fatty acids, glucose, and ketones in patients with septic shock. *Circulation.* 1987;75:533–541.
221. Reilly JM, Cunnion RE, Burch-Whitman C, et al. A circulating myocardial depressant substance is associated with cardiac dysfunction and peripheral hypoperfusion (lactic acidemia) in patients with septic shock. *Chest.* 1989;95:1072–1780.
222. Parrillo JE, Burch C, Shelhamer JH, et al. A circulating myocardial depressant substance in humans with septic shock: septic shock patients with a reduced ejection fraction have a circulating factor that depresses in vitro myocardial cell performance. *J Clin Invest.* 1985;76:1539–1553.
223. Jones SB, Romano RD. Myocardial beta adrenergic receptor coupling to adenylate cyclase during developing septic shock. *Circ Shock.* 1990; 30:51–61.
224. Bristow MR, Ginsburg R, Minobe W, et al. Decreased catecholamine sensitivity and beta adrenergic receptor density in failing human hearts. *N Engl J Med.* 1982;307:205–210.
225. Silverman HJ, Penaranda R, Orens JB, Lee NH. Impaired ß-adrenergic receptor stimulation of cyclic adenosine monophosphate in human septic shock: Association with myocardial hyporesponsiveness to catecholamines. *Crit Care Med.* 1993;21:31–39.
226. Kumar A, Brar R, Wang P, et al. The role of nitric oxide and cyclic GMP in human septic serum-induced depression of cardiac myocyte contractility. *Am J Physiol.* 1999;276:R265–R276.
227. Anel R, Paladugu B, Makkena R, et al. TNFα induces a proximal defect of ß-adrenoreceptor signal transduction in cardiac myocytes. *Crit Care Med.* 1999;27:A95.
228. Gulick T, Chung MK, Pieper SJ, et al. Interleukin-1 and tumor necrosis factor inhibit cardiac myocyte adrenergic responsiveness. *Proc Natl Acad Sci U S A.* 1989;86:6753–6757.
229. Chung MK, Gulick TS, Rotondo RE, et al. Mechanism of cytokine inhibition of beta-adrenergic agonist stimulation of cyclic AMP in rat cardiac myoctyes: impairment of signal transduction. *Circ Res.* 1990;67:753–763.
230. Raper RF, Sibbald WJ, Driedger AA, Gerow K. Relative myocardial depression in normotensive sepsis. *J Crit Care.* 1989;4:9–18.
231. Antonucci E, Fiaccadori E, Donadello K, et al. Myocardial depression in sepsis: from pathogenesis to clinical manifestations and treatment. *J Crit Care.* 2014;29(4):500–511.
232. Kumar A, Schupp E, Bunnell E, et al. Cardiovascular response to dobutamine predicts outcome in severe sepsis and septic shock. *Crit Care.* 2008;12(2):R35–R46.
233. Turner A, Tsamitros M, Bellomo R. Myocardial cell injury in septic shock. *Crit Care Med.* 1999;27(9):1775–1780.
234. ver Elst KM, Spapen HD, Nguyen DN, et al. Cardiac troponins I and T are biological markers of left ventricular dysfunction in septic shock. *Clin Chem.* 2000;46(5):650–657.
235. Mehta NJ, Khan IA, Gupta V, et al. Cardiac troponin I predicts myocardial dysfunction and adverse outcome in septic shock. *Int J Cardiol.* 2004;95(1):13–17.
236. Schrier RW, Wang W, Schrier RW, Wang W. Acute renal failure and sepsis. *N Engl J Med.* 2004;351(2):159–169.
237. Ware LB, Matthay MA, Ware LB, Matthay MA. The acute respiratory distress syndrome. *N Engl J Med.* 2000;342(18):1334–1349.
238. Sevransky JE, Levy MM, Marini JJ, et al. Mechanical ventilation in sepsis-induced acute lung injury/acute respiratory distress syndrome: an evidence-based review. *Crit Care Med.* 2004;32(11 Suppl):S548–S553.
239. The Acute Respiratory Distress Syndrome Network. Ventilation with lower tidal volumes as compared with traditional tidal volumes for acute lung injury and the acute respiratory distress syndrome. *N Engl J Med.* 2000;342(18):1301–1308.
240. Piantadosi CA, Schwartz DA, Piantadosi CA, Schwartz DA. The acute respiratory distress syndrome. *Ann Intern Med.* 2004;141(6):460–470.
241. Hoste EA, Lameire NH, Vanholder RC, et al. Acute renal failure in patients with sepsis in a surgical ICU: predictive factors, incidence, comorbidity, and outcome. *J Am Soc Nephrol.* 2003;14(4):1022–1030.
242. Neveu H, Kleinknecht D, Brivet F, et al. Prognostic factors in acute renal failure due to sepsis. Results of a prospective multicentre study. The French Study Group on Acute Renal Failure. *Nephrol Dialy Transplant.* 1996;11(2):293–299.
243. Bagshaw SM, George C, Bellomo R, ANZICS Database Management Committee. Early acute kidney injury and sepsis: a multicentre evaluation. *Crit Care.* 2008;12(2):R47.
244. Bagshaw SM, Uchino S, Bellomo R, et al. Septic acute kidney injury in critically ill patients: clinical characteristics and outcomes. *Clin J Am Soc Nephrol.* 2007;2(3):431–439.
245. Vincent J-L, Sakr Y, Sprung CL, et al. Sepsis in European intensive care units: results of the SOAP study. *Crit Care Med.* 2006;34(2):344–353.
246. Alobaidi R, Basu RK, Goldstein SL, Bagshaw SM. Sepsis-associated acute kidney injury. *Semin Nephrol.* 2015;35(1):2–11.
247. Astiz ME, Rackow EC, Weil MH. Pathophysiology and treatment of circulatory shock. *Crit Care Clin.* 1993;9:183–203.
248. Deitch E, Bridges W, Baker J, et al. Hemorrhagic shock-induced bacterial translocation is reduced by xanthine oxidase inhibition or inactivation. *Surgery.* 1988;104:191–198.
249. Mainous MR, Deitch EA. Bacterial translocation. In: Schlag G, Redl H, eds. *Pathophysiology of Shock, Sepsis and Organ Failure.* Berlin: Springer-Verlag; 1993:265–278.
250. Lillehei RC, MacLean LD. The intestinal factor in irreversible endotoxin shock. *Ann Surg.* 1958;148:513–519.
251. Meakins JL, Marshall JC. The gut as the motor of multiple organ failure. In: Marston A, Bulkley GB, Fiddian-Green RG, Haglund UH, eds. *Splanchnic Ischemia and Multiple Organ Failure.* London: Edward Arnold; 1989:339.

252. Marrero J, Martinez FJ, Hyzy R, et al. Advances in critical care hepatology. *Am J Resp Crit Care Med.* 2003;168(12):1421–1426.
253. Moseley RH. Sepsis and cholestasis. *Clin Liver Dis.* 1999;3:465–475.
254. Champion HR, Jones RT, Trump BF, et al. A clinicopathologic study of hepatic dysfunction following shock. *Surg Gynecol Obstet.* 1976;142: 657–663.
255. Levi M, ten Cate H. Disseminated intravascular coagulation. *N Engl J Med.* 1999;341(8):586–592.
256. Zeerleder S, Hack CE, Wuillemin WA, et al. Disseminated intravascular coagulation in sepsis. *Chest.* 2005;128(4):2864–2875.
257. Bone RC. Gram positive organisms and sepsis. *Arch Intern Med.* 1994; 154:26–34.
258. ten Cate H. Pathophysiology of disseminated intravascular coagulation in sepsis. *Crit Care Med.* 2000;28(9 Suppl):S9–S11.
259. Woolf PD. Endocrinology of shock. *Ann Emerg Med.* 1986;15:1401–1405.
260. Arnold J, Leinhardt D, Little RA. Metabolic response to trauma. In: Schlag G, Redl H, eds. *Pathophysiology of Shock Sepsis and Organ Failure.* Berlin: Springer-Verlag; 1993:145–160.
261. Bessey PQ, Brooks DC, Black PR, et al. Epinephrine acutely mediates skeletal muscle insulin resistance. *Surgery.* 1983;94:172–179.
262. Brierre S, Kumari R, Deboisblanc BP, et al. The endocrine system during sepsis. *Am J Med Sci.* 2004;328(4):238–247.
263. Mizock B. Metabolic derangments in sepsis and septic shock. *Crit Care Clin.* 2000;16(2):319–336.
264. Naylor JM, Kronfeld DS. In-vivo studies of hypoglycemia and lactic acidosis in endotoxic shock. *Am J Physiol.* 1985;248:E309–E316.
265. Daniel AM, Pierce CH, Shizgal HM, MacLean LD. Protein and fat utilization in shock. *Surgery.* 1978;84:588–594.
266. Bagby GJ, Spitzer JA. Decreased myocardial extracellular and muscle lipoprotein lipase activities in endotoxin-treated rats. *Proc Soc Exp Biol Med.* 1981;168:395–398.
267. Ho HC, Chapital AD, Yu M, et al. Hypothyroidism and adrenal insufficiency in sepsis and hemorrhagic shock. *Arch Surg.* 2004;139(11):1199–1203.
268. Gardelis JG, Hatzis TD, Stamogiannou LN, et al. Activity of the growth hormone/insulin-like growth factor-I axis in critically ill children. *J Pediatr Endocrinol.* 2005;18(4):363–372.
269. Beishuizen A, Thijs LG, Beishuizen A, Thijs LG. Endotoxin and the hypothalamo-pituitary-adrenal (HPA) axis. *J Endotoxin Res.* 2003;9(1):3–24.
270. Heemskerk VH, Daemen MA, Buurman WA, et al. Insulin-like growth factor-1 (IGF-1) and growth hormone (GH) in immunity and inflammation. *Cytokine Growth Factor Rev.* 1999;10(1):5–14.
271. Woods RJ, David J, Baigent S, et al. Elevated levels of corticotrophin-releasing factor binding protein in the blood of patients suffering from arthritis and septicaemia and the presence of novel ligands in synovial fluid. *Br J Rheumatol.* 1996;35(2):120–124.
272. Holmes CL, Patel BM, Russell JA, Walley KR. Physiology of vasopressin relevant to management of septic shock. *Chest.* 2001;120(3):989–1002.
273. Landry DW, Levin HR, Gallant EM, et al. Vasopressin deficiency contributes to the vasodilatation of septic shock. *Circulation.* 1997;95:1122–1125.
274. Marik PE, Zaloga GP. Adrenal insufficiency during septic shock. *Crit Care Med.* 2003;31(1):141–145.
275. Zaloga GP, Marik P. Hypothalamic-pituitary-adrenal insufficiency. *Crit Care Clin.* 2001;17(1):25–42.
276. Annane D, Sebille V, Troche G, et al E. A 3-level prognostic classification in septic shock based on cortisol levels and cortisol response to corticotropin. *JAMA.* 2000;283(8):1038–1045.
277. Manglik S, Flores E, Lubarsky L, et al. Glucocorticoid insufficiency in patients who present to the hospital with severe sepsis: a prospective clinical trial. *Crit Care Med.* 2003;31(6):1668–1675.
278. Marik P, Rotello L, Zaloga G. Secondary adrenal insufficiency is common in critically ill patients. *Crit Care Med.* 2001;29:A163.
279. de Groof F, Joosten KF, Janssen JA, et al. Acute stress response in children with meningococcal sepsis: important differences in the growth hormone/insulin-like growth factor I axis between nonsurvivors and survivors. *J Clin Endocrinol Metab.* 2002;87(7):3118–3124.
280. Felmet KA, Hall MW, Clark RS, et al. Prolonged lymphopenia, lymphoid depletion, and hypoprolactinemia in children with nosocomial sepsis and multiple organ failure. *J Immunol.* 2005;174(6):3765–3772.
281. Medina P, Noguera I, Aldasoro M, et al. Enhancement by vasopressin of adrenergic responses in human mesenteric arteries. *Am J Physiol.* 1997; 272(3 Pt 2):H1087–H1093.
282. Peres BD, Lopes FF, Melot C, Vincent JL. Body temperature alterations in the critically ill. *Intensive Care Med.* 2004;30(5):811–816.
283. Gomez-Jimenez J, Salgado A, Mourelle M, et al. L-arginine: nitric oxide pathway in endotoxemia and human septic shock. *Crit Care Med.* 1995;23(2): 253–258.
284. Kubes P. Nitric oxide affects microvascular permeability in the intact inflamed vasculature. *Microcirculation.* 1995;2(3):235–244.
285. Rackow EC, Kaufman BS, Falk JL, et al. Hemodynamic response to fluid repletion in patients with septic shock: evidence for early depression of cardiac performance. *Circ Shock.* 1987;22:11–22.
286. Parrillo JE, Parker MM, Natanson C, et al. Septic shock in humans: advances in the understanding of pathogenesis, cardiovascular dysfunction, and therapy. *Ann Intern Med.* 1990;113:227–242.
287. Cannon WB. *Traumatic Shock.* New York: Appleton; 1923.
288. Cournand A, Riley RL, Bradley SE, et al. Studies of the circulation in clinical shock. *Surgery.* 1943;13:964–995.
289. Carcillo JA, Davis AL, Zaritsky A. Role of early fluid resuscitation in pediatric septic shock. *JAMA.* 1991;266:1242–1245.
290. Maitland K, Babiker A, Kiguli S, Molyneux E. The FEAST trial of fluid bolus in African children with severe infection. *Lancet.* 2012;379(9816): 613.
291. Levraut J, Ichai C, Petit I, et al. Low exogenous lactate clearance as an early predictor of mortality in normolactatemic critically ill septic patients. *Crit Care Med.* 2003;31(3):705–710.
292. Abramson D, Scalea TM, Hitchcock R, et al. Lactate clearance and survival following injury. *J Trauma Injury Infect Crit Care.* 1993;35(4):584–588.
293. Davis JW, Shackford SR, Mackersie RC, Hoyt DB. Base deficit as a guide to volume resuscitation. *J Trauma Injury Infect Crit Care.* 1988;28(10): 1464–1467.
294. Oud L, Haupt MT. Persistent gastric intramucosal ischemia in patients with sepsis following resuscitation from shock. *Chest.* 1999;115(5):1390–1396.
295. Wo CC, Shoemaker WC, Appel PL, et al. Unreliability of blood pressure and heart rate to evaluate cardiac output in emergency resuscitation and critical illness. *Crit Care Med.* 1993;21(2):218–223.
296. Ward KR, Ivantury RR, Barbee WR. Endpoints of resuscitation for the victim of trauma. *J Intensive Care Med.* 2001;16(2):55–75.
297. Bakker J, Coffemils M, Leon M, et al. Blood lactate levels are superior to oxygen-derived variables in predicting outcome in human septic shock. *Chest.* 1992;99:956–962.
298. Nguyen HB, Rivers EP, Knoblich BP, et al. Early lactate clearance is associated with improved outcome in severe sepsis and septic shock. *Crit Care Med.* 2004;32(8):1637–1642.
299. James JH, Luchette FA, McCarter FD, Fischer JE. Lactate is an unreliable indicator of tissue hypoxia in injury or sepsis. *Lancet.* 1999;354(9177): 505–508.
300. Ernest D, Belzberg AS, Dodek PM. Distribution of normal saline and 5% albumin infusions in septic patients. *Crit Care Med.* 1999;27(1):46–50.
301. Rackow EC, Falk JL, Fein IA, et al. Fluid resuscitation in circulatory shock: a comparison of the cardiorespiratory effects of albumin, hetastarch, and saline solutions in patients with hypovolemic and septic shock. *Crit Care Med.* 1983;11:839–850.
302. Haupt MT, Teerapong P, Green D, et al. Increased pulmonary edema with crystalloid compared to colloid resuscitation of shock associated with increased vascular permeability. *Circ Shock.* 1984;12:213–224.
303. Haupt MT, Rackow EC. Colloid osmotic pressure and fluid resuscitation with hetastarch, albumin, and saline solutions. *Crit Care Med.* 1982;10: 159–162.
304. Wilkes MM, Navickis RJ. Patient survival after human albumin administration: a meta-analysis of randomized, controlled trials. *Ann Intern Med.* 2001;135(3):149–164.
305. Alderson P, Bunn F, Lefebvre C, et al. Human albumin solution for resuscitation and volume expansion in critically ill patients. *Cochrane Database System Rev.* 2002;(1):CD001208.
306. Finfer S, Bellomo R, Boyce N, et al. A comparison of albumin and saline for fluid resuscitation in the intensive care unit. *N Engl J Med.* 2004;350(22):2247–2256.
307. Schierhout G, Roberts I. Fluid resuscitation with colloid or crystalloid solutions in critically ill patients: a systematic review of randomised trials. *Br Med J.* 1998;316(7136):961–964.
308. Caironi P, Tognoni G, Masson S, et al. ALBIOS Study Investigators. Albumin replacement in patients with severe sepsis or septic shock. *N Engl J Med.* 2014;370(15):1412–1421.
309. Zarychanski R, Abou-Setta AM, Turgeon AF, et al. Association of hydroxyethyl starch administration with mortality and acute kidney injury in critically ill patients requiring volume resuscitation: a systematic review and meta-analysis. *JAMA.* 2013;309(7):678–688.
310. Perner A, Haase N, Guttormsen AB, et al. Scandinavian Critical Care Trials Group. Hydroxyethyl starch 130/0.42 versus Ringer's acetate in severe sepsis. *N Engl J Med.* 2012;367(2):124–134.
311. Myburgh J, Finfer S, Bellomo R, et al. Hydroxyethyl starch or saline for fluid resuscitation in intensive care. *N Engl J Med.* 2012;367(20):1901–1911.

312. U.S. Food and Drug Administration. FDA Safety Communication: boxed warning on increased mortality and severe renal injury, and additional warning on risk of bleeding, for use of hydroxyethyl starch solutions in some settings. 2013. Available at: http://www.fda.gov/BiologicsBloodVaccines/SafetyAvailability/ucm358271.htm.
313. Rivers E, Nguyen B, Havstad S, et al. Early goal-directed therapy in the treatment of severe sepsis and septic shock. *N Engl J Med.* 2001; 345(19):1368–1377.
314. Dellinger RP, Carlet JM, Masur H, et al. Surviving sepsis campaign guidelines for management of severe sepsis and septic shock. *Crit Care Med.* 2004;32(3): 858–873.
315. ARISE Investigators; ANZICS Clinical Trials Group, Peake SL, Delaney A, Bailey M, et al. Goal-directed resuscitation for patients with early septic shock. *N Engl J Med.* 2014;371(16):1496–1506.
316. ProCESS Investigators, Yealy DM, Kellum JA, Huang DT, et al. A randomized trial of protocol-based care for early septic shock. *N Engl J Med.* 2014;370(18):1683–1693.
317. Mouncey PR, Osborn TM, Power GS, et al; ProMISe Trial Investigators. Trial of early, goal-directed resuscitation for septic shock. *N Engl J Med.* 2015;372(14):1301–1311.
318. Meehan TP, Fine MJ, Krumholz HM, et al. Quality of care, process, and outcomes in elderly patients with pneumonia. *JAMA.* 1997;278(23): 2080–2084.
319. Ibrahim EH, Sherman G, Ward S, et al. The influence of inadequate antimicrobial treatment of bloodstream infections on patient outcomes in the ICU setting. *Chest.* 2000;118(1):146–155.
320. Kollef MH, Sherman G, Ward S, Fraser VJ. Inadequate antimicrobial treatment of infections: a risk factor for hospital mortality among critically ill patients. *Chest.* 1999;115(2):462–474.
321. Young LS, Martin WJ, Meyer RD, et al. Gram-negative rod bacteremia: microbiologic, immunologic, and therapeutic considerations. *Ann Intern Med.* 1977;86:456–471.
322. Romero-Vivas J, Rubio M, Fernandez C, Picazo JJ. Mortality associated with nosocomial bacteremia due to methicillin-resistant Staphylococcus aureus. *Clin Infect Dis.* 1995;21(6):1417–1423.
323. Nguyen MH, Peacock JE Jr, Tanner DC, et al. Therapeutic approaches in patients with candidemia: evaluation in a multicenter, prospective, observational study. *Arch Intern Med.* 1995;155(22):2429–2435.
324. Vergis EN, Hayden MK, Chow JW, et al. Determinants of vancomycin resistance and mortality rates in enterococcal bacteremia: a prospective multicenter study. *Ann Intern Med.* 2001;135(7):484–492.
325. Byl B, Clevenbergh P, Jacobs F, et al. Impact of infectious diseases specialists and microbiological data on the appropriateness of antimicrobial therapy for bacteremia. *Clin Infect Dis.* 1999;29(1):60–66.
326. Aronin SI, Peduzzi P, Quagliarello VJ. Community-acquired bacterial meningitis: risk stratification for adverse clinical outcome and effect of antibiotic timing. *Ann Intern Med.* 1998;129(11):862–869.
327. Miner JR, Heegaard W, Mapes A, Biros M. Presentation, time to antibiotics, and mortality of patients with bacterial meningitis at an urban county medical center. *J Emerg Med.* 2001;21(4):387–392.
328. Proulx N, Frechette D, Toye B, et al. Delays in the administration of antibiotics are associated with mortality from adult acute bacterial meningitis. *Q J Med.* 2005;98(4):291–298.
329. Ferrer R, Martin-Loeches I, Phillips G, et al. Empiric antibiotic treatment reduces mortality in severe sepsis and septic shock from the first hour: results from a guideline-based performance improvement program. *Crit Care Med.* 2014;42(8):1749–1755.
330. Houck PM, Bratzler DW, Nsa W, et al. Timing of antibiotic administration and outcomes for Medicare patients hospitalized with community-acquired pneumonia. *Arch Intern Med.* 2004;164(6):637–644.
331. Natsch S, Kullberg BJ, Van der Meer JW, Meis JF. Delay in administering the first dose of antibiotics in patients admitted to hospital with serious infections. *EurJ Clin Microbiol Infect Dis.* 1998;17(10):681–684.
332. Ferrer R, Artigas A, Levy MM, et al. Improvement in process of care and outcome after a multicenter severe sepsis educational program in Spain. *JAMA.* 2008;299(19):2294–2303.
333. Bloos F, Thomas-Ruddel D, Ruddel H, et al. Impact of compliance with infection management guidelines on outcome in patients with severe sepsis: a prospective observational multi-center study. *Crit Care.* 2014; 18(2):R42.
334. Kumar A. An alternate pathophysiologic paradigm of sepsis and septic shock: implications for optimizing antimicrobial therapy. *Virulence.* 2014; 5(1):80–97.
335. Pea F, Viale P. Bench-to-bedside review: appropriate antibiotic therapy in severe sepsis and septic shock—does the dose matter? *Crit Care.* 2009; 13(3):214.
336. Drusano GL. Antimicrobial pharmacodynamics: critical interactions of 'bug and drug'. *Nature Rev Microbiol.* 2004;2(4):289–300.
337. Udy AA, Roberts JA, Boots RJ, et al. Augmented renal clearance: implications for antibacterial dosing in the critically ill. *Clin Pharmacokinet.* 2010;49(1):1–16.
338. Pimentel FL, Abelha F, Trigo MA, et al. Determination of plasma concentrations of amikacin in patients of an intensive care unit. *J Chemother.* 1995;7(1):45–49.
339. Whipple JK, Ausman RK, Franson T, Quebbeman EJ. Effect of individualized pharmacokinetic dosing on patient outcome. *Crit Care Med.* 1991;19(12):1480–1485.
340. Joukhadar C, Frossard M, Mayer BX, et al. Impaired target site penetration of beta-lactams may account for therapeutic failure in patients with septic shock. *Crit Care Med.* 2001;29(2):385–391.
341. Franson TR, Quebbeman EJ, Whipple J, et al. Prospective comparison of traditional and pharmacokinetic aminoglycoside dosing methods. *Crit Care Med.* 1988;16(9):840–843.
342. Chelluri L, Jastremski MS. Inadequacy of standard aminoglycoside loading doses in acutely ill patients. *Crit Care Med.* 1987;15(12):1143–1145.
343. Tegeder I, Schmidtko A, Brautigam L, et al. Tissue distribution of imipenem in critically ill patients. *Clin Pharmacol Ther.* 2002;71(5):325–333.
344. Taccone F, Laterre P-F, Dugernier T, et al. Insufficient beta-lactam concentrations in the early phase of severe sepsis and septic shock. *Crit Care.* 2010;14(4):R126.
345. Roger C, Nucci B, Louart B, et al. Impact of 30 mg/kg amikacin and 8 mg/kg gentamicin on serum concentrations in critically ill patients with severe sepsis. *J Antimicrob Chemother.* 2016;71(1):208–212.
346. Moore RD, Smith CR, Lietman PS. The association of aminoglycoside plasma levels with mortality in patients with gram-negative bacteremia. *J Infect Dis.* 1984;149(3):443–448.
347. Moore RD, Smith CR, Lietman PS. Association of aminoglycoside plasma levels with therapeutic outcome in gram-negative pneumonia. *Am J Med.* 1984;77(4):657–662.
348. Forrest A, Nix DE, Ballow CH, et al. Pharmacodynamics of intravenous ciprofloxacin in seriously ill patients. *Antimicrob Agents Chemother.* 1993;37(5): 1073–1081.
349. Preston SL, Drusano GL, Berman AL, et al. Pharmacodynamics of levofloxacin: a new paradigm for early clinical trials. *JAMA.* 1998;279(2): 125–129.
350. Drusano GL, Preston SL, Fowler C, et al. Relationship between fluoroquinolone area under the curve: minimum inhibitory concentration ratio and the probability of eradication of the infecting pathogen, in patients with nosocomial pneumonia. *J Infect Dis.* 2004;189(9):1590–1597.
351. Moore RD, Lietman PS, Smith CR. Clinical response to aminoglycoside therapy: importance of the ratio of peak concentration to minimal inhibitory concentration. *J Infect Dis.* 1987;155(1):93–99.
352. Kashuba AD, Nafziger AN, Drusano GL, Bertino JS Jr. Optimizing aminoglycoside therapy for nosocomial pneumonia caused by gram-negative bacteria. *Antimicrob Agents Chemother.* 1999;43(3):623–629.
353. Schentag JJ, Smith IL, Swanson DJ, et al. Role for dual individualization with cefmenoxime. *Am J Med.* 1984;77(6A):43–50.
354. Craig WA. Pharmacokinetic/pharmacodynamic parameters: rationale for antibacterial dosing of mice and men. *Clin Infect Dis.* 1998;26(1):1–10.
355. Lodise TP, Lomaestro BM, Drusano GL. Piperacillin-tazobactam for Pseudomonas aeruginosa infection: clinical implications of an extended-infusion dosing strategy. *Clin Infect Dis.* 2007;44(3):357–363.
356. Dulhunty JM, Roberts JA, Davis JS, et al. Continuous infusion of beta-lactam antibiotics in severe sepsis: a multicenter double-blind, randomized controlled trial. *Clin Infect Dis.* 2013;56(2):236–244.
357. Craig WA, Ebert SC. Continuous infusion of beta-lactam antibiotics. *Antimicrob Agents Chemother.* 1992;36(12):2577–2583.
358. Craig WA. Once-daily versus multiple-daily dosing of aminoglycosides. *J Chemother.* 1995;7(2 Suppl):47–52.
359. Kashuba AD, Bertino JS Jr, Nafziger AN. Dosing of aminoglycosides to rapidly attain pharmacodynamic goals and hasten therapeutic response by using individualized pharmacokinetic monitoring of patients with pneumonia caused by gram-negative organisms. *Antimicrob Agents Chemother.* 1998;42(7):1842–1844.
360. Bodey GP, Ketchel SJ, Rodriguez V. A randomized study of carbenicillin plus cefamandole or tobramycin in the treatment of febrile episodes in cancer patients. *Am J Med.* 1979;67(4):608–616.
361. Daenen S, Vries-Hospers H. Cure of Pseudomonas aeruginosa infection in neutropenic patients by continuous infusion of ceftazidime. *Lancet.* 1988;1(8591):937.
362. Egerer G, Goldschmidt H, Hensel M, et al. Continuous infusion of ceftazidime for patients with breast cancer and multiple myeloma receiving

high-dose chemotherapy and peripheral blood stem cell transplantation. *Bone Marrow Transplant.* 2002;30(7):427–431.

363. Benko AS, Cappelletty DM, Kruse JA, Rybak MJ. Continuous infusion versus intermittent administration of ceftazidime in critically ill patients with suspected gram-negative infections. *Antimicrob Agents Chemother.* 1996;40(3):691–695.
364. Thalhammer F, Traunmüller F, El Menyawi I, et al. Continuous infusion versus intermittent administration of meropenem in critically ill patients. *J Antimicrob Chemother.* 1999;43(4):523–527.
365. Sfeir T, Saha DC, Astiz M, Rackow EC. Role of interleukin-10 in monocyte hyporesponsiveness associated with septic shock. *Crit Care Med.* 2001; 29(1):129–133.
366. Haupt W, Riese J, Mehler C, et al. Monocyte function before and after surgical trauma. *Digest Surg.* 1998;15(2):102–104.
367. Brandtzaeg P, Osnes L, Ovstebo R, et al. Net inflammatory capacity of human septic shock plasma evaluated by a monocyte-based target cell assay: identification of interleukin-10 as a major functional deactivator of human monocytes. *J Exp Med.* 1996;184(1):51–60.
368. Williams MA, Withington S, Newland AC, Kelsey SM. Monocyte anergy in septic shock is associated with a predilection to apoptosis and is reversed by granulocyte-macrophage colony-stimulating factor ex vivo. *J Infect Dis.* 1998;178(5):1421–1433.
369. Tavares-Murta BM, Zaparoli M, Ferreira RB, et al. Failure of neutrophil chemotactic function in septic patients. *Crit Care Med.* 2002;30(5): 1056–1061.
370. Holzer K, Konietzny P, Wilhelm K, et al. Phagocytosis by emigrated, intra-abdominal neutrophils is depressed during human secondary peritonitis. *Eur Surg Res.* 2002;34(4):275–284.
371. Benjamim CF, Ferreira SH, Cunha FQ. Role of nitric oxide in the failure of neutrophil migration in sepsis. *J Infect Dis.* 2000;182(1):214–223.
372. Barriere SL. Monotherapy versus combination antimicrobial therapy: a review. *Pharmacotherapy.* 1991;11:64S-71.
373. Hughes WT, Armstrong D, Bodey GP, et al. 2002 guidelines for the use of antimicrobial agents in neutropenic patients with cancer. *Clin Infect Dis.* 2002;34(6):730–751.
374. Brunkhorst FM, Oppert M, Marx G, et al. Effect of empirical treatment with moxifloxacin and meropenem vs meropenem on sepsis-related organ dysfunction in patients with severe sepsis: a randomized trial. *JAMA.* 2012;307(22):2390–2399.
375. Paul M, Lador A, Grozinsky-Glasberg S, Leibovici L. Beta lactam antibiotic monotherapy versus beta lactam-aminoglycoside antibiotic combination therapy for sepsis. *Cochrane Database System Rev.* 2014;(1):CD003344.
376. Safdar N, Handelsman J, Maki DG, et al. Does combination antimicrobial therapy reduce mortality in gram-negative bacteraemia? A meta-analysis. *Lancet Infect Dis.* 2004;4(8):519–527.
377. Paul M, Soares-Weiser K, Leibovici L. Beta-lactam monotherapy versus ß-lactam-aminoglycoside combination therapy for fever with neutropenia: systematic review and meta-analysis. *Br Med J.* 2003;326(7399): 1111–1118.
378. Bochud PY, Glauser MP, Calandra T, International SF. Antibiotics in sepsis. *Intensive Care Med.* 2001;27(1 Suppl):S33–S48.
379. Hilf M, Yu VL, Sharp J, et al. Antibiotic therapy for Pseudomonas aeruginosa bacteremia: outcome correlations in a prospective study of 200 patients. *Am J Med.* 1989;87(5):540–546.
380. Chow JW, Fine MJ, Shlaes DM, et al. Enterobacter bacteremia: clinical features and emergence of antibiotic resistance during therapy. *Ann Intern Med.* 1991;115(8):585–590.
381. Korvick JA, Bryan CS, Farber B, et al. Prospective observational study of Klebsiella bacteremia in 230 patients: outcome for antibiotic combinations versus monotherapy. *Antimicrob Agents Chemother.* 1992;36(12): 2639–2644.
382. Anderson ET, Young LS, Hewitt WL. Antimicrobial synergism in the therapy of gram-negative rod bacteremia. *Chemotherapy.* 1978;24(1):45–54.
383. Baddour LM, Yu VL, Klugman KP, et al. Combination antibiotic therapy lowers mortality among severely ill patients with pneumococcal bacteremia. *Am J Resp Crit Care Med.* 2004;170(4):440–444.
384. Waterer GW, Somes GW, Wunderink RG. Monotherapy may be suboptimal for severe bacteremic pneumococcal pneumonia. *Arch Intern Med.* 2001;161(15):1837–1842.
385. Martinez JA, Horcajada JP, Almela M, et al. Addition of a macrolide to a beta-lactam-based empirical antibiotic regimen is associated with lower in-hospital mortality for patients with bacteremic pneumococcal pneumonia. *Clin Infect Dis.* 2003;36(4):389–395.
386. Rodriguez A, Mendia A, Sirvent JM, et al. Combination antibiotic therapy improves survival in patients with community-acquired pneumonia and shock. *Crit Care Med.* 2007;35(6):1493–1498.
387. Kumar A, Zarychanski R, Light B, et al. Early combination antibiotic therapy yields improved survival compared to monotherapy in septic shock: a propensity-matched analysis. *Crit Care Med.* 2010;38(9):1773–1785.
388. Kumar A, Safdar N, Reddy S, Chateau D. The survival benefit of combination antibiotic therapy for serious infections associated with sepsis and septic shock is contingent only on the risk of death: a meta-analytic/meta-regression study. *Crit Care Med.* 2010;38(8):1651–1664.
389. Sprung CL, Finch RG, Thijs LG, Glauser MP. International sepsis trial (INTERSEPT): role and impact of a clinical evaluation committee. *Crit Care Med.* 1996;24(9):1441–1447.
390. Sudarsky LA, Laschinger JC, Coppa GF, Spencer FC. Improved results from a standardized approach in treating patients with necrotizing fasciitis. *Ann Surg.* 1987;206(5):661–665.
391. Moss RL, Musemeche CA, Kosloske AM. Necrotizing fasciitis in children: prompt recognition and aggressive therapy improve survival. *J Pediatr Surg.* 1996;31(8):1142–1146.
392. Azuhata T, Kinoshita K, Kawano D, et al. Time from admission to initiation of surgery for source control is a critical determinant of survival in patients with gastrointestinal perforation with associated septic shock. *Crit Care.* 2014;18(3):R87.
393. Kumar A, Wood K, Gurka D, et al. Outcome of septic shock correlates with duration of hypotension prior to source control implementation. *ICAAC Proc.* 2004:350:K–1222
394. Kumar A, Parrillo JE. Shock: pathophysiology, classification and approach to management. In: Parrillo JE, Dellinger RP, eds. *Critical Care Medicine: Principles of Diagnosis and Management in the Adult.* St Louis, MO: Mosby; 2001:371–420.
395. Bond RF. Peripheral macro- and microcirculation. In: Schlag G, Redl H, eds. *Pathophysiology of Shock, Sepsis and Organ Failure.* Berlin: Springer-Verlag; 1993:893–907.
396. Waechter J, Kumar A, Lapinsky SE, et al. Interaction between fluids and vasoactive agents on mortality in septic shock: a multicenter, observational study. *Crit Care Med.* 2014;42(10):2158–2168.
397. Beck V, Chateau D, Bryson GL, et al. Timing of vasopressor initiation and mortality in septic shock: a cohort study. *Crit Care.* 2014;18(3):R97.
398. Asfar P, Meziani F, Hamel J-F, et al. High versus low blood-pressure target in patients with septic shock. *N Engl J Med.* 2014;370(17):1583–1593.
399. Desjars P, Pinaud M, Potel G, et al. A reappraisal of norepinephrine therapy in human septic shock. *Crit Care Med.* 1987;15(2):134–137.
400. Desjars P, Pinaud M, Bugnon D, Tasseau F. Norepinephrine therapy has no deleterious renal effects in human septic shock. *Crit Care Med.* 1989; 17(5):426–429.
401. Fukuoka T, Nishimura M, Imanaka H, Taenaka N, et al. Effects of norepinephrine on renal function in septic patients with normal and elevated serum lactate levels. *Crit Care Med.* 1989;17(11):1104–1107.
402. Hesselvik JF, Brodin B. Low dose norepinephrine in patients with septic shock and oliguria: effects on afterload, urine flow, and oxygen transport. *Crit Care Med.* 1989;17(2):179–180.
403. Meadows D, Edwards JD, Wilkins RG, Nightingale P. Reversal of intractable septic shock with norepinephrine therapy. *Crit Care Med.* 1988; 16(7):663–666.
404. Redl-Wenzl EM, Armbruster C, Edelmann G, et al. The effects of norepinephrine on hemodynamics and renal function in severe septic shock states. *Intensive Care Med.* 1993;19(3):151–154.
405. De Backer D, Biston P, Devriendt J, et al. Comparison of dopamine and norepinephrine in the treatment of shock. *N Engl J Med.* 2010;362(9):779–789.
406. Neviere R, Mathieu D, Chagnon JL, Lebleu N, Wattel F. The contrasting effects of dobutamine and dopamine on gastric mucosal perfusion in septic patients. *Am J Resp Crit Care Med.* 1996;154(6 Pt 1):1684–1688.
407. Marin C, Eon B, Saux P, Aknin P, Gouin F. Renal effects of norepinephrine used to treat septic shock patients. *Crit Care Med.* 1990;18(3):282–285.
408. Marik PE, Mohedin M. The contrasting effects of dopamine and norepinephrine on systemic and splanchnic oxygen utilization in hyperdynamic sepsis. *JAMA.* 1994;272(17):1354–1357.
409. Ruokonen E, Takala J, Kari A, et al. Regional blood flow and oxygen transport in septic shock. *Crit Care Med.* 1993;21(9):1296–1303.
410. Meier-Hellmann A, Specht M, Hannemann L, et al. Splanchnic blood flow is greater in septic shock treated with norepinephrine than in severe sepsis. *Intensive Care Med.* 1996;22(12):1354–1359.
411. Levy B, Bollaert PE, Charpentier C, et al. Comparison of norepinephrine and dobutamine to epinephrine for hemodynamics, lactate metabolism, and gastric tonometric variables in septic shock: a prospective, randomized study. *Intensive Care Med.* 1997;23(3):282–287.
412. De Backer D, Creteur J, Silva E, Vincent JL. Effects of dopamine, norepinephrine, and epinephrine on the splanchnic circulation in septic shock: which is best? *Crit Care Med.* 2003;31(6):1659–1667.

413. Martin C, Papazian L, Perrin G, et al. Norepinephrine or dopamine for the treatment of hyperdynamic septic shock? *Chest* 1993;103(6):1826–1831.
414. Devins SS, Miller A, Herndon BL, et al. Effects of dopamine on T-lymphocyte proliferative response and serum prolactin in critically ill patients. *Crit Care Med.* 1992;20(12):1644–1649.
415. Annane D, Vignon P, Renault A, et al. Norepinephrine plus dobutamine versus epinephrine alone for management of septic shock: a randomised trial. *Lancet.* 2007;370(9588):676–684.
416. Rhodes A, Lamb FJ, Malagon R, et al. A prospective study of the use of a dobutamine stress test to identify outcome in patients with sepsis, severe sepsis or septic shock. *Crit Care Med.* 1999;27(11):2361–2366.
417. Barton P, Garcia J, Kouatli A, et al. Hemodynamic effects of i.v. milrinone lactate in pediatric patients with septic shock: a prospective, double-blinded, randomized, placebo-controlled, interventional study. *Chest.* 1996;109(5):1302–1312.
418. Gattinoni L, Brazzi L, Pelosi P, et al. A trial of goal-oriented hemodynamic therapy in critically ill patients. SvO2 Collaborative Group. *N Engl J Med.* 1995;333(16):1025–1032.
419. Hayes MA, Timmins AC, Yau EHS, et al. Elevation of systemic oxygen delivery in the treatment of critically ill patients. *N Engl J Med.* 1994;330(24):1717–1722.
420. Bussolino F, Camuss G, Baglioni C. Synthesis and release of platelet activating factor by human vascular endothelial cells treated with tumor necrosis factor or interleukin-1. *J Biol Chem.* 1988;263:11856–11861.
421. Landry DW, Levin HR, Gallant EM, et al. Vasopressin pressor sensitivity in vasodilatory septic shock. *Crit Care Med.* 1997;25:1279–1282.
422. Patel BM, Chittock DR, Russell JA, Walley KR. Beneficial effects of short-term vasopressin infusion during severe septic shock. *Anesthesiology.* 2002;96(3):576–582.
423. Russell JA, Walley KR, Singer J, et al. Vasopressin versus norepinephrine infusion in patients with septic shock. *N Engl J Med.* 2008;358(9):877–887.
424. Serpa Neto A, Nassar AP, Cardoso SO, et al. Vasopressin and terlipressin in adult vasodilatory shock: a systematic review and meta-analysis of nine randomized controlled trials. *Crit Care.* 2012;16(4):R154.
425. Schaer GL, Fink MP, Parrillo JE. Norepinephrine alone versus norepinephrine plus low-dose dopamine: enhanced renal blood flow with combination pressor therapy. *Crit Care Med.* 1985;13:492–496.
426. Hoogenberg K, Smit AJ, Girbes AR. Effects of low-dose dopamine on renal and systemic hemodynamics during incremental norepinephrine infusion in healthy volunteers. *Crit Care Med.* 1998;26(2):260–265.
427. Olson D, Pohlman A, Hall JB. Administration of low-dose dopamine to nonoliguric patients with sepsis syndrome does not raise intramucosal gastric pH nor improve creatinine clearance. *Am J Resp Crit Care Med.* 1996;154(6 Pt 1):1664–1670.
428. Ichai C, Passeron C, Carles M, et al. Prolonged low-dose dopamine infusion induces a transient improvement in renal function in hemodynamically stable, critically ill patients: a single-blind, prospective, controlled study. *Crit Care Med.* 2000;28(5):1329–1335.
429. Bellomo R, Chapman M, Finfer S, et al; Australian and New Zealand Intensive Care Society (ANZICS) Clinical Trials Group. Low-dose dopamine in patients with early renal dysfunction: a placebo-controlled randomised trial. *Lancet.* 2000;356(9248):2139–2143.
430. Marik PE, Iglesias J. Low-dose dopamine does not prevent acute renal failure in patients with septic shock and oliguria. NORASEPT II Study Investigators. *Am J Med.* 1999;107(4):387–390.
431. Mimoz O, Rauss A, Rekik N, et al. Pulmonary artery catheterization in critically ill patients: a prospective analysis of outcome changes associated with catheter-prompted changes in therapy. *Crit Care Med.* 1994;22(4):573–579.
432. Connors AF Jr, McCaffree DR, Gray BA. Evaluation of right-heart catheterization in the critically ill patient without acute myocardial infarction. *N Engl J Med.* 1983;308(5):263–267.
433. Weisel RD, Vito L, Dennis RC, Hechtman HB. Myocardial depression during sepsis. *Am J Surg.* 1977;133:512–521.
434. Cohn JN. Central venous pressure as a guide to volume expansion. *Ann Intern Med.* 1967;66(6):1283–1287.
435. Connors AF Jr, Dawson NV, Shaw PK, et al. Hemodynamic status in critically ill patients with and without acute heart disease. *Chest.* 1990;98(5):1200–1206.
436. Kumar A, Anel R, Bunnell E, et al. Pulmonary artery occlusion pressure and central venous pressure fail to predict ventricular filling volume, cardiac performance, or the response to volume infusion in normal subjects. *Crit Care Med.* 2004;32(3):691–699.
437. Robin ED. The cult of the Swan-Ganz catheter: overuse and abuse of pulmonary flow catheters. *Ann Intern Med.* 1985;103(3):445–449.
438. Dalen JE, Bone RC. Is it time to pull the pulmonary artery catheter? *JAMA.* 1996;276(11):916–918.
439. De Backer D. Ultrasonic evaluation of the heart. *Curr Opin Crit Care.* 2014;20(3):309–314.
440. Romero-Bermejo FJ, Ruiz-Bailén M, et al. Echocardiographic hemodynamic monitoring in the critically ill patient. *Curr Cardiol Rev.* 2011;7(3):146–156.
441. Pronovost PJ, Jenckes MW, Dorman T, et al. Organizational characteristics of intensive care units related to outcomes of abdominal aortic surgery. *JAMA.* 1999;281(14):1310–1317.
442. Carson SS, Stocking C, Podsadecki T, et al. Effects of organizational change in the medical intensive care unit of a teaching hospital: a comparison of 'open' and 'closed' formats. *JAMA.* 1996;276(4):322–328.
443. Pronovost PJ, Angus DC, Dorman T, et al. Physician staffing patterns and clinical outcomes in critically ill patients: a systematic review. *JAMA.* 2002;288(17):2151–2162.
444. Li TC, Phillips MC, Shaw L, et al. On-site physician staffing in a community hospital intensive care unit: impact on test and procedure use and on patient outcome. *JAMA.* 1984;252(15):2023–2027.
445. Pollack MM, Katz RW, Ruttimann UE, Getson PR. Improving the outcome and efficiency of intensive care: the impact of an intensivist. *Crit Care Med.* 1988;16(1):11–17.
446. Reynolds HN, Haupt MT, Thill-Baharozian MC, Carlson RW. Impact of critical care physician staffing on patients with septic shock in a university hospital medical intensive care unit. *JAMA.* 1988;260(23):3446–3450.
447. Hutton P, Dye J, Prys-Roberts C. An assessment of the Dinamap. *Anaesthesia.* 1984;39(3):261–267.
448. Cohn JN. Blood pressure measurement in shock. Mechanism of inaccuracy in ausculatory and palpatory methods. *JAMA.* 1967;199(13):118–122.
449. Gershengorn HB, Wunsch H, Scales DC, et al. Association between arterial catheter use and hospital mortality in intensive care units. *JAMA Intern Med.* 2014;174(11):1746–1754.
450. De Backer D, Fagnoul D. Intensive care ultrasound. VI. Fluid responsiveness and shock assessment. *Ann Am Thorac Soc.* 2014;11(1):129–136.
451. Charron C, Fessenmeyer C, Cosson C, et al. The influence of tidal volume on the dynamic variables of fluid responsiveness in critically ill patients. *Anesthesia Analg.* 2006;102(5):1511–1517.
452. Feissel M, Michard F, Mangin I, et al. Respiratory changes in aortic blood velocity as an indicator of fluid responsiveness in ventilated patients with septic shock. *Chest.* 2001;119(3):867–873.
453. Vieillard-Baron A, Chergui K, Rabiller A, et al. Superior vena caval collapsibility as a gauge of volume status in ventilated septic patients. *Intensive Care Med.* 2004;30(9):1734–1739.
454. De Backer D, Taccone FS, Holsten R, et al. Influence of respiratory rate on stroke volume variation in mechanically ventilated patients. *Anesthesiology.* 2009;110(5):1092–1097.
455. Feissel M, Michard F, Faller J-P, Teboul J-L. The respiratory variation in inferior vena cava diameter as a guide to fluid therapy. *Intensive Care Med.* 2004;30(9):1834–1837.
456. Barbier C, Loubières Y, Schmit C, et al. Respiratory changes in inferior vena cava diameter are helpful in predicting fluid responsiveness in ventilated septic patients. *Intensive Care Med.* 2004;30(9):1740–1746.
457. Connors AF Jr, Speroff T, Dawson NV, et al. The effectiveness of right heart catheterization in the initial care of critically ill patients. *JAMA.* 1996;276(11):889–897.
458. Richard C, Warszawski J, Anguel N, et al. Early use of the pulmonary artery catheter and outcomes in patients with shock and acute respiratory distress syndrome: a randomized controlled trial. *JAMA.* 2003;290(20):2713–2720.
459. Rhodes A, Cusack RJ, Newman PJ, et al. A randomised, controlled trial of the pulmonary artery catheter in critically ill patients. *Intensive Care Med.* 2002;28(3):256–264.
460. Polanczyk CA, Rohde LE, Goldman L, et al. Right heart catheterization and cardiac complications in patients undergoing noncardiac surgery: an observational study. *JAMA.* 2001;286(3):309–314.
461. Sandham JD, Hull RD, Brant RF, et al. A randomized, controlled trial of the use of pulmonary-artery catheters in high-risk surgical patients. *N Engl J Med.* 2003;348(1):5–14.
462. Ivanov RI, Allen J, Sandham JD, Calvin JE. Pulmonary artery catheterization: a narrative and systematic critique of randomized controlled trials and recommendations for the future. *New Horizons.* 1997;5(3):268–276.
463. Connors AF Jr, Dawson NV, McCaffree DR, et al. Assessing hemodynamic status in critically ill patients: do physicians use clinical information optimally? *J Crit Care.* 1987;2:174–180.
464. Michard F, Teboul JL. Predicting fluid responsiveness in ICU patients: a critical analysis of the evidence. *Chest.* 2002;121(6):2000–2008.
465. Marik PE. Pulmonary artery catheterization and esophageal doppler monitoring in the ICU. *Chest.* 1999;116(4):1085–1091.

466. Humphrey H, Hall J, Sznajder I, et al. Improved survival in ARDS patients associated with a reduction in pulmonary capillary wedge pressure. *Chest.* 1990;97(5):1176–1180.
467. Mitchell JP, Schuller D, Calandrino FS, Schuster DP. Improved outcome based on fluid management in critically ill patients requiring pulmonary artery catheterization. *Am Rev Resp Dis.* 1992;145(5):990–998.
468. Zanotti S, Kumar A, Kumar A. Cytokine modulation in sepsis and septic shock. *Exp Opin Invest Drugs.* 2002;11(8):1061–1075.
469. Anel RL, Kumar A. Experimental and emerging therapies for sepsis and septic shock. *Exp Opin Invest Drugs.* 2001;10(8):1471–1485.
470. Alejandria MM, Lansang MA, Dans LF, Mantaring JB. Intravenous immunoglobulin for treating sepsis and septic shock. *Cochrane Database System Rev.* 2002;(1):CD001090.
471. Douzinas EE, Pitaridis MT, Louris G, et al. Prevention of infection in multiple trauma patients by high-dose intravenous immunoglobulins. *Crit Care Med.* 2000;28(1):8–15.
472. Darenberg J, Ihendyane N, Sjolin J, et al. Intravenous immunoglobulin G therapy in streptococcal toxic shock syndrome: a European randomized, double-blind, placebo-controlled trial. *Clin Infect Dis.* 2003;37(3):333–340.
473. Linnér A, Darenberg J, Sjölin J, et al. Clinical efficacy of polyspecific intravenous immunoglobulin therapy in patients with streptococcal toxic shock syndrome: a comparative observational study. *Clin Infect Dis.* 2014;59(6): 851–857.
474. Pitcairn M, Schuler J, Erve PR, Holtzman S, Schumer W. Glucocorticoid and antibiotic effect on experimental gram-negative bacteremic shock. *Arch Surg.* 1975;110(8):1012–1015.
475. Sprung CL, Caralis PV, Marcial EH, et al. The effects of high-dose corticosteroids in patients with septic shock. A prospective, controlled study. *N Engl J Med.* 1984;311(18):1137–1143.
476. Bone RC, Fisher CJ Jr, Clemmer TP, et al. A controlled clinical trial of high-dose methylprednisolone in the treatment of severe sepsis and septic shock. *N Engl J Med.* 1987;317(11):653–658.
477. Luce JM, Montgomery AB, Marks JD, et al. Ineffectiveness of high-dose methylprednisolone in preventing parenchymal lung injury and improving mortality in patients with septic shock. *Am Rev Resp Dis.* 1988;138(1): 62–68.
478. The Veterans Administration Systemic Sepsis Cooperative Study Group. Effect of high-dose glucocorticoid therapy on mortality in patients with clinical signs of systemic sepsis. *N Engl J Med.* 1987;317(11):659–665.
479. Karvellas CJ, Farhat MR, Sajjad I, et al. A comparison of early versus late initiation of renal replacement therapy in critically ill patients with acute kidney injury: a systematic review and meta-analysis. *Crit Care.* 2011;15(1):R72.
480. Schiffl H, Lang SM, Fischer R. Daily hemodialysis and the outcome of acute renal failure. *N Engl J Med.* 2002;346(5):305–310.
481. Ronco C, Bellomo R, Homel P, et al. Effects of different doses in continuous veno-venous haemofiltration on outcomes of acute renal failure: a prospective randomised trial. *Lancet.* 2000;356(9223):26–30.
482. Bellomo R, Cass A, Cole L, et al. Intensity of continuous renal-replacement therapy in critically ill patients. *N Engl J Med.* 2009;361(17):1627–1638.
483. Palevsky P, Zhang J, O'Connor T, et al. VA/NIH Acute Renal Failure Trial Network. Intensity of renal support in critically ill patients with acute kidney injury. *N Engl J Med.* 2008;359(1):7–20.
484. Phu NH, Hien TT, Mai NT, et al. Hemofiltration and peritoneal dialysis in infection-associated acute renal failure in Vietnam. *N Engl J Med.* 2002;347(12):895–902.
485. Krinsley JS. Association between hyperglycemia and increased hospital mortality in a heterogeneous population of critically ill patients. *Mayo Clin Proc.* 2003;78(12):1471–1478.
486. van den Berghe G, Wouters P, Weekers F, et al. Intensive insulin therapy in the critically ill patients. *N Engl J Med.* 2001;345(19):1359–1367.
487. Latham R, Lancaster AD, Covington JF, et al. The association of diabetes and glucose control with surgical-site infections among cardiothoracic surgery patients. *Infect Contr Hosp Epidemiol.* 2001;22(10):607–612.
488. van den Berghe G, Wilmer A, Hermans G, et al. Intensive insulin therapy in the medical ICU. *N Engl J Med.* 2006;354(5):449–461.
489. Finfer S, Chittock DR, Su SY, et al. NICE-SUGAR Study Investigators. Intensive versus conventional glucose control in critically ill patients. *N Engl J Med.* 2009;360(13):1283–1297.
490. Griesdale DE, de Souza RJ, van Dam RM, et al. Intensive insulin therapy and mortality among critically ill patients: a meta-analysis including NICE-SUGAR study data. *Can Med Assoc J.* 2009;180(8):821–827.
491. Wiener R, Wiener DC, Larson RJ. Benefits and risks of tight glucose control in critically ill adults: a meta-analysis. *JAMA.* 2008;300(8):933–944.
492. Cooper MS, Stewart PM. Corticosteroid insufficiency in acutely ill patients. *N Engl J Med.* 2003;348(8):727–734.
493. Annane D, Bellissant E, Sebille V, et al. Impaired pressor sensitivity to noradrenaline in septic shock patients with and without impaired adrenal function reserve. *Br J Clin Pharmacol.* 1998;46(6):589–597.
494. Briegel J, Forst H, Haller M, Schelling G. Stress doses of hydrocortisone reverse byperdynamic septic shock: a prospective randomized, double-blind, single-center study. *Crit Care Med.* 1999;27(4):723–732.
495. Bollaert PE, Charpentier C, Levy B, et al. Reversal of late septic shock with supraphysiologic doses of hydrocortisone. *Crit Care Med.* 1998;26(4): 645–650.
496. Keh D, Boehnke T, Weber-Cartens S, et al. Immunologic and hemodynamic effects of "low-dose" hydrocortisone in septic shock: a double-blind, randomized, placebo-controlled, crossover study. *Am J Resp Crit Care Med.* 2003;167(4):512–520.
497. Annane D, Sebille V, Charpentier C, et al. Effect of treatment with low doses of hydrocortisone and fludrocortisone on mortality in patients with septic shock. *JAMA.* 2002;288(7):862–871.
498. Hamrahian AH, Oseni TS, Arafah BM. Measurements of serum free cortisol in critically ill patients. *N Engl J Med.* 2004;350(16):1629–1638.
499. Sprung C, Annane D, Keh D, et al. Hydrocortisone therapy for patients with septic shock. *N Engl J Med.* 2008;358(2):111–124.
500. Moreno R, Sprung C, Annane D, et al. Time course of organ failure in patients with septic shock treated with hydrocortisone: results of the Corticus study. *Appl Physiol Intensive Care Med.* 2012:423–430.
501. Ranieri VM, Suter PM, Tortorella C, et al. Effect of mechanical ventilation on inflammatory mediators in patients with acute respiratory distress syndrome: a randomized controlled trial. *JAMA.* 1999;282(1):54–61.
502. Tremblay L, Valenza F, Ribeiro SP, Li J, Slutsky AS. Injurious ventilatory strategies increase cytokines and c-fos m-RNA expression in an isolated rat lung model. *J Clin Invest.* 1997;99(5):944–952.
503. International Consensus Conferences in Intensive Care Medicine. Ventilator-associated lung injury in ARDS. This official conference report was cosponsored by the American Thoracic Society, The European Society of Intensive Care Medicine, and The Societé de Réanimation de Langue Française, and was approved by the ATS Board of Directors, July 1999. *Am J Resp Crit Care Med.* 1999;160(6):2118–2124.
504. Ferguson ND, Fan E, Camporota L, et al. The Berlin definition of ARDS: an expanded rationale, justification, and supplementary material. *Intensive Care Med.* 2012;38(10):1573–1582.
505. Futier E, Constantin J-M, Paugam-Burtz C, et al. A trial of intraoperative low-tidal-volume ventilation in abdominal surgery. *N Engl J Med.* 2013;369(5):428–437.
506. Hussain SN, Graham R, Rutledge F, Roussos C. Respiratory muscle energetics during endotoxic shock in dogs. *J Appl Physiol.* 1986;60(2):486–493.
507. Leon A, Boczkowski J, Dureuil B, et al. Effects of endotoxic shock on diaphragmatic function in mechanically ventilated rats. *J Appl Physiol.* 1992;72(4):1466–1472.
508. Marik PE, Zaloga GP. Early enteral nutrition in acutely ill patients: a systematic review. *Crit Care Med.* 2001;29(12):2264–2270.
509. Heyland DK. Nutritional support in the critically ill patients: a critical review of the evidence. *Crit Care Clin.* 1998;14(3):423–440.
510. Heyland DK, MacDonald S, Keefe L, Drover JW. Total parenteral nutrition in the critically ill patient: a meta-analysis. *JAMA.* 1998;280(23):2013–2019.
511. Moore FA, Feliciano DV, Andrassy RJ, et al. Early enteral feeding, compared with parenteral, reduces postoperative septic complications: the results of a meta-analysis. *Ann Surg.* 1992;216(2):172–183.
512. Harvey SE, Parrott F, Harrison DA, et al. Trial of the route of early nutritional support in critically ill adults. *N Engl J Med.* 2014;371(18):1673–1684.
513. Hebert PC, Wells G, Blajchman MA, et al. A multicenter, randomized, controlled clinical trial of transfusion requirements in critical care. *N Engl J Med.* 1999;340(6):409–417.
514. Holst LB, Haase N, Wetterslev J, et al. Lower versus higher hemoglobin threshold for transfusion in septic shock. *N Engl J Med.* 2014;371(15):1381–1391.
515. Leaver SK, Finney SJ, Burke-Gaffney A, Evans TW. Sepsis since the discovery of toll-like receptors: disease concepts and therapeutic opportunities. *Crit Care Med.* 2007;35(5):1404–1410.
516. Van Amersfoort ES, Van Berkel TJ, Kuiper J. Receptors, mediators, and mechanisms involved in bacterial sepsis and septic shock. *Clin Microbiol Rev.* 2003;16(3):379–414.
517. Savva A, Roger T. Targeting toll-like receptors: promising therapeutic strategies for the management of sepsis-associated pathology and infectious diseases. *Frontiers Immunol.* 2013;4:387.

CHAPTER
47

Hemorrhagic Shock

EILEEN M. BULGER and DAVID B. HOYT

INTRODUCTION

The definition of *shock* describes the final common pathway of many disease states: ineffective tissue perfusion, resulting in severe dysfunction of organs vital to survival. The most commonly used classification system for shock includes four categories based on hemodynamic characteristics:

1. *Hypovolemic shock* resulting from a decreased circulating blood volume in relation to the total vascular capacity and characterized by a reduction of diastolic filling pressures and volumes
2. *Cardiogenic shock* related to cardiac pump failure caused by loss of myocardial contractility/functional myocardium or structural/mechanical failure of the cardiac anatomy characterized by elevations of diastolic filling pressures and volumes
3. *Extracardiac obstructive shock* involving obstruction to flow in the cardiovascular circuit and characterized by either impairment of diastolic filling or excessive afterload
4. *Distributive shock* caused by loss of vasomotor control, resulting in arteriolar and venular dilations and characterized by increased cardiac output and decreased systemic vascular resistance after fluid resuscitation

Although the hemodynamic characteristics of the various forms of shock may vary, the final common pathway—inadequate cellular perfusion—must be addressed early to prevent long-term sequelae and death (Fig. 47.1).

Hemorrhagic shock is a form of hypovolemic shock. It is a common, yet complicated, clinical condition that physicians are frequently called upon to evaluate and treat. Etiologies include trauma, postoperative bleeding, medical conditions, and iatrogenic causes. Diagnosis must be accurate and expedient. Therapy must be direct, efficient, and multifactorial in order to avoid the potential multisystem sequelae.

The purpose of this chapter is to review the pathophysiology of hemorrhagic shock, and to focus on the diagnostic and therapeutic approaches to early treatment. Current controversies and new and experimental therapies will also be discussed.

PATHOPHYSIOLOGY

Circulatory Changes

Hemorrhage results in a predictable pattern of events that begins with acute changes in circulating blood volume and culminates in a final common pathway shared by all classifications of shock (see Fig. 47.1). Hemodynamically, hypovolemic shock is characterized by a fall in ventricular preload, resulting in decreased ventricular diastolic filling pressures and volumes. This in turn leads to a decrease in cardiac output and stroke volume (1–4). Following unloading of the cardiac baroreceptors and activation of the sympathetic nervous system, tachycardia ensues in an attempt to compensate for the decrease in cardiac output and stroke volume (5). The sympathetic output also results in vasoconstriction, leading to a decrease in pulse pressure. Greater variations in blood pressure will occur with the respiratory cycle due to an increased sensitivity of the underfilled heart to changes in venous return with varying intrathoracic pressure (6–8). The increased sympathetic tone may prevent a severe drop in arterial blood pressure initially. However, continued blood loss will ultimately result in hypotension and shock. Due to compensatory vasoconstriction, systemic vascular resistance rises early after the development of hypovolemic shock, but may fall in later stages, potentially heralding irreversibility and death (1,9,10).

The response to blood loss is a dynamic process that involves competing adaptive (compensatory) and maladaptive responses at each stage of development. Although intravascular volume replacement is always a necessary component of resuscitation in hypovolemic shock, the complex biologic response to the insult may progress to a point at which such resuscitation is insufficient to reverse the progression of the shock syndrome. Severe hemorrhage leads to a series of inflammatory mediator, cardiovascular, and organ responses that may supersede the injury itself and ultimately drive recovery or death (9,11–14). Furthermore, ongoing blood loss contributes to a progressive coagulopathy and metabolic acidosis that further complicate the resuscitation of the patient.

Oxygen Balance

Shock is characterized by an oxygen deficit in tissues and cells. The significance of the deficit and the extent of cellular injury can be quantified as a function of both the severity and the duration of the deficit—the greater the severity, the longer the duration, the worse the outcome of shock.

Oxygen delivery to tissues is determined by cardiac output and the oxygen content in arterial blood. *Oxygen content* refers to the number of milliliters of oxygen contained in 100 mL of blood (mL/dL) and is a function of the hemoglobin concentration, the oxygen saturation of hemoglobin, and the amount of oxygen dissolved in plasma (the calculation is [Hgb × 1.34 × O_2 saturation] + [PaO_2 × 0.0003]). During hemorrhage, as the cardiac output falls, oxygen delivery to the tissues also falls. Initially, the body will maintain sufficient uptake of oxygen by extracting more from the arterial blood. This will result in a fall in the mixed venous oxygen saturation (SvO_2) with an increase in the arteriovenous oxygen content gradient (CaO_2 – CvO_2). Eventually, this compensatory mechanism also fails, and tissue hypoxia with lactic acidosis ensues. Cerebral and cardiac functions are maintained by diversion of blood flow from other organs (skin, muscle, and kidneys) (14). However, when these compensatory mechanisms are maximized, cardiac function and tissue oxygen delivery deteriorate further, and irreversible shock may develop (15).

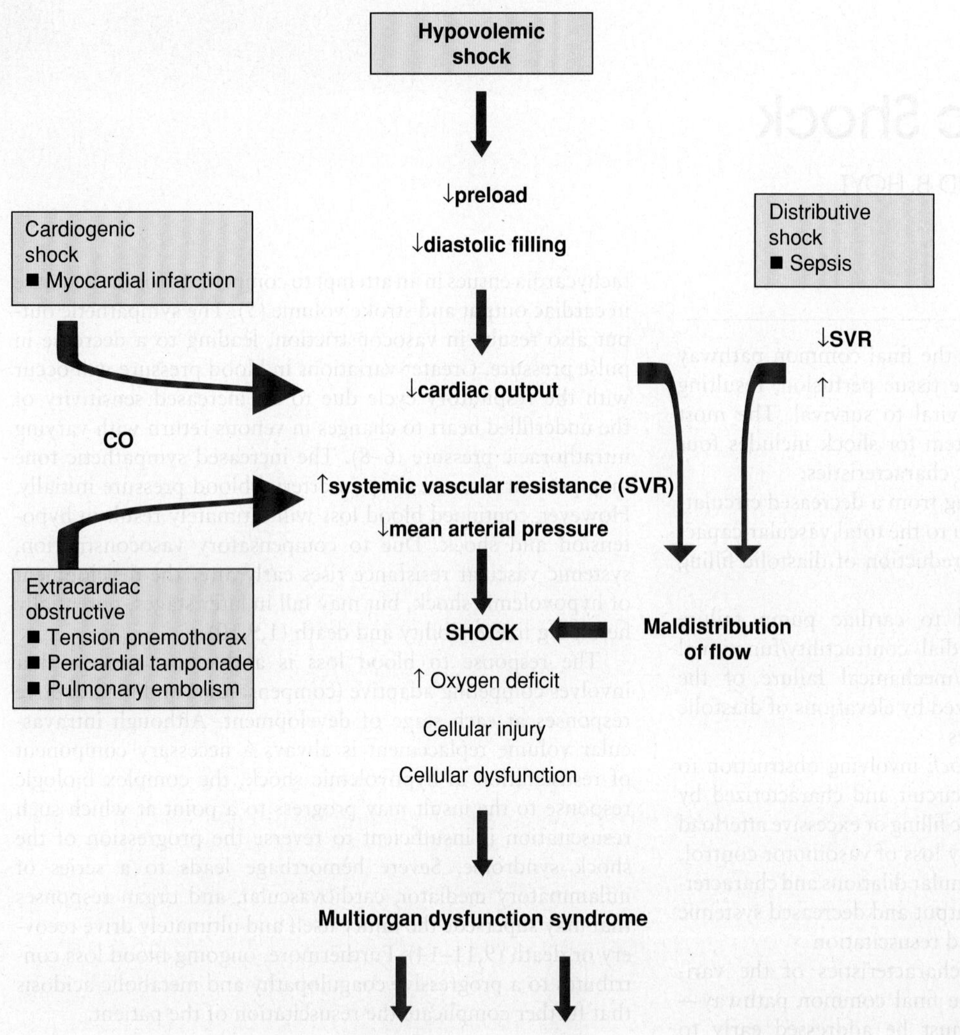

FIGURE 47.1 Final common pathway of shock. Hemorrhagic shock results in acute changes in circulating blood volume that culminates in a final common pathway shared by all classifications of shock.

Critical oxygen delivery is a function of cellular needs for oxygen and the ability of cells to extract oxygen from the arterial blood. Many factors contribute to this equation. During hemorrhage, tissue oxygen needs may increase due to increased respiratory muscle activity and increased catecholamine circulation (16). However, some evidence suggests that catecholamines downregulate the metabolic needs of cells during hypovolemic shock (2,3,17,18). Regional blood flow is modified during hypovolemic shock in an attempt to maintain oxygen delivery to critical tissues (14,19). In addition, the individual needs of various tissues may vary during hemorrhagic shock. For instance, the oxygen needs of the kidney may decline during hemorrhage because a fall in renal perfusion leads to a fall in glomerular filtration and a decrease in energy-consuming tubular absorption (14). In contrast, the gut may experience an increased oxygen debt early due to the high oxygen need of the mucosa, along with redistribution of blood away from the gut to more critical tissues. This is the physiologic basis for gastric tonometry as a means of measuring the adequacy of resuscitation early following hemorrhage (20).

Oxygen extraction in tissues is influenced by the position of the oxyhemoglobin dissociation curve (21–23). Factors that improve the ability of tissues to extract oxygen from hemoglobin (i.e., shift the curve to the right) include acidosis, hypercarbia, hyperthermia, and decreased blood viscosity. However, in any extreme, each of these factors can be overcome by inadequate oxygen delivery and cardiovascular collapse. Interestingly, the oxyhemoglobin curve has been shown to shift to the left in critically ill patients (24). The presence of 2,3-diphosphoglycerate (DPG) in transfused blood has also been associated with a left shift of the oxyhemoglobin dissociation curve (25). Thus, although transfusions may increase the hemoglobin level, theoretically improving oxygen delivery, they may negatively affect the ability of tissues to extract oxygen from the hemoglobin.

The severity of oxygen debt during hypovolemic shock has been shown to be a major determinant of survival in animals and in patients following trauma, hemorrhage, and major surgery (10,15,26,27). A large oxygen debt has been associated with the development of acute respiratory distress syndrome (ARDS) and multiple-organ dysfunction syndrome (MODS) (26,28–30). Conversely, a high oxygen delivery and uptake during resuscitation has been associated with improved survival (15,27,31–33). Whether increasing oxygen delivery to supranormal levels ultimately improves survival during resuscitation in critical illness remains controversial, and the medical literature

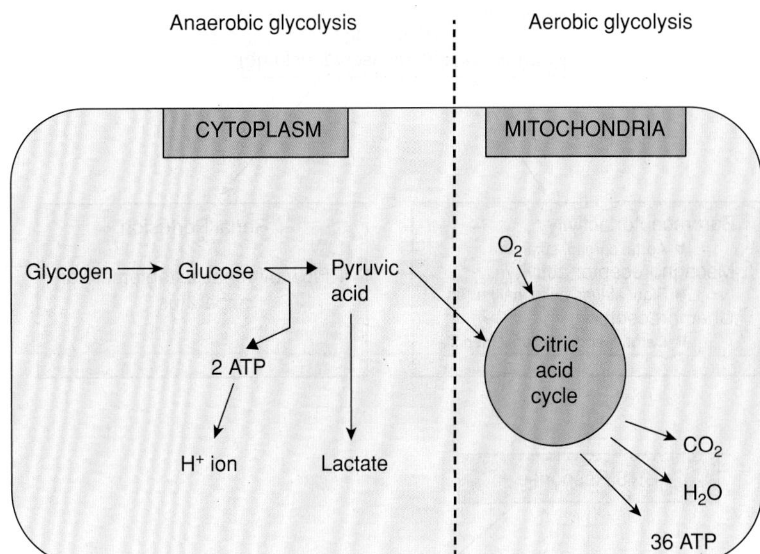

FIGURE 47.2 Cellular mechanisms during anaerobic and aerobic glycolysis. In anaerobic conditions, pyruvic acid cannot enter the citric acid cycle within the mitochondria and is instead shunted to the production of lactate. This process produces only two molecules of ATP, as opposed to the 36 molecules of ATP produced from glucose in the mitochondria during aerobic glycolysis. Hydrolysis of ATP molecules in anaerobic conditions results in the production of hydrogen ions that cannot be cleared, leading to intracellular acidosis. (Adapted from Mizock BA, Falk JL. Lactic acidosis in critical illness. *Crit Care Med.* 1992;20:80–93.)

has produced mixed results (28,34–37) with recent studies suggesting no clear benefit from this approach and concern that overly aggressive fluid resuscitation can lead to abdominal compartment syndrome and other complications (37).

Cellular Response

During hypovolemic shock, the oxygen deficit in the tissues causes a fall in the mitochondrial production and concentration of high-energy phosphates because of greater breakdown than production (38–43). This led many researchers to evaluate the utility of adenosine triphosphate (ATP) in the resuscitation of hemorrhagic shock (44,45). In the presence of sufficient oxygen, aerobic combustion of 1 mol of glucose yields 38 mol of energy-rich ATP. However, in the absence of sufficient oxygen, glucose taken up by the cells cannot be combusted because of insufficient uptake of pyruvate into the mitochondrial tricarboxylic acid cycle. Pyruvate is then converted to lactate within the cytoplasm. Anaerobic glycolysis yields only 2 mol of ATP, which is then hydrolyzed into hydrogen ion, ultimately leading to intracellular and extracellular metabolic acidosis (Fig. 47.2) (38,39,46,47). This process is ultimately a function of the severity and duration of regional hypoperfusion relative to oxygen demand and is more pronounced in some tissues (diaphragm, liver, kidney, gut) than in others (heart, skeletal muscle). Ultimately, a significant fall in the high-energy phosphates for a prolonged duration will lead to irreversible cellular injury and death.

The sequelae of low ATP production are profound. About 60% of the energy produced by respiring cellular mitochondria is needed to fuel the sodium–potassium (Na^+–K^+) pump of the cell. This pump controls the gradient in electrolyte concentrations and electric potential over the cell membrane. In the absence of sufficient ATP, the Na^+–K^+ pump is inhibited, resulting in an influx of sodium into the cell and efflux of potassium out of the cell. This in turn leads to cellular fluid uptake (38,40,48–51). Hyperkalemia may result due to potassium exchange between cells, the interstitial fluid, and vascular space.

Independent of the Na^+–K^+ pump, there may be a selective increase in cell membrane permeability for ions during hemorrhagic shock. Hypovolemic shock has been shown to lead to a rapid decrease in the transmembrane potential (with a less negative inner membrane potential), resulting in rapid electrolyte and fluid shifts across the membrane. Circulating heat shock proteins may also contribute to these changes independent of energy deficit (51–54).

Finally, calcium (Ca^{2+}) influx into cells and their mitochondria inhibits cellular respiration and ultimately contributes to cellular damage and swelling. Plasma levels of free Ca^{2+} may also fall. This may have profound consequences on the function of several organs during shock including the liver, kidney, heart, and vascular smooth muscle (49,50,55–61). Intracellular lysosomes lose their integrity, and proteolytic enzymes are released and contribute to cellular dysfunction and cell death. The sum of the intracellular changes and alterations in signaling transduction pathways described above ultimately leads to the development of cellular dysfunction and MODS, which may be irreversible (61).

Neurohumoral Response

In response to hemorrhage and hypovolemia, a complex neurohumoral response is initiated in an attempt to maintain blood pressure and retain fluid. Decreased intravascular volume stimulates baroreceptors in the carotid body and aortic arch, along with mechanoreceptors in the right atrium. This stimulation leads to several neurohumoral responses (Fig. 47.3). Circulating catecholamines are liberated by activation of the sympathetic nervous system and the adrenal medulla. Direct sympathetic stimulation of the vessel wall leads to vasoconstriction. Angiotensin II is liberated via the renin–angiotensin–aldosterone system. Vasopressin (antidiuretic hormone [ADH]) is released by the pituitary in hypovolemic shock and leads to vasoconstriction. Finally, decreased cardiac filling pressures reduce cardiac secretion of α-atrial natriuretic peptide (ANP), thereby reducing the vasodilatory and diuretic effects of ANP.

Macrocirculation

During loss of circulating blood volume, mechanisms are initiated to counteract the fall in cardiac output and oxygen delivery

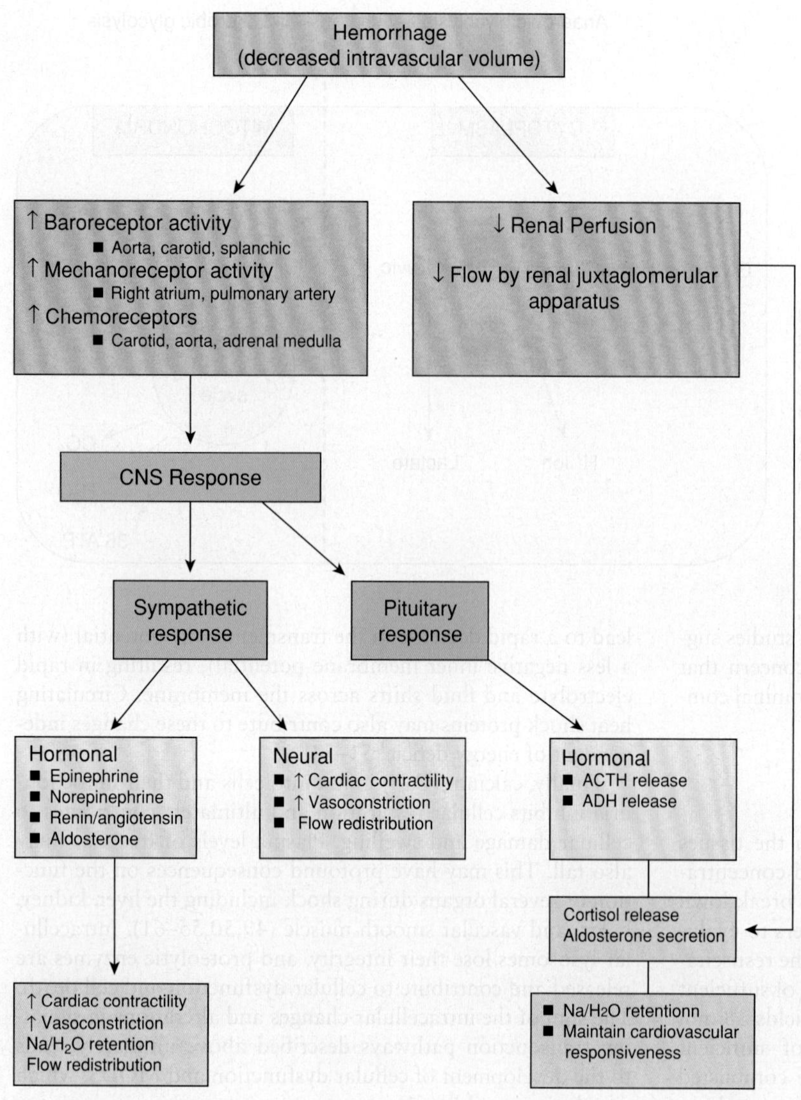

FIGURE 47.3 Neurohormonal response to hemorrhage. Hemorrhage results in a decrease in the circulating intravascular volume, which initiates a complex cascade of compensatory events. CNS, central nervous system; ACTH, adrenocorticotropic hormone; ADH, antidiuretic hormone.

by facilitating a redistribution of peripheral blood flow (14). Regional autoregulation takes place via a delicate balance of endogenous vasodilators and vasoconstrictors. Endothelial cells produce potent vasodilators such as endothelium-derived relaxing factor (nitric oxide [NO]), heme oxygenation–derived carbon monoxide (CO), and metabolic byproducts in tissues, including carbon dioxide (CO_2), potassium, and adenosine (62–69). Some authors describe that inhibition of NO early following hemorrhage ameliorates early hypotension and improves mortality (70–74). Conversely, other authors describe endothelial dysfunction in organs with diminished NO production (75,76). Endothelin is a potent endothelial cell–derived vasoconstrictor that is released upon catecholamine stimulation or hypoxia (77). The overall increase in systemic peripheral vascular resistance is distributed differently among various organs in the body (19). Vasoconstriction also occurs in the venous vasculature, increasing return of available blood to the heart (4,78). The complex interplay of these mechanisms for vasodilation and vasoconstriction ultimately determines the regional redistribution of blood flow to organs following hemorrhagic shock. The redistribution of blood flow results in a greater share of oxygen delivery to organs with high obligatory metabolic demands (heart and brain), and a lesser share to those with fewer demands including the skin, skeletal muscle, kidney, intestine, and pancreas (3,19,66,79).

Microcirculation

One of the most important determinants of tissue perfusion during shock is the response and function of the microvasculature, which is defined as vessels less than 100 to 150 μm in diameter. Although arteries and medium-sized arterioles constrict in response to the extrinsic control mechanisms described above, terminal arterioles, venules, and capillaries remain unaffected and are more controlled by local metabolic factors.

Alterations in microvascular function and flow are affected through precapillary and postcapillary sphincters, which are sensitive to both extrinsic and intrinsic control mechanisms. Exchange of metabolites and compartmental regulation of fluids occur at the capillary level. Therefore, alteration of tone of the pre- and postcapillary sphincters can have significant effects on microcirculatory function (78,80,81). Failure to dilate sphincters supplying metabolically active tissues may result in ischemia and anaerobic metabolism with lactate production. Increased precapillary tone, as seen with sympathetic stimulation, results in increased blood pressure systemically and decreased hydrostatic pressure locally. In fact, the microvascular arterioles may even dilate in response to the above vasoconstriction due to release of metabolic byproducts of underperfusion (carbon dioxide, hydrogen ion, etc.). The decrease in hydrostatic pressure locally then leads to redistribution of fluid from the interstitium to the circulation. Conversely, increased postcapillary tone (relative to precapillary tone) results in vascular pooling of blood and loss of fluid to the interstitium (as a result of increased hydrostatic pressure). This increased hydrostatic pressure may become accentuated in response to crystalloid resuscitation, leading to interstitial edema (81). Finally, hemorrhage and shock have also been shown to induce increased permeability of capillaries, leading to interstitial fluid leak during resuscitation (82,83).

Hypovolemic shock and hemorrhage also induce the expression of endothelial adhesion molecules on neutrophils and endothelium (48,84). This results in neutrophil adherence and "rolling" of cells within the capillary bed (85–87). Capillary flow then diminishes and may also impair red blood cell flow. While this decrease in transit time may augment the ability of tissue to extract oxygen, it may also lead to microvascular thrombosis and further tissue ischemia (88,89).

Metabolic and Hormonal Response

The early hyperglycemic response to trauma/hemorrhage is the combined result of enhanced glycogenolysis, caused by the hormonal response to stress including elevated epinephrine, cortisol, and glucagon levels; increased gluconeogenesis in the liver, partly mediated by glucagon; and peripheral resistance to the action of insulin (38,90). Increased gluconeogenesis in the liver, and to a lesser extent in the kidneys, follows increased efflux of amino acids, such as alanine and glutamine from the muscle to the liver, due to a breakdown of muscle protein. The latter is evidenced by increased urinary losses of nitrogen and a negative nitrogen balance. Lactate produced in muscle can also be converted to glucose in the liver (91). Increased epinephrine also results in skeletal muscle insulin resistance, sparing glucose for use by glucose-dependent organs such as the heart and brain. Later in shock, hypoglycemia may ensue, possibly because of glycogen depletion or hepatic ischemia (38,91,92). Fatty acids are increased early in shock, but later levels fall (90). Without energy for glycolysis, the cell depends on lipolysis and the autodigestion of intracellular protein for energy. Initially, ketone bodies and the branched-chain amino acids are used as alternative fuel sources. Without oxygen, these sources become inefficient, leading to hypertriglyceridemia, increased β-hydroxybutyric acid and acetoacetate levels, and changes in the amino acid concentration pattern. As these metabolic changes occur, set in motion by cellular hypoxia and promoted by systemic hormonal changes, structural changes occur within individual cells (93).

Inflammatory and Immune Response

A detailed discussion of the inflammatory and immune response to trauma and hemorrhage is beyond the scope of this chapter. However, several general concepts can be introduced. Following hemorrhage and resuscitation, macrophages, including lung macrophages and Kupffer cells in the liver, may release pro-inflammatory cytokines such as tumor necrosis factor (TNF)-α and interleukin (IL)-1, -6, and -8. During reperfusion, cytokines may induce and amplify the inflammatory response to ischemia and may further induce local and remote organ damage (94–104). The reperfused gut, for example, may, together with the liver, be a source of systemically circulating cytokines, and possibly endotoxin. Release of mediators into the mesenteric lymph, portal, or systemic circulations during reperfusion may have deleterious effects on remote organs, such as the lungs, due to neutrophil activation and adherence, leading to pulmonary vascular injury with increased permeability (95,98,99). Antigen–antibody complexes activate the complement cascade, and complement fragments thus generated can interact with other cytokines to promulgate the inflammatory response. Complement activation can yield potent vasodilating and leuko-attractant substances (105–108).

Oxygen radicals, such as hydrogen peroxide and superoxide anion, are released by activated neutrophils in response to a variety of stimuli. They are also released when xanthine oxidase is activated after reperfusion in ischemia–reperfusion models. These highly reactive products lead to cell membrane dysfunction, increased vascular permeability, and release of eicosanoids (109–113).

This inflammatory process results in the local accumulation of activated inflammatory cells, which release various local toxins such as oxygen radicals, proteases, eicosanoids, platelet-activating factor, and other substances. When unregulated, such accumulations can cause tissue injury. The initial attachment of neutrophils to the vascular endothelium at an inflammatory site is facilitated by the interaction of adherence molecules on the neutrophil and endothelial cell surfaces (114–119).

Trauma-Induced Coagulopathy

Patients suffering from severe hemorrhagic shock will frequently develop a coagulopathy that can further complicate the control of hemorrhage. Previously, this coagulopathy was thought to be primarily due to loss of clotting factors during hemorrhage combined with dilution during the resuscitation phase. Recent evidence suggests that 25% to 40% of severely injured patients are already manifesting evidence of coagulopathy at the time of hospital admission (120,121). This has been termed trauma-induced coagulopathy. The etiology of trauma-induced coagulopathy is likely multifactorial and six key initiators of coagulopathy have been described (Fig. 47.4). These include tissue trauma, shock, hypothermia, academia, hemodilution, and inflammation (122). Tissue injury leads to exposure of subendothelial type III collagen and tissue factor, which binds von Willebrand factor and platelets inducing coagulation. Hyperfibrinolysis also results from tissue injury due to release of endothelial tissue plasminogen activator and inhibition of plasminogen activator inhibitor-1 in the setting of shock (122). Hypothermia and academia can also directly impair coagulation protease activity. Recent data also suggest that depletion of coagulation factors early after injury may be driven by the protein C system (121). Over time, trauma patients who are initially coagulopathic with increased bleeding will transition to a hypercoagulable state, which increases the risk of thrombotic complications. Additional work is regarded to better understand the timing and mechanism of this transition. Evidence of trauma-induced coagulopathy upon hospital admission has been associated with a fourfold

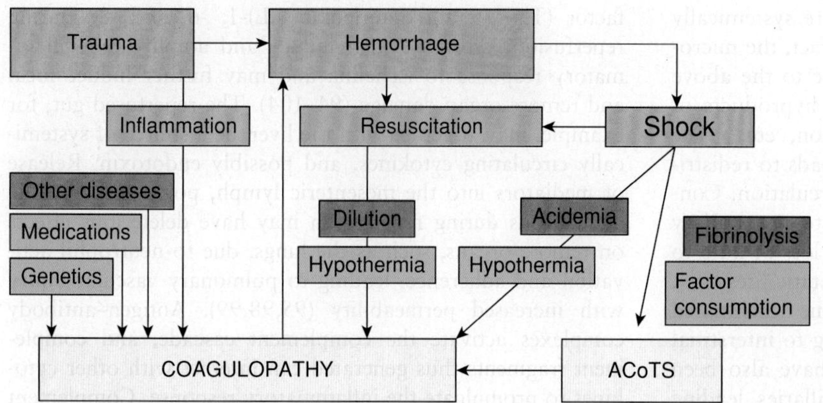

FIGURE 47.4 Mechanisms of trauma-induced coagulopathy. Trauma results in hemorrhage, which leads to resuscitation, which in turn leads to dilution and hypothermia causing coagulopathy and further hemorrhage. This is the classic, "dilutional coagulopathy." Hemorrhage also causes shock, which causes acidosis and hypothermia that also contribute to coagulopathy. Finally, trauma and shock can also cause acute coagulopathy of trauma–shock associated with factor consumption and fibrinolysis. Coagulopathy is further associated with trauma-induced inflammation and modified by genetics, medications and acquired diseases. (With permission from Hess JR, Brohi K, Dutton RP, et al. The coagulopathy of trauma: a review of mechanisms. *J Trauma.* 2008;65:748–754.)

increase in mortality (123,124). Therefore, acute measurement of coagulation parameters during resuscitation from hemorrhagic shock is indicated along with early efforts to address coagulation abnormalities.

DIAGNOSIS

Early diagnosis of hemorrhagic shock is imperative to avoid delay in treatment. However, clinical signs are relatively insensitive for small amounts of blood loss. There is a progressive hemodynamic deterioration with ongoing blood loss. This classic progression is delineated in Table 47.1. Total blood volume is estimated at approximately 70 mL/kg in the average adult, or nearly 5 L for a 70-kg person. The signs and symptoms of hemorrhagic shock vary based on the severity of blood loss. Traditionally, this progression has been defined as four classes of shock.

Class I hemorrhage is marked by a less than 750 mL estimated blood loss, or less than 15% of total circulating blood volume. There are minimal physical signs associated with this volume of blood loss. The patient may not have tachycardia, with a heart rate remaining less than 100 beats per minute; the systolic blood pressure and pulse pressure remain normal; the respiratory rate remains at 14 to 20 breaths per minute; and urine output remains adequate (>30 mL/hr). Only subtle physical signs such as delayed capillary refill and slight anxiety may exist.

Class II hemorrhage is marked by an estimated blood loss of 750 to 1,500 mL (or 15% to 30% of the total circulating blood volume). Physical signs begin to manifest during this stage of hemorrhage. Although the systolic blood pressure may be maintained, the patient usually becomes tachycardic (heart rate greater than 100 beats per minute), the pulse pressure begins to decrease, and capillary refill is delayed. The respiratory rate begins to increase (20 to 30 breaths per minute), urine output becomes diminished (20 to 30 mL/hr), and the patient becomes very anxious.

Class III hemorrhage is marked by an estimated blood loss of >1,500 to 2,000 mL (or >30% to 40% of total circulating blood volume). During this phase, significant hemodynamic compromise becomes apparent. Heart rate increases to >120 beats per minute, systolic blood pressure decreases, pulse pressure decreases, capillary refill decreases, tachypnea worsens with a respiratory rate of 30 to 40 breaths per minute, urine output drops to 5 to 15 mL/hr, and the patient becomes confused, showing further evidence of decreased perfusion of the central nervous system.

Class IV hemorrhage is marked by an estimated blood loss of >2,000 mL (or >40% of total circulating blood volume). During this phase, most compensatory cardiovascular mechanisms have been maximized and total hemodynamic collapse is imminent. Signs of class IV hemorrhage include severe tachycardia with a heart rate >140 beats per minute, a decreased systolic blood pressure, a decreased pulse pressure, delayed capillary refill, significant tachypnea with a respiratory rate of >35 breaths per minute, minimal to no urine output, and severely altered mental status as marked by confusion and/or lethargy.

Another way to classify patients with hemorrhagic shock is based on their response to initial fluid resuscitation. Rapid responders will typically require a limited fluid resuscitation to normalize vital signs. Transient responders will improve following fluid administration but then hypotension will recur. Nonresponders remain hypotensive despite fluid and blood product administration. Generally transient responders and

TABLE 47.1 Clinical Classes of Hemorrhagic Shock

	Class I	Class II	Class III	Class IV
Blood loss	<750 mL	750–1,500 mL	>1,500–2,000 mL	>2,000 mL
	<15%	15–30%	>30–40%	>40%
Heart rate (bpm)	<100	>100	>120	>140
Systolic blood pressure	Normal	Normal	Decreased	Decreased
Pulse pressure	Normal	Decreased	Decreased	Decreased
Capillary refill	Delayed	Delayed	Delayed	Delayed
Respiratory rate (breaths/min)	14–20	20–30	30–40	>35
Urine output (mL/hr)	>30	20–30	5–15	Minimal
Mental status	Slightly anxious	Anxious	Confused	Confused and lethargic

TABLE 47.2 Response to Initial Fluid Resuscitation and Patient Management

	Rapid Response	Transient Response	No Response
Vital signs	Return to normal	Transient response, recurrent hypotension, and/or tachycardia	Remains abnormal
Estimated blood loss	Minimal (10–20%)	Moderate (20–40%)	Severe (>40%)
Additional crystalloid	Unlikely	Yes	Yes
Need for blood transfusion	Unlikely	Moderate to high	Immediate
Blood preparation	Type and cross-match (30–60 min)	Type-specific (10–20 min)	Emergency blood release (immediate type O Rh-negative blood)
Operative intervention	Possible	Likely	Highly likely
Early presence of surgeon	Yes	Yes	Yes

Adapted from American College of Surgeons Committee on Trauma. Shock. In: *Advanced Trauma Life Support.* 7th ed. Chicago, IL: American College of Surgeons; 2004:79.

nonresponders will require additional intervention to obtain hemorrhage control (Table 47.2).

Transient responders can be the most difficult to diagnose. Retrospective studies have shown that patients with field hypotension who become normotensive on arrival to the emergency department have increased morbidity, mortality, need for operation, and admission rate to the intensive care unit (ICU) (125–127). Approximately 15% of these patients will need transfusion, with 37% requiring therapeutic surgery (127). Hence, even a brief episode of hypotension can be a marker for significant underlying injury. Tachycardia is one of the first signs of shock, although some patients may respond to traumatic hemorrhage with bradycardia as a result of a vagal nerve–mediated transient sympathoinhibition due to acute and sudden blood loss (1–3,128,129). Narrowing of the pulse pressure, low end-tidal CO_2, and markers of acidosis (base deficit or lactate) are also useful predictors of compensated shock (130–134).

Special Populations

Geriatrics

Concurrent medication, such as β-blockers, may attenuate the physiologic response to hemorrhage. In the presence of β-blockade, tachycardia may be blunted or may not occur at all. Prior hydration status and use of diuretics can also alter the rate at which these signs present. Elderly patients may have atrial arrhythmias leading to a high ventricular response, making tachycardia less sensitive in this patient population Changes in blood pressure in geriatric patients may also be more difficult to assess. Those with a baseline hypertension may have what appears to be a normal adult blood pressure but may be in compensated shock and have significant organ hypoperfusion (130,135,136).

Pregnant Patients

Pregnant patients have a significantly increased total blood volume, and thus can lose up to 1,000 mL of blood before presenting with any clinical signs of hemorrhage. Blood is diverted from the placenta via vasoconstriction; the mother's total blood circulation is maintained at the expense of the fetus. Fetal distress may be the first sign of shock in the mother (137,138).

Pediatrics

Pediatric patients have extensive compensatory mechanisms, which can result in significant tachycardia before any hypotension is manifested. Hypotension in a pediatric patient is an ominous sign and suggests advanced stages of hemorrhage.

Diagnostic Approach

The first priority in managing a patient with hemorrhagic shock is to identify and control the source of bleeding. If no obvious source of external bleeding is identified, a rapid evaluation should be performed to identify likely occult sources of bleeding. In the trauma patient, significant internal hemorrhage can occur in four defined regions: the thoracic cavity, the peritoneal cavity, the retroperitoneum, and extremity fractures. These areas can be rapidly assessed via chest radiograph, a pelvic radiograph, focused assessment with sonography for trauma (FAST), and physical examination of extremities along with appropriate radiographs. In-depth coverage of the diagnosis of abdominal trauma is provided in a later chapter of this book. In nontrauma patients without clear evidence of bleeding, the gastrointestinal tract should be rapidly evaluated via nasogastric tube, rectal examination, and endoscopy where appropriate. Additional diagnostic tests can be obtained based on clinical history, patient background, and condition. Abdominal aortic aneurysms can be identified on physical examination and bedside ultrasound. In selected instances, angiography may be used to identify and treat sources of hemorrhage not otherwise apparent (pelvic fractures, pancreatitis, lower gastrointestinal bleeding) (139–144). This should only be instituted when a specific source of hemorrhage is highly likely and therapeutic intervention is sought. Computed tomography should be avoided in hemodynamically unstable patients with hemorrhage.

Laboratory Testing

Hematocrit and Hemoglobin

Hemoglobin and hematocrit measurements have long been part of the basic diagnostic workup of patients with hemorrhage and/or trauma. However, in patients with rapid bleeding, a single hematocrit measurement on presentation to the emergency department may not reflect the degree of hemorrhage. In a short transport or presentation time, prior to initiation of resuscitation, the body's compensatory mechanisms for fluid retention and resorption into the vascular space have not taken place, and initial hematocrit levels may remain stable despite significant blood loss. A retrospective study of 524 trauma patients (145) determined that the initial hematocrit had a sensitivity of only 0.50 for detecting patients with an extent of traumatic hemorrhage requiring surgery. The diagnostic value is further confounded by the administration of intravenous fluids and red cell concentrates during resuscitation (146–148).

Two prospective observational studies determined the sensitivity of serial hematocrit measurements for detecting patients with severe injury (148,149). In the first study (148), the authors compared values of hematocrit at admission and 15 and 30 minutes following arrival to the emergency department. A normal hematocrit on admission did not preclude significant injury. The mean change in hematocrit levels between arrival and 15 minutes, and 15 and 30 minutes was not significantly different in patients with or without serious injuries. However, a decrease of hematocrit by over 6.5% at 15 and 30 minutes had a high specificity for injury (0.93 to 1.0), but a low sensitivity (0.13 to 0.16).

Another prospective observational study examined the utility of serial hematocrit measurements during the initial 4 hours following admission (149). A significant limitation to this study is that they removed patients who required a blood transfusion in order to eliminate confounding variables. In the remaining 494 patients, a decrease in hematocrit of more than 10% between admission and 4 hours was highly specific for severe injury (0.92 to 0.96), but again, it was not sensitive (0.09 to 0.27).

Overall, decreasing hematocrit levels over time may reflect continued bleeding. However, patients with significant bleeding may maintain their hematocrit level, especially in the absence of resuscitation. Conversely, hematocrit levels may also be confounded by aggressive fluid resuscitation early during resuscitation (146,147). An initial hematocrit level will help to identify patients who present with pre-existing anemia who may have a lower threshold for hemorrhage. The hematocrit level should be used in conjunction with other measures of perfusion in order to determine the presence of occult hemorrhage.

Measurements of Perfusion

Lactate

Lactate was initially suggested as a diagnostic parameter and prognostic indicator of hemorrhagic shock in the 1960s. Substantial data exist that lactate levels as a marker of tissue oxygen debt can predict outcome in various forms of shock (46,150). Recent studies have suggested that early changes in lactate even in the prehospital environment may be predictive of the need for blood transfusion and hemorrhage control procedures. A recent multicenter trial which enrolled 327 trauma patients with a systolic blood pressure ≤100 mmHg, transported by ground advanced life-support services reported that prehospital lactate ≥2.5 mgmol/L was a better predictor than blood pressure or shock index for the need for resuscitative care (151).

During hemorrhage, not only is the initial lactate level important, but also the rate of clearance (152,153). Two prospective studies confirm this. In one prospective observational study (152), 76 patients with multiple trauma were analyzed with respect to clearance of lactate between survivors and nonsurvivors over 48 hours. If lactate normalized within 24 hours, survival was 100%. Survival decreased to 77.8% if normalization occurred within 48 hours, and to 13.6% in those in whom lactate levels remained elevated above 2 mEq/L for more than 48 hours. This was confirmed in another prospective study of 129 trauma patients (153) in which initial lactate levels were higher in nonsurvivors. A prolonged time to normalization (>24 hours) was associated with the development of posttraumatic organ failure. Finally, venous lactate has been shown to be an excellent approximation for arterial lactate in acute trauma patients and is a useful marker for significant injury (154).

Taken together, these studies suggest that both the initial lactate level and the rate of clearance are reliable indicators of morbidity and mortality following trauma. However, whether lactate should be used as an end point of resuscitation or is merely a marker of tissue ischemia has not been clearly established.

Base Deficit

Base deficit values derived from arterial blood gas analysis have also been shown to provide an indirect estimation of tissue acidosis due to impaired perfusion (155–161). However, base deficit can be affected by resuscitation fluids (hyperchloremic metabolic acidosis) and exogenous administration of sodium bicarbonate. Despite these potential drawbacks, initial base deficit has been shown in several retrospective studies to correlate with transfusion requirements, organ dysfunction, morbidity, and mortality following trauma (26,162–167). The magnitude and severity of the base deficit also correlates to outcome, and is useful in both pediatric and elderly patients (165,166). Base deficit has been shown to be a better predictor of outcome than pH alone following traumatic injury (164).

Lactate versus Base Deficit

Although many studies have shown that both base deficit and serum lactate levels correlate with outcome following trauma and hemorrhage, these two parameters do not always correlate with each other (168,169). In fact, lactate has been found to be a superior predictor of mortality as compared to base deficit in a recent study of patients in the ICU following trauma (168). Both base deficit and lactate have been shown to correlate to outcome in nontraumatic etiologies of hemorrhagic shock (170,171). Given that there are confounding variables following trauma that can affect measured levels of both lactate and base deficit, independent assessment of both parameters along with the patient's clinical condition is recommended for the evaluation of shock in trauma patients.

Measurement of Coagulopathy

Standard Coagulation Studies

Traditional studies of coagulation include prothrombin time (PT), activated partial thromboplastin time (aPTT), fibrinogen level, and platelet count. Although no tightly controlled trials have been performed, current recommendations for therapeutic end points in hemorrhagic shock include maintaining PT and aPTT at less than 1.5 times the normal value, maintaining a platelet count of >100 in patients with active bleeding or traumatic brain injury, and maintaining a fibrinogen level of >1 g/L.

While these laboratory studies are standard, they do present several drawbacks. To begin, *in vivo* coagulation depends on the interaction between platelets and coagulation factor enzymes. Laboratory values of PT and aPTT are performed on platelet-poor plasma and fail to evaluate the cellular interactions of clotting. PT and aPTT measurements also do not take into account hypothermia-induced coagulopathy because samples are warmed prior to measurement. Platelet and fibrinogen assays give numerical values, but fail to assess function. Finally, each of these tests takes time, in most centers up to 30 to 45 minutes. This lag time makes these studies clinically inefficient because when the results become available, they may not truly reflect the patient's clinical condition. During resuscitation, actively bleeding patients are in a constant state of flux. One study has suggested that with efficient laboratory processing and emergency hemorrhage panel which includes PT/INR, platelet count, and fibrinogen can have results available within 20 minutes (172). Alternative point-of-care testing such as the iSTAT handheld analyzer can provide rapid bedside results, but is currently limited to activated clotting time (ACT) and PT/international normalized ratio (INR) (173).

Thromboelastography

The thromboelastograph (TEG) analyzer is a bedside machine that provides a functional evaluation of overall coagulation on whole blood at the same temperature as the patient. The TEG has been shown to be a more sensitive measure of coagulation disorders than standard coagulation measures (174). The TEG assay provides a tracing that measures clotting (R value), clot formation (α angle), clot strength (maximum amplitude [MA]), and clot lysis (LY 30) (Fig. 47.5). Elongation of the R value represents a deficiency in coagulation factors. The α angle represents the rate of fibrin accumulation and cross-linking, which can be affected by fibrinogen function and, to a lesser degree, platelet function. The MA is a measure of clot strength and is affected primarily by platelets and, to a lesser degree, fibrinogen. A recent study investigating the utility of the admission TEG in trauma patients found that the TEG data were superior to conventional coagulation tests at predicting coagulopathy. The TEG data identified patients at increased risk for early transfusion and identified patients with fibrinolysis (175). Several authors have proposed TEG-guided resuscitation strategies for trauma patients with hemorrhagic shock (175,176).

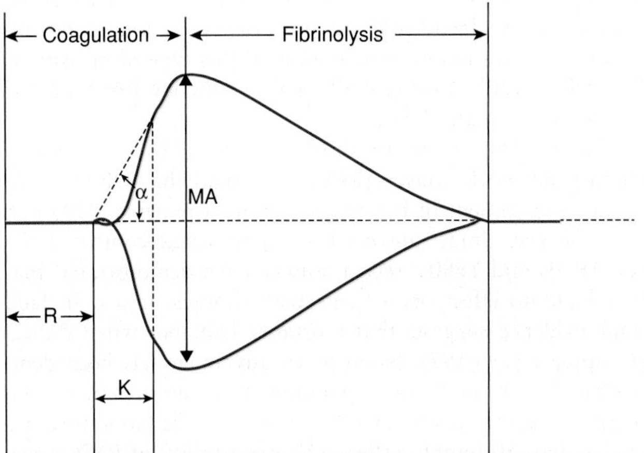

FIGURE 47.5 Thromboelastogram. The thromboelastograph (TEG) analyzer is a bedside machine that provides a functional evaluation of overall coagulation on whole blood at the same temperature as the patient. The thromboelastograph assay provides a tracing that measures time to clot formation (R value), speed to a certain clot strength (K value), rate of clot formation (α angle), overall clot strength (maximum amplitude (MA)) and clot lysis (LY 30).

TREATMENT

Trauma is by far the most common etiology for hemorrhagic shock. While other causes do exist, management priorities are similar regardless of the source of bleeding. Diagnosis, evaluation, and management must often occur simultaneously. A methodical approach is necessary to optimize outcome (Table 47.3). Unique to hemorrhagic shock, as opposed to other forms of shock, is that definitive management frequently requires surgical or procedural intervention to cease bleeding. The diagnostic pathway and interventions pursued become part of the resuscitation pathway. What follows is a summary of the interventions, diagnostic studies, monitoring strategies, and resuscitation techniques for hemorrhagic shock.

Immediate Management

When approaching any patient in shock, the sequence of events should be to address the issues of airway, breathing, and circulation—also known as the "ABCs." Most patients with fully developed shock require tracheal intubation and mechanical ventilation, even if acute respiratory failure has not yet developed. Studies have shown that during shock, the respiratory muscles require a disproportionate percent of the cardiac output (16). Failure to mount a hyperventilatory response to a metabolic acidosis is a significant predictor of the need for subsequent intubation in trauma patients (177). Mechanical ventilation allows flow to be redistributed, lessens the work of breathing, may help reverse lactic acidosis, and supports the patient's airway until other therapeutic measures can be

TABLE 47.3 Key Steps in the Approach to a Patient with Hemorrhagic Shock

1. Early recognition
   a. Signs and symptoms may be subtle.
   b. Astute clinical acumen is necessary to identify hemorrhage prior to hemodynamic collapse.
2. Obtain an accurate patient history
   a. Trauma
   b. Recent surgical procedures
   c. Medical history
      (i) Gastrointestinal disease (peptic ulcer disease, varices, etc.)
      (ii) Atherosclerosis (aneurysmal disease)
      (iii) Coagulation disorders
   d. Medication use
      (i) Antiplatelet therapy
      (ii) Anticoagulants
3. Initiate intervention
   a. "ABCs"—airway, breathing, circulation
   b. Initiate resuscitation
      (i) Crystalloid
      (ii) Blood products
         1. Type O uncross-matched blood if *in extremis*
         2. Cross-matched blood when available
         3. Clotting factors: 1:1:1 ratio of plasma:platelets:red blood cells for those meeting criteria for massive transfusion
4. Directed physical examination
   a. External sources of bleeding (consider tourniquet)
   b. Internal sources of bleeding
5. Expedite definitive treatment
   a. Surgical control
   b. Endoscopic control
   c. Angiographic control
6. Correct coagulopathy (simultaneous with definitive treatment)

effective. Tracheal intubation is also required if there is evidence of mental status changes, such that airway protection is questionable. Evidence of hypoxemia and/or hypoventilation is also an absolute requirement for early intubation.

Perhaps most complex is the patient with evidence of compensated hemorrhagic shock whose mental status is still intact. In this type of patient, clinical acumen is imperative. If the initial response to resuscitation is sustained (i.e., "a responder"), then close observation of the airway may be appropriate while additional workup and treatment are pursued. However, in a patient who is not responsive or has a transient response to fluid resuscitation, control of the airway early is necessary prior to respiratory collapse (177). In addition, if diagnostic and therapeutic interventions, such as angiography and embolization, are required during resuscitation to control hemorrhage, early airway control should be obtained.

Once the airway is secured, it is important to closely monitor techniques of ventilation. Studies have shown that there is a tendency of rescue and medical personnel to hyperventilate patients during resuscitation (178,179). Hyperventilated patients have been shown to have an increased mortality when compared to nonhyperventilated patients in the setting of severe traumatic brain injury (180–182). Animal studies have supported this information, showing that cardiac output increases with hypoventilation and decreases with hyperventilation and positive end-expiratory pressure (PEEP) (183,184). Thus, adequate appropriate ventilator strategies are imperative early in hemorrhagic shock to optimize tissue perfusion and outcome.

The management steps to restore adequate circulation include identifying and controlling the source of hemorrhage and intravenous fluid and blood product resuscitation to restore tissue perfusion. The first step is to control obvious hemorrhage immediately.

Hemorrhage Control

Resuscitation of the bleeding patient requires early identification of potential bleeding sources followed by prompt action to minimize blood loss, restore tissue perfusion, and achieve hemodynamic stability. This is particularly important in the trauma patient where multiple sources may be involved. Wound compression is the initial maneuver to control an exsanguinating wound. For massive soft tissue injuries or major vascular injury to an extremity, placing a tourniquet proximally may decrease hemorrhage and allow resuscitation prior to definitive control (185). Fractures should be splinted or placed in traction. Evidence of pelvic instability or hemorrhage may be temporized by a sheet or a pelvic binder (186,187). In the presence of massive trauma, patients may present with coagulopathy in the emergency department and this should be preemptively addressed. The same principles should be applied to nontraumatic hemorrhagic shock, such as gastrointestinal bleeding and ruptured aortic aneurysms: rapidly identify and attenuate the obvious sources of hemorrhage.

Multiple studies have confirmed that patients in need of emergency surgery for ongoing hemorrhage have a better survival if the elapsed time to definitive care is minimized (188–192). Those patients with unnecessary delays in diagnosis and definitive treatment will have increased morbidity and mortality. A multicenter retrospective review of over 500 deaths in the operating room concluded that delayed transfer to the operating room was a cause of death that could be avoided by shortening the time to diagnosis and resuscitation (193). The development of trauma systems has significantly contributed to improved trauma outcomes by triaging more severely injured patients to hospitals that have systems in place to rapidly diagnose, resuscitate, and definitively treat patients with hemorrhagic shock (188–190). The implementation of trauma systems has resulted in improved outcomes in severely injured patients, decreased time to operating room in hypotensive patients, decreased complications, decreased hospital length of stay, and decreased mortality, especially in patients with severe injury as measured by an ISS of >15 (190). Definitive prompt care is critical to optimize outcomes in patients with trauma and hemorrhage.

Intravenous Access

Access to the bloodstream should be obtained expediently. Two peripheral large-bore intravenous catheters (18 gauge or larger) are necessary. If cannulation of a peripheral vein is difficult due to collapse, then central venous access should be secured. In the presence of trauma to the torso, venous access above and below the diaphragm is preferable. When obtaining intravenous access, it is important to note that the maximal rate of infusion via a catheter is directly proportional to the diameter of the catheter and indirectly proportional to the length. Therefore, a 9 French percutaneous introducer sheath will infuse fluids more rapidly than a 7 French triple-lumen catheter. A large-bore peripheral intravenous catheter will also infuse fluids more rapidly than a 7 French triple lumen catheter due to a shorter length and less resistance. Intraosseus access is an option for both adults and children when i.v. access is difficult. Fluids and blood products can be delivered via this route. However, this should be considered temporary access until better intravenous access can be obtained.

Adjunctive Measures

Historical teachings have been that tilting a patient into head-down position (i.e., Trendelenburg) diverts blood volume into the central circulation and improves venous return, thereby improving stroke volume and cardiac output in hypovolemic shock. However, studies do not show any significant redistribution of blood volume centrally (194). In fact, the head-down position can worsen gas exchange and cardiac function. Therefore, the Trendelenburg position is no longer recommended as a resuscitative technique. If this type of measure is deemed desirable, raising the legs above the level of the heart should be adequate (195).

The use of pneumatic antishock garments (PASGs, previously military antishock trousers [MAST]) currently has a limited role in the management of hypotensive trauma patients. Although their use was almost universal for hemorrhage control in the late 1970s and 1980s, recent studies have demonstrated that they have no effect on patients with thoracic injury. In fact, some evidence suggests that mortality is higher when PASGs are applied (196,197). No survival advantage has been demonstrated in the pediatric population, although there may be a small survival benefit in children with a systolic blood pressure of less than 50 mmHg (198). The main utility of PASGs currently is as a temporizing agent to stabilize pelvic fractures.

Fluid Resuscitation

Careful attention to fluid resuscitation is necessary during management of hemorrhagic shock to optimize outcome. It is still unclear which type of fluid should be employed in the initial treatment of the bleeding patient.

Several meta-analyses have shown an increased risk of death in patients resuscitated with colloids as compared with crystalloids (199–202) during hemorrhagic shock. While three of these studies suggested that the effect was particularly significant in the trauma population, the results of a recent meta-analysis showed no significant difference (203). A trial evaluating 4% albumin versus 0.9% normal saline in nearly 7,000 ICU patients showed that albumin administration was not associated with worse outcome. There was a trend, however, toward higher mortality in the trauma subgroup that received albumin ($p = 0.06$) (204). The difficulty with interpreting these meta-analyses and the individual studies is that they are very heterogeneous. Each evaluates different patient populations and resuscitation strategies, and mortality may not always be a primary end point. However, given these results, crystalloid resuscitation is currently the accepted standard as initial therapy for hemorrhagic shock.

Many synthetic colloid solutions such as hetastarch and dextran have also been associated with coagulopathy. Recent research suggests that hetastarch solutions with a high mean molecular weight and a high C2/C6 ratio suppress coagulation more than solutions with rapidly degradable low-molecular-weight colloids (205–207). This coagulopathy may be produced by one of several potential mechanisms including a reduction in von Willebrand factor, platelet dysfunction, reduced factor VII levels, and an interaction with fibrinogen (173,208).

Crystalloid solutions are not without side effects. Resuscitation with fluids that contain supraphysiologic concentrations of chloride can lead to hyperchloremic acidosis. This can be significant in patients where lactic acidosis may already be present. Lactated Ringer solution contains a more physiologic concentration of chloride (109 mEq/L) than normal saline (NS 154 mEq/L), and therefore may be the preferred choice. Animal studies have also shown that resuscitation with normal saline can lead to more coagulopathy and increased blood loss than resuscitation with lactated Ringer solution (209).

Massive resuscitation with crystalloid fluids alone can lead to several significant complications including cardiac and pulmonary complications, gastrointestinal dysmotility, coagulation abnormalities, and immunologic dysfunction (210). Reports of lactated Ringer solution and normal saline increasing reperfusion injury and leukocyte adhesion suggest that crystalloid resuscitation may worsen acidosis and coagulopathy in severely injured patients and possibly increases the risk of ARDS, systemic inflammatory response syndrome (SIRS), and multi-organ failure (MOF) (210–213). Abdominal compartment syndrome has been clearly associated with excessive use of crystalloid resuscitation (214–218). Recently, there has been increased focus on early use of blood products in order to minimize crystalloid use in the resuscitation of hemorrhagic shock. Finally, resuscitation strategies that focus on early aggressive fluid resuscitation to normalize blood pressure before bleeding is controlled may result in increased hemorrhage and increased mortality. This has led some authors to suggest that "hypotensive resuscitation" should be the goal until the source of hemorrhage is controlled (219–222). However, the exact goals for mean arterial pressure and trigger points for bleeding have not been established. The potential adverse sequelae when used in patients with associated injuries or comorbidities (i.e., severe closed head injury) have not been clearly established.

TABLE 47.4 Damage Control Laparotomy and Damage Control Resuscitation

DAMAGE CONTROL LAPAROTOMY

1. **Abbreviated laparotomy (initial procedure)**
   - Control of bleeding
   - Control of contamination
   - Restitution of blood flow
2. **Resuscitation in the intensive care unit (24–48 hr)**
   - Core rewarming
   - Correction of acidosis
   - Reversal of coagulopathy
   - Optimization of ventilation and hemodynamics
3. **Definitive surgical repair (days to weeks)**
   - Restoration of continuity
   - Completion of resection
   - Removal of packs
   - Closure of abdomen

DAMAGE CONTROL RESUSCITATION

- Hypotensive resuscitation[a]
- Hemostatic resuscitation

[a]Hypotensive resuscitation requires experienced physician oversight and careful patient selection.

Damage Control Resuscitation

Damage control resuscitation (DCR) is a term that has recently been coined to describe a specific strategy during the resuscitation phase of trauma care (173,223–225). It should be initiated within minutes of presentation and is meant to pre-emptively address issues associated with resuscitating critically injured patients: prevention of hypothermia, acidosis, and coagulopathy. DCR involves two components: hypotensive resuscitation and hemostatic resuscitation (Table 47.4).

Hypotensive Resuscitation

Hypotensive resuscitation refers to the concept that fluid should be administered at a rate that returns the systolic blood pressure to a safe but lower than normal pressure until operative control of bleeding can be established. The traditional treatment of hemorrhaging patients has used early and aggressive fluid administration to restore blood volume. However, this approach may increase hydrostatic pressure on the wound or injured vessel, leading to dislodgement of blood clots, a dilution of coagulation factors, and undesirable cooling of the patient. Low-volume fluid resuscitation, or "permissive hypotension," may avoid the adverse effects of early aggressive resuscitation while maintaining a level of tissue perfusion adequate for short periods. This strategy has been suggested historically for the management of ruptured abdominal aortic aneurysm patients (226), and has recently regained attention in the trauma population (220–222,227–230). It has shown promise in animal studies and human trials of penetrating trauma (220,227), but has yet to be confirmed in large-scale prospective randomized human clinical trials in the broader trauma population. A Cochrane database review in 2003 found that there was not conclusive evidence from randomized controlled trials (RCTs) for or against early or larger volumes of intravenous fluid resuscitation in uncontrolled hemorrhage (231). A recent pilot study in the prehospital environment suggested that a controlled resuscitation strategy was safe in blunt trauma patients, but patients with evidence of severe TBI were excluded (221).

Although the concept of permissive hypotension seems promising in some circumstances, further work needs to be done. In addition, it requires extraordinarily tight control by an experienced physician who is guiding fluid resuscitation moment to moment. Hypotensive resuscitation should not be considered in patients with traumatic brain injury and spinal cord injury where adequate cerebral perfusion pressure is crucial to ensure tissue oxygenation (143,232). It should also be carefully considered in elderly patients and may be contraindicated in patients with a history of chronic hypertension (143).

Hemostatic Resuscitation

Conventional resuscitation practice for damage control has focused on rapid reversal of acidosis and prevention of hypothermia. Surgical techniques are aimed at controlling hemorrhage and contamination rapidly, with definitive repair occurring following hemodynamic stabilization. However, early, direct treatment of coagulopathy was previously neglected, and viewed as a byproduct of resuscitation, hemodilution, and hypothermia. Delay in the availability of blood products has also hindered the ability to employ immediate resuscitation with clotting factors.

It has now been demonstrated that *acute traumatic coagulopathy* is present in 25% to 40% of critically injured patients on arrival to the emergency department (120,123,233). The presence of coagulopathy may be even higher in patients with severe closed head injury, with an incidence of 21% to 79% when stratified by ISS (234). It has also been shown that the presence of early coagulopathy is an independent predictor of mortality following trauma (123).

Hemostatic resuscitation employs blood components *early* in the resuscitation process to restore both perfusion and normal coagulation function while minimizing crystalloid use. Several retrospective studies from both the military and civilian communities have suggested that trauma patients who are resuscitated with higher ratios of fresh frozen plasma to packed red blood cells have a higher survival (225,235–239). These studies have all suffered from survival bias in that patients in the high-ratio groups survived long enough to reach the higher ratios. This has led to controversy in the field with some authors suggesting that high-ratio resuscitation leads to greater exposure of patients to blood products and thus increased risk of ARDS and MOFS (240). To address this issue, a recently multicenter clinical trial randomized 680 trauma patients at risk for massive transfusion to received either a 1:1:1 ratio of plasma:platelets:PRBCs versus a 1:1:2 ratio. While there was no significant difference in 24-hour (1:1:1 at 12.7% vs. 1:1:2 at 17%, $p = 0.12$) and 30-day (1:1:1 at 22.4% vs. 1:1:2 at 26.1%, $p = 0.26$) mortality, exsanguination which was the primary cause of death in the first 24 hours was reduced in the 1:1:1 group (9.2% vs. 14.6%, $p = 0.03$). In addition, more patients in the 1:1:1 group achieved hemostasis. There was no difference in subsequent complication in the hospital including the rates of nosocomial infection or organ failure (241).

Massive Transfusion Protocols

Massive transfusion has been traditionally defined as the need for 10 or more units of red cells in the first 24 hours. However, most patients who die from exsanguination die within the first 6 hours and many die before high-volume transfusions can be initiated. This has led to the proposal that massive transfusion be viewed as a rate of bleeding over time rather than an absolute number of blood products administered. In order to employ DCR, it is vital to recognize the patient who is likely to need a massive transfusion early to that blood products can be initiated and crystalloid resuscitation minimized. There have been several scoring systems developed to help identify patients at risk for a massive transfusion (242–246). Many of these scores rely on laboratory data such as PT/INR, base deficit, or hemoglobin, which may not be immediately available. The ABC score has been validated as a simple approach which uses data that are rapidly available upon patient arrival (Table 47.5). The ABC score relies on systolic blood pressure, heart rate, penetrating mechanism, and a positive FAST examination for intraperitoneal fluid (243).

TABLE 47.5 ABC Score to Predict Need for Massive Transfusion

Component	Yes	No
Penetrating mechanism	1	0
SBP ≤90 mmHg	1	0
HR ≥120 beats/min	1	0
Positive FAST examination	1	0

Total score of 2 or greater is predictive of need for massive transfusion in trauma patients in the emergency department (243).
SBP, systolic blood pressure; HR, heart rate; FAST, focused abdominal sonogram for trauma.

Once you have identified a patient in need of a massive transfusion, several studies have shown the benefit of having a structured protocol to ensure good communication with the blood bank so that blood products can be rapidly available at the bedside (247,248). The logistics of rapid access to blood products can be challenging especially in smaller centers with limited blood supply. Prethawed plasma or liquid plasma has been advocated in larger centers to improve rapid access to a balanced resuscitation strategy (249). The results of the PROPPR study discussed above provide compelling evidence to consider a 1:1:1 strategy in the MTP protocol (Table 47.6) (241).

Most authors recommend an empiric resuscitation strategy during the period of active hemorrhage with a fixed ratio of bleed products administered without focusing on the results of traditional coagulation test results due to the inherent delay in receiving these results (250,251). This is an area of controversy with other arguing for a focused factor replacement strategy or a TEG-guided resuscitation utilizing the results of bedside testing (252). Additional study is needed to define the optimal approach. Most authors agree that once hemorrhage control has been achieved, a more targeted correction of residual coagulation abnormalities is a reasonable approach. Once the patient has stabilized and is no longer at risk for ongoing hemorrhage, a restrictive transfusion approach in the ICU is recommended with a target transfusion threshold of hemoglobin of 7 mg/L (253).

TABLE 47.6 Recommended Empiric Massive Transfusion Protocol for Acute Ongoing Hemorrhage

Current Suggested Protocol for Traumatic Hemorrhage
• 6 units of packed red blood cells • 6 units of fresh frozen plasma • 1 platelet pheresis (or 6–10 units of platelets) • Cryoprecipitate as indicated (fibrinogen <100 g/dL)

TABLE 47.7 Noninfectious Transfusion-Associated Complications

Acute (within 24 hr of transfusion)
Hemolytic reactions
Febrile nonhemolytic reactions
Allergic reactions
Transfusion-related acute lung injury (TRALI)
Hypothermia
Hypocalcemia
Hypo- or hyperkalemia
Acid-base derangements
Delayed (more than 24 hr after transfusion)
Alloimmunization
Immunosuppression
Posttransfusion purpura
Graft vs. host disease
Multiple organ dysfunction syndrome

Despite acceptable survival rates, there are several known complications to massive transfusion (Tables 47.7 and 47.8) (254–259). Physicians caring for patients who require massive transfusion must anticipate, identify, and rapidly treat these potential complications in order to optimize outcome.

Adjuncts for Management of Coagulopathy

Several recent studies have explored the use of additional adjuncts for the management of trauma-induced coagulopathy and for the management of patients with coagulopathy secondary to pre-injury treatment with anticoagulant medications such as Coumadin. These adjuncts include activated factor VIIa, tranexamic acid (TXA), prothrombin concentrate complex (PCC), and cryoprecipitate or fibrinogen concentrates. The summary of the current data for each is presented below.

Activated Factor VIIa

Recombinant factor VIIa is a synthesized analog of human factor VII that has been used effectively in the treatment of patients with hemophilia as well as other congenital and acquired coagulopathies. There were subsequently several case series reporting on the off-label use of factor VIIa for management of severely bleeding trauma patients (260,261). Administration of factor VIIa resulted in rapid correction of PT, but its efficacy was unclear. A recent meta-analysis of 29 RCTs of factor VIIa in nonhemophilia patients concluded that there was no evidence of a mortality benefit and while there was a trend toward reduction in the need for blood transfusions, there was also evidence of a increased thrombotic complications (262). It has also been recognized that factor VIIa is not effective in patients who are hypothermic or have severe metabolic acidosis which limits its applicability in the setting of massive transfusion following injury (263).

TABLE 47.8 Infectious Transfusion-Associated Complications (254–257)

Type of Infectious Complication	Incidence Per All Transfused Components
Bacterial contamination (PRBCs + platelets)	1 per 2,000
Hepatitis B transmission	1 per 205,000
PRBC-related bacterial sepsis	1 per 500,000–786,000
Hepatitis A transmission	1 per 1,000,000
Hepatitis C transmission	1 per 1,600,000
HIV transmission	1 per 2,135,000

PRBC, packed red blood cell; HIV, human immunodeficiency virus.

Tranexamic Acid

TXA is an antifibrinolytic agent that acts by inhibiting the binding of plasmin to plasminogen. It remains unclear the optimal assessment for fibrinolysis in trauma patients. Several authors have used TEG analysis and have reported that 2% to 34% of trauma patients have evidence of fibrinolysis on admission (175,264–268). This wide range is due to the heterogeneity of the populations studied. The use of TXA in trauma patients has increased dramatically in response to the CRASH 2 study (28-day mortality 14.5% TXA group vs. 16.0% placebo, RR 0.91, 95% CI 0.85 to 0.97) (269,270). This study demonstrated a survival benefit for patients receiving the drug within 3 hours of injury, but interestingly outcome was worse if the drug was given beyond 3 hours. The greatest benefit also appeared to be in the patients with the greatest risk of hemorrhage (SBP <75 mmHg). Two additional retrospective studies suggest a survival advantage in military casualties receiving TXA in US and UK support hospitals in Afghanistan (271,272). These data have led to a recommendation that TXA be considered for injured soldiers in need of blood transfusion as early as possible but ideally within 3 hours after injury and strongly advocated in patients judged to need a massive transfusion (273).

There remain many questions about the optimal dosing, patient selection, and safety related to the use of TXA in injured patients (273). There are several studies ongoing to address the use of TXA in the prehospital setting and to help clarify the dosing and appropriate patient selection (274). Studies are also underway to evaluate the use of TXA for patients with severe TBI to determine its impact on the progression of intracranial hemorrhage.

Prothrombin Concentrate Complex

Prothrombin complex concentrate (PCC) is a concentrated for of clotting factors used for reversal of vitamin K antagonists such as warfarin in patients with active hemorrhage. It has been particularly advantageous for patients on warfarin with intracranial hemorrhage (275,276). There are three factor (II, IX, X) and four-factor preparations (II, VII, IX, X). The PCC concentration of these factors is approximately 25 times that of plasma (277). Due to the lack of factor VII in the three-factor preparations, some additional plasma may be required. PCC has the advantage of a long shelf life as it is reconstituted for use and can be given in a small volume which results in less risk of fluid overload in elderly patients. It also results more rapid correction of coagulopathy compared to the time delay of thawing frozen plasma. PCC is not advocated for general use in the bleeding patient who is not on warfarin as there is concern for potential prothrombotic complications (277).

Cryoprecipitate/Fibrinogen Concentrates

There is limited clinical data to guide the use of cryoprecipitate or fibrinogen concentrates in trauma patients (278). Cryoprecipitate is a rich source of fibrinogen and has been variably utilized in massive transfusion protocols in the United States. One recent study demonstrated that cryoprecipitate use in trauma patients requiring massive transfusion varied from 7% to 81% among the trauma centers involved (279). One retrospective study from the US military suggested that administration of cryoprecipitate was independently associated with improved survival in critically injured soldiers (271). More studies are needed to clearly define the appropriate use of this product in the setting of a massive transfusion.

Preventing Hypothermia

All fluids during resuscitation from hemorrhagic shock should be warmed to prevent hypothermia. Equipment is now available that allows the rapid infusion of blood and/or crystalloids at warmed temperatures (i.e., up to 750 mL fluid per minute warmed to over 37°C). Other techniques during resuscitation that can be used to prevent hypothermia in the acutely hemorrhaging patient include warming the circuit on the ventilator in ventilated patients, ensuring the patient is covered with warm blankets at all times following exposure and thorough examination, warming the resuscitation and operating rooms, using forced air external warming blankets during resuscitation and in the operating room, and using warm water blankets on the operating room table. Hypothermia is clearly associated with increased mortality following resuscitation from hemorrhagic shock, and every attempt to prevent or minimize its occurrence and severity should be employed (280,281).

CURRENT CONTROVERSIES AND EXPERIMENTAL THERAPIES

Red Cell Substitutes

Although the blood supply in the United States is safe and currently has sufficient capacity to meet most patient needs, there is room for considerable improvement. The current system is dependent on blood donors on a regular basis, and the blood supply is subject to seasonal shortages due to holidays and convenience. The gap between the donor pool and the increasing transfusion requirements of an aging population is narrowing, and shortages are becoming more frequent. The risk of transmission of known infectious diseases still exists (Table 47.8), while the threat of new and emerging infections such as West Nile virus and Creutzfeldt–Jakob disease underscores the risk of a tainted blood supply (282).

The ideal red cell substitute has several characteristics including an ability to deliver (and potentially enhance) oxygen delivery, no risk of disease transmission, no immunosuppressive effects, available in abundant supply, universally compatible, prolonged shelf life, similar *in vivo* half-life to the red blood cell, available at a reasonable cost, easy to administer, able to access all areas of the human body (including ischemic tissues), and effective at room air or ambient conditions (282–284).

The two main types of oxygen carriers that are used as red blood cell substitutes are hemoglobin-based oxygen carriers (HBOCs) and perfluorocarbons (PFCs). Based on previous clinical trials, many obstacles still need to be overcome. Adverse effects associated with HBOCs include severe vasoconstriction due to binding of nitric oxide and dysregulation of endothelin; nephrotoxicity; interference of macrophage function; antigenicity; oxidation on storage; activation of complement, kinin, and coagulation; iron deposition with concerns of hemochromatosis and iron overload; gastrointestinal distress; neurotoxicity free radical generation; and interference with diagnosis of transfusion reaction. Adverse effects of PFCs include limited shelf life, flulike symptoms during infusion, complement and phagocytic activation, and short circulation time (283). The most promising product known as polyheme progressed to a phase III clinical trial for trauma patients in the United States; however, this trial failed to demonstrate benefit and the product is no longer available (285).

Freeze-dried or Lyophylized Plasma

Given the increased use of plasma as a critical component of massive transfusion protocols with the adoption of higher ratios of plasma to red blood cells, there is considerable interest in the development of a plasma product with a prolonged shelf life that could be reconstituted for rapid administration perhaps even in the prehospital environment. There are several promising animal studies of these products in hemorrhagic shock and injury models but clinical trials are still needed (286,287).

Hypertonic Saline

Hypertonic saline (7.5% saline ± 6% dextan-70) has been investigated as an alternative resuscitation strategy in critically injured patients (288). Hypertonic resuscitation evokes an increase in serum osmolarity, which results in the redistribution of fluid from the interstitial and intracellular space to the intravascular space. This leads to a rapid restoration of circulating intravascular volume with a small amount of resuscitation fluid. Hypertonic saline has also been shown to decrease intracranial pressure via its osmotic effects (289,290). This is particularly beneficial in patients with hypovolemic shock and closed head injury due to the ability of hypertonic saline resuscitation to concurrently restore circulating blood volume, improve tissue (including cerebral) perfusion, and lower intracranial pressure (290).

Hypertonic saline resuscitation has also been shown to have significant immunomodulatory effects that could mitigate the dysfunctional inflammatory response seen after traumatic injury (291–298). The hypertonicity associated with hypertonic saline resuscitation is associated with significant effects on the innate and adaptive immune systems.

The most commonly studied dose for resuscitation of shock in trauma patients has been 7.5% saline with or without 6% dextran given as a 250 cc bolus in the prehospital setting. Several early clinical trials and meta-analyses suggested improved outcome in patients resuscitated with hypertonic saline (299–301). However, the largest RCT conducted in the prehospital setting failed to show improved survival in patient with hemorrhagic shock and enrollment was closed early due to a potential safety concern with a higher number of early deaths in the hypertonic saline groups (302). A subsequent meta-analysis concluded that this was due to collider bias in the enrollment and no safety issue was identified (303). Hypertonic fluids have also been studied in patients with severe traumatic brain injury due to their ability to treat intracranial hypertension. Another large prehospital study failed to demonstrate improvement in 6-month neurologic outcome with this approach (304). Various concentrations of hypertonic saline continue to be used in the hospital for ICP management but further study is needed to assess this approach.

Resuscitative Endovascular Balloon Occlusion of the Aorta

A final emerging therapy that warrants discussion is the use of resuscitative endovascular occlusion balloons of the aorta (REBOA) as a temporizing measure for resuscitation of patients in extreme hemorrhagic shock from bleeding in the abdomen or pelvis. Early reports suggest that an intra-aortic balloon can be placed at the bedside via a femoral percutaneous approach to reduce hemorrhage until surgical or angiographic control can be achieved (305–307). For pelvic hemorrhage, the balloon is placed in Zone 3 of the aorta below the renal vessels. For abdominal hemorrhage, the balloon is placed in the distal thoracic aorta (Zone 1). This approach has been suggested as a potential alternative to the traditional cross-clamp on the aorta applied during emergency department thoracotomy. This approach will result in significant tissue ischemia and so must be performed in a setting where rapid hemorrhage control can be achieved to minimize the time of balloon inflation. Current data to support this approach are confined to case series from a limited number of institutions. Further study is warranted to further define the utility of this approach.

SUMMARY

Hemorrhagic shock is a common, yet complicated, clinical condition that physicians are frequently called upon to evaluate and treat. Diagnosis must be accurate and expedient. Therapy must be direct, efficient, and multifactorial in order to avoid the potential multisystem sequelae. Metabolism and function of all organs are altered during hemorrhagic shock. A better understanding of the pathophysiology of hemorrhagic shock has led to improved resuscitation techniques and improved survival over recent years. Damage control laparotomy and DCR have changed the approach to management in patients with multisystem trauma and hemorrhagic shock. Staged resuscitation and operative intervention to avoid irreversible shock are now the mainstays of care. Recognition of acute traumatic coagulopathy has improved the composition of massive transfusion protocols to include the increased use of clotting factors early during resuscitation. New experimental therapies for resuscitation are being evaluated and appear promising. Overall, survival following hemorrhagic shock has improved. Early diagnosis, definitive cessation of bleeding, and comprehensive hemostatic resuscitation are the key elements to successful outcome.

Key Points

- Hemorrhagic shock is a common disorder that requires a high index of suspicion for early recognition and treatment.
- Young patients will compensate for moderate blood loss without major changes in blood pressure, so the clinician must consider other markers of impaired perfusion including the development of metabolic acidosis and coagulopathy.
- Trauma-induced coagulopathy is common in severely injured patients and requires early treatment with blood products.
- Treatment for hemorrhagic shock focuses on rapid control of the source of hemorrhage coupled with fluid and blood product resuscitation.
- For patients requiring a massive transfusion, a balanced resuscitation including plasma, platelets, and red cells is warranted.
- There is no advantage to colloid resuscitation in this setting and excessive crystalloid resuscitation should be avoided.
- Efforts should be made to prevent and treat hypothermia which may exacerbate ongoing bleeding.
- Damage control surgery is preferred in the setting of ongoing coagulopathy, acidosis, and hypothermia.

References

1. Bond RF, Johnson G 3rd. Vascular adrenergic interactions during hemorrhagic shock. *Fed Proc.* 1985;44(2):281–289.
2. Schadt JC, Ludbrook J. Hemodynamic and neurohumoral responses to acute hypovolemia in conscious mammals. *Am J Physiol.* 1991;260(2 Pt 2): H305–H318.
3. Koyama S, Sawano F, Matsuda Y, et al. Spatial and temporal differing control of sympathetic activities during hemorrhage. *Am J Physiol.* 1992; 262(4 Pt 2):R579–R585.
4. Bressack MA, Raffin TA. Importance of venous return, venous resistance, and mean circulatory pressure in the physiology and management of shock. *Chest.* 1987;92(5):906–912.
5. Ludbrook J, Ventura S. Roles of carotid baroreceptor and cardiac afferents in hemodynamic responses to acute central hypovolemia. *Am J Physiol.* 1996; 270(5 Pt 2):H1538–H1548.
6. Westphal G, Garrido Adel P, de Almeida DP, et al. Pulse pressure respiratory variation as an early marker of cardiac output fall in experimental hemorrhagic shock. *Artif Organs.* 2007;31(4):284–289.
7. Magder S, Lagonidis D, Erice F. The use of respiratory variations in right atrial pressure to predict the cardiac output response to PEEP. *J Crit Care.* 2001;16(3):108–114.
8. Rooke GA, Schwid HA, Shapira Y. The effect of graded hemorrhage and intravascular volume replacement on systolic pressure variation in humans during mechanical and spontaneous ventilation. *Anesth Analg.* 1995;80(5):925–932.
9. Zweifach BW, Fronek A. The interplay of central and peripheral factors in irreversible hemorrhagic shock. *Prog Cardiovasc Dis.* 1975;18(2):147–180.
10. Schwartz S, Frantz RA, Shoemaker WC. Sequential hemodynamic and oxygen transport responses in hypovolemia, anemia, and hypoxia. *Am J Physiol.* 1981;241(6):H864–H871.
11. Alyono D, Ring WS, Chao RY, et al. Characteristics of ventricular function in severe hemorrhagic shock. *Surgery.* 1983;94(2):250–258.
12. Sarnoff SJ, Case RB, Waithe PE, Isaacs JP. Insufficient coronary flow and myocardial failure as a complication factor in late hemorrhagic shock. *Am J Physiol.* 1954;176(3):439–444.
13. Rush BF Jr. Irreversibility in the post-transfusion phase of hemorrhagic shock. *Adv Exp Med Biol.* 1971;23(0):215–234.
14. Vatner SF. Effects of hemorrhage on regional blood flow distribution in dogs and primates. *J Clin Invest.* 1974;54(2):225–235.
15. Shoemaker WC. Relation of oxygen transport patterns to the pathophysiology and therapy of shock states. *Intensive Care Med.* 1987;13(4):230–243.
16. Aubier M, Viires N, Syllie G, Mozes R, Roussos C. Respiratory muscle contribution to lactic acidosis in low cardiac output. *Am Rev Respir Dis.* 1982;126(4):648–652.
17. Revelly JP, Gardaz JP, Nussberger J, et al. Effect of epinephrine on oxygen consumption and delivery during progressive hemorrhage. *Crit Care Med.* 1995;23(7):1272–1278.
18. Hannon JP, Wade CE, Bossone CA, et al. Oxygen delivery and demand in conscious pigs subjected to fixed-volume hemorrhage and resuscitated with 7.5% NaCl in 6% dextran. *Circ Shock.* 1989;29(3):205–217.
19. Edouard AR, Degrémont AC, Duranteau J, et al. Heterogeneous regional vascular responses to simulated transient hypovolemia in man. *Intensive Care Med.* 1994;20(6):414–420.
20. Kolkman JJ, Otte JA, Groeneveld AB. Gastrointestinal luminal PCO_2 tonometry: an update on physiology, methodology and clinical applications. *Br J Anaesth.* 2000;84(1):74–86.

21. Riggs TE, Shafer AW, Guenter CA. Acute changes in oxyhemoglobin affinity: effects on oxygen transport and utilization. *J Clin Invest.* 1973;52(10):2660–2663.
22. Malmberg PO, Hlastala MP, Woodson RD. Effect of increased blood-oxygen affinity on oxygen transport in hemorrhagic shock. *J Appl Physiol Respir Environ Exerc Physiol.* 1979;47(4):889–895.
23. Woodson RD. Physiological significance of oxygen dissociation curve shifts. *Crit Care Med.* 1979;7(9):368–373.
24. Myburgh JA, Webb RK, Worthley LI. The P50 is reduced in critically ill patients. *Intensive Care Med.* 1991;17(6):355–358.
25. Herman CM, Rodkey FL, Valeri CR, Fortier NL. Changes in the oxyhemoglobin dissociation curve and peripheral blood after acute red cell mass depletion and subsequent red cell mass restoration in baboons. *Ann Surg.* 1971;174(5):734–743.
26. Sauaia A, Moore FA, Moore EE, et al. Early predictors of postinjury multiple organ failure. *Arch Surg.* 1994;129(1):39–45.
27. Shoemaker WC, Appel PL, Kram HB. Role of oxygen debt in the development of organ failure sepsis, and death in high-risk surgical patients. *Chest.* 1992;102(1):208–215.
28. Kirton OC, Windsor J, Wedderburn R, et al. Failure of splanchnic resuscitation in the acutely injured trauma patient correlates with multiple organ system failure and length of stay in the ICU. *Chest.* 1998;113(4):1064–1069.
29. Abou-Khalil B, Scalea TM, Trooskin SZ, et al. Hemodynamic responses to shock in young trauma patients: need for invasive monitoring. *Crit Care Med.* 1994;22(4):633–639.
30. Bishop MH, Shoemaker WC, Appel PL, et al. Prospective, randomized trial of survivor values of cardiac index, oxygen delivery, and oxygen consumption as resuscitation endpoints in severe trauma. *J Trauma.* 1995;38(5):780–787.
31. Shoemaker WC, Appel PL, Kram HB, et al. Prospective trial of supranormal values of survivors as therapeutic goals in high-risk surgical patients. *Chest.* 1988;94(6):1176–1186.
32. Shoemaker WC, Appel PL, Kram HB. Measurement of tissue perfusion by oxygen transport patterns in experimental shock and in high-risk surgical patients. *Intensive Care Med.* 1990;16(Suppl 2):S135–S144.
33. Chang MC, Mondy JS, Meredith JW, Holcroft JW. Redefining cardiovascular performance during resuscitation: ventricular stroke work, power, and the pressure-volume diagram. *J Trauma.* 1998;45(3):470–478.
34. Kern JW, Shoemaker WC. Meta-analysis of hemodynamic optimization in high-risk patients. *Crit Care Med.* 2002;30(8):1686–1692.
35. Velmahos GC, Demetriades D, Shoemaker WC, et al. Endpoints of resuscitation of critically injured patients: normal or supranormal? A prospective randomized trial. *Ann Surg.* 2000;232(3):409–418.
36. Yu M, Levy MM, Smith P, et al. Effect of maximizing oxygen delivery on morbidity and mortality rates in critically ill patients: a prospective, randomized, controlled study. *Crit Care Med.* 1993;21(6):830–838.
37. Balogh Z, McKinley BA, Cocanour CS, et al. Supranormal trauma resuscitation causes more cases of abdominal compartment syndrome. *Arch Surg.* 2003;138(6):637–642.
38. Chaudry IH. Cellular mechanisms in shock and ischemia and their correction. *Am J Physiol.* 1983;245(2):R117–R134.
39. Mongan PD, Fontana JL, Chen R, Bünger R. Intravenous pyruvate prolongs survival during hemorrhagic shock in swine. *Am J Physiol.* 1999;277(6 Pt 2):H2253–H2263.
40. Amundson B, Jennische E, Haljamäe H. Correlative analysis of microcirculatory and cellular metabolic events in skeletal muscle during hemorrhagic shock. *Acta Physiol Scand.* 1980;108(2):147–158.
41. Ratcliffe PJ, Moonen CT, Holloway PA, Ledingham JG, Radda GK. Acute renal failure in hemorrhagic hypotension: cellular energetics and renal function. *Kidney Int.* 1986;30(3):355–360.
42. Zager RA. Adenine nucleotide changes in kidney, liver, and small intestine during different forms of ischemic injury. *Circ Res.* 1991;68(1):185–196.
43. Salzman AL, Vromen A, Denenberg A, Szabó C. K(ATP)-channel inhibition improves hemodynamics and cellular energetics in hemorrhagic shock. *Am J Physiol.* 1997;272(2 Pt 2):H688–H694.
44. Robinson DA, Wang P, Chaudry IH. Administration of ATP-$MgCl_2$ after trauma-hemorrhage and resuscitation restores the depressed cardiac performance. *J Surg Res.* 1997;69(1):159–165.
45. Kline JA, Maiorano PC, Schroeder JD, et al. Activation of pyruvate dehydrogenase improves heart function and metabolism after hemorrhagic shock. *J Mol Cell Cardiol.* 1997;29(9):2465–2474.
46. Mizock BA, Falk JL. Lactic acidosis in critical illness. *Crit Care Med.* 1992;20(1):80–93.
47. Sjöberg F, Gustafsson U, Lewis DH. Extracellular muscle surface pO_2 and pH heterogeneity during hypovolemia and after reperfusion. *Circ Shock.* 1991;34(3):319–328.
48. Davis JM, Stevens JM, Peitzman A, et al. Neutrophil migratory activity in severe hemorrhagic shock. *Circ Shock.* 1983;10(3):199–204.
49. Sayeed MM. Ion transport in circulatory and/or septic shock. *Am J Physiol.* 1987;252(5 Pt 2):R809–R821.
50. Horton JW. Calcium-channel blockade in canine hemorrhagic shock. *Am J Physiol.* 1989;257(5 Pt 2):R1012–R1019.
51. Eastridge BJ, Darlington DN, Evans JA, Gann DS. A circulating shock protein depolarizes cells in hemorrhage and sepsis. *Ann Surg.* 1994;219(3):298–305.
52. Kiang JG. Inducible heat shock protein 70 kD and inducible nitric oxide synthase in hemorrhage/resuscitation-induced injury. *Cell Res.* 2004;14(6):450–459.
53. Menezes JM, Hierholzer C, Watkins SC, et al. The modulation of hepatic injury and heat shock expression by inhibition of inducible nitric oxide synthase after hemorrhagic shock. *Shock.* 2002;17(1):13–18.
54. Kregel KC. Heat shock proteins: modifying factors in physiological stress responses and acquired thermotolerance. *J Appl Physiol (1985).* 2002;92(5):2177–2186.
55. Zhao Q, Zhao K-S. Inhibition of L-type calcium channels in arteriolar smooth muscle cells is involved in the pathogenesis of vascular hyporeactivity in severe shock. *Shock.* 2007;28(6):717–721.
56. Carlson DE, Nguyen PX, Soane L, et al. Hypotensive hemorrhage increases calcium uptake capacity and Bcl-XL content of liver mitochondria. *Shock.* 2007;27(2):192–198.
57. Zhao K, Liu J, Jin C. The role of membrane potential and calcium kinetic changes in the pathogenesis of vascular hyporeactivity during severe shock. *Chin Med J (Engl).* 2000;113(1):59–64.
58. Maitra SR, Geller ER, Pan W, et al. Altered cellular calcium regulation and hepatic glucose production during hemorrhagic shock. *Circ Shock.* 1992;38(1):14–21.
59. Xu J, Liu L. The role of calcium desensitization in vascular hyporeactivity and its regulation after hemorrhagic shock in the rat. *Shock.* 2005;23(6):576–581.
60. Yang G, Liu L, Xu J, Li T. Effect of arginine vasopressin on vascular reactivity and calcium sensitivity after hemorrhagic shock in rats and its relationship to Rho-kinase. *J Trauma.* 2006;61(6):1336–1342.
61. Jarrar D, Chaudry IH, Wang P. Organ dysfunction following hemorrhage and sepsis: mechanisms and therapeutic approaches (Review). *In J Mol Med.* 1999;4(6):575–583.
62. Thiemermann C, Szabó C, Mitchell JA, Vane JR. Vascular hyporeactivity to vasoconstrictor agents and hemodynamic decompensation in hemorrhagic shock is mediated by nitric oxide. *Proc Natl Acad Sci U S A.* 1993;90(1):267–271.
63. Lieberthal W, McGarry AE, Sheils J, Valeri CR. Nitric oxide inhibition in rats improves blood pressure and renal function during hypovolemic shock. *Am J Physiol.* 1991;261(5 Pt 2):F868–F872.
64. Szabó C, Faragó M, Horváth I, et al. Hemorrhagic hypotension impairs endothelium-dependent relaxations in the renal artery of the cat. *Circ Shock.* 1992;36(3):238–241.
65. Dignan RJ, Wechsler AS, DeMaria EJ. Coronary vasomotor dysfunction following hemorrhagic shock. *J Surg Res.* 1992;52(4):382–388.
66. Bitterman H, Brod V, Weisz G, et al. Effects of oxygen on regional hemodynamics in hemorrhagic shock. *Am J Physiol.* 1996;271(1 Pt 2):H203–H211.
67. Szabó C, Csáki C, Benyó Z, et al. Role of the L-arginine-nitric oxide pathway in the changes in cerebrovascular reactivity following hemorrhagic hypotension and retransfusion. *Circ Shock.* 1992;37(4):307–316.
68. Guarini S, Bini A, Bazzani C, et al. Adrenocorticotropin normalizes the blood levels of nitric oxide in hemorrhage-shocked rats. *Eur J Pharmacol.* 1997;336(1):15–21.
69. Pannen BH, Köhler N, Hole B, et al. Protective role of endogenous carbon monoxide in hepatic microcirculatory dysfunction after hemorrhagic shock in rats. *J Clin Invest.* 1998;102(6):1220–1228.
70. Szabó C, Billiar TR. Novel roles of nitric oxide in hemorrhagic shock. *Shock.* 1999;12(1):1–9.
71. Kiang JG, Bowman PD, Lu X, et al. Geldanamycin inhibits hemorrhage-induced increases in caspase-3 activity: role of inducible nitric oxide synthase. *J Appl Physiol (1985).* 2007;103(3):1045–1055.
72. Ng KC, Moochhala SM, Md S, et al. Preservation of neurological functions by nitric oxide synthase inhibitors following hemorrhagic shock. *Neuropharmacology.* 2003;44(2):244–252.
73. Hierholzer C, Billiar TR, Tweardy DJ, Harbrecht B. Reduced hepatic transcription factor activation and expression of IL-6 and ICAM-1 after hemorrhage by NO scavenging. *Arch Orthop Trauma Surg.* 2003;123(2–3):55–59.
74. Hierholzer C, Menezes JM, Ungeheuer A, et al. A nitric oxide scavenger protects against pulmonary inflammation following hemorrhagic shock. *Shock.* 2002;17(2):98–103.

75. Kobara M, Tatsumi T, Takeda M, et al. The dual effects of nitric oxide synthase inhibitors on ischemia–reperfusion injury in rat hearts. *Basic Res Cardiol.* 2003;98(5):319–328.
76. Adachi T, Hori S, Miyazaki K, et al. Inhibition of nitric oxide synthesis aggravates myocardial ischemia in hemorrhagic shock in constant pressure model. *Shock.* 1998;9(3):204–209.
77. Thompson A, Valeri CR, Lieberthal W. Endothelin receptor A blockade alters hemodynamic response to nitric oxide inhibition in rats. *Am J Physiol.* 1995;269(2 Pt 2):H743–H748.
78. Rothe CF, Drees JA. Vascular capacitance and fluid shifts in dogs during prolonged hemorrhagic hypotension. *Circ Res.* 1976;38(5):347–356.
79. Schlichtig R, Kramer DJ, Pinsky MR. Flow redistribution during progressive hemorrhage is a determinant of critical O2 delivery. *J Appl Physiol (1985).* 1991;70(1):169–178.
80. Zweifach BW. Mechanisms of blood flow and fluid exchange in microvessels: hemorrhagic hypotension model. *Anesthesiology.* 1974;41(2):157–168.
81. Prist R, Rocha e Silva M, Scalabrini A, et al. A quantitative analysis of transcapillary refill in severe hemorrhagic hypotension in dogs. *Shock.* 1994;1(3):188–195.
82. Childs EW, Udobi KF, Hunter FA, Dhevan V. Evidence of transcellular albumin transport after hemorrhagic shock. *Shock.* 2005;23(6):565–570.
83. Schumacher J, Binkowski K, Dendorfer A, Klotz K-F. Organ-specific extravasation of albumin-bound Evans blue during nonresuscitated hemorrhagic shock in rats. *Shock.* 2003;20(6):565–568.
84. Boyd AJ, Rubin BB, Walker PM, et al. A CD18 monoclonal antibody reduces multiple organ injury in a model of ruptured abdominal aortic aneurysm. *Am J Physiol.* 1999;277(1 Pt 2):H172–H182.
85. Pascual JL, Ferri LE, Seely AJ, et al. Hypertonic saline resuscitation of hemorrhagic shock diminishes neutrophil rolling and adherence to endothelium and reduces *in vivo* vascular leakage. *Ann Surg.* 2002;236(5):634–642.
86. Childs EW, Udobi KF, Wood JG, et al. *In vivo* visualization of reactive oxidants and leukocyte-endothelial adherence following hemorrhagic shock. *Shock.* 2002;18(5):423–427.
87. Botha AJ, Moore FA, Moore EE, et al. Early neutrophil sequestration after injury: a pathogenic mechanism for multiple organ failure. *J Trauma.* 1995;39(3):411–417.
88. Barroso-Aranda J, Schmid-Schönbein GW, Zweifach BW, Engler RL. Granulocytes and no-reflow phenomenon in irreversible hemorrhagic shock. *Circ Res.* 1988;63(2):437–447.
89. Connolly HV, Maginniss LA, Schumacker PT. Transit time heterogeneity in canine small intestine: significance for oxygen transport. *J Clin Invest.* 1997;99(2):228–238.
90. Douglas RG, Shaw JH. Metabolic response to sepsis and trauma. *Br J Surg.* 1989;76(2):115–122.
91. Pearce FJ, Connett RJ, Drucker WR. Extracellular–intracellular lactate gradients in skeletal muscle during hemorrhagic shock in the rat. *Surgery.* 1985;98(4):625–631.
92. Alibegovic A, Ljungqvist O. Pretreatment with glucose infusion prevents fatal outcome after hemorrhage in food deprived rats. *Circ Shock.* 1993;39(1):1–6.
93. Barton R, Cerra FB. The hypermetabolism: multiple organ failure syndrome. *Chest.* 1989;96(5):1153–1160.
94. Ramos-Kelly JR, Toledo-Pereyra LH, Jordan JA, et al. Upregulation of lung chemokines associated with hemorrhage is reversed with a small molecule multiple selectin inhibitor. *J Am Coll Surg.* 1999;189(6):546–553.
95. Upperman JS, Deitch EA, Guo W, et al. Post-hemorrhagic shock mesenteric lymph is cytotoxic to endothelial cells and activates neutrophils. *Shock.* 1998;10(6):407–414.
96. Chaudry IH, Ayala A, Ertel W, Stephan RN. Hemorrhage and resuscitation: immunological aspects. *Am J Physiol.* 1990;259(4 Pt 2):R663–R678.
97. Nast-Kolb D, Waydhas C, Gippner-Steppert C, et al. Indicators of the posttraumatic inflammatory response correlate with organ failure in patients with multiple injuries. *J Trauma.* 1997;42(3):446–454.
98. Hierholzer C, Kalff JC, Omert L, et al. Interleukin-6 production in hemorrhagic shock is accompanied by neutrophil recruitment and lung injury. *Am J Physiol.* 1998;275(3 Pt 1):L611–L621.
99. Hierholzer C, Kalff JC, Chakraborty A, et al. Impaired gut contractility following hemorrhagic shock is accompanied by IL-6 and G-CSF production and neutrophil infiltration. *Dig Dis Sci.* 2001;46(2):230–241.
100. Roumen RM, Hendriks T, van der Ven-Jongekrijg J, et al. Cytokine patterns in patients after major vascular surgery, hemorrhagic shock, and severe blunt trauma: relation with subsequent adult respiratory distress syndrome and multiple organ failure. *Ann Surg.* 1993;218(6):769–776.
101. Meng X, Ao L, Song Y, Raeburn CD, et al. Signaling for myocardial depression in hemorrhagic shock: roles of Toll-like receptor 4 and p55 TNF-alpha receptor. *Am J Physiol Regul Integr Comp Physiol.* 2005;288(3):R600–R606.
102. Prince JM, Levy RM, Yang R, et al. Toll-like receptor-4 signaling mediates hepatic injury and systemic inflammation in hemorrhagic shock. *J Am Coll Surg.* 2006;202(3):407–417.
103. Watters JM, Tieu BH, Todd SR, et al. Fluid resuscitation increases inflammatory gene transcription after traumatic injury. *J Trauma.* 2006;61(2):300–308.
104. Lee CC, Chang IJ, Yen ZS, et al. Delayed fluid resuscitation in hemorrhagic shock induces proinflammatory cytokine response. *Ann Emerg Med.* 2007;49(1):37–44.
105. Turnage RH, Kadesky KM, Rogers T, et al. Neutrophil regulation of splanchnic blood flow after hemorrhagic shock. *Ann Surg.* 1995;222(1):66–72.
106. Patel JP, Beck LD, Briglia FA, Hock CE. Beneficial effects of combined thromboxane and leukotriene receptor antagonism in hemorrhagic shock. *Crit Care Med.* 1995;23(2):231–237.
107. Fruchterman TM, Spain DA, Wilson MA, et al. Complement inhibition prevents gut ischemia and endothelial cell dysfunction after hemorrhage/resuscitation. *Surgery.* 1998;124(4):782–791.
108. Spain DA, Fruchterman TM, Matheson PJ, et al. Complement activation mediates intestinal injury after resuscitation from hemorrhagic shock. *J Trauma.* 1999;46(2):224–233.
109. Childs EW, Udobi KF, Hunter FA. Hypothermia reduces microvascular permeability and reactive oxygen species expression after hemorrhagic shock. *J Trauma.* 2005;58(2):271–277.
110. Szabó C. The pathophysiological role of peroxynitrite in shock, inflammation, and ischemia-reperfusion injury. *Shock.* 1996;6(2):79–88.
111. Kapoor R, Prasad K. Role of oxyradicals in cardiovascular depression and cellular injury in hemorrhagic shock and reinfusion: effect of SOD and catalase. *Circ Shock.* 1994;43(2):79–94.
112. Prasad K, Kalra J, Buchko G. Acute hemorrhage and oxygen free radicals. *Angiology.* 1988;39(12):1005–1013.
113. Bulger EM, Maier RV. Antioxidants in critical illness. *Arch Surg.* 2001;136(10):1201–1207.
114. Ahmed N, Christou N. Systemic inflammatory response syndrome: interactions between immune cells and the endothelium. *Shock.* 1996;6(Suppl 1):S39–S42.
115. van Meurs M, Wulfert FM, Knol AJ, et al. Early organ-specific endothelial activation during hemorrhagic shock and resuscitation. *Shock.* 2008;29(2):291–299.
116. Martinez-Mier G, Toledo-Pereyra LH, Ward PA. Adhesion molecules and hemorrhagic shock. *J Trauma.* 2001;51(2):408–415.
117. Horgan MJ, Ge M, Gu J, et al. Role of ICAM-1 in neutrophil-mediated lung vascular injury after occlusion and reperfusion. *Am J Physiol.* 1991;261(5 Pt 2):H1578–H1584.
118. Adams CA, Sambol JT, Xu DZ, et al. Hemorrhagic shock induced up-regulation of P-selectin expression is mediated by factors in mesenteric lymph and blunted by mesenteric lymph duct interruption. *J Trauma.* 2001;51(4):625–631.
119. Xu D-Z, Lu Q, Adams CA, et al. Trauma-hemorrhagic shock-induced up-regulation of endothelial cell adhesion molecules is blunted by mesenteric lymph duct ligation. *Crit Care Med.* 2004;32(3):760–765.
120. Brohi K, Cohen MJ, Ganter MT, et al. Acute traumatic coagulopathy: initiated by hypoperfusion: modulated through the protein C pathway? *Ann Surg.* 2007;245(5):812–818.
121. Cohen MJ, Kutcher M, Redick B, et al. Clinical and mechanistic drivers of acute traumatic coagulopathy. *J Trauma Acute Care Surg.* 2013;75(1 Suppl 1):S40–S47.
122. Hess JR, Brohi K, Dutton RP, et al. The coagulopathy of trauma: a review of mechanisms. *J Trauma.* 2008;65(4):748–754.
123. MacLeod JB, Lynn M, McKenney MG, et al. Early coagulopathy predicts mortality in trauma. *J Trauma.* 2003;55(1):39–44.
124. Maegele M, Lefering R, Yucel N, et al. Early coagulopathy in multiple injury: an analysis from the German Trauma Registry on 8724 patients. *Injury.* 2007;38(3):298–304.
125. Codner P, Obaid A, Porral D, et al. Is field hypotension a reliable indicator of significant injury in trauma patients who are normotensive on arrival to the emergency department? *Am Surg.* 2005;71(9):768–771.
126. Chan L, Bartfield JM, Reilly KM. The significance of out-of-hospital hypotension in blunt trauma patients. *Acad Emerg Med.* 1997;4(8):785–788.
127. Lipsky AM, Gausche-Hill M, Henneman PL, et al. Prehospital hypotension is a predictor of the need for an emergent, therapeutic operation in trauma patients with normal systolic blood pressure in the emergency department. *J Trauma.* 2006;61(5):1228–1233.
128. Victorino GP, Battistella FD, Wisner DH. Does tachycardia correlate with hypotension after trauma? *J Am Coll Surg.* 2003;196(5):679–684.
129. Demetriades D, Chan LS, Bhasin P, et al. Relative bradycardia in patients with traumatic hypotension. *J Trauma.* 1998;45(3):534–539.

130. Zehtabchi S, Baron BJ. Utility of base deficit for identifying major injury in elder trauma patients. *Acad Emerg Med.* 2007;14(9):829–831.
131. Tyburski JG, Collinge JD, Wilson RF, et al. End-tidal CO_2-derived values during emergency trauma surgery correlated with outcome: a prospective study. *J Trauma.* 2002;53(4):738–743.
132. Warner KJ, Cuschieri J, Garland B, et al. The utility of early end-tidal capnography in monitoring ventilation status after severe injury. *J Trauma.* 2009;66(1):26–31.
133. McManus J, Yershov AL, Ludwig D, et al. Radial pulse character relationships to systolic blood pressure and trauma outcomes. *Prehosp Emerg Care.* 2005;9(4):423–428.
134. Holcomb JB, Salinas J, McManus JM, et al. Manual vital signs reliably predict need for life-saving interventions in trauma patients. *J Trauma.* 2005;59(4):821–828.
135. Hashmi A, Ibrahim-Zada I, Rhee P, et al. Predictors of mortality in geriatric trauma patients: a systematic review and meta-analysis. *J Trauma Acute Care Surg.* 2014;76(3):894–901.
136. Jacobs DG. Special considerations in geriatric injury. *Curr Opin Crit Care.* 2003;9(6):535–539.
137. Moise KJ Jr, Belfort MA. Damage control for the obstetric patient. *Surg Clin North Am.* 1997;77(4):835–852.
138. Kaczynski J. Prevention of tissue hypoperfusion in the trauma patient: initial management. *Br J Hosp Med (Lond).* 2013;74(2):81–84.
139. Hagiwara A, Minakawa K, Fukushima H, et al. Predictors of death in patients with life-threatening pelvic hemorrhage after successful transcatheter arterial embolization. *J Trauma.* 2003;55(4):696–703.
140. Hoffer EK, Borsa JJ, Bloch RD, Fontaine AB. Endovascular techniques in the damage control setting. *Radiographics.* 1999;19(5):1340–1348.
141. Shapiro M, McDonald AA, Knight D, et al. The role of repeat angiography in the management of pelvic fractures. *J Trauma.* 2005;58(2):227–231.
142. Gourlay D, Hoffer E, Routt M, Bulger E. Pelvic angiography for recurrent traumatic pelvic arterial hemorrhage. *J Trauma.* 2005;59(5):1168–1173.
143. Spahn DR, Cerny V, Coats TJ, et al. Management of bleeding following major trauma: a European guideline. *Crit Care.* 2007;11(1):R17.
144. Hyare H, Desigan S, Brookes JA, et al. Endovascular management of major arterial hemorrhage as a complication of inflammatory pancreatic disease. *J Vasc Intervent Radiol.* 2007;18(5):591–596.
145. Snyder HS. Significance of the initial spun hematocrit in trauma patients. *Am J Emerg Med.* 1998;16(2):150–153.
146. Greenfield RH, Bessen HA, Henneman PL. Effect of crystalloid infusion on hematocrit and intravascular volume in healthy, nonbleeding subjects. *Ann Emerg Med.* 1989;18(1):51–55.
147. Stamler KD. Effect of crystalloid infusion on hematocrit in nonbleeding patients, with applications to clinical traumatology. *Ann Emerg Med.* 1989;18(7):747–749.
148. Paradis NA, Balter S, Davison CM, et al. Hematocrit as a predictor of significant injury after penetrating trauma. *Am J Emerg Med.*1997;15(3): 224–228.
149. Zehtabchi S, Sinert R, Goldman M, et al. Diagnostic performance of serial haematocrit measurements in identifying major injury in adult trauma patients. *Injury.* 2006;37(1):46–52.
150. Vincent JL, Dufaye P, Berré J, et al. Serial lactate determinations during circulatory shock. *Crit Care Med.* 1983;11(6):449–451.
151. Guyette FX, Meier EN, Newgard C, et al. A comparison of prehospital lactate and systolic blood pressure for predicting the need for resuscitative care in trauma transported by ground. *J Trauma Acute Care Surg.* 2015;78(3): 600–606.
152. Abramson D, Scalea TM, Hitchcock R, et al. Lactate clearance and survival following injury. *J Trauma.* 1993;35(4):584–588.
153. Manikis P, Jankowski S, Zhang H, et al. Correlation of serial blood lactate levels to organ failure and mortality after trauma. *Am J Emerg Med.* 1995;13(6):619–622.
154. Lavery RF, Livingston DH, Tortella BJ, et al. The utility of venous lactate to triage injured patients in the trauma center. *J Am Coll Surg.* 2000; 190(6):656–664.
155. Wilson M, Davis DP, Coimbra R. Diagnosis and monitoring of hemorrhagic shock during the initial resuscitation of multiple trauma patients: a review. *J Emerg Med.* 2003;24(4):413–422.
156. Porter JM, Ivatury RR. In search of the optimal end points of resuscitation in trauma patients: a review. *J Trauma.* 1998;44(5):908–914.
157. Bilkovski RN, Rivers EP, Horst HM. Targeted resuscitation strategies after injury. *Curr Opin Crit Care.* 2004;10(6):529–538.
158. Rixen D, Raum M, Bouillon B, et al. Base deficit development and its prognostic significance in posttrauma critical illness: an analysis by the trauma registry of the Deutsche Gesellschaft fur unfallchirurgie. *Shock.* 2001;15(2):83–89.
159. Rixen D, Siegel JH. Bench-to-bedside review: oxygen debt and its metabolic correlates as quantifiers of the severity of hemorrhagic and posttraumatic shock. *Crit Care.* 2005;9(5):441–453.
160. Dunne JR, Tracy JK, Scalea TM, Napolitano LM. Lactate and base deficit in trauma: does alcohol or drug use impair their predictive accuracy? *J Trauma.* 2005;58(5):959–966.
161. Kaplan LJ, Kellum JA. Initial pH, base deficit, lactate, anion gap, strong ion difference, and strong ion gap predict outcome from major vascular injury. *Crit Care Med.* 2004;32(5):1120–1124.
162. Rutherford EJ, Morris JA Jr, Reed GW, Hall KS. Base deficit stratifies mortality and determines therapy. *J Trauma.* 1992;33(3):417–423.
163. Davis JW, Parks SN, Kaups KL, et al. Admission base deficit predicts transfusion requirements and risk of complications. *J Trauma.* 1996;41(5): 769–774.
164. Davis JW, Kaups KL, Parks SN. Base deficit is superior to pH in evaluating clearance of acidosis after traumatic shock. *J Trauma.* 1998;44(1):114–118.
165. Davis JW, Kaups KL. Base deficit in the elderly: a marker of severe injury and death. *J Trauma.* 1998;45(5):873–877.
166. Randolph LC, Takacs M, Davis KA. Resuscitation in the pediatric trauma population: admission base deficit remains an important prognostic indicator. *J Trauma.* 2002;53(5):838–842.
167. Peterson DL, Schinco MA, Kerwin AJ, et al. Evaluation of initial base deficit as a prognosticator of outcome in the pediatric trauma population. *Am Surg.* 2004;70(4):326–328.
168. Martin MJ, FitzSullivan E, Salim A, et al. Discordance between lactate and base deficit in the surgical intensive care unit: which one do you trust? *Am J Surg.* 2006;191(5):625–630.
169. Mikulaschek A, Henry SM, Donovan R, Scalea TM. Serum lactate is not predicted by anion gap or base excess after trauma resuscitation. *J Trauma.* 1996;40(2):218–222.
170. Singhal R, Coghill JE, Guy A, et al. Serum lactate and base deficit as predictors of mortality after ruptured abdominal aortic aneurysm repair. *Eur J Vasc Endovasc Surg.* 2005;30(3):263–266.
171. Janczyk RJ, Howells GA, Bair HA, et al. Hypothermia is an independent predictor of mortality in ruptured abdominal aortic aneurysms. *Vasc Endovasc Surg.* 2004;38(1):37–42.
172. Chandler WL, Ferrell C, Trimble S, Moody S. Development of a rapid emergency hemorrhage panel. *Transfusion.* 2010;50(12):2547–2552.
173. Tieu BH, Holcomb JB, Schreiber MA. Coagulopathy: its pathophysiology and treatment in the injured patient. *World J Surg.* 2007;31(5):1055–1064.
174. Zuckerman L, Cohen E, Vagher JP, et al. Comparison of thrombelastography with common coagulation tests. *Thromb Haemost.* 1981;46(4): 752–756.
175. Holcomb JB, Minei KM, Scerbo ML, et al. Admission rapid thrombo-elastography can replace conventional coagulation tests in the emergency department: experience with 1974 consecutive trauma patients. *Ann Surg.* 2012;256(3):476–486.
176. Kashuk JL, Moore EE, Sawyer M, et al. Postinjury coagulopathy management: goal directed resuscitation via POC thrombelastography. *Ann Surg.* 2010;251(4):604–614.
177. Daniel SR, Morita SY, Yu M, Dzierba A. Uncompensated metabolic acidosis: an underrecognized risk factor for subsequent intubation requirement. *J Trauma.* 2004;57(5):993–997.
178. Aufderheide TP, Sigurdsson G, Pirrallo RG, et al. Hyperventilation-induced hypotension during cardiopulmonary resuscitation. *Circulation.* 2004;109(16):1960–1965.
179. Davis DP, Hoyt DB, Ochs M, et al. The effect of paramedic rapid sequence intubation on outcome in patients with severe traumatic brain injury. *J Trauma.* 2003;54(3):444–453.
180. Davis DP. Early ventilation in traumatic brain injury. *Resuscitation.* 2008;76(3):333–340.
181. Davis DP, Dunford JV, Poste JC, et al. The impact of hypoxia and hyperventilation on outcome after paramedic rapid sequence intubation of severely head-injured patients. *J Trauma.* 2004;57(1):1–8.
182. Warner KJ, Cuschieri J, Copass MK, et al. The impact of prehospital ventilation on outcome after severe traumatic brain injury. *J Trauma.* 2007;62(6):1330–1336.
183. Pepe PE, Lurie KG, Wigginton JG, et al. Detrimental hemodynamic effects of assisted ventilation in hemorrhagic states. *Crit Care Med.* 2004; 32(9 Suppl):S414–S420.
184. Krismer AC, Wenzel V, Lindner KH, et al. Influence of negative expiratory pressure ventilation on hemodynamic variables during severe hemorrhagic shock. *Crit Care Med.* 2006;34(8):2175–2181.
185. Bulger EM, Snyder D, Schoelles K, et al. An evidence-based prehospital guideline for external hemorrhage control: American College of Surgeons Committee on Trauma. *Prehosp Emerg Care.* 2014;18(2):163–173.

186. Tanizaki S, Maeda S, Matano H, et al. Time to pelvic embolization for hemodynamically unstable pelvic fractures may affect the survival for delays up to 60 min. *Injury.* 2014;45(4):738–741.
187. Giannoudis PV, Pape HC. Damage control orthopaedics in unstable pelvic ring injuries. *Injury.* 2004;35(7):671–677.
188. Hill DA, West RH, Roncal S. Outcome of patients with haemorrhagic shock: an indicator of performance in a trauma centre. *J R Coll Surg Edinb.* 1995;40(4):221–224.
189. Thoburn E, Norris P, Flores R, et al. System care improves trauma outcome: patient care errors dominate reduced preventable death rate. *J Emerg Med.* 1993;11(2):135–139.
190. Peitzman AB, Courcoulas AP, Stinson C, et al. Trauma center maturation: quantification of process and outcome. *Ann Surg.* 1999;230(1):87–94.
191. Bounoua F, Schuster R, Grewal P, et al. Ruptured abdominal aortic aneurysm: does trauma center designation affect outcome? *Ann Vasc Surg.* 2007;21(2):133–136.
192. Salhab M, Farmer J, Osman I. Impact of delay on survival in patients with ruptured abdominal aortic aneurysm. *Vascular.* 2006;14(1):38–42.
193. Hoyt DB, Bulger EM, Knudson MM, et al. Death in the operating room: an analysis of a multi-center experience. *J Trauma.* 1994;37(3):426–432.
194. Reich DL, Konstadt SN, Raissi S, et al. Trendelenburg position and passive leg raising do not significantly improve cardiopulmonary performance in the anesthetized patient with coronary artery disease. *Crit Care Med.* 1989;17(4):313–317.
195. Wong DH, O'Connor D, Tremper KK, et al. Changes in cardiac output after acute blood loss and position change in man. *Crit Care Med.* 1989;17(10):979–983.
196. Mattox KL, Bickell W, Pepe PE, et al. Prospective MAST study in 911 patients. *J Trauma.* 1989;29(8):1104–1111.
197. Mattox KL, Bickell WH, Pepe PE, Mangelsdorff AD. Prospective randomized evaluation of antishock MAST in post-traumatic hypotension. *J Trauma.* 1986;26(9):779–786.
198. Cayten CG, Berendt BM, Byrne DW, et al. A study of pneumatic antishock garments in severely hypotensive trauma patients. *J Trauma.* 1993;34(5): 728–733.
199. Velanovich V. Crystalloid versus colloid fluid resuscitation: a meta-analysis of mortality. *Surgery.* 1989;105(1):65–71.
200. Schierhout G, Roberts I. Fluid resuscitation with colloid or crystalloid solutions in critically ill patients: a systematic review of randomised trials. *BMJ.* 1998;316(7136):961–964.
201. Cochrane Injuries Group Albumin Reviewers. Human albumin administration in critically ill patients: systematic review of randomised controlled trials. *BMJ.* 1998;317(7153):235–240.
202. Choi PT, Yip G, Quinonez LG, Cook DJ. Crystalloids vs. colloids in fluid resuscitation: a systematic review. *Crit Care Med.* 1999;27(1):200–210.
203. Roberts I, Alderson P, Bunn F, et al. Colloids versus crystalloids for fluid resuscitation in critically ill patients. *Cochrane Database Syst Rev.* 2004;18(4):CD000567.
204. Finfer S, Bellomo R, Boyce N, et al. A comparison of albumin and saline for fluid resuscitation in the intensive care unit. *N Engl J Med.* 2004;350(22):2247–2256.
205. Entholzner EK, Mielke LL, Calatzis AN, et al. Coagulation effects of a recently developed hydroxyethyl starch (HES 130/0.4) compared to hydroxyethyl starches with higher molecular weight. *Acta Anaesthesiol Scand.* 2000;44(9):1116–1121.
206. Jamnicki M, Zollinger A, Seifert B, et al. Compromised blood coagulation: an in vitro comparison of hydroxyethyl starch 130/0.4 and hydroxyethyl starch 200/0.5 using thrombelastography. *Anesth Analg.* 1998;87(5): 989–993.
207. Langeron O, Doelberg M, Ang ET, et al. Voluven, a lower substituted novel hydroxyethyl starch (HES 130/0.4), causes fewer effects on coagulation in major orthopedic surgery than HES 200/0.5. *Anesth Analg.* 2001;92(4):855–862.
208. Fenger-Eriksen C, Anker-Møller E, Heslop J, et al. Thrombelastographic whole blood clot formation after ex vivo addition of plasma substitutes: improvements of the induced coagulopathy with fibrinogen concentrate. *Br J Anaesth.* 2005;94(3):324–329.
209. Kiraly LN, Differding JA, Enomoto TM, et al. Resuscitation with normal saline (NS) vs. lactated ringers (LR) modulates hypercoagulability and leads to increased blood loss in an uncontrolled hemorrhagic shock swine model. *J Trauma.* 2006;61(1):57–64.
210. Cotton BA, Guy JS, Morris JA, Abumrad NN. The cellular, metabolic, and systemic consequences of aggressive fluid resuscitation strategies. *Shock.* 2006;26(2):115–121.
211. Rhee P, Wang D, Ruff P, et al. Human neutrophil activation and increased adhesion by various resuscitation fluids. *Crit Care Med.* 2000;28(1):74–78.
212. Rhee P, Koustova E, Alam HB. Searching for the optimal resuscitation method: recommendations for the initial fluid resuscitation of combat casualties. *J Trauma.* 2003;54(5 Suppl):S52–S62.
213. Ayuste EC, Chen H, Koustova E, et al. Hepatic and pulmonary apoptosis after hemorrhagic shock in swine can be reduced through modifications of conventional Ringer's solution. *J Trauma.* 2006;60(1):52–63.
214. Raeburn CD, Moore EE, Biffl WL, et al. The abdominal compartment syndrome is a morbid complication of postinjury damage control surgery. *Am J Surg.* 2001;182(6):542–546.
215. Biffl WL, Moore EE, Burch JM, et al. Secondary abdominal compartment syndrome is a highly lethal event. *Am J Surg.* 2001;182(6):645–648.
216. Maxwell RA, Fabian TC, Croce MA, Davis KA. Secondary abdominal compartment syndrome: an underappreciated manifestation of severe hemorrhagic shock. *J Trauma.* 1999;47(6):995–999.
217. Miller RS, Morris JA Jr, Diaz JJ Jr, et al. Complications after 344 damage-control open celiotomies. *J Trauma.* 2005;59(6):1365–1371.
218. Gracias VH, Braslow B, Johnson J, et al. Abdominal compartment syndrome in the open abdomen. *Arch Surg.* 2002;137(11):1298–1300.
219. Hirshberg A, Hoyt DB, Mattox KL. From "leaky buckets" to vascular injuries: understanding models of uncontrolled hemorrhage. *J Am Coll Surg.* 2007;204(4):665–672.
220. Bickell WH, Wall MJ Jr, Pepe PE, et al. Immediate versus delayed fluid resuscitation for hypotensive patients with penetrating torso injuries. *N Engl J Med.* 1994;331(17):1105–1109.
221. Schreiber MA, Meier EN, Tisherman SA, et al. A controlled resuscitation strategy is feasible and safe in hypotensive trauma patients: results of a prospective randomized pilot trial. *J Trauma Acute Care Surg.* 2015;78(4):687–695.
222. Dutton RP, Mackenzie CF, Scalea TM. Hypotensive resuscitation during active hemorrhage: impact on in-hospital mortality. *J Trauma.* 2002;52(6): 1141–1146.
223. Holcomb JB. Damage control resuscitation. *J Trauma.* 2007;62(6 Suppl): S36–S37.
224. Beekley AC. Damage control resuscitation: a sensible approach to the exsanguinating surgical patient. *Crit Care Med.* 2008;36(7 Suppl):S267–S274.
225. Cotton BA, Reddy N, Hatch QM, et al. Damage control resuscitation is associated with a reduction in resuscitation volumes and improvement in survival in 390 damage control laparotomy patients. *Ann Surg.* 2011;254(4):598–605.
226. Roberts K, Revell M, Youssef H, et al. Hypotensive resuscitation in patients with ruptured abdominal aortic aneurysm. *Eur J Vasc Endovasc Surg.* 2006;31(4):339–344.
227. Owens TM, Watson WC, Prough DS, et al. Limiting initial resuscitation of uncontrolled hemorrhage reduces internal bleeding and subsequent volume requirements. *J Trauma.* 1995;39(2):200–207.
228. Stern SA. Low-volume fluid resuscitation for presumed hemorrhagic shock: helpful or harmful? *Curr Opin Crit Care.* 2001;7(6):422–430.
229. Sondeen JL, Coppes VG, Holcomb JB. Blood pressure at which rebleeding occurs after resuscitation in swine with aortic injury. *J Trauma.* 2003; 54(5 Suppl):S110–S117
230. Wade CE, Holcomb JB. Endpoints in clinical trials of fluid resuscitation of patients with traumatic injuries. *Transfusion.* 2005;45(1 Suppl):4S–8S..
231. Kwan I, Bunn F, Roberts I; WHO Pre-Hospital Trauma Care Steering Committee. Timing and volume of fluid administration for patients with bleeding. *Cochrane Database Syst Rev.* 2003;(3):CD002245.
232. The Brain Trauma Foundation. The American Association of Neurological Surgeons. The Joint Section on Neurotrauma and Critical Care. Resuscitation of blood pressure and oxygenation. *J Neurotrauma.* 2000;17(6–7):471–478.
233. Brohi K, Singh J, Heron M, Coats T. Acute traumatic coagulopathy. *J Trauma.* 2003;54(6):1127–1130.
234. May AK, Young JS, Butler K, et al. Coagulopathy in severe closed head injury: is empiric therapy warranted? *Am Surg.* 1997;63(3):233–236.
235. Ho AM, Karmakar MK, Dion PW. Are we giving enough coagulation factors during major trauma resuscitation? *Am J Surg.* 2005;190(3):479–484.
236. Cinat ME, Wallace WC, Nastanski F, et al. Improved survival following massive transfusion in patients who have undergone trauma. *Arch Surg.* 1999;134(9):964–968.
237. Brown LM, Aro SO, Cohen MJ, et al. A high fresh frozen plasma: packed red blood cell transfusion ratio decreases mortality in all massively transfused trauma patients regardless of admission international normalized ratio. *J Trauma.* 2011;71(2 Suppl 3):S358–S363.
238. Barbosa RR, Rowell SE, Sambasivan CN, et al. A predictive model for mortality in massively transfused trauma patients. *J Trauma.* 2011; 71(2 Suppl 3):S370–S374.
239. Cotton BA, Gunter OL, Isbell J, et al. Damage control hematology: the impact of a trauma exsanguination protocol on survival and blood product utilization. *J Trauma.* 2008;64(5):1177–1182.

240. Fröhlich M, Lefering R, Probst C, et al. Epidemiology and risk factors of multiple-organ failure after multiple trauma: an analysis of 31,154 patients from the TraumaRegister DGU. *J Trauma Acute Care Surg.* 2014;76(4):921–927.
241. Holcomb JB, Tilley BC, Baraniuk S, et al. Transfusion of plasma, platelets, and red blood cells in a 1:1:1 vs a 1:1:2 ratio and mortality in patients with severe trauma: the PROPPR randomized clinical trial. *JAMA.* 2015;313(5):471–482.
242. McLaughlin DF, Niles SE, Salinas J, et al. A predictive model for massive transfusion in combat casualty patients. *J Trauma.* 2008;64(2 Suppl):S57–S63.
243. Nunez TC, Voskresensky IV, Dossett LA, et al. Early prediction of massive transfusion in trauma: simple as ABC (assessment of blood consumption)? *J Trauma.* 2009;66(2):346–352.
244. Mitra B, Rainer TH, Cameron PA. Predicting massive blood transfusion using clinical scores post-trauma. *Vox Sang.* 2012;102(4):324–330.
245. Schreiber MA, Perkins J, Kiraly L, et al. Early predictors of massive transfusion in combat casualties. *J Am Coll Surg.* 2007;205(4):541–545.
246. Callcut RA, Cotton BA, Muskat P, et al. Defining when to initiate massive transfusion: a validation study of individual massive transfusion triggers in PROMMTT patients. *J Trauma Acute Care Surg.* 2013;74(1):59–65, 67–68.
247. Riskin DJ, Tsai TC, Riskin L, et al. Massive transfusion protocols: the role of aggressive resuscitation versus product ratio in mortality reduction. *J Am Coll Surg.* 2009;209(2):198–205.
248. Radwan ZA, Bai Y, Matijevic N, et al. An emergency department thawed plasma protocol for severely injured patients. *JAMA Surg.* 2013;148(2):170–175.
249. Bogert JN, Harvin JA, Cotton BA. Damage control resuscitation. *J Intensive Care Med.* 2016;31(3):177–186.
250. Malone DL, Hess JR, Fingerhut A. Massive transfusion practices around the globe and a suggestion for a common massive transfusion protocol. *J Trauma.* 2006;60(6 Suppl):S91–S96.
251. Hess JR, Dutton RB, Holcomb JB, Scalea TM. Giving plasma at a 1:1 ratio with red cells in resuscitation: who might benefit? *Transfusion.* 2008;48(8):1763–1765.
252. Moore HB, Moore EE, Chin TL, et al. Activated clotting time of thrombelastography (T-ACT) predicts early postinjury blood component transfusion beyond plasma. *Surgery.* 2014;156(3):564–569.
253. Hebert P C, Wells G, Blajchman MA, et al. A multicenter, randomized, controlled clinical trial of transfusion requirements in critical care. Transfusion Requirements in Critical Care Investigators, Canadian Critical Care Trials Group. *N Engl J Med.* 1999;340(6):409–417.
254. Silliman CC, Moore EE, Johnson JL, et al. Transfusion of the injured patient: proceed with caution. *Shock.* 2004;21(4):291–299.
255. Dodd RY, Notari EP 4th, Stramer SL. Current prevalence and incidence of infectious disease markers and estimated window-period risk in the American Red Cross blood donor population. *Transfusion.* 2002;42(8):975–979.
256. McIntyre LA, Hebert PC. Can we safely restrict transfusion in trauma patients? *Curr Opin Crit Care.* 2006;12(6):575–583.
257. Kleinman S, Chan P, Robillard P. Risks associated with transfusion of cellular blood components in Canada. *Transf Med Rev.* 2003;17(2):120–162.
258. Schreiber GB, Busch MP, Kleinman SH, Korelitz JJ. The risk of transfusion-transmitted viral infections: the Retrovirus Epidemiology Donor Study. *N Engl J Med.* 1996;334(26):1685–1690.
259. MacLennan S, Williamson LM. Risks of fresh frozen plasma and platelets. *J Trauma.* 2006;60(6 Suppl):S46–S50.
260. Spinella P C, Perkins JG, McLaughlin DF, et al. The effect of recombinant activated factor VII on mortality in combat-related casualties with severe trauma and massive transfusion. *J Trauma.* 2008;64(2):286–289.
261. Mohr AM, Holcomb JB, Dutton RP, Duranteau J. Recombinant activated factor VIIa and hemostasis in critical care: a focus on trauma. *Crit Care.* 2005;9(Suppl 5):S37–S42.
262. Lin Y, Stanworth S, Birchall J, et al. Recombinant factor VIIa for the prevention and treatment of bleeding in patients without haemophilia. *Cochrane Database Syst Rev.* 2011;(2):CD005011.
263. Knudson MM, Cohen MJ, Reidy R, et al. Trauma, transfusions, and use of recombinant factor VIIa: a multicenter case registry report of 380 patients from the Western Trauma Association. *J Am Coll Surg.* 2011;212(1):87–95.
264. Kashuk JL, Moore EE, Sawyer M, et al. Primary fibrinolysis is integral in the pathogenesis of the acute coagulopathy of trauma. *Ann Surg.* 2010;252(3):434–442.
265. Kutcher ME, Cripps MW, McCreery RC, et al. Criteria for empiric treatment of hyperfibrinolysis after trauma. *J Trauma Acute Care Surg.* 2012;73(1):87–93.
266. Chapman MP, Moore EE, Ramos CR, et al. Fibrinolysis greater than 3% is the critical value for initiation of antifibrinolytic therapy. *J Trauma Acute Care Surg.* 2013;75(6):961–967.
267. Cotton BA, Harvin JA, Kostousouv V, et al. Hyperfibrinolysis at admission is an uncommon but highly lethal event associated with shock and prehospital fluid administration. *J Trauma Acute Care Surg.* 2012;73(2):365–370.
268. Ives C, Inaba K, Branco BC, et al. Hyperfibrinolysis elicited via thromboelastography predicts mortality in trauma. *J Am Coll Surg.* 2012;215(4):496–502.
269. CRASH-2 Trial collaborators; Shakur H, Roberts I, et al. Effects of tranexamic acid on death, vascular occlusive events, and blood transfusion in trauma patients with significant haemorrhage (CRASH-2): a randomised, placebo-controlled trial. *Lancet.* 2010;376(9734):23–32.
270. CRASH-2 collaborators; Roberts I, Shakur H, et al. The importance of early treatment with tranexamic acid in bleeding trauma patients: an exploratory analysis of the CRASH-2 randomised controlled trial. *Lancet.* 2011;377(9771):1096–1101.
271. Morrison JJ, Ross JD, Dubose JJ, et al. Association of cryoprecipitate and tranexamic acid with improved survival following wartime injury: findings from the MATTERs II Study. *JAMA Surg.* 2013;148(3):218–225.
272. Morrison JJ, Dubose JJ, Rasmussen TE, Midwinter MJ. Military Application of Tranexamic Acid in Trauma Emergency Resuscitation (MATTERs) Study. *Arch Surg.* 2012;147(2):113–119.
273. Napolitano LM, Cohen MJ, Cotton BA, et al. Tranexamic acid in trauma: how should we use it? *J Trauma Acute Care Surg.* 2013;74(6):1575–1586.
274. Brown JB, Neal MD, Guyette FX, et al. Design of the Study of Tranexamic Acid during Air Medical Prehospital Transport (STAAMP) trial: addressing the knowledge gaps. *Prehosp Emerg Care.* 2015;19(1):79–86.
275. Joseph B, Hadjizacharia P, Aziz H, et al. Prothrombin complex concentrate: an effective therapy in reversing the coagulopathy of traumatic brain injury. *J Trauma Acute Care Surg.* 2013;74(1):248–253.
276. Le Roux P, Pollack CV Jr, Milan M, Schaefer A. Race against the clock: overcoming challenges in the management of anticoagulant-associated intracerebral hemorrhage. *J Neurosurg.* 2014;121(Suppl):1–20.
277. Ferreira J, DeLosSantos M. The clinical use of prothrombin complex concentrate. *J Emerg Med.* 2013;44(6):1201–1210.
278. Nascimento B, Goodnough LT, Levy JH. Cryoprecipitate therapy. *Br J Anaesth.* 2014;113(6):922–934.
279. Holcomb JB, Fox EE, Zhang X, et al. Cryoprecipitate use in the PROMMTT study. *J Trauma Acute Care Surg.* 2013;75(1 Suppl 1):S31–S39.
280. Reynolds BR, Forsythe RM, Harbrecht BG, et al. Hypothermia in massive transfusion: have we been paying enough attention to it? *J Trauma Acute Care Surg.* 2012;73(2):486–491.
281. Jurkovich GJ, Greiser WB, Luterman A, Curreri PW. Hypothermia in trauma victims: an ominous predictor of survival. *J Trauma.* 1987;27(9):1019–1024.
282. Ness PM, Cushing MM. Oxygen therapeutics: pursuit of an alternative to the donor red blood cell. *Arch Pathol Lab Med.* 2007;131(5):734–741.
283. Jahr JS, Walker V, Manoochehri K. Blood substitutes as pharmacotherapies in clinical practice. *Curr Opin Anaesthesiol.* 2007;20(4):325–330.
284. Moore EE, Johnson JL, Cheng AM, et al. Insights from studies of blood substitutes in trauma. *Shock.* 2005;24(3):197–205.
285. Moore EE, Moore FA, Fabian TC, et al. Human polymerized hemoglobin for the treatment of hemorrhagic shock when blood is unavailable: the USA multicenter trial. *J Am Coll Surg.* 2009;208(1):1–13.
286. Shuja F, Shults C, Duggan M, et al. Development and testing of freeze-dried plasma for the treatment of trauma-associated coagulopathy. *J Trauma.* 2008;65(5):975–985.
287. Spoerke N, Zink K, Cho SD, et al. Lyophilized plasma for resuscitation in a swine model of severe injury. *Arch Surg.* 2009;144(9):829–834.
288. Bulger EM, Hoyt DB. Hypertonic resuscitation after severe injury: is it of benefit? *Adv Surg.* 2012;46:73–85.
289. Freshman SP, Battistella FD, Matteucci M, Wisner DH. Hypertonic saline (7.5%) versus mannitol: a comparison for treatment of acute head injuries. *J Trauma.* 1993;35(3):344–348.
290. Doyle JA, Davis DP, Hoyt DB. The use of hypertonic saline in the treatment of traumatic brain injury. *J Trauma.* 2001;50(2):367–383.
291. Rizoli SB, Kapus A, Parodo J, et al. Hypertonic immunomodulation is reversible and accompanied by changes in CD11b expression. *J Surg Res.* 1999;83(2):130–135.
292. Rizoli SB, Rotstein OD, Parodo J, et al. Hypertonic inhibition of exocytosis in neutrophils: central role for osmotic actin skeleton remodeling. *Am J Physiol Cell Physiol.* 2000;279(3):C619–C633.
293. Junger WG, Liu FC, Loomis WH, Hoyt DB. Hypertonic saline enhances cellular immune function. *Circ Shock.* 1994;42(4):190–196.

294. Junger WG, Coimbra R, Liu FC, et al. Hypertonic saline resuscitation: a tool to modulate immune function in trauma patients? *Shock*. 1997;8(4): 235–241.
295. Junger WG, Rhind SG, Rizoli SB, et al. Prehospital hypertonic saline resuscitation attenuates the activation and promotes apoptosis of neutrophils in patients with severe traumatic brain injury. *Shock*. 2013;40(5):366–374.
296. Coimbra R, Junger WG, Liu FC, et al. Hypertonic/hyperoncotic fluids reverse prostaglandin E2 (PGE2)-induced T-cell suppression. *Shock*. 1995;4(1):45–49.
297. Cuschieri J, Gourlay D, Garcia I, et al. Hypertonic preconditioning inhibits macrophage responsiveness to endotoxin. *J Immunol*. 2002;168: 1389–1396.
298. Bulger EM, Tower CM, Warner KJ, et al. Increased neutrophil adenosine a3 receptor expression is associated with hemorrhagic shock and injury severity in trauma patients. *Shock*. 2011;36(5):435–439.
299. Wade C, Grady J, Kramer G. Efficacy of hypertonic saline dextran (HSD) in patients with traumatic hypotension: meta-analysis of individual patient data. *Acta Anaesthesiol Scand Suppl*. 1997;110:77–79.
300. Wade CE, Kramer GC, Grady JJ, et al. Efficacy of hypertonic 7.5% saline and 6% dextran-70 in treating trauma: a meta-analysis of controlled clinical studies. *Surgery*. 1997;122(3):609–616.
301. Wade CE, Grady JJ, Kramer GC, et al. Individual patient cohort analysis of the efficacy of hypertonic saline/dextran in patients with traumatic brain injury and hypotension. *J Trauma*. 1997;42(5 Suppl):S61–S65.
302. Bulger EM, May S, Kerby JD, et al. Out-of-hospital hypertonic resuscitation after traumatic hypovolemic shock: a randomized, placebo controlled trial. *Ann Surg*. 2011;253(3):431–441.
303. Del Junco DJ, Bulger EM, Fox EE, et al. Collider bias in trauma comparative effectiveness research: the stratification blues for systematic reviews. *Injury*. 2015;46(5):775–780.
304. Bulger EM, May S, Brasel KJ, et al. Out-of-hospital hypertonic resuscitation following severe traumatic brain injury: a randomized controlled trial. *JAMA*. 2010;304(13):1455–1464.
305. Biffl WL, Fox CJ, Moore EE. The role of REBOA in the control of exsanguinating torso hemorrhage. *J Trauma Acute Care Surg*. 2015;78(5): 1054–1058.
306. Brenner ML, Moore LJ, Dubose JJ, et al. A clinical series of resuscitative endovascular balloon occlusion of the aorta for hemorrhage control and resuscitation. *J Trauma Acute Care Surg*. 2013;75(3):506–511.
307. Saito N, Matsumoto H, Yagi T, et al. Evaluation of the safety and feasibility of resuscitative endovascular balloon occlusion of the aorta. *J Trauma Acute Care Surg*. 2015;78(5):897–904.

CHAPTER

48

Neurogenic Shock

RIBAL BASSIL, FIRAS KADDOUH, DAVID M. GREER, and SUSANNE MUEHLSCHLEGEL

INTRODUCTION

Neurologically injured patients frequently experience hypotension and shock. The term *neurogenic shock* refers to a form of circulatory system failure specifically felt to be secondary to acute brain, spinal cord, or peripheral nerve injuries. Neurogenic shock should be considered only after other more common causes of shock have been carefully ruled out. Like other critically ill patients, patients with neurologic injuries are prone to developing systemic conditions resulting in shock, such as hypovolemia, hemorrhage, sepsis, massive pulmonary embolism, or primary cardiac causes of cardiogenic shock, including cardiac ischemia or pericardial tamponade. Herein, we explain the epidemiology, pathophysiology, diagnosis, management strategies, and controversies regarding neurogenic shock.

Contrary to common belief, neurogenic shock is not a single entity due to one pathologic mechanism; rather, there are three mechanisms that can lead to circulatory failure. There can be significant overlap between these mechanisms with different neurologic injuries, and one cannot establish a firm rule by which neurogenic shock occurs. These mechanisms or subtypes are (Fig. 48.1):

- *Vasodilatory (distributive) shock* from autonomic disturbance with interruption of sympathetic pathways and associated parasympathetic excitation, which causes profound vasodilatation and bradycardia, as seen in spinal cord injury or some diseases of the peripheral nervous system (e.g., Guillain–Barré syndrome).
- *Cardiogenic shock* from stunned myocardium after a catecholamine surge, as frequently seen in subarachnoid hemorrhage (SAH) or ischemic stroke, especially those involving the right insula.
- Hypopituitarism/adrenal insufficiency (AI): This form is commonly seen in brain injuries that impact the hypothalamus, pituitary gland, or the pituitary stalk, either in the form of direct injury or due to compression from cerebral edema.

Interestingly, only a minority of patients with neurologic injuries experience true neurogenic shock, and it remains difficult to predict in whom this occurs.

INCIDENCE OF NEUROGENIC SHOCK

Because of the small number of prospective epidemiologic studies, it is difficult to establish the natural incidence of neurogenic shock. In a retrospective review of cervical spinal cord injuries, Bilello et al. (1) reported a 31% incidence of neurogenic shock with hypotension and bradycardia after high cervical spinal cord injury (C1 to C5), and 24% after low cervical spinal cord injury (C6 to C7).

Cardiogenic neurogenic shock has been studied primarily in SAH and ischemic stroke. Banki et al. (2) prospectively studied the incidence of left ventricular (LV) dysfunction in the first week after SAH in 173 patients; 13% had a normal ejection fraction (EF) but had regional wall motion abnormalities that did not correlate with coronary artery territories, and 15% had an LVEF of less than 50%. Others report a 9% incidence of LV wall motion abnormalities, resulting in hypotension requiring vasopressor therapy, as well as pulmonary edema in 80% of these patients (3). The spectrum of injury can range from mild to severe systolic dysfunction—the latter defined as an EF less than 30%. Pollick et al. (4) observed LV abnormalities on transthoracic echocardiogram (TTE) in 4 of 13 patients (31%) studied within 48 hours of SAH. Resolution of these neurologically mediated wall motion abnormalities is usually seen within several days to several months (2,3,5,6).

Hypothalamic–pituitary–AI resulting in neurogenic shock has been studied primarily in traumatic brain injury (TBI). In the largest study to date, AI occurred in about 50% of patients, and 26% of these had hypotension (7). Although it has been documented in other cases of acute brain injury, the exact incidence and relationship to outcome is not clear (8).

PATHOLOGIES OF NEUROGENIC SHOCK

Vasodilatory Neurogenic Shock

This variant of neurogenic shock is commonly seen with spinal cord injuries and acute demyelinating peripheral neuropathy (AIDP, or Guillain–Barré syndrome), but can also occur with TBIs, large hemispheric ischemic strokes, and intracerebral hemorrhages. The hallmark of vasodilatory neurogenic shock is the combination of bradycardia with fluctuating blood pressure and heart rate variability due to interruption of sympathetic output and excitation of parasympathetic fibers.

The sympathetic fibers originate in the hypothalamus, giving rise to neurons projecting to autonomic centers in the brainstem—the periaqueductal gray matter in the midbrain, the parabrachial regions in the pons, and the intermediate reticular formation located in the ventrolateral medulla. From here, neurons project to nuclei in the spinal cord. The sympathetic preganglionic neurons originate in the intermediolateral cell column within the spinal cord gray matter between T1 and L2, and are therefore called the "thoracolumbar branches." From here, they exit the spinal cord and project to 22 pairs of paravertebral sympathetic trunk ganglia next to the spine; the main ganglia within the sympathetic trunk are the cervical and stellate ganglia. The adrenal medulla receives preganglionic fibers and thus is equivalent to a sympathetic ganglion. Blood pressure control depends on tonic activation of the

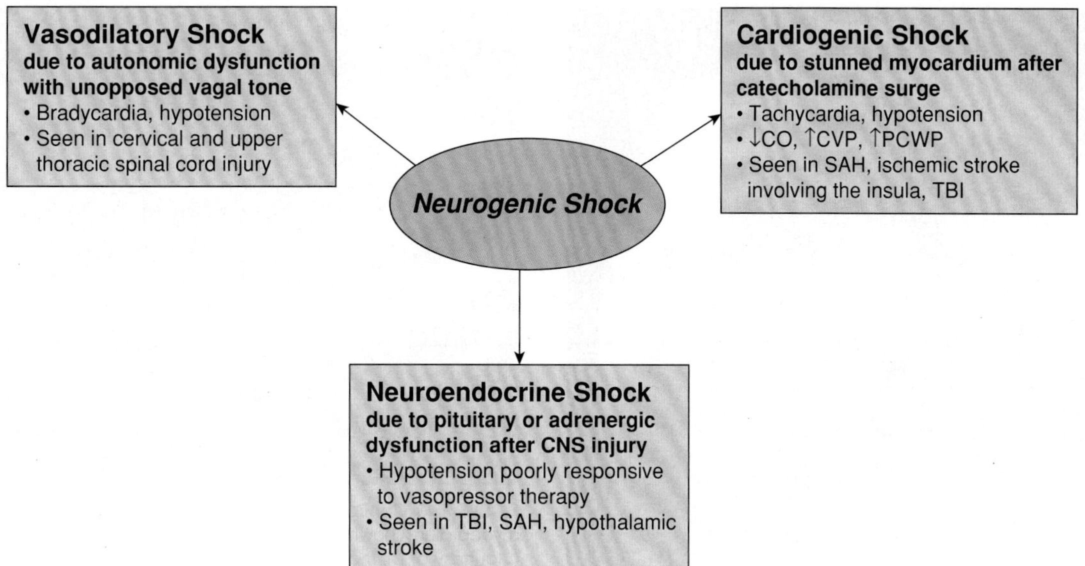

FIGURE 48.1 Neurogenic shock consists of three pathomechanisms. CNS, central nervous system; CO, cardiac output; CVP, central venous pressure; PCWP, pulmonary capillary wedge pressure; SAH, subarachnoid hemorrhage; TBI, traumatic brain injury.

sympathetic preganglionic neurons by descending input from the supraspinal structures (9).

The parasympathetic nervous system consists of cranial and sacral aspects. The cranial parasympathetic neurons originate from the parasympathetic brainstem nuclei of cranial nerves III, VII, IX, X, and XI. The cranial parasympathetic neurons travel along the cranial nerves until they synapse in the parasympathetic ganglia in close proximity to the target organ. The sacral subdivision originates in the sacral spinal cord (S2 to S4), forming the lateral intermediate gray zone where preganglionic neurons travel along the pelvic nerves to the inferior hypogastric plexus and synapse on parasympathetic ganglia within the target organs.

Following a spinal cord injury, the sympathetic pathways are interrupted with resulting loss of the supraspinal sympathetic input above to the level below the injury (10–12). Parasympathetic fibers are usually spared. This leads to unopposed vagal tone with relaxation of vascular smooth muscles below the level of the cord injury, resulting in decreased venous return, decreased cardiac output, hypotension, loss of diurnal fluctuations of blood pressure, reflex bradycardia, and peripheral adrenoreceptor hyperresponsiveness (12,13); the latter is due to upregulation of adrenoreceptors and accounts for the excessive vasopressor response commonly seen in this clinical scenario. Autonomic hyperreflexia with associated hypertension, or hypotension along with bradycardia, has all been observed in humans and in animal models (11,14–16). Autonomic dysreflexia ensues in patients with lesions above T5 (17) and occurs between 2 and 30 days after the spinal cord injury. This state is characterized by sympathetically mediated vasoconstriction in muscular, skin, renal, and presumably gastrointestinal vascular beds, induced by afferent peripheral stimulation below the level of the lesion. For example, stimuli such as urinary catheterization or dressing changes can lead to severe blood pressure spikes out of proportion to the stimulus. In Guillain–Barré syndrome, the autonomic dysregulation is likely caused by acute demyelination not only of sensory and motor fibers but also of autonomic fibers. Patients might also experience a throbbing headache, piloerection, shivering, and diaphoresis above the level of the injury.

Brain injury itself can lead to vasodilatory neurogenic shock. Certain cerebral structures, such as the insular cortex, amygdala, lateral hypothalamus, and medulla, have great influence on the autonomic nervous system. Cortical asymmetry exists and is reflected in a higher incidence of tachycardia, ventricular arrhythmias, and hypertension with lesions of the right insula—resulting in loss of parasympathetic input and thus sympathetic predominance. On the other hand, there is a higher incidence of bradycardia and hypotension with injuries to the left insula—resulting in a loss of sympathetic input and subsequent parasympathetic predominance (Fig. 48.2) (18–20).

Cardiogenic Neurogenic Shock

This form of neurogenic shock is primarily encountered in SAH and TBI, but is also seen in ischemic stroke and intracerebral hemorrhage. Cardiac dysfunction is a well-known complication of ischemic and hemorrhagic stroke, first described over 60 years ago (21). In this setting, electrocardiographic (ECG) changes such as bradycardia, atrial fibrillation, ventricular fibrillation, and tachycardia, T-wave inversions, and prolonged QTc intervals (22–24) can be seen. Studies of SAH and cardiac injury showed that the severity of SAH is an independent predictor of cardiac injury, supporting the hypothesis that cardiac neurogenic shock is a neurally mediated process (25). Studies have also shown that specific ECG changes, for example, prolonged QTc intervals, are predictors of poor survival (26).

Based on the similarities observed between the crises of pheochromocytoma and SAH, the observed cardiovascular changes have been linked to a catecholamine surge; this hypothesis has been confirmed by many studies. Patients with SAH can have a threefold increase in norepinephrine levels that are sustained for 10 days or longer after SAH, but normalize after the acute phase of injury (27). In an animal model,

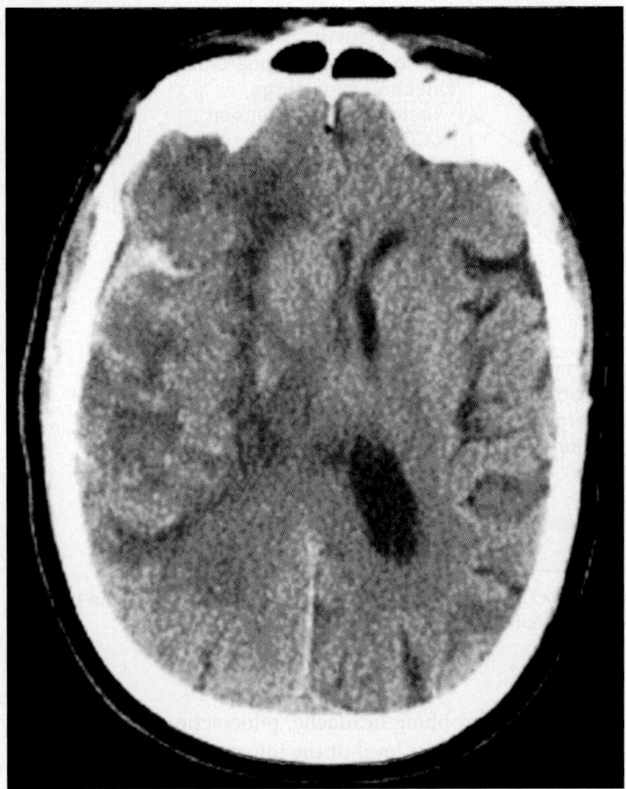

FIGURE 48.2 Example of a right hemisphere ischemic stroke resulting in ventricular dysrhythmias and cardiogenic shock. A 61-year-old man presents with the sudden onset of left hemiparesis affecting his face and arm, left-sided neglect, and a left homonymous hemianopia. He presented outside of any acute treatment window and thus did not undergo thrombolysis or mechanical clot removal. He was admitted to the neurointensive care unit for close monitoring of his cardiac and respiratory function. The noncontrast head CT shows a right middle cerebral artery stroke and incidental hemorrhagic conversion. Electrocardiogram on admission showed diffuse T-wave inversion in all leads. Telemetry revealed frequent premature ventricular complexes and intermittent nonsustained ventricular tachycardia of 4 to 8 beats for the first 72 hours after stroke onset. His systolic blood pressure on admission was elevated at 190 mmHg, but then dropped to 85 mmHg several hours after admission to the neurointensive care unit, requiring vasopressor support for 2 days. Troponin T levels were elevated in the emergency room and peaked 12 hours after stroke onset. Echocardiography showed global hypokinesis and no regional wall motion abnormalities. No other causes for shock were found, so the stroke involving the right insula was felt to be the most likely cause. The shock slowly resolved over 72 hours, and the vasopressor infusion was weaned off successfully. A repeat echocardiogram 2 weeks later showed resolution of the abnormalities.

an increase in plasma catecholamines after experimental SAH causes specific lesions on electron microscopy within 4 hours of SAH (28). Selective myocardial cell necrosis described as focal myocytolysis or myofibrillary degeneration, also known as contraction band necrosis, is the hallmark of catecholamine exposure (Fig. 48.3) (29–31). The same lesions can be found in patients with pheochromocytoma (32) and SAH (33), underlining the pathologic mechanism of cardiac injury in SAH or other neurologic injuries. The cardiac dysfunction is not related to coronary atherosclerosis, as normal coronary arteries have been documented in these patients studied at autopsy or by coronary angiography (5,33–36). In fact, it appears that pre-existing heart disease, such as hypertensive heart disease, might even be *protective* of this form of neurogenic shock (37).

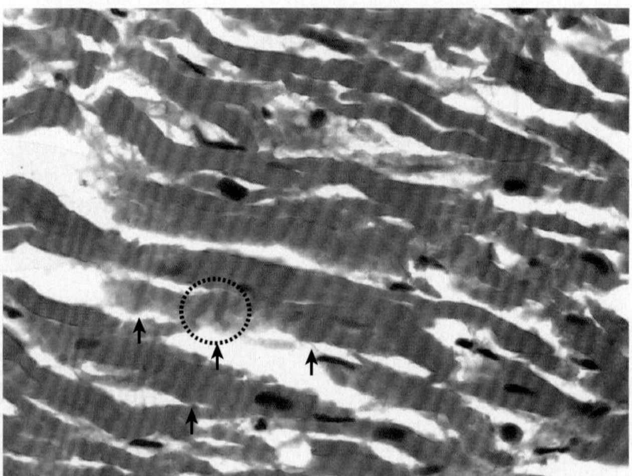

FIGURE 48.3 Contraction band necrosis. Histologic examination of the myocardium showing contraction band necrosis; see *arrows* and *circle*. (Courtesy of Dr. Thomas Smith, MD, Department of Pathology, University of Massachusetts Medical School, Worcester, MA.)

In a case series of 54 consecutive SAH deaths, 42 had myocardial lesions consisting of foci of necrotic muscle fibers, hemorrhages, and inflammatory cells, none of which were found in the control group. Patients with a wider range of heart rate and blood pressure fluctuations were more likely to have myocardial lesions. Pre-existing hypertensive heart disease led to significantly fewer myocardial lesions, possibly reflecting a decreased sensitivity of these patients to the catecholamine surge, probably due to chronic exposure to catecholamines (37).

Pathologic studies link the central catecholamine release to the posterior hypothalamus. Postmortem studies have found microscopic hypothalamic lesions consisting of small hemorrhages and infarctions in those patients with typical myocardial lesions as noted above (33,37–39). However, it appears that raised intracranial pressure (ICP) is not responsible for these hypothalamic changes, as the control group with elevated ICP did not have any hypothalamic injury (37).

Overall, by the described pathomechanism, the catecholamine surge results in direct myocardial injury, leading to decreased inotropy and an increase in cardiac preload due to venous constriction, as well as increased cardiac afterload due to peripheral arterial constriction. As a consequence, stroke volume diminishes, which cannot be compensated by reflex tachycardia, resulting in decreased cardiac output and shock. This transient LV dysfunction with loss of myocardial compliance (myocardial "stunning") is reflected by a characteristic shape of the cardiac silhouette on a ventriculogram and on chest radiograph, which has given this disease entity its other name, "Takotsubo cardiomyopathy," derived from the Japanese word for the Japanese octopus fishing pot, *takotsubo* (Fig. 48.4) (40–42). In a recent retrospective study, Kilbourn (43) reported that neurogenic cardiomyopathy in SAH is associated with higher mortality and poorer long-term outcomes.

Pulmonary edema with concomitant hypoxia is frequently encountered in this context. It may result from the aforementioned acute LV dysfunction, but can occur independently from the cardiac dysfunction as its own entity: neurogenic pulmonary edema (NPE). Massive increases in pulmonary

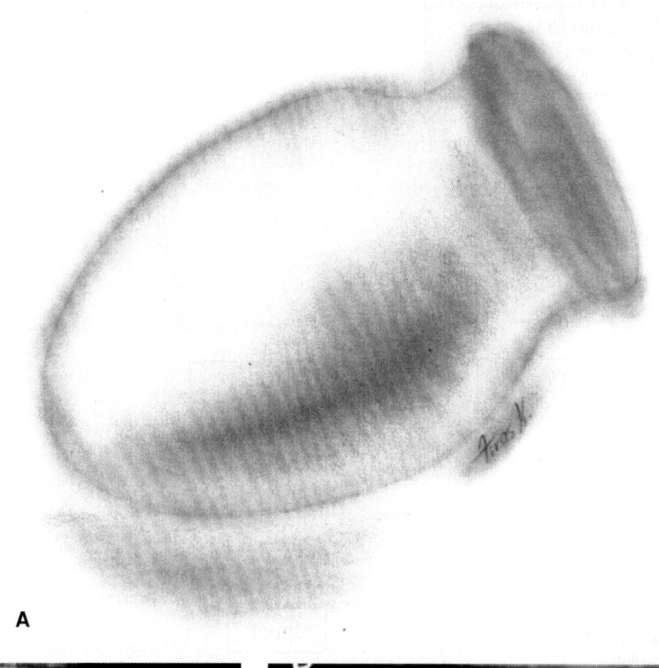

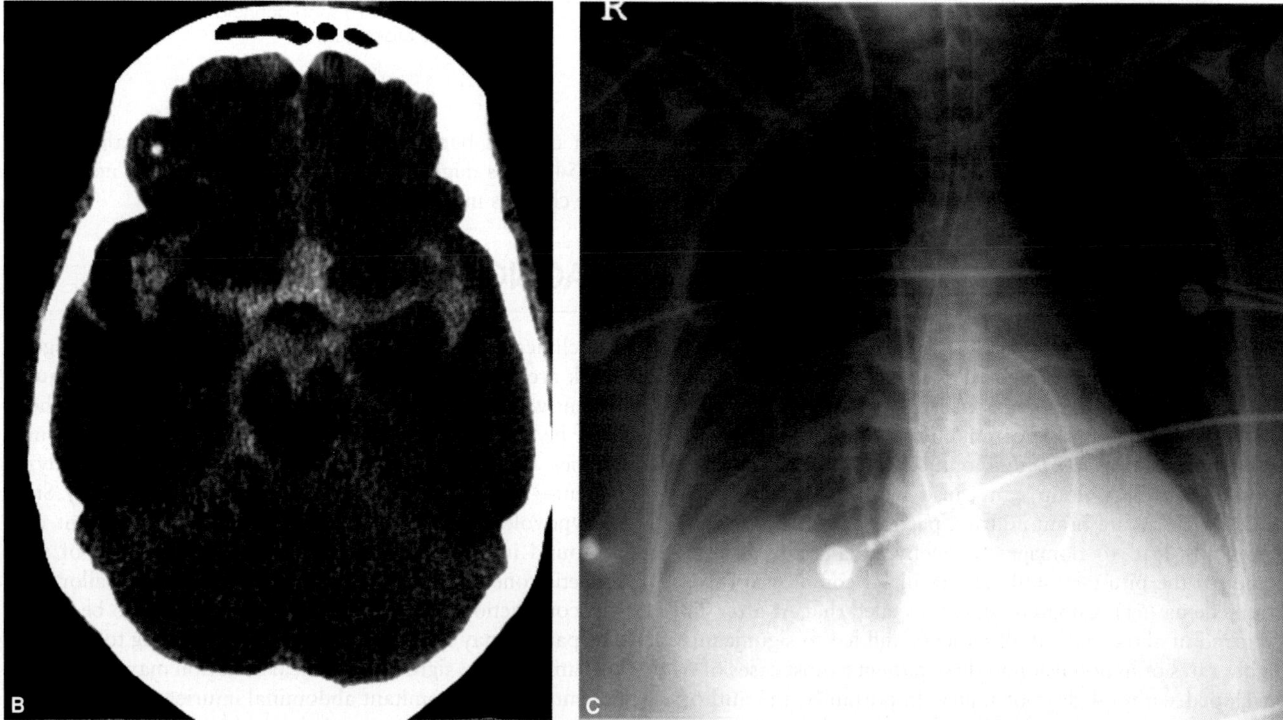

FIGURE 48.4 Takotsubo cardiomyopathy. A: Japanese octopus fishing pot (drawing by Firas Kaddouh, MD.) B: CT brain of a 47-year-old woman with subarachnoid hemorrhage (SAH). C: Chest x-ray view of the same patient with typical cardiac silhouette of Takotsubo cardiomyopathy. An echocardiogram revealed an ejection fraction of 29% with apical ballooning, global hypokinesis, and sparing of the apex. The chest radiograph and echocardiogram became normal within 1 week after her SAH.

capillary pressures lead to pulmonary edema, which in turn decreases the uptake of oxygen in a high demand state, resulting in profound hypoxemia and contributing to hemodynamic instability. The Vietnam war era head injury series (44) reported the rapid onset of acute pulmonary edema after severe head injury. In addition, experimental models as well as multiple human case reports of TBI and SAH have shown massive sympathetic discharge as the primary cause of NPE (45–47). NPE has also been reported in patients with multiple sclerosis, sometimes as the initial presentation, and is believed to be due to demyelination involving the caudal medulla resulting in an increase in hydrostatic pulmonary pressure and the development of pulmonary edema (48–50). Figure 48.5 summarizes the pathophysiology of cardiogenic neurogenic shock.

Overall, cardiac neurogenic shock, with or without NPE, is usually transient, resolving within several days to 2 weeks (2–4). Prevention of secondary brain injury from hypoxia and

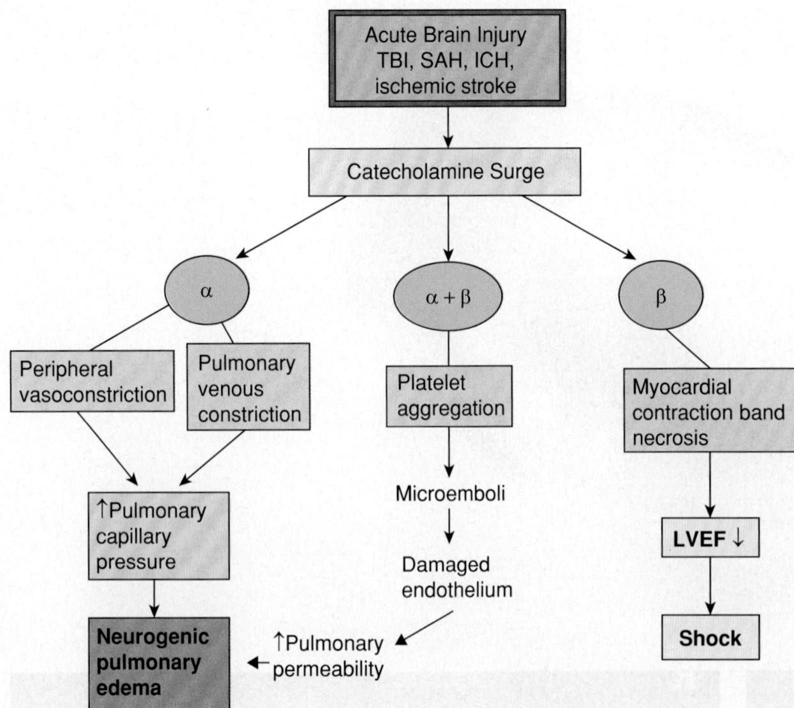

FIGURE 48.5 Summary of the pathophysiology of the cardiogenic type of neurogenic shock. ICH, intracerebral hemorrhage; LVEF, left ventricular ejection fraction; SAH, subarachnoid hemorrhage; TBI, traumatic brain injury.

decreased cerebral perfusion is essential in the management of this neurally mediated complication.

Neuroendocrine Neurogenic Shock

Insufficiency of the hypothalamic–pituitary–adrenal axis has been recognized as an important and easily treatable cause of shock. Inappropriately reduced release of cortisol in stress situations can lead to decreased systemic vascular resistance (SVR), reduced cardiac contractility, hypovolemic shock, or hyperdynamic shock that can mimic septic shock. Secondary adrenal insufficiency (AI) due to injury to the hypothalamic–pituitary feedback loop can cause neuroendocrine neurogenic shock. Acute brain injuries, particularly TBI and SAH, commonly lead to damage to the hypothalamus, pituitary gland, or the pituitary stalk as a result of compression from brain edema (51). Cohan et al. (7) revealed that AI after TBI occurred in about half of all patients and led to significantly higher rates of hypotension in these patients; most cases of AI developed within 4 days of injury. Importantly, the authors defined AI using a low random serum cortisol value, and highlighted the fact that an increase in the cortisol level after a stimulation test does not rule out the presence of AI. This issue is particularly relevant in TBI patients, in whom the hypothalamus and the pituitary gland are the likely affected regions, and the adrenal glands might well be expected to mount an appropriate response when stimulated. In a retrospective study, Pastrana and colleagues (43) also reported that AI was present in 22% of all patients with cervical spinal cord injury who developed shock, and the presence of AI was positively correlated with an increased risk of complications and 30-day mortality; however, further studies to define the underlying pathophysiology are needed.

Few studies in SAH have shown that endogenous vasopressin serum levels are elevated during the first 2 days after the onset of SAH but decrease to subnormal levels after 4 days (52–54). This might provide further evidence for neuroendocrine changes in neurogenic shock.

DIAGNOSIS

The clinical manifestations and symptoms seen in neurogenic shock are noted in Figure 48.6. In any neurologically injured patient with hypotension and shock, systemic causes of shock must be first ruled out. Recognition of other life-threatening injuries can be quite difficult, especially in the paralyzed patient—for example, one with a high spinal cord injury. Signs of hypovolemic shock may be absent, even in a patient with profound internal bleeding, because of the absence of sympathetic tone below the level of injury; the usual pallor from vasoconstriction and reflex tachycardia might also be absent. The patient may be bradycardic while continuing to bleed; for the same reason, signs of peritoneal irritation may be absent in patients with concomitant abdominal injuries.

In the setting of fever and shock, blood cultures must be obtained and the patient appropriately covered with broad-spectrum antibiotics until the cultures result. Furthermore, older and immunosuppressed patients may not mount an appropriate febrile response, and thus sepsis should still be considered in these patients even when they are afebrile, especially in the setting of a rising white blood cell count. Cerebrospinal fluid cultures are very important to consider—when safe and appropriate to obtain—with antibiotic coverage of potential central nervous system (CNS) infections, especially in patients after head trauma with skull fractures or sinus disease, or after instrumentation of the head or spinal canal.

Every patient should undergo serial ECGs, serial cardiac enzyme measurements, and a chest radiograph. As previously

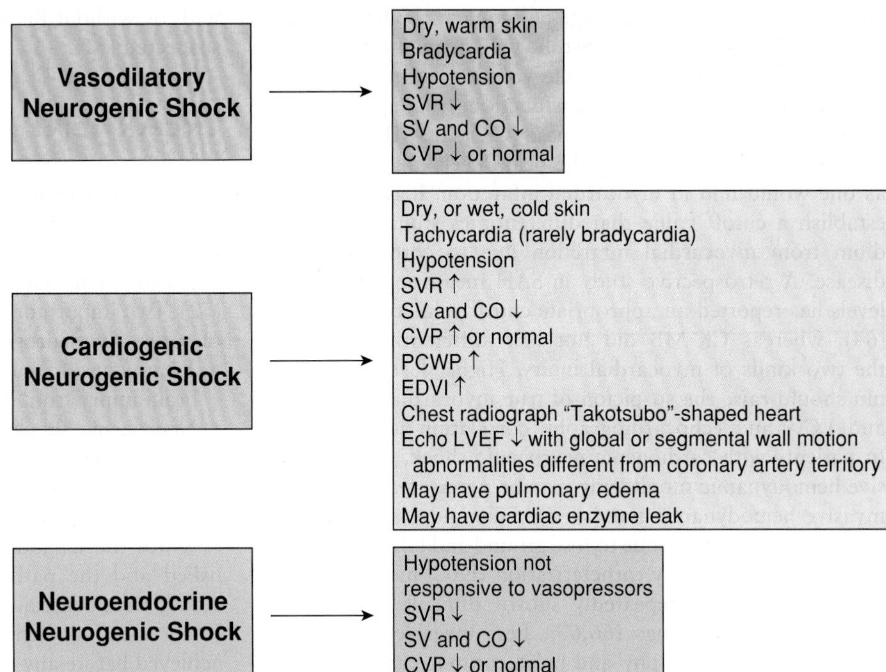

FIGURE 48.6 Clinical manifestations of the different types of neurogenic shock. CO, carbon monoxide; EDVI, end-diastolic volume index; PCWP, pulmonary capillary wedge pressure; SV, stroke volume; SVR, systemic vascular resistance.

mentioned, pulmonary edema and neurocardiogenic injury may occur together or separately, making chest films and echocardiograms important diagnostic tools. In particular, one should look for pulmonary vascular congestion and evaluate the size and shape of the cardiac silhouette. Hemodynamic monitoring with continuous blood pressure measurements should be undertaken. Arteriosclerosis of the upper extremities is common, and should be kept in mind either when there is a large discrepancy between right- and left-sided pressures or when the clinical appearance of the patient does not match the readings from the arterial line. Central venous access is key for administration of fluids and medications, especially vasopressors. The site of the placement of the central venous line may play an important role in the management of shock in a neurologically injured patient. Subclavian venous catheters are the preferred site in patients with elevated ICP, as there is a theoretical risk of venous stasis within the internal jugular vein with congestion and a higher risk for thrombosis, which could result in increased ICP (55). In addition, trauma patients frequently have cervical spine injuries and require cervical collars, making the internal jugular vein accessible only with difficulty. Echocardiography is very important to gain an understanding of the etiology of shock. In most cases, a TTE is sufficient and provides a direct visualization tool to assess myocardial and valvular function, cardiac output, and preload status. The typical echocardiographic appearance is that of apical ballooning, which results from global hypokinesis sparing the apex (56). This part of the heart is devoid of sympathetic nerve terminals, supporting the hypothesis that cardiac injury in SAH is neurally mediated by a sympathetic storm. Segmental wall motion abnormalities not conforming to distinct coronary artery territories is another characteristic of echocardiographic finding. However, myocardial infarction from ischemic coronary disease is frequently seen in brain-injured patients, just as in any critically ill patient, and should always be ruled out first as a cause of shock.

Venous thromboembolism (VTE) is a dreaded complication in the neurocritical care patient, and massive pulmonary embolism can be a cause for shock in this population. The incidence of VTE is believed to be as high as 62% in patients not receiving any prophylaxis (57). With antithrombotic therapy, VTE incidence varies from 1.17% in the ischemic stroke (58,59) to 1.93% in the hemorrhagic stroke population (58,60). Although the incidence of VTE in the spinal cord injury population varies greatly and the data have not been consistent, it has been found to range from 1.6% to 21.7% (61,62).

Vasodilatory neurogenic shock is the consequence of loss of sympathetic tone leading to unopposed parasympathetic effect (63). Acutely, it presents with a "warm and dry" hemodynamic profile. The patient is hypotensive and frequently bradycardic; in fact, in the right clinical setting, bradycardia should raise clinical suspicion for neurogenic shock. The peripheral vessels are dilated, leading to warm limbs and a normal capillary refill time. SVR is always low. Stroke volume and cardiac output are low due to the unopposed vagal tone. When a spinal cord injury is present, a difference in smooth muscle and vasculature tone can be observed between the body parts above and below the level of the injury. For example, in an injury at thoracic level 7 (T7), normal upper limb perfusion might be observed, while vasodilatation below T7 leads to warm and dry lower extremities. Orthostatic hypotension without reflex tachycardia on standing or with reverse Trendelenburg position and autonomic overactivity is common (13,63). When treating this form of neurogenic shock with vasopressors (such as phenylephrine or norepinephrine), extreme caution should be applied, as vasopressor hypersensitivity can lead to severe rebound hypertension, which can be difficult to control.

Cardiogenic neurogenic shock manifests as hypotension and tachycardia, with bradycardia seen rarely. Peripheral vessels are often vasoconstricted, leading to a high SVR and cold and wet skin. Vascular filling, pulmonary capillary wedge pressure (PCWP), and end-diastolic volume index (EDVI) are normal or high, with low stroke volumes and cardiac output due to global myocardial dysfunction. Leaking of cardiac enzymes—troponin, creatine kinase (CK), CK-MB fraction—may be seen, but frequently the peak levels are not as high as one would find in myocardial infarction. It is difficult to establish a cutoff value that differentiates stunned myocardium from myocardial infarction due to coronary artery disease. A retrospective study in SAH measuring troponin-I levels has reported an appropriate cutoff value of 2.8 ng/mL (64), whereas CK-MB did not help differentiate between the two kinds of myocardial injury. Higher levels of troponin should raise the suspicion of true myocardial infarction, and ECG and echocardiography correlation is important. In patients with cardiogenic neurogenic shock, more extensive hemodynamic monitoring may be necessary. Right-heart invasive hemodynamic monitoring techniques, albeit widely used for decades, continue to lose ground and fall out of favor (65). Pulmonary artery catheterization (PAC) measurements, in particular, have repeatedly shown difficult to interpret and inaccurate readings (66,67). Less invasive techniques, such as echocardiography and pulse contour cardiac output (PiCCO), have been shown to be safer, more accurate alternatives (68,69).

Neuroendocrine neurogenic shock presents with hypotension that does not respond well to vasopressor infusion. Hemodynamic signs of this category of neurogenic shock are low SVR, stroke volume, and cardiac output. Low baseline cortisol levels are the hallmark. A cosyntropin stimulation test frequently leads to an appropriate increase in the cortisol level, which *does not* rule out the presence of neuroendocrine neurogenic shock, as the adrenal gland is usually not the primarily affected organ (7). For this reason, we do not find any clinical utility in this test when neuroendocrine neurogenic shock is suspected. Resolution of the hypotension with the use of hydrocortisone clinically confirms the presence of this form of shock. Random serum cortisol levels should be obtained in the early stages of shock, keeping in mind that in some forms of brain injury, low random serum cortisol levels, and thus AI, may be encountered for several days after injury (7). Many neurologically injured patients, especially those with spinal cord injuries, may receive steroids while in the intensive care unit. The doses administered may be high enough to alter the result of a random serum cortisol level, but often the dose is not enough to treat true AI appropriately. In these cases, one could either empirically treat with higher doses of steroids that also treat AI—hydrocortisone, with or without fludrocortisone—or keeping the potential adverse effects of steroids in acute injury in mind, one could withhold the administration of steroids for 12 hours, then obtain a random cortisol level and resume steroid treatment right after the blood draw. However, hypotension is frequently severe enough that immediate treatment is warranted, and withholding steroids often may not be an option. Dexamethasone, which is frequently used in brain-injured patients, is the steroid that interferes the least with the cortisol assay after a corticotropin stimulation test (70,71). In cases of high suspicion, a random cortisol level is often preferred because of its simplicity. The cortisol level should be drawn immediately before the steroid dose. However, given the lack of mineralocorticoid activity of dexamethasone, changing to hydrocortisone with or without fludrocortisone is recommended when AI is suspected (71).

TREATMENT

Identifying patients at risk of developing neurogenic shock has been very difficult, but in SAH it appears that worse neurologic grade, age older than 30 years, and ventricular repolarization abnormalities are risk factors for neurogenic shock (72). Two important reasons for early and proactive treatment of patients in neurogenic shock are:

- Treatment of neurogenic shock helps prevent secondary brain injury from hypoxia and/or hypoperfusion
- Neurogenic shock, especially cardiogenic and neuroendocrine forms, is easily treatable and transient, with potentially good outcomes despite a moribund appearance of the patient in the acute phase

Once the diagnosis of neurogenic shock has been established and the pathophysiology (subtype) has been understood, treatment tailored to the specific subtype is initiated. In all cases, euvolemia is of utmost importance and must be achieved before any other treatment can be successful (73).

Placement of ICP measurement devices does not contribute to the diagnostic workup of shock. While some of the current literature supports the use of ICP monitoring (74–76), other studies did not reveal a benefit (77–79). However, ICP monitoring remains an important tool in the management of neurogenic shock, such as when the goal mean arterial pressure (MAP) is being titrated to the cerebral perfusion pressure (CPP). Furthermore, ICP monitoring remains in the Brain Trauma Foundation and the European Society of Intensive Care Medicine guidelines for the management of severe TBI (80,81). The same controversy applies to cerebral oxygenation monitoring. While more clinical trials are needed, promising data is emerging (82–90). We, therefore, recommend a prudent and judicious use of brain oxygenation guided therapy.

In general, vasopressor treatment as a continuous infusion is initiated and titrated to a goal MAP and/or CPP. As an important management tool, an ICP measurement device is very helpful, allowing the indirect measurement of CPP. The optimal CPP in acute brain injury is not known, and data regarding the minimum tolerable CPP comes from TBI patients, in whom the ICP is often elevated. Several studies have suggested an improved outcome when MAP is maintained greater than 85 mmHg (91,92) or CPP is maintained greater than 70 mmHg (93,94). Other studies using physiologic measurements, such as cerebral blood flow and brain tissue partial pressure of oxygen ($P_{bt}O_2$), indicate that adverse changes do not occur unless the CPP is below 50 to 60 mmHg (95,96). Therefore, CPP targets should be determined on an individual basis using multimodality monitoring. Of note, induced hypertension to improve cerebral perfusion has been associated with an increased incidence of adult respiratory distress syndrome (ARDS), although the benefit of brain tissue perfusion optimization probably outweighs the increased risk of developing ARDS (97,98).

Vasodilatory neurogenic shock can be difficult to treat. In general, vagal tone predominates; however, in this state, patients frequently have peripheral α-adrenoceptor hyperresponsiveness, limiting the use of norepinephrine, epinephrine, ephedrine, and phenylephrine. In fact, sympathomimetics should be avoided as they can lead to severe blood pressure fluctuations. Since arginine vasopressin (AVP) does not affect α- or β-adrenergic receptors but rather acts on V1 receptors, AVP may have an advantage over catecholamines or phenylephrine in this form of neurogenic shock. It has not been studied in neurogenic shock, however, and it remains unclear whether AVP may have adverse effects on neurologically ill patients. This concern is based on animal studies indicating that vasopressin may promote the development of vasospasm in SAH, and indirect experimental studies showing a reduction in brain edema with vasopressin antagonists. No prospective human study has been undertaken to confirm or dismiss this concern, and the only retrospective study on the use of vasopressin in SAH did not show any of these potentially adverse effects (99). In addition to vasopressors, a temporary demand pacemaker and/or atropine may be required in cases of refractory bradycardia and hypotension.

In cardiogenic neurogenic shock, some form of inotropic support may be necessary, either in the form of a dobutamine, milrinone, or norepinephrine infusion. Dopamine is generally avoided because of its prodysrhythmic properties. Dobutamine and milrinone also have vasodilatory effects, frequently leading to more hypotension, requiring additional therapy with an α-receptor agonist, such as phenylephrine or norepinephrine. Afterload increases in the former, and tachycardia in the latter, might be limiting factors and need careful monitoring. Cardiac output monitoring may be undertaken with the guidance of an echocardiogram or PiCCO. Beta-blockade is usually not recommended as, in neurogenic cardiogenic shock, coronary artery disease is typically not present, and compensatory tachycardia is necessary to maintain cardiac output. Afterload reduction with cautious use of angiotensin-converting enzyme (ACE) inhibitors should be attempted, but further hypotension must be avoided in order to maintain tenuous CPPs. Short-acting agents should be used whenever possible. Repeating an echocardiogram several days after the initial one is recommended to monitor the progression/resolution of cardiac dysfunction. The need for an intra-aortic balloon pump to mechanically reduce afterload and improve coronary perfusion pressure may be considered, albeit rarely used (100).

Once diagnosed, neuroendocrine neurogenic shock from primary, or more often secondary, AI is treated with steroid replacement therapy. We use the same dosing as in AI in septic shock: hydrocortisone, 50 mg intravenously every 6 hours. As previously discussed, a cortisol stimulation test is usually not helpful, and empiric treatment after a random cortisol level should be initiated.

CONTROVERSIES

While maintenance of cerebral perfusion and oxygenation is the key principle of management to prevent secondary brain injury and improve outcome, controversies regarding diagnosis and treatment provide abundant material for future studies. Among those controversial topics is the choice of tools for ICP/CCP and tissue oxygenation monitoring, indication and timing of steroid administration, and the use of vasopressin or β-blockers prophylactically in SAH to prevent Takotsubo cardiomyopathy. However, it is important to recognize neurogenic shock as a highly dynamic process associated with multiple complications and comorbidities; therefore, any therapeutic approach should always be tailored on a case-by-case basis.

Key Points

- Neurogenic shock is a form of circulatory failure with three different subtypes in the setting of neurologic injury.
- Neurogenic shock should be considered only after other forms of shock have been ruled out.
- In the right clinical setting, bradycardia with hypotension should raise clinical suspicion of neurogenic shock.
- Treatment is tailored to the specific neurogenic shock subtype and should be determined on an individual basis.

References

1. Bilello JF, Davis JW, Cunningham MA, Groom TF, Lemaster D, Sue LP. Cervical spinal cord injury and the need for cardiovascular intervention. *Arch Surg*. 2003;138(10):1127–1129.
2. Banki N, Kopelnik A, Tung P, et al. Prospective analysis of prevalence, distribution, and rate of recovery of left ventricular systolic dysfunction in patients with subarachnoid hemorrhage. *J Neurosurg*. 2006;105(1):15–20.
3. Mayer SA, Lin J, Homma S, et al. Myocardial injury and left ventricular performance after subarachnoid hemorrhage. *Stroke*. 1999;30(4):780–786.
4. Pollick C, Cujec B, Parker S, Tator C. Left ventricular wall motion abnormalities in subarachnoid hemorrhage: an echocardiographic study. *J Am Coll Cardiol*. 1988;12(3):600–605.
5. Kono T, Morita H, Kuroiwa T, et al. Left ventricular wall motion abnormalities in patients with subarachnoid hemorrhage: neurogenic stunned myocardium. *J Am Coll Cardiol*. 1994;24(3):636–640.
6. Elesber AA, Prasad A, Lennon RJ, et al. Four-year recurrence rate and prognosis of the apical ballooning syndrome. *J Am Coll Cardiol*. 2007; 50(5):448–452.
7. Cohan P, Wang C, McArthur DL, et al. Acute secondary adrenal insufficiency after traumatic brain injury: a prospective study. *Crit Care Med*. 2005;33(10):2358–2366.
8. Dimopoulou I, Tsagarakis S, Douka E, et al. The low-dose corticotropin stimulation test in acute traumatic and non-traumatic brain injury: incidence of hypo-responsiveness and relationship to outcome. *Intensive Care Med*. 2004;30(6):1216–1219.
9. Calaresu FR, Yardley CP. Medullary basal sympathetic tone. *Annu Rev Physiol*. 1988;50:511–524.
10. Osborn JW, Taylor RF, Schramm LP. Determinants of arterial pressure after chronic spinal transection in rats. *Am J Physiol*. 1989;256(3 Pt 2): R666–R673.
11. Maiorov DN, Weaver LC, Krassioukov AV. Relationship between sympathetic activity and arterial pressure in conscious spinal rats. *Am J Physiol*. 1997;272(2 Pt 2):H625–H631.
12. Krassioukov AV, Furlan JC, Fehlings MG. Autonomic dysreflexia in acute spinal cord injury: an under-recognized clinical entity. *J Neurotrauma*. 2003; 20(8):707–716.
13. Teasell RW, Arnold JM, Krassioukov A, Delaney GA. Cardiovascular consequences of loss of supraspinal control of the sympathetic nervous system after spinal cord injury. *Arch Phys Med Rehabil*. 2000;81(4):506–516.
14. Sutters M, Wakefield C, O'Neil K, et al. The cardiovascular, endocrine and renal response of tetraplegic and paraplegic subjects to dietary sodium restriction. *J Physiol*. 1992;457:515–523.
15. Krassioukov AV, Weaver LC. Episodic hypertension due to autonomic dysreflexia in acute and chronic spinal cord-injured rats. *Am J Physiol*. 1995;268(5 Pt 2):H2077–H2083.
16. Osborn JW, Taylor RF, Schramm LP. Chronic cervical spinal cord injury and autonomic hyperreflexia in rats. *Am J Physiol*. 1990;258(1 Pt 2):R169–R174.
17. Karlsson AK. Autonomic dysfunction in spinal cord injury: clinical presentation of symptoms and signs. *Progr Brain Res*. 2006;152:1–8.
18. Lane RD, Wallace JD, Petrosky PP, et al. Supraventricular tachycardia in patients with right hemisphere strokes. *Stroke*. 1992;23(3):362–366.
19. Oppenheimer SM, Gelb A, Girvin JP, Hachinski VC. Cardiovascular effects of human insular cortex stimulation. *Neurology*. 1992;42(9): 1727–1732.
20. Zamrini EY, Meador KJ, Loring DW, et al. Unilateral cerebral inactivation produces differential left/right heart rate responses. *Neurology*. 1990; 40(9):1408–1411.

21. Burch GE, Meyers R, Abildskov JA. A new electrocardiographic pattern observed in cerebrovascular accidents. *Circulation.* 1954;9(5): 719–723.
22. Davies KR, Gelb AW, Manninen PH, et al. Cardiac function in aneurysmal subarachnoid haemorrhage: a study of electrocardiographic and echocardiographic abnormalities. *Br J Anaesth.* 1991;67(1):58–63.
23. Macrea LM, Tramer MR, Walder B. Spontaneous subarachnoid hemorrhage and serious cardiopulmonary dysfunction: a systematic review. *Resuscitation.* 2005;65(2):139–148.
24. Sommargren CE. Electrocardiographic abnormalities in patients with subarachnoid hemorrhage. *Am J Crit Care.* 2002;11(1):48–56.
25. Tung P, Kopelnik A, Banki N, et al. Predictors of neurocardiogenic injury after subarachnoid hemorrhage. *Stroke.* 2004;35(2):548–551.
26. Hjalmarsson C, Bergfeldt L, Bokemark L, et al. Electrocardiographic abnormalities and elevated cTNT at admission for intracerebral hemorrhage: predictors for survival? *Ann Noninvasive Electrocardiol.* 2013; 18(5):441–449.
27. Naredi S, Lambert G, Eden E, et al. Increased sympathetic nervous activity in patients with nontraumatic subarachnoid hemorrhage. *Stroke.* 2000; 31(4):901–906.
28. Elrifai AM, Bailes JE, Shih SR, et al. Characterization of the cardiac effects of acute subarachnoid hemorrhage in dogs. *Stroke.* 1996;27(4):737–741; discussion 741–742.
29. Cowan MJ, Giddens WE Jr, Reichenbach DD. Selective myocardial cell necrosis in nonhuman primates. *Arch Pathol Lab Med.* 1983;107(1): 34–39.
30. Baroldi G, Mittleman RE, Parolini M, et al. Myocardial contraction bands. Definition, quantification and significance in forensic pathology. *Int J Legal Med.* 2001;115(3):142–151.
31. Todd GL, Baroldi G, Pieper GM, et al. Experimental catecholamine-induced myocardial necrosis. I. Morphology, quantification and regional distribution of acute contraction band lesions. *J Mol Cell Cardiol.* 1985; 17(4):317–338.
32. Kline IK. Myocardial alterations associated with pheochromocytomas. *Am J Pathol.* 1961;38:539–551.
33. Hammermeister KE, Reichenbach DD. QRS changes, pulmonary edema, and myocardial necrosis associated with subarachnoid hemorrhage. *Am Heart J.* 1969;78(1):94–100.
34. Koskelo P, Punsar S, Sipilae W. Subendocardial haemorrhage and E.C.G. changes in intracranial bleeding. *Br Med J.* 1964;1(5396):1479–1480.
35. Smith RP, Tomlinson BE. Subendocardial haemorrhages associated with intracranial lesions. *J Pathol Bacteriol.* 1954;68(2):327–334.
36. Boland TA, Lee VH, Bleck TP. Stress-induced cardiomyopathy. *Crit Care Med.* 2015;43(3):686–693.
37. Doshi R, Neil-Dwyer G. A clinicopathological study of patients following a subarachnoid hemorrhage. *J Neurosurg.* 1980;52(3):295–301.
38. Crompton MR. Hypothalamic lesions following the rupture of cerebral berry aneurysms. *Brain.* 1963;86:301–314.
39. Greenhoot JH, Reichenbach DD. Cardiac injury and subarachnoid hemorrhage. A clinical, pathological, and physiological correlation. *J Neurosurg.* 1969;30(5):521–531.
40. Kawai S, Suzuki H, Yamaguchi H, et al. Ampulla cardiomyopathy ('Takotusbo' cardiomyopathy): reversible left ventricular dysfunction: with ST segment elevation. *Jpn Circ J.* 2000;64(2):156–159.
41. Akashi YJ, Nakazawa K, Sakakibara M, et al. Reversible left ventricular dysfunction "takotsubo" cardiomyopathy related to catecholamine cardiotoxicity. *J Electrocardiol.* 2002;35(4):351–356.
42. Akashi YJ, Nakazawa K, Sakakibara M, et al. The clinical features of takotsubo cardiomyopathy. *QJM.* 2003;96(8):563–573.
43. Pastrana EA, Saavedra FM, Murray G, et al. Acute adrenal insufficiency in cervical spinal cord injury. *World Neurosurg.* 2012;77(3–4):561–563.
44. Simmons RL, Martin AM Jr, Heisterkamp CA 3rd, Ducker TB. Respiratory insufficiency in combat casualties. II. Pulmonary edema following head injury. *Ann Surg.* 1969;170(1):39–44.
45. Pender ES, Pollack CV Jr. Neurogenic pulmonary edema: case reports and review. *J Emerg Med.* 1992;10(1):45–51.
46. Hoff JT, Nishimura M, Garcia-Uria J, Miranda S. Experimental neurogenic pulmonary edema. Part 1: the role of systemic hypertension. *J Neurosurg.* 1981;54(5):627–631.
47. Lang SA, Maron MB, Signs SA. Oxygen consumption after massive sympathetic nervous system discharge. *Am J Physiol.* 1989;256(3 Pt 1): E345–E351.
48. van de Beek MT, Taal W, Veldkamp RF, Vecht CJ. A woman with multiple sclerosis and pink saliva. *Lancet Neurol.* 2003;2(4):254–255.
49. Crawley F, Saddeh I, Barker S, Katifi H. Acute pulmonary oedema: presenting symptom of multiple sclerosis. *Mult Scler.* 2001;7(1):71–72.
50. Gentiloni N, Schiavino D, Della Corte F, et al. Neurogenic pulmonary edema: a presenting symptom in multiple sclerosis. *Ital J Neurol Sci.* 1992;13(5):435–438.
51. Aimaretti G, Ambrosio MR, Di Somma C, et al. Traumatic brain injury and subarachnoid haemorrhage are conditions at high risk for hypopituitarism: screening study at 3 months after the brain injury. *Clin Endocrinol (Oxf).* 2004;61(3):320–326.
52. Isotani E, Suzuki R, Tomita K, et al. Alterations in plasma concentrations of natriuretic peptides and antidiuretic hormone after subarachnoid hemorrhage. *Stroke.* 1994;25(11):2198–2203.
53. Huang WD, Yang YM, Wu SD. Changes of arginine vasopressin in elderly patients with acute traumatic cerebral injury. *Chin J Traumatol.* 2003; 6(3):139–141.
54. Barreca T, Gandolfo C, Corsini G, et al. Evaluation of the secretory pattern of plasma arginine vasopressin in stroke patients. *Cerebrovasc Dis.* 2001; 11(2):113–118.
55. Stephens PH, Lennox G, Hirsch N, Miller D. Superior sagittal sinus thrombosis after internal jugular vein cannulation. *Br J Anaesth.* 1991; 67(4):476–479.
56. Zaroff JG, Rordorf GA, Ogilvy CS, Picard MH. Regional patterns of left ventricular systolic dysfunction after subarachnoid hemorrhage: evidence for neurally mediated cardiac injury. *J Am Soc Echocardiogr.* 2000; 13(8):774–779.
57. Geerts WH, Code KI, Jay RM, et al. A prospective study of venous thromboembolism after major trauma. *N Engl J Med.* 1994;331(24):1601–1606.
58. Skaf E, Stein PD, Beemath A, et al. Venous thromboembolism in patients with ischemic and hemorrhagic stroke. *Am J Cardiol.* 2005;96(12):1731–1733.
59. Pongmoragot J, Rabinstein AA, Nilanont Y, et al; Investigators of Registry of Canadian Stroke Network (RCSN) and University of Toronto Stroke Program for Stroke Outcomes Research Canada (SORCan [www.sorcan.ca]) Working Group. Pulmonary embolism in ischemic stroke: clinical presentation, risk factors, and outcome. *J Am Heart Assoc.* 2013; 2(6):e000372.
60. Maramattom BV, Weigand S, Reinalda M, et al. Pulmonary complications after intracerebral hemorrhage. *Neurocrit Care.* 2006;5(2):115–119.
61. Slavik RS, Chan E, Gorman SK, et al. Dalteparin versus enoxaparin for venous thromboembolism prophylaxis in acute spinal cord injury and major orthopedic trauma patients: 'DETECT' trial. *J Trauma.* 2007;62(5): 1075–1081; discussion 1081.
62. Kadyan V, Clinchot DM, Mitchell GL, Colachis SC. Surveillance with duplex ultrasound in traumatic spinal cord injury on initial admission to rehabilitation. *J Spinal Cord Med.* 2003 Fall;26(3):231–235.
63. Mathias CJ. Orthostatic hypotension: causes, mechanisms, and influencing factors. *Neurology.* 1995;45(4 Suppl 5):S6–S11.
64. Bulsara KR, McGirt MJ, Liao L, et al. Use of the peak troponin value to differentiate myocardial infarction from reversible neurogenic left ventricular dysfunction associated with aneurysmal subarachnoid hemorrhage. *J Neurosurg.* 2003;98(3):524–528.
65. Connors AF Jr., Speroff T, Dawson NV, et al. The effectiveness of right heart catheterization in the initial care of critically ill patients. SUPPORT Investigators. *JAMA.* 1996;276(11):889–897.
66. Shah MR, Hasselblad V, Stevenson LW, et al. Impact of the pulmonary artery catheter in critically ill patients: meta-analysis of randomized clinical trials. *JAMA.* 2005;294(13):1664–1670.
67. Sakka SG, Kozieras J, Thuemer O, van Hout N. Measurement of cardiac output: a comparison between transpulmonary thermodilution and uncalibrated pulse contour analysis. *Br J Anaesth.* 2007;99(3):337–342.
68. Belda FJ, Aguilar G, Teboul JL, et al; PICS Investigators Group. Complications related to less-invasive haemodynamic monitoring. *Br J Anaesth.* 2011;106(4):482–486.
69. Donati A, Carsetti A, Tondi S, et al. Thermodilution vs pressure recording analytical method in hemodynamic stabilized patients. *J Crit Care.* 2014;29(2):260–264.
70. Zaloga GP, Marik P. Hypothalamic-pituitary-adrenal insufficiency. *Crit Care Clin.* 2001;17(1):25–41.
71. Asare K. Diagnosis and treatment of adrenal insufficiency in the critically ill patient. *Pharmacotherapy.* 2007;27(11):1512–1528.
72. Mayer SA, LiMandri G, Sherman D, et al. Electrocardiographic markers of abnormal left ventricular wall motion in acute subarachnoid hemorrhage. *J Neurosurg.* 1995;83(5):889–896.
73. Consortium for Spinal Cord Medicine. Early acute management in adults with spinal cord injury: a clinical practice guideline for health-care professionals. *J Spinal Cord Med.* 2008;31(4):403–479.
74. Howells T, Elf K, Jones PA, et al. Pressure reactivity as a guide in the treatment of cerebral perfusion pressure in patients with brain trauma. *J Neurosurg.* 2005;102(2):311–317.

75. Lane PL, Skoretz TG, Doig G, Girotti MJ. Intracranial pressure monitoring and outcomes after traumatic brain injury. *Can J Surg*. 2000;43(6):442–448.
76. Fakhry SM, Trask AL, Waller MA, Watts DD; IRTC Neurotrauma Task Force. management of brain-injured patients by an evidence-based medicine protocol improves outcomes and decreases hospital charges. *J Trauma*. 2004;56(3):492–499; discussion 499–500.
77. Cremer OL, van Dijk GW, van Wensen E, et al. Effect of intracranial pressure monitoring and targeted intensive care on functional outcome after severe head injury. *Crit Care Med*. 2005;33(10):2207–2213.
78. Shafi S, Diaz-Arrastia R, Madden C, Gentilello L. Intracranial pressure monitoring in brain-injured patients is associated with worsening of survival. *J Trauma*. 2008;64(2):335–340.
79. Chesnut RM, Temkin N, Carney N, et al; Global Neurotrauma Research Group. A trial of intracranial-pressure monitoring in traumatic brain injury. *N Engl J Med*. 2012;367(26):2471–2481.
80. Carney N, Totten AM, O' Reilly C, et al. Guidelines for the management of severe traumatic brain injury [Epub ahead of print September 20, 2016]. 4th ed. *Neurosurgery*. PubMed PMID: 27654000.
81. Andrews PJ, Citerio G, Longhi L, et al; Neuro-Intensive Care and Emergency Medicine (NICEM) Section of the European Society of Intensive Care Medicine. NICEM consensus on neurological monitoring in acute neurological disease. *Intensive Care Med*. 2008;34(8):1362–1370.
82. Maloney-Wilensky E, Gracias V, Itkin A, et al. Brain tissue oxygen and outcome after severe traumatic brain injury: a systematic review. *Crit Care Med*. 2009;37(6):2057–2063.
83. Narotam PK, Morrison JF, Nathoo N. Brain tissue oxygen monitoring in traumatic brain injury and major trauma: outcome analysis of a brain tissue oxygen-directed therapy. *J Neurosurg*. 2009;111(4):672–682.
84. Nangunoori R, Maloney-Wilensky E, Stiefel M, et al. Brain tissue oxygen-based therapy and outcome after severe traumatic brain injury: a systematic literature review. *Neurocrit Care*. 2012;17(1):131–138.
85. Spiotta AM, Stiefel MF, Gracias VH, et al. Brain tissue oxygen-directed management and outcome in patients with severe traumatic brain injury. *J Neurosurg*. 2010;113(3):571–580.
86. Martini RP, Deem S, Yanez ND, et al. Management guided by brain tissue oxygen monitoring and outcome following severe traumatic brain injury. *J Neurosurg*. 2009;111(4):644–649.
87. Bohman LE, Heuer GG, Macyszyn L, et al. Medical management of compromised brain oxygen in patients with severe traumatic brain injury. *Neurocrit Care*. 2011;14(3):361–369.
88. McCarthy MC, Moncrief H, Sands JM, et al. Neurologic outcomes with cerebral oxygen monitoring in traumatic brain injury. *Surgery*. 2009;146(4):585–590; discussion 590–591.
89. Stiefel MF, Spiotta A, Gracias VH, et al. Reduced mortality rate in patients with severe traumatic brain injury treated with brain tissue oxygen monitoring. *J Neurosurg*. 2005;103(5):805–811.
90. Haddad S, Aldawood AS, Alferayan A, et al. Relationship between intracranial pressure monitoring and outcomes in severe traumatic brain injury patients. *Anaesth Intensive Care*. 2011;39(6):1043–1050.
91. Vale FL, Burns J, Jackson AB, Hadley MN. Combined medical and surgical treatment after acute spinal cord injury: results of a prospective pilot study to assess the merits of aggressive medical resuscitation and blood pressure management. *J Neurosurg*. 1997;87(2):239–246.
92. Levi L, Wolf A, Belzberg H. Hemodynamic parameters in patients with acute cervical cord trauma: description, intervention, and prediction of outcome. *Neurosurgery*. 1993;33(6):1007–1016; discussion 1016–1017.
93. Eisenberg HM, Frankowski RF, Contant CF, et al. High-dose barbiturate control of elevated intracranial pressure in patients with severe head injury. *J Neurosurg*. 1988;69(1):15–23.
94. Narayan RK, Kishore PR, Becker DP, al. Intracranial pressure: to monitor or not to monitor? A review of our experience with severe head injury. *J Neurosurg*. 1982;56(5):650–659.
95. Bullock R, Chesnut RM, Clifton G, et al; Guidelines for the management of severe head injury. Brain Trauma Foundation. *Eur J Emerg Med*. 1996;3(2):109–127.
96. Czosnyka M, Guazzo E, Iyer V, et al. Testing of cerebral autoregulation in head injury by waveform analysis of blood flow velocity and cerebral perfusion pressure. *Acta Neurochir Suppl (Wien)*. 1994;60:468–471.
97. Contant CF, Valadka AB, Gopinath SP, et al. Adult respiratory distress syndrome: a complication of induced hypertension after severe head injury. *J Neurosurg*. 2001;95(4):560–568.
98. Robertson CS, Valadka AB, Hannay HJ, et al. Prevention of secondary ischemic insults after severe head injury. *Crit Care Med*. 1999;27(10):2086–2095.
99. Muehlschlegel S, Dunser MW, Gabrielli A, et al. Arginine vasopressin as a supplementary vasopressor in refractory hypertensive, hypervolemic, hemodilutional therapy in subarachnoid hemorrhage. *Neurocrit Care*. 2007;6(1):3–10.
100. Lazaridis C, Pradilla G, Nyquist PA, Tamargo RJ. Intra-aortic balloon pump counterpulsation in the setting of subarachnoid hemorrhage, cerebral vasospasm, and neurogenic stress cardiomyopathy: case report and review of the literature. *Neurocrit Care*. 2010;13(1):101–108.

CHAPTER

49

Anaphylactic Shock

BRIGHT I. NWARU and AZIZ SHEIKH

INTRODUCTION

Anaphylaxis has been defined as "a serious life-threatening generalized or systemic hypersensitivity reaction"; it is usually rapid in onset, presenting with a constellation of clinical features, which are potentially fatal (1–5). Activation of mast cell and basophil populations by either IgE-dependent (i.e., anaphylactic reactions) or IgE-independent (i.e., anaphylactoid reactions) mechanisms results in the release of multiple mediators capable of altering vascular permeability and vascular and bronchial smooth muscle tone, as well as recruiting and activating inflammatory cell cascades. Initial sequelae, which typically occur within minutes to an hour after exposure to an inciting stimulus, include generalized hives, tachycardia, flushing, pruritus, faintness, and a sensation of impending doom. Dermatologic (e.g., urticaria and angioedema), respiratory (e.g., dyspnea, wheeze, stridor, bronchospasm, and hypoxemia), and gastrointestinal (e.g., abdominal distension, nausea, emesis, and diarrhea) manifestations are common. Involvement of the cardiovascular and respiratory systems may result in potentially life-threatening manifestations, such as cardiovascular collapse caused by vasodilation and capillary leak, myocardial depression, myocardial ischemia and infarction, atrial fibrillation, and severe bronchospasm (6). Prompt recognition and effective early intervention are essential to prevent anaphylaxis fatalities. Several terms are sometimes used to describe anaphylaxis, including severe allergic reactions, acute IgE-mediated reactions, acute allergic reactions, systemic allergic reactions, anaphylactic shock, and anaphylactic or anaphylactoid reactions. However, for the purposes of this chapter, anaphylaxis will be used throughout. In writing this chapter, we have drawn primarily on key evidence-based guidelines from the UK Resuscitation Council, World Allergy Organization, European Academy of Allergy and Clinical Immunology, the International Consensus (ICON) on anaphylaxis (1–5), and rigorously conducted systematic reviews of the evidence.

Reliable global estimates of the incidence, prevalence, morbidity, and mortality of anaphylaxis are lacking, this being partly explained by variations in definition, underrecognition, underdiagnosis, and underreporting (2). However, recent estimates of the incidence in the United States stand at 50/100,000 person-years and the point prevalence estimated at least 1.6% (7,8). The incidence rate increased from 47 to 59/100,000 person-years between 1999 and 2000 in the United States (7); fatalities stand at 500 to 1,000/year and account for about 1% emergency department visits (1,9,10). Across Europe, the incidence rate of anaphylaxis ranges between 1.5 and 7.9 per 100,000 person-years, while the lifetime prevalence is about 0.3% (11). In the United Kingdom, between 2001 and 2005, a large national database study found that the incidence of anaphylaxis increased from 6.7 to 7.9 per 100,000 person-years; the prevalence rose from 50 to 76/100,000 population; and prescription for epinephrine (adrenaline) auto-injectors increased by 97% (12). It is unclear as to what extent the variations between Europe and the United States in the incidence and prevalence of anaphylaxis might reflect differences in diagnosis and definition.

In children, teenagers, and young adults, foods are the most common triggers of anaphylaxis, while insects and medications are the most common triggers in adults (2,3,7). In the United States and in some countries in Europe and Asia, common food triggers include cow's milk, eggs, peanut, tree nuts, fish, and shellfish; sesame is a common trigger in the Middle East; while in Asia, buckwheat, chickpea, rice, and bird's nest soup are common triggers (3). Overall, shellfish, eggs, nuts, and cow's milk account for one-third of food-induced anaphylactic episodes (Tables 49.1 and 49.2) (13–16). Food-dependent, exercise-induced anaphylaxis (FDEIA) syndrome develops when trigger foods, including seafood, nuts, celery, wheat, and grains, are ingested prior to exercise or exertion (17). Idiopathic anaphylaxis (where no causative agent is identified) accounts for up to two-thirds of patients referred to adult allergy/immunology specialty clinics (13,18).

Anaphylaxis triggered by reactions to stinging or biting insects vary across geographical settings as a result of setting-specific indigenous insects (3,19). While anaphylaxis resulting from stinging insects (such as members of the order Hymenoptera) have been extensively studied in the United States, Europe, and Australia, anaphylaxis triggered by biting insects (such as members of the orders Hemiptera, Diptera, and Acarina) have been less commonly studied (3,19). A positive venom skin test along with a systemic reaction to the insect sting predicts a 50% to 60% risk of reaction to future stings (20). Examples of common medications that trigger anaphylaxis include antimicrobials, anesthetics, and analgesics, which varies across settings depending on the patterns of use (3,19). Among known medications that trigger anaphylaxis, penicillin is one of the most common, with 1 to 5 cases per 10,000 courses of penicillin resulting in allergic reactions and 1 in 50,000 to 1 in 100,000 courses resulting in death (21–23). Nonsteroidal anti-inflammatory drugs (NSAIDs) and aspirin are the second most common class of drugs implicated in anaphylaxis (24,25).

With widespread adoption of universal precautions against infections, latex allergy became a significant problem. The subsequent development of low-protein, powder-free gloves has been associated with reduction in occupational contact urticaria caused by latex rubber gloves (3,26). Despite this, latex allergy is still a concern since latex is found in some gloves, catheters, and tubing (27–29). Iodinated radiocontrast media can also cause anaphylaxis; however, life-threatening reactions are rare (30). A history of a previous reaction to radiocontrast media, asthma or atopic disease, treatment with β-blockers, and cardiovascular disease are risk factors for developing anaphylaxis to radiocontrast media (31–33).

TABLE 49.1 Etiologic Agents for Anaphylaxis (IGE-Mediated)

Haptens
β-Lactam Antibiotics
Sulfonamides
Nitrofurantoin
Demethylchlortetracycline
Streptomycin
Vancomycin
Local anesthetics
Others
Serum Products
γ-Globulin
Immunotherapy for allergic diseases
Heterologous serum
Foods
Nuts (peanuts, brazil nuts, hazelnuts, cashews, pistachios, almonds, soy nuts)
Shellfish
Buckwheat
Egg White
Cottonseed
Cow's Milk
Corn
Potato
Rice
Legumes
Citrus fruits
Chocolate
Others
Venom
Stinging insects, particularly Hymenoptera, fire ants, deer flies, jelly fish, kissing bugs (triatoma), and rattlesnakes
Hormones
Insulin
Adrenocorticotropic hormone
Thyroid-stimulating hormone
Enzymes
Chymopapain
L-Asparaginase
Miscellaneous
Seminal fluid
Others

Boldface: Relatively common causes
Data from Austen KF. Systemic anaphylaxis in man. *JAMA.* 1965;192:108–110; Kaliner M. Anaphylaxis. *NER Allergy Proc.* 1984;5:324.

TABLE 49.2 Etiologic Agents for Anaphylactoid Reactions

Complement-Mediated Reactions
Blood
Serum
Plasma
Plasmate (but not albumin)
Immunoglobins
Nonimmunologic Mast Cell Activators
Opiates and narcotics
Radiocontrast Media
Dextrans
Neuromuscular blocking agents
Arachidonic Acid Modulators
Nonsteroidal anti-inflammatory drugs
Tartrazine (possible)
Idiopathic
Most common conclusion after thorough evaluation
Unknown
Sulfites
Others
Thermoregulatory Mechanism
Cold temperature, exercise

Boldface: Relatively common causes.
Adapted from Kaliner M. Anaphylaxis. *NER Allergy Proc.* 1984;5:324.

PATHOPHYSIOLOGY

The systemic manifestations of anaphylaxis represent sequelae that result from the release of inflammatory mediators by mast cells and basophils, leading to a cascade of mediators, including tryptase, histamine, and platelet-activating factor (34–36). While the classic anaphylactic-type response occurs through allergen-induced cross-linking of IgE tightly bound to the high-affinity FcεR1 receptor constitutively expressed by mast cells (37), other non–IgE mediated immunologic mechanisms and direct mast cell activation have also been found to be important (3,4,19,36). Release of histamine from preformed mast cell granules seems to be the primary pathophysiologic mediator, resulting in systemic vasodilation, increased vascular permeability, bronchoconstriction, pruritus, and increased mucus production. However, a number of other preformed mediators are released, including heparin, serotonin, and mast cell proteases such as chymase and tryptase (36,38). In addition, other important mediators of anaphylaxis are generated by the metabolism of membrane phospholipids. Activation of the 5-lipoxygenase pathway results in the synthesis of leukotrienes, including leukotrienes C_4, D_4, E_4 (termed the slow-reacting substance of anaphylaxis, SRSA), and B_4. Leukotrienes C_4, D_4, and E_4, along with the intermediary products 5-hydroxyeicosatetraenoic acid and 5-hydroperoxyeicosatetraenoic acid, elicit increases in vascular permeability and bronchoconstriction, whereas leukotriene B_4 possesses eosinophil and neutrophil chemotactic properties. Activation of the cyclooxygenase pathway leads to the production of prostaglandin D_2, which produces bronchoconstriction. Platelet-activating factor is also newly synthesized by activated mast cells and can result in bronchoconstriction, increased vascular permeability, platelet aggregation, and neutrophil chemotaxis. It also leads to further production of platelet-activating factor through stimulation of nuclear factor (NF)-κB, a positive feedback mechanism involving the cytokines interleukin-1 (IL-1) and tumor necrosis factor (TNF)-α, and contributes to a biphasic pattern seen in some patients (39). Combined, these primary mediators then facilitate the production of a diverse number of secondary mediators by platelets, neutrophils, eosinophils, and other cells, resulting in activation of the complement, coagulation, and fibrinolytic pathways (40).

Many of these mediators have complicated effects, and their relative roles in mediating anaphylaxis *in vivo* have been difficult to evaluate. Mouse models of anaphylaxis using strains with targeted deletions of specific mediators have been useful in elucidating the importance of different effector molecules, such as the leukotrienes (41–43), and in identifying regulatory pathways, such as IL-10 (44), but have also provided some surprises that may lead to clinically useful information. For example, mice with targeted deletions of either the high-affinity FcεR1 receptor or IgE, not surprisingly, had a markedly decreased susceptibility to IgE-mediated anaphylaxis (38,45). This pathway can also be blocked with targeted deletion of histamine receptor 1 and, to a lesser extent, platelet-activating factor (37,38). However, such mice also revealed the presence of an alternate IgE-independent pathway of anaphylaxis (46). This pathway was mediated largely through platelet-activating factor, which was triggered by the binding of IgG to FcγRIII receptors present on macrophages (37,47). Like the classic IgE-mediated pathway, this alternative pathway required prior exposure to antigen, but differed in that much higher concentrations of antigen were required. The importance of this pathway in humans is as yet unclear (37). However, the administration of biologic agents, such as the anti-TNF antibody infliximab, has been reported to cause an IgE-independent anaphylactic response (48), and may be an example of this alternative pathway (49,50). The use of these biologic agents is expected to continue to increase and they are currently being used for other conditions, such as rheumatoid arthritis, Crohn disease, and inflammatory bowel disease.

DIAGNOSIS

Anaphylaxis is a medical emergency as it is associated with a rapid, critical destabilization of vital organ systems. Signs of anaphylaxis may be clinically indistinguishable and may become rapidly fatal if appropriate therapy is not instituted *immediately.* Initial symptoms can appear within seconds to minutes, but may on rare occasions be delayed by as much as 1—rarely more—hour after exposure to an inciting agent (51), and are often nonspecific (52). Cutaneous manifestations occur in 80% to 90% of patients; absence of skin signs can make it difficult to recognize and diagnose anaphylaxis (3). The clinical features vary from person to person and these reactions can also vary within the same person (3). Common symptoms and signs of anaphylaxis include tachycardia, faintness, cutaneous flushing, urticaria, diffuse or palmar pruritus, and a sensation of impending doom (53). Of these, generalized urticaria is the most common, occurring in approximately 90% of patients (Table 49.3) (54,55). Target organ in anaphylaxis is variable, but common involvement includes the cutaneous system, gastrointestinal tract, respiratory tract, cardiovascular system, and central nervous system (3). Involvement of the cardiovascular and/or respiratory systems is responsible for the fatal complications of anaphylaxis and it is for this reason that these features are particularly emphasized in some definitions (56). An unsettling sensation—including hoarseness, dysphonia, or dyspnea—may precede acute upper airway obstruction secondary to laryngeal edema. Other pulmonary manifestations include acute bronchospasm, intra-alveolar pulmonary hemorrhage, bronchorrhea, and a noncardiogenic, high permeability–type pulmonary edema (21,57). Tachycardia and syncope may precede the development of hypotension and frank cardiovascular collapse (58,59). Anaphylactic shock occurs as a consequence of diminished venous return secondary to systemic vasodilation and intravascular volume contraction caused by capillary leak. Although transient increases in cardiac output may occur at the onset of anaphylaxis, hemodynamic parameters later reveal decreases in cardiac output, systemic vascular resistance, stroke volume, pulmonary artery occlusion, and central venous pressures (60–66). In addition, the acute onset of a lactic acidosis and diminished oxygen consumption has been noticed after anaphylaxis (67). Other potentially serious cardiovascular manifestations are myocardial ischemia and acute myocardial infarction, atrioventricular and intraventricular conduction abnormalities such as prolonged PR interval, transient left bundle branch block, and supraventricular arrhythmias such as atrial fibrillation. Severe, but reversible, myocardial depression also has been reported (59). Hematologic manifestations, such as disseminated intravascular coagulation (DIC) and hemoconcentration secondary to volume contraction, also may complicate anaphylactic and anaphylactoid reactions (53). Gastrointestinal manifestations include nausea, bloating, abdominal cramps, and diarrhea. In 1% to 20% of patients,

TABLE 49.3 Clinical Manifestations of Anaphylaxis

System	Symptom	Frequency	Sign/Clinical Manifestation
Respiratory		60–80%	
Upper	Dyspnea, dysphonia, cough, "lump in throat"		Upper airway obstruction caused by laryngeal edema and spasm; bronchorrhea
Lower	Dyspnea, cyanosis		Noncardiogenic pulmonary edema, bronchospasm, acute hyperinflation, alveolar hemorrhage
Cardiovascular	Palpitations, faintness, weakness	20%	Shock, tachycardia, capillary leak, syncope, supraventricular arrhythmias, conduction disturbances, myocardial ischemia and infarction
Cutaneous	Flushing, pruritus, rash	90%	Urticaria, angioedema, diaphoresis
Gastrointestinal	Abdominal pain, bloating, cramps, nausea	30%	Emesis, diarrhea, hepatosplenic congestion; rarely hematemesis and bloody diarrhea
Neurologic	Dizziness, disorientation, hallucinations, headache, feeling of impending doom	5–10%	Syncope, lethargy, seizures
Nasal	Pruritus, sneezing	16–20%	Rhinorrhea, nasal congestion
Ocular	Conjunctival pruritus, periorbital edema	10–15%	Conjunctival suffusion, lacrimation
Hematologic			Hemoconcentration, DIC

DIC, disseminated intravascular coagulation.

there is a recurrence of symptoms after a period of recovery, termed *biphasic anaphylaxis* (68) and reactions can be prolonged. In most such cases, the clinical features recurred 1 to 8 hours after the initial presentation, although there have been reports of recurrence up to 72 hours later. There are no features of the primary response that reliably predict the occurrence of a secondary response (69).

The diagnosis of anaphylaxis is established primarily on the basis of a detailed clinical history of the specific episode, taking into account the exposures and events preceding onset of symptoms (foods eaten, medications taken, exercise, etc.) and characteristic findings on examination (3,4,19). Expert consensus is that laboratory tests are most often not helpful in diagnosing anaphylaxis upon patient presentation, although serial mast cell tryptase measurements may be helpful in subsequently confirming the diagnosis (3,4,19,56). The mainstay of diagnosis involves careful pattern recognition of the characteristic symptoms and signs, usually rapid in onset and occurring within minutes to a few hours of exposure to a potential trigger (3,4). Fatality can occur within minutes of onset of anaphylaxis (3,4,19). Better symptom recognition requires improved training of health care professionals and standardized application of clinical criteria across settings (19). Sometimes anaphylaxis may be difficult to diagnose, particularly due to the presence of concomitant medical conditions—asthma, chronic obstructive pulmonary disease, or congestive heart failure—use of CNS-active medications such as sedatives, hypnotics, and antidepressants, and concomitant impaired vision, neurologic disease, and psychiatric illnesses (3). Diagnostic difficulty may also occur in the very young and pregnant patients (70,71). For improved diagnosis, the National Institute of Allergy and Infectious Diseases (NIAID), the Food Allergy and Anaphylaxis Network (FAAN), the World Allergy Organization (WAO), and the European Academy of Allergy and Clinical Immunology (EAACI) have provided evidence-based guidelines (1,3,4,19,56). The NIAID and FAAN clinical criteria are shown in Figure 49.1 (1). Because of the multisystem nature of anaphylactic reactions, the list of differential diagnoses that must be considered is extensive. Diagnostic possibilities include cardiac dysrhythmias, myocardial infarction, distributive or hypovolemic shock, vasovagal syncope, asthma, pulmonary embolism, upper airway obstruction secondary to ingestion of a foreign body, hypoglycemia, and the carcinoid syndrome (Table 49.4).

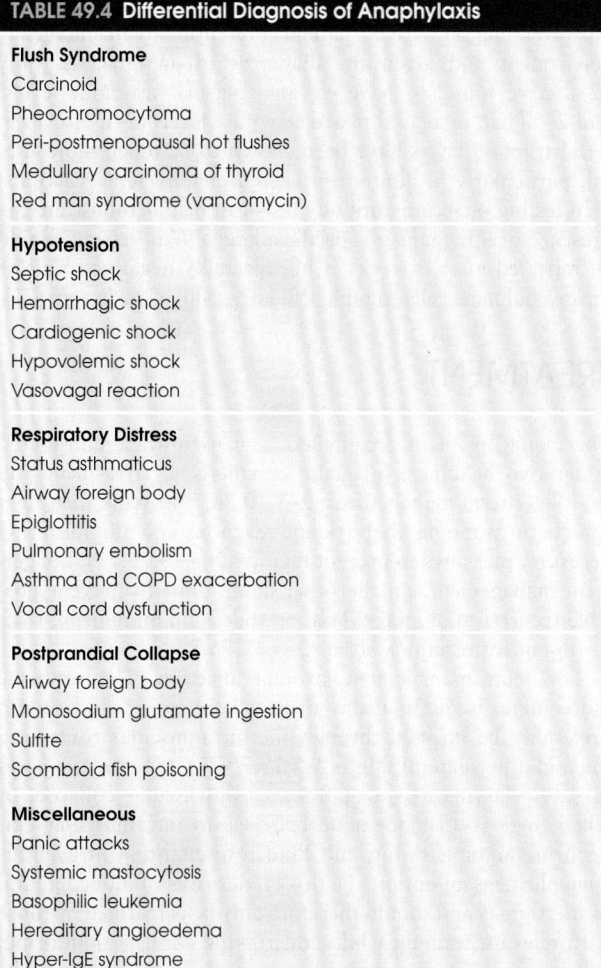

TABLE 49.4 Differential Diagnosis of Anaphylaxis

Flush Syndrome
Carcinoid
Pheochromocytoma
Peri-postmenopausal hot flushes
Medullary carcinoma of thyroid
Red man syndrome (vancomycin)
Hypotension
Septic shock
Hemorrhagic shock
Cardiogenic shock
Hypovolemic shock
Vasovagal reaction
Respiratory Distress
Status asthmaticus
Airway foreign body
Epiglottitis
Pulmonary embolism
Asthma and COPD exacerbation
Vocal cord dysfunction
Postprandial Collapse
Airway foreign body
Monosodium glutamate ingestion
Sulfite
Scombroid fish poisoning
Miscellaneous
Panic attacks
Systemic mastocytosis
Basophilic leukemia
Hereditary angioedema
Hyper-IgE syndrome

IgE, immunoglobulin E; COPD, chronic obstructive pulmonary disorder.

Demonstration of acute elevations of markers specific to mast cell activation such as histamine and tryptase have been

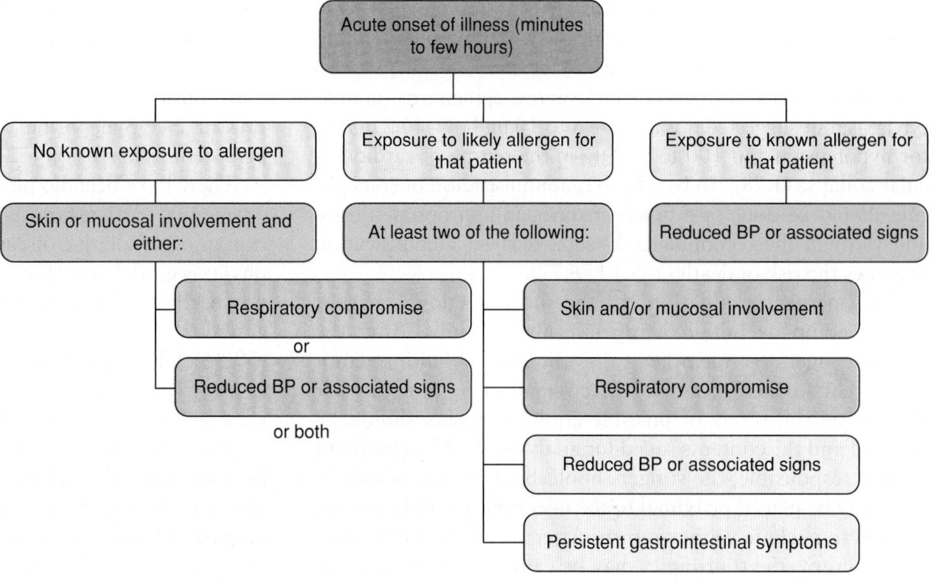

FIGURE 49.1 Clinical criteria for diagnosing anaphylaxis. Fewer signs are required for diagnosis as the history of allergen exposure becomes more certain. **Signs or symptoms of skin involvement:** generalized hives, pruritus, or flushing. **Signs of mucosal involvement:** swollen lips, tongue, and/or uvula. **Signs of respiratory compromise:** dyspnea, wheeze, bronchospasm, stridor, reduced peak expiratory flow, and/or hypoxemia. **Definition of reduced blood pressure (BP):** adults—systolic BP less than 90 mmHg or greater than 30% decrease from that person's baseline; children—systolic BP less than 70 mmHg from 1 month to 1 year, less than (70 mmHg + (2 × age)) from 1 to 10 years, and less than 90 mmHg from 11 to 17 years or **associated signs:** hypotonia, syncope, incontinence. **Persistent gastrointestinal symptoms:** crampy abdominal pain and vomiting.

proposed to help confirm the diagnosis of anaphylaxis (72,73). However, in a series of 97 patients presenting to an emergency department and given the diagnosis of anaphylaxis, only 42% were found to have elevated plasma histamine levels, and 24% had increased plasma tryptase levels (74). However, serial tryptase levels have been shown to be much more useful, particularly in nonfood-triggered anaphylactic reactions. Skin testing or serum antibody tests can help demonstrate the presence of IgE against a specific allergen. Skin testing should be repeated after 4 weeks if unexpectedly negative to allow the dermal mast cells to replenish intracellular mediators (75).

TREATMENT

The management of anaphylaxis can usefully be considered under two headings: (a) acute or emergency treatment and (b) longer-term management (2–5,19,76,77). Acute treatment centers on stopping anaphylactic reactions and administering necessary measures to prevent fatality (2–5,19,76,77). Longer-term management, on the other hand, aims to prevent possible recurrence of anaphylaxis episodes and minimizing risks if subsequent reactions occur (2–5,19,76,77).

For acute management, prompt injection of epinephrine (adrenaline) is the mainstay of initial treatment, and should preferably be injected through the intramuscular route into the mid-anterolateral thigh (2–5,19,76,77). However, in cases of severe laryngospasm or frank cardiovascular collapse, or when there is an inadequate response to intramuscular epinephrine administration and fluid resuscitation, intravenous epinephrine is an option (1); this carries risks of inducing fatal dysrhythmias and should therefore only be performed by those with relevant training while undertaking cardiac monitoring. When epinephrine is administered i.v., the clinician should be aware of the potential adverse consequences of severe tachycardia, myocardial ischemia, hypertension, severe vasospasm, and gangrene—the latter when infused by peripheral venous access (3,4,19,46). Epinephrine decreases mediator synthesis and release by increasing intracellular concentrations of cyclic adenosine monophosphate (cAMP) and antagonizes many of the adverse actions of the mediators of anaphylaxis (63). Aqueous epinephrine, 0.01 mg/kg (maximum dose 0.5 mg in adults; 0.3 mg in children) administered intramuscularly every 5 to 15 minutes as necessary to control symptoms and maintain blood pressure, is recommended (2–5,19,63,78). There is no established dosage regimen for intravenous epinephrine in anaphylaxis, but suggested dosages are 5 to 10 μg bolus (0.2 μg/kg) for hypotension and 100 to 500 μg in the setting of cardiovascular collapse (1,78). To be effective, administration of epinephrine should be done in a timely manner, in appropriate doses, and through the recommended route; delayed administration increases the risk of death (2–5,19,76,77).

An emergent evaluation for the inciting etiologic agent must accompany initial therapeutic interventions. After the etiologic agent is identified, the clinician should attempt to prevent further access to the circulation or limit further absorption. Infusions of possible etiologic agents should be stopped and the contents saved for analysis. If a Hymenoptera sting is responsible, the stinger should be removed. A tourniquet may be placed proximal to the injection site and pressure applied to occlude venous return. After successful pharmacologic therapy, the tourniquet may be cautiously removed and the patient carefully observed for recurrent adverse sequelae. In cases where the offending agent was ingested, consideration may be given to insertion of a nasogastric tube to perform gastric lavage and gastric instillation of activated charcoal.

Blood pressure measurements should be taken frequently, and an indwelling arterial catheter for beat-to-beat measurement of blood pressure should be inserted in cases of moderate to severe anaphylaxis. High-flow oxygen given via endotracheal tube or a nonrebreather mask should be administered to patients experiencing hypoxemia, respiratory distress, or hemodynamic instability (1). Orotracheal intubation may be attempted if airway obstruction compromises effective ventilation despite pharmacologic intervention; however, attempts may be unsuccessful if laryngeal edema is severe. If endotracheal intubation is unsuccessful, then either needle–catheter cricothyroid ventilation, cricothyrotomy, or surgical tracheostomy is required to maintain an adequate airway. Clinicians need to be familiar with at least one of these techniques in the event that endotracheal intubation cannot be accomplished. It has been suggested that inhaled β_2-agonists such as albuterol may be useful for bronchospasm refractory to epinephrine (1,79). Patients should be placed in the recumbent position, with lower extremities elevated to increase fluid return centrally, thereby increasing cardiac output (80). Airway protection should be ensured in the event of vomiting. Cardiopulmonary resuscitation should be initiated as indicated.

Second-line agents include H_1- and H_2-histamine receptor blockers and corticosteroids (1–5). H_1- and H_2-histamine receptor blockers are particularly useful in the treatment of symptomatic urticaria–angioedema and pruritus. Studies suggest that treatment with a combination of H_1- and H_2-histamine receptor blockers may be more effective in attenuating the cutaneous manifestations of anaphylaxis than H_1-blockers alone (74,81). Diphenhydramine hydrochloride (25 to 50 mg i.v. or i.m. for adults and 1 mg/kg, up to 50 mg, for children) and ranitidine (50 mg i.v. over 5 minutes) are sometimes used (82–84). It may, however, be safer to administer these agents via the oral route. However, if hypotension persists despite administration of epinephrine, aggressive volume resuscitation should be instituted and this should precede administration of H_1- and H_2-blockers. Up to 35% of the blood volume may extravasated in the first 10 minutes of a severe reaction, with subsequent reduction in blood volume due to vasodilatation, causing distributive shock (85). Persistent hypotension may require multiple fluid boluses (10 to 20 mL/kg under pressure) as well as colloid and crystalloid infusions (1). Vasopressors such as norepinephrine, vasopressin, Neo-Synephrine, or even metaraminol may be useful in persistent hypotension (52).

There have been no placebo-controlled trials evaluating the efficacy of corticosteroids in anaphylaxis, but their contribution in other allergic diseases has led to their inclusion in anaphylaxis guidelines. Due to their slow onset of action, they are not useful in acute management. However, it has been suggested that they may prevent protracted or biphasic reactions (79,86). The usual dose is 100 mg (maximum for the child) to 200 mg (maximum for the adult) of hydrocortisone orally or i.v. every 6 hours (3,4,19,43).

The management of anaphylaxis in patients receiving β-antagonist medications, such as β-blockers, represents a special circumstance in which the manifestations of anaphylaxis may be exceptionally severe (87). β-blockade increases mediator synthesis and release, as well as end-organ sensitivity. In addition, β-blockade antagonizes the beneficial β-mediated effects of epinephrine therapy, thereby resulting in unopposed α-adrenergic and reflex vagotonic effects: vasoconstriction, bronchoconstriction, and bradycardia. Therapy of anaphylaxis occurring in patients receiving β-antagonist drugs, however, is similar to that of other patients. In addition, atropine may be useful for heart block and refractory bronchospasm, whereas glucagon—which increases cAMP levels through a β-receptor-independent mechanism—have been reported to reverse the cardiovascular manifestations of anaphylaxis in patients receiving β-antagonists (87). Glucagon can be administered as a 1- to 5-mg (20 to 30 μg/kg with maximum dose of 1 mg in children) intravenous infusion over 5 minutes, followed by an infusion of 5 to 15 μg/min titrated to clinical response (1). Furthermore, these patients may require extended periods of observation because of the long duration of action of many β-antagonist medications.

A period of observation should be considered for all patients following treatment of anaphylaxis. On the basis of extant clinical data, the NIAID/FAAN symposium recommends that observation periods be individualized on the basis of severity of initial reaction, reliability of the patient, and access to care. A reasonable time would be 4 to 6 hours for most patients, with prolonged observation or hospital admission for severe or refractory symptoms and patients with reactive airway disease (1). The steps listed below are the therapeutic pearls that are recommended for the emergency management of anaphylaxis:

1. Rapidly assess and maintain the airway, breathing, and circulation. Initiate CPR, if indicated. If airway obstruction is imminent, perform endotracheal intubation; if unsuccessful, consider needle–catheter cricothyroid ventilation, cricothyrotomy, or tracheostomy. Patients should be placed in a recumbent position with the lower extremities elevated, unless precluded by shortness of breath or vomiting.
2. Remove the inciting agent (e.g., remove Hymenoptera stinger, stop the infusion, etc.) and follow with an intramuscular epinephrine injection in the anterior lateral thigh. Consider gastric lavage and administration of activated charcoal if the inciting agent was ingested.
3. Administer aqueous epinephrine, 0.01 mg/kg (maximum dose, 0.5 mg) intramuscularly every 5 to 15 minutes as necessary for controlling symptoms and maintaining blood pressure.
4. Establish intravenous access for hydration and provide high-flow supplemental oxygen.
5. Consider aggressive fluid resuscitation with multiple fluid boluses (10 to 20 mL/kg under pressure), including colloid as well as crystalloid, in patients who remain hypotensive despite epinephrine.
6. Administer histamine antagonists to block vasodilation, capillary leak, and shock (H_1 blockade, 25 to 50 mg of diphenhydramine for adults, and 1 mg/kg—up to 50 mg—for children; H_2 blockade, 50 mg of ranitidine; preferably oral administration) (4).
7. Administer vasopressors for persistent hypotension and titrate to a mean arterial pressure of 60 mmHg.
8. Administer inhaled β_2-agonists such as albuterol or slabutamol for bronchospasm refractory to epinephrine (88).
9. Consider corticosteroid therapy for protracted anaphylaxis or to prevent biphasic anaphylaxis (e.g., 1.0 to 2.0 mg/kg methylprednisolone i.v. every 6 hours). Oral prednisone at 1.0 mg/kg, up to 50 mg, may be used for milder attacks. Corticosteroids are not effective therapy for the acute manifestations of anaphylaxis.
10. Consider glucagon administration (1 to 5 mg i.v. over 1 minute, then 1 to 5 mg/hr by continuous infusion) in the setting of prior β-blockade because of its positive inotropic and chronotropic effects mediated by a β-receptor-independent mechanism.
11. Admission to the intensive care unit is warranted for invasive monitoring with arterial and pulmonary artery catheters, electrocardiography, pulse oximetry, and frequent arterial blood gas measurements.

The aims of longer-term management of patients with anaphylaxis are to minimize the risk of recurrence and to reduce the risk of fatality if a further reaction ensues. This, therefore, entails development of self-management plans for at-risk individuals, including development of guidance on identifying and then avoiding triggers of anaphylactic reactions, preparing for reactions, recognizing reactions when they occur, and initiating appropriate self-management if and when reactions occur (2–5,19,76,77). Along these lines, expert recommendation is that at-risk individuals should, together with the health care practitioners, develop action plans that include regular carriage of epinephrine, required skills to use epinephrine, managing concomitant disease conditions, and regular follow-up assessments (1–5,19,76,77). Consideration should be given to encourage wearing patient identification jewelry (e.g., MedicAlert bracelets/pendants) to help during emergencies, the electronic flagging of records of patients who may be at risk, avoidance of treatments with potential of increasing risk of reactions or reduce the impact of epinephrine (e.g., ACE inhibitors), and establishing contacts with family physicians for regular review and training of patients (89–91). These action plans can reduce the risk of further reactions (1,4). Desensitization (also sometimes known as immunotherapy or allergen immunotherapy) can prove effective in the long-term management of anaphylaxis triggered by venom and drugs, and although trials show it is effective in those with certain food allergies, further work is needed to establish its safety profile (92–94).

Compared to other age groups, the disproportionately greater morbidity and fatality from anaphylaxis among adolescents means that long-term management among this age group requires particular attention (95–101). Transition into adolescence carries with it notable changes in the psychosocial environments of young people, which may increase their risk-taking decisions and can eventually lead to poor adherence to recommended anaphylaxis management approaches (95–101). Current management strategies among adolescents are still those tailored for parents of young children and those directed at adults, and the success rates of these among adolescents has been poor (101). There is, therefore, the need for further work in developing management approaches that are more closely tailored toward adolescents, which take into account the challenges of the developmental transitions they face and the priorities they grapple on a day-to-day basis (101). Recently, a tripartite framework for the management of anaphylaxis has been proposed, which highlights that a more integrated approach is required among adolescents that takes into account three things: the challenges of adolescents' developmental transition, the shortcomings of current clinical management strategies among adolescents, and adolescents' social network (101). Although the effectiveness of the proposed framework has not been evaluated in real life, it provides a new perspective that warrant further exploration (101).

CONTROVERSIES

The key controversies around anaphylaxis center on how to rigorously study and establish the effectiveness of established interventions that are seen by the clinical community as potentially lifesaving. Epinephrine is a particular case in point as it is universally seen as the first-line agent, but its effectiveness has not been established through rigorous randomized controlled trials (84,102,103). There is, more generally, a paucity of high-quality evidence on other supportive and second-line treatment approaches commonly used in the management of anaphylaxis reactions. Well-designed trials of these supportive and second-line treatment approaches should be considered.

Although the effectiveness of immunotherapy has been shown for venom- and drug-triggered anaphylaxis, its safety for food-triggered anaphylaxis remains a source of concern and debate; more work is needed on investigating alternative up-dosing and maintenance schedules, the role of adjuvant therapy in improving safety, and alternative routes (e.g., epicutaneous) and preparations (e.g., peptide immunotherapy). For long-term management of adolescents with anaphylaxis, there is a need to evaluate the effectiveness of holistic strategies which are both cognizant of the barriers and facilitators to effective self-management.

Key Points

- Anaphylaxis most commonly results through a type I immune responses mediated by IgE bound to mast cells or basophils, but other mechanisms are now also recognized. Common triggers include a variety of foods (particularly in children and young people), venom of stinging insects, a range of drugs, latex, radiocontrast media, and exercise. A proportion of reactions are idiopathic, i.e., no clear trigger can be identified.
- Anaphylaxis can become rapidly fatal if appropriate therapy is not instituted immediately. Symptoms appear on the skin in 80% to 90% of patients and can vary from person to person, and within each person unique episodes can differ. Common clinical features include tachycardia, faintness, cutaneous flushing, urticaria, diffuse or palmar pruritus, and a sensation of impending doom. Target organs most commonly affected include the cutaneous system, gastrointestinal tract, respiratory tract, cardiovascular system, and central nervous system. Of these, cardiovascular and respiratory features are the most important as these are often implicated in fatal reactions.
- Diagnosis of anaphylaxis is established primarily on the basis of a detailed clinical history of the specific episode, which takes into account the exposures and events preceding onset of symptoms, e.g., foods eaten, medications taken, and exercise, and the findings on examination. Laboratory tests are not helpful in diagnosing the acute reaction, but may prove helpful in subsequently confirming a reaction. The mainstay of diagnosis involves careful pattern recognition of the characteristic symptoms and signs. Better symptom recognition requires improved training of health care professionals and standardized application of clinical criteria.
- Epinephrine is the initial drug of choice for the management of the acute reaction, supported by a fluid bolus, high-flow oxygen, and inhaled B_2-agonists, as necessary. H_1- and H_2-blocking agents and corticosteroids (104) should be considered as second-line treatments. Long-term management involves the development of tailored self-management plans aimed at preventing future recurrences of reactions, including guidance on avoiding triggers, recognizing reactions, preparing for reactions, and appropriate self-management of reactions if they occur. For adolescents, greater attention is required and management approaches should be tailored to their needs by integrating existing management strategies and their transitional developmental challenges.

ACKNOWLEDGMENTS

We thank Drs Meghavis S. Kosboth and Eric S. Sobel, who prepared the original version of this chapter for the textbook's fourth edition.

References

1. Sampson HA, Munoz-Furlong A, Campbell RL, et al. Second symposium on the definition and management of anaphylaxis: summary report – Second National Institute of Allergy and Infectious Disease/Food Allergy and Anaphylaxis Network symposium. *J Allergy Clin Immunol.* 2006;117:391–397.
2. Simons FE, Ardusso LR, Dimov V, et al; World Allergy Organization. World Allergy Organisation Anaphylaxis Guidelines: 2013 update of the evidence base. *Int Arch Allergy Immunol.* 2013;162:193–204.
3. Simons FE, Ardusso LR, Bilo MB, et al. 2012 Update: World Allergy Organisation Guidelines for the assessment and management of anaphylaxis. *Curr Opin Allergy Clin Immunol.* 2012;12:389–399.
4. Muraro A, Roberts G, Worm M, et al; EAACI Food Allergy and Anaphylaxis Guidelines Group. Anaphylaxis: guidelines from the European Academy of Allergy and Clinical Immunology. *Allergy.* 2014;69:1026–1045.
5. Lieberman P, Nicklas RA, Oppenheimer J, et al. The diagnosis and management of anaphylaxis practice parameter: 2010 update. *J Allergy Clin Immunol.* 2010;126:477–480.
6. Brown SG. Anaphylaxis: clinical concepts and research priorities. *Emerg Med Australas.* 2006;18:155–169.
7. Decker WW, Campbell RL, Manivannan V, et al. The etiology and incidence of anaphylaxis in Rochester, Minnesota: a report from the Rochester Epidemiology Project. *J Allergy Clin Immunol.* 2008;122:1161–1165.
8. Wood RA, Camargo CA Jr, Lieberman P, et al. Anaphylaxis in America: the prevalence and characteristics of anaphylaxis in the United States. *J Allergy Clin Immunol.* 2014;133:461–467.
9. Clark S, Long AA, Gaeta TJ, Camargo CA Jr. Multicenter study of emergency department visits for insect sting allergies. *J Allergy Clin Immunol.* 2005;116:643–649.
10. Neugut AI, Ghatak AT, Miller RL. Anaphylaxis in the United States: an investigation into its epidemiology. *Arch Intern Med.* 2001;161:15–21.
11. Panesar SS, Javad S, de Silva D, et al; EAACI Food Allergy and Anaphylaxis Group. The epidemiology of anaphylaxis in Europe: a systematic review. *Allergy.* 2013;68:1353–1361.
12. Sheikh A, Hippisley-Cox J, Newton J, Fenty J. Trends in national incidence, lifetime prevalence and adrenaline prescribing for anaphylaxis in England. *J R Soc Med.* 2008;101:139–143.

13. Tang AW. A practical guide to anaphylaxis. *Am Fam Physician*. 2003;68: 1325–1332.
14. Thong BY, Cheng YK, Leong KP, et al. Anaphylaxis in adults referred to a clinical immunology/allergy centre in Singapore. *Singapore Med J*. 2005;46:529–534.
15. Novembre E, Cianferoni A, Bernardini R, et al. Anaphylaxis in children: clinical and allergologic features. *Pediatrics*. 1998;101:E8.
16. Kaliner MA. Anaphylaxis. *NER Allergy Proc*. 1984;5:324.
17. Chong SU, Worm M, Zuberbier T. Role of adverse reactions to food in urticaria and exercise-induced anaphylaxis. *Int Arch Allergy Immunol*. 2002;129:19–26.
18. Webb LM, Lieberman P. Anaphylaxis: a review of 601 cases. *Ann Allergy Asthma Immunol*. 2006;97:39–43.
19. Simons FE, Ardusso LR, Bilo MB, et al. International consensus on (ICON) anaphylaxis. *World Allergy Organ J*. 2014;7:9.
20. Graham DM, McPherson H, Lieberman P. Skin testing in the evaluation of Hymenoptera allergy and drug allergy. *Immunol Allergy Clin North Am*. 2001;21:301–320.
21. Delage C, Irey NS. Anaphylactic deaths: a clinicopathologic study of 43 cases. *J Forensic Sci*. 1972;17:525–540.
22. Joint Task Force on Practice Parameters, American Academy of Allergy, Asthma and Immunology, American College of Allergy, Asthma and Immunology, and the Joint Council of Allergy, Asthma and Immunology. The diagnosis and management of anaphylaxis. *J Allergy Clin Immunol*. 1998;101:S465–S528.
23. Idsoe O, Guthe T, Willcox RR, de Weck AL. Nature and extent of penicillin side-reactions, with particular reference to fatalities from anaphylactic shock. *Bull World Health Org*. 1968;38:159–188.
24. Brown AF, McKinnon D, Chu K. Emergency department anaphylaxis: a review of 142 patients in a single year. *J Allergy Clin Immunol*. 2001;108: 861–866.
25. Stevenson DD. Approach to the patient with a history of adverse reactions to aspirin or NSAIDs: diagnosis and treatment. *Allergy Asthma Proc*. 2000;21:25–31.
26. Allmers H, Schmengler J, John SM. Decreasing incidence of occupational contact urticaria caused by natural rubber latex allergy in German health care workers. *J Allergy Clin Immunol*. 2004;114:347–351.
27. Schwartz HA, Zurowski D. Anaphylaxis to latex in intravenous fluids. *J Allergy Clin Immunol*. 1993;92:358–359.
28. Mitsuhata H, Horiguchi Y, Saitoh J, et al. An anaphylactic reaction to topical fibrin glue. *Anesthesiology*. 1994;81:1074–1077.
29. Laxenaire MC, Mata-Bermejo E, Moneret-Vautrin DA, Gueant JL. Life-threatening anaphylactoid reactions to propofol (Diprivan). *Anesthesiology*. 1992;77:275–280.
30. Katayama H, Yamaguchi K, Kozuka T, et al. Adverse reactions to ionic and nonionic contrast media. A report from the Japanese Committee on the Safety of Contrast Media.*Radiology*. 1990;175:621–628.
31. Greenberger PA, Halwig JM, Patterson R, Wallemark CB. Emergency administration of radiocontrast media in high-risk patients. *J Allergy Clin Immunol*. 1986;77:630–634.
32. Enright T, Chua-Lim A, Duda E, Lim DT. The role of a documented allergic profile as a risk factor for radiographic contrast media reaction. *Ann Allergy*. 1989;62:302–305.
33. Bush WH, Swanson DP. Acute reactions to intravascular contrast media: types, risk factors, recognition, and specific treatment. *AJR Am J Roentgenol*. 1991;157:1153–1161.
34. Gill P, Jindal NL, Jagdis A, Vadas P. Platelets in the immune response: Revisiting platelet-activating factor in anaphylaxis. *J Allergy Clin Immunol*. 2015;135:1424–1432.
35. Vadas P, Gold M, Perelman B, et al. Platelet-activating factor, PAF acetylhydrolase, and severe anaphylaxis. *N Engl J Med*. 2008;358:28–35.
36. Simons FE. Anaphylaxis pathogenesis and treatment. *Allergy*. 2011; 66(Suppl 95):31–34.
37. Finkelman FD, Rothenberg ME, Brandt EB, et al. Molecular mechanisms of anaphylaxis: lessons from studies with murine models. *J Allergy Clin Immunol*. 2005;115:449–457; quiz 458.
38. Strait RT, Morris SC, Yang M, et al. Pathways of anaphylaxis in the mouse. *J Allergy Clin Immunol*. 2002;109:658–668.
39. Choi IW, Kim YS, Kim DK, et al. Platelet-activating factor-mediated NF-kappaB dependency of a late anaphylactic reaction. *J Exp Med*. 2003;198:145–151.
40. Kaplan AP, Joseph K, Silverberg M. Pathways for bradykinin formation and inflammatory disease. *J Allergy Clin Immunol*. 2002;109:195–209.
41. Goulet JL, Snouwaert JN, Latour AM, et al. Altered inflammatory responses in leukotriene-deficient mice. *Proc Natl Acad Sci U S A*. 1994;91:12852–12856.
42. Haribabu B, Verghese MW, Steeber DA, et al. Targeted disruption of the leukotriene B(4) receptor in mice reveals its role in inflammation and platelet-activating factor-induced anaphylaxis. *J Exp Med*. 2000;192:433–438.
43. Kanaoka Y, Maekawa A, Penrose JF, et al. Attenuated zymosan-induced peritoneal vascular permeability and IgE-dependent passive cutaneous anaphylaxis in mice lacking leukotriene C4 synthase. *J Biol Chem*. 2001; 276:22608–22613.
44. Mangan NE, Fallon RE, Smith P, et al. Helminth infection protects mice from anaphylaxis via IL-10-producing B cells. *J Immunol*. 2004;173: 6346–6356.
45. Dombrowicz D, Brini AT, Flamand V, et al. Anaphylaxis mediated through a humanized high affinity IgE receptor. *J Immunol*. 1996;157:1645–1651.
46. Oettgen HC, Martin TR, Wynshaw-Boris A, et al. Active anaphylaxis in IgE-deficient mice. *Nature*. 1994;370:367–370.
47. Miyajima I, Dombrowicz D, Martin TR, et al. Systemic anaphylaxis in the mouse can be mediated largely through IgG1 and Fc gammaRIII: assessment of the cardiopulmonary changes, mast cell degranulation, and death associated with active or IgE- or IgG1-dependent passive anaphylaxis. *J Clin Invest*. 1997;99:901–914.
48. Cheifetz A, Mayer L. Monoclonal antibodies, immunogenicity, and associated infusion reactions. *Mt Sinai J Med*. 2005;72:250–256.
49. Leccluse LL, Piskin G, Mekkes JR, et al. Review and expert opinion on prevention and treatment of infliximab-related infusion reactions. *Br J Dermatol*. 2008;159:527–536.
50. Lichtenstein L, Ron Y, Kivity S, et al. Infliximab-related infusion reactions systematic review. *J Crohns Colitis*. 2015;9:806–815.
51. Inomata N, Osuna H, Yanagimachi M, Ikezawa Z. Late-onset anaphylaxis to fermented soybeans: the first confirmation of food-induced, late-onset anaphylaxis by provocation test. *Ann Allergy Asthma Immunol*. 2005;94:402–406.
52. Brown SG. Cardiovascular aspects of anaphylaxis: implications for treatment and diagnosis. *Curr Opin Allergy Clin Immunol*. 2005;5:359–364.
53. Smith PL, Kagey-Sobotka A, Bleecker ER, et al. Physiologic manifestations of human anaphylaxis. *J.Clin Invest*. 1980;66:1072–1080.
54. Kemp SF, Lockey RF, Wolf BL, Lieberman P. Anaphylaxis: a review of 266 cases. *Arch Intern Med*. 1995;155:1749–1754.
55. Kemp SF, Lockey RF. Anaphylaxis: a review of causes and mechanisms. *J Allergy Clin Immunol*. 2002;110:341–348.
56. Soar J, Pumphrey R, Cant A, et al. Working Group of the Resuscitation Council (UK). Emergency treatment of anaphylactic reactions: guidelines for healthcare providers.*Resuscitation*. 2008;77(2):1–50.
57. Carlson RW, Schaeffer RC Jr, Puri VK, et al. Hypovolemia and permeability pulmonary edema associated with anaphylaxis. *Crit Care Med*. 1981;9:883–885.
58. Simon MR. Anaphylaxis associated with relative bradycardia. *Ann Allergy*. 1989;62:495–497.
59. Raper RF, Fisher MM. Profound reversible myocardial depression after anaphylaxis. *Lancet*. 1988;1:386–388.
60. Wasserman SI. The heart in anaphylaxis. *J Allergy Clin Immunol*. 1986; 77:663–666.
61. Nicolas F, Villers D, Blanloeil Y. Hemodynamic pattern in anaphylactic shock with cardiac arrest. *Crit Care Med*. 1984;12:144–145.
62. Serafin WE, Austen KF. Mediators of immediate hypersensitivity reactions. *N Engl J Med*. 1987;317:30–34.
63. Perkin RM, Anas NG. Mechanisms and management of anaphylactic shock not responding to traditional therapy. *Ann Allergy*. 1985;54:202–208.
64. Silverman HJ, Van Hook C, Haponik EF. Hemodynamic changes in human anaphylaxis. *Am J Med*. 1984;77:341–344.
65. Moss J, Fahmy NR, Sunder N, Beaven MA. Hormonal and hemodynamic profile of an anaphylactic reaction in man. *Circulation*. 1981;63:210–213.
66. Hanashiro PK, Weil MH. Anaphylactic shock in man. Report of two cases with detailed hemodynamic and metabolic studies. *Arch Intern Med*. 1967;119:129–140.
67. Fawcett WJ, Shephard JN, Soni NC, Barnes PK. Oxygen transport and haemodynamic changes during an anaphylactoid reaction. *Anaesth Intensive Care*. 1994;22:300–303.
68. Brazil E, MacNamara AF. "Not so immediate" hypersensitivity—the danger of biphasic anaphylactic reactions. *J Accid Emerg Med*. 1998;15: 252–253.
69. Lieberman P. Biphasic anaphylactic reactions. *Ann Allergy Asthma Immunol*. 2005;95:217–226; quiz 226, 258.
70. Simons FE, Sampson HA. Anaphylaxis: unique aspects of clinical diagnosis and management in infants (birth to age 2 years). *J Allergy Clin Immunol*. 2015;135:1125–1131.
71. Simons FE, Schatz M. Anaphylaxis during pregnancy. *J Allergy Clin Immunol*. 2012;130:597–606.

72. Bochner BS, Lichtenstein LM. Anaphylaxis. *N Engl J Med.* 1991;324: 1785–1790.
73. Yocum MW, Khan DA. Assessment of patients who have experienced anaphylaxis: a 3-year survey. *Mayo Clin Proc.* 1994;69:16–23.
74. Lin RY, Schwartz LB, Curry A, et al. Histamine and tryptase levels in patients with acute allergic reactions: An emergency department-based study. *J Allergy Clin Immunol.* 2000;106:65–71.
75. Weiss ME, Adkinson NF. Immediate hypersensitivity reactions to penicillin and related antibiotics. *Clin Allergy.* 1988;18:515–540.
76. Dhami S, Panesar SS, Roberts G, et al; EAACI Food Allergy and Anaphylaxis Guidelines Group. Management of anaphylaxis: a systematic review. *Allergy.* 2014;69:168–175.
77. Simons FE, Sheikh A. Anaphylaxis: the acute episode and beyond. *BMJ* 2013;346:f602.
78. Hepner DL, Castells MC. Anaphylaxis during the perioperative period. *Anesth Analg.* 2003;97:1381–1395.
79. Joint Task Force on Practice Parameters; American Academy of Allergy, Asthma and Immunology; American College of Allergy, Asthma and Immunology; Joint Council of Allergy, Asthma and Immunology. The diagnosis and management of anaphylaxis: an updated practice parameter. *J Allergy Clin Immunol.* 2005;115(Suppl 2):S483–S523.
80. Boulain T, Achard JM, Teboul JL, et al. Changes in BP induced by passive leg raising predict response to fluid loading in critically ill patients. *Chest.* 2002;121:1245–1252.
81. Simons FE. Advances in H1-antihistamines. *N Engl J Med.* 2004;351: 2203–2217.
82. Sheikh A, ten Broek Vm, Brown SG, Simons FE. H1-antihistmines for the treatment of anaphylaxis with and without shock. *Cochrane Database Syst Rev.* 2007;(1):CD006160.
83. Sheikh A, Shehata YA, Brown SG, Simons FE. Adrenaline (epinephrine) for the treatment of anaphylaxis with and without shock. *Cochrane Database Syst Rev.* 2008;4:CD006312.
84. Sheikh A, Simons FE, Barbour V, Worth A. Adrenaline auto-injectors for the treatment of anaphylaxis with and without cardiovascular collapse in the community. *Cochrane Database Syst Rev.* 2012;8:CD008935.
85. Fisher MM. Clinical observations on the pathophysiology and treatment of anaphylactic cardiovascular collapse. *Anaesth Intensive Care.* 1986; 14:17–21.
86. Sampson HA, Mendelson L, Rosen JP. Fatal and near-fatal anaphylactic reactions to food in children and adolescents. *N Engl J Med.* 1992;327:380–384.
87. Thomas M, Crawford I. Best evidence topic report. Glucagon infusion in refractory anaphylactic shock in patients on beta-blockers. *Emerg Med J.* 2005;22:272–273.
88. Sampson HA. Anaphylaxis and emergency treatment. *Pediatrics.* 2003; 111:1601–1608.
89. Worth A, Sheikh A. Prevention of anaphylaxis in healthcare settings. *Expert Rev Clin Immunol.* 2013;9:855–869.
90. Sheikh A, Walker S. Anaphylaxis. *BMJ.* 2005;331:330.
91. Walker S, Sheikh A. Managing anaphylaxis: effective emergency and long-term care are necessary. *Clin Exp Allergy.* 2003;33:1015–1018.
92. Nurmatov U, Devereux G, Worth A, et al. Effectiveness and safety of orally administered immunotherapy for food allergies: a systematic review and meta-analysis. *Br J Nutr.* 2014;111:12–22.
93. Nurmatov U, Venderbosch I, Devereux G, et al. Allergen-specific oral immunotherapy for peanut allergy. *Cochrane Database Syst Rev.* 2012;(9): CD009014.
94. Sheikh A, Nurmatov U, Venderbosch I, Bischoff E. Oral immunotherapy for the treatment of peanut allergy: systematic review of six case series studies. *Prim Care Respir J.* 2012;21:41–49.
95. Monks H, Gowland MH, MacKenzie H, et al. How do teenagers manage their food allergies? *Clin Exp Allergy.* 2010;40:1533–1540.
96. Sampson MA, Mu oz-Furlong A, Sicherer SH. Risk-taking and coping strategies of adolescents and young adults with food allergy. *J Allergy Clin Immunol.* 2006;117:1440–1445.
97. Akeson N, Worth A, Sheikh A. The psychosocial impact of anaphylaxis on young people and their parents. *Clin Exp Allergy.* 2007;37: 1213–1220.
98. Gallagher M, Worth S, Cunningham-Burley S, Sheikh A. Epinephrine auoinjector use in adolescents at risk of anaphylaxis: a qualitative study in Scotland, UK. *Clin Exp Allergy.* 2011;41:869–877.
99. Marrs T, Lack G. Why do few food-allergic adolescents treat anaphylaxis with adrenaline? Reviewing a pressing issue. *Pediatr Allergy Immunol.* 2013;24:222–229.
100. Worth A, Regent L, Levey M, et al. Living with severe allergy: an Anaphylaxis Campaign National Survey of young people. *Clin Transl Allergy.* 2013;3:2.
101. Nwaru BI, Sheikh A. Anaphylaxis in adolescents: a potential tripartite management framework. *Curr Opin Allergy Clin Immunol.* 2015;15: 344–349.
102. Simons FE, Sheikh A. Evidence-based management of anaphylaxis. *Allergy.* 2007;62:827–829.
103. Sheikh A, Shehata YA, Brown SG, Simons FE. Adrenaline for the treatment of anaphylaxis: Cochrane systematic review. *Allergy.* 2009;64: 204–212.
104. Sheikh A. Glucocorticosteroids for the treatment and prevention of anaphylaxis. *Curr Opin Allergy Clin Immunol.* 2013;13:263–267.

CHAPTER

50

Splanchnic Flow and Resuscitation

JOHN W. MAH and ORLANDO C. KIRTON

INTRODUCTION

Ischemia signifies failure to satisfy the metabolic needs of the cell secondary to either impaired oxygen delivery or the impairment of cellular oxygen extraction and utilization. Incomplete splanchnic cellular resuscitation has been associated with the development of multiple organ system failure and increased mortality in the critically ill patient (1,2). For many years, the merits of augmenting systemic oxygen delivery and consumption and attainment of supranormal levels have been examined and debated as primary treatment goals (3–6). There is convincing evidence that systemic hemodynamic and oxygen transport variables fail to accurately portray the complex interaction between energy requirements and the energy supply at the tissue level (7–9), and that achieving supranormal cardiovascular oxygen transport and utilization indices does not reliably confer improved outcome (i.e., decreased mortality rates and diminished multiple organ system failure) in several clinical conditions (e.g., sepsis, acute respiratory distress syndrome [ARDS]) (10–13). These findings have led to the search for monitoring techniques that directly measure changes in regional tissue bioenergetics.

Intestinal tonometry has been proposed as a relatively noninvasive index of the adequacy of aerobic metabolism in organs whose superficial mucosal lining is extremely vulnerable to low flow and hypoxemia, and in which blood flow is sacrificed first in both shock and the cytokine milieu of the systemic inflammatory response (1,14,15). The gastrointestinal tract, therefore, acts like the "canary," displaying early metabolic changes before other indices of adequate oxygen utilization (16). This chapter reviews the fundamental and clinical underpinnings of splanchnic ischemia and resuscitation, intestinal and sublingual tonometry, the potential applications and limitations of these technologies, its use as a prognostic and treatment end point, and, finally, a consideration of potential future directions.

PATHOPHYSIOLOGY

Intestinal Microcirculation

The gastrointestinal tract has three major functions: motility, secretion, and absorption. Blood flow is important for each of these functions, being the highest in the small intestines and the lowest in the colon. The splanchnic circulation contains approximately 30% of the circulating blood volume at any given moment with the bulk of this volume held in the postcapillary venous capacitance vessels (17). Resting blood flow in the intestine is 10 times higher than in skeletal muscle. Most of the blood flow is delivered to the mucosa and submucosa, reflecting the varying demands for oxygen within the intestinal wall, being the highest in the mucosal layer. The arterial supply emanates from an extensive arterial plexus in the submucosa. A *countercurrent* blood flow exchange system exists within the superficial mucosal layer between the arterial and venous circulations, rendering this tissue particularly sensitive to neuronal and systemic vasoconstrictors (18). The arterioles, which run in parallel with the venules in the stalk of the intestinal villus, allow diffusion of oxygen from the arterioles down a concentration gradient to the venules, bypassing the capillary bed at the villus tip; thus, the mucosa at the villus tip is rendered vulnerable to changes in oxygen content. Water also diffuses from arterioles to venules because of an osmotic gradient caused by the absorption of sodium in the capillary bed at the villus tip. Therefore, the sodium concentration is higher in the venules. Plasma water content is then lowered at the villus tip compared with the base of the stalk, predisposing this area to low or absent flow in states of compensated or uncompensated shock when splanchnic circulation is compromised.

Mesenteric vasoconstriction is mediated by α-adrenergic postganglionic sympathetic fibers, but, even more dramatically, by the effects of circulating hormones and peptides (Table 50.1). Endogenous vasoconstrictors known to be released in major injury, sepsis, and other physiologically stressful circumstances include catecholamines, angiotensin, vasopressin, myocardial depressant factor, leukotriene D_4, thromboxane A_2, and serotonin. The high concentration of receptors for these systemically released vasoconstrictors, which affect the splanchnic circulation more than any other tissue beds, has a substantial effect on peripheral (systemic) vascular resistance and, hence, on systemic blood pressure by redistributing blood from the splanchnic organs (as well as the peripheral circulation) to the central circulation (i.e., heart and brain). This effect may be compounded by tissue edema and atheroma in the splanchnic arteries. The peptides, angiotensin II, and vasopressin are the most potent splanchnic vasoconstrictors (14). The splanchnic vasoconstriction induced by these two peptides alone accounts for most of the increase in total vascular resistance recorded in animal models of cardiogenic and hemorrhagic shock. The adequacy of gut mucosal oxygenation cannot be reliably inferred from measurements of tissue oxygenation in the skin or of subcutaneous tissue because of their different response to endogenous vasoconstrictors.

Mesenteric Ischemia

Tissues with a high perfusion-to-extraction (demand) ratio, such as skeletal muscle, have high capillary densities that act as a microvascular reserve to produce an increase in local blood flow. These organs, in situations of low flow, use a disproportionate share of the cardiac output as increased capillary recruitment lowers local vascular resistance. These tissues are characterized by low oxygen extraction ratios and high mixed venous oxygen saturations. Less "fortunate" tissues, including the intestinal tract, possess a lower capillary density

TABLE 50.1 Endogenous Vasoconstrictors Known to Be Released in Stressful Circumstances and Their Actions on Different Tissue Beds

Vasoconstrictor	Gut	Renal	Brain	Coronary	Pulmonary	Muscle	Skin
Catecholamines	+	+	0	+	±	±	+
Angiotensin II	+	+	0	0	0	0	0
Vasopressin	+	+	?0	+	?	?	+
Myocardial depressant factor	+	0	0	0	0	0	0
Leukotriene D_4	+	+	0	+	?	0	0
Thromboxane A_2	+	+	+	+	+	+	+
Serotonin	+	+	?	?	+	–	±

+, vasoconstriction; –, vasodilatation; 0, no effect; ±, effect varies; ?, undefined.
From Fiddian-Green RG. Studies in splanchnic ischemia and multiple organ failure. In: Marston A, Bulkley GR, Fiddian-Green RG, et al., eds. *Splanchnic Ischemia and Multiple Organ Failure*. London: Edward Arnold/St. Louis: CV Mosby; 1989:349.

and are unable to recruit capillaries to augment local blood flow to match increases in metabolic needs. This results in low perfusion-to-oxygen demand ratios and renders this tissue more susceptible to ischemia (15). The gastrointestinal tract is characterized by a high oxygen extraction ratio, high lactate release, and low mixed venous oxygen saturation; it can tolerate severe hypoxemia without a decrease in oxygen consumption but is limited in its ability to respond to decreased blood flow.

Intestinal tissue injury can be induced by the initial ischemia (either from inadequate oxygen content or inadequate flow) or by the generation of oxygen-derived free radicals during reperfusion (1,7). Ischemic injury may be progressive, spanning a spectrum from mild injury characterized by increased capillary permeability with no microscopic changes to transmural infarction, depending on the severity and duration of the ischemia (1,2,19,20). Inadequate oxygen supply results in anaerobic glycolysis and systemic lactic acidosis. In the anoxic cell, uncompensated adenosine triphosphate (ATP) hydrolysis is associated with the intracellular accumulation of adenosine diphosphate (ADP), inorganic phosphate, and hydrogen ions with resultant intracellular acidosis (7,21). These hydrogen ions lead to tissue acidosis as well, with unbound hydrogen ions combining with interstitial bicarbonate to form the weak acid, carbonic acid, that disassociates to produce carbon dioxide (CO_2) plus water.

Intracellular acidosis impairs cellular function by one of several mechanisms: the loss of adenosine nucleotides from mitochondria by the inhibition of the ATP–magnesium/inorganic phosphate carrier; inhibition of sodium–calcium exchange, resulting in the intracellular sequestration of calcium ions; increases in the activity of cyclic adenosine monophosphate (AMP) deaminase and loss of adenine nucleotide precursors from the cell; decreases in the nicotinamide adenine nucleotide pool by the acid-catalyzed destruction of nicotinamide adenine dinucleotide (NAD); and the conversion of intracellular inorganic phosphate to its inhibitory deproteinated form (7).

Hypoxia also results in intracellular calcium overload by inhibiting ATP-driven membrane transport pumps and sodium–calcium exchange. Increases in intracellular calcium are a pivotal event in cellular dysfunction during hypoxia, because calcium-activated proteases can destroy the sarcolemma and the cellular cytoskeleton (7). Cellular membrane degradation seems to be related to calcium influx. Calcium stimulates phospholipase A_2 (PLA_2) and phospholipase C, which are known to degrade membrane phospholipids (22,23). The resultant imbalance between the rate of membrane synthesis and the rate of membrane breakdown results in the accumulation of arachidonic acid, the precursor of thromboxane, prostaglandins, and leukotrienes, substances that produce further cellular damage and profound alterations in microvascular control.

Splanchnic Model of Multiple Organ Failure

Multiple organ failure (MOF) (defined as failure of two or more vital organs or systems, in sequence or simultaneously, irrespective of the primary disease) and sepsis are familiar to surgeons of all specialties (24). Uncompensated or compensated shock leading to progressive oxygen debt, ischemia/reperfusion injury, and cellular dysfunction is the underlying unifying pathophysiologic mechanism (1). Throughout the world, MOF has become the most common cause of death in the intensive care unit (ICU): The reported mortality rates vary from 30% to 100% with a mean of 50%, depending on the number of organ systems involved and consume nearly 40% of all the available ICU days (24–28). Current hypotheses link multiple mechanisms at the cellular level to the development of MOF in animal models; however, none have resulted in any clinically significant targeted therapy (29). Many single-agent attempts (e.g., antibiotics, monoclonal antibodies against cytokines and endotoxin) or combinations of these agents have failed to affect the process. This pathophysiology is likely complex with many redundancies in the initiation and promulgation of MOF, so that attacking a single pathway is ineffective or, perhaps started too late in the sequence of events. For example, bacterial endotoxin in the gut may translocate across the semipermeable mucosa as a result of ischemia/reperfusion. In addition to endotoxins, the products of the damaged mucosa described above contribute to the inflammatory response and subsequent MOF and death of the ICU patient. The translocation of enteric bacteria across the ischemic gut seems to be an important cause of nosocomial infection in the critically ill (14,24). However, reducing the number of nosocomial infections from enteric organisms by selective decontamination does not seem to have a dramatic effect on outcome (30).

The splanchnic model combines the *gut starter* hypothesis popularized by Moore et al. (31) and the *gut motor* hypothesis as described by Deitch (25) and Marshall et al. (26,27). In the gut starter hypothesis, the noxious stimulus leads to a neurohumoral response. High levels of catecholamines cause splanchnic vasoconstriction and a decrease in splanchnic flow. This leads to gut ischemia and, depending on the length of ischemic time, allows various reactions that prime tissue to develop a reperfusion injury once the flow is restored. During reperfusion, PLA_2 is activated, which in turn activates platelet-activating factor (PAF). PAF attracts and primes polymorphonuclear leukocytes (PMNs) in the gut; thereafter, they are released into the systemic circulation, where they undergo activation (the *two-hit* model) and cause end-organ injury (31). Therefore, the PMN is implicated as the major effector of cellular damage attributed to ischemia/reperfusion through its respiratory burst and activation of cytokines and arachidonic acid metabolites.

In the gut motor hypothesis, the steps leading to ischemia are the same. During reperfusion, gut mucosal injury results from the accumulation of intracellular calcium, activation of PLA_2, and generation of free oxygen radicals. This leads to bacterial translocation and initial production and amplification of numerous systemic cytokines (32,33) resulting in MOF.

DIAGNOSIS

Systemic Oxygen Delivery

The determinants of arterial oxygenation include hemoglobin content, inspired oxygen tension, alveolar oxygen tension, pH, temperature, mixed venous oxygen tension, ventilation/perfusion mismatch, physiologic shunting, and cellular–interstitial diffusion abnormalities. Indices of adequacy of systemic perfusion include the following: (a) global systemic parameters, such as blood pressure, heart rate, central venous pressure (CVP) measurements, and urine output (UOP); (b) tissue markers, including arterial pH (pHa), base excess, and serum lactate level; (c) pulmonary artery catheter measurements and derivations, such as cardiac output, oxygen delivery, oxygen consumption, and oxygen extraction; and (d) less invasive monitoring such as arterial pulse contour analysis and esophageal Doppler monitoring. In fact, Rivers et al. demonstrated that goal-directed resuscitation using certain systemic measures (mean arterial pressure [MAP], UOP, CVP) including improving oxygen delivery to an $ScVO_2$ over 70% can improve mortality in patients in severe sepsis and septic shock (34). Nonetheless, the interpretation of oxygen delivery and oxygen consumption measurements is challenging as (a) these parameters are global markers and do not provide any direct information regarding the oxygen requirements of specific tissues; (b) the distribution of oxygen delivery is impacted by local microvascular and neurogenic responses; (c) the effect of cytokines and endogenous peptides is unpredictable; and (d) the disease process may affect cellular metabolism directly (i.e., sepsis and ARDS) (35–37). Several prospective studies suggest that failure to achieve supranormal oxygen delivery and utilization parameters in the acute phase of major injury or physiologic stress is associated with increased mortality and shock-related complications, including multiple organ system dysfunction syndrome. The failure to reverse pathologic flow dependency, tissue hypoxia, and oxygen debt has been inferred as the cause of these adverse outcomes (3–6,38,39). In these prospective studies, both responders and nonresponders achieved normal or hyperdynamic cardiovascular function; however, more cardiovascular interventions were often used in patients who died; so, ultimately, failure of patient response to achieve therapeutic objectives could be considered as the cause of the observed increased mortality. Several reports failed to identify either an optimal or a critical value of oxygen delivery or consumption to distinguish survivors from nonsurvivors in critically ill patients (10–13,40). Adequate or supranormal oxygen delivery may not be tantamount to effective tissue oxygen utilization.

"Critical oxygen delivery" purportedly marks the transition from aerobic to anaerobic metabolism; however, the relationship between oxygen delivery and consumption obtained in critically ill patients with ARDS, sepsis, and heart failure appears to be linear (40). The lack of a clearly defined inflection point in a linear function makes it impossible to determine a critical level of oxygen delivery that aerobically satisfies cellular energy requirements.

Regional Oxygen Delivery

Historical Review of Gastric Tonometry

A tonometer is composed of a semipermeable silicone balloon, which is filled with either air or fluid and allowed to equilibrate with the surrounding tissue. The fluid/air is then accessed and the pressure of CO_2 can be directly measured. Tonometry was first used by Bergofsky (41) and Dawson et al. (42) in 1964 to demonstrate that the gas tension within a hollow viscous approximates that within the mucosa of the viscus. Grum et al. (21) extended this concept to the intestinal tract of adults. Antonsson et al. (43) and Hartmann et al. (44) performed validation studies demonstrating that both the stomach and small intestine could be used as suitable sites to measure intraluminal PCO_2. They confirmed that intraluminal PCO_2 equaled that measured within the intestinal mucosa as well as approximated hepatic vein PCO_2. Moreover, it has been validated that the intramucosal PCO_2 rises and falls in parallel with changes in PCO_2 in arterial blood (45). This indirect method of measuring the pH within the intestinal mucosa (pHi) is based on the fact that CO_2 is a highly permeable gas and on the assumption that this generated CO_2 is the end result of ATP hydrolysis, with neutralization of generated hydrogen ions by intestinal interstitial bicarbonate (46).

The measurement of pHi depends also on the assumption that the bicarbonate concentration in the wall of the organ is the same as that which is delivered to it by arterial blood, and that the dissociation constant (pK) is the same as that in the plasma. Using the Henderson–Hasselbalch equation, pHi is calculated as follows:

$$\text{pHi} = 6.1 + \log(HCO_3^-/0.03 \times PCO_2)$$

where pKa is 6.1, and 0.03 is the solubility coefficient for CO_2. The pK in plasma is not the same as that in the cytosol, but the value 6.1 is the best approximation of the pK within the intestinal fluid of the superficial layers of the mucosa (14,47,48).

Doglio et al. (49) demonstrated that gastric pHi was a predictor of ICU mortality at the time of admission to the ICU and at 12 hours later. Patients admitted with a pHi < 7.36 had a greater ICU mortality rate, 65% versus 44% ($p < 0.04$). Furthermore, patients with persistently low pHi at 12 hours after ICU admission had the highest mortality rate (87%). Maynard et al. (50) repeated the study in patients with acute circulatory failure and found remarkably similar outcomes. In addition, there were significant differences in mean gastric pHi values between survivors and nonsurvivors on admission (7.40 vs. 7.28) and at 24 hours (7.40 vs. 7.24), respectively ($p < 0.001$).

There was no difference in cardiac index, oxygen delivery, and oxygen uptake, suggesting that pHi is a more specific marker of resuscitation than our common global parameters.

Kirton et al. (51) confirmed that failure of splanchnic resuscitation correlated with MOF and increased length of ICU stay in the hemodynamically unstable trauma patient. The relative risk of death in patients whose pHi was less than 7.32 was 4.5-fold higher and the relative risk of developing multiple organ system failure was 5.4 times higher compared with those having a pHi of 7.32 or more. Global parameters of oxygen transport utilization did not distinguish survivors from nonsurvivors nor those patients who developed MOF from those who did not.

Chang et al. (52) then conducted a prospective study of 20 critically ill patients and were able to demonstrate that correction of an abnormal admission pHi correlated with better outcomes. Patients with pHi less than 7.32 on admission, who did not correct within the initial 24 hours, had a higher mortality (50% vs. 0%; $p = 0.03$) and more frequent MOF (2.6 vs. 0.62 organs/patient; $p = 0.02$) than those whose pHi corrected.

Ivatury et al. (53) compared correction of pHi versus supranormal oxygen delivery (as defined by Shoemaker et al. [3] in 27 critically ill trauma patients). Seventy-five percent of the patients who developed MOF had pHi less than 7.3. Interestingly, four of the five patients who died in the supranormal oxygen group achieved supranormal oxygen delivery and consumption goals, but had a pHi less than 7.3 at 24 hours. Moreover, they observed that a late fall in pHi was often associated with a physiologic catastrophe (e.g., intestinal leak, gangrene, bacteremia).

Gutierrez et al. (54) observed that hospital mortality rate was significantly greater in control patients with normal pHi on admission (pHi ≥ 7.35) but developed an abnormal pHi during their ICU stay compared with those with an initial abnormal pHi who received interventions to increase oxygen delivery. Unfortunately, if admission pHi was low, the mortality rates were similar in both treatment and control groups. The authors, however, chose to increase oxygen delivery rather than restore pHi to normal values.

Barquist et al. also specifically studied ICU patients with persistent uncorrected gastric pHi who had pulmonary artery catheters to guide resuscitation (55). They observed a significant reduction in the incidence of MOF per patient (1.9 ± 0.4 to 0.9 ± 0.2; $p = 0.02$), length of ICU stay (35 ± 9 to 18 ± 4 days; $p = 0.03$), and total hospital stay (51 ± 12 to 29 ± 5 days; $p = 0.03$) in patients with persistent gastric intramucosal acidosis who were administered agents that increased splanchnic perfusion. MOF and mortality were increased in those patients whose pHi never corrected (i.e., pHi < 7.25).

Despite the potential benefits of regional monitoring, gastric tonometry has multiple limitations. The monitoring itself is labor intensive and time consuming, often requiring multiple attempts to ensure proper positioning and frequent catheter adjustments, lengthy equilibration times, and need for frequent troubleshooting of abnormal results. Gastric acid must be neutralized (pH > 4.5), requiring pH litmus paper analysis and adjustments to the peptic ulcer prophylaxis regimen in the ICU patient. Tube feedings also must be held. In addition, one must use a dedicated blood gas analyzer for all pHi determinations. Periodic calibration of the analyzer with 10 to 20 ampules at three different PCO_2 levels must be done. The saline sample must be transported immediately on ice because of rapid loss of CO_2 from the sample and overestimation of the pHi.

Sublingual Tonometry

Research progressed more proximally in the gastrointestinal tract in search of a more reliable and efficient place to measure tissue PCO_2, evaluating first the esophagus and finally the sublingual space (56). Weil et al. (57) suggested that the sublingual space would respond similarly to the splanchnic circulation. Marik (58) also demonstrated good correlation of sublingual tonometry with gastric tonometry and more importantly that it was the difference between the sublingual PCO_2 ($slPCO_2$) and arterial PCO_2 (PCO_2 gap) that was more predictive of survival. The device uses a disposable CO_2 sensor that is placed directly under the sublingual space and is kept in place for approximately 60 to 90 seconds. SLC has been used to triage patients with penetrating traumatic injuries showing statistical differences in severe to moderate (>1,500 mL) or minimal to moderate (<1,500 mL) amount of blood loss on admission (59). Our own research supports Marik's findings that the PCO_2 gap and to a lesser degree the absolute SLC value correlates with outcome (60). Our observations of 83 critically ill surgical patients subjected to a standard resuscitation protocol suggest that patients whose PCO_2 gap was not corrected to 9 mmHg or less at 24 hours after admission were 3 times more likely to experience MOF and more than 10 times as likely to die during their hospital stay. Sublingual capnometry is a quick and simple method to directly measure tissue perfusion and is a potential tool for the clinician to help guide goal-directed therapy. The product has unfortunately been recalled in 2003 due to manufacturing problems.

MONITORING PLAN

Intramucosal PCO_2 provides an intermittent direct measure of the ability of tissues to resynthesize high-energy phosphate compounds utilizing aerobic metabolism. In dysoxic states, protons accumulate and pHi falls, indicative of inadequate oxidative metabolism. If this is recognized early and can be reversed, the clinician may be able to prevent or limit the duration of compensated shock. Global measurements of oxygen delivery, oxygen consumption, oxygen extraction ratio, and mixed venous blood hemoglobin oxygen saturation are unsatisfactory for this purpose (47,61). The calculation of pHi can provide clinicians with a metabolic end point that may be used to determine whether the milieu is likely to create a reperfusion injury if resuscitation is successful or whether subclinical maldistribution of blood flow persists—a reflection of a still-active neurohumoral response to stress.

Monitoring all patients likely to have had activation of the neurohumoral response and decreased splanchnic blood flow is probably beneficial because they are at risk for a reperfusion injury, MOF, and a higher mortality rate (47). Outcome can be improved by recognizing compensated shock, preventing ischemia/reperfusion injury, and ensuring that intramucosal acidosis is promptly reversed. Recognize that the window of opportunity for effective therapy is early (61). Both a preemptive intervention to block and modify the ischemia/reperfusion injury and restoration of splanchnic perfusion must be incorporated into a resuscitation algorithm to reduce the incidence of bacterial translocation and systemic white cell priming before the ensuing systemic inflammatory response (1). Because early abnormalities in the gastrointestinal intramucosa act as a marker of mortality and morbidity, efforts to correct them may improve outcome and should diminish resource utilization (62,63).

Concepts in Splanchnic Resuscitation

The limited success thus far that has attended attempts to elevate an already depressed pHi and an understanding of the importance of the ischemia/reperfusion injury as a fundamental part of both the gut starter and gut motor hypotheses suggest that a new perspective is needed. Two separate elements must be combined: a preemptive intervention to prevent the ischemia/reperfusion injury in high-risk patients, and restoration of oxidative high-energy phosphate synthesis as judged by a normalizing pHi. As an approach to preventing intramucosal acidosis and ischemic gut mucosal injury, we suggest the following goals: increase global oxygen delivery, increase splanchnic flow, reduce ischemia/reperfusion injury by stopping the cytokine cascade before it starts, and monitor reversal of ischemia and anaerobic metabolism by restoration of normal pHi or PCO_2 gap (9,19,31–33,64–66).

To increase global oxygen delivery, ensure adequate volume resuscitation with isotonic fluids, albumin solutions, and red blood cells when indicated. Avoid α-agents, which cause splanchnic vasoconstriction. This may require "tolerating" a lower MAP, as long as there is satisfactory end-organ perfusion. Use splanchnic sparing inotropes such as dobutamine when indicated (37,67,68). In theory, vasodilators such as nicardipine, nitroglycerin, nitroprusside, prostaglandin E, or prostacyclin could increase splanchnic flow (69,70) and reperfusion injury could be attenuated by blocking free radical generation with folate or allopurinol and administering free radical scavengers such as albumin, mannitol, vitamin C, vitamin A, and vitamin E (71–73). Injury related to PLA_2 activity has been shown to be suppressed by quinacrine, lidocaine, allopurinol, and steroids (33,74–76). Moreover, vitamin C and vitamin E can stabilize cell membranes and help decrease capillary permeability.

Glutamine has been implicated as sustaining mucosal architecture and function by scavenging free radicals and preventing lipid peroxidation. In addition, glutamine combines with acetyl cystine to form glutathione (77). In the reaction catalyzed by the selenium-containing enzyme glutathione peroxidase, glutathione is transformed to oxidized glutathione. This then combines with hydrogen peroxide and degrades it to water, preventing hydrogen peroxide from reacting with superoxide to produce a hydroxyl radical. *N*-acetyl cystine has been reported to favorably affect indirect indicators of tissue oxygenation (78), perhaps because it is a precursor of glutathione.

Glucocorticoids can re-establish vasomotor tone in patients with critical illness–related corticosteroid insufficiency (CIRCI) but also decrease cytokine release from primed macrophages (79). Although, Annane et al. (80) showed a significant reduction in mortality from 73% to 63% in patients with septic shock who were given low-dose hydrocortisone and fludrocortisone. These results could not be adequately repeated. Nonetheless, steroid therapy still remains a part of the international treatment guidelines for septic shock.

Finally, albumin acts as a free radical scavenger and has been shown to be as effective and safe as saline in a large heterogeneous ICU population. Other investigators have demonstrated improvement in organ function in specific patient populations such as hypoalbuminemic patients and patients with acute lung injury or ARDS (81–83). Activated protein C (APC) had also been proposed to reduce absolute mortality by 6.1% in severely ill patients in septic shock in an attempt to stop parts of the inflammatory cascade before it starts. In theory, APC exerts its effect by modulating the systemic inflammatory response, inhibiting production of TNF-α, interleukin-1, and interleukin-6 (84). Unfortunately, confirmation studies did not support the initial claims and APC was voluntarily withdrawn from the market by the manufacturer in 2011.

FUTURE INVESTIGATIONS

Regional monitoring is preferable to global markers to detect alterations in perfusion at an earlier time point and guide resuscitation with specific tissue-level endpoints. Subsequently, many regional perfusion monitors have been developed including near-infrared resonance spectroscopy (NIRS), laser Doppler flowmetry (LDF), microdialysis, tissue oxygen tension (tPO_2), mitochondrial monitoring, and magnetic resonance spectroscopy. Unfortunately, no standard of care or clinically significant randomized controlled outcome study has been demonstrated in adult patients (85).

Although results of gastric tonometry have been promising and suggestive of improved outcomes in critically ill patients, its practicality in today's ICU remains poor. Sublingual capnometry (if made available again) has good potential as an efficient and effective monitor of "splanchnic" tissue. Sublingual capnometry may be helpful in decisions to both initiate therapy and halt resuscitation at a more appropriate endpoint. In addition, as the existing technology improves, continuous sublingual monitoring may also become feasible, offering real-time monitoring of "splanchnic" tissue perfusion.

Key Points

- The mucosa of the gastrointestinal tract is sensitive to changes in oxygen delivery and is limited in its ability to respond to low blood flow.
- Anoxic intestinal cells develop an intracellular acidosis via multiple mechanisms and subsequent tissue acidosis which can be measured using gastrointestinal tonometers.
- Regional monitoring of perfusion appears to be superior to global parameters in predicting mortality and MOF and correction of low intestinal mucosal pH has improved survival and reduced MOF where normalization of global parameters and empiric supranormal oxygen delivery did not.
- Many regional monitoring devices have been developed; however, few have gained widespread use due to a failure of technology to provide an efficient means of monitoring tissue and lack of clinically significant randomized controlled human outcome studies.

References

1. Fiddian-Green RG. Association between intramucosal acidosis in the gut and organ failure. *Crit Care Med.* 1993;21(2 Suppl):S103–S107.
2. Fiddian-Green RG. Should measurements of tissue pH and PO_2 be included in the routine monitoring of intensive care unit patients? *Crit Care Med.* 1991;19:141–413.
3. Shoemaker W, Appel PL, Kram HB, et al. Prospective trial of supra normal values of survivors as therapeutic goals in high-risk surgical patients. *Chest.* 1988;94:1176–1186.
4. Tuchschmidt J, Fried J, Astiz M, Rackow E. Elevation of cardiac output and oxygen delivery improves outcome in septic shock. *Chest.* 1992;102: 216–220.
5. Moore FA, Haenel JB, Moore EE, Whitehill TA. Incommensurate oxygen consumption in response to maximal oxygen availability predicts post-injury multiple organ failure. *J Trauma.* 1992;33:58–65; discussion 65–67.
6. Boyd O, Grounds M, Bennett ED. A randomized clinical trial of the effect of deliberate perioperative increase of oxygen delivery on mortality in high risk surgical patients. *JAMA.* 1993;270:2699–2707.
7. Gutierrez G. Cellular energy metabolism during hypoxia. *Crit Care Med.* 1991;19:619–626.
8. Gutierrez G, Bismar H, Dantzker DR, Silva N. Comparison of gastric intramucosal pH with measure of oxygen transport and consumption in critically ill patients. *Crit Care Med.* 1992;20:451–457.
9. Fiddian-Green RG, Haglund U, Gutierrez G, Shoemaker WC. Goals for resuscitation of shock. *Crit Care Med.* 1993;21(2 Suppl):S25–S31.
10. Hayes MA, Timmins AC, Yau EH, et al. Elevation of systemic oxygen delivery in the treatment of critically ill patients. *N Engl J Med.* 1994;330: 1717–1722.
11. Steltzer H, Hiesmayr M, Mayer N, et al. The relationship between oxygen delivery and uptake in the critically ill: is there a critical or optimal therapeutic value? *Anesthesia.* 1994;49:229–236.
12. Ronco JJ, Fenwick JC, Tweeddale MG, et al. Identification of the critical oxygen delivery for anaerobic metabolism in critically ill septic and nonseptic humans. *JAMA.* 1993;270:1724–1730.
13. Ronco JJ, Fenwick JC, Wiggs BR, et al. Oxygen consumption is independent of increases in oxygen delivery by dobutamine in septic patients who have normal or increased plasma lactate levels. *Am Rev Respir Dis.* 1993;147:25–31.
14. Fiddian-Green RG. Studies in splanchnic ischemia and multiple organ failure. In: Marston A, Bulkley GR, Fiddian-Green RG, et al., eds. *Splanchnic Ischemia and Multiple Organ Failure.* London: Edward Arnold/St. Louis: CV Mosby; 1989:349–363.
15. Gutierrez G. Regional blood flow and oxygen transport: implications for the therapy of the septic patient. *Crit Care Med.* 1993;21:1263–1264.
16. Dantzker DR. The gastrointestinal tract: the canary of the body? *JAMA.* 1993;270:1247–1248.
17. Hjelmquist B, Teder H, Borgstrom A, Björkman S. Indomethacin and pancreatic blood flow: an experimental study in pigs. *Acta Chir Scand.* 1990;156:543–547.
18. Stephenson RB. The splanchnic circulation. In: Patton HD, Fuchs AF, Hille B, et al., eds. *The Textbook of Physiology.* Vol. 2. No. 46. 21st ed. Philadelphia, PA: WB Saunders; 1989:911.
19. Fink MD, Kaups KL, Wang HL, Rothschild HR. Maintenance of superior mesenteric arterial perfusion prevents increased intestinal mucosal permeability in endotoxic pigs. *Surgery.* 1991;110:154–160; discussion 160–161.
20. Fink MD, Antonsson JB, Wang HL, Rothschild HR. Increased intestinal permeability in endotoxic pigs: mesenteric hypoperfusion on an etiologic factor. *Arch Surg.* 1991;126:211–218.
21. Grum CM, Fiddian-Green RG, Pittenger GL, et al. Adequacy of tissue oxygenation in intact dog intestine. *J Appl Physiol Respir Environ Exerc Physiol.* 1984;56:1065–1069.
22. Otani H, Prasad MR, Jones RM, Das DK. Mechanism of membrane phospholipid degradation in ischemic-reperfused rat hearts. *Am J Physiol.* 1989;257:H252–H258.
23. Otamiri T, Tagesson C. Role of phospholipase A_2 and oxygenated free radicals in mucosal damage after small intestinal ischemia and reperfusion. *Am J Surg.* 1989;157:562–565; discussion 566.
24. Carrico CJ, Meakins JL, Marshall JC, et al. Multiple organ failure syndrome. *Arch Surg.* 1986;121:196–208.
25. Deitch EA. Overview of multiple organ failure: state of the art. *Crit Care Med.* 1993;4:131–168.
26. Marshall JC, Christou NV, Meakins JL. The gastrointestinal tract: the undrained abscess of multiple organ failure. *Am Surg.* 1993;218:111–119.
27. Marshall JC, Christou NV, Horn R, Meakins JL. The microbiology of multiple organ failure. The proximal gastrointestinal tract as an occult reservoir of pathogens. *Arch Surg.* 1988;123:309–315.
28. Meakins JL, Marshall JC. The gut as the monitor of multiple system organ failure. In: Martson A, Bulkley G, Fiddian-Green RG, et al., eds. *Splanchnic Ischemia and Multiple Organ Failure.* London: Edward Arnold/St. Louis: CV Mosby; 1989:339.
29. McConnell KW, Coopersmith CM. Organ failure avoidance and mitigation strategies in surgery. *Surg Clin North Am.* 2012;92:307–319, ix.
30. Cerra FB, Maddaus MA, Dunn DL, et al. Selective gut decontamination reduces nosocomial infection and length of stay but not mortality or organ failure in surgical intensive care patients. *Arch Surg.* 1992;127:163–167; discussion 167–169.
31. Moore EE, Moore FA, Franciose RJ, et al. The post ischemic gut serves as a priming bed for circulating neutrophils that provoke multiple organ failure. *J Trauma.* 1994;37:881–887.
32. Flynn WJ Jr, Hoover EL. Allopurinol plus standard resuscitation preserves hepatic blood flow and function following hemorrhage shock. *J Trauma.* 1994;37:956–961.
33. Xu D, Lu Q, Deitch EA. Calcium and phospholipase A_2 appear to be involved in the pathogenesis of hemorrhagic shock-induced mucosal injury and bacterial translocation. *Crit Care Med.* 1995;23:125–131.
34. Rivers E, Nguyen B, Havstad S, et al.; Early Goal-Directed Therapy Collaborative Group. Early goal-directed therapy in the treatment of severe sepsis and septic shock. *N Engl J Med.* 2001;345:1368–1377.
35. Steffes CP, Dahn MS, Lange MP. Oxygen transport-dependent splanchnic metabolism in the sepsis syndrome. *Arch Surg.* 1994;129:46–52.
36. Marik PE. Gastric intramucosal pH: a better predictor of multiorgan dysfunction syndrome and death than oxygen-derived variables in patients with sepsis. *Chest.* 1993;104:225–229.
37. Marik PE, Mohedin M. The contrasting effects of dopamine and norepinephrine on systemic and splanchnic oxygen utilization in hyperdynamic sepsis. *JAMA.* 1994;272:1354–1357.
38. Bishop MH, Shoemaker WC, Appel PL, et al. Relationship between supranormal circulatory values, time delays, and outcome in severely traumatized patients. *Crit Care Med.* 1993;21:56–63.
39. Abramson D, Scalea TM, Hitchcock R, et al. Lactate clearance and survival following injury. *J Trauma.* 1993;35:584–588; discussion 588–589.
40. Gutierrez G, Pohil RJ. Oxygen consumption is linearly related to O_2 supply in critically ill patients. *J Crit Care.* 1986;1:45–53.
41. Bergofsky EH. Determination of tissue O_2 tensions by hollow visceral tonometers: effect of breathing enriched O_2 mixtures. *J Clin Invest.* 1964;43:193–200.
42. Dawson AM, Trenchard D, Guz A. Small bowel tonometry: assessment of small gut mucosal oxygen tension in dog and man. *Nature.* 1965;206: 943–944.
43. Antonsson JB, Boyle CC, Kruithoff KL, et al. Validation of tonometric measurement of gut intramural pH during endotoxemia and mesenteric occlusion in pigs. *Am J Physiol.* 1990;259:G519–G523.
44. Hartmann M, Montgomery A, Jonsson K, Haglund U. Tissue oxygenation in hemorrhagic shock measured as transcutaneous oxygen tension, subcutaneous oxygen tension and gastrointestinal pH in pigs. *Crit Care Med.* 1991;19:205–210.
45. Stevens MH, Thirlby RC, Feldman M. Mechanism for high pCO_2 in gastric juice: roles of bicarbonate secretion and CO_2 diffusion. *Am J Physiol.* 1987;253:G527–G530.
46. Grum CM. Tissue oxygenation in low flow states during hypoxemia. *Crit Care Med.* 1993;21(2 Suppl):S44–S49.
47. Fiddian-Green RG. Tonometry: theory and applications. *Intensive Care World.* 1992;9:60–65.
48. Rasmussen LB, Haglund U. Early gut ischemia in experimental fecal peritonitis. *Circ Shock.* 1992;38:22–28.
49. Doglio GR, Pusajo JF, Egurrola MA, et al. Gastric mucosal pH as a prognostic index of mortality in critically ill patients. *Crit Care Med.* 1991;19:1037–1040.
50. Maynard N, Bihari D, Beale R, et al. Assessment of splanchnic oxygenation by gastric tonometry in patients with acute circulatory failure. *JAMA.* 1993;270:1203–1210.
51. Kirton OC, Windsor J, Civetta JM, et al. Failure of splanchnic resuscitation in the acutely injured trauma patient correlates with multiple organ system failure and death in the intensive care unit. *Chest.* 1995;108:104S.
52. Chang MC, Cheatham ML, Nelson LD, et al. Gastric tonometry supplements information provided by systemic indicators of oxygen transport. *J Trauma.* 1994;37:488–494.
53. Ivatury RR, Simon RJ, Havriliak D, et al. Gastric mucosal pH and oxygen delivery and consumption indices in the assessment of adequacy of resuscitation after trauma: a prospective, randomized study. *J Trauma.* 1995;39:128–134; discussion 134–136.
54. Gutierrez G, Palizas F, Doglio G, et al. Gastric intramucosal pH as a therapeutic index of tissue oxygenation in critically ill patients. *Lancet.* 1992;339:195–199.

55. Barquist E, Kirton O, Windsor J, et al. The impact of antioxidant and splanchnic-directed therapy on persistent uncorrected gastric mucosal pH in the critically injured trauma patient. *J Trauma.* 1998;44(2):355–360.
56. Sato Y, Weil MH, Tang W, et al. Esophageal PCO_2 as a monitor of perfusion failure during hemorrhagic shock. *J Appl Physiol (1985).* 1997;82: 558–562.
57. Weil M, Nakagawa Y, Tang W, et al. Sublingual capnometry: a new noninvasive measurement for diagnosis and quantitation of severity of circulatory shock. *Crit Care Med.* 1999;27(7):1225–1229.
58. Marik PE. Sublingual capnography: a clinical validation study. *Chest.* 2001; 120(3):923–927.
59. Baron BJ, Sinert R, Zehtabchi S, et al. Diagnostic utility of sublingual PCO_2 for detecting hemorrhage in patients with penetrating trauma. *J Trauma.* 2004;57:69–74.
60. Mah JW, Kirton OC, Keating KP, et al. Utility of sublingual capnometry as a predictor of multi-system organ failure in critically ill surgical patients. *J Trauma.* 2006;61(6):1562.
61. Gutierrez G, Brown SD. Gastric tonometry: a new monitoring modality in the intensive care unit. *J Intensive Care Med.* 1995;10:34–44.
62. Fiddian-Green RG. Tonometry. Part 2: clinical use and cost implications. *Intensive Care World.* 1992;9:130–135.
63. Mythen MG, Webb AR. Intraoperative gut mucosal hypoperfusion is associated with increased postoperative complications and cost. *Intensive Care Med.* 1994;20:99–104.
64. Yee JB, McJames SW. Use of gastric intramucosal pH as a monitor during hemorrhagic shock. *Circ Shock.* 1994;43:44–48.
65. Mythen MG, Webb AR. Perioperative plasma volume expansion reduces the incidence of gut mucosal hypoperfusion during cardiac surgery. *Arch Surg.* 1995;130:423–429.
66. Gutierrez G, Clark C, Brown SD, et al. Effect of dobutamine on oxygen consumption and gastric mucosal pH in septic patients. *Am J Respir Crit Care Med.* 1994;150:324–329.
67. Smithies J, Yee TH, Jackson L, et al. Protecting the gut and the liver in the critically ill: effects of dopexamine. *Crit Care Med.* 1994;22:789–795.
68. Boyd O, Grounds M, Bennet ED. The use of dopexamine hydrochloride to increase oxygen delivery perioperatively. *Anesth Analg.* 1993;76: 372–376.
69. Cullen JJ, Ephgrave KS, Broadhurst KA, Booth B. Captopril decreases stress ulceration without affecting gastric perfusion during canine hemorrhagic shock. *J Trauma.* 1994;37:43–49.
70. Hannemann L, Reinhart K, Meier-Hellmann A, Bredle DL. Prostacyclin in septic shock. *Chest.* 1994;105:1504–1510.
71. Grace RA. Ischemia-reperfusion injury. *Br J Surg.* 1994;81:637–647.
72. Granger DN, McCord JM, Parks DA, Hollwarth ME. Xanthine oxidase inhibition attenuate ischemia-induced vascular permeability changes in the cat intestine. *Gastroenterology.* 1986;90:80–84.
73. Nathens AB, Neff MJ, Jurkovich GJ, et al. Randomized, prospective trial of antioxidant supplementation in critically ill surgical patients. *Ann Surg.* 2002;236:814–822.
74. Boros M, Karacsony G, Kaszaki J, Nagy S. Reperfusion mucosal damage after complete intestinal ischemia in the dog: the effects of antioxidant and phospholipase A2 inhibitor therapy. *Surgery.* 1993;113:184–191.
75. Mikawa K, Maekawa N, Nishina K, et al. Effect of lidocaine pretreatment on endotoxin-induced lung injury in rabbits. *Anesthesiology.* 1994;81:689–699.
76. Sasagawas S. Inhibitory effects of local anesthetics on migration, extracellular release of lysosomal enzyme and superoxide anion production in human polymorphonuclear leukocytes. *Immunopharmacol Immunotoxicol.* 1991;13:607–622.
77. Zimmerman JJ. Therapeutic application of oxygen radical scavengers. *Chest.* 1991;100:189S–192S.
78. Spies CD, Reinhart K, Witt I, et al. Influence of N-acetyl cysteine on indirect indicators of tissue oxygenation in septic shock patients: results from a prospective, randomized double-blind study. *Crit Care Med.* 1994;22:1738–1746.
79. Marik PE, Patores SM, Annane D, et al.; American College of Critical Care Medicine. Recommendations for the diagnosis and management of corticosteroid insufficiency in critically ill adult patients: consensus statements from an international task force by the American College of Critical Care Medicine. *Crit Care Med.* 2008;36(6):1937–1949.
80. Annane D, Sebille V, Charpentier C, et al. Effect of treatment with low doses of hydrocortisone and fludrocortisone on mortality in patients with septic shock. *JAMA.* 2002;288(7):862–871.
81. Finfer S, Bellomo R, Boyce N, et al.; SAFE Study Investigators. A comparison of albumin and saline for fluid resuscitation in the intensive care unit. *N Engl J Med.* 2004;350:2247–2256.
82. Martin GS, Moss M, Wheeler AP, et al. A randomized, controlled trial of furosemide with or without albumin in hypoproteinemic patients with acute lung injury. *Crit Care Med.* 2005;33:1681–1687.
83. Horstick G, Lauterbach M, Kempf T, et al. Early albumin infusion improves global and local hemodynamics and reduces inflammatory response in hemorrhagic shock. *Crit Care Med.* 2002;30:851–855.
84. Bernard G, Vincent JL, Laterre PF, et al.; (PROWESS Study Group). Efficacy and safety of recombinant human activated protein C for severe sepsis. *N Engl J Med.* 2001;344:699–709.
85. Ekbal NJ, Dyson A, Black C, Singer M. Monitoring tissue perfusion, oxygenation, and metabolism in critically ill patients. *Chest.* 2013;143(6):1799–1808.

CHAPTER

51

Cardiopulmonary Resuscitation in the ICU

ARNO L. ZARITSKY

INTRODUCTION

Cardiopulmonary resuscitation (CPR) and advanced life support (ALS) interventions are commonly performed in the intensive care unit (ICU) setting. The recommended CPR and ALS interventions are based on guidelines developed every 5 years by experts from international resuscitation organizations who review the science and weigh new evidence. Members of the International Liaison Committee on Resuscitation (ILCOR, http://www.ilcor.org) developed a Scientific Evidence Evaluation and Review System (SEERS) where interested readers can view the in-depth evidence reviews (https://volunteer.heart.org/apps/pico/Pages/default.aspx). Choose the "PICO Topic" to view the Consensus on Science and Treatment Recommendations (CoSTR) statements, which are freely available.

This chapter is based on the 2015 ILCOR recommendations, which designate the current strength of evidence for interventions by using a range of terms from "may be considered" for consensus recommendations when evidence is very weak or lacking, to "suggest" for weak recommendations based on weak evidence, and "recommend" for those interventions that are supported by good evidence (1). This review includes the science and treatment recommendations for basic life support (BLS) (2,3) and ALS (4,5) for adults and children (6,7), but will not cover neonatal resuscitation (8). Based on the CoSTR evidence evaluation, each of the participating international resuscitation councils will publish resuscitation guidelines in 2016. Of note, the specific interventions may differ among these guidelines because each resuscitation council considers the economic, geographic, and system differences in practice, including the availability of equipment and medications that may vary in different parts of the world.

This chapter reviews the epidemiology of in-hospital cardiac arrest (IHCA), emphasizes the importance of high-quality BLS, reviews recommended ALS interventions, discusses ways to monitor and improve the quality of resuscitation, reviews postresuscitation management, and outcome prediction.

CARDIAC ARREST EPIDEMIOLOGY

Adult

Registry data, such as the American Heart Association's Get-With-The-Guidelines-Resuscitation (GWTG-R; http://www.heart.org/HEARTORG/HealthcareResearch/GetWithThe-Guidelines-Resuscitation/Get-With-The-Guidelines-Resuscitation_UCM_314496_SubHomePage.jsp) and international registries, provide much of our current understanding of the epidemiology and outcome following in-hospital arrests. Annually in the United States, there are an estimated 209,000 treated IHCAs (9). Analysis of the UK National Cardiac Arrest audit from 2011 to 2013 identified an IHCA incidence of 1.6 per 1,000 hospital admissions with an overall unadjusted survival rate of 18.4% (10).

Recent analysis of the GWTG-R data—almost 136,000 IHCAs—observed that 58% were men, 74% were white, and 83% were over 50 years of age. Although ventricular fibrillation (VF) or pulseless ventricular tachycardia (pVT) is common in sudden out-of-hospital CA (OHCA), only 20% of the IHCA cases had VF/pVT as the initial rhythm (11). Overall, 64% of the arrests occurred in the ICU. Of note, half of the reporting hospitals were academic teaching hospitals, 89% were in urban settings and 59% were identified as teaching hospitals, so the GWTG-R data may not accurately represent nationwide epidemiology.

There is substantial variation in the rate of survival by hospital based on analysis of GWTG-R, even after adjusting for 36 predictors (11). Identified significant survival outcome predictors were female gender (OR 1.10, 95% CI: 1.06–1.13), black race (OR 0.93; 95% CI: 0.87–0.99), comorbidities such as dysrhythmia (OR 1.24; 95% CI: 1.20–1.28), a hematology–oncology condition (OR 0.50; 95% CI: 0.47–0.52), and intra-arrest factors including cardiac etiology (OR 1.18; 95% CI: 1.14–1.23). In both the in-hospital and out-of-hospital setting, an initial rhythm of VF/pVT is consistently associated with better outcome; for IHCA, an initial rhythm of VF/pVT was most strongly associated with higher survival (OR 3.14; 95% CI: 3.02–3.27) (11). Arrests occurring at night (OR 0.75; 95% CI: 0.72–0.76) or on the weekend (OR 0.86; 95% CI: 0.83–0.89) were associated with a worse outcome compared with arrests occurring during the day (11). Conversely, being on a monitor (OR 1.72; 95% CI: 1.64–1.81), or in an ICU (OR 1.60; 95% CI: 1.53–1.68) were associated with a better outcome (12).

After adjusting for all of these factors, the analysis demonstrated substantial interhospital variation in outcome following OHCA and IHCA (11). The median adjusted survival to discharge was 11.9% (0%–14.8%, minimum to maximum) in the lowest decile academic hospitals and 22.5% (21.5%–31%) in the top decile. To put this in perspective, the data suggest that there is a 42% greater odds of patients with identical covariates surviving to hospital discharge at one randomly selected high performing hospital compared with another low performing hospital.

The take-home message from these data is that the quality of resuscitation varies across institutions. It is likely that there are other important factors, such as training and team performance in providing rapid defibrillation and high-quality chest compressions that explain some of this variation. In addition, high performing centers may excel in postresuscitation care, which may be very important to survival after IHCA (13,14).

This outcome variation is not restricted to US hospitals. An analysis of data from 144 acute hospitals in the United Kingdom on 22,628 IHCA patients 16 years of age and older also observed significant variation in the rates of survival to hospital discharge (10). Only 16.9% of patients had an initial shockable rhythm of VF/pVT, which again was associated with a much higher rate of hospital survival (49.0%) compared with patients with nonshockable rhythms, asystole, or pulseless electrical activity (PEA), whose mean survival was 10.5% (10). Unlike the United States, over half of the IHCA occurred on the ward in the United Kingdom. Similar to the US data, crude hospital survival rate data suggested worse outcomes for arrests at night or on the weekend compared with weekday.

Analysis of data on over 362,000 ICU admissions from Project IMPACT (Cerner Corporation, Kansas City, MO) provides epidemiologic data on the frequency and outcome following IHCA in the ICU (15). Overall, 1.8% of ICU admissions received CPR; 15.7% survived to hospital discharge. Survival likelihood decreased with increasing age, presence of chronic conditions, diminished functional status on hospital admission, and by admission diagnosis. Patients with sepsis on admission had the lowest post-CPR survival. Conversely, patients with cardiovascular, neurologic, or vascular admitting diagnoses had higher survival. Admission to the ICU from the operating room or recovery room was associated with better survival (22.3% vs. ≤15.5%) for admission from other locations. The type of unit (CTICU, MICU/CCU, MICU/SICU, or SICU/trauma) was not associated with survival to hospital discharge. Multivariate analysis identified four significant poor prognostic factors: having at least one chronic illness, a calculated admission mortality probability of 25% or more, failure of three or more organ systems during the ICU stay, and an admission diagnosis of sepsis/septic shock.

Pediatric

It is estimated that more than 4,000 children in the United States receive in-hospital CPR each year, most in the PICU (16,17). Data from the Virtual PICU Systems (VPS, LLC) database from 2009 to 2013, encompassing almost 330,000 children admitted to 108 PICUs, reported a 2.2% rate for PICU IHCA (18). Overall survival was 65%, which contrasts with 43.4% survival reported from the most recent analysis of the GWTG-R data (19). Both databases collected and entered CA events based on the need for chest compressions or defibrillation, yet the reported survival is markedly different between the two populations. There was no association between center volume and mortality on analysis of the VPS data, after adjusting for known factors affecting arrest outcome. Similar to the adult experience, there were unexplained wide variations in mortality (20), suggesting opportunities for improvement.

A 10-year analysis (2000–2010) of GWTG-R data identified 5,870 pediatric IHCAs from 315 reporting hospitals. A high proportion of pediatric arrests occur in the ICU (93.3%) (21). Over this period, there was a significant increase in the proportion of IHCA occurring in the ICU compared with the wards. Comparison of the rate of return of spontaneous circulation (ROSC) in the 2000 to 2003 period to the 2004 to 2010 period found a concomitant increase in ROSC in association with a higher proportion of the arrests occurring in the ICU (19). Despite the higher ROSC rate, 24-hour survival was significantly higher in ward arrests (62%) compared with ICU arrests (53%), possibly reflecting that the ICU population was more ill. There was an insignificant trend toward better hospital survival in the ward versus ICU population (49% vs. 39%) (21). Analysis of GWTG-R data found the initial CA rhythm was asystole or pulseless electrical activity in 84.8% of children with an increasing frequency of PEA over 10 years. Despite the high rate of nonshockable rhythms, improved survival to discharge over time was not associated with higher rates of neurologic disability among survivors (19).

The explanation for the improved ROSC rate is not clear; it could reflect greater implementation of rapid response teams (RRT) or medical emergency teams (MET) leading to early transfer to the PICU where there is a rapid response to monitored patients; however, as the authors' note, "the limited data in the GWTG-R database and the study design preclude such attributions" (21). These data do suggest that the focus of ALS training should be concentrated on PICU staff as most IHCAs occur there. Since few IHCAs occur on the ward, training ward staff may be best focused on recognizing physiologic deterioration and activation of the RRT/MET (22).

BASIC LIFE SUPPORT

The primary goal of CPR is to generate sufficient oxygen delivery to the coronary and cerebral circulations to maintain cellular viability while attempting to restore a perfusing cardiac rhythm by defibrillation, pharmacologic intervention, or both. Although BLS is often assigned to less experienced health care providers, suggesting that it is easy to perform or relatively unimportant, data show that BLS performance is often suboptimal. In the out-of-hospital setting, the increased focus on high-quality BLS in the 2010 Guidelines (23) improved survival (24), particularly in patients with nonshockable rhythms (25), whereas ALS medications have not been shown to affect outcome. The improvement is even more impressive in children: from 2001 to 2013, rates of ROSC from IHCA increased from 39% to 77% and survival to hospital discharge improved from 24% to 43% (6,19).

The importance of high-quality CPR is illustrated by a recent post hoc analysis of the large OHCA study evaluating the effectiveness of the impedance threshold device (ITD) (26,27). The trial suggested no beneficial effect from the ITD (26), but when only patients who received "acceptable" CPR—defined from electronic recording of compression rate, depth, and compression fraction in 6,199 patients—were evaluated, use of an active ITD was associated with an approximately 50% improvement in the proportion of patients who survived to hospital discharge (9.6% vs. 6.4%) (27).

The fundamental performance metrics of high-quality CPR include the following: ensure chest compressions of adequate rate; ensure chest compressions of adequate, but not excessive, depth; allow full chest recoil between compressions; minimize interruptions in chest compressions; and avoid excessive ventilation. The CoSTR BLS update for adults (2,3) and children (7) focused on the evidence supporting these elements, which are reviewed below.

Starting CPR

After many years of teaching the ABC's of CPR, the emphasis on chest compression led to a recommendation to start with compressions first (compression–airway–breathing, CAB) (23) using a compression-to-ventilation ratio of 30:2 in adults and children for a single rescuer, and 15:2 ratio in children when there are two rescuers in recognition of the importance of ventilation in children. There are no human studies that directly evaluated the impact of this change; manikin studies of low quality reported earlier initiation of chest compressions, leading to the CoSTR suggestion to commence CPR with compressions rather than ventilations (2). It is important to recognize that IHCA, especially in the ICU, is more likely to have multiple rescuers immediately available. Thus, even though BLS algorithms illustrate a stepwise approach, integrated teams of trained rescuers should provide a choreographed simultaneous response where compressions are started, the airway is opened and ventilation is begun, and the rhythm is assessed with shocks provided rapidly if indicated (3).

Chest Compressions

In 1960, Kouwenhoven et al. reported successful resuscitation of dogs and, subsequently, humans with VF cardiac arrest using the combination of closed chest compression, artificial respiration, and electrical defibrillation (28). They hypothesized that the heart was physically squeezed between the sternum and vertebral column, whereby the blood flow generated is similar to the mechanism of spontaneous contraction of the heart; hence, this is called the "cardiac pump" model. This model, however, does not explain several clinical observations that conflict with the cardiac pump theory, such as the ineffectiveness of CPR during flail chest, although theoretically it should be easier to compress the heart in this condition, or the effectiveness of closed chest CPR in patients with a hyperinflated chest due to severe emphysema.

The cardiac pump model was challenged in the 1970s by a report of ROSC with cough during VF (29). In 1980, Rudikoff et al. reported that fluctuations of intrathoracic pressures were primarily responsible for blood flow during CPR (30). These findings supported a noncardiac or "thoracic pump" mechanism for blood flow during CPR. This model proposes that increased intrathoracic pressure during chest compression elevates the pressure of blood located in structures within the thorax, creating the gradient for forward blood flow from intrathoracic to lower-pressure extrathoracic arteries. During relaxation, intrathoracic pressure drops, resulting in refilling of the heart with blood; in this model, the heart acts as a passive conduit. Echocardiographic studies to elucidate the pumping mechanism during cardiac arrest failed to resolve the controversy (31,32). It appears that in adults with thin chest walls, direct cardiac compression does occur, whereas in prolonged resuscitation and in patients with thick chest walls or hyperinflated lungs, the thoracic pump mechanism becomes the predominant flow mechanism; it is also likely that both mechanisms are involved in some cases.

In infants and children, direct cardiac compression is well supported by observation of CPR performed in children while changing the compression position (33,78). Currently, closed chest compression is the standard method of producing blood flow during CPR for both adult and pediatric victims.

In 2015, the evidence for the recommendation to compress over the lower half of the sternum was reevaluated (2,3), as several small clinical studies had yielded conflicting results. One crossover trial in 17 adults with prolonged (>30 minutes) arrest found significant improvements in peak arterial pressure and end-tidal carbon dioxide ($ETCO_2$) with compression over the lower half of the sternum compared with the middle of the chest (34). An out-of-hospital study in intubated CA patients used $ETCO_2$ to monitor the effect of compressing at four different hand positions (35). There was no significant difference with compressing at different locations, but they noted significant interindividual differences, suggesting that using a physiologic feedback tool, such as $ETCO_2$, may help optimize hand position and compression depth during CPR. The lack of new data led to the suggestion to perform chest compressions over the lower half of the sternum (2).

An optimal chest compression rate maximizes cardiac output, recognizing that excessive rates may limit time for diastolic filling, which is a passive process during CPR. Too low a rate leads to low cardiac output. Observational data from large clinical trials—representing 13,469 adults—suggest that the optimal rate is still unknown, but appears to be less than 140 beats/min (36,37). The most recent analysis, after adjusting for compression fraction (defined as compression time ÷ total CPR time) and compression depth, found a significant association between a compression rate of 100 to 119 compressions/min and likelihood for survival (37); higher compression rates were associated with worse outcome.

In 2010, a compression depth of at least 5 cm (2 in) was recommended for all cardiac arrest victims with compressions performed on a firm surface such as backboard (23). There is no evidence, and some concern for harm, for attempting to place a backboard under a patient with multiple vascular lines at risk for dislodgement. Air-filled mattresses are common in the ICU and routinely should be deflated during CPR. Observational studies suggest that survival may improve with increasing compression depth (38,39). Analysis of electronically recorded data from 9,136 adults with OHCA found that optimal ROSC and survival were associated with a compression depth between 40.3 mm and 55.3 mm, with no difference between men and women. Based on data from one relatively small observational study (170 patients) observing injuries in 63% of patients with compression depth of more than 6 cm versus 31% when compression depth was less than 6 cm (40), the 2015 recommendation is to compress approximately 5 cm while avoiding excessive chest compression depths (i.e., ≥6 cm) (2).

Since blood return to the heart during CPR is related to the pressure difference between extrathoracic and intrathoracic venous pressure, it makes sense to limit actions that raise intrathoracic pressure, such as failure to allow full chest recoil. Animal studies show that leaning on the chest precluding full chest recoil reduced the coronary perfusion pressure (CPP) and cardiac index (41,42). These animal data are supported by a clinical study in anesthetized children undergoing cardiac catheterization, which showed that applying sternal pressure comparable to leaning during CPR significantly reduced the CPP (43). These observations support the ILCOR suggestion to avoid leaning on the chest between chest compressions to allow full chest wall recoil (2,7).

One advantage of pausing to check the rhythm and pulse every 2 minutes was to also remind rescuers to change the compressor, since data showed rescuer fatigue resulting in reduced compression depth and frequency after 2 minutes (23). In the ICU, the need to pause chest compressions to provide ventilations should be infrequent since the airway is typically secured, but changing compressors every 2 minutes is still recommended.

Airway management in the hospital is well covered in Chapter 39 and will not be reviewed in this chapter. When a secure airway is in place, continuous chest compressions should be provided along with a ventilation rate of around 6 to 10 breaths/min. If the patient has an arterial line, it is typically unnecessary to pause to check for pulses since ROSC is often visible by the return of a pulsatile arterial pressure wave. Similarly, as discussed in more detail below, continuous monitoring of $ETCO_2$ during CPR may limit the need to interrupt compressions since the $ETCO_2$ typically rises prior to clinical recognition of ROSC (44). There are no data demonstrating the value of pausing every 2 minutes for a pulse check during IHCA, so no treatment recommendation was made regarding the value of a pulse check (2,3).

The emphasis on reducing interruptions of chest compressions is also reflected in the recommendation to immediately resume chest compression after shock delivery (2), which is based on OHCA observational data from three studies enrolling 3,094 OHCA patients showing that pausing to check the rhythm after a shock resulted in harm with respect to discharge from the hospital (45–47). If alternative physiologic evidence suggests ROSC (e.g., arterial waveform or $ETCO_2$), chest compressions can be paused to assess the rhythm. Although some modern defibrillators have electronic filters that attempt to remove motion artifact and potentially permit the monitoring of cardiac rhythm during chest compression, there are no human studies at this time, leading to the ILCOR suggestion against using artifact-filtering algorithms for electrocardiogram (ECG) analysis during CPR unless done as part of a research study (2).

Feedback to Improve CPR Quality

To improve the quality of CPR (compression rate and depth, and ventilation rate), various devices such as metronomes and visual cues have been used. Visual displays on the bedside monitor may guide compression quality, but there is little data from IHCA evaluating the utility of these devices in adults. In OHCA, a sizeable (1,586 patients) cluster-randomized trial of trained EMS providers did not find any difference in survival to hospital discharge or ROSC when using audio and visual feedback on the monitor–defibrillator (48). A small (101 patient) in-hospital study using a CPR-sensing device with feedback showed small improvements in meeting guideline-recommended compression rate and ventilation rate, although the latter was still much higher than recommended (18 ± 8 breaths/min) (49).

The importance of achieving adequate compression depth, rate, and permitting full relaxation was demonstrated in a relatively small study in children in the PICU or ED who were resuscitated using a feedback device applied to the chest (50). Of note, most of the children were older than 8 years, so they were closer in physiology to adults. Both ROSC and 24-hour survival were significantly improved by providing feedback (adjusted odds ratio [aOR] = 10.3; 95% CI: 2.75–38.8) and aOR = 4.21 (95% CI: 1.34–13.2), respectively. Survival to hospital discharge with good neurologic outcome trended higher in those achieving high-quality CPR (18% vs. 5%) but improvement was not significant because of small numbers.

A recent analysis of pediatric OHCA data in the Resuscitation Outcomes Consortium (ROC) Epistry that used an electronic monitoring device noted low compliance with the American Heart Association (AHA) BLS Guidelines (51). Compliance was defined as over 60% of the 1-minute epochs achieving a compression rate of 100 to 120/min, depth of 38 mm or more, and chest compression fraction (CCF) of at least 0.8. Overall, there were 390 children in the registry; 244 were 12 years or older. Overall, only 22% achieved compliance for compression rate and CCF, and 58% for compression depth alone, suggesting there is a need to improve CPR quality. Unfortunately, when adjusting for potential confounders, there was no difference in the rate of ROSC associated with compliance, but if compression depth met the criteria, ROSC was improved (49.4% vs. 29.7%) (51).

Based on these data and data from other observational studies mainly in adults, CoSTR suggests it may be reasonable to use real-time audiovisual feedback and prompt devices during CPR in clinical practice (2,3,7). They emphasize that these devices should not be used in isolation and instead should be part of a comprehensive system that includes team training and individual training on BLS skills. Recording CPR feedback devices can be helpful in debriefing to provide feedback on performance.

ADVANCED LIFE SUPPORT

ALS encompasses a range of interventions from mechanical devices to compress the chest, devices to enhance circulation during CPR including the use of extracorporeal membrane oxygenation (ECMO), and devices to secure the airway, delivery of shocks, physiologic monitoring during CPR, drugs during CPR, and postresuscitation care.

Defibrillation Strategies for VF and pVT

Defibrillation is defined as delivery of electrical energy resulting in termination of VF for at least 5 seconds following the shock (4). The goal is to quickly depolarize the myocardium, terminating the malignant rhythm and hoping that a sinus rhythm will be reinitiated. In most adults, the initial postshock rhythm is asystole or an organized slow rhythm without a pulse (i.e., PEA). This observation is the basis for the recommendation to immediately begin chest compressions after shock delivery. There were no major changes regarding defibrillation between the 2010 (52) and 2015 (4,5) CoSTR conclusions based on the review of available evidence.

Defibrillator Device

Although there are two types of defibrillator devices available, based on the mode and waveform of electrical current delivered—that is, monophasic and biphasic—for more than 10 years newly manufactured defibrillators only produced biphasic waveforms. Although randomized clinical trials have not conclusively documented that biphasic defibrillators save more lives, animal and human data show that biphasic defibrillators have a higher first-shock success in terminating VF compared with monophasic devices and cause less postshock myocardial dysfunction (52,53). Somewhat surprisingly, there is only one study of pulsed biphasic waveforms, in 104 patients, which used a defibrillator that was not impedance adjusted (i.e., the delivered current is not adjusted for chest impedance, which is standard in current defibrillators) (54). In the absence of new data, the 2015 CoSTR recommendation is to use a biphasic waveform defibrillator for both atrial and ventricular arrhythmias in preference to a monophasic defibrillator (4,55). Furthermore, there are no data that define the optimal energy dose, so ILCOR makes a strong recommendation based on weak data to follow the manufacturer's instructions for first and subsequent energy doses.

Biphasic defibrillators can also be further classified based on the delivered waveform into (a) biphasic truncated exponential (BTE) waveform and (b) rectilinear biphasic (RLB) waveform. Based on limited data, the 2010 guidelines recommended a first dose energy of 150 to 200 J for BTE and no lower than 120 J for an RLB waveform defibrillator (52,53). More recent data found single first-shock success of about 88% and first-shock success for recurrent VF of about 84% using 120 J with an RLB defibrillator (56). There was no new data to change the recommendation to use a single shock rather than stacked shocks, and there are no new data evaluating escalating energy doses when the first-shock dose was not successful. In the absence of new data, CoSTR suggests if the first shock is not successful and the defibrillator is capable of delivering higher energy shocks, it is reasonable to increase the energy for subsequent shocks (4).

Recurrent fibrillation after successful defibrillation occurs in the majority of patients (56,57). There are no data showing the need for a different energy dose for recurrent fibrillation; the CoSTR suggestion is to use an escalating energy dose protocol to manage this dysrhythmia. In children with IHCA, VF occurs more often during ALS rather than as the initial dysrhythmia (58). The outcome following late-onset VF is much worse than when VF is the initial rhythm, suggesting that the late occurrence of VF may represent the effects of epinephrine given in the setting of an increasingly hypoxic–ischemic myocardium. It is likely that the same physiologic mechanism may occur in some adults when VF develops during ALS therapy. It is unknown if a different energy dose or waveform may be beneficial in treating refibrillation or late-onset VF/pVT.

Other important elements of safe shock delivery that were not specifically reviewed or updated include a recommendation to use self-adhesive pads rather than defibrillation paddles, avoiding the use of saline-soaked pads as a conductive medium, and avoiding oxygen in the immediate vicinity during shock delivery. When placing electrode pads or paddles, the rescuer should make sure they are not overlapping and are not on top of implanted devices or transdermal medicine patches if present; if the patient is wet, the chest should be wiped dry before placement.

The optimal dose for effective defibrillation in infants and children is not known, with analysis of the GWTG-R IHCA data noting lower first-shock success with 4 J/kg versus 2 J/kg (59). The upper limit for safe defibrillation is also not known, but doses more than 4 J/kg and as high as 9 J/kg have effectively defibrillated children (159,160) and pediatric animal models (161) with no significant reported adverse effects. Recommended manual defibrillation (monophasic or biphasic) doses for children are 2 J/kg for the first attempt and 4 J/kg for subsequent attempts.

Circulatory Support during CPR

This section reviews a range of devices designed to improve blood flow during CPR, including the inspiratory impedance threshold device (ITD), active compression–decompression CPR (ACD-CPR), mechanical devices to enhance chest compressions and reduce the time when compressions are not being delivered, and the use of extracorporeal support (ECMO or cardiopulmonary bypass) during CPR (ECPR). Most of the data on the use of these devices, other than ECPR, is derived from OHCA studies, which may limit its application in the ICU; however, patients may arrive with these devices in place and ICU physicians should be knowledgeable about their indications and use.

Impedance Threshold Device

The impedance threshold device (ITD) was developed to enhance venous return during CPR by reducing the intrathoracic pressure during chest wall recoil. The device is placed between the end of an endotracheal tube or face mask and the resuscitation bag, it then limits air entry into the lungs during chest recoil or when the patient spontaneously breathes; in the latter circumstance, the patient needs to overcome the inspiratory threshold pressure for air flow to occur. The resulting modest reduction in intrathoracic pressure enhances venous return to the heart between chest compressions and, thus, cardiac output. Despite extensive animal data showing that the ITD device enhances venous return, cardiac output, and vital organ blood flow, several randomized controlled trials (RCTs) failed to show a beneficial effect on outcomes, ranging from ROSC to survival to hospital discharge, and 1-year neurologic survival (26,60,61).

Several trials demonstrated a significant improvement in the ROSC rate, survival to hospital discharge, and survival at 1 year with the use of ACD-CPR compared with standard CPR (S-CPR) (26,62,63). ACD-CPR uses a suction cup device placed on the chest to achieve active chest expansion, which lowers intrathoracic pressure, enhancing venous return and, thus, compression-induced cardiac output. The addition of an ITD to ACD-CPR did not improve any of the important outcome measures, but a recent analysis of the quality data from the Resuscitation Outcomes Consortium (https://roc.uwctc.org/) trial (26) found that when the analysis is repeated, looking only at the more than 1,600 patients who had good-quality CPR, use of an active-ITD increased survival to hospital discharge with a modified Rankin Score of at least 3 compared with sham-ITD (7.2% vs. 4.1%; $p = 0.006$) (27). Interestingly, when the quality of CPR was not "acceptable," use of an active-ITD was associated with significantly worse outcome at hospital discharge. Another meta-analysis noted that when the effect of ACD-CPR or the ITD on OHCA outcome is adjusted for whether the arrest was witnessed and for short response time, the ITD device is associated with improved ROSC rates, which are further enhanced by application of ACD-CPR (64). These data illustrate one of the important caveats related to studies evaluating CPR devices—it is often difficult to assure that the quality of CPR is consistent.

Since treatment recommendations are generally not based on post hoc analysis of clinical research data (27), CoSTR recommends against the routine use of an ITD in addition to conventional CPR (4). A consensus recommendation could not be reached for the use of the ITD in combination with ACD-CPR. Furthermore, they note that the optimal compression and ventilation rates using ACD-CPR, with or without an ITD, are unknown. The value of ITD plus ACD-CPR for IHCA also remains to be determined. There is potential utility for the ITD device in spontaneously breathing patients with hypotension to help stabilize their blood pressure and perfusion by enhancing venous return (65,66).

There are no clinical data on the use of ACD-CPR or an ITD device during CPR in children. Pediatric animal studies show that ACD-CPR improves cardiac output and vital organ perfusion, and that the addition of an ITD does not enhance blood flow in this setting (67).

Mechanical CPR Devices

These devices are designed to assure consistent chest compression, sometimes with active decompression, and address the variability observed in clinical trials due to rescuer fatigue and other factors that may affect the depth and rate of chest compression. In theory, these devices would be particularly useful in the OHCA setting when there are relatively few rescuers to provide chest compressions.

The best studied device is the Lund University Cardiac Arrest System (LUCAS), now in a version 2, which is an electrically driven piston with a suction cup designed to provide active decompression as well as compression. The device delivers compressions of 40 to 53 mm in depth, depending on patient size, at a rate of 102 compressions/min with equal time in the compression and relaxation phase. Despite its theoretic benefits, a pragmatic large (4,471 nontraumatic OHCA patients) cluster-randomized trial conducted in four UK Ambulance Services failed to observe any benefit from the use of the LUCAS-2 device over manual CPR in 30-day survival (6% with LUCAS-2 and 7% with manual CPR) (68); ROSC rate was also not different between groups. A meta-analysis of the UK study (68) combined with the two prior RCTs of LUCAS (69,70) failed to show any benefit in 30-day survival, survival to discharge, or neurologic function at 3 months.

An automatic load-distributing band device produces mechanical chest compression without an active relaxation phase. In animal studies, the device produced significantly higher blood flow compared with manual chest compression, but the initial multicenter RCT was halted prematurely because of reduced survival to hospital discharge associated with the use of the device (71). It was thought that higher mortality resulted from the time required to place the device, resulting in less overall chest compressions. A more recent RCT with three US and two European EMS systems compared high-quality manual CPR with an integrated automated load-distributing band. More than 4,000 nontraumatic OHCA patients were included and, again, there was no difference in sustained ROSC, 24-hour survival, or survival to hospital discharge (72).

Based on the current evidence, CoSTR suggests against the routine use of automated chest compression devices in place of high-quality manual chest compression, but they note that these devices may be a reasonable alternative to manual chest compression where maintaining sustained high-quality chest compression may be impractical or puts the rescuer at risk (4). Rescuer risk includes, an unrestrained provider delivering sustained chest compressions in the back of a moving ambulance, or CPR during certain procedures (e.g., coronary angiography or preparing the patient for ECPR); these are situations where mechanical devices have been used successfully (73). There are no data on the use of these devices in children and, based on the ALS recommendations, they should not routinely be used.

Extracorporeal CPR

This refers to the use of ECMO or cardiopulmonary bypass to restore blood flow during CA and provide support until the underlying cause of the arrest is corrected or stabilized. ECPR was first used in children more than 30 years ago as reported in a case series of 33 children with IHCA after open-heart surgery (74). Its use has expanded beyond children to adults for IHCA (75–78) and OHCA (79). Clearly, implementation of ECPR requires a substantial investment in both equipment and manpower with extensive training to reduce the time between request and implementation. This limits its application to major medical centers with appropriate staffing, although the technology continues to evolve making it easier to implement.

There are no RCTs of ECPR; reported studies may reflect reporting bias, but they all note improved survival to hospital discharge, 30-day survival, and intact neurologic survival—defined as cerebral performance category (CPC) score of 1 or 2 (75,77–79). One trial used propensity-matched samples and reported a significantly higher survival with favorable neurologic outcome based on an analysis of 975 patients with IHCA who underwent CPR for more than 10 minutes. Of these, 113 receiving conventional CPR were propensity matched to 59 who received ECPR. The ECPR group had significantly better outcome (RR, 4.67, 95% CI: 1.85–4.26) (78). A more recent trial evaluated ECPR as part of an organized approach to refractory CA. The CHEER trial (mechanical **C**PR, **H**ypothermia, **E**CMO and **E**arly **R**eperfusion) was conducted at a single Australian center. They enrolled patients after either IHCA or OHCA with refractory CA. Recognizing there was likely a selection bias in this high-risk group, they achieved an impressive 54% survival to hospital discharge with intact neurologic recovery (CPC 1–2) in 26 patients (77). Of note, 11 of these patients were OHCA and, overall, 42% of the patients underwent percutaneous coronary intervention (PCI) and one had a pulmonary embolectomy. This rate of good neurologic outcome survival is similar to a report of 32 patients with IHCA of whom 10 were placed on ECPR after ROSC, but with persistent cardiogenic shock; overall 47% survived with CPC 1 to 2 neurologic status (76).

The benefit of ECPR after OHCA is uncertain since there are limited data. A case series of 26 patients at two urban centers who had ECPR implemented in the ED or within 1 hour of arrival reported survival to hospital discharge in four patients (15%), three of whom had CPC scores of 1 to 2 at 6 months (79). A population-based analysis of 320 OHCA patients from 2009 to 2013 who received ECPR in Korea (representing about 1% of eligible OHCA patients) found no significant difference in neurologically favorable survival to discharge after adjusting for covariates (80). Similarly, although cold-water drowning is thought to provide some neurologic protection, an 11-year cohort of ECPR provided to 20 patients with hypothermic (core temperature below 30°C) OHCA associated with drowning found that despite ECMO, only four survived more than 24 hours and two survived to hospital discharge; only one had good neurologic survival (81). It is also noteworthy that cannulation was attempted in 41 patients, but achieved in only about half of them, illustrating the complexity of applying this therapy rapidly. These OHCA data suggest that the role of ECPR for asphyxial OHCA is unclear.

A recent analysis of the GWTG-R data for IHCA in children (<18 years old) who received CPR for 10 minutes or longer compared outcomes of children who also received ECPR to a propensity-matched control group. Over 11 years (2000–2011), there were 3,756 IHCAs that met entry criteria; 591 (16%) received ECPR (82). After adjusting for covariates, patients receiving ECPR were more likely to survive to discharge (40% vs. 27% with conventional CPR), and survive with favorable neurologic outcome (27% vs. 18%); similar findings were observed when the ECPR group was compared with a propensity-matched cohort with significantly better survival to discharge and favorable neurologic outcome, respectively (OR, 1.70; 95% CI: 1.33–2.18) and (OR, 1.78; 95% CI: 1.31–2.41).

Based on the available data, CoSTR suggests ECPR is a reasonable rescue therapy for selected patients with cardiac arrest when conventional CPR fails to achieve ROSC (4,6); implementation is limited by financial and logistical limitations. Moreover, intensivists recognize that ECPR introduces potential ethical issues, such as when a patient's cardiovascular status is stabilized but significant neurologic injury is present. There are also many unknown factors that need to be elucidated to further improve outcome with this technology. These include defining the optimal subgroup of patients who would benefit, the optimal flow rate for ECPR, the duration of ECPR, and the desired target temperature on ECPR.

Physiologic Monitoring during CPR

Physiologic monitoring may provide feedback to guide resuscitation efforts and improve the quality of CPR-induced blood flow and oxygen delivery.

Hemodynamic Monitoring

The focused attention on delivering high-quality chest compressions, limiting excessive ventilation, and using devices to support circulation would be enhanced by monitoring the achievement of explicit hemodynamic goals during CPR. Unfortunately, hemodynamic measurement is often limited during CPR, but ICU patients often have invasive central venous and arterial pressure monitors; once the patients is ventilated, $ETCO_2$ is measured using bedside capnography. Additional sources of potentially valuable data to guide resuscitation efforts include measurement of cerebral oxygen tension by use of near-infrared devices. As Dr. Max Harry Weil—one of the fathers of modern resuscitation—stated 20 years ago, "Performing CPR without measuring the effects is like flying an airplane without an altimeter" (83). The guideline recommendations for depth, rate, and location for compression are just that—guidelines—there is no reason to think that a single compression depth, rate, and location will be optimal for all patients. Similarly, giving epinephrine by the clock rather than based on documented hemodynamic parameters will likely be considered somewhat primitive 10 years from now.

It has long been recognized that CPP is a primary determinant of resuscitation survival since it is a major determinant of myocardial blood flow, which is the parameter we are most interested in restoring and preserving (84,85). Achieving good myocardial blood flow is the main rationale for minimizing the time without effective chest compressions and avoiding excessive ventilations that compromise venous return (86–88). In the ICU, the CPP can be estimated from the difference between the diastolic arterial blood pressure and central venous pressure. Based on animal data, a minimal CPP of 20 mmHg was critical to ROSC (84). More recent animal data showed that using a hemodynamically driven resuscitation approach to achieve a CPP greater than 20 mmHg, rather than using one of two fixed compression depths and epinephrine boluses per AHA Guidelines, resulted in significantly greater ROSC and short-term survival in asphyxial (89) and VF arrest (90). Of note, the animals resuscitated based on hemodynamic monitoring did not receive more epinephrine, suggesting that the improved outcome did not result from more epinephrine, but instead from giving epinephrine at the right time when needed to maintain the CPP.

There are only limited human data at present, and no prospective human study, that show targeting the CPP during resuscitation improves survival. A study in 1990 of 100 OHCA patients who had right atrial and arterial catheters placed after failure of ROSC documented that those who eventually developed ROSC (25 patients) had significantly higher CPPs (91). Only those patients whose CPP was at least 15 mmHg achieved ROSC; there are no data on the optimal CPP for children.

In view of the lack of any clinical data, other than observational studies, describing changes in CPP or diastolic arterial pressure with different CPR techniques (e.g., interposed abdominal compression-CPR and ACD-CPR) CoSTR made no treatment recommendations on using this approach. In the ICU where this monitoring is readily available, it is the author's opinion that this is a reasonable approach to guide BLS and bolus epinephrine administration.

End-Tidal Carbon Monoxide Monitoring

$ETCO_2$ measurement evaluates the partial pressure of CO_2 at the end of an exhaled breath. CO_2 is delivered to the lungs for elimination based on pulmonary blood flow. In low blood flow states, as long as minute ventilation is relatively fixed, the $ETCO_2$ reflects effective pulmonary blood flow (i.e., cardiac output) (92). During CPR, $ETCO_2$ is typically low, characterizing the low cardiac output during CPR and the relatively high minute ventilation relative to pulmonary blood flow. Multiple animal and adult studies show a strong correlation between $ETCO_2$ concentration and interventions that increase cardiac output during CPR in cardiac arrest or in shock models (35,93–96). Similarly, animal models demonstrate that changes in $ETCO_2$ correlate directly with controlled changes in cardiac output (92,97–99). Recently, an analysis of chest compression rate, depth, and $ETCO_2$ in 583 OHCA and IHCA patients showed a linear relationship between chest compression depth and increases in $ETCO_2$ (100). By extrapolation, these data support using $ETCO_2$ monitoring to assess the effect of efforts to increase cardiac output during CPR.

Multiple observational studies performed in adults over more than 25 years, across different countries, both with IHCA and OHCA (101–107) report an association between higher $ETCO_2$ and ROSC, but there is no specific $ETCO_2$ threshold that accurately predicts ROSC. This is partly due to the lack of standardization among studies with analysis of $ETCO_2$ at various time points during resuscitation. Substantial animal and human data (103–105,108,109) and two pediatric prospective cohort studies (93,110) noted an association between persistently low $ETCO_2$ and failure to achieve ROSC, usually after 20 minutes of CPR. Part of the difficulty in identifying a target value of $ETCO_2$ to guide resuscitation or to be used for prognosis is that the value depends on the etiology and duration of the arrest and resuscitation.

Interpretation of $ETCO_2$ concentration during resuscitation is affected by the quality of the measurement, the minute ventilation delivered during resuscitation, the presence of lung disease that increases anatomic dead space, and the presence of right to left shunting, as may occur in children with congenital heart disease (111–113). In addition, therapeutic interventions may affect the reading; specifically, sodium bicarbonate transiently increases $ETCO_2$ concentration since CO_2 is generated as it buffers excess protons (114–116). The time delay between the appearance of increased $ETCO_2$ following sodium bicarbonate administration is directly related to the cardiac output (116), and is consistently observed in ventilated patients, leading to the suggestion to use $ETCO_2$ monitoring to confirm intraoperative central venous line insertion in children (115). Epinephrine, or other vasoconstrictive agents, improves CPP through intense vasoconstriction, which decreases global blood flow; thus, it is not surprising that a transient fall in $ETCO_2$ is observed following epinephrine administration (117–119). The take-home message is to cautiously interpret $ETCO_2$ within 1 to 2 minutes of resuscitation drug administration.

An important limitation of using the *initial* $ETCO_2$ as a prognostic indicator is that there is a significant difference between patients with asphyxial cardiac arrest versus VF/pVT arrest; those with asphyxial arrest are characterized by a period of inadequate ventilation and accumulation of CO_2 (105,108,120). The *initial* $ETCO_2$ concentration in asphyxial arrest is often much higher than the concentration after the first few minutes of CPR. In a relatively small IHCA study of patients with PEA ($n = 50$), the initial $ETCO_2$ was associated with ROSC, but not with survival to discharge (121).

In the absence of high-quality evidence, and in view of the *caveats* in interpretation noted, CoSTR did not suggest using capnography to guide resuscitation efforts. Because of differences in study methodology, emergency response systems, and resuscitation guidelines, the data do not support a specific threshold of $ETCO_2$ to reliably predict failure of ROSC.

It is noteworthy that clinical studies consistently observe a sudden rise of $ETCO_2$ with the onset of ROSC, which often precedes recognition of ROSC by clinical signs (44,104). This observation suggests that continuous monitoring of $ETCO_2$ could replace the need to check for ROSC during CPR in the ICU or other areas where capnography is available. The technology is available, but not consistently used, during CPR in the ICU, since patients are often removed from mechanical ventilation and manually ventilated without capnography being maintained. Even when available, a recent survey found that capnography was used less than half the time to monitor the effectiveness of CPR during IHCA and it was uncommonly used to provide prognostic information (122).

Ultrasound during CPR

Ultrasound (US) is increasingly being used for a wide range of indications as the technology becomes more widely available in the ICU (see Chapter 25) (123). The value of US in identifying a potentially reversible cause of CA such as pericardial tamponade or pulmonary embolus is uncertain since there are only case reports or biased case series. Echocardiography may be helpful to document the effectiveness of mechanical compression devices, such as the LUCAS-2 device, where echocardiography documented ineffective cardiac compression in a recent case report (124).

One observational study suggested that using a focused echocardiographic examination to identify pseudo-PEA during resuscitation ($n = 19$) was helpful in improving ROSC by changing the therapeutic approach to the patients' resuscitation, although it is notable that the comparison group was historical controls (125). An RCT evaluated 100 OHCA patients in a convenience sample randomized to standard care or care with the addition of echocardiography (126). They identified the presence of pseudo-PEA in 78% of the 50 patients who underwent echocardiography during resuscitation and all of the patients with ROSC (43%) were in this group; no patient with absent mechanical cardiac activity had ROSC. Despite the identification of pseudo-PEA, however, there was no difference in the overall rate of ROSC between the groups. A systematic review of focused echocardiography identified 12 trials encompassing 568 patients and found that the absence of cardiac activity is associated with a significantly lower, but not zero, likelihood of ROSC, leading to the CoSTR recommendation that echocardiography should *not* be used alone, but rather as an adjunct with clinical assessment and history to determine if ongoing resuscitation efforts should be discontinued (127).

Based on these limited data, the CoSTR suggestion is that cardiac US may be considered as an additional diagnostic tool to identify potentially reversible causes of CA, provided that it does not interfere with standard ACLS interventions, including limiting the need to interrupt chest compressions (4,5).

Arterial Blood Gas Analysis

The acidosis gradient between arterial and central venous blood—largely determined by PCO_2—reflects the effectiveness of blood flow during low-flow states such as CPR (128). Similarly, animal studies and case reports describe similar arteriovenous differences in PCO_2 between arterial and venous blood at the organ level (e.g., heart) and the entire organism (129,130). These studies suggest that measurement and comparison of a venous blood gas (VBG) and arterial blood gas (ABG) may be predictive during CA. Furthermore, it suggests that the ABG does not accurately reflect the severity of tissue hypoxia, acidosis, or hypercarbia during CPR. Instead, an ABG documents the effectiveness of ventilation during CA, which typically reflects overventilation relative to pulmonary blood flow (i.e., hypocarbia). As expected, both animal and human data show a significant worsening of the ABG values for acidosis and oxygenation with ROSC, representing the washout of built-up tissue acids.

Drugs during CPR

Antidysrhythmics, vasopressors, atropine, sodium bicarbonate, calcium, and magnesium are commonly given in some combination to patients who fail to achieve ROSC with BLS interventions. Although these agents have been used for decades, the value, as well as potential harm, from these agents remains a source of controversy and debate. What is clear is that these medications should be delivered as close to the heart as possible since they have to traverse the pulmonary circulation and be delivered to the systemic circulation to exert their pharmacologic effect. Thus, when a central venous line is available, it is the preferred route over a peripheral venous site. The intraosseous route is an acceptable alternative, but is uncommonly required in the ICU or in-hospital setting.

If IV or IO access cannot be achieved, then several resuscitation medications can be administered via instillation through an endotracheal tube (ET) or tracheostomy. Lipid-soluble medications that can be delivered via ET are lidocaine, epinephrine, atropine, naloxone, and vasopressin. This route, however, results in much lower blood concentrations compared with IV administration. Optimal doses of the medications delivered via the ET route are not known, but it is recommended to administer at least 2 to 2½ times the recommended IV doses. Animal data suggest that using standard IV epinephrine doses via the ET route may not achieve high enough plasma concentrations, and in fact may not only be ineffective, but may be harmful by reducing systemic vascular resistance through a greater β_2-adrenergic effect rather than α-adrenergic effect (131,132).

Epinephrine

This is the most commonly used medication during CPR. Epinephrine's primary action in CA is to increase the CPP through systemic vasoconstriction, mediated by its α-adrenergic effects; the β-adrenergic effects are relatively unimportant. Indeed, even when complete β-adrenergic blockade is used in an animal cardiac arrest model, epinephrine is effective, whereas α-adrenergic blockade completely eliminates epinephrine's effects (133).

Epinephrine is used primarily during CA due to asystole or PEA. It is a second-line agent used for shock-refractory VF or pulseless VT. There is substantial animal data, and anecdotal clinical experience, that epinephrine elevates the CPP and, thus, myocardial blood flow, leading to its effectiveness in various models of CA. But, as reviewed below, the clinical trials suggest that epinephrine may have adverse effects on outcomes that are of significance: that is, survival to hospital discharge with good neurologic outcome.

Since epinephrine's beneficial effect is through systemic vasoconstriction, there was some enthusiasm for using higher doses to produce a greater increase in coronary and cerebral perfusion pressure; this hypothesis was supported by animal data (134), but subsequent clinical trials in OHCA in adults (135–137) showed that high-dose epinephrine (HDE) increased ROSC and survival to hospital admission, but had no beneficial effect on survival to hospital discharge. In an RCT of HDE (0.1 mg/kg) versus standard-dose epinephrine (SDE, 0.01 mg/kg) in 68 children with IHCA who failed to respond to an initial standard dose, the HDE did not result in more ROSC and trended toward a worse 24-hour survival (138).

Since the last evidence review in 2010, there have been two RCTs; both were OHCA studies. One compared no drug to drug administration (139), and the other compared SDE to placebo (140). The former compared outcome in patients with IV access and any drug given in OHCA (139) versus no IV access in a European EMS system; thus, the study was not specific to epinephrine and the outcome may have been impacted by the difference between groups in the time spent obtaining vascular access rather than focusing on providing chest compressions. A subsequent post hoc analysis of just those patients who received epinephrine in this trial observed a higher likelihood of hospital admission if the patient received epinephrine, but there was a nonsignificant trend toward a lower rate of survival to hospital discharge in those patients who received epinephrine and a lower functional outcome, as measured by the CPC score (141).

The Australian RCT of epinephrine versus placebo in OHCA also observed a significantly higher likelihood of ROSC (23.5% vs. 8.4%), and a trend toward higher survival to hospital discharge, which was low in both groups (4.0% vs. 1.9%) (140). Combining the data from these two trials with data from previous publications, including a very large adjusted observational trial in OHCA (142), and a smaller study (143), showed that the use of epinephrine was associated with a lower adjusted likelihood of survival to discharge, and functional survival, when compared with no epinephrine in the OHCA population (144).

Within the hospital, there is limited data, but a recent analysis of more than 25,000 IHCA patients in the GWTG-R database provided an interesting observation that may impact outcome. The patients in this analysis had a nonshockable rhythm and patients were excluded from the analysis if the arrest occurred in the emergency department, ICU, or operating room (145). The primary outcome was survival to hospital discharge. They noted that the median time to the first dose of epinephrine was 3 minutes, and there was a stepwise decrease in survival to discharge with increasing interval of time to epinephrine administration when analyzed in 3-minute increments of time. There also was a significantly higher likelihood of ROSC, 24-hour survival, and neurologically intact survival—defined as CPC score of 1 to 2 at discharge—with early epinephrine administration. An analysis of the GWTG-R database found similar outcomes in 1,558 children with a nonshockable rhythm (146). Longer time to epinephrine administration was associated with lower likelihood of survival to hospital discharge after adjusting for known confounders. When comparing patients with first dose more than 5 minutes after arrest to those who received an epinephrine dose within 5 minutes, survival to discharge was 21.0% versus 33.1% ($p = 0.01$) (146).

These apparently contradictory results within the hospital need to be put into context. In-hospital providers typically arrive at the bedside very quickly whereas OHCA is often associated with a delay of 10 minutes or more before vasoactive drugs may be given. Thus, early in CA, such as within the ICU or hospital, early epinephrine administration appears to be beneficial, leading to the CoSTR recommendation to give epinephrine as soon as feasible for IHCA associated with a nonshockable rhythm in adults, but no recommendation was made for children (4,6).

HDE may be considered in clinical conditions characterized by poor adrenergic responsiveness, such as severe septic shock, β-blocker overdose, neuraxial anesthesia, or systemic bupivacaine overdose. Epinephrine should be given intravascularly whenever possible since intratracheal doses are erratically absorbed as noted above.

Vasopressin

Vasopressin is an endogenous antidiuretic hormone that, when given at high doses, causes vasoconstriction by directly stimulating vascular smooth muscle V_1 receptors (147). Vasopressin improves CPP but, unlike epinephrine, offers theoretical advantages of cerebral vasodilation, possibly improving cerebral perfusion. Its lack of β_1-adrenergic activity potentially avoids unnecessary increases of myocardial oxygen demand, which may reduce the likelihood of developing postresuscitation dysrhythmias. Additionally, unlike epinephrine, vasopressin reduces pulmonary vascular resistance, making it potentially useful in patients with pulmonary hypertension (148,149). Vasopressin has a longer half-life of 10 to 20 minutes compared to the 3 to 5 minutes observed with epinephrine.

Human studies in the early 2000s suggested that vasopressin achieved a comparable rate of ROSC in CA, although no additional benefit was seen, compared with epinephrine (150,151). A single RCT of low quality, because of a 37% rate of postrandomization exclusion, evaluated repeated dose of SDE with multiple doses of standard dose vasopressin (40 IU) in the ED after OHCA (152). A total of 336 patients were randomized; there was no advantage of vasopressin in terms of the rate of ROSC or survival to hospital discharge.

Data from animal models suggested that the combination of vasopressin and epinephrine together may achieve better CPP and myocardial blood flow, leading to a higher rate of ROSC and survival. Several clinical trials, however, failed to show that ROSC, survival to hospital admission for OHCA, and survival to hospital discharge were improved by the combined administration of these two agents (151,153–155). One RCT evaluated the combination of vasopressin (20 IU) with epinephrine (1 mg) every 3 minutes of ongoing CPR in 268 patients with IHCA (156). Additionally, patients in the vasopressin group received 40 mg of methylprednisolone and, if in postresuscitation shock, stress dose hydrocortisone was given for 7 days. Unlike the data on vasopressin during OHCA, this IHCA study reported significantly higher rates of ROSC (83.9% vs. 65.9%) and survival to hospital discharge with CPC score of 1 or 2 (13.9%) versus those treated with epinephrine only (5.1%) (156). These limited data suggest that IHCA is different than OHCA and, just like early administration of epinephrine is associated with improved outcome, the addition of vasopressin and steroids may be beneficial when used for IHCA.

There are little pediatric data on the use of vasopressin. An analysis of GWTG-R data for 1,293 IHCA children found that vasopressin was used infrequently (5% of cases), most often in the ICU with prolonged arrest (157). Its use was associated with a lower rate of ROSC, but no difference in the rate of ultimate survival to hospital discharge when compared with children who did not receive vasopressin. Animal data also do not support the use of vasopressin in pediatric asphyxial CA, where the rate of ROSC was higher in animals who received epinephrine alone compared with vasopressin alone or vasopressin together with epinephrine (158). In a pediatric model of VF arrest, vasopressin either alone or with epinephrine produced better myocardial and cerebral blood flow compared with epinephrine (159).

On review of the available evidence, CoSTR suggests against the use of vasopressin alone in adults and children (4,6). They also suggest against adding vasopressin to SDE during CA. For IHCA, there are too few data to make a recommendation for or against the combined use of vasopressin, epinephrine, and corticosteroids (4). There are no data supporting the combination therapy for OHCA.

Antidysrhythmic Agents

Extensive clinical data emphasize the early administration of shocks in patients with VF/pVT, which has been a major focus of efforts to increase access to AED devices in public locations. Within the hospital, the prevalence of an initial shockable rhythm in IHCA is decreasing. When patients have shock-refractory VF/pVT, antidysrhythmic drugs continue to play an important role. Amiodarone remains the main drug used in this setting, but recent pediatric data resulted in a change regarding the use of lidocaine.

Amiodarone

This complex pharmacologic agent has effects on sodium, potassium, and calcium channels on myocardial cells, as well as α- and β-adrenergic blocking properties. Since the 2005 guidelines, amiodarone has been the preferred agent for both atrial and ventricular dysrhythmias, especially in the presence of impaired cardiac function (160).

Amiodarone is recommended for narrow-complex tachycardias that originate from a reentry mechanism (reentry SVT); ectopic atrial focus; control of hemodynamically stable VT, polymorphic VT with a normal QT interval, or wide-complex tachycardia of uncertain origin; and control of rapid ventricular rate due to accessory pathway conduction in pre-excited atrial arrhythmias with AV nodal blockade in patients with preserved or impaired ventricular function (161). Limited data form the basis for the use of amiodarone over lidocaine in OHCA; a single RCT in 504 shock-refractory patients were randomized to amiodarone (300 mg) or placebo. The rate of ROSC and survival to hospital admission was significantly improved, but there was no impact on survival to hospital discharge (162). A new RCT is underway intending to randomize 3,000 patients, but the results are not yet available (163).

There are no adult clinical trials of amiodarone for IHCA. In children, an analysis of the GWTG-R data in 889 IHCAs with VF/pVT found that 19% received amiodarone, 33% received lidocaine, and 10% received both (164). Interestingly, lidocaine was associated with a higher rate of ROSC and 24-hour survival, but not hospital discharge; amiodarone was not associated with a higher rate of ROSC or 24-hour survival. Since this is a retrospective analysis of IHCA, it does not address potential bias related to the selection of one agent over the other.

Based on the available data, amiodarone is suggested in adults with shock-refractory VF/pVT to improve the rates of ROSC (4), but in children, lidocaine is now recommended as an alternative agent to amiodarone, which is a change from the 2010 guidelines (6).

The major adverse effects of amiodarone are hypotension and bradycardia, which can be minimized by slowing the rate of drug infusion. In addition, amiodarone can increase the QT interval, and therefore its use should be carefully considered when the patient receives other drugs that can prolong the QT interval.

Lidocaine

This is a sodium channel blocker that decreases ectopic electrical myocardial activity by raising the electrical stimulation threshold of the ventricle during diastole. In ischemic myocardial tissue after infarction, it may suppress reentrant dysrhythmias such as VT or VF. There is good evidence that amiodarone is superior to lidocaine in terminating VT (165,166); hence, lidocaine is not considered a first-line agent. As noted, the 2015 Guidelines suggest that lidocaine is an acceptable alternative to amiodarone (4,5).

Procainamide

Procainamide suppresses both atrial and ventricular dysrhythmias with similar mechanisms of action to those of lidocaine. It may suppress an ectopic irritable focus and block reentrant dysrhythmias by slowing electrical conduction. Procainamide may be superior to lidocaine in terminating VT (167). Procainamide is used in the management of PVCs, VT, and persistent VF, but amiodarone is usually preferred.

Procainamide can have profound myocardial depressant effects, especially after myocardial infarction; therefore, continuous ECG and arterial blood pressure monitoring are mandatory. End points limiting therapy include hypotension and a greater than 50% widening of the QRS complex.

Nifekalant

This is a class III antidysrhythmic agent according to the Vaughan Williams classification that selectively blocks the rapid component of the delayed rectifier K^+ current. It is not available in the United States, but has been studied and used in Japan for treatment of dysrhythmias associated with CA. Unlike amiodarone, it has a short half-life and is easily soluble for intravenous administration (168). Unfortunately, it tends to prolong the QT interval, leading to a risk of torsades de pointes. When compared with lidocaine in adults with shock-refractory OHCA, there was a significantly higher 24-hour survival with nifekalant, but the 30-day favorable neurologic outcome was similar. Within the hospital, a relatively small study (55 patients) found that nifekalant more effectively led to termination of shock-resistant VF/pVT than lidocaine (169). A systematic review in 2013 concluded that amiodarone, nifekalant, and lidocaine were effective during initial resuscitation as assessed by ROSC and survival to hospital admission, but there is no evidence these agents change the rate of ultimate hospital survival (170).

In view of the relatively limited data, CoSTR suggested that lidocaine or nifekalant is an alternative to amiodarone in adults with shock-refractory VF/pVT (4,5). They also noted that the early trials of amiodarone may have been biased by the use of polysorbate solvent in the placebo group since this agent is known to reduce blood pressure.

Miscellaneous Drug Therapy

Sodium Bicarbonate

Metabolic and respiratory acidosis develops during CA resulting from anaerobic metabolism, leading to lactic acid generation. Inadequate ventilation along with reduced pulmonary blood flow during CPR leads to inadequate pulmonary delivery of carbon dioxide for elimination. Thus, CA patients have a combined respiratory and metabolic acidosis at the tissue level. Untreated acidosis suppresses spontaneous cardiac activity, decreases the electrical threshold required for the onset of VF, decreases ventricular contractile force, and decreases cardiac responsiveness to catecholamines, such as epinephrine. An elevated PCO_2 tension probably is more detrimental to myocardial function and catecholamine responsiveness than metabolic acidosis. CO_2 readily diffuses across myocardial cell membranes, causing intracellular acidosis; likewise, cerebrospinal fluid acidosis may occur secondary to the diffusion of CO_2 across the blood–brain barrier, producing post–arrest cerebral acidosis.

As noted in the section on $ETCO_2$ monitoring, the action of sodium bicarbonate to buffer excess protons transiently increases CO_2 production and thus the partial pressure of CO_2; sodium bicarbonate administration without sufficient ventilation and circulation to remove the CO_2 that it produces is more detrimental than helpful in animal models of post-hypoxic–ischemic acidosis (171,172). Although acidosis is presumed to be harmful and giving sodium bicarbonate to correct the acidosis seems rationale, clinical studies failed to show any beneficial effect, even when used in prolonged cardiac arrest (173). Since 2005, the Guidelines have not recommended the routine use of sodium bicarbonate except in special circumstances such as the treatment of hyperkalemia, to reverse the effects of hypercalcemia, and in the treatment of tricyclic antidepressant overdose (160,174). A recent analysis of patients with IHCA and hyperkalemia, with serum potassium over 6.5 mEq/L measured during CPR, found that sodium bicarbonate administration was significantly associated with ROSC if the potassium concentration was below 7.9 mEq/L (175). Administration of calcium and sodium bicarbonate together was associated with a higher ROSC rate if serum potassium was below 9.4 mEq/L. Prevalence of hyperkalemia in IHCA patients over a 6-year study period was 12% (109 patients) (175). In this population there was low (3.7%) survival to discharge with 92.7% of the patients having PEA or asystole. This study provides support for bicarbonate in the setting of hyperkalemia, but an accompanying editorial notes that the low rate of survival is not supportive and that insulin–glucose solutions are more effective in lowering serum potassium than bicarbonate and calcium, which have little effect on the serum potassium concentration (176,177).

In pediatric IHCA, a recent analysis of the GWTG-R database over 10 years (2000–2010) examined the association between sodium bicarbonate use and patient outcome in 3,719 events (178). Despite the Guideline recommendation to not use bicarbonate, this agent was given in 68% of the IHCA events, although there was a small decrease in the rate of use comparing the first 5 years to the last 5 years. After adjusting for known confounding factors, sodium bicarbonate use was associated with significantly decreased 24-hour survival and decreased survival to discharge. When the analysis was limited to children with metabolic/electrolyte abnormalities, hyperkalemia, or toxicologic diagnoses, sodium bicarbonate use was not associated with worse outcomes. CoSTR did not update their 2015 evidence review or recommendations on the use of sodium bicarbonate.

Atropine

Atropine was used during CPR for its vagolytic actions, but data showed no benefit, leading to its elimination as a routine agent in adult or pediatric resuscitation. Atropine is used to manage hemodynamically significant bradycardia and has been used to reduce the risk of vagal-induced bradycardia during pediatric intubation. The only new data regarding atropine debunked a long-taught recommendation to use a minimal dose in pediatric patients since small doses in infants were thought to produce paradoxical bradycardia. A study in 60 unpremedicated healthy hospitalized infants used an atropine dose of 0.005 mg/kg while continuously monitoring the ECG; no bradycardia was observed (179). A prospective observational study in 264 neonates and children undergoing emergency intubation was propensity adjusted and noted significantly lower ICU mortality in those children who received atropine (180). Another observational study of atropine use in 327 children undergoing emergency intubation reported a lower rate of dysrhythmias, particularly bradycardia (181). The pediatric CoSTR review could not make a recommendation regarding atropine's use because the available studies are biased, but they did recommend weight-based atropine dosing in infants with no lower dose limit (7). The adult CoSTR review in 2015 did not evaluate the use of atropine.

Calcium

This ion plays a critical role in myocardial contractility and action potential generation, but studies have shown no benefit of calcium administration in CA (182,183), and therefore calcium is not recommended for OHCA or IHCA (160). As reviewed above, it may be considered along with sodium bicarbonate during CA associated with acute hyperkalemia (175). It is also indicated when hypocalcemia is suspected, or calcium channel blockers toxicity or overdose is suspected.

Magnesium

Magnesium is recommended for the treatment of torsades de pointes VT with or without cardiac arrest. Although magnesium is a calcium channel blocker and theoretically may protect ischemic cells from calcium overload, there are no data supporting its routine use in cardiac arrest. The data are limited by small numbers in the available clinical trials as reviewed in the CoSTR statement (4,184). Based on the low-quality evidence and lack of documentation of benefit, they recommended against the routine use of magnesium in adults (4,5). Rapid administration may result in hypotension and bradycardia. Magnesium also should be used cautiously in patients with renal failure.

Advanced Airway Management

Tracheal intubation is indicated when the rescuer is unable to adequately ventilate or oxygenate the arrested or unconscious patient with bag-mask ventilation, or if prolonged ventilation is required and airway protective reflexes are absent in the patient with a perfusing rhythm. A properly placed endotracheal tube (ET) is the gold standard method for securing the airway, although supraglottic airways, such as an LMA or Combitube can be effective. Since there are no unique issues with in-hospital airway management in CA, the reader is referred to Chapter 39 for more details on this topic.

It is important to use an $ETCO_2$ detector in addition to careful auscultation and observing symmetric chest rise following intubation. ICLOR recommends using capnography to confirm tube placement and continuous monitoring during CPR to ensure appropriate position of the tracheal tube (4,5).

POSTRESUSCITATION CARE

Successful ROSC is only the first step toward the goal of complete recovery from cardiac arrest. The complex pathophysiologic processes that occur following whole body ischemia and subsequent reperfusion that characterizes ROSC is called the post–cardiac arrest syndrome (14). Depending upon the cause of the arrest, and the severity of the post–cardiac arrest syndrome, many patients require complex multiple organ support (185). The treatment they receive during this postresuscitation period can significantly influence the overall outcome and particularly the quality of neurologic recovery. The effectiveness of this care in the ICU likely explains some of the observed variation in survival to hospital discharge between different centers (11,20,186,187).

The postresuscitation phase starts at the location where ROSC is achieved; once stabilized, the patient should be transferred to the most appropriate high-care area for continued diagnosis, monitoring, and treatment. Transport should include continuous monitoring of pulse oximetry and $ETCO_2$ in the intubated patient.

Significant improvements in outcome have occurred over the last 20 years so that as many as 40% to 50% of comatose patients admitted to ICUs after cardiac arrest survive to hospital discharge, depending on the cause of arrest, EMS and hospital system, and quality of care. Of the patients who survive to hospital discharge, most are reported to have good neurologic outcome (CPC 1 or 2), although many have subtle cognitive impairment (188–190). The therapeutic approach to management of the postarrest patient includes attention to assuring there is a secure airway, providing appropriate ventilation and oxygenation, rapidly identifying and treating the cause of the arrest, supporting the circulation, protecting the brain from further injury, and monitoring and supporting the function of other organs. These topics are detailed below, but the reader should recognize that this is a rapidly evolving field with little high-quality evidence for many of the postarrest therapies, such as who to cool, and if cooled, to what core temperature and for how long.

Post-Cardiac Arrest Syndrome

Following arrest-induced global hypoxia–ischemia with ROSC, there is often variable reperfusion of all organs, depending on the patient's cause of arrest and underlying cardiac function. This reperfusion syndrome often stimulates a host of inflammatory mediators resulting in a clinical picture that mimics the systemic inflammatory response syndrome (SIRS) (191,192). In addition, the arrest period produces myocardial injury of varying severity depending on the duration of arrest and the effectiveness of CPR to maintain coronary perfusion (193–195). Drugs given during the arrest, such as epinephrine, may add to the myocardial injury. The major components of the post–cardiac arrest syndrome consist of the following:

- Brain injury of varying severity
- Myocardial dysfunction of varying severity
- Systemic ischemia-reperfusion injury in multiple organs (185)
- Diffuse endothelial cell injury with activation of inflammatory and coagulation systems
- Physiologic effects from the precipitating cause of the arrest

The severity of this syndrome varies with the duration and cause of the CA; indeed, it may not occur at all if the CA is brief. Post–cardiac arrest brain injury may manifest as coma, seizures, myoclonus, varying degrees of neurocognitive dysfunction, and/or brain death. Among patients surviving to ICU admission after OHCA but subsequently dying during hospitalization, brain injury is the cause of death in approximately two-thirds; this is the case in approximately 25% after IHCA arrest (196,197). Cardiovascular failure accounts for most deaths in the first 3 days in the ICU after OHCA, while brain injury accounts for most of the later deaths (197). Withdrawal of lifesustaining therapy is the most frequent cause of death—seen in approximately 50%—in patients with a poor prognosis (198), emphasizing the importance of having reliable prognostic indicators (see Prognosis, below). Post–cardiac arrest brain injury may be exacerbated by microcirculatory failure, impaired autoregulation, hypotension, hypercarbia, hypoxemia, hyperoxemia, pyrexia, hypoglycemia, hyperglycemia, and seizures. Significant myocardial dysfunction is common after cardiac arrest, but typically begins to recover 2 to 3 days post-ROSC, although full recovery may take significantly longer (195). The whole body ischemia reperfusion of cardiac arrest activates immune and coagulation pathways, contributing to microcirculatory changes leading to multiple organ failure and increasing the risk of infection. Thus, the post–cardiac arrest syndrome has many features in common with sepsis, including increased vascular permeability leading to intravascular volume depletion, which may be exacerbated by inappropriate vasodilation and maldistribution of blood flow, endothelial injury, and abnormalities of the microcirculation (192,195,199,200).

Airway, Ventilation, and Oxygenation

Patients with a brief cardiac arrest who respond immediately to appropriate treatment may achieve an immediate return of normal cerebral function, and thus do not require tracheal intubation and ventilation, but should be given oxygen via a facemask if their SpO_2 is less than 94%. In patients with diminished consciousness or coma, there is little controversy about the importance of securing the airway and assuring appropriate oxygenation and ventilation. However, maximizing PaO_2 following an ischemic insult is not only *not* helpful but appears to be harmful. The harm is thought to result from cellular exposure to high PaO_2 *following* an ischemic injury, resulting in greater oxygen radical–mediated organ injury (201). Several animal studies indicate that hyperoxemia early after ROSC causes oxidative stress and harms postischemic neurons (202). A metaanalysis of 14 observational studies noted significant heterogeneity across studies, with some studies showing that hyperoxemia was associated with a worse neurologic outcome and others failing to show this association (203). A recent retrospective analysis from an ICU database of 184 patients who survived more than 24 hours following ROSC found a significant association between severe hyperoxemia (>300 mmHg) and increased mortality (204). Limited pediatric data did not find an association between hyperoxemia or hypoxemia and outcome (205,206).

Note that an FiO_2 of 1.0 is still recommended during CPR in adults and children (4–6). Provided that the hemoglobin concentration is adequate, once stable ROSC is achieved, the FiO_2 should be titrated to achieve an oxygen saturation of 94% to 99%, which provides adequate arterial oxygen content and tissue oxygen delivery while assuring that excessive PaO_2 is avoided. If the patient's oxygen saturation is 100%, the provider does not know if the PaO_2 is 110 or 500 mmHg. Since either hypoxemia or hyperoxemia increase the likelihood of a further cardiac arrest, and may contribute to secondary brain injury, they should be avoided by continuous oxygen saturation monitoring.

Ventilation

Hypocarbia causes cerebral vasoconstriction leading to decreased cerebral blood flow (207). After cardiac arrest, hypocapnia induced by hyperventilation causes cerebral ischemia (208). The mechanism may be related to hypocarbia-induced cerebral vasoconstriction, but it also is likely that the increased positive pressure ventilation used to achieve hypocarbia elevates intrathoracic pressure, thus reducing venous return and CO. Observational studies using large cardiac arrest registries document an association between in-ICU hypocapnia and poor neurologic outcome (209,210). Hypercapnia or hypocapnia was also associated with worse outcome based on analysis of a pediatric IHCA registry (206). Conversely, two observational studies documented an association between mild hypercapnia and better neurologic outcome among post–cardiac arrest patients in the ICU (210,211). Until prospective data are available, it is reasonable to adjust ventilation to achieve normocarbia and to monitor this using $ETCO_2$ and ABG analysis. Although there are no specific studies of protective lung ventilation strategies in post–cardiac arrest patients, given that these patients often develop a marked inflammatory response, it is rational to apply protective lung ventilation using tidal volumes of 6 to 8 mL/kg ideal body weight and positive end expiratory pressure of 4 to 8 cm H_2O (212).

To facilitate ventilation, a gastric tube is often needed to decompress the stomach, which may be distended from mouth-to-mouth or bag-mask ventilation. Sedation in the form of benzodiazepines or propofol plus opioids is often used to facilitate ventilation and manage shivering if therapeutic temperature management is used, but the effects of different agents on brain recovery is not known. It seems reasonable to use agents that also have anticonvulsant effects because of the high risk of seizures. Adequate doses of sedatives may also be beneficial by reducing oxygen demand.

Intermittent doses of a neuromuscular blocking agent (NMBA) may be required, particularly if using targeted temperature management (TTM) (see below). Although there is concern about the potential adverse effects of continuous NMBA infusions, limited evidence suggests that short-term infusion (≤48 hours) of short-acting NMBAs given to reduce patient-ventilator dyssynchrony and risk of barotrauma in patients with acute respiratory distress syndrome (ARDS) are not associated with an increased risk of ICU-acquired weakness, and may improve outcome in such patients (213). Furthermore, there are some data suggesting that continuous neuromuscular blockade is associated with decreased mortality in post–cardiac arrest patients (214); however, infusions of NMBAs may mask seizures, and they eliminate the ability to perform neurologic checks. Since status epilepticus (SE) including nonconvulsive status epilepticus (NCSE) may occur in postarrest patients (215–218), continuous electroencephalography (EEG) is recommended to detect seizures in these patients, especially when neuromuscular blockade is used (219–221).

Circulatory Support

Because acute coronary disease is a significant cause of OHCA, once ROSC is established and the patient is stabilized, early identification of coronary obstruction is critical to reverse ongoing myocardial ischemia. Acute coronary syndrome (ACS) is a frequent cause of OHCA as documented in a recent metaanalysis noting the prevalence of an acute coronary artery lesion ranged from 59% to 71% in OHCA patients without an obvious noncardiac etiology (222) (see Chapter 94 for details on ACS and myocardial infarction). Many observational studies showed that emergent cardiac catheterization, including early PCI, is feasible in patients with ROSC after cardiac arrest (223,224). Invasive management—that is, early coronary angiography followed by immediate PCI if deemed necessary—of these patients, particularly those with prolonged resuscitation and nonspecific ECG changes, is controversial because of the lack of high-quality evidence and significant demands on hospital and EMS system resources, including transfer of patients to PCI centers.

In patients with ST segment elevation (STE) or left bundle branch block on the post-ROSC ECG, more than 80% will have an acute coronary lesion (225). Although there are no RCTs, many observational studies reported increased survival and neurologically favorable outcome with early invasive coronary artery management in STE patients (226). Immediate angiography and PCI, when indicated, should be performed in resuscitated OHCA patients whose initial ECG shows ST elevation, even if they remain comatose and ventilated (227,228). Observational studies also indicate that optimal outcomes after OHCA are achieved with a combination of TTM and PCI, which ideally are included in a standardized post–cardiac arrest protocol as part of an overall strategy to improve neurologically intact survival (187,229).

In contrast to the usual presentation of ACS in non–cardiac arrest patients, the standard tools to assess coronary ischemia in cardiac arrest patients are less accurate. Several large observational case series showed that the absence of STE may also be associated with ACS in patients with ROSC following OHCA (230,231). There are conflicting data from observational studies in these non-STE patients regarding the potential benefit of evaluation by emergent cardiac catheterization (230,232,233). CoSTR suggests it is reasonable to discuss and consider emergent cardiac catheterization after ROSC in patients with the highest risk of a coronary cause for their cardiac arrest. Factors such as patient age, duration of CPR, hemodynamic instability, presenting cardiac rhythm, neurologic status upon hospital arrival, and perceived likelihood of a cardiac etiology for the CA can be weighed in making the decision to undertake the intervention in the acute phase or to delay it until later in the hospital stay.

MINIMIZING ORGAN INJURY AND COMPLICATIONS

Hemodynamic Management

Postresuscitation myocardial dysfunction causes hemodynamic instability, which may manifest as low cardiac index, hypotension, and dysrhythmias (195,234,235). To detect the degree of myocardial dysfunction and adequacy of preload, early echocardiography is recommended. Postresuscitation myocardial dysfunction often requires inotropic support, at least transiently. In addition, the systemic inflammatory response that occurs frequently in post-cardiac arrest patients may cause vasoplegia and severe vasodilation, exacerbating hypotension caused by reduced cardiac function (195,235). The optimal agents to use in this setting should balance the adverse effects of stimulating increased myocardial oxygen demand and raising afterload in the context of a poorly contracting ventricle versus maintaining adequate coronary and cerebral perfusion pressure. Currently, norepinephrine, with or without dobutamine, and fluid are usually the most effective treatments for poor cardiac function with or without hypotension. When inappropriate vasodilation is documented or suspected, the controlled infusion of relatively large volumes of fluid is generally tolerated well by patients with post-cardiac arrest syndrome.

Treatment may be guided by achieving target systolic and mean arterial blood pressure, heart rate, urine output, rate of plasma lactate clearance, and central venous oxygen saturation. Traditionally, the targeted mean arterial pressure (MAP) is 65 mmHg with a minimal central venous oxygen saturation of about 70%, but recent data suggest that a higher MAP may produce better outcomes. A recent analysis of 920 patients managed with TTM found an inverse relationship between MAP and mortality (234). A prospective observational study that included simultaneous measurement of cerebral oxygen saturation (CSO_2) by near-infrared spectroscopy with hemodynamic data observed a strong linear relationship between MAP and CSO_2 (236); similarly, there was a strong linear relationship between central venous O_2 saturation and CSO_2 (236). The optimal MAP target is unknown, but excessive vasoconstriction induced by vasopressors is likely to impair cardiac output and cerebral blood flow, especially in the setting of poor ventricular contractile function. This is supported by the observation that an MAP greater than 100 mmHg was associated with a fall in CSO_2 (236).

Maintaining central venous O_2 saturation of 67% to 72% was associated with maximal survival in post-CA patients, suggesting that this can be used as a surrogate marker of adequate tissue oxygen delivery (236). In addition, although a restrictive transfusion policy is often used in the ICU, hemoglobin concentrations less than 10 g/dL were associated with lower CSO_2 and central venous O_2 saturation in postarrest patients, suggesting that a one-size-fits-all approach to transfusion may not be appropriate in all patients (237,238).

Serial echocardiography may also be helpful to assess cardiac function, especially in hemodynamically unstable patients. In the ICU, an arterial line for continuous blood pressure monitoring is essential; cardiac output monitoring may help guide treatment in hemodynamically unstable patients, but there is no evidence that its use affects outcome. The role of supporting the circulation using an intra-aortic balloon pump (IABP) in patients with cardiogenic shock was popular, but the IABP-SHOCK II Trial failed to show that use of the IABP improved 30-day mortality in patients with myocardial infarction and cardiogenic shock (239).

In the absence of definitive data to guide specific hemodynamic targets, it is reasonable to target achieving a MAP that results in an adequate urine output (1 mL/kg/hr), and normal or decreasing plasma lactate values with a central or mixed venous oxygen saturation around 70%. Since pre-existing hypertension may shift the cerebral autoregulatory curve to the right, a higher MAP target may be appropriate in this population (240).

During mild induced hypothermia the normal physiologic response is bradycardia. Recent retrospective studies observed that bradycardia during TTM is associated with a good outcome (241,242). As long as blood pressure, lactate, and urine output are sufficient, a bradycardia of no more than 40 beats/min may be left untreated; the bradycardia is likely tolerated during TTM since oxygen delivery requirements are reduced.

Immediately after a CA there is often a period of hyperkalemia. Subsequent endogenous catecholamine release and correction of metabolic and respiratory acidosis promotes intracellular movement of potassium, often causing hypokalemia. Since hypokalemia may predispose to ventricular dysrhythmias, potassium should be given to maintain the serum potassium concentration between 4.0 and 4.5 mmol/L (219).

Cardiac causes of OHCA have been extensively studied in the last few decades; conversely, little is known about noncardiac causes. The UK Guidelines suggest that early identification of a respiratory or neurologic cause can be achieved by performing a brain and chest CT scan at hospital admission, before or after coronary angiography (219). In the absence of prearrest signs or symptoms suggesting a neurologic or respiratory cause (e.g., headache, seizures, or neurologic deficits for neurologic causes, and shortness of breath or documented hypoxemia in patients suffering from a known and worsening respiratory disease) or if there is clinical or ECG evidence of myocardial ischemia, undertake coronary angiography first, followed by a CT scan in the absence of causative coronary artery lesions (219,243,244).

OPTIMIZING NEUROLOGIC RECOVERY

Cerebral Perfusion

Animal studies show that immediately after ROSC there is a period of hyperemia followed by multifocal cerebral hypoperfusion (245). The pattern of blood flow abnormalities is also determined by the type of arrest, with significant differences seen in models of VF versus asphyxial arrest (246). The initial hyperemia phase is followed by up to 72 hours of cerebral hypoperfusion while the cerebral metabolic rate of oxygen gradually recovers (247,248). After asphyxial cardiac arrest, brain edema may occur transiently after ROSC, but few studies documented whether this is associated with clinically relevant increases in intracranial pressure (ICP) (249). Increased ICP was documented after near drowning in children, and when present, was associated with high mortality (250). It is likely that the occurrence of increased ICP following asphyxial arrest is a marker of more severe cellular injury; there are no data showing that aggressive ICP therapy improves outcome in this setting. As noted above, autoregulation of cerebral blood flow is often impaired (absent or rightshifted) for some time after cardiac arrest, which means that cerebral blood flow may vary with cerebral perfusion pressure instead of being linked to neuronal activity (i.e., metabolic activity) (240). In one study, autoregulation was disturbed in 35% of post–cardiac arrest patients and the majority of these had been hypertensive before their cardiac arrest (251).

Sedation

Although it was common practice to sedate and ventilate patients for at least 24 hours after ROSC, there are no high-level data to support a specified period of ventilation and sedation with or without neuromuscular blockade after cardiac arrest. Patients need to be sedated adequately during treatment with TTM; therefore, the duration of sedation and ventilation is influenced by the duration of this treatment. A combination of opioids and sedative-hypnotics are usually used. Short-acting drugs—propofol, alfentanil, remifentanil—enable more reliable and earlier neurologic assessment and prognostication (252). Adequate sedation reduces oxygen consumption, which may be beneficial, but their use may also increase the need for vasoactive drug infusion to overcome hypotension, which may result from sedation-induced suppression of the patient's endogenous catecholamine stress response (252).

Seizure Control

Seizures are common after CA, occurring in approximately one-third of patients who remain comatose after ROSC. Myoclonus is most common, occurring in 18% to 25%, the remainder having focal or generalized tonic-clonic seizures or a combination of seizure types (253,254). Clinical seizure activity, including myoclonus, may or may not be of epileptic origin. Other motor manifestations could be mistaken for seizures; additionally, there are several types of myoclonus, the majority being nonepileptic (255). In comatose cardiac arrest patients, EEG commonly detects epileptiform activity: post-anoxic SE was detected in 23% to 31% of patients, and epileptic activity was seen in nearly 50% of patients using continuous EEG monitoring (217,256,257).

Seizures increase the cerebral metabolic rate (258) and have the potential to exacerbate brain injury caused by cardiac arrest. Despite that, there are no data showing that prophylactic anticonvulsive therapy improves outcome; furthermore, it is unclear if systematic detection and treatment of EEG epileptic activity improves patient outcome. Routine seizure prophylaxis in post-cardiac arrest patients is not recommended because of the risk of adverse effects and the poor response to antiepileptic drugs among patients with clinical and electrographic seizures (4,5,219). If seizures are documented or suspected, treatment may include sodium valproate, levetiracetam, phenytoin, benzodiazepines, propofol, or a barbiturate, with no documented advantage of one agent over the other; phenytoin therapy is complicated by varying binding to albumin leading to the need to monitor free drug levels. Myoclonus can be particularly difficult to treat. Phenytoin is often ineffective, whereas propofol is often effective to suppress post-anoxic myoclonus (259). Clonazepam, sodium valproate, and levetiracetam are also antimyoclonic drugs that may be effective in post-anoxic myoclonus (260).

Myoclonus and EEG-positive seizure activity, including SE, are associated with a poor prognosis, but individual patients may survive with good outcome, limiting its utility as a single outcome predictor (217,218,254,256). Prolonged patient observation with repeated examination may be necessary after treatment of seizures with sedatives, since they decrease the reliability of a clinical examination (261). Patients with EEG-positive SE may or may not have clinically detectable seizure manifestations (i.e., NCSE), and seizures may be masked by sedation. Because of this, one should consider continuous EEG monitoring of patients, especially if NMBAs are required, or the patient is diagnosed with SE, to monitor the effectiveness of therapy.

Glucose Control

There is a strong association between high blood glucose concentrations after resuscitation from cardiac arrest and poor neurologic outcome (262–264). The exact mechanism is not known, but may reflect a combination of decreased utilization by the brain and other injured organs, and increased epinephrine and endogenous glucocorticoids stimulating gluconeogenesis after the severe stress of a CA. Whether the hyperglycemia is a marker of organ injury or contributes directly to organ injury continues to be debated. Animal and human data suggested that tight glucose control was beneficial in ICU patients; however, in general ICU patients, a large RCT of intensive glucose control (4.5–6.0 mmol/L) versus conventional glucose control (10 mmol/L or less) reported increased 90-day mortality in patients treated with intensive glucose control (265,266). Severe hypoglycemia was more common in the tight glucose control group and is associated with increased mortality in critically ill patients (266); comatose patients are at particular risk from unrecognized hypoglycemia. Irrespective of the target range, variability in glucose values is associated with increased mortality (267). Compared with normothermia, mild induced hypothermia is associated with higher blood glucose values, increased blood glucose variability and greater insulin requirements (268). Increased blood glucose variability also is associated with increased mortality and unfavorable neurologic outcome after cardiac arrest (268). Since efforts to achieve tight glucose control may increase the risk of further brain injury from hypoglycemia, the current ILCOR recommendation is to maintain the blood glucose concentration 10 mmol/L or less and avoid hypoglycemia (219).

Temperature Control

A period of hyperthermia (hyperpyrexia) is common in the first 48 hours after cardiac arrest in adults (269) and children (270). Several studies document an association between post–cardiac arrest fever and poor outcomes (271). The development of hyperthermia after a period of mild induced hypothermia (rebound hyperthermia) is associated with increased mortality and worse neurologic outcome (272,273). There are no RCTs comparing the effect of pyrexia (defined as ≥37.6°C) treatment compared to no temperature control in patients after CA. An elevated post-ROSC temperature may represent a greater SIRS response as well as dysregulation of temperature control due to greater brain injury. Based on recent data from RCTs of hypothermia in adults (274) and children (275), where the control group was maintained at or just below normal temperature and hyperthermia was avoided, the lack of benefit from hypothermia may reflect the beneficial effects of preventing *hyperthermia*. Therefore, it is reasonable to aggressively treat hyperthermia occurring after cardiac arrest with antipyretics and to consider active cooling in unconscious patients (219).

Targeted Temperature Management

The term *targeted temperature management* (TTM) or temperature control is now preferred over the previous term *therapeutic hypothermia*. There was a great deal of enthusiasm for the potential benefits of induced hypothermia after global hypoxia–ischemia based on animal and human data, which demonstrated that mild induced hypothermia is neuroprotective and improves outcome. Cooling suppresses many of the pathways leading to delayed cell death, including apoptosis (276). Hypothermia also decreases the cerebral metabolic rate for oxygen ($CMRO_2$) by about 6% for each 1°C reduction in core temperature and this may reduce the release of excitatory amino acids and free radicals, as well as achieving a better match of oxygen delivery to oxygen demand. Hypothermia blocks the intracellular consequences of excitotoxin exposure—for example, high calcium and glutamate concentrations—and reduces the inflammatory response associated with the post–cardiac arrest syndrome.

To date, all studies of post–cardiac arrest-induced hypothermia only included patients in coma following ROSC. One randomized trial, and a pseudorandomized trial, demonstrated improved neurologic outcome at hospital discharge or at 6 months in comatose patients after OHCA due to VF (277,278). Cooling was initiated within minutes to hours after ROSC and a temperature range of 32° to 34°C was maintained for 12 to 24 hours. In the TTM trial, 950 OHCA patients with any rhythm were randomized to 36 hours of temperature control at either 33°C or 36°C (comprising 28 hours at the target temperature followed by a slow rewarm) (274). There was no difference in mortality and neurologic outcome at 6 months (189,279). With respect to avoidance of hyperthermia, patients in both arms of this trial had their temperature well controlled so that fever was prevented in both groups.

Similar results were recently reported in a large, multicenter RCT of OHCA in children (non-neonates) (275). Within 6 hours of ROSC, comatose children (2 days to 18 years) were randomized to hypothermia (target temperature 33°C) or normothermia (target 36.8°C). The therapeutic target was maintained for 48 hours and then normothermia was actively maintained for a total duration of 120 hours. Survival to hospital discharge and neurologic status at 1-year follow-up was not different between the hypothermia and controlled normothermia groups (275). A simultaneous RCT in children experiencing IHCA completed enrollment and the results from the 1-year follow-up should be available toward the end of 2016 (www.THAPCA.org).

The optimal duration for mild induced hypothermia and TTM is unknown although it is currently most commonly used for 24 hours in adults and 48 hours in children. Previous trials treated patients with 12 to 28 hours of TTM (274,277,278). The TTM trial maintained strict normothermia (<37.5°C) after hypothermia until 72 hours after ROSC (274).

Based on a detailed review of evidence as of early 2015, the various ICLOR ALS committees had the following treatment recommendations regarding TTM (4–6,219,280,281):

- TTM is *recommended* for adults after OHCA with an initial shockable rhythm who remain comatose after ROSC
- TTM is *suggested* for adults after OHCA with an initial nonshockable rhythm who remain comatose after ROSC
- TTM is *suggested* for adults after IHCA who remain comatose after ROSC, regardless of the initial rhythm
- For those patients in whom TTM is used, maintain a target temperature of 32° to 36°C
- If TTM is used, it is suggested that it should be continued for at least 24 hours and then fever should be avoided for at least 72 hours
- In children following OHCA, it is reasonable to either maintain 5 days of continuous normothermia (36° to 37.5°C) or

to provide 2 days of hypothermia (32° to 34°C) followed by 3 days of continuous normothermia (6,280)

- In children after IHCA, there is insufficient evidence to recommend cooling over maintenance of normothermia
- Core temperature should be continuously monitored during TTM

One of the ongoing management controversies regarding TTM is how to best control the patient's temperature. The practical application of TTM is divided into three phases: induction, maintenance, and rewarming (282). External and/or internal cooling techniques can be used to initiate and maintain TTM. Animal data indicate that earlier cooling after ROSC produces better outcome, but this has yet to be demonstrated in humans (283,284). External and/or internal cooling techniques can be used to initiate cooling. If a lower target temperature (e.g., 33°C) is chosen, an infusion of 30 mL/kg of 4°C saline or Hartmann solution decreases core temperature by approximately 1.0 to 1.5°C and is probably safe in a well-monitored environment (285,286). Prehospital cooling using this technique is *not* recommended because of reports of an increased risk of pulmonary edema and rearrest during transport to hospital (287).

Methods of inducing and/or maintaining TTM include:

- Simple ice packs and/or wet towels are inexpensive; however, these methods may be more time consuming for nursing staff, may result in greater temperature fluctuations, and do not enable controlled rewarming. Ice-cold fluids alone cannot be used to maintain hypothermia.
- Cooling blankets or pads
- Water or air-circulating blankets
- Water-circulating gel-coated pads
- Transnasal evaporative cooling—this technique enables cooling before ROSC and is undergoing further investigation in a large multicenter RCT (288)
- Intravascular heat exchanger, placed usually in the femoral or subclavian vein (289)
- Extracorporeal circulation (e.g., cardiopulmonary bypass, ECMO) (77,290)

In most cases, it is easy to cool patients initially after ROSC as the temperature normally decreases within this first hour (269,291). Admission temperature after OHCA is usually between 35°C and 36°C, as seen in adults (274) and children (275). If a target temperature of 36°C is chosen, it is reasonable to allow a slow passive rewarm to 36°C; if a target temperature of 33°C is chosen, initial cooling is facilitated by neuromuscular blockade and sedation, which prevents shivering (292).

In the maintenance phase, a cooling method with effective temperature monitoring that avoids temperature fluctuations is preferred. This is best achieved with external or internal cooling devices that include continuous temperature feedback to achieve a set target temperature (293). The temperature is typically monitored from a thermistor placed in the bladder and/or esophagus. Even though intravascular devices appear to better maintain the target temperature (293,294), as yet, there are no data indicating that any specific cooling technique increases survival when compared with any other cooling technique.

Plasma electrolyte concentrations, effective intravascular volume, and metabolic rate can change rapidly during rewarming, as they do during cooling. Rebound hyperthermia is associated with worse neurologic outcome (272,273), thus, rewarming should be achieved slowly. Although the optimal rate is not known, the consensus is currently about 0.25° to 0.5°C of rewarming per hour (295); choosing a strategy of TTM at 36°C reduces the risk (274).

Physiologic Effects and Complications of Hypothermia

The well-recognized physiologic effects of hypothermia need to be managed carefully (282):

- Shivering increases metabolic demand and heat production, thus reducing cooling rates and strategies to reduce shivering are discussed above. Interestingly, the occurrence of shivering in cardiac arrest survivors who undergo TTM is associated with a good neurologic outcome (296,297); it appears to be a sign of an intact physiologic response. The prevalence of shivering was similar at a target temperature of 33°C or 36°C (274).
- Mild induced hypothermia increases systemic vascular resistance and may cause dysrhythmias (usually bradycardia) (298). Importantly, the bradycardia caused by mild induced hypothermia may be beneficial—similar to the effect achieved by β-blockers—it reduces diastolic dysfunction (299) and its occurrence is associated with good neurologic outcome (241,242).
- Mild induced hypothermia causes a diuresis and may cause electrolyte abnormalities such as hypophosphatemia, hypokalemia, hypomagnesemia, and hypocalcemia (274, 282,300).
- Hypothermia decreases insulin sensitivity and insulin secretion, and therefore may be associated with hyperglycemia (277), which may need treatment with insulin (see glucose control, above).
- Mild induced hypothermia impairs coagulation and may increase bleeding, although this effect seems to be negligible (301) and has not been confirmed in clinical studies (274,278,302).
- Hypothermia can impair the immune system and increase infection rates (282,303). Hypothermia may impair mucociliary clearance and, combined with its immune suppressive effects, is associated with an increased incidence of pneumonia (304,305). However, to date, this has not impacted survival. Although prophylactic antibiotic treatment is typically associated with selection of resistant organisms and more complications in critically ill patients, an observational study noted that the use of prophylactic antibiotics in CA survivors was associated with a reduced incidence of pneumonia (306). In another observational study, of 138 patients admitted to ICU after OHCA, early use of antibiotics was associated with improved survival (307). Like other observational studies, these have intrinsic biases and require prospective randomization to confirm these observations.
- The serum amylase concentration is commonly increased during hypothermia, but its significance is unclear.
- The clearance of sedative drugs and neuromuscular blockers is reduced with the use of TTM (308–310). Clearance of sedative and other drugs will be closer to normal at a temperature closer to 37°C. Delayed clearance of sedative agents needs to be considered when evaluating the neurologic examination of patients who received TTM (308,311).

Contraindications to Hypothermia

Generally recognized contraindications to TTM at 33°C, which are not applied universally, include the following: severe systemic infection or preexisting medical coagulopathy;

fibrinolytic therapy is not a contraindication to mild induced hypothermia.

PROGNOSIS

Evaluating prognosis is often divided into two decision phases: when to stop resuscitation during CA, and when supportive technology should be limited or discontinued in patients with ROSC who remain comatose. With respect to the former, patient-specific IHCA predictors of survival include age (<60 years), and an initial rhythm of VF/VT; with these predictors, there is a 32% survival to discharge compared with only 7.2% in patients with an initial rhythm of asystole, and 4.8% in patients with PEA (312,313). Comorbid risk factors for poor likelihood of survival include hepatic failure, renal insufficiency, sepsis, and malignancy (312). Although these are statistically significant associations, no one factor is considered definitive. The decision to stop CPR requires clinical judgment and knowledge of the patient's wishes; the decision should be openly discussed with the team.

If the patient has a potentially correctable lesion and recurrent VF/VT, there is no specific duration that can be used to decide that ongoing resuscitation efforts are futile. Indeed, more recent data from IHCA registries finds that survival with good outcome is achieved even with prolonged CPR. An analysis of more than 64,000 IHCA from the GWTG-R database found that the median time to achieve ROSC was 12 minutes of CPR. However, when the data were analyzed by centers based on their median duration of CPR, centers in the top quartile of CPR duration (median 25 minutes) had a significantly higher rate of ROSC and survival to discharge, suggesting that decisions to stop efforts earlier may predetermine the outcome (314).

If monitoring of CPR effectiveness, such as capnography, documents good CPR-induced cardiac output, prolonged CPR (>60 minutes) has achieved good outcome (315). Furthermore, if ECPR is available, prolonged resuscitation may lead to good outcome as long as the patient's underlying condition is correctable. Using ECMO in IHCA achieved a nearly two-fold to six-fold improvement in survival and good neurologic outcome based on observational studies and propensity analyses (75,78).

In children, analysis of the GWTG-R data noted that the rate of survival to hospital discharge fell linearly over the first 15 minutes of CPR, with 15.9% of children receiving more than 35 minutes of CPR surviving compared with 44.1% of those who had ROSC with less than 15 minutes of CPR (316). Neurologic outcome was favorable in 70% of those who required less than 15 minutes, but was still favorable in 60% of those survivors who received more than 35 minutes of CPR. This data shows that the previous recommendation to stop CPR for futility if there was no ROSC after 20 minutes is no longer valid. Moreover, a separate analysis of the GWTG-R data found that if ECMO is provided to children even after prolonged CPR, the outcome was significantly better than children who did not receive ECMO, especially if the patient had a surgical cardiac condition (82).

There is an expanding database of evidence regarding prognostic indicators in patients who remain comatose after ROSC. The increasing use of TTM adds new challenges to applying these prognostic indicators. A comprehensive review of neurologic prognostication in comatose survivors of CA was published in 2014 by the European Resuscitation Council and European Society of Intensive Care Medicine (317). Below we delineate highlights of these data as incorporated into the UK Guidelines (219), adding several new references that were not included in that review.

Families expect that advice to limit or withdrawal support will be based on objective and reliable outcome predictors, but few predictors have 100% specificity (i.e., 0% false-positive rate; FPR). Often, a higher degree of prognostic confidence is achieved by combining the results from tests and clinical signs. In most cases, prognostication is not considered to be reliable until at least 72 hours following ROSC or following the completion of TTM (219,317).

Clinical Examination

Bilateral absence of pupillary light reflex at 72 hours from ROSC predicts poor outcome with close to 0% FPR; unfortunately, this test has poor sensitivity as, of those who eventually have a bad outcome, only about 20% have fixed pupils at 72 hours. Similar prognostic performance was documented for bilaterally absent corneal reflexes (318,319).

An absent or extensor motor response to pain at 72 hours from ROSC has a high (about 75%) sensitivity for predicting a poor outcome, but the FPR is also high (about 27%). This sign's high sensitivity suggests it can be used to identify the population with poor neurologic status needing further prognostic testing. Since the corneal reflex and motor response can be suppressed by sedatives or neuromuscular blocking drugs from residual sedation or paralytic agents (261), it is appropriate to prolong the duration of observation of these clinical signs beyond 72 hours from ROSC or normalization of temperature to minimize the risk of obtaining false-positive results (219,317).

A prolonged period of continuous and generalized myoclonic jerks is commonly described as status myoclonus. Although there is no definitive consensus on the duration or frequency of myoclonic jerks required to qualify as status myoclonus, in prognostication studies in comatose survivors of cardiac arrest the minimum reported duration is 30 minutes. While the presence of myoclonic jerks in comatose survivors of cardiac arrest is not consistently associated with poor outcome (FPR 9%), status myoclonus beginning within 48 hours from ROSC is consistently associated with a poor outcome (FPR 0% [95% CI: 0%–5%]; sensitivity 8%–16%). However, there are several case reports of good neurologic recovery despite early onset, prolonged and generalized myoclonus. Patients with post–arrest status myoclonus should be evaluated off sedation whenever possible; in those patients, EEG recording can be useful to identify EEG signs of awareness and reactivity to light or sound stimuli, and to show if there is coexistent epileptiform activity.

There are limited data on the prognostic association of clinical signs in children after CA. Reactive pupils at 24 hours post-ROSC were associated with improved outcome (320). Other cohort studies note higher likelihood of survival with reactive pupils at 24 hours, but there was a high FPR making it an unreliable single sign (16,321,322).

While predictors of poor outcome based on clinical examination are inexpensive and easy to use, their results cannot be concealed and may potentially influence clinical management and cause a self-fulfilling prophecy.

Electrophysiology

Short-Latency Somatosensory Evoked Potentials

In post–arrest comatose patients, bilateral absence of the N20 somatosensory evoked potential (SSEP) wave predicts death or vegetative state (CPC 4–5) with high reliability (FPR 0%–2% with upper 95% CI of about 4%). The few cases of false reports observed in large patient cohorts were due mainly to artifacts. SSEP recording is technically demanding and requires appropriate skills and experience; the utmost care should be taken to avoid electrical interference from muscle artifacts or from the ICU environment. In most prognostication studies, bilateral absence of N20 SSEP was used as a criterion for deciding on withdrawal of lifesustaining treatment, with a consequent risk of becoming a self-fulfilling prophecy.

Electroencephalography

Background reactivity means that there is a change in the EEG in response to a loud noise or a noxious stimulus such as tracheal suction. Absence of EEG background reactivity predicts poor outcome with an FPR of 0% to 2% (upper 95% CI of about 7%). Limitations of EEG reactivity include lack of a standardized stimulus and modest interrater agreement.

Data from two small pediatric observational trials showed that a continuous and reactive EEG performed in the first 7 days after ROSC was associated with a significantly higher likelihood of good neurologic outcome at hospital discharge, whereas a discontinuous or isoelectric tracing was associated with a poor neurologic outcome at discharge (323,324). There are no long-term follow-up studies in children evaluating EEG prediction of outcome after hospital discharge. In TTM-treated patients, the presence of SE is almost invariably, but not always, accompanied by poor outcome (FPR 0%–6%), especially in the presence of an unreactive or discontinuous EEG background.

Burst suppression was recently defined as more than 50% of the EEG record consisting of periods of EEG voltage less than 10 μV, with alternating bursts. However, most prognostication studies do not comply with this definition. In comatose survivors of cardiac arrest, burst suppression is usually a transient finding. During the first 24 to 48 hours after ROSC, burst suppression may be compatible with neurologic recovery, whereas a persistent burst suppression pattern at 72 hours or more from ROSC is consistently associated with poor outcome.

Biomarkers

Neuron-specific enolase (NSE) and S-100B are protein biomarkers that are released following injury to neurons and glial cells, respectively. Their blood concentrations after cardiac arrest are likely to correlate with the extent of hypoxic-ischemic neurologic injury and, therefore, with the severity of neurologic injury. Advantages of biomarkers over both EEG and clinical examination include quantitative results and likely independence from the effects of sedatives. Their main limitation as prognosticators is that it is difficult to identify with a high degree of certainty that a specified threshold is useful to identify patients destined to have a poor outcome. Since the serum concentrations are continuous variables that depend not only on the degree of neuronal injury, but also on the degree of disruption of the blood–brain barrier and maintenance of blood flow to all brain regions, as well as the systemic clearance of the biomarker, it is not surprising that the serum concentrations do not function well as a marker for a dichotomous outcome, especially when a threshold for 0% FPR is desirable.

There is limited data on the value of biomarkers in children. One observational, prospective cohort of 43 children following OHCA or IHCA had repeated measurement of NSE, S-100B, and myelin basic protein over 7 days (320). They found good discrimination, but noted that the concentrations changed over time suggesting that a single sample may not be adequate. Similar variation of concentrations over time was observed in another single center study enrolling 35 children (325).

Imaging

The main CT finding following a global hypoxic-ischemic cerebral insult is cerebral edema, which appears as a reduction in the depth of cerebral sulci (sulcal effacement) and an attenuation of the gray matter/white matter (GM/WM) interface, due to reduced GM density, which is quantitatively measured as the gray:white ratio (GWR) between the GM and the WM densities. The GWR threshold for prediction of poor outcome with 0% FPR in prognostication studies ranged between 1.10 and 1.22. The methods for GWR calculation were inconsistent among studies and quantitative measurements are rarely made in clinical practice.

Brain MRI is more sensitive than CT for detecting global hypoxic-ischemic brain injury caused by cardiac arrest; however, because it is a time-consuming study, its use can be problematic in the most clinically unstable patients. MRI can reveal extensive changes when results of other predictors such as SSEP are normal. All studies on prognostication after cardiac arrest using imaging have small sample sizes with consequent low precision, and very low evidence quality (326). Most studies are retrospective, and did not systematically include all at-risk patients; instead, brain CT or MRI typically is requested at the discretion of the treating physician, which may cause a selection bias and overestimate the tests' performance.

Suggested Prognostication Strategy

A careful clinical neurologic examination remains the foundation for prognostication of the comatose patient after cardiac arrest. The clinical examination should be completed daily to detect signs of neurologic recovery, such as purposeful movements or to identify a clinical picture suggesting that brain death has occurred.

It is thought that brain recovery following a global postanoxic injury is completed, in most patients, within 72 hours of arrest. However, in patients who received sedatives 12 hours or less before the 72-hour post-ROSC neurologic assessment, the reliability of a clinical examination may be reduced (261). Before decisive assessment is performed, major confounders must be excluded (327,328); apart from sedation and neuromuscular blockade, these include hypothermia, severe hypotension, hypoglycemia, and metabolic and respiratory derangements. Sedatives and neuromuscular blocking drugs should be discontinued for long enough to avoid interference with the clinical examination. Short-acting drugs are preferred whenever possible. When residual sedation and/or paralysis is suspected, consider using antidotes to reverse the effects of these drugs.

Neurologic prognosis is typically assessed in all patients who remain comatose with an absent or extensor motor response to pain at 72 hours or more from ROSC. Results of earlier prognostic tests are also considered at this time point. The most robust predictors should be assessed first; these predictors have the highest specificity and precision (FPR <5% with 95% CIs <5% in patients treated with controlled temperature) and were documented in greater than five studies from at least three different groups of investigators. These predictors include bilaterally absent pupillary reflexes at 72 hours or more from ROSC, and bilaterally absent SSEP N20 wave after rewarming; this last sign can be evaluated at 24 hours or more from ROSC in patients who were not treated with controlled temperature. Based on expert opinion, the Guidelines suggest combining the absence of pupillary reflexes with those of corneal reflexes for predicting poor outcome at this time point (219,317). Ocular reflexes and SSEPs maintain their predictive value irrespective of target temperature (329,330).

If none of the preceding signs are present to predict a poor outcome, a group of less accurate predictors can be evaluated, but the degree of confidence in their prediction is lower. These have FPR below 5% but wider 95% CIs than the previous predictors, and/or their definition/threshold is inconsistent in prognostication studies. These predictors include the presence of early status myoclonus (within 48 hours from ROSC), high values of serum NSE at 48 to 72 hours after ROSC, an unreactive malignant EEG pattern (e.g., burst suppression or SE) after rewarming, the presence of a marked reduction of the GWR or sulcal effacement on brain CT within 24 hours after ROSC, or the presence of diffuse ischemic changes on brain MRI at 2 to 5 days after ROSC. Based on expert opinion, the Guidelines suggest waiting at least 24 hours after the first prognostication assessment and confirming unconsciousness with a Glasgow motor score of 1 or 2 before using this second set of predictors (219); the Guidelines also suggest combining at least two of these predictors for prognostication (219).

No specific NSE threshold for prediction of poor outcome with 0% FPR is recommended at present. Ideally, every hospital laboratory assessing NSE should create its own normal values and cutoff concentration based on the test kit used. Sampling at multiple time points is recommended to detect trends in NSE concentrations and to reduce the risk of false-positive results (331); avoid hemolysis when sampling NSE.

Although the most robust predictors showed no false positives in most studies, none of them singularly predicts poor outcome with absolute certainty when the relevant comprehensive evidence is considered. Therefore, the Guidelines recommend that prognostication should be multimodal whenever possible, even in presence of one of these predictors. Apart from increasing safety, limited evidence also suggests that multimodal prognostication increases sensitivity (332–334).

When prolonged sedation and/or paralysis is necessary, for example, because of the need to treat severe respiratory insufficiency, the Guidelines recommend postponing prognostication until a reliable clinical examination can be performed (219). Biomarkers, SSEP, and imaging studies may play a role in this context, since they are insensitive to drug interference.

In view of the limited data and its low quality in children, the CoSTR recommendation is to consider multiple factors when predicting outcome in children after ROSC (6). No specific prognostic variable can be recommended.

When dealing with an uncertain outcome, clinicians should consider prolonged observation; with time, the absence of clinical improvement suggests a worse outcome. If brain death and/or organ donation is being considered, the reader is referred to Chapter 119.

CONTROVERSIES

A detailed list of controversies was included in each section of the 2015 CoSTR statements. The following lists the main controversies related to CPR and postresuscitation management of importance to the ICU clinician:

- Is capnography useful during CPR to guide the quality of BLS interventions, and does it eliminate the need to pause chest compressions to document ROSC (335)?
- Is ACD-CPR, with or without an ITD, helpful to increase the ROSC rate following IHCA?
- What are the appropriate characteristics of candidates for ECPR?
- When ECPR is used, what is the optimal flow rate and MAP to improve organ recovery and protect the brain from further injury? Should TTM be used in all patients or only select patients receiving ECPR?
- Does early epinephrine administration in IHCA patients who fail initial BLS interventions, with or without shocks, improve survival?
- Does a hemodynamically driven approach to the administration of epinephrine and other vasoactive drugs lead to better outcomes compared with time-based epinephrine administration?
- Will targeting CPR interventions to the CPP in patients with invasive arterial and central venous catheters improve outcome?
- Which patients are most likely to benefit from TTM following IHCA?
- When TTM is used, there are numerous questions, such as the best way to cool, the depth and duration of therapy, the duration of actively maintaining a normothermic core temperature after cooling, the rate of rewarming, and the effect of cooling on drug metabolism. Are there outcome predictors that should be used to continue TTM for a longer (or shorter) duration rather than one approach being used in all patients?
- What are the optimal hemodynamic and oxygen delivery (e.g., central venous and/or brain oxygen saturation), hemoglobin concentration, and MAP goals following ROSC? How are these best achieved (i.e., which vasoactive agents are preferable)?
- Does near-infrared oxygen saturation monitoring of the cerebral circulation (or some other method of monitoring brain oxygen delivery) provide useful information to guide therapy during CPR and in the postarrest phase?
- Is continuous EEG monitoring beneficial for all postarrest patients? Does EEG monitoring change outcome by facilitating monitoring of the effects of treatment? If seizures are present, which anticonvulsant agents are optimal to improve outcome?
- The documented variation in outcome across hospitals suggests that there are opportunities for improvement. Similar to efforts to reduce central-line associated blood stream infections, which varied across hospitals, what are the bundles of interventions that are important to optimize outcome?

Key Points

- The importance of high-quality BLS cannot be overemphasized; much of the improved CA outcome observed over the last 10 years is associated with increased attention to achieving an adequate depth and rate of compressions, minimizing interruptions in chest compressions, allowing full chest recoil, and reducing ventilation rate to reduce intrathoracic pressure.
- Coordinated team performance is key to achieving best outcomes. Since IHCA increasingly occurs in the ICU, it is important for all ICU team members to practice good communication skills as well as knowing and demonstrating good psychomotor skills of chest compression, ventilation, vascular access, and drug delivery. Consistent post–arrest team debriefings may significantly improve survival over time (336).
- Capnography is underused as a method both to monitor the quality of chest compression–induced cardiac output and to monitor for ROSC. To help reduce the likelihood of excessive ventilation during CPR in the ICU, it may be helpful to place the patient back on mechanical ventilation with an appropriate ventilator rate and continuous capnography.
- If the IHCA patient has shock-refractory VF/pVT or a nonshockable rhythm, current data suggest it is important to give epinephrine early even though there are concerns about adverse effects from epinephrine.
- The duration of CPR efforts should be driven by knowledge of the underlying condition of the patient and ideally, by monitoring the effectiveness of maintaining good perfusion through monitoring of the CPP and/or $ETCO_2$.
- Following ROSC, it is important to consider the need for urgent cardiac catheterization and PCI based on the suspected etiology of the arrest.
- Postresuscitation management requires careful attention to multiple organ systems—having a protocol likely helps assure that important diagnostic tests and treatment elements are not forgotten.
- Continuous monitoring of core temperature and careful avoidance of hyperthermia is important in the postarrest patient.
- Tight glucose control is *not* helpful and may be harmful in the postarrest patient.

References

1. Morley PT, Lang E, Aickin R, et al. Part 2: Evidence Evaluation and Management of Conflicts of Interest: 2015 International Consensus on Cardiopulmonary Resuscitation and Emergency Cardiovascular Care Science With Treatment Recommendations. *Circulation.* 2015;132:S40–S50.
2. Travers AH, Perkins GD, Berg RA, et al. Part 3: Adult Basic Life Support and Automated External Defibrillation: 2015 International Consensus on Cardiopulmonary Resuscitation and Emergency Cardiovascular Care Science With Treatment Recommendations. *Circulation.* 2015;132:S51–S83.
3. Kleinman ME, Brennan EE, Goldberger ZD, et al. Part 5: Adult Basic Life Support and Cardiopulmonary Resuscitation Quality: 2015 American Heart Association Guidelines Update for Cardiopulmonary Resuscitation and Emergency Cardiovascular Care. *Circulation.* 2015;132:S414–S435.
4. Callaway CW, Soar J, Aibiki M, et al. Part 4: Advanced Life Support: 2015 International Consensus on Cardiopulmonary Resuscitation and Emergency Cardiovascular Care Science With Treatment Recommendations. *Circulation.* 2015;132:S84–S145.
5. Soar J, Callaway CW, Aibiki M, et al. Part 4: Advanced life support: 2015 International Consensus on Cardiopulmonary Resuscitation and Emergency Cardiovascular Care Science with Treatment Recommendations. *Resuscitation.* 2015;95:e71–120.
6. de Caen AR, Berg MD, Chameides L, et al. Part 12: Pediatric Advanced Life Support: 2015 American Heart Association Guidelines Update for Cardiopulmonary Resuscitation and Emergency Cardiovascular Care. *Circulation.* 2015;132:S526–S542.
7. de Caen AR, Maconochie IK, Aickin R, et al. Part 6: Pediatric Basic Life Support and Pediatric Advanced Life Support: 2015 International Consensus on Cardiopulmonary Resuscitation and Emergency Cardiovascular Care Science With Treatment Recommendations. *Circulation.* 2015;132:S177–S203.
8. Perlman JM, Wyllie J, Kattwinkel J, et al. Part 7: Neonatal Resuscitation: 2015 International Consensus on Cardiopulmonary Resuscitation and Emergency Cardiovascular Care Science With Treatment Recommendations. *Circulation.* 2015;132:S204–S241.
9. Merchant RM, Yang L, Becker LB, et al. Incidence of treated cardiac arrest in hospitalized patients in the United States. *Crit Care Med.* 2011;39:2401–2406.
10. Nolan JP, Soar J, Smith GB, et al. Incidence and outcome of in-hospital cardiac arrest in the United Kingdom National Cardiac Arrest Audit. *Resuscitation.* 2014;85:987–992.
11. Merchant RM, Berg RA, Yang L, et al. Hospital variation in survival after in-hospital cardiac arrest. *J Am Heart Assoc.* 2014;3:e000400.
12. Harrison DA, Patel K, Nixon E, et al. Development and validation of risk models to predict outcomes following in-hospital cardiac arrest attended by a hospital-based resuscitation team. *Resuscitation.* 2014;85:993–1000.
13. Peberdy MA, Callaway CW, Neumar RW, et al. Part 9: Post-Cardiac Arrest Care: 2010 American Heart Association Guidelines for Cardiopulmonary Resuscitation and Emergency Cardiovascular Care. *Circulation.* 2010;122:S768–S786.
14. Neumar RW, Nolan JP, Adrie C, et al. Post-cardiac arrest syndrome: epidemiology, pathophysiology, treatment, and prognostication. A Consensus statement from the International Liaison Committee on Resuscitation (American Heart Association, Australian and New Zealand Council on Resuscitation, European Resuscitation Council, Heart and Stroke Foundation of Canada, InterAmerican Heart Foundation, Resuscitation Council of Asia, and the Resuscitation Council of Southern Africa); the American Heart Association Emergency Cardiovascular Care Committee; the Council on Cardiovascular Surgery and Anesthesia; the Council on Cardiopulmonary, Perioperative, and Critical Care; the Council on Clinical Cardiology; and the Stroke Council. *Circulation.* 2008;118:2452–2583.
15. Gershengorn HB, Li G, Kramer A, Wunsch H. Survival and functional outcomes after cardiopulmonary resuscitation in the intensive care unit. *J Crit Care.* 2012;27:421.e9–e17.
16. Meert KL, Donaldson A, Nadkarni V, et al. Multicenter cohort study of in-hospital pediatric cardiac arrest. *Pediatr Crit Care Med.* 2009;10:544–553.
17. Nadkarni VM, Larkin GL, Peberdy MA, et al. First documented rhythm and clinical outcome from in-hospital cardiac arrest among children and adults. *JAMA.* 2006;295:50–57.
18. Gupta P, Tang X, Gall CM, et al. Epidemiology and outcomes of in-hospital cardiac arrest in critically ill children across hospitals of varied center volume: a multi-center analysis. *Resuscitation.* 2014;85:1473–1479.
19. Girotra S, Spertus JA, Li Y, et al. Survival trends in pediatric in-hospital cardiac arrests: an analysis from Get With the Guidelines-Resuscitation. *Circ Cardiovasc Qual Outcomes.* 2013;6:42–49.
20. Jayaram N, Spertus JA, Nadkarni V, et al. Hospital variation in survival after pediatric in-hospital cardiac arrest. *Circ Cardiovasc Qual Outcomes.* 2014;7:517–523.
21. Berg RA, Sutton RM, Holubkov R, et al. Ratio of PICU versus ward cardiopulmonary resuscitation events is increasing. *Crit Care Med.* 2013;41:2292–2297.
22. DeCaen AR, Joffe AR. Ratio of PICU to ward cardiac arrest is increasing: so what? *Crit Care Med.* 2013;41:2438–2439.
23. Sayre MR, Koster RW, Botha M, et al. Part 5: Adult basic life support: 2010 International Consensus on Cardiopulmonary Resuscitation and Emergency Cardiovascular Care Science With Treatment Recommendations. *Circulation.* 2010;122:S298–S324.
24. Lai H, Choong CV, Fook-Chong S, et al. Interventional strategies associated with improvements in survival for out-of-hospital cardiac arrests in Singapore over 10 years. *Resuscitation.* 2015;89:155–161.
25. Kudenchuk PJ, Redshaw JD, Stubbs BA, et al. Impact of changes in resuscitation practice on survival and neurological outcome after out-of-hospital cardiac arrest resulting from nonshockable arrhythmias. *Circulation.* 2012;125:1787–1794.

26. Aufderheide TP, Nichol G, Rea TD, et al. A trial of an impedance threshold device in out-of-hospital cardiac arrest. *N Engl J Med*. 2011;365:798–806.
27. Yannopoulos D, Aufderheide TP, Abella BS, et al. Quality of CPR: An important effect modifier in cardiac arrest clinical outcomes and intervention effectiveness trials. *Resuscitation*. 2015;94:106–113.
28. Kouwenhoven WB, Jude JR, Knickerbocker GG. Closed-chest cardiac massage. *JAMA*. 1960;173:1064–1067.
29. Criley JM, Blaufuss AH, Kissel GL. Cough-induced cardiac compression. *JAMA*. 1976;236:1246–1248.
30. Rudikoff MT, Maughan WL, Effron M, et al. Mechanisms of blood flow during cardiopulmonary resuscitation. *Circulation*. 1980;61:345–351.
31. Deshmukh HG, Weil MH, Gudipati CV, et al. Mechanism of blood flow generated by precordial compression during CPR. I. Studies on closed chest precordial compression. *Chest*. 1989;95:1092–1099.
32. Werner JA, Greene HL, Janko CL, Cobb LA. Two-dimensional echocardiography during CPR in man: implications regarding the mechanism of blood flow. *Crit Care Med*. 1981;9:375–376.
33. Orlowski JP. Optimum position for external cardiac compression in infants and young children. *Ann Emerg Med*. 1986;15:667–673.
34. Cha KC, Kim HJ, Shin HJ, et al. Hemodynamic effect of external chest compressions at the lower end of the sternum in cardiac arrest patients. *J Emerg Med*. 2013;44:691–697.
35. Qvigstad E, Kramer-Johansen J, Tømte Ø, et al. Clinical pilot study of different hand positions during manual chest compressions monitored with capnography. *Resuscitation*. 2013;84:1203–1207.
36. Idris AH, Guffey D, Aufderheide TP, et al. Relationship between chest compression rates and outcomes from cardiac arrest. *Circulation*. 2012; 125:3004–3012.
37. Idris AH, Guffey D, Pepe PE, et al. Chest compression rates and survival following out-of-hospital cardiac arrest. *Crit Care Med*. 2015;43:840–848.
38. Vadeboncoeur T, Stolz U, Panchal A, et al. Chest compression depth and survival in out-of-hospital cardiac arrest. *Resuscitation*. 2014;85:182–188.
39. Stiell IG, Brown SP, Nichol G, et al. What is the optimal chest compression depth during out-of-hospital cardiac arrest resuscitation of adult patients? *Circulation*. 2014;130:1962–1970.
40. Hellevuo H, Sainio M, Nevalainen R, et al. Deeper chest compression: more complications for cardiac arrest patients? *Resuscitation*. 2013;84: 760–765.
41. Yannopoulos D, McKnite S, Aufderheide TP, et al. Effects of incomplete chest wall decompression during cardiopulmonary resuscitation on coronary and cerebral perfusion pressures in a porcine model of cardiac arrest. *Resuscitation*. 2005;64:363–372.
42. Zuercher MMD, Hilwig RWDVMP, Ranger-Moore JP, et al. Leaning during chest compressions impairs cardiac output and left ventricular myocardial blood flow in piglet cardiac arrest. *Crit Care Med*. 2010; 38:1141–1146.
43. Glatz AC, Nishisaki A, Niles DE, et al. Sternal wall pressure comparable to leaning during CPR impacts intrathoracic pressure and haemodynamics in anaesthetized children during cardiac catheterization. *Resuscitation*. 2013;84:1674–1679.
44. Pokorná M, Necas E, Kratochvíl J, et al. A sudden increase in partial pressure end-tidal carbon dioxide (P(ET)CO(2)) at the moment of return of spontaneous circulation. *J Emerg Med*. 2009;8(5):614–621.
45. Kellum MJ, Kennedy KW, Ewy GA. Cardiocerebral resuscitation improves survival of patients with out-of-hospital cardiac arrest. *Am J Med*. 2006; 119:335–340.
46. Bobrow BJ, Clark LL, Ewy GA, et al. Minimally interrupted cardiac resuscitation by emergency medical services for out-of-hospital cardiac arrest. *JAMA*. 2008;299:1158–1165.
47. Rea TD, Helbock M, Perry S, et al. Increasing use of cardiopulmonary resuscitation during out-of-hospital ventricular fibrillation arrest: survival implications of guideline changes. *Circulation*. 2006;114:2760–2765.
48. Hostler D, Everson-Stewart S, Rea TD, et al. Effect of real-time feedback during cardiopulmonary resuscitation outside hospital: prospective, cluster-randomised trial. *BMJ*. 2011;342:d512.
49. Abella BS, Edelson DP, Kim S, et al. CPR quality improvement during in-hospital cardiac arrest using a real-time audiovisual feedback system. *Resuscitation*. 2007;73:54–61.
50. Sutton RM, French B, Niles DE, et al. 2010 American Heart Association recommended compression depths during pediatric in-hospital resuscitations are associated with survival. *Resuscitation*. 2014;85:1179–1184.
51. Sutton RM, Case E, Brown SP, et al. A quantitative analysis of out-of-hospital pediatric and adolescent resuscitation quality: a report from the ROC epistry-cardiac arrest. *Resuscitation*. 2015;93:150–157.
52. Jacobs I, Sunde K, Deakin CD, et al. Part 6: Defibrillation: 2010 International Consensus on Cardiopulmonary Resuscitation and Emergency Cardiovascular Care Science With Treatment Recommendations. *Circulation*. 2010;122:S325–S337.
53. Sunde K, Jacobs I, Deakin CD, et al. Part 6: Defibrillation: 2010 International Consensus on Cardiopulmonary Resuscitation and Emergency Cardiovascular Care Science With Treatment Recommendations. *Resuscitation*. 2010;81 Suppl 1:e71–e85.
54. Didon JP, Fontaine G, White RD, et al. Clinical experience with a low-energy pulsed biphasic waveform in out-of-hospital cardiac arrest. *Resuscitation*. 2008;76:350–353.
55. Morrison LJ, Henry RM, Ku V, et al. Single-shock defibrillation success in adult cardiac arrest: a systematic review. *Resuscitation*. 2013;84:1480–1486.
56. Hess EP, Agarwal D, Myers LA, et al. Performance of a rectilinear biphasic waveform in defibrillation of presenting and recurrent ventricular fibrillation: a prospective multicenter study. *Resuscitation*. 2011;82:685–689.
57. Koster RW, Walker RG, Chapman FW. Recurrent ventricular fibrillation during advanced life support care of patients with prehospital cardiac arrest. *Resuscitation*. 2008;78:252–257.
58. Samson RA, Nadkarni VM, Meaney PA, et al. Outcomes of in-hospital ventricular fibrillation in children. *N Engl J Med*. 2006;354:2328–2339.
59. Meaney PA, Nadkarni VM, Atkins DL, et al. Effect of defibrillation energy dose during in-hospital pediatric cardiac arrest. *Pediatrics*. 2011;127: e16–e23.
60. Plaisance P, Lurie KG, Payen D. Inspiratory impedance during active compression-decompression cardiopulmonary resuscitation: a randomized evaluation in patients in cardiac arrest. *Circulation*. 2000;101:989–994.
61. Plaisance P, Lurie KG, Vicaut E, et al. Evaluation of an impedance threshold device in patients receiving active compression-decompression cardiopulmonary resuscitation for out of hospital cardiac arrest. *Resuscitation*. 2004;61:265–271.
62. Frascone RJ, Wayne MA, Swor RA, et al. Treatment of non-traumatic out-of-hospital cardiac arrest with active compression decompression cardiopulmonary resuscitation plus an impedance threshold device. *Resuscitation*. 2013;84:1214–1222.
63. Wolcke BB, Mauer DK, Schoefmann MF, et al. Comparison of standard cardiopulmonary resuscitation versus the combination of active compression-decompression cardiopulmonary resuscitation and an inspiratory impedance threshold device for out-of-hospital cardiac arrest. *Circulation*. 2003;108:2201–2205.
64. Wang CH, Tsai MS, Chang WT, et al. Active compression-decompression resuscitation and impedance threshold device for out-of-hospital cardiac arrest: a systematic review and metaanalysis of randomized controlled trials. *Crit Care Med*. 2015;43:889–896.
65. Convertino VA, Parquette B, Zeihr J, et al. Use of respiratory impedance in prehospital care of hypotensive patients associated with hemorrhage and trauma: a case series. *J Trauma Acute Care Surg*. 2012;73:S54–S59.
66. Wampler D, Convertino VA, Weeks S, et al. Use of an impedance threshold device in spontaneously breathing patients with hypotension secondary to trauma: an observational cohort feasibility study. *J Trauma Acute Care Surg*. 2014;77:S140–S145.
67. Shih A, Udassi S, Porvasnik SL, et al. Use of impedance threshold device in conjunction with our novel adhesive glove device for ACD-CPR does not result in additional chest decompression. *Resuscitation*. 2013;84:1433–1438.
68. Perkins GD, Lall R, Quinn T, et al. Mechanical versus manual chest compression for out-of-hospital cardiac arrest (PARAMEDIC): a pragmatic, cluster randomised controlled trial. *Lancet*. 2015;385:947–955.
69. Rubertsson S, Lindgren E, Smekal D, et al. Mechanical chest compressions and simultaneous defibrillation vs conventional cardiopulmonary resuscitation in out-of-hospital cardiac arrest: the LINC randomized trial. *JAMA*. 2014;311:53-61.
70. Smekal D, Johansson J, Huzevka T, Rubertsson S. A pilot study of mechanical chest compressions with the LUCAS device in cardiopulmonary resuscitation. *Resuscitation*. 2011;82:702–706.
71. Hallstrom A, Rea TD, Sayre MR, et al. Manual chest compression vs use of an automated chest compression device during resuscitation following out-of-hospital cardiac arrest: a randomized trial. *JAMA*. 2006;295:2620–2628.
72. Wik L, Olsen JA, Persse D, et al. Manual vs. integrated automatic load-distributing band CPR with equal survival after out of hospital cardiac arrest: the randomized CIRC trial. *Resuscitation*. 2014;85:741–748.
73. Larsen AI, Hjornevik A, Bonarjee V, et al. Coronary blood flow and perfusion pressure during coronary angiography in patients with ongoing mechanical chest compression: a report on 6 cases. *Resuscitation*. 2010;81:493–497.
74. del-Nido PJ, Dalton HJ, Thompson AE, Siewers RD. Extracorporeal membrane oxygenator rescue in children during cardiac arrest after cardiac surgery. *Circulation*. 1992;86:II300-II304.

75. Shin TG, Jo IJ, Sim MS, et al. Two-year survival and neurological outcome of in-hospital cardiac arrest patients rescued by extracorporeal cardiopulmonary resuscitation. *Int J Cardiol.* 2013;168:3424–3430.
76. Bednarczyk JM, White CW, Ducas RA, et al. Resuscitative extracorporeal membrane oxygenation for in hospital cardiac arrest: a Canadian observational experience. *Resuscitation.* 2014;85:1713–1719.
77. Stub D, Bernard S, Pellegrino V, et al. Refractory cardiac arrest treated with mechanical CPR, hypothermia, ECMO and early reperfusion (the CHEER trial). *Resuscitation.* 2015;86:88–94.
78. Chen YS, Lin JW, Yu HY, et al. Cardiopulmonary resuscitation with assisted extracorporeal life-support versus conventional cardiopulmonary resuscitation in adults with in-hospital cardiac arrest: an observational study and propensity analysis. *Lancet.* 2008;372:554–561.
79. Johnson NJ, Acker M, Hsu CH, et al. Extracorporeal life support as rescue strategy for out-of-hospital and emergency department cardiac arrest. *Resuscitation.* 2014;85:1527–1532.
80. Choi DS, Kim T, Ro YS, et al. Extracorporeal life support and survival after out-of-hospital cardiac arrest in a nationwide registry: a propensity score-matched analysis. *Resuscitation.* 2016;99:26–32.
81. Champigneulle B, Bellenfant-Zegdi F, Follin A, et al. Extracorporeal life support (ECLS) for refractory cardiac arrest after drowning: an 11-year experience. *Resuscitation.* 2015;88:126–131.
82. Lasa JJ, Rogers RS, Localio R, et al. Extracorporeal-cardiopulmonary resuscitation (E-CPR) during pediatric in-hospital cardiopulmonary arrest is associated with improved survival to discharge: a report from the American Heart Association's Get With the Guidelines®- Resuscitation Registry (GWTG-R). *Circulation.* 2016;133(2):165–176.
83. Sutton RM, Friess SH, Maltese MR, et al. Hemodynamic-directed cardiopulmonary resuscitation during in-hospital cardiac arrest. *Resuscitation.* 2014;85:983–986.
84. Kern KB, Ewy GA, Voorhees WD, et al. Myocardial perfusion pressure: a predictor of 24-hour survival during prolonged cardiac arrest in dogs. *Resuscitation.* 1988;16:241–250.
85. Sanders A, Kern K, Atlas M, et al. Importance of the duration of inadequate coronary perfusion pressure on resuscitation from cardiac arrest. *J Am Coll Cardiol.* 1985;6:113–118.
86. Sigurdsson G, Yannopoulos D, McKnite SH, Lurie KG. Cardiorespiratory interactions and blood flow generation during cardiac arrest and other states of low blood flow. *Curr Opin Crit Care.* 2003;9:183–188.
87. Yannopoulos D, McKnite S, Aufderheide TP, et al. Effects of incomplete chest wall decompression during cardiopulmonary resuscitation on coronary and cerebral perfusion pressures in a porcine model of cardiac arrest. *Resuscitation.* 2005;64:363–372.
88. Kern KB, Hilwig RW, Berg RA, et al. Importance of continuous chest compressions during cardiopulmonary resuscitation: improved outcome during a simulated single lay-rescuer scenario. *Circulation.* 2002;105:645–649.
89. Sutton RM, Friess SH, Bhalala U, et al. Hemodynamic directed CPR improves short-term survival from asphyxia-associated cardiac arrest. *Resuscitation.* 2013;84:696–701.
90. Friess SH, Sutton RM, Bhalala U, et al. Hemodynamic directed cardiopulmonary resuscitation improves short-term survival from ventricular fibrillation cardiac arrest. *Crit Care Med.* 2013;41:2698–2704.
91. Paradis NA, Martin GB, Rivers EP, et al. Coronary perfusion pressure and the return of spontaneous circulation in human cardiopulmonary resuscitation. *JAMA.* 1990;263:1106–1113.
92. Idris AH, Staples ED, O'Brien DJ, et al. End-tidal carbon dioxide during extremely low cardiac output. *Ann Emerg Med.* 1994;23:568–572.
93. Berg RA, Sanders AB, Milander M, et al. Efficacy of audio-prompted rate guidance in improving resuscitator performance of cardiopulmonary resuscitation on children. *Acad Emerg Med.* 1994;1:35–40.
94. Rubertsson S, Karlsten R. Increased cortical cerebral blood flow with LUCAS; a new device for mechanical chest compressions compared to standard external compressions during experimental cardiopulmonary resuscitation. *Resuscitation.* 2005;65:357–363.
95. Ristagno G, Tang W, Chang Y-T, et al. The quality of chest compressions during cardiopulmonary resuscitation overrides importance of timing of defibrillation. *Chest.* 2007;132:70–75.
96. Ornato JP, Gonzalez ER, Garnett AR, et al. Effect of cardiopulmonary resuscitation compression rate on end-tidal carbon dioxide concentration and arterial pressure in man. *Crit Care Med.* 1988;16:241–245.
97. Jin X, Weil MH, Tang W, et al. End-tidal carbon dioxide as a noninvasive indicator of cardiac index during circulatory shock. *Crit Care Med.* 2000;28:2415–2419.
98. Gazmuri RJ, Weil MH, Bisera J, Rackow EC. End-tidal carbon dioxide tension as a monitor of native blood flow during resuscitation by extracorporeal circulation. *J Thorac Cardiovasc Surg.* 1991;101:984–988.
99. Ornato JP, Garnett AR, Glauser FL. Relationship between cardiac output and the end-tidal carbon dioxide tension. *Ann Emerg Med.* 1990; 19:1104–1106.
100. Sheak KR, Wiebe DJ, Leary M, et al. Quantitative relationship between end-tidal carbon dioxide and CPR quality during both in-hospital and out-of-hospital cardiac arrest. *Resuscitation.* 2015;89:149–154.
101. Asplin BR, White RD. Prognostic value of end-tidal carbon dioxide pressures during out-of-hospital cardiac arrest. *Ann Emerg Med.* 1995;25:756–761.
102. Cantineau JP, Lambert Y, Merckx P, et al. End-tidal carbon dioxide during cardiopulmonary resuscitation in humans presenting mostly with asystole: a predictor of outcome. *Crit Care Med.* 1996;24:791–796.
103. Grmec S, Klemen P. Does the end-tidal carbon dioxide (EtCO2) concentration have prognostic value during out-of-hospital cardiac arrest? *Eur J Emerg Med.* 2001;8:263–269.
104. Grmec S, Krizmaric M, Mally S, et al. Utstein style analysis of out-of-hospital cardiac arrest: bystander CPR and end expired carbon dioxide. *Resuscitation.* 2007;72:404–414.
105. Kolar M, Krizmaric M, Klemen P, Grmec S. Partial pressure of end-tidal carbon dioxide successful predicts cardiopulmonary resuscitation in the field: a prospective observational study. *Crit Care.* 2008;12:R115.
106. Eckstein M, Hatch L, Malleck J, et al. End-tidal CO_2 as a predictor of survival in out-of-hospital cardiac arrest. *Prehosp Disaster Med.* 2011;26:148–150.
107. Heradstveit BE, Sunde K, Sunde G-A, et al. Factors complicating interpretation of capnography during advanced life support in cardiac arrest: a clinical retrospective study in 575 patients. *Resuscitation.* 2012;83:813–818.
108. Lah K, Krizmaric M, Grmec S. The dynamic pattern of end-tidal carbon dioxide during cardiopulmonary resuscitation: difference between asphyxial cardiac arrest and ventricular fibrillation/pulseless ventricular tachycardia cardiac arrest. *Crit Care.* 2011;15:R13.
109. Touma O, Davies M. The prognostic value of end tidal carbon dioxide during cardiac arrest: a systematic review. *Resuscitation.* 2013;84: 1470–1479.
110. Bhende MS, Thompson AE. Evaluation of an end-tidal CO_2 detector during pediatric cardiopulmonary resuscitation. *Pediatrics.* 1995;95:395–399.
111. Chuang ML, Chang HC, Lim KE, Vintch JR. Gas exchange detection of right-to-left shunt in dyspneic patients: report of three cases. *Int J Cardiol.* 2006;108:117–119.
112. Matthews IL, Bjornstad PG, Kaldestad RH, et al. The impact of shunt size on lung function in infants with univentricular heart physiology. *Pediatr Crit Care Med.* 2009;10:60–65.
113. Tugrul M, Camci E, Sungur Z, Pembeci K. The value of end-tidal carbon dioxide monitoring during systemic-to-pulmonary artery shunt insertion in cyanotic children. *J Cardiothorac Vasc Anesth.* 2004;18:152–155.
114. Falk JL, Rackow EC, Weil MH. End-tidal carbon dioxide during cardiopulmonary resuscitation. *N Engl J Med.* 1988;318:607–611.
115. Keidan I, Ben-Menachem E, White SE, Berkenstadt H. Intravenous sodium bicarbonate verifies intravenous position of catheters in ventilated children. *Anesth Analg.* 2012;115:909–912.
116. Okamoto H, Hoka S, Kawasaki T, et al. Changes in end-tidal carbon dioxide tension following sodium bicarbonate administration: correlation with cardiac output and haemoglobin concentration. *Acta Anaesthesiol Scand.* 1995;39:79–84.
117. Lindberg L, Liao Q, Steen S. The effects of epinephrine/norepinephrine on end-tidal carbon dioxide concentration, coronary perfusion pressure and pulmonary arterial blood flow during cardiopulmonary resuscitation. *Resuscitation.* 2000;43:129–140.
118. Cantineau JP, Merckx P, Lambert Y, et al. Effect of epinephrine on end-tidal carbon dioxide pressure during prehospital cardiopulmonary resuscitation. *Am J Emerg Med.* 1994;12:267–270.
119. Callaham M, Barton C, Matthay M. Effect of epinephrine on the ability of end-tidal carbon dioxide readings to predict initial resuscitation from cardiac arrest. *Crit Care Med.* 1992;20:337–343.
120. Grmec S, Lah K, Tusek-Bunc K. Difference in end-tidal CO2 between asphyxia cardiac arrest and ventricular fibrillation/pulseless ventricular tachycardia cardiac arrest in the prehospital setting. *Crit Care.* 2003; 7:R139–R144.
121. Pearce AK, Davis DP, Minokadeh A, Sell RE. Initial end-tidal carbon dioxide as a prognostic indicator for inpatient PEA arrest. *Resuscitation.* 2015;92:77–81.
122. Turle S, Sherren PB, Nicholson S, et al. Availability and use of capnography for in-hospital cardiac arrests in the United Kingdom. *Resuscitation.* 2015;94:80–84.
123. Frankel HL, Kirkpatrick AW, Elbarbary M, et al. Guidelines for the appropriate use of bedside general and cardiac ultrasonography in the

evaluation of critically ill patients. Part I: general ultrasonography. *Crit Care Med*. 2015;43:2479–2502.

124. Giraud R, Siegenthaler N, Schussler O, et al. The LUCAS 2 chest compression device is not always efficient: an echographic confirmation. *Ann Emerg Med*. 2015;65:23–26.
125. Prosen G, Krizmaric M, Zavrsnik J, Grmec S. Impact of modified treatment in echocardiographically confirmed pseudo-pulseless electrical activity in out-of-hospital cardiac arrest patients with constant end-tidal carbon dioxide pressure during compression pauses. *J Int Med Res*. 2010;38:1458–1467.
126. Chardoli M, Heidari F, Rabiee H, et al. Echocardiography integrated ACLS protocol versus conventional cardiopulmonary resuscitation in patients with pulseless electrical activity cardiac arrest. *Chin J Traumatol*. 2012;15:284–287.
127. Blyth L, Atkinson P, Gadd K, Lang E. Bedside focused echocardiography as predictor of survival in cardiac arrest patients: a systematic review. *Acad Emerg Med*. 2012;19:1119–1126.
128. Weil M, Rackow E, Trevino R, et al. Difference in acid-base state between venous and arterial blood during cardiopulmonary resuscitation. *N Engl J Med*. 1986;315:153–156.
129. Kette F, Weil MH, Gazmuri RJ, et al. Intramyocardial hypercarbic acidosis during cardiac arrest and resuscitation. *Crit Care Med*. 1993;21:901–906.
130. Tucker KJ, Idris AH, Wenzel V, Orban DJ. Changes in arterial and mixed venous blood gases during untreated ventricular fibrillation and cardiopulmonary resuscitation. *Resuscitation*. 1994;28:137–141.
131. Efrati O, Barak A, Ben-Abraham R, et al. Should vasopressin replace adrenaline for endotracheal drug administration? *Crit Care Med*. 2003; 31:572–576.
132. Manisterski Y, Vaknin Z, Ben-Abraham R, et al. Endotracheal epinephrine: a call for larger doses. *Anesth Analg*. 2002;95:1037–1041.
133. Hilwig RW, Kern KB, Berg RA, et al. Catecholamines in cardiac arrest: role of alpha agonists, beta-adrenergic blockers and high-dose epinephrine. *Resuscitation*. 2000;47:203–208.
134. Chase PB, Kern KB, Sanders AB, et al. Effects of graded doses of epinephrine on both noninvasive and invasive measures of myocardial perfusion and blood flow during cardiopulmonary resuscitation. *Crit Care Med*. 1993;21:413–419.
135. Gueugniaud P-Y, Mols P, Goldstein P, et al. A comparison of repeated high doses and repeated standard doses of epinephrine for cardiac arrest outside the hospital. *N Engl J Med*. 1998;339:1595–1601.
136. Brown CG, Martin DR, Pepe PE, et al. A comparison of standard-dose and high-dose epinephrine in cardiac arrest outside the hospital. *N Engl J Med*. 1992;327:1051–1055.
137. Choux C, Gueugniaud PY, Barbieux A, et al. Standard doses versus repeated high doses of epinephrine in cardiac arrest outside the hospital. *Resuscitation*. 1995;29:3–9.
138. Perondi MBM, Reis AG, Paiva EF, et al. A comparison of high-dose and standard-dose epinephrine in children with cardiac arrest. *N Engl J Med*. 2004;350:1722–1730.
139. Olasveengen TM, Sunde K, Brunborg C, et al. Intravenous drug administration during out-of-hospital cardiac arrest: a randomized trial. *JAMA*. 2009;302:2222–2229.
140. Jacobs IG, Finn JC, Jelinek GA, et al. Effect of adrenaline on survival in out-of-hospital cardiac arrest: a randomised double-blind placebo-controlled trial. *Resuscitation*. 2011;82:1138–1143.
141. Olasveengen TM, Wik L, Sunde K, Steen PA. Outcome when adrenaline (epinephrine) was actually given vs. not given: post hoc analysis of a randomized clinical trial. *Resuscitation*. 2012;83:327–332.
142. Hagihara A, Hasegawa M, Abe T, et al. Prehospital epinephrine use and survival among patients with out-of-hospital cardiac arrest. *JAMA*. 2012;307:1161–1168.
143. Machida M, Miura S, Matsuo K, et al. Effect of intravenous adrenaline before arrival at the hospital in out-of-hospital cardiac arrest. *J Cardiol*. 2012;60:503–507.
144. Patanwala AE, Slack MK, Martin JR, et al. Effect of epinephrine on survival after cardiac arrest: a systematic review and meta-analysis. *Minerva Anestesiol*. 2014;80:831–843.
145. Donnino MW, Salcicciolі JD, Howell MD, et al. Time to administration of epinephrine and outcome after in-hospital cardiac arrest with nonshockable rhythms: retrospective analysis of large in-hospital data registry. *BMJ*. 2014;348:g3028.
146. Andersen LW, Berg KM, Saindon BZ, et al. Time to epinephrine and survival after pediatric in-hospital cardiac arrest. *JAMA*. 2015;314:802–810.
147. Krismer AC, Lindner KH, Wenzel V, et al. The effects of endogenous and exogenous vasopressin during experimental cardiopulmonary resuscitation. *Anesth Analg*. 2001;92:1499–1504.
148. Tayama E, Ueda T, Shojima T, et al. Arginine vasopressin is an ideal drug after cardiac surgery for the management of low systemic vascular resistant hypotension concomitant with pulmonary hypertension. *Interact Cardiovasc Thorac Surg*. 2007;6:715–719.
149. Wang HJ, Wong CS, Chiang CY, et al. Low-dose vasopressin infusion can be an alternative in treating patients with refractory septic shock combined with chronic pulmonary hypertension: a case report. *Acta Anaesthesiol Sin*. 2003;41:77–80.
150. Stiell IG, Hebert PC, Wells GA, et al. Vasopressin versus epinephrine for inhospital cardiac arrest: a randomised controlled trial. *Lancet*. 2001; 358:105–109.
151. Wenzel V, Krismer AC, Arntz HR, et al. A comparison of vasopressin and epinephrine for out-of-hospital cardiopulmonary resuscitation. *N Engl J Med*. 2004;350:105–113.
152. Mukoyama T, Kinoshita K, Nagao K, Tanjoh K. Reduced effectiveness of vasopressin in repeated doses for patients undergoing prolonged cardiopulmonary resuscitation. *Resuscitation*. 2009;80:755–761.
153. Ong ME, Tiah L, Leong BS, et al. A randomised, double-blind, multicentre trial comparing vasopressin and adrenaline in patients with cardiac arrest presenting to or in the emergency department. *Resuscitation*. 2012;83:953–960.
154. Carroll TG, Dimas VV, Raymond TT. Vasopressin rescue for in-pediatric intensive care unit cardiopulmonary arrest refractory to initial epinephrine dosing: a prospective feasibility pilot trial. *Pediatr Crit Care Med*. 2012;13:265–272.
155. Gueugniaud PY, David JS, Chanzy E, et al. Vasopressin and epinephrine vs. epinephrine alone in cardiopulmonary resuscitation. *N Engl J Med*. 2008;359:21–30.
156. Mentzelopoulos SD, Malachias S, Chamos C, et al. Vasopressin, steroids, and epinephrine and neurologically favorable survival after in-hospital cardiac arrest: a randomized clinical trial. *JAMA*. 2013;310:270–279.
157. Duncan JM, Meaney P, Simpson P, et al. Vasopressin for in-hospital pediatric cardiac arrest: results from the American Heart Association National Registry of Cardiopulmonary Resuscitation. *Pediatr Crit Care Med*. 2009;10:191–195.
158. Voelckel WG, Lurie KG, McKnite S, et al. Comparison of epinephrine and vasopressin in a pediatric porcine model of asphyxial cardiac arrest. *Crit Care Med*. 2000;28:3777–3783.
159. Voelckel WG, Lurie KG, McKnite S, et al. Effects of epinephrine and vasopressin in a piglet model of prolonged ventricular fibrillation and cardiopulmonary resuscitation. *Crit Care Med*. 2002;30:957–962.
160. Neumar RW, Otto CW, Link MS, et al. Part 8: Adult Advanced Cardiovascular Life Support: 2010 American Heart Association Guidelines for Cardiopulmonary Resuscitation and Emergency Cardiovascular Care. *Circulation*. 2010;122:S729–S767.
161. Goldschlager N, Epstein AE, Naccarelli GV, et al. A practical guide for clinicians who treat patients with amiodarone: 2007. *Heart Rhythm*. 2007;4:1250–1259.
162. Kudenchuk PJ, Cobb LA, Copass MK, et al. Amiodarone for resuscitation after out-of-hospital cardiac arrest due to ventricular fibrillation. *N Engl J Med*. 1999;341:871–878.
163. Kudenchuk PJ, Brown SP, Daya M, et al. Resuscitation Outcomes Consortium-Amiodarone, Lidocaine or Placebo Study (ROC-ALPS): rationale and methodology behind an out-of-hospital cardiac arrest antiarrhythmic drug trial. *Am Heart J*. 2014;167:653–659.
164. Valdes SO, Donoghue AJ, Hoyme DB, et al. Outcomes associated with amiodarone and lidocaine in the treatment of in-hospital pediatric cardiac arrest with pulseless ventricular tachycardia or ventricular fibrillation. *Resuscitation*. 2014;85:381–386.
165. Somberg JC, Bailin SJ, Haffajee CI, et al. Intravenous lidocaine versus intravenous amiodarone (in a new aqueous formulation) for incessant ventricular tachycardia. *Am J Cardiol*. 2002;90:853–859.
166. Marill KA, Greenberg GM, Kay D, Nelson BK. Analysis of the treatment of spontaneous sustained stable ventricular tachycardia. *Acad Emerg Med*. 1997;4:1122–1128.
167. Gorgels AP, van den Dool A, Hofs A, et al. Comparison of procainamide and lidocaine in terminating sustained monomorphic ventricular tachycardia. *Am J Cardiol*. 1996;78:43–46.
168. Nagao K. Nifekalant hydrochloride for patients with cardiac arrest caused by shockable rhythm. *Circ J*. 2010;74:2285–2287.
169. Shiga T, Tanaka K, Kato R, et al. Nifekalant versus lidocaine for in-hospital shock-resistant ventricular fibrillation or tachycardia. *Resuscitation*. 2010;81:47–52.
170. Huang Y, He Q, Yang M, Zhan L. Antiarrhythmia drugs for cardiac arrest: a systemic review and meta-analysis. *Crit Care*. 2013;17:R173.
171. Graf H, Leach W, Arieff AI. Evidence for a detrimental effect of bicarbonate therapy in hypoxic lactic acidosis. *Science*. 1985;227:754–756.

172. Kette F, Weil MH, Gazmuri RJ. Buffer solutions may compromise cardiac resuscitation by reducing coronary perfusion pressure. *JAMA*. 1991;266:2121–2126.
173. Weng YM, Wu SH, Li WC, et al. The effects of sodium bicarbonate during prolonged cardiopulmonary resuscitation. *Am J Emerg Med*. 2013;31:562–565.
174. Kleinman ME, Chameides L, Schexnayder SM, et al. Part 14: Pediatric Advanced Life Support: 2010 American Heart Association guidelines for cardiopulmonary resuscitation and emergency cardiovascular care. *Circulation*. 2010;122:S876–S908.
175. Wang CH, Huang CH, Chang WT, et al. The effects of calcium and sodium bicarbonate on severe hyperkalaemia during cardiopulmonary resuscitation: a retrospective cohort study of adult in-hospital cardiac arrest. *Resuscitation*. 2016;98:105–111.
176. Alfonzo A. Survival after in-hospital hyperkalaemic cardiac arrest--Does intravenous calcium or sodium bicarbonate influence outcome? *Resuscitation*. 2016;98:A1-A2.
177. Mahoney BA, Smith WA, Lo DS, et al. Emergency interventions for hyperkalaemia. *Cochrane Database Syst Rev*. 2005;(2):CD003235.
178. Raymond TT, Stromberg D, Stigall W, et al. Sodium bicarbonate use during in-hospital pediatric pulseless cardiac arrest: a report from the American Heart Association Get With The Guidelines®-Resuscitation. *Resuscitation*. 2015;89:106–113.
179. Eisa L, Passi Y, Lerman J, et al. Do small doses of atropine (<0.1 mg) cause bradycardia in young children? *Arch Dis Child*. 2015;100:684–688.
180. Jones P, Peters MJ, Pinto da Costa N, et al. Atropine for critical care intubation in a cohort of 264 children and reduced mortality unrelated to effects on bradycardia. *PloS One*. 2013;8:e57478.
181. Jones PB, Dauger S, Denjoy I, et al. The effect of atropine on rhythm and conduction disturbances during 322 critical care intubations. *Pediatr Crit Care Med*. 2013;14:e289–e297.
182. Stueven H, Thompson B, Aprahamian C, et al. The effectiveness of calcium chloride in refractory electromechanical dissociation. *Ann Emerg Med*. 1985;14:626–629.
183. Stueven H, Thompson B, Aprahamian C, et al. Lack of effectiveness of calcium chloride in refractory asystole. *Ann Emerg Med*. 1985;14:630–632.
184. Reis AG, Paiva EFd, Schvartsman C, Zaritsky AL. Magnesium in cardiopulmonary resuscitation: Critical review. *Resuscitation*. 2008;77:21–25.
185. Roberts BW, Kilgannon JH, Chansky ME, et al. Multiple organ dysfunction after return of spontaneous circulation in postcardiac arrest syndrome. *Crit Care Med*. 2013;41:1492–1501.
186. Girotra S, Cram P, Spertus JA, et al. Hospital variation in survival trends for in-hospital cardiac arrest. *JAMA*. 2014;3:e000871.
187. Ewy GA, Bobrow BJ. Cardiocerebral resuscitation: an approach to improving survival of patients with primary cardiac arrest. *J Intensive Care Med*. 2016;31:24–33.
188. Cronberg T, Lilja G. Cognitive decline after cardiac arrest: it is more to the picture than hypoxic brain injury. *Resuscitation*. 2015;91:A3–A4.
189. Lilja G, Nielsen N, Friberg H, et al. Cognitive function in survivors of out-of-hospital cardiac arrest after target temperature management at 33 degrees C versus 36 degrees C. *Circulation*. 2015;131:1340–1349.
190. Sulzgruber P, Kliegel A, Wandaller C, et al. Survivors of cardiac arrest with good neurological outcome show considerable impairments of memory functioning. *Resuscitation*. 2015;88:120–125.
191. Adrie C, Laurent I, Monchi M, et al. Postresuscitation disease after cardiac arrest: a sepsis-like syndrome? *Curr Opin Crit Care*. 2004;10:208–212.
192. Bro-Jeppesen J, Kjaergaard J, Wanscher M, et al. The inflammatory response after out-of-hospital cardiac arrest is not modified by targeted temperature management at 33 degrees C or 36 degrees C. *Resuscitation*. 2014;85:1480–1487.
193. Kern KB. Postresuscitation myocardial dysfunction. *Cardiol Clin*. 2002; 20:89–101.
194. Checchia PA, Sehra R, Moynihan J, et al. Myocardial injury in children following resuscitation after cardiac arrest. *Resuscitation*. 2003;57:131–1317.
195. Laurent I, Monchi M, Chiche JD, et al. Reversible myocardial dysfunction in survivors of out-of-hospital cardiac arrest. *J Am Coll Cardiol*. 2002;40:2110–2116.
196. Laver S, Farrow C, Turner D, Nolan J. Mode of death after admission to an intensive care unit following cardiac arrest. *Intensive Care Med*. 2004;30:2126–2128.
197. Lemiale V, Dumas F, Mongardon N, et al. Intensive care unit mortality after cardiac arrest: the relative contribution of shock and brain injury in a large cohort. *Intensive Care Med*. 2013;39:1972–1980.
198. Dragancea I, Rundgren M, Englund E, et al. The influence of induced hypothermia and delayed prognostication on the mode of death after cardiac arrest. *Resuscitation*. 2013;84:337–342.
199. Fries M, Weil MH, Chang Y-T, et al. Microcirculation during cardiac arrest and resuscitation. *Crit Care Med*. 2006;34:S454–S457.
200. van Genderen ME, Lima A, Akkerhuis M, et al. Persistent peripheral and microcirculatory perfusion alterations after out-of-hospital cardiac arrest are associated with poor survival. *Crit Care Med*. 2012;40:2287–2294.
201. Eastwood GM, Young PJ, Bellomo R. The impact of oxygen and carbon dioxide management on outcome after cardiac arrest. *Curr Opin Crit Care*. 2014;20:266–272.
202. Pilcher J, Weatherall M, Shirtcliffe P, et al. The effect of hyperoxia following cardiac arrest—A systematic review and meta-analysis of animal trials. *Resuscitation*. 2012;83:417-422.
203. Wang CH, Chang WT, Huang CH, et al. The effect of hyperoxia on survival following adult cardiac arrest: a systematic review and meta-analysis of observational studies. *Resuscitation*. 2014;85:1142–1148.
204. Elmer J, Scutella M, Pullalarevu R, et al. The association between hyperoxia and patient outcomes after cardiac arrest: analysis of a high-resolution database. *Intensive Care Med*. 2015;41:49–57.
205. Guerra-Wallace MM, Casey FL III, Bell MJ, et al. Hyperoxia and hypoxia in children resuscitated from cardiac arrest. *Pediatr Crit Care Med*. 2013;14: e143–e148.
206. Del Castillo J, Lopez-Herce J, Matamoros M, et al. Hyperoxia, hypocapnia and hypercapnia as outcome factors after cardiac arrest in children. *Resuscitation*. 2012;83:1456–1461.
207. Skippen P, Seear M, Poskitt K, et al. Effect of hyperventilation on regional cerebral blood flow in head- injured children. *Crit Care Med*. 1997;25:1402–1409.
208. Bouzat P, Suys T, Sala N, Oddo M. Effect of moderate hyperventilation and induced hypertension on cerebral tissue oxygenation after cardiac arrest and therapeutic hypothermia. *Resuscitation*. 2013;84:1540–1545.
209. Roberts BW, Kilgannon JH, Chansky ME, et al. Association between postresuscitation partial pressure of arterial carbon dioxide and neurological outcome in patients with post-cardiac arrest syndrome. *Circulation*. 2013;127:2107–2113.
210. Schneider AG, Eastwood GM, Bellomo R, et al. Arterial carbon dioxide tension and outcome in patients admitted to the intensive care unit after cardiac arrest. *Resuscitation*. 2013;84:927–934.
211. Vaahersalo J, Bendel S, Reinikainen M, et al. Arterial blood gas tensions after resuscitation from out-of-hospital cardiac arrest: associations with long-term neurologic outcome. *Crit Care Med*. 2014;42:1463–1470.
212. Slutsky AS, Ranieri VM. Ventilator-induced lung injury. *N Engl J Med*. 2013;369:2126–2136.
213. Alhazzani W, Alshahrani M, Jaeschke R, et al. Neuromuscular blocking agents in acute respiratory distress syndrome: a systematic review and meta-analysis of randomized controlled trials. *Crit Care*. 2013;17:R43.
214. Salciccioli JD, Cocchi MN, Rittenberger JC, et al. Continuous neuromuscular blockade is associated with decreased mortality in post-cardiac arrest patients. *Resuscitation*. 2013;84:1728–1733.
215. Wijdicks EF, Hijdra A, Young GB, et al. Practice parameter: prediction of outcome in comatose survivors after cardiopulmonary resuscitation (an evidence-based review): report of the Quality Standards Subcommittee of the American Academy of Neurology. *Neurology*. 2006;67:203–210.
216. Oddo M, Rossetti A. Predicting neurological outcome after cardiac arrest. *Curr Opin Crit Care*. 2011;17:254–259.
217. Amorim E, Rittenberger JC, Baldwin ME, et al. Malignant EEG patterns in cardiac arrest patients treated with targeted temperature management who survive to hospital discharge. *Resuscitation*. 2015;90:127–132.
218. Dragancea I, Backman S, Westhall E, et al. Outcome following postanoxic status epilepticus in patients with targeted temperature management after cardiac arrest. *Epilepsy Behav*. 2015;49:173–177.
219. Nolan JP, Soar J, Cariou A, et al. European Resuscitation Council and European Society of Intensive Care Medicine Guidelines for Post-resuscitation Care 2015: section 5 of the European Resuscitation Council Guidelines for Resuscitation 2015. *Resuscitation*. 2015;95:202–222.
220. Herman ST, Abend NS, Bleck TP, et al. Consensus statement on continuous EEG in critically ill adults and children, part I: indications. *J Clin Neurophysiol*. 2015;32:87–95.
221. Feng G, Jiang G, Li Z, Wang X. Prognostic value of electroencephalography (EEG) for brain injury after cardiopulmonary resuscitation. *Neurol Sci*. 2016;37(6):843–849.
222. Larsen JM, Ravkilde J. Acute coronary angiography in patients resuscitated from out-of-hospital cardiac arrest: a systematic review and meta-analysis. *Resuscitation*. 2012;83:1427–1433.
223. Camuglia AC, Randhawa VK, Lavi S, Walters DL. Cardiac catheterization is associated with superior outcomes for survivors of out of hospital cardiac arrest: review and meta-analysis. *Resuscitation*. 2014;85: 1533–1540.

224. Grasner JT, Meybohm P, Caliebe A, et al. Postresuscitation care with mild therapeutic hypothermia and coronary intervention after out-of-hospital cardiopulmonary resuscitation: a prospective registry analysis. *Crit Care.* 2011;15:R61.
225. Garcia-Tejada J, Jurado-Roman A, Rodriguez J, et al. Post-resuscitation electrocardiograms, acute coronary findings and in-hospital prognosis of survivors of out-of-hospital cardiac arrest. *Resuscitation.* 2014;85:1245–1250.
226. Nikolaou NI, Welsford M, Beygui F, et al. Part 5: Acute coronary syndromes: 2015 International Consensus on Cardiopulmonary Resuscitation and Emergency Cardiovascular Care Science With Treatment Recommendations. *Resuscitation.* 2015;95:e121–e146.
227. Harker M, Carville S, Henderson R, et al. Key recommendations and evidence from the NICE guideline for the acute management of ST-segment-elevation myocardial infarction. *Heart.* 2014;100:536–543.
228. O'Gara PT, Kushner FG, Ascheim DD, et al. 2013 ACCF/AHA guideline for the management of ST-elevation myocardial infarction: a report of the American College of Cardiology Foundation/American Heart Association Task Force on Practice Guidelines. *Circulation.* 2013;127:e362–e425.
229. Dumas F, White L, Stubbs BA, et al. Long-term prognosis following resuscitation from out of hospital cardiac arrest: role of percutaneous coronary intervention and therapeutic hypothermia. *J Am Coll Cardiol.* 2012;60:21–27.
230. Hollenbeck RD, McPherson JA, Mooney MR, et al. Early cardiac catheterization is associated with improved survival in comatose survivors of cardiac arrest without STEMI. *Resuscitation.* 2014;85:88–95.
231. Redfors B, Ramunddal T, Angeras O, et al. Angiographic findings and survival in patients undergoing coronary angiography due to sudden cardiac arrest in western Sweden. *Resuscitation.* 2015;90:13–20.
232. Bro-Jeppesen J, Kjaergaard J, Wanscher M, et al. Emergency coronary angiography in comatose cardiac arrest patients: Do real-life experiences support the guidelines? *Eur Heart J Acute Cardiovasc Care.* 2012;1:291–301.
233. Dankiewicz J, Nielsen N, Annborn M, et al. Survival in patients without acute ST elevation after cardiac arrest and association with early coronary angiography: a post hoc analysis from the TTM trial. *Intensive Care Med.* 2015;41:856–864.
234. Bro-Jeppesen J, Annborn M, Hassager C, et al. Hemodynamics and vasopressor support during targeted temperature management at 33 degrees C versus 36 degrees C after out-of-hospital cardiac arrest: a post hoc study of the target temperature management trial. *Crit Care Med.* 2015; 43:318–327.
235. Conlon TW, Falkensammer CB, Hammond RS, et al. Association of left ventricular systolic function and vasopressor support with survival following pediatric out-of-hospital cardiac arrest. *Pediatr Crit Care Med.* 2015;16:146–154.
236. Ameloot K, Meex I, Genbrugge C, et al. Hemodynamic targets during therapeutic hypothermia after cardiac arrest: a prospective observational study. *Resuscitation.* 2015;91:56–62.
237. Ameloot K, Genbrugge C, Meex I, et al. Low hemoglobin levels are associated with lower cerebral saturations and poor outcome after cardiac arrest. *Resuscitation.* 2015;96:280–286.
238. Albaeni A, Eid SM, Akinyele B, et al. The association between post resuscitation hemoglobin level and survival with good neurological outcome following out of hospital cardiac arrest. *Resuscitation.* 2016;99:7–12.
239. Ahmad Y, Sen S, Shun-Shin MJ, et al. Intra-aortic balloon pump therapy for acute myocardial infarction: a meta-analysis. *JAMA.* 2015;175:931–939.
240. Sundgreen C, Larsen FS, Herzog TM, et al. Autoregulation of cerebral blood flow in patients resuscitated from cardiac arrest. *Stroke.* 2001; 32:128–132.
241. Staer-Jensen H, Sunde K, Olasveengen TM, et al. Bradycardia during therapeutic hypothermia is associated with good neurologic outcome in comatose survivors of out-of-hospital cardiac arrest. *Crit Care Med.* 2014;42:2401–2408.
242. Thomsen JH, Hassager C, Bro-Jeppesen J, et al. Sinus bradycardia during hypothermia in comatose survivors of out-of-hospital cardiac arrest: a new early marker of favorable outcome? *Resuscitation.* 2015;89:36–42.
243. Arnaout M, Mongardon N, Deye N, et al. Out-of-hospital cardiac arrest from brain cause: epidemiology, clinical features, and outcome in a multicenter cohort. *Crit Care Med.* 2015;43:453–460.
244. Chelly J, Mongardon N, Dumas F, et al. Benefit of an early and systematic imaging procedure after cardiac arrest: insights from the PROCAT (Parisian Region Out of Hospital Cardiac Arrest) registry. *Resuscitation.* 2012;83:1444–1450.
245. Safar P, Kochanek P. Cerebral blood flow promotion after prolonged cardiac arrest. *Crit Care Med.* 2000;28:3104–3106.
246. Drabek T, Foley LM, Janata A, et al. Global and regional differences in cerebral blood flow after asphyxial versus ventricular fibrillation cardiac arrest in rats using ASL-MRI. *Resuscitation.* 2014;85:964–971.
247. Edgren E, Enblad P, Grenvik A, et al. Cerebral blood flow and metabolism after cardiopulmonary resuscitation: a pathophysiologic and prognostic positron emission tomography pilot study. *Resuscitation.* 2003;57:161–170.
248. Lemiale V, Huet O, Vigue B, et al. Changes in cerebral blood flow and oxygen extraction during post-resuscitation syndrome. *Resuscitation.* 2008;76:17–24.
249. Morimoto Y, Kemmotsu O, Kitami K, et al. Acute brain swelling after out-of-hospital cardiac arrest: pathogenesis and outcome. *Crit Care Med.* 1993;21:104–110.
250. Dean JM, McComb JG. Intracranial pressure monitoring in severe pediatric near-drowning. *Neurosurgery.* 1981;9:627–630.
251. Ameloot K, Genbrugge C, Meex I, et al. An observational near-infrared spectroscopy study on cerebral autoregulation in post-cardiac arrest patients: time to drop 'one-size-fits-all' hemodynamic targets? *Resuscitation.* 2015;90:121–126.
252. Bjelland TW, Dale O, Kaisen K, et al. Propofol and remifentanil versus midazolam and fentanyl for sedation during therapeutic hypothermia after cardiac arrest: a randomised trial. *Intensive Care Med.* 2012;38:959–967.
253. Bouwes A, van Poppelen D, Koelman JH, et al. Acute posthypoxic myoclonus after cardiopulmonary resuscitation. *BMC Neurol.* 2012;12:63.
254. Seder DB, Sunde K, Rubertsson S, et al. Neurologic outcomes and postresuscitation care of patients with myoclonus following cardiac arrest. *Crit Care Med.* 2015;43:965–972.
255. Benbadis SR, Chen S, Melo M. What's shaking in the ICU? The differential diagnosis of seizures in the intensive care setting. *Epilepsia.* 2010;51:2338–2340.
256. Sadaka F, Doerr D, Hindia J, et al. Continuous electroencephalogram in comatose postcardiac arrest syndrome patients treated with therapeutic hypothermia: outcome prediction study. *J Intensive Care Med.* 2015;30:292–296.
257. Mani R, Schmitt SE, Mazer M, et al. The frequency and timing of epileptiform activity on continuous electroencephalogram in comatose post-cardiac arrest syndrome patients treated with therapeutic hypothermia. *Resuscitation.* 2012;83:840–847.
258. Ingvar M. Cerebral blood flow and metabolic rate during seizures: relationship to epileptic brain damage. *Ann NY Acad Sci.* 1986;462:194–206.
259. Thomke F, Weilemann SL. Poor prognosis despite successful treatment of postanoxic generalized myoclonus. *Neurology.* 2010;74:1392–1394.
260. Caviness JN, Brown P. Myoclonus: current concepts and recent advances. *Lancet Neurol.* 2004;3:598–607.
261. Samaniego EA, Mlynash M, Caulfield AF, et al. Sedation confounds outcome prediction in cardiac arrest survivors treated with hypothermia. *Neurocrit Care.* 2011;15:113–119.
262. Mullner M, Sterz F, Binder M, et al. Blood glucose concentration after cardiopulmonary resuscitation influences functional neurological recovery in human cardiac arrest survivors. *J Cereb Blood Flow Metab.* 1997;17:430–436.
263. Daviaud F, Dumas F, Demars N, et al. Blood glucose level and outcome after cardiac arrest: insights from a large registry in the hypothermia era. *Intensive Care Med.* 2014;40:855–862.
264. Nolan JP, Laver SR, Welch CA, et al. Outcome following admission to UK intensive care units after cardiac arrest: a secondary analysis of the ICNARC Case Mix Programme Database. *Anaesthesia.* 2007;62:1207–1216.
265. Nice-Sugar Study Investigators, Finfer S, Chittock DR, et al. Intensive versus conventional glucose control in critically ill patients. *N Engl J Med.* 2009;360:1283–1297.
266. Nice-Sugar Study Investigators, Finfer S, Liu B, et al. Hypoglycemia and risk of death in critically ill patients. *N Engl J Med.* 2012;367:1108–1118.
267. Meyfroidt G, Keenan DM, Wang X, et al. Dynamic characteristics of blood glucose time series during the course of critical illness: effects of intensive insulin therapy and relative association with mortality. *Crit Care Med.* 2010;38:1021–1029.
268. Cueni-Villoz N, Devigili A, Delodder F, et al. Increased blood glucose variability during therapeutic hypothermia and outcome after cardiac arrest. *Crit Care Med.* 2011;39:2225–2231.
269. Zeiner A, Holzer M, Sterz F, et al. Hyperthermia after cardiac arrest is associated with an unfavorable neurologic outcome. *Arch Intern Med.* 2001;161:2007–2012.
270. Hickey RW, Kochanek PM, Ferimer H, et al. Hypothermia and hyperthermia in children after resuscitation from cardiac arrest. *Pediatrics.* 2000;106:118–122.

271. Langhelle A, Tyvold SS, Lexow K, et al. In-hospital factors associated with improved outcome after out-of-hospital cardiac arrest: a comparison between four regions in Norway. *Resuscitation*. 2003;56:247–263.
272. Bro-Jeppesen J, Hassager C, Wanscher M, et al. Post-hypothermia fever is associated with increased mortality after out-of-hospital cardiac arrest. *Resuscitation*. 2013;84:1734–1740.
273. Winters SA, Wolf KH, Kettinger SA, et al. Assessment of risk factors for post-rewarming "rebound hyperthermia" in cardiac arrest patients undergoing therapeutic hypothermia. *Resuscitation*. 2013;84:1245–1249.
274. Nielsen N, Wetterslev J, Cronberg T, et al. Targeted temperature management at 33 degrees C versus 36 degrees C after cardiac arrest. *N Engl J Med*. 2013;369:2197–2206.
275. Moler FW, Silverstein FS, Holubkov R, et al. Therapeutic hypothermia after out-of-hospital cardiac arrest in children. *N Engl J Med*. 2015; 372:1898–1908.
276. Gonzalez-Ibarra FP, Varon J, Lopez-Meza EG. Therapeutic hypothermia: critical review of the molecular mechanisms of action. *Front Neurol*. 2011;2:4.
277. Bernard SA, Gray TW, Buist MD, et al. Treatment of comatose survivors of out-of-hospital cardiac arrest with induced hypothermia. *N Engl J Med*. 2002;346:557–563.
278. The Hypothermia After Cardiac Arrest Study Group. Mild therapeutic hypothermia to improve the neurologic outcome after cardiac arrest. *N Engl J Med*. 2002;346:549–556.
279. Cronberg T, Lilja G, Horn J, et al. Neurologic function and health-related quality of life in patients following targeted temperature management at 33 degrees C vs 36 degrees C After out-of-hospital cardiac arrest: a randomized clinical trial. *JAMA Neurol*. 2015;72:634–641.
280. Maconochie IK, de Caen AR, Aickin R, et al. Part 6: Pediatric basic life support and pediatric advanced life support: 2015 International Consensus on Cardiopulmonary Resuscitation and Emergency Cardiovascular Care Science With Treatment Recommendations. *Resuscitation*. 2015;95:e147–e168.
281. Donnino MW, Andersen LW, Berg KM, et al. Temperature management after cardiac arrest: an advisory statement by the Advanced Life Support Task Force of the International Liaison Committee on Resuscitation and the American Heart Association Emergency Cardiovascular Care Committee and the Council on Cardiopulmonary, Critical Care, Perioperative and Resuscitation. *Resuscitation*. 2016;98:97–104.
282. Polderman KH, Herold I. Therapeutic hypothermia and controlled normothermia in the intensive care unit: practical considerations, side effects, and cooling methods. *Crit Care Med*. 2009;37:1101–1120.
283. Colbourne F, Corbett D. Delayed postischemic hypothermia: a six month survival study using behavioral and histological assessments of neuroprotection. *J Neurosci*. 1995;15:7250–7260.
284. Kuboyama K, Safar P, Radovsky A, et al. Delay in cooling negates the beneficial effect of mild resuscitative cerebral hypothermia after cardiac arrest in dogs: a prospective, randomized study. *Crit Care Med*. 1993;21:1348–1358.
285. Bernard SA, Smith K, Cameron P, et al. Induction of therapeutic hypothermia by paramedics after resuscitation from out-of-hospital ventricular fibrillation cardiac arrest: a randomized controlled trial. *Circulation*. 2010;122:737–742.
286. Bernard SA, Smith K, Cameron P, et al. Induction of prehospital therapeutic hypothermia after resuscitation from nonventricular fibrillation cardiac arrest. *Crit Care Med*. 2012;40:747–753.
287. Kim F, Nichol G, Maynard C, et al. Effect of prehospital induction of mild hypothermia on survival and neurological status among adults with cardiac arrest: a randomized clinical trial. *JAMA*. 2014;311:45–52.
288. Castren M, Nordberg P, Svensson L, et al. Intra-arrest transnasal evaporative cooling: a randomized, prehospital, multicenter study (PRINCE: Pre-ROSC IntraNasal Cooling Effectiveness). *Circulation*. 2010;122:729–736.
289. Deye N, Cariou A, Girardie P, et al. Endovascular versus external targeted temperature management for patients with out-of-hospital cardiac arrest: a randomized, controlled study. *Circulation*. 2015;132:182–193.
290. Nagao K, Kikushima K, Watanabe K, et al. Early induction of hypothermia during cardiac arrest improves neurological outcomes in patients with out-of-hospital cardiac arrest who undergo emergency cardiopulmonary bypass and percutaneous coronary intervention. *Circ J*. 2010;74:77–85.
291. Langhelle A, Tyvold SS, Lexow K, et al. In-hospital factors associated with improved outcome after out-of-hospital cardiac arrest: a comparison between four regions in Norway. *Resuscitation*. 2003;56:247–263.
292. Mahmood MA, Zweifler RM. Progress in shivering control. *J Neurol Sci*. 2007;261:47–54.
293. Gillies MA, Pratt R, Whiteley C, et al. Therapeutic hypothermia after cardiac arrest: a retrospective comparison of surface and endovascular cooling techniques. *Resuscitation*. 2010;81:1117–1122.
294. Hoedemaekers CW, Ezzahti M, Gerritsen A, van der Hoeven JG. Comparison of cooling methods to induce and maintain normo- and hypothermia in intensive care unit patients: a prospective intervention study. *Crit Care*. 2007;11:R91.
295. Arrich J. Clinical application of mild therapeutic hypothermia after cardiac arrest. *Crit Care Med*. 2007;35:1041–1047.
296. Tomte O, Draegni T, Mangschau A, et al. A comparison of intravascular and surface cooling techniques in comatose cardiac arrest survivors. *Crit Care Med*. 2011;39:443–449.
297. Nair SU, Lundbye JB. The occurrence of shivering in cardiac arrest survivors undergoing therapeutic hypothermia is associated with a good neurologic outcome. *Resuscitation*. 2013;84:626–629.
298. Zobel C, Adler C, Kranz A, et al. Mild therapeutic hypothermia in cardiogenic shock syndrome. *Crit Care Med*. 2012;40:1715–1723.
299. Post H, Schmitto JD, Steendijk P, et al. Cardiac function during mild hypothermia in pigs: increased inotropy at the expense of diastolic dysfunction. *Acta Physiol (Oxf)*. 2010;199:43–52.
300. Polderman KH, Peerdeman SM, Girbes AR. Hypophosphatemia and hypomagnesemia induced by cooling in patients with severe head injury. *J Neurosurg*. 2001;94:697–705.
301. Brinkman AC, Ten Tusscher BL, de Waard MC, et al. Minimal effects on ex vivo coagulation during mild therapeutic hypothermia in post cardiac arrest patients. *Resuscitation*. 2014;85:1359–1363.
302. Sunde K, Pytte M, Jacobsen D, et al. Implementation of a standardised treatment protocol for post resuscitation care after out-of-hospital cardiac arrest. *Resuscitation*. 2007;73:29–39.
303. Fries M, Stoppe C, Brucken D, et al. Influence of mild therapeutic hypothermia on the inflammatory response after successful resuscitation from cardiac arrest. *J Crit Care*. 2009;24:453–457.
304. Mongardon N, Perbet S, Lemiale V, et al. Infectious complications in out-of-hospital cardiac arrest patients in the therapeutic hypothermia era. *Crit Care Med*. 2011;39:1359–1364.
305. Perbet S, Mongardon N, Dumas F, et al. Early-onset pneumonia after cardiac arrest: characteristics, risk factors and influence on prognosis. *Am J Resp Crit Care Med*. 2011;184:1048–1054.
306. Gagnon DJ, Nielsen N, Fraser GL, et al. Prophylactic antibiotics are associated with a lower incidence of pneumonia in cardiac arrest survivors treated with targeted temperature management. *Resuscitation*. 2015; 92:154–159.
307. Davies KJ, Walters JH, Kerslake IM, et al. Early antibiotics improve survival following out-of hospital cardiac arrest. *Resuscitation*. 2013;84:616–619.
308. Bjelland TW, Klepstad P, Haugen BO, et al. Effects of hypothermia on the disposition of morphine, midazolam, fentanyl, and propofol in intensive care unit patients. *Drug Metab Dispos*. 2013;41:214–223.
309. Bjelland TW, Klepstad P, Haugen BO, et al. Concentrations of remifentanil, propofol, fentanyl, and midazolam during rewarming from therapeutic hypothermia. *Acta Anaesthesiol Scand*. 2014;58:709–715.
310. Polderman KH. Mechanisms of action, physiological effects, and complications of hypothermia. *Crit Care Med*. 2009;37:S186–S202.
311. Golan E, Barrett K, Alali AS, et al. Predicting neurologic outcome after targeted temperature management for cardiac arrest: systematic review and meta-analysis. *Crit Care Med*. 2014;42:1919–1930.
312. Chan PS, Spertus JA, Krumholz HM, et al. A validated prediction tool for initial survivors of in-hospital cardiac arrest. *Arch Intern Med*. 2012;172:947–953.
313. Cooper S, Janghorbani M, Cooper G. A decade of in-hospital resuscitation: outcomes and prediction of survival? *Resuscitation*. 2006;68:231–237.
314. Goldberger ZD, Chan PS, Berg RA, et al. Duration of resuscitation efforts and survival after in-hospital cardiac arrest: an observational study. *Lancet*. 2012;380:1473–1481.
315. White RD, Goodman BW, Svoboda MA. Neurologic recovery following prolonged out-of-hospital cardiac arrest with resuscitation guided by continuous capnography. *Mayo Clin Proc*. 2011;86:544–548.
316. Matos RI, Watson RS, Nadkarni VM, et al. Duration of cardiopulmonary resuscitation and illness category impact survival and neurologic outcomes for in-hospital pediatric cardiac arrests. *Circulation*. 2013;127: 442–451.
317. Sandroni C, Cariou A, Cavallaro F, et al. Prognostication in comatose survivors of cardiac arrest: an advisory statement from the European Resuscitation Council and the European Society of Intensive Care Medicine. *Resuscitation*. 2014;85:1779–1789.
318. Sandroni C, Cavallaro F, Callaway CW, et al. Predictors of poor neurological outcome in adult comatose survivors of cardiac arrest: a systematic review and meta-analysis. Part 2: patients treated with therapeutic hypothermia. *Resuscitation*. 2013;84:1324–1338.

319. Sandroni C, Cavallaro F, Callaway CW, et al. Predictors of poor neurological outcome in adult comatose survivors of cardiac arrest: a systematic review and meta-analysis. Part 1: patients not treated with therapeutic hypothermia. *Resuscitation*. 2013;84:1310–1323.
320. Fink EL, Berger RP, Clark RS, et al. Serum biomarkers of brain injury to classify outcome after pediatric cardiac arrest. *Crit Care Med*. 2014;42:664–674.
321. Abend NS, Topjian AA, Kessler SK, et al. Outcome prediction by motor and pupillary responses in children treated with therapeutic hypothermia after cardiac arrest. *Pediatr Crit Care Med*. 2012;13:32–38.
322. Moler FW, Donaldson AE, Meert K, et al. Multicenter cohort study of out-of-hospital pediatric cardiac arrest. *Crit Care Med*. 2011;39:141–149.
323. Kessler SK, Topjian AA, Gutierrez-Colina AM, et al. Short-term outcome prediction by electroencephalographic features in children treated with therapeutic hypothermia after cardiac arrest. *Neurocrit Care*. 2011;14:37–43.
324. Nishisaki A, Sullivan J, 3rd, Steger B, et al. Retrospective analysis of the prognostic value of electroencephalography patterns obtained in pediatric in-hospital cardiac arrest survivors during three years. *Pediatr Crit Care Med*. 2007;8:10–17.
325. Topjian AA, Lin R, Morris MC, et al. Neuron-specific enolase and S-100B are associated with neurologic outcome after pediatric cardiac arrest. *Pediatr Crit Care Med*. 2009;10:479–490.
326. Hahn DK, Geocadin RG, Greer DM. Quality of evidence in studies evaluating neuroimaging for neurologic prognostication in adult patients resuscitated from cardiac arrest. *Resuscitation*. 2014;85:165–172.
327. Cronberg T, Brizzi M, Liedholm LJ, et al. Neurological prognostication after cardiac arrest–recommendations from the Swedish Resuscitation Council. *Resuscitation*. 2013;84:867–872.
328. Taccone F, Cronberg T, Friberg H, et al. How to assess prognosis after cardiac arrest and therapeutic hypothermia. *Crit Care*. 2014;18:202.
329. Greer DM, Yang J, Scripko PD, et al. Clinical examination for prognostication in comatose cardiac arrest patients. *Resuscitation*. 2013;84:1546–1551.
330. Dragancea I, Horn J, Kuiper M, et al. Neurological prognostication after cardiac arrest and targeted temperature management 33 degrees C versus 36 degrees C: results from a randomised controlled clinical trial. *Resuscitation*. 2015;93:164–170.
331. Stammet P, Collignon O, Hassager C, et al. Neuron-specific enolase as a predictor of death or poor neurological outcome after out-of-hospital cardiac arrest and targeted temperature management at 33 degrees C and 36 degrees C. *J Am Coll Cardiol*. 2015;65:2104–2114.
332. Lee BK, Jeung KW, Lee HY, et al. Combining brain computed tomography and serum neuron specific enolase improves the prognostic performance compared to either alone in comatose cardiac arrest survivors treated with therapeutic hypothermia. *Resuscitation*. 2013;84:1387–1392.
333. Oddo M, Rossetti AO. Early multimodal outcome prediction after cardiac arrest in patients treated with hypothermia. *Crit Care Med*. 2014;42:1340–1347.
334. Rossetti AO, Oddo M, Logroscino G, Kaplan PW. Prognostication after cardiac arrest and hypothermia: a prospective study. *Ann Neurol*. 2010;67:301–307.
335. Semmons R, Falk J. Predicting a pulse: Can monitoring heart rate and end-tidal carbon dioxide minimize compression pauses and impact outcomes in out-of-hospital cardiac arrest? *Resuscitation*. 2013;84:3-4.
336. Wolfe H, Zebuhr C, Topjian AA, et al. Interdisciplinary ICU cardiac arrest debriefing improves survival outcomes. *Crit Care Med*. 2014;42:1688–1695.

CHAPTER

52

Multiple Organ Dysfunction Syndrome

OYA M. ANDACOGLU and STEPHEN O. HEARD

IMMEDIATE CONCERNS

Major Problems

Progressive dysfunction of multiple organ systems, culminating in the syndrome of multiple organ dysfunction syndrome (MODS), has become a leading cause of death in critically ill and injured patients and is a disease of medical progress. Broader use of intensive care unit (ICU) resources, combined with improvements in single organ–directed therapy, such as mechanical ventilation and renal replacement therapy, has reduced early mortality after major physiologic insults. The result is a longer ICU stay for an increasing number of patients after severe sepsis and trauma, during which inflammation and tissue injury may result in MODS.

MODS represents a systemic disorder of immunoregulation, endothelial dysfunction, and hypermetabolism, with varying manifestations in individual organs. The mortality of MODS will increase as the number of failing organs increases, but organs differ in their host defense functions and sensitivity to host-derived inflammatory mediators or reductions in oxygen delivery ($\dot{D}O_2$). Therefore, diagnosis and therapy focus on preventive measures. Changes in the cellular O_2 supply and metabolism may cause and complicate MODS. Consequences can include direct hypoxic organ damage, secondary ischemia/reperfusion (I/R) injury mediated by neutrophils and reactive O_2 species (ROS), and enhanced injury by activation of cytokines. Initial and subsequent therapy follows a two-tiered approach, targeting systemic factors that contribute to ongoing inflammation and single organ–related problems. Efforts are first directed at stabilizing DO_2 while addressing life-threatening derangements in acid–base balance and gas exchange. Prompt correction of hemodynamic instability minimizes ischemia-related organ damage; time is a critical factor. Delays in completing initial resuscitation, eliminating foci of infection or devitalized tissue, or treating de novo organ-specific problems all worsen outcome. Late-phase (>72 hours) problems involve acquired immunosuppression, predisposition to secondary infection, and hypermetabolism, which impairs wound healing and host defense.

EPIDEMIOLOGY OF MULTIPLE ORGAN DYSFUNCTION SYNDROME

Significant advances have been made in critical care medicine over the past 35 years, particularly in the last decade. Nonetheless, many critically ill patients often suffer the progressive deterioration in the function of one or more organs, a phenomenon that has been termed MODS (1), and is the leading cause of death for ICU patients. In MODS, the death rate remains high even for patients who survive their ICU admission, and the financial costs are significant, with more than 60% of ICU resources consumed by these patients (2).

Individual organ dysfunction may result from a direct insult, such as pulmonary aspiration of gastric contents (primary MODS), or it can be associated with a systemic process such as shock or pancreatitis (secondary MODS) (1). Alterations in organ function seen during MODS are a continuum rather than a discrete, dichotomous event indicating the failure of an organ. A number of organ dysfunction scores have been developed to predict the clinical outcome of these patients (Table 52.1). These scores establish the baseline degree of organ dysfunction and enable the clinician to evaluate the progression or resolution of organ dysfunction over time; in general, an increase in the number of dysfunctional organs increases the risk of death. Examples of early scores of organ failure include those published by Goris et al. (3) and Knaus et al. (4). Refinement of these scores led to the development of the MODS (5) and the sequential organ failure assessment (SOFA) scores (6). In principle, these are based on parameters for six organ systems: Cardiovascular, respiratory, hematologic, renal, central nervous system (CNS), and hepatic (7); the difference in the scores lies in the descriptive parameter for cardiovascular dysfunction. The MOD score describes the degree of cardiovascular dysfunction as a composite of heart rate, central venous pressure, and mean arterial pressure (MAP) (pressure-adjusted heart rate), whereas the SOFA score describes cardiovascular dysfunction by the dose of vasoactive agents administered.

Several trials have evaluated the performance of these scores as descriptors of multiple organ dysfunction and failure, and to assess the incidence of MODS in the intensive care unit. Moreno et al., in a prospective, international multicenter trial composed of 1,449 patients, were able to demonstrate that total maximum SOFA score and change in SOFA score over time (δ) can be used to quantify the degree of organ dysfunction present on ICU admission, the degree of dysfunction or failure that appears during the ICU stay, and the cumulative insult suffered by the patient (7). These findings were subsequently confirmed by Ferreira et al. (10), demonstrating that changes in the SOFA score were a good indicator of prognosis. In their study of 352 consecutive patients, an increase in SOFA score during the first 48 hours of intensive care predicted a mortality rate of at least 50% (10). In a group of patients with acute respiratory distress syndrome (ARDS), the Toronto ARDS Outcomes Group found a significant relationship between the change in MOD score over time of the ICU stay and the distance walked in 6 minutes up to 1 year following discharge from the ICU (11). The European Sepsis Occurrence in Acutely Ill Patients (SOAP) multicenter trial analyzed data from 3,147 adult ICU admissions to determine the incidence of MODS and its associated mortality in mixed medical and surgical ICU populations (12). The overall rate of MODS,

TABLE 52.1 Comparison of the Physiologic and Biochemical Parameters Used by Four Scoring Systems for Organ Dysfunction and Failure

Organ System	Sequential Organ Failure Assessment (SOFA) (6)	Multiple Organ Dysfunction Score (MOD) (5)	Logistic Organ Dysfunction (LOD) (8)	Brussels (9)
Cardiovascular	Blood pressure and vasopressor use	Blood pressure and adjusted heart rate	Blood pressure and heart rate	Blood pressure, fluid responsiveness, and acidosis
Pulmonary	PaO_2/FiO_2 and mechanical ventilation	PaO_2/FiO_2	PaO_2/FiO_2 and mechanical ventilation	PaO_2/FiO_2
Hepatic	Bilirubin	Bilirubin	Bilirubin and prothrombin time	Bilirubin
Hematologic	Platelets	Platelets	Platelets and white blood cell count	Platelets
Renal	Creatinine and urine output	Creatinine	Creatinine, blood urea nitrogen, or urine output	Creatinine
Central nervous system	Glasgow coma score (GCS)	GCS	GCS	GCS

Reprinted from Bernard GR. Quantification of organ dysfunction: seeking standardization. *Crit Care Med.* 1998;26:1767–1768, with permission.

defined as severe acquired dysfunction in two or more organ systems, was 43% for patients without a diagnosis of sepsis and 73% of those with a diagnosis of severe sepsis, a substantially higher incidence than previously reported (4). Like other investigators, they found a direct relationship between the number of organs failing and the ICU mortality (Fig. 52.1). Single organ failure carried an ICU mortality rate of 6%, whereas patients with four or more failing organs had mortality rates of 65%. Although earlier reports have suggested that the increase in mortality associated with an increased number of failed organs is independent of the identity of dysfunctional organ systems (13–15), the SOAP investigators found different results. Organ failure in patients with severe sepsis generally carried a higher mortality than in those patients without a diagnosis of severe sepsis. In the group of patients with severe sepsis, failure of the coagulation system carried the highest mortality (52.9%), followed by the hepatic (45.1%), CNS (43.9%), cardiovascular (42.3%), and renal system (41.2%). Respiratory failure in this analysis was associated with a mortality risk of 34.5%. Certain subsets of patients admitted to the ICU appear to be at greater risk of MODS: patients older than 65 years (older than 55 years in trauma patients) (15), increased severity of illness as assessed by APACHE II scores (20 or more), and diagnosis of sepsis or ARDS on admission. Among the patients with severe sepsis, the SOAP investigators found as independent predictors of mortality the following: "medical" admissions, *Pseudomonas* species infection, SAPS II score on admission, SOFA score at the onset of sepsis, bloodstream infection, cirrhosis, and cumulative fluid balance within the first 72 hours of the onset of sepsis. The latter variable has been identified as an independent predictor of mortality in other studies (16,17) but it remains uncertain whether a positive fluid balance in the ICU is simply a marker of severity of illness or is harmful per se.

PATHOPHYSIOLOGY

MODS usually occurs in patients who exhibit signs of a generalized inflammatory response (systemic inflammatory response syndrome [SIRS]; Table 52.2) (1). Although SIRS is often the result of infection (triggered by microbial products), other conditions such as necrotizing pancreatitis or trauma can release patient-derived factors called danger-associated molecular patterns (DAMPs) that lead to systemic manifestations of inflammation (18). Two or more SIRS criteria due to infection have been defined as sepsis. However, the need for two SIRS criteria to define sepsis will exclude one out of eight patients with sepsis and organ failure (19). Updated guidelines have broadened the diagnostic criteria for sepsis that were originally proposed in 1992 (20). Analysis of these two definitions shows high sensitivity for diagnosing sepsis but with a low specificity (21). For those patients who present with SIRS only, a significant number will progress to sepsis, septic shock, and, ultimately, MODS (22). Although suspected or documented infection is not required for the development of MODS, the syndromes of SIRS, sepsis, and MODS are closely related. Consequently, the review of the pathophysiology of MODS will also include discussions of SIRS and sepsis.

Derangements in Oxygen Delivery and Consumption

In most tissues, oxygen consumption ($\dot{V}O_2$) is determined by metabolic demand and is independent of DO_2. When $\dot{D}O_2$ is

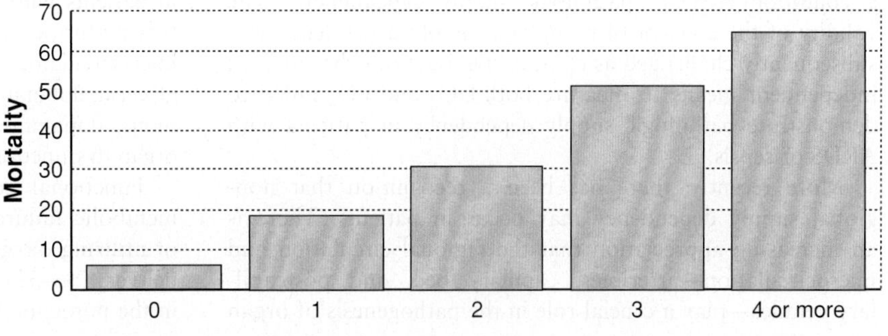

FIGURE 52.1 Relationship between the number of failed organs on admission and intensive care unit mortality. (From Vincent J-L, Sakr Y, Sprung CL, et al. Sepsis in European intensive care units: results of the SOAP study. *Crit Care Med.* 2006;34: 344–353, with permission.)

TABLE 52.2 American College of Chest Physicians/Society of Critical Care Medicine Definitions of Sepsis and Organ Failure

A. Infection
Microbial phenomenon characterized by an inflammatory response to the presence of the microorganism or the invasion of normally sterile host tissue by those organisms

B. Bacteremia
The presence of viable bacteria in the blood

C. Systemic inflammatory response syndrome (SIRS)
The systemic inflammatory response to a variety of severe clinical insults, manifested by any of the following conditions:
1. Temperature greater than 38°C or less than 36°C
2. Heart rate greater than 90 beats/min
3. Respiratory rate more than 20 breaths/min or $PaCO_2$ less than 32 mmHg
4. WBC more than 12,000 cells/μL, less than 4,000 cells/μL, or more than 10% immature (band) forms

D. Sepsis
The systemic response to infection. The manifestations are the same as those enumerated for SIRS.

E. Severe sepsis
Sepsis associated with organ dysfunction, hypoperfusion, or hypotension

F. Septic shock
Sepsis with hypotension, despite adequate fluid resuscitation, and perfusion abnormalities, including but not limited to the following:
1. Lactic acidosis
2. Oliguria
3. Acute alteration in mental status

G. Hypotension
A systolic BP less than 90 mmHg or a reduction of more than 4 mmHg from baseline in the absence of other causes for hypotension

H. Multiple organ dysfunction syndrome
Presence of altered organ function in an acutely ill patient such that homeostasis cannot be maintained without intervention

WBC, white blood cell; BP, blood pressure.
Condensed from American College of Chest Physicians/Society of Critical Care Medicine Consensus Conference. Definitions for sepsis and organ failure and guidelines for the use of innovative therapies in sepsis. *Crit Care Med.* 1992;20:864–874.

reduced, $\dot{V}O_2$ is maintained by increased oxygen extraction by the tissues. If $\dot{D}O_2$ is reduced to the point where the metabolic need cannot be met, $\dot{V}O_2$ becomes "supply dependent" (Fig. 52.2). The point at which $\dot{V}O_2$ decreases is called the critical $\dot{D}O_2$. Although one study (23) suggested that the critical $\dot{D}O_2$ in anesthetized humans is 330 mL/min/m^2, another investigation in which life support was withdrawn in critically ill patients demonstrated that the value is substantially lower (24).

A number of studies from the 1970s, 1980s, and early 1990s seemed to suggest that systemic $\dot{V}O_2$ was supply dependent over a wide range of $\dot{D}O_2$ in patients with sepsis or ARDS, a condition termed "pathologic supply dependency." The validity of the concept of pathologic supply dependency was subsequently challenged as clinical investigations that utilized independent means to measure both $\dot{D}O_2$ and $\dot{V}O_2$ failed to demonstrate pathologic supply dependency in patients with ARDS or sepsis.

More recently, there has been a recognition that nonglobal supply dependency may occur in patients. There is an increasing appreciation that the regional circulation and microcirculation—arterioles, capillary bed, and postcapillary venules—play a crucial role in the pathogenesis of organ

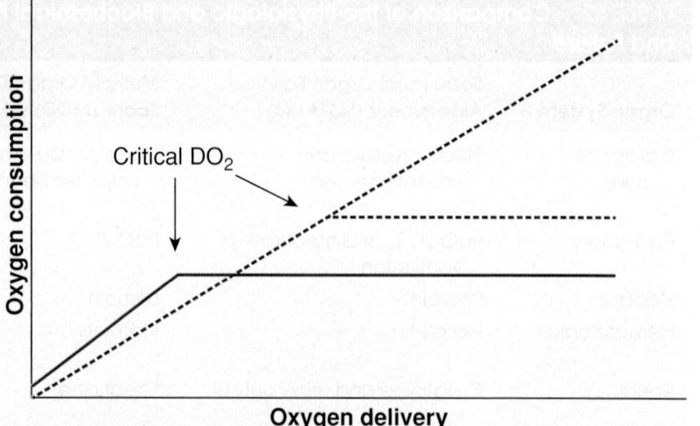

FIGURE 52.2 The relationship between oxygen delivery and consumption. The *solid line* represents the normal relationship. The *dashed line* shows pathologic supply dependency. (From Heard SO, Fink MP. Multiple-organ dysfunction syndrome. In: Murray MJ, Coursin DB, Pearl RG, et al., eds. *Critical Care Medicine. Perioperative Management.* Philadelphia, PA: Lippincott Williams & Wilkins; 2002.)

dysfunction in shock. Heterogeneous microcirculatory abnormalities occur due to changes in the activation state and shape of endothelial cells, alterations in vascular smooth muscle tone, activation of the clotting system, and changes in red and white blood cell deformability. Alterations in microvascular circulation have been demonstrated in congestive heart failure, cardiogenic shock, hemorrhage, and sepsis; in congestive heart failure these include reduced conjunctival microvascular density and attenuated nailfold capillary recruitment during postocclusive reactive hyperemia (25). Animal models of hemorrhagic shock demonstrate attenuated functional capillary perfusion—a measure of the number of capillaries that are actively moving blood—of skeletal muscle and the intestinal villi (26,27). Renal and intestinal regional blood flow is reduced despite resuscitation and return of global hemodynamics back to baseline values (28). Tissue (skeletal muscle) oxygen saturation in septic patients is no different than that observed in healthy controls or postsurgical patients (29); however, microvascular compliance and skeletal muscle oxygen consumption is reduced, and postischemic reperfusion time is increased compared to controls. Sidestream dark field (SDF) imaging is a technique by which perfusion of small and large vessels in the microcirculation of mucosal surfaces can be seen and quantified. Clinical studies (30,31) where SDF imaging has been utilized have shown that the fraction of perfused small vessels in patients with severe heart failure, cardiogenic shock, or sepsis is significantly lower than in those critically ill patients without those conditions (Fig. 52.3). Furthermore, alterations in microvascular perfusion are a strong predictor of poor ICU outcome in patients with severe sepsis (32). Transfusion of packed red blood cells may improve microcirculatory perfusion in patients who are identified as having altered microcirculatory perfusion by SDF imaging. Nonetheless, efforts to improve microcirculatory flow with a variety of agents—including nitroglycerin, dobutamine (33), inhaled nitric oxide (NO) (34), enoximone, dopamine, and corticosteroids—have had no effect on organ dysfunction (35).

Functional cellular hypoxia—"cytopathic hypoxia"—or metabolic failure is a condition where the cell is incapable of utilizing oxygen to produce ATP despite adequate oxygen delivery (36–38). The defect in oxygen utilization likely resides in the mitochondrion. Rapid autopsies of patients dying from

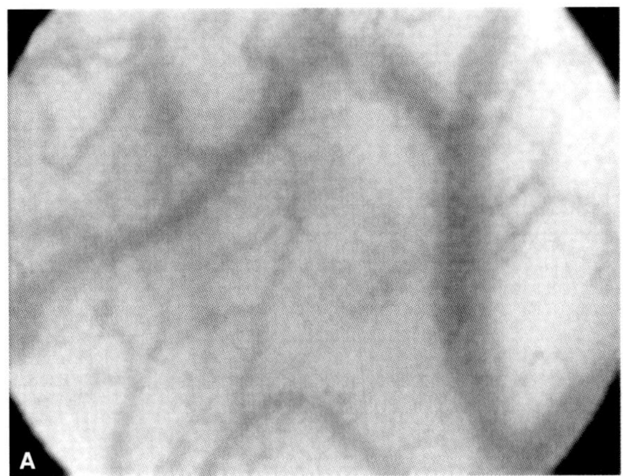

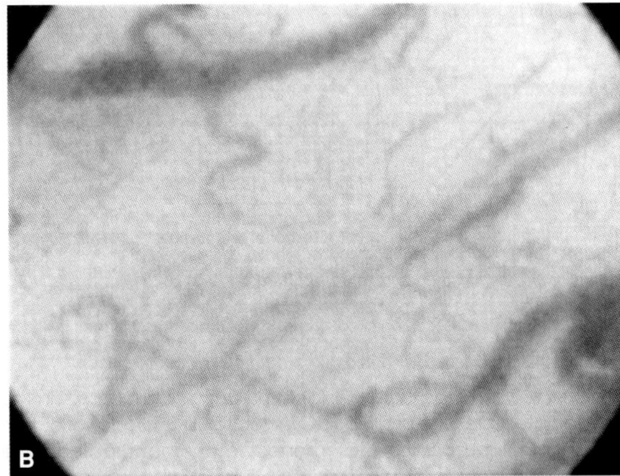

FIGURE 52.3 Sublingual microcirculation as assessed by orthogonal polarization spectral imaging in a healthy volunteer **(A)** and in a patient with early septic shock **(B)**. Normal capillary density is observed in panel A whereas low capillary density is observed in panel B. Real-time images may be viewed at http://www.cooperhealthorg/content/gme_fellowship_shock.htm. (From De Backer D, Creteur J, Preiser J-C, et al. Microvascular blood flow is altered in patients with sepsis. *Am J Respir Crit Care Med.* 2002;166:98–104, with permission.)

sepsis show normal gross histology but significant mitochondrial injury on electron microscopic examination (39). Muscle biopsies from septic patients reveal that skeletal muscle ATP concentrations and respiratory chain activity are lower compared to samples obtained from control patients (40,41). The mechanism by which cytopathic hypoxia or metabolic failure occurs has not been fully elucidated. However, NO and its metabolite, peroxynitrite, are mediators released during sepsis and are inhibitors of the mitochondrial electron transport chain (42). Single-strand breaks in nuclear DNA can occur in sepsis by a variety of endogenously formed oxidants, including peroxynitrite. Poly(ADP-ribose) polymerase (PARP) is a highly energy dependent enzyme that is activated by the formation of these DNA breaks and may cause cellular energy depletion (43,44). Porphyrin-based agents which increase the degradation of peroxynitrite improve cardiovascular function and decrease the incidence of MODS in animal models of septic shock (45). If the reduction in ATP production is sufficient, cell death should occur; however, this does not appear to the overriding cause of MODS. More likely, a new steady state is reached where there is enough ATP production for cell survival but not for all metabolic functions (18).

TABLE 52.3 Inflammatory Mediators Important in the Pathogenesis of Sepsis and the Multiple Organ Dysfunction Syndrome

Complement (C3a, C5a)
Neutrophil products
Proteases
Neutral proteases
Elastase
Cathepsin G
Collagenase
Acid hydrolase
Cathepsins B and D
β-Glucuronidase
Glucosaminase
Oxygen radicals
Superoxide anion
Hydroxyl radical
Hydrogen peroxide
Peroxynitrite
Bradykinin
Lipid mediators
Prostaglandins
Thromboxane A_2
Prostaglandin I_2
Prostaglandin E_2
Leukotrienes (LTB_4, LTC_4, LTD_4, LTE_4)
Platelet-activating factor (PAF)
Cytokines
Tumor necrosis factor α (TNF-α)
Interleukins (IL-1, IL-6, IL-8)
High-mobility group 1 (HMG-1)
Macrophage migration inhibition factor (MIF)
Nitric oxide

Reprinted from Heard SO, Fink MP. Multiple-organ dysfunction syndrome. In: Murray MJ, Coursin DB, Pearl RG, et al., eds. *Critical Care Medicine. Perioperative Management.* Philadelphia, PA: Lippincott Williams & Wilkins; 2002, with permission.

ROLE OF INFLAMMATORY AND VASOACTIVE MEDIATORS

Although early clinical series emphasized the implication of uncontrolled infection in the development of MODS, it is clear that MODS can occur with either extensive tissue injury such as that seen with trauma, pancreatitis, or sepsis. A large amount of evidence is available that implicates the release of inflammatory mediators in the pathogenesis of MODS (Table 52.3).

Complement, Neutrophils, and Reactive Oxygen Metabolites

The complement cascade is activated via three pathways (Fig. 52.4). The *classical pathway* is triggered by antibody-coated targets or antigen–antibody complexes. The *alternative pathway* is activated by aggregated immunoglobulins, products of tissue trauma, lipopolysaccharide (LPS), and other complex polysaccharides. The *lectin-ficolin pathway* is initiated by the binding of organisms to mannose–binding lectin (MBL), a protein important in innate immunity (46). Once MBL is bound to a pathogen, an MBL-associated serine protease is produced, which forms a C3 convertase by cleavage of C4 and C2. Products of the complement pathway activate neutrophils, which can obstruct capillaries and release oxygen radicals and lysosomal enzymes—among other mediators, thereby damaging the endothelium. Furthermore, adhesion molecules, which

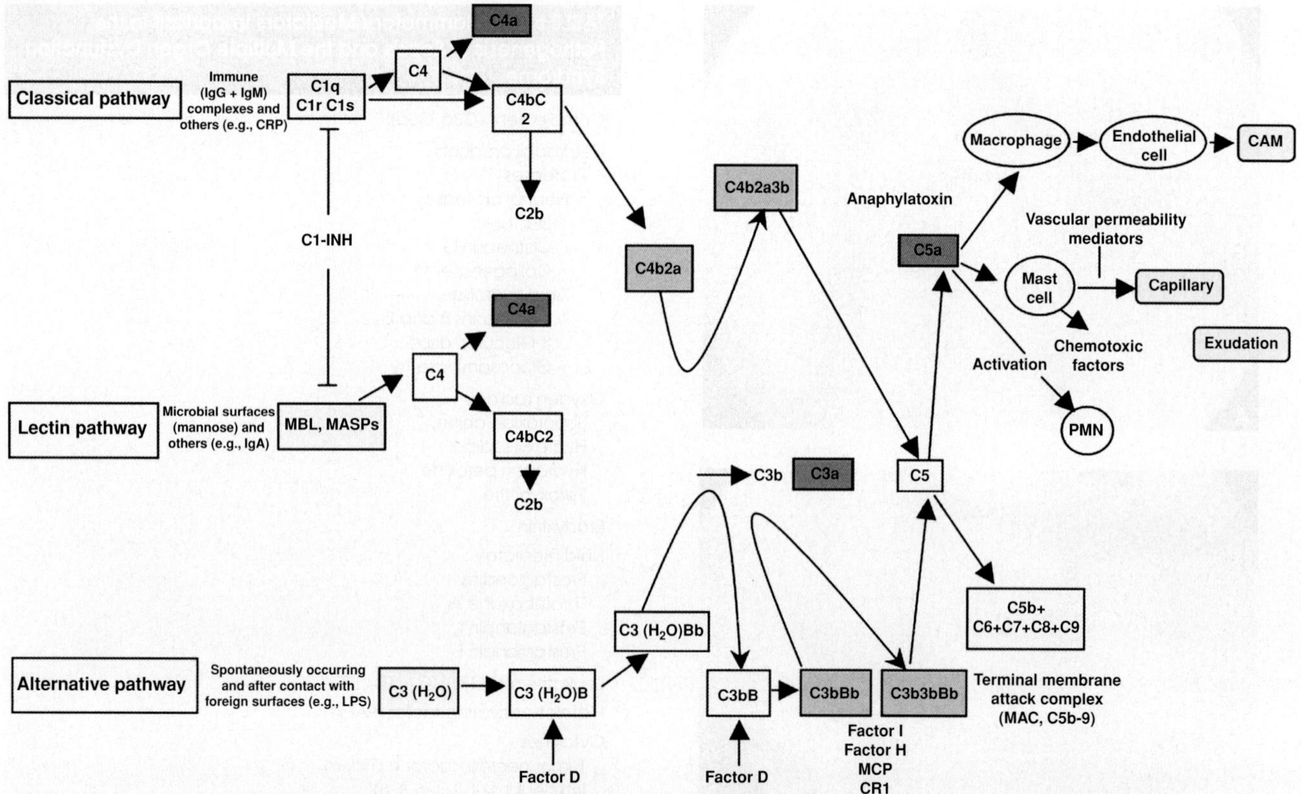

FIGURE 52.4 The three complement activation pathways (classic, alternative, and lectin). IgG, immunoglobulin G; IgM, immunoglobulin M; IgA, immunoglobulin A; CRP, C-reactive protein; MBL, mannose-binding lectin protein; MASP, MBL-associated proteases; C1-INH, C1-inhibitor; LPS, lipopolysaccharide; CAM, cell adhesion molecules; MAC, membrane attack complex; PMN, polymorphonuclear leukocytes; MCP, monocyte chemoattractant protein; CR1, complement component receptor 1. (From Goldfarb RD, Parrillo JE. Complement. *Crit Care Med.* 2005;33:S482–S484, with permission.)

are expressed on both polymorphonuclear leukocytes (PMNs) and vascular endothelium in response to LPS and other inflammatory mediators, facilitate the adherence and diapedesis of PMNs through the endothelium.

A significant amount of animal evidence exists suggesting that complement activation is important in the pathophysiology of MODS (47–50). Clinically, activation of both complement and neutrophils occurs in patients with ARDS or burns (51,52), and circulating plasma levels of C3a correlate with severity of injury and outcome in patients with multiple trauma (53). Evidence of complement and neutrophil activation has also been found in bronchoalveolar lavage (BAL) from patients with ARDS (54). Administration of a C1 inhibitor in patients with severe sepsis and septic shock reduces neutrophil activation (55) and improves renal function and SOFA scores compared to untreated control patients (56).

Reactive oxygen species—superoxide anion, hydrogen peroxide, and the hydroxyl radical—are produced in the mitochondria and released by activated PMNs. They can injure tissues by damaging DNA, cross-linking cellular proteins, and causing peroxidation of membrane lipids (57,58), diminished membrane fluidity and increased membrane permeability, resulting in cellular dysfunction. The conclusion that toxic oxygen radicals are important in the pathophysiology of respiratory dysfunction comes from clinical studies of patients with ARDS where plasma levels of lipid peroxides are elevated, levels of hydrogen peroxide are increased in the expiratory condensate (59), and oxidative damage to proteins in BAL fluid is found (60); ARDS patients have reduced levels of oxygen radical scavengers (e.g., α-tocopherol, ubiquinone, and glutathione), a sign of "oxidant stress" (61,62). Antioxidant therapies, however, have not translated into improved outcome for patients with ARDS or MODS. The OMEGA trial which examined dietary supplementation with omega-3 fatty acids, gamma-linolenic acid, and a number of antioxidants on the outcome of patients with ARDS showed the antioxidant group had fewer ventilator-free days, ICU free days and nonpulmonary organ failure free days (63). Other studies suggest such interventions may improve days "free" of acute lung injury (ALI) (64), mechanical ventilation (65), and incidence of new organ failures (65); decrease SOFA scores (66); and reduce oxidative stress during septic shock (67).

The Kallikrein–Kinin System

The kallikrein–kinin system is part of the contact system, and is composed of complement, coagulation, and kallikrein–kinins, with bradykinin, the end product of this cascade, resulting in vasodilation and increased vascular permeability. Some of these effects are mediated by the release of secondary mediators, such as NO and eicosanoids. A bradykinin receptor antagonist (CP-0127) for the adjuvant therapy of sepsis failed to alter the 28-day mortality (68).

The Coagulation System

LPS and many proinflammatory mediators will activate the coagulation system (Fig. 52.5), primarily by the extrinsic tissue factor–dependent pathway, as these mediators induce the expression of tissue factor (TF) on monocytes and endothelial

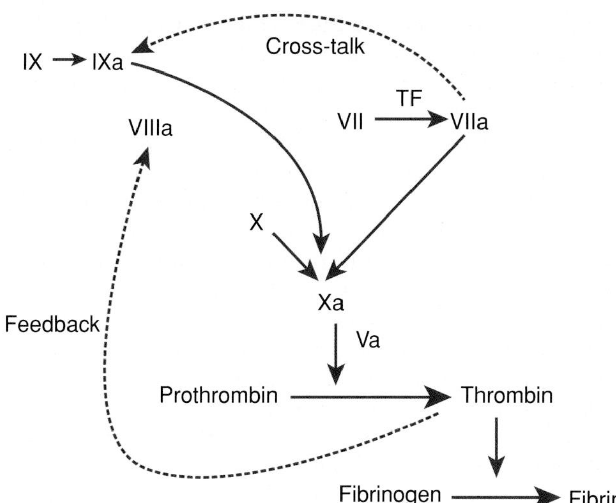

FIGURE 52.5 Revised coagulation scheme. VIIa complex is capable of mediating the conversion of factor IX to IXa directly, thereby establishing a link between the two pathways. Thus, TF appears to have a dual role with respect to coagulation: (i) TF initiates coagulation through activation of factor X, and (ii) through its action on factor IX, TF supports amplification. An additional mechanism that supports the importance of the intrinsic cascade is activation of factor VIII through feedback mechanisms involving thrombin. (From Aird WC. Coagulation. *Crit Care Med.* 2005;33:S485–S487, with permission.)

cells (69). Although these same mediators activate the fibrinolytic system, subsequent increases in plasminogen activator inhibitor-1 (PAI-1) and thrombin-activatable fibrinolysis inhibitor (TAFI) effectively suppress fibrinolysis. Important coagulation inhibitors—antithrombin, tissue factor pathway inhibitor (TFPI), protein C, protein S, and the endothelial-bound modulators heparan sulfate and thrombomodulin—may be downregulated (69), resulting in a net *procoagulant tendency* with potential for the development of disseminated intravascular coagulation (DIC). DIC can cause microvascular thrombosis and organ failure, and/or bleeding from consumption of platelets and clotting factors (70,71). Nonetheless, three clinical trials of anticoagulant therapy failed to showed benefit in patients with severe sepsis (72–74).

Prostaglandins, Leukotrienes, and Platelet-Activating Factor

Prostaglandins (PGs), leukotrienes (LTs), and platelet-activating factor (PAF) are potent lipid mediators formed by the stimulation of a membrane-bound enzyme, phospholipase A_2 (PLA_2), via a variety of mediators including norepinephrine, adenosine, bradykinin, PAF, tumor necrosis factor (TNF), and interleukin (IL)-1β (75). PLA_2 catalyzes membrane phospholipids to lyso-PAF and arachidonic acid (Fig. 52.6). Both experimental and clinical studies support the notion that these mediators play a role in the pathophysiology of sepsis and MODS.

Elevated plasma levels of thromboxane B_2 (TXB_2), the metabolite of the prostaglandin thromboxane A_2 (TXA_2), are observed in animal models of sepsis and are correlated with organ injury and outcome. However, clinical trials of nonselective inhibitors of cyclo-oxygenase (COX) (ibuprofen) showed no effect on survival in sepsis (76) and a trial evaluating the effectiveness of a selective inhibitor of a group IIA secretory phospholipase in patients with suspected sepsis and organ failure showed no effect on organ function (77). Ketoconazole, an imidazole derivative that inhibits thromboxane synthase, prevents the development of ARDS in patients at risk (78,79); established ARDS is not reversed nor is survival improved (80).

Significant data exists supporting the role of PAF in the pathogenesis of sepsis and MODS. In vitro, incubation of macrophages with PAF will lead to an exaggerated release of TNF and TF by these cells after LPS exposure; LPS-induced release of TNF by macrophages is inhibited by PAF receptor antagonists. PAF expression on the surface of endothelial

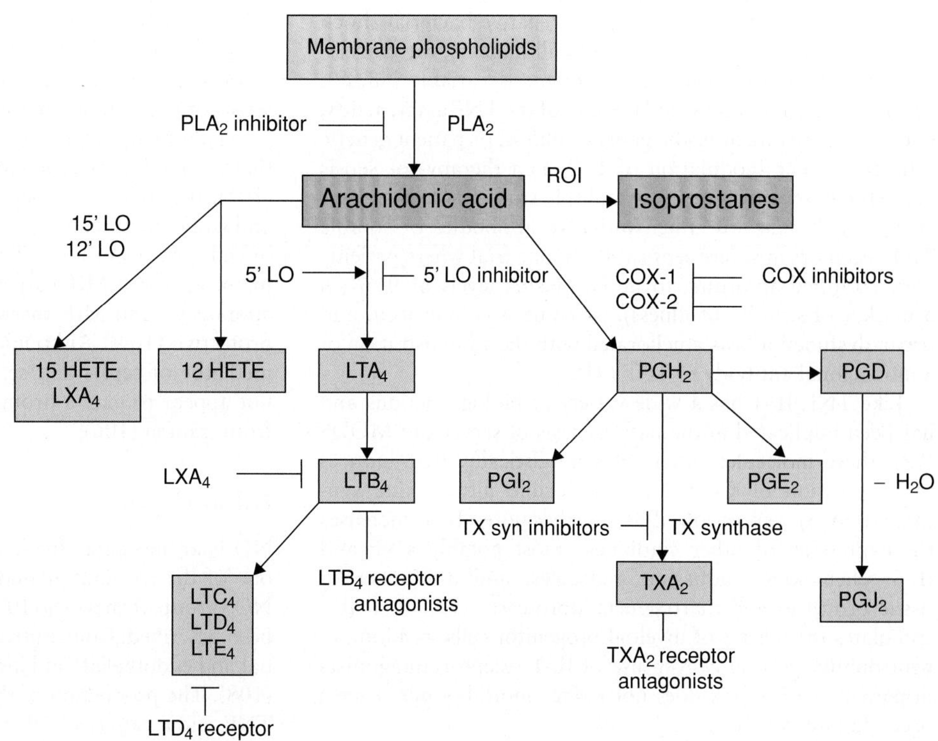

FIGURE 52.6 The eicosanoid pathway. PLA_2, phospholipase A_2; ROI, reactive oxygen intermediates; COX, cyclo-oxygenase; LO, lipo-oxygenase; HETE, hydroxyeicosatetraenoic acid; LT, leukotriene; TX, thromboxane; LX, lipoxin; PG, prostaglandin. (From Cook JA. Eicosanoids. *Crit Care Med.* 2005;33: S488–S491, with permission.)

cells will result in PMN adherence and activation. In addition, stimulation of PAF receptors on the endothelium results in changes in cell shape and cytoskeletal structure. Clinically, depressed plasma levels of PAF acetylhydrolase (PAF-AH), the enzyme responsible for metabolizing PAF, have been observed in critically ill patients and correlate inversely with organ dysfunction. However, a phase III trial of recombinant PAF-AH failed to improve outcome or prevent organ dysfunction (81). A subsequent study of critically ill patients revealed that plasma levels of PAF-AH were variable over time and with severity of illness (82,83), providing a partial explanation for the lack of efficacy of recombinant PAF-AH.

Cytokines

Cytokines are small proteins secreted by nearly all nucleated cells and exhibiting autocrine, paracrine, or endocrine activity (84,85); they are generally classified as proinflammatory or anti-inflammatory. This classification, however, is somewhat arbitrary as an individual cytokine may act in either fashion, depending on the underlying biologic process. Proinflammatory cytokines such as TNF and IL-1 can stimulate the release of other mediators: PAF, NO, LTs, and PGs.

TNF assumes an important role in the pathogenesis of human sepsis, septic shock, and MODS; it is directly cytotoxic to some cell types, will induce the expression of adhesion molecules on neutrophils and endothelial cells to promote the recruitment of these cells to the site of injury or infection and will increase endothelial permeability. Metabolic effects attributable to TNF include activation of the acute-phase response, fever (along with IL-1), skeletal muscle catabolism, and increased peripheral lipolysis and hepatic lipogenesis (85). When injected into normal volunteers, small doses of LPS or recombinant TNF will reproduce many of the metabolic and hemodynamic changes observed in sepsis (83,86). Similar findings are observed in animal studies, and treatment with anti-TNF antibodies will prevent many of the adverse consequences of endotoxic or live gram-negative bacterial shock (87). However, in studies of critically ill patients, the correlation of plasma TNF levels and outcome is variable (88,89), possibly related to timing and method of the TNF assay, acuity, etiology, or treatment of the patient's illness, or patient genetic differences. The modulation of TNF as a therapy for sepsis and MODS remains murky as multiple studies failed to show significant benefit of either anti-TNF antibodies or soluble TNF receptors in severe sepsis (90). In one trial where patients were stratified according to initial plasma levels of IL-6 (as a marker of severity of illness), outcome was improved, and organ dysfunction was ameliorated with the administration of a monoclonal antibody to TNF (91).

Like TNF, IL-1 has a wide variety of biologic actions and has been implicated in the pathogenesis of sepsis and MODS (92); these molecules often act synergistically. IL-1 induces the expression of COX-2 and inducible nitric oxide synthase (iNOS) expression (93). Furthermore, IL-1 increases the expression of other cytokines—most notably TNF and IL-6—chemokines, adhesion molecules, and a number of tissue proteases and matrix metalloproteases (93). IL-1 also stimulates the release of myeloid progenitor cells, resulting in neutrophilia (93). However, use of IL-1 receptor antagonists in patients with sepsis does not reduce mortality nor reverse organ failure (94–96).

Interleukin 6 (IL-6) is another cytokine that has been identified to be important in the response to infection and development of MODS. Small doses of endotoxin administered to normal volunteers will stimulate the release of IL-6 (97). IL-6 will persist for longer periods of time in the blood than other cytokines and may serve as an important marker for the outcome of patients with sepsis or septic shock. Both the IL-6 receptor and the signaling receptor gp130 are required for the biologic activity of IL-6 to be realized (97). Murine models of hemorrhagic shock indicate that IL-6 is important in the development of gut barrier dysfunction (97). In addition, IL-6 may be important in promoting thrombosis during sepsis. Passive immunization with an anti–IL-6 antibody reduces activation of the coagulation cascade in a primate model of endotoxicosis but has no effect on the coagulation abnormalities associated with low-dose LPS in humans (98).

IL-8 is a chemotactic cytokine (chemokine) expressed principally by monocytes and macrophages by stimulation with LPS, bacteria, TNF, and IL-1 (99). IL-8 induces chemotaxis of inflammatory cells, and its presence at sites of inflammation may persist for long periods of time (99). That IL-8 is important in the development of MODS is made by the observation of high IL-8 levels in BAL fluid from patients with ARDS or pneumonia (100). Although neutralizing IL-8 may reduce cardiac ischemia/reperfusion injury in dogs, a reduction in chemokines increases mortality in animal models of pneumonia (99).

High-mobility group box 1 (HMGB1) is a cytokine that was been identified as an inflammatory mediator (Fig. 52.7) (101). HMGB1 is released in a delayed manner from a variety of cells in response to LPS or bacteria (102). Exposure of the lung to HMGB1 increases neutrophil accumulation, edema, and other proinflammatory cytokines, whereas gastrointestinal exposure results in increased gut permeability and translocation of bacteria to mesenteric lymph nodes (102). Administration of this cytokine to animals causes death as a result of epithelial barrier disruption. Treatment of experimental endotoxicosis or sepsis with antibodies to HMGB1 or HMGB1 antagonists improves survival (101–103). There have been no clinical studies to evaluate the efficacy of anti-HMGB1 therapies in sepsis or other inflammatory conditions.

Macrophage migration inhibitory factor (MIF) is a cytokine that is found in macrophages in preformed cytoplasmic pools (104). It is released rapidly in response to bacterial products and works to upregulate and sustain the activation of a variety of cell types to produce TNF, IL-1, IL-6, and IL-8 (104). The major action of MIF may be the regulation of p53-dependent apoptosis. Anti-MIF therapy in animal models of sepsis is protective (104). Although MIF appears to be an important mediator of sepsis and sepsis-induced MODS (105), it does not appear to play a prominent role in tissue injury resulting from trauma (106).

Nitric Oxide

NO is an inorganic free-radical gas, produced by catalysis of one of the terminal guanidine nitrogens of L-arginine by the NOS group of enzymes (107). Two general classes of NOS have been described: Constitutive (calcium-dependent) NOS (neuronal and endothelial) and inducible (calcium-independent) NOS (108). The production of the latter enzyme is induced by LPS, TNF, and a variety of other inflammatory mediators. A variety

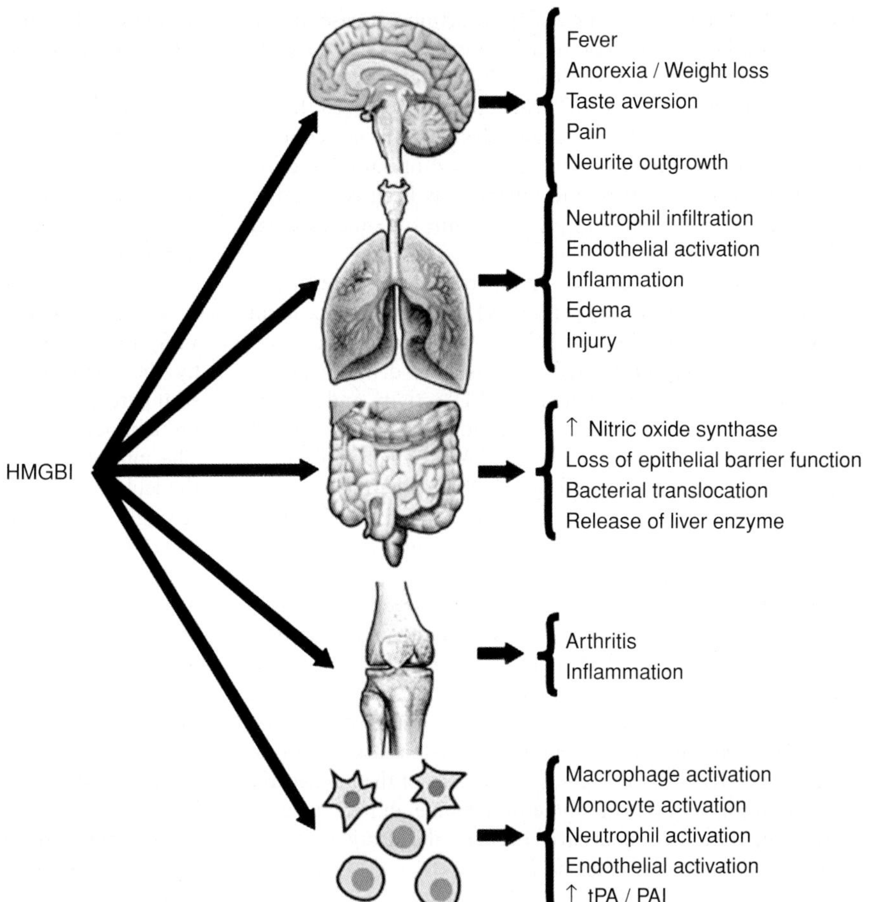

FIGURE 52.7 Inflammatory responses in various areas of the host that are medicated by high-mobility group box 1 (HMGB1). tPA, tissue plasminogen activator; PAI, plasminogen activator inhibitor. (From Wang H, Yang H, Tracey KJ. Extracellular role of HMGB1 in inflammation and sepsis. *J Intern Med.* 2004;255: 320–331, with permission.)

of cells and tissues release NO, including endothelium, vascular smooth muscle, neutrophils, and mononuclear, glial, mast, hepatic, and adrenal medullary cells (108). Vasorelaxation, neurotransmission, and microbicidal activity are some of the important functions that NO possesses. The role that NO plays in the host is a function of the rate and timing of its production and the surrounding environment. Normally, NO acts as a direct signaling molecule (e.g., vasorelaxation and neurotransmission), and low levels of NO (produced by constitutive NOS and at times by inducible NOS) have protective effects (Fig. 52.8) (108). Alternatively, it may function as an indirect cytotoxic agent and induce intestinal barrier dysfunction.

Significant experimental and clinical evidence suggests that NO plays an important role in the pathophysiology of

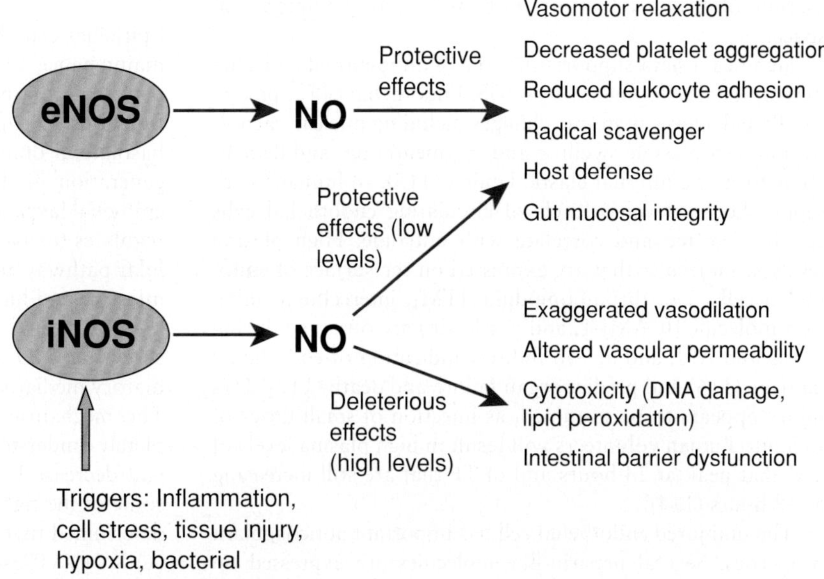

FIGURE 52.8 The divergent effects of nitric oxide (NO) derived from the endothelium (eNOS, endothelial nitric oxide synthase) or as a consequence of inflammation (iNOS, inducible or inflammatory NOS.) (From Levy RM, Prince JM, Billiar TR. Nitric oxide: a clinical primer. *Crit Care Med.* 2005;33:S492–495, with permission.)

sepsis and MODS. iNOS and NO production increase in animals during both endotoxic and hemorrhagic shock. iNOS-deficient mice are protected from LPS-induced hypotension, and have a higher survival following endotoxicosis (109). NO contributes to TNF-induced cardiac dysfunction in a concentration-dependent fashion (110). Increased urinary excretion of NO metabolites (nitrite and nitrate) has been reported in septic patients and correlates inversely with systemic vascular resistance (SVR) (111).

Excess NO in the presence of superoxide anion results in the formation of peroxynitrite (ONOO (–)), a reactive oxidant that causes lipid peroxidation, inhibits mitochondrial respiration, inactivates glyceraldehyde-3-phosphate dehydrogenase, inhibits membrane sodium/potassium ATP activity, and triggers DNA single-strand breakage. As mentioned previously, DNA damage activates the nuclear enzyme, PARP, which can lead to cellular energy depletion and death (109). Furthermore, excessive amounts of NO and peroxynitrite can activate the transcription factor, NFκB, and amplify the inflammatory response (112).

The efficacy of inhibitors of NOS in the treatment of sepsis and MODS is unclear, and the use of some inhibitors may actually be detrimental. Although hypotension, vascular leak, and vasopressor requirements can be reduced with the use of nonspecific NOS inhibitors, microcirculatory blood flow can be altered, resulting in organ injury. Indeed, a large randomized, prospective trial evaluating the efficacy of the nonspecific NOS inhibitor, L-N (G)-monomethylarginine, in patients with septic shock was stopped early because the death rate was higher in the intervention group (113).

THE ENDOTHELIUM

The role of the vascular endothelium is to control the flow of nutrients, blood cells, and a broad array of biologically active molecules to the tissues; this is achieved via membrane-bound receptors for a plethora of molecules and through tight junction proteins and receptors that regulate cell–cell and cell–matrix relationships (114). Endothelial cell injury may well impair the delivery of nutrients to tissues and allow the extravasation of proinflammatory mediators into the interstitial space.

Significant data supports the role of an impaired endothelium in the development of MODS. Endothelial cell exposure to LPS will cause anatomic changes including nuclear vacuolization, cytoplasmic swelling and fragmentation, and detachment from the internal elastic lamina (115). In humans with septic shock, elevated levels of circulating endothelial cells can be detected and correlate with outcome. High plasma levels of molecules that are expressed on the surface of endothelial cells (i.e., thrombomodulin [TM], intercellular adhesion molecule [ICAM]-1, and E-selectin) are observed during sepsis and ALI, and are an indirect indication of endothelial damage (116) and predict organ failure and death (117). This injury appears to be sustained, as injection of small doses of LPS into human volunteers will result in high plasma levels of TM that peak at 24 hours and of TF that are still increasing at 48 hours (114).

The uninjured endothelial cell has important anticoagulant properties. Several heparin-like molecules are expressed on the surface of the cells to accelerate the inactivation of serine proteases of coagulation by antithrombin (114). Thrombomodulin binds thrombin and forms a complex that activates protein C; exposure of the endothelial cells to inflammatory or septic mediators will shift the endothelial cells to a procoagulant state by increasing expression of TF and internalization of TM, and the endothelial cell will have impaired release of tissue plasminogen activator and an increased release of PAI-1. This procoagulant/antifibrinolytic state is associated with fibrin deposition, platelet consumption, microthrombi, tissue ischemia and necrosis, and an increased risk of death (118).

Before leukocytes and monocytes can migrate into tissues, they must adhere to the endothelium, accomplished by the local synthesis of PAF, IL-1, IL-8, and TNF, which stimulates the expression of surface molecules called selectins on leukocytes (L-selectin) and endothelial cells (E-selectin). The interplay between these selectins allows loose binding of the leukocyte to the endothelium. Leukocytes are bound more strongly to the endothelium by the interaction between the CD11/CD18 complex, which is expressed on the leukocyte, and the ICAM-1, which is expressed on the endothelial cell membrane. In animal models of sepsis, endotoxicosis, or ischemia/reperfusion, monoclonal antibodies to the CD11/CD18 integrin or to L-selectin will improve organ dysfunction (119). Knockout animals lacking either ICAM-1 or E-selectin have improved survival during experimental sepsis (120). Clinically, plasma ICAM-1 levels are higher in patients with septic shock than in healthy controls or patients with SIRS (116), and the levels correlate with the severity of shock.

Endothelium-derived relaxation is also impaired in sepsis, and such alteration may contribute to MODS. In normal volunteers, small doses of LPS will also impair endothelium-dependent relaxation for days (121). These data help explain the observations that reactive forearm hyperemia is attenuated in patients with sepsis. In addition, the importance of intact ecNOS in these patients is supported by the observation that treatment of patients with septic shock by nonselective NOS inhibitors is associated with no change or an increase in mortality compared to untreated patients (113).

EPITHELIAL BARRIER DYSFUNCTION

Epithelial cells help maintain normal organ function by the maintenance of distinct compartments. The tight junctions between adjacent epithelial cells serve several important functions: (a) differentiation (122) of the cell into apical and basolateral domains, (b) preservation of cellular polarity, (c) generation of distinct internal environments formed by the epithelial layer, and (d) providing a semipermeable barrier that regulates the passive diffusion of solutes between the paracellular pathway and prevents entry of microbes and toxins (e.g., intestine and lung) (122).

Data from studies using cultured epithelial monolayers show that NO and peroxynitrite, as well as other proinflammatory mediators, increase the permeability of the monolayer. The mechanism for this increase in permeability is incompletely understood; however, some data suggest that there is a decrease in the expression and improper localization of some of the tight junction proteins. Other investigations have determined that inhibition of the epithelial cell membrane Na (+)-K (+)-ATPase pump by these mediators results in cellular swelling and an increase in intracellular sodium concentration, which ultimately impairs the expression and localization of the tight junction proteins. Data from murine models of endotoxemia indicate that LPS will decrease the expression and alter the localization of tight junction proteins in the intestine compared to control animals (123). Furthermore, these animals will have increased number of bacteria recovered from regional mesenteric lymph nodes. NO appears to be important in the disruption of gut barrier function, as neither intestinal permeability nor bacterial translocation is observed when knockout mice lacking iNOS are treated with LPS. Similar alterations in hepatic (124) and pulmonary (125) epithelial barrier function and tight junction protein expression and localization have been shown during murine endotoxicosis.

Derangements in Gut Barrier Function

Although epithelial barrier function in the intestine may be altered during sepsis and other inflammatory states, other components of the gut barrier will prevent the bacteria or bacterial products from gaining access to systemic organs (126). In addition to alterations in the epithelial barrier described previously, other clinical conditions that can contribute to altered gut barrier function include antibiotics, stress ulcer prevention, hypoalbuminemia, vasoactive agents, and use of hyperosmolar feeding preparations. The clinical importance of the disrupted gut barrier function in the pathogenesis of MODS remains ill defined.

APOPTOSIS

Apoptosis (programmed cell death) is the term used to describe a specific method by which cells die; the event is a well-defined, active, and energy-dependent process. There are two primary pathways involved in apoptosis: The intrinsic (mitochondrial and endoplasmic reticulum) pathway and the extrinsic ("death receptor") pathway (127). The latter pathway is activated by receptors such as Fas, with the subsequent activation of two enzymes, caspase-8 or -10. The intrinsic pathway stimulates caspase-9 by loss of the mitochondrial membrane potential and movement of cytochrome c into the cytosol. These initiator caspases cleave effector caspases (e.g., caspase-3 and -7), which result in the cleavage of cellular proteins and DNA and, ultimately, apoptosis (128).

The exact role of apoptosis in the development of MODS is unclear. Data from clinical studies show that upregulation of apoptotic pathways occurs in patients with ARDS (129). Furthermore, widespread apoptosis occurs in splenic and colonic lymphoid populations in patients who die from sepsis and MODS (130,131). The effect of apoptosis on immune function includes loss of various immune cells and impairment of immunity by apoptosis-induced immunosuppression of the remaining immune cells (132). Therapies directed against these programmed pathways are under intense investigation and include inhibition of cytochrome c release, use of RNA interference for gene silencing, and caspase inhibitors (132).

COMPLEX NONLINEAR SYSTEMS

The body may be considered a biologic network that is complex, highly coupled, and nonlinear (133). The host response to trauma, shock, or sepsis—involving metabolic, neural, endocrine, inflammatory, and immune components is such an example (134). The behavior of such a system cannot be predicted with great reliability; however, the system is "attracted" to specific states or stable configurations: "organized variability" (134,135). A large enough perturbation to an organ or mediator network may have unexpected and significant results elsewhere in the host and ultimately lead to MODS (136). In the healthy individual, there is a high degree of heart rate (beat-to-beat) variability; this may be lost and mortality increased in critically ill patients (137). In fact, normal volunteers injected with small doses of LPS exhibit loss of heart rate variability (138). Decreased heart and respiratory rate variability during spontaneous breathing trials predict extubation failure (139). Other examples of increased regularity of rhythms associated with disease include Cheyne–Stokes respiration, parkinsonian gait, neutrophil count in chronic myelogenous leukemia, and fever in Hodgkin disease (135). However, several diseases—acromegaly and Cushing disease—are associated with increased complexity (135). These data suggest that health is determined by "distance" from thermodynamic equilibrium: too much or too little variation (low or high entropy) represents pathologic conditions (135).

GENETIC SUSCEPTIBILITY

Single base variations in DNA—single nucleotide polymorphisms (SNPs)—are commonly used to discern genetic differences among patient populations (140). Approximately 1 in every 1,000 bases in the human genome is different between two unrelated individuals (140). By comparing healthy individuals to patients, SNPs involved in disease can be identified. Indeed, some—but not—all clinical studies have documented an increased risk of death and organ dysfunction in patients suffering from sepsis or ARDS and who are homozygotes for SNPs (141–145); this may have future clinical implications.

PREVENTION AND TREATMENT OF MULTIPLE ORGAN DYSFUNCTION SYNDROME

Prevention and treatment of MODS are nonspecific and include the goals of maintaining adequate tissue oxygenation, finding and treating infection, providing adequate nutrition support, minimizing iatrogenic complications, and when necessary, providing artificial support (e.g., dialysis or mechanical ventilation) for individual dysfunctional organs.

Resuscitation

An episode of circulatory shock is probably the most common event that occurs before the development of MODS. As a result, timely restoration of intravascular volume and oxygen delivery is important in preventing or abrogating MODS in high-risk patients (146).

In the ICU, the use of colloids as resuscitation fluid has been the subject of a number of important recent publications, which culminated in the Food and Drug Administration (FDA) issuing a black box warning on the use of hydroxyethyl starch (HES). The efficacy of volume substitution and insulin therapy in severe sepsis (VISEP) study (147), the Scandinavian starch for severe sepsis/septic shock (6S) trial (148), and the crystalloid versus hydroxyethyl starch (CHEST) trial (149) compared the use of starches with modified Ringer lactate, Ringer acetate, and sodium chloride 0.9%, respectively, for resuscitation. All trials failed to show a survival benefit with the use of starch, but demonstrated an increased risk of AKI. An updated systematic review and meta-analysis on the use of colloid versus crystalloids for fluid resuscitation in critically ill patients concluded that the use of colloids was not associated with an improvement in survival (150). Resuscitation with albumin compared to crystalloid in patients with severe sepsis does not alter 28- or 90-day mortality (151). However, there may be a benefit to the administration of albumin in septic shock as 90-day survival was higher and duration of vasopressor support was shorter in this subgroup (152).

The role of chloride in influencing the adverse effects of colloids or crystalloids on renal function has been recently questioned (153). A prospective, open-label, sequential period pilot study suggested that the use of balanced crystalloid or colloids solutions compared to chloride-rich solutions was associated with a significant decrease in the incidence of AKI and need for renal replacement therapy (154).

Assessing the adequacy of tissue oxygenation can often be difficult. The clinical parameters used most often, including arterial blood pressure, skin color, temperature, urine flow, mixed venous oxygen saturation, and blood lactate concentrations, may be unreliable. Although observational studies found that "supranormal" levels of $\dot{D}O_2$, $\dot{V}O_2$, and cardiac index were associated with higher survival rates, the majority of work over the past 15 years clearly show that resuscitation to these end points in critically ill patients is of no benefit, or actually worsens outcome. Likewise, the use of the pulmonary artery catheter to guide therapy has not been shown to be of benefit in a large number of studies (155–157) and pulmonary capillary wedge pressure does not accurately reflect ventricular volume, even in normal volunteers (158). Less invasive, and probably safer, monitors have been developed for monitoring cardiac output that compare favorably with the accuracy of the thermodilution method. Use of systolic blood pressure variation (SPV), pulse pressure variation (PPV), stroke volume variation (SVV), left ventricular end-diastolic area (as assessed by transesophageal echocardiography) and respiratory variability of the inferior vena cava diameter may be of greater benefit to guide volume resuscitation (159). Whatever monitor is used, resuscitation for severe sepsis or septic shock needs to happen early while avoiding fluid overload (16,17). Protocol-based algorithms do not appear to improve mortality (160–162); initial fluid therapy is 30 mL/kg of crystalloid (146). A higher transfusion threshold in established septic shock does not alter outcome (163). If vasopressor support is needed, norepinephrine is the vasopressor of choice and is titrated to achieve a MAP of 65 mmHg (164). Vasopressin (0.03 units/min) may be added to achieve the MAP goal or to reduce the dose of norepinephrine (146). Dobutamine may be added if signs of hypoperfusion persist and transthoracic or transesophageal echocardiography suggests cardiac dysfunction. Corticosteroids may be administrated if fluids and vasopressors have not restored hemodynamic stability (146). The abdominal compartment syndrome can be the cause of persistent hypotension and should be ruled out by measuring bladder pressure (165).

Mechanical Ventilation

The method by which patients are mechanically ventilated can contribute to organ dysfunction. A plethora of experimental and clinical data indicate that overdistension of the lung through the use of large tidal volumes will cause lung injury, stimulate the release of inflammatory mediators, and effect derangements in organs other than the lung (166–168). Use of small tidal volumes (6 mL/kg) in the care of patients with ALI and ARDS decreases mortality and increase ventilator-free and organ failure–free days (169). Nonetheless, an analysis of data from nine randomized ARDS trials demonstrated a direct correlation between driving pressure and survival (170). In addition, short-term use of cisatracurium (171) (48 hours) and the prone position (172) in patients with severe ARDS will improve outcome.

Cyclic "opening" and "closing" of collapsed airways during tidal ventilation is also thought to cause lung injury (173). A small study of patients with ARDS suggests that the use of positive end-expiratory pressure (PEEP) above the lower inflection point of the respiratory system compliance curve reduces mortality and the number of failed organs compared to control patients (174). Although this concept has been called into question by data demonstrating that efforts to improve recruitment of collapsed lung units with high levels of PEEP do not reduce mortality or duration of mechanical ventilation (175), the experimental protocol in this study was altered in mid-study, making questionable any conclusions drawn from this particular investigation. A systematic review and meta-analysis revealed that higher PEEP compared to lower PEEP in patients with moderate-to-severe ARDS was associated with improved survival (176). A computed tomography (CT) scan investigation of patients with ARDS showed that ventilator-induced hyperinflation rather than cyclic recruitment/derecruitment is associated with a greater release of pulmonary inflammatory mediators (177).

Fluid management is also an important component in the care of the patient with ARDS or ALI. Data show that a restrictive fluid strategy where cumulative fluid balance is kept close to zero in these patients improves the oxygenation index and increases the number of ventilator-free days without increasing the number of other organ failures (178).

Acute Renal Failure

Acute tubular necrosis (ATN) accounts for over 75% of the cases of acute renal failure (ARF) in the ICU (179), with a mortality rate ranging from 40% to 80%. The most common insult that predisposes ICU patients to ATN is persistent prerenal azotemia (179). Furthermore, in the critically ill patient, there is often more than one insult to the kidney: sepsis; exposure to aminoglycosides, amphotericin B, or radiocontrast agents; and the administration of nonsteroidal anti-inflammatory agents. Efforts to minimize these insults to the kidneys should be maximized. Timely resuscitation is important to prevent renal ischemia but targeting oliguria reversal as part of goal-directed management does not reduce renal dysfunction (180). If aminoglycosides must be used to treat infection, once-daily dosing (181) or the use of drug levels to discern pharmacokinetics (182) appears to reduce the risk of nephrotoxicity. Use of liposomal preparations of amphotericin B reduces the risk of renal damage (181). If patients are to receive contrast agents, hydration with sodium bicarbonate solutions have been shown to reduce the risk of subsequent renal dysfunction (183). Although

N-acetylcysteine has been purported to reduce the risk of contrast-induced ARF (184), the observed results may be a reflection of the activation of creatinine kinase or an increase in the tubular secretion of creatinine (181). Medications such as "low-dose" dopamine or fenoldopam, which increase renal blood flow or loop diuretics, have no impact on preserving renal function in high-risk patients and should be avoided (181).

Debridement of Necrotic Tissue and Fracture Stabilization

The presence of dead or devitalized tissue appears to predispose patients to the development of MODS, hence timely debridement of dead tissue is an important component in prevention. Early surgical fixation of major lower extremity fractures will result in a lower incidence of ARDS and pneumonia. However, "damage control" orthopedics has recently gained popularity and is a concept whereby fractures are initially treated with external fixation; definitive therapy occurs later when the patient is more stable. The inflammatory response appears to be attenuated in these patients, and the incidence of organ dysfunction is no higher compared to patients undergoing definitive therapy (185).

Infection

Sepsis is an important cause (or correlate) of MODS, making it imperative to rule out an active source of infection in the critically ill population. Prompt hemodynamic resuscitation and timely administration of antibiotics are crucial, as well as source control (146).

Intra-abdominal Sepsis

There are many diseases presenting with intra-abdominal sepsis treated primarily by surgery (i.e., perforated viscus); these will not be discussed herein. Rather, we will review disease processes those have both medical and surgical aspects requiring ICU care, close monitoring, resuscitation, and possible intervention.

Pancreatitis. Pancreatitis is a common disease among both medical and surgical ICU patients. There have been important changes over the past several decades in the management of pancreatitis: overall there is consensus regarding nonoperative management in the setting of acute severe pancreatitis that mainly includes liberal fluid resuscitation, early enteric nutrition, and avoidance of empiric antibiotics without objective evidence of infection (186). There is less endocrine and exocrine insufficiency in patients managed nonoperatively in severe acute pancreatitis compared to operative management (187). Necrosis of pancreatic parenchyma or extrapancreatic tissue is present in 10% to 20% of patients with acute severe pancreatitis and is associated with high morbidity and mortality rates. Nonoperative management should still be the same as recommended for severe acute pancreatitis.

Urgent endoscopic retrograde cholangiopancreatography (ERCP) is indicated when cholangitis is suspected. A recent Cochrane review showed no benefit of antibiotics in preventing infection of necrotic pancreatic material except when imipenem was considered; in this case a significant decrease in pancreatic infection was found. None of the studies included in the review were adequately powered for mortality (188).

As a result of a shift from early surgical debridement to a staged, minimally invasive, multidisciplinary, step-up approach, outcome following necrotizing pancreatitis has improved substantially (189). Diagnosing infected necrosis is important, as it typically requires invasive intervention. Gas in a necrotic collection demonstrated on imaging investigations is considered proof of infection, occurring in around 40% of patients with infected necrosis. Utilization of fine-needle aspiration (FNA) may be helpful in patients without radiologic evidence of infection. However, there is a clear lack of consensus on the use of FNA to diagnose infected necrotizing pancreatitis (190). Common practice is that FNA must be considered for patients who fail to recover from organ dysfunction and without signs of findings of infection on radiologic studies. Positive FNA result hence documented infection would warrant staged multidisciplinary "step-up" approach (189). Once infection is documented, there is good evidence—and consensus—about the approach to treatment.

The initial step in the "step-up" approach is drainage, either percutaneous or transluminal, by means of cystgastrostomy, or cystduodenostomy, followed by surgical or endoscopic transluminal debridement if needed. The response rate to initial drainage is up to 30%; debridement is delayed until the acute necrotic collection has become encapsulated, typically no earlier than 6 to 8 weeks.

Acute Mesenteric Ischemia. This is another major source of intra-abdominal sepsis, and may occur due to mesenteric arterial thrombus, embolus, or venous thrombus; these are dealt with elsewhere. On the other hand, acute mesenteric ischemia may occur as a secondary problem due to ongoing sepsis, in the setting of underlying mesenteric atherosclerosis. This scenario is the least common type of mesenteric ischemia, also known as "low flow state" ischemia or "nonocclusive mesenteric ischemia"; however, it has higher morbidity and mortality compared to thromboembolic ischemia (191). Essentially, patients become septic from a source other than the abdomen and, if this progresses, the untreated hypotension and hypovolemia can cause ischemia in the gastrointestinal system.

Treatment of nonocclusive mesenteric ischemia relates to optimization of hemodynamics, elimination of vasopressor treatment, and correction of any systemic factors contributing to shock. Patients with peritoneal signs on examination or evidence of bowel necrosis or perforation on CT scan require surgical exploration to remove any source of sepsis; a second-look laparotomy should be performed routinely.

Antibiotic Duration for Intra-abdominal Infections. This has been investigated after successful treatment of intra-abdominal infection. In patients with intra-abdominal infections who have undergone an adequate source-control procedure—via surgical or percutaneous drainage—the outcomes after fixed-duration antibiotic therapy (approximately 4 days) are similar to those after a longer course of antibiotics (approximately 8 days); the latter extending until after resolution of physiologic abnormalities (192).

Pulmonary Sepsis

Ventilator-associated pneumonia (VAP) can play a role in the development and course of MODS. Proven preventive measures include noninvasive positive pressure ventilation, elevation of the head of the bed (193), continuous subglottic suctioning, in-line suctioning systems, weaning protocols, optimization of sedation with daily "wake-ups" or protocolized sedation for the patient (194,195), and chlorhexidine oral rinse.

VAP can be difficult to diagnose because radiographic findings are commonly used to secure the diagnosis and the findings are inaccurate. Recently, a ventilator-associated event (VAE) algorithm has been developed that utilizes duration of mechanical ventilation and new alterations in FiO_2 and PEEP as well as new administration of antibiotics to define complications of mechanical ventilation. At this point it is intended as a surveillance tool but, because most VAEs are associated with pneumonia, ARDS, atelectasis, or congestive heart failure, the tool can provide insight into quality of care at an institution (196).

Selective digestive decontamination (SDD) is a technique by which topical nonabsorbable antibacterial and antifungal agents (usually with a concomitant 3- to 5-day course of systemic antibiotic therapy) are applied to the oropharynx and proximal bowel in mechanically ventilated patients to reduce the incidence of nosocomial infections, organ dysfunction, and mortality. A meta-analysis of 57 randomized controlled trials demonstrated a favorable effect on bloodstream infections and mortality (197,198). Fears concerning the emergence of resistance organisms do not appear to be well founded in ICUs where there is a low level of antibiotics resistance (199) although in one trial, there was a gradual increase in aminoglycoside-resistant gram-negative bacteria (200). SDD may very well reduce the incidence and prevalence of colonization with resistant gram-negative aerobic bacteria (201). However, the use of SDD in the United States does not enjoy widespread popularity for reasons that remain unclear.

Catheter-Related Sepsis

Catheter-related bloodstream infections (CRBSIs) may contribute to the development and propagation of MODS. Proven strategies to reduce the risk of CRBSIs include handwashing prior to catheter insertion, use of maximum barrier precautions (cap, mask, sterile gloves and gown, and a large sterile drape that covers the patient), use of an alcohol-based chlorhexidine skin preparation solution, avoiding the femoral site for catheter insertion, and removing catheters when no longer needed (202,203). If these measures are ineffective in reducing the risk of infection, catheters with antiseptic surfaces (204,205) or impregnated with antibiotics (206) or the use of chlorhexidine dressing sponges can reduce the risk of infection.

Other Sources of Sepsis

Many other inapparent sources of infection in critically ill patients may contribute to the development of MODS. Some of these sources of infection include purulent sinusitis, suppurative thrombophlebitis, otitis media, perirectal abscess, epididymitis, prostatitis, calculous or acalculous cholecystitis, meningitis or brain abscess (particularly after instrumentation of the CNS), prosthetic intravascular graft infection, lower or upper urinary tract infection, and endocarditis. Physical examination and appropriate laboratory and radiographic studies should exclude these conditions.

Nutrition Support

Malnutrition can contribute to the morbidity and mortality of sepsis and MODS. Proteolysis is a prominent finding in sepsis and, although it cannot be suppressed by infusing amino acids, anabolism may be achieved by appropriate nutritional support. Furthermore, catabolism is mediated by endogenous catecholamines, and administration of β-adrenergic blocking agents can reverse the hypermetabolic response and protein catabolism (207). Early nutritional support may be beneficial in patients at risk for developing MODS (208). Data exist to support enteral nutrition (EN) over parenteral nutrition (PN); therefore this should be the choice of feeding unless there is contraindication to use of the GI system. Nutritional support should be initiated within the first 24 to 48 hours following admission (209), although the degree of caloric intake that is required is controversial (see below) (210).

Although current practice supports giving 20 to 25 kcal/kg/day (2 to 5 g/kg/day glucose, 0.5 to 1.0 g/kg/day of fat, and 1.2 to 1.5 g/kg/day of protein) in critically ill patients, a recent prospective randomized demonstrated that permissive "underfed" (moderate nonprotein calories but similar amount of protein compared to standard feeding) resulted in similar 90-day mortality rates and hospital and ICU lengths of stay despite the fact that caloric intake was reduced by 36% in the underfeeding group (211). Protein intake was similar between the two groups. It is to be determined whether current practice will change regarding nonprotein caloric intake in critically ill patients.

Insulin therapy of hyperglycemia has evolved in the critically ill patients. A meta-analysis evaluated 26 trials involving 13,567 patients. Among the 26 trials that reported mortality, the pooled relative risk (RR) of death with intensive insulin therapy (titration of insulin to keep blood glucose between 80 and 110 mg/dL) compared to less "tight" glucose control was not significant. Among the 14 trials that reported hypoglycemia, the pooled RR associated with intensive insulin therapy was significantly higher. The ICU setting was a contributing factor, with patients in surgical ICUs appearing to benefit from intensive insulin therapy whereas patients in the other ICU settings did not. Intensive insulin therapy significantly increased the risk of hypoglycemia and conferred no overall mortality benefit among critically ill patients (212).

Specialty Formulas

A number of enteral nutritional formulas are available that provide specific nutrients: glutamine, peptides, arginine, omega-3 fatty acids, nucleic acids, and antioxidants (e.g., vitamins E and C, β-carotene). Arginine is the substrate for NO synthase and is important in lymphocyte proliferation and wound healing (213). Omega-3 fatty acids change membrane lipid composition and can alter the inflammatory response (214). Nucleic acids assist in the proliferation of lymphocytes and intestinal crypt cells, as well as DNA and RNA synthesis (213). Several enteral nutrition formulas are available that include combinations of these additives. The Canadian Critical Care Clinical Practice Guideline Committee (215) recommends that arginine and other "select" nutrients not be routinely used for enteral nutrition. In patients with ARDS, a formula supplemented with fish oil, borage oil, and antioxidants should be considered (215). Although glutamine should not be used in patients with shock or MODS, enteral glutamine should be considered in trauma and burn patients (215).

SUMMARY

Standard therapy for patients with MODS includes adequate cardiovascular resuscitation, identification and timely treatment of infection, early enteral nutrition, glucose control,

TABLE 52.4 Suggested Strategies for the Prevention of Multiple Organ Dysfunction Syndrome

Prevention of hospital-acquired infection
Prevention of catheter-related bloodstream infections
– Implementation of educational initiatives
– Use of chlorhexidine solution for skin preparation
– Use of maximum barrier precautions
– Avoidance of the femoral insertion site; preference for subclavian site
– Removing catheter as soon as possible when no longer needed
Strict infection control measures and hand hygiene
Metabolic control and support
Strict glucose control
Early enteral nutrition
Early and appropriate treatment of infection and trauma
Early hemodynamic resuscitation for severe sepsis
Early resuscitation of trauma victims with blood products
Prompt eradication of documented sources/foci of infection
Early fracture stabilization in multiple trauma
Appropriate empiric antibiotic therapy according to consensus guidelines where available with earliest possible de-escalation of therapy according to culture results
Prevention of acute lung injury (ALI), acute respiratory distress syndrome (ARDS), and ventilator-associated and aspiration pneumonia
Elevation of the head of bed to 30 degrees in all patients without spine precautions
Stress gastritis prophylaxis according to consensus guidelines
Lung protective ventilation strategies in patients with ALI/ARDS
Implementation of weaning protocols
Daily sedation holidays
Chlorhexidine oral rinse twice daily, oral care every 4 hrs
Selective decontamination of the digestive tract
Use of a subglottic suction endotracheal tube
Prevention of acute renal failure
Normal saline administration to prevent contrast-induced nephropathy with the addition of sodium bicarbonate or *N*-acetylcysteine as indicated
Discontinuation of nephrotoxic drugs whenever possible; consider once-daily dosing regimens for aminoglycoside antibiotics

individualized support for dysfunctional organs, and minimizing iatrogenic complications by following clinical practice guidelines based on evidence-based medicine for mechanical ventilation and prevention of VAP and CRBSIs (Table 52.4). Development of well-functioning ICU teams helps facilitate these paradigms of care. Improved outcome may be realized if patients at high risk for developing the syndrome can be identified earlier so that preventive measures can be instituted when appropriate. Because the pathogenesis of MODS involves numerous mediators, it is doubtful that all patients can be treated with a single agent or mode of therapy.

Key Points

- MODS develops in up to 40% of critically ill patients without a diagnosis of sepsis and up to 70% of those with a diagnosis of severe sepsis. Mortality attributable to MODS rises as the number of failing organ systems increases; mortality rates in patients with one, two, or three failing organs average 30%, 50%, and over 70%, respectively, depending on the etiology of MODS and the organ systems involved.
- Population-based, but not individual, risks of mortality can be predicted with high degrees of precision by several severity-of-illness scoring systems and models.
- MODS may result from "single-hit" insults such as severe infection or trauma, or may evolve through several stages, each having characteristic clinical features.
- An uncontrolled focus of infection, ongoing perfusion deficits resulting in diminished tissue $\dot{D}O_2$, injured or devitalized tissue, and persistent inflammation commonly initiate MODS.
- Fever or hypothermia and leukocytosis are not always the manifestations of sepsis but may represent systemic inflammation.
- TNF-α, IL-1, IL-6, IL-8, platelet-activating factor, ROS, and NO are pivotal early mediators in the host response to infection and have multiple pathophysiologic effects relevant to MODS.
- Inappropriate regulation of the production of cytokines, eicosanoids, ROS, and NO is thought to be of causal significance in MODS, as are pathologic neutrophil–endothelial interactions and cross-talk among elements of the coagulation, complement, and kinin cascades.
- Alterations in microvascular blood flow and mitochondrial dysfunction likely play an important role in the pathogenesis of organ dysfunction in shock. The surface receptors and mediators associated with these alterations include oxidants, lectins, proteases, vasoactive products of iNOS, and altered adrenergic receptor sensitivity.
- Clinically occult dysfunction of the gastrointestinal (GI) mucosal barrier in the ICU is common because of splanchnic ischemia from shock, and may result in endogenous endotoxemia and bacterial translocation.
- Neutrophil- and ROS-mediated intestinal I/R injury in the postresuscitation period is a potential mechanism of remote organ damage. This may lead to a domino-like sequence of organ failures.
- The liver plays a pivotal but clinically inapparent role in systemic host defense through four mechanisms. First, mononuclear phagocytic (Kupffer) cell uptake processes control the magnitude and circulating half-life of endotoxin, bacteria, and vasoactive by-products. Second, production and export of TNF-α with other mediators directly modulate lung function and cardiovascular stability. Third, hepatobiliary clearance is important in the metabolic inactivation and detoxification of such mediators. Fourth, the synthesis of acute-phase reactants regulates several key aspects of metabolism and inflammation.
- Reductions in total hepatic blood flow ($\dot{Q}L$) and $\dot{D}O_2$, or its partitioning between portal venous and hepatic arterial flows, may alter the aforementioned mechanisms, thereby influencing systemic immunoregulation.
- Signs of established MODS are manifested differently in each organ (e.g., ARDS, ARF), yet such changes often reflect generalized endothelial injury and inflammation.
- Diverse medical conditions may mimic sepsis-related MODS and should be excluded when appropriate. These include connective tissue diseases, intoxications, and neoplasms.
- Early rapid resuscitation from shock, irrespective of its etiology, attenuates injury to regional organs and may decrease the incidence of MODS.

References

1. American College of Chest Physicians/Society of Critical Care Medicine Consensus Conference: definitions for sepsis and organ failure and guidelines for the use of innovative therapies in sepsis. *Crit Care Med*. 1992;20:864–874.
2. Garcia Lizana F, Manzano Alonso JL, Gonzalez Santana B, et al. [Survival and quality of life of patients with multiple organ failure one year after leaving an intensive care unit]. *Med Clin (Barc)*. 2000;114:99–103.
3. Goris RJ, te Boekhorst TP, Nuytinck JK, Gimbrere JS. Multiple-organ failure: generalized autodestructive inflammation? *Arch Surg*. 1985;120:1109–1115.
4. Knaus WA, Draper EA, Wagner DP, Zimmerman JE. Prognosis in acute organ-system failure. *Ann Surg*. 1985;202:685–693.
5. Marshall JC, Cook DJ, Christou NV, et al. Multiple organ dysfunction score: a reliable descriptor of a complex clinical outcome. *Crit Care Med*. 1995;23:1638–1652.
6. Vincent JL, Moreno R, Takala J, et al., on behalf of the Working Group on Sepsis-Related Problems of the European Society of Intensive Care Medicine. The SOFA (Sepsis-related Organ Failure Assessment) score to describe organ dysfunction/failure. *Intensive Care Med*. 1996;22:707–710.
7. Moreno R, Vincent JL, Matos R, et al.; Working Group on Sepsis related Problems of the ESICM. The use of maximum SOFA score to quantify organ dysfunction/failure in intensive care: results of a prospective, multicentre study. *Intensive Care Med*. 1999;25:686–696.
8. Le Gall JR, Klar J, Lemeshow S, et al.; ICU Scoring Group. The Logistic Organ Dysfunction system: a new way to assess organ dysfunction in the intensive care unit. *JAMA*. 1996;276:802–810.
9. Russell JA, Singer J, Bernard GR, et al. Changing pattern of organ dysfunction in early human sepsis is related to mortality. *Crit Care Med*. 2000;28:3405–3411.
10. Ferreira FL, Bota DP, Bross A, et al. Serial evaluation of the SOFA score to predict outcome in critically ill patients. *JAMA*. 2001;286:1754–1758.
11. Herridge MS, Cheung AM, Tansey CM, et al. One-year outcomes in survivors of the acute respiratory distress syndrome. *N Engl J Med*. 2003;348:683–693.
12. Vincent JL, Sakr Y, Sprung CL, et al. Sepsis in European intensive care units: results of the SOAP study. *Crit Care Med*. 2006;34:344–353.
13. Bell RC, Coalson JJ, Smith JD, Johanson WG Jr. Multiple organ system failure and infection in adult respiratory distress syndrome. *Ann Intern Med*. 1983;99:293–298.
14. Knaus WA, Wagner DP, Draper EA, et al. The APACHE III prognostic system. Risk prediction of hospital mortality for critically ill hospitalized adults. *Chest*. 1991;100:1619–36.
15. Sauaia A, Moore FA, Moore EE, et al. Early predictors of postinjury multiple organ failure. *Arch Surg*. 1994;129:39–45.
16. Chen C, Kollef MH. Conservative fluid therapy in septic shock: an example of targeted therapeutic minimization. *Crit Care*. 2014;18:481.
17. Kelm DJ, Perrin JT, Cartin-Ceba R, et al. Fluid overload in patients with severe sepsis and septic shock treated with early goal-directed therapy is associated with increased acute need for fluid-related medical interventions and hospital death. *Shock*. 2015;43:68–73.
18. Singer M. The role of mitochondrial dysfunction in sepsis-induced multi-organ failure. *Virulence*. 2014;5:66–72.
19. Kaukonen KM, Bailey M, Pilcher D, et al. Systemic inflammatory response syndrome criteria in defining severe sepsis. *N Engl J Med*. 2015;372:1629–1638.
20. Levy MM, Fink MP, Marshall JC, et al. 2001 SCCM/ESICM/ACCP/ATS/SIS International Sepsis Definitions Conference. *Crit Care Med*. 2003;31:1250–1256.
21. Zhao H, Heard SO, Mullen MT, et al. An evaluation of the diagnostic accuracy of the 1991 American College of Chest Physicians/Society of Critical Care Medicine and the 2001 Society of Critical Care Medicine/European Society of Intensive Care Medicine/American College of Chest Physicians/American Thoracic Society/Surgical Infection Society sepsis definition. *Crit Care Med*. 2012;40:1700–1706.
22. Rangel-Frausto MS, Pittet D, Costigan M, et al. The natural history of the systemic inflammatory response syndrome (SIRS): a prospective study. *JAMA*. 1995;273:117–123.
23. Komatsu T, Shibutani K, Okamoto K, et al. Critical level of oxygen delivery after cardiopulmonary bypass. *Crit Care Med*. 1987;15:194–197.
24. Ronco JJ, Fenwick JC, Tweeddale MG, et al. Identification of the critical oxygen delivery for anaerobic metabolism in critically ill septic and nonseptic humans. *JAMA*. 1993;270:1724–1730.
25. Houben AJ, Beljaars JH, Hofstra L, et al. Microvascular abnormalities in chronic heart failure: a cross-sectional analysis. *Microcirculation*. 2003;10:471–478.
26. Vajda K, Szabo A, Boros M. Heterogeneous microcirculation in the rat small intestine during hemorrhagic shock: quantification of the effects of hypertonic-hyperoncotic resuscitation. *Eur Surg Res*. 2004;36:338–344.
27. Arslan E, Sierko E, Waters JH, Siemionow M. Microcirculatory hemodynamics after acute blood loss followed by fresh and banked blood transfusion. *Am J Surg*. 2005;190:456–462.
28. Cryer HM, Gosche J, Harbrecht J, et al. The effect of hypertonic saline resuscitation on responses to severe hemorrhagic shock by the skeletal muscle, intestinal, and renal microcirculation systems: seeing is believing. *Am J Surg*. 2005;190:305–313.
29. De Blasi RA, Palmisani S, Alampi D, et al. Microvascular dysfunction and skeletal muscle oxygenation assessed by phase-modulation near-infrared spectroscopy in patients with septic shock. *Intensive Care Med*. 2005;31:1661–1668.
30. De Backer D, Creteur J, Dubois MJ, et al. Microvascular alterations in patients with acute severe heart failure and cardiogenic shock. *Am Heart J*. 2004;147:91–99.
31. De Backer D, Creteur J, Preiser J-C, et al. Microvascular blood flow is altered in patients with sepsis. *Am J Respir Crit Care Med*. 2002;166:98–104.
32. De Backer D, Donadello K, Sakr Y, et al. Microcirculatory alterations in patients with severe sepsis: impact of time of assessment and relationship with outcome. *Crit Care Med*. 2013;41:791–799.
33. Hernandez G, Bruhn A, Luengo C, et al. Effects of dobutamine on systemic, regional and microcirculatory perfusion parameters in septic shock: a randomized, placebo-controlled, double-blind, crossover study. *Intensive Care Med*. 2013;39:1435–1443.
34. Trzeciak S, Glaspey LJ, Dellinger RP, et al. Randomized controlled trial of inhaled nitric oxide for the treatment of microcirculatory dysfunction in patients with sepsis. *Crit Care Med*. 2014;42:2482–2492.
35. van der Voort PH, van Zanten M, Bosman RJ, et al. Testing a conceptual model on early opening of the microcirculation in severe sepsis and septic shock: a randomised controlled pilot study. *Eur J Anaesthesiol*. 2015;32:189–198.
36. VanderMeer TJ, Wang H, Fink MP. Endotoxemia causes ileal mucosal acidosis in the absence of mucosal hypoxia in a normodynamic porcine model of septic shock. *Crit Care Med*. 1995;23:1217–1226.
37. Rosser DM, Stidwill RP, Jacobson D, Singer M. Oxygen tension in the bladder epithelium rises in both high and low cardiac output endotoxemic sepsis. *J Appl Physiol*. 1995;79:1878–1882.
38. Boekstegers P, Weidenhofer S, Kapsner T, Werdan K. Skeletal muscle partial pressure of oxygen in patients with sepsis. *Crit Care Med*. 1994;22:640–650.
39. Takasu O, Gaut JP, Watanabe E, et al. Mechanisms of cardiac and renal dysfunction in patients dying of sepsis. *Am J Respir Crit Care Med*. 2013;187:509–517.
40. Brealey D, Brand M, Hargreaves I, et al. Association between mitochondrial dysfunction and severity and outcome of septic shock. *Lancet*. 2002;360:219–223.
41. Svistunenko DA, Davies N, Brealey D, et al. Mitochondrial dysfunction in patients with severe sepsis: an EPR interrogation of individual respiratory chain components. *Biochim Biophys Acta*. 2006;1757:262–272.
42. Singer M. Metabolic failure. *Crit Care Med*. 2005;33:S539–542.
43. Szabo C, Zingarelli B, O'Connor M, Salzman AL. DNA strand breakage, activation of poly (ADP-ribose) synthetase, and cellular energy depletion are involved in the cytotoxicity of macrophages and smooth muscle cells exposed to peroxynitrite. *Proc Natl Acad Sci USA*. 1996;93:1753–1758.
44. Szabo C, Zingarelli B, Salzman AL. Role of poly-ADP ribosyltransferase activation in the vascular contractile and energetic failure elicited by exogenous and endogenous nitric oxide and peroxynitrite. *Circ Res*. 1996;78:1051–1063.
45. Liaudet L, Rosenblatt-Velin N, Pacher P. Role of peroxynitrite in the cardiovascular dysfunction of septic shock. *Curr Vasc Pharmacol*. 2013;11:196–207.
46. Dommett RM, Klein N, Turner MW. Mannose-binding lectin in innate immunity: past, present and future. *Tissue Antigens*. 2006;68:193–209.
47. Nieuwenhuijzen GA, Meyer MP, Hendriks T, Goris RJ. Deficiency of complement factor C5 reduces early mortality but does not prevent organ damage in an animal model of multiple organ dysfunction syndrome. *Crit Care Med*. 1995;23:1686–1693.
48. Ivanovska N, Hristova M, Philipov S. Complement modulatory activity of bisbenzylisoquinoline alkaloids isolated from Isopyrum thalictroides. II. Influence on C3-9 reactions in vitro and antiinflammatory effect in vivo. *Int J Immunopharmacol*. 1999;21:337–347.
49. Harkin DW, Romaschin A, Taylor SM, et al. Complement C5a receptor antagonist attenuates multiple organ injury in a model of ruptured abdominal aortic aneurysm. *J Vasc Surg*. 2004;39:196–206.

50. Hoehlig K, Maasch C, Shushakova N, et al. A novel C5a-neutralizing mirror-image (l-)aptamer prevents organ failure and improves survival in experimental sepsis. *Mol Ther*. 2013;21:2236–2246.
51. Robbins RA, Russ WD, Rasmussen JK, Clayton MM. Activation of the complement system in the adult respiratory distress syndrome. *Am Rev Respir Dis*. 1987;135:651–658.
52. Fosse E, Pillgram-Larsen J, Svennevig JL, et al. Complement activation in injured patients occurs immediately and is dependent on the severity of the trauma. *Injury*. 1998;29:509–514.
53. Hecke F, Schmidt U, Kola A, et al. Circulating complement proteins in multiple trauma patients: correlation with injury severity, development of sepsis, and outcome. *Crit Care Med*. 1997;25:2015–2024.
54. Fowler AA, Hyers TM, Fisher BJ, et al. The adult respiratory distress syndrome: cell populations and soluble mediators in the air spaces of patients at high risk. *Am Rev Respir Dis*. 1987;136:1225–1231.
55. Zeerleder S, Caliezi C, van Mierlo G, et al. Administration of C1 inhibitor reduces neutrophil activation in patients with sepsis. *Clin Diagn Lab Immunol*. 2003;10:529–535.
56. Caliezi C, Zeerleder S, Redondo M, et al. C1-inhibitor in patients with severe sepsis and septic shock: beneficial effect on renal dysfunction. *Crit Care Med*. 2002;30:1722–1728.
57. Saikumar P, Dong Z, Weinberg JM, Venkatachalam MA. Mechanisms of cell death in hypoxia/reoxygenation injury. *Oncogene*. 1998;17:3341–3349.
58. Lindsay TF, Luo XP, Lehotay DC, et al. Ruptured abdominal aortic aneurysm, a "two-hit" ischemia/reperfusion injury: evidence from an analysis of oxidative products. *J Vasc Surg*. 1999;30:219–228.
59. Kietzmann D, Kahl R, Muller M, et al. Hydrogen peroxide in expired breath condensate of patients with acute respiratory failure and with ARDS. *Intensive Care Med*. 1993;19:78–81.
60. Lamb NJ, Gutteridge JM, Baker C, et al. Oxidative damage to proteins of bronchoalveolar lavage fluid in patients with acute respiratory distress syndrome: evidence for neutrophil-mediated hydroxylation, nitration, and chlorination. *Crit Care Med*. 1999;27:1738–1744.
61. Richard C, Lemonnier F, Thibault M, et al. Vitamin E deficiency and lipoperoxidation during adult respiratory distress syndrome. *Crit Care Med*. 1990;18:4–9.
62. Lang JD, McArdle PJ, O'Reilly PJ, Matalon S. Oxidant-antioxidant balance in acute lung injury. *Chest*. 2002;122:314S–20S.
63. Rice TW, Wheeler AP, Thompson BT, et al. Enteral omega-3 fatty acid, gamma-linolenic acid, and antioxidant supplementation in acute lung injury. *JAMA*. 2011;306:1574–1581.
64. Bernard GR, Wheeler AP, Arons MM, et al. A trial of antioxidants N-acetylcysteine and procysteine in ARDS. The Antioxidant in ARDS Study Group. *Chest*. 1997;112:164–172.
65. Gadek JE, DeMichele SJ, Karlstad MD, et al.; Enteral Nutrition in ARDS Study Group. Effect of enteral feeding with eicosapentaenoic acid, gamma-linolenic acid, and antioxidants in patients with acute respiratory distress syndrome. *Crit Care Med*. 1999;27:1409–1420.
66. Fowler AA III, Syed AA, Knowlson S, et al. Phase I safety trial of intravenous ascorbic acid in patients with severe sepsis. *J Transl Med*. 2014;12:32.
67. Ortolani O, Conti A, De Gaudio AR, et al. Protective effects of N-acetylcysteine and rutin on the lipid peroxidation of the lung epithelium during the adult respiratory distress syndrome. *Shock*. 2000;13:14–18.
68. Fein AM, Bernard GR, Criner GJ, et al. Treatment of severe systemic inflammatory response syndrome and sepsis with a novel bradykinin antagonist, deltibant (CP-0127): results of a randomized, double-blind, placebo-controlled trial. CP-0127 SIRS and Sepsis Study Group. *JAMA*. 1997;277:482–748.
69. Levi M. Disseminated intravascular coagulation: what's new? *Crit Care Clin*. 2005;21:449–467.
70. Gando S, Iba T, Eguchi Y, et al. A multicenter, prospective validation of disseminated intravascular coagulation diagnostic criteria for critically ill patients: comparing current criteria. *Crit Care Med*. 2006;34:625–631.
71. Ten Cate H. Trombocytopenia: one of the markers of disseminated intravascular coagulation. *Pathophysiol Haemost Thromb*. 2003;33:413–416.
72. Abraham E, Reinhart K, Opal S, et al. Efficacy and safety of tifacogin (recombinant tissue factor pathway inhibitor) in severe sepsis: a randomized controlled trial. *JAMA*. 2003;290:238–247.
73. Warren BL, Eid A, Singer P, et al. Caring for the critically ill patient. High-dose antithrombin III in severe sepsis: a randomized controlled trial. *JAMA*. 2001;286:1869–1878.
74. Ranieri VM, Thompson BT, Barie PS, et al. Drotrecogin alfa (activated) in adults with septic shock. *N Engl J Med*. 2012;366:2055–2064.
75. Bulger EM, Maier RV. Lipid mediators in the pathophysiology of critical illness. *Crit Care Med*. 2000;28:N27–36.
76. Bernard GR, Wheeler AP, Russell JA, et al.; The Ibuprofen in Sepsis Study Group. The effects of ibuprofen on the physiology and survival of patients with sepsis. *N Engl J Med*. 1997;336:912–918.
77. Abraham E, Naum C, Bandi V, et al. Efficacy and safety of LY315920Na/S-5920, a selective inhibitor of 14-kDa group IIA secretory phospholipase A2, in patients with suspected sepsis and organ failure. *Crit Care Med*. 2003;31:718–728.
78. Slotman GJ, Burchard KW, D'Arezzo A, Gann DS. Ketoconazole prevents acute respiratory failure in critically ill surgical patients. *J Trauma*. 1988;28:648–654.
79. Yu M, Tomasa G. A double-blind, prospective, randomized trial of ketoconazole, a thromboxane synthetase inhibitor, in the prophylaxis of the adult respiratory distress syndrome. *Crit Care Med*. 1993;21:1635–1642.
80. ARDS Network. Ketoconazole for early treatment of acute lung injury and acute respiratory distress syndrome: a randomized controlled trial. *JAMA*. 2000;283:1995–2002.
81. Opal S, Laterre PF, Abraham E, et al. Recombinant human platelet-activating factor acetylhydrolase for treatment of severe sepsis: results of a phase III, multicenter, randomized, double-blind, placebo-controlled, clinical trial. *Crit Care Med*. 2004;32:332–341.
82. Claus RA, Russwurm S, Dohrn B, et al. Plasma platelet-activating factor acetylhydrolase activity in critically ill patients. *Crit Care Med*. 2005;33:1416–1419.
83. Michie HR, Spriggs DR, Manogue KR, et al. Tumor necrosis factor and endotoxin induce similar metabolic responses in human beings. *Surgery*. 1988;104:280–286.
84. Dinarello CA. Proinflammatory and anti-inflammatory cytokines as mediators in the pathogenesis of septic shock. *Chest*. 1997;112:321S–329S.
85. Gosain A, Gamelli RL. A primer in cytokines. *J Burn Care Rehabil*. 2005;26:7–12.
86. Michie HR, Manogue KR, Spriggs DR, et al. Detection of circulating tumor necrosis factor after endotoxin administration. *N Engl J Med*. 1988;318:1481–1486.
87. Tracey KJ, Fong Y, Hesse DG, et al. Anti-cachectin/TNF monoclonal antibodies prevent septic shock during lethal bacteraemia. *Nature*. 1987;330:662–664.
88. Martins GA, Da Gloria Da Costa Carvalho M, Rocha Gattass C. Sepsis: a follow-up of cytokine production in different phases of septic patients. *Int J Mol Med*. 2003;11:585–591.
89. Oberholzer A, Souza SM, Tschoeke SK, et al. Plasma cytokine measurements augment prognostic scores as indicators of outcome in patients with severe sepsis. *Shock*. 2005;23:488–493.
90. Bernard GR, Francois B, Mira JP, et al. Evaluating the efficacy and safety of two doses of the polyclonal anti-tumor necrosis factor-alpha fragment antibody AZD9773 in adult patients with severe sepsis and/or septic shock: randomized, double-blind, placebo-controlled phase IIb study. *Crit Care Med*. 2014;42:504–511.
91. Panacek EA, Marshall JC, Albertson TE, et al. Efficacy and safety of the monoclonal anti-tumor necrosis factor antibody F(ab')2 fragment afelimomab in patients with severe sepsis and elevated interleukin-6 levels. *Crit Care Med*. 2004;32:2173–2182.
92. Oberholzer A, Oberholzer C, Moldawer LL. Cytokine signaling: regulation of the immune response in normal and critically ill states. *Crit Care Med*. 2000;28:N3–12.
93. Dinarello CA. Interleukin-1beta. *Crit Care Med*. 2005;33:S460–462.
94. Vincent JL, Slotman G, Van Leeuwen PA, et al. IL-1ra administration does not improve cardiac function in patients with severe sepsis. *J Crit Care*. 1999;14:69–72.
95. Opal SM, Fisher CJ Jr, Dhainaut JF, et al.; the Interleukin-1 Receptor Antagonist Sepsis Investigator Group. Confirmatory interleukin-1 receptor antagonist trial in severe sepsis: a phase III, randomized, double-blind, placebo-controlled, multicenter trial. *Crit Care Med*. 1997;25:1115–1124.
96. Fisher CJ Jr, Dhainaut JF, Opal SM, et al.; Phase III rhIL-1ra Sepsis Syndrome Study Group. Recombinant human interleukin 1 receptor antagonist in the treatment of patients with sepsis syndrome: results from a randomized, double-blind, placebo-controlled trial. *JAMA*. 1994;271:1836–1843.
97. Song M, Kellum JA. Interleukin-6. *Crit Care Med*. 2005;33:S463–465.
98. Derhaschnig U, Bergmair D, Marsik C, et al. Effect of interleukin-6 blockade on tissue factor-induced coagulation in human endotoxemia. *Crit Care Med*. 2004;32:1136–1140.
99. Remick DG. Interleukin-8. *Crit Care Med*. 2005;33:S466–467.
100. Rodriguez JL, Miller CG, DeForge LE, et al. Local production of interleukin-8 is associated with nosocomial pneumonia. *J Trauma*. 1992;33:74–81.

101. Wang H, Bloom O, Zhang M, et al. HMG-1 as a late mediator of endotoxin lethality in mice. *Science*. 1999;285:248–251.
102. Yang H, Tracey KJ. High mobility group box 1 (HMGB1.) *Crit Care Med*. 2005;33:S472–474.
103. Yang H, Ochani M, Li J, et al. Reversing established sepsis with antagonists of endogenous high-mobility group box 1. *Proc Natl Acad Sci USA*. 2004;101:296–301.
104. Leng L, Bucala R. Macrophage migration inhibitory factor. *Crit Care Med*. 2005;33:S475–S477.
105. Calandra T, Bucala R. Macrophage migration inhibitory factor (MIF): a glucocorticoid counter- regulator within the immune system. *Crit Rev Immunol*. 1997;17:77–88.
106. Joshi PC, Poole GV, Sachdev V, et al. Trauma patients with positive cultures have higher levels of circulating macrophage migration inhibitory factor (MIF.) *Res Commun Mol Pathol Pharmacol*. 2000;107:13–20.
107. Liaudet L, Soriano FG, Szabo C. Biology of nitric oxide signaling. *Crit Care Med*. 2000;28:N37–N52.
108. Levy RM, Prince JM, Billiar TR. Nitric oxide: a clinical primer. *Crit Care Med*. 2005;33:S492–S495.
109. Szabo C, Billiar TR. Novel roles of nitric oxide in hemorrhagic shock. *Shock*. 1999;12:1–9.
110. Horton JW, Maass D, White J, Sanders B. Nitric oxide modulation of TNF-alpha-induced cardiac contractile dysfunction is concentration dependent. *Am J Physiol Heart Circ Physiol*. 2000;278:H1955–1965.
111. Ochoa JB, Udekwu AO, Billiar TR, et al. Nitrogen oxide levels in patients after trauma and during sepsis. *Ann Surg*. 1991;214:621–626.
112. Zingarelli B. Nuclear factor-kappaB. *Crit Care Med*. 2005;33:S414–S416.
113. Lopez A, Lorente JA, Steingrub J, et al. Multiple-center, randomized, placebo-controlled, double-blind study of the nitric oxide synthase inhibitor 546C88: effect on survival in patients with septic shock. *Crit Care Med*. 2004;32:21–30.
114. Vallet B. Bench-to-bedside review: endothelial cell dysfunction in severe sepsis: a role in organ dysfunction? *Crit Care*. 2003;7:130–138.
115. Lee MM, Schuessler GB, Chien S. Time-dependent effects of endotoxin on the ultrastructure of aortic endothelium. *Artery*. 1988;15:71–89.
116. Sessler CN, Windsor AC, Schwartz M, et al. Circulating ICAM-1 is increased in septic shock. *Am J Respir Crit Care Med*. 1995;151:1420–1427.
117. Johansen ME, Johansson PI, Ostrowski SR, et al. Profound endothelial damage predicts impending organ failure and death in sepsis. *Semin Thromb Hemost*. 2015;41:16–25.
118. Vincent JL, De Backer D. Does disseminated intravascular coagulation lead to multiple organ failure? *Crit Care Clin*. 2005;21:469–277.
119. Gardinali M, Borrelli E, Chiara O, et al. Inhibition of CD11-CD18 complex prevents acute lung injury and reduces mortality after peritonitis in rabbits. *Am J Respir Crit Care Med*. 2000;161:1022–1029.
120. Xu H, Gonzalo JA, St Pierre Y, et al. Leukocytosis and resistance to septic shock in intercellular adhesion molecule 1-deficient mice. *J Exp Med*. 1994;180:95–109.
121. Bhagat K, Moss R, Collier J, Vallance P. Endothelial "stunning" following a brief exposure to endotoxin: a mechanism to link infection and infarction? *Cardiovasc Res*. 1996;32:822–829.
122. Fink MP. Intestinal epithelial hyperpermeability: update on the pathogenesis of gut mucosal barrier dysfunction in critical illness. *Curr Opin Crit Care*. 2003;9:143–151.
123. Han X, Fink MP, Yang R, Delude RL. Increased iNOS activity is essential for intestinal epithelial tight junction dysfunction in endotoxemic mice. *Shock*. 2004;21:261–270.
124. Han X, Fink MP, Uchiyama T, et al. Increased iNOS activity is essential for hepatic epithelial tight junction dysfunction in endotoxemic mice. *Am J Physiol Gastrointest Liver Physiol*. 2004;286:G126–136.
125. Han X, Fink MP, Uchiyama T, et al. Increased iNOS activity is essential for pulmonary epithelial tight junction dysfunction in endotoxemic mice. *Am J Physiol Lung Cell Mol Physiol*. 2004;286:L259–267.
126. Magnotti LJ, Deitch EA. Burns, bacterial translocation, gut barrier function, and failure. *J Burn Care Rehabil*. 2005;26:383–391.
127. Perl M, Chung CS, Ayala A. Apoptosis. *Crit Care Med*. 2005;33:S526–S529.
128. Bredesen DE, Rao RV, Mehlen P. Cell death in the nervous system. *Nature*. 2006;443:796–802.
129. Hashimoto S, Kobayashi A, Kooguchi K, et al. Upregulation of two death pathways of perforin/granzyme and FasL/Fas in septic acute respiratory distress syndrome. *Am J Respir Crit Care Med*. 2000;161:237–243.
130. Hotchkiss RS, Schmieg RE Jr, Swanson PE, et al. Rapid onset of intestinal epithelial and lymphocyte apoptotic cell death in patients with trauma and shock. *Crit Care Med*. 2000;28:3207–3217.
131. Hotchkiss RS, Swanson PE, Freeman BD, et al. Apoptotic cell death in patients with sepsis, shock, and multiple organ dysfunction. *Crit Care Med*. 1999;27:1230–1251.
132. Hotchkiss RS, Nicholson DW. Apoptosis and caspases regulate death and inflammation in sepsis. *Nat Rev Immunol*. 2006;6:813–822.
133. Godin PJ, Buchman TG. Uncoupling of biological oscillators: a complementary hypothesis concerning the pathogenesis of multiple organ dysfunction syndrome. *Crit Care Med*. 1996;24:1107–1116.
134. Seely AJ, Christou NV. Multiple organ dysfunction syndrome: exploring the paradigm of complex nonlinear systems. *Crit Care Med*. 2000;28:2193–2200.
135. Seely AJ, Macklem PT. Complex systems and the technology of variability analysis. *Crit Care*. 2004;8:R367–R384.
136. Aird WC. Endothelial cell dynamics and complexity theory. *Crit Care Med*. 2002;30:S180–S185.
137. Haji-Michael PG, Vincent JL, Degaute JP, van de Borne P. Power spectral analysis of cardiovascular variability in critically ill neurosurgical patients. *Crit Care Med*. 2000;28:2578–2583.
138. Godin PJ, Fleisher LA, Eidsath A, et al. Experimental human endotoxemia increases cardiac regularity: results from a prospective, randomized, crossover trial [see comments]. *Crit Care Med*. 1996;24:1117–1124.
139. Seely AJ, Bravi A, Herry C, et al. Do heart and respiratory rate variability improve prediction of extubation outcomes in critically ill patients? *Crit Care*. 2014;18:R65.
140. Villar J, Maca-Meyer N, Perez-Mendez L, Flores C. Bench-to-bedside review: understanding genetic predisposition to sepsis. *Crit Care*. 2004;8:180–189.
141. Stuber F, Petersen M, Bokelmann F, Schade U. A genomic polymorphism within the tumor necrosis factor locus influences plasma tumor necrosis factor-alpha concentrations and outcome of patients with severe sepsis. *Crit Care Med*. 1996;24:381–384.
142. Lorenz E, Mira JP, Frees KL, Schwartz DA. Relevance of mutations in the TLR4 receptor in patients with gram-negative septic shock. *Arch Intern Med*. 2002;162:1028–1032.
143. Gong MN, Zhou W, Williams PL, et al. Polymorphisms in the mannose binding lectin-2 gene and acute respiratory distress syndrome. *Crit Care Med*. 2007;35:48–56.
144. Walley KR, Russell JA. Protein C-1641 AA is associated with decreased survival and more organ dysfunction in severe sepsis. *Crit Care Med*. 2007;35:12–17.
145. Lin MT, Albertson TE. Genomic polymorphisms in sepsis. *Crit Care Med*. 2004;32:569–579.
146. Dellinger RP, Levy MM, Rhodes A, et al. Surviving sepsis campaign: international guidelines for management of severe sepsis and septic shock: 2012. *Crit Care Med*. 2013;41:580–637.
147. Brunkhorst FM, Engel C, Bloos F, et al. Intensive insulin therapy and pentastarch resuscitation in severe sepsis. *N Engl J Med*. 2008;358:125–139.
148. Perner A, Haase N, Guttormsen AB, et al. Hydroxyethyl starch 130/0.42 versus Ringer's acetate in severe sepsis. *N Engl J Med*. 2012;367:124–134.
149. Myburgh JA, Finfer S, Bellomo R, et al. Hydroxyethyl starch or saline for fluid resuscitation in intensive care. *N Engl J Med*. 2012;367:1901–1911.
150. Perel P, Roberts I, Ker K. Colloids versus crystalloids for fluid resuscitation in critically ill patients. *Cochrane Database Syst Rev*. 2013;2:CD000567.
151. Caironi P, Tognoni G, Masson S, et al. Albumin replacement in patients with severe sepsis or septic shock. *N Engl J Med*. 2014;370:1412–1421.
152. Caironi P, Gattinoni L. Proposed benefits of albumin from the ALBIOS trial: a dose of insane belief. *Crit Care*. 2014;18:510.
153. Lobo DN, Awad S. Should chloride-rich crystalloids remain the mainstay of fluid resuscitation to prevent 'pre-renal' acute kidney injury? *Kidney Int*. 2014;86:1096–1105.
154. Yunos NM, Bellomo R, Hegarty C, et al. Association between a chloride-liberal vs chloride-restrictive intravenous fluid administration strategy and kidney injury in critically ill adults. *JAMA*. 2012;308:1566–1572.
155. Richard C, Warszawski J, Anguel N, et al. Early use of the pulmonary artery catheter and outcomes in patients with shock and acute respiratory distress syndrome: a randomized controlled trial. *JAMA*. 2003;290:2713–2720.
156. Harvey S, Harrison DA, Singer M, et al. Assessment of the clinical effectiveness of pulmonary artery catheters in management of patients in intensive care (PAC-Man): a randomised controlled trial. *Lancet*. 2005;366:472–477.
157. Gattinoni L, Brazzi L, Pelosi P, et al.; SvO_2 Collaborative Group. A trial of goal-oriented hemodynamic therapy in critically ill patients. *N Engl J Med*. 1995;333:1025–1032.

158. Kumar A, Anel R, Bunnell E, et al. Pulmonary artery occlusion pressure and central venous pressure fail to predict ventricular filling volume, cardiac performance, or the response to volume infusion in normal subjects. *Crit Care Med.* 2004;32:691–699.
159. Marik PE, Monnet X, Teboul JL. Hemodynamic parameters to guide fluid therapy. *Ann Intensive Care.* 2011;1:1.
160. Mouncey PR, Osborn TM, Power GS, et al. Trial of early, goal-directed resuscitation for septic shock. *N Engl J Med.* 2015;372:1301–1311.
161. Pro CI, Yealy DM, Kellum JA, et al. A randomized trial of protocol-based care for early septic shock. *N Engl J Med.* 2014;370:1683–1693.
162. Investigators A, Group AC, Peake SL, et al. Goal-directed resuscitation for patients with early septic shock. *N Engl J Med.* 2014;371:1496–1506.
163. Holst LB, Haase N, Wetterslev J, et al. Lower versus higher hemoglobin threshold for transfusion in septic shock. *N Engl J Med.* 2014;371: 1381–1391.
164. Asfar P, Meziani F, Hamel JF, et al. High versus low blood-pressure target in patients with septic shock. *N Engl J Med.* 2014;370:1583–1593.
165. Hecker A, Hecker B, Hecker M, et al. Acute abdominal compartment syndrome: current diagnostic and therapeutic options. *Langenbecks Arch Surg.* 2016;401:15–24.
166. Chiumello D, Pristine G, Slutsky AS. Mechanical ventilation affects local and systemic cytokines in an animal model of acute respiratory distress syndrome. *Am J Respir Crit Care Med.* 1999;160:109–116.
167. Ranieri VM, Giunta F, Suter PM, Slutsky AS. Mechanical ventilation as a mediator of multisystem organ failure in acute respiratory distress syndrome. *JAMA.* 2000;284:43–44.
168. Ranieri VM, Suter PM, Tortorella C, et al. Effect of mechanical ventilation on inflammatory mediators in patients with acute respiratory distress syndrome: a randomized controlled trial. *JAMA.* 1999;282:54–61.
169. Ventilation with lower tidal volumes as compared with traditional tidal volumes for acute lung injury and the acute respiratory distress syndrome. The Acute Respiratory Distress Syndrome Network. *N Engl J Med.* 2000; 342:1301–1308.
170. Amato MB, Meade MO, Slutsky AS, et al. Driving pressure and survival in the acute respiratory distress syndrome. *N Engl J Med.* 2015;372:747–755.
171. Papazian L, Forel JM, Gacouin A, et al. Neuromuscular blockers in early acute respiratory distress syndrome. *N Engl J Med.* 2010;363:1107–1116.
172. Guerin C, Reignier J, Richard JC, et al. Prone positioning in severe acute respiratory distress syndrome. *N Engl J Med.* 2013;368:2159–2168.
173. Rouby JJ, Brochard L. Tidal recruitment and overinflation in acute respiratory distress syndrome: yin and yang. *Am J Respir Crit Care Med.* 2007; 175:104–106.
174. Villar J, Kacmarek RM, Perez-Mendez L, Aguirre-Jaime A. A high positive end-expiratory pressure, low tidal volume ventilatory strategy improves outcome in persistent acute respiratory distress syndrome: a randomized, controlled trial. *Crit Care Med.* 2006;34:1311–1318.
175. Brower RG, Lanken PN, MacIntyre N, et al. Higher versus lower positive end-expiratory pressures in patients with the acute respiratory distress syndrome. *N Engl J Med.* 2004;351:327–336.
176. Briel M, Meade M, Mercat A, et al. Higher vs lower positive end-expiratory pressure in patients with acute lung injury and acute respiratory distress syndrome: systematic review and meta-analysis. *JAMA.* 2010;303: 865–873.
177. Terragni PP, Rosboch G, Tealdi A, et al. Tidal hyperinflation during low tidal volume ventilation in acute respiratory distress syndrome. *Am J Respir Crit Care Med.* 2007;175:160–166.
178. Wiedemann HP, Wheeler AP, Bernard GR, et al. Comparison of two fluid-management strategies in acute lung injury. *N Engl J Med.* 2006;354: 2564–2575.
179. Gill N, Nally JV Jr, Fatica RA. Renal failure secondary to acute tubular necrosis: epidemiology, diagnosis, and management. *Chest.* 2005;128: 2847–2863.
180. Egal M, Erler NS, de Geus HR, et al. Targeting oliguria reversal in goal-directed hemodynamic management does not reduce renal dysfunction in perioperative and critically ill patients: a systematic review and meta-analysis. *Anesth Analg.* 2016;122:173–185.
181. Venkataraman R, Kellum JA. Prevention of acute renal failure. *Chest.* 2007; 131:300–308.
182. Rybak MJ, Abate BJ, Kang SL, et al. Prospective evaluation of the effect of an aminoglycoside dosing regimen on rates of observed nephrotoxicity and ototoxicity. *Antimicrob Agents Chemother.* 1999;43:1549–1555.
183. Merten GJ, Burgess WP, Gray LV, et al. Prevention of contrast-induced nephropathy with sodium bicarbonate: a randomized controlled trial. *JAMA.* 2004;291:2328–1334.
184. Duong MH, MacKenzie TA, Malenka DJ. N-acetylcysteine prophylaxis significantly reduces the risk of radiocontrast-induced nephropathy: comprehensive meta-analysis. *Catheter Cardiovasc Interv.* 2005;64: 471–479.
185. Harwood PJ, Giannoudis PV, van Griensven M, et al. Alterations in the systemic inflammatory response after early total care and damage control procedures for femoral shaft fracture in severely injured patients. *J Trauma.* 2005;58:446–452.
186. Tenner S, Baillie J, DeWitt J, Vege SS; American College of Gastroenterology. American College of Gastroenterology guideline: management of acute pancreatitis. *Am J Gastroenterol.* 2013;108:1400–1516.
187. Chandrasekaran P, Gupta R, Shenvi S, et al. Prospective comparison of long term outcomes in patients with severe acute pancreatitis managed by operative and non operative measures. *Pancreatology.* 2015;15:478–484.
188. Villatoro E, Mulla M, Larvin M. Antibiotic therapy for prophylaxis against infection of pancreatic necrosis in acute pancreatitis. *Cochrane Database Syst Rev.* 2010;(5):CD002941.
189. da Costa DW, Boerma D, van Santvoort HC, et al. Staged multidisciplinary step-up management for necrotizing pancreatitis. *Br J Surg.* 2014;101: e65–79.
190. van Grinsven J, van Brunschot S, Bakker OJ, et al.; Dutch Pancreatitis Study Group. Diagnostic strategy and timing of intervention in infected necrotizing pancreatitis: an international expert survey and case vignette study. *HPB (Oxford).* 2016;18(1):49–56.
191. Park WM, Gloviczki P, Cherry KJ Jr, et al. Contemporary management of acute mesenteric ischemia: Factors associated with survival. *J Vasc Surg.* 2002;35:445–452.
192. Sawyer RG, Claridge JA, Nathens AB, et al. Trial of short-course antimicrobial therapy for intraabdominal infection. *N Engl J Med.* 2015;372: 1996–2005.
193. Drakulovic MB, Torres A, Bauer TT, et al. Supine body position as a risk factor for nosocomial pneumonia in mechanically ventilated patients: a randomised trial. *Lancet.* 1999;354:1851–1858.
194. Schweickert WD, Gehlbach BK, Pohlman AS, et al. Daily interruption of sedative infusions and complications of critical illness in mechanically ventilated patients. *Crit Care Med.* 2004;32:1272–1276.
195. Mehta S, Burry L, Cook D; SLEAP Investigators. Sedation interruption for mechanically ventilated patients-reply. *JAMA.* 2013;309:982–983.
196. Bouadma L, Sonneville R, Garrouste-Orgeas M, et al. Ventilator-associated events: prevalence, outcome, and relationship with ventilator-associated pneumonia. *Crit Care Med.* 2015;43:1798–1806.
197. Silvestri L, van Saene HK, Milanese M, et al. Selective decontamination of the digestive tract reduces bacterial bloodstream infection and mortality in critically ill patients: systematic review of randomized, controlled trials. *J Hosp Infect.* 2007;65:187–203.
198. Huang SS, Septimus E, Kleinman K, et al. Targeted versus universal decolonization to prevent ICU infection. *N Engl J Med.* 2013;368:2255–2265.
199. Plantinga NL, Bonten MJ. Selective decontamination and antibiotic resistance in ICUs. *Crit Care.* 2015;19:259.
200. Oostdijk EA, Kesecioglu J, Schultz MJ, et al. Effects of decontamination of the oropharynx and intestinal tract on antibiotic resistance in ICUs: a randomized clinical trial. *JAMA.* 2014;312:1429–1437.
201. de Jonge E, Schultz MJ, Spanjaard L, et al. Effects of selective decontamination of digestive tract on mortality and acquisition of resistant bacteria in intensive care: a randomised controlled trial. *Lancet.* 2003;362:1011–1016.
202. O'Grady NP, Alexander M, Burns LA, et al. Summary of recommendations: guidelines for the prevention of intravascular catheter-related infections. *Clin Infect Dis.* 2011;52:1087–1099.
203. Walz JM, Ellison RT III, Mack DA, et al. The bundle "plus": the effect of a multidisciplinary team approach to eradicate central line-associated bloodstream infections. *Anesth Analg.* 2015;120:868–876.
204. Maki DG, Stolz SM, Wheeler S, Mermel LA. Prevention of central venous catheter-related bloodstream infection by use of an antiseptic-impregnated catheter: a randomized, controlled trial. *Ann Intern Med.* 1997;127:257–266.
205. Ranucci M, Isgro G, Giomarelli PP, et al. Impact of oligon central venous catheters on catheter colonization and catheter-related bloodstream infection. *Crit Care Med.* 2003;31:52–59.
206. Darouiche RO, Raad II, Heard SO, et al. A comparison of two antimicrobial-impregnated central venous catheters. Catheter Study Group. *N Engl J Med.* 1999;340:1–8.
207. Herndon DN, Hart DW, Wolf SE, et al. Reversal of catabolism by beta-blockade after severe burns. *N Engl J Med.* 2001;345:1223–1239.
208. Perel P, Yanagawa T, Bunn F, et al. Nutritional support for head-injured patients. *Cochrane Database Syst Rev.* 2006;(4):CD001530.
209. Martindale RG, McClave SA, Vanek VW, et al. Guidelines for the provision and assessment of nutrition support therapy in the adult critically ill patient: Society of Critical Care Medicine and American Society for

Parenteral and Enteral Nutrition: executive summary. *Crit Care Med*. 2009; 37:1757–1761.

210. Rice TW. Gluttony in the intensive care unit: time to push back from the consensus table. *Am J Respir Crit Care Med*. 2013;187:223–224.
211. Arabi YM, Aldawood AS, Haddad SH, et al. Permissive underfeeding or standard enteral feeding in critically ill adults. *N Engl J Med*. 2015;372: 2398–408.
212. Griesdale DE, de Souza RJ, van Dam RM, et al. Intensive insulin therapy and mortality among critically ill patients: a meta-analysis including NICE-SUGAR study data. *CMAJ*. 2009;180:821–827.
213. Cerra FB, Benitez MR, Blackburn GL, et al. Applied nutrition in ICU patients: a consensus statement of the American College of Chest Physicians. *Chest*. 1997;111:769–778.
214. Endres S, Ghorbani R, Kelley VE, et al. The effect of dietary supplementation with n-3 polyunsaturated fatty acids on the synthesis of interleukin-1 and tumor necrosis factor by mononuclear cells. *N Engl J Med*. 1989;320:265–271.
215. Canadian Critical Care Clinical Practice Guidelines. Summary of Topics and Recommendations. 2015. Available at http://www.criticalcarenutrition.com. Accessed December 23, 2015.

CHAPTER
53

Perioperative Pulmonary Function Testing and Consultation/Preoperative Evaluation of the High-Risk Surgical Patient

BHIKEN I. NAIK and TIMOTHY S. ENG

OVERVIEW

Perioperative morbidity and mortality is a function of both patient and surgery-specific risk factors. It is imperative to have accurate risk estimation models that allow for shared decision making regarding preoperative risk modification, choice of surgical technique, and resource utilization. The American College of Surgeons National Surgical Quality Improvement Program (ACS NSQIP) Surgical Risk Calculator was developed based on data from 1,414,006 patients encompassing 1,557 unique CPT codes (1). The model performs well for estimating mortality/morbidity and as both a universal and procedure-specific risk calculator. The ACS NSQIP Surgical Risk Calculator is available as a web-based, easy to navigate application which further improves its utility in the preoperative evaluation of the surgical patient (2).

This chapter will guide the practitioner on the preoperative evaluation of the high-risk patient presenting for surgery with particular emphasis on the cardiac, pulmonary, renal, and neurologic system.

CARDIOVASCULAR

Noncardiac Surgery

Of the approximately 44 million patients undergoing noncardiac surgery in the United States yearly, 30% either have or are at risk for coronary artery disease (CAD). The presence of CAD increases the incidence of perioperative myocardial ischemia, with a 2.8-fold increase in adverse postoperative cardiac events (3). In an attempt to provide current evidence-based recommendations to manage the cardiac patient presenting for noncardiac surgery, the American College of Cardiology/American Heart Association (ACC/AHA) Task Force on Practice Guidelines convened a panel of experts and published a guideline on the perioperative cardiovascular evaluation and management for noncardiac surgery (4); this was revised in 2014. The important aspects of the guideline are to identify high-risk patients, appropriately stratify them according to their risk category, and perform preoperative testing in a rational and cost-effective manner. The guideline emphasizes that no test should be performed unless it is likely to influence patient treatment.

The ACC/AHA approach to cardiac assessment for CAD is a seven-step algorithm that incorporates clinical predictors based on the patient's history and physical examination, surgery-specific risk, and functional capacity (5). Use of the algorithm must occur within the context of the patient's values and preferences to ensure shared decision making. In the event of emergency surgery, risk assessment should occur, and the patient should be taken to surgery (step 1) with further evaluation, if indicated, performed postoperatively.

The presence of heart failure (HF), significant valvular heart disease, or cardiac dysrhythmias may necessitate further evaluation and management prior to elective or urgent surgery. Among HF patients, those with left ventricular ejection fraction (LVEF) less than 30% have significantly worse survival than those with preserved LVEF; however, HF patients with preserved LVEF still have higher mortality rates than patients without HF. Left-sided stenotic valvular lesions also increase cardiac risk, and patients may require surgical or transcatheter valve replacement or percutaneous balloon dilation prior to noncardiac surgery. It should be noted that while percutaneous aortic valve balloon dilation can be performed safely, mortality and recurrence of stenosis remain high within 6 months of the procedure.

In the absence of an emergent procedure, the decision making proceeds to step 2 of the ACC/AHA algorithm with determination of the presence of an acute coronary syndrome (ACS). The management of these patients should be according to existing guidelines for unstable angina/non–ST-elevation myocardial infarction and ST-elevation myocardial infarction (6,7) and is discussed further in Chapter 94.

In the absence of an ACS, the perioperative risk of major adverse cardiac events (MACE) should be estimated in step 3 by integrating the clinical and surgical risks. Both Goldman et al. (8) and Lee et al. (9) devised cardiac risk indices that have been in use for many years. More recently, Gupta et al. (10) analyzed the 2007 NSQIP database, which included over 200,000 patients from multiple centers, to determine significant risk factors for perioperative myocardial infarction or cardiac arrest (MICA) up to 30 days after surgery. Multivariate analysis demonstrated the following variables to be associated with greater risk: American Society of Anesthesiologist (ASA) physical status (Table 53.1), dependent functional status, increasing age, elevated creatinine (>1.5 mg/dL), and type of surgery. With regard to type of surgery, aortic and

TABLE 53.1 American Society of Anesthesiologists Physical Status Classification

Physical Status	Definition
I	Healthy patient
II	Mild systemic disease; no functional limitation
III	Severe systemic disease; definite functional limitation
IV	Severe systemic disease that is constant threat to life
V	Moribund patient; unlikely to survive 24 hours with or without surgery
VI	Brain-dead patient; organ donor
E	Emergency procedure

peripheral vascular surgeries are generally associated with the highest risk. With the advent of less invasive endovascular approaches, however, this risk is mitigated. Thus, with continually evolving surgical techniques, it has become challenging to assign surgery-specific risk.

The NSQIP risk model (10) had excellent discrimination, or the ability to discern between those who developed MICA and those who did not, with a C-statistic (area under the receiver operating characteristic curve) of 0.88. When the 2008 NSQIP database was assessed, the risk model continued to perform well, with a C-statistic of 0.87. This was compared to the Revised Cardiac Risk Index, developed by Lee et al. (9), which had a C-statistic of 0.75.

Vascular surgery patients represent a unique cohort, as the incidence of CAD in this population group is disproportionately higher than in the general population. Given the deficiencies of the prior cardiac risk indices in patients undergoing major vascular surgery, Gupta et al. (10) applied their risk model to this patient population and found more modest discrimination, with a C-statistic of 0.75. Two risk calculators, the NSQIP MICA and NSQIP Surgical Risk Calculator (2,10), were subsequently developed as additional tools for the surgical decision-making process and can be accessed online. Although the former only estimates the risk of MICA, the latter includes a wider range of potential complications.

Patients at low risk for MACE (<1%) based on the combined clinical and surgical risk may proceed to surgery without further testing (step 4 of the ACC/AHA guideline), whereas patients with elevated risk for MACE (at least 1%) should have an assessment of functional status (step 5). This is most commonly estimated by activities of daily living and functional capacity, which is expressed in metabolic equivalents (METs). One MET is 3.5 mL/kg/min of O_2 consumption in a 70-kg, 40-year-old man at rest. Increasing levels of activity correlate with increasing METs, with activities of daily living or walking at 2 to 3 mph on level ground requiring between 1 and 3 METs and strenuous sports requiring greater than 10 METs. Climbing a flight of stairs or walking uphill is associated with greater than 4 METs. The need for assistance with activities of daily living and inability to perform at least 4 METs are associated with increased perioperative morbidity and mortality (4,11). Therefore, patients with functional capacity of at least 4 METs do not require further testing before surgery.

For those patients with poor (<4 METs) or unknown functional capacity, it should be determined if further testing to delineate cardiac ischemic burden will influence perioperative care (i.e., alter the decision to perform the planned surgery or undergo coronary revascularization if indicated following testing) (step 6). If so, it would be reasonable to order stress testing. If not, it would be appropriate to either proceed to surgery or explore alternate approaches, such as less invasive therapies or palliation (step 7).

Delineation of the ischemic burden can be broadly achieved by two methods. The first method involves coronary vasodilatation and induction of a "steal" phenomenon by pharmacologic agents, followed by a nuclear imaging technique to determine the degree of myocardial ischemia. The second method involves increasing myocardial oxygen demand and evaluating electrocardiographic or echocardiographic data for evidence of ischemia. Myocardial oxygen demand can be increased either by exercise stress testing or pharmacologically with dobutamine or atropine.

Once the degree of myocardial ischemia is quantified, patients can undergo either preoperative medical optimization or revascularization by percutaneous coronary intervention (PCI) or coronary artery bypass graft surgery (CABG). The ACC/AHA guideline emphasizes that patients should only undergo revascularization if otherwise indicated by existing clinical practice guidelines for PCI (12) and CABG (13) and not prior to noncardiac surgery solely to decrease perioperative cardiac events. In the Coronary Artery Revascularization Prophylaxis (CARP) trial (14), patients scheduled for elective vascular surgery who had CAD diagnosed by coronary angiography were randomized to revascularization (CABG or PCI) or no revascularization; there was no difference in 30-day and long-term mortality, MI, or stroke.

For patients in whom PCI is indicated, the process involves balloon angioplasty, which is usually followed by placement of either a bare-metal stent (BMS) or a drug-eluting stent (DES); stents reduce both the acute risk of major complications and long-term restenosis rate. Following placement of a stent, patients require antiplatelet therapy to prevent in-stent thrombosis. Dual antiplatelet therapy (DAPT) is maintained for 1 to 12 months, depending on whether a BMS or DES is placed, respectively. The presence of antiplatelet therapy adds a new dimension of complexity to the patient presenting for noncardiac surgery following PCI. The risk–benefit ratio of preventing thrombosis of the stent versus the risk of catastrophic perioperative bleeding must be carefully weighed. Kaluza et al. (15) reported 7 myocardial infarctions, 11 major bleeding episodes, and 8 deaths in 40 consecutive patients presenting for noncardiac surgery following placement of a stent. All deaths and MIs, as well as 8 of the 11 bleeding episodes, occurred within 2 weeks of coronary stent placement. Wilson et al. (16) reported a 4% incidence of death, MI, or stent thrombosis among 207 patients at the Mayo Clinic; they documented no adverse events in the 39 patients undergoing surgery 7 weeks after stent placement. It appears from these two important studies that the greatest risk of adverse cardiovascular events and bleeding complications occur within 2 weeks of stent placement. According to the ACC/AHA guideline (4), elective surgery should be delayed for at least 14 days after balloon angioplasty and 30 days after BMS implantation to allow for endothelialization of the stent. For patients with a DES, elective noncardiac surgery should ideally be delayed 365 days following DES implantation. Recent data, however, suggest that elective noncardiac surgery may be considered after 180 days following DES implantation (17,18).

Perioperative β-Blockade Therapy

Of the pharmacologic agents that have been used during the perioperative period, β-blockade therapy remains the most studied. β-Blockers have several salutary effects that decrease the risk for cardiovascular morbidity and mortality in a selected cohort of patients. β-Blockers help to correct the imbalance between myocardial oxygen demand and supply. They have additional plaque-stabilizing, antidysrhythmic, anti-inflammatory, and altered gene expression effects (19). Much work has been done to assess their impact on perioperative outcomes; however, this has been accompanied by significant controversy. In particular, the Dutch Echocardiographic Cardiac Risk Evaluation Applying Stress Echocardiography Study Group (DECREASE)-1 (20) and DECREASE-IV randomized controlled trials and other work by Poldermans have been scrutinized due to concerns for scientific misconduct. Moreover, while the PeriOperative ISchemic Evaluation (POISE)-1 (21) trial included over 8,000 patients, it has been criticized for its β-blocker dosing and timing strategy.

To address these concerns and assess the influence of these trials on overall conclusions, in 2014 the ACC/AHA Task Force on Practice Guidelines published a systematic review evaluating perioperative β-blockade in noncardiac surgery (22). This analysis reviewed 17 studies, with all but one being randomized controlled trials. It was determined that perioperative β-blockade led to a decrease in 30-day or in-hospital nonfatal MI, with a relative risk (RR) of 0.68 compared to control. Excluding the DECREASE trials had minimal effect on the RR. However, β-blockade was associated with a greater risk of nonfatal stroke (RR 1.79); this association remained on exclusion of the DECREASE trials (RR 1.86). Conversely, while the DECREASE trials demonstrated a trend toward reduced all-cause mortality, the remaining studies showed a statistically significant increase in all-cause mortality (RR 1.30). Moreover, β-blockade increased the risk of hypotension and bradycardia. Notably, despite concerns with the POISE-1 trial's protocol of starting high-dose extended-release metoprolol merely hours prior to surgery, the POISE-1 findings were overall in agreement with the remaining non-DECREASE trials. Thus, with important questions regarding the safety of longer duration preoperative β-blockade looming after exclusion of the DECREASE trials, the only class I recommendation from the ACC/AHA guideline is to continue β-blockade in patients taking these drugs chronically (4). The guideline recommends against starting β-blockade on the day of surgery.

Cardiac Surgery

Perioperative and long-term risk evaluation in cardiac surgery is complicated by several factors, including procedural and patient factors as well as data collection. Cardiac surgery, with its many confounding variables, requires large patient numbers for studies to be statistically relevant. Appropriate and meaningful data collection has previously been hampered by the reluctance to publish data on high-risk subgroups and the inclusion of data from low-output centers that were not part of a larger data collection network. However, this collection effort has improved, with the Society of Thoracic Surgeons (STS) National Adult Cardiac Surgery Database (NCD) now representing approximately 90% of cardiac surgery providers in the United States (23).

Examining multiple databases, such as the NCD, and large case series, identifies risk factors for cardiac surgery. Unfortunately, many of the assessments of statistical risk are based on odds ratios. In addition, multiple risk factors frequently coexist, making risk profiling for the individual patient difficult. Although patients are presenting cumulatively with more risk factors, the impact of the individual risk factor appears to be decreasing. Data accrued suggest a steady improvement in cardiac surgical outcomes (24). This improvement is attributed to better surgical technique, perioperative care, and patient selection.

Preoperative Evaluation

Cardiac risk profiling begins with a thorough clinical evaluation and a review of the completed special investigations. Additional investigations will be guided by the presence and severity of other organ dysfunction. Cardiac risk evaluation can be performed by risk assessment tools, which are based on large databases, such as the European System for Cardiac Operative Risk Evaluation (EuroSCORE) and the STS NCD (23–26). The value of these databases is that standardized definitions are used to classify patients. The risk assessment tools have two important objectives:

1. Identifying independent risk factors for morbidity and mortality in valvular, coronary, and thoracic aortic surgery.
2. Risk prediction modeling through multivariate logistic regression analysis with goals to assess individual patient risk, compare and audit individual units, and appropriately allocate resources.

Statistical analysis techniques have been used to generate scoring systems. The Parsonnet score, developed in the late 1980s, predicts risk for CABG and valvular surgery based on an additive score of weighted risk factors (27). In 1999, Nashef et al. (24) published an additive-weighted scoring system called EuroSCORE based on and validated using the EuroSCORE database; a logistic model was added in 2003 (28). Given the tendency of EuroSCORE to overestimate perioperative mortality (29), EuroSCORE II was developed in 2012 and is based on a cohort of 22,381 patients (25). In modern practice, EuroSCORE II and the STS risk models (21,24) are commonly used for risk assessment.

Important differences exist between EuroSCORE II and the STS risk models. Although EuroSCORE II only assesses mortality risk, the STS risk models additionally include the following outcomes: permanent stroke, renal failure, prolonged ventilation, deep sternal wound infection, reoperation, prolonged postoperative length of stay, and short postoperative length of stay. Moreover, the STS risk models allow the user to specify the particular surgery being performed (e.g., CABG or combined CABG and aortic valve replacement); EuroSCORE II simply assigns isolated CABG a baseline risk and adds "weight" for non-CABG or combined procedures. On the other hand, unlike the STS risk models, EuroSCORE II provides support for thoracic aortic procedures.

Both systems are well calibrated and provide good discrimination for perioperative mortality. When applied to a validation data set of 5,553 patients, EuroSCORE II predicted in-hospital mortality to be 3.95%, while actual mortality was marginally greater at 4.18% (25). The C-statistic was 0.81, demonstrating good discrimination; however, this was not significantly different from the original EuroSCORE. The STS risk models for CABG, isolated valve, and valve plus CABG surgeries had C-statistics for in-hospital or 30-day mortality of 0.81, 0.80, and 0.75, respectively, when applied to the validation sample (23,26). The performance of the STS risk models varied with regard to the aforementioned morbidity outcomes, but the C-statistics were overall less robust (0.62 to 0.79) than those for mortality.

The strongest risk factors for mortality identified by EuroSCORE II were symptomatic status (i.e., New York Heart Association class IV), prior cardiac surgery, current antibiotic treatment for endocarditis, critical illness preoperatively, decreased LVEF (<31%), emergent or salvage surgery (requiring cardiopulmonary resuscitation prior to anesthetic induction), two or more major cardiac procedures, thoracic aortic surgery, and renal dysfunction. Interestingly, patients on chronic dialysis had lower risk than patients with severe renal dysfunction—creatinine clearance below 50 mL/min—but not yet requiring dialysis.

The important risk factors in the STS risk models were generally consistent with those found in EuroSCORE II, though some definitions were slightly different. Variables with the highest odds ratios for mortality included age of at least 70 years, renal dysfunction—with preoperative dialysis having the greatest risk—severe chronic lung disease, preoperative shock, myocardial infarction within 6 hours, prior cardiac surgery, an emergent or salvage operation, and active infectious endocarditis.

Scoring systems have a role in predicting both perioperative and long-term mortality and intensive care unit (ICU) resource use (30–32). Furthermore, they provide a framework to direct clinical examination and special investigations, thereby facilitating the process of identifying and modifying preoperative risk. These scoring systems can better identify patients with a prohibitive perioperative risk. The EuroSCORE II and STS risk models have been adapted for easy use by clinicians at the bedside and are available online (33,34).

There has been an improvement in the ability to identify and categorize the high-risk patient presenting for cardiac surgery. As more data are accrued, risk profiling is becoming more accurate. This will allow for cost-effective implementation of promising preoperative interventions in the appropriate patient.

PULMONARY SYSTEM

The incidence of postoperative pulmonary complications (PPC) is 5% to 20% for noncardiothoracic surgery (35). The economic burden of perioperative pulmonary complications is significantly higher compared to cardiovascular complications: respiratory (median and IQR): $62,704 ($27,959–135,463) versus cardiovascular: $8,496 ($8,262–56,857) (36). Preoperative identification of the high-risk pulmonary cohort can aid with risk stratification and modification prior to surgery. Currently there exists no standard definition for PPC, which makes risk modeling more variable. Despite the lack of a standard definition, several well-validated studies have been performed that can aid the clinician.

In a systematic review, Smetana et al. (37) identified several important preoperative risk factors associated with PPC after noncardiothoracic surgery. Patient-related factors supported with good evidence include advanced age, ASA Class II, HF, functional dependency, and chronic obstructive pulmonary disease (COPD). Procedure-related factors include vascular, abdominal, thoracic, neurologic, and emergency surgery. Subsequently in a prospective, multicenter observational study, Canet et al. (35) identified low preoperative arterial oxygen saturation, acute respiratory infection during the previous month, preoperative anemia and surgical duration of at least 2 hours as additional risk factors associated with PPC. Finally, Gupta et al. (10), based on a large cohort from the NSQIP database, developed a postoperative respiratory failure risk calculator to facilitate surgical decision making, which can be accessed online (2).

For lung cancer surgery, the STS Database Risk Models developed by Kozower et al. (38) identified pneumonectomy, bilobectomy, ASA rating, Zubrod performance status, renal dysfunction, induction chemoradiation therapy, steroids, age, urgent procedures, male gender, forced expiratory volume 1 (FEV1), and body mass index as risk factors for developing postoperative major morbidity and mortality.

Pulmonary Evaluation

The evaluation of the high-risk pulmonary patient begins with a thorough history and physical examination, which guides further special investigations. Laboratory investigations with good predictive value for PPC include blood urea nitrogen (BUN) greater than 7.5 mMol/L (21 mg/dL), creatinine level greater than 133 μmol/L (1.5 mg/dL) and preoperative anemia (26,35,39,40). In addition, serum albumin below 3.0 g/dL correlates with an increased 30-day perioperative morbidity and mortality (41).

The utility and cost effectiveness of routine preoperative chest radiography has been extensively debated. An abnormal chest radiograph does predict postoperative complications; however, only 4.9% of radiographs in patients younger than 50 years of age will be abnormal. Among routine preoperative chest radiographs ordered, only 0.1% to 3% will alter management (37,42). A focused history and physical examination should identify the patient who is likely to have an abnormal preoperative chest radiograph; this is supported by practice guideline issued by the American College of Physicians suggesting that (37):

1. Only patients with known cardiopulmonary disease should have a *routine* preoperative chest radiograph.
2. Patients older than 50 years undergoing procedures with high pulmonary risk should have a preoperative chest radiograph. These procedures include aortic surgery (thoracic or abdominal), neurosurgery, abdominal surgery, and prolonged surgery.

The factors listed above for both noncardiothoracic and cardiothoracic surgery can assist the perioperative physician in identifying the high-risk cohort and tailor their management to mitigate postoperative complications.

Pulmonary Function Testing

The three most commonly performed pulmonary function tests include spirometry, measurement of lung diffusing capacity, and measurement of lung volumes.

Spirometry and measurement of lung diffusing capacity (DLCO) remain the most commonly utilized pulmonary function tests. For lung resection surgery spirometry, lung diffusing capacity and cardiopulmonary exercise testing form the cornerstone of the evaluation process prior to surgery (43,44). The perioperative risk of morbidity and mortality and eligibility for surgery is directly related to this three-legged physiologic testing algorithm. Based on the guidelines from the American College of Chest Physicians, the preoperative workup for lung resection surgery begins with an estimation of the postoperative FEV_1 (PPO FEV_1) and DL_{CO} (PPO DL_{CO}) (45). Although threshold limits are used to stratify risk, mitigating factors need to be considered in the decision-making process. Although pulmonary function tests are integral to this workup, concomitant cardiac evaluation using the thoracic-revised cardiac risk index is also recommended; this is based on the high prevalence of cardiac disease in this cohort of patients.

When the PPO FEV_1 and PPO DL_{CO} are greater than 60%, with a negative cardiac evaluation, the patient is considered to be low risk. For PPO FEV_1 and PPO DL_{CO} between 30% and 60%, a stair climb or shuttle walk can be performed to stratify the need for formal cardiopulmonary exercise testing (45). A stair climb over 22 m or shuttle walk over 400 m falls in the low-risk group; when the stair climb is less than 22 m or shuttle walk under 400 m, cardiopulmonary exercise testing is recommended. Finally cardiopulmonary exercise testing is also recommended when PPO FEV_1 and PPO DL_{CO} is less than 30% or with a positive high-risk cardiac evaluation. With cardiopulmonary exercise testing VO_2 max of less than 10 mL/kg/min (<35%), 10 to 20 mL/kg/min (35% to 75%), and greater than 20 mL/kg/min (>75%) are classified as high, moderate, and low risk, respectively (45).

Whereas the role of pulmonary function testing prior to cardiothoracic surgery is well defined, its role in the routine preoperative evaluation for noncardiothoracic surgery is controversial and less well defined.

Preoperative Pulmonary Optimization

Strategies to reduce PPC begin prior to surgery with identification of patients with high-risk factors that are potentially modifiable. These include smoking cessation, optimization of nutrition, identification and management of obstructive sleep apnea (OSA) and treating acute exacerbations of COPD.

Smoking is associated with a significant increase in PPC, with rates varying between 4% and 43% based on spirometry findings and the length of prior smoking (46,47). Smoking cessation is associated with a significant reduction (20% to 41%) in postoperative complication rates; however, this is contingent on the duration of abstinence and extent of prior smoking. When surgery is elective, smoking cessation should be initiated 4 weeks prior to surgery (48). As previously reported, low preoperative albumin is associated with a higher PPC. Preoperative enteral nutrition with an immune-repleting diet improves outcomes in malnourished elective gastroenterology oncology patients; they experience a significant decrease in nosocomial sepsis and hospital length of stay (49,50). Enthusiasm for total parenteral nutrition is tempered due to the increased rates of infection associated with long-term central venous access and hyperglycemia (49). The incidence of undiagnosed OSA is reported to be as high 24% (51) and can be associated with significant postoperative respiratory morbidity. Memtsoudis et al. reported a higher incidence of acute respiratory distress syndrome (ARDS), intubation/mechanical ventilation, and aspiration pneumonia in patients with OSA. Minimizing complications related to OSA begins with identification of undiagnosed sleep apnea using tools such as the STOP-BANG (Snore-Tired-Obstruction-Pressure-BMI-Age-Neck-Gender) questionnaire, starting CPAP following confirmation of the diagnosis and optimization of the airway pressure for those patients whose treatment is ineffective.

Obstructive pulmonary disorders are associated with increased risk of PPC, especially when reversible airway obstruction is present (37,52,53). However, Milledge and Nunn (54) demonstrated that even patients with severe airway obstruction—defined as an FEV_1 less than 1 L—can safely undergo an operative intervention without an increase in postoperative complications. The key element in the management of patients with COPD is the identification and appropriate treatment of the reversible component of the airway disease.

β_2-Agonists have a salutary effect on airway hyperreactivity in obstructive airway disease. When symptom-free mild asthmatic volunteers were intubated under local anesthesia, FEV_1 decreased by 50%; in the group pretreated with a β_2-agonist, the FEV_1 decreased by only 20% (55). However, it is important to note that the incidence of postintubation bronchospasm is still significant, even when β_2-agonists are used as monotherapy (56,57).

Preoperative steroid therapy, even of short duration, has been shown to decrease the incidence of wheezing postintubation (57–59). The concern for negative effects on wound healing and increased infection rates have not been borne out (60). With regard to the use of methylxanthines, a Cochrane review in 2001 showed that neither theophylline nor aminophylline offered any advantage over β_2-agonists in the setting of acute bronchospasm (61).

Finally, there is good evidence in adults that upper and lower airway infections increase airway reactivity and result in demonstrable spirometry abnormalities for 6 to 8 weeks postinfection (62). Elective surgery should ideally be delayed in patients with underlying bronchial hyperreactivity and the underlying infection treated.

Intraoperative Mechanical Ventilation

There is well-established evidence that lung protective ventilation strategies that reduce excessive volume/pressure and minimizes atelectasis-related injury in ARDS also reduce postoperative morbidity and mortality (63). However, since the publication of this seminal work, there is compelling evidence supporting the extrapolation of this ventilation strategy in patients without ARDS undergoing intermediate to high-risk surgery. Severgnini et al. (64) demonstrated that a protective ventilation strategy (V_T: 7 mL/kg ideal body weight, 10 cm H_2O PEEP vs. V_T: 9 mL/kg ideal body weight and zero-PEEP) was associated with better postoperative pulmonary function test, higher arterial oxygenation and lower Clinical Pulmonary Infection Score. In a similarly designed study, Futier et al. (65) showed that a protective ventilation strategy (V_T: 6 to 8 mL/kg ideal body weight, 6 to 8 cm H_2O PEEP, recruitment maneuvers) compared to standard therapy (V_T: 10 to 12 mL/kg ideal body weight, 6 to 8 cm H_2O PEEP, no recruitment maneuvers) reduced a composite of major pulmonary and extrapulmonary complications (RR, 0.40; 95% confidence interval [CI], 0.24 to 0.68; $p = 0.001$). Despite the acceptance of protective ventilation strategies in a broader population group, there are still selected cohorts of patients that receive nonprotective ventilation. Using data from the Multicenter Perioperative Outcomes Group database in 330,823 patients undergoing intraoperative mechanical ventilation, Bender et al. (66) reported that females, obese patients and those of short stature still have a high incidence of large tidal volume ventilation (>V_T: 10 mL/kg ideal body weight). These data suggest that all intermediate- and high-risk patients presenting for surgery be managed with lung protective ventilation with careful consideration of the short, obese and female patient sub-population.

NEUROLOGIC SYSTEM

The incidence of perioperative stroke in patients undergoing noncardiac and nonneurologic surgery is 0.1%, but the associated mortality may be as high as 24% (67). Furthermore stroke mortality during the perioperative period is higher than stroke mortality in the community. Previous data on the incidence of perioperative stroke traditionally reported only clinically overt stroke. However, more sensitive tests, such as diffusion-weight MRI (DW-MRI), can detect a much higher incidence of *covert* stroke, which is reported to be as high as 10%. Covert stroke can impair quality of recovery and long-term cognitive function (68,69).

The risk factors associated with perioperative stroke vary based on the type of surgical procedure—cardiac versus noncardiac—and preoperative medical comorbidities. The surgical procedure associated with the highest risk of perioperative neurologic injury is cardiac surgery. Contemporary prospective studies report a 3% incidence of stroke in CABG procedures, 8% in isolated valve surgery, and 11% in combined CABG valve surgery. Advanced age and female gender are additional risk factors for perioperative neurologic injury (70). One of the most important factors for cerebral injury during cardiac surgery is macroembolization of atheromatous debris during aortic manipulation. Every attempt should be made to identify the high-risk patient with a large atheromatous burden by using preoperative CT imaging and epiaortic echocardiography to guide placement of the aortic cannula (71).

Nonsurgical factors associated with perioperative stroke includes a history of previous stroke/TIA, atrial fibrillation, renal disease, history of dialysis, age 62 years or older, female gender, cardiac valvular disease, smoking, COPD, and an elevated body mass index. Based on several well-conducted studies, carotid stenosis does not increase the risk of perioperative stroke (72,73); however the evaluation of the patient with carotid stenosis requires a thorough assessment of the cardiovascular system. Patients with carotid artery stenosis are at an increased risk of CAD. Severe correctable CAD is evident in approximately 26% of patients with cerebrovascular disease, whereas only 9% of patients have normal coronary anatomy (74). Despite the increased incidence of CAD in patients with carotid stenosis, the rate of medical complications in patients undergoing carotid endarterectomy (CEA) is low. Paciaroni et al. (75) reported that medical complications occurred in less than 10% of patients who underwent CEA, and only 0.4% had severe complications. Furthermore perioperative nonfatal and fatal MI occurred in only 1% of the patients and was associated with a mortality rate of approximately 0.2%. For a more detailed discussion on the preoperative evaluation of the cardiac patient presenting for noncardiac surgery refer to the discussion above.

There is some evidence suggesting a possible association between perioperative β-blockade and stroke, as previously discussed in this chapter. In the POISE trial (21), the metoprolol arm had a higher incidence of stroke (41 [1.0%] vs. 19 [0.5%] patients; 2.17, 1.26–3.74; p = 0.0053) and mortality (129 [3.1%] vs. 97 [2.3%] patients; 1.33, 1.03–1.74; p = 0.0317) compared to the placebo arm. The association between β-blockade and stroke also appears to be dependent on the type of β-blocker, with atenolol and metoprolol having a higher incidence of stroke compared to bisoprolol (76,77). With the extensive use of β-blockade in the perioperative period, the risk of stroke must be carefully evaluated based on the other pre-existing risk factors.

Timing of surgery after a recent stroke requires an evaluation of risk based on the urgency of the procedure and the risk of recurrent stroke. Acute stroke impairs autoregulation and cerebral blood flow becomes pressure passive. The restitution of autoregulation is thought to occur at 1 to 3 months and, ideally, elective surgery should be delayed beyond this period. For a more detailed discussion on the perioperative care of patients at high risk for stroke during or after noncardiac, nonneurologic surgery the consensus statement published by the Society for Neuroscience in Anesthesiology and Critical Care is an excellent resource (78).

RENAL SYSTEM

Acute kidney injury (AKI) and chronic kidney disease (CKD) are important medical problems worldwide. Although the incidence of AKI in hospitalized patients ranges from 3.2% to 20%, patients admitted to an ICU have much higher rates, with estimates between 22% and 67% (79). In the United States, the prevalence of CKD has been increasing; in 1988 to 1994, 10.0% of patients had CKD, whereas in 1999 to 2004, this rose to 13.1% (80). This trend can be partially attributed to greater rates of hypertension, diabetes mellitus, and obesity. Consequently, the preoperative evaluation and management of the patient with renal disease is complicated by the coexistence of multiple medical and surgical problems. Therefore a stepwise logical approach to these patients is required to ensure that important data are not omitted.

Risk Evaluation and Stratification

Preoperative renal risk evaluation and stratification are based on the comorbid medical condition of the patient, pre-existing renal function, and the procedure-specific renal risk (Fig. 53.1).

Comorbidity

Comorbid conditions that increase the risk of chronic renal insufficiency include a spectrum of cardiovascular, endocrine, hepatic, autoimmune, and congenital disorders. The severity, duration, and appropriate management of the conditions determine the degree of renal dysfunction a patient will develop. Diabetes mellitus (DM) and hypertension are the leading causes of end-stage renal disease (ESRD) (81), with glomerulonephritis and polycystic kidney disease being other major diagnoses. DM affects the kidney by several mechanisms resulting in albuminuria, the nephrotic syndrome, and progressive renal failure. Therapeutic measures shown to slow

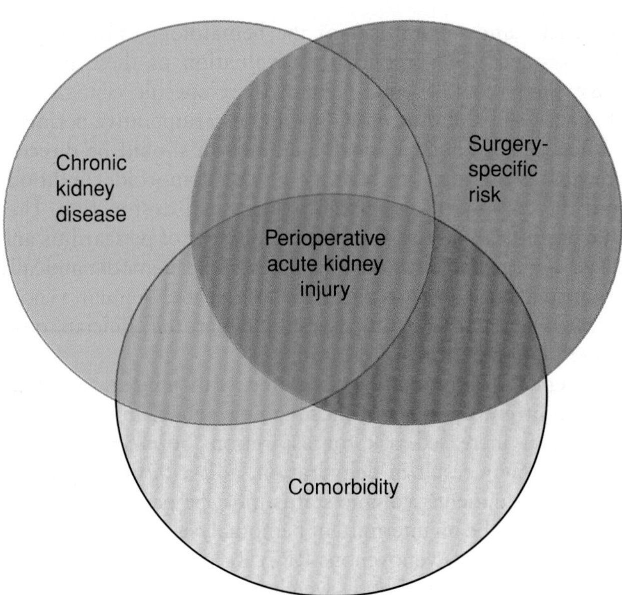

FIGURE 53.1 Triad of factors that collectively increases the risk of perioperative acute kidney injury.

this progression include adequate glycemic control, avoidance of smoking, and treatment of hypertension (82).

Hypertension is both a cause and a consequence of CKD; suboptimal blood pressure control worsens CKD, while the progression of CKD leads to hypertension that is increasingly resistant to therapeutic interventions. The recent 2012 Kidney Disease: Improving Global Outcomes (KDIGO) guideline for the evaluation and management of CKD recommends lowering blood pressure to at least 140/90 mm Hg for patients without albuminuria or 130/80 mm Hg for patients with albuminuria, regardless of the presence of DM (83). Moreover, alteration of the renin-angiotensin-aldosterone system by the introduction of an angiotensin receptor blocker (ARB) or angiotensin-converting enzyme inhibitor (ACE-I) reduces albuminuria and is recommended for patients with albuminuria above 300 mg/24 hours.

Although ESRD is a highly morbid condition, patients with CKD have a greater likelihood of a cardiovascular event, such as an acute myocardial infarction, than progression to ESRD (83). CAD is common in patients with DM and may be asymptomatic due to an associated autonomic neuropathy. A high index of suspicion for untreated CAD should be maintained for patients with diabetic nephropathy. Danaei et al. (84) reported that 21% of deaths from ischemic heart disease and 13% from stroke worldwide are attributable to higher-than-optimum blood glucose concentrations. Therefore, the preoperative workup of the patient with renal dysfunction should be done within the framework of the ACC/AHA algorithm (4) discussed previously. Once comorbid conditions and their related complications are identified, an attempt must be made to quantify the degree of renal dysfunction.

Pre-Existing Renal Dysfunction

The aforementioned KDIGO guideline defines CKD broadly as "abnormalities of kidney structure or function, present for longer than 3 months, with implications for health" (79). The severity of dysfunction can be assessed by quantifying the level of albuminuria and the glomerular filtration rate (GFR). In particular, a cutoff GFR of 60 mL/min has been established, as complications of CKD tend to increase below this value (83). The GFR can be estimated using either mathematical models, or by determining the clearance of inulin or other filtration markers. Historically, either the Cockroft–Gault equation or the formula derived from the Modification of Diet in Renal Disease (MDRD) Study have been used to estimate GFR (85). A more recently developed equation from the Chronic Kidney Disease Epidemiology Collaboration (CKD-EPI) investigators has demonstrated less bias and greater accuracy than the MDRD Study equation (86,87) and is recommended in the KDIGO guideline. These estimates of GFR are based primarily on serum creatinine, however, which limits their utility due to various extra-renal influences on serum creatinine. To address this, the CKD-EPI investigators have incorporated cystatin C, a ubiquitous protein eliminated by glomerular filtration and whose serum level is less dependent on extra-renal factors, into newer equations (88,89). The National Kidney Foundation supports an online calculator for GFR estimation (90). Importantly, assessment of GFR in the perioperative setting is challenging, as significant and rapid changes in GFR will not be reflected immediately by the serum creatinine. Thus, use of the above equations should be limited to situations where steady state has been established.

The presence of pre-existing renal dysfunction has a significant impact on perioperative morbidity and mortality. Mathew et al. (91) performed a systematic review and meta-analysis of 31 studies to assess whether CKD predicts mortality and cardiovascular morbidity in noncardiac surgery; the investigation included a large proportion of studies of vascular procedures. The pooled unadjusted odds ratio of 30-day mortality for patients with CKD compared to those with normal renal function was 2.8. When adjusted for potential confounding factors such as DM, CAD, and HF, the odds ratios remained elevated at over 1.4, though the results were not pooled due to heterogeneity. Cardiovascular events including myocardial infarction, HF, and cardiac arrest were also increased in patients with CKD.

Likewise, Mooney et al. (89) undertook a systematic review and meta-analysis but also included studies of cardiac surgery. The vast majority of studies estimated GFR using either the Cockroft–Gault or MDRD Study equations. At an estimated GFR of less than 60 mL/min/1.73 m^2, patients had an increased risk of postoperative 30-day and long-term mortality, with multivariable adjusted RR of 2.98 and 1.61, respectively. A graded association was discovered between decreasing estimated GFR and increasing odds for 30-day mortality. Recognizing the association between CKD and perioperative mortality and morbidity, various surgical risk prediction scores, including the NSQIP MICA (10), STS risk models (23,26), and EuroSCORE II (25) incorporate an assessment of renal function.

Procedure-Related Risk

Procedure-related renal risk is an important determinant of perioperative renal injury, though risk assessment has been difficult owing to a wide range of definitions for AKI across studies. Cardiac and major vascular procedures are associated with a high risk of AKI, while for patients undergoing noncardiovascular surgery it is much lower. The incidence of AKI following cardiac surgery has been estimated at up to 30%, with approximately 1% of patients requiring renal replacement therapy (RRT) (92,93). The development of AKI is associated with increased mortality and perioperative complications; even relatively small postoperative reductions in estimated GFR (i.e., >25%) confer a fourfold greater risk of death (94).

CPB has several negative effects on renal function, though the exact mechanism of injury has yet to be elucidated (95). Nonpulsatile flow, inadequate renal perfusion pressure, and the induction of an inflammatory response all contribute to renal dysfunction. In a meta-analysis of randomized and observational studies, Nigwekar et al. (96) reported a lower risk of AKI with off-pump CABG compared with on-pump surgery. Although in the observational studies there was a reduced requirement for RRT following off-pump surgery, the randomized trials showed no difference. Furthermore, Chawla et al. (92) reviewed the STS database from 2004 to 2009 and found, in patients with CKD, improved in-hospital mortality and decreased need for RRT with off-pump CABG. This benefit was most pronounced in patients with the lowest baseline estimated GFR. Although off-pump approaches certainly are not feasible for many cardiac operations, this data highlights the positive influence that modification of a surgical technique can have on organ protection.

In open vascular surgery, the location of the arterial reconstruction, the duration of the aortic cross-clamp, and the emergent nature of the procedure are all strong predictors of postoperative renal complications. In a retrospective study of 101 patients who underwent thoracoabdominal aortic aneurysm (AAA) repair, nearly 28% developed postoperative renal dysfunction (97). The rate of renal insufficiency for infrarenal abdominal aortic reconstruction tends to be much lower, and was reported to be 1.7% in one single-center study (98). Unfortunately, the definitions for renal dysfunction in these studies specified high thresholds for postoperative change in serum creatinine, so the true incidence of AKI may be higher using modern definitions. The hypothesized mechanisms of postoperative renal injury are ischemia-reperfusion of the kidneys, atheroembolic injury, intravenous contrast-induced nephropathy, and inflammatory damage.

Measures aimed at modifying surgical technique to reduce the incidence of postoperative renal dysfunction in aortic surgery have been met with mixed success. The most significant advance has been the widespread adoption of endovascular techniques for aortic aneurysm repair. Small studies have suggested that the reduced aortic manipulation and renal ischemia that accompany the endovascular technique are associated with reduced inflammation and postoperative renal injury (99,100). A large retrospective cohort study of 6,614 patients with unruptured AAA discovered lower odds (adjusted odds ratio, 0.42) of acute renal failure associated with endovascular aneurysm repair (EVAR) compared to open repair; however, acute renal failure was identified by diagnostic codes rather than conventional biochemical data (101). Conversely, a cohort study based on NSQIP data (102) and the Dutch Randomized Endovascular Aneurysm Management trial (103) showed no significant differences in renal outcomes between EVAR and open repair; further research will be required to establish whether endovascular techniques are truly renoprotective.

Preoperative Evaluation

AKI and CKD are characterized by retention of nitrogenous waste products, fluid and electrolyte abnormalities, acid–base disorders, and impairment of the hematologic and coagulation systems. The preoperative evaluation of these patients must therefore take into account these specific changes and the increased risk they pose during the perioperative period.

The history and physical examination should be directed toward evaluating the severity of the comorbid conditions and the complications related to the renal dysfunction. Uremic patients are at risk for the development of pericarditis and large pericardial effusions, which can be hemodynamically compromising. The presence of an elevated jugular venous pressure and pulsus paradoxus should alert the clinician to the presence of a pericardial effusion.

Uremia is additionally associated with nausea, vomiting, and recurrent episodes of hiccoughing, which may place the patient at increased risk for aspiration. Severe nausea and vomiting may result in dehydration, and a thorough evaluation of the patient's volume status must be performed. These patients may be on intermittent hemodialysis, peritoneal dialysis, or continuous venovenous RRT. Records of the last dialysis, fluid balance, and body weight must be obtained to help with the assessment of the fluid status.

Anemia in renal failure is multifactorial in nature; bleeding from platelet dysfunction, malnutrition, and decreased erythropoietin production all contribute toward the low red cell mass. Electrolyte abnormalities are common in renal failure; hyperkalemia, hyperphosphatemia, and hypocalcemia are the typical electrolyte profiles seen in renal failure. Inadequately treated hyperkalemia confers the risk of developing malignant cardiac dysrhythmias.

Diagnostic Testing

The diagnostic studies in patients with renal dysfunction are determined by the findings on the history and physical examination. Complete blood count helps to assess the severity of the anemia, morphology of the red blood cells, and the platelet count. Although uremic patients may have normal platelet numbers, they develop an acquired platelet dysfunction that results in an increased risk of bleeding. The pathogenesis of this hemostatic dysfunction is multifactorial and includes the effects of circulating toxins, alteration of the vessel wall, and anemia. To assess the degree of platelet function, a platelet function assay can be performed.

The basic metabolic panel helps to determine the electrolyte profile and allows the anion gap to be calculated. AKI and CKD are commonly characterized by an increased anion gap metabolic acidosis. The BUN can be tracked to assess the efficacy of RRT. Due to the limitations of common parameters such as BUN, serum creatinine, and urine output in diagnosing AKI, significant effort has recently been made in the investigation of various novel biomarkers for detecting kidney damage and predicting AKI. Several molecules have been assessed including interleukin-18, kidney injury molecule-1, liver fatty acid-binding protein, neutrophil gelatinase-associated lipocalin, tissue inhibitor of metalloproteinases-2, and insulin-like growth factor–binding protein 7 (104,105). At present, these are not widely used in the preoperative evaluation of patients but will likely have significant utility in the future.

An electrocardiogram (ECG) should be performed to determine whether ischemia, ventricular hypertrophy, or strain pattern is present. Hyperkalemia is characterized by tall peaked T waves, widened QRS complex, and shortened QT interval.

The ECG of patients with pericardial effusion may demonstrate small QRS complexes and the presence of electrical alternans—change in QRS amplitude with each heartbeat. A chest radiograph may reveal signs of pulmonary edema, cardiomegaly, or a large pericardial effusion.

In conclusion, available data convincingly demonstrate that patients with CKD or who develop AKI have worse outcomes than those with normal renal function. Unfortunately, none of the pharmacologic strategies proposed to protect the kidneys in the perioperative period have shown clear benefit (106). Thus, it is important to identify patients at risk for worsening renal function to be able to appropriately counsel those patients and anticipate complications. With definitions for AKI becoming more standardized, such as the AKI Network and KDIGO (107) definitions, future research should be able to provide more robust findings.

SUMMARY

High-risk surgical patients present a unique challenge to the perioperative physician. Because of their multiple comorbidities and the increasing complexity of surgery being performed, their perioperative risk is disproportionately higher than the general surgical population. To appropriately manage these patients, risk factors must be identified and stratified following completion of the clinical, laboratory, and special investigations. Risk-modification strategies may be implemented preoperatively if they are likely to have a beneficial effect during the operative course. Otherwise, they can be initiated postoperatively as part of the long-term care plan for the patient.

Key Points

- Assessment of the high-risk patient begins with preoperative identification, stratification, and modification of risk factors.
- No preoperative test should be performed unless it is likely to influence patient treatment.
- In noncardiac surgery, the ACC/AHA algorithm provides a structured and cost-effective evaluation strategy.
- Scoring systems in cardiac surgery assist with risk profiling, predicting mortality, and resource use.
- Systematic reviews have now defined patient and surgery-specific risk for PPC.
- It is important to assess and treat reversible airway obstruction in chronic obstructive airway disease.
- Patients with CKD are at elevated risk for perioperative morbidity and mortality irrespective of coexisting medical problems.
- The risk of AKI in patients with chronic renal insufficiency is determined by comorbidities, baseline renal function, and procedure-specific risk.
- Effective interventions to prevent AKI in patients at risk have proven elusive. Strategies should be aimed at optimizing renal perfusion and managing the metabolic and hematologic derangements in patients with CKD.
- The prevention of secondary neuronal injury must be the focus of perioperative intervention.

References

1. Bilimoria KY, Liu Y, Paruch JL, et al. Development and evaluation of the universal ACS NSQIP surgical risk calculator: a decision aid and informed consent tool for patients and surgeons. *J Am Coll Surg.* 2013;217:833–842.
2. *ACS NSQIP surgical risk calculator.* Available at http://riskcalculator.facs.org/ Accessed March 2, 2012.
3. Mangano DT, Browner WS, Hollenberg M, et al. Association of perioperative myocardial ischemia with cardiac morbidity and mortality in men undergoing noncardiac surgery. The Study of Perioperative Ischemia Research Group. *N Engl J Med.* 1990;323:1781–1788.
4. Fleisher LA, Fleischmann KE, Auerbach AD, et al. 2014 ACC/AHA guideline on perioperative cardiovascular evaluation and management of patients undergoing noncardiac surgery: a report of the American College of Cardiology/American Heart Association Task Force on practice guidelines. *J Am Coll Cardiol.* 2014;64:e77–e137.
5. Fleisher LA, Fleischmann KE, Auerbach AD, et al. 2014 ACC/AHA Guideline on Perioperative Cardiovascular Evaluation and Management of Patients Undergoing Noncardiac Surgery. A report of the American College of Cardiology/American Heart Association Task Force on Practice Guidelines. Available at http://circ.ahajournals.org/content/130/24/e278.figures-only. Accessed February 1, 2016.
6. O'Gara PT, Kushner FG, Ascheim DD, et al. 2013 ACCF/AHA guideline for the management of ST-elevation myocardial infarction: a report of the American College of Cardiology Foundation/American Heart Association Task Force on Practice Guidelines. *J Am Coll Cardiol.* 2013;61:e78–e140.
7. Jneid H, Anderson JL, Wright RS, et al. 2012 ACCF/AHA focused update of the guideline for the management of patients with unstable angina/non-ST-elevation myocardial infarction (updating the 2007 guideline and replacing the 2011 focused update): a report of the American College of Cardiology Foundation/American Heart Association Task Force on Practice Guidelines. *J Am Coll Cardiol.* 2012;60:645–681.
8. Goldman L, Caldera DL, Southwick FS, et al. Cardiac risk factors and complications in non-cardiac surgery. *Medicine (Baltimore).* 1978;57:357–370.
9. Lee TH, Marcantonio ER, Mangione CM, et al. Derivation and prospective validation of a simple index for prediction of cardiac risk of major noncardiac surgery. *Circulation.* 1999;100:1043–1049.
10. Gupta H, Gupta PK, Fang X, et al. Development and validation of a risk calculator predicting postoperative respiratory failure. *Chest.* 2011;140:1207–1215.
11. Tsiouris A, Horst HM, Paone G, et al. Preoperative risk stratification for thoracic surgery using the American College of Surgeons National Surgical Quality Improvement Program data set: functional status predicts morbidity and mortality. *J Surg Res.* 2012;177:1–6.
12. Levine GN, Bates ER, Blankenship JC, et al. 2011 ACCF/AHA/SCAI Guideline for Percutaneous Coronary Intervention: a report of the American College of Cardiology Foundation/American Heart Association Task Force on Practice Guidelines and the Society for Cardiovascular Angiography and Interventions. *J Am Coll Cardiol.* 2011;58:e44–e122.
13. Hillis LD, Smith PK, Anderson JL, et al. 2011 ACCF/AHA Guideline for Coronary Artery Bypass Graft Surgery: a report of the American College of Cardiology Foundation/American Heart Association Task Force on Practice Guidelines. Developed in collaboration with the American Association for Thoracic Surgery, Society of Cardiovascular Anesthesiologists, and Society of Thoracic Surgeons. *J Am Coll Cardiol.* 2011;58:e123–e210.
14. McFalls EO, Ward HB, Moritz TE, et al. Coronary-artery revascularization before elective major vascular surgery. *N Engl J Med.* 2004;351:2795–2804.
15. Kaluza GL, Joseph J, Lee JR, et al. Catastrophic outcomes of noncardiac surgery soon after coronary stenting. *J Am Coll Cardiol.* 2000;35:1288–1294.
16. Wilson SH, Fasseas P, Orford JL, et al. Clinical outcome of patients undergoing non-cardiac surgery in the two months following coronary stenting. *J Am Coll Cardiol.* 2003;42:234–240.
17. Hawn MT, Graham LA, Richman JS, et al. Risk of major adverse cardiac events following noncardiac surgery in patients with coronary stents. *JAMA.* 2013;310:1462–1472.
18. Wijeysundera DN, Wijeysundera HC, Yun L, et al. Risk of elective major noncardiac surgery after coronary stent insertion: a population-based study. *Circulation.* 2012;126:1355–1362.
19. Priebe HJ. Perioperative myocardial infarction: aetiology and prevention. *Br J Anaesth.* 2005;95:3–19.
20. Poldermans D, Boersma E, Bax JJ, et al. The effect of bisoprolol on perioperative mortality and myocardial infarction in high-risk patients undergoing vascular surgery. Dutch Echocardiographic Cardiac Risk

Evaluation Applying Stress Echocardiography Study Group. *N Engl J Med.* 1999;341:1789–1794.

21. POISE Study Group, Devereaux PJ, Yang H, et al. Effects of extended-release metoprolol succinate in patients undergoing non-cardiac surgery (POISE trial): a randomised controlled trial. *Lancet.* 2008;371:1839–1847.
22. Wijeysundera DN, Duncan D, Nkonde-Price C, et al. Perioperative beta blockade in noncardiac surgery: a systematic review for the 2014 ACC/AHA guideline on perioperative cardiovascular evaluation and management of patients undergoing noncardiac surgery: a report of the American College of Cardiology/American Heart Association Task Force on practice guidelines. *J Am Coll Cardiol.* 2014;64:2406–2425.
23. Shahian DM, O'Brien SM, Filardo G, et al; Society of Thoracic Surgeons Quality Measurement Task Force. The Society of Thoracic Surgeons 2008 cardiac surgery risk models: part 1—coronary artery bypass grafting surgery. *Ann Thorac Surg.* 2009;88(1 Suppl):S2–22.
24. Nashef SA, Roques F, Michel P, et al. European system for cardiac operative risk evaluation (EuroSCORE). *Eur J Cardio Thorac Surg.* 1999;16:9–13.
25. Nashef SA, Roques F, Sharples LD, et al. EuroSCORE II. *Eur J Cardiothorac Surg.* 2012;41:734–744; discussion 744–745.
26. O'Brien SM, Shahian DM, Filardo G, et al; Society of Thoracic Surgeons Quality Measurement Task Force. The Society of Thoracic Surgeons 2008 cardiac surgery risk models: part 2—solated valve surgery. *Ann Thorac Surg.* 2009;88(1 Suppl):S23–S42.
27. Parsonnet V, Dean D, Bernstein AD. A method of uniform stratification of risk for evaluating the results of surgery in acquired adult heart disease. *Circulation.* 1989;79:I3–12.
28. Roques F, Michel P, Goldstone AR, Nashef SA. The logistic EuroSCORE. *Eur Heart J.* 2003;24:881–882.
29. Bhatti F, Grayson AD, Grotte G, et al; North West Quality Improvement Programme in Cardiac Interventions. The logistic EuroSCORE in cardiac surgery: how well does it predict operative risk? *Heart.* 2006;92:1817–1820.
30. Bernstein AD, Parsonnet V. Bedside estimation of risk as an aid for decision-making in cardiac surgery. *Ann Thorac Surg.* 2000;69:823–828.
31. Biancari F, Kangasniemi OP, Luukkonen J, et al. EuroSCORE predicts immediate and late outcome after coronary artery bypass surgery. *Ann Thorac Surg.* 2006;82:57–61.
32. Nilsson J, Algotsson L, Hoglund P, et al. EuroSCORE predicts intensive care unit stay and costs of open heart surgery. *Ann Thorac Surg.* 2004;78:1528–1534.
33. *Euroscore II.* Available at http://euroscore.org/calc.html. Accessed February 1, 2016.
34. *STS Adult Cardiac Surgery Risk Calculator.* Available at http://riskcalc.sts.org/stswebriskcalc/#./ Accessed February 1, 2016.
35. Canet J, Gallart L, Gomar C, et al; ARISCAT Group. Prediction of postoperative pulmonary complications in a population-based surgical cohort. *Anesthesiology.* 2010;113:1338–1350.
36. Dimick JB, Chen SL, Taheri PA, et al. Hospital costs associated with surgical complications: a report from the private-sector National Surgical Quality Improvement Program. *J Am Coll Surg.* 2004;199:531–537.
37. Smetana GW, Lawrence VA, Cornell JE; American College of Physicians. Preoperative pulmonary risk stratification for noncardiothoracic surgery: systematic review for the American College of Physicians. *Ann Intern Med.* 2006;144:581–595.
38. Kozower BD, Sheng S, O'Brien SM, et al. STS database risk models: predictors of mortality and major morbidity for lung cancer resection. *Ann Thorac Surg.* 2010;90:875–881; discussion 881–883.
39. Arozullah AM, Daley J, Henderson WG, Khuri SF. Multifactorial risk index for predicting postoperative respiratory failure in men after major noncardiac surgery. The National Veterans Administration Surgical Quality Improvement Program. *Ann Surg.* 2000;232:242–253.
40. Arozullah AM, Khuri SF, Henderson WG, Daley J; Participants in the National Veterans Affairs Surgical Quality Improvement Program. Development and validation of a multifactorial risk index for predicting postoperative pneumonia after major noncardiac surgery. *Ann Intern Med.* 2001;135:847–857.
41. Gibbs J, Cull W, Henderson W, et al. Preoperative serum albumin level as a predictor of operative mortality and morbidity: results from the National VA Surgical Risk Study. *Arch Surg.* 1999;134:36–42.
42. Archer C, Levy AR, McGregor M. Value of routine preoperative chest x-rays: a meta-analysis. *Can J Anaesth.* 1993;40:1022–1027.
43. Mazzone PJ, Arroliga AC. Lung cancer: preoperative pulmonary evaluation of the lung resection candidate. *Am J Med.* 2005;118:578–583.
44. Slinger PD, Johnston MR. Preoperative assessment for pulmonary resection. *J Cardiothorac Vasc Anesth.* 2000;14:202–211.
45. Brunelli A, Kim AW, Berger KI, Addrizzo-Harris DJ. Physiologic evaluation of the patient with lung cancer being considered for resectional surgery: Diagnosis and management of lung cancer, 3rd ed. American College of Chest Physicians evidence-based clinical practice guidelines. *Chest.* 2013;143:e166S–e290S.
46. Chalon S, Moreno H Jr, Benowitz NL, et al. Nicotine impairs endothelium-dependent dilatation in human veins in vivo. *Clin Pharmacol Ther.* 2000;67:391–397.
47. Kroenke K, Lawrence VA, Theroux JF, et al. Postoperative complications after thoracic and major abdominal surgery in patients with and without obstructive lung disease. *Chest.* 1993;104:1445–1451.
48. Taylor A, DeBoard Z, Gauvin JM. Prevention of postoperative pulmonary complications. *Surg Clin North Am.* 2015;95:237–254.
49. Braunschweig CL, Levy P, Sheean PM, Wang X. Enteral compared with parenteral nutrition: a meta-analysis. *Am J Clin Nutr.* 2001;74:534–542.
50. Sacks GS, Genton L, Kudsk KA. Controversy of immunonutrition for surgical critical-illness patients. *Curr Opin Crit Care.* 2003;9:300–305.
51. Memtsoudis S, Liu SS, Ma Y, et al. Perioperative pulmonary outcomes in patients with sleep apnea after noncardiac surgery. *Anesth Analg.* 2011;112:113–121.
52. Warner DO, Warner MA, Barnes RD, et al. Perioperative respiratory complications in patients with asthma. *Anesthesiology.* 1996;85:460–467.
53. Warner DO, Warner MA, Offord KP, et al. Airway obstruction and perioperative complications in smokers undergoing abdominal surgery. *Anesthesiology.* 1999;90:372–379.
54. Milledge JS, Nunn JF. Criteria of fitness for anaesthesia in patients with chronic obstructive lung disease. *Br Med J.* 1975;3:670–673.
55. Groeben H, Schlicht M, Stieglitz S, et al. Both local anesthetics and salbutamol pretreatment affect reflex bronchoconstriction in volunteers with asthma undergoing awake fiberoptic intubation. *Anesthesiology.* 2002;97:1445–1450.
56. Maslow AD, Regan MM, Israel E, et al. Inhaled albuterol, but not intravenous lidocaine, protects against intubation-induced bronchoconstriction in asthma. *Anesthesiology.* 2000;93:1198–1204.
57. Silvanus MT, Groeben H, Peters J. Corticosteroids and inhaled salbutamol in patients with reversible airway obstruction markedly decrease the incidence of bronchospasm after tracheal intubation. *Anesthesiology.* 2004;100:1052–1057.
58. Barnes PJ. Mechanisms of action of glucocorticoids in asthma. *Am J Resp Crit Care Med.* 1996;154:S21–S26; discussion S26–S27.
59. Sauder RA, Lenox WC, Tobias JD, Hirshman CA. Methylprednisolone increases sensitivity to beta-adrenergic agonists within 48 hours in Basenji greyhounds. *Anesthesiology.* 1993;79:1278–1283.
60. Pien LC, Grammer LC, Patterson R. Minimal complications in a surgical population with severe asthma receiving prophylactic corticosteroids. *J Allergy Clin Immunol.* 1988;82:696–700.
61. Parameswaran K, Belda J, Rowe BH. Addition of intravenous aminophylline to beta2-agonists in adults with acute asthma. *Cochrane Database System Rev.* 2000:CD002742.
62. Tait AR, Malviya S. Anesthesia for the child with an upper respiratory tract infection: still a dilemma? *Anesth Analg.* 2005;100:59–65.
63. Ventilation with lower tidal volumes as compared with traditional tidal volumes for acute lung injury and the acute respiratory distress syndrome. The Acute Respiratory Distress Syndrome Network. *N Engl J Med.* 2000;342:1301–1308.
64. Severgnini P, Selmo G, Lanza C, et al. Protective mechanical ventilation during general anesthesia for open abdominal surgery improves postoperative pulmonary function. *Anesthesiology.* 2013;118:1307–1321.
65. Futier E, Constantin JM, Paugam-Burtz C, et al; IMPROVE Study Group. A trial of intraoperative low-tidal-volume ventilation in abdominal surgery. *N Engl J Med.* 2013;369:428–437.
66. Bender SP, Paganelli WC, Gerety LP, et al. Intraoperative lung-protective ventilation trends and practice patterns: a report from the Multicenter Perioperative Outcomes Group. *Anesth Analg.* 2015;121:1231–1239.
67. Mashour GA, Shanks AM, Kheterpal S. Perioperative stroke and associated mortality after noncardiac, nonneurologic surgery. *Anesthesiology.* 2011;114:1289–1296.
68. Mashour GA, Woodrum DT, Avidan MS. Neurological complications of surgery and anaesthesia. *Br J Anaesth.* 2015;114:194–203.
69. Ng JL, Chan MT, Gelb AW. Perioperative stroke in noncardiac, nonneurosurgical surgery. *Anesthesiology.* 2011;115:879–890.
70. Taggart DP, Westaby S. Neurological and cognitive disorders after coronary artery bypass grafting. *Curr Opin Cardiol.* 2001;16:271–276.
71. Djaiani GN. Aortic arch atheroma: stroke reduction in cardiac surgical patients. *Semin Cardiothorac Vasc Anesth.* 2006;10:143–157.

72. Evans BA, Wijdicks EF. High-grade carotid stenosis detected before general surgery: is endarterectomy indicated? *Neurology.* 2001;57: 1328–1330.
73. Sonny A, Gornik HL, Yang D, et al. Lack of association between carotid artery stenosis and stroke or myocardial injury after noncardiac surgery in high-risk patients. *Anesthesiology.* 2014;121:922–929.
74. Hertzer NR, Beven EG, Young JR, et al. Coronary artery disease in peripheral vascular patients: a classification of 1000 coronary angiograms and results of surgical management. *Ann Surg.* 1984;199:223–233.
75. Paciaroni M, Eliasziw M, Kappelle LJ, et al. Medical complications associated with carotid endarterectomy. North American Symptomatic Carotid Endarterectomy Trial (NASCET). *Stroke.* 1999;30:1759–1763.
76. Ashes C, Judelman S, Wijeysundera DN, et al. Selective beta1-antagonism with bisoprolol is associated with fewer postoperative strokes than atenolol or metoprolol: a single-center cohort study of 44,092 consecutive patients. *Anesthesiology.* 2013;119:777–787.
77. Mashour GA, Sharifpour M, Freundlich RE, et al. Perioperative metoprolol and risk of stroke after noncardiac surgery. *Anesthesiology.* 2013; 119: 1340–1346.
78. Mashour GA, Moore LE, Lele AV, et al. Perioperative care of patients at high risk for stroke during or after non-cardiac, non-neurologic surgery: consensus statement from the Society for Neuroscience in Anesthesiology and Critical Care. *J Neurosurg Anesthesiol.* 2014;26:273–285.
79. Murugan R, Kellum JA. Acute kidney injury: what's the prognosis? *Nature Rev Nephrol.* 2011;7:209–217.
80. Coresh J, Selvin E, Stevens LA, et al. Prevalence of chronic kidney disease in the United States. *JAMA.* 2007;298:2038–2047.
81. Kiefer MM, Ryan MJ. Primary care of the patient with chronic kidney disease. *Med Clin North Am.* 2015;99:935–952.
82. Ritz E, Orth SR. Nephropathy in patients with type 2 diabetes mellitus. *N Engl J Med.* 1999;341:1127–1133.
83. Stevens PE, Levin A; Kidney Disease: Improving Global Outcomes Chronic Kidney Disease Guideline Development Work Group Members. Evaluation and management of chronic kidney disease: synopsis of the kidney disease: improving global outcomes 2012 clinical practice guideline. *Ann Intern Med.* 2013;158:825–830.
84. Danaei G, Lawes CM, Vander Hoorn S, et al. Global and regional mortality from ischaemic heart disease and stroke attributable to higher-than-optimum blood glucose concentration: comparative risk assessment. *Lancet.* 2006;368:1651–1659.
85. Levey AS, Bosch JP, Lewis JB, et al. . A more accurate method to estimate glomerular filtration rate from serum creatinine: a new prediction equation. Modification of Diet in Renal Disease Study Group. *Ann Intern Med.* 1999;130:461–470.
86. Earley A, Miskulin D, Lamb EJ, et al. Estimating equations for glomerular filtration rate in the era of creatinine standardization: a systematic review. *Ann Intern Med.* 2012;156:785–795.
87. Levey AS, Stevens LA, Schmid CH, et al; CKD-EPI (Chronic Kidney Disease Epidemiology Collaboration). A new equation to estimate glomerular filtration rate. *Ann Intern Med.* 2009;150:604–612.
88. Inker LA, Schmid CH, Tighiouart H, et al; CKD-EPI Investigators. Estimating glomerular filtration rate from serum creatinine and cystatin C. *N Engl J Med.* 2012;367:20–29.
89. Mooney JF, Ranasinghe I, Chow CK, et al. Preoperative estimates of glomerular filtration rate as predictors of outcome after surgery: a systematic review and meta-analysis. *Anesthesiology.* 2013;118:809–824.
90. *National Kidney Foundation. GFR calculator.* Available at https://www.kidney.org/professionals/KDOQI/gfr_calculator. Accessed February 1, 2016.
91. Mathew A, Devereaux PJ, O'Hare A, et al. Chronic kidney disease and postoperative mortality: a systematic review and meta-analysis. *Kidney Int.* 2008;73:1069–1081.
92. Chawla LS, Zhao Y, Lough FC, et al. Off-pump versus on-pump coronary artery bypass grafting outcomes stratified by preoperative renal function. *J Am Soc Nephrol.* 2012;23:1389–1397.
93. Rosner MH, Okusa MD. Acute kidney injury associated with cardiac surgery. *Clin J Am Soc Nephrol.* 2006;1:19–32.
94. Karkouti K, Wijeysundera DN, Yau TM, et al. Acute kidney injury after cardiac surgery: focus on modifiable risk factors. *Circulation.* 2009; 119: 495–502.
95. Thakar CV. Perioperative acute kidney injury. *Adv Chron Kidney Dis.* 2013;20:67–75.
96. Nigwekar SU, Kandula P, Hix JK, Thakar CV. Off-pump coronary artery bypass surgery and acute kidney injury: a meta-analysis of randomized and observational studies. *Am J Kidney Dis.* 2009;54:413–423.
97. Rectenwald JE, Huber TS, Martin TD, et al. Functional outcome after thoracoabdominal aortic aneurysm repair. *J Vasc Surg.* 2002;35:640–647.
98. Hertzer NR, Mascha EJ, Karafa MT, et al. Open infrarenal abdominal aortic aneurysm repair: the Cleveland Clinic experience from 1989 to 1998. *J Vasc Surg.* 2002;35:1145–1154.
99. Sweeney KJ, Evoy D, Sultan S, et al. Endovascular approach to abdominal aortic aneurysms limits the postoperative systemic immune response. *Eur J Vasc Endovasc Surg.* 2002;23:303–308.
100. Wijnen MH, Cuypers P, Buth J, et al. Differences in renal response between endovascular and open repair of abdominal aortic aneurysms. *Eur J Vasc Endovasc Surg.* 2001;21:171–174.
101. Wald R, Waikar SS, Liangos O, et al. Acute renal failure after endovascular vs open repair of abdominal aortic aneurysm. *J Vasc Surg.* 2006; 43:460–466.
102. Hua HT, Cambria RP, Chuang SK, et al. Early outcomes of endovascular versus open abdominal aortic aneurysm repair in the National Surgical Quality Improvement Program-Private Sector (NSQIP-PS). *J Vasc Endovasc Surg.* 2005;41:382–389.
103. Prinssen M, Verhoeven EL, Buth J, et al; Dutch Randomized Endovascular Aneurysm Management (DREAM)Trial Group. A randomized trial comparing conventional and endovascular repair of abdominal aortic aneurysms. *N Engl J Med.* 2004;351:1607–1618.
104. Kellum JA. Diagnostic criteria for acute kidney injury: present and future. *Crit Care Clin.* 2015;31:621–632.
105. Mooney JF, Chow CK, Hillis GS. Perioperative renal function and surgical outcome. *Curr Opin Anaesthesiol.* 2014;27:195–200.
106. Zacharias M, Mugawar M, Herbison GP, et al. Interventions for protecting renal function in the perioperative period. *Cochrane Database System Rev.* 2013;9:CD003590.
107. Khwaja A. KDIGO clinical practice guidelines for acute kidney injury. *Nephron Clin Pract.* 2012;120:c179–c184.

CHAPTER

54

Anesthesia: Physiology and Postanesthesia Problems

SRIKANTH HOSUR and A. JOSEPH LAYON

INTRODUCTION

Modern anesthesia is a complex art and science that involves use of various drugs and procedures in a controlled but safe environment. The overall risk of death from anesthesia is between 1 in 112,000 and 1 in 450,000 (1). Studies show that the most common adverse events are due to respiratory problems, followed by neural injury and damage due to regional anesthesia (2). Over the past years, there is an increase in problems related to cardiovascular issues with a decrease in respiratory events (3). Patients with anesthetic complications may require treatment in the intensive care unit (ICU).

UPTAKE AND DISTRIBUTION OF INHALATIONAL AGENTS

The goal of inhalational anesthesia is to develop a critical partial pressure of the agent within the brain through discrete mechanisms (6) (Table 54.1). The anesthesia system is designed to deliver the anesthetic agent with air, oxygen, nitrous oxide, or a combination achieving a predictable concentration, eliminate carbon dioxide, maintain a predictable FiO_2, while allow monitoring and control of ventilation.

Delivery

Brain tissue partial pressure correlates closely with the end-tidal partial pressure.

Concentration Effect

The inspired concentration directly increases the anesthetic agent concentration in the lung (*concentration effect*). As a rule, a higher initial inspired concentration of the agent results in a higher alveolar level in spite of uptake from the lung.

Second Gas Effect

When a second anesthetic agent is administered, its partial pressure increases more rapidly than when it is administered alone, because it is drawn into the lungs with the first agent.

Alveolar Ventilation

A greater alveolar ventilation ($\dot{V}_A$) increases the rate at which the alveolar partial pressure approaches the inspired partial pressure. It is limited only by lung volume, thus, a larger functional residual capacity (FRC) decreases the "wash-in" rate of the agent.

Uptake from the Lungs

Solubility

The more soluble an inhaled agent is in blood, the more it is dissolved in the pulmonary blood and the longer it takes to reach a necessary partial pressure of agent in the lungs and brain. This is how inhaled agents differ from other commonly used drugs. For example, ampicillin given intravenously is dissolved in blood, carried to the site of infection, and produces the desired pharmacologic effect as its concentration in the blood increases. However the greater the amount of an inhaled agent dissolved in the blood and hence taken away from the alveoli—the longer it takes to develop the necessary alveolar concentration which in turn reflects brain concentration and longer it takes for anesthesia to take effect.

Agents such as nitrous oxide (blood/gas partition coefficient of 0.47), are relatively insoluble, and achieve alveolar partial pressure rapidly compared with that of halothane (blood/gas partition coefficient of 2.36). The speed of induction of a soluble agent can be increased by increasing the inspired fraction to a level well in excess of that required for maintenance of anesthesia (6).

Cardiac Output

High cardiac output increases uptake, decreasing the alveolar partial pressure. It is greater with more soluble inhalational anesthetics resulting in a longer induction time as in thyrotoxicosis. Low cardiac output states result in a rapid induction and possible overdose.

Alveolar–Mixed Venous Anesthetic Partial Pressure Gradient

The alveolar-to-central mixed venous anesthetic partial pressure gradient relates the size of the anesthetic "sink" to the increase or decrease in uptake from the lungs. At the beginning of induction the venous anesthetic partial pressure is much lower than that in the arterial blood, leading to a large uptake of the anesthetic as the venous blood passes through the lungs. However, as the tissue sinks become filled, the alveolar-to-venous anesthetic partial pressure difference decreases, and this effect is minimized. Thus once anesthesia is achieved it is easier to maintain it.

Distribution

Tissue Solubility and Blood Flow

The tissue distribution (delivery) of the anesthetic is dependent on solubility in the tissue and the blood flow to that tissue (Table 54.1). The greater the solubility, the larger the capacity of that tissue for the agent. If the tissue has a large capacity but low blood flow, equilibration takes a long time; for example, fat and a highly fat-soluble agent such as halothane in an

TABLE 54.1 Factors Governing Uptake and Distribution of Inhaled Agents

Delivery
Inspired concentration
Concentration effect
Second gas effect
Ventilation
Uptake from lungs
Solubility
Cardiac output
Alveolar–mixed venous partial pressure gradient
Distribution to tissues
Solubility of agent in tissue
Blood flow to tissue

obese patient, can accumulate but is released after discontinuation of the agent thereby prolonging emergence. If the tissue has a small capacity and large blood flow, equilibration and hence anesthetic induction is rapid (e.g., brain). An intermediate group includes muscle and skin.

Nitrous oxide equilibration with the vessel-rich group occurs within 5 to 15 minutes from the beginning of induction. The muscle group equilibrates within approximately 1 hour, and the vessel-poor group and fat group equilibrate within 2 to 3 hours.

Factors that govern the elimination of the agent from the body are the same as those that govern the uptake and distribution at the beginning. Hypoventilation, increased cardiac output, highly soluble agents, increased alveolar-to-venous anesthetic concentration gradient, all lengthens the period of emergence.

Diffusion Hypoxia

At the end of an anesthetic, large quantities of nitrous oxide diffuse into the alveoli and dilute the oxygen that is present. This lasts for approximately 10 minutes and, if during this time the patient is allowed to breathe room air, hypoxia may ensue.

Changes in Ventilation

For each 1 mmHg decrease in the $PaCO_2$ caused by an increase in $\dot{V}_A$, an approximate 3% to 4% decrease in cerebral blood flow (CBF) occurs. A change in the length of time of anesthetic induction results from three factors: increased $\dot{V}_A$, decreased CBF, and solubility of the inhaled agents. For a moderately soluble agent like halothane the increased $\dot{V}_A$ produces a more rapid rise in end-tidal halothane partial pressure that offsets the decrease in CBF. For a relatively insoluble agent such as nitrous oxide, induction time is increased as the modest increase in end-tidal nitrous oxide partial pressure obtained by hyperventilation is more than offset by the decrease in CBF.

Eventually, no matter what agent is used, the increased end-tidal partial pressure resulting from the decrease in cardiac output and increase in $\dot{V}_A$ is enough to overcome the decrease in CBF.

INHALATION AGENTS AND ORGAN SYSTEM FUNCTION

The minimum alveolar concentration (MAC) is the amount of an inhalational agent that prevents movement in 50% of patients in response to surgical incision. After approximately 31 years of age, the MAC value begins to decrease; theoretically, the value for a patient 100 years of age is only 25% to 50% that of a young adult.

Circulatory Effects

Blood pressure is decreased with all inhalational agents and can be due to decreased contractility (e.g., halothane) or decreased systemic vascular resistance (e.g., isoflurane or desflurane) (6). Isoflurane and desflurane lead to coronary vasodilatation and may cause ischemia. The effect of both isoflurane and desflurane on contractility is less than halothane and enflurane (7).

Cardiac Rhythm

Halothane is the most arrhythmogenic agent while enflurane, desflurane, and sevoflurane are the least. Desflurane at a concentration of 6% led to a significant increase in QTc in children, whereas 2% sevoflurane did not (8).

Hypoxic Pulmonary Vasoconstriction

Hypoxic pulmonary vasoconstriction (HPV) is inhibited in a concentration-dependent fashion (9). However, the clinical significance of the difference between the anesthetic agents in this regard is not clear. When looking at a porcine model of one-lung anesthesia, neither isoflurane nor desflurane was found to have a deleterious effect on oxygenation (10).

Respiratory Effects

All inhalational agents are respiratory depressants. Compensatory responses to both hypoxia and hypercarbia are blunted (11).

Hepatic Effects

Up to 20% of patients may demonstrate mild disturbances in liver function following anesthesia with halothane (6).

Neither desflurane nor sevoflurane seems to have hepatotoxic properties (12).

Renal Effects

All potent inhalation agents result in a dose-dependent decrease in renal blood flow. In patients with preoperative renal impairment, anesthesia with either desflurane or isoflurane did not lead to worsened renal function (13).

INTRAVENOUS AGENTS

Narcotics

General Properties

Morphine sulfate was first isolated from opium in 1803. The use of high-dose narcotics for anesthesia was popularized in the 1970s.

The opiate receptor complex has three major receptor groups: μ, δ, and κ. Pain relief is mediated by the μ-receptor and also affect the respiratory, cardiovascular, gastrointestinal, and neuroendocrine systems (14).

Modern anesthesia practice includes morphine, meperidine, methadone, fentanyl, alfentanil, sufentanil, and, more

TABLE 54.2 Selected Pharmacokinetic Data for Four Opioids

	Morphine	Fentanyl	Sufentanil	Remifentanil
Lipid solubility[a]	1	580	1778	50
t½ π (min)	0.9–2.4	1–3	0.5–2	1
t½ α (min)	10–20	5–20	5–15	6
t½ β (hrs)	2–4	2–4	2–3	0.06
Clearance (mL/kg/min)	10–20	10–20	10–12	40–70
Vd_{ss} (L/kg)	3–5	3–5	2.5	0.2–0.3

[a]Proportional to ease with which agent crosses blood–brain barrier and, hence, potency.
t½ π, rapid redistribution half-life; t½ α, slow redistribution half-life; t½ β, elimination half-life; Vd_{ss}, steady-state volume of distribution.

recently, remifentanil. Morphine is associated with recall, histamine release, respiratory depression, hypertension, and vasodilation. Synthetic drugs related to the phenylpiperidines, such as fentanyl, sufentanil, alfentanil, and remifentanil, do not induce histamine release or vasodilation and thus hemodynamically stable (14). Remifentanil, has a rapid onset, metabolized by plasma esterases, and has a half-life of 8 to 20 minutes independent of liver or renal function thus making it ideal in patients following neurosurgical procedures or head injury who need frequent neurologic assessments. However, narcotic drugs cannot be depended upon to provide complete anesthesia alone.

Pharmacokinetics/Pharmacodynamics

Selected pharmacokinetic data for four commonly used opioids are summarized in Table 54.2. Similarities between the redistribution and elimination half-lives and the clearance and steady-state volume of distribution are noteworthy. The major difference is in lipid solubility, which correlates with potency. The depressant effect from morphine and fentanyl can be seen even after the analgesic effect of that drug has dissipated. Remifentanil has a rapid onset and offset of effect, even after a prolonged infusion.

Hemodynamic Effects

Hypotension is seen with morphine dose of 1 to 4 mg/kg secondary to vagal-induced bradycardia, vasodilation, histamine release, and splanchnic blood sequestration. Hypotension seldom occurs at a rate of 5 mg/min or less.

Treatment with H_1 (diphenhydramine) and H_2 (cimetidine) blockers attenuates the cardiovascular response to histamine. Fentanyl, 30 to 100 μg/kg, rarely causes hypotension, changes in contractility, heart rate, cardiac output, or systemic or pulmonary artery occlusion pressure even in patients with poor left ventricular function, perhaps because it does not cause histamine release. Remifentanil has a beneficial hemodynamic profile, similar to fentanyl (15).

Respiratory Effects

Dose-dependent respiratory depression is seen. Hypoxic and hypercarbic ventilatory drives are decreased. The pontine and medullary centers for respiratory rhythmicity are impaired, resulting in increased irregular and periodic breathing.

With morphine triggering or worsening of bronchospasm due to histamine release is possible but not seen with fentanyl, sufentanil, or remifentanil. Fentanyl and its derivatives can cause chest wall rigidity. The mechanism is not well understood, but may be a result of γ-aminobutyric acid (GABA) receptor stimulation located on interneurons. Treatment is commonly with a muscle relaxant.

Neurologic Effects

Morphine has no effect on CBF, cerebral metabolic rate for oxygen ($CMRO_2$), or cerebral metabolic rate for glucose (CMR_G) in CBF, but autoregulation was better maintained than in the control group (16). Fentanyl, in a model of traumatic brain injury, did not lead to a reduction in CBF despite a decrease in arterial blood pressure (17).

Gastrointestinal Effects

Opioids can cause emesis by stimulation of the chemoreceptor trigger zone in the area postrema of the medulla; increased gastrointestinal secretions; decreased motility that also may affect emetic action; and increased smooth muscle tone of the gastrointestinal tract and the sphincter of Oddi. The effects of opiates on the GIT can be ameliorated by methylnaltrexone which does not cross the blood–brain barrier.

Immune Function

Effects on the immune system are variable but opiates may be associated with suppression of natural killer cells and the immune response in animal studies (18–21).

Barbiturates

Thiobarbiturates (e.g., sodium thiopental and methohexital) are frequently used due to their ultrashort onset and offset action compared with other barbiturates. Methohexital is two to three times more potent than thiopental.

Pharmacokinetics/Pharmacodynamics

Thiopental is highly lipophilic. A dose of 3 to 5 mg/kg induces loss of consciousness within one arm–brain circulation time (10 to 15 seconds). The short duration of action of this drug (5 to 10 minutes) is due to its redistribution from the brain to muscle, skin, and, to a lesser extent, fat. The elimination half-life of the drug is long, making thiopental into a long-acting drug with larger doses.

Methohexital is only slightly less lipid-soluble and the onset and duration of loss of consciousness are approximately the same as with thiopental because of its rapid redistribution, but it is more dependent on hepatic blood flow for clearance.

Neurologic Effects

Barbiturates facilitate inhibitory—GABA—neural transmitters and inhibition of excitatory neural transmitter action and lead an increase in the duration that chloride (Cl^-) ion channels remain open. There is a decrease in $CMRO_2$, CBF, and ICP and hence used for brain protection.

Cardiorespiratory Effects

Contractility is decreased with a 10% to 25% decrease in cardiac output, blood pressure, and stroke volume at clinically relevant doses. A decrease in venous tone decreases preload. The responses to carbon dioxide elevation and hypoxia are impaired.

A continuous barbiturate infusion, affects immune function increasing chances of developing infections (22).

Propofol

Propofol is a sedative–hypnotic agent. The agent is not antianalgesic—as are the thiobarbiturates but has minimal amnestic effects (23). It is insoluble in aqueous media and hence available in a 1% weight/volume (Intralipid) emulsion composed of soybean oil, glycerol, and purified egg phosphatide. No histamine release is seen.

Pharmacokinetics/Pharmacodynamics

Propofol is extensively distributed into vessel-rich tissues, and ultimately redistributed to lean muscle and fat. It has high clearance and the short elimination half-life but affected by age (decreased clearance and dose requirement), obesity (increased clearance and volume of distribution), and type of procedure.

A dose of 2 to 2.5 mg/kg results in loss of consciousness in less than 60 seconds; rapid intravenous injection of 1 to 1.5 mg/kg in the elderly or a patient who has been given narcotic or benzodiazepine premedication is often sufficient for induction. The effective dose in 50% of patients studied (ED_{50}), which is analogous to MAC for potent inhalation agents, is 53.5 μg/kg/min (95% confidence limits; 39.9 to 63 μg/kg/min) (24).

Neurologic Effects

The mechanisms of action of propofol are unclear. At a dosage of more than 150 μg/kg/min results in EEG burst suppression lasting 15 seconds or longer returning to the awake state within 11 minutes of drug discontinuation.

Propofol leads to a dose-related decrease in CBF and $CMRO_2$, and leads to progressive EEG suppression with increasing dose of propofol (25) thus beneficial in patients with intracranial disease and for long-term sedation in the ICU.

Cardiovascular Effects

Propofol is a negative inotrope and produces a dose-dependent decrease in systolic, diastolic, and mean arterial blood pressure; an effect enhanced by narcotic premedication. Profound cardiovascular depression may be seen when propofol is used in elderly or hypovolemic patients and those with impaired ventricular function.

Respiratory Effects

Apnea is seen on induction with propofol and the response to hypoxia is also significantly blunted (26). Adjuvant use of narcotics further depresses respiratory drive.

Propofol Related Infusion Syndrome

First described by Parke et al. (27) propofol related infusion syndrome (PRIS) has been described in adults also (28,29). It is associated usually with high dose (>4 mg/kg/hr) and prolonged infusions (>48 hours) but has also been described after short-term infusions (30). A syndrome characterized by unexplained metabolic acidosis, bradycardia, hypotension, arrhythmias, EKG changes consistent with a brugada-like picture, rhabdomyolysis and renal failure (31). Fatty infiltration of the liver is very common early in the syndrome (Table 54.3).

Propofol increases the activity of malonyl CoA, inhibiting the entry of long chain fatty acids into the mitochondria and uncoupling beta oxidation. This leads to accumulation of fatty acids in muscle and other organ systems. This is more pronounced in a high catecholamine, low carbohydrate state as seen in critically ill malnourished populations such as the extremes of age who are at higher risk of the syndrome (32,33).

TABLE 54.3 Clinical Manifestations of Propofol Related Infusion Syndrome (PRIS)

Unexplained metabolic acidosis
Hypertriglyceridemia
Hypotension
Lactic acidosis
Dysrhythmia – sudden onset
Bradycardia – resistant to treatment
Rhabdomyolysis
Acute renal failure
Hepatomegaly

Treatment is largely supportive. Triglycerides levels should be monitored when patients are on propofol.

Benzodiazepines

The benzodiazepines most commonly employed are diazepam, lorazepam, and midazolam. Diazepam and lorazepam are insoluble in water. Lorazepam is less lipid-soluble than diazepam, and its slow entry into the CNS may be significant to its slower onset of action.

Pharmacokinetics/Pharmacodynamics

Diazepam. Intramuscular injection is painful, and absorption is erratic. Clearance involves oxidation to active metabolites. With hepatic disease, the volume of distribution increases and metabolism decreases, resulting in an increase in the half-life from 40 to 80 hours.

Lorazepam. Lorazepam is unaltered by age or renal disease, but hepatic disease increases the half-life.

Midazolam. Midazolam also can be administered by intramuscular, intravenous, or oral routes. The drug undergoes extensive metabolism to active and inactive metabolites.

Neurologic Effects

Benzodiazepines have dose-dependent effects on the CNS and potentiate inhibitory GABA neurotransmission. They increase the frequency but not the duration of chloride channel opening.

Antegrade amnesia is seen with all of the benzodiazepines, but more so with lorazepam.

Ketamine

Pharmacokinetics/Pharmacodynamics

Ketamine is structurally related to phencyclidine, known in street vernacular as "angel dust." After an intravenous dose of 2 mg/kg, consciousness is lost in little more than one arm–brain circulation time and returns 10 to 15 minutes later secondary to rapid drug redistribution into muscle and other tissues. The most important metabolite is norketamine, and has approximately one-third the potency of ketamine.

Neurologic Effects

The exact mechanism of action of ketamine is not well understood but most likely is NMDA receptor antagonism. It can have hallucinogenic effects including "out of body experiences."

It is a potent analgesic and a dissociative anesthetic, a feeling of indifference to the outside surroundings but preserved muscle tone. Ketamine increases CBF and so must be used with caution in individuals with elevated ICP.

Cardiovascular Effects

Ketamine causes central stimulation of the sympathetic arm of the autonomic nervous system and the cardiovascular effects are primarily related to CNS stimulation with an increase in systemic blood pressure and cerebrovasodilation, resulting in increased ICP. Pulmonary vascular resistance and right ventricular stroke work also are frequently increased.

Respiratory Effects

Ketamine is not a respiratory depressant; the ventilatory response to carbon dioxide is maintained while potentiating the bronchodilatory effects of catecholamines. Ketamine increases oral secretions, necessitating the use of an anticholinergic agent.

Other Effects

The drug has been used safely in patients with malignant hyperthermia (MH). Postanesthetic emergence reactions—nightmares and hallucinations—occur in 5% to 30% of patients and can be attenuated by using a benzodiazepine.

Etomidate

An induction agent that maintains hemodynamic stability, and hence employed for intubation of critically ill patients with hemodynamic instability. It can cause adrenal suppression when used in a prolonged infusion but has also been demonstrated following a single dose (34). However, the benefits of hemodynamic stability may overcome any concerns about adrenal dysfunction and its consequences (35).

Dexmedetomidine

Dexmedetomidine is a highly selective, short-acting central α_2-agonist. It is used in the ICU for providing sedation and some degree of analgesia. It is used primarily for sedation in the ICU. It provides a dose-dependent degree of sedation, analgesia, anxiolysis, and sympatholysis (alpha 2a receptor mediated), inhibits shivering (alpha 2b receptors) and associated with decreased delirium (alpha 2c receptor). When used in postoperative patients in the ICU, dexmedetomidine can provide better sedation with fewer narcotics than propofol (36). It does not cause respiratory depression and hence can be used through an extubation protocol.

It is chemically related to clonidine but has eight times the affinity for alpha 2 receptors.

A biphasic response is seen with initial hypertension and bradycardia followed by a decrease in BP. It can be used perioperatively in cardiac surgery (37) and has some protective effect in brain trauma (38) the MENDS study showed a lower incidence of delirium (39).

ANESTHESIA TECHNIQUES AND SPECIFIC CLINICAL STATES

There is no evidence to conclusively support one anesthetic technique over another in critically ill patients. However, in a hemodynamically unstable patient it is best to avoid potent inhalation agents and prefer an intravenous technique involving either ketamine or one of the phenylpiperidine narcotics. In traumatic brain injury, one can use intravenous benzodiazepines, barbiturates, ketamine and narcotics with isoflurane; while potent-inhaled anesthetic agents are avoided.

Total intravenous anesthesia (TIVA) with short-acting narcotics and propofol allow for an easily titratable anesthesia without the disadvantages of inhalational anesthesia. Closed gas spaces such as pneumothorax, pneumocephalus, or bowel obstruction demand that nitrous oxide be withheld.

Acute Respiratory Distress Syndrome

The development of acute respiratory distress syndrome (ARDS) is hypothesized by a two-hit mechanism. A patient at risk for cytokine release due to various mechanisms (e.g., trauma, sepsis, critical illness, pancreatitis, extensive surgery), if exposed to a second hit such as blood transfusions, high tidal volumes, inappropriate antibiotics can develop lung injury.

ARDS presents with hypoxemia secondary to atelectasis and shunt, thus presenting challenges to mechanical ventilation. Use of low tidal volumes of 6 to 8 mL/kg ideal body weight is preferred (18,40). A higher than normal $PaCO_2$, "permissive hypercapnia" is tolerated. The approach of lung protective strategy has been shown to improve outcome in patients with ARDS and should probably be maintained in patients undergoing surgery (18,41,42). The use of PEEP to prevent derecruitment is important, but the exact amount is still under debate (43–45).

Identifying patients who are at risk for developing lung injury (lung injury predictive score) and avoiding a second trigger such as blood transfusion, high tidal volumes could prevent progression to ARDS (46).

Management of patients with ARDS should be directed at the maintenance of adequate hemodynamics without fluid overload (47,48).

The use of dynamic markers such as pulse pressure variation (PPV) and systolic pressure variation (SPV) may be challenging in a setting of low compliance and low tidal volumes such as ARDS (49). Other techniques such as a response of stroke volume index, cardiac index or increase in end-tidal CO_2 ($ETCO_2$) with passive leg raise (PLR) or an end expiratory occlusion could be employed safely in this setting (50–54).

The Patient with a Head Injury

Optimal cerebral perfusion pressure—generally considered to be "optimized" at 60 to 65 mmHg is the goal. Anesthesia directed at reducing intracerebral pressure, barbiturates, maintenance of normothermia or mild hypothermia, increasing serum osmolarity, and judicious use of diuretics, use of vasopressors and inotropes to improve cardiac output and blood pressure and at times, hyperventilation. The approach is to direct therapy to optimize CBF by improving central perfusion pressure.

The Patient with Shock

In hypovolemic, septic shock patients, it is important to minimize intrathoracic pressures during fluid resuscitation. Drugs that depress contractility and cause vasodilation should be avoided. Sometimes in extreme cases, even drugs that are considered to maintain hemodynamic stability, such as ketamine, can lead to hemodynamic collapse.

In patients with cardiogenic shock, intrathoracic pressure is not detrimental, and may even be beneficial. However, most anesthetics are cardiac depressants and should be used with caution in patients with shock. All patients in shock need invasive hemodynamic monitoring to assess fluid responsiveness (55,56).

POSTOPERATIVE CARE

Postoperative complications have been found to occur in 5% to 30% of patients.

Hypoxemia

Postoperative hypoxemia can result from diverse etiologies (Table 54.4).

Hypoventilation caused by residual anesthetic or muscle relaxant especially in patients who are predisposed such as obesity-hypoventilation syndromes, obstructive sleep apnea (OSA), neuro muscular disorders like myasthenia gravis, amyotrophic lateral sclerosis.

Atelectasis could be secondary to one-lung intubation, upper abdominal and thoracic surgery especially in patients who have pre-existing lung conditions such as COPD, kyphoscoliosis.

Note that closing capacity and FRC alter with age and the older individuals are more predisposed. Early recognition of this condition and application of noninvasive ventilation (NIPPV-CPAP/BiPAP, aggressive incentive spirometry) can prevent the complications such as hypoxia and pneumonia.

Upper airway obstruction due to a decreased level of consciousness is a common reason for hypoxemia and hypercarbia especially in patients with OSA. Pulmonary edema could be cardiogenic or noncardiogenic. Noncardiogenic may be due to aspiration, infection, ARDS, trauma, transfusion-associated lung injury (TRALI) or neurogenic pulmonary edema. Pulmonary vascular permeability index can be measured and can differentiate between cardiogenic and noncardiogenic pulmonary edema. Negative-pressure pulmonary edema can develop after a strenuous inspiratory effort against an obstructed airway and can take up to 10 hours after the episode of airway obstruction. It is most commonly secondary to laryngospasm during anesthetic induction of or emergence from anesthesia.

TABLE 54.4 Etiology of Postoperative Hypercapnia

I. Central respiratory depression
Intravenous (narcotic) anesthetics
Inhaled anesthetic agents
II. Respiratory muscle dysfunction
Site of incision (upper abdominal, thoracic)
Residual neuromuscular blockade
Use of drugs that enhance neuromuscular blockade (gentamicin, clindamycin, neomycin, furosemide)
Physiologic factors that prevent reversal of neuromuscular blockade (hypokalemia, respiratory acidosis) or enhance the blockade (hypothermia, hypermagnesemia)
III. Physical factors
Obesity
Gastric dilation
Tight dressings
Body cast
IV. Increased production of carbon dioxide
Sepsis
Shivering
Malignant hyperthermia
V. Underlying hyperthermia
Chronic obstructive pulmonary disease with CO_2 retention
Neuromuscular—chest cage dysfunction (kyphoscoliosis)
Acute or chronic respiratory failure of any etiology

Data from Feeley TW. The recovery room. In: Miller RD, ed. *Anesthesia*. 2nd ed. New York: Churchill Livingstone; 1986:1921; and Wyngaarden JB, Smith LH Jr, eds. *Cecil Textbook of Medicine*. 18th ed. Philadelphia, PA: WB Saunders; 1988:417, 472, 474.

The pathophysiology is poorly understood. A common explanation is that the massive negative intrapleural pressure generated during airway obstruction shifts the balance in the Starling forces toward a large fluid transudation from the intravascular to the interstitial space.

The radiologic picture in negative-pressure pulmonary edema has been described as alveolar and interstitial edema.

Treatment is mainly supportive and in most cases resolves in 24 hours.

Pulmonary embolism (PE) can result in hypoxia and hypotension. Patients at risk include those with renal cell cancer, hip and knee joint surgery, pelvic trauma, and pelvic malignancies.

PE results in decrease in dead space resulting in a large gradient of CO_2 between the arterial blood gas and $ETCO_2$.

Pneumothorax should be considered especially after thoracic surgery, laparoscopic surgery, trauma, emphysema, and central line placement. Distended neck veins with decreased breath sounds and hypotension are the clinical findings. Emergent needle decompression or placing a chest tube is the treatment. Lately, pneumothorax can be diagnosed with ultrasound techniques.

Pain and Perioperative Stress

Seventy-five percent of patients receiving parenteral narcotics for moderate-to-severe pain have significant residual pain. Sometimes there may be a paradoxical response to opioids known as opioid-induced hyperalgesia (OIH) and can be managed with NMDA receptor antagonist such as ketamine, dextromethorphan, and methadone (57). Uncontrolled pain causes sympathetic nervous system stimulation with elevated plasma catecholamine levels, tachycardia, hypertension, increased systemic vascular resistance, and an increase in myocardial oxygen requirements. In the patient with underlying coronary artery disease, this increased oxygen demand may not be met, resulting in ischemia or infarction.

Surgical procedures on the upper abdomen and thorax can cause splinting and lead to pulmonary complications secondary to a decrease in FRC. These can be minimized by adequate pain relief.

Stress Response

Stress response to surgery has an initial *ebb phase* characterized by a shock state with low cardiac output, and a later *flow phase* characterized by a hyperdynamic state from the endocrine, metabolic, and cardiovascular standpoints.

The endocrine response is evidenced by an increase in catecholamine levels, antidiuretic hormone (ADH) secretion, corticotropin and steroids, and hyperglycemia.

The systemic response to trauma includes an immune depression, which can appear early after the stressful event (58,59) and is mediated through several different pathways (60,61).

Different anesthetic techniques may affect this response in various ways.

General Anesthesia. Roizen et al. (62) have used the acronym MAC-BAR, indicating the minimal alveolar concentration at which the adrenergic response is blocked; it is usually observed at approximately 2 MAC for most inhalational agents. Furthermore, others have shown that graded surgical stress causes minimal endocrine response (63).

In the surgical ICU, patients may begin to mount the metabolic–endocrine response in the postoperative period (64).

Regional Anesthesia. Kehlet et al. (65,66) have studied this relationship extensively and found major differences in levels of corticosteroids, catecholamines, aldosterone, renin, growth hormone, prolactin, and ADH in patients undergoing surgery with epidural anesthesia compared with those given general anesthesia.

Combined Anesthesia. The term coined by Crile in 1921, involves the block of surgical stimulus by a regional technique, combined with loss of consciousness achieved by light general anesthesia (67) and can be used in procedures in lower abdomen and extremities. The benefits of combined over general techniques are controversial (68–70). An extended-release formulation of epidural morphine is available and shown to provide postoperative pain relief for 48 hours with a single dose (71).

Hemodynamic Management

Hypertension: Acute postoperative hypertension is one of the most common complications and can lead to cardiac complications. Causes are usually related to pain and hypoxia.

Hypotension: Hypotension has a varied etiology including hypovolemia secondary to blood loss or an increased SIRS (systemic inflammatory response syndrome) state. The role of fluid responsiveness using dynamic markers has been established (72). Perioperative optimization of such hemodynamics could lead to improved outcomes (73). Use of dynamic markers such as PPV, SPV have been established (55).

However, these techniques have limitations in the spontaneously breathing patients. In such patients, the response to a PLR could be used (74). The response of $ETCO_2$ and cardiac index to PLR has been validated (50–54).

In mechanically ventilated patients, increase in $ETCO_2$ or stroke volume index (SVI) with an end expiratory occlusion of 15 seconds is considered fluid responsive (53).

Supranormal delivery of oxygen (75) although initially promising, did not show benefit with other studies (76,77).

A protocolized treatment with a pulmonary artery catheter found no advantage compared to standard care without invasive monitoring (78). In contrast, Rivers et al. found that, in the early hours of sepsis, goal-directed therapy that is delivered in the emergency room can improve outcome and decrease hospital mortality (79). However the PROCESS, ARISE, and PROMISE studies (80–82) did not show any difference in outcomes with goal-directed therapy. However, early fluid resuscitation was the standard of care in all these trials and should be targeted aggressively.

Postoperative AKI

Acute kidney injury (AKI) could be prerenal, renal, and postrenal. Various classifications have been proposed such as RIFLE AKIN (Acute Kidney Injury Network) and KDIGO Clinical practice guidelines (83). In 2012, the Kidney Disease Improving Global Outcomes (KDIGO) released their clinical practice guidelines for AKI, which build off of the RIFLE criteria and the AKIN criteria (84) (Table 54.5).

TABLE 54.5 Kidney Disease Improving Global Guidelines (KDIGO)

Stage	Serum Creatinine	Urine Output (UO)
1	1–1.9 times baseline or >0.3 mg/dL increase	<0.5 mL/kg/hr for 6–12 hrs
2	2–2.9 times baseline	<0.5 mL/kg/hr >6–12 hrs
3	3 times baseline *or* >4 mg/dL *or* Initiation of renal replacement therapy (RRT) *or* Age <18 yrs, decrease in eGFR <35 mL/min/1.73 m^2	<0.3 mL/kg/hr >12 hrs *or* Anuria >12 hrs

From Clinical Practice Guidelines for Acute Kidney Injury 2012. Available at http://www.kdigo.org/clinical_practice_guidelines/AKI.php.

Type of IV fluids for resuscitation merits some discussion. The SAFE study showed no difference between the use of 4% albumin versus normal saline as a resuscitation fluid with regard to outcome (85). In traumatic brain injury, however, use of albumin was associated with higher mortality rates (86).

The use of hydroxyl ethyl starch (HES) has been shown to have poor renal outcomes as in the 6S and CHEST studies. This is hypothesized to be due to the deposition of starch molecules in the kidney (87,88).

The use of chloride-rich fluids has also been associated with AKI (89).

Postoperative Nausea and Vomiting

Postoperative nausea and vomiting (PONV) is seen in 30% of the general population and as high as 80% in high-risk patients. Patients at risk for PONV are younger females with a previous history of PONV or motion sickness. Exposure to volatile anesthetics, nitrous oxide, and opioids increases the risk of PONV as does procedures like cholecystectomy, laparoscopy, and gynecologic procedures.

The Apfel risk score (90) is based on four predictors and can predict PONV with a 10% risk in those patients with zero and 80% with a score of four (Table 54.6).

The IMPACT study and two other meta-analyses (91–93) showed that avoiding nitrous oxide and using TIVA reduces PONV (Table 54.7).

TABLE 54.6 Apfel Simplified Risk Score

Female sex	1
H/O PONV/motion sickness	1
Nonsmoking	1
Postoperative opioids	1
Score	**Risk of PONV (%)**
0	10
1	21
2	39
3	61
4	78

TABLE 54.7 Factors to Reduce PONV

Avoid nitrous oxide
Avoid volatile anesthetics
Avoid general anesthesia
Use TIVA
Minimize opioids
Adequate hydration

Treatment of PONV involves use of serotonin antagonists such as ondansetron and ramosetron, NK1 receptor antagonists such as aprepitant, rolapitant, corticosteroids, haloperidol, and meclizine. Avoiding postoperative pain can also decrease PONV. Combination antiemetic therapy is preferable to single drug (91).

Delirium

Delirium can be very disturbing for patients and family members and imposes a significant risk to patients. Marcantonio et al. found that postoperative delirium was not related to the type of anesthetic used but intra- and postoperative bleeding and increasing transfusion requirements led to an increase in postoperative delirium (94). Pain, electrolyte abnormalities, and urinary retention can predispose to delirium. Postoperative delirium is not temporally related to emergence from anesthesia. It is associated with increased mortality, cognitive impairment, and dementia in the long term (95,96).

Delirium occurs as a result of inflammatory response and a breakdown of the blood–brain barrier leading to disturbances in the neurotransmitter systems (97).

Risk factors include older age, pre-existing dementia, and use of narcotics/benzodiazepines.

Precipitating factors include use of physical restraints, polypharmacy, malnutrition, presence of urinary bladder catheter, and acute pain (Table 54.8).

Various screening tools are present for diagnosing delirium. The most commonly used are the confusion assessment method for the ICU (CAM-ICU) (98) or intensive care delirium check list (ICDSC) (99) (Table 54.9).

Treatment

Use of antipsychotics is common but the evidence is difficult to interpret because of the heterogeneity of various studies. However, use of antipsychotics reserved only for short term in the agitated patient.

Minimizing sedation, using a daily sedation holiday (100) and a targeted sedation score (101) can minimize delirium.

TABLE 54.8 Risk Factors for Postoperative Delirium

Age >65 yrs
Poor pain control
Cognitive impairment
Sleep deprivation
Severe illness/comorbidities
Hypoxia
Hearing or vision impairment
Hypercarbia
Hip fracture
Electrolyte abnormalities
Infection
Polypharmacy

TABLE 54.9 CAM-ICU (Confusion Assessment Method)

I	Acute onset/fluctuating course
II	Inattention
III	Altered level of consciousness
IV	Disorganized thinking

Delirium = I and II and III or IV.

The use of dexmedetomidine (MENDS study) also showed less delirium (39).

Residual Neuromuscular Blockade

Residual neuromuscular blockade presents in one of three ways: delayed return to consciousness, respiratory difficulty with hypercapnia, or muscle weakness (Table 54.10). It is important to consider it and protect the airway.

Diagnosis

One can monitor the depth of neuromuscular blockade with a twitch-stimulating device or a group of clinical signs. The effect of muscle relaxants can be monitored by applying a supramaximal electrical stimulus to a motor nerve such as the ulnar nerve and monitor the contraction of adductor pollicis brevis.

A single supramaximal stimulus at 50 Hz for 5 seconds that produces contraction without fade correlates with signs of clinical recovery from neuromuscular blockade.

Train-of-four stimulus (four supramaximal stimuli in 2 seconds with each stimulus lasting 0.2 seconds), or double-burst stimulation can also be used. With the train-of-four stimulus, the ratio of the fourth contraction to the first being greater

TABLE 54.10 Etiology of Prolonged Neuromuscular Blockade

Nondepolarizing neuromuscular blocking agents
Intensity of neuromuscular blockade
Renal failure (decreased metocurine and pancuronium excretion)
Hepatic failure (decreased pancuronium and vecuronium excretion)
Residual potent–inhaled anesthetic agent
Inadequate dose of reversal agents
Hypothermia
Acid–base state
Hypokalemia, hypermagnesemia
Drugs
Antibiotics (gentamicin, clindamycin, and multiple other drugs with several mechanisms)
Local anesthetics
Antiarrhythmics (quinidine)
Furosemide
Dantrolene
Trimethaphan (possibly)
Underlying diseases (myasthenia gravis, myasthenic syndrome, familial periodic paralysis)
Depolarizing neuromuscular blocking agents (succinylcholine)
Decreased effective pseudocholinesterase
Phase II block
Hypermagnesemia
Local anesthetics

Modified from Miller RD, Savarese JJ. Pharmacology of muscle relaxants and their antagonists. In: Miller RD, ed. *Anesthesia.* 2nd ed. New York: Churchill Livingstone; 1986:889.

TABLE 54.11 Clinical Signs of Recovery from Neuromuscular Blockade

Awake patient
Opens eyes widely
Coughs effectively
Sustains tongue protrusion
Sustains hand grip
Sustains head lift for more than 5 sec
Vital capacity of ≥15 mL/kg
PNP of ≥20 cm H_2O
Sustained 50-Hz tetanic stimulation for 5 sec
Patient who is asleep or unable to follow commands
Tidal volume of 5–10 mL/kg
PNP of ≥25 cm H_2O
Sustained 50-Hz tetanic stimulation for 5 sec

PNP, peak negative pressure.
Modified from Ali HH, Miller RD. Monitoring of neuromuscular function. In: Miller RD, ed. *Anesthesia*. 2nd ed. New York: Churchill Livingstone; 1986:8.

than 60%, patients and ability to sustain a head lift for 3 seconds or when the ratio is greater than 75%, predicts clinical recovery (Table 54.11).

Treatment

If residual neuromuscular blockade is present, an attempt is made to reverse it. If blockade results from succinylcholine, usually in patients with pseudocholinesterase deficiency, reversal agents will not be of any benefit. The diagnosis can be made by measuring pseudocholinesterase activity in plasma. One can keep the patient mechanically ventilated until neuromuscular recovery or administer fresh-frozen plasma. If a nondepolarizing blocking agent was used, reversal may be attempted with anticholinesterases and anticholinergics (Table 54.12).

Critical Care Illness Neuropathy and Myopathy

Critical illness polyneuropathy and myopathy (CINMA) is a sensory and motor neuropathy associated with weakness, electrophysiologic abnormalities, and respiratory muscle strength weakness.

Prolonged ICU stay, use of vasopressors, renal failure, steroids, and muscle relaxants have been implicated.

Nerve conduction studies reveal mixed axonopathy and can be seen as early as 24 to 48 hours of the critical care illness. Combining protocols for early sedation management while minimizing use of steroids and muscle relaxants can prevent this condition (102–104).

TABLE 54.12 Reversal Agents Used with Neuromuscular Blocking Agents

Anticholinesterase	Anticholinergic
Neostigmine 35–70 µg/kg (maximum, 5 mg)	Atropine 20 µg/kg or
Edrophonium 500–1,000 µg/kg	Glycopyrrolate 10 µg/kg
Pyridostigmine 175–350 µg/kg (maximum, 20 mg)	

Modified from Miller RD, Savarese JJ. Pharmacology of muscle relaxants and their antagonists. In: Miller RD, ed. *Anesthesia*. 2nd ed. New York: Churchill Livingstone; 1986:889.

Glucose Control

Interventions directed at reducing blood glucose showed improved outcomes in some, but not all, studies. After initial studies showing benefit, others, and a metaanalysis of 21 trials, found no benefit from intensive insulin therapy (105,106).

Current evidence suggests that levels between 140 and 180 show benefit in the critically ill populations (107). Targets less than 110 or tight control are not recommended.

The largest trial, the recent NICE–SUGAR study (107) showed an increase in mortality in the group with intensive insulin control (<108 mg/dL).

Current recommendations are not to use intensive insulin therapy in the SICU, MICU patients with or without diabetes mellitus but target a blood glucose of 140 to 180 mg/dL (108).

MALIGNANT HYPERTHERMIA

Manifestations of MH may be divided into early, late, and postcrisis (Table 54.13). MH is a pharmacogenetic clinical syndrome that usually occurs with general anesthesia. Its onset may be delayed for several hours. The hallmark of the syndrome is rapidly increasing temperature caused by uncontrolled skeletal muscle metabolism that can result in rhabdomyolysis and death.

After exposure to a triggering agent, a dramatic increase in aerobic metabolism occurs in the skeletal muscle and oxygen consumption can increase threefold, whereas blood lactate may increase 15- to 20-fold. The mechanism involves myoplasmic calcium accumulation due to a failure of calcium uptake by the sarcoplasmic reticulum.

Susceptibility is increased in those with a family history and an elevated creatine kinase. The definitive test is a muscle biopsy for contracture studies after exposure to halothane, caffeine, halothane plus caffeine, or potassium. A new approach is that of genetic testing—the mutation conferring the susceptibility for MH is recognized and can be mapped. The future of diagnosis of MH susceptibility probably lies in genetic diagnosis (109).

Diagnosis

MH clinical signs overlap with many other conditions. When triggering agents—potent-inhaled anesthetics, succinylcholine—are used, MH must be considered in the presence of unexplained

TABLE 54.13 Signs of Malignant Hyperthermia

Early Signs	Late Signs	Postcrisis Signs
Skeletal muscle rigidity	Hyperpyrexia—may exceed 43°C (109.4°F)	Muscle pain, edema
Tachycardia and hypertension	Cyanosis	Central nervous system damage
Elevated $PetCO_2$	Serum electrolyte abnormalities	Renal failure
Acidosis	Elevated serum creatinine phosphokinase	Continued electrolyte imbalance
Dysrhythmias	Myoglobinuria	
	Coagulopathy	
	Cardiac failure and pulmonary edema	

$PetCO_2$, end-tidal partial pressure of carbon dioxide.

TABLE 54.14 Acute Therapy for Malignant Hyperthermia

Discontinue all anesthetic agents
Hyperventilate with an FiO_2 of 1.0.
CO_2 is increased; so hyperventilate to achieve a normal $PaCO_2$.
Dantrolene
Intravenously 2 mg/kg every 5 min to a total of 10 mg/kg
Effective dosage should be repeated every 10–15 hrs for at least 48 hrs
Sodium bicarbonate
Initial dose (mEq) = (base excess × (body weight in kg))/4
Give half the calculated dose; repeat as determined by arterial blood gas studies.
Control fever
Iced fluids
Surface cooling
Cooling of body cavities with sterile iced saline
Heat exchanger with a pump oxygenator
Dantrolene
Monitor urinary output
At least 0.5 mL/kg/hr
If myoglobinuria is present, at least 1 mL/kg/hr
Further therapy
Guided by blood studies, temperature, and urine output
(Blood studies include blood gases, electrolytes, liver profile, coagulation studies (including DIC studies), serum hemoglobin and myoglobin, and urine hemoglobin and myoglobin.)

DIC, disseminated intravascular coagulation; FiO_2, fraction of inspired oxygen.
Modified from Askanazi J. Principles of nutritional support. In: Barash PG, Deutsch S, Tinker J, eds. *Refresher Courses in Anesthesiology*. Vol. 14. Philadelphia, PA: JB Lippincott; 1986:1.

tachycardia, tachypnea, arrhythmias, mottling, cyanosis, hyperthermia, muscle rigidity, diaphoresis, or hemodynamic instability. Arterial and central venous blood gas analysis show metabolic and respiratory acidosis.

Treatment

The mortality rate of MH has decreased from 70% to less than 5% with improved treatment (Table 54.14). Discontinuing the triggering agent and Dantrolene therapy are recommended along with other supportive measures. The mechanism of action of dantrolene is not completely clear, but it is known to affect the ryanodine receptor, which is a major calcium release channel of the skeletal muscle sarcoplasmic reticulum, thus decreasing the intracellular calcium. Dantrolene is the key to successful MH treatment.

Key Points

- Postoperative acute respiratory failure is uncommon but dramatic and could be secondary to multiple reasons.
- Pulmonary edema in the early postoperative period could be secondary to increased vascular permeability (TRALI, ARDS, aspiration) or increased hydrostatic pressure (left ventricular failure, HTN) or other special situations such as neurogenic stress/negative pressure pulmonary edema/postexpansion edema after large volume thoracentesis.
- Treatment of hypoxemia entails delivering a high fraction of inspired oxygen (FiO_2) via nasal cannula, face mask, high flow devices, Noninvasive positive pressure ventilation or mechanical ventilation. They may need to be closely monitored in the ICU.
- Cardiac complications include arrhythmias, ischemia, dysrhythmias, heart failure, and myocardial infarction are seen usually 3 to 5 days after surgery, but can occur much earlier even on the first postoperative day (4). Monitoring patients at risk for a cardiac complication, for silent ischemia/infarction and earlier interventions can be lifesaving.
- An acute hypertensive crisis in the immediate postoperative period is usually the result of inadequate analgesia and can result in heart failure and cardiac ischemia.
- Goal-directed therapy is more directed toward achieving euvolemia in a timely fashion. Supranormal delivery of oxygen is not helpful and targeting central venous saturation may not be necessary.
- MH can develop at any time after exposure to a triggering agent (e.g., potent inhalational agents or succinylcholine). Treatment is supportive along with administering dantrolene. A malignant hypothermia hotline is available in many countries.

References

1. Brown D. Risk and outcome analysis: myths and truths. In: Kirby RR, Gravenstein N, eds. *Clinical Anesthesia Practice*. Philadelphia, PA: JB Lippincott; 1994:62.
2. Aders A, Aders H. Anaesthetic adverse incident reports: an Australian study of 1,231 outcomes. *Anaesth Intensive Care*. 2005;33(3):336–344.
3. Cheney FW, Posner KL, Lee LA, et al. Trends in anesthesia-related death and brain damage: a closed claims analysis. *Anesthesiology*. 2006;105(6):1081–1086.
4. Badner NH, Gelb AW. Postoperative myocardial infarction (PMI) after noncardiac surgery. *Anesthesiology*. 1999;90(2):644.
5. Ali SZ, Taguchi A, Rosenberg H. Malignant hyperthermia. *Best Pract Res Clin Anaesthesiol*. 2003;17(4):519–533.
6. Evers A, Koblin D. Inhalational anesthetics. In: Evers A, Maze M, eds. *Anesthetic Pharmacology: Physiologic Principles and Clinical Practice*. Philadelphia, PA: Churchill Livingstone; 2004:369–393.
7. Pagel PS, Kampine JP, Schmeling WT, Warltier DC. Comparison of the systemic and coronary hemodynamic actions of desflurane, isoflurane, halothane, and enflurane in the chronically instrumented dog. *Anesthesiology*. 1991;74(3):539–551.
8. Aypar E, Karagoz AH, Ozer S, et al. The effects of sevoflurane and desflurane anesthesia on QTc interval and cardiac rhythm in children. *Paediatr Anaesth*. 2007;17(6):563–567.
9. Loer SA, Scheeren TW, Tarnow J. Desflurane inhibits hypoxic pulmonary vasoconstriction in isolated rabbit lungs. *Anesthesiology*. 1995;83(3):552–556.
10. Schwarzkopf K, Schreiber T, Bauer R, et al. The effects of increasing concentrations of isoflurane and desflurane on pulmonary perfusion and systemic oxygenation during one-lung ventilation in pigs. *Anesth Analg*. 2001;93(6):1434–1438.
11. Groeben H, Meier S, Tankersley CG, et al. Influence of volatile anaesthetics on hypercapnoeic ventilatory responses in mice with blunted respiratory drive. *Br J Anaesth*. 2004;92(5):697–703.
12. Reichle FM, Conzen PF. Halogenated inhalational anaesthetics. *Best Pract Res Clin Anaesthesiol*. 2003;17(1):29–46.
13. Litz RJ, Hubler M, Lorenz W, et al. Renal responses to desflurane and isoflurane in patients with renal insufficiency. *Anesthesiology*. 2002;97(5):1133–1136.

14. Joo HS, Salasidis GC, Kataoka MT, et al. Comparison of bolus remifentanil versus bolus fentanyl for induction of anesthesia and tracheal intubation in patients with cardiac disease. *J Cardiothorac Vasc Anesth.* 2004;18(3):263–268.
15. Ma XD, Hauerberg J, Pedersen DB, Juhler M. Effects of morphine on cerebral blood flow autoregulation CO2-reactivity in experimental subarachnoid hemorrhage. *J Neurosurg Anesthesiol.* 1999;11(4):264–272.
16. Bedell EA, DeWitt DS, Prough DS. Fentanyl infusion preserves cerebral blood flow during decreased arterial blood pressure after traumatic brain injury in cats. *J Neurotrauma.* 1998;15(11):985–992.
17. Shavit Y, Ben-Eliyahu S, Zeidel A, Beilin B. Effects of fentanyl on natural killer cell activity and on resistance to tumor metastasis in rats: dose and timing study. *Neuroimmunomodulation.* 2004;11(4):255–260.
18. Acute Respiratory Distress Syndrome Network. Ventilation with lower tidal volumes as compared with traditional tidal volumes for acute lung injury and the acute respiratory distress syndrome. *N Engl J Med.* 2000; 342(18):1301–1308.
19. Beilin B, Shavit Y, Cohn S, Kedar E. Narcotic-induced suppression of natural killer cell activity in ventilated and nonventilated rats. *Clin Immunol Immunopathol.* 1992;64(2):173–176.
20. McDonough RJ, Madden JJ, Falek A, et al. Alteration of T and null lymphocyte frequencies in the peripheral blood of human opiate addicts: in vivo evidence for opiate receptor sites on T lymphocytes. *J Immunol.* 1980;125(6):2539–2543.
21. Brown SM, Stimmel B, Taub RN, et al. Immunologic dysfunction in heroin addicts. *Arch Intern Med.* 1974;134(6):1001–1006.
22. Frenette AJ, Perreault MM, Lam S, Williamson DR. Thiopental-induced neutropenia in two patients with severe head trauma. *Pharmacotherapy.* 2007;27(3):464.
23. White P. Propofol: pharmacokinetics and pharmacodynamics. *Semin Anesth.* 1988;7(Suppl 1):4.
24. Coates D. Diprivan (propofol) infusion anesthesia. *Semin Anesth.* 1988; 7(Suppl 1):73.
25. Ramani R, Todd MM, Warner DS. A dose-response study of the influence of propofol on cerebral blood flow, metabolism and the electroencephalogram in the rabbit. *J Neurosurg Anesthesiol.* 1992;4(2):110–119.
26. Blouin RT, Seifert HA, Babenco HD, et al. Propofol depresses the hypoxic ventilatory response during conscious sedation and isohypercapnia. *Anesthesiology.* 1993;79(6):1177–1182.
27. Parke TJ, Stevens JE, Rice AS, et al. Metabolic acidosis and fatal myocardial failure after propofol infusion in children: five case reports. *BMJ.* 1992;305(6854):613–616.
28. Corbett SM, Moore J, Rebuck JA, et al. Survival of propofol infusion syndrome in a head-injured patient. *Crit Care Med.* 2006;34(9):2479–2483.
29. Cremer OL. The propofol infusion syndrome: more puzzling evidence on a complex and poorly characterized disorder. *Crit Care.* 2009;13(6):1012.
30. Cravens GT, Packer DL, Johnson ME. Incidence of propofol infusion syndrome during noninvasive radiofrequency ablation for atrial flutter or fibrillation. *Anesthesiology.* 2007;106(6):1134–1138.
31. Smith H, Sinson G, Varelas P. Vasopressors and propofol infusion syndrome in severe head trauma. *Neurocrit Care.* 2009;10(2):166–172.
32. Wolf A, Weir P, Segar P, et al. Impaired fatty acid oxidation in propofol infusion syndrome. *Lancet.* 2001;357(9256):606–607.
33. Vasile B, Rasulo F, Candiani A, Latronico N. The pathophysiology of propofol infusion syndrome: a simple name for a complex syndrome. *Intensive Care Med.* 2003;29(9):1417–1425.
34. Lundy JB, Slane ML, Frizzi JD. Acute adrenal insufficiency after a single dose of etomidate. *J Intensive Care Med.* 2007;22(2):111–117.
35. Ray DC, McKeown DW. Effect of induction agent on vasopressor and steroid use, and outcome in patients with septic shock. *Crit Care.* 2007; 11(3):R56.
36. Gerlach AT, Dasta JF. Dexmedetomidine: an updated review. *Ann Pharmacother.* 2007;41(2):245–252.
37. Wijeysundera DN, Naik JS, Beattie WS. Alpha-2 adrenergic agonists to prevent perioperative cardiovascular complications: a meta-analysis. *Am J Med.* 2003;114(9):742–752.
38. Ma D, Hossain M, Rajakumaraswamy N, et al. Dexmedetomidine produces its neuroprotective effect via the alpha 2A-adrenoceptor subtype. *Eur J Pharmacol.* 2004;502(1-2):87–97.
39. Pandharipande PP, Pun BT, Herr DL, et al. Effect of sedation with dexmedetomidine vs lorazepam on acute brain dysfunction in mechanically ventilated patients: the MENDS randomized controlled trial. *JAMA.* 2007;298(22):2644–2653.
40. Amato MB, Barbas CS, Medeiros DM, et al. Effect of a protective-ventilation strategy on mortality in the acute respiratory distress syndrome. *N Engl J Med.* 1998;338(6):347–354.
41. Futier E, Constantin JM, Paugam-Burtz C, et al. A trial of intraoperative low-tidal-volume ventilation in abdominal surgery. *N Engl J Med.* 2013; 369(5):428–437.
42. Serpa Neto A, Cardoso SO, Manetta JA, et al. Association between use of lung-protective ventilation with lower tidal volumes and clinical outcomes among patients without acute respiratory distress syndrome: a meta-analysis. *JAMA.* 2012;308(16):1651–1659.
43. Meade MO, Cook DJ, Guyatt GH, et al. Ventilation strategy using low tidal volumes, recruitment maneuvers, and high positive end-expiratory pressure for acute lung injury and acute respiratory distress syndrome: a randomized controlled trial. *JAMA.* 2008;299(6):637–645.
44. Brower RG, Lanken PN, MacIntyre N, et al. Higher versus lower positive end-expiratory pressures in patients with the acute respiratory distress syndrome. *N Engl J Med.* 2004;351(4):327–336.
45. Mercat A, Richard JC, Vielle B, et al. Positive end-expiratory pressure setting in adults with acute lung injury and acute respiratory distress syndrome: a randomized controlled trial. *JAMA.* 2008;299(6):646–655.
46. Gajic O, Dabbagh O, Park PK, et al. Early identification of patients at risk of acute lung injury: evaluation of lung injury prediction score in a multicenter cohort study. *Am J Respir Crit Care Med.* 2011;183(4):462–470.
47. Wiedemann HP, Wheeler AP, Bernard GR, et al. Comparison of two fluid-management strategies in acute lung injury. *N Engl J Med.* 2006; 354(24):2564–2575.
48. Nisanevich V, Felsenstein I, Almogy G, et al. Effect of intraoperative fluid management on outcome after intraabdominal surgery. *Anesthesiology.* 2005;103(1):25–32.
49. Teboul JL, Monnet X. Pulse pressure variation and ARDS. *Minerva Anestesiol.* 2013;79(4):398–407.
50. Cavallaro F, Sandroni C, Marano C, et al. Diagnostic accuracy of passive leg raising for prediction of fluid responsiveness in adults: systematic review and meta-analysis of clinical studies. *Intensive Care Med.* 2010;36(9): 1475–1483.
51. Monnet X, Bataille A, Magalhaes E, et al. End-tidal carbon dioxide is better than arterial pressure for predicting volume responsiveness by the passive leg raising test. *Intensive Care Med.* 2013;39(1):93–100.
52. Monnet X, Bleibtreu A, Ferre A, et al. Passive leg-raising and end-expiratory occlusion tests perform better than pulse pressure variation in patients with low respiratory system compliance. *Crit Care Med.* 2012;40(1): 152–157.
53. Monnet X, Osman D, Ridel C, et al. Predicting volume responsiveness by using the end-expiratory occlusion in mechanically ventilated intensive care unit patients. *Crit Care Med.* 2009;37(3):951–956.
54. Monge Garcia MI, Gil Cano A, Gracia Romero M, et al. Non-invasive assessment of fluid responsiveness by changes in partial end-tidal CO2 pressure during a passive leg-raising maneuver. *Ann Intensive Care.* 2012;2:9.
55. Michard F. Changes in arterial pressure during mechanical ventilation. *Anesthesiology.* 2005;103(2):419–428.
56. Michard F, Teboul JL. Predicting fluid responsiveness in ICU patients: a critical analysis of the evidence. *Chest.* 2002;121(6):2000–2008.
57. Chu LF, Angst MS, Clark D. Opioid-induced hyperalgesia in humans: molecular mechanisms and clinical considerations. *Clin J Pain.* 2008;24(6): 479–496.
58. Abraham E. Physiologic stress and cellular ischemia: relationship to immunosuppression and susceptibility to sepsis. *Crit Care Med.* 1991;19(5):613–618.
59. Abraham E, Freitas AA. Hemorrhage in mice induces alterations in immunoglobulin-secreting B cells. *Crit Care Med.* 1989;17(10):1015–1019.
60. Schmand JF, Ayala A, Chaudry IH. Effects of trauma, duration of hypotension, and resuscitation regimen on cellular immunity after hemorrhagic shock. *Crit Care Med.* 1994;22(7):1076–1083.
61. Knoferl MW, Angele MK, Diodato MD, et al. Female sex hormones regulate macrophage function after trauma-hemorrhage and prevent increased death rate from subsequent sepsis. *Ann Surg.* 2002;235(1):105–112.
62. Roizen MF, Horrigan RW, Frazer BM. Anesthetic doses blocking adrenergic (stress) and cardiovascular responses to incision—MAC BAR. *Anesthesiology.* 1981;54(5):390–398.
63. Chernow B, Alexander HR, Smallridge RC, et al. Hormonal responses to graded surgical stress. *Arch Intern Med.* 1987;147(7):1273–1278.
64. Roth-Isigkeit A, Brechmann J, Dibbelt L, et al. Persistent endocrine stress response in patients undergoing cardiac surgery. *J Endocrinol Invest.* 1998;21(1):12–19.
65. Holte K, Kehlet H. Effect of postoperative epidural analgesia on surgical outcome. *Minerva Anestesiol.* 2002;68(4):157–161.
66. Kehlet H, Brandt MR, Hansen AP, Alberti KG. Effect of epidural analgesia on metabolic profiles during and after surgery. *Br J Surg.* 1979;66(8): 543–546.

67. Boltz MG, Krane EJ. Combined regional and light general anesthesia: are the risks increased or minimized? *Curr Opin Anaesthesiol.* 1999; 12(3):321–323.
68. Yeager MP, Glass DD, Neff RK, Brinck-Johnsen T. Epidural anesthesia and analgesia in high-risk surgical patients. *Anesthesiology.* 1987; 66(6):729–736.
69. Baron JF, Bertrand M, Barre E, et al. Combined epidural and general anesthesia versus general anesthesia for abdominal aortic surgery. *Anesthesiology.* 1991;75(4):611–618.
70. Tuman KJ, McCarthy RJ, March RJ, et al. Effects of epidural anesthesia and analgesia on coagulation and outcome after major vascular surgery. *Anesth Analg.* 1991;73(6):696–704.
71. Viscusi ER, Martin G, Hartrick CT, et al. Forty-eight hours of postoperative pain relief after total hip arthroplasty with a novel, extended-release epidural morphine formulation. *Anesthesiology.* 2005;102(5):1014–1022.
72. Marik PE, Cavallazzi R, Vasu T, Hirani A. Dynamic changes in arterial waveform derived variables and fluid responsiveness in mechanically ventilated patients: a systematic review of the literature. *Crit Care Med.* 2009;37(9):2642–2647.
73. Lopes MR, Oliveira MA, Pereira VO, et al. Goal-directed fluid management based on pulse pressure variation monitoring during high-risk surgery: a pilot randomized controlled trial. *Crit Care.* 2007;11(5):R100.
74. Boulain T, Achard JM, Teboul JL, et al. Changes in BP induced by passive leg raising predict response to fluid loading in critically ill patients. *Chest.* 2002;121(4):1245–1252.
75. Shoemaker WC, Appel PL, Kram HB, et al. Prospective trial of supranormal values of survivors as therapeutic goals in high-risk surgical patients. *Chest.* 1988;94(6):1176–1186.
76. Hayes MA, Timmins AC, Yau EH, et al. Elevation of systemic oxygen delivery in the treatment of critically ill patients. *N Engl J Med.* 1994; 330(24):1717–1722.
77. Gattinoni L, Brazzi L, Pelosi P, et al. A trial of goal-oriented hemodynamic therapy in critically ill patients. SvO_2 Collaborative Group. *N Engl J Med.* 1995;333(16):1025–1032.
78. Sandham JD, Hull RD, Brant RF, et al. A randomized, controlled trial of the use of pulmonary-artery catheters in high-risk surgical patients. *N Engl J Med.* 2003;348(1):5–14.
79. Rivers E, Nguyen B, Havstad S, et al. Early goal-directed therapy in the treatment of severe sepsis and septic shock. *N Engl J Med.* 2001;345(19):1368–1377.
80. Yealy DM, Kellum JA, Huang DT, et al. A randomized trial of protocol-based care for early septic shock. *N Engl J Med.* 2014;370(18):1683–1693.
81. Mouncey PR, Osborn TM, Power GS, et al. Trial of early, goal-directed resuscitation for septic shock. *N Engl J Med.* 2015;372(14):1301–1311.
82. Peake SL, Delaney A, Bailey M, et al. Goal-directed resuscitation for patients with early septic shock. *N Engl J Med.* 2014;371(16):1496–1506.
83. Roy AK, Mc Gorrian C, Treacy C, et al. A comparison of traditional and novel definitions (RIFLE, AKIN, and KDIGO) of acute kidney injury for the prediction of outcomes in acute decompensated heart failure. *Cardiorenal Med.* 2013;3(1):26–37.
84. Hoste EA, De Corte W. Implementing the kidney disease: improving global outcomes/acute kidney injury guidelines in ICU patients. *Curr Opin Crit Care.* 2013;19(6):544–553.
85. Finfer S, Bellomo R, Boyce N, et al. A comparison of albumin and saline for fluid resuscitation in the intensive care unit. *N Engl J Med.* 2004;350(22):2247–2256.
86. Myburgh J, Cooper DJ, Finfer S, et al. Saline or albumin for fluid resuscitation in patients with traumatic brain injury. *N Engl J Med.* 2007; 357(9):874–884.
87. Perner A, Haase N, Guttormsen AB, et al. Hydroxyethyl starch 130/0.42 versus Ringer's acetate in severe sepsis. *N Engl J Med.* 2012;367(2):124–134.
88. Myburgh JA, Finfer S, Bellomo R, et al. Hydroxyethyl starch or saline for fluid resuscitation in intensive care. *N Engl J Med.* 2012;367(20):1901–1911.
89. Yunos NM, Bellomo R, Hegarty C, et al. Association between a chloride-liberal vs chloride-restrictive intravenous fluid administration strategy and kidney injury in critically ill adults. *JAMA.* 2012;308(15):1566–1572.
90. Apfel CC, Laara E, Koivuranta M, et al. A simplified risk score for predicting postoperative nausea and vomiting: conclusions from cross-validations between two centers. *Anesthesiology.* 1999;91(3):693–700.
91. Apfel CC, Korttila K, Abdalla M, et al. A factorial trial of six interventions for the prevention of postoperative nausea and vomiting. *N Engl J Med.* 2004;350(24):2441–2451.
92. Tramer M, Moore A, McQuay H. Meta-analytic comparison of prophylactic antiemetic efficacy for postoperative nausea and vomiting: propofol anaesthesia vs omitting nitrous oxide vs total i.v. anaesthesia with propofol. *Br J Anaesth.* 1997;78(3):256–259.
93. Tramer M, Moore A, McQuay H. Omitting nitrous oxide in general anaesthesia: meta-analysis of intraoperative awareness and postoperative emesis in randomized controlled trials. *Br J Anaesth.* 1996;76(2):186–193.
94. Marcantonio ER, Goldman L, Orav EJ, et al. The association of intraoperative factors with the development of postoperative delirium. *Am J Med.* 1998;105(5):380–384.
95. Bickel H, Gradinger R, Kochs E, Forstl H. High risk of cognitive and functional decline after postoperative delirium: a three-year prospective study. *Dement Geriatr Cogn Disord.* 2008;26(1):26–31.
96. Kat MG, Vreeswijk R, de Jonghe JF, et al. Long-term cognitive outcome of delirium in elderly hip surgery patients: a prospective matched controlled study over two and a half years. *Dement Geriatr Cogn Disord.* 2008;26(1):1–8.
97. Rudolph JL, Ramlawi B, Kuchel GA, et al. Chemokines are associated with delirium after cardiac surgery. *J Gerontol A Biol Sci Med Sci.* 2008;63(2):184–189.
98. Ely EW, Margolin R, Francis J, et al. Evaluation of delirium in critically ill patients: validation of the Confusion Assessment Method for the Intensive Care Unit (CAM-ICU). *Crit Care Med.* 2001;29(7):1370–1379.
99. Bergeron N, Dubois MJ, Dumont M, et al. Intensive Care Delirium Screening Checklist: evaluation of a new screening tool. *Intensive Care Med.* 2001;27(5):859–864.
100. Kress JP, Pohlman AS, O'Connor MF, Hall JB. Daily interruption of sedative infusions in critically ill patients undergoing mechanical ventilation. *N Engl J Med.* 2000;342(20):1471–1477.
101. Mehta S, Burry L, Cook D, et al. Daily sedation interruption in mechanically ventilated critically ill patients cared for with a sedation protocol: a randomized controlled trial. *JAMA.* 2012;308(19):1985–1992.
102. Girard TD, Kress JP, Fuchs BD, et al. Efficacy and safety of a paired sedation and ventilator weaning protocol for mechanically ventilated patients in intensive care (Awakening and Breathing Controlled trial): a randomised controlled trial. *Lancet.* 2008;371(9607):126–134.
103. Schweickert WD, Pohlman MC, Pohlman AS, et al. Early physical and occupational therapy in mechanically ventilated, critically ill patients: a randomised controlled trial. *Lancet.* 2009;373(9678):1874–1882.
104. Hopkins RO, Spuhler VJ, Thomsen GE. Transforming ICU culture to facilitate early mobility. *Crit Care Clin.* 2007;23(1):81–96.
105. Kansagara D, Fu R, Freeman M, et al. Intensive insulin therapy in hospitalized patients: a systematic review. *Ann Intern Med.* 2011;154(4):268–282.
106. Brunkhorst FM, Engel C, Bloos F, et al. Intensive insulin therapy and pentastarch resuscitation in severe sepsis. *N Engl J Med.* 2008;358(2):125–139.
107. Finfer S, Chittock DR, Su SY, et al. Intensive versus conventional glucose control in critically ill patients. *N Engl J Med.* 2009;360(13):1283–1297.
108. Qaseem A, Humphrey LL, Chou R, Snow V, Shekelle P. Use of intensive insulin therapy for the management of glycemic control in hospitalized patients: a clinical practice guideline from the American College of Physicians. *Ann Intern Med.* 2011;154(4):260–267.
109. Litman RS, Rosenberg H. Malignant hyperthermia: update on susceptibility testing. *JAMA.* 2005;293(23):2918–2924.

CHAPTER

55

Initial Management of the Critically Ill Trauma Patient

REX T. CHUNG and DANIEL R. MARGULIES

INTRODUCTION

Throughout the years, trauma has consistently been a leading cause of mortality worldwide. According to the World Health Organization (WHO), over 5 million deaths are attributed to traumatic injury annually accounting for 9% of global mortality (1). The largest contributors to these deaths are road traffic injuries, with an estimated 3,500 lives claimed per day. The latest WHO reports cite road traffic injuries as the eighth leading cause of death in all ages and the number one cause of death among those aged 15 to 29 years (2). In the United States, the most deaths occur among those 70 years and older and are primarily due to chronic diseases such as cardiovascular disease, cancer, stroke, COPD, and diabetes (3). However, unintentional injury still remains the fourth leading cause of death for all age groups in the United States and trauma is the leading cause of death in the United States among children, adolescents, and young adults ages 1 to 44 (4). Unlike the above-mentioned chronic diseases, a larger proportion of the overall deaths due to unintentional injury are represented in the younger populations (3).

Not only does trauma account for a large number of deaths, high medical costs and loss of productivity from permanent disability carry further impact on society. When injury is regarded as a category of disease, the economic impact of injury is substantial, with hundreds of billions of dollars in estimated lost wages, medical expenses, property damage, and administrative costs. One estimate by Centers for Disease Control and Prevention (CDC) place the total cost of injuries and violence in the United States in 2013 at $671 billion (5). This estimate is staggering in itself, but one can only imagine the impact on society in terms of lost human potential and the tremendous loss of life-years which is far more difficult to quantify and may be inherently underestimated. This makes trauma a particularly unique and tragic cause of mortality and morbidity.

The fact that trauma and trauma patients have such a significant impact on global society is not surprising. Nobody is immune to trauma and all have been affected directly or indirectly by a traumatic event. The trauma victim can present with a wide range of backgrounds and medical problems that may significantly influence the resiliency of the patient physiology and response to specific therapies. Certain populations require special considerations, including children, pregnant women, the elderly, and the obese. The latter two populations are increasingly prevalent. The baby boomer generation has reached retirement age and now contributes to the general geriatric population. The prevalence of those considered clinically obese is also increasing, recently estimated as one-third of adults and 17% of youth in the United States (6). Furthermore, injuries can involve any area of the body and not uncommonly affect multiple organ systems simultaneously. Adding to this complexity are the multitude of possible mechanisms of injury, each with varying degrees of severity. As will be discussed, it is helpful in the management of trauma to initially categorize these by mechanism: blunt versus penetrating.

Given such a diversity of scenarios and types of victims, major decisions in patient care are often made through a collaboration of various different surgical, medical, and radiologic specialists. Trauma patients first encountered in the field by first responders and the Emergency Medical Services (EMS) are then handed off to the emergency medicine physicians, trauma surgeons, and nurses in the emergency department upon arrival. Depending on the structure of the receiving Trauma Center, the prehospital information received, and the available resources, further members of the team that may be called early on include anesthesiologists, pharmacists, respiratory therapists, social workers, radiology technicians, and radiologists. More serious traumas may require further involvement of those in the blood bank, operating room, interventional radiology suite, intensive care unit, and surgical subspecialties such as neurosurgery, cardiothoracic surgery, and orthopedics. As the complexity of the trauma patient rises, the number of involved care providers also grows, and therefore the potential for miscommunication and error increases. All these variables and pitfalls challenge the provider even further when factoring in the time-sensitive nature of many major injuries. The more rapidly the injuries are identified and treated appropriately, the more likely the preventable death rate from trauma is reduced (7,8).

ADVANCED TRAUMA LIFE SUPPORT

Since the inception of Advanced Trauma Life Support (ATLS) in 1978, the course has become increasingly more widespread and now represents the mainstay of treatment of the acutely injured patient. The course was founded on the assumption that appropriate and timely care could significantly improve outcomes in trauma patients (9). Since then, data exists to demonstrate a positive impact from this approach (10,11). Studies show that ATLS training for doctors in developing countries have resulted in decreased injury mortality (12).

Central to ATLS is the premise of treating the greatest threat to life first, even before the exact diagnosis of the problem is identified, thus forming the basis for the initial assessment and management of the trauma patient. The mnemonic "ABCDE" is not only intentionally simple to remember, it emphasizes that certain patterns of injury kill in systematic time frames and therefore creates an inherent order. Loss of the airway, "A," regardless of mechanism, kills more readily than the loss in ability to breathe, "B." Likewise, loss of the ability to breathe kills more readily than loss of circulating blood volume, "C" (9). The basis for this can be understood at the molecular and cellular level as it relates to preservation of cellular respiration. "D" stands for disability signaling the identification of injuries to the central nervous system (CNS) of which prognosis is generally dependent on good oxygenation and circulation. Finally, "E" represents exposure and environment as a reminder to expose the entire body for general inspection followed by protecting the body from environmental threats, namely hypothermia.

Cells in the human body can survive only a relatively short amount of time without a steady supply of oxygen; resiliency to hypoxia is dependent upon the cell type. Oxygen, the final destination for electrons on the electron transport chain, is the driving force in cellular respiration. Without oxygen, the ATP-generating mitochondria will cease to function and the cell has an abrupt lack of energy to maintain adequate cellular function. Furthermore, the initial insult of hypoxia or associated hypoperfusion triggers a complex physiologic cascade which predisposes tissues to reperfusion injury exacerbating local vasoconstriction, thrombosis, free radical formation, and direct cellular damage. The brain especially has a very limited ability to store energy and therefore is particularly vulnerable to any lapse in supply of oxygen. Cellular injury and death may result from less than 5 minutes of anoxia. Assessing and managing the ABCs can therefore be thought of as prioritizing actions to best facilitate preservation of this vital pathway.

A compromised airway, inadequacies of breathing, and deficient effective circulating volume all further contribute to both metabolic and respiratory acidosis. With hypoxemia, cells resort to anaerobic metabolism in which lactic acid is a byproduct that builds up in the circulation. With hypoventilation, carbon dioxide is not removed from the blood and accumulates to dangerous levels. Hypotension and hypoperfusion to the kidney will result in impaired ability to remove acid from the body. Acidosis in itself will contribute to coagulopathy and multiple organ dysfunction. Severe acidosis will affect heart function and circulation is further impaired.

A major injury affecting the ABCs can thus lead the trauma victim to enter what has traditionally been termed the "lethal triad," consisting of hypothermia, acidosis, and coagulopathy. To successfully resuscitate the critically ill trauma patient, one must understand how elements of the lethal triad propagate one another, as well as how to halt the progression to avoid irreversibility and ultimately death.

PRIMARY SURVEY

The main objective of the primary survey is to identify and manage immediately life-threatening injuries in the most expeditious manner. It is within this critical stage that a heightened awareness and appropriate action can easily make the difference between life and death. Patient outcome is directly related to the time between injury and definitive care. The time-sensitive nature of this critical juncture has been emphasized by past studies demonstrating high mortality attributed to inadequate assessment and resuscitation in the initial phases (7,8).

ATLS advocates simultaneous evaluation and treatment because of the rapidity in which surviving these injuries demand. Having a general algorithm as a guide creates order in situations that are unpredictable and highly stressful and may give a sense of security to the situation. It is helpful to remember in the moment, that there are a limited number of rapidly lethal injury types that may present. Many of these have a rapidly corrective action to take for the best chance at survival. Also important to remember, the primary survey may need to be repeated at any time as trauma is often a dynamic clinical situation. As a general rule, if the patient becomes unstable at any time regardless of prior stability, one should go back and reassess the ABCs.

Airway

Ensuring a stable airway is the initial priority when managing a trauma patient. Regardless of the specific circumstances of the injury, the mechanism of cellular respiration is totally dependent on a secure access to an oxygen supply. When an airway is obstructed, the overall process by which oxygen is delivered to all the tissues of the body halts at the first step and the patient deteriorates quickly. Therefore, the unstable airway must be addressed before continuing on to assessment and treatment of breathing and circulation.

The first step in determining the status of the airway is by eliciting a verbal response from the patient. Patients that are conscious and respond by talking with a normal voice most likely do not have an immediate airway issue. Next, it is important to further assess for an impending airway obstruction or an airway that is at high risk for compromise. In the trauma setting, common examples include massive facial trauma where the airway is at risk for blockage with blood, broken teeth, or edematous soft tissues. Other injuries that threaten the airway are less obvious yet very important to identify early if present. Certain injuries to the neck may risk compromising the airway at the pharyngeal or tracheal level. Examples include penetrating injuries to the neck causing an expanding hematoma or direct tracheal laceration with intraluminal bleeding. Patients that suffer a significant burn must be assessed carefully for signs of an inhalation injury such as singed nasal hairs, soot around the mouth, oral mucosal swelling, anterior neck burn, or dysphonia. The most common situation where an airway may be at risk is in a patient with altered mental status due to severe head injury. Regardless of its etiology, the initial concern comes from the patient's inability to guard against dangers such as obstruction from the tongue, nasopharyngeal bleeding, or aspiration.

In the event that the patient is judged to have an unstable airway, immediate actions need to be taken to obtain a definitive airway; a definitive airway being a cuffed tube within the trachea. Rapid-sequence orotracheal intubation is the preferred method of ensuring airway stability. Although time is limited and tensions are high, it is worthwhile to ensure that equipment, appropriate medications, and ancillary resources are available prior to initiating the act of intubation. It has been demonstrated that the risk of adverse events increases with the number of intubation attempts, therefore it is important to adequately prepare for the intervention (13). Everyone on the team should be aware that the decision has been made to intubate the patient. In this way, one is best able to maintain order and minimize miscommunication. Failure to do so and the "easy" airway can become a "difficult" airway. If adequate oxygenation and ventilation is achieved with Bag-Valve-Mask (BVM), there should be enough time for preparation.

However, it is important to remember that with each assisted ventilation, the stomach becomes more distended with air, and vomiting and aspiration become more likely complications. The coordination of multiple support services is the key to maintaining control over the situation, namely the pharmacist, respiratory therapist, and the involved nurses. Medications for induction and neuromuscular paralysis (typically Etomidate for induction and Succinylcholine for rapid onset transient paralysis) should be drawn and confirmed prior to initiating laryngoscopy and endotracheal intubation.

Simultaneously, the equipment for intubation should be retrieved, checked, and made ready for use. One should assume that a cervical spine injury has not been ruled out prior to the decision to intubate; therefore in-line stabilization must continue throughout the procedure. This is ensured by dedicating one person to manually stabilize the cervical spine while the collar is removed and continue monitoring until the patient is successfully intubated, endotracheal tube (ETT) secured, and collar replaced. The patient should be suctioned and preoxygenated with a high-flow mask or BVM prior to intubation. Often an oropharyngeal airway (OPA) is useful because tongue obstruction is common in the unconscious patient which may only occur after induction and paralysis. Preoxygenation should be attempted; however, times that the instability of the airway is dire or attempts at preoxygenation continue to fail, one should not prolong the situation by waiting for the SaO_2 to rise. Hypotensive patients may not have adequate perfusion such that a pulse oximetry reading is unavailable or inaccurate. In these cases, intubation should proceed without hesitation.

It is advisable to have a second method for intubation immediately available, typically special equipment in the event of a difficult airway. Video laryngoscopy is being more frequently used and has superior visualization to direct laryngoscopy when performed appropriately (14). Confirmation of successful endotracheal intubation is made by direct visualization of the tube passing the vocal cords, capnography, auscultation of bilateral breath sounds with absence of sounds over the epigastrium, and ultimately with a chest radiograph. One should also be prepared for the hemodynamic effects of induction and positive pressure ventilation as hypotension may occur due to increased intrathoracic pressure and subsequent decreased venous return. Volume resuscitation is often needed and it is imperative to obtain a chest x-ray (CXR) soon after intubation to assess for proper tube position and absence of pneumothorax (15).

In less frequent cases, a surgical airway is indicated and appropriate preparation for this contingency should also be made. Situations that may require a surgical airway include massive facial trauma which obscures visualization, repeated failed intubation attempts which may exacerbate vocal cord edema, or direct laryngeal trauma that distorts the anatomy. It is important to have a low threshold to perform a surgical airway when repeated attempts to intubate are failing. A surgical airway may be started while attempts at intubation are ongoing. A generous vertical incision should be made over the cricothyroid membrane to avoid the laterally approaching blood supply and if the need arises to extend the incision superiorly or inferiorly. The thyroid is avoided at this level and there is minimal soft tissue to hinder access to the cricothyroid space. The cricothyroid membrane should then be incised with the scalpel and the opening dilated with a Kelly clamp or scalpel handle. If an appropriately sized tracheostomy tube is available this should be placed; otherwise, using a 6F or larger ETT is acceptable in emergent situations.

Breathing

A stable airway implies a secure and unobstructed path by which oxygenated air can access the lungs. However, this does not necessarily imply that breathing is adequate. Effective breathing involves proper functioning of the mechanical, physiologic, and cellular mechanisms responsible for delivering air through the airway to an alveolar surface for gas exchange. Injuries that may compromise this process to varying degrees of severity include rib fractures, flail chest, pulmonary contusion, pneumothorax, hemothorax, diaphragmatic rupture, and paralysis.

Assessment for effective oxygenation and ventilation begins by looking at the patient even as they are rolling into the trauma bay. All trauma patients that present should be provided supplemental oxygen via nasal cannula and placed on pulse oximetry monitoring. The patient may be awake and talking thereby demonstrating an open airway and the ability to move air. However, the patient may still not be oxygenating and ventilating adequately. Does the patient appear to be short of breath, struggling against restraints to sit up, using accessory muscles, or outright declaring a difficult time breathing?

First, one must globally assess for signs of impending acute respiratory failure including tachycardia, tachypnea, retractions, and diaphoresis. Focus on visually inspecting the neck and chest wall for signs of injury such as contusions, lacerations, chest asymmetry, or splinting. Auscultate the chest over the anterior and lateral lung fields especially taking note of any difference between the breath sounds bilaterally. Finally, palpate over the clavicles, sternum, and rib cage for crepitus, tenderness, chest wall deformity, or flail segment. Unfortunately, the most severely compromised patients are those that are not awake, talking coherently, or moving air at all, making assessment much more difficult.

Two major interventions need to be considered during the breathing assessment of the primary survey prior to moving forward: pleural space decompression with tube thoracostomy and intubation with mechanical ventilatory support.

A tube thoracostomy is the initial management for acute respiratory failure due to pneumothorax or hemothorax. A tension pneumothorax is an extremely dangerous situation which develops when the lung collapses from pleural space violation with reversal of its normal negative pressure state to positive pressure through a one-way valve mechanism. Air enters the pleural space through an injury to the tracheobronchial tree, lung parenchyma, or directly through the chest wall, and becomes trapped in the pleural space. With each breath, the air pressure in the pleural space increases, resulting in further collapse and compression of the lung, affecting both respiratory function and hemodynamics simultaneously and therefore rapidly lethal. A tube thoracostomy should not be delayed to confirm this diagnosis by radiography if suspected. The problem may be temporized by decompressive needle thoracostomy using a large bore angiocath prior to placing the chest tube. This can be performed at the second intercostal space at the midclavicular line. Alternatively, this can be performed at the fifth intercostal space at the midaxillary line, especially in those with a large amount of soft tissue overlying the anterior chest (16). A large hemothorax has a pathophysiology similar to tension pneumothorax but may further be complicated by hemorrhagic shock given the extent of concurrent blood loss. Treatment also starts with placing a chest tube which will relieve the tamponade effect and allow expansion of the lung, but also allows further blood loss and possible worsening hemorrhagic shock.

An open pneumothorax, also termed a sucking chest wound, is also rapidly lethal and occurs when the chest wall is violated from the skin to the level of the pleural space. If the chest wall defect is of comparable size to the tracheal lumen, the negative pressure generated by attempted breathing may cause air to traverse the wound rather than inflate the lungs via the trachea. It often presents with audible air movement and bubbling over a large chest wound. Treatment for this involves immediately covering the defect, preferentially with an occlusive dressing or a gloved hand followed by a chest tube. Definitive closure in the operating room will also be needed.

Other major injuries causing acute respiratory failure that may need to be addressed with intubation and mechanical ventilation include rib fractures, flail chest, pulmonary contusion, and paralysis of the diaphragm or chest wall. Assisted ventilation can be attained manually via face mask, laryngeal mask airway, King tube, or ETT. Once stabilized and a definitive airway is placed, the patient can then be placed on a mechanical ventilator. Arterial blood gas (ABG) analysis should be obtained early and adjustments made accordingly.

Circulation

After addressing the airway and breathing status of the patient, assessment and management of circulation becomes the next priority in the primary survey. Simply, the immediate goal is to ensure delivery of a steady supply of oxygenated blood from the lungs to the rest of the cells in the body. Failure of the body to accomplish this means that the patient is in shock. Shock is defined as the inadequate perfusion of oxygenated blood to the end-organs resulting in tissue death or injury at the cellular level.

Evaluation of circulation begins with palpation of peripheral pulses. Important information gained from this simple act include determining the presence or absence of a pulse, estimating the heart rate and regularity, as well as judging the quality of the pulse, be it bounding or thready. A quick estimate of systolic blood pressure (SBP) based on a pulse examination can be useful at times, especially as an exact blood pressure reading by cuff measurement takes a significantly longer time to attain. Furthermore, a pneumatic cuff will fail to read when a blood pressure is extremely low. Generally, a palpable radial pulse correlates to an SBP of at least 80 mmHg. Likewise, a palpable femoral pulse correlates to SBP of 70 mmHg and a carotid pulse correlates to an SBP of at least 60 mmHg. One should not wait for a cuff pressure reading prior to taking action if a pulse examination suggests blood pressure is low. One must assume that the patient is in shock and proceed with aggressive resuscitation.

Simultaneously with circulation assessment, appropriate intravenous (IV) access should be attained. This is a critical and often underappreciated priority during the primary survey. At times, lack of intravenous access can become the rate-limiting step to providing the needed resuscitation in forms of volume, medications, and blood products. The most frustrating trauma resuscitation situations are those limited by the inability to deliver IV therapy simply because of lack of access. Two large bore angiocaths should be placed, preferably on each of the upper extremities. Two separate access points ensures that blood volume can be delivered twice as fast and that there is a redundancy in place in case an IV becomes dislodged or stops working. Unfortunately, the higher the severity of hemorrhagic shock, the more difficult it is to place IVs as the veins are collapsed and autonomic peripheral vasoconstriction decreases extremity blood flow. In these situations, attention may need to be directed toward attaining more advanced IV access such as a large bore central venous line (CVL), intraosseous (IO) catheter, or a saphenous vein cut down. Intraosseous catheter placement is being used more often in adult patients in shock and can be performed within seconds (17). Once access to the circulation is attained, isotonic fluids infusion should be initiated.

The heart should be auscultated for irregularity, murmurs, or muffled heart sounds, although the noise of the trauma bay makes this difficult at times. A blood pressure cuff should be placed and serial measurements obtained. A useful parameter to note and monitor is the pulse pressure. The pulse pressure will decrease with increasing amounts of blood loss. The loss of effective blood volume causes both a decrease in the SBP and a reflex peripheral vasoconstriction which raises the diastolic blood pressure (DBP). If the automated blood pressure cuff cycles and is unable to provide a measurement, one should be aware that this very well may be due to extreme blood loss with hypotension resulting in equipment error. Hypotension should be assumed until a more accurate reading can be obtained, possibly by obtaining a manual pressure and shifting more reliance on other measurable parameters such as heart rate and pulse character to gauge hemodynamic stability until an accurate measurement can be attained.

There are various types of shock that one may encounter in the critically ill trauma patient including cardiogenic, neurogenic, and septic. However, the most important to rule out early in the setting of trauma is hemorrhagic shock. Hemorrhage is the leading cause of preventable death in the injured patient (7,8). Therefore, identifying bleeding and taking actions to halt it should be the main priority during this stage of the primary survey. Managing the patient in hemorrhagic shock is often, and rightfully so, a stressful situation for the entire team. To maintain a clear focus on the problem, it is helpful to systematically and rapidly consider life-threatening blood loss as coming from five possible sources: the external environment, long bone fractures, the pelvis/retroperitoneum, the thoracic cavity, and the abdominal cavity.

The source of external blood loss is often obvious, such as a large laceration with active bleeding that can be identified readily on physical examination or indicated by the patient's pain. Quickly scan for any sign of a large wound or bloody surfaces on the patient's body and gain immediate control by exposing the area and applying directed point pressure if significant bleeding is detected. At other times, the external bleeding source is less obvious. Significant laceration on the back or perineum may not be initially appreciated until the patient has been logrolled and thoroughly examined. At times, an external injury may already be hemostatic, but starts to bleed again with the onset of resuscitation. The extent of blood loss from an injury may also not be fully appreciated as the blood is "on the floor," meaning it has already been lost in the field or literally on the floor of the trauma bay. A scalp laceration should not be underestimated; a person can fully exsanguinate from an isolated scalp laceration and these injuries may not be easily controlled. Massive bleeding from an extremity may not be adequately controlled with pressure alone and in this situation, a tourniquet would be appropriate to utilize. Recent studies have shown a survival benefit without increase in rates of adverse outcomes or amputations associated with the use of a tourniquet for hemorrhage control in major trauma (18,19).

Long bone fractures that account for life-threatening bleeding as well should be detectable on physical examination as a significant deformity. A person can lose up to 2 L of blood per thigh from a severe associated femur fracture. Thus, bilateral femoral fractures can account for more than half of a patient's total blood volume. Control of bleeding from long bone fractures can be aided by fracture reduction with or without traction splinting. Early consultation with orthopedics can be helpful as they can greatly aid in managing this source of bleeding, especially in the multisystem trauma patients.

The remaining three sources of potentially life-threatening bleeding—thoracic cavity, pelvis/retroperitoneum, and abdominal cavity—are less readily ruled out by physical examination. Therefore the role of adjunctive imaging immediately available in the trauma bay greatly facilitates rapid identification of these bleeding sources.

The thoracic cavity is normally well protected by the sternum, rib cage, and spinal column. However, once violated by either blunt or penetrating trauma, major injury to the residing structures is often fatal. Physical examination of the chest may reveal a penetrating wound, deformity, absence of breath sounds, tenderness, or bony crepitus. An underlying hemothorax can be rapidly fatal as each pleural cavity can hold up to 2 L of blood. A portable CXR is thus an invaluable adjunct to identifying a thoracic source of bleeding. Placing a thoracostomy tube will both confirm suspicion of a hemothorax and act as an immediate treatment by allowing for lung expansion. The hemodynamic response from a chest tube may vary. Relieving tension physiology may allow the component of cardiogenic shock to be relieved. However, allowing an outlet for the bleeding which was somewhat controlled by the confined space of the thorax may exacerbate further bleeding and hypotension and one should pay close attention to the physiologic response to this intervention. Once in place, the thoracostomy tube then provides use as a measuring tool to aid in determining if the patient needs more extensive operative exploration with surgical bleeding control. One should note the initial volume of blood evacuated from the chest, as well as the rate at which blood loss is occurring. Guidelines proposed by ATLS state that an initial output of greater than 1,500 mL of blood or more than 250 mL blood loss per hour should prompt anterolateral thoracotomy and surgical control of bleeding (9). Other important findings on CXR to suggest a thoracic source of bleeding may include a widened mediastinum, spinal fractures, or lung field opacity.

A major pelvic fracture is often a source of bleeding that can be difficult to manage for a variety of reasons. One reason is that the pelvis has three sources of potential bleeding: arterial, venous, and osseous. Another complicating factor is that a pelvic fracture does not necessarily bleed into a discreet cavity, but rather can expand and track along the retroperitoneum, an often underappreciated but considerably large reservoir for blood loss. Many fractures do violate the abdominal cavity where even more bleeding can spill into. Furthermore, 30% of major pelvic fractures are associated with a concomitant intra-abdominal injury (9). When bleeding is suspected to be from either or both the pelvis and abdomen, it may be difficult to determine where to proceed next. During the primary survey, start by scanning the area around the pelvis for signs of a significant injury including deformity and ecchymosis. The pelvis should be handled by palpating the iliac crests bilaterally and then gently adducting to assess for stability, noting if the patient describes pain or if there is any induced movement from this action. The normal pelvis is a strong bony ring and should have no laxity. Care must be taken to avoid applying excessive outward pressure or "rocking the pelvis" as this may exacerbate further bleeding if a fracture is indeed present. More information may be gained by obtaining a pelvic x-ray at this time especially if the patient remains hemodynamically unstable in the trauma bay. Depending on the fracture pattern, temporary pelvic reduction may be helpful in controlling blood loss by using a pelvic binder or wrapping the pelvis with a sheet. Note that certain fracture patterns may actually be worsened by applying a binder and therefore this should not be employed in pelvic fractures indiscriminately. Early consultation with orthopedics is often helpful.

Difficult situations occur when a patient is hypotensive and has an identified pelvic fracture on x-ray. Initial management includes volume resuscitation with or without pelvic reduction. Most pelvic bleeding will be stemmed by these early conservative measures as the tamponade effect of the hematoma and pelvic volume reduction overcomes bleeding from the bone and venous plexus. The question of what to do next arises if the patient remains hypotensive. Approximately 10% of severe pelvic fractures will have bleeding from an arterial source which does not tamponade to a halt readily. Although a CT can often elucidate the source more accurately than an x-ray, it is not appropriate to transport the patient for imaging if the patient is hemodynamically unstable. It is also not necessarily appropriate to venture to the OR in these cases because surgical control of bleeding is extremely difficult considering the inaccessibility of a narrow pelvis, the complex sacral venous plexus, and the retroperitoneal reservoir of blood loss that is not well controlled with simply packing the pelvis intraperitoneally. There is evidence for significant reduction in blood transfusion requirement and trend toward reduction in mortality with preperitoneal pelvic packing in selected high-risk patients (20).

The mainstay of source control for suspected pelvic arterial bleeding in the persistently hypotensive patient is angiography and angioembolization. Several challenges arise when pursuing this avenue of treatment. First and foremost, this modality may not be readily available to the patient. Also, precious time is diverted to notifying and mobilizing the Interventional Radiology team, after which the equipment must then be prepared and the patient needs to be transported to the radiology suite. This location is often separate from the OR and may be a difficult decision if other sources of bleeding are being simultaneously considered. Because of this, some centers are implementing use of hybrid OR/IR suites such that these contingencies can be partially accounted for (21).

The fifth potential source of major bleeding is the abdomen, classically considered the "black box," as it is often the most difficult to rule out. During the primary survey, examination of the abdomen consists of looking for signs such as open wounds, ecchymosis, distention, and abdominal pain. There are many specific sources of bleeding within the abdominal cavity that can account for hemorrhagic shock. Spending valuable time trying to guess which organ is responsible can easily be overwhelming and pointless. Regardless of the specific organ or vessel involved, if the source is deemed intra-abdominal, the next step is to proceed to the operating room for abdominal exploration. Therefore, the crucial step in the algorithm is determining if the bleeding and hemorrhagic shock originates in the abdominal cavity. Two modalities can be employed in the trauma bay for this step: the focused abdominal sonography for trauma (FAST) examination and diagnostic peritoneal lavage (DPL).

With increased utilization of ultrasound technology, FAST examination has largely supplanted DPL as it is rapid, noninvasive, and accurate. The FAST examination includes obtaining four views or windows: the pericardial, perihepatic, perisplenic, and pelvic. For the pericardial window, the probe is placed in the epigastrium and directed cephalad to assess for fluid in the pericardial space that may be indicative of cardiac tamponade. The perihepatic, perisplenic, and pelvic windows are assessed to determine the presence of intra-abdominal fluid, which in a hypotensive trauma patient should be considered blood until otherwise ruled out. Avoid wasting an excessive amount of time reviewing the FAST when a patient is hypotensive. It is either positive for tamponade or not, positive for abdominal fluid or not. Simplifying the assessment and management process in this way is helpful for rapidly proceeding to the next step to resolve the shock state. It is also noteworthy to understand that the window in which the FAST examination is positive does not necessarily correlate with the organ injured (22). Another advantage of the FAST examination being rapid and noninvasive is that it can easily be repeated in cases of refractory or recurrent hypotension.

If the FAST is positive and the patient is hemodynamically unstable, the patient should immediately be taken for an exploratory laparotomy. However, if the FAST is positive and the patient is hemodynamically stable, the patient should be evaluated with a CT abdomen pelvis with contrast to assess for the source of intra-abdominal free fluid.

If the FAST is negative, other sources for hemorrhage should be assessed and the FAST examination should be repeated as sufficient blood volume may not have accumulated. In this situation, another option would be to perform a diagnostic peritoneal lavage (DPL) or a diagnostic peritoneal aspirate (DPA). The DPL involves entering the abdomen via a periumbilical incision and inserting a catheter to aspirate for blood or intestinal contents and infuse a liter of saline. The saline is then allowed to return to the bag and the fluid can be analyzed with specific criteria indicating positivity. As one can imagine, the disadvantages of this technique is that it is invasive, time-consuming, and susceptible to problems with infusion or fluid return. More often it is more expeditious and practical to perform a related procedure, the DPA. This involves accessing the abdominal cavity in the same manner, but relying on the results of simply aspirating for gross blood to determine positivity. If these adjuncts to the primary survey lead one to believe that the source of hemorrhagic shock is the abdominal cavity, the next step is abdominal exploration for control of the bleeding source.

If the reason for shock is indeed hemorrhagic, then halting blood loss is the most crucial step to affect survival. Although often the initial thought is how and when to control this bleeding surgically, it is important to remember the nonsurgical adjuncts that may be employed simultaneously. Tranexamic acid (TXA) is an antifibrinolytic agent that has gained recognition in acute trauma by demonstrating improved survival if given within 3 hours of injury in those with severe blood loss (23,24). Other situations where facilitating hemostasis nonsurgically may be indicated are in patients on antiplatelet medications, such as Aspirin or Plavix, or anticoagulation such as Warfarin. In such cases, platelet transfusion, vitamin K, fresh frozen plasma (FFP), and prothrombin complex concentrate (PCC) may be utilized. Recently, there has been popularity of newer anticoagulant agents for cardiac and thromboembolic disease in the form of direct thrombin inhibitors (e.g., Dabigatran) and direct factor Xa inhibitors (e.g., Rivaroxaban, Apixaban). Unfortunately, no approved reversal agents for these medications have demonstrated efficacy.

Although the identification and control of bleeding is the most important factor determining survival in the setting of hemorrhagic shock, morbidity and mortality can be curtailed by repleting blood volume loss with blood transfusion therapy as well. ATLS continues to promote volume resuscitation in shock with up to 2 L of isotonic IV fluid prior to starting blood transfusion (9). In the event of massive hemorrhage, evidence supports a survival benefit in patients that undergo what is termed the massive transfusion protocol (MTP). MTP involves complementing each packed red blood cell (PRBC) unit transfused with addition of FFP and platelets. Initial studies have utilized a 1:1:1 (PRBC/FFP/platelet) ratio to demonstrate benefit; however, the exact ratio of these components has not been definitively determined. Massive transfusion is defined as needing to receive more than 10 units of PRBC within the first 24 hours (25,26).

Much of the focus in circulation assessment of the primary survey is centered on hemorrhage. However, other causes of shock in the setting of trauma need to be considered, especially if one is unable to determine a source of bleeding. Furthermore, a more severely injured patient may have multiple affected organ systems, and therefore multiple reasons to be in shock. Cardiogenic shock may result from cardiac tamponade, blunt cardiac injury, or acute myocardial infarction. Cardiac tamponade may be suspected in penetrating injury to an area termed the "box," defined by the clavicles superiorly, the nipple lines laterally, and the costal margin inferiorly. Although tamponade may be diagnosed through classic signs described as Beck triad (hypotension, jugular venous distention, and muffled heart sounds), more likely the diagnosis is established during FAST examination. Definitive treatment for this may involve sternotomy or thoracotomy with pericardiotomy and control of bleeding. Blunt cardiac injury may also contribute to shock, though is rarely the sole cause. A more likely scenario for cardiac injury is secondary to myocardial ischemia or infarction secondary to rapid and large volume blood loss. Neurogenic shock is also a consideration when dealing with a major trauma victim. This occurs secondary to a spinal cord injury and concurrent loss of sympathetic tone to the peripheral vessels.

When a trauma patient arrives without a palpable pulse, an emergency department thoracotomy (EDT) may be beneficial in rare cases (27). It is most effective in victims of penetrating trauma that present with recent loss of pulses or signs of life if performed within 15 minutes onset of prehospital CPR (28). However, thoracotomy is rarely of benefit to victims of blunt trauma and overwhelmingly so, with meaningful survival benefits in less than 5% of blunt trauma patients that present in shock and less than 1% of patients that present to the ED without vital signs (29).

Disability

The disability portion of the primary survey involves assessing the neurologic status of the patient once the immediate problems regarding airway, breathing, and circulation have been addressed. This assessment involves determining the Glasgow Coma Score (GCS) of the patient, examining the pupillary size, reactivity to light, and symmetry when compared to each other, as well as noting any obvious sensorimotor deficits and/or lateralizing signs. The key concern with an abnormal neurologic examination is CNS injury, namely traumatic brain injury (TBI) or spinal cord injury. Although nothing can be done to reverse the initial insult or primary CNS injury, avoiding secondary injury to the brain and spinal cord is vital to obtaining the best possible outcome from this type of trauma. The acutely injured brain is especially sensitive to both hypoxia and hypotension. Mortality rates of those patients with severe TBI with hypotension on admission are more than twice that of patients without hypotension. A single hypoxic event documented in TBI patients with concurrent hypotension increases mortality even further (30). Therefore prioritizing the ABCs is the best course of treatment in this population. After hemodynamic stabilization, other important factors to control include minimizing elevations in intracranial pressure (ICP), maintaining normothermia, and decreasing the incidence of posttraumatic seizures. Early consultation with neurosurgical colleagues is advised to help guide medical supportive care in TBI patients, as well as determining which patients are candidates for emergent surgical decompression.

Exposure/Environment

After assuring hemodynamic stability and addressing the neurologic status, the next step in the primary survey is denoted by the letter "E." This should prompt one to think of exposure and environment. The entire patient is exposed by removing all clothing such that one lessens the chance of missing a significant injury that needs to be treated early (31). Although removing layers of clothing contributes to hypothermia somewhat, ongoing blood loss or a large wound from a missed injury is a larger heat sink and a threat to adequate circulation as well. Therefore, full examination should be performed expeditiously and thoroughly prior to covering the patient with warm blankets and obtaining a check of body temperature. Hypothermia contributes to coagulopathy and multiple organ dysfunction syndrome (MODS). In fact, hypothermia is a component of the classically taught Lethal Triad of Trauma: Hypothermia, Coagulopathy, and Acidosis. If hypothermia is severe, one should divert more attention to a variety of methods to counteract this. Options in this arena include using warmed IV fluids or blood, warming the air given through the ventilator, or at the most extreme level, active internal rewarming which may involve irrigating body spaces (e.g., pleura) with warmed fluids or even rewarming through ECMO.

Assessment for Transfer

By the end of the primary survey, the patient should have reached a certain level of stability such that one can take a moment to decide on the best course of definitive management for the patient. If the sustained injuries require definitive management beyond the capacity of the hospital, interhospital consultation with the nearest facility where the patient can receive that care is indicated. Delaying this process is associated with increased mortality (32,33). The facility that can provide the higher level of care should be contacted and physician-to-physician communication detailing the injuries identified and management performed thus far should take place. It is important to remember that the workup does not have to be fully completed prior to transfer as this may delay the patient from receiving definitive care. If a CT scan is necessary to elucidate injuries, this should be deferred as it can be performed at the tertiary care center under the guidance of the accepting physician. Energy and focus should be diverted to arranging appropriate transport, compiling the relevant information to send with the patient, and assessing for any additional interventions needed to guard against clinical deterioration en route. The patient may need intubation for airway protection, a chest tube placement for pneumothorax prior to air transport, or fracture reduction and stabilization to curb bleeding. If there is time while awaiting arrival of transport, then a more thorough history and quick secondary survey may be performed as long as it does not cause further delay to definitive care.

SECONDARY SURVEY

Although the primary survey serves to identify and treat rapidly lethal injuries and ensure that oxygenated blood is delivered to the peripheral tissues, the secondary survey involves a more meticulous and comprehensive review to identify and possibly treat all of the injuries that the patient presents with. Additionally, the background history of the event and prior medical issues come to light at this time. It is worth emphasizing that if the patient clinically deteriorates or becomes hemodynamically unstable at this time, the secondary survey should be aborted and the ABCs reassessed. For example, the patient may have a delayed presentation of intra-abdominal bleeding and need an urgent laparotomy and would therefore be managed in the OR until stability is reassured. The secondary survey may need to be completed after this event.

The secondary survey resembles the more structured H&P that one performs with any new patient but generally more expedient and injury-focused. It is important to acknowledge that other issues seemingly unrelated to the trauma may impact the treatment course for the patient, such as chronic medical problems, past surgeries, social habits, or daily medications.

History

In the acute trauma setting, the history is often pieced together from multiple sources due to the level of distress or impairment the patient is experiencing. The prehospital provider often has the advantage of witnessing the scene of the accident. For example, they may have gained a sense of how much blood was on the ground, how much damage was done to the vehicle, how high the victim fell, or the position the patient was found in. They may have gained information from witnesses of the event, obtained history from the patient prior to deterioration, or observed changes in the patient status from the time of contact to the time of presentation to the ED. Therefore one should consider carefully and deliberately the report given by the prehospital caretaker as it may provide invaluable information. If the clinical status of the patient is such that one cannot receive the initial sign out, the information should be obtained by another member of the team, or the EMS provider may be asked to stay until this can be done.

To aid one in expeditiously obtaining the most relevant information for the situation from the patient, it is helpful to obtain an "AMPLE" history. Each letter correspond the following: "A" for allergies, "M" for medications, "P" for past medical history/past surgical history/pregnancy, "L" for last meal, "E" for events surrounding the trauma (9). Obtaining a list of current medications may be especially relevant and often dictates further management. Beta-blockers are a common medication prescribed and may inhibit a patient from mounting a tachycardic response to traumatic bleeding. Antiplatelet agents are also very commonly encountered and may necessitate actively reversing the effects through platelet transfusion (34). Anticoagulants like warfarin are extremely important to note, especially in those with suspected TBI. Rapid correction of coagulopathy in these case have demonstrated improvement in long-term outcome (35,36).

Physical Examination

Although the physical examination should be performed quickly, it also needs to be meticulous and comprehensive. A head-to-toe assessment is therefore carried out in a standardized manner. By this point, the patient has had all clothing removed during the primary survey and most of the body can be readily examined without delay or disruption in focus. After this is done, it is important to check the back and perineum, which can be areas that hide significant injuries. A dedicated person at the head maintains C-spine precautions and is in charge of verbally directing the log roll. The patient should not assist in moving during this time. At least two additional people are needed to roll the patient in a manner to maintain full spinal precautions. Often a third person assisting with maneuvering the legs is necessary especially with a known lower extremity fracture. Finally, an experienced provider checks the back for any signs of injury from top to bottom, palpates each spinal level for midline tenderness, deformity, or step-offs, and then does a check of the perineum, including a rectal examination if indicated. Findings should be clearly verbalized to the nurse documenting the examination.

Head Trauma and Traumatic Brain Injury

The scalp is checked for lacerations, hematomas, or skull deformities. A thorough palpation of the entire head often finds injuries missed on visual inspection. The posterior aspect of the head is difficult to fully examine and may need to be better assessed when the patient is log-rolled. Large scalp lacerations can bleed significantly and may need to be addressed immediately with staples, suture ligation, or Raney clips. Any sign of injury to the head should increase suspicion for TBI. All patients with altered mental status, loss of consciousness, or significant mechanism should receive a CT scan of the head. This may be deferred only if the patient is neurologically intact with no evidence of posttraumatic amnesia, confusion, or impaired alertness (37).

Facial Trauma

Facial trauma may be obvious upon initial presentation, but in many cases can be subtle and prone to missed detection. It is particularly important to check certain areas that can be occult but very relevant to management. Any abnormality should prompt one to obtain a dedicated CT scan of the face. Aside from the pupillary examination, the eyes are checked more thoroughly for signs of globe injury, extraocular movement abnormality, or visual impairment. An orbital fracture is among the most commonly missed injuries and may be missed on physical examination. The nares should be inspected for deformity, CSF drainage, bleeding, and septal hematoma. The maxilla should be checked for tenderness to movement or instability that may be present in a LeFort fracture. Asking the patient to voluntarily open and close the jaw to assess for abnormal alignment may reveal injury to the maxilla or mandible. The oropharynx should be inspected for tongue lacerations, broken teeth, soft tissue swelling, or signs of inhalation injury. A basilar skull fracture may be detected by noticing periorbital or retroauricular ecchymosis, hemotympanum, or clear fluid from the nose or auditory canal.

Neck Injuries

The neck is a very important area to spend additional attention on during the secondary survey. Injuries to the neck are often missed initially, but have the potential for great morbidity and mortality considering the major vital structures in such a compact space. A cervical collar placed in the field may further hinder a good examination. It is important to stress that the c-spine collar must be removed to perform a thorough examination and that c-spine precautions should be maintained while the collar is removed. It is not acceptable to solely examine the neck through the holes in the collar. If an occult injury is identified, quickly reconsider if the airway needs to be secured as some neck injuries can progress rapidly even if they initially seem minor. Examination of the neck starts with the classification of trauma as penetrating or blunt mechanism.

With penetrating injuries, the examination focuses on if the platysma is violated and where the injury is in regards to the three zones of the neck. Assessment for "hard signs" or "soft signs" will dictate whether to operate immediately or to obtain further investigation. Examples of "hard signs" of neck trauma include pulsatile or expansile masses, active bleeding, stigmata of airway compromise or involvement, hematemesis and neurologic deficits. "Soft signs" of neck trauma include subcutaneous emphysema, difficulty breathing or swallowing, nonexpansile nonpulsatile hematoma, paresthesias. Both Zone I and Zone III injuries in the stable patient need further evaluation of the vascular structures and the aerodigestive tract. This may be with the aid of CT angiography (CTA), laryngoscopy, bronchoscopy, esophagoscopy, and contrast esophagram. In the past, all zone II injuries past the platysma were surgically explored. Nowadays, elective nonoperative management is acceptable for asymptomatic and hemodynamically stable patients in this neck region (38).

Blunt injuries to the neck tend to be even less obvious, but can be equally morbid. The airway may be a concern if a significant hematoma causing airway compression or direct damage to the larynx or trachea is suspected. Blunt esophageal injuries are rare. The neurovascular examination is especially important considering the potential for a cervical spine injury or a blunt cerebrovascular injury (BCVI). Although a somewhat rare occurrence, blunt injury to the carotid or vertebral arteries can have devastating outcomes if not identified and treated early. Risk factors that necessitate screening according to the Western Trauma Association guidelines include: high cervical spine fractures, cervical spine fractures involving the vertebral foramina, basilar skull fractures, LeFort II and III fractures, closed head injury with diffuse axonal injury or GCS less than 6, and hanging injuries. Screening can be performed using CTA (16-slice or greater) which may need a conventional 4-vessel angiogram if findings are equivocal (39). Intervention varies with grade of injury and more severe injuries may need operative or endovascular intervention. Less severe injuries may be managed with antiplatelet agents or anticoagulation. Recent data have demonstrated equal efficacy when retrospectively comparing antiplatelet therapy and therapeutic heparin (40). Typically, treatment decisions are influenced by concurrent injuries and risks of bleeding.

Thoracic Trauma

Much discussion regarding trauma to the chest has been discussed earlier in this chapter while describing the primary survey. This underscores the importance of examining this body region more thoroughly during the secondary survey. Visually inspect for lacerations, gunshot wounds, bruising, deformities, and asymmetry while the patient breathes. Palpate and auscultate each region of the thorax as more subtle injuries may have been missed in the primary survey. The CXR is particularly useful in identifying pneumothoraces, hemothoraces, or rib fractures. It is less useful for more occult injuries and further investigation is often needed with a CT scan. An aortic injury may be suspected if the CXR demonstrates a widened mediastinum, blunting of the aortic knob, or deviation of the NGT. This should be followed up with a CTA of the chest and if found, should be directed to cardiothoracic surgery. Initial management is heart rate and blood pressure control. Definitive surgical treatment may be deferred if other injuries necessitate alternative management such as TBI necessitating emergent operative evacuation or intra-abdominal bleeding needing operative control (41).

Blunt cardiac injury should be suspected in those with significant mechanism to the chest especially those that are found to have a sternal fracture, multiple left-sided or bilateral rib fractures, or chest tenderness. Screening should be performed initially with a 12-lead electrocardiogram (EKG). With a normal EKG, no further evaluation is warranted. Otherwise, the patient may need to be admitted and monitored on telemetry for up to 24 hours. Obtaining serial cardiac enzymes has limited utility in evaluation and management of the patient with suspected cardiac contusion (42,43).

Injury to the tracheobronchial tree can be devastating. This is often identified after a pneumothorax is treated with a chest tube and demonstrates a large airleak, or the pneumothorax does not resolve on repeat CXR, or subcutaneous emphysema is detected on physical examination or imaging. Suspicions may be confirmed via bronchoscopy and operative repair may be considered. If particularly large, the patient may develop worsening respiratory distress after the chest tube is placed and require intubation then operative thoracotomy for definitive repair. As in the neck, esophageal injuries are much more common with a penetrating, as opposed to a blunt, mechanism. If not identified early enough, the consequences are often dire. Any suspicion of esophageal injury necessitates esophagoscopy and contrast esophagram to rule out.

Abdominal Trauma

The abdominal examination is an extremely important part of the trauma evaluation mainly because it may at times be very difficult to ascertain if any significant injury is present therein. Although the abdomen is briefly addressed during the primary survey in regards to a possible bleeding source, the examination in the secondary survey should be more complete and deliberate. One should inspect the abdomen carefully for any external sign of injury such as a laceration, contusion, or a seatbelt sign (44). Palpate for tenderness or signs of peritonitis and document this examination carefully. Injuries to the abdomen are classically indolent and one should be prepared for the abdominal examination to change over time. A patient may have minimal tenderness during the initial period and develop frank peritonitis hours later. Other complicating factors often confound the abdominal examination include head injury, distracting injuries, and drug or alcohol intoxication. The mechanism of injury is among the first steps in the management algorithm. Penetrating injuries to the abdomen most often encountered are stab wounds and gunshot wounds. In regards to anterior abdominal stab wounds, operative intervention is generally advocated if the secondary survey reveals one of three conditions: hemodynamic instability, evisceration, or peritonitis. Selective nonoperative management can be pursued otherwise with admission and serial abdominal examinations (45). Please note, however, that thoracoabdominal stab wounds require special consideration if present due to the chance of an occult diaphragmatic injury. If the injury is below the level of the nipple on the left side, the patient should have a diagnostic laparoscopy or thoracoscopy (46). A CT scan is not adequate to rule this out. Gunshot wounds to the abdomen are given much more consideration due to the high-velocity nature. The statistically high likelihood of injury to the abdominal viscera necessitating surgical repair allows one to readily decide in favor of surgical exploration, although there are a few notable exceptions. For instance, there are recent reports of a single gunshot wound to the right upper quadrant in a hemodynamically stable patient being managed successfully nonoperatively (47). Blunt abdominal trauma is less straightforward in regards to decision for laparotomy. Assessment of hemodynamic stability and the presence of peritonitis in conjunction with available imaging, either FAST or CT, are considered carefully during the decision making process.

The FAST examination has an obvious role in the primary survey, as previously discussed. However, the role of FAST after the primary survey, as well as in the secondary survey and beyond the secondary survey remains as an excellent bedside tool to assess the intra-abdominal compartment, especially in the context of a previously stable patient who has become hemodynamically unstable. If the patient has become hemodynamically unstable, it is worth repeating the primary survey. As in the primary survey, if the FAST is positive and the patient is stable, a CT of the abdomen and pelvis with contrast is recommended. However, if the FAST is positive and the patient is hemodynamically unstable, the patient warrants immediate exploratory laparotomy, as in the initial primary survey. And again, in the hemodynamically stable patient with a positive FAST examination, the patient should proceed to have a CT scan of the abdomen and pelvis with contrast. Free fluid in the setting of solid-organ injury may be managed nonoperatively and monitored depending on the extent of injury or may be amenable to control by interventional radiology. Free fluid without solid-organ injury is concerning for bowel injury and would warrant a lower threshold for operative exploration.

Cases which require abdominal exploration for trauma can vary significantly in regards to indication and urgency. Although certain cases are amenable to definitive repair of injuries and abdominal closure, more recently the standard of care in severe abdominal trauma has evolved toward a damage-control mentality and approach. Once the life-threatening bleeding has been halted and enteric contamination controlled, the patient may be served best globally by temporarily closing the abdomen using a negative-pressure abdominal closure device (e.g., ABThera) or similar contraption. Central to providing the best chance of survival and favorable long-term outcome is to avoid the "lethal triad" mentioned earlier: coagulopathy, acidosis, and hypothermia. The sooner the patient can be transferred to the ICU for resuscitation, warming, and other measures to restore physiologic normalcy, the better the chance for survival. The patient can then be brought back for reexploration and possible fascial closure when more physiologically stable.

Related to the topic of damage-control laparotomy and temporary abdominal closure is the recognition and management of abdominal compartment syndrome (ACS). ACS is characterized by intra-abdominal hypertension (>20 mmHg) as determined by bladder pressure measurements with concurrent end-organ dysfunction (48). Causes of ACS in the setting of trauma most commonly include ischemia and reperfusion of abdominal viscera leading to increased abdominal pressure, massive third spacing of fluids due to the acute response to injury and large volume resuscitation, or ongoing uncontrolled intra-abdominal bleeding occupying space in the peritoneum. Regardless of the cause, the effect of the intra-abdominal hypertension is the compression of inferior vena cava, decrease in venous return, loss of effective cardiac output, and inadequate perfusion to the end-organs. Most commonly affected are the renal system leading to oliguria and the pulmonary system due to impaired tidal volumes. Bladder pressures should be measured serially and conservative measures may be attempted including bowel decompression, sedation, and paralysis; however, ACS that is inadequately treated and progresses to multiorgan failure has a high mortality rate. Therefore one should have a low threshold to proceed to definitive treatment being decompressive laparotomy and temporary abdominal closure.

Pelvic Trauma

The pelvis may be examined physically by looking for any external signs of trauma and then assessing the stability of the pelvic ring. The assessor should attempt to adduct the iliac wings while noting any atypical mobility and to check for patient tenderness. Care must be taken not to be too forceful and to minimize the number of manipulations as this can exacerbate bleeding in an unstable pelvis. A pelvic x-ray can be a useful adjunct to determine the fracture pattern and may be the only opportunity to image the patient if hemodynamically unstable and therefore unable to obtain a CT scan. An open book pelvic fracture should initially be managed by placing a pelvic binder as this help to tamponade venous hemorrhage, decrease pelvic volume, and stem bleeding from the fractured ends of bone. Hemodynamically stable patients should have a CT scan with IV contrast to assess for active extravasation. If an arterial blush is noted, angioembolization is often indicated as this is unlikely to halt spontaneously. In the hemodynamically unstable patient in the setting of significant pelvic fracture, management can be a challenging affair. Often there is significant mechanism to suspect a concurrent abdominal source of hemorrhage as well. With a positive FAST, abdominal exploration should be undertaken; however, pelvic bleeding is notoriously difficult to control intraoperatively. Preperitoneal packing has recently been receiving growing attention in the trauma literature and can be a useful adjunct to aid in hemostasis while arranging for angioembolization (20,21). Packs are placed through a suprapubic extraperitoneal incision in the paravesical space bilaterally. External pelvic stabilization can also be utilized for hemorrhage control. Early involvement of the orthopedic team is often helpful in this decision as well as for long-term definitive care. Aside from bleeding control and definitive fixation, the key issue in management of an unstable pelvic fracture is to assess the surrounding structures for an associated injury such as to the bladder, urethra, rectum, perineum, or genitalia.

Extremity and Peripheral Vascular Trauma

As life-threatening situations are addressed during the primary survey, less attention is typically spent on examining the extremities unless they are a source of major hemorrhage. Often this can be managed with direct pressure and a pressure dressing, but may require a tourniquet and operative exploration if initially uncontrollable. During the secondary survey, a more comprehensive examination of the extremities needs to be undertaken. Lacerations, contusions, deformities should be further evaluated radiologically with careful attention to the joints. Any laceration overlying a fracture should be considered an open fracture and prophylactic antibiotics early on should be administered to reduce long-term morbidity. Each extremity should have a sensory motor examination, range of motion evaluation, and pulse checks. Pulses should be compared with the opposite extremity for any discrepancies and if suspected, an Ankle-Brachial Index should be performed. Extremity compartment syndrome is caused by increased pressure within the fascial compartment leading to venous occlusion which eventually leads to limitation in arterial inflow. If untreated, irreversible nerve and muscle damage may ensue. This should be a consideration in certain injuries such as vascular injuries, crush injuries, tibial-fibular fractures, and cases of ischemia-reperfusion. The treatment for this is decompression via fasciotomy (49).

Back, Spinal Column, and Perineum

The secondary survey physical examination is completed by logrolling while adhering to full spinal precautions as described earlier and taking note of any lacerations, contusions, or deformities. Any midline spinal tenderness should be noted and followed up with the appropriate imaging studies. The perineum is classically neglected during examination and often presents later as a missed injury. The mechanism and associated injuries are important to consider such as a concurrent pelvic fracture. In opposition to traditional teachings, the digital rectal examination (DRE) is not always necessary and should no longer be considered a routine part of the examination (50). It is warranted in selected cases and should always be included in the setting of a pelvic fracture due to a higher risk of associated rectal and urethral injury. When performed, one should note any presence of gross blood, palpable defects in the rectal wall or pelvic bone fragments, a high riding and mobile prostate gland, and abnormal sphincter tone.

Adjuncts to the Secondary Survey

After a complete history and physical examination, often the trauma patient requires additional imaging and laboratory tests to further delineate injuries and conditions. Plain x-rays continue to have value in the evaluation of extremities for fractures and dislocation, evaluation of the thoracic and lumbar spine, and localization of foreign bodies. Multidetector computed tomography (CT) has largely become the imaging modality of choice for trauma patients due to its continually improving speed and resolution. Preferably, the addition of IV contrast is useful in assessing the abdomen and pelvis for bleeding and should be standard. In certain situations, IV contrast with CT angiography protocol is indicated for the head, neck, chest, and extremities if injury to the vasculature is a concern. Although contrast-induced nephropathy is a risk factor, IV contrast should not be withheld in a severely injured trauma patient when hemorrhage is suspected (51). MRI does not have a significant role in acute trauma management and may be utilized in the workup for spinal cord injuries, diffuse axonal injury, and ligamentous injuries. Mostly this can be deferred until after the initial assessment and hemodynamic stability is established.

REASSESSMENT, MISSED INJURIES, AND THE TERTIARY SURVEY

After the secondary survey has been performed and the necessary imaging obtained, it is important to have a planned reevaluation of the patient's condition to assess response to therapy and decide upon appropriate disposition. It is important to stress that if there is a change for the worse noted during reassessment, the primary survey can and should be repeated. If the patient needs to be monitored in the intensive care unit (ICU), plans should be made as early as possible so that the transition of care can be performed in a smooth, safe, and efficient manner. Direct physician-to-physician communication between the trauma team and the ICU providers needs to be performed. As well, one should become familiar with the hospital's system for bed flow and with the key nursing and administrative contacts to optimize this process. Ideally, trauma patients should be move in a unidirectional manner such as from the ED to the Radiology Department to the ICU without diversion back to the ED.

Ideally all injuries should be identified within the context of the primary and secondary survey. However, this is not realistically possible in every situation, especially with the more severe multi trauma patients with complicating factors such as altered mental status due to TBI, distracting injuries, or alcohol intoxication.

Patients that present requiring emergent intubation and perhaps an exploratory laparotomy to control bleeding may end up in the ICU without having completed the remainder of the primary and secondary survey. It is important to implement a system in which ongoing active reassessment once the patient is stabilized becomes the norm to seek out additional injuries. Musculoskeletal injuries, retroperitoneal injuries, and perineal injuries are among the more commonly described missed injuries (31). Many centers have instituted a formal tertiary survey in their trauma systems which have greatly facilitated the decrease in missed injury rates. A tertiary survey should be performed once within 24 hours of admission and additionally in patients who have resolved altered mental status and have become ambulatory.

An additional issue to check for within the initial 24 hours is the existence of "trauma lines," invasive central venous, arterial, or urethral catheters that were placed in the emergent setting. As these devices are often placed under suboptimal conditions due to the urgency of the situation, sterile technique cannot be assumed. This detail is often missed during transition of care from one facility to the next or even between the trauma team and the ICU providers and may contribute to higher rates of avoidable catheter-related infections (52).

Also to be taken into consideration in the trauma population is the very high risk of developing a deep venous thrombosis (DVT). Trauma patients have more than a 50% chance of acquiring a DVT when not receiving prophylaxis. Independent risk factors associated with DVT in trauma patients include lower extremity fractures, pelvic fractures, spinal cord injuries, venous injury requiring repair, femoral CVL, and any major operative intervention. Low-molecular-weight heparin is the preferred agent for prophylaxis and should be considered as early as possible (53). Dosing is based on ideal body weight but may need to be adjusted for reasons which may include obesity and renal failure. Anti-Xa levels are more commonly being used to guide therapy. Many trauma patients present with injuries that are contraindications to DVT prophylaxis, such as intracranial hemorrhage, spinal cord injury, solid-organ injury, coagulopathy, and ongoing hemorrhage. Coordination with consulting services regarding timing of prophylactic low–molecular-weight heparin and the consideration for inferior vena cava filter placement should be a daily discussion.

DOCUMENTATION

The most urgent of trauma cases are fast-paced, dynamic, and often with a degree of diagnostic uncertainty at times. As discussed earlier, management of trauma places more emphasis on identifying and treating the greatest threat to life first, even when the definitive diagnosis remains unclear. As this is the case, there may be a natural tendency for the practitioner to place medical record documentation low on the list of priorities. However, it is also for these very reasons that accurate and timely documentation is critical in providing good patient care. Emphasis should be placed on calling out findings to the recording nurse during the primary and secondary survey to help identify trends and changes as the patient progresses through the hospitalization. An oral discussion between care providers is critical in effective and efficient patient care. However, this should also be supplemented by a written record in the chart. With each instance of a transfer of care, there is a higher chance for miscommunication or inaccuracies to propagate.

Finally, the medical record and documentation is central to the review process after trauma and is a large part of performance improvement. We must never forget that good documentation is a responsibility and essential characteristic of a good physician.

Key Points

- Traumatic injury continues to occupy a large proportion of annual global mortality, which in addition to claiming thousands of lives per day, causes significant long-term morbidity further impacting society in regards to loss of productivity and high medical costs.
- The premise of ATLS is to expeditiously identify and treat the greatest threat to life first even before obtaining a definitive diagnosis or detailed history.
- The primary survey inherently prioritizes the assessment and treatment of a secure airway, intact breathing, and adequate circulation and thus addresses any rapidly lethal injuries prior to performing a more detailed examination, and should be repeated readily with any change in patient status.
- IO access should be considered in the hemodynamically unstable trauma patient that presents with difficult or inadequate intravenous access and can be placed within seconds by a trained practitioner.
- CT has become the imaging modality of choice in trauma patients to readily and accurately identify internal injuries, however the patient must be ascertained to be hemodynamically stable prior to transferring for this diagnostic study.
- MTP, the immediate transfusion of blood products in a 1:1:1 ratio of packed red blood cells (PRBCs), FFP, and platelets, should be activated and administered immediately on recognition of ongoing severe traumatic hemorrhage likely to exceed 10 units of PRBC transfusion in the initial 24 hours.
- The mainstay of treatment for severe TBI focusses on decreasing incidence of secondary injury by maintaining adequate oxygenation and perfusion.
- The lethal triad of trauma includes hypothermia, coagulopathy, and acidosis; the severity of which being manifested in trauma patients requiring surgery should guide one to favor a damage-control approach with temporary abdominal closure and planned reexploration over definitive surgery.

References

1. World Health Organization. *The top 10 causes of death*. Available at http://www.who.int/mediacentre/factsheets/fs310/en./ Accessed May 2014.
2. World Health Organization. *Number of road traffic deaths*. Available at http://www.who.int/gho/road_safety/mortality/number_text/en/. Accessed October 2015.
3. Centers for Disease Control and Prevention. *NCHS Data Brief: Mortality in the United States, 2013*. Available at http://www.cdc.gov/nchs/data/databriefs/db178.htm. Accessed December 2014.
4. Heron M, Centers for Disease Control and Prevention. *Deaths: leading causes for 2011. National Vital Statistics Reports*. http://www.cdc.gov/nchs/data/nvsr/nvsr64/nvsr64_07.pdf. Assessed July 27, 2015.
5. Centers for Disease Control and Prevention. *CDC Newsroom. Injuries cost the US $671 billion in 2013*. Available at http://www.cdc.gov/media/releases/2015/p0930-injury-costs.html. Accessed September 30, 2015.
6. Ogden CL, Carroll MD, Kit BK, Flegal KM. Prevalence of childhood and adult obesity in the United States, 2011–2012. *JAMA*. 2014;311(8):806–814.
7. Acosta JA, Yang JC, Winchell RJ, et al. Lethal injuries and time to death in a level I trauma center. *J Am Coll Surg*. 1998;186(5):528–533.
8. Teixeira PG, Inaba K, Hadjizacharia P, et al. Preventable or potentially preventable mortality at a mature trauma center. *J Trauma*. 2007;63(6):1338–1346; discussion 1346–1347.
9. American College of Surgeons Committee on Trauma. *Advanced Trauma Life Support (ATLS) Student Course Manual*. 9th ed. Chicago, IL: American College of Surgeons; 2012.
10. Mohammad A, Branicki F, Abu-Zidan FM. Educational and clinical impact of Advanced Trauma Life Support (ATLS) courses: a systematic review. *World J Surg*. 2014;38(2):322–329.
11. Navarro S, Montmany S, Rebasa P, et al. Impact of ATLS training on preventable and potentially preventable deaths. *World J Surg*. 2014;38(9):2273–2278.
12. Ali J, Adam R, Butler AK, et al. Trauma outcome improves following the advanced trauma life support program in a developing country. *J Trauma*. 1993;34(6):890–898; discussion 898–899.
13. Sakles JC, Chiu S, Mosier J, et al. The importance of first pass success when performing orotracheal intubation in the emergency department. *Acad Emerg Med*. 2013;20(1):71–78.
14. Sulser S, Ubmann D, Brueesch M, et al. The C-MAC videolaryngoscope compared with conventional laryngoscopy for rapid sequence intubation at the emergency department: study protocol. *Scand J Trauma Resusc Emerg Med*. 2015;23:38.
15. Green R, Hutton B, Lorette J, et al. Incidence of postintubation hemodynamic instability associated with emergent intubations performed outside the operating room: a systematic review. *CJEM*. 2014;16(1):69–79.
16. Inaba K, Ives C, McClure K, et al. Radiologic evaluation of alternative sites for needle decompression of tension pneumothorax. *Arch Surg*. 2012;147(9):813–818.
17. Cooper BR, Mahoney PF, Hodgetts TJ, Mellor A. Intra-osseous access (EZ-IO) for resuscitation: UK military combat experience. *J R Army Med Corps*. 2007;153(4):314–316.
18. Beekley AC, Sebesta JA, Blackbourne LH, et al.; 31st Combat Support Hospital Research Group. Prehospital tourniquet use in Operation Iraqi Freedom: effect on hemorrhage control and outcomes. *J Trauma*. 2008;64(2 Suppl):S28–S37; discussion S37.
19. Kragh JF Jr, Walters TJ, Baer DG, et al. Survival with emergency tourniquet use to stop bleeding in major limb trauma. *Ann Surg*. 2009;249(1):1–7.
20. Cothren CC, Osborn PM, Moore EE, et al. Preperitonal pelvic packing for hemodynamically unstable pelvic fractures: a paradigm shift. *J Trauma*. 2007;62(4):834–839; discussion 839–842.
21. Burlew CC, Moore EE, Smith WR, et al. Preperitoneal pelvic packing/external fixation with secondary angioembolization: optimal care for life-threatening hemorrhage from unstable pelvic fractures. *J Am Coll Surg*. 2011;212(4):628–635; discussion 635–637.
22. Tiling T, Boulion B, Schmid A, et al. Ultrasound in blunt abdominothoracic trauma. In: Border JR, ed. *Blunt Multiple Trauma: Comprehensive Pathophysiology and Care*. New York, NY: Marcel Dekker; 1990:415–433.
23. CRASH-2 trial collaborators, Shakur H, Roberts I, et al. Effects of tranexamic acid on death, vascular occlusive events, and blood transfusion in trauma patients with significant haemorrhage (CRASH-2): a randomised, placebo-controlled trial. *Lancet*. 2010;376(9734):23–32.
24. CRASH-2 collaborators, Roberts I, Shakur H, et al. The importance of early treatment with tranexamic acid in bleeding trauma patients: an exploratory analysis of the CRASH-2 randomised controlled trial. *Lancet*. 2011;377(9771):1096–1101.
25. Holcomb JB, Jenkins D, Rhee P, et al. Damage control resuscitation: directly addressing the early coagulopathy of trauma. *J Trauma*. 2007;62(2):307–310.
26. Como JJ, Dutton RP, Scalea TM, et al. Blood transfusion rates in the care of acute trauma. *Transfusion*. 2004;44(6):809–813.
27. Stockinger ZT, McSwain NE Jr. Additional evidence in support of withholding or terminating cardiopulmonary resuscitation for trauma patients in the field. *J Am Coll Surg*. 2004;198(2):227–231.
28. Cothren CC, Moore EE. Emergency department thoracotomy for the critically injured patient: objectives, indications, and outcomes. *World J Emerg Surg*. 2006;1:4.
29. Rhee PM, Acosta J, Bridgeman A, et al. Survival after emergency department thoracotomy: review of published data from the past 25 years. *J Am Coll Surg*. 2000;190(3):288–298.
30. Stevens RD, Huff JS, Duckworth J, et al. Emergency neurological life support: intracranial hypertension and herniation. *Neurocrit Care*. 2012;17(Suppl 1):S60–S65.
31. Pfeifer R, Pape HC. Missed injuries in trauma patients: a literature review. *Patient Saf Surg*. 2008;2:20.

32. Nirula R, Maier R, Moore E, et al. Scoop and run to the trauma center or stay and play at the local hospital: hospital transfer's effect on mortality. *J Trauma.* 2010;69(3):595–599; discussion 599–601.
33. Sampalis JS, Denis R, Fréchette P, et al. Direct transport to tertiary trauma centers versus transfer from lower level facilities: impact on mortality and morbidity among patients with major trauma. *J Trauma.* 1997;43(2):288–295; discussion 295–296.
34. Ferraris VA, Bernard AC, Hyde B. The impact of antiplatelet drugs on trauma outcomes. *J Trauma Acute Care Surg.* 2012;73(2):492–497.
35. Ivascu FA, Howells GA, Junn FS, et al. Rapid warfarin reversal in anticoagulated patients with traumatic intracranial hemorrhage reduces hemorrhage progression and mortality. *J Trauma.* 2005;59(5):1131–1137; discussion 1137–1139.
36. Ivascu FA, Janczyk RJ, Junn FS, et al. Treatment of trauma patients with intracranial hemorrhage on preinjury warfarin. *J Trauma.* 2006;61(2): 318–321.
37. Cushman JG, Agarwal N, Fabian TC, et al.; EAST Practice Management Guidelines Work Group. Practice management guidelines for the management of mild traumatic brain injury: the EAST practice management guidelines work group. *J Trauma.* 200151(5):1016–1026.
38. Tisherman SA, Bokhari F, Collier B, et al. Clinical practice guideline: penetrating zone II neck trauma. *J Trauma.* 2008;64(5):1392–1405.
39. Berne JD, Reuland KS, Villarreal DH, et al. Sixteen-slice multi-detector computed tomographic angiography improves the accuracy of screening for blunt cerebrovascular injury. *J Trauma.* 2006;60(6):1204–1209; discussion 1209–1210.
40. Biffl WL, Cothren CC, Moore EE, et al. Western Trauma Association critical decisions in trauma: screening for and treatment of bluntcerebrovascular injuries. *J Trauma.* 2009;67(6):1150–1153.
41. Fox N, Schwartz D, Salazar JH, et al. Evaluation and management of blunt traumatic aortic injury: a practice management guideline from the Eastern Association for the Surgery of Trauma. *J Trauma Acute Care Surg.* 2015;78(1): 136–146.
42. Collins JN, Cole FJ, Weireter LJ, et al. The usefulness of serum troponin levels in evaluating cardiac injury. *Am Surg.* 2001;67(9):821–5; discussion 825–826.
43. Biffl WL, Moore FA, Moore EE, et al. Cardiac enzymes are irrelevant in the patient with suspected myocardial contusion. *Am J Surg.* 1994;168(6):523-527; discussion 527–528.
44. Nishijima DK, Simel DL, Wisner DH, Holmes JF. Does this adult patient have a blunt intra-abdominal injury? *JAMA.* 2012;307(14):1517–1527.
45. Zafar SN, Rushing A, Haut ER, et al. Outcome of selective non-operative management of penetrating abdominal injuries from the North American National Trauma Database. *Br J Surg.* 2012;99(Suppl 1):155–164.
46. Berg RJ, Karamanos E, Inaba K, et al. The persistent diagnostic challenge of thoracoabdominal stab wounds. *J Trauma Acute Care Surg.* 2014; 76(2):418–423.
47. Navsaria PH, Nicol AJ, Edu S, et al. Selective nonoperative management in 1106 patients with abdominal gunshot wounds: conclusions on safety, efficacy, and the role of selective CT imaging in a prospective single-center study. *Ann Surg.* 2015;261(4):760–764
48. Vidal MG, Ruiz Weisser J, Gonzalez F, et al. Incidence and clinical effects of intra-abdominal hypertension in critically ill patients. *Crit Care Med.* 2008;36(6):1823–1831.
49. Newton EJ, Love J. Acute complications of extremity trauma. *Emerg Med Clin North Am.* 2007;25(3):751–761, iv.
50. Hankin AD, Baren JM. Should the digital rectal examination be a part of the trauma secondary survey? *Ann Emerg Med.* 2009;53(2):208–212.
51. Inaba K, Branco BC, Lim G, et al. The increasing burden of radiation exposure in the management of trauma patients. *J Trauma.* 2011;70(6):1366–1370.
52. O'Grady NP, Alexander M, Dellinger EP, et al. Guidelines for the prevention of intravascular catheter-related infections. Centers for Disease Control and Prevention. *MMWR Recomm Rep.* 2002;51(RR-10):1–29.
53. Spencer Netto F, Tien H, Ng J, et al. Pulmonary emboli after blunt trauma: timing, clinical characteristics and natural history. *Injury.* 2012;43(9): 1502–1506.

CHAPTER

56

Surgical and Postsurgical Bleeding

POUYA J. BENYAMINI and DANNY M. TAKANISHI, JR.

INTRODUCTION

It is crucial that clinicians who provide care to surgical patients understand the dynamic interplay between the coagulation and fibrinolytic systems. An appreciation for the relevant underlying biologic mechanisms is central to the diagnosis and appropriate management of patients who present with bleeding diatheses in both the operative and the postoperative setting. Surgery provides the most significant challenge to the integrity of the hemostatic system, and the fidelity of the coagulation system serves as the homeostatic defense mechanism that abrogates the proclivity for bleeding in this context. Moreover, with the emergence of novel anticoagulants approved for the ongoing ambulatory management of atrial fibrillation, deep venous thrombosis, and pulmonary embolism in an ever aging population, comes the stipulation for an improved understanding of how these pharmacologic agents complicate the care of the bleeding patient.

PATHOPHYSIOLOGY

It is essential to differentiate between the inherited (primary) coagulation disorders, which are associated with a history of bleeding diatheses, from the more commonly acquired (secondary) coagulation disorders, which are the consequence of pathologic conditions and numerous medications (1–3). This nomenclature (primary vs. secondary) is distinct from, and should not be confused with, the traditional nomenclature used to describe the hemostatic *process* itself. In the formation of a stable clot, the hemostatic process was classically described as comprising two phases, a primary phase (also called *primary hemostasis*) and a secondary phase (also called *secondary hemostasis*). The primary phase of hemostasis involves vascular or tissue injury, initiating platelet adhesion and aggregation to form the platelet plug. The secondary phase involves the activation of the plasmatic coagulation protein cascade (both the extrinsic and the intrinsic systems), which results in formation of the stable fibrin clot. Disorders involving platelet number or function, or vascular interactions, are classified as disorders of primary hemostasis, and disorders involving the plasma coagulation factors are classified as disorders of secondary hemostasis. This serves the purpose of an operational definition, since in vivo these events are highly integrated, not separate processes.

Hemostatic disorders, whether primary (inherited) or secondary (acquired), can both be manifest by diffuse bleeding from the operative site, puncture wounds, vascular access sites, or traumatized tissue outside of the operative field. Surgical and postsurgical bleeding may therefore result from either quantitative (thrombocytopenia) or qualitative (abnormal function) platelet disorders.

Thrombocytopenia, defined as a platelet count less than 140 $\times$ 10^9/L, results from decreased production (aplastic anemia, hypoplastic bone marrow, chemotherapy, space-occupying lesions of the bone marrow as seen with malignancy), ineffective thrombopoiesis (vitamin B_{12} or folic acid deficiency states), sequestration particularly in the spleen (primary or secondary hypersplenism), increased destruction or consumption (microangiopathic processes such as thrombotic thrombocytopenic purpura [TTP], disseminated intravascular coagulation [DIC], or the hemolytic-uremic syndrome [HUS]; immune destruction due to antiplatelet antibodies, such as in posttransfusion purpura or idiopathic thrombocytopenic purpura), and dilution of circulating platelets associated with massive blood transfusion (1,2,4–15). Petechiae, purpura, and mucosal oozing are characteristics of thrombocytopenic states, although these findings may also be observed in qualitative platelet disorders and in conditions associated with increased vascular fragility. Platelet counts of 50 $\times$ 10^9/L or higher are generally considered adequate for surgical hemostasis in the absence of an associated qualitative functional defect, but below 20 $\times$ 10^9/L there is increased risk for spontaneous hemorrhages (1–3,6). Particularly lethal in this regard are those involving the central nervous system.

Cytotoxic chemotherapy and radiation therapy (total body) produce thrombocytopenia by suppression of bone marrow megakaryocytes, the progenitor cell for platelets. Together these are the most common causes of bleeding in patients undergoing therapy for malignancies. Marrow aplasia, hypoplasia, and space-occupying diseases of the bone marrow (e.g., metastatic carcinoma, leukemias, lymphomas) also result in decreased production of platelets. Certain drugs, including alcohol, have been associated with decreased production of platelets via a direct toxic effect on megakaryocytes. Ineffective thrombopoiesis is a characteristic trait of megaloblastic anemia resulting from either vitamin B_{12} or folate deficiency. Although there is an increase in the megakaryocytic mass, platelet production is impaired. Notwithstanding, hemorrhagic diatheses manifest in a few of these individuals (16).

The most frequent cause of thrombocytopenia resulting from increased destruction of circulating platelets is postoperative infection (2,9–12,17). Significantly, thrombocytopenia may be the first presenting sign of an occult infection and may herald impending sepsis. Consequently, in the postoperative setting, thrombocytopenia of unclear cause must promptly direct attention toward uncovering a potential source of occult sepsis.

Thrombocytopenia caused by increased destruction of platelets is also observed in microangiopathic hemolytic states, such as in TTP and HUS (2,18–20). Mechanical injury occurs when platelets traverse the small capillary beds in the peripheral circulation. TTP is characterized by fever, fluctuating neurologic symptoms (headaches, confusion, seizures, or coma), and acute renal failure, in addition to a microangiopathic hemolytic anemia and thrombocytopenia. HUS manifests similarly to TTP, with the notable exceptions that the pediatric population is more commonly affected, neurologic manifestations are minimal, but the renal impairment is more pronounced. Central to the treatment of both these entities is supportive care, with particular attention given to management of the renal dysfunction (18,19). Plasma exchange is often efficacious in treating these diseases, and hemodialysis may also be required in some instances for support of renal failure.

Immune-mediated destruction of platelets is observed in several clinical conditions. Alloimmune antibodies are believed to account for posttransfusion purpura observed primarily in women, who may have been previously immunized by fetal-derived platelets because there is a significant association with a prior history of pregnancy (2,21). Immunizations to a number of candidate alloantigens have been reported in the literature, the most common being the PL^{A1} antigen. The antibodies induced are generally of the IgG class and therefore are also able to cross the placenta, as a described cause of neonatal thrombocytopenia. The purpura becomes apparent approximately 7 to 10 days after blood transfusion, presumably attributed to an anamnestic response, and can last several months. The population at risk has been estimated to be approximately 1% to 3%, and the condition tends to be self-limiting and responds to intravenous immune globulin. Idiopathic thrombocytopenic purpura is one of the more common examples of immune-mediated platelet destruction (2,14,20–23). It tends to occur in otherwise healthy individuals, and both an acute and a chronic form have been described. Mechanistically, platelets coated with autoantibodies are removed by the reticuloendothelial cells in the spleen (and to an extent in the liver). The diagnosis is one of exclusion after other causes of thrombocytopenia have been ruled out. A similar mechanism may account for the thrombocytopenia associated with collagen vascular diseases, such as systemic lupus erythematosus, lymphoreticular diseases, and in some infectious diseases, such as infectious mononucleosis or human immunodeficiency virus infections. It is noteworthy in this regard that the acute form, often observed in the pediatric population, is often preceded by a viral syndrome. Splenectomy is required in a third of patients if immune globulin, corticosteroids, or plasmapheresis is unable to control the condition (2,14,22,23). In this condition, significant bleeding may not occur until platelet counts decrease as low as 10×10^9/L because most of the circulating platelet pool consists of younger, more functionally active platelets. The significance of this impact on the operative approach traditionally adopted during splenectomy. During splenectomy, platelets are hung by the anesthesiologist but not administered until the splenic artery is clamped or splenectomy completed. There is by and large minimal bleeding encountered despite the pronounced degree of thrombocytopenia, and if platelets are infused prior to control of the splenic arterial inflow, the infused platelets will merely be consumed by the spleen and not available for the hemostatic process. Immune-mediated destruction of platelets can also be caused by several drugs that can induce antibodies to platelets via hapten-mediated, or by immune complex–mediated, "innocent bystander" mechanisms. Quinine, amiodarone, sulfa drugs, cimetidine, ranitidine, phenytoin, and semisynthetic penicillins are some examples that may be encountered in the critical care environment (2). Heparin-induced thrombocytopenia is an unusual example of drug-induced thrombocytopenia in this context because a hypercoagulable condition is actually created characterized by thrombotic complications with the manifestation of the "white clot syndrome" (24). This syndrome typically becomes apparent after 1 week of therapy but may present within a few hours after implementing heparin therapy in already sensitized patients. Discontinuation of the offending agent is the appropriate treatment approach central to all causes of drug-induced, immune-mediated thrombocytopenia.

Contrary wise, the qualitative platelet disorders, generally manifesting normal platelet counts with impairment of function, may be inherited (Bernard–Soulier syndrome, abnormal release mechanism, Glanzmann thrombasthenia, storage pool disease, or von Willebrand disease) or acquired.

Acquired disorders are the leading cause of qualitative platelet function abnormalities in the critically ill patient. It is vital to be aware that qualitative bleeding disorders are not measured by the standard battery of coagulation tests described below, with the exception of the template bleeding time.

Ingestion of numerous drugs has been associated with inhibition of platelet function (2,13,25). Among these, aspirin is the most well described and best characterized. Aspirin interferes with cyclo-oxygenase–mediated prostaglandin and thromboxane synthesis and has profound effects at multiple steps in the formation of the hemostatic platelet plug. It decreases the platelet response to aggregation in response to collagen, inhibits the second phase of aggregation in response to adenosine diphosphate (ADP) and epinephrine, and irreversibly injures platelets for the duration of their lifespan.

Another common cause of acquired qualitative defects in platelet function is hypothermia (26–28). Massive blood transfusions or crystalloid infusions without attention to use of blood warmers, lack of attention to maintaining a warm ambient environment in the operating room, especially during long procedures and for individuals at the extremes of age, and prolonged extrications and exposure time in the field in the patient with multiple traumatic injuries are all too familiar causes of hypothermia.

Renal failure is not uncommon in the critical care setting. In its acute form, bleeding is a common manifestation, most often from the gastrointestinal tract. The underlying mechanism is probably multifactorial, as there clearly is a qualitative platelet function defect related to the degree of uremia, in combination with abnormalities in the plasmatic coagulation system (29–31). The presence of acidosis also contributes to both the platelet and coagulation factor dysfunction.

Disorders involving plasmatic coagulation factors are generally caused by either a decrease in production of clotting factors (liver failure, vitamin K deficiency [oral antibiotic usage, which depresses gut flora in the setting of nutritional deficiency; malabsorption syndromes, such as celiac sprue or chronic diarrheal conditions; or obstructive jaundice], and use of warfarin [Coumadin]) (2,15,32) or by an increase in consumption of circulating coagulation factors (such as in DIC) (2,7–12,15,26–28,32).

The most common cause of increased destruction of plasmatic coagulation factors has been variously termed DIC, defibrination syndrome, or consumptive coagulopathy (2,7–12,20,26–28). This syndrome is characterized by a hemorrhagic diathesis with unrestrained clotting and fibrinolysis in the vascular microcirculation, initiated by activation of the intrinsic or the extrinsic system, or both (2,7–12,20,26–28). Release of tissue thromboplastin, from injured tissue or from leukocytes, activates the extrinsic system, whereas damage to vascular endothelium (in addition to releasing tissue thromboplastin) results in activation of the intrinsic system via collagen exposure (7–12). Exposed collagen initiates platelet aggregation with release of platelet factor III and also activates factor XII directly. The net result is deposition of fibrin in the microvasculature. This results in a microangiopathic hemolytic anemia with fragmentation of red blood cells as they traverse these vascular beds. These fragmented red blood cells, or schistocytes, seen on the peripheral blood smear are a classic finding in this syndrome. Additionally, microthrombi cause stasis and ischemia in a number of capillary beds, manifesting as renal insufficiency or failure with kidney involvement, pulmonary insufficiency with lung involvement, mental status changes with brain involvement, or dermal necrosis with skin involvement. Stasis itself can result in further activation of clotting factors. Fibrin deposition and endothelial wall damage both bring about the release of plasminogen activator, which catalyzes the conversion of circulating plasminogen to plasmin. Plasmin proteolytically hydrolyzes both fibrinogen and fibrin (secondary fibrinolysis), resulting in fibrinogen and fibrin degradation (or "split") products. These degradation products then interfere with fibrin polymerization through the formation of complexes, further contributing to the hemorrhagic state. Additionally, these degradation products also interfere with platelet function, impairing both adhesion and aggregation. In the postoperative patient in the ICU, infection is the principle cause for DIC (9–12). Several causative organisms have been implicated, including gram-negative bacteria, such as the Enterobacteriaceae as well as the nonlactose fermenters; gram-positive bacteria; rickettsial organisms (Rocky Mountain spotted fever); mycotic infections, such as disseminated aspergillosis; parasitic agents, such as malaria; and viruses. The underlying pathophysiology has been best elucidated with gram-negative infections, with endotoxin (cell wall lipopolysaccharide) triggering the intrinsic system by activation of factor XII directly and by factor XII exposure to subendothelial collagen, as a result of endotoxin-mediated damage to vascular endothelium. Endotoxin may also trigger the coagulation cascade by inducing expression of procoagulant activity in circulating leukocytes, hepatic macrophages, and endothelial cells, and by activating the extrinsic system mediated by the release of tissue thromboplastin from damaged leukocytes and vascular endothelium (33–35).

Traumatic injuries (particularly involving brain, bone, or liver), thermal injuries, and severe crush injuries, as well as surgical procedures may produce a consumptive coagulopathy (7–12,26–28,36–38). Secondary infection and hemorrhagic shock further serve to aggravate the coagulopathy, especially if acidosis, hypothermia, or tissue ischemia and necrosis develop.

Acute pancreatitis, arising from various causes, may be associated with DIC due to release of enzymes that may directly activate a number of coagulation factors (39). In many instances, there is associated multiorgan dysfunction involving cardiopulmonary, renal, and hepatic function. In addition, pyogenic sequelae, such as the development of infected pancreatic necrosis or abscess formation, may result in DIC attributable to sepsis. Treatment is primarily supportive, with aggressive resuscitation, replacement of deficient coagulation factors if there is associated bleeding, appropriate use of broad-spectrum antibiotics, and surgical debridement and drainage for control of infectious complications.

Obstetric complications can result in some of the most profound and challenging instances of DIC. Well-recognized examples include amniotic fluid embolism, abruptio placentae, retained dead fetus, and eclampsia (9–11). In these circumstances, the culprit is massive systemic release of tissue thromboplastin that generates a fulminant course characterized by bilateral renal cortical necrosis to frank cardiopulmonary collapse, shock, multiorgan failure, and, at times, death even if aggressive attempts are made to treat these individuals.

Both acute and chronic forms of DIC have been identified. In the acute form patients are critically ill, whereas in the chronic form the natural history is more indolent and protracted, and thrombotic complications may be the predominant feature.

Notwithstanding, coagulopathy manifested in the critically ill patient is often a result of a combination of both platelet and plasmatic coagulation factor defects. Well-known examples include obstructive biliary tract disease or chronic liver disease, which results in diminished production of coagulation factors given that the liver is the major site of synthesis of all coagulation factors with the exception of factor VIII. Hepatic parenchymal and biliary obstructive disease results in diverse manifestations of hemostatic abnormalities (15). Extrahepatic biliary obstruction results in diminished absorption of vitamin K due to lack of bile salts necessary for gastrointestinal absorption of lipid soluble vitamins. Decreased synthesis of the vitamin K–dependent factors II, VII, IX, and X occurs with abnormal prolongation of the prothrombin time (PT) and eventually the partial thromboplastin time (PTT). Parenchymal diseases such as cirrhosis, chronic active hepatitis, fulminant hepatic failure, or metastatic carcinoma impact on the hemostatic system in a heterogeneous manner. Most coagulation factors, naturally occurring anticoagulants (such as antithrombin III), fibrinolysin precursors (plasminogen), and inhibitors of the fibrinolytic system (antiplasmins) are synthesized by the liver. In severe liver disease, acquired dysfibrinogenemia has also been reported (15,40). This impairs polymerization of soluble fibrin monomers and is suggested by a prolonged thrombin time (TT) on purified fibrinogen, which is generally done in a research laboratory. The liver also removes activated coagulation factors from the circulation, but it is speculative to conclude that this results in a coagulopathy by itself, despite the fact that this increased consumption of activated factors by the liver lowers coagulation factors already depressed by decreased production in a diseased liver. Clearance of fibrinogen/fibrin degradation products is reduced in chronic liver disease. These breakdown products inhibit both fibrin polymerization and platelet function and thus contribute to a defective hemostatic system, as discussed earlier. Thrombocytopenia occurs secondary to hypersplenism, potentially exacerbated by vitamin deficiencies associated with decreased thrombopoiesis. Additionally, alcohol has a direct toxic effect on megakaryocytes, which contributes to prevailing vitamin deficiencies and decreased bone marrow production of platelets. Massive trauma often results in decreases of both platelets and coagulation factors as a result of consumption secondary to ongoing bleeding or hemorrhage (2,7–11,26–28,37,38). If shock and acidosis develop, there is further decrease in coagulation factor synthesis due to impairment in liver function that results from low perfusion, in addition to impairment of both coagulation factor and platelet function from the acidemic state (26–28,40,41). Additionally, a well-described sequela of massive blood transfusion, often associated with multiple trauma and hemorrhagic shock, is the *development* of a coagulopathy. Major trauma, major orthopedic (spine, hip, or pelvis) or hepatic procedures (major hepatic resections, liver transplantation), or other causes of potentially life-threatening, exsanguinating hemorrhage are often associated with the need for what has been termed *massive blood transfusion*. This term has been variously defined but generally refers to administering the equivalent of one total blood volume or more to a patient in less than a 24-hour period. Due to consumption of coagulation factors and platelets, release of inflammatory mediators, dilution of elements necessary for the optimal function of the coagulation cascade, hypocalcemia, hypothermia, fibrinolysis, and alterations in acid–base homeostasis, a coagulopathy often develops in this scenario (2,5–8,26–28,42–44). Banked blood is a negligible source of viable platelets, which rapidly deteriorate under conditions of cold storage (4–6). Additionally, depending on the age of the unit, plasmatic coagulation factors may also be diminished in activity. The derangement in clotting represents nonlocalized, nonsurgical bleeding that is characterized by sanguineous oozing from all raw surfaces, including any wounds, mucosal or peritoneal surfaces, and percutaneous entry sites. Numerous risk factors for the development of this condition (particularly in the setting of trauma) include high injury severity score, acidosis, hypothermia, and hypotension (7,8,10,26–28,41–43). Last, transient platelet dysfunction, responsive to desmopressin (DDAVP, 1-desamino-8-d-arginine vasopressin), is a well-recognized phenomenon in patients after cardiopulmonary bypass (45–49). To this end, postoperative bleeding is a frequent impediment of cardiopulmonary bypass. Numerous mechanisms are apparently involved, which include contact factor (factors XII and XI) activation, elevations of tissue plasminogen activator level and tissue thromboplastin, dilution of plasmatic coagulation factors, residual effects of systemic heparinization, hypothermia, platelet function defects, and failure of surgical hemostasis (45–50). Some investigations have demonstrated a 30% to 50% decrement in platelet count attributable to the shearing forces that are encountered in the bypass apparatus. The routine use of antiplatelet agents in patients with cardiac disease, such as aspirin and thienopyridine derivatives, also contributes to the increased risk for bleeding. The combined effects of aspirin and a thienopyridine derivative, such as clopidogrel, on bleeding complications are synergistic and not additive. In approximately 4% to 5% of patients, surgical re-exploration of the mediastinum is necessary, which varies based on the original procedure performed (45–50). Several criteria for re-exploration have been proposed that have in common the rate of blood loss from mediastinal or chest tubes. Criteria variably used include blood loss from chest or mediastinal tubes of 300 mL/hr within the first 3 hours; total blood loss of 1,000 mL after 4 hours; a sudden increase in bleeding (>300 mL/hr) in a patient who previously had minimal drainage; or evidence of cardiac tamponade. A coagulopathy must never be presumed to be the cause of bleeding postoperatively unless surgical causes of bleeding have first been excluded. A site of localized bleeding (surgical failure) is identified in more than 50% of patients re-explored based on these types of criteria (45–50). Despite multiple contributing factors to the bleeding that occurs in these patients, the prime offender is collectively believed to be secondary to qualitative platelet function defects (1,2,45–50). The bypass circuitry results in platelet activation with degranulation and aggregation. Although this functional deficit is transient, increased time on bypass, hypothermia, and antiplatelet medications significantly exacerbates this condition. Laboratory analysis reveals a prolongation of the bleeding time with impaired adhesion and aggregation, particularly in the presence of ADP and ristocetin. This latter finding is believed to be linked to low levels of von Willebrand factor (vWF) found in plasma after cardiopulmonary bypass. Hence, some investigators have proposed use of desmopressin in this circumstance (and in patients with a history of preoperative use of aspirin), to increase levels of vWF by stimulating release from endothelial cells, increasing the glycoprotein receptors on platelets, and increasing the level of factor VIII and tissue plasminogen activator. However, others believe that this practice increases the risk of graft thrombosis and coronary occlusion (48–50). Additionally, peer-reviewed, reported outcome data in this circumstance are indeterminate (45–49). Usually the acquired qualitative platelet function defect resolves within 4 hours of completion of cardiopulmonary bypass without any intervention. In instances where there is prolonged nonsurgical postoperative bleeding, platelet transfusions are often beneficial (4,6,49).

Normal physiologic processes (fibrinolytic system) exist to control for unremitting clot formation and are described in several reviews (1,50–52). Impaired function of the coagulation cascade may be the result of various disorders that are characterized by the genesis of circulating anticoagulants, abnormal protein products, or accumulation of proteinaceous breakdown products that affect the normal function of coagulation proteins. Collagen vascular diseases, such as systemic lupus erythematosus, is one example (53,54). In these patients an antibody is produced (lupus anticoagulant) that affects the coagulation cascade at the juncture of the intrinsic and extrinsic systems, resulting in prolongation of both the PT and PTT in vitro. Paradoxically, these patients tend to be hypercoagulable, and if clinically significant bleeding is noted, it is attributable to associated thrombocytopenia and increased vascular fragility. When there are elevated titers of either the lupus anticoagulant or anticardiolipin antibodies, or both, these patients may present with manifestation of the antiphospholipid antibody syndrome with generalized microvascular thrombosis, thrombocytopenia, gangrene of the extremities, multiorgan failure, and death. Plasmapheresis, anticoagulation, and immunosuppressive therapy serve as the foundation of treatment (53,54). Other commonly acquired inhibitors or circulating anticoagulants include factor VIII inhibitors and factor IX inhibitors, related primarily to prior frequency of transfusion with plasma-derived blood concentrates and alloimmunization (55–57). Exogenously administered heparin, the prototype for anticoagulation therapy, binds to circulating antithrombin III and catalyzes its ability to neutralize the action of a number of coagulation factors. The end result is interference with the normal coagulation cascade. Disorders characterized by the production of abnormal globulins, often referred to collectively as the paraproteinemias (associated with multiple myeloma and Waldenstrom macroglobulinemia), also result in interference with coagulation proteins and inhibition of fibrin polymerization. Treatment of the coagulopathy associated with all of these conditions consists of replacement of deficient coagulation factors when bleeding is dominant and definitive treatment directed at the underlying disease process.

DIAGNOSIS

A detailed history and physical examination is the most important preliminary step in elucidating the cause of surgical bleeding and should be done simultaneously with resuscitative efforts (1,2,5,6,8). Collateral history from family members and previous medical records is a helpful adjunct to determine if a primary, congenital defect in the coagulation system is present. A history of easy bruisability, excessive gingival bleeding after brushing of teeth, bleeding diathesis with dental extractions, hypermenorrhagia, frequent spontaneous epistaxis, melenic stools or spontaneous hematuria, petechiae or purpura, hemarthroses, and a family history of bleeding disorders may indicate a congenital or familial coagulation disorder, such as hemophilia A or B or von Willebrand disease. The family pedigree may provide important clues as to the presumptive disease process based on the pattern of inheritance, whether autosomal or sex linked, dominant or recessive. Suspicion for a congenital disorder of coagulation is further raised by a history of blood transfusions required for common ambulatory procedures such as dental extractions, circumcisions, tonsillectomies, or biopsies. Due to differences in gene penetrance, not all individuals afflicted with inherited coagulation disorders are diagnosed at an early age, and clinically latent, attenuated bleeding disorders may be unmasked when confronted by a major surgical procedure or trauma. A past history of liver disease or heavy ethanol consumption should alert the clinician to the possibility of acquired plasmatic factor deficiencies, in addition to thrombocytopenia resulting from secondary hypersplenism with platelet sequestration.

A thorough medication history is essential (including soliciting information on the use of dietary supplements or herbal tonics, and over-the-counter medications), to determine if the patient has been on any medication that interferes with hemostasis (common examples include aspirin, other nonsteroidal anti-inflammatory agents, ticlopidine, clopidogrel, semisynthetic penicillins, and more recently, newer classes of oral anticoagulants such as rivaroxaban, apixaban, and dabigatran) (2–6,13). Popular supplements that may aggravate bleeding are ginkgo, garlic, ginger, ginseng, feverfew, and vitamin E. A history of anticoagulation therapy is equally important in this regard (2,3,32,58). Nutritional assessment is paramount, and careful evaluation for the presence of a vitamin K deficiency is obligatory, as this may occur in patients on parenteral nutrition or with cancer cachexia in those with malignancies. Other variables that may affect the integrity of the coagulation system include previous irradiation, renal failure, and sepsis, which affect the coagulation cascade at multiple points.

Physical examination often provides an index of the severity and the extent of the disease and may provide additional clues that assist in distinguishing localized surgical bleeding from systemic bleeding resulting from a coagulopathy. For example, the presence of petechiae, purpura, and mucosal bleeding is often indicative of thrombocytopenia, a qualitative functional disorder of platelets, or increased vascular fragility. Ecchymoses or spontaneous, nontraumatic hemarthrosis is consistent with plasmatic coagulation factor abnormalities or deficiencies such as hemophilia. Both platelet and plasmatic coagulation disorders are associated with hematomas. Hepatic insufficiency or failure can be presumptively identified by recognizing jaundice, ascites, angiomas, palmar erythema, asterixis, congestive splenomegaly, and testicular atrophy. Splenomegaly itself may also be associated with hematologic dyscrasias and malignancies associated with hemostatic abnormalities (lymphomas and leukemias). Connective tissue or collagen vascular disorders that result in increased vascular fragility may manifest with petechiae, joint abnormalities, and a history of delayed wound healing. These conditions focus attention on the increased risk for a perioperative bleeding complication, which underscores the need for vigilance both intraoperatively and postoperatively. Last, the possibility of sepsis as an underlying cause for the development of a coagulopathy must always be entertained in the postoperative, critically ill patient (12).

The establishment of a definitive diagnosis of a coagulation disorder rests on selective use of a limited battery of laboratory tests guided by information derived from the history and physical examination. These assays are selected to broadly screen the hemostatic system. These tests are, for the most part, automated (except for the bleeding time), readily available, and amenable to point-of-care testing methodology. The tests most commonly used include the template bleeding time, quantitative platelet count, PT, activated PTT, fibrinogen level, and thrombin time (TT). The template bleeding time is the only test that screens for qualitative platelet function abnormalities, a frequent cause of abnormal bleeding. This test is not commonly used, given that it does not lend itself to automation and still requires the laboratory technologist to remain at the patient's bedside. Furthermore, this test has been attended by poor reproducibility, particularly in conditions associated with significant peripheral edema. Nevertheless, when a qualitative platelet function abnormality is suspected, the bleeding time is an appropriate first screening test to guide discriminate use of additional testing to further elucidate the underlying cause. This test also evaluates platelet number and vascular fragility, demonstrating abnormal prolongation in thrombocytopenic states and in conditions associated with increased vascular fragility (examples include connective tissue disorders such as senile purpura, Ehlers–Danlos syndrome, steroid-induced purpura, or Marfan syndrome; scurvy; amyloidosis; or hereditary hemorrhagic telangiectasia/Osler–Weber–Rendu disease). Therefore, if both the platelet count and the template bleeding time are normal, the presumptive differential diagnosis is directed toward a plasmatic coagulation factor abnormality. Measurement of both the PT and PTT will serve to further define the abnormality, given that each test is more sensitive to changes in procoagulants in the initial phases of the extrinsic and intrinsic pathways, respectively. The PTT provides a global measure of the activity of factors XII, XI, IX, and VIII in addition to the common pathway factors shared by the extrinsic system (factors X, V, II, and I) and, therefore, identifies many of the inherited disorders of bleeding, typically a deficiency of factor VIII (hemophilia A), IX (hemophilia B), or vWF (von Willebrand disease). It is worth noting that factor XII deficiency is not associated with any significant bleeding tendency despite abnormal prolongation of the PTT. Enzymatically active vWF is a necessary cofactor for optimum functioning of the factor VIII procoagulant protein. The PT exclusively evaluates factor VII, which is one of the vitamin K–dependent factors (in addition to factors II, IX, and X). Therefore, the PT is prolonged in individuals on warfarin (Coumadin) therapy, and this test is used to measure therapeutic efficacy of this form of oral anticoagulation therapy. Liver disease is another common cause for a prolonged

PT, perhaps most notably because factor VII has the shortest half-life of the plasmatic coagulation factors. Liver disease, by virtue of the diminished synthesis of all plasmatic coagulation factors (with the exception of vWF) also results in prolongation of the PTT in addition to the PT. Due to the sensitivity of factors XII, XI, IX, VIII, and X to the effects of heparin (in the presence of antithrombin III), heparin therapy primarily is reflected by abnormal prolongation of the PTT. In conditions associated with prolongation of both the PT and PTT, quantitative measurement of the fibrinogen (factor I) level may be useful to determine if the coagulation disorder is a result of a defect or deficiency of multiple coagulation factors, which may be associated with liver disease, sepsis, and DIC, or if an inhibitor is present (2,5,6,8,9–12,15,40). Examples of circulating inhibitors include heparin, paraproteinemias associated with monoclonal gammopathies (multiple myeloma or Waldenstrom macroglobulinemia), fibrin/fibrinogen degradation products, or other circulating anticoagulants (such as antibodies to factor VIII or IX, and the lupus anticoagulant). In the case of heparin, paraproteinemias, and fibrin/fibrinogen degradation products the PT, PTT, and TT all are prolonged due to their inhibition of fibrin polymerization. Moreover, factor levels reflect a dynamic equilibrium, and fibrinogen is an acute-phase protein that increases in response to stress. Thus, fibrinogen consumption may not be apparent based solely on measurement of levels because of the propensity for the liver to increase synthesis of this protein in response to the same stressors responsible for fibrinogen consumption. This fact is important to bear in mind for proper interpretation of laboratory results. The TT is a qualitative measure of fibrinogen levels and will be prolonged if the fibrinogen level is less than 100 mg/dL, by the presence of dysfibrinogenemia associated with liver disease, and also by circulating inhibitors similar to the PT and PTT (40). Its most useful role clinically is in the detection of circulating heparin not detectable by changes in the PTT. The laboratory diagnosis of DIC is readily established with routinely available tests. The PT, PTT, and TT are all prolonged, and the platelet count is decreased. Depending on the severity of the disease process, fibrinogen may not be detectable. Fibrinogen/fibrin degradation products are elevated, and the peripheral blood smear often reveals the presence of schistocytes. Factors I (fibrinogen), V, VIII, and XIII tend to be markedly depressed. In milder forms, fibrinogen levels may not be significantly decreased, particularly in the presence of adequate hepatic function. Radioimmunoassays of fibrinopeptide A, a by-product of the action of thrombin on fibrinogen, has been found in research settings to assist in the establishment of the correct diagnosis and management approach, but this assay has not gained widespread clinical acceptance (59). Although rare, primary fibrinolysis differs from DIC (where secondary fibrinolysis occurs) in the following ways. In primary fibrinolysis, platelet count is normal, soluble fibrin monomers are not present (measured by the plasma paracoagulation test), schistocytes (red cell fragments) are not seen, and tests for increased levels of plasmin activity are strongly positive (euglobulin clot lysis time, whole blood clot lysis time). Finally, the diagnostic dilemma associated with the effects of thrombin and factor Xa inhibitor pharmacotherapy is worthy of comment. These agents, such as dabigatran, rivaroxaban, and apixaban, have been Food and Drug Administration-approved for the management of venous and arterial thromboembolic disorders and atrial fibrillation (2,3). These agents offer a number of advantages over warfarin (Coumadin), which include the administration of a fixed dose of drug without a need for routine therapeutic monitoring. Thus, there were no laboratory tests utilized in the clinical trials that evaluated the clinical efficacy of these drugs. Dabigatran, a thrombin inhibitor, may prolong the PTT and TT, while rivaroxaban and apixaban, activated factor X (factor Xa) inhibitors, result in prolongation of the PT (2,3). Measurement of anti-Xa may assist in the quantitation of the plasma levels of these latter two drugs (2,3).

TREATMENT

To expeditiously manage a critically ill patient experiencing life-threatening hemorrhage, it is crucial that a defined approach for prompt recognition of the underlying cause is used. First, attention is directed toward stabilizing the patient. This includes securing an adequate airway, ventilation, vascular access, and restoring intravascular volume. Early recognition of the clinical symptoms and signs attributable to hypovolemia (restlessness, anxiety, shortness of breath, pallor, tachycardia, and oliguria) is compulsory. Adjunctive estimates of intravascular volume status may be obtained using both noninvasive and invasive monitoring, as is common in the critical care setting, described elsewhere in this textbook. Systemic hypotension is a late sign of significant hypovolemia, and expeditious resuscitation is paramount to avert the disastrous consequences of an unrecognized and inappropriately triaged patient with ongoing, potentially life-threatening hemorrhage.

Second, there should be immediate dialogue with individuals involved in the intraoperative management of the patient. This may provide pertinent information regarding the intraoperative course of the patient, specifically regarding any observed characteristics of bleeding that may suggest an underlying coagulation disorder. A generalized slow oozing of blood from raw surfaces (often termed *nonsurgical bleeding*) is often a manifestation of a systemic disorder of hemostasis. On the other hand, bleeding related to technical factors that can be associated with the conduct of any surgical procedure (often termed *surgical bleeding*) is localized and is the most common cause of postoperative bleeding. Although signs of an expanding hematoma or saturated dressings are indicative of localized bleeding, there is considerable overlap, and coagulation system defects may present in a similar fashion postoperatively. Dialogue with the surgical team should include consideration for re-exploration. The evolving coagulopathy may proceed swiftly in critically ill patients. Qualitative abnormalities of platelet function, depletion of both platelets and plasmatic coagulation factors, and hypothermia are major contributors to the underlying pathophysiology responsible for the coagulopathy that manifests in the critical care setting. Moreover, previously undiagnosed, rare, at times clinically latent, congenital coagulation disorders may be unmasked by the physiologic stress resulting from a surgical procedure. Familial coagulation defects that may be encountered in a bleeding postoperative patient include von Willebrand disease, factor VIII deficiency (hemophilia A or classic hemophilia), and factor IX deficiency (hemophilia B or Christmas disease) (4,20,40,55,56,60,61,64).

The therapeutic approach to hemostatic abnormalities must be reasonably guided by the patient's clinical condition and the outcome of appropriately selected laboratory tests (4–6). An important concept is not to fall behind in factor replacement. Due to the lag time in receiving laboratory values, in clinical conditions where the patient is actively bleeding, initiation of fresh-frozen plasma (FFP) and platelets should be started early with red cell transfusion. In patients with known warfarin use and a small bleed in an uncompromising area (skull), FFP should be used *before* patients develop increasing intracranial hemorrhage. In general, FFP is the most commonly used blood component for plasmatic coagulation abnormalities because it provides all necessary coagulation factors in concentrations that approach those found in normal plasma (2–6,40,55–58,60). Despite plasmatic coagulation factor activity deteriorating with storage, dilution of these factors below levels required for adequate hemostasis is rare. Therefore, routine administration of FFP after an arbitrary number of units of banked blood has been transfused is not supported by stringent investigations (5–8,10,26–28,60,62–66). If there is bleeding due to a coagulopathy with concomitant prolongation of the PT and PTT of more than 1.5 times normal, FFP should be infused (to normalize the PTT and achieve a PT international normalized ratio [INR] 1.5). There is emphasis on early correction because timid replacement of coagulation products will lead to more bleeding and being more coagulopathic, leading to a vicious cycle. Cryoprecipitate should be considered if the fibrinogen level is less than 0.8 g/dL.

Cryoprecipitate, a component made from thawing FFP in the cold under specialized conditions, is rich in factors XIII, VIII, I, vWF, and fibronectin. It has been used in factor VIII–deficient states (hemophilia A) if virally inactivated plasma-derived or recombinant factor VIII concentrates are not readily available; in von Willebrand disease recalcitrant to desmopressin and if virally inactivated plasma-derived factor VIII concentrate rich in vWF is not readily available; in hypofibrinogenemic or dysfibrinogenemic conditions; in hemorrhage associated with massive blood transfusions; in DIC; in factor XIII deficiency (FFP is also used); in bleeding uremic patients with qualitative platelet function defects unresponsive to desmopressin therapy; or as a topically applied surgical sealant ("fibrin glue") (67). It should be further highlighted that the number of disorders associated with DIC is substantial, but the unifying approach to management is supportive therapy with replacement of coagulation factors and platelets with attention focused on treating the underlying disease process. In DIC, FFP and platelet concentrates are the two most common blood products used as a temporizing measure (4–6,9–12,60). Stored or banked whole blood is a reasonable source of most clotting factors if the units are less than 24 hours old (4–6,43,60). The biologic half-life of factors V, VII, VIII, and IX are on the order of 24 hours or less; hence whole blood stored for longer than 24 hours may not provide adequate amounts of these coagulation factors. Heparin had been used in the past in a theoretical attempt to abrogate the clotting cascade, but its contemporaneous use for this purpose is at best controversial, may be contraindicated in the perioperative period, and is not supported by evidence-based data (9–12,68). Recombinant activated factor VIIa had demonstrated promise in significantly reducing bleeding and blood transfusion requirements in patients with traumatic injuries, or surgical procedures attended by significant hemorrhage, in addition to liver transplantation. However, a clear survival benefit has not been demonstrated in randomized controlled trials (69–75).

For specific coagulation disorders, such as hemophilia A, hemophilia B (deficiencies of factors VIII and IX, respectively), and von Willebrand disease, virally inactivated plasma-derived factor concentrates are commercially available, as are recombinant products, and these are the blood components of choice if available for use. These concentrates (and the recombinant product) also have a lower risk for virally transmitted disease because of a processing procedure that results in viral inactivation. For deficiencies of the vitamin K–dependent factors (II, VII, IX, X), prothrombin complex concentrates are also commercially available, as is recombinant factor VII for isolated factor VII deficiency states. In these situations, therapy is acutely centered on replacement of coagulation factors, most commonly with use of FFP. Vitamin K can be administered parenterally in patients with deficient states or to reverse the effects of Coumadin, but appreciable effects on coagulation factor synthesis (in the presence of normal hepatic synthetic function) is not generally seen for 24 to 36 hours after administration of parenteral vitamin K (32,58). Treatment of bleeding in liver failure with vitamin K usually is not successful given the lack of hepatic synthetic function. Whole blood both corrects the red blood cell deficit and is as effective as FFP in correcting coagulation factor deficits if the units of blood have not been banked for an extended period of time (4–6,43,60). Platelet transfusions should be judiciously used to raise the platelet count to above 100×10^9/L if bleeding is encountered in this setting, and FFP should be provided to correct deficits in plasmatic coagulation factors (4–6,60). For those patients who have recently (within the prior 24 hours) taken oral activated factor X or thrombin inhibitors, there are no known antidotes in the setting of acute hemorrhage (3). Furthermore, there are no evidence-based guidelines applicable to the use of hemostatic agents. Recombinant activated factor VIIa, and activated and nonactivated prothrombin complex concentrate have all been used clinically, but no outcome-based studies exist to guide management. Studies are underway to evaluate antidote prototypes for this newer class of oral anticoagulants.

Platelet concentrates are used for both quantitative (thrombocytopenias) and qualitative platelet disorders associated with significant bleeding (2,4–6,31). It is generally recommended for patients taking antiplatelet medications, such as aspirin or clopidogrel, that these agents are discontinued approximately 7 to 10 days prior to surgery. For nonsteroidal anti-inflammatory agents other than aspirin, ticlopidine, or clopidogrel, some investigators advocate 2 days of abstinence. It is important to recognize, again, that many over-the-counter medications contain aspirin (e.g., Alka-Seltzer, Ecotrin, Anacin) and many patients are not aware of this, so it is imperative to obtain a comprehensive drug history, specifically querying for use of aspirin-containing products. Discontinuing the antiplatelet drug combined with use of desmopressin and platelet transfusions have been beneficial in treating bleeding encountered in these situations (2,4–6,13). Prophylactic administration of platelets during massive blood transfusion in an attempt to prevent the development of a coagulopathy has been advocated by many centers, but the efficacy of this policy is unproven. Studies have failed to demonstrate conclusively a benefit to this approach (4–6,42,43,62,76,77). It is reasonable, however, to administer platelets to a bleeding patient or one with DIC if the platelet count is less than 50×10^9/L. For those patients with rapid bleeding or with multiple traumatic injuries undergoing surgery or other high-risk procedures, a goal of at least 100×10^9/L has been recommended, albeit in the absence of high-level evidence-based data. One unit of platelet concentrate typically raises the platelet count by 5×10^9/L, whereas one apheresis concentrate raises the platelet count by 20 to 25×10^9/L in an average 70-kg adult.

The fundamental approach to therapy for patients with renal failure attended by qualitative platelet dysfunction centers on dialysis, which results in abatement of the bleeding diathesis. Use of desmopressin and cryoprecipitate, as temporizing measures to transiently stop the bleeding while awaiting institution of dialysis, have been reported to be successful (29–31). Conjugated estrogens have also been used with some success, albeit the effects are not as rapid but more durable, but any positive outcomes are balanced by undesirable consequences of hormonal side effects. In its chronic form, renal failure is still attended by a mild qualitative platelet function defect, but significant impact on hemostatic homeostasis is usually not seen (29–31).

It should be highlighted that patients transfused with any blood component, whether FFP, cryoprecipitate, plasma-derived factor concentrates, or platelet concentrates, incur similar risks of complications attributed to all types of blood component therapy such as febrile and allergic reactions, transmission of blood-borne pathogens (human immunodeficiency virus, hepatitis B and C), immunosuppression, transfusion-related pulmonary injury, and hemolytic transfusion reactions if a substantial volume of ABO-incompatible units are transfused. In the setting of massive blood transfusion, numerous points are warranted. Hemolytic transfusion reactions may occur as a result of ABO incompatibility between the actual units of blood transfused, or potentially because of clerical error, magnified by the volume of units required in a relatively short period of time. Red blood cells are a rich source of tissue thromboplastin, and hemolysis results in a massive release of this extrinsic system activator. This manifests as a generalized oozing from all raw surfaces, similar to the coagulopathy seen with massive blood transfusions, rendering this a difficult diagnosis to make. Hemoglobinuria may be observed due to filtration of plasmafree hemoglobin into the urine. Consistent with other types of transfusion reactions, the coagulation abnormality corrects rapidly once the offending transfusion is terminated. Treatment must be directed toward prevention of hemoglobin casts precipitating in the acidic environment of the collecting tubules, resulting in acute tubular necrosis and acute renal failure. Appropriate fluid resuscitation to maintain intravascular volume and to initiate a diuresis is paramount. Mannitol, an osmotic diuretic and free radical scavenger, may be administered intravenously as an adjunct to maintain urine flow, and intravenous sodium bicarbonate may be considered to alkalinize the urine to avoid further precipitation of hemoglobin in the renal tubules. In essence, judicious use of blood component therapy must always be adhered to.

A few comments on the effects of hypothermia is of merit here. It is important to bear in mind that all enzymatic processes in biologic systems are governed to an extent by the necessity to function in an optimal, typically narrow, temperature range. The coagulation factors are enzymes, and therefore function best under normothermic conditions. Platelets, too, function optimally under normothermic conditions. The implication of this is that the clinician must always remain alert to the effects of hypothermia as the origin of a coagulopathy, particularly in the critical care environment. Reliance solely on the values of the PT, PTT, or TT can be misleading, understanding that these assays are performed by both manual and automated laboratory methods at 37°C and results may thus fall within the reference range in vitro, despite ongoing coagulopathy clinically. External warming measures should include blankets generating heated air, warming of all fluid infusions, heated humidifier in ventilated patients, and warming the ambient environment. In extreme conditions, Gentilello et al. (78) reported that continuous arteriovenous rewarming, which does not require heparinization of the patient and hence does not exacerbate the coagulopathy, improves hemostasis more rapidly than any other method with the exception of cardiopulmonary bypass.

In parallel with the ongoing resuscitation of the bleeding patient, attention must be directed toward expeditiously determining the need for surgical re-exploration. There are certain circumstances where operative re-exploration is obligatory, despite the fact that the bleeding may be self-limiting. Certain surgical procedures are not associated with exsanguinating hemorrhage or hypotension but can nonetheless be life threatening. Prototypic examples include neck operations for endocrine diseases (thyroid, parathyroid surgery), lymphadenectomies (radical neck dissections), major composite resections for tumors of the neck, and carotid surgery. From a pathophysiologic perspective, an expanding neck hematoma results in airway obstruction from both mechanical compression and from mural edema caused by lymphatic obstruction. The cause is frequently venous bleeding, compounded by hypertension and liberal preoperative use of antiplatelet medications in those undergoing carotid surgery. Acutely reopening the incision and evacuating the hematoma is often lifesaving, although endotracheal intubation or cricothyroidotomy may be required as a temporizing measure until the airway edema resolves. In contrast, the natural history of a contained perioperative vascular anastomotic dehiscence is characterized by the evolution of a false aneurysm. In this setting, immediate re-exploration with operative repair is indicated to avert the potentially catastrophic consequence of free rupture and death from exsanguinating hemorrhage. Therefore, nearly all patients who develop neck hematomas require operative re-exploration. It is common practice to place drains in the operative field at the time of surgery prior to closure, and surgical procedural anthologies are replete with instructions substantiating this approach. Caution must be exercised in interpreting drain output as an accurate index of early perioperative bleeding, and it is correspondingly crucial to recognize that placement of a drain is not an appropriate substitute for ensuring meticulous surgical hemostasis (79).

Notwithstanding, all bleeding patients must be considered candidates for reoperation. Postoperative bleeding, often termed local hemostatic failure or surgical bleeding, is a known potential complication of any surgical procedure. When associated with evolving hypovolemia, mental status changes, restlessness, anxiety, tachycardia, dyspnea, and oliguria are commonly associated manifestations. Hypotension is a late finding, and aggressive attempts must be made to avert this serious consequence with expeditious concurrent resuscitation as identification of the source of bleeding is confirmed. The vast majority of patients affected typically present within the immediate perioperative period. Subtle signs may be evident in the postanesthesia care unit, and generally become apparent within the first 8 hours after surgery. A high index of suspicion is necessary to render an early diagnosis of postoperative bleeding, and meticulous attention to look for any evidence of bleeding must be applied, given that many signs of evolving hypovolemia are nonspecific and may also be observed in nonbleeding patients after major thoracic or abdominal procedures (tachycardia associated with postoperative pain, anxiety and restlessness, mental status changes secondary to narcotic analgesic administration, or oliguria resulting from anticipated third-space fluid sequestration after major abdominal surgery). Blood in the peritoneal cavity ordinarily does not result in a significant inflammatory response unless associated with secondary bacterial contamination and therefore is not associated with obvious peritoneal signs. On occasion, localized symptoms may be elicited that are attributable to irritation caused by a collection of blood, exemplified by the Kehr sign. This is referred pain to the right shoulder ascribed to an accumulation of blood under the right hemidiaphragm. Serial hemoglobin and hematocrit levels may assist in determining the degree of bleeding, but isolated, single values can be difficult to interpret. It is difficult to quantitatively account for the effects of isotonic fluid sequestration (third-spacing) after major abdominal procedures that may result in hemoconcentration and elevated hemoglobin and hematocrit levels, or the effects of isotonic fluid administration in the perioperative period that may contribute to hemodilution and lower hemoglobin and hematocrit levels.

Taken collectively, there is no single criterion available to direct re-exploration for control of postoperative bleeding, and this decision is based on considering a number of variables. The timing of the active bleed relative to the operative procedure, its duration, its rate, the potential for additional morbidity, the patient's age as a surrogate for physiologic reserve, and other comorbid diseases (such as underlying cardiac or pulmonary disease, renal disease, diabetes, or obesity) must all be taken into consideration when deciding on the need for reoperation. Timing of re-exploration is of significant concern in conditions associated with limited or poor physiologic reserve as these patients are often quite ill and require judicious resuscitation and expeditious definitive surgical intervention prior to the inception of irreversible shock. The most conservative treatment is to return to the operating room with early control of surgical bleeding. Oftentimes the need to return emergently to the operating room is quite obvious, as in the case of exsanguinating hemorrhage resulting from a coronary artery bypass graft dehiscence attended by brisk bleeding from the mediastinal drain. However, there are two caveats for consideration. First, it is desirable to correct any coagulopathy prior to returning to the operating room, and in some instances with minimal or mild bleeding this may be all that is necessary. It is important to recognize, however, that situations characterized by exsanguinating hemorrhage from failure of local surgical hemostasis may not allow for correction of the coagulopathy because of rapid ongoing consumption of coagulation factors and platelets. In these instances, operative intervention is paramount, and the decision to reoperate must not be unduly delayed while awaiting normalization of coagulation parameters. Second, as stated earlier, some subscribe to the notion that drains placed at the time of surgery are a useful adjunct to alert the surgical team to early signs of postoperative bleeding and to gauge the amount and rate of bleeding when it does occur. Caution with this practice must be promulgated, as it is a well-accepted observation that the absence of blood in a drain is not conclusive evidence that bleeding is not occurring, because the drain tip may be dislodged or may have migrated from its original position and this may not be readily apparent externally, or the drain may be obstructed with clot.

Finally, the surgeon must also be cognizant of the fact that there are some instances where bleeding is optimally addressed without surgical intervention. The prototypic illustration is the severe pelvic fracture with signs of ongoing hemorrhage. In accordance with the Advanced Trauma Life Support protocol, associated injuries and additional sources of obvious bleeding must first be excluded. Once hemoperitoneum and hemothorax have been excluded, the pelvis is stabilized (generally by external fixation), followed by arteriography with embolization of any bleeding pelvic or retroperitoneal blood vessels.

Consequently, a comprehensive assessment must take into account the degree and the duration of active bleeding, the anatomic site of involvement, and the potential for additional morbidity or mortality (e.g., evolving acidosis, myocardial ischemia, diminished mental status, oliguria, or a progressive neck wound hematoma with impending acute airway obstruction). Physiologic reserve is also a compelling variable to consider, for patients with significant comorbidities, such as the elderly, pediatric, obese, and diabetic patients are attended by less reserve. Therefore, vigilant observation to recognize early postoperative bleeding is crucial, before hemodynamic instability and shock become manifest. In these patients, consideration for early operative intervention may be necessary because this cohort may not be able to readily tolerate even mild degrees of anemia, hypovolemia, and hypoperfusion. Consideration of other modalities of hemorrhage control (interventional radiology and embolization) may be entertained in appropriate situations.

It should also be noted that many pharmacologic agents have proven efficacy in the management of nonsurgical bleeding, particularly in the post–cardiopulmonary bypass setting. Desmopressin has already been described. Epsilon aminocaproic acid (EACA) and tranexamic acid are lysine analogs that inhibit binding of plasmin to fibrin (48,50,80,81). EACA appears to have the weakest antifibrinolytic effect compared to tranexamic acid, but nevertheless has been used in the cardiopulmonary bypass patient with some success. Tranexamic acid has met with considerable success in the reduction of postoperative blood loss and the reduced need for red blood cell transfusion in cardiac surgery, total knee arthroplasty, transurethral prostate surgery, and in oral surgery procedures. Neither EACA nor tranexamic acid is associated with thrombotic complications or anaphylactic reactions. The most commonly reported adverse reactions include nausea, diarrhea, and orthostatic reactions (48,50,80).

In conclusion, surgical and postsurgical bleeding requires immediate recognition of early shock, resuscitation, and differentiation between surgical and nonsurgical bleeding. Prudent and meticulous evaluation of the patient, in order to identify primary or secondary coagulation disorders, is paramount. Knowledge of the complexities of the coagulation cascade is essential, in this regard, to ensure timely and precise diagnosis and management of these conditions, with appropriate replacement of blood and blood products, to effect the best patient outcomes.

CONTROVERSIES

Measurement of the viscoelastic properties of clotting blood as a tool to evaluate the integrity of the coagulation system was first described in 1948, prior to the development of the PTT and the activated clotting time (82). Thromboelastography, and thromboelastometry, assays first popularized in Europe, have been used to determine if there is a platelet function abnormality, a deficit in plasmatic coagulation factors, the presence of circulating anticoagulants, or fibrinolysins in patients undergoing cardiopulmonary bypass (6,13,82,83). Not at all surprisingly, in the quest for more enhanced, more dynamic coagulation assays (rather than the static, global measures of coagulation in common use currently), the use of this technology has expanded into the realm of liver transplantation, obstetrics, trauma, sepsis, and therapeutic monitoring of anticoagulation (6,13,82–87). These assays have been touted as having the potential to diagnose early coagulopathies, and subsequently judiciously guide treatment. This technique fundamentally evaluates whole clot formation and dissolution, and continually evaluates clot firmness in an integrated manner, reflecting in vivo hemostasis. Furthermore, it is amenable to point-of-care testing, with short turnaround times, hence its usefulness both intra- and postoperatively. No specific specimen processing is required, and whole blood is used for testing. This technology is rapidly gaining attention as a valuable adjunct to managing complex coagulation disorders (6,82–87). It has been efficacious in decreasing blood transfusion requirements during cardiac surgery and in liver transplantation (82,83). The effect of hypothermia on a patient's coagulation profile can also be determined simply by adjusting the temperature of the apparatus to correspond with the patient's core body temperature. Several automated analyzers are available commercially, now that technical improvements have resulted in improved standardization of the methodology. However, a major disadvantage of these assays is their lack of validation. Systematic reviews of the literature have shown highly variable, heterogeneous study designs, control groups, and reference standards; timing of measurements; and preselected endpoints, all contributing to methodological flaws that have made it challenging to draw conclusive inferences (82–87). Moreover, the predictive value of these assays has not been found to be consistently superior to the coagulation assays currently in use. Taken collectively, adequately powered, stringent randomized controlled trials are needed to validate this technology before it can attain widespread clinical use. Despite its promise, there are currently no universally accepted guidelines that espouse use of this technology (6,82–87).

Key Points

- Hemostatic disorders, whether primary (inherited) or secondary (acquired), can be manifested by diffuse bleeding from the operative site, puncture wounds, vascular access sites, or traumatized tissue outside of the operative field.
- Coagulopathy in the critically ill patient is often a result of a combination of both platelet and plasmatic coagulation factor defects.
- A detailed history and physical examination is the most important preliminary step in elucidating the cause of surgical bleeding and should be done simultaneously with resuscitative efforts.
- Physical examination often provides an index of the severity and the extent of the disease and may provide additional clues that assist in distinguishing localized surgical bleeding from systemic bleeding resulting from a coagulopathy.
- The establishment of a definitive diagnosis of a coagulation disorder rests on selective use of a limited battery of laboratory tests guided by information derived from the history and physical examination.
- To expeditiously manage a critically ill patient experiencing life-threatening hemorrhage, it is crucial that a defined approach for prompt recognition of the underlying cause is used. First and foremost, attention is directed toward stabilizing the patient.
- The therapeutic approach to hemostatic abnormalities must be reasonably guided by the patient's clinical condition and the outcome of appropriately selected laboratory tests. It is important not to fall behind in factor replacement.
- In parallel with the ongoing resuscitation of the bleeding patient, attention must be directed toward expeditiously determining the need for surgical re-exploration.

References

1. Adams GL, Manson RJ, Turner I, et al. The balance of thrombosis and hemorrhage in surgery. *Hematol Oncol Clin North Am.* 2007;21:13–24.
2. Hurwitz A, Massone R, Lopez BL. Acquired bleeding disorders. *Emerg Med Clin North Am.* 2014;32:691–713.
3. Weitz JI, Pollack CV Jr. Practical management of bleeding in patients receiving non-vitamin K antagonist oral anticoagulants. *Thromb Haemost.* 2015;114:1113–1126.
4. Kaufman RM, Djulbegovic B, Gernsheimer T, et al. Platelet transfusion: a clinical practice guideline from the AABB. *Ann Intern Med.* 2015;162: 205–213.
5. Shah A, McKechnie S, Stanworth S. Use of plasma for acquired coagulation factor deficiencies in critical care. *Semin Thromb Hemost.* 2016;42:95–101.
6. Shah A, Stanworth SJ, McKechnie S. Evidence and triggers for the transfusion of blood and blood products. *Anaesthesia.* 2015:70(Suppl 1):10–19.
7. Rossaint R, Cerny V, Coats TJ, et al. Key issues in advanced bleeding care in trauma. *Shock.* 2006;26:322–331.
8. Theusinger OM, Madjdpour C, Spahn DR. Resuscitation and transfusion management in trauma patients: emerging concepts. *Curr Opin Crit Care.* 2012;18:661–670.
9. Dempfle C. Disseminated intravascular coagulation and coagulation disorders. *Curr Opin Anaesthesiol.* 2004;17:125–129.
10. Gando S, Sawamura A, Hayakawa M. Trauma, shock, and disseminated intravascular coagulation: lessons from the classical literature. *Ann Surg.* 2011;254:10–19.
11. Bick RL. Disseminated intravascular coagulation: current concepts of etiology, pathophysiology, diagnosis, and treatment. *Hematol Oncol Clin North Am.* 2003;17:149–176.
12. Zeerleder S, Hack CE, Wuillemin WA. Disseminated intravascular coagulation in sepsis. *Chest.* 2005;128:2864–2875.
13. Shore-Lesserson L. Platelet inhibitors and monitoring platelet function: implications for bleeding. *Hematol Oncol Clin North Am.* 2007;21:51–63.
14. Metjian A, Abrams CS. New insights and therapeutics for immune-mediated thrombocytopenia. *Expert Rev Cardiovasc Ther.* 2008;6:71–84.
15. Pluta A, Gutkowski K, Hartleb M. Coagulopathy in liver diseases. *Adv Med Sci.* 2010;55:16–21.
16. Malara A, Balduini A. Blood platelet production and morphology. *Thromb Res.* 2012;129:241–244.
17. Pongas G, Dasgupta SK, Thiagarajan P. Antiplatelet factor 4/heparin antibodies in patients with gram negative bacteremia. *Thromb Res.* 2013;132:217–220.

18. Shenkman B, Einav Y. Thrombotic thrombocytopenic purpura and other thrombotic microangiopathic hemolytic anemias: diagnosis and classification. *Autoimmun Rev.* 2014;13:584–586.
19. Sadler JE. What's new in the diagnosis and pathophysiology of thrombotic thrombocytopenic purpura. *Hematology Am Soc Hematol Educ Program.* 2015;2015:631–636.
20. Smock KJ, Perkins SL. Thrombocytopenia: an update. *Int J Lab Hematol.* 2014;36:269–278.
21. Gonzalez CE, Pengetze YM. Post-transfusion purpura. *Curr Hematol Rep.* 2005;4:154–159.
22. Koene HR. Critical issues of current and future developments in the treatment of immune thrombocytopenic purpura. *Pediatr Blood Cancer.* 2006;47 (5 Suppl):703–705.
23. Godeau B, Provan D, Bussel J. Immune thrombocytopenic purpura in adults. *Curr Opin Hematol.* 2007;14:535–556.
24. Warkentin TE. Heparin-induced thrombocytopenia in critically ill patients. *Semin Thromb Hemost.* 2015;41:49–60.
25. Mielke CH Jr. Influence of aspirin on platelets and the bleeding time. *Am J Med.* 1983;74:72–78.
26. Duan K, Yu W, Li N. The pathophysiology and management of acute traumatic coagulopathy. *Clin Appl Thromb Hemost.* 2015;21:645–652.
27. Gando S, Hayakawa M. Pathophysiology of trauma-induced coagulopathy and management of critical bleeding requiring massive transfusion. *Semin Thromb Hemost.* 2016;42(2):155–165.
28. Davenport R. Pathogenesis of acute traumatic coagulopathy. *Transfusion.* 2013;53(Suppl 1):23S–27S.
29. Escolar G, Diaz-Ricart M, Cases A. Uremic platelet dysfunction: past and present. *Curr Hematol Rep.* 2005;4:359–367.
30. Boccardo P, Remuzzi G, Galbusera M. Platelet dysfunction in renal failure. *Semin Thromb Hemost.* 2004;30:579–589.
31. Kaw D, Malhotra D. Platelet dysfunction and end-stage renal disease. *Semin Dial.* 2006;19:317–322.
32. Pruthi RK. Review of the American College of Chest Physicians 2012 guidelines for anticoagulation therapy and prevention of thrombosis. *Semin Hematol.* 2013;50:251–258.
33. Thiagarajan P, Niemetz J. Procoagulant-tissue factor activity of circulating peripheral blood leukocytes: results of *in vivo* studies. *Thromb Res.* 1980;17:891–896.
34. Maier RV, Ulevitch RJ. The induction of a unique procoagulant activity in rabbit hepatic macrophages by bacterial lipopolysaccharides. *J Immunol.* 1981;127:1596–1600.
35. Schorer AE, Rick PD, Swaim WR, Moldow CF. Structural features of endotoxin required for stimulation of endothelial cell tissue factor production: exposure of preformed tissue factor after oxidant-mediated endothelial cell injury. *J Lab Clin Med.* 1985;106:38–42.
36. Lavrentieva A. Coagulopathy in burn patients: one part of a deadly trio. *Burns.* 2015;41:419–420.
37. Saggar V, Mittal RS, Vyas MC. Hemostatic abnormalities in patients with closed head injuries and their role in predicting early mortality. *J Neurotrauma.* 2009;26:1665–1668.
38. Risberg B, Medegard A, Heideman M, et al. Early activation of humoral proteolytic systems in patients with multiple trauma. *Crit Care Med.* 1986;14:917–925.
39. Gupta S, Shekhawat VP, Kaushik GG. D-dimer, a potential marker for the prediction of severity of acute pancreatitis. *Clin Lab.* 2015;61:1187–1195.
40. Stevens SM, Woller SC, Bauer KA, et al. Guidance for the evaluation and treatment of hereditary and acquired thrombophilia. *J Thromb Thrombolysis.* 2016;41:154–164.
41. MacLeod JB, Lynn M, McKenney MG, et al. Early coagulopathy predicts mortality in trauma. *J Trauma.* 2003;55:39–44.
42. Levy JH. Massive transfusion coagulopathy. *Semin Hematol.* 2006;43(1 Suppl 1):S59–S63.
43. Levi M, Fries D, Gombotz H, et al. Prevention and treatment of coagulopathy in patients receiving massive transfusion. *Vox Sang.* 2011;101:154–174.
44. Spahn DR. Hypocalcemia in trauma: frequent but frequently undetected and underestimated. *Crit Care Med.* 2005;33:2124–2125.
45. Despotis GJ, Filos KS, Zoys TN, et al. Factors associated with excessive postoperative blood loss and hemostatic transfusion requirements: a multivariate analysis in cardiac surgical patients. *Anesth Analg.* 1996;82: 13–21.
46. Hertfelder HJ, Bos M, Weber D, et al. Perioperative monitoring of primary and secondary hemostasis in coronary artery bypass grafting. *Semin Thromb Hemost.* 2005;31:426–440.
47. Karthik S, Grayson AD, McCarron EE, et al. Reexploration for bleeding after coronary artery bypass surgery: risk factors, outcomes, and the effect of time delay. *Ann Thorac Surg.* 2004;78:527–534; discussion 534.
48. Henry DA, Carless PA, Moxey AJ, et al. Anti-fibrinolytic use for minimizing perioperative allogeneic blood transfusion. *Cochrane Database Syst Rev.* 2011;(3):CD001886.
49. Woodman RC, Harker LA. Bleeding complications associated with cardiopulmonary bypass. *Blood.* 1990;76:1680–1697.
50. Fergusson DA, Hebert PC, Mazer CD, et al.; BART Investigators. A comparison of aprotinin and lysine analogues in high-risk cardiac surgery. *N Engl J Med.* 2008;358:2319–2331.
51. Kwaan HC, Nabhan C. Hereditary and acquired defects in the fibrinolytic system associated with thrombosis. *Hematol Oncol Clin North Am.* 2003;17:103–114.
52. Wolberg AS. Determinants of fibrin formation, structure, and function. *Curr Opin Hematol.* 2012;19:349–356.
53. Galli M, Barbui T. Antiphospholipid syndrome: clinical and diagnostic utility of laboratory tests. *Semin Thromb Hemost.* 2005;31:17–24.
54. Galli M, Luciani D, Bertolini G, Barbui T. Lupus anticoagulants are stronger risk factors for thrombosis than anticardiolipin antibodies in the antiphospholipid syndrome: a systematic review of the literature. *Blood.* 2003;101:1827–1832.
55. Kessler CM, Knobl P. Acquired haemophilia: an overview for clinical practice. *Eur J Haematol.* 2015;95(Suppl 81):36–44.
56. Janbain M, Leissinger CA, Kruse-Jarres R. Acquired hemophilia A: emerging treatment options. *J Blood Med.* 2015;6:143–150.
57. Lusher JM. Inhibitor antibodies to factor VIII and factor IX: management. *Semin Thromb Hemost.* 2000;26:179–188.
58. Dentali F, Ageno W, Crowther M. Treatment of coumarin-associated coagulopathy: a systematic review and proposed treatment algorithms. *J Thromb Haemost.* 2006;4:1853–1863.
59. Leeksma OC, Meijer-Huizinga F, Stoepman-van Dalen EA, et al. Fibrinopeptide A and the phosphate content of fibrinogen in venous thromboembolism and disseminated intravascular coagulation. *Blood.* 1986;67:1460–1467.
60. Contreras M, Ala FA, Greaves M, et al. Guidelines for the use of fresh frozen plasma British Committee for Standards in Haematology, Working Party of the Blood Transfusion Task Force. *Transfus Med.* 1992;2:57–63.
61. Shortt J, Dunkley S, Rickard K, et al. Efficacy and safety of a high purity, double virus inactivated factor VIII/von Willebrand factor concentrate (Biostate) in patients with von Willebrand disorder requiring invasive or surgical procedures. *Hemophilia.* 2007;13:144–148.
62. Gajic O, Dzik WH, Toy P. Fresh frozen plasma and platelet transfusion for nonbleeding patients in the intensive care unit: benefit or harm? *Crit Care Med.* 2006;34(5 Suppl):S170–S173.
63. Desborough M, Stanworth S. Plasma transfusion for bedside, radiologically guided, and operating room invasive procedures. *Transfusion.* 2012;52(Suppl 1):20S–29S.
64. Dara SI, Rana R, Afessa B, et al. Fresh frozen plasma transfusion in critically ill medical patients with coagulopathy. *Crit Care Med.* 2005;33:2667–2671.
65. Gonzalez EA, Moore FA, Holcomb JB, et al. Fresh frozen plasma should be given earlier to patients requiring massive transfusion. *J Trauma.* 2007;62:112–119.
66. Abdel-Wahab OI, Healy B, Dzik WH. Effect of fresh-frozen plasma transfusion on prothrombin time and bleeding in patients with mild coagulation abnormalities. *Transfusion.* 2006;46:1279–1285.
67. MacGillivray TE. Fibrin sealants and glues. *J Card Surg.* 2003;18:480–485.
68. Feinstein DI. Diagnosis and management of disseminated intravascular coagulation: the role of heparin therapy. *Blood.* 1982;60:284–287.
69. Hauser CJ, Boffard K, Dutton R, et al.; CONTROL Study Group. Results of the CONTROL trial: efficacy and safety of recombinant activated Factor VII in the management of refractory traumatic hemorrhage. *J Trauma.* 2010;69:489–500.
70. Levi M, Levy JH, Andersen HF, Truloff D. Safety of recombinant activated factor VII in randomized clinical trials. *N Engl J Med.* 2010;363:1791–1800.
71. Boffard KD, Choong PI, Kluger Y, et al. The treatment of bleeding is to stop the bleeding! Treatment of trauma related hemorrhage. *Transfusion.* 2009;49(Suppl 5);240S–247S.
72. Boffard KD, Riou B, Warren B, et al.; NovoSeven Trauma Study Group. Recombinant factor VIIa as adjunctive therapy for bleeding control in severely injured trauma patients: two parallel randomized, placebo-controlled, double-blind clinical trials. *J Trauma.* 2005;59:8–15; discussion 15–18.
73. Rizoli SB, Boffard KD, Riou B, et al. Recombinant activated factor VII as an adjunctive therapy for bleeding control in severe trauma patients with coagulopathy: subgroup analysis from two randomized trials. *Crit Care.* 2006;10:R178.
74. Coppola A, Windyga J, Tufano A, et al. Treatment for preventing bleeding in people with haemophilia or other congenital bleeding disorders undergoing surgery. *Cochrane Database Syst Rev.* 2015;2:CD009961.
75. Levi M, Peters M, Buller HR. Efficacy and safety of recombinant factor VIIa for treatment of severe bleeding: a systematic review. *Crit Care Med.* 2005;33:883–890.

76. Reed RL 2nd, Ciavarella D, Heimbach DM, et al. Prophylactic platelet administration during massive transfusion: a prospective, randomized, double-blind clinical study. *Ann Surg.* 1986;203:40–48.
77. Segal JB, Dzik WH; Transfusion Medicine/Hemostasis Clinical Trials Network. Paucity of studies to support that abnormal coagulation test results predict bleeding in the setting of invasive procedures: an evidence-based review. *Transfusion.* 2005;45:1413–1425.
78. Gentilello LM, Cortes V, Moujaes S, et al. Continuous arteriovenous rewarming: experimental results and thermodynamic model simulation of treatment for hypothermia. *J Trauma.* 1990;30:1436–1449.
79. Kunkel JM, Gomez ER, Spebar MJ, et al. Wound hematomas after carotid endarterectomy. *Am J Surg.* 1984;148:844–847.
80. McCormack PL. Tranexamic acid: a review of its use in the treatment of hyperfibrinolysis. *Drugs.* 2012;72:585–617.
81. Levy JH. Anti-inflammatory strategies and hemostatic agents: old drugs, new ideas. *Hematol Oncol Clin North Am.* 2007;21:89–101.
82. Hans GA, Besser MW. The place of viscoelastic testing in clinical practice. *Br J Haematol.* 2016;173(1):37–48.
83. Bracey AW, Grigore AM, Nussmeier NA. Impact of platelet testing on presurgical screening and implications for cardiac and noncardiac surgical procedures. *Am J Cardiol.* 2006;98(Suppl 1):25N–32N.
84. Hunt H, Stanworth S, Curry N, et al. Thromboelastography (TEG) and rotational thromboelastometry (ROTEM) for trauma induced coagulopathy in adult trauma patients with bleeding. *Cochrane Database Syst Rev.* 2015;(2):CD010438.
85. Inaba K, Rizoli S, Veigas PV, et al.; Viscoelastic Testing in Trauma Consensus Panel. 2014 consensus conference on viscoelastic test-based transfusion guidelines for early trauma resuscitation: report of the panel. *J Trauma Acute Care Surg.* 2015;78:1220–1229.
86. Da Luz LT, Nascimento B, Shankarakutty AK, et al. Effect of thromboelastography (TEG) and rotational thromboelastometry (ROTEM) on diagnosis of coagulopathy, transfusion guidance and mortality in trauma: descriptive systematic review. *Crit Care.* 2014;18:518.
87. Muller MC, Meijers JC, Vroom MB, Juffermans NP. Utility of thromboelastography and/or thromboelastometry in adults with sepsis: a systematic review. *Crit Care.* 2014;18:R30.

CHAPTER

57

Abdominal Trauma: Nonoperative Management and Postoperative Considerations

CLAY COTHREN BURLEW and ERNEST E. MOORE

INTRODUCTION

Multiply injured patients admitted to the intensive care unit (ICU) have an array of physiologic derangements that may include metabolic failure and cardiopulmonary embarrassment. The intensivist needs to understand the inherent differences in care of the postinjury patient. They should be familiar with the implications of specific injuries including guidelines for nonoperative management, postoperative care, and potential complications. This chapter will focus on the acute resuscitation and ICU management of the trauma patient, rather than the initial evaluation in the emergency department (ED). Initial therapy in the trauma bay, indications for emergent operation, and intraoperative decision making are beyond the scope of this chapter.

INITIAL EVALUATION IN THE INTENSIVE CARE UNIT

Although some patients may arrive in the ICU *in extremis* necessitating continued resuscitation without a thorough history and physical examination, the majority should undergo a complete assessment promptly, and it should not be assumed that the ED evaluation was comprehensive. Such an evaluation may be termed the tertiary survey (1). The evaluation is often more detailed than that performed in the ED, because all diagnostic results should be available, intraoperative findings known, further information is obtained from family members, and the physician has time for a more meticulous physical examination. Key elements include the patient's past medical history, specifically any history of cardiopulmonary disease, past myocardial infarction, use of β-blockers or steroids, chronic hepatic or renal failure, and other elements that may acutely impact the patient's care. Discovering minor injuries on the tertiary survey such as subtle extremity injuries overlooked during the ED evaluation is common (2,3). Documentation of this evaluation, particularly of final imaging results, can be done through a standardized form that facilitates communication among clinicians (Fig. 57.1).

The physical examination is important, even in intoxicated or head injured patients; in addition to external signs of trauma, the patient's reported pain, particularly whether this is increasing or decreasing with time, is paramount. In the intubated patient with a depressed mental status, specific signs of injury such as ecchymosis, abdominal distention, and crepitus are critical to recognize. Similar to the ED, there are clear indications in the ICU for surgeon evaluation for possible laparotomy (Table 57.1).

Some patients will require imaging after ICU admission; patients with emergent operative indications may arrive in the ICU without any computed tomography (CT) scans. These patients, once hemodynamically stable, should undergo CT scanning to delineate additional injuries. Even in patients who undergo exploratory laparotomy, CT of the abdomen may be necessary to diagnose spine fractures and to evaluate the retroperitoneum. Routine postadmission studies include repeat chest radiograph and laboratory studies. A chest radiograph is important to determine central line catheter, tube thoracostomy, nasogastric tube, and endotracheal tube positions, as any of these could become dislodged with transport. The chest radiograph may also show interval change in a patient's hemothorax, pneumothorax, or pulmonary contusion. Based upon physical findings in the tertiary survey, further imaging of extremities may also be indicated.

Once the patient has been fully evaluated by the treating ICU physicians and associated imaging and laboratory results obtained, the therapeutic plan is initiated to optimize the patient's cardiopulmonary, metabolic, and coagulation status. In addition to the patient's resuscitation, there is concurrent treatment of known injuries, ongoing evaluation for missed injuries, and monitoring for the sequelae of recognized injuries.

POSTINJURY RESUSCITATION

ICU management of the trauma patient, either with direct admission from the ED or following emergent operation, is considered in distinct phases with differing priorities. The period of acute resuscitation, typically lasting for the first 12 to 24 hours following injury, combines several principles: optimizing tissue perfusion, ensuring normothermia, and restoring coagulation. There are a multitude of management algorithms aimed at accomplishing these goals—most involve resuscitation with initial volume loading to attain adequate preload, followed by judicious use of inotropic agents or vasopressors (4). Although resuscitation endpoints continue to be debated, most agree that normalizing serum lactate or arterial base deficit within the first 24 hours is a reasonable target. Although the optimal hemoglobin (Hb) level remains debated, during shock resuscitation an Hb over 10 g/dL optimizes oxygen delivery and enhances hemostasis via platelet marginalization (4). A more judicious transfusion trigger of Hb below 7 g/dL in the euvolemic patient after the first 24 hours of resuscitation limits

Name, MR#, Pat#, DOB

DENVER HEALTH MEDICAL CENTER

TERTIARY SURVEY OF THE CRITICALLY ILL PATIENT

Attending: ____ SICU Resident: ____

Date: ____ / ____ / ____ Time: ____
MM DD YY

Injuries Identified:	Operations:
1.	1.
2.	2.
3.	3.
4.	4.
5.	5.

New Information re: PMHx/Comorbidities: ____

Physical Exam

Mental Status: GCS ____ Best exam: ____

HEENT

Scalp: ☐ WNL, or describe: ____

Eyes: ☐ WNL, or describe: ____

Ears: ☐ WNL, or describe: ____

Nose: ☐ WNL, or describe: ____

Mouth/Throat: ☐ WNL, or describe: ____

Facial (step offs, swelling, etc.): ☐ WNL, or describe: ____

Neck: ☐ WNL, or describe: ____

Chest: ☐ WNL, or describe: ____

Abdomen: ☐ WNL, or describe: ____

Back: ☐ WNL, or describe: ____

Pelvis: ☐ WNL, or describe: ____

Extremities:

RUE: ☐ WNL, or describe: ____

LUE: ☐ WNL, or describe: ____

RLE: ☐ WNL, or describe: ____

LLE: ☐ WNL, or describe: ____

radial radial R L L R femoral femoral dorsalis pedis dorsalis pedis

TRAUMA SITES

1. LACERATION / SW	6. DEFORMITY	10. ECCHYMOSIS
2. PUNCTURE / GSW	7. AVULSION	11. HEMATOMA
3. FRACTURE	8. CONTUSION	12. OPEN FX
4. ABRASION	9. CREPITUS	13. PAIN
5. BURN		

A F50-091 (2/05) Pg 1 of 2

Trauma Studies (Big 3 - Plus)		
	Date Completed	Findings
FAST		
Head CT		
Chest CT		
Abdominal CT		
Aortogram		

Diagnostic Studies				
	Ordered	Date Done	WNL	Abnormal - Findings
Repeat Head CT				
4-vessel Angio				
Extremity 1				
Extremity 2				

Status of Spine		
	Radiographically Cleared	Clinically Cleared
Cervical	Name: Date/Time:	Name: Date/Time:
TLS	Name: Date/Time:	Name: Date/Time:

Consultants Involved:
☐ Neurosurgery ☐ Orthopedics ☐ Plastics ☐ GU ☐ Other: ____

Change/New symptoms since ED evaluation: None or describe: ____

Drains (include site): ____

Lines (include site): ____
(Change ED Lines within 24 hours)

Diagnosis	Plan
1.	
2.	
3.	
4.	
5.	
6.	

Resident Signature/Title: ____ ID #: ____ Date: ____ / ____ / ____ Time: ____
MM DD YY

Chief Resident Signature/Title: ____ ID #: ____ Date: ____ / ____ / ____ Time: ____
MM DD YY

Attendings Only Below This Line

Attending Signature/Title: ____ ID #: ____ Date: ____ / ____ / ____ Time: ____
MM DD YY

B F50-091 (2/05) Pg 2 of 2

FIGURE 57.1 A thorough history and physical examination in the intensive care unit including imaging, termed the tertiary survey, can be documented on a standardized form to facilitate communication among care providers.

adverse inflammatory effects and improves mortality (5,6). The resuscitation of the severely injured patient may require an inordinate amount of crystalloid. In fact, this is a challenging aspect of early care—balancing cardiac performance versus promoting an abdominal compartment syndrome (ACS) via tissue edema. Serial base deficit and lactate measurements are helpful; a persistent base deficit of more than 8 mmol/L or lactate over 5 implies ongoing cellular shock (7,8). Evolving technology, such as transesophageal echocardiography may facilitate resuscitation in the patient with cardiac dysfunction (9). During this initial treatment period, a low urine output is usually suggestive of hypovolemia and is not an indication for diuretics. Moreover, the use of diuretics during a patient's initial ICU course should be carefully considered, even if the patient is chronically on such medications. In patients with a challenging resuscitation requiring multiple pressors, one should evaluate for adrenal insufficiency (10,11).

TABLE 57.1 Indications for Surgeon Evaluation in the Intensive Care Unit

- Progressive decline in hemoglobin
- Unexplained leukocytosis and fever
- Hypotension and associated abdominal distension or free fluid on bedside ultrasound
- Diffuse abdominal tenderness
- Computed tomography (CT) scan with evidence of free air or gastrointestinal contrast extravasation
- CT scan with free fluid without associated solid-organ injury
- Intra-abdominal hypertension

Massive transfusion protocols, often initiated in the ED, may be continued in the ICU. Trauma-induced coagulopathy is now well recognized, and underscores the importance of preemptive blood component administration (12). The resurgent interest in viscoelastic hemostatic assays (TEG, ROTEM) has facilitated the appropriate and timely use of clotting adjuncts including the prompt recognition of fibrinolysis. The traditional thresholds for blood component replacement in the patient manifesting a coagulopathy have been INR over 1.5, PTT more than 1.5 normal, platelet count above 50,000/μL, and fibrinogen over 100 mg/dL. However, these guidelines have been replaced by TEG or ROTEM criteria in many trauma centers (Table 57.2). Such guidelines are designed to limit the transfusion of immunologically active blood components and

TABLE 57.2 Transfusion Triggers Using Either Thromboelastography-Based Resuscitation or Traditional Methods

Trigger	Response
TEG-based resuscitation (citrated rapid TEG)	
ACT >128 sec	2 units fresh-frozen plasma
MA <55 mm	1 unit of apheresis platelets
Angle <65 degrees	10 units pooled cryoprecipitate
LY30 >5%	1 g tranexamic acid
Transfusion triggers if TEG is unavailable	
PT, PTT >1.5 control	2 units thawed plasma
Platelet count <50,000/μL	1 unit of apheresis platelets
Fibrinogen <100 mg/dL	10 units pooled cryoprecipitate

decrease the risk of transfusion-associated lung injury and multiple organ failure (12).

Adequate resuscitation is mandatory, and often determines when the surgeon can safely return the patient to the operating room (OR) after initial operative intervention. Specific goals of resuscitation include a core temperature higher than 35°C, base deficit less than −6, and normal coagulation indices. Hyperchloremia associated with normal saline administration and exogenous bicarbonate, occasionally given if the serum pH is below 7.2 to improve cardiovascular function and response to vasoactive agents, obfuscates the acid–base balance and lactate in general is considered a more reliable indicator of adequate tissue perfusion. Although correction of base deficit and lactate values is desirable, how quickly this should be accomplished requires careful consideration. Adverse sequelae of aggressive crystalloid resuscitation include increased intracranial pressure, worsening pulmonary edema, and intra-abdominal visceral and retroperitoneal edema resulting in secondary ACS as well as extremity compartment syndrome (13,14). Therefore, it should be the overall trend of the resuscitation rather than a rapid reduction of the base deficit that is the goal.

NONOPERATIVE MANAGEMENT OF TRAUMA

Blunt Liver and Spleen Injuries

The liver and spleen are the most commonly injured solid organs, occurring in 10% to 15% of all trauma patients (Fig. 57.2). The liver's large size makes it the most susceptible organ injured in blunt trauma, and it is frequently involved in upper torso penetrating trauma. Blunt trauma to the left upper quadrant, often with associated rib fractures, should raise the concern for a splenic injury. Although the liver is more frequently injured, recurrent bleeding from splenic injuries is more common. Nonoperative management of solid-organ injuries is pursued in hemodynamically stable patients who do not have overt peritonitis or other indications for laparotomy (15–25). The clinician should consider the following elements when reviewing the CT scan: the American Association for the Surgery of Trauma (AAST) grade of injury (Table 57.3), the amount of free fluid within the abdomen, the presence of contrast extravasation indicating ongoing arterial bleeding, and

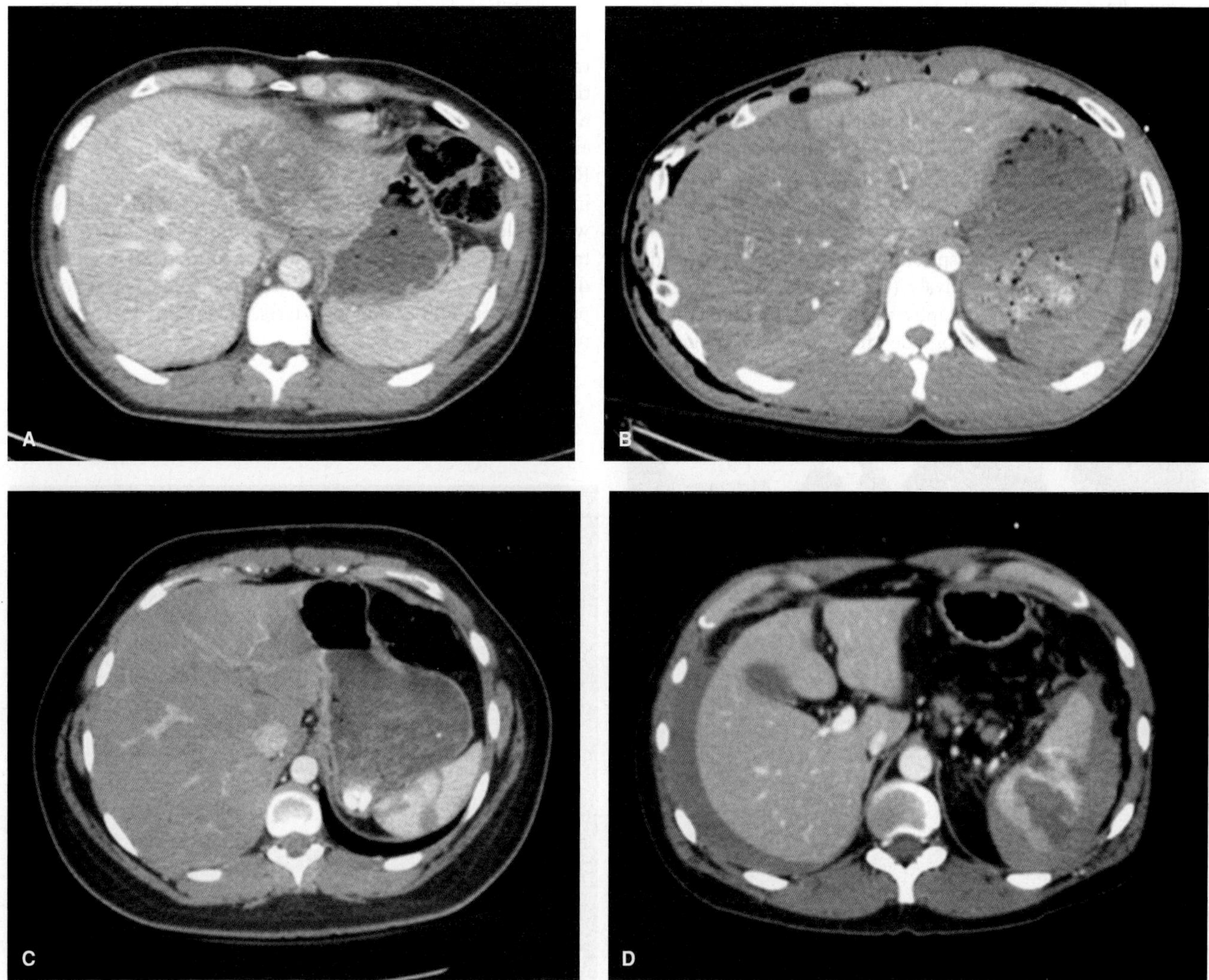

FIGURE 57.2 Representative solid-organ injuries; American Association for the Surgery of Trauma grading includes evidence of grade III and IV hepatic injuries (A, B) and grade III and IV splenic injuries (C, D) and parenchymal lacerations.

TABLE 57.3 American Association for the Surgery of Trauma Solid-Organ Injury Grading Scales

	Subcapsular Hematoma	Laceration
Liver injury grade		
I	<10% surface area	<1 cm in depth
II	10–50% surface area	1–3 cm
III	>50% or >10 cm	>3 cm
IV	25–75% of a hepatic lobe	
V	>75% of a hepatic lobe	
VI	Hepatic avulsion	
Spleen injury grade		
I	<10% surface area	<1 cm in depth
II	10–50% surface area	1–3 cm
III	>50% surface area	>3 cm
IV	>25% devascularization	Hilar injury
V	Shattered spleen	

evidence of pseudoaneurysms (Fig. 57.3). High-grade injuries, a large amount of hemoperitoneum, contrast extravasation, and pseudoaneurysms are not absolute contraindications for nonoperative management; however, these patients are at high risk for failure and are more likely to need angioembolization (26–29). There is no age limit for consideration of nonoperative management for solid-organ injuries, but elderly patients do not tolerate secondary bleeding as well (30–32).

The AAST developed a grading scale to provide a uniform definition of solid-organ injuries based upon the magnitude of anatomic disruption (33–35). The grading of solid-organ injuries permits accurate relay of information between care providers, a predictive value on the incidence of nonoperative failure, and information for appropriate monitoring (Table 57.4). Most patients with liver or spleen injuries, regardless of grade, can be managed nonoperatively (16,23). A multidisciplinary approach including angiography with selective angioembolization and endoscopic retrograde cholangiopancreatography

TABLE 57.4 Appropriate Monitoring and Nonoperative Management Failure Rates for Solid-Organ Injuries by Grade

Grade of Injury	Admission	Monitoring
I	Floor	Exam/Hct every 12 hrs
II	Floor	Exam/Hct every 12 hrs × 4
III	ICU	Exam/Hct every 8 hrs × 6
IV	ICU	Exam/Hct every 4 hrs × 6
V	ICU	Exam/Hct every 4 hrs × 8

Hct, hematocrit; ICU, intensive care unit.

(ERCP) with stenting has resulted in higher rates of successful nonoperative management and improved survival in liver (26,27,36) and splenic injuries (28,29,37–40). Splenic angioembolization has been employed as an adjunct to nonoperative therapy, with reported salvage rates of 98% (40). Patients with contrast extravasation who are hemodynamically stable should likely undergo splenic embolization (28,29,38,39). Additionally, patients with splenic artery pseudoaneurysms or arteriovenous (AV) fistulae within the spleen are also candidates (41). If a patient is going to fail nonoperative management (Fig. 57.4), the time to failure is different for liver versus spleen injuries. Typically liver injuries rebleed within the first hours of admission, while splenic lacerations may have delayed rupture or bleeding weeks following the original injury. With high failure rates reported for grade V splenic injuries, empiric immunization for encapsulated organisms should be considered but may not be mandatory (42). Similarly, patients who undergo angioembolization of the spleen should also receive immunizations. Repeat imaging within 7 days is performed for high-grade injuries (43); hepatic injuries can be evaluated with ultrasound while splenic injuries undergo CT scanning. Patients with liver trauma and evidence of right upper quadrant fluid collections on ultrasound or clinical deterioration (increasing abdominal pain, worsening liver function tests, unexplained fever) should undergo CT scanning.

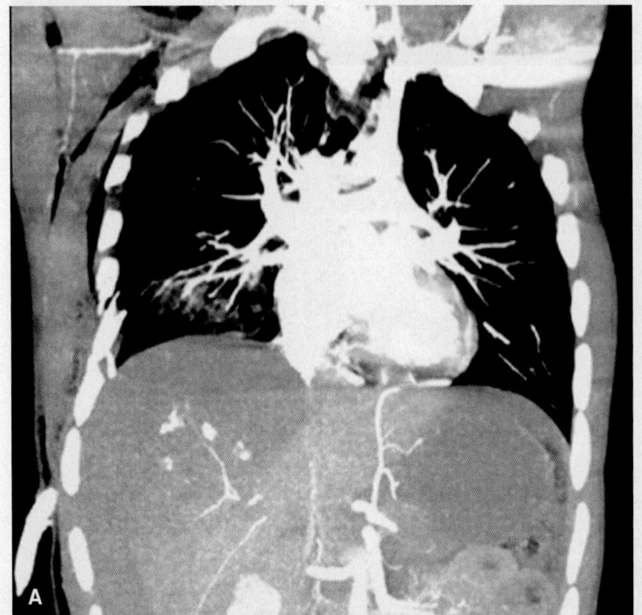

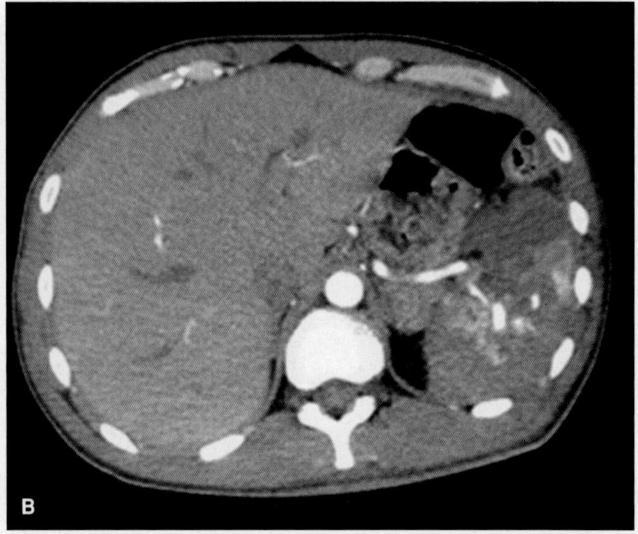

FIGURE 57.3 Contrast blush noted on CT scan imaging of the liver (A) suggestive of active arterial bleeding; postinjury pseudoaneurysms of the spleen are likewise demonstrated with contrasted CT imaging (B).

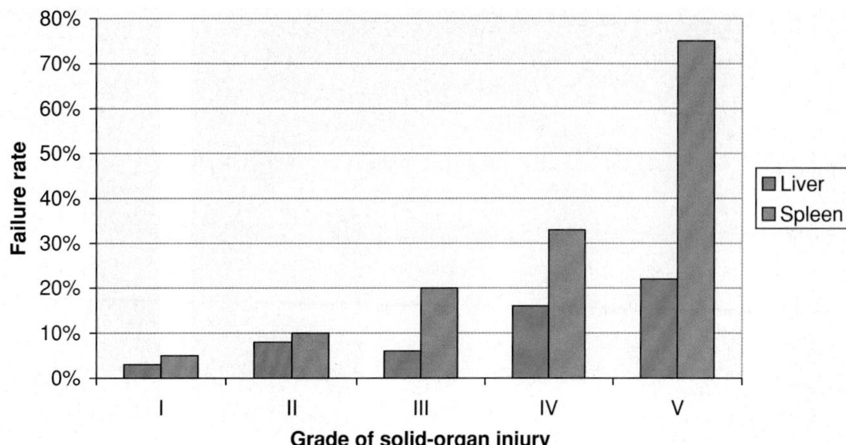

FIGURE 57.4 Rates of nonoperative failure for solid-organ injuries.

Pancreatic Injuries

Historically, injuries to the pancreas were managed with operative intervention (44). With the recent evolution of nonoperative management for solid-organ injuries, a nonresectional management schema has been developed for most pancreatic injuries (45,46). Observation of pancreatic contusions, particularly those in the head of the pancreas that may involve ductal disruption, includes serial examinations and monitoring of serum amylase. Patients with pancreatic injuries involving the major ducts, originally a strict indication for operative intervention, may be managed with ERCP and stenting in selected patients; durability of this approach is currently under investigation (47).

Duodenal Hematomas

Following blunt trauma, patients may develop hematomas in the duodenal wall that obstruct the lumen. Clinical examination findings include epigastric pain associated with either emesis or high nasogastric tube (NGT) output; CT scan imaging with oral contrast failing to pass into the proximal jejunum is diagnostic (Fig. 57.5). Patients with suspected associated perforation, suggested by clinical deterioration or imaging with retroperitoneal free air or contrast extravasation, should be explored operatively. Nonoperative management includes continuous NGT decompression and nutritional support with total parenteral nutrition (TPN) (48,49). A marked drop in NGT output heralds resolution of the hematoma, which typically occurs within 2 weeks. Repeat imaging to document these clinical findings may be helpful before initiating an oral diet. If the patient does not improve clinically or radiographically within 2 to 3 weeks, operative evaluation is warranted.

Penetrating Wounds

Patients with abdominal gunshot wounds (GSWs) violating the peritoneum usually undergo emergent laparotomy due to an approximate 90% visceral injury rate. Selected patients with isolated low-energy GSWs to the right upper quadrant are observed (50); CT scan imaging must delineate the tract of the bullet, which should be confined to the parenchyma of the liver, and the patient must be hemodynamically stable with a benign clinical examination. Recently, several trauma centers have extended this policy to all abdominal GSWs without CT evidence of a hollow visceral injury (51,52). Patients with abdominal stab wounds to the back or flank with negative CT imaging or an isolated kidney injury are also managed nonoperatively (53). Similar to patients with right upper quadrant GSWs, individuals with stab wounds and a CT scan showing the tract of injury confined to the liver are usually observed (53). In some cases, laparoscopy will be done to assess the penetrating liver injury and ensure that hollow viscera are not violated. Regardless of the trauma surgeon's decision for operative versus nonoperative management, it is essential that these patients undergo repeated abdominal examination. Observation for a missed bowel injury is critical; clinical findings in such patients include a rising white blood cell (WBC) count, fever, tachycardia, and increasing abdominal pain or diffuse abdominal tenderness. In patients with isolated liver injuries, complications are similar to those for patients with blunt injuries, namely, bleeding, bile leaks, or biliary sepsis.

COMPLICATIONS OF NONOPERATIVE INJURY MANAGEMENT

Following hepatic injuries, the most common complication is a bile leak or biloma, occurring in up to 20% of patients with major injuries (grade III or higher) (Fig. 57.6) (54,55). Clinical presentation includes abdominal distention, intolerance of enteral feeds, and elevated liver functions tests. CT scanning effectively diagnoses the underlying problem, and the vast majority is treated with percutaneous drainage and ERCP with sphincterotomy. Occasionally, laparoscopy or laparotomy with drainage of biliary ascites is indicated, particularly if the patient fails to resolve their ileus and fever (56). Hemobilia, manifested by the triad of right upper quadrant pain, jaundice, and upper gastrointestinal bleeding, is a rare complication indicative of a communication between a tributary of the hepatic artery and biliary system. Delayed rupture of a subcapsular hematoma with hemorrhage is another infrequent complication but the diagnosis is usually obvious. Patients undergoing angioembolization for liver trauma must be carefully monitored for hepatic necrosis, and

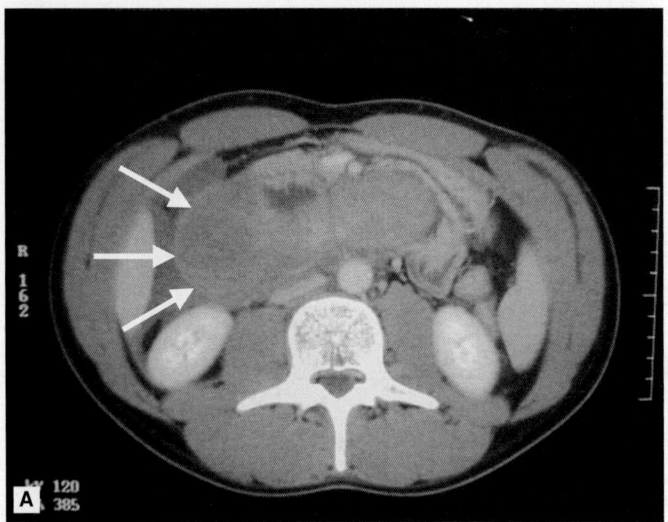

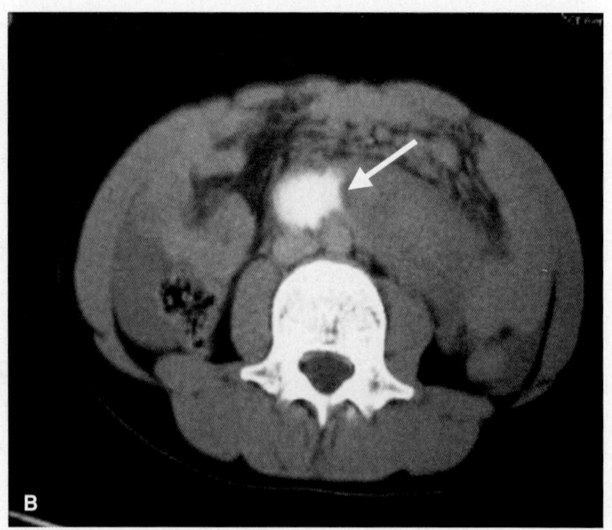

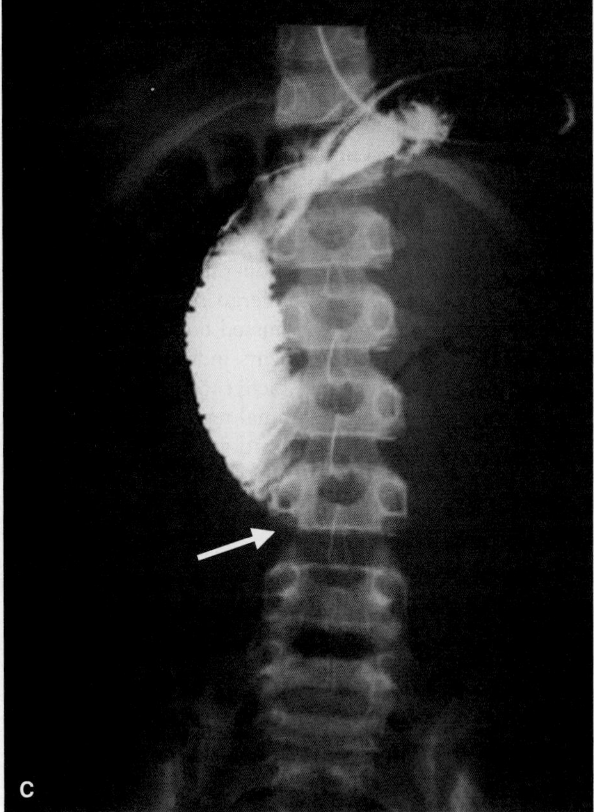

FIGURE 57.5 Duodenal hematomas are diagnosed radiographically by direct identification of a hematoma (A) or failure to pass oral contrast past the third portion of the duodenum on computed tomography scan (B) or upper gastrointestinal series (C).

may occasionally require delayed formal hepatic resection (Fig. 57.7).

The most common problem in patients with splenic injuries is delayed bleeding. Patients undergoing splenic embolization can experience rebleeding, with up to 15% of patients requiring splenectomy (57). Moreover, those undergoing successful angioembolization typically have significant ischemic pain, and some may develop splenic abscesses. In centers that advocate splenic autotransplantation to prevent overwhelming postsplenectomy sepsis (OPSS), recognition of CT scan findings of normal splenic implants versus infected splenic implants is critical in patients with clinical deterioration (58) (see Fig. 57.7).

ONGOING EVALUATION FOR INJURIES: HOW TO AVOID A MISSED INJURY

With the paradigm shift from operative to nonoperative management of trauma, the clinician must have a heightened sense of awareness to identify an occult injury.

Missed bowel injuries are the most commonly pursued injury, not due to their frequency (<5% of blunt trauma) but rather their associated morbidity. Diagnosing a hollow viscus injury is notoriously difficult (59), and even short delays in

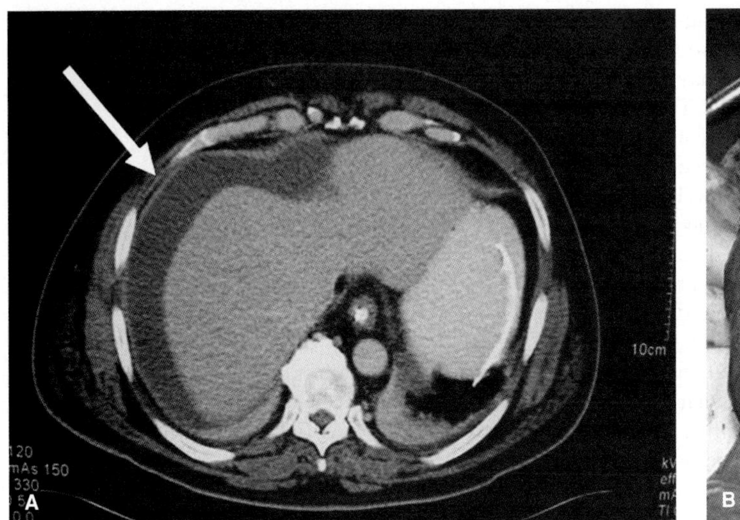

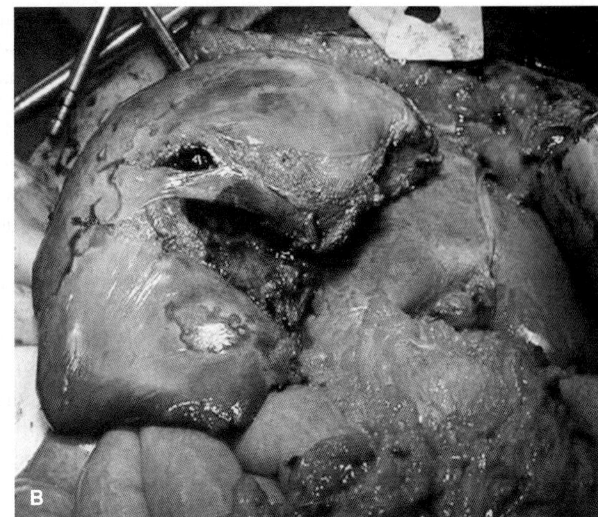

FIGURE 57.6 Bilomas are the most common complication following hepatic trauma (A), while angioembolization for unremitting postinjury liver hemorrhage may result in partial hepatic necrosis (B).

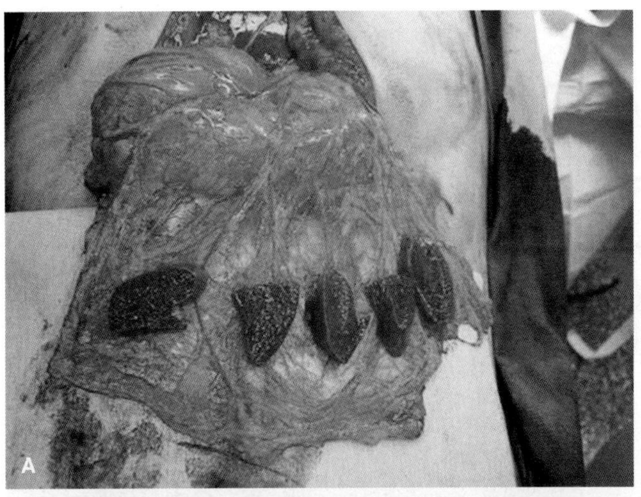

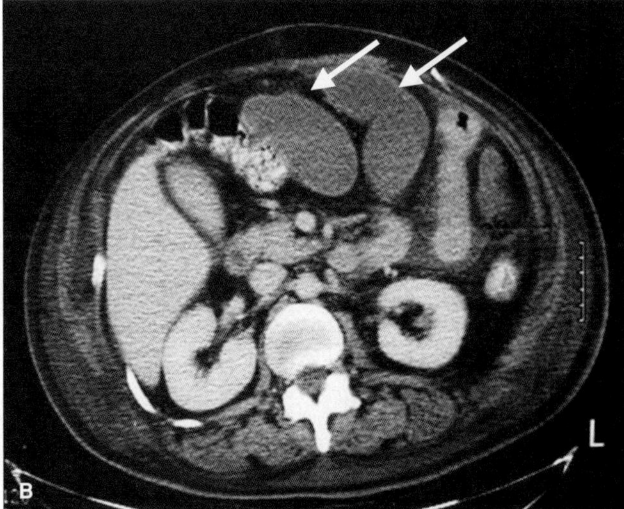

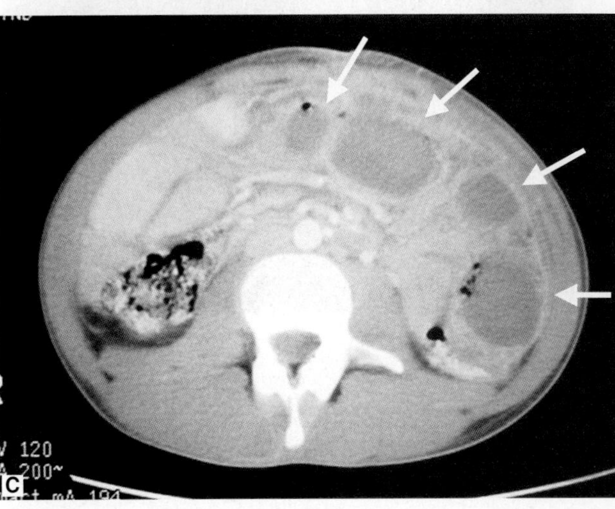

FIGURE 57.7 A: Splenic implants are autotransplanted into the greater omentum to prevent overwhelming postsplenectomy sepsis. Follow-up computed tomography can differentiate between "normal" implants (B) and infected implants (C).

diagnoses result in increased morbidity (60,61). CT scan imaging is not 100% accurate; repeat CT scan imaging, diagnostic peritoneal lavage (DPL), ultrasound, and even laparotomy may be necessary for definitive evaluation. If a patient's initial CT scan of the abdomen shows free fluid without evidence of a solid-organ injury to explain such fluid, patients are monitored closely for evolving signs of peritonitis suggestive of a bowel injury (62–64). If patients have a significant closed head injury or cannot be examined serially, DPL should be performed to exclude bowel injury. DPL should also be considered in a patient if there is increasing intra-abdominal fluid on bedside ultrasound in patients with a solid-organ injury but a stable hemoglobin, and/or in patients with unexplained clinical deterioration. When pursuing a diagnosis of bowel injury using DPL, particular attention should be paid to elevations in bilirubin, alkaline phosphatase, and amylase (65,66) (Table 57.5). The specific type of injury may be either bowel perforation due to ischemia from an avulsed mesentery, a direct antimesenteric blowout injury, or an extensive serosal injury (Fig. 57.8). One should not assume that drugs, alcohol, or their associated withdrawal syndromes are the primary source of a patient's clinical deterioration.

Missing a rectal injury may be life threatening in patients with pelvic fractures. Although some patients have clear findings on physical examination, ranging from hematochezia to overt degloving of the perineum, others may have smaller injuries that are missed on initial evaluation in the trauma bay. In fact, the rectal examination may have been omitted in the trauma bay, so the intensivist should ensure that this has been done. Flexible sigmoidoscopy is the easiest diagnostic procedure for the clinician to perform at the bedside in the ICU; endoscopic evaluation should search for blood within the canal, ischemic mucosa, as well as intestinal perforation (67).

Pancreatic contusions, with or without associated ductal disruption, are difficult to diagnose in patients with blunt

TABLE 57.5 A Positive Diagnostic Peritoneal Lavage Following Blunt Trauma Defined by Specific Laboratory Values

Laboratory Study	Positive Value
White blood cell	>500 cells/μL
Red blood cell	>100,000 cells/μL
Amylase	>19 IU/L
Alkaline phosphatase	>2 IU/L
Bilirubin	>0.1 mg/dL

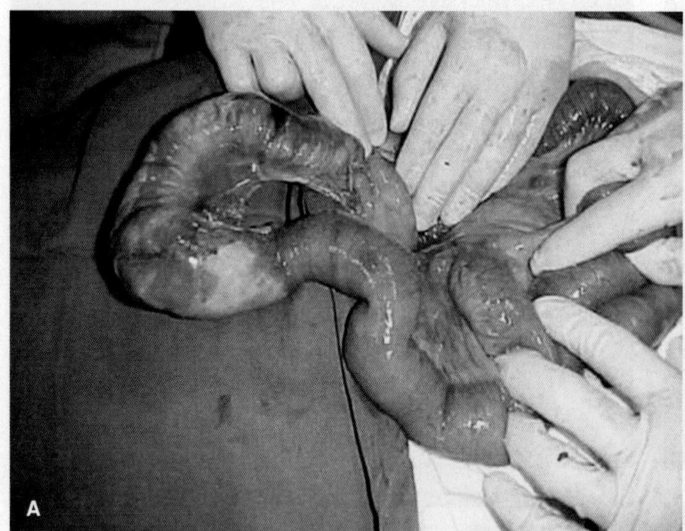

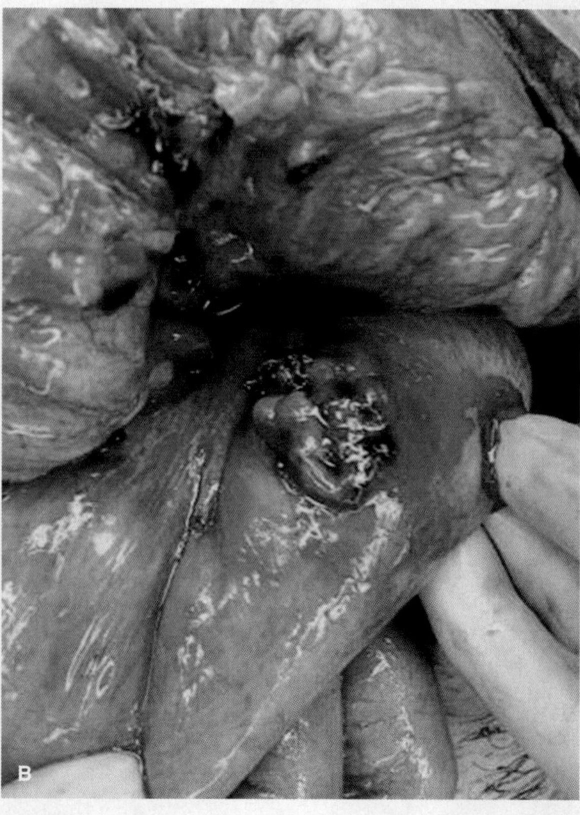

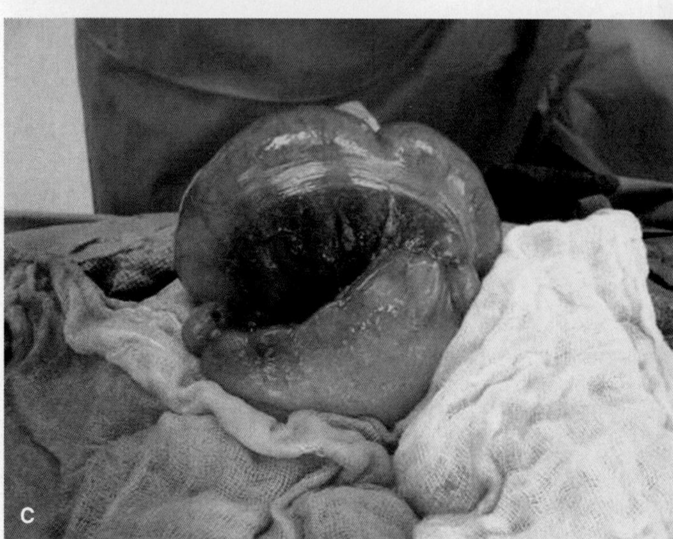

FIGURE 57.8 Bowel injuries following blunt trauma include perforation due to ischemia from an avulsed mesentery (A), a direct antimesenteric blowout injury (B), and a blunt serosal injury (C).

abdominal trauma (68). Patients at risk include those with high-energy mechanisms suggested by a seatbelt sign on physical examination, or a direct blow to the epigastrium (69). The initial CT scan may show nonspecific stranding of the pancreas. Associated fluid around the pancreas should prompt further studies such as ERCP or magnetic resonance cholangiopancreatography (MRCP) to rule out a biliary or pancreatic duct injury. With a tentative diagnosis of a pancreatic contusion, one may consider following serial determinations of amylase/lipase; although these laboratory studies do not have a reliable sensitivity (70), increasing values over time combined with an alteration in clinical examination should prompt a repeat CT scan, a duodenal C-loop study, a DPL, or an ERCP depending upon the suspected lesion.

POSTOPERATIVE MANAGEMENT OF SPECIFIC INJURIES

In addition to resuscitation of the trauma patient, ICU care includes management of injuries found at operative exploration. Communication between the operating surgeon and the intensivist is critical, and should include intraoperative findings and procedures, any tenuous operative repairs, anticipated problems or complications, the need for repeat operative exploration, and location of drains. The intraoperative estimated blood loss (EBL) and associated blood product transfusion requirements are essential data to anticipate events in the postoperative period. The transfusion information should include whether a massive transfusion protocol was initiated, or if evidence of clinical coagulopathy was identified during operative treatment. Finally, all clinicians caring for the patient should remember that injuries can be missed even with prior operative intervention.

Liver and Spleen Injuries

Although the majority of patients with solid-organ injuries are successfully managed nonoperatively, hemodynamically unstable patients or those with associated injuries may require urgent operation. Life-threatening hepatic bleeding is most often controlled with perihepatic packing or sometimes with additional Foley catheter tamponade of deep lacerations (Fig. 57.9). The most immediate concern in the postoperative period is rebleeding; this is heralded by a falling hemoglobin, blood or blood clots accumulating under a temporary abdominal closure dressing, and bloody output from intra-abdominal drains. Substantial hemorrhage is reflected in hemodynamic instability and continued acidosis. Patients with recurrent hemorrhage may be treated with angioembolization or may necessitate repeat operative packing depending on the rate of bleeding (27). Postoperative hepatic ischemia is usually due to either a prolonged intraoperative Pringle maneuver or hepatic artery ligation or embolization; patients with the former should have an elevation but subsequent resolution of their transaminases while those with the latter may have frank hepatic necrosis. Patients are returned to the OR for pack removal 24 to 48 hours after initial injury. Other long-term sources of morbidity are similar to patients undergoing nonoperative management, and include intra-abdominal abscess, biloma, and hemobilia. Although patients should be evaluated for infectious complications, patients with severe liver trauma (grade IV or V) have intermittent "liver fever" for the first 5 postinjury days (71).

Operative intervention for splenic injuries includes splenectomy and splenorrhaphy. Postoperative hemorrhage may be due to the inadequate splenic hilar vessel ligation, a missed short gastric artery, or recurrent bleeding from the spleen if splenic repair was attempted. An early postsplenectomy increase in platelets and WBCs is normal; however, beyond postoperative day 5 a WBC count above 15,000 should prompt a thorough search for underlying infection (72). The role of antiplatelet therapy for thrombocytosis remains controversial; data are lacking on whether aspirin therapy yields a significant outcome benefit, and for which patient population. Therapy may be instituted when the platelet count exceeds 1,000,000/μL, if not contraindicated (e.g., cerebral trauma) due to evidence of platelet hyperactivity of more than 48 hours (73). Additional sources of morbidity include a concurrent but unrecognized iatrogenic injury to the pancreatic tail during splenectomy resulting in pancreatic ascites or fistula. Patients have an increased incidence of intra-abdominal abscesses in the left upper quadrant following splenectomy with concomitant gastrointestinal injury, but presumptive drainage does not prevent this complication. Routine care following splenectomy also includes immunizations for encapsulated organisms (*Streptococcus pneumoniae, Haemophilus influenzae,* and *Meningococcus*) usually just prior to discharge, optimally 2 to 3 weeks after splenectomy (74).

Gastrointestinal Injuries

Operative intervention for either penetrating or blunt gastrointestinal injuries entails primary repair, resection with primary anastomosis, or resection with a stoma diversion. Regardless of the type of operation or the type of anastomosis (stapled vs. sewn) (75), one should await resolution of the patient's expected postoperative ileus before feeding. Return of bowel function is noted by a decrease in gastrostomy or NGT output and the passing of flatus. If an ileostomy or colostomy was required, one should inspect it daily to ensure it is pink without evidence of necrosis. Postoperative complications include anastomotic leak, prolonged ileus, and bowel obstruction. A leak with intra-abdominal contamination or sepsis presents with increasing abdominal pain, fevers, and respiratory compromise in the extubated patient, or persistent fevers and intolerance of enteral feeding in the intubated patient. CT scan is diagnostic and repeat operation is often required.

Important questions for the intensivist following operative intervention for pancreatic injuries include how much of the pancreas was resected, is there a pancreaticoenteric anastomosis, was the pancreatic stump closed securely, was the spleen preserved, and where were drains placed (76). Closed suction drains should remain in place until the patient is tolerating an oral diet or enteral nutrition, with the associated drain output being less than 30 mL/day. Postoperative complications include pancreatic fistula, pseudocyst, abscess, pancreaticoenteric leak, and pancreatitis. The most common of these is a pancreatic fistula, occurring in up to 20% of patients with isolated pancreatic trauma including the major duct, and in up to 35% of patients with combined pancreatic and duodenal injuries. Diagnosis in patients with drains in place is defined as output greater than 30 mL/day with an amylase level three

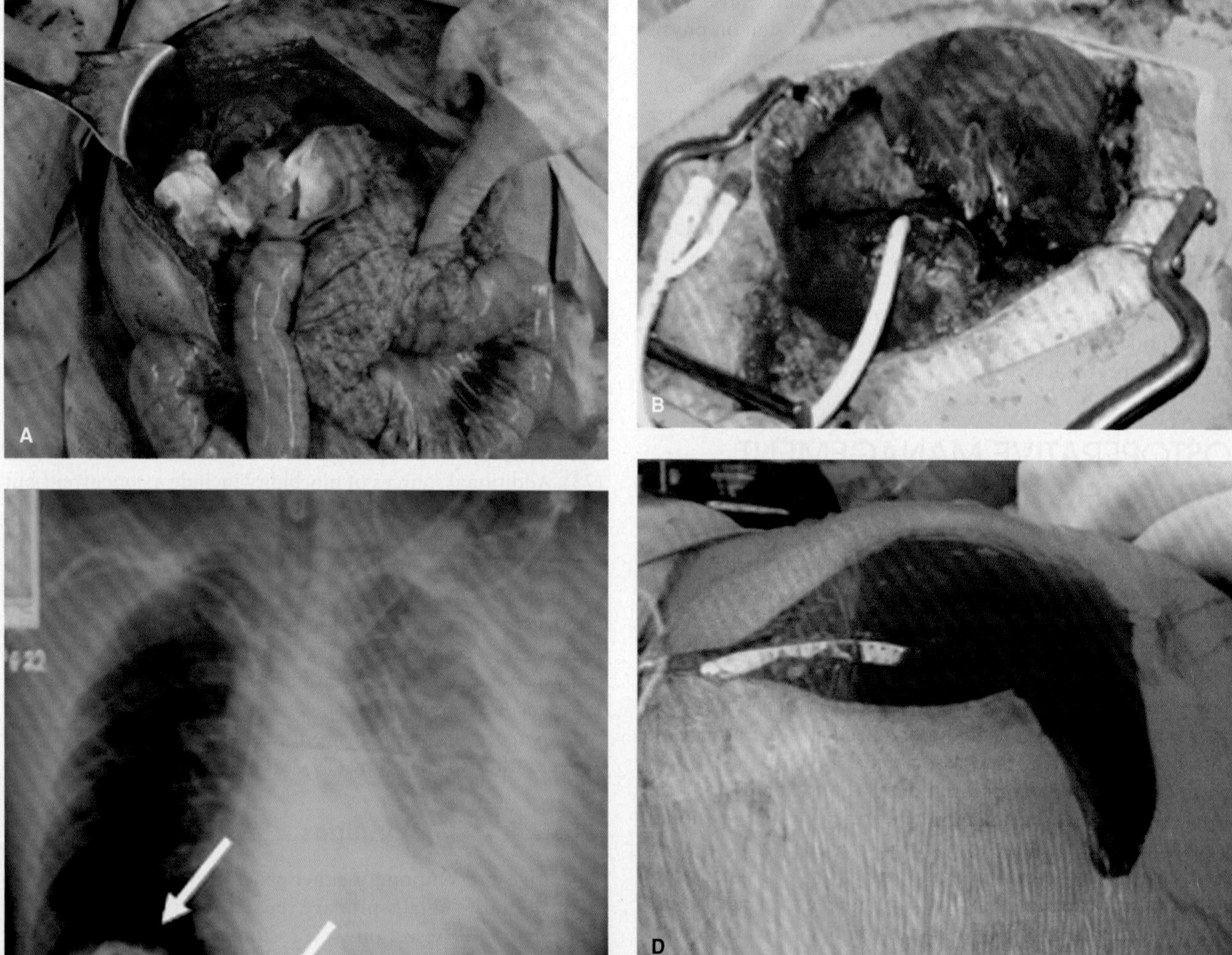

FIGURE 57.9 A,B: Perihepatic liver packing or Foley catheter tamponade of deep lacerations is employed to halt hepatic hemorrhage. C: Subsequent abdominal imaging shows the radiopaque markers of operatively placed laparotomy pads around the liver. D: Accumulation of blood under the temporary abdominal closure heralds recurrent hemorrhage.

times greater than serum value after postoperative day 5 (77). In patients without drains in place who have persistent abdominal pain, fevers, or intolerance of oral intake, CT scan imaging should be performed to evaluate for an intra-abdominal fluid collection. Drainage by interventional radiology (IR) is performed for fistula diagnosis and control. Pancreatic fistulae following trauma are managed in an identical fashion to those occurring following elective pancreatic resection (77).

Abdominal Vascular Injuries

Vascular injuries can produce rapid exsanguination and threaten extremities, or may be a clinically silent time bomb due to temporary retroperitoneal tamponade. Few result in a delayed diagnosis, particularly with CT scanning, and hence the focus of the intensivist is postoperative management. In general, outcome following vascular injuries is related to the technical success of the operation; the main causes of patient morbidity and mortality are associated soft tissue and nerve injuries once the vascular repair has been accomplished. Therefore, optimizing the patient's hemodynamic status, maintaining euthermia, and correcting coagulopathy are critical points of resuscitation. Prosthetic graft infections are rare complications (78) but preventing bacteremia is imperative; administration of perioperative antibiotics and treatment of secondary infections are indicated. Long-term arterial graft complications such as stenosis or pseudoaneurysms are uncommon, and routine graft surveillance is rarely performed. Consequently, long-term antiplatelet agents or antithrombotics are not routine.

There are specific injuries that require additional care. Abdominal aortic injuries are repaired using either a polytetrafluoroethylene (PTFE) patch or interposition graft; the patient's systolic blood pressure should not exceed 120 mm Hg for at least the first 72 hours postoperatively. Patients requiring ligation of an inferior vena cava injury often develop marked bilateral lower extremity edema; to limit the associated morbidity the patient's legs should be wrapped with ACE bandages from the toes to the hips and elevated at a 45- to 60-degree angle. For superior mesenteric vein injuries, either ligation or thrombosis following venorrhaphy results in marked bowel edema; fluid resuscitation should be aggressive and abdominal pressure monitoring routine in these patients. In complex hepatic trauma, the right or left hepatic artery, or in urgent situations, the portal vein may be selectively ligated; persistent elevation in liver transaminases indicates secondary liver parenchymal necrosis and may necessitate delayed resection. Of note, if the right hepatic artery is ligated intraoperatively, cholecystectomy is performed concurrently.

TABLE 57.6 Intraoperative Indications to Perform Damage Control Surgery

Factor	Level
Body temperature	Temperature <35°C
Acid–base status	
Arterial pH	pH <7.2
Base deficit (BD)	BD < −15 mmol/L in patient <55 yrs
	BD < −8 mmol/L in patient >55 yrs
Serum lactate	Lactate >5 mmol/L
Coagulopathy	PT or PTT >50% of normal

PT, prothrombin time; PTT, partial thromboplastin time; BD, base deficit.

Abdominal Wounds

In general, wounds sustained from trauma should be examined daily for progression of healing and signs of infection. Complex soft tissue wounds of the abdomen, such as degloving injuries following blunt trauma (termed *Morel–Lavallee lesions*), shotgun wounds, and other destructive blast injuries, can be particularly difficult to manage. Following initial debridement of devitalized tissue, wound care includes wet-to-dry dressing changes twice daily, or application of the wound vacuum-assisted closure (VAC). One should carefully watch for infection, development of necrotizing fasciitis, subcutaneous abscess, or associated undrained hematoma. Repeated operative debridements may be necessary, and early involvement of the reconstructive surgery service for possible flap coverage is advised for extensive tissue loss.

Midline laparotomy wounds are inspected 48 hours postoperatively by removing the sterile surgical dressing. If the patient develops high-grade fevers, inspection of the wound should be done sooner to exclude an early necrotizing infection. If a wound infection is identified—evidenced by erythema, pain along the wound, or purulent drainage—the wound should be widely opened by removing skin staples. After ensuring that the midline fascia is intact with digital palpation, the wound is managed with wet-to-dry dressing changes.

DAMAGE CONTROL SURGERY

Damage control surgery (DCS) is an abbreviated operation whose goals are to control hemorrhage, limit contamination from enteric sources, and enable rapid transport to the ICU for correction of adverse physiology (79,80). There are standard indications for performing the DCS-abbreviated laparotomy in patients with unresolved metabolic failure (Table 57.6). Intraoperative techniques of DCS include perihepatic packing, balloon tamponade of deep liver lacerations, segmental stapled bowel resection left in discontinuity, ligation of abdominal venous injuries, shunting of abdominal arterial injuries, and external drainage of biliary or urologic injuries.

Following DCS, the surgeon will "close" the abdomen with a temporary closure device. Options for temporary closure include Bogotá bag closure (a 3-L urology irrigation bag), 1010 Steri-Drape (3M Health Care, St. Paul, MN) and Ioban closure, and wound VAC dressing (Fig. 57.10). In most cases, the patient's abdomen is closed with the 1010 Steri-Drape and Ioban closure after the first operation and with the VAC following additional operative explorations. The temporary abdominal closure allows egress of abdominal contents and contains the edematous bowel while providing excellent decompression. Jackson–Pratt (JP) drains are placed under the Ioban covering to control the effluent from third spacing during fluid resuscitation.

Upon transfer to the ICU, aggressive resuscitation of the patient is performed to reverse metabolic failure (81). This includes vigorous rewarming through heating the room, infusion of fluids and blood products through a warming device, and use of a warming device such as the Bair Hugger (Augustine Medical, Inc., Eden Prairie, MN). Invasive rewarming may be warranted for refractory temperatures below 34°C. Restoration of a normal cardiovascular state is attained by infusion of fluids and blood products, as well as judicious use of vasopressor agents. Finally, the patient's coagulopathy must be reversed with appropriate blood products including fresh-frozen plasma, cryoprecipitate, and platelets now usually guided by serial TEG or ROTEM assessments. Ideally, physiologic correction should occur within 24 hours of admission to the ICU, with planned return to the OR for definitive repair by 48 hours. Planned return to the OR includes pack removal, definitive bowel repair, and placement of vascular grafts as indicated.

There are several specific management points of the patient with an open abdomen that deserve mention. Despite a widely open abdomen, patients can develop ACS (82); therefore, bladder pressures should be monitored every 4 hours, with significant increases in pressures alerting the clinician to the possible need for repeat operative intervention and abdominal decompression. Patients with an open abdomen lose between 500 and 2,500 mL/day of abdominal effluent. Appropriate volume compensation for this albumin-rich fluid remains controversial, both in the amount administered (replacement based on clinical indices vs. routine 0.5-mL replacement for every milliliter lost) as well as the type of replacement (crystalloid vs. colloid/blood products). Patients with abdominal packing in place, particularly for liver lacerations, may rebleed from such injuries. In these situations, the patient may begin to exsanguinate from the abdomen through the JP drains placed under the Ioban covering. Rapid blood product resuscitation may provide enough intra-abdominal pressure and subsequent tamponade to stabilize the patient for reoperation. Alternatively, bedside laparotomy with repacking of the liver is an option. Following physiologic restoration, a systematic approach to abdominal closure must be initiated; this aggressive process may include direct peritoneal resuscitation (83), early institution of enteral nutrition (84), careful diuresis, and sequential closure techniques (85).

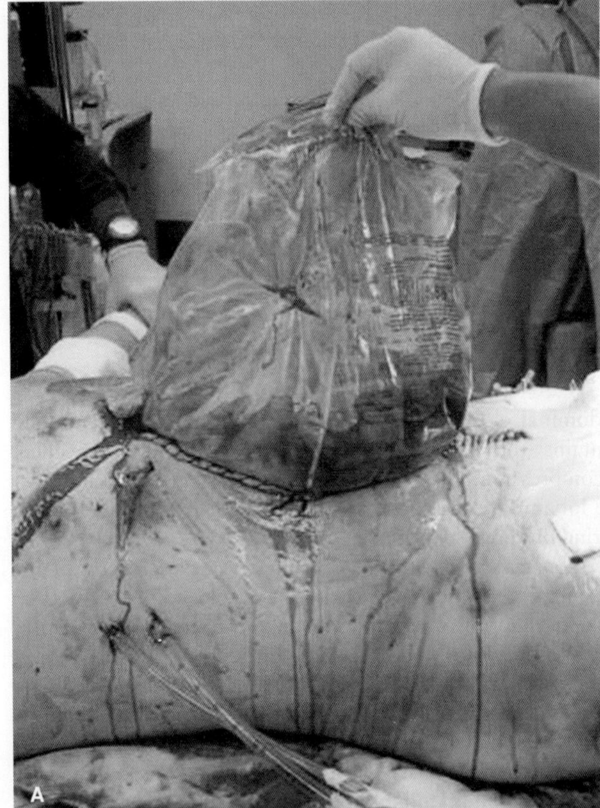

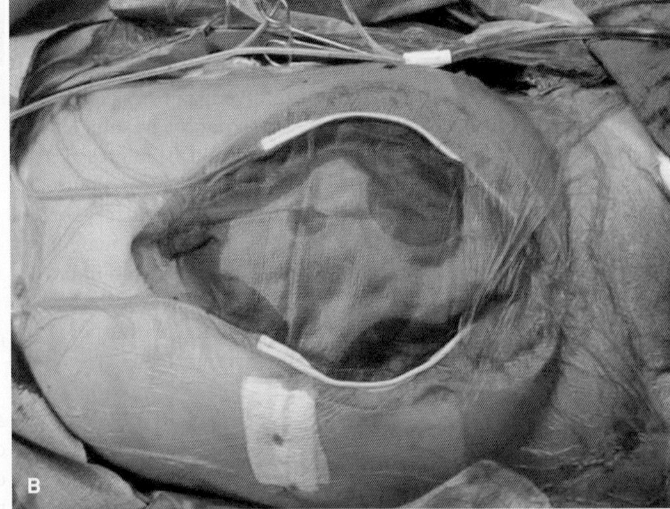

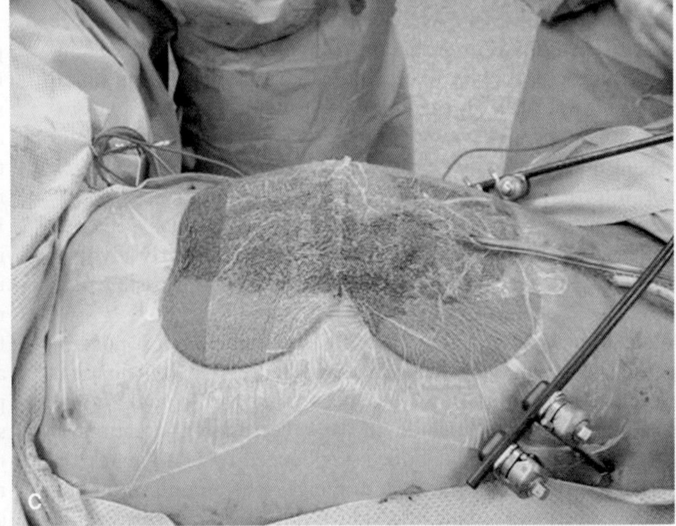

FIGURE 57.10 Methods of temporary abdominal closure following damage control surgery or operative decompression for abdominal compartment syndrome: Bogotá bag closure (A), 1010 Steri-Drape and loban closure (B), and vacuum-assisted closure dressing (C).

ABDOMINAL COMPARTMENT SYNDROME

The ACS represents intra-abdominal hypertension due to either intra-abdominal injury (primary) or following massive resuscitation (secondary) (14,86–88). The large volumes of crystalloid required to manage multiply injured patients results in resuscitation-associated bowel edema, retroperitoneal edema, or large quantities of ascitic fluid. A diagnosis of intra-abdominal hypertension cannot be definitively made by physical examination, but is obtained by measuring bladder pressures (89). Conditions in which the bladder pressure may be unreliable include bladder rupture, external compression from pelvic packing, neurogenic bladder, and adhesive disease.

Increased abdominal pressure affects multiple organ systems (Fig. 57.11). The ACS, however, is defined by intra-abdominal hypertension (bladder pressure higher than 12 mmHg; Table 57.7) causing end-organ sequelae: decreased urine output, increased peak airway pressures, decreased preload, elevated intracranial pressure (ICP), and extremity venous obstruction (86). With morbidity and mortality rates exceeding 50% (82,90), patients at risk for the development of ACS, particularly those receiving large amounts of crystalloid and blood products during shock resuscitation, should be evaluated closely. Development of secondary ACS can be an indolent process. Some clinicians have queried aggressive intervention to prevent the development of ACS. Although perhaps counterintuitive in the acute resuscitation of patients,

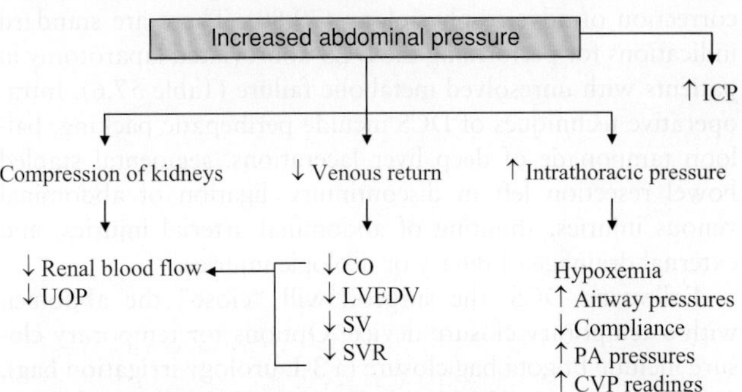

FIGURE 57.11 Physiologic derangements associated with intra-abdominal hypertension leading to abdominal compartment syndrome. ICP, intracranial pressure; UOP, urine output; CO, cardiac output; LVEDV, left ventricular end-diastolic volume; SV, stroke volume; SVR, systemic vascular resistance; PA, pulmonary artery; CVP, central venous pressure.

TABLE 57.7 Abdominal Compartment Syndrome Grading System Based Upon Bladder Pressure Measurements

ACS Grade	Bladder Pressure (cm H_2O)
I	10–15
II	16–25
III	26–35
IV	>35

early administration of vasoactive agents to reduce the volume of crystalloid administered might be a therapeutic alternative in these patients at risk for ACS. In patients with acute renal failure, with minimal to no urine output, judicious fluid administration, early use of pressors, and institution of renal replacement therapy prior to fluid overload may also be warranted.

Organ failure can occur over a wide range of recorded bladder pressures, and, thus, there is not a single measurement of bladder pressure that mandates therapeutic intervention, except >35 cm H_2O. Rather, emergent decompression is warranted in the patient with intra-abdominal hypertension and end-organ dysfunction. Mortality is directly affected by a delay in decompression, with 64% mortality in patients undergoing presumptive decompression, 70% mortality in patients with a delay in decompression, and 89% mortality in those without decompression (91). Decompression for postinjury ACS is usually performed operatively either at the bedside in the ICU if the patient is hemodynamically unstable, or in the operating room. Bedside laparotomy is easily accomplished, eliminates transport in hemodynamically compromised patients, and requires minimal equipment (scalpel, suction, cautery, and abdominal temporary closure dressings).

Patients with significant intra-abdominal fluid as the primary component of their ACS, rather than bowel or retroperitoneal edema, may be candidates for decompression via a percutaneous drain (92,93). Differentiation of those amenable to such drainage is determined by bedside ultrasound, hence obviating a trip to the OR for a critically ill patient.

DCS and the recognition of the ACS have improved patient outcomes but at the cost of an open abdomen. Over 20% of patients with a persistent open abdomen suffer complications that prolong their hospital course. Complications include intra-abdominal abscess, bile leaks, enteric fistula, and anastomotic leaks (Fig. 57.12) (94). Management includes operative or percutaneous drainage of abscesses, ERCP and drainage of bilomas, and control of fistulae and nutritional support for bowel complications. Current research is under way to develop techniques to minimize complications and reduce morbidity in patients with these devastating injuries. All clinicians caring for patients with an open abdomen should understand the potential morbidity and the importance of fascial closure to help mitigate these complications (87).

ANCILLARY CARE ISSUES

Tubes and Drains

Following operative or nonoperative management of abdominal injuries, patients may have a variety of tubes and drains. Intra-abdominal drains are typically closed suction drains such as JP or Blake drains; the amount from the drain should be quantified every 8-hour shift, and the character of the output (bilious, succus, bloody, etc.) from the drains should

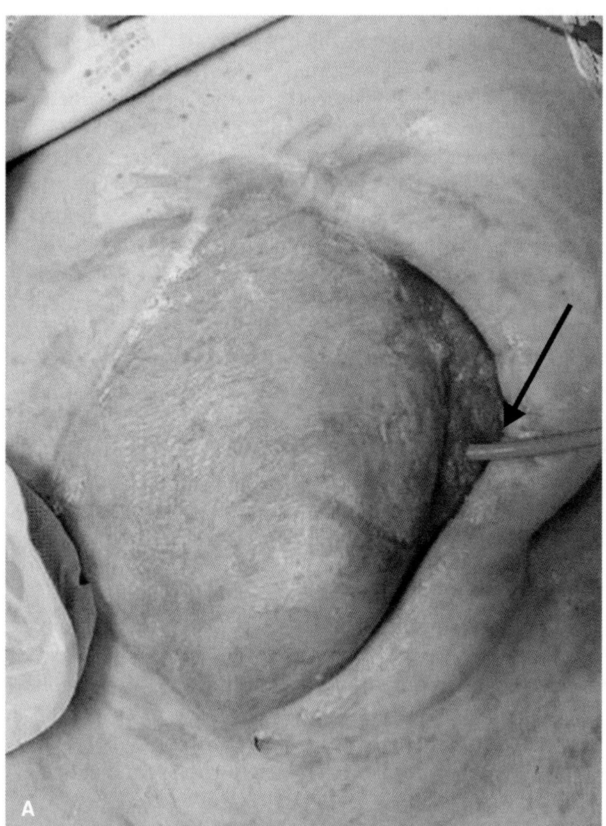

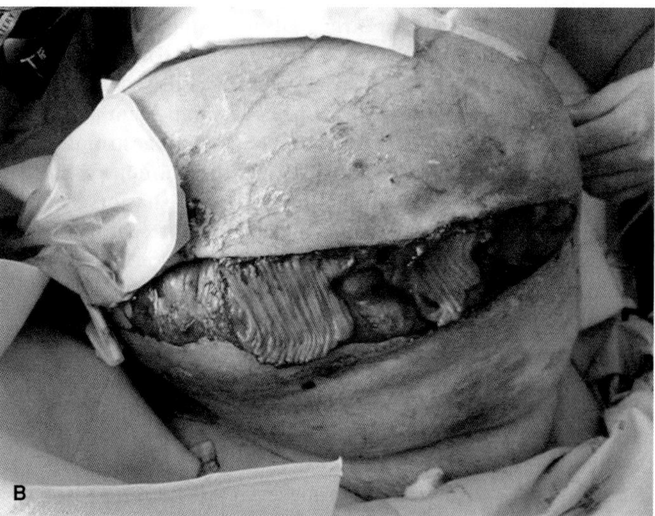

FIGURE 57.12 Complications of the open abdomen include intra-abdominal abscess, bile leaks, enteric fistula (A), and bowel perforations (B).

be monitored daily. Although general guidelines for drain removal are less than 30 to 50 mL/day, one should consult with the surgeon prior to removal because these drains may be difficult to replace. Patients with rectal injuries may have presacral drains placed, which consist of Penrose drains exiting next to the rectum; these are passive drains, and should be covered with ABD pads for appropriate coverage. Patients with open abdomens and temporary abdominal closure will often have drains of some type; again, quantity and quality of the effluent may guide treatment options such as intravenous fluid replacement and need for return to the operating room.

Enteral access for nutrition is acquired through multiple techniques. NGTs, placed for gastric decompression, can be used for enteral nutrition once NGT output decreases. Gastrostomy tubes, either percutaneously or operatively placed, exit the abdominal cavity in the left upper quadrant. These should be placed to gravity for 12 to 24 hours after initial insertion. Dobhoff tubes provide postpyloric access for nutrition, and can be advantageous in patients who have a gastric ileus. Jejunal feeding tubes are usually placed operatively; surgeons may choose to use needle catheter jejunostomy (NCJ) tubes or red rubber catheters. The primary issues with jejunal feeding tubes are those encountered with NCJs. Due to the small caliber of the feeding tube, there is the propensity for clogging. The NCJ should be flushed every 6 hours with saline, and only NCJ compatible enteral formulas should be used. Additionally, no medications should be placed down the NCJ. Nasojejunal tubes, often called nasobiliary feeding tubes, may be placed in the ICU using upper endoscopy for prolonged gastric ileus.

Nutrition

Although the topic of nutrition could encompass an entire textbook, a few issues warrant mention (95). Multiple studies have illustrated the importance of early total enteral nutrition (TEN) in the trauma population, particularly its impact in reducing septic complications (96–99). The route of enteral feedings, stomach versus small bowel, tends to be less important as gut tolerance appears equivalent unless there is upper gastrointestinal pathology (100,101). Although early enteral nutrition is the goal, one should be cognizant of any bowel anastomoses; typically, evidence of bowel function should be present before advancing to goal tube feeds. Overzealous jejunal feeding can lead to small bowel necrosis, a devastating complication (102). Patients undergoing monitoring for nonoperative management of solid-organ injuries should remain NPO in the first 24 to 48 hours in case they require an operation. There is some residual concern about starting TEN in patients with an open abdomen. A recent multicenter trial demonstrated TEN in the postinjury open abdomen is both feasible and advantageous (84); TEN was associated with higher fascial closure rates, decreased complications, and decreased mortality. Once resuscitation is complete, initiation of TEN, even at trophic levels (15 mL/hr), should be considered in all injured patients with an open abdomen unless the bowel remains in discontinuity.

Prophylaxis

A critical component of the ICU care of the multiply injured patient includes prevention of deep venous thrombosis (DVT) and stress gastritis. Administration of heparinoids for the prevention of DVT following trauma or surgical intervention is the current standard of care (103), although the addition of antiplatelet agents appears justified in high-risk patients (73). Issues following abdominal trauma include timing of such administration in patients with either active bleeding from traumatic injury or those with solid-organ injuries. Typically, heparin products are held until patients have resolved their hemorrhagic diathesis or until 24 hours after their hemoglobin has stabilized. Carafate is the current drug of choice for the prevention of stress gastritis (104,105) until enteral feeding is established. In patients who have had specific gastric surgery, H_2 blockers may be used as an alternative.

Key Points

- Systematic management of the multiply injured patient consists of the primary survey, resuscitation, the secondary survey, and definitive care.
- Although some patients may arrive in the ICU in extremis necessitating immediate resuscitation without a thorough history and physical examination, the majority should undergo a complete assessment promptly; it should not be assumed that the evaluation in the ED was comprehensive.
- There are clear indications in the ICU for surgeon evaluation for possible laparotomy: progressive decline in hemoglobin, unexplained leukocytosis and fever, diffuse abdominal tenderness, hypotension and associated abdominal distension or free fluid on bedside ultrasound, CT scan with evidence of free air or gastrointestinal contrast extravasation, CT scan with free fluid without associated solid-organ injury, and intra-abdominal hypertension.
- Even in patients who undergo exploratory laparotomy, CT of the abdomen may be necessary to diagnose spine fractures and to evaluate the retroperitoneum.
- Trauma-induced coagulopathy is now well recognized, and underscores the importance of preemptive blood component administration; the resurgent interest in viscoelastic hemostatic assays (TEG, ROTEM) has facilitated the appropriate and timely use of clotting adjuncts including the prompt recognition of fibrinolysis.
- Adequate resuscitation is mandatory, and often determines when the surgeon can safely return the patient to the OR after initial operative intervention. Specific goals of resuscitation include a core temperature >35°C, base deficit less negative than 6, and normal coagulation indices.
- Nonoperative management of solid-organ injuries is pursued in hemodynamically stable patients who do not have overt peritonitis or other indications for laparotomy. The clinician should consider the following elements when reviewing the CT scan: the AAST grade of injury, the amount of free fluid within the abdomen, the presence of contrast extravasation indicating ongoing arterial bleeding, and evidence of pseudoaneurysms.
- Following hepatic injuries, the most common complication is a bile leak or biloma, occurring in up to 20% of patients with major injuries (grade III or higher). The most common problem in patients with splenic injuries is delayed bleeding.

References

1. Biffl WL, Harrington DT, Cioffi WG. Implementation of a tertiary trauma survey decreases missed injuries. *J Trauma.* 2003;54:38–43.
2. Brooks A, Holroyd B, Riley B. Missed injury in major trauma patients. *Injury.* 2004;35:407–410.
3. Schweitzer G. Re: Buduhan G, McRitchie DI. Missed injuries in patients with multiple trauma. *J Trauma.* 2000;49:600–605.
4. Moore FA, McKinley BA, Moore EE, et al. Inflammation and the Host Response to Injury, a large-scale collaborative project: patient-oriented research core—standard operating procedures for clinical care. III. Guidelines for shock resuscitation. *J Trauma.* 2006;61:82–89.
5. Herbert PC, Wells G, Blajchman MA, et al. A multicenter, randomized, controlled trial of transfusion requirements in critical care. *N Engl J Med.* 1999;340:409–417.
6. Moore FA, Moore EE, Sauaia A. Blood transfusion. An independent risk factor for postinjury multiple organ failure. *Arch Surg.* 1997;132:620–624.
7. Ouellet JF, Roberts DJ, Tiruta C, et al. Admission base deficit and lactate levels in Canadian patients with blunt trauma: are they useful markers of mortality? *J Trauma Acute Care Surg.* 2012;72(6):1532–1535.
8. Callaway DW, Shapiro NI, Donnino MW, et al. Serum lactate and base deficit as predictors of mortality in normotensive elderly blunt trauma patients. *J Trauma.* 2009;66(4):1040–1044.
9. Ferrada P, Evans D, Wolfe L, et al. Findings of a randomized controlled trial using limited transthoracic echocardiogram (LTTE) as a hemodynamic monitoring tool in the trauma bay. *J Trauma Acute Care Surg.* 2014;76(1):31–37.
10. Cooper MS, Stewart PM. Corticosteroid insufficiency in acutely ill patients. *N Engl J Med.* 2003;348:727–734.
11. Offner PJ, Moore EE, Ciesla D. The adrenal response after severe trauma. *Am J Surg.* 2002;184:649–653.
12. Gonzalez E, Moore EE, Moore HB, et al. Trauma-induced coagulopathy: an institution's 35 year perspective on practice and research. *Scand J Surg.* 2014;103(2):89–103.
13. Balogh Z, McKinley BA, Holcomb JB, et al. Both primary and secondary abdominal compartment syndrome can be predicted early and are harbingers of multiple organ failure. *J Trauma.* 2003;54:848–859.
14. Balogh ZJ, Lumsdaine W, Moore EE, Moore FA. Postinjury abdominal compartment syndrome: from recognition to prevention. *Lancet.* 2014;384: 1466–1475.
15. Kozar RA, Moore FA, Moore EE, et al. Western Trauma Association critical decisions in trauma: nonoperative management of adult blunt hepatic trauma. *J Trauma.* 2009;67(6):1144–1148.
16. Polanco PM, Brown JB, Puyana JC, et al. The swinging pendulum: a national perspective of nonoperative management in severe blunt liver injury. *J Trauma Acute Care Surg.* 2013;75(4):590–595.
17. Peitzman AB, Richardson JD. Surgical treatment of injuries to the solid abdominal organs: a 50-year perspective from the Journal of Trauma. *J Trauma.* 2010;69(5):1011–1021.
18. Richardson DJ, Franklin GA, Lukan JK, et al. Evolution in the management of hepatic trauma: a 25-year perspective. *Ann Surg.* 2000;232:324–330.
19. Velmahos GC, Toutouzas KG, Radin R, et al. Nonoperative treatment of blunt injury to solid abdominal organs: a prospective study. *Arch Surg.* 2003;138:844–851.
20. van der Wilden GM, Velmahos GC, Emhoff T, et al. Successful nonoperative management of the most severe blunt liver injuries: a multicenter study of the research consortium of new England centers for trauma. *Arch Surg.* 2012; 147(5):423–438.
21. Moore FA, Davis JW, Moore EE Jr, et al. Western Trauma Association (WTA) critical decisions in trauma: management of adult blunt splenic trauma. *J Trauma.* 2008;65(5):1007–1011.
22. Christmas AB, Wilson AK, Manning B, et al. Selective management of blunt hepatic injuries including nonoperative management is a safe and effective strategy. *Surgery.* 2005;138:606–610.
23. Petrowsky H, Raeder S, Zuercher L, et al. A quarter century experience in liver trauma: a plea for early computed tomography and conservative management for all hemodynamically stable patients. *World J Surg.* 2012;36(2): 247–254.
24. Rojani RR, Claridge JA, Yowler CJ, et al. Improved outcome of adult blunt splenic injury: a cohort analysis. *Surgery.* 2006;140:625–631.
25. Watson GA, Rosengart MR, Zenati MS, et al. Nonoperative management of severe blunt splenic injury: are we getting better? *J Trauma.* 2006;61: 1113–1118.
26. Sivrikoz E, Teixeira PG, Resnick S, et al. Angiointervention: an independent predictor of survival in high-grade blunt liver injuries. *Am J Surg.* 2015; 209(4):742–746.
27. Misselbeck TS, Teicher EJ, Cipolle MD, et al. Hepatic angioembolization in trauma patients: indications and complications. *J Trauma.* 2009;67(4): 769–773.
28. Bhullar IS, Frykberg ER, Siragusa D, et al. Selective angiographic embolization of blunt splenic traumatic injuries in adults decreases failure rate of nonoperative management. *J Trauma Acute Care Surg.* 2012;72(5):1127–1134.
29. Miller PR, Chang MC, Hoth JJ, et al. Prospective trial of angiography and embolization for all grade III to V blunt splenic injuries: nonoperative management success rate is significantly improved. *J Am Coll Surg.* 2014;218(4): 644–648.
30. Siriratsivawong K, Zenati M, Watson GA, Harbrecht BG. Nonoperative management of blunt splenic trauma in the elderly: does age play a role? *Am Surg.*2007;73(6):585–589.
31. Myers JG, Dent DL, Stewart RM, et al. Blunt splenic injuries: dedicated trauma surgeons can achieve a high rate of nonoperative success in patients of all ages. *J Trauma.* 2000;48:801–805.
32. Harbrecht BG, Peitzman AB, Rivera L, et al. Contribution of age and gender to outcome of blunt splenic injury in adults: multicenter study of the Eastern Association for the Surgery of Trauma. *J Trauma.* 2001;51:887–895.
33. Moore EE, Cogbill TH, Jurkovich GJ, et al. Organ injury scaling: spleen and liver (1994 revision). *J Trauma.* 1995;38:323–324.
34. Moore EE, Cogbill TH, Malangoni MA, et al. Organ injury scaling. *Surg Clin North Am.* 1995;75:293–303.
35. Moore EE, Cogbill TH, Malangoni MA, et al. Organ injury scaling, II: pancreas, duodenum, small bowel, colon, and rectum. *J Trauma.* 1990;30:1427–1429.
36. Johnson JW, Gracias VH, Gupta R, et al. Hepatic angiography in patients undergoing damage control laparotomy. *J Trauma.* 2002;52:1102–1106.
37. Haan JM, Biffl WL, Knudson MM, et al. Splenic embolization revisited: a multicenter review. *J Trauma.* 2004;56:542–547.
38. Zarzaur BL, Savage SA, Croce MA, Fabian TC. Trauma center angiography use in high-grade blunt splenic injuries: timing is everything. *J Trauma Acute Care Surg.* 2014;77:666–673.
39. Banerjee A, Duane TM, Wilson SP, et al. Trauma center variation in splenic artery embolization and spleen salvage: a multicenter analysis. *J Trauma Acute Care Surg.* 2013;75(1):69–74.
40. Dent D, Alsabrook G, Erickson BA, et al. Blunt splenic injuries: high nonoperative management rate can be achieved with selective embolization. *J Trauma.* 2004;56:1063–1067.
41. Davis KA, Fabian TC, Croce MA, et al. Improved success in nonoperative management of blunt splenic injuries: embolization of splenic artery pseudoaneurysms. *J Trauma.* 1998;44:1008–1013.
42. Malhotra AK, Carter RF, Lebman DA, et al. Preservation of splenic immunocompetence after splenic artery angioembolization for blunt splenic injury. *J Trauma.* 2010;69(5):1126–1130.
43. Leeper WR, Leeper TJ, Ouellette D, et al. Delayed hemorrhagic complications in the nonoperative management of blunt splenic trauma: early screening leads to a decrease in failure rate. *J Trauma Acute Care Surg.* 2014;76(6):1349–1353.
44. Patton JH Jr, Lyden SP, Croce MA, et al. Pancreatic trauma: a simplified management guideline. *J Trauma.* 1997;43:234–239.
45. Biffl WL, Moore EE, Croce M, et al. Western Trauma Association critical decisions in trauma: management of pancreatic injuries. *J Trauma Acute Care Surg.* 2013;75(6):941–946.
46. Sharpe JP, Magnotti LJ, Weinberg JA, et al. Impact of a defined management algorithm on outcome after traumatic pancreatic injury. *J Trauma Acute Care Surg.* 2012;72(1):100–105.
47. Lin BC, Liu NJ, Fang JF, Kao YC. Long-term results of endoscopic stent in the management of blunt major pancreatic duct injury. *Surg Endosc.* 2006;20:1551–1555.
48. Cogbill TH, Moore EE, Feliciano DV. Conservative management of duodenal trauma: a multicenter perspective. *J Trauma.* 1990;30:1469–1475.
49. Huerta S, Bui T, Porral D, et al. Predictors of morbidity and mortality in patients with traumatic duodenal injuries. *Am Surg.* 2005;71:763–767.
50. Moore EE. When is nonoperative management of a gunshot wound to the liver appropriate? *J Am Coll Surg.* 1999;188:427–428.
51. Navsaria PH, Nicol AJ, Edu S, et al. Selective nonoperative management in 1106 patients with abdominal gunshot wounds: conclusions on safety, efficacy, and the role of selective CT imaging in a prospective single-center study. *Ann Surg.* 2015;261(4):760–764.
52. Inaba K, Branco BC, Moe D, et al. Prospective evaluation of selective nonoperative management of torso gunshot wounds: when is it safe to discharge? *J Trauma Acute Care Surg.* 2012;72(4):884–891.
53. Chiu WC, Shanmuganathan K, Mirvis SE, Scalea TM. Determining the need for laparotomy in penetrating torso trauma: a prospective study using triple-contrast enhanced abdominopelvic computed tomography. *J Trauma.* 2001;51:860–868.

54. Kozar RA, Moore FA, Cothren CC, et al. Risk factors for hepatic morbidity following nonoperative management: multicenter study. *Arch Surg.* 2006;141:451–459.
55. Giss SR, Dobrilovic N, Brown RL, Garcia VF. Complications of nonoperative management of pediatric blunt hepatic injury: diagnosis, management, and outcomes. *J Trauma.* 2006;61:334–339.
56. Goldman R, Zilkowski M, Mullins R, et al. Delayed celiotomy for the treatment of bile leak, compartment syndrome, and other hazards of nonoperative management of blunt liver injury. *Am J Surg.* 2003;185:492–497.
57. Wu SC, Chen RJ, Yang AD, et al. Complications associated with embolization in the treatment of blunt splenic injury. *World J Surg.* 2008; 32(3):476–482.
58. Cothren CC, Biffl WL, Moore EE, et al. Characteristic radiographic findings of post-injury splenic autotransplantation: avoiding a diagnostic dilemma. *J Trauma.* 2004;57(3):537–541.
59. Fakhry SM, Watts DD, Luchette FA; EAST Multi-Institutional Hollow Viscus Injury Research Group. Current diagnostic approaches lack sensitivity in the diagnosis of perforated blunt small bowel injury: analysis from 275,557 trauma admissions from the EAST multi-institutional HVI trial. *J Trauma.* 2003;54:295–306.
60. Fakhry SM, Brownstein M, Watts DD, et al. Relatively short diagnostic delays (<8 hours) produce morbidity and mortality in blunt small bowel injury: an analysis of time to operative intervention in 198 patients from a multicenter experience. *J Trauma.* 2000;48:408–414.
61. Niederee MJ, Byrnes MC, Helmer SD, et al. Delay in diagnosis of hollow viscus injuries: effect on outcome. *Am Surg.* 2003;69:293–298.
62. Ng AK, Simons RK, Torreggiani WC, et al. Intra-abdominal free fluid without solid organ injury in blunt abdominal trauma: an indication for laparotomy. *J Trauma.* 2002;52:1134–1140.
63. Bhagvan S, Turai M, Holden A, et al. Predicting hollow viscus injury in blunt abdominal trauma with computed tomography. *World J Surg.* 2013;37(1):123–126.
64. Rodriguez C, Barone JE, Wilbanks TO, et al. Isolated free fluid on computed tomographic scan in blunt abdominal trauma: a systematic review of incidence and management. *J Trauma.* 2002;53:79–85.
65. McAnena OJ, Marx JA, Moore EE. Peritoneal lavage enzyme determinations following blunt and penetrating abdominal trauma. *J Trauma.* 1991;31:1161–1164.
66. Heneman PL, Marx JA, Moore EE, et al. Diagnostic peritoneal lavage: accuracy in predicting necessary laparotomy following blunt and penetrating trauma. *J Trauma.* 1990;30:1345–1355.
67. Velmahos GC, Gomez H, Falabella A, et al. Operative management of civilian rectal gunshot wounds: simpler is better. *World J Surg.* 2000;24: 114–118.
68. Leppaniemi AK, Haapiainen RK. Risk factors of delayed diagnosis of pancreatic trauma. *Eur J Surg.* 1999;165:1134–1137.
69. Arkovitz MS, Johnson N, Garcia VF. Pancreatic trauma in children: mechanisms of injury. *J Trauma.* 1997;42:49–53.
70. Takishima T, Sugimoto K, Hirata M, et al. Serum amylase level on admission in the diagnosis of blunt injury to the pancreas: its significance and limitations. *Ann Surg.* 1997;226:70–76.
71. Cogbill TH, Moore EE, Feliciano DV, et al. Hepatic enzyme response and hyperpyrexia after severe liver injury. *Am Surg.* 1992;58:395–399.
72. Weng J, Brown CV, Rhee P, et al. White blood cell and platelet counts can be used to differentiate between infection and the normal response after splenectomy for trauma: prospective validation. *J Trauma.* 2005;59:1076–1080.
73. Harr JN, Moore EE, Chin TL, et al. Platelets are dominant contributors to hypercoagulability after injury. *J Trauma Acute Care Surg.* 2013; 74(3):756–762.
74. Howdieshell TR, Heffernan D, Dipiro JT; Therapeutic Agents Committee of the Surgical Infection Society. Surgical infection society guidelines for vaccination after traumatic injury. *Surg Infect (Larchmt).* 2006;7:275–303.
75. Demetriades D, Murray JA, Chan L, et al. Penetrating colon injuries requiring resection: diversion or primary anastomosis? An AAST prospective multicenter study. *J Trauma.* 2001;50:765–775.
76. Conlon KC, Labow D, Leung D, et al. Prospective randomized clinical trial of the value of intraperitoneal drainage after pancreatic resection. *Ann Surg.* 2001;234:487–493.
77. Larsen M, Kozarek R. Management of pancreatic ductal leaks and fistulae. *J Gastroenterol Hepatol.* 2014;29(7):1360–1370.
78. Wolford HY, Cothren CC, Moore EE. Postinjury abdominal aortic graft infection: documentation and successful management. *J Trauma.* 2006;61:1274–1276.
79. Moore EE, Burch JM, Franciose RJ, et al. Staged physiologic restoration and damage control surgery. *World J Surg.* 1998;22:1184–1190.
80. Shapiro MB, Jenkins DH, Schwab CW, Rotondo MF. Damage control: collective review. *J Trauma.* 2000;49(5):969–978.
81. Sagraves SG, Toschlog EA, Rotondo MF. Damage control surgery—the intensivist's role. *J Intensive Care Med.* 2006;21:5–16.
82. Raeburn CD, Moore EE, Biffl WL, et al. The abdominal compartment syndrome is a morbid complication of postinjury damage control surgery. *Am J Surg.* 2001;182:542–546.
83. Smith JW, Garrison RN, Matheson PJ, et al. Direct peritoneal resuscitation accelerates primary abdominal wall closure after damage control surgery. *J Am Coll Surg.* 2010;210:658–667.
84. Burlew CC, Moore EE, Cuschieri J, et al. Who should we feed? A Western Trauma Association multi-institutional study of enteral nutrition in the post-injury open abdomen. *J Trauma Acute Care Surg.* 2012;73:1380–1388.
85. Burlew CC, Moore EE, Johnson JL, et al. 100% Fascial approximation can be achieved in the post-injury open abdomen. *J Trauma.* 2012;72: 235–241.
86. Kirkpatrick AW, Roberts DJ, De Waele J, et al. Intra-abdominal hypertension and the abdominal compartment syndrome: updated consensus definitions and clinical practice guidelines from the World Society of the Abdominal Compartment Syndrome. *Intensive Care Med.* 2013;39(7):1190–1206.
87. Burlew CC. The open abdomen: practical implications for the practicing surgeon. *Am J Surg.* 2012;204(6):826–835.
88. McNelis J, Marini CP, Jurkiewicz A, et al. Predictive factors associated with the development of abdominal compartment syndrome in the surgical intensive care unit. *Arch Surg.* 2002;137:133–136.
89. Kron IL. A simple technique to accurately determine intra-abdominal pressure. *Crit Care Med.* 1989;17:714–715.
90. Biffl WL, Moore EE, Burch JM, et al. Secondary abdominal compartment syndrome is a highly lethal event. *Am J Surg.* 2001;182:645–648.
91. Cheatham ML, White MW, Sagraves SG, et al. Abdominal perfusion pressure: a superior parameter in the assessment of intra-abdominal hypertension. *J Trauma.* 2000;49:621–626.
92. Corcos AC, Sherman HF. Percutaneous treatment of secondary abdominal compartment syndrome. *J Trauma.* 2001;51:1062–1064.
93. Latenser BA, Kowal-Vern A, Kimball D, et al. A pilot study comparing percutaneous decompression with decompressive laparotomy for acute abdominal compartment syndrome in thermal injury. *J Burn Care Rehabil.* 2002;23:190–195.
94. Miller RS, Morris JA Jr, Diaz JJ Jr, et al. Complications after 344 damage-control open celiotomies. *J Trauma.* 2005;59:1365–1371.
95. Jacobs DG, Jacobs DO, Kudsk KA, et al. Practice management guidelines for nutritional support of the trauma patient. *J Trauma.* 2004;57:660–678.
96. Moore FA, Moore EE, Jones TN, et al. TEN versus TPN following major abdominal trauma—reduced septic morbidity. *J Trauma.* 1989;29: 916–922.
97. Moore FA, Feliciano DV, Andrassy RJ, et al. Early enteral feeding, compared with parenteral, reduces postoperative septic complications. The results of a meta-analysis. *Ann Surg.* 1992;216:172–183.
98. Moore FA, Moore EE, Haenel JB. Clinical benefits of early post-injury enteral feeding. *Clin Intensive Care.* 1995;6:21–27.
99. Hasenboehler E, Williams A, Leinhase I, et al. Metabolic changes after polytrauma: an imperative for early nutritional support. *World J Emerg Surg.* 2006;1:29.
100. Neumann DA, DeLegge MH. Gastric versus small-bowel tube feeding in the intensive care unit: a prospective comparison of efficacy. *Crit Care Med.* 2002;30:1436–1438.
101. Reignier J, Bensaid S, Perrin-Gachadoat D, et al. Erythromycin and early enteral nutrition in mechanically ventilated patients. *Crit Care Med.* 2002; 30:1237–1241.
102. Melis M, Fichera A, Ferguson MK. Bowel necrosis associated with early jejunal tube feeding: a complication of postoperative enteral nutrition. *Arch Surg.* 2006;141:701–704.
103. Rogers FB, Cipolle MD, Velmahos G, et al. Practice management guidelines for the prevention of venous thromboembolism in trauma patients: the EAST practice management guidelines work group. *J Trauma.* 2002;53: 142–164.
104. Maier RV, Mitchell D, Gentilello L. Optimal therapy for stress gastritis. *Ann Surg.* 1994;220:353–360.
105. Eddleston JM, Vohra A, Scott P, et al. A comparison of the frequency of stress ulceration and secondary pneumonia in sucralfate- or ranitidine-treated intensive care unit patients. *Crit Care Med.* 1991;19:1491–1496.

CHAPTER
58

Evaluating the Acute Abdomen or Difficult Postoperative Abdomen

PAUL B. MCBETH and TIMOTHY C. FABIAN

INTRODUCTION

The physician caring for surgical patients is often challenged by a variety of problems in the assessment and evaluation of the acute abdomen in critically ill patients. Acute abdominal problems are frequent sources of admission and complications in intensive care units (ICUs) (1). Early diagnosis of the acute abdomen and initiation of resuscitative efforts and surgical therapy often determine outcome. Knowledge of common abdominal problems and having a clinical approach for management are essential to all ICU physicians.

Any surgical procedure carries the risk of postoperative complications and difficult therapeutic management. The difficult postoperative abdomen presents many challenging issues for the ICU physician. Routine surgery may lead to the formation of adhesions leading to recurrent episodes of abdominal pain and partial or complete bowel obstruction. Enterocutaneous, intra-abdominal, or pancreatic fistulas may result from the natural progression of intra-abdominal pathology or the result of invasive procedures. Abdominal catastrophes may result in compartment syndrome leading to temporary abdominal closures and planned ventral hernias.

Herein, we will discuss the evaluation of the acute abdomen and the management of intra-abdominal problems commonly seen in the ICU. Further discussion will also include management of difficult postoperative issues. Considerations will be devoted to a review of etiology, diagnosis, and therapeutic approaches. The core principles of careful surgical technique and meticulous patient management, including wound care, nutritional management, and timing of recurrent interventions, are key in treating these problems.

EVALUATION OF THE ACUTE ABDOMEN

History

Evaluation of the acute abdomen and management of the difficult postoperative abdomen require a careful evaluation of the presenting illness. A detailed history of presenting illness should be obtained from either the patient or a family member. A focused abdominal history should include a review of previous abdominal surgeries and interventions, anesthetic exposure, and family history. The history should also include a review of medications, allergies, immunosuppressive therapies, and the use of drugs, tobacco, and alcohol. Symptomatic complaints should be identified in detail such as nausea and vomiting, hematemesis, hematochezia, diarrhea, and constipation. Characterization of abdominal pain is essential to establish an appropriate differential diagnosis. Location, nature, onset, and radiation of pain are useful in delineating the cause. These details are necessary to help focus diagnostic and therapeutic interventions. Symptoms of biliary disease, especially pain, and jaundice should be noted.

Physical Examination

Physical examination of a critically ill patient is often challenging given they may be sedated, intubated, combative, comatose, or paralyzed. However, thorough examination by inspection, palpation, percussion, and auscultation will usually provide good direction for both definite diagnosis and for appropriate advanced diagnostic investigations. Present and trended vital signs should be carefully evaluated in addition to the intravascular volume status and hemodynamics of a patient. Assessment of end-organ perfusion in critically ill patients is needed to help guide appropriate fluid resuscitation.

A focused examination of the abdomen can also give important clues to underlying pathology. Dilated abdominal wall veins indicate advanced portal hypertension. A pulsating upper abdominal mass in a thin patient may suggest a large abdominal aortic aneurysm. Absent or hypoactive bowel sounds is a nonspecific sign of an ileus. Hyperactive sounds or "rushes" are most common with small bowel obstruction. The presence of bowel sounds, however, does not always correlate with normal bowel function. Guarding or rigidity may indicate peritoneal irritation. Assessment of obese patients is often difficult as the assessment for abdominal wall rigidity is unreliable and specific pathologies such as groin or incisional hernias are difficult to identify. Patients with mesenteric ischemia have pain that is out of proportion to the findings of the physical examination. Serial examination is a useful technique to evaluate for the progression of tenderness, and the overall trend toward improvement or deterioration.

Laboratory Investigations

Laboratory investigations provide useful information in the diagnostic work of a patient. A complete blood count (CBC) including hematocrit, hemoglobin, platelets, and complete white blood cell count is routine, and provides valuable information about bone marrow function, transfusion requirements, and evaluation of infection. Urinalysis, including specific gravity and analysis for bacteria, bile, and reducing substances, should be performed. The serum amylase level is helpful in diagnosing intra-abdominal catastrophe when it is elevated but is not specific. In addition to its elevation in pancreatitis, serum amylase may be increased in ischemic bowel disease, facial trauma, perforated ulcer, or without apparent cause (2). Serum lipase is a specific marker of acute pancreatitis.

Saponification of retroperitoneal fat resulting in hypocalcemia is a helpful marker of severity in pancreatitis. An elevated serum bilirubin level is associated with sepsis, resolving hematoma, hemolysis, and hepatobiliary disease. Likewise, the lactate dehydrogenase (LDH) concentration may be elevated in numerous disease processes. Liver enzymes, including serum glutamate oxaloacetic transaminase (SGOT), serum glutamic pyruvic transaminase (SGPT), and alkaline phosphatase (ALP) may be helpful, but are rarely diagnostic by themselves. Laboratory data are most useful in the management and correction of fluids, electrolytes, and acid–base derangements.

Diagnostic Imaging

Modern diagnostic imaging techniques have become an essential tool in the diagnostic evaluation of critical ill patients. The most common modalities used are plain x-ray, computed tomography (CT) scan, and ultrasound. Each modality has specific applications where it is most useful. Standard x-rays have the benefit of being portable and available at the patient's bedside. Abdominal x-rays are most commonly used to determine the position of intra-abdominal tubes and to evaluate abnormal intra-abdominal gas patterns. The presence of air–fluid levels and bowel distention suggests bowel obstruction, while the absence of gas may be found with ischemic bowel. Free air from a perforated viscus is best seen in an upright chest radiograph.

The CT scan has become the most widely used tool to examine the abdomen for abnormalities. CT can provide greater detail of intra-abdominal organs and pathology than standard abdominal x-rays. In critical ill patients, CT is useful in determining specific diagnostic abnormalities. The utilization of intravenous contrast can help delineate vascular structures and enhancement of intra-abdominal anatomy. However, caution must be utilized in patients with renal dysfunction. In addition, oral and rectally administered contrast can greatly enhance the identification of bowel pathology; a limitation of oral contract is the risk of aspiration. The use of CT also requires transporting the patient to the scanner resulting in logistical challenges and patient safety risk.

Ultrasonography has become an essential adjunctive diagnostic and interventional tool in the emergency department (ED), ICU, and operating room (OR). It can be brought to the bedside and provide diagnostic evaluation of nearly every intra-abdominal organ. It is less invasive and less expensive than CT scan. Ultrasound can also be used as a therapeutic tool to help perform procedures such as percutaneous cholecystostomy.

TREATMENT

Specific Disease States

There are many potential etiologies of the acute abdomen in critical ill patients. The following outlines a selection of conditions commonly seen in the ICU. These include intra-abdominal sepsis/abscess, pneumoperitoneum, biliary disease, pseudo-obstruction of the colon, and acute mesenteric ischemia.

Intra-abdominal Sepsis or Abscess

Intra-abdominal sepsis arises from a variety of sources but is mostly commonly associated with perforated viscous, ischemic bowel, anastomotic failure, or biliary leakage. Intra-abdominal infection should be suspected in any patient deteriorating following abdominal surgery. Peritonitis can develop early or late in the postoperative course. Infected fluid collections typically wall-off to form an abscess after 5 to 7 postoperative days. Peritonitis and abscess formation typically occur as complications of anastomotic leakage from colonic surgery (3). Abscess formation also commonly develops with diverticular disease, appendicitis, inflammatory bowel disease, and malignancy. Initial management of patients with intra-abdominal sepsis is outlined in Figure 58.1 (4).

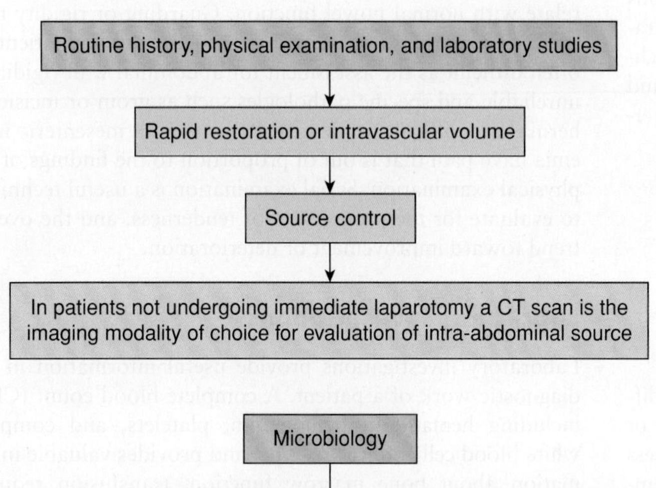

FIGURE 58.1 Initial management of suspected or confirmed intra-abdominal infections. (Adapted from IDSA–Complicated Intra-abdominal Infection—In Adults. http://www.idsociety.org.)

The clinical presentation of an intra-abdominal abscess often requires a high index of suspicion, as the clinical presentation can be subtle. Nonspecific manifestations including leukocytosis, fever, dysuria or urinary retention, unexplained pleural effusion, and change in bowel function (diarrhea) should alert the physician to investigate for an intra-abdominal infection. Investigation should include a CT scan of the abdomen and pelvis with oral and intravenous contrast. Once an abscess is identified, early antibiotic coverage and source control with either surgical or percutaneous drainage are mandated. Clinical factors predicting the failure of source control for intra-abdominal infections are outlined in Table 58.1 (4).

The microbiology of abscesses is dependent on the organ involved and duration of critical illness. Figure 58.2 outlines the antibiotic management guidelines of patients with community-acquired intra-abdominal infections (4). The stomach and duodenum normally have sparse bacterial colonization due to the acid concentration in these segments. The flora is mainly composed of swallowed oral organisms such as *microaerophilic streptococci* and *Streptococcus viridans*, *lactobacillus, fusiform bacteria*, and *Candida*. The concentration of organisms may be altered and significantly increased in patients with acid-suppressive treatment, gastric obstruction, and achlorhydria. The concentration of small bowel flora is variable throughout its length, with greater concentration distally. The normal flora consists primarily of the Enterobacteriaceae, Enterococcus, and anaerobic species. The colon contains a combination of both aerobic and anaerobic bacteria with anaerobes constituting 90% of the bacterial load. Aerobic bacteria are primarily gram-negative rods consisting of the Enterobacteriaceae (*Escherichia coli*, *Klebsiella* spp., *Enterobacter* spp., and *Proteus* spp.), *Pseudomonas*, and gram-positive Enterococci. Anaerobic bacteria include

TABLE 58.1 Clinical Factors Predicting Failure of Source Control for Intra-abdominal Infection

Delay in the initial intervention (>24 hr)
High severity of illness (APACHE II score >5)
Advanced age
Comorbidity and degree of organ dysfunction
Low albumin level
Poor nutritional status
Degree of peritoneal involvement or diffuse peritonitis
Inability to achieve adequate debridement or control of drainage
Presence of malignancy

Modified from Solomkin JS, Mazuski JE, Bradley JS, et al. Diagnosis and management of complicated intra-abdominal infection in adults and children: guidelines by the Surgical Infection Society and the Infectious Diseases Society of America. *Clin Infect Dis.* 2010;50(2):133–164.

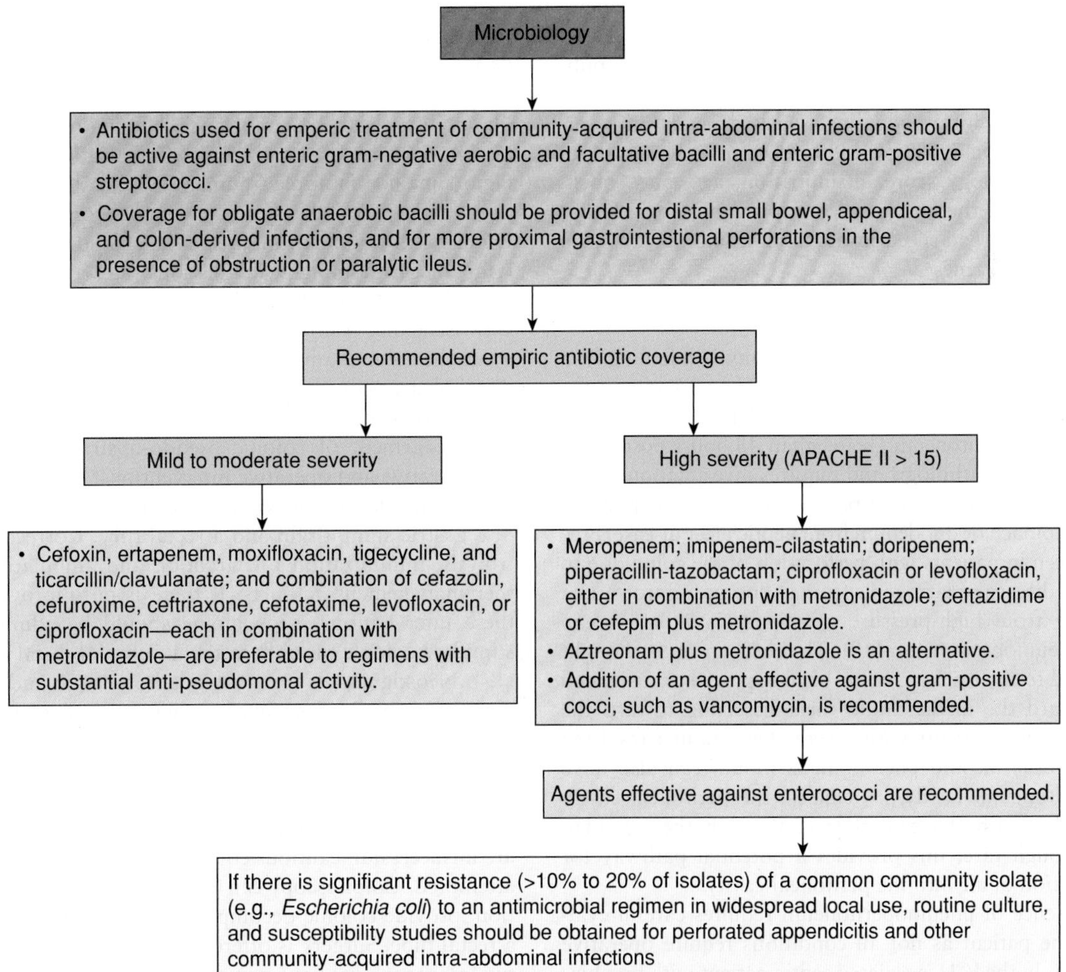

FIGURE 58.2 Microbiology and management of community-acquired intra-abdominal infections in adults. (Adapted from IDSA–Complicated Intra-abdominal Infection—In Adults. http://www.idsociety.org.)

Bacteroides fragilis, *Bacteroides* subspecies, *Clostridium* spp., *Eubacterium* spp., and *Bifidobacterium* spp.; intra-abdominal abscesses are typically polymicrobial.

Patients with generalized peritonitis or hemodynamic instability with suspected intra-abdominal infection require emergent surgical exploration to identify the cause. The primary source of the infection is controlled by repair or resection followed by a thorough washout of the abdominal cavity with warm saline. In some patients with either hemodynamic instability or severe contamination, the abdominal wall may be temporarily left open for additional washout in 24 to 48 hours. Management of the open abdomen is discussed later.

Stable patients with localized peritonitis or suspected intra-abdominal sepsis should undergo a CT scan to identify any abnormal pathology; if a defined abscess or fluid collection is seen on the CT scan, percutaneous drainage is possible using CT or ultrasound image guidance. This technique is well established (5–7) and minimally invasive; re-exploration of the abdomen may be fraught with difficulty (8).

Antibiotic therapy is based on empiric coverage of bacteria normally present within the gut. Antibiotic coverage should include gram-positive, gram-negative, and anaerobic bacteria; therapy can be focused when culture and sensitivities testing is complete. However, due to problems with anaerobic culturing and identification, most patients should receive anaerobic coverage for gut-associated infection, even when anaerobes are not identified. Antifungal agents are not given even if fungi are seen on cultures, unless the patient is immunosuppressed or has recurrent intra-abdominal infection. Guidelines are published elsewhere (4).

Mortality from intra-abdominal sepsis depends on severity and ranges from 7.5% to 43% (9). Mortality correlates with acute physiology score, malnutrition, age, and shock. Early goal-directed therapy targeted at prompt recognition of abdominal sepsis, broad-spectrum antibiotics, and source control will maximize outcomes.

Pneumoperitoneum

The presence of pneumoperitoneum on x-ray is a finding of a perforated viscous until proven otherwise. The exception is the presence of free air less than 48 hours after laparotomy or laparoscopy; pneumoperitoneum greater than 48 hours postoperation is considered pathologic and requires investigation.

The most common cause of pneumoperitoneum is perforation of the stomach or duodenum from peptic ulcer disease. Free air is also seen in patients with perforation of the colon due to diverticular disease or iatrogenic from endoscopy. Barotrauma to the lung from high-pressure mechanical ventilation can result in pneumoperitoneum (10). The mechanism is thought to be related to the tracking of air from ruptured or distended alveoli toward the mediastinum then dissecting toward the peritoneal cavity. Patients with severe chest trauma resulting in a pneumothorax and pneumomediastinum can also have pneumoperitoneum. Lastly, in females, the peritoneal cavity communicates with the genital tract through the fallopian tubes. Although rare, this provides a potential pathway for communication of air into the peritoneal cavity.

The presence of pneumoperitoneum requires careful evaluation of the patient as not all conditions require operative intervention. In the ICU, a sedated septic patient with no obvious source of sepsis, in the presence of pneumoperitoneum, should nearly always prompt an exploratory laparotomy.

Biliary Disease

Pathology related to the biliary system is common in critically ill patients and is typically associated with either calculous or acalculous cholecystitis. Patients with pre-existing calculous disease may present with acute cholecystitis, cholangitis, or pancreatitis. Clinically patients may present with a positive Murphy sign, fever, and increased WBC; local peritonitis is found in only 24% of patients (11). On further investigation, laboratory findings include leukocytosis, elevated bilirubin (65%), and elevated liver enzymes in less than 50% (12). Ultrasound is the most favorable imaging modality of the biliary system. Ultrasonographic findings of acute cholecystitis include dilated gall bladder, gall bladder wall thickening, the presence of gall stones, and evidence of pericholecystic fluid. Acute acalculous cholecystitis is more commonly associated with critically ill surgical and medical patients in the ICU. The development of acalculous cholecystitis is associated with narcotic use, gastric suctioning, prolonged ileus, prolonged mechanical ventilation, intravenous hyperalimentation, and massive transfusion (12,13). Acalculous cholecystitis in critically ill patients carries a 40% mortality rate (11,14).

Drainage of the biliary tree and antibiotics are the mainstay of treatment. Drainage can be achieved by surgically placed cholecystostomy tube or a percutaneous cholecystostomy tube.

Pseudo-obstruction of the Colon

An ileus of the colon without mechanical obstruction is referred to as pseudo-obstruction or Ogilvie syndrome (15). This condition is typically seen in elderly patients with prolonged immobility, electrolyte imbalance (hyponatremia and hypokalemia), narcotic use, and mechanical ventilation. Other risk factors include multiple trauma, abdominal and pelvic operations, orthopedic operations, and spinal cord injuries (15,16). On physical examination, the abdomen appears distended and tympanic. Abdominal x-ray demonstrates a distend colon. As the colon distends, the wall tension increases leading to local wall ischemia, necrosis, and perforation. The highest risk is when the colon diameter exceeds 12 cm. Mechanical causes of distal obstruction should be ruled out using a contrast enema or colonoscopy.

Management of colonic pseudo-obstruction is based on nonoperative and operative interventions. Initial management should include gastrointestinal decompression with placement of a gastric sump drain and a rectal tube. Correction of electrolysis, minimization of narcotics, and ambulation are further management adjuncts. If there is no improvement with these interventions, neostigmine should be administered to stimulate colonic motility in the absence of distal obstruction (17). Neostigmine is a parasympathomimetic and is given as 1 to 2 mg i.v. Bradycardia is a significant side effect of neostigmine; therefore, patients should be in a monitored location. Neostigmine should be avoided in patients with baseline bradycardia, hypotension, heart block, or bronchospasm. If a patient is unable to take neostigmine, or previous measures are unsuccessful, cautious colonoscopic decompression can be attempted. Colonoscopy can evaluate for mechanical obstruction, provide colonic decompression, and guide placement of a rectal tube. Surgery is offered to patients who fail conservative management, have complications, or impending colonic rupture. Depending on the extent of colonic abnormality, the suggested operation is typically a total abdominal colectomy, in which case an ileostomy with mucus fistula should be performed.

Acute Mesenteric Ischemia

Acute mesenteric ischemia is an uncommon condition and often results in significant morbidity and mortality (70% to 80%) (18,19). The etiology of acute mesenteric ischemia is either from arterial or venous pathology. Arterial causes are classified as nonocclusive mesenteric ischemia and occlusive mesenteric arterial ischemia. Occlusive disease is further classified as acute mesenteric arterial embolism and acute mesenteric arterial thrombosis. Acute mesenteric ischemia can also be caused by mesenteric venous thrombosis (20–22). Early clinical recognition, workup, and intervention are needed to improve outcome (19). Death occurs from MSOF secondary to ischemia (65%), sepsis (25%), pulmonary failure (8%), and stroke (2%) (23).

The classic presentation of acute mesenteric ischemia is a patient's complaint of pain out of proportion to physical examination findings. Pain is identified in patients 75% to 90% of the time; nausea, vomiting, and abdominal distention are commonly seen. Leukocytosis (WBC count of 20,000 cells/mm^3) is seen in less than half of patients. As the degree of bowel ischemia progresses toward gangrene, patients will have a worsening clinical presentation. Peritoneal irritation, leukocytosis, elevated hematocrit, unexplained acidosis, and blood-tinged fluid on peritoneal lavage are all signs of advancing intestinal necrosis (24) and are associated with significant mortality.

Early management should include aggressive fluid resuscitation to maintain adequate blood flow in the mesenteric vessels. Gastric decompression with a nasogastric tube and continuous hemodynamic monitoring is required. Heparinization should be used if immediate surgery is not undertaken.

With improved resolution of modern CT scanners, the diagnosis of acute intestinal ischemia can often be made. Multidetector CT angiography can differentiate occlusive from nonocclusive disease. Despite this, selective arteriography remains the gold standard in the diagnostic and therapeutic approach to acute mesenteric ischemia. Acute occlusion is best treated by immediate surgical management with an embolectomy or aorto-superior mesenteric artery bypass. The bowel should be evaluated for ischemia with nonviable segments resected. Segments with questionable viability should be re-evaluated after allowing time for reperfusion. Although second-look operations are frequently used at 24 to 48 hours to determine the viability of remaining bowel, survival is not necessarily improved by this technique (25).

In patients with nonocclusive mesenteric ischemia, an angiogram will demonstrate mesenteric vasoconstriction. Interpretation of the angiogram may be difficult if the patient is in shock and on vasopressors (26). Traditionally, treatment included the administration of papaverine (30 to 60 mg/hr) through a catheter placed selectively in the superior mesenteric artery (SMA) (27). Papaverine is continued until repeat arteriogram after 24 hours. Currently, however, there is a worldwide shortage of papaverine. Therefore, alternative treatment such as nitroglycerin, combined with verapamil, is becoming more commonly used. The presence of peritoneal signs mandates surgical exploration to assess bowel viability. Antibiotics are indicated because of the high incidence of positive blood cultures resulting from compromised bowel.

The Difficult Postoperative Abdomen

The practice of surgery carries risk of postoperative complications and often difficult therapeutic choices to manage these complications. Intra-abdominal surgery will inevitably result in adhesion formation, which may lead to recurrent episodes of abdominal pain and partial or complete bowel obstruction. Fistulae may result from the natural progression of intra-abdominal pathology or from iatrogenic injury. Abdominal catastrophes may result in abdominal compartment syndrome (ACS) and the risk of temporary abdominal closures and planned ventral hernias. Less commonly seen are complications of radiation enteritis and short bowel syndrome. The following sections will review many of these difficult postoperative issues with descriptions of etiology, diagnosis, and therapeutic approaches.

Adhesions

Intra-abdominal surgery will inevitably result in the unavoidable consequence of adhesions. Adhesion formation is a normal physiologic response in postoperative healing. Formation of adhesive tissue protects an anastomosis and prevents leaks, in addition to assisting in the body's attempt to isolate intra-abdominal catastrophes. When adhesive bands become too dense, kink, or encompass loops of bowel, they may result in negative consequences such as bowel obstruction and persistent abdominal pain. Intra-abdominal adhesions are the primary cause for postoperative bowel obstruction, accounting for approximately 75% of cases (28).

The majority (94% to 98%) of abdominal adhesions are acquired from either operative therapy or inflammatory processes. The remaining 2% to 6% of adhesions are congenital. In the reoperative abdomen, adhesions are present in 30% to 40% of patients. The most frequent morbidity in those with postoperative adhesions is small bowel obstruction, which accounts for 12% to 17% of hospital admissions following previous abdominal surgery (29). The degree of morbidity related to adhesion formation is related to the type of surgery performed. Laparoscopic surgeries have a 15% adhesion rate as opposed to open laparotomies, in which 50% result in adhesion formation. Adhesions form more commonly following surgery to the small and large bowels and uterus than with other intra-abdominal organs, especially in surgeries involving bowel distal to the transverse colon or involving gynecologic organs (28). The areas most frequently affected are the undersurface of the midline incision and the operative site. The omentum is the most frequently involved organ (57%). Small and large bowel adhesions continue to result in the highest morbidity (30). Adhesions may result in mechanical fixation points where the bowel may kink, wrap around, or become strangulated, thereby compromising enteric flow and blood supply. Patients with high-grade bowel obstructions require an emergency operation to relieve the obstruction before the adverse sequelae of bowel ischemia.

Given the prevalence and morbidity associated with adhesions extensive research have focused on identifying methods to avoid adhesion formation. Adhesions result from trauma to tissues, tissue ischemia, infection within the abdominal cavity, inflammatory processes, or by the presence of foreign bodies such as suture, talc from gloves, and lint from sponges. To minimize adhesions, gentle tissue handling with strict hemostasis and minimization of intraperitoneal trauma are core principles. In addition, frequent irrigation to dilute or to remove contaminants and the use of small, nonreactive suture material will diminish the contribution to adhesiogenesis. Perhaps the most effective method of preventing serious adhesions is via the use of the omentum. The omentum may be used to wrap anastomoses or to protect abdominal contents from a healing midline incision. Despite the adverse effects of adhesion formation, adhesions are an important part of the wound healing and without adhesions most anastomoses would likely fail.

Fistulae

A fistula is an abnormal communication between two epithelized surfaces. A variety of fistulas can exist within the abdomen, including pancreatic and biliary fistulae, fistulae between two intra-abdominal organs, and enterocutaneous and enteroatmospheric fistulae. The majority of GI fistulae occur as complications of abdominal surgery. The incidence of spontaneous fistula formation is rare and is usually the result of intra-abdominal infection or inflammation. The natural history of a fistula begins as a bowel leak. The type of fistula depends on whether the leak is uncontrolled, partially controlled, or well controlled (31). An uncontrolled leak will result in peritonitis and require surgical exploration for correction of the underlying pathology. A partially controlled leak may result in an intra-abdominal abscess, which will require definitive therapy such as open or percutaneous drainage. Controlled leaks result in fistulae. Management of fistulae can be a long-term challenge for surgeon and patient.

An enterocutaneous fistula is an abnormal communication between the bowel and the skin surface. The majority of these fistulae (71% to 90%) are the result of postoperative iatrogenic complications (29,32). Spontaneous causes of fistulae are uncommon but may include malignancy, inflammatory processes, mechanical obstruction, or vascular insufficiency. Iatrogenic fistulae may result from inadvertent enterotomies, intra-abdominal infections, direct injury or bowel desiccation in the open abdomen, misplaced stitches, or anastomotic breakdown. Impaired tissue perfusion from hypotension or vascular disease may predispose to this complication, as will infections, steroids, and malnutrition. Characterization of the fistula tract and surrounding anatomy is essential, best done with a fistulogram. This is done by injecting gastrografin into the tract and using fluoroscopy to follow the progress of the contrast. A fistulogram is useful to define the length of the tract, tortuosity, tract diameter, and which segment of the gastrointestinal tract is involved. A CT scan is helpful in defining surrounding anatomy such as intra-abdominal abscesses, malignancy, and hernias (33).

A postoperative enterocutaneous fistula typically presents as discolored, watery drainage or frank succus from the midline incision. Palpation along the facial closure suture line will often reveal a local dehiscence. Passage of gas from the midline wound is diagnostic of an enterocutaneous fistula. Patients will usually demonstrate signs of infection characterized by increasing temperature, white blood cell count, and persistent ileus. Some patients may develop profound shock due to electrolyte imbalances and sepsis. In these cases, emergent re-exploration is necessary. However, if the patient presents with drainage or an obvious fistula but is hemodynamically stable, a short-period conservative management is reasonable.

Conservative Management of the Enterocutaneous Fistula. Initial management of enterocutaneous fistulas is based on evaluation and control of sepsis, aggressive fluid resuscitation with correction of electrolytes and nutritional deficiencies, and control and characterization of fistula output with protection of surrounding skin surface. Early and aggressive management of these factors will maximize the potential for spontaneous closure. Patients with enterocutaneous fistulae are prone to malnutrition from protein losses, increased metabolic demands, and limited oral intake; early fluid and electrolyte replacement is needed. Parenteral nutrition is often necessary to provide early nutritional repletion, enable management of electrolyte and protein balances, and to decrease volume transit past the fistula in the gastrointestinal tract. Other methods of reducing volume of enteric content past the fistula is the use of narcotics, loperamide, and somatostatin analogs. The use of octreotide or other somatostatin analogs (100 μg intravenously every 8 hours) may decrease gastrointestinal secretions. Somatostatin inhibits the secretion of most gastrointestinal hormones and enhances fluid and electrolyte absorption, thereby decreasing intraluminal volume and potentially decreasing fistula output. Despite the theoretical benefits of somatostatin use, clinical studies have revealed mixed results on effectiveness. Although some studies have demonstrated a decreased fistula output and higher rate of spontaneous closure, an equivalent literature reveals no statistical difference in output or closure rates (34). As side effects are relatively mild, including gastrointestinal discomfort and increased biliary sludge, we recommend trying a somatostatin analog in conjunction with other conservative therapies while waiting for a fistula to close spontaneously.

Containment and control of fistula output is a significant challenge. Enteric contents are extremely caustic to the skin and surrounding tissues, creating a need to isolate enteric contents from the skin. For a simple enterocutaneous fistula, a stoma appliance is usually sufficient. However, many fistulae present in open wound beds, including on granulating abdomens. These tissue fields are not amenable to the placement of a simple stoma appliance. In these situations, a multidisciplinary approach with the surgeon and wound care nurse/enterostomal therapist is needed to control fistula output. Once initial control is achieved, it may be possible to close fistulae surgically or to skin graft the region.

Spontaneous Fistula Closure. Spontaneous fistula closure is the goal of conservative management. Many fistulae close without operative intervention, and will do so in the first 3 to 6 weeks after appearance. The spontaneous closure of a fistula is dependent on its inherent characteristics. Fistulae with long tracts and narrow mouths are more likely to resolve without intervention. Low-output fistulae (less than 500 mL per day) have a higher likelihood of closure than do high-output ones. A fistula with persistent drainage after 3 months is unlikely to close without surgical therapy. In addition, several patient factors are associated with failure of the fistula closure. These include the presence of a foreign body in the fistula tract, close association with an abscess, presence of malignancy, distal bowel obstruction leading to increased pressure and transit through the fistulous tract, and a short neck with wide fistula mouth. Longstanding fistulae with high outputs are unlikely to close spontaneously. To improve the likelihood of spontaneous fistula closure, optimal nutrition for wound healing and minimization of enteric content should be undertaken. Parenteral nutrition is used to decrease the volume transiting the gastrointestinal tract and through the fistula. A positive nitrogen balance and a transferrin level greater than 200 mg/dL are also associated with successful closure (35).

Surgical Therapy for Enterocutaneous Fistulae. Failure of spontaneous fistula closure is considered after 3 months if the fistula remains open; after this point the likelihood of closure without surgical management is poor. Preoperative management requires characterization of the fistula track and surrounding anatomy, optimization of nutrition, albumin and pre-albumin levels, and wound care. Control of fistula output and maintenance of healthy skin integrity at the time of operation will improve the success of abdominal wall reconstruction (34). With careful planning and delay of operative repair until all criteria are met (nutrition, fistula definition, wound care), the morbidity and mortality may be decreased from 50% mortality and 50% recurrence in early surgeries to 94% successful closure and a 4% mortality rate (29,36).

Surgical management of an enterocutaneous fistula requires a laparotomy. Management of intra-abdominal adhesions from prior surgeries or infection is a challenge. Extensive and dense adhesions may make access to the fistula difficult with the risk of enterotomies. While a common initial impulse is to oversew the fistula primarily, this should be avoided whenever possible as the recurrence rate is high. The preferred method for surgical management remains complete lysis of intra-abdominal adhesions and resection of the involved segment. With this approach, the diseased portion of bowel is removed and the anastomosis is performed between two healthy segments of bowel. The complete lysis of adhesions allows careful inspection of the remaining bowel to rule out downstream obstruction or other pathology. Although time consuming, this approach provides the highest likelihood of recovery without recurrent fistulization.

Enteroatmospheric fistulae communicate with an open granulating abdomen and represent a complex management problem. In particular, managing the fistula drainage on a granulating surface makes it difficult to control contamination. Often a multidisciplinary approach with an enterostomal therapist is necessary to identify a functional solution using a variety of stoma appliance options. A split-thickness skin graft is a favorable option for patients with a fistula in the face of the granulating, open abdomen. The skin graft will decrease the metabolic demands of a granulating abdomen and provides a good base for control of fistula output. At the time of skin grafting, the fistula track should be cannulated with a catheter to allow for preferential drainage of enteric content and to avoid contamination of the skin graft site. Contamination of the graft site often complicated with high rate of graft failure. A vacuum assisted closure (VAC) appliance should be applied to the skin graft site with a specialized porous VAC sponge surrounding the fistula opening to prevent injury to the bowel surface; this should be changed every 2 to 3 days.

The Pancreatic Fistula

The majority of pancreatic fistulae result from trauma or pancreatic resection, with only a small percentage resulting from primary pancreatic diseases. The principles of management are diagnosis of the fistula and wide drainage. Evaluation with a CT scan will provide important information about the pancreatic anatomy, degree of inflammation, and peripancreatic fluid collections. Pancreatic fluid contains a large amount of bicarbonate (70 to 90 mEq/L), and inadequate replacement of bicarbonate may lead to nonanion gap metabolic acidosis. Pancreatic fistulae typically drain between 100 and 1,000 mL of fluid/d. Classification of pancreatic fistulae is outlined in Table 58.2 (37). Pancreatic injury may result in accumulation of pancreatic ascites, resulting in abdominal pain, fever, ileus, and abscess formation. There exists a spectrum of patient clinical presentation from a pancreatic leak: some patients may present in profound shock while others may tolerate large-output pancreatic fistulae with a benign clinical presentation. The source of this variability in clinical presentation is poorly understood but is likely due to the degree of enzymatic activation of the leaking fluid.

For most patients, the initial treatment for a pancreatic fistula is percutaneous drainage. Intraoperative concern for a postoperative pancreatic leak should prompt the surgeon to prove wide drainage with a closed-system drain before closing the patient's abdomen. Wide drainage of pancreatic secretions should allow time for the patient to stabilize and prevent damage to other abdominal organs. Long-term drainage is often needed to enable spontaneous closure of the pancreatic fistula. This conservative approach with drains is generally pursued for up to 6 months and has a success rate of up to 97% in some studies (38). Pancreatic fistulae with persistent drainage should undergo imaging studies to define duct anatomy and determine if an obstructive process is maintaining fistula patency. Magnetic resonance cholangiopancreatography

TABLE 58.2 Criteria for Grading Pancreatic Fistula: ISGPF Classification Scheme

Criteria	No Fistula	Grade A Fistula	Grade B Fistula	Grade C Fistula
Drain amylase	<3x normal serum amylase	>3x normal serum amylase	>3x normal serum amylase	>3x normal serum amylase
Clinical conditions	Well	Well	Often well	Ill appearing
Specific treatment	No	No	Yes/no	Yes
US/CT	Negative	Negative	Negative/positive	Positive
Persistent drainage (>3 wk)	No	No	Usually yes	Yes
Signs of infection	No	No	Yes	Yes
Readmission	No	No	Yes/no	Yes/no
Sepsis	No	No	No	Yes
Reoperation	No	No	No	Yes
Death related to fistula	No	No	No	Yes

From Bassi C, Dervenis C, Butturini G, et al. Postoperative pancreatic fistula: an international study group (ISGPF) definition. *Surgery.* 2005;138:8–13.

(MRCP) and endoscopic retrograde cholangiopancreatography (ERCP) may provide similar information; however, ERCP is generally preferred as it enables characterization of duct anatomy and allows for intervention. Stenting of a proximal obstruction may be adequate to allow prograde drainage of pancreatic secretions and closure of the fistula, thereby avoiding surgical therapy (39). Failure of conservative therapy requires exploratory laparotomy for definitive management of a pancreatic fistula. Surgical management depends on the level of the injury. A fistula resulting from the distal duct is treated by distal pancreatectomy. If the leaking duct is sufficiently large, a pancreaticojejunostomy may be performed to allow for a low-resistance drainage pathway. Pancreatic fistulae involving the proximal duct are most often iatrogenic or related to trauma and are troublesome to deal with, in light of other major structures in the region. For these patients, a pancreaticoduodenectomy will resect the leaking portion of pancreas and allow reconstruction. This procedure should only be performed in patients with good physiologic reserve and nutrition. As noted, an attempt at conservative therapy and complete preoperative imaging and optimization are mandatory as these procedures are a major commitment for surgeon and patient (38).

Adjunctive therapies including parenteral nutrition and octreotide may be helpful in decreasing secretory stimulation to the pancreas. With a low side-effect profile it is reasonable to pursue this therapy for a short course to improve chances of nonoperative resolution.

Abdominal Compartment Syndrome

ACS can be a source of significant patient morbidity and mortality. Since its first description in the 1980s, ACS has become an increasingly recognized clinical entity (40). In current surgical management it is usually seen following a massive fluid resuscitation from trauma, burns, intraoperative resuscitation, pancreatitis, or sepsis. Capillary leak occurs secondary to sepsis or reperfusion injury in the splanchnic circulation and results in massive interstitial edema. As the abdomen is a limited potential space, increasing interstitial edema and free fluid in the abdomen result in increased intra-abdominal pressure, which is transmitted to organs in both the thorax and abdomen; the physiologic effects are seen in almost every organ system. Compression of the inferior vena cava by abdominal contents and fluid results in decreased preload and a subsequent decrease in cardiac output. This ultimately leads to increased systemic vascular resistance and decreased stroke volume. Clinically, patients will become increasingly tachycardic and hypotensive. Increased abdominal volume also places pressure on the diaphragm, limiting intrathoracic space. This results in increasing peak ventilatory pressures (>30 to 35 cm H_2O) and decreased ventilation with hypercapnia and hypoxemia. Compression of the ureters and bladder, as well as renal vein compression, leads to diminished urine output and renal injury (41,42).

Clinically, suspicion is key to diagnosis of ACS. Multiple clinical factors, as noted above, will establish the diagnosis. Measurement of intra-abdominal pressures is evaluated indirectly through measurement of bladder pressure with an indwelling urinary bladder catheter (IUBC); this is illustrated in Figure 58.3. Abdominal pressures greater than 20 mmHg, with new onset organ dysfunction, is indicative of ACS. A classification of ACS is outlined in Figure 58.4. Management of true ACS involves decompressive laparotomy (42,43). A decompressive laparotomy may be indicated at lower intra-abdominal pressures depending on the patient's clinical condition (44). After decompressing the abdominal contents, the abdomen is left open with a temporary abdominal closure until swelling diminishes enough to allow closure.

The Open Abdomen

The open abdomen is an important tool in a surgeon's armamentarium for management of critical ill patients. There are two important management strategies requiring the open abdomen. First is the recognition of primary and secondary ACS allows surgeons to choose the open abdomen as a management strategy for the short term. Second, "damage control laparotomies" have become increasingly common in treating major abdominal trauma. Although the idea of abbreviated laparotomy was first described by Stone et al. in 1983 (45), the formal nomenclature and increasing popularity are credited to Rotondo et al. in 1993 (46). Damage control laparotomy is aimed at limiting intraoperative times by delaying definitive repair and limiting operative intervention to controlling hemorrhage and contamination. The patient's abdomen is

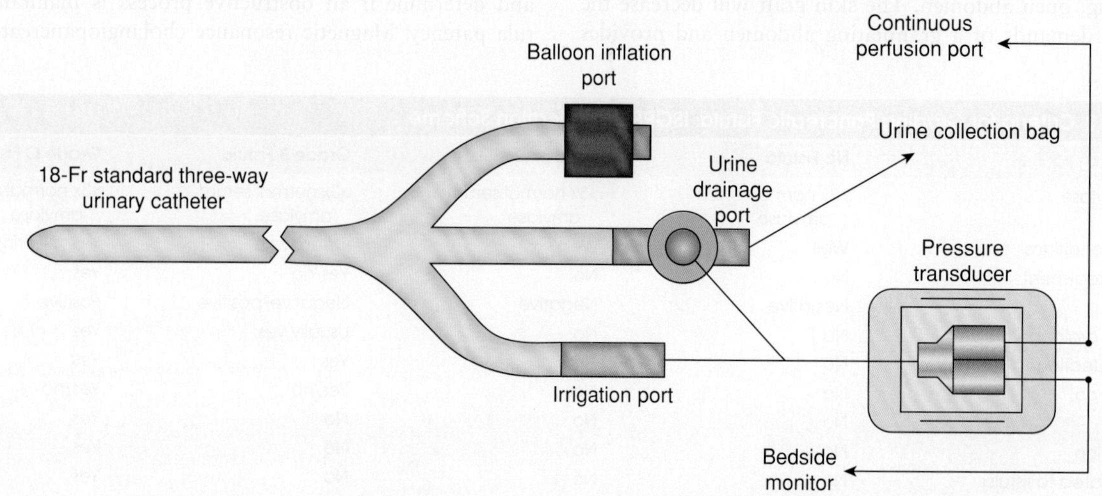

FIGURE 58.3 Intra-abdominal pressure monitoring.

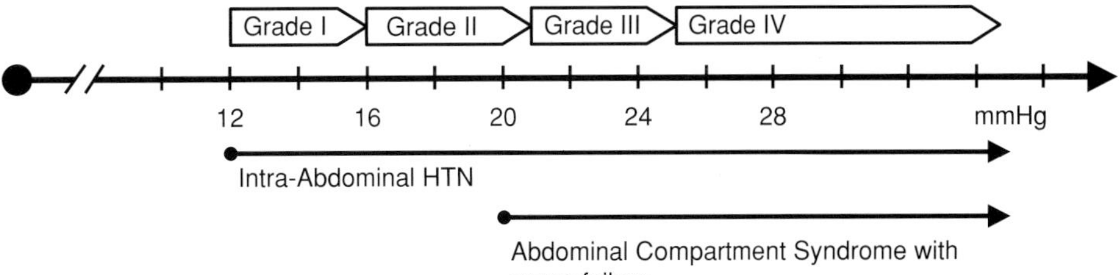

FIGURE 58.4 Classification of abdominal compartment syndrome.

temporary closed with a plan to return when the patient is stable enough to enable definitive repair. Early transfer to the ICU facilitates continued resuscitation and rewarming. Damage control laparotomy remains an aggressive strategy for treatment of patients who develop the deadly triad of coagulopathy, hypothermia, and metabolic acidosis.

The open abdomen represents a complex and challenging management problem involving three decision-making stages: initial operative management (28), decision to close primarily versus a planned ventral hernia (29), and definitive closure of the planned ventral hernia (47). At the conclusion of a damage control laparotomy, the abdominal wall is temporarily closed, using a gusset or negative pressure–type closure devices, to achieve rapid closure with protection of intra-abdominal contents. The original temporary abdominal dressing is known as the Bogota bag. It consists of covering the abdominal contents with a sterile saline bag to protect the bowel until re-exploration; current practice of temporary abdominal wall closure is based on a derivation of the Bogota. A plastic drape, such as a sterile cassette cover, is placed over the bowels to prevent them from injury and to allow drainage of fluid. A sponge or blue towel, with two large Jackson–Pratt drains (Cardinal Health, McGaw Park, IL), is then placed over the plastic drape. The entire system is folded under the fascia to contain the abdominal contents. An adhesive drape is placed over the abdomen to maintain sterility and prevent free drainage of fluid. The drains are placed to suction to allow collection of blood and edema fluid. This dressing is then left intact until return to the operating room (48). Alternatively, vacuum-assisted fascial closure may be used. In this method, the bowels are protected with the plastic drape. A drainage sponge with constant suction is then placed, and the abdomen is covered with an adhesive dressing. The sponge suction provides constant medial tension, without disrupting the fascia, to prevent lateral retraction (48,49). These methods allow for control of abdominal edema and are easily applied in the OR (49).

The patient is returned to the operating room after an appropriate resuscitation period, usually 24 to 48 hours. Once definitive operative repair is complete, the decision to close primarily depends on the degree of intra-abdominal edema and the quality of the fascia. Primary closure of fascia is preferable as long as there is no excessive fascial tension. High-tension closures will elevate intra-abdominal pressures leading to compartment syndrome with cardiopulmonary dysfunction, renal impairment, and risk of dehiscence. In the absence of primary closure, return trips to the OR are indicated to facilitate gradual closure. The goal of temporary closure is to prevent lateral retraction of fascia to facilitate delayed primary closure. Vicryl mesh sewn directly to the fascia is a form of temporary abdominal closure. Daily tightening of the abdominal wall with mesh pleating combined with fluid removal will help improve the likelihood of primary abdominal wall closure (41). Management of the patient's volume status to achieve a net negative balance is important to facilitate re-approximation of the fascia. Achieving a net negative volume balance is often difficult in critically ill trauma patients requiring large-volume resuscitations. Therefore, many of these patients will go on to planned ventral hernias.

Ventral Hernia Repair

A giant ventral hernia is the result of the inability to close an open abdomen. Once it is established that primary closure of the abdominal wall is not possible, the patient is managed with a temporary Vicryl mesh secured across the abdominal wall. After 2 to 3 weeks, the abdominal contents should display a healthy bed of granulation tissue. At this point, a split-thickness skin graft is used to close the surface. Application of skin graft too early or late may result in fistula formation. The patient is then observed for 6 to 12 months while undergoing rehabilitation and nutritional optimization (50).

With the absence of a functional abdominal wall, ventral hernias are debilitating and cosmetically displeasing. Most patients are motivated for definitive closure of the hernia. Consideration of abdominal wall reconstruction requires careful evaluation of the patient's nutritional status, as well as the laxity of the skin graft. Over time, the skin graft and intra-abdominal adhesions will soften, allowing easier graft removal and adhesiolysis. The ideal window for most patients appears to be at 6 to 12 months (51).

The majority of ventral hernias are not amenable to primary closure. As such, the surgeon must decide on the best method of restoring abdominal domain, with options including functional and nonfunctional abdominal wall reconstruction. A functional reconstruction attempts to use the patient's native tissues through a process of component separation. Nonfunctional repairs rely on the placement of synthetic or porcine mesh across the defect. The use of mesh is not possible if enterotomies are made during the lysis stage or if stoma reversal is necessary. Functional abdominal wall reconstruction is based on a component separation technique, which is a type of rectus abdominis muscle advancement flap. After sharply removing the skin graft, small bowel adhesions are freed from the overlying fascia for a distance of 4 to 6 cm. Skin flaps are raised laterally on both sides extending from the iliac crest to the level of the midaxillary line. The component separation technique involves placement of relaxing incisions in the anterior and posterior rectus fascial layers to allow advancement of the abdominal wall to provide a tension-free repair at the abdominal midline. Aggressive closure under tension may lead to postoperative respiratory compromise and complications associated with ACS. Since the original description of this technique by Ramirez (52) in 1990, there have

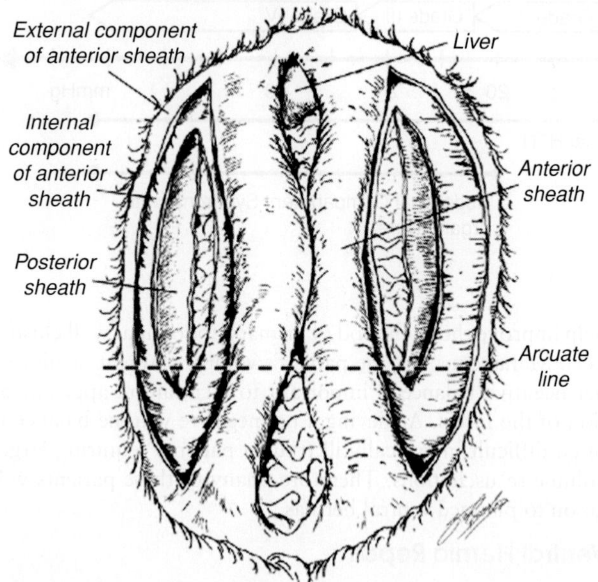

FIGURE 58.5 Abdominal wall reconstruction with component separation. (From DiCocco JM, Fabian TC, Emmett KP, et al. Components separation for abdominal wall reconstruction: the Memphis modification. *Surgery.* 2012;151(1):118–125.)

been many modifications. In some patients, a limited release may be adequate to allow re-approximation of the fascia at the midline. In other patients, further release and translocation of anterior fascia and muscle may be required to bring the abdominal wall together without tension (53); this technique is illustrated in Figure 58.5.

Once the fascia is closed at the midline, four Jackson–Pratt drains are placed, one superior and one inferior bilaterally, and the skin is closed. Postoperatively, nasogastric suction is maintained until output decreases and drains are left in until output drops to less than 20 mL/d. In patients with anterior and posterior fascia release and still unable to close fascia primarily without tension, a mesh interposition may be necessary to achieve closure. Overall, patients tolerate closure well and long-term success is excellent with only a 5% recurrent hernia rate in experienced hands (50,51).

Short Bowel Syndrome

Short bowel is defined as shortening of the gastrointestinal length to less than 200 cm; the etiology is variable and differs between children and adults, but essentially short bowel is the result of an intra-abdominal catastrophe requiring extensive surgical resection of bowel. In children, short gut syndrome is seen in congenital or neonatal processes such as necrotizing enterocolitis, intestinal atresia, volvulus, or gastroschisis. Adults acquire short gut syndrome following extensive surgical resection necessitated by malignancy, trauma, obstruction, or vascular insufficiency. Patient functional outcome is for the most part determined by the length of remaining small bowel and the presence or absence of the colon. Presence of the colon can extend the functional capacity of the remaining bowel. To maintain adequate enteral nutrition, a patient requires at least 150 cm of small bowel, or 60 to 90 cm if the colon is present (54). The ileocecal valve is also important in maintaining hydration and modulating gastrointestinal transit time.

Short gut syndrome is a condition characterized by a short bowel segment and the inability to meet nutritional requirements and dependence on parenteral nutrition. Patients will have significant weight loss, diarrhea, and steatorrhea. Patients often develop gastric emptying abnormalities and rapid transit times due to short intestinal length. Dehydration is a constant problem especially if the colon is absent due to an inability to reabsorb gastrointestinal secretions (approximately 4 L/d). Reduced absorption leads to vitamin deficiencies such as B_{12} and fat-soluble vitamins and bile salts. Short gut patients are also prone to cholelithiasis and nephrolithiasis due to altered absorption of bile salts and oxalate, peptic ulcers due to increased gastric secretions, line sepsis from deep catheters, and liver dysfunction from parenteral nutrition (55).

Surgical management of short bowel requires effort to preserve bowel length and the ileocecal valve. In some cases, limited bowel resection with plan for delayed inspection of marginally viable bowel is necessary to preserve as much bowel as possible. Initial postoperative therapy is often supportive with early administration of parenteral nutrition to prevent malnutrition and optimize would healing. The long-term management of short gut patients then requires a multidisciplinary team involving physicians and nurses, nutritionists, patients, and their families.

Surgical therapy is occasionally required to deal with the sequelae of short gut syndrome. Patients with enteral continuity and increasing oral intake often suffer from rapid transit due to inadequate length for absorption and bowel maladaptation resulting in diarrhea and malnutrition. The initial management should target conservative therapies such as medication and diet modification. Given that surgical therapy for short bowel syndrome is pursued infrequently, patients should be referred to tertiary centers with extensive experience managing these challenging cases.

Radiation Enteritis

Intra-abdominal radiation injury from neoadjuvant or adjuvant oncologic therapy can lead to many challenging problems in the perioperative period. Radiation damages mitotically active cells of the mucosal surface epithelium, leading to cellular injury, and causes production of oxygen free radicals, which further damage cellular function. The incidence of injury is dependent on such factors as volume of irradiated small bowel, total dose and time dose delivered, and type of radiation being delivered (56). Radiation-induced cellular injury results in obliterative arteritis with subsequent bowel ischemia. Acute radiation–associated injury results in transient mucosal atrophy, submucosal edema, and inflammation and infiltration of the lamina propria with leukocytes and plasma cells. The chronic ischemia and inflammation in the affected bowel segment may result in stricture formation, perforation, or fistula formation. Radiation exposure also results in the formation of dense local adhesions. Of patients undergoing abdominal and pelvic radiation, 50% to 75% will have some symptoms related to the therapy in the months to years following treatment; these include, commonly, vague abdominal pain, diarrhea, rectal bleeding, and tenesmus. Up to 15% of patient's symptoms will progress to actual radiation enteritis. Symptoms may occur acutely during therapy or years after treatment. Management of late radiation enteritis should include investigation of recurrence of the initial neoplasm (57,58).

Initial management of radiation enteritis should embrace conservative measures. Sitz baths and stool softeners are effective initial treatments for rectal and anal symptoms. Opiates, antispasmodics, and anticholinergics will prolong transit time if diarrhea is the primary problem. Steroid enemas and sucralfate can diminish irritation of the mucosa, which results in rectal pain and bleeding. If the patient is malnourished, nutritional support may be required, especially if operative intervention is entertained.

Surgical Management of Radiation Enteritis. Perioperative management of radiation enteritis involves both prevention and therapy. If radiation is planned as an adjuvant therapy following surgery, intraoperative goals are to minimize radiation injury. Simple nonsurgical methods to diminish radiation injury include patient positioning, multiple-field techniques, and bladder distention (56). Following pelvic surgery, intraoperative management is aimed to decrease the volume of small bowel included in the radiation field postoperatively. Techniques include reperitonealizing the operative field, the use of a mesh sling for exclusion of small bowel from the pelvis, and using omentum to exclude the pelvis. Small bowel displacement systems have had some success in physically excluding up to 50% of small bowel volume from the radiation field (57).

Surgical intervention is sometimes required in the management of complications related to radiation enteritis. The most common indication for surgery is bowel obstruction, but other indications include bleeding, intractable diarrhea, pain, fistulas, and persistent abscess. Surgical intervention should use the least invasive procedure required to address the problem as excessive handling of radiated tissues and lysis of adhesions commonly results in unplanned enterotomies and may interrupt a tenuous blood supply. Recurrent neoplasm is not uncommon and any suspicious-appearing areas should be biopsied. Diseased segments of bowel should be removed and repaired with an anastomosis in nonradiated bowel. A gastrointestinal bypass may be required if diseased segments of bowel cannot be safely resected (58).

SUMMARY

Acute intra-abdominal pathology is commonly seen in critically ill patients. As such physicians must maintain a high level of suspicion of an abdominal problem in a deteriorating patient. History and physical examination are used to guide further laboratory and diagnostic imaging tests, and surgical consultation should be obtained early in a patient's course, as treatment frequently requires surgical intervention.

Early goal-directed fluid resuscitation, antibiotic administration, and source control should be the priority for the health care team. Perioperative management of even the most routine abdominal surgery has the potential to be difficult. When the anticipated progress of a postoperative patient deviates from the expected, a high index of suspicion is important for rapid diagnosis and treatment. Careful evaluation of the patient's operative details, postoperative course, and clinical evaluation will dictate appropriate management. Interventions may vary from the addition of antibiotics to percutaneous drainage of an abscess to surgical re-exploration. The critical care surgeon must be adept in a multitude of complex postoperative issues to provide appropriate therapy.

Key Points

- Patients presenting with abdominal pain, fever, evidence of multi-organ failure, unexplained acidosis, or jaundice should be evaluated for an intra-abdominal source of infection.
- Early goal-directed resuscitation, antibiotic administration, and source control is required for patients with acute abdominal problems.
- Common postoperative abdominal problems include abscess, leak from anastomoses or perforated bowel, acalculous cholecystitis, and ileus.
- Abdominal distension in combination with organ dysfunction suggests evaluation of abdominal compartment pressures and surgical consult.
- Routes to provide enteral feedings should be considered at the time of surgery for patients in whom oral intake is not anticipated for some time.
- All tubes and drains must be labeled secured to minimize inadvertent dislodgement. Loss of carefully placed tubes and drains can lead to significant morbidity.
- Carefully assess the patient's general condition before entering a hostile abdomen. Cardiovascular and pulmonary status, nutritional support, blood sugar control, and coagulation profile should be optimized if possible.

References

1. Brewer RJ, Golden GT, Hitch DD, et al. Abdominal pain: an analysis of 1,000 consecutive cases in a university hospital emergency room. *Am J Surg*. 1976;131:219.
2. Weaver DW, Busuito MJ, Bouwman DL, et al. Interpretation of serum amylase levels in the critically ill patient. *Crit Care Med*. 1985;13:532.
3. Deveney CW, Lurie K, Deveny KE. Improved treatment of intra-abdominal abscess. *Arch Surg*. 1988;123:1126.
4. Solomkin JS, Mazuski JE, Bradley JS, et al. Diagnosis and management of complicated intra-abdominal infection in adults and children: guidelines by the Surgical Infection Society and the Infectious Diseases Society of America. *Clin Infect Dis*. 2010;50(2):133.
5. Levison MA. Percutaneous versus open operative drainage of intra-abdominal abscesses. *Infect Dis Clin N Am*. 1992;6:25.
6. Wright HK, Dunn E, MacArthur JD, et al. Specific but limited role of new imaging techniques in decision-making intra-abdominal abscesses. *Am J Surg*. 1982;143:456.
7. Montgomery RS, Wilson SE. Intra-abdominal abscesses: image-guided diagnosis and therapy. *Clin Infect Dis*. 1996;23:8.
8. Sahai A, Belair M, Fianfelice D, et al. Percutaneous drainage of intra-abdominal abscesses in Crohn's disease: short and long term outcome. *Am J Gastroenterol*. 1997;92:75.
9. Dellinger EP, Wertz MJ, Meakins JL, et al. Surgical infection stratification system for intra-abdominal infection: multicenter trial. *Arch Surg*. 1985:120:21.
10. Macklin MT, Macklin CC. Malignant interstitial emphysema of the lungs and mediastinum as an important occult complication in many respiratory diseases and other conditions: an interpretation of the clinical literature in the light of laboratory experiment. *Medicine*. 1944;23:281.
11. Long TN, Heimbach DM, Carrico CJ. Acalculous cholecystitis in critically ill patients. *Am J Surg*. 1978;136:31.
12. Savino JA, Scalea TM, Del Guercio LR. Factors encouraging laparotomy in acalculous cholecystitis. *Crit Care Med*. 1985;13:377.
13. Petersen SR, Sheldon GF. Acute acalculous cholecystitis: a complications of hyperalimentation. *Am J Surg*. 1979;138:814.
14. Longmaid HE, Bassett JG, Gottlieb H. Management of gallbladder perforation by percutaneous cholecystostomy. *Crit Care Med*. 1985;13:686.
15. Ogilvie H. Large intestine colic due to sympathetic deprivation: a new clinical syndrome. *Br J Med*. 1948;2:671.
16. Jetmore AB, Timmcke AE, Gathright JB, et al. Ogilvie's syndrome: colonoscopic decompression and analysis of predisposing factors. *Dis Colon Rectum*. 1992;35:1135.

17. Ponec RJ, Saunders MD, Kimmey MB. Neostigmine for the treatment of acute colonic pseudo-obstruction. *N Engl J Med.* 1999;341:137.
18. Edwards MS, Cherr GS, Craven TE, et al. Acute occlusive mesenteric ischemia: surgical management and outcomes. *Ann Vasc Surg.* 2003;17:72.
19. Birnabaum W, Rudy L, Wylie EJ. Colonic and rectal ischemia following abdominal aneurysmectomy. *Dis Colon Rectum.* 1964;7:293.
20. Stoney RJ, Cunningham CG. Acute mesenteric ischemia. *Surgery.* 1993; 114:489.
21. Safioleas MC, Moulakakis KG, Papavassiliou VG, et al. Acute mesenteric ischaemia, a highly lethal disease with a devastating outcome. *Vasa.* 2003;35:106.
22. Endean ED, Barnes SL, Kwolek CJ, et al. Surgical management of thrombotic acute intestinal ischemia. *Ann Surg.* 2001;233:801.
23. Edwards MS, Cherr GS, Craven TE, et al. Acute occlusive mesenteric ischemia: surgical management and outcomes. *Ann Vasc Surg.* 2003;17:72.
24. Boley SJ, Brandt LJ, Veith FJ. Ischemic disorders of the intestine. *Curr Probl Surg.* 1978;15:1.
25. Kaminsky O, Yampolski I, Aranovich D, et al. Does a second-look operation improve survival in patients with peritonitis due to acute mesenteric ischemia? A five-year retrospective experience. *World J Sur.* 2005;29:645.
26. Ottinger LW. The surgical management of acute occlusion of the superior mesenteric artery. *Ann Surg.* 1978;188:721.
27. Nishida A, Fukui K. Transcatheter treatment of thromboembolism in the superior mesenteric artery. *N Engl J Med.* 2005;353:4.
28. Fazio VW, Cohen Z, Fleshman JW, et al. Reduction in adhesive small-bowel obstruction by seprafilm adhesion barrier after resection. *Dis Colon Rectum.* 2006;49(1):1–11.
29. Cameron JL, ed. *Current Surgical Therapy.* 7th ed. St. Louis, MO: Mosby; 2001.
30. Johns A. Evidence based prevention of postoperative adhesions. *Hum Reprod Update.* 2001;7(6):577–579.
31. Owen RM, Love TP, Perez SD, et al. Definitive surgical treatment of enterocutaneous fistula: outcomes of a 23-year experience. *AMA Surg.* 2013;148(2):118–126.
32. Memon AS, Siddiqui FG. Causes and management of postoperative enterocutaneous fistulas. *J Coll Physicians Surg Pak.* 2004;14(1):25–28.
33. Maconi G, Parente F, Porro GB. Hydrogen peroxide enhanced ultrasound-fistulography in the assessment of enterocutaneous fistulas complicating Crohn's disease. *Gut.* 1999;45(6):874–878.
34. Gray M, Jacobson T. Are somatostatin analogues (octreotide and lanreotide) effective in promoting healing of enterocutaneous fistulas? *J Wound Ostomy Contin Nurs.* 2002;29(5):228–233.
35. Li J, Ren J, Zhu W, et al. Management of enterocutaneous fistulas: 30-year clinical experience. *Chinese Med J.* 2003;116(2):171–175.
36. Draus JM Jr, Huss SA, Harty NJ, et al. Enterocutaneous fistula: are treatments improving? *Surgery.* 2006;140(4):570–578.
37. Bassi C, Dervenis C, Butturini G, et al. Postoperative pancreatic fistula: an international study group (ISGPF) definition. *Surgery.* 2005;138:8–13.
38. Pannegeon V, Pessaux P, Sauvanet A, et al. Pancreatic fistula after distal pancreatectomy: predictive risk factors and value of conservative treatment. *Arch Surg.* 2006;141(11):1071–1076.
39. Kaman L, Behera A, Singh R, et al. Internal pancreatic fistulas with pancreatic ascites and pancreatic pleural effusions: recognition and management. *ANZ J Surg.* 2001;71(4):221–225.
40. Kron IL, Harman PK, Nolan S. The measurement of intra-abdominal pressure as a criterion for abdominal reexploration. *Ann Surg.* 1984; 199(1):28–30.
41. Maxwell RA, Fabian TC, Croce MA, et al. Secondary abdominal compartment syndrome: an underappreciated manifestation of severe hemorrhagic shock. *J Trauma.* 1999;47(6):995.
42. Crandall M, West MA. Evaluation of the abdomen in the critically ill patient: opening the black box. *Curr Opin Crit Care.* 2006;12(4):333–339.
43. Ivatury RR. Abdominal compartment syndrome: a century later, isn't it time to accept and promulgate? *Crit Care Med.* 2006;34(9):2494.
44. DeWaele JJH, Malbrain EA, Lng M. Decompressive laparotomy for abdominal compartment syndrome—a critical analysis. *Crit Care.* 2006;10(2):R51.
45. Stone HH, Strom PR, Mullins RJ. Management of the major coagulopathy with onset during laparotomy. *Ann Surg.* 1983;197:532–535.
46. Rotondo M, Schwab CW, McGonigal MD, et al. Damage control: an approach for improved survival in exsanguinating penetrating abdominal injury. *J Trauma.* 1993;35:375–383.
47. ten Raa S, van den Tol MP, Sluiter M, et al. The role of neutrophils and oxygen free radicals in postoperative adhesions. *J Surg Res.* 2006;136(1):45–52.
48. Stone PA, Hass SM, Flaherty SK, et al. Vacuum-assisted fascial closure for patients with abdominal trauma. *J Trauma.* 2004;57(5):1082–1086.
49. James C, Stawicki SP, Hoff WS, et al. A proposed algorithm for managing the open abdomen. *Am Surg.* 2005;71(3):202–207.
50. Jernigan TW, Fabian TC, Croce MA, et al. Staged management of giant abdominal wall defects: acute and long-term results. *Ann Surg.* 2003;238(3): 349–357.
51. Fabian TC. Damage control in trauma: laparotomy wound management acute to chronic. *Surg Clin North Am.* 2007;87:73–93.
52. Ramirez OM1, Ruas E, Dellon AL. "Components separation" method for closure of abdominal-wall defects: an anatomic and clinical study. *Plast Reconstr Surg.* 1990;86(3):519–526.
53. DiCocco JM, Fabian TC, Emmett KP, et al. Components separation for abdominal wall reconstruction: the Memphis modification. *Surgery.* 2012;151(1):118–125.
54. DiBaise JK, Matarese LE, Messing B, et al. Strategies for parenteral nutrition weaning in adult patients with short bowel syndrome. *J Clin Gastroenterol.* 2006;40(Suppl 2):S94–S98.
55. Nightingale J, Woodward JM. Guidelines for management of patients with a short bowel. *Gut.* 2006;55(Suppl 4):1–12.
56. Thompson JS. Surgical aspects of the short bowel syndrome. *Am J Surg.* 1995;170(6):532–536.
57. Park W, Huh SJ, Lee JE, et al. Variation of small bowel sparing with small bowel displacement system according to the physiological status of the bladder during radiotherapy for cervical cancer. *Gynecol Oncol.* 2005;99(3):645–651.
58. Onodera H, Nagayama S, Mori A, et al. Reappraisal of surgical treatment for radiation enteritis. *World J Surg.* 2005;29(4):459–463.

CHAPTER

59

Critical Care Implications in Acute Care Surgery

STEPHANIE N. LUECKEL and KIMBERLY A. DAVIS

INTRODUCTION

As many things in medicine, the evolution and development of acute care surgery was born out of necessity and innovation. Over the past two decades, it has been recognized that there have been an insufficient number of physicians participating in emergency call panels (1). In 2005, nearly half of all hospital emergency departments reported that they were routinely at or beyond capacity resulting in ambulance diversion (2). The Institute of Medicine highlighted this crisis in a report entitled "Hospital Based Emergency Care at the Breaking Point" (3).

Compounding this crisis in access to emergency care is a growing workforce shortage of general surgeons. The American Association of Medical Colleges estimates that a 35% increase in the number of surgeons will be necessary to meet clinical demands by 2025 (4). An aging surgical workforce and increasing surgical subspecialization driven in part by technologic advances have compounded these shortages (3). As a result, there are fewer general surgeons available to take emergency department call, and to care for patients with time-sensitive general surgical conditions. A survey conducted by the American College of Emergency Physicians in 2005 demonstrated that nearly 75% of emergency department medical directors believed that they had inadequate on-call surgical specialist coverage, up from 66% in 2005 (5).

Just as the needs of the injured patient drove the development of the field of trauma surgery, so did the needs of the emergency general surgery patient drive the development of the acute care surgery paradigm (6). The Acute Care Surgery (ACS) training paradigm was developed by the leadership of the American Association for the Surgery of Trauma (AAST) to meet patients' needs. This specialty enhances the training of young surgeons in the areas of trauma, surgical critical care, and time-sensitive general surgery. This chapter will describe the crises that exist in general surgery, explain how an acute care surgery model might address these crises, define the curriculum for the training of an acute care surgeon, and discuss how this model has affected the delivery of emergency surgical care and the training of future physicians so far.

GENERAL SURGERY WORKFORCE SHORTAGES

Over 50 years ago, there were concerns about physician shortage, prompting a deliberate expansion of medical school enrollment and eventual increase in the physician workforce (7). In 1991, Congress authorized an evaluation of the surgical workforce. This report predicted a 15% shortage of general surgeons, citing considerable workload increases in both inpatient and outpatient procedures by the year 2010, predominantly due to the growing geriatric population (8). In 2008, the Association of American Medical Colleges (AAMC) reported on supply and demand discrepancies existing in the US health care work force and predicted a shortage of almost 160,000 physicians (Fig. 59.1) (9). In response, available medical school positions were increased by 30% as were the number of graduate medical education (GME) positions. However, these changes were not expected to solve the supply problem but rather diminish it. It is anticipated that the shortage will increase steeply over time with the growing and aging population.

Although workforce shortages exist across a range of medical disciplines, they are generally more significant for surgical disciplines. While the workforce in nonsurgical specialties has grown steadily over time, the number of surgeons trained in our nation's GME system has remained stable for more than 20 years (Fig. 59.2). The rate of growth of the US population has outpaced the supply of general surgeons. Over the 25-year period between 1981 and 2006, the US population grew 31%, while the number of general surgeons grew by 4% (9). The American Association of Medical Colleges estimates that a 35% increase in the number of surgeons will be necessary to meet clinical demands by 2025 (Fig. 59.3). An aging surgical workforce is compounded these shortages (1). As of 2012, 43% of general surgeons were aged 55 or older, compared to only 36% of internal medicine physicians (9). Changes in the field of surgery, particularly those regarding reimbursement, may make early retirement more attractive. Mid-career surgeons indicate that the most important factor in choosing to retire early, restrict practice, and/or change career has been an unfavorable work environment (7). This unfavorable environment has been fostered primarily by the commoditization of medicine, which includes decreased reimbursement, managed care with its ever-changing rules, and the lack of professional liability reform (10). The increased out-migration of surgeons from the field is exacerbating workforce shortages.

Further impairing workforce shortages are the increased subspecialization of surgeons after completing a general surgery residency, driven in part by technologic advances. General surgery has been seen as too rigorous with little time devoted to other interests. The advent of the resident 80-hour work week in 2003 has alleviated some of the concern regarding lifestyle but the discrepancies in those choosing general surgery continues. Almost 80% of general surgery residents finishing from Accreditation Council for Graduate Medical Education (ACGME)–approved programs pursue fellowships and become specialists (10). A study by Yeo et al. (11) reported survey results on resident opinion regarding surgical resident training. Over 4,402 residents, in 248 of the 249 surgical residency programs, participated in the survey, representing 82%

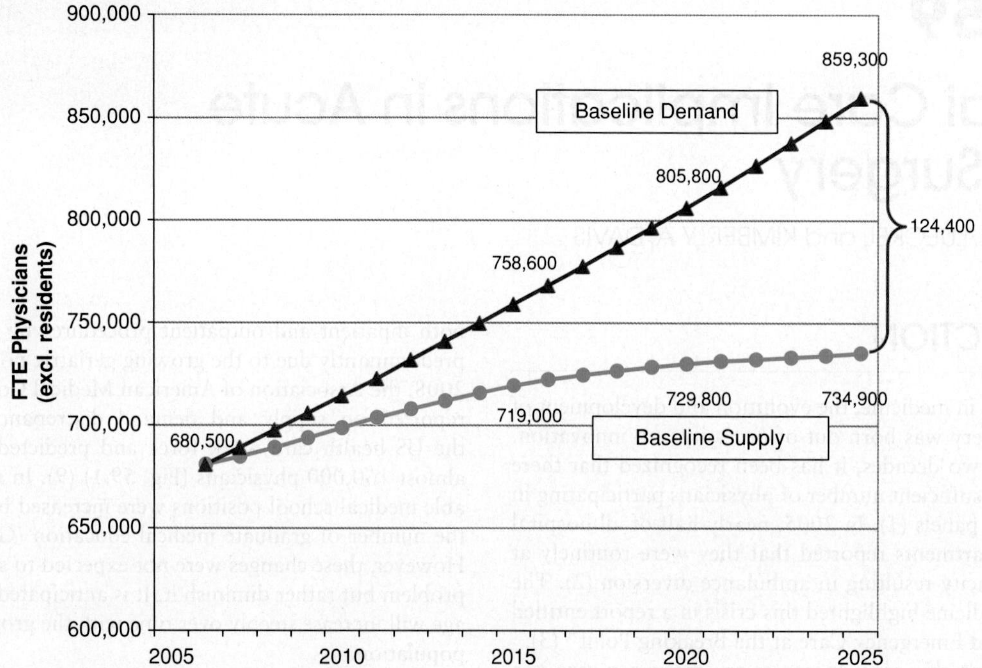

FIGURE 59.1 Baseline physician FTE supply and demand projections, 2006–2025. (From Center for Workforce Studies. *The Complexities of Physician Supply and Demand: Projections Through 2025.* Available at: https://members.aamc.org/eweb/upload/The%20Complexities%20of%20Physician%20Supply.pdf. Accessed August 12, 2015.)

of all categorical residents at the time. The findings demonstrated that residents believed fellowship training to be necessary in order for them to be successful, competitive, and to have a better lifestyle and income (Fig. 59.4). With an average debt from medical school of $175,000 and an accruing interest due to forbearance or deferment, residents cater their future endeavors to best fit an imagined lifestyle as well as pay off college and medical school debt (12).

Though the majority of residents choose to further specialize with fellowship training, they have not traditionally chosen to specialize in trauma and/or surgical critical care. Reasons behind this are complex and include the additional time commitment, nonoperative nature of a trauma surgery practice, a perception of a higher percentage of unfunded and underfunded patients, payment for effort/services that rely more heavily on evaluation and management coding and less on

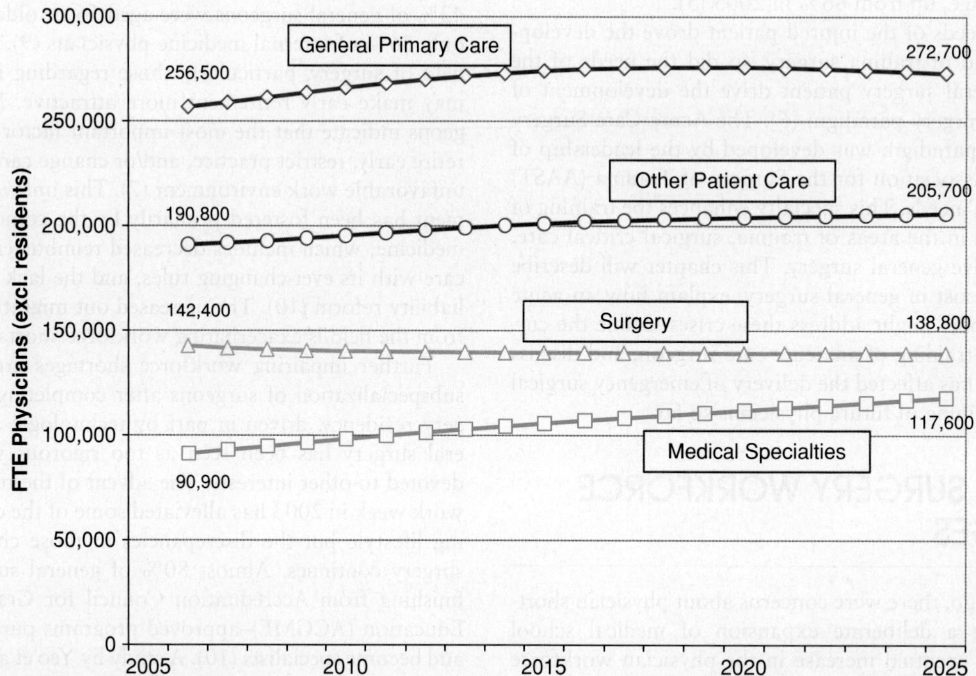

FIGURE 59.2 Projections of physicians by specialty group. (From Center for Workforce Studies. *The Complexities of Physician Supply and Demand: Projections Through 2025.* Available at: https://members.aamc.org/eweb/upload/The%20Complexities%20of%20Physician%20Supply.pdf. Accessed August 12, 2015.)

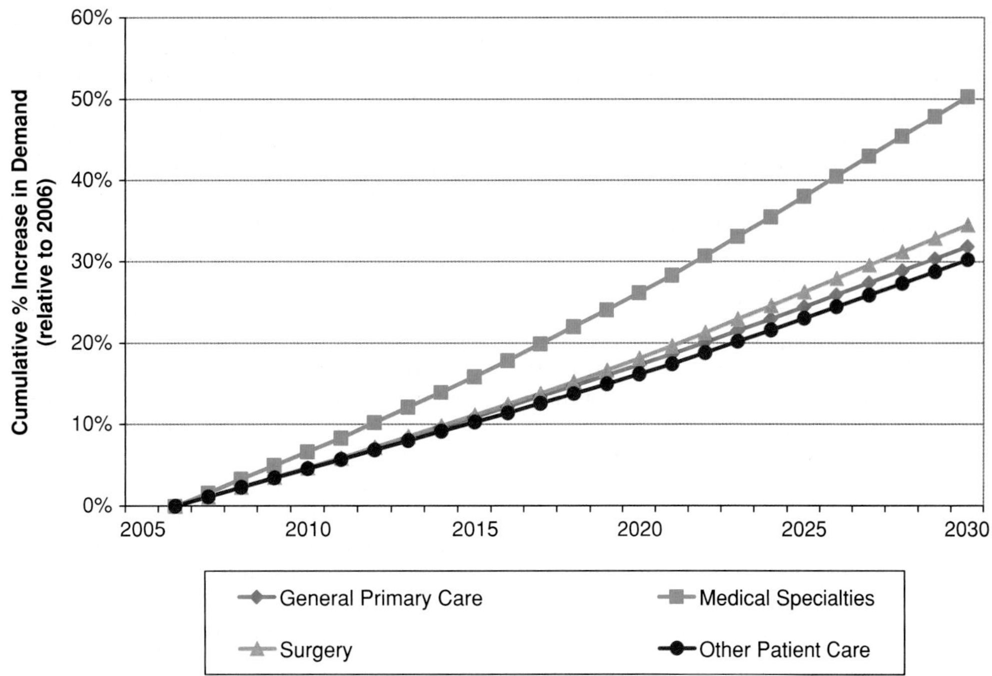

FIGURE 59.3 Cumulative percent growth in demand by specialty group. (From Center for Workforce Studies. *The Complexities of Physician Supply and Demand: Projections Through 2025.* Available at: https://members.aamc.org/eweb/upload/The%20Complexities%20of%20Physician%20Supply.pdf. Accessed August 12, 2015.)

procedure-based coding, and a possible interference with elective operative schedule given the unscheduled nature of critical illness. More specifically, surgical residents' opinion of trauma surgery is double-sided. Residents describe trauma surgery as clinically rewarding and recognize its importance but also recognize the nonoperative nature, high levels of stress and long hours without expected financial compensation (11). Additionally, trauma surgeons are viewed as being dissatisfied, a perception that resulted in 44% of the Surgical Critical Care fellowship positions going unfilled in 2011 (2). As a result, there are fewer general surgeons and even less trauma surgeons. With this, there are fewer persons available to take emergency department call and care for patients with time-sensitive general surgical conditions.

EMERGENCY SURGICAL CARE AT THE BREAKING POINT

The provision of care to critically ill and injured patients challenges not only health care providers and medical centers, but is straining the health care system nationwide (13,14). According

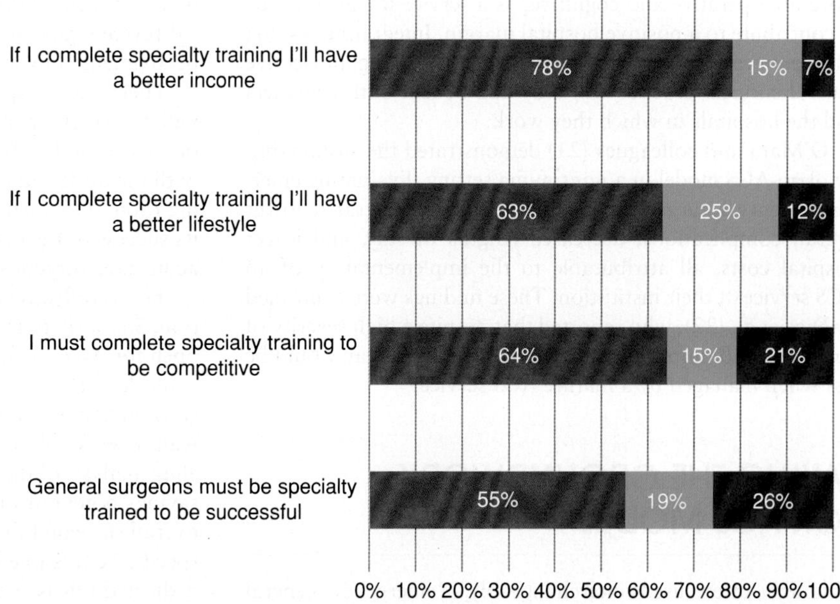

FIGURE 59.4 Survey results on resident opinion regarding surgical resident training. (From Yeo H, Bucholz E, Ann Sosa J, et al. A national study of attrition in general surgery training: which residents leave and where do they go? *Ann Surg.* 2010;252(3):529–534; Davis KA. EAST 2015 Presidential address: look both ways. *J Trauma Acute Care Surg.* 2015;79:1–9.)

to the National Center for Health Statistics, 36 million people or 11.5% of the population had no health insurance in 2014 (15). From 1993 to 2013, there has been an increase of approximately 44% in the number of patients receiving care in emergency rooms across the country, while the number of emergency departments decreased by 558 (16). Nearly half of all hospital emergency departments reported that they were at or beyond capacity in 2005, resulting in ambulance diversion (5). This problem is more severe for major teaching institutions, with 79% of their emergency rooms at or exceeding capacity (17). The nation's emergency medical system as a whole is overburdened, underfunded, and highly fragmented. As result, ambulances are turned away from emergency departments once every minute on average and patients in many areas may wait hours or even days for a hospital bed (2).

Concurrently, the trend in patient care has shifted to the outpatient setting whenever possible in an effort to reduce costs. Consequently, hospitals have noted an increased acuity of inpatients, while simultaneously dealing with the demands for improved clinical efficiency and quality improvement. Operating rooms (ORs) are run at maximal efficiency with little slack in the system. Surgeons are increasingly pressured to maximize their productivity as a method of maintaining reimbursement (18). Almost all of surgical specialties contribute positively to the hospital margin, and therefore to the hospital's overall financial stability (19). Therefore, it is in the hospital's financial benefit to support surgical activity and utilize a model that will increase that activity such as an ACS model. Davis et al. (20) compared the hospital contribution margin over two time frames, before and after the implementation a practice paradigm where all trauma patients were admitted to an ACS team for at least 24 hours. With more trauma team oversight, there was a 10% increase in charges between the two time periods and the overall contribution model became positive were it had previously been negative. Additionally, collections and revenues markedly increased with trauma team oversight and a focus on billing capture. These financial benefits, both to physicians and to hospitals, are further support for the ACS model. Despite the fact that trauma has become more nonoperative and cognitive, as a service it can continue to contribute to a positive hospital margin. Integrating trauma into acute care surgery and perhaps incorporating an elective general surgical practice will only add benefit both providers and the hospitals in which they work.

O'Mara and colleagues (21) demonstrated the sustainability of an ACS model in a nontrauma setting. Evaluating emergency general surgery cases only, they demonstrated lower overall complications, decreased lengths of stay, and lower hospital costs, all attributable to the implementation of an ACS service at their institution. These findings were confirmed by Diaz et al. (22), who reported that despite a high severity of illness, overall mortality and hospital lengths of stay would be less when managed by a mature ACS service.

LAYING THE GROUNDWORK FOR ACS MODEL

Although often used interchangeably, "emergency general surgery" and "acute care surgery" have different meanings. Whereas *emergency general surgery* refers to acute general surgical disorders, *acute care surgery* includes surgical critical care and the surgical management of acutely ill patients with a variety of conditions including trauma, burns, surgical critical care, or an acute general surgical condition. The challenges in caring for these patients include around-the-clock readiness for the provision of comprehensive care, the often constrained time for preoperative optimization of the patient, and the greater potential for intraoperative and postoperative complications due to the emergent nature of care. In managing these patients, acute care surgeons are fulfilling a huge patient care demand as the number of patients with acute surgical disorders is on the rise (2). Doubling as surgical intensivists, acute care surgeons provide not only a much needed service but a continuity of care, both operating on the acute surgical disorder as well as caring for the critically ill postoperatively, that is not matched in any other field.

The unscheduled nature of critical illness and injury, combined with the significant resources required to treat these diseases, continues to challenge health care providers and medical centers. The introduction of operative emergencies is inherently inefficient and disruptive to the smooth running of an OR schedule thereby adding stress to an already strained system, and increasing frustration of the surgeons and the staff. Additionally, the off-hours nature of most surgical emergencies requires that very costly resources be available 24 hours a day, regardless of utilization (23).

Sweeting et al. (24) evaluated at the change in relative value units (RVUs) before and after the implementation of an ACS program. This article compared an ACS program to the preexisting elective surgery model. They showed that operative volume increased by 25% but it tended to be smaller cases with less RVUs per case (colectomy vs. incision and drainage of an abscess, for example). With this, overall RVUs were only up 21%. Additionally, the ACS division showed an increased percentage of uncompensated care relative to the department of surgery as a whole. There was also an increased write-off to bad debt and a worse net reimbursement as compared to the pre-ACS model. The authors calculated that the loss of clinical income due to lower RVU procedures and a declining payer mix meant that salaries could not be supported solely on clinical revenue generation and that fixed support would need to be augmented by about 28% to remain revenue neutral.

Therefore, hospital-based financial support and resources will be necessary in order to implement and maintain a rigorous ACS model. Wanis et al. (25) showed a positive impact with the initiation of an ACS model (decreased time to operating room (OR), length of stay); however, they attribute part of its success to the dedicated OR that was available daily to the acute care surgeons. Having this dedicated room contributed to the overall success of the model as well as surgeon satisfaction. Similarly to the trauma model, leaving an OR completely open for ACS means that room does not generate revenue and could lead to other case delays. However, Anantha et al. (26) showed that allocating an OR to the ACS service did not affect wait times for elective cancer surgeries. Additionally, cost modeling analysis of the ACS model, with a dedicated OR, has cost savings potential for the health care system without reducing overall surgeon billing (27). Having dedicated surgeons to this specific field is one hurdle, however, baseline resources, like a dedicated OR is critical.

ACS services must be staffed in such a way to assure continuity of patient. A cohesive group of surgeons dedicated to the service will assure accurate handoffs and consistency in patient throughput. There are various ways to implement the ACS model. Given the tripartite missions of acute care surgery, surgeons are often dedicated to either the ICU or a "floor" service, comprising either trauma, emergency general surgery, or some combination thereof. In busier institutions, elective cases are generally reserved for weeks when the ACS surgeon is "off-service," depending on their average volume of emergency and urgent surgery. Some models may incorporate non-ACS surgeons so as to spread the call-out over a larger number of surgeons. This model is attractive to those surgeons who are interested in maintaining their "acute" surgical skills, as well as those who wish to augment their elective practice volumes with emergency room referrals.

Infancy of ACS Fellowship Training

In the early years of the 21st century, the leadership at the AAST responded to the crisis in access to emergency surgeons with the foundation for the training of surgeons in acute care surgery. The paradigm for ACS capitalized on the already existing training of trauma critical care surgeons while also enhancing their operative experience. Although the field of trauma surgery has become increasingly nonoperative over the last two decades, trauma surgeons remain among the few who can operate in multiple anatomic regions as well as care for the most critically ill patients. In 2008, the first AAST-approved ACS fellowship started. Since this time, there have been constant evaluations as to how to implement and improve the program (Table 59.1).

The core components of ACS are trauma, surgical critical care, and emergency general surgery with the training designed to create a versatile surgeon able to confront a host of acute surgical disease processes. The suggested curriculum includes focusing on clinical experience but also operative expectations of a trainee in an accredited program. An initial list of "essential and desirable" cases was created, which focused on a broad range of predominantly trauma case types divided into anatomic regions. This design attempts to ensure that a fully trained acute care surgeon is comfortable with a wide variety of anatomic exposures across all body regions (28).

The first draft of the curriculum dictated mandatory components while also allowing some flexibility for the fellows in terms of rotations. With some creativity, programs could capitalize on not only the individual's strengths but address the weaknesses as well. Rotations in thoracic surgery, transplant/hepatobiliary/pancreatic, and vascular were encouraged but not required by the curriculum (28). The goal of the ACS fellowship was to master complex operative procedures in addition to completing an ACGME-approved Surgical Critical Care fellowship. The original fellowship program was approved in 2008. Since then, 20 additional programs have been approved by the AAST. Similar to general surgery residency, a case log system (Infotech, San Diego, CA) was created and used to track the operative experience of the fellows. So far, 59 fellows have graduated from AAST-approved ACS fellowships (Table 59.2).

The case log data were used to determine if the fellows were receiving the intended operative experience. Dente et al. (28) reviewed the initial year of case log data and showed that the ACS fellows were averaging over 200 cases during their fellowship. There was a high variability in the case mix, with approximately 50% of fellows not meeting the goals laid out in the initial curriculum. Duane et al. (29) confirmed these findings when looking at a case log spanning 2 years. Overall, these two studies concluded that the ACS trainees lacked adequate exposure to head/neck surgery, thoracic, and vascular surgery as defined by the ACS curriculum. In order to adjust for this, the authors suggested including elective surgeries that might provide for similar exposures or organ-based management. The incorporation of urgent and elective cases into the experience would allow the fellow to learn the appropriate

TABLE 59.1 Historical Timeline of the AAST Acute Care Surgery Fellowship Development

Date	Advance
2003	Joint meeting of ACS, AAST, WEST, and EAST addressing problems of access to emergency surgical care and the future of trauma surgery. AAST forms ad hoc committee to develop the reorganized specialty of trauma, surgical critical care, and emergency surgery.
2005	ACEP surveys nearly 75% emergency departments identify inadequate on-call specialty coverage. AAST renames previous ad hoc committee the Acute Care Surgery Committee.
2006	IOM report: Future of Emergency Care confirms shortage of on call specialists
2007	Development of curriculum, competency tools, case registry, certification criteria, site visits during an AAST retreat
July 2008	First formal AAST Acute Care Surgery Fellowship program begins.
2014	Refinement of operative case requirements

ACS, American College of Surgeons; AAST, American Association for the Surgery of Trauma; WEST, Western Trauma Association; EAST, Eastern Association for the Surgery of Trauma.

Adapted from Historical timeline. TraumaSource. American Association for the Surgery of Trauma website. http://www.aast.org/AcuteCareSurgery.aspx. Accessed August 12, 2015.

TABLE 59.2 Approved AAST ACS Fellowship Training Programs

University of Arizona, Tucson, Arizona
University of California, San Francisco–Fresno, Fresno, California
University of Colorado School of Medicine, Denver, Colorado
Hartford Hospital/University of Connecticut, Hartford, Connecticut
Yale University, New Haven, Connecticut
University of Florida-Gainesville, Gainesville, Florida
Orlando Regional Medical Center, Orlando, Florida
Emory University Medical School, Atlanta, Georgia
Indiana University Medical School, Indianapolis, Indiana
University of Maryland/R. Adams Cowley Shock Trauma Center, Baltimore, Maryland
Massachusetts General Hospital, Boston, Massachusetts
Baystate Medical Center, Springfield, Massachusetts
University of Nevada School of Medicine, Las Vegas, Nevada
UMDNJ–Robert Wood Johnson Medical School, New Brunswick, New Jersey
East Carolina University/Viadent Medical Center, Greenville, North Carolina
Wake Forest Baptist Medical Center, Winston-Salem, North Carolina
Wright State University, Dayton, Ohio
University of Pittsburgh Medical Center, Pittsburgh, Pennsylvania
Vanderbilt Univeristy, Nashville, Tennessee
University of Texas Health Science Center, Houston, Texas

Adapted from Approved sites. TraumaSource. American Association for the Surgery of Trauma website. http://www.aast.org/AcuteCareSurgery.aspx. Accessed August 12, 2015.

exposure and handling of anatomy via a more elective procedure in the same anatomic region.

Next Generation of ACS Fellowship Training

In light of the aforementioned concerns regarding case volumes, the operative curriculum for the ACS fellowship was restructured. Suggested elective rotations were identified as required for the ACS fellows (Table 59.3). Curricular changes included the identification of a minimum number of operative cases needed in specific body regions, in a manner similar to defined case volumes in general surgery. The desired case volume provides guidance to the fellows, program directors, and subspecialty colleagues as to the types of cases deemed important for the fellows' training (30). In an effort to distinguish the surgical training in the fellowship from that obtained in surgical residency, metrics regarding patient comorbidity as defined by the AAST emergency general surgery disease grading scales (31) and the technical difficulty of the operative case were added to the case log system. These changes were implemented in 2015.

The AAST and ACS fellowships will continue to build on the strong foundation of process and structure that already exists. Future plans include the creation of a comprehensive core curriculum that would potentially offer state-of-the-art media dedicated to complex surgical exposures, and technical tricks needed when doing complex operative procedures on patients who, due to severity of illness, do not have the luxury of preoperative optimization. A second priority for ACS training will remain the development and maturation of a secure end-of-fellowship examination, with psychometrics to demonstrate that we are testing what we are training. Finally, the acute care surgery community needs to arrive at several research questions that we wish to answer regarding not only the training of acute care surgeons, but also about the value delivered by our specialty to our patients and the medical community at large (32).

TABLE 59.3 Required and Elective Clinical Rotations for the AAST ACS Fellowship

Required Clinical Rotation	Length
Surgical critical care including:	
• Trauma/surgical critical care, including other relevant critical care rotations	12 mo
• This portion of the fellowship must comply with ACGME requirements for a surgical critical care residency	
Emergency and elective surgery, including:	12 mo
• Trauma/emergency surgery	2–3 mo
• Thoracic	1–2 mo
• Transplant/hepatobiliary/pancreatic	1–2 mo
• Vascular/interventional radiology	1–2 mo
Total	24 mo
Suggested Clinical Rotations	**Length**
Orthopedic surgery	1 mo
Neurologic surgery	1 mo
Electives:	1–3 mo
• Recommended: burn surgery and pediatric surgery	
• Also include endoscopy, imaging, plastic surgery, etc.	

Adapted from Curriculum. TraumaSource. American Association for the Surgery of Trauma website. http://www.aast.org/AcuteCareSurgery.aspx. Accessed August 12, 2015.

The goals of training ACS surgeons would be to demonstrate mastery in the field of acute care surgery, above and beyond that learned in a general surgery residency. Those trained in the ACS fellowships are eligible for board certification in surgical critical care through the American Board of Surgery. Added certification in acute care surgery is currently offered through the AAST. Currently, there are 20 approved acute care surgery programs. Unlike most specialty training, this paradigm strives to create a broad-based surgical specialist, specifically trained in the treatment of acute surgical disease across as a wide array of anatomic regions (30).

Impact of ACS Fellowships

As with the addition of any surgical fellowship, there is always a concern for how the current general surgery residents will be impacted. Dinan et al. (33) sought to determine if the addition of an ACS fellow negatively impacted the training of the current general surgery residents, comparing case volume among the general surgery residents before and after the initiation of the AAST-approved ACS fellowship at a Level I trauma center. The study examined ACGME case log data, both before and after the initiation of the ACS fellowship and found that there was no significant change in the number of cases performed by the chief residents. Furthermore, residents were queried about the added value of the ACS fellow. Overall, there was a positive opinion of the fellows as teachers and most agreed that the fellow did not detract from the residents' experience.

Several studies have focused on surgeon productivity since the implementation of an acute care surgery model. Barnes et al. (18) compared operative productivity before and after the implementation of acute care surgery and demonstrated a 66% increase in operative volume with an ACS division in place. Similarly, there was an increase in Evaluation and Management (E&M) work Relative Value Unit (wRVU) production as well as a rise in procedural wRVU production for both ACS and nontrauma surgeons (19). Other studies have also shown an increase in OR cases and billing as well as an increase in surgeon satisfaction after the implementation of ACS (20).

Additional studies have focused mainly on resident and surgeon interest and satisfaction with acute care surgery. Recruitment into the field of trauma and critical care surgery was traditionally poor, as demonstrated by approximately 18% of fellowship positions unfilled in 2011. In 2015, this has improved to only 10% of positions going unfilled (34). In 2012, Coleman et al. (35) surveyed residents regarding a career path in acute care surgery, which yielded a greater interest and understanding of acute care surgery as a career. Overall, these studies showed a much greater interest and understanding of acute care surgery as a career choice, encompassing surgical critical care and emergency surgery.

A Canadian study looked at surgeons' satisfaction within an ACS model compared to those with a traditional call schedule. Those within the model, on average, had higher satisfaction scores than those surgeons not using an ACS model (22). In Barnes' paper, both ACS surgeons and non-ACS surgeons reported improved job satisfaction with the implementation of an ACS service, stating they would prefer to work in a department that incorporated an ACS model (18). As the fellowship matures and acute care surgeons enter the workforce, this will hopefully become a more attractive option for rising surgical residents.

In addition to improved productivity, interest, and satisfaction, other studies have emphasized the ACS model as improving patient throughput. Multiple studies in the North America, Australia, and Asia have demonstrated the efficiency and utility of an ACS model. The majority of these studies looked at the effectiveness of an ACS model as it pertained to appendectomies, cholecystectomies with some also looking at small bowel obstructions as these are the most common ACS operations performed. Cubas et al. (36) showed a statistically significant decrease in time to surgical consultation, time to the OR, fewer complications, and a reduced length of stay for appendectomies performed within an ACS model. Again looking at appendectomies, Fu et al. (37) showed a decreased amount of time in the Emergency Department by approximately 7 hours in Taiwan, and Pillai et al. (38) in Australia demonstrated an increase in the proportion of daytime procedures. Michailidou et al. (39) showed similar results when looking exclusively at cholecystectomies with 75% of patients undergoing an operation within 24 hours in the ACS group as compared to 59% in the non-ACS group.

With a slightly different perspective, Khalil et al. (40) compared the ACS model between ACS-approved Level 1 trauma centers (ACS-TCs), Level 1 trauma centers (TC), and nontrauma centers (NTCs). This study showed that patients managed in ACS-TCs had shorter hospital stay, lower complication rate, and lower overall hospital costs when compared with patients managed in both TCs and NTCs with statistical significance. With the most recent evidence, the acute care surgery model provides an efficient 24-hour coverage for surgical emergencies, providing not only surgical care but postoperative critical care in a timely and efficient fashion. Proven benefit in patient care combined with cost-effective management should lead to further adoption of the ACS model, more approved fellowships in the training of these surgeons, and attract trainees to a career that is vibrant and satisfying.

CONCLUSION

The combination of surgeon shortage and poor access to emergency surgical care drove the creation of the ACS model. Creation of ACS services allow the time-critical delivery of emergent and urgent surgical care, in the face of an identified surgeon workforce shortage. Potential pitfalls and initial concerns regarding the implementation of this model and introduction of this fellowship have not come to fruition. Specifically, resident education and nontrauma surgeons' operative logs have not been negatively impacted. However, our most critically ill surgical patients have benefited, with improved outcomes, more efficient care, and decreased mortality. The ACS practice model will continue to be interpreted differently among various hospitals. Just as the needs of the injured patient drove the development of the field of trauma surgery, so did the needs of the emergency general surgery patient drive the development of the acute care surgery paradigm. The training paradigm for the ACS fellows will continue to ensure that fully trained acute care surgeons are comfortable with a wide variety of anatomic exposures across all body regions. Acute care surgeons are uniquely positioned to impact health care cost containment and improve care in the United States as mandated by the Affordable Care Act of 2010. Cost savings can be actualized, and the system for care delivery can be optimized by focusing on throughput and the use of standardized, evidence-based, consistent care. Acute care surgeons stand at the front line of care delivery for the patients who are most critically ill and for the injured surgical patients with time-sensitive diseases. Getting the right patient to the right venue at the right time is the paramount skill that the acute care surgeon, through training and experience, adds to the value equation (41).

Key Points

- Acute care surgery was born out of necessity, addressing the crisis in emergency services.
- Acute care surgeons should feel comfortable operating in multiple anatomic locations.
- The ACS fellow will be board certified in surgical critical care.

References

1. Division of Advocacy and Health Policy. A growing crisis in patient access to emergency surgical care. *Bull Am Coll Surg.* 2006;91:8–19.
2. Napolitano LM, Fulda JG, Davis KA, et al. Challenging Issues in surgical critical care, trauma and acute care surgery: a report from the Critical Care Committee of the American Association for the Surgery of Trauma. *J Trauma.* 2010;69:1619–1633.
3. Institute of Medicine. *The Future of Emergency Care in the United States Health System. Hospital based care at the breaking point.* 2006; National Academies Press, Washington DC.
4. Association of American Medical Colleges. Physician Supply and Demand Through 2025: Key Findings. Available at: https://www.aamc.org/download/426260/data/physiciansupplyanddemandthrough2025keyfindings.pdf. Accessed July 2, 2015.
5. American College of Emergency Physicians On-Call Specialist in U.S. Emergency Departments, ACEP Survey of Emergency Department Directors, April 2006; American College of Emergency Physicians, Irving, TX.
6. Davis KA, d Jurkovich GJ. An update on acute care surgery: emergence of acute care surgery. *ACS Surgery News,* June 11, 2015.
7. Jonasson O, Kwakwa MA, Sheldon GF. Calculating the workforce in general surgery. *JAMA.* 1995;274(9):731–734.
8. Abt Associates. *Reexamination of the Adequacy of Physicians Supply Made in 1980 by the Graduate Medical Education National Advisory Committee for Selected Specialties: Final Report.* Springfield, VA: National Technical Information Service, US Department of Commerce; 1991. Publication HSRA: 240–89–0041.
9. Association of American Medical Colleges. The Complexities of Physician Supply and Demand: Projections from 2013 to 2025. Final Report. Available at: https://www.aamc.org/download/426242/data/ihsreportdownload.pdf?cm_mmc = AAMC-_-ScientificAffairs-_-PDF-_-ihsreport. March 2015. Accessed August 12, 2015.
10. Fischer JF. The impending disappearance of the general surgeon. *JAMA.* 2007;298(18):2191–2193.
11. Yeo H, Bucholz E, Ann Sosa J, et al. A national study of attrition in general surgery training: which residents leave and where do they go? *Ann Surg.* 2010;252(3):529–534.
12. Association of American Medical Colleges. AAMC Medloans® Organizer and Calculator. Available at: https://apps.aamc.org/first-gloc-web/#/landing. Accessed July 15, 2015.
13. Jurkovich GJ; Committee to Develop the Reorganized Specialty of Trauma, Surgical Critical Care, Emergency Surgery. Acute care surgery: trauma, critical care, and emergency surgery. *J Trauma.* 2005;58(3):614–616.
14. Moore EE, Maier RV, Hoyt DB, et al. Acute care surgery: Eraritjaritjaka. *J Am Coll Surg.* 2006;202(4):698–701.
15. Centers for Disease Control and Prevention. Nation at a Glance: Uninsured Americans. Available at: http://www.cdc.gov/nchs/features/nation_jun2015/nation_at_a_glance_jun2015.htm. Published June 25, 2015. Accessed July 3, 2015.
16. American Hospital Association. Trendwatch Chartbook 2015. Available at: http://www.aha.org/research/reports/tw/chartbook/2015/table3–3.pdf. Accessed July 3, 2015.
17. American Hospital Association. *Hospital Statistics 2006.* Health Forum LLC; 2006; Chicago, IL.

18. Barnes SL, Cooper CJ, Coughenour JP, et al. Impact of acute care surgery to departmental productivity. *J Trauma.* 2011;71(4):1027–1034.
19. Resnick AS, Corrigan D, Mullen JL, Kaiser LR. Surgeon contribution to hospital bottom line not all are created equal. *Ann Surg.* 2005;242(4):530–539.
20. Davis KA, Cabbad NC, Schuster KM, et al. Trauma team oversight of patient management improves efficiency of care and augments clinical and economic outcomes. *J Trauma.* 2008;65(6):1236–1242.
21. O'Mara MS, Scherer L, Wisner D, Owens LJ. Sustainability and success of the acute care surgery model in the nontrauma setting. *J Am Coll Surg.* 2014;219(1):90–98.
22. Diaz JJ, Norris PR, Gunter OL, et al. Does regionalization of acute care surgery decrease mortality? *J Trauma.* 2011;71(2):442–446.
23. Kaplan LJ, Frankel H, Davis KA, Barie PS. Pitfalls of implementing acute care surgery. *J Trauma.* 2007;62(5):1264–1270.
24. Sweeting RS, Carter JE, Meyer AA, et al. The price of acute care surgery. *J Trauma Acute Care Surg.* 2013;74(5):1239–1242; discussion 1242–1245.
25. Wanis KN, Hunter AM, Harington MB, Groot G. Impact of an acute care surgery service on timeliness of care and surgeon satisfaction at a Canadian academic hospital: a retrospective study. *World J Emerg Surg.* 2014;9(1):4.
26. Anantha RV, Paskar D, Vogt K, et al. Allocating operating room resources to an acute care surgery service does not affect wait-times for elective cancer surgeries: a retrospective cohort study. *World J Emerg Surg.* 2014;9(1):21.
27. Anantha RV, Parry N, Vogt K, et al. Implementation of an acute care emergency surgical service: a cost analysis from the surgeon's perspective. *Can J Surg.* 2013;57(2):E9–E14.
28. Dente CJ, Duane TM, Jurkovich GJ, et al. How much and what type: analysis of the first year of the acute care surgery operative case log. *J Trauma Acute Care Surg.* 2014;76(2):329–339.
29. Duane TM, Dente CJ, Fildes JJ, et al. Defining the acute care surgery curriculum. *J Trauma Acute Care Surg.* 2015;78(2):259–263; discussion 263–264.
30. Davis KA, Dente CJ, Burlew CC, et al. Refining the operative curriculum of the acute care surgery fellowship. *J Trauma Acute Care Surg.* 2014;78(1):192–196.
31. Shafi S, Aboutanos M, Brown CV, et al. Measuring anatomic severity of disease in emergency general surgery. *J Trauma Acute Care Surg.* 2014; 76(3):884–887.
32. Davis KA. EAST 2015 Presidential address: look both ways. *J Trauma Acute Care Surg.* 2015;79:1–9.
33. Dinan KA, Davis JW, Wolfe MM, et al. An acute care surgery fellowship benefits a general surgical residency. *J Trauma Acute Care Surg.* 2014; 77(2):209–212.
34. National Resident Matching Program. Results and Data: 2015 Main Residency Match. Available at: http://www.nrmp.org/.
35. Coleman JJ, Esposito TJ, Rozycki GS, Feliciano DV. Acute care surgery: now that we have built it, will they come? *J Trauma Acute Care Surg.* 2013; 74(2):463–469.
36. Cubas RJ, Gomez NR, Rodriguez S, et al. Outcomes in the management of appendicitis and cholecystitis in the setting of a new acute care surgery service model: impact on timing and cost. *J Am Coll Surg.* 2012;215:715–721.
37. Fu CY, Huang HC, Chen RJ, et al. Implementation of the acute care surgery model provides benefits in the surgical treatment of the acute appendicitis. *Am J Surg.* 2014;208:794–799.
38. Pillai S, Hsee L, Pun A, et al. Comparison of appendicectomy outcomes: acute surgical versus traditional pathway. *ANZ J Surg.* 2013;83:739–743.
39. Michailidou M, Kulvatunyou N, Friese RS, et al. Time and cost analysis of gallbladder surgery under the acute care surgery model. *J Trauma Acute Care Surg.* 2014;76(3):710–714.
40. Khalil M, Pandit V, Rhee P, et al. Certified acute care surgery programs improve outcomes in patients undergoing emergency surgery: a nationwide analysis. *J Trauma Acute Care Surg.* 2015;79(1):60–64.
41. Frankel HL, Butler KL, Cuschieri J, et al. The role and value of surgical critical care, an essential component of acute care surgery, in the affordable care act: a report from the Critical Care Committee and Board of Managers of the American Association for the Surgery of Trauma. *J Trauma Acute Care Surg.* 2012;73(1):20–26.

CHAPTER

60

Critical Care of Hepatopancreaticobiliary Surgery Patients

KRISTIN L. MEKEEL, OYA M. ANDACOGLU, and ALAN W. HEMMING

INTRODUCTION

Patients are admitted to the intensive care unit (ICU) for a variety of reasons following hepatopancreaticobiliary (HPB) surgery, including maintenance, or restoration, of normal physiology immediately after extensive surgery and the subsequent management of complications that develop. Many of the issues that require ICU management are common to all ICU patients and will not be discussed in this chapter; however, there are recurring issues that are relatively specific to HPB surgery patients that will be discussed. The role of normal liver physiology and its alteration during HPB surgery and disease states will be discussed as well as the management of common problems that arise after HPB surgery.

HPB surgery is a surgery of the liver, bile duct, and pancreas, and may include portal decompressive procedures for complications of portal hypertension. Surgical procedures on the pancreas and bile duct alone generally do not require care in a critical care setting immediately after leaving the operating room unless complications occur. Liver resections, particularly when extensive, can require admission to a critical care unit immediately following surgery due to the alterations in normal physiology that occur during the procedure itself. An understanding of normal liver physiology and the alterations it undergoes during liver surgery is important when managing these patients.

LIVER ANATOMY AND PHYSIOLOGY

The liver is approximately 2% of total body weight and has multiple complex functions. The anatomy of the liver has been described using various methods (1–5); however, surgical anatomy is based on the segmental nature of vascular and bile duct distribution. The liver receives a dual blood supply from both the portal vein and hepatic artery that run, along with the bile duct, within the Glissonian sheath or main portal pedicle. The portal pedicle divides into right and left branches and then supplies the liver in a segmental fashion. Venous drainage is via the hepatic veins, which drain directly into the inferior vena cava. Hepatic segmentation is based on the distribution of the portal pedicles and their relation to the hepatic veins (Fig. 60.1). The three hepatic veins run in the portal scissurae and divide the liver into four sectors, which are in turn divided by the portal pedicles running in the hepatic scissurae. The liver is divided into right and left hemi-livers by the middle hepatic vein. The right lobe is divided by the right hepatic vein into anterior and posterior sectors. The anterior sector is divided by the plane of the portal pedicle into an inferior segment 5 and a superior segment 8. The posterior sector is divided by the plane of the portal pedicle into an inferior segment 6 and a superior segment 7. The left lobe lies to the left of the middle hepatic vein and is divided into anterior and posterior sectors by the left hepatic vein. The anterior sector is divided by the umbilical fissure into segment 4 medially and segment 3 laterally. The segment posterior to the left hepatic vein is segment 2. Segment 4 can be divided by the plane of the portal pedicle into a superior segment 4a and an inferior segment 4B. Segment 1 is the caudate lobe which lies between the inferior vena cava and the hepatic veins. The caudate lobe has variable portal venous, hepatic arterial, and biliary anatomy, and is essentially independent of the portal pedicle divisions and hepatic venous drainage. Segmental anatomy becomes important in considering surgical resection when essentially any segment or combination of segments can be resected if attention is paid to maintaining vascular and biliary continuity to remaining segments. Common liver resections that are performed that might require ICU admission after surgery are left or right hepatectomies in which approximately 50% of liver volume is removed or more extensive procedures such as right or left trisectionectomy in which up to 80% of the liver is removed (see Fig. 60.1). If less than 40% of the liver is resected in patients with normal underlying liver function, relatively little derangement of liver physiology is noted.

The liver performs many functions, including uptake, storage, and eventual distribution of nutrients from the blood or gastrointestinal (GI) tract and synthesis metabolism and elimination of a variety of endogenous and exogenous substrates and toxins (including narcotics and other drugs). Although the liver is only 4% to 5% of body weight, it is responsible for 20% to 25% of body oxygen consumption and 20% of total energy expenditure (6). The liver receives a dual blood supply with 75% of flow from the portal vein and 25% from the hepatic artery. Total blood flow to the liver is approximately 1.5 L/min/1.73 m^2 (7). Decreasing portal venous flow causes a subsequent increase in hepatic arterial flow; however with complete portal occlusion or diversion, hepatic arterial flow does not completely compensate and total liver blood flow is diminished (8). The opposite is not true, however. That is, decreasing flow in the hepatic artery does not increase flow in the portal vein; there is autoregulation of hepatic arterial flow but not the portal venous system. Portal flow is increased by food intake, bile salts, secretin, pentagastrin, vasoactive intestinal peptide (VIP), glucagon, isoproterenol, prostaglandin E1 and E2, and papaverine. Portal flow is decreased by serotonin, angiotensin, vasopressin, nitrates, and somatostatin.

Bile, composed of inorganic ions and organic solutes, is formed at the canalicular membrane of the hepatocyte as well as in the bile ductules and is secreted by an active process that is relatively independent of blood flow (9). The major organic

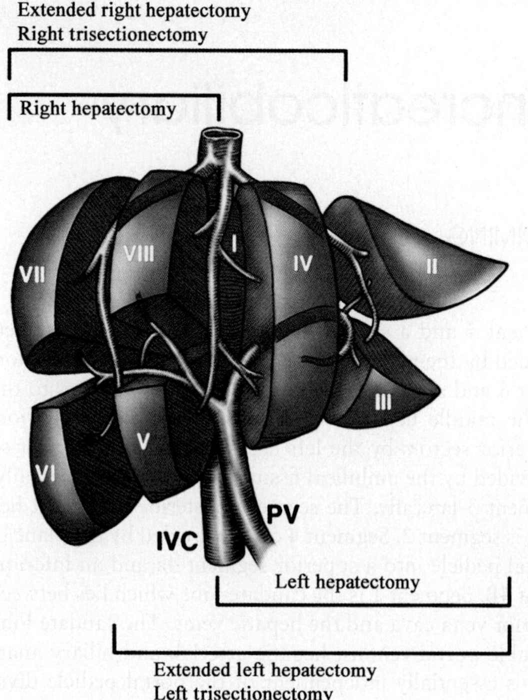

FIGURE 60.1 Diagrammatic representation of liver segments with standard liver resections demonstrated.

components of bile are the conjugated bile acids, cholesterol, phospholipid, bile pigments, and protein. Under normal conditions, 600 to 1,000 mL of bile is produced daily (10). Bile secretory pressure is approximately 10 to 20 cm H_2O, with maximal secretory pressures of 30 to 35 cm H_2O in the presence of complete biliary obstruction.

Bilirubin is a degradation product of heme and is eliminated almost entirely in the bile. It circulates bound to albumin and is removed from the plasma by the liver by a carrier mediated transport system. In the hepatocyte, bilirubin is bound to glucuronic acid before being secreted in bile. While the liver maintains the ability to clear bilirubin with partial duct obstruction, complete obstruction of one of the right or left hepatic ducts alone will cause marked liver enzyme abnormalities, but rarely causes jaundice.

The liver synthesizes many of the major human plasma proteins including albumin, gamma globulin and many of the coagulation proteins. Liver dysfunction can have a profound effect on coagulation by decreased production of coagulation proteins or, in the case of obstructive jaundice, a decreased activity of factors II, V, VII, IX, and X secondary to a lack of vitamin K–dependent posttranslational modification. Reversal of coagulation abnormalities by exogenous administration of vitamin K differentiates between synthetic dysfunction and lack of vitamin K absorption secondary to obstructive jaundice.

After hepatic resection, liver function is altered through both a reduction in functional liver mass as well as potential ischemia/reperfusion injury to the liver remnant. With extensive liver resection in patients with normal underlying liver function, reduction of functional liver volume below 25% has been associated with increased risk of both liver failure and mortality (11). To reduce the risk of liver failure in this setting, preoperative portal vein embolization (PVE) has been developed. During PVE the portal vein of the side of the liver to be resected is embolized percutaneously. Diversion of portal flow and its hepatotrophic factors to the future liver remnant (FLR) causes growth and hypertrophy of the FLR of about 30% (Fig. 60.2) over a 6-week period and has been shown to reduce the complications associated with subsequent extended liver resections (12).

Patients with biliary obstruction may require preoperative drainage prior to surgery. For patients with obstruction of the common hepatic duct or bifurcation, scheduled to undergo a major liver resection (most commonly diagnosed with cholangiocarcinoma [CCC]), we recommend preoperative percutaneous drainage of the remnant liver until the total bilirubin is less than 2 mg/dL; this decreases the risk of postoperative liver dysfunction (13), although this is controversial. For patients with obstruction of the distal common bile duct, intrapancreatic bile duct, or ampulla (most commonly diagnosed with a pancreatic malignancy), drainage is only recommended for severe jaundice, cholangitis, or severe malnutrition (14,15).

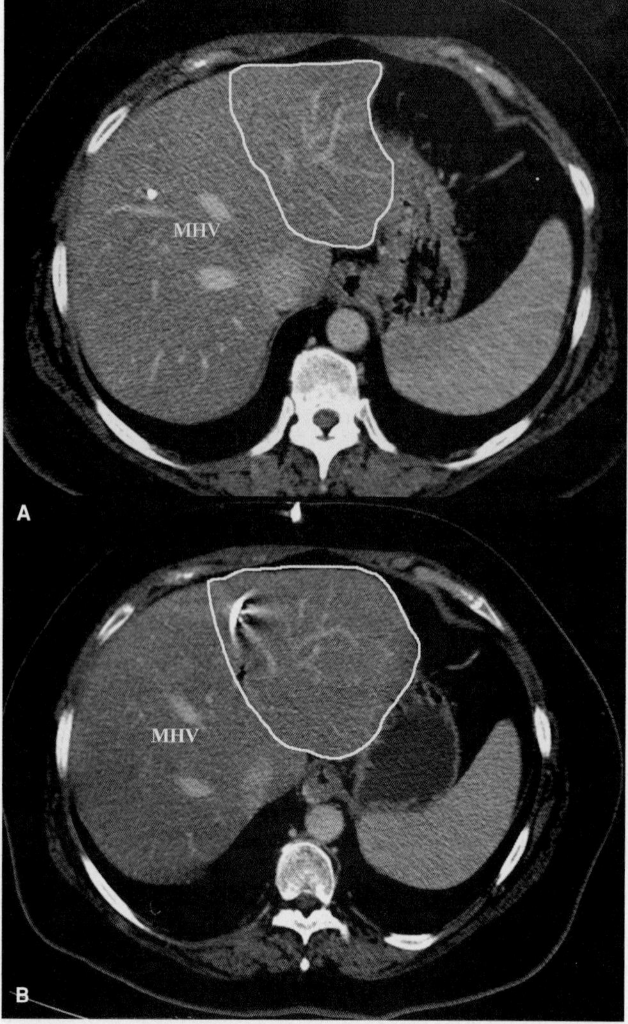

FIGURE 60.2 Portal vein embolization of the right portal vein preoperatively allows an increase of functional liver remnant of approximately 30% from prior to embolization (A) to postembolization (B). (Reproduced with permission from Hemming AW, Reed AI, Howard RJ, et al. Preoperative portal vein embolization for extended hepatectomy. *Ann Surg.* 2003;237(5):686–691.)

SURGICAL PROCEDURES

Liver Resection

As the liver is a tremendously vascular organ, intraoperative or postoperative complications are often related to excessive blood loss (16); thus a number of techniques have been developed to achieve preresection vascular control and decreased bleeding. While liver resection can often be performed without the need for interruption of blood flow to the liver, in many cases some degree of reduction of flow is required to prevent excessive blood loss.

Selective inflow control can be established by division or occlusion of the vascular structures supplying the segment(s) of liver to be removed. The right or left portal pedicle containing the respective portal vein, hepatic artery, and bile duct are controlled with a vascular clamp. This technique has the advantage of preserving blood flow to the segment of the liver being preserved but is generally only useful in smaller resections.

Total inflow occlusion (Pringle maneuver) results from clamping the entire inflow of the liver at the hepatoduodenal ligament; this has been shown to reduce blood loss during the parenchymal transection phase of the resection (17). While there is some concern regarding warm ischemic injury, abundant data shows that the normal liver can tolerate inflow occlusion for up to 1 hour, and there are reports suggesting that some cirrhotic livers can safely tolerate 60 minutes of inflow occlusion as well (18). We use total inflow occlusion when selective occlusion provides insufficient control. Clamp times are expected to be less than 30 minutes for formal hepatectomies, but may be higher for more complex parenchymal transections. In such cases, total occlusion is carried out in 15-minute increments with 5-minute reperfusion intervals. An alternative to the intermittent clamping technique is to use ischemic preconditioning, during which the liver inflow is occluded for 10 minutes, after which it is allowed to reperfuse for 15 minutes prior to clamping again for a sustained time period up to 1 hour. Intermittent clamping is associated with more blood loss than ischemic preconditioning; however, the protective results of ischemic preconditioning in ischemia reperfusion injury have not been uniform across age groups and may not be as effective in livers that have been exposed to preoperative chemotherapy (19).

Total vascular isolation of the liver, with both inflow occlusion and occlusion of the supra- and infrahepatic vena cava, can be useful for technically demanding cases where the vena cava or proximal hepatic veins are involved with tumor (Fig. 60.3). Total isolation has been shown to be safe for up to 60 minutes in normal liver, but can be accompanied by varying degrees of hemodynamic instability (20). In cases where this is required, we carry out as much of the operation as possible prior to isolation of the liver to reduce the ischemic time and the period of hemodynamic instability.

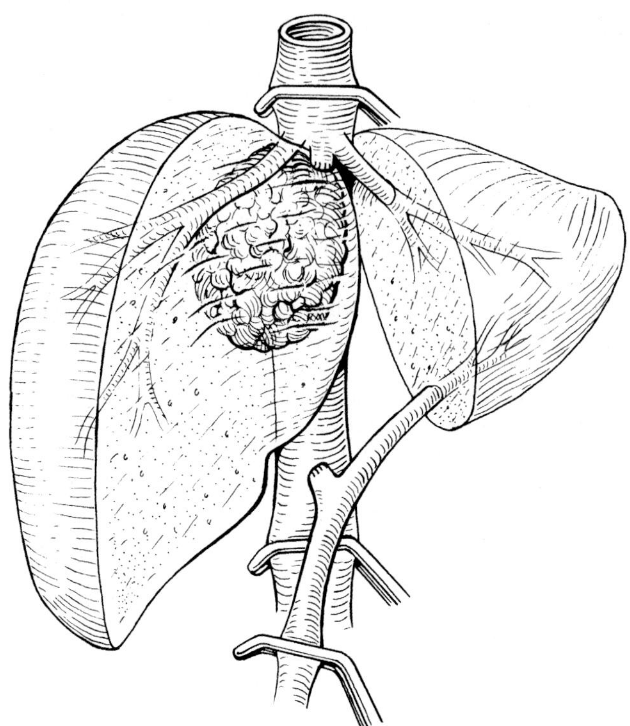

FIGURE 60.3 Tumors that involve the inferior vena cava or hepatic veins may require total vascular isolation of the liver. Both the infra- and suprahepatic inferior vena cava are clamped along with the portal vein and hepatic artery. (Reproduced with permission from Hemming AW, Reed AI, Howard RJ, et al. Preoperative portal vein embolization for extended hepatectomy. *Ann Surg.* 2003;237(5):686–691.)

Hemodynamic Monitoring during Liver Resection

Central venous pressure (CVP) monitoring has traditionally been used to minimize blood loss during hepatectomy. During liver resection, hepatic vein pressure and blood loss are linearly related to CVP, with a CVP of 2 to 3 mmHg optimal for hepatic resections (21,22). The most troublesome bleeding during liver resection is usually from branches of the hepatic vein; this can be minimized by maintaining the CVP of 5 mmHg or less during the period of hepatic transection. Cooperation of the anesthesiologist in minimizing volume loading, and occasionally using pharmacologic agents to reduce CVP is essential. However, if total vascular isolation is to be used, volume loading prior to caval clamping is required to avoid an acute decrease in cardiac output at the time the clamps are applied. Low CVP anesthesia can result in significant volume depletion postoperatively and needs to be considered as part of the differential of hypotension and low urine output in the ICU after liver resection.

Knowledge of the details of intraoperative conduct of the operation is, therefore, important to the physicians that are to manage the postoperative care of the liver resection patient in the ICU setting. Was inflow occlusion or vascular isolation required and for how long? Prolonged clamp times are associated with greater liver dysfunction. Was the patient maintained with a low CVP throughout the course of the surgery? If so then the patient may need volume expansion on arrival to the ICU. How much liver remains and is it normal? If the percentage of liver is less than 25% in normal livers, or less than 40% in cirrhotic livers or livers with bile duct obstruction, the chance of liver failure and the need for its management is higher. Was there significant blood or fluid requirements? Patients may need a period of ventilation while fluid shifts and equilibrates.

Pancreatic and Bile Duct Surgery

The majority of patients undergoing pancreatic or bile duct surgeries do not require admission to an ICU setting immediately postoperatively because of issues specific to the pancreaticobiliary surgery itself. In general, procedures on the pancreas or biliary tree should not be associated with major intraoperative hemodynamic changes or alterations in physiology. Tumors of the head of the pancreas or bile duct may involve the portal vein or cause extensive fibrotic reaction in the area. Technical difficulties can arise in which damage occurs to, or resection is required of, the portal vein (Fig. 60.4). If portal vein resection or repair is required, it is more likely that the patient will require ICU care. Portal vein resection, when planned, requires variable durations of portal venous outflow obstruction from the gut, which are usually short and well tolerated, but can increase the amount of fluid third spaced in the bowel wall. Portal vein injury, however, can lead to massive transfusion requirements and hypotension that can require postoperative ICU care. The more common indications for admission to the ICU after pancreatic or biliary surgery are either an underlying medical condition or the development of a complication postoperatively. Pancreatic or bile leaks can lead to sepsis but will be discussed later in the chapter.

Portal Decompressive Procedures

Surgical portal decompressive procedures are becoming a rarity since the introduction of transjugular intrahepatic portosystemic shunt (TIPS) procedures. Decompressive procedures do, however, remain indicated in select patients with variceal bleeding with preserved liver function that have failed medical management and who are not transplant candidates. The myriad technical variations of surgical portosystemic shunts are beyond the scope of this chapter but certain commonalities exist.

Whether total or partial shunts, selective or nonselective patients will have had the high-pressure portal system surgically connected to the low-pressure caval circulation to lower the pressure in the portal venous system and stop variceal bleeding. Reduction of portal flow in patients that have borderline liver function can precipitate liver dysfunction or failure. Additionally, the fraction of portal flow diverted into the systemic circulation through the shunt is not cleared by the liver until it returns to the liver via the arterial circulation. This may induce encephalopathy, and shunts that divert most or all of the portal flow into the systemic circulation are more likely to induce encephalopathy than do those shunts that are selective or partial. One special case scenario is Budd–Chiari syndrome in which the hepatic venous outflow is obstructed, usually due to thrombosis secondary to a hypercoagulable state. In this disorder, blood flow perfuses the hepatic sinusoids from both hepatic artery and portal vein, but cannot exit through the blocked hepatic veins. A functional side-to-side shunt is performed (portacaval, mesocaval) that allows hepatic arterial blood to flow into the sinusoids and then exit via the portal vein, and through the shunt into the systemic circulation. It is not uncommon for liver function to deteriorate initially after the shunt is performed with subsequent gradual improvement and liver regeneration. Support of liver function may be required immediately after the shunt while liver function stabilizes. In some cases the shunt may precipitate acute liver failure making urgent liver transplantation the only option.

Immediate Postoperative Management

Postoperative fluid management is important in the care of patients after major hepatobiliary surgery. In particular, fluid shifts in patients who have had major liver resection can be difficult to manage after surgery. Intraoperatively, most liver resections are performed with low CVP and low intravascular volume. This practice minimizes bleeding during the hepatic parenchymal transection phase of the procedure, but may pose some difficulty in postoperative management. Postoperatively,

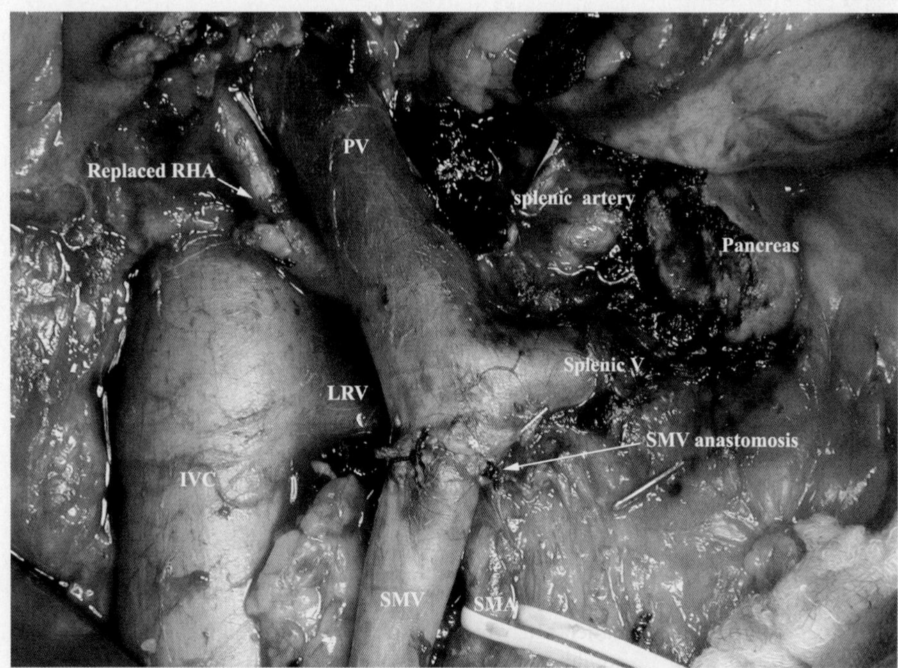

FIGURE 60.4 Pancreaticoduodenectomy demonstrating resection of the portal vein. IVC, inferior vena cava; LRV, left renal vein; PV, portal vein; RHA, right hepatic artery; SMA, superior mesenteric artery; SMV, superior mesenteric vein; splenic V, splenic vein. (Reproduced with permission from Hemming AW, Reed AI, Howard RJ, et al. Preoperative portal vein embolization for extended hepatectomy. *Ann Surg.* 2003;237(5):686–691.)

patients that have had a major liver resection may have signs of hypovolemia with low urine output and low blood pressure. Volume re-expansion should be gentle, as partial liver resection leads to hypoalbuminemia, and pulmonary edema and ascites can develop with aggressive resuscitation. Although the use of albumin infusions is generally frowned upon in critical care medicine, albumin and fresh frozen plasma (FFP) may be useful in the resuscitation of patients after liver resection as the physiology is similar to patients with cirrhosis. We will use albumin containing fluids for volume expansion if the serum albumin is less than 2.9 mg/dL. FFP can be used for volume expansion; however, it is generally reserved for abnormalities in coagulation. Serial lactate levels are helpful in the postoperative management of patients after liver resection. Elevated lactic acid levels may be a sign of hypovolemia, but the lack of response to volume can indicate liver dysfunction.

After liver resections, glucose metabolism is altered, due to both a reduction in functional liver mass and relative dysfunction of the remaining liver secondary to ischemia reperfusion injury, especially if vascular control has been used during the procedure. As glycogen stores are depleted, the liver uses gluconeogenesis to provide glucose. As a result, patients may become hypoglycemic, although lethal hypoglycemia is rare. It has become standard practice in most critical care units to tightly control blood glucose levels. While the advantages of this approach, particularly regarding reduced risk of sepsis, remains for patients after major liver resection, aggressive blood glucose control with insulin infusions requires closer monitoring and may require reduced insulin dosing to prevent hypoglycemia.

Patients who have undergone shunt surgery need a different approach than patients undergoing other hepatobiliary surgery. Patients need more aggressive fluid management immediately postoperatively to maintain circulating intravascular volume and reduce the risk of shunt thrombosis. Maintenance fluid should be D5 0.45% saline solution to provide the liver with carbohydrate. After the immediate postoperative period, patients are also at risk for ascites formation, hence excessive sodium should be minimized. Additional volume expansion should be with albumin or FFP. Diuretics can be reinstituted after the immediate postoperative period. A general rule is to use furosemide and spironolactone in combination with 100 mg of spironolactone for every 40 mg of furosemide. Antibiotics should be administered for 24 hours postoperatively to minimize infection.

While encephalopathy is rare in patients after liver resection, unless they present in liver failure or have pre-existing liver disease, the presence of asterixis can be an early sign of encephalopathy. Encephalopathy is treated with lactulose and dietary protein restriction, as in other patients with end-stage liver disease. Infection, dehydration, and bleeding, as well as narcotic use, must be evaluated as they can trigger encephalopathy.

Hypophosphatemia

After liver resection, care must be taken to aggressively replace low serum phosphate.

The exact mechanism of the hypophosphatemia remains unclear, as both increased utilization during liver regeneration and renal wasting mechanism have been proposed (23).

Regardless of the etiology, the clinical consequences of hypophosphatemia are well established, and include respiratory depression, diaphragmatic insufficiency, seizures, and cardiac irritability. Additionally, hepatocellular regeneration is dependent on ATP and, after liver resection, regeneration may be impaired if phosphate is not repleted (24). In a series of 35 liver resections, 21% had significant postoperative hypophosphatemia (less than 2.5 mg/dL). This group had a significant increase in complications (80%) compared with the normophosphatemic group (28%) (25). Phosphate should be replaced with potassium or sodium phosphate preparations, or added to parenteral nutrition solutions. Recent studies in living donor right hepatic lobectomies suggest that replacement up to two times the recommended daily allowance (60 mmol) is necessary to replete severe hypophosphatemia and prevent its complications (26).

Liver Function: Assessment and Support

Liver function should be carefully monitored after major liver resections and shunt surgery, as liver failure is a risk in any major hepatobiliary surgery. The risk of liver failure increases with the extent of hepatectomy and in patients with preoperative liver disease or cirrhosis (27,28). Although standard liver function tests are helpful after major liver resection or shunt surgery, they may not show elevation until the patient has significant liver failure. Transaminases are frequently elevated in the 200 to 300 units/dL range postresection due to the direct effect of mechanical injury to the liver during transection, as well as to partial devascularization of areas of the liver. Measurements of liver function, including the prothrombin time and lactate, are more helpful in evaluating for early postoperative liver dysfunction.

Elevated total and indirect bilirubin are also useful indicators of postoperative liver dysfunction; however, isolated elevation of total bilirubin in the presence of normal liver function can have other etiologies. Perioperative blood transfusions can lead to hemolysis and hyperbilirubinemia with a predominance of direct hyperbilirubinemia, and can be diagnosed with a standard hemolytic workup. Bile leaks or obstruction can also lead to an elevated serum bilirubin. The diagnosis and treatment of bile leaks are covered later in this chapter. Many popular anesthetics, antibiotics, and other drugs can cause hepatotoxicity and elevation of the serum bilirubin, and need to be reduced or stopped if liver failure occurs.

When postoperative liver dysfunction does develop, it is important to exclude sepsis and anatomic causes of liver failure. A postoperative ultrasound can evaluate for portal vein, hepatic arterial, or hepatic vein thrombosis or obstruction, which may be amenable to surgical intervention. If the patient does not have sepsis, drug toxicity, biliary obstruction or leak, or vascular occlusion, the liver failure is likely related to a pre-existing liver disease and/or the extent of resection. Treatment is then supportive, with correction of coagulopathy, encephalopathy, and ascites, as above. Systemic antibiotics, or gut decontamination may be beneficial since the liver Kupffer cells play a role in decreasing bacterial translocation from the portal blood flow, and patients with liver failure or biliary leak or obstruction, may have an increased risk of bacteremia and sepsis. In some patients postoperative liver failure is fatal.

N-acetylcysteine has been shown to decrease liver injury after acetaminophen overdose (29) and lessen hepatic ischemia reperfusion injury (30). Intravenous infusions of prostaglandin have also been linked to improvement of ischemia reperfusion injury and liver damage (31). Although definitive clinical data are lacking, both *N*-acetylcysteine and PGE1 have been used to ameliorate postoperative damage in both liver resection and transplant patients. *N*-acetylcysteine is given over 16 hours as a continuous infusion of 40 mL of 10% solution mixed in 250 mL of D5W. Prostaglandin is also given as a continuous intravenous infusion, starting at 0.15 mcg/kg/hr. It is titrated up to 1 mcg/kg/hr based on systemic hypotension.

Coagulation Disorders

The liver synthesizes both procoagulant and anticoagulant proteins and, with liver dysfunction after liver resection, patients may be hypercoaguable, hypocoagulable, or both. Coagulopathy is more commonly associated with liver resection and dysfunction and can be particularly significant in the immediate postoperative period when excessive coagulopathy can lead to surgical bleeding and reoperation. Several studies have demonstrated and increase in prothrombin time directly proportional to the extent of liver resection (32,33). This coagulopathy has been attributed to impaired synthesis and clearance of clotting factors, inhibitors, and regulatory proteins (34,35). Patients with underlying liver disease and cirrhosis also often have thrombocytopenia and qualitative platelet defects. In addition, intraoperative hypothermia and perioperative transfusions, which, while not routine, are not uncommon during major hepatobiliary surgery, and can contribute to postoperative coagulopathy.

Serial hemoglobin and prothrombin levels should be measured. Because of the vascular nature of hepatobiliary surgery combined with postoperative coagulopathy from decreased liver function, as well as the frequent need for intravascular volume expansion, serial hemoglobin levels should be followed to watch for postoperative bleeding. In general, we would obtain a hematocrit and international normalized ratio (INR) on ICU arrival and then repeat about 6 hours later. The surgeon should be notified of excessive bloody output from the drains, increasing abdominal distention, or hemodynamic instability. In the immediate postoperative period or if bleeding is suspected, the INR should be corrected if it goes above 2.0, unless specified otherwise by the surgeon (36). Vitamin K should be given in addition to FFP. Any patient who is bleeding should have their coagulopathy completely corrected. For severe bleeding, both aprotinin and activated factor VII or 4-factor prothrombin complex are safe in patients during and after liver resection (35,37). A thromboelastogram may be helpful in these situations to determine the exact cause of the coagulopathy and is now routinely used in liver transplantation and hepatobiliary surgery. Patients who fail to stop bleeding after correction of their coagulopathy require return to the operating room. The surgical team should be made aware of any patient immediately postsurgery that requires transfusion.

There is a common perception that patients post liver resection have some degree of auto-anticoagulation from physiologic liver dysfunction that is protective against venous thromboembolism (VTE) (38). In reality, patients undergoing major liver resection are considered at moderate to high risk for thromboembolic complications according to 2012 American College of Chest Physician (ACCP) guideline (39). It is imperative to start prophylaxis for VTE once the acute risk of hemorrhage has passed, especially in patients with malignancies. At our institution, we prefer low–molecular-weight heparin unless the patient has renal insufficiency or another contraindication to VTE prophylaxis. There are data suggesting VTE rate actually is increased in proportion to the extent of hepatectomy. Additionally, advanced age, higher BMI, male gender, high ASA classification (3 or higher), postoperative organ space infection, longer procedure times, as well as higher postoperative INR (1.5 or higher vs. less than 1.5), all increase the risk of postoperative VTE (38,40).

Pain Management and Sedation

The large subcostal incision needed for major hepatobiliary surgery can result in significant pain after surgery. However, altered pharmacokinetics and coagulopathy in particular after partial liver resection or shunt surgery can make postoperative pain management challenging. Patients with liver failure or compromised liver function secondary to hepatectomy have altered metabolism of many common medications, in particular, narcotics and sedatives that require clearance via the liver.

One of the more common problems that arises in the ICU after liver resection is oversedation of patients. A standard dose of narcotics given to a patient who has had 80% of the liver resected may well cause prolonged respiratory depression and signs and symptoms of encephalopathy. Narcotics and benzodiazepines should be used at the minimum dose required to achieve pain control/sedation. After liver resection, it is recommended that basal rates on patient-controlled anesthesia pumps be avoided, as metabolism of narcotics is difficult to forecast. Benzodiazepines also have altered clearance after liver resection, and thus should be dosed at lower levels or avoided altogether, if possible. In patients who require ongoing intubation we have found it useful to use sedative agents such as propofol, rather than narcotics, since the level of sedation can be more easily titrated and reversed.

Epidural pain management may be optimal after liver resection; however, it is contraindicated in many patients because of postoperative coagulopathy. Unfortunately, that includes many hepatic resections and shunt surgery. Recent literature has examined the use of epidural catheters in patients undergoing living donor partial hepatic resection. In one review of eight patients, good pain control was achieved with only one case of oversedation requiring naloxone. Although postoperative coagulopathy did occur, it was not to the extent that factor transfusion was needed prior to catheter removal, and there were no cases of hemorrhage (41). Epidural analgesia may be useful in select patients who do not have underlying liver disease and who are not undergoing extended resections.

Nutrition

Although nutrition plays an important role in the care of any critically ill patient, the role of the liver in protein and carbohydrate metabolism makes proper postoperative nutrition imperative in the management of patients after major hepatobiliary surgery, in particular, after partial liver resection when liver function is temporarily reduced. Patients with preoperative biliary obstruction, malignancy, and cirrhosis are at higher risk for nutrition-related complications after major liver or bile duct surgery. Preoperative nutritional risk factors that are associated with postoperative complications in hepatobiliary surgery include weight loss of over 14% lean body mass over 6 months, serum albumin less than 3 g/dL, hematocrit less than 30%, total body potassium less than 85% normal, less than 25th percentile for mid-arm circumference, and skin test anergy (42). Preoperative bilirubin, albumin, prealbumin, prothrombin time, transferring, and vitamin and trace mineral deficits may also be important preoperatively.

As with most critically ill patients, early enteral nutrition has been associated with improved outcomes. In hepatobiliary surgery, both enteral and parenteral nutrition have been associated with improved outcomes, especially in high-risk patients (42,43). However, parenteral nutrition has been clearly associated with an increased risk of infection (44). Enteral nutrition has been shown to improve gut flora, preventing gastrointestinal atrophy and loss of immunocompetence. A review of five prospective randomized trials on enteral and parenteral nutrition in patients after liver resection found a decrease in wound infection and line sepsis in patients on enteral nutrition (45). There were no differences in mortality.

In patients who have undergone routine liver resection or shunt surgery, low-volume enteral feeds can be started almost immediately postoperatively. In patients who have had hepaticojejunostomies or pancreatic surgery, return of bowel function is necessary prior to starting feeds, unless the feeding tube is placed distal to the anastomosis. It is best to consult with the operating surgeon before starting enteral feeds in any patient, in particular those with enteric reconstruction. Patients with major pancreatic surgery (pancreaticoduodenectomy [PD], subtotal or total pancreatectomy) may require pancreatic enzyme supplementation with enteral feeds or when resuming oral intake.

Patients with chronic liver disease or cirrhosis often have severe metabolic derangements that make nutritional management difficult. The depletion of the fat-soluble vitamins, in particular a loss of vitamin K, leads to coagulopathy and diminished antioxidant response. Chronic liver disease also stimulates a catabolic state with proteolysis and cachexia; protein loss can be exacerbated by dietary restriction to help decrease encephalopathy. Branched-chain amino acids, initially thought to reduce the development of encephalopathy in catabolic patients with advanced liver failure, have not borne out in clinical trials. Patients with cirrhosis also have abnormal glucose tolerance and insulin levels, along with elevated ammonia levels, hypophosphatemia, and hypoalbuminemia, all of which influence perioperative nutrition. All Child's B or C cirrhotic patients should be fed enterally when hospitalized. Caloric needs of the patients are increased to a goal of 25 to 25 kcal/kg/d; protein requirements are 1 to 1.5 g/kg dry weight in those not encephalopathic, with a minimum of 0.5 g/kg dry weight if encephalopathy has ensued (45). Patients with ascites require sodium restriction of 2 g/d and a fluid restriction of 1 to 1.5 L/d, in combination with diuretics, if tolerated.

Patients with preoperative obstructive jaundice often have chronic, low-grade endotoxemia and sepsis. This can lead to weight loss and anorexia, often due to malabsorption of fat and fat-soluble vitamins related to the obstruction, which itself leads to coagulopathy and a diminished antioxidant response. Endotoxemia also results in decreased hepatic protein synthesis and catabolism (46). Patients with biliary obstruction require a low-fat diet, as absorption is impaired, as well as replacement of the fat-soluble vitamins. Medium-chain triglycerides may be helpful, because their absorption is not bile salt dependent and these may avoid diarrhea until bile flow is re-established.

Partial liver resections also cause metabolic abnormalities secondary to the regenerating liver. Hepatic mitochondria switch to fat from glucose as their preferred energy source in hepatic regeneration (47). As a result, hypertonic glucose and insulin infusions should be avoided immediately after resection, as hyperglycemia and insulinemia suppress fatty acid release and decrease ketone body production by the liver. Some investigators have advocated administering fat and/or ketone bodies after liver resection to accelerate regeneration; conclusive evidence that this is beneficial is lacking. Similarly, infusions of glucose and insulin directly into the portal vein have also been looked at to improve regeneration although, again, conclusive evidence is lacking. Adequate liver regeneration is dependent on protein and calories; postoperative parenteral nutrition should be protein and fat supplemented, but low on glucose, to improve hepatic regeneration. General goals are 30 kcal/kg/d, with 1.0 to 1.5 g protein, glucose not to exceed 5 mg/kg/min, and fat making up 30% of the calories. Patients with cancer may need an increase of up to 35 kcal/kg/d and 2 g protein.

Well-nourished patients need no postoperative support, while malnourished patients will benefit from early enteral nutrition when possible, or parenteral nutrition until they are capable of taking enteral nutrition.

Renal Failure

Acute renal failure occurs after major hepatobiliary surgery in 10% of patients (48) and, similar to other critically ill patients, significantly increases postoperative mortality (49). Risk factors for perioperative renal failure include postoperative sepsis, preoperative uremia, preoperative anemia, malignant disease, and preoperative jaundice (48,50,51). In particular, preoperative obstructive jaundice appears to be a significant risk factor, with an estimated 10% of patients developing postoperative renal failure (52). Both dehydration and endotoxin production from bile duct obstruction have been postulated to cause renal failure in these patients (53). Many studies have been performed trying to decrease this risk, including using mannitol, bile salts, hydration, and lactulose (52–55).

In all patients with acute renal failure, adequate hydration, treatment of sepsis, and avoidance of nephrotoxic drugs are mandatory. However, in patients with obstructive jaundice, lactulose and bile salts may decrease endotoxin absorption, and have been shown in some studies to be beneficial in the prevention of renal failure (51,52). Preoperative biliary drainage to help lessen the perioperative inflammatory response is also an important adjunct to prevent postoperative renal failure. Once acute renal failure does occur, supportive care and dialysis are needed until renal function returns.

Patients with advanced cirrhosis or postoperative liver failure may develop hepatorenal syndrome (HRS). This is more significant in the acute care of patients with liver failure or after liver transplantation. HRS is a diagnosis of exclusion, based on urine sodium less than 10 mEq/L combined with a urine osmolality greater than that of plasma osmolality that does not respond to volume. The cause of HRS is likely multifactorial, but is primarily related to circulatory disturbances in patients with advanced liver disease, reduced liver function, and portal hypertension. Systemic vasodilatation and low mean arterial pressure results in afferent renal arterial vasoconstriction and a reduction in glomerular filtration rate

(56). Although liver transplantation remains the only cure for HRS, vasoconstrictors, albumin infusions, and transhepatic portosystemic shunts are able to reduce HRS, and may prevent its development in patients with spontaneous bacterial peritonitis (57).

Postoperative Complications

Complications Following Liver Resection

The morbidity associated with liver resection is reported to be between 30.7% and 47.7% (57–60). In addition to the standard complications associated with all major operations, liver resection is associated with specific problems including bleeding, bile leaks, liver insufficiency, ascites, pleural effusions, and infections.

Risk factors of complications following liver resection include increased blood loss, increased number of segments resected, increased preoperative bilirubin, increased prothrombin time, prolonged operative time, resection of segment 8, diabetes, and concomitant surgical procedures (60–65).

Mortality. In-hospital mortality due to liver resection has decreased over the past two decades and high-volume centers have reported rates of 0% to 5% (57,59,60,66–68). The decrease in mortality is attributed to improved surgical technique, intraoperative anesthesia management, and perioperative care. These changes have helped decrease in-hospital mortality in liver resection patients despite their increased mean age and comorbidities (57).

Risk factors associated with increased mortality include hypoalbuminemia, thrombocytopenia, preoperative total bilirubin greater than 6 mg/dL, elevated serum creatinine greater than 1.5 mg/dL, cholangitis, major hepatic resection, increased number of segments resected, synchronous abdominal procedure, major comorbid illness, diabetes, and blood transfusion requirements (57,59,62,68–71).

Specific surgical strategies to decrease mortality include minimizing blood loss and transfusions, and avoiding ischemic injury to the remnant liver. Specific posthepatectomy strategies include minimizing ongoing liver injury by maintaining tissue oxygenation, early support to facilitate liver regeneration by early feeding, and replenishing phosphate levels (66).

Bleeding. Bleeding, once the Achilles heel of liver resection surgery, has decreased dramatically over the last two decades due to a better appreciation of liver anatomy, surgical technique, and improved anesthetic management (66). As a result, centers routinely performing liver resections have noted a decrease in estimated blood loss of from 300 to 750 mL, and perioperative transfusion rates of 17.3% to 28.3% (57,59,68).

Risk factors for increased bleeding from liver resection include cirrhosis, portal hypertension, increased segments resected, coagulopathy, thrombocytopenia, and elevated CVP during resection (62,72). Strategies to minimize blood loss during liver resection include appropriate patient selection (especially avoiding resection in patients with portal hypertension), maintenance of CVP under 6 mmHg, Pringle maneuver, preoperative correction of coagulopathy and thrombocytopenia, use of fibrin sealant on raw liver surfaces, use of intraoperative ultrasound to locate the hepatic venous branches, and utilization of selective hepatic vascular exclusion (72–76).

Bile Leak

Biliary leaks occur in 3.6% to 17% of liver resections (77–80) and are associated with increased mortality and concomitant complications (78,79,81). Risk factors associated with biliary leaks following liver resection include older age, preoperative leukocytosis, left-sided hepatectomy, prolonged operative time, resection for peripheral CCC, and resection of segment 4 (77,79). When liver resection is performed for hepatocellular carcinoma (HCC), risk factors for bile leaks include central tumor location, and preoperative transarterial chemoembolization (TACE) (78).

Various strategies have been described to prevent bile leaks following resection. A few groups have shown that the use of fibrin glue on the cut surface of the liver reduces bile leaks (77). Others have combined fibrin glue with bioabsorbable polyglycolic acid to significantly reduce bile leaks (82). While these small studies may indicate some effect of fibrin glue in reducing biliary leaks, there are at least as many studies that show no difference in bile leak rate when fibrin glue is employed.

Most bile leaks following liver resections without biliary reconstructions are small and can be managed nonoperatively. A percutaneous drain is placed—if a drain placed at surgery is not present—to prevent abdominal sepsis from an undrained biloma and to control the leak (79) and broad-spectrum antibiotics initiated for fevers, leukocytosis, or positive bile cultures. Persistent drainage for 2 to 3 days of more than 100 mL of bilious fluid confirms an active leak, and is managed with endoscopic retrograde cholangiopancreatography (ERCP), sphincterotomy, and stent placement. This procedure may define the location of the leak and facilitate enteric biliary drainage and leak closure. When leaks are at the resected hepatic duct stump, a stent traversing the leak may further facilitate leak closure, although the main principle of treatment is to reduce the pressure in the biliary tree and allow spontaneous closure (79). Early endoscopic management of biliary leaks can minimize hospital length of stay and are not associated with late biliary complications (80). Others have used endoscopically placed nasobiliary tubes to decompress the biliary system as it allows easy repeat cholangiograms and later removal (80,83). Although most leaks will close with time with these measures, they may persist for months (28).

From 10% to 32% of patients ultimately require reoperation because the leak cannot be controlled, and these procedures are associated with a high mortality rate (79,80,83). Biliary enteric drainage is performed on patients in whom ERCP cannot be performed for technical reasons, or who persist on leaking despite ERCP. Important factors contributing to a good outcome are early reoperation, control of the biliary fistula before surgery, and utilization of healthy bile duct edges for enteric anastomosis.

Hemobilia may complicate either bile leaks, liver resection, or occur secondary to trauma. Open communication from a branch of the hepatic artery to the biliary tree occurs and leads to intermittent and sometimes exsanguinating GI bleeding. Identification is made when blood is seen exiting the ampulla during endoscopy for upper GI bleeding. While CT scanning with arterial phase contrast can localize the bleeding within the liver, management is by angiographic embolization.

Liver Failure/Dysfunction. Liver failure complicates liver resection in up to 12% of cases (61), and occurs when inadequate functional liver volume is left after resection. This complication occurs primarily in patients undergoing resection for HCC with underlying liver disease, and is often a consequence of patient selection and choice of operation.

Risk factors for hepatic insufficiency in cirrhotics include major resection—especially right lobectomy—portal hypertension, longstanding jaundice, Childs–Pugh–Turcotte (CPT) score greater than A, and hepatic steatosis (57). More recently, preoperative chemotherapy has become routine in patients with colorectal cancer metastatic to the liver. While there is no doubt that the addition of newer agents such as irinotecan, oxaliplatin, and bevacizumab have improved long-term results, they also cause an increase in hepatic steatosis as well as steatohepatitis, which can contribute to postoperative liver dysfunction.

By assessing the patient's functional liver status, the surgeon can estimate the maximum amount of liver mass that can be resected while preserving adequate functional liver volume. In patients with normal livers, up to 75% of total liver volume can be resected safely. It is patients with abnormal livers, such as cirrhotics, that need careful assessment. In general, Child–Pugh class C is a contradiction to any sort of resection. Early Child's class B patients without portal hypertension may undergo minor resections from wedge resection to a single segmentectomy; however, these patients may be better served by nonoperative local ablation techniques. Child–Pugh class A patients being considered for major hepatectomy (resection of 4 or more segments) should undergo assessment of both liver and physiologic status (84,85). Others have found that a model for end-stage liver disease (MELD) equal to or greater than 11 predicts liver failure following HCC resection (86). Portal hypertension, defined as a hepatic vein pressure gradient (HVPG) greater than 10 mmHg and suggested by signs such as esophageal varices, anatomic portosystemic shunts, and ascites (87), has been associated with increased morbidity and mortality following major resection (88). Thrombocytopenia with platelet counts less than 100,000 cells/µL is one laboratory indicator of portal hypertension and has been associated with in-hospital mortality following liver resection (84).

Although various tests exist to assess liver function in Child–Pugh classes A and B patients before possible major liver resection (greater than or equal to four segments), none have been uniformly adopted. The indocyanine green (ICG) clearance test, commonly used in Asia, is one method of quantifying liver function (66,89,90). Early studies have shown that an ICG retention at 15 minutes (ICGR15) of less than 20% allows safe limited liver resection, and a value of less than 14% is associated with near-zero operative mortality (91–93).

In Child–Pugh class A patients with right-sided lesions curable by major resection but whose liver reserve may be inadequate, preoperative ipsilateral PVE increases the remnant contralateral liver volume (92). Portal vein embolization is generally performed in patients with a predicted function liver remnant of less than 25% in noncirrhotics or less than 40% in patients with significant fibrosis and/or cirrhosis.

Liver failure following liver resection presents clinically with encephalopathy and asterixis. In severe cases, patients appear similar to fulminant liver failure patients with marked acidosis, jaundice, and hemodynamic instability. The patient ultimately succumbs to multiorgan failure and sepsis. In mild cases, treatment is supportive with judicious fluid management, optimizing tissue oxygenation, infection prophylaxis, and nutritional support if recovery is prolonged. The goal in the mild and salvageable cases is to promote immediate liver functional recovery from the insults inherent to liver resection, to promote liver regeneration with nutritional and electrolyte repletion (particularly phosphate), and to minimize the change of infections complications. With early studies demonstrating significantly improved hepatic oxygen delivery and extraction in patients receiving *N*-acetylcysteine for nonacetominophen-induced liver failure (94,95), subsequent conflicting studies have failed to support a definite role in patient following liver resection (96). Nonetheless, many centers—including our own—selectively administer *N*-acetylcysteine in patients with marginal liver function following resection mainly based on favorable small-series and anecdotal benefits (97). This practice may be reasonable because of the sheer number of favorable outcome reports and the good drug safety profile, but controlled trials are needed.

Ascites and Pleural Effusion. Ascites occurs in up to 9% of liver resections (61) and is associated with decreased survival as it is a surrogate marker of liver insufficiency and because of its potential contribution to prerenal insufficiency (81). Pleural effusion usually occurs on the right side and frequently accompanies ascites. Pleural effusion following liver resection occurs in 3.8% to 21% of cases (61,98), is usually asymptomatic, and most often requires no treatment. Effusion may develop from underlying ascites that crosses the diaphragm. In addition, the same pathophysiologic processes of fluid overload and hypoproteinemia that cause ascites also contribute to the development of pleural effusion.

Risk factors for both ascites and pleural effusion include right lobectomy, diabetes, poor nutritional status, and hypoalbuminemia, left-sided cardiac insufficiency, liver and renal insufficiency (57,99). In addition, risk factors specifically associated with pleural effusion have been found to include resection for HCC with underlying liver disease, subphrenic collections, postoperative liver insufficiency with ascites, and duration of inflow occlusion (98).

Strategies to prevent postresection ascites and pleural effusion include avoiding overhydration (including gentle diuresis), preventing renal insufficiency by avoiding nephrotoxic drugs and hypotension, early detection and treatment of infection, maintaining adequate nutrition, and the use of perioperative drains (99). The appropriate selection of patients and resection to maintain adequate liver function, especially in patients with hepatomas and underlying liver disease, will minimize the risk of liver failure and subsequent ascites.

Complications Following Bile Duct Resection/Reconstruction

Perhaps the most extensive hepatobiliary operations are performed for proximal extrahepatic CCCs. With mounting evidence demonstrating significantly improved survival following extended liver and bile duct resections and reconstructions versus local bile duct resections, centers with experienced hepatobiliary surgeons are presenting series with improved outcomes (100–103). Nonetheless, significant complications remain associated with these procedures.

Perioperative mortality following extended liver and biliary resections ranges from 1.3% to 16% (102,104–106). Complications following these procedures occur in 51% to 81%, and many patients have multiple complications (100,102,105,106).

Complications include bile duct leaks, bleeding, liver failure, pleural effusions, wound infection, and sepsis (104,106–108). Each of these complications can also be found in liver resections alone and share the same risk factors. In addition, each complication can be approached with the same preventative strategy and treatment.

Liver failure following extended resections for obstructive CCC may have a unique pathophysiology and hence preventative strategy. Prolonged biliary obstruction causes significant hepatocellular dysfunction, and liver failure occurs in up to 27.6% of patients who undergo extended liver and biliary resections and reconstructions for CCC and is frequently fatal (106,108). Resection of up to 75% of the liver along with possible vascular reconstruction that requires an increased duration of ischemic injury to the liver is often necessary to resect hilar CCC and in the setting of pre-existing liver dysfunction liver failure can be problematic. Strategies to optimized functional liver volume prior to extended liver resections for hilar CCCs are essential to preventing postoperative liver failure. One strategy is to promote hepatocellular functional recovery by preoperatively decompressing the biliary tree using percutaneous transhepatic cholangiocatheterization. This practice is somewhat controversial as it may introduce infection into an otherwise sterile biliary tree, and so may be avoided in patients who can undergo surgery within 2 to 3 weeks after the onset of jaundice. Another strategy is to perform contralateral PVE to increase the remnant liver volume prior to resection. A number of centers have demonstrated decreased liver failure rates when these strategies are employed (103,104,109).

Complications Following Pancreatic Surgery

The mortality rate following PD ranges between 2.7% and 6.9% (109–114). Risk factors for perioperative mortality include elevated serum bilirubin, diameter of pancreatic duct, increased intraoperative blood loss, pancreatic fistulas, and older age (113).

Complications occur in between 22.1% and 30.2% of PDs, and include pancreatic fistulae, delayed gastric emptying, bleeding, abdominal abscesses, and wound infections (112,113).

Pancreatic fistulae are a dreaded complication of PD, occurring in 12% to 18% of patients (110–112,115–118). Pancreatic fistulae are associated with a mortality rate of 0% to 19% (104,111,112). These patients often die secondary to massive erosive *bleeding* from sepsis and pancreatic enzyme accumulation. These bleeding episodes occur in 1% to 8.8% of PD patients and carry a mortality rate of 47% to 50% (114,119,120).

Risk factors for pancreatic fistulae include small duct size, soft pancreas texture, duration of surgery greater than 8 hours, diabetes, lower creatinine clearance, preoperative jaundice, and increased intraoperative blood loss (112,116,118,121).

Despite numerous studies evaluating potential strategies to prevent pancreatic fistulae following PD, including the use of octreotide, fibrin sealants, pancreatic stents, different methods, and sites of pancreatic anastomosis, none have proven effective (117,122–125). Pancreatic fistulae are initially detected on postoperative day 6, presenting with abdominal pain, fever, nausea/vomiting, and leukocytosis. Fistulae are then confirmed by CT scan which often demonstrates a fluid collection behind the pancreatic anastomosis, elevated serum amylase, drain output greater than 50 mL/d, and drain amylase 10-fold greater than serum amylase (117,122). Management is initially conservative with bowel rest, total parenteral nutrition, antibiotics, and monitoring of clinical signs and symptoms and drain output. If repeat imaging demonstrates increased accumulation of fluid and the patient does not respond to conservative measures, another drain may be placed percutaneously to prevent progression of abdominal sepsis. Eighty percent to 90% of patients seal pancreatic fistulae with these measures (110,115). However, those patients who develop uncontrolled leaks and abdominal sepsis may require surgery, usually for completion pancreatectomy. In addition, a smaller group of patients with fistulae will suffer life-threatening erosive intra-abdominal bleeding, usually from the stump of the gastroduodenal artery, small arterial branches to the pancreas, or rarely from the portal vein. These patients will present with signs and symptoms of sepsis and hypovolemia, such as fever, abdominal pain, hypotension, anemia, and bloody drain output; they are treated by rapid resuscitation and angiography for potential embolization of the bleeding arterial branch. If arterial bleeding cannot be controlled in this manner, or if the bleeding is venous, the patient is surgically explored for hemostasis and completion pancreatectomy. Surgery in this setting is associated with a high mortality: up to 36% of patients requiring surgery after PD for bleeding will not survive (114,120,123).

Key Points

- After hepatic resection, liver function is altered through both a reduction in functional liver mass as well as potential ischemia/reperfusion injury to the liver remnant.
- With extensive liver resection in patients with normal underlying liver function, reduction of functional liver volume below 25% has been associated with increased risk of both liver failure and mortality.
- Preoperative PVE diverts portal flow from the side of the liver to be resected to the FLR allowing for growth and hypertrophy over a 6-week period. This has been shown to reduce the complications associated with extended liver resections.
- A CVP of 5 mmHg or less during hepatic transection has been shown to decrease blood loss and improve outcomes, and can lead to hypovolemia postresection.
- Patients at an increased risk for liver insufficiency or complications post liver resection include liver remnant of less than 40%, cirrhosis, bile duct obstruction, vascular reconstruction, total vascular isolation or prolonged inflow occlusion, and significant intraoperative blood loss.
- Patients can develop significant hypophosphatemia post liver resection and need aggressive phosphorous replacement to facilitate liver regeneration and prevent the clinical consequences of low phosphate.
- PT/INR and lactate are the best postoperative indicators of liver function. AST and ALT are measurements of parenchymal damage and commonly elevated after major resection.
- Patients undergoing major liver resection are considered at moderate to high risk for thromboembolic complications and it is imperative to start prophylaxis

for VTE once the acute risk of hemorrhage has passed, especially in patients with malignancies.
- Pancreatic fistula is a common and dreaded complication after PD. Most fistulae are managed nonoperatively with drainage, antibiotics, and bowel rest. A small percentage of patients develop uncontrolled leaks that lead to hemorrhage, sepsis, and death.

References

1. Bismuth H. Surgical anatomy and anatomical surgery of the liver. *World J Surg*. 1982;6(1):3–9.
2. Couinaud C. [Surgical anatomy of the liver. Several new aspects]. *Chirurgie*. 1986;112(5):337–342.
3. McClusky DA III, Skandalakis LJ, Colborn GL, Skandalakis JE. Hepatic surgery and hepatic surgical anatomy: historical partners in progress. *World J Surg*. 1997;21(3):330–342.
4. Strasberg SM. Terminology of liver anatomy and liver resections: coming to grips with hepatic Babel. *J Am Coll Surg*. 1997;184(4):413–434.
5. Botero AC, Strasberg SM. Division of the left hemiliver in man: segments, sectors, or sections. *Liver Transpl Surg*. 1998;4(3):226–231.
6. Baldwin R, Smith NE. Molecular control of energy metabolism. In: Sink, ed. *The Control of Metabolism*. University Park: Pennsylvania State University Press; 1974.
7. Bradley EL 3rd. Measurement of hepatic blood flow in man. *Surgery*. 1974;75(5):783–789.
8. Kock NG, Hahnloser P, Roding B, Schenk WG Jr. Interaction between portal venous and hepatic arterial blood flow: an experimental study in the dog. *Surgery*. 1972;72(3):414–419.
9. Brauer R. Hepatic blood supply and the secretion of bile. In: RW T, ed. *The Biliary System*. Oxford: Blackwell Scientific Publishers; 1965.
10. Prandi D. Canalicular bile production in man. *Eur J Clin Invest*. 1975; 5(1):1–6.
11. Abdalla EK, Barnett CC, Doherty D, et al. Extended hepatectomy in patients with hepatobiliary malignancies with and without preoperative portal vein embolization. *Arch Surg*. 2002;137(6):675–680.
12. Hemming AW, Reed AI, Howard RJ, et al. Preoperative portal vein embolization for extended hepatectomy. *Ann Surg*. 2003;237(5):686–691.
13. Nimura Y. Radical surgery: vascular and pancreatic resection for cholangiocarcinoma. *HPB (Oxford)*. 2008;10(3):183–185.
14. Arkadopoulos N, Kyriazi MA, Papanikolaou IS, et al. Preoperative biliary drainage of severely jaundiced patients increases morbidity of pancreaticoduodenectomy: results of a case-control study. *World J Surg*. 2014;38(11):2967–2972.
15. Sun C, Yan G, Li Z, Tzeng CM. A meta-analysis of the effect of preoperative biliary stenting on patients with obstructive jaundice. *Medicine (Balt)*. 2014;93(26):e189.
16. Takenaka K, Kanematsu T, Fukuzawa K, Sugimachi K. Can hepatic failure after surgery for hepatocellular carcinoma in cirrhotic patients be prevented? *World J Surg*. 1990;14(1):123–127.
17. Man K, Fan ST, Ng IO, et al. Prospective evaluation of Pringle maneuver in hepatectomy for liver tumors by a randomized study. *Ann Surg*. 1997;226(6):704–711; discussion 711–713.
18. Nagasue N, Yukaya H, Suehiro S, Ogawa Y. Tolerance of the cirrhotic liver to normothermic ischemia: a clinical study of 15 patients. *Am J Surg*. 1984;147(6):772–775.
19. Clavien PA, Selzner M, Rudiger HA, et al. A prospective randomized study in 100 consecutive patients undergoing major liver resection with versus without ischemic preconditioning. *Ann Surg*. 2003;238(6):843–850.
20. Huguet C, Addario-Chieco P, Gavelli A, et al. Technique of hepatic vascular exclusion for extensive liver resection. *Am J Surg*. 1992;163(6):602–605.
21. Guo Y, Lin CX, Lau WY, et al. Hemodynamics and oxygen transport dynamics during hepatic resection at different central venous pressures in a pig model. *Hepatobiliary Pancreat Dis Int*. 2011;10(5):516–520.
22. Lin CX, Guo Y, Lau WY, et al. Optimal central venous pressure during partial hepatectomy for hepatocellular carcinoma. *Hepatobiliary Pancreat Dis Int*. 2013;12(5):520–524.
23. Salem RR, Tray K. Hepatic resection-related hypophosphatemia is of renal origin as manifested by isolated hyperphosphaturia. *Ann Surg*. 2005;241(2):343–348.
24. Campbell KA, Wu YP, Chacko VP, Sitzmann JV. In vivo 31P NMR spectroscopic changes during liver regeneration. *J Surg Res*. 1990;49(3): 244–247.
25. Buell JF, Berger AC, Plotkin JS, et al. The clinical implications of hypophosphatemia following major hepatic resection or cryosurgery. *Arch Surg*. 1998;133(7):757–761.
26. Pomposelli JJ, Baxter JK III, Babineau TJ, et al. Early postoperative glucose control predicts nosocomial infection rate in diabetic patients. *J Parenter Enteral Nutr*. 1998;22(2):77–81.
27. Midorikawa Y, Kubota K, Takayama T, et al. A comparative study of postoperative complications after hepatectomy in patients with and without chronic liver disease. *Surgery*. 1999;126(3):484–491.
28. Nanashima A, Yamaguchi H, Shibasaki S, et al. Comparative analysis of postoperative morbidity according to type and extent of hepatectomy. *Hepatogastroenterology*. 2005;52(63):844–848.
29. Riordan SM, Williams R. Fulminant hepatic failure. *Clin Liver Dis*. 2000; 4(1):25–45.
30. Glantzounis GK, Yang W, Koti RS, et al. The role of thiols in liver ischemia-reperfusion injury. *Curr Pharm Des*. 2006;12(23):2891–2901.
31. Hossain MA, Wakabayashi H, Izuishi K, Okano K, Yachida S, Maeta H. The role of prostaglandins in liver ischemia-reperfusion injury. *Curr Pharm Des*. 2006;12(23):2935–2951.
32. Suc B, Panis Y, Belghiti J, Fekete F. "Natural history" of hepatectomy. *Br J Surg*. 1992;79(1):39–42.
33. Vishnevskii VA, Titova MI, Sivkov VV, Saidov SS, Guseinov EK. [Hemostasis disorders after resection of liver and approaches to their prevention and correction]. *Klin Med (Mosk)*. 1996;74(8):32–34.
34. Borromeo CJ, Stix MS, Lally A, Pomfret EA. Epidural catheter and increased prothrombin time after right lobe hepatectomy for living donor transplantation. *Anesth Analg*. 2000;91(5):1139–1141.
35. Silva MA, Muralidharan V, Mirza DF. The management of coagulopathy and blood loss in liver surgery. *Semin Hematol*. 2004;41(Suppl 1): 132–139.
36. Martin RC II, Jarnagin WR, Fong Y, et al. The use of fresh frozen plasma after major hepatic resection for colorectal metastasis: is there a standard for transfusion? *J Am Coll Surg*. 2003;196(3):402–409.
37. Shao YF, Yang JM, Chau GY, et al. Safety and hemostatic effect of recombinant activated factor VII in cirrhotic patients undergoing partial hepatectomy: a multicenter, randomized, double-blind, placebo-controlled trial. *Am J Surg*. 2006;191(2):245–249.
38. Tzeng CW, Katz MH, Fleming JB, et al. Risk of venous thromboembolism outweighs post-hepatectomy bleeding complications: analysis of 5651 National Surgical Quality Improvement Program patients. *HPB*. 2012;14(8):506–513.
39. Gould MK, Garcia DA, Wren SM, et al. Prevention of VTE in nonorthopedic surgical patients: Antithrombotic Therapy and Prevention of Thrombosis, 9th ed. American College of Chest Physicians evidence-based clinical practice guidelines. *Chest*. 2012;141(2 Suppl):e227S–e277S.
40. Nathan H, Weiss MJ, Soff GA, et al. Pharmacologic prophylaxis, postoperative INR, and risk of venous thromboembolism after hepatectomy. *J Gastrointest Surg*. 2014;18(2):295–302.
41. Schumann R, Zabala L, Angelis M, et al. Altered hematologic profiles following donor right hepatectomy and implications for perioperative analgesic management. *Liver Transpl*. 2004;10(3):363–368.
42. Fan ST, Lo CM, Lai EC, et al. Perioperative nutritional support in patients undergoing hepatectomy for hepatocellular carcinoma. *N Engl J Med*. 1994;331(23):1547–1552.
43. Richter B, Schmandra TC, Golling M, Bechstein WO. Nutritional support after open liver resection: a systematic review. *Dig Surg*. 2006;23(3): 139–145.
44. Gramlich L, Kichian K, Pinilla J, et al. Does enteral nutrition compared to parenteral nutrition result in better outcomes in critically ill adult patients? A systematic review of the literature. *Nutrition*. 2004;20(10):843–848.
45. McCullough AJ, Tavill AS. Disordered energy and protein metabolism in liver disease. *Semin Liver Dis*. 1991;11(4):265–277.
46. Curran RD, Billiar TR, Stuehr DJ, et al. Multiple cytokines are required to induce hepatocyte nitric oxide production and inhibit total protein synthesis. *Ann Surg*. 1990;212(4):462–469.
47. Nakatani T, Ozawa K, Asano M, et al. Changes in predominant energy substrate after hepatectomy. *Life Sci*. 1981;28(3):257–264.
48. Thompson JN, Edwards WH, Winearls CG, et al. Renal impairment following biliary tract surgery. *Br J Surg*. 1987;74(9):843–847.
49. Schroeder RA, Marroquin CE, Bute BP, et al. Predictive indices of morbidity and mortality after liver resection. *Ann Surg*. 2006;243(3):373–379.
50. Dixon JM, Armstrong CP, Duffy SW, Davies GC. Factors affecting morbidity and mortality after surgery for obstructive jaundice: a review of 373 patients. *Gut*. 1983;24(9):845–852.
51. Uslu A, Cayci M, Nart A, et al. Renal failure in obstructive jaundice. *Hepatogastroenterology*. 2005;52(61):52–54.

52. Pain JA, Cahill CJ, Gilbert JM, et al. Prevention of postoperative renal dysfunction in patients with obstructive jaundice: a multicentre study of bile salts and lactulose. *Br J Surg*. 1991;78(4):467–469.
53. Evans HJ, Torrealba V, Hudd C, Knight M. The effect of preoperative bile salt administration on postoperative renal function in patients with obstructive jaundice. *Br J Surg*. 1982;69(12):706–708.
54. Cahill CJ, Pain JA, Bailey ME. Bile salts, endotoxin and renal function in obstructive jaundice. *Surg Gynecol Obstet*. 1987;165(6):519–522.
55. Gubern JM, Sancho JJ, Simo J, Sitges-Serra A. A randomized trial on the effect of mannitol on postoperative renal function in patients with obstructive jaundice. *Surgery*. 1988;103(1):39–44.
56. Gines P, Guevara M, Arroyo V, Rodes J. Hepatorenal syndrome. *Lancet*. 2003;362(9398):1819–1827.
57. Poon RT, Fan ST, Lo CM, et al. Improving perioperative outcome expands the role of hepatectomy in management of benign and malignant hepatobiliary diseases: analysis of 1222 consecutive patients from a prospective database. *Ann Surg*. 2004;240(4):698–708.
58. Imamura H, Seyama Y, Kokudo N, et al. One thousand fifty-six hepatectomies without mortality in 8 years. *Arch Surg*. 2003;138(11):1198–1206.
59. Vauthey JN, Pawlik TM, Abdalla EK, et al. Is extended hepatectomy for hepatobiliary malignancy justified? *Ann Surg*. 2004;239(5):722–730.
60. Benzoni E, Cojutti A, Lorenzin D, et al. Liver resective surgery: a multivariate analysis of postoperative outcome and complication. *Langenbecks Arch Surg*. 2007;392(1):45–54.
61. Shimada M, Matsumata T, Akazawa K, et al. Estimation of risk of major complications after hepatic resection. *Am J Surg*. 1994;167(4):399–403.
62. Fan ST, Lo CM, Liu CL, et al. Hepatectomy for hepatocellular carcinoma: toward zero hospital deaths. *Ann Surg*. 1999;229(3):322–330.
63. Pol B, Campan P, Hardwigsen J, et al. Morbidity of major hepatic resections: a 100-case prospective study. *Eur J Surg*. 1999;165(5):446–453.
64. Wu CC, Yeh DC, Lin MC, et al. Improving operative safety for cirrhotic liver resection. *Br J Surg*. 2001;88(2):210–215.
65. Jarnagin WR, Gonen M, Fong Y, et al. Improvement in perioperative outcome after hepatic resection: analysis of 1,803 consecutive cases over the past decade. *Ann Surg*. 2002;236(4):397–406.
66. Miyagawa S, Makuuchi M, Kawasaki S, Kakazu T. Criteria for safe hepatic resection. *Am J Surg*. 1995;169(6):589–594.
67. Belghiti J, Hiramatsu K, Benoist S, et al. Seven hundred forty-seven hepatectomies in the 1990s: an update to evaluate the actual risk of liver resection. *J Am Coll Surg*. 2000;191(1):38–46.
68. Melendez J, Ferri E, Zwillman M, et al. Extended hepatic resection: a 6-year retrospective study of risk factors for perioperative mortality. *J Am Coll Surg*. 2001;192(1):47–53.
69. Little SA, Jarnagin WR, DeMatteo RP, et al. Diabetes is associated with increased perioperative mortality but equivalent long-term outcome after hepatic resection for colorectal cancer. *J Gastrointest Surg*. 2002;6(1):88–94.
70. Wei AC, Tung-Ping Poon R, Fan ST, Wong J. Risk factors for perioperative morbidity and mortality after extended hepatectomy for hepatocellular carcinoma. *Br J Surg*. 2003;90(1):33–41.
71. Smyrniotis V, Kostopanagiotou G, Theodoraki K, et al. The role of central venous pressure and type of vascular control in blood loss during major liver resections. *Am J Surg*. 2004;187(3):398–402.
72. Nakajima Y, Shimamura T, Kamiyama T, et al . Control of intraoperative bleeding during liver resection: analysis of a questionnaire sent to 231 Japanese hospitals. *Surg Today*. 2002;32(1):48–52.
73. Lo CM, Fan ST, Liu CL, Lai EC, Wong J. Biliary complications after hepatic resection: risk factors, management, and outcome. *Arch Surg*. 1998; 133(2):156–161.
74. Schwartz M, Madariaga J, Hirose R, et al. Comparison of a new fibrin sealant with standard topical hemostatic agents. *Arch Surg*. 2004;139(11): 1148–1154.
75. Frilling A, Stavrou GA, Mischinger HJ, et al. Effectiveness of a new carrier-bound fibrin sealant versus argon beamer as haemostatic agent during liver resection: a randomised prospective trial. *Langenbecks Arch Surg*. 2005;390(2):114–120.
76. Wang WD, Liang LJ, Huang XQ, Yin XY. Low central venous pressure reduces blood loss in hepatectomy. *World J Gastroenterol*. 2006;12(6): 935–939.
77. Yamashita Y, Hamatsu T, Rikimaru T, et al. Bile leakage after hepatic resection. *Ann Surg*. 2001;233(1):45–50.
78. Bhattacharjya S, Puleston J, Davidson BR, Dooley JS. Outcome of early endoscopic biliary drainage in the management of bile leaks after hepatic resection. *Gastrointest Endosc*. 2003;57(4):526–530.
79. Lee CC, Chau GY, Lui WY, et al. Risk factors associated with bile leakage after hepatic resection for hepatocellular carcinoma. *Hepatogastroenterology*. 2005;52(64):1168–1171.
80. Capussotti L, Ferrero A, Vigano L, et al. Bile leakage and liver resection: where is the risk? *Arch Surg*. 2006;141(7):690–694; discussion 695.
81. Hayashibe A, Sakamoto K, Shinbo M, et al. New method for prevention of bile leakage after hepatic resection. *J Surg Oncol*. 2006;94(1): 57–60.
82. Tanaka S, Hirohashi K, Tanaka H, et al. Incidence and management of bile leakage after hepatic resection for malignant hepatic tumors. *J Am Coll Surg*. 2002;195(4):484–489.
83. Reed DN Jr, Vitale GC, Wrightson WR, et al. Decreasing mortality of bile leaks after elective hepatic surgery. *Am J Surg*. 2003;185(4):316–318.
84. Llovet JM, Schwartz M, Mazzaferro V. Resection and liver transplantation for hepatocellular carcinoma. *Semin Liver Dis*. 2005;25(2):181–200.
85. Cucchetti A, Ercolani G, Vivarelli M, et al. Impact of model for end-stage liver disease (MELD) score on prognosis after hepatectomy for hepatocellular carcinoma on cirrhosis. *Liver Transpl*. 2006;12(6):966–971.
86. Llovet JM. Updated treatment approach to hepatocellular carcinoma. *J Gastroenterol*. 2005;40(3):225–235.
87. Bruix J, Castells A, Bosch J, et al. Surgical resection of hepatocellular carcinoma in cirrhotic patients: prognostic value of preoperative portal pressure. *Gastroenterology*. 1996;111(4):1018–1022.
88. Poon RT, Fan ST. Assessment of hepatic reserve for indication of hepatic resection: how I do it. *J Hepatobiliary Pancreat Surg*. 2005;12(1):31–37.
89. Hemming AW, Scudamore CH, Shackleton CR, et al. Indocyanine green clearance as a predictor of successful hepatic resection in cirrhotic patients. *Am J Surg*. 1992;163(5):515–518.
90. Takayama T, Sekine T, Makuuchi M, et al. Adoptive immunotherapy to lower postsurgical recurrence rates of hepatocellular carcinoma: a randomised trial. *Lancet*. 2000;356(9232):802–807.
91. Fan ST, Lai EC, Lo CM, et al. Hospital mortality of major hepatectomy for hepatocellular carcinoma associated with cirrhosis. *Arch Surg*. 1995;130(2):198–203.
92. Sugawara Y, Yamamoto J, Higashi H, et al. Preoperative portal embolization in patients with hepatocellular carcinoma. *World J Surg*. 2002;26(1): 105–110.
93. Poon RT, Fan ST. Hepatectomy for hepatocellular carcinoma: patient selection and postoperative outcome. *Liver Transpl*. 2004;10(Suppl 1): S39–S45.
94. Devlin J, Ellis AE, McPeake J, et al. N-acetylcysteine improves indocyanine green extraction and oxygen transport during hepatic dysfunction. *Crit Care Med*. 1997;25(2):236–242.
95. Sklar GE, Subramaniam M. Acetylcysteine treatment for non-acetaminophen-induced acute liver failure. *Ann Pharmacother*. 2004;38(3):498–500.
96. Ben-Ari Z, Vaknin H, Tur-Kaspa R. N-acetylcysteine in acute hepatic failure (non-paracetamol-induced). *Hepatogastroenterology*. 2000;47(33): 786–789.
97. Bilimoria MM, Chaoui AS, Vauthey JN. Postoperative liver failure. *J Am Coll Surg*. 1999;189(3):336–338.
98. Matsumata T, Taketomi A, Kawahara N, et al. Morbidity and mortality after hepatic resection in the modern era. *Hepatogastroenterology*. 1995; 42(5):456–460.
99. Hemming AW, Reed AI, Fujita S, Foley DP, Howard RJ. Surgical management of hilar cholangiocarcinoma. *Ann Surg*. 2005;241(5):693–699; discussion 9–702.
100. Jarnagin WR, Fong Y, DeMatteo RP, et al. Staging, resectability, and outcome in 225 patients with hilar cholangiocarcinoma. *Ann Surg*. 2001;234(4):507–517.
101. Kawarada Y, Das BC, Naganuma T, et al. Surgical treatment of hilar bile duct carcinoma: experience with 25 consecutive hepatectomies. *J Gastrointest Surg*. 2002;6(4):617–624.
102. Zervos EE, Pearson H, Durkin AJ, et al. In-continuity hepatic resection for advanced hilar cholangiocarcinoma. *Am J Surg*. 2004;188(5):584–588.
103. Shimada K, Sano T, Sakamoto Y, Kosuge T. Safety and effectiveness of left hepatic trisegmentectomy for hilar cholangiocarcinoma. *World J Surg*. 2005;29(6):723–727.
104. Meunier B, Lakehal M, Tay KH, Malledant Y, Launois B. Surgical complications and treatment during resection for malignancy of the high bile duct. *World J Surg*. 2001;25(10):1284–1288.
105. Kawasaki S, Imamura H, Kobayashi A, et al. Results of surgical resection for patients with hilar bile duct cancer: application of extended hepatectomy after biliary drainage and hemihepatic portal vein embolization. *Ann Surg*. 2003;238(1):84–92.
106. Ijitsma AJ, Appeltans BM, de Jong KP, et al. Extrahepatic bile duct resection in combination with liver resection for hilar cholangiocarcinoma: a report of 42 cases. *J Gastrointest Surg*. 2004;8(6): 686–694.
107. Nagino M, Kamiya J, Uesaka K, et al. Complications of hepatectomy for hilar cholangiocarcinoma. *World J Surg*. 2001;25(10):1277–1283.

108. Sano T, Shimada K, Sakamoto Y, et al. One hundred two consecutive hepatobiliary resections for perihilar cholangiocarcinoma with zero mortality. *Ann Surg*. 2006;244(2):240–247.
109. Yang YM, Tian XD, Zhuang Y, et al. Risk factors of pancreatic leakage after pancreaticoduodenectomy. *World J Gastroenterol*. 2005;11(16):2456–2461.
110. Cullen JJ, Sarr MG, Ilstrup DM. Pancreatic anastomotic leak after pancreaticoduodenectomy: incidence, significance, and management. *Am J Surg*. 1994;168(4):295–298.
111. Rumstadt B, Schwab M, Korth P, et al. Hemorrhage after pancreatoduodenectomy. *Ann Surg*. 1998;227(2):236–241.
112. Bottger TC, Engelmann R, Junginger T. Is age a risk factor for major pancreatic surgery? An analysis of 300 resections. *Hepatogastroenterology*. 1999;46(28):2589–2598.
113. Grobmyer SR, Rivadeneira DE, Goodman CA, et al. Pancreatic anastomotic failure after pancreaticoduodenectomy. *Am J Surg*. 2000;180(2):117–120.
114. Hashimoto N, Yasuda C, Ohyanagi H. Pancreatic fistula after pancreatic head resection; incidence, significance and management. *Hepatogastroenterology*. 2003;50(53):1658–1660.
115. Yeh TS, Jan YY, Jeng LB, et al. Pancreaticojejunal anastomotic leak after pancreaticoduodenectomy: multivariate analysis of perioperative risk factors. *J Surg Res*. 1997;67(2):119–125.
116. Srivastava S, Sikora SS, Pandey CM, et al. Determinants of pancreaticoenteric anastomotic leak following pancreaticoduodenectomy. *Austral NZ J Surg*. 2001;71(9):511–515.
117. Aranha GV, Aaron JM, Shoup M, Pickleman J. Current management of pancreatic fistula after pancreaticoduodenectomy. *Surgery*. 2006;140(4):561–568.
118. Koukoutsis I, Bellagamba R, Morris-Stiff G, et al. Haemorrhage following pancreaticoduodenectomy: risk factors and the importance of sentinel bleed. *Dig Surg*. 2006;23(4):224–228.
119. Santoro R, Carlini M, Carboni F, et al. Delayed massive arterial hemorrhage after pancreaticoduodenectomy for cancer: management of a life-threatening complication. *Hepatogastroenterology*. 2003;50(54):2199–2204.
120. Tien YW, Lee PH, Yang CY, et al. Risk factors of massive bleeding related to pancreatic leak after pancreaticoduodenectomy. *J Am Coll Surg*. 2005;201(4):554–559.
121. Lillemoe KD, Cameron JL, Kim MP, et al. Does fibrin glue sealant decrease the rate of pancreatic fistula after pancreaticoduodenectomy? Results of a prospective randomized trial. *J Gastrointest Surg*. 2004;8(7):766–772.
122. Lowy AM, Lee JE, Pisters PW, et al. Prospective, randomized trial of octreotide to prevent pancreatic fistula after pancreaticoduodenectomy for malignant disease. *Ann Surg*. 1997;226(5):632–641.
123. Mansueto G, D'Onofrio M, Iacono C, et al. Gastroduodenal artery stump haemorrhage following pylorus-sparing Whipple procedure: treatment with covered stents. *Dig Surg*. 2002;19(3):237–240.
124. Barnett SP, Hodul PJ, Creech S, et al. Octreotide does not prevent postoperative pancreatic fistula or mortality following pancreaticoduodenectomy. *Am Surg*. 2004;70(3):222–226.
125. Levy MJ, Chari S, Adler DG, et al. Complications of temporary pancreatic stent insertion for pancreaticojejunal anastomosis during pancreaticoduodenectomy. *Gastrointest Endosc*. 2004;59(6):719–724.

CHAPTER 61

Critical Care of Thoracic Surgery Patients

THOMAS L. HIGGINS, GARY M. HOCHHEISER, and ROSE B. GANIM

INTRODUCTION

Thoracic surgical patients are among the most complicated admissions to the intensive care unit (ICU), due to challenging preoperative status, the variety of possible operative procedures, airway and pleural appliances, and requirement for postoperative interventions, including airway management, mechanical ventilation, and pain control. Information transfer is key: the ICU physicians and nurses must have a clear understanding of the operative procedure accomplished, the patient's expected medical course, and the predictable potential complications. More time than usual must be allotted for briefing of the ICU team by the operative team.

Immediate concerns include assessment of oxygenation, cardiovascular support to ensure adequate oxygen delivery, provision of ventilation support if needed, and transferring monitors and drains that accompany the patient from the operating room. Special concerns apply to fluid management (discussed in detail below) and pain control, which is especially important as pain will limit respiratory effort and can precipitate delirium and agitation. Table 61.1 provides a checklist for immediate interventions.

In operations where the pleural space has been opened, the patient will arrive with at least one, and usually two or more chest tubes. Complete lung expansion helps force out any remaining extrapleural air. The apical chest tube should demonstrate evidence of removing air from the thorax with bubbling seen in the water seal bottle. The posterior/inferior tube(s) should be draining blood; and some clots are expected. However, large quantity of clot suggests continued bleeding is occurring. An immediate chest radiograph will confirm the absence of significant pneumothorax or effusions, and confirm proper invasive line and chest tube placement.

PREOPERATIVE CONSIDERATIONS: IDENTIFYING THE HIGH-RISK PATIENT

The patient undergoing thoracic surgery is frequently older with concurrent medical problems, and often debilitated due to cancer and associated malnutrition. Pulmonary abnormalities commonly arise from prior occupational exposure, tobacco use, or a primary disease process. Prior history of asthma, wheezing, or allergic airway responses are risk factors and serve to identify patients in whom bronchodilator management may be needed in the postoperative period.

Many thoracic surgical patients have preoperative pulmonary function tests (PFTs), particularly if lung resection is contemplated. However, these tests by themselves are not reliable predictors of postoperative pulmonary function. The FEV_1 (forced expiratory volume in 1 second) provides a reasonable indicator of a patient's postoperative ability to cough effectively and clear secretions. A patient's postoperative FEV_1 is affected by inspiratory muscle strength, elastic recoil, and degree of obstructive air trapping, as well as any surgical removal of lung tissue. However, the decrease in FEV_1 after lung resection for cancer is not necessarily a simple proportional relationship if an obstructed lobar or mainstem bronchus was present. A cutoff value for postpneumonectomy FEV_1 of 800 mL is commonly used as a criterion of resectability, since this amount is required to generate a cough adequate to clear secretions.

Surgical entry to the chest cavity, even if tissue is not resected, produces substantial changes in lung function, with lateral thoracotomy producing greater postoperative impairment than median sternotomy or thoracoscopy. Following thoracotomy, forced vital capacity and functional residual capacity (FRC) can fall to less than 60% of their preoperative values on the first postoperative day. Subsequent return to baseline can take up to 14 days. Any decline in FRC is especially important, because the resulting atelectasis contributes to physiologic shunting and hypoxemia.

Diffusion capacity for carbon monoxide (DLCO) is routinely measured prior to lung resection and can be useful as a predictor of postoperative pulmonary morbidity and mortality. DLCO has been found to be more predictive of postoperative mortality than FEV_1. With preoperative DLCO below 80%, postoperative pulmonary complications are increased, and DLCO below 60% is associated with increased mortality (1); DLCO can be further compromised by chemotherapy and radiation. PFTs can be combined with pulmonary perfusion scanning to determine a predicted postoperative DLCO (ppoDLCO) to estimate the amount of capacity that will be present after resection.

In patients with severe chronic obstruction, the best predictors of postoperative ventilation requirements are arterial pO_2 less than 70% of that predicted for age, and the presence of dyspnea at rest (2). Factors associated with postoperative pneumonia after elective surgery include low preoperative serum albumin values, high ASA physical status classification, smoking history, prolonged preoperative stay, longer operative procedure, and thoracic or upper abdominal site for surgery (3).

Advanced age is frequently cited as a surgical risk factor, although frailty may be more discriminating than chronologic age (4). Elderly patients have a number of age-related changes in pulmonary function, including decreased elastic recoil and progressive stiffening of the chest wall, increased ratio of FRC to total lung capacity, and diminished vital capacity and FEV_1 (5). The activity of upper airway reflexes is blunted, which may result in impaired clearance of secretions and ability to protect the airway. The loss of elasticity and compliance can result in compromised vital capacity and increased residual volume. Elderly patients also have a decreased response to hypoxia and hypercapnia, and the decline in muscular reserve can affect

TABLE 61.1 Immediate ICU Considerations in the Thoracic Surgical Patient

Preparation
- Supplemental oxygen or mechanical ventilator ready
- Bedside monitoring: ECG, pulse oximetry; possible arterial, central or PA line
- Infusion pumps if inotropes, vasopressors or vasodilators in use
- Wall suction to connect to pleural drainage system

On arrival in ICU
- Connect patient to bedside monitors and ventilator (if needed)
- Check and secure all connections to chest tubes and assess function
- Auscultate breath sounds and observe chest excursion; suction if necessary
- Assess adequacy of circulation (BP, HR, pulse oximetry)
- Assess adequacy of oxygenation and ventilation (via ABG or noninvasive devices)
- Consider need for lung-protective ventilation if trauma/sepsis/operative issues
- Fluid management: confirm need for continued maintenance fluid; generally keep "dry"
- Monitor input and output; label all chest tubes and chart outputs
- Pain control with intravenous analgesics and/or regional anesthetics/analgesics
- Order any necessary laboratory studies and chest radiograph

Information to be obtained from operating room team
- Patient name, age, gender, and brief history
- Operation performed and any major problems encountered
- Circulatory and ventilatory requirements as determined in OR
- Current drug infusions and titration plans; timing and dose antibiotics
- Anesthetic agents given and plans for awakening/extubation (if relevant)
- Fluids and blood products given; urine output during case
- Estimated blood loss, assessment of hemostasis at closing and blood products available (including surgical salvage if any)
- Laboratory results (e.g., ABGs, Hct) obtained during operating room

TABLE 61.2 Respiratory Failure Risk Index

Preoperative Predictor	Point Value
Type of Surgery	
Abdominal aortic aneurysm	27
Thoracic procedure	21
Neurosurgery, upper abdominal, or peripheral vascular	14
Neck procedure	11
Emergency surgery	11
Albumin (<30 g/L)	9
BUN (>30 mg/dL)	8
Partially or fully dependent functional status	7
History of chronic obstructive pulmonary disease	6
Age (yr)	
≥70	6
60–69	4

Adapted from Arozullah AM, Daley J, Henderson WG, et al. Multifactorial risk index for predicting postoperative respiratory failure in men after major noncardiac surgery. *Ann Surg.* 2000;332:242–253.

FEV_1 (6). Obesity results in decreases in FRC and expiratory reserve volume (ERV), causing the ERV to drop below closing volume, resulting in perfused, unventilated segments of lung and a widened alveolar–arterial (A-a) O_2 gradient. Obese patients are more likely to cough poorly, retain secretions and develop basilar atelectasis.

Cigarette smoking is well recognized for its contribution to perioperative morbidity via effects on the cardiovascular system, mucus secretion and clearance, and small airway narrowing. Although patients are invariably counseled to stop smoking prior to elective surgery, data from coronary artery bypass patients suggests this should occur at least 8 weeks prior to surgery, because smoking cessation just prior to surgery may actually increase the risk of postoperative pulmonary complications (7), probably due to transient increases in sputum volume. In the case of cancer, however, surgery is rarely delayed and aggressive pulmonary toilet including liberal use of bronchoscopy may be employed.

Major operations such as lobectomy and many pleural procedures are now accomplished without thoracotomy and the use of rib retraction. Video-assisted thoracic surgery (VATS) has become a more standard approach in major lung resection. The physiologic insult created using this technique has changed the acceptable risk profile for patients undergoing thoracic procedures. VATS lobectomy has been shown to have decreased morbidity, lower narcotic requirement, and quicker recovery time, as well as less delirium in the elderly and an earlier return to ambulation (8–12). This decrease in postoperative morbidity has allowed for these operations to be performed on patients with preoperative functional status that would be unacceptable for thoracotomy.

Expectations as to the duration of postoperative respiratory failure allow the caregiver to heighten his or her awareness if the patient behaves in unanticipated ways. A very large patient population from the Veterans Affairs Medical Centers provided a database for researchers to learn what factors play a role in predicting postoperative respiratory failure (13). Factors negatively influencing outcome included the type of surgery, emergency surgery, low preoperative albumin, high preoperative BUN, partial or full dependent status, COPD, and age greater than 60 years (7). These factors are all assigned a point status (Table 61.2); more points increase the probability of postoperative respiratory failure (Table 61.3). It is important to realize women were excluded from data collection in this study but the factors noted do not have gender specificity.

OPERATING ROOM EVENTS IMPACTING ICU CARE

The pace of postoperative recovery depends on the amount and types of anesthetic agents given as premedication and during the operative procedure. Anesthetic delivery is constrained by patient factors. For example, the need for high FiO_2, particularly during one-lung anesthesia, limits the ability to use nitrous oxide (N_2O). In general, the FiO_2 should be minimized due to concerns for oxygen-induced pulmonary toxicity, particularly in patients who have received neoadjuvant radiation and/or chemotherapy (14). A goal of early extubation limits the use of opioids. Regional techniques—spinal, epidural—can supplement general anesthesia but are generally not applicable to operative anesthesia for open thoracic procedures because of the difficulty in providing a high-enough spinal level. Controlled ventilation is necessary to sustain respiration during open-thorax procedures. For most procedures, the plan is to have the patient awake, comfortable, and extubated at the end

TABLE 61.3 Respiratory Failure Risk Index Scores and Outcomes

Class	Point Total	*N* (%)[a]	Predicted Probability of Postoperative Respiratory Failure	Observed Phase I[a] (% Respiratory Failure)	PRF Phase II[a] (% Respiratory Failure)
1	≤10	39,567 (48%)	0.5%	0.5%	0.5%
2	11–19	18,809 (23%)	2.2%	2.1%	1.8%
3	20–27	13,865 (17%)	5.0%	5.3%	4.2%
4	28–40	7,976 (10%)	11.6%	11.9%	10.1%
5	>40	1,502 (2%)	30.5%	30.9%	26.6%

[a]Phase I indicates patients enrolled between October 1, 1991, and December 31, 1993, and phase II indicates patients enrolled between January 1, 1994, and August 31, 1995.
Adapted from Arozullah AM, Daley J, Henderson WG, et al. Multifactorial risk index for predicting postoperative respiratory failure in men after major noncardiac surgery. *Ann Surg*. 2000;332:242–253.

of the procedure, thus avoiding the potential stress on fresh suture lines from positive-pressure ventilation and coughing or bucking on the endotracheal tube.

Selective endobronchial intubation with isolation of the right and left lungs permits the surgeon to operate on a quiet, collapsed lung, while the contralateral side is ventilated. Disposable polyvinyl double-lumen tubes are available in odd sizes between 35 and 41 French in both right-sided and left-sided configurations. The nonoperative bronchus is usually chosen for selective intubation in lobectomies and pneumonectomies, so that surgical manipulation does not displace the tube, and to allow resection of the mainstem bronchus if necessary. When selective endobronchial intubation is impossible—as in pediatric patients, very small adults, laryngectomy patients—a bronchial blocker can be placed under fiberoptic guidance to selectively occlude a bronchus.

One-lung ventilation alters the ventilation–perfusion relationship as blood passing through the unventilated lung effectively causes a right-to-left shunt, reducing arterial saturation. Perfusion of the unventilated lung will be reduced somewhat by physical collapse of the lung and hypoxic pulmonary vasoconstriction. The double-lumen endotracheal tube (DLETT) is large and has the potential to cause airway trauma and edema, may shift its position, and is a more challenging suction portal. The DLETT is generally removed at the end of the operation and replaced by a single-lumen tube when continued mechanical ventilation is required. Specific indications for continued postoperative selective endobronchial intubation include the need to protect the lung against soilage—pus or blood—and provision of different levels of positive end-expiratory pressure (PEEP) to differentially compliant lungs in emphysematous patients undergoing single-lung transplantation. A fiberglass resin tube-changer and a pediatric (small diameter) fiberoptic bronchoscope are essential tools, which should be available in the ICU for placement and adjustment of double-lumen tubes.

Minimally invasive techniques have been used with increasing frequency in thoracic surgery. These include VATS for major anatomic lung resection, pleural space procedures, and minimally invasive esophagectomy; robotic-assisted surgical procedures are performed through similar incisions. The benefit to smaller incisions, with no retraction placed on ribs or abdominal musculature, has improved the postoperative complication and recovery profile for these operations. The use of VATS in the resection of early-stage lung cancer has resulted in a decrease in overall complications, pulmonary complications, atrial dysrhythmias, and need for transfusion (15).

The choice of location for postoperative recovery depends on the degree of patient illness, and the ability of a particular nursing unit to deal with postoperative ventilation and/or hemodynamic monitoring. At many hospitals, patients undergoing bronchoscopy, mediastinoscopy, esophageal dilatation, esophagoscopy, gastrostomy, jejunostomy, laryngoscopy, pleuroscopy, or scalene node biopsy can spend a short time in the postanesthesia recovery unit (PACU) and then be transferred to a step-down or general nursing floor, or even sent home. Patients undergoing lobectomy, segmental or wedge pulmonary resections, hiatal hernia repairs, or Heller myotomy can generally be recovered in PACU and then sent to a step-down unit if there are no complications. Patients undergoing esophagectomy, esophagogastrectomy, and pneumonectomy are likely to have ongoing monitoring or postoperative ventilation needs, and generally are managed in an ICU.

IMMEDIATE POSTOPERATIVE ISSUES

Usual postoperative monitoring includes intermittent blood pressure determinations, continuous electrocardiography, and pulse oximetry. In selected patients, assessing intravascular volume status and cardiopulmonary function may be facilitated with central venous pressure or pulmonary artery catheters but is rarely necessary.

Chest tubes are usually inserted to drain the surgical site at the end of the procedure, except with pneumonectomy patients where standard practice is to avoid a chest tube unless there is the need to monitor the pneumonectomy space postoperatively. Chest tubes should never be clamped during patient transport, because of the dangers of unrecognized bleeding and tension pneumothorax. Chest tubes, except for those in pneumonectomy spaces, are usually connected to a vacuum regulator to provide negative 20 cm H_2O suction. A chest radiograph will confirm endotracheal, nasogastric, and chest tube placement, and identify any pneumothorax, mediastinal shift, or significant atelectasis. Routine chest x-rays are not necessary after uncomplicated removal of chest tubes and the decision to reinsert a chest tube is usually based on clinical appearance rather than radiologic findings (16).

Commercially available chest tube systems vary in their appearance, but all provide calibrated drainage chambers, a method to release excess positive pressure, and regulated amounts of negative pressure. Air bubbles are normally expected in the chamber that limits the amount of applied suction; air bubbles in the water seal chamber represent an active leak.

Thoracic drain devices have been developed to quantitatively measure air flow through the system as a measurement of the size of an air leak. This allows for greater confidence in the determination of when a leak has sealed. Data is collected and stored locally which can be visualized in a graph format allowing visual assessment of the trend of air flow (Thopaz drain, Medela Switzerland). Use of this system has allowed for earlier chest tube removal (17).

Hourly output from chest tubes should be recorded, and the operative team notified if drainage is greater than 100 mL/hr for more than 4 hours, or if greater than 200 mL of drainage is recorded in any 1-hour observation period. Expected chest tube drainage from major procedures in the first 24 hours is roughly 300 to 600 mL, tapering to less than 200 mL by the second day. Daily chest radiographs are usually obtained while chest tubes are in place. The level of fluid in the water seal chamber should fluctuate with each respiration (assuming no air leak) and serves as confirmation of chest tube patency. Most pulmonary resection patients will return with mild-to-moderate air leaks, which become problematic only if the underlying lung parenchyma does not completely expand to fill the pleural space, or if a significant percentage of tidal volume is lost through the chest tubes with mechanical ventilation. Additional pleural drainage may then be required, or changes in ventilation made to minimize the air leak and optimize ventilation. Leaks may occur only above a given inflation pressure, and ventilation techniques such as smaller volumes at higher rates, pressure-controlled inverse ratio ventilation (IRV), or high-frequency oscillation (HFO) can minimize leaks and allow a seal to develop. Once all air leaks resolve and drainage is minimal—less than 100 mL/24 hr—chest tubes may be removed during the expiratory phase of ventilation or while the patient performs a Valsalva maneuver.

Prophylactic PEEP is sometimes used in an effort to decrease postoperative drain output, especially from mediastinal drains in cardiac surgery patients. The evidence, however, suggests higher PEEP levels do not affect chest tube output or transfusion requirements (18).

Extubation and Airway Concerns

Extubation can often be accomplished in the operating room, but continued ventilation may be necessary with concurrent cardiac illness, inability to protect airway, malnutrition, or coexisting lung disease. Silent aspiration of gastric contents is an important complication following pulmonary resections, and maintenance of endotracheal intubation for 24 hours postoperatively has been shown to decrease the occurrence of pneumonia and the operative mortality rate (19) in high-risk patients.

Measurement of maximal inspiratory pressure (MIP)—often called negative inspiratory force (NIF)—is helpful in determining respiratory muscle strength, particularly in patients recovering from thymectomy for myasthenia gravis, and in those who received long-acting neuromuscular blocking agents in the operating room. Residual neuromuscular blockade can be assessed using a train-of-four monitor and reversed, if necessary, with small doses of neostigmine plus vagolytic agents such as atropine or glycopyrrolate. Ideally, the patient should be awake and following instructions, and have an adequate gag reflex—signifying airway protection—and cough—for secretion clearance. Measured parameters suggesting readiness for extubation include a respiratory rate to tidal volume (f/Vt) ratio of <100, an MIP of greater than 25 cm H_2O and adequate oxygen saturation (≥92%) on FiO_2 ≤50% at PEEP ≤5 cm H_2O. Although many patients will not strictly meet these criteria for extubation, it is usually best to attempt weaning and extubation rather than risk of the complications of continued ventilation. Specific indications to delay extubation are in Table 61.4.

TABLE 61.4 Selected Indications for Continued Postoperative Ventilation

- Airway compromise due to edema or bleeding
- Inadequate pulmonary reserve postsurgery
- Compromised myocardial function, especially with perioperative infarction
- Expected large fluid shifts with thoracoabdominal procedures
- Severe neurologic impairment
- Continued bleeding with likelihood of return to operating room
- Esophageal surgery patients (risk for reflux and aspiration; delay extubation until airway reflexes have fully recovered as for "full-stomach" intubation)

Laryngeal and glottic edema frequently occurs after airway manipulation or intubation with a large DLETT. The presence of serious laryngeal edema can be detected—after first suctioning the posterior pharynx—by deflating the endotracheal tube cuff, and occluding the endotracheal tube and watching for evidence of airway obstruction. Endotracheal intubation may need to be maintained while edema resolves; racemic epinephrine and corticosteroids are traditionally used, although the literature support for this is sparse. If there is any doubt about airway patency, the endotracheal tube should be removed only under direct laryngoscopic or fiberoptic observation, with a percutaneous tracheostomy set immediately at hand to provide airway access should re-intubation be impossible because of airway swelling.

Only a minority of thoracic surgery patients require postoperative ventilation and, in these, reduction of barotrauma becomes an additional consideration. Mechanical ventilation is associated with cytokine production, and even conventional tidal volumes may contribute to lung injury in critically ill patients (20). Low tidal volumes (6 mL/kg) are recommended in patients at risk for ARDS (21), but more research is needed to conclude whether a lung-protective strategy benefits all patients (22). The normal inspiratory to expiratory ratio is about 1:2, and inspiratory times longer than 1 second are poorly tolerated in awake patients. Longer inspiratory times reduce peak airway pressure, but often require addition of sedative agents and in patients with significant airway obstruction may not allow sufficient time for exhalation, resulting in auto-PEEP with consequent hemodynamic compromise.

Assist control, intermittent mandatory ventilation, or continuous positive airway pressure with pressure support can be employed. Evidence is insufficient to conclude whether pressure-controlled ventilation is superior or inferior to volume-controlled ventilation with acute lung injury (23). The FiO_2 in the early postoperative period is generally set at 0.5 to 0.6, and then reduced as clinically appropriate. The combination of pulse oximetry and end-tidal carbon dioxide monitoring will reduce the need for frequent arterial blood gas sampling. Controversy still exists as to the optimal level of PEEP in the thoracic surgery patient. Low levels of PEEP (3 to 5 cm H_2O) may be helpful in restoring FRC and substituting for the "physiologic PEEP" of the glottis.

Airway pressure release ventilation (APRV) is a pressure-controlled mode of ventilation; exhalation occurs when the inflating pressure is released from a sustained high level. With the majority of time spent in the high-pressure phase, it is thus a form of IRV. Because it allows spontaneous breathing, it is often better tolerated, with less sedation, than pressure-controlled IRV (PC-IRV). The higher mean airway pressures may be a concern with air leaks, but APRV has been shown to improve oxygenation, particularly in thoracic trauma patients (24).

Neurally adjusted ventilator assist (NAVA) is emerging as a method to better match ventilator assistance to patient needs, by assessing diaphragmatic electrical activity via an esophageal probe (25). As diaphragmatic activity occurs before airway flow or pressure changes, synchrony between the patient and the ventilator may be improved using NAVA, although more clinical studies are presently needed.

HFO ventilation is the logic extension of the "open lung" concept; cyclic exchange of tidal volume is replaced by sustained inflation with air exchange taking place by a variety of mechanisms including convection and diffusion stimulated by oscillations in the range of 3 to 7 Hz (equivalent to 180 to 420 breaths/min). While long employed in neonatal critical care, HFO has been widely adopted for adults with ARDS; recent literature suggests no advantage and possible harm in a subset of patients where HFO was applied early in adults with moderate to severe ARDS (26). HFO requires a specialized ventilator (Sensormedics 3100B, Viasys Healthcare, Yorba Linda, CA). High-frequency jet ventilation (HFJV), which involves rapid pulses of air entraining additional volume, has a role in the operating room during "shared airway" procedures (i.e., laryngoscopy, bronchoscopy, microlaryngeal procedures, and airway surgery). The role of HFJV in the ICU, particularly for management of hypoxemic respiratory failure, is poorly defined; the one exception being ventilation of a patient with a bronchopleural fistula. In theory, HFJV allows ventilation at lower airway pressures than conventional ventilation. The reduction in ventilation pressure will minimize the amount of air passing through the fistula and may promote healing by allowing adjacent tissues to approximate and possibly seal the fistula. In the face of decreased pulmonary compliance, the beneficial effect of HFJV in lowering airway pressure may be lost (27).

Noninvasive ventilation (NIV) has been shown to improve survival in acute care patients, particularly when applied early rather than as a rescue treatment. A recent review summarizes 178 studies, including the use of NIV for prevention and treatment of postextubation and postoperative acute respiratory failure (28).

Postoperative Fluid Management

Thoracic surgery patients present unique issues in terms of fluid management in the postoperative period due to the heightened potential for pulmonary edema. Postpneumonectomy pulmonary edema occurs in approximately 4% to 27% of patients (29,30) and pulmonary edema from all causes in 27% of pneumonectomy patients (14). Understanding the contribution of insensible—600 to 1200 mL/d in a 70-kg adult—and measured fluid loss during the surgical procedure provides valuable information when anticipating the patient's needs in the postoperative period. Thoracic surgery patients may also have operative losses of 6 to 8 mL/kg/hr of "third-space" fluid to the interstitial space and intracavitary areas (31). The choice of fluid for resuscitation is left to the discretion of the caregiver as there is no known difference in outcome with the use of either isotonic crystalloid or colloid.

During their procedures, patients are exposed to intraoperative handling of the lung, fresh frozen plasma (FFP), prolonged one-lung ventilation, collapse and re-expansion of the lung, as well as increases in postresection pulmonary artery pressures (32). These factors all contribute to the lung parenchyma being primed for a more profound inflammatory response and potential fluid accumulation. Patients undergoing procedures involving the mediastinum, such as esophagectomies or tumor excision, experience even more profound fluid shifts and pose a greater management challenge in the postoperative period.

There is no formula applicable across the broad spectrum of patient types seen in this population to adequately predict fluid needs. Traditional markers of perfusion help determine if a patient is adequately volume resuscitated. These include urine output—usually over 0.5 mL/kg/hr—mental status, blood pressure, heart rate, blood lactate level, capillary refill time, venous oxygen saturation, and filling pressures and cardiac performance. Pulse pressure and stroke volume variation (SVV) can be helpful in assessing preload in mechanically ventilated patients; PPV and SVV are less useful in the operating room when the chest is open (33).

Resection patients, especially if a right-sided pneumonectomy and experiencing high ventilatory pressures during surgery (14), require greater scrutiny when determining fluid needs due to the increased risk for postpneumonectomy pulmonary edema. Ideally, the clinician will limit crystalloid infusion to 20 mL/kg for the first 24 hours in this cohort (13). If a state of poor perfusion persists, then invasive devices allowing for precise hemodynamic monitoring and oxygen consumption need consideration in an effort to accurately establish goals of therapy.

Pain Management

The pain associated with thoracotomy is considered one of the most intense of any surgical procedures (34); adequate pain control is important not only to ensure patient comfort but also avoid potential cardiac and pulmonary complications. Early pain management is also important in an effort to reduce the chances of developing long-term postthoracotomy pain (35). The reasons for pain in this setting are many and include the skin incision, dissection of the intercostal muscles and pleura, pleural irritation, chest tube insertion, and prolonged rib retraction leading to ligamentous and muscle injury (15). Without satisfactory pain relief the patient is exposed to adverse effects, including an inability to breathe deeply which decreases vital capacity and FRC. Splinting also occurs making it more difficult to clear secretions. These factors increase the likelihood of developing respiratory failure in the postoperative period. The cardiovascular system is at risk, as pain is associated with elevated circulating levels of catecholamines, which act on the myocardium to increase oxygen consumption.

A variety of options exist for pain management, including systemic analgesics, neuraxial opioids, and local anesthetics via the epidural or intrathecal route, regional anesthesia such as intercostal and paravertebral nerve blocks, and adjuvant therapies such as transcutaneous electrical nerve stimulation (TENS) or applied heat.

The mainstay of postoperative pain control is systemic analgesics in the form of opioids. Agents such as morphine, fentanyl, and hydromorphone are frequently used and can be administered intravenously, subcutaneously, or intramuscularly, with the intravenous route providing the most predictable responses; barring an emergency, intramuscular injections would be considered less than optimal. Opioid side effects remain the greatest issue with respiratory depression, nausea, vomiting, and ileus being a few examples. Nonopiate medications such as nonsteroidal anti-inflammatory agents, including the parenteral prostaglandin inhibitor ketorolac (36), are reasonable adjuncts to the opioids. It is necessary to exercise caution when using NSAIDs in the face of underlying renal insufficiency as their use may exacerbate the renal dysfunction. Additionally, NSAIDs may pose a risk with postoperative healing; one animal model demonstrated less effective pleural adhesions following pleurodesis (37).

Neuraxial opioids and local anesthetics via the epidural or intrathecal route provide excellent regional pain control. Epidural catheters have been the preferred route, and when local anesthetics, either with or without opioids, are infused in this manner the incidence of pulmonary complications decrease relative to systemic opioids (38). The initiation of epidural catheters prior to the operation appears to be the ideal approach as it allows for better management of pain in the postoperative setting (39). Hypotension due to sympathetic blockade is a potential side effect when local anesthetics, such as bupivicaine, are administered. Therefore, it may be necessary to either decrease the dose or eliminate the local anesthetic completely from the infusion and utilize opioids exclusively.

Intercostal and paravertebral nerve blocks provide for regional pain control; these may be performed either intraoperatively or postoperatively, provide relief lasting up to 12 hours, may need repetitive dosing, and can even be accomplished with cryoablation of the intercostal nerves during the surgery (40). Chest tube insertion sites are potential sites of discomfort and may be blocked either directly or proximally. Intercostal nerve blocks are relatively contraindicated in post-pneumonectomy patients due to the risks of entering and contaminating the empty chest cavity.

ON-Q Pain Relief System

The On-Q® system (On-Q, Lake Forest, CA) consists of an elastomeric ball reservoir for local anesthetic such as bupivacaine or ropivacaine, connected to a long fine catheter. The catheter can be tunneled to provide a multilevel paraspinal block and may be placed at the bedside or in the operating room at thoracotomy (41). These long paraspinal blocks are a viable alternative to an epidural catheter for the management of both rib fracture and postthoracotomy pain; the local anesthetics provide an opioid-sparing effect (42,43).

The described methods are some of the traditional modalities utilized when controlling pain in the thoracic surgery patient. TENS, heat and cold application, music therapy, and relaxation techniques are additional means of providing a comfortable setting (23). In addition, patients requiring prolonged postoperative mechanical ventilation may benefit from the centrally acting alpha adrenergic agonist dexmedetomidine, which reduces the amount of narcotic needed for pain control (44) and is associated with less delirium than other agents.

SPECIFIC PATIENT POPULATIONS

Thoracic Trauma

Trauma patients are typically evaluated and treated for acute, life-threatening injuries prior to ICU arrival. The critical care physicians' role is to understand the nature of the injuries, whether blunt or penetrating, and the anticipated clinical course. In addition, maintaining a high degree of vigilance is paramount for diagnosing potential missed injuries.

Typical blunt injuries to the chest include rib fractures, flail chest, hemothorax, pneumothorax, tension pneumothorax, pulmonary contusion, cardiac contusion, and aortic disruption. Penetrating traumas such as gunshots and stabbings are less predictable in terms of the injuries generated and therefore require a case-by-case assessment in terms of management issues. Uncontrolled hemoptysis or cavitary lesions following penetrating injury require emergent surgical intervention.

Mortality increases in thoracic trauma with increasing age, lower Glasgow Coma Scale scores, liver injury, splenic injury, >5 rib fractures, and long-bone fractures. Mortality rates typically are between 9% and 20% in the United States (45). If the patient suffers an out-of-hospital cardiac arrest in relation to their trauma, the chances of survival diminish even further, with less than 10% of patients in this group surviving to hospital discharge (46).

Rib fractures are the most common type of chest trauma with ribs five through nine the most susceptible; while this injury is rarely life-threatening, rib fractures may serve as indicators for more severe intrathoracic or intra-abdominal injuries. Pain may be significant, leading to splinting, hypoventilation, atelectasis, and potentially pneumonia as pulmonary toilet is compromised. First and/or second rib fractures indicate a large transfer of energy to the thoracic cage and should raise further suspicion for other intrathoracic problems, such as aortic rupture or tear (47). Patients aged 65 and older pose a particular problem when faced with these types of injuries as, with each rib fracture, mortality increases by 19% and the risk of pneumonia by 27% (48). The implications of age begin at 45 years as those with four or more rib fractures in this group show more in-hospital complications, such as increased ventilator and ICU days (49).

Flail chest (Fig. 61.1) is defined as three or more adjacent ribs fractured at two or more sites creating a segment of paradoxical wall motion; any large number of rib fractures can similarly impair respiratory mechanics, especially, as is often

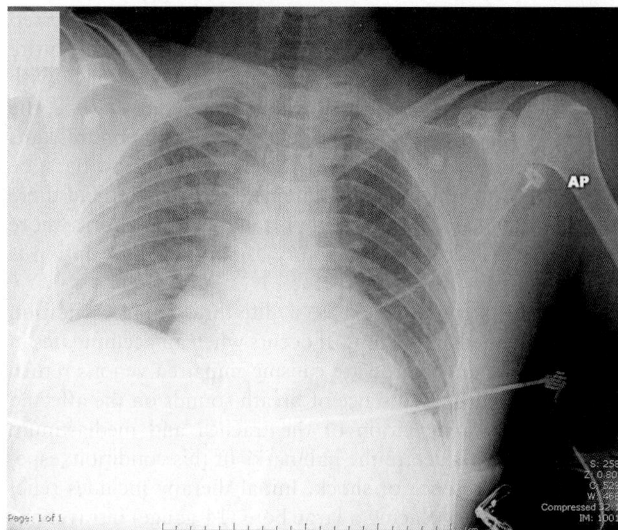

FIGURE 61.1 There are multiple fractured ribs on the right with several fractured in more than one place. This leads to a flail segment with inspiration.

the case, there is associated pulmonary contusion. Mainstays of management include aggressive pain control (including the use of either an epidural catheter or On-Q device), aggressive pulmonary toilet, and both invasive and noninvasive mechanical ventilation. Stabilization of rib fractures through surgical internal fixation has demonstrated both reduced pain and increased pulmonary function with subsequent earlier separation from mechanical ventilation. In some patients at risk for respiratory decompensation, mechanical ventilation may be avoided altogether (50).

Hemothorax is a collection of blood in the pleural cavity. Patients potentially experience chest pain, dyspnea, and tachycardia along with dullness to percussion and decreased or absent breath sounds to auscultation on the affected side. Chest x-ray helps to confirm the diagnosis if the collection of blood is large enough (i.e., >200 mL) to be seen radiographically. The mainstays of therapy are ensuring adequate circulating blood volume and tube thoracostomy to drain blood from the pleural space. Thoracotomy is required if bleeding continues at a significant rate, defined as 1,500 mL of blood output with initial tube placement or continuous bleeding of at least 250 mL/hr for 4 hours or if the patient's vital signs suddenly decompensate (28). Failure to adequately drain the hemothorax potentially leads to a condition of retained clot; this is problematic as it may progress toward empyema or fibrothorax. Options for therapy include further tube thoracostomy, open thoracotomy, VATS, or intrapleural fibrinolytic therapy. Further, tube thoracostomy likely has a limited role as it will not consistently liberate clotted blood products, while early surgical drainage with VATS decreases duration of tube drainage, length of hospital stay, and hospital cost (51). VATS is the surgical intervention of choice as it is less invasive than open thoracotomy and just as effective unless there are extensive adhesions (52). Fibrinolytic therapy offers a possible alternative to thoracoscopy or decortication, especially if the time from injury to therapy is delayed, with a response rate of up to 92% in terms of resolution (53).

Pneumothorax is the accumulation of air, originating from the lung, between the visceral and parietal pleura and is the most common intrathoracic finding following blunt or penetrating trauma. The size of the pneumothorax is expressed as a percentage, determined by its size relative to the entire lung on an anterior–posterior chest x-ray film. Treatment with tube thoracostomy is indicated when the size is over 20%, the patient is on positive-pressure ventilation, or there are signs and symptoms of hypoxia and dyspnea. If, following tube placement, the lung does not completely re-expand and there is a persistent air leak, it is important to search for a more severe tracheal or bronchial injury as surgical intervention is then required.

Tension pneumothorax is a life-threatening condition requiring immediate therapy. It occurs when air accumulates in a hemithorax under pressure causing impaired venous return and cardiac output. Absence of breath sounds on the affected side along with deviation of the trachea and mediastinum away from that side are the hallmarks of this condition, especially in the presence of shock. Initial therapy includes relief of the pressure by placing a large bore (14-gauge) intravenous catheter into the second intercostal space in the midclavicular line on the affected side followed by tube thoracostomy to treat the pneumothorax.

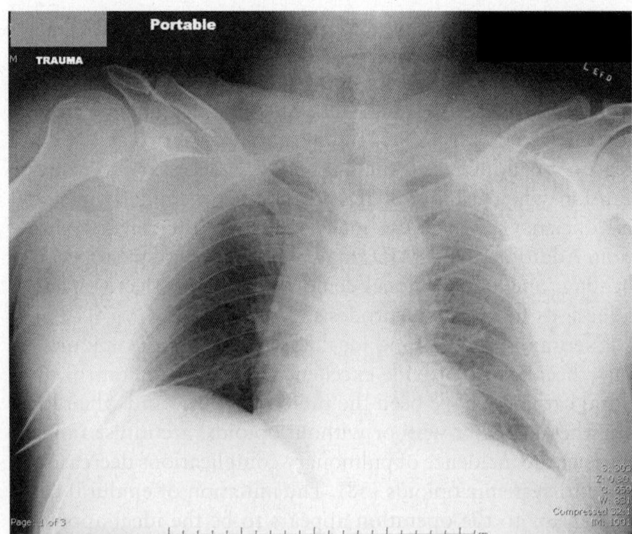

FIGURE 61.2 Diffuse infiltrative pattern on the left side is consistent with findings seen following pulmonary contusion.

Pulmonary contusion (Fig. 61.2) is a result of blunt force transmitted across the thorax. The mechanism for its development is not completely understood but is felt to be related to compression and re-expansion of the lung tissue leading to capillary disruption with interstitial and intra-alveolar edema, decreased compliance, and hypoxemia due to shunt physiology (28). Care is largely supportive in this population with close attention to pain management and pulmonary toilet.

Cardiac contusion is a potential complication of blunt chest trauma; its exact incidence is unclear as different studies utilized varying criteria to make the diagnosis (35). It is typically well tolerated in mildly injured patients, but may lead to fatal dysrhythmias or cardiogenic shock if severe. Rapid deceleration, as occurs in motor vehicle accidents, is the most common cause as the heart is able to move freely and strike the internal sternum with a substantial amount of force (54). Electrocardiographic findings of cardiac contusion are summarized in Table 61.5. Biomarkers, such as creatine kinase (CK) or troponin

TABLE 61.5 Electrocardiographic Findings in Cardiac Contusion

Nonspecific abnormalities
Pericarditis-like ST segment elevation or PTa depression
Prolonged QT interval
Myocardial injury
New Q wave
S-T segment elevation or depression
Conduction disorders
Right bundle branch block
Fascicular block
AV nodal conduction disorders (1-, 2- and 3-degree AV block)
Dysrhythmias
Sinus tachycardia
Atrial and ventricular extrasystoles
Atrial fibrillation
Ventricular tachycardia
Ventricular fibrillation
Sinus bradycardia
Atrial tachycardia

AV, atrioventricular.

Adapted from Sybrandy KC, Cramer MJM, Burgersdijk C. Diagnosing cardiac contusion: old wisdom and new insights. *Heart.* 2003;89:485–489.

TABLE 61.6 Echocardiographic Findings in Acute Cardiac Contusion

Transthoracic echocardiography
- Regional wall motion abnormalities
- Pericardial effusion
- Valvular lesions
- Right and left ventricular enlargement
- Ventricular septum rupture
- Intracardiac thrombus

Transesophageal echocardiography
- Aortic endothelial laceration or aortic dissection
- Aortic rupture

I and T, are potentially helpful in the diagnosis as the histologic changes associated with contusion are similar to those seen with infarction. Troponin I and T are specific to the myocardium and may allow avoidance of false positives by relying solely on CK as trauma patients often have diffused muscular damage leading to massive CK release from many tissues. Electrocardiography may show nonspecific findings, such as sinus tachycardia and premature atrial or ventricular systoles, and not offer further clarification of the diagnosis (35). Echocardiography, whether transthoracic (TTE) or transesophageal (TEE), offers the best insight into cardiac damage from contusion as wall motion abnormalities are directly visualized (Table 61.6). Treatment involves cardiac monitoring and stabilization of the traumatically induced injuries, supporting blood pressure and cardiac output as indicated.

Aortic disruption leads to a high mortality, as less than 15% of these patients reach the hospital alive. Those surviving to reach the hospital have a 30% chance of subsequent rupture and death (55). Diagnostic modalities include chest x-ray showing a widened mediastinum, aortography (the gold standard), CT scanning, and TEE. Treatment is immediate surgery by a cardiothoracic surgeon to repair the injury.

Posttraumatic empyema occurs in up to 2% of the thoracic trauma population and is most often caused by *Staphylococcus aureus* (56). Factors increasing the likelihood of developing empyema include retained hemothorax, pulmonary contusion, and multiple chest tube placements (57). Treatment includes removal of the infected fluid collection which may be accomplished by guided drainage, VATS, or open thoracotomy.

Lung Volume Reduction Surgery

Lung volume reduction surgery (LVRS) is used in an effort to improve pulmonary dynamics of patients with severe emphysema by palliating dyspnea and improving functional status. Along with supplemental oxygen, this is the only intervention associated with reduced mortality in these patients. This population is prone to more postsurgical complications than most other thoracic surgery patients due to their underlying fragility—loss of physiologic reserve. Anticipated complications include dysrhythmias, prolonged respiratory failure, prolonged air leaks, pneumonia, and ICU readmission. Air leaks occur in 90% of patients and rarely benefit from pulmonary reoperation (58). The prevalence of air leaks correlate with a more prolonged, complicated hospital course, and severity is predicted by patient characteristics such as worse pulmonary function, use of inhaled steroids, distribution of disease (lower lobe disease less frequent and shorter duration), and presence of adhesions (40). Management involves chest tube drainage with efforts to minimize or eliminate suction, so the tissue has the greatest chance to heal. These leaks may be ameliorated by bronchoscopic placement of intrabronchial one-way valves (such as the investigational Spiration IBV, Olympus Respiratory, Tokyo, Japan) that allow clearance of secretions and the exhalation of air, but prevent further escape to the pleural space (59).

Esophageal Surgery

Esophageal surgery patients undergo procedures that traumatize the lung, the interposed stomach, and the diaphragm. Patients undergoing esophageal resection for carcinoma tend to be malnourished and are often compromised by preoperative neoadjuvant chemotherapy and radiation therapy. Pulmonary complications including atelectasis, pneumonia, aspiration, and retained secretions are seen. Up to 29% of patients experience respiratory complications (60), with increasing patient age and decreasing performance on spirometry predictive of increased risk (61). Aspiration risk is minimized by having patients undergo a thorough swallowing evaluation, including radiographic testing, prior to initiating oral intake.

The most dangerous complication of esophageal surgery is surgical site leak. Anastomotic leak occurs in as many as 11% of patients, and factors impacting the incidence include high estimated intraoperative blood loss, cervical location of the anastomosis, and the development of postoperative ARDS (62). Interestingly, the use of thoracic epidural analgesia is associated with a decreased occurrence of anastomotic leakage (55). Mortality associated with anastomotic leaks is historically high, but with improved surgical technique patients now have a more promising outcome. One center showed a reduction in mortality with intrathoracic leaks from 43% to 3.3% over a 34-year period (63). Early identification is important; endoscopy provides a safe method for evaluating the integrity of the graft and whether surgery is necessary to avoid its loss (64).

Minimally invasive techniques are also being used in the treatment of esophageal disease, including major esophageal resection for malignancy. The advantages of minimally invasive techniques for lung procedures are also seen with patients undergoing minimally invasive esophagectomy. Postoperative pulmonary complications, length of ICU stay, and intraoperative blood loss have been found to be decreased with the minimally invasive approach (65). Esophagectomy can be performed with these techniques either through an abdominal and thoracic approach with either a thoracic or cervical anastamosis.

RESPIRATORY THERAPY

Thoracic surgical patients often have significant underlying COPD, impaired mucociliary clearance, excessive secretions, and/or increased closing volumes, all of which predispose to atelectasis. The respiratory therapist plays an important role in providing secretion management and chest physiotherapy, including percussion and vibration. Other modalities supporting recovery include adequate hydration, aerosolized bronchodilators, humidified oxygen, and early identification and treatment of infection of the tracheobronchial tree. Chest physiotherapy should begin as soon as the patient has recovered sufficiently from anesthesia to cooperate. Mucolytic agents,

TABLE 61.7 Postoperative Complications following Any Thoracic Procedure

Airway edema/stridor
Arytenoid dislocation
Aspiration of gastric contents
Atelectasis
Bronchospasm
Bronchopleural fistula
Chylothorax
Congestive heart failure
Deep venous thrombosis
Dysrhythmias (especially atrial fibrillation, multifocal atrial tachycardia)
Empyema
Hemorrhage
Hemothorax
Infection (superficial, deep)
Lobar collapse
Lobar torsion
Myocardial infarction
Pain and splinting
Pleural effusion
Pneumothorax
Pulmonary embolus
Re-expansion pulmonary edema
Respiratory failure
Retaining secretions
Subcutaneous emphysema
Tension pneumothorax

From Higgins TL. Selected issues in postoperative management. In: *The ACCP Critical Care Board Review*. Northbrook, IL: American College of Chest Physicians; 1998:323–334, with permission.

such as *N*-acetylcysteine, are helpful in solubilizing thick secretions, and are usually given in conjunction with a bronchodilator since they may cause bronchospasm. Oral or nasotracheal suctioning is utilized in selected extubated patients, but discomfort and the possibility of complications—hypoxemia, vagal-mediated bradycardia or cardiac arrest—limit routine use. A minitracheostomy (bedside percutaneous cricothyroidotomy for suctioning) can provide access to the lower airway in patients with thick secretions. Inadequate clearance of secretions often requires flexible bronchoscopy, which is of greatest benefit in the extubated patient who cannot adequately be suctioned. If pulmonary parenchymal involvement is confined to one lung, altering body position can improve gas exchange by changing the relationships between ventilation and perfusion. The lateral decubitus position, with the *uninvolved* lung "down," allows maximal blood flow to ventilated areas during spontaneous ventilation. This relationship may be altered with mechanical breaths and application of PEEP. Specialized beds can be set to supine, lateral, or rotating modes to optimize oxygenation (66).

COMPLICATIONS

Complications common to all thoracic surgical patients are listed in Table 61.7; those more likely to occur following specific procedures are listed in Table 61.8.

Airway complications can be precipitated by prolonged intubation with large or DLETTs, passage of bronchial blockers, use of rigid bronchoscopes, or frequent reintubation. Edema of the larynx or trachea can substantially narrow the cross-sectional area of the airway. Assessing the patient for an

TABLE 61.8 Complications of Specific Thoracic Procedures

Procedure	Complications
Anterior mediastinotomy (Chamberlain)	Damage to recurrent laryngeal nerve (particular left)
Bronchoscopy/mediastinoscopy	Bleeding from major vessels if torn, air leak with biopsy of bronchus
Bronchopleural fistula repair	Persistent leak, dehiscence
Bronchopulmonary lavage	Respiratory distress/contralateral spillage
Bullectomy	Tension pneumothorax; air leak
Chest wall reconstruction	Blood loss, altered chest wall compliance, unstable chest, infection prosthetic material
Clagett window	Air leak
Collis Belsey	Gastric leak, splenic injury
Decortication	Blood loss, air leak(s)
Esophageal dilatation	Esophageal perforation, pleural effusion, airway obstruction
Esophagoscopy	Esophageal perforation
Esophagogastrectomy	"Third-spacing" of fluids, anastomotic leak, gastric devascularization, splenic injury, gastric torsion
Heller myotomy	Esophageal tear
Lobectomy	Bronchial leak, lobar collapse, lobar torsion
Mediastinal tumor excision	Airway obstruction with sedation/anesthesia; damage to recurrent laryngeal nerve
Nissen fundoplication	Esophageal obstruction (with tight wrap), splenic injury
Pectus repair	Costrochondritis, unstable sternum
Pleuroscopy	Pharyngeal laceration, air leak
Pneumonectomy	Atrial dysrhythmias (atrial fibrillation, MAT), mediastinal shift, cardiac torsion, air embolism, disrupted bronchus)
Thoracic aortic aneurysm	Paraplegia, bleeding, aortobronchial fistula, esophageal injury
Thymectomy	In myasthenics, possible weakness and respiratory failure
Lung transplant	Rejection (day 5), reperfusion injury, infection, overdistension of native lung, dehiscence
Tracheal resection	Fixed neck flexion postoperatively; dehiscence, air leak

From Higgins TL. Selected issues in postoperative management. In: *The ACCP Critical Care Board Review*. Northbrook, IL: American College of Chest Physicians; 1998:323–334, with permission.

air leak around an occluded endotracheal tube just prior to extubation may identify significant laryngeal and supraglottic edema. Upright or sitting position, intravenous corticosteroids (67), and racemic epinephrine respiratory treatments are the mainstay of edema reduction. A critical airway may be converted to an adequate airway by the administration of Heliox, a helium and oxygen mixture (68); helium, being less dense and less viscous than nitrogen, allows maintenance of laminar flow through a critically swollen upper airway. Prolonged endotracheal intubation or temporary tracheostomy may be required to allow resolution of airway edema.

The recurrent laryngeal nerves branch from the vagus nerves as they enter the chest. The right recurrent laryngeal nerve arises high in the apex of the right chest and loops around the right subclavian artery to travel back to the larynx in the tracheoesophageal groove. The left recurrent laryngeal nerve, which is more susceptible to injury, wraps around the aortic arch in the left chest before it enters the tracheoesophageal groove. Injury can result from excessive traction, aggressive dissection about these nerves, or the operative sacrifice of these nerves. Mediastinoscopy, anterior mediastinotomy, left pulmonary resection with subaortic exenteration, and resections of mediastinal tumors are common operations in which the recurrent laryngeal nerve may be damaged. Associated airway and laryngeal edema may allow for adequate coaptation of the vocal cords for the first days postextubation often preventing identification of cord injury until after discharge from the ICU, when ineffective cough or aspiration of secretions will become apparent. If there is permanent damage or division of the recurrent laryngeal nerve, injection of the vocal cord with a long-lasting substance such as Teflon may be considered. In many instances, aggressive chest physiotherapy, careful airway management, and temporary avoidance of oral feeding may eliminate the need for any intervention until recovery of the nerve function has occurred. Intermittent noisy inspiration and painful swallowing suggest arytenoid dislocation, an uncommon cause of postextubation respiratory failure (69). Treatment consists of surgical reduction which must be accomplished before the cricoarytenoid joint becomes fibrosed in poor position.

Retained secretions and blood in the airway are especially common if the airway was opened, as during a bronchoplastic procedure or closure of a bronchial stump. Mechanical airway obstruction secondary to secretions may be aggravated by bronchospasm, and preoperative bronchodilators should be continued in patients with reactive airways as secretions can precipitate coughing and bronchospasms.

Postoperative air leaks most often result from very distal fistulae between tiny bronchioles or respiratory units and the pleural cavity. One of the main functions of the chest tube is to evacuate air from these small air leaks to assure complete expansion of the lung and coaptation of the cut surface of the lung to the parietal pleura, which will seal these leaks. Repositioning of the chest tubes or insertion of further chest tubes into undrained spaces, adequate suction applied to the pleural cavity, and full expansion of the lung with vigorous chest physiotherapy help to close these small distal fistula. A substantial persistent air leak from the chest tube or incomplete expansion of the lung suggests a significant bronchopleural fistula. Major proximal airway problems such as failure of the anastomosis, disruption of a bronchial closure, or retained secretions or foreign bodies can be identified by bronchoscopy. Within the first 7 postoperative days, any fistula is likely to be due to a technical problem. More than 1 week after the operation, but usually within the first 6 weeks, fistulae are more often due to an empyema or local peribronchial abscess. Late occurrence of a bronchopleural fistula—more than 6 months after the operation—is frequently due to recurrent lung carcinoma.

Early postoperative bronchopleural fistula in a pneumonectomy patient is a surgical emergency. The typical presentation is sudden expectoration of copious amounts of pink, frothy sputum, which may be misdiagnosed as pulmonary edema. The patient should be positioned with the operated or pneumonectomy side down, to trap remaining fluid in the pneumonectomy space and prevent drowning. A chest x-ray will show loss of fluid from the pneumonectomy space. Further management will likely include bronchoscopy to assess the stump closure, and likely immediate reoperation.

Postpneumonectomy empyema is initially treated with closed tube drainage and antibiotic therapy. After the patient has been stabilized then definitive surgical management will be required. This may include decontamination of the space through antimicrobial irrigation, drainage, and subsequent space filling and closure (Claggett procedure) or the creation of an open window thoracostomy (Claggett window, or Eloesser flap). A vacuum-assisted closure (VAC) device may be used to assist in infection control and wound closure in this very difficult patient population (70).

Postoperative hypoxemia is common, and may be due to sepsis, ARDS, pneumonia, or pulmonary embolization. If pulmonary emboli are suspected, ventilation/perfusion scanning, spiral computed tomography, and pulmonary angiography should be done, and treatment initiated with anticoagulation or lytic therapy, depending on timing and indications. If these measures are contraindicated, then an inferior vena caval filter should be placed. Systemic tumor emboli, though uncommon, may be seen after pulmonary resections for primary bronchogenic carcinomas or metastatic sarcomas.

Massive postoperative hemorrhage can present as significant shock, occasionally as the patient is transferred to the recovery room or ICU. This potentially lethal condition can be the result of a slipped tie from the pulmonary vein, or less commonly, the pulmonary artery, and requires emergent reoperation. Slower postoperative hemorrhage usually results from small bleeding arteries or veins in the mediastinum or chest wall. Reoperation is required for control of bleeding, and to evaluate the hemothorax to prevent future fibrothorax or restrictive lung disease.

Pulmonary Parenchymal Complications

Tracheoesophageal Fistula

A communication may occur between the anterior esophageal wall and membranous (posterior) wall of the trachea following prolonged intubation due to pressure exerted from the cuff of the endotracheal or tracheostomy tube potential tissue necrosis. Tracheoesophageal fistula should be suspected when feedings are aspirated from the airway. While surgical revision of the damaged area is the definitive therapy, it may not be practical in patients still requiring positive-pressure ventilation and is often delayed until the patient has been weaned off mechanical ventilation (71). Stenting of the esophagus, performed at the bedside in the ICU, allows for temporary sealing of the fistula until the patient is a suitable candidate for final surgical repair (72).

Tracheoinnominate Fistula

Bleeding seen 48 hours or more following tracheostomy raises concern about the presence of a tracheoinnominate fistula. Even though this occurs rarely, it is a life-threatening complication and requires urgent action. The majority of cases arise when pressure necrosis on the posterior aspect of the blood vessel occurs due to overinflation of the tracheostomy cuff. Initial steps include hyperinflation of the tracheostomy cuff or direct arterial compression with a finger to tamponade the bleeding. Classically, bronchoscopy is the diagnostic procedure of choice followed by surgery to divide the innominate artery with subsequent buttressing of the trachea from the divided artery by viable tissue (73). CT angiography and stent grafting are increasingly described as a less invasive option in these tenuous patients (74).

Atelectasis

The most common complication following thoracic surgery is atelectasis. Potential contributors include hypoventilation, splinting, bronchospasm, poor cough, retained secretions, pneumothorax, and trauma to the lung during the surgical procedure. The majority of patients in the ICU will tolerate some degree of atelectasis with symptoms including fever, tachypnea, dysrhythmias, hypoxia, or respiratory failure. More severe atelectasis, or a compromised host, can present with respiratory failure requiring mechanical ventilation. Auscultation of the lungs may identify the impaired areas due to diminished air movement, and chest x-ray may further highlight the portions of collapsed lung. Atelectasis is not limited to the lung on the operative side, although it is more likely to occur in that parenchyma. Likely influenced by the ARDSnet study (22), clinicians are now routinely using lower tidal volumes than in the past, contributing to an increased incidence of atelectasis (75). Recruitment maneuvers and increasing PEEP may counteract the atelectasis created by lung-protective ventilation strategies (76).

Efforts to avoid atelectasis include frequent suctioning of the tracheobronchial tree, chest percussion and postural drainage, humidification of inspired gases, frequent patient rotation, bronchodilators, pain control, coughing, deep breathing, bronchoscopy for removal of mucus plugs or secretions, and early ambulation (15). Chest physiotherapy uses physical therapy such as clapping and vibration to stimulate coughing and thereby move secretions out of the lungs. Incentive spirometry, often employed following surgical procedures, does not provide the same benefit as chest physiotherapy in the recovery phase; the latter potentially decreases hospital costs due to shorter lengths of stay (77).

Lobar Collapse and Torsion

Lobar collapse most commonly occurs in the right upper lobe following surgery utilizing a DLTT due to bronchial occlusion. It may be due to kinking due to upward rotation of the airway, particularly in the right middle lobe after right upper lobectomy, and in the left lower lobe after upper lobectomy. Retained secretions may be managed with liberal bronchoscopy and usually diminish with the resolution of airway edema and acute inflammation.

Lobar torsion occurs as the result of a lung segment twisting about its hilar structures. This twisting occludes the bronchial, arterial, and venous supply to the affected segment, with infarction occurring if the process is not recognized and treated. Right middle lobe torsion is most common after upper lobectomy; however, any lobe can be at risk (15). The patient initially presents with atelectasis, but a high level of suspicion should prompt early diagnostic bronchoscopy; this is a surgical emergency. Prompt reoperation should follow, with reduction of the torsion and either pexy or lobectomy as appropriate.

Pleural Complications

Pneumothorax is the second most frequent postoperative complication after atelectasis (15). Signs and symptoms of pneumothorax range from subtle to severe, and include increased work of breathing, decreased breath sounds and chest movement, wheezing, hypoxia, increased airway pressures if still on the ventilator, and hemodynamic instability if tension pneumothorax occurs. Chest x-ray is the first test used in the diagnosis of pneumothorax save for the instance when tension is present and chest tube placement must occur immediately to prevent further clinical deterioration of the patient. If a pneumothorax develops on the surgical side and chest tubes are already present, it is necessary to ensure the tubes are functioning properly. This involves inspecting the entire system for any evidence of leaks, inadequate suction, or loss of tubing patency due to blood clots. It is possible to declot chest tubes with vigorous "stripping" or placing a balloon occlusion catheter to physically remove the obstruction.

Pleural effusions persisting in the postoperative period should be evaluated via thoracentesis to determine if there is intrathoracic or extrathoracic cause. If the fluid is transudative, the underlying etiology needs to be addressed; if exudative, a high suspicion for empyema must be maintained. If pleural effusions and pneumothoraces do not resolve over time, the decision for more definitive therapy, such as pleurodesis, needs be entertained.

Thoracic duct injury is a known complication following any surgery involving dissection in the posterior mediastinum and may result in chylothorax. Confirmation of the diagnosis includes testing the pleural fluid which will be high in triglycerides and chylomicrons. Initial management includes thoracostomy tube drainage and parenteral nutrition. Octreotide may assist in decreasing the volume of chyle. High-volume (1,000 mL/d) chyle loss is predictive of failure of conservative management and prompt surgical ligation of the thoracic duct can decrease morbidity (78). In select centers, this may be accomplished with lymphangiography and embolization (79).

Other Complications

Atrial Fibrillation

Atrial fibrillation occurs in up to 30% of thoracic surgical patients and is likely due to a combination of factors such as local inflammation, volume changes, and adrenergic stimulation. Unfortunately, this is associated with increased hospital stay, morbidity, and mortality. For these reasons, all patients undergoing major thoracic surgery, who do not have a contraindication, should receive prophylaxis. In patients already on beta-blocker therapy, it should be continued without interruption. Other effective options include magnesium supplementation, calcium channel blockers, and amiodarone (80,81); some attempt to keep the serum K^+ level at 4 to 4.5 mEq/L and the Mg^{++} level at 2 to 2.5 mg/dL. Preoperative administration of statins is also associated with reduced incidence of atrial fibrillation in noncardiac thoracic surgery (82).

Postoperative Infections

The incidence of developing nosocomial infection following lung surgery increases with a history of COPD, duration of surgery (with an increased risk for each additional minute), and ICU admission (83). Surgical site infection occurs rarely due to the richly vascular muscle closures of the thorax, and the use of prophylactic perioperative antibiotics. Factors increasing the risk of an infection at the incision site include emergent thoracotomy in the trauma patient, and procedures for treatment of empyema, lung abscess, mediastinitis, or perforated esophagus. Any unexplained fever requires careful inspection of the surgical site.

When air tracks into the subcutaneous space via the path of least resistance, it generates subcutaneous emphysema. The air is forced along these pathways with positive-pressure ventilation and instances of increased intrathoracic pressure during spontaneous breathing: coughing and forced exhalation are two examples. Subcutaneous air may be striking in appearance but rarely affects patient outcome in a detrimental way. If the collection of air is massive enough to compromise the airway, endotracheal intubation may be indicated, recognizing the pitfalls of instituting positive-pressure ventilation in such a situation. Historically, small skin incisions loosely packed with saline-soaked gauze or angiocath sheaths can be placed at the top of the shoulders to allow the evacuation of air. More effective treatment is establishing control of the pleural space, usually with the placement of an (additional) thoracostomy tube. In a complex pleural space, this can most effectively be accomplished with CT guidance.

SUMMARY

The thoracic patient presents unique management issues due to the complexities of fluid management, preoperative morbidities, the need for specialized pain control to preserve respiratory function, and nature of drainage devices left in place postoperatively. As a critical care physician, it is important to understand the interplay of these circumstances when anticipating the patient's postoperative needs in the ICU. The pulmonary system is more susceptible to adverse events if fluid management is not judiciously managed. Patients undergoing thoracotomies for lung or esophageal surgery tend to have an impaired functional status and nutrition at baseline, negatively impacting their postoperative course. If pain control is inadequate, the patient will have impaired pulmonary function, which potentially delays their recovery. Chest tubes require extra vigilance due to the potential complications should they malfunction. As with all ICU patients, early mobilization can be helpful in reducing ICU and hospital length of stay, as well as reducing the need for sedation and incidence of delirium (84). With a well thought–out care plan, the outcome for thoracic surgery patients will be positive and the road to recovery smooth.

Key Points

- Risk should be assessed preoperatively and at ICU admission:
  - PFTs and DLCO
  - Age and fragility
  - Comorbid conditions, especially renal and cardiac
  - Operating room events reducing or increasing risk
- Immediate ICU concerns
  - Monitor BP, EKG, pulse oximetry; CVP or PAC monitoring rarely needed
  - Mechanical ventilation if not extubated; lung protection if at risk for ARDS
  - Preload assessment and fluid resuscitation if indicated; otherwise minimize fluids
  - Understand chest tubes, air leaks, expected levels of bloody drainage
- Routine for uncomplicated patients
  - Pain management: systemic and local; minimize sedation
  - Early extubation or conversion to non-invasive ventilation
  - Early mobilization to reduce delirium, length-of-stay, and costs
  - ICU safety and prophylaxis against stress ulcers, DVT, infection
- Common complications and their management
  - Respiratory insufficiency, atelectasis, secretions, ARDS
  - Airway edema (especially after double-lumen intubation)
  - Air leaks, pneumothorax, and hemothorax
  - Atrial fibrillation and role of prophylaxis
  - Recognition of surgical emergencies such as lobar torsion and tension pneumothorax

References

1. Ferguson MK, Little L, Rizzo L, et al. Diffusing capacity predicts morbidity and mortality after pulmonary resection. *J Thorac Cardiovasc Surg*. 1988; 96:894–900.
2. Nunn JF, Miledge S, Chen D, Dore C. Respiratory criteria for fitness for surgery and anesthesia. *Anaesthesia*. 1988;43:543–611.
3. Garibaldi RA, Britt MR, Coleman ML, et al. Risk factors for postoperative pneumonia. *Am J Med*. 1981;70:677–680.
4. Makary MA, Segev DL, Pronovost PJ, et al. Frailty as a predictor of surgical outcomes in older patients. *J Am Coll Surg*. 2010;210:901–908.
5. Wahba WM. Influence of aging on lung function: clinical significance of changes from age twenty. *Anesth Analg*. 1983;62:764–776.
6. Janssens JP, Pache JC, Nicod LP. Physiological changes in respiratory function associated with ageing. *Eur Respir J*. 1999;13:197–205.
7. Warner MA, Offord KP, Warner ME, et al. Role of preoperative cessation of smoking and other factors in postoperative pulmonary complications: a blinded, prospective study of coronary artery bypass patients. *Mayo Clin Proc*. 1989;64:609–616.
8. Decamp MM Jr, Jaklitsch MT, Mentzer SJ, et al. The safety and versatility of video-thoracoscopy: a prospective analysis of 895 cases. *J Am Coll Surg*. 1995;181:113–120.
9. McKenna R. Thoracoscopic lobectomy with mediastinal sampling in 80 year old patients. *Chest*. 1994;106:1902–1904.
10. Landreneau RL, Hazelrigg SR, Mack MJ, et al. Postoperative pain-related morbidity: video-assisted thoracic surgery versus thoracotomy. *Ann Thorac Surg*. 1993;56:1285–1289.
11. Jaklitsch MT, Decamp MM Jr, Liptay MJ, et al. Video-assisted thoracic surgery in the elderly: a review of 307 cases. *Chest*. 1996;110(3):751–758.
12. Cattaneo SM, Park BJ, Wilton AS, et al. Use of video-assisted thoracic surgery for lobectomy in the elderly results in fewer complications. *Ann Thorac Surg*. 2008;85(1):231-235.

13. Arozullah AM, Daley J, Henderson WG, et al. Multifactorial risk index for predicting postoperative respiratory failure in men after major noncardiac surgery. *Ann Surg*. 2000;332:242–253.
14. Grocott HP. Oxygen toxicity during one-lung ventilation: is it time to re-evaluate our practice? *Anesthesiol Clin*. 2008;26:273–280.
15. Boffa DJ, Dhamija A, Kosinski AS, et al. Fewer complications result from a video-assisted approach to anatomic resection of clinical stage I lung cancer. *J Thorac Cardiovasc Surg*. 2014;148(2):637–643.
16. Palesty JA, McKelvey AA, Dudrick SJ. The efficacy of x-rays after chest tube removal. *Am J Surg*. 2000;179:13–16.
17. Pompilli C, Detterbeck FC, Papagiannopoulos K, et al. Multicenter international randomized comparison of objective and subjective outcomes between electronic and traditional chest drainage systems. *Ann Thorac Surg*. 2014; 98(2):490–496.
18. Collier B, Kolff J, Devineni R, Gonzalez LS. Prophylactic positive end-expiratory pressure and reduction of postoperative blood loss in open-heart surgery. *Ann Thorac Surg*. 2002;74(4):1191–1194.
19. DeHaven CB Jr, Hurst JM, Branson RD. Evaluation of two different extubation criteria: attributes contributing to success. *Crit Care Med*. 1986;14:92–94.
20. Determann RM, Royakkers A, Wolthius EK, et al. Ventilation with lower tidal volumes as compared with conventional tidal volumes for patients without acute lung injury: a preventive randomized controlled trial. *Crit Care*. 2010;14:R1.
21. The Acute Respiratory Distress syndrome Network. Ventilation with lower tidal volumes as compared with traditional tidal volumes for acute lung injury and the acute respiratory distress syndrome. *N Engl J Med*. 2000;342:1301–1308.
22. Neto AS, Nagtzaam L, Schultz MJ. Ventilation with lower tidal volumes for critically ill patients without the acute respiratory distress syndrome: a systematic translational review and meta-analysis. *Curr Opin Crit Care*. 2014; 20:25–32.
23. Chacko B, Peter JV, Tharyan P, et al. Pressure-controlled versus volume-controlled ventilation for acute respiratory failure due to acute lung injury (ALI) or acute respiratory distress syndrome (ARDS). *Cochrane Database Syst Rev*. 2015;14(1):CD008807.
24. Dart BW 4th, Maxwell RA, Richart CM, et al. Preliminary experience with airway pressure release ventilation in a trauma/surgical intensive care unit. *J Trauma*. 2005;59:71–76.
25. Terzi N, Piquilloud L, Roze H, et al. Clinical review: update on neurally adjusted ventilator assist: report of a round-table conference. *Crit Care*. 2012;16:225.
26. Ferguson ND, Cook DJ, Guyatt GH, et al. High frequency oscillation in early acute respiratory distress syndrome. *N Engl J Med*. 2013; 368. 795–805.
27. Baumann MH, Sahn SA. Medical management and therapy of bronchopleural fistulas in the mechanically ventilated patient. *Chest*. 1990;97:721–728.
28. Cabrini L, Landoni G, Oriani A, et al. Noninvasive ventilation and survival in acute care settings: a comprehensive systematic review and meta-analysis of randomized controlled trials. *Crit Care Med*. 2015; 43:880–888.
29. Slinger PD. Perioperative fluid management for thoracic surgery: the puzzle of postpneumonectomy pulmonary edema. *J Cardiothorac Vasc Anesth*. 1995; 9(4):442–451.
30. van der Werff YD, van der Houwen HK, Heijmans P, et al. Postpneumonectomy pulmonary edema: a retrospective analysis of incidence and possible risk factors. *Chest*. 1997;111:1278-1284.
31. Amini S, Gabrielli A, Caruso LJ, et al. The thoracic surgical patients: initial postoperative care. *Semin Cardiothorac Vasc Anesth*. 2002;6(3):169–188.
32. Jordan S, Mitchell JA, Quinlan GJ, et al. The pathogenesis of lung injury following pulmonary resection. *Eur Respir J*. 2000;15:790–799.
33. de Waal EEC, Rex S, Kruitwagen CJLL, et al. Dynamic preload indicators fail to predict fluid responsiveness in open-chest conditions. *Crit Care Med*. 2009;37:510–515.
34. Loan WB, Morrison JD. The incidence and severity of postoperative pain. *Br J Anaesth*. 1967;39:695–698.
35. Katz J, Jackson M, Kavanagh BP. Acute pain relief after thoracic surgery predicts long term post-thoracotomy pain. *Clin J Pain*. 1996;12(1):50–55.
36. Yee JP, Koshiver JE, Allbon C, et al. Comparison of intramuscular ketorolac tromethemine and morphine sulfate for analgesia of pain after major surgery. *Pharmacotherapy*. 1986;6(5):253-261.
37. Lardinois D, Vogt P, Yang L, et al. Non-steroidal anti-inflammatory drugs decrease the quality of pleurodesis after mechanical pleural abrasion. *Eur J Cardiothorac Surg*. 2004;25(5):865–871.
38. Ballantyne JC, Carr DB, deFerranti S, et al. The comparative effects of postoperative analgesic therapies on pulmonary outcome: cumulative meta-analyses of randomized, controlled trials. *Anesth Analg*. 1998;86:598–612.
39. Yegin A, Erdogan A, Kayacan N, et al. Early postoperative pain management after thoracic surgery; pre and postoperative versus postoperative epidural anesthesia: a randomized study. *European J Cardiothoracic Surg*. 2003;24(3):420–424.
40. Peeters-Asdourian C, Gupta S. Choices in pain management following thoracotomy. *Chest*. 1999;115:122S–124S.
41. Chelly JE, Ghisi D, Fanelli A. Continuous peripheral nerve blocks in acute pain management. *Br J Anaesth*. 2010;105(S1):86–96.
42. Ried M, Schilling C, Potzger T, Ittner KP, et al. Prospective, comparative study of the On-Q® PainBuster® postoperative pain relief system and thoracic epidural analgesia after thoracic surgery. *J Cardiothorac Vasc Anesth*. 2014;28:985–990.
43. Truitt MS, Mooty RC, Amos J, et al. Out with the old, in with the new: a novel approach to treating pain associated with rib fractures. *World J Surg*. 2010;34:2359–2362.
44. Herr DL, Sum-Ping ST, England M. ICU sedation after coronary artery bypass graft surgery: dexmedetomidine-based versus propofol-based regimens. *J Cardiothoracic Vasc Anesth*. 2003;17(5):576–584.
45. Kulshrestha P, Munshi I, Wait R. Profile of chest trauma in a level I trauma center. *J Trauma*. 2004;57:576–581.
46. Lockey D, Crewsdon K, Davies G. Traumatic cardiac arrest. who are the survivors? *Ann Emerg Med*. 2006;48(3):240–244.
47. Munshi IA. Thoracic trauma. In: Higgins TL, ed. *Cardiopulmonary Critical Care*. Oxford: BIOS Scientific Publishers Ltd; 2002:363–379.
48. Bulger EM, Arneson MA, Mock CN, et al. Rib fractures in the elderly. *J Trauma*. 2000;48(6):1040–1046.
49. Holcomb JB, McMullin NR, Kozar RA, et al. Morbidity from rib fractures increases after age 45. *J Am Coll Surg*. 2003;196(4):549–555.
50. Doben AR, Eriksson EA, Denlinger CE, et al. Surgical rib fixation for flail chest deformity improves liberation from mechanical ventilation. *J Crit Care*. 2014 29:139–143.
51. Meyer DM, Jessen ME, Wait MA, et al. Early evacuation of traumatic retained hemothoraces using thoracoscopy: a prospective, randomized trial. *Ann Thorac Surg*. 1997;64:1396–1400.
52. Navsaria PH, Vogel RJ, Nicol AJ. Thoracoscopic evacuation of retained posttraumatic hemothorax. *Ann Thorac Surg*. 2004;78:282–285.
53. Inci I, Ozcelik C, Ulku R, et al. Intrapleural fibrinolytic treatment of traumatic clotted hemothorax. *Chest*. 1998;114:160–165.
54. Sybrandy KC, Cramer MJM, Burgersdijk C. Diagnosing cardiac contusion: old wisdom and new insights. *Heart*. 2003;89:485–489.
55. Fabian TC, Richardson JD, Croce MA, et al. Prospective study of blunt aortic injury: multicenter trial of the American Association for the Surgery of Trauma. *J Trauma*. 997;42(3):1128–1143.
56. Mandal AK, Thadepalli H, Chettipalli U. Posttraumatic empyema thoracis: a 24-year experience at a major trauma center. *J Trauma Inj Infect Crit Care*. 1997;43(5):764–771.
57. Aguilar MM, Battistella FD, Owings JT, Su T. Posttraumatic empyema: risk factor analysis. *Arch Surg*. 1997;132(6):647–650.
58. DeCamp MM, Blackstone EH, Naunheim KS, et al. Patient and surgical factors influencing air leak after lung volume reduction surgery: lessons learned from the national Emphysema Treatment Trial. *Ann Thorac Surg*. 2006;82:197–207.
59. Gillespie CT, Sterman DH, Cerfolio RJ, et al. Endobronchial valve treatment for prolonged air leaks of the lung. a case series. *Ann Thorac Surg*. 2011; 91:270–273.
60. Atkins BZ, Shah AS, Hutcheson KA, et al. Reducing hospital morbidity and mortality following esophagectomy. *Ann Thorac Surg*. 2004;78(4): 1170–1176.
61. Ferguson MK, Durkin AE. Preoperative prediction of the risk of pulmonary complications after esophagectomy for cancer. *J Thorac Cardiovasc Surg*. 2002;123(4):661–669.
62. Michelet P, D'Journo KB, Roch A, et al. Perioperative risk factors for anastomotic leakage after esophagectomy: influence of thoracic epidural analgesia. *Chest*. 2005;128(5):3461–3466.
63. Martin LW, Swisher SG, Hofstetter W, et al. Intrathoracic leaks following esophagectomy are no longer associated with increased mortality. *Ann Surg*. 2005;242:392–402.
64. Maish MS, DeMeester SR, Choustoulakis E, et al. the safety and usefulness of endoscopy for evaluation of the graft and anastomosis early after esophagectomy and reconstruction. *Surg Endosc*. 2005;19(8):1093–1102.
65. Sihaq S, Wright CD, Wain JC, et al. comparison of perioperative outcomes following open versus minimally invasive Ivor-Lewis oesophagectomy at a single, high-volume centre. *Eur J Cardiothoracic Surg*. 2012; 42:430–437.
66. Dickinson S, Park PK, Napolitano LM. Prone positioning therapy in ARDS. *Crit Care Clin*. 2011; 27:511–523.

67. Cheng K-C, Hou C-C, Huang H-C, et al. Intravenous injection of methylprednisone reduces the incidence of postextubation stridor in intensive care unit patients. *Crit Care Med.* 2006;34:1345–1350.
68. Skrinskas GJ, Hyland RH, Hutcheon MA. Using helium-oxygen mixtures in the management of acute upper airway obstruction. *Can Med Assoc J.* 1983;128:555–558.
69. Castella X, Gilabert J, Perez C. Arytenoid dislocation after tracheal intubation: an unusual cause of acute respiratory failure? *Anesthesiology.* 1991; 74:613–615.
70. Perentes JY, Abdelnour-Berchtold E, Blatter J, et al. Vacuum-assisted closure device for the management of infected postpneumonectomy chest cavities. *J Thorac Cardiovasc Surg.* 2015;149(3):745–750.
71. Athanassiadi K, Gerazounis M. Repair of postintubation tracheoesophageal fistula in polytrauma patients. *Injury.* 2005;36(8):897–899.
72. Eleftheriadis E, Kotzampassi K. Temporary stenting of acquired benign tracheoesophageal fistulas in critically ill ventilated patients. *Surg Endosc.* 2005;19(6):811–815.
73. Allan JS, Wright CD. Tracheoinnominate fistula: diagnosis and management. *Chest Surg Clin North Am.* 2003;13(2):331–341.
74. Troutman DA, Dougherty MJ, Spivack AI, Calligaro KD. Stent graft placement for a tracheoinnominate artery fistula. *Ann Vasc Surg.* 2014;28: 1037.e21–e24.
75. Wongsurakiat P, Pierson DJ, Rubenfeld GD. Changing patterns of ventilator settings in patients without acute lung injury. *Chest.* 2004;126:1281–1291.
76. Richard JC, Maggiore SM, Jonson B, et al. Influence of tidal volume on alveolar recruitment. *Am J Respir Crit Care Med.* 2001;163:1609–1613.
77. Varela G, Ballesteros E, Jimenez MF, et al. Cost-effectiveness of prophylactic respiratory physiotherapy in pulmonary lobectomy. *Eur J Cardiothorac Surg.* 2006;29:216–220.
78. Cerfolio RJ, Allen MS, Deschamps C, et al. Postoperative chylothorax. *J Thorac Cardiovasc Surg.* 1996;112:1361–1365.
79. Chen E, Itkin M. Thoracic duct embolization for chylous leaks. *Semin Intervent Radiol.* 2011;28:63–74.
80. Riber LP, Larsen TB, Christensen TD. Postoperative atrial fibrillation prophylaxis after lung surgery: systematic review and meta-analysis. *Ann Thorac Surg.* 2014;98:1989–1997.
81. Fernando HC, Jaklitsch MT, Walsh GL, et al. The Society of Thoracic Surgeons practice guideline on the prophylaxis and management of atrial fibrillation associated with general thoracic surgery: executive summary. *Ann Thorac Surg.* 2011;92:1144–1152.
82. Amar D, Zhang H, Heerdt PM, et al. Statin use is associated with a reduction in atrial fibrillation after noncardiac thoracic surgery independent of C-reactive protein. *Chest.* 2005;128:3421–3427.
83. Nan DN, Fernandez-Ayala M, Farinas-Alvarez C, et al. Nosocomial infection after lung surgery. *Chest.* 2005;128:2647–2652.
84. Engel HJ, Needham DM, Morrise PE, Gropper MA. ICU early mobilization: from recommendation to implementation at three medical centers. *Crit Care Med.* 2013;41:S69–S80.

CHAPTER

62

Postoperative Management of Adult Cardiovascular Surgery Patients

HOWARD K. SONG and MATTHEW S. SLATER

INTRODUCTION

Adult patients undergoing cardiovascular surgery procedures all pass through a period of critical illness during their recovery. These patients present intensivists with unique critical care management challenges because of the hemodynamic changes that occur as a result of the surgery itself and the broad inflammatory aftereffects of cardiopulmonary bypass (CPB). The specialized nature of the critical care of adult cardiovascular surgery patients is apparent in the proliferation of heart centers, specialized units, treatment protocols, and pathways designed to optimize patient outcomes by standardizing care and focusing provider expertise. Optimal outcomes for adult cardiovascular surgery patients are most likely to occur where critical care systems are designed to support this specific patient population and practitioners have strong familiarity with normal recovery milestones and complications that can interrupt this process.

Cardiopulmonary Bypass

The majority of adult cardiovascular surgery procedures are performed with the use of CPB. The development of the heart lung machine over the past 60 years represents one of the major achievements of modern medicine and has made complex repairs of intracardiac structures and the great vessels feasible. CPB techniques allow the surgeon to interrupt blood flow through the heart and lungs, providing a relatively bloodless and motionless field for the conduct of the operation. The most basic components of a CPB system are a venous cannula, a venous reservoir, a pump, an oxygenator, a heat exchanger, a filter, and an arterial cannula (Fig. 62.1). Other components that are commonly used are a cardioplegia delivery system, an ultrafiltration unit, a cardiotomy suction system, a left ventricular vent, and a cell saver system.

While CPB is an indispensable tool for the intraoperative care of the cardiovascular surgery patient, it incites a broad inflammatory cascade that can have far-reaching consequences on the subsequent intensive care unit (ICU) course of the patient. The primary trigger for this inflammatory cascade is the interaction between the patient's blood components and the large plastic surface area represented by the CPB circuit (1). This interaction activates plasma enzyme systems and blood cells, dilutes plasma proteins, causes coagulopathy, produces emboli, and leads to the release of an array of vasoactive mediators that affect vascular motor tone and endothelial permeability (Table 62.1). Because of the systemic nature of this response, nearly every end organ is susceptible to at least temporary inflammatory-mediated dysfunction in the postoperative period.

Fortunately, the post-CPB inflammatory cascade is typically self-limited (Fig. 62.2). Circulating levels of vasomotor mediators peak within 24 hours of surgery and subside over ensuing days (2). Although cardiovascular surgery patients frequently have temporary mild end-organ dysfunction postoperatively, rates of major complications for elective routine cases are low. Much of the critical care of cardiovascular surgery patients is oriented toward supporting patients through the early period during which they are subject to the temporary effects of CPB.

Immediate Concerns

The patient's admission to the ICU is a hectic transition period during which the patient is physically transported, monitoring and mechanical ventilation is re-established, intravenous medications are titrated, diagnostic tests are performed, and patient information is transferred from providers on the perioperative team to providers on the postoperative ICU team. In the midst of all these activities, almost all patients arriving in the ICU after cardiovascular surgery are in a state of controlled shock because of fluid shifts and changes in vascular tone. Cardiovascular surgery patients are, therefore, especially vulnerable to lapses in monitoring or distractions that divert the attention of providers at the bedside. A checklist is useful to assure that essential tasks are accomplished within the first 30 minutes of a patient's arrival in the ICU (Table 62.2).

The first step on the patient's arrival to the ICU should be to transfer arterial pressure monitoring from the portable unit accompanying the patient to the ICU monitor. The systemic arterial pressure waveform allows you to assess adequate systemic perfusion pressure and provides a means to detect arrhythmias while the electrocardiogram (ECG) and other pressure measurement catheters are connected and calibrated. Next, connect the hemodynamic monitoring catheters that provide some measure of central circulatory volume status, including the central venous pressure (CVP) catheter, pulmonary artery catheter, or both. The ECG leads are then switched from the transport unit to the ICU system. After these monitors are established, others can be connected and calibrated including the mixed venous oxygen saturation (SO_2) and pulse oximetry waveform.

Mechanical ventilation is continued using the ICU ventilator. Significant arterial–alveolar (A-a) gradients are common following CPB, so patients should routinely be given high concentrations of oxygen (70% to 80%) until adequate oxygenation is confirmed. Tidal volume in the absence of acute lung injury is set at 8 cc/kg of predicted body weight and respiratory rate is set at 14 breaths/min. If the patient is not synchronized with the ventilator, analgesia and sedation are assessed for adequacy.

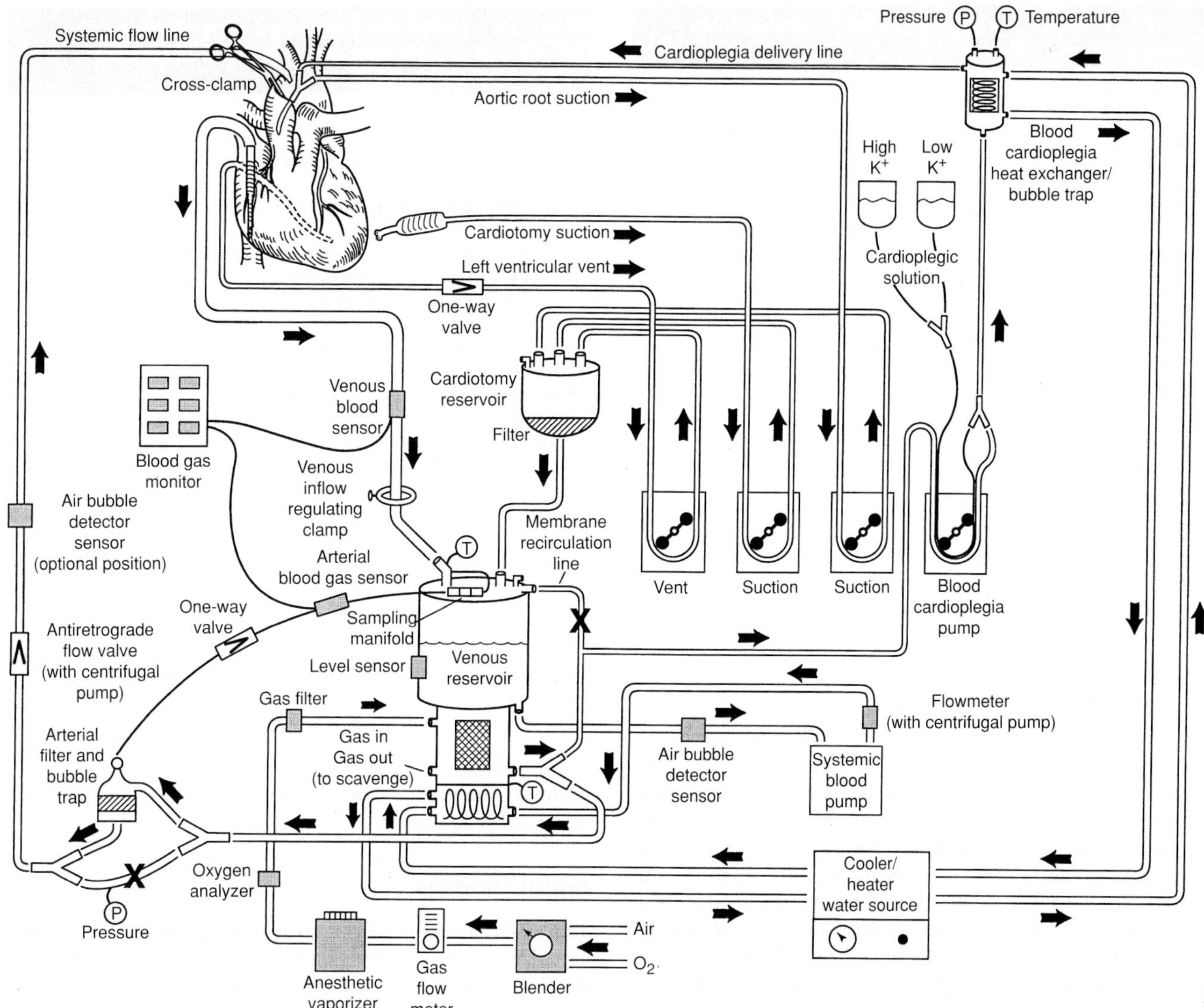

FIGURE 62.1 Detailed schematic diagram of the arrangement of a typical cardiopulmonary bypass circuit using a membrane oxygenator with integral hard-shell venous reservoir (**lower center**) and external cardiotomy reservoir. Venous cannulation is by a cavoatrial cannula and arterial cannulation is in the ascending aorta. Some circuits do not incorporate a membrane recirculation line; in these cases, the cardioplegia blood source is a separate outlet connector built into the oxygenator near the arterial outlet. The systemic blood pump may be either a roller or centrifugal type. The cardioplegia delivery system (**right**) is a one-pass combination blood/crystalloid type. The cooler–heater water source may be operated to supply water to both the oxygenator heat exchanger and cardioplegia delivery system. The air bubble detector sensor may be placed on the line between the venous reservoir and systemic pump, between the pump and membrane oxygenator inlet, or between the oxygenator outlet and arterial filter (neither shown), or on the line after the arterial filter (optional position on drawing). One-way valves prevent retrograde flow (some circuits with a centrifugal pump also incorporate a one-way valve after the pump and within the systemic flow line). Other safety devices include an oxygen analyzer placed between the anesthetic vaporizer (if used) and the oxygenator gas inlet and a reservoir level sensor attached to the housing of the hard-shell venous reservoir (on the left). Arrows, directions of flow; X, placement of tubing clamps; P and T (within circles), pressure and temperature sensors, respectively. Hemoconcentrator (described in text) not shown. (From Hessel EA II. Circuitry and cannulation techniques. In: Gravlee GP, Davis RF, Stammers AF, Ungerleider RM, eds. *Cardiopulmonary Bypass: Principles and Practice.* Philadelphia, PA: Lippincott Williams & Wilkins; 2008:63–113.)

Once stable hemodynamic function is confirmed, pressure monitoring can be interrupted to obtain blood samples for various tests, including arterial blood gas, complete blood count, serum potassium, ionized calcium, hematocrit, platelet count, and coagulation studies. Re-zeroing of all pressure monitors and calibration of the venous saturation monitor should be performed. For patients with a pulmonary artery catheter, baseline measurements of cardiac output and calculations of systemic vascular resistance (SVR) and pulmonary vascular resistance (PVR) are obtained.

A directed physical examination is performed. Particular attention is given to adequacy of airway control and ventilation. Assessment of peripheral pulses in all extremities is extremely important within the first hour and thereafter. Although affected sometimes by the presence of severe atherosclerosis, skin temperature, pulse amplitude, and capillary refill time provide essential clinical information about the adequacy of cardiac output. Palpable peripheral pulses are an excellent indicator of systemic perfusion.

A portable chest radiograph is obtained to determine the proper placement of the endotracheal tube, monitoring catheters, and nasogastric tube. Examine this radiograph closely for evidence of a pneumothorax, hemopneumothorax, and areas of collapse or atelectasis.

TABLE 62.1 Vasoactive Substances Released Following Cardiopulmonary Bypass

Aldosterone
Angiotensin II
Atrial natriuretic peptide
Complement: C3a, C4a, C5a, C5b-9
Electrolytes: Ca^{2+}, Mg^{2+}, K^{+}
Endothelin-1
Epinephrine
Glucagon
Histamine
Interleukins: IL-1, IL-6, IL-8, IL-10
Leukotrienes: LTB_4, LTC_4, LTD_4
Lysozomal enzymes
Nitric oxide
Norepinephrine
Oxygen free radicals
Platelet-activating factor
Prostacyclins
Prostaglandin E_2
Proteases
Renin
Serotonin
Thromboxane A_2
Thyroid hormones: T_3, T_4
Vasopressin

TABLE 62.2 Tasks to Be Completed within the First 30 Minutes of a Patient's Arrival to the ICU Following Cardiovascular Surgery

- Establish monitoring
  - Arterial waveform
  - Central venous and pulmonary artery waveforms
  - ECG
  - Mixed venous oxygen saturation
  - Pulse oxymetry
  - Mark and record urimeter and mediastinal drains
- Re-establish mechanical ventilation
  - Assess airway control and bilateral air entry
  - 70% to 100% FIO_2
  - Tidal volume = 8 cc/kg of predicted body weight
  - Respiratory rate 14 breaths/min
- Directed physical examination
  - Airway
  - Ventilation
  - Adequacy of blood pressure and cardiac output
  - Abdomen
  - Peripheral pulse exam
- Studies
  - ABG, serum potassium, ionized calcium, hematocrit, platelet count, coagulation studies
  - Chest x-ray
  - Transfer responsibility of patient care from perioperative team to ICU team
  - Verbal sign out of patient's clinical history and perioperative course

A word of caution is necessary about obtaining chest radiographs immediately after the patient arrives in the ICU, particularly if the body temperature is below 35.5°C and hemodynamic instability is present. In this situation, the chest radiograph should be deferred until the temperature rises above 35.5°C to avoid the occurrence of life-threatening arrhythmias during placement of the film cassette. Sudden movement may induce ventricular tachycardia or fibrillation resulting from the reduced fibrillation threshold caused by hypothermia and electrolyte imbalance, especially hypokalemia.

As the physical process of patient admission to the ICU is taking place, a transfer of responsibility for the patient's care is also occurring. This usually involves a verbal sign-out of patient information from providers on the perioperative team to providers on the ICU team. The patient's clinical history is reviewed and the perioperative course is described. This information is particularly important to assure the safe transition from perioperative to postoperative care. Important details may include information on ease of intubation, perioperative ventricular function, inotropic and vasopressor requirement, optimal volume status, completeness of revascularization, and suspected coagulopathy.

Initial Therapy

The first hour after admission to the ICU following cardiovascular surgery is a critical and unstable time. The goals in this first hour are to maintain adequate systemic perfusion, establish adequate oxygenation and respiration, and control cardiac rate and rhythm. Patients who experience intravascular volume shifts during transport to the ICU require intravascular volume expansion, bolus dosages of intravenous calcium chloride, or both to maintain adequate systemic blood pressure and flow during the crucial 15 to 30 minutes required to settle the patient in the ICU.

In this early period of stabilization, especially when the patient is mildly to moderately hypothermic, serum potassium levels should be assessed rapidly and supplemented to maintain levels in the 4.5 to 5.0 mMol/L range. This intervention helps protect the heart against ventricular irritability. At times, patients arrive to the ICU in an acidemic state.

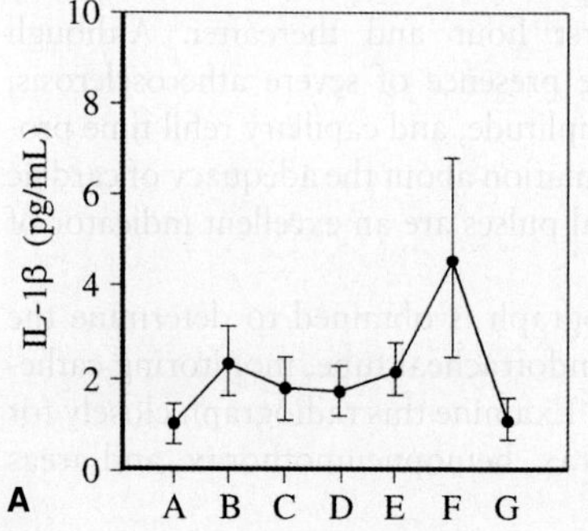

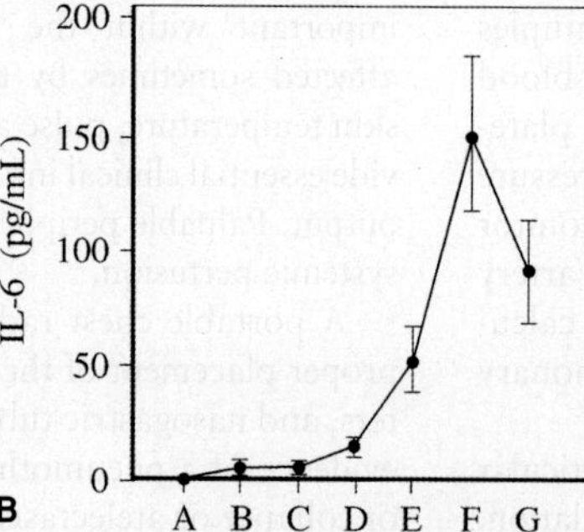

FIGURE 62.2 Changes in IL-1β (A) and IL-6 (B) in 30 patients who had elective first-time myocardial revascularization. Letters on x-axis represent the following events: A, induction of anesthesia; B, 5 minutes after heparin; C, 10 minutes after starting CPB; D, end of CPB; E, 20 minutes after protamine; F, 3 hours after CPB; G, 24 hours after CPB. (Adapted from Steinberg JB, Kapelanski DP, Olson JD, Weiler JM. Cytokine and complement levels in patients undergoing cardiopulmonary bypass. *J Thorac Cardiovasc Surg.* 1993;106:1008.)

Avoid attempting to correct acidosis with rapid intravenous infusions of sodium bicarbonate. Serum potassium can be acutely lowered, which may increase ventricular irritability. Once the potassium level is adequate, moderate to severe metabolic acidosis (base deficit > 5 mMol/L) can be corrected with sodium bicarbonate.

Urine output is monitored closely to detect inappropriate diuresis, which occurs commonly in patients after CPB. Patients exhibiting this may require especially rapid replacement of crystalloid and electrolyte losses. Mediastinal drain output is also closely observed to detect excessive blood loss. If rapid hemorrhage is suspected, transfusion therapy is initiated early to replace red blood cell mass and correct coagulopathy as directed by postoperative studies and clinical findings. The operating team should be made aware of any patient who has massive hemorrhage so that mediastinal exploration can be undertaken expeditiously when indicated.

The First 8 Hours after Cardiopulmonary Bypass

After initial stabilization, a period frequently follows when the patient's hemodynamics are adequate and the patient is relatively stable. This period of time is designated the *golden period* and lasts for approximately 8 hours after cessation of CPB. Pay careful attention to optimizing cardiac function, because the subsequent 8 to 14 hours are characterized by decreasing cardiac function. The nadir of this decline occurs approximately 12 hours after CPB. Particularly notable is a decrease in ventricular compliance leading to reduced cardiac output at any given filling pressure. This condition generally persists over the next 12 to 24 hours, followed by a gradual improvement in cardiopulmonary performance over the next 48 hours. In the golden period, the goal is to optimize cardiorespiratory performance so that the ensuing decrease in cardiac function from 8 to 24 hours after CPB does not jeopardize end-organ system function. Caution should be used in weaning inotropes rapidly during this period despite adequate hemodynamics in anticipation of the deterioration that typically follows.

Despite this caution, stable patients undergoing nonemergent cardiovascular surgery can usually be extubated safely during this period. The major criteria for proceeding with extubation during this early period are adequate central nervous system function, stable hemodynamics without malignant arrhythmias, normothermia, low A-a gradient, adequate pulmonary mechanics, and no ongoing mediastinal hemorrhage. If these screening criteria are met, patients can be observed for a brief period on minimal ventilatory support followed by extubation if this is successful. Intravenous narcotics are useful to treat incisional pain during the period that sedative drugs are weaned just prior to extubation. Anesthetic technique should also be tailored to allow patients who can reasonably be expected to be extubated early to emerge from the effects of anesthesia during this period. In our institution, the majority of patients undergoing nonemergent cardiovascular surgery are extubated within the first 6 hours of admission to the ICU using this strategy. Patients who have undergone a period of deep hypothermic circulatory arrest or long CPB periods, patients with poor ventricular function or unstable hemodynamics, and patients with hemorrhage or coagulopathy and large anticipated transfusion requirement are not suitable for early extubation.

The Next 16 Hours after Cardiopulmonary Bypass

The next 16 hours is probably the most challenging time, especially for the patients whose cardiac performance was not optimized during the golden period. The cause of the slump in cardiac performance during this time period is unclear. It is notable that many of the vasoactive factors that are released after CPB reach their peak concentrations during this period (2). The effects of cardiac reperfusion injury are also maximized during this period in patients who have had aortic cross-clamping and obligatory global myocardial ischemia during their operation (3).

Changes in Heart Compliance

Clinically, the heart seems to become noncompliant or "stiff." In this situation, one usually observes a rise in pulmonary artery pressure and pulmonary artery capillary wedge pressure (PACWP), and a reduction in the systemic arterial pressure, cardiac output, and mixed venous oxygen saturation (4). If the patient is doing extremely well before the onset of compliance changes, alterations in these parameters may go unnoticed. However, patients with a low cardiac output syndrome before the onset of changes in compliance often develop hemodynamic instability.

Time Course

The usual time course is a steady deterioration in cardiac performance between the 8th and 12th hours following CPB. This condition seems to stabilize near the 12th hour and remains stable for the next 6 to 8 hours. Avoid unnecessary manipulations of the determinants of cardiac performance during this period. Once a patient becomes unstable, far more interventions are required to return to a steady state than if problems are anticipated and appropriate changes made to help maintain stability. Even if patients remain in a relatively low cardiac output state during these 16 hours, they tolerate this condition better than those who are subjected to marked swings in hemodynamics.

Optimizing the Determinants of Cardiac Output

As patients enter this period, all parameters of cardiac performance should be evaluated individually. A strategy of optimizing cardiac rate and rhythm, preload, afterload, and contractility is useful. Heart rate and rhythm play a particularly important role in determining cardiac output in post-CPB patients. This is because the ventricles are stiff and noncompliant with limited capacity to increase stroke volume. Contrary to other ICU settings, slower heart rates do not necessarily lead to increased filling and improved stroke volume. Rates of 90 to 110 beats/min are typically necessary to optimize this component of cardiac output. In addition, atrial fibrillation may also be poorly tolerated during this period as the noncompliant ventricles may be dependent on atrial contraction to be adequately filled. Measures such as those described below should be taken to maintain sinus rhythm and restore it if atrial arrhythmias occur.

During this period, volume loading to achieve a PACWP beyond 12 to 14 mmHg is unlikely to lead to significant increases in stroke volume due to noncompliance. Therefore, once a PACWP in this range is achieved, attention should be turned to other determinants of cardiac output to improve cardiac performance.

Afterload reduction is an efficient way to improve cardiac performance without increasing myocardial oxygen consumption (MO_2) (5). Afterload reduction should be instituted cautiously during this period to avoid hypotension. Renal function in older patients may be particularly sensitive to decreases in perfusion pressure. Patients with recent right ventricular infarcts and right ventricular stunning are also sensitive to hypotension.

Patients with a relatively normal cardiac output before surgery often poorly tolerate a cardiac index below 2.0 L/min/m^2, a venous PO_2 below 30 mmHg, or an SO_2 below 50% after surgery. Although costly to the heart in terms of MO_2, enhancement of cardiac contractility is an effective method to augment cardiac output by increasing the ejection fraction. In this period, inotropic support is a useful and frequently necessary means to achieve an adequate cardiac output until reversible cardiac dysfunction related to CPB and reperfusion effects have resolved. Moderate doses of inotropes are generally well tolerated by patients with ischemic heart disease who have been completely revascularized and by patients with valvular heart disease. Inotropes can cause myocardial ischemia in patients with ischemic heart disease who have been incompletely revascularized and should be used with caution in this setting.

Myocardial Ischemia

Increases in heart rate, filling pressures, and contractility to support patients during this period may cause myocardial ischemia. An ECG should be obtained immediately after surgery and as clinically indicated thereafter. Continuous telemetry should be monitored closely for ischemic changes in the ST segment. Cardiac enzymes are usually not helpful in diagnosing myocardial ischemia during this early period because they typically rise in all cardiovascular surgery patients postoperatively. An unusually high enzyme level or a sudden change in the usual pattern of enzyme leak may be useful, however. If acute graft closure is suspected following a coronary artery bypass procedure, echocardiography should show a new segmental wall motion abnormality. Comparison with intraoperative transesophageal studies, if performed, is particularly useful. If bypass graft failure of a large myocardial territory is suspected, coronary angiography with either percutaneous or open surgical re-intervention may be indicated. In the absence of ischemia, cardiac performance will stabilize, usually by the 12th post-CPB hour.

The Second 24 Hours after Cardiopulmonary Bypass

During the second 24 postoperative hours, cardiovascular function typically improves. Small increases in the SO_2 and cardiac output, together with a noticeable decrease in fluid requirements, herald this recovery phase. Patients who preoperatively have normal systolic ventricular function usually tolerate having their inotropes weaned off or to low levels. In these patients, the amount of active intervention is largely determined by the function of other organ systems such as the lungs and kidneys. If supraphysiologic cardiac output is desired to facilitate diuresis and optimize lung and kidney function, moderate inotropic support may be continued. For patients who preoperatively have decompensated left ventricular function, weaning of inotropic support should be done in a slow, stepwise fashion. During this process, active diuresis and substitution of oral afterload-reducing drugs, particularly ACE inhibitors, may be useful.

Invasive monitoring with arterial and pulmonary artery catheters should be maintained until patients demonstrate they are on a recovery trajectory. If a patient has not been extubated in the early postoperative period, he should be continuously re-evaluated for extubation to limit their risk for ventilator-associated complications. For patients who have undergone straightforward elective procedures, transfer to a step-down telemetry ward may be considered. Important criteria for transfer include adequate CNS function, no or trivial requirement for inotropes, no dependence on temporary pacemaker leads, and good pulmonary toilet. On the other hand, patients who have required maximum support during the first 24 hours after surgery may require an additional 24 hours before any progress is realized.

The Third 24 Hours after Cardiopulmonary Bypass

During this period, patient care is focused on the transition from ICU care to ward care. Compliance in the left ventricle should improve rapidly, accompanied by a decrease in interstitial pulmonary water. Lower pulmonary artery pressures and improved cardiac performance at lower filling pressure can be anticipated. Mobilization of third-spaced fluid occurs and active diuresis should be instituted. Oral medications oriented more toward long-term cardiovascular risk reduction, such as β-blockers, aspirin, and statins, are started. ACE inhibitors are favored in patients with valvular heart disease, particularly those who have had adverse left ventricular remodeling preoperatively. Physical rehabilitation with emphasis on pulmonary toilet and early ambulation is instituted. Intravenous insulin protocols are transitioned to long-acting subcutaneous regimens. Most patients who have undergone elective surgical procedures are able to be transferred to the step-down telemetry unit by the third postoperative day.

Catheters and Tubes

Mediastinal drains, pacing wires, arterial lines, Foley catheters, and pulmonary artery catheters often can be removed. If continuous invasive cardiac monitoring is still considered necessary, a CVP catheter positioned in the superior vena cava will provide a measurement of right ventricular filling pressure. Venous saturation readings from the superior caval–atrial junction correlate closely with the SO_2 in the absence of a left-to-right shunt (6,7). The association of the CVP and PACWP will be known by this point, and left heart filling pressures can thus be estimated.

Arrhythmias

Despite rapid improvements in the third 24-hour period, this is a time when atrial arrhythmias are prominent, including atrial flutter and atrial fibrillation. These may be significant problems because the atrial contribution to cardiac output remains high and a rapid heart rate may not be well tolerated.

Prophylaxis and treatment strategies for atrial fibrillation vary from institution to institution (8–12). Patients undergoing elective cardiovascular procedures frequently are already on β-blockers preoperatively. At our institution, β-blockers are instituted the week prior to surgery if patients are not already on them. Amiodarone and atorvastatin have also shown promise for prophylaxis against atrial fibrillation (9,11,12). Postoperatively, all patients are begun on low-dose metoprolol as soon as inotropes are discontinued. The dose of metoprolol is uptitrated as the patient's blood pressure and heart rate permit. For patients with depressed left ventricular function who require prolonged inototropic support, amiodarone may be used for arrhythmia prophylaxis.

The mainstays of atrial fibrillation treatment in the hemodynamically stable patient include diuresis, aggressive repletion of serum potassium and magnesium, intravenous amiodarone loading, and intravenous β-blockers. β-Blockers should be used with caution in patients still requiring inotropic support. Intravenous calcium channel blockers and procainamide are used occasionally in certain circumstances. For instance, procainamide is useful in heart transplant recipients who are still on inotropic support because of the desire to avoid long-acting agents such as amiodarone which may have a prolonged slowing effect on sinus and atrioventricular (AV) node function. Of course, patients who deteriorate hemodynamically with the onset of atrial fibrillation should be treated with synchronized direct-current cardioversion. Whenever feasible, rapid atrial pacing should be attempted to overdrive suppress atrial flutter with a 2:1 block.

Monitoring and Managing Cardiovascular Performance

No single physiologic parameter reliably predicts adequacy of a patient's hemodynamic performance early in the postoperative course after cardiovascular surgery. We therefore rely on several physiologic measurements and clinical signs to assess hemodynamic performance and end-organ perfusion.

Arterial Blood Pressure

For all critically ill patients, a minimum arterial blood pressure is required for overall systemic perfusion and especially for cerebral and renal perfusion. Most adults require a mean arterial pressure of at least 50 to 55 mmHg (13). Older patients, particularly those with severe atherosclerotic disease, may require a mean arterial pressure of 65 mmHg or greater.

Pulse pressure is a useful indicator of systemic perfusion. We recommend display of the arterial waveform at full scale on the patient monitor. Determination of the systolic, diastolic, and mean pressures, as well as the height of the dicrotic notch provides an indication of left ventricular ejection volume. Poorer ventricular ejection is observed when the dicrotic notch is at the base of the arterial pressure trace. Better ventricular output is found when the dicrotic notch is located midway up the down slope of the tracing, resulting in a greater area under the arterial pressure curve (14). The arterial pressure waveform also provides an indication of peripheral vascular tone. Harmonic augmentation in peripheral arteries suggests an increase in peripheral vascular tone and is characterized by a sharp, spiked arterial pressure tracing with virtually no dicrotic notch.

Normally, the arterial blood pressure is continuously monitored in a peripheral vessel such as the radial artery. However, any doubt concerning the pressure waveform from a peripheral artery should lead to measurement in a more central vessel, such as the femoral artery. A central arterial pressure reading provides better and more reliable assessment of overall hemodynamic function and cardiac output.

Heart Rate and Rhythm

Sinus rhythm is extremely important in the first 24 hours, and efforts should be focused on maintaining sequential AV activity for better loading of the ventricles and optimal cardiac output. Normally, the atrial contraction or atrial "kick" contributes approximately 5% of the cardiac output. However, in the postoperative patient, the atrial contribution to cardiac output may be as high as 30%. Minimizing the incidence of atrial fibrillation using prophylaxis regimens as described above is an important component of rhythm management after cardiovascular surgery.

Pacemakers. Temporary epicardial atrial and ventricular pacing wires are commonly placed at the completion of cardiovascular procedures and can be invaluable both diagnostically and therapeutically. Heart rates of 90 to 110 beats/min are generally well tolerated, even in patients who have undergone revascularization procedures. This is an important strategy to optimize cardiac output because of the poor compliance of the ventricles immediately following cardiovascular surgery. In addition, premature ventricular beats can frequently be suppressed by pacing to this heart rate range. Patients with temporary heart block following surgery can have A-V synchrony restored with DDD mode pacing.

In certain situations, an atrial pacing wire may be needed to determine the cardiac rhythm and differentiate supraventricular tachycardia. To perform an atrial ECG, simply connect the atrial pacing wire to the right arm ECG limb lead and observe the rhythm of leads I, II, or III on the patient monitor. Observation of the contour of the left and right atrial waveforms is another useful way of determining sinus rhythm.

Ventricular Preload

Ventricular preload, the load on the muscle that determines resting muscle length, is primarily manipulated in the postoperative period by fluid administration. Generally, we try to maintain cardiac preload at an adequate but not excessive level. For the left ventricle, this means maintaining the left ventricular end diastolic pressure between 12 and 14 mmHg as assessed by PACWP.

Fluid Administration. A common tendency is the desire to increase right and left ventricular filling pressures to their upper limits (16 to 20 mmHg) to assure adequate volume resuscitation. This approach exacerbates several problems that are difficult to manage later in the postoperative period, especially pulmonary dysfunction. Immediately after CPB, colloid oncotic pressure is reduced by as much as 50% and returns to normal over a 2-week period of time (15). In addition, neutrophil and endothelial activation following CPB increases pulmonary vascular permeability resulting in a higher loss of intravascular fluids at lower hydrostatic pressures, promoting increased pulmonary interstitial water accumulation and pulmonary edema (16). We therefore caution against trying to maximize cardiac output by moving toward the upper pressure–volume limits along the Starling curve. Attempts to reach venous pressures greater than 16 mmHg result in administration of excess fluids accompanied by increased pulmonary interstitial water.

Crystalloids and Colloids. Controversy persists concerning which types of fluids are most effective for volume resuscitation in post-CPB patients. The focus of this debate concerns the administration of crystalloid versus colloid (blood products, albumin, or hydroxyethyl starch) solutions (17). We have employed multiple fluid combinations for maintaining adequate preload, all of which have advantages and disadvantages. Sole reliance on crystalloid solutions such as Ringer's lactate for volume expansion may result in an inordinate amount of fluid administration to maintain adequate preload. Our current practice for volume resuscitation in patients without ongoing hemorrhage is to use up to 2 L of crystalloid solution after which 5% albumin may be used.

When the hematocrit is low (<22%) and the patient is bleeding or hemodynamically unstable, blood products are indicated. If red cell mass is adequate but coagulation factors are abnormal and bleeding continues, fresh frozen plasma and platelets should be considered. The threshold to give blood is lowered in patients with incomplete revascularization, low cardiac output, and signs of inadequate oxygen delivery such as low SO_2.

Ventricular Afterload

Afterload reduction offers the most efficient means to improve cardiac output at little or no expense to myocardial oxygen demand. Following afterload reduction, ventricular volume, wall tension, and MO_2 usually are not increased. In some patients, the ejection fraction can be dramatically improved by a reduction in SVR and PVR. Afterload reduction should be performed after judicious volume loading to avoid hypotension and hemodynamic collapse. Afterload reduction typically begins in the operating room after the cessation of CPB with the release of vasoactive mediators and with systemic rewarming. The extent of afterload reduction that is necessary greatly depends on ventricular performance. Patients with severely depressed systolic ventricular function benefit the most from afterload reduction.

Vasodilators. Nicardipine hydrochloride, a peripheral acting calcium channel blocker, acts as a direct systemic arterial vasodilator. Its dose range is 1 to 15 mg/hr. It is our primary afterload-reducing agent because it is reasonably evanescent and avoids problems with cyanide toxicity associated with sodium nitroprusside. In our experience, it is less associated with pulmonary artery shunting and resulting ventilation–perfusion (V-Q) mismatch than sodium nitroprusside as well.

Sodium nitroprusside remains as an alternative agent for afterload reduction. It increases venous capacitance and directly vasodilates the systemic and pulmonary arterioles. Its advantage is its fast onset of action (15 to 20 seconds), allowing rapid titration (0.3 to 10 μg/kg/min). It can be associated with cyanide toxicity as well as pulmonary artery shunting and V-Q mismatch.

Nitroglycerin is a venous and arterial vasodilator. It is primarily a preload-reducing agent but does have mild afterload-reducing effects, including on the coronary arterial tree. An additional advantage in patients with right ventricular failure is its vasodilatory effects on the pulmonary vasculature. The intravenous dosage of NTG ranges between 0.5 and 2 μg/kg/min. It decreases myocardial oxygen consumption and may be especially useful in patients with incomplete revascularization.

Pulmonary Artery Vasodilators. Certain patients benefit from vasodilators that act specifically on the pulmonary artery tree. Right ventricular failure is common in patients who have suffered right ventricular myocardial infarction and in patients who have undergone orthotopic heart transplantation as the implanted organ adjusts to its new setting of increased pulmonary artery vascular resistance. Patients who have had pulmonary endarterectomy may have reactive pulmonary artery constriction. Patients with a long-standing history of congestive heart failure also may have a component of reactive pulmonary artery hypertension following CPB in addition to fixed changes. In these scenarios, isolated right ventricular failure may be the primary cause of low cardiac output because of inadequate left ventricular filling.

The inhaled prostacyclin analog ileoprost is our preferred specific pulmonary artery vasodilator. An important advantage is its ease of administration. It can be delivered intermittently via a nebulizer to either intubated or extubated patients. Inhaled nitric oxide also has vasodilatory activity restricted to the pulmonary artery tree because of its short half-life. It requires continuous delivery via a specialized system and can only be used in intubated patients.

It is important to keep in mind the pulmonary vasoconstrictive effects of hypercapnea and hypoxia when managing patients with severe right ventricular dysfunction. Hypercapnea and hypoxia should be strictly avoided in patients with marginal right ventricular function, even if this requires prolonging the period of intubation. High FIO_2 can be considered a form of pulmonary vasodilator in this subset of patients.

Vasoconstrictors. CPB causes release of numerous vasoactive substances, many of which have vasodilatory effects (1). Vasodilation following cardiovascular surgery is especially common in patients who have had prolonged CPB, a period of circulatory arrest, or who have been treated with ACE inhibitors preoperatively (18,19). Various agents, including steroids and methylene blue, have been studied for the treatment of vasoplegic shock following CPB (20). Vasoconstrictors remain the first-line treatment for patients with low SVR and adequate volume status and contractile state, however (21). It is crucial that prior to instituting vasoconstrictor treatment, the patient be adequately volume resuscitated and that their hypotension is determined to be related to vasodilation rather than pump failure. Treatment of hypotension related to pump failure with a pure vasoconstrictor can lead to permanent end-organ damage. Patients ideally treated with vasoconstrictors are in a high cardiac output state with low SVR.

Phenylephrine hydrochloride, an α-specific catecholamine, acts as a pure peripheral vasoconstrictor. Its dose range is 20 to 180 μg/min. It has a relatively short half-life and its primary advantage is that it can be easily titrated for goal parameters, such as mean arterial blood pressure.

Vasopressin also acts as a pure peripheral vasoconstrictor. Because of its longer half-life, it is less suited for minute-to-minute changes in response to blood pressure changes. It may be particularly useful in patients treated preoperatively with ACE inhibitors. Its usual dose range is 1 to 10 units/hr. Its mechanism of action is synergistic with norepinephrine. Vasopressin in combination with norepinephrine is therefore useful in patients who have profound vasodilatory shock.

Contractility

The contractile state of the heart is a determinant of cardiac output and patients with reversible myocardial stunning after aortic cross-clamping and CPB or preexisting decompensated left ventricular function frequently benefit from a period of inotropic support. When required, inotropes are usually begun in the operating room at the time of weaning from CPB under guidance of intraoperative transesophageal echocardiography, and are continued into the postoperative period. In the ICU, if cardiac performance is marginal and does not respond to other measures, we quickly institute inotropes and continue them throughout the first 24 to 48 hours. Remember that the specific conditions under which the operation was conducted, including repairs performed, completeness of revascularization, length of CPB, and quality of myocardial preservation can profoundly influence postoperative myocardial contractility in the postoperative period.

Inotropes. Few pharmacologic agents affect only one determinant of cardiac performance and this is especially true of inotropes. When selecting drugs, individually or in combination, bear in mind that a major goal after CPB is to gain cardiac output with as little increase in myocardial oxygen consumption as possible.

Epinephrine, in the 0.01 to 0.10 μg/kg/min range, is our principle choice. These dosage levels are not exceeded unless absolutely necessary to maintain an acceptable mean arterial perfusion pressure. Epinephrine also has vasoconstrictor and chronotropic effects; however, its inotropic effects predominate in this dose range. Epinephrine can be particularly useful when used to support right ventricular function.

Norepinephrine, also in the 0.01 to 0.10 μg/kg/min range, is also frequently used. Because of increased α-agonism, norepinephrine has stronger vasoconstrictor effects in this range and has been associated with improved coronary and splanchnic blood flow (22,23). Because of its vasoconstrictor properties, it can be especially useful in patients with vasodilatation after CPB who also require inotropic support.

Isoproterenol is a relatively weak inotrope with primarily chronotropic properties. In our ICU, its primary use is in heart transplant recipients in whom we are trying to cause relative tachycardia because of the normal coronary arteries, diastolic dysfunction, and right ventricular distension commonly encountered in this population. It can be used in dosages between 0.005 and 0.02 μg/kg/min to drive heart rates into the 100 to 120 beats/min range.

Milrinone is a phosphodiesterase inhibitor with potent inotropic and vasodilatory effects. It is commonly used in patients with preexisting ventricular systolic dysfunction. It is given as a loading dose of 50 μg/kg followed by a continuous infusion of 0.1 to 0.75 μg/kg/min. Because of its vasodilatory properties, it is important that patients be adequately volume resuscitated prior to its use. It frequently is given in combination with agents that have vasoconstrictor properties, such as norepinephrine, phenylephrine, or vasopressin.

Dopamine hydrochloride at dosages between 3 and 5 μg/kg/min can be used to decrease SVR and augment cardiac contractility when a more potent catecholamine is not required. In this dosage range, dopamine also stimulates dopaminergic receptors in the kidney, thereby enhancing renal perfusion.

Dobutamine in dosages between 3 and 5 μg/kg/min has inotropic and vasodilatory effects similar to milrinone. At higher doses, it has α-stimulatory effects and acts as a vasoconstrictor. Our practice has increasingly relied on epinephrine and milrinone as first-line inotropes rather than dopamine and dobutamine because of their perceived proarrhythmic effects. When selecting an inotropic regimen, remember that catecholamines at varying doses stimulate both β- and α-receptors. When we wish to avoid α-receptor activity, multiple catecholamines are used synergistically to increase β-receptor activity without stimulating α-receptor activity.

Cardiac Output and Cardiac Index

A pulmonary artery catheter allows cardiac output measurement by the thermodilution method as well as facilitates calculation of SVR and PVR, pulmonary and intracardiac shunts, and estimation of LVEDP by PACWP. Cardiac output readings should always be normalized by conversion to cardiac index (cardiac output divided by the body surface area). This adjusts cardiac output for the size of the individual patient and therefore is a better estimate of adequacy of tissue perfusion. A cardiac index of 2.0 L/min/m^2 or greater is usually sufficient to maintain end-organ performance. Exceptions exist in certain pathologic condition, however. For example, patients with long-standing mitral valve disease and in a low cardiac output state preoperatively may well tolerate a cardiac index of less than 2.0 L/min/m^2 in the immediate postoperative period. In contrast, higher body temperature and agitation may lead to cardiac index requirements of greater than 2.0 L/min/m^2. Bear in mind that these indices are at the lower limits for providing adequate organ function and that postoperative stress normally produces cardiac indices approaching 3.5 to 4.0 L/min/m^2. Cardiac output should not be the sole criterion used to determine adequacy of end-organ oxygen delivery.

Mixed Venous Saturation

Continuous display of the SO_2 affords one the opportunity to observe acute as well as gradual changes in cardiac performance, increasing oxygen consumption (O_2), or both. Based on the Fick method of determining cardiac output, changes in the SO_2 reflect changes in systemic blood flow as long as O_2 remains stable. Acute changes in O_2 and cardiac performance are especially demonstrable during episodes of agitation, tracheal suctioning, and rapid extracellular volume shifts. SO_2 monitoring is particularly helpful in tracking the gradual deterioration of cardiac performance during the second 8-hour period after CPB.

Equipment used to measure physiologic parameters such as the arterial pressure and SO_2 must be calibrated regularly. SO_2 monitors are calibrated using venous saturation readings from a mixed venous blood sample from the pulmonary artery. The accuracy of any single measure of cardiac performance should always be evaluated in the context of other measures. For example, if the arterial pressure waveform is dampened, it may be compared against readings from an oscillometric, Doppler, or return-to-flow technique. Incongruent readings should always be evaluated with a suspicion for the accuracy of measurement.

Serum Lactate

As an indicator of anaerobic metabolism, serum lactate can provide information about the adequacy of cardiac performance in meeting the body's oxygen requirement. Several problems, however, limit the usefulness of serum lactate as a means to assess cardiac performance. On arrival to the ICU, lactate values may range between normal (<2.0 mMol/L) to as high as 8 to 9 mMol/L. As body temperature rises to normal, serum lactate may actually rise despite improving hemodynamics, because underperfused vascular beds open and release lactate into the systemic circulation. The difficulty in this situation is whether to attribute a rise in serum lactate to a "washout" phenomenon or to a diminution of cardiac performance. Evaluation of the cardiac index, SO_2, and SVR in conjunction with serial serum lactate determinations helps to resolve this dilemma. Lactate levels should decrease after 8 hours if perfusion is adequate.

Serum Ionized Calcium and Potassium

Rapid access (5 to 10 minutes) to laboratory determinations is essential for guiding therapy, especially in the first 24 hours. Important serum values include ionized calcium (Ca^{2+}), potassium, hematocrit, glucose, and sodium. Serial measurement of Ca^{2+} is especially helpful when solutions containing protein such as blood, fresh frozen plasma, albumin, or plasma protein solutions are administered. Protein binds calcium and may diminish that which is available for myocardial function. Clinically, this phenomenon can be recognized during the rapid infusion of protein-containing solutions by noting a rise in cardiac filling pressures, a drop in blood pressure, and a drop in the SO_2, all indicative of worsening performance despite volume resuscitation. In certain situations, particularly in hemodynamically unstable patients, simultaneous infusion of calcium chloride markedly improves cardiac performance.

Postoperative maintenance of adequate serum potassium is crucial, especially after the usually brisk diuresis following CPB and in conjunction with diuretic therapy. Potassium chloride should be considered a first-line agent for prevention and treatment of arrhythmias after cardiovascular surgery. Potassium chloride should be given as a standing medication to actively diuresing patients with normal renal function and serum potassium values should be measured frequently to guide replacement therapy toward a normal to high normal range (4.5 to 5 mMol/L).

Urine Output

In the initial postoperative period, urine output is typically brisk but then diminishes dramatically between the 8th and 12th post-CPB hours. Initially, urine output alone should not be relied upon to judge cardiac performance, because it is influenced by a number of variables including high serum glucose, denatured plasma protein fractions, and diuretics such as furosemide and mannitol used during CPB. In later stages of the postoperative period, urine output may be influenced by various stress hormones such as antidiuretic hormone, aldosterone, and cortisol, which generally cause conservation of intravascular volume. Similarly, conservation of intravascular volume occurs in patients who enter surgery with high ventricular end-diastolic filling pressures but return to the ICU after surgery with lower filling pressures. In patients who are conditioned to higher filling pressures, the sudden reduction in atrial pressure usually sets off a strong antidiuretic hormone–mediated response designed to correct perceived hypovolemia.

Almost all patients return from the operating room with excess total body water because of the hemodilution and obligate volume load caused by the bypass circuit. These effects have been partially ameliorated by cell saver systems and ultrafiltration units which reconcentrate red cell mass. Despite the usual excess in total body water, intravascular volume status is variable, because of third spacing related to increased capillary permeability and post-CPB inflammation. Diuretic therapy should therefore be guided by cardiac filling pressures. Our practice is to diurese patients to low normal filling pressures as long as hemodynamics are not compromised in order to minimize interstitial lung water and improve pulmonary function. Diuresis should be performed cautiously during the early postoperative period when ventricular compliance is poor and cardiac function may be especially preload dependent. This is particularly true in patients with concentric ventricular hypertrophy, such as those with long-standing hypertension or aortic stenosis.

Special Concerns

Bleeding

Bleeding after cardiovascular operations with CPB is a major destabilizing complication. Severe postoperative bleeding occurs in 3% to 5% of patients who undergo CPB (24). Significant progress has been made in understanding its causes and optimal treatment.

Causes. While inadequate surgical hemostasis should always be suspected, at least half of patients with severe postoperative bleeding have acquired hemostatic defects (25,26). These include activation of fibrinolysis, decreased levels of clotting factors due to dilution and consumption, and transient platelet dysfunction. Therapeutic protocols may influence postoperative bleeding. For example, chronic preoperative use of antiplatelet agents such as clopidogrel and aspirin is associated with increased postoperative transfusion requirement.

Treatment. Antifibrinolytic agents, such as epsilon aminocaproic acid and aprotinin, have been shown to decrease the need for transfusion in high-risk subpopulations (27,28). These agents are begun intraoperatively and discontinued shortly upon arrival to the ICU. There is no evidence supporting initiation of their use in the postoperative period. When bleeding does occur, blood component replacement is guided by laboratory studies. Red blood cell transfusions should be initiated promptly when massive hemorrhage is suspected. Clotting factor deficiencies demonstrated by prolonged prothrombin and activated partial thromboplastin times are treated with fresh frozen plasma. Cryoprecipitate is usually reserved for patients with low fibrinogen levels. Factor replacement therapy with recombinant clotting factors such as activated factor VII and factor XIII is an emerging strategy (29,30). Prothrombin complex concentrates also have been used with some efficacy to rescue patients with life-threatening hemorrhage that is refractory to conventional treatment by transfusion (31).

Isolated elevation of the activated partial thromboplastin time may indicate heparin rebound and should be reversed with protamine sulfate administration (25). Circulating heparin levels are also useful in guiding protamine administration (32).

Platelet counts of greater than 100,000 may seem reassuring; however, the function of these platelets is frequently inadequate in patients with clinical coagulopathy. Point-of-care platelet function assays may be useful for directing platelet transfusion in patients without thrombocytopenia.

Our threshold for returning the patient to the operating room is a blood loss rate through the chest tubes of greater than 3 mL/kg/hr for several consecutive hours. Patients who experience bleeding at this rate cannot be stabilized hemodynamically, irrespective of the amount of volume replacement. Patients with brisk hemorrhage should be returned to the operating room even before coagulopathy is corrected in order to stop presumed surgical bleeding prior to development of cardiac tamponade and hemodynamic collapse. Even when no source of surgical bleeding is identified upon mediastinal re-exploration, clinical coagulopathy frequently improves after evacuation of the mediastinal hematoma.

Cardiac Tamponade. Mediastinal drains may fail to adequately evacuate blood after cardiovascular surgery, leading to cardiac tamponade. Abrupt cessation of bleeding from the mediastinal drains warrants close attention to the cardiac filling pressures and to overall cardiac performance. When flexible drains have been used, they should be periodically milked to prevent clotting off.

Two fairly reliable signs of cardiac tamponade are (1) increased or exaggerated cycling of the systolic blood pressure during positive-pressure ventilation, and (2) equalization of right and left atrial and pulmonary artery diastolic pressures. A reduction in SO_2 and a decrease in urine output will also be observed. The diagnosis may be confirmed by echocardiography.

In cardiac tamponade, equalization of the atrial pressures does not always occur. Blood clots on the acute margin of the right ventricle may substantially affect cardiac performance without atrial pressure equalization. In severe low-output states, cardiac tamponade must be ruled out by either mediastinal exploration in the operating room or a limited opening of the lower portion of the chest incision at the beside. Percutaneous drainage is not useful in the immediate postoperative period because the hematoma is generally clotted.

Thrombocytopenia

Thrombocytopenia is common following cardiovascular surgery (25). Causes include platelet activation and consumption during CPB, mechanical destruction by intravascular devices including prosthetic heart valves and intra-aortic balloon pumps (IABPs), inadequate production caused by malnutrition and drugs such as milrinone, and heparin-induced thrombocytopenia. Platelet counts of less than 100,000/μL are quite typical and are generally managed conservatively by removal of offending agents as soon as is feasible. If the platelet count falls by greater than 50% or a thrombotic event occurs between 4 and 14 days of heparin exposure, a diagnosis of HIT should be excluded by testing for HIT antibody seroconversion. If HIT is diagnosed or is strongly suspected, anticoagulation with a nonheparin anticoagulant such as lepirudin or bivalirudin should be considered because of the risk of thrombotic complications (33). Patients should be screened for deep vein thrombosis (DVT) with ultrasonography. For patients who require long-term anticoagulation for DVT, warfarin can be started once platelet levels return to a normal range. Warfarin is not recommended for initial therapy of HIT due to the risk of thrombotic complications.

Ventilatory Management

Ventilatory management after cardiac surgery is directed toward optimizing pulmonary function without compromising hemodynamics. On patient admission to the ICU in our institution, the synchronous intermittent mandatory ventilation (SIMV) rate is set at 14 breaths/min with a tidal volume of 8 mL/kg of predicted body weight. We do not pressure-limit the ventilator, and we carefully monitor hemodynamic function throughout the period of assisted ventilation. Acute hemodynamic changes may be indicative of patient distress, a blocked endotracheal tube, the need for suctioning, or a bronchodilator such as albuterol. Patient dyssynchrony with the ventilator should prompt assessment of the patient's level of sedation and analgesia.

Caution is advised when using positive-end expiratory pressure (PEEP) above 8 to 10 cm H_2O, because chamber filling may be affected causing cardiac performance to decrease. When high PEEP is used, intravascular volume augmentation may be necessary to raise the effective LVEDP. As a rule of thumb, one-half of the PEEP subtracted from the PACWP is the effective LVEDP.

Administration of nitroprusside and to a lesser extent nicardipine to patients who are heavy smokers or have severe chronic lung disease may increase the amount of pulmonary shunting and cause hypoxia due to V-Q mismatch. Bronchodilators and PEEP as high as 15 to 20 cm H_2O are of little use to correct this problem. In such cases, these vasodilators should be discontinued and substituted with another drug such as nitroglycerin (3 to 5 μg/kg/min) or hydralazine.

The appearance of the acute respiratory distress syndrome (ARDS) after cardiac surgery is much less frequent due, in part, to shorter CPB times and the use of membrane oxygenators. Unfortunately, when ARDS does occur in the postoperative period, it may be accompanied by multiple organ dysfunction syndrome or sepsis (34).

Diuretics

Diuresis is desirable during the recovery period to reverse hemodilution and improve pulmonary function, but should always be closely monitored and excessive urine output is to be avoided. Excessive diuretic therapy rapidly depletes intravascular volume if the renal response to these drugs is brisk. Forced diuresis that results in a urine output of 500 to 1,500 mL over several hours may significantly reduce cardiac performance and promote increased SVR.

Smaller and more frequent doses of diuretics produce a more constant diuresis and the ability to maintain a gradual negative fluid balance throughout the second 24-hour postoperative period. A sustained diuresis that prevents large hourly urine loss spares the patient rapid volume shifts. To accomplish a stable diuresis in patients with normal ventricular and renal function, our practice is to use frequent doses of relatively small doses of furosemide (10 to 20 mg) every 4 to 8 hours. In patients with marginal ventricular or renal function, particularly those who have been treated with furosemide chronically, more aggressive treatment is necessary. In this situation we use a continuous furosemide infusion at doses of 0 to 20 mg/hr. We state a 24-hour diuresis goal and titrate the infusion to meet this goal over the course of the day. Intermittent doses of thiazide diuretics are a useful adjunct in patients who have an inadequate response to the infusion.

Renal Failure

Patients who experience an extremely low cardiac output or hypotension during the first 24 hours after CPB may develop acute tubular necrosis. Most respond to diuretic therapy and can be maintained in a nonoliguric renal failure. However, some, especially those with a preoperative creatinine clearance of less than 50 mL/min, experience oliguric or anuric renal failure.

Diuretics. Patients with oliguria should be given a test bolus of both furosemide (60 to 20 mg) and then be evaluated for a urine response of greater than 50 mL/hr. A continuous furosemide infusion at doses of 0 to 20 mg/hr can then be maintained with intermittent doses of thiazide diuretics as necessary. This regimen usually maintains urine output and avoids gross volume overload after surgery, even if acute tubular necrosis is present.

Ultrafiltration. Patients with renal failure manifest primarily by volume overload may be candidates for ultrafiltration in order to remove excess salt and water (35). There are a number of advantages to this approach for patients who fail initial diuretic therapy. Commercially available systems are highly automated and allow device-based removal of salt and water from the circulation without clinically significant effects on hemodynamics or electrolyte balance. Standard central or peripheral venous catheters can be used for access, frequently avoiding the need for invasive procedures to place specialized hemodialysis catheters. We reserve this approach for patients with adequate electrolyte and urea clearance who require removal of excess water in the interval prior to anticipated return of renal function.

Dialysis. Intravascular volume overload and inadequate clearance of potassium levels are the principal indications for dialyzing a patient with acute renal failure in the immediate postoperative period. The overall goal of dialysis is to remove excess water and solutes while maintaining cardiovascular stability. For the postoperative cardiovascular surgery patient, this is best achieved with the use of continuous venovenous hemodialysis (CVVHD). This technique is easily initiated, offers good clearance, and allows accurate control of ultrafiltration that is adaptable to the patient's hemodynamic requirements. Fluid removal can therefore usually be accomplished while maintaining stable hemodynamics. CVVHD does require placement of a dedicated double-lumen central venous catheter. If postoperative bleeding is not a concern, heparin should be administered to prolong filter life. Without heparin, the average filter life ranges from 16 to 24 hours.

Patients should only be transitioned to conventional hemodialysis after a significant period of myocardial recovery. Conventional hemodialysis requires blood flow rates of at least 200 cc/hr and results in large volumes of fluid removal over a several hour period. The fluid shifts associated with this technique are inappropriate for patients early in their recovery from CPB.

Central Nervous System Complications

After operations with CPB, the historical incidence of cerebrovascular accidents (CVAs) with focal neurologic sequelae is 2% to 5% (36). The contemporary rate may be lower because of advancements in intraoperative technique including routine use of epiaortic ultrasound (37). Advanced age, history of CVA, peripheral vascular disease, valvular heart surgery, and procedures requiring a period of circulatory arrest are associated with a higher incidence of central nervous system events. Patients with a history of CVA whose focal deficits have resolved prior to operation may have "unmasking" of their old symptoms in the immediate postoperative period. Untoward psychological and cognitive sequelae are more prevalent than focal CVAs (38,39). The precise etiology of neuropsychological complications remains unclear; however, recent data suggest that microemboli, especially air, are related to both severe and subtle postoperative neuropsychological deficits (40,41).

Patients should be continuously monitored for the appearance of neuropsychological complications in the postoperative period. From the time of their emergence from anesthesia, patients should be assessed for focal motor deficits and the ability to comprehend and follow simple commands. Focal deficits should be evaluated promptly with noncontrast computed tomography (CT) of the brain to rule out hemorrhagic mass lesions that may require intervention. Magnetic resonance imaging (MRI) may be useful to identify smaller embolic foci that are not apparent on head CT. Fresh post-CPB patients are usually poor candidates for thrombolysis because of their risk for bleeding. The treatment for major embolic CNS events is usually supportive. Higher blood pressures may lead to greater perfusion via collaterals in patients with severe occlusive cerebrovascular disease.

Delirium. Postcardiotomy delirium is typically preceded by a lucid interval, usually 36 to 48 hours from the time patients awaken from anesthesia. This syndrome is characterized by confusion, disorientation, and disordered thinking and perception (38). Severe manifestations may include visual and auditory illusions, hallucinations, and paranoid ideation (42). Treatment consists of undisturbed rest, frequent reorientation, assuring patient safety, reassurance to both the patient and family, and treatment with haloperidol. It is our practice to avoid the use of benzodiazepines in this situation because of their paradoxical excitatory response seen occasionally in the elderly population. Subtle changes in mentation and thinking processes occur frequently during the first few weeks after surgery. They may be frightening to the patient and may interfere with the immediate recovery process. However, most of these problems are temporary and usually resolve by the sixth postoperative month (38,39,43).

Sedation and Paralysis

In addition to the pain and discomfort characteristic of any major surgical procedure, several conditions occurring after cardiac operation warrant sedation, and, in rare instances, complete paralysis. As the patient emerges from anesthesia, a perceived reduction in cardiac performance may result, in part, from shivering, agitation, or both. Shivering can produce a marked increase in O_2, a reduction in SO_2, and an overall imbalance of oxygen supply and demand in the body, especially in low cardiac output states. Once gross neurologic function is assessed (e.g., movement and sensation in the extremities and the ability to follow simple commands), shivering or agitation in the immediate postoperative period is best treated with narcotic agents. Our preference is to use a fentanyl to control shivering or agitation, although these conditions can be managed with morphine or other narcotics. Meperidine is particularly efficacious, although the mechanism by which it acts is unknown.

For patients who have undergone elective procedures and are expected to be extubated early in the postoperative course, a propofol infusion is started soon upon arrival to the ICU. This agent is useful in this setting because once hemodynamics and bleeding are assessed and the patient is warm, the patient's sedation can be stopped quickly because of the agent's short half-life. The patient's neurologic function can be assessed and the patient can be extubated after a brief spontaneous breathing trial.

When a patient is expected to require a prolonged period of mechanical ventilation, we typically use a combination of narcotic and benzodiazepine infusions. Fentanyl is our preferred narcotic because of its limited effects on myocardial contractility and the peripheral vasculature. In rare instances, such as severe pulmonary artery hypertension and right heart failure, a paralytic agent may be indicated to prevent any respiratory effort by the patient which can trigger increased pulmonary artery pressures and precipitate hemodynamic collapse. Because of their association with critical illness neuropathy, we prefer to avoid paralytic agents and treat these patients with deep sedation. When paralytics are required, our practice is to use vecuronium, which has a lesser chronotropic effect than pancuronium.

Mechanical Circulatory Support

Mechanical circulatory support devices include IABPs, centrifugal blood pumps, ventricular assist devices (VADs), and total artificial hearts. In some cases, extracorporeal membrane oxygenation (ECMO) is indicated for profound cardiorespiratory failure.

Intra-aortic Balloon Pumps. An IABP should be considered when patients fail to respond to moderately high-dose inotropic drug combinations such as epinephrine and milrinone. The IABP improves cardiac performance primarily by afterload reduction and augmentation of systemic diastolic pressure, thereby increasing coronary artery perfusion pressure. IABP therapy should be considered earlier rather than late, and can be instituted quickly at the bedside via a percutaneous technique. Its main contraindications are aortic insufficiency and aortoiliac occlusive disease. Complications and adverse effects include platelet consumption, catheter sepsis, and lower extremity ischemic complications.

Ventricular Assist Devices and Total Artificial Hearts. VADs replace or augment the pumping function of the right or left ventricle, or both. Because left heart failure is more common, usually only the left ventricle requires mechanical support with a left (L)VAD. Occasionally patients presenting with a right coronary infarction require implant of a right (R) VAD for support. Biventricular (Bi)VAD implant also is occasionally necessary in cardiomyopathy patients presenting with biventricular failure. A number of different VAD systems are FDA-approved and marketed for these various applications. Table 62.3 lists some commonly used VAD systems that are commercially available in the United States, separated by short-term or long-term indication.

There are a number of scenarios in which a short-term VAD may be implanted. A short-term VAD may be implanted in a patient with critical coronary anatomy so that a percutaneous coronary intervention can be performed without the patient suffering cardiovascular collapse. In this situation, the patient is supported with the VAD only in the immediate periprocedural period. Short-term VADs may be implanted in patients presenting with cardiogenic shock, either from a large myocardial infarction or from an acute chronic heart failure exacerbation in a patient with cardiomyopathy. In this setting, the patient may be supported for a period of time to allow stabilization, end-organ recovery, and myocardial recovery. If sufficient myocardial recovery does not occur, the patient may undergo implant of a long-term VAD before the short-term VAD can be safely removed.

TABLE 62.3 Commonly Used Ventricular Assist Device Systems in the United States

Short-term devices for stabilization or bridge to recovery
CentriMag (Thoratec Corporation)
Impella (Abiomed)
TandemHeart (CardiacAssist, Inc.)
Long-term devices for destination therapy or bridge to transplantation
HeartMate II (Thoratec Corporation)
Thoratec PVAD™ (Thoratec Corporation)
HeartWare Ventricular Assist System (HeartWare Inc.)

Long-term VADs were initially developed to support patients with chronic heart failure who were awaiting heart transplantation. This indication became known as bridge to transplantation. Because of the success with long-term LVADs used for the bridge to transplantation indication, their use was extended to patients who are not candidates for heart transplantation. This therapy is known as destination therapy because the LVAD is the only advanced treatment that the patient is eligible to receive.

For patients with severe biventricular failure awaiting heart transplantation, implant of BiVADs or a total artificial heart may be necessary to support the patient until a suitable donor heart becomes available. There is currently only one total artificial heart commercially available in the United States (Syncardia Systems, Inc.).

Extracorporeal Membrane Oxygenation. In specialized centers, ECMO may be used for the treatment of patients presenting with biventricular failure and respiratory failure related to pulmonary edema and volume overload.

Patients who have received mechanical circulatory support devices present a special challenge to the critical care team because of their underlying heart failure and their typical acute presentation with cardiogenic shock. Their neurologic status may be uncertain if they present with a period of cardiac arrest. They may have associated respiratory failure because of left heart failure and volume overload. They may have renal failure related to hypoperfusion and hypotension. Patients with right ventricular failure may present with liver failure related to hepatic congestion. Patients may present with malnutrition and cachexia if they have had chronic congestive heart failure.

For patients presenting with cardiogenic shock who are supported with a short-term device such as an IABP or VAD, the main goal of treatment is to maintain end-organ function until a definitive cardiovascular procedure such as revascularization can be performed or myocardial function has recovered. Mechanical ventilation and dialysis are frequently necessary because of the frequent associated conditions of respiratory and renal failure in patients presenting with shock. If myocardial recovery and function are not restored, the patient should be evaluated for implant of a long-term VAD, either as destination therapy or bridge to transplantation.

Complications related to mechanical circulatory support devices are common. CVAs, infections, and bleeding complications are particularly troublesome and can limit successful outcomes in these patients. Best practices, clinical pathways, and certification programs have been developed to optimize outcomes in this challenging patient population (44).

Blood Glucose Control

There has been increasing emphasis on maintaining tight blood glucose control in critically ill patients because of demonstrated reductions in morbidity and mortality. The benefits of tight glucose control have been demonstrated in cardiac surgery patients specifically (45–47). Maintenance of tight glucose control reduces the incidence of mediastinitis, atrial fibrillation, ischemia, length of stay, hospital costs, and mortality, and has been shown to benefit both diabetic and nondiabetic patients following cardiovascular surgery. In our practice, we have instituted an intensive intravenous insulin therapy protocol with a goal of maintaining normoglycemia (blood glucose 80 to 110 mg/dL). A continuous insulin infusion is typically started intraoperatively, and we have found all adult patients to require intravenous insulin at least through the immediate postoperative period if normoglycemia is to be maintained.

The requirement for intravenous insulin is reduced as inotropes, particularly epinephrine, are weaned. Once patients begin taking an oral diet, we supplement the intravenous insulin infusion with a fast-acting insulin formulation such as insulin aspart given subcutaneously. The dose of insulin aspart is based upon the patient's oral intake and intravenous insulin requirement over the preceding 12 hours. Patients are subsequently transitioned to a long-acting insulin formulation, such as NPH, given subcutaneously three times a day to cover basal needs in addition to fast-acting insulin which is still based on the percentage of meals consumed. Nondiabetic patients typically have a progressively decreasing insulin requirement during their hospital recovery and are not discharged on any insulin. We have found this regimen to provide improved blood glucose control while also decreasing the frequency and severity of episodes of hypo- and hyperglycemia.

Catheter Sepsis

Blood stream infections have particularly significant implications in cardiovascular surgery patients as prosthetic intravascular devices, such as heart valves and arterial conduits, are frequently implanted during surgery. Patients typically return from the operating room following cardiovascular surgery with multiple invasive monitoring catheters including central lines, pulmonary artery catheters, arterial lines, and urinary catheters. The incidence of sepsis increases when invasive monitoring catheters are left in place for longer than 72 hours (48). For straightforward cases, our goal is to have all monitoring catheters removed by this time. All peripheral intravenous lines are also removed at the time of the patient's transfer to the intermediate care floor and a new peripheral intravenous line is placed. If a patient remains critically ill and still requires invasive monitoring, we observe the patient closely for signs of sepsis such as fever and leukocytosis, and have a low threshold to remove old lines. We avoid rewiring catheters and prefer to insert new catheters at a different site. Cultures are drawn at this time and vancomycin is started if clinical suspicion for catheter sepsis is high. Antibiotic coverage is narrowed or discontinued based on subsequent culture results.

Clinical Pathways

Clinical pathways have been increasingly used by health care systems to improve the continuity and coordination of care for patients being treated for many diseases. They frequently are developed around procedures, and patients undergoing CABG procedures were among the first to benefit from their implementation. CABG procedures are common, usually elective, have typical recovery milestones, and require coordination of multidisciplinary provider teams. These characteristics make CABG pathways extremely useful to support both clinical and administrative management.

Many institutions have implemented clinical pathways for other cardiovascular procedures as well, including heart valve repair or replacement and heart transplantation. Clinical pathways typically are based around a timeline, categories of care such as nursing and physical therapy, and a variance record which allows deviations to be incorporated. When successfully implemented, they encourage the use of clinical guidelines, improve multidisciplinary teamwork, reduce variations in patient care, and improve clinical outcomes. It is important that clinical pathways not discourage personalized care and that they function well even in the face of unexpected changes in a patient's condition.

Cardiac Surgery Databases

Institutional and multi-institutional databases are useful tools with which to track outcomes following cardiovascular operations, conduct clinical research, and guide continuous quality improvement. This data is also used by various regulatory bodies and third party payers to monitor health care quality and costs. It will also be used for pay-for-performance initiatives in the future. The data collected in these databases is clinical, administrative, or a combination of both. The Society of Thoracic Surgeons Cardiac Database is the largest clinical cardiothoracic surgery database in the world and currently has more than 500 participating sites. The large volume of clinical information collected allows risk modeling for common procedures and provides individual institutions with comparative outcomes data and national benchmarks. All cardiac databases are limited by the variable quality of collected data, which in many instances is self-reported. Comparison of outcomes is also subject to selection bias not corrected by imprecise risk models.

Special Clinical Scenarios

Off-pump Coronary Artery Bypass Surgery

Over the last 10 years, there has been increasing interest in performing CABG surgery without the use of CPB. This growth has been largely driven by the increasing recognition of the deleterious effects of CPB and the desire to avoid the diffuse inflammatory response, multiorgan dysfunction, and neurocognitive complications that may follow (see Table 62.4) (49–57). Approximately 25% of CABGs performed in the United States are performed off-pump, and some centers report a significantly higher percentage of off-pump coronary artery bypass procedures (OPCABs). Even among surgeons not routinely performing coronary revascularization off-pump, there are newly recognized clinical scenarios, such as a patient with severe atherosclerosis of the ascending aorta, for whom the use of OPCAB techniques is strongly favored. OPCAB itself

TABLE 62.4 Benefits of Off-pump Coronary Artery Bypass Grafting Demonstrated in Prospective, Randomized Studies

Myocardial protection
- Reduced release of cardiac enzymes
- Decreased need for inotropic support
- Fewer postoperative arrhythmias

Pulmonary function
- Decreased requirement for mechanical ventilation

Renal protection
- Improved preservation of glomerular filtration and renal tubular function

Coagulation
- Decreased coagulopathy
- Decreased transfusion requirement

Inflammation
- Reduced release of cytokines
- Reduced complement activation
- Decreased incidence of postoperative infections

Neurocognitive function

Improved early postoperative neurocognitive function

Resource utilization
- Decreased total resource utilization

From Song HK, Puskas JD. Off-pump coronary artery bypass surgery. In: Kaiser LR, Kron IL, Spray TL, eds. *Mastery of Cardiothoracic Surgery*. 2nd ed. Philadelphia, PA: Lippincott Williams & Wilkins; 2007:305–314.

is a facilitating technology for surgeons developing minimally invasive approaches to coronary revascularization. OPCAB has therefore evolved into a requisite component of modern cardiovascular surgery practice.

The postoperative care of patients who have undergone OPCAB surgery does not differ in many respects from that of patients undergoing conventional CABG surgery. There are a number of important differences, however, that providers must be aware of to take advantage of the opportunity for expedited care that OPCAB surgery can offer. Patients who have undergone OPCAB surgery have a decreased need for inotropic support in the postoperative period, most likely because of avoidance of global ischemia and reduced myocardial stunning. The intravenous fluid requirement for patients who have undergone OPCAB surgery is also reduced because the systemic inflammatory response and capillary leak related to CPB is avoided. Massive volume resuscitation in the early postoperative period should be avoided in favor of low-dose vasopressors that may be necessary secondary to intravenous sedation. OPCAB patients typically are volume loaded intraoperatively and are more likely to be euvolemic in the immediate postoperative period than conventional CABG patients.

Postoperative hemorrhage and transfusion requirements are reduced in OPCAB patients because of reduced fibrinolytic pathway activation and coagulation factor and platelet consumption. We do not routinely check platelet counts or clotting times in these patients in the immediate postoperative period for this reason. Persistent or massive hemorrhage in the postoperative period should prompt early evaluation for surgical bleeding because this is unlikely to be related to factor or platelet deficiency in an OPCAB patient.

Patients who have undergone OPCAB surgery are in a relatively hypercoagulable state as opposed to manifesting the coagulopathy that is typical after CPB. This state has the potential to adversely affect graft patency in the postoperative period. After surgery, we continue aspirin administration daily as with patients undergoing conventional CABG surgery. In addition, we start clopidogrel 75 mg/d in the immediate postoperative period once chest tube drainage has been low for 3 consecutive hours.

One of the major benefits of OPCAB surgery to the health care system is the potential for OPCAB patients to have reduced resource utilization. An area where this advantage can be exploited is in reducing the length of mechanical ventilation and ICU stay. To realize this benefit for the patient and the health system, providers should be cognizant of this and be immediately prepared to wean and extubate patients as their need for mechanical assistance is diminished. With appropriate anesthesia planning and staffing, patients can generally be extubated in the operating room after an OPCAB procedure or within 30 minutes of arrival in the ICU. When this is not feasible, clinical pathways that set objective criteria and goals facilitate the timely progression of ventilator weaning and extubation that minimizes patient exposure to ventilator-related complications and maximizes efficiency and cost-effectiveness.

Thoracic Aortic Surgery

Patients undergoing surgery for disorders of the thoracic aorta present critical care providers with several unique challenges, including neurologic complications, hemodynamic disturbances, and malperfusion syndromes. Several of these conditions are caused by the period of circulatory arrest that the patient undergoes during the conduct of the surgical repair while others are caused by the specific anatomy of the underlying thoracic aortic pathology.

Circulatory Arrest Sequelae

Patients undergoing aortic arch procedures usually have a period of circulatory arrest during their operation. This increases their risk for neurologic complications, particularly psychological and cognitive disorders. It is typical for elderly patients who require prolonged hypothermic circulatory arrest (greater than 30 minutes) to have neurologic dysfunction resulting in agitation and delirium. Although this finding is usually transient, it may necessitate a several-day period of supportive care during which the patient requires mechanical ventilation.

Circulatory arrest is also associated with increased bleeding and transfusion requirement related to profound coagulopathy (58,59). Profound coagulopathy is especially problematic in this patient group because of the long suture lines used in large vessel surgery. Patients presenting with acute aortic dissections have attenuated and friable aortic tissue making vascular anastomoses potentially tenuous. Coagulopathy following emergency thoracic aortic surgery for dissection should be treated aggressively as described earlier in this chapter. Surgical bleeding should always be suspected in patients with brisk hemorrhage. Avoidance of hypertension is desirable in patients with long suture lines and friable aortic tissue.

Patients who have undergone complex vascular repairs with long bypass times and circulatory arrest also may develop profound vasodilatory shock that is recalcitrant to combination therapy with multiple vasopressors. The cause for this is unclear but may be related to bacterial translocation of intestinal flora (60–62). Patients who exhibit this should be adequately volume resuscitated and supported with vasopressors and inotropes if poor myocardial contractility is contributing to the hypotension. We have also used intravenous steroids and methylene blue in patients with profound vasodilation (20,63–65). Addition of these agents has allowed reduction of high doses of vasopressors that can lead to ischemic complications.

Spinal Cord Ischemia

Spinal cord ischemia and paralysis is a particularly devastating complication following thoracoabdominal aneurysm repair. Spinal cord ischemia occurs at the time of thoracoabdominal aneurysm repair and is exacerbated by postoperative hypoperfusion, particularly when the variable origin of the artery of Adamkiewicz is not adequately reconstituted. This results in an anterior spinal artery syndrome with impaired lower extremity motor function and to a lesser degree impaired sensory function. Patients should be monitored closely for these findings in the immediate postoperative period. When spinal cord ischemia is suspected, a lumbar drain should be placed if one was not already placed intraoperatively. Cerebrospinal fluid (CSF) should be drained for a CSF pressure of 10 mmHg or greater and the mean arterial blood pressure should be raised to 85 to 100 mmHg using vasopressors in order to increase the perfusion pressure to the spinal cord. These maneuvers have led to reversal of acute lower extremity neurologic findings in patients following thoracoabdominal aneurysm repair. MRI is useful for confirming the diagnosis of spinal cord ischemia. Treatment as outlined above should not be delayed until after MRI scanning, if spinal cord ischemia is suspected.

Malperfusion Syndromes

Malperfusion syndromes occur in patients with aortic dissection as a result of obstruction of arterial branch orifices by the dissected intimal flap or inadequate perfusion via the false lumen of the aorta. Patients presenting with aortic dissection can develop malperfusion of virtually any limb or end organ, depending on the anatomic extent of the dissection. Patients with ascending aorta involvement (Stanford Type A) typically undergo emergency surgery while patients with only descending aorta involvement (Stanford Type B) are treated initially with medical therapy. Even patients who have undergone repair of ascending aortic dissection are frequently left with residual dissection involving the descending aorta; therefore, providers must remain vigilant for the development of malperfusion syndromes in both patient groups. Patients admitted to the ICU with dissection should undergo serial peripheral pulse, neurologic, and abdominal examinations for evidence of malperfusion. Serial arterial blood gases, liver enzymes, and lactate levels are useful when visceral malperfusion is suspected.

We have a low threshold for performing angiography when malperfusion is suspected. If confirmed by this study, interventional techniques such as fenestration or stenting can frequently be used to treat malperfusion during the same procedure. Laparotomy may be occasionally required for patients with visceral malperfusion who progress to bowel infarction.

Transcatheter Aortic Valve Replacement

The development of transcatheter aortic valve replacement (TAVR) has been an important advance in the treatment of patients with aortic stenosis. It allows the aortic valve replacement procedure to be performed percutaneously via femoral artery puncture or through a transapical approach via left minithoracotomy. The procedure is performed without the use of CPB. In the United States, the TAVR procedure is restricted for use in patients who are at high or prohibitive risk for surgical aortic valve replacement. Although TAVR patients benefit from undergoing a less invasive procedure and avoidance of CPB, they still present a challenge to the critical care team because of their comorbid conditions that make them eligible for the TAVR procedure in the first place (66). TAVR patients typically are older, more frail, and have more serious comorbid conditions such as chronic obstructive pulmonary disease and renal insufficiency compared to patients undergoing surgical aortic valve replacement.

Embolic stroke is a relatively common complication of TAVR. Heart block requiring pacemaker implantation is common, especially after implant of a self-expanding TAVR device. A condition known as suicidal left ventricle is seen exclusively in TAVR patients. Some patients with hyperdynamic left ventricles secondary to chronic aortic stenosis may develop interventricular gradients after acute removal of left ventricular outflow obstruction by TAVR implantation. Inotropes given to treat the resulting hypotension may exacerbate this problem, leading to the spiraling condition known as suicidal left ventricle. These patients may be successfully managed similar to patients with hypertrophic obstructive cardiomyopathy with volume expansion, avoidance of inotropes, and judicious use of vasoconstrictors.

Paravalvar leak remains an important challenge in patients undergoing TAVR. It can occur in up to 21% of patients undergoing TAVR (67). A significant paravalvar leak is associated with poorer long-term survival and occasionally a large paravalvar leak can complicate the perioperative care of patients undergoing TAVR. Large leaks are typically identified intraoperatively with the use of transesophageal echocardiography but occasionally develop or worsen in the postoperative period. In patients with recalcitrant CHF after TAVR implant, paravalvar leaks should be sought. Large leaks may necessitate re-ballooning of the TAVR device to achieve greater expansion or percutaneous closure with a vascular plug.

Key Points

- All patients undergoing major cardiovascular surgery procedures pass through a period of critical illness during their recovery.
- The management of cardiovascular surgery patients is complicated by the hemodynamic changes related to the cardiovascular repair itself as well as the broad aftereffects of CPB and myocardial reperfusion.
- CPB leads to the systemic release of an inflammatory cascade that affects the function of virtually every organ system.
- Cardiovascular surgery patients pass through phases in the immediate postoperative period where issues such as organ dysfunction, inflammation, changes in vasomotor tone, ventricular compliance, and fluid shifts typically occur. Vigilance for these critical care management problems is necessary to achieve optimal outcomes.
- Cardiovascular surgery patients benefit from standardized critical care protocols implemented by providers with strong familiarity of normal recovery milestones and complications seen in this unique patient population.

References

1. Hall RI, Smith MS, Rocker G. The systemic inflammatory response to cardiopulmonary bypass: pathophysiological, therapeutic, and pharmacological considerations. *Anesth Analg*. 1997;85:766–782.
2. Steinberg JB, Kapelanski DP, Olson JD, Weiler JM. Cytokine and complement levels in patients undergoing cardiopulmonary bypass. *J Thorac Cardiovasc Surg*. 1993;106:1008–1016.
3. Miller BE, Levy JH. The inflammatory response to cardiopulmonary bypass. *J Cardiothorac Vasc Anesth*. 1997;11:355–366.
4. Lobato EB, Gravenstein N, Martin TD. Milrinone, not epinephrine, improves left ventricular compliance after cardiopulmonary bypass. *J Cardiothorac Vasc Anesth*. 2000;14:374–377.
5. Kouchoukos NT, Karp RB. Management of the postoperative cardiovascular surgical patient. *Am Heart J*. 1976;92:513–531.
6. Reinhart K, Kersting T, Fohring U, Schafer M. Can central-venous replace mixed-venous oxygen saturation measurements during anesthesia? *Adv Exp Med Biol*. 1986;200:67–72.
7. Reinhart K, Rudolph T, Bredle DL, et al. Comparison of central-venous to mixed-venous oxygen saturation during changes in oxygen supply/demand. *Chest*. 1989;95:1216–1221.
8. Halonen J, Hakala T, Auvinen T, et al. Intravenous administration of metoprolol is more effective than oral administration in the prevention of atrial fibrillation after cardiac surgery. *Circulation*. 2006;114:I1–I4.
9. Katariya K, DeMarchena E, Bolooki H. Oral amiodarone reduces incidence of postoperative atrial fibrillation. *Ann Thorac Surg*. 1999;68:1599–1603.
10. Kurz DJ, Naegeli B, Kunz M, et al. Epicardial, biatrial synchronous pacing for prevention of atrial fibrillation after cardiac surgery. *Pacing Clin Electrophysiol*. 1999;22:721–726.
11. Patti G, Chello M, Candura D, et al. Randomized trial of atorvastatin for reduction of postoperative atrial fibrillation in patients undergoing cardiac surgery: results of the ARMYDA-3 (Atorvastatin for Reduction of Myocardial Dysrhythmia After cardiac surgery) study. *Circulation*. 2006; 114:1455–1461.
12. Stamou SC, Hill PC, Sample GA, et al. Prevention of atrial fibrillation after cardiac surgery: the significance of postoperative oral amiodarone. *Chest*. 2001;120:1936–1941.
13. Spaan JA, Piek JJ, Hoffman JI, Siebes M. Physiological basis of clinically used coronary hemodynamic indices. *Circulation*. 2006;113:446–455.
14. Kouchoukos NT, Sheppard LC, McDonald DA, Kirklin JW. Estimation of stroke volume from the central arterial pressure contour in postoperative patients. *Surg Forum*. 1969;20:180–182.
15. Webber CE, Garnett ES. The relationship between colloid osmotic pressure and plasma proteins during and after cardiopulmonary bypass. *J Thorac Cardiovasc Surg*. 1973;65:234–237.
16. Ng CS, Wan S, Yim AP, Arifi AA. Pulmonary dysfunction after cardiac surgery. *Chest*. 2002;121:1269–1277.
17. Gallagher JD, Moore RA, Kerns D, et al. Effects of colloid or crystalloid administration on pulmonary extravascular water in the postoperative period after coronary artery bypass grafting. *Anesth Analg*. 1985;64: 753–758.
18. Morales DL, Garrido MJ, Madigan JD, et al. A double-blind randomized trial: prophylactic vasopressin reduces hypotension after cardiopulmonary bypass. *Ann Thorac Surg*. 2003;75:926–930.
19. Weis F, Kilger E, Beiras-Fernandez A, et al. Association between vasopressor dependence and early outcome in patients after cardiac surgery. *Anaesthesia*. 2006;61:938–942.
20. Shanmugam G. Vasoplegic syndrome: the role of methylene blue. *Eur J Cardiothorac Surg*. 2005;28:705–710.
21. Masetti P, Murphy SF, Kouchoukos NT. Vasopressin therapy for vasoplegic syndrome following cardiopulmonary bypass. *J Card Surg*. 2002;17: 485–489.
22. Di Giantomasso D, Morimatsu H, May CN, Bellomo R. Increasing renal blood flow: low-dose dopamine or medium-dose norepinephrine. *Chest*. 2004;125:2260–2267.
23. Nikolaidis LA, Trumble D, Hentosz T, et al. Catecholamines restore myocardial contractility in dilated cardiomyopathy at the expense of increased coronary blood flow and myocardial oxygen consumption (MvO2 cost of catecholamines in heart failure). *Eur J Heart Fail*. 2004;6:409–419.
24. Eagle KA, Guyton RA, Davidoff R, et al. ACC/AHA 2004 guideline update for coronary artery bypass graft surgery: summary article: a report of the American College of Cardiology/American Heart Association Task Force on Practice Guidelines (Committee to Update the 1999 Guidelines for Coronary Artery Bypass Graft Surgery). *Circulation*. 2004;110:1168–1176.
25. Linden MD. The hemostatic defect of cardiopulmonary bypass. *J Thromb Thrombolysis*. 2003;16:129–147.
26. Woodman RC, Harker LA. Bleeding complications associated with cardiopulmonary bypass. *Blood*. 1990;76:1680–1697.
27. Slaughter TF, Faghih F, Greenberg CS, et al. The effects of epsilon-aminocaproic acid on fibrinolysis and thrombin generation during cardiac surgery. *Anesth Analg*. 1997;85:1221–1226.
28. Smith PK, Datta SK, Muhlbaier LH, et al. Cost analysis of aprotinin for coronary artery bypass patients: analysis of the randomized trials. *Ann Thorac Surg*. 2004;77:635–642.
29. Bishop CV, Renwick WE, Hogan C, et al. Recombinant activated factor VII: treating postoperative hemorrhage in cardiac surgery. *Ann Thorac Surg*. 2006;81:875–879.
30. Halkos ME, Levy JH, Chen E, et al. Early experience with activated recombinant factor VII for intractable hemorrhage after cardiovascular surgery. *Ann Thorac Surg*. 2005;79:1303–1306.
31. Song HK, Tibayan FA, Kahl EA, et al. Safety and efficacy of prothrombin complex concentrates for the treatment of coagulopathy after cardiac surgery. *J Thorac Cardiovasc Surg*. 2014;147:1036–1040.
32. Hayward CP, Harrison P, Cattaneo M, et al. The Platelet Physiology Subcommittee of the Scientific and Standardization Committee of the International Society on Thrombosis and H. Platelet function analyzer (PFA)-100 closure time in the evaluation of platelet disorders and platelet function. *J Thromb Haemost*. 2006;4:312–319.
33. Holmes-Ghosh E. Heparin-induced thrombocytopenia and thrombosis syndrome after cardiopulmonary bypass. *Am J Crit Care*. 2000;9:276–278.
34. Asimakopoulos G, Smith PL, Ratnatunga CP, Taylor KM. Lung injury and acute respiratory distress syndrome after cardiopulmonary bypass. *Ann Thorac Surg*. 1999;68:1107–1115.
35. Jaski BE, Miller D. Ultrafiltration in decompensated heart failure. *Curr Heart Fail Rep*. 2005;2:148–154.
36. Gardner TJ, Horneffer PJ, Manolio TA, et al. Stroke following coronary artery bypass grafting: a ten-year study. *Ann Thorac Surg*. 1985;40:574–581.
37. Hogue CW Jr, Palin CA, Arrowsmith JE. Cardiopulmonary bypass management and neurologic outcomes: an evidence-based appraisal of current practices. *Anesth Analg*. 2006;103:21–37.
38. Gao L, Taha R, Gauvin D, et al. Postoperative cognitive dysfunction after cardiac surgery. *Chest*. 2005;128:3664–3670.
39. O'Brien DJ, Bauer RM, Yarandi H, et al. Patient memory before and after cardiac operations. *J Thorac Cardiovasc Surg*. 1992;104:1116–1124.
40. Clark RE, Brillman J, Davis DA, et al. Microemboli during coronary artery bypass grafting: genesis and effect on outcome. *J Thorac Cardiovasc Surg*. 1995;109:249–257.
41. Stump DA. Embolic factors associated with cardiac surgery. *Semin Cardiothorac Vasc Anesth*. 2005;9:151–152.
42. Vasquez E, Chitwood WR Jr. Postcardiotomy delirium: an overview. *Int J Psychiatry Med*. 1975;6:373–383.
43. Townes BD, Bashein G, Hornbein TF, et al. Neurobehavioral outcomes in cardiac operations: a prospective controlled study. *J Thorac Cardiovasc Surg*. 1989;98:774–782.
44. Slaughter MS, Pagani FD, Rogers JG, et al. Clinical management of continuous-flow left ventricular assist devices in advanced heart failure. *J Heart Lung Transplant*. 2010;29:S1–S39.
45. Ouattara A, Lecomte P, Le Manach Y, et al. Poor intraoperative blood glucose control is associated with a worsened hospital outcome after cardiac surgery in diabetic patients. *Anesthesiology*. 2005;103:687–694.
46. Rassias AJ, Givan AL, Marrin CA, et al. Insulin increases neutrophil count and phagocytic capacity after cardiac surgery. *Anesth Analg*. 2002;94: 1113–1119.
47. Shann KG, Likosky DS, Murkin JM, et al. An evidence-based review of the practice of cardiopulmonary bypass in adults: a focus on neurologic injury, glycemic control, hemodilution, and the inflammatory response. *J Thorac Cardiovasc Surg*. 2006;132:283–290.
48. Eggimann P, Sax H, Pittet D. Catheter-related infections. *Microbes Infect*. 2004;6:1033–1042.
49. Angelini GD, Taylor FC, Reeves BC, Ascione R. Early and midterm outcome after off-pump and on-pump surgery in Beating Heart Against Cardioplegic Arrest Studies (BHACAS 1 and 2): a pooled analysis of two randomised controlled trials. *Lancet*. 2002;359:1194–1199.
50. Ascione R, Lloyd CT, Gomes WJ, et al. Beating versus arrested heart revascularization: evaluation of myocardial function in a prospective randomized study. *Eur J Cardiothorac Surg*. 1999;15:685–690.
51. Ascione R, Lloyd CT, Underwood MJ, et al. Economic outcome of off-pump coronary artery bypass surgery: a prospective randomized study. *Ann Thorac Surg*. 1999;68:2237–2242.
52. Ascione R, Williams S, Lloyd CT, et al. Reduced postoperative blood loss and transfusion requirement after beating-heart coronary operations: a prospective randomized study. *J Thorac Cardiovasc Surg*. 2001;121:689–696.

53. Puskas JD, Williams WH, Duke PG, et al. Off-pump coronary artery bypass grafting provides complete revascularization with reduced myocardial injury, transfusion requirements, and length of stay: a prospective randomized comparison of two hundred unselected patients undergoing off-pump versus conventional coronary artery bypass grafting. *J Thorac Cardiovasc Surg*. 2003;125:797–808.
54. Puskas JD, Williams WH, Mahoney EM, et al. Off-pump vs conventional coronary artery bypass grafting: early and 1-year graft patency, cost, and quality-of-life outcomes: a randomized trial. *JAMA*. 2004;291:1841–1849.
55. Van Dijk D, Jansen EW, Hijman R, et al. Cognitive outcome after off-pump and on-pump coronary artery bypass graft surgery: a randomized trial. *JAMA*. 2002;287:1405–1412.
56. van Dijk D, Nierich AP, Jansen EW, et al. Early outcome after off-pump versus on-pump coronary bypass surgery: results from a randomized study. *Circulation*. 2001;104:1761–1766.
57. Zamvar V, Williams D, Hall J, et al. Assessment of neurocognitive impairment after off-pump and on-pump techniques for coronary artery bypass graft surgery: prospective randomised controlled trial. *BMJ*. 2002;325:1268.
58. Westaby S. Coagulation disturbance in profound hypothermia: the influence of anti-fibrinolytic therapy. *Semin Thorac Cardiovasc Surg*. 1997;9:246–256.
59. Wilde JT. Hematological consequences of profound hypothermic circulatory arrest and aortic dissection. *J Card Surg*. 1997;12:201–206.
60. Rossi M, Sganga G, Mazzone M, et al. Cardiopulmonary bypass in man: role of the intestine in a self-limiting inflammatory response with demonstrable bacterial translocation. *Ann Thorac Surg*. 2004;77:612–618.
61. Ryan T, Mc Carthy JF, Rady MY, et al. Early bloodstream infection after cardiopulmonary bypass: frequency rate, risk factors, and implications. *Crit Care Med*. 1997;25:2009–2014.
62. Tsunooka N, Maeyama K, Hamada Y, et al. Bacterial translocation secondary to small intestinal mucosal ischemia during cardiopulmonary bypass: measurement by diamine oxidase and peptidoglycan. *Eur J Cardiothorac Surg*. 2004;25:275–280.
63. Callister ME, Evans TW. Haemodynamic and ventilatory support in severe sepsis. *J R Coll Phys Lond*. 2000;34:522–528.
64. Maslow AD, Stearns G, Batula P, et al. The hemodynamic effects of methylene blue when administered at the onset of cardiopulmonary bypass. *Anesth Analg*. 2006;103:2–8.
65. Sparicio D, Landoni G, Zangrillo A. Angiotensin-converting enzyme inhibitors predispose to hypotension refractory to norepinephrine but responsive to methylene blue. *J Thorac Cardiovasc Surg*. 2004;127:608.
66. Tomey MI, Gidwani UK, Sharma SK. Cardiac critical care after transcatheter aortic valve replacement. *Cardiol Clin*. 2013;31:607–618.
67. Sinning JM, Vasa-Nicotera M, Chin D, et al. Evaluation and management of paravalvular aortic regurgitation after transcatheter aortic valve replacement. *J Am Coll Cardiol*. 2013;62:11–20.

CHAPTER
63

Burn Injury: Thermal and Electrical

WINSTON T. RICHARDS, DAVID J. HALL, MARTIN D. ROSENTHAL, and DAVID W. MOZINGO

INTRODUCTION

Burn injury accounts for 40,000 hospital admissions/year, including 30,000 admissions to hospitals with specialized burn centers. More than 60% of the 40,000 hospitalizations for burn injuries in the United States each year are now admitted to 127 hospitals with specialized burn centers. Thirty-eight percent of the admissions exceeded 10% total body surface area (TBSA), and 10% exceeded 30% TBSA involvement. Most included severe burns of such vital body areas as the face, hands, and feet; interestingly, 69% of burn patients were male. Data from the National Hospital Discharge survey of 2010, as well as the National Inpatient Sample 2012, and the American Burn Association National Burn Repository 2013 report suggest that the causes of the burns include fire (43%), scald (34%), contact with a hot object (9%), electrical (4%), and chemical (3%) (1).

Burn injury has a systemic effect on the patient, and each organ system responds to this injury in a predictable manner proportional to the extent of burn. The current literature supports the following physiologic responses in each organ system.

BURN PHYSIOLOGY AND THE EFFECTS ON ORGAN SYSTEMS

Cardiovascular System

Immediately after a burn injury cardiac output (CO) becomes depressed, systemic vascular resistance (SVR) increases, and the patient's capillary permeability increases. Each of these occurs in a burn size- and time-dependent fashion.

During the late 1960s and early 1970s, animal studies by Moncrief, Asch, and Wilmore clearly defined the physiologic response of the heart and systemic and pulmonary vasculature to burn injury (3–4). These experiments showed a burn size- and severity-dependent depression in CO, which resolved over time, and could be altered with fluid resuscitation and the addition of vasoactive medications. They also showed a time-dependent increase in SVR and pulmonary vascular resistance (PVR), which resolved with fluid resuscitation as well as with the administration of vasoactive medication.

Burn injury causes loss of the skin's fluid barrier function. These resultant fluid losses, as well as increased capillary permeability, lead to hypovolemia and burn shock. The loss of fluid leads to decreased cardiac preload and ultimately, decreased CO. Integumentary fluid losses and tissue edema drive the cardiovascular response to burn injury, but improvement in cardiac function parameters achieved by fluid resuscitation do not fully resolve this deficit; there is evidence linking a myocardial depressant factor to multiple inflammatory mediators (5–8).

Cardiac depression after a thermal injury is mediated by the interaction of multiple inflammatory and anti-inflammatory molecular signals. Early and late inflammatory mediators influence myocardial contraction and relaxation in the first 24 to 48 hours after burn injury (9,10). Factors including tumor necrosis factor-α (TNF-α), Fas ligand, interleukin (IL)-1, IL-18, IL-6, macrophage migration inhibitory factor (MIF), high mobility group box 1 (HMGB-1) chemokines, and caspase-1 have been implicated in the loss of cardiac contractility as well as myocardial relaxation, leading to decreased CO after injury. By contrast, the anti-inflammatory pathways involving IL-10, transforming growth factor (TGF)-β, and soluble TNF receptor lead to the resolution of the initial myocardial depression.

Resuscitation of the burn patient addresses the cardiac depression, with administered fluid bolstering the intravascular volume by replacing losses and anticipating future deficits. Multiple resuscitation strategies exist for fluid management in the burn patient, which are discussed separately below. Myocardial depression can be marginally supported pharmacologically with the use of inotropic agents. Further research toward more direct management of the decreased contractility could target the inflammatory mediators released after burn injury (8).

Pulmonary System

Burn injury has multiple effects on the pulmonary system. Depending on the mode of injury, including inhalation and direct burns to the chest wall, these effects may be manifest as alterations in respiratory rate, tidal volume, gas exchange, and even long-term effects on pulmonary function. Burn injury not only affects the lungs in a direct manner, but complications of these injuries may add to further dysfunction. Pneumonia and tracheal irritation from prolonged intubation are some of the complicating factors that affect the burn patient (2).

The pulmonary response to burn injury is characterized by transient pulmonary hypertension, decreased lung compliance, and hypoxia. These functional changes are mediated by multiple factors including inflammation, acid–base imbalance, airway injury, and chest wall restriction. The body's pH balance highlights the close interaction between the pulmonary and renal systems in addressing disturbances caused by burn injury. Studies of anti-inflammatory treatment prior to burn injury altered the pattern of decreased compliance, pulmonary hypertension, and hypoxia, suggesting a cause-and-effect relationship (11).

With relatively small TBSA burns, respiratory rates increased, peaking by postburn day 8 and returning to control levels by about 3 weeks postburn. Along with these respiratory rate changes, an increase in tidal volume and minute ventilation were also recorded; these returned to control levels in approximately 3 weeks (11).

Chest burns with their concurrent edema formation showed notable restrictive effects on pulmonary function during the first 3 days postinjury; these effects resolved over time. During the patient's initial resuscitation, decreased chest wall compliance may lead to restricted ventilation and increased airway pressures; burn wound escharotomy of the chest wall is indicated in these situations to improve chest wall compliance.

Further effects of burn injury on pulmonary function have been attributed to burn wound infection, which may lead to lung dysfunction secondary to inflammatory mediator release from around the burned tissue, possibly mediated by thromboxane A2; management of the inflammatory process initiated by burn injury may prove to be helpful in modulating this effect (12).

Complications associated with intubation after burn injuries include ventilator-associated pneumonia (VAP) and tracheal stenosis. Protocols for the reduction/prevention of VAP have been extensively reviewed and are currently being used in many hospitals. The judicious management of ventilator support and endotracheal intubation addresses postinjury tracheal stenosis. Tracheal decannulation at the earliest opportunity afforded by the patient's physiology is important in reducing this complication. Presently, a generalized benefit from the VAP bundle has not been clearly defined in the burn patient population, and requires further study (13–15).

Smoke inhalation injury affects between 10% and 30% of burn patients. This injury is caused by the inhalation of hot gases and products of incomplete combustion; when present, an inhalation injury is associated with increased mortality up to 20% over that predicted by age and extent of burn alone. Although in the past, increased fluid resuscitation was advocated for patients with inhalation injury, this did not correlate well with fluid requirements during resuscitation; interestingly, a low initial PaO_2/FiO_2 ratio does so correlate. An increased TBSA injury is associated with increased pneumonia rates, and the presence of pneumonia in patients with an inhalation injury results in a higher mortality rate. Pneumonia and inhalation injury increase length of stay over inhalation injury alone; this is discussed further below (16).

In the late 1980s, high-frequency percussive ventilation (HFPV) was used to treat patients with severe inhalation injury; the results were promising, and further studies followed. By 2007, it had been noted that HFPV for inhalation injury did not change mean ventilator days, intensive care unit (ICU) length of stay, hospital length of stay, or incidence of pneumonia. Despite the similarities in the HFPV and conventional ventilator groups, a decrease in both overall morbidity and mortality in a subset of patients with less than or equal to 40% TBSA burned was noted. This finding led to the recommendation for further study in a randomized and controlled fashion (17–28).

Renal System

Renal failure has been reported in up to 20% of burn injury patients, with a clinical picture related to the size and severity of burn injury. Multifactorial in nature, the time course of renal failure falls into early or late categories. The mortality of patients developing severe renal failure with burn injury approaches 80%. Early acute renal failure appears to be directly associated with clinical events such as delayed resuscitation, under-resuscitation, hypotension, and rhabdomyolysis.

Increased burn severity is associated with a higher incidence of acute renal failure. Rhabdomyolysis, a rare consequence of flame burns, but often associated with electrical injury, has a direct association with renal failure. Late episodes of acute renal failure are more commonly associated with sepsis, toxic drugs, and pre-existing medical conditions.

Treatment of acute renal failure in the burn patient and other patient populations involves multiple steps. Adequate fluid resuscitation initiated as early as possible during the time course of the burn injury will reduce the presentation of early acute renal failure. Monitoring urine output as a measure of renal perfusion allows the clinician to maintain adequate fluid input. Late episodes of acute renal failure can be addressed by treating the underlying cause. Sepsis from invasive vascular access, wounds, pneumonia, or urinary tract should be controlled by replacing the lines, excising the burn wound, and providing adequate antibiotic therapy for pneumonia and urinary tract infection. When needed, renal replacement therapy should be instituted and has shown benefit. The application of CVVH in adult patients with severe burns and acute kidney injury was associated with a decrease in 28-day and hospital mortality (29).

Gastrointestinal Tract and Liver

Ileus presents in patients with burns exceeding 20% TBSA. Despite this problem, using the gut with some—even minimal—level of feeding is advocated early after injury, and is usually well tolerated. Tube feeding should be instituted for patients with large burns where the patient is unable to tolerate sufficient intake by mouth to sustain the markedly increased nutritional requirements (30).

Gastroduodenal stress ulceration has been a hallmark of early burn care, with significant bleeding or perforation complicating the care of extensively burned individuals. This complication markedly decreased with the use of antacids, H_2-antagonists, and proton pump inhibiting medications; their use has become routine in the management of the thermally injured patient (31).

Perforation

Poor perfusion of the gut during resuscitation may lead to segmental ischemia in the watershed areas of the intestine. With this condition, there is a risk for developing necrosis and subsequent perforation; vasoactive medications used during burn resuscitation or during prolonged septic events may increase this risk (32). Clinicians may use physical examinations, laboratory studies, and x-rays to monitor this complication.

Normal gut flora has been identified as an infection source in the burn patient as well as in other critically injured patients (33–35). Maintaining gut integrity with nutritional support in the form of glutamine supplementation has been proposed and studied in the burn patient. A second approach to this problem, selective gut decontamination, has been proposed and tested in animal models (36–38). Selective gut decontamination has been shown to reduce bacterial translocation from the gut in burned rats (39). With this reduction in translocation, immunosuppression was reduced and the cardiac response to subsequent septic challenge was improved. Clinical success with this approach is not well documented (40–44).

Intra-abdominal hypertension, as defined by a bladder pressure of 30 mmHg or greater is the precursor to the abdominal compartment syndrome. Respiratory compromise with increasing peak airway pressures, renal compromise with decreased renal perfusion and urine output, and increased mortality among burn patients are the features of this syndrome (45). Burn patients with 30% or greater TBSA injury, requiring fluid resuscitation over and above the standard calculated rates are at risk for this complication (46). We recommend monitoring bladder pressures in each patient with burns greater than 30% and initiating therapeutic maneuvers for those patients with pressures of greater than 30 mmHg (47).

Therapy for intra-abdominal hypertension follows a graded response. Reduced fluid administration, sedation, and neuromuscular blocking agent (NMBA) use for the patient are the initial treatments. Escharotomies and peritoneal drainage make up the next most invasive line of management and, ultimately, abdominal decompression through a laparotomy incision may be needed to relieve the symptoms. In the severely burned population, abdominal compartment syndrome has a high mortality rate and should be addressed urgently when recognized (48–50).

Central Nervous System

Burn injury and resuscitation in an ovine model showed that cerebral autoregulation adjusted to the hemodynamic changes caused by burn injury. Autoregulation of cerebral blood flow was effective to a point and then began to fail as resuscitation proceeded, suggesting that the cerebrovascular system has a limited reserve to tolerate the effects of burn injury (51–53).

Endocrine System

There is a graded response of the endocrine system after burn injury. Hormone levels are directly related to the TBSA involved; these levels rise and fall in a time-dependent fashion from the onset of injury. Burn injury is characterized by a painful incident followed by a significant inflammatory response, with fluid losses and shifts occurring both near the burn wound itself and systemically. Each part of the endocrine system reacts to regain or maintain its preburn state.

The hypothalamus responds by secreting antidiuretic hormone (ADH) which acts on the collecting ducts of the kidney to facilitate the reabsorption of water into the blood. This reduces the volume of urine formed while retaining water in response to losses of fluid from the intravascular space. The anterior pituitary releases adrenal corticotropic hormone (ACTH), which stimulates the release of the mineralocorticoid aldosterone and glucocorticoid cortisol. Aldosterone acts on the kidney to promote retention of sodium ions in the blood. Water follows the salt and helps maintain normal blood volume and pressure. Glucocorticoids increase blood sugar levels through the stimulation of gluconeogenesis. This elevation in blood glucose levels is thought necessary to supply the increased metabolic demand of the injured body. Cortisol and other glucocorticoids also have a potent anti-inflammatory effect on the body (54–62). They depress the immune response, especially cell-mediated immune responses.

The adrenal medulla releases the tyrosine-derived neurotransmitters adrenaline and noradrenaline into the blood. This response is associated with the autonomic nervous system—sometimes called the fight or flight response—and leads to multiple effects, some of which are an increase in the rate and strength of the heartbeat, resulting in increasing blood pressure, and the shunting of blood from the skin to the skeletal muscles, coronary arteries, liver, and brain. With the release of adrenaline and noradrenaline, blood sugar rises and the metabolic rate is increased; bronchial dilation occurs; pupils dilate; and blood clotting time is decreased. This autonomic response also leads to increased ACTH secretion from the anterior lobe of the pituitary.

The elevations in stress-related hormones are noted in a time- and burn size–dependent manner after injury. This hormone response follows a pattern associated with the ebb and flow of the burn injury process. An initial increase in the hormone levels in response to fluid shifts and inflammation resolves over time as the patient's fluid balance returns to normal, and the burn wounds close.

Several medications are available that can modify the endocrine response to burn injury. A recent prospective, double-blind, randomized single-center study on the effect of oxandrolone on the endocrine, inflammatory, and hypermetabolic responses during the acute phase of burn injury suggested that this treatment shortened the length of acute hospital stay, maintained lean body mass, and improved body composition and hepatic protein synthesis while having no adverse effects on the endocrine axis postburn. This study, and another using beta-blockade to modify the metabolic response after burn injury, are at the heart of attempts to improve the outcome of patients after a severe burn injury (63,64).

Hematopoietic System

Typically, the red blood cell (RBC) mass in the burn patient declines in a burn size- and severity-dependent fashion. This is initially related to the burn injury itself and thereafter decreased RBC production, increased RBC damage, and RBC losses from therapeutic interventions. Although surgery and phlebotomy account for the iatrogenic loss of RBCs, several possible causes have been explored for the injury-related loss of blood in the burn patient. Initial heat injuries to the RBCs, as well as sequestration of blood in the burn eschar, are early factors in the loss of RBCs and the decline in hemoglobin and hematocrit. Damage to RBCs secondary to the inflammatory response to the burn wound is a later developing cause for blood loss in these patients (65–70).

In 1973, Loebl (69) described studies of RBC half-life in burn victims and healthy volunteers. RBCs from the burn patient had a normal half-life when transfused into healthy volunteers. The same RBCs had a decreased half-life in the burn victim and, when normal RBCs were transfused into a burn victim, they acquired a similar decrease in their half-life; this study suggested a humoral or inflammatory process driving the loss of red cells.

Later studies have linked this loss in RBCs to a process mediated by inflammation and the release of toxic oxygen–free radicals, representing a nonspecific mechanism for the destruction of red cells. Immune system–mediated processes for the destruction of RBCs in burn patients have also been postulated, but Coombs testing in these patients has failed to reveal a definite link to immune-mediated blood loss. Studies by Posluszny et al. in a mouse model show a decrease in bone marrow hematopoetic commitment to erythroid cells and an increase in myeloid cells. This accounted for a decrease in RBC production after burn injury. Further study is needed to identify the same patterns in burn patients (71,72).

Immune System

Infection remains a major complicating factor of burn injury (73–76). Burned skin loses its barrier function against the environment, and normal skin flora and environmental pathogens are able to gain access to the system. Risk of infection and its complications are directly related to the size of the burn injury and additional factors, such as inhalation injury and pre-existing medical conditions. Burn injury leads to compromised immune function, resulting in increased susceptibility to sepsis and multiple organ system failure.

Immune system dysfunction occurs on the cellular and humoral levels. Multiple avenues for this effect have been investigated. Currently, macrophages, T cells, other lymphocyte subpopulations, and humoral factors such as opsonins, immunoglobulins, protease inhibitors, toll-receptors, and chemotactic factors have been implicated in the process. Some combination of all of the above factors, related to their natural interaction, produces a weakened immune system susceptible to infection entering through multiple avenues (77–79).

In general, burn patients are assailed by bacteria from multiple directions. Damaged skin, its barrier function destroyed, is the most obvious portal. Burn-related hypotension and peripheral vasoconstriction may permit intestinal hypoperfusion, with normal gastrointestinal flora becoming a source of proinflammatory mediators, pathogens, and toxins that contribute to multi-organ failure. Other clinically relevant pathways include cannulation of the respiratory, vascular, and genitourinary systems, providing ready access for bacteria into the compromised host; these are considered nosocomial infections (80).

Musculoskeletal System

Loss of muscle mass and bone are notable in severely burned patients. Bone loss is, in part, due to an increase in glucocorticoids that inhibit bone formation and osteoblast differentiation, hypercalciuria secondary to hypoparathyroidism, and vitamin D deficiency. Muscle loss is secondary to an intense catabolic state initiated by the inflammatory response to burn injury and is fueled by the need to repair the surface injury suffered. Propranolol administration in pediatric patients reduces thermogenesis, cardiac work, resting energy expenditure, and peripheral lipolysis; it also increases skeletal muscle protein anabolism. These effects are being studied in adult burn patients (81–86). A randomized, double-blinded, placebo-controlled study by Klein and Herndon (82) suggested that intravenous pamidronate administration may help preserve bone mass in children with over 40% TBSA burns. Follow-up to that study 2 years later showed a sustained improvement in bone mineral content as measured by dual-energy radiograph absorptiometry (83). This effect was attributed to a decrease in the glucocorticoid-mediated effect on bone mass.

FLUID RESUSCITATION

Fluid resuscitation addresses the clinical picture of burn shock. Multiple resuscitation regimens have been developed to overcome the cardiac depression, vasoconstriction, and hypovolemia associated with acute burn injury. Most, if not all, of the current formulae have been developed through retrospective review of the fluid requirements of burn patients. Aided by the use of the rule of nines and Lund-Browder charts, a patient's TBSA burn and weight measurements are used to determine their initial fluid requirement. One-half of the fluid requirements calculated are given in the first 8 hours after the burn injury, with the remaining amount administered over the subsequent 16 hours. A slight variation in the composition of the resuscitation fluid is present in the different formulae; there are also differences in the addition of colloid to the initial resuscitation scheme (87–98); the most commonly used formulae are noted in Table 63.1.

TABLE 63.1 The Common Resuscitation Formulae

	Evans Formula	Brooke Formula	Parkland Formula
Colloid	1.0 mL/kg/%	0.5 mL/kg/%	None
Crystalloid	1.0 mL/kg/%	1.5 mL/kg/%	4.0 mL/kg/%
Free water	2,000 mL	2,000 mL	None

Colloid infusion during the resuscitation of acutely injured patients has been debated for some time. Acute burn injury leads to capillary permeability, which allows loss of intravascular albumin into the interstitial spaces of the acutely injured patient. Currently, the application of albumin or fresh-frozen plasma is considered after the initial 8-hour period postburn in an attempt to avoid loss of the colloid secondary to capillary permeability (99–102).

Adequate resuscitation is measured by end-organ perfusion. Currently, exact measures of end-organ perfusion are being developed and tested. A surrogate measure of the success of fluid administration is the measurement of urine output. Renal function is highly dependent on renal blood flow, which can be adequately assessed by the rate of urine output. Most practitioners view a urine production rate of 0.5 to 1.0 mL/kg ideal (or adjusted) body weight per hour as adequate. Secondary measures of perfusion are also important in the resuscitation plan. The combination of blood pressure, heart rate, oxygenation, and central venous pressure are used in tandem to determine the adequacy of treatment.

Measures of adequate resuscitation, such as blood pressure, heart rate, and central venous pressure used alone, must be monitored cautiously. Postburn tissue edema will decrease the accuracy of cuff blood pressure measurements, and the vasoconstriction caused by catecholamine release will adversely affect the accuracy of indwelling arterial lines. Central venous pressure measurements require the interaction of multiple physiologic and environmental parameters to provide the practitioner with meaningful measurements.

Patients who begin to lag in their urine output during resuscitation should have their fluid rates adjusted. Urinary rates of less than one third the predicted value based on the patient body weight over two consecutive hours should prompt an increase in intravenous fluid administration. On the other hand, patients running one third or more over their expected urine output may benefit from decreased fluid administration. A graded increase or decrease of the intravenous fluid rate of 20% per hour is a measured and conservative response to these situations. Those patients who do not respond as expected to calculated fluid administration or who require more than 6 mL/kg per percent TBSA fluid administration should be considered for more invasive monitoring, such as pulse-waveform analysis (FlowTrack, PICCO, LiDCO, and bedside Echo) or pulmonary artery catheter monitoring. With measurements obtained through this more advanced monitoring, a decision can be made to either support the CO or reduce the SVR, or both. Small doses of hydralazine may be used to reduce peripheral resistance in situations where the CO remains low. Hydralazine doses on the order of 0.5 mg/kg have been shown to be effective when used in this situation. In animal models of burn injury, sodium nitroprusside and verapamil decreased SVR and supported CO with good effect. This approach should be used with caution in the severely burn-injured patient to avoid further tissue hypoperfusion, which may exacerbate the condition of the partially burned tissues, increase fluid creep, worsen tissue edema, and may precipitate abdominal compartment syndrome (103).

At-risk patients for volume over-resuscitation include pediatric patients with an increased TBSA to weight, patients with inhalation injuries, electrical injuries, intoxication, and delayed fluid resuscitation. Fluid creep during resuscitation is worsened by exceeding the Parkland formula early or pushing high urine output during goal-directed therapy. Other factors that contribute to increased fluid administration include sedation and pain management with opioids, propofol, and benzodiazepines, or patient factors like morbid obesity (104–106).

Insensible water losses become more significant with larger TBSA burns. Evaporative water losses from the open wounds/burns usually peak on the third day postburn and then trail off until the wounds are completely closed. An estimation of insensible water losses may be calculated as follows:

$$\text{Insensible water loss (in mL/h)} = (125 + \%\text{TBSA burned}) \times \text{BSA (in m}^2).$$

The body surface area may be estimated using the formula of DuBois and DuBois as follows:

$$\text{BSA} = (W^{0.425} \times H^{0.725}) \times 0.007184$$

where W is the weight in kilograms and H is the height in centimeters. Initially, the replacement fluid is free water initially and then it is altered based on electrolyte measurements (107,108).

ELECTRICAL INJURY

Electrical injuries can be divided into those due to low voltage (<1,000 volts) and those due to high voltage (≥1,000 volts) (109). These injuries have varying patterns: Low-voltage injuries range from the circumoral injuries noted in children who have bitten home electrical cables to deaths caused by dropping electrical appliances in a bathtub full of water; high-voltage injuries have a range that includes the more severe episodes of instant death, massive tissue loss, and secondary clothing ignition. Some of the less dramatic injuries include thermal injury, central nervous system–related trauma, and fractures. With high-voltage injuries, there is a high ratio of limb amputations, highlighting the danger of this modern-day source of power. Herein, we will concentrate on high-voltage injuries.

Electrical energy interacts with human anatomy following the basic principles of physics. Current flowing through tissue is related to the voltage drop across the resistance of that tissue. Heat produced by this current can be represented mathematically as follows:

$$\text{J (heat in Joules)} = I^2 \times R \times T$$

where I is the current, R is the resistance, and T is the time in seconds. Body tissues have differing electrical resistances. Given the above equation, it appears that differing tissues would create varying degrees of heat and subsequent damage; interestingly, clinical findings do not wholly support this concept. The highest resistance is found in the bone, fat, and tendons, whereas the lowest resistance has been identified in the muscles, blood, and nerves; skin has an intermediate resistance. Clinical findings in electrically injured patients support the idea that the body represents a volume conductor with a resistance on the order of 500 to 1,000 ohms. In this model, the relative differences in tissue resistance are small enough that the body is considered a single resistor. Heat generated by the current flowing through the resistor is related to the cross-sectional area of the entry or exit wound and the local anatomy.

Contact wounds on the hands and feet are common. Each of the contact areas might have a low cross section, releasing more heat in that area; as the current crosses the "bottleneck" areas of the ankles and wrists, there may be more tissue damage generated at those sites. At its most extreme, heat released by high-voltage injuries produces coagulation necrosis of the tissues and varying other effects on the organs as the electricity passes through.

Arc injuries are less common, but just as destructive. Electricity can travel 2 to 3 cm/10,000 volts, and may travel 10 ft or more to its target. Temperatures at the contact points range from 2,000 to 4,000°C, with spikes of up to 20,000°C; this intense temperature leads to severe and deep tissue damage.

Electrical injuries have specific organ effects in addition to the thermal injury described above. With high-voltage injuries, cardiac standstill and ventricular fibrillation are the most lethal cardiac injuries. Other electrocardiographic (ECG) findings and rhythm changes that have been reported include atrial fibrillation, focal ectopic arrhythmias, supraventricular tachycardia, right bundle branch block, and nonspecific ST-T segment changes. These clinical findings are thought to be associated with direct myocardial muscle damage, coronary vasospasm, and coronary endarteritis.

Renal injury may be direct, although this is rare, or may take on the more familiar form of acute renal failure secondary to rhabdomyolysis. Large quantities of muscle protein, hemoglobin, and other tissue proteins released from the tissues coagulated by high voltage and current are filtered into the renal tubules, causing acute renal failure with oliguria or polyuria. Up to 15% of patients injured in high-voltage accidents will suffer from this type of renal injury.

Central nervous system injury ranges from the devastating effect of high voltage and current on the brain and brainstem, leading to instant death or to more subtle findings. Altered levels of consciousness with varying degrees of recovery have been reported, while progressive neurologic deterioration has been noted in both the central and the peripheral nervous systems. With high-voltage injuries, progressive deterioration of the microvascular nutrient vessels to the nerves has been identified, and is thought to lead to ischemia, necrosis, and fibrosis of the injured nerve; progressive loss of function can be seen as a late developing problem (110).

Other organ systems may be directly affected by the passage of current through them. Each is susceptible to both the current and the resistance-induced production of high temperatures and tissue damage. Cataracts may form in the eyes of a patient who has had an electrical injury in which the current pathway is through the orbits; this complication has been reported in up to 30% of patients suffering from this injury (111,112).

INHALATION INJURY

The pathophysiology associated with smoke inhalation injury falls into three broad categories: (i) upper airway injury; (ii) asphyxiant gases and hypoxic environments; and (iii) carbonaceous particle deposition (113–116).

The diagnosis of inhalation injury is based on several site-specific and clinical findings surrounding each burn patient. For example, closed space injuries or explosions are some of the circumstances surrounding inhalation injury. Noxious fumes noted at the scene by the scene responders, as well as facial burns noted on the patient, are other findings consistent with inhalation injury. Clinical findings on examination, such as large burns, carbonaceous sputum, hoarseness, or an abnormal lung examination, are associated with this injury, and elderly patients are more susceptible to inhalation injury.

Once inhalation injury is suspected, upper airway pathology should be expected. Heated smoke or ambient air may injure the supraglottic airway from the lips to the vocal cords. This injury may occur abruptly, leading to significant edema and swelling of the face and oropharynx, as well as affecting the region around the vocal cords.

True heat injury below the cords is rare, with the exception of steam injuries or ignition of flammable gases in the airway. Signs and symptoms of a true airway burn injury include hoarseness; stridor and/or wheezing; carbonaceous sputum; singed nasal hair, eyebrows, or facial hair; and edema or inflammatory changes in the upper airway. The resultant upper airway edema formation can threaten the airway and the patient's breathing.

Asphyxiant gases and hypoxic environments lead to the second area of pathology associated with inhalation injury. In fires involving structures, the ambient oxygen level markedly decreases; this lack of oxygen may lead to carbon monoxide generation, as this molecule is a byproduct of incomplete combustion in the burning structure. Carbon monoxide binds tightly to hemoglobin, reducing the amount of oxygen delivered to end organs, which may cause a hypoxic injury. Aside from carbon monoxide, other toxic gases can be released by the flames. Cyanide generation is associated with burning plastics; this molecule is highly lethal. Treatment of carbon monoxide intoxication includes a high concentration of oxygen and, sometimes, hyperbaric oxygen. Cyanide poisoning treatment includes delivery of oxygen, as well as a three-part regimen to bind the cyanide compound in the blood.

The third broad area of pathology associated with smoke inhalation injury is related to the deposition of carbonaceous particles in the airway. The flame-generated toxins that are bound to the carbon particles will slowly be released after the latter are deposited in the lungs, inducing a chemical tracheal bronchitis. This effect is manifested by impaired ciliary function and edema, significant inflammation, and ulceration or necrosis of the respiratory epithelium. The clinical sequelae of tracheal bronchial injury include bronchorrhea, bronchospasm, distal airway obstruction, and atelectasis, as well as pneumonia. Epithelial injury leads to sloughing of the mucosa and blockage of the airways with this cellular debris. Air trapping in this situation leads to atelectasis and the development of barotrauma and pneumonia.

Treatment for each area of pathology is based on standard clinical practice. When presented with a patient who is suspected of having an inhalation injury and upper airway edema, endotracheal intubation to protect the airway should be performed early to avoid the consequences of airway compromise. Patients suffering from carbon monoxide exposure, and showing clinical signs of intoxication, should be treated with 100% oxygen to displace the molecule from hemoglobin. If immediately available, and if the patient is stable, high levels of carboxyhemoglobin and severe neurologic symptoms should be treated with hyperbaric oxygen therapy. The tracheal-bronchial injury associated with inhalation injury and carbonaceous particle deposition should be treated with humidified oxygen by face mask, and frequent examination of the airway should be performed to evaluate for signs of compromise that may require endotracheal intubation.

Cyanide toxicity presents clinically with lethargy, nausea, headache, weakness, and coma. Cyanide combines with cytochrome oxidase, thereby blocking oxygen use and inhibiting high-energy phosphate compound production. Cyanide toxicity begins at 0.1 μg/mL of serum and quickly leads to death at concentrations of 1 μg/mL. Laboratory studies show a decreased arteriovenous oxygen difference with severe metabolic acidosis; this acidosis is unresponsive to fluids and oxygen administration.

S-T segment elevations may be seen on the patient's electrocardiogram, mimicking a myocardial infarction. Treatment of this condition includes the administration of 100% oxygen and a three-part medication regimen. Initially, the administration of amyl nitrate pearls, by inhalation for 15 to 30 seconds every minute, is followed by 10 mL 3% sodium nitrate solution (300 mg) intravenously over 3 minutes, repeated at one-half the dosage in 2 hours if symptoms persist or recurrent signs of toxicity are present. Sodium thiosulfate is the final medication, given in a dose of 50 mL of a 25% solution (12.5 g) intravenously over 10 minutes, repeated at half the dosage in 2-hour intervals if persistent or recurrent signs of toxicity are present.

INFECTION CONTROL

Historically, mortality from burn injury was associated with burn shock (117–119); the loss of fluid through the burned and damaged skin, as well as fluid shifts related to the release of inflammatory mediators, led to hypovolemia and unrecoverable end-organ failure. As our understanding of the injury suffered during burns improved, so did the survivability of these injuries. Currently, burn shock is well controlled by our fluid resuscitation regimens. The new challenge in burn injury is the concurrent development of infection in a compromised host. Burn injury is associated with a burn size–dependent depression in the immune system in which bacterial, fungal, and viral elements are better able to breach the defense mechanisms of the body, thereby worsening the injury.

As fluid resuscitation techniques advanced, wound colonization and sepsis became a leading factor in morbidity and mortality. The advent of topical antibiotic/anti-infective agents addressed this new area of pathology. Subsequent movement toward early wound excision and skin grafting led to improvements in the rates of wound sepsis and its complications. Although the burn wound has become less of a risk for infection, other portals of entry have persisted in plaguing the burn patient. With our current methods of intubating the respiratory, vascular, and genitourinary systems, we expose the burn patient to other portals of entry for pathogens.

NUTRITION

Burn patients present to the ICU in a severe inflammatory state. This state, along with a wide variety of prehospital factors and premorbid conditions, provides the practitioner with a challenging nutritional problem. Nutritional support for the burn patient can be addressed in several steps: first, an assessment of the patient's initial nutritional status, and second, monitoring of his or her nutritional status throughout the hospital course, and adjustments based on the monitoring measures. By using a combination of variables, including burn size and severity, time from injury, physical parameters such as age, weight, and the presence of other medical factors, nutrition support can be tailored to each burn patient.

Nutritional assessment begins with measurement of the patient's weight, estimation of the patient's calorie and protein needs, measurement of the patient's serum albumin, prealbumin, and C-reactive protein levels (120–133). Pre-existing illnesses should prompt the practitioner to make adjustments in the rate of feeding, use of additional medications, and the need for additional nutrient support.

Glutamine supplementation has been shown to improve morbidity and mortality when administered to critically ill patients. This response appears to improve with increasing doses of the amino acid, and parenteral administration appears to have an improved response over enteral administration. Not all of the trials reported to date have shown a definitive benefit, and the general consensus is that a large randomized controlled trial would be needed to confirm or refute the benefits of glutamine administration (134,135).

Physiologically, glutamine affects the immune system, the anti-oxidant status, glucose metabolism, and heat shock protein response. These physiologic effects appear to provide benefit with regard to gastrointestinal mucosal integrity, wound healing, gram-negative bacteremia and infection—including with *Pseudomonas*—as well as a reduction in mortality, and possibly cost savings to burn patients. At the time of this writing, a consensus has not been reached on the length of time for glutamine therapy, the optimal dose, and definite safety aspects of the supplementation of glutamine in critically ill and burn patients. Most studies suggest that clinically important differences appear to commence at doses over 0.2 g/kg body weight per day, and most trials have used 15 to 30 g/day glutamine supplementation.

WOUND MANAGEMENT

With the exception of chemical burns, for which prompt water irrigation to remove the offending agent is required, no specific treatment of the thermal burn wound is needed in the prehospital setting (113,136,137). The patient should be covered with a clean sheet and blanket to conserve body heat and minimize burn wound contamination during transport to the hospital. The application of ice or cold-water soaks, when initiated within 10 minutes after burning, may reduce tissue heat content and lessen the depth of thermal injury. If cold therapy is used, care must be taken to avoid causing hypothermia; this is accomplished by limiting this form of therapy to 10% or less of the body surface and only for the time required to produce analgesia.

Following admission to the burn center, definitive care of the burn wound can begin. Daily wound care involves cleansing, debridement, and dressing of the burn wound. On the day of injury, the burn wound is best cleansed by means of hydrotherapy, a practice that has been used in the treatment of burn patients for many years and remains an integral part of current treatment plans. Hydrotherapy is accomplished by means of showering or use of a spray table. Showering is often used for ambulatory patients who remain capable of independent, or near-independent, wound care. Patients who are near to discharge are encouraged to use the shower, especially if showering is to be used at home.

Use of a spray table is generally reserved for newly admitted patients, those with limited mobility, or those with large open wounds. The patient is placed on the table, and the wounds are washed and rinsed with running water. As an alternative, a stretcher or plinth can be placed over a Hubbard tank. The patient is placed on the stretcher, and the wounds are washed and rinsed as described previously.

Wound debridement involves the removal of all loose tissue, wound debris, and eschar (nonviable tissue); debridement of a burn wound is accomplished through mechanical, chemical (enzymatic), or surgical means.

Surgical, or sharp, debridement requires the use of scalpels and scissors to debride wounds of loose, necrotic tissue. Care must be taken to avoid excessive debridement that results in bleeding and pain. Bleeding may indicate injury to the healthy underlying tissue. In most instances, sharp debridement should be carried out in the operating room to ensure adequate debridement and hemostasis. Definitive management of third-degree burn wounds and deep second-degree injuries may require tangential excision of the eschar or necrotic tissue followed by wound closure with skin grafts or other wound closure adjuncts. This process will not be reviewed here.

Multiple topical antimicrobial agents are used in burn wound care. Mafenide acetate (Sulfamylon), silver sulfadiazine (Silvadene), and silver nitrate are the three most commonly used topical antimicrobial agents for burn wound care. Each agent has specific limitations and advantages with which the physician must be familiar to ensure patient safety and optimal benefit. Mafenide acetate and silver sulfadiazine are available as topical creams to be applied directly to the burn wound, whereas silver nitrate is applied as a 0.5% solution in occlusive dressings. Either cream is applied in a half-inch (about one-third of a centimeter) layer to the entire burn wound in an aseptic manner after initial debridement, and reapplied at 12-hour intervals or as required to maintain continuous topical coverage. Once daily, all of the topical agents should be cleansed from the patient using a surgical detergent disinfectant solution and the burn wounds examined by the attending physician. Silver nitrate is applied as a 0.5% solution in multilayered occlusive dressings that are changed twice daily.

Mafenide acetate burn cream is an 11.1% suspension in a water-soluble base. This compound diffuses freely into the eschar, owing to its high degree of water solubility. Mafenide is the preferred agent if the patient has heavily contaminated burn wounds or has had burn wound care delayed by several days. This agent has the added advantage of being highly effective against gram-negative organisms, including most *Pseudomonas* species. Physicians using this agent must be aware of several potential clinical limitations associated with its use. Hypersensitivity reactions occur in 7% of patients, and pain or discomfort of 20 to 30 minutes duration is common when it is applied to partial-thickness burn wounds. This agent is also an inhibitor of carbonic anhydrase, and a diuresis of bicarbonate is often observed after its use. The resultant metabolic acidosis may accentuate postburn hyperventilation, and significant acidemia may develop if compensatory hyperventilation is impaired. Inhibition of this enzyme rarely persists for more than 7 to 10 days, and the severity of the acidosis may be minimized by alternating applications of mafenide with silver sulfadiazine cream every 12 hours (138).

Silver sulfadiazine burn cream is a 1% suspension in a water-miscible base. Unlike mafenide, silver sulfadiazine has limited solubility in water and, therefore, limited ability to penetrate into the eschar. The agent is most effective when applied to burns soon after injury to minimize bacterial proliferation on the wound's surface. This agent is painless on application, and serum electrolytes and acid–base balance are not affected by its use. Hypersensitivity reactions are uncommon; an erythematous maculopapular rash sometimes seen subsides on discontinuation of the agent. Silver sulfadiazine occasionally induces neutropenia by a mechanism thought to involve direct bone marrow suppression; white blood cell counts usually return to normal following discontinuation. With continual use, resistance to the sulfonamide component of silver sulfadiazine is common, particularly in certain strains of *Pseudomonas* and many *Enterobacter* species. However, the continued sensitivity of microorganisms to the silver ion of this compound has maintained its effectiveness as a topical antimicrobial agent.

A 0.5% silver nitrate solution has a broad spectrum of antibacterial activity imparted by the silver ion. This agent does not penetrate the eschar, because the silver ions rapidly precipitate on contact with any protein or cationic material. Use of this agent is not associated with more intense wound pain, except from the mechanical action required for dressing changes. The dressings are changed twice daily and moistened every 2 hours with the silver nitrate solution to prevent evaporation from increasing the silver nitrate concentration to cytotoxic levels within the dressings. Transeschar leaching of sodium, potassium, chloride, and calcium should be anticipated, and these chemical constituents should be appropriately replaced. Hypersensitivity to silver nitrate has not been described. Mafenide acetate, silver sulfadiazine, and 0.5% silver nitrate are effective in the prevention of invasive burn wound infection; however, because of their lack of eschar penetration, silver nitrate soaks and silver sulfadiazine burn cream are most effective when applied soon after burn injury.

PAIN MANAGEMENT

Because burn pain is variable in its degree and time course, reliance on a single analgesic regimen is unreliable at best and unsuccessful at worst. Conversely, the diverse spectrum of burn patients—adult versus children, large burns versus small, ICU nursing versus ward setting—makes the routine individualization of analgesic plans overwhelming and impractical. Our recommendation is to determine an analgesic regimen for each individual patient based on two broad categories: the assessed clinical need for analgesia and the limitations imposed by the patient.

The first step is to address background, procedural, postoperative, and breakthrough pain treatment separately, and then consider individual drug choices based on patient limitations. To reinforce this type of approach to analgesic management, detailed institutional guidelines to help physicians and nurses choose and administer specific analgesics are recommended.

Background Pain

In general, because it is a pain of continuous nature, background pain is best treated with mild-to-moderately potent, longer-acting analgesics administered so that plasma drug concentrations remain relatively constant throughout the day. Examples include the continuous IV infusion of fentanyl or morphine (with or without patient-controlled analgesia [PCA]), oral administration of long-acting opioids with prolonged elimination (methadone) or prolonged enteral absorption (sustained-release morphine, sustained-release oxycodone), or oral administration on a regular schedule of short-acting oral analgesics (oxycodone, hydromorphone, codeine, acetaminophen). Such analgesics should almost never be administered on an as-needed (PRN) basis during the early and middle phases of hospitalization.

Procedural Pain

In contrast, procedural pain is significantly more intense but shorter in duration; therefore, analgesic regimens for procedural pain are best composed of more potent opioids that have a short duration of action. Intravenous access is helpful in this setting, with short-acting opioids (fentanyl) offering a potential advantage over more longer-acting agents (morphine, hydromorphone). When intravenous access is not present, orally administered opioids (morphine, hydromorphone, oxycodone, codeine) are commonly used, although their relatively long duration of action (2 to 6 hours) may potentially limit postprocedure recovery for other rehabilitative or nutritional activities. Oral transmucosal fentanyl and nitrous oxide are useful agents when IV access is not present due to their rapid onset and short duration of action.

Postoperative Pain

Postoperative pain deserves special mention because increased analgesic needs should be anticipated following burn wound excision and grafting. This is particularly true when donor sites have been harvested, as these are often the source of increased postoperative pain complaints. In contrast, pain from excised/grafted burns may increase, decrease, or not change postoperatively compared to preoperatively. Typically, this increased analgesic need in the postoperative period is limited to 1 to 4 days following surgery before returning to, or falling below, preoperative levels.

Breakthrough Pain

Breakthrough pain occurs at rest when background analgesic therapy is inadequate. Breakthrough pain occurs commonly in burn patients, particularly in early stages of hospitalization until a stable, appropriate, and individualized pharmacologic regimen can be determined for each patient. Analgesia for breakthrough pain can be provided with IV or oral opioids. When breakthrough pain occurs repeatedly, it is an indication to re-evaluate and likely increase the patient's background pain analgesic regimen, as it may be inadequate in terms of analgesic dose and/or frequency. Tolerance develops rapidly in these patients and may initially manifest as breakthrough pain.

Patient Limitations

As stated above, the presence of intravenous access directly influences analgesic drug choice, particularly in children. Similarly, patients who are endotracheally intubated and ventilated are somewhat protected from the risk of opioid-induced respiratory depression; thus, opioids may be more generously administered in these individuals, as is often required for painful burn debridements. Also, individual differences in opioid efficacy should be considered in all patients, including opioid tolerance in patients requiring prolonged opioid analgesic therapy or in those with pre-existing substance abuse histories.

An appropriate rationale is to titrate the drug dose to the desired effect, rather than to rely on a particular textbook dose for all patients. Because of the development of drug tolerance with prolonged medical use or recreational abuse of opioids (i.e., increasing drug doses are required to attain adequate levels of analgesia), opioid analgesic doses needed for burn analgesia may exceed those recommended in standard dosing guidelines. Furthermore, because of cross-tolerance, tolerance to one opioid analgesic usually implies tolerance to all opioid analgesics. One clinically relevant consequence of drug tolerance is the potential for opioid withdrawal to occur during inpatient burn treatment. Thus, the period of inpatient burn care is not an appropriate time to institute deliberate opioid withdrawal or detoxification measures in tolerant patients, because such treatment ignores the very real analgesic needs—background pain and procedural pain—of these patients. Similarly, when reductions in analgesic therapy are considered as burn wounds close, reductions should occur by careful tapering, rather than abrupt discontinuation of opioids, to prevent the acute opioid withdrawal syndrome.

Anxiolysis in the Treatment of Burn Pain

Current aggressive therapies for cutaneous burns, together with the qualities of background and wound care pain, make burn care an experience that normally induces anxiety in a large proportion of adult and pediatric patients. Anxiety, in itself, can exacerbate acute pain. This has led to the common practice in many burn centers of using anxiolytic drugs in combination with opioid analgesics. Intuitively, this practice seems particularly useful in premedicating patients for wound care, to diminish the anticipatory anxiety experienced by these patients prior to and during debridement. Low-dose benzodiazepine administration significantly reduces burn wound care pain scores and narcotic requirements. It appears that the patients most likely to benefit from this therapy are not those with *high trait* or premorbid anxiety, but rather those with *high state* or the time of the procedure anxiety, or those with high baseline pain scores. Other nonpharmacologic anxiolysis techniques, such as hypnosis and behavioral therapy, could also be considered.

TEAM APPROACH TO BURN PATIENTS

The management of the burned patient is a multidisciplinary effort of burn care professionals to provide optimal care to the burn patient. This multidisciplinary care spans the early resuscitative phases of care through the long-term rehabilitation and reconstructive phases. The Burn Center Director coordinates all activities of the multidisciplinary care of the critically ill burn patients. Team members include burn surgeons, plastic and reconstructive surgeons, critical care specialists, anesthesiologists, critical care burn nurses, physical therapists, occupational therapists, clinical nutritional specialists, psychologists, social workers, and pastoral care support personnel. This multidisciplinary approach affords the patients and their families state-of-the-art resources for optimal outcome, education, and rehabilitation. This concept of team care, originating in the 1950s when the first burn centers opened, has persisted to this day and is a model of coordinated, interdisciplinary, outcome-driven patient care.

Key Points

- Role of inflammation and inflammatory mediators in the depression of cardiac function and increase in capillary permeability.
- Smoke inhalation and its effect on mortality from burn injury.
- Renal replacement therapy and its potential role in modulating the inflammatory effects of burn injury.
- Modulating the hypermetabolic response to burn injury medically as well as reducing the loss of bone density in patients with severe burn injuries.
- Addressing the effects of burn injury on the immune system and reducing the incidence of infection through VAP bundles, catheter management, and improving the rate of wound closure. Further study in supporting the immune system despite the burn injury.

References

1. Bessey PQ, Phillips BD, Lentz CW, et al. Synopsis of the 2013 annual report of the national burn repository. *J Burn Care Res.* 2014;35 Suppl 2: S218–S234.
2. Moncrief JA. Effect of various fluid regimens and pharmacologic agents on the circulatory hemodynamics of the immediate postburn period. *Ann Surg.* 1966;164(4):723–750.
3. Asch MJ, Feldman RJ, Walker HL, et al. Systemic and pulmonary hemodynamic changes accompanying thermal injury. *Ann Surg.* 1973;178(2): 218–221.
4. Wilmore DW, Aulick LH, Mason AD, Pruitt BA. Influence of the burn wound on local and systemic responses to injury. *Ann Surg.* 1977;186(4):444–456.
5. Kuntscher MV, Germann G, Hartmann B. Correlations between cardiac output, stroke volume, central venous pressure, intra-abdominal pressure and total circulating blood volume in resuscitation of major burns. *Resuscitation.* 2006;70(1):37–43.

6. Cioffi WG, DeMeules JE, Gamelli RL. Vascular reactivity following thermal injury. *Circ Shock*. 1988;25(4):309–317.
7. Lund T, Reed RK. Acute hemodynamic effects of thermal skin injury in the rat. *Circ Shock*. 1986;20(2):105–114.
8. Hilton JG. Effects of verapamil on the thermal trauma depressed cardiac output in the anaesthetized dog. *Burns Incl Therm Inj*. 1984;10(5):313–317.
9. Carlson DL, Horton JW. Cardiac molecular signaling after burn trauma. *J Burn Care Res*. 2006;27:669–675.
10. Horton JW, Sanders B, White DJ, Maass DL. The effects of early excision and grafting on myocardial inflammation and function after burn injury. *J Trauma*. 2006;61(5):1069–1077.
11. Tripathi FM, Pandey K, Paul PS, et al. Blood gas studies in thermal burns. *Burns Incl Therm Inj*. 1983;10(1):13–16.
12. Iglesias G, Zeigler ST, Lentz CW, et al. Thromboxane synthetase inhibition and thromboxane receptor blockade preserve pulmonary and circulatory function in a porcine burn sepsis model. *J Am Coll Surg*. 1994;179(2):187–192.
13. Shi Z, Xie H, Wang P, et al. Oral hygiene care for critically ill patients to prevent ventilator-associated pneumonia. *Cochrane Database System Rev*. 2013;8:CD008367.
14. Wang L, Li X, Yang Z, et al. Semi-recumbent position versus supine position for the prevention of ventilator-associated pneumonia in adults requiring mechanical ventilation. *Cochrane Database System Rev*. 2016;1:CD009946.
15. Tokmaji G, Vermeulen H, Müller MC, et al. Silver-coated endotracheal tubes for prevention of ventilator-associated pneumonia in critically ill patients. *Cochrane Database System Rev*. 2015;8:CD009201.
16. Shirani KZ, Pruitt BA Jr, Mason AD Jr. The influence of inhalation injury and pneumonia on burn mortality. *Ann Surg*. 1987;205(1):82–87.
17. Nieminen S, Fraki J, Niinikoski J, et al. Acute effects of burn injury on tissue gas tensions in the rabbit. *Scand J Plast Reconstr Surg*. 1977;11(1):69–74.
18. Mlcak R, Desai MH, Robinson E, et al. Lung function following thermal injury in children: an 8-year follow up. *Burns*. 1998;24(3):213–216.
19. Whitener DR, Whitener LM, Robertson KJ, et al. Pulmonary function measurements in patients with thermal injury and smoke inhalation. *Am Rev Respir Dis*. 1980;122(5):731–739.
20. Tripathi FM, Pandey K, Paul PS, et al. Respiratory functions in thermal burns. *Burns Incl Therm Inj*. 1983;9(6):401–408.
21. Demling RH, Wenger H, Lalonde CC, et al. Endotoxin-induced prostanoid production by the burn wound can cause distant lung dysfunction. *Surgery*. 1986;99(4):421–431.
22. Demling RH, Wong C, Jin LJ, et al. Early lung dysfunction after major burns: role of edema and vasoactive mediators. *J Trauma*. 1985; 25(10):959–966.
23. Demling RH. Effect of early burn excision and grafting on pulmonary function. *J Trauma*. 1984;24(9):830–834.
24. Tasaki O, Goodwin CW, Saitoh D, et al. Effects of burn on inhalation injury. *J Trauma*. 1997;43(4):603–607.
25. Teixidor HS, Novick G, Rubin E. Pulmonary complications in burn patients. *J Can Assoc Radiol*. 1983;34(4):264–270.
26. Pruitt BA Jr, Erickson DR, Morris A. Progressive pulmonary insufficiency and other pulmonary complications of thermal injury. *J Trauma*. 1975;15(5):369–379.
27. Endorf FW, Gamelli RL. Inhalation injury, pulmonary perturbations, and fluid resuscitation. *J Burn Care Res*. 2007;28(1):80–83.
28. Petroff PA, Hander EW, Mason AD Jr. Ventilatory patterns following burn injury and effect of sulfamylon. *J Trauma*. 1975;15(8):650–656.
29. Chung KK, Lundy JB, Matson JR, et al. Continuous venovenous hemofiltration in severely burned patients with acute kidney injury: a cohort study. *Crit Care*. 2009;13(3):R62.
30. McDonald WS, Sharp CW Jr, Deitch EA. Immediate enteral feeding in burn patients is safe and effective. *Ann Surg*. 1991;213(2):177–183.
31. Alhazzani W, Alenezi F, Jaeschke RZ, et al. Proton pump inhibitors versus histamine 2 receptor antagonists for stress ulcer prophylaxis in critically ill patients: a systematic review and meta-analysis. *Crit Care Med*. 2013;41(3):693–705.
32. Moore LJ, Kowal-Vern A, Latenser BA. Cecal perforation in thermal injury: case report and review of the literature. *J Burn Care Rehabil*. 2002;23(6):371–374.
33. Manson WL, Klasen HJ, Sauer EW, Olieman A. Selective intestinal decontamination for prevention of wound colonization in severely burned patients: a retrospective analysis. *Burns*. 1992;19(2):98–102.
34. Mackie DP, van Hertum WA, Schumburg TH, et al. Reduction in *Staphylococcus aureus* wound colonization using nasal mupirocin and selective decontamination of the digestive tract in extensive burns. *Burns*. 1994;20 (Suppl 1):S14–S17.
35. Mackie DP, van Hertum WA, Schumburg T, et al. Prevention of infection in burns: preliminary experience with selective decontamination of the digestive tract in patients with extensive injuries. *J Trauma*. 1992;32(5):570–575.
36. Horton JW, Maass DL, White J, Minei JP. Reducing susceptibility to bacteremia after experimental burn injury: a role for selective decontamination of the digestive tract. *J Appl Physiol*. 2007;102(6):2207–2216.
37. Yao YM, Lu LR, Yu Y, et al. Influence of selective decontamination of the digestive tract on cell-mediated immune function and bacteria/endotoxin translocation in thermally injured rats. *J Trauma*. 1997;42(6):1073–1079.
38. Yao YM, Yu Y, Sheng ZY, et al. Role of gut-derived dedotoxaemia and bacterial translocation in rats after thermal injury: effects of selective decontamination of the digestive tract. *Burns*. 1995;21(8):580–585.
39. Baron P, Traber LD, Traber DL, et al. Gut failure and translocation following burn and sepsis. *J Surg Res*. 1994;57(1):197–204.
40. Taylor N, van Saene HK, Abella A, et al. Selective digestive decontamination. why don't we apply the evidence in the clinical practice? *Med Intensiva*. 2007;3193:136–145.
41. de La Cal MA, Cerda E, Garcia-Hierro P, et al. Survival benefit in critically ill burned patients receiving selective decontamination of the digestive tract: a randomized, placebo-controlled, double-blind trial. *Ann Surg*. 2005;241(3):424–430.
42. Szanto Z, Pulay I, Kotsis L, Dinka T. Selective bowel decontamination. *Orv Hetil*. 2006;147(14):643–647.
43. Barrett JP, Jeschke MG, Herndon DN. Selective decontamination of the digestive tract in severely burned pediatric patients. *Burns*. 2001; 27(5):439–445.
44. Verwaest C, Verhaegen J, Ferdinande P, et al. Randomized, controlled trial of selective digestive decontamination in 600 mechanically ventilated patients in a multidisciplinary intensive care unit. *Crit Care Med*. 1997;25(1):63–71.
45. Tuggle D, Skinner S, Garza J, et al. The abdominal compartment syndrome in patients with burn injury. *Acta Clin Belg Suppl*. 2007;(1):136–140.
46. Oda J, Yamashita K, Inoue T, et al. Resuscitation fluid volume and abdominal compartment syndrome in patients with major burns. *Burns*. 2006;32(2):151–154.
47. Meldrum DR, Moore FA, Moore EE, et al. Prospective characterization and selective management of the abdominal compartment syndrome. *Am J Surg*. 1997;174(6):667–672.
48. Hobson KG, Young KM, Ciraulo A, et al. Release of abdominal compartment syndrome improves survival in patients with burn injury. *J Trauma*. 2002;53(6):1129–1133.
49. Hershberger RD, Hunt JL, Arnoldo BD, Purdue GF. Abdominal compartment syndrome in the severely burned patient. *J Burn Care Res*. 2007; 28(5):708–714.
50. Wise R, Jacobs J, Pilate S, et al. Incidence and prognosis of intra-abdominal hypertension and abdominal compartment syndrome in severely burned patients: Pilot study and review of the literature. *Anaesthesiol Intensive Ther*. 2016;48(2):95–109.
51. Khedr EM, Khedr T, El-Oteify MA, Hassan HA. Peripheral neuropathy in burn patients. *Burns*. 1997;23(7–8):579–583.
52. Shin C, Kinsky MP, Thomas JA, et al. Effect of cutaneous burn injury and resuscitation on the cerebral circulation in an ovine model. *Burns*. 1998;24(1):39–45.
53. Maybauer DM, Maybauer MO, et al. Effects of severe smoke inhalation injury and septic shock on global hemodynamics and microvascular blood flow in sheep. *Shock*. 2006;26(5):489–495.
54. Finfer S. Corticosteroids in septic shock. *N Engl J Med*. 2008;358(2):188–190.
55. Jeschke MG, Boehning EF, Finnerty CC, Herndon DN. Effect of insulin on the inflammatory and acute phase response after burn injury. *Crit Care Med*. 2007;35(9 Suppl):S519–523.
56. Matsui M, Kudo T, Kudo M, et al. The endocrine response after burns. *Agressologie*. 1991;32(4):233–235.
57. Murton SA, Tan ST, Prickett TCR, et al. Hormone responses to stress in patients with major burns. *Br J Plast Surg*. 1998;51:388–392.
58. Smith A, Barclay C, Quaba A, et al. The bigger the burn, the greater the stress. *Burns*. 1997;23(4):291–294.
59. Sprung CL, Annane D, Keh D, et al, for the CORTICUS Study Group. Hydrocortisone therapy for patients with septic shock. *N Engl J Med*. 2008;358(2):111–124.
60. Sedowofia K, Barclay C, Quaba A, et al. The systemic stress response to thermal injury in children. *Clin Endocrinol*. 1998;49:335–341.
61. Jeschke MG, Finnerty CC, Suman OE, et al. The effect of xyandrolone on the endocrinologic, inflammatory, and hypermetabolic responses during the acute phase postburn. *Ann Surg*. 2007;246(3):351–362.
62. Wick S. Endocrinology: hormone effects. University of Nebraska at Omaha, Human Physiology and Anatomy Laboratories, August 1997.

63. Jeschke MG, Norbury WB, Finnerty CC, et al. Propranolol does not increase inflammation, sepsis, or infectious episodes in severely burned children. *J Trauma*. 2007;62(3):676–681.
64. Norbury WB, Jesche MG, Herndon DN. Metabolism modulators in sepsis: propranolol. *Crit Care Med*. 2007;35(9 Suppl):S616–620.
65. Wong CH, Song C, Heng KS, et al. Plasma free hemoglobin: a novel diagnostic test for assessment of the depth of burn injury. *Plast Reconstruct Surg*. 2006;117(4):1206–1213.
66. Lawrence C, Atac B. Hematologic changes in massive burn injury. *Crit Care Med*. 1992;20(9):1284–1288.
67. Endoh Y, Kawakami M, Orringer EP, et al. Causes and time course of acute hemolysis after burn injury of the rat. *J Burn Care Rehab*. 1992;13 (2 Pt 1):203–209.
68. Hatherill JR, Till GO, Bruner LH, Ward P. Thermal injury, intravascular hemolysis, and toxic oxygen products. *J Clin Invest*. 1986;78:629–636.
69. Loebl EC, Baxter CR, Curreri PW. The mechanism of erythrocyte destruction in the early post-burn period. *Ann Surg*. 1973;178(6):681–686.
70. Kawakami EY, Orringer EP, Peterson HD, Meyer AA. Causes and time course of acute hemolysis after burn injury in the rat. *J Burn Care Rehabil*. 1992;12(2 Pt 1):203–209.
71. Posluszny JA Jr, Muthumalaiappan K, Kini AR, et al. Burn injury dampens erythroid cell production through reprioritizing bone marrow hematopoietic response. *J Trauma*. 2011;71(5):1288–1296.
72. Howell K, Posluszny J, He LK, et al. High MafB expression following burn augments monocyte commitment and inhibits DC differentiation in hemopoietic progenitors. *J Leukoc Biol*. 2012;91(1):69–81.
73. Griswold JA. White blood cell response to burn injury. *Semin Nephrol*. 1993;13(4):409–415.
74. Oberbeck R, Schmitz D, Wilsenack K, et al. Adrenergic modulation of survival and cellular immune functions during polymicrobial sepsis. *Neuroimmunomodulation*. 2004;11(4):214–223.
75. Schmitz D, Wilsenack K, Lendemanns S, et al. Beta-adrenergic blockade during systemic inflammation: impact on cellular immune functions and survival in a murine model of sepsis. *Resuscitation*. 2007; 72(2):286–294.
76. Alexander M, Chaudry IH, Schwacha MG. Relationships between burn size, immunosuppression, and macrophage hyperactivity in a murine model of thermal injury. *Cell Immunol*. 2002;220(1):63–69.
77. Schwacha MG, Chaudry IH. The cellular basis of post-burn immunosuppression: macrophages and mediators. *Int J Mol Med*. 2002;10(3):239–243.
78. Kobayashi M, Jeschke MG, Shigematsu K, et al. M2b monocytes predominated in peripheral blood of severely burned patients. *J Immunol*. 2010;185(12):7174-7179.
79. Schwacha MG, Zhang Q, Rani M, et al. Burn enhances toll-like receptor induced responses by circulating leukocytes. *Int J Clin Exp Med*. 2012;5(2):136–144.
80. Moore FA. The role of the gastrointestinal tract in postinjury multiple organ failure. *Am J Surg*. 1999;178(6):449–453.
81. Klein GL. Burn-induced bone loss: importance, mechanisms, and management. *J Burns Wounds* 2006;5:32–38.
82. Klein GL, Herndon DN, Goodman WG, et al. Histomorphometric and biochemical characterization of bone following acute severe burns in children. *Bone*. 1995;17(5):455–460.
83. Przkora R, Herndon DN, Sherrard DJ, et al. Pamidronate preserves bone mass for at least 2 years following acute administration for pediatric burn injury. *Bone*. 2007;41:279–302.
84. Klein GL, Wimalawansa SJ, Kulkarni G, et al. The efficacy of acute administration of pamidronate on the conservation of bone mass following severe burn injury in children: a double-blind, randomized, controlled study. *Osteoporos Int*. 2005;16(6):631–635.
85. Núñez-Villaveirán T, Sánchez M, Millán P, García-de-Lorenzo A. Systematic review of the effect of propanolol on hypermetabolism in burn injuries. *Med Intensiva*. 2015;39(2):101–113.
86. Finnerty CC, Herndon DN. Is propranolol of benefit in pediatric burn patients? *Adv Surg*. 2013;47:177–197.
87. Tanaka H, Matsuda T, Miyagantani Y, et al. Reduction of resuscitation fluid volumes in severely burned patients using ascorbic acid administration. *Arch Surg*. 2000;135:326–331.
88. Klein MB, Hayden D, Elson C, et al. The association between fluid administration and outcome following major burn. *Ann Surg*. 2007;245(4):622–628.
89. Hoskins SL, Elgjo GI, Lu J, et al. Closed-loop resuscitation of burn shock. *J Burn Care Res*. 2006;27(3):377–385.
90. Berger MM, Bernath MA, Chiolero RL. Resuscitation, anesthesia and analgesia of the burned patient. *Curr Opin Anaesthesiol*. 2001;14:431–435.
91. Mansfield MD. Resuscitation and monitoring. *Ballieres Clin Anesthesiol*. 1997;11(3):369–384.
92. Demling RH. The burn edema process: current concepts. *J Burn Care Rehab*. 2005;26:207–277.
93. Bert J, Gyenge C, Bowen B, et al. Fluid resuscitation following a burn injury: implications of a mathematical model of microvascular exchange. *Burns*. 1997;23(2):93–105.
94. Ampratwum RT, Bowen BD, Lund T, et al. A model of fluid resuscitation following burn injury: formulation and parameter estimation. *Comput Methods Programs Biomed*. 1995;47:1–19.
95. Lund T, Bert JL, Onarheim H, et al. Microvascular exchange during burn injury. I. A review. *Circ Shock*. 1989;28(3):179–197.
96. Bert JL, Bowen BD, Gu X, et al. Microvascular exchange during burn injury: ii. formulation and validation of a mathematical model. *Circ Shock*. 1989;28(3):199–219.
97. Bowen BD, Bert JL, Gu X, et al. Microvascular exchange during burn injury. III. Implications of the model. *Circ Shock*. 1989;28(3):221–233.
98. Bert JL, Bowen BD, Reed RK, Onarheim H. Microvascular exchange during burn injury: iv, fluid resuscitation model. *Circ Shock*. 1991;34(3):285–297.
99. O'Mara MS, Slater H, Goldfarb IW, Caushaj PF. A prospective, randomized evaluation of intra-abdominal pressures with crystalloid and colloid resuscitation in burn patients. *J Trauma*. 2005;58(5):1011–1018.
100. Tricklebank S. Modern trends in fluid therapy for burns. *Burns*. 2009;35(6):757–767.
101. Cochran A, Morris SE, Edelman LS, Saffle JR. Burn patient characteristics and outcomes following resuscitation with albumin. *Burns*. 2007;33(1):25–30.
102. Lawrence A, Faraklas I, Watkins H, et al. Colloid administration normalizes resuscitation ratio and ameliorates "fluid creep". *J Burn Care Res*. 2010;31(1):40–47.
103. Lavrentieva A, Palmieri T. Determination of cardiovascular parameters in burn patients using arterial waveform analysis: a review. *Burns*. 2011;37(2):196–202.
104. Greenhalgh DG. Burn resuscitation. *J Burn Care Res*. 2007;28(4):555–565.
105. Saffle JI. The phenomenon of "fluid creep" in acute burn resuscitation. *J Burn Care Res*. 2007;28(3):382–395.
106. Sullivan SR, Friedrich JB, Engrav LH, et al. "Opioid creep" is real and may be the cause of "fluid creep." *Burns*. 2004;30(6):583–590.
107. Cancio LC, Chávez S, Alvarado-Ortega M, et al. Predicting increased fluid requirements during the resuscitation of thermally injured patients. *J Trauma*. 2004;56(2):404–413.
108. Namdar T, Stollwerck PL, Stang FH, et al. Transdermal fluid loss in severely burned patients. *Geriatr Med Sci*. 2010;8:Doc28.
109. Remensnyder JP. Acute electrical injuries. In: Martyn JAJ, ed. *Acute Management of the Burned Patient*. Philadelphia, PA: WB Saunders Company, 1990:66–86.
110. Kwon KH, Kim SH, Minn YK. Electrodiagnostic study of peripheral nerves in high-voltage electrical injury. *J Burn Care Res*. 2014;35(4): e230–e233.
111. Korn BS, Kikkawa DO. Images in clinical medicine. Ocular manifestation of electrical burn. *N Engl J Med*. 2014;370(4):e6.
112. Boozalis GT, Purdue GF, Hunt JL, McCulley JP. Ocular changes from electrical burn injuries: a literature review and report of cases. *J Burn Care Rehab*. 1991;12(5):458–462.
113. Mozingo DW, Cioffi WG Jr, Pruitt BA Jr. Burns. In: Bongard FS, Sue DY, eds. *Current Critical Care Diagnosis & Treatment*. 2nd ed. New York: Lange Medical Books/McGraw-Hill, 2002:799–828.
114. Elderman DA, Khan N, Kempf K, White MT. Pneumonia after inhalation injury. *J Burn Care Res*. 2007;28(2):241–246.
115. Cioffi WB, Graves TA, McManus WF, Pruitt BA Jr. High-frequency percussive ventilation in patients with inhalation injury. *J Trauma*. 1989; 29(3):350–354.
116. Hall JJ, Hunt JL, Arnoldo BD, Purdue GF. Use of high-frequency percussive ventilation in inhalation injuries. *J Burn Care Res*. 2007;28(3):396–400.
117. O'grady NP, Alexander M, Dellinger EP, et al. Healthcare infection control practices advisory committee: guidelines for the prevention of intravascular catheter-related infections. *Am J Infect Control*. 2002;30(8): 476–489.
118. Tompkins RG, Burke JF, Schoenfeld DA, et al. Prompt eschar excision: a treatment system contributing to reduced burn mortality. *Ann Surg*. 1986;204(3):272–280.
119. Gastmeier P, Geffers C. Prevention of ventilator-associated pneumonia: analysis of studies published since 2004. *J Hosp Infect*. 2007;67(1):1–8.
120. Purdue GF. American Burn Association presidential address 2006 on nutrition: yesterday, today, and tomorrow. *J Burn Care Res*. 2006;28(1):1–5.
121. Juang P, Fish DN, Jung R, MacLaren R. Enteral glutamine supplementation in critically ill patients with burn injuries: a retrospective case-control evaluation. *Pharmacotherapy*. 2007;27(1):11–19.

122. Peng YZ, Yuan ZQ, Ciao GX. Effects of early enteral feeding on the prevention of enterogenic infection in severely burned patients. *Burns*. 2001;27(2):145–149.
123. Chen Z, Wang S, Yu B, Li A. A comparison study between early enteral nutrition and parenteral nutrition in severe burn patients. *Burns*. 2007;33(6):708–712.
124. Prelack K, Dylewski M, Sheridan RL. Practical guidelines for nutritional management of burn injury and recovery. *Burns*. 2007;33:14–24.
125. Berger MM, Shenkin A. Trace element requirements in critically ill burned patients. *J Trace Elements*. 2007;SI:44–48.
126. Wolf SE. Nutrition and metabolism in burns: state of the science, 2007. *J Burn Care Res*. 2007;28(4):572–576.
127. Windle EM. Glutamine supplementation in critical illness: evidence, recommendations, and implications for clinical practice in burn care. *J Burn Care Res*. 2006;27(6):764–772.
128. Bongers T, Griffiths RD, McArdle A. Exogenous glutamine: the clinical evidence. *Crit Care Med*. 2007;35(9):S545–S552.
129. Druml W. Protein metabolism in acute renal failure. *Miner Electrolyte Metab*. 1998;24(1):47–54.
130. Druml W. Nutritional management of acute renal failure. *Am J Kidney Dis*. 2001;37(1 Suppl 2):S89–94.
131. Chan L. Nutritional support in acute renal failure. *Curr Opin Clin Nutr Metab Care*. 2004;7:207–212.
132. Cynober L. Amino acid metabolism in thermal burns. *J Parenter Enteral Nutr*. 1989;12(2):196–205.
133. Windle EM. Glutamine supplementation in critical illness: evidence, recommendations, and implications for clinical practice in burn care. *J Burn Care Res*. 2006;27(6):764–772.
134. Tao KM, Li XQ, Yang LQ, et al. Glutamine supplementation for critically ill adults. *Cochrane Database Systemat Rev*. 2014;9:CD010050.
135. Tan HB, Danilla S, Murray A, et al. Immunonutrition as an adjuvant therapy for burns. *Cochrane Database Systemat Rev*. 2014;12: CD007174.
136. Nguyen TT, Gilpin DA, Meyer NA, Herndon DN. Current treatment of severely burned patients. *Ann Surg*. 1996;223(1):14–25.
137. Murphy KD, Lee JO, Herndon DN. Current pharmacotherapy for the treatment of severe burns. *Exp Opin Pharmacother*. 2003;4(3):369.
138. Brown TP, Cancio LC, McManus AT, Mason AD Jr. Survival benefit conferred by topical antimicrobial preparations in burn patients: a historical perspective. *J Trauma*. 2004;56(4):863-866.

CHAPTER

64

Vascular Surgery

ROBERT J. FEEZOR and TIMOTHY C. FLYNN

Patients requiring vascular intervention—whether open surgery or endovascular procedures—typically are elderly and have comorbidities that make their overall care complicated. To achieve a successful outcome, the perioperative care of the vascular surgery patient requires meticulous attention to detail and knowledge about the possible pitfalls these patients can encounter. Even the most seemingly innocuous clinical symptom must be thoroughly investigated and potentially treated in order to achieve acceptable perioperative outcomes. Despite meticulous attention to detail, vascular patients often fall victim to their comorbidities or succumb to failure of the primary intervention.

In general, vascular problems are defects in plumbing, and in that regard, the "pipes" (arteries) can either clog or burst. Despite the focalized anatomic defect that drives the presentation and surgical therapy, it is imperative that clinicians recognize vascular pathology as a systemic disease and not just a focal anatomic problem. The nature of atherosclerosis is that it affects the blood vessels of all circulatory beds: cardiac, peripheral, renal, and cerebral. Thus, patients who present with leg ischemia are at significantly higher risk than the general population for having myocardial infarctions, renal dysfunction, and cerebrovascular accidents. In fact, the average patient with critical limb ischemia has an estimated mortality rate of 50% at 5 years, with the predominant cause of death being cardiovascular (1). Furthermore, there is progressing evidence that the vascular occlusive process is proinflammatory in nature. These patients have elevated levels of C-reactive protein (CRP), interleukin (IL)-6, and soluble intercellular adhesion molecule-1. Elevated CRP has recently been shown to be a predictor of cardiovascular events among patients with peripheral artery disease (PAD) (2). Upregulation of inflammatory mediators may contribute to complications in the ICU.

In most series, patients with vascular occlusive disease have a high incidence of chronic obstructive pulmonary disease, evident or occult cardiac disease, diabetes, and renal insufficiency. The adverse pulmonary sequelae of arterial revascularization are frequently related to the ravages of smoking. In most reports of operative repair of PAD, the incidence of tobacco use among patients exceeds 50%, and often approaches 90%. In a study looking at femoral atherosclerosis using duplex ultrasound, smoking was the largest risk factor, more influential than exercise tolerance, hypertension, or hypercholesterolemia (3). We may choose a potentially less durable endovascular therapy for patients based on their condition and ability to tolerate general anesthesia. Although general endotracheal anesthesia (GETA) is still the most common type of anesthesia used in vascular patients, increasing evidence suggests that spinal or epidural anesthesia may be more appropriate. In a review of 14,788 patients in the National Surgical Quality Improvement Program (NSQIP) of the Department of Veterans Affairs, GETA was associated with a higher incidence of cardiac, pulmonary, and graft complications when compared to spinal or epidural anesthesia (4).

Patients with known vascular disease are assumed to have associated coronary artery disease, even though they may be asymptomatic. In a landmark study by Hertzer et al., over 90% of patients undergoing peripheral vascular reconstruction had coronary artery disease evident by cardiac catheterization, and nearly one-third had multivessel disease (5). The goals of the American Heart Association/American College of Cardiology should be targeted, including a blood pressure less than 140/90 mmHg, serum low-density lipoprotein (LDL) <100 mg/dL, and hemoglobin A_{1C} less than 7% (6). To achieve these goals, patients should potentially be on an aspirin, a β-blocker dosed to a target heart rate of 70 to 75, an angiotensin-converting enzyme (ACE) inhibitor or other antihypertensive therapy, and probably a statin (independent of baseline cholesterol levels). Earlier recommendations of widespread β-blocker usage have been since refuted, and at present, perioperative efforts should focus on avoidance of excessive hypotension or bradycardia may still be reasonable (7). Initiation of β-blockers in patients not previously on such medications likely should be avoided.

There is increasing evidence that patients with vascular disease should all be treated with a statin regardless of cholesterol levels (8). Statins have numerous effects other than reduction of cholesterol including anti-inflammatory, immunomodulatory, and anticoagulant effects. Moreover, abrupt discontinuation may lead to a rebound effect and possibly increase cardiovascular complications (9). It is our practice to routinely start patients on a statin preoperatively and continue it throughout the postoperative period. The antiplatelet drug clopidogrel is frequently used in vascular patients. Preoperatively we review the indications for this drug, and if the indications are compelling, such as the patient with a recent coronary stent placement, we will continue the drug through the perioperative period, recognizing that there may be a slightly increased incidence of wound complications. We do not hesitate to start the drug in patients who exhibit cardiac ischemia in the postoperative period.

The electrocardiogram (ECG) should be monitored continuously for any changes suggestive of ischemia. For the diabetic population, angina may present as nausea and must be interpreted as signs of myocardial ischemia until proven otherwise. Finally, cardiac dysrhythmias are often caused by ischemia, electrolyte disturbances, or fluid shifts in the postoperative period, and patients should be monitored closely for such events.

In order to decrease the risk of perioperative cardiac events in the vascular surgery patient population, much attention has been given to preoperative risk stratification. In the surgical and anesthesia literature, most vascular surgery procedures for occlusive or aneurysmal disease are placed in the high-risk category. The question is how to minimize the risk of perioperative cardiac complications. Data from several randomized, multicenter trials have shown that coronary revascularization (percutaneous or open) before elective major vascular surgery does not decrease the overall mortality (10). Nevertheless, many clinicians request preoperative cardiology consultation to help determine existing cardiac function, usually with an ECG, an echocardiogram, or a chemical cardiac stress test.

Even without prior known elevated serum creatinine, many vascular patients have renal insufficiency as determined by creatinine clearance. Nephrotoxic effects of the IV contrast commonly used in revascularization procedures make postoperative renal dysfunction a constant threat. Moreover, perioperative mortality after most vascular procedures is significantly increased in patients with renal failure (11). Strict monitoring of fluid balance, maintenance of serum electrolytes, appropriate dosing of nephrotoxic medications, adequate hydration, and resumption of chronic diuretics will all help to minimize the chance of postoperative renal dysfunction.

A majority of vascular patients have diabetes mellitus and this group is at higher risk for postoperative complications, both vascular and nonvascular. From a vascular perspective, patients with diabetes have a higher rate of postoperative amputations after peripheral bypass surgery for tissue loss (11). Diabetics are also at risk for other postoperative morbidities including postoperative wound infections. They should be maintained euglycemic, even if that requires a constant intravenous infusion of insulin, with target blood glucose of 80 to 110 mg/dL.

There is a subset of patients with vascular disease with underlying hypercoagulable states. The concern for a hypercoagulable state should be raised with patients with seemingly advanced atherosclerotic disease at a younger age. A careful history can assist with determining these patients, but when identified, they should be started on appropriate anticoagulation. Hematology consultation should be obtained, but may be of somewhat limited value in the setting of the acute thrombotic event. A growing concern in this population is the rapidly expanding number of anticoagulants that are available. More of them require less intensive monitoring as an outpatient and are less affected by dietary modifications than the traditional warfarin. The significant drawback is the inability to rapidly and reliably reverse their hematologic effects in the event of the need for emergency surgery.

VASCULAR CARE IN THE INTENSIVE CARE UNIT

All patients in an ICU have a propensity for developing venous thromboembolic events. Virchow's triad dictates that patients at risk include those with stasis, endothelial injury, and a hypercoagulable state. In the postsurgical population, venous stasis is inevitably due to the patients' relative immobility. Endothelial injury occurs during the course of the surgical procedure. It is our practice that all patients receive chemical and/or mechanical prophylaxis; we routinely use low–molecular-weight or unfractionated heparin and/or sequential compression devices when there is no existing contraindication. We avoid lower extremity sequential compression devices in patients with severe peripheral arterial occlusive disease, although the data for this practice are anecdotal. The incidence of heparin-induced thrombocytopenia is relatively rare, and when suggested by a decline in platelet count, we promptly cease all systemic or local heparin and transition to mechanical prophylaxis and use an alternate anticoagulant. In these instances, hematologic consultation proves quite insightful.

Stress gastritis is a constant threat in the vascular ICU patient and frequently manifests as blood-tinged nasogastric aspirate or frank hematemesis. Patients are routinely placed on either histamine-receptor blockers or proton pump inhibitors, irrespective of any clinically detected gastrointestinal hemorrhage. Opponents of this practice suggest that in doing so, one of the body's natural defense mechanisms (gastric acidity) is altered, but we find that the risk of stress gastritis exceeds the diminution in host defenses.

Ventilator-associated pneumonia has been well documented to increase in-hospital mortality, length of stay, and overall cost of hospitalization. Early extubation and mobilization seem to be key preventative strategies to minimize this risk. We employ routine suctioning, aggressive bronchoscopy to control secretions, and head elevation for all our intubated patients. Once extubated, activity is encouraged and adequate pain control is important for patients with an abdominal or a thoracic incision.

The routine assessment of the vascular ICU patient includes not only all the usual cardiovascular, pulmonary, and metabolic parameters, but also frequent and detailed physical examinations. All incisions should be inspected for signs of early wound complications such as infection, separation, or hematoma. Objective assessment of distal perfusion should be performed regularly, even hourly, in the immediate postoperative period. This assessment includes looking at the extremity for cutaneous signs of malperfusion, assessing motor function, and palpating the major muscle groups for tenseness, which may signify compartment syndrome in patients who are too sedated to relate the classic "pain with passive motion." The best examination, in our opinion, is to elevate the lower extremity by placing the hand behind the Achilles tendon and palpating the anterior calf compartment with the posterior leg off the bed. A patient should be alert enough to follow commands of simple dorsiflexion, again ensuring that the posterior knee is off the bed. (Dorsiflexing the foot with the heel resting on the bed can be achieved with flexion of the quadriceps muscles, thereby not testing the anterior calf compartment, which is the muscle group of interest.)

Some centers have advocated use of pressure monitoring devices to measure compartment pressures, but it has been our practice that if compartment syndrome is even suspected, it is imperative to perform fasciotomies emergently. This is best accomplished by either a one- or two-incision technique. All four calf compartments should be incised and released. Fasciotomies can be performed in the ICU setting using Bovie electrocautery and sterile scissors. The underlying muscle should bulge when released, thereby confirming the diagnosis. The wound should be left open and treated with routine dressing changes with subsequent closure in several days to weeks when the swelling abates. The metabolic sequelae of compartment syndrome may consist of cellular lysis with release of potassium and myoglobin that may cause systemic hyperkalemia and possibly acute renal failure. We routinely check urine myoglobin and administer aggressive intravenous fluids to ensure brisk urine output of at least 100 mL/hr. Electrolytes are checked frequently and continuous telemetric cardiac monitoring is employed. The data supporting alkalinization are weak and probably less imperative than fluid resuscitation, but on occasion, clinicians may choose to employ it.

The distal perfusion of the critically ill vascular patient should receive the same attention as the cardiopulmonary status. Clearly, adequacy of perfusion should be assessed in patients who have undergone distal revascularization, but even for aortic reconstructive procedures, the risk of limb ischemia is not insignificant, and missing an acutely ischemia extremity in a patient who is sedated and intubated can have catastrophic consequences. Each extremity should be assessed by checking for palpable pulses; if none are found, Doppler signals must be auscultated to assess the perfusion. Ample quantity of Doppler gel should be used and the Doppler probe should be positioned at 60 degrees from the long axis of blood flow to maximize the signal. Normal Doppler signals are described as triphasic: the initial forward flow of blood is due to left ventricular systolic ejection; the second (reversal) flow is due to the intrinsic resistance of the arterioles in the circulation; the third phase again is forward-directed flow, and is largely attributed to the elasticity of the aorta. Doppler signals distal to an obstruction may be characterized as biphasic or monophasic signals with the latter suggesting significantly diminished blood flow. Sometimes it is difficult to tell if the sound is venous or arterial. If the sound disappears with gentle pressure on the Doppler probe, it is likely a venous sound. Also, if the sound in one of the pedal pulses disappears with gentle compression around the forefoot, it may be a venous and not arterial sound. At the conclusion of any vascular procedure, extremity perfusion is assessed prior to leaving the operating room (OR). The operating surgeon should relay to the ICU team of physicians and nurses the quality and location of each Doppler signal or palpable pulse, as well as the frequency that he or she wants the perfusion assessed. Any change in the examination or inability of the examiner to detect the signal may potentially constitute an emergent trip back to the OR to restore perfusion. Loss of a palpable pulse even if the pulse remains by Doppler should always be cause for alarm and the operating team should be alerted.

All vascular surgery wounds should be examined daily for signs of infection. Of particular difficulty are the incisions made in the groins. The incidence of groin wound complications in the vascular surgery patient has been estimated to be up to 44% in some series (12,13). Although most surgeons try to close groin wounds with several layers of suture, any breakdown of the wound can be a significant complication. Groin wound breakdown is especially common in obese patients and efforts should be directed toward keeping this area dry and covered with sterile gauze. Most breakdowns can be treated with local therapy, usually routine dressing changes at the bedside with the possible addition of enzymatic debridement agents. On occasion, patients require surgical debridement either at the bedside or if more extensive, in the OR.

Although there has been a great deal of interest in new techniques and agents to expedite wound healing, few advances have impacted the overall rate of wound complications, possibly owing to the patient's underlying systemic illnesses that translate into slow healing. The most disastrous complication of groin, or any other wound, breakdown is the exposure of the underlying vascular graft or anastomosis with the devastating potential for anastomotic disruption. When the bypass graft is noted to be exposed, patients should be scheduled for the OR for exploration and attempted reclosure of the wound, preferably with autogenous tissue such as a sartorius or rectus flap. Until the patient can go back to the OR, it is imperative that all health care personnel treating the patient be aware of exposed vasculature. We have instituted a "blowout precaution" protocol wherein patients are kept at bedrest and blood typed and crossed, and a large easily read sign is placed at the head of the bed. Any bleeding from the wound is a potential emergency. Immediate pressure should be held on the wound, the patient stabilized, and the operating team notified. We have on occasion had to rush back to the OR with a member of the team holding direct pressure on the wound until the patient is intubated and anesthetized, the surgeon scrubbed in, and the operative field prepped (even if this includes the team member's gloved hand being prepped into the field).

For the vascular patient, meticulous care of the skin is mandatory, and even modest duration of pressure on the heel by the bed mattress can lead to skin breakdown and turn a successful revascularization into an amputation. Because a significant number of vascular patients have compromised distal perfusion, we try to keep patients' heels off of the bed by placing the calves on pillows, which allows the weight of the leg to be borne over a larger atraumatic surface area. There is no substitute for frequent inspection of all pressure-sensitive areas and this should be part of the clinician's and nurse's practice.

Pharmacologic prophylaxis against thromboembolic events is the routine. However, many patients require systemic anticoagulation after vascular surgical procedures (14) such as with distal bypasses when there is compromised outflow or less than ideal conduit. The need for systemic anticoagulation must be balanced with the risk of bleeding complications, and usually we hold off full anticoagulation until postoperative day 2 or 3. We readily employ our institution's "low-intensity" protocols balancing the need for anticoagulation with the risk of postoperative hemorrhage. As a matter of protocol, warfarin or similar longer-acting anticoagulants are not initiated until patients leave the ICU because of the frequent need for central lines or similar procedures. Any patient on systemic or prophylactic heparin is monitored for any decline in platelet count, and if seen, a heparin antibody panel is sent and all heparin products are discontinued. Regardless of the agent chosen, it is imperative that the anticoagulation be monitored closely, ideally with protocol-driven therapy (15).

As stated earlier, acute limb ischemia in the ICU setting can have disastrous consequences. Given the nature of patients in the modern ICU, this can happen in vascular patients and nonvascular patients alike. The pathologic differential includes embolic events (usually from cardiac, aortic, or rarely, venous sources) or in situ thrombosis of pre-existing atherosclerotic lesions that likely is a consequence of plaque instability and the aggregation of platelets, which then occludes the vessel. If identified acutely, there may be a role for intra-arterial thrombolysis, although in the setting of the postsurgical patient, this role is limited due to excessive bleeding risk. When an ischemic extremity is identified, patients should immediately be fully anticoagulated if tolerated while resources are being mobilized to further evaluate the problem. More aggressive intervention, either catheter-based therapy or open surgical thrombectomy, should be entertained. However, if the acute arterial occlusion is associated with motor or sensory deficits, then an emergent exploration is indicated. On rare occasions, patients present with acute lower extremity paralysis secondary to acute infrarenal aortic occlusion. There is often a delay in diagnosis owing to an investigation of neurologic causes of the paraplegia. Absence of femoral pulses is a clue to the vascular nature of the paralysis. These patients typically require emergent procedures, often direct aortic reconstruction or extra-anatomic bypass, and despite operative success, the perioperative mortality rate exceeds 50% (16).

The acutely ischemic limb often is the upper extremities as well. In this setting, common ICU causes of arterial occlusion include sequelae of invasive monitoring, usually intra-arterial lines. In a recent review of brachial artery cannulations for cardiac catheterizations, the overall complication rate was an astonishing 36% (17). Not infrequently we are called to assess lack of distal perfusion in an extremity with an indwelling arterial line. The first step is to remove the catheter and to observe for restoration of perfusion. The collateral blood supply should also be assessed (usually the ulnar pulse in the event of radial artery occlusion) as well as the distal perfusion, including motor and sensory assessment. Choices of therapy include observation, systemic anticoagulation, local thrombolysis, and operative thrombectomy with the potential for bypass. As with lower extremity acute arterial occlusion, any motor dysfunction should be treated with emergent surgical exploration, arterial reconstruction, and consideration of fasciotomies. A brachial sheath hematoma that is associated with mild sensory deficits is also best treated with expeditious surgical exploration, decompression, and arterial reconstruction to avoid permanent damage to the median nerve that is enclosed in the brachial sheath, juxtaposed to the antecubital brachial artery.

The choice of invasive arterial and venous monitoring can represent a continuous challenge in any ICU patient, but in particular the vascular ICU patient. Lower extremity intravenous and arterial lines are contraindicated in patients with peripheral arterial occlusive disease. In patients who have a functional arteriovenous fistula or graft for hemodialysis, every effort should be made to avoid the use of ipsilateral extremity noninvasive blood pressure cuffs, IVs, arterial lines, or central venous catheters. If a patient is identified as likely to require permanent vascular access in the future, duplex ultrasonography should be used to identify a potential extremity for future dialysis access, and the identified extremity should be preserved.

Various bleeding complications can occur in the postoperative vascular wound. These can range from simple "skin edge" bleeding to frank exsanguination from an exposed anastomosis. Skin edge bleeding may be a nuisance, and may be treated with manual compression, application of silver nitrate, or a simple suture. Hematomas are monitored closely. Recurrent blood transfusion requirements, overlying skin or wound compromise, deleterious mass effects, and hemodynamic instability are all indications for operative evacuation of the hematoma. Patients who have had percutaneous interventions (usually through the groin at the common femoral artery) should also be monitored for hematomas, and in these instances, simple manual compression may be adequate. Attempted femoral artery punctures that are aimed more cephalad may in fact be external iliac artery punctures. Compression for hemostasis may be ineffective due to the retroperitoneal location of the arteriotomy. A progressive hematoma in such a location more often requires surgical repair (open or endovascular). Additionally, patients with transient or sustained hypotension, or a decline in hematocrit, should be assessed for a retroperitoneal hematoma, usually with a CT scan using intravenous contrast in the arterial phase.

SPECIFIC CONDITIONS

Aneurysmal Disease

Infrarenal Abdominal Aortic Aneurysm

Approximately 90% of the extracranial aneurysms found in the human body involve the infrarenal aorta. The natural history of aneurysms of the aorta is to expand and rupture. The tension of the thinning aortic wall can be estimated by the law of Laplace, which describes the relationship between aortic diameter and wall tension. The results of randomized trials and observational studies have led vascular surgeons to recommend operative repair when the diameter of the aorta reaches 5.5 cm in asymptomatic men (18), but the numeric value varies, especially with female patients. Most aneurysms are asymptomatic and many are discovered during radiographic workup of other problems. Patients who have symptomatic aneurysms generally complain of back or abdominal pain. Unless definitively attributable to other pathologies, these symptoms should be interpreted as a sign of impending rupture necessitating urgent repair. We no longer place pulmonary artery catheters routinely, but all patients have arterial lines and Foley catheters and most have central lines. All patients get a single dose of preoperative antibiotics, which are not continued postoperatively in the absence of ongoing infection. It is our routine to obtain preoperative transthoracic echocardiography, but mostly as a means of assisting perioperative care, as rarely do patients have correctable cardiomyopathies. Cardiology consultation is not routinely employed because all patients are assumed to have concomitant coronary artery disease and are medically treated appropriately as such.

Endovascular Repair. Depending on patient anatomy and patient/physician preference, abdominal aortic aneurysm (AAA) repair can be performed either via an open or endovascular approach. The endovascular approach holds great appeal in terms of reduced physiologic insult to the patient. Typically, both common femoral arteries are accessed either percutaneously or via an open groin exposure, and the device is placed from within the arterial lumen using fluoroscopic guidance. The weakened arterial wall is bolstered from within with stents made of a malleable metal alloy and a woven fabric. At our institution, these patients rarely require admission to the ICU but are monitored for hematomas and lower extremity pulses. The devices used to deploy endovascular stents can be as large as 26 French, and these are introduced through femoral or external iliac arteries. There is a possibility of local arterial damage or dislodging of plaque that may embolize distally. Again, patients are assessed intraoperatively, and any change in the hard signs of distal perfusion postoperatively may reflect a surgical emergency. The likely pathologic culprits for acute limb ischemia after endovascular AAA repair include access site (common femoral artery) occlusion/dissection or endovascular stent limb thrombosis.

Open Repair. Open aneurysms, on the other hand, require surgical ICU monitoring postoperatively. The overall perioperative mortality is approximately 5% (19). Because a prosthetic graft has been sewn to the abdominal aorta, the main concern is bleeding, and a recent review of over 20,000 Medicare beneficiaries reported a 1.2% incidence of reintervention for bleeding. Furthermore, because the blood supply to the lower extremities is occluded intraoperatively during the aortic repair, it is vital to objectively assess and document lower extremity perfusion. Lower extremity ischemic events after open AAA repairs occur in 2% to 5% of patients (20). As stated earlier, any inability to detect a Doppler signal or palpate a pulse when there previously was one is a potential surgical emergency.

A major complication of open AAA surgery is gastrointestinal problems. A large retrospective study estimated the incidence of postoperative prolonged ileus to be 11% and nonischemic diarrhea to be 7.1% (20). All patients will have a brief period of postoperative ileus that may be shortened by use of a retroperitoneal approach to aneurysmorrhaphy (21). However, the dreaded complication is colonic ischemia with an estimated prevalence of 0.6% (20), but a mortality of 55% to 90% depending on the severity, recognition and management, and patient reserve. Most instances present as bloody stools 3 to 5 days postoperatively but may occur as early as the first 24 hours after surgery and are cause for considerable concern. Warning signs include fever, abdominal pain, thrombocytopenia, unexplained leukocytosis, or lactic acidosis. Any suspicion of colonic ischemia should prompt endoscopic evaluation, with the obvious caveat that endoscopy will only view the mucosal changes, and cannot evaluate for transmural ischemia. However, in the appropriate clinical setting, mucosal ischemia may justify operative exploration with possibly colon resection and end colostomy. These patients require intensive invasive ICU monitoring, as they often progress to multisystem organ failure as a result of their colonic ischemia. Routine broad-spectrum antibiotics to include gram-negative and anaerobic coverage are used.

Other potential gastrointestinal complications known to occur include cholecystitis and pancreatitis. The latter is probably related to direct surgical trauma during aortic exposure and is usually self-limited. Cholecystitis may be ischemia-related or may be a variant of acalculous cholecystitis seen in ICU patients. Treatment options range from percutaneous cholecystostomy to surgical cholecystectomy. Much like the problem of colon ischemia in the setting of an aortic graft, an infected gallbladder should not be overlooked or minimized.

The incidence of postoperative renal dysfunction can be as high as 5.4% after open infrarenal aortic surgery, but dialysis requirement is much less at 0.6% (20). Renal dysfunction is significantly lower in patients who have undergone infrarenal aortic cross-clamp, thereby avoiding the obligate renal ischemia-reperfusion. The exact etiology of the renal dysfunction after infrarenal clamping is largely speculative, but may involve migration of atheroemboli leading to acute tubular necrosis or hypotension-induced renal dysfunction. In the early postoperative period, oliguria is most frequently due to intravascular depletion and not intrinsic renal dysfunction. However, patients with baseline renal insufficiency, those more than 2 days postoperative, or those who do not respond appropriately to intravenous fluid challenges should be investigated for acute tubular necrosis or other intrinsic (nonprerenal) cause of oliguria. The initial management includes assessment of volume resuscitation, urine and serum electrolytes, and a renal artery duplex.

In the absence of other causes (e.g., colon ischemia), patients may experience postoperative thrombocytopenia. Although an inciting event or agent is not always identifiable, there are several likely etiologies. Before occluding the aorta in the OR, all patients are systemically heparinized, and although our practice is to reverse the anticoagulant effects of heparin toward the end of the case, the drug's side effects (i.e., thrombocytopenia) may persist. Unless there is evidence of ongoing bleeding, mild thrombocytopenia is usually well tolerated.

The cohort of patients who get abdominal aneurysms may have coronary artery disease and are at risk for postoperative myocardial infarctions, dysrhythmias, and episodes of congestive heart failure. Johnston reported an incidence of myocardial infarctions (5.2%), heart failure (8.9%), and dysrhythmia requiring treatment (10.5%). The overall incidence of any perioperative cardiac event was 15.1% (20). Unless contraindicated, patients undergoing open aneurysm repair should be on a medical regimen consisting of a β-blocker with a target heart rate of less than 70, a statin (independent of serum cholesterol levels), and some form of antiplatelet therapy, usually aspirin.

Ruptured Aortic Aneurysms

Whereas surgical repair of intact aneurysms is a prophylactic procedure, repair of ruptured aneurysms is an attempt at life-saving surgery. A meta-analysis found the operative mortality rate of ruptured AAA to be 48%, with a small decline in mortality for each decade from the 1950s to the 1990s (22) (much higher than an elective AAA repair of <5% mortality). With ruptured AAA, there are impressive fluid shifts that transpire during such an emergent operation, independent of overt blood loss. These fluid shifts, associated with the hypotension and the physiologic strain of an emergent procedure, contribute to a tenuous postoperative course. The incidence of colonic ischemia is significantly higher after ruptured aneurysm repair compared to elective open aneurysmorrhaphy, and some authors recommend empiric and routine endoscopic evaluation of the colonic mucosa.

Juxtarenal or Suprarenal Aortic Aneurysms

Most aortic aneurysms are infrarenal, meaning that the proximal extent of the dilated segment of aorta is caudal to the lowest renal artery. Therefore, operative repair usually can be performed with infrarenal aortic occlusion in the OR. If the aneurysm extends to the level of the renal arteries, or involves the paravisceral aorta, the repair becomes technically more challenging, and the postoperative complications escalate dramatically due to renal and possibly mesenteric ischemia-reperfusion. Depending on the length of intraoperative ischemia, there is a resultant release of pro- and anti-inflammatory cytokines that drives a systemic inflammatory reaction resulting in multisystem organ failure (23). There is considerable third spacing of fluid in the first 24 hours as edema collects in the interstitial spaces. Attempts to improve mortality and morbidity by a hybrid approach involving multiple visceral bypasses and endovascular repair of the aneurysm have met with mixed results (24).

If the thoracic cavity is violated as a part of the aneurysm repair, the patient will have an even greater risk of pulmonary complications. Routinely a chest tube is placed intraoperatively to drain any pleural fluid that may accumulate. Adequate pain control is key in these patients.

Infected Aortic Graft

One of the more dreaded complications of aortic surgery is infection of the prosthesis, which happens in less than 2% of aortic surgery. This rarely happens in the early postoperative period, and the majority occurs months to years later with unexplained fevers and malaise, occult or clinically evident gastrointestinal bleeding, and a computed tomography (CT) scan that shows fluid around an aortic graft. These are serious, life-threatening surgical problems, and patients should be treated aggressively. Broad-spectrum antibiotics, appropriate intravenous resuscitation, and close hemodynamic monitoring should be undertaken. Patients should be medically optimized and prepared for a significant surgical challenge. The classic surgical remedy was a staged procedure of extravascular bypass (axillobifemoral) with subsequent aortic graft explantation and oversewing of the infrarenal aortic stump. Although it remains debated, more often we elect to perform a single-stage aortic replacement using autogenous tissue (syndactylized bilateral femoral veins), antibiotic-soaked prosthesis, or cadaveric vessels. Explantation of an infected surgical graft remains among the most challenging cases performed by a vascular surgeon, and likely should be done only at institutions with significant local expertise and systematic resources. Each case is a balance of underlying pathology with patient physiologic reserve. Nevertheless, these patients are routinely sent to the ICU because some may become floridly septic after manipulation of the infected retroperitoneum. Compared to virginal aortic replacement surgery, excision and replacement of an infected aortic graft is associated with more profound fluid shifts postoperatively, an elevated incidence of organ dysfunction, and an overall higher rate of complications such as prolonged ventilator support, renal dysfunction, and bleeding. Local infection control proves to be particularly difficult with patients whose infected extends up to the level of the renal arteries or in whom the offending organism is a gram-negative pathogen, particularly *Pseudomonas*.

Arterial Occlusive Disease

Unlike aneurysmal disease, which tends to occur in certain segments of the arterial tree, occlusive disease can occur almost anywhere. Aortoiliac occlusive disease can be detected by the absence of a palpable femoral pulse and symptoms of lower extremity vascular compromise: claudication, tissue loss, or ischemic rest pain. The specific diagnosis and management of these problems are beyond the scope of this chapter. The most durable surgical solution for aortoiliac occlusive disease is an aortobifemoral (ABF) bypass. This is accomplished using a celiotomy incision as well as two groin incisions. The prosthetic graft (usually Dacron) is sewn to the aorta just below the renal arteries with similar complications as with open aneurysmorrhaphy (i.e., bleeding, postoperative ileus, colonic ischemia, renal dysfunction, lower extremity ischemia, cholecystitis, pancreatitis). The limbs of the bifurcated graft are then tunneled beneath the ureters and sewn into the femoral bifurcation, usually hooded onto the profunda femoris arteries. The groin incisions, similar to those used for infrainguinal bypasses, should be monitored for wound breakdown, infection, and drainage. Wound complications and the intrinsic diminished sterility of groin incisions as opposed to abdominal incisions have been implicated in the elevated risk of aortic graft infections seen with ABF reconstruction compared to aortic reconstructions performed without concomitant groin incisions. Peripheral pulses are regularly monitored and any deviation from the immediate postoperative result is a potential emergency as it may represent a graft thrombosis. Another complication is distal embolization with ischemia of the toes (trash foot). Management is expectant and most often this resolves with minimal or no permanent tissue loss.

As endovascular technology has evolved, many iliac lesions are being treated with angioplasty and possible stent placement. Although better tolerated by patients because of the less invasive nature of the procedure, the stents may not be as durable as surgical bypass. A small subset of patients, namely patients under the age of 55, are believed to have better long-term vascular durability for infrarenal aortic reconstruction with autogenous tissue rather than Dacron (25). Femoral veins can be harvested and syndactylized to be used as aortic replacement. This requires more extensive operations with longer OR times and larger leg incisions, which can be a cause of significant morbidity.

As with any surgical procedure, redo aortic surgery is fraught with intraoperative and postoperative complications. Patients generally require longer recovery periods. If the decision is made to avoid operating in the same surgical field (abdomen and retroperitoneum), extra-anatomic bypasses may be performed, usually axillobifemoral. These procedures are considered to be less invasive but less durable and still require the same vascular monitoring as any other bypass procedures. Although abdominal complications are not seen, patients still require groin and axillary incisions and there is significant subcutaneous tunneling for the graft placement. With rehabilitation, trapeze devices are contraindicated to avoid undue stress on a fresh arterial axillary anastomosis.

Infrainguinal Bypasses

Infrainguinal bypasses are commonly performed to alleviate symptoms of vascular compromise. The principles for vascular surgery are simple: the patient must have adequate inflow (usually inflow to the femoral artery), adequate outflow (of the popliteal, tibial, peroneal, or pedal arteries), and conduit ("pipe" to perform the bypass). The incisions that are made are often significant, and may not only be located on the extremity being reperfused, but also may be on either leg or either arm as a site of vein harvest. We are particularly aggressive about harvesting autogenous tissue for vein conduit as the patency of infrainguinal bypass grafts using autogenous tissue, especially the great saphenous vein, is clearly superior to that using prosthetic tissue (e.g., polytetrafluoroethylene [PTFE]) (26), and for bypasses to infrageniculate arteries, the patency is much better with even autogenous spliced conduit is superior to nonautogenous conduit. Furthermore, efforts at endoscopic vein harvest have shown worse long-term patency than standard vein harvest techniques, and as a result, distal bypass, although a "skin operation," is associated with significant incision and hence the potential for wound complications. Other than wounds, predominant sources of morbidity from these procedures are arterial occlusion (which can be detected with routine close pulse/Doppler monitoring), bleeding, and cardiopulmonary systemic complications. The mortality from peripheral bypasses is estimated to be between 2% and 8%, and the cause of mortality is primarily cardiac, so aggressive cardiac medical management, judicious use of antiplatelet therapy, and careful fluid status monitoring are essential (27,28).

Any revascularization procedure is associated with a reperfusion syndrome that is usually mild and well tolerated.

However, the reperfused extremity should always be monitored for compartment syndrome and acted upon early. Details about the technique of detecting compartment syndrome and fasciotomies have been described above. Electrolytes and cardiac rhythm should be monitored, and the urine assessed for myoglobinuria, even if that means a simple visual inspection of the urine color. Again, as a clinical rule, if compartment syndrome is suspected, it should be treated.

A major complication of any revascularization procedure is graft thrombosis with the highest risk in the immediate postoperative period most likely due to technical failure and/or platelet aggregation on a surgically damaged endothelium. Patients with "high-risk" grafts (i.e., multiple segments of vein sewn together as a conduit, small distal target arteries, or poor-quality arteries) are routinely systemically anticoagulated postoperatively with heparin (14). At our institution, there has been a slight increase in the incidence of postoperative wound hematomas, but the fraction that needs operative evacuation is small. In addition to full anticoagulation, patients with endovascular stents are routinely placed on clopidogrel to decrease the incidence of in-stent restenosis, although the data for this are limited and largely anecdotal. All patients should be on aspirin unless otherwise contraindicated.

Carotid Endarterectomy

Carotid endarterectomy (CEA) has been shown to decrease the chance of a future cerebrovascular accident in certain patients with carotid stenosis. The procedure involves a neck incision along the anterior border of the sternocleidomastoid muscle, and occlusion of the carotid artery to attain vascular control. Once occluded, the operating surgeon then may place a plastic shunt to reroute blood flow and allow distal perfusion while the endarterectomy is being performed. Although there are many intraoperative variables in technique (mode of anesthesia, whether or not to shunt, and type of shunt), the key outcome variable is perioperative stroke related to disruption of cerebral blood flow or embolic event from clamping an atherosclerotic vessel. Aspirin should be continued in the recovery phase, but full anticoagulation is seldom indicated unless carotid occlusion has occurred. Neurologic deficit may manifest itself upon awakening or occur in the early postoperative period. Any change in neurologic function that occurs after awakening with a normal neurologic examination should be reported to the operating team. Opinions vary whether to investigate with imaging or return directly to the OR depending on where in the recovery phase the patient is upon recognition of the alteration and whether the deficit is transient or seems to be dense and progressive.

Because of the baroreceptors in the carotid bulb, patients often experience large fluctuation in blood pressures, which should be targeted to the "normal systolic range" of 120 to 140 mmHg. Additionally, any wound hematoma, because the neck is a relative closed space, can cause carotid compression and resultant bradycardia or potentially airway compression. The operating team should be alerted if hematoma is suspected. Because the field of dissection is intimately associated with the cranial nerves, a detailed head and neck examination is mandatory at regular intervals. Particular attention should be paid to assessing the function of the marginal mandibular nerve and the hypoglossal nerve, which usually is mobilized and gently retracted cephalad during the course of a CEA. Headache and even seizure activity may be a manifestation of cerebral reperfusion syndrome. This is rarely seen in the immediate postoperative period, but may cause readmission for blood pressure control in the weeks after carotid endarterectomy. These patients should also have a CT scan because of the incidence of intracranial bleeding that accompanies these symptoms.

Mesenteric Revascularization

Mesenteric ischemia, whether acute or chronic, can have lethal consequences. The restoration of intestinal perfusion sets in motion a cascade of inflammatory cytokines that frequently progresses to the systemic inflammatory response syndrome, multisystem organ failure, and even death. After restoration of blood flow, patients typically have a period of hemodynamic stability for 24 to 48 hours after the procedure, but then progress to retaining more fluid and show signs of systemic inflammation, most often manifesting in pulmonary dysfunction. Subtle early changes such as a diminution in platelet count should elicit concern. To date, despite numerous anticytokine therapies, the treatment of the systemic inflammation is largely supportive (29). As this response is not uniform, efforts to predict which patient will progress to clinical deterioration have been unsuccessful. As with any other revascularization bypass, the patency of the mesenteric graft should be assessed objectively. Duplex ultrasound is noninvasive and is highly sensitive. Despite all the usual supportive measures, the average postoperative length of stay is over 3 weeks (30).

VASCULAR TRAUMA

The care of the trauma patient with vascular injuries shares many of the same principles as care of other vascular surgery patients with the exception that this cohort frequently, but not always, lacks the systemic comorbidities of the typical atherosclerotic vascular patient. Most extremity vascular injuries are associated with orthopedic fractures and dislocations; some injuries are nearly synonymous with vascular injuries, such as a posterior knee dislocation and popliteal artery injury. In the secondary survey as part of the Advanced Trauma Life Support (ATLS) evaluation of the trauma patient, extremity pulses should be assessed and clearly documented. For any patient recovering from an orthopedic procedure, the same attention to distal perfusion is merited. Any change in pulse examination or hard sign of vascular injury mandates radiographic evaluation, usually with an arteriogram, although a CT angiogram is occasionally sufficient.

Although most surgeons no longer explore extremities when a penetrating injury is in proximity to a vessel, penetrating trauma associated with hard signs of vascular injury (decreased distal perfusion, active arterial hemorrhage, or a rapidly expanding hematoma) should be evaluated immediately after life-saving measures are undertaken. Often, the area of interest is operatively explored and the vessel visually inspected. If injured, it is either repaired or blood is rerouted around the "blast field" (e.g., an external iliac artery injury in a contaminated field may be repaired with vessel ligation and a femoral–femoral bypass to perfuse the ipsilateral leg). Venous injuries are ligated unless easily repaired. Revascularization of an extremity that has been malperfused for greater than 6 hours increases the likelihood of a reperfusion syndrome and at the least, compartment syndromes should be considered and treated liberally. Naturally, vascular injury to an extremity that has too extensive musculoskeletal damage to be salvageable can be treated with simple ligation and amputation. The mangled extremity is a challenging problem facing vascular surgeons, but in general the combination of multiple orthopedic injuries, nerve injury, and arterial injury leads to a higher likelihood of a nonuseful extremity. It remains a significant challenge to primarily perform amputation unless the patient's life is immediately threatened by the presence of the extremity. Most vascular surgeons elect to perform a bypass, tunneled in a relatively spared tissue plane, and then wait to assess the neurologic function over time.

Finally, trauma to an artery and adjacent vein can result in a traumatic arteriovenous fistula. This can occur even months after the inciting trauma, and unexplained extremity swelling, distal ischemic symptoms, heart failure, or an audible bruit over an extremity should alert the clinician to the presence of a fistula. Most often, it is of little consequence unless it is very proximal and/or the patient has limited cardiopulmonary reserve.

The perceived incidence of aortic trauma is increasing, possibly due to the increased use of CT scans in trauma management. In the abdomen, any central periaortic hematoma should be operatively evaluated. With the resolution of the current scanners we are seeing a number of intimal injuries and short segments of dissection in the infrarenal aorta, mesenteric and iliac vessels that previously were not detected. In the absence of hemodynamic compromise most of these can be observed. Our typical protocol is to repeat CT imaging in 48 to 72 hours, or to obtain a dedicated arterial duplex in the event of mesenteric or renal abnormalities. Thoracic aortic injuries are nearly uniformly treated with endovascular devices. Initial care is directed toward treating the urgent life-threatening injuries and controlling blood pressure with β-blockers. Open surgical repair is still a viable option, though in most series the morbidity is clearly greater.

Penetrating neck trauma can involve the carotid artery, which can be exposed readily in certain locations (zone 2) or require more extensive operations to expose adequately (zones 3 and 1). Our current management of neck trauma in the stable patient with a zone 2 injury is to cover the wound in the trauma bay, perform the global assessment of the patient including abdominal sonography and intravenous resuscitation, and then take the patient to the OR for exploration. Only then is the injury exposed because unroofing a clot and losing hemostasis is best done with good exposure in the OR. For more proximal or distal injuries, angiography (standard contrast angiography or CT angiography) plays a vital role in both diagnosing and planning either open or endovascular treatment.

Blunt trauma to the head can result in injury to the carotid or vertebral arteries. Because these injuries are relatively rare (<1% of blunt trauma patients), controversy remains about the best way to diagnose and treat these patients. The Eastern Association for the Surgery of Trauma (EAST) has recently published practice management guidelines on blunt cerebrovascular injury (31). They recommended screening, preferably with angiography, for blunt trauma patients who present with or develop an unexplained neurologic deficit or who have cervical spine fractures, LeFort II or III fractures, petrous bone fracture, or fracture through the foramen transversum, and for those with a Glasgow coma scale score <8 or diffuse axonal injury. Although CT angiography has been reportedly used as screening, some have questioned its sensitivity, although it is likely that the newest generation of devices may eventually be accurate enough for diagnosis in this situation (32). The most common lesion discovered is a dissection or intramural hematoma. Our preference is that these lesions should be treated with either full anticoagulation or an antiplatelet agent that should continue for 3 to 6 months, and reimaging at some interval to ensure no aneurysmal degeneration. Occasionally pseudoaneurysms are seen and endovascular repair seems to be the evolving treatment modality for this lesion. Morbidity from this lesion remains high because many patients present with a deficit. In one large series there was a 26% mortality and only 31% of patients were discharged to home. However, in the asymptomatic group that was treated with either anticoagulation or antiplatelet therapy, the failure rate was only 9% (33).

Traumatic amputations, although grossly impressive, typically are not life threatening. Traumatic amputations of a major extremity (digits not included) should be wrapped with warm gauze, and manual pressure applied while the protocol-driven trauma evaluation proceeds. Once other life-threatening injuries have been evaluated, the amputated stump may be examined. The treatment priority should be hemostasis and local debridement to remove large debris. Patients should be given tetanus toxoid if there are no other contraindications. Dressing changes should be initiated, and when stabilized, a formal, closed amputation can be undertaken, with an emphasis on leaving a functional stump for the patient to use.

HEMODIALYSIS

Although the annual mortality of patients on hemodialysis approaches 25%, many patients in the ICU are on chronic hemodialysis with functional fistulae or tunneled catheters. The extremity with the fistula should be preserved from invasive and noninvasive monitoring devices, and all IVs and central lines should be placed away from that extremity unless there are no other options. Because of the presence of the fistula, the extremity distal to it is at risk of ischemic events, and should be monitored closely. Additionally, tunneled catheters already in place should not be routinely used as a convenient intravenous line except in dire circumstances. These lines can often be a source of infection, and limiting their use to their intended purpose will decrease the chance of infection. When they are accessed for dialysis purposes, it is routine practice to "lock" the catheter with concentrated heparin to minimize the chance of a mechanical catheter complication. Flushing this heparin "lock" will systemically anticoagulate the patient, even if transiently.

Key Points

- Peripheral vascular disease is one manifestation of a systemic process that is proinflammatory in nature and affects the coronary, cerebral, and peripheral vasculature.
- Ninety-three percent of patients undergoing the most common vascular procedures (AAA repair, carotid endarterectomy, peripheral bypass) have documented coronary artery disease; all patients should be medically

managed accordingly. As a rule, coronary revascularization is not indicated for patients with stable coronary disease prior to major vascular reconstruction.
- Patients with diabetes can manifest angina as nausea, diaphoresis, or "indigestion."
- Any objective change in the assessment of distal perfusion—either by palpation of pulses or auscultation of Doppler signals—is a potential surgical emergency.
- All patients with obstructive or aneurysmal vascular disease should be continued on a β-blocker, an aspirin, and a statin, unless otherwise contraindicated. Starting β-blockade may be deleterious if done immediately preoperatively.
- Compartment syndrome may be subtle, especially in the sedated ICU patient. The disappearance of pulses is a late finding. Clinicians should have a low threshold to perform fasciotomies.
- Colon ischemia after aortic surgery may present as hematochezia or melena, or may be more insidious: leukocytosis, thrombocytopenia, or fevers.

References

1. Muluk SC, Muluk VS, Kelley ME, et al. Outcome events in patients with claudication: a 15-year study in 2,777 patients. *J Vasc Surg*. 2001;33: 251–257.
2. Rossi E, Biasucci LM, Citterio F, et al. Risk of myocardial infarction and angina in patients with severe peripheral vascular disease: predictive role of C-reactive protein. *Circulation*. 2002;105:800–803.
3. Leng GC, Papacosta O, Whincup P, et al. Femoral atherosclerosis in an older British population: prevalence and risk factors. *Atherosclerosis*. 2000;152: 167–174.
4. Singh N, Sidawy AN, Dezee K, et al. The effects of the type of anesthesia on outcomes of lower extremity infrainguinal bypass. *J Vasc Surg*. 2006;44: 964–968.
5. Hertzer NR, Beven EG, Young JR, et al. Coronary artery disease in peripheral vascular patients: a classification of 1,000 coronary angiograms and results of surgical management. *Ann Surg*. 1984;199:223–233.
6. Smith SC Jr, Allen J, Blair SN, et al. AHA/ACC guidelines for secondary prevention for patients with coronary and other atherosclerotic vascular disease: 2006 update: endorsed by the National Heart, Lung, and Blood Institute. *Circulation*. 2006;113:2363–2372.
7. Perioperative ischemia evaluation (POISE). Available at http://www.cardiosource.com/clinicaltrials/trial.asp?trialID=1629. Accessed December 4, 2007.
8. Durazzo AE, Machado FS, Ikeoka DT, et al. Reduction in cardiovascular events after vascular surgery with atorvastatin: a randomized trial. *J Vasc Surg*. 2004;39:967–975.
9. Weant KA, Cook AM. Potential roles for statins in critically ill patients. *Pharmacotherapy*. 2007;27:1279–1296.
10. McFalls EO, Ward HB, Moritz TE, et al. Coronary-artery revascularization before elective major vascular surgery. *N Engl J Med*. 2004;351:2795–2804.
11. Seeger JM, Pretus HA, Carlton LC, et al. Potential predictors of outcome in patients with tissue loss who undergo infrainguinal vein bypass grafting. *J Vasc Surg*. 1999;30:427–435.
12. Kent KC, Bartek S, Kuntz KM, et al. Prospective study of wound complications in continuous infrainguinal incisions after lower limb arterial reconstruction: incidence, risk factors, and cost. *Surgery*. 1996;119:378–383.
13. Wengrovitz M, Atnip RG, Gifford RR, et al. Wound complications of autogenous subcutaneous infrainguinal arterial bypass surgery: predisposing factors and management. *J Vasc Surg*. 1990;11:156–161.
14. Sarac TP, Huber TS, Back MR, et al. Warfarin improves the outcome of infrainguinal vein bypass grafting at high risk for failure. *J Vasc Surg*. 1998;28:446–457.
15. Baird RW. Quality improvement efforts in the intensive care unit: development of a new heparin protocol. *Proc (Bayl Univ Med Cent)*. 2001;14:294–296.
16. Babu SC, Shah PM, Nitahara J. Acute aortic occlusion–factors that influence outcome. *J Vasc Surg*. 1995;21:567–572.
17. Hildick-Smith DJ, Khan ZI, Shapiro LM, et al. Occasional-operator percutaneous brachial coronary angiography: first, do no arm. *Catheter Cardiovasc Interv*. 2002;57:161–165.
18. Lederle FA, Wilson SE, Johnson GR, et al. Immediate repair compared with surveillance of small abdominal aortic aneurysms. *N Engl J Med*. 2002;346:1437–1444.
19. Johnston KW, Scobie TK. Multicenter prospective study of nonruptured abdominal aortic aneurysms. I. Population and operative management. *J Vasc Surg*. 1988;7:69–81.
20. Johnston KW. Multicenter prospective study of nonruptured abdominal aortic aneurysm. Part II. Variables predicting morbidity and mortality. *J Vasc Surg*. 1989;9:437–447.
21. Cinar B, Goksel O, Kut S, et al. Abdominal aortic aneurysm surgery: retroperitoneal or transperitoneal approach? *J Cardiovasc Surg (Torino)*. 2006;47:637–641.
22. Bown MJ, Sutton AJ, Bell PR, et al. A meta-analysis of 50 years of ruptured abdominal aortic aneurysm repair. *Br J Surg*. 2002;89:714–730.
23. Welborn MB, Oldenburg HS, Hess PJ, et al. The relationship between visceral ischemia, proinflammatory cytokines, and organ injury in patients undergoing thoracoabdominal aortic aneurysm repair. *Crit Care Med*. 2000;28:3191–3197.
24. Lee WA, Brown MP, Martin TD, et al. Early results after staged hybrid repair of thoracoabdominal aortic aneurysms. *J Am Coll Surg*. 2007;205:420–431.
25. Jackson MR, Ali AT, Bell C, et al. Aortofemoral bypass in young patients with premature atherosclerosis: is superficial femoral vein superior to Dacron? *J Vasc Surg*. 2004;40:17–23.
26. Gentile AT, Lee RW, Moneta GL, et al. Results of bypass to the popliteal and tibial arteries with alternative sources of autogenous vein. *J Vasc Surg*. 1996;23:272–279.
27. Abou-Zamzam AM Jr, Lee RW, Moneta GL, et al. Functional outcome after infrainguinal bypass for limb salvage. *J Vasc Surg*. 1997;25:287–295.
28. Nicoloff AD, Taylor LM Jr, McLafferty RB, et al. Patient recovery after infrainguinal bypass grafting for limb salvage. *J Vasc Surg*. 1998;27:256–263.
29. Huber TS, Gaines GC, Welborn MB III, et al. Anticytokine therapies for acute inflammation and the systemic inflammatory response syndrome: IL-10 and ischemia/reperfusion injury as a new paradigm. *Shock*. 2000;13: 425–434.
30. Rectenwald JE, Huber TS, Martin TD, et al. Functional outcome after thoracoabdominal aortic aneurysm repair. *J Vasc Surg*. 2002;35:640–647.
31. Bromberg WJ, Collier BC, Diebel LN, et al. Blunt cerebrovascular injury practice management guidelines: the Eastern Association for the Surgery of Trauma. *J Trauma*. 2010;68:471–477.
32. Malhotra AK, Camacho M, Ivatury RR, et al. Computed tomographic angiography for the diagnosis of blunt carotid/vertebral artery injury: a note of caution. *Ann Surg*. 2007;246:632–642.
33. Edwards NM, Fabian TC, Claridge JA, et al. Antithrombotic therapy and endovascular stents are effective treatment for blunt carotid injuries: results from longterm followup. *J Am Coll Surg*. 2007;204:1007–1013.

CHAPTER

65

Orthopedic Critical Care

DEBORAH M. STEIN, ANDREW N. POLLAK, and THOMAS M. SCALEA

INTRODUCTION

Bony and soft tissue injuries often complicate trauma. Optimal treatment of these injuries is essential for good overall patient care. Patients treated suboptimally are at risk for myriad complications, such as fat embolism syndrome, pulmonary embolus, soft tissue infection, and multiple organ failure. While there is little prospective randomized data to guide treatment decisions in patients with bony injuries, certain treatment principles have emerged. These must, of course, be interpreted in the context of the total patient.

Fracture stabilization is an operative procedure of significance. Some patients may be too critically ill or injured at the time of initial presentation to tolerate definitive fracture fixation. The critical care staff must be well versed in the management principles that govern musculoskeletal injuries as they will often have important roles to play in decision making. Orthopedic surgeons and/or anesthesiologists may not have sufficient information on total patient physiology in order to make these decisions without input from the critical care staff.

DIAGNOSING MUSCULOSKELETAL INJURY

Patients presenting after injury should typically have either signs or symptoms to guide diagnosis of their injuries. Pain, swelling, and soft tissue discoloration often accompany musculoskeletal injury, particularly in badly displaced or comminuted fractures. However, the initial presentation of many fractures may be far more subtle. Patients who have fractures that are not significantly displaced may actually have only modest soft tissue swelling and discoloration or none-at-all at the time of presentation. Patients who are multiply injured often undergo endotracheal intubation at the time of emergency department presentation and are unable to complain of pain. Multiply injured patients may have other injuries that distract them from the pain of a minor fracture; patients with brain injury and/or intoxication may also not complain of pain. The authors are constantly impressed how the signs and symptoms of fractures can be subtle or completely absent initially. As with any injury, fractures are dynamic; it is not simply that a bone is broken. Radiographic images are static and will not allow the clinician to appreciate the degree of energy transfer at the time of impact. Bones may be substantially displaced at the time of impact and then be spontaneously reduced or be reduced by actions of the local muscle and appear relatively undisplaced in the emergency department. Fractures are also a source of significant bleeding, either from the fracture fragments themselves, muscle bleeding, or accompanied major vascular injury. Physical examination should be able to identify blood loss in the extremity. The generally accepted rule is that closed long bone fractures can bleed up to 2 units of blood. Thus, bilateral femur fractures and a tibia fracture in a 70-kg person may result in a 3-L blood loss, which can produce class III hemorrhage.

Fractures missed at the time of initial presentation can cause significant morbidity both in the long and short term. Estimates are that fractures are missed up to 10% of the time in multiply injured patients (1,2); several options exist to try to reduce that incidence. One option is to perform a "tertiary survey" somewhere between 12 and 24 hours postadmission (1). Patients with fractures that have been missed generally develop some signs or symptoms in the ensuing hours after admission. The tertiary survey is a careful head-to-toe physical examination attempting to identify areas of missed injuries. Diagnostic imaging can be obtained to diagnose injuries that had been initially missed.

Careful neurovascular examination directed by patient complaints should pick up virtually every injury in patients who are awake and alert. The same is not true for intubated multiply injured patients in the intensive care unit (ICU). In addition, neurovascular injury may evolve over time. For instance, nerve contusion can progress to neurapraxia or paralysis. Swelling around the fracture site can progress and compress the nerve, producing neurologic dysfunction. Compartment syndrome often occurs 6 to 24 hours postinjury as a result of muscular swelling within the noncompliant fascial envelope following crush injuries and/or fractures. Partial-thickness vascular injuries can go on to vascular thrombosis hours or even days after injury, producing limb-threatening ischemia.

Critical care practitioners must be cognizant of all of these. Careful ongoing assessment is critical in order to make these diagnoses as early as possible. A delayed diagnosis can produce substantial disability that is lifelong. Even worse, unrecognized ischemia and/or compartment syndrome can place a limb at jeopardy, requiring amputation later. Either can also produce life-threatening electrolyte abnormalities such as hyperkalemia and/or be the source of multiple organ failure, which can obviously prove to be fatal.

TREATMENT OPTIONS FOR FRACTURES

Clearly, simple fractures that are not associated with life-threatening bleeding are not the highest priority upon initial patient presentation. However, all long bone fractures should be splinted as part of the initial management. Every time the patient is transferred or moved in any way, unsplinted fractures are displaced, producing additional blood loss, inflammation and pain, and risking secondary nerve or vascular injury. Splinting can be accomplished simply by utilizing several IV boards and some rolled gauze to fashion a makeshift splint. There are commercially available molded metal splints that can also be used short term. These two methods can lead to skin breakdown if applied for long periods of time. Once time permits, more definitive, lightweight plaster splints can be made to restore stability and decrease the risk of skin breakdown.

It is also important for the critical care practitioner to understand the various options for more definitive fracture fixation. Rigid fracture fixation is generally obtained via open reduction/internal fixation (ORIF) or closed intramedullary (IM) nail fixation. ORIF involves directly exposing the fracture fragments. They are then manually reduced and rigid fixation is achieved utilizing a number of techniques such as plates and screws or rods. Overlying muscles must often be divided in order to obtain adequate exposure. This also allows for debridement of nonviable and/or contused muscle and irrigation of the fracture hematoma. Studies have demonstrated that nonviable muscle and/or the fracture itself is metabolically active and can activate the inflammatory cascade causing multiple organ failure (3). However, depending on the particular fracture, ORIF can be a substantial operative procedure with significant soft tissue injury and blood loss from the procedure itself. Fractures often treated with ORIF include proximal and distal tibial fractures, acetabular fractures, periarticular humerus, elbow fractures, and distal radius fractures (Fig. 65.1).

Approximately 75 years ago, the technique of closed IM nailing was developed. This technique involves making a small incision proximally or distally in the extremity. The fracture

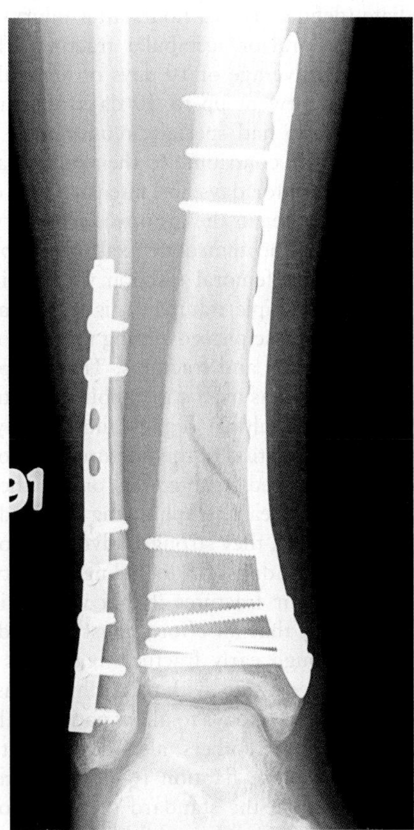

FIGURE 65.1 This 17-year-old girl sustained a high-energy distal tibial fracture as a result of a motorcycle crash. Open reduction with plate fixation offers the best chance of achieving anatomic restoration of articular congruity and reduction of the risk of posttraumatic arthritis.

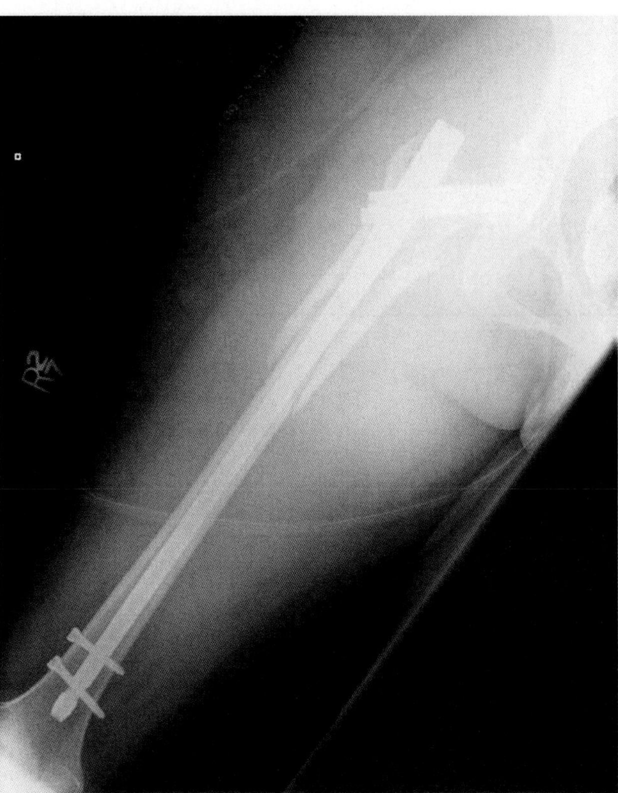

FIGURE 65.2 The fracture was treated with early intramedullary nail fixation. With early fixation of femoral fractures in multiply injured patients, many pulmonary problems can be avoided. Stable fixation of even complex, comminuted injuries can allow early weight bearing and facilitate functional rehabilitation despite polytrauma.

fragments are then reduced manually under fluoroscopic visualization. The medullary canal is accessed and a guidewire is placed across the fracture. A nail is then driven up the medullary canal over the guidewire to sterilize the bone. If desired, the canal can be reamed before the nail is placed. The nail can be locked in place by placing several screws in the very proximal or distal portion of the nail through a secondary small incision. These screws are placed under fluoroscopic control (Fig. 65.2).

IM nailing does not typically require direct exposure of the fracture fragment. Theoretically, there is less soft tissue injury and less blood loss associated with IM nailing as compared to ORIF of fractures. However, the fracture fragments and injured muscle remain in situ. Passage of a nail through the medullary canal is also associated with liberation of a number of mediators and/or fat globules into the systemic circulation; these—alone or in combination—can produce systemic inflammatory response syndrome (SIRS) and/or acute lung injury (ALI). In addition, driving the nail through the medullary canal can produce significant bleeding around the fracture itself, which may not be appreciated as it is not directly visualized in the operative field. IM nailing is generally used for most midshaft femur and tibia fractures. It is necessary to have adequate bone on either side of the fracture in order to achieve sufficient fixation to restore stability.

External fixation involves placing an external frame that spans the fracture, limiting fracture movement (Fig. 65.3). External fixation achieves relatively good fracture stabilization, though it may not produce optimal fracture reduction,

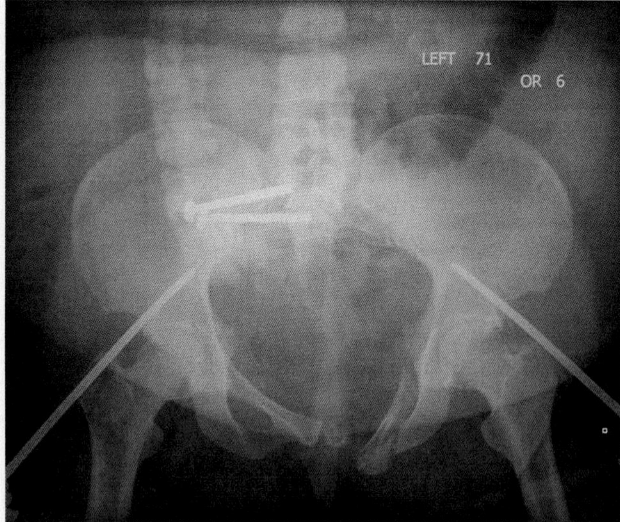

FIGURE 65.3 This patient's pelvic ring injury was treated with posterior screw fixation and an anterior external fixator.

particularly with periarticular injuries. It can be rapid and noninvasive and result in substantially less blood loss than ORIF or IM nailing. Pins are placed into the bone on either side of the fracture connected to a frame. This can be used as definitive fixation for some fractures if acceptable restoration of length, alignment, and stability has been achieved.

Open fractures require an initial debridement and irrigation of the fracture fragments as a minimum. This is done to reduce the rate of early soft tissue infection and late osteomyelitis. Although ideal operative therapy of fractures involves irrigation, debridement, and definitive fracture fixation, this is not always the wisest course. Options include irrigation and debridement which can be followed by temporary external fixation. In some cases, irrigation and debridement can be followed by simple splinting of the fractures if there are more immediate patient care priorities. This technique is ideally performed in the operating room and involves debridement followed by pulse lavage. Irrigation and debridement can be performed in the ICU and emergency department if patients are too physiologically unstable to go to the operating room. Patients can be temporized with a bedside procedure if that is all they are able to tolerate initially or if there are other more urgent priorities. Although the data supporting any treatment algorithm are not definitive, most studies suggest that rates of infection are similar provided operative debridement is accomplished within 24 hours of injury (4).

OPTIMAL TIMING OF FRACTURE FIXATION

There are a significant number of advantages to early definitive fracture fixation. Ideally, this should take place as soon as possible following patient presentation. Although the definition of early fracture fixation has varied over the years, most would agree that fracture fixation within 24 hours is considered early. The advantages of early fixation may be most pronounced in patients with multiple system injury. Obviously, these are also the patients most at risk for systemic complications from a significant operative procedure. Thus, experienced judgment must be used in weighing the various risks and benefits to early fracture fixation.

Patients who are initially managed nonoperatively are often treated in some type of balanced traction, particularly for femoral and acetabular fractures. This requires that the patient remain supine in bed. Patients in this position, however, are at risk for developing dependent atelectasis resulting in worsening respiratory failure; these patients may also be at increased risk for aspiration. Patients with traumatic brain injury and intracranial hypertension may have worsening of their intracranial pressures (ICPs) if they cannot have the head of the bed elevated with this positioning. Even though the fracture is somewhat reduced by the traction apparatus or by a splint, as with any fracture, motion at the fracture site worsens bleeding and produces pain and such motion is only reduced by traction and splinting, not eliminated. Either bleeding or pain can increase the systemic inflammatory response. Any immobilized patient is at risk for thromboembolic complications such as deep vein thrombosis or pulmonary embolus, and those in traction may be at particular risk. Patients kept at bed rest in traction cannot be rolled from side to side, producing pressure ulcerations on areas in contact with the bed. Finally, the incidence of fat embolism syndrome (FES) may be higher in patients who undergo delayed fracture repair.

In 1985, Seibel et al. published a prospective nonrandomized cohort study of patients with femoral shaft fractures or acetabulum fractures who also had additional injury (5). All aspects of care of the patients were reportedly standardized except fracture management. The patient population in this study was divided into four groups. The first group underwent immediate (defined as <24 hours after injury) operative fixation of their femoral or acetabular fracture. The second group underwent an average of 10 days of femoral traction. The third group underwent up to 30 days of femoral traction. The fourth group had special circumstances that were predicted to potentially contribute to their pulmonary failure and septic state. Ventilator days and intensive care days were both substantially greater in the groups that underwent prolonged traction than in the immediate fixation group, supporting the conclusion that femoral traction was detrimental in the setting of blunt multiple trauma. This led the authors to propose a number of principles governing the care of patients with multisystem trauma and fractures. They proposed that the fracture hematoma was itself a metabolically active organ, capable of producing multiple organ failure. Early fracture fixation allowed for irrigation of the fracture hematoma. They also included the orthopedic surgeon as one of the frontline members of the trauma team, emphasizing the need for early consultation. In addition, they strongly advocated for fracture repair on the night of admission including using two teams to simultaneously repair fractures if that was available and prudent. They argued that all efforts must be made to support the patient through early fracture fixation as they had demonstrated far better results with this technique as opposed to delaying repair for some days to allow patient stabilization.

Following this report, others also demonstrated better results with early fracture fixation (6–8). Fracture fixation within 24 hours became the standard of care. However, in the early 1990s, data began being published that suggested that not every patient benefited from early fracture fixation. In fact, these studies strongly suggested that patient outcome was much more a function of underlying injury and not so much the timing of fracture fixation. Poole et al. published a series of patients with long bone fracture and traumatic brain injury (9). They were unable to demonstrate any advantage to early fracture fixation, and instead argued that the severity of the brain injury was the ultimate determinate of final outcome. Rogers et al. addressed the cost of performing early fracture fixation, particularly on off hours in hospitals that did not have in-house operating room resources (10). Outcomes were the same when femur fractures were repaired in the middle of the night as compared to a group of patients who were placed on the operating room schedule for the next day; the cost, however, was significantly higher in patients who underwent emergency fracture fixation.

It is unclear as to why these authors were unable to substantiate the findings that seemed to show clear benefit to early operative fixation. One possibility is that the care during the critical care phase of these multiply injured patients improved over the late 1980s and early 1990s. End points of resuscitation were defined (11) and the role of invasive monitoring was clarified (12). Specific needs for patient populations such as geriatric trauma patients were defined (13). Thus, it is possible that the time taken to stabilize the patient in the ICU preoperatively was now, in fact, time well spent.

In the mid- to late 1990s, several papers were published that strongly suggested that early fracture fixation was, in fact, dangerous, particularly in patients who sustained traumatic brain injury. The group from Yale reported on 32 patients treated over a 5-year period with brain injury and long bone fractures (14). Those who underwent early fracture fixation, defined as within the first 24 hours of admission, had statistically significant worse neurologic outcome at the time of discharge. This was thought to be secondary to the increased rate of intraoperative hypotension and hypoxia seen in patients with early fracture fixation. Townsend et al. observed similar findings (15). In their study, episodes of intracranial hypertension were more common in patients who underwent early fracture fixation. They also noted an increased rate of intraoperative hypotension and hypoxia; this risk seemed to persist for approximately 24 hours.

Scalea et al., however, reported different findings. They studied over 180 patients with long bone fracture and traumatic brain injury over the same 5-year period as studied by the group at Yale (16). They found no difference in neurologic outcome in the group of patients treated with early fracture fixation.

How, then, should a critical care physician decide when a patient ought to have fracture fixation? It would seem reasonable to address a number of issues. The first would be to assess the risk of anesthesia and the magnitude of the operative procedure. There certainly are scoring systems that can be applied to assess perioperative risk; careful clinical assessment may be equally good. The second issue would be to examine operative options. For instance, does the patient have a reasonable nonoperative option? Would a lesser procedure, while perhaps not ideal, at least be adequate? This obviously would require a discussion between the critical care service and the orthopedic surgeons, trauma team, and anesthesiologist. Finally, one must ask whether the patient is in optimal condition. Can we reduce perioperative risk with a reasonable period of preoperative optimization? Can cardiac performance be improved with volume and/or inotropes? Will 1 to 2 days allow ventilatory requirements to be reduced? Would a delay improve renal function? Only when all of these questions are answered can an intelligent decision about the optimal time and fracture fixation be made.

DAMAGE CONTROL ORTHOPEDICS

Damage control is a technique developed in the late 1980s and early 1990s in early urban American trauma centers. This shift in approach coincided with a period of time when rates of penetrating trauma were increasing. Not only was penetrating trauma more common, but also multiple high-velocity missiles became the norm, rather than the exception. Traditional teaching had been to repair all injuries at the time of initial surgical procedure. Unfortunately, this often required prolonged operative care. In the operating room undergoing lengthy operative procedures, patients developed what was termed the lethal triad of acidosis, coagulopathy, and hypothermia, only to arrive in the ICU and die of acute organ failure, usually 6 to 24 hours postoperatively (Table 65.1).

Many trauma centers began using a staged approach with encouraging results. In 1993, Rotondo et al. published the series that named the technique "damage control," and demonstrated statistically significant better outcomes in a group of patients treated with the staged care as opposed to definitive care at the index operation (17). When damage control is used for abdominal injuries, only life-saving procedures are performed at the time of the initial procedure. Important but non–life-threatening injuries such as gastrointestinal injuries are simply temporized. Nonsurgical bleeding is controlled with packing and the fascia left open to avoid the potential of developing abdominal compartment syndrome. A vacuum dressing, either one that is commercially available or homemade is often used. Some data exist suggesting the type of dressing used may affect the degree of inflammation stemming from the abdominal cavity (18). The patient is then admitted to the ICU and resuscitated. When physiologically stable, the patient can be brought back to the operating room for reexploration, gastrointestinal reconstruction, and an attempt at fascial closure. The same principles can be applied to bony injuries. Fractures are common and occur in over 75% of multiply injured patients. There are clear advantages to early fracture fixation. Yet, some patients may not be best served by such technique. A technique that would achieve many of the advantages of fracture fixation without the disadvantages of definitive surgery would be advantageous for some patients.

Remote organ dysfunction occurs not only in association with, but also as a direct consequence of, long bone fractures. In addition to the fracture itself, soft tissue injury, compartment syndrome, infection, and extremity ischemia-reperfusion injury can all be associated with release of toxic mediators that can cause remote endothelial cell damage. The primary target of this remote organ injury appears to be the lungs,

TABLE 65.1 Principles of Damage Control

- It is easy to miss an injury if you rush.
- Hypothermia, acidosis, and coagulopathy only lead to more of the same.
- The best place for a sick person is in the ICU.
- Only blood loss kills early.
- GI injuries cause problems much later.
- Everything takes longer than you think.

but secondary targets include the gut, kidney, and brain. The resultant injury is progressive and can lead to multiple organ dysfunction syndrome (MODS). This understanding led to the development of the concept of damage control orthopedics (DCO). DCO is the process by which temporary stabilization of long bone fractures is accomplished using techniques not associated with secondary systemic injury. Secondary definitive stabilization is delayed until after physiologic stabilization has been achieved (Fig. 65.4 to 65.6). The goal of damage control therefore is to provide the patient with the benefits of early stabilization of long bones without exposing him or her to the risks associated with definitive stabilization procedures.

Several groups of surgeons have engaged in the process of temporary stabilization of long bone fractures in polytrauma patients using techniques associated with minimal systemic consequences. Scalea et al. published their experience with external fixation as a temporary tool for stabilization of long bone fractures in polytrauma patients in 2000 and coined the now commonly used term DCO (19). They concluded that external fixation was an alternative mechanism of achieving temporary stabilization in multiply injured patients and that it was rapid, associated with minimal blood loss, and safely convertible to better definitive fixation after appropriate delayed physiologic stabilization of the patient. Other authors have expanded on the DCO concept and have reported more specifically on its efficacy (20).

The physiologic rationale for DCO is based upon the timing and extent of the initial inflammatory response that follows

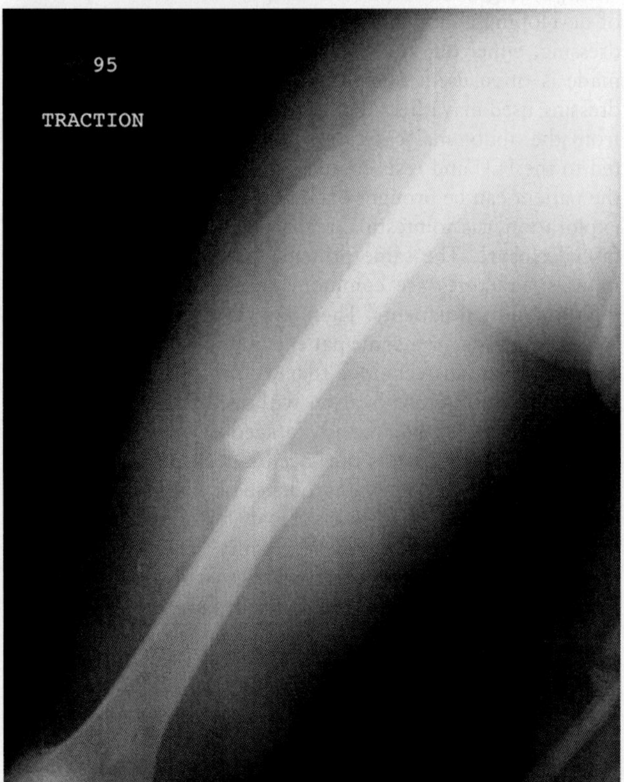

FIGURE 65.4 Damage control orthopedics case example. This 27-year-old motorcyclist sustained multiple injuries including an open right femoral shaft fracture. He presented in physiologic extremis. Laparotomy demonstrated a grade 5 hepatic injury and a retrohepatic caval injury. Right hepatic lobectomy and repair of a vena caval laceration were performed as part of a damage control laparotomy procedure.

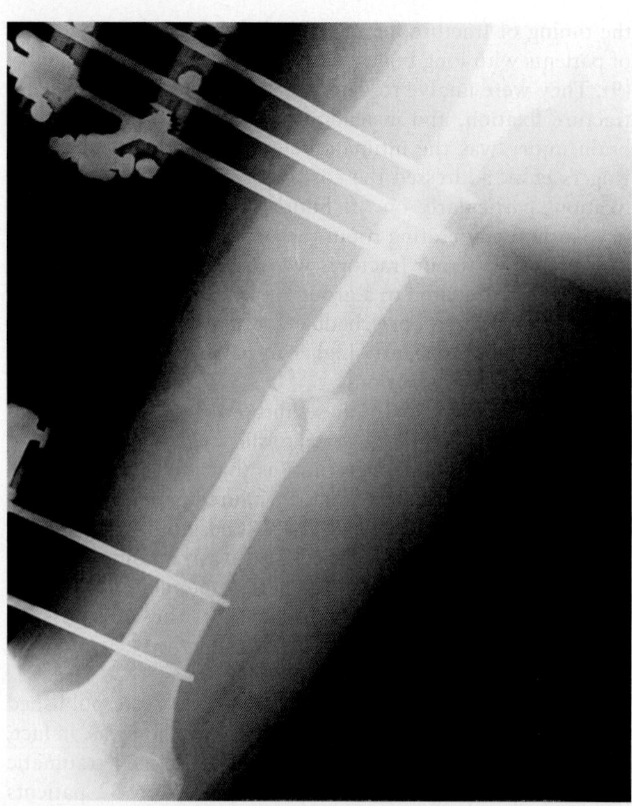

FIGURE 65.5 Damage control orthopedics consisted of rapid debridement of the open femoral fracture plus temporizing external fixation to achieve restoration of femoral length and alignment and decrease ongoing injury secondary to release of inflammatory mediators.

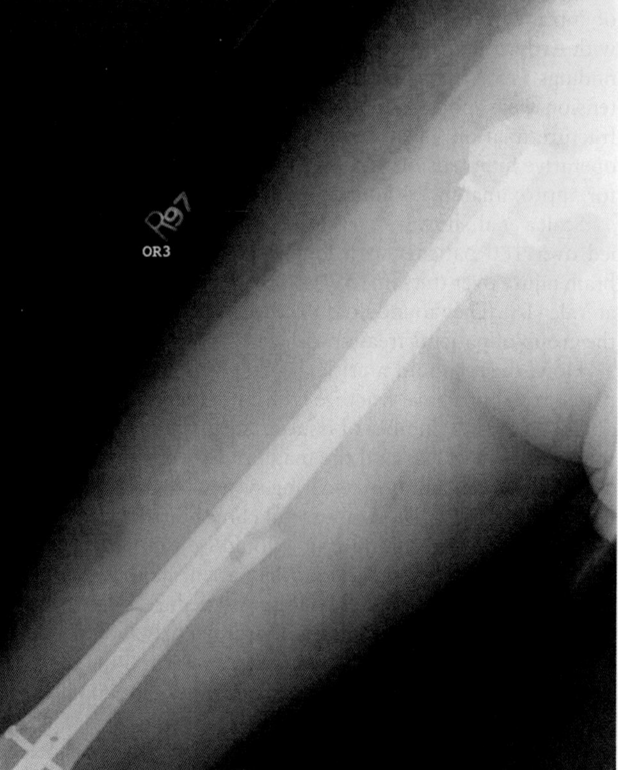

FIGURE 65.6 On postinjury day 5, after adequate restoration of physiologic stability, the patient underwent removal of the temporary external fixator and definitive fixation of the femoral fracture using a reamed intramedullary nail. He was discharged to a rehabilitation facility 19 days after injury.

a major injury. In most individuals, that initial inflammatory response is followed by a counterregulatory anti-inflammatory response that leads to spontaneous recovery. In situations where the initial inflammatory response is excessive, secondary remote organ injury such as ALI related to increased pulmonary capillary membrane permeability can occur. The likelihood of this secondary remote organ injury developing may be increased in situations associated with substantial ischemia-reperfusion injury—such as prolonged shock—continued loss of body temperature, tourniquet-mediated ischemia-reperfusion injury, surgical blood loss with failure of resuscitation, and embolization of fat and marrow contents secondary to instrumentation of the femoral or tibial canal. This secondary remote organ injury is characterized by increased capillary membrane permeability, ALI, gut bacterial translocation, and acute tubular necrosis. It can be mediated by cytokines, complement, activated neutrophils, eicosanoids, and reactive oxygen products (21). Thus, both early total care and ongoing long bone instability can serve as second hits that lead to the development of severe secondary remote organ injury. In the "at-risk" patient population, early DCO can limit ongoing release of inflammatory mediators and allow for further physiologic stabilization prior to proceeding with definitive stabilization (22).

The issues that led to the use of this damage control strategy have been debated for some time. In 1989, Bone et al. published a prospective randomized trial of early (<24 hours after injury) versus late (>72 hours after injury) nail fixation of femoral shaft fractures (23). They found that in patients with an overall Injury Severity Score (ISS) of greater than 18 (indicative of polytrauma), intensive care days and pulmonary complications were reduced with early fixation as compared to late fixation. They concluded that stabilization of femoral fractures within 24 hours of injury in multiply injured patients decreased pulmonary morbidity as compared to stabilization after 72 hours. The study was flawed in that it was not blinded, that parameters of resuscitation were not defined, and that very few patients with severe pulmonary injury were included in the early fixation group.

In 1993, Pape et al. published a worrisome report implicating primary nail fixation of reamed femoral shaft fractures as a potential cause of posttraumatic acute respiratory distress syndrome (ARDS) (24). They reviewed patients admitted over a period of 10 years with an ISS greater than 18 and midshaft femoral fractures. Those with and without chest injury and those who underwent femoral nailing less than 24 hours and greater than 24 hours after injury were compared. They found a higher incidence of ARDS and death in patients with severe chest trauma who were treated with early reamed nailing as compared to those with severe chest trauma treated with delayed reamed nailing. They concluded that early reamed nail stabilization of femoral shaft fractures in "borderline" patients may increase the risk of secondary pulmonary injury and development of ARDS. They recommended that definitive fracture fixation be delayed in these patients and that temporizing techniques such as external fixation be employed. The criticism of Pape's study was that the early nailing group included eight patients with pulmonary contusions as compared to only two in the late nailing group. Both Pape et al. (24) and Bone et al. (23) failed to report on any parameters of resuscitation within their patient populations.

In a prospective randomized trial, Pape et al. compared nailing to DCO with regard to immunoinflammatory parameters in patients with tibial or femoral shaft fractures, and ISS greater than 16 (25). Patients with a thoracic abbreviated injury scale (AIS) score greater than 3, ongoing shock, or elevated ICP were excluded. They found that primary femoral nailing was associated with significantly higher systemic interleukin (IL)-6 and IL-8 levels for 48 hours postoperatively compared to either initial DCO procedures or secondary femoral nailing after initial damage control. This suggested that the secondary release of inflammatory mediators associated with femoral nailing can be effectively mitigated by initial DCO with delayed femoral nailing. O'Toole et al. looked at the effect of resuscitation prior to femoral nailing on the development of ARDS in multiply injured patients (26). They utilized a resuscitation protocol that included normalization of lactate prior to IM nailing, resulting in rare need of DCO. The rate of ARDS was also quite low, even in polytrauma patients with serious chest injury.

For that subset of patients whose physiologic condition precludes primary definitive operative stabilization of fractures (early total care), external fixation is a useful technique for temporary stabilization of long bone fractures. Such external fixation is advantageous because it can be applied rapidly, with minimal blood loss, and with sufficient restoration of stability to prevent ongoing soft tissue injury and to prevent ongoing release of inflammatory mediators. Effective limitation of secondary effects of shock has been demonstrated with this type of initial DCO approach (27).

The disadvantages to employing DCO in all patients with even questionable polytrauma are at least twofold. First, employing temporizing external fixation techniques necessitates a return to the operating room for delayed definitive fixation, thus exposing the patient to two separate operative interventions/anesthetics. This is obviously warranted if the benefit is prevention of a serious secondary consequence such as ARDS. In the absence of a clear decrease in the risk of ARDS, it is harder to justify exposing polytrauma patients to a need for secondary surgical procedures. A second major disadvantage to external fixation (a temporary device) is the risk of complications with conversion from external fixation to IM nailing or other definitive treatment. Experience with tibial fractures has suggested that if external fixation is in place for less than 2 weeks, the risk of infection with definitive fixation is lower, particularly if there is no history of pin tract infection at any point (28). In the femur, conversion from external fixation to definitive nailing appears safe within the first 4 weeks following application of the initial frame (29).

Hildebrand et al. evaluated the association between the timing of secondary definitive surgical intervention, inflammatory changes, and systemic outcome (30). They reviewed a prospective cohort of patients treated with DCO. They compared those treated with early secondary surgery (2 to 4 days after initial injury) to those treated with late secondary surgery (5 to 8 days after initial injury). They found that early secondary surgery was associated with a higher incidence of organ dysfunction and concluded that there was no particular advantage to early secondary surgery. They recommended that if DCO is selected, secondary surgery should be delayed more than 5 days after the initial DCO procedure.

The operative procedure of IM stabilization of long bone fractures, both femoral and tibial shaft fractures, is associated with some component of pulmonary injury (31,32). Although fracture fixation–associated pulmonary injury appeared to be well tolerated in the majority of patients, including those with polytrauma, certain susceptible polytrauma patients seemed to be at risk for worsening lung injury. Paradoxically, these are likely the same patients who are at greatest risk for developing secondary pulmonary injury from a nonoperative management of their long bone fractures and the most in need of early fracture stabilization.

DCO, the practice of utilizing temporary external fixation to limit ongoing injury secondary to long bone fractures in situations where definitive operative stabilization is contraindicated, may be effective in patients with polytrauma and lung or brain injury. For the majority of patients with femoral shaft fractures, including most polytrauma patients, primary reamed femoral nailing within 24 hours of injury remains the gold standard of treatment (31). Defining the "at-risk" patients who are unable to tolerate early reamed nailing is difficult, but if adequate resuscitation and normalization of serum lactate is achieved, damage control should rarely be necessary (26). In borderline patients who are physiologically unstable because of severe chest or head injury or inadequate resuscitation, temporizing external fixation and DCO may be advantageous.

FRACTURES IN GERIATRIC PATIENTS

As the US population ages, there is an increasing volume of injured geriatric patients. Injury is now the seventh leading cause of death for those over age 64 (33). Geriatric trauma is increasing both in absolute number and as a proportion of volume presenting to trauma centers each year. Based upon the National Trauma Data Bank, the proportion of trauma patients aged 65 years or older in Level I and II trauma centers increased from 23% in 2003 to 30% in 2009. These numbers are likely underestimates as many injured geriatric patients are treated at non-trauma centers and community hospitals (34,35). There are a number of unique considerations for this patient population that are exceptionally important for those caring for the geriatric patient with orthopedic injuries to recognize.

Elderly patients sustain all the same injuries as the younger trauma patient. Unfortunately, aging is associated with a decrease in the physiologic reserve that many younger trauma patients have. Under normal circumstances, the elderly compensate to meet their needs. However, during times of increased physiologic demand many elderly are unable to compensate effectively. Additionally, pre-existing medical conditions in the elderly limit their ability to tolerate the increased physiologic demands associated with acute trauma. It has been demonstrated that elderly patients have substantially worse outcomes than younger trauma patients (36–38). The cause of this is clearly multifactorial; in addition to decreased physiologic reserve, referred to as fragility (39), comorbid medical conditions, and poorer baseline functional status, osteopenia, and sarcopenia may result in a higher severity of injury (40).

As a general rule, the aim of treatment of geriatric fractures is to obtain a fixation that both reduces pain and permits early mobilization (41). The decision for surgical intervention should be based primarily on the injury pattern and not solely on the age of the patient (42), but it is well recognized that in addition to increased risk of mortality and major morbidity following trauma, geriatric patients also may be at risk of orthopedic-specific complications following orthopedic injuries. Some have demonstrated that advanced age is associated with poor fracture healing due to an increased risk of nonunion due to an inability to achieve mechanical stability in osteopenic bone and overall poorer fracture biology (41,43). However, others have demonstrated that patient age alone at the time of surgery is not independently associated with poorer nonunion of fractures (44,45).

When managing the geriatric patient with orthopedic injuries, although operative fixation is often preferred for many fractures, the risks of perioperative morbidity and mortality from comorbid conditions must be carefully weighed against the benefit of operative stabilization. Careful perioperative risk assessment is appropriate in which the patient undergoes a risk stratification that weighs the patient's operative risk against the benefit of operative intervention. Patients may be stratified into low, medium, or high risk of events based on history, baseline exercise tolerance, and the absence or presence of active cardiac conditions as well as EKG and echocardiographic findings. This risk can then be balanced against the magnitude of the procedure—high-risk procedures such as large blood loss procedures or complex revisional joint replacement, moderate-risk procedures such as femoral ORIF, and low-risk procedures such as simple upper extremity fracture fixation—and the emergent (such as compartment syndrome or an acutely threatened limb) or urgent (acetabular fracture with an unstable joint or ankle/talus fracture with threatened skin) nature of the procedure.

Although elective surgery in the elderly provides an opportunity to optimize health preoperatively, those having emergency orthopedic procedures are not afforded time for optimization, and may present malnourished, dehydrated, and acutely ill. In geriatric polytrauma patients, this becomes a particular concern as these patients may have competing priorities of care and often will require large volume resuscitation with the goal of oxygen delivery to balance tissue oxygen demand.

Pre- and postoperative monitoring of geriatric patients with orthopedic injuries is essential, although there is some controversy about the optimal way to accomplish this. Fluid management, for example, can be challenging in this patient population. Underlying cardiac and renal dysfunction predisposes elderly patients to volume overload and pulmonary edema but this must be balanced against the need to maintain adequate organ perfusion. Scalea et al. demonstrated significant hemodynamic compromise in elderly patients, clinically stable after initial trauma evaluation, using invasive monitoring (13). The authors demonstrated an increase in survival from 7% to 53% with the use of early optimization of patients with volume, inotropes, and afterload reduction. The authors concluded that emergent invasive monitoring identifies occult shock early and improves outcome. Since this early work, demonstrating the benefit of aggressive and invasive monitoring in geriatric trauma patients, newer monitoring devices including continuous central venous oximetry ($ScvO_2$) and stroke volume variance (SVV) have been introduced that may be used to help guide resuscitation in the elderly trauma patient. Noninvasive hemodynamic monitoring in the elderly, high-risk surgical patient has been shown to be as effective as traditional invasive thermodilution techniques using a pulmonary artery catheter (46,47). Additionally, transthoracic (TTE) or transesophageal echocardiography (TEE) may provide important information regarding volume status and cardiac function to help guide resuscitation.

In addition to the unique challenges facing providers caring for geriatric patients with orthopedic injuries related to poor outcomes due to increased morbidity and mortality, there are also a few important types of fractures relatively unique to this population.

Fractures of the proximal humerus are very common in geriatric population and remain a difficult problem; when associated with rotator cuff injury these can lead to poor functional outcome (41). Fractures of the distal radius are exceptionally common in elderly females and, while most fractures of the distal radius can be treated conservatively, unstable distal radius fractures require surgical fixation. Spine fractures are also quite common in geriatric patients, ranging from vertebral compression fractures that can result in kyphosis to devastating spinal cord injuries, associated with significant mortality (48).

Geriatric hip fractures are also exceptionally common and, whether treated in a trauma center or community hospital, present a significant source of both short-term and long-term pain and disability. Additionally, in elderly patients with hip fractures, mortality of up to 10% at 1 month, 20% at 4 months, and 30% at 1 year are seen (49). Optimal management of these patients is somewhat debated, but two large systematic reviews of thousands of patients have concluded that early surgery—typically within 48 hours of admission—after a hip fracture reduces hospital stay, complications, and mortality (50,51). Optimizing these patients preoperatively can be difficult, however, as many have significant comorbidities. As hip repair surgery is largely considered an intermediate-risk surgery, there is little preoperative intervention that should be performed at the risk of delaying intervention. Medical optimization is appropriate for uncontrolled hypertension, dysrhythmias, and active myocardial ischemia. However, these interventions should not delay surgery beyond 24 to 48 hours given the known risks of increased complication rates in patients in whom surgery is delayed (52).

COMPARTMENT SYNDROME

Compartment syndrome occurs when there is increased tissue pressure within a confined osseofascial space. This increased pressure compromises blood flow and subsequently results in tissue damage if left untreated. The fascia of muscle compartments is stiff and does not expand to accommodate significant swelling. Increases in compartment volume and subsequent pressure can be caused by fractures, soft tissue crush injury, hemorrhage, reperfusion following arterial revascularization, and increased capillary permeability as may occur in the setting of burns or shock states.

Compartment syndrome was first recognized as a causative factor in ischemia of the hand by Richard von Volkmann in 1881 (53). Other investigators subsequently described and confirmed that ischemia of muscle in a fascial compartment was caused by an increase in pressure from compromised venous outflow and edema secondary to reperfusion (54,55). Although most typically found in the leg, compartment syndrome of the arm and hand is well recognized, as is compartment syndrome of the buttock, thigh, and foot (56–59). The reported incidence of compartment syndrome varies widely. Rates of 6% in patients with open tibial fractures and 1% in patients with closed fractures have been reported, but much higher percentages have been published in association with concomitant vascular injury (60,61). In children, rates of up to 20% have been reported with open forearm fractures (56).

Any increase in compartment volume elevates compartment pressures, which, in turn, compromises lymphatic and venous outflow; this leads to additional edema and ultimately arterial insufficiency. Compromised arterial inflow causes tissue ischemia and cellular edema, which only serves to increase compartment pressures further (62,63). Experimental studies have shown that the longer pressure remains elevated, the more severe the muscle and nerve damage (63). Additionally, episodes of hypotension increase the extent of muscle ischemia.

External restriction of an extremity may also lead to compartment syndrome. Compartment syndrome has been described as a result of constrictive casting or dressings and with the use of pneumatic antishock garments (military antishock trousers) (64). Regardless of the underlying cause, if left untreated, the end result of compartment syndrome is muscle and nerve injury from infarction and necrosis.

The clinical diagnosis of compartment syndrome can be elusive, as symptoms may often be ascribed to other causes (65,66). In the alert patient, pain is typically the first symptom. Pain is typically worsened with palpation of the affected compartment and ameliorated with passive stretch of the muscle group. Pain or physical findings are frequently attributed to the associated fracture, however. Sensory deficits may occur late and are typically in the distribution of the sensory nerve traversing the affected compartment. The classic description of sensory loss is in the first web space of the foot secondary to elevated anterior leg compartment pressures and the effect on the deep peroneal nerve. Motor weakness is a late and ominous sign. Loss of palpable pulses is typically associated with vascular injury and is a very late and rare finding in the extremity with compartment syndrome.

In the patient who is not awake and alert, the diagnosis of compartment syndrome requires extreme vigilance and a high degree of clinical suspicion. The diagnosis in these patients requires frequent physical examination and tissue pressure measurements. Tissue pressure measurements are typically accomplished via accessing the affected compartment with a needle or catheter and recording pressure measurements via manometry or pressure transduction. Many techniques have been described, but the simplest and most widely used is the STIC Device (Stryker Corporation, Kalamazoo, MI). The handheld STIC catheter utilizes a disposable syringe and needle and, after zeroing the monitor, insertion of the needle through the fascia of the compartments. It allows for rapid and reliable assessment of compartment pressures (67). Alternatively, a 16-gauge needle attached to a transduction system also can produce reliable measurements (68). Some have advocated continuous pressure monitoring using systems designed specifically for that purpose, although recent data do not support the use of continuous monitoring in the alert patient (69,70). Several researchers have attempted to develop noninvasive methods of compartment pressure measurements with limited success in the setting of acute compartment syndrome (71,72).

There is some debate in the literature concerning the measured pressure at which the diagnosis of compartment syndrome should be made and fasciotomy performed. Many advocate the use of absolute values of greater than 30 to 35 mmHg as an indication for fasciotomy (69,73). Others have stressed the importance of the difference between systemic diastolic pressure and measured compartment pressure (74,75). This difference in pressures has been shown to be a more reliable indicator of impending compartment syndrome. A Δp of less than 30 mmHg is used by many as an indication for fasciotomy. This highlights the concern that patients who are hypotensive are at significantly greater risk of compartment syndrome than normotensive patients with comparable absolute compartment pressure measurements. Therefore, intraoperative Δp should be calculated based on the preoperative diastolic blood pressure and compartment pressures should be measured early in the postoperative period (75).

In the patient who is at risk of compartment syndrome, there are some steps that can be taken that may minimize the development of compartment syndrome. First, tight casts, splints, and dressings should be avoided and promptly removed if the patient complains of pain out of proportion to the underlying injury or fracture. There is some controversy about the optimal extremity position in patients at risk for compartment syndrome. Elevation of the extremity may lead to a reduction of arterial perfusion pressure and subsequent blood flow (52,76). Alternatively, placing the limb in a dependent position may exacerbate edema and reduce venous outflow. The optimal position for the patient at risk of compartment syndrome is to place the affected extremity at the level of the heart to optimize both arterial and venous flow.

Surgical decompression is the treatment of compartment syndrome. Care must be taken to ensure that all affected osseofascial compartments are widely opened. The fasciotomy wounds should be left open, as any attempt to provide tissue coverage over the at-risk muscle may lead to additional muscle injury. A variety of techniques have been described for fasciotomy of the various compartments of the extremities.

In the patient at high risk for the development of compartment syndrome, prophylactic fasciotomy may be appropriate. If the patient will be unexaminable, unable to complain of symptoms or unavailable for serial or continuous measurements of compartment pressures, prophylactic fasciotomy may be indicated to prevent the morbid sequelae of untreated compartment syndrome. In patients with prolonged hypotension or arterial vascular repairs, prophylactic fasciotomy should be performed if the affected extremity was poorly vascularized or unvascularized for more than a few hours. In the setting of concomitant venous injury, fasciotomy should not be delayed because venous insufficiency may exaggerate edema and increase the risk of the development of compartment syndrome.

Once fasciotomies are performed, sterile dressings or a closed vacuum suction device should be applied and the wounds re-examined in about 48 hours. If fasciotomy was done late in the course of compartment syndrome, frankly necrotic muscle should be debrided at the time of decompression. Muscle with borderline or questionable viability should be left and re-examined in 24 to 48 hours. Patients who develop hyperkalemia or signs of sepsis early after fasciotomy should be re-explored in the OR to examine muscle viability. Extensive and potentially functionally unacceptable debridement and/or amputation be necessary to salvage life over limb in a patient who is critically ill.

There are a number of techniques available for delayed muscle coverage following fasciotomy that have been described. Closure by secondary intention is an option, as is split-thickness skin grafting. Other techniques of delayed coverage include the "Op-Site roller," the "shoelace technique," the STAR (suture tension adjustment reel) method, and vacuum-assisted closure (77–80).

Complications of untreated compartment syndrome include muscle necrosis, irreparable nerve damage, and limb loss (81,82). Delay in therapy may also result in these morbid sequelae (74,81,82). When irreversible ischemia in an affected extremity occurs, there is a depreciable decrease in functional recovery (83,84). Additionally, delay in fasciotomy causes an increase in infection rates, which may lead to sepsis and multiple organ system failure (81,84). When treatment is delayed more than 12 hours, amputation rates may be over 20%.

Massive necrosis of muscle also has significant systemic effects. Myonecrosis can result in the release of large amounts of myoglobin. Myoglobin is also released from damaged muscle, particularly during the reperfusion phase following fasciotomy, causing rhabdomyolysis. Myoglobin can precipitate renal failure via three mechanisms: decreased renal perfusion, renal tubular obstruction due to cast formation, and direct toxic effects of myoglobin on the kidney (85,86). The incidence of renal failure in the setting of rhabdomyolysis is estimated at 4% to 33% and carries a mortality of 3% to 50% (86,87). Early diagnosis is critical to prevention of renal failure, and all patients who have compartment syndrome should be monitored with serial creatine kinase (CK) levels. Generally, CK levels of greater than 5,000 U/L are diagnostic of rhabdomyolysis, although renal failure is usually seen at higher levels (87). The mainstay of treatment of rhabdomyolysis is aggressive hydration and maintenance of high-volume urine output. Some have advocated the use of mannitol and urine alkalinization with bicarbonate-containing solutions, although others have demonstrated no benefit of these therapies over high-volume normal saline hydration alone. Continuous renal replacement therapies can also be used to clear myoglobin from the blood and are advantageous if renal failure occurs due to greater hemodynamic stability and tolerance in critically ill patients.

In addition to poor long-term functional recovery following late or untreated compartment syndrome, a Volkmann contracture may occur. A Volkmann contracture is the chronic limb deformity arising from untreated compartment syndrome causing muscular ischemia and subsequent fibroblastic proliferation, contraction, and adhesion formation. Additionally, nerve ischemia leads to loss of denervation of the muscle, muscle paresis, and paralysis. A Volkmann contracture causes significant long-term morbidity and may lead to a need for amputation or extensive reconstruction to regain function of the affected extremity.

FAT EMBOLISM SYNDROME

FES has been reported to occur in bone marrow transplant, pancreatitis, fatty liver, and liposuction (88,89); however, FES is most commonly associated with long bone fractures. Although fat embolism may occur in up to 90% of trauma patients, FES occurs in only 2% to 5% of patients with long bone fractures (90,91). FES is characterized by both pulmonary and systemic fat embolism and includes a spectrum from subclinical to mild and fulminate presentations (89,92,93). Clinical FES typically involves multiple organ systems; however, involvement of the pulmonary, neurologic, hematologic, and dermatologic systems is the most common.

Fat embolization can occur at the time of fracture. Long bone fixation may result in additional embolization and FES. Elevated pressures during reaming of the IM canal appear to be temporally associated with embolization to the pulmonary circulation when studied with echocardiography (94). Once fat is liberated into the circulation and embolizes, the pulmonary microvasculature becomes occluded. Depending on the size of fat globules, smaller globules may traverse the pulmonary microvasculature and reach the systemic circulation, leading to the common neurologic manifestation of FES. Although the pulmonary, cerebral, retinal, and skin microcirculations are typical clinical manifestations of FES, fat embolization can affect any microcirculatory bed.

ALI and ARDS may result from fat emboli occluding pulmonary capillaries, and biochemical alterations directly damage the pulmonary capillary endothelium (89,95–97). Although many patients with long bone fractures develop fat embolism, far fewer develop FES, suggesting that additional factors may be necessary in the development of lung injury. Biochemical fat embolization is associated with the release of free fatty acids (FFAs) (98). FFAs in the lung are locally hydrolyzed in pulmonary circulation by lipoprotein lipase, which releases toxic substances that injure the capillary endothelium. The release of FFAs increases vascular permeability, producing alveolar hemorrhage, edema, and inactivation of the surfactant molecules (99,100). Ultimately, these pulmonary alterations lead to ALI and ARDS. As fat accumulates in the pulmonary microcirculation and lipoprotein lipase liberates FFAs, disseminated intravascular coagulation (DIC) and platelet aggregation further compound capillary disruption and systemic inflammation.

Fat emboli that pass through the pulmonary vasculature result in systemic embolization, most commonly in the brain and kidneys (101). Cerebral FES is a rare, yet potentially lethal, complication of long bone fractures. Neurologic symptoms vary from confusion to encephalopathy with coma and seizures. A clinical diagnosis may be difficult as cerebral FES may be masked by other clinical scenarios (102). Diffuse encephalopathy, petechial hemorrhages, localized cerebral edema, and white matter changes have also been seen in patients diagnosed with FES. Magnetic resonance imaging (MRI) may show the characteristic cerebral lesions of the acute state of FES as opposed to a computed tomography (CT) scan, which often may appear normal (103).

A specific treatment for FES does not currently exist. Treatments with heparin, dextran, and corticosteroids have not been shown to reduce the morbidity or mortality (88,104). However, when given prophylactically, corticosteroids (methylprednisolone) may have beneficial effects (105,106). The mainstay of treatment for FES is supportive; therefore, prevention, early diagnosis, and adequate symptom management are paramount. Although long bone fracture fixation is the main cause of fat embolism and FES, early fracture fixation may be critical in reducing recurrent liberation of fat into the circulation as a result of fracture movement and decreases the incidence of FES (107).

Patients with polytrauma are at risk of other forms of respiratory failure (atelectasis, pneumonia) and multiple system organ failure (MSOF). Early fixation and patient mobilization may reduce those complications (108). Methods to reduce IM pressure and embolization during reaming have been developed, which include venting or applying a vacuum during reaming to limit the elevation of IM pressure and thus reduce the incidence of fat embolization (109,110).

Respiratory failure from FES is characterized as permeability edema with decreased compliance similar to oleic acid lung injury. Gas exchange abnormalities include shunt and increased dead space from atelectasis and alveolar flooding comparable to ALI and ARDS from other causes (111,112). The general goals of ALI and ARDS management focus on maintaining acceptable gas exchange while limiting ventilator-associated lung injury (VALI).

Patients with FES may develop cerebral edema, leading to rapid deterioration (113). In such cases, ICP monitoring may be beneficial (114). In general, trauma patients should not have their neurologic examination obscured by excessive sedation or neuromuscular blocking agents in order to allow them to tolerate mechanical ventilation (115).

The outcome in patients with FES who receive supportive care is generally favorable, with mortality rates of less than 10% (116). Pulmonary, neurologic, and retinal abnormalities generally resolve completely. General management is supportive in nature and focuses on early fixation and mobilization. Organ support includes shock resuscitation and gas exchange support, which balances lung recruitment and limits the potential for VALI. Ideally, neurologic support would include the ability to conduct a clinical neurologic examination.

PELVIC FRACTURES

Pelvic fractures occur from high impact trauma and are usually associated with mortality rates ranging from 10% to 15% (117). Initial care of patients with suspected pelvic fractures is not different from any other trauma patient. Signs of hemorrhage must be identified and resuscitation initiated; as with other patients, limiting crystalloid is wise. Blood, plasma, and platelets used early and in rates that approximate 1:1 may be helpful in patients with profound hemorrhage (118).

The pelvic retroperitoneum is almost an infinite space and patients can easily exsanguinate into it. The most important initial step in managing pelvic fracture hemorrhage is to reduce the bony pelvis to a normal alignment. This can be accomplished with something as simple as a bed sheet that is wrapped around the patient's pelvis and tied. In most trauma centers, commercially available binders are now commonly used as the initial hemostatic maneuver.

Angiographic embolization is mainstay of definitive hemostasis. A flush aortic pelvic aortogram often identifies major vascular injuries. Smaller vascular injuries can be identified by selective hypogastric angiography. Once identified, vascular injuries can be occluded with the use of stainless steel coils, gel foam, or a combination of the two. Early embolization is key to prevent coagulopathy and hypothermia. Older patients have a higher likelihood of arterial bleeding with more transfusion requirements (119,120). Some patients require more than one embolization procedure to control hemorrhage (121). CT scanning can be helpful, as it may identify vascular injuries which appear as contrast blush in the pelvis.

In patients who are bleeding too quickly to tolerate the time it takes to mobilize angiographic resources, several other options exist. Extraperitoneal pelvic packing can be helpful.

This is a procedure generally performed in the operating room. The pelvic hematoma is entered and evacuated. Small vessel bleeding can be controlled by tightly packing the pelvis with a number of laparotomy pads. This has been shown to be effective but is unlikely to control major hemorrhage (122).

Resuscitative endovascular balloon occlusion of the aorta (REBOA) is a new technique that can be especially useful in patients with pelvic fractures (123,124). A transfemoral catheter is inserted into the common femoral artery via a 12-French sheath. In the case of pelvic fracture hemorrhage, it is inflated just above the aortic bifurcation. This limits pelvic fracture hemorrhage and most patients generally stabilize. This can be left inflated for some time to allow for additional imaging studies, such as CT scanning, as well as time to mobilize angiographic resources, obviating the need for extraperitoneal pelvic packing in some patients. Early work with the REBOA in patients with pelvic fractures has been encouraging (125). At the authors' center, pelvic fracture hemorrhage is the most common indications for deployment of the REBOA.

Key Points

- Patients presenting after injury should typically have either signs or symptoms to guide diagnosis of their injuries.
- Fractures missed at the time of initial presentation can cause significant morbidity both in the long and short term. Estimates are that fractures are missed up to 10% of the time in multiply injured patients.
- All long bone fractures should be splinted as part of the initial management. Every time the patient is transferred or moved in any way, unsplinted fractures are displaced, producing additional blood loss, inflammation and pain, and risking secondary nerve or vascular injury.
- The physiologic rationale for Damage Control Orthopaedics is based upon the timing and extent of the initial inflammatory response that follows a major injury.
- A difference (Δp) between the systemic diastolic and compartment pressures of 30 mmHg or less is a reliable indicator of impending compartment syndrome and is used by many as an indication for fasciotomy.
- Resuscitative endovascular balloon occlusion of the aorta (REBOA) is a new technique that can be especially useful in patients with pelvic fractures.

References

1. Enderson BL, Reath DB, Meadors J. The tertiary trauma survey: a prospective study of missed injury. *J Trauma*. 1990;30:666–670.
2. Giannakopoulos GF, Saltzherr TP, Beenen LF, et al. Missed injuries during the initial assessment in a cohort of 1124 level-1 trauma patients. *Injury*. 2012;43(9):1517–1521.
3. Strecker W, Gebhard F, Rager J, et al. Early biochemical characterization of soft-tissue trauma and fracture trauma. *J Trauma*. 1999;47:358–364.
4. Pollak A. Timing of debridement of open fractures. *J Am Acad Orthopaed Surg*. 2006;14:548–551.
5. Seibel R, LaDuca J, Hassett JM, et al. Blunt multiple trauma (ISS 36), femur traction, and the pulmonary failure-septic state. *Ann Surg*. 1985; 202:283–295.
6. Charash WE, Fabian TC, Croce MA. Delayed surgical fixation of femur fractures is a risk factor for pulmonary failure independent of thoracic trauma. *J Trauma*. 1994;37:663–672.
7. Behrman SW, Fabian TC, Kudsk KA, et al. Improved outcome with femur fractures: early versus delayed fixation. *J Trauma*. 1994;37:667–672.
8. Johnson KD, Cadambi A, Seibert B. Incidence of adult respiratory distress syndrome in patients with multiple musculoskeletal injuries: effect of early operative stabilization of fractures. *J Trauma*. 1985;25:375–384.
9. Poole GV, Miller JD, Agnew SG, et al. Lower extremity fracture fixation in head-injured patients. *J Trauma*. 1992;32:654–659.
10. Rogers FB, Shackford SR, Vane DW, et al. Prompt fixation of isolated femur fractures in a rural trauma center: a study examining the timing of fixation and resource allocation. *J Trauma*. 1994;36:774–777.
11. Abrahamson D, Scalea T, Hitchcock R, et al. Lactate clearance and its effects on survival. *J Trauma*. 1992;32:951.
12. Abou-Khalil B, Scalea T, Trooskin S. Hemodynamic responses to shock in young trauma patients. The need for invasive monitoring. *J Trauma*. 1991;31:1713.
13. Scalea TM, Simon HM, Duncan AO, et al. Geriatric blunt trauma: improved survival with early invasive monitoring. *J Trauma*. 1990;30:129–136.
14. Jaicks RR, Cohn SM, Moller BA. Early fracture fixation may be deleterious after head injury. *J Trauma*. 1997;42P:1–6.
15. Townsend RN, Lheureau T, Protetch J, et al. Timing fracture repair in patients with severe brain injuries. *J Trauma*. 1998;44:977–981.
16. Scalea TM, Scott JD, Brumback RJ, et al. Early fracture fixation may be "just fine" after head injury: no difference in central nervous system outcomes. *J Trauma*. 1999;46:839–846.
17. Rotondo M, Schwab CW, McGonigal M, et al. Damage control: an approach for improved survival in exsanguinating penetrating abdominal injury. *J Trauma*. 1993;35:375–382.
18. Shah SK, Jimenez F, Letourneau PA. Strategies for modulating the inflammatory response after decompression from abdominal compartment syndrome. *Scand J Trauma Resusc Emerg Med*. 2012;20:25.
19. Scalea TM, Boswell SA, Scott JD, et al. External fixation as a bridge to intramedullary nailing for patients with multiple injuries and with femur fractures: damage control orthopaedics. *J Trauma*. 2000;48:613–623.
20. Pape HC, Hildebrand F, Pertschy S, et al. Changes in the management of femoral shaft fractures in polytrauma patients. From early total care to damage control orthopedic surgery. *J Trauma*. 2002;53:452–462.
21. Giannoudis PV, Smith RM, Bellamy MC, et al. Stimulation of the inflammatory system by reamed and unreamed nailing of femoral fractures: an analysis of the second hit. *J Bone Joint Surg Br*. 1999;81(2):356–361.
22. Roberts CS, Pape HC, Jones AL, et al. Damage control orthopaedics: evolving concepts in the treatment of patients who have sustained orthopaedic trauma. *J Bone Joint Surg*. 2005;2:434–449.
23. Bone LB, Johnson KD, Weigelt J, et al. Early versus delayed stabilization of femoral fractures—a prospective randomized study. *J Bone Joint Surg*. 1989;3:336–340.
24. Pape HC, Auf m'Koolk M, Paffrath T, et al. Primary intramedullary femur fixation in multiple trauma patients with associated lung contusion: a cause of posttraumatic ARDS? *J Trauma*. 1993;34:540–548.
25. Pape HC, Grimme K, Van Griensven M, et al; EPOFF study group. Impact of intramedullary instrumentation versus damage control for femoral fractures on immunoinflammatory parameters: prospective randomized analysis by the EPOFF study group. *J Trauma*. 2003;55:7–13.
26. O'Toole R, O'Brien M, Habashi N, et al. Resuscitation prior to stabilization of femoral shaft fractures limits ARDS in polytrauma patients despite low utilization of damage control orthopaedics. *J Trauma*. 2009; 67(5):1013–1021.
27. Pape HC, Rixen D, Morley J, et al; EPOFF study group. Impact of the method of initial stabilization for femoral shaft fractures in patients with multiple injuries at risk for complications (borderline patients). *Ann Surg*. 2007;246(3):491–501.
28. Bhandari M, Zlowodzki M, Tornetta P, et al. Intramedullary nailing following external fixation in femoral and tibial shaft fractures. *J Orthop Trauma*. 2005;19:140–144.
29. Nowotarski PJ, Turen CH, Brumback RJ, et al. Conversion of external fixation to intramedullary nailing for fractures of the shaft of the femur in multiply injured patients. *J Bone Joint Surg*. 2000;6:781–787.
30. Hildebrand F, Giannoudis PV, Griensven M, et al. Management of polytraumatized patients with associated blunt chest trauma: a comparison of two European countries. *Injury*. 2005;36:293–302.
31. Bosse MJ, MacKenzie EJ, Riemer BL, et al. Adult respiratory distress syndrome, pneumonia and mortality following thoracic injury and a femoral fracture treated either with intramedullary nailing with reaming or with a plate. *J Bone Joint Surg*. 1997;6:799–809.
32. Pape HC, Regel G, Dwenger A, et al. The risk of early intramedullary nailing of long bone fractures in multiply traumatized patients. *Complications Orthop*. 1995;15–23.

33. Injury prevention and control: data and statistics (WISQARS®). Available at http://www.cdc.gov/injury/images/lc-charts/leading_causes_of_death_age_group_2014_1050w760h.gif. Accessed May 2, 2016.
34. Gage AM, Traven N, Rivara FP, et al. Compliance with Centers for Disease Control and Prevention field triage guidelines in an established trauma system. *J Am Coll Surg* 2012;215(1):146–148.
35. Garwe T, Cowan LD, Neas BR, et al. A propensity score analysis of prehospital factors and directness of transport of major trauma patients to a level I trauma center. *J Trauma* 2011;70(1):120–129.
36. Davidson GH, Hamlat CA, Rivara FP, et al. Long-term survival of adult trauma patients. *JAMA*. 2011;305(10):1001–1007.
37. Labib N, Nouh T, Winocour S, et al. Severely injured geriatric population: morbidity, mortality, and risk factors. *J Trauma* 2011;71(6):1908–1914.
38. Bergeron E, Clement J, Lavoie A, et al. A simple fall in the elderly: not so simple. *J Trauma*. 2006;60(2):268–273.
39. Clegg A, Trust DM. CME Geriatric medicine:AS the frailty syndrome. 2011;11(1):72–75.
40. Hanrahan RB, Layde PM, Zhu S, et al. The association of driver age with traffic injury severity in Wisconsin. *Traffic Inj Prev*. 2009;10(4):361–367.
41. Pesce V, Speciale D, Sammarco G, et al. Surgical approach to bone healing in osteoporosis. *Clin Cases Mineral Bone Metab*. 2009;6(2):131–135.
42. Herscovici D, Scaduto JM. Management of high-energy foot and ankle injuries in the geriatric population. *Geriatr Orthop Surg Rehabil*. 2012;3(1):33–44.
43. Bishop JA, Palanca AA, Bellino MJ, Lowenberg DW. Assessment of compromised fracture healing. *Am Acad Orthop Surg*. 2012; 20(5):273–282.
44. Taormina DP, Shulman BS, Karia R, et al. Older age does not affect healing time and functional outcomes after fracture nonunion surgery. *Geriatr Orthop Surg Rehab*. 2014;5(3):116–121.
45. Egol KA, Bechtel C, Spitzer AB, et al. Treatment of long bone nonunions: factors affecting healing. *Bull NYU Hosp Joint Dis*. 2012;70(4):224–231.
46. Brown CV, Shoemaker WC, Wo CC, et al. Is noninvasive hemodynamic monitoring appropriate for the elderly critically injured patient. *J Trauma*. 2005;58:102–107.
47. Shoemaker WC, Wo CC, Bishop MH, et al. Noninvasive physiologic monitoring in high-risk surgical patients. *Arch Surg*. 1996;131:732–737.
48. Fassett DR, Harrop JS, Maltenfort M, et al. Mortality rates in geriatric patients with spinal cord injuries. *J Neurosurg Spine*. 2007;7(3):277–281.
49. Roberts SE, Goldacre MJ. Time trends and demography of mortality after fractured neck of femur in an English population, 1968–98: database study. *BMJ*. 2003;327:771–775.
50. Moja L, Piatti A, Pecoraro V, et al. Timing matters in hip fracture surgery: patients operated within 48 hours have better outcomes: a meta-analysis and meta-regression of over 190,000 patients. *PLoS One*. 2012;7:e46175.
51. Khan SK, Kalra S, Khanna A, et al. Timing of surgery for hip fractures: a systematic review of 52 published studies involving 291,413 patients. *Injury*. 2009;40:692–697.
52. Beaupre LA, Jones CA, Saunders LD, et al. Best practices for elderly hip fracture patients: a systematic overview of the evidence. *J Gen Intern Med*. 2005;20(11):1019–1025.
53. Volkmann R. Die ischaemischen muskellahmungen und kontrakturen. *Zentrabl Chir*. 1881;8:801–803.
54. Murphy JB. Myositis. *JAMA*. 1914;63:1249–1255.
55. Brooks B, Johnson JS, Kirtley JA. Simultaneous vein ligation. *Surg Gynecol Obstet*. 1934;59:496.
56. Haasbeek JF, Cole WG. Open fractures of the arm in children. *J Bone Joint Surg*. 1995;77:576–581.
57. Hayden G, Leung M, Leong J. Gluteal compartment syndrome. *ANZ J Surg*. 2006;76:668–670.
58. Schwartz JT, Brumback RJ, Lakatos R, et al. Acute compartment syndrome of the thigh. *J Bone Joint Surg*. 1989;71:392.
59. Meyerson M. Acute compartment syndromes of the foot. *Bull Hosp J Dis Orthop*. 1987;47:251.
60. DeLee JC, Stiehl JB. Open tibia fracture with compartment syndrome. *Clin Orthop*. 1981;160:175–184.
61. Rorabeck CH, Clarke KM. The pathophysiology of the anterior tibial compartment syndrome: an experimental investigation. *J Trauma*. 1978; 18:299.
62. Heppenstall RB, Scott R, Sapiga A, et al. A comparative study of the tolerance of skeletal muscle to ischemia. *J Bone Joint Surg*. 1986;68:820.
63. Geary N. Late surgical decompression for compartment syndrome of the forearm. *J Bone Joint Surg*. 1984;66:745.
64. Kunkel JM. Thigh and leg compartment syndrome in the absence of lower extremity trauma following MAST application. *Am J Emerg Med*. 1987;5:118–120.
65. Rorabeck CH. The treatment of compartment syndromes of the leg. *J Bone Joint Surg*. 1984;66:93–97.
66. Boody AR, Wongworawat MD. Accuracy in the measurement of compartment pressures: a comparison of three commonly used devices. *J Bone Joint Surg*. 2005;87:2415–2422.
67. Wilson SC, Vrahas MS, Berson L, et al. A simple method to measure compartment pressures using an intravenous catheter. *Orthopedics*. 1997; 20:403.
68. Rorabeck CH, Castle GSP, Hardie R, et al. Compartment pressure measurements: an experimental investigation using the slit catheter. *J Trauma*. 1981;21:446.
69. Harris IA, Kadir A, Donald G. Continuous compartment pressure monitoring for tibia fractures: does it influence outcome? *J Trauma*. 2006;60:1330–1335.
70. Abraham P, Leftheriotis G, Saumet JL. Laser Doppler flowmetry in the diagnosis of chronic compartment syndrome. *J Bone Joint Surg*. 1998; 80:365.
71. Weimann JM, Ueno T, Leek BT, et al. Noninvasive measurements of intramuscular pressure using pulsed phase-locked loop ultrasound for detecting compartment syndrome. *J Orthop Trauma*. 2006;20:458–463.
72. Amendola A, Twaddle BC. Compartment syndrome. In: *Browner: Skeletal Trauma: Basic Science, Management and Reconstruction*. 3rd ed. WB Saunders St. Louis, MO; 2003.
73. McQueen JMM, Court-Brown CM. Compartment monitoring in tibial fractures. *J Bone Joint Surg*. 1995;78:99.
74. Whitesides TE, Haney TC, Morimoto K, et al. Tissue perfusion measurements as a determinant for the need for fasciotomy. *Clin Orthop*. 1975;113:43.
75. Kakar S, Firoozabadi R, McKean J, et al. Diastolic blood pressure in patients with tibia fractures under anaesthesia: implications for the diagnosis of compartment syndrome. *J Orthop Trauma*. 2007;21:99–103.
76. Matsen FA, Wyss CR, Krugmire RB, et al. The effects of limb elevation and dependency on local arteriovenous gradients in normal human limbs with particular reference to limbs with increased tissue pressure. *Clin Orthop*. 1980;150:187.
77. Bulstrode CK, King JB, Worpole R, et al. A simple method for closing fasciotomies. *Ann R Coll Surg*. 1985;67:119.
78. Bermann SS, Schnilling JD, McIntyre KE, et al. Shoelace technique for delayed primary closure of fasciotomies. *Am J Surg*. 1994;167:435–436.
79. McKenney MG, Nir I, Fee T, et al. A simple device for closure of fasciotomy wounds. *Am J Surg*. 1995;172:275.
80. Yang CC, Chang DS, Webb LX. Vacuum-assisted closure of fasciotomy following compartment syndrome of the leg. *J Surg Orthop Adv*. 2006;15:19–23.
81. Frink M, Klaus AK, Kuther G, et al. Long term results of compartment syndrome of lower limb in polytraumatized patients. *Injury Int J Care Injured*. 2007;38:607–613.
82. Mithoefer K, Lhowe DW, Vrahas MS, et al. Functional outcome after acute compartment syndrome of the thigh. *J Bone Joint Surg*. 2006;88:729–737.
83. Bradley EL. The anterior tibial compartment syndrome. *Surg Gynecol Obstet*. 1973;136:289–297.
84. Sheridan GW, Matsen FA. Fasciotomy in the treatment of the acute compartment syndrome. *J Bone Joint Surg*. 1976;58:112–115.
85. Slater M, Mullins R. Rhabdomyolysis and myoglobinuric renal failure in trauma and surgical patients. A review. *J Am Coll Surg*. 1998;186:693–716.
86. Ward MM. Factors predictive of acute renal failure in rhabdomyolysis. *Arch Intern Med*. 1998;148:1553–1557.
87. Homsi E, Barreiro MF, Orlando JM, et al. Prophylaxis of acute renal failure in patients with rhabdomyolysis. *Ren Fail*. 1997;19:283–288.
88. Dudney TM, Elliott CG. Pulmonary embolism from amniotic fluid, fat and air. *Prog Cardiovasc Dis*. 1994;36:447–474.
89. Levy D. The fat embolism syndrome: a review. *Clin Orthop Relat Res*. 1990;261:281–286.
90. Riska EB, Myllynen P. Fat embolism in patients with multiple injuries. *J Trauma*. 1982;22:891–894.
91. Glover P, Worthley L. Fat embolism. *Crit Care Resus*. 1999;1:276–284.
92. Peltier LF. Fat embolism. *A perspective. Clin Orthop Relat Res*. 1988;232: 263–207.
93. Fabian TC, Hoots AV, Stanford DS, et al. Fat embolism syndrome: prospective evaluation in 92 fracture patients. *Crit Care Med*. 1990;18:42–26.
94. Mellor A, Soni N. Fat embolism. *Anesthesia*. 2001;56:145–154.
95. Riseborough EJ, Herndon JH. Alterations in pulmonary function, coagulation and fat metabolism in patients with fractures of the lower limbs. *Clin Orthop Relat Res*. 1976;115:248–267.
96. Fonte DA, Hausberger FX. Pulmonary free fatty acids in experimental fat embolism. *J Trauma*. 1971;11:668–672.
97. Hofmann S, Huemer G, Slazer M. Pathophysiology and management of the fat embolism syndrome. *Anaesthesia*. 1998;2:35–37.

98. Nakata Y, Tanaka H, Kuwagata Y, et al. Triolein-induced pulmonary embolization and increased microvascular permeability in isolated perfused rat lungs. *J Trauma*. 1999;47:111–119.
99. Brow PJ, Toung T, Margolis S, et al. Pulmonary injury caused by free fatty acid: evaluation of steroid and albumin therapy. *Surgery*. 1981;89: 582–587.
100. Gemer M, Dunegan LJ, Lehr JL, et al. Pulmonary insufficiency induced by oleic acid in the sheep: a model for investigation of extracorporeal oxygenation. *J Thorac Cardiovasc Surg*. 1975;69:793–799.
101. Richards RR. Fat embolism syndrome. *Can J Surg*. 1997;40:334–339.
102. Parizel PM, Demey HE, Veeckmans G, et al. Early diagnosis of cerebral fat embolism syndrome by diffusion-weighted MRI (starfield pattern). *Stroke*. 2001;32:2942–2944.
103. Satoh H, Kurisu K, Ohtani M, et al. Cerebral fat embolism studied by magnetic resonance imaging, transcranial Doppler sonography, and single photon emission computed tomography: case report. *J Trauma*. 1997;43: 345–348.
104. Worthley LI, Fisher MM. The fat embolism syndrome treated with oxygen, diuretics, sodium restriction and spontaneous ventilation. *Anaesth Intensive Care*. 1979;7:136–142.
105. Alho A, Saikku K, Eerola P, et al. Corticosteroids in patients with a high risk of fat embolism syndrome. *Surg Gynecol Obstet*. 1978;147: 358–362.
106. Shier MR, Wilson RF, James RE, et al. Fat embolism prophylaxis: a study of four treatment modalities. *J Trauma*. 1977;17:621–629.
107. Gossling HR, Donohue TA. The fat embolism syndrome. *JAMA*. 1979; 241:2740–2742.
108. Brundage SI, McGhan R, Jurkovich GJ, et al. Timing of femur fracture fixation: effect on outcome in patients with thoracic and head injuries. *J Trauma*. 2002;52:299–307.
109. Pitto RP, Schramm M, Hohmann D, et al. Relevance of the drainage along the linea aspera for the reduction of fat embolism during cemented total hip arthroplasty: a prospective, randomized clinical trial. *Arch Orthop Trauma Surg*. 1999;119:146–150.
110. Pitto RP, Koessler M, Kuehle JW. Comparison of fixation of the femoral component without cement and fixation with use of a bone-vacuum cementing technique for the prevention of fat embolism during total hip arthroplasty. A prospective, randomized clinical trial. *J Bone Joint Surg Am*. 1999;81:831–843.
111. Peltier LF. Fat embolism. III. The toxic properties of neutral fat and free fatty acids. *Surgery*. 1956;40:665–670.
112. Gossling Hr, Pellegrini VD Jr. Fat embolism syndrome: a review of the pathophysiology and physiological basis of treatment. *Clin Orthop Relat Res*. 1982;165:68–82.
113. Meeke RI, Fitzpatrick GJ, Phelan DM. Cerebral edema and the fat embolism syndrome. *Intensive Care Med*. 1987;15:147–148.
114. Sie MY, Toh KW, Rajeev K. Cerebral fat embolism: an indication for ICP monitor? *J Trauma*. 2003;55:1185–1186.
115. Habashi N. Other approaches to open-lung ventilation: airway pressure release ventilation. *Crit Care Med*. 2005;33:228–240.
116. Fulde GW, Harrison P. Fat embolism: a review. *Arch Emerg Med*. 1991; 8:233–239.
117. Durkin A, Sagi HC, Durham R, Flint L. Contemporary management of pelvic fractures. *Am J Surg*. 2006;192:211–223.
118. Holcomb JB, Tilley BC, Baraniuk S, et al. Transfusion of plasma, platelets, and red blood cells in a 1:1:1 vs a 1:1:2 ratio and mortality in patients with severe trauma: the PROPPR randomized clinical trial. *JAMA*. 2015;313(5):471–482.
119. Kimbrell BJ, Velhamos GC, Chan LS, Demetriades D. Angiographic embolization for pelvic fractures in older patients. *Arch Surg*. 2004;139:728–732; discussion 732–733.
120. Henry, SM, Pollak AN, Jones AL, et al. Pelvic fractures in geriatric patients: a distant clinical entity. *J Trauma*. 1012;53:15–20.
121. Gourlay D, Hoffer E, Routt M, et al. Pelvic angiography for recurrent traumatic pelvic arterial hemorrhage. *J Trauma*. 2005;59:1168–1173; discussion 1173–1174.
122. Cothren CC, Osborn PM, Moore EE, et al. Preperitoneal pelvic packing for hemodynamically unstable pelvic fractures: a paradigm shift. *J Trauma*. 2007;62:834–839; discussion 839–842.
123. Brenner ML, Moore LJ, DuBose JJ, et al. A clinical series of resuscitative endovascular balloon occlusion of the aorta for hemorrhage control and resuscitation. *J Trauma Acute Care Surg*. 2013;75(3):506–511.
124. Moore LJ, Brenner M, Kozar RA, et al. Implementation of resuscitative endovascular balloon occlusion of the aorta as an alternative to resuscitative thoracotomy for noncompressible truncal hemorrhage. *J Trauma Acute Care Surg*. 2015;79(4):523–530; discussion 530–532.
125. Martinelli T, Thony F, Decléty P, et al. Intra-aortic balloon occlusion to salvage patients with life-threatening hemorrhagic shock from pelvic fractures. *J Trauma* 2010;68(4):942–948.

CHAPTER

66

Urologic Surgery and Trauma

MICHAEL COBURN

INTRODUCTION

From the critical care perspective, urologic surgical emergencies that may require urgent assessment and intervention include hemorrhagic, obstructive, infectious, ischemic, and traumatic processes, in addition to a wide variety of general urologic surgical and postoperative difficulties. Various oncologic emergencies also arise in urology and may require urgent critical care management. Urologic trauma—addressed in a separate section, below—encompasses a wide variety of injuries that may vary from immediately life-threatening issues to those requiring specialized reconstructive surgical capability, often impacting long-term functional outcomes. The ability to identify emergency urologic conditions for which time-sensitive action is needed is of paramount importance. A close, collaborative team effort between the urologic surgeon, the critical care specialist, and other specialty services, is important in the successful management of urologic emergencies.

PATHOPHYSIOLOGY

Gross Hematuria

This is an alarming symptom to both the patient and the medical practitioner, and may mandate immediate critical care intervention, depending on the magnitude of the hematuria and details of the individual case (1). Patients presenting with gross hematuria to the emergency department or in the hospital or postoperative setting may have a defined cause (e.g., diagnosed radiation cystitis, recurrent benign prostatic hypertrophy [BPH]-related bleeding, postoperative hemorrhage) or may represent a new sign not previously evaluated. In the posturologic surgery setting, troublesome gross hematuria may occur following transurethral surgery (prostate or bladder tumor resection) or following renal surgery. Immediate urologic intervention is necessary if the patient has clot retention, that is, unable to void or empty adequately due to the presence of clots in the bladder; is bleeding severely (which may be difficult to measure); has significant pain; is infected; has coagulopathy; or has other underlying medical factors leading to an increased risk of further complications. Vital sign measurement, physical examination, and basic laboratory studies including complete blood count (CBC), coagulation functions, electrolyte and renal function testing, urinalysis, and culture will often shed light on the above issues and determine the need for immediate intervention. Palpation and percussion of the bladder may reveal distention with or without tenderness; bladder ultrasound units (BladderScan) or other readily available ultrasound instruments may rapidly answer the question of whether the bladder is distended. In the setting of gross hematuria and a distended bladder, drainage is needed and a catheter must be inserted. Often a small-caliber catheter is initially placed; this will not allow for adequate drainage or irrigation of clots. Clots must first be fully evacuated to allow proper catheter drainage as well as to determine the presence and degree of ongoing bleeding. Small clots may be evacuated via an 18- to 20-French catheter; large clots require a larger-bore catheter (22 to 24 French) for satisfactory evaluation. The catheter should be irrigated to and fro with a piston syringe using 60 to 120 mL of normal saline. When no further clot can be retrieved, the irrigation efflux should become clear if bleeding is not ongoing. If the efflux remains bloody despite complete clot evacuation, or if new clots continue to form, there is ongoing bleeding and input from the urologist is needed. One can change to a three-way catheter in the setting of continuing bleeding, and regulate the rate of saline inflow in order to keep the catheter patent, but this decision is best made along with urologic consultation. There are risks involved in the implementation of continuous bladder irrigation, including bladder rupture if the inflow of irrigant continues while the outflow lumen becomes occluded without recognition. It is desirable to seek early determination of the cause of troublesome gross hematuria, as definitive intervention via cystoscopic examination and fulguration may solve the problem with less morbidity and less blood replacement than more conservative approaches. Gross hematuria in the urologic postoperative setting will be addressed in more detail below.

Other hemorrhagic urologic problems requiring immediate critical care intervention include renal or perirenal bleeding (e.g., spontaneous hematoma in the anticoagulated patient or the renal tumor patient, surgical bleeding following intrarenal surgery) or scrotal hematoma. Bleeding in these sites is often trauma related (see below Penetrating and Blunt Trauma to the Genitourinary System).

Urosepsis

This process is another major concern in the urology patient. Sepsis arising from the urinary tract may present in a precipitous and potentially life-threatening manner, or may be indolent (2–5). It is essential to understand the precarious nature of the combination of infection and obstruction in producing a dangerous septic state. A common scenario is the patient presenting with an obstructing ureteral calculus. Typical symptoms of ureteral colic include flank pain—often radiating to the lower quadrant, and ipsilaterally to the genitalia with distal stones—irritative voiding symptoms (when the stone is distal in the intramural ureter), nausea, vomiting, or distention, due to ileus. These symptoms can be extremely distressing and require urgent medical attention, but the most critical emergency seen in such a setting occurs when these symptoms are accompanied by infection and sepsis. The combination of infection and obstruction of the urinary tract (upper or lower) is a veritable surgical emergency requiring immediate action. Severe sepsis and septic shock may unfold rapidly in such situations with a significant mortality rate, even in the otherwise healthy host. *We teach our residents that the sun should never set on an undrained, infected obstructed urinary tract.*

Other infectious states requiring urgent critical care intervention include renal or perirenal abscess, scrotal abscess, acute epididymo-orchitis, and Fournier gangrene (see below).

Obstruction of the Urinary Tract and Urinary Retention

Obstruction may require critical care intervention, independent of the presence or absence of hematuria or infection, in order to avoid or limit acute renal injury and persistent functional damage to the bladder. Upper or lower tract obstruction can result in acute or chronic renal failure, mandating prompt drainage to control metabolic instability. Acute urinary retention with bladder distention is a miserable experience for the patient, and must be promptly relieved by introduction of a catheter into the bladder, preferably by a transurethral route, or alternatively by a suprapubic (SP) route if the urethra is impassable.

Ischemic States

These represent another form of pathology for which immediate intervention is essential (6,7). The classic example in urology is that of testicular torsion; delayed diagnosis of torsion is a common cause of unnecessary testicular loss, as well as avoidable litigation. After 8 hours of torsion, the likelihood of testicular salvage decreases significantly. A high index of suspicion is necessary when addressing "the acute scrotum," with accurate history and physical examination forming the core of this assessment, and diagnostic imaging—mainly scrotal ultrasound, occasionally computed tomography (CT) scanning when extension from an intra-abdominal process is suspected—as appropriate. When clinical suspicion of acute testicular torsion is high, surgical exploration should not be delayed if confirmatory imaging is not readily and rapidly available; the outcome with regard to testicular salvage is critically time sensitive. The occasional negative exploration or the finding of some other cause of the acute scrotum is appropriate, similar to the principles of exploration for the acute abdomen and for acute appendicitis. Naturally, proper patient education is important preoperatively in addressing the differential diagnosis and the possibility of finding a lesion, which might have been manageable without surgery, as well as the possibility of orchiectomy. The differential diagnosis of the acute scrotum includes incarcerated or strangulated inguinal hernia for which urgent surgical management is also critical. Physical and sonographic findings are usually diagnostic preoperatively.

Other ischemic states of critical care relevance in urology include the ischemic kidney due to atherosclerotic or embolic disease or pedicle injury from trauma. The kidney begins to undergo irreversible loss of function following approximately 30 minutes of warm ischemia time; thus, rapid action is necessary.

Oncologic Emergencies

In urology these often involve hemorrhagic, obstructive, and infectious problems due to the effects of the primary tumor. Other emergencies include neurologic compromise and pain management issues. Prostate cancer may preferentially metastasize to the skeletal system, and sudden neurologic compromise from spinal cord compression due to prostate cancer is occasionally seen. Sensory loss, paralysis, and loss of urinary, bowel, and sexual function may be manifestations of neurologic compromise from malignant involvement of the central nervous system. When observed, immediate neurosurgical consultation should be obtained to determine if corticosteroids, emergency radiation therapy, or decompressive laminectomy are indicated; in addition, the input of a medical oncologist is valuable. Commencing androgen blockade therapy emergently may be of great value when prostate cancer patients present with complications such as neurologic or urinary obstructive compromise. Intramuscular luteinizing hormone–releasing hormone (LH-RH) agonists such as leuprolide acetate may be started immediately; to prevent transient worsening from the androgen flare that accompanies the initiation of such regimens, an antiandrogen drug such as bicalutamide should be commenced simultaneously or prior to the LH-RH analog.

POSTOPERATIVE MANAGEMENT

Both major and minor urologic surgery may present critical care issues that require rapid and accurate assessment and intervention. While the postoperative considerations following major retroperitoneal or pelvic surgery will be familiar to the surgical critical care specialist, as they present challenges similar to those seen in general and vascular surgery, there are special considerations in urologic patients. Patients undergoing endoscopic urologic surgery and genital surgery may present with postoperative issues less familiar to the critical care team, and it is important to understand the anatomy and the issues that may require expeditious intervention. Currently, many urologic procedures that had traditionally been performed through open surgical approaches are now commonly being approached via laparoscopic, robotic, and other minimally invasive surgical (MIS) techniques, bringing with them their own set of postoperative challenges. We will address the more common and important types of urologic procedures with relevance to the critical care provider.

Upper Abdominal Surgery

In urology this usually involves extirpative procedures on the adrenal gland, kidney, or ureter and/or reconstructive procedures on these structures.

Patient position during surgery and selection of incision are relevant to the postoperative management. While the anterior midline incision is often favored by general surgeons for open abdominal and intraperitoneal procedures, urologists often prefer to operate through the flank or through other incisional approaches to the upper abdomen. Large renal tumors are often approached through a subcostal or thoracoabdominal incision, which may penetrate the chest through the bed of the 8th to 11th rib through a rib resection or intercostal technique. Smaller or lower pole tumors renal are commonly approached through a subcostal flank or anterior incision, which generally does not enter the thoracic cavity. Such incisions may be developed as extraperitoneal exposure or through a transperitoneal route. The critical care provider in these postoperative patients should know how the patient was positioned, what kind of incision was made, and whether it was transthoracic and intra- or extraperitoneal. These details allow one to anticipate the types of problems that may arise postoperatively. In flank surgery, postoperative atelectasis may involve the lung positioned downward against the operating table, particularly when the operation is prolonged and the patient is large. Occasionally lobar or complete lung atelectasis may be noted and may require bronchoscopic intervention. If a tube thoracostomy is placed following urologic surgery, the standard problems typical of the use of such tubes can occur, including air leak or postoperative intrathoracic bleeding. Excellent pulmonary toilet is critical following upper abdominal and flank urologic surgery and, ideally, should be initiated preoperatively, with patients being medically optimized and taught to use an incentive spirometer, and then being closely monitored for pulmonary difficulties with early intervention as indicated. Postoperative pain from flank surgery can be a major problem and may require expert pain management intervention, continuous epidural analgesic strategies, subcutaneous pain pumps, and patient-controlled intravenous analgesic. Appropriate pain control is also key to minimizing pulmonary complications by aiding respiratory and coughing efforts.

Following surgery that involves removal or manipulation of the adrenal gland, the possibility of an early postoperative hypoadrenal state should be considered, including the potential for Addisonian crisis. These entities may be unsuspected and may be missed or noted with a delay in diagnosis when assessing postoperative electrolyte and hemodynamic abnormalities and other nonspecific signs that may be consistent with acute adrenal dysfunction or deficiency. The critical care specialist should know if the adrenal was removed along with a nephrectomy procedure, and whether there is any reason to suspect hypofunction or absence of the contralateral gland. These challenges are more common when the opposite adrenal gland has been manipulated or is absent.

Acute renal insufficiency may occur following any major surgery, and is of particular concern following renal surgery. Partial nephrectomies may be performed using warm or cold ischemia techniques, and through open, laparoscopic, or robotic techniques. While the objective in such surgery is to minimize the negative impact on the function of the operated kidney, some degree of postoperative acute tubular necrosis (ATN) and acute kidney injury (AKI) may still occur. Whether this is clinically noted, or even relevant, depends largely on the state of the contralateral kidney; standard management principles for acute renal insufficiency are applicable.

Postoperative bleeding following renal surgery may be manifested by gross hematuria; hemodynamic instability; acute anemia; physical findings such as palpable flank hematoma or ecchymosis; or radiologic findings of blood in the renal fossa, chest (after a transthoracic procedure), or peritoneal cavity (after a transperitoneal procedure). If a drain is left in place following surgery, elevated output of bloody fluid is important to monitor. Following a partial nephrectomy, significant postoperative bleeding most commonly arises from arterial branch vessels within the renal parenchyma at the resection site. An effort is made intraoperatively to suture significant parenchymal bleeding points, whether the surgery is performed through open surgical or a MIS approach, often supplemented by the use of additional hemostatic agents, and coagulation instruments. If significant bleeding occurs following renal surgery, expectant management with transfusion and correction of any coagulopathy, return to the operating room (OR) for reexploration, angiographic embolization, or CT scanning—to assess the specific anatomic site of bleeding and judge the size of the hematoma—are options to consider. The choice between these measures is individualized based on the severity of the bleeding, patient condition and physiologic reserve, and access to imaging, interventional radiologic, and surgical resources. If there is evidence of major, early postoperative bleeding, rapid surgical reexploration is the best approach. If bleeding occurs in a delayed fashion and renal parenchymal bleeding is suspected, interventional radiology (IR) is usually favored. The patient should be maintained in a fluid-resuscitated state when a renal bleeding issue is evolving, with the hemoglobin at a level that would allow the patient to tolerate continued blood loss without catastrophic decompensation.

Urinary extravasation following upper urinary tract surgery may be manifested by increased drainage from suction drains, for which creatinine determination confirms the fluid's identity as urine. Alternatively, urinary extravasation may present as intra-abdominal sepsis or with a mass effect from urinoma formation. Urologic input should be sought as to whether the region is well drained, whether the leak is expected, and whether intervention versus observation is indicated.

Pelvic Surgery

These procedures, frequently requiring postoperative critical care support, include exenterative interventions for malignancies (radical prostatectomy or cystectomy), simple open prostatectomy for benign prostatic hyperplasia, and reconstructive pelvic or perineal surgeries for obstruction or incontinence. Critical care issues typically relate to standard postoperative abdominal surgical concerns such as pain, bleeding, and ileus. Specifically with pelvic urologic procedures, management of tubes and drains, and recognizing when urinary extravasation arising in the postoperative period requires urgent attention, or can be managed expectantly, is important. Patients that have undergone major surgery involving an open bladder (open prostatectomy, bladder stone removal, etc.) may have significant bladder spasm postoperatively, requiring antispasmodic or anticholinergic medication. Bleeding following major urologic pelvic surgery may result in Foley (indwelling urinary bladder catheter [IUBC]) catheter occlusion with clot; it should be established with the urologist how much hematuria is acceptable and what measures should be taken if failure of IUBC drainage develops. Catheter manipulation should be pursued only with the input of the urologist, as aggressive IUBC irrigation after lower urinary tract surgery may damage the surgical closure or reconstruction site. Significant bleeding from the IUBC is relatively uncommon following radical prostatectomy, while dramatic hematuria is much more common following an open simple prostatectomy performed for BPH, in which the adenoma is enucleated from the prostatic capsule by finger dissection, leaving a raw, vascular tissue bed; urologic input is needed for problematic bleeding in such patients.

The possibility of anastomotic leakage or a missed injury to the ureter exists in the pelvic surgical patient. If inordinately high pelvic suction drainage is noted, the fluid should be sent for creatinine level to determine if a urine leak is present. If well drained, no immediate intervention may be necessary, but radiographic studies may be indicated to localize the site of extravasation and plan definitive management.

Following radical cystectomy for bladder cancer, complications may include urinary extravasation from the urinary diversion reconstruction, pelvic bleeding, ileus, bowel obstruction or anastomotic leak, and pelvic lymphocele. Cystectomy patients invariably require initial stays in the intensive care unit (ICU) postoperatively, due to the length and complexity of the surgery, potential for postoperative bleeding, and general comorbidity management. Patients undergoing major urologic surgery, and especially patients undergoing cystectomy and urinary diversion, may require nutritional support. These patients, who have had both a major exenterative procedure as well as complex bowel surgery, may have a prolonged ileus, develop partial small bowel obstruction, and be depressed, often requiring aggressive nutritional supplementation, which should be initiated early when a prolonged recovery is anticipated, to avoid the healing problems seen with development of a progressive catabolic state.

Deep venous thrombosis (DVT) and pulmonary embolism (PE) are risks of many urologic surgical procedures, and urologists are acutely aware of the issues related to DVT prophylaxis. Practice guidelines have been developed to support DVT prophylaxis and treatment decision making in urologic surgery (8). Because major retroperitoneal or pelvic surgery also presents significant risks for postoperative bleeding, a judicious approach to postoperative anticoagulation is applied, with careful assessment of DVT risk factors and risk–benefit analysis. Radical cystectomy is the procedure with the greatest DVT risk of the urologic operations, as an extensive pelvic lymphadenectomy is typically included, and many urologic oncologists will start medical prophylaxis regimens prior to, or early following surgery if there are no bleeding issues.

Other pelvic surgical procedures the intensivist may encounter include the wide range of pelvic floor reconstructive operations performed for management of prolapse or stress incontinence, as well as reconstructive procedures for obstructive lower urinary tract entities. The traditional pubovaginal sling or retropubic bladder neck suspension procedures, and particularly some of the newer procedures that involve passage of artificial tape and mesh materials either via the retropubic space, through a transobturator foramen approach, or through other transvaginal techniques, may introduce risk of enteric pelvic injury or major pelvic vascular or nerve injury. If major bleeding occurs following these types of procedures, either via the surgical incisions or resulting in large pelvic hematomata and hemodynamic instability, pelvic exploration or angiographic study and control may be indicated, and vascular surgical expertise may be necessary.

Endoscopic Upper and Lower Urinary Tract Surgery

This encompasses a wide variety of commonly performed procedures, including diagnostic cystoscopy (rigid or flexible), cystoscopic surgery (bladder biopsy, transurethral resection of prostate or bladder tumor [TURP, TURBT]), ureteroscopy (rigid or flexible, diagnostic alone, or with stone manipulation or biopsy/fulguration), and percutaneous renal access surgery (percutaneous nephrostolithotripsy [PCNL]). Each of these forms of urologic instrumentation can be simple or complicated, and may present challenges for the critical care provider (9–11).

Lower tract endoscopy for diagnostic purposes is usually performed in an office setting, typically using a flexible cystoscope; lidocaine jelly is usually used as a local anesthetic, typically instilled with a prepackaged applicator (Uro-Jet). While the procedure causes minimal discomfort, postprocedure infection can occur, but the risk is small if the urine is sterile or bacteriuria is appropriately treated preprocedure. Prophylactic oral or IV antibiotics are often administered for endourologic procedures to minimize the infection risk, but it is important to appreciate that the potential for postprocedural urinary infection and urosepsis cannot be entirely eliminated, even with judicious use of antibiotics. Gross hematuria can occur following even simple diagnostic cystoscopy, but is usually self-limiting and minimal. More involved cystoscopic surgery, on the other hand, is generally performed under regional or general anesthesia, and specific potential postoperative problems may occur following such procedures.

When endoscopic cutting or resection is required, a resectoscope is used which is a rigid instrument employing a cutting loop or blade. Until recently, the most common irrigant used for TURP in the United States was 1.5% glycine, which is nonelectrolyte and isotonic to plasma. This irrigant would allow the electroresection system to function properly while avoiding hemolysis if intravascular extravasation occurs, a problem seen historically when sterile water was used as the irrigant. Cystoscopic surgery using glycine irrigation may result in significant hyponatremia if major absorption occurs, either directly into the vasculature (as with cutting into a periprostatic venous sinus during a TURP) or into interstitial tissues (as with fluid entering the retropubic space or infiltrating under the bladder trigone). If hyponatremia develops, one may observe altered mental status, bradycardia, hypertension, and respiratory compromise. Severe hyponatremia may result in cerebral edema and seizures. If this problem occurs and is recognized intraoperatively, the procedure is prematurely terminated. Diuretics with normal saline or hypertonic saline administered intravenously may be indicated, depending on the clinical manifestations. In most centers, the use of glycine irrigation and monopolar resection systems has now been replaced with bipolar systems that utilize normal saline irrigation, largely eliminating the problems seen with glycine irrigation. It is, however, important for the intensivist to understand the issues with the use of nonsaline irrigants, as such systems remain in use in some regions. In general, sterile water is avoided as an irrigant for extensive operative cystoscopy, confining its use to simple diagnostic cystoscopy.

If bladder perforation occurs during TURBT or bladder biopsy procedures, there is the potential for significant irrigant extravasation to occur rapidly. If extraperitoneal, management with catheter drainage will suffice and the fluid is usually reabsorbed without sequelae unless the volume is very large, in which case placing a drain in the retropubic space to evacuate the fluid may be indicated. Minimal intraperitoneal resectoscopic injuries may be manageable with catheter drainage alone. If problems arise—such as abdominal distention, persistent extravasation—with this nonoperative approach to intraperitoneal bladder perforation, laparoscopic or open surgical repair should be performed. This situation is, of course, very different from the intraperitoneal bladder rupture due to blunt trauma, which typically results in a large defect in the bladder dome, consistently requiring suture repair to prevent urinary ascites and sepsis.

Bleeding may be a problem following either TURP or TURBT. Urologists are well trained to deal with this problem and distinguish arterial bleeding, which will likely warrant return to the OR for a second look and fulguration attempt, from acceptable venous bleeding, which is self-limiting. Often, continuous bladder irrigation via a three-way catheter is employed in the postoperative period to maintain catheter patency and prevent clot formation. While these devices are valuable adjuncts in our management of such patients, they introduce the potential for postoperative difficulties with occlusion of the outflow channel from clot, while irrigant inflow continues, as discussed above; bladder distention and bladder rupture can result in this situation. When managing any continuous bladder irrigation system, the intensivist must closely monitor the inflow and output, and palpate the lower abdomen on a regular basis to be certain that catheter occlusion with bladder distention does not occur. If uncertain as to whether the three-way catheter is draining properly, the inflow should be turned off while the catheter is irrigated or urologic assistance is obtained. Only normal saline should be used as irrigant for continuous bladder irrigation systems. For TURP procedures, maintaining gentle catheter traction may help control bleeding from within the prostatic fossa; only the urologist should implement or adjust the traction system. For TURBT procedures, catheter traction is of no value, as most bladder wall bleeding cannot be compressed with traction on the catheter balloon; a lower threshold to take the patient back to surgery for a second look is safer for troublesome post-TURBT bleeding. If a catheter needs to be changed in the early postoperative period following a TURP or TURBT, it is best done by the operating urologist's team or on their specific order, as catheter reinsertion may be challenging or require a particular type of catheter or technique. In addition to the advent of the saline-based bipolar resection systems, other newer technologies for TURP and TURBT employing laser energy to ablate, vaporize, or coagulate tissue endoscopically, have gained popularity; these approaches usually result in less bleeding than the traditional electroresection approaches. Complications may relate to obstruction following catheter removal or to iatrogenic injury from misdirection of the laser energy.

Upper tract endoscopy—ureteroscopy, percutaneous nephroscopy—has progressed greatly in recent years, with the current instrumentation usually allowing complex upper tract procedures to be performed with low morbidity. Ureteroscopy is often performed for hematuria evaluation, treatment of ureteral or renal stones, endoscopic assessment, and treatment of upper tract urothelial neoplasms, and for addressing obstructive lesions with laser or other incision procedures. Normal saline is used for most such procedures, although glycine or sterile water may be needed when electrofulguration in the upper tract is planned. Problems that the intensivist may encounter usually relate to ureteral perforation, gross hematuria with stent occlusion or "clot colic," obstructive problems related to retained stone fragments, or postoperative urinary infection or urosepsis. Percutaneous renal surgery may be accompanied by problems related to prone-position surgery, a high percutaneous access site traversing or affecting the lower chest, postoperative bleeding, or infection. Percutaneous nephrostolithotomy or nephrolithotomy involves gaining access to the collecting system through the flank with the patient in the prone position. A needle, guidewire, and balloon or other dilating system is utilized to place a hollow plastic working sheath through the flank and renal parenchyma into the collecting system, through which a flexible or rigid working nephroscope can be advanced. Laser, electrohydraulic, ultrasonic, or pneumatic devices are used to fragment and remove stones, or resection, incision, or fulguration instruments can be introduced to deal with neoplastic or obstructive lesions. Depending on the task to be accomplished, the access for percutaneous renal surgery may be obtained by the interventional radiologist or by the urologist. If entry into the upper pole calyx is needed for stone access, a supracostal puncture, above the 12th rib, may be required. Traversing the chest, the risk exists that a pneumothorax or hydrothorax may result, requiring tube thoracostomy postoperatively. If elevated airway pressures and difficulty with ventilation occur intraoperatively, these possibilities should be entertained and managed acutely. As the kidney is a highly vascular organ and the access traverses the renal parenchyma, significant bleeding can occur intraoperatively, perioperatively, or even days or weeks postoperatively at the time of nephrostomy removal. Occasionally, angiographic embolization may be necessary for major renal bleeding associated with PCNL. If brisk bleeding with hemodynamic instability occurs via an indwelling nephrostomy tube, the tube can be clamped while urologic input is urgently obtained. When removing a nephrostomy tube following PCNL, it is desirable to have a balloon tamponade catheter immediately available to place into the tract and inflate if significant bleeding ensues following tube removal.

For stone management, an alternative to endoscopic surgery that the intensivist may encounter is extracorporeal shock wave lithotripsy (ESWL). This approach involves the noninvasive fragmentation of renal or ureteral calculi with a shock wave generator system under fluoroscopic or ultrasound guidance. The procedure commonly produces transient gross hematuria, which is rarely troublesome, as ESWL does result in some mild blunt trauma to the kidney. The typical procedure involves focally administering approximately 3,000 shocks to the stone(s). Following ESWL, colic can occur due to obstruction from passage of fragments. Whether manageable expectantly with hydration and analgesics, or requiring stent insertion, depends on the stone burden, the amount of debris created, the size of residual fragments, the degree of symptoms, and whether there are signs of infection with obstruction.

Laparoscopy and Robotic Surgery

In urologic surgery in recent years, these techniques have become common and are now a major—if not the primary—modality for a wide range of surgical tasks that were previously performed solely through major open approaches. In many centers, the open radical retropubic prostatectomy (RRP) has been nearly replaced by the robotic-assisted laparoscopic prostatectomy (RALP), and kidney surgery done through a flank incision has been largely replaced by laparoscopic/robotic approaches, both for partial and total nephrectomy. The same special considerations that are relevant to all laparoscopic surgeries are important to urologic laparoscopy. Such common issues include postoperative ileus, CO_2 retention, venous CO_2 embolism, postoperative bleeding, unrecognized intraoperative iatrogenic injury, and trochar and port-site complications (12).

In laparoscopy for renal surgery, there are two potential major sites of postoperative bleeding: the renal pedicle and the renal parenchyma, the latter relevant for partial nephrectomy. The traditional means of controlling vessels in open surgery, using suturing and ligation, is often replaced in laparoscopic surgery with vascular stapling devices and instruments like the harmonic scalpel. The technology has advanced rapidly with these tools, and they are generally reliable and secure. There are, however, user-dependent factors and a learning curve involved in mastering the use of these devices. Bleeding can occur intraoperatively, immediately postoperatively or in a more delayed fashion, and manifest by hemodynamic and laboratory changes, or visible bleeding from instrument ports or incisions. When precipitous and life threatening, a quick return to the OR with either laparoscopic or open reexploration or, if rapidly available, angiographic control may be the most appropriate course. When less emergent and when the luxury of "further evaluation" is appropriate, postoperative CT scanning to determine if there is a renal or perirenal hematoma may be appropriate prior to a surgical intervention. If bleeding occurs from the cut surface of the kidney following either open or laparoscopic partial nephrectomy, angiography with subselective embolization is often the preferred approach.

Drains left within the abdomen, at the anticipated site of blood or urine drainage, following laparoscopic procedures are often placed intraperitoneally, as opposed to the case in extraperitoneal flank surgery, where the drain is often not within the peritoneal cavity. As such, intraperitoneal drains may at times evacuate retained irrigant, peritoneal or lymphatic fluid in variable amounts following surgery. If there is uncertainty as to the significance of increased drain output, fluid may be sent for chemical analysis: creatinine to determine if fluid is urine, amylase to rule out pancreatic fluid leak. Leakage of urine following laparoscopic urologic surgery may not require immediate intervention if the leak is well drained. If action is needed, postoperative ureteral stent insertion, along with an IUBC for optimal drainage or in some cases nephrostomy insertion, will often allow the collecting system to heal without sequelae. In general, drains should be removed as early as possible, as they may potentially allow the entry of bacteria into the abdominal cavity.

In the course of dissection during laparoscopic or robotic urologic surgery, especially if electrocautery is extensively utilized, the risk of unrecognized bowel or other visceral injury must be appreciated. The presentation of such complications may be subtle, with low-grade fever; minimal diffuse tenderness, which may be consistent with the expected postsurgical state; or delayed return of bowel function or persistent anorexia. A high degree of suspicion is important when patients fail to thrive following laparoscopic surgery, and postoperative CT scanning may demonstrate a fluid collection in an unexpected location or inflammatory changes in or near the intestine that would not be otherwise anticipated.

As robotic surgery for radical prostatectomy has now become standard and commonplace, the intensivist may encounter such patients in the postoperative period. The same considerations noted above apply to the RALP patient with regard to suspecting and identifying inadvertent injuries. Gross hematuria causing catheter occlusion is important to recognize, as the vesicourethral anastomosis in these patients is quite delicate and usually performed with a running suture. Clot retention from catheter occlusion can result in bladder distention, which may strain, or cause dehiscence of, the anastomosis. Clear instructions from the urologist should be noted regarding catheter management, what to expect regarding volume and appearance of efflux, and appropriate interventions. If a catheter fails to drain following RALP, cautious irrigation with normal saline is generally safe, using no more than 60 mL. If a small clot is present and this maneuver results in normal clear efflux, no further action is necessary. Otherwise, the urologist should be informed and should provide specific intervention instructions or deal with the situation personally. Under no circumstances should anyone but the operating urologist remove and/or attempt replacement of an IUBC during the early perioperative period following major lower tract urologic surgery, especially when a fresh anastomosis or reconstructive site is present such as post-RALP for after cystectomy with orthotopic urinary diversion; such manipulation without direct visualization may disrupt the reconstruction site and cause major additional complications.

Genital Surgery

Issues that may arise with these procedures, in the ICU, relate to urologic prosthetic devices such as penile, artificial sphincter, testicular prostheses; neurologic stimulator implants; or complications of the wide range of other genital and perineal procedures urologists perform. Dressings on the genitalia should be inspected for bleeding or excessive tightness, which can cause vascular compromise, especially if applied circumferentially around the penis. Paraphimosis, persistently retracted foreskin, must be promptly recognized and corrected. Any major local complaint by a patient following genital surgery should be referred to the urologic surgeon for input. It is important for the intensivist to know that a genitourinary prosthesis has been implanted. Obviously, there should never be any needle placement or incisional procedure performed by a nonurologist in the region of the genitalia in the setting of a prosthetic implant, as the fluid-filled components are prone to damage. If a patient with an artificial urinary sphincter (AUS) device needs an IUBC inserted, it is important that the device be deactivated (i.e., cycled and appropriately locked in an open position with the urethral cuff deflated). Forcibly passing a Foley catheter into the urethra of an AUS patient risks damage to the urethra and erosion of the device. Infection and erosion can occur with any of the urologic prostheses, occasionally resulting in abscess formation and/or major soft tissue infections and, potentially, sepsis; explantation and drainage procedures may be necessary, which require urologic surgical expertise. If uncertain as to how to approach any genitourinary prosthesis, it is best to seek urologic consultation. Other genital surgery procedures such as vasectomy, testicular biopsy, reconstructive microsurgery for fertility treatment, and orchiectomy for tumor or benign disease can be complicated by bleeding or infection. If marked swelling occurs following genital surgery, the urologist should be immediately made aware. Orchiectomy for tumor is performed through an inguinal incision and involves removing the testis, its investing tunics, and the spermatic cord to the level of the internal inguinal ring. If bleeding occurs from the stump of the spermatic cord, hematoma can develop in the retroperitoneum and require high exploration for control.

UROLOGIC TRAUMA

Trauma centers vary markedly with regard to the role played by the urologist in trauma management. Some highly respected centers utilize the urologist's expertise routinely for assistance with the management of genitourinary injuries, while others include the urologist only selectively. At our trauma center, the urology service plays a central role in the assessment and management of urologic injuries, participating in the selection and interpretation of imaging studies, the decision of when to operate, and the operative intervention itself (13). As such, we have achieved a high level of cooperation between our service and the trauma surgery and critical care medicine services.

Herein, we will address the basic approach to the diagnosis and management of urologic trauma, with a recommendation that the urologist be included whenever feasible in management decisions (14). We will address management of iatrogenic urinary tract trauma, followed by trauma from external violence for renal, ureteral, bladder, urethral, and genital injuries with regard to assessment and management, and discuss the relevance of damage control strategies in urologic trauma. The urologist's experience in elective urologic surgery; endoscopic, radiologic, and open surgical intervention; reconstructive approaches; and management of complications may be very helpful to the trauma and critical care teams when faced with the multiply injured patient or one with solitary urologic organ trauma. When no urologist is available, however, or when critical care decisions need to be made in the absence of urologic input, the intensivist or the acute care/trauma or general surgeon must have a working knowledge of the approach to the most common and important types of urologic trauma.

Evidenced-based Urologic Trauma guidelines have recently been published through both the U.S. and international urologic professional organizations; those with an interest in this specialized area of trauma care may find these reports of particular interest (11,15).

Iatrogenic Injury Management

The concern for, or recognition of, the occurrence of an iatrogenic urologic injury provokes significant anxiety in the surgical team. Having a basic concept of the common forms of injury, the procedures introducing significant injury risk, and the standard approach to management is essential in maintaining a focus on prompt resolution of the problem (16–19).

For uncomplicated bladder injuries, simple suture closure is feasible as long as the injury involves the upper bladder segment, the trigone is uninvolved, and there is not significant tissue loss. A running, two-layer closure using heavy absorbable suture is standard. A generously sized IUBC should be used—20 French or larger—to allow drainage of bloody efflux and allow efficient irrigation when needed. If the bladder wall surrounding the injury is markedly abnormal (fibrotic, friable, irradiated), a two-layer closure may not be feasible. In these cases, we prefer a one-layer, interrupted closure with heavy suture, with a plan to leave the bladder catheterized for a longer period of time.

If there is involvement of the trigone, ureteral orifices, or intramural ureters, the situation is more complex, and ureteral stent insertion or ureteral reimplantation may be needed. This is best accomplished with urologic support, and may involve placing an externalized single-J or internalized double-J ureteral stent, then suturing the bladder injury. If a stricture ultimately forms, endoscopic management or delayed elective ureteral reimplantation is always an option. Feeding tubes may also be temporarily passed up the ureters during the bladder repair to identify and protect the ureters, and support performing a safe cystorrhaphy (bladder repair). Prophylactic insertion of externalized ureteral catheters prior to complex pelvic or retroperitoneal surgery may be helpful in avoiding surgical injury to the ureter, though their efficacy in reducing the risk of ureteral injury is not universally accepted (20).

For iatrogenic ureteral injuries, the approach for repair depends on the level of injury, whether there is loss of ureteral length, the condition of the ureter and surrounding tissue, and the comfort of the surgeon. Traditional urologic teaching states that if the ureter is transected caudal to the crossing of the internal iliac artery, a reimplantation rather than a primary anastomosis should be performed. This policy reflects the concern for the viability of the distal ureteral stump in the setting of abnormal pelvic anatomy and surgical insult. The reimplantation can be performed with or without a "psoas hitch"—suturing the upper bladder segment to the ipsilateral psoas muscle fascia—depending on ureteral length and bladder status. For injuries in the mid or upper ureter, primary, spatulated anastomosis performed over an indwelling stent is the preferred solution. As long as one is dissecting outside the ureteral adventitial sheath, substantial length can be gained by mobilizing the ureter toward the kidney and deep into the pelvis with devascularization unlikely. If primary ureteral repair is not possible, the options include ligation followed by nephrostomy insertion and planned delayed reconstruction, transureteroureterostomy, renal autotransplantation, or ileal ureteral replacement, neither of which is usually appropriate in the acute care surgery setting.

When dissecting in the groin, especially in the setting of a redo hernia, the spermatic cord is at risk for injury. If there is injury to cord vasculature, precise suture ligation of bleeding points should occur, as a hematoma around the cord is very problematic. If there is concern for devascularization of the testis, use of a fine-tipped Doppler probe to detect an arterial pulse distal to the area of dissection or over the testis itself is helpful. Even if one is quite concerned that most of the cord vasculature has been lost, we would generally recommend leaving the testis in place and observing it, as the testis has redundant blood supplies—internal spermatic, external spermatic, and vasal arteries, which come from aortic, external iliac, and internal iliac sources, respectively—and may survive on collateral blood supply. The status of the testis can be addressed postoperatively.

Penetrating and Blunt Trauma to the Genitourinary System

General Evaluation

Diagnosis of urinary tract injury is typically based on history and mechanism of injury, physical examination, laboratory assessment, and the findings on imaging studies (21). Any patient with a history of gross hematuria following trauma should be imaged, unless of course he or she is unstable and/or must be taken directly to surgery (22). In addition, current literature supports obtaining contrast imaging studies for patients with microscopic hematuria and hypotension at any time following trauma, as well as those patients with significant deceleration mechanisms of injury and other injury factors that portend a high risk of urinary tract injury, such as lower posterior rib fracture, transverse spinal process fracture, or pelvic or femur fracture. The contrast-enhanced CT scan of the abdomen and pelvis has become the standard study of choice for assessment of hematuria, for staging of injuries in the trauma setting, and for the evaluation of renal or ureteral injuries. The "shock room intravenous pyelogram (IVP)" has fallen out of favor, provides much less information than the CT scan, and is uncommonly utilized. Bladder injuries may be suspected based on the presence of gross hematuria following pelvic trauma, with confirmation by either standard radiographic or CT cystography. Adequate bladder filling must be accomplished to demonstrate extravasation and minimize false-negative studies. When urethral injury is suspected following pelvic fracture or perineal or genital trauma, especially when blood is exiting from the urethra or present at the urethral meatus, retrograde urethrography should be performed prior to any attempt at urethral catheterization, to avoid exacerbating a partial urethral rupture. For genital trauma, scrotal ultrasonography may be of great value in diagnosing testicular rupture from blunt forces; in penetrating genital trauma, surgical exploration is usually necessary and one can often forego genital imaging studies.

Urethral Injuries

These are suspected in cases of pelvic fracture, particularly with severe pubic diastasis and vertical shear injuries. A urethrogram that demonstrates contrast extravasation is diagnostic (23). Some urologists may be comfortable with a careful attempt at catheter insertion under cystoscopic guidance, or a fluoroscopically and endoscopically guided catheter realignment procedure, though whether this approach provides outcome advantages over traditional SP diversion remains controversial (24,25). The standard approach remains immediate postinjury SP tube insertion. Certainly any nonurologist should handle such injuries with placement of an SP catheter, obtaining urologic consultation when available. SP cystostomy insertion may be accomplished using trochar-based percutaneous systems if the bladder is adequately distended and the required kit is available. If not, or if most expeditious—as for a patient undergoing an emergent laparotomy—an open surgical approach in the OR is preferable. Blunt trauma to the perineum with crush injury and complete bulbar urethral rupture is also best handled with SP diversion. Penetrating injuries to the urethra can be managed in a delayed fashion with SP diversion or, if the injury is readily apparent and accessible, direct suture repair with fine absorbable suture may be attempted in the stable patient. All such injuries can be managed in a delayed fashion as long as proximal urinary diversion is achieved acutely. In the absence of advanced specialty expertise, temporary SP tube diversion and referral to a reconstructive urology center is a wise strategy.

Bladder Injuries

These are most often diagnosed on cystography (26) or by gross intraoperative observation. Many blunt injuries to the bladder can be managed with catheter drainage alone, if the injury is uncomplicated and *extraperitoneal*; this type of bladder trauma is often related to pelvic fracture. An adequate-bore IUBC—20 French or larger—is preferable to evacuate grossly bloody efflux. If there is failure of catheter management, such as continued profuse hematuria with repeated occlusion of the catheter or continued urinary extravasation, surgical repair may be necessary. If it is necessary to surgically repair such an injury, a high midline cystotomy should be made to avoid entering into a fresh retropubic hematoma, the result of which could result in problematic bleeding. The laceration may be sutured in a single layer transvesically by placing retractors into the bladder and exposing the injury. Other variants of extraperitoneal bladder injury that benefit from surgical repair, as opposed to catheter drainage alone, include those which involve communication with a vaginal or rectal injury, or are in communication with an open pelvic fracture. An SP tube, in addition to the urethral IUBC, may be left indwelling in cases in which the repair is tenuous or prolonged tube drainage is anticipated, such as in closed head or spinal cord injuries. In uncomplicated cases, performing a contrast cystogram via the IUBC at approximately 10 to 14 days post injury, and prior to catheter removal, ensures complete healing before stressing the bladder.

For *intraperitoneal* bladder injuries direct suture repair is required. Such injuries result in entry of urine directly into the peritoneal cavity, which must be controlled to avoid urinary ascites, sepsis, azotemia, and other complications. These injuries typically result from sudden compression of the full bladder—such as from a blow to the lower abdomen, or seatbelt compression in a motor vehicle crash—causing a large bladder dome laceration. Transabdominal suture repair is straightforward; under appropriate circumstances, such repair may be performed laparoscopically with success. We generally place a urethral IUBC and do not use SP tubes in such cases.

Ureteral Injury

These are usually noted upon abdominal exploration in the penetrating trauma setting, or may be noted by observing urinary extravasation on preoperative CT scanning (27). It is necessary to obtain a delayed excretory phase on the CT, such that the excreted contrast column has transited the entire ureter, or the risk of missing a ureteral injury is significant. Injuries from penetrating trauma are managed similarly to the approach described above for iatrogenic injuries, or by applying damage control techniques when necessary (see below). For gunshot wounds to the mid and upper ureter, limited debridement to the viable ureter, careful extra-adventitial mobilization, and spatulated suture anastomosis is appropriate. For distal ureteral injuries, reimplantation into the bladder (ureteroneocystostomy) is a more dependable approach, as the problem of the distal stump having impaired vascularity is avoided. Ureteral injuries from blunt trauma are rare; exceptions would include the pediatric population, where ureteropelvic avulsion injuries or renal pelvic lacerations may occur following blunt injuries. When major injury occurs to the urinary tract following seemingly trivial trauma, one should be suspicious of the presence of previously existent underlying pathology of the urinary tract such as neoplasm or congenital ureteropelvic junction obstruction.

Renal Injuries

These are typically staged by contrast-enhanced CT using the American Association for the Surgery of Trauma (AAST) Organ Injury Scaling system (28,29). Renal injuries are managed according to a multifactorial decision process that considers injury grade, whether due to blunt or penetrating forces, patient clinical status and hemodynamic stability, and the presence of other nonurologic injuries (30,31). In general, for *blunt renal injury*, grade I, II, and III injuries are routinely managed nonoperatively. *Grade IV* injuries, which involve deeper, significant parenchymal injury and laceration to the collecting system, or branch renal vessel injuries, require a selective approach, largely influenced by hemodynamic parameters and degree of progressive blood loss, and often warrant ICU monitoring to address whether continued bleeding or urinoma formation occurs, which may warrant delayed intervention (32). The majority of such injuries in most series do not require early exploration, and the observation of extravasation from the collecting system is not, in itself, an absolute indication for surgical exploration. If there is extensive medial extravasation on CT, retrograde pyelography may be indicated to exclude a major injury to the renal pelvis or proximal ureter. *Grade V* injuries from blunt trauma routinely require surgical exploration and often nephrectomy; most reported results of attempts to manage true grade V injuries nonoperatively have not resulted in favorable outcomes. Renal pedicle injuries, considered in both the grade IV and V groups, require careful consideration to select appropriate management. When the kidney suffers a pedicle stretch injury from deceleration trauma, resulting in arterial intimal disruption, the artery can thrombose, resulting in renal devascularization (33); this can be diagnosed on CT scan with the finding of renal nonperfusion. If the vessels are thrombosed but not avulsed or lacerated, the decision of whether to operate to revascularize the kidney depends on how much time has elapsed—which predicts renal salvage—as well as the patient's other injuries and ability to tolerate a laparotomy. After 30 minutes of warm ischemia, irreversible renal damage begins; by 3 hours, the kidney is probably not retrievable. If there is a pedicle avulsion injury, surgery is mandatory to prevent early or delayed catastrophic bleeding.

For *penetrating renal trauma*, the standard approach has traditionally been surgical exploration and repair, or nephrectomy. This view has evolved over the past two decades, however, with reports demonstrating favorable outcomes from nonoperative management of carefully selected penetrating injuries. It has been reported that up to 50% of renal stab wounds and over 20% of renal gunshot wounds may be successfully managed nonoperatively. When comparing the approach to blunt versus penetrating trauma, one must consider the high likelihood of there being associated injuries in penetrating trauma. Still, a fully staged penetrating kidney injury—based on CT—may be appropriately managed nonoperatively if certain conditions are met. These include, in my view, a lateral or polar parenchymal injury, which spares the renal sinus or deep central region of the kidney; a hemodynamic stable patient; a low suspicion of injury to the extrarenal collecting system or ureter. The larger the renal hematoma, the less comfortable I am with nonoperative management of a penetrating renal injury. Proactive angiography may be considered when weighing the safety of a nonoperative approach to the penetrating renal injury in selected cases; admission to the ICU is essential to monitor for renewed bleeding. It should be stated for the intensivist that the default mode for penetrating trauma to genitourinary organs is operative exploration and repair; departure from this approach is appropriate when complete staging information is available that predicts a favorable outcome for a specific injury with a nonoperative approach, the patient is hemodynamically stable, and careful monitoring for failure of nonoperative management can be carried out. Criteria and a plan for changing to an operative strategy should exist.

Genital Injuries

These require specialized care and should be handled by practitioners experienced in genital surgery. As a general principle, a very conservative approach to genital debridement should be maintained, with tissues of questionable viability reassessed in a delayed fashion. Nearly all penetrating genital injuries should be acutely surgically explored, assuming the patient is sufficiently stable to undergo a reconstructive effort. Penetrating penile injuries are repaired surgically by closing lacerations to the tunica albuginea of the corpus cavernosum, urethral repair, and skin and soft tissue reconstruction. Penetrating testicular injuries can usually be repaired by closing the tunica albuginea of the testis after debriding nonviable testicular parenchyma. Blunt fracture of the penis, which results from forcible flexing of the penile shaft during erection—often due to trauma during intercourse—should be explored and repaired acutely upon presentation, to achieve the most favorable cosmetic and functional outcome. For blunt scrotal injury, it is often useful to assess the patient with scrotal ultrasonography to determine if testicular rupture is present; it may be difficult to determine this on physical examination if there is scrotal wall swelling, which makes identification of internal structures difficult. Ultrasound is quite accurate for detecting testicular rupture: loss of capsular continuity or marked heterogeneity of testicular parenchyma is predictive of rupture. Testicular salvage is enhanced by early exploration and repair.

Damage Control Strategies for the Management of Urologic Injury in the Unstable Patient

Damage control approaches to the management of the unstable trauma patient have become well accepted in the trauma center setting. This concept refers to abbreviating the initial operative effort in order to minimize the effects of prolonged surgery, which results in progressive metabolic deterioration. Critical injuries—surgical bleeding, fecal contamination sources—are addressed, while noncritical injuries are handled in a delayed fashion, on a subsequent visit to the OR after ICU stabilization. This approach avoids development of the "lethal triad" of progressive acidosis, hypothermia, and coagulopathy, which occurs in critically injured patients when initial surgical efforts are prolonged. Many urologic injuries are quite amenable to initial management by applying damage control strategies (34). With the exception of severe renal or bladder bleeding cases, urinary tract injuries rarely directly result in early mortality. When, in the surgeon's judgment, the patient would not tolerate the magnitude of reconstructive effort needed to deal definitively with a urologic injury at initial laparotomy—due to pattern of injury, hypothermia, acidosis, coagulopathy, or other parameters that mandate a damage control approach—certain temporary solutions may be very desirable (35). We have gained substantial experience with such approaches in our center, and have achieved an effective working relationship with the trauma surgeons in patient selection and technical approach for such cases.

Renal injuries that are incompletely staged, or unstaged, may be approached with delayed assessment and exploration, as long as a determination is made that early exsanguinating bleeding from the injury is unlikely. In the absence of significant bleeding from the renal fossa into the peritoneal cavity, a large midline hematoma, or an expanding or pulsatile renal hematoma, one can elect to leave the perinephric hematoma undisturbed and either obtain postoperative imaging during the resuscitation phase following initial laparotomy, or explore at the time of a second-look procedure. If the kidney is already surgically exposed, hemostasis for major bleeding from parenchyma or branch renal vessels can be rapidly obtained. If a major reconstructive effort is still needed in the unstable patient, packing the kidney and returning for reconstructive interventions later is also an option.

Ureteral injuries may be initially managed with externalized stenting, ligation, or simple local drainage. Of these options, we favor externalized stenting, as it allows control of the urinary output, minimizes ongoing urinary extravasation, and can be maintained for several days until the patient is stable enough to return to surgery for definitive reconstruction. A 7-French or 8.5-French single-J urinary diversion stent can be placed into the ureter through the injury site and advanced proximally into the kidney, then externalized through the abdominal wall. The stent should be tied to the very end of the injured ureter at the injury site, so as not to lose ureteral length by ligating it more proximally and making later reconstruction more challenging. The distal ureteral limb is best left undisturbed; ligating it requires subsequent debridement and causes further tissue loss.

A similar approach can be utilized for extensive bladder injuries: the ureteral orifices can be catheterized, the catheters externalized, and the pelvis packed, leaving bladder reconstruction to be performed at a more suitable time, following appropriate resuscitation. Urethral and genital injuries are also amenable to damage control approaches, generally involving tube urinary diversion, placement of moistened dressings, and tissue preservation until definitive reconstruction following appropriate resuscitation.

UROLOGIC TUBES AND DRAINS FOR THE INTENSIVIST

Tube drainage and diversion of the urinary tract and adjacent areas constitute important and commonly employed strategies in urologic care and urologic surgery. The safe insertion, maintenance, and management of such tubes are essential to avoid preventable morbidity and support appropriate medical and surgical management. The frequently utilized tubes that may be encountered by the critical care provider include nephrostomy, SP cystostomy, IUBC (urethral Foley catheter), and internal ureteral stents. In addition, externalized drains are often placed near the site of urologic surgery or injuries and employed for various purposes including drainage of blood, infectious fluid, lymph, or extravasated urine. The general principles behind urologic tube drainage along with specific management considerations for the different types of tube mentioned above will be addressed in this section (36,37).

Tubes placed within the urinary tract may be intended as temporary or permanent solutions to various urologic problems, including bladder muscle failure and obstructive upper or lower tract lesions. Patients with detrusor muscle failure require regular bladder emptying, which may be managed by intermittent catheterization—typically utilizing a clean/nonsterile technique—or by an indwelling catheter; in the case of indwelling catheters, the options include an IUBC or an SP cystostomy tube. In the male, due to the potential morbidity of a long-term IUBC—including urethral erosion, periurethral abscess, epididymitis, and traumatic hypospadias—the SP tube is often favored. Nearly all patients with indwelling bladder catheters of either variety will become bacteriuric, but patients with SP tubes are less likely to develop the list of urethral catheter-related complications noted above. In women, long-term urethral catheters are better tolerated, though the urethra may gradually become dilated and capacious, resulting in troublesome leakage around the tube.

Urethral Catheters

Urethral catheter placement techniques are well known. If a standard IUBC is needed but resistance is met during placement, it is important not to force the catheter into the urethra, which risks urethral mucosal perforation, creation of a false passage, and bleeding, greatly complicating further catheterization attempts; this principle is relevant both to the trauma and nontrauma setting. The catheter balloon should not be inflated until urine return is assured; if no urinary drainage occurs upon catheter insertion, aspiration of the catheter using a piston syringe should occur before balloon inflation. In general, most catheter balloons should be inflated with a full 10 mL of saline or water to avoid inadvertent distal balloon migration into the urethra. Some balloons are rated to 30-mL inflation volume or greater; this information is clearly printed on the catheter inflation hub. If a standard catheter will not advance into the bladder, options include trying a smaller catheter, using a Coudé catheter, or requesting urologic consultation. If obstruction is met deep in the urethra in the male, the Coudé catheter is particularly helpful, as the curved tip will often navigate over an enlarged prostate and bladder neck and solve the problem. If resistance is met more distally in the penile or distal bulbar urethra, a stricture may be present for which a smaller catheter may be of benefit. Beyond these measures, the safest approach is to seek urologic expertise to assist with bladder access.

In the female, urethral catheter insertion is seldom difficult; true urethral strictures are uncommon—seen occasionally following radiation therapy or local surgery—as the urethra is generally straight and short. At times, due to atrophic changes, the female urethral meatus may be difficult to identify visually. In such cases, the meatus is often retracted onto the distal anterior vaginal wall. We can typically palpate it with a gloved fingertip and guide a catheter into the appropriate location. Problems in placing a female urethral catheter not solved by the above technique or by using a smaller tube may indicate significantly abnormal anatomy and should prompt urologic consultation.

In the hospital setting, patients often arrive in the ICU with an indwelling catheter in place. It is important to verify that, on arrival, the catheter is properly positioned and is draining properly. It is remarkable how often we are consulted for a mysteriously malfunctioning catheter only to find that most of the catheter shaft length is outside the meatus, and the balloon is easily palpable in the perineum or penis, plainly indicative of malposition. If a catheter appears properly positioned but fails to drain, it should be irrigated with 60 to 120 mL of normal saline or water; it should be possible to infuse and withdraw the instilled irrigant. If the catheter is not draining spontaneously and one can infuse but not withdraw fluid, the catheter may be malpositioned and will likely require repositioning or replacement. When changing a chronic indwelling catheter for routine purposes (generally monthly is advised), choose a convenient time when help is readily available in case difficulty is encountered, not in the middle of the night shift. If a patient forcibly removes a catheter with the balloon inflated, dramatic urethral bleeding often occurs. Catheter replacement is typically necessary, and may be difficult due to deep laceration of the urethral mucosa. We would recommend trying to pass a Coudé catheter with the tip pointed cephalad; if not successful, obtain urologic assistance. The cost of iatrogenic urinary catheter-related trauma is considerable; this common procedure should be carried out with due respect and caution, with a liberal approach to urologic consultation when challenges arise (38).

Suprapubic Cystostomy Tubes

SP cystostomy tubes are straightforward devices that may be used as a temporary bladder drain or as a permanent strategy as noted above. SP tubes can be placed in the awake patient under local anesthesia using trochar-based kits, or can be placed through an open surgical approach under anesthesia in the OR. If placed percutaneously, it is essential that the bladder be well distended prior to insertion. If this is not the case, the trochar—over which the catheter is advanced—can penetrate fully through the bladder lumen and pierce the posterior bladder wall, causing bladder injury and potentially injuring the vagina or rectum, or can injure intraperitoneal structures; signs of such adjacent organ injury should prompt immediate surgical and urologic consultation. Once in place, an SP tube should generally be left indwelling for at least a week so that an established track forms between the skin and the bladder lumen. If an SP tube is intended to remain indwelling for an extended period, we prefer to perform the first tube change after at least a month, so that a mature track will be present. If prematurely removed, extravasation of urine into the retropubic and perivesical space may occur, which can result in urine absorption, azotemia, or urosepsis. A long-term indwelling SP tube through an established track is usually easy to change by simple removal and replacement with the same caliber and type of tube. Occasionally the track may be oblique or tortuous and direct visualization with a flexible cystoscope by a urologist and placement of the new tube over a guidewire may be necessary. If an SP tube is inadvertently removed or displaced, the track may close within a matter of hours, certainly over the course of a day or so, even when the tube has been in place long term. It is important that tube replacement be accomplished promptly to avoid track closure and the need to reestablish access in a more invasive manner.

It is important to realize, as noted above, that nearly all indwelling urinary tract tubes that communicate with the external environment will result in bacteriuria, often within about 10 days of tube placement (39). In most cases this is a harmless process and does not result in clinical infection. If, however, urinary tract manipulation or an invasive urinary tract procedure is planned, instrumentation in the face of such bacteriuria may precipitate urosepsis, as the tissues are vulnerable to intravasation of bacteria when a chronic catheter has been present. It is beneficial to obtain urine culture data and institute therapy with culture-specific agents prior to significant instrumentation of the chronically catheterized urinary tract, to minimize the risk of iatrogenically induced clinical infection or urosepsis.

The same principle applies when considering removal of an indwelling bladder tube, especially when there is the potential for the patient failing a voiding trial and developing urinary retention following catheter removal, as in BPH patients with episodic retention who may or may not pass a voiding trial. If a patient with catheter-related bacteriuria develops urinary retention upon catheter removal, the risk of clinical infection or urosepsis is significant. These patients, as well, should have coverage with culture-specific antibiotics whenever possible, or at least have the provision of empiric broad-spectrum urinary antibiotics—fluoroquinolone or extended-spectrum penicillin derivative—prior to a voiding trial. Such patients are likely to have resistant organisms, as they have often been in the hospital environment.

Nephrostomy Tubes

Nephrostomy tubes are placed directly through the renal parenchyma into the collecting system to provide proximal ipsilateral urinary tract drainage and diversion. They may be placed percutaneously under fluoroscopic, CT, or ultrasound guidance in an IR suite, or in the OR as part of a urologic surgical procedure through radiologic, endoscopic, or open techniques. Several types of tube are available and intensivists should know what type of tube they are dealing with. Most commonly used are the loop nephrostomy tubes, which have some type of retention system, usually consisting of a pull-string that is deployed upon tube placement to allow it to be retained effectively within the collecting system. Percutaneously placed tubes are usually in the range of 8 to 12 French in size and are attached to drainage bags with connector tubing. Tubes placed as part of percutaneous stone or other upper tract surgical procedures may be larger; often IUBCs ranging from 16 to 24 French in size are employed. In such cases the tube is usually sutured to the skin for retention, as inflating the balloon is problematic in the renal collecting system and may impair drainage or stress or tear the delicate collecting system wall. Intensivists should be entirely clear as to what is expected with regard to such tubes under their care; a conversation with the urologist or whomever is responsible for the tube insertion and familiar with its specific purpose is desirable: Is it expected to drain continuously? What action should be taken if it fails to drain? How should bloody efflux be interpreted or acted upon? The purposes of these tubes may vary from providing a large-bore drain after a bloody percutaneous lithotripsy to a small tube placed only to drain urine for an obstructed ureter. It may be safe to irrigate nephrostomy tubes if they fail to drain, but again, this should be arranged by specific order, and assumptions regarding the purpose and management approach to such tubes introduce unnecessary risk. When irrigating a nephrostomy after determining that doing so is safe and appropriate, a small volume of saline—5 to 10 mL—should be utilized. If, in the postoperative urologic surgery setting, a nephrostomy tube begins to drain blood at an alarming rate, the best course of action may be to clamp the tube, address hemodynamics urgently, and rapidly call the urologist for instructions. As for other tubes mentioned above, the collecting system will become colonized with bacteria after being indwelling for a week or so, and clamping trials, manipulation, or tube removal is best done following provision of culture-specific or at least empiric antibiotics (37,40).

Internal Ureteral Stents

Internal ureteral stents are commonly used in urology, often for the purpose of relieving ureteral obstruction, but also following urologic surgery or trauma to allow low-pressure drainage or provide urinary diversion while the trauma of surgery or local edema or inflammatory changes are allowed to resolve. The most common variety of stent is the internal double-J stent; these stents have a loop in the bladder and a loop in the kidney. They are placed either retrograde via cystoscopy or antegrade during open or percutaneous surgery, over a guidewire. The proximal and distal coils form upon removal of the guidewire. Typical sizes in adults are 6- to 7-French caliber and 22 to 28 cm length, depending on the patient's height and ureteral length and tortuosity. Some stents include a pull-string on the distal coil, which, at the urologist's discretion, may be either cut short or allowed to exit the external urethral meatus to aid in subsequent removal without requiring repeat cystoscopy. Patient care personnel should be instructed as to the presence of a pull-string and should be aware of the importance of not pulling on it or allowing the patient to do so. Stents are of great value in urologic surgery but they do have their pitfalls, mainly related to their small caliber and proneness to obstruction, the potential for them to migrate and become malpositioned, their tendency to cause unpleasant flank or bladder symptoms, and the risk that they may be forgotten and lost to follow-up. In the ICU, the major issues relate to obstruction, migration, or infection. Significant flank pain, chills or fever, or a change in stent position on serial abdominal radiographs should prompt urologic consultation to address these stent-related complications. Stent occlusion with resultant ureteral obstruction, in the setting of proximal infection, is a surgical emergency that may result in sepsis, and require immediate urologic intervention in the form of endoscopic stent replacement or urgent nephrostomy insertion. Many stents are certified for a 3- to 6-month maximum indwelling time, after which they need to be changed to avoid calcification and obstruction. Some stents are specifically designed for long indwelling times—used for persistent obstructive states such as benign or malignant retroperitoneal fibrosis or postradiation strictures—of up to 12 months. There are stents that combine the function of an externalized nephrostomy and an internal stent; these are usually termed nephrostents or "universal stents." They can be capped at the flank entry point and made to drain internally, or may be uncapped to drain as an externalized nephrostomy tube. Nephrostomy change or removal and stent change or removal should only be performed by a urologist or interventional radiologist or upon his or her specific direction.

For a patient presenting with symptomatic upper tract obstruction, such as for an obstructing ureteral calculus, the option often exists to observe, or provide relief with stent insertion or nephrostomy placement (41), depending on the details of the clinical situation. The decision of how to manage such patients acutely depends on the ability to get the patient to either the cystoscopy suite or the IR suite more expeditiously, the expertise available, and the clinical picture. For acutely ill patients with an obstructed, infected upper tract, many urologists prefer to have IR place a nephrostomy tube percutaneously, control the infection, and then reserve any retrograde instrumentation or definitive stone management for an elective setting. If the patient is coagulopathic or anticoagulated, a retrograde cystoscopic approach may be safer, as the radiologist will be quite reticent to enter the kidney percutaneously when the coagulation functions are abnormal for fear of creating a major hemorrhagic complication.

Closed Suction Drains or Penrose Drains

These drains may be left in place following urologic surgery to allow external drainage of blood, urine, lymph, or infectious fluid. From the intensivist viewpoint, the urologist should be asked specifically what should be expected regarding appropriate function of the drain and exactly what parameters should be a cause for concern: Is significant blood output expected? Is continuous drainage important? Under what circumstances should the surgeon be informed urgently? Urine leaks following certain types of urologic surgery, such as some partial nephrectomies for trauma, may be expected, and if adequately drained externally, seldom constitute an emergency. Elevated blood output may be an indication of internal bleeding and should prompt a call to the surgeon if there is any doubt as to whether the situation is acceptable.

As a general statement to the ICU team, urologic drainage tubes have widely varying purposes and specifications and should be managed in concert with the surgeon who placed them or is responsible for them to avoid confusion and preventable complications.

URINARY DIVERSION MANAGEMENT FROM THE ICU PERSPECTIVE

Beyond the considerations regarding tube diversion or drainage, some patients under the critical care team's care may have undergone, either acutely or remotely, a surgical urinary diversion procedure, most commonly utilizing a bowel segment. The variety of such diversions is considerable, and the ICU team deserves a full explanation of the patient's anatomy and how to deal with any problems that may arise. Urinary outflow obstruction, intra-abdominal urinary extravasation, infectious complications, and problems with the intestinal anastomosis may occur with any type of urinary diversion. One can divide urinary diversion procedures into conduits and reservoirs, and reservoirs may be subdivided into cutaneous and orthotopic.

Conduits are simple surgical reconstructions that allow urine to exit to the outside and do not involve an internal urinary reservoir (42). An *ileal conduit* is one of the most commonly encountered urinary diversions, often performed following cystectomy for lower urinary tract cancer, but also at times for neurogenic or inflammatory disease or devastating pelvic trauma. In this procedure, a segment of distal ileum is isolated from the fecal stream, followed by a small bowel anastomosis to reestablish intestinal continuity. The proximal end of the isolated segment is closed and the distal end is brought to the skin of the abdominal wall as a stoma. The ureters are sutured into the conduit intra-abdominally to route the urinary stream externally. Most ileal conduits seen acutely by the ICU team in the immediate post-surgical period have indwelling tube drainage present—often externalized stents that enter the stoma, travel up each ureter to allow the ureteroileal anastomosis to heal, and avoid obstruction or urinary extravasation in the early postoperative period. A second tube, often a simple straight catheter segment, may also be placed from outside the stoma to inside the conduit beneath the abdominal wall fascia to allow conduit drainage.

Other conduits employed in urologic surgery may utilize other bowel segments, including jejunum and descending or transverse colon, especially when there has been extensive pelvic irradiation that has damaged the ileum and lower small intestine.

Reservoirs (neobladders) involve the use of larger segments of intestine to fashion a neobladder reservoir internally, along with some form of urinary efflux mechanism, often designed to create a continent diversion that the patient can catheterize—and not wear a urinary collection appliance—or that is sutured to the native urethra, in either the male or female, to allow restoration of voiding (an "orthotopic neobladder").

While conduits may be complicated by obstruction or urinary leakage as noted above, and the same issues can arise in neobladder reservoirs, the reservoir urinary diversions can develop certain other potentially serious problems including "pouchitis," pouch rupture, and formation of pouch calculi. These issues require specialty input and prompt urologic consultation. The issue of pouch rupture, however, deserves specific mention as this must be promptly recognized. Any patient with signs of abdominal infection, peritonitis or sepsis who has a neobladder should raise the suspicion of pouch rupture. This entity can also be seen in patients who have had an augmentation cystoplasty, in which a segment of bowel is added to the native bladder to increase capacity or deal with severe and intransigent overactive bladder symptoms. Such patients should have urgent urologic assessment, which may involve contrast imaging studies—CT or "pouchography"—to rule out urinary leakage intra-abdominally. Broad-spectrum antibiotics should be instituted early in such cases, as the urine is often colonized and intra-abdominal infection may develop. Many such cases of minimal or contained rupture can be managed with tube drainage of the neobladder alone although, in some cases, surgical exploration and repair, and/or evacuation of infectious fluid from the abdominal cavity are necessary.

Depending on the type of urinary diversion and the specific segment of the gastrointestinal tract used for the reconstruction, these patients may be at risk for dehydration, and specific electrolyte and metabolic disturbances may be seen (43,44). The significance of these problems is related to the portion of the gastrointestinal tract utilized for the diversion and the length of time the urine is exposed to the bowel surface. Jejunal conduits may result in hyponatremic, hypochloremic metabolic acidosis; this process may be clinically manifested by nausea, vomiting, anorexia, and muscular weakness. When ileum and colon are utilized for the urinary diversion, hyperchloremic metabolic acidosis may also be seen. Clinically this may produce weakness, anorexia, vomiting, or Kussmaul breathing, and may progress to coma; this process was seen more commonly in the past when ureterosigmoidostomy was a commonly used form of diversion. With appropriate metabolic management, it is much less commonly noted with contemporary conduit or continent diversions. When gastric segments are utilized for urinary diversion, dehydration and hyponatremic metabolic alkalosis may occur, requiring replacement of sodium and chloride through intravenous salt administration.

Other metabolic abnormalities seen with urinary diversion procedures may include altered bile salt metabolism following ileal resection, which can affect fat digestion and uptake of vitamins A and D; malabsorption and steatorrhea and a propensity to develop cholelithiasis may also be associated with ileal resection; and gastric or ileal resection may cause vitamin B_{12} deficiency, which can lead to megaloblastic anemia and peripheral nerve dysfunction, for which B_{12} nutritional supplementation may be indicated.

Other complications include stomal stenosis, recurrent upper tract urinary infection and deteriorating renal function, and calculus formation in the upper tract or within the diversion conduit or reservoir. Stomal stenosis may cause obstructive uropathy requiring catheterization and stomal revision. Catheter insertion into a conduit or reservoir construct may be challenging; if difficulty is encountered, a small-bore Coudé catheter may be useful, as may use of fluoroscopy to guide catheter positioning. Stomal bleeding is usually superficial and manageable with local compression or minimal cautery when necessary. Parastomal hernias may occasionally become incarcerated requiring urgent surgical intervention. Azotemia and upper tract dilation may be problematic, especially when more than 10 years have elapsed since the diversion. Upper tract deterioration is seen in at least 50% of patients who have undergone urinary diversion during childhood or young adult years, and the risk of developing chronic renal insufficiency is increased in such patients. Calculi occur in roughly 8% to 10% of urinary diversion or bladder substitution patients, where urease-producing organisms—*Proteus, Pseudomonas, Klebsiella,* etc.—are the bacteria commonly seen.

UROSEPSIS AND COMPLEX UROGENITAL INFECTION IN THE ICU

Urosepsis has been addressed in several sections within this chapter, related to trauma, urologic tubes and drains, and below in renal failure management. It is also addressed elsewhere in this text (Chapters 46, 84, 87–92) with regard to general management principles for sepsis and septic shock (2,3,45–50). In addition, there are several specific urologic infectious disease phenomena that warrant specific mention.

Specific Infectious Processes of the Upper and Lower Urinary Tract

The combination of obstruction and infection of the upper and lower urinary tract requires urgent drainage, antibiotic therapy, and supportive care. Initial empiric antibiotic therapy for possible urosepsis must address the likely offending organisms and must consider the "worst-case scenario" from the bacteriologic standpoint. While awaiting culture data, Gram stain findings can also be very helpful in selecting initial therapy. Broad-spectrum antibiotics that cover aerobic gram-negative rods and the typical gram-positive cocci that appear as uropathogens are critical. If the patient has been recently instrumented, has been recently hospitalized, or has other risk factors for having sepsis due to atypical or resistant pathogens, coverage should be expanded accordingly. The newer-generation cephalosporins, imipenem, meropenem and related drugs, aminoglycosides, and vancomycin are commonly used in such circumstances. It may be necessary in certain situations to consider the presence of anaerobic infections of the genitourinary system. Sepsis following transrectal prostate biopsy procedures—typically ultrasound-guided and office-based—may introduce the risk of anaerobic infection. I am aware of deaths where a patient presented with urosepsis and retroperitoneal cellulitis following a needle biopsy of the prostate, in which anaerobic coverage was not provided and, ultimately, death from *Bacteroides fragilis* infection occurred. Anaerobic infection of the urinary tract has also been described outside the setting of iatrogenic rectal violation, both with enteric fistula and without identifiable anaerobic source, so this uncommon scenario is worth bearing in mind (51). Staphylococcal infections of the urinary system do also occur, particularly in the elderly or immunocompromised population, and in patients who have iatrogenic manipulation—percutaneous lithotripsy or SP cystostomy tube presence—which may result in the entry of skin flora into the urinary system. When a gram-positive coccus is noted on stained urine or infected fluid, vancomycin is an appropriate empiric choice for sepsis of urinary tract origin, as both *Enterococcus* and *Staphylococcus* species are usually covered. With the emergence of vancomycin-resistant *Enterococcus* (VRE) and other more resistant gram-positive cocci, the advisability of providing coverage for such resistant pathogens pending culture and sensitivity data should be considered. Fungal organisms should be considered, especially in the diabetic patient and in the patient who has had extensive antibiotic therapy; fluconazole is an appropriate initial empiric coverage agent pending culture results. With the wide variations in organism sensitivity patterns among institutions and clinical environments, a close collaboration with the locally knowledgeable infectious disease specialists is advisable in selecting empiric and specific treatment regimens.

In addition to supportive care and antibiotic management, prompt drainage of the urinary tract is critical in certain conditions of urinary infection and urosepsis (52). When either upper or lower tract obstruction is suspected with urosepsis, prompt imaging of the urinary tract should be obtained, either noncontrast CT of the abdomen and pelvis, or renal and bladder ultrasound to exclude retention (50,53). Rapid decline in clinical status may ensue if there is a delay in instituting prompt drainage of an infected, obstructed system (54). I encourage our medical colleagues to practice the principle that the "sun never sets" on an obstructed, infected urinary tract. Uncertainty occasionally arises when there is incomplete obstruction, as evidenced by contrast passing beyond a stone on an imaging study, and the patient is clinically stable. The goal is to provide low-pressure drainage of the infected system because the patient can still deteriorate even when some urine is progressing beyond the point of obstruction. Whether to drain the upper tract through cystoscopy and stent placement versus percutaneous nephrostomy, or the lower tract through IUBC placement or SP tube insertion, reflects a set of clinical judgments that varies from case to case, as discussed above. The available facilities and expertise, promptness of access to resources, coagulation status, and clinical instability and mobility all come into play in selecting the best approach to draining the urinary tract emergently. One major potential diagnostic pitfall occurs when a patient has complete unilateral upper tract obstruction with a negative urinalysis, as no urine from the obstructed system enters the bladder, and the urinary tract origin of sepsis is therefore not suspected. From the urologic perspective, routine abdominal imaging of septic patients with an unknown source is a wise approach, as it minimizes the potential for missing upper tract obstruction, potentially with a preventable poor outcome.

Certain specific infectious processes of the urinary tract deserve mention with regard to their relevance to the critical care provider (55,56). Emphysematous pyelonephritis and cystitis are infections of the kidney and bladder, respectively, which result in gas formation within the tissues (57,58). The presence of gas in the urinary tract may be due to gas-forming infection, previous instrumentation, or fistula. The clinical situation will usually lead to identification of the correct etiology. Gas-forming infections in the upper tract may represent a range of infectious processes: emphysematous pyelitis describes infection that results in gas within the collecting system, whereas emphysematous pyelonephritis describes gas within the renal parenchyma, which may progress into the perinephric space or other sites in the retroperitoneum. The most commonly seen organism in such infections is not the classic gas-forming anaerobes, but *Escherichia coli*, which may enter into a state of facultative anaerobic metabolism, especially in a diabetic when severe hyperglycemia is present. These patients may become severely ill and require aggressive resuscitation and sometimes drainage procedures or occasionally urgent nephrectomy; urologic consultation is essential. Emphysematous cystitis reflects the same bacteriologic basis and propensity for the diabetic patient as for the renal counterpart. IUBC drainage and aggressive antibiotic management will usually correct the process.

Acute papillary necrosis may also be seen in a diabetic due to microvascular renal disease that affects the vasculature of the renal papillae and pyramids, though other underlying conditions include excessive use of certain analgesics. When accompanied by infection, these patients behave like those with ureteral colic from calculous disease, as the sloughed papilla may obstruct the ureter, and will often require drainage and decompression of the urinary tract along with aggressive medical management. Sloughed papillae may dwell within the renal collecting system and undergo surface calcification, often resembling typical calculous disease, though the changes in the appearance of the calyces due to the sloughed papilla are indicative.

Renal and perinephric abscesses are important causes of urosepsis, and one must have a high index of suspicion in the setting of incomplete resolution of upper tract urinary infection with standard antibiotic regimens, prompting imaging to detect an undrained source of relapsing or persistent infection. CT scanning is significantly superior to ultrasound for imaging the perinephric space, and is preferable when an abscess is suspected. Small renal parenchymal abscesses not causing a septic picture may resolve with antibiotic treatment alone. Large parenchymal abscesses or perinephric collections usually require drainage, which in most cases can be carried out by a CT- or ultrasound-guided percutaneous approach. When multiloculated or an abscess inadequately drained by the percutaneous route is encountered, an open surgical drainage procedure may be necessary.

Acute prostatitis may be categorized by etiology—bacterial, abacterial—or clinical course and manifestations, acute or chronic (59,60). Acute bacterial prostatitis can present with a septic picture. Common symptoms include dysuria, frequency, urgency, chills and fever, elevated white blood count on CBC, and infected urine. Some urologists believe that urethral catheterization and instrumentation should be avoided in such patients due to concern of worsening sepsis. If the patient is emptying adequately, antibiotic administration is usually adequate without catheter drainage. If the patient is in acute urinary retention, bladder drainage is needed; one can proceed either with a gentle attempt at IUBC passage via the urethra or with percutaneous SP cystostomy placement. My view is that urethral catheterization is usually preferable and is certainly less invasive. For patients presenting with acute prostatitis or other complex lower tract infection who do not respond appropriately to antibiotic therapy, or for those with suspicious findings on a digital rectal examination, prostatic abscess should be suspected. The findings of concern on digital rectal examination would include unusual tenderness and/or an area of fluctuance on prostatic palpation. One should avoid an aggressive prostate examination on such patients, and it is generally ill advised to put significant digital pressure on the tender, acutely infected prostate to obtain a sample of expressed prostatic secretion as is often done in the chronic prostatitis patient. Acute prostatitis patients usually have infected urine and culture information from prostatic secretions is usually not necessary. Transrectal ultrasound or CT scanning of the pelvis will usually confirm the presence of a prostatic abscess, when present, and can also guide therapy by revealing whether the abscess cavity may be best drained through a transurethral, transperineal, or transrectal route. I usually prefer the transurethral approach if the cavity is abutting the prostatic urethral lumen. A transperineal drainage procedure can be performed under ultrasound guidance if the abscess is deep and a transurethral approach is deemed too risky. Unless the abscess has already started to drain spontaneously into the rectal lumen, this approach to prostatic abscess drainage is not favored. Acute infectious complications following transrectal prostate biopsy are well described and require aggressive antibiotic therapy and supportive care (61–63).

Acute infectious conditions involving the genitalia and perineum are important both with regard to the challenges sometimes faced in differential diagnosis, such as epididymitis versus torsion, trauma, or incarcerated hernia, and systemic management as in some conditions, for example, Fournier gangrene. Acute epididymitis or epididymo-orchitis may be due to standard enteric bacteria—more common in patients over 35 years of age and those with obstructive urethral or prostatic disease—or to venereal transmission of Chlamydial or Gonococcal infection. Mild epididymitis can be treated on an ambulatory basis with antibiotics. A fluoroquinolone often is acceptable if enteric infection is suspected; a tetracycline derivative is more appropriate if venereal transmission is likely, or a combination of two drugs if coverage for both entities is desired while awaiting culture data. Severe epididymo-orchitis is manifested by global enlargement of the hemiscrotal contents and loss of palpable anatomic landmarks, often with skin fixation and marked redness and tenderness. Such patients find it very painful to walk or stand, and may be best managed by hospitalization, bedrest, scrotal elevation, anti-inflammatory drugs, and broad-spectrum antibiotics until improvement is observed. Scrotal ultrasound examination may be useful for clarifying the diagnosis and excluding the presence of abscess formation, which may require surgical drainage and sometimes orchiectomy, and late torsion with testicular necrosis, which may have a similar clinical appearance.

Urologic Involvement in Complex Soft Tissue Infectious Processes

Urologic participation in the management of such entities as perirectal abscess or Fournier gangrene is common. Fournier gangrene, or necrotizing fasciitis involving the genital and perineal soft tissues, may be idiopathic with no identifiable point of origin, or may be due to extension from primary rectal, urinary, intra-abdominal, or retroperitoneal processes. Diabetics are at increased risk for this disease. When there is genital, perineal, or groin involvement in such processes, several applicable management principles may be of value to the critical care provider or acute care surgeon. Such patients should be treated with broad-spectrum antimicrobial regimens that cover gram-positive and gram-negative aerobes and anaerobes, as polymicrobial infection is common. These patients require a combination of aggressive antibiotic therapy, metabolic and fluid resuscitation, and prompt and aggressive surgical debridement and drainage (see Chapter 85). These infectious processes can progress very rapidly, and delays in bringing the patient to surgery may result in loss of otherwise salvageable tissues, progression of sepsis, and increased mortality.

The surgical approach for this entity in our institution is based on the areas of involvement and typically includes the urology and general surgery teams in a close collaboration to address relevant areas of anatomic specialty expertise, with surgery performing proctoscopy and addressing debridement of involved abdominal wall, rectal, ischiorectal fossa, thigh, or buttock tissues, and urology performing cystoscopy as indicated and addressing genital and perineal debridement. The advantages of this combined specialty collaboration assists in functional and organ preservation, and subsequent reconstructive efforts. When an abscess or necrotizing process extends into the region of the perineum or genital soft tissues, incision or debridement of scrotal or penile skin and underlying dartos fascia may be necessary. In the scrotum, a dissection plane just superficial to the parietal tunica vaginalis is established in order to keep this membrane, which surrounds the testes, intact. The testes are rarely involved in these soft tissue infections, and not directly exposing the testes to the wound will aid in subsequent wound management and avoid the pain and desiccation that occurs when the testis is exposed externally. On the penis, necrotic skin and dartos may be debrided up to the coronal sulcus when necessary, taking care to stay superficial to the deep (Buck) fascial layer of the penis, to avoid injury to the corpora and the dorsal neurovascular bundle, which lies in a wide band across the center on the top of the penis, and to the urethra, which lies ventrally. Fournier gangrene may occasionally arise from a urethral source, such as a periurethral abscess or perforated stricture or diverticulum. Debridement of urethral tissue should be avoided unless it is grossly necrotic, as a superficial exudate may create the appearance of marginally perfused tissue; such changes can be reassessed upon OR take-back and allowed to declare themselves further into the course of the disease. If the surgeon must enter the scrotal wall for drainage of a local abscess, it is best to avoid deep incision into the tunica vaginalis compartment to avoid preventable injury to the scrotal contents.

As general considerations for the patient with urosepsis, there is the potential that the patient's hemodynamics and degree of severity of sepsis may transiently worsen following needed urinary tract drainage or manipulation. A low threshold to have such patients in the ICU is appropriate, even if they are not so critically ill that, initially, they are in need of ICU management. For example, in our institution, if we perform percutaneous nephrostomy insertion or ureteral stent placement in a patient with infection, an obstructing stone, tachycardia, and fever, especially when a pyonephrosis is encountered, we arrange overnight ICU observation to ensure that any deterioration is promptly recognized and managed. When culture data become available, broad-spectrum empiric antibiotic regimens should be simplified based upon bacteriologic identification and sensitivities. Tubes that are placed into the urinary tract to drain infected spaces must be appropriately secured to the patient to avoid inadvertent malposition or removal, and observed to avoid kinking or occlusion of outflow systems, which may prevent low-pressure drainage and exacerbate sepsis.

UROLOGIC CAUSES OF RENAL FAILURE

The urologist's view of renal failure is usually focused on "postrenal" factors, as this is the setting in which we are typically consulted. At times, however, it is unclear whether a patient with acute renal failure (ARF) is suffering from an obstructive process, whether the process is remediable, and how best to approach therapy.

Assessment and management of ARF are covered in detail in Chapter 132. The urologist is typically consulted when there is suspicion or evidence that the state of renal failure is due to a mechanical or vascular etiology, usually manifested by significant oliguria and distention of some level of the urinary tract.

If an IUBC is in place in a patient with impaired urine output, palpation of the lower abdomen to detect bladder distention, ultrasound assessment of bladder volume, and/or irrigation of the catheter to ensure patency are appropriate initial steps. Management of catheter-related dysfunction is discussed in detail above. If uncertainty remains as to the appropriate positioning or function of an indwelling catheter, urologic consultation should be obtained.

If lower tract or bladder catheter malfunction has been excluded, one must exclude upper urinary tract obstruction. Renal ultrasound or noncontrast CT scanning is commonly employed for this purpose. The findings of hydronephrosis or ureteral dilatation raise concerns about the possibility of postrenal failure. It is important to appreciate that ureteral obstruction can exist without significant collecting system dilation in some cases, particularly if the obstructive process is of very recent onset. Patients with two normally functioning kidneys should not develop renal failure in the face of unilateral upper tract obstruction; in fact, complete obstruction of one ureter often causes little or no change in serum creatinine if the contralateral kidney is functionally normal. Unilateral upper tract obstruction involving a solitary kidney—or marked hypofunction of the contralateral kidney—may result in anuria and renal failure. In most of these cases, radiographic evidence of underlying inadequacy of the contralateral kidney is evident in that atrophy, long-standing obstruction with hydronephrosis and marked parenchymal thinning are present. In entities that can cause asymmetric and asynchronous development of obstructive uropathy—advancing prostate cancer with trigonal invasion, progressive pelvic lymphadenopathy, asymmetric retroperitoneal fibrosis with extrinsic ureteral compression—unrecognized loss of function of one kidney may result from obstruction without symptoms or a significant change in serum creatinine. Only when the remaining kidney becomes obstructed and renal failure ensues is the entire process recognized.

When evidence of upper tract obstruction is noted, one must expeditiously implement a strategy to determine definitively if postrenal obstruction is present, and choose the least morbid means of relieving it. The gold standard for such determination is to perform cystoscopy and retrograde pyelography. This procedure can be performed in the OR setting using static or fluoroscopic imaging capability, or at the bedside in the ICU. I have successfully performed flexible cystoscopy, retrograde pyelography, guidewire insertion and manipulation past a point of obstruction, and internal or externalized stent placement in the ICU. This approach is especially applicable in the hemodynamically unstable patient for whom movement to the OR may be hazardous. The newer digital x-ray units are ideally suited for such procedures, as the digital plate is placed beneath the patient once, allowing multiple images to be obtained and viewed on the monitor almost immediately. If an obstructed or tortuous ureter is encountered, the area of difficulty may often be navigated using a 5 French open-ended catheter through which an angle-tipped guidewire is advanced. Rotating the guidewire may allow passage across an area of ureter that is not possible using straight wires or catheters. Once a guidewire has been advanced past the complex ureter into the kidney, either an open-ended catheter or a double-J type internal stent may be inserted over the wire. Open-ended catheters may be tied to an IUBC for stability and attached to an external drainage appliance.

An alternative to achieving upper tract drainage cystoscopically is to have a percutaneous nephrostomy tube placed through IR techniques. It is important that the patient's coagulation functions be normal when pursuing such an approach, and it is also important to verify, as best as possible that there is, in fact, upper tract obstruction present before introducing the risk of a percutaneous puncture. In the appropriate clinical setting, where there is certainty that upper tract drainage is needed, PCNL is an important option, and may be preferable to achieving drainage through lower tract instrumentation when dealing with urosepsis or challenging lower tract anatomy where manipulation may be difficult, as when gross hematuria, some cases of prior lower tract surgery, or permanent urinary diversion states exist. It is usually necessary for the patient to be prone on the radiology table to accomplish PCNL placement, and one must determine if such a position is safe or advisable. Respiratory compromise, recent abdominal surgery, or body habitus may create major challenges in placing the patient prone for such a procedure.

When lower or upper tract drainage is achieved in the setting of postrenal failure, one must observe the patient closely for transient worsening of urosepsis and for the possibility of pathologic postobstructive diuresis. Worsening of sepsis can result from instrumenting the infected urinary tract, and supportive measures may be necessary, including the institution of pressor support. Adequate hydration prior to urinary tract manipulation and provision of prophylactic antibiotics will minimize the risk of worsening sepsis with instrumentation. Pathologic postobstructive diuresis may occur when there is a major solute load and severe obligatory water loss occurs following relief of obstruction. This can be seen with lower tract or bilateral upper tract obstruction. Fluid and electrolyte monitoring and judicious fluid replacement may be necessary during the diuresis period.

Acute papillary necrosis may result in ARF. Papillary necrosis may develop as a gradually progressive, indolent process, recognized by the classic cavitary appearance of the renal calyces on contrast studies, or may present as a fulminant, infectious course with urosepsis and obstruction from sloughed papillae. Relief of obstruction, treatment of infection, and supportive care are indicated.

Other entities for which urologic input may be valuable when ARF occurs include vasculogenic renal failure, due to renal artery or renal vein thrombosis, and abdominal compartment syndrome–related renal failure. An important pitfall in diagnosis occurs when a patient presents with abrupt onset of flank pain, nonfunction of the ipsilateral kidney is noted in intravenous pyelography, and the presumptive diagnosis of renal colic from stone is declared. In fact, complete nonfunction is uncommon as an IVP finding from ureteral obstruction; more commonly, a persistent nephrogram with delayed excretion is observed. Complete nonfunction may be due to vascular compromise of the kidney either from primary arterial occlusion or renal vein thrombosis, which leads to microvascular occlusion and nonfunction. One should be suspicious of renovascular compromise whenever acute onset of flank pain occurs. Contrast-enhanced CT scanning is diagnostic, as the affected kidney will fail to opacify. When vascular compromise of the kidney occurs, urgent vascular surgical and IR consultation should be obtained to determine if immediate revascularization is feasible and warranted.

SUMMARY

Critical care issues in urology are many and varied. The intensivist must be familiar with the anatomic and physiologic factors that are relevant to urologic disease, and must have a low threshold to request urologic consultation when specialty expertise may be of value to the patient. Recognition of obstructive, infectious, and ischemic entities for which time-sensitive intervention is important is most essential for the critical care provider. In the postoperative setting, issues common to other surgical specialties are relevant to urology patients, and various specialty-specific problems may also arise, often related to renal dysfunction, the complexities of endoscopic and reconstructive surgery, and perioperative infection. Urologic residency training in the United States provides a strong background in critical care knowledge and skills, as all urology residents spend 1 to 2 years in general surgery and related specialties, including exposure to surgical ICU experience. The field of critical care requires an enormous breadth of knowledge and capability, however, and the practicing urologist and his or her patients may benefit greatly from the input and expertise of those specializing in the care of critical care patients. A close collaboration between these specialties greatly enhances the quality of urologic patient care.

Key Points

- Urologic surgery represents a diverse and complex set of interventions, involving upper and lower tracts and genital procedures, and open, endoscopic, laparoscopic, and robotic approaches. The intensivist must be familiar with the significant variety of management challenges and potential complications that may ensue when caring for urologic surgical patients in the ICU setting.
- Potentially immediately life-threatening issues in urology include severe bleeding and urosepsis. The intensivist must be able to rapidly assess the patient to exclude and when present, effectively manage these serious conditions. The magnitude and rate of urologic hemorrhage and the presence of a source of sepsis in the urinary tract must be expeditiously addressed.
- Minimally invasive approaches to urologic surgery have progressed significantly in recent years, changing the mode of presentation of urologic surgical complications and requiring a high index of suspicion for effective diagnosis. Laparoscopic and endoscopic surgery can result in significant morbidity which must be promptly diagnosed and treated.
- The combination of infection and obstruction of the urinary tract represents a surgical emergency, whether it occurs in the setting of an obstructing ureteral calculus, or an obstructed urinary drainage catheter in a colonized urinary tract. Rapid diagnosis with prompt decompression of the infected, obstructed urinary tract is essential to limit the morbidity and mortality of such surgical emergencies.
- Urologic trauma can occur in the setting of iatrogenic surgical procedures, or due to external violence. Urologic consultation should be obtained early when urologic trauma is suspected, so that the patient may benefit from the anatomic knowledge and management expertise of the urologist. Preventing further complications of the initial urologic injury, such as by avoiding injudicious urinary catheter placement when there is evidence of a pelvic fracture–related posterior urethral injury, is important in urologic trauma management.

References

1. Hicks D, Li CY. Management of macroscopic haematuria in the emergency department. *Emerg Med J*. 2007;24:385–390.
2. Coburn M, Zimmerman JL. Sepsis and septic shock in the urology patient. *Am Urol Assoc Update Series*. 2002;21(14).
3. Wagenlehner FM, Alidjanov J, Pilatz A. [Urosepsis. Update on diagnosis and treatment]. *Urologe A*. 2016;55(4):454–459.
4. Søgaard KK, Thomsen RW, Schønheyder HC, Søgaard M. Positive predictive values of the International Classification of Diseases, 10th revision. Diagnoses of gram-negative septicemia/sepsis and urosepsis for presence of gram-negative bacteremia. *Clin Epidemiol*. 2015;7:195–199.
5. Ramanathan R, Duane TM. Urinary tract infections in surgical patients. *Surg Clin North Am*. 2014;94 (6):1351–1368.
6. Cummings JM, Boullier JA, Sekhon D, Bose K. Adult testicular torsion. *J Urol*. 2002;167:2109–2110.
7. Marcozzi D, Suner S. The nontraumatic acute scrotum. *Emerg Med Clin North Am*. 2001;19:547–568.
8. Geerts WH, Bergqvist D, Pineo GF, et al; American College of Chest Physicians. Prevention of venous thromboembolism. American College of Chest Physicians Evidence-Based Clinical Practice Guidelines (8th Edition). *Chest*. 2008;133:381S–543S.
9. Chew BH, Flannigan R, Kurtz M, et al. A single dose of intraoperative antibiotics is sufficient to prevent urinary tract infection during ureteroscopy. *J Endourol*. 2016;30(1):63–68.
10. Motamedinia P, Korets R, Badalato G, Gupta M. Perioperative cultures and the role of antibiotics during stone surgery. *Transl Androl Urol*. 2014;3(3):297–301.
11. Morey AF, Brandes S, Dugi DD III, et al; American Urological Assocation. Urotrauma: AUA guideline. *J Urol*. 2014;192(2):327–335.
12. Philips P, Amaral J. Abdominal access complications in laparoscopic surgery. *J Am Coll Surg*. 2001;192:525–536.

13. Coburn M. Genitourinary trauma. In: Moore EE, Feliciano DV, Mattox KL, eds. *Trauma*. 5th ed. New York: McGraw-Hill; 2004.
14. Coburn M, Guerriero WG. Complications in genitourinary trauma. In: Mattox KL, ed. *Complications of Trauma*. New York: Churchill Livingstone; 1994.
15. Bryk DJ, Zhao LC. Guideline of guidelines: a review of urological trauma guidelines. *BJU Int*. 2016;117(2):226–234.
16. Zinman LN, Vanni AJ. Surgical management of urologic trauma and iatrogenic injuries. *Surg Clin North Am*. 2016;96(3):425–439.
17. Sharp HT, Adelman MR. Prevention, recognition, and management of urologic injuries during gynecologic surgery. *Obstet Gynecol*. 2016;127(6):1085–1096.
18. Dassel MW, Adelman MR, Sharp HT. Recognition and management of urologic injuries with laparoscopic hysterectomy. *Clin Obstet Gynecol*. 2015;58(4): 805–811.
19. Metcalf M, Broghammer JA. Genitourinary trauma in geriatric patients. *Curr Opin Urol*. 2016;26(2):165–170.
20. Kuno K, Menzin A, Kauder HH, et al. Prophylactic ureteral catheterization in gynecologic surgery. *Urology*. 1998;52:1004–1008.
21. Zaid UB, Bayne DB, Harris CR, et al. Penetrating trauma to the ureter, bladder, and urethra. *Curr Trauma Rep*. 2015;1(2):119–124.
22. Ahn JH, Morey AF, McAninch JW. Workup and management of traumatic hematuria. *Emerg Med Clin North Am*. 1998;15:145–164.
23. Chapple CR, Png D. Contemporary management of urethral trauma and post-traumatic stricture. *Curr Opin Urol*. 1999;9:253–260.
24. Bhattar R, Priyadarshi S, Yadav SS, et al. Re: primary endoscopic realignment of urethral disruption injuries-a double-edged sword? *J Urol*. 2016;195(5): 1626–1627.
25. Rios E, Martinez-Piñeiro L. Re: primary endoscopic realignment of urethral disruption injuries-a double-edged sword? *Eur Urol*. 2016;69(3):536–537.
26. Gomez RG, Ceballos L, Coburn M, et al. Consensus statement of bladder injuries. *Br J Urol Int*. 2004;94:27–32.
27. Brandes S, Coburn M, Armenakas N, et al. Diagnosis and management of ureteric injury: an evidenced-based analysis. *Br J Urol Int*. 2004;94:277–289.
28. Kawashima A, Sandler CM, Corl FM, et al. Imaging of renal trauma: a comprehensive review. *Radiographics*. 2001;21:557–574.
29. Moore EE, Shackford SR, Pachter HL, et al. Organ injury scaling: spleen, liver, kidney. *J Trauma*. 1989;29:1664–1666.
30. Dangle PP, Fuller TW, Gaines B, et al. Evolving mechanisms of injury and management of pediatric blunt renal trauma: 20 years of experience. *Urology*. 2016;90:159–163.
31. Chouhan JD, Winer AG, Johnson C, et al. Contemporary evaluation and management of renal trauma. *Can J Urol*. 2016;23(2):8191–8197.
32. Santucci RA, McAninch JW. Grade IV renal injuries: evaluation, treatment and outcome. *World J Surg*. 2001;25:1562.
33. Knudson MM, Harrison PB, Hoyt DB, et al. Outcome after major renovascular injuries: a Western Trauma Association multicenter report. *J Trauma*. 2000;49:1116–1122.
34. Coburn M. Damage control for urologic injuries. *Surg Clin North Am*. 1997;77:821–834.
35. Coburn M. Genitourinary trauma—minimally invasive alternatives. In: Moore RG, Bischoff JT, Loening S, et al, eds. *Minimally Invasive Urologic Surgery*. New York: Taylor & Francis Group; 2005.
36. Bloom DA, McGuire EJ, Lapides J. A brief history of urethral catheterization. *J Urol*. 1994;151:317–325.
37. Benson AD, Juliano TM, Miller NL. Infectious outcomes of nephrostomy drainage before percutaneous nephrolithotomy compared to concurrent access. *J Urol*. 2014;192(3):770–774.
38. Bhatt NR, Davis NF, Addie D, et al. Evaluating the cost of iatrogenic urethral catheterisation injuries. *Ir J Med Sci*. 2016:1–5. doi: 10.1007/s11845-016-1451-5.
39. Bjerklund TE, Cek M, Naber K, et al. Prevalence of hospital-acquired urinary tract infections in urology departments. *Eur Urol*. 2007;51: 1100–1111.
40. Lai WS, Assimos D. The role of antibiotic prophylaxis in percutaneous nephrolithotomy. *Rev Urol*. 2016;18(1):10–14.
41. Lopez Cubillana P. What is the best method for urgent urinary diversion in patients with obstruction and infection due to ureteral colic? *Urol Int*. 2001;66:178.
42. Bloom DA, Grossman HB, Konnak JW. Stomal construction and reconstruction. *Urol Clin North Am*. 1986;13:275–283.
43. Hall MC, Koch MO, McDougal WS. Metabolic consequences of urinary diversion through intestinal segments. *Urol Clin North Am*. 1991; 18:725–735.
44. Stein R, Lotz J, Andreas J, et al. Long-term metabolic effects in patients with urinary diversion. *World J Urol*. 1998;16:292–297.
45. Nicolle L. AMMI Canada Guideline Committee: complicated urinary tract infection in adults. *Can J Infect Dis Med Microbiol*. 2005;16:349–360.
46. Wagenlehner FM, Weidner W, Naber KG. Optimal management of urosepsis from the urological perspective. *Int J Antimicrob Agents*. 2007;30: 390–397.
47. Qiang XH, Yu TO, Li YN, Zhou LX. Prognosis risk of urosepsis in critical care medicine: a prospective observational study. *Biomed Res Int*. 2016:9028924.
48. Wagenlehner FM, Pilatz A, Weidner W, Naber KG. Urosepsis: overview of the diagnostic and treatment challenges. *Microbiol Spectr*. 2015;3(5). doi: 10.1128/microbiolspec.UTI-0003-2012.
49. Schneeberger C, Holleman F, Geerlings SE. Febrile urinary tract infections: pyelonephritis and urosepsis. *Curr Opin Infect Dis*. 2016;29(1):80–85.
50. Sørensen SM, Schønheyder HC, Nielsen H. The role of imaging of the urinary tract in patients with urosepsis. *Int J Infect Dis*. 2013;17(5):e299–e303.
51. Brook I. Urinary tract and genito-urinary suppurative infections due to anaerobic bacteria. *Int J Urol*. 2004;11:133–141.
52. Watson RA, Esposito M, Richter F, et al. Percutaneous nephrostomy as adjunct management in advanced upper urinary tract infection. *Urology*. 1999;54:234–239.
53. Rubenstein JN, Schaeffer AJ. Managing complicated urinary tract infections: the urologic view. *Infect Dis Clin North Am*. 2003;17:333–351.
54. Abramson S, Walders N, Applegate KE, et al. Impact in the emergency department of unenhanced CT on diagnostic confidence and therapeutic efficacy in patients with suspected renal colic: a prospective study. *Am J Roentgenol*. 2000;175:1689–1695.
55. Stapleton A. Urinary tract infections in patients with diabetes. *Am J Med*. 2002;113(Suppl 1A):80S–84S.
56. Wan YL, Lo SK, Bullard MJ, et al. Predictors of outcome in emphysematous pyelonephritis. *J Urol*. 1998;159:369–373.
57. Fatima R, Jha R, Muthukrishnan J, et al. Emphysematous pyelonephritis: a single center study. *Indian J Nephrol*. 2013;23(2):119–124.
58. Sharma R, Mitra SK, Choudhary A, Majee P. Emphysematous cystitis-gas in bladder: a rare urological emergency. *BMJ Case Rep*. 2015. pii: bcr2015210836.
59. Ludwig M. Diagnosis and therapy of acute prostatitis, epididymitis and orchitis. *Andrologia*. 2008;40:76–80.
60. Barozzi L, Pavlica P, Menchi I, et al. Prostatic abscess: diagnosis and treatment. *Am J Roentgenol*. 1998;170:753–757.
61. Toner L, Bolton DM, Lawrentschuk N. Prevention of sepsis prior to prostate biopsy. *Invest Clin Urol*. 2016;57(2):94–99.
62. Taylor AK, Murphy AB. Preprostate biopsy rectal culture and postbiopsy sepsis. *Urol Clin North Am*. 2015;42(4):449–458.
63. Lee SJ. Infection after transrectal ultrasound-guided prostate biopsy. *Korean J Urol*. 2015;56(5):346–350.

CHAPTER
67
Facial Trauma

EMMANUEL KYEREME-TUAH and M. BARBARA HONNEBIER

INTRODUCTION

Facial trauma is any injury of the midface, including the maxillary complex. Panfacial injuries involve trauma to the upper, middle, and lower facial bones. Traditionally, mandibular fractures and injuries to the frontal bone and frontal sinuses are discussed as separate entities even when accompanying other facial fractures. These distinctions, based on anatomic boundaries (1), are used for the sake of organization, as injuries to the nasal cavity or sinuses, orbits, and ethmoids may also involve violations of the cranium and cranial space. The Arbeitsgemeinschaft für Osteosynthesefragen (AO) classifies fractures in the adult craniomaxillofacial (CMF) skeleton using anatomic modules in a precision three-level hierarchy, with each level accounting for an increasing complexity and details. Level 1 is most elementary and identifies no more than the presence of fractures in four separate anatomical units: the mandible, midface, skull base, and cranial vault (2). Level 2 relates the detailed topographic location of the fractures in the defined areas of the mandible, midface, and internal orbits. Level 3 is a more refined topographic measurement focusing on the morphology: fragmentation, displacement, and defects within levels 1 and 2 (2).

Facial trauma may be due to penetrating or blunt trauma, and may present clinically either singly or as a combination of lacerations of skin and soft tissues, obstruction of the nasal cavities or sinuses, problems with vision, and occlusion, which often are more outward manifestations of underlying facial fractures. Comprehensive management and treatment of facial trauma involves airway control, control of bleeding, reduction of swelling, prevention of infection, repair of soft tissue lacerations, and repair of bone fractures to restore function and esthetic form to the face. The aim of this chapter is to discuss the potential pitfalls and problems that facial injuries may create. The operative management of facial fractures has undergone many changes in the last few years. With the advent of rigid fixation and continued new technologies, detailed discussions of methods of operative reconstruction of different types of facial fractures are best discussed in specialty textbooks.

PATHOPHYSIOLOGY

In the treatment of a patient with multiple maxillofacial injuries, it is critical to differentiate injuries that require immediate operative intervention from those for which operation can be deferred. A complete evaluation, including radiologic evaluation, is paramount and technologies like three-dimensional imaging, angiography, CT, and MRI/MRA help to risk-stratify patients. The surgeon must be cognizant of neurologic, ophthalmologic, and cervical spine injuries as well as associated vascular insults or injury (3,4); however, immediate intervention may be indicated for stabilization. Procedures that require an extensive workup are delayed until the patient is clinically stable. Reconstruction consists of three stages: initial stabilization, definitive reconstruction, and potential secondary refinement; in gunshot wounds, contemporary practice is definitive immediate reconstruction (5).

The most essential component of initial care begins with the ABCs (airway, breathing, circulation), as well as cervical spine assessment. As with any other trauma patient, the facial trauma patient should be evaluated in a systematic and comprehensive fashion in cooperation with the trauma team. Although rare, isolated facial trauma may be severe and life threatening. Critical facial injuries are usually obvious upon presentation (e.g., gunshot wound to the face, profuse bleeding from orifices). Abdominal, thoracic, cervical spine, and neurosurgical emergencies take priority over maxillofacial injury. If possible, a detailed history of the event and past medical history should be obtained from the patient, paramedics, and/or family members. Dental records are typically difficult to obtain but can be very helpful in diagnosis and treatment planning. The force required for fracture of the facial bones varies by anatomic segment (Table 67.1), but it is notable that the mandible is more sensitive to lateral forces than frontal (6).

Particularly in the facial trauma patient, early airway control and neurologic assessment of a potential head injury are critical because the eyes and oropharynx are the "shock organs" of the face and development of facial edema will obscure the pupils and obstruct the upper airway. Immediate treatment of maxillofacial trauma patients is indicated in the following situations: airway compromise, severe hemorrhage, large open wounds, superior orbital fissure and orbital apex syndrome, mandibular condylar impaction into the cranial fossa, and if urgent surgical procedures need to be performed by other services.

CONTRAINDICATIONS

Definitive treatment of maxillofacial injuries is delayed if the patient has severe, concomitant, and/or undetermined systemic trauma. Definitive treatment of facial fractures can be delayed as much as 2 weeks after injury as long as the fractures do not violate the cranial space (7); patients with neurologic or cranial injury are operated on when stable. Blood volume, electrolytes, and acid–base problems should all be addressed prior to the surgical intervention. In addition, the resolution of facial edema and perineural contusion during this period of time allows for a much more accurate evaluation and simplifies surgical planning and operative treatment.

TABLE 67.1 Forces Required to Fracture Facial Bones

Bone	Force (lb)
Nasal bones	25–75
Maxilla	140–445
Zygomatic arch	208–475
Body of zygoma	200–450
Frontal bones	800–1,600
Mandible	425–925, depending on site and angle of force

From Pappachan B, Alexander M. Biomechanics of cranio-maxillofacial trauma. *J Maxillofac Oral Surg.* 2012;11(2):224–230.

EPIDEMIOLOGY: CAUSES, INCIDENCE, AND RISK FACTORS

The etiology of facial trauma is multifactorial ranging from sports injuries, falls, penetrating injuries (projectiles), assaults and violence, to motor vehicle accidents. The incidence and frequency of any specific etiology varies with culture and within geographic regions. In Europe, a large case series showed assaults and falls were the most common etiologic factors, outweighing motor vehicle accidents (8). Urban trauma centers evaluate and treat many facial trauma patients on a daily basis. Many university hospitals are well known for their high volume of facial fracture management (9). Oral and maxillofacial surgery, plastic surgery, and otolaryngology services are heavily consulted by the emergency department (ED) and trauma team to assist with management of facial injuries. A large body of research has focused on data collection regarding types of facial trauma and studies on the outcome and morbidity associated with the treatment of facial fractures. Data regarding age, race, gender, social habits, mechanism of injury, and incidence of previous facial trauma are available from many centers in many countries (10). In most urban areas, mandibular fractures account for the majority of injuries, followed by lacerations and miscellaneous facial injuries. Half of the patients who experience facial injuries as victims of assault are likely to have interpersonal violence and have a high likelihood for a future injury. Men outnumber women in facial injuries. Personal assaults and motor vehicle accidents still account for the majority of facial injuries worldwide though pan-facial injuries are less frequent (11–15).

Airway Management

The possibility of cervical spine injury makes airway management more complex in the facial trauma patient. Spinal injuries are increased fourfold if there is a clinically significant head injury (Glasgow coma scale [GCS] score ≤8). A cervical spine injury should be suspected in all patients involving forced blunt trauma. Cervical spine injury may be occult, in which case secondary injury to the spinal cord must be avoided. Immobilization of the cervical spine must be instituted immediately until a complete clinical and radiologic evaluation has excluded injury (16,17).

A fully conscious, coherent patient will maintain his/her airway; as overall status may deteriorate at any time, the ABCs must constantly be reassessed. The following subsets of patients require that the airway be immediately secured to prevent respiratory failure: (a) patients with GCS scores of 8 or less; (b) patients with sustained seizure activity; (c) patients with unstable midface trauma; (d) patients with direct injuries to the airway; (e) patients with aspiration risk or unable to maintain an airway; and (f) patients with oxygenation problems.

Hutchison et al. (18) identified six specific maxillofacial trauma situations, which could have adverse effects on the airway:

1. Posteroinferior displacement of a fractured maxilla blocking the nasopharyngeal airway. This is managed by pulling maxilla forward with index and middle fingers to disimpact;
2. A bilateral fracture of the anterior mandible may cause the fractured symphysis and the tongue to slide posteriorly and block the oropharynx in the supine patient. This is managed by placing a 0-silk suture transversely through dorsum of tongue and pulling the tongue forward using a towel clip/pulling mandible forward;
3. Obstruction of oropharynx, larynx and trachea/bronchi by teeth, bone fragments vomitus, hematoma, or other foreign bodies. This is managed by manual clearing of debris with a hooked gloved finger/using large bore suction with adequate illumination (e.g., laryngoscope) to examine and clear oropharynx and larynx;
4. Hemorrhage from distinct vessels in open wounds or severe nasal bleeding from anterior/posterior ethmoidal vessels or terminal portion of maxillary artery. This is managed by packing or putting occlusive pressure on the area, with definitive treatment to follow;
5. Soft tissue swelling and edema resulting from trauma of the oral cavity leading to delayed airway compromise. This is managed by being cognizant of potential for delayed airway compromise and early airway securement;
6. Trauma of the larynx and trachea causing swelling and displacement of structures, such as the epiglottis, arytenoid cartilages, and vocal cords, thereby increasing the risk of airway obstruction. This is managed by having high index of suspicion especially if mechanism of injury suggests trauma to the aforesaid areas, monitoring for alarm features such as surgical emphysema, tenderness, or tracheal or laryngeal crepitus. Bronchoscopy can be performed to seek the site of injury.

In an emergent situation, the clinical situation may dictate that the quickest way to secure the airway, rather than the safest and most appropriate way, be used.

The airway should be cleared of debris, foreign bodies (teeth), blood, and secretions. The classic "chin lift" or "jaw thrust" maneuvers are commonly employed for assessment of airway patency and to remove obstruction of the tongue base. However, jaw thrust and chin lift may cause distraction of at least 5 mm in a cadaver with C5–6 instability, unaffected by the use of a rigid collar (16). Manual in-line axial stabilization must therefore be maintained throughout. Bag-mask ventilation may also produce significant degrees of cervical spine movement at zones of instability. The "sniffing" position for standard endotracheal intubation should, similarly, be avoided as it flexes the lower cervical spine and extends the occiput on the atlas. As atlanto-occipital extension is necessary to visualize the vocal cords, patients with unstable C1 or C2 injuries might be at more risk from this technique. Although the hard C-collar may interfere with intubation efforts, the front part of the collar may be removed to facilitate intubation as long as manual stabilization remains in effect.

In this situation, the safest method of securing an endotracheal tube remains debatable. Advanced Trauma Life Support (ATLS) recommends a nasotracheal tube in the spontaneously breathing patient, and orotracheal intubation in the apneic patient. Orotracheal intubation is the fastest and surest method of intubating the trachea and therefore the more commonly used method. At the University of Maryland–Shock Trauma in Baltimore, Maryland, more than 3,000 patients were intubated orally with a modified rapid sequence induction technique with preoxygenation (actually denitrogenation of the alveoli) and cricoid pressure. Ten percent of these patients were found to have cervical spine injury and none deteriorated neurologically following intubation (19). Blind nasal intubation is ultimately successful in 90% of patients, but requires multiple attempts in up to 90% of these. Nasotracheal intubation is (relatively) contraindicated in patients with potential skull base fractures or unstable midface injuries that typically involve the naso-orbito-ethmoid (NOE) complex. The same holds true for the use of nasogastric tube placement. Any paranasal manipulation may notoriously produce or recreate local hemorrhage, making airway manipulations difficult or impossible. Inadvertent placement and contamination/violation of the cranial space is a theoretical possibility. Submental orotracheal/endotracheal intubation is a possibility for patients whom may need maxillomandibular repair or with NOE injury (19–21).

Nasotracheal intubation in nontrauma patients is often accomplished by rotating or flexing the neck to align the tube correctly; in the trauma patient, this requires prior cervical spine clearance. Local anesthetic preparation of the airway is also time consuming and might increase the risk of aspiration. Laryngeal mask airway (LMA) does not protect the airway from aspiration, and by acting as a bolus in the pharynx, may increase esophageal reflux. The need for a surgical airway should be recognized and obtained without delay. A percutaneous needle cricothyroidotomy with high-flow oxygen is indicated in emergency situations when standard tracheotomy is not feasible or advisable. The potential for carbon dioxide retention with this technique must be remembered and the levels in arterial samples monitored. Studies on movement of the neck during cricothyroidotomy, ease of cricothyroidotomy with neck immobilization, or neurologic deterioration following cricothyroidotomy are lacking. If identification of anatomic landmarks is ambiguous, one should proceed with standard tracheotomy or the needle cricothyroidotomy, especially if time is of the essence. Cricothyroidotomy is contraindicated in laryngeal or tracheal trauma, cervical infection, and young children, but unfortunately is necessary if unable to intubate. A standard tracheotomy is essential in unstable patients who require prolonged maxillomandibular fixation (MMF) for fracture stabilization and management.

Life-Threatening Hemorrhage and Bleeding from Facial Fractures

In the multisystem-injured patient, hemorrhage is the most common cause of hypovolemia. Hemorrhage can be external or internal, into body cavities. Because the face and neck have a rich vascular supply, injuries in these areas can lead to substantial blood loss leading to hemorrhagic shock. Major hemorrhage can result from large scalp wounds, nasal or midface fractures, and penetrating wounds. As opposed to bleeding into body cavities, hemorrhage in the head and neck area is almost always immediately detectable in the trauma bay on clinical examination and is most often external in nature. Direct pressure to wounds or to major arteries proximal to wounds often is effective in staunching the flow of blood. Scalp wounds are notorious for large amounts of blood loss in a short time if the galea is involved. Scalp wounds can be rapidly approximated with 2-0 nonabsorbable sutures (nylon, Prolene) or staples, if available. Sutures should be placed away from the wound edge to ensure hemostasis, as the galea tends to retract. The patient should be stabilized prior to continuing with further diagnostic studies.

Nasal and midface fractures can result in tearing of the ethmoidal arteries. Most of these can be controlled with direct pressure or packing. Nasal packing can be made of gauze, foam, or cotton. It may be commercial, preformed specifically for the purpose, or adapted to the task. Packings may be made by cutting the fingers of a sterile examination glove and stuffing with gauze. Nasal packing may be coated with petrolatum, antibiotic ointment, or agents such as lidocaine and thrombin that aid in hemostasis and clot formation. Preformed foam nasal packs may have small tubes in the center of the pack to allow nasal breathing while the packing is in place, as nasal packing usually prevents air exchange through the nose. Nonintubated patients with nasal packing in place should have the head of the bed elevated 30 degrees and be observed for respiratory distress. Continued bleeding may not be apparent on the nasal side of the packing. Nasal packing easily slips posteriorly with swallowing or out with movement or sneezing. The posterior oropharynx should be checked regularly.

Fractures of the posterior maxillary wall, as in LeFort I and II fractures, may be associated with profuse bleeding from the internal maxillary artery. Bleeding from this artery can be very difficult to control by gauze packing. Epinephrine and liquid thrombin can be added to the packing and the head elevated to help achieve hemostasis. However, a postnasal pack has to be used to treat the bleeding in the postnasal area; this is a difficult area to pack. A balloon catheter can be passed through the nose and pulled out through the mouth. The safety and length of nasal packing is not evidence based. In rhinoplasty surgery, nasal stents and packs are routinely left in place for 7 to 10 days. The role of systemic antibiotics routinely in patients with nasal packing is still controversial, but current evidence seems to suggest topical, rather than systemic, antimicrobials should be used in epistaxis, with preoperative antibiotics sufficing for maxillofacial trauma, as infections are quite rare in maxilla, condylar and zygoma fractures, and seen in less than 10% in those of the mandible (22–24).

Complications can be packing related. The most common complication of nasal packing is that removal of the packing dislodges healing tissue and causes recurrent hemorrhage. Hypoxemia and hypercarbia can cause respiratory and cardiac complications. Airway obstruction and asphyxiation can occur if the nasal packing slips back into the airway, particularly during sleep. Complications may occur if a pack compresses the eustachian tube. Rarely, infections can develop in the nose, sinus, or middle ear after nasal packing and lead to toxic shock syndrome (TSS). Risk factors for TSS include any wound and respiratory infections, such as sinusitis, sore throat (pharyngitis), laryngitis, tonsillitis, or pneumonia. Foul odor is alarming as the nasal pack ages over 48 hours from insertion. Bruising or swelling of the eyelids secondary to nasal packing may develop. Therefore, packing is best removed within 24 to 48 hours following placement, provided the patient's clinical condition has stabilized.

When tight nasal/oral packing fails in unstable patients, supraselective arteriography and embolization is the treatment of choice, if this modality is available (25). Ligation of the external carotid artery is a last resort in the unstable multitrauma patient who cannot be transported. However, due to collateral circulation of the face, ligation is seldom truly effective. The best control of hemorrhage is obtained by exploratory surgery and fracture fixation. In patients with isolated LeFort fractures, open reduction/internal fixation (ORIF) is the first line of treatment (26).

Wound Management

The management of facial soft tissue injuries depends on the area of injury. However, there are some basic rules that apply in treating these injuries. Soft tissue injuries are only properly evaluated after the wound is cleaned of dirt, foreign bodies, debris, and dry blood. A local anesthetic is usually necessary to properly clean the wound and perform a thorough examination. In the awake patient, most local infiltrative anesthetics cause great discomfort, which may compromise spinal precautions. Very slow injection using a fine needle (30 gauge) as well as adding bicarbonate in a 1:10 ratio may help. Facial nerve function should be assessed in all patients with facial lacerations and nerve function should be documented *prior* to anesthetic use. Anatomic landmarks are of great importance: if facial nerve paralysis results from a laceration anterior to a line perpendicular to the lateral canthus of the eye, the terminal nerve branches are involved. If facial nerve paralysis results from a laceration posterior to this imaginary line, the facial nerve should be explored. Ideally, repair of the facial nerve should occur as soon as possible, but no later than 72 hours, unless the wound is heavily contaminated. In this case, the nerve endings are tagged with a permanent suture and repair is performed when the wound is clean. In patients with deep lacerations of the cheek, the wound should also be explored for injury to the parotid (Stensen) duct. One may see saliva in the wound if the duct is lacerated. The parotid duct is repaired over a stent to prevent stenosis. Lacerations and contusions of specialized three-dimensional structures such as the eyelid, nasal alae, and ear are often best referred to a specialist, especially if flaps show signs of devascularization.

Optimum timing of facial laceration repair is a topic of some debate. After tetanus prophylaxis, soft tissue repair can be performed within 12 to 24 hours, provided the wounds are irrigated, cleaned, and kept moist. Because of the abundant blood supply, definite wound closure can be delayed and, in general, requires minimal debridement. "Traumatic tattooing" is a greater problem in the face than skin loss. A perfect repair is difficult to obtain in the acute setting as areas of contusion have to declare themselves and often leave irregularities later on. As long as important anatomic landmarks are aligned (e.g., vermillion border of the lip, gray line of the eyelid) and like tissues are approximated (mucosa to mucosa, muscle to muscle, cartilage to cartilage, and skin to skin), revisions can be done later. Deep sutures are used to close dead space to avoid hematomas and to remove tension from the skin closure, preventing an unsightly scar. Good esthetic results depend less on suture technique than on proper redraping of tissues. Scars are noticeable as a result of reflection of light and creation of shadow. For cosmesis, it is of importance to create an "even" closure and, if possible, to place scars in areas of shadow and along lines perpendicular to facial muscle pull. Photographic documentation is important so that the patient may later realize the extent of the original injury, to follow healing, to document subsequent revisions, and for medical-legal reasons.

PATIENT EXAMINATION

Cranial Nerve Examination

Olfaction (Cranial Nerve (CN) I)

Olfaction is typically not examined in the acute trauma bay setting but reserved for later trauma surveys (e.g., tertiary survey). Damage to CN I should be considered with NOE fractures and frontal sinus fractures if disruption of the cribriform plate is present.

Pupillary Responses (CN II, III)

Examine the pupil size and shape at rest. This can be difficult in patients with extensive orbital trauma as the eyelid swells rapidly and is difficult to open. Next, examine with a flashlight. Note the direct constriction of the illuminated pupil, as well as the consensual constriction of the opposite pupil. In an afferent pupillary defect there is decreased direct response in the affected eye. This can be demonstrated by moving the flashlight back and forth between the two eyes, with a lag of 2 to 3 seconds. The afferent defect becomes evident when the flashlight is moved from the normal to the affected eye because the affected eye will dilate in response to light. Brief pupillary oscillations of the stimulated pupil (hippus) are normal and should be distinguished from pathologic response. Finally, test the pupillary response to accommodation, by moving an object (e.g., finger) from far to near. The pupils should constrict. The direct response of the ipsilateral pupil is absent in lesions to the ipsilateral optic nerve, the pretectal area, the ipsilateral sympathetic nerves traveling with CN III, or the pupillary constrictor muscle of the iris. The consensual response is impaired (contralateral pupil illuminated) in lesions of the contralateral optic nerve, the pretectal area, the sympathetic nerves, or the pupillary constrictor of the iris. Accommodation is affected for the same reasons and in pathways from optic nerve to the visual cortex. Accommodation is spared in injury to the pretectal area (27).

Extraocular Movements (CN III, IV, VI)

Extraocular movement is readily checked by asking patients to look in all directions without moving their head and asking them if they experience any diplopia in any direction. Test "smooth pursuit" by slowly moving an object or finger up and down and sideways. Test convergence by asking the patient to fixate on an object that is moved toward a point between the eyes. During these tests, look closely for nystagmus and dysconjugate gaze.

Facial Sensation and Muscles of Mastication (CN V)

Test facial sensation using a soft object or finger in the forehead, cheek, and lower jaw line to capture all three branches of the nerve. Test the masseter muscles during jaw clench. In facial fractures, the most commonly affected nerve is the Vb branch, which may indicate maxillary, orbital, or zygomaticomaxillary complex (ZMC) fractures.

Muscles of Facial Expression and Taste (CN VII)

Look for asymmetries in spontaneous facial expressions and blinking, smiling, and squinting. Taste testing is usually not performed. Facial weakness can be caused by lesions of upper motor neuron in the contralateral cortex or in descending nerve pathways (ipsilateral). Upper motor neurons to the upper face cross over to both facial nuclei so in intracranial injury or stroke, motor functions of the upper face remain intact. Lower motor neuron lesions typically cause weakness to the entire ipsilateral face.

Hearing and Vestibular Sense (CN VIII)

Hearing and vestibular sense are seldom checked in the acute setting. Vestibular sense is typically not tested except in patients with vertigo.

Palate Elevation and Gag Reflex (CN IX, X)

Perform an intraoral examination and observe palatal motion when the patient says "aaah." Observe the gagging motion when the posterior pharynx is touched. The gag reflex is usually checked in patients with suspected brainstem pathology.

Sternocleidomastoid and Trapezius Muscles (CN XI)

These muscles are examined by asking the patient to shrug the shoulders and turn the head from side to side. Of note is that bilateral upper motor neuron projections control the sternocleidomastoid, analog to the bilateral CN VII projections controlling the upper face.

Tongue (CN XII)

The tongue will deviate toward the weak side. Lesions of the motor cortex cause contralateral tongue weakness as opposed to lower motor lesions or lesions of the tongue muscles.

SPECIFIC SIGNS AND SYMPTOMS OF FACIAL FRACTURES

Nasal Bones

The clinical features of an isolated nasal fracture are noted in Table 67.2. Because of the prominence of the nose, nasal injuries are fairly common and the nose is the most commonly fractured bone in the facial skeleton. Nasal fracture diagnosis is often a clinical, and not a radiologic, diagnosis. External nasal deformities are usually obvious during examination. Crepitus will distinguish recent trauma from a nasal deformity due to a previous injury. Septal hematoma must be ruled out in every patient. A septal hematoma forms between the septal cartilage and perichondrium from which it gets its blood supply. It appears as edema and ecchymosis of the septum with narrowing of the nasal airway on speculum examination. Septal hematoma is treated with incision and drainage. Failure to treat can lead to a septal abscess, intracranial complications, or delayed saddle nose deformity due to cartilage loss.

Leakage of cerebrospinal fluid (CSF) indicates a fracture through the cribriform plate of the ethmoid bone. Although this potentially carries a risk of meningitis, there remains controversy on the use of prophylactic antibiotics; our practice is to prophylax. Epistaxis is treated by packing the nose as discussed above. If this is not successful, an epistaxis catheter can be inserted to control bleeding from branches of the anterior ethmoidal artery. Treatment of most noncomminuted nasal fractures is closed reduction. Manipulation is required to restore an obstructed nasal airway and for restoration of facial cosmesis. The ideal timing for manipulative treatment varies. If reduction is not performed within the first few hours following injury, treatment is delayed 3 to 5 days for swelling to resolve. After a prolonged period (7 to 14 days), manipulation becomes increasingly difficult as the nasal bones will be difficult to move into place without osteotomies and a formal rhinoplasty may be required.

NASO-ORBITO-ETHMOID FRACTURES

The clinical features of a nasoethmoidal fracture are noted in Table 67.3. With true nasoethmoidal fractures, a CSF leak should be assumed, even if not clinically evident. Classically, an increased intercanthal distance (>35 mm) and depression of the nasal root are unequivocal clinical signs of traumatic telecanthus. Closed manipulation of NOE injuries notoriously gives a poor result, with a high incidence of persistent or recurrent deformity postoperatively. The results of secondary surgery of this deformity are seldom satisfactory. ORIF, often with bone grafting to the nose, is usually necessary as the NOE complex is a very difficult area of the facial skeleton to reconstruct. Access to the nasoethmoidal region can be obtained through an existing laceration, if present, or through a coronal incision for adequate access to the frontal bone, nasal root, and orbits (28).

TABLE 67.2 Clinical Features of an Isolated Nasal Fracture
• Tenderness over nasal bones
• Mobility
• Swelling
• Flattened or deviated nose
• Epistaxis
• Septal deviation
• Septal hematoma
• Mouth breathing

TABLE 67.3 Clinical Features of a Nasoethmoidal Fracture
• Flat nasal bridge with splaying of nasal complex and crepitus
• Saddle-shaped deformity of nose ("punched-in" look)
• Telecanthus (increased distance between the medial canthi)
• Circumorbital edema and ecchymosis ("raccoon eyes")
• Subconjunctival hemorrhage
• Epistaxis
• CSF rhinorrhea
• Supraorbital/supratrochlear nerve paresthesia

The evaluation of the stability of the medial canthal ligament forms an integral part of the clinical assessment. The clinical classification of status of the medial canthal ligament and its attachment to underlying bone can be classified according to Gruss et al. (29) or Markowitz et al. (30). The medial canthus must be stabilized, usually by wiring to the opposite anterior lacrimal crest (transnasal canthopexy). If both canthal ligaments are detached, then the telecanthus can be addressed by means of wiring the two medial canthal ligaments to each other (transnasally).

Orbital Blowout Fracture

The term *orbital blowout fracture* is reserved for a fracture of the bones of the orbit. This may involve the orbital floor, walls, or roof. The majority of cases involve the orbital floor and medial wall, as these areas comprise the thinnest bone of the orbit. An isolated orbital blowout fracture is usually secondary to a blunt blow. Smith and Regan demonstrated that when an object with a diameter slightly greater than that of the orbital rim strikes the orbit and incomprehensible eyeball, a middle orbital fracture may occur secondary to increased intra-orbital pressure (31). Often, the thin bone of the floor displaces downward into the maxillary antrum, remaining attached to the orbital periosteum as one fragment ("trap door"). The periorbital fat herniates through the defect, thereby interfering with the inferior rectus and inferior oblique muscles, which are contained within the same fascia sheath. This prevents upward movement and outward rotation of the eye and the patient experiences diplopia on upward gaze. This clinical finding should be distinguished from true "entrapment," which indicates impingement of the ocular muscles. Those patients will present with pain, tenderness around the eye, swelling, and subjective diplopia in all outer fields of gaze. Painful eye movement is common with significant swelling and hemorrhage in the orbit, and restriction of eye motility and double vision are not necessarily an indication for surgical repair of the fracture. Ophthalmologic evaluation is advised if significant eye trauma is detected. If the patient is unresponsive, an afferent pupillary defect may uncover occult visual loss. If indicated clinically, tonometry may be used to assess intraocular pressure. This may serve as a baseline for serial examinations. Also, forced duction testing can be done to check extraocular movements. This is done by grasping the sclera in the fornix and mechanically moving the globe. To test inferior rectus entrapment, the globe is moved superiorly. Inhibition of this motion would indicate need for exploration. A computed tomography (CT) scan will determine the presence or absence, and size, of the fracture. Surgical repair of orbital fractures depends on symptoms and largely on the size of the fracture itself. Small fractures (<50% of the floor or <2 cm^2), even if associated with double vision, can be observed for 1 to 2 weeks to assess for the need to repair, if symptoms do not resolve repair is indicated. Patients are instructed to avoid blowing their nose and to use nasal decongestants. Should symptoms persist and/or if the fracture is large, surgical intervention is required to return the orbital contents to their correct position and to restore orbital volume. This is done by placement of a graft in the orbital floor. Many different graft materials can be used, but autologous bone remains the gold standard and may be required if the defect is large enough, especially in a young patient (32). Complications of unrecognized orbital floor fracture are noted in Table 67.4.

TABLE 67.4 Complications of Unrecognized Orbital Floor Fracture

- Posttraumatic persistent enophthalmos
- Hypoglobus (inferior displacement of the orbit)
- Persistent diplopia
- Lower eyelid retraction (ectropion) and scleral show
- Persistent edema of the lower eyelid

Zygoma Fractures

Clinical features of ZMC fractures are noted in Table 67.5. Zygomatic fractures usually result from high-impact trauma; the leading causes include assault, motor vehicle or motorcycle accidents, sports injuries, and falls. The ZMC is both a functional and esthetic unit of the facial skeleton and the prominent zygoma is the second most commonly fractured facial bone. The majority of zygomatic fractures occur in men in the third decade of life. The zygoma separates the orbit from the maxillary sinus and temporal fossa. Because the zygoma articulates superficially with the maxilla, frontal, and temporal bones, zygomatic fractures in the past have been referred to as tripod or trimalar fractures; however, the fourth articulation with the sphenoid really makes it a quadripod fracture. The ZMC can be defined by two arcs: a vertical arc from the zygomaticofrontal suture down to the lateral antrum, and a horizontal arc from the zygomatic arch to the inferior orbital rim. The intersection of these two arcs defines the malar prominence (1). The zygoma itself is a relatively strong bone, and isolated fractures of the body of the zygoma are rare unless it receives a direct blow. Due to traction on the infraorbital nerve, patients often complain of upper lip/tooth numbness. Trismus may be present as the masseter muscle pulls the malar fragment down, which impinges on the mandible. Radiologic imaging remains an important step in the evaluation of orbito-zygomatico-maxillary fractures. CT scanning offers advantages over plain films that justify the increased cost. Important areas to evaluate on CT scanning include the buttresses, the orbital walls, the zygomatic arch, the palate, and the mandibular condyles (33).

The timing of zygomal repair is 5 to 7 days postinjury to allow tissue edema and swelling to subside. After 10 days, masseter contracture may complicate closed reduction of the zygoma. If the zygomatic arch is minimally displaced and there is no comminution, the patient is a candidate for "simple" reduction. If there is moderate displacement or comminution of the maxillary wall, the maxilla will have to be plated for stability. For true ZMC fractures, ORIF is typically necessary at the lateral maxilla, the inferior orbital rim, the zygomatico-frontal

TABLE 67.5 Clinical Features of Zygomatic Fractures

- Swelling and bruising over the cheek/flattening
- Step-off deformity at the orbital rim
- Periorbital ecchymosis
- Subconjunctival hemorrhage
- Paresthesia/anesthesia of the infraorbital nerve
- Trismus and restricted lateral excursion
- Paresthesia/anesthesia of zygomatic or facial/temporal nerves

(ZF) suture, the zygomatic arch, and commonly the orbital floor as well. Full access to the arch unfortunately requires a coronal approach (34).

The Midfacial Skeleton: LeFort Fractures

LeFort fractures tend to result from anterior forces. The fracture possibilities and combinations thereof are numerous; hence, classification schemes fail to describe them all. The original fracture patterns described by LeFort in 1901 are based on experimentally induced midface trauma. LeFort established that midface fractures tend to occur in reproducible patterns along weaker areas of the craniofacial skeleton. The LeFort I fracture essentially separates the lower maxilla, including the alveolar ridge and teeth, from the rest of the midface. The fracture classically travels through the inferior portion of the piriform aperture across the maxilla to the pterygoid fissure. This fracture pattern may occur as a single entity, or in association with LeFort II and III fractures. The LeFort II fracture is a pyramidal fracture that includes the entire piriform aperture in the distracted midface. The fracture line includes the frontonasal suture, passes through the inferomedial orbit, and runs between the zygoma and maxilla for a larger area of dissociation. The LeFort III fracture is a suprazygomatic fracture through the lateral orbit. The fracture line extends from the dorsum of the nose and the cribriform plate along the medial and lateral wall of the orbit to the ZF suture line. This is also known as craniofacial dissociation as the bones of the midface are essentially completely disarticulated from the cranium (35).

Signs and Symptoms of LeFort Fractures

All complete LeFort fractures will create mobility of the maxilla, especially the upper alveolus (tooth-bearing portion of the maxilla). Hence, all will lead to subjective (and objective) malocclusion in varying degrees of severity. Infraorbital nerve paresthesia may be present. There can be palpable crepitus in the upper buccal sulcus from the fracture line; an intraoral hematoma or ecchymosis is likely. In LeFort II and III fractures, the nose is often involved and epistaxis common. In LeFort III fractures, this should be distinguished from CSF rhinorrhea. Periorbital ecchymosis and edema, subconjunctival hemorrhage, and visual disturbance occur only in LeFort III fractures.

Management of Maxillary Fractures

Minimally displaced fractures can be clinically observed provided no malocclusion is present. The patient is allowed oral intake, but only full liquid/soft foods as load bearing (chewing) may displace fracture fragments. Comminuted fractures and fractures with malocclusion are treated with MMF and/or by ORIF. Truly rigid fixation of the midface, unlike the mandible, is unattainable due to the thin bones and correspondingly thin plates but bone grafting can be done (5).

For comminuted or displaced fractures, the status of the mandible is critical for management. If the mandible is intact, it serves as a guide for placing the upper dentition into occlusion. MMF is placed, and then the midface is treated with appropriate ORIF. Intraoperatively used MMF can be released after fracture fixation and the patient allowed range of motion (soft diet only). If the mandible is also fractured, the patient is placed in MMF for 2 to 3 weeks (36).

SUMMARY

Evaluating the patient with facial trauma can be challenging. The basics of ATLS apply to this patient population as well as those with general trauma. Stabilizing and securing the airway may be difficult in the presence of extensive facial trauma with the possibility of basilar skull base injury; where endotracheal intubation is relatively contraindicated one must consider a surgical airway. Any patient who has sustained forces adequate to cause facial fractures must be assumed to have a cervical spine injury until proven otherwise. Epistaxis can be troublesome and hemodynamically significant. In the clinical evaluation of facial fractures, subjective data that the patient is able to provide offer clues to facial fracture diagnosis and include: pain, malocclusion, numbness in portions of the face, trismus, and diplopia. Malocclusion is a very sensitive indicator of injury due to the high sensitivity of the periodontal ligaments. Numbness often indicates disruption or compression of a peripheral nerve. Trismus may result from mandibular trauma or from an impacted zygoma impinging on the temporalis muscle. Diplopia may result from entrapment of the extraocular muscles or gross globe malposition. Of special note, monocular diplopia indicates an intrinsic globe problem and mandates prompt ophthalmologic evaluation.

Unfortunately, many trauma patients are obtunded or intoxicated and unable to provide any subjective information. Although physical examination alone is inconclusive in the majority of cases, the examiner should note presence and location of lacerations, ecchymoses, and gross asymmetry. Palpation is done to assess instability, crepitus, tenderness, bony stepoffs, and canthal tendon disruption. The trigeminal nerve should be tested. Ophthalmologic examination deserves special mention. Many authors believe that it is impractical to expect ophthalmologic consultation on every patient with facial injury (32). Most physicians are able to test visual acuity (subjective and objective), pupillary function, ocular motility, anterior chamber examination (to look for hyphema), and funduscopic examination; ophthalmologic consultation should then be obtained as indicated. Last but not least, although cosmesis is not an immediate concern, it is of great concern to patients, especially once the acute trauma experience has worn off. Long-term goals and appearance outcomes should therefore be discussed with every patient on an individual basis to avoid misunderstandings and misconceptions. Facial fracture management aims to restore facial height, width, and projection. Newer techniques of rigid fixation are constantly being developed to optimize treatment outcomes for facial fracture management. Bioresorbable plates have come onto the market, with particular utility in the pediatric population, where there is concern that rigid fixation with hardware may get incorporated in growing bone and inhibit facial growth. However, the behavior of the soft tissue envelope is much more difficult to predict depending on age, gender, race, and soft tissue trauma sustained at the injury. In general, the abatement of swelling and soft tissue adjustment takes at least 3 months, and neurapraxia substantially longer. In general, patients should be told that it takes about a year before final settling and a stable end result. This helps dissuade requests for interventions as the tissues continue to improve (37).

Key Points

- It is critical to differentiate injuries requiring immediate operative intervention from those that can be deferred for a later time period.
- Patient should be stabilized initially by using the ABCs of ATLS in conjunction with the trauma or emergency team.
- Cervical spine injury must be sought for and addressed by immobilization of cervical spine and active exclusion of cervical spine injury by physical and neurologic examinations with imaging adjuncts as necessary.
- In emergency situations secure the airway by the quickest way not necessarily the safest.
- Systemic antibiotic use is still controversial but current evidence suggests topical antibiotic use with usual perioperative antibiotics should suffice.

References

1. Frost DE, Kendell BD. Applied surgical anatomy of the head and neck. In: Fonseca RJ, Walker RV, eds. *Oral and Maxillofacial Trauma*. 3rd ed. Philadelphia, PA: WB Saunders; 2005.
2. Cornelius CP, Kunz C, Neff A, et al. *The Comprehensive AOCMF Classification System: Fracture Case Collection, Diagnostic Imaging Work Up, AOCOIAC Iconography and Coding in Craniomaxillofac Trauma Reconstruct*. 2014;7(Suppl 1):S131–S135.
3. Sharabi SE, Koshy JC, Thornton JF, Hollier LH Jr. Facial fractures. *Plast Reconstr Surg*. 2011;127(2):25e–34e.
4. Mundinger GS, Dorafshar AH, Gilson MM, et al. Blunt-mechanism facial fracture patterns associated with internal carotid artery injuries: recommendations for additional screening criteria based on analysis of 4,398 patients. *J Oral Maxillofac Surg*. 2013;71(12):2092–2100.
5. Kaufman Y, Cole P, Hollier LH Jr. Facial gunshot wounds: trends in management. *J Craniomaxillofac Trauma Reconstr*. 2009;2(2):85–90.
6. Pappachan B, Alexander M. Biomechanics of cranio-maxillofacial trauma. *J Maxillofac Oral Surg*. 2012;11(2):224–230.
7. Hohlrieder M, Hinterhoelzl J, Ulmer H, et al. Traumatic intracranial hemorrhages in facial fracture patients: review of 2,195 patients. *Intensive Care Med*. 2003;29(7):1095–1100.
8. Litschel R, Tasman AJ. Contemporary management of facial trauma. *Facial Plast Surg*. 2015;31(4):317–318.
9. Clark N, Birely B, Manson PN, et al. High-energy ballistic and avulsive facial injuries: classification, patterns, and an algorithm for primary reconstruction. *Plastic Reconstr Surg*. 1996;98(4 Suppl 1):583–601.
10. Sahlin GF, Guimaraes-Ferreira J, Lauritzen C. Orbital fractures in craniofacial trauma in Goteborg: trauma scoring, operative techniques, and outcome. *Scand J Plast Reconstr Surg Hand Surg*. 2003;37:69–74.
11. Ford K. A hospital-based violence prevention intervention reduced hospital recidivism for violent injury and arrests for violent crimes. *Evid Based Med*. 2007;12(4):110.
12. Hollier LH Jr, Sharabi SE, Koshy JC, Stal S. Facial trauma: general principles of management. *J Craniofac Surg*. 2010;21(4):1051–1053.
13. Mundinger GS, Dorafshar AH, Gilson MM, et al. Analysis of radiographically confirmed blunt-mechanism facial fractures. *J Craniofac Surg*. 2014;25(1):321–327.
14. Boffano P, Roccia F, Zavattero E, et al. European Maxillofacial Trauma (EURMAT) project: a multicentre and prospective study. *J Craniomaxillofac Surg*. 2015;43(1):62–70.
15. Boffano P, Kommers SC, Karagozoglu KH, Forouzanfar T. Aetiology of maxillofacial fractures: a review of published studies during the last 30 years. *Br J Oral Maxillofac Surg*. 2014;52(10):901–906.
16. Manoach S, Paladino L. Manual in-line stabilization for acute airway management of suspected cervical spine injury: historical review and current questions. *Ann Emerg Med*. 2007;50(3):236–245.
17. Bellamy JL, Mundinger GS, Flores JM, et al. Facial fractures of the upper craniofacial skeleton predict mortality and occult intracranial injury after blunt trauma: an analysis. *J Craniofac Surg*. 2013;24(6):1922–1926.
18. Hutchison I, Lawlor M, Skinner D. ABC of major trauma. Major maxillofacial injuries. *BMJ*. 1990;301(6752):595–599.
19. Kwok H, McCormack J, Cece R, et al. Controlled trial of oronasal versus nasal mask ventilation in the treatment of acute respiratory failure. *Crit Care Med*. 2003;31(2):468–473.
20. Barak M, Bahouth H, Leiser Y, et al. Airway management of the patient with maxillofacial trauma: review of the literature and suggested clinical approach. *Biomed Res Int*. 2015;724032.
21. Biglioli F, Mortini P, Goisis M, et al. Submental orotracheal intubation: an alternative to tracheotomy in transfacial cranial base surgery. *Skull Base*. 2003;13(4):189–195.
22. Biggs TC, Nightingale K, Patel NN, Salib RJ. Should prophylactic antibiotics be used routinely in epistaxis patients with nasal packing. *Ann R Coll Surg Engl*. 2013;95(1):40–42.
23. Kreutzer K, Storck K, Weitz J. Current evidence regarding prophylactic antibiotics in head and neck and maxillofacial surgery review. *Biomed Res Int*. 2014;2014:879437.
24. Campos GB, Lucena EE, da Silva JS, et al. Efficacy assessment of two antibiotic prophylaxis regimens in oral and maxillofacial trauma surgery: preliminary results. *Int J Clin Exp Med*. 2015;8(2):2846–2852.
25. Chen CC, Jeng SF, Tsai HH, et al. Life threatening bleeding of bilateral maxillary arteries in maxillofacial trauma: report of two cases. *J Trauma Inj*. 2006;61:1–5.
26. Janus SC, MacLeod SP, Odland R. Analysis of results in early versus late midface fracture repair. *Otolaryngol Head Neck Surg*. 2008;138(4):464–467.
27. Wang BH, Robertson BC, Girotto JA, et al. Traumatic optic neuropathy: a review of 61 patients. *Plastic Reconstr Surg*. 2001;107(7):1655–1664.
28. Sargent LA. Nasoethmoid orbital fractures: diagnosis and treatment. *Plastic Reconstr Surg Craniofac Trauma*. 2007;120(7 Suppl 2):16S–31S.
29. Gruss JS, Hurwitz JJ, Nik NA, Kassel EE. The pattern and incidence of nasolacrimal injury in naso-orbital-ethmoid fractures: the role of delayed assessment and dacryocystorhinostomy. *Br J Plast Surg*. 1985;38:116–121.
30. Markowitz BL, Manson PN, Sargent L, et al. Management of the canthal tendon in nasoethmoid orbital fractures: the importance of the central fragment in classification and treatment. *Plast Reconstr Surg*. 1991;87:843–853.
31. Smith B, Regan WF Jr. Blow-out fracture of the orbit; mechanism and correction of internal orbital fracture. *Am J Ophthalmol*. 1957;44(6):733–739.
32. Cole P, Boyd V, Banerji S, Hollier LH Jr. Comprehensive management of orbital fractures. *Plast Reconstr Surg Craniofac Trauma*. 2007;120(7 Suppl 2):57S–63S.
33. Ellis E. Fractures of the zygomatic complex and arch. In: Fonseca RJ, Walker RV, eds. *Oral and Maxillofacial Trauma*. 3rd ed. Philadelphia, PA: WB Saunders; 2005:569.
34. Stanley RB Jr. The zygomatic arch as a guide to reconstruction of comminuted malar fractures. *Arch Otolaryngol Head Neck Surg*. 1989;115:1459–1462.
35. Manson PN, Clark N, Robertson B, et al. Subunit principles on midface fractures: the importance of sagittal buttresses, soft-tissue reductions, and sequencing treatment of segmental fractures. *Plastic Reconstr Surg*. 1999;103(4):1287–1306; quiz 1307.
36. Lew D, Sinn DP. Diagnosis and treatment of midface fractures. In: Fonseca RJ, Walker RV, eds. *Oral and Maxillofacial Trauma*. Philadelphia, PA: WB Saunders; 1991.
37. Girotto JA, MacKenzie E, Fowler C, et al. Long-term physical impairment and functional outcomes after complex facial fractures. *Plastic Reconstr Surg*. 2001;108(2):312–327.

CHAPTER
68

Temperature-Related Injuries

TAKERU SHIMIZU and TARO MIZUTANI

Human body temperature is maintained within tight limits by a balance between heat production and dissipation. Heat is normally generated by muscular activity and metabolic reactions, the latter mainly by the liver. It is dissipated by a combination of radiation, convection, conduction, and evaporation. This balance between heat generation and dissipation is the key to maintaining optimal body temperature. Under normal circumstances, body temperature is 37°C under the tongue, 38°C in the rectum, 32°C at the skin, and 38.5°C in the central liver. Significant deviation from normal body temperature is a critical condition that requires prompt diagnosis, treatment, and normalization of the temperature alteration. Herein, we discuss hypothermia, hyperthermia, and malignant hyperthermia (MH) and the neuroleptic malignant hyperthermia (NMH).

HYPOTHERMIA

Hypothermia is generally defined as a core temperature below 35°C (95°F) (1–3). In a more detailed manner, the literature classifies hypothermia as mild, moderate, or severe: mild hypothermia is the temperature above 34°C (93.2°F), moderate hypothermia between 30°C and 34°C (86° and 93.2°F), and severe hypothermia below 30°C (86°F) (4). Table 68.1A outlines the classification of severe and clinical manifestations. However, it is not always possible to readily measure the core temperature. Therefore, the use of Swiss staging system (Table 68.1B) of hypothermia, which stages clinically on the basis of vital signs (stages HT I to HT IV) is favored over traditional staging (5,6). Yet, measurement of the core temperature is necessary to confirm staging and management decisions (5). When measurement is performed, it should be taken into consideration that the recorded temperature can vary depending on the body site, perfusion, and environmental temperature (5).

Hypothermia may be precipitated by various acute and chronic medical conditions, environmental exposure, or drugs. Hypothermia caused without exposure to the extreme temperatures is generally limited to mild to moderate in degree. Interestingly, however, with equivalent body temperature, patients found indoors were more severely affected and died more frequently than those found outdoors (7).

Hypothermia is considered to be an underrecognized condition, especially in the aged (2,3). Elderly patients who develop hypothermia are more likely to live alone, have other intercurrent diseases, to have their home heating turned off or inadequate home heating, and to wear inappropriate clothing for actual ambient temperatures (8).

Several confounding factors can further impair temperature control. Intoxicants, medications, extremes of age, and the general state of health—including intercurrent diseases—can modify the heat loss. Hypothermia occurs in various clinical settings. Table 68.2 outlines the clinical causes and disorders associated with this finding.

Accidental hypothermia is defined as a spontaneous decrease in core temperature. It is often caused by a cold environment and associated with an acute problem, but without any primary disorder of the temperature regulatory center. This is most commonly observed in neonates; the elderly; unconscious, immobile, or drugged persons; and workers in an extremely cold environment. Mortality rates for accidental hypothermia have been reported to range between 10% and 80%. A multicenter review of 428 cases of accidental hypothermia reported an overall mortality of 17% (9–11). Intercurrent diseases or infection seem to contribute to most deaths, as it was shown that patients with sepsis had a markedly worse mortality rate when they presented with hypothermia, as opposed to fever (12).

Temperature Regulation and Mechanism of Heat Loss

Hypothermia presents when heat generation cannot keep up with heat dissipation. Heat generation depends on the metabolic process at rest and on skeletal muscle metabolism during exercise. Humans have a high capacity to dissipate heat, with four primary means of heat dissipation or transmission. It is important to know these mechanisms to prevent hypothermia and to develop effective rewarming strategies.

1. *Conduction:* Conduction is the transfer of heat between two masses in contact with one another. The rate of heat transfer depends on the temperature gradient at the interface and the size of the contact area. It is also determined by the thermal conductivity of the materials. Metals and liquids are most conductive, and gases are most insulating. For example, water has a 25- to 30-fold larger conductivity than air. This means that contacting a wet surface is one of the fastest ways to dissipate body temperature.
2. *Convection:* Convection is the transfer of heat due to the flow of liquids or gases over a surface. Convective heat loss occurs when air around a patient is continuously swept away, and it is directly proportional to the body surface area, the temperature gradient, and the air velocity.
3. *Radiation:* Transfer of radiant energy is due to electromagnetic transmission.
4. *Evaporation:* Evaporation is the process whereby atoms or molecules in a liquid state gain sufficient energy to enter the gaseous state. Evaporation proceeds more quickly at higher temperature and/or at higher flow rates between the gaseous and liquid phase. Therefore, the heat loss by this mechanism is proportional to the change of the vapor pressure from the surface to ambient air and the velocity of air movement. Approximately 30% of evaporative heat loss occurs in the lung, and the rest is from the skin surface at usual room temperature.

TABLE 68.1A Classification of Hypothermia

Core Temperature	Consciousness	Shivering	Heart Rate	ECG	Respiration
Mild (35–33°C)	Normal	+	Normal	Normal	Normal
Moderate (33–30°C)	Depressed (stupor)	–	Slight decrease	Prolongation	Depressed
Severe (30–25°C)	Confusion	–	Decreased	Osborne J-wave	Apneic/agonal
25–20°C	Coma	Muscle rigidity	Decreased	Atrial fibrillation	Apneic
Below 20°C	Coma	Muscle rigidity	Asystole	Ventricular fibrillation	Apneic

TABLE 68.1B Staging and Management of Accidental Hypothermia

Stage	Clinical Symptoms	Typical Core Temperature (°c)	Treatment
HT I	Conscious, shivering	35 to 32	Warm environment and clothing, warm sweet drinks, and active movement (if possible)
HT II	Impaired consciousness, not shivering	<32 to 28	Cardiac monitoring, minimal and cautious movements to avoid arrhythmias, horizontal position and immobilization, full-body insulation, active external and minimally invasive rewarming techniques (warm environment; chemical, electrical, or forced-air heating packs or blankets; warm parenteral fluids)
HT III	Unconscious, not shivering, vital signs present	<28 to 24	HT II management plus airway management as required; ECMO or CPB in cases with cardiac instability that is refractory to medical management
HT IV	No vital signs	<24	HT II and III management plus CPR and up to three doses of epinephrine (at an intravenous or intraosseous dose of 1 mg) and defibrillation, with further dosing guided by clinical response; rewarming with ECMO or CPB (if available) or CPR with active external and alternative internal rewarming

Adopted from Brown DJ, et al. Accidental hypothermia. *N Engl J Med.* 367;20, 2012
Hypothermia may be determined clinically on the basis of vital signs with the use of the Swiss staging system.
Measurement of body core temperature is helpful but not mandatory.
CPB: cardiopulmonary bypass, CPR: cardiopulmonary resuscitation, ECMO: extracorporeal membrane oxygenation

Evaporation accounts for 10% to 15% of total body heat loss. The heat of evaporation of water is 0.58 kcal/g H_2O. Given that 30 g of water is lost during the breathing of dry room air per hour, about 18 kcal, which is nearly half of an anesthetized patient's hourly heat production, is lost.

TABLE 68.2 Causes of Hypothermia

Clinical Cause	Associated Disorders
Central nervous system	Head trauma, tumor, stroke, Wernicke encephalopathy, Shapiro syndrome, Parkinson disease, multiple sclerosis, sarcoidosis, acute spinal cord transection, paraplegia
Metabolic	Hypoglycemia, hypothyroidism, hypoadrenalism, panhypopituitarism, diabetic ketoacidosis, anorexia nervosa
Integument	Burns, erythroderma, ichthyosis, psoriasis, exfoliative dermatitis
Infection	Sepsis
Chronic diseases	Chronic heart failure, chronic renal failure, chronic hepatic insufficiency, advanced age
Environmental exposure	Outdoor activities and physical or metabolic exhaustion, cold water immersion, inadequate indoor heating (particularly in the elderly and infirm), operating room
Pharmaceuticals/ drugs	Ethanol, muscle relaxants, phenothiazines, barbiturates, tricyclic antidepressants, lithium (toxic dose), α-adrenergic agonist (clonidine), anticholinergic drugs, β-adrenergic blocker

Clinical Syndromes

Cardiovascular

A sympathetic response increases myocardial oxygen consumption and causes tachycardia and peripheral vasoconstriction—that is, diminished pulses, pallor, acrocyanosis, and cold extremities—in patients with mild hypothermia. Blood pressure and heart rate are initially increased, followed by bradycardia, which further deteriorates at 32°C, and consequently, cardiac output, myocardial contractility, and arterial pressure fall.

Electrocardiographic (ECG) findings include the Osborne J-wave after the QRS complex as hypothermia becomes more severe (Fig. 68.1). The Osborne J-wave is an important diagnostic feature, which can be observed in other pathologic conditions such as central nervous system lesions and sepsis, but it is frequently absent (3,13). Atrial and ventricular fibrillation are common, and electrical defibrillation during hypothermia is often ineffective. It is important to remember that the hypothermic myocardium is irritable, making placement of pulmonary artery or other central catheters dangerous.

Respiratory System

Respiratory rate falls. The patient becomes apneic or has an agonal respiratory pattern when the body temperature is less than 28°C.

Central Nervous System

The electroencephalogram (EEG) becomes flat at 19° to 29°C (14). Cerebrovascular autoregulation remains intact until the core temperature falls to below 25°C, but mentation starts to

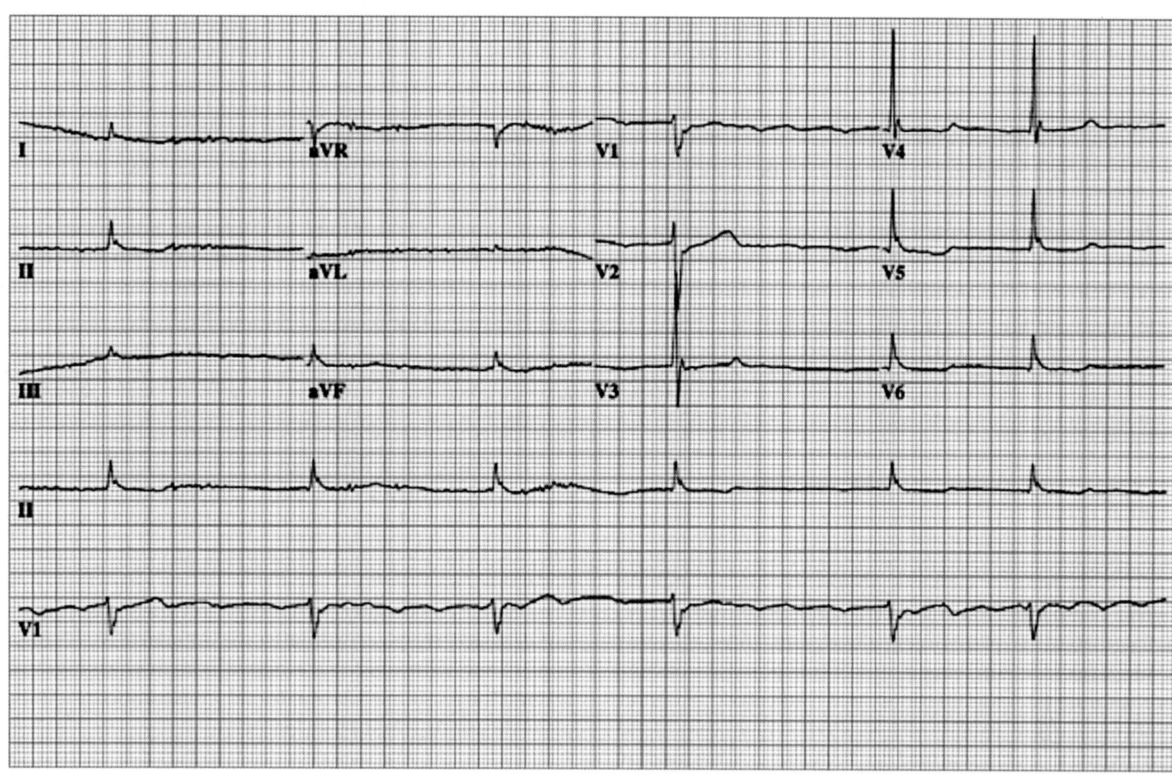

FIGURE 68.1 The electrocardiogram (ECG) shows atrial fibrillation with a very slow ventricular response, prominent J (Osborne) waves (late, terminal upright deflection of QRS complex; best seen in leads V3–V6), and nonspecific QRS widening. (Adapted from O'Keefe J, Hammill S, Freed M, et al. *The Complete Guide to ECGs.* 2nd ed. Royal Oak, MI: Physicians' Press; 2002.)

drop at 30°C. Dysarthria and hyperreflexia occur below 35°C, and hyporeflexia occurs below 32°C.

Coagulation

Hypothermia produces coagulopathy via three major mechanisms (15,16). First, the enzymatic coagulation cascade is impaired; second, platelet dysfunction occurs; and third, plasma fibrinolytic activity is enhanced. Because coagulation tests, such as prothrombin time (PT) or partial thromboplastin time (PTT), are performed at 37°C in the laboratory, a major disparity between clinical coagulopathy and the reported values is frequently observed (17). A disseminated intravascular coagulation (DIC) type of syndrome is also reported (18). Clinically significant coagulopathies occur and are often associated with trauma (19,20).

Renal System

Exposure to cold induces a diuresis irrespective of the state of hydration. Centralization of the blood volume—due to the initial peripheral vasoconstriction—stimulates the diuresis. Hypothermia depresses renal blood flow by 50% at 27° to 30°C, and the renal cellular basal metabolic rate decreases (2). As a result, renal tubular cell reabsorptive function decreases and the kidney excretes a large amount of dilute urine. This is termed *cold diuresis,* resulting in a decreased blood volume and progressive hemoconcentration (21).

Glucose Metabolism

Blood glucose concentration commonly increases because pancreatic function, insulin activity, and/or response to insulin decrease, along with activated function of the autonomic nervous system in hypothermia. At the same time, hemoconcentration results in elevated serum glucose concentration.

Therapeutic Approach

While rewarming is the common goal in the clinical treatment of the hypothermic patient, it is both difficult and controversial to treat. At the same time as treatment is initiated, a search for and discovery of the mechanism of heat loss will play a key role in achieving a better outcome. Clinical management includes prehospital treatment as well as in-hospital critical care.

Prehospital Treatment

Hypothermia is often combined with mental and physical exhaustion. Even if a patient is found down, cold, stiff, and cyanotic, the patient is not necessarily dead and may make a recovery even when signs of life are initially absent. Thus, rescue efforts should not be given up while the patient is cold. Since ventricular fibrillation or asystole may be induced by any stimuli, such as tracheal intubation, comatose patients should be treated with extreme care.

The initial primary focus of prehospital treatment is to avoid further loss of heat. Removal of wet clothing and applying dry insulating covers such as blankets, pads, coats, and sleeping bags are effective in treating all the mechanisms of heat loss described above. During transportation, an aluminized space blanket may be used. To make the most of its effect, the patient should be carefully wrapped with additional blankets. The patient should be kept horizontal to minimize the circulatory and sympathetic change. Vigorous rubbing should be avoided because it induces vasodilation, which may be followed by hypotension or "rewarming shock." Hot water bottles or hot packs may be used if available but should be used cautiously to avoid burn injury.

If the hypothermic patient has no signs of life, CPR should be begun without delay (4). Warmed (42° to 46°C), humidified oxygen during bag/mask ventilation (22) and warmed intravenous fluids should be given if possible. Death should not be declared below 32°C. Defibrillation may be attempted at any temperature though the specific algorithm has not been established. If the ventricular arrhythmia is refractory, it may be reasonable to perform further defibrillation attempts according to the standard BLS algorithm concurrent with rewarming strategies (4).

In-hospital Treatment

Indicated monitoring includes an ECG, Doppler evaluation of pulses, and temperature. General laboratory studies include electrolytes, complete blood count, coagulation studies (PT and partial thromboplastin time), blood urea nitrogen, creatinine, amylase, calcium, magnesium, and glucose concentrations. Radiologic examinations are indicated. Patients with hypothermia are usually dehydrated, which should be corrected with IV fluids warmed to 43°C (22). The use of glucose-containing solutions should be used with caution as hypothermic patients are usually hyperglycemic due to hypoactivity of insulin.

The various options for therapeutic approaches can be considered, and rewarming should be performed along with other supportive therapy depending upon the severity of hypothermia. Techniques of rewarming include active and passive methods, and external and internal (core) methods (Table 68.3). In a patient with hypothermia and stable circulation, active external and minimally invasive rewarming is indicated, because of the increased risk of complications, including hemorrhage or thrombosis, as well as the absence of evidence that these methods improve the outcome (5). In patients with hypothermia and cardiac instability who do not have a response to medical management, ECMO or cardiopulmonary bypass (CPB) should be considered (23–32). When patients are in stage HT IV where signs of life and vital signs are absent, there is consensus that treatment with ECMO or CPB is safe and efficient (2–5,29,31,32). Although there are some reports on successful management with warm-water lavage of the thoracic cavity (32–36), this technique is indicated for patients in stage HT IV when ECMO or CPB is not available (5,32,36).

Bronchopneumonia secondary to aspiration is a common complication. Oral intake of warm or hot drink should be avoided because obtunded, hypothermic patients may have suppressed airway protective mechanisms, including cough or gag reflexes. Prophylactic tracheal intubation may be considered if suppression of these reflexes is present or patients are in arrest as recommended in the standard ACLS guidelines (4). When the trachea is intubated, warmed (42° to 46°C), humidified oxygen should be administered (22).

Previous guidelines suggest withholding IV drugs during CPR if the patient's core body temperature is <30°C (86°F) because it has been conventionally indicated that the hypothermic heart may be unresponsive to cardiovascular drugs, pacemaker stimulation, and defibrillation. However, it may be reasonable to consider administration of a vasopressor during cardiac arrest according to the standard ACLS algorithm concurrent with aggressive active core rewarming strategies though the recommendation for administration or withholding of medications is not clear yet (4).

HYPERTHERMIA

There are many conditions that elevate the body temperature. Table 68.4 outlines the major causes, which may be classified as hyperthermia or fever. In this section, we discuss environmental hyperthermia as well as MH and the neuroleptic malignant syndrome (NMS).

Environmental Hyperthermia—Heat Stroke

Heat stroke is a medical emergency, characterized by a high body temperature, altered mental status, and hot dry flushed skin (37). It may lead to multisystem organ dysfunction with hemorrhage and necrosis in the lungs, heart, liver, kidneys, brain, and intestines (38). Heat stroke is thought to be relatively uncommon in

TABLE 68.3 Rewarming Methods

Classification		Methods	Effects
Passive	External	Adding an insulating layer (e.g., blanket, sleeping bag)	0.1–0.7°C increase/hr
		Increasing ambient temperature	Effective when body temperature is above 32°C
Active	External	Hot water bottles Heating blanket Infrared lamp	1–4°C increase/hr Internal rewarming should be applied to avoid rewarming shock
		Submersion in a warm water tank	5–7°C increase/hr
	Internal (core)	Warmed crystalloid fluids or blood transfusion	1.5–2°C increase/hr
		Gastric lavage Rectal lavage Cystic lavage Airway rewarming	Warmed fluids administration required due to loss of circulatory blood volume caused by cold diuresis
	(invasive)	Peritoneal dialysis Thoracic cavity lavage Hemodialysis Cardiopulmonary bypass Percutaneous cardiopulmonary support	3–15°C increase/hr

TABLE 68.4 Hyperthermia and Fever

HYPERTHERMIA
Environmental exposure
Malignant hyperthermia
Neuroleptic malignant syndrome
Thyroid storm
Pheochromocytoma
Serotonin syndrome
Iatrogenic hyperthermia
Brainstem/hypothalamic injury
Drugs
Diuretics
Antidepressants
Ethanol
Anticholinergics
Lithium
Salicylates
Phenothiazines
Antihistamines
β-Adrenergic blockers
FEVER
Inflammatory disorders
Infection
Allergic reactions
Collagen diseases
Neoplasm
Inherited and metabolic diseases
Factitious fever

temperate climates. However, extreme heat events are expected to become more common in such areas as the climate continues to change. In addition, urban areas are more affected because of the "urban heat island effect" (39). The documented body temperature with this disorder is 41.1°C or more. There has been no obvious decrease in mortality in the last 50 years, which is variably quoted as ranging between 10% and 50% (38).

There are several heat-related illnesses, which may take the form of heat syncope, heat cramps, heat exhaustion, and heat stroke. Heat stroke may be further classified as exertional and nonexertional (classic heatstroke). Table 68.5 outlines the syndromes.

- *Heat syncope:* Heat syncope is fainting due to peripheral vasodilation secondary to high ambient temperature.
- *Heat cramp:* Heat cramp refers to muscular cramping occurring during exercise in heat, which is related to electrolyte deficiency; it is usually benign.
- *Heat exhaustion:* This is often referred to as heat prostration. Heat exhaustion occurs when the individual becomes dehydrated and weak. The patient collapses from dehydration, salt depletion, and hypovolemia. Anorexia, nausea, and vomiting frequently occur. Excessive sweating leads to a loss of water and/or electrolytes. There are two mechanisms for this disorder: salt-depletion and water-depletion heat exhaustion. Salt-depletion heat exhaustion usually occurs when an unacclimatized person exercises and replaces only water. Water-depletion heat exhaustion is usually observed in an acclimatized person who has inadequate water intake during exposure to extreme heat. Serum sodium concentration may be normal or mildly elevated. The core temperature may or may not be raised (usually mild to moderate, <38°C) and tissue damage does not occur.
- *Heat stroke:* Heat stroke occurs when the core body temperature rises against a failing thermoregulatory system (37). The core temperature most often quoted is a rectal temperature exceeding 40.6°C (40). Heat stroke may be divided into exertional and nonexertional (classic) heat stroke (40). Exertional heat stroke occurs in previously healthy young people exercising in hot and humid climates without being acclimatized. Nonexertional heat stroke occurs during extreme heat waves, the elderly being particularly vulnerable (Table 68.6).

TABLE 68.5 Heat Syndromes

Syndrome	Temperature	Manifestation
Heat syncope	Normal	Faintness
Heat cramps	Normal	Muscle cramps
Heat exhaustion	Normal to 39°C	Faintness, weakness
Heat stroke	>40.6°C	Gross neurologic impairment

TABLE 68.6 Exertional and Nonexertional Heat Stroke Syndromes

	Exertional	Nonexertional
Age	Young	Elderly
Precipitating event	Heat, strenuous activity	Heat
Underlying process	None	Medical illness, drug therapy
Onset	Rapid	Slow
Sweating	Present	Absent

Temperature Regulation

Normal heat production is primarily due to metabolic activity in the liver and skeletal muscle, with the liver generating most body heat at rest and muscle being the major source with exercise or shivering. Skeletal muscle heat production ranges from 65 to 85 kcal/hr at basal level, but it may increase up to 900 kcal/hr (41). Heat elimination occurs by four major mechanisms as we have discussed in hypothermia. Convection and radiation are normally the most important mechanisms for heat elimination. Evaporation becomes a major mechanism for heat dissipation with incremental skeletal muscle metabolic activity. If the ambient temperature exceeds body temperature, heat loss may depend only on evaporation. However, sweating produces only 400 to 650 kcal/hr of heat dissipation. Therefore, blood flow regulation to skin and sweat gland activity are critical in maintaining thermal balance. There is a distinction made between exertional and nonexertional heat stroke at this point; failure of thermoregulation (lack of sweating) may be more important in nonexertional (classic) heat stroke and less so in exertional heat stroke (42).

The process of thermoregulation consists of three parts: (i) afferent thermal sensing, (ii) hypothalamic processing, and (iii) efferent responses through the sympathetic system. Heat stimuli are carried by C fibers from the skin to the spinal cord. Central temperature sensors in the abdominal and thoracic viscera, spinal cord, and brain may play a significant role in preventing hyperthermia, although peripheral sensors in the skin seem to be most important. The hypothalamus integrates all afferent temperature input to alter body temperature by regulating vasomotor tone to the skin and inducing sweat formation. Neural output to the cerebral cortex is also important in modifying behavior to compensate for changes in temperature. The efferent hypothalamic response to heat consists of cutaneous vasodilation, sweat formation, and inhibition of muscle tone. Vasomotor tonic changes result in cutaneous dilation and shunting of blood away from the liver and splanchnic circulation, facilitating heat transfer from the core to skin. Sweat formation is under cholinergic sympathetic control. Removing clothes, limiting physical activity, and moving to a cooler place are important behaviors.

Acclimatization is a physiologic process whereby an individual adapts to work in a hot environment (41). Acclimatization to sustained increases in body temperature is slow and requires 1 to 2 weeks for peak effect. Sweat volume increases from 1.5 L/hr up to 4 L/hr. The sweating threshold decreases over an extended period of time. Sweat sodium concentration decreases from 30 to 60 mEq/L to about 5 mEq/L. Plasma antidiuretic hormone, growth hormone, and aldosterone levels increase. Cardiovascular mechanisms include a 10% to 25% increase in plasma volume and an increased stroke volume and cardiac output with a slowing of heart rate.

Clinical Syndrome

Heat stroke is mostly defined as a core temperature above 40.6°C, but neurologic impairment may occur at lower temperatures in some cases; indeed, neurologic dysfunction is a cardinal feature of heat stroke (43). Neurologic manifestations include slurred speech, delirium, stupor, lethargy, coma, and seizures (44). Seizures occur more commonly at temperatures above 41°C. Ataxia, dysmetria, and dysarthria may also be observed.

The cardiovascular system is commonly compromised in the presence of heat stroke. Tachydysrhythmia and hypotension frequently occur (44). Hypotension may result from translocation of blood from the central circulation to the periphery to dissipate heat, or the increased production of nitric oxide may result in vasodilation (43,45). A study of Doppler and echocardiographic findings in patients with classic heat stroke and heat exhaustion reported a circulation that was hyperdynamic, with tachycardia, resulting in high cardiac output (40). It also reported that hypovolemia was more pronounced in heat stroke patients with signs of peripheral vasoconstriction. Heat exhaustion patients were more likely to demonstrate peripheral vasodilation.

Metabolic acidosis associated with hyperlactatemia may occur. Since patients in heat stroke are in shock, the mechanism by which lactate is cleared by the liver and converted to glucose is less effective, and restoration of the circulating volume may lead to worsening metabolic acidosis as skeletal muscle is reperfused and the elevated lactate cleared. Patients typically hyperventilate to compensate for the acute acidosis with an acute respiratory alkalosis. This may lead to heat-induced tetany. After several hours, a mixed acid–base disorder may occur because of sustained tissue damage.

Significant dehydration is noted in most patients with exertional heat stroke and may be reflected as elevated blood urea nitrogen and creatinine levels or hemoconcentration. Sodium, potassium, phosphate, calcium, and magnesium serum concentrations are frequently low in the early period (41,46–50). Sodium, potassium, and magnesium are lost through increased sweating. Hypokalemia may be as a result of catecholamine release or may occur secondary to hyperventilation. Hypokalemia decreases sweat secretion and skeletal muscle blood flow, which may impair heat dissipation. Cellular death begins to occur throughout the body at temperatures above 42°C. Hyperkalemia may occur if significant skeletal muscle damage or cellular lysis develops. If significant rhabdomyolysis develops, injured cells release phosphate, which reacts with serum calcium and may lead to hypocalcemia.

Renal dysfunction is well documented in exertional heat stroke, with the incidence of acute renal failure approximately 25% (51). The cause is usually multifactorial, including direct thermal injury, the prerenal insults of volume depletion, and renal hypotension, rhabdomyolysis, and DIC (39).

Liver damage is very frequently seen and is probably related to splanchnic redistribution (52,53). Elevated liver enzymes are common.

Hemorrhagic complications may be observed. These may be petechial hemorrhages and ecchymoses, which may represent direct thermal injury or may be related to the development of DIC. Damatte et al. (44) reported that 45% of patients had laboratory evidence of DIC. This consumption coagulopathy may be further compounded by hepatocellular damage.

Complications

Cardiac complications include myocardial pump failure, tachydysrhythmia, high cardiac output, and myocardial infarction. ECG abnormalities are also observed (54). Sinus tachycardia and QT prolongation are followed by nonspecific ST-T wave changes, suggesting cardiac ischemia.

Neurologic complications include seizures, cerebral edema, and localized brain hemorrhages. Irreversible brain damage occurs above 42°C. Cerebellar impairment may persist after recovery.

Pulmonary edema may be caused by a limited cardiac function or may develop secondary to the acute respiratory distress syndrome (ARDS) (55). Pulmonary aspiration may be observed in obtunded patients.

Acute renal failure may be caused by direct heat damage, renal hypoperfusion, or rhabdomyolysis. The incidence of renal failure is about 35% with exertional heat stroke and about 5% in classic nonexertional heat stroke, with which rhabdomyolysis is less likely to coexist.

Liver damage and dysfunction occur in most patients with heat stroke. Cholestasis and centrilobular necrosis elevate bilirubin and liver enzymes, which may not be apparent until 48 to 72 hours after injury (50).

Hematologic complications include hemolysis, thrombocytopenia, and DIC (55). DIC is triggered by diffuse endothelial and organ damage, has an onset delay of 2 to 3 days after the initiating event, and is associated with high mortality.

Therapeutic Approach

Heat stroke requires prompt and effective treatments. Oxygen therapy, rapid cooling, and cautious hydration should be immediately instituted to avoid complications and achieve recovery. Tracheal intubation should be considered if the patient is obtunded or in respiratory distress. Oxygen delivery is often less than normal, and pulmonary shunt fraction is increased (56).

Rapid cooling is accomplished by external techniques. These include immersion in ice water or application of cooling blankets above and below the patient (conductive cooling technique), and wetting the skin with water or alcohol, followed by the use of fans to facilitate evaporation and heat dissipation (evaporative-convective cooling technique) (57). Both techniques usually reduce core temperature below 40°C in 1 hour. A significant disadvantage of immersion is impairment of access to the patient and limited monitoring. Another disadvantage of immersion is that intense vasoconstriction can slow the rate of heat loss (58). Vasoconstriction may also have adverse cardiovascular effects in patients with limited cardiac function because it increases cardiac afterload. Vasoconstriction may be reduced by skin massage, which prevents dermal stasis of cooled blood. More aggressive cooling techniques include gastric lavage with iced saline, cold hemodialysis, and cardiopulmonary bypass. They are only rarely required, being used in cases of refractory temperature elevation or malignant hyperthermia, in which thermogenesis is ongoing. In addition, the efficacy of rapid infusion of large-volume ice-cold intravenous fluid (LVICF)—using either lactated Ringer solution or normal saline—has been implicated in clinical trials of induced hypothermia. Bernard et al. (59) showed that 30 mL/kg of LVICF (lactated Ringer solution at 4°C) over 30 minutes decreased core temperature by 1.7°C immediately after infusion, with improvements in acid–base and renal function.

Core body temperature should be monitored closely at the rectum, bladder, or tympanic membrane. Vital signs, neurologic functions, urine output, and laboratory measurements should also be monitored closely. Laboratory measurements include arterial blood gas and serum electrolyte concentrations, especially potassium, which may increase significantly and result in life-threatening hyperkalemia. Glucose–insulin therapy should be instituted emergently in patients with ECG changes.

Intravenous volume repletion should be individualized. Volume deficit is not a prominent feature in classic nonexertional heat stroke. Central venous catheter and pulmonary artery catheter placement may be invaluable to assess volume depletion, peripheral vascular vasodilation, or primary myocardial dysfunction, especially in patients with limited cardiac reserve. Hypotension usually responds to intravenous fluids, but if an inotropic drug is needed, dobutamine is the drug of choice for heat stroke.

Seizures occur commonly in heat stroke patients and should be treated with intravenous diazepam or other benzodiazepines. The efficacy or clinical rationale for the administration of dehydrating drugs is uncertain, but these drugs may be potentially beneficial for some patients at risk of acute renal failure secondary to rhabdomyolysis, as acute renal failure can be a major cause of patient morbidity. This may be prevented by prompt repletion of intravascular volume and restabilizing adequate renal perfusion pressure. Hemodialysis may be required if hyperkalemia or other metabolic disturbances exist.

DIC may be treated with continuous infusion heparin therapy. Although this therapy brings some benefit, its utility seems uncertain (46,48,50).

TABLE 68.7 Drugs Associated with Malignant Hyperthermia and the Neuroleptic Malignant Syndrome

Classification	Associated Drugs
MALIGNANT HYPERTHERMIA	
Volatile anesthetics	Halothane, cyclopropane, enflurane, methoxyflurane, isoflurane, sevoflurane, desflurane, diethyl ether
Depolarizing muscle relaxants	Succinylcholine, decamethonium
Antidysrhythmics	Lidocaine
NEUROLEPTIC MALIGNANT SYNDROME	
Phenothiazines	Fluphenazine, chlorpromazine, levomepromazine, thioridazine, trimeprazine, methotrimeprazine, trifluoperazine, prochlorperazine, promethazine, alimemazine
Butyrophenones	Haloperidol, bromperidol, droperidol
Thioxanthenes	Thiothixene, zuclopenthixol
Dibenzazepines	Loxapine
Dopamine-depleting drugs	Alpha-methyltyrosine, tetrabenazine, amoxapine
Dopamine agonist withdrawal	Levodopa, levodopa/carbidopa, amantadine
Serotonin dopamine antagonists	Risperidone
Serotonin-depleting drugs	Paroxetine

Malignant Hyperthermia and the Neuroleptic Malignant Syndrome

MH and the NMS are disorders of rising body temperature related to an imbalance between heat production and heat dissipation. MH was not clearly described as a syndrome until 1960 (60,61). NMS was first described by Delay et al. (62) after the introduction of neuroleptics in 1960. These disorders are uncommon but life-threatening complications related to the administration of anesthetic or neuroleptic drugs. Their main features include hyperthermia, muscle rigidity, metabolic acidosis, and autonomic disturbances. Endogenous heat production resulting from impaired physiologic heat-dissipating mechanisms and hypothalamic temperature regulation is responsible for elevation of core body temperature in NMS. On the other hand, it usually appears intact in MH (63). Both of them are uniquely characterized by their association with various drugs, although they are distinctive from each other; associated drugs are listed in Table 68.7 (63–72). An additive in commercial succinylcholine, chlorocresol, has been reported as an additional trigger in MH (73). The in vitro halothane–caffeine contracture test on skeletal muscle helps to identify susceptible individuals and to establish with certainty the genetic nature of the disorder in most individuals (74). Similar to NMS, use of serotonergic drugs including selective serotonin reuptake inhibitors (SSRIs) is known to cause the serotonin syndrome (SS) (75). Serotonin, a neurotransmitter in the central nervous system, is involved in neuronal circuits that control sleep–wakefulness cycles, mood, and thermoregulation. SS, which presents a combination of mental status changes, autonomic hyperactivity, and neuromuscular abnormalities, is caused by overstimulation of serotonin receptors. The differential diagnosis of the symptoms may be confusing in severe SS. Serotonergic drugs that may produce SS is listed in Table 68.8 (76).

Incidence

The overall incidence of MH is between 1 in 50,000 and 1 in 100,000 patients receiving general anesthesia (77–79). The incidence of fulminant MH was reported to be 1 case per 62,000 anesthetics administered when triggering agents were not used, but the incidence of suspected cases was 1 in 4,500

TABLE 68.8 Drugs That Can Produce the Serotonin Syndrome

Mechanism of Action	Related Drugs
Increased serotonin synthesis	L-triptophan
Decreased serotonin breakdown	MAOIs (including linezolide), ritonavir
Increased serotonin release	Amphetamines, MDMA, cocaine, fenfluramine
Decreased serotonin reuptake	SSRIs, TCAs, dextrometho-rphan, meperidine, fentanyl, tramadol
Serotonin receptor agonist	Lithium, sumitriptan, buspirone, LSD

anesthetics administered when triggering agents including potent volatile agents and succinylcholine (78). Incidence rates of MH reported vary by country. A Danish survey indicates an incidence of fulminant MH of 1 in 250,000 patients (77). The incident rates in Japanese people was calculated to be between 1 in 60,000 to 1 in 73,000 (80,81). The mortality rate was initially 60%; earlier diagnosis and use of dantrolene have reduced it to less than 1.4% (82).

The incidence of NMS ranges from 0.07% to 2.2% among patients receiving neuroleptic agents (83–85). A decrease in mortality has been reported; NMS has had a 76% mortality before 1970, a 22% mortality from 1970 to 1980, and a 15% mortality since 1980 (86).

Temperature Regulation

Most patients with an episode of MH have a history of relatives with a similar episode or an abnormal response to the halothane–caffeine contracture test. Genetic inheritance patterns reflect the complexity of the responsible genes of MH. Genes on chromosomes 1, 3, 5, 7, 17, and 19 (1q32, 3q13, 5p, 7q21–24, 17q21–24) have been indicated (87–89). The exact mechanisms of MH are poorly understood. The initial focus was on an abnormal calcium channel receptor, ryanodine RYR1 receptor, in patients with MH, which is responsible for calcium release from the sarcoplasmic reticulum and plays a critical role in muscle depolarization. Further studies have shown that many patients with MH have a normal ryanodine receptor. However, mutations in RYR1 occur in at least 50% of susceptible subjects and almost all families. More than 30 missense mutations and one deletion have been associated with a positive contracture test result or clinical MH (90). Other than RYR1, CACNA1S is implicated (91). For practical purposes, it seems the RYR1 gene remains the target for genetic analysis (91).

Resultant from this mutation, free inbound ionized calcium can be released from the storage sites, which normally maintain skeletal muscle relaxation by sequestering calcium from the muscle contractile apparatus (63). The administration of anesthetics may unpredictably trigger rapid calcium release into the myoplasm, followed by the development of muscle contracture, rigidity, and increased muscle metabolic activity. This process can cause core body temperature to rise vigorously at a rate of 1°C every 5 minutes.

The administration of certain neuroleptic drugs may induce a similar elevation of body core temperature. A common pathophysiology of NMS and MH has been suggested (92,93). This suggestion is based mainly on three points: (i) NMS and MH have clinical features in common, such as hyperthermia, rigidity, an elevated creatine kinase (CK) concentration, and a mortality rate of 10% to 30%; (ii) sodium dantrolene has been used successfully in both syndromes; and (iii) abnormal findings have been observed in in vitro contractility tests in patients with either of the syndromes. Caroff et al. (94) suggested that patients with a genetic predisposition for MH might also be at risk for developing NMS. However, Adnet et al. (95) reported that abnormal sarcolemmal calcium permeability was not shared in the pathogenesis of these disorders. The mechanism of hyperthermia and muscle rigidity is not yet defined, but two major theories have been postulated, which are central dopamine receptor blockade and the direct toxic effect of skeletal muscle induced by neuroleptics. Hypothalamic thermoregulation involves noradrenergic, serotoninergic, cholinergic, and central dopaminergic pathways (96). Dopamine plays a role in central thermoregulation in mammals. A dopamine injection into the hypothalamus causes a reduction in core temperature (97). Since neuroleptics block dopamine receptors, the hyperthermia associated with NMS may result from a blockade of hypothalamic dopamine sites. In addition, the blockade of dopamine receptors in the corpus striatum is thought to cause muscular rigidity and heat generation. Muscle contracture has been induced in vitro by chlorpromazine (98), which is reported to influence calcium ion transport across the sarcoplasmic reticulum and the contractile system (99). However, other studies that do not support the mechanism have also been reported (94,95).

Clinical Syndrome

MH may occur shortly after induction of anesthesia, at any time during the administration of anesthetics, or postoperatively. Trismus is the initial event in 50% of patients, and other early signs are tachycardia and hypercapnia due to increased metabolism (100). These are followed by whole-body rigidity and a marked increase in core body temperature. Trismus may occur in up to 1% of normal patients, and it has been also reported that fewer than 50% of patients prove to be susceptible to MH by muscle testing (101). Tachypnea is obvious when muscle relaxants are not administered. Sympathetic system overactivity produces tachycardia, hypertension, and mottled cyanosis. These symptoms precede hyperthermia, hyperkalemia, hypercalcemia, and lactic acidosis. Capnography may provide an early warning, since carbon dioxide production is remarkably increased while MH is in progress (102). Core body temperature can rise at a rate of 1°C every 5 minutes when hyperthermia occurs. Hypertension may be rapidly followed by hypotension as cardiac depression occurs, and cardiac arrest may occur (103). Anesthesia should be aborted if these signs appear or if MH is suspected. Laboratory evaluation reveals increased serum myoglobin, creatine kinase (CK >20,000 U/L), lactate dehydrogenase, and aldolase levels. Dark urine reflects myoglobinemia and myoglobinuria. However, elevation of both myoglobin and CK levels can be observed in some normal patients after succinylcholine administration without MH. The recent most significant study on a clinical grading scale for the prediction of MH was reported and is summarized in Tables 68.9 and 68.10 (100).

NMS should be suspected in patients given any neuroleptic drugs who subsequently develop signs of muscular rigidity, dystonia, or unexplained catatonic behavior, followed by hyperpyrexia. Other symptoms include unstable blood pressure, confusion, coma, and delirium. Although laboratory

TABLE 68.9 Scoring Rules for the Malignant Hyperthermia (MH) Clinical Grading Scale

MH INDICATORS

Review the list of clinical indicators. If any indicator is present, add the points applicable for each indicator while observing the double-counting rule below, which applies to multiple indicators representing a single process.

If no indicator is present, the patient's MH score is zero.

DOUBLE-COUNTING

If more than one indicator represents a single process, *count only the indicator with the highest score.* Application of this rule prevents double-counting when one clinical process has more than one clinical manifestation.

Exception: The score for any relevant indicators in the final category of Table 68.1B ("other indicators") *should* be added to the total score without regard to double-counting.

MH SUSCEPTIBILITY INDICATORS

The italicized indicators listed below apply only to MH susceptibility. Do not use these indicators to score an MH event. To calculate the score for MH susceptibility, add the score of the italicized indicators below to the score for the highest-ranking MH event.

Positive family history of MH in relative of first degree

Positive family history of MH in relative not of first degree

Resting elevated serum creatinine kinase

Positive family history of MH together with another indicator from the patient's own anesthetic experience other than elevated serum creatine kinase

INTERPRETING THE RAW SCORE: MH RANK AND QUALITATIVE LIKELIHOOD

Raw Score Range	MH Rank	Description of Likelihood
0	1	Almost never
3–9	2	Unlikely
10–19	3	Somewhat less than likely
20–34	4	Somewhat greater than likely
35–49	5	Very likely
50+	6	Almost certain

TABLE 68.10 Clinical Indicators for Use in Determining the Malignant Hyperthermia (MH) Raw Score

Process	Indicator	Points
Process I: Rigidity	Generalized muscular rigidity (in the absence of shivering due to hypothermia, or during or immediately following emergence from inhalational general anesthesia)	15
	Masseter spasm shortly following succinylcholine administration	15
Process II: Muscle breakdown	Elevated creatine kinase >20,000 IU after anesthetic that included succinylcholine	15
	Elevated creatine kinase >10,000 IU after anesthetic without succinylcholine	15
	Cola-colored urine in perioperative period	10
	Myoglobin in urine >60 μg/L	5
	Myoglobin in serum >170 μg/L	5
	Blood/plasma/serum K >6 mEq/L (in the absence of renal failure)	3
Process III: Respiratory acidosis	$PETCO_2$ >55 mmHg with appropriately controlled ventilation	15
	$PaCO_2$ >60 mmHg with appropriately controlled ventilation	15
	$PETCO_2$ >60 mmHg with spontaneous ventilation	15
	$PaCO_2$ >65 mmHg with spontaneous ventilation	15
	Inappropriate hypercarbia (in anesthesiologist's judgment)	15
	Inappropriate tachypnea	10
Process IV: Temperature increase	Inappropriately rapid increase in temperature (in anesthesiologist's judgment)	15
	Inappropriately increased temperature >38.8°C (101.8°F) in the preoperative period (in anesthesiologist's judgment)	10
Process V: Cardiac involvement	Inappropriate sinus tachycardia	3
	Ventricular tachycardia or ventricular fibrillation	3
Process VI: Family history (used to determine MH susceptibility only)	Positive MH family history in relative of first degree[a]	15
	Positive MH family history in relative not of first degree[a]	5
Other indicators that are not part of a single process[b]	Arterial base excess more negative than −8 mEq/L	10
	Arterial pH <7.25	10
	Rapid reversal of MH signs of metabolic and/or respiratory acidosis with IV dantrolene	5
	Positive MH family history together with another indicator from the patient's own anesthetic experience other than elevated resting serum creatine kinase[a]	10
	Resting elevated serum creatine kinase[a] (in patient with a family history of MH)	10

[a]These indicators should be used only for determining MH susceptibility.

[b]These should be added without regard to double-counting.

TABLE 68.11 Criteria for Guidance in the Diagnosis of Neuroleptic Malignant Syndrome

Category	Manifestations
Major	Fever, rigidity, elevated creatine kinase concentration
Minor	Tachycardia, abnormal arterial pressure, tachypnea, altered consciousness, diaphoresis, leukocytosis

data may vary, a raised CK may be observed in patients who develop rhabdomyolysis. Some authors incline to make a diagnosis of NMS if certain signs are present. Levenson (104), for example, suggested that the presence of all three major signs, or two major and four minor signs (Table 68.11), indicates a high probability of NMS. These criteria are commonly used in clinical research studies (94,95).

The onset of SS is usually abrupt, and over half of the cases are evident within 6 hours after the responsible drug administration (75). The clinical symptoms include mental status changes (confusion, delirium, coma), autonomic hyperactivity (mydriasis, tachycardia, hypertension, hyperthermia, diaphoresis), and neuromuscular abnormalities (hyperkinesis, hyperactive deep tendon reflexes, clonus, and muscle rigidity) (75).

Complications

Complications arising from MH and NMS are in general parallel to those of heat stroke syndrome, but complications associated with MH may be more severe because of extreme elevation of temperature. Rhabdomyolysis and hepatic necrosis may be fulminant, and DIC is more common (63). Renal failure is seen almost exclusively in patients with severe rhabdomyolysis. Ventricular fibrillation can occur, and cerebral edema with seizures is uncommon but may be seen. Patients with NMS are at risk for aspiration pneumonia because of dystonia and the inability to handle secretions (105).

Therapeutic Approach

Successful treatment of MH and NMS depend on early clinical recognition and prompt withdrawal of the suspected drugs. In MH, discontinuation alone is effective if the syndrome is not well established (63). NMS may be similarly aborted with discontinuation of the drugs. It may take 5 to 7 days to return to the patient's baseline (100) because neuroleptics cannot be removed by dialysis and blood concentrations decline slowly. General symptomatic treatment, such as hydration, nutrition, and reduction of fever, is essential.

Dantrolene should be administered emergently to prevent further release of calcium from the sarcoplasmic reticulum. The dose is 2 mg/kg intravenously every 5 minutes to a total dose of 10 mg/kg until the episode terminates (106). Dantrolene also decreases temperature in NMS and thyroid storm. However, dantrolene is also known to cause complications. Therefore, close observation should be done (107).

Acidosis should be treated aggressively with intravenous administration of bicarbonate, 2 to 4 mEq/kg. Hyperkalemia should be treated with insulin and glucose infusion, and diuresis.

Fever should be controlled by iced fluids, surface cooling, and cooling of body cavities with sterile iced fluids. Cold dialysis and CPB may also be applicable if other measures fail.

Mannitol infusion—0.5 g/kg—with or without furosemide should be used to establish a diuresis and prevent the onset of acute renal failure from myoglobinuria.

Further therapy is guided by blood gases, electrolytes, temperature, arrhythmia, muscle tone, and urinary output. Blood chemical analyses include electrolytes, CK concentrations, liver enzymes, blood urea nitrogen, lactate, glucose, serum hemoglobin and myoglobin, and urine hemoglobin and myoglobin. Coagulation studies also should be done.

In the management of SS, removal of the responsible drug is the most important element, and this will work within 24 hours after commencement (76). Benzodiazepines (108) and a serotonin antagonist cyproheptadine (109) are considered to be effective.

SUMMARY

In general, when significant deviation from normal body temperature exists, prompt diagnosis, treatment, and normalization of the temperature alteration are required immediately, followed by careful review of each patient's condition. Therapeutic approaches vary from conservative to invasive methods, and thus risk–benefit balance always should be taken into consideration for a better outcome.

Key Points

- To make a diagnosis for adequate therapies for hypothermia, Swiss staging system, which stages clinically on the basis of vital signs, is favored.
- If the patient is severely hypothermic, external and invasive rewarming including ECMO or CPB should be considered. If the hypothermic patient has no signs of life, CPR should be given without delay.
- Prehospital treatments are important in both situations (hypothermia and hyperthermia) to facilitate in-hospital treatments.
- MH and neuroleptic malignant syndrome (NMH) are uncommon but life-threatening complications related to the administration of anesthetic or neuroleptic drugs. Therefore, physicians should keep these disorders in mind when in use of related drugs.
- Early clinical recognition and prompt withdrawal of the suspected drugs are important for successful treatment of MH and NMH. Emergent administration of dantrolene should be considered.
- The SS is also described recently, and it should be distinguished from other hyperthermic disorders.
- Removal of the responsible drug is the most important element, and benzodiazepines and a serotonin antagonist cyproheptadine are considered to be effective.

References

1. Moss J. Accidental severe hypothermia. *Surg Gynecol Obstet.* 1986;162:501–513.
2. Larach MG. Accidental hypothermia. *Lancet.* 1995;345:493–498.
3. Danzl DF, Pozos RS. Accidental hypothermia. *N Engl J Med.* 1994;331:1756–1760.
4. Vanden Hoek TL, Morrison LJ, Shuster M, et al. Part 12: Cardiac arrest in special situations. Hypothermia. 2010 American Heart Association guidelines for cardiopulmonary resuscitation and emergency cardiovascular care. *Circulation.* 2010;122(18 Suppl 3):S829–S861.

5. Brown DJ, Brugger H, Boyd J, Paal P. Accidental hypothermia. *N Engl J Med.* 2012;367:1930–1938.
6. Durrer B, Brugger H, Syme D; International Commission for Mountain Emergency Medicine. The medical on-site treatment of hypothermia: ICAR-MEDCOM recommendation. *High Alt Med Biol.* 2003Spring;4:99–103.
7. Megarbane B, Axler O, Chary I, et al. Hypothermia with indoor occurrence is associated with a worse outcome. *Intensive Care Med.* 2000;26:1843–1849.
8. Woodhouse P, Keatinge WR, Coleshaw SR. Factors associated with hypothermia in patients admitted to a group of inner city hospitals. *Lancet.* 1989;2:1201–1205.
9. Fox RH, Brooke OG, Collins JC, et al. Measurement of deep body temperature from the urine. *Clin Sci Mol Med.* 1975;48:1–7.
10. Miller JW, Danzl DF, Thomas DM. Urban accidental hypothermia: 135 cases. *Ann Emerg Med.* 1980;9:456–461.
11. Koutsavlis AT, Kosatsky T. Environmental-temperature injury in a Canadian metropolis. *J Environ Health.* 2003;66:40–45.
12. Clemmer TP, Fisher CJ Jr, Bone RC, et al. Hypothermia in the sepsis syndrome and clinical outcome. The Methylprednisolone Severe Sepsis Study Group. *Crit Care Med.* 1992;20:1395–1401.
13. Solomon A, Barish RA, Browne B, Tso E. The electrocardiographic features of hypothermia. *J Emerg Med.* 1989;7:169–173.
14. Ehrmantraut WR, Fazekas JF, Ticktin HE. Cerebral hemodynamics and metabolism in accidental hypothermia. *AMA Arch Intern Med.* 1957; 99:57–59.
15. Ferrara A, MacArthur JD, Wright HK, et al. Hypothermia and acidosis worsen coagulopathy in the patient requiring massive transfusion. *Am J Surg.* 1990;160:515–518.
16. Ferraro FJ Jr, Spillert CR, Swan KG, Lazaro EJ. Cold-induced hypercoagulability in vitro: a trauma connection? *Am Surg.* 1992;58:355–357.
17. Rohrer MJ, Natale AM. Effect of hypothermia on the coagulation cascade. *Crit Care Med.* 1992;20:1402–1405.
18. Patt A, McCroskey BL, Moore EE. Hypothermia-induced coagulopathies in trauma. *Surg Clin North Am.* 1988;68:775–785.
19. Kashuk JL, Moore EE, Millikan JS, Moore JB. Major abdominal vascular trauma—a unified approach. *J Trauma.* 1982;22:672–679.
20. Cosgriff N, Moore EE, Sauaia A, et al. Predicting life-threatening coagulopathy in the massively transfused trauma patient: hypothermia and acidoses revisited. *J Trauma.* 1997;42:857–861; discussion 861–862.
21. Cupples WA, Fox GR, Hayward JS. Effect of cold water immersion and its combination with alcohol intoxication on urine flow rate of man. *Can J Physiol Pharmacol.* 1980;58:319–321.
22. American Heart Association. Hypothermia. 2005 American Heart Association (AHA) guidelines for cardiopulmonary resuscitation (CPR) and emergency cardiovascular care (ECC). *Circulation.* 2005;112:IV136–IV138.
23. Gregory JS, Bergstein JM, Aprahamian C, et al. Comparison of three methods of rewarming from hypothermia: advantages of extracorporeal blood warming. *J Trauma.* 1991;31:1247–1251; discussion 1251–1252.
24. Wong PS, Pugsley WB. Partial cardiopulmonary bypass for the treatment of profound accidental hypothermic circulatory collapse. *J R Soc Med.* 1992;85:640.
25. Gentilello LM, Cobean RA, Offner PJ, et al. Continuous arteriovenous rewarming: rapid reversal of hypothermia in critically ill patients. *J Trauma.* 1992;32:316–325; discussion 325–327.
26. Vretenar DF, Urschel JD, Parrott JC, Unruh HW. Cardiopulmonary bypass resuscitation for accidental hypothermia. *Ann Thorac Surg.* 1994;58:895–898.
27. Antretter H, Dapunt OE, Mueller LC. Portable cardiopulmonary bypass: resuscitation from prolonged ice-water submersion and asystole. *Ann Thorac Surg.* 1994;58:1786–1787.
28. Mair P, Schwarz B, Komberger E, Balogh D. Case 5-1997. Successful resuscitation of a patient with severe accidental hypothermia and prolonged cardiocirculatory arrest using cardiopulmonary bypass. *J Cardiothorac Vasc Anesth.* 1997;11:901–904.
29. Dobson JA, Burgess JJ. Resuscitation of severe hypothermia by extracorporeal rewarming in a child. *J Trauma.* 1996;40:483–485.
30. Roeggla G, Wagner A, Roeggla M, Hoedl W. Immediate use of cardiopulmonary bypass in patients with severe accidental hypothermia in the emergency department. *Eur J Emerg Med.* 1994;1:155.
31. Gilbert M, Busund M, Skagseth A, et al. Resuscitation from accidental hypothermia of 13.7°C with circulatory arrest. *Lancet.* 2000;355:375–376.
32. Althaus UL, Aeberhard PE, Schupbach P, et al. Management of profound accidental hypothermia with cardiorespiratory arrest. *Ann Surg.* 1982;195:492–495.
33. Hall KN, Syverud SA. Closed thoracic cavity lavage in the treatment of severe hypothermia in human beings. *Ann Emerg Med.* 1990;19:204–206.
34. Walters DT. Closed thoracic cavity lavage for hypothermia with cardiac arrest. *Ann Emerg Med.* 1991;20:439–440.
35. Winegard C. Successful treatment of severe hypothermia and prolonged cardiac arrest with closed thoracic cavity lavage. *J Emerg Med.* 1997;15:629–632.
36. Plaisier BR. Thoracic lavage in accidental hypothermia with cardiac arrest: report of a case and review of the literature. *Resuscitation.* 2005;66: 99–104.
37. Duthie DJ. Heat-related illness. *Lancet.* 1998;352:1329–1330.
38. Bouchama A. Heatstroke: a new look at an ancient disease. *Intensive Care Med.* 1995;21:623–625.
39. Simpson C, Abelsohn A. Heat-induced illness. *C M A J.* 2012;184:1170.
40. Shahid MS, Hatle L, Mansour H, Mimish L. Echocardiographic and Doppler study of patients with heatstroke and heat exhaustion. *Int J Card Imaging.* 1999;15:279–285.
41. Porter AM. Heat illness and soldiers. *Mil Med.* 1993;158:606–609.
42. Knochel JP. Exertional heat stroke: pathophysiology of heat stroke. In: Hopkins PM, Ellis FR, eds. *Hyperthermic and Hypermetabolic Disorders.* Cambridge, UK: Cambridge University Press; 1996:42–46.
43. Alzeer AH, Al-Arifi A, Warsy AS, et al. Nitric oxide production is enhanced in patients with heat stroke. *Intensive Care Med.* 1999;25:58–62.
44. Dematte JE, O'Mara K, Buescher J, et al. Near-fatal heat stroke during the 1995 heat wave in Chicago. *Ann Intern Med.* 1998;129:173–181.
45. Howorth PJ. The biochemistry of heat illness. *J R Army Med Corps.* 1995; 141:40–41.
46. Knochel JP. Environmental heat illness. An eclectic review. *Arch Intern Med.* 1974;133:841–864.
47. Hart GR, Anderson RJ, Crumpler CP, et al. Epidemic classical heat stroke: clinical characteristics and course of 28 patients. *Medicine (Baltimore).* 1982;61:189–197.
48. O'Donnell TF Jr. Acute heat stroke. Epidemiologic, biochemical, renal, and coagulation studies. *JAMA.* 1975;234:824–828.
49. Tucker LE, Stanford J, Graves B, et al. Classical heatstroke: clinical and laboratory assessment. *South Med J.* 1985;78:20–25.
50. Hassanein T, Razack A, Gavaler JS, Van Thiel DH. Heatstroke: its clinical and pathological presentation, with particular attention to the liver. *Am J Gastroenterol.* 1992;87:1382–1389.
51. Yu FC, Lu KC, Lin SH, et al. Energy metabolism in exertional heat stroke with acute renal failure. *Nephrol Dial Transplant.* 1997;2087–2092.
52. Giercksky T, Boberg KM, Farstad IN, et al. Severe liver failure in exertional heat stroke. *Scand J Gastroenterol.* 1999;34:824–827.
53. Saissy JM. Liver transplantation in a case of fulminant liver failure after exertion. *Intensive Care Med.* 1996;22:831.
54. Akhtar MJ, al-Nozha M, al-Harthi S, Nouh MS. Electrocardiographic abnormalities in patients with heat stroke. *Chest.* 1993;104:411–414.
55. el Kassimi FA, Al-Mashhadani S, Abdullah AK, Akhtar J. Adult respiratory distress syndrome and disseminated intravascular coagulation complicating heat stroke. *Chest.* 1986;90:571–574.
56. Dahmash NS, al-Harthi SS, Akhtar J. Invasive evaluation of patients with heat stroke. *Chest.* 1993;103:1210–1214.
57. Bouchama A, Dehbi M, Chaves-Carballo E. Cooling and hemodynamic management in heatstroke: practical recommendations. *Crit Care.* 2007;11:R54.
58. Gonzalez-Alonso J, Mora-Rodriguez R, Below PR, Coyle EF. Dehydration markedly impairs cardiovascular function in hyperthermic endurance athletes during exercise. *J Appl Physiol (1985).* 1997;82:1229–1236.
59. Bernard S, Buist M, Monteiro O, Smith K. Induced hypothermia using large volume, ice-cold intravenous fluid in comatose survivors of out-of-hospital cardiac arrest: a preliminary report. *Resuscitation.* 2003;56:9–13.
60. Denborough MA, Lovell RR. Anaesthetic deaths in a family. *Lancet.* 1960;2:45.
61. Denborough MA, Forster JF, Lovell RR, et al. Anaesthetic deaths in a family. *Br J Anaesth.* 1962;34:395–396.
62. Delay J, Pichot P, Lemperiere T, et al. A non-phenothiazine and non-reserpine major neuroleptic, haloperidol, in the treatment of psychoses. *Ann Med Psychol (Paris).* 1960;118:145–152.
63. Urwyler A, Censier K, Kaufmann MA, Drewe J. Genetic effects on the variability of the halothane and caffeine muscle contracture tests. *Anesthesiology.* 1994;80:1287–1295.
64. Gronert GA. Malignant hyperthermia. *Anesthesiology.* 1980;53:395–423.
65. Neuroleptic malignant syndrome. *Lancet.* 1984;1:545–546.
66. Smego RA Jr, Durack DT. The neuroleptic malignant syndrome. *Arch Intern Med.* 1982;142:1183–1185.
67. Morris HH 3rd, McCormick WF, Reinarz JA. Neuroleptic malignant syndrome. *Arch Neurol.* 1980;37:462–463.
68. Guze BH, Baxter LR Jr. Current concepts: neuroleptic malignant syndrome. *N Engl J Med.* 1985;313:163–166.

69. Kemperman CJ. Zuclopenthixol-induced neuroleptic malignant syndrome at rechallenge and its extrapyramidal effects. *Br J Psychiatry.* 1989;154:562–563.
70. van Maldegem BT, Smit LM, Touw DJ, Gemke RJ. Neuroleptic malignant syndrome in a 4-year-old girl associated with alimemazine. *Eur J Pediatr.* 2002;161:259–261.
71. Webster P, Wijeratne C. Risperidone-induced neuroleptic malignant syndrome. *Lancet.* 1994;344:1228–1229.
72. Heinemann F, Assion HJ, Hermes G, Ehrlich M. Paroxetine-induced neuroleptic malignant syndrome [in German]. *Nervenarzt.* 1997;68:664–666.
73. Tegazzin V, Scutari E, Treves S, Zorzato F. Chlorocresol, an additive to commercial succinylcholine, induces contracture of human malignant hyperthermia-susceptible muscles via activation of the ryanodine receptor Ca^{2+} channel. *Anesthesiology.* 1996;84:1380–1385.
74. Rosenberg H, Reed S. In vitro contracture tests for susceptibility to malignant hyperthermia. *Anesth Analg.* 1983;62:415–420.
75. Boyer EW, Shannon M. The serotonin syndrome. *N Engl J Med.* 2005:17: 1112–1120.
76. Hyperthermia and hypothermia syndromes. In: *The ICU Book.* 3rd ed. Philadelphia, PA; 2007:705–707.
77. Ording H. Incidence of malignant hyperthermia in Denmark. *Anesth Analg.* 1985;64:700–704.
78. Ording H. Investigation of malignant hyperthermia susceptibility in Denmark. *Dan Med Bull.* 1996;43:111–125.
79. Halliday NJ. Malignant hyperthermia. *J Craniofac Surg.* 2003;14:800–802.
80. Suyama H, Kawamoto M, Yuge O. Prevention and treatment of malignant hyperthermia in certified training hospitals in Japan: a questionnaire. *J Anesth.* 2002;16:207–210.
81. Sumitani M, Uchida K, Yasunaga H, et al. Prevalence of malignant hyperthermia and relationship with anesthetics in Japan: data from the diagnosis procedure combination database. *Anesthesiology.* 2011;114:84–90.
82. Lerman J. Perioperative management of the paediatric patient with coexisting neuromuscular disease. *Br J Anaesth.* 2011;107 (Suppl 1):i79–i89.
83. Gelenberg AJ, Bellinghausen B, Wojcik JD, et al. A prospective survey of neuroleptic malignant syndrome in a short-term psychiatric hospital. *Am J Psychiatry.* 1988;145:517–518.
84. Hermesh H, Aizenberg D, Lapidot M, Munitz H. Risk of malignant hyperthermia among patients with neuroleptic malignant syndrome and their families. *Am J Psychiatry.* 1988;145:1431–1434.
85. Hermesh H, Aizenberg D, Weizman A, et al. Risk for definite neuroleptic malignant syndrome. A prospective study in 223 consecutive in-patients. *Br J Psychiatry.* 1992;161:254–257.
86. Adnet P, Lestavel P, Krivosic-Horber R. Neuroleptic malignant syndrome. *Br J Anaesth.* 2000;85:129–135.
87. Fletcher JE, Tripolitis L, Hubert M, et al. Genotype and phenotype relationships for mutations in the ryanodine receptor in patients referred for diagnosis of malignant hyperthermia. *Br J Anaesth.* 1995;75:307–310.
88. Wallace AJ, Wooldridge W, Kingston HM, et al. Malignant hyperthermia–a large kindred linked to the RYR1 gene. *Anaesthesia.* 1996;51:16–23.
89. Serfas KD, Bose D, Patel L, et al. Comparison of the segregation of the RYR1 C1840T mutation with segregation of the caffeine/halothane contracture test results for malignant hyperthermia susceptibility in a large Manitoba Mennonite family. *Anesthesiology.* 1996;84:322–329.
90. McWilliams S, Nelson T, Sudo RT, et al. Novel skeletal muscle ryanodine receptor mutation in a large Brazilian family with malignant hyperthermia. *Clin Genet.* 2002;62:80–83.
91. Larach MG, Brandom BW, Allen GC, et al. Malignant hyperthermia deaths related to inadequate temperature monitoring, 2007–2012: a report from the North American malignant hyperthermia registry of the malignant hyperthermia association of the United States. *Anesth Analg.* 2014;119:1359–1366.
92. Denborough MA, Collins SP, Hopkinson KC. Rhabdomyolysis and malignant hyperpyrexia. *Br Med J (Clin Res Ed).* 1984;288:1878.
93. Tollefson G. A case of neuroleptic malignant syndrome: in vitro muscle comparison with malignant hyperthermia. *J Clin Psychopharmacol.* 1982;2: 266–270.
94. Caroff SN, Rosenberg H, Fletcher JE, et al. Malignant hyperthermia susceptibility in neuroleptic malignant syndrome. *Anesthesiology.* 1987; 67:20–25.
95. Adnet PJ, Krivosic-Horber RM, Adamantidis MM, et al. The association between the neuroleptic malignant syndrome and malignant hyperthermia. *Acta Anaesthesiol Scand.* 1989;33:676–680.
96. Bligh J, Cottle WH, Maskrey M. Influence of ambient temperature on the thermoregulatory responses to 5-hydroxytryptamine, noradrenaline and acetylcholine injected into the lateral cerebral ventricles of sheep, goats and rabbits. *J Physiol.* 1971;212:377–392.
97. Cox B, Kerwin R, Lee TF. Dopamine receptors in the central thermoregulatory pathways of the rat. *J Physiol.* 1978;282:471–483.
98. Kelkar VV, Doctor RB, Jindal MN. Chlorpromazine-induced contracture of frog rectus abdominis muscle. *Pharmacology.* 1974;12:32–38.
99. Takagi A. Chlorpromazine and skeletal muscle: a study of skinned single fibers of the guinea pig. *Exp Neurol.* 1981;73:477–486.
100. Larach MG, Localio AR, Allen GC, et al. A clinical grading scale to predict malignant hyperthermia susceptibility. *Anesthesiology.* 1994;80:771–779.
101. O'Flynn RP, Shutack JG, Rosenberg H, Fletcher JE. Masseter muscle rigidity and malignant hyperthermia susceptibility in pediatric patients. An update on management and diagnosis. *Anesthesiology.* 1994;80:1228–1233.
102. Meier-Hellman A, Romer M, Hannemann L, et al. Early recognition of malignant hyperthermia using capnometry. *Anaesthesist.* 1990;39: 41–43.
103. Larach MG, Brandom BW, Allen GC, et al. Cardiac arrests and deaths associated with malignant hyperthermia in North America from 1987 to 2006: a report from the North American malignant hyperthermia registry of the malignant hyperthermia association of the United States. *Anesthesiology.* 2008;108:603–611.
104. Levenson JL. Neuroleptic malignant syndrome. *Am J Psychiatry.* 1985;142: 1137–1145.
105. Wedel DJ, Quinlan JG, Iaizzo PA. Clinical effects of intravenously administered dantrolene. *Mayo Clin Proc.* 1995;70:241–246.
106. Brandom BW, Larach MG. The North American malignant hyperthermia registry. Reassessment of the safety and efficacy of dantrolene. *Anesthesiology.* 2002;96:A1199.
107. Brandom BW, Larach MG, Chen MS, Young MC. Complications associated with the administration of dantrolene 1987 to 2006: a report from the North American Malignant Hyperthermia Registry of the Malignant Hyperthermia Association of the United States. *Anesth Analg.* 2011;112: 1115–1123.
108. Hick JL, Smith SW, Lynch MT. Metabolic acidosis in restraint-associated cardiac arrest: a case series. *Acad Emerg Med.* 1999;6:239–243.
109. Graudins A, Stearman A, Chan B. Treatment of the serotonin syndrome with cyproheptadine. *J Emerg Med.* 1998;16:615–619.

CHAPTER

69

The Morbidly Obese Patient in the Critical Care Unit

MARY JANE REED, ANGELA M. DEANTONIO, ADRIAN ALVAREZ, and JUAN C. CENDAN

Obesity, as defined by the World Health Organization (WHO), is the "abnormal or excessive fat accumulation that may impair health." Body mass index (BMI), weight in kilograms divided by the square of height in meters (kg/m^2), has been the most commonly used scale of obesity. The WHO classifies weight by BMI into the following ranges:

- Normal weight: BMI > 18.5–24.9 kg/m^2
- Overweight: BMI > 25–29.9 kg/m^2
- Obesity: BMI > 30–39.9 kg/m^2
- Severe (morbid) obesity BMI > 40 kg/m^2

Other terms used in the description of BMI classes include severe obesity to include BMI over 35 kg/m^2 in the presence of comorbidities or super obese when BMI is above 50 kg/m^2. More valid measures of obesity have been proposed rather than the BMI. Waist to hip ratio, sagittal abdominal diameter, and dual energy x-ray absorptiometry may reflect body composition and distribution better than BMI (1).

Globally, the prevalence of obesity has significantly increased over the last decades. More than a third of the population of the United States are obese with severe or morbid obesity greater than 5%. Although the prevalence of obesity may have plateaued in some developed nations (2), authors note a projected faster rise in the prevalence of morbid obesity in the next decade (3). Therefore, care of the obese especially the morbidly obese has become part of all aspects of health care including critical care. The prevalence of obesity and morbid obesity in the intensive care population reflects the general population distribution (4,5).

CELLULAR PATHOPHYSIOLOGY

Obesity has been shown to be a state of chronic inflammation and hypercoagulapathy. White adipose tissue especially visceral adipose tissue is an active immunoendocrine organ. Adipocytes of the obese have up to a fourfold increase in the density of macrophages (6). Adipose tissue macrophages produce and secrete proinflammatory cytokines including but not limited to tumor necrosis factor alpha (TNF-alpha), interleukin-6, interleukin-8, and monocyte chemoattractant protein-1 (MCP-1) (7). The blood levels of these inflammatory protein increase as adiposity rises (8). Adipocytes produce signaling molecules known as adipokines. Leptin, adiponectin, and plasminogen activator inhibitor-1 (PAI-1) are such molecules. Leptin is an upregulator of cell-mediated immune response. Leptin is increased in obesity, and its proinflammatory properties have been linked to obesity-associated disease states such as cardiovascular disease, diabetes, and cancer (9). Adiponectin is a protective, anti-inflammatory cytokine that is important in insulin-sensitization, antiatherogenisis, and antithrombus formation. Adiponectin is depressed in the obese patient contributing to the development of cardiovascular disease, metabolic syndrome, and venous thrombosis (10). PAI-1 increased in obesity causes hypercoagulable state by decreasing fibrinolysis and increasing platelet aggregation. Angiotensinogen levels are elevated in obesity increasing angiotensin II thus contributing to obesity-induced hypertension and toxic effects on the myocardium (11).

Adipose tissue inflammation disrupts the normal functions of the adipocytes and leads to dyslipidemia. This increase in circulating lipid levels leads to the heterotopic deposit of lipids within liver, pancreas, and heart. Local toxic effects of visceral fat deposits can induce organ pathology. Obesity especially central or abdominal obesity leads to changes in cellular, organ, and system levels. The pathophysiologic consequences of obesity involve all major organ systems. Diabetes mellitus, elevated fasting glucose, hypertension, and hyperlipidemia are associated with central obesity and collectively known as the metabolic syndrome or syndrome X. These conditions contribute to chronic morbidity in the obese. Cardiopulmonary concerns are the most often encountered by the intensivists (12). A summary of adipokines effects is given in Table 69.1.

CARDIOVASCULAR CONSIDERATIONS IN THE MORBIDLY OBESE

Cardiovascular diseases are common in obese individuals and manifest as ischemic heart disease, hypertension, and cardiac failure. Obesity has been observed to be an independent risk factor for the development of these conditions (13).

The relationship between the increase in blood pressure and the risk of cardiovascular disease is considered to be independent of other risk factors. The chances of myocardial infarction, heart failure, stroke, and kidney disease are all greater as a patient's blood pressure increases. Obesity is also well recognized as a risk factor for ischemic heart disease. Many obese individuals also suffer from metabolic syndrome, which has a strong association with being a precursor to the development of diabetes, cardiovascular disease, and increased mortality rates from cardiovascular disorders. There is also a 5% to 7% risk of heart failure associated with each 1% increase in body mass (14).

Pathophysiology

There is an increase in stroke volume as weight increases resulting in higher cardiac output. Total blood volume also increases thought to be due to polycythemia and sodium retention from adipose-produced angiotensinogen thus increasing preload. These changes manifest clinically as arterial hypertension,

TABLE 69.1 Adipokines in Obesity and Effect

Leptin	↑ in obesity	Proinflammatory	↑ in CV disease, ↑ BP, ↑ LVH
Angiotensinogen	↑ in obesity	↑ angiotensin II, ↑aldosterone	↑ vasoconstriction, ↑ blood volume, ↑ BP, cardiac myocyte toxicity
PAI-1	↑ in obesity	↓ fibrinolysis	↑ hypercoagulable state, ↑ thrombosis
Adiponectin	↓ in obesity	Anti-inflammatory, cardioprotective	↑ myocardial hypertrophy, insulin resistance, cell death

increased left ventricular mass, and hypertrophy. Both eccentric and concentric hypertrophy is seen in obese individuals. This can result in left ventricular and diastolic dysfunction with atrial enlargement. It is the complex interaction of hypertension, ischemic heart disease, and pulmonary hypertension that contribute to the development of global cardiac dysfunction and exacerbates congestive heart failure. This clinical situation is referred to as "obesity cardiomyopathy" (15).

RESPIRATORY CONSIDERATIONS IN THE MORBIDLY OBESE

Morbidly obese patients have significant anatomic and pathophysiologic changes of the pulmonary system. Reduced lung volumes, increased work of breathing, respiratory muscle inefficiency, and alterations in control of breathing and gas exchange can complicate the care of the morbidly obese. Many factors are involved including, but not limited to, BMI, patient's age, duration of obesity, fat distribution (central or peripheral), and the strong association of certain sleep-related breathing disorders such as obstructive sleep apnea (OSA) and obesity hypoventilation syndrome (OHS) (16).

Morbidly obese patients have the lower functional residual capacity (FRC), expiratory reserve volume (ERV) and to a lesser extent total lung capacity (TLC). Forced vital capacity (FVC), forced expiratory volume in 1 second (FEV_1), and maximum voluntary ventilation (MVV) are also reduced in the morbidly obese suggesting small airway remodeling and decrease in caliber. These changes are worsened by supine positioning, in which diaphragmatic movement is hampered by the increased abdominal pressure. The increased adipose tissue around the rib cage decreases chest wall compliance, which also reduces FRC. As the FRC decreases it approaches the closing capacity, which can lead to airway closure within the range of tidal breathing. Areas of the lung may be underventilated leading to intrapulmonary shunting and hypoxemia. Respiration can also be comprised by early airway closure resulting in air trapping and auto-PEEP, which increases work of breathing (17). This loss of FRC with resultant smaller airway collapse and atelectasis decreases pulmonary compliance. Increased blood volume within the pulmonary circulation also contributes to the diminished pulmonary compliance and is exponentially related to BMI. These changes result in increased work of breathing, which is compounded by decreased diameter of the upper airway caused by parapharangeal fat (18).

As with nonobese individuals, lower lung segments in the obese are well perfused, but because of the closure of small airways in these areas, ventilation is shifted to the upper lung segments resulting in increased V/Q mismatch and hypoxemia. Chronic hypoxemia contributes to persistent increased pulmonary vascular resistance and right heart failure. The level of hypoxemia is worse in OHS. Respiratory muscle endurance is also decreased in the obese patient and to a greater degree in OHS with a marked increase in oxygen consumption of the respiratory muscles. This decline in respiratory muscle endurance leads to earlier fatigue and respiratory failure (18).

Obese patients require higher minute ventilation to match the oxygen consumption and metabolic demands, which result in increased respiratory rate and shallower volumes. In OHS, the neural drive fails resulting in hypercapnia and hypoxia. There is not a linear association between these respiratory changes and degree of obesity. However, the cumulative effect can result in lower pulmonary reserve and increase the risk of respiratory failure in obese patients (17).

Obstructive sleep apnea syndrome (OSAS) is more prevalent in the morbidly obese than OHS and is often underdiagnosed. This can lead to difficulties in the management of morbidly obese patients in stressed situations such as perioperative or in acute disease states where OSAS pathophysiology may not be recognized. OSAS is associated with increased risk of postoperative cardiac events, respiratory failure, and intensive care admissions. OSAS is associated with difficult mask ventilation and intubation. OSAS patients are more susceptible to sedation effect of hypnotics and opioids. OSAS is also associated with increased overall mortality (19). Use of empiric positive airway pressure in patients who are high risk for OSA but undiagnosed may be of use in the management of the morbidly obese for perioperative care, acute respiratory failure, and bridge after extubation (20–22). In patients with OHS, noninvasive continuous positive airway pressure may improve upper airway patency, increase FRC, offset auto-PEEP, augment respiratory muscles, and oxygenation. However, the additional inspiratory component of bilevel positive airway pressure helps ameliorate the hypercapnia of OHS. Noninvasive positive pressure ventilation (NIPPV) does not appear to impact the need for endotracheal intubation in acute hypoxic respiratory failure due to ARDS in this population, however so close monitoring of these patients is warranted preferably in an intensive care setting where difficult airways can be managed if intubation is warranted (16).

It is still a debatable issue whether or not morbid obesity should be considered a risk factor for difficult airway management especially in the elective situation such as in the operating room. More important was consideration of Mallampati score of 3 or greater, previous documented difficult airway, limited mouth opening or cervical mobility, and history of OSA. There is also some data to suggest that patients intubated in the intensive care unit are more likely to have difficult airways and complications related to intubation than those patients in an operating room setting (23). Whether or not morbid obesity is considered a risk factor for intubation, issues related specifically to the patient's BMI that impact airway management should be considered.

Less cardiopulmonary reserve in the morbidly obese from pathophysiologic changes described previously results in more rapid desaturation during intubation. Supine positioning increases V/Q mismatch thereby worsening hypoxemia. Obesity alters upper airway anatomy. Increased fat deposition in pharyngeal tissues increases the likelihood of pharyngeal wall collapse and also decreases the cross-sectional area of the upper trachea. These changes, as well as increased airway resistance from decreased pulmonary and chest wall compliance, makes bag mask ventilation more difficult. Obese patients have increased the risk of aspiration pneumonitis resulting from increased intra-abdominal pressure (IAP) and increase in gastric volumes (23).

The key to maximizing intubation success and decreasing complications is preparation if possible with the following important points preoxygenation, positioning, and resources. Preoxygenation with 100% oxygen by mask or by NIPPV with the patient in the 30- to 45-degree head up or reverse Trendelenburg position. This positioning helps unload the abdominal contents from the diaphragm. Before induction of sedation, the obese patient should be placed in a ramped position. In the ramped position, blankets or commercially available tools or beds are used to elevate the head and torso such that the external auditory meatus and the sternum are horizontally aligned. Essential equipment and personnel should be gathered. The exact list of equipment needed may vary slightly depending on the intubating individual's preference, but endotracheal tubes with stylets, functioning suction, a bag-valve device connected to an oxygen source, laryngoscope (direct or video) and blades, oral/nasal airways, and a device to detect end-tidal carbon dioxide are essential. Continued oxygen delivery via high-flow nasal cannula during laryngoscopy may extend safe apnea time. All providers who are responsible for intubation of critically ill morbidly obese should be familiar with an accepted difficult airway guideline (Table 69.2) (24–27).

Obesity is associated with more severe asthma and increased risk of adult respiratory distress syndrome (ARDS). Recent viral pandemics such as H1N1 showed obesity as a risk factor for ARDS and multi-system organ failure. However, BMI alone is not associated with increased mortality from ARDS (28). Morbidly obese patients often require longer ventilatory support in their normal weight counterpart. The mechanically ventilated morbidly obese patient presents the critical care physician with unique challenges. There is no clear optimum mode of ventilation in the critically ill, mechanically ventilated morbidly obese patient. Much of the literature on ventilation in this population is from elective surgical patients undergoing bariatric surgery. Positioning the patient in a 70-degree sitting position rather than a semi-Fowler position where the head of the bed is at 30 to 45 degrees has been reported to improve expiratory flow and decrease auto-PEEP (29). Recent studies suggest that intensivists underestimate appropriate PEEP needed to optimize end-expiratory lung volumes in the intubated morbidly obese patient. Utilization of pressure–volume curve to determine lower inflection point (where alveoli collapse) or utilization of esophageal balloon manometry as a surrogate for transpleural pressure may be a better guide to determining the optimal level of PEEP in these patients. Some authors suggest routine recruitment maneuvers shortly after intubation (i.e., PEEP 30 cm H_2O for 30 seconds) in addition to PEEP guided by transpleural pressure monitoring or equivalent (30). If estimating, empiric PEEP of 10 to 15 cm H_2O has been suggested as optimal for the morbidly obese mechanically ventilated patient (31). Ideal body weight should be used to determine tidal volume and monitoring of acid–base status as a guide to appropriate minute ventilation.

TABLE 69.2 Summary of Endotracheal Intubation Concerns in Morbidly Obese Patients

- Pulmonary aspiration of gastric contents
- Difficult mask ventilation and tracheal intubation
- Rapid development of hypoxemia after apnea
- Pulmonary atelectasis
- Hemodynamic instability
- Decreased ability to deal with the physiologic responses to stressful situations (i.e., hyperglycemia, hypertension, cardiac failure, arrhythmias, and myocardial ischemia)
- Delayed recovery
- Postoperative respiratory dysfunction
- Deep venous thrombosis

TABLE 69.3 Vital Measures to Prevent or Reduce the Severity and Duration of Atelectasis in the Obese Patient

- Place patients in the semirecumbent position and, if possible, out of bed in a chair as tolerated, as this maneuver may increase functional residual capacity.
- Provide effective analgesia, which will allow early and effective mobilization, cough, and excellent tolerance to physiotherapy.
- Institute aggressive incentive spirometry.
- During the first 3 postoperative days, deliver humidified "supplemental oxygen," but avoid inspired fractions higher than 0.8. Supplemental humidified oxygen will not reduce atelectasis, but will facilitate respiratory secretion clearance, and will prevent hypoxemic episodes in efforts to improve the host's defenses against bacterial infections.
- During surgery or postoperatively in intubated patients, instituting positive end-expiratory pressure is probably effective in increasing functional residual capacity via recruitment of atelectatic regions of the lung. Applying vital capacity maneuvers (also known as recruitment maneuvers) may also reduce the incidence and/or severity of atelectasis while improving the quality and effective time of alveoli recruitment.
- Noninvasive positive pressure ventilation can be used to avoid intubation in selected patients.

When preparing to extubate the morbidly obese patient, one must take into consideration the underlying lung mechanics. Decreasing PEEP to 5 cm H_2O or use of T-piece during weaning may result in loss of recruited end-expiratory volume. Keeping PEEP above the level of lower inflection point during weaning may prevent derecruitment. Postextubation bridging with NIPPV at the same level of PEEP used during weaning should be considered. NIPPV helps overcome upper airway resistance, decreases respiratory muscle fatigue and prevents atelectasis (32). Keeping the patient in a more upright position will also help optimize lung mechanics (Table 69.3).

IMPORTANCE OF COUPLED CARDIORESPIRATORY FUNCTION

It is vital to maintain the best possible ventilation/perfusion (V/Q) balance because V/Q mismatch is a prominent mechanism that can trigger respiratory and subsequent cardiac dysfunction in the morbidly obese patient. In mechanically ventilated, morbidly obese patients, airway pressure may be elevated. Additionally, morbid obesity is associated with volume and pressure overload. Volume load conditions may fluctuate according to patient positioning. For example, changing position from the "physiologically ideal" reverse Trendelenburg to the supine position can significantly increase venous blood return to the heart and, as a result, augment cardiac output, pulmonary capillary wedge pressure, and mean pulmonary artery pressure, potentially increasing the risk of acute heart failure; one would expect this maneuver to increase airway pressure as well due to the increased weight of the chest.

Compression of the inferior vena cava may reduce venous return to the heart, and is thus a possible mechanism of hypotension. This can be avoided by placing a wedge under the patient. Considering that the reverse Trendelenburg position or semi-Fowler position significantly improves cardiac and respiratory performance, it should be maintained unless there is a particular contraindication (33).

RENAL CONSIDERATIONS

Morbid obesity is a risk factor for chronic kidney disease (CKD). Comorbidities such as hypertension and diabetes contribute to decrease in kidney function as well as the increased glomerular filtration rate (GFR) from morbid obesity itself. Obesity-related glomerulopathy is manifested as glomerulomegaly, mesangial expansion, and secondary focal and segmental glomerulosclerosis. CKD is a risk factor for acute kidney injury (AKI). The critically ill morbidly obese patient increased GFR might mask underlying renal insufficiency predisposing these patients to AKI from inappropriate drug dosing, exposure to nephrotoxins such as IV contrast dye, overestimation of intravascular volume, and failure to recognize abdominal compartment syndrome (ACS) (34).

AKI increases mortality in the critically morbidly obese patient. Strategies to avoid AKI in the critically ill morbidly obese patient include recognition of the risk of underlying kidney pathology. Class III obesity and above have been shown to be an independent risk factor in developing AKI in the perioperative population. Obtaining euvolemia while maintaining renal perfusion pressure with minimum vasopressors is a logical goal. Management of dynamic fluid responsiveness should avoid suspected nephrotoxins, such as starch based colloids (35).

GASTROINTESTINAL CONSIDERATIONS

There is an increased prevalence of gastroesophageal reflux in the morbidly obese. Coupled with increased gastric volume, increased IAP and decreased lower esophageal sphincter, the obese patient is at risk for aspiration during critical illness and endotracheal intubation. Several studies have shown an association between increases in BMI and intra-abdominal hypertension (defined as IAP >12 mmHg). This baseline increase in IAP can predispose obese individuals to develop ACS. ACS occurs when the IAP exceeds 20 mmHg with evidence of organ dysfunction, such as oliguria, decreased cardiac output from impedance on venous return, decreased pulmonary compliance, increased intracranial pressure, and lactic acidosis. Disorders such as ascites, intra-abdominal hemorrhage, visceral edema, bowel distension, or large abdominal tumors can lead to ACS. Treatment is usually focused on the cause (i.e., paracentesis for massive ascites) and sometimes may require surgical decompression.

Nonalcoholic fatty liver disease (NAFLD) is more prevalent in the obese patient. The NAFLD covers a spectrum of disease, from asymptomatic elevations of alanine transaminase to steatosis with lobular inflammation and ballooning degeneration, termed nonalcoholic steatohepatitis (NASH) to liver fibrosis and cirrhosis. Some patients diagnosed with NAFLD may have NASH or cirrhosis, which could lead to complications, particularly prolonged drug metabolism and relative immune suppression of liver disease, and worse outcomes in the intensive care unit (36).

DRUG DOSING

The distribution, metabolism, protein binding, and clearance of many drugs are altered by the physiologic changes associated with obesity as reviewed in the previous sections. Also, obesity-associated comorbidities may substantially influence the pharmacokinetic properties of a drug. Although data on effects of morbid obesity on pharmacokinetics is increasing, there is still a paucity of well-powered studies. This clinician should be aware of weight-based dosing is complicated by which value one uses: ideal body weight, adjusted body weight, or actual body weight. Many drugs used in the intensive care setting can be titrated to obvious effect such as vasoactive medications. Although sedation and pain medications can also be titrated to effect, the lipophilic nature of commonly used benzodiazepines may prolong elimination of these drugs. Sedation and opiates in the nonintubated seriously ill morbidly obese patient requires heightened awareness as this population may have undiagnosed sleep-disordered breathing and may have increased hypercapnia and hypoxia (37). Some drugs can be monitored in steady state by drug levels or laboratory values. However, often it is imperative to have adequate initial or loading dosing for many drugs in the critically ill. For example, underdosing antimicrobials by providers has been shown to be common in the morbidly obese which may lead to treatment failure and resistance (38). Drugs with narrow therapeutic windows such as anticoagulants should be monitored closely. Consultation with critical care pharmacists and development of protocols can help achieve early adequate dosing (39).

VENOUS THROMBOEMBOLISM

Obesity is a risk factor for venous thromboembolic disease. Literature suggests relative risk for deep vein thrombosis (DVT) of 2.50 in obese versus nonobese patients and relative risk for pulmonary embolus (PE) of 2.21 (40).

There are several proposed mechanisms for the increased risk of VTE in obese patients in the intensive care unit. Because of limitations of body habitus, these patients are often less ambulatory and assisted mobilization in the hospital may also be limited. Also, prophylactic measures may be inadequate. Compression devices are less likely to fit properly, and the limited data on appropriate pharmacologic prophylaxis dosing in the obese may result in subtherapeutic levels. Increased procedural complications exist in this patient population, and limited intravenous access may increase the duration of central access, which can lead to thrombosis.

Diagnosis of VTE may also be compromised. Studies have shown that clinical signs of a DVT are often absent. Entities involved in critical illness such as peripheral edema–decreased sensorium, surgical dressing, and adiposity further impair clinical signs of DVT (41).

The best regimen for thromboprophylaxis in this high-risk group is not single armed. The risk of bleeding should be balanced with the risk of thrombosis. In patients with low risk of bleeding, chemoprophylaxis should be used in conjunction with mechanical prophylactic devices such as intermittent pneumatic compression boots. If the bleeding risk is high, mechanical prophylactic devices should be used until chemoprophylaxis can be instituted. Prophylactic inferior vena cava filters can be considered, but not recommended for primary prophylaxis. Unfractionated or low–molecular-weight heparins are both viable options though precise dosing regimens and duration of dosage have emerged largely from uncontrolled trials. There are reports in the bariatric literature that 40 mg of enoxaparin every 12 hours may provide better thromboprophylaxis than 30 mg every 12 hours. Weight-based dosing of 0.5 mg/kg with weights over 150 kg following anti-factor Xa levels after the third dose with the goal of 0.2 to 0.5 IU/mL is suggested by many authors (42).

VASCULAR ACCESS

Venous access is difficult in this population. Peripheral venous access is often limited. Use of ultrasound can be very helpful in gaining peripheral access in this population. When central access is needed peripherally inserted central catheters (PICCs) should be considered as central catheters may remain in place longer in the obese patient than nonobese patients and may cause increased risk of infection (43). Ultrasound guidance has been particularly helpful in the placement of central venous catheters in the morbidly obese patient. Ultrasound guidance can overcome the limitation of altered surface anatomic landmarks in the obese patient. Many authors suggest internal jugular over other sites due to the ability to visualize the vessels easier with ultrasound guidance in this population. Arterial access is recommended as noninvasive blood pressure cuffs can give inaccurate measurements in this patient population. When accessing a vessel in this population, longer equipment may be needed. Catheters placed in left internal jugular may not be of adequate length to reach the distal superior vena cava. Greater care should be taken when securing the catheter. Excess adipose tissue can shift when the patient is in an upright position thereby pulling the distal catheter out of the vessel without evidence of movement on the skin surface.

When using a noninvasive blood pressure cuff, the bladder size should be at least 80% of the arm circumference in length with a width of at least half of the arm length.

Nutrition

Obese critically ill patient may have increased protein catabolism. In addition, many obese patients are paradoxically malnourished. Early enteral feedings should be instituted if possible. Estimation of nutritional needs done by indirect calorimetry if available or by resting energy expenditure equations. There is some literature that suggests hypocaloric feeding while maintaining high protein intake in the obese critically ill patient to avoid overfeeding. General goals of nutrition are 20 to 25 kcal/kg of ideal body weight per day with 2.0 g/kg ideal body weight of protein. Obese patients have also been found to have significant micronutrient deficiencies. These deficiencies of vitamin D, thiamine, copper, zinc, selenium among others can be made worse by bariatric surgical procedures and should be supplemented when low (44–46).

OUTCOMES

There is no consensus whether obesity confers a survival advantage or disadvantage in critical illness. This disparity may reflect the difficulty in defining obesity only based on a measure of weight and not the complex tissue and system effect of adiposity. Obese patients present the entire critical care team with obstacles to overcome. From acute illness and resuscitation to mobilization and rehabilitation; the morbidly obese critically ill patient requires an understanding of the pathophysiology at a cellular, tissue, and system level.

Key Points

- Obesity is a worldwide epidemic in which the morbidly obese is rapidly increasing.
- In the morbidly obese, adipose tissue is immunologically active and through a multitude of inflammatory pathways causes pathology on cellular, tissue, and system levels.
- Changes to the cardiopulmonary system, lead to little reserve during critical illness. Obese patients have increased blood volume.
- Increase in body mass leads to increase oxygen demand, and results in chronic stress on myocardium coupled with increase in arterial resistance can lead to left ventricular systolic and diastolic dysfunction.
- FRC is chronically decreased in the morbidly obese leading to V/Q mismatch and hypoxia. This coupled with decreased excursion of diaphragms and decreased chest wall compliance can lead to rapid desaturation during critical illness and intubation.
- Anatomical alterations from fat deposits of the upper airway and increased resistance from narrowed trachea and bronchioles can be additive, making the morbidly obese patient a "difficulty airway."
- Intensivists underestimate the amount of peep to recruit collapsed alveoli in the ventilated morbidly obese. Levels of at least 10 cm H_2O should be a started point.
- Consideration of extubating to NIPPV even in recent thoracic and bowel surgery should be strongly considered. There has been no evidence that NIPPV in postoperative patient disrupts anastomosis except for possibly the pharyngeal and oral surgeries.
- Drug dosing in the morbidly obese is complex and maybe unique in each patient. Underdosing antibiotics and anticoagulation has been shown to be as serious a problem as overdosing. Expert consultation with critical care pharmacist is imparitive.
- Many morbidly obese patients are malnourish both macro and micronutrients. Adequate protein should be given.
- Morbidly obese patients should not be ridiculed, or disparaged.
- Equipment should be made available to morbidly obese patient that can safely handle extreme weight safely.

References

1. Schneider HJ, Friedrich N, Klotsche J, et al. The predictive value of different measures of obesity for incident cardiovascular events and mortality. *J Clin Endocrinol Metab.* 2010;95(4):1777–1785.
2. Ng M, Fleming T, Robinson M, et al. Global, regional and national prevalence of overweight and obesity in children and adults during 1980–2013: a systematic analysis for the Global Burden of Disease Study 2013. *Lancet.* 2014;384:766–781.
3. Finkelstein EA, Khavjou OA, Thompson H, et al. Obesity and severe obesity forecasts through 2030. *Am J Prev Med.* 2012;42:563–570.
4. Honiden S, McArdle JR. Obesity in the intensive care unit. *Clin Chest Med.* 2009;30:581–599.
5. Akinnusi ME, Pineda LA, El Solh AA. Effect of obesity on intensive care morbidity and mortality: a meta-analysis. *Crit Care Med.* 2008;36:151–158.
6. Weisberg SP, McCann D, Desai M, et al. Obesity is associated with macrophage accumulation in adipose tissue. *J Clin Invest.* 2003;112:1796–1808.
7. Craft M, Reed MJ. Immunologic changes in obesity. *Crit Care Clin.* 2010; 26:629–631.
8. Derosa G, Fogari E, D'Angelo A, et al. Adipocytokine levels in obese and nonobese subjects: an observational study. *Inflammation.* 2013;36:914–920.
9. Trivedi V, Bavishi C, Jean R. Impact of obesity on sepsis mortality: a systematic review. *J Crit Care.* 2015;30:518–524.
10. Paz-Filho G, Mastronardi C, Franco CB, et al. Leptin: molecular mechanisms, systemic pro-inflammatory effects and clinical implications. *Arq Bras Endocrinol Metabol.* 2012;56:597–607.
11. Zhang C. The role of inflammatory cytokines in endothelial dysfunction. *Basic Res Cardiol.* 2008;103(5):398–406.
12. Gharib M, Kaul S, LoCurto J, et al. The obesity factor in critical illness: between consensus and controversy. *Trauma Acute Care Surg.* 2015;78(4): 866–873.
13. Roger VL, Go AS, Lloyd-Jones DM, et al. Heart disease and stroke statistics—2012 update: a report from the American Heart Association. *Circulation.* 2012;125:e2–e220.
14. Kenchaiah S, Evans JC, Levy D. Obesity and the risk of heart failure. *N Engl J Med.* 2002;347:305–313.
15. Wong C, Marwick TH. Obesity cardiomyopathy: pathogenesis and pathophysiology. *Nat Clin Pract Cardiovasc Med.* 2007;4:436–443.
16. Bahammam AS, Al-Jawder SE. Managing acute respiratory decompensation in the morbidly obese. *Respiratory.* 2012;17:759–771.
17. Shashaty M, Stapleton RD. Physiological and management implications of obesity in critical illness. *Ann Am Thorac Soc.* 2014;11:1286–1297.
18. Ashburn DD, DeAntonio A, Reed MJ. Pulmonary system and obesity. *Crit Care Clin.* 2010;26:597–602.
19. Hai F, Porhomayon J, Vermont L, et al. Postoperative complications in patients with obstructive sleep apnea: a meta-analysis. *J Clin Anesth.* 2014; 26:591–600.
20. O'Gorman SM, Gay PC, Morgenthaler TI. Does auto titrating positive airway therapy improve postoperative outcome in patients as risk for obstructive sleep apnea syndrome? A randomized controlled clinical trial. *Chest.* 2013;144:72–80.
21. Neligan PJ, Malhotra G, Fraser M, et al. Continuous positive airway pressure via the Bossignac system immediately after extubation improves lung function in morbidly obese patients with obstructive sleep apnea undergoing laparoscopic bariatric surgery. *Anesthesiology.* 2009;110:878–884.
22. Mutter TC, Chateau D, Moffatt M, et al. A matched cohort study of postoperative outcomes in obstructive sleep apnea: could preoperative diagnosis and treatment prevent complications. *Anesthesiology.* 2014;121:707–718.
23. De Jong A, Molinari N, Pouzeratte Y, et al. Difficult intubation in obese patients: incidence, risk factors, and complications in the operating theatre and in intensive care units. *Br J Anaesth.* 2015;114:297–306.
24. Ramachandran SK, Cosnowski A, Shanks A, Turner CR. Apneic oxygenation during prolonged laryngoscopy in obese patients: a randomized, controlled trial of nasal oxygen administration. *J Clin Anesth.* 2010;22: 164–168.
25. Apfelbaum JL, Hagberg CA, Caplan RA, et al. Practice guidelines for management of the difficult airway: an updated report by the American Society of Anesthesiologists Task Force on management of the difficult airway. *Anesthesiology.* 2013;118:251–270.
26. Aceto P, Perilli V, Modesti C, et al. Airway management in obese patients. *Surg Obes Relat Dis.* 2013;9:809–815.
27. Frerk C, Mitchell VS, McNarry AF, et al. Difficult airway society 2015 guidelines for management of unanticipated difficult intubation in adults. *Br J Anaesth.* 2015;115:827–848.
28. Soubani AO, Chen W, Jang H. The outcomes of acute respiratory distress syndrome in relation to body mass index and diabetes mellitus. *Heart Lung.* 2015;44:441–447.
29. Lemyze M, Mallat J, Duhamel A, et al. Effects of sitting position and applied positive end expiratory pressure on respiratory mechanics of the critically ill obese patients receiving mechanical ventilation. *Crit Care Med.* 2013;41:2592–2599.
30. Pirrone M, Fisher D, Chipman D, et al. Recruitment maneuvers and positive end-expiratory pressure titration in morbidly obese ICU patient. *Crit Care Med.* 2016;44:300–307.
31. Calvo-Ayala E, Marik P. Noninvasive ventilation after extubation obese critically ill subjects. In: Esquinas AM, ed. *Noninvasive Mechanical Ventilation and Difficult Weaning in Critical Care: Key Topics and Practical Approaches.* Norfolk, VA: Springer International Publishing; 2016:241–245.
32. El-Solh AA, Aquilina A, Pineda L, et al. Noninvasive ventilation for prevention of post-extubation respiratory failure in obese patients. *Eur Respir J.* 2006;28:588–595.
33. Brodsky JB. Positioning the morbid obese patient for surgery. In: Alvarez A, ed. *Morbid Obesity Perioperative Management.* Cambridge: Cambridge University Press; 2004:274–283.
34. Bucaloiu ID, Perkins RM, DiFilippo W, et al. Acute kidney injury in the critically ill morbidly obese patient: diagnostic and therapeutic challenges in a unique patient population. *Crit Care Clin.* 2010;26:607–624.
35. Sanuja M, Kumar A. Obesity and perioperative acute kidney injury: a focused review. *J Crit Care.* 2014;29:694.e1–e6.
36. Ashburn DD, Reed MJ. Gastrointestinal system and obesity. *Crit Care Clin.* 2010;26:625–627.
37. Jain SS, Dhand R. Perioperative treatment of patients with obstructive sleep apnea. *Curr Opin Pulm Med.* 2004;10:482–488.
38. Al-Dorzi HM, Al Harbi SA, Arabi YM. Antibiotic therapy of pneumonia in the obese: dosing and delivery. *Curr Opin Infect Dis.* 2014;27:165–173.
39. Russell JM, Nick-Dart RL, Nornhold BD. Development of a pharmacist driven protocol for automatic medication dosage adjustments in obese patients. *Am J Health Syst Pharm.* 2015;72;1656–1663.
40. Stein P, Goldman J. Obesity and thromboembolic disease. *Clin Chest Med.* 2009;30:489–493.
41. Craft M, Reed MJ. Venous thromboembolic disease and hematologic considerations in obesity. *Crit Care Clin.* 2010;26:637–640.
42. Gould MK, Garcia DA, Wren SM, et al. Prevention of VTE in nonorthopedic surgical patients. *Chest.* 2012;141:e227S–e277S.
43. Dossett LA, Dageforde LA, Swenson BR, et al. Obesity and site-specific nosocomial infection risk in the intensive care unit. *Surg Infect.* 2009;10: 137–142.
44. Choban P, Dickerson R, Malone A, et al.; American Society for Parenteral and Enteral Nutrition. A.S.P.E.N. Clinical guidelines: nutrition support of hospitalized patients with obesity. *J Parenter Enteral Nutr.* 2013;37:714–744.
45. Winfield RD. Caring for the critically ill morbidly obese patient: challenges and opportunities. *Nutr Clin Pract.* 2014;29:747–750.
46. Pickkers P, de Keizer N, Dusseljee J, et al. Body mass index is associated with hospital mortality in critically ill patients: an observational cohort study. *Crit Care Med.* 2013;41:1878–1883.

CHAPTER
70

The Geriatric Patient

CARL W. PETERS

INTRODUCTION

The elderly population in the United States is growing at a remarkable rate, with considerable implications for delivery of intensive care to those in the later years of life. The numbers tell the story: in the 2000 US census, those 62 years of age and older represented 14.7% of the population. Between 2000 and 2010, the population 65 years and older increased at a faster rate (15.1%) than the total US population (9.7%). In fact, the 85- to 94-year-old group experienced the fastest growth between 2000 and 2010, increasing in size by 29.9%, from 3.9 to 5.1 million (1). As of 2013, remaining life expectancy for 65-year-old men was 18 more years, and for 65-year-old women, it was over 20 years (2).

At the dawn of the 20th century, the elderly population of the United States was a small percentage of its total, 3.1 million people (4% of the population); presently, the corresponding value is 35 million people (11.3%). Based on revolutionary advances in public health and the development of medications and techniques of acute medical care provided to those born in the 20 years after World War II, 70,000,000 individuals will find themselves in the population subgroup known as "elderly" by 2030 (3). At that time, those 65 years and older are forecast to compose 26% of the population of Florida, which recently passed New York to become the third most populous state behind California and Texas (4). By virtue of the diseases and natural organ aging and deterioration that accompany 65—and more—years of living and working, those who advance into this age range become increasingly voracious consumers of medical care resources, including the specialized capabilities of the intensive care unit (ICU). In 2013, spending by Medicare for those older than 65 years totaled approximately $420 billion of the $2.9 trillion spent nationwide for health care (5). The US Census Bureau predicts that, by 2025, of the nearly 75,000,000 individuals of 65 years or older living in the United States, about 119,000 will be centenarians (6). Intensive care consumes 4% of national health care expenditures (7). During the last 6 months of their lives, 11% of Medicare recipients spend 8 or more days in the ICU; various studies documenting ICU occupancy by those older than 65 years note that this use consumes from one-quarter to one-half of available ICU beds (8,9). The financial implications of these statistics are significant, as a portion of this care will be provided in the ICU; in 2011, the mean cost of hospitalization that included ICU care was 2.5 times as expensive as that which did not include the ICU: $61,800 versus $25,200 (10). The level of these expenditures, projected to continue their slow but exponential growth, has resulted in the argument being made that, in the context of *increasing* demand for *limited* health care resources—an economically unsustainable situation—blanket cost-cutting actions such as limiting scarce ICU availability to those who would "most benefit" society and themselves in later life should be instituted. The geriatric population, in the minds of some, does not qualify for this category of expenditure. The logic of this position, however, belies reality. Although functionality diminishes with advancing age in a bell-curve like manner, many individuals continue to perform both complex physical and intellectual tasks well into their eighth or ninth decades of life, bringing to bear resources of experience and problem solving not yet acquired by their descendants. The tactic of cost savings through measures that "cut out the expensive waste" in the ICU care of the elderly is both misleading and inaccurate (11–13). Furthermore, at least in the United States, while increasingly alarmed by the financial implications of medical care costs associated with an aging population, we continue to postpone in-depth reckoning with the consequences and management of this information, just as we continue to postpone end-of-life (EOL) discussions. Until we are ready to deal with these issues, one must maximize use of the resources available, while being mindful of the individual patient's expectations and likelihood of recovery.

The response of the human body to physiologic insult evolves with age. A parallel with outdoor activity is useful in understanding this evolution. Imagine that a man is placed on a long ridgetop that is quite wide and smooth, and that man is told to walk down the middle of the ridge with his eyes closed. Unknown to him, as he walks, the ridge slowly becomes strewn with larger and larger rocks and other impediments to ambulation, and narrows inexorably as he approaches the end. Initially, the man walks quickly, with little risk of tripping or nearing the edge. As he advances further, however, his drifting excursions off the centerline each take him closer to the treacherous rocky edge, increasing the risk of a fall. If he is careful and walks slowly, he hears the wind blowing near the cliff and is able to redirect himself away from the danger. Eventually, however, the narrowed ridgetop is completely covered with loose rocks to the very edges, and no step is possible without catastrophe. By analogy, one can think of the human body as possessing a certain amount of physiologic reserve that sustains it through times of stress brought on by disease or injury, with the maximum amount of reserve being present in young adulthood. With age, baseline organ function declines at a generally predictable rate, leaving the aging person with progressively less and less capacity to respond fully and expeditiously to stressful demands. Furthermore, there is the accumulation of permanent detrimental consequences of lifestyle decisions, such as tobacco use and lack of exercise, and of only partially controllable genetic influences, such as familial hypercholesterolemia or essential hypertension, with which the aging individual must contend, thereby increasing the likelihood of succumbing to a stressful physiologic insult. This progressive loss of physiologic reserve has come to be termed *frailty*, a syndrome of vulnerability involving domains of functional status, deficit accumulation, and biologic indices, separate from direct effects of age, comorbidity, and disability (14) and generally increasing the likelihood of poorer outcome from physiologically stressful events (15). The progressive impairment of physiologic vigor is exemplified by the *exponential* increase in the death rate from sepsis with age, although the incidence of sepsis increases only *linearly* (16), reflecting the compromised physiologic vigor accessible to the critically ill elder. Quantification of frailty to assist in assessment and management of elderly patients that have sustained traumatic injuries is an area of investigation among acute care surgeons (17,18).

CARDIOVASCULAR DISEASE IN THE ELDERLY

Approximately 35% of all deaths in the United States are attributable to one of several manifestations of cardiovascular (CV) pathophysiology, namely coronary artery disease and other conditions that involve the myocardium, hypertension, and arteriosclerosis of the central and peripheral arterial tree and cerebral vascular system, with three-fourths of these deaths directly attributable to a cardiac cause (19). This proportion is higher in the elderly population, with CV disease manifesting itself as a complicating cofactor in the management of *any* older person's serious illness. For example, although only 6% of the US population is 75 years of age or older, individuals in this age group account for 30% of all myocardial infarctions and 60% of the infarction-related deaths (20).

Aging and the CV System

Studying the effect of the natural aging process on CV physiology is quite complex. From the epidemiologic standpoint, it is difficult to differentiate the basis of decline in CV function of the well-conditioned octogenarian who exercises aggressively from that of his sedentary twin who has led a life of excess, because some features and consequences of natural aging resemble those seen with disease. Although degenerative CV processes are most often looked on as "what happens as you grow old," these have been demonstrated not to be the obligatory sequence of events in human aging (21,22). The common causative elements within modern civilized existence, such as diet, minimal demands for aerobic exercise, and recurrent and ubiquitous emotional and physical stress are so intimately associated with mere existence that they may be looked on as inevitable and unchangeable. The clinical consequences to these apparently unalterable processes may be perceived by the clinician or investigator as the natural process of CV aging, but the accuracy of this perception may be compromised. The rapidity of deterioration seen in aging is increased by both a sedentary lifestyle and by the CV disease processes that are epidemic in western society's geriatric populations.

A degenerative process that occurs in most elderly individuals is that of stiffening of the central arterial tree. Although the consequences of this process do not manifest in acute ways that are within the direct purview of the intensivist, they induce chronic progressive conditions that complicate critical illness in the elderly. Oxygen- and nutrient-bearing blood is carried to organs via the arterial tree. In doing so, distensible large arteries perform transport and cushioning functions, transforming pulsatile flow into a steady stream of blood to the periphery (23). Release of the potential energy stored with each heartbeat within the stretched arterial wall elastin fibers propels the column of blood smoothly toward the muscular arterioles and capillary bed (23). With age—likely related to both replacement of deteriorating, nonregenerating structural elastin fibers with nondistensible collagen, and to the progressive calcification of wall structural components (24)—vascular remodeling causes the progressive slow dilation and stiffening of the arterial wall, transforming the robust, pliant central vasculature typical of youth to that commonly seen in the elderly, more akin to a thick-walled, stiff, nondistensible garden hose (25,26). Augmented tensile and shear stresses, related to the nonlaminar flow characteristic of fluid flow through vessels with impaired compliance contribute to progressive occlusive disease (27), typically found at turbulent areas of narrowing, bending, and bifurcation (28). The prominent manifestation of this progressive central arterial stiffening is that of the so-called systolic hypertension syndrome—the gradual increase in systolic blood pressure with simultaneous diastolic decline or maintenance at the same level (29). In years past, the transmission velocity of the cardiac-generated pressure impulse was discovered to change with patient age and to vary as a function of central arterial stiffness (30–33). With increased central arterial elastance—stiffness—comes an increased velocity of impulse transmission in both the forward and backward (i.e., reflected) directions. In the young, with distensible central arteries, the arrival of the reflected wave coincides with diastole, thereby augmenting coronary perfusion and modulating the magnitude of the disease-inducing tensile shear forces on the vasculature. Youthful vessels have little disease, and thus seldom display the wide pulse pressure (PP) that is the hallmark of central thickening. Aging and stiff central arteries transmit the cardiac impulse outward more rapidly and turbulently such that its reflected return arrives at the end or even the height of systole (33). In those with such vessels—the elderly—isolated *systolic* hypertension is noted. Although this term seems to imply a benignity that was previously thought to be true, with opinion further generalized that sustained *diastolic* pressure elevation was the lethal culprit (34); this is no longer thought to be the case. The insidiously destructive nature of the *augmentation index*—the reflected augmentation of systolic pressure at the expense of diastolic coronary perfusion, yielding an easily observed increased PP (35)—has been recognized as the true contribution of central vascular stiffness to the morbidity and mortality among the elderly. Indeed, the speed with which the cardiac impulse is propelled outward, known as pulse wave velocity (PWV), and PP are recognized as factors strongly associated with all forms of CV disease:

$$PP = SBP - DBP$$

where SBP is systolic blood pressure and DBP is diastolic blood pressure. These measurements, when elevated over time, strongly predict mortality and are indicative of vascular and cardiac pathology, even if the patient's blood pressure measurements and examination findings at a given moment appear benign (27,34,36,37).

Other specific processes within the CV system change with age, even in healthy elderly. With myocardial aging, there is a predictable loss of myocytes, possibly from apoptosis (38,39). Because cardiac myocytes are unable to regenerate, functional "replacement" of these contractile cells occurs by hypertrophy of the remaining myocytes, with only slight overall loss of myocardial mass. As cardiac fibroblast synthetic function is maintained, cardiac tissue becomes infiltrated with an increasing proportion of noncompliant connective tissue, causing the gradual thickening and stiffening of the ventricular wall and impairment of left ventricular diastolic relaxation and filling. This appears similar to the fibrosis seen in pathologic left ventricular hypertrophy leading to congestive heart failure (HF) (40). Diastolic relaxation is an energy-requiring process, consuming ATP to recover calcium back into the sarcoplasmic reticulum after its release during systole (41). Development of impaired diastolic relaxation with age, resulting from age-related malfunction of the calcium-sequestering mechanism involving a dysfunctional SERCA (smooth endoplasmic reticulum calcium) pump, is partially responsible for the increased percentage of geriatric HF who display lusitropic dysfunction (42). Consequently, the filling process is delayed, with a smoother—though steeper—slope of passive diastolic ventricular filling (43) into a more slowly relaxing ventricle that ends diastole with lower volume. The ventricle thereby becomes more dependent on the contribution of atrial contraction to ventricular filling for optimum systolic function. In other words, as the aging ventricle becomes progressively more and more lusitropically impaired, it fills progressively less well by virtue of thickening from age-related myocyte depletion and incomplete relaxation from SERCA pump dysfunction. The resulting dependence on volume repletion, control of heart rate, and the robust synchronous atrial contribution to ventricle filling assume increasing importance in managing geriatric cardiac issues. In the critically ill elderly patient in whom there is a very high chance of harboring occult diastolic dysfunction if not overt congestive HF, the strictest attention must be paid to maintenance of both sinus rhythm and volume repletion within a narrow range. Furthermore, preserved ejection fraction viewed on echocardiogram may be deceptive, because systolic function is preserved in the normal healthy geriatric heart (44) and can be maintained at greater than 50% in a very high proportion of those whose cardiac status has deteriorated to the point of being symptomatic from lusitropically deficient congestive HF (45,46).

Equally important is recognition of the progressive decrease in the responsiveness of myocardial and vascular tissue to adrenergic stimulation (47–49). This phenomenon manifests itself as an age-associated lowering of exercise-induced maximal heart rate, with a gradual shift to augmented ventricular filling to meet exercise-related demands. The stressed or exercising younger adult musters additional cardiac output by increasing contractility and heart rate and by vasodilation in the areas of maximum demand—in the case of exercise, the skeletal muscles—in response to increased levels of norepinephrine and epinephrine, with unchanged or reduced end systolic volume as output is ejected into a dilated vascular tree. The elderly, by comparison, with reduced myocardial and vasodilatory responsiveness to exercise-induced beta-1 and beta-2 stimulus (49) have increased reliance on *ventricular filling* (the Frank–Starling mechanism) to achieve augmented cardiac output (50,51).

Optimal care requires clinical awareness of age-related CV differences such as diastolic dysfunction. The clinician must contend with the challenge of managing the stiff, hypertrophied ventricle perfusing a nondistensible vascular tree. With the fraction of elderly patients who harbor CV disease being as large as it is in western society, clinical manifestations of this condition may complicate the management of virtually every older patient. Because the elderly may not display the "usual, common" symptoms of HF, one *must* maintain a level of suspicion to recognize the more subtle presentations of age-related lusitropic pathophysiology. The phenomenon of lusitropic insufficiency that is termed *diastolic dysfunction* has recently been recognized as part of a constellation of cardiac and systemic symptoms and pathology, associated with advancing age, that is more accurately named *h*eart *f*ailure with *p*reserved *e*jection *f*raction (HFpEF), and it is exceedingly sensitive to the impact of common elderly comorbidities on cardiac function (52). Accurate diagnosis of HFpEF by the most common noninvasive modality, echocardiography, can be a difficult and complex task to accomplish (53).

Acute Coronary Syndrome in the Elderly

Acute coronary syndrome (ACS) presents a particular challenge from the standpoints of recognition and management. Optimal management of myocardial ischemia and infarction in the elderly population is less well defined than in younger populations, because those older than 75 years are less commonly included in ischemia-related studies (54). Further, elderly patients are, unfortunately, less likely to be managed according to evidence-based guidelines (55), or to be admitted under the care of a cardiologist (56). The ACS mortality rate of the elderly exceeds that found in younger individuals (57) but the former benefit most in mortality reduction from intervention (58). In the young, acute ischemic processes are often associated with onset of classic angina or one of its common equivalents; in the elderly, symptoms may be much more subtle and nondistinguishing, but the condition is more likely to be fatal (59). Therefore, proper identification of myocardial ischemia and infarction must occur in a timely manner, as aggressive management is warranted. The diagnostic picture can be further complicated by the postoperative sedated state, when hypotension or arrhythmias may easily be attributed to hydration or electrolyte disturbances rather than to coronary insufficiency. ICU patients often have contraindications to intervention, and the risks of reperfusion therapy must be weighed thoughtfully against the benefits; the intensivist must remember that only a small percentage of elderly patients warranting reperfusion therapy actually receive it (60), even when no absolute contraindication exists. This is attributable to two misperceptions: the magnitude of risk to the geriatric patient, and the likelihood of benefit (58). The cardiology literature contains studies covering enormous numbers of patients evaluating the strategies of treatment to optimize the restoration of coronary blood flow, and in-depth discussion is beyond the scope of this chapter. Nonetheless, a few generalities focusing on the management of the elderly patient can be made.

As mentioned above, few elderly individuals have been included in many of the large trials (61), especially considering the prevalence of coronary disease in this group; for this reason, optimal management strategies may not be as well defined as those that address ACS within a younger population. ACS must be identified correctly, nonetheless, because treatment strategies of the patient subgroups within this very large category differ (62). One of the underpinnings of any strategy is that of expeditious implementation, in that the more quickly the intervention is begun, the greater the mass of myocardial tissue preserved and the greater number of lives saved (63). Rapid restoration of coronary blood flow is the major goal of the treatment for STEMI (ST-segment elevation myocardial infarction). A decrease in mortality of 25% with reperfusion therapy has been demonstrated (64). From identification of STEMI, it is recommended that the infusion of thrombolytics begin within 30 minutes, or that the dilating balloon be inflated within 90 minutes (65). In general, percutaneous coronary intervention (PCI) is the preferred mode of treatment for STEMI, as long as the time constraints are met (66). Again, extrapolation of this analysis to the elderly population is done with some trepidation, because only small numbers of elderly patients were included in the studies covered by this meta-analysis (66). Nevertheless, it appears that elderly patients in the situation of evolving myocardial infarction, in which the risk of death is particularly high by virtue of the risk factors associated with advanced age (67) and by the emergent nature of the situation, are best served by PCI (57,68). PCI yielded lower mortality in the elderly population than did thrombolysis, with more benefit found as age progressively advanced, although possibly at the risk of a slightly increased rate of major bleeding events.

In non-STEMI, early invasive strategy with catheterization and revascularization (when warranted) significantly benefits those older than 65 years of age (69); early invasive strategy, however, led to a significant increase in in-hospital major bleeding (16.6% vs. 6.5%; $p = 0.009$) and blood transfusion (20.9% vs. 7.9%; $p = 0.002$) in the patients older than 75 years of age. There were no significant increases in minor bleeding or stroke in any study group. The potential benefits of PCI in the elderly patient in the elective and emergent arenas must be weighed closely against the risks incurred by this group of individuals in the form of increased bleeding and vascular complications (70). Over the past decade, the use of PCI in the management of ACS in the elderly has been increasing (71).

Cardiomyopathy

In the United States, 5,000,000 persons suffer from HF, with more than 50,000 new cases diagnosed yearly; over 80% of the individuals with HF are older than 65 years of age (72–74). Symptomatic HF *by itself* carries a dismal prognosis, with a median survival of 1.7 years for men and 3.2 years for women (75). Critical illness superimposed on decompensated HF is challenging for even the most adept clinician. Common causes for HF in the elderly include coronary artery disease and hypertension, followed by diabetes mellitus, valvular disease (especially aortic stenosis and mitral regurgitation) and cardiomyopathies other than ischemic (76). The incidence of HF increases with age; Framingham Study data reveal a doubling in incidence with each decade after 45 to 54 years of age (77). Factors in the critical care arena that may precipitate HF decompensation abound; these include ischemia and infarction, which is more often "silent" and subtly manifested in the elderly (78), dysrhythmias and extremes of heart rate, fever and infection, medication side effects, and rapid fluid shifts such as with bleeding and aggressive fluid resuscitation. Suspicion of CV decompensation warrants aggressive, timely investigation. Marginal coronary reserve should be presumed and investigated with measurement of cardiac enzymes and documentation of electrocardiogram (ECG) patterns. An echocardiogram is usually readily available and may be useful in separating those suffering from lusitropic dysfunction from those with inotropic insufficiency. Particular points of interest to be investigated include systolic ejection fraction, lusitropic state (i.e., diastolic "relaxability" between contractions, reflecting preload), valvular integrity, and wall motion abnormalities. Over the last several years, it has been recognized that an increasing predominance of instances of HF in the elderly are those with preserved ejection fraction (HFpEF), especially in women and increasing in prevalence with progressively older individuals (52). HFpEF, which can be challenging to manage successfully (79) seems to be a manifestation of a systemic global disorder of associated with aging and multiple comorbidities seen in older patients. The initial diagnosis of HF is clinical; early clarification of ventricular function can be provided by echocardiogram which may reveal a nearly normal ejection fraction despite the patient's clinical decompensation. The intensivist should maintain a low threshold to advance to invasive monitoring to clarify an uncertain hemodynamic state and guide infusion of vasoactive medications. In the elderly patient with HF, an eroded reserve may not allow more than a trivial aberration beyond the margins of physiologic compensation.

Dysrhythmias

Dysrhythmias are frequent in the elderly patient (80,81), including those who manifest no other overt CV abnormalities, although 20% to 45% of those with atrial fibrillation (AF) harbor coronary artery disease (82). With advancing age, sinus node and conduction system integrity deteriorate, with gradual replacement of cardiac pacemaker cells by collagen and elastic tissue (83–87). Such triggering events as autonomic tone disruption (88,89), ischemia or infarction (which portends worse outcome) (90,91), anatomic alterations such as fluid overload or cardiac surgery (92,93), and a host of other cardiac conditions (including strong correlation with the presence of diastolic dysfunction) (94,95) may initiate potentially injurious tachydysrhythmic events, the most common of which is AF.

The occurrence of AF increases with age (96), carrying an increased risk of stroke and death (97) in those older than 60 years, even in the absence of other cardiac abnormalities. Several issues remain unsettled in the optimal management of AF (98). Of these, the two that receive the most attention are rate control versus rhythm control, and management of anticoagulation. The AFFIRM investigators (99) found no clear survival advantage to either rate or rhythm control in AF, but the rate control strategy did appear to manifest some advantages in the area of medication side effects. All choices for chemical control of rate and rhythm in the elderly population must be made within the skewed context of the high percentage of these patients who harbor comorbid conditions, especially HF; as choices for immediate rate control include beta-blockers and calcium channel blockers, the clinician must remain mindful of their impact on the state of HF compensation. Amiodarone or digoxin may be used in those with HF in the absence of an accessory pathway. Digoxin is not recommended in such patients, as it may precipitate *profound* tachycardia via the accessory pathway, with heart rate nearing 300 beats per minute (bpm), leading to CV collapse. In the case of acute hemodynamic instability, recovery of sinus rhythm with biphasic DC cardioversion after sedation is appropriate. Digoxin or amiodarone can provide rate control, but the former is *not* recommended for chemical cardioversion, and several medications primarily used by cardiologists surpass the latter in class of recommendation for this purpose (100).

There is no "one size fits all" solution to the question of anticoagulation in AF, although it has been well demonstrated (101) to reduce the incidence of AF-related stroke, a *major* avoidable comorbidity in the elderly. Equally well demonstrated (102,103) is the extent to which anticoagulation is *under* used in the elderly, presumably because of concern for bleeding risk in this accident- and fall-prone population, and inadequate awareness of the extent to which AF warrants anticoagulation to minimize the risk of AF-associated stroke. Oral anticoagulation therapy (OAC) is warranted in those with AF to decrease embolic stroke, reducing its instance in nonvalvular AF by 60% when warfarin is utilized (104). A variety of non-vitamin K antagonist oral anticoagulants (NOACs) have come to market recently, offering the benefit of reduced testing frequency—as is required with warfarin therapy—at the expense of very limited reversibility. Target international normalized ratio (INR) of 2.0 to 3.0 is recommended for those receiving vitamin K antagonists (105). The final anticoagulant medication decision must take into account bleeding risk, presence of CAD, renal and hepatic function, the frailty of the patient, other medications, and the patient's risk of an embolic event (106). Clearly, maintenance of long-term anticoagulant regimens has limited applicability to the patient who suffers a critical injury or illness, and rapid normalization of INR may be warranted. Quickly reversible heparin may be a better choice in such a situation if continued anticoagulation is, in any event, warranted. AF that persists beyond 48 hours mandates anticoagulation for 2 weeks (100,105) or transesophageal echocardiogram evaluation by a cardiologist—with particular attention to the left atrium and its appendage—for the presence of clot prior to conversion to sinus rhythm. The most complete and recent American College of Cardiology/American Heart Association guidelines for the management of all issues relating to AF appear in the references to this chapter (107).

Complex ventricular dysrhythmias and ventricular tachycardia (VT) present a difficult management problem in the elderly. Sudden cardiac death (SCD) is, to a large extent, a product of untreated VT degenerating into ventricular fibrillation (VF), followed by asystole (108,109). In the elderly population as a whole, ambulatory monitoring reveals a very high instance of ventricular dysrhythmias, including VT (110,111). Therefore, there is a high likelihood that any given elderly ICU patient will have worrisome ventricular ectopy, with a significant number displaying VT (112–114). Despite the high prevalence of ventricular ectopy in this population, only those patients with underlying heart disease have a poorer long-term prognosis by virtue of the ectopy (115). Underlying HF and left ventricular hypertrophy (116) associated with increased ectopy are prognostic of an increased likelihood of subsequent adverse cardiac events, including myocardial infarction and sudden death (117). Pulseless cardiac arrest due to VF or VT warrants management following current advanced cardiac life support (ACLS) guidelines, using cardiopulmonary resuscitation (CPR) with chest compressions and immediate defibrillation (118). The timely recognition of these lethal dysrhythmias and initiation of most recent ACLS protocols is crucial for patient welfare, because survival is a direct function of the immediacy of electrical resynchronization therapy (119); defibrillation for VF provides the optimal chance of survival if provided within 3 minutes (120). The frequency of ventricular ectopy is increased in the geriatric ICU population where several factors, including ischemia, sepsis, extremes of heart rate, hypoxia, electrolyte imbalance, and autonomic disruption associated with recent surgery, can aggravate cardiac irritability and induce lethal dysrhythmias in a marginally compensated individual. These inciting factors should be readily recognized and reversed in the constantly vigilant ICU environment. Empiric treatment of ventricular ectopy per se, however, has been demonstrated to be more prodysrhythmic than beneficial (121,122), often increasing mortality and/or inducing drug-related side effects. Nonetheless, certain medications warrant closer attention; beta-blockers after myocardial infarction have been demonstrated to reduce subsequent total mortality and SCD (123). After initial enthusiasm, amiodarone has not, in a recent study of cardiomyopathy patients, proven to be beneficial in reducing SCD when given prophylactically to patients with ejection fraction ≤35% and New York Heart Association (NYHA) class II or III HF, as compared to that achieved with a single-lead automatic implantable cardiac defibrillator (AICD) (124). With the emergence of AICD technology, there has been a gradual reduction in mortality from SCD in elderly patients, in whom there is a higher incidence than in the general population of coronary artery disease. In this situation, the AICD appears superior to medications in preventing SCD (125). Elderly individuals accrue an equal or greater benefit from AICD placement compared to younger individuals, with minimal risk involved in the actual placement of the device (126). The indications for AICD placement continue to evolve (127–130). Clearly, the expertise of a cardiac electrophysiologist is indicated when medications or AICD placement are considered in the management of a patient at risk for or who has survived SCD.

With advancing age comes a parallel increase in conduction system disease, often mandating permanent pacemaker (PPM) placement. In 1990, the implantation rate for cardiac pacemakers was 329 devices per million patients; by 2002, the rate had risen to 612 per million (131); the mean age of implanted patients was 75.1 years (131), and the commonest reason for implantation of a pacemaker is sick sinus syndrome (SSS), a cardiac rhythm irregularity that affects 1 in 600 patients over the age of 65 (132). Such statistics make it likely that an elderly person with a PPM will at some time arrive in the ICU for a noncardiac ailment. Furthermore, advances in engineering and microcircuitry have allowed the development of single devices that incorporate PPM and AICD capability. Although management of issues directly referable to these increasingly complex machines is more within the purview of the cardiologist, certain data can be gathered quickly that will expedite investigation of such a device's performance, as is well detailed in the recent literature (133–135). Considerable guidance can be formulated from information on the PPM manufacturer's card that is carried by the patient, from a chest radiograph showing lead position and integrity, and from an ECG with rhythm strip. Details of electrical patterns should be apparent from the rhythm strip and interrogation findings. Any ICD discharge should be investigated with interrogation.

In the instance of withdrawal or termination of unwanted medical care from a terminally ill patient, the intervention of a normally functioning ICD or PPM is directly contrary to the natural process of dying, analogous to instituting CPR when "Do Not Resuscitate" orders exist. In such an instance, deactivation is indicated (136).

PULMONARY DISEASE

Human pulmonary function deteriorates with age, yet quantification of this age-induced deterioration is quite difficult. Measurement solely of the effects of aging on the respiratory system would require exclusion of all factors that influence respiratory function other than those relating directly to breathing and gas exchange, namely chest wall mechanics, lung histologic structure, and neural/muscular respiratory control. The list of such influencing factors includes environmental pollution and tobacco smoke exposure, occult disease, and effects of previous nutritional deficiencies. Furthermore, these factors complicate contemporaneous comparison between different generations because of the variability of their impacts on these generations. The alternative is the longitudinal study of a rigorously screened cohort of subjects, which has been performed in a few cases (137,138). Analytic difficulties notwithstanding, it is possible, in some instances, to identify the predictable alterations in respiratory physiology that occur with age, so as to prepare the intensivist to contend with a common form of critical illness pathophysiology in the elderly—that of profound respiratory insufficiency.

Microscopic examination of tissue samples from young and older individuals reveals the basis of age-related changes in pulmonary physiology. One sees alveoli from older patients to be less fully surrounded by the elastin/collagen network (139,140), each less robustly tethered open by one another—less *radial traction*—yielding an increasingly compliant lung with diminished recoil (141). Loss of cartilaginous supporting tissue in the small airways further contributes to loss of lung elasticity. The concepts of first, airway collapse, worsened in the patient with advanced emphysema, and second, the progressive stiffening of the chest wall with age allow one to forecast and better understand the evolution of geriatric respiratory function: alterations in lung volume due to gas trapping at higher residual volumes and deterioration of gas exchange. In addition, neural factors alter responsiveness to changes in $PaCO_2$ and PaO_2 (142,143); the magnitude of these changes varies from person to person.

Geriatric flow–volume curves reveal "scooping" of the expiratory limb, implying early closure of airways, and increased residual volume as seen in obstruction from airway collapse in emphysema, a similar phenomenon (144,145). Furthermore, chest wall compliance decreases from calcification of the cartilaginous rib and thoracic spine joints, with kyphotic changes stiffening the thoracic spine itself (146). Compromised compliance results in a substantial increase in the work of breathing, to be provided by deconditioned, aging muscles, likely in the face of low cardiac output and poor nutrition. Such factors yield the respiratory pattern displayed by a significant percentage of the elderly: rapid, shallow breathing at rest, with little exertional reserve. A diagram of lung volumes versus age reveals a slight increase in functional residual capacity (FRC) and residual volume, with a steep rise in *closing capacity,* the volume at which airway collapse takes place in the dependent airways. Thus, airway closure occurs in the upright person *without pulmonary disease* at a lung volume that exceeds FRC (147). In other words, airway collapse can take place in the upright healthy elderly lung even during quiet resting tidal volume during spontaneous breathing, with ventilation/perfusion (V/Q) mismatch increasing shunt fraction and alveolar–arterial partial pressure of oxygen (PO_2) gradient, with relative hypoxemia for a given inspired fraction of oxygen (FiO_2). Subjecting the supine elderly patient with compromised FRC to controlled positive pressure ventilation demands that meticulous attention must be paid to ventilator management to correct V/Q mismatch. The complex details of mechanical ventilation are addressed elsewhere in this textbook (see Chapter 103). In general, one must use PEEP (positive end-expiratory pressure) while administering the lowest FiO_2 possible, avoiding overdistention of the better inflated (more superior, nondependent) alveoli, and providing sufficient expiratory time to avoid auto-PEEP and breath stacking, as well as sufficient tidal volume into the restricted thoracic cage without exceeding peak pressure limits.

It is commonly held that healthy elderly individuals have a significantly lower PaO_2 for a given FiO_2, compared to equally healthy younger counterparts. Traditional teaching has proposed the following formulae (148,149):

$$PaO_2\ (\text{mmHg}) = 104.2 - (0.27 \times \text{age})$$
$$PaO_2 = 100.1 - 0.325 \times \text{age (years)}$$
$$PaO_2 = 109 - 0.43\ (\text{age})$$

More recent studies have yielded varying results (150,151), certainly not confirmatory of a pronounced "predestined" decline in oxygenation with age, and questioning the hypothesis that progressive disruption of the matching of ventilation and perfusion in the elderly is actually the cause of whatever decline actually occurs (152). The related questions of rise in (A–a) gradient with age, and "normal" age-related decline in PaO_2 are, similarly, quantified by different investigators (148,149,153,154).

NUTRITIONAL ISSUES

Malnutrition, also known as undernutrition, is a common companion of elderly individuals and frequently a complicating factor in the efficient and successful management of an elderly ICU patient. The natural decline in energy expenditure with age begins at about age 30 and accompanies the age-related increase in body fat-to-protein ratio (155–157). The evolution of nutritional intake with age is one of decline that exceeds the decrease in energy expenditure (158,159) for various reasons. Thus, even the healthy individual will eat less and lose weight with time, and will be at risk for malnutrition if illness occurs or social support wanes. For example, in elderly nursing home patients, a population in whom initially minor medical problems can quickly blossom into life-threatening conditions, the incidence of undernutrition can approach 85% (160,161). Malnutrition at the onset of critical illness portends poor outcome, as does insufficient nutritional support during the course of the illness (162,163). Mortality is considerably higher in the malnourished elderly patient, compared to those who are nutritionally replete (162). Undernutrition has several common causes: (i) functional decline and social isolation from family and other support systems, (ii) anorexia associated with older age—the so-called *anorexia of aging*—or chronic illness, (iii) anatomic or gustatory impediments to mastication or swallowing, (iv) abuse or neglect, and (v) insufficient financial resources (164–167). Therefore, the prevalence of undernutrition in hospitalized, geriatric patients is relatively high (168,169) and is often unrecognized unless sought specifically (170).

Identification of malnutrition in the elderly patient (170) may be facilitated by the routine employment of easily used physical examination and laboratory screening tools as part of an organized, proactive nutrition screening program (171). There is little literature addressing nutrition in the geriatric ICU patient per se, and the principles set forth below are generally applicable to any ill elderly patient.

Undernutrition imposes a considerable burden on the marginally compensated geriatric patient. The conditions known as protein–energy malnutrition (PEM) and micronutrient deficiency complicate the treatment of several conditions seen in the ICU. These include the contribution of gastrointestinal (GI) tract nonintegrity to multiorgan system failure (172,173), and other common CV (174,175), pulmonary (176–178), and infectious issues (179). Wound healing is impeded by a poor nutritional state (180–182); in particular, development of decubitus ulcers is more common in malnourished elderly individuals, and successful management is decidedly more difficult (181). Patients with PEM are at increased risk for serious complications while in the hospital (182), with slower recovery (183), poorer functional status at discharge, and higher rates of mortality after discharge (184–187).

Malnutrition is a disorder of body composition in which macronutrient and/or micronutrient deficiencies occur when nutrient intake is insufficient, resulting in reduced organ function, abnormal blood chemistry studies, and suboptimal clinical outcomes (188). Nutritional deficiency is found in 35% to 65% of elderly hospitalized patients (189). Of the available screening techniques reflecting nutritional status, one of the most revealing is the dietary and weight loss history, as found in such structured nutritional questionnaires as the Mini Nutritional Assessment (MNA) and other tools (190,191) and nutrition evaluation steps taken on admission (192). Although probably more applicable to the long-term outpatient setting, certain pieces of information gathered from the patient or family via the MNA are helpful in providing a "snapshot" of the patient's nutritional status as the initial steps in the continuing attention that must be paid to nutritional integrity (193). Obtaining the patient's weight *immediately on admission* is an obvious step in assessing nutritional condition. Because of the various types of body habitus found in ICU patients, a calculation of the Quetelet body mass index (BMI) is helpful to standardize weight to height, providing a relatively standardized estimate of body fat (194):

$$\text{BMI} = \text{weight (in kg) divided by height (in m}^2\text{)}$$

The Department of Health and Human Services defines normal BMI as being within the range of 18 to 24.9, with those with BMIs less than 18 being underweight, the overweight range being 25 to 29.5, and those displaying a BMI above 30 being obese (195). These data, however, cover—in the United States—the adult population as a whole. The picture in a unique subset such as the elderly is more complex. In the geriatric population, BMI less than 20 is predictive of nearly 50% 1-year mortality (196), a stronger predictor of mortality than is diagnosis; similar results were found among critically ill adults with a BMI less than or equal to the 15th percentile (197). Such data lead researchers to suggest that the optimal BMI lies higher in the elderly than in the general population (198); this supposition has been supported by a large study demonstrating that the detrimental effect on mortality of excess body weight declines with age (199). Furthermore, the BMI calculation does not differentiate between differences in body morphology; obese, malnourished individuals whose BMIs fall within the normal range may go unidentified using this formula (200). Because an age-associated loss of height can be significant in the geriatric population, especially in kyphotic individuals, substitution of arm span as the denominator of the BMI calculation has been suggested to give a more accurate comparison of an individual patient's BMI to the standards that were originally established in younger persons (201,202). Arm span is identical to height in younger years; although height may decline with age, arm span remains unchanged, providing more accuracy within the previously determined younger age frame of BMI reference. Knee height, as measured from plantar surface to top of patella with the ankle at 90 degrees, is another measurement (203) that can be substituted in corrected BMI calculations in those with diminished stature who are unsuitable for arm span measurement. Triceps skin fold thickness and mid-arm circumference can also provide an idea of body fat content (204).

In general, however, use of the BMI in the elderly is suspect, regardless of the height measurement used, as there are few normal BMI data that specifically describe those older than 65 years. The ages of geriatric patients included in nutrition studies vary, anthropometric characteristics vary in different advanced decades, and incidence of weight-changing diseases and conditions—such as cancer or the anorexia of aging—increases with age (205). These factors make the formulation of accurate statements and recommendations addressing ideal weight and BMI in the elderly difficult to formulate (156). Although the percentage of older Americans falling into the definition of obese continues to climb (206), one should not make the assumption of nutritional integrity. Age-related redistribution of caloric stores may disguise the overweight elderly patient with severe PEM (200) as one who is obese in the mind of the unwary clinician who is not familiar with the metabolism of geriatric patients and the pathophysiologic implications of these changes (207). Misguided hypocaloric feeding, directed at mobilizing excess fat stores in the obese, but malnourished, elderly patient may worsen the situation by leaving the ongoing catabolic protein breakdown associated with critical illness uncorrected (208). Several easily measured laboratory parameters are reflective of nutritional status on admission, and some can be followed periodically to assess the success of nutritional support. Albumin is a product of hepatic metabolism, synthesized ultimately from ingested or infused nitrogenous precursors in the presence of adequate caloric support. Although it is held that the serum albumin level is reflective of the nutritional state, various factors influencing serum albumin levels make it only vaguely reflective of overall nutritional status (209), with an ROC (receiver operating characteristic) curve rating of 0.58 compared to the clinical subjective global assessment tool. Serum albumin level does decline somewhat with age—0.8 g/L per decade for individuals older than 60 years of age—but generally remains within the numerical normal range. Significantly reduced albumin concentration, therefore, should be attributed to disease processes (210,211) and be aggressively investigated. A substantial decline in serum albumin concentration is accurately predictive of mortality and worse outcome among the elderly, both in the setting of apparent health and illness (212–216), possibly reflective of the presence of chronic disease- or inflammation-induced mediators that simultaneously suppress albumin gene expression (217). The half-life of albumin, 18 to 19 days (218–220), makes its use less than optimal in monitoring metabolic and synthetic functions, in which rapid change is significant. The reliability of previously favorite nutritional indicators such as prealbumin and retinol-binding protein in demonstrating the adequacy of nutritional support in critically ill patients has recently been called into question (221).

As critical illness induces substantial catabolism (220,222,223), resting energy expenditure (REE) rises during the first 2 weeks of this state, with mobilization of nitrogen stores as a component of the associated inflammatory response to physiologic insult. Total energy expenditure (TEE) may rise dramatically in critically ill, septic, or trauma patients, repletion of which is most difficult without correcting the underlying inciting process (224,225). In the elderly individual with marginal nutritional reserve at the onset of critical illness, early provision of caloric and protein support is warranted. Catabolic processes characteristic of critical illness are not reversible by nutrient supplementation alone; they are incited by inflammatory mediators rather than by pre-existing deficiency or inadequate repletion and are thus not forestalled by aggressive nutritional support. Traditional guidance recommends 25 kcal/kg/day of nutritional support, with an additional protein supply of 1.2 to 1.5 g/kg/day (188,226) based on *actual* body weight. Obese individuals, defined as above (227,228), warrant feeding based on *ideal,* rather than actual, body weight (IBW):

$$\text{Men: IBW (kg)} = 50 + 2.3 \text{ kg per inch over 5 ft}$$
$$\text{Women: IBW (kg)} = 45.5 + 2.3 \text{ kg per inch over 5 ft}$$

Greater accuracy can be achieved using one of several formulas to calculate REE (229) the Harris–Benedict equation is commonly used (230):

$$\textbf{Men: REE} = 66.5 + (13.75 \times \text{weight in kg}) + (5.003 \times \text{height in cm}) - (6.775 \times \text{age in years})$$
$$\textbf{Women: REE} = 655.1 + (9.563 \times \text{weight in kg}) + (1.850 \times \text{height in cm}) - (4.676 \times \text{age in years})$$

This may be insufficient in the critically ill geriatric patient in the throes of the inflammatory response, unless the higher stress and activity factor is used (231). Resting metabolic rate may be nearly double in the critically ill or injured individual (224) compared to the healthy uninjured person. Protein supplementation for the most critically ill ranges from 1.2–1.5 g/kg to 2.0–2.5 g/kg (232–234) although, in the initial stages of such a condition, the rate of catabolism may just not be ameliorable despite aggressive support in appropriate quantities (235). Initial empiric dosages should subsequently be adjusted based on indirect calorimetry and nitrogen balance studies if there is suspicion of inadequate nutritional support (236–240). Enthusiastic overprovision of macronutrients in a misguided and vain attempt to thwart and correct inflammatory catabolism, on the other hand, leads to a host of complications and considerable morbidity (241) for which the geriatric patient may be unable to compensate. Most recently, it appears that the optimal outcome attributable to nutritional support is achieved only when both the energy (as determined by indirect calorimetry) and protein requirements are reached within 1 to 2 days (242); the wisdom of "permissive underfeeding" of predicted energy requirements has recently also been documented (243). The confounding factor of obesity sometimes seen in the nutritionally deficient geriatric patient makes the recipe that provides optimal nutritional support frustratingly difficult to determine. In such situations, measurements of energy expenditure performed at frequent intervals are even more strongly advisable, because energy requirements fluctuate with time and medical condition, and vary significantly from those of younger patients on whose metabolism nutritional recommendations are often based. In general, most, although not all, studies show that enteral nutrition is preferred because of the purported preservative effects on intestinal mucosal integrity, cost issues, and a lesser degree of risk exposure to the patient, both infectious and mechanical, associated with placement of flexible nasointestinal feeding tube versus central line for parenteral nutrition (188,244–249). This statement, however, is the source of endless controversy and the basis of considerable investigation (249–251). The optimal site of delivery of the enteral solution, gastric versus postpyloric, surprisingly, remains controversial (252,253) as does the importance of gastric residual volume (GRV) measurement and its impact on outcome (254,255). The risks and benefits of the common routes of nutritional support have been reviewed in considerable detail (256,257).

One additional point that is critical to remember is that of the possibility of development of potentially fatal ***refeeding syndrome*** in a critically ill patient who is already nutritionally deficient, as many elderly people are. Meticulous attention to the introduction of nutrients in those at risk, with frequent monitoring and generous replenishment of electrolytes, is very important to avoid this morbid complication (258).

Renal Considerations

Deterioration of renal function in a critically ill patient has a dramatic impact on survival. Despite this, it is often not recognized in a timely manner, is managed poorly or incompletely, and is often preventable or able to be ameliorated by suitable intervention (259). Acute kidney injury (AKI, the name given to what was previously known as acute renal failure [ARF]) carries a mortality of nearly 30% in a general ICU population; a decline of renal function of even lesser severity also impacts mortality significantly (260), more so in the geriatric population. An elderly patient with compromised renal function will often succumb to the added insult of renal failure after a complex surgical intervention or traumatic injury. The chance for at least partial renal functional recovery after critical illness-related AKI is greater than 90% among those alive a year after their illness (261). Presently there is little available for treatment of renal insufficiency or failure other than identification of the etiology with certainly so as to administer the correct theraputic medications when warranted (e.g. steroids, imuran, etc.), optimization of hemodynamics, prevention of further renal damage by removal of any nephrotoxic medications or processes, aggressive management of complications such as hyperkalemia, and initiation of renal replacement therapy if indicated and deemed appropriate within the patient's wishes. The intensivist holds a pivotal role in the understanding of renal physiology and the principles of renal protection to minimize the impact of critical illness on renal function and its influence on outcome.

Just as in other physiologic systems, there is a gradual deterioration of renal function with age, beginning at age 30 years

(262,263). It is well described that renal blood flow declines after the fourth decade (264,265). When the sixth decade is reached, this deterioration *generally* continues, although with a very wide bell curve of distribution (266). There is loss of renal—primarily cortical—mass (267) and the onset of glomerular sclerosis and involution, causing a decrease in the number of functional glomeruli (268), in turn causing a decrease in glomerular filtration rate (GFR) of 30% to 40% by the age of 80 years (262,269). Deterioration of tubular function parallels that of the glomerulus (270). In the elderly patient, factors other than age-related deterioration may complicate renal function, including pre-existing renovascular disease, hypertensive nephrosclerosis, or hypotension associated with trauma or neglect. Laboratory measurement of serum blood urea nitrogen (BUN) and creatinine (S_{cr}), used individually or in a ratio, act as surrogates of renal function; they are, however, less accurately reflective of renal function in the elderly than in a younger person. BUN rises slightly with age over 60 years, paralleling the gradual decline in renal function; S_{cr} reflects muscle mass and, while completely filtered (and only minimally secreted) into the tubule and therefore generally reflective of GFR, may not climb as expected despite age-related falling renal filtration (271). The age-related muscle mass diminution, frequently paralleling deterioration of renal function, generates less creatine (and thus, creatinine), leading to what may erroneously be looked upon as a normal baseline S_{cr}. Assessment of GFR should be individualized by using the Cockcroft–Gault formula (272) to generate a more accurate estimate of function based on weight, age, and serum creatinine:

$$\text{Creatinine clearance} = [(140 - \text{age})\ (\text{weight in kg})]/(72 \times \text{Scr})$$
$$(\text{arithmetic result} \times 0.85 = \text{clearance for female patients})$$

This formula provides a "snapshot" of function at a given time and is most useful if calculated on ICU arrival and daily thereafter. Other laboratory surrogates of GFR have been devised, such as the measurement of cystatin C (273–275) and MDRD (modification of diet in renal disease) equations (276), but the ease with which the Cockcroft–Gault calculation is performed, especially when performed daily to "trend" the result rather than depend on one individual number, makes its routine replacement unlikely. The CKD-EPI formula (277) has been found to be more accurate in some circumstances. One must be mindful that any assessment of renal function utilizing S_{cr} to infer creatinine clearance as reflective of GFR is limited by the nonlinear rise in S_{cr} as renal function declines (278,279) in that a small change in a close-to-normal value S_{cr} represents an insignificant change in GFR, while a similar numerical change in an already-elevated S_{cr} likely represents further compromise of already impaired renal function. If GFR remains uncertain, urine collection for measurement of creatinine clearance can be done with fair accuracy using at least an 8-hour urine collection period (280,281); 24-hour collection is preferred in critically ill patients and is easily done in patients with indwelling urinary catheters. A variety of methods exist to assess renal function, both by measurement and by estimation (282,283).

Fluid and electrolyte handling is altered in the aging kidney, related to tubular dysfunction which is proportional to the GFR decline. Although baseline electrolyte values and fluid status are likely within normal range in the previously healthy geriatric patient, age-related tubular dysfunction narrows the limits of correction of water and sodium aberrations that the elderly kidney can readily accomplish. Sodium excretion and reabsorption declines in efficiency, with those older than 60 years requiring considerably more time to achieve homeostasis in the face of sodium overload or deprivation (284). Similarly, the range of specific gravity and osmolarity achievable in the face of water excess or deficit is narrowed in comparison to that of a younger individual (285); rectification of acid–base perturbations is similarly deficient (286). The stresses of critical illness or injury typical of the elderly ICU patient intensify the effects of these functional deficiencies, and must be foreseen and addressed aggressively to forestall the profound effects of deterioration of renal function on morbidity and mortality. These stresses include volume depletion from GI bleeding, severe dehydration, diarrhea, aggressive diuresis, insensible losses in burn patients or those with drainage from wounds or fistulas, and disruption of renal blood flow from sepsis, shock, or surgical causes such as complex renovascular surgery. Management of deteriorating renal function requires accurate diagnosis of the inciting cause, while addressing complicating or resultant metabolic derangements and preventing further insult. The details of the diagnosis of renal pathology are not specific to the geriatric patient and are addressed elsewhere in this text (see Chapter 132).

It is important to recognize that AKI occurs in as many as 67% of ICU admissions (260), as identified by RIFLE (risk, injury, failure, loss, end-stage) criteria (287), and that the effect of renal deterioration is quite detrimental to the elderly individual. Initial evaluation must include performance of a physical examination that may reveal an occluded urinary catheter causing an enlarged bladder; bladder scanning can be performed on those in whom an enlarged bladder might not be palpable. Hypovolemia, both absolute, as in severe dehydration, and relative, as in sepsis, must be aggressively corrected with appropriate fluid and blood products; invasive monitoring is warranted in this population of patients with limited reserve. Dosage adjustment of potentially nephrotoxic medications is mandatory, using assessment of GFR as a guide. Antimicrobials such as cephalosporins and aminoglycosides, nonsteroidal anti-inflammatory medications, certain chemotherapeutic medications, and angiotensin-converting enzyme inhibitors are common offenders (288). The use of "protective" medications such as N-acetylcysteine, dopamine, mannitol, or loop diuretics to minimize the detrimental impact of contrast material on renal function has generally been demonstrated to be ineffective (289,290). On the other hand, pre-procedure isotonic fluid loading, mindful of the possibility of occult HF in elderly patients, is the strategy most likely to benefit postcontrast renal function (291). The use of isotonic bicarbonate solution, while possibly decreasing the incidence of CIN compared to isotonic saline, does not decrease the subsequent incidence of dialysis or in-hospital mortality (292,293).

Beyond awareness of medications that impact renal function, there is the effect of age-related diminished renal function on drug metabolism and excretion (294). Recall again that common indicators of renal function, BUN and S_{cr}, although appearing normal in the elderly, may mask a compromised GFR, risking medication-induced complications if this fact is overlooked, and mandating more specific assessment of GFR (see above) if question arises. Early nephrology consultation is encouraged when RIFLE criteria suggest compromised renal function; similarly, a critical care pharmacologist can assist in clarifying renal-active medication issues in these complex patients.

ASSESSMENT AND MANAGEMENT OF TRAUMATIC INJURIES

Elderly individuals suffer a significant number of severe and often lethal traumatic injuries, the analysis and management of which can be frustratingly complex (295). In the 55- to 64-year-old age group, unintentional injury was the *THIRD* leading cause of death in 2013; in those older than 65 years of age, 45,942 deaths were attributed to trauma (296) compared with 35,000 in 2003 (297). Most serious injuries are caused by falls, the occurrence rising dramatically as age advances into the 60s and beyond (298). This predominance continued to be seen through 2015 (299). Falls from a standing or even sitting position, imparting an apparently trivial amount of kinetic energy to frail tissue, may result in fatal injury, accounting for half the trauma-related deaths as compared to those of younger people (300). Most remaining significant traumatic injuries to the elderly involve motor vehicles, either as vehicle occupants or as pedestrians (301), while there is a small but persistent incidence of injury and death from penetrating trauma in the geriatric population, declining to less than 1% in those older than 75 years (299,302,303).

Evaluation and management of the injured elderly requires familiarity with characteristic injury patterns and knowledge of comorbid diseases and particulars of geriatric physiology that impact treatment (304). Practice management guidelines for geriatric trauma (305) are helpful in this situation. Triage of injured geriatric patients to more experienced trauma centers improves outcomes, to such an extent that some practitioners in the field of trauma management advocate the hyperspecialization of some centers to be the location of management of seriously injured elders (306).

Immediate assessment of the resuscitation status of any patient arriving in the ICU, whether from the operating room, emergency department, or elsewhere in the hospital, is imperative. The paucity of overt physical findings of intravascular fluid deficiency seen in the elderly patient adds additional urgency to its accurate analysis, while the lusitropic compromise that typifies the geriatric patient mandates avoidance of overgenerous fluid repletion. Although standard protocols may serve as a guide to ensure that all systems are evaluated, one must remain mindful that standard and acceptable initial hemodynamic measurements may actually conceal unsuspected injury or bleeding in the confused elderly trauma patient who may be taking medications that affect vital signs. Airway management in the elderly carries its own set of difficulties. Age-associated arthritic spinal, mandibular, and arytenoid deformities, and an increased incidence of occult cervical spinal injuries (307–309) may be seen; marginal respiratory drive and compromised airway reflexes may warrant securing the airway preemptively, avoiding a later "crash" difficult airway emergency. A thorough and detailed physical examination is fundamental. Timely sequential measurement of routine hematology tests, even in the stable geriatric patient, may reveal unsuspected hemorrhage. Arterial blood gas analysis is a convenient tool because it is quickly performed and allows frequent measurement of hemoglobin, base deficit, and lactate. The latter two values are powerful indicators of resuscitation status and, when elevated, predict increased mortality in the elderly population (310,311). In one study of elderly trauma patients, mortality was decreased from 54% to 34% ($p < 0.003$) by institution of a protocol of trauma team activation and early noninvasive and subsequently invasive monitoring for resuscitation of all patients older than age 70 years with an injury severity score (ISS) greater than 15, even for those with nonworrisome initial vital signs and fairly minor injuries (311). This supports the precept that achieving adequate tissue perfusion *early,* while often difficult to accomplish, is fundamental to successful trauma management. One must be mindful, furthermore, that while invasive monitoring carries its own risks, judicious use of these tools can improve outcome and survival in the elderly trauma patient (312–314).

Certain patterns of injury are found in geriatric patients. Traumatic brain injury (TBI) afflicts the elderly with extraordinary severity. High mortality leaves fewer survivors, most of whom suffer debilitating sequelae (315). A large meta-analysis revealed an overall mortality of 38.3% in patients 60 years and older with moderate and severe TBI (316). In 2003, there were 90,000 emergency department visits involving TBI in those older than 65 years, of whom 38.4% died (317); some series document mortality rates for severe TBI in those older than 55 years of age as high as 80% (318). Initial neurologic examination of an elder with significant intracranial injury may be deceptively normal (319); the reliability of the Glasgow Coma Scale in identifying elders with severe TBI is not as great as in younger individuals (320). A high index of suspicion for the presence of an occult central nervous system (CNS) injury must be maintained if such individuals arrive in the ICU without radiologic evaluation having been performed, warranting frequent, sequential neurologic evaluations by the same examiner and a conservative approach to ordering a cranial CT scan. Those elderly whose cause of TBI is a fall—nearly 50%, from 1988 to 1998—are likely to have three or more significant comorbid conditions complicating ICU management (321,322). Outcome after TBI is optimized by using meticulous clinical assessment, timely radiologic re-evaluation, and aggressive invasive monitoring to facilitate immediate recognition of worsening status, such as that due to recurrent intracranial hemorrhage, while minimizing secondary injury. Elderly patients taking anticoagulant medications and antiplatelet (ACAP) agents experience higher TBI-related in-hospitality mortality (323). Secondary injury may occur when even transient episodes of hypoxia or hypotension affect cerebral perfusion pressure (CPP) (324) and, in the setting of elevated intracranial pressure (325), with hyperglycemia (326), hyperthermia (327), or aggressive hyperventilation (328,329). Infusion of hypertonic saline (330) may supplement the management of elevated intracranial pressure that resists control by the usual initial measures. The cornerstone of TBI treatment is the maintenance of cerebral oxygenation by ensuring adequate oxygen content and CPP, guided by data derived via invasive intracranial monitoring devices that are inserted based on specific indications (331). Little, however, has been written specifically addressing geriatric CPP requirements. Although ~60 mmHg is considered the threshold below which the CPP should not be allowed to drop (332), this has not been rigorously studied specifically in the geriatric population. Cerebral autoregulation in the elderly is subject to the same influences as those that affect the younger individual. In this population, the abundance of comorbidities, such as untreated hypertension, may have acclimated the cerebral vasculature to a new baseline, making invasive cerebral monitoring even more critical in ensuring adequate perfusion for the aging brain. The profound influence of even mild TBI (316,332–335) on short- and long-term outcome in the elderly patient mandates aggressive monitoring, optimization of cerebral perfusion, and meticulous attention to hemodynamic parameters. The impact on long-term survival of severe head-injured elderly trauma patients, compared to other multi-trauma patients *without* TBI is considerable (336).

Cervical spine injury is common in the geriatric trauma patient (337); plain radiographs (307,338) may be unrevealing of fracture or difficult to interpret because of age-related boney changes obscuring acute pathology (308). Fracture of the upper cervical spine is more common in the elderly than in younger individuals, especially in those who have fallen (309), and is more likely to be unstable (339). There is a very high incidence of odontoid fracture in the very elderly, with significant associated mortality (340,341). Helical CT is superior to plain radiographs to identify cervical spine injury in this population (338,339,342,343). Cervical spine pathology may exist in totally asymptomatic individuals with unremarkable examination findings, only to be discovered by a diligent clinician who takes extra steps to search for such an injury (344,345). In the geriatric patient with a cervical injury, the likelihood of coincident painful injury—a *distracting injury* in which the pain from another injury distracts the patient's attention from the perception of neck pain or a condition such as altered mental status—that would affect the examiner's decision to forgo radiographic evaluation is so high as to make such an evaluation imperative in nearly all cases. Again, one must be mindful of the greater likelihood that cervical injuries in the elderly often occur in the arthritis-prone superior vertebrae, which are notoriously difficult to depict on plain films (346), and consider CT evaluation of virtually all geriatric trauma patients in whom even subtle symptoms, history, or mechanism of injury suggest cervical injury, regardless of the initial examination findings or any comforting results of a protocol-based decision-assisting algorithm that suggest the safety of less aggressive investigation.

Traumatic rib fractures impose substantial morbidity; those older than 45 years with more than four fractures are particularly affected (347). In a study of patients traditionally defined as *elderly*—those older than 64 years—rib fractures profoundly affected morbidity and mortality, with longer length of stay (LOS) in the ICU, more frequent pneumonia, and overall mortality rate of 22% compared to 10% ($p < 0.001$) in those less seriously injured (348). Of note in this study was that rates of mortality and pneumonia both increased with each additional rib fracture. Epidural analgesia would appear to be the ideal technique to alleviate the pain associated with rib fractures to optimize pulmonary status and, indeed, has been found to be successful in nongeriatric adults (349,350). In one recent study, however, the opposite has been demonstrated in an elderly population when compared to parenteral analgesia (351).

The management of abdominal trauma follows pathways similar to those for younger patients, with certain caveats: findings on physical examination indicating serious abdominal pathology can be subtle, especially when complicated by distracting orthopedic or mild head injury. Liberal use of CT scanning is strongly recommended if mechanism of injury, external abdominal findings such as a seat belt mark, or laboratory evidence of hypoperfusion (elevated base deficit or serum lactate) suggest visceral injury. Nonoperative management of certain radiologically well-characterized injuries of solid organs—namely the spleen, the liver, and the pancreas—in the hemodynamically stable elderly patient is becoming increasingly accepted as evidence of the success of this approach accumulates (352–354).

Serious orthopedic injuries frequently befall older victims of polytrauma, and portend a substantial risk of mortality (355). Decrease in bone mineral density (BMD) in patients older than about 30 years heightens the risk of fracture in general; this phenomenon is observed in varying degrees in both genders and all races, but is particularly severe in postmenopausal Caucasian women (356,357). Pelvic fracture in the aged is associated with a greater likelihood of significant blood volume transfusion and mortality ($p < 0.005$) (358). Open pelvic fracture often has substantial associated bleeding, which is seldom treatable, with the exception of arterial bleeding, in any way other than with early stabilization, aggressive transfusion, and correction of coagulopathy in hopes of eventual tamponade of the retroperitoneal bleeding source. Arterial bleeding from lacerated pelvic vessels warrants embolization (359). The more typical scenario, however, is that of diffuse venous oozing, which, nonetheless, may render the elderly patient hemodynamically unstable, requiring large-volume transfusion of blood products as a temporizing measure until anatomic stabilization can be achieved (359,360). The presence of an open pelvic fracture, with frequent associated visceral injuries (361,362), further worsens outcome (358). Hemodynamic consequences of large-volume transfusion and frequent septic complications can drive the mortality in both younger and older adults to nearly 80% (363). Long-bone fractures, in general, warrant early immobilization and stabilization to minimize ongoing hemorrhage and generation of fat emboli; such fixation improves mortality significantly (364). Optimal timing of surgical stabilization of these quite morbid fractures, however, is a complex issue to resolve when they occur in the larger setting of the patient with severe head, chest, or abdominal injuries (365). Although postponing the operative stabilization of a femur or complex pelvic fracture to allow time to achieve hemodynamic stability in a traumatized patient has benefit, it is also not without risks (366,367). Prolonged immobilization of the elderly patient with such a fracture prior to stabilization results in compromised respiratory status, likely exposing the patient to extended intubation, pulmonary thromboembolism, and infection.

Studies of elderly trauma patients have consistently documented the increase in mortality in this population (302,313,367,368). The mortality rate begins to climb for those in their sixth decade, even for less severe injuries (369) when compared to younger individuals. For those with moderate injuries, the mortality curves steepen beginning in the fifth decade, with another even steeper turn in the seventh. With advancing age, trauma-related mortality rates for those in the seventh decade and above range as high as 47% for those with an ISS more than 30, compared to those 45 years old or younger (20.1%) (370). Identification of parameters which might predict mortality in the individual patient is an important area of study (371). Within the context to which allusion was earlier made—that of future payoff in return for resource use—the complexity and enormity of the issue grows as health care costs rise, and as the percentage of the population represented by the elderly increases. As these rising numbers of individuals cease working, and, thereby, are no longer able to generate an income that can be taxed to finance public health care funding programs such as Medicare, or be used to pay for personal private health insurance to cover costs of traumatic injuries, the costs of providing that trauma—and, indeed, all—care will have to be borne by a source other than the patients themselves. It is clear that focusing the resources of the modern ICU on the management of elderly trauma patients improves outcome (372), so the skills associated with successful management of elderly trauma patients are improving with experience. Based on the size of these costs and the likelihood of marginally or poorly acceptable outcomes among a substantial minority of geriatric trauma patients (3,370,373–375), investigations have tried to answer two important trauma outcome-related questions. These are as follows: (1) is it possible to identify an elderly trauma patient who will certainly die later, even if the patient survives the initial period of resuscitation, surgery, and further stabilization, and (2) to what level of functioning will the elderly survivor of trauma-related intensive care return on discharge? For many elderly individuals, the prospect of lingering in the netherworld of prolonged posttrauma multi-organ system failure with the certainty of death pushed back "only as long as the machines keep me running," or existing debilitated in a non-home environment where even bowel function and bathing are at the behest of another, is worse than death itself, not really living at all, and is the basis of much concern among the elderly.

There are, however, grounds for hope. In one study of victims of penetrating trauma more than 60 years old, 91% were discharged home, most without assistance (303). The postdischarge level of functioning in elderly patients surviving blunt trauma varies widely, as would be expected in a population whose baseline physiologic attributes are so diverse. Clearly, even the healthiest octogenarian is not the physiologic equal of a two-sets-of-tennis 65-year-old and will have a significantly decreased likelihood of returning to premorbid functionality, although both individuals may be described as elderly. Nonetheless, even after significant traumatic injuries, a substantial percentage of recovering geriatric patients, even the very old, will be able to live relatively independently, albeit for some patients, in a protected environment with assistance. Many will be able to return home with or without periodic professional assistance (373,376–378). In one retrospective study of 38,707 elderly trauma patients with a mean ISS of 11.7 ± 0.05 (standard error of mean), in which 10.3% died in hospital, 52.2% of the survivors went home. The percentage of patients returning home after serious traumatic injuries, many requiring prolonged intensive care, varied considerably with age, from 66.7% of those 65 to 74 years to 30.5% of those 85 years of age or older (378). With aggressive rehabilitation, improvement in function and independence can continue for substantial periods of time after discharge, including in those who have suffered TBI (379,380). In another study, recovery of elderly trauma patients was improved by early involvement of physicians from a geriatric trauma consult service, who assisted in recognition and treatment of medical issues, and in advanced care and disposition planning (381). Additionally, determining the optimal destination for posthospitalization rehabilitation can be facilitated by employment of assessment tools that include such parameters as the 15-item Trauma Specific Frailty Index, the Barthel Index, and others (382). The likelihood of leaving the hospital after a trauma-related ICU admission can be improved from the outset, as noted earlier, by aggressive attention to adequate resuscitation to rectify suboptimal perfusion, by attention to maintenance of acceptable CPP in TBI, and by recognition and treatment of the early subtle signs of cardiac and respiratory decompensation. Finally, trauma care outcome must be scrutinized within the context of profound personal and social issues, beyond those solely of medical success, that are integral to ICU care in patients in this age group.

OUTCOME AFTER A CRITICAL ILLNESS IN THE GERIATRIC POPULATION

Life expectancy in the United States is presently 78.8 years (383), and while it is greater at any given age now than it was even 15 years ago, objective evaluation must be made of the appropriateness—and likelihood of successful outcome—of aggressive critical care medical services provided to geriatric patients. Presently, geriatric patients represent between 25% and 50% of all ICU admissions (9,11). In 2000, ICU costs represented 13.3% of hospital costs, 4.2% of health care expenditures, and 0.56% of the US gross domestic product (384). By 2005, the latter value had increased to 0.66%, with Critical Care expenditures representing 13.4% (~ $82 billion) of hospital expenditures (385). As of this writing in 2016, expenditure for CCM services represents approximately 1% of the US GDP. The enormous expense associated with ICU care has prompted some analysts to raise the subject of limits on expenditures for the elderly (386,387), because, for example, an 80-year-old who is supported through a 3-week bout of sepsis is not likely to return to the revenue-generating work force. Indeed, the literature dealing with geriatric medical issues is liberally populated with articles addressing ageism in the context of delivery of services to the elderly (388–390), raising the concept of providing less aggressive or intensive levels of acute care to an elderly person on the basis of age, the inference being that such care provides a less robust postillness benefit to the patient and to society as a whole. Meaningful discussions addressing the more philosophical issues of critical care such as the correct level of aggressiveness of care and appropriateness of withdrawal of care, to say nothing of the financial issues, simply cannot be addressed in any rational way without an accurate picture of what critical care accomplishes in these elderly patients.

A successful ICU admission is certainly defined within cultural and social, as well as personal, contexts. Although the family member's "do *everything* for Granddad" dictum is familiar, it often represents an unrealistic appraisal of the possible benefit from certain modalities of care that can be, but possibly should not be, carried out. Although the ICU is designed as a temporary environment that allows support of body functions during recovery, the complicated technology and meticulous attention to detail that characterize that environment are not the basis for such "magical" accomplishments as saving the life of a patient who has a lethal condition, despite the expectations and exhortations of some. Indeed, death can often skillfully be forestalled with polished and professional ICU care to such a degree that it may occur immediately after a de-escalation of such care, or later while the patient is on the general ward, in a step-down unit or rehabilitation facility, or after returning home (either early or late) (391). Meaningful discussions with elderly patients and their families, whether prior to complex morbid surgical procedures or as an ICU stay extends past the first few days, *must* include accurate outcome data, so as to facilitate informed decisions regarding the specifics and suitability of continued care. Studies addressing outcome in the critically ill geriatric population have produced various results that vary with the metric employed, the duration over which the outcome is monitored and broad intrapopulation patient variability. The latter category highlights differences in age, premorbid physical status, statements of preference regarding aggressiveness of long-term medical care, and patient and family declarations addressing such subjective concepts as posthospitalization quality of life (QOL). As the numbers of geriatric patients admitted to ICUs increased with the growing geriatric population, some more meaningful data identifying which elderly patients are likely to survive and return to *meaningful* posthospitalization lives is becoming available (392). In one recent study from Canada, 25% of elderly ICU patients 80 years of age and older survived and had returned to their premorbid levels of functioning by 1 year later (393).

The term *geriatric population* encompasses a quite heterogeneous group of individuals from the standpoint of age, premorbid general medical health as a reflection of functional status, the severity of the event justifying ICU admission, and cultural mores as they impact interaction with the modern health care structure of the country in question. Studies assessing the results of care delivered to the elderly may or may not reflect this diversity (394), making interpretation of individual study conclusions and their application to individual clinical situations suspect. Furthermore, the term *outcome* must be specifically defined as to the ***depth of support required by the post-ICU elder and its correspondence with that autonomous person's preferences*** which, again, may vary widely based on cultural, religious, national, and other parameters. Although many elders prefer a less aggressive care regimen designed around EOL comfort at the expense of duration of remaining life, some may desire life extension in the face of critical illness by use of complex technology despite a vanishingly small or nonexistent expectation of recovery (9,395,396). Furthermore, the clinician's perceptions of the patient's desires may not be accurate, and thus may lead to withdrawal of care or withholding of a modality of treatment in a manner that would not be considered in the care of a younger patient (395). It is important to remember that while age may be associated with worse outcome from critical illness, numerous investigations have demonstrated that age, in and of itself, is less a factor than is the severity of the specific condition that warrants intensive care or the general medical condition (i.e., frailty) (397) of the patient prior to the institution of intensive care (398–403). Despite being subjected to procedures that are potentially morbid, the otherwise healthy elderly patient may fare quite as well as a younger individual (400,404). In one study of outcome after intensive care in octogenarians, postdischarge survival was more accurately forecast by care dependency at the time of discharge, as a reflection of premorbid condition and severity of illness, rather than solely by LOS (405). The subjective term *Quality of Life* in the post-ICU elder does not necessarily imply inferiority to that of younger individuals (406); indeed, overall QOL has been demonstrated to be similarly good across age groups ranging from middle aged to very old (above 80 years) (407,408). It must be remembered, however, when evaluating outcome data in elderly ICU patients, that while ICU survival is less a function of age than of premorbid condition or severity of illness (36,405,406,409,410), when the aggressive ICU support is de-escalated with recovery, physiologic reserve may no longer suffice to forestall death in the few months after discharge, and thus may not be reflected in ICU outcome statistics. With the wide variability of desires for aggressiveness of care displayed by the elderly and the inaccuracy with which they are analyzed by many physicians (411), the most important function of the geriatric intensivist may be that of conducting a thorough discussion at the outset of care with the patient and involved family members so as to tailor intensiveness of care to the patient's educated and informed preferences. Fluency in initiating and conducting EOL discussions with patient and family is important for intensivists to possess, and can be learned with clear guidance and polished with experience (412). Depending on the intensivist's point of view and experience, some modalities of available ICU treatment may be viewed as "futile"—or possibly more objectively spoken as "medically inappropriate." Although this may lead to strong differences of opinion regarding the depth of and extent to which intensive care plans are formulated and should be executed (413,414), it is incumbent upon the ICU practitioner to expend all possible effort to resolve the differences equitably and objectively; the assistance of Ethics Consultative services may be beneficial (415).

DRUG DOSING IN THE ELDERLY

As more patients live longer and are placed on a larger number of medications, it is necessary for health care providers to understand the risks, benefits, and consequences of drug therapy in older patients. Several important pharmacologic and nonpharmacologic issues influence the safety and effectiveness of drug therapy in this population. *Pharmacokinetics,* the study of the action of a drug in the body over a period of time, changes with age. The physiologic changes accompanying aging affect the pharmacologic processes of absorption, distribution, metabolism, and excretion (Table 70.1). The effects of these age-related changes are variable and difficult to predict; some changes are related solely to aging, whereas others are most likely due to the combined effects of age, disease, and the environment. Although increasing age is often accompanied by decreased physiologic reserve in many organ systems independent of the effects of disease, this change is not uniform. The alterations in pharmacokinetics and pharmacodynamics that occur with increasing age suggest a pharmacologic basis for concern about the vulnerability of the elderly to the effects of medications. Unfortunately, the results of epidemiologic studies that explore these relationships are unclear, in part due, in this area of medical investigation as in many others (416), to the small number of older people included in premarketing studies relative to the patient population most likely to be exposed to the drug. The oldest—those aged 80 years or older—have not generally been included in clinical

TABLE 70.1 Age-Related Changes Relevant to Drug Pharmacology

Pharmacologic Process	Physiologic Change	Clinical Significance
Absorption	Decreased absorptive surface Decreased splanchnic blood flow Increased gastric pH Altered gastrointestinal motility	Little change in absorption with age
Distribution	Decreased total body water Decreased lean body mass Increased body fat Decreased serum albumin Altered protein binding	Higher concentration of drugs that distribute in body fluids; increased distribution and often prolonged elimination half-life of fat-soluble drugs Increased free fraction in plasma of some highly protein-bound acidic drugs
Metabolism	Reduced hepatic mass Reduced hepatic blood flow Decreased phase I metabolism	Often decreased first-pass metabolism and decreased rate of biotransformation of some drugs
Elimination	Reduced renal plasma flow Reduced glomerular filtration rate Decreased tubular secretion function	Decreased renal elimination of drugs and metabolites; marked interindividual variation
Tissue sensitivity	Alterations in receptor number Alterations in receptor affinity Alterations in second-messenger function Alteration in cellular and nuclear responses	Patients are more sensitive or less sensitive to an agent

trials of investigational drugs, and those older subjects who do participate in such trials tend to be healthy "young-old" people. Thus, the results of these trials and the side effects reported often have limited application to the older patient with multiple illnesses, taking several medications. In general, consideration of the individual patient, his or her physiologic status—hydration, nutrition, and cardiac output, and how this status affects the pharmacology of a particular drug—are more important in prescribing that drug than any specific age-related changes.

Absorption of drugs, which occurs mainly by passive diffusion, changes little with advancing age; the changes listed in Table 70.1 could potentially affect drug absorption. More important changes result from concurrent administration of several medications. For example, antacids decrease the oral absorption of cimetidine, and alcohol accelerates the absorption of chloral hydrate.

Unlike absorption, drug distribution is affected by age in clinically meaningful ways. In older persons, the relative increase in body fat and the decrease in lean body mass alter drug distribution so that fat-soluble drugs are distributed more widely and water-soluble drugs less so (Table 70.2) (417). The increased distribution of fat-soluble drugs can delay elimination and may result in prolonged duration of action of a single

TABLE 70.2 Volume of Distribution of Commonly Prescribed Drugs

Increased Volume	Decreased Volume[a]
Acetaminophen	Cimetidine
Chlordiazepoxide	Digoxin
Diazepam	Ethanol
Oxazepam	Gentamicin
Prazosin	Meperidine
Salicylates	Phenytoin
Thiopental	Quinine
Tolbutamide	Theophylline

[a]If the volume of distribution is decreased, drug levels tend to be higher.

dose. This effect is especially important for drugs such as hypnotics and analgesics, which may be given in single doses on an intermittent basis. For example, the volume of distribution of diazepam is increased almost twofold in older patients, and the elimination half-life is prolonged from 24 hours in young patients to approximately 90 hours in the elderly. By way of contrast, the volume of distribution of water-soluble compounds, such as digoxin, is decreased in older patients, and thus the dose required to reach a target plasma concentration is decreased. Likewise, due to the decreased volume of distribution, the loading dose of aminoglycosides is decreased in older patients.

For drugs that bind to serum proteins, equilibrium exists between the bound or ineffective portion and the unbound (free), or effective, portion. For acidic drugs that are highly bound to albumin, the free plasma concentration may correlate best with pharmacologic effect. Although albumin concentration decreases only slightly with age, it may decrease dramatically during periods of critical illnesses; this can result in elevated levels of unbound acidic drugs in older persons during episodes of illnesses, and thus in an increased potential for toxicity. These changes can be significant for drugs such as thyroid hormone, digoxin, warfarin, and phenytoin. On the other hand, some basic drugs, such as lidocaine and propranolol, bind mainly to alpha-1 acid glycoprotein, an acute phase–reactant protein; the concentration of this protein tends to rise as a person ages and is elevated following myocardial infarction and in chronic inflammatory diseases and malignant conditions (418). The plasma binding of these drugs is increased in older patients, but because these age-related changes are not great, their exact clinical relevance is uncertain.

Overall, changes in protein binding are an important consideration initially when a drug is being started, when the dosage is changed, when serum protein levels change, or when a newly administered drug displaces another protein-bound agent. Because the free portion of the drug is generally smaller than the bound portion, the normal mechanisms of metabolism and excretion ultimately eliminate the free drug. If either hepatic or renal function is impaired due to age or disease, this elimination may be slowed.

Although in vitro studies of drug-metabolizing enzyme activity from human liver biopsy samples have not demonstrated any changes with aging, some investigators speculate that the decline in liver size with age may result in decreased metabolic capacity. A significant decline in hepatic blood flow occurs with age, reductions of 25% to 47% being reported in persons between the ages of 25 and 90 years. This decrease in hepatic blood flow is clinically important because hepatic metabolism is the rate-limiting step that determines the clearance of most metabolized drugs. This change is especially relevant for drugs that undergo rapid hepatic metabolism (e.g., propranolol); drugs that undergo extensive first-pass metabolism are likely to reach higher blood levels if hepatic blood flow is decreased.

The liver metabolizes drugs through two distinct systems: phase I metabolism, involving drug oxidation, reduction and hydrolysis; and phase II metabolism, involving glucuronidation, sulfation, acetylation, and methylation. Phase I metabolism is catalyzed primarily by the cytochrome P-450 system in the smooth endoplasmic reticulum of hepatocytes; this enzyme system is a superfamily of microsomal drug-metabolizing enzymes important in the biosynthesis and degradation of endogenous compounds such as steroids, lipids, and vitamins, as well as the metabolism of most commonly used drugs (419). Phase I metabolism activity decreases substantially with age, so drugs that are metabolized through phase I enzymatic activity have prolonged half-lives. Examples of some drugs whose metabolism is slowed because of these age-related changes in hepatic metabolism include meperidine, phenytoin, diazepam, propranolol, theophylline, labetalol, lidocaine, and quinidine. Age-related changes in phase I metabolism, coupled with the use of multiple medications, place older patients at increased risk for adverse drug reactions; these occur due either to inhibition or induction of cytochrome P-450 enzymes, especially CYP3A, which is thought to be involved in the metabolism of more than half of the currently prescribed drugs (420). Clinical outcomes are determined by the potency of the CYP3A inhibitor (moderate vs. potent), the availability of alternative pathways, and the seriousness of the symptoms. A drug is considered a potent CYP3A inhibitor if it causes more than a fivefold increase in the plasma concentration of another drug that is primarily dependent on CYP3A for its metabolism (421). Thus, clinicians should be cognizant of potential drug interactions when they prescribe drugs from classes that include potent or moderate inhibitors of CYP3A. If a potent CYP3A inhibitor or inducer and substrate must be taken together, dosage adjustment and close clinical monitoring are warranted to avoid adverse reactions.

Phase II hepatic metabolism involves the conjugation of drugs or their metabolites to organic substrates. The elimination of drugs that undergo phase II metabolism by conjugation is generally altered less with age. Thus, drugs that require only phase II metabolism for excretion (e.g., triazolam) do not have a prolonged half-life in older people. These drugs contrast with agents such as diazepam that undergo both phases of metabolism and have active intermediate metabolites. Although the effect of aging on hepatic drug metabolism is variable, phase I metabolism is the process that is most likely to decrease in older persons. The apparent variable effect of age on drug metabolism is probably due to the fact that age is only one of many factors that affect drug metabolism. For example, cigarette smoking, alcohol intake, dietary modification, drugs, viral illness, caffeine intake, and other unknown factors also affect the rate of drug metabolism. Induction of drug metabolism can occur in older persons. The rate of elimination of theophylline is increased by smoking and by phenytoin in both young and older persons (422). Not all metabolizing isoenzymes are induced equally in the young and the old. For example, antipyrine elimination is increased after pretreatment with dichloralphenazone in younger patients but not in older patients.

An important pharmacokinetic change that occurs in persons of advanced age is that of reduced renal elimination of drugs. This change results from the age-related decline in both GFR and tubular function. Drugs that depend on glomerular function (e.g., gentamicin) and/or on tubular secretion (e.g., penicillin) for elimination both exhibit reduced elimination in older patients. Because drug elimination is correlated with creatinine clearance, measurement of creatinine clearance is helpful in determining the maintenance dose. As noted earlier, the average creatinine clearance declines by 50% from age 25 to 85 despite a serum creatinine level that remains unchanged at approximately 1.0 mg/dL. The Cockcroft–Gault formula (see above) is useful in the accurate assessment of renal function when planning administration of medications excreted by the kidneys. Although helpful in adjusting for age, weight, and the measured serum creatinine level, it does not account for individual variation.

Altered renal clearance leads to two clinically relevant consequences: the half-lives of renally excreted drugs are prolonged, and the serum levels of these drugs are increased. For drugs with large therapeutic indices (e.g., penicillin), this is of little clinical importance, but for drugs with a narrower therapeutic index (e.g., digoxin, cimetidine, aminoglycosides), side effects may occur in older patients if dose reductions are not made. Thus, it is not surprising that digoxin is the drug that most often causes side effects in the elderly, especially if the dose exceeds 0.125 mg daily (423). To define dose requirements further, therapeutic drug monitoring should be performed for drugs with a low therapeutic index.

In addition to the factors that determine the drug concentration at the site of action—the *pharmacokinetics*—the effect of a drug also depends on the sensitivity of the target organ to the drug. The biochemical and physiologic effects of drugs and their mechanisms of action—*pharmacodynamics*—and the effects of aging are not clearly known. Pharmacodynamics has been even less extensively studied in older patients than has been pharmacokinetics. Accurate generalizations are very difficult to make, and the effect of age on sensitivity to drugs varies with the drug studied and the response measured. These differences in sensitivity occur in the absence of marked reductions in the metabolism of the drug and its related compounds. Thus, sensitivity to drug effects may either increase or decrease with increasing age. For example, older patients seem to be more sensitive to the sedative effects of given blood levels of benzodiazepine drugs (e.g., diazepam) but less sensitive to the effects of drugs mediated by beta-adrenergic receptors (e.g., isoproterenol, propranolol). Although an age-related decline in hormone receptor affinity or number (e.g., in beta-adrenergic receptors) is suspected, definitive data demonstrating such an alteration are sparse. Other possible explanations offered for these differences are alterations in second-messenger function and alterations in cellular and nuclear responses.

Because the response of older patients to any given medication is variable and cannot be foreseen, all drugs should be used judiciously in older patients. The physician should resist the temptation to apply protocol-based strategies to administration of medicines in the elderly. In general, knowledge of the pharmacology of the drugs prescribed, limits on the number used, determination of the preparation and dosage based on the patient's general condition and ability to handle the drug, combined with downward adjustment of the dose in the presence of known hepatic or renal impairment in concert with surveillance for untoward effects, will minimize the risks of medication use in elderly patients.

SPECIFIC ISSUES

Neurologic Disorders

Neurologic problems common among older adults in the critical care setting include delirium, stroke, and sleep disorders.

Delirium

Background and Risk Factors

Delirium is an acute mental disorder common among elderly patients; a recent review noted that 29% to 64% of the hospitalized elderly develop delirium (424) increasing the 6-month mortality rate among these patients to 10% to 26% (425,426). Recognition is difficult, with only 25% of cases being diagnosed using standard screening tools (427,428). Delirium-associated morbidity complicates the hospitalization of 2.3 million older people annually, adding 17.5 million inpatient days and $4 billion to Medicare expenditures to cover increased lengths of stay and greater need for postdischarge institutionalization, rehabilitation, and home care (429–432). Of note, delirium is associated with increased in-hospital mortality even after correction for severity of disease, as documented in a meta-analysis of 42 studies covering 16,595 patients (433,434). Older adults with multiple comorbidities, particularly pre-existing cognitive deficits, are predisposed to delirium (434–436), with a prevalence rate surpassing 50% during intensive care; symptoms persist in nearly that number after ICU departure (437). Particularly at risk are those with a history of hypertension, smoking, elevated bilirubin level, recent epidural analgesia, and recent administration of morphine (435,436,438). Other predictors of delirium include respiratory disease, infection, fever, hypotension, hypocalcemia, and hyperamylasemia (439). Invasive devices, sensory alteration, and inadequate or overaggressive pain control likely aggravate delirium-inducing medication effects in the critically ill patient (435,438,440). Among the many other factors, some *particularly* predictive factors include smoking more than 10 cigarettes per day, consuming three or more alcoholic drinks per day, or living alone; these all substantially increase the odds ratio of developing delirium during hospitalization (441). Most studies show that among the most critically ill, comatose patients, those with high APACHE II scores, "poly-trauma" patients that undergo emergency surgery, and those with metabolic acidosis are additionally at risk for falling into a delirious state (442).

Pathophysiology

Specific pathophysiologic mechanisms are not well understood. The phenomenon can be viewed as a final pathway of various causes of acute brain dysfunction. These include the following: (a) direct brain injury from trauma, cerebrovascular disease (443), or CNS infection; (b) systemic disturbances such as hypoxemia, hypotension, renal failure, hepatic failure, sepsis, and endocrine dysfunction; (c) effects of toxic or pharmacologic agents such as anticholinergics, narcotics, and sedative-hypnotics; and (d) the consequences of withdrawal of substances to which the brain has developed tolerance (e.g., alcohol or benzodiazepines). Delirium is more likely to occur when these factors coexist in patients with pre-existing comorbidities (444–456). Those elderly patients that enter the delirious state with pre-existing dementia, a condition commonly found in older patients, have less chance of full recovery of mental faculties and greater chance of dying than those without pre-existing dementia (457). Current theory proposes alteration of CNS neurotransmitter levels and metabolism by age, medication, or illness as paramount in producing the mental status that characterizes delirium, particularly the acetylcholine and dopamine pathways, serotonin, GABA, histamine, glutamine, and norepinephrine systems (458–461); rapid advances in neuroimaging may allow additional insight into microanatomic bases of delirium (462).

Diagnosis

Criteria defining delirium are detailed in the *Diagnostic and Statistical Manual of Mental Disorders* (DSM-5) of the American Psychiatric Association, specifically: (a) a disturbance in attention and awareness; (b) the disturbance develops over a short period of time, represents an acute change from baseline attention and awareness, and tends to fluctuate in severity during the course of a day; (c) there is an additional disturbance in cognition; (d) the disturbances in Criteria A and C are not better explained by a pre-existing, established or evolving neurocognitive disorder and do not occur in the context of a severely reduced level of arousal such as coma; and (e) there is evidence from the history, physical examination, or laboratory findings that the disturbance is a direct physiologic consequence of another medical condition, substance intoxication or withdrawal (i.e., due to a drug of abuse or to a medication), or exposure to a toxin, or is due to multiple etiologies (463). Additional features include alteration of sleep/wake cycle and psychomotor activities. Various screening tools and protocols have been developed that allow accurate and timely diagnosis using these criteria (436,464–468) when the diagnosis is specifically sought. Patterns of psychomotor symptoms are termed *hyperactive* and *hypoactive* (469–471). Patients occasionally display features of both types, termed *mixed. Hyperactive* patients are agitated and combative, with loud, inappropriately boisterous outbursts and motor activity that can be harmful to self or caregiver. Those termed *hypoactive* alternate between calm, possibly appropriate behavior and a minimally interactive, withdrawn state with flat affect, making this variant easy to overlook. *Mixed* delirious patients' symptoms fluctuate between agitated and apathetic (472); more than half of the delirious patients older than 65 years display the *mixed* subtype (473). Delirium may erroneously be attributed to such conditions as dementia or depression—the three may coexist—or simply not be recognized (474), delaying the diagnosis. Delays may be explained by the following: (a) the fluctuating nature of the signs and symptoms; (b) inadequate or insufficiently detailed scheduled neurologic and cognitive assessments of patients at risk for delirium; (c) avoidance of interactions with patients displaying altered mental status; or (d) misperception of mental status changes "expected" in critically ill patients (475,476). Altered mental status in any patient suggests delirium; an organized approach to its investigation (477) that focuses on known risk factors is paramount to avoid overlooking the condition. Of particular interest to the intensivist who manages elderly patients are alterations of mental status temporally related to a surgical procedure, specifically delirium developing within the immediate (minutes to days) postoperative period, and the more indolent neurocognitive decline that may appear days to weeks to months later, termed *postoperative cognitive dysfunction* (POCD); the uniqueness of these conditions lies in their association with the postoperative period. Emergence delirium, the transitory restlessness and disorientation often apparent in the postanesthesia care unit or an ICU that receives patients directly from the operating room, is seen in up to 30% of adults after operation, most often manifests with hypoactive signs of delirium, may portend worse outcome in the postoperative period but generally clears without sequelae (478). More worrisome is interval delirium, appearing 2 to 7 days after operation, the patient manifesting disorientation and agitation, and being at risk for postoperative complications and suboptimal outcome (including increased mortality) (479) by virtue of its appearance. Risk factors for postoperative delirium are additive to those menacing the nonoperative elderly patient such as preexisting mental compromise, age over 70 years, consumption of substances such as tobacco, alcohol, and sedatives, and renal compromise (480). Procedure-related factors include perioperative hypoxemia and hypotension, exposure to anesthesia-related medications—anticholinergics such as atropine, volatile inhalational anesthetics, neuromuscular blocking agents, and potent opioids—and high-volume blood transfusion and rapid fluid shifts associated with surgery. Procedures using cardiopulmonary bypass raise the possibility of microscopic atheromatous or air emboli as contributors, although investigators have found that the incidence of postoperative cognitive dysfunction at the 6-year milestone is similar for on- and off-pump coronary artery bypass graft (CABG) (481). The incidence of postoperative delirium may not even be related to the anesthetic technique employed (482). The incidence of postoperative delirium ranges from 0% to 74%, varying with age group, surgical procedure, variability of diagnostic criteria, and pre- and postoperative cognitive status (483).

POCD was first identified in 1955 (484), characterized by the appearance weeks to months after a surgical procedure of impairment of memory, concentration, comprehension of language, and social integration (485). Although seldom charged with management of POCD, the intensivist is instrumental in its recognition in that delirium in the early postoperative period may forecast its later reappearance (486). One well-designed investigation of elderly patients undergoing noncardiac surgery reported the incidence of delirium to be 25% at 1 week after operation, with symptoms of POCD being present in 9.9% of patients at 3 months, significantly worse than controls at both intervals (485), and revealing advancing age as the only factor significantly predictive of POCD. More recently, it has been recognized that, in the postsurgical patient, in addition to age over 60, those with previous CVA (even without residua), lower level of education, and POCD at the time of discharge are all predictive of much longer duration of cognitive dysfunction, and of a higher likelihood of dying within 3 months of major noncardiac surgery (487). Similarly, abundant literature (488–491) exists addressing this syndrome in cardiac surgery patients following both on- and off-pump procedures, most of whom were older than 60 years. Although most cardiac surgery patients suffer various concurrent confounding medical conditions that make the specific effects solely of cardiac surgery on subsequent mental status difficult to isolate, meticulous attention to statistical and study control issues allows identification of a substantial incidence (53%) of CABG patients (average age, 60.9 ± 10.6 years) showing cognitive deterioration consistent with POCD at the time of discharge, and 42% at 5 years (491), with age being a univariate predictor of decline. The specific cause of POCD is obscure; suggested causes are those noted above as well as more abstract considerations such as brain inflammation, genetic factors, cerebral edema, and blood–brain barrier dysfunction (492–496), and possibly direct toxic effects of some general anesthesics, and effects of disordered postoperative sleep patterns on brain chemistry (495). Timely recognition of the onset of delirium is required for optimal treatment, facilitating rapid identification of reversible precipitating factors. Beyond that, treatment is supportive, with aggressive treatment of symptoms and protection of the patient from the sequelae of their delirious state. Prevention is central, requiring a multicomponent approach that includes modification of environmental factors and provision of supportive measures, as demonstrated in a prospective—although nonrandomized—study of 852 patients over 70 years old admitted to a general medicine service in which a multicomponent delirium prevention strategy achieved a one-third reduction in the incidence of delirium, compared to those who received standard care (429). Although this study included patients in a general ward, one may extrapolate the findings to profoundly at-risk ICU patients. A skilled geriatrician can help decrease the incidence of postoperative delirium (POD) by assisting in utilizing delirium intervention programs (496). Symptomatic treatment uses both pharmacologic and nonpharmacologic strategies. Instrumental are the use of repeated reorientation, cognitive stimulating activities, promotion of adequate sleep on a normal sleep/wake cycle, physical therapy and mobilization, early removal of catheters and physical restraints, and provision of eyeglasses and hearing aids, combined with the judicious use of medications particularly targeted at calming agitation. All potentially neuroactive medications such as benzodiazepines, opioids, or those with anticholinergic effects that are not absolutely fundamental to the patient's treatment plan and improvement should be discontinued (436,438,439). Beware, however, of withholding benzodiazepine medications from delirious patients in situations in which they are appropriate such as alcohol withdrawal (497). Nonbenzodiazepine medications are recommended for intubated patients requiring sedation, after sufficient analgesia is achieved (498). It appears that dexmedetomidine, the centrally acting alpha-agonist, has a lower associated incidence of delirium than benzodiazepines when sedation is needed (499). Additionally, this medication allows smoother arousal from the sedated state and earlier extubation in some patients, but at the expense of a greater instance of bradycardia and hypotension (500). The butyrophenone haloperidol is often used in the management of delirium-induced agitation, having few active metabolites and minimal anticholinergic, sedative, and hypotensive effects (501). A recent retrospective analysis suggested that haloperidol use was independently associated with lower mortality in 989 critically ill patients (502). More recently, the so-called *atypical* antipsychotic medications have been utilized in the treatment of delirium in the elderly, with varying results (503). For POCD, there is no management other than prevention; no therapy has been identified that is curative once the syndrome had developed. In all cases, contributing problems must be identified and corrected and the patient protected. Support must also be provided to family members, who likely will be affected by their loved one's distressing symptoms and by the prospect of additional responsibilities for caring for that person.

Stroke

Incidence and Risk Factors

Stroke is the third leading cause of death and the *leading cause of disability* in the elderly. Compared to the 40 to 59 age group, the prevalence of stroke quadruples between 60 and 79 years of age, and nearly doubles again above 80 years of age (504). The stroke incidence similarly increases dramatically with age > 55 years, especially in women (504). Each year, nearly 800,000 individuals suffer strokes in the United States, corresponding to one event every 45 seconds and leading to one death every 3 minutes. Among those ≥ 55 years old, the incidence of stroke doubles with each additional decade of life (504), despite a decline in the United States, Canada, and Western Europe through the later part of the 20th century to the present, attributable to improved management of modifiable risk factors. Among these factors, hypertension is by far the most powerful; aggressive blood pressure control can reduce the risk of stroke by 40% (504). Coronary atherosclerosis, left ventricular hypertrophy, and AF contribute to stroke risk; diabetes mellitus may increase likelihood of stroke by a factor of two to four, but tight glucose control significantly reduces this risk, and may postpone such vascular complications as retinopathy and nephropathy (505,506). Modifiable factors also include cigarette smoking, hyperlipidemia, lack of physical activity, and excessive alcohol consumption (507).

Classification

Stroke classification can be based on location, cause, and time course. Prior to routine availability of CT, history and clinical findings provided the sole method of neurologic lesion identification. Today, rapid CT localization supplemented by the time-sensitive history and clinical examination findings allow much more rapid formulation of a treatment plan. Although the details of stroke syndromes are addressed elsewhere in this textbook (see Chapter 124), discussion of some issues as they affect the elderly are warranted.

Location

The most common location in which a stroke occurs, representing approximately two-thirds of ischemic strokes (508) is in the distribution of the middle cerebral artery (MCA). Findings include contralateral hemiplegia and hemianesthesia. Proximal MCA occlusion produces profound symptoms: contralateral homonymous hemianopsia with deviation of the head and eyes toward the side of the lesion. Involvement of the dominant MCA distribution may cause aphasia, either expressive, receptive, or both. Dominant hemisphere MCA lesions may induce depression in the elderly, whereas those in the nondominant hemisphere produce visuospatial deficits, unilateral neglect, and emotional lability that can mimic depression, sometimes delaying correct diagnosis. Anterior cerebral artery (ACA) stroke, the least common variety accounting for about 2% of ischemic infarcts (508), most profoundly affects the contralateral leg and foot, generally with lesser impact on the arm and little involvement of the face. Very proximal ACA occlusion, however, may affect the entire contralateral side. Abundant collateral flow in ACA territory yields various symptoms associated with anterior circulation stroke. One may observe frontal lobe features such as emotional lability, mood impairment, personality changes, and intellectual deficits; aphasia is uncommon. Stroke-related paraplegia and incontinence may leave the elderly victim wheelchair-bound and unable to control critical body functions, greatly complicating rehabilitation and subsequent independent living. Strokes in the distribution of the posterior cerebral artery (PCA) manifest a diversity of findings due to the variability of anatomic origin, namely partial or complete origin from the basilar artery or internal carotid arteries. Neurologic consequences of PCA stroke include contralateral hemianesthesia and hemianopsia with sparing of central macular vision, difficulty with reading and calculations, and hemiballismus from subthalamic involvement (508). With vertebrobasilar atherothrombotic disease, cerebellar dysfunction predominates. Common symptoms include vomiting, dizziness, ataxia, nystagmus, and double vision. Vertigo can be profound, causing an already tenuously balanced elderly person to sustain a fatal fall. Other symptoms include weakness of the face and the contralateral body, with dysarthria or dysphasia; facial numbness may occur. Brain stem involvement may be revealed by altered mental status or quadriplegia (508). Lacunar stroke, caused by occlusions of the small penetrating and subcortical arteries, tend to occur in the basal ganglia, internal capsule, thalamus, or pons. Depending on the specific sites of lesions, a wide variety of presentation may occur, including pure motor or sensory findings, symptoms that appear parkinsonian, or a mixture of presenting abnormalities.

Cause

Strokes are either ischemic or hemorrhagic, the distribution being approximately 87% and 13%, respectively. Ischemic events involve occlusion of the cerebral vessel by embolus or thrombosis; the remaining include hemorrhage into the brain parenchyma (10%) or its surrounding spaces (subarachnoid hemorrhage, 3%) (504). Rapid identification of the specific cause of the stroke is fundamental to its management, because modalities of treatment vary with cause. Embolic phenomena most often originate from the heart, commonly associated with atrial fibrillation, which is frequent in the elderly population. Atherosclerotic disease of the aortic arch is emerging as an increasingly important and recognized risk factor for recurrent stroke when the wall thickness exceeds 4 mm (509). Atheroma-associated clot formation may produce neurologic syndromes known as thrombotic stroke. Subintimal vascular disease is the ultimate inciting event, inducing arterial narrowing with ulcerated plaque formation in areas of more turbulent flow, such as the carotid bifurcation, leading ultimately to symptoms ranging from a temporary deficit (i.e., a transient ischemic attack [TIA]) to complete arterial occlusion caused by clot formation.

Time Course

Stroke phases are termed acute, subacute, and chronic, each with its unique needs and goals of care. Time spans are generally said to extend from symptom onset to 48 hours, 48 hours to 3 months, and past 3 months, respectively. The intensivist is little involved in direct management of stroke-related symptoms after the first few days, although elderly patients who fall within the later stages of recovery may certainly require intensive care for recurrent stroke, a stroke-related complication, or other critical illness.

Acute Phase of Stroke (Admission to 48 hours). Management of the acute phase involves, first and foremost, ensuring airway and hemodynamic stability. Thereafter, the goals of care are (a) identification of the stroke as ischemic or hemorrhagic; (b) initiation of thrombolytic therapy when indicated; and (c) recognition and treatment of medical or neurologic complications. The first goal is most easily achieved by obtaining a non–contrast-enhanced CT scan of the brain as quickly as possible when stroke is suspected; hemorrhage is usually obvious on this scan. Early in the course of ischemic stroke there may be no visible abnormality. Early CT may reveal one of the many mimics of stroke: subdural hematoma, neoplasm, or hydrocephalus; contrast enhancement may improve yield if tumor or infection are likely. Recall that comorbid conditions abound in the elderly; cardiac dysrhythmias or infarction may provoke or result from a cerebrovascular event, mandating 12-lead ECG and continuous cardiac monitoring in all stroke patients. Questions of the numerous other causes of altered mental status in the geriatric patient must be investigated and settled quickly. For those in whom, with the assistance of expert consultation, it is decided that ischemic stroke is present, the risks and benefits of thrombolytic therapy must be weighed. Current recommendations for management include initiation of intravenous thrombolytic therapy with recombinant tissue plasminogen activator (rt-PA) as soon as possible, within 180 minutes of onset of stroke, in the absence of contraindications (510). Thrombolysis between 3 and 4.5 hours is associated with improved 90-day outcome, but with a higher risk of intracranial hemorrhage (511). Intra-arterial thrombolysis may be an option for those with occlusion of the MCA. Of note is that rt-PA is approved by the Food and Drug Administration (FDA) for intravenous administration, but not for intra-arterial use. None-the-less, the use of rt-PA improves outcome from stroke at 3 months (512).

There is a relative paucity of data documenting treatment of older stroke patients compared to those in younger age groups (a situation similar to those studies addressing thrombolysis in myocardial infarction), although there is presently an ongoing study in Italy investigating the use of rt-PA in patients older than 80 years (513). It does appear, however, that while there may be poorer outcome from stroke in the elderly population *in general,* there is no increased likelihood of rt-PA–induced severe intracranial hemorrhage (514–517). This was more recently confirmed in a publication from Australia in a study of 206 patients over 80 years to whom rt-PA was administered for acute stroke, and in which there was no increase in the instance of hemorrhagic transformation after thrombolysis (518). A number of stroke scales, including the National Institutes of Health Stroke Scale (NIHSS), have been devised to assist in quantification of severity of stroke-related symptoms as a guide to optimal management. Important issues such as blood pressure management and anticoagulation are best addressed in concert with expert consultation (510,511,519).

Subacute and Chronic Phases of Stroke Management. The acute events and aggressive treatment related to stroke often stabilize within 48 hours; thereafter, close attention to complications or neurologic decompensation is warranted. With meticulous attention to the return of intact airway reflexes and sufficient recovery of mental status, early extubation of the trachea is advisable. Otherwise, early tracheostomy for airway protection allows withdrawal of sedation, early mobilization, and more robust participation in physical and occupational therapy, with the long-term goal of rehabilitation to maximal recovery. During the period from 2 to 5 days after the stroke, the risk of acute complications continues, including such events as hemorrhagic transformation, the onset of catastrophic cerebral edema warranting aggressive monitoring and management, deep venous thrombosis, hyperglycemia, and elevated temperature, all of which must be recognized and treated aggressively to optimize outcome (520). The common complications associated with compromised mental status, namely pulmonary aspiration, skin breakdown, infections, and limitation of extremity range of movement, can be ameliorated by aggressive rehabilitation efforts. Early nutritional support via feeding tube is sometimes overlooked in the flurry of initial management activity but must be initiated as early as possible. Formal rehabilitation programs may be organized in the setting of the acute inpatient rehabilitation unit, or in long-term rehabilitation hospitals, skilled nursing facilities, outpatient rehabilitation centers, or home. Optimal programs incorporate comprehensive assessment and treatment by a multidisciplinary team that includes physical, occupational, and speech therapists, and a geriatrician, physiatrist, psychologist, nurse, and social worker in the first few months during which most neurologic recovery occurs. A pre-existing state of debilitation, however, may limit the 3-hour period of active participation traditional to inpatient environments, mandating alternate plans. General goals of rehabilitation include restoration of motor and sensory function, and strengthening of intact functions to facilitate compensation for residual deficits. Beyond the first few months, while neurologic function likely plateaus, functional recovery continues when encouraged and supported by family presence, social interaction, and adequate nutrition. The stroke recurrence rate of 30% within 10 years warrants continued attention to chronic medical conditions. The Framingham Study data document survival in stroke victims of 50% in 5 years (521–523). Preservation of functional gains, avoidance of complications, and aggressive management of contributing comorbid conditions may well forestall the decline that often follows a stroke in an elderly patient.

Sleep Disorders

Background

Insomnia plagues the elderly, afflicting nearly 50% of older adults (524). The genders are generally equally affected, although sleepless men predominate after 85 years of age. Prevalence increases in the elderly with the number of coincident medical conditions (525,526). Common sleep complaints among the community-dwelling elderly are difficulty in initiation of sleep, and nighttime and early morning awakening (527). Sequelae of insomnia include physical and mental fatigue, anxiety, and irritability, which worsen as bedtime approaches and personal worries re-emerge without the protective diversion of normal daytime activities (528). Chronic dysfunctional sleep induces a state of endless fatigue, affecting memory and concentration (525,529). The elderly are particularly affected, with steepened cognitive decline and risk of falls, with associated morbidity and mortality (530–532). Hospitalization amplifies the morbidity of sleep disturbances; ICU admission likely subverts any semblance of a normal sleep pattern. Sedation to facilitate mechanical ventilation subdues consciousness but disrupts normal variation in sleep stages, preventing rest. Circadian rhythms are disrupted, with dyssynchrony in anticipated light/dark time cycles and inadequate daily morning exposure to sufficient bright light (533,534). Many elderly patients become disoriented at night. Exhaustion and confusion from constant alarms, noises, dressing changes, and unscheduled diagnostic procedures, and the impact of acute severe illness may all produce delirium in nearly two-thirds of elderly ICU patients. Dementia contributes to this problem.

Identification and Management of Sleep Disorders

The sleep/wake cycle is regulated by a complex neurochemical interaction subserved by the brainstem, hypothalamus, pons, and preoptic areas of the brain (534). Aberrations of sleep patterns produce dysfunctional sleep (535), disrupting daytime functioning. Sleep architecture is determined for an individual by performance of a sleep study displayed on a hypnogram. Normal sleep architecture displays three segments: light sleep (stages one and two); deep (delta or slow wave) sleep (stages three and four), which is the most restorative segment; and rapid eye movement, or REM, sleep (stages one and four) (536). In nonelderly adults, typical cycle time between REM and non-REM sleep is 90 to 120 minutes (537). Advanced age alters sleep by shortening sleep latency and total sleep time, preserving REM sleep, decreasing the delta segment, and advancing the natural onset of sleepiness to an earlier time in the evening (527). Nocturnal sleep fragmentation worsens with age, with daytime somnolence and frequent napping being commonplace, sometimes causing reversal of the sleep/wake cycle. Acute insomnia in the geriatric patient may be precipitated by a host of issues, including the critical illness itself. Metabolic derangements related to sepsis or trauma, recent exposure to potent anesthetic agents, and the unfamiliar ICU environment filled with off-schedule and frequent disruptions effectively prevent restful sleep. Although not generally within the purview of the intensivist, investigation of the cause of insomnia may be initiated for the ICU patient by meticulous history gathering, discussion with family members, use of sleep-related questionnaires such as the Multiple Sleep Latency Test (535) and the Epworth sleepiness scale screening too (537), and observation of the patient for evidence of any of the primary sleep disorders that respond to specific treatment modalities. These include a spectrum of conditions collectively termed sleep-disordered breathing (SDB), periodic limb movements in sleep/restless legs syndrome, and REM sleep behavior disorder. Some causes of SDB (obstructive sleep apnea, specifically) respond to continuous positive airway pressure (CPAP) (538), and the latter two respond to medications (539,540). Secondary causes of disordered sleep are legion, including medications, sleep-disruptive behavioral habits (such as prolonged daytime naps, sedentary lifestyle, overindulgence in tobacco or alcohol, late evening meals), numerous medical conditions (HF with orthopnea, incomplete bladder emptying with nocturia, gastric reflux, dementia), or environmental deficiencies (insufficient daytime sunlight exposure, inadequate climate control) (536).

In the ICU, it is unlikely that a patient will experience a normal sleep cycle, and the consequences of disrupted sleep may be consequential. In the adult ICU patient, sleep architecture is typically disrupted, with decrease in REM sleep and redistribution of bouts of fragmented sleep into unusual patterns of time distribution (541). Examination of schedules of care during the 12-hour "night shift" time period has revealed that the typical ICU patient likely experiences an astounding number of potential sleep interruptions—42 in 12 hours, or *3.5 per hour* (542); is it any wonder that our patients are at risk for delirium while in our ICUs? Circadian rhythm patterns are altered in the critically ill, associated with disrupted melatonin and cortisol secretion, and altered 24-hour cyclic temperature and other vital sign patterns (543,544), all of which contribute to aberrant sleep patterns. In those with age-related Circadian Rhythm compromise (545), the impact of sleep disruption on the onset of delirium and associated worsening of outcome can be profound; effective treatment obviously requires accurate diagnosis. Evidence of primary causes should be relayed to the patient, family members, and the physician responsible for long-term management of the patient after transfer. All possible accommodations should be made to minimize interruption of the older patient's restful nighttime sleep periods, minimizing noise, procedures, and cycling of lights on and off. Daily exposure to bright sunlight through nearby windows is beneficial (546,547). Pharmacologic treatments are best addressed on an individual basis, and within certain guidelines (548). Various medications are available (536); each, however, may provoke delirium in elderly patients. The use of benzodiazepines and opioids to promote sleep in the elderly, with their impact on the occurrence of delirium, is discouraged (549). In-depth guidelines for the evaluation and treatment of sleep disorders are available (529,550–556).

REHABILITATION AFTER ACUTE ILLNESS

The impact of critical illness on the lives of elderly patients is profound. Beyond the associated death rates, level of functioning is compromised in a substantial percentage of survivors (557), and increasing vulnerability to long-term dependence increases with age (558). Medical intervention in the critically ill or injured patient has evolved to a level of sophistication and capability that allows a previously unsalvageable patient to survive. Thoughtful and comprehensive discharge planning, initiated at the time of admission, can shorten LOS (559) and provide the springboard for return to a reasonable, though often compromised, level of functional autonomy (560). Many of these elderly individuals, after considerable improvement, may nevertheless linger for a prolonged period, requiring a single isolated critical intervention such as mechanical ventilation, and thus further risking the decline of inactivity, and subsequently find themselves after hospital discharge confined to a non-home location (561). The deleterious effects of such a prolonged hospital confinement can be ameliorated by early use of the expertise of rehabilitation professionals. Additionally, optimal recovery from common medical occurrences and conditions simply is not possible without active patient participation, which can be assisted and promoted by the physical medicine team. It is being increasingly recognized that *early* institution of rehabilitation planning and execution by such a team of specialists can reduce health care costs, LOS, and severity of disability after discharge (562). Shortening of hospitalization decreases the exposure of the marginally compensated patient to its debilitating risks (563). Avoidance of postillness disability is of paramount importance in that it is associated with higher mortality and greater dependence on family and other caregivers (564,565) (see Chapter 12).

Rehabilitation, as a general concept, encompasses several basic tenets that meld smoothly with the critical care frame of reference (566). Fundamental to any rehabilitation plan is stabilization and treatment of the primary inciting disorder; such a precept is the essence of the practice of critical care medicine, and thus is accomplished by virtue of the provision of critical care services. The unique jeopardy in which the elderly exist by virtue of their frailty and vulnerability to complications warrants the most meticulous attention to routine ICU precautions, which must be recognized by the intensivist (567). These include frequent turning, early nutrition, appropriate deep venous thrombosis (DVT) prophylaxis, semi-recumbent positioning, and maintenance of day–night cycle of auditory and visual stimulation. Early evaluation by a multidisciplinary team of specialists facilitates identification of evolving and anticipated functional deficits that are amenable to treatment, whether preventive or corrective. Integrated rehabilitation treatment and planning should occur in both the immediate and long-term settings by involvement of the physiatry team. Attention by the intensivist to ICU occurrences that are predictors of disability after critical illness—delirium and immobility—can assist in minimizing subsequent disability that would warrant institutionalization (568). Admission of a frail elder to a specialized unit designed around and attentive to specific features of geriatric pathophysiology has been demonstrated to improve functional outcomes (569). A number of evaluation tools have been devised to assess an individual's frailty that may be used in rehabilitation planning after illness; they appear to be useful primarily in *excluding* rather than identifying frailty (570).

The fundamental tool available to the geriatrician with which to organize the management and treatment of medical issues, including problems warranting formal rehabilitation, is the Comprehensive Geriatric Assessment (CGA) (571). The integrated, patient-centered concept of treatment implicit in CGA is often accomplished in specialized hospital units or within the framework of treatment considerations peculiar to the elderly, managed by a devoted multidisciplinary team. Such units include the geriatric evaluation and management (GEM) unit, as is found in some Veterans Administration hospitals, a specifically formulated management plan termed Acute Care for Elders (ACE) (572), or a construct of aggressive hospital-wide screening and treatment for at-risk patients by specialists and volunteers in an organization such as the Hospital Elder Life Program (HELP) (573). An alternative for the intensivist, whose patients are clearly unavailable for transfer to such a location remote from the ICU, is consultation by an in-patient geriatric consultation service team including individuals knowledgeable in rehabilitation issues (574). To date, the success of CGA in improving functionality and decreasing disability in the elderly after discharge seems clear (569,575), and has been validated as an effective tool to decrease morbidity and mortality in acutely ill elderly patients (576).

Several specific medical issues mandating ICU admission require active rehabilitation measures to achieve successful treatment. These include cardiac events related both to ACS and cardiac surgery, stroke, serious traumatic injury, various debilitating musculoskeletal conditions, and such morbid orthopedic procedures as lower extremity amputation and hip fracture repair. Large studies and reviews (577) document the success of aggressive rehabilitation after acute myocardial infarction and cardiac surgery in reducing cardiac mortality; over recent years, the benefit of this treatment is beginning to be documented (578) in the elderly population as well. It appears that an aggressive program of cardiac rehabilitation conducted for elderly patients, although often limited by arthritis or coexistent peripheral vascular or pulmonary disease, is safe, able to improve aerobic capacity, and favorably affects body fat percentage, lipid profiles, and physical function scores (579–581). A variety of issues may explain lower participation among elderly cardiac patients, especially women, compared to younger people (582–585).

Recovery from acute stroke presents a complex challenge to victim and physician alike. Whereas the cardiac patient may see improvement after surgery that continues during rehabilitation, the stroke patient often must endure impaired mental status and motor/sensory capabilities from the initial insult, often yielding a debilitated depressed individual (586) with little motivational reserve to assist recovery, an occurrence that impacts mortality after discharge (587). Survival beyond the first few days likely mandates prolonged assistance that may be required for months to achieve optimal improvement. Stroke rehabilitation targets improvement of impaired movement and function to minimize disability and optimize recovery to the premorbid state (588); this rehabilitation process hopefully will be initiated while the patient is still confined to the ICU. The extent of improvement hinges on several issues. These include age (589), the nature and severity of the initial deficit (590,591), presence of intracranial hemorrhage-related, rather than infarction-related, stroke as a with the former improves more than one with the latter for a given initial severity (592), and early initiation of the rehabilitation activities, preferably within 7 days (593), this period possibly including the ICU period. The plasticity of injured and unaffected normal brain tissue may allow gradual improvement over the subsequent several months (594). Specific stroke-related rehabilitation issues include the following: (a) optimal location for therapy; (b) speech and swallowing; (c) recovery of upper extremity function; (d) balance and walking; and (e) strengthening exercises (590). Evaluation tools such as the Barthel Index and the Stroke Impact Scale (595) are used to quantify a stroke patient's recovery, which may continue for as long as 6 months of recovery in the absence of another complication (596,597). Success of recovery from stroke varies over a large population (598) based on aforementioned variables and, to some extent, social status (599).

Rehabilitation of an injured elderly patient often involves continued long-term supportive therapy of conditions from which a younger individual may well recover quickly, namely mild TBI and/or extremity fracture. Indeed, continuity of specialized geriatrician involvement may facilitate continued attention to several issues during a prolonged trauma-ICU admission. These include comorbid problems, functional abilities and family support, formulation and continuous assessment of an itemized management plan toward realistic goals, and early initiation of planning for discharge and follow-up care (600,601). Of particular concern to intensivists managing elderly patients is hip fracture, of which more than 250,000 occur annually (602), with most patients being older than 50 years of age. Such fractures increase mortality—compared to that of similar patients without fracture—in those older than 65 years of age by 12% to 36% (603), as well as the likelihood of subsequent institutionalization (604) and functional dependence (605,606). A patient with pre-existing cognitive dysfunction or delirium will likely fare worse (604,606). Successful management requires identification and correction/stabilization of comorbid conditions, appropriate surgical treatment, and early initiation of important precepts of rehabilitation (602,607). These include early mobilization, initially to chair, followed by standing and walking with weight bearing; prolonged bed rest fosters deconditioning and is to be avoided. The intensivist who manages a particularly ill elder must address the potential for thromboembolic complications by encouraging early mobilization to minimize venous stasis, and by using prophylactic anticoagulant medication; regimens differ according to the exact situation (608–611). Functionality can be profoundly affected after hip fracture (612,613) and is further impacted by a high level of comorbidity (614). Although more men than women die initially after hip fracture, those who survive after the first year experience comparable functional recovery equally (615). Very advanced age is not necessarily a contraindication to hip fracture surgery in the absence of a prohibitive comorbidity; those older than 90 years often do quite well, returning, with aggressive rehabilitation and social support, to independent living (616).

About 50,000 amputations are performed annually in the United States, most on patients who are older than 60 years (617). Rates of lower extremity amputation declined from the 1980s to the mid-1990s, paralleling the improvement in arterial bypass and angioplasty techniques and the heightened attention to control of risk factors for vascular disease; rates since then seem to have stabilized (618). Eighty percent of amputations are performed as a result of arteriosclerotic occlusive disease and complications of diabetes mellitus (619), coincident with common comorbidities that may direct an elderly patient to the ICU. Nearly half of lower extremity amputees die within 2 years (620); a substantial percentage of survivors go on to lose the other leg (621) within a few years. Despite the attention paid to morbid consequences of amputation during the immediate postoperative period, this procedure profoundly impacts the patient's remaining life span. Optimal therapy for the amputee is achievable only with the early involvement and assistance of a rehabilitation team of physicians, technologists, and therapists skilled specifically in the management of amputation-related issues and familiar with prosthetic devices. Level of amputation varies with severity of lower extremity involvement; although medically sound judgement is the preeminent guide in this decision, it is important to note that the more joints and muscles replaced by prostheses, the greater the associated forfeiture of mobility and increase in energy cost of ambulation. The transmetatarsal amputee requires fairly trivial energy supplement to return to ambulation; the similar requirement for a transfemoral amputation patient can balloon by nearly 100% (619–622). Such CV and energy demands are considerable, even in an otherwise healthy amputee (622,623), and may not be achievable in the debilitated geriatric vascular or traumatized patient without risk of further decompensation. Although there is little definitive information documenting improvement in mobility after lower limb amputation in the elderly (624), early mobilization is to be encouraged. Prolonged bed rest further compromises balance and endurance, inviting the onset of contractures and loss of strength in compensatory muscle groups during prosthesis introduction. In the past, elderly amputees were seldom offered prosthesis; this picture has reversed with the more modern approach to elderly amputee care (625), in which such an offering is made to nearly 90% of elderly. An early visit from the physiatrist to the amputee's ICU bedside facilitates initiation of an organized rehabilitation care plan to formulate future prosthetic, physical therapy, wound care, and emotional support needs. Parts of these recovery plan components may be initiated by the intensivist while the patient is still critically ill and more fully conducted on a regular hospital ward, a specialty rehabilitation facility, or even at home. Follow-up must be long term; medical, emotional, and physical needs continue long after the amputee's surgical stump has completely healed (626,627); the amputation obviously effects the patient's self-image and dependence on others (628).

SUMMARY

The health care needs of elderly patients represent enormous challenges to all members of the medical profession. The aspirations and personal convictions of such individuals are as fundamental to the well-being and fruitfulness of their lives as are those of any other segment of the population. Although years of living bring elderly patients with the most complex illnesses and comorbid conditions to the hospital and ICU, it is to be remembered that the elderly often recover fully, or almost so, from profoundly serious illness despite numerous worrisome impediments that would discourage all but the most optimistic clinician. In general, vigilance and dispatch in investigations and treatment of critically ill geriatric patients, using the guidelines listed in this chapter, will facilitate recognition of the subtleties of such conditions. Although a substantial percentage of the elderly cannot be brought back to an independent level of functioning, every effort should be expended to achieve accurate diagnosis and expeditious treatment, providing full intensive support to conditions that are correctable and recognition when reasonable limits have been reached.

Key Points

- The number of elderly individuals is increasing, both in actual numbers and as a percentage of the population, with important implications in the management of critical care resources over the next 20 to 40 years.
- Physiologic reserve diminishes inexorably with age as part of aging, independent of the impact of comorbidities common in the elderly, with significant importance in managing the medical conditions in the elderly.
- The desire to continue aggressive critical medical care in the face of likely marginal chance of recovery varies widely in the elderly population, so it is critically important to generate an accurate plan of care early in the course of treatment in the elderly critically ill.
- CV compromise, often occult, affects most elderly individuals, just from the effects of less compliant vasculature and restructuring of myocardial architecture associated with age; addition of comorbidities of HFpEF, hypertension, and coronary disease explain the high morbidity and mortality from cardiac events in the elderly.
- Virtually all other body systems in the elderly, such as the pulmonary, neurologic, and renal systems, are at risk for sudden pathologic deterioration, similar to that seen in the CV system, when a disease process is imposed upon a system that is less robust by virtue of aging.
- Acute interventions involving intravascular interventions, both chemical and mechanical, to relieve vascular occlusion in the elderly should not be bypassed solely on the basis of age, because the elderly often benefit greatly from such interventions.
- Drug administration must be scrutinized closely in the elderly because of altered medication kinetics seen in geriatric physiology.

ACKNOWLEDGMENT

We thank Rebecca J. Byeth and Miho K. Bautista for their contribution to previous editions of this chapter, on which this revision is based.

References

1. U.S. Census Bureau. The older population: 2010; 2010 census briefs. U.S. Department of Commerce, Economics and Statistics Administration website. Available at https://www.census.gov/prod/cen2010/briefs/c2010br-09.pdf. Issued November 2011. Accessed January 2016.
2. National Center for Health Statistics. *Health, United States, 2014: with special feature on adults aged 55–64*. Centers for Disease Control and Prevention website. Available at http://www.cdc.gov/nchs/data/hus/hus14.pdf#015. Accessed January 2016.
3. Rice DP, Fineman N. Economic implications of increased longevity in the United States. *Annu Rev Public Health*. 2004;25:457–473.
4. U.S. Census Bureau. Florida passes New York to become the nation's third most populous state. Census Bureau reports press release CB14-232, December 23, 2014. Available at http://www.census.gov/newsroom/press-releases/2014/cb14-232.html. Accessed February 2016.
5. U.S. Department of Health and Human Services. *Centers for Medicare and Medicaid Services website*. Available at www.cms.hhs.gov/NationalHealthExpendData. Accessed October 2015.
6. U.S. Census Bureau. 2014 national population projections: summary tables Available at http://www.census.gov/population/projections. Accessed February 2016.
7. Alsarraf AA, Fowler R. Health, economic evaluation, and critical care. *J Crit Care*. 2005;20:194–197.
8. Angus DC, Kelley MA, Schmitz RJ, et al; Committee on Manpower for Pulmonary and Critical Care Societies (COMPACCS). Caring for the critically ill patient: current and projected workforce requirements for care of the critically ill and patients with pulmonary disease: can we meet the requirements of an aging population? *JAMA*. 2000;284:2762–2770.
9. Rockwood K, Noseworthy TW, Gibney RT, et al. One-year outcome of elderly and young patients admitted to intensive care units. *Crit Care Med*. 1993;21:687–691.
10. Barrett ML, Smith MW, Elixhauser A, Leah S, et al. *Utilization of intensive care services, 2011. Agency for Healthcare Research and Quality Statistical Brief #185*. Available at http://www.hcup-us.ahrq.gov/reports/statbriefs/sb185-Hospital-Intensive-Care-Units-2011.pdf. Published December 2014. Accessed January 2016.
11. Luce JM, Rubenfeld GD. Can health care costs be reduced by limiting intensive care at the end of life? *Am J Respir Crit Care Med*. 2002;165:750–754.
12. Fries JF, Koop CE, Beadle CE, et al. Reducing health care costs by reducing the need and demand for medical services. The Health Project Consortium. *N Engl J Med*. 1993;329:321–325.
13. Emanuel EJ, Emanuel LL. The economics of dying. The illusion of cost savings at the end of life. *N Engl J Med*. 1994;330:540–544.
14. Adams SD, Holcomb JB. Geriatric trauma. *Curr Opin Crit Care*. 2015;21(6):520–526.
15. Joseph B, Pandit V, Zangbar B et al. Superiority of frailty over age in predicting outcomes among geriatric trauma patients: a prospective analysis. *JAMA Surg*. 2014;149(8):766–772.
16. Martin GS, Mannino DM, Moss M. The effect of age on the development and outcome of adult sepsis. *Crit Care Med*. 2006;34:15–21.
17. Fairchild B, Webb TP, Xiang Q, et al. Sarcopenia and frailty in elderly trauma patients. *World J Surg*. 2015;39(2):373–379.
18. Joseph B, Pandit V, Zangbar B, et al. Validating trauma-specific frailty index for geriatric trauma patients: a prospective analysis. *J Am Coll Surg*. 2014;219(1):10–17.
19. National Center for Health Statistic. Cardiovascular disease in the elderly. Centers for Disease Control and Prevention website. Available at http://www.cdc.gov/nchs/fastats/heart-disease.htm. Accessed February 2016.
20. Crispell KA. Common cardiovascular issues encountered in geriatric critical care. *Crit Care Clin*. 2003;19:677–691.
21. Timio M. Blood pressure trend and psychosocial factors: the case of the nuns in a secluded order. *Acta Physiol Scand Suppl*. 1997;640:137–139.
22. Poulter NR, Khaw KT, Mugambi M, et al. Blood pressure patterns in relation to age, weight and urinary electrolytes in three Kenyan communities. *Trans R Soc Trop Med Hyg*. 1985;79:389–392.
23. Nichols WW, O'Rourke MF. *McDonald's Blood Flow in Arteries*. London, England: Edward Arnold Publishers; 1990.
24. Greenwald SE. Ageing of the conduit arteries. *J Pathol*. 2007;211:157–172.
25. London GM, Marchais SJ, Guerin AP, et al. Arterial stiffness: pathophysiology and clinical impact. *Clin Exp Hypertens*. 2004;26:689–699.
26. Dao HH, Essalihi R, Bouvet C, Moreau P. Evolution and modulation of age-related medial elastocalcinosis: impact on large artery stiffness and isolated systolic hypertension. *Cardiovasc Res*. 2005;66:307–317.
27. Avolio A, Jones D, Tafazzoli-Shadpour M. Quantification of alterations in structure and function of elastin in the arterial media. *Hypertension*. 1998;32:170–175.
28. O'Rourke M. Mechanical principles in arterial disease. *Hypertension*. 1995;26:2–9.
29. Izzo JL Jr. Arterial stiffness and the systolic hypertension syndrome. *Curr Opin Cardiol*. 2004;19:341–352.
30. Bramwell JC, Hill AV. Velocity of tansmission of the Pulse Wave. *Lancet*. 1922;1:891–892.
31. O'Rourke MF, Blazek JV, Morreels CL Jr, Krovetz LJ. Pressure wave transmission along the human aorta: changes with age and in arterial degenerative disease. *Circ Res*. 1968;23:567–579.
32. Nichols WW, O'Rourke MF, Avolio AP, et al. Effects of age on ventricular-vascular coupling. *Am J Cardiol*. 1985;55:1179–1184.
33. Nichols WW, Edwards DG. Arterial elastance and wave reflection augmentation of systolic blood pressure: deleterious effects and implications for therapy. *J Cardiovasc Pharmacol Ther*. 2001;6:5–21.
34. Strandberg TE, Pitkala K. What is the most important component of blood pressure: systolic, diastolic or pulse pressure? *Curr Opin Nephrol Hypertens*. 2003;12:293–297.
35. Nichols WW, Singh BM. Augmentation index as a measure of peripheral vascular disease state. *Curr Opin Cardiol*. 2002;17:543–551.
36. Safar ME. Systolic blood pressure, pulse pressure and arterial stiffness as cardiovascular risk factors. *Curr Opin Nephrol Hypertens*. 2001;10:257–261.

37. Franklin SS, Gustin W 4th, Wong ND, et al. Hemodynamic patterns of age-related changes in blood pressure. The Framingham Heart Study. *Circulation.* 1997;96:308–315.
38. Olivetti G, Melissari M, Capasso JM, Anversa P. Cardiomyopathy of the aging human heart. Myocyte loss and reactive cellular hypertrophy. *Circ Res.* 1991;68:1560–1568.
39. Wei JY. Age and the cardiovascular system. *N Engl J Med.* 1992;327: 1735–1739.
40. Weber KT, Brilla CG. Structural basis for pathologic left ventricular hypertrophy. *Clin Cardiol.* 1993;16(5 Suppl 2):II10–14.
41. Kass DA, Bronzwaer JG, Paulus WJ. What mechanisms underlie diastolic dysfunction in heart failure? *Circ Res.* 2004;94:1533–1542.
42. Periasamy M, Kalyanasundaram A. SERCA pump isoforms: their role in calcium transport and disease. *Muscle Nerve.* 2007;35:430–442.
43. Aurigemma GP, Gaasch WH. Clinical practice: diastolic heart failure. *N Engl J Med.* 2004;351:1097–1105.
44. Mandinov L, Eberli FR, Seiler C, Hess OM. Diastolic heart failure. *Cardiovasc Res.* 2000;45:813–825.
45. Kitzman DW, Gardin JM, Gottdiener JS, et al; Cardiovascular Health Study Research Group. Importance of heart failure with preserved systolic function in patients > or = 65 years of age. CHS Research Group. Cardiovascular Health Study. *Am J Cardiol.* 2001;87:413–419.
46. Brucks S, Little WC, Chao T, et al. Contribution of left ventricular diastolic dysfunction to heart failure regardless of ejection fraction. *Am J Cardiol.* 2005;95:603–606.
47. Lakatta EG. Diminished beta-adrenergic modulation of cardiovascular function in advanced age. *Cardiol Clin.* 1986;4:185–200.
48. Lakatta EG, Sollott SJ. Perspectives on mammalian cardiovascular aging: humans to molecules. *Comp Biochem Physiol A Mol Integr Physiol.* 2002; 132:699–721.
49. Lakatta EG. Catecholamines and cardiovascular function in aging. *Endocrinol Metab Clin North Am.* 1987;16:877–891.
50. Rodeheffer RJ, Gerstenblith G, Becker LC, et al. Exercise cardiac output is maintained with advancing age in healthy human subjects: cardiac dilatation and increased stroke volume compensate for a diminished heart rate. *Circulation.* 1984;69:203–213.
51. Stratton JR, Levy WC, Cerqueira MD, et al. Cardiovascular responses to exercise: effects of aging and exercise training in healthy men. *Circulation.* 1994;89:1648–1655.
52. Upadhya B, Taffet GE, Cheng CP, Kitzman DW. Heart failure with preserved ejection fraction in the elderly: scope of the problem. *J Mol Cell Cardiol.* 2015;83:73–87.
53. Gupta DK, Solomon SD. Imaging in heart failure with preserved ejection fraction. *Heart Fail Clin.* 2014;10(3):419–434.
54. Mehta RH, Granger CB, Alexander KP, et al. Reperfusion strategies for acute myocardial infarction in the elderly: benefits and risks. *J Am Coll Cardiol.* 2005;45:471–478.
55. Zaman MJ, Stirling S, Shepstone L, et al. The association between older age and receipt of care and outcomes in patients with acute coronary syndromes: a cohort study of the Myocardial Ischaemia National Audit Project (MINAP). *Eur Heart J.* 2014;35(23):1551–1558.
56. Gale CP, Cattle BA, Woolston A, et al. Resolving inequalities in care? Reduced mortality in the elderly after acute coronary syndromes. The Myocardial Ischaemia National Audit Project 2003-2010. *Eur Heart J.* 2012;33(5):630–639.
57. Goldberg RJ, McCormick D, Gurwitz JH, et al. Age-related trends in short- and long-term survival after acute myocardial infarction: a 20-year population-based perspective (1975–1995). *Am J Cardiol.* 1998;82:1311–1317.
58. Angeja BG, Gibson CM, Chin R, et al. Use of reperfusion therapies in elderly patients with acute myocardial infarction. *Drugs Aging.* 2001; 18:587–596.
59. Canto JG, Shlipak MG, Rogers WJ, et al. Prevalence, clinical characteristics, and mortality among patients with myocardial infarction presenting without chest pain. *JAMA.* 2000;283:3223–3229.
60. Giugliano RP, Camargo CA Jr, Lloyd-Jones DM, et al. Elderly patients receive less aggressive medical and invasive management of unstable angina: potential impact of practice guidelines. *Arch Intern Med.* 1998; 158:1113–1120.
61. Lee PY, Alexander KP, Hammill BG, et al. Representation of elderly persons and women in published randomized trials of acute coronary syndromes. *JAMA.* 2001;286(6):708–713.
62. Kumar A, Cannon CP. Acute coronary syndromes: diagnosis and management, parts I & II. *Mayo Clin Proc.* 2009;84(10, 11):917–938,1021–1036.
63. Gersh BJ, Anderson JL. Thrombolysis and myocardial salvage. Results of clinical trials and the animal paradigm: paradoxic or predictable? *Circulation.* 1993;88(1):296–306.
64. Fibrinolytic Therapy Trialists' (FTT) Collaborative Group. Indications for fibrinolytic therapy in suspected acute myocardial infarction: collaborative overview of early mortality and major morbidity results from all randomised trials of more than 1000 patients. *Lancet.* 1994;343(8893):311–322.
65. O'Gara PT, Kushner FG, Ascheim DD, et al. 2013 ACCF/AHA guideline for the management of ST-elevation myocardial infarction: executive summary: a report of the American College of Cardiology Foundation/ American Heart Association Task Force on Practice Guidelines. *Circulation.* 2013;127(4):529–555.
66. Keeley EC, Boura JA, Grines CL. Primary angioplasty versus intravenous thrombolytic therapy for acute myocardial infarction: a quantitative review of 23 randomised trials. *Lancet.* 2003;361(9351):13–20.
67. Guagliumi G, Stone GW, Cox DA, et al. Outcome in elderly patients undergoing primary coronary intervention for acute myocardial infarction: results from the Controlled Abciximab and Device Investigation to Lower Late Angioplasty Complications (CADILLAC) trial. *Circulation.* 2004;110(12):1598–1604.
68. Zahn R, Schiele R, Schneider S, et al. Primary angioplasty versus intravenous thrombolysis in acute myocardial infarction: can we define subgroups of patients benefiting most from primary angioplasty? Results from the pooled data of the Maximal Individual Therapy in Acute Myocardial Infarction Registry and the Myocardial Infarction Registry. *J Am Coll Cardiol.* 2001;37(7):1827–1835.
69. Bach RG, Cannon CP, Weintraub WS, et al. The effect of routine, early invasive management on outcome for elderly patients with non-ST-segment elevation acute coronary syndromes. *Ann Intern Med.* 2004;141(3):186–195.
70. Assali AR, Moustapha A, Sdringola S, et al. The dilemma of success: percutaneous coronary interventions in patients > or = 75 years of age-successful but associated with higher vascular complications and cardiac mortality. *Catheter Cardiovasc Interv.* 2003;59(2):195–199.
71. De Luca L, Olivari Z, Bolognese L, et al. A decade of changes in clinical characteristics and management of elderly patients with non-ST elevation myocardial infarction admitted in Italian cardiac care units. *Open Heart.* 2014;1:1–10.
72. Hunt SA, Abraham WT, Chin MH, et al. 2009 focused update incorporated into the ACC/AHA 2005 Guidelines for the Diagnosis and Management of Heart Failure in Adults: a report of the American College of Cardiology Foundation/American Heart Association Task Force on Practice Guidelines: developed in collaboration with the International Society for Heart and Lung Transplantation. *Circulation.* 2009;119(14):e391–e479.
73. Masoudi FA, Havranek EP, Krumholz HM. The burden of chronic congestive heart failure in older persons: magnitude and implications for policy and research. *Heart Fail Rev.* 2002;7(1):9–16.
74. Kannel WB, Belanger AJ. Epidemiology of heart failure. *Am Heart J.* 1991;121(3 Pt 1):951–957.
75. Kannel WB, Ho K, Thom T. Changing epidemiological features of cardiac failure. *Br Heart J.* 1994;72(2 Suppl):S3–S9.
76. Aronow WS. Epidemiology, pathophysiology, prognosis, and treatment of systolic and diastolic heart failure in elderly patients. *Heart Dis.* 2003;5(4):279–294.
77. Kannel WB. Incidence and epidemiology of heart failure. *Heart Fail Rev.* 2000;5(2):167–173.
78. Aronow WS, Tresch DD. Management of the older patient with acute myocardial infarction: difference in clinical presentations between older and younger patients. *J Am Geriatr Soc.* 1998;46(9):1157–1162.
79. Alagiakrishnan K, Banach M, Jones LG, et al. Update on diastolic heart failure or heart failure with preserved ejection fraction in the older adults. *Ann Med.* 2013;45(1):37–50.
80. Marinchak RA, Friehling TD, Kowey PR. Diagnosis and treatment of cardiac rhythm disorders in the elderly. *Clin Geriatr Med.* 1988;4(1):83–110.
81. Rials SJ, Marinchak RA, Kowey PR. Arrhythmias in the elderly. *Cardiovasc Clin.* 1992;22(2):139–157.
82. AFFIRM Investigators. Atrial Fibrillation Follow-up Investigation of rhythm management: baseline characteristics of patients with atrial fibrillation: the AFFIRM Study. *Am Heart J.* 2002;143(6):991–1001.
83. Falk RH. Etiology and complications of atrial fibrillation: insights from pathology studies. *Am J Cardiol.* 1998;82(8A):10N–17N.
84. Fujino M, Okada R, Arakawa K. The relationship of aging to histological changes in the conduction system of the normal human heart. *Jpn Heart J.* 1983;24(1):13–20.
85. Lev M. Aging changes in the human sinoatrial node. *J Gerontol.* 1954;9(1): 1–9.
86. Roberts WC. The aging heart. *Mayo Clin Proc.* 1988;63(2):205–206.
87. Thery C, Gosselin B, Lekieffre J, et al. Pathology of sinoatrial node: correlations with electrocardiographic findings in 111 patients. *Am Heart J.* 1977;93(6):735–740.

88. Tai CT, Chiou CW, Chen SA. Interaction between the autonomic nervous system and atrial tachyarrhythmias. *J Cardiovasc Electrophysiol.* 2002; 13(1):83–87.
89. Coumel P. Autonomic influences in atrial tachyarrhythmias. *J Cardiovasc Electrophysiol.* 1996;7(10):999–1007.
90. Wong CK, White HD, Wilcox RG, et al. Significance of atrial fibrillation during acute myocardial infarction, and its current management: insights from the GUSTO-3 trial. *Card Electrophysiol Rev.* 2003;7(3):201–207.
91. Wong CK, White HD, Wilcox RG, et al. New atrial fibrillation after acute myocardial infarction independently predicts death: the GUSTO-III experience. *Am Heart J.* 2000;140(6):878–885.
92. Kailasam R, Palin CA, Hogue CW Jr. Atrial fibrillation after cardiac surgery: an evidence-based approach to prevention. *Semin Cardiothorac Vasc Anesth.* 2005;9(1):77–85.
93. McMurry SA, Hogue CW Jr. Atrial fibrillation and cardiac surgery. *Curr Opin Anaesthesiol.* 2004;17(1):63–70.
94. Chatap G, Giraud K, Vincent JP. Atrial fibrillation in the elderly: facts and management. *Drugs Aging.* 2002;19(11):819–846.
95. Gersh BJ, Tsang TS, Seward JB. The changing epidemiology and natural history of nonvalvular atrial fibrillation: clinical implications. *Trans Am Clin Climatol Assoc.* 2004;115:149–160.
96. Hersi A, Wyse DG. Management of atrial fibrillation. *Curr Probl Cardiol.* 2005;30(4):175–233.
97. Kopecky SL, Gersh BJ, McGoon MD, et al. Lone atrial fibrillation in elderly persons: a marker for cardiovascular risk. *Arch Intern Med.* 1999;159(10): 1118–1122.
98. Nattel S, Opie LH. Controversies in atrial fibrillation. *Lancet.* 2006;367 (9506):262–272.
99. Wyse DG, Waldo AL, DiMarco JP, et al; Atrial Fibrillation Follow-up Investigation of Rhythm Management (AFFIRM) Investigators. A comparison of rate control and rhythm control in patients with atrial fibrillation. *N Engl J Med.* 2002;347(23):1825–1833.
100. Psotka MA, Lee BK. Atrial fibrillation: antiarrhythmic therapy.*Curr Probl Cardiol.* 2014;39(10):351–391.
101. Snow V, Weiss KB, LeFevre M, et al; AAFP Panel on Atrial Fibrillation; ACP Panel on Atrial Fibrillation. Management of newly detected atrial fibrillation: a clinical practice guideline from the American Academy of Family Physicians and the American College of Physicians. *Ann Intern Med.* 2003;139(12):1009–1017.
102. Monette J, Gurwitz JH, Rochon PA, Avorn J. Physician attitudes concerning warfarin for stroke prevention in atrial fibrillation: results of a survey of long-term care practitioners. *J Am Geriatr Soc.* 1997;45(9):1060–1065.
103. Vasishta S, Toor F, Johansen A, Hasan M. Stroke prevention in atrial fibrillation: physicians' attitudes to anticoagulation in older people. *Arch Gerontol Geriatr.* 2001;33(3):219–226.
104. Hart RG, Pearce LA, Aguilar MI. Meta-analysis: antithrombotic therapy to prevent stroke in patients who have nonvalvular atrial fibrillation. *Ann Intern Med.* 2007;146(12):857–867.
105. Singer DE, Albers GW, Dalen JE, et al. Antithrombotic therapy in atrial fibrillation: the Seventh ACCP Conference on Antithrombotic and Thrombolytic Therapy. *Chest.* 2004;126(3 Suppl):429S–456S.
106. Turagam MK, Velagapudi P, Flaker GC. Stroke prevention in the elderly atrial fibrillation patient with comorbid conditions: focus on non-vitamin K antagonist oral anticoagulants. *Clin Interv Aging.* 2015;10:1431–1444.
107. January CT, Wann LS, Alpert JS, et al; ACC/AHA Task Force Members. 2014 AHA/ACC/HRS guideline for the management of patients with atrial fibrillation: executive summary: a report of the American College of Cardiology/American Heart Association Task Force on practice guidelines and the Hearth Rhythm Society. *Circulation.* 2014;130(23):2071–2104.
108. Zipes DP, Wellens HJ. Sudden cardiac death. *Circulation.* 1998;98(21): 2334–2351.
109. Bayes de Luna A, Coumel P, Leclercq JF. Ambulatory sudden cardiac death: mechanisms of production of fatal arrhythmia on the basis of data from 157 cases. *Am Heart J.* 1989;117(1):151–159.
110. Fleg JL, Kennedy HL. Cardiac arrhythmias in a healthy elderly population: detection by 24-hour ambulatory electrocardiography. *Chest.* 1982;81(3): 302–307.
111. Fleg JL, Kennedy HL. Long-term prognostic significance of ambulatory electrocardiographic findings in apparently healthy subjects greater than or equal to 60 years of age. *Am J Cardiol.* 1992;70(7):748–751.
112. Sajadieh A, Nielsen OW, Rasmussen V, et al. Ventricular arrhythmias and risk of death and acute myocardial infarction in apparently healthy subjects of age > or = 55 years. *Am J Cardiol.* 2006;97(9):1351–1357.
113. Manolio TA, Furberg CD, Rautaharju PM, et al. Cardiac arrhythmias on 24-h ambulatory electrocardiography in older women and men: the Cardiovascular Health Study. *J Am Coll Cardiol.* 1994;23(4):916–925.
114. Hedblad B, Janzon L, Johansson BW, et al. Survival and incidence of myocardial infarction in men with ambulatory ECG-detected frequent and complex ventricular arrhythmias. 10-year follow-up of the 'Men born 1914' study in Malmo, Sweden. *Eur Heart J.* 1997;18(11):1787–1795.
115. Kennedy HL, Whitlock JA, Sprague MK, et al. Long-term follow-up of asymptomatic healthy subjects with frequent and complex ventricular ectopy. *N Engl J Med.* 1985;312(4):193–197.
116. Kahan T, Bergfeldt L. Left ventricular hypertrophy in hypertension: its arrhythmogenic potential. *Heart.* 2005;91(2):250–256.
117. Aronow WS, Epstein S, Koenigsberg M, Schwartz KS. Usefulness of echocardiographic left ventricular hypertrophy, ventricular tachycardia and complex ventricular arrhythmias in predicting ventricular fibrillation or sudden cardiac death in elderly patients. *Am J Cardiol.* 1988;62(16):1124–1125.
118. ECC Committee, Subcommittees and Task Forces of the American Heart Association. 2005 American Heart Association guidelines for cardiopulmonary resuscitation and emergency cardiovascular care. *Circulation.* 2005;112(24 Suppl):IV1–203.
119. Valenzuela TD, Roe DJ, Nichol G, et al. Outcomes of rapid defibrillation by security officers after cardiac arrest in casinos. *N Engl J Med.* 2000; 343(17):1206–1209.
120. Eisenberg MS, Mengert TJ. Cardiac resuscitation. *N Engl J Med.* 2001; 344(17):1304–1313.
121. Teo KK, Yusuf S, Furberg CD. Effects of prophylactic antiarrhythmic drug therapy in acute myocardial infarction: an overview of results from randomized controlled trials. *JAMA.* 1993;270(13):1589–1595.
122. Aronow WS, Mercando AD, Epstein S, Kronzon I. Effect of quinidine or procainamide versus no antiarrhythmic drug on sudden cardiac death, total cardiac death, and total death in elderly patients with heart disease and complex ventricular arrhythmias. *Am J Cardiol.* 1990;66(4):423–428.
123. Hilleman DE, Bauman AL. Role of antiarrhythmic therapy in patients at risk for sudden cardiac death: an evidence-based review. *Pharmacotherapy.* 2001;21(5):556–575.
124. Bardy GH, Lee KL, Mark DB, et al. Sudden Cardiac Death in Heart Failure Trial (SCD-HeFT) Investigators. Amiodarone or an implantable cardioverter-defibrillator for congestive heart failure. *N Engl J Med.* 2005;352(3): 225–237.
125. Siddiqui A, Kowey PR. Sudden death secondary to cardiac arrhythmias: mechanisms and treatment strategies. *Curr Opin Cardiol.* 2006;21(5): 517–525.
126. Tresch DD, Troup PJ, Thakur RK, et al. Comparison of efficacy of automatic implantable cardioverter defibrillator in patients older and younger than 65 years of age. *Am J Med.* 1991;90(6):717–724.
127. Goldberger Z, Lampert R. Implantable cardioverter-defibrillators: expanding indications and technologies. *JAMA.* 2006;295(7):809–818.
128. Epstein AE, DiMarco JP, Ellenbogen KA, et al. American College of Cardiology/American Heart Association Task Force on Practice Guidelines (Writing Committee to Revise the ACC/AHA/NASPE 2002 Guideline Update for Implantation of Cardiac Pacemakers and Antiarrhythmia Devices); American Association for Thoracic Surgery; Society of Thoracic Surgeons ACC/AHA/HRS 2008 Guidelines for Device-Based Therapy of Cardiac Rhythm Abnormalities: a report of the American College of Cardiology/American Heart Association Task Force on Practice Guidelines (Writing Committee to Revise the ACC/AHA/NASPE 2002 Guideline Update for Implantation of Cardiac Pacemakers and Antiarrhythmia Devices) developed in collaboration with the American Association for Thoracic Surgery and Society of Thoracic Surgeons. *J Am Coll Cardiol.* 2008;51(21):e1–e62.
129. Prystowsky EN. Prevention of sudden cardiac death. *Clin Cardiol.* 2005; 28(11 Suppl 1):I12–I18.
130. Tracy CM, Epstein AE, Darbar D, et al; American College of Cardiology Foundation; American Heart Association Task Force on Practice Guidelines; Heart Rhythm Society. 2012 ACCF/AHA/HRS focused update of the 2008 guidelines for device-based therapy of cardiac rhythm abnormalities: a report of the American College of Cardiology Foundation/American Heart Association Task Force on Practice Guidelines and the Heart Rhythm Society. [corrected]. *Circulation.* 2012;126(14):1784–1800.
131. Birnie D, Williams K, Guo A, et al. Reasons for escalating pacemaker implants. *Am J Cardiol.* 2006;98(1):93–97.
132. Monfredi O, Boyett MR. Sick sinus syndrome and atrial fibrillation in older persons: a view from the sinoatrial nodal myocyte. *J Mol Cell Cardiol.* 2015;83:88–100.
133. McPherson CA, Manthous C. Permanent pacemakers and implantable defibrillators: considerations for intensivists. *Am J Respir Crit Care Med.* 2004;170(9):933–940.
134. Stone KR, McPherson CA. Assessment and management of patients with pacemakers and implantable cardioverter defibrillators. *Crit Care Med.* 2004;32(4 Suppl):S155–S165.

135. Trohman RG, Kim MH, Pinski SL. Cardiac pacing: the state of the art. *Lancet.* 2004;364(9446):1701–1719.
136. Mueller PS, Hook CC, Hayes DL. Ethical analysis of withdrawal of pacemaker or implantable cardioverter-defibrillator support at the end of life. *Mayo Clin Proc.* 2003;78(8):959–963.
137. Ware JH, Dockery DW, Louis TA, et al. Longitudinal and cross-sectional estimates of pulmonary function decline in never-smoking adults. *Am J Epidemiol.* 1990;132(4):685–700.
138. van Pelt W, Borsboom GJ, Rijcken B, et al. Discrepancies between longitudinal and cross-sectional change in ventilatory function in 12 years of follow-up. *Am J Respir Crit Care Med.* 1994;149(5):1218–1826.
139. Lang MR, Fiaux GW, Gillooly M, et al. Collagen content of alveolar wall tissue in emphysematous and non-emphysematous lungs. *Thorax.* 1994;49(4):319–326.
140. Andreotti L, Bussotti A, Cammelli D, et al. Connective tissue in aging lung. *Gerontology.* 1983;29(6):377–387.
141. Turner JM, Mead J, Wohl ME. Elasticity of human lungs in relation to age. *J Appl Physiol.* 1968;25(6):664–671.
142. Kronenberg RS, Drage CW. Attenuation of the ventilatory and heart rate responses to hypoxia and hypercapnia with aging in normal men. *J Clin Invest.* 1973;52(8):1812–1819.
143. Brischetto MJ, Millman RP, Peterson DD, et al. Effect of aging on ventilatory response to exercise and CO2. *J Appl Physiol Respir Environ Exerc Physiol.* 1984;56(5):1143–1150.
144. Babb TG, Rodarte JR. Mechanism of reduced maximal expiratory flow with aging. *J Appl Physiol.* 2000;89(2):505–511.
145. Fowler RW, Pluck RA, Hetzel MR. Maximal expiratory flow-volume curves in Londoners aged 60 years and over. *Thorax.* 1987;42(3):173–182.
146. Mittman C, Edelman NH, Norris AH, et al. Relationship between chest wall and pulmonary compliance and age. *J Appl Physiol.* 1965;20:1211–1216.
147. Levitzky MG. Effects of aging on the respiratory system. *Physiologist.* 1984;27(2):102–107.
148. Mellemgaard K. The alveolar-arterial oxygen difference: its size and components in normal man. *Acta Physiol Scand.* 1966;67(1):10–20.
149. Sorbini CA, Grassi V, Solinas E, Muiesan G. Arterial oxygen tension in relation to age in healthy subjects. *Respiration.* 1968;25(1):3–13.
150. Cardus J, Burgos F, Diaz O, et al. Increase in pulmonary ventilation-perfusion inequality with age in healthy individuals. *Am J Respir Crit Care Med.* 1997;156(2 Pt 1):648–653.
151. Delclaux B, Orcel B, Housset B, et al. Arterial blood gases in elderly persons with chronic obstructive pulmonary disease (COPD). *Eur Respir J.* 1994;7(5):856–861.
152. Janssens JP. Aging of the respiratory system: impact on pulmonary function tests and adaptation to exertion. *Clin Chest Med.* 2005;26(3):469–484.
153. Knudson RJ. How aging affects the normal lung. *J Respir Dis.* 1981;2:74–84.
154. Skorodin MS. Respiratory disease and A-a gradient measurement. (Letter) *JAMA.* 1984;252:1344.
155. Prentice AM, Jebb SA. Beyond body mass index. *Obes Rev.* 2001;2(3):141–147.
156. Ritz P. Factors affecting energy and macronutrient requirements in elderly people. *Public Health Nutr.* 2001;4(2B):561–568.
157. Steen B. Body composition and aging. *Nutr Rev.* 1988;46(2):45–51.
158. Wurtman JJ, Lieberman H, Tsay R, et al. Calorie and nutrient intakes of elderly and young subjects measured under identical conditions. *J Gerontol.* 1988;43(6):B174–B180.
159. Rolls BJ, Dimeo KA, Shide DJ. Age-related impairments in the regulation of food intake. *Am J Clin Nutr.* 1995;62(5):923–931.
160. Mowe M, Bohmer T. The prevalence of undiagnosed protein-calorie undernutrition in a population of hospitalized elderly patients. *J Am Geriatr Soc.* 1991;39(11):1089–1092.
161. Visvanathan R. Under-nutrition in older people: a serious and growing global problem! *J Postgrad Med.* 2003;49(4):352–360.
162. Cederholm T, Jagren C, Hellstrom K. Outcome of protein-energy malnutrition in elderly medical patients. *Am J Med.* 1995;98(1):67–74.
163. Constans T, Bacq Y, Brechot JF, Guilmot JL, et al. Protein-energy malnutrition in elderly medical patients. *J Am Geriatr Soc.* 1992;40(3):263–268.
164. Brownie S. Why are elderly individuals at risk of nutritional deficiency? *Int J Nurs Pract.* 2006;12(2):110–118.
165. Deschamps V, Astier X, Ferry M, et al. Nutritional status of healthy elderly persons living in Dordogne, France, and relation with mortality and cognitive or functional decline. *Eur J Clin Nutr.* 2002;56(4):305–312.
166. Pearson JM, Schlettwein-Gsell D, Brzozowska A, et al. Life style characteristics associated with nutritional risk in elderly subjects aged 80–85 years. *J Nutr Health Aging.* 2001;5(4):278–283.
167. Hays NP, Roberts SB. The anorexia of aging in humans. *Physiol Behav.* 2006;88(3):257–266.
168. Omran ML, Morley JE. Assessment of protein energy malnutrition in older persons. Part I: history, examination, body composition, and screening tools. *Nutrition.* 2000;16(1):50–63.
169. Omran ML, Morley JE. Assessment of protein energy malnutrition in older persons. Part II: laboratory evaluation. *Nutrition.* 2000;16(2):131–140.
170. van Bokhorst-de van der Schueren MA, Klinkenberg M, Thijs A. Profile of the malnourished patient. *Eur J Clin Nutr.* 2005;59(10):1129–1135.
171. Harris D, Haboubi N. Malnutrition screening in the elderly population. *J R Soc Med.* 2005;98(9):411–414.
172. Schmidt H, Martindale R. The gastrointestinal tract in critical illness. *Curr Opin Clin Nutr Metab Care.* 2001;4(6):547–551.
173. Nieuwenhuijzen GA, Deitch EA, Goris RJ. Infection, the gut and the development of the multiple organ dysfunction syndrome. *Eur J Surg.* 1996;162(4):259–273.
174. Witte KK, Nikitin NP, Parker AC, et al. The effect of micronutrient supplementation on quality-of-life and left ventricular function in elderly patients with chronic heart failure. *Eur Heart J.* 2005;26(21):2238–2244.
175. Webb JG, Kiess MC, Chan-Yan CC. Malnutrition and the heart. *CMAJ.* 1986;135(7):753–758.
176. Creutzberg EC, Wouters EF, Mostert R, et al. Efficacy of nutritional supplementation therapy in depleted patients with chronic obstructive pulmonary disease. *Nutrition.* 2003;19(2):120–127.
177. Schols AM. Nutrition in chronic obstructive pulmonary disease. *Curr Opin Pulm Med.* 2000;6(2):110–115.
178. Schols AM. Pulmonary cachexia. *Int J Cardiol.* 2002;85(1):101–110.
179. Lesourd B. Nutrition: a major factor influencing immunity in the elderly. *J Nutr Health Aging.* 2004;8(1):28–37.
180. Hollington P, Mawdsley J, Lim W, et al. An 11-year experience of enterocutaneous fistula. *Br J Surg.* 2004;91(12):1646–1651.
181. Demling RH. The incidence and impact of pre-existing protein energy malnutrition on outcome in the elderly burn patient population. *J Burn Care Rehabil.* 2005;26(1):94–100.
182. Witte MB, Barbul A. Repair of full-thickness bowel injury. *Crit Care Med.* 2003;31(8 Suppl):S538–S546.
183. Mathus-Vliegen EM. Old age, malnutrition, and pressure sores: an ill-fated alliance. *J Gerontol A Biol Sci Med Sci.* 2004;59(4):355–360.
184. Sullivan DH, Bopp MM, Roberson PK. Protein-energy undernutrition and life-threatening complications among the hospitalized elderly. *J Gen Intern Med.* 2002;17(12):923–932.
185. Johansen N, Kondrup J, Plum LM, et al. Effect of nutritional support on clinical outcome in patients at nutritional risk. *Clin Nutr.* 2004;23(4):539–550.
186. Covinsky KE, Martin GE, Beyth RJ, et al. The relationship between clinical assessments of nutritional status and adverse outcomes in older hospitalized medical patients. *J Am Geriatr Soc.* 1999;47(5):532–538.
187. Giner M, Laviano A, Meguid MM, et al. In 1995 a correlation between malnutrition and poor outcome in critically ill patients still exists. *Nutrition.* 1996;12(1):23–29.
188. Cerra FB, Benitez MR, Blackburn GL, et al. Applied nutrition in ICU patients: a consensus statement of the American College of Chest Physicians. *Chest.* 1997;111(3):769–778.
189. Sullivan DH, Sun S, Walls RC. Protein-energy undernutrition among elderly hospitalized patients: a prospective study. *JAMA.* 1999;281(21):2013–2019.
190. Guigoz Y, Vellas B, Garry PJ. Assessing the nutritional status of the elderly: the Mini Nutritional Assessment as part of the geriatric evaluation. *Nutr Rev.* 1996;54(1 Pt 2):S59–S65.
191. Omran ML, Salem P. Diagnosing undernutrition. *Clin Geriatr Med.* 2002;18(4):719–736.
192. Reid MB, Allard-Gould P. Malnutrition and the critically ill elderly patient. *Crit Care Nurs Clin North Am.* 2004;16(4):531–536.
193. Hiesmayr M. Nutrition risk assessment in the ICU. *Curr Opin Clin Nutr Metab Care.* 2012;15(2):174–180.
194. Garrow JS, Webster J. Quetelet's index (W/H2) as a measure of fatness. *Int J Obes.* 1985;9(2):147–153.
195. US Department of Health and Human Services. National Institutes of Health website. http://www.nhlbi.nih.gov/health/public/heart/obesity/lose_wt/risk.htm. Accessed February 2016.
196. Flodin L, Svensson S, Cederholm T. Body mass index as a predictor of 1 year mortality in geriatric patients. *Clin Nutr.* 2000;19(2):121–125.
197. Galanos AN, Pieper CF, Kussin PS, et al; SUPPORT Investigators. Relationship of body mass index to subsequent mortality among seriously ill hospitalized patients: the study to understand prognoses and preferences for outcome and risks of treatments. *Crit Care Med.* 1997;25(12):1962–1968.

198. Beck AM, Ovesen L. At which body mass index and degree of weight loss should hospitalized elderly patients be considered at nutritional risk? *Clin Nutr.* 1998;17(5):195–198.
199. Stevens J, Cai J, Pamuk ER, et al. The effect of age on the association between body-mass index and mortality. *N Engl J Med.* 1998;338(1):1–7.
200. Davidson I, Smith S. Nutritional screening: pitfalls of nutritional screening in the injured obese patient. *Proc Nutr Soc.* 2004;63(3):421–425.
201. Kalliomaki JL, Siltavuori L, Virtama P. Stature and aging. *J Am Geriatr Soc.* 1973;21(11):504–506.
202. Dequeker JV, Baeyens JP, Claessens J. The significance of stature as a clinical measurement of aging. *J Am Geriatr Soc.* 1969;17(2):169–179.
203. Han TS, Lean ME. Lower leg length as an index of stature in adults. *Int J Obes Relat Metab Disord.* 1996;20(1):21–27.
204. Noppa H, Andersson M, Bengtsson C, et al. Body composition in middle-aged women with special reference to the correlation between body fat mass and anthropometric data. *Am J Clin Nutr.* 1979;32(7):1388–1395.
205. Rossner S. Obesity in the elderly: a future matter of concern? *Obes Rev.* 2001;2(3):183–188.
206. Villareal DT, Apovian CM, Kushner RF, et al. Obesity in older adults: technical review and position statement of the American Society for Nutrition and NAASO, The Obesity Society. *Am J Clin Nutr.* 2005;82(5):923–934.
207. Zamboni M, Mazzali G, Zoico E, et al. Health consequences of obesity in the elderly: a review of four unresolved questions. *Int J Obes (Lond).* 2005;29(9):1011–1029.
208. Liu KJ, Cho MJ, Atten MJ, et al. Hypocaloric parenteral nutrition support in elderly obese patients. *Am Surg.* 2000;66(4):394–399.
209. Covinsky KE, Covinsky MH, Palmer RM, et al. Serum albumin concentration and clinical assessments of nutritional status in hospitalized older people: different sides of different coins? *J Am Geriatr Soc.* 2002; 50(4):631–637.
210. Campion EW, deLabry LO, Glynn RJ. The effect of age on serum albumin in healthy males: report from the Normative Aging Study. *J Gerontol.* 1988;43(1):M18–M20.
211. Cooper JK, Gardner C. Effect of aging on serum albumin. *J Am Geriatr Soc.* 1989;37(11):1039–1042.
212. Fuhrman MP, Charney P, Mueller CM. Hepatic proteins and nutrition assessment. *J Am Diet Assoc.* 2004;104(8):1258–1264.
213. Goldwasser P, Feldman J. Association of serum albumin and mortality risk. *J Clin Epidemiol.* 1997;50(6):693–703.
214. Don BR, Kaysen G. Serum albumin: relationship to inflammation and nutrition. *Semin Dial.* 2004;17(6):432–437.
215. Sung J, Bochicchio GV, Joshi M, et al. Admission serum albumin is predictive of outcome in critically ill trauma patients. *Am Surg.* 2004; 70(12):1099–1102.
216. Corti MC, Guralnik JM, Salive ME, et al. Serum albumin level and physical disability as predictors of mortality in older persons. *JAMA.* 1994;272(13):1036–1042.
217. Chojkier M. Inhibition of albumin synthesis in chronic diseases: molecular mechanisms. *J Clin Gastroenterol.* 2005;39(4 Suppl 2):S143–S146.
218. Nicholson JP, Wolmarans MR, Park GR. The role of albumin in critical illness. *Br J Anaesth.* 2000;85(4):599–610.
219. Rothschild MA, Oratz M, Schreiber SS. Albumin synthesis. 1. *N Engl J Med.* 1972;286(14):748–757.
220. Rothschild MA, Oratz M, Schreiber SS. Albumin synthesis (second of two parts). *N Engl J Med.* 1972;286(15):816–821.
221. Ferrie S, Allman-Farinelli M. Commonly used "nutrition" indicators do not predict outcome in the critically ill: a systematic review. *Nutr Clin Pract.* 2013;28(4):463–484.
222. Cerra FB. Hypermetabolism, organ failure, and metabolic support. *Surgery.* 1987;101(1):1–14.
223. Wernerman J, Hammarqvist F, Gamrin L, et al. Protein metabolism in critical illness. *Baillieres Clin Endocrinol Metab.* 1996;10(4):603–615.
224. Plank LD, Hill GL. Energy balance in critical illness. *Proc Nutr Soc.* 2003; 62(2):545–552.
225. Uehara M, Plank LD, Hill GL. Components of energy expenditure in patients with severe sepsis and major trauma: a basis for clinical care. *Crit Care Med.* 1999;27(7):1295–1302.
226. Singer P, Berger MM, Van den Berghe G, et al. ESPEN Guidelines on Parenteral Nutrition: intensive care. *Clin Nutr.* 2009;28(4):387–400.
227. Heiat A, Vaccarino V, Krumholz HM. An evidence-based assessment of federal guidelines for overweight and obesity as they apply to elderly persons. *Arch Intern Med.* 2001;161(9):1194–1203.
228. Executive summary of the clinical guidelines on the identification, evaluation, and treatment of overweight and obesity in adults. *Arch Intern Med.* 1998;158(17):1855–1867.
229. Walker RN, Heuberger RA. Predictive equations for energy needs for the critically ill. *Respir Care.* 2009;54(4):509–521.
230. Harris J, Benedict F. *A Biometric Study of Basal Metabolism in Man.* Washington, DC: Carnegie Institute of Washington; 1919.
231. Cheng CH, Chen CH, Wong Y, et al. Measured versus estimated energy expenditure in mechanically ventilated critically ill patients. *Clin Nutr.* 2002;21(2):165–172.
232. Ishibashi N, Plank LD, Sando K, Hill GL. Optimal protein requirements during the first 2 weeks after the onset of critical illness. *Crit Care Med.* 1998;26(9):1529–1535.
233. Ziegler TR. Parenteral nutrition in the critically ill patient. *N Engl J Med.* 2009;361(11):1088–1097.
234. Hoffer LJ, Bistrian BR. Appropriate protein provision in critical illness: a systematic and narrative review. *Am J Clin Nutr.* 2012;96(3):591–600.
235. Frankenfield DC, Smith JS, Cooney RN. Accelerated nitrogen loss after traumatic injury is not attenuated by achievement of energy balance. *JPEN J Parenter Enteral Nutr.* 1997;21(6):324–329.
236. Long CL, Schaffel N, Geiger JW, et al. Metabolic response to injury and illness: estimation of energy and protein needs from indirect calorimetry and nitrogen balance. *JPEN J Parenter Enteral Nutr.* 1979;3(6):452–456.
237. McClave SA, Martindale RG, Kiraly L. The use of indirect calorimetry in the intensive care unit. *Curr Opin Clin Nutr Metab Care.* 2013; 16(2):202–208.
238. Schlein KM, Coulter SP. Best practices for determining resting energy expenditure in critically ill adults. *Nutr Clin Pract.* 2014;29(1):44–55.
239. Lev S, Cohen J, Singer P. Indirect calorimetry measurements in the ventilated critically ill patient: facts and controversies: the heat is on. *Crit Care Clin.* 2010;26(4):e1–e9.
240. Haugen HA, Chan LN, Li F. Indirect calorimetry: a practical guide for clinicians. *Nutr Clin Pract.* 2007;22(4):377–388.
241. Klein CJ, Stanek GS, Wiles CE 3rd. Overfeeding macronutrients to critically ill adults: metabolic complications. *J Am Diet Assoc.* 1998;98(7):795–806.
242. Weijs PJ, Stapel SN, de Groot SD, et al. Optimal protein and energy nutrition decreases mortality in mechanically ventilated, critically ill patients: a prospective observational cohort study. *JPEN J Parenter Enteral Nutr.* 2012;36(1):60–68.
243. Arabi YM, Aldawood AS, Haddad SH, et al. PermiT Trial Group. Permissive Underfeeding or Standard Enteral Feeding in Critically Ill Adults. *N Engl J Med.* 2015;372(25):2398–2408.
244. Heyland DK, Dhaliwal R, Drover JW, et al; Canadian Critical Care Clinical Practice Guidelines Committee. Canadian clinical practice guidelines for nutrition support in mechanically ventilated, critically ill adult patients. *JPEN J Parenter Enteral Nutr.* 2003;27(5):355–373.
245. Woodcock NP, Zeigler D, Palmer MD, et al. Enteral versus parenteral nutrition: a pragmatic study. *Nutrition.* 2001;17(1):1–12.
246. Heyland DK, Dhaliwal R, Day A, et al. Validation of the Canadian clinical practice guidelines for nutrition support in mechanically ventilated, critically ill adult patients: results of a prospective observational study. *Crit Care Med.* 2004;32(11):2260–2266.
247. Wernerman J. Guidelines for nutritional support in intensive care unit patients: a critical analysis. *Curr Opin Clin Nutr Metab Care.* 2005; 8(2):171–175.
248. Kreymann KG, Berger MM, Deutz NE, et al; ESPEN (European Society for Parenteral and Enteral Nutrition). ESPEN Guidelines on Enteral Nutrition: intensive care. *Clin Nutr.* 2006;25(2):210–223.
249. Bistrian BR, McCowen KC. Nutritional and metabolic support in the adult intensive care unit: key controversies. *Crit Care Med.* 2006;34(5): 1525–1531.
250. Griffiths RD, Bongers T. Nutrition support for patients in the intensive care unit. *Postgrad Med J.* 2005;81(960):629–636.
251. Griffiths RD. Is parenteral nutrition really that risky in the intensive care unit? *Curr Opin Clin Nutr Metab Care.* 2004;7(2):175–181.
252. Wernerman J. Feeding the gut: how, when and with what: the metabolic issue. *Curr Opin Crit Care.* 2014;20(2):196–201.
253. Deane AM, Dhaliwal R, Day AG, et al. Comparisons between intragastric and small intestinal delivery of enteral nutrition in the critically ill: a systematic review and meta-analysis. *Crit Care.* 2013;17(3):R125.
254. Alhazzani W, Almasoud A, Jaeschke R, et al. Small bowel feeding and risk of pneumonia in adult critically ill patients: a systematic review and meta-analysis of randomized trials.*Crit Care.* 2013;17(4):R127.
255. Kuppinger DD, Rittler P, Hartl WH, Rüttinger D. Use of gastric residual volume to guide enteral nutrition in critically ill patients: a brief systematic review of clinical studies. *Nutrition.* 2013;29(9):1075–1079.
256. Debaveye Y, Van den Berghe G. Risks and benefits of nutritional support during critical illness. *Annu Rev Nutr.* 2006;26:513–538.

257. Mahanna E, Crimi E, White P, et al. Nutrition and metabolic support for critically ill patients. *Curr Opin Anaesthesiol.* 2015;28(2):131–138.
258. Byrnes MC, Stangenes J. Refeeding in the ICU: an adult and pediatric problem. *Curr Opin Clin Nutr Metab Care.* 2011;14(2):186–192.
259. Lewington AJ, Cerdá J, Mehta RL. Raising awareness of acute kidney injury: a global perspective of a silent killer. *Kidney Int.* 2013;84(3):457–467.
260. Hoste EA, Clermont G, Kersten A, et al. RIFLE criteria for acute kidney injury are associated with hospital mortality in critically ill patients: a cohort analysis. *Crit Care.* 2006;10(3):R73.
261. Schiffl H. Renal recovery from acute tubular necrosis requiring renal replacement therapy: a prospective study in critically ill patients. *Nephrol Dial Transplant.* 2006;21(5):1248–1252.
262. Lindeman RD. Overview: renal physiology and pathophysiology of aging. *Am J Kidney Dis.* 1990;16(4):275–282.
263. Epstein M. Aging and the kidney. *J Am Soc Nephrol.* 1996;7(8):1106–1122.
264. Lindeman RD, Goldman R. Anatomic and physiologic age changes in the kidney. *Exp Gerontol.* 1986;21(4–5):379–406.
265. Davies DF, Shock NW. Age changes in glomerular filtration rate, effective renal plasma flow, and tubular excretory capacity in adult males. *J Clin Invest.* 1950;29(5):496–507.
266. Lindeman RD, Tobin J, Shock NW. Longitudinal studies on the rate of decline in renal function with age. *J Am Geriatr Soc.* 1985;33(4):278–285.
267. Hollenberg NK, Adams DF, Solomon HS, et al. Senescence and the renal vasculature in normal man. *Circ Res.* 1974;34(3):309–316.
268. Cortes P, Zhao X, Dumler F, et al. Age-related changes in glomerular volume and hydroxyproline content in rat and human. *J Am Soc Nephrol.* 1992;2(12):1716–1725.
269. Meyer BR. Renal function in aging. *J Am Geriatr Soc.* 1989;37(8):791–800.
270. Wharton WW 3rd, Sondeen JL, McBiles M, et al. Measurement of glomerular filtration rate in ICU patients using 99mTc-DTPA and inulin. *Kidney Int.* 1992;42(1):174–178.
271. Tietz NW, Shuey DF, Wekstein DR. Laboratory values in fit aging individuals: sexagenarians through centenarians. *Clin Chem.* 1992;38(6): 1167–1185.
272. Cockcroft DW, Gault MH. Prediction of creatinine clearance from serum creatinine. *Nephron.* 1976;16(1):31–41.
273. Burkhardt H, Bojarsky G, Gretz N, et al. Creatinine clearance, Cockcroft-Gault formula and cystatin C: estimators of true glomerular filtration rate in the elderly? *Gerontology.* 2002;48(3):140–146.
274. Hoek FJ, Kemperman FA, Krediet RT. A comparison between cystatin C, plasma creatinine and the Cockcroft and Gault formula for the estimation of glomerular filtration rate. *Nephrol Dial Transplant.* 2003;18(10): 2024–2031.
275. Dharnidharka VR, Kwon C, Stevens G. Serum cystatin C is superior to serum creatinine as a marker of kidney function: a meta-analysis. *Am J Kidney Dis.* 2002;40(2):221–226.
276. Kuan Y, Hossain M, Surman J, et al. GFR prediction using the MDRD and Cockcroft and Gault equations in patients with end-stage renal disease. *Nephrol Dial Transplant.* 2005;20(11):2394–2401.
277. Levey AS, Stevens LA, Schmid CH, et al. A new equation to estimate glomerular filtration rate. *Ann Intern Med.* 2009;150(9):604–612.
278. Fesler P, Mimran A. Estimation of glomerular filtration rate: what are the pitfalls? *Curr Hypertens Rep.* 2011;13(2):116–121.
279. Martin JH, Fay MF, Udy A, et al. Pitfalls of using estimations of glomerular filtration rate in an intensive care population. *Intern Med J.* 2011;41(7):537–543.
280. O'Connell MB, Wong MO, Bannick-Mohrland SD, et al. Accuracy of 2- and 8-hour urine collections for measuring creatinine clearance in the hospitalized elderly. *Pharmacotherapy.* 1993;13(2):135–142.
281. Baumann TJ, Staddon JE, Horst HM, et al. Minimum urine collection periods for accurate determination of creatinine clearance in critically ill patients. *Clin Pharm.* 1987;6(5):393–398.
282. Traynor J, Mactier R, Geddes CC, Fox JG. How to measure renal function in clinical practice. *BMJ.* 2006;333(7571):733–737.
283. Fliser D. Assessment of renal function in elderly patients. *Curr Opin Nephrol Hypertens.* 2008;17(6):604–608.
284. Luft FC, Weinberger MH, Fineberg NS, et al. Effects of age on renal sodium homeostasis and its relevance to sodium sensitivity. *Am J Med.* 1987;82(1B):9–15.
285. Rowe JW, Shock NW, DeFronzo RA. The influence of age on the renal response to water deprivation in man. *Nephron.* 1976;17(4):270–278.
286. Agarwal BN, Cabebe FG. Renal acidification in elderly subjects. *Nephron.* 1980;26(6):291–295.
287. Bellomo R, Ronco C, Kellum JA, et al; Acute Dialysis Quality Initiative workgroup. Acute renal failure: definition, outcome measures, animal models, fluid therapy and information technology needs: the Second International Consensus Conference of the Acute Dialysis Quality Initiative (ADQI) Group. *Crit Care.* 2004;8(4):R204–R212.
288. Taber SS, Mueller BA. Drug-associated renal dysfunction. *Crit Care Clin.* 2006;22(2):357–374.
289. Leblanc M, Kellum JA, Gibney RT, et al. Risk factors for acute renal failure: inherent and modifiable risks. *Curr Opin Crit Care.* 2005;11(6):533–536.
290. Tao SM, Wichmann JL, Schoepf UJ, et al. Contrast-induced nephropathy in CT: incidence, risk factors and strategies for prevention. *Eur Rad iol.*2016;26(9):3310–3318.
291. Weisbord SD, Palevsky PM. Prevention of contrast-induced nephropathy with volume expansion. *Clin J Am Soc Nephrol.* 2008;3(1):273–280.
292. Brar SS, Hiremath S, Dangas G, et al. Sodium bicarbonate for the prevention of contrast induced-acute kidney injury: a systematic review and meta-analysis. *Clin J Am Soc Nephrol.* 2009;4(10):1584–1592.
293. Hoste EA, De Waele JJ, Gevaert SA, et al. Sodium bicarbonate for prevention of contrast-induced acute kidney injury: a systematic review and meta-analysis. *Nephrol Dial Transplant.*2010;25(3):747–758.
294. Muhlberg W, Platt D. Age-dependent changes of the kidneys: pharmacological implications. *Gerontology.* 1999;45(5):243–253.
295. Lonner JH, Koval KJ. Polytrauma in the elderly. *Clin Orthop Relat Res.* 1995;(318):136–143.
296. 10 Leasing causes of death by age group in the United States: 2013. Centers for Disease Control and Prevention web site. Available at http://www.cdc.gov/injury/images/lc-charts/leading_causes_of_death_by_age_group_2013-a.gif. Accessed December 2015.
297. National Center for Injury Control and Prevention. CDC injury fact book. Center for Disease Control website. Available at http://www.cdc.gov/ncipc/fact_book/factbook.htm. Updated September 26, 2014. Accessed January 2016.
298. Hogue CC. Injury in late life: part I. Epidemiology. *J Am Geriatr Soc.* 1982;30(3):183–190.
299. NationalTraumadatabank2014annualreport.AmericanCollegeofSurgeons website. Available at https://www.facs.org/~/media/files/quality%20programs/trauma/ntdb/ntdb%20annual%20report %202015.ashx. Accessed January 2016.
300. Mosenthal AC, Livingston DH, Elcavage J, et al. Falls: epidemiology and strategies for prevention. *J Trauma.* 1995;38(5):753–756.
301. Spaite DW, Criss EA, Valenzuela TD, et al. Geriatric injury: an analysis of prehospital demographics, mechanisms, and patterns. *Ann Emerg Med.* 1990;19(12):1418–1421.
302. Hannan EL, Waller CH, Farrell LS, Rosati C. Elderly trauma inpatients in New York state: 1994–1998. *J Trauma.* 2004;56(6):1297–1304.
303. Nagy KK, Smith RF, Roberts RR, et al. Prognosis of penetrating trauma in elderly patients: a comparison with younger patients. *J Trauma.* 2000;49(2):190–193.
304. McMahon DJ, Shapiro MB, Kauder DR. The injured elderly in the trauma intensive care unit. *Surg Clin North Am.* 2000;80(3):1005–1019.
305. Calland JF, Ingraham AM, Martin N, et al. Eastern Association for the Surgery of Trauma, Evaluation and management of geriatric trauma: an Eastern Association for the Surgery of Trauma practice management guideline. *J Trauma Acute Care Surg.* 2012;73(5 Suppl 4):S345–S350.
306. Zafar SN, Obirieze A, Schneider EB, et al. Outcomes of trauma care at centers treating a higher proportion of older patients: the case for geriatric trauma centers. *J Trauma Acute Care Surg.* 2015;78(4):852–859
307. Mann FA, Kubal WS, Blackmore CC. Improving the imaging diagnosis of cervical spine injury in the very elderly: implications of the epidemiology of injury. *Emerg Radiol.* 2000;7(1):36–41.
308. Ehara S, Shimamura T. Cervical spine injury in the elderly: imaging features. *Skel Radiol.* 2001;30(1):1–7.
309. Prasad VS, Schwartz A, Bhutani R, et al. Characteristics of injuries to the cervical spine and spinal cord in polytrauma patient population: experience from a regional trauma unit. *Spinal Cord.* 1999;37(8):560–568.
310. MacLeod J, Lynn M, McKenney MG, et al. Predictors of mortality in trauma patients. *Am Surg.* 2004;70(9):805–810.
311. Davis JW, Kaups KL. Base deficit in the elderly: a marker of severe injury and death. *J Trauma.* 1998;45(5):873–877.
312. Demetriades D, Karaiskakis M, Velmahos G, et al. Effect on outcome of early intensive management of geriatric trauma patients. *Br J Surg.* 2002;89(10):1319–1322.
313. McKinley BA, Marvin RG, Cocanour CS, et al. Blunt trauma resuscitation: the old can respond. *Arch Surg.* 2000;135(6):688–693.
314. Scalea TM, Simon HM, Duncan AO, et al. Geriatric blunt multiple trauma: improved survival with early invasive monitoring. *J Trauma.* 1990;30(2):129–134.

315. Flanagan SR, Hibbard MR, Riordan B, et al. Traumatic brain injury in the elderly: diagnostic and treatment challenges. *Clin Geriatr Med.* 2006;22(2):449–468.
316. McIntyre A, Mehta S, Aubut J, et al. Mortality among older adults after a traumatic brain injury: a meta-analysis. *Brain Inj.* 2013;27(1):31–40.
317. Rutland-Brown W, Langlois JA, Thomas KE, et al. Incidence of traumatic brain injury in the United States, 2003. *J Head Trauma Rehabil.* 2006;21(6):544–548.
318. Thompson HJ, McCormick WC, Kagan SH. Traumatic brain injury in older adults: epidemiology, outcomes, and future implications. *J Am Geriatr Soc.* 2006;54(10):1590–1595.
319. Rathlev NK, Medzon R, Lowery D, et al. Intracranial pathology in elders with blunt head trauma. *Acad Emerg Med.* 2006;13(3):302–307.
320. Kehoe A, Rennie S, Smith JE. Glasgow Coma Scale is unreliable for the prediction of severe head injury in elderly trauma patients. *Emerg Med J.* 2015;32(8):613–615.
321. Adekoya N, Thurman DJ, White DD, Webb KW. Surveillance for traumatic brain injury deaths—United States, 1989–1998. *MMWR Surveill Summ.* 2002;51(10):1–14.
322. Coronado VG, Thomas KE, Sattin RW, et al. The CDC traumatic brain injury surveillance system: characteristics of persons aged 65 years and older hospitalized with a TBI. *J Head Trauma Rehabil.* 2005;20(3):215–228.
323. Peck KA, Calvo RY, Schechter MS, et al. The impact of preinjury anticoagulants and prescription antiplatelet agents on outcomes in older patients with traumatic brain injury. *J Trauma Acute Care Surg.* 2014;76(2):431–436.
324. Stocchetti N, Furlan A, Volta F. Hypoxemia and arterial hypotension at the accident scene in head injury. *J Trauma.* 1996;40(5):764–767.
325. Eisenberg HM, Frankowski RF, Contant CF, et al. High-dose barbiturate control of elevated intracranial pressure in patients with severe head injury. *J Neurosurg.* 1988;69(1):15–23.
326. Jeremitsky E, Omert LA, Dunham CM, et al. The impact of hyperglycemia on patients with severe brain injury. *J Trauma.* 2005;58(1):47–50.
327. Cairns CJ, Andrews PJ. Management of hyperthermia in traumatic brain injury. *Curr Opin Crit Care.* 2002;8(2):106–110.
328. Coles JP, Fryer TD, Coleman MR, et al. Hyperventilation following head injury: effect on ischemic burden and cerebral oxidative metabolism. *Crit Care Med.* 2007;35(2):568–578.
329. Muizelaar JP, Marmarou A, Ward JD, et al. Adverse effects of prolonged hyperventilation in patients with severe head injury: a randomized clinical trial. *J Neurosurg.* 1991;75(5):731–739.
330. Doyle JA, Davis DP, Hoyt DB. The use of hypertonic saline in the treatment of traumatic brain injury. *J Trauma.* 2001;50(2):367–383.
331. Brain Trauma Foundation; American Association of Neurological Surgeons; Congress of Neurological Surgeons; Joint Section on Neurotrauma and Critical Care, AANS/CNS; Bratton SL, Chestnut RM, Ghajar J, et al. Guidelines for the management of severe traumatic brain injury. IX. Cerebral perfusion thresholds. *J Neurotrauma.* 2007;24(Suppl 1):S59–S64.
332. Mosenthal AC, Lavery RF, Addis M, et al. Isolated traumatic brain injury: age is an independent predictor of mortality and early outcome. *J Trauma.* 2002;52(5):907–911.
333. LeBlanc J, de Guise E, Gosselin N, Feyz M. Comparison of functional outcome following acute care in young, middle-aged and elderly patients with traumatic brain injury. *Brain Inj.* 2006;20(8):779–790.
334. Hukkelhoven CW, Steyerberg EW, Rampen AJ, et al. Patient age and outcome following severe traumatic brain injury: an analysis of 5,600 patients. *J Neurosurg.* 2003;99(4):666–673.
335. McIntyre A, Mehta S, Janzen S, et al. A meta-analysis of functional outcome among older adults with traumatic brain injury. *Neurorehabilitation.* 2013;32(2):409–414.
336. Grossman MD, Ofurum U, Stehly CD, Stoltzfus J. Long-term survival after major trauma in geriatric trauma patients: the glass is half full. *J Trauma Acute Care Surg.* 2012;72(5):1181–1185.
337. Hu R, Mustard CA, Burns C. Epidemiology of incident spinal fracture in a complete population. *Spine.* 1996;21(4):492–499.
338. Gale SC, Gracias VH, Reilly PM, Schwab CW. The inefficiency of plain radiography to evaluate the cervical spine after blunt trauma. *J Trauma.* 2005;59(5):1121–1125.
339. Lomoschitz FM, Blackmore CC, Mirza SK, Mann FA. Cervical spine injuries in patients 65 years old and older: epidemiologic analysis regarding the effects of age and injury mechanism on distribution, type, and stability of injuries. *AJR Am J Roentgenol.* 2002;178(3):573–577.
340. Ryan MD, Henderson JJ, The epidemiology of fractures and fracture-dislocations of the cervical spine. *Injury.* 1993;23:38–40.
341. Harris MB, Reichmann WM, Bono CM, et al; Mortality in elderly patients after cervical spine fractures. *J Bone Joint Surg Am.* 2010;92(3):567–574.
342. Widder S, Doig C, Burrowes P, et al. Prospective evaluation of computed tomographic scanning for the spinal clearance of obtunded trauma patients: preliminary results. *J Trauma.* 2004;56(6):1179–1184.
343. Schenarts PJ, Diaz J, Kaiser C, et al. Prospective comparison of admission computed tomographic scan and plain films of the upper cervical spine in trauma patients with altered mental status. *J Trauma.* 2001;51(4):663–668.
344. Mace SE. The unstable occult cervical spine fracture: a review. *Am J Emerg Med.* 1992;10(2):136–142.
345. Barry TB, McNamara RM. Clinical decision rules and cervical spine injury in an elderly patient: a word of caution. *J Emerg Med.* 2005;29(4):433–436.
346. Heffernan DS, Schermer CR, Lu SW. What defines a distracting injury in cervical spine assessment? *J Trauma.* 2005;59(6):1396–1399.
347. Holcomb JB, McMullin NR, Kozar RA, et al. Morbidity from rib fractures increases after age 45. *J Am Coll Surg.* 2003;196(4):549–555.
348. Bulger EM, Arneson MA, Mock CN, et al. Rib fractures in the elderly. *J Trauma.* 2000;48(6):1040–1046.
349. Karmakar MK, Critchley LA, Ho AM, et al. Continuous thoracic paravertebral infusion of bupivacaine for pain management in patients with multiple fractured ribs. *Chest.* 2003;123(2):424–431.
350. Bulger EM, Edwards T, Klotz P, Jurkovich GJ. Epidural analgesia improves outcome after multiple rib fractures. *Surgery.* 2004;136(2):426–430.
351. Kieninger AN, Bair HA, Bendick PJ, Howells GA. Epidural versus intravenous pain control in elderly patients with rib fractures. *Am J Surg.* 2005;189(3):327–330.
352. Falimirski ME, Provost D. Nonsurgical management of solid abdominal organ injury in patients over 55 years of age. *Am Surg.* 2000;66(7):631–635.
353. Krause KR, Howells GA, Bair HA, et al. Nonoperative management of blunt splenic injury in adults 55 years and older: a twenty-year experience. *Am Surg.* 2000;66(7):636–640.
354. Franklin GA, Casos SR. Current advances in the surgical approach to abdominal trauma. *Injury.* 2006;37(12):1143–1156.
355. Keller JM, Sciadini MF, Sinclair E, O'Toole RV. Geriatric trauma: demographics, injuries, and mortality. *J Orthop Trauma.* 2012;26:e161–e165.
356. Looker AC, Johnston CC Jr, Wahner HW, et al. Prevalence of low femoral bone density in older U.S. women from NHANES III. *J Bone Miner Res.* 1995;10(5):796–802.
357. Wehren LE. The epidemiology of osteoporosis and fractures in geriatric medicine. *Clin Geriatr Med.* 2003;19(2):245–258.
358. Henry SM, Pollak AN, Jones AL, et al. Pelvic fracture in geriatric patients: a distinct clinical entity. *J Trauma.* 2002;53(1):15–20.
359. Dyer GS, Vrahas MS. Review of the pathophysiology and acute management of haemorrhage in pelvic fracture. *Injury.* 2006;37(7):602–613.
360. Pohlemann T, Bosch U, Gansslen A, Tscherne H. The Hannover experience in management of pelvic fractures. *Clin Orthop Relat Res.* 1994;(305):69–80.
361. Perry JF Jr. Pelvic open fractures. *Clin Orthop Relat Res.* 1980;(151):41–45.
362. Hanson PB, Milne JC, Chapman MW. Open fractures of the pelvis. Review of 43 cases. *J Bone Joint Surg Br.* 1991;73(2):325–329.
363. Dente CJ, Feliciano DV, Rozycki GS, et al. The outcome of open pelvic fractures in the modern era. *Am J Surg.* 2005;190(6):830–835.
364. Bone LB, McNamara K, Shine B, et al. Mortality in multiple trauma patients with fractures. *J Trauma.* 1994;37(2):262–264.
365. Dunham CM, Bosse MJ, Clancy TV, et al; EAST Practice Management Guidelines Work Group. Practice management guidelines for the optimal timing of long-bone fracture stabilization in polytrauma patients: the EAST Practice Management Guidelines Work Group. *J Trauma.* 2001;50(5):958–967.
366. Crowl AC, Young JS, Kahler DM, et al. Occult hypoperfusion is associated with increased morbidity in patients undergoing early femur fracture fixation. *J Trauma.* 2000;48(2):260–267.
367. Grossman MD, Miller D, Scaff DW, Arcona S. When is an elder old? Effect of preexisting conditions on mortality in geriatric trauma. *J Trauma.* 2002;52(2):242–246.
368. Perdue PW, Watts DD, Kaufmann CR, Trask AL. Differences in mortality between elderly and younger adult trauma patients: geriatric status increases risk of delayed death. *J Trauma.* 1998;45(4):805–810.
369. Morris JA Jr, MacKenzie EJ, Damiano AM, Bass SM. Mortality in trauma patients: the interaction between host factors and severity. *J Trauma.* 1990;30(12):1476–1482.
370. Taylor MD, Tracy JK, Meyer W, et al. Trauma in the elderly: intensive care unit resource use and outcome. *J Trauma.* 2002;53(3):407–414.
371. Hashmi A, Ibrahim-Zada I, Rhee P, et al. Predictors of mortality in geriatric trauma patients: a systematic review and meta-analysis. *Trauma Acute Care Surg.* 2014;76(3):894–901.

372. Lerolle N, Trinquart L, Bornstain C, et al. Increased intensity of treatment and decreased mortality in elderly patients in an intensive care unit over a decade. *Crit Care Med.* 2010;38(1):59–64.
373. McKevitt EC, Calvert E, Ng A, et al. Geriatric trauma: resource use and patient outcomes. *Can J Surg.* 2003;46(3):211–215.
374. Ross N, Timberlake GA, Rubino LJ, Kerstein MD. High cost of trauma care in the elderly. *South Med J.* 1989;82(7):857–859.
375. Young JS, Cephas GA, Blow O. Outcome and cost of trauma among the elderly: a real-life model of a single-payer reimbursement system. *J Trauma.* 1998;45(4):800–804.
376. Grossman M, Scaff DW, Miller D, et al. Functional outcomes in octogenarian trauma. *J Trauma.* 2003;55(1):26–32.
377. van Aalst JA, Morris JA Jr, Yates HK, et al. Severely injured geriatric patients return to independent living: a study of factors influencing function and independence. *J Trauma.* 1991;31(8):1096–1101.
378. Carrillo EH, Richardson JD, Malias MA, et al. Long term outcome of blunt trauma care in the elderly. *Surg Gynecol Obstet.* 1993;176(6):559–564.
379. Richmond TS, Kauder D, Strumpf N, Meredith T. Characteristics and outcomes of serious traumatic injury in older adults. *J Am Geriatr Soc.* 2002;50(2):215–222.
380. Mosenthal AC, Livingston DH, Lavery RF, et al. The effect of age on functional outcome in mild traumatic brain injury: 6-month report of a prospective multicenter trial. *J Trauma.* 2004;56(5):1042–1048.
381. Fallon WF Jr, Rader E, Zyzanski S, et al. Geriatric outcomes are improved by a geriatric trauma consultation service. *J Trauma.* 2006;61(5):1040–1046.
382. Biffl WL, Biffl SE. Rehabilitation of the geriatric surgical patient: predicting needs and optimizing outcomes. *Surg Clin North Am.* 2015;95(1):173–190.
383. National Center for Health Statistics. Deaths and mortality. Centers for Disease Control and Prevention website. Available at http://www.cdc.gov/nchs/fastats/deaths.htm. Updated April 27, 2016. Accessed January 2016.
384. Halpern NA, Pastores SM, Greenstein RJ. Critical care medicine in the United States 1985–2000: an analysis of bed numbers, use, and costs. *Crit Care Med.* 2004;32(6):1254–1259.
385. Halpern NA, Pastores SM. Critical care medicine in the United States 2000-2005: an analysis of bed numbers, occupancy rates, payer mix, and costs. *Crit Care Med.* 2010;38(1):65–71.
386. Callahan D. Old age and new policy. *JAMA.* 1989;261(6):905–906.
387. Levinsky NG. Age as a criterion for rationing health care. *N Engl J Med.* 1990;322(25):1813–1816.
388. Hubbard RE, Lyons RA, Woodhouse KW, et al. Absence of ageism in access to critical care: a cross-sectional study. *Age Ageing.* 2003;32(4):382–387.
389. Nuckton TJ, List ND. Age as a factor in critical care unit admissions. *Arch Intern Med.* 1995;155(10):1087–1092.
390. Attitudes of critical care medicine professionals concerning distribution of intensive care resources. The Society of Critical Care Medicine Ethics Committee. *Crit Care Med.* 1994;22(2):358–362.
391. Somme D, Maillet JM, Gisselbrecht M, et al. Critically ill old and the oldest-old patients in intensive care: short- and long-term outcomes. *Intensive Care Med.* 2003;29(12):2137–2143.
392. Orsini J, Butala A, Salomon S, et al. Prognostic factors associated with adverse outcome among critically ill elderly patients admitted to the intensive care unit. *Geriatr Gerontol Int.* 2015;15(7):889–894.
393. Heyland DK, Garland A, Bagshaw SM, et al. Recovery after critical illness in patients aged 80 years or older: a multi-center prospective observational cohort study. *Intensive Care Med.* 2015;41(11):1911–1920.
394. Hennessy D, Juzwishin K, Yergens D, et al. Outcomes of elderly survivors of intensive care: a review of the literature. *Chest.* 2005;127(5):1764–1774.
395. Hamel MB, Teno JM, Goldman L, Lynn J, et al. Patient age and decisions to withhold life-sustaining treatments from seriously ill, hospitalized adults. SUPPORT Investigators. Study to Understand Prognoses and Preferences for Outcomes and Risks of Treatment. *Ann Intern Med.* 1999;130(2):116–125.
396. Somogyi-Zalud E, Zhong Z, Hamel MB, Lynn J. The use of life-sustaining treatments in hospitalized persons aged 80 and older. *J Am Geriatr Soc.* 2002;50(5):930–934.
397. McDermid RC, Stelfox HT, Bagshaw SM. Frailty in the critically ill: a novel concept. *Crit Care.* 2011;15(1):301.
398. Hamel MB, Davis RB, Teno JM, et al. Older age, aggressiveness of care, and survival for seriously ill, hospitalized adults. SUPPORT Investigators. Study to Understand Prognoses and Preferences for Outcomes and Risks of Treatments. *Ann Intern Med.* 1999;131(10):721–728.
399. Kleinpell RM. Exploring outcomes after critical illness in the elderly. *Outcomes Manag.* 2003;7(4):159–169.
400. Layon AJ, George BE, Hamby B, et al. Do elderly patients overutilize healthcare resources and benefit less from them than younger patients? A study of patients who underwent craniotomy for treatment of neoplasm. *Crit Care Med.* 1995;23(5):829–834.
401. Bagshaw SM, McDermid RC. The role of frailty in outcomes from critical illness. *Curr Opin Crit Care.* 2013;19(5):496–503.
402. Baldwin MR, Reid MC, Westlake AA, et al. The feasibility of measuring frailty to predict disability and mortality in older medical intensive care unit survivors. *J Crit Care.* 2014;29(3):401–408.
403. Zeng A, Song X, Dong J, et al. Mortality in relation to frailty in patients admitted to a specialized geriatric intensive care unit. *J Gerontol A Biol Sci Med Sci.* 2015;70(12):1586–1594.
404. Blair SL, Schwarz RE. Advanced age does not contribute to increased risks or poor outcome after major abdominal operations. *Am Surg.* 2001;67(12):1123–1127.
405. Rady MY, Johnson DJ. Hospital discharge to care facility: a patient-centered outcome for the evaluation of intensive care for octogenarians. *Chest.* 2004;126(5):1583–1591.
406. Wehler M, Geise A, Hadzionerovic D, et al. Health-related quality of life of patients with multiple organ dysfunction: individual changes and comparison with normative population. *Crit Care Med.* 2003;31(4):1094–1101.
407. Kleinpell RM, Ferrans CE. Quality of life of elderly patients after treatment in the ICU. *Res Nurs Health.* 2002;25(3):212–221.
408. Eddleston JM, White P, Guthrie E. Survival, morbidity, and quality of life after discharge from intensive care. *Crit Care Med.* 2000;28(7):2293–2299.
409. Chelluri L, Pinsky MR, Donahoe MP, Grenvik A. Long-term outcome of critically ill elderly patients requiring intensive care. *JAMA.* 1993;269(24):3119–3123.
410. Wu AW, Rubin HR, Rosen MJ. Are elderly people less responsive to intensive care? *J Am Geriatr Soc.* 1990;38(6):621–627.
411. Teno JM, Fisher E, Hamel MB, et al. Decision-making and outcomes of prolonged ICU stays in seriously ill patients. *J Am Geriatr Soc.* 2000;48 (5 Suppl):S70–S74.
412. Levin TT, Moreno B, Silvester W, Kissane DW. End-of-life communication in the intensive care unit. *Gen Hosp Psychiatry.* 2010;32(4):433–442.
413. Wilkinson DJ, Savulescu J. Knowing when to stop: futility in the ICU. *Curr Opin Anaesthesiol.* 2011;24(2):160–165.
414. Niederman MS, Berger JT. The delivery of futile care is harmful to other patients. *Crit Care Med.* 2010;38(10 Suppl):S518–S522.
415. Fawole OA, Dy SM, Wilson RF, et al. A systematic review of communication quality improvement interventions for patients with advanced and serious illness. *J Gen Intern Med.* 2013;28(4):570–577.
416. Herrera AP, Snipes SA, King DW, et al. Disparate inclusion of older adults in clinical trials: priorities and opportunities for policy and practice change. *Am J Public Health.* 2010;100(Suppl 1):S105–S112.
417. Vestal RE, Norris AH, Tobin JD, et al. Antipyrine metabolism in man: influence of age, alcohol, caffeine, and smoking. *Clin Pharmacol Ther.* 1975;18(4):425–432.
418. Abernethy DR, Kerzner L. Age effects on alpha-1-acid glycoprotein concentration and imipramine plasma protein binding. *J Am Geriatr Soc.* 1984;32(10):705–708.
419. Wilkinson GR. Drug metabolism and variability among patients in drug response. *N Engl J Med.* 2005;352(21):2211–2221.
420. Nebert DW, Russell DW. Clinical importance of the cytochromes P450. *Lancet.* 2002;360(9340):1155–1162.
421. CYP3A and drug interactions. *Med Lett Drugs Ther.*2005;47(1212):54–55.
422. Crowley JJ, Cusack BJ, Jue SG, et al. Aging and drug interactions. II. Effect of phenytoin and smoking on the oxidation of theophylline and cortisol in healthy men. *J Pharmacol Exp Ther.* 1988;245(2):513–523.
423. Nolan L, O'Malley K. Prescribing for the elderly. Part I: Sensitivity of the elderly to adverse drug reactions. *J Am Geriatr Soc.* 1988;36(2):142–149.
424. Inouye SK, Westendorp RG, Saczynski JS. Delirium in elderly people. *Lancet.* 2014;383(9920):911–922.
425. Kakuma R, du Fort GG, Arsenault L, et al. Delirium in older emergency department patients discharged home: effect on survival. *J Am Geriatr Soc.* 2003;51(4):443–450.
426. O'Keeffe S, Lavan J. The prognostic significance of delirium in older hospital patients. *J Am Geriatr Soc.* 1997;45(2):174–178.
427. Cameron DJ, Thomas RI, Mulvihill M, Bronheim H. Delirium: a test of the Diagnostic and Statistical Manual III criteria on medical inpatients. *J Am Geriatr Soc.* 1987;35(11):1007–1010.
428. Foreman MD, Wakefield B, Culp K, Milisen K. Delirium in elderly patients: an overview of the state of the Science. *J Gerontol Nurs.* 2001;27(4):12–20.
429. Inouye SK, Bogardus ST Jr, Charpentier PA, et al. A multicomponent intervention to prevent delirium in hospitalized older patients. *N Engl J Med.* 1999;340(9):669–676.
430. Inouye SK, Viscoli CM, Horwitz RI, et al. A predictive model for delirium in hospitalized elderly medical patients based on admission characteristics. *Ann Intern Med.* 1993;119(6):474–481.

431. McCusker J, Cole MG, Dendukuri N, et al. Does delirium increase hospital stay? *J Am Geriatr Soc.* 2003;51(11):1539–1546.
432. Cole MG, Primeau FJ. Prognosis of delirium in elderly hospital patients. *CMAJ.* 1993;149(1):41–46.
433. Salluh JI, Wang H, Schneider EB, et al. Outcome of delirium in critically ill patients: systematic review and meta-analysis. *BMJ.* 2015;350:h2538.
434. Cole MG. Delirium in elderly patients. *Am J Geriatr Psychiatry.* 2004;12(1):7–21.
435. Cole MG, Primeau FJ, Elie LM. Delirium: prevention, treatment, and outcome studies. *J Geriatr Psychiatry Neurol.* 1998;11(3):126–137.
436. Ely EW, Shintani A, Truman B, et al. Delirium as a predictor of mortality in mechanically ventilated patients in the intensive care unit. *JAMA.* 2004;291(14):1753–1762.
437. McNicoll L, Pisani MA, Zhang Y, et al. Delirium in the intensive care unit: occurrence and clinical course in older patients. *J Am Geriatr Soc.* 2003;51(5):591–598.
438. Dubois MJ, Bergeron N, Dumont M, et al. Delirium in an intensive care unit: a study of risk factors. *Intensive Care Med.* 2001;27(8):1297–1304.
439. Aldemir M, Ozen S, Kara IH, et al. Predisposing factors for delirium in the surgical intensive care unit. *Crit Care.* 2001;5(5):265–270.
440. Morrison RS, Magaziner J, Gilbert M, et al. Relationship between pain and opioid analgesics on the development of delirium following hip fracture. *J Gerontol A Biol Sci Med Sci.* 2003;58(1):76–81.
441. Van Rompaey B, Elseviers MM, Schuurmans MJ, et al. Risk factors for delirium in intensive care patients: a prospective cohort study. *Crit Care.* 2009;13(3):R77.
442. Zaal IJ, Devlin JW, Peelen LM, Slooter AJ. A systematic review of risk factors for delirium in the ICU. *Crit Care Med.* 2015;43(1):40–47.
443. Mesulam MM, Waxman SG, Geschwind N, Sabin TD. Acute confusional states with right middle cerebral artery infarctions. *J Neurol Neurosurg Psychiatry.* 1976;39(1):84–89.
444. Teasdale E, Cardoso E, Galbraith S, Teasdale G. CT scan in severe diffuse head injury: physiological and clinical correlations. *J Neurol Neurosurg Psychiatry.* 1984;47(6):600–603.
445. Noldy NE, Carlen PL. Acute, withdrawal, and chronic alcohol effects in man: event-related potential and quantitative EEG techniques. *Ann Med.* 1990;22(5):333–339.
446. van Sweden B, Mellerio F. Toxic ictal delirium. *Biol Psychiatry.* 1989;25(4):449–458.
447. Trzepacz PT, Sclabassi RJ, Van Thiel DH. Delirium: a subcortical phenomenon? *J Neuropsychiatry Clin Neurosci.* 1989;1(3):283–290.
448. Woods JC, Mion LC, Connor JT, et al. Agitation among ventilated medical intensive care unit patients: frequency, characteristics and outcomes. *Intensive Care Med.* 2004;30(6):1066–1072.
449. Konsman JP, Parnet P, Dantzer R. Cytokine-induced sickness behaviour: mechanisms and implications. *Trends Neurosci.* 2002;25(3):154–159.
450. Allan SM. The role of pro- and antiinflammatory cytokines in neurodegeneration. *Ann N Y Acad Sci.* 2000;917:84–93.
451. Young GB, Bolton CF, Austin TW, et al. The encephalopathy associated with septic illness. *Clin Invest Med.* 1990;13(6):297–304.
452. Sprung CL, Peduzzi PN, Shatney CH, et al. Impact of encephalopathy on mortality in the sepsis syndrome. The Veterans Administration Systemic Sepsis Cooperative Study Group. *Crit Care Med.* 1990;18(8):801–806.
453. Moller K, Strauss GI, Qvist J, et al. Cerebral blood flow and oxidative metabolism during human endotoxemia. *J Cereb Blood Flow Metab.* 2002;22(10):1262–1270.
454. Wong ML, Bongiorno PB, Rettori V, et al. Interleukin (IL) 1beta, IL-1 receptor antagonist, IL-10, and IL-13 gene expression in the central nervous system and anterior pituitary during systemic inflammation: pathophysiological implications. *Proc Natl Acad Sci U S A.* 1997;94(1):227–232.
455. Sharshar T, Gray F, Poron F, et al. Multifocal necrotizing leukoencephalopathy in septic shock. *Crit Care Med.* 2002;30(10):2371–2375.
456. Sharshar T, Annane D, de la Grandmaison GL, et al. The neuropathology of septic shock. *Brain Pathol.* 2004;14(1):21–33.
457. Cole MG, Bailey R, Bonnycastle M, et al. Partial and no recovery from delirium in older hospitalized adults: frequency and baseline risk factors. *J Am Geriatr Soc.* 2015;63(11):2340–2348.
458. van der Mast RC, Fekkes D. Serotonin and amino acids: partners in delirium pathophysiology? *Semin Clin Neuropsychiatry.* 2000;5(2):125–131.
459. Mussi C, Ferrari R, Ascari S, et al. Importance of serum anticholinergic activity in the assessment of elderly patients with delirium. *J Geriatr Psychiatry Neurol.* 1999;12(2):82–86.
460. Tune LE, Egeli S. Acetylcholine and delirium. *Dement Geriatr Cogn Disord.* 1999;10(5):342–344.
461. Roche V. Southwestern Internal Medicine Conference. Etiology and management of delirium. *Am J Med Sci.* 2003;325(1):20–30.
462. Choi SH, Lee H, Chung TS, et al. Neural network functional connectivity during and after an episode of delirium. *Am J Psychiatry.* 2012;169(5):498–507.
463. American Psychiatric Association. *Diagnostic and Statistical Manual of Mental Disorders.* 5th ed. Washington DC: American Psychiatric Association; 2013.
464. Trzepacz PT, Mittal D, Torres R, et al. Validation of the Delirium Rating Scale-revised-98: comparison with the delirium rating scale and the cognitive test for delirium. *J Neuropsychiatry Clin Neurosci.* 2001;13(2):229–242.
465. Bergeron N, Dubois MJ, Dumont M, et al. Intensive Care Delirium Screening Checklist: evaluation of a new screening tool. *Intensive Care Med.* 2001;27(5):859–864.
466. Inouye SK, van Dyck CH, Alessi CA, et al. Clarifying confusion: the confusion assessment method. A new method for detection of delirium. *Ann Intern Med.* 1990;113(12):941–948.
467. Gusmao-Flores D, Salluh JI, Chalhub RÁ, Quarantini LC. The confusion assessment method for the intensive care unit (CAM-ICU) and intensive care delirium screening checklist (ICDSC) for the diagnosis of delirium: a systematic review and meta-analysis of clinical studies. *CritCare.* 2012;16(4):R115.
468. Kuczmarska A, Ngo LH, Guess J, et al. Detection of delirium in hospitalized older general medicine patients: a comparison of the 3D-CAM and CAM-ICU. *J Gen Intern Med.* 2016;31(3):297–303.
469. Meagher DJ, O'Hanlon D, O'Mahony E, et al. Relationship between symptoms and motoric subtype of delirium. *J Neuropsychiatry Clin Neurosci.* 2000;12(1):51–56.
470. Lipowski ZJ. Delirium in the elderly patient. *N Engl J Med.* 1989;320(9):578–582.
471. Ross CA, Peyser CE, Shapiro I, et al. Delirium: phenomenologic and etiologic subtypes. *Int Psychogeriatr.* 1991;3(2):135–147.
472. Mistraletti G, Pelosi P, Mantovani ES, et al. Delirium: clinical approach and prevention. *Best Pract Res Clin Anaesthesiol.* 2012;26(3):311–326.
473. Peterson JF, Pun BT, Dittus RS, et al. Delirium and its motoric subtypes: a study of 614 critically ill patients. *J Am Geriatr Soc.* 2006;54(3):479–484.
474. Francis J, Martin D, Kapoor WN. A prospective study of delirium in hospitalized elderly. *JAMA.* 1990;263(8):1097–1101.
475. Ely EW, Siegel MD, Inouye SK. Delirium in the intensive care unit: an under-recognized syndrome of organ dysfunction. *Semin Respir Crit Care Med.* 2001;22(2):115–126.
476. Ely EW, Stephens RK, Jackson JC, et al. Current opinions regarding the importance, diagnosis, and management of delirium in the intensive care unit: a survey of 912 healthcare professionals. *Crit Care Med.* 2004;32(1):106–112.
477. Inouye SK. Delirium in older persons. *N Engl J Med.* 2006;354(11):1157–1165.
478. Card E, Pandharipande P, Tomes C, et al. Emergence from general anaesthesia and evolution of delirium signs in the post-anaesthesia care unit. *Br J Anaesth.* 2015;115(3):411–417.
479. Morandi A, Jackson JC. Delirium in the intensive care unit: a review. *Neurol Clin.* 2011;29(4):749–763.
480. Deiner S, Silverstein JH. Postoperative delirium and cognitive dysfunction. *Br J Anaesth.* 2009;103(Suppl 1):i41–i46.
481. Selnes OA, Grega MA, Bailey MM, et al. Do management strategies for coronary artery disease influence 6-year cognitive outcomes? *Ann Thorac Surg.* 2009;88(2):445–454.
482. Evered L, Scott DA, Silbert B, Maruff P. Postoperative cognitive dysfunction is independent of type of surgery and anesthetic. *Anesth Analg.* 2011;112(5):1179–1185.
483. Dyer CB, Ashton CM, Teasdale TA. Postoperative delirium: a review of 80 primary data-collection studies. *Arch Intern Med.* 1995;155(5):461–465.
484. Bedford PD. Adverse cerebral effects of anaesthesia on old people. *Lancet.* 1955;269(6884):259–263.
485. Moller JT. Cerebral dysfunction after anaesthesia. *Acta Anaesthesiol Scand Suppl.* 1997;110:13–16.
486. Rogers MP, Liang MH, Daltroy LH, et al. Delirium after elective orthopedic surgery: risk factors and natural history. *Int J Psychiatry Med.* 1989;19(2):109–121.
487. Monk TG, Weldon BC, Garvan CW, et al. Predictors of cognitive dysfunction after major noncardiac surgery. *Anesthesiology.* 2008;108(1):18–30.
488. Selnes OA, Goldsborough MA, Borowicz LM Jr, et al. Determinants of cognitive change after coronary artery bypass surgery: a multifactorial problem. *Ann Thorac Surg.* 1999;67(6):1669–1676.
489. Selnes OA, Royall RM, Grega MA, et al. Cognitive changes 5 years after coronary artery bypass grafting: is there evidence of late decline? *Arch Neurol.* 2001;58(4):598–604.

490. Stroobant N, Van Nooten G, Van Belleghem Y, Vingerhoets G. Relation between neurocognitive impairment, embolic load, and cerebrovascular reactivity following on- and off-pump coronary artery bypass grafting. *Chest.* 2005;127(6):1967–1976.
491. Newman MF, Kirchner JL, Phillips-Bute B, et al; Neurological Outcome Research Group and the Cardiothoracic Anesthesiology Research Endeavors Investigators. Longitudinal assessment of neurocognitive function after coronary-artery bypass surgery.. *N Engl J Med.* 2001;344(6):395–402.
492. Dodds C, Allison J. Postoperative cognitive deficit in the elderly surgical patient. *Br J Anaesth.* 1998;81(3):449–462.
493. Bryson GL, Wyand A. Evidence-based clinical update: general anesthesia and the risk of delirium and postoperative cognitive dysfunction. *Can J Anaesth.* 2006;53(7):669–677.
494. Bekker AY, Weeks EJ. Cognitive function after anaesthesia in the elderly. *Best Pract Res Clin Anaesthesiol.* 2003;17(2):259–272.
495. Krenk L, Rasmussen LS, Kehlet H, New insights into the pathophysiology of postoperative cognitive dysfunction. *Acta Anaesthesiol Scand.* 2010;54(8):951–956.
496. Marcantonio ER, Flacker JM, Wright RJ, Resnick NM. Reducing delirium after hip fracture: a randomized trial. *J Am Geriatr Soc.* 2001; 49(5):5165–5122.
497. Sachdeva A, Choudhary M, Chandra M. Alcohol withdrawal syndrome: benzodiazepines and beyond. *J Clin Diagn Res.* 2015;9(9):VE01–VE07.
498. Barr J, Fraser GL, Puntillo K, et al. Clinical practice guidelines for the management of pain, agitation, and delirium in adult patients in the intensive care unit. *Crit Care Med.* 2013;41(1):263–306.
499. Nelson S, Muzyk AJ, Bucklin MH, et al. Defining the role of dexmedetomidine in the prevention of delirium in the intensive care unit. *Biomed Res Int.* 2015;2015:635737.
500. Jakob SM, Ruokonen E, Grounds RM, et al. Dexmedetomidine vs midazolam or propofol for sedation during prolonged mechanical ventilation: two randomized controlled trials. *JAMA.* 2012;307(11):1151–1160.
501. Jacobi J, Fraser GL, Coursin DB, et al; Task Force of the American College of Critical Care Medicine (ACCM) of the Society of Critical Care Medicine (SCCM), American Society of Health-System Pharmacists (ASHP), American College of Chest Physicians. Clinical practice guidelines for the sustained use of sedatives and analgesics in the critically ill adult. *Crit Care Med.* 2002;30(1):119–141.
502. Milbrandt EB, Kersten A, Kong L, et al. Haloperidol use is associated with lower hospital mortality in mechanically ventilated patients. *Crit Care Med.* 2005;33(1):226–229.
503. Ford AH, Almeida OP. Pharmacological interventions for preventing delirium in the elderly. *Maturitas.* 2015;81(2):287–292.
504. Roger VL, Go AS, Lloyd-Jones DM, et al; American Heart Association Statistics Committee and Stroke Statistics Subcommittee. Heart disease and stroke statistics: 2011 update: a report from the American Heart Association. *Circulation.* 2011;123(4):e18–e209.
505. Sacco RL. Risk factors, outcomes, and stroke subtypes for ischemic stroke. *Neurology.* 1997;495(Suppl 4):S39–S44.
506. Sacco RL. Reducing the risk of stroke in diabetes: what have we learned that is new? *Diabetes Obes Metab.* 2002;4(Suppl 1)S27–S34.
507. Sherzai AZ, Elkind MS. Advances in stroke prevention. *Ann N Y Acad Sci.* 2015;1338:1–15.
508. Pulsinelli WA. Pathophysiology and management of major neurological symptoms. In: Bennett JC, Plum F, eds. *Cecil Textbook of Medicine.* 20th ed. Philadelphia, PA: WB Saunders; 1996:2063–2073.
509. Atherosclerotic disease of the aortic arch as a risk factor for recurrent ischemic stroke. The French Study of Aortic Plaques in Stroke Group. *N Engl J Med.* 1996;334(19):1216–1221.
510. Jauch EC, Saver JL, Adams HP Jr, et al. Guidelines for the early management of patients with acute ischemic stroke: a guideline for healthcare professionals from the American Heart Association/American Stroke Association. *Stroke.* 2013;44(3):870–947.
511. Hacke W, Kaste M, Bluhmki E, et al. Thrombolysis with alteplase 3 to 4.5 hours after acute ischemic stroke. *N Engl J Med.* 2008;359(13):1317–1329.
512. Lees KR, Bluhmki E, von Kummer R, et al. Time to treatment with intravenous alteplase and outcome in stroke: an updated pooled analysis of ECASS, ATLANTIS, NINDS, and EPITHET trials. *Lancet.* 2010; 375(9727):1695–1703.
513. Lorenzano S, Toni D; TESPI trial Investigators TESPI (Thrombolysis in Elderly Stroke Patients in Italy. A randomized controlled trial of alteplase (rt-PA) versus standard treatment in acute ischaemic stroke in patients aged more than 80 years where thrombolysis is initiated within three hours after stroke onset. *Int J Stroke.* 2012;7(3):250–257.
514. Berrouschot J, Rother J, Glahn J, et al. Outcome and severe hemorrhagic complications of intravenous thrombolysis with tissue plasminogen activator in very old (> or = 80 years) stroke patients. *Stroke.* 2005;36(11):2421–2425.
515. Tissue plasminogen activator for acute ischemic stroke. The National Institute of Neurological Disorders and Stroke rt-PA Stroke Study Group. *N Engl J Med.* 1995;333(24):1581–1587.
516. Engelter ST, Bonati LH, Lyrer PA. Intravenous thrombolysis in stroke patients of > or = 80 versus < 80 years of age: a systematic review across cohort studies. *Age Ageing.* 2006;35(6):572–580.
517. Pundik S, McWilliams-Dunnigan L, Blackham KL, et al. Older age does not increase risk of hemorrhagic complications after intravenous and/or intra-arterial thrombolysis for acute stroke. *J Stroke Cerebrovasc Dis.* 2008;17(5):266–272.
518. Costello CA, Campbell BC, Perez de la Ossa N, et al. Age over 80 years is not associated with increased hemorrhagic transformation after stroke thrombolysis. *J Clin Neurosci.* 2012;19(3):360–363.
519. Kasner SE. Clinical interpretation and use of stroke scales. *Lancet Neurol.* 2006;5(7):603–612.
520. Finley Caulfield A, Wijman CA. Management of acute ischemic stroke. *Neurol Clin.* 2008;26(2):345–371.
521. Gresham GE, Fitzpatrick TE, Wolf PA, et al. Residual disability in survivors of stroke–the Framingham study. *N Engl J Med.* 1975;293(19):954–956.
522. Kelly-Hayes M, Wolf PA, Kannel WB, et al. Factors influencing survival and need for institutionalization following stroke: the Framingham Study. *Arch Phys Med Rehabil.* 1988;69(6):415–418.
523. Sacco RL, Wolf PA, Kannel WB, et al. Survival and recurrence following stroke. The Framingham study. *Stroke.* 1982;13(3):290–295.
524. Cooke JR, Ancoli-Israel S. Sleep and its disorders in older adults. *Psychiatr Clin North Am.* 2006;29(4):1077–1093.
525. Foley DJ, Monjan A, Simonsick EM, et al. Incidence and remission of insomnia among elderly adults: an epidemiologic study of 6,800 persons over three years. *Sleep.* 1999;22(Suppl 2):S366–S372.
526. Foley D, Ancoli-Israel S, Britz P, et al. Sleep disturbances and chronic disease in older adults: results of the 2003 National Sleep Foundation Sleep in America Survey. *J Psychosom Res.* 2004;56(5):497–502.
527. Neubauer DN. Sleep problems in the elderly. *Am Fam Physician.* 1999; 59(9):2551–2558, 2559–2560.
528. Vgontzas AN, Kales A. Sleep and its disorders. *Annu Rev Med.* 1999; 50:387–400.
529. Schubert CR, Cruickshanks KJ, Dalton DS, et al. Prevalence of sleep problems and quality of life in an older population. *Sleep.* 2002;25(8):889–893.
530. Brassington GS, King AC, Bliwise DL. Sleep problems as a risk factor for falls in a sample of community-dwelling adults aged 64–99 years. *J Am Geriatr Soc.* 2000;48(10):1234–1240.
531. Cricco M, Simonsick EM, Foley DJ. The impact of insomnia on cognitive functioning in older adults. *J Am Geriatr Soc.* 2001;49(9):1185–1189.
532. Manabe K, Matsui T, Yamaya M, et al. Sleep patterns and mortality among elderly patients in a geriatric hospital. *Gerontology.* 2000;46(6):318–322.
533. Shochat T, Martin J, Marler M, Ancoli-Israel S. Illumination levels in nursing home patients: effects on sleep and activity rhythms. *J Sleep Res.* 2000;9(4):373–379.
534. Espana RA, Scammell TE. Sleep neurobiology for the clinician. *Sleep.* 2004;27(4):811–820.
535. Feinsilver SH. Sleep in the elderly. What is normal? *Clin Geriatr Med.* 2003;19(1):177–188, viii.
536. Kamel NS, Gammack JK. Insomnia in the elderly: cause, approach, and treatment. *Am J Med.* 2006;119(6):463–469.
537. Johns MW. A new method for measuring daytime sleepiness: the Epworth sleepiness scale. *Sleep.* 1991;14(6):540–545.
538. Shochat T, Pillar G. Sleep apnoea in the older adult: pathophysiology, epidemiology, consequences and management. *Drugs Aging.* 2003; 20(8):551–560.
539. Olson EJ, Boeve BF, Silber MH. Rapid eye movement sleep behaviour disorder: demographic, clinical and laboratory findings in 93 cases. *Brain.* 2000;123(Pt 2):331–339.
540. Littner MR, Kushida C, Anderson WM, et al; Standards of Practice Committee of the American Academy of Sleep Medicine. Practice parameters for the dopaminergic treatment of restless legs syndrome and periodic limb movement disorder. *Sleep.* 2004;27(3):557–559.
541. Friese RS, Diaz-Arrastia R, McBride D, et al. Quantity and quality of sleep in the surgical intensive care unit: are our patients sleeping? *J Trauma.* 2007;63(6):1210–1214.
542. Tamburri LM, DiBrienza R, Zozula R, Redeker NS. Nocturnal care interactions with patients in critical care units. *Am J Crit Care.* 2004; 13(2):102–112.
543. Chan MC, Spieth PM, Quinn K, et al. Circadian rhythms: from basic mechanisms to the intensive care unit. *Crit Care Med.* 2012;40(1):246–53.

544. Oldham MA, Lee HB, Desan PH. Circadian rhythm disruption in the critically ill: an opportunity for improving outcomes. *Crit Care Med.* 2016;44(1):207–217.
545. Nakamura TJ, Nakamura W, Yamazaki S, et al. Age-related decline in circadian output. *J Neurosci.* 2011;31(28):10201–10205.
546. Kobayashi R, Kohsaka M, Fukuda N, et al. Effects of morning bright light on sleep in healthy elderly women. *Psychiatry Clin Neurosci.* 1999;53(2):237–238.
547. Fetveit A, Skjerve A, Bjorvatn B. Bright light treatment improves sleep in institutionalised elderly—an open trial. *Int J Geriatr Psychiatry.* 2003;18(6):520–526.
548. Kupfer DJ, Reynolds CF 3rd. Management of insomnia. *N Engl J Med.* 1997;336(5):341–346.
549. Pisani MA, Murphy TE, Araujo KL, et al. Benzodiazepine and opioid use and the duration of intensive care unit delirium in an older population. *Crit Care Med.* 2009;37(1):177–183.
550. Chesson A Jr, Hartse K, Anderson WM, et al. Practice parameters for the evaluation of chronic insomnia. An American Academy of Sleep Medicine report. Standards of Practice Committee of the American Academy of Sleep Medicine. *Sleep.* 2000;23(2):237–241.
551. Howes JB, Ryan J, Fairbrother G, et al. Benzodiazepine prescribing in a Sydney teaching hospital. *Med J Aust.* 1996;165(6):305–308.
552. Kripke DF. Chronic hypnotic use: deadly risks, doubtful benefit. REVIEW ARTICLE. *Sleep Med Rev.* 2000;4(1):5–20.
553. Morin CM, Colecchi C, Stone J, et al. Behavioral and pharmacological therapies for late-life insomnia: a randomized controlled trial. *JAMA.* 1999;281(11):991–999.
554. Obermeyer WH, Benca RM. Effects of drugs on sleep. *Neurol Clin.* 1996;14(4):827–840.
555. Smith MT, Perlis ML, Park A, et al. Comparative meta-analysis of pharmacotherapy and behavior therapy for persistent insomnia. *Am J Psychiatry.* 2002;159(1):5–11.
556. Zdanys KF, Steffens DC. Sleep Disturbances in the Elderly. *Psychiatr Clin North Am.* 2015;38(4):723–741.
557. Sager MA, Franke T, Inouye SK, et al. Functional outcomes of acute medical illness and hospitalization in older persons. *Arch Intern Med.* 1996;156(6):645–652.
558. Covinsky KE, Palmer RM, Fortinsky RH, et al. Loss of independence in activities of daily living in older adults hospitalized with medical illnesses: increased vulnerability with age. *J Am Geriatr Soc.* 2003;51(4): 451–458.
559. Nasraway SA, Button GJ, Rand WM, et al. Survivors of catastrophic illness: outcome after direct transfer from intensive care to extended care facilities. *Crit Care Med.* 2000;28(1):19–25.
560. Montuclard L, Garrouste-Orgeas M, Timsit JF, et al. Outcome, functional autonomy, and quality of life of elderly patients with a long-term intensive care unit stay. *Crit Care Med.* 2000;28(10):3389–3395.
561. Robinson TN, Wallace JI, Wu DS, et al. Accumulated frailty characteristics predict postoperative discharge institutionalization in the geriatric patient. *J Am Coll Surg.*2011;213(1):37–42.
562. Stucki G, Stier-Jarmer M, Grill E, et al. Rationale and principles of early rehabilitation care after an acute injury or illness. *Disabil Rehabil.* 2005;27(7–8):353–359.
563. Creditor MC. Hazards of hospitalization of the elderly. *Ann Intern Med.* 1993;118(3):219–223.
564. Manton KG. A longitudinal study of functional change and mortality in the United States. *J Gerontol.* 1988;43(5):S153–S161.
565. Gill TM, Allore HG, Holford TR, Guo Z. Hospitalization, restricted activity, and the development of disability among older persons. *JAMA.* 2004;292(17):2115–2124.
566. Brummel-Smith K. Rehabilitation. In: Cassel CK, Leipzig RM, Cohen HJ, et al, eds. *Geriatric Medicine: An Evidence-Based Approach.* New York: Springer-Verlag; 2003:259–277.
567. Hoenig H, Nusbaum N, Brummel-Smith K. Geriatric rehabilitation: state of the art. *J Am Geriatr Soc.* 1997;45(11):1371–1381.
568. Brummel NE, Balas MC, Morandi A, et al. Understanding and reducing disability in older adults following critical illness. *Crit Care Med.* 2015;43(6):1265–1275.
569. Landefeld CS, Palmer RM, Kresevic DM, et al. A randomized trial of care in a hospital medical unit especially designed to improve the functional outcomes of acutely ill older patients. *N Engl J Med.* 1995; 332(20):1338–1344.
570. Pijpers E, Ferreira I, Stehouwer CD, Nieuwenhuijzen-Kruseman AC. The frailty dilemma: review of the predictive accuracy of major frailty scores. *Eur J Intern Med.* 2012;23(2):118–123.
571. Ellis G, Langhorne P. Comprehensive geriatric assessment for older hospital patients. *Br Med Bull.* 2005;71:45–59.
572. Counsell SR, Holder CM, Liebenauer LL, et al. Effects of a multicomponent intervention on functional outcomes and process of care in hospitalized older patients: a randomized controlled trial of Acute Care for Elders (ACE) in a community hospital. *J Am Geriatr Soc.* 2000;48(12):1572–1581.
573. Inouye SK, Bogardus ST Jr, Baker DI, et al. The Hospital Elder Life Program: a model of care to prevent cognitive and functional decline in older hospitalized patients. Hospital Elder Life Program. *J Am Geriatr Soc.* 2000;48(12):1697–1706.
574. Winograd CH. Inpatient geriatric consultation. *Clin Geriatr Med.* 1987; 3(1):193–202.
575. Stuck AE, Siu AL, Wieland GD, et al. Comprehensive geriatric assessment: a meta-analysis of controlled trials. *Lancet.* 1993;342(8878):1032–1036.
576. Ellis G, Whitehead MA, Robinson D, et al. Comprehensive geriatric assessment for older adults admitted to hospital: meta-analysis of randomised controlled trials. *BMJ.* 2011;343:d6553.
577. Jolliffe JA, Rees K, Taylor RS, et al. Exercise-based rehabilitation for coronary heart disease. *Cochrane Database Syst Rev.* 2000;4:CD001800.
578. Hammill BG, Curtis LH, Schulman KA, Whellan DJ. Relationship between cardiac rehabilitation and long-term risks of death and myocardial infarction among elderly Medicare beneficiaries. *Circulation.* 2010;121(1):63–70.
579. Pasquali SK, Alexander KP, Peterson ED. Cardiac rehabilitation in the elderly. *Am Heart J.* 2001;142(5):748–755.
580. Lavie CJ, Milani RV, Littman AB. Benefits of cardiac rehabilitation and exercise training in secondary coronary prevention in the elderly. *J Am Coll Cardiol.* 1993;22(3):678–683.
581. Kreizman IJ, Allen D. Aging with cardiopulmonary disease: the rehab perspective. *Phys Med Rehabil Clin North Am.* 2005;16(1):251–265.
582. Lavie CJ, Milani RV. Effects of cardiac rehabilitation programs on exercise capacity, coronary risk factors, behavioral characteristics, and quality of life in a large elderly cohort. *Am J Cardiol.* 1995;76(3):177–179.
583. Ades PA, Waldmann ML, Polk DM, Coflesky JT. Referral patterns and exercise response in the rehabilitation of female coronary patients aged greater than or equal to 62 years. *Am J Cardiol.* 1992;69(17):1422–1425.
584. Cottin Y, Cambou JP, Casillas JM, et al. Specific profile and referral bias of rehabilitated patients after an acute coronary syndrome. *J Cardiopulm Rehabil.* 2004;24(1):38–44.
585. Menezes AR, Lavie CJ, Milani RV, et al. Cardiac rehabilitation and exercise therapy in the elderly: Should we invest in the aged? *J Geriatr Cardiol.* 2012;9(1):68–75.
586. Donnellan C, Hickey A, Hevey D, O'Neill D. Effect of mood symptoms on recovery one year after stroke. *Int J Geriatr Psychiatry.* 2010; 25(12):1288–1295.
587. Kouwenhoven SE, Kirkevold M, Engedal K, Kim HS. Depression in acute stroke: prevalence, dominant symptoms and associated factors: a systematic literature review. *Disabil Rehabil.* 2011;33(7):539–556.
588. Brewer L, Horgan F, Hickey A, Williams D. Stroke rehabilitation: recent advances and future therapies. *QJM.* 2013;106(1):11–25.
589. Arboix A, Garcia-Eroles L, Massons J, et al. Acute stroke in very old people: clinical features and predictors of in-hospital mortality. *J Am Geriatr Soc.* 2000;48(1):36–41.
590. Dobkin BH. Clinical practice. Rehabilitation after stroke. *N Engl J Med.* 2005;352(16):1677–1684.
591. Macciocchi SN, Diamond PT, Alves WM, et al. Ischemic stroke: relation of age, lesion location, and initial neurologic deficit to functional outcome. *Arch Phys Med Rehabil.* 1998;79(10):1255–1257.
592. Kelly PJ, Furie KL, Shafqat S, et al. Functional recovery following rehabilitation after hemorrhagic and ischemic stroke. *Arch Phys Med Rehabil.* 2003;84(7):968–972.
593. Musicco M, Emberti L, Nappi G, Caltagirone C; Italian Multicenter Study on Outcomes of Rehabilitation of Neurological Patients. Early and long-term outcome of rehabilitation in stroke patients: the role of patient characteristics, time of initiation, and duration of interventions. *Arch Phys Med Rehabil.* 2003;84(4):551–558.
594. Hallett M. Plasticity of the human motor cortex and recovery from stroke. *Brain Res Brain Res Rev.* 2001;36(2–3):169–174.
595. Duncan PW, Wallace D, Lai SM, et al. The Stroke Impact Scale version 2.0: evaluation of reliability, validity, and sensitivity to change. *Stroke.* 1999;30(10):2131–2140.
596. Lai SM, Studenski S, Duncan PW, Perera S. Persisting consequences of stroke measured by the Stroke Impact Scale. *Stroke.* 2002;33(7):1840–1844.
597. Jorgensen HS, Nakayama H, Raaschou HO, et al. Outcome and time course of recovery in stroke. Part II: time course of recovery. The Copenhagen Stroke Study. *Arch Phys Med Rehabil.* 1995;76(5):406–412.
598. Jorgensen HS, Nakayama H, Raaschou HO, et al. Outcome and time course of recovery in stroke. Part I: outcome. The Copenhagen Stroke Study. *Arch Phys Med Rehabil.* 1995;76(5):399–405.

599. Weir NU, Gunkel A, McDowall M, Dennis MS. Study of the relationship between social deprivation and outcome after stroke. *Stroke.* 2005;36(4):815–819.
600. Barnes MP. Rehabilitation after traumatic brain injury. *Br Med Bull.* 1999;55(4):927–943.
601. Horan MA, Clague JE. Injury in the aging: recovery and rehabilitation. *Br Med Bull.* 1999;55(4):895–909.
602. Zuckerman JD. Hip fracture. *N Engl J Med.* 1996;334(23):1519–1525.
603. Richmond J, Aharonoff GB, Zuckerman JD, Koval KJ. Mortality risk after hip fracture. *J Orthop Trauma.* 2003;17(1):53–56.
604. Cree M, Soskolne CL, Belseck E, et al. Mortality and institutionalization following hip fracture. *J Am Geriatr Soc.* 2000;48(3):283–288.
605. Cree M, Carriere KC, Soskolne CL, et al. Functional dependence after hip fracture. *Am J Phys Med Rehabil.* 2001;80(10):736–743.
606. Marcantonio ER, Flacker JM, Michaels M, Resnick NM. Delirium is independently associated with poor functional recovery after hip fracture. *J Am Geriatr Soc.* 2000;48(6):618–624.
607. Koval KJ, Sala DA, Kummer FJ, Zuckerman JD. Postoperative weight-bearing after a fracture of the femoral neck or an intertrochanteric fracture. *J Bone Joint Surg Am.* 1998;80(3):352–356.
608. Handoll HH, Farrar MJ, McBirnie J, et al. Heparin, low molecular weight heparin and physical methods for preventing deep vein thrombosis and pulmonary embolism following surgery for hip fractures. *Cochrane Database Syst Rev.* 2002;4:CD000305.
609. Bergqvist D, Benoni G, Bjorgell O, et al. Low-molecular-weight heparin (enoxaparin) as prophylaxis against venous thromboembolism after total hip replacement. *N Engl J Med.* 1996;335(10):696–700.
610. Dahl OE, Bergqvist D. Current controversies in deep vein thrombosis prophylaxis after orthopaedic surgery. *Curr Opin Pulm Med.* 2002;8(5):394–397.
611. Freedman KB, Brookenthal KR, Fitzgerald RH Jr, et al. A meta-analysis of thromboembolic prophylaxis following elective total hip arthroplasty. *J Bone Joint Surg Am.* 2000;82A(7):929–938.
612. Rosell PA, Parker MJ. Functional outcome after hip fracture: a 1-year prospective outcome study of 275 patients. *Injury.* 2003;34(7):529–532.
613. Lin PC, Chang SY. Functional recovery among elderly people one year after hip fracture surgery. *J Nurs Res.* 2004;12(1):72–82.
614. Press Y, Grinshpun Y, Berzak A, et al. The effect of co-morbidity on the rehabilitation process in elderly patients after hip fracture. *Arch Gerontol Geriatr.* 2007; 45(3):281–294.
615. Hawkes WG, Wehren L, Orwig D, et al. Gender differences in functioning after hip fracture. *J Gerontol A Biol Sci Med Sci.* 2006;61(5):495–499.
616. Shah MR, Aharonoff GB, Wolinsky P, et al. Outcome after hip fracture in individuals ninety years of age and older. *J Orthop Trauma.* 2001;15(1):34–39.
617. Cutson TM, Bongiorni DR. Rehabilitation of the older lower limb amputee: a brief review. *J Am Geriatr Soc.* 1996;44(11):1388–1393.
618. Feinglass J, Brown JL, LoSasso A, et al. Rates of lower-extremity amputation and arterial reconstruction in the United States, 1979 to 1996. *Am J Public Health.* 1999;89(8):1222–1227.
619. Esquenazi A. Geriatric amputee rehabilitation. *Clin Geriatr Med.* 1993; 9(4):731–743.
620. Cruz CP, Eidt JF, Capps C, et al. Major lower extremity amputations at a Veterans Affairs hospital. *Am J Surg.* 2003;186(5):449–454.
621. Waters RL, Perry J, Antonelli D, Hislop H. Energy cost of walking of amputees: the influence of level of amputation. *J Bone Joint Surg Am.* 1976;58(1):42–46.
622. Fisher SV, Gullickson G Jr. Energy cost of ambulation in health and disability: a literature review. *Arch Phys Med Rehabil.* 1978;59(3):124–133.
623. Pagliarulo MA, Waters R, Hislop HJ. Energy cost of walking of below-knee amputees having no vascular disease. *Phys Ther.* 1979;59(5):538–543.
624. Fortington LV, Rommers GM, Geertzen JH, et al. Mobility in elderly people with a lower limb amputation: a systematic review. *J Am Med Dir Assoc.* 2012;13(4):319–325.
625. Harris KA, van Schie L, Carroll SE, et al. Rehabilitation potential of elderly patients with major amputations. *J Cardiovasc Surg (Torino).* 1991;32(4):463–467.
626. Legro MW, Reiber G, del Aguila M, et al. Issues of importance reported by persons with lower limb amputations and prostheses. *J Rehabil Res Dev.* 1999;36(3):155–163.
627. Esquenazi A, DiGiacomo R. Rehabilitation after amputation. *J Am Podiatr Med Assoc.* 2001;91(1):13–22.
628. Frieden RA. The geriatric amputee. *Phys Med Rehabil Clin North Am.* 2005;16(1):179–195.

CHAPTER
71

Lung and Heart Transplantation

J. EMANUEL FINET, SEBASTIAN FERNANDEZ-BUSSY, ZUBAIR A. HASHMI, and MAHER A. BAZ

LUNG TRANSPLANTATION

Lung transplantation has become a therapeutic option for patients with end-stage lung diseases who have severe functional impairment and limited life expectancy. Lung transplantation thus offers the possibility of improving the quality of, and prolonging, life in a select recipient population. It has been applied with success to most advanced lung diseases, with the exception of lung cancers. Nonetheless, complications are frequent with a median survival of 5.6 years. The purpose of this chapter is to give the reader an overview of lung transplantation, its application, benefits, and potential complications.

PRETRANSPLANT CONSIDERATIONS AND CANDIDATE SELECTION

Waiting Lists, Donor Availability, and Donor Management and Suitability

The number of lung diseases successfully treated by transplantation has increased, resulting in an increase in the number of eligible candidates and in the number of lung transplant operations in the last decade (1). Moreover, the number of lungs procured yearly has also significantly increased in the last decade (Fig. 71.1), likely due to increased experience of transplant centers as well as improved collaboration between transplant centers and the organ procurement organizations (OPOs) in managing potential organ donors. The previous waiting list system was based purely on the waiting time, with list seniority going to patients with the longest waiting time, regardless of their level of illness or potential benefit from lung transplantation. A new lung allocation system (LAS) score was implemented in the United States on May 4, 2005. A score is calculated based on the probability of surviving 1 year on the waiting list minus the probability of surviving the first year post transplant, hence using the principle of "maximal benefit" (2). The proportion of patients transplanted with interstitial lung diseases (ILDs), which historically accounted for the highest proportion of deaths on the waiting list, has progressively increased since the implementation of the LAS score (Fig. 71.2). The implementation of LAS has resulted in the reduction of deaths on the waiting list and in the ability to prioritize patients based on medical urgency (3); there are currently approximately 1,700 patients waiting for lung transplantation in the United States. The LAS system has recently been adopted by Eurotransplant.

All hospitals in the United States are obligated to report all deaths to their local OPOs. Each OPO covers several counties—and sometimes a whole state. The OPO reviews and identifies potential organ donors (brain death with consenting families). Once a suitable donor is identified, the OPO offers the lungs first to the transplant centers located within the geographic boundaries of their working area. The local recipient list is organized first by blood type and height; patients on the waiting list with the highest LAS score will be offered the lungs first. The list is then run by compatible blood types if no recipients with identical blood types match in the OPO's region. If the transplant center(s) within the geographic boundaries of the OPO does not accept the lungs, the procurement agency will widen the search to include transplant centers within a radius of 500 miles—as determined by ZIP codes—with lungs offered to patients with the highest LAS score in those areas. Since lungs can tolerate a 6- to 8-hour period of ischemia, travel time limitations are also a factor for accepting lungs.

Most organ donors are procured from patients declared brain dead, whose families consent to donation. The most common causes of brain death are from head trauma (gunshot wounds, car accidents), followed by cerebrovascular accidents. Historically, lung(s) were procured only from about 15% to 20% of potential solid organ donors; in contrast, about 80% of donors have kidneys and livers procured. Unique factors affecting the suitability of lungs for organ donation are donor smoking history, potential of aspiration at the time of death, and fluid overload from resuscitation of the donor. Potential lung donors are managed by the OPOs prior to procurement, with the goal of maximizing organ function and suitability. The medical management is ideally geared toward keeping the donor lungs "dry," using hormone replacement therapy and administering broad-spectrum antibacterial therapy to the donor. This strategy has seemingly resulted in increased organ availability and increased the lung procurement to between about 24% and 28% of potential donors (4–7). Although Table 71.1 has criteria for "ideal" donors, other lungs with less ideal characteristics have been successfully transplanted with reasonable short-term outcomes (8,9). Recently, some "unacceptable donors" have been rehabilitated by ex vivo lung perfusion with good reported short-term outcomes (10,11).

Timing of Referrals

Patients should be referred to a lung transplant center when the projected 2-year survival is about 50%, especially when they have failed medical therapy. The patient's report

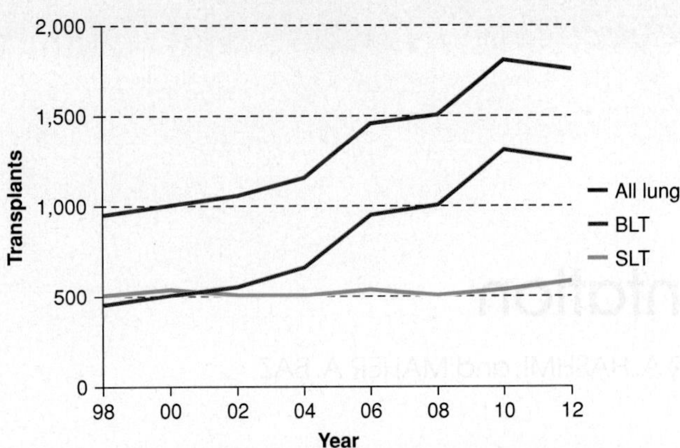

FIGURE 71.1 Volume of lung transplants in the United States. There has been significant increase in the volume of lung transplantation in the past decade, mostly due to increase in the number of bilateral lung transplant operations. (From U.S. Organ Procurement and Transplantation Network and the Scientific Registry of Transplant Recipients.)

TABLE 71.1 Criteria for "Ideal" Lung Donors

- PaO_2 >300 mmHg on FiO_2 = 1.0 and 5 cm H_2O continuous positive airway pressure (CPAP)
- <20 pack-years' smoking history
- Clear chest radiograph
- Minimal secretions on bronchoscopy
- Negative viral serology (HIV, hepatitis B and C infections)
- <60–65 years old

of an unacceptable quality of life is an important factor to consider in evaluating their candidacy for lung transplantation, but the life expectancy must be the overriding impetus for listing. An anticipated waiting time of 12 to 24 months, during which the candidate's condition must remain functionally suitable for transplantation, must be integrated into the decision process for referring and listing patients. Disease-specific guidelines for referral are listed in Table 71.2 (12).

Selection Criteria for Suitable Candidates

Although transplantation has been successful in most lung diseases, not all patients with advanced lung diseases are suitable candidates. The patient's medical records are screened carefully prior to the initial clinic visit. Patients are often declined at the initial clinic visit if there is any history of cigarette smoking in the last 6 months or if there is evidence of irreversible extrapulmonary end-organ damage. Patients are also screened for their insurance coverage, as lung transplantation is an expensive endeavor. Medicare and most state Medicaid and private insurers provide coverage (Table 71.3). After an initial screening of the patient's records, the potential lung recipients are seen in the lung transplant clinic. A detailed discussion of lung transplantation, its outcome, and potential complications occurs with the patient if there are no obvious contraindications identified during the clinic visit. If the patient consents to the transplant procedure, he or she is then referred for a more detailed transplant evaluation and testing. Lung transplant evaluation and the guidelines for the selection of recipients are listed in Tables 71.3, 71.4, and 71.5 respectively (12). A body mass index (BMI) greater than 30 has been identified as an independent predictor of mortality in the first 12 months post transplantation (13,14). However, BMI greater than 30 is a relative contraindication and must be considered in the context of muscle strength, as more recent data shows that BMI up to 34.9 has no effect on survival (15). Chronic obstructive pulmonary disease (COPD) patients are likely to be scrutinized the closest for BMI and muscle strength, as improvement in quality of life is the indication in the majority of patients in this disease category. Patients who are suitable for lung transplantation are listed with the United Network for Organ Sharing (UNOS).

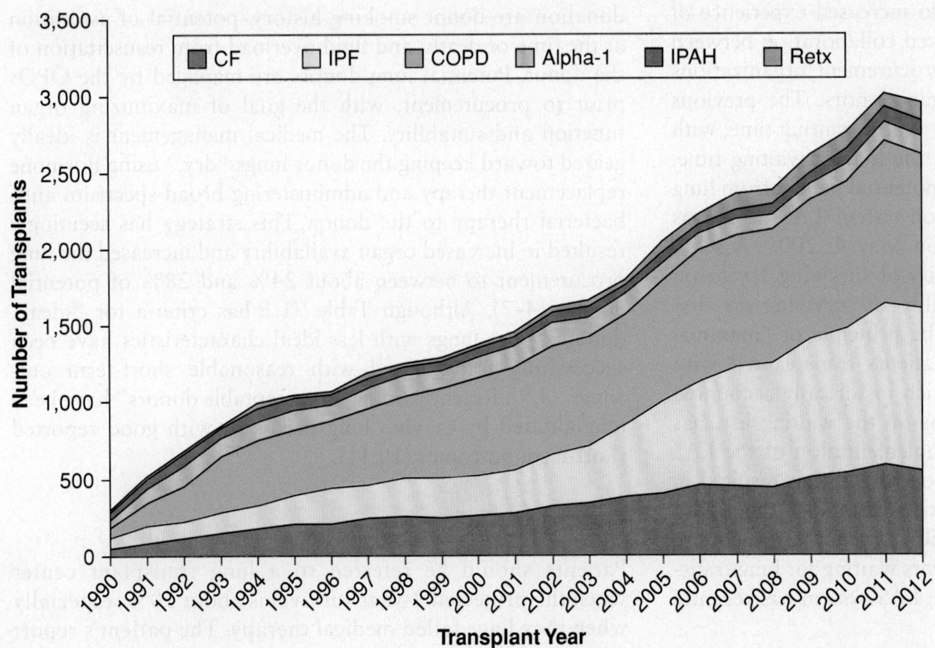

FIGURE 71.2 Worldwide adult lung transplants major indications by year. There has been a significant increase in the volume of lung transplant in the United States and worldwide. The number and proportion of patients with ILD has also increased since the implementation of the LAS score in 2005. (From the International Society of Heart Lung Transplantation, with permission.)

TABLE 71.2 Disease-Specific Guidelines for Referral

Chronic Obstructive Pulmonary Disease (COPD)

- FEV_1 <25% of predicted
- Three or more severe exacerbations during the preceding year
- One severe exacerbation with acute hypercapnia respiratory failure
- Mild to moderate pulmonary hypertension
- BODE index of 6–7

Cystic Fibrosis (CF)

- FEV_1 <30% of predicted
- $PaCO_2$ >50 mmHg
- Frequent severe exacerbations
- Rapid decline in lung function (especially in women)

Idiopathic Pulmonary Fibrosis (IPF)

- Vital capacity (VC) <65% of predicted
- 10% decline in VC or in diffusion capacity in the last 12 mo
- Initiation of oxygen therapy

Idiopathic Pulmonary Arterial Hypertension (iPAH)

- NYHA (New York Heart Association) functional class III or IV
- Cardiac index <2 L/min/m^2
- Mean right atrial pressure >15 mmHg
- Failure of medical therapy to improve hemodynamic indexes or functional class

Eisenmenger Syndrome

- NYHA functional class III or IV despite optimal medical therapy (especially if patients are discontented with their current quality of life)

TABLE 71.3 Primary Payers of Adult Lung Transplant Recipients in the United States in 2012

Primary Payer	
Private	51.5%
Medicare	38.7%
Other government	7.8%
Other	1.9%
Costs of Medicare patients for care for 1 yr after lung transplantation	
No. of patients	885
Total costs Part A	$162,982,412
Total costs Part B	$22,723,606

(Data from U.S. Organ Procurement and Transplantation Network and Scientific Registry of Transplant Recipients.)

TABLE 71.4 Transplant Evaluation Testing

- Chest radiograph, electrocardiogram
- Computed tomography (CT) scan of chest
- Pulmonary function tests, arterial blood gas
- Differential ventilation/perfusion scan
- Two-dimensional echocardiography
- Coronary angiography (in patients >45 yrs)
- Right heart catheterization (in all candidates)
- 24-hr pH study and esophageal manometry
- Abdominal imaging (ultrasound or CT scan)
- Bone density (if indicated)
- Sputum culture (in patients with suppurative lung disease)
- Laboratory studies: Viral serologies (human immunodeficiency virus, hepatitis B and C, cytomegalovirus, herpes simplex virus, Epstein–Barr virus), ABO blood typing, human leucocyte antigen typing, reactive antibodies panel, complete blood count, liver and chemistry batteries
- Consults: Physical therapy (6-min walk test, musculoskeletal strength assessment, rest and exercise oxygen requirements); social work; psychology; nutritional services; transplant thoracic surgeon; transplant pulmonologist

TABLE 71.5 General Guidelines for Selection of Recipients

Indications

- End-stage lung disease with average life expectancy <2 yrs and >80% likelihood of surviving at least 90 days post lung transplantation
- Failed medical and/or surgical therapy
- Severe functional limitation, but ambulatory with good muscle strength
- Upper age limit (at some centers) ≤74 yrs

Absolute Contraindications

- Significant extrapulmonary end-organ active disease or damage
- Acute evolving critical illness
- History of cancer in the last 2–5 yrs (depending on type of cancer)
- Active psychosis or history of noncompliance with therapy
- Cigarette smoking in the last 6 mo
- History of substance abuse with risk factors for recidivism
- Nonambulatory, with poor rehabilitation potential
- Inadequate social support
- Extrapulmonary infections (human immunodeficiency virus, hepatitis B, C active infections)
- Body mass index >35

Relative Contraindications

- Mechanical ventilation or extracorporeal life support
- Extensive pleural adhesions from previous surgical procedures (especially talc)
- Airway colonization with bacteria panresistant to all antibacterials
- Body mass index 30–35

SURGICAL TECHNIQUES FOR LUNG TRANSPLANTATION

Isolated Lung Transplant

Dr. James Hardy from University of Mississippi reported the first lung transplantation in a human in 1963. Many failed attempts thereafter were mainly due to infections and anastomotic dehiscence from the high doses of steroids used for immunosuppression. The introduction of cyclosporine, in the early 1980s, allowed for reduction of steroid doses. Dr. Joel Cooper from University of Toronto reported successful lung transplantation in 1983. Points to remember include lung recruitment maneuvers upon visualization, as well as adequate heparinization, steroid, and prostaglandin administration. After discussions with the heart procurement team, it is important to retrieve pulmonary artery and vein of appropriate length.

Recipients are usually listed with a height range of ±20%, as height and gender are the primary determinant for lung volumes. Lung transplant centers usually prefer to implant lungs from taller donors into recipients with obstructive lung diseases (COPD, cystic fibrosis [CF]), and lungs from shorter donors into recipients with restrictive lung diseases (idiopathic pulmonary fibrosis [IPF]). Bilateral lung transplantation (BLT) is performed in approximately 75% of COPD patients, 60% of ILD patients, 99% of CF patients, and in 95% of idiopathic pulmonary artery hypertension (iPAH) patients.

There are four lung transplant surgical procedures: single-lung transplantation (SLT), bilateral sequential lung transplantation (BLT), combined heart–lung transplantation (HLT), and bilateral lobar transplantation from living-related donors. Higher rates of intrathoracic bleeding, reexploration, and renal dysfunction are to be expected in patients with previous chest procedures, mainly due to longer time in explanting the native lung. These conditions may be exacerbated if patients require cardiopulmonary bypass (CPB). However, a history of previous chest surgeries is not felt to be an absolute contraindication to lung transplantation. Historically, SLT used to be the most applied technique, but lately BLT has become more prevalent. The advantages of SLT include a shorter waiting time for the recipient, technical ease, and the fact that lungs from one donor can be potentially used for two recipients. With the exception of suppurative lung diseases, SLT has been applied to all lung diseases.

There are different approaches for transplantation depending upon whether single or double lung transplant is considered: posterolateral thoracotomy, anterolateral thoracotomy, sternotomy, or clamshell incision. Procedures can be performed on CPB or extracorporeal membrane oxygenation (ECMO), depending on perfusion mismatch and pulmonary artery pressures. Patients with moderate to severe pulmonary hypertension are more likely to need bypass. Pulmonary artery pressure always increases when the pulmonary artery is clamped. Nitric oxide or inhaled epoprostenol can be used to assist in lowering pulmonary pressures.

Once donor lungs are visualized and determined to be suitable for transplantation, recipient surgery is begun. To avoid hypoxemia due to shunting through the deflated lung during dissection, the pulmonary artery may be clamped first. The recipient pneumonectomy is performed, and the hilum is prepared for anastomosis, providing enough length to clamp pulmonary artery and vein, and still be able to perform anastomosis. This anastomosis can be done without clamping if CPB is used. The main stem bronchus is transected just proximal to upper lobe takeoff, taking care to achieve hemostasis with not only dissected lymph nodes, but bronchial arteries. The phrenic, vagus, and recurrent laryngeal nerves must be spared.

The donor lung hilum is fashioned for transplant on the back table and the pulmonary vasculature is flushed retrograde to remove any emboli. The bronchus staple line is removed and airways are suctioned free. The donor lung is then brought up to be implanted. The three anastomoses are hand sewn in their posterior-to-anterior anatomic sequence: bronchus, pulmonary artery, and pulmonary veins—left atrium. The bronchial blood supply to the donor lung is disrupted during transplantation, so the donor bronchus is dependent upon retrograde bronchial blood flow through the pulmonary circulation, unless direct bronchial revascularization is performed. Most centers do not perform bronchial revascularization due to technical difficulty in anastomosing the bronchial arteries.

Mannitol and high-dose methylprednisolone are given once all anastomoses are completed. Prior to clamps being removed, de-airing maneuvers are performed via steep Trendelenburg positioning, CO_2 flooded on the field, and visualization via echocardiogram. The implanted lung is then ventilated as it is being perfused.

Function is confirmed via blood gas, hemostasis is achieved, and chest tubes are placed, followed by closure. Intraoperative bronchoscopy is performed at the end to visualize not only anastomosis, but to clear secretions, evaluate for torsion, and assess for development of primary graft dysfunction (PGD) manifested with severe pulmonary edema. Postoperative pulmonary vein thrombosis, a rather uncommon complication, may manifest as persistent pulmonary edema (in spite of adequate diuresis).

Heart–Lung Transplant

In 1981, the first HLT was performed in a patient with pulmonary arterial hypertension. The only absolute indication for this procedure is Eisenmenger syndrome associated with complex congenital heart disease. Other indications are patients with concurrent significant LV dysfunction and advanced lung disease, and idiopathic pulmonary hypertension with severe right ventricular failure. The latter is an uncommon indication for this type of surgery as the majority of RV dysfunction recovers after isolated BLT (Fig. 71.3). The implantation itself is *en bloc* on CPB, either via sternotomy or clamshell incision. Tracheal anastomosis is performed first, followed by bicaval anastomosis, then aorta. Techniques can be inferred from individual organ implantation.

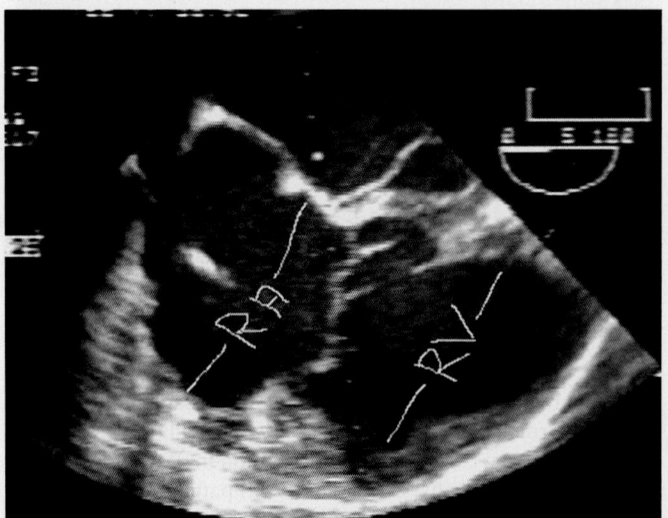

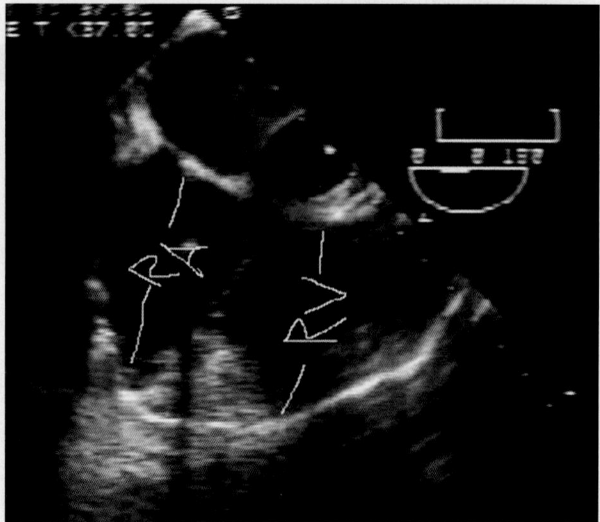

FIGURE 71.3 Intraoperative transesophageal echocardiogram (TEE) in a patient with iPAH undergoing BLT. Note the reduction of the size of the right atrium (RA) and right ventricle (RV) at end systole about 1 hour after reperfusion of the lungs.

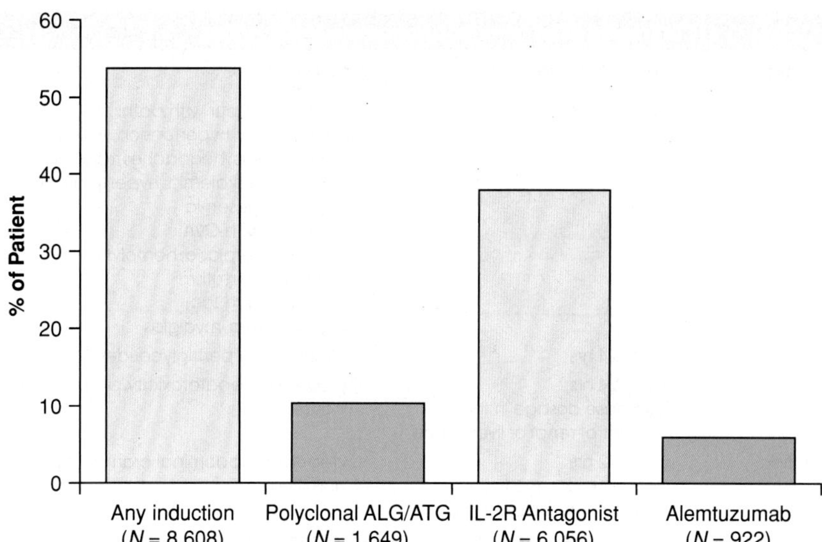

FIGURE 71.4 Induction immunosuppression. Use of induction immunosuppression (in addition to intraop pulse methylprednisolone) in adult lung transplant recipients. Data from January 2002 to June 2013. (From the International Society of Heart Lung Transplantation, with permission.)

Living-Related Lobar Transplant

About 130 of these transplantations have been performed in the United States since 1991. This technique is generally reserved for patients who meet all the criteria for lung transplantation, but have a minimal chance of surviving the waiting time on the lung transplant waiting list. Donors are typically family members who undergo full evaluation for thoracotomy. Because this procedure presents risks to two individuals, appropriate recipient and donor selection, and timing of transplantation, are critical to minimize the morbidity to the donor and maximize the chance of a successful outcome in the recipient.

IMMUNOSUPPRESSION

Induction therapy is intensive immunosuppressant therapy given at the time of transplant to reduce the risk of acute rejection and to delay initiation of maintenance immunosuppression. An intravenous bolus of 500 to 1,000 mg of methylprednisolone is given in the operating room. Most centers use another agent for induction, with the interleukin-2 receptor antagonists (basiliximab) being most common, followed by antilymphocyte antibody (thymoglobulin, alemtuzumab) (Fig. 71.4). Some studies have shown a survival benefit with induction therapy (16) as well as significant decrease in acute rejection early after transplant without significant increase in infection rates (17,18) (Fig. 71.5).

Maintenance immunosuppression is lifelong therapy given to prevent acute and chronic rejection. Doses and medications are changed and adjusted to minimize their side effects. Table 71.6 details the numerous side effects, interactions, and dosing of the immunosuppressive medications. Triple immunosuppression with calcineurin inhibitor, antiproliferative agent, and corticosteroids is the rule for maintenance immunosuppression. The most commonly used agents in the last 5 years are: tacrolimus (Tac), mycophenolate mofetil (MMF),

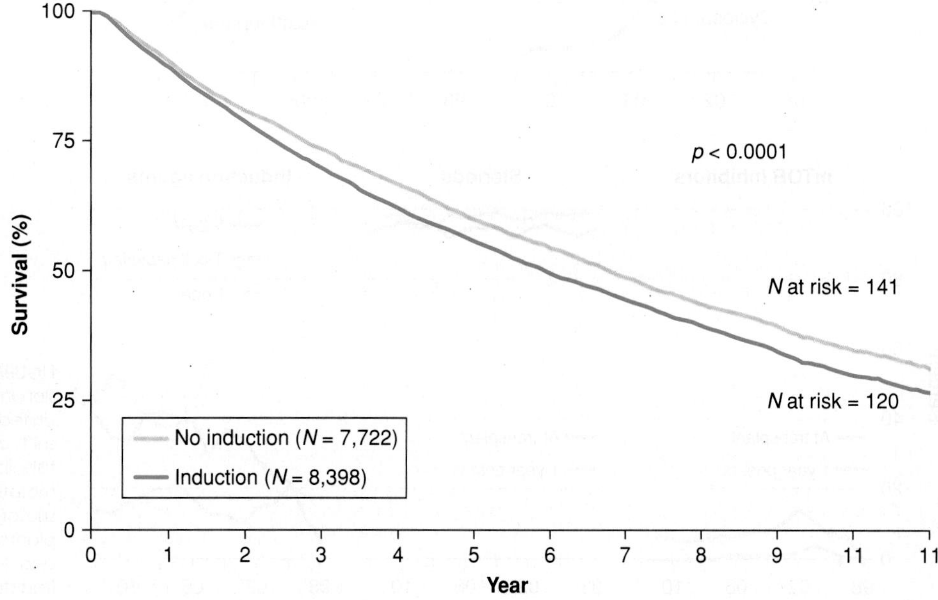

FIGURE 71.5 Survival was calculated using the Kaplan–Meier method, which incorporates information from all transplants for whom any follow-up has been provided. Survival rates were compared using the log-rank test statistic. (From the International Society of Heart Lung Transplantation, with permission.)

TABLE 71.6 Commonly Used Immunosuppressive Medications

Drug	Dosing & Adjustments	Side Effects	Drug Interactions
CyA & Tac	Every 12 hrs	Commonly occur with both: Nephrotoxicity, hypertension, neurotoxicity (tremors, headaches, rarely seizures), hyperkalemia, hyperlipidemia, hypomagnesemia Occur only with CyA: Gingival hyperplasia, hemolytic-uremic syndrome, hirsutism Occur only with Tac: Hyperglycemia, myalgias	Blood levels are increased with all macrolide antibiotics (except azithromycin), azole antifungals, calcium channel blockers (except nifedipine). Blood levels are decreased by Dilantin, barbiturates, and rifampin
Sirolimus	Every 24 hrs	Cytopenias, hypertriglyceridemia	Same as CyA and Tac
Aza	Every 24 hrs Decrease dosage in the event of renal or liver failure	Cytopenias, hepatotoxicity, pancreatitis, nausea	Increased bone marrow suppression with allopurinol, ganciclovir, and thymoglobulin
MMF	Every 12 hrs Decrease dosage in the event of renal or liver failure	Cytopenias, abdominal cramps, diarrhea, vomiting	Increased bone marrow suppression with allopurinol, ganciclovir, and thymoglobulin
Prednisone	0.3–0.5 mg/kg/d in the first 3 mo, then tapered afterward	Hypertension, hyperglycemia, weight gain, myopathy, osteoporosis, cataracts, mood swings, hyperlipidemia	No significant interactions

and prednisone (Fig. 71.6). Tac has been shown to reduce the incidence of bronchiolitis obliterans syndrome (BOS) when compared to cyclosporine, but without any differences in acute rejection incidence, or survival, after 3 years (19). However, another study compared a triple immunosuppression maintenance therapy containing CyA to tacrolimus and found that the number of episodes of acute rejection per 100 patient days was lower in the tacrolimus group (20). In two prospective trials comparing azathioprine and MMF, Palmer et al. showed no difference in acute rejection rates in the first 6 months while McNeil et al. showed no difference in acute or chronic rejection at 3 years (21,22).

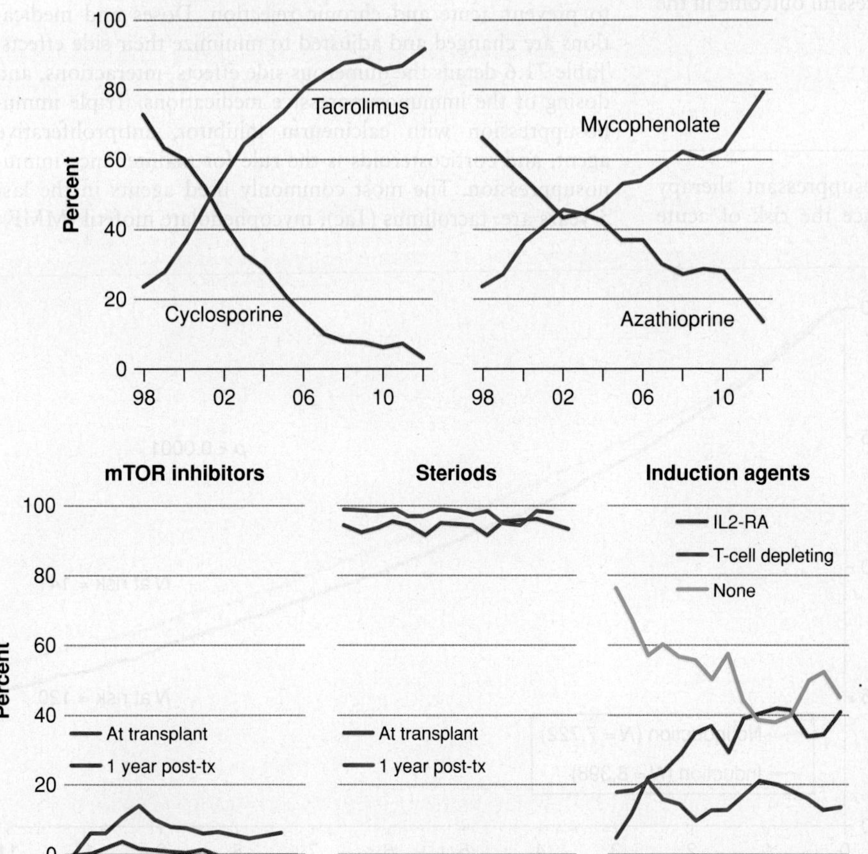

FIGURE 71.6 Maintenance immunosuppression in adult lung transplant recipients in the United States. Note in the last decade the shift of calcineurin inhibitors and antimetabolites to tacrolimus and mycophenolate mofetil, respectively. Also note the increased use of induction agents at the time of transplantation. (From U.S. Organ Procurement and Transplantation Network and Scientific Registry of Transplant Recipients.)

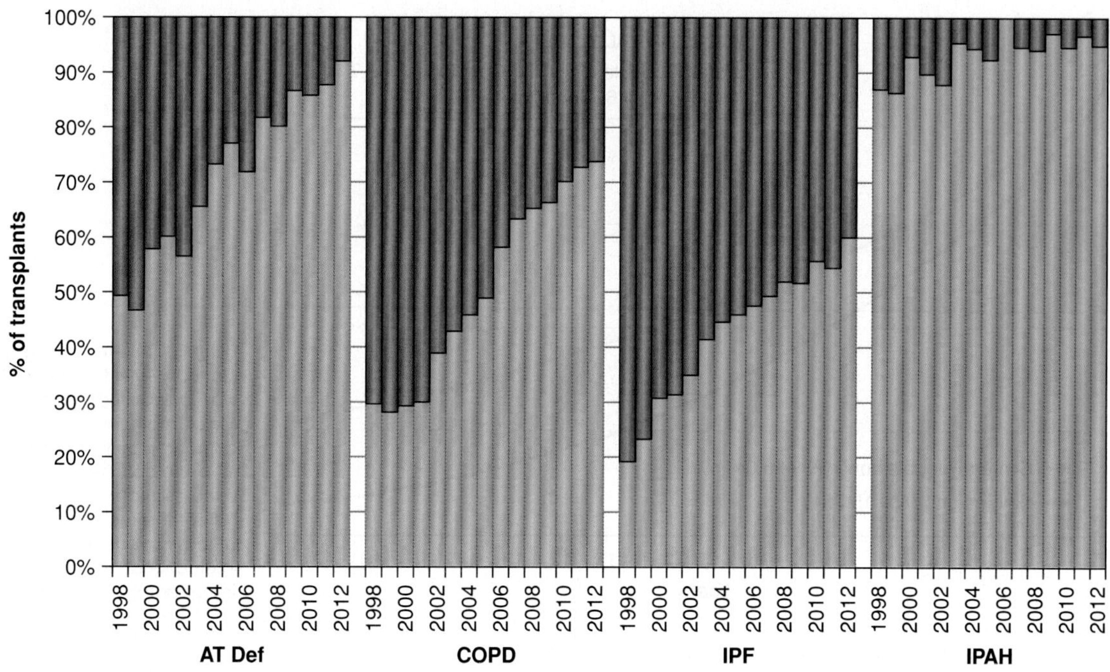

FIGURE 71.7 Adult lung transplants.Procedure type within indication, by year, from 1998 to 2012. Blue indicated bilateral double lung transplant; red indicates single lung transplant. (From the International Society of Heart Lung Transplantation, with permission.)

The calcineurin inhibitor cyclosporine A (CyA) is sometimes substituted for Tac or azathioprine for MMF in patients intolerant of their side effects (especially GI symptoms). Sirolimus is substituted for calcineurin inhibitors in some patients with kidney injury with amelioration of kidney injury and seemingly preserved lung function (23).

OUTCOMES FOLLOWING LUNG TRANSPLANTATION

Survival

The median survival after lung transplantation is 5.6 years. The 1-, 3-, 5-, and 10-year actuarial survivals after lung transplantation are 80%, 69%, 53%, and 30%, respectively (1). BLT is being applied much more frequently than SLT in the last decade (Fig. 71.7). BLT has significantly higher survival compared to SLT (Fig. 71.8). The survival is also significantly better in lung transplant programs doing higher volumes (Fig. 71.9) (13,24). However, these survival rates lag considerably behind those of liver or kidney transplant recipients, for whom the 5-year actuarial survival approximates 80%. In the absence of prospective randomized trials, it is difficult to ascertain whether lung transplantation truly increases survival over the natural history of the lung disease. Hosenpud et al. (25) made a disease-specific comparison of survival after transplantation and found that patients with CF and IPF benefit from transplantation. No such advantage has yet been demonstrated for patients with COPD, a disease that typically follows a protracted course with a 5-year survival of 40% to 50% for patients with forced expiratory volume in 1 second (FEV_1) less than 20% of predicted (26). Thus, the main indication for lung transplantation in patients with COPD is to improve quality of life in patients with FEV_1 in the 15% to 25% range, rather than prolonging survival. BODE index (body mass index [B], airflow obstruction [O], dyspnea [D], and exercise capacity [E]) has been identified as a predictor of survival and rehospitalization in COPD patients (27).

There have been a few risk factors identified by multivariate analysis that are associated with risk of death 1 year after transplantation: diagnosis of iPAH or IPF, increased severity of recipient illness at the time of transplantation (i.e., ventilator dependence, ICU care), transplant volume less than 30 per year, older recipient age at the time of transplant (especially above 60 years of age), higher pretransplant supplemental oxygen, lower cardiac index, and retransplantation (1). However, it is important to remember that those statistics are aggregate data, reported by multiple centers to the International Society for Heart and Lung Transplantation (ISHLT). Since different centers have different expertise and experience, those risk factors may not be uniform among centers. For example, in carefully selected ventilator-dependent patients who are not critically ill, mechanical ventilation did not influence the 1-year outcome after transplantation (28,29). The leading causes of death in the first 30 days after transplantation are primary allograft failure and bacterial pneumonia, with infection being the leading cause of death in the first year (Fig. 71.10) (1). Chronic lung rejection is the most common cause of death in patients surviving past the first year after transplantation and occurs in 50% of recipients surviving 5 years after transplantation (Fig. 71.11).

Pulmonary Function and Gas Exchange

Both SLT and BLT patients result in significant improvement in pulmonary function tests (PFTs) and in gas exchange post transplantation. The peak improvement in PFTs is achieved at 1 to 3 months after SLT and in 4 to 6 months after BLT. The factors associated with the delay in achieving peak values are reperfusion injury, postoperative pain, altered chest wall mechanics, and respiratory muscle

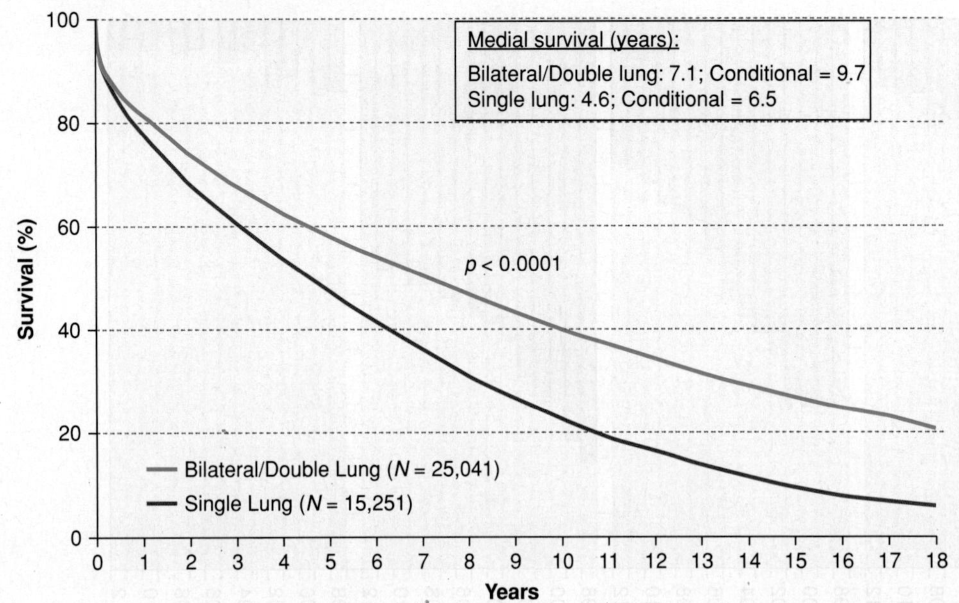

FIGURE 71.8 Adult lung transplants (January 1994 to June 2012). Survival was calculated using the Kaplan–Meier method. Survival rates were compared using the log-rank test statistic. The conditional median survival is the estimated time point at which 50% of the recipients who survive to at least 1 year have died. (From the International Society of Heart Lung Transplantation, with permission.)

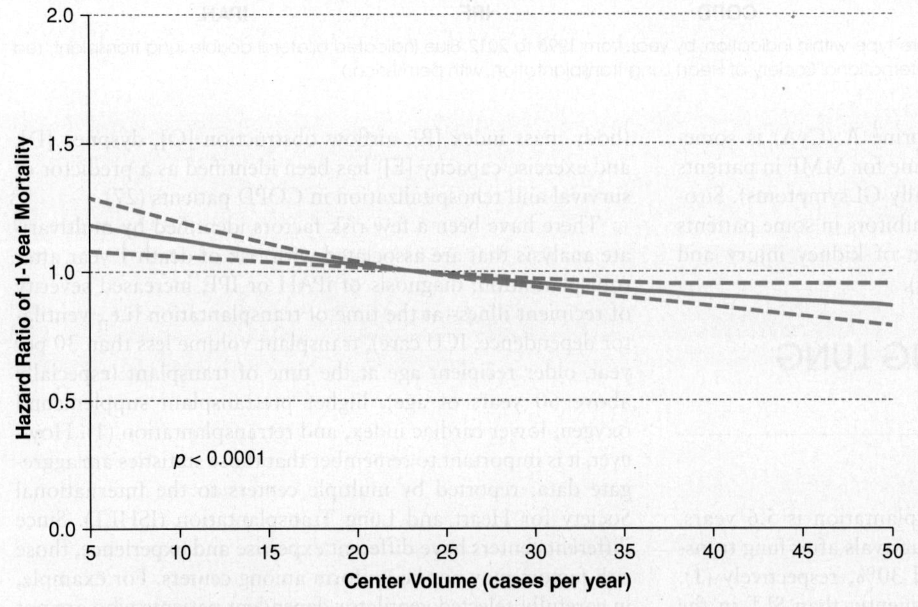

FIGURE 71.9 Adult lung transplant center volume and hazard ratio for mortality within the first posttransplant year (January 2000 to June 2012). Dashed lines are 95% confidence intervals. (From the International Society of Heart Lung Transplantation, with permission.)

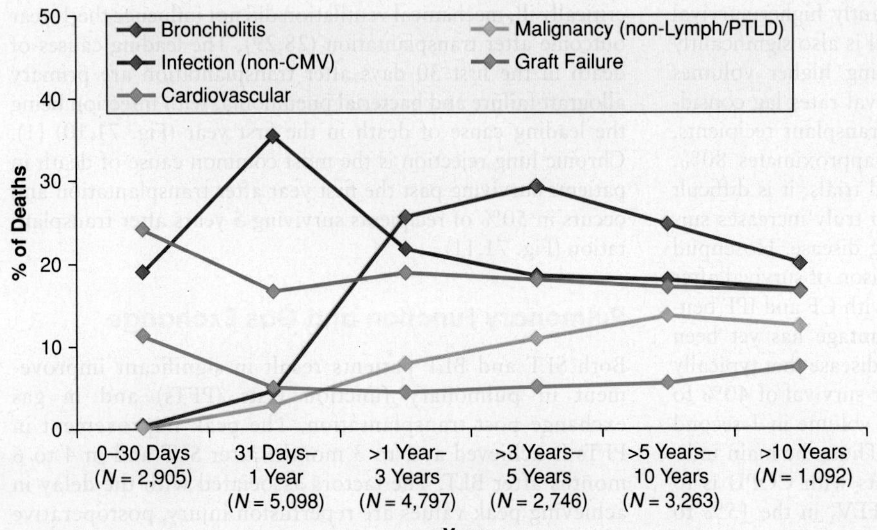

FIGURE 71.10 Infection is the leading cause of death in the first year, while chronic lung rejection is the leading cause of death in patients who live past the first year, data collected 1992–2013. Most of Graft failure is due to PGD in the first year, and due to chronic lung rejection beyond the first year. Bronchiolitis is chronic lung rejection. (From the International Society of Heart Lung Transplantation, with permission.)

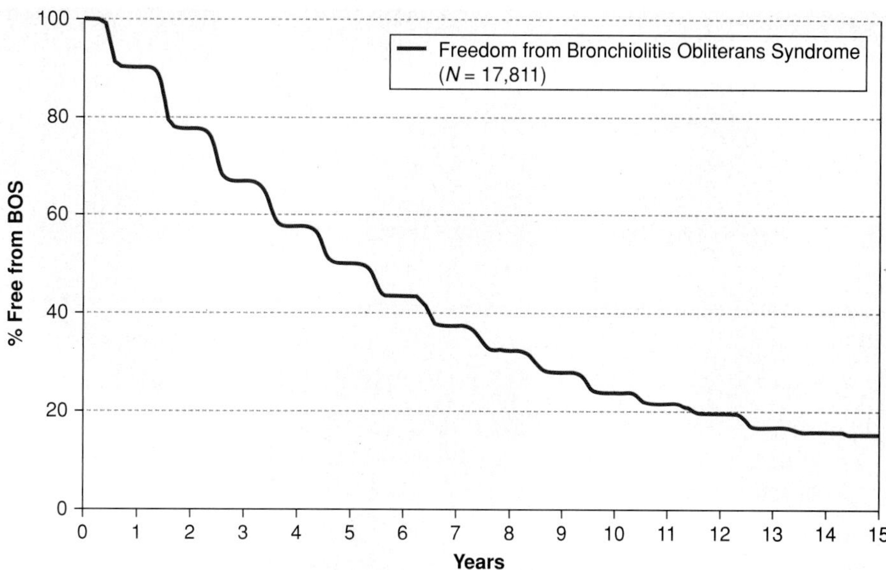

FIGURE 71.11 Freedom from bronchiolitis obliterans syndrome (BOS) rates were computed using the Kaplan–Meier method. Data from 1994 to 2012, conditional on patients surviving 14 days. (From the International Society of Heart Lung Transplantation, with permission.)

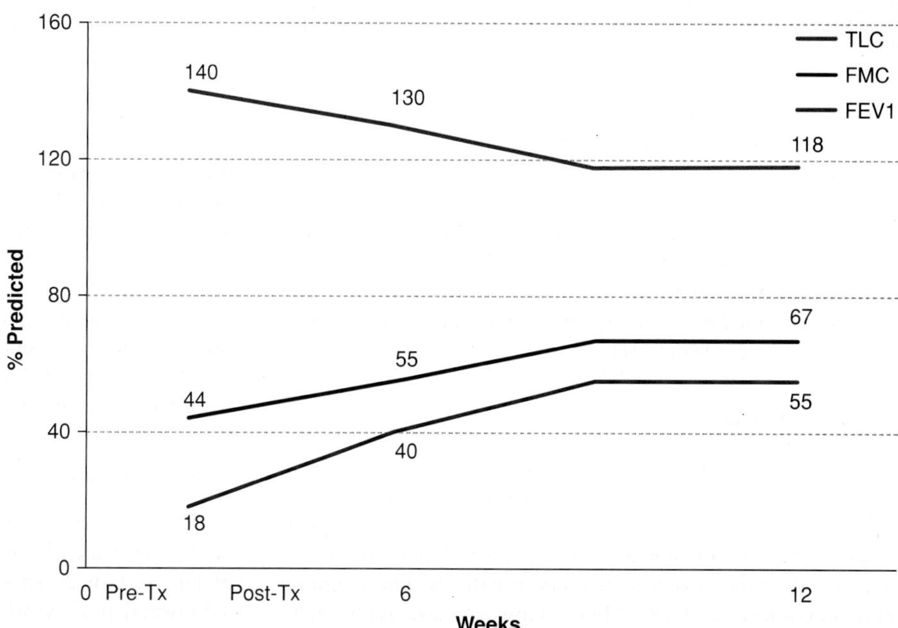

FIGURE 71.12 FEV_1, FVC, and TLC in six COPD patients before and after single lung transplantation. Note the significant improvement in FEV_1 and in the decline in TLC.

dysfunction after transplant surgery. After SLT in patients with COPD, the FEV_1 significantly improves to 45% to 60% of the predicted value and lung volumes approach the normal predicted values, with associated midline shift on chest radiograph (Figs. 71.12 and 71.13) (30). After SLT in patients with IPF, the vital capacity improves to about 70% to 80% of the predicted value, with associated midline shift of the allograft into native chest cavity (Figs. 71.14 and 71.15) (30). After BLT, the spirometry values approximate predicted values for the recipient's chest cavity size and the chest radiograph will show normal lung fields (Figs. 71.16 and 71.17).

After lung transplantation, in allografts with minimal or no injury immediately post transplant, arterial oxygenation and hypercapnia return to normal within a few days. Supplemental oxygen is unnecessary for most patients at the time of hospital discharge.

Hemodynamics

In patients with significant pulmonary hypertension (iPAH, or pulmonary hypertension associated with ILD), BLT has been adopted as the procedure of choice in most centers. Between 1995 and 2008, 714 patients have undergone BLT, and 94 patients SLT, according to the ISHLT registry report. BLT results in immediate and sustained normalization of pulmonary artery pressures in this population, barring significant reperfusion injury. This is associated with total or near-total resolution of the associated tricuspid valve insufficiency and is accompanied by an immediate increase of the cardiac output with a gradual remodeling of the right ventricle (see Fig. 71.3). The right ventricle decreases in size and regains normal function over the next few days to weeks. This hemodynamic improvement is sustained after successful transplantation. The advantage of BLT over SLT for patients with pulmonary vascular disease is

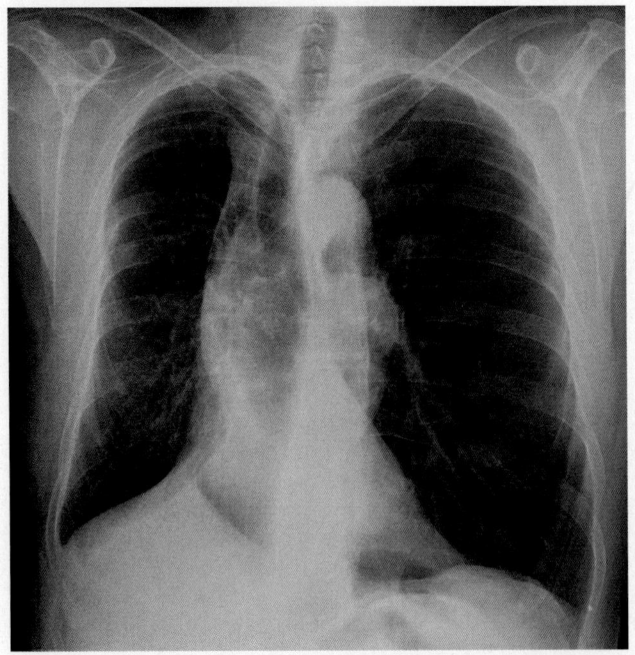

FIGURE 71.13 Chest radiograph after right single lung transplant in a patient with COPD. Note the more compliant hyperinflated native COPD lung with flat diaphragm and (clinically asymptomatic) shift across the midline into the right allograft side.

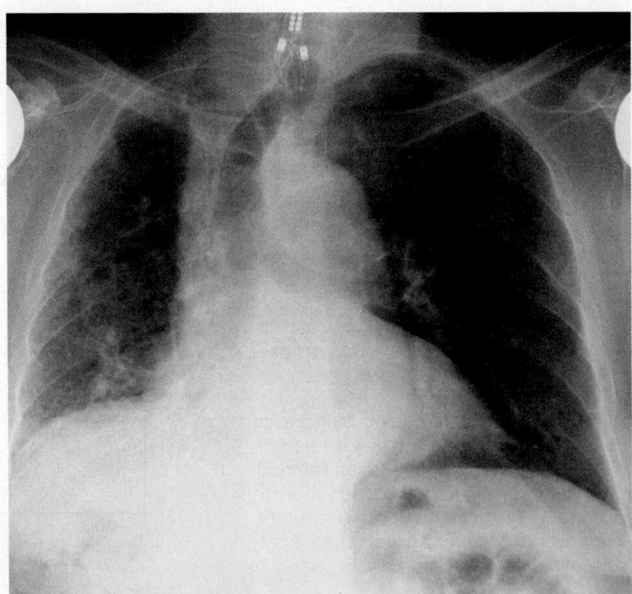

FIGURE 71.15 Chest radiograph in a patient with IPF who underwent single left lung transplantation. Note the mild midline shift (clinically asymptomatic) of the more compliant left allograft into the right chest cavity containing the native lung.

that airway injury is better tolerated in BLT. Due to the resultant severe ventilation/perfusion mismatch, airway injury after SLT (caused by pneumonia, or acute or chronic rejection) may result in profound hypoxemia, especially in patients with severe pulmonary hypertension (31).

Quality of Life

Several studies show a dramatic, global improvement in all measures of quality of life (physical, social, and psychological) in most recipients as early as 3 months after transplantation. These improvements are maintained or continue to improve over the next several years in patients who maintain lung function (Fig. 71.18) (32–35). However, because bronchiolitis obliterans (BO) causes progressive deterioration of lung function, any newly acquired improvement in the quality of life deteriorates if BO occurs after transplantation (36). Only approximately one-third of recipients return to work after transplantation. Factors that may contribute to this relatively low reemployment rate include potential reluctance to hire employees with complex medical conditions, potential loss of income or medical benefits as a result of returning to work, and the change of priorities and goals of recipients after recovering from their previous incapacitating condition (Fig. 71.19) (37).

Exercise Capacity

Peak exercise performance, as measured by cycle ergometry, is characteristically reduced in both SLT and BLT recipients as late as 1 or 2 years after the surgery. These patients have subnormal peak work rate, peak oxygen consumption, and

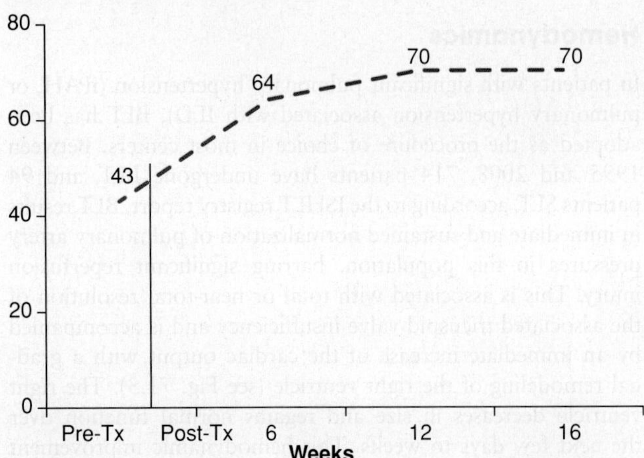

FIGURE 71.14 Vital capacity in patients with IPF undergoing SLT, resulting in a significant improvement in lung volumes.

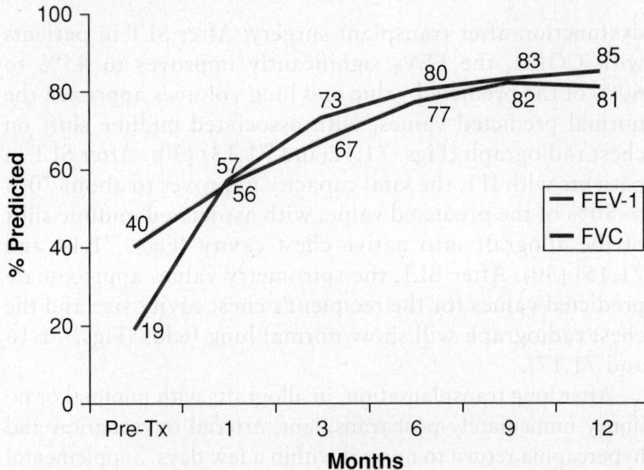

FIGURE 71.16 FEV-1 and FVC in five patients with cystic fibrosis before and after transplant. Values are percentage of predicted.

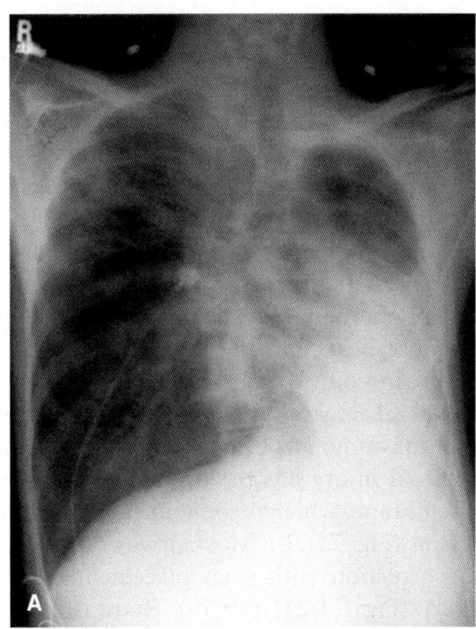

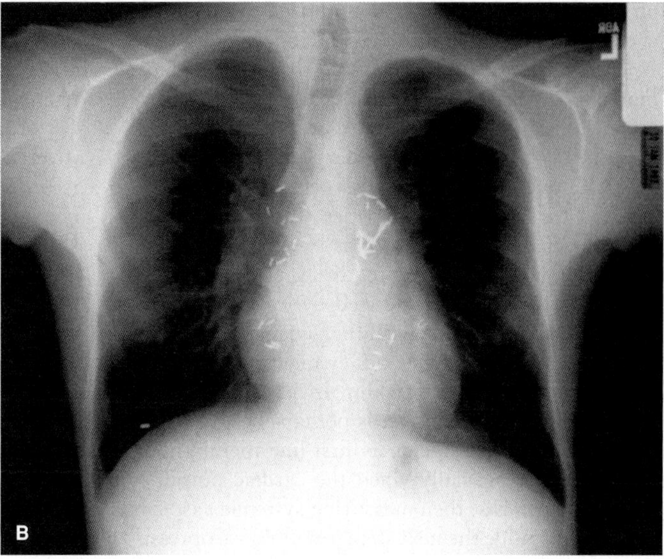

FIGURE 71.17 A: Pretransplant chest radiograph in a patient with CF showing bilateral bronchiectasis, severe left lower lobe necrosis and volume loss with shift of the heart into the left hemithorax. B: Three months after bilateral lung transplant.

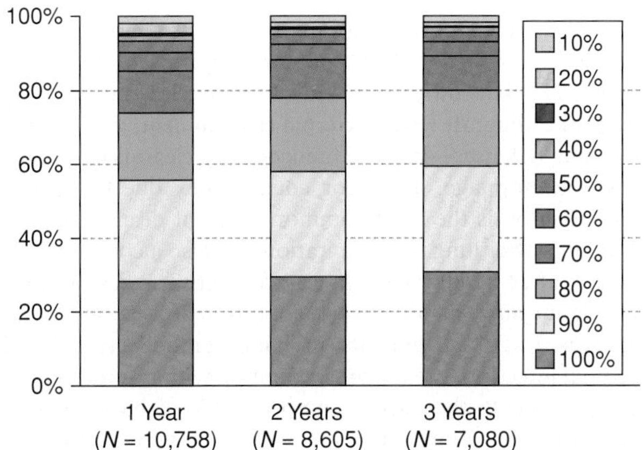

FIGURE 71.18 Functional status is collected using Karnofsky score for adult recipients and Lansky score for pediatric recipients. This figure shows the functional status reported on the 1-year, 2-year, and 3-year annual follow-ups. Because all follow-ups between March 2005 and June 2013 were included, the bars do not include the same patients. (From the International Society of Heart Lung Transplantation, with permission.)

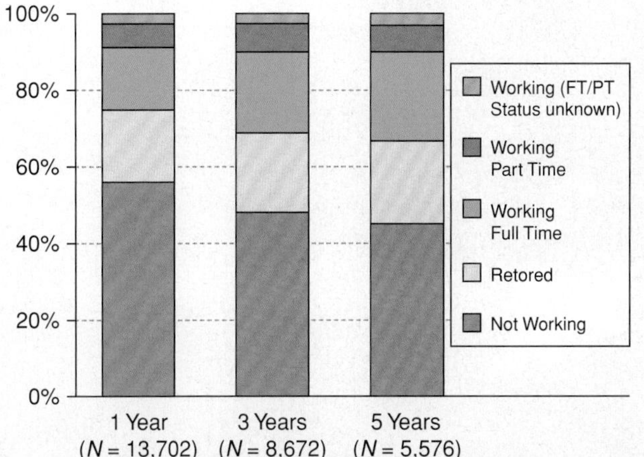

FIGURE 71.19 Employment status reported on the 1-year, 3-year, and 5-year annual follow-ups. Because all follow-ups between April 1994 and June 2013 were included, the bars do not include the same patients. (From the International Society of Heart Lung Transplantation, with permission.)

early lactate threshold on incremental exercise testing. Maximal oxygen consumption is significantly increased after lung transplantation, but it typically is 40% to 60% of the maximal predicted value. Interestingly, the limitation to exercise is not cardiac or ventilatory in nature, and, surprisingly, the maximal oxygen consumption attained during exercise testing is similar whether the recipients are of SLT or BLT (38). Reduced mitochondrial oxidative capacity and peripheral oxygen use in the skeletal muscles of lung transplant recipients (39–41) may be secondary to the deconditioning associated with chronic lung diseases or to impairment in skeletal muscle mitochondrial respiration associated with calcineurin inhibitors (42–44).

COMMON COMPLICATIONS AFTER LUNG TRANSPLANTATION

Primary Graft Dysfunction

PGD is a form of acute lung injury occurring in the first few days after lung and is due to a spectrum of diseases (45). PGD represents a spectrum of diseases characterized to variable degree by fever, hypoxemia, pulmonary hypertension, hypotension, pulmonary edema, and acute kidney injury. The incidence of severe PGD is about 15% and is a common cause of mortality within the first posttransplant year. Severe PGD leads to increased duration of mechanical ventilation and intensive care unit length of stay, poor functional outcomes, and increased risk of BOS. The differential diagnosis includes ischemia–reperfusion injury, hyperacute rejection, donor-related bacterial pneumonia, pulmonary vein thrombosis, or edema from acute kidney injury. The chest radiograph and clinical scenario are almost identical in all these etiologic factors, that is, all have widespread interstitial and alveolar infiltrates in the allograft(s) and hypoxemia. Severity of PGD is graded by PaO_2/FiO_2 ratio and chest radiographic abnormalities at 24 and 72 hours. The diagnosis of reperfusion injury is established by excluding other causes of graft dysfunction. An algorithm for the workup of reperfusion injury is summarized in the article by Zander et al. (46). Inhaled nitric oxide, independent lung ventilation, and extracorporeal membrane oxygenation have been attempted with variable success for patients with severe PGD. The clinical course in survivors of severe PGD is protracted, but some of the survivors are able to ultimately attain normal allograft function. Variables associated with severe PGD are related to donor characteristics (such as smoking history), recipient characteristics (such as presence of pulmonary hypertension), and in patients requiring prolonged CPB runs (47). As PGD is often characterized by leaky capillaries and decreased cardiac output, medical management should be aimed at preserving and optimizing kidney function in the first 72 hours; this is best achieved by avoiding nephrotoxic agents and avoiding hypotension. The latter is perhaps best achieved by using low-dose inotropic agents as first-line therapy (i.e., low-dose epinephrine) especially when the cardiac output is low. If hypotension persists, then measuring systemic vascular resistance (SVR) will guide the next step: low-dose vasopressin if SVR is low, or judicious use of intravenous fluids or blood products if SVR is high. This strategy aims to minimize fluid overload and maximize kidney perfusion without using high dose of vasoconstrictors or large volumes of intravenous fluids. Retransplantation has been attempted for patients with severe PGD with variable success.

Airway Complications

Airway complications requiring intervention occur in 7% to 15% of bronchial anastomosis (48). This reflects both improved surgical techniques that occurred with the advent of bronchial telescoping and relatively lower steroid doses compared to those used with transplantation in the 1970s and early 1980s. Complete dehiscence of the bronchial anastomosis, rare at present, is an emergency situation that requires immediate surgical intervention. Anastomotic stenosis is the most common airway complication, followed by bronchomalacia. Most airway complications manifest in the first 100 days after transplantation. They may present as wheezing, exertional dyspnea, or decline in FEV_1. As the bronchial arteries are not reconnected at the time of transplantation, the bronchial mucosa distal to the anastomosis could be affected by bronchial artery reperfusion injury. This manifests as bronchial mucosal injury with ischemic mucosal surface. The mucosal injury may heal with minimal sequelae, thereby resulting in airway stricture, or, if the bronchial artery ischemia injures the underlying cartilaginous support of the bronchus, it may cause bronchomalacia. Alternatively, bronchial stenosis may be caused by overgrowth of the scar tissue at the site of the bronchial anastomosis. Thus, airway complications may be at the anastomotic site or a few centimeters distally. Bronchial mucosal injury has the bronchoscopic appearance of a pseudomembrane, which is sometimes superinfected with fungal organisms (Fig. 71.20). Most airway complications are amenable to correction with stent placement, balloon dilation, or cautery (Fig. 71.21) (49,50). Retransplantation has been attempted for this complication with variable success.

Infections

The rate of infection among lung transplant recipients is two to three times higher than that for recipients of other solid organs (51). This difference is most likely related to the exposure of the allograft to the external environment, and impaired local lung defenses—impaired mucociliary clearance, impaired lymphatic drainage, and poor cough reflex due to denervation. Infection is the most common cause of death in the first 12 months after lung transplantation and also a common cause of death after the first year. In a retrospective review at a lung transplant center, the rate of freedom from at least one episode of infection is 32% in patients surviving 12 months (Fig. 71.22). Bacterial infections are the most common with respiratory tract pathogens being the most common source of bacterial infections. Microbes from donor lungs cause a significant number

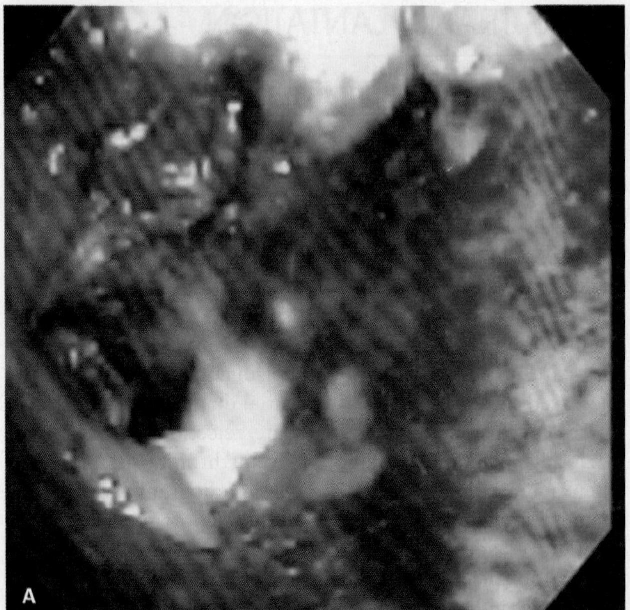

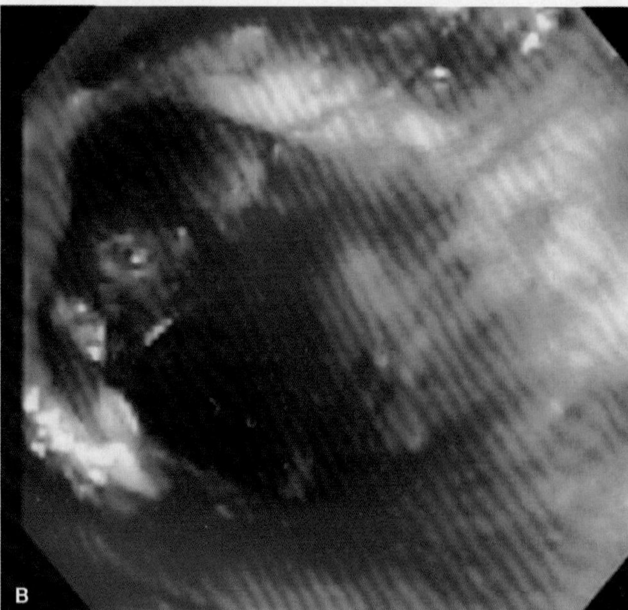

FIGURE 71.20 Bronchial mucosal reperfusion injury and *Aspergillus* infection of RUL orifice and bronchus intermedius before (A) and after debridement and right bronchus intermedius stent placement (B).

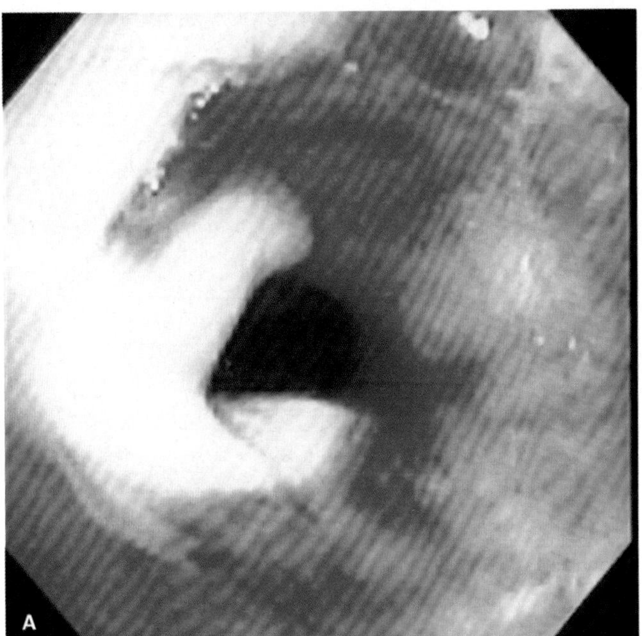

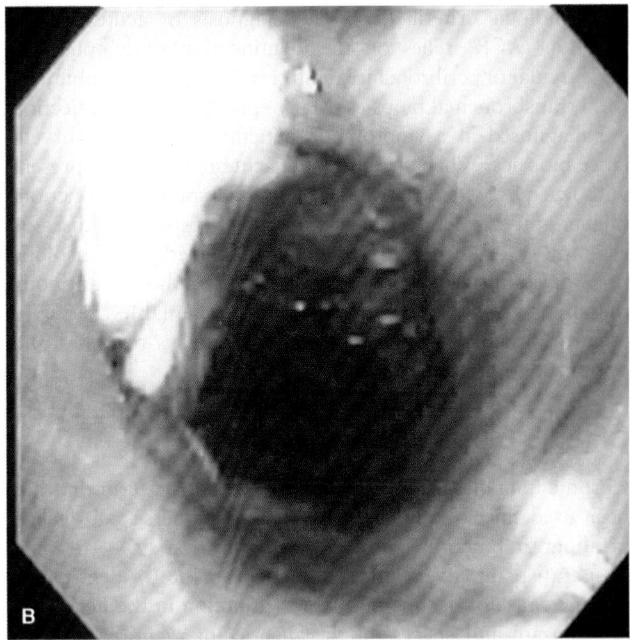

FIGURE 71.21 Bronchus intermedius showing pseudomembrane formation and severe bronchostenosis (at medial edge, **A**) prior to stent placement; and after 10- × 20-mm Ultraflex stent placement (**B**).

of early episodes of bacterial pneumonia, but the incidence has decreased because antibacterial prophylaxis is used at the time of transplantation. A prospective, multicenter trial from Spain noted an incidence of 72 pneumonic episodes per 100 lung transplant recipients per year, with *Pseudomonas aeruginosa* being the most common, followed by *Staphylococcus aureus* (52). Viral infections are the second most common cause of infections; cytomegalovirus (CMV) infection is the most common among the viral etiologies. Patients at highest risk of infection and morbidity are CMV-seronegative recipients from a seropositive lung donor. The case fatality rate of CMV infection is reported to be about 5%. Extended CMV prophylaxis has resulted in significant decline of risk of CMV reactivation (53). Herpes simplex (HSV) and varicella zoster (VZ) infections are also quite common, and are mostly caused by reactivation of a latent viral infection. Acquired respiratory viral infections are mostly secondary to respiratory syncytial virus (RSV), influenza, and parainfluenza viruses. These viral infections may cause cough, wheezing or, in extreme cases, acute respiratory distress syndrome (ARDS). Parvovirus has been reported to cause refractory anemia in recipients of solid organ transplants. The most common cause of fungal infection is *Candida albicans,* likely due to central lines. Aspergillus also commonly infects the lung; the spectrum of disease ranges from necrotic bronchitis to invasive fungal pneumonia (54). The incidence of *Pneumocystis jirovecii* is probably 5% to 10% since the institution of long-term prophylaxis.

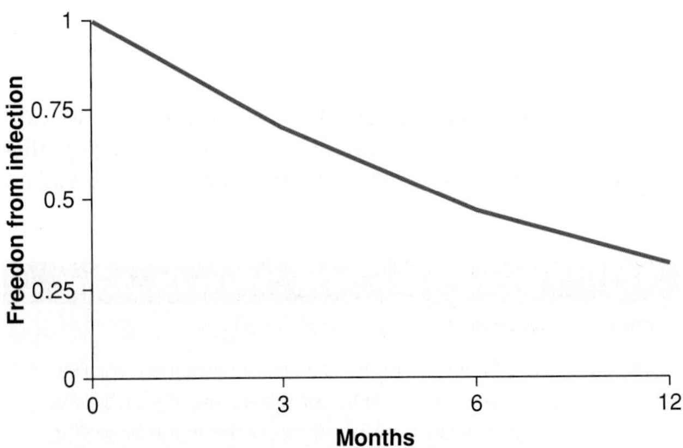

FIGURE 71.22 The 12-month freedom from any infection is 32% after lung transplantation in patients surviving 12 months (*N* = 110). (Data from University of Florida database.)

Acute Rejection

The lung is characterized by the highest rates of rejection among the commonly transplanted solid organs, with 20% to 25% freedom from acute rejection in the first year (55,56). Acute rejection denotes the infiltration of the allograft by lymphocytes (Fig. 71.23); severity of the rejection is classified

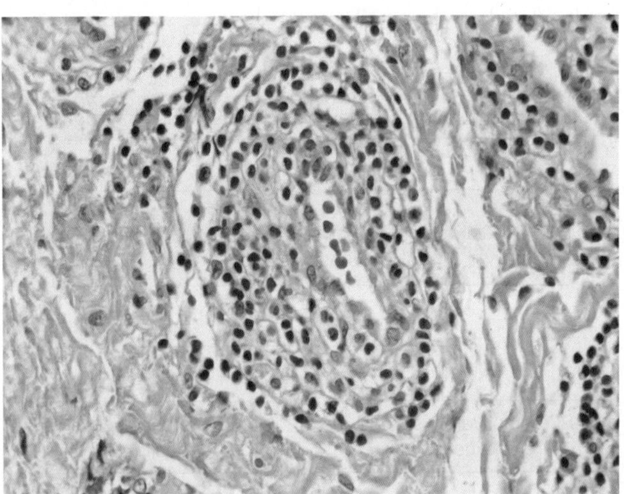

FIGURE 71.23 Perivascular cuffing of a blood vessel is diagnostic of acute rejection. Transbronchial biopsy specimen.

by pathologic criteria (57). The diagnosis of acute cellular rejection (ACR) relies on the identification of lymphocytic perivascular or peribronchiolar infiltrates in lung tissue obtained from transbronchial biopsies. Many episodes of acute rejection are diagnosed in asymptomatic patients undergoing surveillance biopsies. When symptomatic, acute rejection can present with fever, hypoxemia, dyspnea, cough, or sputum production. Higher-grade rejection can lead to acute respiratory distress. Therapy of acute rejection is daily pulse methylprednisolone for 3 days. In steroid-resistant cases, antilymphocyte antibody therapy is given (thymoglobulin or alemtuzumab). The maintenance immunosuppression regimen is always reviewed and optimized to prevent recurrence.

Chronic Lung Allograft Dysfunction

Chronic lung allograft dysfunction (CLAD) is a term that has been used since about 2010 to describe the persistent decline in allograft function compared with the best FEV_1 attained post transplant. Every effort should be made to identify the specific cause of decline in allograft function in the hope that appropriate and successful therapeutic interventions can be undertaken to restore and optimize graft function. However, patients who have persistent allograft dysfunction without an identifiable cause are labeled as having CLAD (Fig. 71.24) (58). Most insults to the allograft bronchial epithelium have been identified as potential risk factors for CLAD: severe PGD, recurrent ACR, antibody-mediated rejection (AMR), gastroesophageal (GE) reflux, and possibly respiratory viral infection (59–63). Approximately 66% of cases of CLAD are due to obstructive lung disease, synonymous with BOS; and 34% is due to restrictive lung disease, synonymous with restrictive allograft syndrome (RAS). BOS and RAS are two distinct phenotypes that are characterized by different chest radiographs and prognoses (64). Moreover, BOS is divided into distinct stages based on spirometry, with each lower stage carrying a poorer prognosis (65,66). In patients with decline in lung function, the CLAD diagnosis is made once reversible causes have been excluded. Bronchoscopy and transbronchial biopsy is performed to exclude the potentially reversible causes such as anastomotic complications, infections, acute rejection, or disease recurrence in the allograft. Unlike acute lung rejection, pathologic diagnosis of CLAD by transbronchial biopsy is difficult related to the small size of the lung sample obtained.

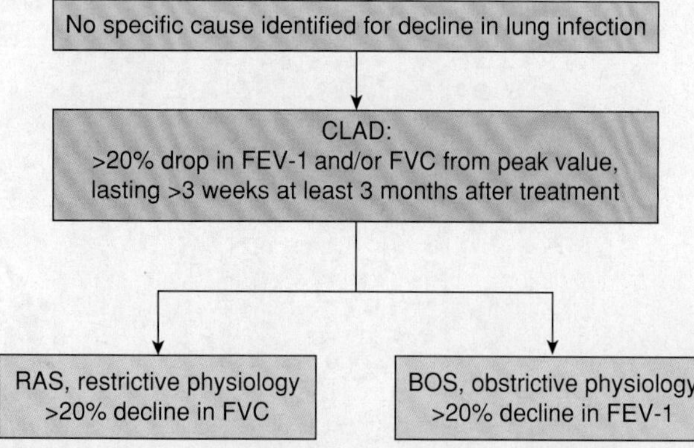

FIGURE 71.24 Chronic lung allograft dysfunction could be of obstructive or restrictive physiology, with different prognosis in each category. FEV_1, forced expiratory pressure in 1 second; FVC, forced vital capacity.

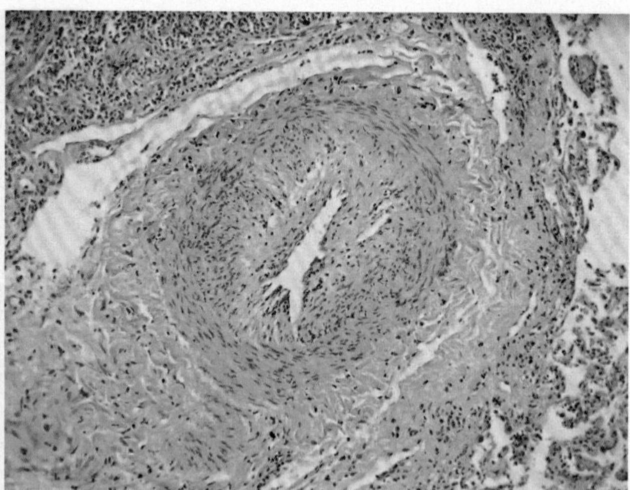

FIGURE 71.25 Open lung biopsy sample showing obliteration of a bronchiolar lumen with granulation tissue, diagnostic of obliterative bronchiolitis.

Patients are also carefully assessed for GE reflux as treatment may stop the decline in spirometry.

BO is the histologic equivalent of chronic lung rejection. BO is characterized by initial lymphocytic-mediated cytotoxicity directed at the epithelial cells lining the respiratory bronchioles. The lymphocytes initially infiltrate the submucosa of the airways and migrate through the basement membrane into the epithelial layer. At this site, epithelial cell necrosis occurs, resulting in a secondary cascade of inflammatory mediators and cytokines attracting neutrophils, fibroblasts, and myofibroblasts. This results in formation of granulation tissue obliterating the bronchiolar lumen, airway obstruction, and proximal bronchiectasis (Fig. 71.25). BOS occurs in approximately 50% of recipients 5 years after transplantation (see Fig. 71.11). It is the most common cause of death in patients surviving more than 1 year; the median survival after the diagnosis of BOS approximates 2 years. In most patients, BOS is characterized by a relentless decline in airflows (Table 71.7), albeit at variable rates in different patients, and ultimately results in respiratory failure. In BOS, the chest radiograph is initially clear, but in the advanced stages will show bronchiectasis and interstitial infiltrates. The chest radiograph in RAS shows interstitial infiltrates with restrictive spirometric changes. Retransplantation has been attempted for this complication but with variable success.

Cancers

Solid organ transplant recipients have elevated risk of cancers (67). Skin cancers are the most common form of malignancies, affecting more than half of solid organ transplant

TABLE 71.7 Staging of Bronchiolitis Obliterans Syndrome

Stage	Description
BOS-p	10–19% decline in FEV_1 compared with the peak FEV_1
1	20–33% decline in FEV_1 compared with the peak FEV_1
2	33–50% decline in FEV_1 compared with the peak FEV_1
3	>50% decline in FEV_1 compared with the peak FEV_1

BOS-p, potential bronchiolitis obliterans syndrome; FEV_1, forced expiratory volume in 1 second.

recipients during their long-term course. Several studies have shown that after a first cutaneous squamous cell carcinoma, the majority will develop subsequent skin cancers within 3 years. A decrease in cutaneous carcinogenesis after the reduction of immunosuppression has been reported. Moreover, sirolimus has been shown to reduce the rate of secondary recurrence of squamous cell carcinoma (68). Bronchogenic carcinomas have been reported in the native lung months-years after SLT. A transplant-related malignancy posttransplant lymphoproliferative disorder (PTLD), has also been reported in 1% to 5% of recipients in the first 5 years. The presentation and pattern of organ involvement is related to the time of onset, with intrathoracic predominance in the first year and extrathoracic predominance after the first year. The incidence of PTLD increases in proportion to the intensity of immunosuppression, especially when antilymphocyte antibodies are used. Most PTLD falls under the spectrum of non-Hodgkin lymphoma, and it is predominantly B-cell lymphocyte in lineage. Epstein–Barr virus (EBV) reactivation or infection is a major risk factor, with the majority showing EBV infection in lymphoma tissue. Decreasing the intensity of immunosuppression is the mainstay of therapy, but carries the risk of allograft rejection. Antiviral therapy, anti-CD20 monoclonal antibody therapy, combination chemotherapy, and radiation therapy have all been used, with variable success; an optimal treatment protocol has yet to be determined. Many patients die of the side effects of treatment rather than from disease progression (69).

Recurrence of Native Lung Diseases

Sarcoidoses, giant cell pneumonitis, lymphangiomyomatosis, diffuse panbronchiolitis and, most recently, polymyositis-associated ILD have each been documented to recur in the allograft (70–74). Due to the small number of recipients with these diagnoses, and the relatively short follow-up time, the recurrence rate and its impact on the allograft function is not known with certainty. Additionally, the transplant community continues to transplant these diseases.

CONCLUSION

Lung transplantation has become an acceptable therapeutic option for patients with end-stage lung diseases who have failed all possible medical and surgical interventions. Patients should be referred for transplantation when projected 2-year survival is about 50% and transplantation is expected to increase the probability of survival. The patient's perception of an unacceptable quality of life associated with the end-stage lung disease is an important additional consideration, but the life expectancy must be the overriding impetus for referral. In addition, since the waiting time may be up to 12 months, the patient's health must remain stable during this time so that the patient will be able to endure transplantation, as well as the pulmonary rehabilitation that follows. The use of relatively stringent criteria is important in identifying candidates for whom transplantation is likely to be successful; it is important to avoid selecting poor candidates simply because of the desperate nature of their situation. Patients should be functionally disabled but ambulatory. They should also be free of clinically significant cardiac, renal, or hepatic impairment. Lung transplantation has been proven to prolong the 2- and 4-year survival in advanced stage IPF and CF patients, but not in patients with COPD. In COPD patients, we generally wait until the patient has a projected 2-year survival—with or without transplantation—before performing transplantation, with improvement in the quality of life being the most important factor to consider as the justification.

HEART TRANSPLANTATION

Heart failure affects 20 million people worldwide, 5.8 million are in the United States, where 550,000 cases are diagnosed yearly (75). With the exception of that caused by reversible etiologies, heart failure continues to progress over time, resulting in markedly decreased survival and quality of life (76). End-stage heart failure carries a dramatic 1-year mortality of 50% to 80% despite optimal medical therapy (77). Soon after its inception, orthotopic heart transplantation was shown to dramatically improve both survival and quality of life (78). However, despite the increasing number of patients in need of this life-changing therapy, the number of heart transplants has remained relatively steady in the last 20 years (79). Therefore, ISHLT has been diligent in developing registries and guidelines to optimize the application and management of this life-changing therapy (79–85).

OVERVIEW

As of June 30th, 2013, 104,027 adult heart transplants have been performed worldwide, and reported to the ISHLT; approximately 3,300 of these have occurred in last year (79). Advanced heart failure with reduced ejection fraction is the most common condition leading to cardiac transplantation; both nonischemic cardiomyopathy and ischemic cardiomyopathy account for 49% and 43% of all heart transplants, respectively. Other diagnoses leading to cardiac transplantation include valvular heart disease, congenital heart disease, retransplantation, and intractable ventricular arrhythmias. Multiorgan transplantation, generally resulting from end-stage heart failure leading to severe end-organ dysfunction, continues to progressively increase in the form of heart–kidney, heart–liver, and heart–lung transplants (79).

ORGAN ALLOCATION

The rate of heart donation has remained stable over the past decade; only 3.5 hearts per 1,000 patient deaths are recovered and transplanted in the United States (86). In order to ensure equitable distribution of organs, the UNOS, the entity responsible for the procurement and distribution of cadaveric organs in the United States, has developed an organ allocation system, the OPTN (Organ Procurement and Transplantation Network), based on blood type compatibility, geographical distance, severity of illness, and time accrued on the wait list. It operates through 11 geographic regions of the country, with each region further divided into many OPOs. The OPOs' main responsibility is the identification and screening of potential donors, and coordination of the transplant process. In general, the allocation of hearts is first done within the OPO, and then outside it, in 500 nautical mile concentric zones from the donor hospital.

DONOR SELECTION

After consent for organ donation is obtained, the initial donor screening consists of confirmation of brain death, age, gender, height, weight, and ABO blood type. The OPO also investigates the circumstances leading to death, presence of active malignancies, time of severe hypotension and cardiopulmonary resuscitation, and other cardiovascular risk factors. Routine laboratory and serologic tests are performed (human immunodeficiency virus [HIV], hepatitis B [HBV], and C viruses [HCV], CMV, EBV, syphilis testing [RPR/VDRL], and human T-lymphotropic viruses [HTLV I/II]), as well as a succinct cardiovascular workup (electrocardiogram, chest x-ray, and a transthoracic echocardiogram; coronary angiography is usually done for donors older than 40 to 50 years old, and occasionally a right heart catheterization is justified). Class I and II HLA genotyping is also performed for prospective virtual cross-matching. Once the evaluation is complete, the donor is entered into the UNOS database and OPTN rank list for organ allocation. The vitality of the donor organs is maintained by the OPO, ensuring appropriate ventilation and organ perfusion; intravenous vasopressin, levothyroxine, and glucocorticoids are used to preserve the allograft function after brain death (87). The final evaluation is done in situ by the cardiovascular surgeon at the time of recovery.

Suitable donor characteristics include: Age less than 55 years, projected ischemic time less than 4 hours, left ventricular wall thickness less than 12 to 14 mm, LVEF more than 40% to 45%, no CAD (or single vessel CAD amenable to surgical revascularization), none or low-dose active inotropic agents, donor body weight no greater than 30% below that of the recipient, among others. Height matching is also of paramount importance; undersized hearts will be eventually insufficient to maintain the needs of the body, and oversized hearts will develop constrictive-like physiology and congestive heart failure symptoms (82).

The median donor age is currently 34 years, and it has been progressively rising in recent years; in the United States, only about 8% of donors are older than 50 years of age (79). Additionally, donors continue to be mostly males (about 69%), with an average BMI of 25. Comorbidities have become progressively more prevalent in the most recent era: 25% of donors have diabetes mellitus, 44% have hypertension, and 6% have had a previous malignancy (84).

RECIPIENT SELECTION

Due to the limited availability of donor hearts, and the increasing prevalence of patients in need of cardiac transplantation, the process of recipient selection and organ allocation continues to grow in importance. The expected survival of patients with end-stage heart failure is markedly reduced compared with healthy individuals of similar age; heart transplantation results in a remarkable improvement in survival and quality of life in appropriately selected patients (81).

The most common indications for cardiac transplantation are cardiogenic shock, end-stage heart failure despite optimal medical therapy, life-threatening refractory ventricular arrhythmias, and intractable angina (81). Ambulatory end-stage heart failure patients amenable to cardiac transplantation, are preferably evaluated with a cardiopulmonary exercise stress test (CPET) to assess their exercise performance; a peak VO_2 of less than 12 mL/kg/min (while on optimal beta-blocker therapy), or less than 50% of predicted VO_2, or a V_E/V_{CO_2} slope greater than 35, are all markers of high short-term mortality on standard medical therapy alone, and eligible candidates for cardiac transplantation. Additionally, combining the Heart Failure Survival Score (HFSS) (88) and the Seattle Heart Failure Model (SHFM) (89) improves the predictive ability for HF risk stratification in patients referred for transplantation (90).

Potential recipients undergo a thorough evaluation (81) to identify any condition or situation that could adversely affect the recipient's survival or quality of life after cardiac transplantation (Tables 71.8, 71.9) (91). Once the evaluation is complete, the patient is given a UNOS status based on the severity of illness (Table 71.10) (86). The overall goal is to list a patient for transplantation after all the standard medical and surgical options have been maximized, but before the patient develops significant impairment of end-organ function to preclude this therapy.

TABLE 71.8 Evaluation Work-up Prior to Heart Transplantation: Anamnesis and Physical Examination

- Immunocompatibility evaluation: ABO blood type and antibody screen, HLA genotyping, panel of reactive antibodies (PRA) screen
- Heart failure severity evaluation: ECG, echocardiogram, CXR, CPET, RHC, LHC
- Multiorgan function evaluation: Laboratory data (CBC, BMP, 24-hr CrCl, TSH, LFT, HbA1c, UA, lipid panel, PT/INR, microalbuminuria), vascular data (carotid duplex, abdominal ultrasound, eye examination, ABIs), dental examination (panoramic dental x-ray), DEXA scan, PFTs
- Infectious and vaccination evaluation: HBV, HCV, HIV, HSV I/II, CMV, EBV, RPR/VDRL, HTLV I/II, *Toxoplasma*, VZV, PPD
- Preventive evaluation: PSA, colonoscopy, PAP, mammography
- Psychosocial and financial evaluation: Psychiatric, neurocognitive, financial, and social work consultations

TABLE 71.9 Contraindications for Heart Transplantation

- Systemic illness with a life expectancy of <2 yrs
- Active or recent malignancy within 5 yrs
- AIDS with frequent opportunistic infections
- Active systemic disease with severe multiorgan dysfunction
- Severe single organ dysfunction (liver, kidney, lung) if being considered for heart-only transplantation
- Pulmonary hypertension
  - PASP >60 mmHg
  - Mean TPG >15 mmHg
  - PVR >6 WU
- Other relative contraindications
  - Age >65–70 yrs
  - Active infection
  - Active PUD
  - Severe PVD
  - Morbid obesity (BMI >35 kg/m^2)
  - Cachexia (BMI <18 kg/m^2)
  - Pulmonary infarction <6 wks
  - Irreversible neuromuscular disorder
  - Severe neurocognitive impairment
  - Drug, tobacco, or alcohol abuse <6 mo

TABLE 71.10 UNOS Status Definitions

Status	Description
1A	LVAD/RVAD (initial 30 days), IABP, ECMO, TAH, LVAD with device-related complication, mechanical ventilation, continuous high-dose IV inotrope or multiple continuous IV inotropes and a pulmonary catheter in place
1B	Continuous IV inotrope, LVAD/RVAD after expiration of initial 30 days of 1A status
2	Eligible for transplantation, but not meeting 1A or 1B criteria
7	Temporarily ineligible for heart transplantation

Based on the latest ISHLT registry report (79), the median adult recipient age is 54 years and has remained constant for the last 25 years; however, the proportion of patients transplanted more than 70 years old continues to increase. An increasingly lower percentage of recipients are hospitalized, on inotropes, or on mechanical ventilation at the time of transplant; whereas an increasing higher percentage, currently 40% of all recipients, are using mechanical circulatory support devices (largely left ventricular assist devices [LVADs]) as a bridge to transplant. This phenomenon is likely driven by the increasing number of potential recipients in need of transplantation, and the scarcity of available organs. Based on registry data, the posttransplant survival of patients bridged to transplant with continuous flow devices is similar to that of patients without LVADs and on inotropic support at the time of transplant; this is not the case of patients requiring biventricular support, in which the posttransplant survival is significantly less (79).

SURGICAL TECHNIQUE

The principles of orthotopic heart transplantation techniques were first described by Norman Shumway in the 1960s (92). In December of 1967, Christiaan Barnard performed the first human heart transplant in Cape Town, South Africa (93); however, many posttransplant complications led to a dismal survival, and the excitement was short lived. Stanford University was one of the few programs in the world that continued exploring this therapeutic option, at that time uncertain. Many of the surgical techniques utilized today in heart and lung transplantation were developed at this institution in the 1970s and 1980s (94–97).

Essential factors to ensure a successful heart procurement include proper heparinization prior to clamping, prevention of left or right heart distention, proper cooling and preservation of the organ during transport, and close monitoring of the donor allograft prior to harvest while other organs are being dissected to prevent ischemic injury. Recipient surgery usually begins once the donor surgical team confirms the suitability of the donor heart by direct visualization. After adequate anesthesia and placement of hemodynamic monitoring catheters, the recipient is prepped and draped from chin down, giving exposure to femoral vessels, if needed, for CPB in redo sternotomy (or LVAD explants). Once the mediastinum is exposed after median sternotomy, systemic heparin is given, followed by CPB via bicaval venous and ascending aorta arterial cannulation (axillary or femoral artery can be used, as well); subsequently, the recipient is cooled. As the donor heart arrives to the operating room, the ascending aorta is clamped and the native heart is explanted, leaving a cuff for anastomosis of inferior vena cava, superior vena cava, pulmonary artery, aorta, and left atrium. The donor heart is prepared on the back table, fashioning anastomotic edges, and closing the patent foramen ovale, if extant. With longer ischemic times, cardioplegia can be given once or multiple times during implantation. The sequence of end-to-end anastomosis varies from surgeon to surgeon. Generally, all connections are hand sewn with suture; the left atrium is anastomosed first, followed by the aorta, allowing for subsequent rewarming and removal of cross clamp. Alternatively, the cross clamp can be removed after all five anastomoses have been completed. Once the heart regains contractile function, de-airing maneuvers are performed via steep Trendelenburg position with CO_2 flooding the field, left heart venting, and transesophageal echocardiogram imaging. Inotrope and vasoconstrictor support is then begun and CPB is weaned off. Temporary mechanical support (intra-aortic balloon pump [IABP], right ventricular assist device [RVAD], or ECMO) may be indicated at this time if ventricular failure ensues. If a flow-limiting coronary artery disease lesion had been identified in the donor heart prior to implantation, a suitable aortocoronary bypass graft can be implanted at this time. Arterial and venous cannulae are removed after the patient has been weaned from CPB. Subsequently, anticoagulation is reversed, hemostasis is obtained at all surgical sites, temporary pacing wires and chest tubes are placed, the sternum is reapproximated with steel wires, and the chest incision is ultimately closed in planes.

ACUTE CARDIAC ALLOGRAFT DYSFUNCTION

The immediate dysfunction of the cardiac allograft has been recently consensually classified into "primary" (idiopathic) and "secondary," where there is an identifiable etiology (98). Primary cardiac allograft dysfunction can be biventricular, or affect the left or right ventricle in isolation; its severity has been further classified based on the degree of hemodynamic compromise (Table 71.11). Secondary cardiac allograft dysfunction is usually attributable to pulmonary hypertension,

TABLE 71.11 Primary Cardiac Allograft Dysfunction

Type	Severity	Definition
LV or BiV	Mild	LVEF ≤40% *or* abnormal hemodynamics (RA >15 mmHg, PCWP >20 mmHg, CI <2.0 L/min/m^2) lasting >1 hr, *and* requiring low-dose inotropic agents
	Moderate	LVEF ≤40% *or* abnormal hemodynamics (RA >15 mmHg, PCWP >20 mmHg, CI <2.0 L/min/m^2, MAP <70 mmHg) lasting >1 hr, *and* requiring high-dose inotropic agents or newly placed IABP
	Severe	Dependence on left or biventricular mechanical support, including ECMO, LVAD, BiVAD, or percutaneous LVAD. Excludes requirement for IABP
RV		Abnormal hemodynamics (RA >15 mmHg, PCWP <15 mmHg, CI <2.0 L/min/m^2) and TPG <15 mmHg and/or PASP <50 mmHg, *or* need for RVAD

Adapted from Kobashigawa J, Zuckermann A, Macdonald P, et al. Report from a consensus conference on primary graft dysfunction after cardiac transplantation. *J Heart Lung Transplant.* 2014;33(4):327–340.

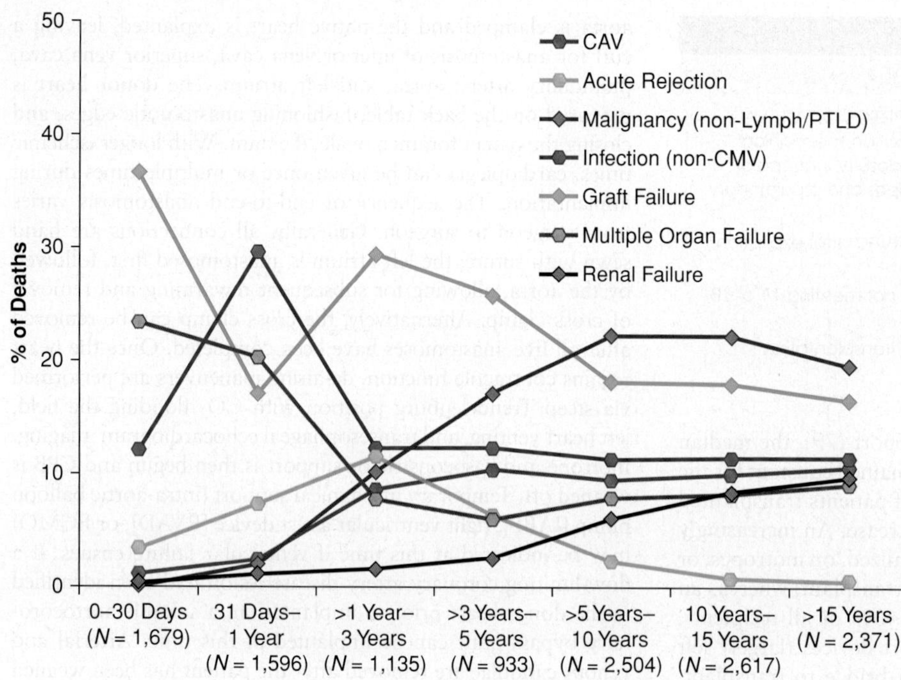

FIGURE 71.26 Relative incidence of leading causes of death after adult heart transplantation (January 2006 to June 2013). Early after cardiac transplantation, primary allograft failure, infections, and multiple organ failure are the most common causes of death. Beyond 3 years, malignancy, cardiac allograft vasculopathy, and renal failure, become additionally important fatal comorbidities. (Adapted from Lund LH, Edwards LB, Kucheryavaya AY, et al. The registry of the International Society for Heart and Lung Transplantation: thirty-first official adult heart transplant report—2014. Focus theme: retransplantation. *J Heart Lung Transplant.* 2014;33(10):996–1008.)

poor allograft preservation leading to ischemia–reperfusion injury, or known surgical complications. The automation of ABO and HLA compatibility during organ allocation has dramatically decreased the incidence of hyperacute allograft rejection. Acute cardiac allograft dysfunction accounts for about 35% of overall 30-day mortality after cardiac transplantation; it is the leading condition leading to early retransplantation (Fig. 71.26) (79).

Primary Cardiac Allograft Dysfunction

The ISHLT recently published a consensus statement on this devastating complication, broadly defined as idiopathic early systolic ventricular dysfunction or abnormal cardiac hemodynamics, requiring various degrees of hemodynamic support to maintain life (Table 71.11) (98). Prior to this consensus, multiple reports have identified risk factors, potential etiologies, and management strategies; however, the lack of a standard definition has made this devastating complication difficult to characterize and prognosticate (99–106). In 2011, Segovia et al. (107) described the RADIAL score, a nonimmunologic risk prediction model that incorporates recipient (right atrial pressure ≥10 mmHg, age ≥60 years, diabetes mellitus, preoperative inotrope dependence), donor (age ≥30 years), and procedural (ischemic time ≥240 minutes) variables. This score was validated in a single center (107), and in a contemporary multicenter prospective cohort (108), with good correlation between the actual and predicted incidences of primary cardiac allograft dysfunction. Some reports have also suggested that mechanical circulatory support prior to cardiac transplantation is a risk factor for primary allograft dysfunction (104,109), although this has not been unequivocally established (79). The use of "suboptimal" donor organs (>55 years of age, mild left ventricular hypertrophy, CAD, CDC high-risk donors, etc.), now common in many centers due to the limited donor pool and increasing number of potential recipients (110–112), has been also proposed as a risk factor for primary allograft dysfunction; this perception, however, remains yet to be verified (104,112). Additionally, the changing demographics of recipients (higher status, older age, frailer condition, more comorbidities) and increasing surgical challenges (explantation of ventricular assist devices, recurrent cardiothoracic surgeries, etc.) may also be likely contributors of this condition (113). It has been well established that several inflammatory (TNF-α, IL-6 (114,115)) and hormonal (thyroid hormones (116) and vasopressin (117)) factors significantly affect the function of the heart after brain death ensues; inadvertent omission of glucocorticoid (118), levothyroxine (119), and vasopressin (120) infusion prior to organ recovery may have deleterious effects (87,121).

Secondary Cardiac Allograft Dysfunction

Cardiac allograft dysfunction secondary to treatable conditions such as severe pulmonary hypertension, and surgical complications (massive hemorrhage, cardiac tamponade, kinking of the pulmonary artery, coronary artery embolism, etc.) must be suspected and addressed immediately before irreversible myocardial damage ensues (Fig. 71.27). Severe pulmonary hypertension has been historically considered a risk factor for isolated right ventricular failure, and seems to be clinically evident in everyday practice; interestingly however, recent studies have failed to statistically validate this clinical perception (107).

Severe acute cardiac allograft dysfunction can also result from ischemia–reperfusion injury and/or prolonged cold ischemic time (i.e., time from cross clamping the donor, with subsequent excision and immersion of the heart in iced saline, to removal of the cross clamp after implantation in the recipient) (104). This phenomenon can produce transient myocardial stunning, lasting for 12 to 24 hours after transplantation (122), or irreversible myocardial damage of varying degree of severity. Ischemic-related inflammation is characterized

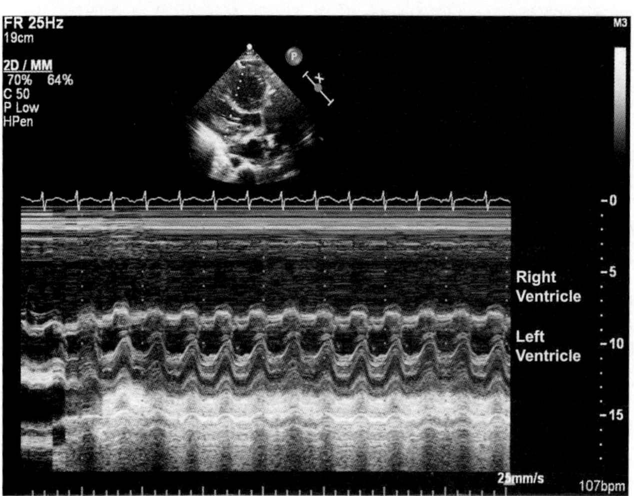

FIGURE 71.27 Acute right ventricular failure after heart transplantation secondary to severe pulmonary hypertension. M-mode echocardiogram of a recently transplanted heart, parasternal long view, at the level of the papillary muscle. There is enlargement and akinesis of the right ventricle. The left ventricle is hyperkinetic and the left ventricular cavity is small ("empty") due to decreased transpulmonary flow. (Courtesy of J. Emanuel Finet, MD, Indiana University, Indianapolis, Indiana.)

by predominantly polymorphonuclear and histiocytic cellular infiltrates, with a paucity of lymphocytes, and significant amounts of contraction-band necrosis, and eventual fibrosis (Fig. 71.28) (123). Cold ischemic times longer than 4 to 5 hours have been associated with a higher incidence of allograft dysfunction and decreased survival (104,124). The type of preservation solution also seems to have a significant role in the incidence of ischemia–reperfusion injury; for example, the University of Wisconsin solution has been associated with less necrosis than Celsior in early biopsy specimens (125).

Management

The management of acute cardiac allograft dysfunction is based on the severity of the hemodynamic compromise and the underlying causes leading to it. Certainly, surgical complications need to be addressed as soon as possible, based on their risk/benefit balance, and probability of success. Additionally, hemodynamic stability is to be maintained with appropriate volume or blood product repletion, and inotropic and vasoactive agents, to prevent the development of multiorgan failure. Pulmonary vasodilators, such as inhaled nitric oxide (126), inhaled prostacyclin (127), and oral sildenafil (128), have been shown to safely and effectively reduce pulmonary hypertension and improve right ventricular function. Albeit not yet approved in the United States, levosimendan, a new calcium-sensitizer inotrope, has been shown to be a useful adjunctive agent (129). Additionally, several case studies have been published on the effectiveness of mechanical circulatory support in addition to standard therapy, with moderately good outcomes (99–108,130,131). For example, surviving patients after posttransplant ECMO support have the same 1-year conditional survival rates as unaffected patients (109). Ultimately, retransplantation can be reserved for refractory cases; however, reported outcomes have been uniformly poor (79,132).

ACUTE CARDIAC ALLOGRAFT REJECTION

Hyperacute Cardiac Allograft Rejection

Hyperacute rejection is the most dreadful cause of acute cardiac allograft rejection, usually occurring within the first 24 hours after transplantation, but many times evident soon after the cardiac allograft is reperfused. Hyperacute rejection is caused by the presence of preformed recipient antibodies that bind to endothelial epitopes on the allograft (133). Widespread endothelial damage leads to leaky capillaries, endothelial swelling, microthrombosis, and rapid polymorphonuclear infiltrates. Despite therapy, global ischemia and catastrophic allograft failure develop soon after, irreversibly leading to allograft loss and, many times, death (134). The incidence of this devastating complication has declined dramatically due

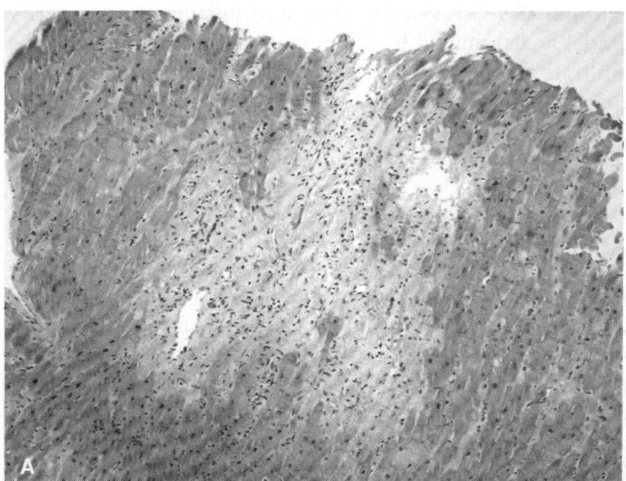

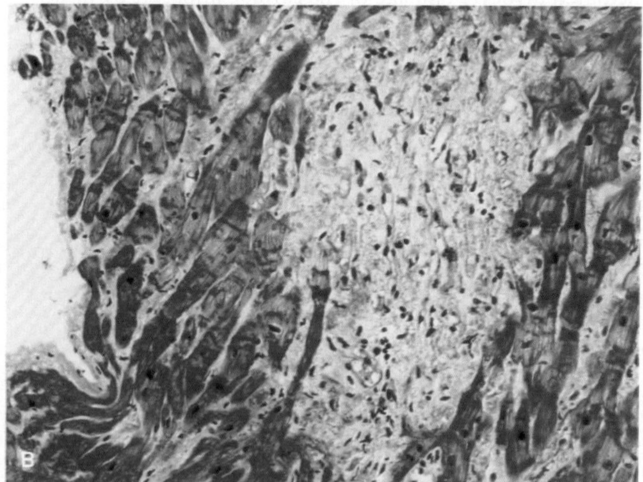

FIGURE 71.28 Myocardial ischemia. **A:** Areas of ischemic cell necrosis are generally zonal, with comparatively little inflammation, in contrast with necrosis secondary to rejection. In this example, the ischemia is associated with early fibrosis and is seen in a biopsy that is 3 weeks after transplantation. **B:** Masson trichrome stain demonstrates minimal fibrosis in the area. (From Burke A, Tavora F. Cellular rejection. In: *Practical Cardiovascular Pathology*. Philadelphia, PA: Lippincott Williams & Wilkins; 2011:286.)

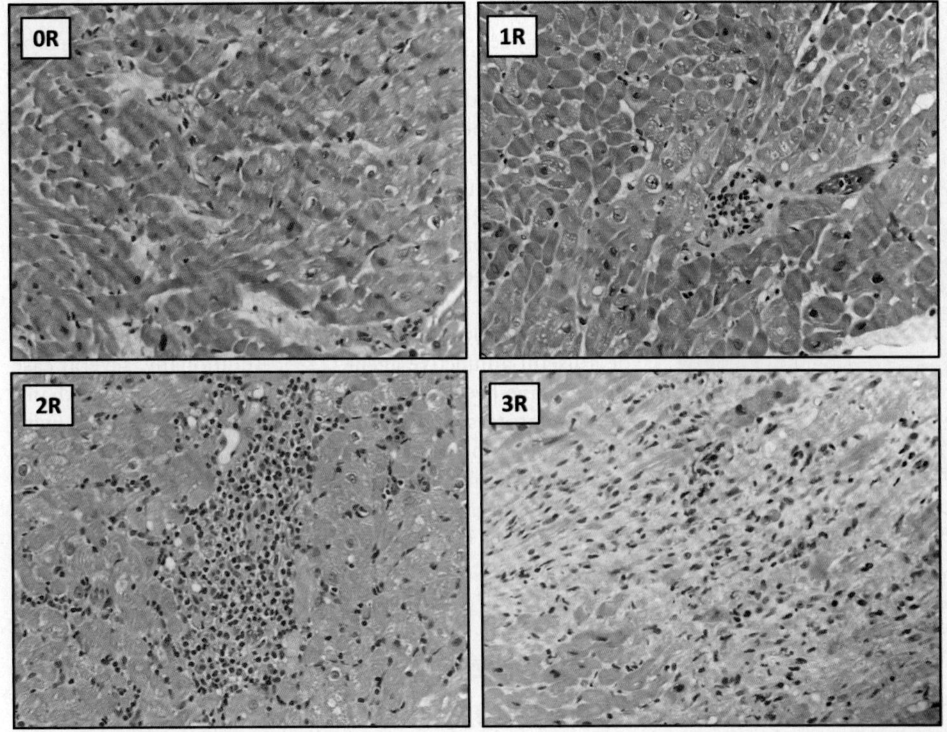

FIGURE 71.29 Acute cellular cardiac allograft rejection. **0R**: Normal myocardial biopsy without myocyte necrosis or an inflammatory cell infiltrate. There is no endothelial swelling. **1R**: Mild acute cellular rejection with one small perivascular infiltrate of lymphocytes without myocyte necrosis. There is no endothelial swelling. The infiltrate may be interstitial instead of perivascular. **2R**: Moderate acute cellular rejection with a dense inflammatory cell infiltrate and focal myocyte necrosis. Several similar foci were present in the same biopsy (not shown). **3R**: Severe acute cellular rejection with extensive myocyte necrosis and a mixed inflammatory cell infiltrate. This can also be complicated with hemorrhage, vasculitis, and extensive tissue edema. (Courtesy of Oscar W. Cummings, MD, Indiana University. Indianapolis, Indiana.)

to the systematic prospective ABO and HLA virtual cross-matching of the donor and the recipient prior to cardiac transplantation.

Acute Cellular Cardiac Allograft Rejection

Acute rejection per se accounts for about 11% of deaths in the first 3 years after cardiac transplantation; however, acute and chronic immune injury are likely important contributors to overall cardiac allograft failure, which remains the leading cause of death after cardiac transplantation (see Fig. 71.26) (84). ACR generally occurs within weeks to months after cardiac transplantation. It is characterized by cellular-mediated myocyte damage of the cardiac allograft by means of specific HLA allorecognition and induction of donor cell apoptosis by the recipient's cytotoxic T cells (80). Most commonly, clinical presentation resembles that of an acute heart failure syndrome (dyspnea, lower extremity edema, tachycardia, etc.), but it can quickly progress to cardiogenic shock and multiorgan failure if not properly treated. The concomitant presence of arrhythmias, general malaise, and fever increases the diagnostic likelihood of inflammatory-mediated allograft failure (135). Although many noninvasive diagnostic modalities have been proposed to screen and diagnose ACR, the endomyocardial biopsy remains the gold-standard modality to reliably assess the severity of myocardial damage and guide therapy (82). The diagnosis of ACR is confirmed by the interstitial and/or perivascular aggregate of CD4+ and CD8+ T lymphocytes ("infiltrate") in the myocardium (Fig. 71.29). The degree of inflammation (severity grade) is determined by the number and morphology of the infiltrate, presence or absence of necrosis, macrophages and eosinophils, hemorrhage, vasculitis, or interstitial edema (Table 71.12) (80).

TABLE 71.12 Acute Cellular Cardiac Allograft Rejection

ISHLT 1990 Grade	Histologic Features	ISHLT 2004 Grade
0	No infiltrates or necrosis	0R
1A	Focal (perivascular or interstitial) infiltrate without necrosis	1R, mild
1B	Diffuse, sparse infiltrate without necrosis	
2	Single focus of aggressive infiltration and/or myocyte damage	
3A	Multifocal aggressive infiltration and/or myocyte damage	2R, moderate
3B	Diffuse inflammatory process with necrosis	3R, severe
4	Diffuse aggressive polymorphous infiltrate with edema, hemorrhage, vasculitis, and myocyte necrosis	

ISHLT, International Society for Heart and Lung Transplantation.

Acute Antibody-Mediated Cardiac Allograft Rejection

AMR is distinct from cellular rejection by its biology and histologic findings; however, it leads to identical clinical features, such as acute heart failure, arrhythmias, and cardiogenic shock (136). It is characterized by the antibody-mediated endothelial damage of the cardiac allograft, by means of activation of the classical pathway of the complement cascade, with minimal lymphocytic response (85). The first episode of AMR can usually occur within the first month after cardiac transplantation, and may recur many months or years after (137). The prevalence of AMR is 7% to 18%, and AMR associated to ACR can be detected in 23% of patients (136). Similarly to ACR,

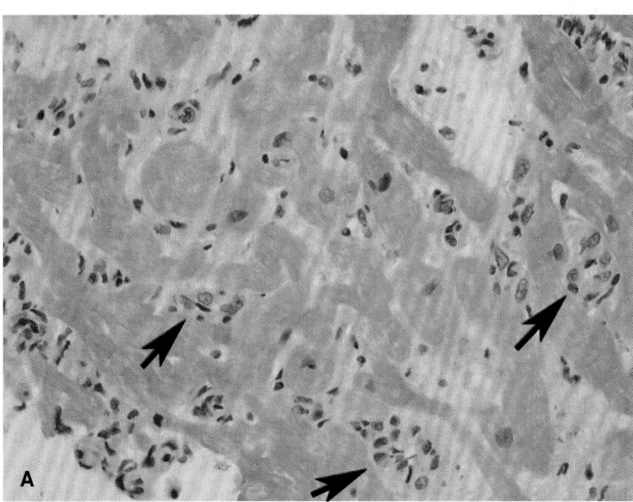
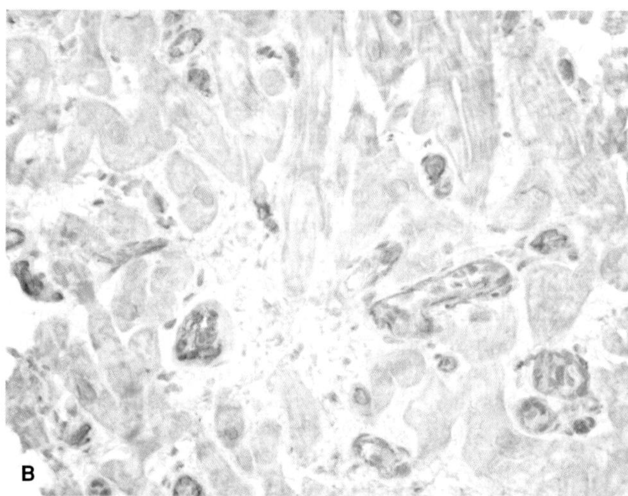

FIGURE 71.30 Acute antibody-mediated cardiac allograft rejection. **A:** Antibody-mediated rejection. Capillaries are prominent with swollen endothelial cells (*arrows*). **B:** Anti-C4d immunohistochemical staining. Note diffuse endothelial capillary positivity. (From Burke A, Tavora F. Antibody-mediated cardiac allograft rejection. In: *Practical Cardiovascular Pathology*. Philadelphia, PA: Lippincott Williams & Wilkins; 2011:290–291.)

AMR can also be detected in asymptomatic patients by routine endomyocardial biopsy, and it is always a predictor of poor outcomes due to an increased risk of cardiac allograft vasculopathy (CAV) and accelerated graft failure (138). The histologic diagnosis of AMR is based on the presence of endothelial cell swelling, intravascular macrophages, and neutrophils in and around capillaries, along with the deposition of complement proteins (C4d or C3d) (Fig. 71.30). The severity of the inflammatory reaction is determined by the presence or absence of interstitial hemorrhage, capillary fragmentation, mixed inflammatory infiltrates, endothelial cell pyknosis and/or karyorrhexis, and marked edema (Table 71.13) (85).

Surveillance of Acute Cardiac Allograft Rejection

The percutaneous transvenous endomyocardial biopsy technique was developed in Stanford University in the early 1970s, and allowed clinicopathologic correlation between patient's syndrome and the histopathology of the transplanted heart (139–141); to this day it remains the "gold-standard" diagnostic test of acute allograft rejection (80). Other proposed methodologies such as ECG parameters, echocardiography, cardiac magnetic resonance imaging, and biomarkers (brain natriuretic peptide, troponin, inflammatory markers, etc.), have not yielded consistent results and are not recommended (82).

Currently, the majority of endomyocardial biopsies are done through the right internal jugular vein or right femoral vein. The middle and apical portions of the right ventricular septum are sampled with the assistance of echocardiography or fluoroscopy. It is recommended to sample at least three separate myocardial pieces from the right ventricular septum, devoid of thrombus or scar tissue; the pieces should be immediately fixed in formalin, and paraffin-embedded for standard processing and H&E staining (see Fig. 71.29). Occasionally, the slides can be also stained with Masson trichrome to aid the pathologic diagnosis of fibrosis (see Fig. 71.28). An additional myocardial piece can be obtained and frozen for immunofluorescence studies (e.g., C4d, C3d) (see Fig. 71.30).

Typical endomyocardial biopsy protocols involve frequent biopsies in the first 6 to 12 months after cardiac transplantation, when acute cardiac allograft rejection is most common, being progressively tapered beyond 12 months, to the point that many programs stop performing biopsies altogether beyond 5 years (82). Interestingly, severe acute rejection can still be found late after cardiac transplantation, and its incidence is not predicted by early rejection episodes (142). However, the utility of biopsy surveillance in stable patients beyond 5 years is thought to provide no clinical benefit (143).

TABLE 71.13 Acute Antibody-Mediated Cardiac Allograft Rejection

pAMR Grade	Definition	Substrates
0	Negative for pathologic AMR	Histologic and immunopathologic studies are both negative
1 (H+)	Histopathologic AMR alone	Histologic findings are present and immunopathologic findings are negative (endothelial cell swelling, intravascular macrophages, vascular neutrophils, endothelialitis)
1 (I+)	Immunopathologic AMR alone	Histologic findings are negative and immunopathologic findings are positive (CD68+ and/or C4d+)
2	Pathologic AMR	Histologic and immunopathologic findings are both present
3	Severe pathologic AMR	Interstitial hemorrhage, capillary fragmentation, mixed inflammatory infiltrates, endothelial cell pyknosis, and/or karyorrhexis, and marked edema and immunopathologic findings are present

Adapted from Berry GJ, Burke MM, Andersen C, et al. The 2013 International Society for Heart and Lung Transplantation Working Formulation for the standardization of nomenclature in the pathologic diagnosis of antibody-mediated rejection in heart transplantation. *J Heart Lung Transplant.* 2013;32(12):1147–1162.

Also, the initial biopsy schedule may be altered to evaluate the response to maintenance immunosuppression changes, or antirejection therapy (143). In a recent analysis, the overall complication rate was found to be less than 1%, including tricuspid valve regurgitation (due to chordae rupture), right bundle branch block, supraventricular arrhythmias, and cardiac tamponade due to RV-free wall perforation, many times requiring immediate pericardiocentesis (135,144). Gene expression profiling of mononuclear cells from peripheral blood has been recently validated as an alternative to surveillance endomyocardial biopsy to detect ACR 2R or greater after cardiac transplantation in patients with no signs of clinical rejection, yielding comparable outcomes (145,146). A score of less than 30 at 6 to 12 months and of less than 34 beyond 12 months offers an excellent negative predictive value for ACR; recent data has validated its use as early as 2 months after transplantation (146).

IMMUNOSUPPRESSION

The development of cyclosporine A and its use in cardiac transplant recipients in the beginning of the 1980s initiated the modern era of cardiac transplantation (147,148). Current immunosuppressive strategies can be categorized into induction, maintenance, and antirejection (149,150).

Induction

Historically, the concept of "induction" was developed as a strategy to diminish long-term allograft rejection, by means of near-complete elimination of all immune responses during the early posttransplant period, subsequent exposure to the donor antigens, and eventual generation of immune tolerance in the recipient (151). Additionally, their use has shown to allow the delayed initiation of cyclosporine A and preserve renal function after cardiac transplantation (152). However, routine immunosuppressive induction in all patients has not definitely been shown to translate into significantly superior outcomes (82), likely due to higher infection and malignancy rates (153). Currently, most transplant programs generally reserve induction strategies for those patients with high risk of long-term rejection, and those with early postoperative kidney dysfunction, as to delay the initiation of calcineurin inhibitors.

Agents used for inductive immunosuppression are classified into lymphocyte depleting, such as antithymocyte globulin (ATG) and alemtuzumab, or lymphocyte nondepleting, like basiliximab. ATG are rabbit- or horse-derived polyclonal antibodies directed against multiple T-cell (CD2, CD3, CD4, CD8) and B-cell (CD19, CD20, CD21) surface antigens, and to other myeloid forms, leading to cell depletion. Generally, after an initial dose (e.g., 1.5 mg/kg), absolute CD3 cell counts are used for dose adjustment and efficacy monitoring during therapy (goal of <25 cells/microL) (154,155); the length of therapy is variable, from 3 to 10 days depending on the center (156). Serious complications include the cytokine release syndrome (fever, rigors, and hypotension), myelosuppression, and increased risk of infections, especially CMV, and of posttransplant lymphoproliferative disorder (PTLD). A combination of glucocorticoids, antihistamines, and acetaminophen is usually given to prevent the cytokine-induced complications; their severity will determine the reduction or termination of therapy. The chimeric anti–IL-2R (CD25) monoclonal antibody basiliximab (30% murine, 70% human) selectively inhibits T-cell proliferation by preventing activation and clonal expansion. The advantages over its polyclonal counterpart are its ease of use (20 mg IV at posttransplant day 0 and day 4), lack of cytokine release syndrome, and alleged superior safety profile (157). It has been suggested that ATG may be superior to basiliximab in preventing long-term allograft rejection (158) and it seems to reduce the production of de novo circulating antibodies during the first year after heart transplantation (151). Basiliximab, on the contrary, seems to offer improved tolerability than ATG, with lower risk of lethal infections (157,159). A novel strategy of adjusting ATG dosing based on recipient's immunologic risk has been recently shown to be safe, and effective in decreasing both cellular and humoral allograft rejection (160). Alemtuzumab, a humanized murine anti-CD52 monoclonal antibody, has lately gained momentum in the cardiac transplantation world. Its use as an induction agent results in a comparable 1-year survival, but with a greater freedom from rejection, despite lower maintenance immunosuppression doses (161), and a similar safety profile than that of ATG or IL-2R antagonists (162). Based on the latest ISHLT registry analysis, slightly over 50% of transplanted patients receive immunosuppressive induction; basiliximab is the most commonly used agent in primary transplantation (about 59% of those receiving induction), followed by ATG (79).

Maintenance

Maintenance immunosuppressive agents are used to prevent the occurrence of rejection episodes that threaten the function of the cardiac allograft and shorten its lifespan. Advances in immunosuppression therapy have resulted in a marked decrease in the incidence of acute rejection in the last 20 years (84). Currently used maintenance immunosuppressive agents are summarized in Table 71.14. Most transplant centers initiate a triple immunosuppressive strategy, consisting of a glucocorticoid (prednisone), a calcineurin inhibitor (cyclosporine A or tacrolimus), and a cell cycle inhibitor (MMF, mycophenolic acid, or azathioprine), to target different pathways of T-cell activation and achieve effective immunosuppression (163).

Glucocorticoids are overall effective immunosuppressants; their safety profile, however, limits their long-term use. They have been used clinically since the 1920s, affecting multiple steps in immune activation, such as antigen presentation, cell migration, cell recognition, cytokine production, proliferation of lymphocytes (164,165), and in particular, T-cell responses to antigen presentation (166–168). After a series of initial IV high-dose infusions at the time of transplant (e.g., 125 mg every 8 hours for four doses), oral prednisone (e.g., 0.5 mg/kg BID) is started with the goal of progressively weaning it by 3 to 12 posttransplant months; the continuation of a very low maintenance dose (e.g., 5–2.5 mg daily) is alternatively acceptable (82). According to the latest ISHLT registry analysis, more than half of patients are "steroid-free" at 5 years after transplant (79).

Calcineurin inhibitors, such as tacrolimus and cyclosporine A, are another immunosuppressive pillar after cardiac transplantation. They exert their effect by binding first to cytosolic immunophilins (FKBP-12 and cyclophilin, respectively), and subsequently to calcineurin, inhibiting its downstream

TABLE 71.14 Maintenance Immunosuppressive Agents

Class/Drug	Target Level (ng/mL)	Common Toxicities
Glucocorticoid		
Prednisone	Not measured	Adrenal insufficiency Diabetes mellitus Cataracts Osteopenia Myopathy Hirsutism Cushing syndrome Hypertension Psychosis Infections
Calcineurin inhibitor		
Cyclosporine A	250–350 (0–2 m) 200–300 (2–4 m) 100–150 (4–6 m) 75–100 (6–12 m) 50–75 (>12 m)	Nephrotoxicity Hypertension Hypertrichosis Gingival hyperplasia Gout
Tacrolimus	10–15 (0–3 m) 8–12 (3–12 m) 5–10 (>12 m)	Neurotoxicity Diabetes mellitus Hyperlipidemia Hypomagnesemia Hyperkalemia Alopecia Infections
Cell cycle inhibitors		
Mycophenolate mofetil Mycophenolic acid Azathioprine	Not recommended (Keep WBC >3,000 cells/μL)	Diarrhea Myelosuppression Infections
mTOR inhibitors		
Sirolimus	4–12	Hyperlipidemia diarrhea Impaired wound healing Myelosuppression Infections
Everolimus	3–8	

transcriptional regulation effects on T-cell activation and proliferation (169). Tacrolimus is about 100 times more potent than cyclosporine A, and shares a similar toxicity profile. Most recent studies have shown significant superiority of tacrolimus over cyclosporine A in terms of efficacy (170,171) and safety (172), and the effectiveness of replacing cyclosporine A with tacrolimus in cases of refractory rejection (173). These findings best explain the declining use of cyclosporine over the last 10 years, and the simultaneous increase in the use of tacrolimus as the primary calcineurin inhibitor in cardiac transplantation (79). However, no differences in survival between the two agents have been categorically demonstrated to date (82).

Antiproliferative agents, such as azathioprine and MMF, exert their main immunosuppressant effect by blocking the purine nucleotide synthesis, impairing DNA metabolism, and hence suppressing both B-cell and T-cell cloning and proliferation. Specifically, MMF is a prodrug of mycophenolic acid, an inosine monophosphate dehydrogenase type II inhibitor; this enzyme is the main rate-limiting enzyme in the de novo synthesis pathway of purine nucleotides of activated T-cell and B-cell lymphocytes (174). Given this relative "target specificity," in contrast to azathioprine, mycophenolic acid has a preferentially more potent effect on activated lymphocytes than any other cell, leading to a safer profile (175). Additionally, MMF has been shown to be superior to azathioprine in reducing mortality and rejection at 1 and 3 years after cardiac transplantation (176,177). Consequently, the use of azathioprine has significantly declined over the last decade, having been replaced by MMF or mycophenolic acid (79). Interestingly, however, tacrolimus monotherapy versus tacrolimus plus MMF seem to result in comparable incidences of rejection in the first year after heart transplantation, in the context of early glucocorticoid withdrawal (178). Since mycophenolic acid drug levels do not clearly correlate with the likelihood of rejection, the ISHLT guidelines advice against the routine monitoring of drug levels, except in situations of suspected medication uncompliance (82).

The mTOR (mammalian Target of Rapamycin) inhibitors, such as sirolimus and everolimus, are a variant of antiproliferative agents that are becoming increasingly important in heart transplantation; their worldwide use has doubled over the last 10 years (79). The mTOR inhibitors form a complex with FKBP-12 upon entering the cell, to subsequently bind and inactivate the cytoplasmic mTOR enzyme. This enzyme naturally transduces cell surface signals (e.g., IL-2R activation) into cell cycle activation, advancing the G1 phase to S phase, via the cyclin-dependent kinases (CDK) pathway, ultimately inducing T-cell proliferation and growth (179,180). Sirolimus was naturally discovered in 1975 (181), whereas everolimus is a synthetic derivative of sirolimus that possesses shorter half-life (about 30 vs. 60 hours for sirolimus) and increased bioavailability (182). Both sirolimus and everolimus were shown to be more efficacious than azathioprine in reducing the severity and incidence of CAV (183), as well as decreasing the incidence of acute rejection, when added to a standard therapy regimen of cyclosporine A and steroids (184). Moreover, substituting the calcineurin inhibitor with sirolimus as primary immunosuppressant–in conjunction with steroids and antiproliferative agents–leads to an improvement in short-term and long-term renal function, without compromising the cardiac allograft function or incidence of rejection (185,186). This substitution has also been shown to attenuate CAV progression (187), and even improve cardiac-related events, and long-term survival (188). Interestingly, when analyzed by virtual histology–intravascular ultrasound (VH-IVUS), sirolimus was found to attenuate coronary artery plaque progression in heart transplant recipients who were substituted early (up to 2 years posttransplant) from a calcineurin inhibitor (189). However, those with late substitution (at least 6 years posttransplant) had increases in the necrotic core and dense calcium volume of the coronary plaque, advocating for the early, rather than late, initiation of mTOR inhibitors (189). It is worth noting, that the concomitant use of both agents at standard doses can intensify the calcineurin inhibitor-induced nephrotoxicity; however, both the trough levels and the dosage of calcineurin inhibitors can be significantly reduced when used in combination with mTOR inhibitors, without higher rejection rates (190). Confirming these findings, it was recently shown that everolimus 1.5 mg with reduced-dose cyclosporine offers similar efficacy to MMF with standard-dose cyclosporine and reduces intimal proliferation at 12 months in de novo heart transplant recipients (191).

Antirejection

Approximately 25% of patients develop some form of rejection within the first year posttransplant (79), but only 13%

require treatment, given the more widely accepted view that mild forms of ACR might be self-limited and that treatment does not increase the likelihood of resolution (192). Once acute allograft rejection is clinically suspected or confirmed with an endomyocardial biopsy, the therapeutic options will be based on the severity of myocardial inflammation and graft dysfunction (Tables 71.11 and 71.12).

Low-grade ACR rejection (1R) is usually not treated, but warrants optimization of maintenance immunosuppression (82). Interestingly however, grade 1R/2 has been suggested as the strongest predictor of subsequent 2R or greater rejection (193), and if recurrent, may warrant the initiation of additional immunosuppressive agent such as low-dose methotrexate. Moderate-grade rejection (2R) merits a high-dose steroid pulse in addition to optimization of maintenance therapy; a typical regimen is oral prednisone or IV methylprednisolone 0.5 to 1 mg/day for 3 days (194,195), and subsequent return to maintenance therapy with a steroid taper. High-grade rejection (3R), or any rejection grade with concomitant allograft systolic dysfunction, warrants the use of lymphocyte-depleting agents (ATG 1.5 mg/kg for 3–5 days, based on CD3 cell counts), and high-dose IV steroids (methylprednisolone 0.5–1 mg/day for 3–5 days), and subsequent optimization of maintenance immunosuppressive therapy. Of note, maintenance therapy should be either lowered or stopped completely during the ATG course to prevent an increased incidence of infective complications. Additionally, and if required by the degree of hemodynamic instability, inotropic, vasoactive, and mechanical circulatory support strategies should be employed to maintain proper hemodynamics during antirejection treatment.

In a similar manner, the treatment of AMR is tailored to the degree of inflammation and allograft systolic dysfunction (137); this is less well defined, however. Optimization of the maintenance immunosuppressive therapy, high-dose IV glucocorticoids, ATG, plasmapheresis to acutely remove pathogenic donor-specific antibodies (196), infusion of antilymphocyte B or antiplasma cell agents, such as rituximab (anti-CD20) (197) or bortezomib (26S proteasome inhibitor) (198), and intravenous immunoglobulin (IVIG) to acutely block pathogenic antibodies, or to replete circulating antibodies after plasmapheresis or antilymphocyte B agents (199), are some of the strategies currently used, in various combinations. Depending on the severity of the clinical presentation, treatment may also involve that of ACR, given their occasional coexistence. Allosensitized patients—those with circulating donor-specific antibodies, particularly those able to bind complement—are at increased risk of developing AMR; regimens that include IVIG, rituximab, and bortezomib comprise the current armamentarium to decrease allosensitization (200,201). Additionally, photophoresis (202) and total lymphoid irradiation (203) have been shown to be effective in decreasing rejection, but these are costly and time consuming, with no significant survival benefit.

Cardiac Allograft Vasculopathy

CAV is a major cause of morbidity and mortality after cardiac transplantation (204), and remains the main limitation of its long-term success. Approximately 10% of heart transplant recipients are diagnosed with CAV within 1 year after transplant, and more than 50% after 10 years (84).

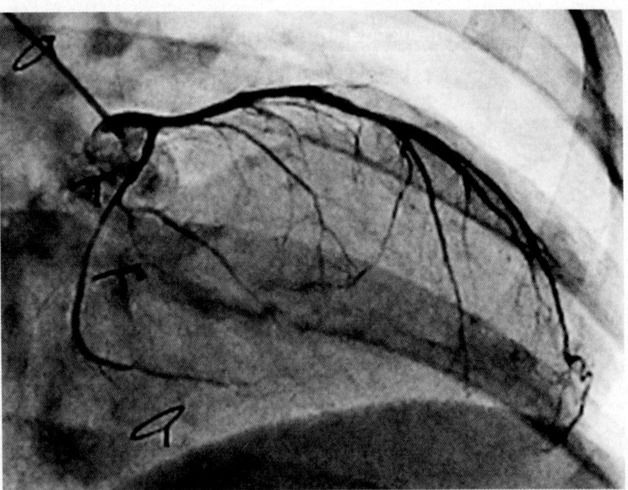

FIGURE 71.31 Cardiac allograft vasculopathy. Coronary angiography of the left coronary artery, 15 years after cardiac transplantation. There is severe diffuse narrowing of the vessel lumen, paucity of small vessels, and sudden "cut-off" endings of small branches (pruning). This leads to chronic allograft ischemia, and severe restrictive physiology. (Courtesy of J. Emanuel Finet, MD. Indiana University.)

CAV is a chronic form of allograft rejection, characterized by diffuse intimal hyperplasia of the cardiac allograft vasculature, eventually compromising blood flow, and causing myocardial ischemia. It is believed to be mediated by the indirect allorecognition pathway of cell-mediated response. Antigens from the donor are processed by host dendritic cells and presented as peptides, which in turn trigger multiple iterations of lymphocyte activation and a subsequent healing response to vessel injury (205). This repetitive process leads to accelerated diffuse atherosclerosis, concentric intimal thickening (proliferation of smooth muscle cells, myofibroblasts, and matrix), and progressive vessel narrowing (Figs. 71.31 and 71.32).

Common risk factors associated with CAV include increasing donor age and donor hypertension; immunosuppressive regimens utilizing azathioprine and cyclosporine A instead of MMF and tacrolimus are less protective against

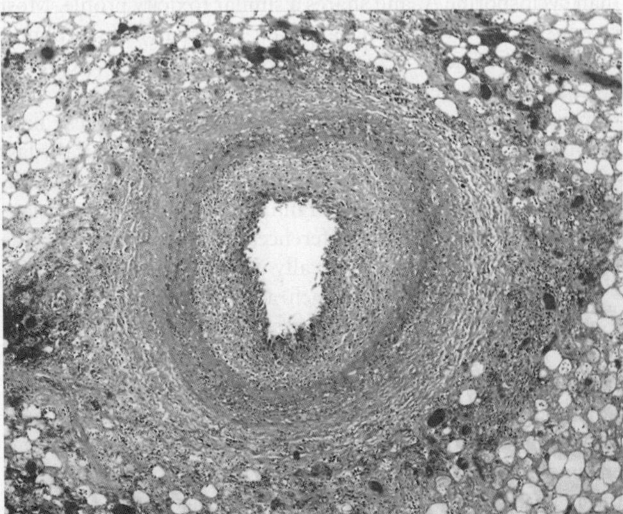

FIGURE 71.32 Cardiac allograft vasculopathy. Epicardial coronary artery shows concentric thickening; there are no lipid pools. (From Burke A, Tavora F. Cardiac allograft vasculopathy. In: *Practical Cardiovascular Pathology*. Philadelphia, PA: Lippincott Williams & Wilkins; 2011:294.)

CAV (79). CMV mismatch status (CMV R-/D+) has been associated with higher risk of developing CAV (206,207), and the presence of circulating donor-specific antibodies to class II HLA antigens has also been associated with accelerated CAV (208).

Due to allograft denervation after transplantation, the chronic myocardial ischemia ensuing from progressive CAV is generally silent. Instead, clinical CAV commonly presents as acute congestive heart failure, usually secondary to restrictive physiology, ventricular arrhythmias, and sudden cardiac death. Coronary angiography is one of the most widely used diagnostic modalities to screen for CAV; annual or biannual screening is recommended for the first 3 to 5 years, and less frequently afterward if there is freedom from disease. An ISHLT consensus has recently proposed a CAV classification based on angiographic imaging and presence of restrictive physiology (83). Despite the widespread use of coronary angiography for CAV screening, VH-IVUS (204,209) and optical coherence tomography (OCT) (210) have been proven more sensitive invasive diagnostic modalities. Common noninvasive modalities, such as perfusion-gated SPECT (211) and dobutamine echocardiography stress testing (212), are also widely used for CAV screening, prior to coronary angiography, with an acceptable negative predictive value (82). Coronary computer tomographic angiography is a newer noninvasive technique, recently suggested to be a reliable alternative to the invasive intracoronary counterparts (213).

Beyond 3 years after cardiac transplantation, at least 10% of all deaths are attributed to CAV; this number is likely an underestimation, given that a large percentage of "graft failure" is also caused by CAV (see Fig. 71.26). The survival of patients affected by CAV has been progressively improving in recent years; this trend may be the result of newer established therapeutic strategies, such as statins (214,215), mTOR inhibitors (187,188), and drug-eluting coronary stents (216,217). Current management strategies are focused mainly on primary prevention, controlling risk factors such as hypertension, hyperlipidemia, smoking, among others; as well as prevention and treatment of CMV infection (82).

NONCARDIAC COMPLICATIONS

Infections

It is well known that a chronic immunosuppressed state is more prone to bacterial, viral, fungal, and protozoal infections (153); there is no exception after cardiac transplantation, as infections account for up to 30% of overall mortality during the first years, and 10% thereafter (see Fig. 71.26) (79).

During the first 30 days after transplantation, bacterial and fungal (especially *Candida* spp) infections account for more than 95% of all nosocomial infections, which are for the most part related to surgical wounds and indwelling catheters in the immediate postoperative period (Fig. 71.33). In contrast, infections occurring in the subsequent few months, when most immunosuppressive regimens are strong, are most often composed of opportunistic organisms such as CMV, *P. jirovecii, Aspergillus* spp, *Nocardia asteroides, Listeria monocytogenes, Toxoplasma gondii,* and EBV (218). Beyond 6 months, the intensity of immunosuppression therapy usually wanes, and the infectious risk becomes closer to that of the general population.

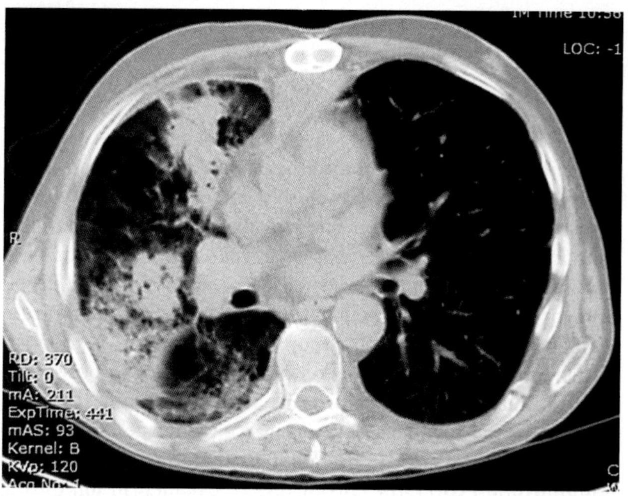

FIGURE 71.33 Bacterial pneumonia after heart transplantation. Chest CT scan of a patient days after cardiac transplantation and immunosuppressive induction with ATG. Extensive infiltrates in the left lung are consistent with severe pneumonia; *Pseudomonas aeruginosa* was isolated from the blood and bronchoalveolar lavage. (Courtesy of J. Emanuel Finet, MD. Indiana University.)

Because of this phenomenon, heart transplant patients require antiviral, antibacterial, antiprotozoal, and antifungal prophylaxis for 6 to 12 months after transplantation (219); this antimicrobial regimen is tailored to the recipient's viral immunization, and the donor's seropositivity, particularly in the case of CMV. Additionally, a similar regimen of antimicrobial prophylaxis is employed after antirejection therapy. A typical antimicrobial prophylaxis regimen after cardiac transplantation would include variations of the following: vancomycin 1 g IV twice daily and cefuroxime 1.5 g IV three times daily for 4 days immediately after transplant (especially if the chest is left open after the procedure); amphotericin B nebulization 100 mg daily for 4 days, and 50 mg weekly for 2 months; nystatin 500,000 units (5 mL) swish and swallow four times daily; trimethoprim–sulfamethoxazole (TMP–SMX) 80 to 400 mg daily for 12 months; valganciclovir 900 mg daily for 6 months (if CMV D+/R–, or CMV R+) or valaciclovir 1 gm daily for 6 months (if CMV D–/R–, HSV +).

Malignancies

Malignancies are responsible for more than 20% of all deaths 5 years after cardiac transplantation (see Fig. 71.26) (84). Skin tumors and PTLDs are considered the most common types of malignancies after cardiac transplantation (79). Both increasing recipient age and chronic immunosuppressive therapy are considered the strongest predictors of occurrence. Skin cancer, in particular, has a large preponderance, accounting for nearly 40% of all de novo malignancies after cardiac transplantation (220). PTLD is a unique type of B-cell lymphoma, 90% of the time associated with EBV, which occurs in 3.4% of heart transplant recipients; it is most frequently intra-abdominally localized, and its severity ranges from benign to highly malignant (221). Particular risk factors include EBV D+/R–, preceding CMV infection, and the type and level of immunosuppression. The first step in managing these patients is the marked decrease of immunosuppressant doses—both calcineurin inhibitor and cell cycle inhibitor—which can lead to lymphoma regression in up to 50% of cases (221); additionally, standard cancer therapies should be applied. Yearly dermatologic screening is highly recommended.

Chronic Renal Failure

Chronic renal dysfunction after transplantation of a nonrenal organ is very frequent, and is closely associated with late posttransplant mortality (222). The prevalence of severe renal dysfunction is approximately 6% at 1 year posttransplant, and 16% at 5 years posttransplant (84). Risk factors for the development of severe renal dysfunction early after transplantation include nonischemic cardiomyopathy, dialysis prior to posttransplant discharge, pacemaker placement prior to posttransplant discharge, VAD placement after transplant, diabetes mellitus in the recipient, increasing recipient age, and recipient pretransplant creatinine, among others (84). In terms of immunosuppression, the chronic use of calcineurin inhibitors, cyclosporine even more so than tacrolimus, has been also associated with the development of acute (functional) and chronic (structural) renal insufficiency. The early form of nephrotoxicity occurs via acute vasoconstriction of afferent arterioles, resulting in decreased glomerular filtration rate. In contrast, the late form of calcineurin inhibitor–induced nephrotoxicity is thought to arise from direct injury to the renal tubular epithelial cells, leading to atrophy and replacement fibrosis (223). Substituting the calcineurin inhibitor with sirolimus as primary immunosuppressant leads to an improvement in short-term and long-term renal function (185,186). Kidney transplantation should be considered for end-stage dysfunction.

Other Complications of Immunosuppression

Hypertension, diabetes mellitus, hyperlipidemia, gout, osteoporosis, and electrolyte abnormalities are some of the common additional complications arising from chronic immunosuppression, depending of the agent used (Table 71.14). Therapeutic options are focused on drug discontinuation or dose lowering, based on the severity, and initiation of specific therapies for the respective conditions: antihypertensives, insulin and oral hypoglycemic agents, statins, fibrates, allopurinol, vitamin D supplementation, biphosphonates, and potassium and magnesium supplementation.

OUTCOMES AND SURVIVAL

Heart transplantation is associated with dramatic improvements in survival, functional status, and quality of life, when compared with previous end-stage heart disease (81). Current 1 year posttransplant survival is about 85%, well contrasted to the 25% survival of those patients managed with optimal standard medical therapy (Fig. 71.34) (79,224). At 1 to 3 years after transplantation, 90% of survivors are capable of normal activity, achieving Karnofsky scores of 80 to 100; these outcomes have remained steady for the last 10 years (79). Early after cardiac transplantation, acute allograft failure, infection, and multiple organ failure account for the majority of deaths; beyond 3 to 5 years, malignancy, CAV, and renal failure become the major contributors of mortality (see Fig. 71.26) (79). Based on the latest ISHLT registry, multivariate risk factors for short-term mortality after cardiac transplantation are those related to the severity of illness immediately leading to cardiac transplantation, such as hospitalized state, ventilator support, temporary mechanical circulatory support, renal replacement therapy, blood product transfusions, and retransplantation, among others. Variables such as older donor age, allograft ischemic time less than 200 minutes, recipient serum creatinine or need for hemodialysis, and bilirubin are also associated with linear increases in risk (79). Risk factors for long-term mortality include those related to recipient comorbidities, such as diabetes mellitus, panel reactive antibody, and elevated BMI, with the exception of retransplantation, which

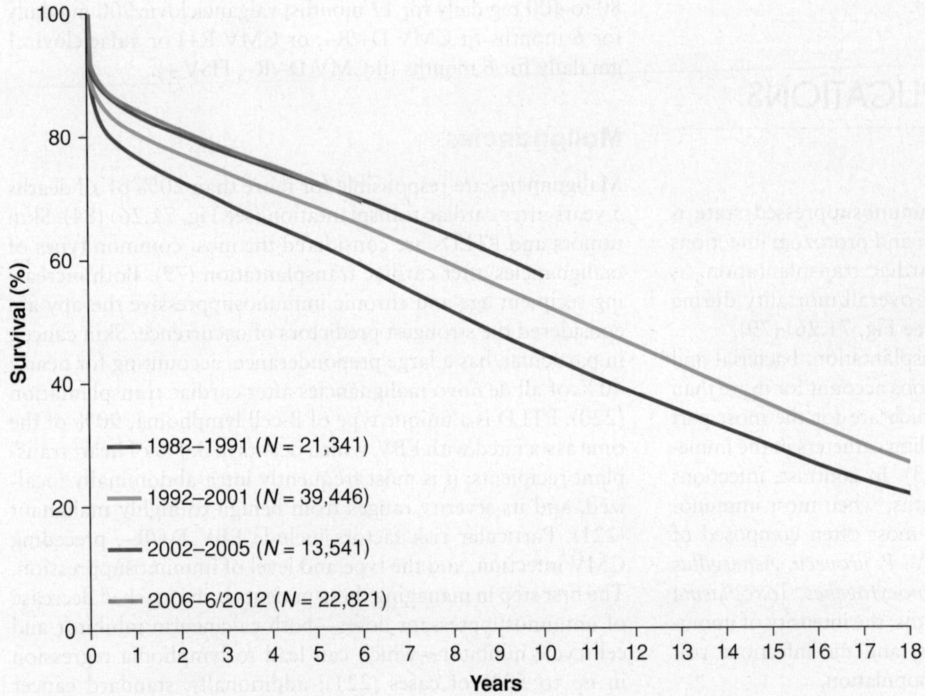

FIGURE 71.34 Survival after adult heart transplantation (Kaplan–Meier survival by era (January 1982 to June 2012)). There has been a consistent increase in overall survival beyond 1 year from 1982 to 2002. However, survival has remained steady for the last 13 years, approximately 85% at 1 year. (Adapted from Lund LH, Edwards LB, Kucheryavaya AY, et al. The registry of the International Society for Heart and Lung Transplantation: thirty-first official adult heart transplant report—2014. Focus theme: retransplantation. *J Heart Lung Transplant.* 2014;33(10):996–1008.)

remains the single strongest predictor of long-term mortality (79). In addition, a number of factors affecting donor-recipient immunologic interactions, such as PRA level above 10%, higher number of HLA mismatches, and recipient pregnancy status, have been also shown to decrease long-term survival.

RETRANSPLANTATION

The incidence of retransplantation has remained constant for the last 30 years, about 2% to 4% of all adult heart transplants (79). Primary cardiac allograft dysfunction is the dominant condition leading to retransplantation in the first month after primary transplant, whereas CAV is the major determinant beyond 1 year (79). Survival after retransplantation is 70% at 1 year and 38% at 10 years, and has remained constant over the past 15 years. CAV has the best prognosis, especially due to favorable survival during the first year; patients retransplanted following primary cardiac allograft dysfunction, on the contrary, have the highest mortality over the first year, reaching 46% (79,132).

References

1. Yusen RD, Edwards LB, Kucheryavaya AY, et al. The registry of the International Society for Heart and Lung Transplantation: thirty-first adult lung and heart-lung transplant report–2014; focus theme: retransplantation. *J Heart Lung Transplant.* 2014;33(10):1009–1024.
2. Egan TM, Murray S, Basmati RT, et al. Development of the new lung allocation system in the United States. *Am J Transplant.* 2006;6(5 Part 2): 1212–1227.
3. McShane PJ, Garrity ER. Impact of lung allocation score. *Semin Respir Crit Care Med.* 2013;34(3):275–280.
4. Van Raemdonck D, Neyrinck A, Verleden GM, et al. Lung donor selection and management. *Proc Am Thorac Soc.* 2009;6:28–38.
5. Callahan DS, Kim D, Bricker S, et al. Trends in organ donor management: 2002–2012. *J Am Coll Surg.* 2014;219:752–756.
6. Miñambres E, Pérez-Villares JM, Chico-Fernández M, et al. Lung donor treatment protocol in brain dead-donors: a multicenter study. *J Heart Lung Transplant.* 2015;34(6):773–780.
7. Pilcher DV, Scheinkestel CD, Snell GI, et al. High central venous pressure is associated with prolonged mechanical ventilation and increased mortality after lung transplantation. *J Thorac Cardiovasc Surg.* 2005;129:912–918.
8. Orens JB, Boehler A, de Perrot M, et al. A review of lung transplant donor acceptability criteria. *J Heart Lung Transplant.* 2003;22(11):1182–1200.
9. Aigner C, Winkler G, Peter Jaksch P, et al. Extended donor criteria for lung transplantation: a clinical reality. *Eur J Cardiothorac Surg.* 2005; 27:757–761.
10. Cypel M, Yeung JC, Liu M, et al. Normothermic ex vivo lung perfusion in clinical lung transplantation. *N Engl J Med.* 2011;364:1431–1440.
11. Cypel M, Keshavjee S. Extending the donor pool: rehabilitation of poor organs. *Thorac Surg Clin.* 2015;25:27–33.
12. Weill D, Benden C, Corris PA, et al. A consensus document for the selection of lung transplant candidates: 2014—an update from the Pulmonary Transplantation Council of the ISHLT. *J Heart Lung Transplant.* 2015;34:1–15.
13. Trulock EP, Edwards LB, Taylor DO, et al.; International Society for Heart and Lung Transplantation. Registry of the International Society for Heart and Lung Transplantation: twenty-third official adult lung and heart–lung transplantation report—2006. *J Heart Lung Transplant.* 2006;25(8):880–891.
14. Kanasky WF, Anton SD, Rodrigue JR, et al. Impact of body weight on long- term survival after lung transplantation. *Chest.* 2002;121:401–406.
15. Singer JP, Peterson ER, Snyder ME, et al. Body composition and mortality after adult lung transplantation in the United States. *Am J Resp Crit Care Med.* 2014;190(9):1012–1021.
16. Jaksch P, Ankersmit J, Scheed A, et al. Alemtuzumab in lung transplantation: an open-label, randomized, prospective single center study. *Am J Transplant Am.* 2014;14:1839–1845.
17. Bhorade SM, Stern E. Immunosuppression for lung transplantation. *Proc Am Thorac Soc.* 2009;6:47–53.
18. Whited L, Latran M, Hashmi Z, et al. Evaluation of alemtuzumab versus basiliximab induction; a retrospective cohort study in lung transplant recipients. *Transplantation.* 2015;99(10):2190–2195.
19. Treede H, Glanville AR, Kleptko W, et al; European and Australian Investigators in Lung Transplantation. Tacrolimus and cyclosporine have differential effects on the risk of development of bronchiolitis obliterans syndrome: results of prospective, randomized international trial in lung transplantation. *J Heart Lung Transplant.* 2012;31:797–804.
20. Treede H, Klepetko W, Reichenspurner H, et al; Munich and Vienna Lung Transplant Group. Tacrolimus versus cyclosporine after lung transplantation: a prospective, open, randomized two-center trial comparing two different immunosuppressive protocols. *J Heart Lung Transplant.* 2001;20:511–517.
21. Palmer SA, Baz MA, Sanders L, et al. Results of a randomized, prospective, multicenter trial of mycophenolate mofetil versus azathioprine in the prevention of acute lung allograft rejection. *Transplantation.* 2001;71:1772–1776.
22. McNeil K, Glanville AR, Wahlers T, et al. Comparison of mycophenolate mofetil and azathioprine for prevention of bronchiolitis obliterans in de novo lung transplant recipients. *Transplantation.* 2006;81:998–1003.
23. Hunt J, Lerman M, Magee MJ, et al. Improvement of renal dysfunction by conversion from calcineurin inhibitors to sirolimus after heart transplantation. *J Heart Lung Transplant.* 2005;24:1863–1867.
24. Kilic A, George T, Beaty CA, et al. The effect of center volume on the incidence of postoperative complications and their impact on survival after lung transplantation. *J Thorac Cardiovasc Surg.* 2012;144:1502–1508.
25. Hosenpud JD, Bennett LE, Ked BM, et al. Effect of diagnosis on survival benefit of lung transplantation for end-stage lung disease. *Lancet.* 1998;351:24–27.
26. Anthonisen NR. Prognosis in chronic obstructive pulmonary disease: results from multicenter clinical trials. *Am Rev Respir Dis.* 1989;140: S95–S99.
27. Celli BR, Cote CG, Marin JM, et al. The body-mass index, airflow obstruction, dyspnea, and exercise capacity index in chronic obstructive pulmonary disease. *N Engl J Med.* 2004;350(10):1005–1012.
28. Baz MA, Palmer SM, Staples ED, et al. Lung transplantation after long-term mechanical ventilation: results and 1 year follow up. *Chest.* 2001;119:224–227.
29. Meyers BF, Lynch JP, Battafarano RJ, et al. Lung transplantation is warranted for stable, ventilator-dependent recipients. *Ann Thorac Surg.* 2000;70:1675–1678.
30. Chacon RA, Corris PA, Dark JH, Gibson GJ. Comparison of the functional results of single lung transplantation for pulmonary fibrosis and chronic airway obstruction. *Thorax.* 1998;53:43–49.
31. Gammie JS, Keenan RJ, Pham SM, et al. Single- versus double-lung transplantation for pulmonary hypertension. *J Thorac Cardiovasc Surg.* 1998;115:397–402 ; discussion 402–403.
32. Lanuza DM, Lefaiver CA, Brown R, et al. A longitudinal study of patients' symptoms before and during the first year after lung transplantation. *Clin Transplant.* 2012;26(6):E576–E589.
33. Singer JP, Singer LG. Quality of life in lung transplantation. *Semin Respir Crit Care Med.* 2013;34(3):421–430.
34. Fox KR, Posluszny DM, DiMartini AF, et al. Predictors of post-traumatic psychological growth in the late years after lung transplantation. *Clin Transplant.* 2014;28(4):384–393.
35. Rodrigue JR, Baz MA, Kanasky WF Jr, MacNaughton KL. Does lung transplantation improve health-related quality of life? The University of Florida experience. *J Heart Lung Transplant.* 2005;24(6):755–763.
36. van den Berg JW, Geertsma A, van der BIJ W, et al. Bronchiolitis obliterans syndrome after lung transplantation and health-related quality of life. *Am J Respir Crit Care Med.* 2000;161:1937–1941.
37. Paris W, Diercks M, Bright J, et al. Return to work after lung transplantation. *J Heart Lung Transplant.* 1998;17:430–436.
38. Schwaiblmair M, Reichenspurner H, Muller C, et al. Cardiopulmonary exercise testing before and after lung and heart-lung transplantation. *Am J Respir Crit Care Med.* 1999;159:1277–1283.
39. Tirdel GB, Girgis R, Fishman RS, Theodore J. Metabolic myopathy as a cause of the exercise limitation in lung transplant recipients. *J Heart Lung Transplant.* 1998;17:1231–1237.
40. Lands LC, Smountas AA, Mesiano G, et al. Maximal exercise capacity and peripheral skeletal muscle function following lung transplantation. *J Heart Lung Transplant.* 1999;18:113–120.
41. Wang XN, Williams TJ, McKenna MJ, et al. Skeletal muscle oxidative capacity, fiber type, and metabolites after lung transplantation. *Am J Respir Crit Care Med.* 1999;160:57–63.

42. Pantoja JG, Andrade FH, Stoki DS, et al. Respiratory and limb muscle function in lung allograft recipients. *Am J Respir Crit Care Med.* 1999;160:1205–1211.
43. Krieger AC, Szidon P, Kesten S. Skeletal muscle dysfunction in lung transplantation. *J Heart Lung Transplant.* 2000;19:392–400.
44. Walsh JR, Chambers DC, Davis RJ, et al. Impaired exercise capacity after lung transplantation is related to delayed recovery of muscle strength. *Clin Transplant.* 2013;27:E504–E511.
45. Diamond J, Carby M, Bag R, et al. Report of the ISHLT Working Group on Primary Lung Graft Dysfunction. Part II: definition. A consensus statement of the International Society for Heart and Lung Transplantation. *J Heart Lung Transplant.* 2005;14:1454–1459.
46. Zander DS, Baz MA, Visner GA, et al. Analysis of early deaths after isolated lung transplantation. *Chest.* 2001;120:225–232.
47. Diamond JM, Lee JC, Kawut SM, et al. Clinical risk factors for primary graft dysfunction after lung transplantation. *Am J Respir Crit Care Med.* 2013;187(5):527–534.
48. Santacruz JF, Mehta AC. Airway complications and management after lung transplantation: ischemia, dehiscence, and stenosis. *Proc Am Thorac Soc.* 2009;6:79–93.
49. Fernández-Bussy S, Majid A, Caviedes I, et al. Treatment of airway complications following lung transplantation. *Arch Bronconeumol.* 2011; 47(3):128–133.
50. Machuzak M, Santacruz JF, Gildea T, Murthy SC. Airway complications after lung transplantation. *Thorac Surg Clin.* 2015;25:55–75.
51. Speich R, van der Bij W. Epidemiology and management of infections after lung transplantation. *Clin Infect Dis.* 2001;33:S58–S65.
52. Aquilar-Guisado M, Givalda J, Ussetti P, et al; RESITRA cohort. Pneumonia after lung transplantation in the RESITRA Cohort: a multicenter prospective study. *Am J Transplant.* 2007;7:1989–1996.
53. Palmer SM, Limaye AP, Banks M, et al. Extended valganciclovir prophylaxis to prevent cytomegalovirus after lung transplantation: a randomized, controlled trial. *Ann Intern Med.* 2010;152(12):761–769.
54. Remund KF, Best M, Egan JJ. Infections relevant to lung transplantation. *Proc Am Thorac Soc.* 2009;6:94–100.
55. Baz MA, Layish DT, Govert JA, et al. Diagnostic yield of bronchoscopies after isolated lung transplantation. *Chest.* 1996;110(1):84–88.
56. Garrity ER, Villanueva J, Bhorade SM, et al. Low rate of acute lung allograft rejection after the use of daclizumab, an interleukin 2 receptor antibody. *Transplantation.* 2001;71:773–777.
57. Stewart S, Fishbein MC, Snell GI, et al. Revision of the 1996 working formulation for the standardization of nomenclature in the diagnosis of lung rejection. *J Heart Lung Transplant.* 2007;26:1229–1242.
58. Verleden GM, Raghu G, Meyer KC, et al. A new classification system for chronic lung allograft dysfunction. *J Heart Lung Transplant.* 2014; 33:127–133.
59. Huang HJ, Yusen RD, Meyers BF, et al. Late primary graft dysfunction after lung transplantation and bronchiolitis obliterans syndrome. *Am J Transplant.* 2008;8(11):2454–6242.
60. Burton CM, Iversen M, Carlsen J, et al. Acute cellular rejection is a risk factor for bronchiolitis obliterans syndrome independent of post-transplant baseline FEV1. *J Heart Lung Transplant.* 2009;28:888–893.
61. Hachem R. Antibody-mediated lung transplant rejection. *Curr Respir Care Rep.* 2012;1(3):157–161.
62. Gulack BC, Meza JM, Lin SS, et al. Reflux and allograft dysfunction: Is there a connection? *Thorac Surg Clin.* 2015;25:97–105.
63. Vua DL, Bridevaux PO, Aubert JD, et al. Respiratory viruses in lung transplant recipients: a critical review and pooled analysis of clinical studies. *Am J Transplant.* 2011;11:1071–1078.
64. Verleden GM, Vos R, Verleden SE, et al. Survival determinants in lung transplant patients with chronic allograft dysfunction. *Transplantation.* 2011;92:703–708.
65. Sato M, Ohmori-Matsuda K, Saito T, et al. Time-dependent changes in the risk of death in pure bronchiolitis obliterans syndrome (BOS). *J Heart Lung Transplant.* 2013;32:484–491.
66. Barker AF, Bergeron A, Rom WN, Hertz MI. Obliterative bronchiolitis. *N Engl J Med.* 2014;370:1820–1828.
67. Hall EC, Pfeiffer RM, Segev DL, Engels EA. Cumulative incidence of cancer after solid organ transplantation. *Cancer.* 2013;119(12):2300–2308.
68. Euvrard S, Morelon E, Rostaing L, et al. Sirolimus and secondary skin-cancer prevention in kidney transplantation. *N Engl J Med.* 2012;367:329–339.
69. Muchtar E, Kramer MR, Vidal L, et al. Posttransplantation lymphoproliferative disorder in lung transplant recipients: a 15-year single institution experience. *Transplantation.* 2013;96(7):657–663.
70. Johnson BA, Duncan SR, Ohmori NP, et al. Recurrence of sarcoidosis in pulmonary allograft recipients. *Am Rev Respir Dis.* 1993;148:1373–1377.
71. Frost AE, Keller CA, Brown RW, et al. Giant cell interstitial pneumonitis: disease recurrence in the transplanted lung. *Am Rev Respir Crit Care Med.* 1993;148:1401–1404.
72. O'Brien JD, Lium JH, Parosa JF, et al. Lymphangiomyomatosis recurrence in the allograft after single-lung transplantation. *Am J Respir Crit Care Med.* 1995;151:2033–2036.
73. Baz MA, Kussin PS, VanTrigt P, et al. Recurrence of diffuse panbronchiolitis after lung transplantation. *Am J Respir Crit Care Med.* 1995; 151:895–898.
74. Arboleda R, Gonzalez O, Cortes M, Perez-Cerda F. Recurrent polymyositis-associated lung disease after lung transplantation. *Interact Cardiovasc Thorac Surg.* 2015;20(4):560–562.
75. Bui AL, Horwich TB, Fonarow GC. Epidemiology and risk profile of heart failure. *Nature Rev Cardiol.* 2011;8(1):30–41.
76. Juenger J, Schellberg D, Kraemer S, et al. Health related quality of life in patients with congestive heart failure: comparison with other chronic diseases and relation to functional variables. *Heart.* 2002;87(3):235–241.
77. Roger VL, Weston SA, Redfield MM, et al. Trends in heart failure incidence and survival in a community-based population. *JAMA.* 2004; 292(3):344–350.
78. Hunt SA, Rider AK, Stinson EB, et al. Does cardiac transplantation prolong life and improve its quality? An updated report. *Circulation.* 1976;54(6 Suppl):III56–60.
79. Lund LH, Edwards LB, Kucheryavaya AY, et al. The registry of the International Society for Heart and Lung Transplantation: thirty-first official adult heart transplant report—2014. Focus theme: retransplantation. *J Heart Lung Transplant.* 2014;33(10):996–1008.
80. Stewart S, Winters GL, Fishbein MC, et al. Revision of the 1990 working formulation for the standardization of nomenclature in the diagnosis of heart rejection. *J Heart Lung Transplant.* 2005;24(11):1710–1720.
81. Mehra MR, Kobashigawa J, Starling R, et al. Listing criteria for heart transplantation: International Society for Heart and Lung Transplantation guidelines for the care of cardiac transplant candidates—2006. *J Heart Lung Transplant.* 2006;25(9):1024–1042.
82. Costanzo MR, Dipchand A, Starling R, et al. The International Society of Heart and Lung Transplantation Guidelines for the care of heart transplant recipients. *J Heart Lung Transplant.* 2010;29(8):914–956.
83. Mehra MR, Crespo-Leiro MG, Dipchand A, et al. International Society for Heart and Lung Transplantation working formulation of a standardized nomenclature for cardiac allograft vasculopathy-2010. *J Heart Lung Transplant.* 2010;29(7):717–727.
84. Stehlik J, Edwards LB, Kucheryavaya AY, et al. The Registry of the International Society for Heart and Lung Transplantation: 29th official adult heart transplant report—2012. *J Heart Lung Transplant.* 2012;31(10):1052–1064.
85. Berry GJ, Burke MM, Andersen C, et al. The 2013 International Society for Heart and Lung Transplantation Working Formulation for the standardization of nomenclature in the pathologic diagnosis of antibody-mediated rejection in heart transplantation. *J Heart Lung Transplant.* 2013;32(12):1147–1162.
86. Colvin-Adams M, Smith JM, Heubner BM, et al. OPTN/SRTR 2013 Annual Data Report: Heart. *Am J Transpl.* 2015;15(Suppl 2):1–28.
87. McKeown DW, Bonser RS, Kellum JA. Management of the heartbeating brain-dead organ donor. *Br J Anaesth.* 2012;108(Suppl 1):i96–i107.
88. Aaronson KD, Schwartz JS, Chen TM, et al. Development and prospective validation of a clinical index to predict survival in ambulatory patients referred for cardiac transplant evaluation. *Circulation.* 1997;95(12):2660–7266.
89. Mozaffarian D, Anker SD, Anand I, et al. Prediction of mode of death in heart failure: the Seattle Heart Failure Model. *Circulation.* 2007;116(4):392–398.
90. Goda A, Williams P, Mancini D, Lund LH. Selecting patients for heart transplantation: comparison of the Heart Failure Survival Score (HFSS) and the Seattle heart failure model (SHFM). *J Heart Lung Transplant.* 2011;30(11):1236–1243.
91. Mancini D, Lietz K. Selection of cardiac transplantation candidates in 2010. *Circulation.* 2010;122(2):173–183.
92. Lower RR, Shumway NE. Studies on orthotopic homotransplantation of the canine heart. *Surg Forum.* 1960;11:18–19.
93. Barnard CN. The operation. A human cardiac transplant: an interim report of a successful operation performed at Groote Schuur Hospital, Cape Town. *S Afr Med J.* 1967;41(48):1271–1274.
94. Griepp RB, Stinson EB, Clark DA, et al. A two-year experience with human heart transplantation. *Calif Med.* 1970;113(2):17–26.
95. Copeland JG, Griepp RB, Bieber CP, et al. Successful retransplantation of the human heart. *J Thorac Cardiovasc Surg.* 1977;73(2):242–247.

96. Reitz BA, Bieber CP, Raney AA, et al. Orthotopic heart and combined heart and lung transplantation with cyclosporin-A immune suppression. *Transplant Proc.* 1981;13(1 Pt 1):393–396.
97. Jamieson SW, Baldwin J, Reitz BA, et al. Combined heart and lung transplantation. *Lancet.* 1983;1(8334):1130–1132.
98. Kobashigawa J, Zuckermann A, Macdonald P, et al. Report from a consensus conference on primary graft dysfunction after cardiac transplantation. *J Heart Lung Transplant.* 2014;33(4):327–340.
99. Kavarana MN, Sinha P, Naka Y, et al. Mechanical support for the failing cardiac allograft: a single-center experience. *J Heart Lung Transplant.* 2003;22(5):542–547.
100. Huang J, Trinkaus K, Huddleston CB, et al. Risk factors for primary graft failure after pediatric cardiac transplantation: importance of recipient and donor characteristics. *J Heart Lung Transplant.* 2004;23(6):716–722.
101. Leprince P, Aubert S, Bonnet N, et al. Peripheral extracorporeal membrane oxygenation (ECMO) in patients with posttransplant cardiac graft failure. *Transplant Proc.* 2005;37(6):2879–2880.
102. Marasco SF, Esmore DS, Negri J, et al. Early institution of mechanical support improves outcomes in primary cardiac allograft failure. *J Heart Lung Transplant.* 2005;24(12):2037–2042.
103. Aubert S, Leprince P, Bonnet N, et al. Limited mechanical circulatory support following orthotopic heart transplantation. *Interact Cardiovasc Thorac Surg.* 2006;5(2):88–89.
104. Lima B, Rajagopal K, Petersen RP, et al. Marginal cardiac allografts do not have increased primary graft dysfunction in alternate list transplantation. *Circulation.* 2006;114(1 Suppl):I27–I32.
105. Ibrahim M, Hendry P, Masters R, et al. Management of acute severe perioperative failure of cardiac allografts: a single-centre experience with a review of the literature. *Can J Cardiol.* 2007;23(5):363–367.
106. Russo MJ, Iribarne A, Hong KN, et al. Factors associated with primary graft failure after heart transplantation. *Transplantation.* 2010;90(4):444–450.
107. Segovia J, Cosio MD, Barcelo JM, et al. RADIAL: a novel primary graft failure risk score in heart transplantation. *J Heart Lung Transplant.* 2011;30(6):644–651.
108. Cosio Carmena MD, Gomez Bueno M, Almenar L, et al. Primary graft failure after heart transplantation: characteristics in a contemporary cohort and performance of the RADIAL risk score. *J Heart Lung Transplant.* 2013;32(12):1187–1195.
109. D'Alessandro C, Golmard JL, Barreda E, et al. Predictive risk factors for primary graft failure requiring temporary extra-corporeal membrane oxygenation support after cardiac transplantation in adults. *Eur J Cardiovasc Surg.* 2011;40(4):962–969.
110. Jeevanandam V, Furukawa S, Prendergast TW, et al. Standard criteria for an acceptable donor heart are restricting heart transplantation. *Ann Thorac Surg.* 1996;62(5):1268–1275.
111. Marelli D, Laks H, Fazio D, et al. The use of donor hearts with left ventricular hypertrophy. *J Heart Lung Transplant.* 2000;19(5):496–503.
112. Samsky MD, Patel CB, Owen A, et al. Ten-year experience with extended criteria cardiac transplantation. *Circ Heart Fail.* 2013;6(6):1230–1238.
113. Isaac D. Primary cardiac graft failure-defining, predicting, preventing. *J Heart Lung Transplant.* 2013;32(12):1168–1169.
114. Birks EJ, Burton PB, Owen V, et al. Elevated tumor necrosis factor-alpha and interleukin-6 in myocardium and serum of malfunctioning donor hearts. *Circulation.* 2000;102(19 Suppl 3):III352–III358.
115. Birks EJ, Owen VJ, Burton PB, et al. Tumor necrosis factor-alpha is expressed in donor heart and predicts right ventricular failure after human heart transplantation. *Circulation.* 2000;102(3):326–331.
116. Novitzky D, Cooper DK, Reichart B. Hemodynamic and metabolic responses to hormonal therapy in brain-dead potential organ donors. *Transplantation.* 1987;43(6):852–854.
117. Chen JM, Cullinane S, Spanier TB, et al. Vasopressin deficiency and pressor hypersensitivity in hemodynamically unstable organ donors. *Circulation.* 1999;100(19 Suppl):II244–II246.
118. Baan CC, Niesters HG, Balk AH, et al. The intragraft cytokine mRNA pattern reflects the efficacy of steroid antirejection therapy. *J Heart Lung Transplant.* 1996;15(12):1184–1193.
119. Jeevanandam V, Todd B, Regillo T, et al. Reversal of donor myocardial dysfunction by triiodothyronine replacement therapy. *J Heart Lung Transplant.* 1994;13(4):681–687.
120. Pennefather SH, Bullock RE, Mantle D, Dark JH. Use of low dose arginine vasopressin to support brain-dead organ donors. *Transplantation.* 1995;59(1):58–62.
121. Salim A, Vassiliu P, Velmahos GC, et al. The role of thyroid hormone administration in potential organ donors. *Arch Surg.* 2001;136(12):1377–1380.
122. Appleyard RF, Cohn LH. Myocardial stunning and reperfusion injury in cardiac surgery. *J Cardiac Surg.* 1993;8(2 Suppl):316–324.
123. Garcia-Poblete E, Fernandez H, Alvarez L, et al. Structural and ultrastructural study of the myocardium after 24-hour preservation in University of Wisconsin solution. *Histol Histopathol.* 1997;12(2):375–382.
124. Jahania MS, Sanchez JA, Narayan P, et al. Heart preservation for transplantation: principles and strategies. *Ann Thorac Surg.* 1999;68(5):1983–1987.
125. George TJ, Arnaoutakis GJ, Beaty CA, et al. A novel method of measuring cardiac preservation injury demonstrates University of Wisconsin solution is associated with less ischemic necrosis than Celsior in early cardiac allograft biopsy specimens. *J Heart Lung Transplant.* 2012;31(4):410–418.
126. Girard C, Fargnoli JM, Godin-Ribuot D, et al. Inhaled nitric oxide: effects on hemodynamics, myocardial contractility, and regional blood flow in dogs with mechanically induced pulmonary artery hypertension. *J Heart Lung Transplant.* 1996;15(7):700–708.
127. Theodoraki K, Tsiapras D, Tsourelis L, et al. Inhaled iloprost in eight heart transplant recipients presenting with post-bypass acute right ventricular dysfunction. *Acta Anaesthesiol Scand.* 2006;50(10):1213–1217.
128. De Santo LS, Mastroianni C, Romano G, et al. Role of sildenafil in acute posttransplant right ventricular dysfunction: successful experience in 13 consecutive patients. *Transplant Proc.* 2008;40(6):2015–2018.
129. Weis F, Beiras-Fernandez A, Kaczmarek I, et al. Levosimendan: a new therapeutic option in the treatment of primary graft dysfunction after heart transplantation. *J Heart Lung Transplant.* 2009;28(5):501–504.
130. Radovancevic B, Nakatani T, Frazier OH, et al. Mechanical circulatory support for perioperative donor heart failure. *ASAIO Trans.* 1989;35(3):539–541.
131. Sweeney MS, Lammermeier DE, Frazier OH, et al. Extension of donor criteria in cardiac transplantation: surgical risk versus supply-side economics. *Ann Thorac Surg.* 1990;50(1):7–10.
132. John R, Chen JM, Weinberg A, et al. Long-term survival after cardiac retransplantation: a twenty-year single-center experience. *J Thorac Cardiovasc Surg.* 1999;117(3):543–555
133. Mullerworth MH, Lixfeld W, Rachkewich RA, et al. Hyperacute rejection of heterotopic heart allografts in dogs. *Transplantation.* 1972;13(6):570–575.
134. Weil R 3rd, Clarke DR, Iwaki Y, et al. Hyperacute rejection of a transplanted human heart. *Transplantation.* 1981;32(1):71–72.
135. Pickham D, Hickey K, Doering L, et al. Electrocardiographic abnormalities in the first year after heart transplantation. *J Electrocardiol.* 2014;47(2):135–139.
136. Michaels PJ, Espejo ML, Kobashigawa J, et al. Humoral rejection in cardiac transplantation: risk factors, hemodynamic consequences and relationship to transplant coronary artery disease. *J Heart Lung Transplant.* 2003;22(1):58–69.
137. Olsen SL, Wagoner LE, Hammond EH, et al. Vascular rejection in heart transplantation: clinical correlation, treatment options, and future considerations. *J Heart Lung Transplant.* 1993;12(2):S135–S142.
138. Wu GW, Kobashigawa JA, Fishbein MC, et al. Asymptomatic antibody-mediated rejection after heart transplantation predicts poor outcomes. *J Heart Lung Transplant.* 2009;28(5):417–422.
139. Caves PK, Stinson EB, Billingham ME, et al. Diagnosis of human cardiac allograft rejection by serial cardiac biopsy. *J Thorac Cardiovasc Surg.* 1973;66(3):461–466.
140. Caves PK, Stinson EB, Graham AF, et al. Percutaneous transvenous endomyocardial biopsy. *JAMA.* 1973;225(3):288–291.
141. Rider AK, Copeland JG, Hunt SA, et al. The status of cardiac transplantation, 1975. *Circulation.* 1975;52(4):531–539.
142. Gradek WQ, D'Amico C, Smith AL, et al. Routine surveillance endomyocardial biopsy continues to detect significant rejection late after heart transplantation. *J Heart Lung Transplant.* 2001;20(5):497–502.
143. Stehlik J, Starling RC, Movsesian MA, et al. Utility of long-term surveillance endomyocardial biopsy: a multi-institutional analysis. *J Heart Lung Transplant.* 2006;25(12):1402–1409.
144. Saraiva F, Matos V, Goncalves L, et al. Complications of endomyocardial biopsy in heart transplant patients: a retrospective study of 2117 consecutive procedures. *Transplant Proc.* 2011;43(5):1908–1912.
145. Pham MX, Teuteberg JJ, Kfoury AG, et al.; IMAGE Study Group. Gene-expression profiling for rejection surveillance after cardiac transplantation. *N Engl J Med.* 2010;362(20):1890–900.
146. Kobashigawa J, Patel J, Azarbal B, et al. Randomized pilot trial of gene expression profiling versus heart biopsy in the first year after heart transplant: early invasive monitoring attenuation through gene expression trial (EIMAGE). *Circ Heart Fail.* 2015;8(3):557–564.
147. Jamieson SW, Burton NA, Bieber CP, et al. Cardiac-allograft survival in primates treated with cyclosporin A. *Lancet.* 1979;1(8115):545.
148. Reitz BA, Wallwork JL, Hunt SA, et al. Heart-lung transplantation: successful therapy for patients with pulmonary vascular disease. *N Engl J Med.* 1982;306(10):557–564.

149. Lindenfeld J, Miller GG, Shakar SF, et al. Drug therapy in the heart transplant recipient: part I: cardiac rejection and immunosuppressive drugs. *Circulation.* 2004;110(24):3734–3740.
150. Lindenfeld J, Miller GG, Shakar SF, et al. Drug therapy in the heart transplant recipient: part II: immunosuppressive drugs. *Circulation.* 2004;110(25):3858–3865.
151. Rafiei M, Kittleson M, Patel J, et al. Anti-thymocyte gamma-globulin may prevent antibody production after heart transplantation. *Transplant Proc.* 2014;46(10):3570–3574.
152. Rosenberg PB, Vriesendorp AE, Drazner MH, et al. Induction therapy with basiliximab allows delayed initiation of cyclosporine and preserves renal function after cardiac transplantation. *J Heart Lung Transplant.* 2005;24(9):1327–1331.
153. Mazimba S, Tallaj JA, George JF, et al. Infection and rejection risk after cardiac transplantation with induction vs. no induction: a multi-institutional study. *Clin Transplant.* 2014;28(9):946–952.
154. Krasinskas AM, Kreisel D, Acker MA, et al. CD3 monitoring of antithymocyte globulin therapy in thoracic organ transplantation. *Transplantation.* 2002;73(8):1339–1341.
155. Uber WE, Uber LA, VanBakel AB, et al. CD3 monitoring and thymoglobulin therapy in cardiac transplantation: clinical outcomes and pharmacoeconomic implications. *Transplant Proc.* 2004;36(10): 3245–3249.
156. Goland S, Czer LS, Coleman B, et al. Induction therapy with thymoglobulin after heart transplantation: impact of therapy duration on lymphocyte depletion and recovery, rejection, and cytomegalovirus infection rates. *J Heart Lung Transplant.* 2008;27(10):1115–1121.
157. Carrier M, Leblanc MH, Perrault LP, et al. Basiliximab and rabbit anti-thymocyte globulin for prophylaxis of acute rejection after heart transplantation: a non-inferiority trial. *J Heart Lung Transplant.* 2007;26(3):258–263.
158. Flaman F, Zieroth S, Rao V, et al. Basiliximab versus rabbit anti-thymocyte globulin for induction therapy in patients after heart transplantation. *J Heart Lung Transplant.* 2006;25(11):1358–1362.
159. Mattei MF, Redonnet M, Gandjbakhch I, et al. Lower risk of infectious deaths in cardiac transplant patients receiving basiliximab versus anti-thymocyte globulin as induction therapy. *J Heart Lung Transplant.* 2007;26(7):693–699.
160. Czer LS, Phan A, Ruzza A, et al. Antithymocyte globulin induction therapy adjusted for immunologic risk after heart transplantation. *Transplant Proc.* 2013;45(6):2393–2398.
161. Teuteberg JJ, Shullo MA, Zomak R, et al. Alemtuzumab induction prior to cardiac transplantation with lower intensity maintenance immunosuppression: one-year outcomes. *Am J Transpl.* 2010;10(2):382–388.
162. Chivukula S, Shullo MA, Kormos RL, et al. Cancer-free survival following alemtuzumab induction in heart transplantation. *Transplant Proc.* 2014;46(5):1481–1488.
163. Denton MD, Magee CC, Sayegh MH. Immunosuppressive strategies in transplantation. *Lancet.* 1999;353(9158):1083–1091.
164. O'Malley BW. Mechanisms of action of steroid hormones. *N Engl J Med.* 1971;284(7):370–377.
165. Fauci AS, Dale DC, Balow JE. Glucocorticosteroid therapy: mechanisms of action and clinical considerations. *Ann Intern Med.* 1976;84(3):304–315.
166. Gillis S, Crabtree GR, Smith KA. Glucocorticoid-induced inhibition of T cell growth factor production. I. The effect on mitogen-induced lymphocyte proliferation. *J Immunol.* 1979;123(4):1624–1631.
167. Gillis S, Crabtree GR, Smith KA. Glucocorticoid-induced inhibition of T cell growth factor production. II. The effect on the in vitro generation of cytolytic T cells. *J Immunol.* 1979;123(4):1632–1638.
168. Larsson EL. Cyclosporin A and dexamethasone suppress T cell responses by selectively acting at distinct sites of the triggering process. *J Immunol.* 1980;124(6):2828–2833.
169. Fruman DA, Klee CB, Bierer BE, et al. Calcineurin phosphatase activity in T lymphocytes is inhibited by FK 506 and cyclosporin A. *Proc Natl Acad Sci U S A.* 1992;89(9):3686–3690.
170. Reichart B, Meiser B, Vigano M, et al. European Multicenter Tacrolimus (FK506) Heart Pilot Study: one-year results– European Tacrolimus Multicenter Heart Study Group. *J Heart Lung Transplant.* 1998;17(8): 775–781.
171. Grimm M, Rinaldi M, Yonan NA, et al. Superior prevention of acute rejection by tacrolimus vs. cyclosporine in heart transplant recipients: a large European trial. *Am J Transplant.* 2006;6(6):1387–1397.
172. Taylor DO, Barr ML, Radovancevic B, et al. A randomized, multicenter comparison of tacrolimus and cyclosporine immunosuppressive regimens in cardiac transplantation: decreased hyperlipidemia and hypertension with tacrolimus. *J Heart Lung Transplant.* 1999;18(4):336–345.
173. Onsager DR, Canver CC, Jahania MS, et al. Efficacy of tacrolimus in the treatment of refractory rejection in heart and lung transplant recipients. *J Heart Lung Transplant.* 1999;18(5):448–455.
174. Taylor DO, Ensley RD, Olsen SL, et al. Mycophenolate mofetil (RS-61443): preclinical, clinical, and three-year experience in heart transplantation. *J Heart Lung Transplant.* 1994;13(4):571–582.
175. Allison AC, Eugui EM. Mycophenolate mofetil and its mechanisms of action. *Immunopharmacology.* 2000;47(2–3):85–118.
176. Kobashigawa JA. Mycophenolate mofetil in cardiac transplantation. *Curr Opin Cardiol.* 1998;13(2):117–121.
177. Hosenpud JD, Bennett LE. Mycophenolate mofetil versus azathioprine in patients surviving the initial cardiac transplant hospitalization: an analysis of the Joint UNOS/ISHLT Thoracic Registry. *Transplantation.* 2001;72(10):1662–1665.
178. Baran DA, Zucker MJ, Arroyo LH, et al. Randomized trial of tacrolimus monotherapy: tacrolimus in combination, tacrolimus alone compared (the TICTAC trial). *J Heart Lung Transplant.* 2007;26(10):992–997.
179. Brown EJ, Albers MW, Shin TB, et al. A mammalian protein targeted by G1-arresting rapamycin-receptor complex. *Nature.* 1994;369(6483): 756–758.
180. Abraham RT, Wiederrecht GJ. Immunopharmacology of rapamycin. *Annu Rev Immunol.* 1996;14:483–510.
181. Vezina C, Kudelski A, Sehgal SN. Rapamycin (AY-22,989), a new antifungal antibiotic. I. Taxonomy of the producing streptomycete and isolation of the active principle. *J Antibiot (Tokyo).* 1975;28(10):721–726.
182. Nashan B. Early clinical experience with a novel rapamycin derivative. *Therap Drug Monit.* 2002;24(1):53–58.
183. Eisen HJ, Tuzcu EM, Dorent R, et al. Everolimus for the prevention of allograft rejection and vasculopathy in cardiac-transplant recipients. *N Engl J Med.* 2003;349(9):847–858.
184. Keogh A, Richardson M, Ruygrok P, et al. Sirolimus in de novo heart transplant recipients reduces acute rejection and prevents coronary artery disease at 2 years: a randomized clinical trial. *Circulation.* 2004;110(17):2694–2700.
185. Kushwaha SS, Khalpey Z, Frantz RP, et al. Sirolimus in cardiac transplantation: use as a primary immunosuppressant in calcineurin inhibitor-induced nephrotoxicity. *J Heart Lung Transplant.* 2005;24(12):2129–2136.
186. Gustafsson F, Ross HJ, Delgado MS, et al. Sirolimus-based immunosuppression after cardiac transplantation: predictors of recovery from calcineurin inhibitor-induced renal dysfunction. *J Heart Lung Transplant.* 2007;26(10):998–1003.
187. Raichlin E, Bae JH, Khalpey Z, et al. Conversion to sirolimus as primary immunosuppression attenuates the progression of allograft vasculopathy after cardiac transplantation. *Circulation.* 2007;116(23):2726–2733.
188. Topilsky Y, Hasin T, Raichlin E, et al. Sirolimus as primary immunosuppression attenuates allograft vasculopathy with improved late survival and decreased cardiac events after cardiac transplantation. *Circulation.* 2012;125(5):708–720.
189. Matsuo Y, Cassar A, Yoshino S, et al. Attenuation of cardiac allograft vasculopathy by sirolimus: relationship to time interval after heart transplantation. *J Heart Lung Transplant.* 2013;32(8):784–791.
190. Schweiger M, Wasler A, Prenner G, et al. Everolimus and reduced cyclosporine trough levels in maintenance heart transplant recipients. *Transplant Immunol.* 2006;16(1):46–51.
191. Eisen HJ, Kobashigawa J, Starling RC, et al. Everolimus versus mycophenolate mofetil in heart transplantation: a randomized, multicenter trial. *Am J Transplant.* 2013;13(5):1203–1216.
192. Lloveras JJ, Escourrou G, Delisle MB, et al. Evolution of untreated mild rejection in heart transplant recipients. *J Heart Lung Transplant.* 1992;11(4 Pt 1):751–756.
193. Brunner-La Rocca HP, Sutsch G, Schneider J, et al. Natural course of moderate cardiac allograft rejection (International Society for Heart Transplantation grade 2) early and late after transplantation. *Circulation.* 1996;94(6):1334–1338.
194. Hosenpud JD, Norman DJ, Pantely GA. Low-dose oral prednisone in the treatment of acute cardiac allograft rejection not associated with hemodynamic compromise. *J Heart Transplant.* 1990;9(3 Pt 2):292–296.
195. Park MH, Starling RC, Ratliff NB, et al. Oral steroid pulse without taper for the treatment of asymptomatic moderate cardiac allograft rejection. *J Heart Lung Transplant.* 1999;18(12):1224–1227.
196. Berglin E, Kjellstrom C, Mantovani V, et al. Plasmapheresis as a rescue therapy to resolve cardiac rejection with vasculitis and severe heart failure: a report of five cases. *Transplant Int.* 1995;8(5):382–387.
197. Bierl C, Miller B, Prak EL, et al. Antibody-mediated rejection in heart transplant recipients: potential efficacy of B-cell depletion and antibody removal. *Clin Transpl.* 2006:489–496.

198. Eckman PM, Thorsgard M, Maurer D, et al. Bortezomib for refractory antibody-mediated cardiac allograft rejection. *Clin Transpl.* 2009: 475–478.
199. Leech SH, Lopez-Cepero M, LeFor WM, et al. Management of the sensitized cardiac recipient: the use of plasmapheresis and intravenous immunoglobulin. *Clin Transplant.* 2006;20(4):476–484.
200. John R, Lietz K, Burke E, et al. Intravenous immunoglobulin reduces anti-HLA alloreactivity and shortens waiting time to cardiac transplantation in highly sensitized left ventricular assist device recipients. *Circulation.* 1999;100(19 Suppl):II229–II235.
201. Patel J, Everly M, Chang D, et al. Reduction of alloantibodies via proteasome inhibition in cardiac transplantation. *J Heart Lung Transplant.* 2011;30(12):1320–1326.
202. Barr ML, Meiser BM, Eisen HJ, et al. Photopheresis for the prevention of rejection in cardiac transplantation. Photopheresis Transplantation Study Group. *N Engl J Med.* 1998;339(24):1744–1751.
203. Salter MM, Kirklin JK, Bourge RC, et al. Total lymphoid irradiation in the treatment of early or recurrent heart rejection. *J Heart Lung Transplant.* 1992;11(5):902–911.
204. Kobashigawa JA, Tobis JM, Starling RC, et al. Multicenter intravascular ultrasound validation study among heart transplant recipients: outcomes after five years. *J Am Coll Cardiol.* 2005;45(9):1532–1537.
205. Lechler R, Ng WF, Steinman RM. Dendritic cells in transplantation: friend or foe? *Immunity.* 2001;14(4):357–368.
206. Petrakopoulou P, Kubrich M, Pehlivanli S, et al. Cytomegalovirus infection in heart transplant recipients is associated with impaired endothelial function. *Circulation.* 2004;110(11 Suppl 1):II207–II212.
207. Potena L, Holweg CT, Chin C, et al. Acute rejection and cardiac allograft vascular disease is reduced by suppression of subclinical cytomegalovirus infection. *Transplantation.* 2006;82(3):398–405.
208. Topilsky Y, Gandhi MJ, Hasin T, et al. Donor-specific antibodies to class II antigens are associated with accelerated cardiac allograft vasculopathy: a three-dimensional volumetric intravascular ultrasound study. *Transplantation.* 2013;95(2):389–396.
209. Torres HJ, Merello L, Ramos SA, et al. Prevalence of cardiac allograft vasculopathy assessed with coronary angiography versus coronary vascular ultrasound and virtual histology. *Transplant Proc.* 2011;43(6):2318–2321.
210. Garrido IP, Garcia-Lara J, Pinar E, et al. Optical coherence tomography and highly sensitivity troponin T for evaluating cardiac allograft vasculopathy. *Am J Cardiol.* 2012;110(5):655–661.
211. Manrique A, Bernard M, Hitzel A, et al. Diagnostic and prognostic value of myocardial perfusion gated SPECT in orthotopic heart transplant recipients. *J Nucl Cardiol.* 2010;17(2):197–206.
212. Sade LE, Sezgin A, Eroglu S, et al. Dobutamine stress echocardiography in the assessment of cardiac allograft vasculopathy in asymptomatic recipients. *Transplant Proc.* 2008;40(1):267–270.
213. Wever-Pinzon O, Romero J, Kelesidis I, et al. Coronary computed tomography angiography for the detection of cardiac allograft vasculopathy: a meta-analysis of prospective trials. *J Am Coll Cardiol.* 2014;63(19):1992–2004.
214. Kobashigawa JA, Katznelson S, Laks H, et al. Effect of pravastatin on outcomes after cardiac transplantation. *N Engl J Med.* 1995;333(10):621–627.
215. Kobashigawa JA, Moriguchi JD, Laks H, et al. Ten-year follow-up of a randomized trial of pravastatin in heart transplant patients. *J Heart Lung Transplant.* 2005;24(11):1736–1740.
216. Lee MS, Kobashigawa J, Tobis J. Comparison of percutaneous coronary intervention with bare-metal and drug-eluting stents for cardiac allograft vasculopathy. *JACC Cardiovasc Interv.* 2008;1(6):710–715.
217. Agarwal S, Parashar A, Kapadia SR, et al. Long-term mortality after cardiac allograft vasculopathy: implications of percutaneous intervention. *JACC Heart Fail.* 2014;2(3):281–288.
218. Nishi SP, Valentine VG, Duncan S. Emerging bacterial, fungal, and viral respiratory infections in transplantation. *Infect Dis Clin North Am.* 2010;24(3):541–555.
219. Olsen SL, Renlund DG, O'Connell JB, et al. Prevention of Pneumocystis carinii pneumonia in cardiac transplant recipients by trimethoprim sulfamethoxazole. *Transplantation.* 1993;56(2):359–362.
220. Taylor DO, Edwards LB, Boucek MM, et al. The Registry of the International Society for Heart and Lung Transplantation: twenty-first official adult heart transplant report—2004. *J Heart Lung Transplant.* 2004;23(7):796–803.
221. Cockfield SM. Identifying the patient at risk for post-transplant lymphoproliferative disorder. *Transpl Infect Dis.* 2001;3(2):70–78.
222. Ojo AO, Held PJ, Port FK, et al. Chronic renal failure after transplantation of a nonrenal organ. *N Engl J Med.* 2003;349(10):931–940.
223. Issa N, Kukla A, Ibrahim HN. Calcineurin inhibitor nephrotoxicity: a review and perspective of the evidence. *Am J Nephrol.* 2013;37(6):602–612.
224. Rose EA, Gelijns AC, Moskowitz AJ, et al.; Randomized Evaluation of Mechanical Assistance for the Treatment of Congestive Heart Failure (REMATCH) Study Group. Long-term use of a left ventricular assist device for end-stage heart failure. *N Engl J Med.* 2001;345(20):1435–1443.

CHAPTER

72

Liver Transplantation

LAURA HAMMEL, ZOLTAN G. HEVESI, and DOUGLAS B. COURSIN

INTRODUCTION

Liver failure or end-stage liver disease (ESLD) is the fourth leading cause of death in the United States in patients 45 to 54 years of age, and 12th among all age groups (1). Liver transplantation (LT) is the only definitive cure for irreversible liver failure. The first successful transplant was performed in 1967, but it remained a difficult procedure with suboptimal outcomes until the early 1980s when patient survival rates more than doubled. Improvements in surgical and anesthetic techniques, the introduction of the University of Wisconsin solution, which extended cold preservation time, and advancements in immunosuppressive drugs have resulted in even lower graft failure rates and improved patient and graft survival rates since the early 1980s (Figs. 72.1 and 72.2). Currently, 1- and 5-year survival rates exceed 85% and 74%, respectively, according to the Scientific Registry of Transplant Recipients (2). In 2012, 6,256 liver transplants were performed and more than 65,000 liver transplant recipients were alive in the United States (Fig. 72.3). According to the Organ Procurement and Transplantation Network (OPTN) there were 15,275 patients wait listed for LT at 165 liver transplant centers in the United States as of April, 2015; only about 25% of these centers perform more than 70 transplants annually (2). It is important for intensive care unit (ICU) physicians to understand the process of LT, including preoperative assessment, organ allocation, and the postoperative ICU course as they care for patients with ESLD and acute liver failure (ALF) being considered for LT.

PRESURGICAL PROCESS, ISSUES, AND EVALUATION

Patients with decompensation of chronic liver disease or ALF are often admitted to an ICU. In some cases this may be their first contact with the transplant system and pretransplant evaluation may be initiated during their ICU stay. A multidisciplinary approach to the evaluation of these patients should include hepatology, transplant surgery, transplant anesthesiology and, if the clinical situation warrants, the expertise of nephrology, cardiology, and pulmonology.

Organ Allocation

The appropriate assignment and prioritization of solid organs remains a challenge for organizations, such as United Network for Organ Sharing (UNOS) and the American Society of Transplantation (AST), that strive to achieve optimal and fair distribution for transplantation. Since 2002, the MELD (Model for End-Stage Liver Disease) scoring system has been the method of liver allocation and its accuracy of predicting 3-month mortality on the transplant waiting list has been validated (3–5); it is calculated as shown in Table 72.1[1] using easily obtained serum indices: bilirubin, international standardized ratio (INR) for prothrombin time (PT), and creatinine. Any patient who is on dialysis receives an automatic 4 mg/dL for creatinine score. An exception to the MELD scoring system is made for LT candidates who present with acute fulminant liver failure without history of chronic liver disease; they receive first priority (4,5). An increasing score predicts increasing likelihood of 30-day mortality. For example, a MELD of 10 indicates a 3-month mortality rate of nearly 0% and a score of 40 approaching 90% (Fig. 72.4); UNOS has modified the system to an upper limit cap of 40 for the purpose of allocation for LT (4).

There are still subsets of patients at higher risk for mortality than predicted by their MELD score. Periodically, the system is adjusted to make allocation fair for all patients with ESLD. OPTN continuously monitors wait-list dropouts and reviews patient scores to maintain impartiality. For example, studies reveal a higher wait-list mortality rate in patients with hyponatremia compared to those with a normal serum sodium at the same MELD (6,7). The proposal to add serum sodium to the MELD score calculation was approved with an amendment by the OPTN board in June of 2014. Upon implementation by 2016, approximately 34% of candidates will have a different MELD score and will receive 1 to 13 additional MELD points depending on the serum sodium level. A survival benefit has been shown for earlier transplantation in patients with hyponatremia and a baseline MELD of at least 12 (7).

Other subsets of patients who are at higher risk of death than predicted by their MELD score include, but are not limited to, those with portopulmonary hypertension (PoPH), hepatopulmonary syndrome (HPS), hereditary hemorrhagic telangiectasias, and hepatocellular carcinoma. These patients are assigned a "MELD exception" score based on the expected mortality predictions related to the associated condition. An in-depth discussion of the conditions for which a MELD exception may be assigned and the evidence supporting these decisions is available online (8). Other patients may be considered on a case-by-case basis for exception as published by the MELD exception study group (9).

Cardiovascular Issues and Pretransplantation Evaluation

Hemodynamic Physiology

The classic hemodynamic physiology of ESLD is characterized by a hyperdynamic profile with a high cardiac output (CO) state and low systemic vascular resistance (SVR); as the liver

[1]A calculator for the MELD score can also be found at the OPTN website: http://optn.transplant.hrsa.gov/converge/resources/MeldPeld Calculator.asp?index=98.

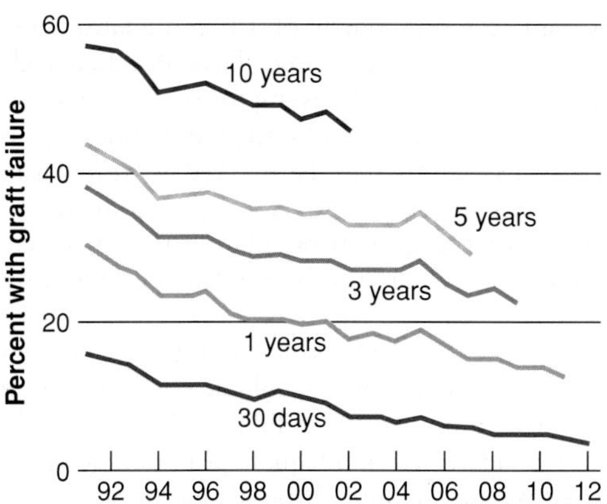

FIGURE 72.1 Graft failure among adult recipients of livers transplanted from deceased donors, 2012. (Adapted from 2012 Annual Report of the U.S. Organ Procurement and Transplantation Network and the Scientific Registry of Transplant Recipients: Transplant Data 1994–2003. Department of Health and Human Services, Health Resources and Services Administration, Healthcare Systems Bureau, Division of Transplantation, Rockville, MD; United Network for Organ Sharing, Richmond, VA; University Renal Research and Education Association, Ann Arbor, MI. http://optn.transplant.hrsa.org.)

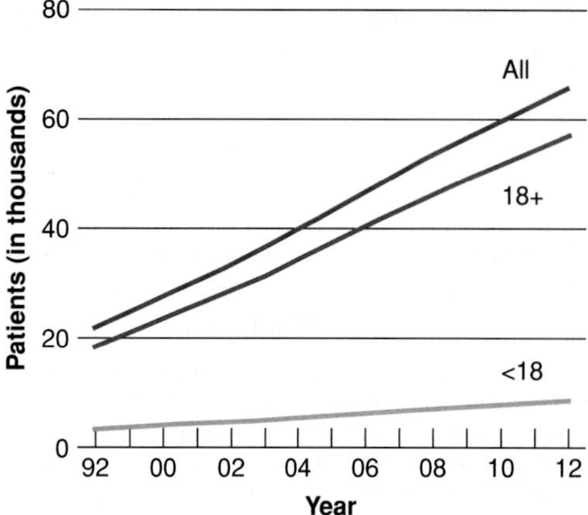

FIGURE 72.3 Recipients alive and with a functioning liver transplant as of June 30, 2012. (From 2012 Annual Report of the U.S. Organ Procurement and Transplantation Network and the Scientific Registry of Transplant Recipients: Transplant Data 1994–2003. Department of Health and Human Services, Health Resources and Services Administration, Healthcare Systems Bureau, Division of Transplantation, Rockville, MD; United Network for Organ Sharing, Richmond, VA; University Renal Research and Education Association, Ann Arbor, MI. http://optn.transplant.hrsa.org.)

disease progresses so too does the degree of the hyperdynamic circulation. A growing body of evidence supports the proposition that systemic vasodilation is due to an increase in nitric oxide (NO) production. Additionally, vascular endothelial growth factor (VGEF) stimulates angiogenesis and the development of portosystemic collaterals (10). In combination, these processes increase intravascular capacity and vascular endothelial surface area. Despite an elevated blood volume in cirrhosis, there is a relative intravascular volume deficit; the distribution of volume between central and noncentral vascular compartments is unbalanced. Central and arterial blood volume is decreased, whereas the splanchnic circulation may be congested. The high pressure present in the hepatic sinusoids, in concert with low oncotic forces due to hypoalbuminemia common in ESLD, increases the translocation of fluid to the abdominal cavity, which results in total body volume overload secondary to ascites and interstitial edema. High output cardiac failure may be present, as defined by a high CO and elevated left ventricular (LV) end-diastolic pressure. These collective processes decrease end-organ perfusion and predispose to complications such as the hepatorenal syndrome (HRS) (discussed below), peritonitis, and bacteremia due to intestinal bacterial translocation (10–12).

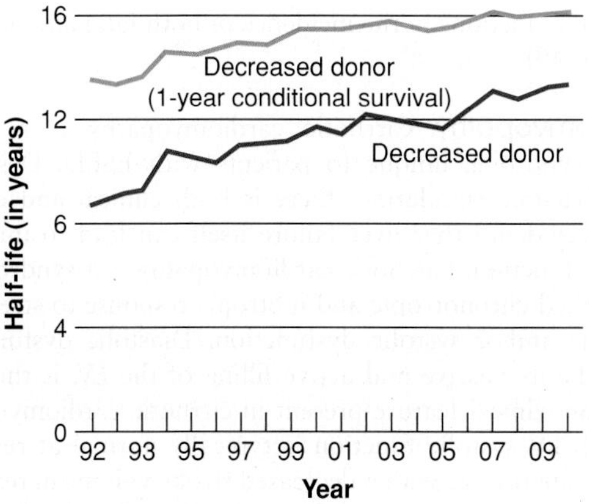

FIGURE 72.2 Half-lives for adult recipients of livers transplanted from deceased donors, 2012. (Adapted from 2012 Annual Report of the U.S. Organ Procurement and Transplantation Network and the Scientific Registry of Transplant Recipients: Transplant Data 1994–2003. Department of Health and Human Services, Health Resources and Services Administration, Healthcare Systems Bureau, Division of Transplantation, Rockville, MD; United Network for Organ Sharing, Richmond, VA; University Renal Research and Education Association, Ann Arbor, MI. http://optn.transplant.hrsa.org.)

Cardiovascular complications are the leading cause of non–graft-related mortality and morbidity following LT in the acute transplant period and remain the number one cause of 1-year mortality (13). Therefore, an important element of the pretransplant evaluation is the assessment of the cardiovascular system. LT is a hemodynamically challenging procedure and individuals must have adequate cardiovascular reserve to tolerate the surgery.

Essentials of the Cardiac Evaluation

In addition to a thorough history and physical examination, adult patients undergoing evaluation for LT should have an ECG, looking for findings that suggest the presence of underlying ischemic, conductive, or structural cardiac disease; if present, this should prompt further testing. Transthoracic echocardiography (TTE) is an excellent noninvasive test that

TABLE 72.1 Model for End-Stage Liver Disease (MELD) Scoring System[a]

3.78 × log$_e$ serum bilirubin in mg/dL
+
11.20 × log$_e$ INR
+
9.57 × log$_e$ serum creatinine in mg/dL[b]
+
6.43, which is a constant for liver disease

INR, international normalized ratio.
[a]Use 1 for any value less than 1 to prevent scores below 0.
[b]If the patient has undergone dialysis twice within the previous 7 days, use 4.0 as the serum creatinine value.
(Adapted from Wiesner R, Edwards E, Freeman R, et al. Model for end-stage liver disease (MELD) and allocation of donor livers. *Gastroenterology.* 2003;124:91–96.)

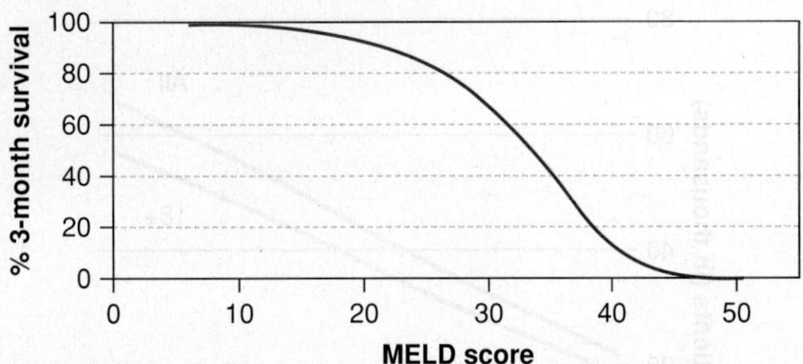

FIGURE 72.4 Estimated 3-month survival as a function of MELD score. (Adapted from Wiesner R, Edwards E, Freeman R, et al; The United Network for Organ Sharing Liver Disease Severity Score Committee. Model for end-stage liver disease (MELD) and allocation of donor liver. *Gastroenterology*. 2003;124(1):91–96.)

should be considered in all patients under consideration for LT. Much information can be garnered from a TTE including, but not limited to, diastolic and systolic ventricular function, presence of cardiomyopathies, structural defects, valvular abnormalities, evidence of an intrapulmonary shunt on the bubble contrast study, and the presence of pulmonary artery (PA) hypertension. There are several significant cardiopulmonary conditions associated with ESLD outlined below which can be safely ruled out on a screening TTE.

Coronary Artery Disease. It has been reported that the prevalence of CAD in patients with ESLD approaches 30%, clearly exceeding that of the general population (14,15). This is at least in part due to the increasing age of patients receiving LT combined with comorbidities considered risk factors for CAD. In fact, the number of recipients older than 65 years has more than doubled from 2002 to 2012 (11,16). Chronic HCV infection is also independently associated with presence of metabolic conditions—insulin resistance, type 2 diabetes mellitus, and hypertension—which are established risk factors for CAD (17). Patients with nonalcoholic steatohepatitis (NASH), in particular, are more likely to be older, obese, hypertensive, diabetic, have chronic kidney disease, and have hyperlipidemia or metabolic syndrome, all risk factors for CAD, and to suffer posttransplant cardiovascular events (18,19). In fact, growing evidence suggests that NASH itself is an independent risk factor for cardiovascular disease (20). LT candidates with two or more of the following traditional cardiac risk factors (21) are more likely to have obstructive CAD (11,19,22–25):

- Age: male 45 or older, female 55 or older or premature menopause without estrogen replacement therapy
- Family history of premature coronary disease: definite myocardial infarction or sudden death before age 55 years in male first-degree relative and before age 65 in female first-degree relative
- Current cigarette smoking
- Hypertension: blood pressure over 140/90 mmHg, or an antihypertensive medication
- HDL cholesterol below 40 mg/dL (1.03 mmol/L)

The presence of even nonobstructive CAD has been shown to negatively impact short and long-term mortality outcomes in LT (26–31). Therefore, it is important to identify and treat patients at risk for CAD prior to LT given the risk of perioperative cardiac complications (29,32,33); in some cases the burden of CAD may be severe enough to prohibit LT.

Approximately one-fourth of LT candidates with traditional coronary risk factors may have developed clinically significant CAD even while asymptomatic. As patients with ESLD often are sedentary and encephalopathic, typical signs of myocardial ischemia may be masked. Extrapolating from currently accepted preoperative, cardiac evaluation guidelines created for the general population that place emphasis on symptomatology may not be prudent in the setting of LT (34,35).

The evaluation for the presence of inducible ischemia with noninvasive exercise or pharmacologic stress testing has limited predictive value in LT candidates (36). The inability to achieve target heart rate or adequate peak double product due to impaired adrenergic and chronotropic responses is associated with an increased risk of postoperative cardiovascular events (37). In the ICU setting, hemodynamic instability, use of vasopressors, mechanical ventilation (MV), and kidney injury make noninvasive stress testing impractical and unlikely to yield findings worthy of interpretation. The decision to pursue stress testing should be based on individualized evaluation of the candidate's pretest probability for having CAD.

Coronary angiography (CA) should be considered for LT candidates with high pretest probability of CAD (two or more traditional coronary risk factors) those who cannot undergo stress testing, have suboptimal response to pharmacologic stress testing, or who have inducible ischemia on stress imaging. CA can be performed safely in LT candidates even with renal dysfunction and elevated bleeding risk (38–40). CA via the transradial approach, if possible, is the preferred method in LT candidates, to improve hemostasis and reduce periprocedural complications (41–43).

Revascularization of obstructive CAD may be pursued in order to improve symptoms and cardiovascular mortality per ACC/AHA guidelines, and in cases where the burden of obstructive CAD would prohibit LT in an otherwise appropriate surgical candidate (36,44–46). There is evidence suggesting revascularization will improve post-LT outcomes (47,48). Increases in the frequencies of CA and percutaneous coronary intervention (PCI) corresponded to significant reductions in postoperative MIs and 1-year all-cause mortality rates in LT through reductions in the incidence of both fatal and nonfatal MIs (36,49).

Cardiomyopathy. Cirrhotic cardiomyopathy is a physiologic syndrome unique to patients with ESLD. Despite a hyperdynamic circulation, there is both clinical and experimental evidence that liver failure itself can lead to impaired cardiac function. Cirrhotic cardiomyopathy is a syndrome of diminished chronotropic and inotropic response to stress and diastolic and/or systolic dysfunction. Diastolic dysfunction, which limits passive and active filling of the LV, is the most common clinical feature present in cirrhotic cardiomyopathy (50,51). LV systolic function is typically normal at rest, but inadequate reserve with a decreased stroke volume in response to stress is the hallmark of this entity (51–57). This impaired inotropic response, combined with the diminished capacity for a chronotropic response in patients with ESLD limits cardiac reserve during times of stress.

A common electrophysiologic abnormality associated with cirrhotic cardiomyopathy is a prolonged QT interval on ECG. A rate-corrected QT interval of greater than 440 ms has been estimated to be present in 30% to 60% of patients with cirrhotic cardiomyopathy (58). However, the incidence of sudden cardiac death in patients with cirrhosis who develop a pronged QT interval does not seem to be elevated (59–61). The clinical significance of a prolonged QT interval associated with cirrhotic cardiomyopathy remains unknown, but drugs that prolong ventricular repolarization should be avoided.

There is no standard treatment for cirrhotic cardiomyopathy. Down regulation of β-adrenergic receptors and attenuation of response to chronotropic and inotropic drugs is a common feature of this entity and, therefore, β-agonists may not elicit the expected response (62–64). β-Blockers may be beneficial as they improve QTc interval prolongation and may oppose the downregulation of adrenoreceptor density. However, it is unknown if they have an effect on long-term contractile function in cirrhotic cardiomyopathy (65–68). Mineralocorticoid antagonists (aldosterone) and angiotensin-converting enzyme (ACE) inhibitors have not shown long-term benefit in cirrhotic cardiomyopathy (65,69). Fortunately, there is strong evidence that LT reverses the majority of cirrhotic cardiomyopathy (70–73). After LT, heart function parameters improve and the QT interval normalizes in the majority of patients (74). Nonetheless, immediate perioperative stresses may precipitate myocardial dysfunction in the perioperative period (75).

Cardiomyopathies are myocardial diseases presenting as structural or functional disorders of the heart. The prevalence of secondary causes of cardiomyopathy is significantly higher in LT candidates compared with the general population. Certain indications for LT, such as alcoholism, hemochromatosis, and amyloidosis, may also have both direct and indirect toxic myocardial effects. In fact, alcohol is the main cause of nonischemic, dilated cardiomyopathy in the western world (76,77). Careful pretransplant cardiac evaluation is essential and diagnosis of cardiac involvement in these disorders requires a high index of clinical suspicion and coordinated multidisciplinary evaluation for LT candidacy. Decompensated congestive heart failure can be difficult to appreciate as peripheral edema, dyspnea, orthopnea, and elevated jugular venous pressure are frequent findings of ESLD.

The presence of preoperative LV dysfunction is not an absolute contraindication to LT per se, but is a risk factor for perioperative cardiovascular complications and mortality. Most centers restrict LT to those with LV ejection fraction (EF) over 40%; there is general consensus that patients with worse function do not have the reserve to withstand the rigorous hemodynamic insults associated with LT (78). As the typical pretransplant hemodynamic profile is one of low SVR, cirrhotics are considered to be "auto-afterload reduced" and LV systolic dysfunction may be masked or under appreciated. With successful transplantation there is an abrupt increase in SVR and afterload, and patients may develop decompensated congestive heart failure. A decrease in cardiac index (CI) or CO is seen in most recipients after LT acutely, but nonsurvivors typically have lower EF prior to transplant than the survivors indicating poorer cardiac reserve (13,79–81).

Pulmonary Issues and Pretransplantation Evaluation

There are several reasons for pulmonary disease to co-exist with liver failure. Some are related to the cause of liver failure itself, such as emphysema in α-1 antitrypsin deficiency and fibrosing alveolitis associated with primary biliary cirrhosis. Additionally, complications of portal hypertension, regardless of etiology of liver failure, can affect lung function. Ascites and hepatic hydrothorax cause physiologic restriction and decreased functional residual capacity. However, the pulmonary issues that receive the most attention include the vascular abnormalities of HPS and PoPH (82).

Hepatopulmonary Syndrome

The term hepatopulmonary syndrome (HPS) was first used in 1977 and was preceded by autopsy descriptions of marked pulmonary vascular vasodilation correlating with clinical findings of hypoxemia. Enhanced NO production has been implicated as the key factor for the development of pulmonary vascular vasodilation leading to a ventilation–perfusion mismatch and hypoxemia. NO-synthase (NOS) activity in the endothelium and intravascular macrophages appears to be responsible for the enhanced NO production in the lungs (83). Data from multiple liver transplant centers suggest that the incidence of HPS, including mild stages, ranges from 5% to 32% (84). Even after the adjustment for severity of liver disease, the presence of HPS infers a worse survival rate with a median survival of 24 months and 5-year mortality rate of 28% without LT; for patients with severe HPS, the mortality is much worse (Table 72.2) (84–86).

Dyspnea, resting or exertional, is the primary but nonspecific symptom in HPS. Platypnea, dyspnea that increases in the upright position and improves when supine, is a somewhat more specific complaint encountered in HPS. Physical findings of clubbing, cyanosis, hypoxemia, and spider nevi are suggestive of HPS. Severe hypoxemia (PaO_2 below 60 mmHg) without another cause and orthodeoxia (a decrease in PaO_2 by 5% or more with change from supine to upright position) are strongly suggestive of HPS (84).

The gold standard and most practical method in the diagnosis of HPS is contrast echocardiogram demonstrating intrapulmonary shunting. Microbubble opacification of the left atrium following three to six cardiac cycles after its appearance in the right atrium indicates passage through an abnormally dilated pulmonary vascular bed; microbubbles will not pass through normal capillaries (<8–15 μm) (84,87,88). A more invasive

TABLE 72.2 Diagnostic Criteria for Hepatopulmonary Syndrome

Variable	Criterion
Oxygenation defect	Partial pressure of oxygen <80 mmHg or Aa oxygen gradient ≥15 mmHg while breathing ambient air
Pulmonary vascular dilatation	Positive findings on contrast-enhanced echocardiography or abnormal uptake in the brain (>6%) with radioactive lung-perfusion scanning
Liver disease	Portal hypertension (most common) with or without cirrhosis
Degree of severity	
Mild	Aa oxygen gradient ≥15 mmHg, paO_2 ≥80 mmHg
Moderate	Aa oxygen gradient ≥15 mmHg, paO_2 ≥60 to <80 mmHg
Severe	Aa oxygen gradient ≥15 mmHg, paO_2 ≥50 to <60 mmHg
Very severe	Aa oxygen gradient ≥15 mmHg, partial paO_2 <50 mmHg <300 mmHg while the patient is breathing 100% oxygen)

Aa, alveolar–arterial; paO_2, partial pressure of oxygen.

and less sensitive approach is a technetium-99m–labeled, microaggregated albumin lung scan with quantitative uptake in the brain (84).

LT is the only therapy for HPS and results in resolution in 85% of patients transplanted, but there remains an inability to predict reversibility (82,84,85,89). The duration of time after LT until improvement can be quite variable, ranging from a few days to 2 years. The overall 5-year survival rate of all stages of HPS following LT is 76%. The duration of time to improvement and postoperative mortality are both increased in those with severe pretransplantation HPS (84). Because of the high mortality without LT in those with HPS and a PaO_2 below 60 mmHg, LT should be considered in these patients who are otherwise adequate candidates for transplantation. A room air PaO_2 of at least 50 mmHg is the greatest predictor of posttransplant mortality; most centers choose a transplantation cut-off of a PaO_2 somewhere between 40 and 50 mmHg (84,85).

Identification of HPS on pretransplant evaluation requires a multidisciplinary approach to evaluation and management. Consultation with a pulmonologist who is familiar with the syndrome is recommended. In patients with severe HPS who are not considered to be candidates for LT, referral to palliative care is a reasonable option.

Portopulmonary Hypertension

PoPH is a condition involving the pulmonary circulation in cirrhotic patients with portal hypertension (90–92). The definition of PoPH consists of three essential elements:

1. Mean pulmonary arterial pressure (mPAP) greater than 25 mmHg
2. Pulmonary vascular resistance (PVR) greater than 240 dynes·sec·cm^{-5}
3. Pulmonary arterial occlusion pressure (PAOP) less than or equal to 15 mmHg (93,94)

About 8% of patients on the wait list for LT have PoPH and its presence profoundly impacts survival. Patients with PoPH are candidates for a MELD exception to expedite LT (Table 72.3). A retrospective study from the Mayo Clinic composed of PoPH patients from 1994 until 2007 revealed a median survival of 15 months and a 5-year survival of 14% in those not treated with pulmonary vasodilators (95). For individuals who received pulmonary vasodilators, the median survival improved to 46 months with a 5-year survival of 45%. The perioperative mortality of LT in patients with untreated PoPH is profound. An early study by Krowka et al. (96) revealed an mPAP greater than 50 mmHg to be associated with 100% mortality, while a mPAP between 35 and 50 mmHg with a PVR above 250 dynes·sec·cm^{-5} had a 50% mortality rate.

TABLE 72.3 Criteria for MELD Exception

Initial abnormal mPAP and PVR Documentation of pulmonary vasodilator treatment Posttreatment achievement of mPAP <35 mmHg and PVR <400 dynes·sec·cm^{-5} Transpulmonary gradient (mPAP – PAOP) ≥12 mmHg to correct for volume overload
MELD score of 22 if above met
MELD score increases by 10% every 3 mo if hemodynamic parameters are maintained by right ventricular catheterization

(From Organ Procurement and Transplantation Network. Policy 9: allocation of livers and livers-intestines. http://optn.transplant.hrsa.gov/ContentDocuments/OPTN_Policies.pdf#nameddest = Policy_09. Accessed May 1, 2014.)

All potential LT recipients should be screened for PoPH, given the associated mortality; PoPH is reported present in up to 16% of patients with cirrhosis and refractory ascites, but 4% or less in those without refractory ascites (97). Mild PoPH may be asymptomatic and the symptoms associated with more severe PoPH, such as peripheral edema, ascites, and dyspnea on exertion, mimic those of ESLD and are easily overlooked or misinterpreted (94). An ECG with findings of right atrial or right ventricular (RV) enlargement or RBBB and chest radiographic findings of enlarged pulmonary arteries and cardiomegaly should raise suspicion for PoPH, but both CXR and ECG have low sensitivity for the diagnosis. TTE is an excellent screening tool, with a sensitivity of 98% and specificity of 96% when using a cutoff value for the RV systolic pressure of 40 mmHg; the diagnosis of pulmonary hypertension is confirmed by right heart catheterization (94).

In the past the presence of PoPH was considered a contraindication to LT given the profound perioperative mortality rates. Now, most centers treat these patients with pulmonary vasodilators. LT may commence if there is adequate response to treatment based on improved mPAP and RV function. This is a laborious and costly undertaking; it requires close follow-up with frequent echocardiography and/or right heart catheterization to monitor the response to treatment. The medical regimens are intense and require close attention to detail and unfailing compliance by the patient. The treatment may require an infusion pump and continuous supply of a refrigerated drug such as epoprostenol. Ideally, a pulmonologist or other expert in pulmonary vascular disorders should manage these patients. Many centers will proceed with LT if mPAP is reduced below 35 mmHg and RV function improves. Adequate RV function is likely the best predictor of operative survival, although no studies are available to support assertion (97–100). In some patients LT reverses PoPH and they are eventually weaned from the pulmonary vasodilators over a period of time. Currently, there are no means to predict who will respond and who will need continued treatment for PoPH for life (94,97).

Compliance with the pulmonary vasodilator therapy before, during, and after surgery is essential. These drugs have varying half-lives and abrupt cessation or changes in dosing can cause a precipitous decline in RV systolic function, serious systemic hypotension, and death. Close consultation with the prescribing physician may be necessary during the acute perioperative period or during any ICU stay for patients with PoPH who are on these therapies.

Hepatorenal Syndrome

HRS is a functional renal impairment that occurs in 11.4% of patients with liver failure within 5 years of the first episode of significant ascites (101). There are two types, both potentially reversible with LT. HRS 1 is rapidly progressive, with doubling of initial creatinine to above 2.5 mg/dL, oliguria, or 50% reduction of creatinine clearance to less than 20 mL/min occurring in less than 2 weeks. HRS 2 is associated with a more moderate, steady decline in renal function and ascites refractory to diuretics (102). Criteria for the diagnosis of HRS include the following (103):

- Cirrhosis with ascites
- Serum creatinine over 1.5 mg/dL

- No improvement in serum creatinine after 2 days of treatment with diuretics and volume expansion with albumin (1 g/kg to a maximum of 100 g/day)
- Absence of shock
- No current or recent exposure to nephrotoxic agents
- Absence of signs of parenchymal renal disease as suggested by proteinuria or hematuria or abnormal renal ultrasound results

Arterial vasodilation in the splanchnic circulation caused by portal hypertension plays a primary role in the pathogenesis of HRS. As liver failure progresses, despite the increases in CO and decreased SVR, there are local increases in renal vascular resistance due to the activation of the renin–angiotensin system, followed by a further decline in renal perfusion and glomerular filtration rate (GFR) and impaired sodium and water excretion. It is important to bear in mind that the true reduction in GFR may be disguised by a relatively normal serum creatinine as muscle mass in patients with long-standing liver disease and cirrhosis is usually significantly reduced (102,104).

Without the recovery of hepatic function, the prognosis for patients with HRS is very poor overall, with an approximate survival rate of 50% in 1 month even with dialysis (102,105,106). Kidney function may recover if liver failure resolves or LT is performed. The potential for renal recovery, however, is difficult to predict and is negatively impacted the longer dialysis is needed. Deciding which patients will require a combined liver/kidney transplant remains in evolution and requires a multidisciplinary approach (107).

Patients with HRS 1 are often managed in an ICU setting as they are likely to deteriorate. In most cases diuretics should be stopped, particularly potassium-sparing diuretics. Early management may include large volume paracentesis if the abdomen is tense, followed by albumin infusion of 8 g for each liter of ascitic fluid removed. Early paracentesis may improve intra-abdominal pressure and renal perfusion and allow assessment for peritonitis (79). Maintenance of euvolemia, preferably with albumin, and vasoconstrictor therapy to improve mean arterial pressure (MAP) is the mainstay of treatment (102,108). Terlipressin, a vasopressin analogue, is the treatment of choice in some countries, but is not approved in the United States or Canada (102,109–111). The efficacy of treating HRS with terlipressin versus norepinephrine appears similar, but adverse events (particularly abdominal pain, chest pain, ischemic events, and arrhythmias) are more frequently encountered with terlipressin. The cost of terlipressin is more than threefold that of norepinephrine (112,113). Norepinephrine is the vasopressor of choice in the United States for the treatment of HRS in the ICU. Oral midodrine, a selective α-1 adrenergic agonist, may be used in patients not considered critically ill. Octreotide, a somatostatin analogue, inhibits endogenous vasodilator release and increases splanchnic vasoconstriction. Octreotide, combined with a vasoconstrictor, theoretically improves renal and splanchnic hemodynamics. There is limited evidence that supports the efficacy and safety of octreotide use in combination with a vasoconstrictor for patients with HRS (114,115).

In select patients with HRS who fail to respond to medical therapy, placement of a transjugular intrahepatic portosystemic shunt (TIPS) is a possible therapeutic option (103,116). Some patients appear to benefit exhibiting improvement in creatinine clearance, reduction in serum creatinine, and increased urinary sodium excretion. Patients in the ICU may be too ill to tolerate placement of TIPS and there are complications that occur following TIPS placement, including hepatic encephalopathy, worsened hepatic function, further renal injury from the use of IV contrast agents during TIPS placement, and death. Mortality rates from HRS are still substantial following TIPS without LT or return of hepatic function (116).

Early consultation with nephrologists knowledgeable about HRS is recommended. Renal replacement therapy (RRT) is an option for appropriate patients who fail medical therapy. In the ICU continuous renal replacement therapy (CRRT) is often required due to concomitant hemodynamic instability. Patients who have the potential to recover from acute hepatic failure or those on the LT waiting list are more likely to benefit. Benefit is less clear in patients with HRS who do not have recoverable liver failure and who are not transplant candidates (102). Since recovery of liver function is the greatest hope for survival in HRS, urgent assessment for possible LT should transpire in appropriate patients. In those patients with non-recoverable liver failure who are deemed not to be candidates for LT, realistic expectations and outcomes should be communicated to the patient and family; palliative care is a reasonable approach to treatment in this situation.

OBESITY IN LIVER TRANSPLANTATION

Obesity is a global pandemic; patients presenting for consideration of LT are no exception. This has made NASH one of the fastest growing indications for LT. Currently, it is the third most common etiology of liver disease in patients who have had LT in the United States (2,117) and the second most common etiology of liver failure on the transplant waiting list (118). It has been predicted that NASH may exceed hepatitis C and alcohol as the most common reason for LT within the next decade (117–119). NASH is the hepatic manifestation of metabolic syndrome, which is a combination of increased abdominal girth, hypertension, hyperglycemia, and hyperlipidemia. Patients with NASH have increased risk for early postoperative and delayed morbidity and mortality, particularly cardiovascular events (18,19,117). The impact of obesity itself on mortality following LT remains uncertain; early analyses and reviews suggest that obese patients have worse survival outcomes. However, the findings of more recent single-center and multicenter reviews contradict the earlier findings (119–121). Given that obese patients are more likely to have comorbid conditions such as metabolic syndrome, obstructive sleep apnea, diabetes mellitus, and coronary artery disease, and are often less functional than nonobese candidates, it is not surprising that they appear to be at increased risk for postoperative morbidity and increased resource utilization. These are evidenced by longer ICU and hospital stays, operative times, transfusion needs, wound complications, infectious complications, cardiovascular events, and biliary complications requiring interventions (19,120,121). Hence, LT in the morbidly obese is not a trivial undertaking. But, given that patient and graft survival appear to be similar to that in nonobese patients, obesity itself should not be considered an absolute contraindication (117,121). Preoperative LT assessment of obese patients should include a thorough evaluation for cardiac, pulmonary, endocrine, and nutritional disturbances commonly associated with obesity. Sustained weight loss through diet and exercise is the most effective strategy for NASH and a multidisciplinary approach to the pretransplantation and posttransplantation weight management should be utilized (117).

COAGULOPATHY OF LIVER FAILURE AND TRANSFUSION

Patients with cirrhosis have a true bleeding–clotting diathesis. Several pathophysiologic abnormalities, other than low levels of procoagulants, may promote bleeding complications in ESLD. The vascular phase of hemostasis is impaired by vasodilation and a reduced vascular constrictive response to injury. Hemodynamic alterations of portal hypertension cause vascular congestion, especially of the mesenteric vessels. This, combined with the fragility of esophageal varices, explains the proclivity of these patients to present with gastrointestinal bleeding rather than a coagulopathy. Other factors may promote bleeding, including thrombocytopenia, which is secondary to hypersplenism, bone marrow suppression, and decreased thrombopoietin production in ESLD. Fibrinolysis may be poorly regulated due to elevated levels of tissue plasminogen activator (tPA), as well as poor hepatic clearance and increased extravascular production of tPA (122–124).

Historically, it was suggested that patients with liver failure are "auto-anticoagulated." This old dogma was based on abnormal findings of traditional tests of coagulation, such as PT, international normalized ratio (INR), platelet count, and partial thromboplastin time (PTT) suggesting risk for bleeding and poor coagulation. The emerging model of coagulation in patients with ESLD is one of "rebalanced hemostasis" (Fig. 72.5). This theory takes into account that procoagulant and anticoagulant factors are decreased in parallel, since most are manufactured by the liver (122–124). In ESLD, the INR does not accurately predict the need for transfusion or the risk of bleeding during invasive procedures (125–130). Furthermore, there is a lack of supportive evidence that transfusion with FFP for the purpose of normalizing the INR prior to an invasive procedure reduces transfusion needs and bleeding risk. In fact, it may actually increase the risk of bleeding by increasing central venous pressure (CVP) and vascular congestion (127–129,131,132,133). Blood from patients with ESLD generates as much thrombin as normal controls when methods of dynamic testing, such as thromboelastography (TEG), are used; this represents the activity of both procoagulants and anticoagulants (122,125,134–138). TEG is an accepted alternative to traditional tests of coagulation to assess coagulation and guide transfusion in ESLD, as most serum component markers of coagulation are reflected in the intricate dynamics of whole blood clotting.

Even more interesting, patients with cirrhosis have a nearly twofold increased risk for spontaneous venous thromboembolism (VTE) compared to age-matched population controls (139). There are several mechanisms that tip the hemostatic balance in favor of coagulation and thrombin generation (122,123,134–139). Important contributors include elevated levels of factor VIII and Von Willebrand factor in ESLD. Activated protein C downregulates thrombin formation, and thrombomodulin is the primary activator of protein C; levels of both are low in ESLD. ADAMTS 13, which normally limits the function of VWF on platelets, is present at lower levels than normal in ESLD. This elevated level of VWF and the greater affinity of VWF for platelets may explain why platelet adhesion to injured vascular endothelium is maintained, despite lower platelet counts. Factor VIII plays a key role in thrombin generation, and circulating levels actually increase as the severity of liver disease progresses (122–124,135). Given the tendency toward increased VTE risk, consideration should be given to the use of antithrombotic prophylaxis for patients with ESLD in the ICU.

FULMINANT HEPATIC FAILURE

ALF may be defined as the abrupt loss of liver function, characterized by hepatic encephalopathy and coagulopathy within 26 weeks of the onset of symptoms—classically jaundice—in a patient without previous liver disease. Although ALF frequently results in death, many will recover with supportive medical therapy. In the past 20 years, improved critical care management has substantially improved survival in ALF without LT (140). When LT for ALF transpires, the burden of neurologic and infectious complications of ALF extend into the posttransplant period, resulting in inferior survival rates compared to those of elective LT. This combination of improved survival without LT and suboptimal survival after LT makes accurate identification of those patients who will actually benefit from LT complex (141–143).

The prognosis of fulminant liver failure is determined by four key elements (144):

- Etiology
- Rate of progression
- Age of the patient
- Laboratory markers of disease severity

Since the pace of the evolution of ALF has important implications on mortality, it may be subdivided based on the jaundice-to-encephalopathy interval. With hyperacute liver failure the interval is 7 days or less; ALF has an interval of 8 to 28 days; and subacute liver failure more than 28 days. In general, patients with hyperacute liver failure have a more favorable rate of spontaneous survival without LT. This group is more likely to have acetaminophen (APAP) overdose or acute hepatitis A as the etiology of ALF, but are also more likely to have cerebral edema; in contrast, subacute liver failure patients have a worse rate of spontaneous survival. APAP overdose constitutes nearly 50% of the cases of ALF in the United States (Fig. 72.6) (140).

Infection occurs in 80% of patients with fulminant hepatic failure. The use of prophylactic antibiotics may increase the risk of fungal infections, often fatal, which occur in roughly one-third of patients with ALF. Encephalopathy inversely correlates with prognosis; Table 72.4 summarizes the four stages of encephalopathy that are seen in FHF. Cerebral edema occurs in most cases that progress to stage 4. Typical symptoms of severe cerebral edema are the Cushing reflex, decerebrate rigidity, disconjugate eye movements, and a loss of pupillary reflexes (145).

The King's College Hospital criteria, described in 1989, were the first to differentiate between APAP-induced ALF and other causes; Table 72.5 summarizes the King's College criteria for LT (146). The sensitivity and specificity of the King's College criteria for LT in ALF have been evaluated in

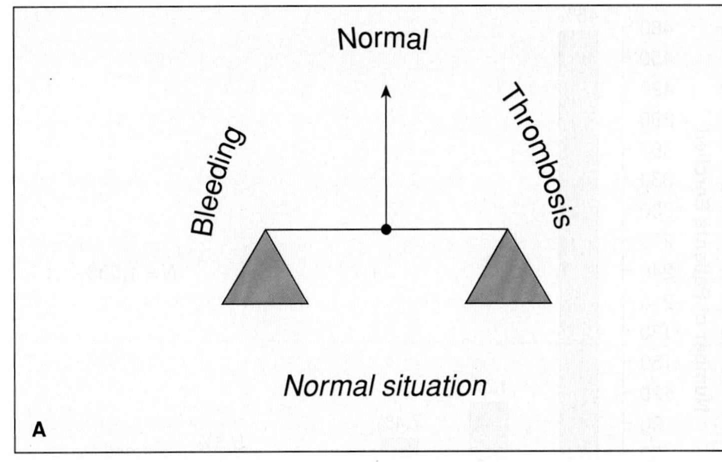

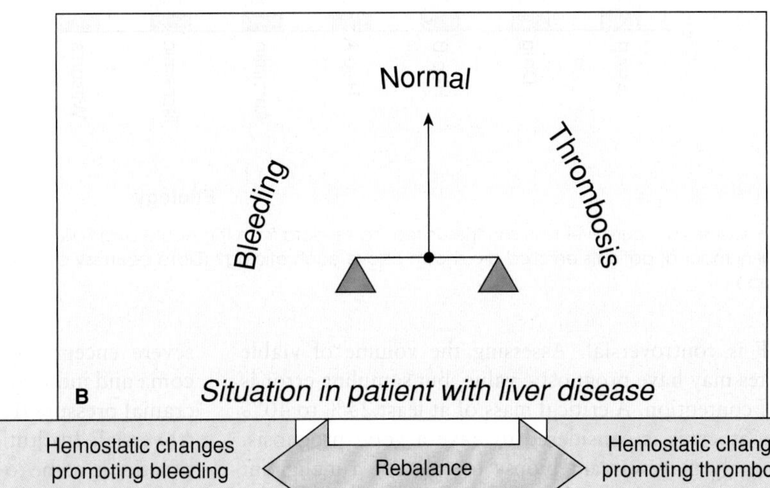

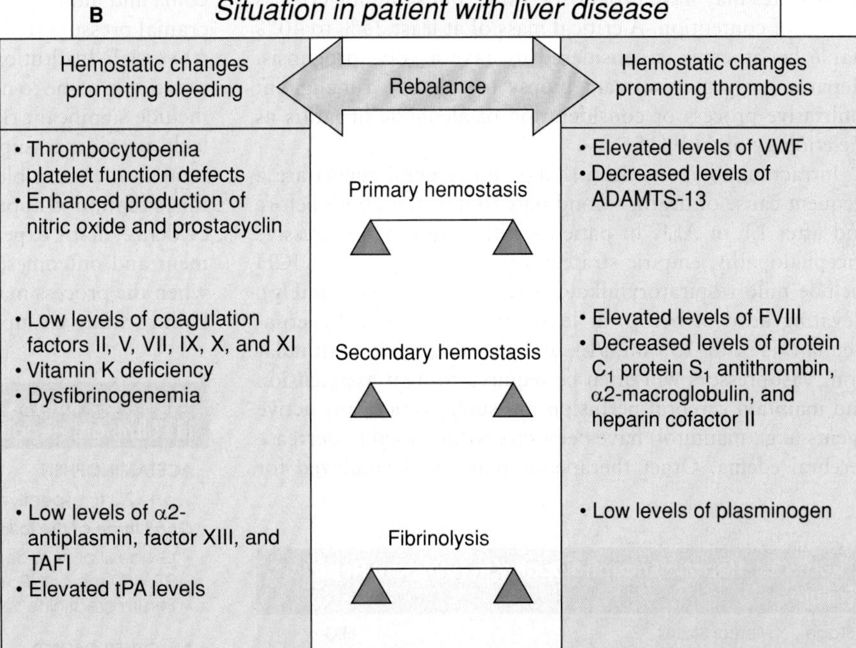

FIGURE 72.5 Schematic presentation of the balance between procoagulant and anticoagulant factors in patients with liver disease. Both sides of the balance are functionally reduced, resulting in a more or less rebalancing of the hemostatic system in these patients, although at a lower level with smaller margins. FVIII, factor VIII; YTAFI, thrombin activatable fibrinolysis inhibitor; tPA, tissue plasminogen activator; VWF, von Willebrand factor. (Adapted from Warnaar N, Lisman T, Porte R. The two tales of coagulation in liver transplantation. *Curr Opin Organ Transplant.* 2008;13(3):298–303.)

several meta-analysis and systematic reviews, with reported overall specificity of 82% for non-APAP etiologies and 92% to 95% for APAP-induced ALF (144,146–149). When considering whether or not to proceed with LT, reduced sensitivity leads to failure to transplant a patient with ALF who will die without LT, but reduced specificity carries the risk of unnecessary transplantation in a patient likely to recover spontaneously. In this setting, the MELD score has a high sensitivity and negative predictive value, but a low specificity. Use of the MELD score in conjunction with King's College criteria may be beneficial to the decision-making process (144,150). One of the main components of both scores is the INR, hence unnecessary correction of the INR may affect prognostication. The use of liver biopsy for prognostication in patients

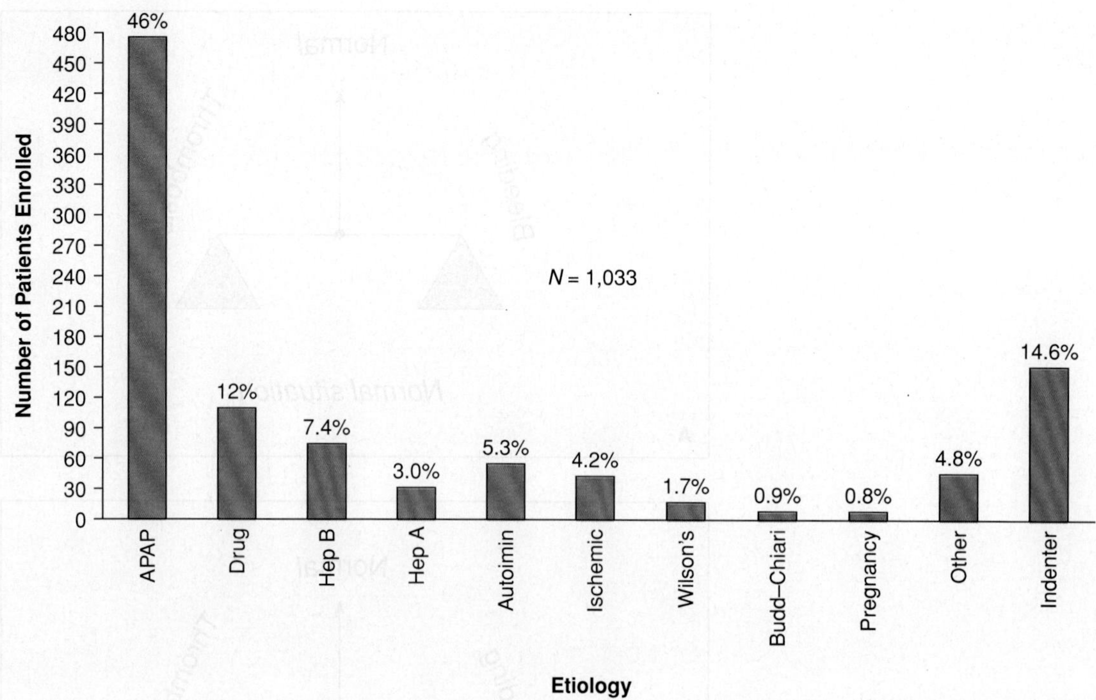

FIGURE 72.6 Causes of acute liver failure in the United States: data from the Acute Liver Failure Study Group Registry, from 1998 to 2007. Percentages of the total number of patients enrolled are shown above each etiology. (Data courtesy of W.M. Lee, Principal Investigator, the Acute Liver Failure Study Group.)

with ALF is controversial. Assessing the volume of viable hepatocytes may have prognostic value, but sampling error is a point of contention. A critical mass of at least 25% to 40% viable hepatocytes is considered to have a good prognosis. Hepatomegaly may warrant biopsy to rule out a malignant infiltrative process or consideration of alcoholic hepatitis as the etiology of ALF (151).

Intracranial hypertension (ICH) and cerebral edema are a frequent cause of death, second only to infection, both before and after LT in ALF. In patients with severe or progressive encephalopathy, empiric strategies to prevent or reduce ICH include mild respiratory alkalosis ($PaCO_2$ of 30–35 mmHg), elevating head of bed to at least 30 degrees, mild hypernatremia (Na^+ 145–155 mEq/L), and avoiding noxious stimulation. Vasopressors will often be required to treat hypotension and maintain cerebral perfusion pressure. Osmotically active agents (e.g., mannitol) have been successfully used to decrease cerebral edema. Other therapeutic maneuvers employed for severe encephalopathy and ICH have included barbiturate coma and induced hypothermia (140). The utilization of intracranial pressure (ICP) monitors to manage ICH in ALF is controversial. Institutional practices vary widely from standard practice in some to never in others. Major points of contention include significant risk of associated intracranial bleeding and lack of evidence supporting improved outcomes. The rate of fatal intracranial bleeding associated with ICP placement in this situation is approximately 3.5% (140). Despite a lack of evidence, many experts believe ICP monitors improve management and outcomes, but may also provide information as to when the process may not be recoverable. The US Acute Liver Failure Study Group has supported the use of ICP for patients

TABLE 72.4 Hepatic Encephalopathy in Fulminant Hepatic Failure

Stage	Mental Status	EEG
I	Confusion, slow mentation and affect, slurred speech, disordered sleep	Normal
II	Accentuation of stage I, drowsy, inappropriate, loss of sphincter control	Slowing
III	Marked confusion, sleeps mostly but arousable, incoherent	Abnormal
IV	Not arousable; may or may not respond to painful stimuli	Abnormal

EEG, electroencephalograph.
(From Sass DA, Shakil AO. Fulminant hepatic failure. *Liver Transplant.* 2005;11(6):594–605, with permission.)

TABLE 72.5 King's College Criteria for Liver Transplantation in Fulminant Hepatic Failure

ACETAMINOPHEN
- pH <7.3 (irrespective of encephalopathy)

Or all three of the following:
- Grade III or IV encephalopathy
- PT >100 sec or INR >6.5
- Serum creatinine >3.4 mg/dL

ALL OTHER CAUSES
- PT >100 sec or INR >6.5 (irrespective of encephalopathy)

Or any three of the following:
- Age <10 or >40 yrs
- Cause: non–A, non–B hepatitis; halothane; idiosyncratic drug reaction; Wilson disease
- Length of time from jaundice to encephalopathy >7 days
- PT >50 sec or INR >3.5
- Serum bilirubin >17.5 mg/dL

PT, prothrombin time; INR, international normalized ratio.
(From O'Grady JG, Alexander GJ, Hayllar KM, et al. Early indications of prognosis in fulminant hepatic failure. *Gastroenterology.* 1989;97:439–445, with permission.)

with ALF, particularly in those with severe encephalopathy who will go on to LT or who have a high likelihood of spontaneous recovery (140,152).

Due to improved ICU management, the past two decades have witnessed improved outcomes of ALF with and without transplantation. There is now some doubt about the benefit of LT in patients with APAP-induced ALF, the prompt recognition of which is critical, since a specific antidote, *N*-acetylcysteine (NAC), effectively limits hepatocellular injury by replenishing glutathione, the putative scavenger of the reactive APAP metabolite (*N*-acetyl-*p*-benzoquinoneimine), and preventing its binding to hepatocellular proteins. King's College Hospital treated 3,300 patients with ALF between 1973 and 2008, with overall survival rate increasing from 16.7% to 62.2%. This improvement followed the introduction of NAC and LT as treatment for APAP-induced ALF; more notably, survival without transplantation improved to 48% (144). A prospective study of 275 APAP-related ALF carried out by the US Acute Liver Failure Group included 72 patients who were placed on the waiting list for transplantation. The overall survival rate was 73%, increasing to only 78% after LT; more remarkable, over half of the patients placed on the wait list recovered without being transplanted. There was no statistically significant difference in survival after listing for transplantation based on whether or not a transplant took place (149). In both European (ELTR) and US (UNOS) transplant databases, neurologic complications account for 13% of post-transplant mortality in ALF. Both databases attribute death to infection in 18% to 24% of cases of which approximately 25% are fungal infections (141–143).

There are few more difficult decisions in critical care than the determination as to whether a patient with ALF should be listed for LT. In ALF the clinical condition can change significantly within short time intervals. The implication is that their clinical status may markedly improve or deteriorate from the time of their placement on the wait list to organ allocation, making LT irrelevant, either because they are now recovering with supportive care or too ill to proceed with LT. Defining the point when the anticipated outcome no longer justifies the utilization of the organ is difficult from an evidence-based standpoint. An outline of some indicators of when to proceed to transplantation, pause to consider, or abandon a plan to transplant is presented in Table 72.6 (144). A multidisciplinary decision-making process should include a thorough psychosocial evaluation, and consultations by hepatology, transplant surgery, the intensivist and the patient or their proxy.

TABLE 72.6 Kings College Criteria Guidelines for Urgent Liver Transplantation in Acute Liver Failure

PROCEED
- Criteria of poor prognosis persist
- Absence of comorbidity independent of liver failure that precludes transplant
- Absence of complications related to liver transplant that reduce survival
- Absence of psychosocial profile suggestive of poor graft or patient survival following transplant

WAIT
- Evidence of sustained clinical improvement suggesting favorable prognosis without transplant
- Acetaminophen-induced acute liver failure without grade III-IV encephalopathy regardless of coagulopathy
- Acetaminophen-induced acute liver failure with severe lactic acidosis that responds rapidly to resuscitative measures
- Allocated liver is steatotic, from an advanced age donor, non-ABO compatible or otherwise marginal

STOP
- Evidence of compromised brainstem function
- Invasive fungal infection
- Rapidly escalating vasopressor and inotrope requirements
- Severe pancreatitis

(From O'Grady J. Timing and benefit of liver transplantation in acute liver failure. *J Hepatol.* 2014;60:663–670.)

SURGICAL AND ANESTHETIC MANAGEMENT

LT is one of the most complex surgical procedures, requiring intensive resources and multidisciplinary care. However, in the past two decades improved outcomes have reached levels that would have been inconceivable previously. This success has been achieved through enhancements of care by all involved in LT including:

- Enhanced donor management
- Improved surgical techniques
- Advances in anesthetic management
- Superior immunosuppressive medications

Surgical Management

As described by Starzl, the original surgical procedures were prolonged and required complete cross-clamping of the portal vein (PV) and the inferior vena cava (IVC) above and below the liver. Venovenous bypass (VVB) was introduced to combat the hemodynamic challenges and mesenteric congestion created by the interruption of the IVC and PV. However, VVB carries complications of its own including vascular and nerve injury, fatal air- or thromboembolism, hemothorax, lymphedema, prolongation of ischemic times of the graft, hypothermia, and infections. In the late 1980s, the piggyback technique, a caval-sparing technique, with end-to-side or side-to-side caval anastomosis was introduced and is generally the procedure of choice for most primary liver transplants today (Fig. 72.7). It spares the IVC and results in improved outflow of the allograft. This technique has resulted in shortened operative and ischemic times and diminished transfusion needs (153,154). A few centers still use VVB routinely, but many feel the shortened anhepatic time of the piggyback technique and partial, rather than complete, clamping of the IVC minimizes mesenteric congestion. VVB may be used occasionally for select, high-risk cases, such as redotransplantations or transplantation for ALF.

Anesthetic Management

Dramatic improvements in anesthetic management have positively impacted outcomes in LT at least equal to that of surgical advancements. These changes include improvements in clinical care as well as evidenced-based administrative practices.

Massive intraoperative blood loss and transfusion requirements were nearly insurmountable prior to the last two decades. Now, bloodless LT is a reality and many transplants transpire with few or no blood products transfused. This is of paramount significance in improving LT outcomes as transfusion is linked increased complication rates, morbidity, and

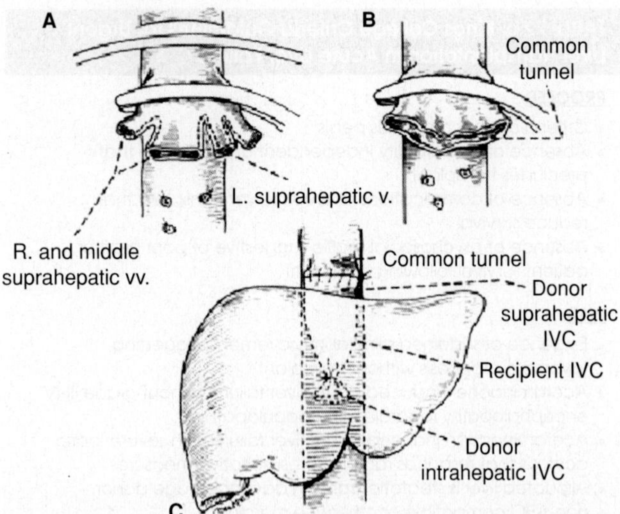

FIGURE 72.7 Piggyback technique and creation of a common confluence for hepatic venous outflow. (From Eghtesad B, Kadry Z, Fung J. Technical considerations in liver transplantation: what a hepatologist needs to know (and every surgeon should practice). *Liver Transpl.* 2005;11(8):861–871.)

mortality (155,156). Several anesthetic practices have been credited in the reduction of transfusion needs. Lower CVP and fluid restriction during hepatic dissection reduces hepatic and vascular congestion and, consequently, bleeding (157). In addition, avoiding excess intravenous fluid also prevents dilutional coagulopathy and hypothermia, and results in a less edematous allograft with improved function. Using vasopressors to maintain adequate MAP rather than fluids is now standard management in LT. Normovolemic hemodilution, another method utilized to decrease both bleeding and allogeneic transfusion needs in patients with adequate hematocrit, is used successfully in donor hepatectomies for live donor LT to prevent unnecessary transfusions in this otherwise healthy population (158). Anesthesiologists are vigilant in preventing and treating hypothermia and correcting hypocalcemia to further minimize intraoperative bleeding (159,160).

Understanding the rebalanced hemostasis of ESLD and avoiding "prophylactic" transfusion with FFP, platelets and cryoprecipitate to unnecessarily correct abnormal tests of coagulation is key. Transfusion begets more transfusion, due at least in part to increased CVP, splanchnic congestion, and increased serum citrate concentration (124,129). Accepting lower transfusion thresholds, using point of care testing, such as TEG, and clinical assessment of hemostasis on the surgical field to guide transfusion should have become standard of care in LT.

Antifibrinolytic drugs have been used successfully to improve hemostasis in LT in the past, but controversy surrounds this practice, given the risk of thrombosis. Although there is no conclusive evidence to link the use of antifibrinolytics to thrombosis in LT, when thrombosis occurs it is associated with a high mortality rate (161). Logic dictates empiric use be avoided when there is a history of VTE, evidence of hypercoagulability on tests such as TEG or the patient has a condition with a predisposition to thrombosis such as cancer or primary biliary cirrhosis. Use on demand when there is excess bleeding and evidence of thrombolysis by TEG may be a more acceptable approach.

Mannitol is often administered just prior to, or during, the anhepatic stage of the procedure to increase CVP and improve hemodynamic tolerance during IVC clamp. Its oxygen radical scavenging properties may protect the allograft and the kidney from ischemia–reperfusion injury, and its osmotic effects have the added benefit of preventing or reducing mesenteric edema, unlike crystalloid solutions. Furthermore, mannitol appears to temper postreperfusion syndrome, the marked hemodynamic instability that occurs immediately after initial perfusion of the new allograft (162).

The marked intraoperative circulatory challenges require a comprehensive evaluation of preload, afterload, and cardiac function by the anesthesiologist. At a minimum, this includes standard American Society of Anesthesiology (ASA) monitors, an arterial catheter for invasive blood pressure monitoring, and a large-bore central venous catheter for CVP monitoring. The latter also allows optimal access for volume resuscitation and vasopressors. The use of PA catheters for LT has been largely replaced by transesophageal echocardiography (TEE) in many transplant centers; risk of hemorrhage from variceal injury during placement is minimal. TEE allows for direct visualization and assessment of preload, volume status, and cardiac contractility. It offers the added benefit of rapid diagnosis of intracardiac thrombosis which is an uncommon, but often catastrophic, event unique to LT. Air embolism, tension pneumothorax, and large pericardial effusions or tamponade can be also detected immediately (163). As absolute values cannot be calculated with TEE, one indication for PA catheters may be PoPH; the PA pressure measurement often drives management decisions in this scenario. More over, TEE allows visual assessment of function of the right ventricle (RV) which is crucial, not only in PoPH, but during massive transfusion. Pressure and volume overload of the RV can lead to overstretching of the ventricle and ischemia; using TEE to guide preload and volume may prevent RV failure in this instance.

Traditionally, patients who had LT remained intubated after surgery for 1 or 2 days or longer. This practice was founded in the belief that remaining intubated reduced physiologic stress. In the last decade, there has been a movement toward early, or "fast-track" extubation. Patients are now extubated immediately in the operating suite or within a few hours of ICU admission if they meet criteria, such as adequate oxygenation, adequate mental status, and hemodynamic stability. This practice has shortened ICU and hospital stays (164). While "fast-tracking" facilitates decreased cost and resource utilization, it may also help to prevent complications, such as nosocomial infections and others associated with longer ICU stays and hospitalizations.

In 2008, Hevesi et al. (165) reported on the benefits of a dedicated liver transplant anesthesia team at the University of Wisconsin. This team included a small, core group of anesthesiologists who provided anesthesia for all LT and a director who worked closely with the transplant surgery department in many of the administrative and clinical duties associated with LT. This was the first such description of a collaboration between two disciplines that substantially improved outcomes (165). Prior to this, there was enormous institutional variation in practices and resource utilization. The core team of anesthesiologists employed consistent clinical practices that resulted in less transfusion, decreased MV time, and shorter ICU stays. The director also became intimately involved in the preoperative evaluation to insure selection of recipients able to tolerate LT, which is tantamount to appropriate organ allocation. This approach to care yielded improved communication and professional partnership between the surgeons and anesthesiologists. Although an unmeasurable element, this type of collaboration and satisfaction likely leads to improved quality of care. The success of this program led the ASA and UNOS to adopt this model as the standard for institutions that provide LT.

POSTOPERATIVE ICU MANAGEMENT

Physiologic perturbations of the preoperative and intraoperative periods accompany the patient into the acute postoperative phase. In most cases, the patient will be admitted to the ICU following LT for continued resuscitation, ongoing transfusion and hemostasis, hemodynamic monitoring, support of organ systems, and close monitoring of the graft function. The approach to the postoperative care of the liver transplant patient should include coordination between the intensivists, transplant surgeons, and hepatologists, along with other subspecialty management as necessary.

Cardiovascular Management

Hypotension and hemodynamic instability in the immediate posttransplant phase have multiple causes, including surgical bleeding, underresuscitation, baseline infiltrative disease, ischemic cardiomyopathy, new dilated cardiomyopathy, bleeding due to coagulopathy, abdominal hypertension, heart failure, dysrhythmias, infection, inflammatory response, electrolyte and acid/base derangements, and graft failure, to name some (166). The patient will usually arrive to the ICU following transplantation with hemodynamic monitors in place, including central venous and arterial catheters and, occasionally, a PA catheter. Utilization of these or other devices, such as continuous CO monitors and bedside ultrasound, in conjunction with clinical examination, evaluation of drain output, vital signs, assessment of fluid responsiveness, urine output, and targeted laboratory tests will aid the intensivist in establishing the etiology of hemodynamic instability. Useful laboratory studies may include mixed venous O_2 saturation, pH, electrolytes, hematocrit, and dynamic tests of coagulation (Fig. 72.8) (166). Identifying the correct cause of hemodynamic instability avoids inappropriate therapies that can negatively impact outcome and graft function, not to mention failing to treat the true problem. For example, volume resuscitation in a nonfluid responsive state can cause pulmonary edema and vascular congestion of the graft, mesentery and abdominal hypertension, which will worsen allograft function. Alternatively, treatment of hypotension with vasopressors in a nonvasodilatory state may worsen graft perfusion due to splanchnic vasoconstriction. In the case of a failing left ventricle (LV) increasing SVR will further compromise CO. Therefore, it is crucial for patient and graft survival to methodically assess hypotension for cardiac, hypovolemic, and distributive causes.

Volume Resuscitation, Electrolyte, and Acid–Base Management

Hypovolemia in the immediate postoperative phase of LT is commonly encountered. Ongoing bleeding, either surgical or coagulopathic, continued production of ascites, fluid shifts, and inadequate intraoperative resuscitation are a few of the causes. Treatment of hypovolemia is necessary to maintain adequate perfusion of the allograft. In a stable situation compensatory responses will allow for a 25% to 30% loss of blood volume without a decrease in systemic blood pressure, but the splanchnic vasculature and, therefore, the liver are compromised by a 10% reduction (167). It is imperative that close observation of hematocrit and tests of coagulation accompany hemodynamic monitoring in the first 48 to 72 hours after LT. The goal of volume resuscitation is euvolemia, while avoiding excess volume administration leading to elevated CVP, portal hypertension, and hepatic and pulmonary edema.

Several options are available for the treatment of hypovolemia. Crystalloids are cost-effective, readily available, and do not carry the risks of blood product transfusion. Conventional wisdom and evidence support minimizing transfusion; however, the newly transplanted liver patient presents different challenges and is not represented well in standard transfusion practice guidelines. Vascular barrier permeability in the allograft has been compromised by ischemia–reperfusion injury. Crystalloids in the early posttransplant period rapidly exit the intravascular space causing edema and congestion of the sinusoids. Extravasation of fluid also increases abdominal compartment pressure further compromising allograft perfusion. Fluid and protein shifts in the allograft are less when

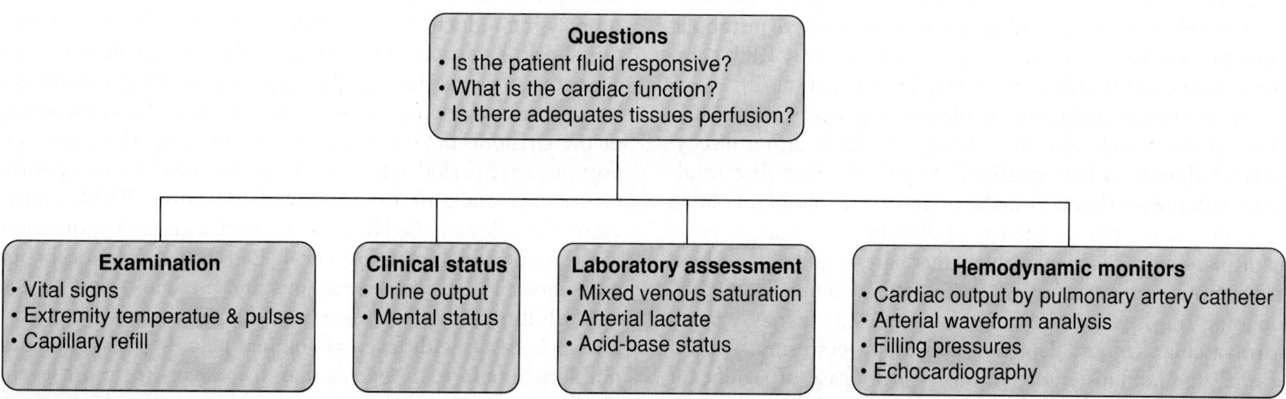

FIGURE 72.8 Initial hemodynamic and perfusion assessment to establish the cause of hemodynamic instability. (Adapted from Hastie J, Moitra V. Routine postoperative care in liver transplantation. In: Wagener G, ed. *Liver Anesthesiology and Critical Care Medicine*. New York: Springer Science; 2012:355–369.)

using blood products, as opposed to crystalloids, for volume expansion (168). Colloids may be considered during attempts at fluid resuscitation as they have a more sustained effect than crystalloids, but the effects are still transient and colloids are also prone to causing edema of the graft (169). Given that hypovolemia is frequently due to bleeding from coagulopathy, blood products have the added benefit of correcting these, whereas, crystalloids may worsen coagulopathy by dilution. Colloid starch solutions are best used judiciously, if at all, during this phase of care given the inherent risks associated with them. It is important to prevent and treat hypothermia during volume resuscitation as it will worsen coagulopathy. Active warming of the patient, blood products, and fluids along with the room are measures that can be utilized for this purpose.

Abnormal levels of all electrolytes are commonly encountered after LT. Sodium, potassium, calcium, phosphorous, and magnesium should be monitored closely and corrected judiciously. It is reasonable to follow these serum values three or four times a day in the first 48 to 72 hours. Hypocalcemia is a frequent occurrence. To prevent clots, citrate is often used in CRRT systems and blood banking. Between the amount of citrate administered during CRRT and that from blood products, hypocalcemia may develop with resultant hypotension; serum ionized calcium should be monitored closely and replaced accordingly.

Hyponatremia occurs in many LT recipients and represents another cause for caution when considering crystalloid administration after LT given the risk of central pontine myelinolysis (CPM), discussed in further detail below. Normal saline is hypernatremic to serum and may raise sodium levels inappropriately in patients with hyponatremia. Albumin also contains sodium and caution is advised with infusion of it as well (170,171).

Metabolic acidosis is frequently encountered in the LT perioperative period. It is important to treat the underlying cause of the acidosis. The new graft may have reduced ability to metabolize lactate, particularly in times of increased production. Poor tissue oxygenation and perfusion due to hypotension, poor CO, hypovolemia and severe anemia, complications of infection, and intestinal ischemia are common causes of lactate production. Acute kidney injury (AKI) and chronic renal failure cause further metabolic acidosis. During volume resuscitation excessive use of normal saline solutions should be avoided as this may lead to worsened acidosis due to hyperchloremia. Severe metabolic acidosis may be encountered in delayed or poor graft function. It is important to optimize hemodynamic parameters and minute ventilation in the face of metabolic acidosis. Severe metabolic acidosis may require sodium bicarbonate or tromethamine (THAM) administration. Correction of severe metabolic acidosis may be faster and safer with the use of CRRT compared to sodium bicarbonate or THAM infusions (172).

Attempting to maintain euvolemia in patients with ESLD particularly acutely after liver transplant leads into a discussion of diuretic administration. Despite the fact that total-body volume overload is usually present, intravascular volume depletion is the norm. The use of diuretics in the acute posttransplant period is inadvisable if there are ongoing fluid shifts from intra- to extravascular spaces, hemodynamic instability, ongoing transfusion, or vasopressor needs as it may worsen intravascular volume depletion and organ perfusion. Diuretics may be administered cautiously in the case of significant intravascular volume overload in a patient who is otherwise hemodynamically stable. If diuresis is considered necessary, the concomitant use of diuretics or CRRT and transfusion or colloid infusion can improve preload and splanchnic perfusion while minimizing allograft edema.

Cardiogenic Shock

The incidence of new heart failure following LT has been reported in several series to be between 7% and 31% (80). In the posttransplant setting, findings of hypotension and poor end-organ perfusion should prompt an assessment of cardiac function. As discussed previously, cirrhotic physiology is one of an "auto-afterload" reduced state. Abrupt increases in SVR following transplantation, the surgical stresses, and myocardial ischemia can lead to depressed systolic function or unmask previously unrecognized myocardial dysfunction. This is usually a temporary or reversible state, but if severe heart failure occurs within the first 12 hours of LT, death and multiorgan failure have been described (173). Bedside echocardiography is a valuable, noninvasive tool in establishing the diagnosis of myocardial dysfunction. A PA catheter may also be useful if parameters suggesting cardiac failure are present. A mixed venous oxygen saturation below 60% is also indicative of a poor CO. Inotropes, adequate preload, and lowered afterload are the mainstay of care for a failing LV. Cardiology assistance in the management of these patients is frequently necessary and valuable.

Hemodynamic instability in the perioperative period is a complex issue in patients with PoPH. Right heart failure can lead to cardiogenic shock and inotropic agents should be considered the mainstay of therapy. Lowering of the PVR with inhaled NO or prostacyclins to achieve afterload reduction of the RV may also be beneficial. Perioperatively, close attention to fluid management is critical. It is essential to optimize preload while avoiding volume overload and RV wall stress (98,99,173). Some patients will have been prescribed pulmonary vasodilators prior to LT and these should be continued perioperatively without fail. TEE or TTE and PA catheters may be useful in guiding intraoperative and postoperative LT management in patients with PoPH.

Vasodilatory Hypotension

Vasodilation and vasopressor responsive hypotension are also encountered after LT and have multiple etiologies in this setting. Hypocalcemia, infections/sepsis, and inflammatory responses are common causes of vasodilation and hypotension following LT. Adrenal crisis is an unlikely cause as patients receive large doses of corticosteroids as part of their immunosuppression induction. The mainstay of treatment for distributive shock is vasopressor administration. Vasodilation creates a relative increase in vascular capacity, so attention should be given to achieving normovolemia as well. The persistence of the cirrhotic physiology, high CO and low SVR, into the postoperative period may be a concerning indicator of a poorly functioning allograft or primary nonfunction (PNF). Graft-versus-host disease (GvHD) is an unusual cause of hypotension in the immediate, posttransplant ICU setting. GvHD occurs in only about 1% of liver transplants and presents 1 to 6 weeks after LT. Rarely, it may present in a fulminant fashion that mimics septic shock with fever, abdominal pain, hypotension, and multiorgan failure. Cytopenia may accompany the most severe cases and severe neutropenia is an indicator of poor prognosis. Treatment is high-dose corticosteroids with modifications or decrease in other immunosuppressive medication dosages.

If suspected, the transplant team should be consulted to assist with management of the immunosuppression regimen. Short tandem repeat (STR) levels of over 20% for CD3+ donor lymphocytes in the peripheral blood is confirmatory. Skin biopsy, if a rash is present, or intestinal biopsy may also aid in the diagnosis. Risk factors include a discrepancy between the age of the donor and the recipient. Younger donors have a greater number of lymphocytes in the liver. Older recipients (>65 years) are less able to reject the donor lymphocytes. The risk of severe GvHD increases when the age difference is over 40 years (174).

Certain drugs received in the peritransplant period may also cause vasodilation and refractory hypotension. Antithymocyte globulin (ATG) is an immunosuppressive agent that is more often used in kidney transplant recipients, but is used occasionally in liver transplant recipients considered at high risk for rejection. ATG is known to cause a systemic response that mimics septic shock due to cytokine release syndrome (CRS). This syndrome is particularly likely to occur when infusions are administered too rapidly. Fever, chills, hypotension, shock, pulmonary edema, or even death may occur from CRS in patients receiving ATG. Patients receiving ATG should be monitored closely during infusions.

General Postoperative ICU Care

Mechanical Ventilation and Extubation

Traditionally, patients remained intubated and on MV in the ICU following LT, often for over 48 hours. Although there is variability in practice among centers, early extubation or "fast tracking" has increased over the past decade. Many patients are now extubated safely in the OR immediately following LT, or within hours of admission to the ICU. This practice has been associated with decreased cost and ICU length of stay. It has also been suggested that avoiding the positive pressure of MV has beneficial effects on splanchnic and liver perfusion (164,175). For many reasons, this practice is not feasible in all patients. Hemodynamic instability, ongoing bleeding, a complicated or prolonged intraoperative course, massive transfusion, pulmonary edema, need for repeat laparotomies, and nonfunction of the allograft are some of the circumstances leading to a need for continued MV. Patient-specific factors limiting early extubation include obesity, pretransplant encephalopathy, prolonged hospitalization, prolonged ICU stay, severe malnutrition, hydrothorax, underlying lung disease, and severe deconditioning. HPS or PoPH may also delay liberation from MV. Patient selection is key to the success of early extubation.

Management of MV in this population is no different from others in the ICU. While patients are ventilated, standards of care for stress ulcer prophylaxis with either an H_2-blocker or proton pump inhibitor therapy should be maintained. Strategies to prevent ventilator-associated pneumonia should be adhered to, including keeping the head of bed elevated to at least 30 degrees, oropharyngeal decontamination with chlorhexidine, secretion management, and high-volume, low-pressure endotracheal tube cuffs. Daily sedation holidays and spontaneous breathing trials should be practiced in this population. Use of PAD bundles (pain, agitation, and delirium protocols) to direct sedation and analgesia have been shown to be effective in decreasing time on MV when paired with daily sedation holidays. It may be prudent to limit the use of benzodiazepines, particularly long-acting formulations, as hepatic clearance may be limited in liver transplant recipients. Early mobility and early enteral nutrition have also been associated with decreased complications, improved outcomes, and decreased time to extubation and ICU days (176,177).

A central concern is the development of acute respiratory distress syndrome (ARDS) following LT. Inflammatory responses related to the surgery, massive transfusion, organ failure, and infections are all risks for ARDS. Fundamental MV management requires lung-protective ventilatory strategies for all liver recipients, given this concern and, particularly, in patients exhibiting hypoxia or evidence of ARDS. In severe cases of refractory hypoxemia, rescue strategies include prone positioning, inhaled NO, inhaled prostaglandin, or extracorporeal membrane oxygenation. There is an overall lack of evidence that these maneuvers will improve survival, but there are supportive case reports (177,178).

Successful weaning and freedom from the ventilator may take hours to weeks depending on the clinical situation as outlined above. Parameters for extubation are no different for LT recipients than other ICU patients. In general, the patient should be oxygenating adequately on lower levels (<50%–60%) of inspired oxygen, hemodynamically stable, have adequate mental status, ability to manage secretions and airway, satisfactory cough and gag reflex, and adequate capacity to meet their minute ventilation requirements (166,177). Furthering their chance of successful extubation, their overall clinical status should be one of steady improvement without evidence of impending or ongoing deterioration such as new bleeding, untreated or refractory infection, and worsening AKI.

Glycemic Management

Because of the presence of cirrhosis-induced insulin resistance, the increase in stress hormones during surgery, and the use of high-dose steroids, patients may become quite hyperglycemic even if there were no glucose control issues prior to surgery (179). Hyperglycemia is a marker of poorer outcomes in LT. It has been related to sepsis, poor wound healing, and wound infection and suboptimal graft function (166). Hyperglycemia in the perioperative period can enhance ischemia–reperfusion injury and certain inflammatory mediators, leading to increased risk of rejection and poorer graft function (180). The ideal management of glucose in the ICU is a matter of debate; hyperglycemia has many negative consequences, but tight glucose control was associated with increased mortality in the NICE-SUGAR trial (181). A rational plan may be to avoid hypoglycemia with a glucose goal of 100 to 150 mg/dL. This will require frequent glucose measurements and, often, an insulin infusion while in the ICU. Hypoglycemia may be encountered when poor graft function occurs following transplant and may require treatment with glucose-containing solutions and enhanced glucose monitoring.

Nutrition

Early initiation of enteral nutrition is an important part of ICU care, perhaps more so in LT recipients. Early enteral nutrition in critically ill patients appears to lower mortality and infection. Nutrition plays an important role in recovery following LT, as the stresses of LT result in a catabolic state. Many patients presenting for LT have nutritional deficiencies at baseline, so early intervention is even more crucial. The ability to achieve adequate oral intake may be impacted by prolonged MV, encephalopathy, prolonged ileus, or poor appetite. Early consideration should be given to placement of an enteral feeding tube for nutritional purposes in select patients (180).

In such patients this will have the added benefit of allowing enteral access for medications, reducing the need for intravenous catheters and, therefore, catheter-related septicemia.

ACUTE POSTTRANSPLANT COMPLICATIONS

Acute Kidney Injury

AKI is an all too common phenomenon following LT, with estimates of 20% to 80%, frequently presenting within the first 48 hours post transplant. AKI after LT requiring RRT impacts mortality negatively, with early reports of 30-day mortality at 40% to 50% (182). As defined by the Acute Kidney Injury Network (AKIN), AKI is an abrupt (within 48 hours) reduction in kidney function presenting with an absolute increase in serum creatinine of at least 0.3 mg/dL (26.4 mmol/L), a percentage increase in serum creatinine of 50% or higher (1.5-fold from baseline), or a reduction in urine output (documented oliguria of less than 0.5 mL/kg/hr for more than 6 hours) (183). Severe chronic kidney disease will develop in approximately 4% of LT recipients who survive 1 year and with at least half requiring RRT (184). Predictors of posttransplant AKI include pretransplant renal dysfunction, diabetes mellitus, allograft dysfunction or PNF, intraoperative hypotension, intraoperative prolonged caval and PV cross clamp, massive transfusion, abdominal hypertension, sepsis, exposure to intravenous contrast, and acute cardiogenic shock. Hemolytic uremic syndrome (HUS) has also been described acutely in the posttransplant recipient in the ICU, triggered by calcineurin inhibitors (CNIs).

Early recognition of AKI is crucial to prevent further injury and initiate treatment. The most common etiology of post-LT AKI is acute tubular necrosis (ATN). The cause is usually multifactorial due to any combination of the previously described risk factors. Initial treatment should include optimization of volume status, CO, and renal perfusion. Abdominal hypertension that compromises renal perfusion may require paracentesis or laparotomy for decompression. Avoidance of nephrotoxins and contrast dye is principal to the recovery of AKI. Consultation with transplant surgery or hepatology regarding immunosuppression management and adjustment of dosages is essential. Early consultation with nephrology for assistance in evaluation and management is vital to care, as well. Loop diuretics may be administered in an effort to stimulate urine output, but if the patient does not respond and renal failure progresses these should be discontinued to avoid further renal injury. RRT will be required when severe oliguria or anuria, volume overload, severe uremia, electrolyte derangements, or acidosis is present. Intermittent hemodialysis may be adequate for patients who are hemodynamically stable. CRRT, such as continuous venovenous hemodialysis, is more appropriate for patients with hemodynamic instability who cannot tolerate intermittent hemodialysis (166,180). Patients who required RRT pretransplant for AKI or HRS will most likely continue to require treatment posttransplant for an indefinite period while awaiting the return of renal function. In patients who have not been maintained on RRT for a prolonged period, most will undergo liver-only transplantation in hopes of reversal of AKI, but the degree is unpredictable. In time, if kidney failure persists then consideration may be given to kidney transplantation. In patients who have been on RRT for a longer period of time prior to LT, the likelihood of reversal is diminished and consideration may be given to a combined liver–kidney transplant. However, there is not an accurate model to predict recovery of pretransplant HRS or AKI following LT (102,104,105,107).

Infection

Infection is one of the most common causes of shock and of mortality and morbidity in LT recipients, despite advances in techniques and antimicrobial prophylaxis. Infectious complications are more common in LT recipients than in any other organ recipient, and mortality from infection is currently below 10%, significantly lower than in earlier days of LT when it approached 50% to 60% (185). Infections are most common in the first 6 months, but may occur at any time following LT. Discussion here will be limited to infections in the acute, posttransplant period.

Risk factors for posttransplant infections start in the pretransplant phase. Fulminant hepatic failure, renal failure, ICU status, MV, high MELD score, pre-existing infections, diabetes mellitus, and malnutrition are all risk factors for infection following transplant. Latent infections, such as cytomegalovirus and tuberculosis, may reactivate in the face of induction immunosuppression following LT. Surgical and intraoperative events that increase the likelihood of infection include prolonged surgical time, massive transfusion, disruption of the gastrointestinal tract, vascular complications that lead to tissue necrosis, and repeat laparotomy; rarely, infections may be acquired from the donor liver. Retransplantation, prolonged ICU stay, protracted MV, renal failure, CRRT, antimicrobial pressure, vascular catheters, colonization with resistant flora, and immunosuppression after LT further increase the likelihood of infection in the recipient (185–187).

The locale of the infection, such as central line–associated blood stream infection (CLA-BSI), pneumonia, intra-abdominal wound or urinary tract infection, may be predictive of the microorganisms that are isolated. Intra-abdominal infections are frequently polymicrobial and may include fungi. In the early posttransplant period (<1 month) most infections are bacterial, followed by fungal. Common bacterial pathogens in this setting include methicillin-sensitive and methicillin-resistant *Staphylococcus aureus* (respectively, MSSA, and MRSA), coagulase-negative staphylococci, *Enterococcus faecalis,* Enterobacteriaceae, and *Pseudomonas aeruginosa.* The occurrence of bacteremia from gram-positive organisms and gram-negative bacilli in the early transplant period is nearly equal, with a slight predisposition toward gram-positive pathogens (185,186). Vancomycin-resistant enterococci (VRE) infections and colonization are on the rise in liver transplant patients; invasive infections carry a poor prognosis in this population with mortality reported to be 60% to 80%. VRE is more commonly seen in patients with prolonged hospital and ICU stays, renal failure, repeat laparotomies, intensive antimicrobial pressure, and the presence of other infections (188).

Fungal infections occur in approximately 10% of LT recipients; indeed, liver recipients have the highest incidence of fungal infection of all organ recipients. Ninety percent of all invasive fungal infections occur in the first 2 months after transplant, with most being a *Candida* species. *Aspergillus* is the second most common fungal infection, compromising about 10% to 20% of fungal infections; unfortunately, invasive *Aspergillus* infections are frequently fatal, and *Aspergillus* infections of the central nervous system are nearly universally fatal (185,186,189,190).

Viral infections are much less common in the acute posttransplant phase, although herpes simplex virus (HSV) may be encountered occasionally, despite prophylaxis. HSV infection most commonly presents as a mucosal infection, involving the oropharynx or esophagus, but hepatitis, encephalitis, or disseminated herpes are reported as well (191).

When sepsis is suspected adequate empirical therapy should be instituted, with haste, guided by suspected site of infection, probable flora, prior pathogens isolated, institutional microorganism susceptibility patterns, and the presence of renal insufficiency. A thorough examination is necessary along with cultures of the blood, lower respiratory tract, and urine to identify the source of the infection. The need for other studies, such as computed tomography of the abdomen or examination of the cerebrospinal fluid or ascites, are indicated *based on the differential diagnosis* garnered from the initial assessment. Once the source and organisms have been identified, then specific therapy can begin. Source control is vital in cases that require evacuation or surgical debridement of a discrete infectious collection. Removal of infected catheters and devices are necessary to abolish the infection. Infections in LT patients have become increasingly complex with complicated resistance patterns. Assistance from an infectious disease consultant, particularly one experienced in the care of transplant recipients and knowledgeable regarding institutional patterns, is instrumental in delivering appropriate antimicrobial regimens, both empiric and specific.

Neurologic Complications

Neurologic complications occur in about 25% of LT recipients, with CPM a particularly serious and dreaded neurologic complication. Fortunately the incidence is below 1% following LT despite the frequent presence of hyponatremia in ESLD; when it does occur, however, CPM can be devastating (192). Symptoms include paralysis, depressed consciousness, dysarthria, and dysphagia; pre-existing hepatic encephalopathy may mask symptoms of CPM acutely. Care is supportive and primarily preventative by avoiding rapid changes in serum sodium in patients with hyponatremia. Reality dictates that this can be extremely difficult during periods of rapid fluid and blood losses, such as during the transplant surgery. There is not a definitive serum sodium level that is a contraindication to LT. However, levels below 125 mEq/L are associated with an increased risk of CPM (192). Correction of severe or symptomatic hyponatremia in the ICU should occur slowly with close monitoring. A universally accepted, established rate of correction which insures prevention of CPM does not exist, but many experts consider an increase of less than 12 mEq/L/day (0.5 mEq/L/hr) to be a reasonably safe therapeutic goal. Diagnosis of CPM is made when magnetic resonance imaging of the head shows areas of T2 signal intensity in the pons in conjunction with clinical suspicion; there are no therapies to reverse the syndrome (180,192).

Encephalopathy is a frequent complication of cirrhosis and will often persist into the posttransplant phase. Although transplant usually improves encephalopathy, poor graft function will delay resolution. Medications such as benzodiazepines and narcotics may have impaired metabolism and complicate, or prolong, encephalopathy as well. Uremia and persistent hyperbilirubinemia may also worsen or delay recovery of encephalopathy. Care is supportive with close attention to neurologic examination, correction of metabolic disturbances, such as uremia, and avoidance of drugs that will further suppress consciousness (180).

CNIs are associated with several neurologic complications. Posterior reversible encephalopathy syndrome (PRES) is one such complication. PRES may present as altered mentation or coma. PRES is more likely to occur when CNIs are administered to patients with more severe, pre-existing encephalopathy; blood–brain barrier defects are present and increase the susceptibility to PRES when CNIs are administered (193,194).

Seizures are another adverse effect of CNIs. Seizures may also result from infection, hyponatremia, alkalosis, substance withdrawal, and cerebrovascular accidents. In addition to determining the cause of the seizure, all potential neurotoxic substances should be withheld. Basic care includes airway protection, ventilation, reversal of electrolyte and metabolic derangements, and antiepileptic medications. Acutely, benzodiazepines may be required for refractory or recurrent seizures; levetiracetam is usually the drug of choice for suppression of seizures. Imaging studies or sampling of the CSF may be warranted to determine the cause of the seizures. Electroencephalography (EEG) may be necessary to assess for the presence of subclinical seizures or a seizure focus (180,194).

Cerebrovascular complications or strokes are uncommonly reported following LT but, when they occur, are associated with significant morbidity and mortality. Several recent investigations of LT cohorts report incidence rates for stroke within the first 30 days of LT ranging from 0.6% to 4% (193–196). Perioperative stroke in LT is associated with an in-hospital mortality of up to 10%. More compelling is of the remaining survivors, 33% will die within a year and less than 50% will make full recovery and gain independence; more than half are institutionalized (194).

Perioperative hemorrhagic strokes appear to be more common than ischemic strokes in LT, compared with other types of surgery (196). Global hypoperfusion of the central nervous system occurs in LT during periods of sustained blood and fluid loss, hypotension, and anemia. Patients with ESLD are known to have abnormalities in cerebral perfusion and cerebral edema, which may increase the risk of injury from central nervous system hypoperfusion and, thereby, intracranial hemorrhage. The presence of a patent foramen ovale (PFO) may theoretically increase the risk of paradoxical embolic stroke due to events inherent in LT, particularly following reperfusion of the new liver graft (193,194,196).

When cerebrovascular accidents occur in the setting of LT, treatment is generally supportive. Correction of coagulopathy is important in hemorrhagic CVAs. Adequate airway protection and ventilation should be established along with optimization of the blood pressure and CO to ensure adequate cerebral perfusion while avoiding increase of the ICP. Craniotomy for management of intracranial hemorrhage in this population has been reported to be universally futile (197).

Graft-Related Complications

Primary Nonfunction and Delayed Function

Some degree of allograft dysfunction immediately following transplantation is not uncommon, but resolution is expected, given the regenerative capacity of the liver. Some patients, however, may develop graft failure or PNF. Although no formal definition of PNF exists, it is generally accepted as total graft failure that results in death or retransplantation within the first 7 days after transplantation without a definite technical or immunologic cause. In the post-MELD era of allocation, the incidence of PNF is about 5% (198). Fulminant hepatic failure as manifested by high levels of aminotransferases, hyperbilirubinemia, prolonged PT, hepatic encephalopathy, hypoglycemia, and lactic acidosis is the usual presentation (199). The diagnosis of PNF is usually made within the first 3 days after transplant, but can be recognized as early as during the transplant surgery itself. Intraoperative signs include increasing vasopressor requirements, worsening metabolic and lactic acidosis, hypothermia, hypoglycemia, and severe coagulopathy after reperfusion that does not resolve. A combination of clinical, laboratory, and histologic findings are used to make the diagnosis of PNF following transplant. Steadily increasing serum transaminases or peak AST levels over 5,000 to 10,000 units/L imply severe organ injury and decreased likelihood of recovery of function.

Risk factors implicated in PNF include cold ischemic time of more than 12 hours, retransplantation, and use of high-dose vasopressors. Possible donor-related factors include donation after cardiac death (DCD), advanced age, macrovesicular steatosis below 30%, sodium level above 155 mEq/L, CVA as cause of death, and prolonged ICU stay (199,200). It is imperative that other causes of graft failure such as vascular occlusion, acute rejection, or cardiac failure be excluded.

Clinical evidence of multiorgan failure, including encephalopathy, cerebral edema, AKI, and respiratory failure are inescapable consequences of PNF. PNF requires intensive support of all organ systems in the ICU until retransplantation, which is the only definitive treatment for PNF. In the most severe cases, a total allograft hepatectomy with portocaval shunting may be performed for stabilization purposes, but a new graft must become available within a critically short time period or death is likely. Even when retransplantation occurs within 72 hours of total hepatectomy, survival is as low as 35% (199).

Vascular Occlusions

The most common occlusive vascular complications following LT involve the hepatic artery. Hepatic artery thrombosis (HAT) is reported in 4% to 15% of transplantations and hepatic artery stenosis in 5% to 13% (201). Both may exist concomitantly as stenosis may lead to HAT. HAT usually occurs in the first month following transplant, often within 72 hours, but can also have a delayed presentation. Clinical manifestations of HAT and stenosis are similar and vary with the most severe of these usually presenting early after transplant. The worst complications of HAT are hepatic necrosis and fulminant failure, which are associated with a high mortality rate and often require retransplantation. Significantly elevated transaminases, fever and new abdominal pain should prompt urgent investigation. Delayed presentations include ischemic cholangiopathy with necrosis of bile ducts, bile leak, peritonitis, and sepsis, also with a high mortality rate. Recurrent cholangitis and bacteremia carry a mortality rate of 30% and often requires retransplantation (202).

Although angiography is historically the gold standard for diagnosis of HAT and hepatic artery stenosis, Doppler ultrasonography has become the primary technique. It is noninvasive and has a high sensitivity (75%–100%) with the added convenience of its ability to be performed at the bedside. CT angiography (CTA) and magnetic resonance angiography (MRA) have also been established as accurate diagnostic tools to identify HAT (201).

The treatment of HAT and stenosis depends upon the severity of the clinical presentation. Those with fulminant failure require aggressive support in the ICU and, often, retransplantation. Alternative management including surgical reconstruction of the hepatic artery or thrombectomy; vascular interventions such as angioplasty and stenting or thrombolysis may be appropriate for less symptomatic patients with the intent of graft salvage (201,202). However, about 50% of patients in this scenario will still require retransplantation. There is insufficient data to evaluate the efficacy of such procedures and long-term patency rates remain a problem (203). In the least severe or asymptomatic cases expectant management and systemic anticoagulation are considered adequate (201).

Portal vein thrombosis (PVT) is present in about 12% of patients at the time of transplant. Pre-existing PVT makes surgery more challenging and increases the risk of rethrombosis after transplantation, but it has not been shown to alter mortality (204). The incidence of PVT presenting after transplantation is 2% to 7%, with most occurrences early after transplant (202). In addition to a prior history of PVT, risk factors include a hypercoagulable state, perioperative hypotension, and allograft cirrhosis. PVT may also result from technical complications due to stricture at the anastomotic site, malalignment, and vascular kinks. Acutely, it can lead to hepatic failure, but chronically it has is a more insidious presentation involving portal hypertension with ascites and varices (199). Transaminases are typically elevated; diagnosis is made by Doppler ultrasonography or magnetic resonance venogram (204).

Hepatic vein thrombosis (HVT) is very unusual following LT; usually related, when it occurs, to technical complications such as kinking of the hepatic veins, small allografts that rotate, or a hypercoagulable state. Patients who have undergone transplantation for Budd–Chiari syndrome and have subtherapeutic anticoagulation are also at risk for HVT. Diagnosis is often made by Doppler ultrasonography; hepatic venography is confirmatory. Treatment depends on the severity of the presentation. Extensive thrombosis can result in graft failure. Options for treatment include surgical reconstruction and repositioning, thrombectomy, stenting, anticoagulation, or expectant management (202).

Rejection

Not only is rejection less common in LT than in other solid organ transplants, but less rejection occurs in the latter group when performed in the setting of a concurrent or previous liver transplant (205). In addition, rejection that occurs early after the liver is transplanted does not necessarily affect overall graft survival (206). This effect is not due to antigenic indifference, but instead to an active immune system process for which there are several theoretical causes. Microchimerism is one such hypothesis where donor hematopoietic cells persist in the recipient, producing tolerance through a balance of graft-versus-host and host-versus-graft reactions (205). Nonetheless, transplantation tolerance is not attainable consistently, and complete cessation of immune suppression is associated with about a 30% incidence of rejection (206).

In most institutions, high-dose corticosteroids are typically used for induction immunosuppression. Many patients can be tapered off corticosteroid immune suppression after transplantation with CNIs as the mainstay of therapy. In those with

TABLE 72.7 Immunosuppressive Drugs and their Common Side Effects

Drug	Adverse Effects
Tacrolimus	Nephrotoxicity, *neurotoxicity, diabetes*, hyperkalemia, metabolic acidosis, hypertension, hyperlipidemia
Cyclosporine	Nephrotoxicity, neurotoxicity, diabetes, *hyperlipidemia, hypertension*, hyperkalemia, metabolic acidosis, gingival hyperplasia, hypertrichosis
MMF	Myelosuppression, gastrointestinal side effects, viral infections (CMV, HSV), spontaneous abortions in pregnant women
Sirolimus	Hyperlipidemia, myelosuppression, proteinuria, poor wound healing, pneumonitis, skin rash
Corticosteroid	Diabetes, hypertension, obesity, osteoporosis, avascular necrosis, growth retardation, Cushingoid features, psychosis, poor wound healing, adrenal suppression, cataracts

Effects in italics are common in respective agent.
MMF, mycophenolate mofetil; CMV, cytomegalovirus; HSV, herpes simplex virus.
(From Pillai AA, Levitsky J. Overview of immunosuppression in liver transplantation. *World J Gastroenterol.* 2009;15(34):4225–4233.)

renal insufficiency, an antimetabolite such as a mycophenolate compound combined with a low-dose CNI or corticosteroid may be used as maintenance (206,207). The immunosuppressives commonly used in LT and their side effects are listed in Table 72.7 (206); side effects will result in the alteration of which medications are used (205–207).

Acute rejection occurs within the first 5 to 15 days after transplantation, manifested by fever, graft enlargement, tenderness, leukocytosis with increased eosinophils, and reduced bile production. Biopsies are done only when symptoms are present because the morphologic features consistent with acute rejection can be present in a significant percentage of patients in the early posttransplant period (208). Treatment for acute rejection is 3 to 5 days of 500 to 1,000 mg of methylprednisolone daily, resulting in about 75% resolution; a second course is sufficient for treatment in an additional 10%. The rest require an antilymphocyte therapy, with the rare case requiring retransplantation (209). Patients who develop rejection in the setting of complete immune suppressive cessation have been shown to have an increased risk of steroid-resistant rejection (206).

Biliary Complications

Despite the increased use of organs donated after cardiac death, biliary complications following LT have decreased from early estimates of 50% to currently reported 5% to 25% (210). However, they are still a significant cause of mortality and morbidity. There are a wide range of types and presentations of biliary complications, with biliary leaks and strictures being the most common. About two-thirds will present within the first 3 months following LT; complaints of abdominal pain, anorexia, ileus, and fever may be associated with biliary tract disorders. The serum markers, total bilirubin and γ-glutamyltransferase, are the most sensitive indicators of biliary complications (211). Initial imaging for diagnosis is usually Doppler ultrasonography; abnormalities can be further followed up with CT, cholangiography (direct via T tube or endoscopic), or magnetic resonance cholangiography (MRCP).

Biliary complications can often be managed with endoscopic or percutaneous stenting or strategic placement of a drain, and require surgery only if a major leak is present (212). The transplant surgeons will be intimately involved with the treatment and evaluation of potential biliary complications. A very rare syndrome of diffuse biliary necrosis may require retransplantation; in this scenario, patients present with a combination of sepsis, cholestasis, and bile leakage in which temporizing measures are useless. However, most cases of biliary dysfunction are not a cause for retransplantation or mortality (212).

Living Donor Liver Transplantation and Small-for-Size Syndrome

For the most part, the recipient receives essentially the same measures, however, there is an increased risk of vascular and biliary problems postoperatively. Unique to this type of transplantation is small-for-size syndrome. Although, this syndrome can occur in whole-organ grafts, it is a feared complication of living donor partial grafts. Small-for-size syndrome is defined as dysfunction during the first posttransplant week and requires the presence of two of the following findings on 3 consecutive days: total bilirubin over 5.8 mg/dL, INR above 2, and grade III or IV encephalopathy (213). Essentially, the patient develops jaundice, coagulopathy, delayed synthetic function, encephalopathy, and ascites in the first week. These patients are at risk for sepsis and have increased mortality (213). A similar situation may affect patients who receive a split liver from deceased donors as well. The mechanism of this syndrome appears to be acute, severe portal hypertension combined with an overwhelmed metabolic capacity of the allograft; sinusoidal injury occurs from portal pressures that exceed sinusoidal compliance. Experimental evidence supports this theory and suggests these events cause failure of graft regeneration (214).

SUMMARY

The patient undergoing LT has a significantly altered physiology and undergoes specific management to ensure optimal outcome. Coordinated care from the perioperative physician, surgeon, hepatologist, and anesthesiologist can minimize the risks from this procedure so the intensivist is in the position to positively affect prognosis.

Key Points

- Understand the presurgical selection, allocation, and evaluation of potential liver transplant recipients
- Identify the comorbidities and physiology associated with liver failure
- Understand the complex coagulopathy and transfusion decisions in ESLD
- An update of the advances in surgical and anesthetic management of LT
- Standard ICU management and practices following LT
- Defining and recognizing of the complications of LT

References

1. Steadman RH. Anesthesia for liver transplant surgery. *Anesthesiol Clin North Am.* 2004;22:687–711.
2. Department of Health and Human Services, Health Resources and Services Administration, Healthcare Systems Bureau, Division of Transplantation. *2012 Annual Report of the U.S. Organ Procurement and Transplantation*

Network and the Scientific Registry of Transplant Recipients: Transplant Data 1994–2003. Rockville, MD; United Network for Organ Sharing; Richmond, VA; University Renal Research and Education Association; Ann Arbor, MI. http://optn.transplant.hrsa.org.

3. Durand F, Valla D. Assessment of the prognosis of cirrhosis. *Semin Liver Dis*. 2008;28:110–122.
4. Khwaja K, Pomfret E. Organ allocation: the US model. In: Busuttil R, Klintmalm G, eds. *Transplantation of the Liver*. 3rd ed. Philadelphia, PA: Elsevier Saunders; 2015:64–71.
5. United Network for Organ Sharing. MELD/PELD calculator documentation. Available at: www.unos.org/resources. Accessed Oct 12, 2007.
6. Heuman DM, Abou-Assi SG, Habib A, et al. Persistent ascites and low serum sodium identify patients with cirrhosis and low MELD scores who are at high risk for early death. *Hepatology*. 2004;40:802–810.
7. Sharma P, Schaubel D, Goodrich N, Merion RM. Serum sodium and survival benefit of liver transplantation. *Liver Transpl*. 2015;21:308–313.
8. Liver and Intestinal Organ Transplantation Committee. Introduction to proposal for standard guidelines for MELD/PELD exceptions. Organ Procurement and Transplantation network website. Available at: https://optn.transplant.hrsa.gov/.../adult-meld-exception-review-guidance/. Accessed June 23, 2017.
9. Freeman RB, Gish RG, Harper A, et al. Model for end-stage liver disease (MELD) exception guidelines: results and recommendations from the MELD Exception Study Group and Conference (MESSAGE) for the approval of patients who need liver transplantation with diseases not considered by the standard MELD formula. *Liver Transpl*. 2006;12(12,S3):S128–S136.
10. Møller S, Henriksen J. Haemodynamic profile of patients with end-stage liver disease. In: Milan Z, ed. *Cardiovascular Diseases and Liver Transplantation*. Hauppauge, NY: Nova Science Publishers; 2011:1–30.
11. Tiukinhoy-Laing SD, Rossi JS, Bayram M, et al. Cardiac hemodynamic and coronary angiographic characteristics of patients being evaluated for liver transplantation. *Am J Cardiol*. 2006;98(2):178–181.
12. Blei TA, Mazhar S, Davidson CJ, et al. Hemodynamic evaluation before liver transplantation: insights into the portal hypertensive syndrome. *J Clin Gastroenterol*. 2007;41(S3):S323–S329.
13. Smith A, Therapondos G, Fouad T, et al. Cardiovascular profile and cardiac complications following liver transplantation. In: Milan Z, ed. *Cardiovascular Diseases and Liver Transplantation*. Hauppauge, NY: Nova Science Publishers; 2011:259–274.
14. Safadi A, Homsi M, Maskoun W, et al. Perioperative risk predictors of cardiac outcomes in patients undergoing liver transplantation surgery. *Circulation*. 2009;129: 1189–1194.
15. Keeffe BG, Valantine H, Keeffe EB. Detection and treatment of coronary artery disease in liver transplant candidates. *Liver Transpl Surg*. 1996;7: 755–761.
16. Xia VW, Taniguchi M, Steadman RH. The changing face of patients presenting for liver transplantation. *Curr Opin Organ Transplant*. 2008;13(3):280–284.
17. Younossi ZM, Stepanova M, Nader F, et al. Associations of chronic hepatitis C with metabolic and cardiac outcomes. *Aliment Pharmacol Ther*. 2013;37:647–652.
18. Watt K. Extrahepatic implications of metabolic syndrome. *Liver Transpl*. 2013;19:S56–S61.
19. VanWagner LB, Bhave M, Te HS, et al. Patients transplanted for nonalcoholic steatohepatitis are at increased risk for postoperative cardiovascular events. *Hepatology*. 2012;56:1741–1750.
20. Lazo M, Hernaez R, Bonekamp S, et al. Non-alcoholic fatty liver disease and mortality among US adults: prospective cohort study. *BMJ*. 2011;343:d6891.
21. Expert Panel on Detection, Evaluation, and Treatment of High Blood Cholesterol in Adults. Data from Executive Summary of the Third Report of the National Cholesterol Education Program (NCEP) Expert Panel on Detection, Evaluation, and Treatment of High Blood Cholesterol in Adults (Adult Treatment Panel III). *JAMA*. 2001;285:2486–2497.
22. Kadayifci A, Tan V, Ursell PC, et al. Clinical and pathologic risk factors for atherosclerosis in cirrhosis: a comparison between NASH-related cirrhosis and cirrhosis due to other aetiologies. *J Hepatol*. 2008;49(4):595–599.
23. Targher G, Bertolini L, Padovani R, et al. Increased prevalence of cardiovascular disease in Type 2 diabetic patients with non-alcoholic fatty liver disease. *Diabet Med*. 2006;23(4):403–409.
24. Targher G, Arcaro G. Non-alcoholic fatty liver disease and increased risk of cardiovascular disease. *Atherosclerosis*. 2007;191(2):235–240.
25. Targher G, Day CP, Bonora E. Risk of cardiovascular disease in patients with nonalcoholic fatty liver disease. *N Engl J Med*. 2010;363(14):1341–1350.
26. Johnston SD, Morris JK, Cramb R, et al. Cardiovascular morbidity and mortality after orthotopic liver transplantation. *Transplantation*. 2002; 73(6):901–906.
27. Appleton CP, Hurst RT. Reducing coronary artery disease events in liver transplant patients: moving toward identifying the vulnerable patient. *Liver Transpl*. 2008;14(12):1691–1693.
28. Carey WD, Dumot JA, Pimentel RR, et al. The prevalence of coronary artery disease in liver transplant candidates over age 50. *Transplantation*. 1995;59(6):859–864.
29. Plotkin JS, Johnson LB, Rustgi V, Kuo PC. Coronary artery disease and liver transplantation: the state of the art. *Liver Transpl*. 2000;6(4 Suppl 1): S53–S56.
30. Yoo HY, Thuluvath PJ. The effect of insulin-dependent diabetes mellitus on outcome of liver transplantation. *Transplantation*. 2002;74(7):1007–1012.
31. Yong CM, Sharma M, Ochoa V, et al. Multivessel coronary artery disease predicts mortality, length of stay, and pressor requirements after liver transplantation. *Liver Transplant*. 2010;16(11):1242–1248.
32. Diedrich DA, Findlay JY, Harrison BA, Rosen CB. Influence of coronary artery disease on outcomes after liver transplantation. *Transplant Proc*. 2008;40(10):3554–3557.
33. Plotkin JS, Scott VL, Pinna A, et al. Morbidity and mortality in patients with coronary artery disease undergoing orthotopic liver transplantation. *Liver Transpl Surg*. 1996;2(6):426–430.
34. Lentine KL, Costa SP, Weir M, et al. Cardiac disease evaluation and management among kidney and liver transplantation candidates: a scientific statement from the American Heart Association and the American College of Cardiology Foundation. *Circulation*. 2012;126:617–663.
35. Fleisher L, Fleischmann K, Auerbach A, et al. 2014 ACC/AHA Guideline on perioperative cardiovascular evaluation and management of patients undergoing noncardiac surgery. A report of the American College of Cardiology/American Heart Association Task Force on Practice Guidelines. *J Am Coll Cardiol*. 2014;130:e278–e233.
36. Raval Z, Harinstein ME, Flaherty JD. Role of cardiovascular intervention as a bridge to liver transplantation. *World J Gastroenterol*. 2014;20: 10651–10657.
37. Umphrey LG, Hurst RT, Eleid MF, et al. Preoperative dobutamine stress echocardiographic findings and subsequent short-term adverse cardiac events after orthotopic liver transplantation. *Liver Transpl*. 2008;14(6): 886–892.
38. MacDonald LA, Beohar N, Wang NC, et al. A comparison of arterial closure devices to manual compression in liver transplantation candidates undergoing coronary angiography. *J Invasive Cardiol*. 2003;15(2):68–70.
39. Sharma M, Yong C, Majure D, et al. Safety of cardiac catheterization in patients with end-stage liver disease awaiting liver transplantation. *Am J Cardiol*. 2009;103(5):742–746.
40. Azarbal B, Poommipanit P, Arbit B, et al. Feasibility and safety of percutaneous coronary intervention in patients with end-stage liver disease referred for liver transplantation. *Liver Transpl*. 2011;17(7):809–813.
41. Rao SV, Cohen MG, Kandzari DE, et al. The transradial approach to percutaneous coronary intervention: historical perspective, current concepts, and future directions. *J Am Coll Cardiol*. 55(20):2187–2195.
42. Jacobs E, Singh V, Damluji A, et al. Safety of transradial cardiac catheterization in patients with end-stage liver disease. *Catheter Cardiovasc Interv*. 2014;83:360–366.
43. Huded CP, Blair JE, Sweis RN, Flaherty JD. Transradial cardiac catheterization in liver transplant candidates. *Am J Cardiol*. 2014;113(10): 1634–1638.
44. Ehtisham J, Altieri M, Salame E, et al. Coronary artery disease in orthotopic liver transplantation: pretransplant assessment and management. *Liver Transpl*. 2010;16(5):550–557.
45. Axelrod D, Koffron A, Dewolf A, et al. Safety and efficacy of combined orthotopic liver transplantation and coronary artery bypass grafting. *Liver Transpl*. 2004;10(11):1386–1390.
46. Benedetti E, Massad MG, Chami Y, et al. Is the presence of surgically treatable coronary artery disease a contraindication to liver transplantation? *Clin Transplant*. 1999;13(1 Pt 1):59–61.
47. Russo MW, Pierson J, Narang T, et al. Coronary artery stents and antiplatelet therapy in patients with cirrhosis. *J Clin Gastroenterol*. 2012; 46(4):339–344.
48. Wray C, Scovotti JC, Tobis J, et al. Liver transplantation outcome in patients with angiographically proven coronary artery disease: a multi-institutional study. *Am J Transplant*. 2013;13(1):184–191.
49. Maddur H, Bourdillon PD, Liangpunsakul S, et al. Role of cardiac catheterization and percutaneous coronary intervention in the preoperative assessment and management of patients before orthotopic liver transplantation. *Liver Transpl*. 2014;20(6):664–672.
50. Finucci G, Desideri A, Sacerdoti D, et al. Left ventricular diastolic function in liver cirrhosis. *Scand J Gastroenterol*. 1996;31:279–284.

51. Pozzi M, Carugo S, Boari G, et al. Evidence of functional and structural cardiac abnormalities in cirrhotic patients with and without ascites. *Hepatology.* 1997;26:1131–1137.
52. Ma Z, Lee SS. Cirrhotic cardiomyopathy: getting to the heart of the matter. *Hepatology.* 1996;24:451–459
53. Liu H, Lee SS. Cardiopulmonary dysfunction in cirrhosis. *J Gastroenterol Hepatol.* 1999;14:600–608.
54. Myers RP, Lee SS. Cirrhotic cardiomyopathy and liver transplantation. *Liver Transpl.* 2000;6(4 Suppl 1):S44–S52.
55. Kelbaek H, Eriksen J, Brynjolf I, et al. Cardiac performance in patients with asymptomatic alcoholic cirrhosis of the liver. *Am J Cardiol.* 1984;54: 852–855.
56. Grose RD, Nolan J, Dillon JF, et al. Exercise-induced left ventricular dysfunction in alcoholic and non-alcoholic cirrhosis. *J Hepatol.* 1995;22: 326–332.
57. Wong F, Girgrah N, Graba J, et al. The cardiac response to exercise in cirrhosis. *Gut.* 2001;49:268–275.
58. Bernardi M, Calandra S, Colantoni A, et al. Q-T interval prolongation in cirrhosis: prevalence, relationship with severity, and etiology of the disease and possible pathogenetic factors. *Hepatology.* 1998;27:28–34.
59. Trevisani F, Merli M, Savelli F, et al. QT interval in patients with non-cirrhotic portal hypertension and in cirrhotic patients treated with transjugular intrahepatic porto-systemic shunt. *J Hepatol.* 2003;38:461–467.
60. Bal JS, Thuluvath PJ. Prolongation of QTc interval: relationship with etiology and severity of liver disease, mortality and liver transplantation. *Liver Int.* 2003;23:243–248.
61. Zambruni A, Trevisani F, Caraceni P, Bernardi M. Cardiac electrophysiological abnormalities in patients with cirrhosis. *J Hepatol.* 2006;44:994–1002.
62. Møller S, Hove JD, Dixen U, Bendtsen F. New insights into cirrhotic cardiomyopathy. *Int J Cardiol.* 2013;167:1101–1108.
63. Mikulic E, Munoz C, Puntoni LE, Lebrec D. Hemodynamic effects of dobutamine in patients with alcoholic cirrhosis. *Clin Pharmacol Ther.* 1983;34:56–59.
64. Ramond MJ, Comoy E, Lebrec D. Alternations in isoprenaline sensitivity in patients with cirrhosis: evidence of abnormality of the sympathetic nervous activity. *Br J Clin Pharmacol.* 1986;21:191–196.
65. Wong F. Cirrhotic cardiomyopathy. *Hepatol Int.* 2009;3:294–304.
66. Moller S, Henricksen JH. Cirrhotic cardiomyopathy: a pathophysiologic review of circulatory dysfunction in liver disease. *Heart.* 2002;87(9):42.
67. Zardi EM, Abbate A, Zardi DM, et al. Cirrhotic cardiomyopathy. *J Am Coll Cardiol.* 2010;56:539–549.
68. Ma Z, Lee SS, Meddings JB. Effects of altered cardiac membrane fluidity on beta-adrenergic receptor signalling in rats with cirrhotic cardiomyopathy. *J Hepatol.* 1997;26:904–912.
69. Pozzi M, Grassi G, Ratti L, et al. Cardiac, neuroadrenergic, and portal hemodynamic effects of prolonged aldosterone blockade in postviral child A cirrhosis. *Am J Gastroenterol.* 2005;100:1110–1116.
70. Liu H, Lee SS. What happens to cirrhotic cardiomyopathy after liver transplantation? *Hepatology.* 2005;42:1203–1205.
71. Torregrosa M, Aguade S, Dos L, et al. Cardiac alterations in cirrhosis: reversibility after liver transplantation. *J Hepatol.* 2005;42:68–74.
72. Garcia-Tsao G, Lim JK; Members of Veterans Affairs Hepatitis C Resource Center Program. Management and treatment of patients with cirrhosis and portal hypertension: recommendations from the Department of Veterans Affairs Hepatitis C Resource Center Program and the National Hepatitis C Program. *Am J Gastroenterol.* 2009;104:1802–1829.
73. Acosta F, De La Morena G, Villegas M, et al. Evaluation of cardiac function before and after liver transplantation. *Transplant Proc.* 1999;31:2369–2370.
74. Moller S, Henriksen JH. Cirrhotic cardiomyopathy: a pathophysiological review of circulatory dysfunction in liver disease. *Heart.* 2002;87:9–15.
75. Gayowski T, Marino IR, Singh N, et al. Orthotopic liver transplantation in high-risk patients: risk factors associated with mortality and infectious morbidity. *Transplantation.* 1998;65:499–504.
76. Lazarevic AM, Nakatani S, Neskovic AN, et al. Early changes in left ventricular function in chronic asymptomatic alcoholics: relation to the duration of heavy drinking. *J Am Coll Cardiol.* 2000;35:1599–1606.
77. Piano MR. Alcoholic cardiomyopathy: incidence, clinical characteristics, and pathophysiology. *Chest.* 2002;121:1638–1650.
78. Kittleson MM. Pretransplantation evaluation: cardiac. In: Busuttil R, Klintmalm G, eds. *Transplantation of the Liver.* 3rd ed. Philadelphia, PA: Elsevier Saunders; 2015:411–418.
79. Nasraway S, Klein R, Spanier T, et al. Hemodynamic correlates of outcome in patients undergoing orthotopic liver transplantation: evidence for early postoperative myocardial depression. *Chest.* 1995;107:218–224.
80. Eimer M, Wright J, Wang E, et al. Frequency and significance of acute heart failure following liver transplantation. *Am J Cardiol.* 2008;101:242–244.
81. Silvestro O. Early-onset and late-onset heart failure after liver transplantation. *Liver Transpl.* 2014;20:122.
82. Fallon MB, Abrams GA. Pulmonary dysfunction in chronic liver disease. *Hepatology.* 2000;32(4):859–865.
83. Fallon MB, Abrams GA, Luo B, et al. The role of endothelial nitric oxide synthase in the pathogenesis of a rat model of hepatopulmonary syndrome. *Gastroenterology.* 1997;113:606–614.
84. Rodriguez-Roisin R, Krowka MJ. Hepatopulmonary syndrome: a liver-induced lung vascular disorder. *N Engl J Med.* 2008;358:2378–2387.
85. Swanson KL, Wiesner RH, Krowka MJ. Natural history of hepatopulmonary syndrome: impact of liver transplantation. *Hepatology.* 2005;41(5): 1122–1129.
86. Schiffer E, Majno P, Mentha G, et al. Hepatopulmonary syndrome increases the postoperative mortality rate following liver transplantation: a prospective study in 90 patients. *Am J Transplant.* 2006;6:1430–1437.
87. Krowka MJ, Tajik AJ, Dickson ER, et al. Intrapulmonary vascular dilatations (IPVD) in liver transplant candidates: screening by two-dimensional contrast-enhanced echocardiography. *Chest.* 1990;97:1165–1170.
88. Abrams GA, Jaffe CC, Hoffer PB, et al. Diagnostic utility of contrast echocardiography and lung perfusion scan in patients with hepatopulmonary syndrome. *Gastroenterology.* 1995;109:1283–1288.
89. Lange PA, Stoller JK. The hepatopulmonary syndrome. *Clin Chest Med.* 1996;17(1):115–123.
90. Krowka MJ, Swanson KL, Frantz RP, et al. Portopulmonary hypertension: results from a 10-year screening algorithm. *Hepatology.* 2006;44(6): 1502–1510.
91. Kawut SM, Taichman DB, Ahya VN, et al. Hemodynamics and survival of patients with portopulmonary hypertension. *Liver Transpl.* 2005;11(9): 1107–1111.
92. Colle IO, Moreau R, Godinho E, et al. Diagnosis of portopulmonary hypertension in candidates for liver transplantation: a prospective study. *Hepatology.* 2003;37(2):401–409.
93. Rodríguez-Roisin R, Krowka MJ, Hervé P, Fallon MB; ERS Task Force Pulmonary-Hepatic Vascular Disorders (PHD) Scientific. Pulmonary-hepatic vascular disorders (PHD). *Eur Respir J.* 2004;24(5):861–880.
94. Swanson KL, Krowka MJ. Screen for portopulmonary hypertension, especially in liver transplant candidates. *Cleve Clin J Med.* 2008;75:121–132, 125–130.
95. Swanson KL, Wiesner RH, Nyberg SL, et al. Survival in portopulmonary hypertension: Mayo Clinic experience categorized by treatment subgroups. *Am J Transplant.* 2008;8(11):2445–2453.
96. Krowka MJ, Plevak DJ, Findlay JY, et al. Pulmonary hemodynamics and perioperative cardiopulmonary-related mortality in patients with portopulmonary hypertension undergoing liver transplantation. *Liver Transpl.* 2000;6(4):443–450.
97. Sussman N, Kaza V, Barshes N, et al. Successful liver transplantation following medical management of portopulmonary hypertension: a single-center series. *Am J Transplant.* 2006;6(9):2177–2182.
98. Krowka MJ, Mandell MS, Ramsay MA, et al. Hepatopulmonary syndrome and portopulmonary hypertension: a report of the multicenter liver transplant database. *Liver Transpl.* 2004;10(2):174–182.
99. Ashfaq M, Chinnakotla S, Rogers L, et al. The impact of treatment of portopulmonary hypertension on survival following liver transplantation. *Am J Transplant.* 2007;7(5):1258–1264.
100. Hollatz TJ, Musat A, Westphal S, et al. Treatment with sildenafil and treprostinil allows successful liver transplantation of patients with moderate to severe portopulmonary hypertension. *Liver Transpl.* 2012;18:686–695.
101. Planas R, Montoliu S, Balleste B, et al. Natural history of patients hospitalized for management of cirrhotic ascites. *Clin Gastroenterol Hepatol.* 2006;4(11):1385–1394.
102. Ginès P, Schrier RW. Renal failure in cirrhosis. *N Engl J Med.* 2009;361: 1279–1290.
103. Salerno F, Gerbes A, Gines P, et al. Diagnosis, prevention and treatment of hepatorenal syndrome in cirrhosis. *Gut.* 2007;56:1310–1318.
104. Solà E, Ginès P. Renal and circulatory dysfunction in cirrhosis: current management and future perspectives. *J Hepatol.* 2010;53:1135–1145.
105. Schepke M, Appenrodt B, Heller J, et al. Prognostic factors for patients with cirrhosis and kidney dysfunction in the era of MELD: results of a prospective study. *Liver Int.* 2006;26:834–839.
106. Alessandria C, Ozdogan O, Guevara M, et al. MELD score and clinical type predict prognosis in hepatorenal syndrome: relevance to liver transplantation. *Hepatology.* 2005;41:1282–1289.
107. Marik PE, Wood K, Starzl TE. The course of type 1 hepato-renal syndrome post liver transplantation. *Nephrol Dial Transplant.* 2006;21:478–482.
108. Wadei HM, Mai ML, Ahsan N, et al. Hepatorenal syndrome: pathophysiology and management. *Clin J Am Soc Nephrol.* 2006;1:1066–1079.

109. US Food and Drug Administration. For health professionals. FDA website. Available at: http://www.fda.gov/ForHealthProfessionals/default.htm. Updated April 20, 2016.
110. Solanki P, Chawla A, Garg R, et al. Beneficial effects of terlipressin in hepatorenal syndrome: a prospective, randomized placebo-controlled clinical trial. *J Gastroenterol Hepatol.* 2003;18:152–156.
111. Gluud LL, Christensen K, Christensen E, Krag A. Terlipressin for hepatorenal syndrome. *Cochrane Database Syst Rev.* 2012;9:CD005162.
112. Nassar Junior AP, Farias AQ, D' Albuquerque LA, et al. Terlipressin versus norepinephrine in the treatment of hepatorenal syndrome: a systematic review and meta-analysis. *PLoS One.* 2014;9:e107466.
113. Singh V, Ghosh S, Singh B, et al. Noradrenaline vs. terlipressin in the treatment of hepatorenal syndrome: a randomized study. *J Hepatol.* 2012;56:1293–1298.
114. Kalambokis G, Economou M, Fotopoulos A, et al. The effects of chronic treatment with octreotide versus octreotide plus midodrine on systemic hemodynamics and renal hemodynamics and function in nonazotemic cirrhotic patients with ascites. *Am J Gastroenterol.* 2005;100:879–885.
115. Angeli P, Volpin R, Gerunda G, et al. Reversal of type 1 hepatorenal syndrome with the administration of midodrine and octreotide. *Hepatology.* 1999;29:1690–1697.
116. Malinchoc M, Kamath PS, Gordon FD, et al. A model to predict poor survival in patients undergoing transjugular intrahepatic portosystemic shunts. *Hepatology.* 2000;31:864–871.
117. Said A. Non-alcoholic fatty liver disease and liver transplantation: outcomes and advances. *World J Gastroenterol.* 2013;19(48):9146–9155.
118. Wong RJ, Aguilar M, Cheung R, et al. Nonalcoholic steatohepatitis is the second leading etiology of liver disease among adults awaiting liver transplantation in the United States. *Gastroenterology.* 2015;148:547–555.
119. Burke A, Lucey MR. Non-alcoholic fatty liver disease, non-alcoholic steatohepatitis and orthotopic liver transplantation. *Am J Transplant.* 2004;4:686–693.
120. Saab S, Lalezari D, Pruthi P, et al. The impact of obesity on patient survival in liver transplant recipients: a meta-analysis. *Liver Int.* 2014;14:1–7.
121. LaMattina JC, Foley DP, Fernandez LA, et al. Complications associated with liver transplantation in the obese recipient. *Clin Transplant.* 2012;26:910–918.
122. Tripodi A, Mannucci PM. The coagulopathy of chronic liver disease. *N Engl J Med.* 2011;365:147–156.
123. Tripodi A, Primignani M, Chantarangkul V, et al. An imbalance of pro- vs anti-coagulation factors in plasma from patients with cirrhosis. *Gastroenterology.* 2009;137:2105–2111.
124. Kang Y, Audu P. Coagulation and liver transplantation. *Int Anesthesiol Clin.* 2006;44:17–36.
125. Hendriks HG, Meijer K, de Wolf JT, et al. Effects of recombinant activated factor VII on coagulation measured by thromboelastography in liver transplantation. *Blood Coag Fibrinolysis.* 2002;13:309–313
126. McGill DB, Rakela J, Zinsmeister AR, Ott BJ. A 21-year experience with major hemorrhage after percutaneous liver biopsy. *Gastroenterology.* 1990;99:1396–1400.
127. Diaz LK, Teruya J. Liver biopsy. *N Engl J Med.* 2001;344:2030.
128. Terjung B, Lemnitzer I, Dumoulin FL, et al. Bleeding complications after percutaneous liver biopsy: an analysis of risk factors. *Digestion.* 2003;67:138–145.
129. Segal JB, Dzik WH; Transfusion Medicine/Hemostasis Clinical Trials Network. Paucity of studies to support that abnormal coagulation test results predict bleeding in the setting of invasive procedures: an evidence-based review. *Transfusion.* 2005;45:1413–1425.
130. Ewe K. Bleeding after liver biopsy does not correlate with indices of peripheral coagulation. *Dig Dis Sci.* 1981;26:388–393.
131. Stanworth S. The evidence-based use of FFP and cryoprecipitate for abnormalities of coagulation tests and clinical coagulopathy. *Am Soc Hematol Educ Program.* 2007;1:179–186.
132. Youssef WI, Salazar F, Dasarathy S, et al. Role of fresh frozen plasma infusion in correction of coagulopathy of chronic liver disease: a dual phase study. *Am J Gastroenterol.* 2003;98:1391–1394.
133. Kor D, Stubbs J, Gajic O. Perioperative coagulation management-fresh frozen plasma. *Best Pract Res Clin Anesthesiol.* 2010;24:51–64.
134. Tripodi A, Primignani M, Lemma L, et al. Detection of imbalance of procoagulant versus anticoagulant factors in cirrhosis by a simple laboratory method. *Hepatology.* 2010;52:249–255.
135. DeSancho MT, Pastores S. Synthetic function. In: Rodes J, Benhamou JP, Reichen J, Rizetto M, eds. *Textbook of Hepatology: From Basic Science to Clinical Practice.* 3rd ed. New York: Blackwell; 2008:255–263.
136. Tripodi A, Salerno F, Chantarangkul V, et al. Evidence of normal thrombin generation in cirrhosis despite abnormal conventional coagulation tests.*Hepatology.* 2005;41:553–558.
137. Lisman T, Bakhtiari K, Pereboom IT, et al. Normal to increased thrombin generation in patients undergoing liver transplantation despite prolonged conventional coagulation tests. *J Hepatol.* 2010;52:355–361.
138. Gatt A, Riddell A, Calvaruso V, et al. Enhanced thrombin generation in patients with cirrhosis-induced coagulopathy. *J Thromb Haemost.* 2010;8:1994–2000.
139. Soogard KK, Horváth-Puhó E, Grønbæk H, et al. Risk of venous thromboembolism in patients with liver disease: a nationwide population-based, case-control study. *Am J Gastroenterol.* 2009;104:96–101.
140. Stravitz RT. Critical management decisions in patients with acute liver failure. *Chest.* 2008;134:1092–1102.
141. Germani G, Theocharidou E, Adam R, et al. Liver transplantation for acute liver failure in Europe: outcomes over 20 years from the ELTR database. *J Hepatol.* 2012;57:288–296.
142. Barshes NR, Lee TC, Balkrishnan R, et al. Risk stratification of adult patients undergoing orthotopic liver transplantation for fulminant hepatic failure. *Transplantation.* 2006;81:195–201.
143. Bernal W, Cross TJ, Auzinger G, et al. Outcome after wait-listing for emergency liver transplantation in acute liver failure: a single centre experience. *J Hepatol.* 2009;50:306–313.
144. O'Grady J. Timing and benefit of liver transplantation in acute liver failure. *J Hepatol.* 2014;60:663–670.
145. Sass DA, Shakil AO. Fulminant hepatic failure. *Liver Transpl.* 2005;11(6):594–605.
146. McPhail MJ, Wendon JA, Bernal W. Meta-analysis of performance of King's College Hospital Criteria in prediction of outcome in non-paracetamol-induced acute liver failure. *J Hepatol.* 2010;53:492–499.
147. Bailey B, Amre DK. Gaudreault P. Fulminant hepatic failure secondary to acetaminophen poisoning: a systematic review of the meta-analysis of prognostic criteria determining the need for liver transplantation. *Crit Care Med.* 2003;31:299–305.
148. Ichai P, Legeal C, Froncoz C, et al. Patients with acute liver failure listed for super-urgent liver transplantation in France: reevaluation of the Clichy-Villejuif criteria. *Liver Transpl.* 2015;21:512–523.
149. Larson AM, Polson J, Fontana RJ, et al. Acetaminophen-induced acute liver failure: results of a United States multicenter prospective study. *Hepatology.* 2005;42:1364–1372.
150. Zaman MB, Hoti E, Qasim A, et al. MELD score as a prognostic model for listing acute liver failure patients for liver transplantation. *Transplant Proc.* 2006;38(7):2097–2098.
151. O'Grady J. Transplantation for fulminant hepatic failure. In: Busuttil R, Klintmalm G, eds. *Transplantation of the Liver.* 3rd ed. Philadelphia, PA: Elsevier Saunders; 2015:153–158.
152. Stravitz RT, Kramer AH, Davern T, et al. Intensive care of patients with acute liver failure: recommendations of the US Acute Liver Failure Study Group. *Crit Care Med.* 2007;35:2498–2508.
153. Parrilla P, Sanchez-Bueno F, Figueras J, et al. Analysis of the complications of the piggy-back technique in 1,112 liver transplants. *Transplantation.* 1999;67(9):1214–1217.
154. Belghiti J, Panis Y, Sauvanet A, et al. A new technique of side to side caval anastomosis during orthotopic hepatic transplantation without inferior vena caval occlusion. *Surg Gynecol Obstet.* 1992;175(3):270–272.
155. de Boer MT, Christensen MC, Asmussen M, et al. The impact of intraoperative transfusion of platelets and red blood cells on survival after liver transplantation. *Anesth Analg.* 2008;106(1):32–44.
156. Massicotte L, Sassine M-P, Lenis S, et al. Survival rates change with transfusion of blood products during liver transplantation. *Can J Anesth.* 2005;52:148–155.
157. Massicotte L, Lenis S, Thibeault L, et al. Effect of low central venous pressure and phlebotomy on blood product transfusion requirements during liver transplantations. *Liver Transpl.* 2006;12(1):117–123.
158. Segal JB, Blasco-Colmenares E, Norris EJ, Guallar E. Preoperative acute normovolemic hemodilution: a meta-analysis. *Transfusion.* 2004;44:632–644.
159. Trzebicki J, Flakiewicz E, Kosieradzki M, et al. The use of thromboelastometry in the assessment of hemostasis during orthotopic liver transplantation reduces the demand for blood products. *Ann Transpl.* 2010;15(3):19–24.
160. Coakley M, Reddy K, Mackie I, Mallet S. Transfusion triggers in orthotopic liver transplantation: a comparison of the thromboelastometry analyzer, the thromboelastogram, and conventional coagulation tests. *J Cardiothorac Vasc Anesth.* 2006;20(4):548–553.
161. Molenaar IQ, Warnaar N, Groen H, et al. Efficacy and safety of antifibrinolytic drugs in liver transplantation: a systematic review and meta-analysis. *Am J Transpl.* 2007;7:185–194.
162. Vater Y, Levy A, Martay K, et al. Adjuvant drugs for end-stage liver failure and transplantation. *Med Sci Monit.* 2004;10(4):RA77–RA88.

163. Burtenshaw AJ, Isaac JL. The role of trans-oesophageal echocardiography for perioperative cardiovascular monitoring during orthotopic liver transplantation. *Liver Transpl.* 2006;12(11):1577–1583.
164. Mandell MS, Lezotte D, Kam I, Zamudio S. Reduced use of intensive care after liver transplantation: influence of early extubation. *Liver Transpl.* 2002;8:676–681.
165. Hevesi Z, Lopukhin L, Mezrich J, et al. Dedicated liver transplant anesthesia team reduces blood transfusion, need for mechanical ventilation, and duration of intensive care. *Liver Transpl.* 2009;15:460–465.
166. Hastie J, Moitra V. Routine postoperative care in liver transplantation. In: Wagener G, ed. *Liver Anesthesiology and Critical Care Medicine.* New York: Springer Science; 2012:355–369
167. Pearse R, Dawson D, Fawcett J, et al. Early goal-directed therapy after major surgery reduces complications and duration of hospital stay: a randomized controlled trial. *Crit Care.* 2005;9:R687–R693.
168. Strunden MS, Heckel K, Goetz AE, Reuter DA. Perioperative fluid and volume management: physiological basis, tools and strategies. *Am Intensive Care.* 2011;1:2–8.
169. Romanelli RG, La Villa G, Barletta G, et al. Long-term albumin infusion improves survival in patients with cirrhosis and ascites: an unblended randomized trial. *World J Gastroenterol.* 2006;12(9):1403–1407.
170. Abbasoglu O, Goldstein RM, Vodapally MS, et al. Liver transplantation in hyponatremic patients with emphasis on central pontine myelinolysis. *Clin Transplant.* 1998;12:263–269.
171. Lampl C, Yazdi K. Central pontine myelinolysis. *Eur Neurol.* 2002;47:3–10.
172. Heering P, Ivens K, Thumer O, et al. Acid-base balance and substitution fluid during continuous hemofiltration. *Kidney Int Suppl.* 1999;56(S72):S37–S40.
173. Raval Z, Harinstein M, Skaro A, et al. Cardiovascular risk assessment of the liver transplant candidate. *J Am Coll Cardiol.* 2011;58:223–231.
174. Chinnakotla S, Eghtesad B, Klintmalm G. Graft-versus-host-disease. In: Busuttil R, Klintmalm G, eds. *Transplantation of the Liver.* 3rd ed. Philadelphia, PA: Elsevier Saunders; 2015:1257–1261.
175. Glanemann M, Langrehr J, Kaisers U, et al. Postoperative tracheal extubation after orthotopic liver transplantation. *Acta Anaesth Scand.* 2001;45:333–339.
176. Schweickert W, Kress J. Implementing early mobilization interventions in mechanically ventilated patients in the ICU. *Chest.* 2011;140:1612–1617.
177. Feltracco P, Barbieri S, Galligioni H, et al. Intensive care management of liver transplanted patients. *World J Hepatol.* 2011;3:61–71.
178. Choi ND, Hwang S, Kim KW, et al. Intensive pulmonary support using extracorporeal membrane oxygenation for adult liver transplant recipients. *Hepatogastroenterology.* 2012;59:1189–1191.
179. Shangraw RE. Metabolic issues in liver transplantation. *Int Anesthesiol Clin.* 2006;44(3):1–20.
180. McKenna G, Klintmalm GB. Postoperative intensive care management in adults. In: Busuttil R, Klintmalm G, eds. *Transplantation of the Liver.* 3rd ed. Philadelphia, PA: Elsevier Saunders; 2015:866–894.
181. The NICE-SUGAR Study Investigators, Finfer S, Chittock DR, Su SY, et al. Intensive versus conventional glucose control in critically ill patients. *N Engl J Med.* 2009;360:1283–1297.
182. Ishitani M, Wilkowski M, Stevenson W, Pruett T. Outcome of patients requiring hemodialysis after liver transplantation. *Transplant Proc.* 1993;25(2):1762–1763.
183. Mehta RL, Kellum JA, Shah SV. Acute Kidney Injury Network: report of an initiative to improve outcomes in acute kidney injury. *Crit Care.* 2007;11(2):R31.
184. Fisher NC, Nightengale PG, Gunson BK, et al. Chronic renal failure following liver transplantation. *Transplantation.* 1998;66:59–66.
185. Winston DJ, Emmanouilides C, Busuttil RW. Infections in liver transplant recipients. *Clin Infect Dis.* 1995;21:2077–2091.
186. Romero FA, Razonable RR. Infections in liver transplant recipients. *World J Hepatol.* 2011;3:83–92.
187. Sun HY, Caccierelli TV, Singh N. Identifying a targeted population at high risk for infections after liver transplantation in the MELD era. *Clin Transpl.* 2011;25:420–425.
188. Bakir M, Bova JL, Newell KA, et al. Epidemiology and clinical consequences of vancomycin-resistant enterococci in liver transplant patients. *Transplantation.* 2001;72:1032–1037.
189. Singh N. Fungal infections in the recipients of solid organ transplantation. *Infect Dis Clin North Am.* 2003;17:113–134, viii.
190. Kuback BM, Pegues DA, Holt CD, et al. Changing pattern of fungal infections in transplantation. *Curr Opin Organ Transplant.* 2000;5:176.
191. Haagsma EB, Klompmaker U, Grond J, et al. Herpes virus infections after orthotopic liver transplantation. *Transplant Proc.* 1987;19:4054–4056.
192. Lee EM, Kang JK, Yun SC, et al. Risk factors for central pontine and extrapontine myelinolysis following orthotopic liver transplantation. *Eur Neurol.* 2009;62:362–368.
193. Saner FH, Sotiropoulos GC, Gu Y, et al. Severe neurological events following liver transplantation. *Arch Med Res.* 2007;38:75–79.
194. Zivkovic SA. Neurologic complications after liver transplantation. *World J Hepatol.* 2013;5:409–416.
195. Bronster DJ, Emre S, Boccagni P, et al. CNS complications in liver transplant recipients: incidence, timing and long term follow up. *Clin Transplant.* 2000;14:1–7.
196. Ling L, He X, Zeng J, Liang Z. In-hospital cerebrovascular complications following orthotopic liver transplantation: a retrospective study. *BMC Neurol.* 2008 8:52.
197. Wang WL, Yang ZF, Lo CM, et al. Intracerebral hemorrhage after liver transplantation. *Liver Transpl.* 2000;6:345–348.
198. Johnson SR, Alexopoulos S, Curry M, Hanto DW. Primary nonfunction (PNF) in the MELD era: an SRTR database analysis. *Am J Transplant.* 2007;7:1003–1009.
199. Burton JR, Rosen HR. Diagnosis and management of allograft failure. *Clin Liver Dis.* 2006;10:407–435, x.
200. Petrowsky H, Busuttil R. Graft failure. In: Busuttil R, Klintmalm G, eds. *Transplantation of the Liver.* 3rd ed. Philadelphia, PA: Elsevier Saunders; 2015:960–974.
201. Cheaito A, Bussattil R. Arterial complications after liver transplantation. In: Busuttil R, Klintmalm G, eds. *Transplantation of the Liver.* 3rd ed. Philadelphia, PA: Elsevier Saunders; 2015:997–1005.
202. Duffy JP, Hong JC, Farmer DG, et al. Vascular complications of orthotopic liver transplantation: experience in more than 4200 patients. *J Am Coll Surg.* 2009;208:896–903.
203. Stange BJ, Glanemann M, Nuessler NC, et al. Hepatic artery thrombosis after adult liver transplantation. *Liver Transplant.* 2003;9(6):612–620.
204. Llado L, Fabregat J, Castellote J, et al. Management of portal vein thrombosis in liver transplantation: influence on morbidity and mortality. *Clin Transplant.* 2007;21(6):716–721.
205. Benseler V, McCaughan GW, Schlitt HJ, et al. The liver: a special case in transplantation tolerance. *Semin Liver Dis.* 2007;27(2):194–213.
206. Pillai AA, Levitsky J. Overview of immunosuppression in liver transplantation. *World J Gastroenterol.* 2009;15(34):4225–4233.
207. Hirose R, Vincenti F. Immunosuppression: today, tomorrow and withdrawal. *Semin Liver Dis.* 2006;26(3):201–210.
208. Gornicka B, Ziarkiewicz-Wroblewska M, Bogdanska U, et al. Pathomorphological features of acute rejection in patients after orthotopic liver transplantation: own experience. *Transplant Proc.* 2006;38:221–225.
209. Encke J, Waldemar U, Stremmel W, et al. Immunosuppression and modulation in liver transplantation. *Nephrol Dial Transplant.* 2004;19(Suppl 4):iv22–iv25.
210. Akamatsu N, Suguwara Y, Hashimoto D. Biliary reconstruction, its complications and management of biliary complications after adult liver transplantation: a systematic review of the incidence, risk factors and outcome. *Transpl Int.* 2011;24:379–392.
211. Dunham DP, Aran PP. Receiver operating characteristic analysis for biliary complications in liver transplantation. *Liver Transpl Surg.* 1997;3:374–378.
212. Moser MA, Wall WJ. Management of biliary problems after liver transplantation. *Liver Transpl.* 2001;11(S1):S46–S52.
213. Dahm F, Georgiev P, Clavien PA. Small-for-size syndrome after partial liver transplantation: definition, mechanisms of disease and clinical implications. *Am J Transpl.* 2005;7:2605–2610.
214. Shimamura T, Tanaguchi M, Jin MB, et al. Excessive portal venous inflow as a cause of allograft dysfunction in small-for-size syndrome in living donor liver transplantation. *Transplant Proc.* 2001;33:1331.

CHAPTER

73

Pancreatic Transplantation

ANGELIKA C. GRUESSNER, RAJA KANDASWAMY, KHALID M. KHAN, DAVID E. R. SUTHERLAND, and RAINER W. GRUESSNER

INTRODUCTION

The treatment options for insulin-dependent diabetes mellitus are either exogenous insulin administration or β-cell replacement by pancreas or islet transplantation. Exogenous insulin administration is burdensome to the patient and gives imperfect glycemic control, predisposing to secondary complications of the eyes, nerves, kidneys, and other systems. On the other hand, β-cell replacement, when successful, establishes a constant euglycemic state but requires major surgery (a pancreas transplant) and immunosuppression to prevent rejection, predisposing to complications, often compounded by comorbidities from pre-existing diabetes.

The Diabetes Control and Complications Trial (1) showed that intensive insulin therapy (multiple injections per day with dose adjusted by frequent blood sugar determinations) decreased (although rarely normalized) glycosylated hemoglobin ($HgbA_{1c}$) levels and reduced the rate of secondary complications (2). The threshold for totally eliminating the risks of secondary diabetic complications is perfect glycemic control, an objective that can be achieved by the most sophisticated exogenous insulin delivery devices unfortunately at the cost of frequent hypoglycemic episodes. This may change in the future with real-time glucose monitoring systems combined with insulin pumps (3,4). Pancreas transplantation induces insulin independence in diabetic recipients without the risk of hypoglycemia and can ameliorate secondary complications. With major advances in the management of pancreas transplantation, the success rate of pancreas transplants has progressively increased during the past two decades (5,6). Today's recipients have a high probability of being insulin independent for years, if not indefinitely.

Historically, islet transplants have been less successful for a variety of reasons. In the late 1990s at the University of Alberta, insulin independence was achieved in several consecutive recipients by sequential grafting of islets from multiple donors and the use of a steroid-free nondiabetogenic immunosuppressive regimen (7). In another series from the University of Minnesota with a similar regimen, single-donor islet transplants induced insulin independence (8). In the Minnesota series, the donors had a high body mass index and the recipients had a low body mass index. Thus, the net number of islets transplanted per unit weight was similar in the Alberta and Minnesota series. Islet transplants can succeed with stringent donor and recipient selections, but is not yet able to supersede pancreas transplants as the mainstay of β-cell replacement. Until islet transplants can consistently succeed from a single donor, regardless of size or recipient insulin requirements, an integrated approach is preferable (9): low-risk patients should undergo a surgically more challenging pancreas transplant, high-risk patients an islet transplant.

Although short-term islet graft survival appears promising (even with single donors) (10), long-term graft function after islet transplants (even with multiple donors) continues to be a major impediment to rapid progress. In the University of Alberta series, only 10% of islet transplant recipients were insulin independent at 5 years posttransplant (11).

The main tradeoff for recipients of β-cell allografts is the need for immunosuppression. A successful graft makes the recipient euglycemic and normalizes $HgbA_{1c}$ levels (11,12), but the combined risks of immunosuppression and pancreas transplant surgery must be weighed against the long-term risks of imperfect glycemic control and of development of secondary complications with exogenous insulin. A randomized prospective trial has not been done to weigh these risks. The burden of day-to-day management of diabetes, with need for multiple needlesticks to inject insulin and monitor blood sugar levels tilts the balance in favor of a transplant for many diabetic patients. Furthermore, antirejection strategies are continually being developed to decrease the side effects of immunosuppression. Nevertheless, only a few institutions perform pancreas transplants soon after the onset of the disease (13).

The main indications for a pancreas transplant in patients with normal kidney function has been labile diabetes with frequent insulin reactions and hypoglycemic unawareness, a syndrome that may emerge years after the onset of diabetes, particularly in patients with autonomic neuropathy (14). However, even for nonlabile diabetic patients who attempt tight control by intensive glucose monitoring, literature shows a high rate of secondary complications that are just as morbid as (15), if not more so than, chronic immunosuppressive complications in organ allograft recipients (16,17). Thus, for a patient who wishes to avoid a lifetime of insulin injections and glucose monitoring and who prefers the risks of immunosuppressive complications to the secondary complications of diabetes, a pancreas transplant can be performed with good results (18). This also applies to type 2 diabetics who are obligatory insulin dependent. About 5% of pancreas transplants are performed in selected type 2 diabetics (19).

In the past, most pancreas transplant candidates had advanced diabetic nephropathy and required a kidney transplant also. As the risks of immunosuppression are assumed because of the kidney transplant, a simultaneous or sequential pancreas transplant does not pose any additional risks other than surgery (13). Indeed, pancreas transplants have been done in renal allograft recipients who meet the criteria for type 2 diabetes with elimination of the need for exogenous insulin (20).

RECIPIENT CATEGORIES

Diabetic pancreas transplant candidates are divided into three categories: uremic (need a kidney transplant), posturemic (have a functioning kidney transplant), and nonuremic (do not need a kidney transplant). For candidates who are uremic, the options are to receive kidney and pancreas transplants either simultaneously in one operation or sequentially in separate operations. The decision as to which option to take is usually based on the availability and suitability of living and cadaveric donors for one or both organs (5). Accordingly, there are three broad categories of recipients: simultaneous pancreas–kidney (SPK), pancreas after kidney (PAK), and pancreas transplants alone (PTA).

PK Transplants

Most SPK transplants have been done with both organs coming from the same cadaveric donor. Because a large number of patients are waiting for a kidney, unless priority is given to SPK candidates, waiting times tend to be long (years). Thus, to avoid two operations and a long wait, a simultaneous kidney and segmental pancreas transplant from a living donor can be done (20–22). Only a few centers offer this option (23,24). There has been a report from Japan of a successful islet transplantation from a live donor (25). Therefore, a simultaneous living-donor islet kidney transplant may become a viable option in the future (26,27). If a living donor is suitable for or only willing to give a kidney, another option is a simultaneous living-donor kidney and cadaveric pancreas transplant (23,24). For these options, the living kidney donor usually must be available on a moment's notice (the same as for the recipient), as the cadaveric pancreas must be transplanted soon after procurement. Alternatively, a recipient of a scheduled living-donor kidney transplant could also receive a cadaveric pancreas simultaneously if one became available fortuitously. If not, and only a kidney is transplanted, the recipient becomes a PAK candidate.

PAK Transplants

For nephropathic diabetic patients who have already undergone a kidney transplant from a living or a cadaveric donor, a PAK transplant can be performed. Most PAK transplants today are done in patients who previously received a living-donor kidney because suitable uremic diabetic patients without a living donor will undergo a cadaveric pancreas transplant. Although a PAK means a uremic diabetic patient requires two operations to achieve both a dialysis-free and insulin-independent state, the two transplants done separately are smaller procedures than a combined transplant. The interval between the living-donor kidney and cadaveric pancreas transplant depends on several factors, including recipient recovery from the kidney transplant and donor availability, but the outcome is similar for all intervals more than 1 month. PAK is the largest pancreas transplant category at the University of Minnesota (28,29).

PTA Transplants

For recipients with adequate kidney function, a solitary pancreas transplant can be performed from either a living or a cadaveric donor. Because the waiting time for a cadaveric pancreas is relatively short at the present time, living-donor pancreas transplants are done infrequently, but are particularly indicated if a candidate has a high panel-reactive antibody and a negative cross-match to a living donor. Most PTA candidates have problems with glycemic control, hypoglycemic unawareness, and frequent insulin reactions. A successful PTA not only obviates these problems, but also improves the quality of life, and may ameliorate secondary complications, thus increasing the applicability of PTA (28–30).

EVOLUTION AND IMPROVEMENTS

The first clinical pancreas transplant was performed at the University of Minnesota in 1966 (31). The number of transplants remained low during the 1970s, but progressively increased in the 1980s, following the introduction of cyclosporine. By the end of 2014, almost 50,000 pancreas transplants had been performed in 55 countries around the world (Fig. 73.1), including almost 30,000 in the United States (Fig. 73.2) (6).

The history of pancreas transplants involves many different techniques and eras (32). The first series of pancreas transplants at the University of Minnesota used enteric drainage (ED) (32). Urinary drainage was first done into the ureter by Gliedman in the early 1970s (33,34), then via duct injection by Dubernard et al. (35) in 1974, and then via direct bladder drainage (BD) by Sollinger et al. (36) in 1982. During the 1980s, BD became the predominant technique (Fig. 73.3) with good results (37). ED was still used (38), although sparingly, but since the late 1990s it has become the most frequent (Fig. 73.4) technique, especially in SPK transplants.

Venous drainage of the pancreas has also evolved over the years. Portal drainage was used with segmental grafts in the 1980s (32,39–42). For whole-organ pancreas transplants, systemic drainage was the norm until the 1990s, when portal drainage gained popularity, especially with ED (43,44), as opposed to BD (45). Between 1996 and 2000, about one-fifth of all SPKs used portal drainage, by anastomosis either to the recipient splenic vein (40) or, more commonly, to the superior mesenteric vein (Fig. 73.5) (46). Over the past decade, systemic drainage has reestablished itself as the most common technique (5,6).

Before techniques were developed to procure both liver and pancreas grafts with intact blood supply (47,48), segmental pancreas grafts were commonly used. Since the early 1990s, whole-organ pancreaticoduodenal grafts predominate (49), although segmental grafts are still used for living-donor pancreas transplants (28). The first living-donor pancreas transplant was performed at the University of Minnesota in 1979 (50). The early series of living-donor pancreas transplants consisted of solitary pancreases because the rejection rate of cadaveric pancreases was high (23). In the 1990s, living-donor pancreas transplants were predominantly performed in combination with a kidney from the same donor (Fig. 73.6) (22,51–53). Living-donor segmental pancreatectomy are now performed laparoscopically (54). Another approach, as previously mentioned, is to perform a living-donor kidney transplant simultaneously with a cadaveric pancreas transplant (24).

Immunosuppressive regimens have made great strides over the years. Today, there are more than 100 pancreas transplant centers in the United States (55). Some centers have reported extensive experience. For example, more than 1,000 SPK transplants have been performed at the University of Wisconsin (UW) (56), and more than 2,000 pancreas transplants of all categories have been performed at the University of Minnesota (28). The International Pancreas Transplant Registry, formed in 1980, collects data from all centers in the world (57) and is the best resource for outcome analysis.

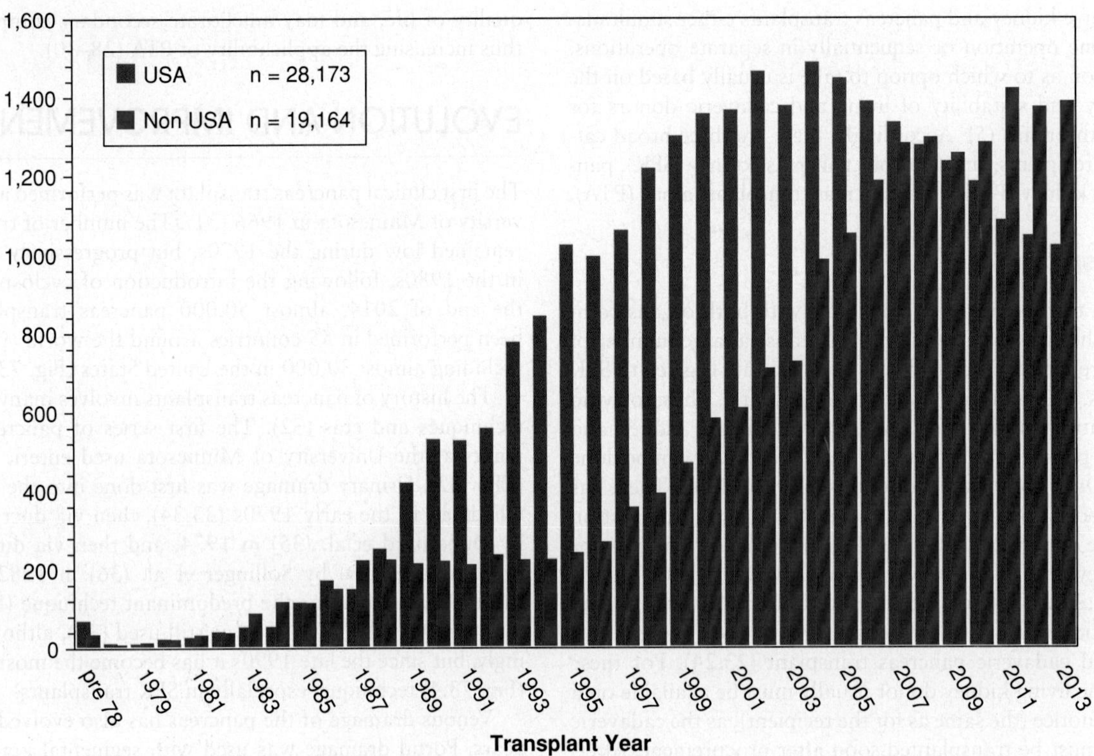

FIGURE 73.1 Number of pancreas transplants worldwide tabulated by the International Pancreas Transplant Registry from 1966 to 2013.

RESULTS

Outcomes after pancreas transplants have consistently improved over the years (5,6). The latest report from the International Pancreas Transplant Registry (6) outlined recent results, focusing on U.S. transplants from 2009 through 2013, including more than 3,900 SPK, more than 500 PAK, and 389 PTA cases. Patient survival rates for all three categories was more than 95% at 1 year posttransplant (Fig. 73.7). Primary pancreas graft survival rates at 1 year posttransplant were higher for SPK (88.9%) than for PAK (84.4%) and PTA (81.5%) recipients (Fig. 73.8). Graft loss from rejection was low at 1 year in all three categories (1.7% SPK, 4.4% PAK, 5.5% PTA). In the majority of all transplants, ED was used for duct management, and of the ED transplants, portal venous drainage was used in about 20% of SPK and 10% of solitary transplants. Although overall graft function did not vary with ED or BD, the PTA group had a higher immunologic graft loss rate in ED versus BD cases. BD may result in earlier diagnosis of rejection because of the ability to monitor for a decline in urine amylase activity as a marker (28). Nevertheless, the late rejection rate is higher in the PTA than in other categories.

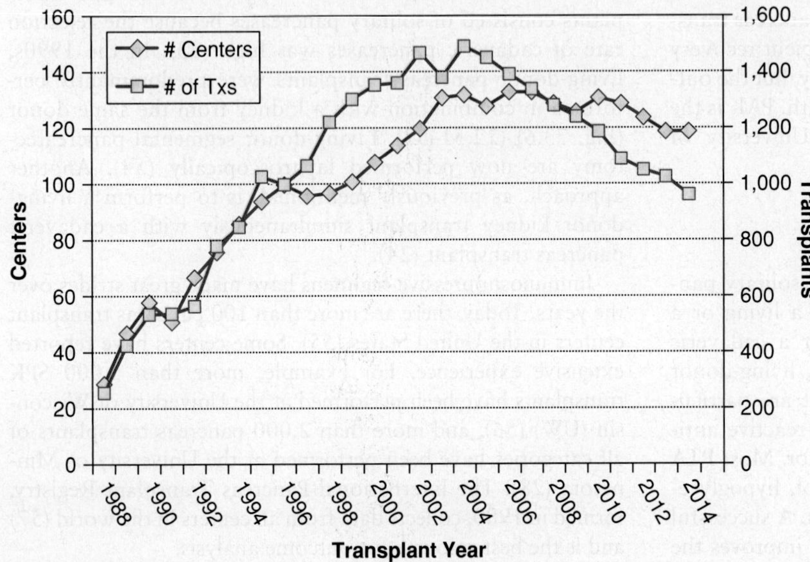

FIGURE 73.2 Number of US transplant centers tabulated by the International Pancreas Transplant Registry from 1966 to 2014. Tx, transplant.

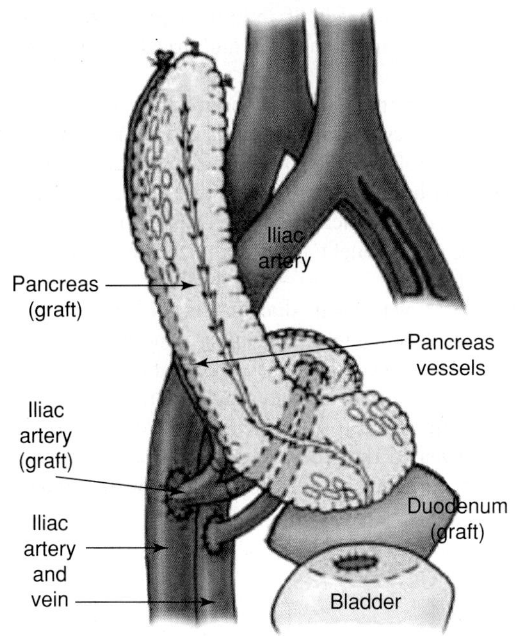

FIGURE 73.3 Bladder-drained (BD) pancreaticoduodenal transplant alone (PTA) from a cadaver donor.

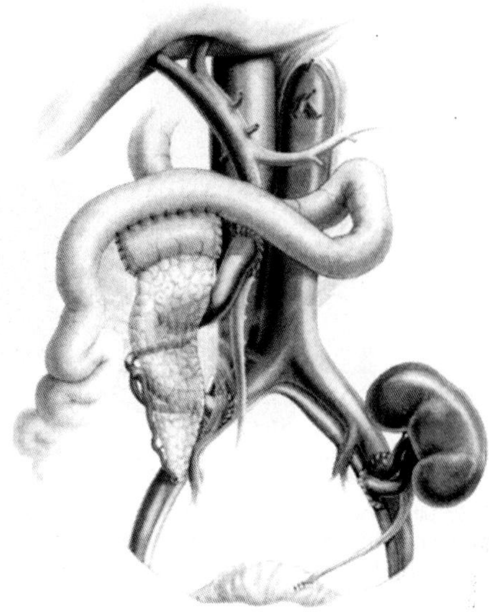

FIGURE 73.5 Enteric drainage (ED) simultaneous pancreas and kidney (SPK) transplants with portal venous drainage of the pancreas graft via the superior mesenteric vein.

INDICATIONS AND CONTRAINDICATIONS

The indications for a pancreas transplant have evolved and expanded over the years as the results have improved. The position statement of the American Diabetes Association (58) on indications for a pancreas transplant (Table 73.1) is conservative. A pancreas transplant is also indicated for patients who have developed secondary complications of diabetes. The progression of complications is halted by a functioning pancreas graft. In fact, even an improvement in neuropathy has been documented (5,22,34,59,60). In addition to improvement in glomerular architecture, a recent study shows that interstitial expansion is reversible, and atrophic tubules can be reabsorbed (61). Advanced retinopathy and vascular disease, however, are unaffected (62). Atherosclerotic risk factors decrease and endothelial function improves posttransplant (63). A pancreas transplant should be offered early, before the onset of complications of diabetes, to interested patients

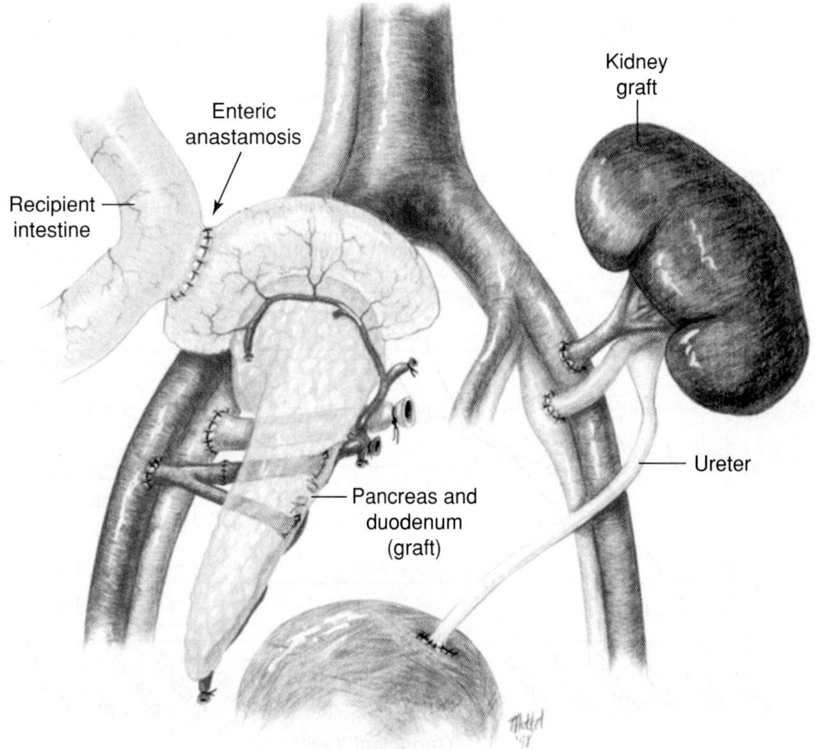

FIGURE 73.4 Enteric-drained (ED) simultaneous pancreas and kidney (SPK) transplant from a cadaver donor with systemic venous drainage.

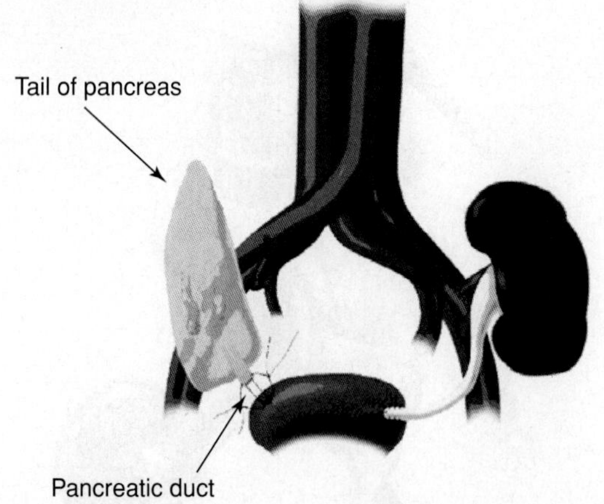

FIGURE 73.6 Simultaneous segmental pancreas and kidney transplant from a living donor (LD). Either bladder drainage (BD) or enteric drainage (ED) can be used, but the BD technique has a lower complication rate and is illustrated.

who understand the risk of immunosuppression versus the benefit of insulin independence and freedom from diabetic complications.

Contraindications include those for any other transplant, such as malignancy, active infections, noncompliance, serious psychosocial problems, and prohibitive cardiovascular risk. Candidates with advanced vascular disease have an increased risk of surgical complications, yet those who do well post-transplant greatly benefit from stabilization of their cardiovascular risk.

Although it was clear that insulin-dependent recipients with renal failure benefited from a pancreas transplant in addition to the kidney, the survival benefit for pancreas transplant in patients with preserved renal function was questioned by at least one study (64). However, a more comprehensive reanalysis revealed that there was no increased mortality for solitary pancreas transplant recipients over wait-listed patients (65,66).

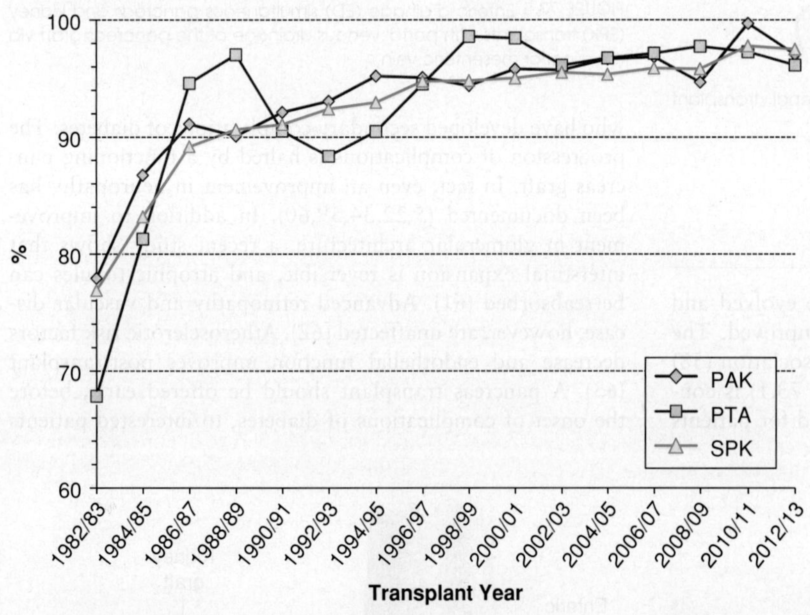

FIGURE 73.7 Patient survival after primary deceased donor pancreas transplants in the United States from 1980 to 2013 by the International Pancreas Transplant Registry. PAK, pancreas after kidney; PTA, pancreas transplant alone; SPK, simultaneous pancreas–kidney.

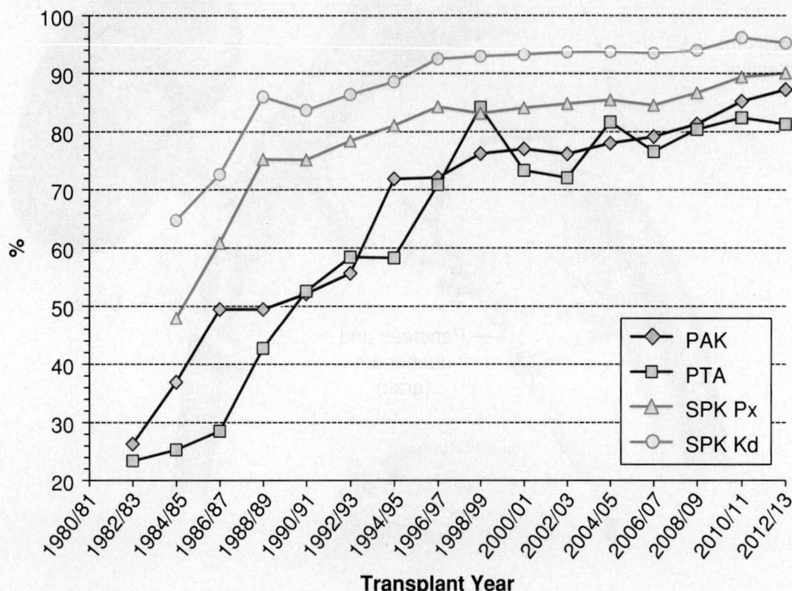

FIGURE 73.8 Pancreas graft survival after primary deceased donor pancreas transplants in the United States from 1980 to 2013 by International Pancreas Transplant Registry. PAK, pancreas after kidney; PTA, pancreas transplant alone; SPK, simultaneous pancreas–kidney.

TABLE 73.1 Summary of American Diabetes Association (ADA) Recommendations for Indications for Pancreas Transplants

1. Established end-stage renal disease (ESRD) in patients who have had, or plan to have, a kidney transplant.
2. History of frequent, acute, and severe metabolic complications (e.g., hypoglycemia, hyperglycemia, ketoacidosis).
3. Incapacitating clinical and emotional problems with exogenous insulin prescription.
4. Consistent failure of insulin-based management to prevent acute complications.

PRETRANSPLANT EVALUATION

The pretransplant workup should include a detailed medical and psychosocial evaluation. Cardiac risk assessment is mandatory because diabetes is a major risk factor for coronary artery disease (CAD). Cardiologists vary on the type of test to screen for CAD in pretransplant diabetic patients. Coronary angiograms are performed in most candidates. Noninvasive tests are not very sensitive for CAD and poorly predictive for subsequent postoperative events in long-standing diabetic patients (67,68). With the use of iso-osmolar radio contrast, there does not seem to be an increased risk of contrast-induced nephropathy in patients with chronic kidney disease (69). In selected patients (i.e., young, healthy patients with short-duration diabetes), dobutamine stress echocardiograms are used for cardiac evaluation with good results (70). Once significant CAD is detected, aggressive treatment by revascularization, angioplasty, or stenting is recommended. In one study, revascularized transplant candidates had significantly fewer postoperative cardiac events, as compared with those who received medical therapy alone (71).

A detailed vascular examination must be done to rule out significant vascular insufficiency. If such insufficiency is found, it may need correction pretransplant because the transplant surgery, involving an anastomosis to the iliac artery, may further diminish lower-extremity blood flow. Pulmonary function tests are indicated in chronic smokers and patients with a history of chronic pulmonary disease. Postoperative intensive care unit monitoring and perioperative bronchodilator therapy may be indicated in some patients. Liver function tests should be done to rule out hepatic insufficiency and viral hepatitis. The diagnosis of viral hepatitis (either B or C) is associated with worse long-term outcome after extrahepatic transplantation (72). Abnormal liver function tests or the diagnosis of viral hepatitis should be followed up with a liver biopsy to rule out cirrhosis. The presence of cirrhosis is a contraindication for pancreas transplant. A gastrointestinal evaluation must be done to rule out autonomic dysfunction. Some immunosuppressive medications may worsen gastrointestinal dysfunction. A prokinetic agent may be indicated to treat gastroparesis. A urologic examination is especially important for BD recipients because bladder dysfunction predisposes to graft pancreatitis.

DECEASED DONOR SELECTION

Pancreas donor selection criteria are not standardized, but instead vary from center to center. Absolute contraindications are the obvious ones applied to most solid organs: active hepatitis B, C, and non A–non B; human immunodeficiency virus; non–central nervous system (CNS) malignancy; surgical or traumatic damage to the pancreas; history of diabetes mellitus; pancreatitis; and extremes of age (younger than 10 or older than 60 years). Prolonged intensive care unit stay and duration of brain death have been associated with an increased risk of graft failure (73). Other studies have shown that donor age is important; even middle-aged donors (older than 40 years) are associated with increased complications and graft failure (73–75). However, the so-called marginal donor organs are associated with good outcome if the pancreas, on inspection, is found to be "healthy" in appearance (76,77).

Donors after cardiac death (DCD) are being used increasingly to expand the donor pool. However, there may be a higher rate of early organ dysfunction with these donors (78). A recent survey showed equivalent patient and graft survival at 1, 3, and 5 years in SPK transplant recipients from DCD compared with donors after brain death (78).

PANCREAS PRESERVATION

UW solution was first used for pancreas preservation in a preclinical model in 1987 (79). As with most solid organs, in vivo flush followed by simple storage in cold UW solution is the standard for pancreas preservation. In the original model, pancreases were preserved for up to 96 hours (80). In clinical transplantation, pancreas cold preservation exceeding 24 hours has been associated with increased graft dysfunction (81). Even when there is less than 24 hours, it has been shown that the longer the cold ischemia time, the greater the technical complication rate (82). Therefore, every effort should be made to minimize the cold ischemia time in order to optimize graft function and to lower complication rates. Recent data suggest a new method of preservation that may be advantageous: the two-layer method using UW solution and perfluorochemical (83). This method allows for longer preservation time while providing a mechanism for repair of ischemic damage due to cold storage (84–86). More clinical trials are needed before the two-layer method becomes routine.

Recently, histidine-tryptophan ketoglutarate solution has been increasingly used in pancreas transplantation (87). Advantages include lower viscosity, less potassium, and lower cost. Early outcome studies do not show inferiority compared to the more expensive UW solution (88,89).

HUMAN LEUKOCYTE ANTIGEN MATCHING

The impact of human leukocyte antigen (HLA) matching on outcome varies. It is generally accepted that HLA matching has little effect on graft outcome for the SPK category (90,91), although higher rejection rates have been reported with poor matches (92–94). For solitary pancreas transplants (PAK and PTA), the data are mixed, ranging from studies showing no impact (95) to registry data showing that HLA A and B matches have a significant impact (91). At the University of Minnesota, SPKs are done regardless of HLA match; for PAKs, generally at least one antigen in the B locus matches, and for PTAs, at least one antigen in each of the A, B, and DR loci matches.

ANESTHETIC CONSIDERATIONS

A patient with brittle diabetes and secondary complications (e.g., CAD, autonomic neuropathy) can pose special problems for the anesthesiologist. Dysautonomic response to drugs or hypoxia can lead to significant morbidity and even death (96). It has also been documented that long-standing diabetes poses a challenge to the anesthesiologist during intubation (97). Awareness of these risks and employment of an experienced anesthesiology team might help decrease the risks or morbidity. A major operation such as a pancreas transplant or combined kidney–pancreas transplant is often prolonged and can be associated with significant blood loss. Prompt replacement with blood or colloids should be instituted to avoid hypoperfusion after significant blood loss. Before and after revascularization of the pancreas, careful blood glucose monitoring, along with continuous intravenous (IV) insulin therapy to maintain tight control of blood glucose levels, is essential. Perioperative β-blockade should be considered for long-standing diabetic patients with a cardiac history.

BACK-TABLE PREPARATION OF THE DONOR PANCREAS

Once the donor pancreas has been opened in the recipient operating room, some back-table work is necessary to prepare it for the transplant, including these steps (98):

1. Donor splenectomy (taking care to avoid injury to the pancreatic tail)
2. Trimming down of the donor duodenum to the shortest length without damage to the main or accessory duct (especially important with BD to minimize bicarbonate loss)
3. Oversewing or individual vessel ligation of the mesocolic and mesenteric stumps on the anterior aspect of the pancreas
4. Excision of lymphatic and ganglionic tissue in the periportal area
5. Reconstruction of the splenic and superior mesenteric arteries with a Y graft of the donor iliac A bifurcation (to provide for a single arterial anastomosis in the recipient).

RECIPIENT OPERATION

Several techniques have been described for the recipient operation (32,99). The techniques vary based on whether a solitary pancreas transplant (PTA, PAK) or a combined transplant (SPK) is done.

Solitary Pancreas Transplant

Choice of Exocrine Secretion of the Pancreas—Drainage of Bowel or Bladder?

Currently, for pancreas transplants in the United States, 86% of PAK, 79% of PTA, and 87% of SPK transplants are drained enterically (5,6). ED is more physiologic and does away with the complications of BD (e.g., acidosis, pancreatitis, urinary infections, hematuria). Between 10% and 20% of BD recipients are ultimately converted to ED because of such complications once they are 6 to 12 months posttransplant and their rejection risk is lower. BD, however, allows for direct measurement of urinary amylase as a marker of exocrine function. A decrease in urine amylase is sensitive, but not very specific, for acute rejection of the pancreas (100,101). Hyperglycemia is a late event in the rejection, and a decrease in urine amylase occurs early. Thus, rejection episodes are detected early with BD, and the rejection loss rate is lower with BD than with other techniques (55). In clinical practice, the choice of exocrine drainage varies. Some groups always use ED, while some always use BD (101,102). Others base it on the individual recipient's immunologic risk versus the risk of urologic complications (28). The surgical risks and short-term outcome with both techniques are comparable (74,103). ED is likely to predominate as the major technique in the future as immunologic strategies to eliminate rejection are developed (102).

Choice of Venous Drainage—Portal or Systemic?

Currently in the United States, of all ED transplants, 20% of SPK, 10% of PAK, and 12% of PTA cases are drained to the portal vein (5,6). Portal drainage is more physiologic than systemic drainage (104,105). Theoretically, portal drainage preserves the first-pass metabolism of insulin in the liver. Therefore, portally drained recipients will have lower systemic insulin levels (106). However, there is no evidence of any detrimental effect on lipid levels (107) or on risk of vascular disease (62) as seen in de novo hyperinsulinemia (syndrome X). Portal venous drainage is difficult to perform with exocrine BD (45). Portal drainage had gained in popularity after initial reports that rejection rates are lower in this category (103,108). It appears, however, based on registry data (5,6) that the immunologic advantage is much smaller than initially found. Recent modifications include a retroperitoneal portal-ED technique (109).

Transplantation Portion—Whole Organ or a Segment?

Almost all cadaveric pancreas transplants performed today use whole-organ grafts. Segmental grafts have little role to play in this group, except when a rare anatomic abnormality is noted such that the head of the pancreas cannot be used. A rare instance of a split cadaveric pancreas transplanted into two different recipients has been described (110). All living-donor pancreas transplants use segmental grafts (body and tail); doing so maintains normoglycemia in the recipient (12).

Simultaneous Pancreas-Kidney

SPK transplants have a lower rejection rate than do solitary pancreases. Further, rejection episodes are rarely isolated to the pancreas alone. Most pancreas rejection episodes can be indirectly detected by monitoring serum creatinine as a marker for kidney rejection. Therefore, most SPK transplants are done using ED, as advocated by the Stockholm group (111) (Fig. 73.5). With ED, the risk of acute technical complications is slightly higher, but the chronic complication rate is lower (112). Choice of venous drainage varies by center. Because ED is the choice for exocrine drainage, there is no impediment to performing portal venous drainage.

POSTOPERATIVE CARE

After an uncomplicated pancreas transplant, the recipient is transferred to the postanesthesia care unit (PACU) or the surgical intensive care unit (SICU). Centers that have a specialized monitored transplant unit (with central venous and arterial monitoring capabilities) transition the postoperative recipients through the PACU to the transplant unit. Others transfer directly to the SICU for the first 24 to 48 hours. Care during the first few hours after transplant is similar to care after any major operative procedure. Careful monitoring of vital signs, central venous pressure, oxygen saturation, and hematologic and laboratory parameters is crucial. The factors below are unique to pancreas recipients and should be attended to.

Blood Glucose Levels

Any sudden, unexplained increase in glucose levels should raise the suspicion of graft thrombosis. An immediate ultrasound examination must be done to assess blood flow to the graft. Maintenance of tight glucose control (<150 mg/dL) using an IV insulin drip is important to "rest" the pancreas in the early postoperative period.

Intravascular Volume

Because the pancreas is a "low-flow" organ, intravascular volume must be maintained to provide adequate perfusion to the graft. Central venous pressure monitoring is used to monitor intravascular volume status. In some cases, such as patients with depressed cardiac function, pulmonary artery catheter monitoring may be required during the first 24 to 48 hours. If the hypovolemia is associated with low hemoglobin levels, then washed packed red blood cell transfusions should be given. Otherwise, colloid or crystalloid replacement can be used.

Maintenance IV Fluid Therapy

The choice of IV fluid is usually 5% dextrose in 0.45% saline solution. The use of dextrose is not contraindicated and may be of benefit, as long as IV insulin is used to maintain good blood glucose control. In SPK recipients, whose IV rate is based on urine output, dextrose should be eliminated if the urine output is high (>500 mL/hr). Maintenance solution for BD recipients should include 10 mEq of HCO_3 added to each liter to account for the excess HCO_3 loss (113,114); sodium lactate can be used as an alternative (115).

Antibiotic Therapy

Broad-spectrum antibiotic therapy (with strong gram-negative coverage) and antifungal therapy are instituted before the incision is made in the operating room, then continued for 3 (for antibiotics) and 7 days (for antifungal). At the University of Minnesota, since the introduction of this protocol, we have noted a decrease in postoperative abdominal infections (74). Cytomegalovirus (CMV) and antiviral prophylaxis are similar to that for other solid organs.

Octreotide

The use of octreotide in pancreas recipients helps reduce the incidence of technical complications (116). This benefit should be weighed against evidence from rat studies that shows decreased pancreatic islet blood flow with octreotide use (117), although clinically no detrimental effects of octreotide use have been documented. A dose of 100 to 150 μg IV or subcutaneously three times a day is administered for 5 days posttransplant. Dose adjustments may be made for nausea, which is the predominant side effect.

Anticoagulation

The use of low-dose heparin in the early postoperative period (days 0 to 5) decreases the risk of graft thrombosis (118). An intraoperative dose of 70 units/kg is given, followed by an IV infusion of 3 units/kg started at 4 hours postoperatively and gradually increased up to 7 units/kg (depending on hemodynamic stability and hemoglobin levels). Enteric-coated aspirin (80 mg) is started on day 1 and continued for 6 months. At the University of Minnesota, this protocol decreased the thrombosis rate from about 12% to 6%, but increased the relaparotomy rate due to bleeding from 4% to 6%. Segmental pancreas transplants (as in living-donor transplants) have a higher thrombosis risk and therefore therapeutic heparinization (with a target-activated partial thromboplastin time [aPTT] of 50 seconds) for 5 days and Coumadin therapy (with a target international normalized ratio [INR] of 2 to 2.5) are recommended for 6 months. The higher risk of thrombosis is due to the smaller vessels in a segmental graft (119,120).

IMMUNOSUPPRESSION

Immunosuppression is essential to thwart rejection in all allotransplant recipients (17). Before the advent of cyclosporine in the early 1980s (121), azathioprine and prednisone were the mainstays of immunosuppression. From the early 1980s to the mid-1990s, cyclosporine was added to the mix and resulted in significant improvement in immunologic outcomes (122). Since the mid-1990s, tacrolimus and mycophenolate mofetil have replaced cyclosporine and azathioprine as the main drugs, resulting in even better pancreas graft survival rates (122–124). In addition, steroids have been successfully withdrawn from some pancreas recipients (125) and, in some cases, avoided (126). With a recently introduced drug, rapamycin, used in combination with tacrolimus, steroids have been successfully avoided in some pancreas recipients (127,128).

Anti–T-cell therapy has always remained a part of the induction protocol for pancreas recipients. With the recent emphasis on steroid withdrawal or avoidance, anti–T-cell therapy has taken on added importance to avoid rejection. Anti-CD25 antibodies are also used frequently as induction therapy (129). Avoidance of calcineurin inhibitors has been attempted in pancreas transplantation. When combined with steroid avoidance, this required prolonged anti–T-cell therapy, which increases the risk of infection without adequately controlling rejection (130). Table 73.2 presents the immunosuppressive protocol for pancreas transplant recipients at the University of Minnesota.

For PTA recipients, whose rejection rates are the highest of all categories, pretransplant immunosuppression has decreased rejection rates and graft loss from rejection (31).

TABLE 73.2 University of Minnesota Standard Immunosuppression Pancreas Program

SPK	PAK and SPLK	PTA	Rejection
Antithymocyte globulin 1.25 mg/kg [a]5 doses First dose intraoperative Give methylprednisolone 500 mg, 250 mg, and 100 mg before first, second, and third doses, respectively	**Antithymocyte globulin** 1.25 mg/kg [a]7 doses First dose intraoperative Give methylprednisolone 500 mg, 250 mg, and 100 mg before first, second, and third doses, respectively	**Antithymocyte globulin** 1.25 mg/kg [a]7–10 doses First dose intraoperative Give methylprednisolone 500 mg, 250 mg, and 100 mg before first, second, and third doses, respectively	**Methylprednisolone** Day #0: 500 mg IV Day #1: 250 mg IV Day #2: 125 mg IV **Antithymocyte globulin** 1.25 mg/kg IV[a] × 5–7 d Give premedication Monitor ALC *Resistant rejection*
Tacrolimus 2 mg orally, twice daily Start when creatinine less than 3 mg/dL or postoperative day #5, whichever is later If tacrolimus is delayed continue TMG until tacrolimus levels are therapeutic Levels 8–10 ng/mL for 3 mo, then 5–8 ng/mL	**Tacrolimus** 2 mg orally, twice daily Start postoperative If tacrolimus is delayed continue TMG until tacrolimus levels are therapeutic Levels 8–10 ng/mL for 3 mo, then 5–8 ng/mL	**Tacrolimus** 2 mg orally, twice daily Start postoperative If tacrolimus is delayed continue TMG until tacrolimus levels are therapeutic Levels 8–10 ng/mL for 3 mo, then 5–8 ng/mL	
Mycophenolate Start postoperative 1 g orally, twice daily	**Mycophenolate** Start postoperative 1 g orally, twice daily	**Mycophenolate** Start postoperative 1 g orally, twice daily	**Note:** Kidney rejections on the kidney steroid avoidance study should be treated with ALG, ATG, or other antibody preparations

SPK, simultaneous pancreas kidney; PAK, pancreas after kidney; SPLK, simultaneous cadaver pancreas living-donor kidney; TMG, antithymocyte globulin; ALC, absolute lymphocyte count; mo, month.
[a]Round up antithymocyte globulin dose to the nearest 25.
ALC levels: If zero, hold antithymocyte globulin; if 0.1 give half-dose antithymocyte globulin; if 0.2 or above give full dose.
Antithymocyte globulin and other antibody preparations require "premedication."

Heavy use of immunosuppression may increase the infection rate, but effective antimicrobial prophylaxis has helped ameliorate this problem (131,132).

INTRAVENOUS IMMUNOGLOBULIN AND PLASMAPHERESIS

IV immunoglobulin has many applications in transplantation. It has been used successfully to decrease anti-HLA antibodies in transplant recipients on the waiting list and to shorten their waiting times (133,134). It can also be used to control acute humoral rejection in kidney and heart allograft recipients (135). Plasmapheresis has been used to decrease humoral antibody titers in ABO-incompatible liver and kidney recipients (136,137). It has also been used to control hyperacute and accelerated acute rejection in positive cross-match kidney recipients (138,139) and lung (140) recipients. At the University of Minnesota, for ABO-incompatible (A2 to O, B, or AB) or positive cross-match (T-cell) pancreas recipients, the treatment protocol consists of intraoperative IV immunoglobulin (0.5 mg/kg) followed by a course of 5 to 7 days in combination with daily plasmapheresis. For B-cell positive cross-match recipients, IV immunoglobulin may be used without plasmapheresis.

SURGICAL COMPLICATIONS

Bleeding

Postoperative bleeding is a frequent reason for early relaparotomy in pancreas recipients. The incidence ranges from 6% to 8% (74,141). This risk is increased by the use of anticoagulation in the immediate postoperative period. Frequent physical examinations and monitoring of hemoglobin help detect bleeding early. Heparin may be temporarily suspended to stabilize the patient. If bleeding continues, early operative intervention is indicated. If bleeding stops or slows down, heparin should be restarted at a lower rate and judiciously increased as tolerated.

Thrombosis

The incidence of thrombosis posttransplant ranges from 5% to 13% (118,141). The risk is increased after segmental pancreas transplants because of the small caliber of vessels (51). Most thromboses are due to technical reasons. A short portal vein (requiring an extension graft) or atherosclerotic arteries in the pancreas graft increases the risk for thrombosis. In the recipient, a narrow pelvic inlet with a deeply placed iliac vein, atherosclerotic disease of the iliac artery, a technically difficult vascular anastomosis, kinking of the vein by the pancreas graft, significant hematoma formation around the vascular anastomosis, and a hypercoagulable state are some of the factors that increase the risk for thrombosis. The most common form of hypercoagulable state is factor V Leiden mutation in the Western population. The incidence ranges from 2% to 5% but may be as high as 50% to 60% in patients with a history (self or family) of thrombosis (142). Other causes of hypercoagulable state include antithrombin deficiency, protein C or S deficiency, activated protein C resistance, and anticardiolipin antibodies (143).

Duodenal Leaks

The incidence of duodenal leaks ranges from 4% to 6% (74,141). A leak from the anastomosis of the duodenum to the bowel almost always leads to a relaparotomy. Gross peritoneal contamination due to an enteric leak necessitates a graft pancreatectomy. The diagnosis is made by elevated pancreatic enzymes associated with acute abdomen. The differential diagnosis is pancreatitis, abdominal infection, or acute severe rejection. A Roux-en-Y anastomosis to the pancreatic duodenum may be preferred if the risk of leak is thought to be increased during intraoperative inspection of the pancreas. Other novel techniques such as a venting jejunostomy (Roux-en-Y) have been used in selected recipients (144). Duodenal leaks in BD recipients are usually managed nonoperatively with prolonged catheter decompression of the urinary bladder. The diagnosis is made using plain or computed tomography (CT) cystography. The size and extent of the leak cannot always be assessed by the imaging studies. Large leaks may require operative intervention, such as a repair or enteric conversion (145).

Major Intra-Abdominal Infections

The incidence of intra-abdominal infections requiring reoperation ranges from 4% to 10% (74,141). Opening the duodenal segment intraoperatively, with associated contamination, predisposes to this high rate; fungal and gram-negative infections predominate. With the advent of advanced interventional radiologic procedures to drain intra-abdominal abscesses, the incidence of reoperations is fast decreasing. If the infection is uncontrolled or widespread, then graft pancreatectomy followed by frequent washouts may be necessary.

Renal Pedicle Torsion

Torsion of the kidney has been reported after the SPK transplants (146,147). The intraperitoneal location of the kidney (allowing for more mobility) predisposes to this complication. Additional risk factors are a long renal pedicle (>5 cm) and a marked discrepancy between the length of artery and vein. Prophylactic nephropexy to the anterior or lateral abdominal wall is recommended in intraperitoneal transplants to avoid this problem.

Others

Other surgical complications that may require laparotomy also decreased from 9% to 1%. Improved anti-infective prophylaxis, surgical techniques, immunosuppression, and advances in interventional radiology have all contributed to this disease (74).

NONSURGICAL COMPLICATIONS

Pancreatitis

The incidence of posttransplant pancreatitis varies based on the type of exocrine drainage. BD recipients with abnormal bladder function are at increased risk secondary to incomplete bladder emptying or urine retention causing resistance to the flow of pancreatic exocrine secretions. Other causes of pancreatitis include drugs (corticosteroids, azathioprine, cyclosporine), hypercalcemia, viral infections (CMV or hepatitis C), and reperfusion injury after prolonged ischemia. Pancreatitis is usually manifested by an increase in serum amylase and lipase with or without local signs of inflammation. The treatment usually consists of catheter decompression of the bladder for a period of 2 to 6 weeks, depending on the severity. In addition, octreotide therapy may be used to decrease pancreatic secretions. The underlying urologic problem, if any, should be treated. If repeated episodes of pancreatitis occur, an enteric conversion of exocrine drainage may be indicated (148–150).

Rejection

The incidence of rejection is discussed in the Results section earlier in this chapter. The diagnosis is usually based on an increase in serum amylase and lipase and a decrease in urine amylase in BD recipients. A sustained significant drop in urinary amylase from baseline should prompt a pancreas biopsy to rule out rejection (151). In ED recipients, one has to rely on serum amylase and lipase only. A rise in serum lipase has recently shown to correlate well with acute pancreas rejection (149). Other signs and symptoms include tenderness over the graft, unexplained fever, and hyperglycemia (usually a late finding). Diagnosis can be confirmed by a percutaneous pancreas biopsy (152–154). In cases in which percutaneous biopsy is not possible due to technical reasons, empiric therapy may be started. Rarely, open biopsy is indicated. Transcystoscopic biopsy, which was used in the past, has been largely abandoned.

Others

Other findings include infectious complications such as CMV, hepatitis C, extra-abdominal bacterial or fungal infections, posttransplant malignancy such as posttransplant lymphoproliferative disorder, and other rare complications such as graft-versus-host disease that occur in pancreas transplantation. The diagnosis and management of these complications are similar to those of other solid-organ transplants.

FUTURE DIRECTIONS

In diabetic patients with kidney dysfunction, SPK or PAK transplant is the standard of care. A PTA, however, is less common because the long-term risks of diabetes are pitted against the long-term risks of immunosuppression. A successful transplant can improve existing neuropathy (62) in diabetic recipients, and the survival after a solitary pancreas transplant is better than remaining on the waiting list (65). As the risks of immunosuppression decrease with novel methods of tolerance and immunomodulation (102), the balance will tilt in favor of an early transplant. The limiting factor will then be the organ shortage, which could be alleviated if xenotransplantation is able to overcome its current barrier of hyperacute rejection (155).

The application of islet transplants is rapidly growing. Recent successes (7,8) suggest that islet transplants can provide all the benefits of pancreas transplants without the risks of major surgery. Xenotransplantation of islets may be more readily achievable using encapsulation (156) than with other organs. Prolonged diabetes reversal after intraportal xenotransplant in primates has been documented (157) and may pave the way for human xenotransplant trials. Also, stem cells that are manipulated to differentiate into islets may provide a rich supply for transplantation (158). Islet transplants can be combined with immunomodulation and tolerogenic strategies to minimize or avoid immunosuppression (159). This combination would provide for minimally invasive cellular (islet) transplants for all type 1 diabetic patients without the need for long-term immunosuppression. But unless the results of clinical islet transplantation continue to substantially improve, pancreas transplantation remains the best treatment option long-term for (labile) type 1 diabetic patients with or without uremia.

Key Points

1. Pancreas transplantation remains the most reliable treatment option for insulin-dependent patients with diabetes that offers freedom from insulin administration long-term and achieves normoglycemia.
2. Pancreas transplantation can hold or even reverse some of the secondary complications of diabetes mellitus.
3. Pancreas transplants can be performed in (a) nonuremic, brittle diabetic patients, (b) uremic diabetic patients, and (c) posturemic diabetic patients who underwent a previous kidney transplant.
4. One-year patient survival rates after pancreas transplantation are over 95%, graft survival rates are above 80%.
5. Quality of life is markedly improved in previously diabetic patients after successful pancreas transplantation.
6. Graft loss from technical or immunologic complications is less than 5% each at 1 year.

References

1. The effect of intensive treatment of diabetes on the development and progression of long-term complications in insulin-dependent diabetes mellitus. The Diabetes Control and Complications Trial Research Group. *N Engl J Med.* 1993;329:977–986.
2. Lifetime benefits and costs of intensive therapy as practiced in the diabetes control and complications trial. The Diabetes Control and Complications Trial Research Group. *JAMA.* 1997;277:372.
3. Diabetes Research in Children Network (DirecNet) Study Group, Buckingham B, Beck RW, et al. Continuous glucose monitoring in children with type 1 diabetes. *J Pediatr.* 2007;151:388–393.
4. Cobry E, Chase HP, Burdick P, et al. Use of CoZmonitor in youth with type 1 diabetes. *Pediatr Diabetes.* 2008;9:148–151.
5. Gruessner RW, Gruessner AC. The current state of pancreas transplantation. *Nat Rev Endocrinol.* 2013;9:555–562.
6. Gruessner AC, Gruessner RW. Pancreas transplant outcomes for United Stated and non United States cases as reported to the United Network for Organ Sharing and the International Pancreas Transplant Registry as of December 2011. *Clin Transpl.* 2012:23–40.
7. Shapiro AM, Lakey JR, Ryan EA, et al. Islet transplantation in seven patients with type 1 diabetes mellitus using a glucocorticoid-free immunosuppressive regimen. *N Engl J Med.* 2000;343:230–238.
8. Hering BJ, Kandaswamy R, Harmon J. Insulin independence after single-donor islet transplantation in type I diabetes with hOKT3-1 (ala-ala), sirolimus, and tacrolimus therapy. *Am J Transplant.* 2001;1:180.
9. Gruessner RW, Gruessner AC. What defines success in pancreas and islet transplantation:insulin independence or prevention of hypoglycemia. *Transplant Proc.* 2014;46:1898–1899.
10. Hering BJ, Kandaswamy R, Ansite JD, et al. Single-donor, marginal-dose islet transplantation in patients with type 1 diabetes. *JAMA.* 2005; 293:830–835.
11. Ryan EA, Paty BW, Senior PA, et al. Five-year follow-up after clinical islet transplantation. *Diabetes.* 2005;54:2060–2069.
12. Gruessner AC, Sutherland DE, Gruessner RW. Long-term outcome after pancreas transplantation. *Curr Opin Organ Transplant.* 2012;17:100–105.
13. Sutherland DE, Stratta RJ, Gruessner AC. Pancreas transplant outcome by recipient category: single pancreas versus combined kidney-pancreas. *Curr Opin Organ Transplant.* 1998;3:231–241.
14. Gruessner RW, Sutherland DE, Najarian JS, et al. Solitary pancreas transplantation for nonuremic patients with labile insulin-dependent diabetes mellitus. *Transplantation.* 1997;64:1572–1577.
15. Krolewski AS, Warram JH, Freire MB. Epidemiology of late diabetic complications: a basis for the development and evaluation of preventive programs. *Endocrinol Metab Clin North Am.* 1996;25:217–242.
16. Syndman DR. Infection in solid organ transplantation. *Transplant Infect Dis.* 1999;1:21–28.
17. First MR. Immunosuppressive agents and their actions. *Transplant Proc.* 2002;34:1369–1371.
18. Gruessner RW, Sutherland DE, Kandaswamy R, Gruessner AC. Over 500 solitary pancreas transplants in nonuremic patients with brittle diabetes mellitus. *Transplantation.* 2008;85:42–47.
19. Nath DS, Gruessner AC, Kandaswamy R, et al. Outcomes of pancreas transplants for patients with type 2 diabetes mellitus. *Clin Transplant.* 2005;19:792–797.
20. Light JA, Sasaki TM, Currier CB, Barhyte DY. Successful long-term kidney-pancreas transplants regardless of C-peptide status or race. *Transplantation.* 2001;71:152–154.
21. Benedetti E, Dunn T, Massad MG, et al. Successful living related simultaneous pancreas-kidney transplant between identical twins. *Transplantation.* 1999;67:915–918.
22. Gruessner RW, Kendall DM, Drangstveit MB, et al. Simultaneous pancreas-kidney transplantation from live donors. *Ann Surg.* 1997;226:471–480 discussion 480–482.
23. Sutherland DE, Gores PF, Farney AC, et al. Evolution of kidney, pancreas, and islet transplantation for patients with diabetes at the University of Minnesota. *Am J Surg.* 1993;166:456–491.
24. Farney AC, Cho E, Schweitzer EJ, et al. Simultaneous cadaver pancreas living-donor kidney transplantation: a new approach for the type 1 diabetic uremic patient. *Ann Surg.* 2000;232:696–703.
25. Matsumoto S, Okitsu T, Iwanaga Y, et al. Insulin independence after living-donor distal pancreatectomy and islet allotransplantation. *Lancet.* 2005;365:1642–1644.
26. Matsumoto S, Okitsu T, Iwanaga Y, et al. Follow-up study of the first successful living donor islet transplantation. *Transplantation.* 2006;82: 1629–1633.
27. Iwanaga Y, Matsumoto S, Okitsu T, et al. Living donor islet transplantation, the alternative approach to overcome the obstacles limiting transplant. *Ann N Y Acad Sci.* 2006;1079:335–339.
28. Sutherland DE, Gruessner RW, Dunn DL, et al. Lessons learned from more than 1,000 pancreas transplants at a single institution. *Ann Surg.* 2001;233:463–501.
29. Gruessner AC, Sutherland DE, Dunn DL, et al. Pancreas after kidney transplants in posturemic patients with type I diabetes mellitus. *J Am Soc Nephrol.* 2001;12:2490–2499.
30. Gruessner RW, Gruessner AC. Pancreas transplant alone: a procedure coming of age. *Diabetes Care.* 2013;36:2440–2447.
31. Kelly WD, Lillehei RC, Merkel FK, et al. Allotransplantation of the pancreas and duodenum along with the kidney in diabetic nephropathy. *Surgery.* 1967;61:827–837.
32. Gruessner RWG. Recipient procedures. In: Gruessner RW, Sutherland DE, eds. *Transplantation of the Pancreas.* New York: Springer-Verlag; 2004:150–178.
33. Gold M, Whittaker JR, Veith FJ, Gliedman ML. Evaluation of ureteral drainage for pancreatic exocrine secretion. *Surg Forum.* 1972;23:375–377.
34. Gliedman ML, Natale DL, Riflan H, et al. Clinical segmental pancreatic transplantation with ureter-to-pancreatic duct anastomosis for exocrine drainage. *Bull Soc Int Chir.* 1975;34:15–20.
35. Dubernard JM, Traeger J, Neyra P, et al. A new method of preparation of segmental pancreatic grafts for transplantation: trials in dogs and in man. *Surgery.* 1978;84:633–639.
36. Sollinger HW, Cook K, Kamps D, et al. Clinical and experimental experience with pancreaticocystostomy for exocrine pancreatic drainage in pancreas transplantation. *Transplant Proc.* 1984;16:749–751.
37. Nghiem DD, Corry RJ. Technique of simultaneous renal pancreatoduodenal transplantation with urinary drainage of pancreatic secretion. *Am J Surg.* 1987;153:405–406.
38. Groth CG, Collste H, Lundgren G, et al. Successful outcome of segmental human pancreatic transplantation with enteric exocrine diversion after modifications in technique. *Lancet.* 1982;2:522–524.
39. Calne RY. Paratopic segmental pancreas grafting: a technique with portal venous drainage. *Lancet.* 1984;1:595–597.
40. Gil-Vernet JM, Fernandez-Cruz L, Caralps A, et al. Whole organ and pancreaticoureterostomy in clinical pancreas transplantation. *Transplant Proc.* 1985;17:2019–2022.

41. Sutherland DE, Goetz FC, Moudry KC, et al. Use of recipient mesenteric vessels for revascularization of segmental pancreas grafts: technical and metabolic considerations. *Transplant Proc.* 1987;19:2300–2304.
42. Tyden G, Lundgren G, Ostman J. Grafted pancreas with portal venous drainage. *Lancet.* 1984;1:964–965.
43. Rosenlof LK, Earnhardt RC, Pruett TL, et al. Pancreas transplantation. An initial experience with systemic and portal drainage of pancreatic allografts. *Ann Surg.* 1992;215:586–595; discussion 596–597.
44. Shokouh-Amiri MH, Gaber AO, Gaber LW, et al. Pancreas transplantation with portal venous drainage and enteric exocrine diversion: a new technique. *Transplant Proc.* 1992;24:776–777.
45. Muhlbacher F, Gnant MF, Auinger M, et al. Pancreatic venous drainage to the portal vein: a new method in human pancreas transplantation. *Transplant Proc.* 1990;22:636–637.
46. Gaber AO, Shokouh-Amiri MH, Hathaway DK, et al. Results of pancreas transplantation with portal venous and enteric drainage. *Ann Surg.* 1995;221:613–622; discussion 622–624.
47. Marsh CL, Perkins JD, Sutherland DE, et al. Combined hepatic and pancreaticoduodenal procurement for transplantation. *Surg Gynecol Obstet.* 1989;168:254–258.
48. Delmonico FL, Jenkins RL, Auchincloss H Jr, et al. Procurement of a whole pancreas and liver from the same cadaveric donor. *Surgery.* 1989; 105:718–723.
49. Stratta RJ, Taylor RJ, Gill IS. Pancreas transplantation: a managed cure approach to diabetes. *Curr Probl Surg.* 1996;33:709–808.
50. Sutherland DE, Goetz FC, Najarian JS. Living-related donor segmental pancreatectomy for transplantation. *Transplant Proc.* 1980;12:19–25.
51. Gruessner RW, Sutherland DE. Simultaneous kidney and segmental pancreas transplants from living related donors: the first two successful cases. *Transplantation.* 1996;61:1265–1268.
52. Sutherland DE, Najarian JS, Gruessner R. Living versus cadaver donor pancreas transplants. *Transplant Proc.* 1998;30:2264–2266.
53. Gruessner RW, Sutherland DE, Drangstveit MB, et al. Pancreas transplants from living donors: short- and long-term outcome. *Transplant Proc.* 2001;33:819–820.
54. Gruessner RW, Kandaswamy R, Denny R. Laparoscopic simultaneous nephrectomy and distal pancreatectomy from a live donor. *J Am Coll Surg.* 2001;193:333–337.
55. Gruessner AC, Sutherland DE. Pancreas transplant outcomes for United States (US) and non-US cases as reported to the United Network for Organ Sharing (UNOS) and the International Pancreas Transplant Registry (IPTR) as of October 2002. In: Cecka JM, Terasaki PI, eds. *Clinical Transplants 2002.* Los Angeles: UCLA Immunogenetics Center; 2003.
56. Sollinger HW, Odorico JS, Knechtle SJ, et al. Experience with 500 simultaneous pancreas-kidney transplants. *Ann Surg.* 1998;228:284–296.
57. Sutherland DE. International human pancreas and islet transplant registry. *Transplant Proc.* 1980;12(4 Suppl 2):229–236.
58. Pancreas transplantation for patients with type 1 diabetes: American Diabetes Association. *Diabetes Care.* 2000;23:117.
59. Kennedy WR, Navarro X, Goetz FC, et al. Effects of pancreatic transplantation on diabetic neuropathy. *N Engl J Med.* 1990;322:1031–1037.
60. Solders G, Tyden G, Persson A, Groth CG. Improvement of nerve conduction in diabetic neuropathy: a follow-up study 4 yr after combined pancreatic and renal transplantation. *Diabetes.* 1992;41:946–951.
61. Fioretto P, Sutherland DE, Najafian B, Mauer M. Remodeling of renal interstitial and tubular lesions in pancreas transplant recipients. *Kidney Int.* 2006;69:907–912.
62. Stratta RJ. Impact of pancreas transplantation on complications of diabetes. *Curr Opin Organ Transplant.* 1998;3:258–273.
63. Fiorina P, La Rocca E, Venturini M, et al. Effects of kidney-pancreas transplantation on atherosclerotic risk factors and endothelial function in patients with uremia and type 1 diabetes. *Diabetes.* 2001;50:496–501.
64. Venstrom JM, McBride MA, Rother KI, et al. Survival after pancreas transplantation in patients with diabetes and preserved kidney function. *JAMA.* 2003;290:2817–2823.
65. Gruessner RW, Sutherland DE, Gruessner AC. Mortality assessment for pancreas transplants. *Am J Transplant.* 2004;4:2018–2026.
66. Gruessner RW, Sutherland DE, Gruessner AC. Survival after pancreas transplantation. *JAMA.* 2005;293:675; author reply 675–676.
67. Vandenberg BF, Rossen JD, Grover-McKay M, et al. Evaluation of diabetic patients for renal and pancreas transplantation: noninvasive screening for coronary artery disease using radionuclide methods. *Transplantation.* 1996;62:1230–1235.
68. Herzog CA, Marwick TH, Pheley AM, et al. Dobutamine stress echocardiography for the detection of significant coronary artery disease in renal transplant candidates. *Am J Kidney Dis.* 1999;33:1080–1090.
69. Tadros GM, Malik JA, Manske CL, et al. Iso-osmolar radio contrast iodixanol in patients with chronic kidney disease. *J Invasive Cardiol.* 2005;17:211–215.
70. Bates JR, Sawada SG, Segar DS, et al. Evaluation using dobutamine stress echocardiography in patients with insulin-dependent diabetes mellitus before kidney and/or pancreas transplantation. *Am J Cardiol.* 1996;77:175–179.
71. Manske CL, Wang Y, Rector T, et al. Coronary revascularisation in insulindependent diabetic patients with chronic renal failure. *Lancet.* 1992;340:998–1002.
72. Legendre C, Garrigue V, Le Bihan C, et al. Harmful long-term impact of hepatitis C virus infection in kidney transplant recipients. *Transplantation.* 1998;65:667–670.
73. Douzdjian V, Gugliuzza KG, Fish JC. Multivariate analysis of donor risk factors for pancreas allograft failure after simultaneous pancreas-kidney transplantation. *Surgery.* 1995;118:73–81.
74. Humar A, Kandaswamy R, Granger D, et al. Decreased surgical risks of pancreas transplantation in the modern era. *Ann Surg.* 2000;231:269–275.
75. Humar A, Harmon J, Gruessner A, et al. Surgical complications requiring early relaparotomy after pancreas transplantation: comparison of the cyclosporine and FK 506 eras. *Transplant Proc.* 1999;31:606–607.
76. Kapur S, Bonham CA, Dodson SF, et al. Strategies to expand the donor pool for pancreas transplantation. *Transplantation.* 1999;67:284–290.
77. Bonham CA, Kapur S, Dodson SF, et al. Potential use of marginal donors for pancreas transplantation. *Transplant Proc.* 1999;31:612–613.
78. Salvalaggio PR, Davies DB, Fernandez LA, Kaufman DB. Outcomes of pancreas transplantation in the United States using cardiac-death donors. *Am J Transplant.* 2006;6:1059–1065.
79. Wahlberg JA, Love R, Landegaard L, et al. 72-hour preservation of the canine pancreas. *Transplantation.* 1987;43:5–8.
80. Kin S, Stephanian E, Gores P, et al. Successful 96-Hr cold-storage preservation of canine pancreas with UW solution containing the thromboxane A2 synthesis inhibitor OKY046. *J Surg Res.* 1992;52:577–582.
81. D'Alessandro AM, Kalayoglu M, Sollinger HW, et al. Current status of organ preservation with University of Wisconsin solution. *Arch Pathol Lab Med.* 1991;115:306–310.
82. Humar A, Kandaswamy R, Drangstveit MB, et al. Surgical risks and outcome of pancreas retransplants. *Surgery.* 2000;127:634–640.
83. Matsumoto S, Kandaswamy R, Sutherland DE, et al. Clinical application of the two-layer (University of Wisconsin solution/perfluorochemical plus O_2) method of pancreas preservation before transplantation. *Transplantation.* 2000;70:771–774.
84. Kuroda Y, Kawamura T, Suzuki Y, et al. A new, simple method for cold storage of the pancreas using perfluorochemical. *Transplantation.* 1988;46:457–460.
85. Fujita H, Kuroda Y, Saitoh Y. The mechanism of action of the two-layer cold storage method in canine pancreas preservation–protection of pancreatic microvascular endothelium. *Kobe J Med Sci.* 1995;41:47–61.
86. Tanioka Y, Kuroda Y, Saitoh Y. Amelioration of rewarming ischemic injury of the pancreas graft during vascular anastomosis by increasing tissue ATP contents during preservation by the two-layer cold storage method. *Kobe J Med Sci.* 1994;40:175–189.
87. Agarwal A, Murdock P, Pescovitz MD, et al. Follow-up experience using histidine-tryptophan ketoglutarate solution in clinical pancreas transplantation. *Transplant Proc.* 2005;37:3523–3526.
88. Englesbe MJ, Moyer A, Kim DY, et al. Early pancreas transplant outcomes with histidine-tryptophan-ketoglutarate preservation: a multicenter study. *Transplantation.* 2006;82:136–139.
89. Becker T, Ringe B, Nyibata M, et al. Pancreas transplantation with histidine-tryptophan-ketoglutarate (HTK) solution and University of Wisconsin (UW) solution: is there a difference? *JOP.* 2007;8:304–311.
90. Mancini MJ, Connors AF Jr, Wang XQ, et al. HLA matching for simultaneous pancreas-kidney transplantation in the United States: a multivariable analysis of the UNOS data. *Clin Nephrol.* 2002;57:27–37.
91. Gruessner AC, Sutherland DE, Gruessner RW. Matching in pancreas transplantation—a registry analysis. *Transplant Proc.* 2001;33:1665–1666.
92. Malaise J, Berney T, Morel P, et al; EUROSPK Study Group. Effect of HLA matching in simultaneous pancreas-kidney transplantation. *Transplant Proc.* 2005;37:2846–2847.
93. Lo A, Stratta RJ, Alloway RR, Hodge EE; PIVOT Study Group. A multicenter analysis of the significance of HLA matching on outcomes after kidney-pancreas transplantation. *Transplant Proc.* 2005;37:1289–1290.
94. Berney T, Malaise J, Morel P; Euro-SPK Study Group. Impact of HLA matching on the outcome of simultaneous pancreas-kidney transplantation. *Nephrol Dial Transplant.* 2005;20(Suppl 2):ii48–53, ii62.
95. Gruber SA, Katz S, Kaplan B, et al. Initial results of solitary pancreas transplants performed without regard to donor/recipient HLA mismatching. *Transplantation.* 2000;70:388–391.

96. Page MM, Watkins PJ. Cardiorespiratory arrest and diabetic autonomic neuropathy. *Lancet.* 1978;1:14–16.
97. Hogan K, Rusy D, Springman SR. Difficult laryngoscopy and diabetes mellitus. *Anesth Analg.* 1988;67:1162–1165.
98. Gruessner RW. Donor procedures. In: Gruessner RW, Sutherland DE, eds. *Transplantation of the Pancreas.* New York, NY: Springer-Verlag; 2004:126–142.
99. Krishnamurthi V, Philosophe B, Bartlett ST. Pancreas transplantation: contemporary surgical techniques. *Urol Clin North Am.* 2001;28:833–838.
100. Gruessner RW, Sutherland DE: Clinical diagnosis in pancreas allograft rejection. In: Solez K, Racusen LC, Billingham ME, eds. *Solid Organ Transplant Rejection: Mechanisms, Pathology and Diagnosis.* New York, NY: Marcel Dekker; 1996:455–499.
101. Benedetti E, Najarian JS, Gruessner AC, et al. Correlation between cystoscopic biopsy results and hypoamylasuria in bladder-drained pancreas transplants. *Surgery.* 1995;118:864–872.
102. Kirk AD. Immunosuppression without immunosuppression? How to be a tolerant individual in a dangerous world. *Transplant Infect Dis.* 1999;1:65–75.
103. Stratta RJ, Shokouh-Amiri MH, Egidi MF, et al. A prospective comparison of simultaneous kidney-pancreas transplantation with systemic-enteric versus portal-enteric drainage. *Ann Surg.* 2001;233:740–751.
104. Bagdade JD, Ritter MC, Kitabchi AE, et al. Differing effects of pancreas-kidney transplantation with systemic versus portal venous drainage on cholesteryl ester transfer in IDDM subjects. *Diabetes Care.* 1996;19:1108–1112.
105. Carpentier A, Patterson BW, Uffelman KD, et al. The effect of systemic versus portal insulin delivery in pancreas transplantation on insulin action and VLDL metabolism. *Diabetes.* 2001;50:1402–1413.
106. Diem P, Abid M, Redmon JB, et al. Systemic venous drainage of pancreas allografts as independent cause of hyperinsulinemia in type I diabetic recipients. *Diabetes.* 1990;39:534–540.
107. Konigsrainer A, Foger BH, Miesenbock G, et al. Pancreas transplantation with systemic endocrine drainage leads to improvement in lipid metabolism. *Transplant Proc.* 1994;26:501–502.
108. Philosophe B, Farney AC, Schweitzer EJ, et al. Superiority of portal venous drainage over systemic venous drainage in pancreas transplantation: a retrospective study. *Ann Surg.* 2001;234:689–696.
109. Boggi U, Vistoli F, Signori S, et al. A technique for retroperitoneal pancreas transplantation with portal-enteric drainage. *Transplantation.* 2005;79:1137–1142.
110. Sutherland DE, Morel P, Gruessner RW. Transplantation of two diabetic patients with one divided cadaver donor pancreas. *Transplant Proc.* 1990;22:585.
111. Tyden G, Tibell A, Sandberg J. Improved results with a simplified technique for pancreaticoduodenal transplantation with enteric exocrine drainage. *Clin Transplant.* 1996;10:306.
112. Becker YT, Collins BH, Sollinger HW. Technical complications of pancreas transplantation. *Curr Opin Organ Transplant.* 1998;3:253.
113. Elkhammas EA, Henry ML, Tesi RJ, et al. Control of metabolic acidosis after pancreas transplantation using acetazolamide. *Transplant Proc.* 1991;23:1623–1624.
114. Schang T, Timmermann W, Thiede A, et al. Detrimental effects of fluid and electrolyte loss from duodenum in bladder-drained pancreas transplants. *Transplant Proc.* 1991;23:1617–1618.
115. Peltenburg HG, Mutsaerts KJ, Hardy EL, van Hooff JP. Sodium lactate as an alternative to sodium bicarbonate in the management of metabolic acidosis after pancreas transplantation. *Transplantation.* 1992;53:225–226.
116. Benedetti E, Coady NT, Asolati M, et al. A prospective randomized clinical trial of perioperative treatment with octreotide in pancreas transplantation. *Am J Surg.* 1998;175:14–17.
117. Carlsson PO, Jansson L. The long-acting somatostatin analogue octreotide decreases pancreatic islet blood flow in rats. *Pancreas.* 1994;9:361–364.
118. Kandaswamy R, Humar A, Gruessner AC, et al. Vascular graft thrombosis after pancreas transplantation: comparison of the FK 506 and cyclosporine eras. *Transplant Proc.* 1999;31:602–603.
119. Humar A, Gruessner RW, Sutherland DE. Living related donor pancreas and pancreas-kidney transplantation. *Br Med Bull.* 1997;53:879–891.
120. Benedetti E, Rastellini C, Sileri P, et al. Successful simultaneous pancreas-kidney transplantation from well-matched living-related donors. *Transplant Proc.* 2001;33:1689.
121. Calne RY, Rolles K, White DJ, et al. Cyclosporin A initially as the only immunosuppressant in 34 recipients of cadaveric organs: 32 kidneys, 2 pancreases, and 2 livers. *Lancet.* 1979;2:1033–1036.
122. Stratta RJ. Simultaneous use of tacrolimus and mycophenolate mofetil in combined pancreas-kidney transplant recipients: a multi-center report. The FK/MMF Multi-Center Study Group.*Transplant Proc.* 1997;29:654–655.
123. Gruessner AC, Sutherland DE. Analysis of United States (US) and non-US pancreas transplants as reported to the International Pancreas Transplant Registry (IPTR) and to the United Network for Organ Sharing (UNOS). *Clin Transpl.* 1998;53–73.
124. Gruessner RW, Sutherland DE, Drangstveit MB, et al. Mycophenolate mofetil and tacrolimus for induction and maintenance therapy after pancreas transplantation. *Transplant Proc.* 1998;30:518–520.
125. Gruessner RW, Sutherland DE, Parr E, et al. A prospective, randomized, open-label study of steroid withdrawal in pancreas transplantation-a preliminary report with 6-month follow-up. *Transplant Proc.* 2001;33:1663–1664.
126. Kaufman DB, Leventhal JR, Gallon LG. Pancreas transplantation in the prednisone-free era. *Am J Transplant.* 2003;3:322.
127. Salazar A, McAlister VC, Kiberd BA, et al. Sirolimus-tacrolimus combination for combined kidney-pancreas transplantation: effect on renal function. *Transplant Proc.* 2001;33:1038–1039.
128. Kaufman DB, Leventhal JR, Koffron AJ, et al. A prospective study of rapid corticosteroid elimination in simultaneous pancreas-kidney transplantation: comparison of two maintenance immunosuppression protocols: tacrolimus/mycophenolate mofetil versus tacrolimus/sirolimus. *Transplantation.* 2002;73:169–177.
129. Stratta RJ, Alloway RR, Lo A, Hodge E. A multicenter trial of two daclizumab dosing strategies versus no antibody induction in simultaneous kidney-pancreas transplantation: interim analysis. *Transplant Proc.* 2001;33:1692–1693.
130. Gruessner RW, Kandaswamy R, Humar A, et al. Calcineurin inhibitor- and steroid-free immunosuppression in pancreas-kidney and solitary pancreas transplantation. *Transplantation.* 2005;79:1184–1189.
131. Rubin RH. A new beginning. *Transplant Infect Dis.* 1999;1:1.
132. Villacian JS, Paya CV. Prevention of infections in solid organ transplant recipients. *Transplant Infect Dis.* 1999;1:50–64.
133. Tyan DB, Li VA, Czer L, et al. Intravenous immunoglobulin suppression of HLA alloantibody in highly sensitized transplant candidates and transplantation with a histoincompatible organ. *Transplantation.* 1994;57:553–562.
134. Glotz D, Haymann JP, Niaudet P, et al. Successful kidney transplantation of immunized patients after desensitization with normal human polyclonal immunoglobulins. *Transplant Proc.* 1995;27:1038–1039.
135. Jordan SC, Quartel AW, Czer LS, et al. Posttransplant therapy using high-dose human immunoglobulin (intravenous gammaglobulin) to control acute humoral rejection in renal and cardiac allograft recipients and potential mechanism of action. *Transplantation.* 1998;66:800–805.
136. Watanabe H, Misu K, Kobayashi T, et al. ABO-incompatible auxiliary partial orthotopic liver transplant for late-onset familial amyloid polyneuropathy. *J Neurol Sci.* 2002;195:63–66.
137. Shishido S, Asanuma H, Tajima E, et al. ABO-incompatible living-donor kidney transplantation in children. *Transplantation.* 2001;72:1037–1042.
138. Montgomery RA, Zachary AA, Racusen LC, et al. Plasmapheresis and intravenous immune globulin provides effective rescue therapy for refractory humoral rejection and allows kidneys to be successfully transplanted into cross-match-positive recipients. *Transplantation.* 2000;70:887–895.
139. Takeda A, Uchida K, Haba T, et al. Acute humoral rejection of kidney allografts in patients with a positive flow cytometry crossmatch (FCXM). *Clin Transplant.* 2000;14(Suppl 3):15–20.
140. Bittner HB, Dunitz J, Hertz M, et al. Hyperacute rejection in single lung transplantation–case report of successful management by means of plasmapheresis and antithymocyte globulin treatment. *Transplantation.* 2001;71:649–651.
141. Reddy KS, Stratta RJ, Shokouh-Amiri MH, et al. Surgical complications after pancreas transplantation with portal-enteric drainage. *J Am Coll Surg.* 1999;189:305–313.
142. Wuthrich RP. Factor V Leiden mutation: potential thrombogenic role in renal vein, dialysis graft and transplant vascular thrombosis. *Curr Opin Nephrol Hypertens.* 2001;10:409–414.
143. Friedman GS, Meier-Kriesche HU, Kaplan B, et al. Hypercoagulable states in renal transplant candidates: impact of anticoagulation upon incidence of renal allograft thrombosis. *Transplantation.* 2001;72:1073–1078.
144. Zibari GB, Aultman DF, Abreo KD, et al. Roux-en-Y venting jejunostomy in pancreatic transplantation: a novel approach to monitor rejection and prevent anastomotic leak. *Clin Transplant.* 2000;14:380–385.
145. Eckhoff DE, Ploeg RJ, Wilson MA, et al. Efficacy of 99mTc voiding cystourethrogram for detection of duodenal leaks after pancreas transplantation. *Transplant Proc.* 1994;26:462–463.
146. Roza AM, Johnson CP, Adams M. Acute torsion of the renal transplant after combined kidney-pancreas transplant. *Transplantation.* 1999;67:486–488.
147. West MS, Stevens RB, Metrakos P, et al. Renal pedicle torsion after simultaneous kidney-pancreas transplantation. *J Am Coll Surg.* 1998;187:80–87.
148. Del Pizzo JJ, Jacobs SC, Bartlett ST, Sklar GN. Urological complications of bladder-drained pancreatic allografts. *Br J Urol.* 1998;81:543–547.
149. Kaplan AJ, Valente JF, First MR, et al. Early operative intervention for urologic complications of kidney-pancreas transplantation. *World J Surg.* 1998;22:890–894.

150. Troppmann C, Gruessner AC, Dunn DL, et al. Surgical complications requiring early relaparotomy after pancreas transplantation: a multivariate risk factor and economic impact analysis of the cyclosporine era. *Ann Surg.* 1998;227:255–268.
151. Gruessner RW. Immunobiology, diagnosis, and treatment of pancreas graft rejection. In: Gruessner RW, Sutherland DE, eds. *Transplantation of the Pancreas.* New York, NY: Springer-Verlag; 2004:349–380.
152. Papadimitriou JC, Drachenberg CB, Wiland A, et al. Histologic grading of acute allograft rejection in pancreas needle biopsy: correlation to serum enzymes, glycemia, and response to immunosuppressive treatment. *Transplantation.* 1998;66:1741–1745.
153. Klassen DK, Weir MR, Cangro CB, et al. Pancreas allograft biopsy: safety of percutaneous biopsy-results of a large experience. *Transplantation.* 2002;73:553–555.
154. Malek SK, Potdar S, Martin JA, et al. Percutaneous ultrasound-guided pancreas allograft biopsy: a single-center experience. *Transplant Proc.* 2005; 37:4436–4437.
155. Auchincloss H Jr, Sachs DH. Xenogeneic transplantation. *Ann Rev Immunol.* 1998;16:433–470.
156. Lanza RP, Chick WL. Transplantation of encapsulated cells and tissues. *Surgery.* 1997;121:1–9.
157. Hering BJ, Wijkstrom M, Graham ML, et al. Prolonged diabetes reversal after intraportal xenotransplantation of wild-type porcine islets in immunosuppressed nonhuman primates. *Nat Med.* 2006;12:301–303.
158. Shapiro AM, Lakey JR. Future trends in islet cell transplantation. *Diabetes Technol Ther.* 2000 Autumn;2:449–452.
159. Cooke A, Phillips JM, Parish NM. Tolerogenic strategies to halt or prevent type 1 diabetes. *Nat Immunol.* 2001;2:810–815.

CHAPTER

74

Small Bowel Transplantation

KHALID M. KHAN, CHIRAG S. DESAI, and RAINER W. GRUESSNER

INTRODUCTION

The development of parenteral nutrition (PN) was instrumental in the mitigation of intestinal failure as a life-threatening illness. Unfortunately administration of PN is not without consequences. In particular, PN-associated liver disease (PNALD); central venous line–related sepsis and loss of vascular access pose severe limitation to survival of patients on PN. Transplantation of the small bowel would appear to be the natural next step. However, historically the large lymphoid presence in the small bowel (SB) and the complex role it plays in immune tolerance was considered a barrier to small bowel transplantation (SBTx) as a treatment option for intestinal failure. Despite these concerns, major strides have been achieved in the development of SBTx over the past 5 decades. Although the immunologic role of the SB remains the most challenging management problem among abdominal solid organ transplants, SBTx is the acknowledged treatment option for adults and children with intestinal failure who develop problems on intravenous nutrition (1).

PATHOPHYSIOLOGY OF INTESTINAL FAILURE

Organ failure that necessitates SBTx is either from disease or as a consequence of removal or loss of a critical length of SB. The term *short bowel syndrome* (SBS) is used to describe an anatomical reduction of SB length and, more specifically, the mucosal surface area. A disease of the intestine, therefore, may result in primary intestinal failure or the patient may develop SBS as a result of anatomical or mucosal loss.

Short Bowel Syndrome

A reduction in the bowel length that constitutes SBS is the most common scenario for intestinal failure in both adults and children (Fig. 74.1) (2). Although specific patterns to the loss of SB are dependent on the underlying etiology, the actual length of SB lost is variable and determines whether intestinal failure will occur. In infants, for instance, necrotizing enterocolitis typically involves the distal SB and cecum, while midgut volvulus in a malrotated bowel is demarked by the SB arterial vasculature in the mesentery. Both of these pathologies may result in sufficient loss of SB to cause SBS-related intestinal failure. Intestinal atresia and gastroschesis are the other most common causes of SBS in infants, where the length of bowel lost can be variable and segmental.

Volvulus related to malrotation is also a cause of SBS in adults, although vascular insufficiency from thrombosis or emboli is much more commonly seen. Additionally, and primarily in adults, loss of SB from trauma or as a consequence or complication of surgery—in particular, the Roux-en-Y gastric bypass procedure—may be extensive enough to develop intestinal failure from SBS. Radiation therapy represents a treatment where loss of intestinal function can be expected and does, rarely, result in intestinal failure.

Mucosal Disease

Primary disorders that result in intestinal failure in children include congenital enteropathies, while Crohn disease is the most common cause of intestinal failure in adults. The mechanism involves loss of absorptive function, shortening of the bowel, and resection of diseased bowel.

Neuromuscular Disease

Failure of function is the natural sequel to neuromuscular disease of the SB; the best known example of this is the total aganglionic form of Hirschsprung disease in infants. In children and adults, hollow visceral myopathy or neuropathy, presents clinically as pseudo-obstruction. Though pseudo-obstructive disorders are still not well understood from an etiopathologic perspective, they may accompany more systemic morphologic anomalies and familial cases of pseudo-obstruction presenting in childhood and adulthood are known to occur.

Malignancy

Primary or secondary malignances of the intestine do not cause intestinal failure in the majority of cases due to the localized nature of tumor at the time of diagnosis. While removal of the colon is a necessity for widespread disease related to hereditary polyposis, resection of the SB is usually limited though malabsorption may be a feature of extensive involvement. Desmoid tumors are unique in that while the SB mucosal surface is not involved, the SB may be encased by the tumor and cannot be resected.

Indication for a Liver Graft in Addition to a Small Bowel Graft

In the absence of a functional intestine, PN is the only method to deliver adequate nutrition. Although a life-saving therapy, there are clear consequences to the use of PN. Apart from those related to delivery of PN, hepatic steatosis or cholestasis may develop. In particular, the latter form of PNALD may progress to hepatic fibrosis and eventually result in portal hypertension. Cholestatic liver disease is multifactorial and historically most often seen in infants. It is associated with an extremely short SB, a bowel that is not in continuity and in a severely diseased short bowel where enteral feeding is not possible (3). Severe dysmotility may give rise to bacterial overgrowth, and repeated bouts of sepsis are precipitants of liver failure. Similarly, the length of the remnant SB necessary to

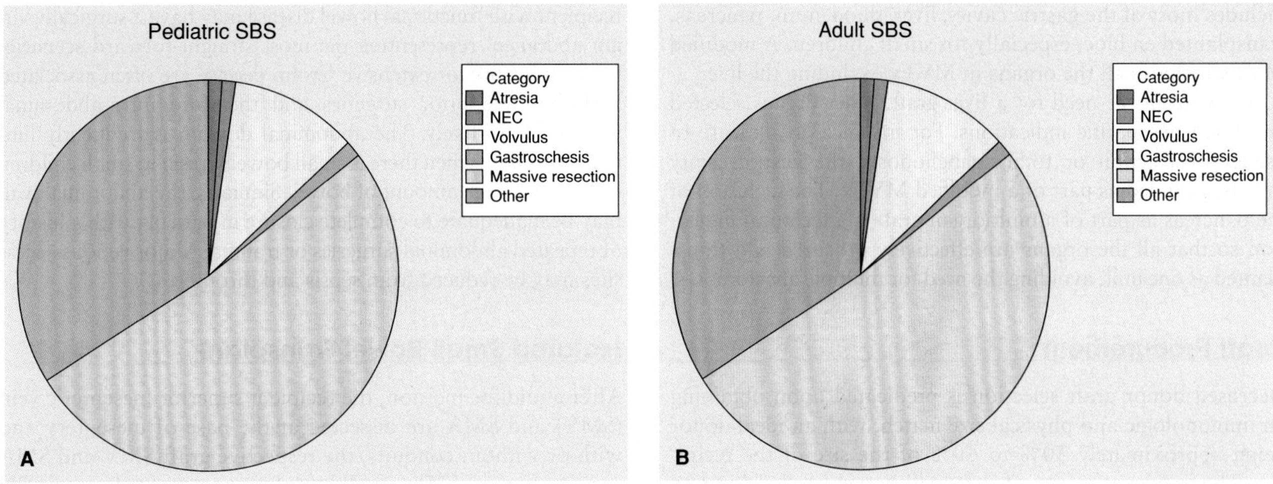

FIGURE 74.1 Causes of short bowel syndrome (SBS) leading to intestinal transplantation in children (**A**) and adults (**B**).

maintain adequate nutrition is much smaller with the preservation of the ileocecal valve (4). The contents of PN and particularly the lipid component has been regarded as a potential etiologic agent in the progression of cholestatic liver disease and, recently, limiting the lipid content and using an omega-3 rich formula based on fish oil have been shown to reduce the potential for cholestatic disease (5).

There are no clear definitions of intestinal failure that allow patient status quantification. The use of PN can potentially be tracked; short-term PN, whether in the hospital or ambulatory, is commonly used for nutritional support, but it does not necessarily imply intestinal failure. Furthermore SBS does not, in every case, necessarily result in intestinal failure. Patients may be on PN for a prolonged period, only to reestablish enteral nutrition after rehabilitation that may include surgery. Although population data is lacking in the United States, the Dutch registry recently reported a prevalence (per million) of 12.24 for adults and 9.56 for children with intestinal failure (6). If we were to apply these data to the United States United Network of Organ Sharing (UNOS) wait-list, data indicate that only a small proportion of patients with intestinal failure are wait-listed (2). In a multicenter study of children on continuous PN for more than 60 days, 29% were referred for SBTx (7).

TRANSPLANTATION

Patient Selection

Broadly similar to the use of dialysis for renal failure, PN is the immediate therapy for intestinal failure. In general, transplantation of the kidney is the preferred option for end-stage kidney disease so that patients, though on dialysis, will be wait-listed for kidney transplant.

Patients with intestinal failure have specific features that determine a poor outcome, including loss of central venous line access, recurrent episodes of dehydration while on intravenous therapy, systemic bacterial and fungal infection, and progressive liver disease. Not surprisingly these features have been determined by the United States Centers for Medicare and Medicaid Services to be indications for SBTx.

Evaluation of SBTx candidates for suitability for transplantation has developed over time as with other abdominal organ transplant recipients, and the necessity for a liver graft in a proportion of these patients puts them in competition with those on the liver transplant (alone) wait-list. Contraindications to transplant include the presence of a systemic infection; a history of malignancy is also a contraindication to transplantation, at least until a designated follow-up period has determined a state of cure; unstable cardiac status and primary immune deficiency present challenges to the success of operative and early post-transplant outcome and therefore may be deemed as relative contraindications. Patients with static neurologic injury are candidates and transplantation may simplify their overall care by reducing the need for support with PN and intravenous fluids. Age is not a usual limitation, but the general health of patients and their ability to tolerate the rigors of transplant are of importance. It has been noted that individuals with intestinal failure transplanted from home, as compared to inpatients, have a better outcome and is a statement on the importance of the patient's condition and the lack of reserve in more severely ill patients (1).

Malnutrition is a factor in poor perioperative outcome in general so that, in *all* SBTx candidates, nutritional deficiency must be addressed. Detailed imaging of the intra-abdominal vascular and enteric anatomy with computed tomography (CT) or magnetic resonance imaging (MRI) is a prerequisite, as is assessment for patency of central venous access sites. A liver biopsy and evaluation for portal hypertension will determine whether a patient is a candidate for a simultaneous liver graft. Additionally, SBTx candidates with a history of vascular thrombosis should be evaluated thoroughly for an underlying hypercoagulability disorder.

Graft Selection

The operative procedure of SBTx is still performed according to the "cluster" concept originally proposed by Thomas Starzl (8). The SB can be combined with the liver or with any of the abdominal viscera, including the abdominal wall if necessary. Isolated SBTx is the basic graft necessary to reconstitute primary SB function and comprises the SB from jejunum to ileum. The liver-small bowel transplant (L-SBTx) includes part or all of the liver. In practice, most of these transplants are a composite that includes the duodenum and the pancreas primarily to avoid the need for bile duct reconstruction. In a similar fashion, a multivisceral transplant (MVTx) of the small bowel includes most of the gastric cavity, liver, duodenum, pancreas, transplanted en bloc, especially for small children. A modified MVTx includes all the organs in MVTx excluding the liver.

Apart from the need for a liver graft, other organs selected are based on specific indications. For instance, in the case of pseudo-obstruction or total aganglionosis, the gastric cavity may be included as part of a modified MVTx. The inclusion of the pancreas as part of a multiorgan graft is a technical indication so that all the organs are effectively procured and transplanted as one unit, avoiding the need for multiple anastomoses.

Graft Procurement

Deceased donor graft selection is predicated upon obtaining an immunologic and physical size match, with an ideal donor being approximately 50% to 60% of the size of the recipient. The immunogenicity of the small bowel has led some to advocate antithymocyte treatment of the donor. Technically this may be a challenge given that multiple organs are usually procured from the youngest donors; the quality of the graft for SBTx is highly critical, and procurements after "brain death"—and not after "cardiac death"—are the ones most often considered suitable for Tx. A clinical history of gastrointestinal disease or bowel surgeries in the donor may be clues to inadequacy of the bowel as a graft.

Cannulation of the distal abdominal aorta to set up for the University of Wisconsin (UW) solution flush is the initial step in the donor operation. In preparation for cross-clamping, the supraceliac aorta is circumscribed, taking care that it should be as proximal as possible in pediatric donors in order to use the descending thoracic aorta for necessary conduits. *Isolated small bowel graft* procurement proceeds with dissection of the base of the mesentery followed by dissection of the portal vein and superior mesenteric artery (SMA) just below the pancreatic uncinate process; thereby facilitating pancreatic and small intestinal grafts from the same donor. In these cases, the inferior pancreatico-duodenal artery stays with the simultaneously procured donor pancreas. The small bowel is stapled just below the ligament of Treitz, and distally the colon is stapled at the level of left branch of middle colic vessel. The SMA is dissected free and looped at its origin and the pancreatic neck is then divided to remove the small bowel graft.

The *liver-small bowel and multivisceral graft* procurement commences as for an isolated small bowel graft. The tail of the pancreas and spleen is dissected, and the proximal duodenum is dissected and divided at the level of the pylorus. A patch containing the origins of the celiac axis and SMA is included with the potential of creating an aortic conduit if necessary. The graft is then removed *en bloc* including the pancreas, spleen, small bowel, liver, an intact inferior vena cava and duodenum. For a multivisceral graft, modified or otherwise, the stomach is included. A similar dissection is performed for the modified multivisceral graft with the exception that the liver is not included. The distal pancreas is resected or stapled off to the right of the mesenteric vessels. The left gastric artery and splenic arteries are ligated while the gastroduodenal and inferior pancreatico-duodenal arteries are preserved.

The Recipient Operative Procedure

The recipient procedure comes with challenges that depend on the underlying disorder that caused the intestinal failure. A recipient with functional bowel disease may have a surgically virgin abdomen, representing the most straight-forward scenario. Conversely, SBS or extensive Crohn disease are often associated with multiple prior surgeries and therefore intra-abdominal adhesions are likely. The abdominal domain is frequently limited, especially when there is small bowel atresia in small children or loss of a large amount of bowel. Similarly, the abdominal wall may be inadequate to complete closure in patients with a history of repeated abdominal surgeries or trauma. Major venous access sites may be reduced from sepsis and thrombosis.

Isolated Small Bowel Transplant

After a midline incision, the recipient superior mesenteric vein (SMV) and SMA are dissected at the base of mesentery and with or without conduits, the respective graft SMV and SMA are anastomosed. The small bowel is anastomosed proximally end-to-side or side-to-side to the recipient jejunum or distal duodenum (Fig. 74.2). A stoma, "chimney" or loop ileostomy is created and distal intestinal continuity is established either end-to-end or side-to-end with the recipient colon. If the mesentery is scarred and primary portal drainage is not possible, the portal flow is drained systemically; the SMV is anastomosed end-to-side to the inferior vena cava, similarly the SMA may be anastomosed end-to-side to the infrarenal aorta.

Liver-Small Bowel Transplant

A midline incision is performed with bilateral subcostal extensions facilitating dissection of the liver hilum, and ligation of the hepatic artery and common bile duct. The portal vein is then dissected and prepared for construction of a native portocaval shunt to the infrahepatic vena cava. This is followed by dissecting the liver from the cava as for a "piggyback" liver transplant exposing the infrarenal aorta for anastomosis. A thoracic aortic donor conduit is then placed on the infrarenal aorta to facilitate inflow to the graft; in some cases the supraceliac aorta is used. The hepatic veins are now clamped and the liver removed. An end-to-side, "native," portocaval shunt is constructed. The graft is then brought into the field and the suprahepatic caval anastomosis is performed in a piggyback fashion. In children, the entire aorta with the origin of celiac

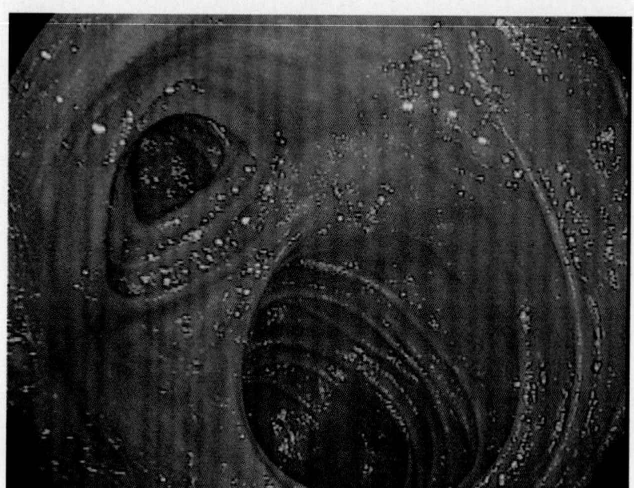

FIGURE 74.2 Endoscopic view of the proximal small bowel graft anastomosis (side-to-side).

and SMA is used for inflow. In adults, an iliac-Y-graft can be used to establish inflow. Enteral continuity is reestablished with a side-to-side graft duodeno-jejunal junction anastomosis with the recipient distal duodenum or proximal jejunum depending on the recipient anatomy. The distal anastomosis is as with an isolated SBTx; a gastrostomy or a gastrojejunostomy tube is placed to facilitate nutrition.

Multivisceral Transplant

Radical surgery is performed to remove the entire splanchnic circulation with associated viscera including the pancreas and spleen, the root of the small bowel mesentery, the stomach, and the liver. The celiac and SMA are ligated, and the organs are removed together, preserving the inferior vena cava for piggyback liver transplant. Vascular anastomoses and enteral continuity is reestablished as for liver-small bowel graft implantation. A pyloroplasty is usually performed to improve gastric emptying.

Operative Caveats

Size-matched organ availability is an issue for small children, and the use of larger donors may be necessary. In adults and children, loss of abdominal domain may result in an inability to obtain primary closure of the abdominal wall. Alternatives for abdominal closure include abdominal expansion, nonbiologic or biologic mesh, acellular dermal matrix, human skin, a rotational flap, and/or a donor abdominal wall graft implanted into the recipient's iliac or epigastric vessels (9–11).

Living Donor Small Bowel Transplant

Early attempts at living donor (LD) SBTx were not successful long-term because of technical issues and/or ongoing need for TPN. In the 1990s, a successful, standardized technique was developed by Rainer Gruessner at the University of Minnesota, using 150 to 200 cm of the distal jejunum and ileum, leaving 40 cm of prececal ileum and the ileocecal valve; the arterial supply was limited to only one artery and vein of the superior mesenteric vessels (12). Using this technique, Enrico Benedetti, at the University of Illinois, subsequently reported the combination of LD liver and small bowel grafts (13). Apart from the obvious advantages of human leukocyte antigen (HLA) matching, there is shorter graft ischemia time, reduction in wait-list numbers and avoidance of a simultaneous liver graft if advanced PNALD is not yet present. Selection of the *donor* for LD is not dissimilar to other solid organs with particular attention to the arterial supply a necessity (14).

Posttransplant Management

The general issues related to global care of the postoperative patient after major surgery apply to the SBTx patient. The common issues include respiratory support, fluid balance and nutrition, and pain relief. Initial nutritional rehabilitation of the donor small bowel in the recipient is based on the premise that the small bowel is in a denervated state and that lymphatic channels will take several weeks to form. A low fat, predigested formula is therefore standard for adults and children and antimotility drugs are necessary to reduce fluid and electrolyte losses. Anticipatory management of the SBTx patient in the posttransplant period is centered on certain areas that are discussed below.

Posttransplant surgical complications require vigilance in the first several days after transplantation and include the possibility of thrombosis of vascular conduits, dehiscence of anastomoses and perforation of the graft from loss of integrity or from indwelling feeding tubes. Surveillance for arterial vascular compromise with frequent visual examination of the ostomy site and regular Doppler ultrasound evaluation are routine. Similarly, abdominal ultrasound is performed for the examination of hepatic vessels.

The second potential source of morbidity in the early posttransplant period is infection, either bacterial or fungal; prophylaxis for both is routine for the first several days. As noted, hospitalized patients at the time of transplant have the highest morbidity in the posttransplant period, in part related to control of sepsis in the peritransplant period, and will be further dependent on complications during surgery. Tailoring the antimicrobial regimen to specific pathogens based on laboratory findings may be necessary under these circumstances.

The third major issue is acute cellular rejection (Fig. 74.3). Not surprisingly, immunosuppressive regimens are more aggressive in this group of patients as compared to other abdominal organ transplants. In order to preempt the development of severe rejection, serial small bowel biopsies are taken routinely through the distal stoma. Acute rejection is typically heralded by the onset diarrhea or increased ostomy output. The presentation is the same for enteric viral infections, particularly with adenovirus, rotavirus and norovirus; these must be differentiated from acute rejection.

Immunosuppression

Current induction regimens consist of high-dose steroids along with interleukin (IL)-2 receptor blockade and/or antithymocyte globulin (1); maintenance immunosuppression is based on tacrolimus. A second agent is considered by most to be necessary for several months and often much longer. Commonly used agents include mycophenolate and sirolimus (15,16). Alemtuzumab has also been an induction agent historically though it has been less commonly used in children (17). Consistent with the notion that the small bowel is a highly immunogenic organ, acute cellular rejection after SBTx has been shown to occur more aggressively than rejection of any other abdominal organ and is seen in up to 70% of recipients (18). However, more recent data indicate that rates of acute cellular rejection have improved with current regimens. Treatment regimens for established acute cellular rejection are based on the same agents as used for induction. Apart from severe acute cellular rejection, graft loss occurs from chronic allograft dysfunction, the nature and precise etiology of which remains to be elucidated (19). Monoclonal antibodies to tumor necrosis factor (TNF)-α have been shown to be effective for treating acute rejection especially for intractable cases (20). Antibody-mediated acute rejection is a risk in patients with high circulating levels of antibody as determined by panel-reactive antibody (PRA) testing (21). Similar to renal transplant patients, a high PRA level is of great concern in retransplant cases. Our center has previously demonstrated that mutations in the gene coding for nucleotide-binding oligomerization domain containing 2 (NOD2) may also have a role in rejection (22). This finding may be of significance given the relationship of the mutation and Crohn disease and may also explain the response to anti–TNF-α treatment.

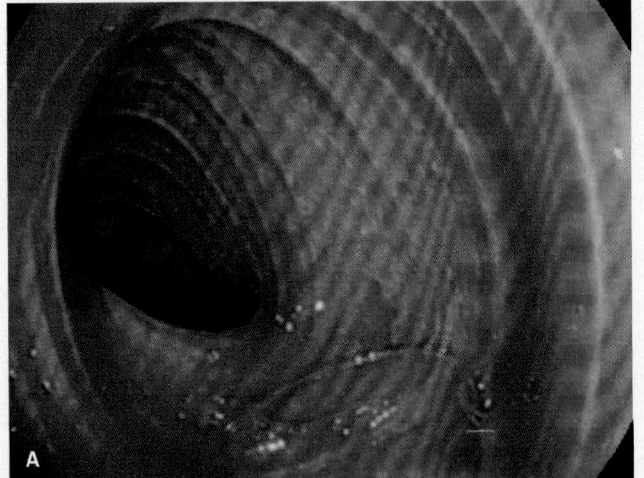

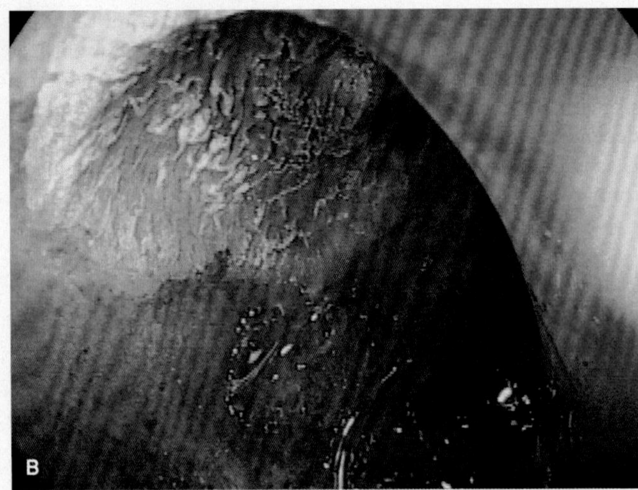

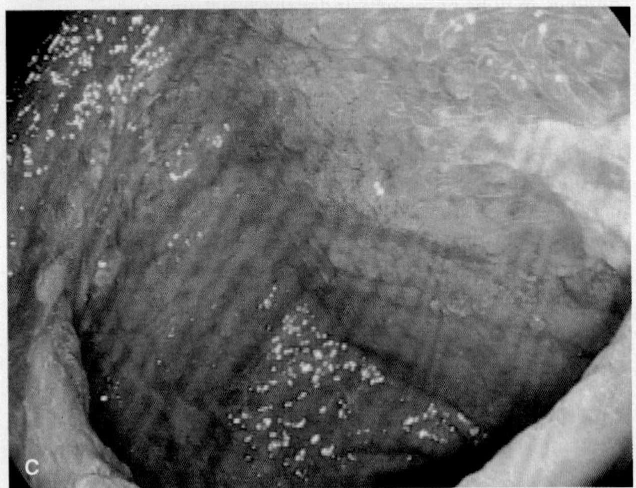

FIGURE 74.3 A: Severe acute rejection of the small bowel graft. B: Early regeneration after treatment of severe acute rejection of the small bowel graft. C: Hyperplastic mucosa typical of almost complete regeneration of the small bowel graft.

Posttransplant Viral Infections

Viral infections are a concern in the posttransplant period, especially in younger children and infants who have not had sufficient exposure to seroconvert. Titers for cytomegalovirus (CMV) and Epstein–Barr virus (EBV) DNA by polymerase chain reaction are checked weekly and CMV prophylaxis is routine for the first several months. Development of DNAemia of EBV raises concerns for the potential to develop posttransplant lymphoproliferative disease (PTLD).

The inability to control viral elements under potent immunosuppression is a common problem among different transplant groups. Historically, CMV was a common occurrence in the early posttransplant period and remains a major risk in CMV-negative recipients of CMV-positive donors. Fortunately, current anti-CMV prophylaxis regimens are largely successful in preventing CMV viremia. There is, however, no specific treatment for EBV and the potential for PTLD remains especially in the SBTx population. There has also been a reduction in the number of cases of PTLD and outcome of PTLD has improved with more diligent use of immunosuppressive agents and rituximab (23).

Viruses that affect the GI tract directly are of particular concern in the posttransplant period. Adenovirus, norovirus, and rotavirus are a source of morbidity for SBTx patients especially early in the posttransplant period. Not insignificant is the impact of common viral infections such as respiratory syncytial virus (RSV) that may result in respiratory failure. Beyond drastically lowering immune suppression and supportive care effective anti-viral therapies are yet to be developed for most viruses.

Patient and Graft Outcomes

Outcome of patients following SBTx have improved over the past two decades (1,18). We have previously reported a dichotomy in the patient outcome of transplants with those needing a liver-inclusive graft having a high rate of attrition in the immediate posttransplant period (18,19). This is largely explained in that patients with liver failure are much sicker at the time of transplant. Patient survival at 1 year can be expected to be around 90% with current practices. Patient and graft survival rates at 5 years have been around 50% to 60%, and there has also been a gradual increase over time. Early deaths are mainly caused by sepsis and rejection. Later deaths are also related to sepsis and rejection, along with PTLD.

Solid organ transplantation has matured to the point that retransplantation of organs is well established in certain circumstances. The small bowel recipient is at greatest risk for graft failure from severe ACR with the potential of mucosa deprived small bowel to be the portal for immediate translocation of microorganisms. Under such circumstances, the graft may have to be removed to save the patient. Unfortunately when this involves L-SBTx or MVTx, removal of the small bowel is obviously not an option (18). This may account for the differences in early patient and graft outcome between L-SBTx and MVTx versus SBTx (19).

Long-term complications are yet to be defined in this population. Another complicating factor is the use of calcineurin inhibitors and, probably is an even greater issue than in other transplant populations. The most significant side effect is chronic renal impairment and the need for dialysis, or even kidney transplantation, in a proportion of these patients (24).

Social and Financial Outcomes

Patients with intestinal failure on PN typically struggle with day-to-day issues. A successful transplant without the need for parenteral support and gastrointestinal symptoms clearly improves quality of life for these patients. Although the cost of SBTx is not insignificant, as compared to other solid organ transplants, improved survival beyond the immediate post-transplant period makes it much more cost effective as compared to long-term PN (25). The comparison itself is of little significance because only patients with complications on long-term PN are considered for transplantation. As yet, there are no data available to compare transplant to the newer modalities applied to the treatment of intestinal failure (see below).

RECENT TRENDS

Composition of Multiorgan Transplant Grafts

The inclusion of the colon along with the small bowel has not been a standardized part of the intestinal graft. We have noted, however, that there is a tendency toward terminal ileal inflammation in patients with a native colon and graft ileal anastomosis. This inflammation is most often amenable to antibiotics, indicating that the backwash of organisms from the native colon is the likely cause. At our center, it has become routine to include the colon graft where possible, with the result that, with this procedural modification, ileal inflammatory problems have not been a problem. More importantly there has been no increase in the rate of complications from adding the colon as a graft.

The Wait-List

Historically, mortality on the transplant wait-list was highest for patients awaiting SBTx. Infants with an extremely short small bowel were at greatest risk for the development of liver failure and comprised the major patient population. In the last decade, these compelling observations resulted in a change in the prioritization of organs by UNOS. We have shown that, more recently, there has been a marked reduction in the numbers of pediatric patients on the wait-list, especially those requiring a liver graft. There were no corresponding changes in adults or children waiting for an isolated SBTx. Our findings are an indication of the improvements in the management of intestinal failure in infants and in particular PNALD. As it is the common practice now, reducing the component of soy-based lipid in the PN or using a fish oil–based emulsion that has a greater omega-3/omega-6 long-chain fatty acid component has impacted the numbers of infants with progressive cholestatic PNALD (26). Although less quantifiable, the routine use of the serial transverse enteroplasty (STEP) for infants with a dilated small bowel remnant may also have had an impact. The glucagon like polypeptide-2 (GLP2) analog teduglutide (Gattex, Shire pharmaceuticals) is now used in adult patients although it is not clear whether this will reduce the number of patients that eventually require SBTx.

Transplant Outcomes and Inclusion of the Liver

We have also reported that a liver-inclusive graft may confer a benefit to other transplants, including lung transplant (27). This is consistent with the general consensus that the liver adds an immunologic advantage that improves the recipients tolerance to other organs transplanted simultaneously. Conversely it has also been reported in pediatric patients that food allergy may be increased after transplantation of solid organs; the majority of reports involve liver transplant patients. The liver is known to process antigen that arrives through the portal circulation so that increased tendency to food allergy after liver transplant may be related to immune dysregulation. Furthermore we have demonstrated an increase in prevalence of food allergy and eosinophilic esophagitis in children after SBTx as compared to children in the community (28). We speculate that abnormal uptake of food antigens by the small bowel graft may be implicated in the development of food allergy in children after SBTx.

FUTURE DIRECTIONS

There is clearly a role for SBTx in children and adults with intestinal failure facing possible death from recurrent septicemia, loss of central venous access, and PNALD. There appears to be less need for SBTx for pediatric patients, however it is not clear how many patients that remain stable or wean off intravenous nutrition will eventually need transplantation (29). Therefore, individuals who remain stable on long-term PN need careful monitoring. There are future prospects for new immunosuppressive regimens, especially immune-modulating biologic medications, of which there are a number in development. Current challenges include a better understanding of the mechanisms involved in chronic graft loss and safe transplantation of highly sensitized patients. Newly discovered avenues in the mechanism of rejection such as the T helper cell (TH)17 pathway may be of future relevance (30). There are also nontransplant options that continue to evolve, such as tissue engineering and the impact of GLP2 treatment; their impact on the wait-list remains to be seen.

Key Points

- Persistent cholestasis in patients on PN is predictor of mortality and an indication for small bowel transplantation.
- Thrombosis of central venous access sites in the upper limbs and neck are an indication for small bowel transplantation.
- Increased ostomy output or diarrhea is the typical presentation of acute rejection and needs to be differentiated from viral causes of diarrhea.

References

1. Fishbein TM. Intestinal transplantation. *N Engl J Med.* 2009;361:998–1008.
2. Khan KM, Desai CS, Mete M, et al. Developing trends in the intestinal transplant waitlist. *Am J Transplant.* 2014;14(12):2830–2837.
3. Spencer AU, Neaga A, West B, et al. Pediatric short bowel syndrome: redefining predictors of success. *Ann Surg.* 2005;242:403–409; discussion 409–412.
4. Khan FA, Squires RH, Litman HJ, et al; Pediatric Intestinal Failure Consortium. Predictors of enteral autonomy in children with intestinal failure: a multicenter cohort study. *J Pediatr.* 2015;167(1):29–34.
5. Diamond IR, Sterescu A, Pencharz PB, et al. Changing the paradigm: omegaven for the treatment of liver failure in pediatric short bowel syndrome. *J Pediatr Gastroenterol Nutr.* 2009;48(2):209–215.
6. Neelis EG, Roskott AM, Dijkstra G, et al. Presentation of a nationwide multicenter registry of intestinal failure and intestinal transplantation. *Clin Nutr.* 2016;35(1):225–229.
7. Squires RH, Duggan C, Teitelbaum DH, et al; Pediatric Intestinal Failure Consortium. Natural history of pediatric intestinal failure: initial report from the Pediatric Intestinal Failure Consortium. *J Pediatr.* 2012;161(4):723–728.
8. Starzl TE, Todo S, Tzakis A, et al. The many faces of multivisceral transplantation. *Surg Gynecol Obstet.* 1991;172:335–344.
9. Levi DM, Tzakis AG, Kato T, et al. Transplantation of the abdominal wall. *Lancet.* 2003;361:2173–2176.
10. DiBenedetto F, Lauro A, Masetti M, et al. Use of prosthetic mesh in difficult abdominal wall closure after small bowel transplantation in adults. *Transplant Proc.* 2005;37:2272–2274.
11. Asham E, Uknis ME, Rastellini C, et al. Acellular dermal matrix provides a good option for abdominal wall closure following small bowel transplantation: a case report. *Transplant Proc.* 2006;38:1770–1771.
12. Gruessner RW, Sharp HL. Living related intestinal transplantation: first report of a standardized surgical technique. *Transplantation.* 1997;11: 271–274.
13. Tzvetanov IG, Oberholzer J, Benedetti E. Current status of living donor small bowel transplantation. *Curr Opin Organ Transplant.* 2010;15(3):346–348.
14. Testa G, Panaro F, Schena S, et al. Living related small bowel transplantation: donor surgical technique. *Ann Surg.* 2004;240:779–784.
15. Fishbein TM, Florman S, Gondolesi G, et al. Intestinal transplantation before and after the introduction of sirolimus. *Transplantation.* 2002;73: 1538–1542.
16. Vianna RM, Mangus RS, Fridell JA, et al. Induction immunosuppression with thymoglobulin and rituximab in intestinal and multivisceral transplantation. *Transplantation.* 2008;85:1290–1293.
17. Tzakis AG, Kato T, Nishida S, et al. Alemtuzumab (Campath-1H) combined with tacrolimus in intestinal and multivisceral transplantation. *Transplantation.* 2003;75:1512–1517.
18. Desai CS, Gruessner AC, Khan KM, et al. Isolated intestinal transplants vs. liver-intestinal transplants in adult patients in the United States: 22 yr of OPTN data. *Clin Transplant.* 2012;26(4):622–628.
19. Desai CS, Khan KM, Gruessner AC, et al. Intestinal retransplantation: analysis of organ procurement and transplantation network database. *Transplantation.* 2012;93(1):120–125.
20. Pascher A, Radke C, Dignass A, et al. Successful infliximab treatment of steroid and OKT3 refractory acute cellular rejection in two patients after intestinal transplantation. *Transplantation.* 2003;76:615–618.
21. Hawksworth JS, Rosen-Bronson S, Island E, et al. Successful isolated intestinal transplantation in sensitized recipients with the use of virtual crossmatching. *Am J Transplant.* 2012;12(Suppl 4):S33–S42.
22. Fishbein T, Novitskiy G, Mishra L, et al. NOD2-expressing bone marrow-derived cells appear to regulate epithelial innate immunity of the transplanted human small intestine. *Gut.* 2008;57(3):323–330.
23. Nishida S, Kato T, Burney T, et al. Rituximab treatment for posttransplantation lymphoproliferative disorder after small bowel transplantation. *Transplant Proc.* 2002;34:957.
24. Pironi L, Lauro A, Soverini V, et al. Renal function in patients on long-term home parenteral nutrition and in intestinal transplant recipients. *Nutrition.* 2014;30(9):1011–1014.
25. Roskott AM, Groen H, Rings EH, et al. Cost-effectiveness of intestinal transplantation for adult patients with intestinal failure: a simulation study. *Am J Clin Nutr.* 2015;101(1):79–86.
26. Cowles RA, Ventura KA, Martinez M, et al. Reversal of intestinal failure-associated liver disease in infants and children on parenteral nutrition: experience with 93 patients at a referral center for intestinal rehabilitation. *J Pediatr Surg.* 2010;45(1):84–87; discussion 87–88.
27. Desai CS, Gruessner A, Habib S, et al. Survival of cystic fibrosis patients undergoing liver and liver-lung transplantations. *Transplant Proc.* 2013; 45(1):290–292.
28. Khan KM, Desai CS, Fishbein TM, Kaufman SS. Esophageal eosinophilic disease after intestinal transplantation in children. *Transplantation.* 2014;98(3):e25–e28.
29. Matsumoto CS, Kaufman SS, Island ER, et al. Hepatic explant pathology of pediatric intestinal transplant recipients previously treated with omega-3 fatty acid lipid emulsion. *J Pediatr.* 2014;165(1):59–64.
30. Yang JJ, Feng F, Hong L, et al. Interleukin-17 plays a critical role in the acute rejection of intestinal transplantation. *World J Gastroenterol.* 2013; 19(5):682–691.

CHAPTER
75
Renal Transplantation

LINDA L. WONG, KIMI R. UEDA, and V. RAM PEDDI

INTRODUCTION

Because of advances in critical care and medical treatment, more patients are living with end-stage renal disease (ESRD). By the end of 2009, more than 398,000 patients in the United States received some form of renal replacement therapy for ESRD. The economic burden of ESRD is staggering, with $42.5 billion spent in the United States in public and private funds in 2009. The annual cost for treating a patient on hemodialysis is approximately $70,000 which is about three times the cost of caring for a transplant patient (1). Renal transplantation is clearly the most cost-effective treatment option for ESRD when compared to all other forms of renal replacement therapy (2,3). The improvement in outcome after renal transplantation has resulted in a more liberal selection of patients. Unfortunately, the demand for kidney transplants far exceeds the supply of available organs. Although nearly 110,000 patients currently await renal transplantation in the United States, only 17,106 renal transplant procedures were performed in 2014 (4). As a result, patients on the deceased donor organ transplant waiting list wait prolonged periods and suffer the consequences of chronic disease and associated comorbidities before finally undergoing transplantation. This serious shortage of donor kidneys has prompted many institutions to expand their donor criteria. In an attempt to increase the utilization of suboptimal kidneys, transplantation of both kidneys (dual transplant) with intent to increase the nephron-mass into a single recipient has been performed at some centers with good short-term results (5). There has been increase in the use of organs from donors after cardiac death (non–heart-beating donors) also with good results (6,7). Another innovative strategy to increase living-donor transplantation includes "kidney paired exchange programs" in which incompatible living-donor/recipient pairs are enrolled in a registry in hopes of finding a compatible pair by exchange. This can sometimes result in complicated chains of exchange and these kidneys now travel to distant centers. Although this can potentially increase the opportunity for kidney transplant, it can also increase the ischemic times of living-donor kidneys, which traditionally had little, if any, cold ischemia time, as the procurement and transplant procedures were previously done within the same institutions. For these reasons, the result of which may lead to an increase in the incidence of delayed or slow graft function, the critical care management of these patients has become increasingly important. Furthermore, advances in transplant management now allows for long-term survival after transplantation. There are now over 140,000 patients living on chronic immunosuppression after renal transplant in the United States, some of whom may present to the critical care unit for unique problems and complications long after they have undergone transplant surgery (8).

EVALUATION OF POTENTIAL TRANSPLANT CANDIDATE

Before undergoing renal transplantation, each patient must undergo thorough evaluation, as not all ESRD patients are appropriate candidates for transplantation. Although each center has a specific protocol for candidate evaluation, the main purpose of any evaluation is to identify major contraindications to transplantation including active malignancy, advanced cardiopulmonary disease, active infection, substance abuse, and noncompliance with medical therapy. With most malignancies, a waiting period before transplantation is recommended (time period varies with the type of malignancy) and patients should be thoroughly evaluated for any recurrence or metastasis, which would contraindicate transplantation. There is no completely reliable algorithm for evaluating patients for cardiac disease for renal transplant surgery. General recommendations include noninvasive cardiac stress testing for the following population: diabetics, males older than 45 years, females older than 55 years, a family history of premature cardiac disease (myocardial infarction [MI] or sudden death in first-degree male relative younger than 55 years or first-degree female relative younger than 65 years), current cigarette smoking, hypertension, total cholesterol above 200 mg/dL, and high–density-lipoprotein cholesterol below 35 mg/dL. For those with positive stress testing, coronary angiography may be indicated. Some centers routinely advocate coronary angiography for all diabetics, as the incidence of ischemic heart disease is high in this population (9).

Patients undergoing evaluation should be screened for hepatitis B and C viruses, and HIV; any active infection should be treated. Although hepatitis B and C viruses and HIV positivity are not absolute contraindications, patients with advanced forms of these infections are generally not candidates for transplantation.

Other potential relative contraindications to transplantation include obesity, severe peripheral vascular/cerebrovascular disease, and advanced age. Although obesity is not an absolute contraindication, U.S. data on over 27,000 patients have indicated that those with morbid obesity (body mass index [BMI] >35) have a higher rate of delayed graft function, acute rejection, and worse overall survival, as well as longer hospitalizations (10). Thrombophilia, prostatic disease, high immunologic sensitization, psychosocial problems, and renal diseases with a high recurrence rate such as focal and segmental glomerulosclerosis should be identified during this transplant evaluation. Potential anatomic abnormalities such as severe iliac arterial disease and genitourinary anomalies should also be delineated before transplantation.

Candidates on the deceased donor waiting list should be reassessed periodically for any changes in the status of their medical and psychosocial problems. Potential recipients with diabetes mellitus should be evaluated annually as they often have associated ischemic heart disease. As patients wait longer for deceased organ donors, they will need to be monitored carefully as significant changes in their medical status may occur during the waiting period.

TYPES OF DONORS

Kidneys are transplanted from deceased donors after brain death or cardiac death, and from living donors. Brain death is defined by the Uniform Determination of Death Act of 1981 as follows: "an individual is dead if there is irreversible cessation of circulatory and respiratory functions or if there is irreversible cessation of all brain functions of the entire brain, including the brainstem." A brain-dead donor has suffered head trauma, cerebrovascular accident, cerebral anoxia, or a nonmetastasizing brain tumor. Physicians caring for the patient can diagnose brain death with the assistance of physical examination findings and a confirmatory study: an apnea test, a nuclear brain flow scan, or—less commonly—an electroencephalogram, though none of these tests is specifically required. It is the responsibility of all health professionals, and especially critical care medicine physicians, to report all patients with brain death and impending brain death to the local organ procurement organization (OPO). Once family members have accepted that their relative is brain dead, the trained donation coordinator may approach the family to discuss organ donation.

Because of the disparity between organ demand and supply, kidneys that traditionally would not have been used are now being considered. These deceased donors were previously defined by the United Network for Organ Sharing (UNOS), the national organization that coordinates organ allocation, as "expanded donors." Expanded criteria donors (ECDs) included all kidneys procured from donors of age older than 60, or aged between 50 and 59 years with at least two of the following: hypertension, serum creatinine over 1.5 mg/dL, or death due to a cerebrovascular accident. Some studies have shown that recipients of kidneys with expanded donor criteria have slightly diminished graft function, but comparable long-term graft and patient survival (11). Use of ECD kidneys may offer survival advantages to those on dialysis and were previously offered principally to recipients older than 60 years or perhaps allocated to OPOs with longer waiting times (12). As of late 2014, a new kidney allocation scheme (KAS) was implemented. The primary goal of this scheme was to extend the length of time kidney recipients have a functioning transplant by better allocating kidneys to the appropriate recipient. Each donor kidney is now assigned a Kidney Donor Profile Index (KDPI) score, which ranges from 0% to 100% based upon donor factors: age, weight, creatinine, race, hypertension, diabetes, and hepatitis C status. Those kidneys with a KDPI over 85% are comparable to the ECD kidneys and are considered to be of higher risk. The true outcome and long-term consequences of this allocation system will be more evident in the next few years.

In donation after cardiac death (DCD), death is determined by the usual cardiopulmonary criteria, that is, the absence of circulation, and can be used in clinical scenarios in which the donor does not meet brain death criteria. Conditions that may warrant consideration of DCD include irreversible brain injury, end-stage musculoskeletal disease, and high spinal cord injury. Early reports suggest that the time between extubation of the donor and the initiation of cold perfusion of the organs (warm ischemia) should be less than 60 minutes for successful kidney removal and function, though this does vary somewhat between centers (13).

Living donors are people who have been evaluated extensively both medically and psychosocially for possible donor nephrectomy. Medical evaluation should include thorough history and physical examination, laboratory studies (chemistry panel, complete blood count, hepatitis B and C viruses, and HIV testing, ABO typing, tissue typing, cross-match testing), 24-hour urine for creatinine clearance and protein, chest radiograph, computed tomography (CT), or magnetic resonance imaging (MRI) to evaluate both kidneys. Psychosocial evaluation is done to determine the emotional relation of the donor to the potential recipient and to ensure that the donor truly desires to donate and for altruistic reasons (not financial or other gain). An individual should be considered as a potential living donor only if the following basic requirements have been fulfilled:

- Donor and recipient are ABO blood group compatible.
- The warm T-lymphocyte cross-match is negative.
- The person is in excellent physical condition, emotionally stable, and well motivated.
- The individual is willing to undergo donor nephrectomy, is fully informed about the procedure, and is not under pressure from family members to donate a kidney.

The cytotoxic T-cell cross-match must be negative immediately before transplantation in order to proceed with surgery. A positive high-titer B-cell cross-match is also a contraindication to transplantation; however, transplantation may proceed in the presence of a low-titer B-cell cross-match, provided that the T-cell cross-match and the flow cytometry cross-match are negative (14).

IMMEDIATE PREOPERATIVE MANAGEMENT

Appropriate recipients are selected based on a list that is generated by UNOS. This list takes into account the following factors: ABO blood type, human leukocyte antigen (HLA) matching, antibody testing, and waiting time. Although potential recipients are familiar to the transplant center physicians, they are carefully evaluated for recent infection or illness with blood tests, chest radiograph, and electrocardiogram (ECG). Because waiting lists are long and patients may have been waiting for several years, other illnesses may have developed in the interim that may contraindicate transplant surgery. Patients may require a treatment of hemodialysis or peritoneal dialysis prior to transplant surgery if there is evidence of hyperkalemia or fluid overload.

IMMEDIATE POSTTRANSPLANT MANAGEMENT

Renal transplantation is carried out in the standard fashion through an incision that exposes the iliac fossa. The donor renal vessels are sutured in an end-to-side fashion to the external iliac artery and vein and a ureteroneocystostomy is created. Patients are monitored with continuous ECG and central venous pressure in the immediate postoperative period. Blood pressures are carefully monitored, as most patients have underlying hypertension and administration of immunosuppressive medications such as corticosteroids can affect blood pressure control. In addition, pain, catecholamine release, and fluid status may contribute to difficulties with blood pressure control. Although adequate blood pressure control is important for the integrity of the renal arterial anastomosis, it is equally important to avoid hypotension and therefore prevent renal hypoperfusion and graft thrombosis.

Urine output is carefully monitored on an hourly basis via an indwelling urinary catheter. This urinary catheter also serves to protect the ureteroneocystostomy during the early postoperative period. Any increase in intravesical pressure due to incomplete emptying of the bladder could compromise the newly created anastomosis between the ureter and bladder. Hematuria occurring early posttransplant may be due to bleeding at the ureteral anastomosis, in the bladder, or along the urethra. This can be managed with gentle flushing of the urinary catheter with 20 to 30 mL of sterile saline; changing the urinary catheter to one of a larger caliber may also help remove clots. Three-way urinary catheters are also used to facilitate continuous bladder irrigation should other measures fail to treat the hematuria.

Blood glucose monitoring is also done on a regular basis. Many transplant recipients have underlying diabetes mellitus and all patients may have hyperglycemia exacerbation related to administration of steroids and other immunosuppressive agents. Use of continuous insulin infusion and frequent blood glucose monitoring may be necessary to maintain good glycemic control. Optimal control of hyperglycemia in the postoperative period and in critically ill patients has been shown to decrease morbidity and mortality (15,16).

Particular attention should be paid to the volume and electrolyte status as the urine output in the immediate posttransplant period can vary from oliguria (frequently due to delayed graft function) to several liters as a result of generous fluid replacement during the surgery and also due to solute-induced osmotic diuresis. Living-donor allografts typically have excellent immediate function and may have prompt and marked diuresis. Most transplant centers utilize a center-specific protocol with a fixed-rate maintenance of intravenous fluids usually with 0.9% normal saline at 50 to 100 mL/hr together with replacement fluid at two-thirds or one-half of previous hour urine output. Some recipients may need hourly fluid replacement on a milliliter-for-milliliter basis in order to keep up with fluid losses. Kidneys from expanded donors or DCD or with longer cold ischemia times may not have immediate function due to acute tubular necrosis (ATN). These recipients should be kept on a maintenance volume of intravenous fluids and the central venous pressure can be used to guide fluid status (Fig. 75.1). Other factors to consider would include the timing of the last dialysis and the amount of urine produced by the patient before transplant. Hemodialysis treatment shortly before the transplant surgery may render a recipient relatively hypovolemic during the perioperative period. Patients who have not yet been started on renal replacement therapy or who make a normal amount of urine may not have issues with hypovolemia.

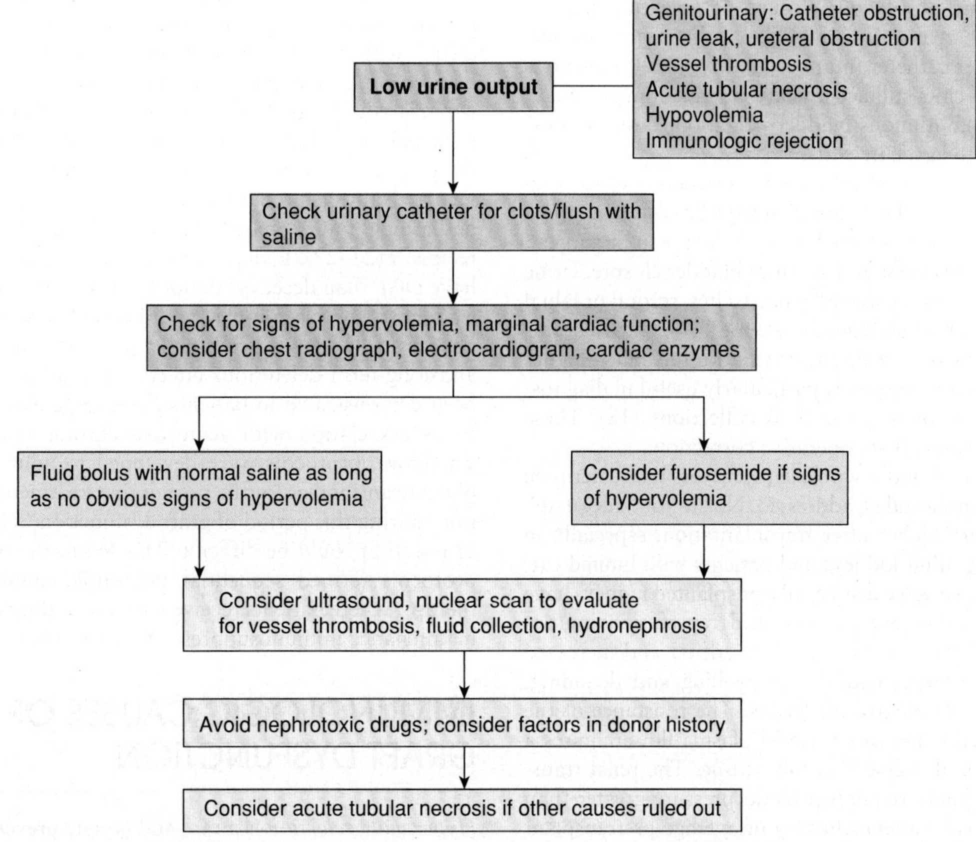

FIGURE 75.1 Algorithm for the management of low urine output following renal transplant.

Postoperative evaluation of electrolytes should include monitoring of serum sodium, potassium, bicarbonate, calcium, magnesium, and phosphorous. Although some patients require bicarbonate supplements, potassium supplements are usually not necessary. However, supplementation may be required in patients with large-volume posttransplant diuresis.

Prophylaxis with subcutaneous heparin to prevent deep venous thrombosis and with H_2 receptor blockers or proton pump inhibitors to prevent gastric and/or duodenal ulcers is often administered. Patients should be evaluated for the need for dialysis based on their electrolyte, metabolic, and volume status.

EARLY COMPLICATIONS

The most common complication early posttransplant is an inappropriately low urine output. The differential diagnosis includes obstruction of urine flow anywhere between the renal pelvis and the collection bag; graft hypoperfusion; urinary leak; renal parenchymal disease, usually ATN; and acute rejection in immunologically sensitized patients. If a brisk diuresis was observed in the operating room or has been recorded in previous hours, a sudden reduction in urine flow should immediately raise suspicion of a mechanical problem.

Frequently, blood clots obstruct the urinary catheter. The patient complains of a sense of fullness and need to urinate. "Milking" the urinary catheter tubing poses no risk of contaminating the closed system and usually dislodges the clots. If catheter irrigation is necessary, meticulously sterile technique is used. Sterile saline, 20 to 30 mL, should be instilled retrograde to facilitate mechanically breaking up the clot. Avoid overdistention of the bladder, which risks rupture of the ureteroneocystostomy or bladder closure. If irrigation fails to evacuate the clot, removal of the Foley catheter and replacement with a larger catheter (number 18 through 20 French) is recommended. If clots still accumulate, a triple-lumen urinary catheter permits continuous bladder irrigation; rarely, cystoscopy is required to evacuate clots.

Other mechanical problems include obstruction of the ureter or urine leak (17). These should always be suspected when there has been a history of brisk urine flow noted at surgery, but little or none has been noticed since bladder closure. Urine leak can present as severe wound pain, ascites, scrotal or labial edema, and fluid draining from the wound or operative drains with urea nitrogen and creatinine concentrations much higher than serum. Ultrasonography is particularly useful in diagnosing hydroureter or perinephric fluid collections (18). These problems require immediate operative correction.

After exclusion of outflow problems, factors that determine allograft perfusion should be addressed. Norms for "adequate" blood pressure are higher after transplantation, especially in children receiving adult kidneys and patients with limited cardiac contractility. To some degree, all transplanted kidneys have sustained predonation procurement and reperfusion injuries (19). There is an increase in interstitial edema and increased venocapillary resistance, endothelial swelling and denuding, and activation of vasoactive mediators. The resistance of the renal vascular bed is increased. Renal plasma flow requires a higher mean arterial pressure in this setting. The renal transplant recipient usually requires a blood pressure greater than 120/80 mmHg. The patient's history of average pretransplant pressures is valuable in targeting perfusion pressure.

Unless there is clear evidence of intravascular volume overload, fluid boluses with normal saline are usually required. A transient response may justify further volume expansion. Most dialysis-dependent patients have total-body fluid overload. Their "dry weight," used to calculate an end point on dialysis, is always in excess of the dry weight they reach with normal renal function. Several centers use low-dose dopamine (2.5 μg/kg/min) in an attempt to improve renal perfusion, although it is most unlikely that any increased perfusion actually occurs. In rare circumstances, the intrarenal vascular resistance may be excessively high, and adequate perfusion pressures do not produce sufficient intrarenal blood flow. This problem dramatically increases the risk of further ischemic injury or even thrombosis. Grafts from pediatric donors, especially those younger than 4 years, are prone to thrombosis. As an additional safeguard, in recipients of pediatric en bloc kidneys, low-dose aspirin therapy immediately after surgery to minimize the risk of thrombosis should be considered. Graft thrombosis is rare, but any hope of graft salvage requires immediate return to the operating room.

DELAYED GRAFT FUNCTION AND ACUTE TUBULAR NECROSIS

Delayed graft function (DGF) or acute renal dysfunction in the immediate posttransplant period has been a serious and frequent problem in cadaveric renal transplantation, occurring in up to 30% of the recipients (20), and in up to 35% to 40% in ECD and DCD kidney recipients, respectively. However, this diagnosis should be considered only after all other causes are eliminated. ATN is the most common histologic feature in patients with DGF. The risk factors associated with an increased incidence of DGF include donor hypovolemia or hypotension, particularly in the presence of nephrotoxic drugs or vasopressors; prolonged cold or warm ischemia times; kidneys procured from older donors and from donors with hypertension or vascular occlusive disease; injury incurred during procurement, preservation, or implantation; and a high (>50%) panel reactive antibody (PRA) level in the recipient (21–23). Living-donor kidneys are much less likely to have DGF than deceased donor kidneys. The pathophysiology leading to DGF is complex and incompletely understood, but appears to be due to ischemia–reperfusion injury. The short- and long-term deleterious effects on graft survival that have been demonstrated in patients developing this disorder relate to its association with acute and chronic rejection (23,24). Therefore, protocols were developed to administer antilymphocyte antibodies for the preemptive treatment of acute rejection, during this period of graft dysfunction, when a diagnosis of rejection could be difficult. This led to the development of protocols termed sequential quadruple immunosuppressive therapy, where patients receive antibody induction followed by maintenance immunosuppression, usually with three agents.

IMMUNOLOGIC CAUSES OF EARLY GRAFT DYSFUNCTION

Hyperacute rejection is a rare and largely preventable cause of immediate graft failure. It is caused by preformed antibodies present in the recipients' serum at the time of transplantation against donor antigens. These antibodies are the consequence of previous exposure to donor antigens due to blood transfusions, prior transplantation, or pregnancy. It also occurs when transplantation is attempted across ABO-incompatible barriers. The events that lead to hyperacute rejection may occur with such rapidity that the kidney becomes visibly ischemic while the patient is still on the operating table. It always occurs within 24 hours of transplantation. Renal histology shows fibrin thrombi occluding the glomerular capillaries and small vessels with extensive tissue necrosis. Although plasmapheresis and anticoagulation have been advocated, there is no established effective treatment and interventions are seldom successful. A kidney with hyperacute rejection should always be removed promptly. The current cross-match techniques, because of their increased sensitivity, have greatly diminished the incidence of hyperacute rejection.

Antibody-mediated (C4D⁺) acute rejection is another form of early rejection that can occur in previously sensitized patients, but who have an initial negative cross-match. This form of acute rejection is potentially reversible if diagnosed early and treated aggressively with plasmapheresis and intravenous immunoglobulin (25). Eculizumab a humanized monoclonal antibody that specifically binds to the complement protein C5, thereby inhibiting its cleavage to C5a and C5b and preventing the generation of the terminal complement complex C5b-9 is currently in studies for the prevention of antibody mediated rejection (AMR) in renal transplant recipients. Eculizumab is approved for the treatment of patients with paroxysmal nocturnal hemoglobinuria (PNH) and another rare disease, atypical hemolytic uremic syndrome (aHUS) and currently available commercially. It is being evaluated in Phase 2 clinical studies in kidney transplant recipients for prophylaxis of AMR and also for the prevention of DGF (26). Patients receiving eculizumab may have increased susceptibility to infections, especially those with encapsulated bacteria. Life-threatening and fatal meningococcal infections have been reported. Children treated with eculizumab may also be at increased risk of developing serious infections due to *Streptococcus pneumoniae* and *Haemophilus influenzae* type b (Hib) (27).

IMMUNOSUPPRESSION

The different phases of immunosuppressive therapy after transplantation are as follows:

1. Induction immunosuppression in the immediate post-transplantation period when potent therapy is required to prevent rejection.
2. Maintenance immunosuppression for long-term therapy to prevent allograft rejection, but at the same time preserving host defense mechanisms against infections.
3. Intensification of the immunosuppressive therapy for the treatment of an acute rejection episode.

Antilymphocyte antibodies—available as immunosuppressive agents since the late 1960s—are ideally suited for use as induction immunosuppressive agents and, to some extent, for the treatment of acute rejection. All early forms of antilymphocyte antibodies were polyclonal, made by injecting human lymphocytes into horses, goats, rabbits, or sheep. In contrast to polyclonal antibodies, a monoclonal antibody is highly specific, and recognizes a single antigen epitope. They have a greater potency at lower doses, and have a more predictable and consistent effect. Monoclonal antibodies that have been approved for use in transplantation are directed either at cell surface receptors such as the CD3/T-cell receptor (TCR) complex (OKT3), or the interleukin-2 (IL-2) receptor (IL-2R; daclizumab and basiliximab). OKT3 and daclizumab have been withdrawn and are no longer available. These immunosuppressive agents are classified as depleting-antibody or nondepleting antibody, depending on their ability to deplete lymphocytes from the peripheral circulation.

Current maintenance immunosuppression protocols often use the combination of a calcineurin inhibitor, an antimetabolite, and corticosteroids. However, the principles of the different regimens are similar: more intense immunosuppression in the induction phase with gradual reduction in immunosuppression in the maintenance phase. The immunosuppression protocol an institution implements should provide a balance between preventing rejection and avoiding the consequences of overimmunosuppression such as infection and malignancy.

Induction Agents

Depleting Antibodies

Rabbit antithymocyte globulin (thymoglobulin), a polyclonal antilymphocyte antibody, is produced by the immunization of rabbits with human thymocytes. Several mechanisms of action have been proposed to explain the immunosuppressive effect of thymoglobulin. These include complement-mediated cell lysis, clearance of lymphocytes by opsonization and subsequent phagocytosis by macrophages, and antibody-dependent cell-mediated cytolysis (28).

Polyclonal antibody treatment induces marked lymphocyte depletion that persists during the entire treatment period. The number of circulating T cells will gradually increase after the cessation of treatment and reach pretreatment levels in several weeks, with significant variability among patients. Each polyclonal antilymphocyte preparation varies in its constituent antibodies. Due to this unpredictable antibody mixture and batch-to-batch variability, treatment responses and side effects are variable between the different preparations (29).

Thymoglobulin (antithymocyte globulin) is the only polyclonal agent currently available for use in the United States. Thymoglobulin consists of antibodies specific for T-cell epitopes, including CD2, CD3, CD4, CD8, CD11a, CD18, CD25, HLA-DR, and HLA class I. An uncommon, but serious, side effect of thymoglobulin treatment is the cytokine release syndrome, which usually occurs after the administration of the first few doses. This syndrome includes the development of skin rashes, hypotension, acute respiratory distress, and anaphylaxis. Polyclonal antibodies often cross-react with antigens on unrelated cells, resulting in such side effects as granulocytopenia, thrombocytopenia, arthralgia, serum sickness, phlebitis, and immune complex glomerulonephritis. Because these agents severely impair cell-mediated immunity, patients are prone to develop opportunistic infections and posttransplantation malignancies, especially posttransplantation lymphoproliferative disorders (PTLDs).

Thymoglobulin is dosed at 1.5 mg/kg/day for a total dose of 6 mg/kg. It is administered as an IV infusion over a period of about 6 hours. Premedication is recommended using high-dose methylprednisolone, an antihistamine, and acetaminophen 1 hour prior to its administration.

Alemtuzumab (Campath-1H) is a humanized monoclonal antibody directed against the CD52 antigen (30,31); it is not approved by the Food and Drug Administration for use in kidney transplant patients but is used off-label in approximately 15% of these recipients. Targeting of CD52 with antibody has shown to be exceptionally lytic of lymphocytes. The mechanism of action of alemtuzumab includes complement-mediated lysis, cell-mediated killing (antibody-dependent cellular cytotoxicity [ADCC]), and induction of apoptosis of targeted cells. Alemtuzumab is a relatively low-affinity antibody, requiring 20 to 50 μg/mL to saturate its receptors (32). Because of the humanization of alemtuzumab, the first-dose effect is relatively mild; there is an associated tumor necrosis factor (TNF)-α and interferon-γ (IFN-γ) release that can be reduced with steroids. First infusion reactions such as fever, rash, nausea, vomiting, headache, and rigors due to a cytokine release syndrome have been reported with alemtuzumab treatment; however, these effects have been of a low-grade nature and limited with steroid pretreatment (32,33). Alemtuzumab effectively depletes immune cells, namely T and B lymphocytes, some natural killer (NK) cells, and some monocyte/macrophage lineage. Results from a number of single-center trials (34,35) and a multicenter trial (36) comparing alemtuzumab induction with that of basiliximab in low–immunologic-risk recipients and with thymoglobulin for high–immunologic-risk recipients have confirmed the efficacy of alemtuzumab as an induction agent.

Rituximab (Rituxan) antibody is a genetically engineered chimeric (human and mouse) monoclonal antibody directed against the CD20 antigen found on the surface of normal and malignant B lymphocytes (37). Rituximab is approved for the treatment of patients with relapsed or refractory, low-grade or follicular, CD20-positive, B-cell, non-Hodgkin lymphoma (38,39). Because of its effects on the B lymphocytes, rituximab is believed to be effective in the treatment of patients with antibody-mediated (humoral) acute rejection and is also thought to have a role in decreasing the PRA level in sensitized patients. However, it is not FDA approved for the latter indications and has not gained widespread support for use in transplant recipients, except for treatment in patients with PTLD (40).

Nondepleting Antibody

Basiliximab is an anti–interleukin-2α receptor antibody that is currently used as an induction agent in kidney transplant recipients that are unsensitized and are immunologically at a lower risk for acute rejection. IL-2 is a cytokine responsible for the growth and proliferation of activated T cells. During an immune response, IL-2 exerts its effects by binding to the IL-2R on the surface of the antigen-activated T cell; anti–interleukin-2α receptor antibodies are monoclonal antibodies directed against the IL-2R on activated T cells. These antibodies are used as induction agents for prophylaxis against acute rejection in renal transplant recipients (41).

Basiliximab (Simulect) is a chimeric (human and mouse) $IgG_1\kappa$ monoclonal antibody that is administered as an IV infusion of two doses of 20 mg each. The first dose is given within 2 hours before transplantation, and the second dose is administered 4 days after transplantation. Adverse effects of the IL-2R antibodies are minimal and equivalent to placebo in controlled trials; hypersensitivity reactions have been reported.

Maintenance Agents

Calcineurin Inhibitors

Calcineurin inhibitors are currently considered to be the mainstay of immunosuppression regimens following transplantation. They are potent immunosuppressants, inhibiting T-cell activation by inhibiting calcineurin phosphatase, a key step in the regulation of cytokine expression. The introduction of calcineurin inhibitors in the mid-1980s revolutionized the field of transplantation by dramatically reducing acute rejection rates and improving short-term allograft survival (42).

Cyclosporine A (CsA), the first calcineurin inhibitor approved for use in transplant recipients for maintenance immunosuppression, binds to cyclophilin in the T cell. The CsA/cyclophilin complex, in turn, inhibits calcineurin phosphatase, which is responsible for the transcription of IL-2. CsA is highly lipophilic and water insoluble. Early formulations (Sandimmune) were administered orally as an oil-based solution. In this form, bioavailability was erratic, highly variable, and bile dependent for its absorption. This erratic absorption profile led to the development of a microemulsion formulation (modified cyclosporine, Neoral) that demonstrated a more reliable and predictable absorption. These two formulations are not bioequivalent and are thus not interchangeable. CsA is available in an IV formulation, as an oral solution, and in a capsule form. The IV formulation should be administered as a continuous infusion and should be limited to patients unable to take CsA orally; the patient should be monitored closely during the infusion process. The CsA dosage should be titrated based on whole blood concentration; the recommended starting dose of oral solution or capsules is 10 to 14 mg/kg/day for the nonmodified CsA and 6 to 12 mg/kg/day of the modified CsA, administered 12 hours apart in divided doses. In the United States, use of CsA has been superseded by that of tacrolimus in the majority of kidney transplant recipients and in almost all pancreas transplant recipients.

Tacrolimus (Prograf, FK-506) is a macrolide agent that inhibits IL-2 production in a similar fashion as CsA in the T lymphocyte. However, instead of binding to cyclophilin, tacrolimus binds to the FK-binding protein 12 (FKBP-12), with the resulting complex inhibiting calcineurin phosphatase. Tacrolimus is available in IV injection and oral capsule dosage forms. The IV form of tacrolimus is also administered as a continuous infusion and, because of the risk of neurotoxicity, should be limited to select patients unable to take tacrolimus orally. Tacrolimus is readily absorbed in the stomach and should be given orally or through nasogastric tube whenever feasible. The recommended starting dose of oral tacrolimus is 0.2 mg/kg/day administered 12 hours apart in divided doses.

Astagraf XL is an extended-release formulation of tacrolimus capsule that is indicated for the prevention of rejection in kidney transplant recipients. It shares the same efficacy and side-effect profile as that of immediate-release tacrolimus. It provides a once-daily dosing option and, as a result, may improve compliance (43,44).

Envarsus is also an extended-release formulation of tacrolimus utilizing the proprietary MeltDose drug-delivery technology that significantly increases the bioavailability of tacrolimus; it is designed for once a day administration. In a large-phase III study it showed comparable efficacy to that of immediate-release twice a day tacrolimus. Because of its improved absorption, patients required lower doses of

Envarsus than immediate-release tacrolimus (45). Envarsus is currently available for use in Europe. Final regulatory approval and marketing of this agent in the United States are currently pending and is expected to be available for use soon.

Adverse Effects of the Calcineurin Inhibitors

Both calcineurin inhibitors have a narrow therapeutic window, multiple side effects, and drug interactions. Both drugs are metabolized by the cytochrome P450–3A4 enzyme system; their blood concentrations are affected by drugs that block or induce this cytochrome enzyme system. These drugs interact with some of the commonly used antibiotics, antifungal agents, and antihypertensive agents (Table 75.1).

Both drugs cause acute and chronic nephrotoxicity; the acute nephrotoxicity is due in part to hemodynamic changes secondary to their vasoconstrictor effects on the afferent arteriole of the glomerulus. This results in a reduction in the glomerular filtration rate, manifested by an increase in the serum creatinine concentration. This acute change is dose related and reversible. However, the lesions associated with calcineurin inhibitor–induced chronic nephropathy may lead to end-stage renal failure. These lesions, which consist of tubulointerstitial-striped fibrosis, tubular atrophy, afferent arteriolopathy, and global or focal glomerular sclerosis or collapse, have been well demonstrated in patients with autoimmune diseases treated with cyclosporine, as well as in the various organ transplant recipients: heart, liver, renal, and bone marrow (46,47). The other reported adverse effects of CsA and tacrolimus include hypertension, hyperkalemia, hyperlipidemia, and headache. Adverse effects unique to CsA include hirsutism and gingival hyperplasia, whereas those unique to tacrolimus include alopecia, fine tremor, and hyperglycemia. The adverse-effect profiles of both CsA and tacrolimus are compared in Table 75.2.

TABLE 75.1 Common Drug Interactions with Cyclosporine and Tacrolimus

Decreases blood concentrations

Phenytoin
Carbamazepine
Phenobarbital
Rifampin
Rifabutin
St. John wort

Increases blood concentrations

Diltiazem
Nicardipine
Nifedipine
Verapamil
Ketoconazole
Fluconazole
Itraconazole
Clarithromycin
Erythromycin
Cimetidine
Metoclopramide
Oral contraceptives
Prednisone
Protease inhibitors
Grapefruit juice
Amiodarone

TABLE 75.2 Adverse Effect Profile of Cyclosporine A and Tacrolimus

Adverse Event	Cyclosporine A (%)	Tacrolimus (%)	p
Hypertension	52.2	49.8	
Hyperlipidemia	38.2	30.7	
Nephrotoxicity	41.5	45.4	
Hyperglycemia	4.0	19.9	<0.001
Headache	37.7	43.9	
Tremors	33.8	54.1	<0.001
Alopecia	1.0	10.7	<0.001
Hirsutism	8.7	0.5	<0.001
Gingival hyperplasia	5.3	0.5	0.004
Gingivitis	8.7	1.5	<0.001

From Pirsch JD, Miller J, Deierhoi MH, et al., for the FK506 kidney transplant study group. A comparison of tacrolimus (FK506) and cyclosporine for immunosuppression after cadaveric renal transplantation. *Transplantation.* 1997;63:977–983.

Dose modifications of both CsA and tacrolimus are based on whole blood trough concentrations. Monitoring of the respective drug concentrations is an essential aid in the management of a transplant recipient for the evaluation of rejection, toxicity, dose adjustments, drug interactions, and compliance. Two methods for monitoring CsA levels in whole blood include high-pressure liquid chromatography (HPLC) and radioimmunoassay, or TDx. For tacrolimus, a microparticle enzyme immunoassay (MEIA) or an enzyme-linked immunosorbent assay (ELISA)-based IMx assay are utilized. Target levels of either drug vary, based on the type of assay used, the type of monitoring (trough vs. C2 [drug level 2 hours postdose] vs. AUC [area under the curve]), transplant center standards, time posttransplantation, and the recipients' risk for acute rejection.

Antimetabolites

Mycophenolate mofetil (MMF) (CellCept) and enteric-coated mycophenolate sodium (MPS) (Myfortic) contain the active moiety mycophenolic acid (MPA), a reversible inhibitor of inosine monophosphate dehydrogenase (IMPDH), a key, rate-limiting step in the de novo pathway of guanosine nucleotide synthesis. Depletion of the guanosine nucleotides inhibits T- and B-cell proliferation as they are dependent on the de novo pathway of purine synthesis rather than salvage pathways.

The recommended dose of MMF is 1,000 mg orally or IV twice daily, divided 12 hours apart. MMF is the prodrug of MPA and allows for increased oral bioavailability. Some centers monitor MPA drug levels for dose adjustments. The MPS equivalent is 720 mg orally twice daily, 12 hours apart, although due to differences in absorption, these two formulations are not interchangeable. MPS is not available for IV infusion and the enteric-coated tablets should not be cut, crushed, or chewed.

Adverse effects of MPA include gastrointestinal effects (dyspepsia, nausea, vomiting, diarrhea, and constipation) and bone marrow suppression (leukopenia and thrombocytopenia). Diarrhea, leukopenia, and thrombocytopenia are often dose limiting requiring dose reduction to ameliorate the toxic effects. These patients, however, should be monitored closely, as a relationship exists between an increased incidence of acute rejection and decreased MPA doses (48,49).

Azathioprine (Imuran)—a purine analog that inhibits DNA and RNA production in the T cell—is an imidazole derivative of 6-mercaptopurine. The initial recommended dose of azathioprine is 3 to 5 mg/kg/day, administered orally or IV once daily. Adverse effects of azathioprine include hematologic toxicities (pancytopenia, macrocytic anemia, thrombocytopenia, and leukopenia), alopecia, pancreatitis, and hepatotoxicity. Dose reductions may be required for myelosuppressive toxicities. A potent drug interaction may be seen with the coadministration of azathioprine and allopurinol (a xanthine oxidase inhibitor). Although it is recommended that the dose of azathioprine should be reduced by 75% when coadministered with allopurinol, it is more prudent to avoid the use of these two agents together.

mTOR Inhibitors

Sirolimus (Rapamune) is a macrolide antibiotic produced by *Streptomyces hygroscopicus* and is structurally similar to tacrolimus. Like tacrolimus, sirolimus also binds to FKBP-12. However, unlike tacrolimus, this complex binds to and inhibits the activation of the mammalian target of rapamycin (mTOR). This interferes with biochemical signal transductions from the cell membrane to the nucleus by inhibiting the stimulation of T cells by IL-2, -4, and -6 and by blocking the CD28 costimulatory signal. Sirolimus is available in oral tablets and solution. The recommended initial dose of sirolimus is approximately 6-mg (5 to 10 mg) loading dose, followed by 2-mg once-daily maintenance dose. Dose adjustments are made based on weekly or biweekly trough level monitoring ($t_{1/2}$ = 62 hours).

Adverse effects of sirolimus include anemia, leukopenia, thrombocytopenia, hyperlipidemia, prolongation of delayed graft function, impaired wound healing, pneumonitis, arthralgia, aphthous mouth ulcers, lymphocele, and diarrhea. The advantage of sirolimus is due to its lack of nephrotoxicity (50,51). However, when coadministered with CsA, the nephrotoxic effect of CsA can be potentiated (52). Sirolimus is metabolized by the cytochrome P450–3A4 enzyme system and has a similar drug interaction profile as that of the calcineurin inhibitors.

Everolimus (Zortress) is a rapamycin derivative with increased oral bioavailability and a shorter half-life. The recommended initial dose of everolimus is 0.75 mg orally twice daily with dose adjustments made weekly or biweekly to target trough levels between 3 and 8 ng/mL. Everolimus shares some of the same advantages and adverse effects associated with sirolimus; everolimus is used in combination with cyclosporine or tacrolimus and appears to be efficacious even with lower tacrolimus doses (53).

Costimulation Blockade

Belatacept represents a new class of immunosuppressive therapy for renal transplantation. It is a selective costimulation blocker that binds to the B7 receptors on the surface of antigen-presenting cells and provides effective immunosuppression while avoiding the toxicities associated with calcineurin inhibitors. It is administered intravenously at monthly intervals in the long term. Although there is a trend toward higher rates of early rejection episodes in patients treated with belatacept, longer-term data have shown superior graft function and reduction of death or graft loss with belatacept (54). A safety issue that must be considered when using belatacept is the potential for increased risk of posttransplant lymphoproliferative disease (PTLD), especially in Epstein–Barr virus (EBV) seronegative recipients or patients treated with lymphocyte-depleting agents. Therefore, belatacept is contraindicated in kidney transplant recipients who are EBV seronegative or serologic status is unknown.

Corticosteroids

Corticosteroids exert their immunosuppressive effects through multiple pathways, the most important of which is through their ability to inhibit cytokine and cytokine receptor transcription. Corticosteroids inhibit the expression of various cytokines responsible for the activation of T cells including IL-1, -2, -3, -6, TNF-α, and IFN-γ. Corticosteroids function as both induction and maintenance immunosuppressive agents, as well as for the treatment of acute rejection episodes. Typical induction protocols call for high-dose methylprednisolone, the first dose administered intraoperatively prior to organ perfusion with tapering doses for the first few days posttransplantation. This is followed by oral prednisone with continued tapering to a baseline maintenance dose. Corticosteroids are typically administered once a day in the morning concurrent with intrinsic cortisol release.

Adverse effects of corticosteroids are numerous and include cosmetic changes, avascular necrosis, cataracts, osteoporosis, impaired wound healing, glucose intolerance, hypertension, hyperlipidemia, increased appetite, hypothalamic–adrenal axis (HPA) suppression, and mood swings.

Corticosteroids were the first immunosuppressants used when renal transplants were done in the 1960s. Because of numerous adverse effects, steroid withdrawal has been attempted, but only with moderate success because of increased acute rejection. However, with the advent of newer and more effective immunosuppressive therapy, there has been a renewed interest in early withdrawal or complete elimination of corticosteroids. Short-term success has been achieved in several small single-center trials and a few larger multicenter trials. Early corticosteroid withdrawal has also been associated with a more favorable cardiovascular risk profile, as evidenced by less hypertension, posttransplant diabetes mellitus (PTDM), and hyperlipidemia (55).

MINIMIZING OPPORTUNISTIC INFECTIONS IN THE TRANSPLANT

Recipient

Within the first month following transplantation, surgical wound-related and nosocomial infections are the most common infections observed in renal allograft recipients. As a result, bacterial infections involving the urinary tract, the respiratory tract, the surgical wound, and/or intravenous lines are the ones frequently encountered. In a few instances, infections may be due to reactivation of pre-existing infection in the recipient such as subclinical bacterial infections, especially urinary tract infections (UTIs) and tuberculosis, or transmission of infections from the donor to the recipient.

Infections in the 1- to 6-month period after transplantation are due to opportunistic organisms, most notably viruses belonging to the herpes group, especially cytomegalovirus (CMV), and due to *Candida* species and *Pneumocystis jiroveci.* Antimicrobial prophylaxis specific to these opportunistic organisms should be given to all renal allograft recipients

TABLE 75.3 Cytomegalovirus (CMV) Risk Stratification and Treatment Options

Risk Status	Donor CMV IgG Serostatus	Recipient CMV IgG Serostatus	Usual Drug of Choice	Dose	Duration (days)
High	Positive	Negative	Valganciclovir	450–900 mg daily	180
Moderate	Positive	Positive	Valganciclovir	450–900 mg daily	90
	Negative	Positive	Valganciclovir	450–900 mg daily	90
Low	Negative	Negative	Valacyclovir	500 mg twice or thrice daily	30

From Razonable R, Humar A. Cytomegalovirus. In: Kumar D, Humar A, eds. *The AST Handbook of Transplant Infections*. Chichester, West Sussex, UK: Wiley-Blackwell; 2011:35–41.

early posttransplantation. Prophylaxis protocols differ among centers in antimicrobial selection and duration of therapy. Prophylaxis with antifungals such as clotrimazole, nystatin, or fluconazole may be used against *Candida* infections of the mouth and throat (thrush). Prophylaxis against *P. jiroveci* pneumonia (PCP) includes sulfamethoxazole/trimethoprim; for those patients with a sulfa allergy, monthly inhaled pentamidine or oral dapsone will provide adequate prophylaxis against PCP. Drug and dose selection of antiviral prophylaxis against CMV infection can be stratified by infection risk based on previous CMV exposure, or the presence of anti-CMV antibodies in the recipient (Table 75.3). Valganciclovir is currently the drug of choice for antiviral prophylaxis against CMV.

Several antimicrobial agents adversely interact with cyclosporine and tacrolimus, and careful consideration should be given to the choice of the antimicrobial agent.

"STABLE" ALLOGRAFT RECIPIENTS READMITTED TO THE INTENSIVE CARE UNIT

Successful transplantation restores patients to an active and functional life, but it does not prevent subsequent occurrence of atherosclerotic cardiovascular disease, cancer, trauma, infections, and other major problems. Furthermore, the care of transplant patients with other diseases demands an awareness of the long-term problems that are unique to this patient population, and these are also discussed below.

INFECTIONS

Viral Infections

Cytomegalovirus

CMV is the most important viral infection affecting transplant recipients. CMV infection risk is highest in patients who are CMV IgG-seronegative and received an allograft from a CMV-seropositive donor (see Table 75.3) or who have received CMV-positive blood transfusion. CMV infection often presents clinically with fever after cessation of anti-CMV prophylaxis and in some instances may present as disseminated or tissue invasive CMV disease affecting the gastrointestinal tract, liver, kidney, or lungs with organ-specific symptoms (i.e., pneumonitis). CMV is diagnosed by identification and quantification of the viral DNA in the blood by polymerase chain reaction (PCR). Tissue-invasive disease may be diagnosed by the identification of the characteristic *owl-eye* inclusions on tissue biopsy (56). Treatment of CMV viremia and tissue-invasive CMV disease should be initiated promptly with oral valganciclovir or intravenous ganciclovir. Concomitant treatment with CMV immune globulin may be required in some patients with severe tissue disease. Duration of treatment depends on the extent of the disease and continued positivity of the CMV-DNA by PCR.

Polyoma (BK Virus) Infection

With the increased use of potent immunosuppressive agents, there has been an emergence of opportunistic infections such as polyomavirus infection in renal transplant recipients. Polyomavirus is a member of the papovavirus family. The two sub-types—BK and JC virus—were first described in 1971 and named after the initials of the original patients. BK virus is associated with interstitial nephritis and ureteral stenosis in the transplant kidney and with hemorrhagic cystitis in bone marrow transplant recipients. So far, there is no evidence linking polyomavirus infection to any particular immunosuppressive agent. Tissue injury due to recurrent episodes of acute rejection and treatment with potent immunosuppressive agents appears to potentiate polyomavirus infection. Notably, this infection is rarely seen in solid organ transplants other than the kidney. Recent studies have shown that polyomavirus has been implicated as a cause of interstitial nephritis in 5% of renal transplant recipients with subsequent graft failure in as many as 45% of the affected patients. The time from transplantation to the diagnosis of polyomavirus infection is variable, with a range of 2 to 60 months (median 9 months). PCR for polyomavirus DNA in the urine and blood is a sensitive and specific method for detecting the agent; at the present time, there is no specific therapy for polyomavirus infection. Screening with urine and/or blood PCR for polyomavirus prospectively and reduction in immunosuppression in the presence of increasing or high viral loads is indicated and is the most effective option currently available. Many protocols include discontinuation/reduction of antimetabolites such as MMF and/or substitution of tacrolimus with cyclosporine; m-TOR inhibitors are being used increasingly because of their antiviral properties (57–59).

Other viral infections that may occur in the immunosuppressed renal allograft recipient include EBV, which may lead to the development of EBV-positive lymphomas; herpes simplex virus (types I and II); hepatitis B and C viruses; varicella-zoster virus; and the influenza virus. Treatment of viral infections depends on the type of virus and the extent of the disease. All transplant recipients should receive an annual influenza immunization.

Fungal Infections

Fungal infections are a major concern in the immunosuppressed renal allograft recipient. As with the general population,

Candida albicans infections resulting from endogenous flora are common. However, with immunosuppression, these infections can rapidly become more serious. Other fungal pathogens seen in transplant recipients include nocardiosis, aspergillosis, *Cryptococcus,* histoplasmosis, coccidiomycosis, blastomycosis, and mucormycosis. Treatment of fungal infections include the use of antifungals specific to the organism, surgical excision—especially in the case of mucormycosis—and reduction in the overall immunosuppression. Careful consideration should be given to the choice of the antimicrobial agent because of drug interactions (azole antifungals) or additive nephrotoxicity (amphotericin B) in the presence of immunosuppressant agents. Invasive fungal infections in transplant recipients are associated with a high risk of graft loss and mortality. Early diagnosis and aggressive treatment can preserve organ function and can be lifesaving.

Other Opportunistic Infections

UTIs are a frequent complication of renal transplantation. Although UTIs are frequently asymptomatic, they constitute the major source of bacteremia in this patient population. Therefore, all UTIs, even asymptomatic ones, should be treated appropriately. Fortunately, renal dysfunction is an uncommon complication of UTIs in the transplant recipient. It usually occurs with severe pyelonephritis involving the allograft, usually in the setting of ureteral obstruction or vesicoureteral reflux. Chronic UTIs may require daily prophylactic antibiotic administration.

Renal allograft recipients, especially patients with poor allograft function with a background of intensive acute and chronic immunosuppressive therapy for recurrent rejection episodes, are susceptible to a large range of infections. Empiric treatment should be initiated at the first sign of infection as infections can be aggressive and worsen rapidly.

GASTROINTESTINAL COMPLICATIONS

A wide variety of gastrointestinal complications may occur after transplantation due to infections with organisms such as CMV, *Candida* sp., and *Clostridium difficile;* adverse effects associated with immunosuppressive agents; posttransplantation complications of pre-existing conditions such as diverticulitis; and other complications such as acute appendicitis, gastrointestinal bleeding, colonic or small bowel perforations, pancreatitis, and ischemic colitis. Diarrhea is a common problem in transplant recipients and may be related to the immunosuppressive drugs, due to opportunistic infections, or due to pre-existing autonomic dysfunction often related to diabetes mellitus.

Peptic Ulcer Disease

Gastroduodenal ulcers account for most of the gastrointestinal complications posttransplantation and often occur soon after renal transplantation or acute rejection therapy. Gastroduodenal ulcers presenting posttransplantation can be attributed to a variety of causes including pre-existing ulcer history, viral pathogens (CMV in 15%, herpes simplex in 2%), and immunosuppressive agents, mainly corticosteroids (60–63). The treatment of posttransplantation gastroduodenal ulcers is the same as with the general population. Proton pump inhibitors and H_2-receptor blocking agents may be used for both therapy and prophylaxis. Intermittent therapy with calcium, aluminum, or magnesium salts can provide immediate relief; however, coadministration of these agents with MMF (CellCept) may inhibit absorption of the active moiety of this drug in the intestinal tract. All kidney transplant recipients diagnosed with gastroduodenal ulcers should be evaluated for *Helicobacter pylori* and CMV infection. Clarithromycin (Biaxin), commonly used for the treatment of *H. pylori,* interacts with CsA and tacrolimus (see Table 75.1); therefore, under ideal circumstances, an alternate antibiotic regimen should be used. For CMV-related gastrointestinal lesions, ganciclovir or valganciclovir treatment should be initiated promptly.

Bowel Perforation

Colonic perforation should be suspected in the presence of one or more of the following: abdominal pain, fever, increased white blood cell count, tenderness, and pneumoperitoneum. These clinical criteria may be blunted in the presence of poor renal function, use of high-dose corticosteroids, or based upon the overall state of immunosuppression. A plain abdominal radiograph, CT scan, or colonoscopy may help in the diagnosis. Mortality rates after colonic perforation can be reduced with minimal delay in time to surgery, broad-spectrum antibiotic therapy, and reduction of immunosuppression. Operative intervention has been shown to improve patient survival significantly (64). Screening for colonic diverticula before transplantation should be applied to all patients older than age 50 years, and a segmental colectomy may be required in patients who have experienced clinical symptoms of diverticulitis (60,64).

Acute Pancreatitis

Acute pancreatitis is an infrequent but severe complication following renal transplantation. A review of the literature has documented an incidence of 2.3%, with a mortality rate of 61.3% in 3,253 renal transplant recipients (65). Several etiologic factors have been considered in the etiology of this process. Azathioprine has been reported to cause pancreatitis with rapid improvement after cessation and with recurrence of symptoms with reinstitution (66). Corticosteroids and cyclosporine have also been reported to cause pancreatitis; however, this association is not as convincing as is that of azathioprine. Other causes of pancreatitis include hyperparathyroidism, CMV infection, biliary tract disease, alcoholism, and hyperlipidemia (65). Although the diagnosis of pancreatitis depends largely on an increase in the serum amylase and/or serum lipase levels, ultrasonography and CT scan may be useful. Intensive medical management with particular attention to volume replacement, electrolyte balance, and nutrition is essential.

Severe diarrhea with ensuing dehydration and acidosis, gastrointestinal bleeding, cholecystitis, and diverticulitis are other commonly encountered gastrointestinal problems in the transplant recipient. Advances in the management of peptic ulcer disease, prophylaxis against CMV disease, and better preparation of recipients prior to transplantation have reduced the overall morbidity and mortality. Several of the gastrointestinal problems may be related to the side effects of the immunosuppressive drugs or due to the net state of overimmunosuppression. Careful consideration should be given to the change in the immunosuppressive agent and to decrease in the dosages of these medications.

Hematologic Complications

Neutropenia is a frequent complication posttransplantation, often as a result of the adverse effects of immunosuppressive medications. Antithymocyte globulin can cause transient decreases in neutrophils that often rebound after cessation of therapy. Maintenance immunosuppression with mycophenolic acid, mTOR inhibitors, and prophylaxis with ganciclovir and sulfamethoxazole/trimethoprim contribute to the development of neutropenia due to their myelosuppressive effects. Careful dose reduction of these agents and/or use of granulocyte-stimulating factors are often required for persistent neutropenia. Of particular importance is that neutropenia can be a sign of CMV infection, and therefore this should always be excluded in transplant recipients with persistent neutropenia.

Anemia is a frequent occurrence in the early posttransplantation period as a result of pre-existing anemia of ESRD, surgical blood loss, and immunosuppressive medications. Patients with slow or DGF may have a more pronounced and prolonged anemia. Anemia in the late posttransplantation phase can be attributed to a combination of immunosuppressive medications, renal allograft dysfunction, use of angiotensin-converting enzyme (ACE) inhibitors or angiotensin II receptor blockers, and/or iron deficiency (67). As cardiovascular disease is the leading cause of morbidity and mortality in kidney transplant recipients, it is important to manage anemia aggressively in this patient population with the use of erythropoietin. Furthermore, given the high incidence of coexisting cardiovascular disease in this patient population, blood transfusions should not be withheld for acute indications.

Thrombocytopenia is also a frequent occurrence in renal allograft recipients and often is caused by the immunosuppressive medications. Antithymocyte globulin, valganciclovir, and dapsone can cause transient decreases in platelets. Withholding doses or dose adjustments of the responsible agent may be required for the treatment of thrombocytopenia. Platelet recovery is rapid, often returning to baseline within days. In rare circumstances, thrombocytopenia may be due to HUS that is caused by immunosuppressive drugs (calcineurin inhibitors, mTOR inhibitors), severe acute vascular rejection, transmission from donor, recurrence of previous HUS, or causes similar to those in nontransplant recipients.

CARDIAC AND VASCULAR DISEASES

Coronary Artery Disease

Atherosclerotic vascular disease is the major cause of late morbidity and mortality in transplant recipients, and coronary artery disease is the principal cause of death (68–72). In transplant recipients, risk factors for posttransplantation coronary artery disease include increased age, male gender, history of diabetes mellitus, hypercholesterolemia, smoking history, acute renal allograft rejection episodes, and greater cumulative dose of steroids (73). The key to the early detection of significant coronary artery disease in renal transplant recipients without coronary symptoms is repeated evaluation for the known risk factors. The management of transplant patients with coronary artery disease is similar to that of other patients and should include noninvasive exercise or resting diagnostic testing, coronary arteriography, or both. However, some noninvasive screening tests have been shown to be less useful, especially in the presence of diabetes, uremia, and left ventricular hypertrophy (74). With the increasing number of transplantations performed in the elderly and in patients with diabetes mellitus, cardiovascular disease will continue to be a major cause of posttransplantation morbidity. Of particular note, during cardiac catheterization, femoral arterial puncture on the ipsilateral side to the renal transplant should be avoided whenever feasible to reduce the risks of mechanical injury and atheroembolization to the renal allograft.

Cerebrovascular and Peripheral Vascular Disease

Cerebrovascular disease occurs in 1% to 3% of all renal allograft recipients (68,75). There is also an increased risk of peripheral vascular disease (68,71,76,77). A thorough history to elicit symptoms associated with cerebrovascular and peripheral vascular disease and examination of the carotid arteries and peripheral circulation should be performed annually, and the presence of a carotid bruit should be further investigated with duplex ultrasonography and magnetic resonance angiography (MRA). In the presence of more than 60% stenosis of the carotid artery, the patient should be referred to the neurovascular surgeon for further evaluation (78).

Successful transplantation does not reduce the rate of atherosclerosis initiated in renal failure. Factors contributing to the high incidence of vascular disease include hypertension, hyperlipidemia, obesity, cigarette smoking, and the presence of pre-existing diabetes mellitus or the development of posttransplantation diabetes mellitus (68). The mortality rate from coronary artery disease was increased 25-fold to that of age-matched and gender-matched controls in an Australian study (79), was increased 10-fold in a study from Stockholm (80), and was increased 3- to 4-fold in a Minneapolis study (73). By actuarial analysis, 15% of patients who survived with a functioning allograft for 15 years developed peripheral vascular disease (76).

HYPERTENSION

Hypertension is a common complication of renal transplantation and remains an important risk factor for mortality from cardiovascular disease. Posttransplantation hypertension is a major risk factor for graft survival. It is unclear, however, whether this is because of the deleterious effects of hypertension on the structure and function of the renal allograft, or whether hypertension is a marker of underlying renal disease (81,82). The causes of hypertension in renal transplant recipients include acute and/or chronic allograft rejection; recurrent or de novo transplant glomerulonephritis; transplant renal artery stenosis; high renin output state from diseased native kidneys; immunosuppressive agents such as steroids, cyclosporine, and tacrolimus; obesity; hypercalcemia; and new-onset essential hypertension (83).

HYPERLIPIDEMIA

As discussed earlier, cardiovascular disease is the most common cause of posttransplantation morbidity and mortality among long-term renal transplant survivors. As in the general population, posttransplantation lipoprotein abnormalities contribute to the development of cardiovascular and peripheral vascular disease in renal transplant recipients (70,76,84,85). The prevalence of posttransplantation hyperlipidemia ranges from 16% to 78% of recipients (68), depending at which time point posttransplantation serum lipid levels were obtained. Elevations in triglycerides, low-density lipoproteins (LDLs), apolipoprotein B, and total cholesterol levels are common (86–94). The pathogenesis of hyperlipidemia in renal transplant recipients is poorly understood and appears to be multifactorial. The numerous factors that have been shown to be associated with hyperlipidemia after renal transplantation are age, body weight, gender, pretransplantation lipid levels, renal dysfunction, proteinuria, concomitant use of diuretics or β-blockers, diabetes, steroid use, and cyclosporine, everolimus, and sirolimus use (84,86–92,95,96).

NEW-ONSET DIABETES AFTER TRANSPLANTATION

New-onset diabetes after transplantation (NODAT) has been reported in 3% to 40% of transplant recipients with an even higher incidence occurring in African Americans, Hispanics, and patients with a family history of diabetes mellitus, increasing with recipient age and weight (68,69,72,75,97–99). NODAT has been attributed to the use of immunosuppressive agents, especially with tacrolimus and corticosteroids; however, cyclosporine has also been implicated (99–102). Patients with NODAT have a poor outcome in terms of patient and graft survival, with increased mortality resulting from cardiovascular and possibly infectious complications (98,103).

Insulin treatment may be required in patients with NODAT who do not respond to lifestyle modification and oral hypoglycemic agents. About half of patients in whom NODAT develops require insulin. Aggressive treatment with either intravenous or subcutaneous insulin may also be indicated during periods of intercurrent illness and stress.

GRAFT DYSFUNCTION AND GRAFT FAILURE

The differential diagnosis of acute allograft dysfunction can be divided into (a) early, occurring less than 90 days posttransplantation, and (b) late, occurring more than 90 days after transplantation. It can be further differentiated into medical and surgical problems as outlined in Table 75.4. Some of the more common medical and surgical problems are discussed below.

Acute Rejection

Although acute allograft rejection is a common cause of graft dysfunction both in the early and late periods, it most commonly occurs during the first 90 days posttransplantation. Recipients of transplants from living donors have a significantly lower incidence of rejection episodes. Factors significantly associated with the development of acute rejection are HLA mismatch, donor-specific anti-HLA antibodies, retransplantation, African-American race, and recipient age under 16 (104,105). The classic clinical features associated with acute rejection are fever, oliguria, weight gain, edema, hypertension, and the presence of an enlarged, tender graft. However, these features are frequently absent, and the most common presentation may be an asymptomatic rise in serum creatinine. An increase in serum creatinine above 20% is often the cardinal feature of rejection. Percutaneous needle biopsy of the allograft is the most reliable method of diagnosis of acute rejection. Acute rejection is classified histologically using the Banff 07 classification of renal allograft pathology depending on the severity of lymphocytic infiltration of tubules (tubulitis), arterioles (arteritis), and the renal interstitium and the presence of C4d deposition which can indicate the presence of AMR (106).

The principles and the management of acute rejection include rapid diagnosis, accurate classification, and prompt administration of antirejection therapy. Currently, corticosteroids and antilymphocyte antibodies represent the main components of antirejection treatment protocols. The decision on treatment of acute rejection is based on histologic severity. One approach is to treat mild acute cellular rejection with a course of 250 to 500 mg of intravenous methylprednisolone administered daily for 3 or 4 days, and moderate and severe acute cellular rejection and acute vascular rejection are treated

TABLE 75.4 Causes of Graft Dysfunction and Failure

	Early (0–90 Days Posttransplantation)	Late (>90 Days Posttransplantation)
Medical	Hyperacute rejection	Acute rejection
	Delayed graft function	Calcineurin inhibitor toxicity
	Acute rejection	Chronic rejection
	Acute calcineurin inhibitor nephrotoxicity	Dehydration
	Dehydration	Other drug toxicities
	Other drug toxicities	Infection
	Infection	BK virus nephropathy
	De novo/recurrent disease	De novo/recurrent disease
Mechanical	Lymphocele	Renal artery stenosis
	Ureteric obstruction	Ureteric obstruction
	Urine leak	Urine leak
	Vascular thrombosis	Vascular thrombosis

with a 4- to 7-day course of lymphocyte depleting antibody (thymoglobulin).

Chronic Rejection

Chronic rejection is characterized clinically by a progressive decline in renal function, persistent proteinuria, and hypertension; the course of chronic rejection is slow and insidious. Chronic rejection often occurs in conjunction with other histologic causes of allograft dysfunction, namely, acute rejection, calcineurin inhibitor nephrotoxicity, and recurrent or de novo glomerular diseases. The diagnosis of chronic rejection should, therefore, be based on morphologic characteristics of allograft histology and the clinical observation of a gradual decline in renal allograft function. The pathophysiology of chronic rejection is not completely understood, but most likely involves both immune and nonimmune factors. Risk factors for the development of chronic rejection include delayed graft function, ischemia–reperfusion injury, degree of HLA mismatching, histoincompatibility, acute rejection episodes, inadequate renal mass, hypertension, hyperlipidemia, and CMV infection (107). There is no treatment for chronic rejection at the present time.

UROLOGIC COMPLICATIONS

Urologic problems have been reported in between 2% and 20% of all renal transplants. These complications can include urinary retention, urine leak, and ureteral stenosis. Urinary retention can occur because of a neurogenic bladder (related to diabetes or a congenital neurologic disorder) or perhaps to undetected prostatic hypertrophy. These can be managed with an initially longer period of urinary catheterization and use of α-antagonists (tamsulosin, terazosin, prazosin) to improve bladder emptying. More extreme cases may require long-term intermittent self-catheterization or surgical urinary diversion. Urine leak or stenosis can occur both early and later after renal transplant and will be manifested by a rising serum creatinine. Urine leaks may also result in increased fluid through an operative drain or fluid leakage through the wound. This fluid can be sent for creatinine level to confirm the presence of a urine leak. Ultrasound studies may demonstrate a fluid collection around the allograft or hydronephrosis in the case of ureteral stenosis. Nuclear medicine scans can also be obtained to confirm the presence of a ureteral stenosis or urine leak. Mild cases of ureteral stenosis/leakage can be managed with percutaneous methods including insertion of ureteral stents and transluminal balloon dilation. Many of these stenoses/leaks will require operative management to reimplant the ureter or a more complex urologic procedure using the recipient's native ureter or bladder (108–112).

URINARY STONES

Urinary calculi are a relatively uncommon complication of renal transplantation. Calculi may have been present in the donor kidney or may develop after transplantation. Predisposing factors include obstruction, recurrent UTI, hypercalciuria, hyperoxaluria, internal stents, and nonabsorbable suture material (113). Open removal of a calculus from the transplanted kidney is rarely necessary. Complete stone removal is usually possible by standard urologic techniques.

VASCULAR COMPLICATIONS

Vascular complications including vessel thrombosis or stenosis have been reported in 2% to 12% of all renal transplants. Vascular complications in general are significantly associated with ATN and graft loss. Early graft dysfunction should be evaluated for vascular complications with Doppler ultrasound (114). Patients with underlying thrombophilia are at a higher risk for early allograft loss without appropriate anticoagulation. Screening for thrombophilia in those ESRD patients with a history of a thromboembolic event may be appropriate to prevent this complication. Those patients with graft loss due to vascular thrombosis in the absence of an obvious technical problem should undergo a thrombophilia evaluation before retransplant (115).

LYMPHOCELE

A lymphocele is a collection of lymphatic fluid around the allografted kidney that can occur due to leakage of small lymphatic channels around the iliac vessels at the time of the transplant. The incidence of lymphoceles has been reported from as low as 0.02% up to 26% following renal transplant (116–118). Consequences of lymphoceles can include distention due to the fluid collection as well as venous or ureteral obstruction and graft compromise. Treatment of lymphoceles can include percutaneous techniques with drainage and sclerosis of the cavity or may include operative marsupialization via the laparoscopic or open technique. Laparoscopic techniques are less invasive, have less morbidity, and are generally the first line of therapy (118).

POSTTRANSPLANT MALIGNANCIES

Prolonged and intensive immunosuppression impairs the ability of the body to cope with cancers caused by carcinogens such as sunlight or oncogenic viruses, and may lead to the development of an unusual assortment of malignancies (119,120). Infections with potentially oncogenic viruses are common in immunosuppressed patients, including EBV-related B-cell PTLD, human papillomavirus, hepatitis B and C viruses—related hepatocellular carcinoma, and the human herpes virus 8 (Kaposi sarcoma) (120). Malignancies that occur in transplant recipients have a pattern that is very different from that of the general population. The frequency of the cancers that are common in the general population, such as carcinomas of the lung, prostate, breast, and colon, and invasive carcinomas of the uterine cervix, are not increased among transplant recipients (119). Most patients who develop malignancies posttransplant have received multiple immunosuppressive drugs and no single agent can be implicated. The natural history of tumors associated with immunosuppression used for renal transplantation may be more aggressive than would be expected in patients without immunosuppression or transplantation. Cancers of the lip and skin are the most common malignancies. In contrast to the general population, squamous cell carcinoma outnumbers basal cell carcinoma and occurs at a much younger age.

PTLDs are the second most common malignancies found in renal transplant recipients, with the bulk being non-Hodgkin lymphomas. The EBV genome has been isolated from many lymphomas in transplant recipients and causes a variety of lesions that range from benign polyclonal B-cell hyperplasia to frank monoclonal B-cell lymphomas (119,121). Risk factors for PTLD include the overall extent of immunosuppression of the patient. The use of monoclonal/polyclonal antibodies for induction and repeated treatments for acute rejection will significantly increase the risk for PTLD (119,122). The clinical symptoms of PTLD may be extremely variable, and a high index of suspicion is required for accurate diagnosis; PTLD may present in the lymph nodes or extranodally. There are two basic clinical patterns with some overlap. The first, occurring in the early (usually <90 days) posttransplantation period, most often manifests with widespread lesions in an EBV-susceptible patient. The second pattern occurs in patients who received long-term immunosuppression and may present several years after transplantation, with lesions confined to a single organ (123,124).

Treatment of PTLD consists of partial or complete withdrawal of immunosuppression. Such treatment carries the risk of allograft rejection and return of the renal allograft recipient to dialysis. Treatment with prednisone may be continued, however, because it is an important component of many cancer chemotherapy protocols. If EBV infection is suspected, treatment with acyclovir, ganciclovir, or valacyclovir should be initiated pending documentation of EBV infection. Other treatment options include IFN-γ therapy to enhance the immune attack on the lymphoma cells; surgical excision or local radiotherapy to localized tumors; and in advanced cases, chemotherapy. Rituximab (Rituxan; Genentech), a monoclonal antibody directed against the CD20 antigen, has been used successfully to treat CD20-positive tumors (125–127).

Key Points

- Increasing numbers of patients are living with ESRD on renal replacement therapy.
- Renal transplantation is the most effective and cost-effective option for patients with ESRD, but is limited by the number of available kidneys for transplant.
- Immediate posttransplant care involves careful management of fluids and electrolytes in patients who frequently have multiple underlying medical comorbidities.
- Management of renal transplant patients is a balance between preventing acute/chronic rejection with use of immunosuppression and avoiding complications such as infection and malignancy with long-term use of these medications.

References

1. *Kidney and Urologic Diseases Information Clearinghouse. A service of the National Institute of Diabetes and Digestive Diseases and Kidney Diseases, National Institutes of Health.* Available at http://kidney.niddk.nih.gov/kudiseases/pubs/kustats/index.htm. Accessed January 21, 2015.
2. Winkelmayer WC, Weinstein MC, Mittleman MA, et al. Health economic evaluations: the special case of end-stage renal disease treatment. *Med Decis Making.* 2002;22:417–430.
3. Loubeau PR, Loubeau JM, Jantzen R. The economics of kidney transplantation versus hemodialysis. *Prog Transplant.* 2001;11:291–297.
4. National transplant statistics, 2005. *United Network for Organ Sharing.* Available at www.unos.org. Accessed March 21, 2015.
5. Remuzzi G, Grinyo J, Ruggenenti P, et al. Early experience with dual kidney transplantation in adults using expanded donor criteria. Double Kidney Transplant Group (DKG). *J Am Soc Nephrol.* 1999;10:2591–2598.
6. Gok MA, Buckley PE, Shenton BK, et al. Long-term renal function in kidneys from non-heart beating donors: a single-center experience. *Transplantation.* 2002;74:664–669.
7. Sanchez-Fructuoso A, Prats Sanchez D, Marqués Vidas M, et al. Non-heart beating donors. *Nephrol Dial Transplant.* 2004;19(Suppl 3):iii26–iii31.
8. U.S. Organ Procurement and Transplantation Network/Scientific Registry of Transplant Recipients. Annual Report 2012.
9. Kasiske BL, Cangro CB, Hariharan S, et al. The evaluation of renal transplant candidates: clinical practice guidelines. *Am J Transplantation.* 2001; 2(Suppl 1):5–95.
10. Gore JL, Pham PT, Danovitch GM, et al. Obesity and outcome following renal transplantation. *Am J Transplant.* 2006;6:357–363.
11. Stratta RJ, Rohr MS, Sundberg AK et al. Intermediate-term outcomes with expanded criteria deceased donors in kidney transplantation: a spectrum or specter of quality. *Ann Surg.* 2006;243:594–601; discussion 601–603.
12. Merion RM, Ashby VB, Wolfe RA, et al. Deceased-donor characteristics and the survival benefit of kidney transplantation. *JAMA.* 2005;294: 2726–2733.
13. Bernat JL, D'Alessandro AM, Port FK, et al. Report of a national conference on donation after cardiac death. *Am J Transplant.* 2006;6:281–291.
14. Ting A, Welsh K. HLA matching and crossmatching in renal transplantation. In: Morris PJ, ed. *Kidney Transplantation: Principles and Practice.* 4th ed. Philadelphia, PA: WB Saunders; 1994:109.
15. Furnary AP, Wu Y, Bookin SO. Effect of hyperglycemia and continuous intravenous insulin infusions on outcomes of cardiac surgical procedures: the Portland Diabetic Project. *Endocr Pract.* 2004;10:21–33.
16. Finney SJ, Zekveld C, Elia A, Evans TW. Glucose control and mortality in critically ill patients. *JAMA.* 2003;290:2041–2047.
17. Starzl TE, Broth CG, Putnam CW, et al. Urologic complications in 216 human recipients of renal transplants. *Ann Surg.* 1973;172:609.
18. Petrek J, Tilney NL, Smith EH, et al. Ultrasound in renal transplantation. *Ann Surg.* 1977;185:441–447.
19. Hoshino T, Maley WR, Bulkley GB, Williams GM. Ablation of free radical-medicated reperfusion injury for the salvage of kidneys taken from non-heartbeating donors. A quantitative evaluation of the proportion of injury caused by reperfusion following periods of warm, cold, and combined warm and cold ischemia. *Transplantation.* 1988;45:284–289.
20. Sola R, Alarcon A, Jimenez C, Osuna A. The influence of delayed graft function. *Nephrol Dial Transplant.* 2004;19(Suppl 3):iii32–iii37.
21. Boom H, Mallat MJ, deFijter JW, et al. Delayed graft function influences renal function, but not survival. *Kidney Int.* 2000;58:859–866.
22. Irish WD, McCollum DA, Tesi RJ, et al. Nomogram for predicting the likelihood of delayed graft function in adult cadaveric renal transplant recipients. *J Am Soc Nephrol.* 2003;14:2967–2974.
23. Shoskes DA, Halloran PF. Delayed graft function in renal transplantation: etiology, management and long-term significance. *J Urol.* 1996;155: 1831–1840.
24. Ojo AO, Wolfe RA, Held PJ, et al. Delayed graft function: risk factors, and implications for renal allograft survival. *Transplantation.* 1997;63:968–974.
25. Rocha PN, Butterly DW, Greenberg A, et al. Beneficial effect of plasmapheresis and intravenous immunoglobulin on renal allograft survival of patients with acute humoral rejection. *Transplantation.* 2003;75:1490–1495.
26. Clinical trials. *A service of the U.S. National Institutes of Health.* Available at https://clinicaltrials.gov. Accessed May 18, 2015.
27. Legendre C, Sberro-Soussan R, Zuber J, et al. Eculizumab in renal transplantation. *Transplant Rev (Orlando).* 2013;27:90–92.
28. SOLIRIS (eculizumab) [package insert]. Cheshire, CT: Alexion Pharmaceuticals. Revised April 2014.
29. Bonnefoy-Berard N, Revillard JP. Mechanisms of immunosuppression induced by antithymocyte globulins and OKT3. *J Heart Lung Transplant.* 1996;15:435–442.
30. Rossi SJ, Schroeder TJ, Hariharan S, First MR. Prevention and management of the adverse effects associated with immunosuppressive therapy. *Drug Saf.* 1993;9:104–131.
31. Riechmann L, Clark M, Waldmann H, Winter G. Reshaping human antibodies for therapy. *Nature.* 1988;332:323–327.
32. Hale G, Xia MQ, Tighe HP, et al. The CAMPATH-1H antigen (CDw52). *Tissue Antigens.* 1990;35:118–127.

33. Hale G. CD52 antigen as a target for immunotherapy. *Transpl Rev.* 2003;17:S8.
34. Waldmann H. Development and clinical use of CAMPATH 1H. *Transpl Rev.* 2003;17:S5.
35. Kaufman DB, Leventhal JR, Axelrod D, et al. Alemtuzumab induction and prednisolone-free maintenance immunotherapy in kidney transplantation: comparison with basiliximab induction. Long-term results. *Am J Transpl.* 2005;78:426.
36. Shapiro R, Basu A, Tan H, et al. Kidney transplantation under minimal immunosuppression after pretransplant lymphoid depletion with Thymoglobulin or Campath. *J Am Coll Surg.* 2005;200:505–515; quiz A59–A61.
37. Hanaway MJ, Woodle ES, Mulgaonkar S, et al. Alemtuzumab induction in renal transplantation. *N Engl J Med.* 2011;364:1909–1919.
38. Nadler LM, Ritz J, Hardy R, et al. A unique cell surface antigen identifying lymphoid malignancies of B-cell origin. *J Clin Invest.* 1981;67:134–140.
39. Maloney D, Liles T, Czerwinski D, et al. Phase I clinical trial using escalating single dose infusion of chimeric anti-CD 20 monoclonal antibody in patients with recurrent B-cell lymphoma. *Blood.* 1994;84:2457–2466.
40. Coiffier B, Haioun C, Ketterer N, et al. Rituximab for the treatment of patients with relapsing or refractory aggressive lymphoma: a multicenter phase II study. *Blood.* 1998;92:1927–1932.
41. Blaes AH, Peterson BA, Bartlett N, et al. Rituximab therapy is effective for post transplant lymphoproliferative disorders after solid organ transplantation: results of a phase II trial. *Cancer.* 2005;104:1661–1667.
42. Nashan B, Moore R, Amlot P, et al., for the CH1B 201 International Study Group. Randomized trial of basiliximab versus placebo for control of acute cellular rejection in renal allograft recipients. *Lancet.* 1997;350:1193–1198.
43. Rosenthal JT, Hakala TR, Iwatsuki S, et al. Cadaveric renal transplantation under cyclosporine-steroid therapy. *Surg Gynecol Obstet.* 1983;157:309–315.
44. Hougardy JM, de Jonge H, Kuypers D, Abramowicz D. The once-daily formulation of tacrolimus: a step forward in kidney transplantation? *Transplantation.* 2012;93:241–243.
45. Budde K, Bunnapradist S, Grinyo JM, et al. Novel once-daily extended release tacrolimus (LCPT) versus twice-daily tacrolimus in de novo kidney transplants: one-year results of Phase III, double-blind, randomized trial. *Am J Transplant.* 2014;14:2796–2806.
46. Myers BD, Newton L, Oyer P. The case against the indefinite use of cyclosporine. *Transplant Proc.* 1991;23:41–42.
47. Bennett WM, DeMattos A, Meyer MM, et al. Chronic cyclosporine nephropathy: the Achilles' heel of immunosuppressive therapy. *Kidney Int.* 1996;50:1089–1100.
48. Hardinger KL, Brennan DC, Mutinga N, et al. Long-term outcome and cost of gastrointestinal complications in renal transplant patients treated with mycophenolate mofetil (MMF). Poster presented at American Society of Transplantation, May 30–June 4, 2003; Washington DC.
49. Knoll GA, MacDonald I, Khan A, Van Walraven C. Mycophenolate mofetil dose reduction and the risk of acute rejection after renal transplantation. *J Am Soc Nephrol.* 2003;14:2381–2386.
50. Morales JM, Wramner L, Kreis H, et al. Sirolimus does not exhibit nephrotoxicity compared to cyclosporine in renal transplant recipients. *Am J Transplant.* 2002;2:436–442.
51. Reitamo S, Spuls P, Sassolas B, et al. Efficacy of sirolimus (rapamycin) administered concomitantly with a subtherapeutic dose of cyclosporine in the treatment of severe psoriasis: a randomized controlled trial. *Br J Dermatol.* 2001;145:438–445.
52. Shihab FS, Bennett WM, Yi H, et al. Sirolimus increases transforming growth factor-beta1 expression and potentiates chronic cyclosporine nephrotoxicity. *Kidney Int.* 2004;65:1262–1271.
53. Shihab F, Christians U, Smith L, et al. Focus on mTOR inhibitors and tacrolimus in renal transplantation: pharmacokinetics, exposure-response relationships, and clinical outcomes. *Transpl Immunol.* 2014;31:22–32.
54. Wojciechowski D, Vincenti F. Belatacept in kidney transplantation. *Curr Opin Organ Transplant.* 2012;17:640–647.
55. Matas AJ, Kandaswamy R, Humar A, et al. Long-term immunosuppression, without maintenance prednisone, after kidney transplantation. *Ann Surg.* 2004;240:510–516; discussion 516–517.
56. Ulrich W, Schlederer MP, Buxbaum P, et al. The histopathologic identification of CMV infected cells in biopsies of human renal allografts: an evaluation of 100 transplant biopsies by in situ hybridization. *Pathol Res Pract.* 1986;181:739–745.
57. Pham PT, Schaenman J, Pham PC. BK virus infection following kidney transplantation: an overview of risk factors, screen strategies, and therapeutic interventions. *Curr Opin Organ Transplant.* 2014;19:401–412.
58. Costa C, Cavallo R. Polyomavirus-associated nephropathy. *World J Transplant.* 2012;2:84–94.
59. Hirsch HH, Randhawa P; AST Infectious Diseases Community of Practice. BK polyomavirus in solid organ transplantation. *Am J Transplant.* 2013;13 (Suppl 4):179–188.
60. Benoit G, Moukarzel M, Verdelli G, et al. Gastrointestinal complications in renal transplantation. *Transpl Int.* 1993;6:45–49.
61. Troppmann C, Papalois BE, Chiou A, et al. Incidence, complications, treatment, and outcome of ulcers of the upper gastrointestinal tract after renal transplantation during the cyclosporine era. *J Am Coll Surg.* 1995;180:433–443.
62. Gianello P, Squifflet JP, Pirson Y, et al. Gastroduodenal complications after transplantation. *Clin Transplant.* 1988;2:221.
63. Hadjiyannakis EJ, Smellie WA, Evans DB, Calne RY. Gastrointestinal complications after renal transplantation. *Lancet.* 1971;2:781–785.
64. Carson SD, Krom RA, Uchida K, et al. Colon perforation after kidney transplantation. *Ann Surg.* 1978;188:109–113.
65. Fernandez-Cruz L, Targarona EM, Cugat E, et al. Acute pancreatitis after renal transplantation. *Br J Surg.* 1989;76:1132–1135.
66. Kawanishi H, Rudolph E, Bull FE. Azathioprine-induced acute pancreatitis. *N Engl J Med.* 1973;289:357.
67. Vanrenterghem Y, Ponticelli C, Morales JM, et al. Prevalence and management of anemia in renal transplant recipients: a European survey. *Am J Transplant.* 2003;3:835–845.
68. First MR. Long-term complications after transplantation. *Am J Kidney Dis.* 1993;22:477–486.
69. Kirkman RL, Strom TB, Weir MR, Tilney NL. Late mortality and morbidity in recipients of long-term renal allografts. *Transplantation.* 1982;34:347–351.
70. Hill MN, Grossman RA, Feldman HI, et al. Changes in causes of death after renal transplantation, 1966 to 1987. *Am J Kidney Dis.* 1991;5:512–518.
71. Rao KV, Andersen RC. Long-term results and complications in renal transplant recipients: observations in the second decade. *Transplantation.* 1988;45:45–52.
72. Braun WE. Long-term complications of renal transplantation. *Kidney Int.* 1990;37:1363–1378.
73. Kasiske BL. Risk factors for accelerated atherosclerosis in renal transplant recipients. *Am J Med.* 1988;84:985–992.
74. Braun WE, Marwick TH. Coronary artery disease in renal transplant recipients. *Cleve Clin J Med.* 1994;61:370–385.
75. Keown PA, Shackleton CR, Ferguson BM. Long-term mortality, morbidity, and rehabilitation in organ transplant recipients. In: Paul LC, Solez K, eds. *Organ Transplantation: Long-Term Results.* New York: Marcel Dekker; 1992:57–84.
76. Kasiske BL, Guijjaro C, Massy ZA, et al. Cardiovascular disease after renal transplantation. *J Am Soc Nephrol.* 1996;7:158–165.
77. Vanrenterghem Y, Roels L, Lerut T, et al. Long-term prognosis after cadaveric kidney transplantation. *Transplant Proc.* 1987;19:3762–3764.
78. Brott T, Toole JF. Medical compared with surgical treatment of asymptomatic carotid artery stenosis. *Ann Intern Med.* 1995;123:720–722.
79. Ibels LS, Stewart JH, Mahony JF, Sheil AG. Deaths from occlusive arterial disease in renal allograft recipients. *BMJ.* 1974;3:552–554.
80. Gunnarsson R, Lofmark R, Nondlander R, et al. Acute myocardial infarction in renal transplant recipients: incidence and prognosis. *Eur Heart J.* 1984;5:218–221.
81. Held PJ, Port FK, Blagg CR, Agodoa LY. Survival and mortality: excerpts from United States Renal Data System 1990 Annual Report. *Am J Kidney Dis.* 1990;16(Suppl 2):44.
82. Luke RG. Pathophysiology and treatment of posttransplant hypertension. *J Am Soc Nephrol.* 1991;2(Suppl 1):S37–S44.
83. Luke RG. Hypertension in renal transplant recipients. *Kidney Int.* 1987;31:1024–1037.
84. Abdulmassih Z, Chevalier A, Bader C, et al. Role of lipid disturbances in the atherosclerosis of renal transplant patients. *Clin Transplant.* 1992;6:106–113.
85. Summary of the second report of the National Cholesterol Education Program (NCEP) expert panel on detection, evaluation, and treatment of high blood cholesterol in adults (adult treatment panel II). *JAMA.* 1993;269:3015–3023.
86. Cattran DC, Steiner G, Wilson DR, Fenton SA. Hyperlipidemia after renal transplantation: natural history and pathophysiology. *Ann Intern Med.* 1979;91:554–559.
87. Vathsala A, Weinberg RB, Schoenberg L, et al. Lipid abnormalities in cyclosporine-prednisone-treated renal transplant recipients. *Transplantation.* 1989;48:37–43.

88. Kasiske BL, Umen AJ. Persistent hyperlipidemia in renal transplant recipients. *Medicine (Baltimore)*. 1987;66:309–316.
89. Divaker D, Bailey RR, Frampton CM, et al. Hyperlipidemia in stable renal transplant recipients. *Nephron*. 1991;59:423–428.
90. Massy ZA, Kasiske BL. Post-transplant hyperlipidemia: mechanisms and management. *J Am Soc Nephrol*. 1996;7:971–977.
91. Duerke TB, Abdulmassih Z, Lacour B, et al. Atherosclerosis and lipid disorders after renal transplantation. *Kidney Int Suppl*. 1991;39:S24–S28.
92. Raine AE, Carter R, Mann JI, Morris PJ. Adverse effect of cyclosporin on plasma cholesterol in renal transplant recipients. *Nephrol Dial Transplant*. 1988;3:458–463.
93. Jung K, Neumann R, Scholz D, Nugel E. Abnormalities in the composition of serum high density lipoprotein in renal transplant recipients. *Clin Nephrol*. 1982;17:191–194.
94. Averna MR, Barbagallo CM, Sparacino V, et al. Follow-up of lipid and apoprotein levels in renal transplant level in renal transplant recipients. *Nephron*. 1991;58:255–256.
95. Kasiske BL, Tortorice KL, Heim-Duthoy KL, et al. The adverse impact of cyclosporine on serum lipids in renal transplant recipients. *Am J Kidney Dis*. 1991;17:700–707.
96. Bittar AE, Ratcliffe PJ, Richardson AJ, et al. The prevalence of hyperlipidemia in renal transplant recipients associations with immunosuppressive and antihypertensive therapy. *Transplantation*. 1990;50:987–992.
97. Roth D, Milgrom M, Esquenazi V, et al. Posttransplant hyperglycemia increased incidence in cyclosporine-treated renal allograft recipients. *Transplantation*. 1989;47:278–281.
98. Sumrani NB, Delaney V, Ding ZK, et al. Diabetes mellitus after renal transplantation in the cyclosporine era: an analysis of risk factors. *Transplantation*. 1991;51:343–347.
99. Jindal RM. Posttransplant diabetes mellitus: a review. *Transplantation*. 1994;58:1289–1298.
100. Pirsch JD, Miller J, Deierhoi MH, et al. A comparison of tacrolimus (FK506) and cyclosporine for immunosuppression after cadaveric renal transplantation. FK506 Kidney Transplant Study Group. *Transplantation*. 1997;63:977–983.
101. A comparison of tacrolimus (FK506) and cyclosporine for immunosuppression in liver transplantation. The U.S. Multicenter FK506 Liver Study Group. *N Engl J Med*. 1994;331:1110–1115.
102. Randomised trial comparing tacrolimus (FK506) and cyclosporin in prevention of liver allograft rejection. European FK506 Multicentre Liver Study Group. *Lancet*. 1994;344:423–428.
103. Sumrani N, Delaney V, Ding Z, et al. Posttransplant diabetes mellitus in cyclosporine-treated renal transplant recipients. *Transplant Proc*. 1991;23: 1249–1250.
104. Koyama H, Cecka JM. Rejection episodes. *Clin Transpl*. 1992;391–404.
105. Peddi VR, First MR. Early posttransplant care of renal transplant recipients. *Semin Dial*. 1999;12:320–328.
106. Solez K, Colvin RB, Racusen LC, et al. Banff 07 Classification of renal allograft pathology: updates and future directions. *Am J Transplant*. 2008; 8:753–760.
107. Monaco AP, Burke JF Jr, Ferguson RM. Current thinking on chronic renal allograft rejection: issues, concerns, and recommendations from a 1997 round table discussion. *Am J Kidney Dis*. 1999;33:150–160.
108. Hernandez D, Rufino M, Armas S, et al. Retrospective analysis of surgical complications following cadaveric kidney transplantation in the modern transplant era. *Nephrol Dial Transplant*. 2006;10:2908–2815.
109. Dalgic A, Boyvat F, Karakayali H, et al. Urologic complications in 1523 renal transplantations: the Baskent University experience. *Transplant Proc*. 2006;38:543–547.
110. Juaneda B, Alcaraz A, Bujons A, et al. Endourological management is better in early-onset ureteral stenosis in kidney transplantation. *Transplant Proc*. 2005;37:3825–3827.
111. Pisani F, Iaria G, D'Angelo M, et al. Urologic complications in kidney transplantation. *Transplant Proc*. 2005;37:2521–2522.
112. Praz V, Leisinger HJ, Pascual M, Jichlinski P. Urological complications in renal transplantation from cadaveric donor grafts: a retrospective analysis of 20 years. *Urol Int*. 2005;75:144–149.
113. Yigit B, Aydin C, Titiz I, et al. Stone disease in kidney transplantation. *Transplant Proc*. 2004;36:187–189.
114. Osman Y, Shokeir A, Ali-el Dein B, et al. Vascular complications after live donor renal transplantation: study of risk factors and effects of graft and patient survival. *J Urol*. 2003;169:859–862.
115. Morrissey PE, Ramirez PJ, Gohh RY, et al. Management of thrombophilia in renal transplant patients. *Am J Transplant*. 2002;2:872–876.
116. Smyth GP, Beitz G, Eng MP, et al. Long-term outcome of cadaveric renal transplant after treatment of symptomatic lymphocele. *J Urol*. 2006;176:1069–1072.
117. Atray NK, Moore F, Zaman F, et al. Post-transplant lymphocele: a single centre experience. *Clin Transplant*. 2004;18:46–49.
118. Bailey SH, Mone MC, Holman JM, Nelson EW. Laparoscopic treatment of post renal transplant lymphoceles. *Surg Endosc*. 2003;17: 1896–1899.
119. Penn I. Cancers complicating organ transplantation. *N Engl J Med*. 1990; 323:1767–1769.
120. Penn I. Tumors in the transplant. In: Jacobson HR, Striker GF, Klahr S, eds. *The Principles and Practice of Nephrology*. Philadelphia, PA: Mosby; 1995:833.
121. Hanto DW. Polyclonal and monoclonal posttransplant lymphoproliferative diseases (PTLD). *Clin Transpl*. 1992;6:227–234.
122. Penn I. The changing pattern of posttransplant malignancies. *Transplant Proc*. 1991;23:1101–1103.
123. Renoult E, Aymard B, Gregoire MJ, et al. Epstein-Barr virus lymphoproliferative disease of donor origin after kidney transplantation: a case report. *Am J Kidney Dis*. 1995;26:84–87.
124. Alfrey EJ, Friedman AL, Grossman RA, et al. Two distinct patterns of post-transplantation lymphoproliferative disorder (PTLD): early and late onset. *Clin Transpl*. 1992;6:246–248.
125. Penn I. Immunosuppression: a contributory factor in lymphoma formation. *Clin Transpl*. 1992;6:214–219.
126. Milpied N, Vasseur B, Parquet N, et al. Humanized anti-CD20 monoclonal antibody (rituximab) in post transplant lymphoproliferative disorder: a retrospective analysis on 32 patients. *Ann Oncol*. 2000;1(Suppl 1): S113–S116.
127. Faye A, Van Den Abeele T, Peuchmaur M, et al. Anti-CD20 monoclonal antibody for post-transplant lymphoproliferative disorders. *Lancet*. 1998; 352:1285.

CHAPTER

76

Critical Care Aspects of Stem Cell Transplantation

AMIN RAHEMTULLA and ROBERT PETER GALE

INTRODUCTION

Bone marrow and blood cell transplants are widely used to treat aplastic anemia, leukemias, lymphomas, myeloma, and immune deficiency disorders. Increasingly, transplants are used to treat other bone marrow disorders such as sickle cell disease and thalassemia. Morbidity and mortality associated with transplants usually result from regimen-related toxicity, such as adverse effects of drugs and radiation given pretransplant, complications of graft-versus-host disease (GvHD), as well as infections resulting from bone marrow failure. Morbidity and mortality of transplants has steadily decreased over the past four decades because of better supportive care. Recently, there is increased use of reduced-intensity conditioning allotransplants. Although this is associated with less immediate toxicity, treatment-related mortality by 1 year seems similar to conventional transplants. There are also increased transplants from partially HLA-matched related and unrelated donors. These transplants are associated with increased treatment-related morbidity and mortality for diverse reasons.

Pretransplant evaluation of recipients typically includes the following (1–9):

- Measurement of the left ventricular ejection fraction (LVEF), which should be at least 40% and a check for arrhythmias. This is arbitrarily chosen as an eligibility criteria as some studies have shown an association between poor cardiac function and the risk of developing posttransplant cardiotoxicity while others have not. Several recent studies also suggest that these are low-yield procedures (10)
- Pulmonary function tests, including carbon monoxide diffusing capacity (DL_{CO}), and forced vital capacity (FVC_1), which should be more than 50% of predicted.
- Liver function tests which should be in the acceptable range.
- Creatinine clearance, which should be more than 50 mL/min/1.73 m^2 body surface area
- A pretransplant performance score consistent with an independent life.

Because the risk of GvHD increases with age, allotransplants are typically done in subjects younger than 55 years (11). However, with the increased use of reduced-intensity conditioning regimens, allotransplants are increasingly being performed in older persons. Autotransplant recipients, on the other hand, are at risk for fewer treatment-related complications such as GvHD, so older transplant recipients are not excluded (12). The risk of infection is minimized by various preventative or isolation procedures (see below). Transplants are typically delayed in subjects with active infections until the infection resolves (13,14). The 100-day transplant-related mortality after autotransplants is 2% to 5%; after related allotransplants, it is 15% to 20%; and after alternative (unrelated) allotransplants, it is about 30% (13,14).

IMMEDIATE CONCERNS: THE FIRST 30 DAYS

Pretransplant Conditioning Regimens

In the setting of allotransplants, the pretransplant conditioning regimen needs to moderate or eliminate recipient immunity to prevent graft rejection (15,16). When the allotransplant recipient has cancer, the pretransplant conditioning regimen may also play an important anticancer role. Most allotransplant conditioning regimens contain cyclophosphamide and busulfan or total-body radiation (17,18). Antilymphocyte antibodies, such as antilymphocyte globulin (ALG), antithymocyte globulin (ATG), or alemtuzumab (anti-CD52), are often used in reduced-intensity conditioning regimens or in alternative donor transplants. In immune deficiency disorders such as severe combined immune deficiency (SCID), pretransplant conditioning is not necessary, as the host is already immune deficient.

For autotransplants, the choice of pretransplant conditioning regimen is based entirely on anticancer effect, a steep dose–response curve, lack of cross-resistance with other drugs, and low non–bone marrow dose-limiting toxicities. In general, these regimens contain alkylating drugs, such as melphalan or cyclophosphamide, combined with two or three other drugs. Immune suppression is unnecessary and an unwanted side effect of the conditioning regimen; radiation is not typically used in autotransplants.

Pretransplant conditioning regimens are typically empirically determined, as there are few large randomized trials. Consequently, it is difficult to determine which regimen, if any, is best (19). The choice of a pretransplant conditioning regimen depends not only on effectiveness of the regimen in a specific disease and the need for immune suppression but also on avoiding toxicity from prior therapy or current organ dysfunction. For example, prior mantle radiation or exposures to radiosensitizers, such as bleomycin or carmustine (BCNU), increase the pulmonary toxicity of total-body radiation, whereas prior therapy of testicular cancer patients with cisplatin increases the renal toxicity of platinum-based conditioning regimens. In some diseases and disease states, data from large observational databases, and occasionally from randomized trials suggest superiority of one regimen over another. Examples include total-body radiation regimens in persons with acute lymphoblastic leukemia (20) and cyclophosphamide and busulfan rather than total-body radiation in acute myeloid leukemia (21). Non–bone marrow dose-limiting toxicities of

TABLE 76.1 Toxicity of Conditioning Regimen Drugs

Drug/Dose	Extramedullary Dose-Limiting Toxicity	Other Toxicities
BCNU	Interstitial pneumonitis	Renal insufficiency, encephalopathy, nausea, vomiting, sinusoidal obstruction syndrome/veno-occlusive disease (SOS/VOD)
Busulfan	Mucositis, SOS/VOD	Seizures, rash, hyperpigmentation, nausea, vomiting, pneumonitis
CCNU (lomustine)	Interstitial pneumonitis	Renal insufficiency, encephalopathy, nausea, vomiting, SOS/VOD
Cyclophosphamide	Heart failure	Hemorrhagic cystitis, syndrome of inappropriate antidiuretic hormone (SIADH), nausea, vomiting, pulmonary edema, interstitial pneumonitis
Cytarabine	Mucositis, cerebellar ataxia	Pulmonary edema, conjunctivitis, rash, fever, hepatitis, toxic epidermal necrolysis
Cisplatin	Renal insufficiency, peripheral neuropathy	Nausea, vomiting, renal tubular acidosis, hypomagnesemia
Carboplatin	Ototoxicity, hepatitis	Renal insufficiency, hypomagnesemia, peripheral neuropathy
Etoposide	Mucositis	Nausea, vomiting, hemorrhagic cystitis, pneumonia, hepatitis
Ifosfamide	Encephalopathy, renal insufficiency	Hemorrhagic cystitis, renal tubular acidosis
Melphalan	Mucositis	Nausea, vomiting, hepatitis, SIADH, pneumonitis, renal insufficiency
Mitoxantrone	Cardiotoxicity	Mucositis
Paclitaxel	Mucositis	Peripheral neuropathy, bradycardia, anaphylaxis
Thiotepa	Mucositis	Intertriginous rash, hyperpigmentation, nausea, vomiting

drugs in commonly used pretransplant conditioning regimens are listed in Table 76.1.

Bone Marrow and Blood Cell Collection

Cells used for transplants are most often collected from the blood, but may also be collected from the bone marrow or umbilical cord blood (22–27). Collection of blood cells is an outpatient procedure accomplished with an apheresis device, such as the Cobe Spectra. In the context of autotransplants, recipients often receive chemotherapy and/or hematopoietic growth factors to increase numbers of circulating blood cells and therefore blood cells collected. Normal allotransplant donors often receive only hematopoietic growth factors. The timing of apheresis correlates with the method used to increase numbers of cells collected: apheresis is usually done for 1 to 3 days, starting 4 days after beginning hematopoietic growth factor therapy. In contrast, when chemotherapy is used, apheresis is usually done for 1 to 3 days when neutrophils are present at a level of greater than or equal to 1×10^9 cells/L; this is usually 10 to 16 days after induction of chemotherapy. The advantages of collecting blood rather than bone marrow cells include: no need for anesthesia; use in subjects with hypocellular, fibrotic, or cancer-infiltrated bone marrow; and a more rapid posttransplant bone marrow recovery. A disadvantage of using blood as opposed to bone marrow cells is an increased incidence and severity of chronic GvHD, likely because blood contains 10-fold more T cells, the cells causing chronic GvHD (26). The cost of blood cell collection is similar to collecting bone marrow cells. Complications of blood cell collection are rare, but include infection, anaphylaxis, and hypocalcemia.

Bone marrow cells are collected in the operating room under general, epidural, spinal, or caudal anesthesia. The donor may be admitted on the day of the procedure and discharged the next day. Sometimes, an autologous unit of red blood cells (RBCs) unit is collected 3 to 4 weeks before the procedure for autotransfusion. Complications of bone marrow collection are rare but include the risks of anesthesia: hypotension, nausea, vomiting, cardiac arrest, pulmonary emboli, pain, hemorrhage, and infection.

Cord blood cells are obtained from the umbilical cord and placental blood at the time of birth. The target is to collect 2 to 4×10^7 nucleated cells/kg recipient weight. This is more than 10-fold less than the 2 to 4×10^8 nucleated cells/kg recipient weight collected from the bone marrow. Cord blood cell transplants are often restricted to children because of the small number of cells collected. The potential advantages of cord blood are a higher proportion of progenitor cells compared to bone marrow and possibly less GvHD from fewer T cells. Recently, adults have been transplanted with double umbilical cord blood cells with some success (28).

Bone Marrow and Blood Cell Infusion

Bone marrow and blood cells may be frozen in dimethyl sulfoxide (DMSO) for later use (29,30). The intracellular contents of cells destroyed in the freezing and thawing processes—and DMSO itself—may cause hypotension, anaphylaxis, or dysrhythmias, including transient heart block (31). To avoid complications, subjects are premedicated with diphenhydramine hydrochloride (Benadryl) and methylprednisolone sodium succinate (Solu-Medrol). Intubation equipment and epinephrine should be available at the bedside when cells are infused. If hypotension occurs, the infusion is slowed or temporarily interrupted until the blood pressure stabilizes. If the bone marrow or blood cells have not been frozen, the risk of anaphylaxis is similar to a standard blood transfusion, and premedication is unnecessary.

Bone marrow and blood cell collections are routinely analyzed for quality control at various times during collection, processing, storage, and infusion. Approximately 1.2% of cultures obtained during these processes are found to contain bacteria (32). Most cultures show coagulase-negative *Staphylococcus sp.*, which colonize the skin; pathogenic gram-negative bacteria are occasionally present. Bone marrow and blood cell collections inconvenience the donor and cost approximately $16,000. Thus, despite positive culture results, most centers infuse the cells after appropriate antibiotic coverage; although controversial, this approach has generally been without adverse effects.

Fluids and Hypotension

High-dose chemotherapy and radiation damage vascular endothelial cells, resulting in extravascular leakage of fluids. Furthermore, GvHD and cytokines such as tumor necrosis factor (TNF), interleukin 2 (IL-2), and interferon-gamma (IFN-γ) contribute to a posttransplant capillary leak syndrome (33–36). In addition, subjects often receive large volumes of intravenous (IV) fluids from drug infusions, parenteral nutrition, and prophylaxis for hemorrhagic cystitis. Consequently, all transplant recipients gain weight, with the result that diuretics are frequently given to maintain baseline weight and mitigate fluid retention. If hypotension develops, emphasis should be placed on early invasive cardiovascular monitoring, inotropic support, and irradiated packed RBC transfusion to maintain intravascular oncotic pressure. Aggressive hydration may precipitate pulmonary and peripheral edema, even with normal pulmonary artery wedge pressure and right atrial pressure.

Electrolyte Balance

Electrolyte abnormalities are common in transplant recipients, resulting from the underlying disease, prophylactic hydration for hemorrhagic cystitis, diarrhea, parenteral nutrition, renal insufficiency, diuretics, and other medications. Ifosfamide, especially when combined with carboplatin, causes a Fanconi syndrome–like renal tubular acidosis 3 to 7 days after the pretransplant conditioning regimen (37,38). The resulting normal anion gap acidosis may be treated with sodium bicarbonate. Other drugs associated with renal tubular wasting of electrolytes are amphotericin, foscarnet, and aminoglycosides. The syndrome of inappropriate secretion of antidiuretic hormone (SIADH) may result from high-dose cyclophosphamide and/or ifosfamide. Cyclosporine may cause hypomagnesemia and hypokalemia or hyperkalemia; hypomagnesemia increases the risk of cyclosporine-associated seizures. Tumor lysis syndrome is rare, as most transplant recipients have relatively few cancer cells and receive intensive hydration. Finally, uric acid, a major blood antioxidant, is markedly decreased soon after a transplant, independent of allopurinol, which is often given (39).

Blood Product Transfusions

Subjects receiving transplants are immune compromised and at risk for transfusion-associated GvHD. All cellular blood products contain white blood cells (WBCs), including immune-competent T cells, and should be irradiated to 25 Gy (40).

Cytomegalovirus (CMV) infection is another risk. Allotransplant recipients should receive CMV-negative blood product transfusions, especially when the recipient is CMV seronegative (41–44). If CMV seronegative blood is unavailable, removal of contaminating WBC with an inline microfilter is an alternative (45,46). When an allotransplant recipient is CMV seropositive, no special CMV-related precautions are needed. Because autotransplant recipients do not develop GvHD or receive posttransplant immune suppression, the risk of CMV-related infection is low (47), and no special CMV-related precautions are needed.

Special consideration is needed regarding ABO-compatibility between recipient and donor (48–50). As engraftment occurs, there is a gradual switch of RBCs to the donor ABO type with a transition period when RBCs with recipient and donor ABO types are present in the blood. When there is A and/or B incompatibility between recipient and donor, there is the possibility that residual anti-A or -B recipient antibodies may react against donor RBCs. Also, B cells in the graft may produce anti-A or -B antibodies against residual recipient RBCs. This complexity of blood product transfusion support should be viewed in terms of whether there is major or minor ABO incompatibility between the recipient and the donor (Tables 76.2 and 76.3). A major ABO incompatibility occurs when the recipient has antibodies to the donor RBC phenotype, for example, recipient group O, donor group A. To prevent immediate RBC destruction by pre-existing recipient antibodies, RBCs should be removed from the graft. Posttransplant, the recipient should receive recipient ABO-type or O-type RBC transfusions from which plasma and platelets are removed. With a minor ABO incompatibility, the donor has anti-A and/or anti-B antibodies to the recipient's RBC ABO type, for example, donor O type, and recipient A or B type. Donor anti-A and/or anti-B antibodies should be removed from the graft. Posttransplant, the recipient should receive O-type RBC transfusions and recipient ABO-type plasma and platelets. When recipient and donor have anti-A and/or anti-B antibodies to each other's ABO type, for example, recipient A

TABLE 76.2 Donor–Recipient ABO Incompatibility

Major ABO Incompatibility	Minor ABO Incompatibility	Major and Minor ABO Incompatibility
Recipient has antibody to donor	Donor has antibody to recipient	Recipient has antibody to donor and donor has antibody to recipient
IMMEDIATE HEMOLYSIS		
Prevent by RBC depletion of marrow	Prevent by plasma depletion of marrow	Prevent by RBC and plasma depletion of marrow
DELAYED HEMOLYSIS		
Occurs 2–4 weeks after SCT	Occurs Day 9 to Day 16 after SCT	+ Direct antiglobulin test
+ Direct antiglobulin test	+ Direct antiglobulin test	
Risk increased with high recipient isohemagglutinin titer	Risk increased with T-cell depleted marrow	
DELAYED ERYTHROPOIESIS		
Plasma exchange, erythropoietin, steroids		Plasma exchange, erythropoietin, steroids

RBC, red blood cell; SCT, stem cell transplantation; +, positive.

TABLE 76.3 ABO Type of Blood Components Used in Patients Who Have Received an ABO-Incompatible Transplant

Donor	Recipient	Red Cells	Platelets[a]	FFP
MAJOR ABO INCOMPATIBILITY				
A	O	O	A	A
B	O	O	B	B
AB	O	O	A	AB
AB	A	A	A	AB
AB	B	B	B	AB
MINOR ABO INCOMPATIBILITY				
O	A	O	A	A
O	B	O	B	B
O	AB	O	A	AB
A	AB	A	A	AB
B	AB	B	B	AB
MAJOR AND MINOR ABO INCOMPATIBILITY				
A	B	O	B	AB
B	A	O	A	AB

[a]Occasionally, due to nonavailability of platelets of the requested group, group O platelets (labeled as "low titer," i.e., low titer of anti-A and anti-B) may be used for patients of any group.

When full ABO conversion has taken place, all patients receive products of their new ABO group.

type and donor B type, there is a combined major/minor ABO incompatibility. In this instance, RBC and plasma should be removed from the graft. Posttransplant, the recipient should receive O-type RBC transfusions and AB-type platelets and plasma.

Despite using ABO-compatible platelets, many subjects fail to respond to platelet transfusions early posttransplant. Causes include fever, hepatic sinusoidal obstruction syndrome/veno-occlusive disease (SOS/VOD), drugs, infection, disseminated intravascular coagulation (DIC), and microangiopathic hemolytic anemia related to cyclosporine and/or GvHD (51).

Infection Prevention

Tactics to prevent bacterial, viral, and fungal infections vary considerably between centers (52–54), reflecting the absence of definitive studies and frequent availability of new drugs. Types of infections in transplant recipients correlate with the interval posttransplant. Tactics to prevent bacterial infections early posttransplant are based on two considerations: most infections arise from endogenous microorganisms; and in studies of neutropenic animals, the oral inoculum of gram-negative bacteria required to cause death is increased by colonization of the gastrointestinal tract with anaerobic bacteria. This has led to selective aerobic gastrointestinal decontamination, first, with nonabsorbable antibiotics such as gentamicin, vancomycin, and nystatin, and later, with absorbable antimicrobials selective for aerobes such as oral quinolones (55–57).

Standards for prevention of infection vary from complete isolation in laminar airflow (LAF) rooms to none. In LAF rooms, the subject is in a sterile environment; persons entering must be gloved and gowned, and food is sterilized or has a low microbial content because it is autoclaved or microwaved (58–61). Prophylactic oral antibiotics are given to destroy enteric pathogens, which not only are reservoirs for infection, but also may function as super-antigens that increase the severity of GvHD (62). The minimal standards to prevent bacterial infections include the following:

- A transplant unit set aside from general hospital, patients, and visitor traffic.
- High-efficiency particulate air (HEPA) filtration to prevent iatrogenic *Aspergillus* sp. infection (63,64).
- Careful handwashing before entering a patient's room.
- A diet without fresh salads, vegetables, or fruits, as these may be contaminated with gram-negative bacteria, or without pepper, as this may be contaminated with an *Aspergillus* spp (65).

Other measures, such as shoe covers, gloves, masks, and gowns and low microbial diets and anterooms are also commonly used but their effectiveness is debatable. Bacterial prophylactic measures are generally discontinued when granulocytes exceed 0.5×10^9 cells/L.

Tactics to prevent fungal infections include the use of oral triazoles, such as itraconazole, voriconazole, posaconazole, or fluconazole, given orally or intravenously for the first month posttransplant (66). The azole antifungals are effective against most *Candida* spp; in transplant recipients, fluconazole is ineffective and itraconazole, voriconazole, and posaconazole are more effective against *Aspergillus* spp. Most *Aspergillus* spp infections are iatrogenic and preventable by HEPA filtration of rooms. Subjects with prior aspergillus infection are at high risk of recurrence (67), especially when there is:

- Prolonged postransplant neutropenia
- Advanced cancer
- A brief interval from beginning systemic antifungal therapy to the transplant
- Severe acute GvHD

Persons with prior aspergillosis should receive amphotericin, voriconazole, posaconazole, or caspofungin early posttransplant (68).

Herpes simplex reactivation is usually prevented by using intravenous or oral aciclovir for the first month posttransplant (69,70). Treatment thereafter results in frequent aciclovir resistance and delays the development of natural immunity.

Fever and Neutropenia

Transplant recipients are immune compromised because of neutropenia, breakdown in mucosal barriers (e.g., mucositis), invasive therapies (e.g., indwelling urinary bladder [IUBC, Foley] catheter or central venous lines), immune suppressive drugs (e.g., cyclosporine, corticosteroids, and methotrexate), and GvHD. Lymphocyte function is also affected by thymic involution, weak proliferative responses to T- or B-cell mitogens, and inverted CD4+/CD8+ ratios for 6 months after autotransplants and more than 1 year after allotransplants (71, 72). When an allotransplant is complicated by chronic GvHD, normal lymphocyte function may never return (73). The risk of infection depends on the genetic link between the donor and the recipient, graft type, and posttransplant immune suppression.

In transplant recipients with fever—temperature greater than or equal to 38°C—and granulocytes less than 0.5×10^9 cells/L (74), one should try to identify a possible infection source using a chest radiograph, blood, and urine cultures and physical examination with emphasis on intravenous catheter sites, the perineal and, oropharyngeal regions and the sinuses. Often no source is identified and broad-spectrum antibiotics are begun. The choice of antibiotics may include an antipseudomonal penicillin, aminoglycoside and vancomycin, or a third-generation antipseudomonal cephalosporin or carbapenem. Transplant recipients commonly receive loop diuretics such as furosemide, which can additively increase ototoxicity. Allotransplant recipients receive cyclosporine, whose nephrotoxicity is increased by aminoglycosides. Recurrent or persistent fever for 3 to 5 days without source in a person with granulocytes less than 0.5×10^9 cells/L is an indication for empiric antifungal therapy with amphotericin. The renal toxicity of amphotericin is enhanced by cyclosporine and aminoglycosides.

Mucositis

The severity of mucositis depends on the components of the preconditioning regimen. The non–bone marrow dose-limiting toxicity of etoposide, busulfan, cytarabine, thiotepa, and paclitaxel is mucositis; radiation also contributes to mucositis. Not surprisingly, conditioning regimens containing these drugs and/or radiation are associated with severe mucositis. Other risk factors include posttransplant methotrexate and pretransplant IFN-γ. Methotrexate should be withheld if severe mucositis develops, whereas IFN-γ should be discontinued at least 2 to 4 weeks before giving radiation.

Management of mucositis includes good oral hygiene, using, for example, saline, chlorhexidine, and nystatin rinses, and topical analgesics (75,76). Opioids are often needed, and should be given intravenously on a schedule—as opposed to PRN (as needed)—or using patient-controlled analgesia (PCA). Severe mucositis may require prophylactic intubation for airway protection. Ultimately, the resolution of mucositis generally correlates with recovery of blood granulocytes. New drugs, such as palifermin (recombinant human keratinocyte growth factor-1) reduce the incidence and severity of oral mucositis (77).

Diarrhea

Diarrhea in transplant recipients may be caused by high-dose drugs and radiation, antibiotics, bacterial and/or viral infections, GvHD, and other factors (78–80). The pretransplant conditioning regimen is the most common cause of diarrhea within 2 to 3 weeks posttransplant. Nevertheless, an infectious cause should always be considered, including *Clostridium difficile* and *Escherichia coli* (0157:H7), CMV, herpes simplex, adenoviruses, rotaviruses, echoviruses, astroviruses, Norwalk virus, Coxsackie virus, *Strongyloides* spp, *Giardia* spp, and *Cryptosporidium* spp. GvHD also causes diarrhea; the diagnosis can be confirmed by intestinal biopsy showing loss of crypts, vacuolization of crypt epithelium, karyorrhectic apoptotic debris, microabscesses, and, in severe cases, ulceration and denudation of the epithelium. Therapy is directed toward appropriate antibiotics for infections and immune suppression for GvHD. Conditioning regimen- and GvHD-associated diarrhea may respond to octreotide, a somatostatin analog whose mechanism of action is partly through the inhibition of secretory hormones (81). Some viral infections, such as CMV, respond to ganciclovir, foscarnet, or cidofovir (82).

Hemorrhagic Cystitis

Hemorrhagic cystitis, occurring 2 to 3 weeks posttransplant, usually results from drugs in the pretransplant conditioning regimen, such as cyclophosphamide, ifosfamide, or etoposide (83–85). Prophylaxis for hemorrhagic cystitis includes hydration and diuretics to maintain urine output at 2 mL/Kg per hour (86,87). Sodium mercaptoethane sulfate (Mesna) is often used, especially with high-dose cyclophosphamide or ifosfamide (88). Mesna is inert in plasma but is hydrolyzed in the urine to reactive monomers that conjugate alkylating drugs. It has a short half-life and is therefore given by continuous intravenous infusion. Complications of hemorrhagic cystitis are uncontrolled bleeding and clotting of the ureters or urethra, resulting in acute kidney failure. Obstruction of the ureters by clots may be asymptomatic or cause kidney colic from ureteral spasm. Severe pain may occur in the back or flank and radiate into the groin or genitals; occasionally it is necessary to insert ureteral stents or a ureterostomy.

Therapy of hemorrhagic cystitis consists of using a Foley catheter to irrigate the bladder with normal saline at 250 mL/hr to prevent intravesicular clotting. Platelets should be maintained at more than 50×10^9 cells/L with platelet transfusions and RBC transfusion should be given to replace blood loss. Discomfort from local bladder spasm can be treated with antispasmodic agents such as oxybutynin chloride (Ditropan). In severe cases, arterial embolization or cystectomy may be necessary.

Hemorrhagic cystitis seen more than 2 weeks posttransplant can result from pretransplant conditioning or viral infection due to, for example, adenovirus, CMV, JC, or BK viruses of the bladder epithelium (89–91); except for CMV, there are no effective antiviral drugs.

Sinusoidal Obstruction Syndrome/ Veno-Occlusive Disease of the Liver

SOS/VOD of the liver is caused by drugs and/or radiation in the pretransplant conditioning regimen within 1 to 3 months posttransplant (92). Unlike the Budd–Chiari syndrome with thrombosis of the large hepatic veins, SOS/VOD arises from thrombosis of the central venule. High-dose therapy damages endothelial cells throughout the body. However, metabolism or activation of drugs by hepatocytes results in a high local concentration. Histologically, the central venule is occluded by concentric fibrosis best shown by a trichrome Masson stain. Lesions are composed initially of von Willebrand factor, soon replaced by collagen (93). Obliteration of the central venule results in intrahepatic hypertension, diminished or reversal of portal blood flow, and ascites.

SOS/VOD, with a reported incidence of 1% to 56%, is a clinical diagnosis suggested by elevated bilirubin, weight gain, ascites, and tender hepatomegaly (94–96) (Table 76.4). The incidence variability results partly from different pretransplant conditioning regimens and the clinical criteria used to diagnose SOS/VOD. For instance, although diagnostic criteria from Johns Hopkins and Seattle seem similar, a retrospective comparison showed SOS/VOD incidence rates of 32% versus 8% (97). Risk factors for SOS/VOD include increased pretransplant liver transaminases, conditioning regimen intensity, prolonged fever, and age (95). Prior hepatitis virus exposure does not increase the risk of SOS/VOD if pretransplant liver function tests are normal. Altered drug metabolism is probably responsible for the decreased incidence of SOS/VOD in children and increased risk for SOS/VOD in persons with abnormal pretransplant liver function. Cytokines that cause fever also damage endothelial cells and probably cause the

TABLE 76.4 Clinical Criteria for Veno-Occlusive Disease of the Liver

McDonald Criteria—Seattle	Jones Criteria—Johns Hopkins
Before day 30: Any two of the following:	*Before day 21: Any two of the following:*
Bilirubin >27 μmol/L = 1.7 mg/dL	Bilirubin >34 μmol/L = 2.0 mg/dL
Hepatomegaly	Hepatomegaly
Ascites or weight gain	Ascites
	Weight gain

increased risk of SOS/VOD in persons with prolonged fever. In general, SOS/VOD incidence is not significantly different in recipients of allo- versus autotransplants.

Clinical symptoms of SOS/VOD are also associated with many common but unrelated transplant complications. For instance, jaundice may result from hemolysis—for example, ABO incompatibility, bacterial sepsis, hepatic candidiasis, parenteral nutrition, drugs such as cyclosporine and methotrexate, or GvHD. Initial evaluation for SOS/VOD should include ultrasound of the liver, with Doppler measurement of portal vein blood flow. Reversal or diminished portal flow is consistent with intrahepatic obstruction of blood flow secondary to SOS/VOD (98); ultrasonographic findings are generally present only in overt clinical disease (99). Although uncertain cases may require liver biopsy, a percutaneous biopsy is contraindicated because of ascites, coagulopathy, and low platelets. Transjugular biopsy may, in general, be performed safely and provides an opportunity to measure the hepatic venous pressure gradient, which, if greater than 10 mmHg, is consistent with SOS/VOD (100).

Therapy for SOS/VOD is predominantly supportive. Emphasis should be on avoiding hepatotoxic drugs that will further damage the liver. Persons with severe SOS/VOD may develop hepatorenal syndrome, marked by renal insufficiency and a low fractional sodium excretion. Therapy includes diuretics to maintain baseline weight and oral ursodeoxycholic acid to lower the bilirubin and prevent further liver injury from free radicals generated by bile acids (101). Some centers attempt to maintain intravascular volume and renal perfusion with RBC transfusions, aiming for a hemoglobin of 12 to 15 g/dL. Early studies of defibrotide, a single-stranded polydeoxyribonucleotide with fibrinolytic, antithrombotic, and anti-ischemic properties, in severe SOS/VOD, suggested activity with complete response rates of 36% to 55% (102–104). No severe hemorrhage or other serious toxicity related to defibrotide was reported.

The prognosis of SOS/VOD is poor when bilirubin is more than 15 to 20 mg/dL. Thrombolytic therapy with tissue plasminogen activator and heparin has been used successfully but may be complicated by severe bleeding (105,106). Once the thrombus is replaced by fibrin and collagen, thrombolytic therapy is probably ineffective. However, in late SOS/VOD, another option is a transjugular, intrahepatic portosystemic shunt to decompress the portal vein (107–109). If there is engraftment without severe GvHD or recurrence of the underlying disorder prompting the transplant, consideration should also be given to a liver transplant (110–112).

Respiratory Failure

Transplant recipients who develop respiratory failure and require mechanical ventilation have a poor prognosis (113,114). Once endotracheally intubated, 80% of recipients are never able to be liberated from mechanical ventilation and, at 6 months, only 3% of subjects who required intubation survive. Except for procedures performed as a prelude to surgery, the reason for intubation is not correlated with a likelihood of survival, but age younger than 40 years and intubation being performed more than 100 days posttransplant correlated with better survival.

Respiratory failure within the first 30 days is usually caused by pretransplant conditioning, regimen-related epithelial cell damage, and/or infection (115–118). Early posttransplant radiotherapy and chemotherapy releases free radicals and cytokines, resulting in damage to pulmonary epithelial cells. This leads to blebs in the cell membranes, separation of junctions between cells, and necrosis, the end result being pulmonary edema, occasionally with focal or diffuse pulmonary alveolar hemorrhage (119). This may occur without an increase in pulmonary artery occlusion pressure (PAOP). Median time to the onset of alveolar hemorrhage posttransplant is about 4 months, but it may occur as late as 1 to 2 years. Symptoms are nonspecific and include dyspnea, hypoxia, and diffuse infiltrates; although hemoptysis is rare, bronchoalveolar lavage often shows intrapulmonary hemorrhage. Early in the course of respiratory distress, efforts should be directed to preventing intubation. Although not evaluated in prospective studies, and therefore of unproven benefit, management may include early invasive hemodynamic monitoring, RBC transfusions to maintain hemoglobin more than 12 g/dL, ultrafiltration to decrease intravascular volume, and anticytokine monoclonal antibodies or cytokine receptor antagonists. Use of high-dose corticosteroids is controversial but, in theory, inhibits generation of free radicals, decreases cytokine release, and decreases inflammation.

The repair process after high-dose chemotherapy and radiation may further interfere with gas exchange by causing interstitial fibrosis. Further, infection aggravates parenchymal inflammation and protracts the repair of the interstitium. Transplant recipients are especially susceptible to pulmonary infections because of bone marrow failure, immune suppressive drugs, mucositis, aspiration, and bronchial epithelial cell damage with impaired ciliary motility. Gram-negative and gram-positive pneumonias are common in the first 30 days posttransplant. Fungal infections of the lung also occur early posttransplant, and isolation of *Aspergillus* spp in a nasal or sputum culture should prompt initial therapy with amphotericin, voriconazole, or caspofungin. Risk factors for aspergillosis are long-term duration of impaired immunity pretransplant, for example, aplastic anemia or SCID; centers without HEPA filters to prevent inhalation of aerosolized spores; and prior invasive aspergillosis. Viral pneumonia is rare early posttransplant; the most common etiologic agent when this does occur is herpes simplex.

Heart Failure

Heart failure may result from volume overload or impairment of left ventricular function from sepsis or toxicity from pretransplant conditioning regimen drugs such as cyclophosphamide, ifosfamide, and/or anthracyclines (120–124). Pretransplant risk factors for cardiac failure are a prior history of heart failure or a low resting LVEF of less than 40% (4). Prior mediastinal radiation or a high cumulative anthracycline dose is not independent risk factors, provided the ejection fraction is normal. High-dose cyclophosphamide causes hemorrhagic myocarditis; transient ST-segment depression and T-wave inversions are common during cyclophosphamide infusion but are not a reason to alter therapy. Cyclophosphamide damages cardiac capillary endothelial cells, leading to hemorrhage between, and separation of, myocytes. The end result is loss of voltage, heart failure, and/or pericardial effusion. Unlike anthracycline-related heart damage arising from myocyte damage, even severe cyclophosphamide-induced left ventricular dysfunction is reversible after an interval of weeks to months.

Renal Failure

Renal insufficiency is usually multifactorial. Cause includes the underlying disease—for example, cast nephropathy in myeloma, prerenal decrease in glomerular filtration, intrinsic renal dysfunction or postrenal obstruction. The most common reason for renal insufficiency early in the posttransplant period is drug related, especially with use of aminoglycosides, cyclosporine, and amphotericin (125,126). Mortality in persons requiring dialysis is about 85% (127). Prerenal causes of azotemia include hepatic SOS/VOD, diarrhea, diuretics, third-spacing from sepsis, hypoalbuminemia, and a capillary leak syndrome from high-dose drugs and radiation. Hepatic SOS/VOD, like other causes of prerenal azotemia, is marked by decreased fractional excretion of sodium (FeNa+) in the urine.

Azotemia from intrinsic renal failure may result from acute tubular necrosis (ATN), glomerulonephritis, interstitial nephritis, or renal vascular damage. Causes of ATN in transplant recipients include sepsis, hypovolemia, and drugs such as aminoglycosides, amphotericin, platinums, foscarnet, and cyclosporine. In ATN, the FeNa+ is high, and the urine has muddy hyaline casts. Renal insufficiency from glomerulonephritis usually results from streptococcal or staphylococcal bacteremia. In glomerulonephritis, FeNa+ is low, and the urine sediment contains RBC casts and increased protein. Interstitial nephritis arising in the early stem cell transplantation (SCT) period is usually drug induced. Causes of allergic interstitial nephritis are penicillins, cephalosporins, sulfamethoxazole-trimethoprim, and fluoroquinolones. In allergic interstitial nephritis, the urine FeNa+ is high, and urine sediment contains WBCs, WBC casts, and eosinophils. Renal insufficiency from renovascular damage is usually caused by drugs such as cyclosporine or from hemolytic uremic syndrome (HUS), which is marked by schistocytes, thrombocytopenia, and azotemia. HUS arises from endothelial cell damage, which may be related to cyclosporine, GvHD, or high-dose drugs and radiation.

Postrenal kidney failure in transplant recipients may result from hemorrhagic cystitis with ureteral or urethral obstruction due to blood clots, retroperitoneal hemorrhage, urate nephropathy, or drugs that undergo intratubular crystallization and obstruction such as aciclovir ciprofloxacin, and triamterene. Regardless of the cause, posttransplant renal insufficiency may require a dose reduction of prophylactic immune suppressive drugs such as cyclosporine or methotrexate; this may increase GvHD.

Engraftment

Definition of graft failure is controversial. After a bone marrow graft, there is usually a rise in the WBC count by 3 weeks. After a blood cell transplant the WBC count usually rises by about 2 weeks. Platelet recovery, defined as more than 20×10^9 cells/L without transfusions typically occurs 2 to 3 weeks later. Occasionally, recipients require platelet transfusions for months posttransplant. Generally, graft failure is defined as a neutrophil count less than or equal to 0.5×10^9 cells/L by day 28. Causes of graft failure include too few normal hematopoietic cells, damage to the bone marrow microenvironment, immune-mediated graft rejection, or drug- or virus-related immune suppression (128,129).

The minimal number of bone marrow or blood cells needed for sustained engraftment is unknown. There are several reasons for this:

- It is not known which hematopoietic cell(s) are responsible for sustained engraftment.
- Different hematopoietic cells may operate under different circumstances and in different persons.
- After autotransplants there is no need for sustained *engraftment* because of autologous bone marrow recovery.
- There is no routinely used technique to identify the hematopoietic cell(s) responsible for sustained engraftment (130,131).

Because of these limitations, surrogate markers are used to assess the hematopoietic-restoring functionality of grafts. For instance, CD34 is a surface membrane marker of immature hematopoietic cells. In animals and humans, retrovirus-transduced CD34+ cells sometimes contribute to long-term engraftment but are not a necessary condition (132). To ensure sustained engraftment in humans, most data suggest a threshold of 2 to 4×10^8 mononuclear cells or 2×10^6 CD34+ cells/kg of recipient body weight. Autotransplant recipients receiving extensive prior chemotherapy and/or radiation frequently have fewer CD34+ cells. It may be difficult to obtain large numbers of CD34+ cells from these persons, and recipients generally recover bone marrow function later than after grafts from normal or less extensively treated donors. This may reflect decreased numbers and/or function of CD34+ cells and/or damage to the bone marrow microenvironment.

Immune-mediated graft failure is theoretically impossible after an autotransplant but it is the most common cause of graft failure for allotransplants. Risk of immune-mediated graft failure correlates with the degree of HLA-disparity between the donor and the recipient. Graft failure occurs in less than 1% after HLA-identical sibling allotransplants, 6% to 8% after unrelated HLA-matched allotransplants and in up to 20% after HLA-haplotype–matched allotransplants (133–135) (Tables 76.5 and 76.6). Immunity to non-HLA antigens, such as H-Y and KIR, also operates to increase risk of immune-mediated graft failure. Other variables influencing the risk of immune-mediated graft failure are transfusion-induced sensitization to HLA and non-HLA antigens, intensity of the pretransplant conditioning regimen and quantity of T cells in the graft. In persons with aplastic anemia, the volume of pretransplant RBC or platelet transfusions correlates with a higher rate of graft failure. This is presumed to result from sensitization of the recipient to disparate HLA and non-HLA antigens. These observations were made before microfilters were available to deplete WBC from transfused blood products. Whether this risk still operates is unknown. However, because of these considerations, potential allotransplant recipients should avoid unnecessary transfusions or receive microfiltered blood products. Removal of donor T cells from

TABLE 76.5 Graft-Versus-Host Disease, Graft Failure, and Disease-Free Survival for Transplants with Sibling-Matched or Unrelated Donors

Degree of HLA Match	Acute GvHD Grade III or IV (%)	Chronic GvHD (%)	Graft Failure (%)	DFS-AML or ALL in Remission (%)	DFS-CML in Chronic Phase (%)	DFS-AML or ALL in Relapse (%)	DFS-CML in Transformation (%)	DFS-AA (%)
Sibling 6/6	7–15	30–35	<2	50–60	60–80	20	10–35	78–90
Related 5/6	25–30	50	7–9	40–60	60–80	20	10–35	25–40
Related 4/6	45–50	50	21	10–40	—	10	10–30	—
Haploidentical	50–100	>50	20	10–40	—	10	10–30	—
Unrelated 6/6	45–50	55	6	45	40	20	20	30–40

GvHD, graft-versus-host disease; DFS, disease-free survival; AML, acute myelogenous leukemia; CML, chronic myelogenous leukemia; ALL, acute lymphoblastic leukemia; AA, aplastic anemia.

the bone marrow graft to prevent GvHD also increases the risk of graft failure; compensation may be possible by more intensive pretransplant immune suppression (136,137). Graft-failure risk is also increased after male grafts to parous and/or transfused female recipients. Here, the recipient is presumed to be sensitized to donor H-Y antigens (138,139).

Several bone marrow suppressive drugs commonly used posttransplant may delay and/or reverse engraftment, for example, methotrexate and sulfamethoxazole-trimethoprim. Viruses, especially herpes simplex, parvovirus, HHV-6, parvovirus-B19, and CMV, cause bone marrow suppression, possibly because they infect bone marrow stroma cells. A decline in the WBC and/or platelets after recovery posttransplant should prompt a search for a drug- or virus-related cause. Declines are also temporarily associated with tapering immune suppression; whether these are related phenomena is unclear. The effect, if any, of acute GvHD on bone marrow function is poorly understood. However, there is a clear association of decreased bone marrow function and chronic GvHD (see below). The response of chronic GvHD to immune suppression is often correlated with improved bone marrow function.

Treatment for graft failure includes using molecularly cloned hematopoietic growth factors (G- or GM-CSF), a second graft, and/or increased immune suppression. Subjects with primary graft failure (i.e., no engraftment) have a poor prognosis, whereas those with secondary or late graft failure (unsustained engraftment) do better. When graft failure is associated with reemergence of host T cells, repeat pretransplant conditioning is usually given before the second graft based on the assumption that graft failure is immune mediated; this may be incorrect in some instances. Consequently, early or late bone marrow failure should be referred to as such and not as graft rejection.

Acute Graft-Versus-Host Disease

The principal manifestations of acute GvHD are rash, diarrhea, and jaundice, present individually or in combination (140,141). Histologically, there is involvement of the basal cell layer of the skin, biliary ductules of the liver, and crypts of the distal gastrointestinal tract. Symptoms occur close to the time of engraftment but may occur earlier or at any time within the first 100 days posttransplant. Acute GvHD is an allogeneic response mediated by donor T cells, which recognizes recipient tissues as foreign. The incidence and severity of acute GvHD increase with increasing recipient age and HLA and non-HLA disparity between the recipient and the donor (142,143) (see Tables 76.5 and 76.6).

The major HLA genes are inherited from both paternal and maternal chromosome 6. The classic HLA class-1 genes are A, B, and C, and more HLA molecules are being characterized. The classical HLA class-1 molecules are present on the surface of all cells and function to present small intracellular peptides to T cells. HLA class-2 molecules are DR, DP, and DQ. These surface molecules present extracellular peptides that result from endocytosis of extracellular protein and degradation of these proteins into smaller peptides (144,145). Even after an HLA genotypically matched allotransplant, acute GvHD invariably develops when—usually inadvertently—no posttransplant immune suppression is given. This likely arises because of recognition of host-derived peptides presented by HLA molecules and recognized as foreign by donor T cells (146).

Skin involvement in acute GvHD results in a maculopapular, erythematous rash, often beginning on the palms and soles and which may become systemic. In severe cases, acute GvHD with skin involvement may be pruritic with bullae. The skin involvement in acute GvHD may be precipitated by exposure to sunlight and/or drugs. Histologically, one can see the dermal–epidermal border disrupted by vacuolar degeneration of epithelial cells, dyskaryotic bodies, acantholysis (i.e., separation of cell–cell contact), epidermolysis (separation of the epidermal and dermal layers), and lymphocytic infiltration. These clinical and histologic findings are not unique to acute GvHD and may occur from drug allergy or the effects of the high-dose chemotherapy and radiation used in the pretransplant conditioning regimen.

Gastrointestinal involvement with acute GvHD results in diarrhea, often accompanied by cramping abdominal pain. In severe cases, the diarrhea may be bloody or associated with a paralytic ileus. Histologically, lymphocytes and apoptotic cells are present and intestinal crypts are lost, which leads to epithelial denudation. Evaluation of gastrointestinal tract signs and symptoms should include stool cultures for bacteria, fungi, and viruses, especially CMV. Sigmoidoscopy with biopsy may be helpful if the diagnosis is in doubt and platelet levels are

TABLE 76.6 Incidence of Grade III–IV Acute Graft-Versus-Host Disease in CML According to the Number of Mismatched Class I and Class II Alleles

	0 Class I (%)	1 Class I (%)	≥2 Class I (%)	Total (%)
0 Class II	32	29	36	32
1 Class II	45	31	55	45
≥2 Class II	67	67	86	74
Total	34	30	44	35

There were 467 chronic myeloid leukemia unrelated donor–recipient pairs.

sufficient. Acute GvHD with hepatic involvement presents as jaundice and an elevated alkaline phosphatase with or without elevated transaminases. The differential diagnosis includes SOS/VOD or infections with CMV or *Candida* spp and may require a transjugular liver biopsy for accurate diagnosis. In acute GvHD, the liver biopsy may show T-cell infiltration of the portal triad, with apoptosis of epithelial cells lining the biliary tree.

Acute GvHD and infections from immune suppression are major causes of early death after allotransplant. Consequently, acute GvHD prophylaxis is needed for all allotransplant recipients. One effective method to prevent acute GvHD is a 2- to 3-log depletion of T cells from the graft (147–149). However, benefits from preventing acute GvHD are offset by increased graft failure and leukemia relapse. Increased graft failure is presumed to result from immune-mediated graft rejection but may also reflect loss of the interaction of donor T cells and hematopoietic cells. Increased leukemia relapse is presumed to result from decreased T-cell–mediated antileukemia effects, sometimes referred to as *graft-versus-leukemia* or GvL. Experimental approaches to retain GvL while decreasing acute GvHD include selective T-cell depletion or adding back subsets of T cells or natural killer (NK) cells to the graft, use of cytokines, and modulation of costimulatory T-cell or chemokine pathways (150).

Pharmacologic approaches to prevent acute GvHD are simpler and more widely used than T-cell depletion. Cyclosporine and methotrexate given on days 1, 3, 6, and 11 posttransplant are the most common preventative regimens (151). Other regimens include cyclosporine and prednisolone or cyclosporine, methotrexate, and methylprednisolone (152). In HLA-identical sibling transplants, weekly intravenous immunoglobulin (IVIG) until day 100 results in a lower incidence of acute GvHD but the effect size is small and this approach is not often used, especially because of substantial cost (153). GvHD is associated with a lower leukemia relapse rate, and, therefore, the aim should not be to completely eliminate acute GvHD, but rather to balance the risk of acute GvHD against the risk of a leukemia relapse. Thus, more intensive immune suppressive regimens are used when GvHD risk is high, for instance, in HLA-mismatched transplants, and when the leukemia relapse risk is low, whereas less intensive regimens are used when the leukemia relapse risk is high such as in advanced leukemia and when acute GvHD risk is least. Convincing data supporting these approaches are lacking.

Clinical staging of acute GvHD considers individual tissue/organ involvement scores, which are combined for an overall grade (Tables 76.7 and 76.8). Grade 1 acute GvHD is not clinically important and requires no specific therapy. Grades 2 through 4 acute GvHD are typically treated with corticosteroids such as methylprednisolone, 1 to 2 mg/kg/day, with or without cyclosporine. Acute GvHD unresponsive to this approach has a poor prognosis. Further therapies include monoclonal or polyclonal antibodies to T cells, such as ATG or alemtuzumab (anti-CD52), or cytokines such as daclizumab or infliximab. Daclizumab binds to the high-affinity IL-2 receptor found on activated T cells, whereas infliximab binds to TNF-α, a cytokine involved in acute GvHD (154). Several reports suggest that giving IVIG, typically used for CMV-infection prevention (see below), is associated with less acute GvHD, but these data are inconsistent.

TABLE 76.7 Grading of Acute Graft-Versus-Host Disease

Organ	Grade	Severity of Individual Organ Involvement Description
Skin	+1	A maculopapular eruption involving <25% of the body surface
	+2	A maculopapular eruption involving 25–50% of the body surface
	+3	Generalized erythroderma
	+4	Generalized erythroderma with bullous formation and often with desquamation
Liver	+1	Moderate increase of AST (150–750 IU) and bilirubin (2.0–3.0 mg/dL)
	+2	Bilirubin rise (3.1–6.0 mg/dL) with or without an increase in AST
	+3	Bilirubin rise (6.1–15 mg/dL) with or without an increase in AST
	+4	Bilirubin rise (>5 mg/dL) with or without an increase in AST
Gut		Diarrhea, nausea, and vomiting graded +1 to +4 in severity. The severity of gut involvement is assigned to the most severe involvement noted.
	+1	Diarrhea more than 500 mL/day
	+2	Diarrhea more than 1,000 mL/day
	+3	Diarrhea more than 1,500 mL/day
	+4	Diarrhea more than 2,000 mL/day; or severe abdominal pain with or without ileus

AST, aspartate transaminase.

INTERMEDIATE CONCERNS (DAYS 30 TO 100)

CMV Prophylaxis

Prophylaxis for CMV infection after autotransplants is unnecessary. In allotransplants, ganciclovir is often given when a surveillance blood culture or bronchoalveolar lavage (BAL) is CMV-positive by quantitative polymerase chain reaction (PCR). Subjects with CMV viremia and CD4+ T cells less than 0.1×10^9 cells/L are at greatest risk of developing CMV disease (155). Surveillance CMV-PCR is started 2 weeks before transplantation and continued until day 100 postprocedure. A positive CMV-PCR usually prompts giving full-dose ganciclovir for 2 weeks or until the CMV-PCR becomes negative, and then for another 2 weeks at one-half dose (156–159). Valganciclovir is then given as prophylaxis until day 100. G-CSF may be given if there is bone marrow

TABLE 76.8 Overall Grade of Graft-Versus-Host Disease[a]

Grade	Skin	Gut		Liver	ECOG Performance
I	+1 to +2	0		0	0
II	+1 to +3	+1 to +2	And/or	+1 to +2	0 to 1
III	+2 to +4	+2 to +4	And/or	+2 to +4	2 to 3
IV	+2 to +4	+2 to +4	And/or	+2 to +4	3 to 4

ECOG, Eastern Cooperative Oncology Group. AST, aspartate transaminase.
[a]If no skin disease, the overall grade is the higher single organ grade.
Adapted from Glucksberg H, Storb R, Fefer A, et al. Clinical manifestations of graft versus host disease in human recipients of marrow from HL-A-matched sibling donors. *Transplantation*. 1974;18:295–304.

suppression, or therapy may be changed to foscarnet, which is associated with less bone marrow suppression.

Pneumonitis

Between 30% and 50% of early posttransplant deaths are associated with respiratory failure (160,161). Although bacterial and fungal pulmonary infections can occur, the two most common causes are idiopathic and CMV-related interstitial pneumonia.

Interstitial pneumonia is more common after an allotransplant (40%) compared with an autotransplant (10%). Risk factors include a radiation-based pretransplant conditioning regimen, severe GvHD, older age, and posttransplant use of methotrexate. The median time to onset of interstitial pneumonia is about 50 days posttransplant, with only rare cases developing after 6 months. Affected persons are hypoxic and/or hypocapnic; physical examination often shows basilar crackles; and the chest roentgenogram shows an interstitial reticular-nodular infiltrate; between 40% and 65% of cases of interstitial pneumonia are CMV related. Diagnosis is usually by bronchoscopy with BAL. Early intervention with combined IVIG and ganciclovir has reduced mortality of CMV pneumonia to about 50% (162,163). It is very rare for a subject to develop CMV pneumonia when routine screening for CMV activation by PCR is carried out and appropriate interventions taken. Adoptive immunotherapy, giving CMV-specific cytotoxic T cells has also been used to treat CMV pneumonia (164). Other opportunistic infections causing interstitial pneumonia, such as *Chlamydia trachomatis* and *Legionella pneumophila*, are less common. Prophylaxis for *Pneumocystis carinii* pneumonia with sulfamethoxazole-trimethoprim (Bactrim) is usually begun after engraftment and continued for 1 year.

The cause(s) of 30% to 50% of posttransplant interstitial pneumonias are unknown (165–167). Etiologies are complex and poorly understood; likely contributors include the toxicity of the pretransplant conditioning regimen, chronic GvHD, and unidentified infectious organisms such as human herpes virus-6 (HHV-6) and respiratory syncytial virus (RSV) (168). Carmustine (BCNU)-related interstitial pneumonia may respond to corticosteroids, but most cases of idiopathic pneumonia syndrome do not.

Epstein–Barr Virus Posttransplant Lymphoproliferative Disease

Infection of B cells by Epstein–Barr virus (EBV) results in B-cell proliferation. In a normal person, infection-induced, EBV-specific cytotoxic T cells prevent uncontrolled B-cell proliferation. In immune-deficient allotransplant recipients, failure of immune surveillance by EBV-specific cytotoxic T cells results in a polyclonal or, less often, monoclonal proliferation of donor or recipient B cells (169). EBV-lymphoproliferative syndrome (EBV-LPS) occurs in about 0.5% of allotransplant recipients. Risk factors include T-cell–depleted grafts and the use of ATG or anti-CD3 antibodies posttransplant to prevent acute GvHD. EBV-LPS typically develops 45 days to 1.5 years posttransplant; the median time to onset is 70 to 80 days. Presenting features of early-onset EBV-LPS include fever and extranodal involvement; the course is typically unfavorable. Later-onset EBV-LPS generally has a more indolent course, manifested by fever and lymph node enlargement. Antiviral therapy of EBV-LPS is generally ineffective. Rituximab (anti-CD20 monoclonal antibody) has been used and is very effective (170). Giving donor EBV-specific cytotoxic T cells sometimes results in prompt remission of polyclonal and monoclonal EBV-LPS (171).

LATE CONCERNS (BEYOND DAY 100)

Chronic GvHD

Chronic GvHD usually occurs after day 100 posttransplant. Chronic disease may seemingly develop de novo without prior clinically diagnosed acute GvHD, or after a quiescent interval following resolution of acute GvHD. Most often, acute GvHD evolves into the chronic process (172,173). The most important risk factors for developing chronic GvHD are older recipient age and severity of acute GvHD. Whereas acute GvHD is predominately an alloimmune disorder, chronic GvHD has features of alloimmunity and autoimmunity.

Skin involvement in chronic GvHD involves scleroderma-like changes with hypopigmentation and hyperpigmentation, loss of hair follicles, thickened skin, and joint contractures. Mucosal involvement manifests by dryness, pain, ulceration, and lacy white buccal mucosal membranes. Ocular features include sicca conjunctivitis, ectropion, and, in severe cases, corneal ulceration. In contrast to acute GvHD of the gastrointestinal tract, which is marked by watery or bloody diarrhea, chronic gastrointestinal GvHD manifests as nausea, anorexia, malabsorption, dysphagia, and weight loss. Ulcerations, strictures, and narrowing may occur at any site along the gastrointestinal tract. Hepatic involvement in chronic GvHD presents similarly to acute GvHD with predominance of cholestasis—that is, increased bilirubin and alkaline phosphatase.

Chronic GvHD may have various autoimmune features, including antibodies to DNA, mitochondria, smooth muscle, or connective tissue. Autoimmune syndromes associated with chronic GvHD include polymyositis, myasthenia gravis, systemic lupus erythematosus, rheumatoid arthritis, primary biliary cirrhosis, and thyroiditis. Chronic GvHD of the lung presents with cough and dyspnea caused by progressive obstructive small airway disease with hyperinflated lungs and reduced midexpiratory flows; histologically, the process resembles bronchiolitis obliterans. Chronic GvHD results from underlying immune dysregulation, which also causes immune deficiency that predisposes to infection independent of the immune suppressive drugs used to treat GvHD.

Chronic GvHD may be limited or extensive (Table 76.9). Limited-stage chronic GvHD has a favorable prognosis and

TABLE 76.9 Chronic Graft-Versus-Host Disease Grades

Limited	Disease localized only to skin involvement or hepatic involvement
Extensive	1. Generalized skin involvement
	2. Limited skin involvement or hepatic involvement and
	a. Liver histologic features showing chronic progressive hepatitis, bridging necrosis, or cirrhosis
	b. Eye involvement (Schirmer test with <5 mm wetting)
	c. Involvement of minor salivary glands or oral mucosa
	d. Involvement of any other organ

requires no therapy. Extensive-stage chronic GvHD has a poor prognosis; therapy is needed (174). Adverse prognostic variables in persons with extensive-stage GvHD include thrombocytopenia (<100 × 10^9 cells/L) and poor performance status. Standard therapy of extensive-stage chronic GvHD is alternate day corticosteroids. Other options include thalidomide, extracorporeal photophoresis, psoralen, and ultraviolet irradiation (PUVA) for chronic cutaneous GvHD, and ursodeoxycholic acid for chronic hepatic GvHD (175). Clinical trials with thalidomide analogs, such as pomalidomide, are beginning. The natural history of chronic GvHD is to "burn out" or for subjects to die from an opportunistic infection. The therapy paradox here is that one is forced to use immune suppression to treat a disease that kills subjects because of intrinsic immune suppression.

Herpes Zoster

Varicella zoster occurs in 20% of autotransplant (176) and 20% to 50% of allotransplant recipients, usually 100 days to 1 year posttransplant (177,178). Infection may present with cutaneous or visceral involvement. Persons with visceral involvement may present with severe acute abdominal pain from virus reactivation in the celiac plexus, which spreads to the pancreas and small bowel. If cutaneous or visceral herpes varicella zoster is suspected, the subject should be hospitalized, placed in isolation, and given IV aciclovir.

New Cancers

Transplant recipients are at increased risk to develop cancer (179–181). Autotransplants are associated with increased clonal cytogenetic changes in bone marrow cells posttransplant. Some of these abnormalities are typical of therapy-related myelodysplastic syndrome (MDS), including monosomy 5 or 7 (del[5] and del[7]), and translocations involving 11q23. These abnormalities are reported in up to 9% of recipients at 3 years posttransplant and are likely related to the effects of exposing the bone marrow to drugs and radiation as part of disease therapy and as part of pretransplant conditioning. Allotransplant recipients have a four- to sixfold age-adjusted risk of developing cancer. Risk factors include pretransplant conditioning with radiation and acute GvHD equal to or greater than grade 2. The 10-year cumulative incidence of solid cancers after allotransplants is about 3%, whereas the 15-year probability is about 6% for persons not receiving radiation versus 20% for persons receiving radiation.

Relapse

Relapse of disease after autotransplants or allotransplants may be treated with a second auto- or allotransplant (182–185). If the first pretransplant conditioning regimen included radiation, it should not be used prior to the second transplant; if, however, the first pretransplant conditioning regimen lacked radiation, it should be considered for the second transplant if this is disease appropriate. If the first transplant was an autotransplant, it is unlikely that a second autotransplant will succeed, and thus, an allotransplant is preferred.

Subjects relapsing less than 1 year after autotransplant or allotransplant are often not reasonable candidates for a second transplant because of substantial transplant-related morbidity and mortality and a low likelihood of leukemia control. Subjects retransplanted less than 6 months after a first transplant have done particularly poorly. Sometimes leukemia relapse can be reversed by discontinuing posttransplant immune suppression or by giving donor lymphocytes, or both (186–188). Donor lymphocyte infusions are effective in many subjects with recurrent chronic phase chronic myelogenous leukemia provided they are done in early relapse (189). In acute myeloid leukemia, about 30% of subjects with relapse respond; the interval to remission after donor lymphocyte infusion is 1 to 3 months. Complications include bone marrow failure and worsening of acute GvHD. Mixed chimeras have a lower risk of bone marrow failure than persons with only recipient hematopoiesis. The risk of acute GvHD after donor lymphocyte infusion is about 80% with a tendency to cause hepatic acute GvHD. Attempts to modulate precipitating acute GvHD by genetically engineering donor lymphocytes to express herpes simplex virus thymidine kinase (HSVTK) and treating with ganciclovir if acute GvHD develops are reported (190).

Hypothyroidism

For the first 3 to 6 months, posttransplant recipients may have a "euthyroid sick syndrome" with decreased tri-iodothyronine (T3), decreased thyroxine (T4), and low thyroid-stimulating hormone (TSH) (191,192). As in other nonthyroid diseases associated with a euthyroid sick syndrome, these abnormalities are reversible and probably are normal physiologic responses to decreased protein catabolism. Replacement therapy with thyroxine is unnecessary.

Primary hypothyroidism posttransplant is caused by high-dose radiation in the pretransplant conditioning regimen (193–195). Primary hypothyroidism—elevated TSH and low T4—occurs in less than 2% of recipients not receiving radiation (196), but in about 10% of radiation recipients. A greater proportion of subjects have compensated primary hypothyroidism with increased TSH but normal T4. The time interval to onset of primary hypothyroidism is 6 to 41 months posttransplant, with a median of 13 months. The risk of primary hypothyroidism is greater after single-dose than fractionated radiation. Whereas overt hypothyroidism is treated with hormone replacement, compensated disease may be treated with close follow-up or hormone replacement.

Growth and Development

Child and adolescent transplant recipients have delayed or interrupted growth and development; the composition of the pretransplant conditioning regimen is a major determinant (194,197). Other risk factors for growth retardation are central nervous system (CNS) radiation, single-dose radiation pretransplant, chronic GvHD, corticosteroid use, and age. Children receiving only high-dose cyclophosphamide do not, in general, have growth retardation. Radiation regimens, on the other hand, adversely affect the rate of height and growth. Radiation may also inhibit normal dental and facial skeletal development, especially in children younger than 6 years. Although chemotherapy regimens were originally not thought to alter growth, combined busulfan and cyclophosphamide pretransplant conditioning causes growth retardation comparable to that of cyclophosphamide combined with fractionated radiation (198). How pretransplant conditioning regimens cause growth retardation is incompletely understood but includes direct injury to the growth plates, decreased pituitary and hypothalamic growth hormone production, and primary gonadal failure with decreased estrogens and testosterone, as well as elevated luteinizing hormone and follicle-stimulating hormone. In premenopausal transplant recipients, secondary sexual characteristics and menarche are usually delayed. Growth hormone therapy may improve final height in children younger than 10 years at transplant but has no impact on older children (199).

Fertility

Primary gonadal failure, for example, hypergonadotropic hypogonadism, is common posttransplant (194,197,200,201). Recovery of gonadal function depends on recipient age and pretransplant conditioning regimen. In postmenopausal women receiving cyclophosphamide only, gonadal dysfunction is usually transitory. Gonadal failure occurs in about one-half of recipients of busulfan and cyclophosphamide (201), whereas almost all recipients of radiation-containing pretransplant conditioning regimens develop gonadal failure. The return of menstruation within 10 years after radiation occurs in more than 90% of recipients who were younger than 18 years at the time of transplant and in 10% to 15% of recipients older than 18 years at the time of transplant. Posttransplant gonadal failure is often associated with symptoms of estrogen deficiency, including hot flashes, dyspareunia, dysuria, and vaginal dryness, which may be helped by hormone replacement therapy (202). Cases have been reported of cryopreservation and orthotopic transplantation of ovarian tissue that has resulted in recovery of ovarian function and subsequent pregnancy (203,204).

Cataracts

Corticosteroids and radiation cause cataracts within a median of 2.5 to 5 years posttransplant (205–208). The incidence of cataracts, both subclinical and clinical, is 85% to 100% for unfractionated radiation recipients, 30% to 50% for fractionated radiation recipients, and 5% to 20% for persons not receiving radiation. Eye shielding decreases the cataract risk but is not generally done because of the concern of increasing leukemia relapse, as blood cells in the eye would escape irradiation.

Late Renal Effects

Reversible renal dysfunction is common early posttransplant, with causes that are multifactorial including, but not limited to, drugs and infections (209,210). Although long-term complications are rare, there are occasional reports of late-onset renal dysfunction consistent with radiation nephropathy occurring after multidrug and radiation-containing pretransplant conditioning regimens. Onset is typically 3 to 7 months posttransplant and is characterized by hypertension, edema, uremia, and occasionally hemolytic uremic syndrome (HUS). Cyclosporine may cause a similar picture of hypertension, renal insufficiency, and HUS that can be confused with or complicate transplant-related renal failure.

Late Lung Effects

Late-onset noninfectious pulmonary complications (LONIPC) occur in 10% to 25% of subjects (211–213). These are further classified as bronchiolitis obliterans, bronchiolitis obliterans with organizing pneumonia, interstitial pneumonia, and diffuse alveolar disease. These abnormalities are thought to result from the pretransplant conditioning regimen, especially radiation. Chronic GvHD and pretransplant pulmonary function are the main determinants predicting worsening pulmonary function in long-term survivors posttransplant (213). Bronchiolitis obliterans presents as cough and wheezing. Studies typically show severe obstructive lung disease with a hyperinflated thorax resulting from obliteration of small bronchioles. This typically occurs 3 months to 2 years posttransplant. Although usually associated with allotransplants complicated by chronic GvHD, bronchiolitis obliterans occurs rarely after autotransplants. Corticosteroids are usually used to treat bronchiolitis obliterans, but the results, at best, are poor. Lymphocytic interstitial pneumonia is characterized by a lymphocytic interstitial infiltrate that may progress to fibrosis. The cause is not clear but is thought to be immune mediated, and is also treated with corticosteroids. Survival of persons with LONIPC is poor; death usually results from respiratory failure and/or infections.

IMMUNE SUPPRESSIVE DRUGS

Antiproliferative Drugs

Mycophenolate mofetil (MPA), used to modify GvHD in allotransplants, is metabolized to mycophenolic acid, a potent, reversible noncompetitive inhibitor of inosine monophosphate dehydrogenase (IMPDH). IMPDH is the first of two enzymes that convert inosine monophosphate (IMP) to guanosine monophosphate (GMP). GMP is normally converted to GDP, GTP, and dGTP. IMPDH is not involved in the salvage pathway of purine biosynthesis. MPA treatment decreases GTP and dGTP in lymphocytes that inhibit DNA synthesis and GTP-dependent metabolic events resulting in immune suppression (214).

Cyclophosphamide is a common component of pretransplant conditioning. It is a cyclic phosphamide ester of mechlorethamine, inactive in its native form. Cyclophosphamide is converted in the liver to active alkylating metabolites, acrolein, and phosphoramide mustard, which prevent cell division by cross-linking DNA strands. High-dose cyclophosphamide, if given without mesna, results in hemorrhagic cystitis via acrolein formation. Prior pelvic radiation also increases the risk of cyclophosphamide-related hemorrhagic cystitis.

Corticosteroids and Other Immune Suppressive Drugs

Prednisone is widely used in oncology for anticancer and immune suppression effect. The agent is highly active in acute lymphoblastic leukemia and lymphomas. Prednisone is also used to palliate symptomatic advanced cancers where it enhances appetite and produces a sense of well-being. Corticosteroids are also powerful immune suppressive drugs used to prevent and/or treat GvHD. The relatively high mineralocorticoid activity of cortisone and hydrocortisone with resultant fluid retention makes them unsuitable for long-term immune suppression. Prednisone has predominantly glucocorticoid activity, and is the corticosteroid most commonly used for long-term immune suppression in chronic GvHD. The maintenance dose of prednisone in this setting should be kept as low as possible to minimize adverse effects, including peptic ulcers, proximal myopathy, osteoporosis, kidney suppression, hirsutism, weight gain, susceptibility to infections, euphoria, depression, cataracts, impaired healing, among others.

Cyclosporine, a calcineurin inhibitor, is a potent immune suppressive drug that adversely affects the kidney but not the bone marrow. Cyclosporine is widely used to prevent and/or treat GvHD.

Tacrolimus is also a calcineurin inhibitor. Although not chemically related to cyclosporine, tacrolimus has a similar mode of action and side-effect profile. The incidences of neural and renal toxicity are greater with tacrolimus than cyclosporine. Additionally, cardiomyopathy and glucose intolerance are reported; hypertrichosis is less a problem with tacrolimus than cyclosporine. Tacrolimus is not commonly used in bone marrow and blood cell allotransplants.

IL-2 and its receptor (IL-2R) are important in T-cell–mediated immunity. Monoclonal antibodies to these moieties, basiliximab and daclizumab, are used to treat corticosteroid-resistant GvHD (215). Rare side effects include hypersensitivity reactions. Infliximab is also used in the treatment of corticosteroid-refractory GvHD (154,216).

Thalidomide, a member of a class of immune modulating compounds, termed ImiDs, has been used to prevent and/or treat chronic GvHD (217). It is also used, combined with other drugs, to treat multiple myeloma. Thalidomide causes drowsiness, constipation, thrombosis, and neuropathy. Because of its teratogenic effects, it should not be given to sexually active persons without proper precautions. Lenalidomide, a thalidomide analog, is also used to treat bone marrow disorders, including MDS and multiple myeloma. Clinical trials of lenalidomide and pomalidomide, a third ImiD, in chronic GvHD are beginning.

Alemtuzumab (Campath-1H) directed at the CD52 molecule on the surface of all lymphocytes is sometimes used to remove T cells from allografts. Alemtuzumab is also sometimes used to treat corticosteroid-resistant, acute GvHD (218). Infusion-related adverse effects may occur, including fever, chills, nausea and vomiting, and allergic reactions. There is also increased susceptibility to infections, particularly with fungi, viruses, and protozoa.

Key Points

- Pretransplant assessment of a person's fitness for a transplant is essential.
- Different pretransplant conditioning regimens have different risks and benefits.
- Posttransplant complications may arise from effects of the conditioning regiment, graft failure, GvHD, or posttransplant suppression.
- Bacterial, fungal, and viral infections are common.
- Chronic GvHD is common and has considerable morbidity. Incidence and severity may be reduced with ATG.
- Complications are common in many long-term survivors. Regular medical surveillance is needed.

References

1. Ghalie R, Szidon JP, Thompson L, et al. Evaluation of pulmonary complications after bone marrow transplantation: the role of pretransplant pulmonary function tests. *Bone Marrow Transplant.* 1992;10:359–365.
2. Milburn HJ, Prentice HG, du Bois RM. Can lung function measurements be used to predict which patients will be at risk of developing interstitial pneumonitis after bone marrow transplantation? *Thorax.* 1992;47:421–425.
3. Crawford SW, Fisher L. Predictive value of pulmonary function tests before marrow transplantation. *Chest.* 1992;101:1257–1264.
4. Hertenstein B, Stefanic M, Schmeiser T, et al. Cardiac toxicity of bone marrow transplantation: predictive value of cardiologic evaluation before transplant. *J Clin Oncol.* 1994;12:998–1004.
5. Fujimaki K, Maruta A, Yoshida M, et al. Severe cardiac toxicity in hematological stem cell transplantation: predictive value of reduced left ventricular ejection fraction. *Bone Marrow Transplant.* 2001;27:307–310.
6. Chien JW, Madtes DK, Clark JG. Pulmonary function testing prior to hematopoietic stem cell transplantation. *Bone Marrow Transplant.* 2005;35: 429–435.
7. Parimon T, Au DH, Martin PJ, et al. A risk score for mortality after allogeneic hematopoietic cell transplantation. *Ann Intern Med.* 2006;144: 407–414.
8. Singh AK, Karimpour SE, Savani BN, et al. Pretransplant pulmonary function tests predict risk of mortality following fractionated total body irradiation and allogeneic peripheral blood stem cell transplant. *Int J Radiat Oncol Biol Phys.* 2006;66:520–527.
9. Savani BN, Montero A, Srinivasan R, et al. Chronic GVHD and pretransplantation abnormalities in pulmonary function are the main determinants predicting worsening pulmonary function in long-term survivors after stem cell transplantation. *Biol Blood Marrow Transplant.* 2006;12:1261–1269.
10. Bearman SI, Petersen FB, Schor RA, et al. Radionuclide ejection fractions in the evaluation of patients being considered for bone marrow transplantation: risk for cardiac toxicity. *Bone Marrow Transplant.* 1990;5:173–177.
11. Ditschkowski M, Elmaagacli AH, Trenschel R, et al. Myeloablative allogeneic hematopoietic stem cell transplantation in elderly patients. *Clin Transplant.* 2006;20:127–131.
12. Klepin HD, Hurd DD. Autologous transplantation in elderly patients with multiple myeloma: are we asking the right questions? *Bone Marrow Transplant.* 2006;38:585–592.
13. Klingemann HG, Shepherd JD, Reece DE, et al. Regimen-related acute toxicities: pathophysiology, risk factors, clinical evaluation and preventive strategies. *Bone Marrow Transplant.* 1994;14(Suppl 4):S14–18.
14. Reece DE, Bredeson C, Perez WS, et al. Autologous stem cell transplantation in multiple myeloma patients <60 vs ≥60 years of age. *Bone Marrow Transplant.* 2003;32:1135–1143.
15. Barrett AJ. Immunosuppressive therapy in bone marrow transplantation. *Immunol Lett.* 1991;29:81–87.
16. Storb R, Yu C, Deeg HJ, et al. Current and future preparative regimens for bone marrow transplantation in thalassemia. *Ann N Y Acad Sci.* 1998; 850:276–287.
17. Thomas ED, Buckner CD, Banaji M, et al. One hundred patients with acute leukemia treated by chemotherapy, total body irradiation, and allogeneic marrow transplantation. *Blood.* 1977;49:511–533.
18. Santos GW, Tutschka PJ, Brookmeyer R, et al. Marrow transplantation for acute nonlymphocytic leukemia after treatment with busulfan and cyclophosphamide. *N Engl J Med.* 1983;309:1347–1353.
19. Socie G, Clift RA, Blaise D, et al. Busulfan plus cyclophosphamide compared with total-body irradiation plus cyclophosphamide before marrow transplantation for myeloid leukemia: long-term follow-up of 4 randomized studies. *Blood.* 2001;98:3569–3574.
20. Bunin N, Aplenc R, Kamani N, et al. Randomized trial of busulfan vs total body irradiation containing conditioning regimens for children with acute lymphoblastic leukemia: a Pediatric Blood and Marrow Transplant Consortium study. *Bone Marrow Transplant.* 2003;32:543–548.
21. Copelan EA. Better leukemia-free and overall survival in AML in first remission following cyclophosphamide in combination with busulfan compared with TBI. *Blood.* 2013;122:3863–3870.
22. Montgomery M, Cottler-Fox M. Mobilization and collection of autologous hematopoietic progenitor/stem cells. *Clin Adv Hematol Oncol.* 2007;5:127–136.
23. Saraceni F, Shem-Tov N, Olivieri A, Nagler A. Mobilized peripheral blood grafts include more than hematopoietic stem cells: the immunological perspective. *Bone Marrow Transplant.* 2015;50(7):886–891.
24. Jantunen E, Varmavuo V. Plerixafor for mobilization of blood stem cells in autologous transplantation: an update. *Expert Opin Biol Ther.* 2014;14:851–861.

25. Duong HK, Savani BN, Copelan E, et al. Peripheral blood progenitor cell mobilization for autologous and allogeneic hematopoietic cell transplantation: guidelines from the American Society for Blood and Marrow Transplantation. *Biol Blood Marrow Transplant.* 2014;20:1262–1273.
26. Group SCTC. Allogeneic peripheral blood stem-cell compared with bone marrow transplantation in the management of hematologic malignancies: an individual patient data meta-analysis of nine randomized trials. *J Clin Oncol.* 2005;23:5074–5087.
27. Gluckman E. Milestones in umbilical cord blood transplantation. *Blood Rev.* 2011;25:255–259.
28. Brunstein CG, Gutman JA, Weisdorf DJ, et al. Allogeneic hematopoietic cell transplantation for hematologic malignancy: relative risks and benefits of double umbilical cord blood. *Blood.* 2010;116:4693–4699.
29. Berz D, McCormack EM, Winer ES, et al. Cryopreservation of hematopoietic stem cells. *Am J Hematol.* 2007;2(6):463–472.
30. Watt SM, Austin E, Armitage S. Cryopreservation of hematopoietic stem/progenitor cells for therapeutic use. *Methods Mol Biol.* 2007;368:237–259.
31. Shu Z, Heimfeld S, Gao D. Hematopoietic SCT with cryopreserved grafts: adverse reactions after transplantation and cryoprotectant removal before infusion. *Bone Marrow Transplant.* 2014;49:469–476.
32. Klein MA, Kadidlo D, McCullough J, et al. Microbial contamination of hematopoietic stem cell products: incidence and clinical sequelae. *Biol Blood Marrow Transplant.* 2006;12:1142–1149.
33. Mackie FE, Umetsu D, Salvatierra O, et al. Pulmonary capillary leak syndrome with intravenous cyclosporin A in pediatric kidney transplantation. *Pediatr Transplant.* 2000;4:35–38.
34. Woywodt A, Haubitz M, Buchholz S, et al. Counting the cost: markers of endothelial damage in hematopoietic stem cell transplantation. *Bone Marrow Transplant.* 2004;34:1015–1023.
35. Schots R, Kaufman L, Van Riet I, et al. Proinflammatory cytokines and their role in the development of major transplant-related complications in the early phase after allogeneic bone marrow transplantation. *Leukemia.* 2003;17:1150–1156.
36. Carreras E, Diaz-Ricart M. The role of the endothelium in the short-term complications of hematopoietic SCT. *Bone Marrow Transplant.* 2011;46:1495–1502.
37. Hanly L, Chen N, Rieder M et al. Ifosfamide nephrotoxicity in children: a mechanistic base for pharmacological prevention. *Expert Opin Drug Saf.* 2009;8:155–168.
38. Skinner R. Chronic ifosfamide nephrotoxicity in children. *Med Pediatr Oncol.* 2003;41:190–197.
39. Durken M, Agbenu J, Finckh B, et al. Deteriorating free radical-trapping capacity and antioxidant status in plasma during bone marrow transplantation. *Bone Marrow Transplant.* 1995;15:757–762.
40. Treleaven J, Gennery A, Marsh J et al. Guidelines on the use of irradiated blood components prepared by the British Committee for Standards in Haematology Blood Transfusion Task Force. *Br J Haematol.* 2011;152:35–51.
41. Ljungman P, Perez-Bercoff L, Jonsson J, et al. Risk factors for the development of cytomegalovirus disease after allogeneic stem cell transplantation. *Haematologica.* 2006;91:78–83.
42. Takami A, Mochizuki K, Asakura H, et al. High incidence of cytomegalovirus reactivation in adult recipients of an unrelated cord blood transplant. *Haematologica.* 2005;90:1290–1292.
43. Boeckh M, Fries B, Nichols WG. Recent advances in the prevention of CMV infection and disease after hematopoietic stem cell transplantation. *Pediatr Transplant.* 2004;8(Suppl 5):19–27.
44. Gentile G, Picardi A, Capobianchi A, et al. A prospective study comparing quantitative cytomegalovirus (CMV) polymerase chain reaction in plasma and pp65 antigenemia assay in monitoring patients after allogeneic stem cell transplantation. *BMC Infect Dis.* 2006;6:167.
45. Blajchman MA. The clinical benefits of the leukoreduction of blood products. *J Trauma.* 2006;60:S83–90.
46. van Prooijen HC, Visser JJ, van Oostendorp WR, et al. Prevention of primary transfusion-associated cytomegalovirus infection in bone marrow transplant recipients by the removal of white cells from blood components with high-affinity filters. *Br J Haematol.* 1994;87:144–147.
47. Rossini F, Terruzzi E, Cammarota S, et al. Cytomegalovirus infection after autologous stem cell transplantation: incidence and outcome in a group of patients undergoing a surveillance program. *Transpl Infect Dis.* 2005;7:122–125.
48. Heal JM, Liesveld JL, Phillips GL, et al. What would Karl Landsteiner do? The ABO blood group and stem cell transplantation. *Bone Marrow Transplant.* 2005;36:747–755.
49. Seebach JD, Stussi G, Passweg JR, et al. ABO blood group barrier in allogeneic bone marrow transplantation revisited. *Biol Blood Marrow Transplant.* 2005;11:1006–1013.
50. Stussi G, Muntwyler J, Passweg JR, et al. Consequences of ABO incompatibility in allogeneic hematopoietic stem cell transplantation. *Bone Marrow Transplant.* 2002;30:87–93.
51. Benson K, Fields K, Hiemenz J, et al. The platelet-refractory bone marrow transplant patient: prophylaxis and treatment of bleeding. *Semin Oncol.* 1993;20:102–109.
52. Trifilio S, Verma A, Mehta J. Antimicrobial prophylaxis in hematopoietic stem cell transplant recipients: heterogeneity of current clinical practice. *Bone Marrow Transplant.* 2004;33:735–739.
53. Nichols WG. Combating infections in hematopoietic stem cell transplant recipients. *Expert Rev Anti Infect Ther.* 2003;1:57–73.
54. Neumann S, Krause SW, Maschmeyer G, et al.; Infectious Diseases Working Party (AGIHO); German Society of Hematology and Oncology (DGHO). Primary prophylaxis of bacterial infections and Pneumocystis jirovecii pneumonia in patients with hematological malignancies and solid tumors : guidelines of the Infectious Diseases Working Party (AGIHO) of the German Society of Hematology and Oncology (DGHO). *Ann Hematol.* 2013;92:433–442.
55. Bow EJ. Fluoroquinolones, antimicrobial resistance and neutropenic cancer patients. *Curr Opin Infect Dis.* 2011;24:545–553.
56. Reuter S, Kern WV, Sigge A, et al. Impact of fluoroquinolone prophylaxis on reduced infection-related mortality among patients with neutropenia and hematologic malignancies. *Clin Infect Dis.* 2005;40:1087–1093.
57. Gafter-Gvili A, Paul M, Fraser A, et al. Effect of quinolone prophylaxis in afebrile neutropenic patients on microbial resistance: systematic review and meta-analysis. *J Antimicrob Chemother.* 2007;59:5–22.
58. Buckner CD, Clift RA, Sanders JE, et al. Protective environment for marrow transplant recipients: a prospective study. *Ann Intern Med.* 1978; 89:893–901.
59. Fenelon LE. Protective isolation: who needs it? *J Hosp Infect.* 1995;30(Suppl): 218–222.
60. Passweg JR, Rowlings PA, Atkinson KA, et al. Influence of protective isolation on outcome of allogeneic bone marrow transplantation for leukemia. *Bone Marrow Transplant.* 1998;21:1231–1238.
61. Hayes-Lattin B, Leis JF, Maziarz RT. Isolation in the allogeneic transplant environment: how protective is it? *Bone Marrow Transplant.* 2005; 36:373–381.
62. Beelen DW, Elmaagacli A, Muller KD, et al. Influence of intestinal bacterial decontamination using metronidazole and ciprofloxacin or ciprofloxacin alone on the development of acute graft-versus-host disease after marrow transplantation in patients with hematologic malignancies: final results and long-term follow-up of an open-label prospective randomized trial. *Blood.* 1999;93:3267–3275.
63. Cornet M, Levy V, Fleury L, et al. Efficacy of prevention by high-efficiency particulate air filtration or laminar airflow against *Aspergillus* airborne contamination during hospital renovation. *Infect Control Hosp Epidemiol.* 1999;20:508–513.
64. Sherertz RJ, Belani A, Kramer BS, et al. Impact of air filtration on nosocomial *Aspergillus* infections. Unique risk of bone marrow transplant recipients. *Am J Med.* 1987;83:709–718.
65. Moody K, Charlson ME, Finlay J. The neutropenic diet: what's the evidence? *J Pediatr Hematol Oncol.* 2002;24:717–721.
66. Fleming S, Yannakou CK, Haeusler GM, et al. Consensus guidelines for antifungal prophylaxis in haematological malignancy and haemopoietic stem cell transplantation, 2014. *Intern Med J.* 2014;44:1283–1297.
67. Martino R, Parody R, Fukuda T, et al. Impact of the intensity of the pretransplantation conditioning regimen in patients with prior invasive aspergillosis undergoing allogeneic hematopoietic stem cell transplantation: a retrospective survey of the Infectious Diseases Working Party of the European Group for Blood and Marrow Transplantation. *Blood.* 2006;108: 2928–2936.
68. Richard C, Romon I, Baro J, et al. Invasive pulmonary aspergillosis prior to BMT in acute leukemia patients does not predict a poor outcome. *Bone Marrow Transplant.* 1993;12:237–241.
69. Hann IM, Prentice HG, Blacklock HA, et al. Acyclovir prophylaxis against herpes virus infections in severely immunocompromised patients: randomised double blind trial. *Br Med J (Clin Res Ed).* 1983;287: 384–388.
70. Saral R, Burns WH, Laskin OL, et al. Acyclovir prophylaxis of herpes-simplex-virus infections. *N Engl J Med.* 1981;305:63–67.
71. Bosch M, Khan FM, Storek J. Immune reconstitution after hematopoietic cell transplantation. *Curr Opin Hematol.* 2012;19:324–335.
72. Bemark M, Holmqvist J, Abrahamsson J, et al. Translational Mini-Review Series on B cell subsets in disease. Reconstitution after haematopoietic stem cell transplantation: revelation of B cell developmental pathways and lineage phenotypes. *Clin Exp Immunol.* 2012;167:15–25.

73. Friedrich W, O'Reilly RJ, Koziner B, et al. T-lymphocyte reconstitution in recipients of bone marrow transplants with and without GVHD: imbalances of T-cell subpopulations having unique regulatory and cognitive functions. *Blood*. 1982;59:696–701.
74. Freifeld AG, Bow EJ, Sepkowitz KA et al. Clinical practice guideline for the use of antimicrobial agents in neutropenic patients with cancer: 2010 Update by the Infectious Diseases Society of America. *Clin Infect Dis*. 2011; 52:427–431.
75. Scully C, Sonis S, Diz PD. Oral mucositis. *Oral Dis*. 2006;12:229–241.
76. Silverman S, Jr. Diagnosis and management of oral mucositis. *J Support Oncol*. 2007;5:13–21.
77. Spielberger R, Stiff P, Bensinger W, et al. Palifermin for oral mucositis after intensive therapy for hematologic cancers. *N Engl J Med*. 2004;351: 2590–2598.
78. Cox GJ, Matsui SM, Lo RS, et al. Etiology and outcome of diarrhea after marrow transplantation: a prospective study. *Gastroenterology*. 1994;107:1398–1407.
79. Schiller GJ, Gale RP. A critical reappraisal of gastrointestinal complications of allogeneic bone marrow transplantation. *Cell Transplant*. 1992; 1:265–269.
80. Schulenburg A, Turetschek K, Wrba F, et al. Early and late gastrointestinal complications after myeloablative and nonmyeloablative allogeneic stem cell transplantation. *Ann Hematol*. 2004;83:101–106.
81. Ippoliti C, Champlin R, Bugazia N, et al. Use of octreotide in the symptomatic management of diarrhea induced by graft-versus-host disease in patients with hematologic malignancies. *J Clin Oncol*. 1997;15: 3350–3354.
82. Meijer E, Boland GJ, Verdonck LF. Prevention of cytomegalovirus disease in recipients of allogeneic stem cell transplants. *Clin Microbiol Rev*. 2003;16:647–657.
83. Cheuk DK, Lee TL, Chiang AK, et al. Risk factors and treatment of hemorrhagic cystitis in children who underwent hematopoietic stem cell transplantation. *Transpl Int*. 2007;20:73–81.
84. Giraud G, Bogdanovic G, Priftakis P, et al. The incidence of hemorrhagic cystitis and BK-viruria in allogeneic hematopoietic stem cell recipients according to intensity of the conditioning regimen. *Haematologica*. 2006;91:401–404.
85. Hale GA, Rochester RJ, Heslop HE, et al. Hemorrhagic cystitis after allogeneic bone marrow transplantation in children: clinical characteristics and outcome. *Biol Blood Marrow Transplant*. 2003;9:698–705.
86. Meisenberg B, Lassiter M, Hussein A, et al. Prevention of hemorrhagic cystitis after high-dose alkylating agent chemotherapy and autologous bone marrow support. *Bone Marrow Transplant*. 1994;14:287–291.
87. Turkeri LN, Lum LG, Uberti JP, et al. Prevention of hemorrhagic cystitis following allogeneic bone marrow transplant preparative regimens with cyclophosphamide and busulfan: role of continuous bladder irrigation. *J Urol*. 1995;153:637–640.
88. Hows JM, Mehta A, Ward L, et al. Comparison of mesna with forced diuresis to prevent cyclophosphamide induced haemorrhagic cystitis in marrow transplantation: a prospective randomised study. *Br J Cancer*. 1984;50:753–756.
89. Spach DH, Bauwens JE, Myerson D, et al. Cytomegalovirus-induced hemorrhagic cystitis following bone marrow transplantation. *Clin Infect Dis*. 1993;16:142–144.
90. Hale GA, Heslop HE, Krance RA, et al. Adenovirus infection after pediatric bone marrow transplantation. *Bone Marrow Transplant*. 1999;23: 277–282.
91. Erard V, Storer B, Corey L, et al. BK virus infection in hematopoietic stem cell transplant recipients: frequency, risk factors, and association with postengraftment hemorrhagic cystitis. *Clin Infect Dis*. 2004;39:1861–1865.
92. Bearman SI. Veno-occlusive disease of the liver. *Curr Opin Oncol*. 2000;12: 103–109.
93. McDonald GB, Hinds MS, Fisher LD, et al. Veno-occlusive disease of the liver and multiorgan failure after bone marrow transplantation: a cohort study of 355 patients. *Ann Intern Med*. 1993;118:255–267.
94. Shulman HM, Gown AM, Nugent DJ. Hepatic veno-occlusive disease after bone marrow transplantation: immunohistochemical identification of the material within occluded central venules. *Am J Pathol*. 1987;127: 549–558.
95. Mohty M, Malard F, Abecassis M, et al. Sinusoidal obstruction syndrome/ veno-occlusive disease: current situation and perspectives-a position statement from the European Society for Blood and Marrow Transplantation (EBMT). *Bone Marrow Transplant*. 2015;50:781–789.
96. Jones RJ, Lee KS, Beschorner WE, et al. Venoocclusive disease of the liver following bone marrow transplantation. *Transplantation*. 1987;44: 778–783.
97. Blostein MD, Paltiel OB, Thibault A, et al. A comparison of clinical criteria for the diagnosis of veno-occlusive disease of the liver after bone marrow transplantation. *Bone Marrow Transplant*. 1992;10:439–443.
98. Herbetko J, Grigg AP, Buckley AR, et al. Venoocclusive liver disease after bone marrow transplantation: findings at duplex sonography. *AJR Am J Roentgenol*. 1992;158:1001–1005.
99. Hommeyer SC, Teefey SA, Jacobson AF, et al. Venocclusive disease of the liver: prospective study of US evaluation. *Radiology*. 1992;184:683–686.
100. Shulman HM, Gooley T, Dudley MD, et al. Utility of transvenous liver biopsies and wedged hepatic venous pressure measurements in sixty marrow transplant recipients. *Transplantation*. 1995;59:1015–1022.
101. Essell JH, Schroeder MT, Harman GS, et al. Ursodiol prophylaxis against hepatic complications of allogeneic bone marrow transplantation. A randomized, double-blind, placebo-controlled trial. *Ann Intern Med*. 1998;128:975–981.
102. Chopra R, Eaton JD, Grassi A, et al. Defibrotide for the treatment of hepatic veno-occlusive disease: results of the European compassionate-use study. *Br J Haematol*. 2000;111:1122–1129.
103. Kornblum N, Ayyanar K, Benimetskaya L, et al. Defibrotide, a polydisperse mixture of single-stranded phosphodiester oligonucleotides with lifesaving activity in severe hepatic veno-occlusive disease: clinical outcomes and potential mechanisms of action. *Oligonucleotides*. 2006;16:105–114.
104. Richardson PG, Murakami C, Jin Z, et al. Multi-institutional use of defibrotide in 88 patients after stem cell transplantation with severe veno-occlusive disease and multisystem organ failure: response without significant toxicity in a high-risk population and factors predictive of outcome. *Blood*. 2002;100:4337–4343.
105. Bearman SI, Lee JL, Baron AE, et al. Treatment of hepatic venocclusive disease with recombinant human tissue plasminogen activator and heparin in 42 marrow transplant patients. *Blood*. 1997;89:1501–1506.
106. Schriber J, Milk B, Shaw D, et al. Tissue plasminogen activator (tPA) as therapy for hepatotoxicity following bone marrow transplantation. *Bone Marrow Transplant*. 1999;24:1311–1314.
107. Fried MW, Connaghan DG, Sharma S, et al. Transjugular intrahepatic portosystemic shunt for the management of severe venoocclusive disease following bone marrow transplantation. *Hepatology*. 1996;24:588–591.
108. Azoulay D, Castaing D, Lemoine A, et al. Transjugular intrahepatic portosystemic shunt (TIPS) for severe veno-occlusive disease of the liver following bone marrow transplantation. *Bone Marrow Transplant*. 2000;25:987–992.
109. Zenz T, Rossle M, Bertz H, et al. Severe veno-occlusive disease after allogeneic bone marrow or peripheral stem cell transplantation–role of transjugular intrahepatic portosystemic shunt (TIPS). *Liver*. 2001;21:31–36.
110. Hagglund H, Ringden O, Ericzon BG, et al. Treatment of hepatic venoocclusive disease with recombinant human tissue plasminogen activator or orthotopic liver transplantation after allogeneic bone marrow transplantation. *Transplantation*. 1996;62:1076–1080.
111. Nimer SD, Milewicz AL, Champlin RE, et al. Successful treatment of hepatic venoocclusive disease in a bone marrow transplant patient with orthotopic liver transplantation. *Transplantation*. 1990;49:819–821.
112. Rapoport AP, Doyle HR, Starzl T, et al. Orthotopic liver transplantation for life-threatening veno-occlusive disease of the liver after allogeneic bone marrow transplant. *Bone Marrow Transplant*. 1991;8:421–424.
113. Huynh TN, Weigt SS, Belperio JA, et al. Outcome and prognostic indicators of patients with hematopoietic stem cell transplants admitted to the intensive care unit. *J Transplant*. 2009;2009:917294.
114. Martin PL. To stop or not to stop: how much support should be provided to mechanically ventilated pediatric bone marrow and stem cell transplant patients? *Respir Care Clin North Am*. 2006;12:403–419.
115. Ho VT, Weller E, Lee SJ, et al. Prognostic factors for early severe pulmonary complications after hematopoietic stem cell transplantation. *Biol Blood Marrow Transplant*. 2001;7:223–229.
116. Khurshid I, Anderson LC. Non-infectious pulmonary complications after bone marrow transplantation. *Postgrad Med J*. 2002;78:257–262.
117. Sharma S, Nadrous HF, Peters SG, et al. Pulmonary complications in adult blood and marrow transplant recipients: autopsy findings. *Chest*. 2005;128:1385–1392.
118. Yen KT, Lee AS, Krowka MJ, et al. Pulmonary complications in bone marrow transplantation: a practical approach to diagnosis and treatment. *Clin Chest Med*. 2004;25:189–201.
119. Afessa B, Tefferi A, Litzow MR, et al. Diffuse alveolar hemorrhage in hematopoietic stem cell transplant recipients. *Am J Respir Crit Care Med*. 2002;166:641–645.
120. Gottdiener JS, Appelbaum FR, Ferrans VJ, et al. Cardiotoxicity associated with high-dose cyclophosphamide therapy. *Arch Intern Med*. 1981;141: 758–763.

121. Hochster H, Wasserheit C, Speyer J. Cardiotoxicity and cardioprotection during chemotherapy. *Curr Opin Oncol.* 1995;7:304–309.
122. Murdych T, Weisdorf DJ. Serious cardiac complications during bone marrow transplantation at the University of Minnesota, 1977–1997. *Bone Marrow Transplant.* 2001;28:283–287.
123. Tang WH, Thomas S, Kalaycio M, et al. Clinical outcomes of patients with impaired left ventricular ejection fraction undergoing autologous bone marrow transplantation: can we safely transplant patients with impaired ejection fraction? *Bone Marrow Transplant.* 2004;34:603–607.
124. Morandi P, Ruffini PA, Benvenuto GM, et al. Cardiac toxicity of high-dose chemotherapy. *Bone Marrow Transplant.* 2005;35:323–334.
125. Parikh CR, Coca SG. Acute renal failure in hematopoietic cell transplantation. *Kidney Int.* 2006;69:430–435.
126. Kersting S, Koomans HA, Hene RJ, et al. Acute kidney failure after allogeneic myeloablative stem cell transplantation: retrospective analysis of incidence, risk factors and survival. *Bone Marrow Transplant.* 2007;39:359–365.
127. Lane PH, Mauer SM, Blazar BR, et al. Outcome of dialysis for acute kidney failure in pediatric bone marrow transplant patients. *Bone Marrow Transplant.* 1994;13:613–617.
128. Mattsson J, Ringdén O, Storb R. Graft failure after allogeneic hematopoietic cell transplantation. *Biol Blood Marrow Transplant.* 2008;14(1 Suppl 1): 165–170.
129. Woodard P, Tong X, Richardson S, et al. Etiology and outcome of graft failure in pediatric hematopoietic stem cell transplant recipients. *J Pediatr Hematol Oncol.* 2003;25:955–959.
130. Shizuru JA, Negrin RS, Weissman IL. Hematopoietic stem and progenitor cells: clinical and preclinical regeneration of the hematolymphoid system. *Annu Rev Med.* 2005;56:509–538.
131. van Os R, Kamminga LM, de Haan G. Stem cell assays: something old, something new, something borrowed. *Stem Cells.* 2004;22:1181–1190.
132. Engelhardt M, Lubbert M, Guo Y. CD34(+) or CD34(-): which is the more primitive? *Leukemia.* 2002;16:1603–1608.
133. Petersdorf EW. HLA matching in allogeneic stem cell transplantation. *Curr Opin Hematol.* 2004;11:386–391.
134. Davies SM, Ramsay NK, Haake RJ, et al. Comparison of engraftment in recipients of matched sibling of unrelated donor marrow allografts. *Bone Marrow Transplant.* 1994;13:51–57.
135. Bearman SI, Mori M, Beatty PG, et al. Comparison of morbidity and mortality after marrow transplantation from HLA-genotypically identical siblings and HLA-phenotypically identical unrelated donors. *Bone Marrow Transplant.* 1994;13:31–35.
136. Holler E. Risk assessment in haematopoietic stem cell transplantation: GvHD prevention and treatment. *Best Pract Res Clin Haematol.* 2007;20:281–294.
137. Champlin R, Giralt S, Gajewski J. T cells, graft-versus-host disease and graft-versus-leukemia: innovative approaches for blood and marrow transplantation. *Acta Haematol.* 1996;95:157–163.
138. Goulmy E, Termijtelen A, Bradley BA, et al. Y-antigen killing by T cells of women is restricted by HLA. *Nature.* 1977;266:544–545.
139. Gahrton G. Risk assessment in haematopoietic stem cell transplantation: impact of donor-recipient sex combination in allogeneic transplantation. *Best Pract Res Clin Haematol.* 2007;20:219–229.
140. Deeg HJ, Antin JH. The clinical spectrum of acute graft-versus-host disease. *Semin Hematol.* 2006;43:24–31.
141. Holtan SG, Pasquini M, Weisdorf DJ. Acute graft-versus-host disease: a bench-to-bedside update. *Blood.* 2014;124:363–373.
142. Hansen JA, Petersdorf E, Martin PJ, et al. Hematopoietic stem cell transplants from unrelated donors. *Immunol Rev.* 1997;157:141–151.
143. Petersdorf EW, Anasetti C, Martin PJ, et al. Tissue typing in support of unrelated hematopoietic cell transplantation. *Tissue Antigens.* 2003; 61:1–11.
144. Shastri N, Cardinaud S, Schwab SR, et al. All the peptides that fit: the beginning, the middle, and the end of the MHC class I antigen-processing pathway. *Immunol Rev.* 2005;207:31–41.
145. Villadangos JA, Schnorrer P, Wilson NS. Control of MHC class II antigen presentation in dendritic cells: a balance between creative and destructive forces. *Immunol Rev.* 2005;207:191–205.
146. Ferrara JL, Reddy P. Pathophysiology of graft-versus-host disease. *Semin Hematol.* 2006;43:3–10.
147. Ringden O, Pihlstedt P, Markling L, et al. Prevention of graft-versus-host disease with T cell depletion or cyclosporin and methotrexate: A randomized trial in adult leukemic marrow recipients. *Bone Marrow Transplant.* 1991;7:221–226.
148. Chao NJ, Chen BJ. Prophylaxis and treatment of acute graft-versus-host disease. *Semin Hematol.* 2006;43:32–41.
149. Bacigalupo A, Palandri F. Management of acute graft versus host disease (GvHD). *Hematol J.* 2004;5:189–196.
150. Fowler DH. Shared biology of GVHD and GVT effects: potential methods of separation. *Crit Rev Oncol Hematol.* 2006;57:225–244.
151. Storb R, Deeg HJ, Whitehead J, et al. Methotrexate and cyclosporine compared with cyclosporine alone for prophylaxis of acute graft versus host disease after marrow transplantation for leukemia. *N Engl J Med.* 1986;314:729–735.
152. Leelasiri A, Greer JP, Stein RS, et al. Graft-versus-host-disease prophylaxis for matched unrelated donor bone marrow transplantation: comparison between cyclosporine-methotrexate and cyclosporine-metho-trexate-methylprednisolone. *Bone Marrow Transplant.* 1995;15: 401–405.
153. Sullivan KM, Kopecky KJ, Jocom J, et al. Immunomodulatory and antimicrobial efficacy of intravenous immunoglobulin in bone marrow transplantation. *N Engl J Med.* 1990;323:705–712.
154. Jacobsohn DA, Vogelsang GB. Anti-cytokine therapy for the treatment of graft-versus-host disease. *Curr Pharm Des.* 2004;10:1195–1205.
155. Einsele H, Ehninger G, Steidle M, et al. Lymphocytopenia as an unfavorable prognostic factor in patients with cytomegalovirus infection after bone marrow transplantation. *Blood.* 1993;82:1672–1678.
156. Mori T, Okamoto S, Matsuoka S, et al. Risk-adapted pre-emptive therapy for cytomegalovirus disease in patients undergoing allogeneic bone marrow transplantation. *Bone Marrow Transplant.* 2000;25:765–769.
157. Matthes-Martin S, Lion T, Aberle SW, et al. Pre-emptive treatment of CMV DNAemia in paediatric stem cell transplantation: the impact of recipient and donor CMV serostatus on the incidence of CMV disease and CMV-related mortality. *Bone Marrow Transplant.* 2003;31:803–808.
158. Ng AP, Worth L, Chen L, et al. Cytomegalovirus DNAemia and disease: incidence, natural history and management in settings other than allogeneic stem cell transplantation. *Haematologica.* 2005;90:1672–1679.
159. Razonable RR, Emery VC. Management of CMV infection and disease in transplant patients. 27–29 February 2004. *Herpes.* 2004;11:77–86.
160. Scaglione S, Hofmeister CC, Stiff P. Evaluation of pulmonary infiltrates in patients after stem cell transplantation. *Hematology.* 2005;10:469–481.
161. Panoskaltsis-Mortari A, Griese M, Madtes DK et al. American Thoracic Society Committee on Idiopathic Pneumonia Syndrome. An official American Thoracic Society research statement: noninfectious lung injury after hematopoietic stem cell transplantation: idiopathic pneumonia syndrome. *Am J Respir Crit Care Med.* 2011;183:1262–1279.
162. Ljungman P, Hakki M, Boeckh M. Cytomegalovirus in hematopoietic stem cell transplant recipients. *Infect Dis Clin North Am.* 2010;24:319–337.
163. Travi G, Pergam SA. Cytomegalovirus pneumonia in hematopoietic stem cell recipients. *J Intensive Care Med.* 2014;29:200–212.
164. Nicholson E, Peggs KS. Cytomegalovirus-specific T-cell therapies: current status and future prospects. *Immunotherapy.* 2015;7:135–146.
165. Bilgrami SF, Metersky ML, McNally D, et al. Idiopathic pneumonia syndrome following myeloablative chemotherapy and autologous transplantation. *Ann Pharmacother.* 2001;35:196–201.
166. Keates-Baleeiro J, Moore P, Koyama T, et al. Incidence and outcome of idiopathic pneumonia syndrome in pediatric stem cell transplant recipients. *Bone Marrow Transplant.* 2006;38:285–289.
167. Wong R, Rondon G, Saliba RM, et al. Idiopathic pneumonia syndrome after high-dose chemotherapy and autologous hematopoietic stem cell transplantation for high-risk breast cancer. *Bone Marrow Transplant.* 2003;31:1157–1163.
168. Taplitz RA, Jordan MC. Pneumonia caused by herpesviruses in recipients of hematopoietic cell transplants. *Semin Respir Infect.* 2002;17: 121–129.
169. Singavi AK, Harrington AM, Fenske TS. Post-transplant lymphoproliferative disorders. *Cancer Treat Res.* 2015;165:305–327.
170. Trappe R, Oertel S, Leblond V et al.; German PTLD Study Group; European PTLD Network. Sequential treatment with rituximab followed by CHOP chemotherapy in adult B-cell post-transplant lymphoproliferative disorder (PTLD): the prospective international multicentre phase 2 PTLD-1 trial. *Lancet Oncol.* 2012;13:196–206.
171. Bollard CM, Rooney CM, Heslop HE. T-cell therapy in the treatment of post-transplant lymphoproliferative disease. *Nat Rev Clin Oncol.* 2012;9:510–519.
172. Linhares YP, Pavletic S, Gale RP. Chronic GVHD: Where are we? Where do we want to be? Will immunomodulatory drugs help? *Bone Marrow Transplant.* 2013;48:203–209.
173. Socié G, Ritz J. Current issues in chronic graft-versus-host disease. *Blood.* 2014;124:374–384.
174. Flowers ME, Martin PJ. How we treat chronic graft-versus-host disease. *Blood.* 2015;125:606–615.

175. Beuers U, Trauner M, Jansen P, et al. New paradigms in the treatment of hepatic cholestasis: From UDCA to FXR, PXR and beyond. *J Hepatol.* 2015;62:S25–S37.
176. Offidani M, Corvatta L, Olivieri A, et al. A predictive model of varicella-zoster virus infection after autologous peripheral blood progenitor cell transplantation. *Clin Infect Dis.* 2001;32:1414–1422.
177. Leung TF, Chik KW, Li CK, et al. Incidence, risk factors and outcome of varicella-zoster virus infection in children after haematopoietic stem cell transplantation. *Bone Marrow Transplant.* 2000;25:167–172.
178. Koc Y, Miller KB, Schenkein DP, et al. Varicella zoster virus infections following allogeneic bone marrow transplantation: frequency, risk factors, and clinical outcome. *Biol Blood Marrow Transplant.* 2000;6:44–49.
179. Majhail NS. Secondary cancers following allogeneic haematopoietic cell transplantation in adults. *Br J Haematol.* 2011;154:301–310.
180. Bilmon IA, Ashton LJ, Le Marsney RE, et al.; CAST study group. Second cancer risk in adults receiving autologous haematopoietic SCT for cancer: a population-based cohort study. *Bone Marrow Transplant.* 2014;49:691–698.
181. Lenz G, Dreyling M, Schiegnitz E, et al. Moderate increase of secondary hematologic malignancies after myeloablative radiochemotherapy and autologous stem-cell transplantation in patients with indolent lymphoma: results of a prospective randomized trial of the German Low Grade Lymphoma Study Group. *J Clin Oncol.* 2004;22:4926–4933.
182. Meshinchi S, Leisenring WM, Carpenter PA, et al. Survival after second hematopoietic stem cell transplantation for recurrent pediatric acute myeloid leukemia. *Biol Blood Marrow Transplant.* 2003;9:706–713.
183. Eapen M, Giralt SA, Horowitz MM, et al. Second transplant for acute and chronic leukemia relapsing after first HLA-identical sibling transplant. *Bone Marrow Transplant.* 2004;34:721–727.
184. Qazilbash MH, Saliba R, De Lima M, et al. Second autologous or allogeneic transplantation after the failure of first autograft in patients with multiple myeloma. *Cancer.* 2006;106:1084–1089.
185. Yoshimi A, Mohamed M, Bierings M, et al. Second allogeneic hematopoietic stem cell transplantation (HSCT) results in outcome similar to that of first HSCT for patients with juvenile myelomonocytic leukemia. *Leukemia.* 2007;21:556–560.
186. Dazzi F, Goldman J. Donor lymphocyte infusions. *Curr Opin Hematol.* 1999;6:394–399.
187. Loren AW, Porter DL. Donor leukocyte infusions after unrelated donor hematopoietic stem cell transplantation. *Curr Opin Oncol.* 2006;18:107–114.
188. Slavin S, Morecki S, Weiss L, et al. Immunotherapy of hematologic malignancies and metastatic solid tumors in experimental animals and man. *Crit Rev Oncol Hematol.* 2003;46:139–163.
189. Chalandon Y, Passweg JR, Guglielmi C, et al. Chronic Malignancies Working Party of the European Group for Blood and Marrow Transplantation (EBMT). Early administration of donor lymphocyte infusions upon molecular relapse after allogeneic hematopoietic stem cell transplantation for chronic myeloid leukemia: a study by the Chronic Malignancies Working Party of the EBMT. *Haematologica.* 2014;99:1492–1498.
190. Ciceri F, Bonini C, Gallo-Stampino C, et al. Modulation of GvHD by suicide-gene transduced donor T lymphocytes: clinical applications in mismatched transplantation. *Cytotherapy.* 2005;7:144–149.
191. Toubert ME, Socie G, Gluckman E, et al. Short- and long-term follow-up of thyroid dysfunction after allogeneic bone marrow transplantation without the use of preparative total body irradiation. *Br J Haematol.* 1997;98:453–457.
192. Vexiau P, Perez-Castiglioni P, Socie G, et al. The 'euthyroid sick syndrome': incidence, risk factors and prognostic value soon after allogeneic bone marrow transplantation. *Br J Haematol.* 1993;85:778–782.
193. Sklar CA, Kim TH, Ramsay NK. Thyroid dysfunction among long-term survivors of bone marrow transplantation. *Am J Med.* 1982;73:688–694.
194. Shalitin S, Phillip M, Stein J, et al. Endocrine dysfunction and parameters of the metabolic syndrome after bone marrow transplantation during childhood and adolescence. *Bone Marrow Transplant.* 2006;37:1109–1117.
195. Faraci M, Barra S, Cohen A, et al. Very late nonfatal consequences of fractionated TBI in children undergoing bone marrow transplant. *Int J Radiat Oncol Biol Phys.* 2005;63:1568–1575.
196. Slatter MA, Gennery AR, Cheetham TD, et al. Thyroid dysfunction after bone marrow transplantation for primary immunodeficiency without the use of total body irradiation in conditioning. *Bone Marrow Transplant.* 2004;33:949–953.
197. Sanders JE. Endocrine complications of high-dose therapy with stem cell transplantation. *Pediatr Transplant.* 2004;8(Suppl 5):39–50.
198. Wingard JR, Plotnick LP, Freemer CS, et al. Growth in children after bone marrow transplantation: busulfan plus cyclophosphamide versus cyclophosphamide plus total body irradiation. *Blood.* 1992;79:1068–1073.
199. Sanders JE, Guthrie KA, Hoffmeister PA, et al. Final adult height of patients who received hematopoietic cell transplantation in childhood. *Blood.* 2005;105:1348–1354.
200. Tauchmanova L, Selleri C, Rosa GD, et al. High prevalence of endocrine dysfunction in long-term survivors after allogeneic bone marrow transplantation for hematologic diseases. *Cancer.* 2002;95:1076–1084.
201. Bakker B, Oostdijk W, Bresters D, et al. Disturbances of growth and endocrine function after busulphan-based conditioning for haematopoietic stem cell transplantation during infancy and childhood. *Bone Marrow Transplant.* 2004;33:1049–1056.
202. Chiodi S, Spinelli S, Cohen A, et al. Cyclic sex hormone replacement therapy in women undergoing allogeneic bone marrow transplantation: aims and results. *Bone Marrow Transplant.* 1991;8(Suppl 1):47–49.
203. Demeestere I, Simon P, Buxant F, et al. Ovarian function and spontaneous pregnancy after combined heterotopic and orthotopic cryopreserved ovarian tissue transplantation in a patient previously treated with bone marrow transplantation: case report. *Hum Reprod.* 2006;21:2010–2014.
204. Donnez J, Dolmans MM, Demylle D, et al. Restoration of ovarian function after orthotopic (intraovarian and periovarian) transplantation of cryopreserved ovarian tissue in a woman treated by bone marrow transplantation for sickle cell anaemia: case report. *Hum Reprod.* 2006;21:183–188.
205. Tichelli A, Gratwohl A, Egger T, et al. Cataract formation after bone marrow transplantation. *Ann Intern Med.* 1993;119:1175–1180.
206. Benyunes MC, Sullivan KM, Deeg HJ, et al. Cataracts after bone marrow transplantation: long-term follow-up of adults treated with fractionated total body irradiation. *Int J Radiat Oncol Biol Phys.* 1995;32:661–670.
207. van Kempen-Harteveld ML, Struikmans H, Kal HB, et al. Cataract after total body irradiation and bone marrow transplantation: degree of visual impairment. *Int J Radiat Oncol Biol Phys.* 2002;52:1375–1380.
208. Zierhut D, Lohr F, Schraube P, et al. Cataract incidence after total-body irradiation. *Int J Radiat Oncol Biol Phys.* 2000;46:131–135.
209. Miralbell R, Bieri S, Mermillod B, et al. Kidney toxicity after allogeneic bone marrow transplantation: the combined effects of total-body irradiation and graft-versus-host disease. *J Clin Oncol.* 1996;14:579–585.
210. Tarbell NJ, Guinan EC, Niemeyer C, et al. Late onset of kidney dysfunction in survivors of bone marrow transplantation. *Int J Radiat Oncol Biol Phys.* 1988;15:99–104.
211. Sakaida E, Nakaseko C, Harima A, et al. Late-onset noninfectious pulmonary complications after allogeneic stem cell transplantation are significantly associated with chronic graft-versus-host disease and with the graft-versus-leukemia effect. *Blood.* 2003;102:4236–4242.
212. Afessa B, Litzow MR, Tefferi A. Bronchiolitis obliterans and other late onset non-infectious pulmonary complications in hematopoietic stem cell transplantation. *Bone Marrow Transplant.* 2001;28:425–434.
213. Savani BN, Montero A, Srinivasan R, et al. Chronic GVHD and pretransplantation abnormalities in pulmonary function are the main determinants predicting worsening pulmonary function in long-term survivors after stem cell transplantation. *Biol Blood Marrow Transplant.* 2006;12:1261–1269.
214. Ransom JT. Mechanism of action of mycophenolate mofetil. *Ther Drug Monit.* 1995;17:681–684.
215. Bordigoni P, Dimicoli S, Clement L, et al. Daclizumab, an efficient treatment for steroid-refractory acute graft-versus-host disease. *Br J Haematol.* 2006;135:382–385.
216. Bruner RJ, Farag SS. Monoclonal antibodies for the prevention and treatment of graft-versus-host disease. *Semin Oncol.* 2003;30:509–519.
217. Flowers ME, Martin PJ. Evaluation of thalidomide for treatment or prevention of chronic graft-versus-host disease. *Leuk Lymphoma.* 2003;44:1141–1146.
218. Chakrabarti S, Hale G, Waldmann H. Alemtuzumab (Campath-1H) in allogeneic stem cell transplantation: where do we go from here? *Transplant Proc.* 2004;36:1225–1227.

CHAPTER 77

The Obstetric Patient

MICHAEL A. FRÖLICH and MALI MATHRU

INTRODUCTION

Major scientific advances have occurred in virtually all areas of patient care. One of the major changes in obstetrics has been the recognition of the specialty nature of medical complications related to pregnancy. The physiologic alterations that accompany pregnancy may have profound effects on a variety of pathologic conditions. In addition, maternal disease or its therapy may adversely affect the fetus, which makes these considerations unique to the obstetric patient.

The intensivist must be knowledgeable of the considerations specific to pregnant women and should also understand the pathophysiologic alterations associated with high-risk conditions such as preeclampsia. Obstetricians have done a remarkably good job in managing common diseases such as diabetes, asthma, and chronic hypertension with great sophistication. Nevertheless, life-threatening emergencies during pregnancy challenge the knowledge and skills of anyone who works with this group of patients. Clinicians have acquired considerable information about the management of critically ill obstetric patients; however, this information is not geared toward the critical care provider in most textbooks. This chapter is intended to fill this gap and provide the essential information about the most severe critical conditions that might arise during pregnancy.

An extensive review of all maternal high-risk conditions would go beyond the scope of this chapter. Therefore, we will limit our review to the discussion of physiologic changes of pregnancy that clearly have to be recognized when managing the critically ill pregnant woman. This review is focused mainly on the most life-threatening pathophysiologic processes, including thrombosis and thromboembolism, hypertensive disease of pregnancy, hemorrhage, and amniotic fluid embolism (Tables 77.1 and 77.2), but is inclusive of other more common pregnancy-related problems that come to the attention of the intensivist, such as peripartum cardiomyopathy (PPCM) and pulmonary edema.

PHYSIOLOGY

Several physiologic changes are associated with normal pregnancy. These adaptations are necessary to meet the demands of the growing fetus, and have to be considered when evaluating and managing pregnant patients.

Body Constitution

Optimal weight gain in pregnancy is currently a matter of debate (1–3). In general, an approximate weight gain of 6 kg is attributed to the fetus, placenta, and uterus, with the remainder of the weight gain due to an increase in maternal blood, interstitial fluid volume, and fat. A gestational weight gain of more than 12 kg in women of normal prepregnant weight puts her into an augmented risk category—even though the lowest one—for complications during delivery. Thorsdottir et al. (4) studied the relationship between gestational weight gain and complications during pregnancy, comparing pregnant women with normal weight gain with other higher gestational weight gain. They found that women who exceeded 18 kg of weight gain during pregnancy are at greater risk for maternal (preeclampsia, gestational diabetes) and fetal (increased incidence of operative delivery) complications.

Changes in maternal physiology occur normally during pregnancy, and have the potential to alter the absorption, distribution, and elimination of drugs used therapeutically in pregnant women (5).

Metabolism and Respiration

Key physiologic changes of respiration that occur in pregnancy are an increased minute ventilation, which is caused by increased respiratory center sensitivity and drive; a compensated respiratory alkalosis; and a low expiratory reserve volume (ERV) (6,7). Vital capacity and forced expiratory measurements are well preserved. Patients who have severe lung diseases tolerate pregnancy well, with the exception of those with pulmonary hypertension or chronic respiratory insufficiency from parenchymal or neuromuscular disease.

Lung volumes have been measured in several case series, where pregnant women were compared to nonpregnant women or those in the postpartum state (8), with body plethysmography being the preferred technique of measurement (9); volumes were found to be well preserved in the majority of cases. The *residual volume* tends to decrease slightly, leading to no change or a small increase in the vital capacity (8,10–13). The most consistent change in static lung volumes with pregnancy is the reduction in the *functional residual capacity* (FRC) and ERV. As the uterus enlarges, FRC decreases by 10% to 25% of the previous value, starting about the 12th week of pregnancy (8); this decrement is accentuated further in the supine position (14). The reduction in FRC is due to a decrease in chest wall compliance of from 35% to 40% (15). The lung compliance

TABLE 77.1 Direct Maternal Deaths, 1991–2008[a]

Cause of Death	1991–93	1994–96	1997–99	2000–02	2003–05	2006–08
Thrombosis and thromboembolism	35	48	35	30	18	26
Hypertensive disease of pregnancy	20	20	15	14	18	19
Hemorrhage	15	12	7	17	41	18
Amniotic fluid embolism	10	17	8	5	17	13
Deaths in early pregnancy total	18	15	17	15	14	11
Ectopic	8	12	13	11	10	6
Spontaneous miscarriage	3	2	2	1	1	5
Legal termination	5	1	2	3	2	0
Other	2	0	0	0	1	0
Genital tract sepsis	9[b]	14[c]	14[c]	11[c]	14	9
Other direct total	14	7	7	8	6	7
Genital tract trauma	4	5	2	1	4	4
Fatty liver	2	2	4	3	3	0
Other	8	0	1	4	1	3
Anaesthetic	8	1	3	6	0	1
Total number of deaths	128	134	106	106	132	107

[a]Deaths reported to the Enquiry only and excluding other deaths identified by ONS.
[b]Excluding early pregnancy deaths due to sepsis.
[c]Including early pregnancy deaths due to sepsis.
From Centre for Maternal and Child Enquiries (CMACE). *Publication 2011: Saving Mothers' Lives 2006–2008*. London, UK; 2011.

remains normal during pregnancy, whereas expiratory muscle strength is in the low-normal range (10). The decreased chest wall compliance is the result of the enlarging uterus increasing abdominal pressure, leading to a reduction in FRC (16); the diaphragm elevates about 4 cm and the circumference of the lower rib cage increases about 5 cm (17). The lower end-expiratory lung volume leads to an increased area of apposition of the diaphragm to the chest wall, which improves the coupling of the diaphragm and chest wall. Thus, the increased tidal volume of pregnancy is achieved without an increase in the respiratory excursions of the diaphragm.

The rib cage undergoes structural changes during pregnancy (18). Progressive relaxation of the ligamentous attachments of the ribs causes the subcostal angle of the rib cage to increase early in pregnancy, persisting for months into the postpartum period. The increased elasticity of the rib cage is mediated by the polypeptide hormone, relaxin, which is increased during pregnancy and is responsible for the softening of the cervix and relaxation of the pelvic ligaments (19,20). Changes in pulmonary function during pregnancy are summarized in Figure 77.1.

Changes in Arterial Blood Gases

The hormonal changes of pregnancy lead to remarkable respiratory changes throughout its course. The resulting changes of arterial blood gas values have been measured by Sheldon (21) and Templeton and Kelman (22), who obtained serial measurements of maternal blood gases during pregnancy. The same investigators also measured serial alveolar-to-arterial oxygen tension differences ($PAO_2 - PaO_2$), and calculated the pulmonary venous admixture (physiologic shunt), dead space-to-tidal volume ratio (V_D/V_T), and respiratory minute volume (Table 77.3). The mean arterial PO_2 was found to be consistently greater than 100 mmHg throughout pregnancy, with no alterations of dead space-to-tidal volume ratio (V_D/V_T) and shunt.

Cardiovascular System

Management of pregnancy, especially for women with heart disease, requires an understanding of gestational hemodynamic stress. The most important hemodynamic change in the maternal circulation during pregnancy is an increase in the cardiac output up to 45% (23), which can be primarily attributed to an increase in stroke volume, while heart rate and blood pressure do not change significantly (Fig. 77.2).

This alteration has several unique features: (a) the augmentation occurs relatively early in pregnancy (20 to 24 weeks); (b) it cannot be explained entirely on the basis of fetal needs; and (c) fluctuations in cardiac output occur with changes in body position as the gravid uterus impinges, to varying degrees, on the inferior vena cava, thus altering systemic venous return (25). Electrocardiographic (ECG) changes observed, but are

TABLE 77.2 Indirect Maternal Deaths, 2000–2002[a]

Causes of Indirect Deaths	1991–93	1994–96	1997–99	2000–02	2003–05	2006–08
Cardiac	37	39	35	44	48	53
Psychiatric	N/A	9	15	16	37	36
Other indirect	63	86	75	90	18	13
Indirect malignancies	N/A	N/A	11	5	10	3
Total number of indirect deaths	100	134	136	155	50	49

[a]Deaths reported to the Enquiry only and excluding other deaths identified by ONS.
From Confidential Enquiry into Maternal and Child Health (CEMACH). Publication 2004: Why Mothers Die 2000–2002. London, UK; 2004.

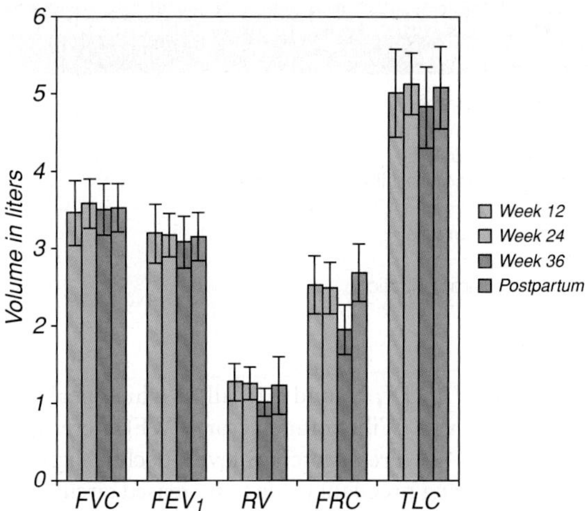

FIGURE 77.1 Pulmonary changes of pregnancy (9). FVC, forced vital capacity; FEV_1, forced expiratory volume in 1 second; RV, plethysmographic residual volume; FRC, plethysmographic functional residual capacity; TLC, plethysmographic total lung capacity.

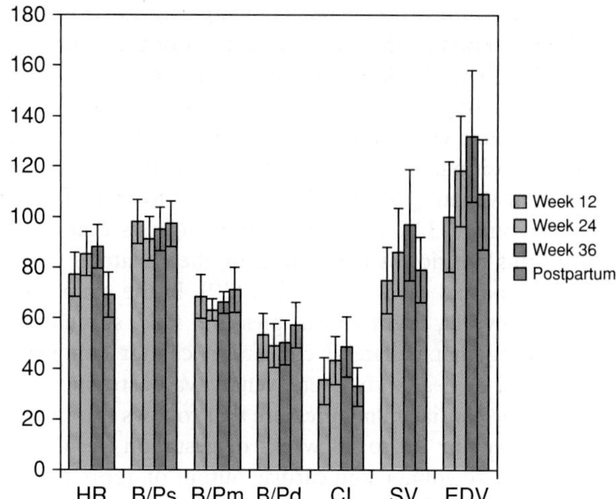

FIGURE 77.2 Cardiovascular changes of pregnancy (24). HR, heart rate (bpm); B/Ps, systolic blood pressure (mmHg); B/Pm, mean blood pressure (mmHg); B/Pd, diastolic blood pressure (mmHg); CI, cardiac index (L/min/m²); SV, stroke volume (mL); EDV, end-diastolic volume (mL).

of no clinical significance, include: sinus tachycardia, left axis deviation, ectopic beats, inverted or flattened T waves, and a Q wave in lead III (26).

Red Blood Cell, Plasma, and Blood Volume

An increase of plasma volume is evident by the sixth week of gestation, reaching a value by the end of the first trimester of 15% above that of the nongravid state. There is subsequently a steep increase of this parameter until 28 to 30 weeks of gestation, followed by a more gradual rise, to a final volume at term of 55% above the nonpregnant level (27). Red blood cell mass decreases during the first 8 weeks of gestation due to a decrease in the life span of erythrocytes (23), but increases to nearly 30% above the nonpregnant level at term. These physiologic changes result in a 45% increase of total blood volume and a reduction of the hemoglobin concentration and hematocrit to values of approximately 11.6 g/dL and 35.5 volume %, respectively (Fig. 77.3). Estrogens, progesterone, and placental lactogen elevate aldosterone production either directly or indirectly, and are responsible for the increase of plasma volume during pregnancy. The hyperaldosteronism of pregnancy can result in retention up to 500 to 900 mEq of sodium and an increase of 6,000 to 8,000 mL of total body water, 70% of which is extracellular. The elevated red blood cell volume after 8 to 12 weeks can be attributed to increased serum erythropoietin. Erythropoiesis may also be stimulated by prolactin, progesterone, and placental lactogen. Changes of blood counts during pregnancy are summarized in Figure 77.3.

Plasma Proteins, Colloid Osmotic Pressure, and GFR

The total serum protein concentration decreases from the nonpregnant value of 7.3 to 6.5 g/dL at term gestation. The change is due primarily to a decline of the albumin concentration, which decreases from a nonpregnant level of 4.4 to 3.4 g/dL at term. Although the concentration of globulins declines by 10% during the first trimester, the level rises subsequently to a value at term that is 5% to 10% above the nonpregnant level. These changes result in a progressive decrease in the albumin-to-globulin ratio from approximately 1.5 during pregnancy to 1.1 at term gestation. Maternal colloid osmotic pressure decreases in parallel with the decline in serum albumin concentration from nonpregnant values of 25 to 26 mmHg to approximately 22 mmHg at term. During pregnancy, the glomerular filtration rate (GFR) increases 50% as compared to pregravid levels (28).

TABLE 77.3 Blood Gas Analysis in Late Pregnancy[a] (22)

pH	7.44	HCO_3^- (mMol/L)	20
PaO_2 (mmHg)	103	BE (mMol/L)	2.5
$PaCO_2$ (mmHg)	30		

[a]Averages.

Aortocaval Compression

Angiographic studies show that the aorta and inferior vena cava can be significantly compressed by the gravid uterus when the woman is in the supine position. In fact, Kerr et al. (29) observed a complete obstruction of the inferior vena cava at

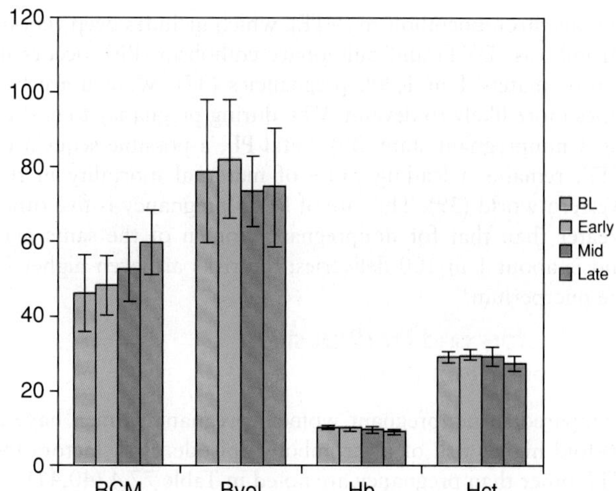

FIGURE 77.3 Changes of blood count during pregnancy (27). RCM, red cell mass in mL/10; Bvol, blood volume in mL/kg; Hb, hemoglobin in g/100 mL; Hct, hematocrit in %; BL, prepregnant data; early, 8th week of pregnancy; mid, 14th week of pregnancy; late, 20th week of pregnancy.

the level of the bifurcation in 80% of women in late pregnancy. Partial obstruction of the aorta at the level of the lumbar lordosis (L3–L5) has also been demonstrated in patients between the 27th week of pregnancy and term gestation (30,31).

The pregnant woman at term, when placed in the lateral decubitus position, exhibits a right ventricular filling pressure (central venous pressure [CVP]) similar to that of a nonpregnant woman (32). This observation suggests that venous return in this position is maintained by the collateral circulation despite partial caval obstruction (29). In the plain supine position, however, right atrial pressure falls substantially, demonstrating that collateral circulation cannot compensate for complete, or nearly complete, vena cava obstruction (30). The fall in the cardiac filling pressure that follows this position change, evident by 20 to 28 weeks of gestation, results in a decreased stroke volume and cardiac output of approximately 25%, and a 20% reduction of uterine blood flow (33); these are reliably improved by a tilt to the left of at least 25 degrees (34).

Despite the reduction of cardiac output and stroke volume, a position change from lateral to supine can be associated with elevation of blood pressure, resulting from an increase of systemic vascular resistance due to compression of the aorta by the gravid uterus and enhanced sympathetic nervous system outflow (35). In approximately 5% of women, however, a substantial drop in blood pressure occurs ("supine hypotensive syndrome"), which is associated with bradycardia (usually following a transient tachycardia) and maternal symptoms of low systemic perfusion, such as of pallor and sweating, possibly followed by cardiocirculatory collapse. This occasional, but profound, drop of venous return may be exacerbated by neuraxial block, the preferred method of providing anesthesia in pregnant women (36). In conclusion, and based on the observations above, the intensivist should always consider in his or her emergency treatment plan the proper positioning of the pregnant patient and its influence on hemodynamics.

DIAGNOSIS AND TREATMENT

Thrombosis and Thromboembolism in Pregnancy

Venous thromboembolism (VTE), which includes deep venous thrombosis (DVT) and pulmonary embolism (PE), occurs in approximately 1 in 1,000 pregnancies (37). Women are five times more likely to develop VTE during pregnancy than during a nonpregnant state (38). Fatal PE, a possible sequela of VTE, remains a leading cause of maternal mortality in the Western world (39). The rate of PE in pregnancy is five times greater than that for nonpregnant women of the same age, and is about 1 in 100 deliveries; the risks are even higher in the puerperium.

Risk Factors and Predisposition to Venous Thrombosis

Compared to nonpregnant women, pregnant women have a 10-fold higher risk of a thrombotic episode. Risk factors for VTE other than pregnancy are noted in Table 77.4 (40,41).

TABLE 77.4 Risk Factors for Venous Thromboembolism (VTE) During Pregnancy

- Cesarean delivery
- History of prior VTE
- Family history of VTE
- Inherited or acquired thrombophilia
- Obesity
- Older maternal age
- Higher parity
- Prolonged immobilization

Pregnancy is associated with an increased clotting potential, decreased anticoagulant properties, and decreased fibrinolysis. Pregnancy is accompanied by a two- to threefold increased concentration of fibrinogen and a 20% to 1,000% increase in factors VII, VIII, IX, X, and XII, all of which peak at term (42). Levels of von Willebrand factor (vWF) increase up to 400% at term (42). Free protein S levels decline significantly (up to 55%) during pregnancy due to increased circulating levels of its carrier molecular, complement 4 binding protein (42). As a consequence, pregnancy is associated with an increase in resistance to activated protein C (42,43). Levels of plasminogen activation inhibitor-1 (PAI-1) increase three- to fourfold during pregnancy, while plasma PAI-2 values, negligible before pregnancy, reach concentrations of 160 mg/L at delivery (35).

Pregnancy is also associated with venous stasis in the lower extremities, due to compression of the inferior vena cava and pelvic veins by the enlarging uterus and hormone-mediated increases—in circulating levels of estrogen and local production of prostacyclin and nitric oxide—in deep vein capacitance secondary. Important hereditary risk factors that can increase DVT risk are antithrombin III deficiency, protein S and C deficiency, a G1691A mutation of the factor V gene (44), and a G20210A mutation of the factor II gene (45).

Diagnosis of Venous Thromboembolism during Pregnancy

Bates and Ginsberg have recently addressed the diagnosis of VTE during pregnancy in detail (49). In pregnant women presenting with lower extremity edema, back pain, and/or chest pain, the prevalence of VTE is less than in the general population because of the high frequency of these complaints related to pregnancy. D-dimer assays, which can be used to exclude VTE in healthy nonpregnant individuals, usually become positive late in pregnancy, which decreases the utility of this assay (47). Radiologic studies used to diagnose VTE in the nonpregnant woman have not been validated in pregnancy, and potential risks to the fetus, particularly in terms of ionizing radiation exposure, need to be considered (48). Compression ultrasonography (CUS) of the proximal veins has been recommended as the initial test for suspected DVT during pregnancy (46). When results are equivocal or an iliac vein thrombosis is suspected, magnetic resonance venography (MRV) can be used. MRV does not carry the radiation risk of contrast venography, and is becoming increasingly available in the United States.

The approach to the diagnosis of PE is similar in the pregnant and nonpregnant individual. Ventilation/perfusion (V/Q) scanning confers relatively low radiation exposure to the fetus, a risk less than that of missing a diagnosis of PE in the mother. However, when a V/Q study is indeterminate in a pregnant woman without demonstrated lower extremity thrombosis, it is usually followed by angiography. A brachial approach carries less radiation exposure to the fetus than spiral computed tomography (CT).

Prevention of Thrombosis during Pregnancy

The optimal anticoagulation regimen has not been established. Low–molecular-weight heparins (LMWHs) have become the anticoagulant of choice because, like unfractionated heparin (UFH), they do not cross the placenta, have better bioavailability, and carry less risk of osteoporosis and heparin-induced thrombocytopenia than UFH (49,50). A recent review of published data on the use of LMWHs in pregnancy supports their use as safe alternatives to UFH as anticoagulants during pregnancy (51). A more recent practice trend, especially in the United States, has been to switch patients to the longer-acting, subcutaneous UFH a few weeks before delivery to allow the use of activated partial thromboplastin time (aPTT) as a diagnostic test to assess anticoagulation pre- and postlabor (52).

Another means of providing VTE prophylaxis is with elastic compression stockings, which may be used for the entire pregnancy. Elastic stockings are appropriate for in-hospital patients at increased risk of VTE, and may be combined with the use of LMWH. Vena cava filter placement represents a potentially important, but poorly evaluated, therapeutic modality in the prevention of pulmonary emboli. Randomized trials to establish the appropriate role of vena cava filters in the treatment of venous thromboembolic disease are lacking (53).

Thrombolytic Therapy for Pulmonary Embolism

The indications for thrombolytic therapy for PE remain controversial. The incidence of intracranial hemorrhage may be as high as 2% to 3% with systemic thrombolytic therapy (54), although rates were lower in a recent trial (55). Fatality rates in patients with PE presenting in cardiogenic shock may be as high as 30% (54); thrombolytic therapy should be considered in this circumstance, although evidence for this subgroup is limited (56). Approximately 10% of symptomatic pulmonary emboli are rapidly fatal (57,58). The International Cooperative Pulmonary Embolism Registry, established to ascertain PE mortality, reported that 2% of patients were first diagnosed with PE at autopsy (59). Of patients diagnosed with PE before death, 5% to 10% have shock at presentation, which is associated with a mortality of 25% to 50% (59–61). Echocardiographic evidence of right ventricular dysfunction at presentation also has been suggested as an indication for thrombolytic therapy (55); however, a recent randomized trial failed to demonstrate a survival benefit with thrombolysis in patients with this finding (55), and mortality rates with conventional therapy are conflicting (54). At the time of this writing, routine thrombolysis cannot be justified in all patients.

Hemorrhage

Peripartum hemorrhage (PPH) remains a significant cause of maternal and fetal morbidity and mortality. In the United States and other industrialized nations, massive obstetric hemorrhage has generally ranked among the top three causes of maternal death despite modern improvements in obstetric practice and transfusion services.

PPH includes a wide range of pathophysiologic events. Antepartum bleeding occurs in nearly 4% of pregnant women (62). The causes of serious antepartum bleeding are abnormal implantation (placenta previa, placenta accreta), placental abruption, or uterine rupture. The latter is often caused by a dehiscence of a pre-existing uterine scar. The main reason for postpartum bleeding is uterine atony when myometrial contraction is inadequate. It is not surprising that uterine bleeding may be fatal when considering the massive amount of blood flow perfusing the uterus at term (up to 600 mL/min).

TABLE 77.5 Management of Severe Postpartum Hemorrhage

Conservative Management
General Measures
• Administration of supplemental oxygen
• Placement of adequate intravenous access lines
• Intravenous hydration
• Blood typing and cross-matching
• Placement of arterial line for repeated blood sampling
Pharmacologic Measures
• Oxytocin
• Methylergonovine
• 15-Methyl prostaglandin F_2-α
Surgical Management
Vascular Ligation
• Uterine artery
• Hypogastric artery
• Ovarian artery
Hysterectomy
• Supracervical
• Total

Patients with hemodynamic instability or massive hemorrhage require prompt resuscitative measures, including the administration of supplemental oxygen, placement of at least two large bore* intravenous lines, intravenous hydration with isotonic crystalloid, and blood typing and cross-matching for the replacement of packed red blood cells (Table 77.5). A delay in the correction of hypovolemia, diagnosis and treatment of impaired coagulation, or surgical control of bleeding are the avoidable factors in most maternal mortality cases caused by hemorrhage. If a transfusion must be given before full cross-matching is finished, type-specific uncross-matched blood can be used (63); alternatively, if there is no cross-matched blood, type O, Rh negative blood may be used in an emergency. Several recent studies suggest that fibrinogen is an important predictor of severe PPH (64,65). Standard coagulation screening tests such as the prothrombin time, partial thromboplastin time, and fibrinogen concentration have been supplemented or replaced by global coagulation tests such as thromboelastography (TEG) or rotational thrombelastography (ROTEM) (66).

There is virtually unanimous agreement from professional societies on the need of multidisciplinary hemorrhage protocols for management of both trauma and PPH (67–69). Such protocols ensure rapid availability of prepared blood products and a concomitant reduction in the time to transfusion and resuscitation. If the placenta has not been delivered when hemorrhage begins, it should be removed, if necessary by manual exploration of the uterine cavity. Placenta accreta is diagnosed if the placental cleavage plane is indistinct. In this situation, the patient should be prepared by the intensivist or the anesthesiologist for probable urgent hysterectomy. Firm bimanual

*Remember that resistance to flow is proportional to the fourth power of the radius of an orifice. Thus a shorter, larger catheter is preferred, whether peripheral or central. A 14-gauge 1.25-in peripheral IV or a 7-French (Fr) peripheral introducer may be used, as may a 9- to 12-Fr 15 cm (length) central introducer.

compression of the uterus (with one hand in the posterior vaginal fornix and the other on the abdomen) can limit hemorrhage until help can be obtained. Hemorrhage after placental delivery should prompt vigorous fundal massage while the patient is rapidly given 10 to 30 units of oxytocin in 1 L of intravenous crystalloid. Uterotonic agents such as oxytocin are routinely used in the management of uterine atony (70). This synthetic nonpeptide is a first-line therapeutic agent because of the paucity of side effects and the absence of contraindications. If the fundus does not become firm, uterine atony is the presumed (and most common) diagnosis. Although fundal massage continues, the patient may be then given 0.2 mg of methylergonovine (Methergine) intramuscularly, with this dose to be repeated at 2- to 4-hour intervals if necessary. Methylergonovine, an ergot alkaloid, is used as a second-line uterotonic agent in the setting of massive obstetric hemorrhage due to uterine atony. It may cause undesirable adverse effects such as cramping, headache, and dizziness. Coexisting severe hypertension is an absolute contraindication to its use.

Injectable prostaglandins may also be used when oxytocin fails. Both prostaglandin E and prostaglandin F2 stimulate myometrial contractions, and have been used intramuscularly or intravenously for refractory hemorrhage due to uterine atony. In particular, carboprost (Hemabate), 15-methyl prostaglandin F2-α, may be administered intramuscularly or intramyometrially in a dosage of 250 μg every 15 to 90 minutes, up to a maximum dosage of 2 mg. Sixty-eight percent of patients respond to a single carboprost injection; 86% respond to a second dose (71). Because oxygen desaturation has been reported with the use of carboprost (72), patients should be monitored by pulse oximetry.

The use of a hydrostatic balloon has been advocated as an alternative to uterine packing for controlling hemorrhage due to uterine atony (73). The inflated Rusch balloon can conform to the contour of the uterine cavity and provides an effective tamponade. Life-threatening hemorrhage can also be treated via arterial embolization by interventional radiology (74). Finally, in cases of continuing hemorrhage, a variety of surgical techniques can be used to avoid a hysterectomy, such as bilateral uterine artery ligation or internal iliac artery ligation (75).

Amniotic Fluid Embolism

Although the entry of amniotic fluid into the maternal circulation was already recognized as early as 1926 (76), Morgan published the first major review on the topic in 1979 (77). He reviewed 272 cases reported in the English language literature to that date. Although the true incidence of this disease entity is not known, most authors estimate it to be between 1 in 8,000 and 1 in 80,000 pregnancies.

Clinical Presentation

The classic presentation of amniotic fluid embolism is described as a sudden, profound, and unexpected cardiovascular collapse followed, in many cases, by irreversible shock and death (78). The only known predisposing factor to this life-threatening complication of pregnancy appears to be multiparity, seen with 88% of cases (77). In a smaller percentage of cases (51%), the presenting symptom is respiratory related. Hypotension is present in 27% of surviving cases, with coagulopathy comprising 12% and seizures 10%. Fetal bradycardia (17%) and hypotension (13%) are the next most common presenting features (Table 77.6).

TABLE 77.6 Clinical Presentation of Amniotic Fluid Embolism

- Acute cardiorespiratory collapse
- Acute respiratory distress
- Hypotension
- Hemorrhage/coagulopathy
- Seizures
- Fetal distress

Etiology and Pathophysiology

A common misperception in the literature is that the entry of amniotic fluid into maternal circulation is routine. This belief arises from the recognized presence of squamous cells in the pulmonary vasculature as a marker signaling the entry of amniotic fluid into the maternal circulation. Studies have now shown that squamous cells can appear in the pulmonary blood of heterogeneous populations of both pregnant and nonpregnant patients who have undergone pulmonary artery (PA) catheterization (79–83); the presence of these cells is probably the result of contamination by epithelial cells derived from the cutaneous entry site of the device (79,80). Because it is difficult to differentiate adult from fetal epithelial cells, the isolated finding of squamous cells in the pulmonary circulation of pregnant patients, with or without coexisting thrombotic PE, should be seen as a contaminant and not indicative of maternal exposure to amniotic fluid (84–86).

It has been hypothesized that amniotic fluid could act as a direct myocardial depressant. In vitro observation shows that amniotic fluid can cause a decrease in myometrial contractility (87). Other humoral factors, including proteolytic enzymes, histamine, serotonin, prostaglandins, and leukotrienes, may contribute to the hemodynamic changes and consumptive coagulopathy associated with amniotic fluid embolus, with a pathophysiologic mechanism similar to distributive or anaphylactic shock (87,88).

Diagnosis and Management

Amniotic fluid embolus syndrome is a diagnosis of exclusion (Table 77.7), and the treatment is essentially supportive. Hemodynamic instability should be treated with optimization of preload by rapid volume infusion. An α-receptor agonist, such as phenylephrine, may be useful to maintain adequate aortic perfusion pressure (90 mmHg systolic) while volume is infused. Coagulopathy associated with amniotic fluid embolus should be treated with aggressive administration of blood component therapy. If maternal cardiopulmonary resuscitation (CPR) must be initiated, and the fetus is sufficiently mature and is undelivered at the time of the cardiac arrest, a perimortem cesarean section should be immediately instituted (88–90).

TABLE 77.7 Differential Diagnosis of Amniotic Fluid Embolus

- Thrombosis
- Air embolus
- Septic shock
- Acute myocardial infarction
- Peripartum cardiomyopathy
- Anaphylaxis
- Aspiration
- Placental abruption
- Transfusion reaction
- Local anesthetic toxicity

Peripartum Cardiomyopathy

PPCM, a rare disease of unknown cause that strikes women in the childbearing years, is associated with a high mortality rate. PPCM is defined by the development of left ventricular or biventricular failure in the last month of pregnancy or within 5 months of delivery in the absence of other identifiable cause (91). In the United States, PPCM can affect women of various ethnic backgrounds at any age, but is more common in women 30 years of age or older. The strong association of PPCM with gestational hypertension and twin pregnancy should raise the level of suspicion for this condition in pregnant patients who develop symptoms of congestive heart failure (92).

Etiology and Diagnosis

A number of possible causes have been proposed for PPCM, including myocarditis (93), abnormal immune response to pregnancy, maladaptive response to the hemodynamic stresses of pregnancy (94), stress-activated cytokines, and prolonged tocolysis. A genetic tract is probable, as there have been reported few cases of familial PPCM. The diagnosis of PPCM requires the exclusion of more common causes of cardiomyopathy, and should be confirmed by standard echocardiographic assessment of the left ventricular systolic dysfunction, including depressed fractional shortening and ejection fraction documentation (95,96). PPCM shows many clinical characteristics of dilated cardiomyopathy (DCM) (97). Although the two conditions likely share part of their pathogenesis, such as predisposing mutations, increased oxidative stress, impaired microvasculature, and damaged sarcomere integrity, the exact underlying pathways might be differently altered in PPCM and DCM.

Treatment and Prognosis

Therapy should be initiated using standard clinical protocols for heart failure, although angiotensin-converting enzyme inhibitors should be avoided prenatally. Long-term clinical prognosis is usually defined within 6 months after delivery (98). In one study, approximately half of 27 women studied had persistent left ventricular dysfunction beyond 6 months, with a cardiac mortality rate of 85% over 5 years, as compared with the group in whom cardiac size returned to normal by the same time interval, with no mortality (91). The identification of the underlying cause of heart failure in the pregnant woman is another important factor that influences long-term survival (99). It is critical to note that the risk of recurrence with future pregnancies is particularly high in women with persistent left ventricular dysfunction prior to their subsequent pregnancy (100).

Hypertensive Disease of Pregnancy

Diagnosis

Preeclampsia complicates around 5% of pregnancies and, worldwide, hypertensive disorders of pregnancy are responsible for over 60,000 maternal deaths annually (101). Hypertensive disorders of pregnancy include chronic hypertension, preeclampsia/eclampsia, preeclampsia superimposed on chronic hypertension, and gestational hypertension (102). Preeclampsia is a pregnancy-specific, multisystem disorder that is characterized by the development of hypertension and proteinuria after 20 weeks of gestation (103). The disorder complicates approximately 5% to 7% of pregnancies (104), with an incidence of 23.6 cases per 1,000 deliveries in the United States (105). Chronic hypertension is defined by elevated blood pressure that predates the pregnancy, and is documented before 20 weeks of gestation or is present 12 weeks after delivery. Eclampsia, a severe complication of preeclampsia, is a new onset of seizures in women with preeclampsia.

TABLE 77.8 Physical Examination of the Severely Preeclamptic Patient

Funduscopic

- Arteriolar spasm (focal or diffuse)
- Retinal edema
- Retinal hemorrhages (superficial and flame shaped, or deep and punctate)
- Retinal exudates (hard or "cotton wool")
- Papilledema

Cardiovascular

- Heart failure (rales, elevated jugular venous pressure, S_3) or aortic dissection
- New or increased murmur of mitral regurgitation
- Bruits

Neurologic

- Hypertensive encephalopathy: Disorientation
- Depressed consciousness (Glasgow coma scale score <13)
- Focal deficits, generalized or focal seizures

Abdominal

- Palpation for liver tenderness or increase in size

Fetal

- Assessment of fetal well-being (fetal heart rate strip, biophysical profile)

Diagnostic criteria for preeclampsia include new onset of elevated blood pressure and proteinuria after 20 weeks of gestation. Severe preeclampsia is indicated by more substantial blood pressure elevations and a greater degree of proteinuria. Other features of severe preeclampsia include oliguria, cerebral or visual disturbances, and pulmonary edema or cyanosis (Table 77.8) (102,106).

Therapy

A major goal toward improving antenatal management of preeclampsia is to develop accurate prediction models that identify women at high risk of disease. Initial therapeutic goals during labor are focused on preventing seizures and controlling hypertension (106). Magnesium sulfate is the medication of choice to prevent eclamptic seizures for either preeclampsia or eclamptic seizures (107). Magnesium sulfate has been shown to be superior to phenytoin (Dilantin) and diazepam (Valium) for the treatment of eclamptic seizures, although magnesium does not prevent the progression of the disorder (108,109). Women with systolic blood pressures of 160 to 180 mmHg, or higher diastolic blood pressures of 105 to 110 mmHg should receive immediate antihypertensive therapy. The treatment goal is to lower systolic pressure to 140 to 150 mmHg and diastolic pressure to 90 to 100 mmHg. Hydralazine (Apresoline) and labetalol (Normodyne, Trandate) are the antihypertensive drugs most commonly used. Nifedipine (Procardia) and sodium nitroprusside (Nitropress) are potential alternatives, but their use is associated with significant adverse effects and risk of overdose. Similarly, labetalol should not be used in women with asthma or congestive heart failure. Angiotensin-converting enzyme inhibitors are also contraindicated in this group of patients as they may cause birth defects (110). In women with preeclampsia, blood pressure usually normalizes within a few hours after delivery but may remain elevated for 2 to 4 weeks (111).

Care and Management of the Hypertensive Parturient

Some patients with severe preeclampsia will require intensive care unit (ICU) admission for invasive monitoring and close supervision. Typical indications include (a) a severe increase in blood pressure, with diastolic blood pressures greater than 115 to 120 mmHg or a systolic blood pressure greater than 200 mmHg, refractory to initial antihypertensive therapy; (b) oliguria refractory to repeated fluid challenges; (c) eclamptic seizures; or (d) respiratory insufficiency. The initial physical examination should include a neurologic assessment, fundoscopic examination, auscultation of the heart and lungs, and palpation of the abdomen (see Table 77.8). If magnesium sulfate is given, it should be continued for 24 hours following delivery or for at least 24 hours after the last seizure. Regular assessment of urine output, maternal reflexes, respiratory rate, and oxygen saturation is paramount while magnesium is infused. A loading dose of 4 g should be given by infusion pump over 5 to 10 minutes, followed by a further infusion of 1 g/hr maintained for 24 hours after the last seizure. Gradual antihypertensive therapy can be accomplished with a 25% reduction of mean arterial pressure within minutes to 2 hours, to 160/100 mmHg (Table 77.9) (112).

Most patients satisfying the criteria for ICU admission should be monitored with central venous access and an arterial catheter. The use of invasive monitoring facilitates therapeutic goals and can clarify the suspected diagnosis. Although, occasionally, the use of a PA catheter facilitates cardiovascular management by monitoring cardiac output and systemic oxygen delivery while gradually reducing systemic vascular resistance and restoring preload, recent advances in noninvasive cardiac output measurement devices have been validated and may be used to monitor the effect of therapeutic interventions (113).

Fetal Monitoring in the Intensive Care Setting

Electronic fetal monitoring (EFM) is used in the management of labor and delivery in nearly three of four pregnancies in the United States. The apparent contradiction between the widespread use of EFM and expert recommendations to limit its routine use indicates that a reassessment of this practice is warranted (114). Even more difficult is the question of whether fetal monitoring is of any substantial use in the critically ill mother or the mother undergoing surgery. Continuous cardiotocography (CTG) during labor is associated with a reduction in neonatal seizures, but no significant differences in cerebral palsy, infant mortality, or other standard measures of neonatal well-being. On the contrary, this monitoring technique was associated with an increase in cesarean sections and instrument-aided vaginal births. When considering the use of EFM, the intensivist should consider the effects of many sedative, hypnotic, or analgesic drugs routinely used in the critical care setting on fetal heart rate variability (115–117). At this time, no systematic studies have been performed concerning the value of CTG during general anesthesia for nonobstetric surgery; it is assumed that uneventful sedation and analgesia provide adequate oxygenation and circulatory stability without having any influence on the fetus (115–117).

TABLE 77.9 Antihypertensive Therapy in Preeclampsia

Labetalol (Normodyne, Trandate)

IV bolus, 20–40 mg IV. May repeat in 10 min. Usual effective dose is 50–200 mg, or continuous infusion of 2 mg/min (this regimen avoids reflex tachycardia)

Nitroglycerin

Start at 10 μg/min (6 mL/hr). Titrate by 10–20 μg/min to 400 μg/min until desired effect

Hydralazine (Apresoline)

Initial dose: 5 mg IV. Maintenance: 5–10 mg IV q20–30min

Other antihypertensive options

Nicardipine, nitroprusside, phentolamine, fenoldopam, diazoxide

Pulmonary Edema in Pregnancy

Pulmonary edema is a rare, but well-documented, complication of tocolytic therapy in pregnant women (118–120). The incidence of pulmonary edema related to β-mimetic tocolysis is estimated to be 0.15% (121). The etiology of the pulmonary edema is unclear, but is likely multifactorial (122), and both cardiogenic and noncardiogenic mechanisms have been proposed. Possible cardiogenic causes include fluid overload, catecholamine-related myocardial necrosis, cardiac failure secondary to reduced diastolic compliance, and down-regulation of β-receptors (121–125).

Treatment

Immediate recognition and appropriate therapy can ameliorate the course of respiratory insufficiency in patients who develop pulmonary edema during tocolytic treatment. Therapy involves discontinuing the medication, ensuring adequate ventilation and oxygenation, correcting fluid imbalance and hypotension, and maintaining adequate cardiac output. Continuous assessment of the fetus' well-being is necessary.

Tocolytic Therapy

The development of pulmonary edema during the course of β-adrenergic agonist treatment for preterm labor is an indication for discontinuing the treatment and either switching to a different type of labor-inhibiting drug or terminating all efforts to prevent preterm delivery. Magnesium sulfate, calcium channel blockers, or oxytocin antagonists are the most frequently used alternatives.

Ventilatory Support

This topic is reviewed extensively in other sections of the book. Mechanical ventilation principles are not different for the pregnant woman, and are being standardized by evidence-based medicine and consensus conferences (125–127).

Fetal Considerations

Fetal well-being must be interpreted within the context of maternal respiratory failure. Minimally, intermitted fetal monitoring is indicated. If refractory maternal hypoxemia and acidosis presents, and results in fetal distress, cesarean delivery to salvage the fetus should be considered.

Cardiopulmonary Resuscitation in Pregnancy

The major causes of maternal cardiac arrest are due to trauma, cardiac conditions, and embolism. Other causes are sepsis, magnesium overdose, complications of eclampsia, or the result of an unanticipated difficult intubation. The general treatment of the pregnant woman in cardiac arrest is no different than any other patient, including drug dosages and defibrillation settings. Chest compressions and ventilations should be performed with the recommended sequence. Because a slight left tilt of the pregnant patient during CPR enhances venous return after 24 weeks of gestation, this position is recommended (90,128,129). Because of reduced pulmonary reserve, pregnant women do not tolerate hypoxia well. IV fluid should be running wide open on pressure bags, and blood products should be considered if hemorrhage is suspected. Once the age of the fetus is determined, a decision can be made whether to proceed with a perimortem cesarean section. The fetus can tolerate hypoxia longer than normal, but the decision to proceed with a cesarean delivery should be made within 4 minutes (126). In a recent retrospective review on CPR with perimortem cesarean section, authors found 35 reports with 20 potentially resuscitable causes, of which 13 women survived (127). Although this recent review fell short of proving that perimortem cesarean delivery within 4 minutes of maternal cardiac arrest improves maternal and neonatal outcomes, it provided additional support for this procedure. An extensive review of this topic is also available on the American Society of Anesthesiologists (ASA) website (130).

Anesthesiologists have recognized that the management of the airway in the obstetric patient may be especially challenging. According to the closed claims analysis of the ASA, the main mechanisms for airway problems are inadequate ventilation, esophageal intubation, and difficult intubation (131). If the anesthesiologist encounters an unanticipated difficult airway, alternative airway management attempts may include the laryngeal mask airway (LMA) or the Combitube. If cricothyrotomy becomes necessary, this maneuver should be initiated in a timely fashion to minimize the chance of maternal hypoxic brain damage.

SUMMARY

The obstetric patient poses exceptional challenges to the ICU team. Knowledge of the physiologic changes of pregnancy and specific pregnancy-related disorders is necessary for optimal management. The critically ill obstetric patient is unique in terms of medical management and often requires the input of several specialties. These patients require specialized nursing care and aggressive monitoring of both mother and fetus, and often include invasive monitoring of the mother. ICU diagnoses may include preeclampsia, including the HELLP (Hemolysis, Elevated Liver enzymes, Low Platelets) syndrome, pulmonary embolic disease, amniotic fluid embolism, status asthmaticus, respiratory infection, acute respiratory distress syndrome, and sepsis. Although there is little doubt that intensivists in an ICU can best treat these patients, the maternal–fetal medicine physician should be included in the treatment team. The management of mechanical ventilation is based on modern principles of avoiding lung injury, while hypercapnia may be tolerated even during the pregnancy. Care must include the consideration of pregnancy-induced physiologic changes, normal laboratory alterations, and continued fetal well-being if antepartum. Ultimately, the goal of this interdisciplinary approach is to ensure cohesive coordinated care for the pregnant woman.

Key Points

- The pregnant woman undergoes important physiologic changes: minute ventilation increases leading to a compensated respiratory alkalosis. The ERV is decreased and the time to desaturation with apnea decreases. Cardiac output increases up to 45%, which can be primarily attributed to an increase in stroke volume. The aorta and inferior vena cava can be significantly compressed by the gravid uterus in the supine position resulting in supine hypotension in up to 5% of term pregnant women.
- Compared to nonpregnant women, pregnant women have a 10-fold risk of a thrombotic episode and thromboembolic events are the leading causes of death in developed countries.
- Other important diagnoses leading to an intensive care admission are eclampsia, congenital or acquired cardiac diseases or pulmonary edema.

References

1. Lederman SA. Pregnancy weight gain and postpartum loss: avoiding obesity while optimizing the growth and development of the fetus. *J Am Med Womens Assoc.* 2001;56(2):53–58.
2. Abrams B, Altman SL, Pickett KE. Pregnancy weight gain: still controversial. *Am J Clin Nutr.* 2000;71(5 Suppl):1233S–1241S.
3. Feig DS, Naylor CD. Eating for two: are guidelines for weight gain during pregnancy too liberal? *Lancet.* 1998;351(9108):1054–1055.
4. Thorsdottir I, Torfadottir JE, Birgisdottir BE, et al. Weight gain in women of normal weight before pregnancy: complications in pregnancy or delivery and birth outcome. *Obstet Gynecol.* 2002;99(5 Pt 1):799–806.
5. Frederiksen MC. Physiologic changes in pregnancy and their effect on drug disposition. *Semin Perinatol.* 2001;25(3):120–123.
6. Tan EK, Tan EL. Alterations in physiology and anatomy during pregnancy. *Best Pract Res Clin Obstet Gynaecol.* 2013;27:791–802.
7. Hegewald MJ, Crapo RO. Respiratory physiology in pregnancy. *Clin Chest Med.* 2011;32:1–13, vii.
8. Cugell DW, Frank NR, Gaensler EA, et al. Pulmonary function in pregnancy. I. Serial observations in normal women. *Am Rev Tuberc.* 1953;67(5):568–597.
9. Garcia-Rio F, Pino-Garcia JM, Serrano S, et al. Comparison of helium dilution and plethysmographic lung volumes in pregnant women. *Eur Respir J.* 1997;10(10):2371–2375.
10. Gee JB, Packer BS, Millen JE, et al. Pulmonary mechanics during pregnancy. *J Clin Invest.* 1967;46(6):945–952.
11. Gazioglu K, Kaltreider NL, Rosen M, et al. Pulmonary function during pregnancy in normal women and in patients with cardiopulmonary disease. *Thorax.* 1970;25(4):445–450.
12. Baldwin GR, Moorthi DS, Whelton JA, et al. New lung functions and pregnancy. *Am J Obstet Gynecol.* 1977;127(3):235–239.
13. Alaily AB, Carrol KB. Pulmonary ventilation in pregnancy. *Br J Obstet Gynaecol.* 1978;85(7):518–524.
14. Blair E, Hickam JB. The effect of change in body position on lung volume and intrapulmonary gas mixing in normal subjects. *J Clin Invest.* 1955;34(3):383–389.
15. Marx GF, Murthy PK, Orkin LR. Static compliance before and after vaginal delivery. *Br J Anaesth.* 1970;42(12):1100–1104.
16. Contreras G, Gutierrez M, Beroiza T, et al. Ventilatory drive and respiratory muscle function in pregnancy. *Am Rev Respir Dis.* 1991;144(4):837–841.
17. Field SK, Bell SG, Cenaiko DF, et al. Relationship between inspiratory effort and breathlessness in pregnancy. *J Appl Physiol.* 1991;71(5):1897–1902.

18. Oddoy A, Merker G. Lung mechanics and blood gases in pregnant guinea pigs. *Acta Physiol Hung*. 1987;70(2–3):311–315.
19. Sherwood OD, Downing SJ, Guico-Lamm ML, et al. The physiological effects of relaxin during pregnancy: studies in rats and pigs. *Oxf Rev Reprod Biol*. 1993;15:143–189.
20. Goldsmith LT, Weiss G, Steinetz BG. Relaxin and its role in pregnancy. *Endocrinol Metab Clin North Am*. 1995;24(1):171–186.
21. Sheldon CP. Studies on the physiology of respiration in pregnancy: effects of barbiturates administered during labor. *J Clin Invest*. 1939;18(1):157–164.
22. Templeton A, Kelman GR. Maternal blood-gases, PAo2–Pao2, physiological shunt and VD/VT in normal pregnancy. *Br J Anaesth*. 1976;48(10): 1001–1004.
23. Sanghavi M, Rutherford JD: Cardiovascular physiology of pregnancy. *Circulation*. 2014;130:1003–1008.
24. Katz R, Karliner JS, Resnik R. Effects of a natural volume overload state (pregnancy) on left ventricular performance in normal human subjects. *Circulation*. 1978;58(3 Pt 1):434–441.
25. Chesley LC, Duffus GM. Posture and apparent plasma volume in late pregnancy. *J Obstet Gynaecol Br Commonw*. 1971;78(5):406–412.
26. Pedersen H, Finster M. Anesthetic risk in the pregnant surgical patient. *Anesthesiology*. 1979;51:439–451.
27. Metcalfe J, Ueland K. Maternal cardiovascular adjustments to pregnancy. *Prog Cardiovasc Dis*. 1974;16(4):363–374.
28. Cheung KL, Lafayette RA: Renal physiology of pregnancy. *Adv Chronic Kidney Dis*. 2013;20:209–214.
29. Kerr MG, Scott DB, Samuel E. Studies of the inferior vena cava in late pregnancy. *BMJ*. 1964;1(5382):532–533.
30. Abitbol MM. Aortic compression by pregnant uterus. *N Y State J Med*. 1976;76(9):1470–1475.
31. Bieniarz J, Branda LA, Maqueda E, et al. Aortocaval compression by the uterus in late pregnancy. 3. Unreliability of the sphygmomanometric method in estimating uterine artery pressure. *Am J Obstet Gynecol*. 1968;102(8):1106–1115.
32. Clark SL, Cotton DB, Lee W, et al. Central hemodynamic assessment of normal term pregnancy. *Am J Obstet Gynecol*. 1989;161(6 Pt 1):1439–1442.
33. Ueland K, Novy MJ, Peterson EN, et al. Maternal cardiovascular dynamics. IV. The influence of gestational age on the maternal cardiovascular response to posture and exercise. *Am J Obstet Gynecol*. 1969;104(6):856–864.
34. Newman B, Derrington C, Dore C. Cardiac output and the recumbent position in late pregnancy. *Anaesthesia*. 1983;38(4):332–335.
35. Milsom I, Forssman L. Factors influencing aortocaval compression in late pregnancy. *Am J Obstet Gynecol*. 1984;148(6):764–771.
36. Mendonca C, Griffiths J, Ateleanu B, et al. Hypotension following combined spinal-epidural anaesthesia for Caesarean section: left lateral position vs. tilted supine position. *Anaesthesia*. 2003;58(5):428–431.
37. Phillips OP. Venous thromboembolism in the pregnant woman. *J Reprod Med*. 2003;48(11 Suppl):921–929.
38. Prevention of venous thrombosis and pulmonary embolism. NIH Consensus Development. *JAMA*. 1986;256(6):744–749.
39. Confidential Enquiry into Maternal and Child Health. Saving Mothers' Lives 2000–2002: reviewing maternal deaths to make motherhood safer: 2006–2008. *BJOG*. 2011;118:S1.
40. Marshall AL. Diagnosis, treatment, and prevention of venous thromboembolism in pregnancy. *Postgrad Med*. 2014;126:25–34.
41. Greer IA. Thrombosis in pregnancy: updates in diagnosis and management. *Hematology Am Soc Hematol Educ Program*. 2012;2012:203–207.
42. Bremme KA. Haemostatic changes in pregnancy. *Best Pract Res Clin Haematol*. 2003;16(2):153–168.
43. Ku DH, Arkel YS, Paidas MP, et al. Circulating levels of inflammatory cytokines (IL-1 beta and TNF-alpha), resistance to activated protein C, thrombin and fibrin generation in uncomplicated pregnancies. *Thromb Haemost*. 2003;90(6):1074–1079.
44. Bertina RM, Koeleman BP, Koster T, et al. Mutation in blood coagulation factor V associated with resistance to activated protein C. *Nature*. 1994;369(6475):64–67.
45. Poort SR, Rosendaal FR, Reitsma PH, et al. A common genetic variation in the 3-untranslated region of the prothrombin gene is associated with elevated plasma prothrombin levels and an increase in venous thrombosis. *Blood*. 1996;88(10):3698–3703.
46. Hart RG, Halperin JL. Atrial fibrillation and thromboembolism: a decade of progress in stroke prevention. *Ann Intern Med*. 1999;131(9):688–695.
47. Albers GW, Dalen JE, Laupacis A, et al. Antithrombotic therapy in atrial fibrillation. *Chest*. 2001;119(1 Suppl):194S–206S.
48. Mok CK, Boey J, Wang R, et al. Warfarin versus dipyridamole-aspirin and pentoxifylline-aspirin for the prevention of prosthetic heart valve thromboembolism: a prospective randomized clinical trial. *Circulation*. 1985;72(5):1059–1063.
49. Bates SM, Ginsberg JS. How we manage venous thromboembolism during pregnancy. *Blood*. 2002;100(10):3470–3478.
50. Gandara E, Carrier M, Rodger MA: Intermediate doses of low-molecular-weight heparin for the long-term treatment of pregnancy thromboembolism. A systematic review. *Thromb Haemost*. 2014;111:559–561.
51. Sanson BJ, Lensing AW, Prins MH, et al. Safety of low-molecular-weight heparin in pregnancy: a systematic review. *Thromb Haemost*. 1999;81(5): 668–672.
52. Anderson DR, Ginsberg JS, Burrows R, et al. Subcutaneous heparin therapy during pregnancy: a need for concern at the time of delivery. *Thromb Haemost*. 1991;65(3):248–250.
53. Streiff MB. Vena caval filters: a comprehensive review. *Blood*. 2000; 95(12):3669–3677.
54. Dalen JE. The uncertain role of thrombolytic therapy in the treatment of pulmonary embolism. *Arch Intern Med*. 2002;162(22):2521–2523.
55. Konstantinides S, Geibel A, Heusel G, et al. Heparin plus alteplase compared with heparin alone in patients with submassive pulmonary embolism. *N Engl J Med*. 2002;347(15):1143–1150.
56. Jerjes-Sanchez C, Ramirez-Rivera A, de Lourdes Garcia M, et al. Streptokinase and heparin versus heparin alone in massive pulmonary embolism: a randomized controlled trial. *J Thromb Thrombolysis*. 1995;2(3):227–229.
57. Stein PD, Henry JW. Prevalence of acute pulmonary embolism among patients in a general hospital and at autopsy. *Chest*. 1995;108(4):978–981.
58. Bell WR, Simon TL. Current status of pulmonary thromboembolic disease: pathophysiology, diagnosis, prevention, and treatment. *Am Heart J*. 1982;103(2):239–262.
59. Goldhaber SZ, Visani L, De Rosa M. Acute pulmonary embolism: clinical outcomes in the International Cooperative Pulmonary Embolism Registry (ICOPER). *Lancet*. 1999;353(9162):1386–1389.
60. Grifoni S, Olivotto I, Cecchini P, et al. Short-term clinical outcome of patients with acute pulmonary embolism, normal blood pressure, and echocardiographic right ventricular dysfunction. *Circulation*. 2000;101(24):2817–2822.
61. Goldhaber SZ, Haire WD, Feldstein ML, et al. Alteplase versus heparin in acute pulmonary embolism: randomised trial assessing right-ventricular function and pulmonary perfusion. *Lancet*. 1993;341(8844):507–511.
62. Fong J, Gadalla F, Pierri MK, et al. Are Doppler-detected venous emboli during cesarean section air emboli? *Anesth Analg*. 1990;71(3):254–257.
63. Gervin AS, Fischer RP. Resuscitation of trauma patients with type-specific uncrossmatched blood. *J Trauma*. 1984;24(4):327–331.
64. Butwick AJ. Postpartum hemorrhage and low fibrinogen levels: the past, present and future. *Int J Obstet Anesth*. 2013;22:87–91.
65. Levy JH, Welsby I, Goodnough LT. Fibrinogen as a therapeutic target for bleeding: a review of critical levels and replacement therapy. *Transfusion*. 2014;54:1389–1405.
66. Afshari A, Wikkelso A, Brok J, et al. Thrombelastography (TEG) or thromboelastometry (ROTEM) to monitor haemotherapy versus usual care in patients with massive transfusion. *Cochrane Database Syst Rev*. 2011;3:CD007871.
67. Ducloy-Bouthors AS, Susen S, Wong CA, et al. Medical advances in the treatment of postpartum hemorrhage. *Anesth Analg*. 2014;119:1140–1147.
68. Kacmar RM, Mhyre JM, Scavone BM, et al. The use of postpartum hemorrhage protocols in United States academic obstetric anesthesia units. *Anesth Analg*. 2014;119:906–910.
69. Mhyre JM, D'Oria R, Hameed AB, et al. The maternal early warning criteria: a proposal from the national partnership for maternal safety. *Obstet Gynecol*. 2014;124:782–786.
70. Dildy GA III. Postpartum hemorrhage: new management options. *Clin Obstet Gynecol*. 2002;45(2):330–344.
71. Hayashi RH, Castillo MS, Noah ML. Management of severe postpartum hemorrhage with a prostaglandin F2 alpha analogue. *Obstet Gynecol*. 1984;63(6):806–808.
72. Hankins GD, Berryman GK, Scott RT Jr, et al. Maternal arterial desaturation with 15-methyl prostaglandin F2 alpha for uterine atony. *Obstet Gynecol*. 1988;72(3 Pt 1):367–370.
73. Johanson R, Kumar M, Obhrai M, et al. Management of massive postpartum haemorrhage: use of a hydrostatic balloon catheter to avoid laparotomy. *BJOG*. 2001;108(4):420–422.
74. Pelage JP, Le Dref O, Mateo J, et al. Life-threatening primary postpartum hemorrhage: treatment with emergency selective arterial embolization. *Radiology*. 1998;208(2):359–362.
75. B-Lynch C, Coker A, Lawal AH, et al. The B-Lynch surgical technique for the control of massive postpartum haemorrhage: an alternative to hysterectomy? Five cases reported. *Br J Obstet Gynaecol*. 1997;104(3):372–375.

76. Masson RG. Amniotic fluid embolism. *Clin Chest Med.* 1992;13(4):657–665.
77. Morgan M. Amniotic fluid embolism. *Anaesthesia.* 1979;34(1):20–32.
78. Steiner PE, Lushbaugh CC. Landmark article, Oct. 1941. Maternal pulmonary embolism by amniotic fluid as a cause of obstetric shock and unexpected deaths in obstetrics. *JAMA.* 1986;255(16):2187–2203.
79. Clark SL, Pavlova Z, Greenspoon J, et al. Squamous cells in the maternal pulmonary circulation. *Am J Obstet Gynecol.* 1986;154(1):104–106.
80. Giampaolo C, Schneider V, Kowalski BH, et al. The cytologic diagnosis of amniotic fluid embolism: a critical reappraisal. *Diagn Cytopathol.* 1987;3(2):126–128.
81. Lee W, Ginsburg KA, Cotton DB, et al. Squamous and trophoblastic cells in the maternal pulmonary circulation identified by invasive hemodynamic monitoring during the peripartum period. *Am J Obstet Gynecol.* 1986;155(5):999–1001.
82. Masson RG, Ruggieri J. Pulmonary microvascular cytology: a new diagnostic application of the pulmonary artery catheter. *Chest.* 1985;88(6):908–914.
83. Lee KR, Catalano PM, Ortiz-Giroux S. Cytologic diagnosis of amniotic fluid embolism. Report of a case with a unique cytologic feature and emphasis on the difficulty of eliminating squamous contamination. *Acta Cytol.* 1986;30(2):177–182.
84. Dib N, Bajwa T. Amniotic fluid embolism causing severe left ventricular dysfunction and death: case report and review of the literature. *Cathet Cardiovasc Diagn.* 1996;39(2):177–180.
85. Clark SL, Cotton DB, Gonik B, et al. Central hemodynamic alterations in amniotic fluid embolism. *Am J Obstet Gynecol.* 1988;158(5):1124–1126.
86. Vanmaele L, Noppen M, Vincken W, et al. Transient left heart failure in amniotic fluid embolism. *Intensive Care Med.* 1990;16(4):269–271.
87. Clark SL. New concepts of amniotic fluid embolism: a review. *Obstet Gynecol Surv.* 1990;45(6):360–368.
88. Dudney TM, Elliott CG. Pulmonary embolism from amniotic fluid, fat, and air. *Prog Cardiovasc Dis.* 1994;36(6):447–474.
89. Clark SL, Hankins GD, Dudley DA, et al. Amniotic fluid embolism: analysis of the national registry. *Am J Obstet Gynecol.* 1995;172(4 Pt 1):1158–1167.
90. Drukker L, Hants Y, Sharon E, et al. Perimortem cesarean section for maternal and fetal salvage: concise review and protocol. *Acta Obstet Gynecol Scand.* 2014;93:965–972.
91. Demakis JG, Rahimtoola SH. Peripartum cardiomyopathy. *Circulation.* 1971;44(5):964–968.
92. Elkayam U, Akhter MW, Singh H, et al. Pregnancy-associated cardiomyopathy: clinical characteristics and a comparison between early and late presentation. *Circulation.* 2005;111(16):2050–2055.
93. Midei MG, DeMent SH, Feldman AM, et al. Peripartum myocarditis and cardiomyopathy. *Circulation.* 1990;81(3):922–928.
94. Mone SM, Sanders SP, Colan SD. Control mechanisms for physiological hypertrophy of pregnancy. *Circulation.* 1996;94(4):667–672.
95. Hilfiker-Kleiner D, Haghikia A, Nonhoff J, Bauersachs J. Peripartum cardiomyopathy: current management and future perspectives. *Eur Heart J.* 2015;36:1090–1097.
96. Hilfiker-Kleiner D, Sliwa K. Pathophysiology and epidemiology of peripartum cardiomyopathy. *Nat Rev Cardiol.* 2014;11:364–370.
97. Bollen IA, Van Deel ED, Kuster DW, Van Der Velden J. Peripartum cardiomyopathy and dilated cardiomyopathy: different at heart. *Front Physiol.* 2014;5:531.
98. Fett JD, Markham DW. Discoveries in peripartum cardiomyopathy. *Trends Cardiovasc Med.* 2014;25(5):401–406.
99. Felker GM, Thompson RE, Hare JM, et al. Underlying causes and long-term survival in patients with initially unexplained cardiomyopathy. *N Engl J Med.* 2000;342(15):1077–1084.
100. Elkayam U. Risk of subsequent pregnancy in women with a history of peripartum cardiomyopathy. *J Am Coll Cardiol.* 2014;64:1629–1636.
101. Duhig KE, Shennan AH. Recent advances in the diagnosis and management of pre-eclampsia. *F1000Prime Rep.* 2015;7:24.
102. Report of the National High Blood Pressure Education Program Working Group on High Blood Pressure in Pregnancy. *Am J Obstet Gynecol.* 2000;183(1):S1–S22.
103. Lo JO, Mission JF, Caughey AB. Hypertensive disease of pregnancy and maternal mortality. *Curr Opin Obstet Gynecol.* 2013;25:124–132.
104. Witlin AG, Sibai BM. Magnesium sulfate therapy in preeclampsia and eclampsia. *Obstet Gynecol.* 1998;92(5):883–889.
105. Samadi AR, Mayberry RM, Zaidi AA, et al. Maternal hypertension and associated pregnancy complications among African-American and other women in the United States. *Obstet Gynecol.* 1996;87(4):557–563.
106. ACOG practice bulletin. Diagnosis and management of preeclampsia and eclampsia. Number 33, January 2002. *Obstet Gynecol.* 2002;99(1):159–167.
107. Altman D, Carroli G, Duley L, et al. Do women with pre-eclampsia, and their babies, benefit from magnesium sulphate? The Magpie Trial: a randomised placebo-controlled trial. *Lancet.* 2002;359(9321):1877–1890.
108. Scott JR. Magnesium sulfate for mild preeclampsia. *Obstet Gynecol.* 2003;101(2):213.
109. Sibai BM. Diagnosis and management of gestational hypertension and preeclampsia. *Obstet Gynecol.* 2003;102(1):181–192.
110. Cooper WO, Hernandez-Diaz S, Arbogast PG, et al. Major congenital malformations after first-trimester exposure to ACE inhibitors. *N Engl J Med.* 2006;354 (23):2443–2451.
111. Ferrazzani S, De Carolis S, Pomini F, et al. The duration of hypertension in the puerperium of preeclamptic women: relationship with renal impairment and week of delivery. *Am J Obstet Gynecol.* 1994;171(2):506–512.
112. Chobanian AV, Bakris GL, Black HR, et al. Seventh report of the Joint National Committee on Prevention, Detection, Evaluation, and Treatment of High Blood Pressure. *Hypertension.* 2003;42(6):1206–1252.
113. Marik PE. Noninvasive cardiac output monitors: a state-of the-art review. *J Cardiothorac Vasc Anesth.* 2013;27:121–134.
114. Alfirevic Z, Devane D, Gyte GM. Continuous cardiotocography (CTG) as a form of electronic fetal monitoring (EFM) for fetal assessment during labour. *Cochrane Database Syst Rev.* 2006;3:CD006066.
115. Liu PL, Warren TM, Ostheimer GW, et al. Foetal monitoring in parturients undergoing surgery unrelated to pregnancy. *Can Anaesth Soc J.* 1985;32(5):525–532.
116. Katz JD, Hook R, Barash PG. Fetal heart rate monitoring in pregnant patients undergoing surgery. *Am J Obstet Gynecol.* 1976;125(2):267–269.
117. Caforio L, Draisci G, Ciampelli M, et al. Rectal cancer in pregnancy: a new management based on blended anesthesia and monitoring of fetal well being. *Eur J Obstet Gynecol Reprod Biol.* 2000;88(1):71–74.
118. Karaman S, Ozcan O, Akercan F, et al. Pulmonary edema after ritodrine therapy during pregnancy and subsequent cesarean section with epidural anesthesia. *Clin Exp Obstet Gynecol.* 2004;31(1):67–69.
119. Kayacan N, Dosemeci L, Arici G, et al. Pulmonary edema due to ritodrine. *Int J Clin Pharmacol Ther.* 2004;42(6):350–351.
120. Paternoster DM, Manganelli F, Fantinato S, et al. Maternal complications from tocolytic treatment with ritodrine: three cases of pulmonary edema. *Minerva Ginecol.* 2004;56(5):491–492.
121. Gyetvai K, Hannah ME, Hodnett ED, et al. Tocolytics for preterm labor: a systematic review. *Obstet Gynecol.* 1999;94(5 Pt 2):869–877.
122. Lamont RF. The pathophysiology of pulmonary oedema with the use of beta-agonists. *BJOG.* 2000;107(4):439–444.
123. Kleinman G, Nuwayhid B, Rudelstorfer R, et al. Circulatory and renal effects of beta-adrenergic-receptor stimulation in pregnant sheep. *Am J Obstet Gynecol.* 1984;149(8):865–874.
124. Senzaki H, Fetics B, Chen CH, et al. Comparison of ventricular pressure relaxation assessments in human heart failure: quantitative influence on load and drug sensitivity analysis. *J Am Coll Cardiol.* 1999;34(5):1529–1536.
125. Tatara T, Morisaki H, Shimada M, et al. Pulmonary edema after long-term beta-adrenergic therapy and cesarean section. *Anesth Analg.* 1995;81(2):417–418.
126. Katz VL, Dotters DJ, Droegemueller W. Perimortem cesarean delivery. *Obstet Gynecol.* 1986;68(4):571–576.
127. Atta E, Gardner M. Cardiopulmonary resuscitation in pregnancy. *Obstet Gynecol Clin North Am.* 2007;34(3):585–597.
128. Jeejeebhoy F, Windrim R. Management of cardiac arrest in pregnancy. *Best Pract Res Clin Obstet Gynaecol.* 2014;28:607–618.
129. McGregor AJ, Barron R, Rosene-Montella K. The pregnant heart: cardiac emergencies during pregnancy. *Am J Emerg Med.* 2015;33(4):573–579.
130. American Society of Anesthesiologists Task Force on Obstetric Anesthesia. Practice Guidelines for Obstetrical Anesthesia. An Updated Report by the American Society of Anesthesiologists Task Force on Obstetrical Anesthesia. *Anesthesiology.* 2007;106:843–863.
131. Cheney FW. The American Society of Anesthesiologists Closed Claims Project: what have we learned, how has it affected practice, and how will it affect practice in the future? *Anesthesiology.* 1999;91(2):552–556.

CHAPTER

78

Cardiac Disease and Hypertensive Disorders in Pregnancy

KENNETH K. CHEN, NIHARIKA MEHTA, ERICA J. HARDY, SRILAKSHMI MITTA, and RAYMOND O. POWRIE

HYPERTENSIVE DISORDERS OF PREGNANCY

Hypertension during pregnancy has been classified by the American College of Obstetricians and Gynecologists into four distinct categories: (a) preeclampsia and eclampsia, (b) chronic hypertension (hypertension that was present before pregnancy), (c) chronic hypertension with superimposed preeclampsia or eclampsia, and (d) gestational hypertension (1). Most chronic hypertensive pregnant patients have essential hypertension, which has no appreciable effect during pregnancy unless end-organ damage is present. Chronic hypertension is seen in a critical care unit typically only when a patient has a hypertensive urgency/emergency unrelated to pregnancy, or if the patient has a secondary cause of hypertension that represents a short-term risk to maternal health. Similarly, latent or transient hypertension is also relatively benign, occurring in the last trimester or the immediate postpartum period, with a return of normotension by the first 3 weeks after delivery. It is preeclampsia or eclampsia—whether occurring de novo or superimposed on pre-existing hypertension—that is most likely to require critical care support, and therefore will be the focus of this section.

Preeclampsia and Eclampsia

Preeclampsia is a multisystem disorder unique to human pregnancies. Its pathophysiology is not well understood, and its cause is unknown. It is associated with an increased risk of fetal loss, intrauterine growth restriction, and preterm birth, and remains a leading cause of maternal death worldwide. Eclampsia refers to preeclampsia that is complicated by seizures, but it is our present understanding that the underlying condition is the same (2).

Although much of the care of the preeclamptic patient will fall into the domain of the obstetrician, familiarity with the manifestations and management of preeclampsia is important for any critical care physician. Primary obstetric disorders—of which, preeclampsia and its complications constitute the majority—account for 50% to 80% of ICU admissions during pregnancy and the puerperium in all parts of the world (3).

Risk Factors for Preeclampsia

Five percent to 8% of all pregnancies are complicated by preeclampsia, typically occurring in the final weeks prior to the due date and very rare prior to 20 weeks of gestation. The risk factors for preeclampsia are listed in Table 78.1. The diverse nature of the risk factors suggests that preeclampsia may be a common end point for a variety of processes related to placental dysfunction (4,5).

Etiology and Pathophysiology

Preeclampsia is believed to be an abnormal vascular response to the formation of the placenta. It is associated with endothelial cell dysfunction, activation of the coagulation system, enhanced platelet aggregation, and increased systemic vascular resistance. The maternal effects of these changes are manifest in the cardiovascular system, kidneys, lungs, and brain. Pathologic examination of affected maternal organs reveals areas of edema, endothelial swelling, microinfarctions, and microhemorrhages. The cardiovascular features of preeclampsia include decreased plasma volume—despite an increase in total-body water and salt retention—and colloid osmotic pressure, largely due to a drop in serum albumin (6). Generalized arteriolar vasospasm accounts for the hypertension in preeclampsia, which is often very labile.

Our understanding of the etiology of preeclampsia is evolving. The condition is felt to begin early in pregnancy, long before it becomes clinically apparent as the maternal syndrome. Three distinct, sequential phases occur in its evolution (4,7,8). The first phase is incomplete invasion of the trophoblast into the endometrium, perhaps due to a maladaptive immune response in the mother, followed by inadequate "placentation"—formation of the placenta—which leads to the second phase in which decreases in the levels of angiogenic growth factors and increased placental debris is found in the maternal circulation. This stage of the development of preeclampsia is not associated with any clinical symptoms or signs, however, decreases in placental growth factor (PlGF) and elevations of soluble FMS-like tyrosine kinase 1 (sFlt-1) and endoglin can be detected (9–11); these changes then incite a maternal inflammatory response. The third phase is the response of the maternal endothelium and cardiovascular system to these stressors, which is modulated by the woman's own level of metabolic and cardiovascular health and then leads to the clinical presentation of the maternal preeclamptic syndrome. Although this response is manifested predominantly as hypertension and proteinuria, less common manifestations of cardiac, pulmonary, hematologic, neurologic, and hepatic complications can lead to admission in the intensive care unit.

Clinical Features

Clinically preeclampsia can have a highly variable presentation. It can manifest as a fetal syndrome (abnormal fetal oxygenation, reduced amniotic fluid, and fetal growth restriction), a maternal syndrome (proteinuria and hypertension with or without other multisystem abnormalities), or a combination of both. In most patients, both the fetal and maternal syndrome will be apparent, however one or the other will often predominate in an individual case. This chapter will focus on the maternal manifestations.

TABLE 78.1 Risk Factors for Preeclampsia

Maternal
- First pregnancy
- New partners
- Age younger than 18 or older than 35 yr
- Chronic hypertension
- Prior history of preeclampsia
- Family history of preeclampsia
- Pregestational diabetes
- Obesity
- Thrombophilias
- Antiphospholipid antibody syndrome
- Systemic lupus erythematosus
- Renal disease

Fetal
- Multiple gestations
- Molar pregnancies (can cause preeclampsia at <20 wk gestation)
- Fetal hydrops
- Triploidy

Preeclampsia is defined by the maternal manifestations of hypertension and proteinuria occurring in the second half of pregnancy. The presentation and diagnostic features of preeclampsia are reviewed in Tables 78.2 and 78.3 (12–17). Although hypertension above 140/90 mmHg and proteinuria over 300 mg/24 hr are required for the diagnosis of preeclampsia, some cases may present initially without these features, or may present—as in the case of postpartum eclampsia—after some of these features have already resolved.

Preeclampsia is defined to be severe by the presence of one or more of the following (1):

- Hypertension: systolic above 160 mmHg or diastolic above 110 mmHg on two occasions at least 4 hours apart while the patient is on bed rest
- Thrombocytopenia (platelet count <100,000 cells/µL)
- Impaired liver function (elevated blood levels of liver transaminases to twice the normal concentration)
- Severe persistent right upper quadrant or epigastric pain unresponsive to medication and not accounted for by alternative diagnoses
- New development of renal insufficiency (elevated serum creatinine >1.1 mg/dL, or doubling of serum creatinine in the absence of other renal disease)
- Pulmonary edema
- New-onset cerebral or visual disturbances

Eclampsia results when seizures occur that are not related to other underlying disorders. These features describe a group of patients with an increased risk of fetal and maternal morbidity for whom delivery should be strongly considered. Preeclamptic patients who lack any of the features of severe preeclampsia may have to be observed without moving toward delivery if the fetus is significantly premature and the mother remains under close observation; however, such patients are rarely seen in intensive care settings.

Life-threatening maternal complications of preeclampsia such as severe hypertension, seizure, cerebral hemorrhage, pulmonary edema, disseminated intravascular coagulation (DIC), acute renal failure (ARF), and hepatic failure and/or

TABLE 78.2 Clinical Features of Preeclampsia

Feature	Description
Symptoms	
Headache	The headache that characterizes preeclampsia is typically frontal in location, throbbing in character, persistent, and not responsive to mild analgesia.
Visual phenomena	The visual disturbances that characterize preeclampsia are presumed to be due to cerebral vasospasm and are typically scintillations or scotomas. Longer-lasting visual field deficits and rarely transient blindness can result from edema, posterior reversible encephalopathic syndrome, and even infarction in the occipital region of the brain.
	Serous retinal detachments can also occur in preeclampsia and are related to retinal edema. Magnesium, which is commonly used to prevent seizures in preeclamptic women, can cause mild visual blurring or double vision, but should not cause scotomas, scintillations, or visual loss.
Epigastric pain	The epigastric or right upper quadrant discomfort that occurs in preeclampsia can be marked, and may be out of proportion to the degree of liver enzyme abnormalities. It is believed to be caused by edema in the liver that stretches the hepatic capsule. In rare cases, it may be caused by hepatic infarction or rupture.
Edema	Edema is present in more than 30% of normal pregnancies, and is thus not a reliable sign of preeclampsia. Rapid weight gain (more than 1 lb per week in the third trimester) or edema in the hands or facial area (nondependent edema) is best viewed as a sign that should lead the clinician to evaluate the patient for other, more specific, evidence of preeclampsia.
Signs	
Hypertension >140/90 mmHg	Hypertension in preeclampsia is due to vasospasm and can be very labile. Ideally, blood pressure should be measured in the sitting position with a manual cuff, with the brachial artery at the level of the heart. There is a literature suggesting that some automated blood pressure cuffs may be less reliable in preeclampsia and that either a manual cuff or arterial line should be used to verify blood pressure in preeclamptic patients with severe hypertension (13).
Epigastric or right upper quadrant tenderness	Abdominal pain in preeclampsia is attributed to hepatic capsular stretching from edema. The degree of tenderness is often out of proportion to the degree of elevation of liver function tests. Epigastric tenderness is suggestive of severe preeclampsia, and is associated with an increased risk of both maternal and fetal adverse outcomes.
Hyperreflexia	Clonus is an important sign of preeclampsia but should be distinguished from the very brisk reflexes commonly seen in normal pregnancies.
Retinal artery vasospasm on funduscopy	Retinal vasospasm, retinal edema (in the form of soft exudates), hemorrhage, and exudative retinal detachment are uncommon findings in preeclampsia. Papilledema is rare.

TABLE 78.3 Laboratory Features of Preeclampsia

Feature	Description
Complete blood count with elevated hemoglobin and/or thrombocytopenia	The "elevation of hemoglobin" seen with preeclampsia (which may manifest as a hemoglobin of 12 g/dL at 37 wk, when it would be expected to be closer to 10 g/dL because of the physiologic dilutional anemia that is seen in pregnancy) is due to hemoconcentration. Much less commonly, hemoglobin may fall with preeclampsia due to a microangiopathic hemolytic anemia.
	Platelet consumption in preeclampsia can cause an increased mean platelet volume and thrombocytopenia, and is an important manifestation of severe disease (14).
	In severe cases of preeclampsia or HELLP (a subset of preeclampsia), schistocytes (fragmented red cells) may be seen on peripheral smear and can lead to a mild drop in hemoglobin. Brisk hemolysis is rare, however, and should lead to the consideration of HUS or TTP.
Elevated serum creatinine	Typically serum creatinine is <0.8 mg/dL (70 μmol/L) in pregnancy and values greater than this are considered abnormal.
	Renal function impairment is caused by decreased renal blood flow and glomerular filtration rate secondary to swelling of intracapillary glomerular cells, fibrin deposition along the basement membranes, and afferent arteriolar spasm.
Elevated serum uric acid	Typically, serum uric acid is <5.0 mg/dL (280 μmol/L) in pregnancy. Uric acid is the most sensitive test for identifying preeclampsia but it is still only elevated in approximately 80% of cases of preeclampsia. Uric acid rises in this setting due to impaired excretion of uric acid in the renal tubules that is caused by preeclampsia-related changes in the renal microcirculation (14). Although an important sign of preeclampsia, the elevated uric acid level is distinct from an elevated creatinine, AST, or decreased platelet count in that the uric acid level is not generally believed to have any direct clinical consequences and should not be used as a marker of disease severity.
Elevated liver enzymes	Mild elevations of AST, typically <100 U/L, suggest hepatic involvement. Greater levels may be due to severe preeclampsia, HELLP syndrome, hepatic infarction, hepatic rupture, or superimposed acute fatty liver of pregnancy.
Proteinuria	Proteinuria is an essential diagnostic feature of preeclampsia. Urine dipsticks are routinely used to screen for proteinuria in asymptomatic patients. However, dipsticks lack the needed sensitivity and specificity to make them a reliable test for proteinuria in patients in whom the diagnosis of preeclampsia is suspected because of the presence of other features of this disease. When preeclampsia is suspected, a 24-hour urine test for proteinuria with creatinine and creatinine clearance should be obtained. Proteinuria is present if there is more than 300 mg of protein excreted over 24 hours. Total urinary creatinine should be measured to assess the adequacy of urine collection. The creatinine clearance can be used in conjunction with the serum creatinine as a measure of renal function.
	The use of a random spot urinary protein-to-creatinine ratio to diagnose proteinuria in pregnancy has had many advocates, but it remains unclear at this time whether this test can replace the 24-hour urine in pregnant patients with suspected preeclampsia (15,16).
DIC screen	Severe preeclampsia can rarely cause DIC, but it is almost always seen in association with thrombocytopenia. Checking INR, PTT, and fibrinogen degradation products is usually only done if the patient with preeclampsia has thrombocytopenia or is undergoing an invasive procedure.

HUS, hemolytic uremic syndrome; TTP, thrombotic thrombocytopenic purpura; AST, aspartate aminotransferase; DIC, dissemination intravascular coagulation; INR, international normalized ratio; PTT, partial thromboplastin time.

rupture, occur in a minority of cases of preeclampsia. However, these conditions are most likely to require intensive care and are therefore reviewed here in more detail.

Severe Hypertension

A single blood pressure threshold that would absolutely necessitate treatment in the setting of preeclampsia is not established. Expert opinion favors urgent treatment of blood pressures greater than 180 mmHg (systolic) and 110 mmHg (diastolic) and, in the setting of obvious hypertensive end-organ damage (retinal hemorrhage, papilledema, pulmonary edema, severe headache, or renal failure), the blood pressure should be kept under 160/100 mmHg; beyond this consensus, opinions vary considerably (18,19).

Although no evidence suggests that treating blood pressures between 160/100 and 180/110 mmHg in the setting of preeclampsia improves maternal or fetal outcomes, many experts believe that the risks for seizure, placental abruption, stroke, and cerebral hemorrhage are decreased by bringing blood pressures down into the normal or mildly hypertensive range (20). Because preeclampsia is felt to be a dynamic vasospastic disorder with associated target-organ ischemia, some experts suggest letting blood pressures run in a moderately severe range to avoid worsening ischemia in areas of regional vasospasm. In the absence of direct evidence of end–target-organ damage from severe hypertension, it is our practice to treat all blood pressures over 160/105 mmHg. However, although we treat these blood pressures urgently, we are careful to avoid any severe, sudden decreases in maternal blood pressure that may adversely affect uteroplacental and cerebral perfusion.

If urgent blood pressure reduction is required, intravenous labetalol or intravenous hydralazine can be used. Increasing evidence indicates that labetalol may be the better choice of the two; it is our preferred agent, although both agents are still acceptable (20). Hydralazine has been associated with an increased risk of an emergency cesarean in women who receive it while still pregnant and with lower Apgar scores in the infants of mothers who have been given this agent prior to delivery. Short-acting oral nifedipine is also used at some centers as an alternative to labetalol or hydralazine for the acute treatment of severe hypertension. Although its use in medical patients is now discouraged, its use for control of blood pressure in young pregnant or postpartum women without coronary artery disease remains an acceptable practice. Previous concerns about a drug interaction between magnesium and calcium channel blockers appear to be ill-founded (21). Diuretics should not be used in this setting unless pulmonary edema is present because, despite the edema that is so common in preeclamptic patients, most hemodynamic studies of preeclamptic women suggest that they are actually intravascularly volume depleted.

Once the patient has delivered, any antihypertensive agent can be used for blood pressure control. At that point, nitroprusside and nitroglycerin are excellent choices because of their very short half-lives.

Seizures

Seizures are the most well-known severe manifestation of preeclampsia. The risk of an eclamptic seizure in a patient with untreated preeclampsia is estimated to be about 1 in 200. Because of early identification of preeclampsia and the widespread use of magnesium prophylaxis, the incidence of eclampsia in the United States ranges from 1 in 1,000 to 1 in 20,000 deliveries; when it does occur, eclampsia is associated with a maternal mortality rate of 5% and a perinatal mortality rate between 13% and 30%.

Eclamptic seizures are typically of the grand mal variety, with clonic–tonic muscular activity followed by a postictal period. However, focal, jacksonian-type and absence seizures have been described. Most eclamptic seizures occur in the setting of established preeclampsia with hypertension and proteinuria. Classically, they are preceded by evidence of neuromuscular irritability such as tremulousness, agitation, nausea, vomiting, and/or clonus. However, some patients will present with seizure as their first manifestation of preeclampsia, usually occurring in the absence of hypertension or proteinuria.

The onset of eclamptic convulsions can be antepartum (38% to 53%), intrapartum (18% to 36%), or postpartum (11% to 44%). Postpartum eclamptic seizures generally occur in the first 48 hours after delivery, but it is not unusual to see them occur anytime in the first week after delivery; eclamptic seizures have been reported as late as 23 days postpartum.

The underlying pathophysiology of the eclamptic seizure is unclear. They cannot be attributed simply to severe hypertension, because eclampsia can be seen in patients with only mild elevations in blood pressure. Electroencephalograms may show epileptiform abnormalities, but usually show only a nonspecific diffuse slowing that may persist for weeks after delivery. Computed tomography (CT) and magnetic resonance imaging (MRI) of the eclamptic patient can be normal, or may show findings ranging from diffuse edema to focal areas of hemorrhage or infarction. Symmetrical white matter edema in the posterior cerebral hemispheres, particularly the parieto-occipital regions is characteristic for reversible posterior leukoencephalopathy syndrome (RPLS). Some suggest that RPLS could be considered an indicator of eclampsia, even when the other features of eclampsia (proteinuria, hypertension) are not present. MRI is more sensitive in detecting abnormalities in eclamptic patients, but both CT and MRI of the brain can be normal, particularly if done in the first 24 hours after the seizure. When radiologic changes are present, some—but not all—of these changes usually resolve with time (22).

Management of Eclamptic Seizures

Even when delivery is impending, a preeclamptic woman should still receive an anticonvulsant to prevent eclamptic seizures; magnesium sulfate is the medication of choice for this purpose (23). It halves the risk of eclampsia in patients with preeclampsia and lowers the risk of recurrent seizures and maternal death in women with eclampsia. It is superior to phenytoin and benzodiazepines in preventing further seizures. Magnesium is typically given as an intravenous bolus of 4 to 6 g, followed by a continuous intravenous infusion of 1 to 4 g/hr. Either monitoring plasma concentrations (which should run between 4 and 7 mmol/L), or observing the patient closely for symptoms and signs of toxicity (hypotension, hypotonia, muscular weakness, and respiratory depression) are reasonable options. Carefully monitoring for toxicity is important, particularly in patients with worsening renal function. Severe respiratory depression in a patient on magnesium should be treated with intravenous calcium. The only role of magnesium in preeclampsia is that of an anticonvulsant. Despite the possibility of a transient decrease in blood pressure with its initial administration, magnesium has no significant sustained effect on blood pressure. Its mechanism of action remains unclear, but it does not seem to have any intrinsic anticonvulsant effect, and may actually prevent seizures through its action as a cerebral vasodilator.

If the woman does have an acute eclamptic seizure, intravenous benzodiazepine is indicated to acutely stop the seizure, and magnesium should then be initiated if this has not already occurred. If an eclamptic convulsion occurs while a patient is receiving magnesium, most clinicians will add phenytoin to the regimen. Continued seizures should warrant the involvement of neurology and consideration of the use of other antiepileptic drugs. Anticonvulsant therapy can generally be stopped once postpartum diuresis has begun and the manifestations of preeclampsia have started to improve.

Neuroimaging with CT or MRI is recommended for most patients with eclamptic seizures to rule out an intracerebral hemorrhage. The timing of these neuroimaging tests should be determined by the level of clinical suspicion for this diagnosis, and should not substantially delay delivery.

Cerebrovascular Accidents

Cerebrovascular accidents are three to seven times more common in pregnancy. Preeclampsia accounts for over a third of the strokes that do occur during pregnancy, and at least half of the deaths from preeclampsia in the developed world are due to stroke. Most of the strokes in patients with preeclampsia will be related to intracerebral hemorrhage, but can also occur due to vasospastic ischemia (24). Preeclampsia-related stroke is often, but not always, associated with severe hypertension and/or eclamptic convulsions. Sudden onset or worsening of a headache, a change in mental status, or any focal neurologic complaint occurring in the context of preeclampsia should lead to consideration of this diagnosis and urgent neuroimaging.

Pulmonary Edema

Pulmonary edema occurs in about 3% of cases of preeclampsia, and can cause significant maternal morbidity (25–27). It occurs as a result of the interplay of preeclampsia-related pulmonary endothelial damage and the low plasma oncotic pressure seen in all pregnancies; excessive intravenous fluid is also, typically, a contributing factor. It is often seen in the postpartum period after a patient has received a substantial amount of intravenous fluid in labor (or with cesarean delivery) and when mobilization of fluid from the involuting uterus begins. Pulmonary edema in this setting is often amenable to gentle diuresis but may be severe enough to warrant mechanical ventilation.

Echocardiographic studies demonstrate that transient systolic or diastolic ventricular dysfunction is present in up to one-third of preeclampsia cases associated with pulmonary edema. This preeclampsia-related myocardial dysfunction is believed to be a manifestation of vasospastic coronary ischemia, and usually resolves rapidly with resolution of the preeclampsia. We consider this to be a distinct entity from peripartum cardiomyopathy (PPCM) and do not believe there is a substantial recurrence risk of cardiac disease for these patients in a subsequent pregnancy.

Prevention and Treatment of Pulmonary Edema

It is important to avoid excessive fluid administration to patients with preeclampsia because of their propensity for pulmonary edema. Ideally, one individual should be designated to approve and monitor all fluid administration in these patients. Regular auscultation of the lungs and use of transcutaneous pulse oximetry in patients with severe preeclampsia will help identify cases of pulmonary edema as they evolve. This careful observation should be continued in the postpartum period because pulmonary edema often occurs as late as 2 to 3 days after delivery. Acute treatment of pulmonary edema should involve supplemental oxygen, low-dose furosemide, and, if needed, morphine (27,28). Blood pressure control may help treat pulmonary edema by decreasing afterload. An echocardiogram should be obtained to look for an underlying cardiac contribution. Intubation and mechanical ventilation may become necessary if the above measures do not improve the patient's oxygenation.

Disseminated Intravascular Coagulation

Disseminated intravascular coagulation (DIC) can occur as a late and severe complication of preeclampsia or eclampsia (29). Because most patients with preeclampsia-related DIC have low platelet counts or elevated transaminase levels, DIC screening in the absence of these abnormalities is generally not necessary (30). However, a DIC screen should be ordered in all preeclamptic patients with rising liver enzymes, dropping platelet counts, and/or any abnormal bleeding. This is particularly important if there is a possibility of an operative delivery.

Acute Renal Failure

Preeclampsia is often associated with a mild degree of renal impairment manifesting as a slightly elevated creatinine or a decreased urine output. This is due to a combination of intravascular volume depletion, renovascular vasospasm, and a preeclampsia-related glomerular lesion known as glomerular endotheliosis. This mild renal impairment usually resolves rapidly after delivery.

Acute renal failure in preeclampsia is not common. If it does occur, acute tubular necrosis (ATN) and partial or total cortical necrosis are the most likely underlying lesions, and are thought to be caused by preeclampsia-related, vasospasm-induced renal ischemia. A history of transient hypotension is also typically present in these cases. The differential diagnosis includes ATN from sepsis or hemorrhage, or renal failure from causes unassociated with pregnancy such as hemolytic uremic syndrome, medication effects, or acute glomerulonephritis.

Most renal failure in the setting of preeclampsia is rapidly reversible, but if significant hypotension has occurred (as may happen with placental abruption or DIC-related hemorrhage), ATN or renal cortical necrosis may result and necessitate dialysis. In persons with sustained oliguria in the setting of preeclampsia, fluid challenges should be given cautiously because of the risk of pulmonary edema. Poor outcomes in preeclampsia are far more commonly related to pulmonary edema than they are to decreased urine output. Diuretics to improve urine output should be avoided in the absence of pulmonary edema because of the intravascular volume depletion present in most patients with preeclampsia.

If the patient is unresponsive to small fluid boluses, the use of central venous pressure (CVP) monitoring may be a helpful, if not completely reliable, guide. The role of the pulmonary artery catheter in this context is unproven, and should only be used by nurses and physicians who are trained and experienced in its use. Increasing data from randomized control trials have shown that pulmonary artery catheters are of less benefit than previously believed in nonpregnant patients, and there is little reason to believe this tool has a uniquely beneficial role in the pregnant population.

Sustained oliguria in preeclampsia is unusual, and therefore significant and rapid peripartum renal deterioration should also lead to consideration of differential diagnoses that include the hemolytic uremic syndrome (HUS), thrombotic thrombocytopenic purpura (TTP), and renal cortical necrosis. It is therefore advisable to perform careful microscopic examination of urinary sediment and a peripheral smear in all pregnant or postpartum patients with oliguria (31).

HELLP Syndrome

A distinct clustering of the manifestations of preeclampsia is the HELLP syndrome (*h*emolysis, *e*levated *l*iver enzymes, and *l*ow *p*latelet counts). This constellation of findings represents a particularly severe form of preeclampsia with significant risk for maternal illness and fetal injury or death (32,33). HELLP occurs in up to 20% of cases of severe preeclampsia. The hemolysis is microangiopathic, and therefore schistocytes (fragmented erythrocytes) are seen on peripheral smears of the blood. Lactate dehydrogenase levels are usually increased and liver enzyme elevation may be two- to threefold. The thrombocytopenia can be precipitous and severe. High-dose dexamethasone is often given to treat patients with HELLP, but it is not clear that this intervention has clinically significant effects on outcomes, and the treatment remains supportive care coupled with delivery (34,35).

Hepatic Rupture, Infarction, or Hemorrhage

Epigastric or right upper quadrant pain and elevation of hepatic enzymes due to preeclampsia are common. When these factors are present, it suggests severe disease and preeclampsia-related hepatic edema and ischemia. It generally is associated with no more than a two- to fourfold increase in aspartate aminotransferase (AST) or alanine aminotransferase (ALT). When pain is severe and/or hepatic enzymes rise above this level, preeclampsia-related hepatic infarction, hemorrhage, and rupture should be considered and investigated with a hepatic ultrasound or CT (36). Acute fatty liver of pregnancy (AFLP) is also part of the differential diagnoses in these cases.

Diabetes Insipidus

Diabetes insipidus is a rare complication of preeclampsia with significant hepatic involvement. It can also be seen with AFLP. It has been hypothesized that the acute liver dysfunction in these patients reduces the degradation of vasopressinase (an enzyme which itself degrades vasopressin), and results in a state of relative vasopressin deficiency (37). The course of the condition follows that of the underlying disorder and can be treated with additional vasopressin until it resolves.

The Role of Arterial Lines, Central Venous Pressure Monitors, and Pulmonary Artery Catheters in Preeclamptic Patients

Most severe preeclamptic patients have normal or hyperdynamic left ventricular function with normal pulmonary artery pressure. Thus, a CVP monitor usually is adequate to assess volume status and left ventricular function. However, severely preeclamptic patients may develop cardiac failure, progressive and marked oliguria, or pulmonary edema. In such cases, some authors suggest that a pulmonary artery (PA) catheter may be helpful for proper diagnosis and treatment, because right and left ventricular pressures may not correlate (38,39). Given that evidence has evolved that the routine use of pulmonary artery catheters may not be as beneficial in the care of nonobstetric patients as once believed, the rather limited literature about their use in obstetric populations cannot help but be questioned (40–42). No clear consensus exists as to their role in the management of preeclampsia (43). We rarely employ them in any obstetric patients, as the risks—especially on labor and delivery units where the personnel have less experience in their placement and interpretation—seem to outweigh the evidence justifying their use. When questions arise as to whether cardiac dysfunction is contributing to a preeclamptic patient's pulmonary edema and/or renal failure, we obtain an urgent bedside echocardiogram to guide our care and, in the absence of a significant cardiac cause, manage these patients clinically.

An intra-arterial catheter monitor may be indicated for protracted severe hypertension during therapy with potent antihypertensive agents or when there is a significant disparity between automated and manual cuff measurements of blood pressure.

CARDIAC DISEASE

Cardiac disease during pregnancy has an incidence rate of 0.4% to 4%, and is associated with a maternal mortality of 0.4% to 6%, depending on the cardiac lesion being discussed (44). Indeed, it is now the leading cause of maternal mortality in North America (45). Although rheumatic heart disease is far less of a concern in the West than it was several decades ago, it remains a problem, along with peripartum cardiomyopathy, pulmonary hypertension, adult congenital heart disease, and myocardial ischemia. These conditions will be the focus of this section. Although many of the patients with cardiac disease who end up under the care of a critical care physician will have cardiac disease that was identified prior to pregnancy, a significant portion of patients will also have their cardiac disease present for the first time during pregnancy. The physiologic changes of pregnancy may exacerbate, and thereby unmask, previously undiagnosed cardiac disease, and pregnancy can predispose patients to the onset of certain cardiac diseases such as PPCM or ischemic heart disease. Some of the physiologic changes associated with pregnancy are reviewed below and are summarized in Table 78.4.

Physiologic Changes

Maternal blood volume gradually increases during pregnancy to 150% of nonpregnant levels (46). The increase in plasma volume (45% to 55%) is greater than the increase in red blood cell volume (20% to 30%), resulting in a relative anemia of pregnancy. This increase in blood volume is associated with an increase in cardiac output (CO), which begins early in gestation and peaks at levels 30% to 40% over nonpregnant values between 20 and 30 weeks (46); the increase then plateaus until term. CO in a twin pregnancy is 15% higher than that of a singleton pregnancy (47).

The increase in CO with gestation is dependent on heart rate and stroke volume. Heart rate gradually increases throughout pregnancy, starting as early as 4 weeks of gestation, with a 10% to 15% increase by term. Stroke volume, in contrast, peaks during the second trimester, with a 20% to 40% increase over the nonpregnant state.

During labor, CO rises another 15% to 45% above prelabor values with an additional increase of 10% to 25% during uterine contractions. The increase in CO in labor during contractions versus that seen between contractions is greater late in the first stage (34%) versus early in the first stage (16%) (48).

Oxygen consumption increases 20% during pregnancy, and may increase as much as 40% to 100% during active labor. In

TABLE 78.4 Hemodynamic Changes in Pregnancy

	% Change[a]		
	Pregnancy	Labor and Delivery	Postpartum
Cardiac output	+30–50	+50–65[b]	+60–80
Heart rate	+10–15	+10–30[b]	−10–15
Stroke volume	+20–30	+40–70	+60–80
Blood volume	+20–80	—	+0–10
Plasma volume	+44–55	—	+0–30
Red cell volume	+20–30	—	−10
Oxygen consumption	+20	+40–100[b]	−10–15
Systemic vascular resistance	−10–25	—	—
Systemic blood pressure			
Systolic	−5	+10–30[b]	+10
Diastolic	−10	+10–30[b]	+10
Pulmonary vascular resistance	−30	—	—
Pulmonary artery occlusion pressure (PAOP)	0	—	—
Colloid oncotic pressure (COP)	−10	—	—
COP–PAOP	−25	—	—

[a]Percentage change from nonpregnant state.
[b]Percentage change without regional anesthesia (local anesthetic).

the immediate postpartum period, CO increases 30% to 40% over the labor period or 60% to 80% over the nonpregnant state, with the increased blood volume shifting to the central circulation from the contracted uterus, as well as alleviation of aortocaval compression and a slight decrease in total peripheral resistance.

CO and other hemodynamic parameters are thought to return to their baseline prepregnant state by 6 weeks after delivery. However, CO may remain elevated for up to 12 weeks (49).

Systemic arterial pressure decreases by 10 to 15 mmHg over the first two trimesters and then gradually returns to baseline by term. Systemic vascular resistance decreases 10% to 20% during pregnancy. Moreover, systemic vascular resistance may remain decreased for at least 12 weeks postpartum.

Venous pressure in the lower extremities increases and peaks near term as the gravid uterus compresses the inferior vena cava—especially when the patient is supine—while CVP remains unchanged. Total-body water increases by about 2 kg throughout pregnancy.

Invasive PA catheterization in low-risk, near-term pregnant patients (36 to 38 weeks) reveals a significant decrease in pulmonary vascular resistance, colloid oncotic pressure (COP), and COP–pulmonary artery occlusion pressure (PAOP) gradient, with no change in PAOP or left ventricular stroke work index (50).

With a significant increase in oxygen consumption, especially during labor, along with a decrease in functional residual capacity, the importance of adequate preoxygenation (***denitrogenation***) before rapid sequence induction of anesthesia cannot be overemphasized. Morbidity and mortality statistics from England and Wales reveal that anesthetic-related maternal mortality is predominantly caused by the inability to intubate the trachea or by pulmonary aspiration during general anesthesia (51). Thus, an awake orotracheal intubation should be considered when airway patency is suspect. The most experienced person available should typically be the individual who intubates pregnant women on a regular basis.

Despite an average 200- to 500-mL blood loss for routine, uncomplicated vaginal deliveries and an 800- to 1,000-mL blood loss for cesarean section deliveries, blood transfusions are seldom necessary because of the increased blood volume and the autotransfusion of approximately 500 mL of blood from the contracted uterus in the postpartum period. Although this increase in blood volume protects against blood loss at delivery, pulmonary congestion and cardiac failure can result in patients with underlying cardiac dysfunction.

Pregnant women have a predisposition to pulmonary edema. Physiologic changes in pregnancy that favor the development of pulmonary edema include an increase in intravascular volume, decreased blood viscosity ("physiologic anemia of pregnancy"), decreased COP, and fluid shifts, especially in the immediate postpartum period.

Patients with minimal cardiac reserve may tolerate early pregnancy, and subsequently decompensate from increasing blood volume and the need for an increased CO in the late second trimester and early third trimester. Patients with moderate cardiac reserve may tolerate pregnancy well until labor and delivery or the puerperium. Thus, cardiac patients should continue to be closely monitored in the postpartum period because cardiac decompensation most frequently occurs during this time; the prepregnant baseline state may not be reached for as long as 12 weeks after delivery.

The enlarging uterus in the third trimester predisposes to aortocaval compression and decreased CO in supine patients. Inferior vena cava compression occurs in up to 90% of near-term parturients in the supine position. However, only about 10% to 15% of patients manifest the supine hypotensive syndrome because of shunting of venous blood away from the caval system to the azygos system by the intervertebral plexus of veins. Patients most susceptible to supine hypotension are those with polyhydramnios and multiple gestation. However, in most patients in the lateral position, CO is maintained. Turning from the supine to the lateral decubitus position increases CO from 8% at 20 to 24 weeks to as much as 30% near term (52). Therefore, to avoid aortocaval compression, measures such as uterine displacement by maternal position (lateral decubitus), bed position (left lateral tilt), or uterine displacement devices are imperative, especially in the last trimester. Moreover, maternal hypotension and placental hypoperfusion from aortocaval compression can be compounded by regional anesthesia that interferes with compensatory sympathetic nervous system mechanisms (53).

As a consequence of these cardiovascular changes, normal symptoms of pregnancy can include fatigue, dyspnea, decreased exercise capacity, and lightheadedness. Cardiac signs that may be seen in normal pregnancies include distended neck veins, peripheral edema, loud first heart sound, loud third heart sound, systolic ejection murmurs, and continuous murmurs (cervical venous hums and mammary souffle). Fourth heart sounds and diastolic murmurs occur rarely in normal pregnancy and should be considered pathologic unless proven otherwise. These changes are reviewed in Table 78.5. Therefore, the normal signs and symptoms of pregnancy may simulate pathologic disease states, thereby rendering the diagnosis of heart disease difficult.

TABLE 78.5 Normal Cardiac Symptoms and Signs in Pregnancy

SYMPTOMS
Fatigue
Dyspnea
Decreased exercise tolerance
Lightheadedness
Syncope
SIGNS
General
Distended neck veins
Peripheral edema
Hyperventilation
Heart
Loud S_1; increased split S_1
Loud S_3
Systolic ejection murmur
Continuous murmurs (venous hums, mammary souffle)
Chest radiograph
Increased pulmonary vasculature
Horizontal position of heart
Electrocardiogram
Left axis deviation
Nonspecific ST-T–wave changes
Mild sinus tachycardia

Normal chest radiographic findings demonstrate increased lung markings (prominent pulmonary vasculature partly due to both increased blood volume and increased breast shadow). Electrocardiographic (ECG) changes may include a left QRS axis deviation and nonspecific ST-segment and T-wave changes.

Who Is Most at Risk and When Is That Risk Greatest?

Table 78.6 classifies the risk of various cardiac lesions in pregnancy. When we speak about "risk" for these patients, we refer to congestive heart failure, arrhythmias, stroke, and death. Overall, about 13% of cardiac patients will suffer one of these outcomes in pregnancy. The presence of pulmonary hypertension is always associated with an increased risk, and this risk is commensurate to its degree of severity. Other factors associated with an increased risk of cardiac complications in pregnancy include the following (54):

- New York Heart Association (NYHA) functional class. This is perhaps the most important predictor of pregnancy outcome. Patients with NYHA class I and II cardiac disease generally have a good prognosis during pregnancy. Patients with NYHA class III and IV are more likely to experience complications and may require special management around the time of delivery.
- Left-sided obstructive cardiac lesions. Patients with lesions such as aortic stenosis may have difficulty accommodating the increased blood volume and CO seen in pregnancy, and become increasingly symptomatic. Interestingly, patients with regurgitant valvular lesions may have less difficulty in pregnancy, as CO in these cases may benefit from the decrease in systemic vascular resistance seen in pregnancy.
- Cyanosis
- Left ventricular systolic dysfunction
- Prior cardiac events or previous dysrhythmia

TABLE 78.6 Peripartum Risk of Various Cardiac Lesions

Risk Category	Lesion
Lower-risk lesion	Mitral valve prolapse
	Mitral valve prolapse with regurgitation
	Atrial septal defect
	Ventricular septal defect with normal pulmonary pressures
	Trace to mild valvular regurgitation
	NYHA class I
	History of SVT with recent good control
	Presence of an implanted pace maker
Intermediate-risk lesion	Stable ischemic heart disease
	Mild to moderate pulmonary hypertension
	Moderate to severe valvular insufficiency
	NYHA class II
	Cardiomyopathy with ejection fraction 30–50%
	Poorly controlled SVT
High-risk lesion	Unstable ischemic heart disease
	Moderate to severe left ventricular obstruction (e.g., aortic <1.5 cm^2 or mitral valvular stenosis <2 cm^2, peak gradient LV outflow tract of >30 mmHg)
	NYHA class III
	Cardiomyopathy with ejection fraction <30%
	Dilated aortic root, Marfan syndrome, Ehlers–Danlos syndrome
	Moderate pulmonary hypertension
	History of ventricular tachycardia with or without AICD
	Mechanical prosthetic heart valve
	History of TIA or CVA
Highest-risk lesion	Pulmonary hypertension >80 mmHg
	Eisenmenger syndrome
	NYHA class IV
	Cyanosis

NYHA, New York Heart Association; SVT, supraventricular tachycardia; AICD, automated implantable cardioverter-defibrillator; TIA, transient ischemic attack; CVA, cerebrovascular accident.

Items above can be used to calculate a risk index with 1 point being assigned for each and 0, 1, and >1 points being associated with a risk of some cardiac event during the entire pregnancy of 5%, 27%, and 75%, respectively.

Risk calculation adapted from Siu S, Sermer M, Colman JM, et al. Prospective multicenter study of pregnancy outcomes in women with heart disease. *Circulation.* 2001;104:515.

Although pregnant women with cardiac disease may experience complications at any point during pregnancy, there are three periods of particular risk:

1. At the end of the second trimester, when CO has increased to its peak
2. At the time of labor and delivery, when cardiac work may be increased dramatically by both pain and the autotransfusion of blood from the placenta and uterus with each contraction
3. In the first 72 hours following delivery, when the uterine involution and resolution of pregnancy-related edema leads to mobilization of large amounts of fluid

General Management of Cardiac Patients During Pregnancy

Management of patients with cardiac disease in pregnancy should, in general, include good preconception counseling to assess and inform the patient of the risks associated with a pregnancy. Although no woman should be told that she "should never get pregnant," a clear discussion of the risk is essential. With cases such as severe pulmonary hypertension or Eisenmenger syndrome, the patient should be strongly cautioned against pursuing a pregnancy. Women with congenital heart disease need also be informed that they are at increased risk of giving birth to a child with congenital heart disease. If a woman with cardiac disease decides to pursue a pregnancy after a clear discussion of risk, the cardiologist should ensure that her cardiac status is clearly delineated and optimized. Ideally, any necessary investigations or interventions should be carried out prior to conception. Once a woman is pregnant, regular visits with a medical specialist and an obstetrician trained in the care of high-risk pregnancies to watch for evidence of heart failure and arrhythmias are essential. Consultation with an obstetric anesthesiologist prior to delivery is also prudent.

As stated earlier, most cardiac medications can be used in pregnancy when indicated. Table 78.7 lists many common cardiac medications, and classifies them as to which drugs we know the most about regarding their safe use during pregnancy and which drugs we know the least. However, it should be emphasized that among the more commonly used cardiac

TABLE 78.7 Commonly Used Cardiac Medications and Their Safety in Pregnancy

	Use Generally Justifiable for This Indication in Pregnancy	Use Justifiable in Special Circumstances for This Indication in Pregnancy	Use Almost Never Justifiable for This Indication in Pregnancy
Dysrhythmia	Digoxin β-Blockers (all probably safe but most avoid propranolol and atenolol, which may cause intrauterine growth restriction) Calcium channel blockers, especially verapamil and diltiazem (less known about amlodipine) Adenosine Quinidine Procainamide Lidocaine	Amiodarone Disopyramide, mexiletine, and flecainide (less is known about these agents in pregnancy but there is no evidence at this point of human teratogenesis; they should generally be considered second-line agents in pregnancy)	
Ischemia	Nitrates Low-dose (<100 mg) ASA β-Blockers Heparin (unfractionated or low molecular weight) Tissue plasminogen activator Streptokinase	HMG-coA reductase inhibitors ("statins") have concerning animal pregnancy data, but very limited reported human experiences thus far have been encouraging; should only be used in pregnancy when short-term benefits are clear Abciximab (and other glycoprotein IIb/IIIa inhibitors) dipyridamole, ticlopidine, and clopidogrel lack published human data; they are probably safe but should only be used in pregnancy when short-term benefits are clear	Warfarin
Heart failure	Furosemide Digoxin Hydralazine β-Blockers Dopamine Dobutamine	Nitroprusside (fetal cyanide toxicity possible at high doses)	ACE inhibitors Angiotensin II receptor blockers
Hypertension	Labetalol β-Blockers Nifedipine Hydralazine Methyldopa	Thiazide diuretics (in this category for the treatment of hypertension because of effects of blood volume in pregnancy) Clonidine, prazosin, verapamil, diltiazem, and amlodipine (in this category for the treatment of hypertension because of limited data on safety and the availability of many good alternatives with more data) Nitroprusside (fetal cyanide toxicity possible at high doses)	ACE inhibitors Angiotensin II receptor blockers

ASA, acetylsalicylic acid; ACE, angiotensin-converting enzyme.

medications, only angiotensin-converting enzyme inhibitors, angiotensin receptor blockers, and warfarin are known or strongly suspected to be human teratogens. Amiodarone has had mixed data with respect to its safety in pregnancy, with some reports of congenital hypothyroidism, goiter, prematurity, hypotonia, and bradycardia (55,56). Although use in an acute setting is appropriate, it is not a first-line agent for maintenance therapy in pregnancy. Angiotensin-converting enzymes and angiotensin receptor blockers both have been associated with fetal anomalies, fetal loss, oligohydramnios, cranial ossification abnormalities, and neonatal renal failure. Although their use in the first trimester was once supported, recent evidence suggests they should not be used at any time in gestation (57). Warfarin is associated with a high risk of miscarriage and anomalies of the eyes, hands, neck, and central nervous system (58). Again, the guiding principle of managing critical illness in pregnancy should be that, because fetal well-being depends on maternal well-being, medications that are of benefit to maternal health should also be considered to be in the fetus' best interest. Useful sources for reviewing the available safety data for medications during pregnancy and with breastfeeding are found in references (59–65).

For any structural cardiac lesion, we typically will obtain an echocardiogram as a baseline early in pregnancy, in the third trimester, and with any change in clinical status. Additional investigations and interventions should be dictated by the patient's clinical status, and no needed test or procedure should be withheld during gestation. In particular, pregnancy should not limit necessary diagnostic testing (66). Ultrasound has a long history of safe use in pregnancy. The radiation exposure associated with plain film radiographs, nuclear medicine scans, angiography, and CT scans are all well below what is deemed acceptable during pregnancy. Contrast agents appear to be well tolerated by the fetus. MRI has not been associated with any ill effects in human pregnancies. Because fetal well-being is dependent on maternal well-being, more harm will generally be caused to a mother and her fetus by withholding necessary investigations than by obtaining them.

Women with congenital heart disease should undergo a detailed fetal ultrasound in the early second trimester to allow early diagnosis of congenital heart disease in the fetus. This will allow informed decision-making by the mother, and will prepare the neonatology team should a problem be present.

Labor and delivery and the first 72 hours postpartum warrant special consideration with respect to assembling the appropriate team and determining what monitoring will be needed. For most cardiac patients, a multidisciplinary patient care conference should be assembled well in advance of the anticipated time of delivery and a written care plan developed for the peripartum management of the patient. This team should generally include representation from critical care, nursing, anesthesia, obstetrics, and cardiology. The plans that are developed should be explicit and detailed and recognize that the labor and delivery room is a place where cardiac care is not commonly provided. Even the best-trained obstetricians and obstetric nurses will lack the volume of experience in the management of cardiac cases that is common among cardiac and critical care providers. It is our conviction that joint nursing of such patients by obstetric and cardiac-trained nurses during labor and delivery, followed by postpartum care in a cardiac or critical care unit, seems the ideal approach when possible. Table 78.8 offers a comprehensive checklist of parameters to be considered and addressed in a multidisciplinary patient care conference dedicated to developing a labor and delivery plan for a cardiac patient.

The mode of delivery should not generally be determined by medical concerns. The need for cesarean deliveries is generally dictated by obstetric concerns, and vaginal deliveries should generally be viewed as the safest and best option for cardiac patients. The choice between spontaneous labor and elective induction of labor should be made both on the likelihood of successful induction and the availability of medical expertise and resources should a cardiac patient go spontaneously into labor during the off hours and weekends.

Most patients should be kept in neutral fluid balance over the course of their delivery period, and careful monitoring of both input and output will be essential. Early and good anesthesia is important to decrease the cardiac work of delivery, and most patients should receive regional anesthesia in a manner that will minimize the need for the fluid boluses typically given to decrease the hypotension associated with establishing regional anesthesia. It is also important to consider that certain lesions, such as an aortic stenosis, may be highly volume dependent and require this additional fluid support.

Intra-arterial lines are advisable for cardiac lesions for which moment-to-moment monitoring of blood pressure might be desirable, such as severe aortic stenosis. The role of the pulmonary artery catheter in the laboring patient remains unclear and, in the absence of clear benefit, it is this author's opinion that their use during delivery should be limited to the most severe cardiac cases, if it is used at all.

Bacterial endocarditis prophylaxis is no longer recommended by the American Heart Association for vaginal or cesarean deliveries because the bacteremia associated with delivery is unlikely to cause endocarditis (67). If done at all, endocarditis prophylaxis should be reserved for patients with prosthetic heart valves, a prior history of subacute bacterial endocarditis, complex cyanotic congenital heart disease, or surgically constructed systemic pulmonary shunts or conduits, and an agent active against enterococci such as penicillin, ampicillin, or vancomycin should be utilized.

It is critical that all team members recognize that the cardiac patient remains at risk for at least 72 hours postpartum, so despite the sense of completion that comes with a successful delivery, caregivers need to remain vigilant for early signs of deterioration in the days following the birth.

Specific Lesions

Mitral Stenosis. Rheumatic heart disease remains a potential form of heart disease in pregnancy despite its declining incidence in the developed world. Mitral stenosis (MS) accounts for approximately 90% of the rheumatic valvular lesions in pregnancy. It often presents for the first time in pregnancy; complications include atrial fibrillation, pulmonary edema, and thromboembolic stroke. The normal physiologic cardiac changes in pregnancy are poorly tolerated in MS. Most patients will experience some worsening of symptoms during pregnancy, and the risk continues during labor and delivery as the increased blood volume after delivery of the placenta may worsen pulmonary edema (68). Complication rates were found in one study to be 38% in moderately severe MS and 67% in severe cases (69). Avoidance of tachycardia (which decreases time available for ventricular filling), increased PA pressure, decreased systemic vascular resistance, and increased central blood volume are essential to patient management. For this reason, many patients will benefit from β-blockade to improve left ventricular filling time during pregnancy (70). Echocardiograms should be done once every trimester and with any change in status in these patients. Careful attention should be focused on pulmonary pressures (although echocardiography may provide a less reliable estimate of pulmonary pressures in pregnancy). Pulmonary edema should be treated with diuretics and β-blockade. If severe symptoms persist despite optimal medical management, percutaneous mitral balloon valvuloplasty, commissurotomy, or even valve replacement may be warranted; all have been successfully performed in pregnancy (71–73). Open procedures may be associated with a higher risk of miscarriage, fetal loss, and preterm labor, and thus balloon valvuloplasty may be preferable at centers experienced with this procedure. Although surgery can be performed at any point in the pregnancy, the risk to the fetus is lowest in the second trimester.

If atrial fibrillation occurs, it should be treated promptly to decrease tachycardia and the associated risk of a low CO state or degeneration into more malignant dysrhythmias. Rate control, full anticoagulation with heparin, and consideration of either medical or electrical cardioversion remain the core management principles in pregnant women with atrial fibrillation as they are for nonpregnant women.

For labor and delivery (vaginal or cesarean), excellent pain control is important and is best achieved with early establishment of regional anesthesia. Control of pain will limit the undesirable effects of labor on heart rate and blood pressure (which are tachycardia and increased systemic vascular resistance). A conservatively dosed lumbar epidural anesthetic with special attention to fluid status, left uterine displacement, and careful use of α-adrenergic agents to treat hypotension is often helpful. These patients are dependent on high left ventricular

(text continues on page 14)

TABLE 78.8 Cardiac Patient Delivery Plan Checklist

PRIOR TO HOSPITALIZATION	
Is additional testing needed to assess risk or guide peripartum therapy? • Baseline ECG done in third trimester • Echocardiogram at any time in the past for lowest-risk lesions, in this pregnancy for moderate-risk lesions, and in the third trimester for high- and highest-risk lesions • Stress testing (exercise echo or dobutamine echo in past year for patients with known or suspected ischemic heart disease or more recently if they are symptomatic) • EP testing for life-threatening dysrhythmia (investigation often deferred until postpartum but can be done in pregnancy if warranted)	Consider for all levels of risk.
Has the patient's cardiac status been optimized? • Is medical therapy optimized and have appropriate dose adjustments been made for the changes of pharmacokinetics in pregnancy? • Are there interventions that would be done if the woman was not pregnant that should be done while she is pregnant to optimize patient's status for delivery (e.g., diagnostic or therapeutic cardiac catheterization (angioplasty, stent), valvuloplasty, valve replacement, diagnostic or therapeutic EP studies, AICD or pacemaker placement or adjustment)?	Consider for all levels of risk.
• Multidisciplinary team meeting needed and arranged (generally should have occurred by 34 wk). Team should include: • Nursing (LDR and postpartum care RN +/– ICU/CCU nursing)__________ • Maternal fetal medicine__________ • Anesthesia (ideally obstetric anesthesia, also consider cardiac anesthesia for high- and highest-risk cases)__________ • Cardiology__________ • ICU/CCU doctor__________	Consider having meeting of RN/MFM/Anesthesia for moderate-risk patients and all of the listed providers for high- and highest-risk patients.
• Written delivery plan should be generated and distributed and made available to all relevant parties including nursing (should include who to call and how to do so when the patient comes in)	Consider for all levels of risk.
• Case-specific nursing education should occur in advance of delivery.	Consider for all levels of risk. For lowest-risk lesions it may be adequate to have a standardized nursing care plan or the written delivery plan.
INTRAPARTUM	
Determine mode and timing of delivery: • Planned induction at what gestation/cervical status • Planned cesarean delivery at what gestation • Spontaneous delivery	Decision to be made on the basis of obstetric factors and the need to ensure availability of necessary members of the care team. Planned delivery may be advisable for high- and highest-risk patients.
Delivery location: • Standard LDR • Specialized LDR • Obstetric ICU • MICU • CCU	Decision to be made on the basis of local facilities and expertise. In general, care during delivery is best provided in LDR and afterward in medical setting.
Delivery personnel who should be notified of admission (make sure needed parties available on day of any planned delivery)	Consider having both LDR nurse and critical care nurse for high- and highest-risk patients.
Medical Attendants: • Obstetrician • Cardiologist • Anesthesia (ideally obstetric anesthesia; also consider cardiac anesthesia for high- and highest-risk cases) • Intensivist	
Nursing (Consider need for team approach of ICU/CCU/RR/ER nurse with LDR nurse. Define necessary nurse-to-patient ratio): • LDR nurse • LDR nurse with ACLS training • LDR nurse with ACLS and special critical care training • Critical care nurse (ICU/CCU/RR/ER) nurse	Consider required response time of ACLS trained personnel if nursing team caring for patient is not ACLS certified/experienced
	This question is particularly important for free-standing obstetric centers.
EDUCATION • Verify written care plan is available to all team members • Is a "recap" in-service for care team advisable on day of delivery?	Consider summary in-service on day of delivery for high- and highest-risk patients and any patient for whom medications may be required urgently that are not routinely used on obstetric floors.

TABLE 78.8 Cardiac Patient Delivery Plan Checklist (*Continued*)

MONITORING • Cardiac monitor options (choose one) • Not necessary • To be in room but does not need to be on if patient asymptomatic • To be on patient at all times but not continuously observed • To be on patient at all times and should be continually observed by ACLS-trained individual • To be on patient at all times and should be observed at all times by critical care nurse/MD/PA/RNP	Most cardiac patients, aside from the highest-risk patients or those with a history of life-threatening hemodynamically unstable arrhythmias, will not need continuous monitoring by ACLS-trained personnel. Low-risk lesions may warrant one of the first two approaches. Moderate- and high-risk lesions may warrant only option 3.
Pulse oximeter (choose one) • Not necessary • Readily available but use only with symptoms • In room and check hourly • In room and on continuously	Pulse oximeter may provide evidence of CHF but should always be interpreted in view of strength of pulse signal. Option 2 is probably adequate for most cardiac patients aside from those with cyanotic heart disease or those in CHF, who probably warrant option 4.
Fetal monitoring	Obtain explicit plan from obstetric team including who will read the fetal monitoring strips and the plan of action should they be concerning.
Defibrillator • On the unit with ready access to defibrillator pads • Defibrillator and defibrillator pads in the room • Defibrillator pads on patient but machine not hooked up • Patient to be monitored using defibrillator with defibrillator pads	Option 1 is generally adequate. Consider other options in highest-risk patients.
IV access • No IV necessary • Single peripheral IV lines needed • Two peripheral IV lines needed • Central line • Central line with CVP • Central line with pulmonary artery catheter	Option 2 is enough for most patients. Consider central line in highest-risk lesions.
FLUID BALANCE	
All patients need strict ins and outs measured throughout hospitalization. Most cardiac patients we will want to keep in a neutral fluid balance during hospitalization.	Make sure to add in all fluids given with medications and for regional anesthesia.
Fluid to be run:________	
Rate:________	
Arterial line • No arterial line needed • Arterial line warranted	Arterial line advisable when hemodynamics make moment-to-moment monitoring of blood pressure useful (e.g., aortic stenosis)

MEDICATIONS
• Need for SBE prophylaxis (SBE prophylaxis for high-risk lesions only and even then not absolutely necessary)
• Special issues related to interactions with commonly used obstetric medications
• Possibly necessary cardiac medications not routinely used on obstetric units________
  • Need for RN/MD education regarding these medications
  • Need for written instructions with respect to preparation and administration of this medication
  • Need for medication to be at bedside
  • Pharmacy notified in advance of request (especially if free-standing obstetrics hospital)
	May be given for prosthetic heart valves, prior SBE, complex cyanotic congenital heart disease, surgically constructed systemic pulmonary shunts or conduits but not necessary for the rest
	• Standard dosing: Ampicillin 2 g IV plus gentamicin 1.5 mg/kg within 30 min of delivery; ampicillin 1 g IV 6 h after delivery
	• Penicillin allergy: Vancomycin 1 g IV over 1–2 h plus gentamicin 1.5 mg/kg IV within 30 min of delivery

Anesthetic concerns • Special issues related to anesthesia • Special issues with respect to cautery for cesarean delivery	Anesthesia will determine preferred modality of anesthesia timing and precautions in technique. Implanted defibrillators may need to be turned off prior to surgery because of interference from cautery.
Thromboprophylaxis • Intermittent compression stockings • Heparin 5,000 units SQ q12h • Heparin 5,000 units SQ q8h • Enoxaparin 40 units SQ daily • Enoxaparin 30 units SQ q12h • Full anticoagulation necessary in peripartum period (please see peripartum anticoagulation protocol)	Options 1 and 2 compatible with epidural anesthesia. Options 3–6 should only be done after the epidural catheter is removed. Consider option 1 or 2 antepartum and option 2, 3, 4, or 5 for most patients postpartum while in hospital.

(*Continued*)

TABLE 78.8 Cardiac Patient Delivery Plan Checklist (*Continued*)

POSTPARTUM	
How long postpartum will patient require special observation? • Usual period of postpartum observation • 6 h • 12 h • 24 h • 48 h • 72 h • 96 h	Low-risk patients probably only warrant the usual period of observation given all patients. Moderate-risk patients warrant 6 h. High-risk patients warrant between 6 and 48 h and highest-risk patients 72–96 h.
Location of special postpartum observation • Room on regular postpartum floor • Room on high-risk antenatal floor • Standard LDR/postop CS area • Specialized LDR/postop CS area • Obstetric ICU • MICU • CCU • Other__________	Option 1, 2, or 3 for low-risk; 2, 3, or 4 for moderate-risk; and 4, 5, 6, or 7 for high- and highest-risk patients
MONITORING Cardiac monitor options (choose one) • Not necessary • To be in room but does not need to be on if patient asymptomatic • To be on patient at all times but not continuously observed • To be on patient at all times and should be continually observed by ACLS-trained individual • To be on patient at all times and should be observed at all times by critical care nurse/MD/PA/RNP	Option 1 or 2 for low-risk; 2 or 3 for moderate-risk; 3 for high-risk; and 3, 4, or 5 for highest-risk patients
Postpartum monitoring/interventions recommended and for how long • Peripheral IV__________ • Central line__________ • CVP__________ • Arterial line__________ • Pulmonary artery catheter__________	No special monitoring or interventions for low-risk patients; 1 for 24 h for moderate-risk patients; and 1 or 2 for 48–72 h for high- and highest-risk patients
All patients need strict ins and outs measured throughout hospitalization. Most cardiac patients we will want to keep in a neutral fluid balance during hospitalization. Fluid to be run:__________ Rate:__________	Make sure to add in all fluids given with medications and for regional anesthesia.
Pulse oximeter in room and checked how often • Not necessary • In room but use only with symptoms • In room and check hourly • In room and on continuously	Pulse oximeter may provide evidence of CHF but should always be interpreted in view of strength of pulse signal. Option 2 probably adequate for most cardiac patients aside from those with cyanotic heart disease and those in CHF, who probably warrant option 4.
Availability of ACLS trained physician/PA/RNP: • Special availability not necessary • Special availability necessary with what maximum response time	
Postpartum care team: Identify the care team and circle who will be the initial contact should medical problems arise. Make sure the person's name and contact number are clearly documented in the chart. Medical attendants: • Obstetrician • Cardiologist • Anesthesia (ideally obstetric anesthesia; also consider cardiac anesthesia for high- and highest-risk cases) • General internist • ICU team • CCU team • Medical ICU vs. LDR with cardiac nursing (consider need for team approach and necessary nurse-to-patient ratio) • LDR nurse • LDR nurse with ACLS training • LDR nurse with ACLS and special critical care training • Critical care (ICU/CCU/RR/ER) nurse	Consider required response time of ACLS-trained personnel if not present
Defibrillator • On the floor • In the room • Pads on patient • Patient to be monitored with defibrillator pads on • Special issues related to interactions with commonly used obstetric medications	Option 1 is generally adequate. Consider other options in highest-risk patients.

TABLE 78.8 Cardiac Patient Delivery Plan Checklist (*Continued*)

Thromboprophylaxis
START________
DURATION________

- Intermittent compression stockings
- Heparin 5,000 units SQ q 2h
- Heparin 5,000 units SQ q8h
- Enoxaparin 40 units SQ daily
- Enoxaparin 30 units SQ q12h
- Full anticoagulation will be needed postpartum: See peripartum anticoagulation protocol
- Possibly necessary cardiac medications not routinely used on obstetric units________
  - Need for RN/MD education regarding these medications
  - Need for written instructions with respect to preparation and administration of this medication
  - Need for medication to be at bedside
  - Pharmacy notified in advance of request (especially if free-standing obstetric hospital)

DISCHARGE PLANNING

Will there be any adjustments to medication necessary postpartum (e.g., resumption/replacing of medications stopped/started because of pregnancy OR dosing adjustments necessary in postpartum period because of increases made during pregnancy)?

Who will follow the patient after discharge and when will patient need to be seen (letter or phone call should be sent/made to receiving MD):

- Cardiology________
- Primary care doctor________
- Obstetrics________

ECG, electrocardiogram; EP, electrophysiologic; AICD, automatic implantable cardioverter-defibrillator; LDR, labor and delivery room; RN, registered nurse; ICU, intensive care unit; CCU, critical care unit; MFM, maternal–fetal medicine; MICU, medical intensive care unit; RR, recovery room; ER, emergency room; ACLS, Advanced Cardiac Life Support; MD, doctor; PA, physician assistant; RNP, registered nurse practitioner; CHF, congestive heart failure; CVP, central venous pressure; SBE, subacute bacterial endocarditis; CS, cesarean section.

filling pressures for their CO (74,75). Obstetricians will generally try to limit the second stage of delivery (the "pushing" stage) and assist a prolonged second stage through the use of vacuum extractors or forceps to decrease maternal work. The role of pulmonary artery catheters and intra-arterial lines for cardiac patients in labor was discussed previously and remains unclear. If there is a group who benefits from these interventions, it will likely be those patients with severe obstructive lesions or very poor ejection fractions. If the pulmonary artery catheter is used for patients with MS, it will be important to remember that the PAOP may overestimate left ventricular end-diastolic pressure.

Aortic Stenosis

Aortic stenosis is a valvular lesion rarely seen during pregnancy, and can be of rheumatic or congenital origin. Although bicuspid aortic valves are common, they are unlikely to be associated with significant stenosis in the childbearing years. They may be associated with an increased risk of both coarctation and dissection. Although mild to moderate aortic stenosis is generally well tolerated in pregnancy, severe stenosis (defined as <1.0 cm^2) carries a significant fetal and maternal risk. The rate of complication varies from 10% to 31%, depending on the severity of the lesion (76–78). Ideally, symptomatic aortic stenosis should be repaired prior to pregnancy. If the patient is classified as NYHA functional class III or IV while pregnant, consideration should be given to percutaneous valvuloplasty, surgical repair, or valve replacement. Ideally, such procedures are best done in the middle of the pregnancy but, if necessary, can be done at any time. When severe disease is identified after the first trimester, it is important to be aware that both labor and delivery and a late termination are associated with significant risks. Due to the fixed outflow obstruction, these patients will not tolerate sudden drops in volume or preload, and their peripartum period should be managed in such a way as to minimize the risk of such events and ensure the ability to respond rapidly if and when they do occur. Arterial lines are strongly advised, and the use of pulmonary artery catheters, while not proven, may be of benefit.

In the past, with severe stenotic lesions of the aorta, regional anesthesia has been avoided because of the resulting local anesthetic–induced sympathectomy, which can lead to bradycardia and decreased venous return. However, good results have been obtained in patients with severe aortic stenosis managed during labor with a carefully titrated epidural anesthetic (78,79).

Mitral and Aortic Insufficiency

Mitral insufficiency is the second most common valvular lesion seen in pregnancy, and is typically due to rheumatic heart disease (75). Aortic insufficiency is less common, and may be due to rheumatic, infectious, or rheumatologic conditions. These lesions, when found in isolation, tend to do well in pregnancy unless there is associated ventricular decompensation. Treatments when symptomatic may include diuretics, β-blockers, or vasodilators, but angiotensin receptor blockers should not be used despite the benefits of afterload reduction. Increases in systemic vascular resistance, decreased heart rate, atrial dysrhythmias, and myocardial depressants may be poorly tolerated. Perhaps the most important peripartum issue for these patients is early regional anesthesia to prevent pain-associated increases in systemic vascular resistance.

Congenital Heart Disease

Approximately 25% of heart disease in pregnancy is congenital. It can be categorized as left-to-right shunt, right-to-left shunt, and aortic lesions.

Left-to-Right Shunt

The most common congenital heart lesions are atrial septal defects (ASDs) and ventricular septal defects (VSDs), which are usually well tolerated in pregnancy. The risk of cardiac complications is greatest in patients with large defects. Congestive heart failure (due to increased blood volume in pregnancy leading to cardiac decompensation), atrial dysrhythmias, shunt reversal (occurring due to sudden systemic hypotension), and thromboembolic disease are all possible complications seen with ASD and VSD in pregnancy. Ideally, hemodynamically significant septal defects should be repaired prior to pregnancy. However, when symptomatic septal defects present in pregnancy, the principles of management include (a) acetylsalicylic acid (ASA) 81 mg daily to prevent thromboembolism, (b) use of diuretics and digoxin to treat heart failure, (c) avoidance of hypotension with epidural administration or postpartum blood loss, and (d) rapid rate control with any arrhythmia.

Right-to-Left Shunt and Pulmonary Hypertension

The high-risk congenital disorders in pregnancy include right-to-left shunts, as seen in Eisenmenger syndrome (any congenital heart lesion with a bidirectional or right-to-left shunt at the atrial, ventricular, or aortic level), and any other lesions associated with significant pulmonary hypertension. Patients with uncorrected cyanotic heart disease have increased spontaneous abortion rates, pulmonary embolization, congestive heart failure, and incidence for congenital heart defects in the fetus. A high hematocrit (≥65%) is not only an indication of the severity of the cardiac disease, but also in itself has a poorer prognosis secondary to complications from hyperviscosity (decreased CO, organ hypoperfusion, and thrombosis).

During pregnancy, right-to-left shunting is increased because of decreased systemic vascular resistance, resulting in decreased pulmonary artery perfusion and hypoxia. A review on maternal and fetal outcome in patients with Eisenmenger syndrome reveals maternal mortality rates of 25% to 52% and fetal loss as high as 44% (80–82). Because of the grim prognosis for these pregnancies, these women should be strongly warned about the dangers of pursuing a pregnancy and, if they do become pregnant, should be offered the opportunity for an early termination. If they continue with the pregnancy, they may warrant hospitalization from 20 weeks onward. Oxygen should be administered for dyspnea, and prophylactic heparin should be considered throughout pregnancy and for 6 weeks postpartum. The mode of delivery should be determined on the basis of obstetric indications. Pulmonary artery catheterization can carry additional risks in patients with significant pulmonary hypertension, and should probably be avoided in these patients. Active efforts should be made to avoid sudden decreases in systemic vascular resistance, blood volume, and venous return. Increased pulmonary vascular resistance promotes right-to-left shunting; therefore, hypercapnia and hypoxia are to be avoided. How best to provide peripartum anesthesia to these patients is not clear, and discussion of this matter is beyond the scope of this chapter. What *is* clear is that if regional anesthesia is used, care must be taken to prevent precipitous drops in venous return. Patients with pulmonary hypertension and/or Eisenmenger syndrome should be observed for 72 hours postpartum in a cardiac setting, as many of the maternal deaths associated with these conditions will occur during this period.

Aortic Disease

Coarctation of the aorta and aortic manifestations of Marfan syndrome pose significant problems in pregnancy (83–85). The physiologic changes during pregnancy, including increased blood volume and increased blood pressure during labor and delivery, may promote aortic dissection in either of these conditions. Patients with coarctation of the aorta may also suffer from worsening hypertension or congestive heart failure in pregnancy.

Marfan syndrome is often associated with aortic dilation, aortic valve regurgitation, and mitral valve disease. Aortic dissection occurs in about 10% of patients with Marfan syndrome who undergo a pregnancy, and is most likely to occur if the aortic root measures beyond 4.5 cm in diameter (86,87). Ideally, women with this severity of aortic root dilation should have their aorta repaired prior to pregnancy. However, if they have not, serial echocardiography during pregnancy to watch for worsening dilation should be performed. If the root is increasing in size, aortic repair should be considered. The activity of patients with significant aortic dilation in pregnancy should be limited, and they should be placed on β-blockers to decrease shear stresses upon the vessel wall (88,89). Although we generally teach that the indications for cesarean delivery are obstetric and not medical, it is common practice to deliver women with aortic roots dilated beyond 4.0 cm by cesarean to avoid additional stress on the aorta associated with the pain and pushing of a vaginal delivery. However, it is worth noting that the majority of aortic dissections in these patients occur prior to the onset of labor.

Aortic coarctation in pregnancy is associated with an increased risk of worsening hypertension and, less commonly, congestive heart failure or preeclampsia (90). It is much less likely to be associated with aortic dissection than Marfan syndrome, but dissection can and does occur. Blood pressure should be kept less than 160/100 mmHg in these patients but not brought below 120/70 mmHg, as there may be a significant gradient between blood pressure measurement in the arm and the estimated blood pressure of the placenta circulation that is distal to the aortic narrowing. β-Blockers are the preferred antihypertensives for these patients. Patients with coarctation can undergo a vaginal delivery but should have a limited second stage (i.e., prolonged pushing should be avoided by the use of vacuum extractor or forceps).

Tetralogy of Fallot

Tetralogy of Fallot is the most common cyanotic congenital heart disease. It consists of a VSD, an overriding aorta, infundibular pulmonary stenosis, and secondary right ventricular hypertrophy. Patients with uncorrected tetralogy have significant complications in pregnancy including biventricular failure, dysrhythmias, stroke, and risk of shunt reversal with worsening cyanosis. Preconception surgical repair should be undertaken if at all possible. If these patients do proceed with a pregnancy unrepaired, they should be managed in a manner similar to patients with Eisenmenger syndrome.

Patients with a surgically corrected tetralogy of Fallot who enter a pregnancy with a good functional status generally tolerate pregnancy well. The main risks are right-sided heart failure and dysrhythmias. Their volume status should be monitored throughout pregnancy and complaints of palpitations or syncope investigated with a Holter or an event monitor. Delivery should include cardiac monitoring (91–94).

Other Repaired Congenital Heart Conditions

An increasing number of women with congenital heart problems that were repaired in childhood are reaching adulthood and undergoing pregnancy. In general, these patients' course in pregnancy is readily predictable by the parameters outlined earlier in this chapter. The majority will have a good pregnancy outcome for both themselves and their offspring if they enter the pregnancy with a good functional status (75,95).

Peripartum Cardiomyopathy

The National Heart, Lung, and Blood Institute (NHLBI) defines PPCM as the new onset of systolic dysfunction occurring in the absence of other plausible causes anytime between the final month of pregnancy up to 5 months postpartum. The incidence is between 1 in 2,000 to 1 in 15,000 pregnancies, and may be increasing (96–98). Multiparity, twin gestation, maternal age greater than 30 years, presence of preeclampsia/eclampsia and black race are all known to be risk factors, but causality is not yet proven. Precise mechanisms that lead to PPCM remain poorly defined. Many etiologic processes have been suggested (99) including abnormal immune response to pregnancy, maladaptive response to the hemodynamic changes of pregnancy, prolonged tocolysis, increased concentration of inflammatory cytokines, angiogenic imbalance mediated via prolactin and its fragments (100), and possible genetic mechanisms, though a specific genetic mutation causally associated with PPCM is yet to be identified. Generally, patients with PPCM have a greater recovery of LV function and a better prognosis than patients with other forms of dilated cardiomyopathy. Most women with PPCM will have complete or at least partial recovery within 6 months of onset while women with depressed LV function beyond 6 months of diagnosis have worse clinical outcomes and higher 5-year mortality rates (101). Mortality can be due to end-stage heart failure, arrhythmia, or thromboembolism.

Pathologic findings include four-chamber enlargement with normal coronary arteries and valves. Light microscopic findings include myocardial hypertrophy and fibrosis with scattered mononuclear infiltrates. Clinical signs include symptoms of ventricular failure with possible associated dysrhythmias and/or pulmonary emboli. Treatment includes bed rest, sodium restriction, diuresis, and preload/afterload reduction with a calcium channel blocker and hydralazine while pregnant and an angiotensin-converting enzyme inhibitor postpartum. Because pregnancy is associated with increased risk of thrombosis, patients with an ejection fraction less than 35% should be considered for anticoagulation with low–molecular-weight heparin (LMWH) while pregnant and warfarin postpartum. Antidysrhythmics should be used in a manner similar to what would be done for any patient with an idiopathic cardiomyopathy. Although the exact risk remains unclear, there is evidence that PPCM may recur or worsen with subsequent pregnancies (102).

Hypertrophic Cardiomyopathy

During pregnancy, the course of hypertrophic cardiomyopathy is variable because while the normal increase of blood volume is beneficial, the decrease in systemic vascular resistance and the increase in heart rate may be detrimental. Several large case series have highlighted the risks for these patients during pregnancy (103–106). The risks are inherently greater for those women who are symptomatic before pregnancy or in those with severe left ventricular outflow tract obstruction. Complications are not common, but include congestive heart failure, chest pain, supraventricular tachycardias (SVTs), ventricular tachycardia, and sudden death. Complications can occur at any point in the pregnancy or during labor as a result of stress, pain, and increased circulating catecholamines. Moreover, the immediate postpartum period can increase risk due to blood loss and decrease in systemic vascular resistance. Atrial fibrillation and SVTs are a common feature of this cardiac anomaly; thus, cardioselective β-blockers and verapamil are usually administered to these patients. Tocolytics, sympathomimetic agents, and digoxin should be avoided in these patients, as they may increase the risk of dysrhythmia. The peripartum period should include cardiac monitoring and use of forceps or vacuum extractor so that the mother has to do little or no pushing. If regional anesthesia is employed, it should be done incrementally and with agents that minimize the risk of a sudden drop in preload.

Ischemic Heart Disease in Pregnancy

Although myocardial infarction in pregnancy is uncommon, with an incidence estimated at between 1 in 10,000 and 1 in 35,700, it does appear to be increasing. Risk factors include advancing age, preeclampsia, multiparity, chronic hypertension, obesity, and diabetes. Myocardial infarctions associated with pregnancy can occur at any time during gestation, with one report finding that 38% occurred antepartum, 21% intrapartum, and 41% in the first 6 weeks postpartum. Maternal mortality rate ranges from 7% to 35%, with a disproportionate number of deaths occurring among the antenatal cases (107–109). A large portion of pregnancy-associated myocardial infarctions are not due to atherosclerotic heart disease but instead due to coronary artery in situ thrombus formation, dissection, or spasm.

Diagnosis of ischemic heart disease in pregnancy does require considering it as part of the differential diagnosis, even in the absence of traditional risk factors. Clinicians should also be aware that creatine phosphokinase (CPK) and creatine kinase-MB (CK-MB) can be mildly elevated following a cesarean delivery and that troponin is a more specific marker of cardiac disease in the peripartum period. All forms of stress testing can be safely carried out in pregnancy, including nuclear imaging, although many centers prefer exercise echocardiography for this population. Diagnostic coronary angiography can and should be performed on pregnant women for the same indications as for nonpregnant patients.

Treatment of coronary artery disease remains largely unchanged in pregnancy. None of the medications commonly used to treat ischemic heart disease have been shown to cause adverse effects in the fetus. There is broad experience with low-dose aspirin, nitrates, β-blockers, and heparins in pregnancy. The paucity of data regarding the use of clopidogrel and the platelet glycoprotein IIb/IIIa inhibitors should limit their use in pregnancy to clinical scenarios with proven benefits. Statins were previously considered to be teratogenic but a recent systematic review suggests that the doses which are commonly prescribed do not in fact increase any adverse fetal outcomes (110). Coronary angiography, angioplasty and stenting, and thrombolysis have been and can be carried out safely throughout pregnancy (111–114).

The management of laboring patients with ischemic heart disease should be the same for other cardiac patients as discussed in the section above on general principles of management of cardiac disease at the time of delivery, and has strong parallels with the management of the cardiac patient undergoing general surgery.

Cardiac Dysrhythmias in Pregnancy

Dysrhythmias during gestation, and especially labor and delivery, appear to be more common than in the nonpregnant population (115). Hormonal changes, stress, and anxiety are contributing factors; however, most dysrhythmias are not serious unless they are associated with organic heart disease.

Atrial Fibrillation

Atrial fibrillation occurring in pregnancy is usually associated with underlying disease such as MS, peripartum cardiomyopathy, hypertensive heart disease, thyroid disease, or ASDs. Patients with acute atrial fibrillation and significant hemodynamic changes—such as hypotension or loss of consciousness—require direct current cardioversion. Cardioversion appears to have no adverse effects on the fetus. Most patients, however, will require only medical management with rate-controlling or rhythm-restoring antidysrhythmics. β-Adrenergic blockers such as metoprolol, calcium channel blockers such as diltiazem or verapamil, and agents such as procainamide or digoxin can all be used safely during pregnancy. Amiodarone would not be considered a first-line agent for hemodynamically stable atrial fibrillation because of its possible effects on the fetal thyroid, but its use in pregnancy is not absolutely contraindicated and the risks of potential use must be weighed against the potential benefits and seriousness of the indication. Anticoagulation for atrial fibrillation in pregnancy has the same indications as in nonpregnant patients, but the agent that must be used is heparin—usually in the form of subcutaneous LMWH—because warfarin is associated with adverse fetal effects throughout gestation.

Supraventricular Tachycardia

SVTs during pregnancy can occur with or without organic heart disease. Four percent of women with SVT report that their condition was first identified in pregnancy, and up to 22% state that pregnancy exacerbated their condition (116). In the absence of underlying cardiac disease, these tachycardias are not usually associated with increased morbidity. However, in patients with underlying structural cardiac disease or cardiomyopathy, SVT can lead to heart failure and death. Treatment protocols for SVT remain unchanged in pregnancy and include carotid sinus massage, adenosine, calcium channel blockers, β-blockers, and direct current cardioversion (117,118).

Ventricular Dysrhythmias

Ventricular dysrhythmia during pregnancy may be associated with cocaine use, peripartum or any other form of cardiomyopathy, ischemic heart disease, and digitalis toxicity. Antidysrhythmic agents for which we have the most pregnancy data are lidocaine, β-blockers, and procainamide. Amiodarone is associated with an increased risk of fetal thyroid disease and, although its use in pregnancy is permissible, it should not be considered a first-line agent. Implantable defibrillators can and should be used when indicated in pregnancy, although they will need to be turned off during surgical procedures that require the use of cautery.

Bradycardia

Bradydysrhythmias during pregnancy are rare and may result from infection such as Lyme disease (which can cause heart blocks of varying degrees), hypothyroidism, myocarditis, drug-induced, or congenital or acquired heart blocks. Permanent pacemakers are indicated for hemodynamically significant bradycardia. Patients with pre-existing pacemakers may need to have their baseline rate increased during pregnancy to mimic the normal physiologic changes of pregnancy.

Antidysrhythmic Drugs

Table 78.7 classifies the commonly used antidysrhythmic agents on the basis of what is known about their safety in pregnancy. Although there are obviously agents that we know more about than others, it is important to reemphasize here that both mother and fetus benefit from the use of the best agent to control cardiac symptoms in pregnancy, and treatment should never be withheld from a pregnant woman based on theoretic fears of fetal harm.

Cardiac Surgery During Pregnancy

As in other semielective nonobstetric surgery during pregnancy, if nonurgent cardiac surgery is necessary, it should ideally take place during the second trimester. Deferring when possible until after the first trimester avoids the period of organogenesis and the risk of miscarriage. Third-trimester surgery carries the risk of precipitating preterm labor. However, surgery that is important to a patient's short-term well-being and survival should be done at any point in gestation as required. Coronary artery bypass grafts, valvuloplasties, valvular replacements, and aortic root replacements have all been done in pregnancy with good outcomes for mother and baby. When medical management can ameliorate the disease process, surgery may be postponed until the patient has recovered at least 4 to 6 weeks postpartum; however, such decisions should be based on the best plan of action for the mother's safety rather than a cultural discomfort related to performing surgery in pregnancy.

Special intraoperative considerations in pregnant patients include fetal monitoring during and after surgery, maintenance of high flow and systemic mean arterial pressure (during cardiopulmonary bypass), and uterine displacement devices if the patient is in the supine position for a median sternotomy. Although the pregnant patient has fared well with open heart procedures, fetal mortality rate can be high. Generally, better results are seen in closed heart procedures. Postoperatively, fetal monitoring should be continued and maternal analgesia maintained to avoid precipitating labor from accelerated postoperative pain.

Pregnancy After Prosthetic Valve Surgery

Patients with mechanical heart valve prostheses pose a significantly increased risk for thromboembolic events during pregnancy. Fewer maternal and fetal complications occur with bioprosthetic valves but the need for reoperation on these valves for degenerative changes means they are not commonly used in women of reproductive age.

Heparin, typically LMWH, is the anticoagulant agent of choice during pregnancy because its molecular weight prevents placental crossover, and it is not teratogenic. It is now well established as the anticoagulant of choice in pregnancy for all indications except for mechanical heart valves. Questions still remain as to whether LMWH provides the same level of protection against mechanical valve thrombosis as warfarin. Although warfarin and its derivatives are associated with an increased risk of central nervous system anomalies and warfarin embryopathy, it may be that the risk is worth taking to prevent the catastrophic consequences of valve thrombosis (119–121). Some experts therefore recommend that women with mechanical heart valves use LMWH during the period of organogenesis, switch to warfarin for the majority of the pregnancy, and then switch back to LMWH close to term to avoid both fetal and maternal bleeding associated with delivery. Other experts would use LMWH but carry out frequent testing of the peak and trough heparin levels—anti-Xa levels—to ensure that the patient is adequately anticoagulated.

Cardiac Transplant Patients

With the increasing number and survival of heart transplant recipients, increasing numbers of women who have undergone this procedure have become pregnant (122,123). The pregnancy experience with solid tissue transplant patients in general has found a 25% risk of maternal complications (with over half of these complications being hypertension), a 29% risk of miscarriage, and a 41% risk of prematurity (123). The best data specific to cardiac transplantation describe 32 US pregnancies in women who had undergone cardiac transplantation, and found a 44% rate of hypertension, a 22% risk of rejection, and a 13% risk of worsening renal function. Neonatal complications were similar to the data described above for all solid tissue transplants (124). In light of these data, women who have undergone cardiac transplantation are warned of the possible risks of a pregnancy, and are encouraged to wait 2 years after transplantation before becoming pregnant to ensure that the transplant has been a success. Drugs used to prevent rejection should be continued during pregnancy; evidence of their safety is accumulating. If antirejection treatment is continued, pregnancy does not appear to increase the risk of rejection (123,124). The peripartum management should be dictated by the quality of left ventricular function in a manner similar to that discussed previously in this chapter.

Cardiopulmonary Resuscitation

Pregnancy poses some unique problems during cardiopulmonary resuscitation (CPR). In the third trimester and particularly near term, the gravid uterus impairs venous return. Thus, during CPR, the uterus should be displaced (i.e., left uterine tilt). Moreover, if defibrillation is required, the left breast needs to be displaced because of marked enlargement during pregnancy. The unlikely but theoretical possibility that there may be electrical arcing between a defibrillator and any fetal monitoring devices means that fetal monitoring devices should be removed prior to defibrillation. Otherwise, the Advanced Cardiac Life Support (ACLS) protocols, including medications and the use of the defibrillator, should be followed as done in a nonpregnant patient. Some experts would suggest that the use of amiodarone should be deferred in cardiac resuscitation until alternative appropriate agents have failed. However, in the context of a cardiac arrest, the authors would support the use of any recommended ACLS medication, as the one-time use of any of these agents is very unlikely to be of any harm, and may be of great benefit to both mother and fetus.

Data about the risk and benefits of an emergency cesarean delivery in the context of maternal resuscitation are very limited. The present-day view is that if the fetus has reached a point in the pregnancy where survival after delivery is possible (typically more than 24 weeks of gestation), emergency cesarean should be considered a part of the resuscitative efforts. Evacuation of the gravid uterus, with the concomitant release of pressure on the inferior vena cava and removal of the low-resistance circulatory unit that is the placenta, may improve the efficacy of chest compressions and improve the outcome for both mother and baby. Present recommendations are for consideration of cesarean delivery in pregnant women greater than 24 of weeks gestation who have had a cardiac arrest and failed to respond to 4 minutes of aggressive and appropriate resuscitative efforts (125). Consensus statements have been published by both the American Heart Association (126) and Society of Obstetric Anesthesia and Perinatology (127) on this topic.

Key Points

- Preeclampsia complicates 5% to 8% of all pregnancies, can occur at any time in the second half of pregnancy and the postpartum period, and is related to placental insufficiency.
- The following are all life-threatening maternal complications of preeclampsia: severe hypertension, eclamptic seizures, cerebral hemorrhage, pulmonary edema, disseminated intravascular coagulation, acute renal failure, hepatic failure and/or rupture, and diabetes insipidus.
- A particularly severe form of preeclampsia is the HELLP syndrome (hemolysis, elevated liver enzymes, and low platelet counts).
- Magnesium sulfate is the drug of choice to prevent eclamptic seizures, but careful monitoring for toxicity (hypotension, muscular weakness, respiratory depression) is important particularly in patients with worsening renal dysfunction.
- Cardiac disease during pregnancy has an incidence rate of 0.4% to 4%, and is now the leading cause of maternal mortality in the developed world.
- Factors associated with an increased risk of cardiac complications in pregnancy are: premorbid New York Heart Association (NYHA) functional class III or IV status, cyanosis, presence of pulmonary hypertension, left-sided obstructive cardiac lesions, left ventricular systolic dysfunction, prior cardiac events and/or previous arrhythmias.
- Three periods of particular risks are: end of second trimester, time of labor and delivery, immediate postpartum period (first 72 hours).

- Among the more commonly used cardiac medications, only angiotensin-converting enzyme inhibitors, angiotensin receptor blockers, and warfarin are absolutely contraindicated in pregnancy.
- The radiation exposure associated with all plain film radiographs, CT scans, nuclear scans, and angiography are all well below what is deemed acceptable during pregnancy. None of the contrast agents used have been associated with any fetal complications.
- For most cardiac patients, it is recommended that a multidisciplinary patient care conference be assembled well in advance of the anticipated time of delivery.
- The need for cesarean deliveries is generally dictated by obstetric concerns, and vaginal deliveries should generally be viewed as the safest and best options for cardiac patients.
- For either mode of delivery, early establishment of regional anesthesia is recommended to reduce the undesired effects of labor on heart rate (tachycardia) and blood pressure (increased systemic vascular resistance).
- PPCM is defined as the new onset of systolic dysfunction occurring in the absence of other plausible causes anytime between the final month of pregnancy up to 5 months postpartum.
- Emergency cesarean delivery should be strongly considered in pregnant women beyond 24 weeks of gestation who have had a cardiac arrest and failed to respond to 4 minutes of aggressive and appropriate resuscitative efforts.

References

1. Roberts JM, August PA, Bakris G, et al. Hypertension in pregnancy. Report of the American College of Obstetricians and Gynecologists' Task Force on Hypertension in Pregnancy. *Obstet Gynecol.* 2013;122(5):1122–1131.
2. Powrie RO. A 30-year-old woman with chronic hypertension trying to conceive. *JAMA.* 2007;298(13):1548–1558.
3. Soubra SH, Guntupalli KK. Critical illness in pregnancy: an overview. *Crit Care Med.* 2005;33:S248–S255.
4. Sibai B, Dekker G, Kupferminc M. Preeclampsia. *Lancet.* 2005;365(9461): 785–799.
5. ACOG Committee on Practice Bulletins-Obstetrics. ACOG practice bulletin: diagnosis and management of preeclampsia and eclampsia. *Obstet Gynecol.* 2002;99(1):159–167.
6. Bletka M, Hlavatj V, Tenkova M, et al. Volume of whole blood and absolute amount of serum proteins in the early stages of late toxemia of pregnancy. *Am J Obstet Gynecol.* 1970;106:10.
7. Redman CW, Sargent IL. Latest advances in understanding preeclampsia. *Science.* 2005;308(5728):1592–1594.
8. Lain KY, Roberts JM. Contemporary concepts of the pathogenesis and management of pre-eclampsia. *JAMA.* 2002;287:3183–3186.
9. Levine RJ, Lam C, Qian C, et al. Soluble endoglin and other circulating antiangiogenic factors in preeclampsia. *N Engl J Med.* 2006;355(10):992–1005.
10. Levine RJ, Maynard SE, Qian C, et al. Circulating angiogenic factors and the risk of preeclampsia. *N Engl J Med.* 2004;350(7):672–683.
11. Levine RJ, Thadhani R, Qian C, et al. Urinary placental growth factor and risk of preeclampsia. *JAMA.* 2005;293(1):77–85.
12. Powrie RO, Miller MA. Hypertension in pregnancy. In: Rosene-Montella K, Lee R, Keely EJ, et al., eds. *Medical Care of the Pregnant Patient.* Philadelphia, PA: American College of Physicians; 2007:153–162.
13. Natarajan P, Shennan AH, Penny J, et al. Comparison of auscultatory and oscillometric automated blood pressure monitors in the setting of preeclampsia. *Am J Obstet Gynecol.* 1999;181(5 Pt 1):1203–1210.
14. von Dadelszen P, Magee LA, Devarakonda RM, et al. The prediction of adverse maternal outcomes in preeclampsia. *J Obstet Gynaecol Can.* 2004; 26(10):871–879.
15. Lam C, Lim KH, Kang DH, et al. Uric acid and preeclampsia. *Semin Nephrol.* 2005;25(1):56–60.
16. Rodriguez-Thompson D, Lieberman ES. Use of a random urinary protein-to-creatinine ratio for the diagnosis of significant proteinuria during pregnancy. *Am J Obstet Gynecol.* 2001;185(4):808–811.
17. Durwald C, Mercer B. A prospective comparison of total protein/creatinine ratio versus 24-hour urine protein in women with suspected preeclampsia. *Am J Obstet Gynecol.* 2003;189(3):848–852.
18. Martin JN Jr, Thigpen BD, Moore RC, et al. Stroke and severe preeclampsia and eclampsia: a paradigm shift focusing on systolic blood pressure. *Obstet Gynecol.* 2005;105:246–254.
19. Committee on Obstetric Practice. Committee opinion No. 514: emergent therapy for acute-onset, severe hypertension with preeclampsia or eclampsia. *Obstet Gynecol.* 2011;118:1465–1468.
20. Magee LA, Cham C, Waterman EJ, et al. Hydralazine for treatment of severe hypertension in pregnancy: meta-analysis. *BMJ.* 2003;327(7421):955–960.
21. Magee LA, Miremadi S, Li J, et al. Therapy with both magnesium sulfate and nifedipine does not increase the risk of serious magnesium-related maternal side effects in women with preeclampsia. *Am J Obstet Gynecol.* 2005;193(1):153–163.
22. Sibai BM. Diagnosis, prevention, and management of eclampsia. *Obstet Gynecol.* 2005;105(2):402–410.
23. Duley L. Evidence and practice: the magnesium sulphate story. *Best Pract Res Clin Obstet Gynaecol.* 2005;19(1):57–74.
24. Jeng JS, Tang SC, Yip PK. Stroke in women of reproductive age: comparison between stroke related and unrelated to pregnancy. *J Neurol Sci.* 2004;221(1–2):25–29.
25. Engelhardt T, MacLennan FM. Fluid management in preeclampsia. *Int J Obstet Anesth.* 1999;8(4):253–259.
26. Sibai BM, Mabie BC, Harvey CJ, et al. Pulmonary edema in severe preeclampsia-eclampsia: analysis of thirty-seven consecutive cases. *Am J Obstet Gynecol.* 1987;156(5):1174–1179.
27. Bandi VD, Munnur U, Matthay MA. Acute lung injury and acute respiratory distress syndrome in pregnancy. *Crit Care Clin.* 2004;20(4):577–607.
28. Powrie RO, Levy M. Pulmonary edema in pregnancy. In: Rosene-Montella K, Lee R, Keely EJ, et al, eds. *Medical Care of the Pregnant Patient.* Philadelphia, PA: American College of Physicians; 2007:383–394.
29. Letsky EA. Disseminated intravascular coagulation. *Best Pract Res Clin Obstet Gynaecol.* 2001;15(4):623–644.
30. Kramer RL, Izquierdo LA, Gilson GJ, et al. Preeclamptic labs for evaluating hypertension in pregnancy. *J Reprod Med.* 1997;42:223–228.
31. Gammil HS, Jeyabalan A. Acute renal failure in pregnancy. *Crit Care Med.* 2005;33(10 Suppl):S372–S384.
32. Dotsch J, Hohmann M, Kuhl PG. Neonatal morbidity and mortality associated with maternal hemolysis elevated liver enzymes and low platelets syndrome. *Eur J Pediatr.* 1997;156:389–391.
33. Baxter JK, Weinstein L. HELLP syndrome: the state of the art. *Obstet Gynecol Surv.* 2004;59(12):838–845.
34. van Runnard Heimel PJ, Franx A, Schobben AF. Corticosteroids, pregnancy, and HELLP syndrome a review. *Obstet Gynecol Surv.* 2005;60(1):57–70.
35. Katz L, de Amorim MM, Figueiroa JN, et al. Postpartum dexamethasone for women with hemolysis, elevated liver enzymes, and low platelets (HELLP) syndrome: a double-blind, placebo-controlled, randomized clinical trial. *Am J Obstet Gynecol.* 2008;198(3):283.e1–283.e8.
36. Sheikh RA, Yasmeen S, Pauly MP, et al. Spontaneous intrahepatic hemorrhage and hepatic rupture in the HELLP syndrome: four cases and a review. *J Clin Gastroenterol.* 1999;28(4):323–328.
37. Kalelioglu I, Kubat Uzum A, Yildirim A, et al. Transient gestational diabetes insipidus diagnosed in successive pregnancies: review of pathophysiology, diagnosis, treatment, and management of delivery. *Pituitary.* 2007;10(1):87–93.
38. Strauss RG, Keefer JR, Burke T, et al. Hemodynamic monitoring of cardiogenic pulmonary edema complicating toxemia of pregnancy. *Obstet Gynecol.* 1980;55:170–174.
39. Benedetti TJ, Cotton DB, Read JC, et al. Hemodynamic observations in severe preeclampsia with a flow-directed pulmonary artery catheter. *Am J Obstet Gynecol.* 1980;136:465–470.
40. Young P, Johanson R. Haemodynamic, invasive and echocardiographic monitoring in the hypertensive parturient. *Best Pract Res Clin Obstet Gynaecol.* 2001;15(4):605–622.
41. Fujitani S, Baldisseri MR. Hemodynamic assessment in a pregnant and peripartum patient. *Crit Care Med.* 2005;33(10 Suppl):S354–S361.
42. Gilbert WM, Towner DR, Field NT, Anthony J. The safety and utility of pulmonary artery catheterization in severe preeclampsia and eclampsia. *Am J Obstet Gynecol.* 2000;182(6):1397–1403.
43. Young PF, Leighton NA, Jones PW, et al. Fluid management in severe preeclampsia (VESPA): Survey of members of ISSHP. *Hypertens Pregnancy.* 2000;19(3):249–259.

44. Elkayam U, Gleicher N. *Cardiac Problems in Pregnancy: Diagnosis and Management of Maternal and Fetal Heart Disease*. New York: Wiley-Liss; 1998.
45. Berg CJ, Callaghan WM, Syverson C, Henderson Z. Pregnancy-related mortality in the United States, 1998 to 2005. *Obstet Gynecol*. 2010;116:1302–1309.
46. James CF, Banner T, Levelle JP, et al. Noninvasive determination of cardiac output throughout pregnancy. *Anesthesiology*. 1985;63(Suppl 3A):A434.
47. Hunter S, Robson SC. Adaptation of the maternal heart in pregnancy. *Br Heart J*. 1992;68:540–543.
48. Robson SC, Dunlop W, Boys RJ, et al. Cardiac output during labour. *BMJ*. 1987;295:1169–1172.
49. Capeless EL, Clapp JF. When do cardiovascular parameters return to their preconception values? *Am J Obstet Gynecol*. 1991;165:883–886.
50. Clark SL, Cotton DG, Lee W, et al. Central hemodynamic assessment. *Am J Obstet Gynecol*. 1989;161:1439–1442.
51. Munnur U, de Boisblanc B, Suresh MS. Airway problems in pregnancy. *Crit Care Med*. 2005;33(10 Suppl):S259–S268.
52. Ueland K, Hansen JM. Maternal cardiovascular dynamics. II, Posture and uterine contractions. *Am J Obstet Gynecol*. 1969;103(1):1–7.
53. Gogarten W. Spinal anaesthesia for obstetrics. *Best Pract Res Clin Anaesthesiol*. 2003;17(3):377–392.
54. Siu SC, Sermer M, Colman JM, et al. Prospective multicenter study of pregnancy outcomes in women with heart disease. *Circulation*. 2001;104:515–521.
55. Pradhan M, Manisha M, Singh R, et al. Amiodarone in treatment of fetal supraventricular tachycardia: a case report and review of literature. *Fetal Diagn Ther*. 2006;21(1):72–76.
56. Lomenick JP, Jackson WA, Backeljauw PF. Amiodarone-induced neonatal hypothyroidism: a unique form of transient early-onset hypothyroidism. *J Perinatol*. 2004;24(6):397–399.
57. Cooper WO, Hernandez-Diaz S, Arbogast PG, et al. Major congenital malformations after first-trimester exposure to ACE inhibitors. *N Engl J Med*. 2006;354(23):2443–2451.
58. Schaefer C, Hannemann D, Meister R, et al. Vitamin K antagonists and pregnancy outcome: a multi-centre prospective study. *Thromb Haemost*. 2006;95(6):940–957.
59. Briggs GG, Freeman RK. *Drugs in Pregnancy and Lactation*. 10th ed. Philadelphia, PA: Wolters Kluwer; 2014.
60. Shepard TH, Lemire RS. *Shepard's Catalog of Teratogenic Agents*. 13th ed. Baltimore, MD: Johns Hopkins University Press; 2010.
61. Coustan DR, Michizuki TK. *Handbook for Prescribing Medications in Pregnancy*. 3rd ed. Philadelphia, PA: Lippincott Williams & Wilkins; 1998.
62. Friedman JM, Polifka JE. *Teratogenic Effects of Drugs: A Resource for Clinicians*. 2nd ed. Baltimore, MD: Johns Hopkins University Press; 2000.
63. Hale TW, Rowe HE. *Medications and Mothers' Milk: A Manual of Lactational Pharmacology*. 16th ed. Plano, TX: Hale Publishing; 2014.
64. Reprotox website. www.REPROTOX.org.
65. TERIS: clinical teratology web. University of Washington website. http://depts.washington.edu/~terisweb/teris/.
66. Patel SJ, Reede DL, Katz DS, et al. Imaging the pregnant patient for nonobstetric conditions: algorithms and radiation dose considerations. *Radiographics*. 2007;27(6):1705–1722.
67. Wilson W, Taubert KA, Gewitz M, et al. Prevention of infective endocarditis: guidelines from the American Heart Association. *Circulation*. 2007;116:1736–1754.
68. Hameed A, Karaalp IS, Tummala PP, et al. The effect of valvular heart disease on maternal and fetal outcome of pregnancy. *J Am Coll Cardiol*. 2001;37:893–899.
69. Silversides CK, Colman JM, Sermer M, et al. Cardiac risk in pregnant women with rheumatic mitral stenosis. *Am J Cardiol*. 2003;91:1382–1385.
70. al Kasab SM, Sabag T, al Zaibag M, et al. Beta-adrenergic receptor blockade in the management of pregnant women with mitral stenosis. *Am J Obstet Gynecol*. 1990;163:37–40.
71. Esteves CA, Ramos AL, Braga SL. Effectiveness of percutaneous balloon mitral valvotomy during pregnancy. *Am J Cardiol*. 1991;68:930–934.
72. de Souza JAM, Martinez EE, Ambrose JA, et al. Percutaneous balloon mitral valvuloplasty in comparison with open mitral valve commissurotomy for mitral stenosis during pregnancy. *J Am Coll Cardiol*. 2001;37:900.
73. Sullivan HJ. Valvular heart surgery during pregnancy. *Surg Clin North Am*. 1995;75:59–75.
74. Oakley C, Child A, Jung B. Expert consensus document on management of cardiovascular disease during pregnancy. *Eur Heart J*. 2003;24:761.
75. Elkayam U, Bitar F. Valvular heart disease and pregnancy. *J Am Coll Cardiol*. 2005;46:223–230.
76. Silversides CK, Colman JM, Sermer M, et al. Early and intermediate-term outcomes of pregnancy with congenital aortic stenosis. *Am J Cardiol*. 2003;91(11):1386–1389.
77. Tzemos N, Silversides CK, Colman JM, et al. Late cardiac outcomes after pregnancy in women with congenital aortic stenosis. *Am Heart J* 2009;157(3):474–480.
78. Easterling TR, Chadwick HS, Otto CM, et al. Aortic stenosis in pregnancy. *Obstet Gynecol*. 1988;72:113–118.
79. Graham TP. Ventricular performance in adults after operation for congenital heart disease. *Am J Cardiol*. 1982;50:612–620.
80. Gleicher N, Midwall J, Hochberger D, et al. Eisenmenger's syndrome and pregnancy. *Obstet Gynecol Surv*. 1979;34:721–741.
81. Avila WS, Grinberg M, Snitcowsky R, et al. Maternal and fetal outcome in pregnant women with Eisenmenger's syndrome. *Eur Heart J*. 1995;16:460–464.
82. Yentis SM, Steer PJ, Plaat F. Eisenmenger's syndrome in pregnancy; maternal and fetal mortality in the 1990s. *Br J Obstet Gynaecol*. 1998;105:921–922.
83. Elkayam U, Ostzega A, Shotan A, et al. Cardiovascular problems in pregnant women with the Marfan syndrome. *Ann Intern Med*. 1995;123:117–122.
84. Lipscomb KJ, Smith JC, Clarke B, et al. Outcome of pregnancy in women with Marfan's syndrome. *BJOG*. 1997;104:201–206.
85. Lind J, Wallenburg HC. The Marfan syndrome and pregnancy: a retrospective study in a Dutch population. *Eur J Obstet Gynecol Reprod Biol*. 2001;98:28–35.
86. Rossiter JP, Repke JT, Morales AJ, et al. A prospective longitudinal evaluation of pregnancy in the Marfan syndrome. *Am J Obstet Gynecol*. 1995;173:1599–1606.
87. Carabello BA, Chatterjee K, de Leon AC, et al. ACC/AHA 2006 guidelines for the management of patients with valvular heart disease. *J Am Coll Cardiol*. 2006;48(3):e1–e148.
88. Beauchesne LM, Connolly HM, Ammash NM, et al. Coarctation of the aorta; outcome of pregnancy. *J Am Coll Cardiol*. 2001;38(6):1728–1733.
89. Vriend JW, Drenthen W, Pieper PG, et al. Outcome in pregnancy in patients after repair of aortic coarctation. *Eur Heart J*. 2005;26(20):2173–2178.
90. Fishburne JI Jr, Dormer KJ, Payne GG, et al. Effects of amrinone and dopamine on uterine blood flow and vascular responses in the gravid baboon. *Am J Obstet Gynecol*. 1988;158:829–837.
91. Meijer JM, Pieper PG, Drenthen W, et al. Pregnancy, fertility and recurrence risk in corrected Tetralogy of Fallot. *Heart*. 2005;91:801–805.
92. Singh H, Bolton PJ, Oakley CM. Pregnancy after surgical correction of tetralogy of Fallot. *BMJ*. 1982;285:168–170.
93. Presbitero P, Somerville J, Stone S, et al. Pregnancy in cyanotic congenital heart disease: outcome of mother and fetus. *Circulation*. 1994;89:2673–2676.
94. Patton DE, Lee W, Cotton DB, et al. Cyanotic maternal heart disease in pregnancy. *Obstet Gynecol Surv*. 1990;45:594–600.
95. Nunley WC, Kolp LA, Dabinett LN, et al. Subsequent fertility in women who undergo cardiac surgery. *Am J Obstet Gynecol*. 1989;161:573–576.
96. Bernstein PS, Magriples U. Cardiomyopathy in pregnancy: a retrospective study. *Am J Perinatol*. 2001;18:163–168.
97. Gunderson EP, Croen LA, Chiang V, et al. Epidemiology of peripartum cardiomyopathy: incidence, predictors, and outcomes. *Obstet Gynecol*. 2011;118(3):583–591.
98. Sliwa K, Fett J, Elkayam U. Peripartum cardiomyopathy. *Lancet*. 2006; 368(9536):687–693.
99. Johnson-Coyle L, Jensen L, Sobey A. Peripartum cardiomyopathy. *Am J Crit Care*. 2012;21(2):89–98.
100. Hilfiker-Kleiner D, Sliwa K. Pathophysiology and epidemiology of peripartum cardiomyopathy. *Nature Rev Cardiol*. 2014;11:364–370.
101. Elkayam U. Clinical characteristics of peripartum cardiomyopathy in the United States: diagnosis, prognosis, and management. *J Am Col Cardiol*. 2011;58(7):659–670.
102. Elkayam U, Tummala PP, Rao K. Maternal and fetal outcomes of subsequent pregnancies in women with peripartum cardiomyopathy. *N Engl J Med*. 2001;344(21):1567–1571.
103. Autore C, Conte MR, Piccininno M, et al. Risk associated with pregnancy in hypertrophic cardiomyopathy. *J Am Coll Cardiol*. 2002;40:1864–1869.
104. Thaman R, Varnava A, Hamid MS, et al. Pregnancy related complications in women with hypertrophic cardiomyopathy. *Heart*. 2003;89:752–756.
105. Wigle ED, Rakowski H, Kimball BP, et al. Hypertrophic cardiomyopathy: clinical spectrum and treatment. *Circulation*. 1995;92:1680–1692.
106. Avila WS, Amaral FM, Ramires JA, et al. Influence of pregnancy on clinical course and fetal outcome of women with hypertrophic cardiomyopathy. *Arq Bras Cardiol*. 2007;88:423–428.
107. James AH, Jamison MG, Biswas MS, et al. Acute myocardial infarction in pregnancy: a United States population-based study. *Circulation*. 2006;113:1564–1571.

108. Badin E, Enciso R. Acute myocardial infarction during pregnancy and puerperium: a review. *Angiology*. 1996;47:739–756.
109. Ladner HE, Danielsen B, Gilbert WM. Acute myocardial infarction in pregnancy and the puerperium: a population-based study. *Obstet Gynecol*. 2005;105:480–484.
110. Kusters DM, Hassani Lahsinoui H, van de Post JA, et al. Statin use in pregnancy: a systematic review & meta-analysis. *Expert Rev Cardiovasc Ther*. 2012;10(3):363–378.
111. Turrentine MA, Braems G, Ramirez MM. Use of thrombolytics for the treatment of thromboembolic disease during pregnancy. *Obstet Gynecol Surv*. 1995;50:534–541.
112. Cowan NC, deBelder MA, Rothman MT. Coronary angioplasty in pregnancy. *Br Heart J*. 1988;59:588–592.
113. Giudici MC, Artis AK, Webel RR, et al. Postpartum myocardial infarction treated with balloon coronary angioplasty. *Am Heart J*. 1989;118:614.
114. Saxena R, Nolan TE, von Dohlen T, et al. Postpartum myocardial infarction treated by balloon coronary angioplasty. *Obstet Gynecol*. 1992;79:810–811.
115. Shotan A, Ostrzega E, Mehra A, et al. Incidence of arrhythmias in normal pregnancy and relation to palpitations, dizziness, and syncope. *Am J Cardiol*. 1997;79:1061–1064.
116. Lee SH, Chen SA, Chiang CE, et al. Effects of pregnancy on first onset and symptoms of paroxysmal supraventricular tachycardia. *Am J Cardiol*. 1995;76:675–678.
117. Tawan M, Levine J, Mendelson M, et al. Effect of pregnancy on paroxysmal supraventricular tachycardia. *Am J Cardiol*. 1993;72:838.
118. Silversides CK, Harris L, Haberer K, et al. Recurrence rates of arrhythmias during pregnancy in women with previous tachyarrhythmia and impact on fetal and neonatal outcomes. *Am J Cardiol*. 2006;97:1206–1212.
119. Chan WS, Anand S, Ginsberg JS. Anticoagulation of pregnant women with mechanical heart valves: a systematic review of the literature. *Arch Intern Med*. 2000;160:191–196.
120. Maxwell CV, Poppas A, Dunn E, et al. Pregnancy, mechanical heart valves and anticoagulation: navigating the complexities of management during gestation. In: Rosene-Montella K, Keely EJ, Lee RV, et al., eds. *Medical Care of the Pregnant Patient*. 2nd ed. Philadelphia, PA: American College of Physicians; 2007:344–355.
121. Bonow RO, Carabello BA, Chatterjee K, et al. ACC/AHA 2006 guidelines for the management of patients with valvular heart disease: a report of the American College of Cardiology/American Heart Association Task Force on Practice Guidelines. (Writing Committee to revise the 1998 Guidelines for the Management of Patients With Valvular Heart Disease). Developed in collaboration with the Society of Cardiovascular Anesthesiologists: endorsed by the Society for Cardiovascular Angiography and Interventions and the Society of Thoracic Surgeons. *Circulation*. 2006;114(5):e84–e231.
122. Miniero R, Tardivo I, Curtoni ES, et al. Outcome of pregnancy after organ transplantation: a retrospective survey in Italy. *Transplant Int*. 2005;17:724.
123. Wagoner L, Taylor D, Olson S, et al. Immunosuppressive therapy, management and outcomes of heart transplant recipients during pregnancy. *J Heart Lung Transplant*. 1993;12:993.
124. Branch KR, Wagoner LE, McGrory CH, et al. Risk of subsequent pregnancies on mother and newborn in female heart transplant recipients. *J Heart Lung Transplant*. 1998;17:698.
125. Hui D, Morrison LJ, Windrim R, et al. The American Heart Association 2010 guidelines for the management of cardiac arrest in pregnancy: consensus recommendations on implementation strategies. *J Obstet Gynaecol Can*. 2011;33:858–863.
126. Vanden Hoek TL, Morrison LJ, Shuster M, et al. Part 12. Cardiac arrest in special situations. 2010 American Heart Association Guidelines for Cardiopulmonary Resuscitation and Emergency Cardiovascular Care. *Circulation*. 2010;122:S829–S861.
127. Lipman S, Cohen S, Einav S, et al. The Society for Obstetric Anesthesia and Perinatology Consensus Statement on the management of cardiac arrest in pregnancy. *Anesth Analg*. 2014;118(5):1003–1016.

CHAPTER

79

Hemorrhagic and Liver Disorders of Pregnancy

ERICKA DOMALAKES, GENE T. LEE, and CARL P. WEINER

INTRODUCTION

Maternal mortality is defined as "The death of a woman while pregnant or within 42 days of termination of pregnancy, irrespective of the duration and the site of the pregnancy, from any cause related to or aggravated by the pregnancy or its management, but not from accidental or incidental causes" (Internal Classification of Diseases, 10th Revision, code O95). During the past century, the maternal mortality ratio in the United States significantly fell from 850 deaths per 100,000 deliveries in 1900, to 7.5 deaths per 100,000 in 1982, and then increased to 17.8 deaths per 100,000 live births in 2009 (1); unfortunately, this ratio has continued increasing. The National Center for Health Statistics has reported that the maternal mortality ratio increased by 62% between 1990 and 2006, from 8.2 to 13.3 per 100,000 (2). There are currently renewed efforts focusing on hospital safety, early warning signs, and improved training for perinatologists to address maternal mortality and morbidity (3–5).

Hemorrhage and hypertensive disorders are the major contributors to maternal death rates (6). Placental abruption, placenta previa, and accreta/increta/percreta disorders can become life threatening, and quickly pose a challenge for even an experienced obstetrician. Preeclampsia with severe features, including HELLP, can cause multiorgan failure including widespread coagulopathy. Appropriate care requires an efficient plan with the understanding of the unique complications associated with pregnancy and the gravid uterus. This chapter will focus on these conditions as well as imitators that are frequently equally morbid such as thrombotic thrombocytopenia purpura (TTP), atypical hemolytic uremic syndrome (aHUS), and acute fatty liver of pregnancy.

BACKGROUND PHYSIOLOGY CHANGES

Coagulation Changes

In pregnancy, if factors are measured, one will note an increase in factors I (fibrinogen), VII, VIII, IX, and X. Functional tests, such as the prothrombin time (PT), partial thromboplastin time (PTT), and bleeding times (BT) should not change in normal pregnancy. There is a relatively common disorder in pregnancy, gestational thrombocytopenia, that elicits an asymptomatic low platelet count. Most of these women have platelet values greater than 70,000 cells/μL, and two-thirds of them fall between 130,000 and 150,000 cells/μL (7). This diagnosis is used for women with no previous history of thrombocytopenia with occurrence during the third trimester. There is no fetal thrombocytopenia seen, and the disorder spontaneously resolves after delivery.

The reader is referred to Chapter 143 for a detailed description on coagulation disorders.

Liver Changes

Pregnancy-related hormones and fetal enzymes significantly affect the maternal liver. Known changes in the liver profile reveal a decrease in serum albumin, which is secondary to the dilutional effect of a 50% increase in maternal plasma volume. There is also an increase in serum alkaline phosphatase due to placental/fetal production. Markers of liver injury, such as aspartate aminotransferase, alanine aminotransferase, and lactate dehydrogenase, will not change in normal pregnancy. Bilirubin and gamma-glutamyl transpeptidase are both significantly lowered (8).

One of the main hormones causing alterations in the hepatic physiology is estrogen, which produces an increase in the hepatic rough endoplasmic reticulum, thereby increasing the production of proteins. The approximate sevenfold increase in estradiol—related to multiple factors, from changes in the binding hormones, to changes in metabolism and production—in the first trimester and a further fivefold increase by term, stimulates an approximate sixfold increase in the production of the sex hormone–binding globulin (9). Estrogen also has an inverse relationship with bile salt production and bile flow. There is a change in both composition of the bile and in the rate of cholesterol and phospholipid production; these changes produce increase in lithogenicity (10).

Progesterone, another hormone known to cause significant hepatic changes, mainly affects an increase of smooth endoplasmic reticulum and an increase in cytochrome P-450. Additionally, there is notable smooth muscle relaxation of the gallbladder and biliary ductal system. Progesterone can also produce slow-wave dysrhythmia in the gastrointestinal tract (11).

It is now thought that there are genetic influences specifically related to MDR3 gene mutations in liver diseases in pregnancy. Refer to Chapter 17 for more detailed description of essential physiologic concerns related to the liver.

Hemorrhagic Concerns

Significant bleeding in the pregnancy can be quantified by the total amount or by amount and time period over which the bleeding occurred (12,13). Generally, postpartum hemorrhage—defined by the total estimated blood loss—is established when there is greater than 500 mL for vaginal deliveries and more than 1 L for cesarean deliveries. Additionally, clinical symptoms and signs with respect to the blood loss are considered in the management. Postpartum hemorrhage can quickly become an emergent situation. There are many hospital systems that utilize a massive transfusion protocol; the main objective of these is to administer blood products early in the resuscitation process. These protocols involve a series of blood products and serum tests, which are automatically supplied based on the initiation of the protocol, without waiting for lab results. There are nuances seen, but many centers focus on a ratio of 1:1:1 for packed red blood cells, fresh frozen plasma, and platelets (14).

PLACENTAL COMPLICATIONS

Placental Abruption

Placental abruption (abruption placentae) is a condition in which the placenta separates from the implantation site of the uterus prior to the delivery of the fetus. The area of hemorrhage along the decidua basalis expands as the bleeding progresses. This hematoma may be concealed or present clinically with vaginal bleeding. The underlying mechanism may be related to vascular damage caused by preeclampsia, trauma, cocaine/alcohol use, or chorioamnionitis. Risk factors for abruption include either maternal or paternal (second-hand) smoking, multiparity, prior cesarean delivery, and African-American ethnicity (15,16). The incidence ranges between 0.4% and 0.8%, and there is a 15% recurrence rate for a subsequent pregnancy and a 20% recurrence rate after two previous episodes (17). Morbidity and mortality of both the mother and fetus can be significant with this process if the hemorrhage is significant.

Classic clinical manifestations include vaginal bleeding, abdominal pain/uterine irritability, and fetal heart rate abnormalities or fetal distress; of note, however, is that none or all of these symptoms may be present. It is important to have a high index of suspicion, because ultrasound has limited usefulness for diagnosis. It reveals a retroplacental blood clot in only 15% of cases, thus giving a high false-negative rate (15).

Treatment with fluid resuscitation, adequate oxygenation, and close fetal monitoring is critical. With evidence of significant hemorrhage or fetal distress, delivery must be expedited. It is critical to anticipate additional postpartum complications, such as uterine atony, to limit further hemorrhage.

Placenta Previa

Placental previa occurs with improper implantation of the placenta such that it overlies the internal os of the cervix during the third trimester. The incidence of placenta previa is noted to be approximately 0.5% (18). Risk factors include prior placenta previa, a history of cesarean delivery, a history of suction curettage, maternal age older than 35 years, African-American or non-Caucasian ethnicity, and cigarette smoking.

Clinical symptoms include painless vaginal bleeding beginning in the second or third trimester. Ultrasound is then performed to confirm or rule out the diagnosis. Management is expectant unless maternal bleeding or fetal heart rate abnormalities/fetal distress necessitate imminent delivery via cesarean section. If the patient is stable—meaning no bleeding—and the fetal surveillance is reassuring, the patient is closely monitored on pelvic rest until fetal lung maturity or 37 weeks' gestation, at which time a cesarean delivery is

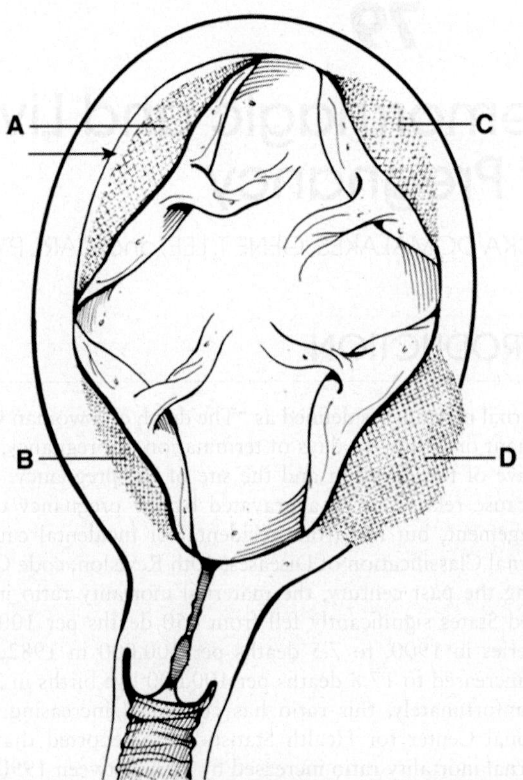

FIGURE 79.1 Forms of placenta accreta. A: Normal placenta. Nitabuch's layer is the clear space indicated by the *arrow*. B: Placenta accrete; note the lack of the Nitabuch's layer. C: Placenta increta, with deeper invasion into the myometrium. D: Placenta percreta, penetrating the uterine serosa. (From Lee RH, Grover J. Placenta accreta. In: Beall MH, Ross MG, eds. *Lippincott's Obstetrics Case-based Review*. Philadelphia, PA: Wolters Kluwer Health and Pharma; 2011:166.)

performed. Risks of placenta previa include other placental implantation abnormalities, such as placenta accreta, placenta increta, and placenta percreta (Fig. 79.1). The physician must be aware of these risks at the time of delivery and be prepared for a possible cesarean hysterectomy (hysterectomy performed at the time of a cesarean delivery) if necessary.

Placenta Accreta, Increta, Percreta

The issue of abnormal placentation can involve not only the specific location, but also how it is attached to the endometrial layer. Placenta accreta is a term for implantation in which there is abnormally firm adherence to the uterus. This is caused by abnormalities in the decidua basalis and Nitabuch layer (19). More specifically, placenta accreta, involves direct attachment between the placental villi and myometrium. Whereas placenta increta describes the villi invading the myometrium, percreta refers to a complete penetration through the myometrium, and may invade surrounding organs.

The overall incidences of the above placental problems has increased. This is thought to be due to the increasing rates of cesarean deliveries (20). Often, after a surgical procedure involving the lower uterine segment, the healing surgical site becomes an abnormal placentation attachment area. There is a noted significant increased risk with increasing cesarean deliveries, especially when considered at the time of a placenta previa. Early suspicion and detection are crucial for preventing significant morbidity and mortality. Antenatal diagnosis using ultrasound in conjunction with Doppler imaging may be helpful (21).

Abnormal placental attachment is an emergent issue facing clinicians today. There are more women presenting with increasing numbers of repeat cesarean sections, and many clinicians are not adequately prepared for the possible emergency at hand. Oftentimes, a placenta accreta/increta/percreta requires a cesarean hysterectomy; without proper antenatal diagnosis and preparation, this can become a dire situation. When diagnosed antenatally, there is the necessary time to plan for multidisciplinary management inputs. These may include uterine artery balloon occlusion by interventional radiology, urologic stent placement, additional surgical expertise from gynecologic oncology or general surgery, and early activation of massive transfusion protocols. While studies often do not show a significant difference in mortality or even total amount of blood products transfused for urologic stents or balloon occlusion of iliac arteries, many tertiary and quarternary centers nevertheless include these preparatory steps in their approach (22–24).

OTHER CONDITIONS ASSOCIATED WITH DISSEMINATED INTRAVASCULAR COAGULATION IN PREGNANCY

HELLP Syndrome

The topic of preeclampsia and eclampsia is discussed in Chapter 78, Cardiac Disease and Hypertensive Disorders in Pregnancy.

The acronym HELLP, for the syndrome consisting of hemolysis, elevated liver enzymes, and low platelets, was first used by Weinstein in 1982 (25). It is currently thought to be a distinct variant, rather than a progression, of the preeclampsia/eclampsia continuum. The incidence is rare, with Bhattacharya and Campbell (26) noting 13 cases of HELLP in a population of 4,188 patients with preeclampsia (310 cases/100,000 patients). Although much speculated, the true cause is unclear. Currently there are numerous genes thought to play a role in the development of HELLP syndrome, each of which seem to also interact in a complicated mechanism. In current research, near 200 genes have been identified in relation to preeclampsia or HELLP syndrome (27). We have also seen that the Fas receptor, Vascular Endothelial Growth Factor gene, and Factor V Leiden mutation are associated with an increased risk of HELLP when compared to healthy women (28). Although hundreds of possibilities have been discussed, there is no practical application for this information yet. Risk factors for this syndrome have been shown to include African Americans (29) and a history of prior pregnancies with HELLP. The recurrence rate has been reported at 14% (30).

HELLP is a disease with significant morbidity and mortality, both maternal and perinatal. In a prospective study of 442 pregnancies with HELLP, the risk of maternal death was found to be 1.1% (31). Significant maternal morbidity included DIC (21%), placental abruption (16%), acute renal failure (7.7%), pulmonary edema (6%), and rare occurrences of subcapsular liver hematoma and retinal detachment (32). Additionally, case reports of hepatic rupture (33–36) have been documented. Fetal outcome is typically related to the necessity to proceed with preterm delivery. Neonatal outcomes include risk of intensive care requirements, mechanical ventilation, sepsis, and intraventricular hemorrhage (37).

The clinical features and laboratory evaluation of HELLP have not been firmly defined. Generally, the findings reflect the disease process on the vascular supply of the maternal liver. The hemolysis can be noted by an abnormal peripheral smear, elevated serum bilirubin, low serum haptoglobin levels, elevated lactate dehydrogenase (LDH) of subtypes LDH1/LDH2, or a fall in the hemoglobin (32). Elevated liver enzymes, generally aspartate transaminases (AST), alanine transferase (ALT), and/or bilirubin are present; however, there is no strict definition of the degree of elevation, although many use a value roughly twice the upper limit of normal. There is also great variability in establishing the criteria for low platelets, varying from 150,000 to less than 50,000 cells/μL. Patients with HELLP will also have altered vascular reactivity (38), and methods of prediction by Doppler ultrasound have been examined, revealing a decrease in dual hepatic blood supply preceding the onset of HELLP (39,40). Objective parameters for disseminated intravascular coagulation (DIC) include prolonged prothrombin time (PT) and activated partial thromboplastin time (aPTT), elevated fibrinogen degradation products, and elevated D-dimers. It is important to note fibrinogen is increased in a normal pregnancy, so the value indicative of DIC may decrease to "normal" (nonpregnant) values; thus it is not used as an objective parameter.

Treatment of HELLP includes supportive care in a facility suited for such high-level care. Prompt delivery of the fetus is indicated if the patient is beyond 34 gestational weeks or sooner if the disease has progressed to multiorgan dysfunction, DIC, liver infarction or hemorrhage, renal failure, suspected placental abruption, or a nonreassuring fetal status (32). There has been debate regarding the management of a patient diagnosed with HELLP under 34 weeks gestation. There was a randomized controlled trial exploring expectant management for severe preeclamptic patients between 28 and 32 weeks, which had some positive outcomes; however, they excluded any patient with abnormal lab values (41), which is a diagnostic factor for HELLP. When making the decision to continue with pregnancy or expedite delivery, maternal morbidity/mortality is weighed against the risk of fetal prematurity and its associated morbidities. Many clinicians recommend treating with antenatal steroids for fetal lung maturity with subsequent delivery 24 to 48 hours later, if the patient is stable enough to delay delivery (31,42).

There is significant debate over the use of steroids for the treatment of the laboratory abnormalities of HELLP. Some studies have shown clinical benefit (32,33); whereas others (34) found insufficient evidence of beneficial effect. In 1990, a study performed at the University of Mississippi Medical Center found the use of glucocorticoids, antenatally or postpartum, demonstrated disease stabilization and accelerated recovery (43,44). Additionally, Eculizumab, a targeted inhibitor of complement protein C5, was utilized in a case report for the treatment of preeclampsia and HELLP syndrome. This resulted in a normalization of laboratory parameters and delayed delivery for 17 days, thus reducing neonatal morbidity (45). Although there are several promising possibilities for treatment, when HELLP syndrome progresses, management of DIC must address the underlying cause (46); transfusion of both packed red cells and component therapy as indicated, as well as fluid replacement and oxygenation, are critical.

Thrombotic Thrombocytopenic Purpura

When faced with thrombocytopenia in pregnancy, it is crucial to differentiate the cause so that the correct treatment may be utilized. Thrombotic thrombocytopenic purpura (TTP) is associated with low platelets and the formation of platelet thrombi in the microvasculature. Oftentimes, these are the only two signs present. However, the classic pentad includes microangiopathic hemolytic anemia, thrombocytopenic purpura, renal disease, neurologic abnormalities, and fever. It is often difficult to differentiate TTP from HELLP syndrome but, in general, with TTP the platelet counts will be lower and the LDH will be higher (47). The cause of TTP is a deficiency of ADAMTS13, a plasma metalloprotease, whose job is to cleave large von Willebrand factor multimers into smaller, more compact ones. There are a variety of reasons as to why plasma ADAMTS13 concentrations may be decreased in a pregnant patient, including genetic deficiency, autoimmune disorders, infection, DIC, pancreatitis, and pregnancy itself (48).

It is often necessary to make a presumptive diagnosis of TTP, based upon presentation and initial laboratory testing. Initial testing should include a CBC (thrombocytopenia), peripheral blood smear, complete metabolic profile (creatinine may be normal or increased), LDH (markedly elevated), bilirubin (elevated), haptoglobin level, coagulation testing (usually normal), Coombs test (negative), and ADAMTS13 activity and inhibitor. ADAMTS13 testing is only performed at specialized laboratories; therefore, treatment should be initiated when TTP suspected, even without confirmatory results. The mainstay treatment is plasma exchange therapy with glucocorticoids. With TTP, platelet transfusions are contraindicated, unless they are addressing an immediate life-threatening bleed (47). Platelet transfusion may actually worsen the condition by providing more material that will accumulate, then thrombose in the microvasculature (49). Because of this major difference in treatment, it is extremely important to differentiate between TTP and HELLP syndrome.

Atypical Hemolytic Uremic Syndrome

Hemolytic uremic syndrome (HUS) is defined as microangiopathic hemolytic anemia, thrombocytopenia, and acute kidney injury. aHUS, also referred to as complement-mediated HUS, is due to gene mutations on complement factors (48,49). aHUS is a rare condition, quoted to occur one-third to one-half as frequent as TTP; however, TTP and aHUS can be difficult to differentiate. There are clinical features which may help distinguish between the two, such as focal deficits are more common in TTP, and abdominal symptoms such as nausea, vomiting, and pain are more frequently seen with aHUS (48). Treatment for aHUS often involves supportive care along with plasma exchange; there has been promising research and outcomes with the addition of the drug Eculizumab (48).

ACUTE FATTY LIVER DISEASE IN PREGNANCY

Acute fatty liver disease of pregnancy (AFLP) is an extremely rare but potentially fatal disease that occurs in the third trimester. Mean gestational ages vary between 34.5 (50,51) and 37 weeks of gestation (52). Incidence has been documented as 1 in 6,659 births (53) to 1 in 15,900 births (53). It is characterized by significant malaise, nausea/vomiting, anorexia, abdominal pain, and jaundice (54). Clinical signs include hypertension, jaundice, elevated serum transaminases, coagulopathies, thrombocytopenia, and hypoglycemia. A high index of suspicion should be maintained if evidence of these signs and symptoms are noted (55). Imaging studies are often performed, but have limited usefulness in making the diagnosis; ultrasound may show nonspecific findings (55). Computed tomography (CT) has a high false-negative rate (51). Liver biopsy is the gold standard in confirming the diagnosis; however, it is rarely necessary and carries significant maternal risks in the setting of DIC.

This disease is noted to have significant risks with respect to morbidity and mortality. Older research reported maternal and perinatal mortality rates as high as 75% and 85%, respectively (55). Although the maternal mortality rate has fallen significantly, fetal mortality has remained as high as 66% (55). Maternal morbidity includes coagulopathies (specifically DIC) (56), hepatic encephalopathy (51), respiratory compromise (pulmonary edema or respiratory arrest) (51), and renal insufficiency (53). Research has shown that AFLP is more common if a woman is pregnant with a fetus homozygous for an inherited enzyme deficiency in mitochondrial beta-oxidation of fatty acids, long-chain 3-hydroxyacyl CoA dehydrogenase (LCHAD) deficiency. Presence of this deficiency increases the mother's risk 18-fold for developing AFLP (57).

Treatment of this disease is supportive, with management in a higher-level setting, specifically an ICU. Delivery is recommended as efficiently as possible. Debates regarding prolonged inductions and surgical risks of cesarean are common. The decision should be individualized, and should include the patient and her family. Hypoglycemia should be treated with dextrose-containing solutions. Elevated ammonia levels can be decreased with neomycin. Blood transfusions and replacement of clotting factors should be considered as appropriate. AFLP generally resolves within 7 to 10 days postpartum; however, cases of permanent hepatic failure requiring liver transplantation have been reported (58).

LIVER CONCERNS

Hyperemesis Gravidarum

Hyperemesis gravidarum (HG) is a condition characterized by serious and persistent vomiting that limits fluid intake and adequate nutrition. Clinical manifestations include weight loss greater than 5% of prepregnancy weight, weakness, dehydration, ketosis, and muscle wasting. HG occurs in approximately 0.3% to 2.0% of pregnancies, seems to affect a diverse population with multiple risk factors, and can be associated with a range of outcomes. Studies have associated HG to various hormone levels, including those of human chorionic gonadotropin, estrogen (59), prolactin (60), thyroxine (61), androgens (61), cortisol (62), and maternal prostaglandins (63). Other factors identified include a prior history of HG with previous pregnancies (64), female fetal gender (65,66), maternal age, maternal weight (67), and smoking (68). *Helicobacter pylori* may (69–71) or may not (72) have a role. Chronic medical conditions such as history of gastritis, allergies, and gallbladder disease (62) contribute to the risk. Additionally, the interpregnancy interval and paternity (65) have been examined; although the cause cannot be established, the relationship is being studied.

A complete differential diagnosis includes multiple systems. Obstetric and gynecologic conditions such as a molar pregnancy, degenerating uterine leiomyoma, or ovarian torsion should be considered. Gastrointestinal causes could include gastroenteritis, gastroparesis, achalasia, biliary tract disease, hepatitis, intestinal obstruction, peptic ulcer disease, pancreatitis, and appendicitis. The patient needs to be evaluated for urinary tract conditions, including pyelonephritis, uremia, and kidney stones. Metabolic diseases, including hyperthyroidism, diabetic ketoacidosis, porphyria, and Addison disease, should be ruled out. Neurologic disorders, drug reactions, and psychiatric conditions are other considerations.

Some studies have found HG to be protective against adverse outcomes (73), whereas more recent studies have failed to prove this relationship (74). Current research shows a relationship between HG and low birth weight that is mostly attributed to poor maternal weight gain (75–77). In addition to potentially compromised fetal outcomes, a worsened maternal morbidity and mortality are also noted. Cases of Wernicke encephalopathy (78–81), central pontine myelinolysis (82–84), severe liver injury (85), splenic avulsion (86) pneumomediastinum following esophageal rupture (87), and acute renal failure (88) have been reported.

Treatment for HG is primarily supportive, with antiemetics, fluid therapy, and electrolyte replacement. Natural remedies such as pyridoxine (vitamin B6) and ginger (89) have been shown to be effective. Additionally, behavior modification with avoidance of strong odors/scents and adjustment of diet may be tried. However, if these measures are inadequate, hospitalization and treatment with steroids (90–92) and parenteral nutrition may be necessary.

INTRAHEPATIC CHOLESTASIS OF PREGNANCY

Intrahepatic cholestasis of pregnancy (ICP) is the most frequent of the pregnancy-related liver diseases (93), occurring in approximately 1% of pregnancies (94). It is a condition characterized by the progressive pruritus of cholestasis, with elevated fasting bile salts—specifically chenodeoxycholic acid, deoxycholic acid, and cholic acid elevations more than 10 μmol/L—and elevated aminotransferases. Clinical manifestations begin in the late second or third trimester and most often will resolve spontaneously within 2 to 3 weeks postpartum. Although the direct cause is unknown, research has shown a strong familial component. Nonetheless, ICP affects specific populations at different rates. For example, ICP occurs in less than 0.2% of pregnancies in women of North American and Central/Western European descent, whereas Scandinavian and Baltic populations show a rate of 1% to 2%, and Chilean and Bolivian populations have shown rates of 5% to 15% (94). The severe form of ICP—bile acid levels above 40 μmol/L—in the Swedish population is associated with a frame shift mutations in the gene coding for the ATP-binding cassette transporter, specifically the ABCB4_5 gene variant (formerly known as multidrug resistance gene 3, MDR3) (95–97). Mutations in the bile salt export pump (BSEP) can also predispose a patient to ICP (98). Other possible causes relate to "leaky gut" theories (99). This theory is based on the increased absorption of bacterial endotoxins and the enterohepatic circulation of cholestatic metabolites of sex hormones and bile salts. Research has also shown an association with low maternal serum estrogen (100,101).

Fetal complication rates are directly related to maternal serum bile acids (102). Bile acid levels greater than 40 μmol/L are associated with preterm delivery, fetal asphyxia events, and meconium staining (103). Additionally, case reports of neonatal respiratory distress syndrome (103) and fetal death (104) are noted; on the other hand, maternal morbidity and mortality are low.

Supportive measures for pruritus with antihistamine are inadequate, as this agent has limited effectiveness and fails to address the bile acid elevation and fetal concerns. Cholestyramine, S-adenosylmethionine, and dexamethasone were the treatments of choice (105). However, newer research is advocating the use of ursodeoxycholic acid, which is a tertiary bile acid. Initial use of ursodeoxycholic acid was with bear bile in traditional Chinese medicine for the treatment of liver disease (106). Recent research has shown ursodeoxycholic acid to be more effective in reducing bile acids and bilirubin (107–110). Fetal risks are decreased, but not eliminated. Because of this, careful fetal monitoring and delivery at 36 to 37 weeks should be considered (111). Earlier delivery at fetal lung maturity has also been advocated (105).

Key Points

- Maternal mortality has been increasing in the United States over the last decade due to a lapse in attention and training regarding critical conditions in pregnancy.
- Placenta previa and accreta are disorders which require multidisciplinary teamwork involving interventional radiology, urology, gynecology oncology, and blood bank.
- HELLP syndrome requires prompt delivery, with delay reserved for administration of antenatal steroids, and supportive therapy in a critical care setting.
- TTP and atypical HUS are imitators of HELLP syndrome. Diagnosis should include assessment of ADAMTS13 levels for TTP and complement levels for aHUS.
- Fetal death is associated with cholestasis of pregnancy. It is infrequent but unpredictable, and earlier delivery is advocated due to this.

References

1. Creanga AA, Berg CJ, Ko JY, et al. Maternal mortality and morbidity in the United States: where are we now? *J Womens Health (Larchmt)*. 2014;23(1):3–9.
2. Heron M, Hoyert DL, Murphy SL, et al. Deaths: final data for 2006. *Natl Vital Stat Rep*. 2009;57:1–136.
3. Mhyre JM, D'Oria R, Hameed AB, et al. The maternal early warning criteria: a proposal from the national partnership for maternal safety. *Obstet Gynecol*. 2014;124(4):782–786.
4. D'Alton ME. Where is the "M" in maternal-fetal medicine? *Obstet Gynecol*. 2010;116(6):1401–1404.
5. D'Alton ME, Bonanno CA, Berkowitz RL, et al. Putting the "M" back in maternal-fetal medicine. *Am J Obstet Gynecol*. 2013;208(6):442–448.
6. Khan KS, et al. WHO analysis of causes of maternal death: a systematic review. *Lancet*. 2006. 367(9516):1066–1074.

7. George JN, Knudson EJ. Thrombocytopenia in pregnancy. UpToDate. Avaible at: http://www.uptodate.com/contents/thrombocytopenia-in-pregnancy?source=search_result&search=thrombocytopenia+in+pregnancy&selectedTitle=1~150. Updated November 13, 2015; accessed March 4, 2016.
8. Bacq Y, Zarka O, Bréchot JF, et al. Liver function tests in normal pregnancy: a prospective study of 103 pregnant women and 103 matched controls. *Hepatology*. 1996;23(5):1030–1034.
9. O'Leary P, Boyne P, Flett P, et al. Longitudinal assessment of changes in reproductive hormones during normal pregnancy. *Clin Chem*. 1991;37(5):667–672.
10. Lynn J, Williams L, O'Brien J, et al. Effects of estrogen upon bile: implications with respect to gallstone formation. *Ann Surg*. 1973;178(4):514–524.
11. Walsh JW, Hasler WL, Nugent CE, Owyang C. Progesterone and estrogen are potential mediators of gastric slow-wave dysrhythmias in nausea of pregnancy. *Am J Physiol*. 1996;270(3 Pt 1):G506–G514.
12. Sobieszczyk S, Breborowicz G. Management recommendations for postpartum hemorrhage. *Arch Perinat Med*. 2004;10(4):1–4.
13. Macphail S, Talks K. Massive post-partum haemorrhage and management of disseminated intravascular coagulation. *Curr Obstet Gynaecol*. 2004;14(2):123–131.
14. Pacheco LD, Saade GR, Constantine MM, et al. An update on the use of massive transfusion protocols in obstetrics. *Am J Obstet Gynecol*. 2016; 214(3):340–344.
15. Tikkanen M, Nuutila M, Hiilesmaa V, et al. Clinical presentation and risk factors of placental abruption. *Acta Obstet Gynecol Scand*. 2006;85(6):700–705.
16. Getahun D, Oyelese Y, Salihu HM, Ananth CV. Previous cesarean delivery and risks of placenta previa and placental abruption. *Obstet Gynecol*. 2006;107(4):771–778.
17. Rasmussen S, Irgens LM, Dalaker K. The effect on the likelihood of further pregnancy of placental abruption and the rate of its recurrence. *Br J Obstet Gynaecol*. 1997;104(11):1292–1295.
18. Iyasu S, Saftlas AK, Rowley DL, et al. The epidemiology of placenta previa in the United States, 1979 through 1987. *Am J Obstet Gynecol*. 1993;168(5):1424–1429.
19. Placental Abnormalities. In: Cunningham FG, Leveno KJ, Bloom SL, et al., eds. Williams Obstetrics, 24th ed. New York, NY: McGraw-Hill; 2013. Available at: http://accessmedicine.mhmedical.com/content.aspx?bookid=1057§ionid=59789142; accessed April 06, 2017.
20. Silver RM, Landon MB, Rouse DJ, et al. Maternal morbidity associated with multiple repeat cesarean deliveries. *Obstet Gynecol*. 2006;107(6):1226–1232.
21. Shetty MK, Dryden DK. Morbidly adherent placenta: ultrasound assessment and supplemental role of magnetic resonance imaging. *Semin Ultrasound CT MR*. 2015;36(4):324–331.
22. Shrivastava V, Nageotte M, Major C, et al. Case-control comparison of cesarean hysterectomy with and without prophylactic placement of intravascular balloon catheters for placenta accreta. *Am J Obstet Gynecol*. 2007;197(4):402.e1–5.
23. Eller AG, Porter TF, Soisson P, Silver RM. Optimal management strategies for placenta accreta. *BJOG*. 2009;116(5):648–654.
24. Sentilhes L, Goffinet F, Kayem G. Management of placenta accreta. *Acta Obstet Gynecol Scand*. 2013;92(10):1125–1134.
25. Weinstein L. Syndrome of hemolysis, elevated liver enzymes, and low platelet count: a severe consequence of hypertension in pregnancy. *Am J Obstet Gynecol*. 1982;142(2):159–167.
26. Bhattacharya S, Campbell DM. The incidence of severe complications of preeclampsia. *Hypertens Pregnancy*. 2005;24(2):181–190.
27. Jebbink J, Wolters A, Fernando F, et al. Molecular genetics of preeclampsia and HELLP syndrome: a review. *Biochim Biophys Acta*. 2012; 1822(12):1960–1969.
28. Haram K, Mortensen JH, Nagy B. Genetic aspects of preeclampsia and the HELLP syndrome. *J Pregnancy*. 2014;2014:910751.
29. Haddad B, Barton JR, Livingston JC, et al. Risk factors for adverse maternal outcomes among women with HELLP (hemolysis, elevated liver enzymes, and low platelet count) syndrome. *Am J Obstet Gynecol*. 2000;183(2):444–448.
30. Hupuczi P, Rigó B, Sziller I, et al. Follow-up analysis of pregnancies complicated by HELLP syndrome. *Fetal Diagn Ther*. 2006;21(6):519–522.
31. Sibai BM. Diagnosis, controversies, and management of the syndrome of hemolysis, elevated liver enzymes, and low platelet count. *Obstet Gynecol*. 2004;103(5 Pt 1):981–991.
32. Sibai BM, Ramadan MK, Usta I, et al. Maternal morbidity and mortality in 442 pregnancies with hemolysis, elevated liver enzymes, and low platelets (HELLP syndrome). *Am J Obstet Gynecol*. 1993;169(4):1000–1006.
33. Hafeez, M, S Hameed, Hellp syndrome and subcapsular liver haematoma. *J Coll Physicians Surg Pak*. 2005;15(11):733–735.
34. Herring CS, Heywood SG, Hatjis CG. The multiple challenges in the management of a patient with HELLP syndrome, liver rupture and eclampsia. *W V Med J*. 2005;101(6):261–262.
35. Shrivastava VK, Imagawa D, Wing DA. Argon beam coagulator for treatment of hepatic rupture with hemolysis, elevated liver enzymes, low platelets (HELLP) syndrome. *Obstet Gynecol*. 2006;107(2 Pt 2):525–526.
36. Araujo AC, Leao MD, Nobrega MH, et al. Characteristics and treatment of hepatic rupture caused by HELLP syndrome. *Am J Obstet Gynecol*. 2006;195(1):129–133.
37. Kim HY, Sohn YS, Lim JH, et al. Neonatal outcome after preterm delivery in HELLP syndrome. *Yonsei Med J*. 2006;47(3):393–398.
38. Fischer T, Schneider MP, Schobel HP, et al. Vascular reactivity in patients with preeclampsia and HELLP (hemolysis, elevated liver enzymes, and low platelet count) syndrome. *Am J Obstet Gynecol*. 2000;183(6):1489–1494.
39. Oosterhof H, Voorhoeve PG, Aarnoudse JG. Enhancement of hepatic artery resistance to blood flow in preeclampsia in presence or absence of HELLP syndrome (hemolysis, elevated liver enzymes, and low platelets). *Am J Obstet Gynecol*. 1994;171(2):526–530.
40. Kawabata I, Nakai A, Takeshita T. Prediction of HELLP syndrome with assessment of maternal dual hepatic blood supply by using Doppler ultrasound. *Arch Gynecol Obstet*. 2006;274(5):303–309.
41. Sibai BM, Mercer BM, Schiff E, Friedman SA. Aggressive versus expectant management of severe preeclampsia at 28 to 32 weeks' gestation: a randomized controlled trial. *Am J Obstet Gynecol*. 1994;171(3):818–822.
42. Magee LA, Yong PJ, Espinosa V, et al. Expectant management of severe preeclampsia remote from term: a structured systematic review. *Hypertens Pregnancy*. 2009;28(3):312–347.
43. Magann EF, Perry KG Jr, Meydrech EF, et al. Postpartum corticosteroids: accelerated recovery from the syndrome of hemolysis, elevated liver enzymes, and low platelets (HELLP). *Am J Obstet Gynecol*. 1994;171(4):1154–1158.
44. Magann EF, Bass D, Chauhan SP, et al. Antepartum corticosteroids: disease stabilization in patients with the syndrome of hemolysis, elevated liver enzymes, and low platelets (HELLP). *Am J Obstet Gynecol*. 1994;171(4):1148–1153.
45. Burwick RM, Feinberg BB. Eculizumab for the treatment of preeclampsia/HELLP syndrome. *Placenta*. 2013;34(2):201–203.
46. Labelle CA, Kitchens CS. Disseminated intravascular coagulation: treat the cause, not the lab values. *Cleve Clin J Med*. 2005;72(5):377–378.
47. Guntupalli KK, Hall N, Karnad DR, et al. Critical illness in pregnancy: part I: an approach to a pregnant patient in the ICU and common obstetric disorders. *Chest*. 2015;148(4):1093–1104.
48. Tsai HM, Untying the knot of thrombotic thrombocytopenic purpura and atypical hemolytic uremic syndrome. *Am J Med*. 2013;126(3):200–209.
49. Kappler S, Ronan-Bentle S, Graham A. Thrombotic microangiopathies (TTP, HUS, HELLP). *Emerg Med Clin North Am*. 2014;32(3):649–671.
50. Usta IM, Barton JR, Amon EA, et al. Acute fatty liver of pregnancy: an experience in the diagnosis and management of fourteen cases. *Am J Obstet Gynecol*. 1994;171(5):1342–1347.
51. Mjahed K, Charra B, Hamoudi D, et al. Acute fatty liver of pregnancy. *Arch Gynecol Obstet*. 2006;274(6):349–353.
52. Castro MA, Fassett MJ, Reynolds TB, et al. Reversible peripartum liver failure: a new perspective on the diagnosis, treatment, and cause of acute fatty liver of pregnancy, based on 28 consecutive cases. *Am J Obstet Gynecol*. 1999;181(2):389–395.
53. Reyes H, Sandoval L, Wainstein A, et al. Acute fatty liver of pregnancy: a clinical study of 12 episodes in 11 patients. *Gut*. 1994;35(1):101–106.
54. Bacq Y. Acute fatty liver of pregnancy. *Semin Perinatol*. 1998;22(2):134–140.
55. Kaplan MM. Acute fatty liver of pregnancy. *N Engl J Med*. 1985;313(6):367–370.
56. Yucesoy G, Ozkan SO, Bodur H, et al. Acute fatty liver of pregnancy complicated with disseminated intravascular coagulation and haemorrhage: a case report. *Int J Clin Pract Suppl*. 2005;(147):82–84.
57. Goel A, Jamwal KD, Ramachandran A, et al. Pregnancy-related liver disorders. *J Clin Exp Hepatol*. 2014;4(2):151–162.
58. Ockner SA, Brunt EM, Cohn SM, et al. Fulminant hepatic failure caused by acute fatty liver of pregnancy treated by orthotopic liver transplantation. *Hepatology*. 1990;11(1):59–64.
59. Lagiou P, Tamimi R, Mucci LA, et al. Nausea and vomiting in pregnancy in relation to prolactin, estrogens, and progesterone: a prospective study. *Obstet Gynecol*. 2003;101(4):639–644.
60. Panesar NS, Li CY, Rogers MS. Are thyroid hormones or hCG responsible for hyperemesis gravidarum? A matched paired study in pregnant Chinese women. *Acta Obstet Gynecol Scand*. 2001;80(6):519–524.
61. Carlsen SM, Vanky E, Jacobsen G. Nausea and vomiting associate with increasing maternal androgen levels in otherwise uncomplicated pregnancies. *Acta Obstet Gynecol Scand*. 2003;82(3):225–228.

62. Jarnfelt-Samsioe A, Samsioe G, Velinder GM. Nausea and vomiting in pregnancy: a contribution to its epidemiology. *Gynecol Obstet Invest.* 1983;16(4):221–229.
63. Gadsby R, Barnie-Adshead A, Grammatoppoulos D, Gadsby P. Nausea and vomiting in pregnancy: an association between symptoms and maternal prostaglandin E2. *Gynecol Obstet Invest.* 2000;50(3):149–152.
64. Trogstad LI, Stoltenberg C, Magnus P, et al. Recurrence risk in hyperemesis gravidarum. *BJOG.* 2005;112(12):1641–1645.
65. del Mar Melero-Montes M, Jick H. Hyperemesis gravidarum and the sex of the offspring. *Epidemiology.* 2001;12(1):123–124.
66. Schiff MA, Reed SD, Daling JR. The sex ratio of pregnancies complicated by hospitalisation for hyperemesis gravidarum. *BJOG.* 2004;111(1):27–30.
67. Depue RH, Bernstein L, Ross RK, et al. Hyperemesis gravidarum in relation to estradiol levels, pregnancy outcome, and other maternal factors: a seroepidemiologic study. *Am J Obstet Gynecol.* 1987;156(5):1137–1141.
68. Zhang J, Cai WW. Severe vomiting during pregnancy: antenatal correlates and fetal outcomes. *Epidemiology.* 1991;2(6):454–457.
69. Kuscu NK, Koyuncu F. Hyperemesis gravidarum: current concepts and management. *Postgrad Med J.* 2002;78(916):76–79.
70. Lee RH, Pan VL, Wing DA. The prevalence of *Helicobacter pylori* in the Hispanic population affected by hyperemesis gravidarum. *Am J Obstet Gynecol.* 2005;193(3 Pt 2):1024–1027.
71. Verberg MF, Gillott DJ, Al-Fardan N, Grudzinskas JG. Hyperemesis gravidarum, a literature review. *Hum Reprod Update.* 2005;11(5):527–539.
72. Jacobson GF, Autry AM, Somer-Shely TL, et al. *Helicobacter pylori* seropositivity and hyperemesis gravidarum. *J Reprod Med.* 2003;48(8):578–582.
73. Weigel RM, Weigel MM. Nausea and vomiting of early pregnancy and pregnancy outcome: a meta-analytical review. *Br J Obstet Gynaecol.* 1989;96(11):1312–1318.
74. Weigel MM, Reyes M, Caiza ME, et al. Is the nausea and vomiting of early pregnancy really feto-protective? *J Perinat Med.* 2006;34(2):115–122.
75. Bailit JL. Hyperemesis gravidarium: epidemiologic findings from a large cohort. *Am J Obstet Gynecol.* 2005;193(3 Pt 1):811–814.
76. Dodds L, Fell DB, Joseph KS, et al. Outcomes of pregnancies complicated by hyperemesis gravidarum. *Obstet Gynecol.* 2006;107(2 Pt 1):285–292.
77. Fell DB, Dodds L, Joseph KS, et al. Risk factors for hyperemesis gravidarum requiring hospital admission during pregnancy. *Obstet Gynecol.* 2006;107(2 Pt 1):277–284.
78. Chiossi G, Neri I, Cavazzuti M, et al. Hyperemesis gravidarum complicated by Wernicke encephalopathy: background, case report, and review of the literature. *Obstet Gynecol Surv.* 2006;61(4):255–268.
79. Rastenyte D, Obelieniene D, Kondrackiene J, Gleizniene R. (Wernicke's encephalopathy induced by hyperemesis gravidarum (case report)). *Medicina (Kaunas).* 2003;39(1):56–61.
80. Indraccolo U, Gentile G, Pomili G, et al. Thiamine deficiency and beriberi features in a patient with hyperemesis gravidarum. *Nutrition.* 2005;21(9):967–968.
81. Togay-Isikay C, Yigit A, Mutluer N. Wernicke's encephalopathy due to hyperemesis gravidarum: an under-recognised condition. *Aust N Z J Obstet Gynaecol.* 2001;41(4):453–456.
82. Tonelli J, Zurrú MC, Castillo J, et al. (Central pontine myelinolysis induced by hyperemesis gravidarum). *Medicina (B Aires).* 1999;59(2):176–178.
83. Burneo J, Vizcarra D, Miranda H. [Central pontine myelinolysis and pregnancy: a case report and review of literature]. *Rev Neurol.* 2000; 30(11):1036–1040.
84. Valiulis B, Kelley RE, Hardjasudarma M, London S. Magnetic resonance imaging detection of a lesion compatible with central pontine myelinolysis in a pregnant patient with recurrent vomiting and confusion. *J Neuroimag.* 2001;11(4):441–443.
85. Vitoratos N, Botsis D, Detsis G, Creatsas G. Severe liver injury due to hyperemesis gravidarum. *J Obstet Gynaecol.* 2006;26(2):172–173.
86. Nguyen N, Deitel M, Lacy E. Splenic avulsion in a pregnant patient with vomiting. *Can J Surg.* 1995;38(5):464–465.
87. Liang SG, Ooka F, Santo A, Kaibara M. Pneumomediastinum following esophageal rupture associated with hyperemesis gravidarum. *J Obstet Gynaecol Res.* 2002;28(3):172–175.
88. Hill JB, Yost NP, Wendel GB Jr. Acute renal failure in association with severe hyperemesis gravidarum. *Obstet Gynecol.* 2002;100(5 Pt 2):1119–1121.
89. Jewell D, Young G. Interventions for nausea and vomiting in early pregnancy. *Cochrane Database Syst Rev.* 2003;(4):CD000145.
90. Moran P, Taylor R. Management of hyperemesis gravidarum: the importance of weight loss as a criterion for steroid therapy. *QJM.* 2002;95(3): 153–158.
91. Nelson-Piercy C, Fayers P, de Swiet M. Randomised, double-blind, placebo-controlled trial of corticosteroids for the treatment of hyperemesis gravidarum. *BJOG.* 2001;108(1):9–15.
92. Bondok RS, El Sharnouby NM, Eid HE, Abd Elmaksoud AM. Pulsed steroid therapy is an effective treatment for intractable hyperemesis gravidarum. *Crit Care Med.* 2006;34(11):2781–2783.
93. Lammert F, Marschall HU, Glantz A, Matern S. Intrahepatic cholestasis of pregnancy: molecular pathogenesis, diagnosis and management. *J Hepatol.* 2000;33(6):1012–1021.
94. Ropponen A, Sund R, Riikonen S, et al. Intrahepatic cholestasis of pregnancy as an indicator of liver and biliary diseases: a population-based study. *Hepatology.* 2006;43(4):723–728.
95. Dixon PH, Weerasekera N, Linton KJ, et al. Heterozygous MDR3 missense mutation associated with intrahepatic cholestasis of pregnancy: evidence for a defect in protein trafficking. *Hum Mol Genet.* 2000;9(8):1209–1217.
96. Floreani A, Carderi I, Paternoster D, et al. Intrahepatic cholestasis of pregnancy: three novel MDR3 gene mutations. *Aliment Pharmacol Ther.* 2006;23(11):1649–1653.
97. Wasmuth HE, Glantz A, Keppeler H, et al. Intrahepatic cholestasis of pregnancy: the severe form is associated with common variants of the hepatobiliary phospholipid transporter ABCB4 gene. *Gut.* 2007;56(2):265–270.
98. Kubitz R, Keitel V, Scheuring S, et al. Benign recurrent intrahepatic cholestasis associated with mutations of the bile salt export pump. *J Clin Gastroenterol.* 2006;40(2):171–175.
99. Reyes H, Zapata R, Hernández I, et al. Is a leaky gut involved in the pathogenesis of intrahepatic cholestasis of pregnancy? *Hepatology.* 2006; 43(4):715–722.
100. Reyes H, Simon FR. Intrahepatic cholestasis of pregnancy: an estrogen-related disease. *Semin Liver Dis.* 1993;13(3):289–301.
101. Leslie KK, Reznikov L, Simon FR, et al. Estrogens in intrahepatic cholestasis of pregnancy. *Obstet Gynecol.* 2000;95(3):372–376.
102. Glantz A, Marschall HU, Mattsson LA. Intrahepatic cholestasis of pregnancy: relationships between bile acid levels and fetal complication rates. *Hepatology.* 2004;40(2):467–474.
103. Zecca E, De Luca D, Marras M, et al. Intrahepatic cholestasis of pregnancy and neonatal respiratory distress syndrome. *Pediatrics.* 2006;117(5): 1669–1672.
104. Sentilhes L, Verspyck E, Pia P, Marpeau L. Fetal death in a patient with intrahepatic cholestasis of pregnancy. *Obstet Gynecol.* 2006;107(2 Pt 2): 458–460.
105. Lammert F, Marschall HU, Matern S. Intrahepatic cholestasis of pregnancy. *Curr Treat Options Gastroenterol.* 2003;6(2):123–132.
106. Hagey LR, Crombie DL, Espinosa E, et al. Ursodeoxycholic acid in the Ursidae: biliary bile acids of bears, pandas, and related carnivores. *J Lipid Res.* 1993;34(11):1911–1917.
107. Brites D. Intrahepatic cholestasis of pregnancy: changes in maternal-fetal bile acid balance and improvement by ursodeoxycholic acid. *Ann Hepatol.* 2002;1(1):20–28.
108. Copaci I, Micu L, Iliescu L, Voiculescu M. New therapeutical indications of ursodeoxycholic acid. *Rom J Gastroenterol.* 2005;14(3):259–266.
109. Glantz A, Marschall HU, Lammert F, Mattsson LA. Intrahepatic cholestasis of pregnancy: a randomized controlled trial comparing dexamethasone and ursodeoxycholic acid. *Hepatology.* 2005;42(6):1399–1405.
110. Zapata R, Sandoval L, Palma J, et al. Ursodeoxycholic acid in the treatment of intrahepatic cholestasis of pregnancy: a 12-year experience. *Liver Int.* 2005;25(3):548–554.
111. Geenes V, Chappell LC, Seed PT, et al. Association of severe intrahepatic cholestasis of pregnancy with adverse pregnancy outcomes: a prospective population-based case-control study. *Hepatology.* 2014;59:1482–1491.

CHAPTER

80

Acute Abdomen and Trauma during Pregnancy

SCOTT ALEXANDER HARVEY

INTRODUCTION

Pregnancy induces different physiologic and anatomic factors that make evaluation and treatment of a pregnant woman different than that of the nonpregnant individual. The clinician has the opportunity to care for two (or more) patients, as the survival of the fetus will be dependent on instituting normal maternal physiology or delivering the fetus, depending on the gestational age. This chapter summarizes the approach to evaluate, diagnose, and treat the gravid patient with a surgical or traumatic process within the abdomen, highlighting the key differences owing to maternal physiology.

Of women aged 12 to 44 years old, 102.1 per 1,000 women are pregnant at any given time, with the highest rate of pregnancy in ages 20s to 30s (1). The incidence of a pregnant woman developing a disease requiring nonobstetric surgery is approximately 0.2% to 0.75% (2). The American College of Obstetricians and Gynecologists (ACOG) has released multiple guidelines to help guide surgical and obstetrical management with recommendations for disease conditions as they relate to the pregnant woman. Some foundational facts regarding surgery during pregnancy are found in Table 80.1, with the knowledge that no woman should be declined *indicated* surgery based on pregnancy status or gestational age (3).

In addition to acute surgical conditions, trauma affects 5% to 8% of pregnant women and is the leading cause of nonobstetric death in the United States (4–7). The scope of trauma could be as minor as bumping the abdomen into a table to a pregnant woman falling, as pregnant women are more prone to falls (8), to a motor vehicle passenger ejection, victim of domestic violence, or other major traumatic event. Clinical knowledge that the patient is pregnant is an integral part of the trauma assessment, either in the primary survey (based on history or physical examination), or the secondary survey as an incidental finding from an ultrasound examination or pregnancy test. In one trauma center, "incidental pregnancy" found on routine screening during the trauma assessment in 11% of women of reproductive age, where 8% of those patients were unaware of their gravid state (9); this warrants routine pregnancy screening during trauma assessment of all women age 12 to 50 years old. Resuscitation, evaluation, and monitoring algorithms are altered in pregnancy; nonetheless, these management principles will involve the mother primarily. Improvements in fetal and neonatal management allow better administration of medical care to save the life of the fetus, despite a higher incidence of fetal mortality with surgical disease (around 2% to 20%, depending on disease [10]). Of note, motor vehicle crashes still are the leading cause of fetal death due to maternal trauma (11,12). When evaluating pregnant women for a surgical or traumatic process, it is important to understand the basics of their altered physiology.

MATERNAL PHYSIOLOGY AND LABORATORY VALUES

Maternal adaptations in physiologic and anatomic parameters are paramount for fetal growth and maternal protection during parturition. A full explanation of maternal adaptations with pregnancy is beyond the scope of this chapter, but understanding the basics of cardiopulmonary, gastrointestinal, renal, and hematologic changes are important for management and resuscitation of these patients. Selected physiologic laboratory parameters are displayed in Table 80.2.

The maternal blood volume increases by 40% to 50%, starting at about 8 weeks of gestational age (wGA), to peak around 32 wGA. A physiologic anemia is induced by estrogen's effects on the renal–angiotensin–aldosterone system as blood plasma increases in greater proportion than that of the red blood cell mass (13–15). Placental factors to include progesterone and placental chorionic somatotropin increase erythropoietin production and bone marrow stimulation of red blood cell synthesis (16). Blood vessels are more prone to vasodilation causing a reflex tachycardia, and in conjunction with a higher blood volume and cardiac preload, cardiac output increases by about 1.5% (17,18). There is a higher oxygen consumption that increases with gestational age as blood flow to the uterus increases from 2% in the nonpregnant uterus to about 17% at term.

With anatomic compression of the abdominal contents by the uterus, there is a reduction in total lung capacity, residual volume, and expiratory reserve volume. Tidal volume and respiratory rate increase to create a higher minute ventilation, a respiratory alkalosis, relative hypocarbia, and a compensatory reduced bicarbonate (19). With the increase in 2,3-diphosphoglycerate, there is a relatively unchanged hemoglobin–oxygen dissociation curve, while the partial pressure of oxygen (PaO_2) reduces slightly due to lung atelectasis and intrapulmonary shunting (20,21). Of note, fetal oxygenation is the best with a PaO_2 above 70 mmHg and oxygen saturation over 95% (21).

There is increased renal blood flow and glomerular filtration with a resultant reduction in blood urea nitrogen and creatinine (22). The normalized hemoglobin is reduced and white blood cells are slightly increased, with an unchanged platelet count. In order to prevent exsanguination at delivery, maternal adaptations increase fibrinogen by about 50%, reduce fibrinolysis, and increase excretion of Protein S, creating a hypercoagulable state and increasing the risk of deep vein thrombosis and pulmonary embolism. Lastly, there is reduced gut motility,

TABLE 80.1 ACOG Statement and Recommendations for Nonobstetric Surgery

- No current anesthetics have been shown for teratogenic effects at standard concentrations at any gestational age
- Fetal monitoring
  - May aid in intraoperative maternal positioning
  - Previable fetus: preoperative and postoperative fetal doptones
  - Viable fetus
    - At least preoperative and postoperative fetal monitoring is recommended
    - Intraoperative monitoring is advised if it is physically possible during the procedure, an obstetric provider is available and able to intervene during the procedure for fetal indications, the nature of surgery can safely accommodate an emergency delivery, and when possible, the woman has given informed consent for cesarean delivery
  - Surgery to be performed at an institution with obstetric and neonatal/pediatric care
- A pregnant woman should not be denied indicated surgery, regardless of trimester of gestation
- Avoidance of elective surgery in pregnancy
- If able, avoidance of surgery until the second trimester

From American College of Obstetrics and Gynecology. Nonobstetric surgery during pregnancy. *ACOG Committee Opinion*. Feb 2011, No 474.

increased insulin resistance, and maternal hyperglycemia to improve nutrition to the fetus (19). These and many more maternal adaptations are pivotal for fetal development, and normalization of maternal physiology to these parameters is recommended as endpoints of resuscitation.

PRETERM LABOR

A preterm birth is defined as a delivery between 20 0/7 and 36 6/7 weeks of gestation (23) and is the second leading cause to neonatal mortality in the United States (second to birth defects) (24). Advancements in neonatal medicine have reduced mortality, but there is still a strikingly high rate of disability in periviable neonates that survive (23). As preterm labor is the highest risk factor for a preterm birth, it is crucial for the clinician to recognize the syndrome and employ appropriate counseling and management in conjunction with the consultative services of the Obstetrician and Neonatologist and/or Pediatrician.

TABLE 80.2 Normal Laboratory Values during Pregnancy

Value	Change	Range
WBC	Increased	5,000–15,000 cells/mm^3
Hemoglobin	Decreased	10.5–13.5 g/dL
Hematocrit	Decreased	30.5–39%
Platelet	Unchanged	150–380 × 103/µL
Fibrinogen	Increased	265–615 mg/dL
D-Dimer	Frequently positive	—
HCO_3^-	Compensatory acidosis	18–22 mEq/L
BUN	Decreased	3–4 mg/dL
Creatinine	Decreased	0.4–0.7 mg/dL
Albumin	Decreased	2.7–3.7 g/dL
AST, ALT	Unchanged	12–38 U/L
Bilirubin	Unchanged	0.2–0.6 mg/dL
Alkaline phosphatase	Increased	60–140 IU/L

ALT, alanine aminotransferase; AST, aspartate aminotransferase; BUN, blood urea nitrogen; HCO_3^-, bicarbonate; WBC, white blood cell count.
From Lockitch G. The effect of normal pregnancy on common biochemistry and hematology tests. In: Barron WM, Lindheimer MD, eds. *Medical Disorders During Pregnancy*. 3rd ed. St. Louis, MO: Mosby; 2000.

Preterm Labor Evaluation

Preterm labor is defined as regular uterine contractions in conjunction with cervical dilation and/or effacement (25). Multiple risk factors for preterm labor include nonwhite race, age less than 17 or more than 35 years old, low socioeconomic status, low prepregnancy weight, history of preterm birth, vaginal bleeding during pregnancy, and smoking (26). The pathophysiology of preterm labor relates to activation of the labor process that is similar, but prior, to a term gestation. There is a physiologic activation of the "common labor pathway," with anatomical, biochemical, immunologic, and endocrinologic events that dilate the cervix, rupture amniotic membranes, and cause uterine contractions to evacuate the fetus. The preterm activation of this "common labor pathway" is considered pathologic and may relate to a multitude of diseases to include underlying uterine infections, systemic infections and microbial induced inflammation, uterine distention, placental dehiscence, and even maternal stress (27). Both surgical syndromes and trauma may induce the activation of preterm labor, making it critical to recognize and employ treatment when appropriate. Preterm labor is frequent among surgical interventions. In one series of 77 patients undergoing nonobstetric surgery, preterm labor was seen in 26% of patients in the second trimester and in 82% of those in the third trimester. Preterm labor leading to preterm delivery was most common after appendicitis and adnexal surgery, where preterm birth was seen in 16% of the patients. However, only 5% of surgical cases demonstrated a clear established link to the surgical procedure (10). Another study showed 18% of 62 pregnant subjects with nonobstetric abdominal surgery delivered preterm, again associating abdominal surgery to preterm birth (28).

The evaluation of preterm labor may include imaging and laboratories in addition to the history and physical examination. Fetal monitoring should begin to assess the frequency of patient perceived and nonperceived contractions and to evaluate fetal status by the fetal heart rate pattern. In general, patients with pregnancies beyond 34 wGA are monitored for contractions and cervical change, evaluated for rupture of membranes (ROM) and urinary tract infections, hydrated, and if the fetal heart rate is reactive (reassuring), then the patient is expectantly managed in an observed environment. A re-examination will determine the presence of preterm labor and for appropriate disposition (25). For those patients between 24 and 34 wGA, additional diagnostic modalities may include an ultrasound for cervical length, fetal fibronectin screen (FFN), vaginitis swab, and culture for Gonorrhea or Chlamydia for those at risk for the disease (25,29). The cervical length is performed by an intravaginal ultrasound that measures the external os distance from the internal os and presenting fetal part in the lower uterine segment over a 5-minute period. Cervical lengths of more than 3 cm indicate a low likelihood of preterm labor, while lengths of 1.5 to 3 cm require further diagnostic intervention or monitoring, usually in conjunction with FFN. Lengths less than 1.5 cm have a high incidence of preterm labor. The detection of the biomarker fetal fibronectin in the vaginal vault can be used independently or in conjunction with cervical length screening, and if negative, carries a 98% negative predictive value (NPV) for subsequent delivery in the next 7 days and rules against preterm labor (30). FFN has a poor positive predictive value (PPV), so if the test is positive, further diagnostic workup should ensue. A limited abdominal ultrasound (US) documenting fetal number and position, amniotic fluid (maximum vertical pocket or amniotic fluid index), and location and characterization of the placenta is performed. The underlying cause of preterm labor should be aggressively sought after and treated, especially in cases of acute abdomen and/or trauma.

Evaluating if the patient has ROM is paramount in every preterm labor evaluation. In addition to the patient history, this can be diagnosed by a sterile speculum examination and visualization of pooling amniotic fluid from the cervix, or in the use of adjuvant laboratories evaluating for alkaline fluid in the vagina (i.e., Nitrazine), biomarker detection of amniotic fluid containing PAMG-1 (i.e., AmniSure) (31), or the presence of ferning on a microscopic slide. The gold standard detection of ruptured membranes in equivocal cases is the tampon dye test, involving an infusion of inert dye (at the time of amniocentesis) into the uterine cavity and evaluating a vaginally placed tampon for colored dye 1 hour after. In the event of membrane rupture, the diagnosis of preterm premature ROM indicates immediate hospital admission and specific management protocols as these patients have higher risks of labor, placental abruption, and intrauterine infection (32).

Preterm Labor Management

Patients with preterm labor after 34 wGA usually are managed expectantly, that is, without attempts to stop the labor process. In most patients between 24 and 34 wGA, there is indication for antenatal corticosteroid administration for neonatal benefit to reduce neonatal acute respiratory distress, necrotizing enterocolitis, intraventricular hemorrhage, and other disabling neonatal diseases (33,34). Two common regimens include either two doses of intramuscular betamethasone 12 mg given 24 hours apart or four doses of intramuscular dexamethasone 6 mg 6 hours apart (34). To quell the uterine contractions for the full administration and effect of corticosteroid administration, it is common to utilize a tocolytic regimen such as indomethacin PO, nifedipine i.v. or PO, or magnesium sulfate i.v. drip for approximately 48 hours. The choice of drug is determined by the maternal condition and gestational age. Contraindications to tocolytic medications include intrauterine fetal demise, lethal fetal anomalies, nonreassuring fetal status, severe preeclampsia or eclampsia, maternal bleeding and hemodynamic instability, preterm premature ROM (in most cases), and maternal intolerance of the tocolytic (25). Finally, there is recent evidence that administration of magnesium sulfate i.v. drip within hours of delivery for neonates less than 32 wGA can reduce cerebral palsy in the survivors, commonly termed as "magnesium for fetal neuroprotection" (35).

Consultants

The recognition, management, and treatment of preterm labor or preterm premature ROM should be in conjunction with an obstetrician and neonatology/pediatric consultation at a hospital that provides such services. These consultants will be able to provide consultation on the labor and postpartum course for the mother and fetus and help the general surgeon or intensivist with specifics of management. In the event of a surgical procedure, ACOG has stated, "it is important for a physician to obtain an obstetric consultation before performing nonobstetric surgery and some invasive procedures (e.g., cardiac catheterization or colonoscopy) because obstetricians are uniquely qualified to discuss aspects of maternal physiology and anatomy that may affect intraoperative maternal–fetal well-being" (3). In addition, the obstetrician may provide information to help distinguish the acute abdomen from pregnancy related conditions and give recommendations on timing and route of delivery, appropriate medication and diagnostic imaging usage in pregnancy, and updates on fetal status. The neonatologist consultant works closely with the obstetrician to provide continued care for the neonate after delivery, educate families regarding neonatal aspects of care, and whether to perform a cesarean section and/or neonatal resuscitation on an individualized basis. Although the overall prognosis for premature infants has steadily improved, the morbidity and mortality for extremely low–birth-weight infants remains high. The mean survival rates for infants born between 23 and 25 wGA increase from 30%, to 52%, to 76% with each additional week of development. Likewise, the survival for infants weighing 401 to 800 g ranges from 11% in those under 500 g to 74% in those over 701 g. Severe disability is common among survivors in this group of vulnerable neonates and noninitiation of resuscitation for newborns under 23 wGA or 400 g birth weight is appropriate (36).

DIAGNOSTIC IMAGING IN PREGNANCY

Several modalities are available for diagnostic imaging to aid in the evaluation of surgical diseases in the gravid patient. Medically necessary diagnostic tests should not be withheld solely on the basis of pregnancy, but one should contemplate the potential advantages and disadvantages when selecting a particular testing method. Ultrasound (US) uses sound waves and thus does not expose the patient and fetus to ionizing radiation and is typically considered the first-line imaging tool to image the abdomen in pregnancy (37). Magnetic resonance imaging (MRI) makes use of the altered energy state of protons to create imaging and also does not expose the patient to ionizing radiation. MRI provides good sensitivity and specificity for surgical disorders in the *stable* pregnant patient. Although time consuming and more expensive, an MRI can evaluate placental abnormalities (placenta accreta) and characterize fetal central nervous system (CNS) malformations in addition to surgical processes in the abdomen. To date, MRI and ultrasound has been used safely during pregnancy are consistent with American College of Radiology guidelines. Radiography and computed tomography (CT) involve ionizing radiation, and for this reason, need to be used judiciously in gravid patients (38). Radiation and fetal teratogenicity has a dose-dependent relationship, with risk malformation and damage with fetal doses 150 to 200 mGy and 500 mGy, respectively (37,39). In perspective, a fetal dose of 100 mGy carries a 1% risk of organ malformation or childhood cancer (39), and an unshielded abdominopelvic CT provides about 25 mGy (38). Exposure to 50 to 100 mGy during the preimplantation period may cause blastocyst implantation failure and spontaneous abortion (37). Given the above information, it is paramount to image the pregnant abdomen with the appropriate imaging technique, with preferred use of nonionizing techniques of US and MRI.

Ultrasound

Obstetric US serves to assess fetal number, viability, size, gestational age, position, anatomy, as well as amniotic fluid volume, uterine mapping, and placental location and characterization (38). Obstetric US studies can be limited to evaluate basic pregnancy information or provide comprehensive information on detailed anatomy or even fetal echocardiography.

In the trauma setting, surgeon-performed focused assessment with sonography for trauma (FAST) is a useful screening tool for intra-abdominal bleeding and has similar sensitivity in the pregnant and nonpregnant individuals (40). The finding of free fluid in blunt trauma in pregnancy indicates a higher intra-abdominal injury rate, noting that free fluid is not necessarily a normal or physiologic finding of pregnancy (41). At one institution, FAST was additionally used as a screen for pregnancy where 18 of 144 (11%) of female patients were newly diagnosed with pregnancy prior to a pregnancy test (42). With diagnosis of pregnancy, FAST contributed to a significant decrease in fetal radiation exposure when compared to other trauma patients diagnosed with pregnancy by serum human chorionic gonadotropin (HCG) screening (42). However, FAST and US are of limited value in the diagnosis of placental abruption after trauma and may provide false-negative results in up to 50% to 58% of cases. The vascular nature of the placenta may have the same echogenicity as blood, so identification of retroplacental bleeding is not always possible (43,44).

Graded compression ultrasonography (GCUS) is still the initial test of choice in the assessment of appendicitis during pregnancy, despite a low sensitivity for diagnosis of 20% to 36% (45). Imaging is approximated on the self-reported area of maximal pain as McBurney's point changes based on the size of the uterus (46) with diagnostic criteria of a dilated (≥7 mm), fluid-filled, noncompressible, blind-ending tubular structure (45). MRI is the second preferred modality for evaluating appendicitis in pregnancy with sensitivity of 96.8%, specificity of 99.2, accuracy of 99%, PPV of 92.4%, NPV of 99.7% (47). CT scan is reserved for those patients for which a rapid and accurate diagnosis is required, to prevent the potential dangerous sequelae of appendix rupture.

Imaging of the biliary tract is similar to that of the nonpregnant patient. Acute cholecystitis detection using US with findings of cholelithiasis, gallbladder wall thickening, pericholecystic fluid, and Murphy's sign confers a 94% PPV compared to 88% when gallstones are present in isolation (45). Magnetic resonance cholangiopancreatogram (MRCP) is the appropriate second-line agent to evaluate for biliary disease approaching 98% sensitivity and 94% specificity for biliary tract disorders. Endoscopic retrograde cholangiopancreatography (ERCP) typically is utilized only if therapeutic intervention is expected or necessary, as it does expose the patient to ionizing radiation and is associated with several potential complications (45).

Magnetic Resonance Imaging

MRI has become a useful tool to identify the source abdominal pain in clinically stable pregnant patients. It is considered a safe modality in all trimesters of pregnancy, but due to thermal increases of imaging tissue during the MRI, there is a theoretical fetal teratogenic risk during the first trimester (37). Additionally, paramagnetic contrast agents such as gadolinium can cross through the placenta and enter the fetal circulation, and have proven higher rates of spontaneous abortion, skeletal abnormalities, and visceral abnormalities in animals when given as a dose two to seven times the normal dose. There have not been any reports of human teratogenicity. This agent should be used in pregnancy only if it provides substantial benefit over potential risk (38,48). Given the theoretical fetal risks, it is recommended to consent for this procedure (48). A clinician should use MRI with the knowledge that it is time consuming and challenging to evaluate an unstable patient while undergoing the examination and is reserved for clinically stable patients (38). MRI has been a useful imaging technique for appendicitis, inflammatory bowel disease, pancreatitis, intussusception, hydronephrosis and pyelonephritis, fibroids (and fibroid degeneration), adnexal masses (49), and placental abnormalities (accreta, perceta, increta) (49). MRI studies confirm that the appendix and cecum are superiorly displaced as pregnancy advances (46) and more reliably identifies the appendix than does US, with a sensitivity approaching 100% (49–51).

Computed Tomography

CT may be considered for evaluation of the abdomen if other studies are equivocal or unavailable, for blunt trauma, or as a triaging tool to prevent delays in treatment. The radiation dose can be reduced to limit excessive ionizing radiation exposure to the fetus, and as the doses are cumulative, it is suggested to avoid repeated studies if clinically appropriate (45,52,53).

Angiography

Ionizing radiation with fluoroscopy presents at about 100 mGy/min (24) and should be used with caution in pregnancy, particularly in the use of evaluating and treating pelvic bleeding. Abdominal shielding and limiting fluoroscopy time should be considered when performing this procedure. It is currently not recommended to use embolization techniques directly to the pregnant uterus (6). Alternatives to treat pelvic bleeding include laparotomy and preperitoneal packing with possible external fixation of the pelvis (54).

SPECIFIC ABDOMINAL SYNDROMES

Trauma

Trauma complicates 1 in 12 pregnancies and is the leading cause of nonobstetric death under 40 years of age, accounting for 46% of maternal deaths in the United States. The mean age for trauma is 24 years old with a mean gestation of 25.9 wGA and is caused by motor vehicle accidents (55%), falls (23%), assaults (22%), and burns (1%) (6,55). Sequelae can lead to significant maternal morbidity with higher incidence of spontaneous abortion, preterm premature ROM, preterm birth, uterine rupture, cesarean delivery, placental abruption, and stillbirth. Approximately 5% to 24% of patients admitted for trauma will deliver during the same admission, suggesting

TABLE 80.3 Trauma Team Personnel for the Pregnant Individual

- Trauma surgeon
- Surgical intensivist
- Emergency room physician
- Emergency room nurse
- Emergency room recorder/scribe
- Blood bank representative and laboratory
- Respiratory technician
- Obstetrician
- Obstetric nurse
- Anesthesiologist
- Pediatrician or neonatologist
- Neonatal intensive care nurse
- Operating room team on standby

that these patients should be transported to a center that provides trauma, obstetric, and neonatal service lines (5,6,56). Identified risk factors for traumatic accidents include younger women (<25 years old), African Americans, Hispanics, underinsured (5), use of illicit drugs or alcohol, history of domestic violence, and noncompliance to seatbelt use (6) (Table 80.3).

The immediate goal for a pregnant trauma patient is to stabilize the mother first, as fetal outcomes are dependent on early and aggressive maternal resuscitation (56). The primary survey includes the evaluation and prompt treatment of the maternal airway, ensuring adequate ventilation and oxygenation, and effective circulatory volume. In the event of cardiac arrest, prompt initiation of advanced cardiac life support (ACLS) should be performed with slight alterations described below. It is important to note that the maternal physiologic manifestation of increased plasma volume and red blood cell mass will allow more blood loss prior to changes in the maternal vital signs, but fetal perfusion may be impaired. Uterine compression of the vena cava can reduce blood return to, and preload of, the heart. Therefore, in gestations beyond 20 wGA the uterus needs to be displaced *upward and leftward* by either a 15- to 30-degree left lateral tilt or manual displacement upon its recognition. Spinal precautions and C-spine mobilization should be maintained through the uterine displacement process if indicated. An assessment of disability and exposure of the patient for a full primary survey is paramount prior to approaching the fetal status, which is typically performed in the secondary survey (except for in instances of obvious uterine hemorrhage, then prompt measures to correct the circulatory volume and address the bleeding is in the primary survey) (57).

The secondary survey (Table 80.4) immediately follows the primary survey, the initial resuscitation, and initial adjuncts to care such as cardiac monitoring, blood pressure monitoring, pelvic binding or shock trousers, and pulse oximetry. During the secondary survey, pregnancy should be assessed by history, physical examination, HCG (urine or blood) in women of childbearing age, and possibly by the FAST. The entire trauma team should be made aware of pregnancy status, have placement of intravenous access *above* the diaphragm as pelvic compression may limit resuscitative medications and fluids to the circulatory volume. All indicated traumatic bedside procedures can be performed as indicated with consideration to alter technique (57). A diagnostic peritoneal lavage can be preferably performed above the umbilicus and fundus in a pregnancy beyond 20 wGA to avoid uterine instrumentation, usually performed after gastric decompression. Additionally, chest tubes should be placed one to two rib spaces above its

TABLE 80.4 Trauma's Secondary Assessment in the Pregnant Woman

Positioning and preparation
- Fundus at umbilicus? (displace uterus upward and leftward)
- IV's placed above diaphragm
- Prepared for a perimortem cesarean delivery
- Neonatal warmer/resuscitation equipment available
- Appropriate consultations (obstetrics, neonatology, pediatrics, anesthesia)

Diagnosis of pregnancy
- B-HCG (urine or blood)
- FAST

Obstetric ultrasound
- Fetal heart tones
- Number of fetuses
- Assessment of gestational age/weight
- Evaluation uterus, placenta location and appearance, amniotic fluid volume assessment

Speculum exam and cervical examination (if indicated)
Fetal monitoring (>20 wGA)
- Fetal heart tones (continuously if viable)
- Tocometry

Laboratory tests
- Indicated trauma labs
- Complete blood count
- Type and screen (Rh status and possible rhogam)
- Kleihauer–Betke test

Disposition
- Monitoring
- Antenatal corticosteroid course

normal placement of above the fifth rib, to prevent abdominal entry (56). A limited obstetric US should be performed by an experienced provider to determine fetal number, viability, size and gestational age, position, and evaluation of placenta for abruption and uterus for rupture. Continuous fetal monitoring should ensue if the gestation is beyond 20 wGA by means of a fetal cardiotocometry (heart rate monitor and monitor for contractions). An assessment of labor and ROM should be performed by history, physical examination, sterile speculum examination, cervical examination, and other adjunctive tests as indicated. Consultants may include an obstetrician, anesthesiologist, neonatologist, and/or pediatrician (57).

Treatment of the pregnant trauma patient should be virtually identical to a non-pregnant patient with several specific alterations. Usage of all diagnostic modalities, including CT scan should be performed if indicated. Placing abdominal shielding and attenuating the dose of radiation may help reduce unnecessary radiation exposure to the fetus if feasible to achieve the appropriate image. CT of the head and neck involves very low fetal exposure and should be performed as per routine hospital protocols (58). If avoidance of ionizing radiation (CT and radiography) is plausible, then alternative methods to diagnosis should be employed. In addition to the aforementioned consultants, a pharmacist should review medications prescribed to prevent unnecessary administration to the fetus. However, there are very few medications that need to be withheld for treatment of the pregnant woman. In case of the need for an emergent delivery for fetal or maternal indications, the medical center should ensure that clinicians have easy and prompt access to a neonatal warmer and resuscitation kit, cesarean section surgical kit, and fetal monitoring system. These items should be with the patient at all times (intensive care unit, operating room, imaging suite, etc.).

The obstetrician as a consultant should remark on the following:

1. If the patient is Rh negative, a Kleihauer–Betke (KB) test and 300 μg of Rh-D immunoglobin (Rh-D Ig) should be administered within 72 hours of the trauma. An additional dose of Rh-D Ig 300 μg should be given to all Rh-women for every additional 30 mL of fetal blood found on KB testing, to prevent isoimmunization of the mother that can have deleterious effects on a subsequent pregnancy (12).
2. If the patient is between 24 and 34 wGA and a preterm birth is anticipated in the next 7 days, consideration for administration of antenatal corticosteroids and tocolysis may be indicated.
3. There should be comments on fetal status, indicated length of monitoring, appropriate positioning to monitor of the fetus and patient, and determination for further fetal evaluation with ultrasound.
4. Depending on the maternal and fetal conditions, the consultant should comment on timing and recommended route of delivery, patient disposition, and outpatient follow-up.
5. The consultant should obtain records or directly obtain routine prenatal labs, cultures, and diagnostics, as well as group B streptococcal screening and treatment if indicated. Of note, routine KB tests have been widely adopted in the trauma assessment; however, it has a poor predictive value of fetal distress or death, preterm birth, placental abruption, and typically does not alter management (12,56). Its utility has remained in aiding the calculated amount of Rh-D Ig to administer.

Duration of fetal monitoring recommendations after minor and major trauma is still controversial, and there is a lack of level I evidence for management guidelines. However, the EAST Practice Management in 2010 developed several level II and III guidelines to guide the clinician for appropriate duration of monitoring: "All women >20 week gestation who suffer trauma should have cardiotocographic monitoring for a minimum of 6 hours. Monitoring should be continued (for 24–48 hours) and further evaluation should be carried out if uterine contractions (>1 contraction per 10 minutes), a nonreassuring fetal heart rate pattern, vaginal bleeding, significant uterine tenderness or irritability, serious maternal injury (Injury Severity Score [ISS] >9, ejection from motor vehicle, motorcycle or pedestrian accident), or ROM is present" (59).

The rationale for extended fetal monitoring in the above criteria is that screening modalities such as history, physical examination, and obstetrical ultrasound are poor predictors for placental abruption, preterm labor, and fetal death. In a retrospective study, there was a higher rate of placental abruption for patients in motor vehicle accident ejections, maternal tachycardia above 110 beats/min, ISS over 9, or fetal bradycardia or tachycardia, suggesting a minimum of 24 hours of monitoring in this cohort of patients (43). Older studies have noted that placental abruption did not occur in trauma patients with less than one contraction every 10 minutes when monitored for a 4-hour period (12,44,60). Many hospitals follow the guideline for a minimum of 4 to 6 hours of cardiotocographic monitoring for patients who do not meet the above criteria for extended monitoring.

Five percent to 24% of pregnant patients admitted for trauma deliver during that hospitalization and usually within 24 hours of the trauma. This is likely a result of placental abruption causing uteroplacental insufficiency and fetal distress, activating the labor process (6). In studies that include route of delivery after trauma, about 75% of all deliveries are performed by cesarean section (5,6). The route of delivery is decided by routine obstetric guidelines in addition to the following conditions. Pelvic fracture is not an absolute contraindication to vaginal delivery, even in highly displaced pelvic fractures or hardware placement. However, large dislocating or unstable fractures may prohibit an attempt at vaginal delivery, and may require a cesarean delivery (12,61). Delivery induction is recommended for patients suffering burns over 40% of the body because of the high fetal mortality rate, aggressive fluid resuscitation, high need for ventilatory support, and high suspicion for thrombosis and/or sepsis (62,63). In burns, an early delivery may improve maternal condition and prevent fetal death (Fig. 80.1).

Fortunately, severe trauma requiring admission to the ICU is infrequent (3 in 1,000 pregnancies). It is estimated that 1,300 to 3,900 fetuses are lost due to maternal trauma each year. Mild maternal injuries carry a 1% to 5% fetal loss rate, whereas life-threatening trauma is associated with loss rates up to 40% to 50%. Because mild trauma is more prevalent, most fetal loss is due to minor maternal injury (12). Pregnant patients with pelvic or acetabular fractures are associated higher maternal and fetal death rates, 9% and 35%, respectively (64). The high fetal mortality rate is likely due to concentration of force enough to break the maternal pelvis, which is likely to also impact the fetus directly. As such, in penetrating abdominal injuries at the level of the uterus has a higher fetal mortality rate, but actually has a reduced maternal mortality rate, presumably as the uterus shields other vital maternal organs (7,65). Population-based data indicate that motor vehicle crashes account for 82% of fetal deaths after trauma, with an overall rate of 3.7 per 100,000 live births. The highest rate of fetal death due to trauma is seen in patients between 15 and 19 years of age (11,66).

Acute Abdomen

Acute abdominal pain in the pregnant female is a very common complaint. Although most times it can be attributed to labor, round ligament pain, constipation, urinary tract infection, or gastrointestinal reflux, it is important to obtain an appropriate history and physical examination to screen for life-threatening disease. The diagnosis can be difficult as some complaints may start with vague symptomatology, compounded with the hesitancy of a clinician to perform invasive or radiologic procedures due to fear of fetal safety. The most common diagnosis yielded from "abdominal pain" nearing a term gestation is labor that typically presents with regular and increasing frequency of abdominal cramping, pelvic pressure, bloody or fluid vaginal discharge. Although it not characteristic to have rebound abdominal tenderness in labor, syndromes such as chorioamnionitis and placental abruption may cause exquisite fundal tenderness, further disguising an underlying surgical disease. Another confounding factor is that both term and preterm labor can be *precipitated* from these acute abdominal processes, necessitating the clinician to recognize an abdominal illness in addition to labor (67).

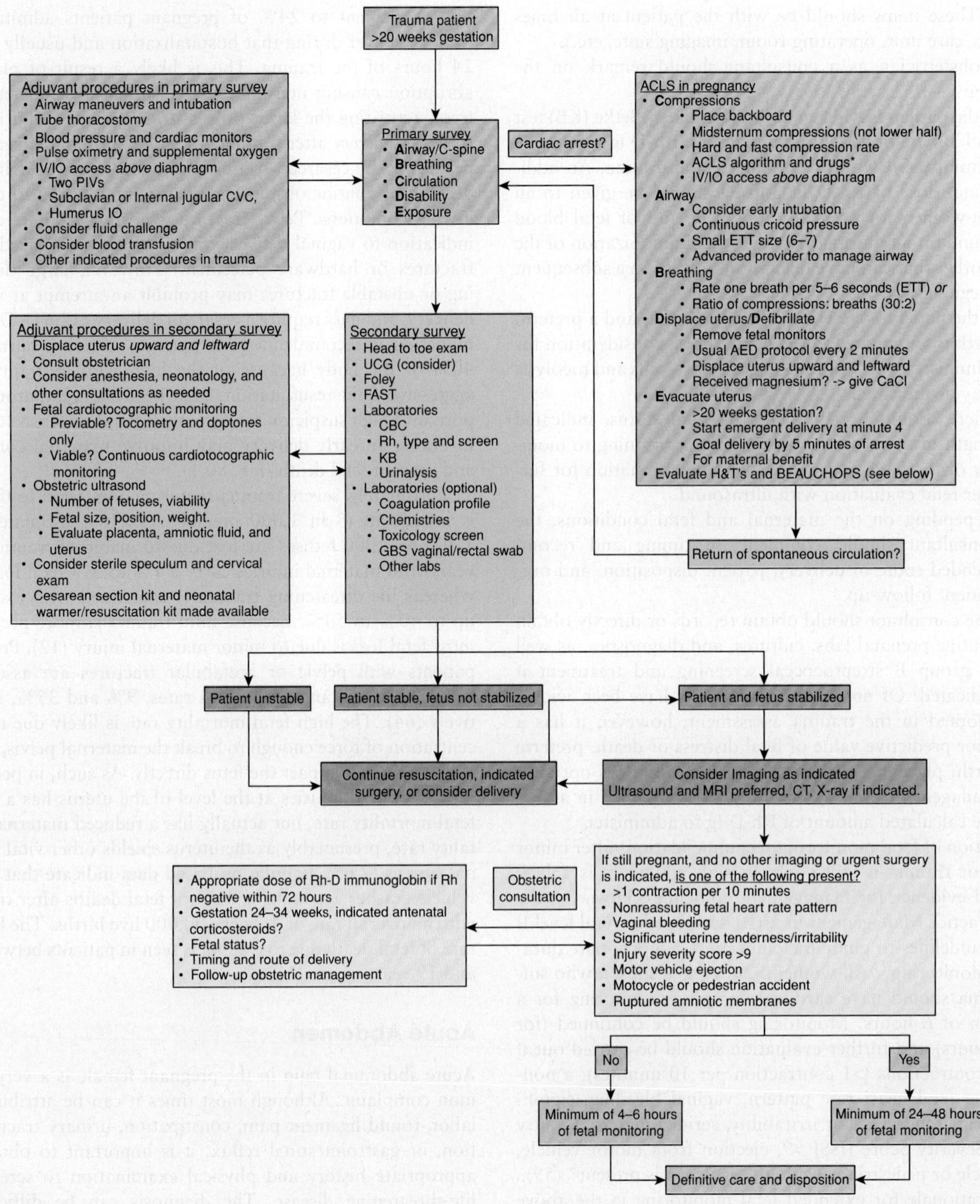

FIGURE 80.1 Advanced trauma life-support algorithm for trauma in pregnancy. *Use of lidocaine i.v. 1 to 1.5 mg/kg is recommended over amiodarone for refractory ventricular fibrillation and ventricular tachycardia. ACLS, advanced cardiac life support; AED, automated electronic defibrillator; C-spine, cervical spine; CaCl, calcium chlorie 10 mg in 10% solution; CBC, complete blood count; CT, computed tomography; CVC, central venous catheter; ETT, endotracheal tube; FAST, focused assessment of sonography for trauma; GBS, group B streptococci; IO, intraosseous; IV, intravenous; KB, Kleihauer-Betke; MRI, magnetic resonance imaging; PIV, peripheral intravenous line; UCG, urine β-human chorionic gonadotropin.

In a recent patient survey and chart review, the highest nonobstetric complaints lead to diagnoses of biliary ascariasis (28%), peptic ulcer disease (24%), lower urinary tract infection (10%), acute pyelonephritis (6%), acute gastroenteritis (6%), acute cholecystitis (6%), acute appendicitis (6%), renal colic (4%), choledocolithiasis (3%), acute pancreatitis (2%), ovarian solid mass (2%), torsed ovarian mass (2%), and renal calculus (1%) (68). This section will focus on surgical diseases of the abdomen in pregnancy, which is estimated to occur in about 1 per 635 pregnancies (67).

Acute Appendicitis

Acute appendicitis complicates approximately 1 in 1,500 pregnancies, most commonly in the second trimester, and appendectomy is the most common nonobstetric procedure performed in pregnancy (69–71). Appendicitis can be difficult to diagnose as the signs and symptoms, as well as normal pregnancy-induced physiologic leukocytosis, can obscure the diagnostic picture. It is more common for the presentation to be subsequent to a perforation as there is a reluctance to perform appropriate diagnostic imaging examinations and/or operate on a pregnant women. Clinical features of appendicitis include periumbilical abdominal pain that migrates to McBurney's point, which is more cephalic from the right lower quadrant the uterus enlarges. Anorexia, nausea, vomiting, fever over 38.5°C may subsequently develop. Occasionally, pain on rectal or vaginal examination and microscopic hematuria and leukocyturia can be present if the inflamed appendix is adjacent to the ureter or bladder. There is usually an elevated leukocytosis, C-reactive protein, and erythrocyte sedimentation rate, but these are all nonspecific for appendicitis (71). In a typical presentation, a compression abdominal US at the point of maximal pain is the first-line imaging technique of the appendix. If the US is equivocal and the patient is clinically stable, an MRI without contrast is the next best imaging study to evaluate the abdomen and appendix. A CT scan is reserved for cases where an urgent diagnosis is needed to prevent morbidity or to evaluate other abdominal structures as the potential cause of abdominal pain as it does confer ionizing radiation to the fetus (38,45,71). Acute appendicitis is a histologic diagnosis where prompt surgical resection within 24 hours is recommended in pregnancy, despite recent literature of antibiotic therapy alone in nonpregnant patients. Preoperative antibiotics to cover gram-positive and gram-negative bacteria, and anaerobic bacteria are recommended in conjunction to surgery. A delay in diagnosis of more than 24 hours has lead to a higher prevalence of perforated appendix (14% to 43%) (72), which usually occurs in the third trimester of pregnancy. The risk of fetal loss in perforated appendicitis is about 36% versus the nonperforated appendicitis to be 1.5%, a higher rate of preterm delivery (11% vs. 4%), suggesting that there should not be any delay in operative treatment in suspected acute appendicitis (73). Given the dangerous sequelae of delayed treatment, a higher "negative appendectomy rate" of 20% to 35% is acceptable. The negative appendectomy rate may be reduced with the use of MRI diagnostic imagery in selected stable patients. The surgical technique can be by laparoscopic approach (preferred), infraumbilical vertical laparotomy, or by transverse laparotomy over the suspected location of the appendix in all trimesters in pregnancy. The prognosis for the patient is good, and despite lacking data on the ultimate fetal outcomes, studies to date have reported normal child development (71,74). An appendectomy during pregnancy is not an indication for cesarean delivery, and route/timing of delivery may be decided on by obstetric and fetal indications.

Acute Cholecystitis

Acute cholecystitis with gallstones affects almost 20% of women by age 40 (75). It has a predilection to women as estrogen increases cholesterol secretion and progesterone reduces soluble bile acids and gallbladder mobility promoting stone formation and subsequent inflammation (76). Other risk factors include race, weight, diet, physical activity, obesity, serum lipids, and family history. A reported incidence of 1% to 4% of pregnant women have asymptomatic cholelithiasis, and 0.1% become symptomatic during pregnancy (70,77). Symptoms of biliary colic include bloating, nausea, and heartburn with eating. Acute cholecystitis may be diagnosed with right upper quadrant (RUQ) pain and tenderness (Murphy's sign), fever, tachycardia, leukocytosis, hyperbilirubinemia, transaminitis, and have ultrasonographic signs of gallbladder thickening over 5 mm, pericholecystic fluid, calculi, and possibly a dilated biliary duct on imaging (45,70). As mentioned above, MRCP is the next best imaging tool, and ERCP can be used if there is a need for an endoscopic removal of ductal stones. CT does not offer utility in diagnosis during pregnancy.

The first-line treatment is conservative therapy of intravenous hydration, pain control, bowel rest, and for those with systemic symptoms, antimicrobial therapy. Studies have demonstrated reduction of inflammation of the gallbladder with a short course of indomethacin prior to 32 wGA without fetal complications (70,77). Ursodeoxycholic acid, which can dissolve hepatic calculi, does not have safety data in pregnancy and is not recommended for treatment of cholelithiasis in pregnancy. Surgical therapy is indicated when acute cholecystitis is associated with sepsis, ileus, perforation, gallstone pancreatitis, refractory pain, and choledocolithiasis (78).

The surgical management of symptomatic cholelithiasis is less clear. Recent studies suggest performance of a laparoscopic cholecystectomy with a skilled provider. The rationale for surgery is that risks are low with few complications noted in its performance in all three trimesters, and it will lead to a reduction of short- and long-term morbidity to include recurrent hospitalizations for the disease (79,80), parenteral nutrition during pregnancy, induction of labor, lost to follow-up, and recurrent symptoms in subsequent pregnancy (79,81). This negates the prior dictum of waiting to perform surgery until the postpartum period. Lastly, there are several case reports of image guided catheterization of the gallbladder for decompression without fetal or neonatal complications, but research is lacking in this modality of treatment.

Adnexal Masses

With the increase in early pregnancy evaluations by transvaginal or abdominal ultrasound, there is an increasing incidence of adnexal masses diagnosed during pregnancy. The prevalence of adnexal masses range from 2.3% to 5.3% (82–84), and most (>90%) resolve spontaneously. The adnexal mass can range from benign ovarian or fallopian tube tissue or cyst, to oncologic processes involving the fallopian tube, ovary, or metastasized tissue from a different organ. Occasionally, the adnexal mass identified is of a different organ tissue (i.e., uterine fibroid or loop of bowel). Despite the majority of masses being benign, up to 5% may represent a malignant process, most commonly a borderline ovarian tumor (84). US is the imaging of choice for an adnexal mass that can help discern its histopathologic morphology by evaluating size, location, laterality, presence of ascites, morphology of tumor, and blood flow within the mass (85). Characterization of the adnexal mass will lead the clinician to offer expectant management, additional and/or follow-up imaging, blood draw for tumor markers, or surgical management. Most masses will resolve spontaneously and require a follow-up image at a 4- to 8-week interval to document resolution. For masses that appear concerning for malignancy, tumor markers (cancer antigen-125, alpha fetoprotein, carcinoembrionic antigen, cancer antigen 19-9, beta-HCG, lactate dehydrogenase, human epididymis protein 4, inhibin B, serum testosterone) may be drawn with caution as other pregnancy variables may cause elevations in these markers. Additional imaging with MRI may offer more detailed information regarding the mass and other organ involvement. CT imaging may determine cancer staging if suspicion of a high stage of cancer is suggested by US, MRI, or tumor markers (86). Positron emission tomography is currently not recommended in preoperative evaluation adnexal masses in pregnancy.

Most adnexal masses are asymptomatic, but occasionally can cause tremendous discomfort in the occurrence of adnexal torsion. Torsion is considered a surgical emergency for the viability of the fallopian tube and ovary. It is characterized by a sudden onset of immense right or left lower quadrant pain with nausea and vomiting. Demonstration of lack of blood flow on Doppler US does *not* preclude that the adnexa is not torsed, but typically demonstrates a 5- to 10-cm mass on the side of maternal pain (84). Suspicion of ovarian torsion is an indication for emergent laparotomy or laparoscopic procedure for removal of the mass and detorsion.

If the adnexal mass is likely a malignancy based on laboratory and imaging examinations, an individualized plan devised by a multidisciplinary team approach of obstetricians, gynecology oncologists, oncologists, neonatologist, and psychologists should be performed (87). Neoadjuvent or adjuvant chemotherapy can generally be performed after the 12th week of gestation to avoid complications of teratogenesis, but is associated with preterm birth and intrauterine growth restriction, and still carries a low risk of malformation (88). Surgical removal of a cyst, mass, or cancer is generally safe during pregnancy (89). However, care needs to be taken not to remove ovarian masses in pregnancies before 12 wGA without progesterone supplementation, as the mass may be the corpus luteum supporting the pregnancy and will cause a spontaneous abortion if removed.

Other Abdominal Syndromes and Abdominal Sepsis

Surgery on the maternal appendix, biliary tree, adnexal masses, and for trauma are the most frequent nonobstetric indications for abdominal surgery in pregnancy. There are multiple other indications for abdominal surgery in pregnancy and require a multidisciplinary team approach for management. Abdominal sepsis may be another indication for surgical procedures where there is no standardized approach for treatment (other than chorioamnionitis). It should be mentioned that interventional radiologic procedures are increasing in efficacy to remove collections of infectious material in the abdomen and should be considered in pregnancy to additionally compliment laparoscopy and laparotomy. Septic etiologies should be considered in pregnancy with fever, leukocytosis, and labor or preterm labor. A common septic cause worth reviewing is an intra-amniotic infection, or chorioamnionitis.

Chorioamnionitis is a histopathologic diagnosis, typically resulting from bacterial infection of the amniotic membranes and fluid, as well as the placenta. As pathologic specimens are not available prior to delivery, physicians need a high index of suspicion for chorioamnionitis which can be diagnosed clinically by a maternal fever over 38°C, absence of other sources of infection including the urinary tract, and one of the following: uterine tenderness, foul-smelling leucorrhea, leukocytosis higher than 15,000 cells/mm (3), maternal tachycardia, or fetal tachycardia. An amniocentesis can be performed and the presence of a micro-organism (Gram stain and culture), glucose below 20 mg/dL, elevated interleukins-1 and -6, and high white blood cell count in the amniotic fluid are all sensitive predictors for chorioamnionitis. Chorioamnionitis is an indication for prompt antibiotic administration cover aerobic gram-positive and gram-negative microbes and for delivery of the fetus, regardless of gestational age (90).

PERIOPERATIVE MANAGEMENT

Anesthesia

Anesthesia for a nonobstetric surgery requires a skilled technician knowledgeable in adult and fetal medicine, usually requiring anesthesia consultation prior to surgery. Regional or local anesthetics are thought to be safer than general anesthesia in most cases. Regional anesthesia for abdominal surgery has the advantage of minimal fetal local anesthetic drug exposure and is less likely to be associated with maternal airway complications. Local anesthetics are not known to be teratogenic when used in this clinical setting (91).

Due to the risk of aspiration from gastroesophageal (GE) reflux and delayed gastric emptying, it is customary to administer a nonparticulate antacid or H_2 blocker as well as medication to improve GE sphincter tone preoperatively. If general anesthesia is planned, pre-oxygenation and rapid-sequence intubation are typically performed. Care should be taken to avoid hyperventilation, as uterine blood flow is impaired. Inhalational agents, such as isoflurane and others, decrease uterine tone and can effectively inhibit labor during surgery.

Agents used for general anesthesia during pregnancy, including a single dose of benzodiazepines, nitrous oxide, and inhalational agents, do cross the placenta but have not been shown to be teratogenic (91). Nonobstetric surgery during pregnancy denotes a low maternal mortality of less than 1 in 10,000, did not increase the rate of birth defects, and does have an increased incidence of low–birth-weight nor preterm labor (92).

Fetal Monitoring

Intraoperative fetal monitoring is advised for viable pregnancies if it is plausible for an emergent delivery for fetal indications. This includes having the appropriate measures for delivery to include cesarean section operative equipment, personnel to evaluate fetal cardiotocography, an obstetric provider, and when possible, consent to perform a cesarean delivery. In addition, having a neonatologist or pediatrician and a neonatal resuscitation warmer, equipment, and resources available are recommended if delivery is indicated. In a previable fetus, preoperative and postoperative fetal doptones are appropriate (see Table 80.1) (3).

Laparoscopy in Pregnancy

Guidelines for the general surgeon regarding laparoscopy in pregnancy have been reviewed by the Society of American Gastrointestinal and Endoscopic Surgeons with the following consensus guidelines. Surgical laparoscopy for the acute abdomen has the same indications in all trimesters of pregnancy when compared to nonpregnant women, which has a good record of safety during pregnancy. Special considerations for laparoscopy during pregnancy might include the use of an open technique (Hassan) or alternate placement of optical trochars/veress needle for access into the abdominal cavity, direct visualization for additional trochar placement, lower insufflation pressures (10 to 15 mmHg), and positioning the patient in a leftward lateral recumbent position. Intraoperative monitoring of CO_2 levels by using end-tidal capnography and/or episodic arterial blood gasses may help prevent maternal acid base disturbances and fetal acidemia. Laparoscopy is of additional benefit over laparotomy to reduce postoperative narcotic requirements, lower risk of wound complications, reduced respiratory splinting and hypoventilation, offer shorter hospital stays, and reduced thromboembolic events because of early ambulation. Use of abdominal shielding to prevent fetal exposure of intraoperative ionizing radiation is recommended. The consensus guidelines further evaluate specific procedures as to be able to be performed in pregnancy as well as remarks on venous thromboembolism prophylaxis (93,94).

MATERNAL CARDIAC ARREST

Maternal cardiac arrest is a devastating occurrence that puts a woman and her baby's life in extremis. Although this event is rare, the rate has risen almost 2.5 times in the past 10 years, as the maternal death rate is now 14.5 per 100,000 pregnancies (95). Typical ACLS courses do not devote instructional time to the specifics about maternal cardiac arrest and obstetric teams lack experience in its management, which may create a very chaotic maternal code situation. Recently, the Society for Obstetric Anesthesia and Perinatology created a consensus statement on cardiac arrest during pregnancy to highlight unique aspects on management (96).

In the event of a maternal code, initiation of usual ACLS with chest compressions and ventilation, early automated external defibrillator (AED) use, and activating the hospital-specific "obstetric code" are paramount. This specific code team should assemble an obstetrician and neonatal resuscitation team, in additional to intensivists, respiratory technicians, pharmacists, and code nurses. In addition to the ACLS algorithm (Fig. 80.1), there are several pregnancy-specific recommendations for resuscitation for patients beyond 20 wGA (Table 80.5) (96):

1. Perform compressions on the midsternum instead of the "lower half of the sternum." The gravid abdomen displaces the diaphragm and heart orientation to a more superior and lateral position than nonpregnant women.
2. All intravenous access should be *above* the diaphragm (i.e., peripheral i.v., subclavian and internal jugular central venous catheters, midlines, or humeral head intraosseous access) to adequately access the central circulation.
3. Give typical ACLS medications and AED doses. There are no contraindicated medications for pregnant patients in extremis.
4. Assess for hypovolemia and give fluid boluses as indicated.
5. Due to the progesterone effect of slowed gastric emptying during pregnancy and common occurrence of laryngeal edema, the provider should anticipate a difficult airway and consider early placement of an advanced airway with a slightly smaller endotracheal tube than one would use for a nonpregnant woman. Also, continuous cricoid pressure is recommended during intubation during a maternal code.

TABLE 80.5 Causes for Maternal Cardiac Arrest: H&T's and BEAUCHOPS

H&T's
- Hypovolemia
- Hypoxia
- Hydrogen ion (acidosis)
- Hypokalemia
- Hyperkalemia
- Hypothermia
- Tension pneumothorax
- Tamponade, cardiac
- Thrombosis, pulmonary
- Thrombosis, coronary
- Toxins

BEAUCHOPS
- Bleeding, disseminated intravascular coagulopathy
- Embolism: coronary, pulmonary, amniotic fluid
- Anesthesia complications (epidural/spinal)
- Uterine atony
- Cardiac disease (myocardial infarction, cardiomyopathy
- Hypertension (preeclampsia, eclampsia)
- Other H&T's
- Placenta abruption/previa
- Sepsis

(Adapted from Lipman S, Cohen S, Einav S, et al. The Society for Obstetric Anesthesia and Perinatology consensus statement on the management of cardiac arrest in pregnancy. *Anesth Analg.* 2014;118(5):1003–1016.)

6. If the patient has received recent magnesium sulfate infusions, stop the infusion and give calcium chloride 10 mL in 10% solution upon code initiation, which will empirically reverse a magnesium toxic dose.
7. Remove all fetal monitors. If the patient cannot perfuse her own heart and brain, she is not likely perfusing the fetus, and *the fetal heart rate tracing will not change management during a cardiac arrest.*
8. Prevent aortocaval compression by tilting the patient 15 to 30 degrees in the left lateral decubitus position or manually displace the uterus leftward and upward to improve blood return to the heart from the lower extremities.
9. If there is no return of spontaneous circulation (ROSC) by 4 minutes in a pregnancy beyond 20 wGA, start an emergent cesarean delivery (known as a resuscitative hysterotomy in this case) with the goal of delivery by 5 minutes of the cardiac arrest for *maternal benefit* of improving perfusion.
10. Continue all maternal resuscitation during and after the perimortem cesarean delivery (PMCD).
11. In addition to the "H&T's" that are considered in the 2010 American Heart Association guidelines for ACLS, consider using the pneumonic BEAUCHOPS to aid in the recollection of the most common reasons for a pregnant patient to have a cardiac arrest.

Perimortem Cesarean Delivery

During a maternal cardiac arrest, the recorder should prompt the team when 4 minutes have occurred in the undelivered pregnant woman beyond 20 wGA. If ROSC has not been achieved, the team should promptly perform a PMCD within 1 minute and goal delivery within 5 minutes of maternal cardiac arrest (97). If feasible for an operative vaginal delivery (assisted with a fetal vacuum or forceps), an obstetrician should perform this prior to the 5-minute time from the initial cardiac arrest. As mentioned above, a PMCD is performed for *maternal benefit* with improved venous return to the heart by an auto-transfusion from the uterine blood flow and relief of caval compression, reduced oxygen demand from removal of the fetus and placenta, and improved pulmonary function with the reduction of abdominal/uterine compression (96–98). This may be lifesaving for the fetus. In a case series including 38 women undergoing PMCD, no cases of cesarean delivery worsened maternal condition and of the 20 women who had ROSC, 12 occurred immediately after delivery (10). In over 50% of maternal cardiac arrests does ROSC occur, and neonatal survival was based on in-hospital or in-community maternal arrest (99).

Maternal Brain Death

On rare occasions maternal brain death is identified in a pregnant woman while somatic support has been maintained and the fetus remains alive. Under these circumstances, a determination must be made as to whether to deliver the fetus immediately, to initiate supportive care to allow further fetal maturation, or to allow the fetus to die as the mother is removed from mechanical ventilation. Immediate delivery when gestational age is consistent with neonatal survival is usually preferred. However, if the mother's condition permits, it is possible to support the mother and previable fetus until fetal maturation allows for neonatal survival. This somatic support can be provided for extended periods with no apparent neonatal or pediatric sequelae with 2-year follow-up reported (100,101).

Ethical Decision-Making

There is a potential for conflicts in decision-making between the clinician and the pregnant woman. Patients may be asked to consent to procedures that carry some risk to the fetus. Alternatively, interventions proposed for fetal benefit may present a risk to maternal health. Principle-based ethics, based on the concepts of autonomy, beneficence, and justice, have been used to aid choices. Providers also need to take into account the social and cultural contexts within which the patient is making her choices. According to the ACOG Ethical Guidelines, "Every reasonable effort should be made to protect the fetus, but the pregnant woman's autonomy should be respected.... Intervention against the wishes of a pregnant woman is rarely, if ever, acceptable" (102).

In the case of a patient who is incapacitated, state laws vary with respect to who may serve as a surrogate decision-maker. The designees should base their decisions on the values and wishes of the patient, which may or may not have previously been stated in writing. Clinicians should try to anticipate such scenarios and attempt to adhere to the woman's wishes regarding treatment for herself and/or her fetus. If there is no consensus about who should be designated, the advice of an ethics committee should be considered.

INJURY PREVENTION AND REDUCTION

Thromboembolism Prevention

Pregnancy induces a prothrombotic state and increases the risk of both venous and arterial thromboembolism to an incidence of 0.1% to 0.2% of pregnant women, with a higher propensity to affect the venous system (103,104) and occurrence during the postpartum period (105). Pulmonary thromboembolism (PE) has been reported to be the cause of death of 10.2% of maternal deaths between 1998 and 2005 and occurs in 0.6 to 1.8 per 1,000 deliveries (106). Placental factors increase protein S excretion and increase fibrinogen, cause mechanical compression iliac and caval venous vessels (especially the left iliac vein as it traverses the pelvis longer than the right iliac vein) that both injures the endothelium and causes blood stasis. Each risk factor of Virchow's triad is elevated, which explains the propensity for thromboembolism in pregnancy. Firm guidelines are yet to be established in the United States, but the Royal College of Obstetricians and Gynecologists (RCOG) have recommended that all women undergo risk assessment for venous thromboembolism during early pregnancy. Those at high risk should be counseled for using chemoprophylaxis during pregnancy. Approved prophylactic agents in pregnancy include low–molecular-weight heparins and unfractionated heparin during the antepartum course, transitioning to unfractionated heparin during labor as it is more readily reversible with protamine sulfate in the case of bleeding. Coumadin is a longer-acting drug that has teratogenic effects and should be avoided during pregnancy, but is acceptable for administration postpartum (after postpartum day 3) as it does not get secreted in breast milk. If there is suspicion of a venous thrombus, a compression venous duplex US should be performed and treatment with therapeutic unfractionated heparin should ensue. If suspicious of a PE, empiric treatment with therapeutic unfractionated heparin should ensue while diagnostic tests are completed. A compression venous duplex US is first line in diagnosis as the treatment for a venous thrombus and pulmonary embolism includes supportive therapy and therapeutic anticoagulation. This will avoid ionizing radiation of a CT scan of the chest during pregnancy. If the compression venous duplex is not remarkable for a thrombus, and a high suspicion for PE still exists, then a CT for pulmonary angiography or V/Q scan should be performed. If thrombus or pulmonary embolism is confirmed, treatment to therapeutic anticoagulation and clinical endpoints are the same in pregnant women when compared to non-pregnant women. During parturition, discontinuing or using reversal agents to negate the effects of anticoagulation is necessary until approximately 6 to 12 hours after delivery. Treatment should ensue for 3 to 6 months postpartum for most patients with thromboembolic disease (106).

Restraints and Motor Vehicle Accidents

Lack of seatbelt use has been shown to contribute to the severity of maternal and fetal injuries. Knowledge of proper seatbelt use is low among some patients, especially teens and those with low education levels. In one survey of 450 pregnant women, only 72.5% reported using the seatbelt in the proper location. Women who always wore restraints were more likely to report correct placement. Sixty percent of respondents thought restraints would protect their baby, whereas 11.6% thought restraints caused injury to the baby, and 37% were unsure. The most common reasons for lack of use were lack of comfort (52.8%) and forgetting (42.5%). However, only 36.9% of women reported receiving information about seatbelt use during that pregnancy (107). Another survey of 807 women revealed that although 79% of women used safety restraints, only 52% of them did so correctly, and only 21% were educated on proper use during pregnancy (108). Proper restraint use protects against ejection in a motor vehicle accident, lowering the maternal Injury Severity Score and also lowering the fetal risk of death (43). Educational interventions during prenatal care and emergency room visits can improve the proper use of seatbelts. As the majority of vehicles now install airbags as a safety feature, some literature is emerging on its deployment in pregnancy. Although nonsignificant, there were trends toward a reduction of preterm labor and fetal death in passengers or drivers of vehicles that did not have airbags in comparison to vehicles that would have had airbag deployment if installed in the vehicle. There were no adverse effects from airbag deployment in this study (109).

Intimate Partner Violence

Intimate partner violence occurs when an intimate partner displays controlling behavior that may include physical, psychological, or sexual abuse. Abusive patterns have a wide range of presentation, from constant threats and intimidation to financial and physical coercive techniques that result in the patient's dependence on the partner (110). Estimations of about one-third of women in the United States have experienced rape or physical violence, or have had an intimate partner stalk them (111). This may be an underestimate as women may be afraid of disclosing these events for fear of repercussions from the partner. The female gender, adolescents, immigrants, disabled, and elderly women are all at increased risk for intimate partner violence. The effects can lead to a multiple sequelae of psychological, physical, and sexual syndromes, as well as specific pregnancy risks of poor weight gain, tobacco use, pelvic fracture, placental abruption, preterm delivery, stillbirth, postpartum depression, and low birth weight (112). ACOG endorses the screening for intimate partner violence at well woman, family planning (contraception), and pregnancy clinical visits and for ongoing care. Screening is by conducted by history, physical examination, and observation of the partner–patient relationship, ensuring that patient disclosure of violence is held confidential. Most states do not mandate abuse reporting, but providing resource information and developing a safety plan are initial steps to aid these patients. Individualized plans of care should be made for these patients using community resources (110). Two 24-hour toll-free hotlines to provide more information in the United States on intimate partner violence are: National Domestic Violence Hotline (800) 799-SAFE and Rape Abuse & Incest National Network (RAINN) (800) 656-HOPE.

Key Points

- Pregnancy induces different physiologic variables when compared to nonpregnant women.
- The primary survey in the trauma assessment for pregnant women is the same for nonpregnant women. There are multiple modifications in maternal positioning, diagnosis, and treatment within the secondary survey.
- Imaging of the acute abdomen in pregnancy usually consists of US, then MRI if the US is equivocal in stable patients. CT is reserved for patients who require immediate evaluation due to risk of delayed diagnosis or hemodynamically instability, due to the fetal risk of ionizing radiation.
- Surgical indications for the acute abdomen in the pregnant woman are virtually identical for that of the nonpregnant woman, but specific alterations in ascertaining diagnosis, treatment, and surgical technique should be considered.
- There are several alterations in maternal ACLS, including prompt delivery in any gestation beyond 20 weeks by 5 minutes time after arrest for maternal benefit.

ACKNOWLEDGMENTS

I thank the Queen's Medical Center Surgical Intensive Care Unit nurses, staff, and physicians for my continual educational support in surgical critical care. Above all, I want to thank Dr. Mihae Yu for her continual mentorship, teachings, and guidance.

References

1. Curtin SC, Abma JC, Ventura SJ, Henshaw SK. Pregnancy rates for U.S. women continue to drop. *NCHS Data Brief.* 2013;(136):1–8.
2. Stewart MK, Terhune KP. Management of pregnant patients undergoing general surgical procedures. *Surg Clin North Am.* 2015;95(2):429–442.
3. ACOG Committee on Obstetric Practice. The American College of Obstetricians and Gynecologists. ACOG Committee Opinion No. 474: nonobstetric surgery during pregnancy. *Obstet Gynecol.* 2011;117(2 Pt 1): 420–421.
4. Van Hook JW. Trauma in pregnancy. *Clin Obstet Gynecol.* 2002;45(2): 414–424.
5. Ikossi DG, Lazar AA, Morabito D, et al. Profile of mothers at risk: an analysis of injury and pregnancy loss in 1,195 trauma patients. *J Am Coll Surg.* 2005;200(1):49–56.
6. Oxford CM, Ludmir J. Trauma in pregnancy. *Clin Obstet Gynecol.* 2009; 52(4):611–629.
7. Mirza FG, Devine PC, Gaddipati S. Trauma in pregnancy: a systematic approach. *Am J Perinatol.* 2010;27(7):579–586.
8. Cakmak B, Ribeiro AP, Inanir A. Postural balance and the risk of falling during pregnancy. *J Matern Fetal Neonatal.* 2015:1–3.
9. Bochicchio GV, Napolitano LM, Haan J, et al. Incidental pregnancy in trauma patients. *J Am Coll Surg.* 2001;192(5):556–569.
10. Visser BC, Glasgow RE, Mulvihill KK, Mulvihill SJ. Safety and timing of nonobstetric abdominal surgery in pregnancy. *Dig Surg.* 2001;18(5): 409–417.
11. Weiss HB, Songer TJ, Fabio A. Fetal deaths related to maternal injury. *JAMA.* 2001;286(15):1863–1868.
12. American College of Obstetricians and Gynecologists. ACOG educational bulletin. Obstetric aspects of trauma management. Number 251, September 1998 (replaces Number 151, January 1991, and Number 161, November 1991). *Int J Gynaecol Obstet.* 1999;64:87–94.
13. Pritchard JA. Changes in the blood volume during pregnancy and delivery. *Anesthesiology.* 1965;26:393–399.
14. Lund CJ, Donovan JC. Blood volume during pregnancy: significance of plasma and red cell volumes. *Am J Obstet Gynecol.* 1967;98(3): 394–403.
15. Wilson M, Morganti A, Zervoudakis I, et al. Blood pressure, the renin-aldosterone system and sex steroids throughout normal pregnancy. *Am J Med.* 1980;68(1):97–104.
16. Jepson JH. Endocrine control of maternal and fetal erythropoeisis. *Can Med Assoc J.* 1968;98(18):844–847.
17. Burg JR, Dodek A, Kloster FE, Metcalfe J. Alterations of systolic time intervals during pregnancy. *Circulation.* 1974;49(3):560–564.
18. Gilson GJ, Samaan S, Crawford MH, et al. Changes in hemodynamics, ventricular remodeling, and ventricular contractility during normal pregnancy: a longitudinal study. *Obstet Gynecol.* 1997;89(6):957–962.
19. Monga M. Maternal cardiovascular, respiratory, and renal adaptation to pregnancy. In: *Creasy and Resnik's Maternal-Fetal Medicine: Principles and Practice.* 6th ed. Philadelphia, PA: Saunders/Elsevier; 2009:101–109.
20. Bille-Brahe NE, Rorth M. Red cell 2,3-diphosphoglycerate in pregnancy. *Acta Obstet Gynecol Scand.* 1979;58(1):19–21.

21. Awe RJ, Nicotra MB, Newsom TD, Viles R. Arterial oxygenation and alveolar-arterial gradients in term pregnancy. *Obstet Gynecol.* 1979;53(2):182–186.
22. Jeyabalan A, Lain KY. Anatomic and functional changes of the upper urinary tract during pregnancy. *Urol Clin North Am.* 2007;34(1):1–6.
23. Jarjour IT. Neurodevelopmental outcome after extreme prematurity: a review of the literature. *Pediatr Neurol.* 2015;52(2):143–152.
24. The American College of Obstetricians and Gynecologists. Risk factors for preterm birth. *ACOG Practice Bulletin.* 2000, No 31.
25. ACOG Committee on Practice Bulletins–Obstetrics. ACOG Practice Bulletin. Management of preterm labor. Number 43,May 2003. *Int J Gynaecol Obstet.* 2003;82:127–135.
26. Committee on Practice Bulletins—Obstetrics, The American College of Obstetricians and Gynecologists. Practice bulletin no. 130: Prediction and prevention of preterm birth. *Obstet Gynecol.* 2012;120:964–973.
27. Romero R, Dey SK, Fisher SJ. Preterm labor: one syndrome, many causes. *Science.* 2015;345(6198):760–765.
28. Gerstenfeld TS, Chang DT, Pliego AR, Wing DA. Nonobstetrical abdominal surgery during pregnancy in Women's Hospital. *J Matern Fetal Med.* 2002;9(3):170–172.
29. van Baaren GJ, Vis JY, Wilms FF, et al. Predictive value of cervical length measurement and fibronectin testing in threatened preterm labor. *Obstet Gynecol.* 2014;123(6):1185–1192.
30. Foster C, Shennan AH. Fetal fibronectin as a biomarker of preterm labor: a review of the literature and advances in its clinical use. *Biomark Med.* 2014;84(4):471–484.
31. Cousins LM, Smok DP, Lovett SM, Poeltler DM. AmniSure placental alpha microglobulin-1 rapid immunoassay versus standard diagnostic methods for detection of rupture of membranes. *Am J Perinatol.* 2005;22(6):317–320.
32. The American College of Obstetricians and Gynecologists. Premature rupture of membranes. *ACOG Practice Bulletin.* Oct 2013, No 139.
33. Ballard PL, Ballard RA. Scientific basis and therapeutic regimens for use of antenatal glucocorticoids. *Am J Obstet Gynecol.* 1995;173(1):254–262.
34. Brownfoot FC, Gagliardi DI, Bain E, et al. Different corticosteroids and regimens for accelerating fetallung maturation for women at risk of preterm birth. *Cochrane Database Syst Rev.* 2013(8):1–91.
35. Reeves SA, Gibbs RS, Clark SL. Magnesium for fetal neuroprotection. *Am J Obstet Gynecol.* 2011;204(3):202.e1–e4.
36. MacDonald H. Perinatal care at the threshold of viability. *Pediatrics.* 2002;110:1024–1027.
37. Wang PI, Chong ST, Kielar AZ, et al. Imaging of pregnant and lactating patients: part 1, evidence-based review and recommendations. *AJR Am J Roentgenol.* 2012;198(4):778–784.
38. The American College of Obstetricians and Gynecologists. Guidelines for diagnostic imaging during pregnancy. *Obstet Gynecol.* 2004;104 reaffirmed 2014, No 299:647–651.
39. McCollough CH, Schueler BA, Atwell TD, et al. Radiation exposure and pregnancy: when should we be concerned? *Radiographics.* 2007;27(4):909–917; discussion 917–918.
40. Goodwin H, Holmes JF, Wisner DH. Abdominal ultrasound examination in pregnant blunt trauma patients. *J Trauma.* 2001;50(4):689–693.
41. Ormsby EL, Geng J, McGahan JP, Richards JR. Pelvic free fluid: clinical importance for reproductive age women with blunt abdominal trauma. *Ultrasound Obstet Gynecol.* 2005;26(3):271–278.
42. Bochicchio GV, Haan J, Scalea TM. Surgeon-performed focused assessment with sonography for trauma as an early screening tool for pregnancy after trauma. *J Trauma.* 2002;52(6):1125–1128.
43. Curet MJ, Schermer CR, Demarest GB, et al. Predictors of outcome in trauma during pregnancy: identification of patients who can be monitored for less than 6 hours. *J Trauma.* 2000;49(1):18–24; discussion 24–25.
44. Reis PM, Sander CM, Pearlman MD. Abruptio placentae after auto accidents: a case-control study. *J Reprod Med.* 2000;45(1):6–10.
45. Wang PI, Chong ST, Kielar AZ, et al. Imaging of pregnant and lactating patients. Part 2: evidence-based review and recommendations. *AJR Am J Roentgenol.* 2012;198(4):785–792.
46. Oto A, Srinivasan PN, Ernst RD, et al. Revisiting MRI for appendix location during pregnancy. *AJR Am J Roentgenol.* 2006;186(3):883–887.
47. Burke LM, Bashir MR, Miller FH, et al. Magnetic resonance imaging of acute appendicitis in pregnancy: a 5-year multi-institutional study. *Am J Obstet Gynecol.* 2015;213(5):693.e1–e6.
48. Kanal E, Borgstede JP, Barkovich AJ, et al.; American College of Radiology. American College of Radiology White Paper on MR Safety. *AJR Am J Roentgenol.* 2002;178:1335–1347.
49. Birchard KR, Brown MA, Hyslop WB, et al. MRI of acute abdominal and pelvic pain in pregnant patients. *AJR Am J Roentgenol.* 2004;184:452–458.
50. Cobben LP, Groot I, Haans L, et al. MRI for clinically suspected appendicitis during pregnancy. *AJR Am J Roentgenol.* 2004;183:671–675.
51. Pedrosa I, Levine D, Eyvazzadeh AD, et al. MR imaging evaluation of acute appendicitis in pregnancy. *Radiology.* 2006;238(3):891–899.
52. Damilakis J, Perisinakis K, Voloudaki A, Gourtsoyiannis N. Estimation of fetal radiation dose from computed tomography scanning in late pregnancy: depth-dose data from routine examinations. *Invest Radiol.* 2000;35(9):527–533.
53. Woussen S, Lopez-Rendon X, Vanbeckevoort D, et al. Clinical indications and radiation doses to the conceptus associated with CT imaging in pregnancy: a retrospective study. *Eur Radiol.* 2016;26(4):979–985.
54. Amorosa LF, Amorosa JH, Wellman DS, et al. Management of pelvic injuries in pregnancy. *Orthop Clin North Am.* 2013;44(3):301–315, viii.
55. Hill CC, Pickinpaugh J. Trauma and surgical emergencies in the obstetric patient. *Surg Clin North Am.* 2008;88(2):421–440, viii.
56. Mendez-Figueroa H, Dahlke JD, Vrees RA, Rouse DJ. Trauma in pregnancy: an updated systematic review. *Am J Obstet Gynecol.* 2013;209(1):1–10.
57. ATLS Subcommittee; American College of Surgeons' Committee on Trauma; International ATLS working group. Advanced trauma life support (ATLS®): the ninth edition. *J Trauma Acute Care Surg.* 2013;74(5):1363–1366.
58. Bailitz J, Starr F, Beecroft M, et al. CT should replace three-view radiographs as the initial screening test in patients at high, moderate, and low risk for blunt cervical spine injury: a prospective comparison. *J Trauma.* 2009;66(6):1605–1609.
59. Barraco RD, Chiu WC, Clancy TV, et al.; EAST Practice Management Guidelines Work Group. Practice management guidelines for the diagnosis and management of injury in the pregnant patient: the EAST Practice Management Guidelines Work Group. *J Trauma.* 2010;69(1):211–214.
60. Pearlman MD, Tintinallli JE, Lorenz RP. A prospective controlled study of outcome after trauma during pregnancy. *Am J Obstet Gynecol.* 1990;162(6):1507–1510.
61. Vallier HA, Cureton BA, Schubeck D. Pregnancy outcomes after pelvic ring injury. *J Orthop Trauma.* 2012;26(5):302–307.
62. Guo SS, Greenspoon JS, Kahn AM. Management of burn injuries during pregnancy. *Burns.* 2001;27(4):394–397.
63. Maghsoudi H, Samnia R, Garadaghi A, Kianvar H. Burns in pregnancy. *Burns.* 2006;32(2):246–250.
64. Leggon RE, Wood GC, Indeck MC. Pelvic fractures in pregnancy: factors influencing maternal and fetal outcomes. *J Trauma.* 2002;53(4):796–804.
65. Muench MV, Canterino JC. Trauma in pregnancy. *Obstet Gynecol Clin North Am.* 2007;34(3):555–583.
66. Horon IL, Cheng D. Enhanced surveillance for pregnancy-associated mortality—Maryland. 1993–1998. *JAMA.* 2001;285(11):1455–1459.
67. Baldwin EA, Borowski KS, Brost BC, Rose CH. Antepartum nonobstetrical surgery at ≥23 weeks' gestation and risk for preterm delivery. *Am J Obstet Gynecol.* 2015;212(2):232.e1–e5.
68. Haque M, Kamal F, Chowdhury S, et al. Non obstetric causes and presentation of acute abdomen among the pregnant women. *J Family Reprod Health.* 2014;8(3):117–122.
69. Andersen B, Nielsen TF. Appendicitis in pregnancy: diagnosis, management and complications. *Acta Obstet Gynecol Scand.* 1999;78:758–762.
70. Gilo NB, Amini D, Landy HJ. Appendicitis and cholecystitis in pregnancy. *Clin Obstet Gynecol.* 2009;52(4):586–596.
71. Franca Neto AH, Amorim MM, Nobrega BM. Acute appendicitis in pregnancy: literature review. *Rev Assoc Med Bras.* 2015;61(2):170–177.
72. Bickell NA, Siu AL. Why do delays in treatment occur? Lessons learned from ruptured appendicitis. *Health Serv Res.* 2001;36(1):1–5.
73. Silvestri MT, Pettker CM, Brousseau EC, et al. Morbidity of appendectomy and cholecystectomy in pregnant and nonpregnant women. *Obstet Gynecol.* 2011;118(6):1261–1270.
74. Viktrup L, Hée P. Fertility and long-term complications four to nine years after appendectomy during pregnancy. *Acta Obstet Gynecol Scand.* 1998;77(7):746–750.
75. Ramin KD, Ramsey PS. Disease of the gallbladder and pancreas in pregnancy. *Obstet Gynecol Clin North Am.* 2001;28(3):571–580.
76. Everson GT, McKinley C, Kern F Jr. Mechanisms of gallstone formation in women. Effects of exogenous estrogen (Premarin) and dietary cholesterol on hepatic lipid metabolism. *J Clin Invest.* 1991;87(1):237–246.
77. Dietrich CS, Hill CC, Hueman M. Surgical diseases presenting in pregnancy. *Surg Clin North Am.* 2008;88(2):403–419.
78. Cosenza CA, Saffari B, Jabbour N, et al. Surgical management of biliary gallstone disease during pregnancy. *Am J Surg.* 1999;178(6):545–548.
79. Dhupar R, Smaldone GM, Hamad GG. Is there a benefit to delaying cholecystectomy for symptomatic gallbladder disease during pregnancy? *Surg Endosc.* 2010;24(1):108–112.

80. Jorge AM, Keswani RN, Veerappan A, et al. Non-operative management of symptomatic cholelithiasis in pregnancy is associated with frequent hospitalizations. *J Gastrointest Surg.* 2015;19(4):598–603.
81. Jelin EB, Smink DS, Vernon AH, Brooks DC. Management of biliary tract disease during pregnancy: a decision analysis. *Surg Endosc.* 2008;22(1):54–60.
82. Glanc P, Brofman N, Salem S, et al. The prevalence of incidental simple ovarian cysts ≥3 cm detected by transvaginal sonography in early pregnancy. *J Obstet Gynaecol Can.* 2007;29(6):502–506.
83. Goh WA, Rincon M, Bohrer J, et al. Persistent ovarian masses and pregnancy outcomes. *J Matern Fetal Neonatal Med.* 2013;26(11):1090–1093.
84. Goh W, Bohrer J, Zalud I. Management of the adnexal mass in pregnancy. *Curr Opin Obstet Gynecol.* 2014;26(2):49–53.
85. Zanetta G. A prospective study of the role of ultrasound in the management of adnexal masses in pregnancy. *BJOG.* 2003;110(6):578–583.
86. The American College of Obstetricians and Gynecologists. Management of adnexal masses. *ACOG Practice Bulletin.* No 83. Jul 2007.
87. Minig L, Otano L, Diaz-Padilla I, et al. Therapeutic management of epithelial ovarian cancer during pregnancy. *Clin Transl Oncol.* 2013;15(4):259–264.
88. Van Calsteren K, Heyns L, De Smet F, et al. Cancer during pregnancy: an analysis of 215 patients emphasizing the obstetrical and the neonatal outcomes. *J Clin Oncol.* 2010;28(4):683–689.
89. Horowitz NS. Management of adnexal masses in pregnancy. *Clin Obstet Gynecol.* 2011;54(4):519–527.
90. Duff P, Sweet R, Edwards R. Maternal and fetal infections. In: *Creasy and Resnik's Maternal-Fetal Medicine: Principles and Practice.* 6th ed. Philadelphia, PA: Saunders/Elsevier; 2009:739–795.
91. The American College of Obstetricians and Gynecologists. Obstetric analgesia and anesthesia. *ACOG Practice Bulletin.* 2002, No 36.
92. Cheek TG, Baird E. Anesthesia for nonobstetric surgery: maternal and fetal considerations. *Clin Obstet Gynecol.* 2009;52(4):535–545.
93. Guidelines Committee of the Society of American Gastrointestinal and Endoscopic Surgeons, Yumi H. Guidelines for diagnosis, treatment, and use of laparoscopy for surgical problems during pregnancy: this statement was reviewed and approved by the Board of Governors of the Society of American Gastrointestinal and Endoscopic Surgeons (SAGES), September 2007. It was prepared by the SAGES Guidelines Committee. *Surg Endosc.* 2008;22(4):849–861.
94. Soper NJ. SAGES' guidelines for diagnosis, treatment, and use of laparoscopy for surgical problems during pregnancy. *Surg Endosc.* 2011;25: 3477–3478.
95. D'Alton ME, Main EK, Menard MK, Levy BS. The National Partnership for Maternal Safety. *Obstet Gynecol.* 2014;123(5):973–977.
96. Lipman S, Cohen S, Einav S, et al.; Society for Obstetric Anesthesia and Perinatology. The Society for Obstetric Anesthesia and Perinatology consensus statement on the management of cardiac arrest in pregnancy. *Anesth Analg.* 2014;118(5):1003–1016.
97. Katz V, Balderston K, DeFreest M. Perimortem cesarean delivery: were our assumptions correct? *Am J Obstet Gynecol.* 2005;192(6):1916–1920.
98. Katz VL. Perimortem cesarean delivery: its role in maternal mortality. *Semin Perinatol.* 2012;36(1):68–72.
99. Einav S, Kaufman N, Sela HY. Maternal cardiac arrest and perimortem caesarean delivery: evidence or expert-based? *Resuscitation.* 2012;83(10): 1191–1200.
100. Bernstein IM, Watson M, Simmons GM, et al. Maternal brain death and prolonged fetal survival. *Obstet Gynecol.* 1989;74(3):434–437.
101. Powner DJ, Bernstein IM. Extended somatic support for pregnant women after brain death. *Crit Care Med.* 2003;31(4):1241–1249.
102. American College of Obstetricians and Gynecologists. Patient choice and the maternal-fetal relationship. Number 214, April 1999 (replaces number 55, October 1987). Committee on Ethics. *Int J Gynecol Obstet.* 1999;65(2):213–215.
103. Melnick DM, Wahl WL, Dalton VK. Management of general surgical problems in the pregnant patient. *Am J Surg.* 2004;187(2):170–180.
104. James AH. Pregnancy and thrombotic risk. *Crit Care Med.* 2010; 38(2 Suppl):S57–63.
105. Heit JA, Kobbervig CE, James AH, et al. Trends in the incidence of venous thromboembolism during pregnancy or postpartum: a 30-year population-based study. *Ann Intern Med.* 2005;143(10):697–706.
106. Donnelly JC, D'Alton ME. Pulmonary embolus in pregnancy. *Semin Perinatol.* 2013;37(4):225–233.
107. McGwin G, Russell SR, Rux RL, et al. Knowledge, beliefs, and practices concerning seat belt use during pregnancy. *J Trauma Inj Infect Crit Care.* 2004;56(3):670–675.
108. McGwin G Jr, Willey P, Ware A, et al. A focused educational intervention can promote the proper application of seat belts during pregnancy. *J Trauma Inj Infect Crit Care.* 2004;56(5):1016–1021.
109. Schiff MA, Mack CD, Kaufman RP, et al. The effect of air bags on pregnancy outcomes in Washington State: 2002–2005. *Obstet Gynecol.* 2010; 115(1):85–92.
110. The American College of Obstetricians and Gynecologists. ACOG Committee Opinion No. 518: Intimate partner violence. *Obstet Gynecol.* 2012; 119:412–417.
111. Black MC, Basile KC, Breidig MJ, et al. *The National Intimate Partner and Sexual Violence Survey (NISVS): 2010 Summary Report.* Atlanta, GA: National Center for Injury Prevention and Control, Centers for Disease Control and Prevention; 2011;75.
112. El Kady D, Gilbert WM, Xing G, Smith LH. Maternal and neonatal outcomes of assaults during pregnancy. *Obstet Gynecol.* 2005;105(2):357–363.

CHAPTER
81

Fetal Monitoring Concerns

SARAH B. ANDERSON and RODNEY K. EDWARDS

INTRODUCTION

The care of a pregnant woman poses a special set of challenges due to the fact that one is really caring for two separate patients—the woman and her fetus. To further complicate matters, one of these patients, the fetus, cannot be assessed directly. The needs of one are often congruent with the needs of the other. However, this may not always be the case. In many situations, fetal status will improve with stabilization of maternal status. However, fetal status may sometimes necessitate preterm delivery.

Immediate issues to address that are unique to caring for a pregnant woman include assessing the gestational age, whether the fetus is alive and, if alive, assessing the fetal condition. A diagnosis of fetal demise eliminates the fetus as a confounding factor in decisions regarding maternal treatment. In contrast, confirmation of a live fetus indicates a need to avoid teratogenic agents and optimize oxygen delivery to the fetus via the placenta. In either case, one should consider the physiologic changes that occur during pregnancy when formulating a plan of care.

Estimation of gestational age is an important factor to establish. If the pregnancy is near term and nonobstetric surgical treatment is indicated, delivery of the fetus prior to such treatment may be warranted. The earliest gestational age at which neonatal survival may occur is around 23 weeks. However, survival, particularly without significant morbidity, becomes more likely at later gestational ages. Even prior to the time when *ex utero* survival is possible, some treatments may better be avoided for the sake of the fetus, but as gestational age advances, discussion regarding delivery of the fetus may be appropriate to maximize treatment to the woman without placing the fetus at unnecessary risk.

Finally, fetal assessment is dependent on gestational age. At early gestational ages, simply documenting fetal cardiac activity is sufficient. At later gestational ages, the goal of fetal assessment and monitoring is determination of the adequacy of fetal oxygenation, and, when necessary, alerting the physician to potential hypoxia and/or fetal compromise. These indirect assessments of the fetal condition (discussed later in this chapter) allow for intervention, with the aim of improving fetal oxygenation or effecting delivery if improvement does not occur. If the gestational age is 23 weeks or more (or if the woman is visibly pregnant), maternal evaluation should be undertaken with left lateral displacement of the uterus (1); oxygen can be given to the mother while awaiting fetal evaluation (2).

When instituting therapies for a pregnant woman, the effect of such therapies on the fetus must be considered. Many treatments provided to pregnant women are also in the best interest of the fetus. Optimal maternal oxygenation, blood pressure, temperature, and electrolyte balance benefit both the mother and the fetus. Some therapies, however, may be detrimental to the fetus. Imaging studies that are necessary for maternal diagnosis should not be avoided due to pregnancy; of note, MRI without contrast has not been associated with fetal adverse effects (3). Ionizing radiation, if the calculated fetal dose is less than 5 rad, is considered safe during pregnancy. This threshold of radiation is far higher than the fetal exposure from a CT scan of the abdomen/pelvis or CT angiogram assessing for pulmonary embolism. Consultation with an obstetrician or maternal–fetal medicine specialist will provide appropriate recommendations regarding the effects of the physiologic changes of pregnancy on the planned treatment and which medications and other agents to avoid.

PATHOPHYSIOLOGY

Anatomy and Function of the Placenta

The placenta develops from trophoblastic cells called the syncytiotrophoblast. As these cells proliferate, the intervillous space is created. This space is where maternal blood bathes the fetal chorionic villi and where fetal–maternal and maternal–fetal exchanges occur (4). Although the intervillous space is an area characterized by low pressure, a pressure differential does exist and ensures adequate circulation; the maternal arteriolar pressure exceeds the pressure in the intervillous space, which exceeds the pressure in the maternal veins. The placenta itself is a low-resistance organ, and, accordingly, the pressure differential across the intervillous space is small. Therefore, the vascular resistance of the maternal arteries governs the rate of flow into and across the intervillous space. During uterine contractions, the intrauterine pressure exceeds the pressure in the intervillous space, and flow temporarily stops. However, the intervillous space becomes somewhat dilated during a contraction, allowing for continued contact with maternal blood and continued gas exchange, although with reduced efficiency.

The placenta has a high rate of oxygen consumption. It serves as the main organ of gas and nutrient exchange for the fetus (5). However, oxygen extracted at the fetal–maternal interface serves not only the fetus, but the placenta as well. This highly metabolic organ uses as much, and possibly more, of the total oxygen and nutrients as the fetus in order to maintain its own growth and metabolism (6).

Fetal–Placental Respiration

Fetal oxygen consumption remains constant over a wide range of changes in oxygen delivery and will decrease only when extraction is maximal and delivery is further reduced (7). A 50% reduction in uterine blood flow is compensated by an increase in umbilical blood flow and an increase in oxygen extraction to maintain oxygen delivery (8). This compensatory mechanism remains adequate only with short-term reductions in uterine blood flow. A critical point exists below which oxygen uptake becomes dependent on oxygen delivery (9). Long-term reductions result in decreased consumption secondary to the decrease in delivery. Below this threshold, tissue hypoxia occurs, there is an inability to maintain oxidative metabolism, and fetal acidemia results (10). A chronic decrease in oxygen consumption also will lead to decreases in both fetal growth and fetal activity in an effort to conserve oxygen for cellular homeostasis (11).

Oxygenated blood is carried to the fetus via the umbilical vein, while deoxygenated blood is carried back to the placenta via the two umbilical arteries. The human fetal umbilical venous PO_2 is low compared to postnatal standards—around 30 mmHg. Despite this low PO_2, adequate amounts of oxygen can be delivered to the fetal tissues. This delivery is facilitated by the high fetal cardiac output, relative to body size, and the affinity of fetal hemoglobin for oxygen (12). Fetal hemoglobin's high affinity for oxygen ensures that virtually all of the fetal hemoglobin is maximally saturated, even at the low PO_2 of the fetal umbilical venous blood. This affinity can be altered by factors such as acidosis and temperature. An increase in pH or a decrease in temperature causes a shift of the hemoglobin oxygen dissociation curve to the left, indicating a higher oxygen affinity.

At baseline, a healthy fetus has twice as much placental respiratory function as is needed to maintain its normal oxygen consumption (13). However, if placental function, even temporarily, deteriorates beyond that threshold, the fetus has very few adaptations available to deal with acute hypoxia. There are no short-term homeostatic mechanisms to alter placental respiratory gas exchange (13–17). The fetus is also unable to further increase its combined ventricular output from its high baseline level. However, the fetus does respond to hypoxia by preferentially redistributing blood to the brain, adrenal glands, and heart, and decreasing blood flow to other organs in an attempt to limit the adverse effects of hypoxia to the most vital organs.

Once the reduction in O_2 content in the peripheral tissues reaches a level where anaerobic metabolism is required, the fetus quickly becomes acidotic, because it has difficulty metabolizing lactic acid. Accumulation of lactic acid decreases the oxygen tension in the umbilical vein further by shifting the fetal oxyhemoglobin dissociation curve to the right and therefore decreasing hemoglobin saturation and total oxygen uptake in the placenta.

Hypoxemia results in decreases in fetal breathing movements, rapid eye movements, general muscle tone and activity, and baseline heart rate (18). These changes minimize the fetus's consumption of oxygen and allow a greater proportion of the cardiac output to be used for maintaining the oxygen supply to the brain (19). Resumption of these activities will occur after several hours, even in the presence of continued hypoxia, as the fetus begins to adapt to a chronic hypoxic condition (20). Therefore, fetal heart rate monitoring or ultrasound observation of the fetus is limited in its ability to predict poor outcome in cases when significant hypoxic episodes occurred prior to the monitoring period. For example, the fetal heart rate has been noted to return to baseline 12 to 16 hours after a hypoxemic event that was not associated with prolonged acidosis (21).

Maternal hypercarbia can also contribute to fetal acidosis. Usually transfer of carbon dioxide from the fetal to maternal circulation occurs readily, because the placenta is highly permeable to carbon dioxide. In fact, CO_2 transfer across the chorionic villi is accomplished faster than the transfer of oxygen. Also, favoring the transfer of carbon dioxide is the higher affinity that maternal blood has for carbon dioxide compared to fetal blood. Finally, the mild respiratory alkalosis that is normally present in pregnant women results in a lower PCO_2, further enhancing the transfer of carbon dioxide from the fetus to the maternal blood. However, if maternal PCO_2 is abnormally elevated, fetal transfer is hindered and will result in elevations of fetal PCO_2 and fetal acidosis (22).

DIAGNOSIS

Regulation of the fetal heart rate is governed by a complex interplay of the sympathetic and parasympathetic nervous systems (23). The sympathetic nervous system exerts influence through the release of norepinephrine, which accelerates the heart rate and increases inotropy; the parasympathetic nervous system decreases the heart rate. Fetal heart rate variability results from the constant "push–pull" of these two systems. Gestational age has some effect on the fetal heart rate, with a general decrease in the baseline heart rate occurring with advancing gestation.

Electronic fetal monitoring, introduced in the 1960s, has become ubiquitous in labor and delivery units in developed countries. This type of fetal monitoring typically is used at any gestational age at which *ex utero* survival is possible, that is when cesarean delivery would be considered for the indication of an abnormal fetal heart rate tracing. Electronic fetal monitoring requires very little in preparation or maintenance but does require an experienced interpreter. This technique results in a continuous tracing of the fetal heart rate, coupled with a tracing of uterine activity. Monitoring may be used during labor or may be used as a way to evaluate for fetal well-being during the antepartum period. The goal for electronic fetal monitoring is twofold: to avoid stillbirth, and to avoid neonatal encephalopathy and cerebral palsy. The efficacy of the currently available techniques is controversial and further research is needed in this area. Continuous fetal monitoring during labor does decrease the likelihood of stillbirth but has not impacted the rate of neonatal encephalopathy or cerebral palsy (24–26).

Antenatal Fetal Testing

Given the limited evidence of efficacy, antenatal testing is only recommended in high-risk patients. Conditions that might indicate antenatal fetal testing include but are not limited to diabetes, hypertension, fetal growth restriction, multiple gestations, oligohydramnios, prior stillbirths, preterm premature rupture of membranes, and decreased fetal movement.

Nonstress Test

The most commonly used antenatal test is the nonstress test (NST), which utilizes the same cardiotocography technology as continuous fetal monitoring during labor. An NST involves fetal heart rate monitoring for a period of 20 to 40 minutes. The underlying premise for this test relates to the fact that a nonacidotic, neurologically intact fetus will have fetal heart rate accelerations in response to fetal movement. The NST is

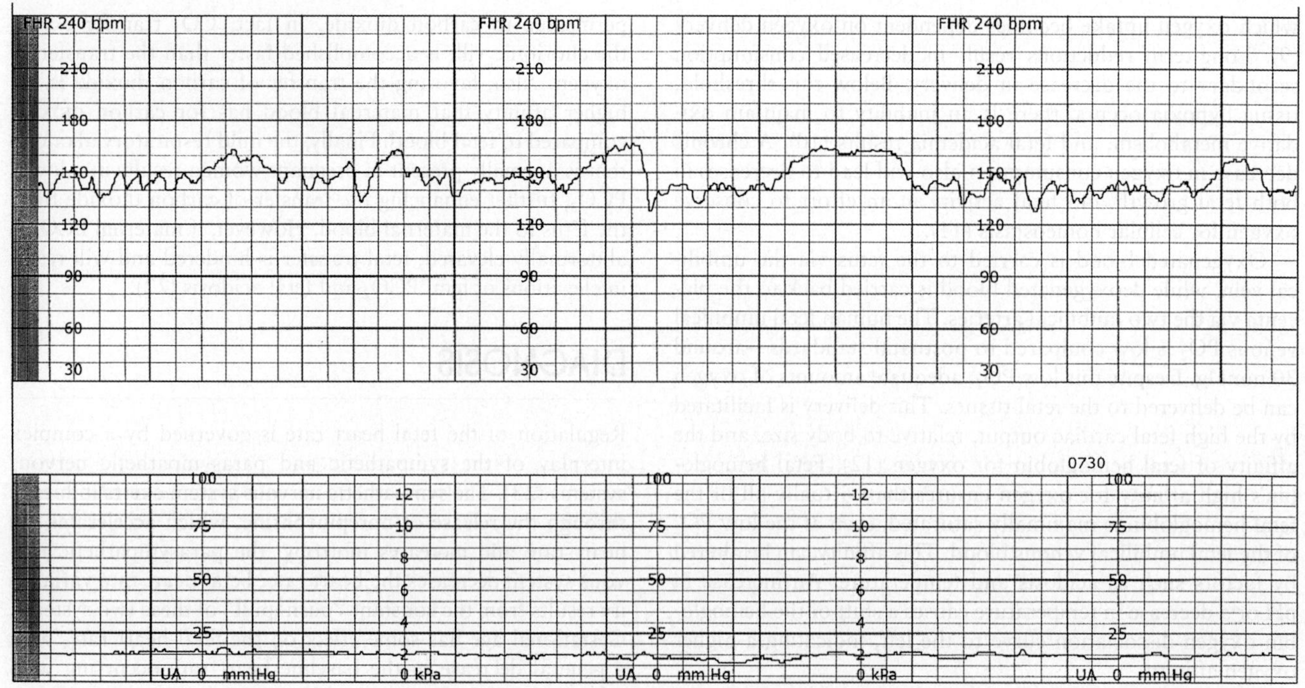

FIGURE 81.1 Reactive nonstress test. This nonstress test is reassuring, indicating fetal well-being.

described as reactive or nonreactive. The presence within a 20-minute window of two fetal heart rate accelerations lasting at least 15 seconds, that peak at least 15 beats per minute (bpm) above the baseline, characterizes a "reactive" NST (Fig. 81.1). A reactive test is highly reassuring, with a false-negative (i.e., fetal death within the next week) rate of 1.9 per 1,000 (27). However, the normal fetus periodically has episodes of decreased heart rate variability and no accelerations for 30 to 40 minutes due to sleep, and this is the most common reason for a "nonreactive" test result. A nonreactive NST often only requires further testing. Due to immaturity of the sympathetic and parasympathetic nervous systems, fetuses at less than 32 weeks gestational age may not have a reactive NST despite the absence of compromise (28).

Fetal heart rate decelerations can also be appreciated on an NST or during continuous fetal monitoring during labor. Decelerations occur when the fetal heart rate falls below the baseline heart rate; they are classified according to their appearance and location in relation to uterine contractions. Different types of decelerations are caused by different mechanisms. Therefore, each type of deceleration has different implications for fetal status.

- **Early decelerations:** Early decelerations begin at the onset of uterine contractions and appear to mirror the contraction (Fig. 81.2) (29). They are believed to be caused by pressure on the fetal head. This pressure results in an alteration in cerebral blood flow and stimulation of the vagal center, causing parasympathetic stimulation and a subsequent decrease in the fetal heart rate. Early decelerations are thought to be benign and generally are not associated with fetal hypoxia, acidosis, or low Apgar scores.
- **Variable decelerations:** Variable decelerations are abrupt decreases in the fetal heart rate at least 15 bpm below baseline with the onset to nadir lasting less than 30 seconds. Variable decelerations do not necessarily correlate with contractions (Fig. 81.3) (29). They are thought to be caused by intermittent umbilical cord compression. "Shoulders" can be seen both preceding and following these variable decelerations, and should not be considered accelerations, as they are a manifestation of the increase in sympathetic nervous system stimulation during fetal heart rate decelerations. Mild or isolated variable decelerations are benign. Repetitive moderate or severe variable decelerations may indicate fetal compromise.
- **Late decelerations:** Late decelerations occur late in relation to the uterine contraction. Their onset begins after the contraction begins, and they resolve after the resolution of the contraction (29) (Fig. 81.4). These decelerations occur as a result of decreased uteroplacental oxygen delivery to the fetus, but they may not necessarily signify poor placental function—late decelerations may be caused by maternal hypotension or decreased uterine blood flow. Persistence of late decelerations, especially in the absence of baseline fetal heart rate variability, is an ominous sign of fetal compromise.
- **Prolonged decelerations:** A prolonged deceleration is any deceleration at least 15 bpm below the baseline that lasts for 2 to 10 minutes (29). Repetitive prolonged decelerations are cause for concern for fetal compromise. Any deceleration lasting longer than 10 minutes is considered a change in baseline if the new rate is greater than 110 bpm, or bradycardia if the new heart rate is less than 110 bpm.

The last aspect of the fetal heart rate tracing analyzed on an NST is heart rate variability, or the fluctuations in the fetal heart rate seen outside of accelerations or decelerations (29). Variability is described as absent (no fluctuation), minimal (<5 bpm), moderate (5 to 15 bpm), or marked (>25 bpm) (29). In addition to causing the NST to be nonreactive, fetal sleep can be a reason for decreased variability, but persistently minimal or absent fetal heart rate variability is *the* most significant sign of fetal compromise (30). When evaluating all of these aspects of an NST, a normal result is a reactive NST with a

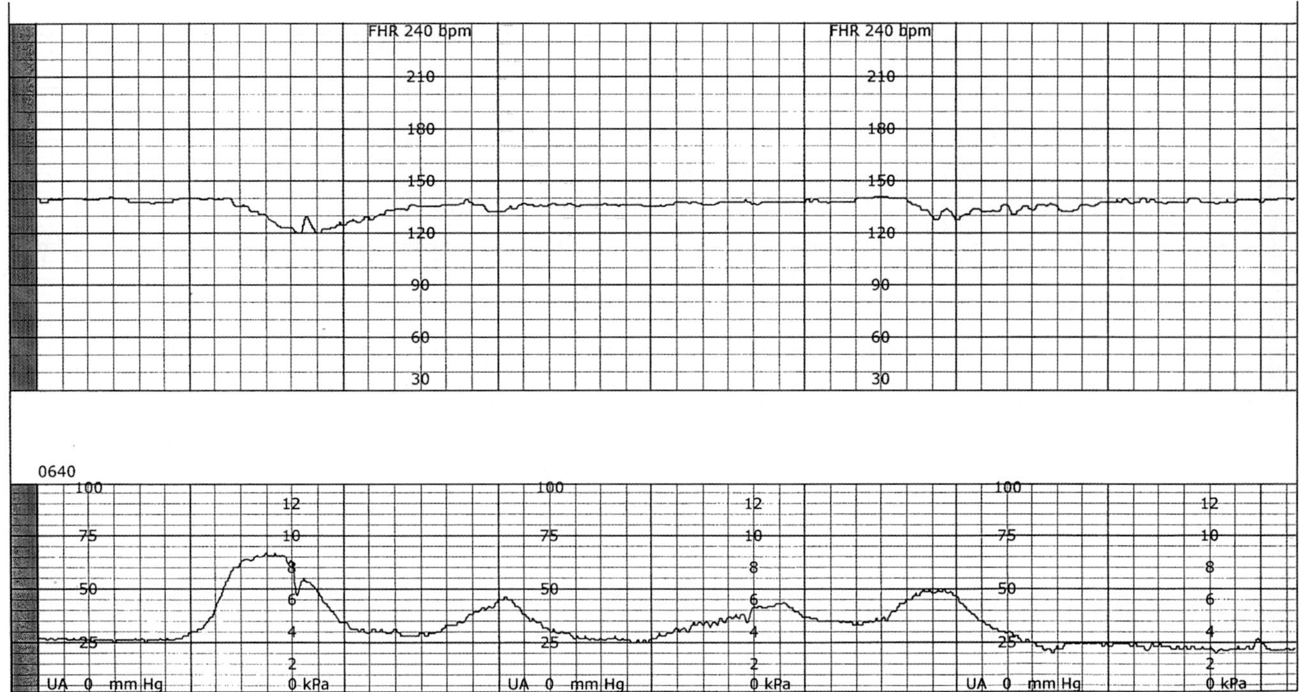

FIGURE 81.2 Early decelerations. Early decelerations mirror the contraction and are not associated with fetal compromise.

baseline between 110 and 160 bpm, no decelerations, and moderate variability.

The other (bottom panel) line on the NST represents the tocodynamometer, a strain gauge placed on the maternal abdomen used to measure uterine contractions. Though frequency and duration of contractions can be assessed with a tocodynamometer, the strength of a contraction cannot be assessed without an intrauterine pressure catheter (IUPC), placement of which requires ruptured amniotic membranes.

Contraction Stress Test

The contraction stress test (CST) is cardiotocography evaluated during spontaneous or induced contractions. It may be used as a follow-up to a nonreactive NST. The test requires at least three contractions during a 10-minute window and evaluates the fetal heart rate response to these contractions. Because of the necessity of uterine contractions, this test is contraindicated in various situations, including significantly

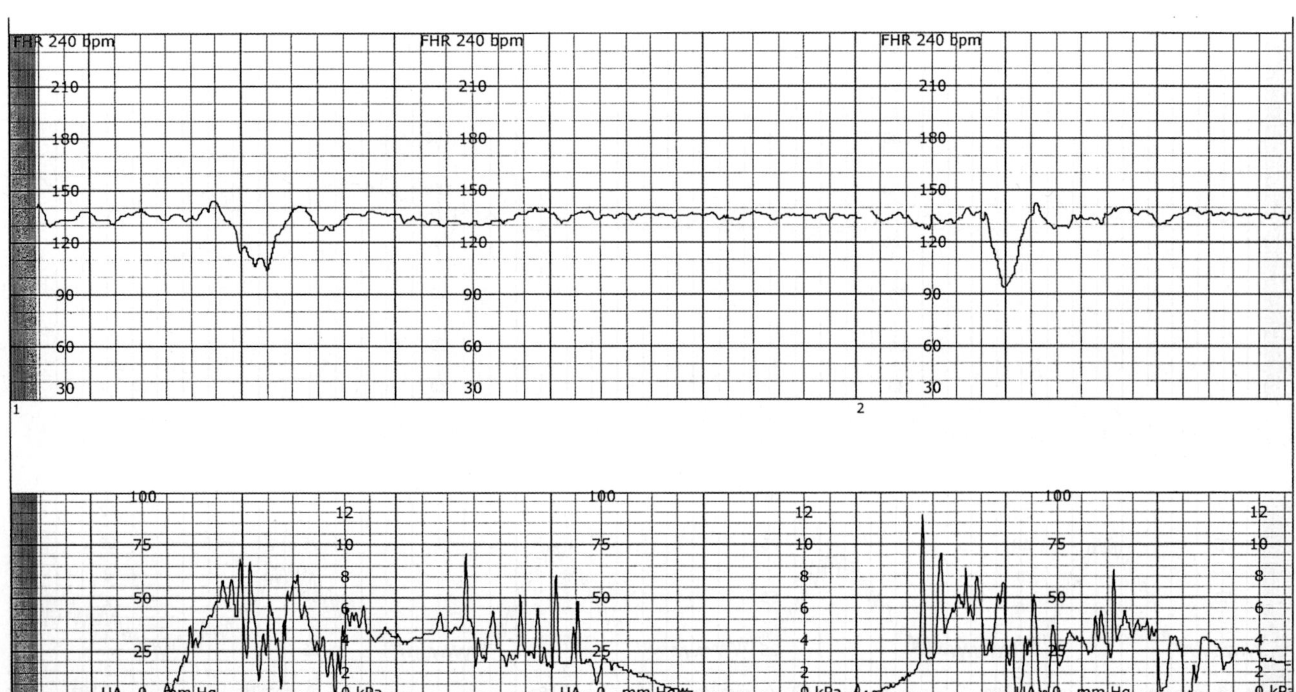

FIGURE 81.3 Variable decelerations occur at various times in relation to the contraction and are a result of transient umbilical cord compression.

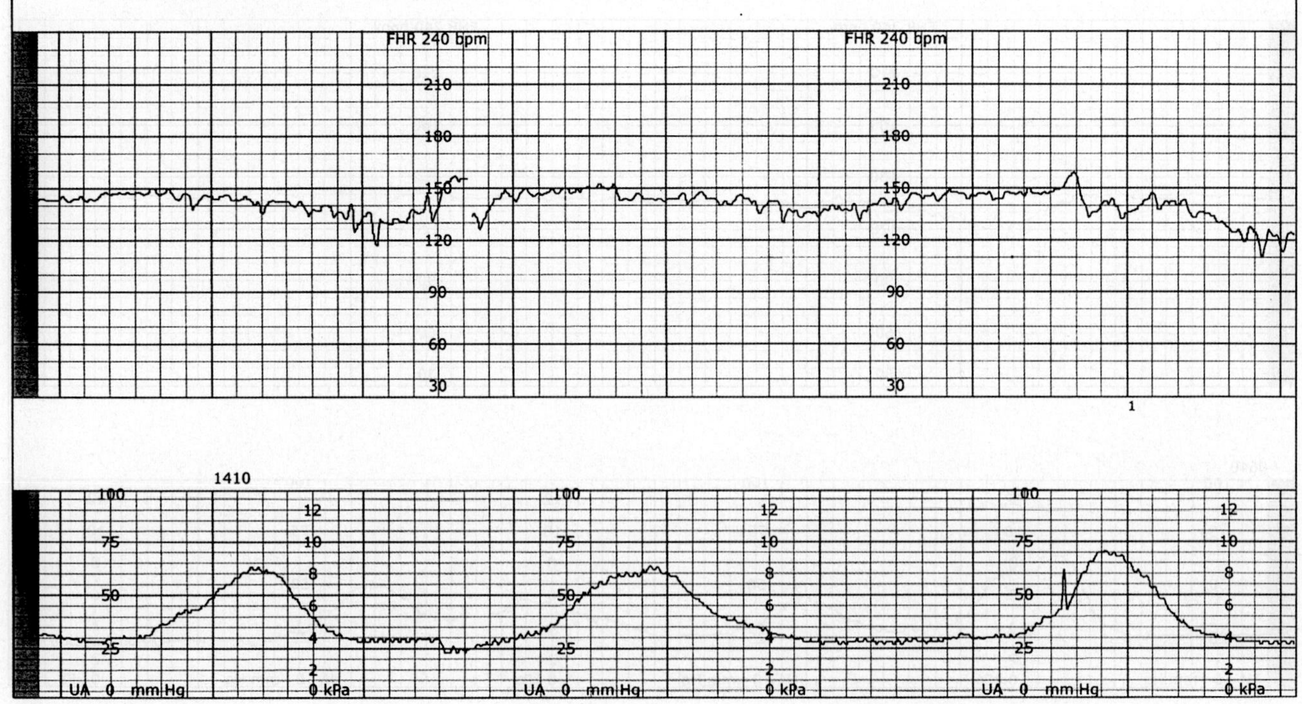

FIGURE 81.4 Late decelerations occur late in relation to the contraction and may be a sign of fetal compromise.

preterm gestations and those in whom labor is contraindicated. The underlying premise for this test involves the idea that fetal oxygenation will transiently worsen in the presence of uterine contractions. In the already-compromised fetus, this will result in late decelerations. The CST is interpreted based on the presence or absence of late decelerations. A positive CST is one in which late decelerations occur with at least 50% of contractions and generally indicates that delivery is warranted. A negative test result (with no late decelerations) is highly reassuring, with a false-negative rate of only 0.3 in 1,000 (27) (Fig. 81.5). In practice, CST is infrequently utilized today, because the test is resource intensive and has more frequent contraindications than other forms of antenatal testing.

Biophysical Profile

The biophysical profile (BPP) consists of an NST and an ultrasound examination. This test can be performed as a

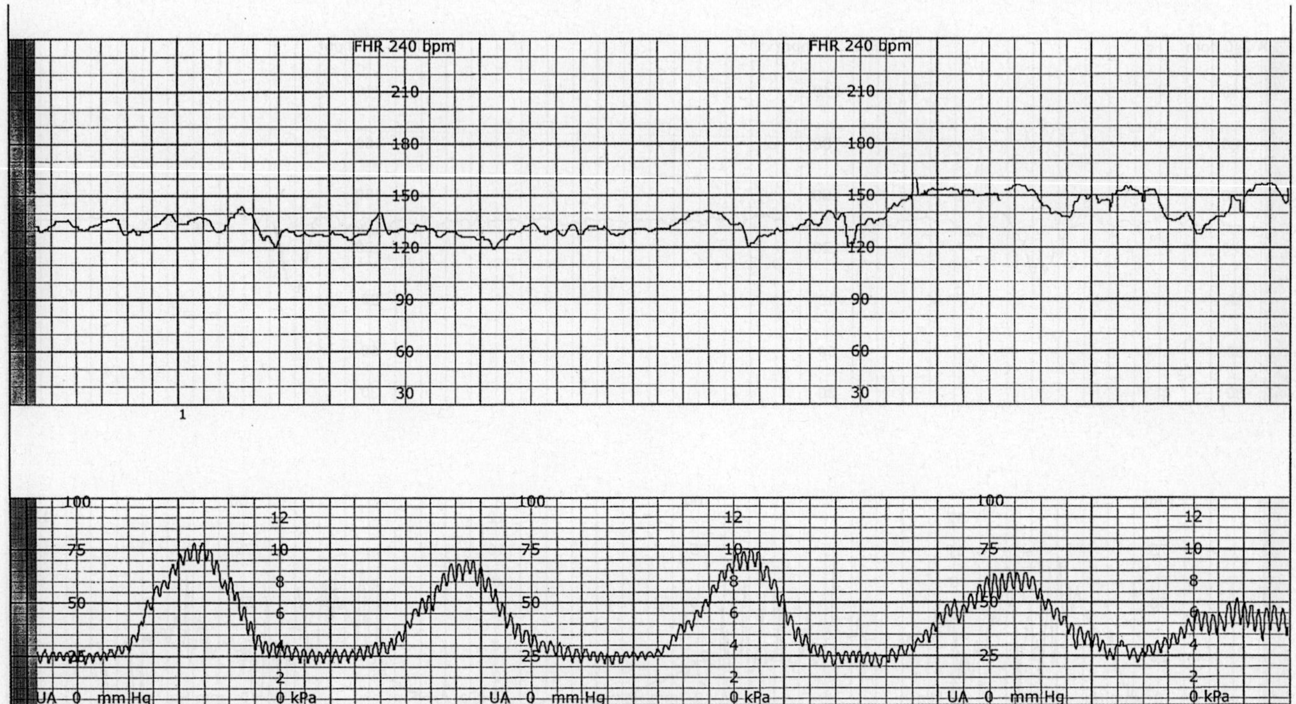

FIGURE 81.5 Negative contraction stress test. This contraction stress test is negative, indicating good fetal reserve.

TABLE 81.1 Components and Scoring of the Biophysical Profile[a]

Parameter	Score = 2	Score = 0
Nonstress test	Reactive	Nonreactive
Fetal breathing	≥1 episode of fetal breathing for ≥30 s	<30 s of breathing
Fetal tone	≥1 episode of active extension and flexion	No flexion/ extension
Gross movement	≥3 movements	<3 movements
Amniotic fluid	Single pocket ≥2 cm	Largest pocket <2 cm

[a]Score is 2 or 0 for each parameter. The maximum duration of the test is 30 minutes.

follow-up test to a nonreactive NST or can be used as a primary form of surveillance. Ultrasound is used to evaluate fetal tone, gross body movements, breathing movements, and amount of amniotic fluid present. The score is derived from these various assessments (Table 81.1). The false-negative rate of a BPP of 8/10 or 10/10 is 0.8 per 1,000 (27). However, as with all antenatal testing, many factors may alter the results of the BPP including maternal sedation, drug use, or hypoglycemia.

Doppler

As an adjunct to antenatal testing with NST, CST, or BPP, Doppler ultrasound is used to address specific concerns in fetuses at high risk for stillbirth. In growth-restricted fetuses, Doppler evaluation of flow in the umbilical artery is utilized. Diminished diastolic flow signifies placental insufficiency and increased resistance to flow in the placenta. Absent end-diastolic flow indicates the need for delivery if the gestational age is 34 weeks or more. Reversed end-diastolic flow signifies even more critical resistance to flow and is an indication for delivery even earlier (31).

The other clinical situation in which Doppler is routinely used is for evaluation of fetuses at high risk for anemia. In this situation, elevated peak systolic velocity in the middle cerebral artery correlates with fetal anemia, and assessment of middle cerebral artery Doppler is used to help determine the need for percutaneous umbilical blood sampling. Umbilical blood sampling directly assesses fetal hematocrit and, if anemia is confirmed, intrauterine fetal blood transfusion can be done (32,33). Current recommendations are to plan for fetal blood sampling and possible transfusion when the peak systolic velocity is more than 1.55 multiples of the median for the given gestational age (34). Amniocentesis, to assess indirectly the bilirubin concentration in amniotic fluid, previously was the mainstay for monitoring fetuses at risk for anemia; middle cerebral artery Doppler interrogation has almost completely replaced amniocentesis for that indication.

Intrapartum Fetal Surveillance

Intrapartum fetal surveillance is cardiotocography during labor. The same parameters evaluated on an NST are used in an ongoing fashion for intrapartum fetal surveillance. However, fetal heart rate tracings in the intrapartum period are described according to three categories (35):

- Category I: Baseline fetal heart rate 110 to 160 bpm; moderate fetal heart rate variability accelerations may be present or absent; no late or variable decelerations; may have early decelerations
- Category II: All fetal heart rate patterns that are not category I or category III
- Category III: *Absent* variability with recurrent late decelerations, absent variability with recurrent variable decelerations, or bradycardia

These categories were developed to help determine the need for treatment. However, because most tracings are category II, utility of this classification system is limited, and some authors have advocated further stratification of category II (36,37). Consideration should also be given to the tocodynamometer (or IUPC tracing) during labor. Tachysystole is the term for more than five contractions in 10 minutes, averaged over 30 minutes. Tachysystole may occur as a result of oxytocin administered to stimulate contractions during labor inductions or augmentation of spontaneous labor. If tachysystole occurs spontaneously, it may signify placental abruption.

TREATMENT

Abnormal Antenatal Testing

All tests used for antenatal testing (NST, CST, BPP) have low positive predictive values and high negative predictive values. That is, they all have a low rate of false-negative results but a high rate of false-positive results. Therefore, if antenatal testing is concerning, repeat testing is appropriate. Generally, an alternative test is used as the method of repeat testing. For example, if the NST was nonreactive, a BPP would be performed (Table 81.2). If the second test is reassuring, the likelihood of fetal acidemia is low, and repeat testing would be scheduled within the next few days to a week. However, if repeat testing also is nonreassuring, the approach generally would be to proceed with delivery. The mode of delivery would be determined by the degree of concern caused by antenatal testing results and obstetric factors. However, in some cases, fetal testing will be abnormal due to maternal disease, and these fetal testing abnormalities may resolve with maternal stabilization. Some specific examples of maternal situations where special consideration is required in interpreting fetal testing are addressed below:

- Maternal fever: Maternal fever, regardless of cause, generally causes fetal tachycardia. In this situation, fetal tachycardia may not be an indication for delivery but rather treatment of maternal infection and ongoing fetal monitoring.
- Sickle cell crisis: Sickle cell crisis can cause fetal hypoxia due to the decreased maternal oxygen–carrying capacity, and maternal treatment with oxygen, intravenous fluid resuscitation and blood transfusion will frequently improve fetal testing.
- Maternal hypoxia: Once maternal hypoxia is corrected, the fetus will frequently resuscitate *in utero* with return to reassuring fetal testing over an hour or two.

TABLE 81.2 Biophysical Score and Recommended Interventions

BPP Score	Intervention
8/10 or 10/10	Normal; continue care as indicated
6/10 or 8/10 with low amniotic fluid	Repeat within 24 hr
0/10, 2/10, 4/10	Delivery is usually indicated

- Maternal hypotension: Maternal hypotension will frequently cause uteroplacental insufficiency and late decelerations on the fetal heart rate tracing. However, upon resolution of maternal hypotension, the fetal tracing usually improves.
- Maternal acidosis without hypoxemia: Metabolic acidosis (seen in diabetic ketoacidosis and some drug toxicities) will take longer than maternal hypoxia to affect the fetus. However, *in utero* fetal resuscitation after maternal stabilization will take longer as well.
- Seizures: During a grand mal seizure, the pregnant woman becomes hypoxic. A resultant fetal bradycardia most often occurs. In cases of short-duration seizures such as is seen in patients with eclampsia, this bradycardia will usually resolve when maternal respiration resumes and should not be an indication for emergent delivery. Maternal stabilization should be achieved prior to consideration of fetal delivery.
- Cardiac arrest: The presence of an enlarged uterus, especially in the third trimester, compromises maternal cardiopulmonary resuscitation. Therefore, left lateral displacement of the uterus is essential from the beginning of any cardiopulmonary resuscitation of a pregnant woman in the second half of pregnancy. *In addition, perimortem cesarean delivery should be begun by 4 minutes into an unsuccessful resuscitation* or the likelihood that the infant will be alive and neurologically intact will be low (38).

Abnormal Intrapartum Testing

A category I tracing is considered normal, and no treatment is required. A category III tracing is considered to represent a high probability of abnormal fetal acid–base status, and efforts should be made to expeditiously resolve the underlying cause or deliver the fetus. A category II tracing requires continued surveillance, reevaluation, and actions to try to resolve the underlying cause (29).

The response to category II or category III tracings initially should consist of maneuvers aimed at "intrauterine resuscitation." These maneuvers include turning the pregnant woman to left lateral position, providing supplemental oxygen, stopping any exogenous augmentation of uterine contractions, and increasing the rate of intravenous fluid delivery. The left lateral (and also right lateral) position decreases the pressure exerted on the IVC by the gravid uterus and allows for improved maternal venous return (1). Minimizing contractions allows for more continuous flow of oxygenated maternal blood to the intervillous space. The administration of supplemental oxygen has no effect on uterine or umbilical blood flow but may increase fetal venous PO_2.

CONTROVERSIES

As discussed previously, though the use of electronic fetal monitoring has been associated with a decrease in intrapartum stillbirth rates, hopes that it would decrease the likelihood of cerebral palsy have not been realized. Furthermore, the low positive predictive value of intrapartum monitoring is thought to have contributed significantly to an increase in the cesarean delivery rate in the United States from 5% in 1970 to 32% today (39). Likewise, the low positive predictive value of tests used for antenatal fetal testing can lead to iatrogenic preterm delivery, an argument for testing only high-risk patients.

The currently advocated intrapartum fetal heart rate categories were created because intrainterpreter and interinterpreter variations in fetal heart rate tracing interpretation are high, and therefore, responses to the same fetal heart rate tracing varied widely (29). The current three-tier category system was an effort to more objectively stratify tracings. However, there are continued concerns that the current categories do not sufficiently stratify patients, and we agree with others that it is likely that subcategories of category II tracings will emerge (40). Such technologies as fetal pulse oximetry and analysis of the ST segment of the fetal electrocardiogram have been evaluated (41–43). However, these technologies have not been shown to improve on current monitoring.

Key Points

- Whether or not the gestational age is compatible with the possibility of extrauterine survival significantly affects how to care for a critically ill pregnant woman;
- Diagnostic testing and treatment should not be withheld due to concerns about fetal effects. Consultation with an obstetrician or maternal–fetal medicine specialist can facilitate tailoring treatment for pregnant women;
- Physiologic changes occur in pregnancy that maximize oxygen delivery to the fetus and carbon dioxide transfer back to the maternal circulation;
- Antenatal fetal testing is indicated to evaluate a potentially viable fetus when there is concern for fetal hypoxia or death;
- The negative predictive value of all tests used for fetal surveillance is high, but the positive predictive value of all tests of fetal well-being is low.

References

1. Lees MM, Scott DB, Kerr MG, Taylor SH. The circulatory effects of recumbent postural change in late pregnancy. *Clin Sci.* 1967;32:453–465.
2. Battaglia FC, Meschia G, Makowski EL, Bowes W. The effect of maternal oxygen inhalation upon fetal oxygenation. *J Clin Invest.* 1968;47:548–555.
3. ACOG Committee on Obstetric Practice. ACOG committee opinion. Number 299, September 2004 (replaces No. 158, September 1995). Guidelines for diagnostic imaging during pregnancy. *Obstet Gynecol.* 2004;104:647–651.
4. Ramsey EM, Martin CB Jr, Donner MW. Fetal and maternal placental circulations. Simultaneous visualization in monkeys by radiography. *Am J Obstet Gynecol.* 1967;98:419–423.
5. Hay WW Jr. Placental transport of nutrients to the fetus. *Horm Res.* 1994;42:215–222.
6. Bell AW, Hay WW Jr, Ehrhardt RA. Placental transport of nutrients and its implications for fetal growth. *J Reprod Fertil Suppl.* 1999;54:401–410.
7. Jensen A, Garnier Y, Berger R. Dynamics of fetal circulatory responses to hypoxia and asphyxia. *Eur J Obstet Gynecol Reprod Biol.* 1999;84:155–172.
8. Anderson DF, Parks CM, Faber JJ. Fetal O_2 consumption in sheep during controlled long-term reductions in umbilical blood flow. *Am J Physiol.* 1986;250:H1037–H1042.
9. Carter AM. Factors affecting gas transfer across the placenta and the oxygen supply to the fetus. *J Dev Physiol.* 1989;12:305–322.
10. Carter AM. Placental oxygen consumption. Part I: in vivo studies–a review. *Placenta.* 2000;21(Suppl A):S31–S37.
11. Peebles DM. Fetal consequences of chronic substrate deprivation. *Semin Fetal Neonatal Med.* 2004;9:379–386.
12. Hellegers AE, Schruefer JJ. Nomograms and empirical equations relating oxygen tension, percentage saturation, and pH in maternal and fetal blood. *Am J Obstet Gynecol.* 1961;81:377–384.

13. Wilkening RB, Meschia G. Fetal oxygen uptake, oxygenation, and acid–base balance as a function of uterine blood flow. *Am J Physiol.* 1983;244: H749–H755.
14. Wilkening RB, Meschia G. Effect of umbilical blood flow on transplacental diffusion of ethanol and oxygen. *Am J Physiol.* 1989;256:H813–H820.
15. Battaglia FC, Bowes W, McGaughey HR, et al. The effect of fetal exchange transfusions with adult blood upon fetal oxygenation. *Pediatr Res.* 1969; 3:60–65.
16. Rankin JH, Meschia G, Makowski EL, Battaglia FC. Relationship between uterine and umbilical venous PO2 in sheep. *Am J Physiol.* 1971;220:1688–1692.
17. Wilkening RB, Boyle DW, Meschia G. Fetal neuromuscular blockade: effect on oxygen demand and placental transport. *Am J Physiol.* 1989;257: H734–H738.
18. Weismann DN, Robillard JE. Renal hemodynamic responses to hypoxemia during development: relationships to circulating vasoactive substances. *Pediatr Res.* 1988;23:155–162.
19. Giussani DA, Spencer JA, Moore PJ, et al. Afferent and efferent components of the cardiovascular reflex responses to acute hypoxia in term fetal sheep. *J Physiol.* 1993;461:431–449.
20. Bocking AD, Gagnon R, Milne KM, White SE. Behavioral activity during prolonged hypoxemia in fetal sheep. *J Appl Physiol.* 1988;65:2420–2426.
21. Bocking AD, White S, Gagnon R, Hansford H. Effect of prolonged hypoxemia on fetal heart rate accelerations and decelerations in sheep. *Am J Obstet Gynecol.* 1989;161:722–727.
22. Blechner JN. Maternal-fetal acid-base physiology. *Clin Obstet Gynecol.* 1993;36:3–12.
23. Dalton KJ, Dawes GS, Patrick JE. The autonomic nervous system and fetal heart rate variability. *Am J Obstet Gynecol.* 1983;146:456–462.
24. Signore C, Freeman RK, Spong CY. Antenatal testing: a reevaluation: executive summary of a Eunice Kennedy Shriver National Institute of Child Health and Human Development Workshop. *Obstet Gynecol.* 2009;113:687–701.
25. Haws RA, Yakoob MY, Soomro T, et al. Reducing stillbirths: screening and monitoring during pregnancy and labour. *BMC Pregnancy Childbirth.* 2009;9(Suppl 1):S5.
26. Pattison N, McCowan L. Cardiotocography for antepartum fetal assessment. *Cochrane Database Syst Rev.* 2000:CD001068.
27. Practice Bulletin No. 145: Antepartum fetal surveillance. *Obstet Gynecol.* 2014;124:182–192.
28. Smith CV, Phelan JP, Paul RH. A prospective analysis of the influence of gestational age on the baseline fetal heart rate and reactivity in a low-risk population. *Am J Obstet Gynecol.* 1985;153:780–782.
29. American College of Obstetricians and Gynecologists. ACOG Practice Bulletin No. 106: Intrapartum fetal heart rate monitoring: nomenclature, interpretation, and general management principles. *Obstet Gynecol.* 2009;114:192–202.
30. Williams KP, Galerneau F. Intrapartum fetal heart rate patterns in the prediction of neonatal acidemia. *Am J Obstet Gynecol.* 2003;188: 820–823.
31. Society for Maternal–Fetal Medicine, Berkley E, Chauhan SP, Abuhamad A. Doppler assessment of the fetus with intrauterine growth restriction. *Am J Obstet Gynecol.* 2012;206:300–308.
32. Mari G, Adrignolo A, Abuhamad AZ, et al. Diagnosis of fetal anemia with Doppler ultrasound in the pregnancy complicated by maternal blood group immunization. *Ultrasound Obstet Gynecol.* 1995;5:400–405.
33. Mari G, Deter RL, Carpenter RL, et al. Noninvasive diagnosis by Doppler ultrasonography of fetal anemia due to maternal red-cell alloimmunization. Collaborative Group for Doppler Assessment of the Blood Velocity in Anemic Fetuses. *N Engl J Med.* 2000;342:9–14.
34. Society for Maternal-Fetal Medicine(SMFM); Berry SM, Stone J, Norton ME, et al. Fetal blood sampling. *Am J Obstet Gynecol.* 2013;209: 170–180.
35. Macones GA, Hankins GD, Spong CY, et al. The 2008 National Institute of Child Health and Human Development workshop report on electronic fetal monitoring: update on definitions, interpretation, and research guidelines. *Obstet Gynecol.* 2008;112:661–666.
36. Blackwell SC, Grobman WA, Antoniewicz L, et al. Interobserver and intraobserver reliability of the NICHD 3-Tier Fetal Heart Rate Interpretation System. *Am J Obstet Gynecol.* 2011;205:378.e1–e5.
37. Gyamfi Bannerman C, Grobman WA, Antoniewicz L, et al. Assessment of the concordance among 2-tier, 3-tier, and 5-tier fetal heart rate classification systems. *Am J Obstet Gynecol.* 2011;205:288.e1–e4.
38. Vencken PM, van Hooff MH, van der Weiden RM. Cardiac arrest in pregnancy: increasing use of perimortem caesarean section due to emergency skills training? *BJOG.* 2010;117:1664–1665.
39. American College of Obstetricians and Gynecologists (College); Society for Maternal-Fetal Medicine, Caughey AB, Cahill AG, Guise JM, Rouse DJ. Safe prevention of the primary cesarean delivery. *Am J Obstet Gynecol.* 2014; 210:179–193.
40. Clark SL, Nageotte MP, Garite TJ,, et al. Intrapartum management of category II fetal heart rate tracings: towards standardization of care. *Am J Obstet Gynecol.* 2013;209:89–97.
41. Saade G. 1: Fetal ECG analysis of the ST segment as an adjunct to intrapartum fetal heart rate monitoring: a randomized clinical trial. *Am J Obstet Gynecol.* 2015;1(212):S2.
42. Belfort MA, Saade GR. ST segment analysis (STAN) as an adjunct to electronic fetal monitoring, Part II: clinical studies and future directions. *Clin Perinatol.* 2011;38:159–167, vii.
43. East CE, Begg L, Colditz PB, Lau R. Fetal pulse oximetry for fetal assessment in labour. *Cochrane Database Syst Rev.* 2014;(10):CD004075.

CHAPTER
82

The Febrile Patient

PAUL E. MARIK

INTRODUCTION

Fever is a common problem in the intensive care unit (ICU). A prospective observational study in a general ICU reported fever (core temperature over 38.3°C) in 70% of patients, caused equally by infective and noninfective processes (1). In a large retrospective cohort study (24,204 ICU admissions), Laupland et al. (2) reported that 44% of patients experienced a temperature higher than 38.2°C during their ICU stay; 17% of these patients had positive cultures. The discovery of fever in an ICU patient has significant impact on health care costs, as blood cultures, radiologic imaging, and antibiotics routinely follow. It is, therefore, important to have a good understanding of the mechanisms and etiology of fever in ICU patients, how and when to initiate a diagnostic workup, and when initiation of antibiotics is indicated.

The *Society of Critical Care Medicine* and the *Infectious Disease Society of America* considers a temperature of 38.3°C or greater (101°F) a fever in an ICU patient which warrants further evaluation (3). This does not necessarily imply that a temperature below 38.3°C (101°F) does not require further investigation, as many variables determine a patient's febrile response to an insult. In addition, it should be recognized that there is a daily fluctuation of temperature by 0.5° to 1.0°C, with women having wider variations in temperature than men. Furthermore, with aging, the maximal febrile response decreases by about 0.15°C per decade.

Accurate and reproducible measurement of body temperature is important in detecting disease and in monitoring patients with an elevated temperature. A variety of methods are used to measure body temperature, combining different sites, instruments, and techniques (4,5). Infrared ear thermometry has been demonstrated to provide values that are a few tenths of a degree below the temperature in the pulmonary artery and brain. Rectal temperatures obtained with a mercury thermometer or electronic probe are often a few tenths of a degree higher than core temperatures. However, patients perceive having rectal temperatures taken as unpleasant and intrusive. Furthermore, access to the rectum may be limited by patient position with an associated risk of rectal trauma. Many tachypneic patients are unable to keep their mouth closed to obtain an accurate oral temperature. Axillary measurements *substantially underestimate* core temperature and lack reproducibility. Body temperature is, therefore, most accurately measured by an intravascular thermistor; however, measurement by infrared ear thermometry or with an electronic probe in the rectum is an acceptable alternative.

PATHOGENESIS OF FEVER

Cytokines released by monocytic cells play a central role in the genesis of fever (6,7). The cytokines primarily involved in the development of fever include interleukin-1 (IL-1), interleukin-6 (IL-6), and tumor necrosis factor-α (TNF-α). These cytokines bind to their own specific receptors located in close proximity to the preoptic region of the anterior hypothalamus. Here the cytokine receptor interaction activates phospholipase A2, resulting in the liberation of plasma membrane arachidonic acid as substrate for the cyclooxygenase pathway.

Fever appears to be a preserved evolutionary response within the animal kingdom (8,9). With few exceptions, reptiles, amphibians, fish, and several invertebrate species have been shown to manifest fever in response to challenge with micro-organisms. Increased body temperature has been shown to enhance the resistance of animals to infection. Although fever has some harmful effects, it appears to be an adaptive, evolved response that helps rid the host of invading pathogens. Temperature elevation has been shown to enhance several parameters of immune function including antibody production, T-cell activation, production of cytokines, and enhanced neutrophil and macrophage function. Furthermore, some pathogens such as *Streptococcus pneumoniae* are inhibited by febrile temperatures.

CAUSES OF FEVER IN THE INTENSIVE CARE UNIT

Any disease process that results in the release of the pro-inflammatory cytokines IL-1, IL-6 and TNF-α will result in the development of fever. While infections are common causes of fever in ICU patients, many noninfectious inflammatory conditions cause the release of the pro-inflammatory cytokines and induce a febrile response. Similarly, it is important to appreciate that not all patients with infections are febrile. Approximately 10% of septic patients are *hypothermic,* and 35% *normothermic* at presentation. Septic patients who fail to develop a fever have a significantly higher mortality than febrile septic patients. The reason that patients with established infections fail to develop a febrile response is unclear; however, it appears that this aberrant response is not due to diminished cytokine production (10). The approach to a patient who presents to hospital with a fever is different from that of a patient who develops a fever in the ICU; this chapter reviews fever that develops in the ICU.

Fever Patterns

Attempts to derive reliable and consistent clues from evaluation of a patient's fever pattern is fraught with uncertainly and is not likely to be helpful diagnostically (11–13). Most patients have remittent or intermittent fever, which, when due to infection, usually follow a diurnal variation. Sustained fevers have been reported in patients with gram-negative pneumonia or CNS damage. The appearance of fever at different time points in the course of a patient's illness may, however, provide some diagnostic clues. Fevers that arise more than 48 hours after institution of mechanical ventilation may be secondary to a developing pneumonia. Fevers that arise 5 to 7 days postoperatively may be related to abscess formation. Fevers that arise 10 to 14 days postinstitution of antibiotics for intra-abdominal abscess may be due to fungal infections.

Infectious Causes

Hospital-acquired infections (HAIs) are infections developing in the hospital setting and are a worldwide problem occurring both in developed and in developing countries. The greatest percentage of HAIs are acquired in the ICU, with the most important being central line–associated bloodstream infection (CLABSI), catheter-associated urinary tract infections (CA-UTI), hospital/ventilator-associated pneumonia (VAP), *Clostridium difficile* enterocolitis, and nosocomial rhinosinusitis (NS). The infectious causes of fever in the ICU are listed in Table 82.1. It was estimated that, in 2002, a total of 1.7 million HAIs (4.5 per 100 admissions) occurred in the United States and that almost 99,000 deaths resulted from or were associated with a HAIs; similar data have been reported from Europe (14–16). These facts have been widely publicized in the lay press and attracted the attention of hospital administrators and governmental agencies. It is, however, likely that these estimates are inflated. More recent data suggests that there are approximately 440,000 to 640,000 HAIs annually in the United States (17,18). In a recent point prevalence study conducted in 183 acute care hospitals in 10 "geographically diverse states" in the United States, 4% of patients developed one or more HAIs (18). In this study, the most common infections were pneumonia (21.8%), surgical site infections (21.8%) and gastrointestinal infections (17.1%); *C. difficile* was the most commonly reported pathogen, causing 12.1% of all HAIs. Device-associated infections (CLABSI, CA-UTI, and VAP), which have traditionally been the major focus of infection control programs, accounted for only 25.6% of HAIs.

TABLE 82.1 Most Common Infectious Causes of Fever in the ICU

Clostridium difficile colitis
Surgical site or wound infection
Catheter-related bloodstream infection
Ventilator-associated pneumonia
Primary septicemia
Urinary tract infection (including catheter related)
Sinusitis
Cellulitis or infected decubitus ulcer
Suppurative thrombophlebitis
Endocarditis
Diverticulitis
Septic arthritis
Abscess or empyema

TABLE 82.2 Noninfectious Causes of Fever in the ICU

Drug-related
Drug fever
Neuroleptic malignant syndrome
Malignant hyperthermia
Serotonin syndrome
Drug withdrawal (including alcohol and recreational drugs)
IV contrast reaction
Posttransfusion fever
Neurologic
Intracranial hemorrhage
Cerebral infarction
Subarachnoid hemorrhage
Seizures
Endocrine
Hyperthyroidism
Pheochromocytoma
Adrenal insufficiency
Rheumatologic
Crystal arthropathies
Vasculitis
Collagen vascular diseases
Hematologic
Phlebitis
Hematoma
Gastrointestinal or hepatic
Acalculous cholecystitis
Ischemic bowel
Cirrhosis
Hepatitis
Gastrointestinal bleed
Pancreatitis
Pulmonary
Aspiration pneumonitis
Acute respiratory distress syndrome
Thromboembolic disease
Fat embolism syndrome
Cardiac
Myocardial infarction
Dressler's syndrome
Pericarditis
Oncologic
Neoplastic syndromes

Noninfectious Causes

A large number of noninfectious conditions result in tissue injury with inflammation and a febrile reaction. Those noninfectious disorders which should be considered in ICU patients are listed in Table 82.2. For reasons that are not entirely clear, most noninfectious disorders usually do not lead to a fever in excess of 38.9°C (102°F); therefore, if the temperature increases above this threshold, the patient should be considered to have an infectious etiology as the cause of the fever (19). However, patients with drug fever may have a temperature >102°F. Similarly, fever secondary to blood transfusion may exceed 102°F. In patients with a temperature above 40°C (104°F), neuroleptic malignant syndrome, malignant hyperthermia, the serotonin syndrome, and subarachnoid hemorrhage must always be considered. The most common noninfectious causes of a fever in ICU patients include drug fever, transfusion of blood and blood products, alcohol withdrawal, postoperative fever, and thromboembolic disease. Acalculous cholecystitis is a relatively uncommon cause of fever in ICU patients. However, as it may be associated with severe morbidity and mortality, it should always be considered in the differential diagnosis. Most of the clinical conditions listed in Table 82.2 are clinically obvious and do not require additional diagnostic tests to confirm their presence. However, a few of these disorders require special consideration.

Drug Fever

Most ICU patients receive numerous medications; all drugs have side effects, including fever. It is estimated that about 10% of inpatients develop drug fever during their hospital stay (20). The diagnosis of drug fever in ICU patients is challenging as the onset of fever can occur immediately after the administration of the drug or it can occur days, weeks, months, or even years after the patient has been on the offending medication. Furthermore, once the implicated medication is discontinued, the fever can persist in excess of 4 or 5 days. Associated rashes and leukocytosis occur in less than 20% of cases; an eosinophilia is suggestive of drug fever. Penicillins, cephalosporins, anticonvulsants, heparin, and histamine 2-blockers are commonly used ICU medications that are associated with drug fever.

Postoperative Fever

Surgery alone can cause a self-limited and spontaneously resolving fever (21–23). In the early postoperative period, a patient's temperature may increase up to 1.4°C, with the peak occurring approximately 11 hours after surgery (21). Fifty percent of postoperative patients will develop a fever greater than or equal to 38°C, with 25% reaching 38.5°C or higher; the fever typically lasts for 2 to 3 days. Postoperative fever is believed to be caused by tissue injury and inflammation with associated cytokine release (21). The invasiveness of the procedure, as well as genetic factors, influences the degree of cytokine release and the febrile response. A good physical examination and history of the timing and sequence of events are crucial to help to differentiate postoperative fever from other infectious and noninfectious causes of fever. Reactions to medications (especially anesthesia), blood products, and infections that might have existed prior to the surgery should also be considered during a patient's early postoperative course. Nosocomial and surgical site infections usually develop 3 to 5 days after surgery.

Atelectasis is commonly implicated as a cause of postoperative fever (22). Standard ICU texts list atelectasis as a cause of fever, although they provide no primary source. Indeed a major surgery text states that "fever is almost always present (in patients with atelectasis)" (24). During rounds, many medical students and house staff have been taught that atelectasis is one of the "five" main causes of postoperative fever. However, there is very little data to support this widely held belief (myth). Engeron (25) studied 100 postoperative cardiac surgery patients and was unable to demonstrate a relationship between atelectasis and fever. Furthermore, when atelectasis is induced in experimental animals by ligation of a main-stem bronchus, fever does not occur (26). The role of atelectasis as a cause of fever is unclear; however, atelectasis probably does not cause fever in the absence of pulmonary infection.

Blood Transfusions

A large number of patients in the ICU will receive transfusions of blood products. Febrile nonhemolytic transfusion reactions are common following transfusion of blood and blood products. This is likely mediated by the transfusion of cytokines such as IL-1, IL-6, IL-8, and TNF-α, which accumulate with increasing length of blood storage (27,28). Febrile nonhemolytic reactions normally present within the first 6 hours after transfusion, are self-limiting, and may present with chills and rigors in addition to fever. It is crucial to differentiate these from febrile acute hemolytic transfusion reactions which can be life threatening. Leukoreduction has been shown to reduce the risk of febrile nonhemolytic transfusion reactions.

Thromboembolic Disease

Fever has been reported in 18% to 60% of patients with thromboembolic disease. Typically the fever is low grade (37.5° to 38°C); however, fever up to 39°C has been reported (29,30).

Acalculous Cholecystitis

Acute acalculous cholecystitis (AAC) is an inflammatory condition of the gallbladder in the absence of calculi (31). AAC most commonly complicates surgery, multiple trauma, or burn injuries. However, this disease is not uncommon in medical patients undergoing mechanical ventilation. AAC is a disease with significant morbidity and mortality as it can lead to empyema, gangrenous gallbladder, and gallbladder perforation. A high index of suspicion is required as this can be a difficult diagnosis to make, especially in the endotracheally intubated and sedated patient. While initial presentation may be subtle, clinical features include fever, leukocytosis, abnormal liver function tests, a palpable right upper quadrant mass, vague abdominal discomfort, and jaundice. Untreated, bacterial superinfection may occur and this can progress to empyema, peritonitis, and septic shock.

Malignant Hyperthermia

Malignant hyperthermia is a rare genetic disorder of the muscle membrane causing an increase of calcium ions in the muscle cells. This can cause a variety of clinical problems, most commonly a dangerous hypermetabolic state after the use of agents such as the depolarizing neuromuscular blocking agent succinylcholine and inhaled anesthetic agents. This reaction typically occurs within 1 hour of anesthesia, but can be delayed for up to 10 hours. Patients' presentation is with continually increasing fevers, muscle stiffness, and tachycardia, and can rapidly develop hemodynamic instability with progression into multiorgan failure. Since the introduction of dantrolene, the mortality of malignant hyperthermia has decreased from 80% in the 1960s to less than 10% today.

Neuroleptic Malignant Syndrome

Neuroleptic malignant syndrome is characterized by high fevers, a change in mental status, muscle rigidity, extrapyramidal symptoms, autonomic nervous system disturbances, and altered levels of consciousness. Symptoms usually begin within days to weeks of starting the offending drug, and patients typically have very high creatinine kinase levels. Neuroleptic malignant syndrome is caused by excessive dopaminergic blockade causing dopamine deficiency in the central nervous system (CNS). Agents most commonly implicated include neuroleptic medications and certain antiemetics. Treatment includes discontinuing the offending drug, aggressive supportive care, and close hemodynamic monitoring. Drug treatment of neuroleptic malignant syndrome is controversial. A case-controlled analysis and a retrospective analysis of published cases suggested that dantrolene, bromocriptine, and amantadine may be beneficial.

Serotonin Syndrome

Serotonin syndrome is characterized by the triad of neuromuscular hyperactivity, autonomic hyperactivity, and change in mental status (32,33). It is not an idiosyncratic drug reaction but is a predictable response to serotonin excess in the CNS. It can occur from an overdose, drug interaction, or adverse drug effect involving serotonergic agents. Most severe cases result from a drug combination especially the combination of selective serotonin reuptake inhibitors (SSRIs) and monoamine oxidase inhibitors (MAOIs). It occurs in approximately 15% of patients with SSRI overdose, with hyperthermia developing in approximately half of cases, resulting from increased muscle activity due to agitation and tremor. A core temperature as high as 40°C is common in moderate to severe cases. Tachycardia, hypertension, mydriasis, hyperactive bowel sounds, myoclonus, and ocular clonus are common; however, not all of these symptoms are present in every patient. Hyperreflexia, clonus, and hypertonicity are greater in lower extremities than in upper extremities. Sustained clonus is usually found at the ankles. Most of the laboratory abnormalities are a consequence of poorly treated hyperthermia and include elevated CPK, serum creatinine, and aminotransferases, as well as a metabolic acidosis. The most important step in the treatment of the serotonin syndrome is removal of the offending drug. Control of agitation with a benzodiazepine is an essential step in the management. 5-HT_{2A} antagonists (cyproheptadine and chlorpromazine) have been used in moderate to severe cases. There are no randomized clinical trials demonstrating the effectiveness of 5-HT_{2A} antagonists.

APPROACH TO THE FEBRILE ICU PATIENT

The diagnostic workup of an ICU patient who develops a fever can be a daunting task. Frequently, the presence of a fever in the ICU patient triggers a battery of diagnostic tests that are costly, expose the patient to unnecessary risks, and often produce misleading or inconclusive results. It is, therefore, important that fever in ICU patients be evaluated in a systematic, prudent, clinically appropriate, and cost-effective manner (Fig. 82.1).

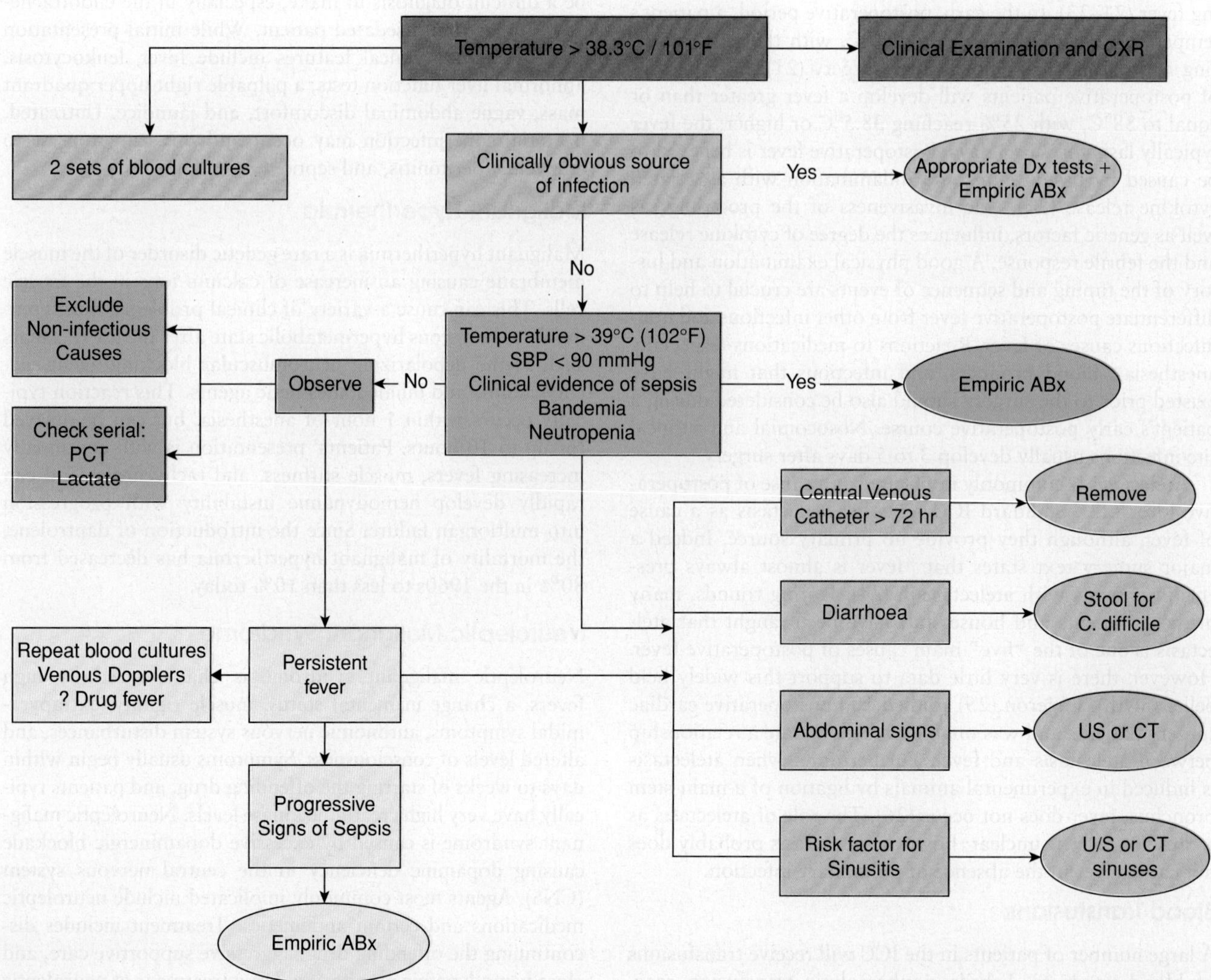

FIGURE 82.1 Suggested algorithm for the management of fever.

The signs and symptoms of systemic inflammation are not useful in distinguishing infectious from noninfectious causes of the systemic inflammatory response syndrome (SIRS). Furthermore, despite exhaustive microbiologic tests, a pathogen is not isolated in about 25% of patients with suspected sepsis (34). While blood cultures are considered to provide the clinical gold standard for the diagnosis of bacterial infections, only about 20% to 30% of patients with sepsis have positive cultures; moreover, it takes 2 to 3 days before the results become available. Although molecular methods based on polymerase chain reaction (PCR) technology hold promise for the early diagnosis of bacterial infection and for pathogen identification, these are not in common clinical use.

Currently, a number of biomarkers have been evaluated as more specific indicators of infection. Procalcitonin (PCT) has, to date, been the most useful biomarker to aid in the diagnosis of sepsis. PCT, a propeptide of calcitonin, is normally produced in the C-cells of the thyroid. In healthy individuals, PCT levels are very low (below 0.01 ng/mL). In patients with sepsis, however, PCT levels increase dramatically, sometimes to more than several hundred nanograms per milliliter. The use of PCT for the diagnosis of sepsis and in determining the duration of antibiotics is controversial. The test is not perfect and should always be interpreted in the clinical context together with other diagnostic tests. Wacker (35) performed a meta-analysis to evaluate the diagnostic accuracy of PCT. In this meta-analysis, the sensitivity was 0.77 (95% CI 0.72–0.81), the specificity was 0.79 (95% CI 0.74–0.84), and the area under the ROC curve was 0.85 (95% CI 0.81–0.88). This diagnostic accuracy is better than any other single test to diagnose sepsis. A PCT above 0.5 ng/mL is highly suggestive of a bacterial infection, while a level below 0.1 ng/mL makes this diagnosis less likely (36). However, the optimal diagnostic threshold is unclear and has been reported to vary from 0.25 to 1.4 ng/mL (36,37). This variation in diagnostic threshold may be partly explained by the case-mix of each study and by the fact that patients' with gram-negative infection have significantly higher PCT levels than those with gram-positive infections (38–40). Infection with a gram-negative pathogen is highly likely in a patient with a PCT level above 5 ng/mL. It should be noted that patients with fungal infections often have much lower or "normal" PCT level (38).

The following approach is suggested in patients who develop a fever in the ICU, with two temperature recordings above 38.3°C, a single temperature above 38.3°C with signs of sepsis or a single temperature above 39°C (see Fig. 82.1). A comprehensive physical examination and review of the chest radiograph is essential to identify infectious causes of a fever. In patients with a high fever and a high white cell count *C. difficile* infection should always be excluded. Because of the frequency, excess morbidity and mortality associated with bacteremia, blood cultures—two sets from different sites—are recommenced in all febrile ICU patients. In patients with a central venous catheter (including PICCs), a CLABSI should always be considered. The catheter insertion site should be closely examined for signs of infection and consideration made for the removal of the device if no source of fever is identified. The urinary tract of patients with an indwelling urinary bladder catheter (IUBC) rapidly becomes colonized with gram-negative bacteria and candida species. Urinalysis and urine culture cannot adequately distinguish urinary tract colonization from urinary tract infection. It is widely quoted that CA-UTIs are the most common HAI in the ICU, accounting for approximately 23% of HAI infections among US adult ICU patients (41). It is, however, likely that these data are wrong and that most ICU patients who are treated for CA-UTIs have "asymptomatic" bacteriuria which does not require treatment. CA-UTI–related sepsis is exceedingly uncommon in general ICU patients. Consequently, unless the patient has had urologic surgery, has stents or stones routine *culture of the urine should be avoided* in ICU patients who develop a fever; removal of the IUBC is the first line of therapy in potential CA-UTI. Similarly, routine culture of sputa cannot distinguish respiratory tract colonization from infection and should not be performed as a routine in ICU patients who develop a fever.

Noninfectious causes of fever should be excluded; these include consideration of drug fever, alcohol or drug withdrawal, and venous thromboembolism. In patients with an obvious focus of infection (e.g., purulent nasal discharge, abdominal tenderness, profuse green diarrhea), a focused diagnostic workup is required. If there is no clinically obvious source of infection, and unless the patient is clinically deteriorating, it may be prudent to perform blood cultures and then observe the patient before embarking on the further diagnostic tests and commencing empiric antibiotics. However, the following features suggest bacterial infection and should prompt the immediate initiation of broad spectrum antibiotics pending further diagnostic workup:

- Temperature greater than 39°C (102°F);
- Fall in blood pressure or SBP to less than 90 mmHg
- Heart rate higher than 120 beats/min
- An increasing lactate or lactate over 2.0 mEq/L
- PCT greater than 0.5 ng/mL
- Bandemia over 5%
- Lymphocytopenia less than 0.5×10^3 cells/µL
- Fall in platelet count or platelet count less than 150×10^3 cells/µL
- Neutropenia with a neurophil count less than 0.5×10^3 cells/µL
- WBC count greater than 20,000 cells/µL.

In patients whose clinical picture is consistent with infection and in whom no clinically obvious source has been documented, removal of all central lines greater than 72 hours old is recommended, stool for *C. difficile* toxin (in those patients with loose stools and *not* on stool softeners), and an ultrasound examination, CT, or plain films of the maxillary sinuses are recommended. If the patient is at risk of abdominal sepsis or has any abdominal signs (tenderness, distension, unable to tolerate enteral feeds), a CT scan of abdomen is indicated. Patients with right upper quadrant tenderness require an abdominal ultrasound or CT examination. An IUBC should be removed as soon as it is no longer indicated.

Treatment of Fever

Data from a retrospective study of 636,051 patients showed that, although the presence of fever in the first 24 hours after ICU admission was associated with an increased risk of mortality in patients without infection, it was associated with a decreased risk of mortality in those with an infection (42). In this study, the adjusted in-hospital mortality risk progressively decreased with increasing peak temperature in patients with infection. Similarly, Weinstein and colleagues (43) reported that patients with spontaneous bacterial peritonitis had improved survival if they had a temperature greater than 38°C. While fever is generally regarded as a beneficial response to infection, up to 70% of ICU patients with a fever are treated with antipyretic agents (44). Yet, the preponderance of data suggests that treating a fever in this setting is harmful. Schulman et al. (45) investigated the benefit of fever control in patients admitted to a trauma ICU. Patients were randomized to an active treatment group in which acetaminophen and cooling blankets were used to aggressively cool patients, as compared to a permissive group in which fever was only treated once it reached 40°C. In this study, there was a strong trend toward increased mortality in the active treatment group; all the patients who died in the aggressive treatment group had an infectious etiology as the cause of the fever. Lee et al. (46) performed a prospective observational study to determine the association between antipyretic treatment of fever and mortality in 1,425 critically ill patients with and without sepsis. These authors demonstrated that treatment with nonsteroidal anti-inflammatory drugs or acetaminophen independently increased 28-day mortality for septic patients (odds ratio (OR): NSAIDs: 2.61, $p = 0.028$, acetaminophen: 2.05, $p = 0.01$), but not for nonseptic patients. Against this background of convincing evidence demonstrating the harm of antipyretic agents in patients with sepsis, Schortgen and colleagues (47) performed a multicenter, RCT in which vasopressor-dependent febrile patients with septic shock were randomized to external cooling to achieve normothermia for 48 hours or no external cooling. In this study, there was a greater reduction of pressor use, more rapid shock reversal, and a lower mortality at 14 days (19% vs. 34%; $p = 0.013$) in the cooling group. However, the difference in mortality was no longer significant at ICU or hospital discharge. Based on the results of this single study and the fact that fever is widely believed to be beneficial in the setting of infection, external cooling cannot be recommended at this time. This study, however, does raise the possibility that external cooling may be beneficial in vasodilatory shock. The HEAT trial randomized 700 patients with fever (body temperature, ≥ 38°C) and known or suspected infection to receive either 1 g of intravenous acetaminophen or placebo every 6 hours until ICU discharge, resolution of fever, cessation of antimicrobial therapy, or death (48). The number of ICU-free days, the primary outcome of the study, did not differ between groups. Similarly, there was no difference in 90-day mortality between the groups. However, it should be noted that open-label acetaminophen was administered to 30% of patients assigned to acetaminophen and 29.4% assigned to placebo. Furthermore, the mean daily peak body temperature between the groups differed by only 0.25°C with the mean body temperature on day 1 being 37.5°C in the acetaminophen group and 37.0°C in the placebo group. While this study does not definitively answer the question of the role of fever control in ICU patients with infections, it does suggest that in this setting acetaminophen may not be harmful. Treatment of fever with acetaminophen may, therefore, be appropriate in patients who are highly symptomatic or have decreased cardiovascular reserve. However, it should be recognized that fever is an important vital sign that can be used to indicate resolution of the infectious process; treatment with antipyretics can mask nonresolution of infection.

In contrast to patients with infectious disorders, patients with acute cerebral insults (ischemic stroke, hemorrhagic stroke, SAH, head injury, after cardiac arrest) have worse outcomes with increased temperature. For these patients, the current recommendation is to maintain the patient's temperature in the normothermic range. Antipyresis must always include an antipyretic agent, as external cooling alone increases heat generations and catecholamine production (49). Furthermore, acute hepatitis may occur in ICU patients with reduced glutathione reserves (e.g., alcoholics, malnourished) who have received regular therapeutic doses of acetaminophen.

CONCLUSION

Fever is a common finding in ICU patients, caused equally by infective and noninfective processes. A systematic and evidence-based approach should be followed in the diagnostic workup of ICU patients with fever. All ICU patients with a temperature greater than 38.3°C (101°F) require blood cultures and a clinical evaluation to determine the source of fever. Urine and sputum should not be routinely cultured in ICU patients with a fever. Contrary to common teaching, atelectasis does not cause a fever. Antipyretic agents should not be used to control fever in patients with an infection but are indicated in many noninfectious causes of fever.

Key Points

- Fever defined as a temperature of 38.3°C or greater (101°F) is common in ICU patients and warrants a diagnostic workup.
- In ICU patients a fever is caused equally by infective and noninfective causes.
- Body temperature is most accurately measured by an intravascular thermistor; however, measurement by infrared ear thermometry or with an electronic probe in the rectum is an acceptable alternative.
- Fever is an evolutionary preserved adaptive host response in reaction to invading pathogens that serves to enhance the immune response against the pathogen.
- HAIs are infections developing in the hospital setting. The most important HAIs in ICU patients include CLABSI, HAP/VAP, and *C. difficile* enterocolitis.
- The most common noninfectious causes of a fever in ICU patients include drug fever, transfusion of blood and blood products, alcohol withdrawal, and postoperative fever. Although widely quoted as a cause of fever, atelectasis alone does not cause fever.
- Aggressive treatment of fever is indicated in patients with acute cerebral insults.
- Treatment of fever with acetaminophen may be appropriate in patients with infections who are highly symptomatic or have decreased cardiovascular reserve.
- External cooling should be reserved to patients who have failed treatment with antipyretic agents, as external cooling alone may paradoxically increase heat production.

References

1. Circiumaru B, Baldock G, Cohen J. A prospective study of fever in the intensive care unit. *Intensive Care Med.* 1999;25:668–673.
2. Laupland KB, Shahpori R, Kirkpatrick AW, et al. Occurrence and outcome of fever in critically ill adults. *Crit Care Med.* 2008;36:1531–1535.

3. O'Grady NP, Barie PS, Bartlett JG, et al. American College of Critical Care Medicine; Infectious Diseases Society of America. Guidelines for evaluation of new fever in critically ill adult patients: 2008 update from the American College of Critical Care Medicine and the Infectious Diseases Society of America. *Crit Care Med.* 2008;36:1330–1349.
4. Sund-Levander M, Forsberg C, Wahren LK. Normal oral, rectal, tympanic and axillary body temperature in adult men and women: a systematic literature review. *Scand J Care Sci.* 2002;16:122–128.
5. Erickson RS, Kirklin SK. Comparison of ear-based, bladder, oral, and axillary methods for core temperature measurement. *Crit Care Med.* 1993; 21:1528–1534.
6. Saper CB, Breder CD. The neurologic basis of fever. *N Engl J Med.* 1994;330:1880–1886.
7. Kluger MJ, Kozak W, Leon LR, Conn CA. The use of knockout mice to understand the role of cytokines in fever. *Clin Exp Pharmacol Physiol.* 1998;25:141–144.
8. Kluger MJ, Ringler DH, Anver MR. Fever and survival. *Science.* 1975; 188:166–168.
9. Kluger MJ, Kozak W, Conn CA, et al. The adaptive value of fever. *Infect Dis Clin North Am.* 1996;10:1–20.
10. Marik PE, Zaloga GP. Hypothermia and cytokines in septic shock. Norasept II Study Investigators. North American study of the safety and efficacy of murine monoclonal antibody to tumor necrosis factor for the treatment of septic shock. *Intensive Care Med.* 2000;26:716–721.
11. Musher DM, Fainstein V, Young EJ, Pruett TL. Fever patterns. Their lack of clinical significance. *Arch Intern Med.* 1979;139:1225–1228.
12. Mackowiak PA, Bartlett JG, Borden EC, et al. Concepts of fever: recent advances and lingering dogma. *Clin Infect Dis.* 1997;25:119–138.
13. Mackowiak PA. Concepts of fever. *Arch Intern Med.* 1998;158:1870–1881.
14. Klevens RM, Edwards JR, Richards CL Jr, et al. Estimating health care-associated infections and deaths in U.S. hospitals, 2002. *Public Health Rep.* 2007;122:160–166.
15. Kung HC, Hoyert DL, Xu J, Murphy SL. Deaths: final data for 2005. *Natl Vital Stat Rep.* 2008;56:1–120.
16. Chopra I, Schofield C, Everett M, et al. Treatment of health-care-associated infections caused by gram-negative bacteria: a consensus statement. *Lancet Infect Dis.* 2008;8:133–139.
17. Zimlichman E, Henderson D, Tamir O, et al. Health care-associated infections. A meta-analysis of costs and financial impact on the US health care system. *JAMA Intern Med.* 2013;173:2039–2046.
18. Magill SS, Edwards JR, Bamberg W, et al; Emerging Infections Program Healthcare-Associated Infections and Antimicrobial Use Prevalence Survey Team. Multistate point-prevalence survey of health care-associated infections. *N Engl J Med.* 2014;370:1198–1208.
19. Marik PE. Fever in the ICU. *Chest.* 2000;117:855–869.
20. Johnson DH, Cunha BA. Drug fever. *Infect Dis Clin North Am.* 1996;10: 85–91.
21. Frank SM, Kluger MJ, Kunkel SL. Elevated thermostatic setpoint in postoperative patients. *Anesthesiology.* 2000;93:1426–1431.
22. Dionigi R, Dionigi G, Rovera F, Boni L. Postoperative fever. *Surg Infect (Larchmt).* 2006;7(Suppl 2):S17-S20.
23. Lenhardt R, Negishi C, Sessler DI, et al. Perioperative fever. *Acta Anaesthesiol Scand Suppl.* 1997;111:325–328.
24. Hiyama DT, Zinner MJ. Surgical complications. In: Schwartz SI, Shires GT, Sencer FC, Cowles Husser W, eds. *Principles of Surgery.* 6th ed. New York, NY: McGraw-Hill; 1994:455–487.
25. Engoren M. Lack of association between atelectasis and fever. *Chest.* 1995;107:81–84.
26. Shields RT. Pathogenesis of postoperative pulmonary atelectasis an experimental study. *Arch Surg.* 1949;48:489–503.
27. Snyder EL. The role of cytokines and adhesive molecules in febrile nonhemolytic transfusion reactions. *Immunol Invest.* 1995;24:333–339.
28. Hendrickson JE, Hillyer CD. Noninfectious serious hazards of transfusion. *Anesth Analg.* 2009;108:759–769.
29. Stein PD, Afzal A, Henry JW, Villareal CG. Fever in acute pulmonary embolism. *Chest.* 2000;117:39–42.
30. Murray HW, Ellis GC, Blumenthal DS, Sos TA. Fever and pulmonary thromboembolism. *Am J Med.* 1979;67:232–235.
31. Kalliafas S, Ziegler DW, Flancbaum L, Choban PS. Acute acalculous cholecystitis: incidence, risk factors, diagnosis, and outcome. *Am Surg.* 1998;64:471–475.
32. Boyer EW, Shannon M. The serotonin syndrome. *N Engl J Med.* 2005;352: 1112–1120.
33. Isbister GK, Buckley NA, Whyte IM. Serotonin toxicity: a practical approach to diagnosis and treatment. *Med J Aust.* 2007;187:361–365.
34. Ranieri VM, Thompson BT, Barie PS, et al; PROWESS-SHOCK Study Group. Drotrecogin Alfa (activated) in adults with septic shcok. *N Engl J Med.* 2012;366:2055–2064.
35. Wacker C, Prkno A, Brunkhorst FM, Schlattmann P. Procalcitonin as a diagnostic marker for sepsis: a systematic review and meta-analysis. *Lancet Infect Dis.* 2013;13:426–435.
36. Schuetz P, Chiappa V, Briel M, Greenwald JL. Procalcitonin algorithms for antibiotic therapy decisions: a systematic review of randomized controlled trials and recommendations for clinical algorithms. *Arch Intern Med.* 2011;171: 1322–1331.
37. Tromp M, Lansdorp B, Bleeker-Rovers CP, et al. Serial and panel analyses of biomarkers do not improve the prediction of bacteremia compared to one procalcitonin measurement. *J Infect.* 2012;65:292–301.
38. Brodska H, Malickova K, Adamkova V, et al. Significantly higher procalcitonin levles could differentiate Gram-negative sepsis from Gram-positive and fungal sepsis. *Clin Exp Med.* 2014;13:165–170.
39. Feezor RJ, Oberholzer C, Baker HV, et al. Molecular characterization of the acute inflammatory response to infections with gram-negative versus gram-positive bacteria. *Infect Immun.* 2003;71:5803–5813.
40. Charles PE, Ladoire S, Aho S, et al. Serum procalcitonin elevation in critically ill patients at the onset of bacteremia caused by either Gram negative or Gram positive bacteria. *BMC Infect Dis.* 2008;8:38.
41. Shuman EK, Chenoweth CE. Recognition and prevention of healthcare-associated urinary tract infections in the intensive care unit. *Crit Care Med.* 2010;38:S373–S379.
42. Young PJ, Saxena M, Beasley R, et al. Early peak temperature and mortality in critically ill patients with or without infection. *Intensive Care Med.* 2012;38:437–444.
43. Weinstein MP, Iannini PB, Stratton CW, Eickhoff TC. Spontaneous bacterial peritonitis: a review of 28 cases with emphasis on improved survival and factors influencing prognosis. *Am J Med.* 1978;64:592–598.
44. Young P, Saxena M, Eastwood GM, et al. Fever and fever management among intensive care patients with known or suspected infection: a multicentre prospective cohort study. *Crit Care Resus.* 2011;13:97–102.
45. Schulman CI, Namias N, Doherty J, et al. The effect of antipyretic therapy upon outcomes in critically ill patients: a randomized, prospective study. *Surg Infect (Larchmt).* 2005 Winter;6:369–375.
46. Lee BH, Inui D, Suh GY, et al; Fever and Antipyretic in Critically ill patients Evaluation (FACE) Study Group. Association of body temperature and antipyretic treatments with mortality of critically ill patients with and without sepsis: multi-centered prospective observational study. *Crit Care.* 2012;16:R33.
47. Schortgen F, Clabault K, Katsahian S, et al. Fever control using external cooling in septic shock: a randomized controlled trial. *Am J Respir Crit Care Med.* 2012;185:1088–1095.
48. Young P, Saxena M, Bellomo R, et al; HEAT Investigators; Australian and New Zealand Intensive Care Society Clinical Trials Group. Acetaminophen for fever in critically ill patients with suspected infection. *N Engl J Med.* 2015; 373:2215–2224.
49. Lenhardt R, Negishi C, Sessler DI, et al. The effects of physical treatment on induced fever in humans. *Am J Med.* 1999;106:550–555.

CHAPTER

83

Antibiotics in the Management of Serious Hospital-Acquired Infections

MOLLIE GOWAN, JENNIFER BUSHWITZ, and MARIN H. KOLLEF

INTRODUCTION

As antimicrobial resistance spreads and new antimicrobial agents are developed, designing an empiric antibiotic regimen for patients in the intensive care unit (ICU) has become increasingly complex. In order to ensure that the initial antibiotic agents chosen are appropriate, clinicians must consider a variety of risk factors for infection with resistant pathogens that are specific to the patient, hospital, and community, as well as drug-specific properties that affect efficacy at the site of infection. Although recently developed rapid diagnostic techniques and biomarkers may aid in optimizing antimicrobial therapy, these technologies are not currently widely available. This chapter not only reviews factors predisposing patients to infection with resistant organisms and available diagnostic tests to streamline antibiotic therapy, but also discusses strategies to improve antimicrobial stewardship and limit the spread of resistance.

PATHOPHYSIOLOGY

Clinical Factors That Affect Initial Antimicrobial Selection

When developing an empirical antimicrobial regimen, choice of agents should be based on multiple factors, including likely causative pathogens, local pathogen distribution, resistance patterns, and patient-specific risk factors for resistance. Reports from the National Nosocomial Infections Surveillance (NNIS) System describe hospital and ICU infection rates in participating acute care general hospitals throughout the United States. A 2005 publication also reported pathogen distribution by site of infection and compared data from 1975 and 2003, as shown in Table 83.1. Overall, the occurrence of hospital-acquired infections caused by potentially resistant bacteria, such as *Staphylococcus aureus* and *Pseudomonas aeruginosa,* is increasing. In hospital-acquired pneumonia, gram-negative aerobes remain the most frequently reported pathogens; however, *S. aureus* was the most frequently reported *single* species (1,2). A 2013 report published by the National Healthcare Safety Network (NHSN) demonstrated that *S. aureus* was, overall, the pathogen isolated most frequently in hospital-acquired infections from 2009 to 2010. *S aureus* was also the predominant pathogen in ventilator-associated pneumonia (VAP), followed by *P. aeruginosa* and *Klebsiella* species (3).

One of the most concerning trends reported in the NNIS data is the increasing isolation of *Acinetobacter* species in urinary tract infections, pneumonia, and surgical site infections (1,2,5). Although overall numbers of isolates of *Acinetobacter* are still relatively small (approximately 2.0%), the percentage increase is significant. Similarly, the NHSN report showed that *Acinetobacter* was the fifth most common pathogen isolated in VAP (3). Even more concerning is the recent report of community-acquired pneumonia (CAP) now attributed to *Acinetobacter* species, suggesting that this pathogen is extending its area of influence outside of the health care setting (6).

Also disconcerting is the observation made by the NNIS report that for each of the antibiotic–pathogen combinations tested, there was a significant increase in resistance between study periods. Most impressive were trends in carbapenem- and cephalosporin-resistant *P. aeruginosa* and *Acinetobacter* species (1,2). The NHSN data demonstrate that over 60% of tested *Acinetobacter* isolates in VAP were resistant to imipenem and meropenem, and an even greater percentage met the definition of multidrug resistant (MDR) (3). Many isolates lack effective treatment options and represent a serious public health concern (2,7). Rates of carbapenem resistance, up to 30% in *P. aeruginosa* isolates and 12.8% in *Klebsiella* species, are concerning as these organisms are often MDR and have very limited treatment options in hospitals in the United States (3,4).

The prevalence of MDR pathogens varies by patient population, hospital, and type of floor or unit in which the patient resides, underscoring the need for local surveillance data. MDR pathogens are more commonly isolated from patients with severe, chronic underlying disease—for example, those with risk factors for health care–associated infection (Table 83.2) and patients with late-onset hospital-acquired infections. Specifically, in patients with VAP, prolonged ventilation and recent antibiotic exposure have been identified as significant risk factors for infection with MDR organisms (8).

Distribution of MDR pathogens has been shown to be highly variable not only between cities and countries but also among different ICUs within the same hospital (9–11). These data suggest that consensus guidelines for antimicrobial therapy will need to be modified at the local level (e.g., according to county, city, hospital, and ICU) to take into account local patterns of antimicrobial resistance. Additionally, it is helpful for clinicians to appreciate local specific resistance rates of certain gram-negative pathogens such as extended-spectrum β-lactamase (ESBL)-producing *Klebsiella pneumoniae* or *Escherichia coli,* fluoroquinolone-resistant *P. aeruginosa,* or carbapenem-resistant *Acinetobacter baumannii.* When risk of these pathogens is identified, empirical therapy must be tailored accordingly.

In addition to local or regional variance, numerous patient-specific factors affect the risk of isolation of a resistant pathogen. Therefore, the choice of empiric antibiotic agents should be based on local patterns of antimicrobial susceptibility and must also take into account patient-specific characteristics that may influence the risk of infection with a resistant pathogen. Patients of particular concern are those at risk for

TABLE 83.1 Relative Percentage by Site of Infection of Pathogens Associated with Nosocomial Infection (2,4)

Pathogen	Pneumonia				BSI				SSI				UTI			
Year	1975	1989–1998	2003	2009–2010[a]	1975	1989–1998	2003	2009–2010[b]	1975	1989–1998	2003	2009–2010	1975	1989–1998	2003	2009–2010[c]
Number	4,018	65,056	4,365	6,632	1,054	50,091	2,351	27,766	7,848	22,043	2,984	16,019	16,434	47,502	4,109	19,058
Staphylococcus aureus	13.4	16.8	27.8	24.1	16.5	10.7	14.3	12.3	18.5	12.6	22.5	30.4	1.9	1.6	3.6	2.1
Pseudomonas aeruginosa	9.6	16.1	18.1	16.6	4.8	3	3.4	3.8	4.7	9.2	9.5	5.5	9.3	10.6	16.3	11.3
Enterococcus subspecies	3	1.9	1.3	0.9	8.1	10.3	14.5	18.1	11.9	14.5	13.9	11.6	14.2	13.8	17.4	15.1
Enterobacter subspecies	9.6	10.7	10	8.6	6	4.2	4.4	4.5	4.6	8.8	9	4	4.7	5.7	6.9	4.2
Escherichia coli	11.8	4.4	5	5.9	15	2.9	3.3	4	17.6	7.1	6.5	9.4	33.5	18.2	26	26.8
Klebsiella subspecies	8.4	6.5	7.2	10.1	4.5	2.9	4.2	7.9	2.7	3.5	3	4	4.6	6.1	9.8	11.2
Serratia subspecies	2.2	—	4.7	4.6	2.6	—	2.3	2.5	0.5	—	2	1.8	1.4	—	1.6	1
Acinetobacter species	1.5	—	6.9	6.6	1.8	—	2.4	2.1	0.5	—	2.1	0.6	0.6	—	1.6	0.9

[a]Ventilator-associated pneumonia
[b]Catheter-associated bloodstream infection
[c]Catheter-associated urinary tract infection
BSI, bloodstream infection; SSI, surgical site infection; UTI, urinary tract infection; —, not reported.

TABLE 83.2 Definitions of Infection Categories (with Focus on Bacterial Pathogens)

Infection Category	Definition
Community-acquired infection	Patients with a first-positive bacterial culture obtained within 48 hrs of hospital admission lacking risk factors for health care–associated infection
Hospital-acquired infection	Patients with a first-positive bacterial culture >48 hrs after hospital admission
Health care–associated infection	Patients with a first-positive bacterial culture within 48 hrs of admission and any of the following: • Admission source indicates a transfer from another health care facility (e.g., hospital, nursing home) • Receiving hemodialysis, wound, or infusion therapy as an outpatient • Prior hospitalization for ≥3 days within 90 days • Immunocompromised state due to underlying disease or therapy (human immunodeficiency virus, chemotherapy)

hospital-acquired infections caused by *S. aureus, P. aeruginosa,* and *Acinetobacter species* due to the high frequency with which they cause infection, their resistance to numerous antibiotics, and their associated high mortality rates. Infections with these potentially antibiotic-resistant bacteria have occurred primarily among hospitalized patients and/or among patients with an extensive hospitalization history and other predisposing risk factors like indwelling catheters, past antimicrobial use, decubitus ulcers, postoperative surgical wound infections, or treatment with enteral feedings or dialysis.

Antimicrobial Resistance: Risk Factors and Influence on Outcome

Although several factors contribute to the emergence of antimicrobial resistance, antibiotic use is the key driver for its development in both gram-positive and gram-negative bacteria (8,12,13). Prolonged hospitalization, invasive devices such as endotracheal tubes and intravascular catheters, residence in long-term treatment facilities, and inadequate infection control practices also promote resistance (12). Furthermore, the emergence of new bacterial strains in the community setting, such as community-associated methicillin-resistant *S. aureus,* has created additional stressors favoring the entry of resistant microorganisms into the hospital setting (14). However, the prolonged administration of antimicrobial therapy appears to be the most important factor associated with the emergence of resistance that is potentially amenable to intervention (8,15,16).

It is critical to maintain awareness of risk factors associated with the development of antimicrobial resistance as clinical investigations have repeatedly demonstrated that inappropriate initial antimicrobial therapy is associated with greater in-hospital mortality (17–22). When initial therapy is *inadequate,* adjusting treatment regimens once antimicrobial sensitivity data is available has not been shown to improve patient outcomes (23). Antimicrobial resistance is also associated with excess costs. While most of this is associated with the acquisition of a nosocomial infection, the presence of antibiotic resistance may confer additional morbidity and further increase cost (8,24,25). For these reasons, local antibiograms, both within individual hospitals and ICUs, should be updated frequently to guide clinicians in choosing appropriate therapy.

DIAGNOSIS

A thorough diagnostic assessment is essential to ensure initiation of appropriate antimicrobial therapy and allow for de-escalation. Data from a patient history, physical examination, and imaging are combined to create an initial antimicrobial regimen. The development of rapid molecular diagnostics has added a new element to the clinician's arsenal that may improve the likelihood of covering all possible pathogens early in the course of therapy. Cultures from likely infectious sources enable the clinician to streamline initial antimicrobial regimens. The use of such targeted therapies minimizes the risk of medication adverse effects, decreases the risk of selecting for new, resistant pathogens, and reduces cost.

Rapid Microbiologic Diagnostics

Conventional microbiologic procedures are time consuming and often delay identification of resistant bacteria resulting in inadvertent administration of inappropriate initial antimicrobial therapy. Recently, several molecular diagnostic platforms for the rapid identification of infectious organisms and their accompanying resistance genes have been introduced and evaluated.

Matrix-Assisted Laser Desorption/Ionization Time-of-Flight Mass Spectrometry (MALDI-TOF MS)

Mass spectrometry was first utilized for bacterial identification in the 1970s (26). This technique has evolved significantly in recent years and has the potential to revolutionize the way pathogens are identified in clinical practice. Following organism isolation from a clinical specimen, MALDI-TOF MS utilizes mass spectrometry to rapidly identify pathogens. The use of this technique has been reported to decrease time to bacterial identification by up to 48 hours compared to conventional techniques (27). Further, when combined with interventions from an antimicrobial stewardship team, MALDI-TOF has been shown to decrease not only time to bacterial identification but also time to effective antibiotic therapy, mortality, ICU length of stay, and recurrent bacteremia compared to conventional microbiologic methods (28). While most research has focused on the identification of bacterial isolates, MALDI-TOF has also been investigated for the identification of fungi and viruses. Practical hurdles to the wide spread adaptation of this evolving technology exist including a large upfront investment in the instrument and a current lack of clarity regarding how to best utilize MALDI-TOF when dealing with specimens other than blood (29). As this technology continues to evolve however it is likely to become a prominent feature of infectious disease management in the future.

Peptide Nucleic Acid Fluorescent In Situ Hybridization (PNA-FISH)

PNA-FISH allows for rapid identification of bacteria and yeast from positive blood cultures. Compared to conventional methods, PNA-FISH has been shown to decrease time to organism identification by nearly 72 hours and has been associated with decreased mortality and antibiotic use (30,31). Compared with other rapid diagnostics, PNA-FISH has the advantage of a relatively small investment in equipment up front and comparative ease of use. A major limitation of this technology currently is the lack of probes for some clinically relevant organisms. However, this technology has evolved rapidly in recent years and will likely continue to grow and expand its place in therapy.

Microarrays

Compared to the previously discussed rapid diagnostic techniques, DNA-probe–based assays, or microarrays, have the comparative advantage of being able to simultaneously identify organisms and resistance markers from positive blood cultures. Probes for commonly encountered resistance mechanisms, such as *mecA, vanA/vanB,* and a number of genes responsible for production of extended-spectrum β-lactamases and carbapenemases exist (32–34). To date, microarrays have been predominantly studied clinically in gram-positive bloodstream infections. In this setting, time to organism and resistance identification has been shown to be decreased by up to 48 hours compared to conventional techniques (32). As the role of microarrays for the treatment of gram-positive infections becomes more established, it is likely that its role will continue to expand to gram-negative infections as well.

Quantitative Cultures and Assessment of Infection Risk

Pneumonia is the most common hospital-acquired infection among mechanically ventilated patients. A meta-analysis of four randomized trials demonstrated that the use of quantitative bacterial cultures obtained from the lower respiratory tract may, in theory, facilitate de-escalation of empiric broad-spectrum antibiotics and reduce drug-specific antibiotic days of treatment (35). Another study found that patients with a clinical suspicion for VAP and culture-negative bronchoalveolar lavage (BAL) results for a major pathogen could have antimicrobial therapy safely discontinued within 72 hours (36). Interestingly, the mean modified clinical pulmonary infection scores (CPISs) of these patients was approximately six, suggesting that this quantitative clinical assessment of the risk for VAP could have been used to discontinue antibiotics as previously suggested (37). Regardless of whether quantitative culture methods are used, the results of microbiologic testing should be used to routinely modify or discontinue antibiotic treatment in the appropriate clinical setting.

TREATMENT

Antibiotics, Their Mode of Action, Clinical Indications for Use, and Associated Toxicities

Most antimicrobial agents used for the treatment of infections may be categorized according to their principal mechanism of action. For antibacterial agents, the major modes of action are the following (38):

- Interference with cell wall synthesis
- Disruption of the bacterial cell membrane
- Inhibition of protein synthesis
- Interference with nucleic acid synthesis
- Inhibition of a metabolic pathway

Tables 83.3 to 83.5 review the major pathogens, the antimicrobials of choice by pathogen, and the major toxicities of specific agents, respectively.

Cell Wall Active Antibiotics

Antibacterial drugs that work by inhibiting bacterial cell wall synthesis include the β-lactams—such as the penicillins, cephalosporins, carbapenems, and monobactams—and the glycopeptides, including vancomycin and teicoplanin. β-Lactam agents inhibit the synthesis of the bacterial cell wall by interfering with the enzymes required for the synthesis of the peptidoglycan layer. Vancomycin and teicoplanin also interfere with cell wall synthesis by preventing the cross-linking steps required for stable cell wall synthesis.

Disruption of Bacterial Cell Membrane

Disruption of the bacterial membrane is a less well characterized mechanism of action. Polymyxin antibiotics appear to exert their inhibitory effects by increasing bacterial membrane permeability, causing leakage of bacterial contents. The cyclic lipopeptide, daptomycin, appears to insert its lipid tail into the bacterial cell membrane, causing membrane depolarization and eventual death of the bacterium.

Inhibition of Bacterial Protein Synthesis

Macrolides, aminoglycosides, tetracyclines, chloramphenicol, streptogramins, and oxazolidinones produce their antibacterial effects by inhibiting protein synthesis. Bacterial ribosomes differ in structure from their counterparts in eukaryotic cells. Antibacterial agents take advantage of these differences to selectively inhibit bacterial growth. Macrolides, aminoglycosides, and tetracyclines bind to the 30S subunit of the ribosome, whereas chloramphenicol binds to the 50S subunit. Linezolid is a gram-positive antibacterial oxazolidinone that binds to the 50S subunit of the ribosome on a site that has not been shown to interact with other classes of antibiotics.

Inhibition of Nucleic Acid Synthesis

Fluoroquinolones exert their antibacterial effects by disrupting DNA synthesis and causing lethal double-strand DNA breaks during DNA replication.

Inhibition of a Metabolic Pathway

Sulfonamides and trimethoprim block the pathway for folic acid synthesis, which ultimately inhibits DNA synthesis. The common antibacterial drug combination of trimethoprim, a folic acid analogue, plus sulfamethoxazole (a sulfonamide) inhibits two steps in the enzymatic pathway for bacterial folate synthesis.

Mechanisms of Resistance to Antibacterial Agents

Most antimicrobial agents exert their effect by influencing a single step in bacterial reproduction or bacterial cell function. Therefore, resistance can emerge with a single point mutation aimed at bypassing or eliminating the action of the antibiotic. Some species of bacteria are innately resistant to at least one class of antimicrobial agents, with resulting resistance to all

TABLE 83.3 Most Common Pathogens Associated with Sites of Serious Infection Commonly Seen in the Adult Intensive Care Unit Setting

Infection Site	Pathogens
Pneumonia	
1. Community-acquired pneumonia (nonimmunocompromised host)	*Streptococcus pneumoniae* *Haemophilus influenzae* *Moraxella catarrhalis* *Mycoplasma pneumoniae* *Legionella pneumophila* *Chlamydia pneumoniae* Methicillin-resistant *Staphylococcus aureus (MRSA)* Influenza virus
2. Health care–associated pneumonia	MRSA *Pseudomonas aeruginosa* *Klebsiella pneumoniae* *Acinetobacter* species *Stenotrophomonas* species *Legionella pneumophila*
3. Pneumonia (immunocompromised host)	
a. Neutropenia	Any pathogen listed above *Aspergillus* species *Candida* species
b. HIV	Any pathogen listed above *Pneumocystis jirovecii* *Mycobacterium tuberculosis* *Histoplasma capsulatum* Other fungi Cytomegalovirus
c. Solid organ transplant or bone marrow transplant	Any pathogen listed above (Can vary depending on timing of infection to transplant)
d. Cystic fibrosis	*Haemophilus influenzae* (early) *Staphylococcus aureus* *Pseudomonas aeruginosa* *Burkholderia cepacia*
4. Lung abscess	*Bacteroides* species *Peptostreptococcus* species *Fusobacterium* species *Nocardia* (in immunocompromised patients) *Amebic* (when suggestive by exposure)
5. Empyema	*Staphylococcus aureus*, *Streptococcus pneumoniae*, Group A *Streptococci*, *Haemophilus influenzae* } Usually acute Anaerobic bacteria, *Enterobacteriaceae*, *Mycobacterium tuberculosis* } Usually subacute or chronic
Meningitis	*Streptococcus pneumoniae* *Neisseria meningitidis* *Listeria monocytogenes* *Haemophilus influenzae* *Escherichia coli*, Group B streptococci } Neonates *Staphylococcus aureus*, *Enterobacteriaceae*, *Pseudomonas aeruginosa* } Postsurgical or posttrauma
Brain abscess	Streptococci *Bacteroides* species *Enterobacteriaceae*, *Staphylococcus aureus* } Postsurgical or posttrauma *Nocardia*, *Toxoplasma gondii* } Immunocompromised or HIV infected

TABLE 83.3 Most Common Pathogens Associated with Sites of Serious Infection Commonly Seen in the Adult Intensive Care Unit Setting (*Continued*)

Infection Site	Pathogens	
Encephalitis	West Nile virus	
	Herpes simplex	
	Arbovirus	
	Rabies	
	Cat-scratch disease	
Endocarditis	*Streptococcus viridans*	
	Enterococcus species	
	Staphylococcus aureus	
	Streptococcus bovis	
	MRSA	Intravenous drug user, prosthetic valve
	Candida species	Prosthetic valve
Catheter-associated bacteremia	*Candida* species	
	Staphylococcus aureus	
	Enterococcus species	
	Enterobacteriaceae	
	Pseudomonas aeruginosa	
Pyelonephritis	*Enterobacteriaceae*	
	Escherichia coli	
	Enterococcus species	
	Pseudomonas aeruginosa	Catheter-associated, postsurgical
	Acinetobacter species	
Peritonitis		
1. Primary or spontaneous	*Enterobacteriaceae*	
	Streptococcus pneumoniae	
	Enterococcus species	
	Anaerobic bacteria (rare)	
2. Secondary (bowel perforation)	*Enterobacteriaceae*	
	Bacteroides species	
	Enterococcus species	
	Pseudomonas aeruginosa (uncommon)	
3. Tertiary (bowel surgery, hospitalized on antibiotics)	*Pseudomonas aeruginosa*	
	MRSA	
	Acinetobacter species	
	Candida species	
Skin structure infections		
1. Cellulitis	Group A streptococci	
	Staphylococcus aureus	
	Enterobacteriaceae	Diabetics
2. Decubitus ulcer	Polymicrobial	
	Streptococcus pyogenes	
	Enterococcus species	
	Enterobacteriaceae	
	Anaerobic streptococci	
	Pseudomonas aeruginosa	
	Staphylococcus aureus	
	Bacteroides species	
3. Necrotizing fasciitis	*Streptococcus* species	
	Clostridia species	
	Mixed aerobic/anaerobic bacteria	
Muscle infection		
1. Myonecrosis (gas gangrene)	*Clostridium perfringens*	
	Other *Clostridium* species	
2. Pyomyositis	*Staphylococcus aureus*	
	Group A streptococci	
	Anaerobic bacteria	
	Gram-negative bacteria (rare)	

(*Continued*)

TABLE 83.3 Most Common Pathogens Associated with Sites of Serious Infection Commonly Seen in the Adult Intensive Care Unit Setting (*Continued*)

Infection Site	Pathogens
Septic shock	
1. Community-acquired	*Streptococcus pneumoniae*
	Neisseria meningitidis
	Haemophilus influenzae
	Escherichia coli
	Capnocytophaga (DF-2 with splenectomy)
2. Health care—associated	MRSA
	Pseudomonas aeruginosa
	Acinetobacter species
	Candida species
3. Toxic shock syndrome	*Staphylococcus aureus*
	Streptococci species
4. Regional illness or special circumstances	Rickettsial species
	Ehrlichiosis
	Babesiosis
	Cat-scratch disease (immunocompromised hosts)
	Yersinia pestis
	Francisella tularensis
	Leptospira
	Salmonella enteritidis
	Salmonella typhi

HIV, human immune deficiency virus.

the members of those antibacterial classes. However, the emergence and spread of acquired resistance due to the selective pressure to use specific antimicrobial agents is of greater concern due to the spread of such resistance. Several mechanisms of antimicrobial resistance are readily transferred to various bacteria.

First, the organism may acquire genes encoding enzymes, such as β-lactamases, that destroy the antibacterial agent before it can have an effect. Second, bacteria may acquire efflux pumps that extrude the antibacterial agent from the cell before it can reach its target site and exert its effect. Third, bacteria may acquire several genes for a metabolic pathway that ultimately produces altered bacterial cell walls that no longer contain the binding site of the antimicrobial agent, or bacteria may acquire mutations that limit access of antimicrobial agents to the intracellular target site via downregulation of porin genes. Susceptible bacteria can also acquire resistance to an antimicrobial agent via new mutations such as are noted above.

New Antimicrobial Agents

Most new antibiotics have been developed for the treatment of gram-positive bacteria. Until recently, the glycopeptides, vancomycin and teicoplanin, were the only antibacterial compounds available to which MRSA strains remained uniformly susceptible. In 1996, the first clinical isolate of *S. aureus* with reduced susceptibility to vancomycin (vancomycin-intermediate *S. aureus*, or VISA) was reported in Japan and, since then, similar cases have been reported around the world. Only a few years later, clinical isolates of *S. aureus* that were fully resistant to vancomycin were reported in South Africa and Michigan. The emergence of MRSA strains with reduced vancomycin susceptibility has limited the treatment options and increased the incidence of treatment failure (39); infection with one of these strains may be an independent predictor of mortality (40). More concerning are the observations that upward drift in the minimum inhibitory concentrations (MICs) for vancomycin in MRSA are associated with an increased risk of clinical treatment failures (41). As a result of this upsurge in MRSA resistance, most of the recent advances in the development of new antibiotic agents have predominantly occurred for gram-positive bacteria.

Unfortunately, gram-negative antibiotic development has lagged behind. In an effort to encourage development and marketing of new antimicrobials against resistant bacteria, the FDA began offering a Qualified Infections Disease Product (QIDP) designation as a part of the Generating Antibiotic Incentives Now (GAIN) act in 2012. This designation allows priority review and an extended period of market exclusivity for qualifying products (42). All of the following antimicrobials marketed after 2012 were granted QIDP status.

Dalbavancin (Dalvance)

Approved by the FDA in 2014, dalbavancin is a lipoglycopeptide antimicrobial that has been studied in the treatment of complicated skin and skin structure infections and catheter-related bloodstream infection. Dalbavancin is a bactericidal agent whose long-terminal plasma half-life (8.5 days) allows for the unique dosing of 1,000 mg given on day 1 and 500 mg given on day 8. The long half-life may turn out to be the strength of the drug, allowing for more convenient treatment options in patients requiring prolonged antibiotic therapy (e.g., right-sided infective endocarditis or osteomyelitis). However, the impact of this prolonged half-life on adverse reactions also needs further evaluation.

Oritavancin (Orbactiv)

Oritavancin is a lipoglycopeptide antibacterial that gained FDA approval in 2014. It has demonstrated in vitro bactericidal

TABLE 83.4 Drugs of Choice in Serious Infections[a]

Organism	Drug of Choice	Alternative Drugs
GRAM-POSITIVE COCCI		
Staphylococcus aureus[b] or		
Staphylococcus epidermidis		
Penicillin-sensitive	Penicillin G	Cephalosporin, vancomycin, or clindamycin[c]
Penicillinase-producing[d]	Oxacillin or nafcillin	Cephalosporin, vancomycin, or clindamycin
Methicillin-resistant[e]	Vancomycin (linezolid for pneumonia)	Quinolone, TMP/SMX, minocycline, clindamycin, linezolid, ceftaroline, daptomycin (unless pneumonia)
Nonenterococcal streptococci	Penicillin G	Cephalosporin, vancomycin, or clindamycin
Enterococcus	Penicillin or ampicillin + gentamicin	Vancomycin + gentamicin
Streptococcus pneumoniae[f]	Penicillin G	Cephalosporin, vancomycin, macrolide, or clindamycin
GRAM-POSITIVE BACILLI		
Actinomyces israelii	Penicillin G	Tetracycline
Bacillus anthracis	Penicillin G	Tetracycline, macrolide
Clostridium difficile	Metronidazole	Oral vancomycin
Clostridium perfringens	Penicillin[g]	Clindamycin, metronidazole, tetracycline, imipenem
Clostridium tetani	Penicillin[h]	Tetracycline
Corynebacterium diphtheriae	Macrolide[g]	Penicillin
Corynebacterium JK	Vancomycin	Penicillin G + gentamicin, erythromycin
Listeria monocytogenes	Ampicillin gentamicin	TMP/SMX
Nocardia asteroides	TMP/SMX	carbapenem + amikacin
Propionibacterium sp.	Penicillin	Clindamycin, erythromycin
GRAM-NEGATIVE COCCI		
Moraxella catarrhalis	TMP/SMX	Amoxicillin/clavulanic acid, ceftriaxone, macrolide, tetracycline
Neisseria gonorrhoeae	Ceftriaxone	Penicillin G, quinolone
Neisseria meningitidis	Penicillin G	Ceftriaxone
ENTERIC GRAM-NEGATIVE BACILLI		
Bacteroides		
Oral source	Penicillin	Clindamycin, cefoxitin, metronidazole, cefotetan
Bowel source	Metronidazole	Cefoxitin, cefotetan, imipenem, ampicillin/sulbactam ticarcillin/clavulanate, piperacillin/tazobactam, clindamycin
Citrobacter	Cefepime or imipenem/meropenem	Aminoglycoside, quinolone, piperacillin, aztreonam
Enterobacter sp.[i]	Cefepime or imipenem/meropenem	Ciprofloxacin, aminoglycoside, aztreonam
Escherichia coli[j]	3rd-generation cephalosporin	Aminoglycoside, carbapenem, cefepime, ß-lactam/ß-lactamase inhibitor, ciprofloxacin, TMP/SMX
Klebsiella[j]	3rd-generation cephalosporin	As for *E. coli*
Proteus mirabilis	Ampicillin	Aminoglycoside, quinolone, cephalosporin, piperacillin, ticarcillin, TMP/SMX
Proteus, nonmirabilis	3rd-generation cephalosporin	Aminoglycoside, quinolone, piperacillin, aztreonam, imipenem
Providencia	2nd- or 3rd-generation cephalosporin	Gentamicin, amikacin, piperacillin, aztreonam, imipenem, ticarcillin, mezlocillin, TMP/SMX
Salmonella typhi	Ceftriaxone or quinolone	Ampicillin, TMP/SMX
Salmonella, nontyphi[k]	Cefotaxime, ceftriaxone, or quinolone	Ampicillin, TMP/SMX
Serratia	Cefepime or imipenem/meropenem	Aminoglycoside, aztreonam piperacillin, TMP/SMX, quinolone
Shigella	Quinolone	Ampicillin, TMP/SMX, ceftriaxone, cefixime
Yersinia enterocolitica	TMP/SMX	Aminoglycoside, tetracycline, 3rd-generation cephalosporin, quinolone
OTHER GRAM-NEGATIVE BACILLI		
Acinetobacter	Imipenem	Cefepime, aminoglycoside, TMP/SMX, colistin, sulbactam
Eikenella corrodens	Ampicillin	Penicillin G, erythromycin, tetracycline, ceftriaxone
Francisella tularensis	Streptomycin, gentamicin	Tetracycline
Fusobacterium	Penicillin	Clindamycin, metronidazole, cefoxitin
Haemophilus influenzae	3rd-generation cephalosporin	Ampicillin, imipenem, quinolone, cefuroxime[l], quinolone, macrolide, TMP/SMX

(Continued)

TABLE 83.4 Drugs of Choice in Serious Infections[a] (Continued)

Organism	Drug of Choice	Alternative Drugs
Legionella	Erythromycin (1 g q6h) + rifampin	
Pasteurella multocida	Penicillin G	Tetracycline, cephalosporin, ampicillin/sulbactam
Pseudomonas aeruginosa	Antipseudomonal penicillin[m] + aminoglycoside	Aztreonam, cefepime, imipenem, quinolone
Pseudomonas cepacia	TMP/SMX	Ceftazidime
Spirillum minus	Penicillin G	Tetracycline, streptomycin
Streptobacillus moniliformis	Penicillin G	Tetracycline, streptomycin
Vibrio cholerae[n]	Tetracycline	TMP/SMX, quinolone
Vibrio vulnificus	Tetracycline	Cefotaxime
Xanthomonas maltophilia	TMP/SMX	Quinolone, minocycline, ceftazidime
Yersinia pestis	Streptomycin	Tetracycline, gentamicin
CHLAMYDIAE		
Chlamydia pneumoniae (TWAR)	Macrolide	Tetracycline
Chlamydia psittaci	Tetracycline	Chloramphenicol
Chlamydia trachomatis	Macrolide	Sulfonamide, tetracycline
MYCOPLASMA sp.	Macrolide	Tetracycline
	Tetracycline	Quinolone
SPIROCHETES		
Borrelia burgdorferi	Doxycycline, amoxicillin	Penicillin G, macrolide, cefuroxime, ceftriaxone, cefotaxime
Borrelia sp.	Tetracycline	Penicillin G
Treponema pallidum	Penicillin	Tetracycline, ceftriaxone
VIRUSES		
Cytomegalovirus	Ganciclovir[o]	Foscarnet, cidofovir
Herpes simplex	Acyclovir	Foscarnet, ganciclovir
HIV	See Centers for Disease Control Web site	
Influenza	Amantadine	Rimantadine, oseltamivir, zanamivir
Respiratory syncytial	Ribavirin	
Varicella zoster	Acyclovir	Famciclovir[p]
FUNGI		
Aspergillus	Voriconazole	Amphotericin B, echinocandin, Itraconazole[r]
Blastomyces	Amphotericin B or itraconazole	Ketoconazole
Candida[q]		
Mucosal	Fluconazole, echinocandin[s]	Ketoconazole, itraconazole
Systemic	Fluconazole, echinocandin	Amphotericin B
Coccidioides	Amphotericin B or fluconazole	Itraconazole, ketoconazole
Cryptococcus	Amphotericin	Fluconazole, itraconazole
Histoplasma	Itraconazole or Amphotericin B	
Pseudallescheria	Ketoconazole or itraconazole	
Zygomycosis ("mucor")	Amphotericin B	Posaconazole

[a]This table does not consider minor infections that may be treated with oral agents, single-agent therapy, or less toxic drugs. Sensitivity testing must be done on bacterial isolates to confirm the sensitivity pattern.
[b]Some authorities recommend clindamycin as the first choice for susceptible toxin-producing staphylococci, streptococci, or clostridia.
[c]First-generation cephalosporins are most active. If endocarditis is suspected, do not use clindamycin. Some authorities recommend the addition of gentamicin for endocarditis caused by nonenterococcal streptococci or tolerant staphylococci.
[d]Penicillinase-producing staphylococci are also resistant to ampicillin, amoxicillin, carbenicillin, ticarcillin, mezlocillin, and piperacillin.
[e]Methicillin-resistant staphylococci should be assumed to be resistant to all cephalosporins and penicillins, even if disk testing suggests sensitivity. Dalbavancin and oritavancin may be alternatives for specific types of methicillin-resistant infection pending future studies and indications.
[f]Some strains show intermediate- or high-level penicillin resistance. Highly resistant strains are treated with vancomycin, or rifampin, or both. In regions with high prevalence of resistant pneumococcus, ceftriaxone or vancomycin should be considered until sensitivity is known.
[g]Use as an adjunct to debridement of infected tissues.
[h]Use as an adjunct to active and passive immunization.
[i]Because of rapid development of resistance, cephalosporins not recommended even if initial tests indicate susceptibility.
[j]*Klebsiella sp.* and *E. coli* producing extended-spectrum β-lactamase (ESBL) should be preferentially managed with a carbapenem.
[k]Uncomplicated *Salmonella* enteritis should not be treated with antibiotics.
[l]Should not be used in meningitis because of poor CNS penetration.
[m]Antipseudomonal penicillins include ticarcillin, mezlocillin, and piperacillin.
[n]Primary therapy is fluid and electrolyte repletion.
[o]Oral form should be used only in maintenance therapy of retinal cytomegalovirus.
[p]Approved only for mild herpes zoster in immunocompetent hosts.
[q]*Candida krusei* and *Torulopsis glabrata* may be resistant to azole therapy, *Candida parapsilosis* may be resistant to echinocandins.
[r]In multidrug combinations.
[s]Echinocandins include caspofungin, micafungin, and anidulafungin.

TABLE 83.5 Toxicities Associated with Antimicrobials

Antimicrobial	Serious Toxicities, Uncommon	Common Toxicities[a]
Penicillins Ampicillin Penicillin	Anaphylaxis, seizures, hemolytic anemia, neutropenia, thrombocytopenia, drug fever	Diarrhea, nausea, vomiting
Antistaphylococcal penicillins Nafcillin Oxacillin	Anaphylaxis, neutropenia, thrombocytopenia, acute interstitial nephritis, hepatotoxicity	Diarrhea, nausea, vomiting
β-Lactam/β-lactamase inhibitors Amoxicillin/clavulanate Ampicillin/sulbactam Piperacillin/tazobactam Ticarcillin/clavulanate	Anaphylaxis, seizures, hemolytic anemia, neutropenia, thrombocytopenia *Clostridium difficile* colitis, cholestatic jaundice, drug fever	Diarrhea, nausea, vomiting
Cephalosporins	Anaphylaxis, seizures, neutropenia, thrombocytopenia, drug fever	Diarrhea, nausea, vomiting
Carbapenems Imipenem Meropenem Ertapenem Doripenem	Anaphylaxis, seizures (imipenem > meropenem, ertapenem, doripenem) *C. difficile* colitis, drug fever	Diarrhea, nausea, vomiting
Glycopeptides Vancomycin	Ototoxicity, nephrotoxicity (unlikely without concomitant nephrotoxins), thrombocytopenia	Red-man syndrome
Oxazolidinones Linezolid	*More common with long-term use:* Peripheral and optic neuropathy, myelosuppression *Possible with short-term use:* Lactic acidosis, myopathy anemia	Diarrhea
Lipopeptides Daptomycin		Diarrhea, constipation, vomiting
Streptogramin Quinupristin/dalfopristin		Arthralgia, myalgia, inflammation, pain, edema at infusion site, hyperbilirubinemia
Aminoglycosides Amikacin Gentamicin Tobramycin		Nephrotoxicity, ototoxicity
Fluoroquinolones 2nd generation Ciprofloxacin 3rd generation Levofloxacin 4th generation Gatifloxacin Moxifloxacin Gemifloxacin	Anaphylaxis, dysglycemia QTc prolongation, joint toxicity in children	Nausea, vomiting, diarrhea, photosensitivity, rash CNS stimulation, dizziness, somnolence
Macrolides Erythromycin Azithromycin Clarithromycin	QTc prolongation (erythromycin > clarithromycin > azithromycin), cholestasis	Nausea, vomiting, diarrhea, abnormal taste
Ketolides Telithromycin	Acute hepatic failure QTc prolongation	Nausea, vomiting, diarrhea
Clindamycin	*C. difficile* colitis	Nausea, vomiting, diarrhea, abdominal pain, rash
Tetracyclines Tetracycline Doxycycline Minocycline pseudotumor cerebri	Tooth discoloration and retardation of bone growth (in children), renal tubular necrosis, dizziness, vertigo	Photosensitivity, diarrhea
Glycylcyclines Tigecycline		Nausea, vomiting, diarrhea
Trimethoprim/sulfamethoxazole	Myelosuppression Stevens–Johnson syndrome, hyperkalemia, aseptic meningitis, hepatic necrosis	Rash, nausea, vomiting, diarrhea
Metronidazole	Seizures, peripheral neuropathy	Nausea, vomiting, metallic taste, disulfiram-like reaction

(Continued)

TABLE 83.5 Toxicities Associated with Antimicrobials (*Continued*)

Antimicrobial	Serious Toxicities, Uncommon	Common Toxicities[a]
Nitrofurantoin	Pulmonary toxicity, peripheral neuropathy	Urine discoloration, photosensitivity
ANTIFUNGAL AGENTS		
Azoles Fluconazole Itraconazole Voriconazole Posaconazole	Hepatic failure, increased AST/ALT, cardiovascular toxicity, hypertension, edema	Nausea, vomiting, diarrhea, rash, visual disturbances, phototoxicity
Amphotericin B products Amphotericin B deoxycholate ABLC ABCD Liposomal amphotericin B	Acute liver failure, myelosuppression	Nephrotoxicity (less common with lipid formulations), acute infusion-related reactions, hypokalemia, hypomagnesemia
Echinocandins Caspofungin Micafungin Anidulafungin	Hepatotoxicity, infusion-related rash, flushing, itching	
Flucytosine	Myelosuppression, hepatotoxicity, confusion, hallucinations, sedation	Nausea, vomiting, diarrhea, rash
ANTIVIRAL AGENTS		
Nucleoside analogues Acyclovir Valaciclovir Ganciclovir Valganciclovir	Nephrotoxicity, rash, encephalopathy, inflammation at injection site, phlebitis	Bone marrow suppression, headache, nausea, vomiting, diarrhea (with oral forms)
Amantadine **Rimantadine**	CNS disturbances (amantadine > rimantadine)	Nausea, vomiting, anorexia, xerostomia
Neuraminidase inhibitors Oseltamivir Zanamivir	Anaphylaxis, bronchospasm	Nausea, vomiting, cough, local discomfort
Cidofovir	Anemia, neutropenia, fever, rash	Nephrotoxicity, uveitis/iritis, nausea, vomiting
Foscarnet	Seizures, anemia, fever	Nephrotoxicity, electrolyte abnormalities (hypocalcemia, hypomagnesemia, hypokalemia, hypophosphatemia), nausea, vomiting, diarrhea, headache

[a]Toxicities were classified as "common" relative to the other toxicities that agent is known to cause. Because toxicities are classified as "common" does not imply they are not serious.

activity against a variety of gram-positive organisms including methicillin-resistant, vancomycin-intermediate, and vancomycin-resistant, *S. aureus* and vancomycin-resistant VanA and VanE strains of *Enterococcus faecalis* and *Enterococcus faecium* (43,44). Oritavancin has been investigated chiefly for the treatment of skin and skin structure infections. It has been observed to have a terminal half-life of approximately 10 days allowing for single-dose administration to treat most infections (45).

Tedizolid (Sivextro)

Tedizolid is an oxazolidinone antibacterial that gained FDA approval in 2014. Tedizolid has a similar spectrum of activity to linezolid with the added advantage of having activity against linezolid-resistant strains of MRSA (46). Tedizolid has a similar side effect profile to linezolid and is available in both oral and IV dosage forms (47).

Ceftaroline (Teflaro)

Ceftaroline is an intravenous, broad-spectrum, cephalosporin antibiotic that gained FDA approval in 2010. Ceftaroline has activity against gram-positive organisms, oral anaerobes, and a variety of *Enterobacteriaceae.* It is the only antibiotic in the cephalosporin class with activity against methicillin-resistant, vancomycin-intermediate, and vancomycin-resistant *S. aureus.* Its activity against *Enterobacteriaceae,* though, is limited to organisms that do not produce Amp-C β-lactamase. Additionally, most nonfermenting gram-negative bacilli, such as *P. aeruginosa,* are inherently resistant to ceftaroline (48). The adverse effects of ceftaroline are similar to those observed with other cephalosporins (49). Originally approved for the treatment of skin and skin structure infections and community-acquired pneumonia, clinical experience with ceftaroline has expanded to a variety of infectious processes and is likely to continue to expand based on its spectrum of activity and favorable side effect profile.

Ceftolozane/Tazobactam (Zerbaxa)

This intravenous combination product was approved by the FDA in 2014 and contains ceftolozane, a new cephalosporin antibiotic, and tazobactam, a β-lactamase inhibitor. Ceftolozane alone is a broad-spectrum, bactericidal antibiotic that closely resembles ceftazidime. Ceftolozane has activity against a variety of resistant gram-negative bacilli including some ESBL producing strains. The addition of tazobactam extends this spectrum of activity to include many ESBL organisms, MDR strains of *P. aeruginosa,* and some anaerobes (50,51).

Ceftazidime/Avibactam (Avycaz)

This intravenous combination product was approved by the FDA in 2015 and contains the cephalosporin ceftazidime with a new synthetic β-lactamase inhibitor, avibactam. The addition of avibactam expands the gram-negative spectrum of ceftazidime to include activity against a variety of otherwise resistant organisms. Notably ceftazidime/avibactam has demonstrated activity against a variety of carbapenemase producing *Enterobacteriaceae* and MDR *P. aeruginosa.* The addition of avibactam does not appear however to enhance the activity of ceftazidime against *Acinetobacter spp* or enhance its gram-positive spectrum (52,53).

Initial Antimicrobial Therapy

An initial appropriate antibiotic regimen should be prescribed with adequate activity against all pathogens likely to be responsible for the infection. Inappropriate initial antibiotic therapy has been associated with a very high risk of mortality in patients with septic shock attributable to a variety of bacterial and fungal pathogens from numerous sources (17,19,21,54–58). Patient history, including drug intolerances, recent receipt of antibiotics, underlying disease, the clinical syndrome, and susceptibility patterns of pathogens in the community and hospital should be utilized when making decisions regarding initial antimicrobial regimen selection. However, given the severity of illness for patients with severe sepsis and septic shock, erring on the side of initial overtreatment may be preferable to the administration of an inappropriately narrow initial antibiotic regimen. Balancing these competing interests is at the core of antimicrobial stewardship in the ICU; methods for refining this balance are described below.

STRATEGIES THAT OPTIMIZE THE EFFICACY OF ANTIBIOTICS WHILE MINIMIZING ANTIBIOTIC RESISTANCE

Hospital and System Level Interventions

Formal Protocols and Guidelines

Antibiotic practice guidelines or protocols have emerged as a means of both avoiding unnecessary antibiotic administration and increasing the effectiveness of prescribed antibiotics. Automated antimicrobial utilization guidelines have been successfully used to identify and minimize the occurrence of adverse drug effects and improve antibiotic selection (12). Their use has also been associated with stable antibiotic susceptibility patterns for both gram-positive and gram-negative bacteria, possibly as a result of promoting antimicrobial heterogeneity and specific end points for antibiotic discontinuation. Automated and nonautomated guidelines have also been employed to reduce overall antibiotic use and limit inappropriate antimicrobial exposure, both of which could affect the development of antibiotic resistance (59). One way these guidelines limit the unnecessary use of antimicrobial agents is by recommending that therapy be modified when initial empiric broad-spectrum antibiotics are prescribed and the culture results reveal that narrow-spectrum antibiotics can be used.

Hospital Formulary Restrictions

Restricted use of specific antibiotics or antibiotic classes from the hospital formulary has been used to reduce resistance, minimize adverse drug reactions, and reduce cost. However, not all experiences have been uniformly successful, and the homogeneous use of a single or limited number of drug classes may actually promote the emergence of resistance (12). Restricted use of specific antibiotics has generally been applied to those drugs with a broad spectrum of action (e.g., carbapenems), rapid emergence of antibiotic resistance (e.g., cephalosporins), and readily identified toxicity (e.g., aminoglycosides). To date, it has been difficult to demonstrate that restricted hospital formularies are effective in curbing the overall emergence of antibiotic resistance. While this may be due in large part to methodologic problems, their use has been successful in specific outbreaks of infection with antibiotic-resistant bacteria, particularly in conjunction with infection control practices and antibiotic educational activities.

Formalized Antimicrobial Stewardship Programs

Formally implemented antimicrobial stewardship programs (ASPs) have been associated not only with reduced infection rates but also significant cost savings associated with reductions in the defined daily doses of the antimicrobials targeted by the ASP (60,61). ASPs have been shown to increase the appropriateness of therapy and increase the number of infectious diseases consultations, which may improve patient outcomes including mortality, hospital lengths of stay, and readmission rates by providing more precise antibiotic prescription (60,62–65). These attributes of ASPs account for why they are now recognized as mandatory components of hospital quality improvement efforts. Formalized ASPs not only restrict the use of unnecessary antibiotics but also insure that antimicrobials are employed in an effective manner to optimize patient outcomes.

Antimicrobial Exposure

Use of Narrow-Spectrum Antibiotics

Another proposed strategy to curtail the development of antimicrobial resistance, in addition to the judicious overall use of antibiotics, is to use drugs with a narrow antimicrobial spectrum. Several investigations have suggested that infections such as CAP can usually be successfully treated with narrow-spectrum antibiotic agents, especially if the infections are not life threatening. Similarly, the avoidance of broad-spectrum antibiotics, especially those associated with rapid emergence of resistance (cephalosporins, quinolones), and the reintroduction of narrow-spectrum agents (penicillin, trimethoprim, gentamicin), along with infection control practices have been successful in reducing the occurrence of specific infections in the hospital setting (12). Unfortunately, ICU patients often have already received prior antimicrobial treatment, making it more likely that they will be infected with an antibiotic-resistant pathogen (8). Therefore, initial empiric treatment with broad-spectrum agents is often initially necessary for hospitalized patients to avoid inappropriate treatment until culture results become available and de-escalation can occur (Fig. 83.1) (18).

Step 1: Initial suspicion of serious infection in critically ill patient:

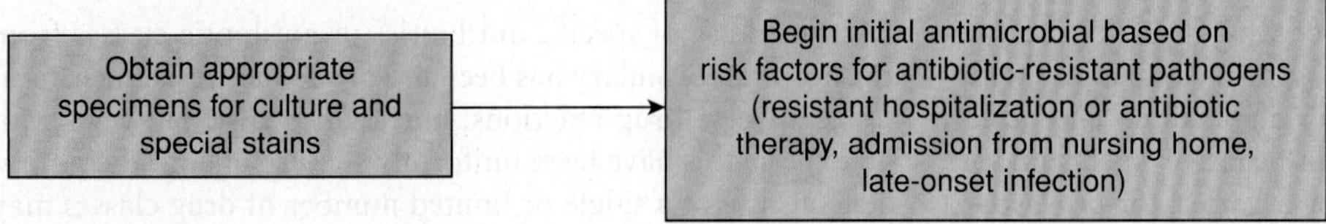

Step 2: Subsequent evaluation of clinical and microbiologic date:

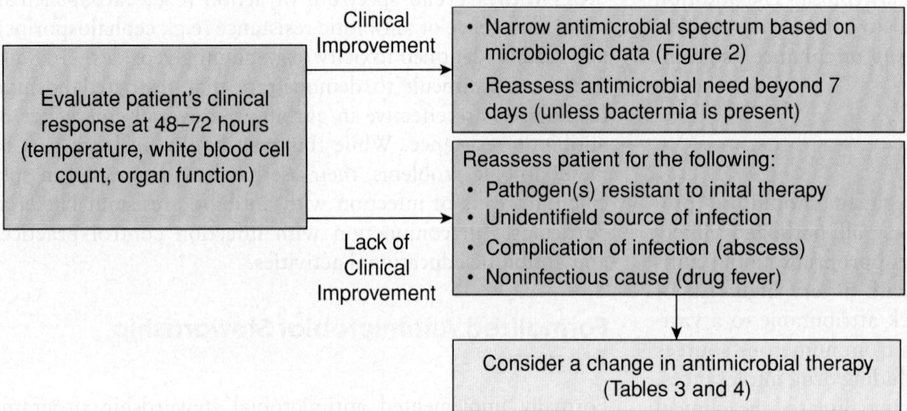

FIGURE 83.1 Clinical algorithm for the de-escalation approach to antibiotic treatment of serious infections in patients with risk factors for multidrug-resistant pathogens. Optimally, de-escalation of antimicrobial treatment would always occur once the pathogen causing infection and its antimicrobial susceptibility are known.

Combination Antibiotic Therapy

Several meta-analyses recommend the use of monotherapy with a β-lactam antibiotic, as opposed to combination therapy including an aminoglycoside, for the definitive treatment of severe sepsis once antimicrobial susceptibilities are known (66,67). Additionally, there is no definitive evidence that the emergence of antibiotic resistance is reduced by the use of combination antimicrobial therapy. However, empiric combination therapy directed against high-risk pathogens such as *P. aeruginosa* should be encouraged until the results of antimicrobial susceptibility become available. Such an approach to empiric treatment can increase the likelihood of providing appropriate initial antimicrobial therapy with improved outcomes (19).

Shorter Courses of Antibiotic Treatment

Prolonged administration of antibiotics to hospitalized patients has been shown to be an important risk factor for the emergence of colonization and infection with antibiotic-resistant bacteria (8,16). Therefore, attempts have been made to reduce the duration of antibiotic treatment for specific bacterial infections. Several clinical trials have found that 7 to 8 days of antibiotic treatment is acceptable for most nonbacteremic patients with VAP (15,37). Similarly, shorter courses of antibiotic treatment have been successfully used in patients at low risk for VAP (36,37,59), with pyelonephritis (68), and for CAP (69). In general, the shorter-course treatment regimens have been associated with a significantly lower risk for the emergence of antimicrobial resistance and several guidelines for the antibiotic management of nosocomial pneumonia and severe sepsis currently recommend the discontinuation of empiric antibiotic therapy after 48 to 72 hours if cultures are negative or the signs of infection have resolved (70,71). There are clinical scenarios in which shorter durations of therapy may not be appropriate, including fungemia, endocarditis, osteomyelitis, meningitis, and VAP caused by *P. aeruginosa* or other nonfermenters. In ICU patients, all antimicrobials should be reviewed on a daily basis to ensure they are needed (59).

De-escalation Approach for the Antibiotic Treatment of Serious Infection in the Hospitalized Patient

After an initial, appropriately broad-spectrum, antibiotic regimen is prescribed, modification of the regimen using a de-escalation strategy should occur based on the results of the patient's clinical response and microbiologic testing (Fig. 83.2). Based on the de-escalation strategy, modification of the initial antibiotic regimen should include decreasing the number and/or spectrum of antibiotics, if possible based on culture and sensitivity results, shortening the duration of therapy in patients with uncomplicated infections who are demonstrating signs of clinical improvement, or discontinuing antibiotics altogether in patients who have a noninfectious cause identified accounting for the patient's signs and symptoms. A number of strategies have been used to promote de-escalation including the use of computer decision support systems, protocol-guided therapies, and clinical pharmacist–supported guidelines (60,72–74).

PHARMACOKINETIC CONSIDERATIONS

Optimizing Pharmacokinetic/Pharmacodynamic (Pk/Pd) Principles

Antibiotic concentrations that are sublethal can promote the emergence of resistant pathogens. Optimization of antibiotic regimens on the basis of pharmacokinetic/pharmacodynamic principles could play a role in the reduction of antibiotic resistance (13). The duration of time the serum drug concentration remains above the MIC of the antibiotic (T > MIC) enhances bacterial eradication with β-lactams, carbapenems, monobactams, glycopeptides, and oxazolidinones (Fig. 83.3). Frequent dosing, prolonged infusion times, or continuous infusions can increase the T greater than MIC and improve clinical and microbiologic cure rates. To maximize the bactericidal

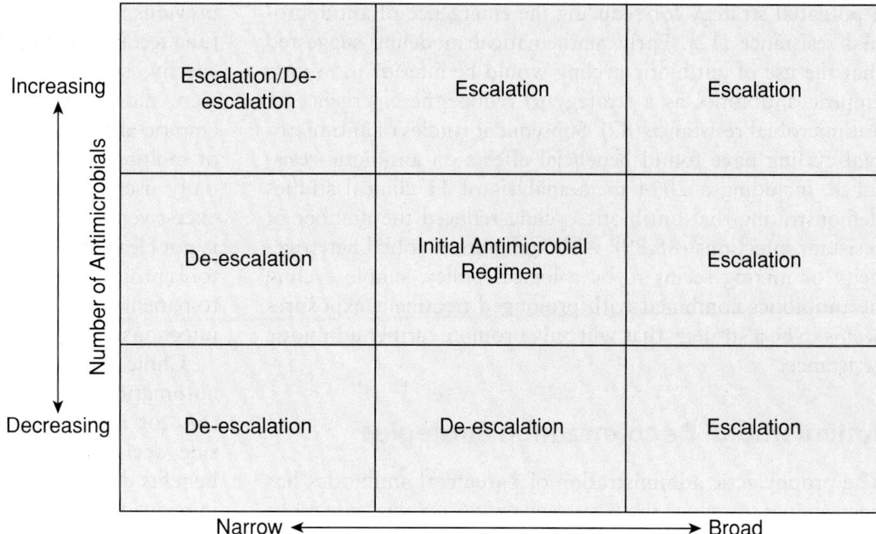

FIGURE 83.2 Antimicrobial de-escalation promotes initial administration of broad-spectrum antibiotics to patients at risk for infection with multidrug-resistant pathogens, followed by the reduction of the number of antimicrobials used and/or their spectrum of activity based on subsequent pathogen identification and antimicrobial susceptibility testing.

effects of aminoglycosides, clinicians must optimize the maximum drug concentration (C_{max})-to-MIC ratio. A C_{max}:MIC ratio of at least 10:1 using once-daily aminoglycoside dosing (5–7 mg/kg) has been associated with preventing the emergence of resistant organisms, improving clinical response to treatment, and avoiding toxicity. The 24-hour area under the antibiotic concentration curve-to-MIC ratio (AUIC) is correlated with fluoroquinolone efficacy and prevention of resistance development. An AUIC value higher than 100 has been associated with a significant reduction in the risk of resistance development while on therapy. As a general rule, clinicians should use the *maximum approved dose* of an antibiotic for a potentially life-threatening infection to optimize tissue concentrations of the drug and killing of pathogens.

Augmented Renal Clearance

Augmented renal clearance (ARC) is defined as an 8-hour creatinine clearance more than or equal to 130 mL/min/1.73 m^2 (39). It has been suggested that a large proportion of ICU patients experience at least one occasion of ARC during the first 7 days of their critical illness (75). ARC has been linked with subtherapeutic β-lactam (76) and glycopeptide concentrations (77), as well

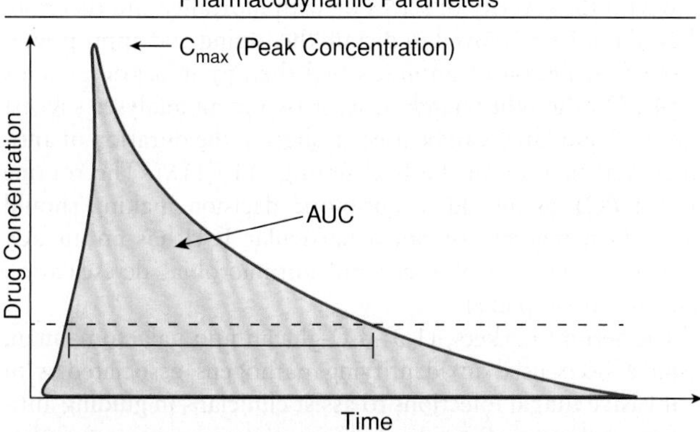

FIGURE 83.3 Pharmacodynamic parameters found to be important for the efficacy of antimicrobial agents. AUC, area under the concentration–time curve; C_{max}, maximum concentration; MIC, minimum inhibitory concentration; T, time.

as increased therapeutic failures in patients receiving antimicrobial therapy resulting in adverse patient outcomes (78,79). Additionally, data suggest that shorter durations of therapy among patients with ARC, and thus lower circulating antibiotic levels, may contribute to excess mortality (80).

A scoring system to identify patients at high risk for ARC has been developed (81) and validated with a 100% sensitivity and 71.4% specificity (82). The following factors were included: age of 50 years or younger (6 points), trauma (3 points), and SOFA score of 4 or less (1 point). Monte Carlo pharmacokinetic simulations demonstrated increased time at therapeutic antibiotic levels with the use of extended infusion dosing in the setting of ARC at a drug cost savings of up to 66.7% over multiple intermittent dosing regimens. In addition to ARC, the use of renal replacement therapies can also result in under exposure of antibiotics at the site of infection requiring careful dosing adjustments (83).

Therapeutic Drug Monitoring

The use of therapeutic drug monitoring (TDM) for antibiotics other than vancomycin, aminoglycosides, and voriconazole has not become a routine or standard practice in most ICUs. TDM for β-lactams and carbapenems can be accomplished by several methodologies (84,85). Unfortunately, at the present time, large variations exist in the type of β-lactams tested, the patients selected for TDM, drug assay methodologies, Pk/Pd targets, and dose-adjustment strategies employed in the critically ill (86). Further studies are needed to determine which patients should receive TDM and how best to perform it, to include robustly defining Pk/Pd targets and dosing adjustments for optimizing β-lactam and carbapenem delivery.

CONTROVERSIES

Antibiotic Cycling and Scheduled Antibiotic Changes

The concept of antibiotic class cycling, in which a class of antibiotics or a specific drug is withdrawn from use for a defined period of time and later reintroduced, has been suggested as a potential strategy for reducing the emergence of antimicrobial resistance (12). Early mathematical modeling suggested that the use of antibiotic cycling would be inferior to mixing empiric antibiotics as a strategy to reduce the emergence of antimicrobial resistance (87). Subsequent studies of antimicrobial cycling have found beneficial effects on antibiotic resistance, including a 2014 meta-analysis of 11 clinical studies demonstrating that antibiotic cycling reduced the number of resistant infections (88,89). Although antimicrobial heterogeneity or mixing seems to be a logical policy, simple cycling of antibiotics combined with prolonged treatment exposures seems to be a strategy that will only promote further antibiotic resistance.

Antimicrobial Decolonization Strategies

The prophylactic administration of parenteral antibiotics has been shown to reduce the occurrence of nosocomial infections in specific high-risk patient populations requiring intensive care (90). Similarly, selective digestive decontamination with topical antibiotics, with or without concomitant parenteral antibiotics, has also been shown to be effective at reducing nosocomial infections caused by the targeted organism(s) (91,92). However, the routine use of selective digestive decontamination has also been linked to the emergence of antimicrobial resistance (93). Similarly, selective oropharyngeal decontamination has also produced mixed results (93–96). Based on these studies, antimicrobial and non-antimicrobial agents should be considered for oral decontamination only in *appropriate high-risk ICU* patients or to assist in the containment of outbreaks of MDR bacterial infections in conjunction with established infection control practices.

Use of Antibiotic Resistance Prediction Tools

Knowledge of patient risk factors for the presence of infection with antibiotic-resistant pathogens should be a routine part of antibiotic decision making and can be used in a de-escalation algorithm. For example, antibiotic-resistant pathogens are more commonly found in patients with CAP who have health care–associated risk factors (recent hospitalization, admission from a nursing home, recent antibiotic treatment). Shorr et al. examined patients admitted with pneumonia and found four variables predictive of antibiotic-resistant pneumonia: recent hospitalization, nursing home residence, hemodialysis, and ICU admission (97). A scoring system assigning 4, 3, 2, and 1 points, respectively, for each variable had moderate predictive power for segregating those with and without resistant bacteria. Among patients with fewer than 3 points, the prevalence of resistant pathogens was less than 20% compared with 55% and more than 75% in persons with scores ranging from 3 to 5 and more than 5 points, respectively ($p < 0.001$). In an independent population, this score better identified patients infected with resistant bacteria than the definition of HCAP (98). Similarly, a 2014 meta-analysis also found that the current definition of HCAP did not accurately identify infections caused by antibiotic-resistant pathogens, further underscoring the need for more objective criteria to determine patients' risk for resistant infections (99).

Independent risk factors for antibiotic-resistant bacteria have been demonstrated in both patients diagnosed with CAP and HCAP including prior hospitalization, immunosuppression, previous antibiotic use, use of gastric acid–suppressive therapy, tube feeding, and nonambulatory status (100). In another prospective study of CAP and HCAP patients, MDR pathogens were more common in patients with HCAP (101). Basing empiric antibiotic therapy on disease severity and the presence of multiple risk factors for MDR pathogens may be a potentially useful approach that achieves good outcomes without excessive use of broad-spectrum antibiotic therapy. However, it is not clear that clinicians can effectively apply such prediction tools prospectively in order to target broad-spectrum antibiotics to patients at greatest risk for infection with antibiotic-resistant infections.

Clinical decision support systems represent one way of automating informatics data, to include potential risk factors for infection with antibiotic-resistant bacteria, for bedside decision making (74,102). Other specific examples of benefits derived from the use of computerized systems include improvements in the efficiency and costs of existing stewardship programs, improvements in clinicians' knowledge regarding the treatment of infectious diseases, and improvements in pathogen prediction (102–108). These data suggest that an opportunity exists to employ hospital informatics systems to improve the identification of patients infected with antibiotic-resistant bacteria in order to prescribe more appropriate initial therapy.

Biomarker Guidance of Antibiotic Therapy

When prescribing antimicrobial therapy, clinicians frequently look for objective indicators that antibiotic treatment is appropriate and to determine duration of treatment. Procalcitonin (PCT), a precursor of calcitonin that is rapidly released into the bloodstream in the presence of an infection, has demonstrated utility in guiding decisions regarding antimicrobial therapy (109–111). However, not all experiences with PCT-guided decision making have shown reductions in duration of antibiotic exposure (112,113). A recent comprehensive literature review of PCT-guided antibiotic management in critically ill patients found that the diagnostic value of serum PCT concentrations to discriminate among systemic inflammatory response syndrome (SIRS), sepsis, severe sepsis, and septic shock was unestablished (114). Moreover, although higher PCT concentrations suggest the presence of a systemic bacterial infection as opposed to a viral, fungal, or inflammatory etiology of sepsis, serum PCT concentrations did not correlate with the severity of sepsis or with mortality and therefore should not be employed to dictate the timing and appropriateness of escalation of antimicrobial therapy in septic patients (114). On the other hand, at least two meta-analyses suggest that PCT guidance can be used to shorten the duration of antimicrobial therapy in the ICU setting (115,116). The routine use of PCT as an aid in antibiotic decision making should depend on whether or not a particular ICU has an already established culture of successful antimicrobial de-escalation and stewardship (59).

- The serum markers, (1,3)-β-D-glucan and galactomannan, have been used in identifying pathogens associated with invasive fungal infections to assist clinicians in guiding antifungal therapy. Fungal infections often present a considerable diagnostic challenge to clinicians, and mere suspicion of these infections often leads to liberal and prolonged antimicrobial use. Based on their high negative predictive value in the appropriate clinical setting, the most suitable use of these markers seems to be in excluding the presence of invasive fungal infections (117,118). However, one study suggests that (1,3)-β-D-glucan may be the most rapid method for the identification of intra-abdominal candidiasis in order to provide timely therapy in such patients (119). In addition, an investigation that measured galactomannan levels in BAL fluid obtained from ICU patients lends support to its use in pathogen identification and early treatment of pulmonary infection (120). Nonetheless, a more recent study only showed modest agreement between galactomannan in BAL fluid and validated clinical diagnostic criteria for invasive fungal disease (121). These markers of infection certainly have the potential to enhance stewardship—primarily through de-escalation once a fungal infection has been excluded—and future clinical experience with these markers will determine if this potential can be fully realized.

Key Points

- Initial treatment with an appropriate antibiotic regimen is one of the most important factors influencing the outcome of critically ill patients with infection.
  - Infection with antibiotic-resistant microorganisms increases the likelihood that inappropriate initial antibiotic therapy will be prescribed to critically ill patients.
  - The prevalence of antibiotic resistance varies locally and regionally.
  - Host factors influence the likelihood that a patient will be infected with antibiotic-resistant pathogens (e.g., prior hospitalization or antibiotic treatment, admission from a nursing home or other high-risk environment).
- Efforts should be made to rapidly identify the source and site of infection and to obtain specimens for culture, antimicrobial susceptibility testing, and rapid diagnostic tests. Obtaining these specimens should not delay initial empiric therapy in a critically ill patient.
- Avoidance of unnecessary antibiotic exposure in the ICU setting is important to reduce the emergence of and subsequent infection with antibiotic-resistant microorganisms.
- Optimization of antibiotic regimens using pharmacokinetic and pharmacodynamic principles to minimize organism exposure to sublethal antimicrobial concentrations could play a role in the reduction of antibiotic resistance.

References

1. National Nosocomial Infections Surveillance (NNIS) system report, data summary from January 1992-April 2000, issued June 2000. *Am J Infect Control.* 2000;28:429–448.
2. Gaynes R, Edwards JR. National Nosocomial Infections Surveillance System. Overview of nosocomial infections caused by gram-negative bacilli. *Clin Infect Dis.* 2005;41:848–854.
3. Dudeck MA, Weiner LM, Allen-Bridson K, et al. National Healthcare Safety Network (NHSN) report, data summary for 2012: device-associated module. *Am J Infect Control.* 2013;41:1148–1166.
4. Sievert DM, Ricks P, Edwards JR, et al. National Healthcare Safety Network (NHSN) Team and Participating NHSN Facilities. Antimicrobial-resistant pathogens associated with healthcare-associated infections: summary of data reported to the National Healthcare Safety Network at the Centers for Disease Control and Prevention, 2009–2010. *Infect Control Hosp Epidemiol.* 2013;34:1–14.
5. Richards MJ, Edwards JR, Culver DH, Gaynes RP. Nosocomial infections in combined medical-surgical intensive care units in the United States, 1. *Infect Control Hosp Epidemiol.* 2000;21:510–515.
6. Leung WS, Chu CM, Tsang KY, et al. Fulminant community-acquired *Acinetobacter baumannii* pneumonia as a distinct clinical syndrome. *Chest.* 2006;129:102–109.
7. Paterson DL, Bonomo RA. Extended-spectrum beta-lactamases: a clinical update. *Clin Micro Rev.* 2005;18:657–686.
8. Trouillet JL, Chastre J, Vuagnat A, et al. Ventilator-associated pneumonia caused by potentially drug-resistant bacteria. *Am J Respir Crit Care Med.* 1998;157:531–539.
9. Rello J, Sa-Borges M, Correa H, et al. Variations in etiology of ventilator-associated pneumonia across four treatment sites: implications for antimicrobial prescribing practices. *Am J Respir Crit Care Med.* 1999;160:608–613.
10. Masterton RG, Kuti JL, Turner PJ, et al. The OPTIMA programme: utilizing MYSTIC (2002) to predict critical pharmacodynamic target attainment against nosocomial pathogens in Europe. *J Antimicrob Chemother.* 2005;55:71–77.
11. Namias N, Samiian L, Nino D, et al. Incidence and susceptibility of pathogenic bacteria vary between intensive care units within a single hospital: implications for empiric antibiotic strategies. *J Trauma.* 2000;49:638–645.
12. Kollef MH, Fraser VJ. Antibiotic resistance in the intensive care unit. *Ann Intern Med.* 2001;134:298–314.
13. Kollef MH, Micek ST. Strategies to prevent antimicrobial resistance in the intensive care unit. *Crit Care Med.* 2005;33:1845–1853.
14. Kollef MH, Micek ST. Methicillin-resistant *Staphylococcus aureus:* a new community-acquired pathogen. *Curr Opin Infect Dis.* 2006;19:161–168.
15. Chastre J, Wolff M, Fagon JY, et al; PneumA Trial Group. Comparison of 15 vs. 8 days of antibiotic therapy for ventilator-associated pneumonia in adults: a randomized trial. *JAMA.* 2003;290:2588–2598.
16. Dennesen PJ, van der Ven AJ, Kessels AG, et al. Resolution of infectious parameters after antimicrobial therapy in patients with ventilator-associated pneumonia. *Am J Respir Crit Care Med.* 2001;163:1371–1375.
17. Ibrahim EH, Sherman G, Ward S, et al. The influence of inadequate antimicrobial treatment of bloodstream infections on patient outcomes in the ICU setting. *Chest.* 2000;118:146–155.
18. Kollef MH. Inadequate antimicrobial treatment: an important determinant of outcome for hospitalized patients. *Clin Infect Dis.* 2000;31:S131–S138.
19. Micek ST, Lloyd AE, Ritchie DJ, et al. Pseudomonas aeruginosa bloodstream infection: importance of appropriate initial antimicrobial treatment. *Antimicrob Agents Chemother.* 2005;49:1306–1311.
20. Dhainaut JF, Laterre PF, LaRosa S, et al. The clinical evaluation committee in a large multicenter phase 3 trial of drotrecogin alfa (activated) in patients with severe sepsis (PROWESS): role, methodology, and results. *Crit Care Med.* 2003;31:2291–2301.
21. Harbarth S, Garbino JK, Pugin J, et al. Inappropriate initial antimicrobial therapy and its effects on survival in a clinical trial of immunomodulating therapy for severe sepsis. *Am J Med.* 2003;115:529–535.
22. Garnacho-Montero J, Garcia-Garmendia JL, Barrero-Almodovar A, et al. Impact of adequate empirical antibiotic therapy on the outcome of patients admitted to the intensive care unit with sepsis. *Crit Care Med.* 2003;31:2742–2751.
23. Kollef MH, Ward S. The influence of mini-BAL cultures on patient outcomes: implications for the antibiotic management of ventilator-associated pneumonia. *Chest.* 1998;113:412–420.
24. Rello J, Ollendorf DA, Oster G, et al. Epidemiology and outcomes of ventilator-associated pneumonia in a large US database. *Chest.* 2002;122:2115–2121.
25. Shorr AF, Combes A, Kollef MH, Chastre J. Methicillin-resistant *Staphylococcus aureus* prolongs intensive care unit length of stay in ventilator-associated pneumonia—despite initially appropriate antibiotic therapy. *Crit Care Med.* 2006;34:700–706.
26. Anhalt JP, Fenselau C. Identification of bacteria using mass spectrometry. *Anal Chem.* 1975;47(2):219–225.
27. La Scola B, Raoult D. Direct identification of bacteria in positive blood culture bottles by matrix-assisted laser desorption ionization time-of-flight mass spectrometry. *PLoS One.* 2009;4(11):e8041.
28. Huang A, Newton D, Kunapuli A, et al. Impact of rapid organism identification via matrix-assisted laser desorption/ionization time-of-flight combined with antimicrobial stewardship team intervention in adult patients with bacteremia and candidemia. *Clin Infect Dis.* 2013;57(9):1237–1245.
29. Croxatto A, Prod'hom G, Greub G. Application of MALDI-TOF mass spectrometry in clinical diagnostic microbiology. *FEMS Mircrobiol Rev.* 2012;36:380–407.

30. Harris DM, Hata DJ. Rapid identification of bacteria and *Candida* using PNA-FISH from blood and peritoneal fluid cultures: a retrospective clinical study. *Ann Clin Microbiol Antimicrob.* 2013;22:2–9.
31. Ly T, Gulia J, Pyrgos V, et al. Impact upon clinical outcomes of translation of PNA FISH-generated laboratory data from the clinical microbiology bench to bedside in real time. *Ther Clin Risk Manag.* 2008;4(3):637–640.
32. Samuel LP, Tibbetts RJ, Agotesku A, et al. Evaluation of a microarray-based assay for rapid identification of positive organisms and resistance markers in positive blood cultures. *J Clin Microbiol.* 2013;51(4):1188–1192.
33. Fishbain JT, Sinyavskiy O, Riederer K, et al. Detection of extended-spectrum beta-lactamase and *Klebsiella pneumoniae* carbapenemase genes directly from blood cultures by use of a nucleic acid microarray. *J Clin Microbiol.* 2012;50(9):2901–2904
34. Cleven BE, Palka-Santini M, Gielen J, et al. Identification and characterization of bacterial pathogens causing bloodstream infections by DNA microarray. *J Clin Microbiol.* 2006;44(7):2389–2397.
35. Shorr AF, Sherner JH, Jackson WL, et al. Invasive approaches to the diagnosis of ventilator-associated pneumonia: a meta-analysis. *Crit Care Med.* 2005;33:46–53.
36. Kollef MH, Kollef KE. Antibiotic utilization and outcomes for patients with clinically suspected ventilator-associated pneumonia and negative quantitative BAL culture results. *Chest.* 2005;128:2706–2713.
37. Singh N, Rogers P, Atwood CW, et al. Short-course empiric antibiotic therapy for patients with pulmonary infiltrates in the intensive care unit: a proposed solution for indiscriminate antibiotic prescription. *Am J Respir Crit Care Med.* 2000;162:505–511.
38. Tenover FC. Mechanisms of antimicrobial resistance in bacteria. *Am J Med.* 2006;119:s3–s10.
39. Howden BP, Ward PB, Charles PG, et al. Treatment outcomes for serious infections caused by methicillin-resistant *Staphylococcus aureus* with reduced vancomycin susceptibility. *Clin Infect Dis.* 2004;38:521–528.
40. Fridkin SK, Hageman J, McDougal LK, et al. Epidemiological and microbiological characterization of infections caused by *Staphylococcus aureus* with reduced susceptibility to vancomycin, United States, 1997–2001. *Clin Infect Dis.* 2003;36:429–439.
41. Sakoulas G, Moellering RC, Eliopoulos GM. Adaptation of methicillin-resistant *Staphylococcus aureus* in the face of vancomycin therapy. *Clin Infect Dis.* 2006;42:S40–S50.
42. H.R. 2182—112th Congress: Generating Antibiotic Incentives Now Act of 2011. Available at: https://www.govtrack.us/congress/bills/112/hr2182. Accessed March 19, 2015.
43. Arhin FF, Draghi DC, Pillar CM, et al. Comparative in vitro activity profile of oritavancin against recent gram-positive clinical isolates. *Antimicrob Agents Chemother.* 2009;53(11):4762–4771.
44. Mendes RE, Farrell DJ, Sader HS, Jones RN. Oritavancin microbiologic features and activity results from the surveillance program in the United States. *Clin Infect Dis.* 2012;54(Suppl 3):S203–S213.
45. Orbactiv® [package insert]. Parsippany, NJ: The Medicines Company; 2014.
46. Shaw KJ, Poppe S, Schaadt R, et al. In vitro activity of TR-700, the antibacterial moiety of the prodrug TR-701, against linezolid-resistant strains. *Antimicrob Agents Chemother.* 2008;52(12):4442–4447.
47. Prokocimer P, De Anda C, Fang E, et al. Tedizolid phosphate vs linezolid for treatment of acute bacterial skin and skin structure infections: the ESTABLISH-1 randomized trial. *JAMA.* 2013;309(6):559–569.
48. Saravolatz LD, Stein GE, Johnson LB. Ceftaroline: a novel cephalosporin with activity against methicillin-resistant *Staphylococcus aureus*. *Clin Infect Dis.* 2011;52(9):1156–1163.
49. Lim L, Sutton E, Brown J. Ceftaroline: a new broad-spectrum cephalosporin. *Am J Health Syst Pharm.* 2011;68(6):491–498.
50. Craig WA, Andes DR. In vivo activities of ceftolozane, a new cephalosporin, with and without tazobactam against Pseudomonas aeruginosa and Enterobacteriaceae, including strains with extended-spectrum β-lactamases, in the thighs of neutropenic mice. *Antimicrob Agents Chemother.* 2013;57(4):1577–1582.
51. Zhanel GG, Chung P, Adam H, et al. Ceftolozane/tazobactam: a novel cephalosporin/β-lactamase inhibitor combination with activity against multidrug-resistant gram-negative bacilli. *Drugs.* 2014;74(1):31–51.
52. Sader HS, Castanheira M, Flamm RK, et al. Antimicrobial activity of ceftazidime-avibactam against gram-negative organisms collected from U.S. medical centers in 2012. *Antimicrob Agents Chemother.* 2014;58(3):1684–1692.
53. Keepers TR, Gomez M, Celeri C, et al. Bactericidal activity, absence of serum effect, and time-kill kinetics of ceftazidime-avibactam against β-lactamase–producing Enterobacteriaceae and Pseudomonas aeruginosa. *Antimicrob Agents Chemother.* 2014;58(9):5297–5305.
54. Vardakas KZ, Rafailidis PI, Konstantelias AA, Falagas ME. Predictors of mortality in patients with infections due to multi-drug resistant gram negative bacteria: the study, the patient, the bug or the drug? *J Infect.* 2013;66(5):401–414.
55. Kollef MH, Sherman G, Ward S, et al. Inadequate antimicrobial treatment of infections: a risk factor for hospital mortality among critically ill patients. *Chest.* 1999;115(2):462–474.
56. Labelle AJ, Micek ST, Roubinian N, Kollef MH. Treatment-related risk factors for hospital mortality in Candida bloodstream infections. *Crit Care Med.* 2008;36(11):2967–2972.
57. Kollef M, Micek S, Hampton N, et al. Septic shock attributed to *Candida* infection: importance of empiric therapy and source control. *Clin Infect Dis.* 2012;54(12):1739–1746.
58. Bassetti M, Righi E, Ansaldi F, et al. A multicenter study of septic shock due to candidemia: outcomes and predictors of mortality. *Intensive Care Med.* 2014;40(6):839–845.
59. Micek ST, Ward S, Fraser VJ, et al. A randomized controlled trial of an antibiotic discontinuation policy for clinically suspected ventilator-associated pneumonia. *Chest.* 2004;125:1791–1799.
60. Jenkins TC, Knepper BC, Sabel AL, et al. Decreased antibiotic utilization after implementation of a guideline for inpatient cellulitis and cutaneous abscess. *Arch Intern Med.* 2011;171(12):1072–1079.
61. Malani AN, Richards PG, Kapila S, et al. Clinical and economic outcomes from a community hospital's antimicrobial stewardship program. *Am J Infect Control.* 2013;41(2):145–148.
62. Ambroggio L, Thomson J, Murtagh Kurowski E, et al. Quality improvement methods increase appropriate antibiotic prescribing for childhood pneumonia. *Pediatrics.* 2013;131(5):e1623–e1631.
63. Morrill HJ, Gaitanis MM, LaPlante KL. Antimicrobial stewardship program prompts increased and earlier infectious diseases consultation. *Antimicrob Resist Infect Control.* 2014;3:12.
64. Pasquale TR, Trienski TL, Olexia DE, et al. Impact of an antimicrobial stewardship program on patients with acute bacterial skin and skin structure infections. *Am J Health Syst Pharm.* 2014;71(13):1136–1139.
65. Wenisch JM, Equiluz-Bruck S, Fudel M, et al. Decreasing Clostridium difficile infections by an antimicrobial stewardship program that reduces moxifloxacin use. *Antimicrob Agents Chemother.* 2014;58(9):5079–5083.
66. Paul M, Benuri-Silbiger I, Soares-Weiser K, Leibovici L. Beta-lactam monotherapy versus beta-lactam-aminoglycoside combination therapy for sepsis in immunocompetent patients: systematic review and meta-analysis of randomized trials. *BMJ.* 2004;328:668.
67. Safdar N, Handelsman J, Maki DG. Does combination antimicrobial therapy reduce mortality in gram-negative bacteraemia? A meta-analysis. *Lancet Infect Dis.* 2004;4:519–527.
68. Talan DA, Stamm WE, Hooton TM, et al. Comparison of ciprofloxacin (7 days) and trimethoprim-sulfamethoxazole (14 days) for acute uncomplicated pyelonephritis in women: a randomized trial. *JAMA.* 2000;283:1583–1590.
69. Dunbar LM, Wunderink RG, Habib MP, et al. High-dose, short-course levofloxacin for community-acquired pneumonia: a new treatment paradigm. *Clin Infect Dis.* 2003;37:752–760.
70. Dellinger RP, Carlet JM, Masur H, et al. Surviving Sepsis Campaign Management Guidelines Committee. Surviving Sepsis Campaign guidelines for management of severe sepsis and septic shock. *Crit Care Med.* 2004;32:858–873.
71. American Thoracic Society, Infectious Diseases Society of America. Guidelines for the management of adults with hospital-acquired, ventilator-associated, and healthcare-associated pneumonia. *Am J Respir Crit Care Med.* 2005;171:388–416.
72. Rello J, Vidaur L, Sandiumenge A, et al. De-escalation therapy in ventilator-associated pneumonia. *Crit Care Med.* 2004;32(11):2183–2190.
73. Ibrahim EH, Ward S, Sherman G, et al. Experience with a clinical guideline for the treatment of ventilator-associated pneumonia. *Crit Care Med.* 2001;29(6):1109–1115.
74. Thursky KA, Buising KL, Bak N, et al. Reduction of broad-spectrum antibiotic use with computerized decision support in an intensive care unit. *Int J Qual Health Care.* 2006;18(3):224–231.
75. Udy AA, Baptista JP, Lim NL, et al. Augmented renal clearance in the ICU: results of a multicenter observational study of renal function in critically ill patients with normal plasma creatinine concentrations. *Crit Care Med.* 2014;42(3):520–527.
76. Carlier M, Carrette S, Roberts JA, et al. Meropenem and piperacillin/tazobactam prescribing in critically ill patients: Does augmented renal clearance affect pharmacokinetic/ pharmacodynamic target attainment when extended infusions are used? *Crit Care.* 2013;17(3):R84.

77. Baptista JP, Sousa E, Martins PJ, Pimentel JM. Augmented renal clearance in septic patients and implications for vancomycin optimisation. *Int J Antimicrob Agents.* 2012;39(5):420–423.
78. Roberts JA, Paul SK, Akova M, et al. DALI: defining antibiotic levels in intensive care unit patients: Are current β-lactam antibiotic doses sufficient for critically ill patients? *Clin Infect Dis.* 2014;58(8):1072–1083.
79. Claus BO, Hoste EA, Colpaert K, et al. Augmented renal clearance is a common finding with worse clinical outcome in critically ill patients receiving antimicrobial therapy. *J Crit Care.* 2013;28(5):695–700.
80. Kollef MH, Chastre J, Clavel M, et al. A randomized trial of 7-day doripenem versus 10-day imipenem-cilastatin for ventilator-associated pneumonia. *Crit Care.* 2012;16(6):R218.
81. Udy AA, Roberts JA, Shorr AF, et al. Augmented renal clearance in septic and traumatized patients with normal plasma creatinine concentrations: identifying at-risk patients. *Crit Care.* 2013;17(1):R35.
82. Akers KS, Niece KL, Chung KK, et al. Modified Augmented Renal Clearance score predicts rapid piperacillin and tazobactam clearance in critically ill surgery and trauma patients. *J Trauma Acute Care Surg.* 2014;77 (3 Suppl 2):S163–S170.
83. De Waele JJ, Carlier M. Beta-lactam antibiotic dosing during continuous renal replacement therapy: How can we optimize therapy? *Crit Care.* 2014;18(3):158.
84. Barco S, Bandettini R, Maffia A, et al. Quantification of piperacillin, tazobactam, meropenem, ceftazidime, and linezolid in human plasma by liquid chromatography/tandem mass spectrometry. *J Chemother.* 2015;27(6):343–347.
85. Zander J, Maier B, Suhr A, et al. Quantification of piperacillin, tazobactam, cefepime, meropenem, ciprofloxacin and linezolid in serum using an isotope dilution UHPLC-MS/MS method with semi-automated sample preparation. *Clin Chem Lab Med.* 2015;53(5):781–791.
86. Wong G, Brinkman A, Benefield RJ, et al. An international, multicentre survey of β-lactam antibiotic therapeutic drug monitoring practice in intensive care units. *J Antimicrob Chemother.* 2014;69(5):1416–1423.
87. Bergstrom CT, Lo M, Lipsitch M. Ecological theory suggests that antimicrobial cycling will not reduce antimicrobial resistance in hospitals. *Proc Natl Acad Sci USA.* 2004;101:13285–13290.
88. Sarraf-Yazdi S, Sharpe M, Bennett KM, et al. A 9-year retrospective review of antibiotic cycling in a surgical intensive care unit. *J Surg Res.* 2012; 176(2)e73–e78.
89. Abel zur Wiesch P, Kouyos R, Abel S, et al. Cycling empirical antibiotic therapy in hospitals: meta-analysis and models. *PLoS Pathogens.* 2014;10(6):e1004225.
90. Sirvent JM, Torres A, El-Ebiary M, et al. A protective effect of intravenously administered cefuroxime against nosocomial pneumonia in patients with structural coma. *Am J Respir Crit Care Med.* 1997;155:1729–1734.
91. Krueger WA, Lenhart FP, Neeser G, et al. Influence of combined intravenous and topical antibiotic prophylaxis on the incidence of infections, organ dysfunctions, and mortality in critically ill surgical patients: a prospective, stratified, randomized, double-blind, placebo-controlled clinical trial. *Am J Respir Crit Care Med.* 2002;166:1029–1037.
92. de Smet AM, Kluytmans JA, Cooper BS, et al. Decontamination of the digestive tract and oropharynx in ICU patients. *N Engl J Med.* 2009; 360:20–31.
93. Oostdijk EA, Kesecioglu J, Schultz MJ, et al. Effects of decontamination of the oropharynx and intestinal tract on antibiotic resistance in ICUs. *JAMA.* 2014;312(14):1429–1437.
94. Kollef MH, Pittet D, Sánchez García M, et al. A randomized, double-blind, placebo-controlled, multinational phase III trial of iseganan in prevention of ventilator-associated pneumonia. *Am J Respir Crit Care Med.* 2006;173:91–97.
95. Fourrier F, Dubois D, Pronnier P, et al. Effect of gingival and dental plaque antiseptic decontamination on nosocomial infections acquired in the intensive care unit: a double-blind placebo-controlled multicenter study. *Crit Care Med.* 2005;33:1728–1735.
96. Koeman M, van der Van A, Hak E, et al. Oral decontamination with chlorhexidine reduces the incidence of ventilator-associated pneumonia. *Am J Respir Crit Care Med.* 2006;173:1348–1355.
97. Shorr AF, Zilberberg MD, Micek ST, Kollef MH. Prediction of infection due to antibiotic-resistant bacteria by select risk factors for health care-associated pneumonia. *Arch Intern Med.* 2008;168(20):2205–2210.
98. Shorr AF, Zilberberg MD, Reichley R, et al. Validation of a clinical score for assessing the risk of resistant pathogens in patients with pneumonia presenting to the emergency department. *Clin Infect Dis.* 2012;54(2):193–198.
99. Chalmers JD, Rother C, Salih W, Ewig S. Healthcare-associated pneumonia does not accurately identify potentially resistant pathogens: a systematic review and meta-analysis. *Clin Infect Dis.* 2014;58(3):330–339.
100. Shindo Y, Ito R, Kobayashi D, et al. Risk factors for drug-resistant pathogens in community-acquired and healthcare-associated pneumonia. *Am J Respir Crit Care Med.* 2013;188(8):985–995.
101. Maruyama T, Fujisawa T, Okuno M, et al. A new strategy for healthcare-associated pneumonia: a 2-year prospective multicenter cohort study using risk factors for multidrug-resistant pathogens to select initial empiric therapy. *Clin Infect Dis.* 2013;57(10):1373–1383.
102. Micek ST, Heard KM, Gowan M, Kollef MH. Identifying critically ill patients at risk for inappropriate antibiotic therapy: a pilot study of a point-of-care decision support alert. *Crit Care Med.* 2014;42(8): 1832–1838.
103. Evans RS, Pestotnik SL, Classen DC, et al. A computer-assisted management program for antibiotics and other anti-infective agents. *N Engl J Med.* 1998;338(4):232–238.
104. Pestotnik SL, Classen DC, Evans RS, Burke JP. Implementing antibiotic practice guidelines through computer-assisted decision support: clinical and financial outcomes. *Ann Intern Med.* 1996;124(10):884–890.
105. Paul M, Nielsen AD, Goldberg E, et al. Prediction of specific pathogens in patients with sepsis: evaluation of TREAT, a computerized decision support system. *J Antimicrob Chemother.* 2007;59(6):1204–1207.
106. McGregor JC, Weekes E, Forrest GN, et al. Impact of a computerized clinical decision support system on reducing inappropriate antimicrobial use: a randomized controlled trial. *J Am Med Inform Assoc.* 2006; 13(4):378–384.
107. Bochicchio GV, Smit PA, Moore R, et al. Pilot study of a web-based antibiotic decision management guide. *J Am Coll Surg.* 2006;202(3): 459–467.
108. Thiel SW, Asghar MF, Micek ST, et al. Hospital-wide impact of a standardized order set for the management of bacteremic severe sepsis. *Crit Care Med.* 2009;37(3):819–824.
109. Stolz D, Smyrnios N, Eggimann P, et al. Procalcitonin for reduced antibiotic exposure in ventilator-associated pneumonia: a randomised study. *Eur Respir J.* 2009;34(6):1364–1375.
110. Bouadma L, Luyt CE, Tubach F, et al; PRORATA Trial Group. Use of procalcitonin to reduce patients' exposure to antibiotics in intensive care units (PRORATA trial): a multicentre randomised controlled trial. *Lancet.* 2010;375(9713):463–474.
111. Hochreiter M, Köhler T, Schweiger AM, et al. Procalcitonin to guide duration of antibiotic therapy in intensive care patients: a randomized prospective controlled trial. *Crit Care.* 2009;13(3):R83.
112. Jensen JU, Hein L, Lundgren B, et al. Procalcitonin and Survival Study (PASS) Group. Procalcitonin-guided interventions against infections to increase early appropriate antibiotics and improve survival in the intensive care unit: a randomized trial. *Crit Care Med.* 2011;39(9):2048–2058.
113. Shehabi Y, Sterba M, Garrett PM, et al. Procalcitonin algorithm in critically ill adults with undifferentiated infection or suspected sepsis: a randomized controlled trial. *Am J Respir Crit Care Med.* 2014;190(10):1102–1110.
114. Sridharan P, Chamberlain RS. The efficacy of procalcitonin as a biomarker in the management of sepsis: slaying dragons or tilting at windmills? *Surg Infect (Larchmt).* 2013;14(6):489–511.
115. Prkno A, Wacker C, Brunkhorst FM, Schlattmann P. Procalcitonin-guided therapy in intensive care unit patients with severe sepsis and septic shock: a systematic review and meta-analysis. *Crit Care.* 2013;17(6):R291.
116. Soni NJ, Samson DJ, Galaydick JL, et al. Procalcitonin-guided antibiotic therapy: a systematic review and meta-analysis. *J Hosp Med.* 2013; 8(9):530–540.
117. Maertens J, Deeren D, Dierickx D, Theunissen K. Preemptive antifungal therapy: still a way to go. *Curr Opin Infect Dis.* 2006;19(6):551–556.
118. Pfeiffer CD, Fine JP, Safdar N. Diagnosis of invasive aspergillosis using a galactomannan assay: a meta-analysis. *Clin Infect Dis.* 2006;42(10): 1417–1427.
119. Tissot F, Lamoth F, Hauser PM, et al. β-Glucan antigenemia anticipates diagnosis of blood culture-negative intraabdominal candidiasis. *Am J Respir Crit Care Med.* 2013;188(9):1100–1109.
120. Meersseman W, Lagrou K, Maertens J, et al. Galactomannan in bronchoalveolar lavage fluid: a tool for diagnosing aspergillosis in intensive care unit patients. *Am J Respir Crit Care Med.* 2008;177(1):27–34.
121. Affolter K, Tamm M, Jahn K, et al. Galactomannan in bronchoalveolar lavage for diagnosing invasive fungal disease. *Am J Respir Crit Care Med.* 2014;190(3):309–317.

CHAPTER

84

Surgical Infections

MICHAELA A. WEST and MICHAEL W. CRIPPS

INTRODUCTION

Critical care practitioners should be familiar with unique aspects of surgical patients that make diagnosis and management of infections challenging in these individuals. In addition, the epidemiology of perioperative and postoperative infections is often qualitatively different than other patients in the intensive care unit (ICU). Surgical infections are traditionally considered to be infections that require surgical therapy (e.g., complicated intra-abdominal and soft tissue infections). Intra-abdominal and soft tissue infections are considered in detail elsewhere in this textbook. Surgical patients are also especially vulnerable to nosocomial infection, so a more expansive definition should include any infection that affects surgical patients (Table 84.1). In this chapter, we will review the pathophysiology of infection in surgical and trauma patients, expound on the principles of surgical antibiotic prophylaxis, explain the approach to workup of surgical patients with a possible infection, discuss common infectious conditions and syndromes, and describe the tenets of treatment.

BACKGROUND

There are many reasons why surgical patients are at particular risk of infection. Any surgical intervention is inherently invasive, breaching natural epithelial barriers and thereby allowing microbes to gain access to areas of the body that are normally sterile. Surgical patients are also uniquely afflicted by infections of incisions and surgical procedures may involve postoperative catheters and a longer need for intravenous access than nonsurgical ICU patients. Many conditions that require surgical interventions are immunosuppressive (e.g., trauma, burns, malignant tumors) as are surgical interventions themselves. Therapeutic immunosuppression is also needed following solid organ transplantation. Nosocomial pneumonia occurs more frequently among surgical patients than comparably ill medical patients. General anesthesia almost always means a period of mechanical ventilation and reduced consciousness during emergence from anesthesia that poses a risk of pulmonary aspiration of gastric contents and impaired mucociliary clearance, increasing the risk of pneumonia.

Development of a postoperative infection has a negative impact on surgical outcomes; recognizing risk, minimizing it, and taking an aggressive approach to the diagnosis and treatment of such infections is crucial to improve surgical outcomes.

Surgical Source Control

Surgical "source control" can be defined as the operative or interventional measures taken to eliminate a source of infection. Several basic principles apply to surgical source control:

- Nonviable or infected tissue needs to be removed (debrided).
- Openings in the GI tract need to be repaired or controlled.
- Macroscopic abscesses need to be drained.

Debridement

Debridement is the removal of nonviable tissue using basic surgical techniques and principles. The extent of tissue necrosis or the severity of infection will dictate whether this requires a minor or a very major surgical intervention. Antimicrobial agents and host defense cells are delivered via the bloodstream and infection control requires viable, well-perfused tissue. Nonviable or poorly perfused tissue that is infected tissue should be debrided to prevent infection and minimize the inflammatory response arising from necrotic tissue (see Approach to Surgical Patient with Suspected Infection, below). The guiding principle is that *all* nonviable or necrotic tissue must be removed.

Repair or Control of the Primary Source of Infection

In many cases, primary source control requires resection, repair, or percutaneous control of the primary source of infection (1). The Surviving Sepsis Guideline places a high priority on identification and control of the source of infection (Table 84.2) (2). Ultrasound and computer tomography (CT) imaging are important adjuncts for identification of the source of surgical infections. Once identified, several possible surgical/radiologic interventions can be considered depending on the clinical condition of the patient, comorbidities, attributes of the specific infection, and the resources available.

Drain (Macroscopic) Abscesses

An abscess is a collection of bacteria, tissue, and host immune cells. Because abscesses contain very high numbers of bacteria, little or no blood supply, and very low pH, host defense cells (e.g., neutrophils and macrophages) cannot eradicate the infection (3). When very small abscesses are identified, it may be possible for them to resolve without formal drainage procedures, but almost all larger (macroscopic) abscesses will need to be drained. Drainage of an abscess removes a significant volume of fluid and bacteria, allows the walls to collapse, improves perfusion and oxygen levels in the residual cavity, thereby allowing antibiotics and host cells to control the infection.

Identification of Surgical Patients at Risk for Infection

When a surgical or injured patient is admitted to the ICU, it is always important to discuss with the surgeon what transpired before and during the operation. It's also useful to ascertain if the surgeon has particular concerns for postoperative complications, including infection. For example, it is well established that intraoperative shock, or the need for blood transfusion,

TABLE 84.1 Health Care–Associated Infections in the Intensive Care Unit

Pneumonia
Ventilator-associated events
Ventilator-associated pneumonia
Central line–associated bloodstream infections
Intra-abdominal infections
Intra-abdominal abscess
Secondary peritonitis
Tertiary peritonitis
Catheter-associated urinary tract infections
Skin and soft tissue infections
Superficial surgical site infections
Decubitus ulcers
Burn wound sepsis
Clostridium difficile–associated disease
Empyema
Sinusitis
Perianal infections

is associated with an increased risk of postoperative infection and/or anastomotic breakdown. Did the surgeons have concerns about the quality of tissue or presence of necrotic tissue requiring debridement? Did they place drains, and if so why were they placed, where are they located, and how long will they need to be in place? Drainage catheters of any sort (including nasogastric tubes and urinary catheters) increase

TABLE 84.2 Surviving Sepsis Guidelines for Initial Resuscitation and Infection Control Priorities for Septic Shock and Severe Sepsis

Diagnosis of Infection
Obtain appropriate cultures prior to start antibiotics (but do not delay antibiotic administration) (1C)
≥2 blood culture samples
≥1 blood percutaneous culture
Culture all vascular access device present >48 hr
Culture other sites as indicated
Perform imaging studies promptly to identify source of infection (UG)
Antibiotic Therapy
Choice of antibiotics
Broad-spectrum activity
≥1 agent active against likely pathogens (1B)
Good penetration for presumed source (1B)
Begin IV antibiotics ≤1 hr after recognition septic shock (1B) or severe sepsis (1C)
Reassess antibiotics daily for de-escalation (1B)
Duration typically 7–10 days (2C)
Infection Source Identification and Control
Evaluate patient for infection focus amenable to source control (1C)
Establish anatomic site of infection ASAP (1C) and ≤6 hr of presentation (1D)
Implement source control measures ASAP after successful initial resuscitation (1C)
Choose means of source control that maximizes efficacy and minimizes physiologic impact (1D)
Remove potentially infected intravascular access devices (1C)
GRADE criteria (139) in parentheses reflect strength of recommendation and quality of evidence.

Adapted from Dellinger RP, Levy MM, Rhodes A, et al. Surviving sepsis campaign: international guidelines for management of severe sepsis and septic shock: 2012. *Crit Care Med.* 2013;41(2):580–637.

the risk of infection. That said, the vast majority of surgeons have strong feelings about drains placed during an operation and ICU practitioners should not remove drains without consulting with the operative surgeon.

PATHOPHYSIOLOGY OF SURGICAL INFECTIONS

In many respects, the diagnosis and treatment of a surgical infections is fundamentally different than diagnosis of "medical infections." With nonsurgical infections the diagnostic principles center upon *identification* of the infecting organism. Generally, there is only one microbial species responsible for "medical" infections. Once identified, the appropriate treatment involves selection of the antimicrobial agent(s) needed to treat this organism. In contrast, the organisms responsible for surgical infections are frequently known, at least in a general sense, based on the anatomic location of the surgical intervention or infection, and knowledge of the organisms present. In the ICU setting, clinicians caring for surgical patients must consider the entire range of surgical, "medical," and hospital-acquired infectious etiologies in this population.

Resident endogenous bacteria are always present on the skin and throughout the gut. Following admission to the hospital or ICU, the composition of the endogenous flora changes significantly, with a greater proportion of drug-resistant species. Despite the presence of bacteria, humans normally do not become infected because a balance of three factors exists: First, the preponderance of organisms, especially outside the hospital, are nonvirulent bacteria; second, the major reservoirs of micro-organisms (skin and GI tract) are intact; third, host defense mechanisms destroy bacteria that gain access to sterile areas of the body. However, any or all of these factors may be altered by the pre-existing conditions, surgical interventions, nosocomial colonization, indwelling catheters, or prior antibiotic treatment. Knowledge of the community and ICU bacterial flora and the polymicrobial nature of surgical infections informs the selection of antimicrobial agents.

Under normal circumstances, the overwhelming numbers of nonpathogenic bacteria constitute a robust "defense" against infection, because infection is proportionately less likely if >99% of the inoculum is incapable of producing infection. This concept of adherent resident bacteria preventing invasion has been termed *colonization resistance* (4). As mentioned above, not all microbes are pathogenic, that is, capable of initiating invasion of the body. For example, *Escherichia coli* (gram-negative aerobe) and *Bacteroides fragilis* (gram-negative anaerobe) are frequently cultured from intra-abdominal infections (IAIs), yet they constitute 0.01% and 1% of the colonic flora, respectively. These organisms cause infection because they possess virulence factors that favor growth, invasion, or prevent their eradication. This knowledge forms the basis for the selection of empiric antimicrobial therapy, which must have activity against the anticipated pathogens. It has been shown that more than 99% of the colonic microflora are "nonpathogenic" anaerobes on admission to the ICU, but within 3 days the microflora shifts to a much higher proportion of aerobic pathogens (5). Changes in the gut flora within the ICU are harmful in two ways (6): (1) There are a greater proportion of pathogenic and/or resistant bacteria; and (2) there are far fewer nonpathogenic bacteria, organisms which ordinarily suppress overgrowth of aerobic pathogens.

Surgical patients in the ICU have additional factors that put them at increased risk for infection. Postoperative pain and limited mobility, coupled with the lingering effects of general anesthesia, increase the risk for respiratory complications and pneumonia. Vigorous pulmonary toilet, early mobilization (if possible), and adequate analgesia will mitigate, but unfortunately cannot eliminate, this increased risk. Suboptimal nutrition can impair host defenses and innate immunity, and surgical patients often have pre-existing nutritional deficiencies (e.g., in the context of cancer). Postoperative nutritional support is more difficult in surgical patients because of slow return of bowel function coupled with the increased metabolic demand imposed by healing. Patients admitted to the ICU after solid organ transplantation have overt immunosuppression. Immunosuppression and an increased risk of infection have also been well documented in trauma and burn patients, especially those requiring blood transfusions.

The general principles of surgical care, critical care, and infection control cannot be overemphasized. Resuscitation must be rapid, yet precise. Infection prevention measure must sometimes be sacrificed under the chaotic conditions of acute resuscitation, but every attempt should be made so that this is not the case. If central venous catheters (CVCs) were inserted under nonsterile conditions, they must be removed and, if necessary, replaced by a fresh puncture at a new site as soon as the patient's condition permits. Detailed evidence-based guidelines for the general prevention of infection (7,8) and the prevention of ventilator-associated pneumonia have been published (9). All who provide critical care must be familiar with the guidelines and adhere to them insofar as possible.

APPROACH TO SURGICAL PATIENT WITH SUSPECTED INFECTION

Identification of an ICU infection in surgical and trauma patients is challenging for several reasons. All postoperative and injured patients have a baseline degree of inflammatory response as part of the endogenous reaction to the physiologic insult of surgery and/or the underlying process that required a surgical intervention. Diagnosis of infection is also complicated by the presence of potential signs of infection, such as tachycardia, tachypnea that arise from pain, immobility, or fluid shifts. Elevated temperatures and leukocytosis are also seen commonly for the first few days (<96 hours) after surgery. In the vast majority of new surgical ICU admissions, such early signs and symptoms are not associated with infection. These signs will tend to dissipate with time after the surgical intervention or injury. That said, development of a new fever more than 4 days postoperatively should warrant an investigation for an infectious etiology. A rare, but important, exception to this approach is a very high fever associated with significant systemic toxicity arising in the immediate (<24 hours) postoperative period. Such a presentation can arise from group A β-hemolytic *Streptococci* or *Staphylococcus aureus* (toxic shock syndrome); in such a setting it's important to examine the surgical incisions—which can be diagnostic.

The presence of a new temperature elevation can be a very useful clinical sign in identifying patients with infection. Fever is an elevated temperature above baseline and rises when the hypothalamic "set point" is altered in response to physiologic stimuli. A patient with a core temperature ≥38.3°C (≥101°F) is considered to be febrile and such patients may warrant further evaluation to determine if infection is present. However, the mere presence of fever has a relatively poor positive- and negative-predictive value. It can often be difficult to determine if an abnormal temperature is a reflection of a physiologic process, a drug, or an environmental influence (Table 84.3). It has been noted that fever is due to a noninfectious cause in more than 50% of surgical patients (10,11), and it is now clear that factors released from damaged or ischemic tissue activate the identical toll-like receptors (TLRs) and induce an identical innate immune response with elaboration of pro- and anti-inflammatory cytokines (12,13) as do infectious agents. This may explain why the presence of large amounts of damaged tissue from trauma, burns, acute vascular insufficiency, etc. result in a clinical syndrome that can be indistinguishable from the host response to microbial infection (13). Finally, a minority of patients with impaired immune responsiveness may not manifest fever in response to infection. As a general rule, greater temperature elevations are more likely to arise from a new infection or infectious complication.

TABLE 84.3 Noninfectious Causes of Fever
Acalculous cholecystitis
Acute myocardial infarction
Adrenal insufficiency
Blood product transfusion
Cytokine-related fever
Pericardial injury syndrome
Drug fever
Fat emboli
Fibroproliferative phase of acute respiratory distress syndrome
Gout
Heterotopic ossification
Immune reconstitution inflammatory syndrome
Intracranial bleed
Jarisch–Herxheimer reaction
Pancreatitis
Pulmonary infarction
Pneumonitis without infection
Stroke
Thyroid storm
Transplant rejection
Tumor lysis syndrome
Venous thrombosis

From O'Grady NP, Barie PS, Bartlett JG, et al. Guidelines for evaluation of new fever in critically ill adult patients: 2008 update from the American College of Critical Care Medicine and the Infectious Diseases Society of America. *Crit Care Med.* 2008;36:1330–1349.

Performing a careful and focused history and physical examination will assist immeasurably in terms of diagnosing surgical infections. Laboratory tests or imaging studies to search for infection should be performed only *after* a clinical assessment (history and physical examination) indicates that infection might be present. In postoperative patients, surgical wounds and incisions should be examined. A careful assessment of the respiratory system, including recent alterations in oxygenation or character of sputum, should be done. Examination should focus on identifying the most frequent ICU-acquired infections; catheter-associated urinary tract infection (CA-UTI), pneumonia, and central line–associated blood stream infections (CLABSI), and eliminating noninfectious causes of fever, such as deep vein thrombosis or pulmonary embolism.

Blood cultures should be obtained from patients with a new fever when clinical evaluation suggests an infectious cause (11,14). The site of venipuncture should be cleaned with either 2% chlorhexidine gluconate in 70% isopropyl alcohol, or 1% to 2% tincture of iodine, and the site allowed to dry for at least 30 seconds (15). A 20 to 30 mL sample of blood per culture should be drawn from each single site. Paired blood cultures should always be obtained to avoid false-positive cultures arising from contamination. It is also critical to always try to obtain blood cultures before the initiation of antimicrobial therapy (3). The sensitivity of blood culturing for detection of true bacteremia or fungemia is related to many factors, most importantly, the volume of blood drawn and obtaining the cultures before initiation of anti-infective therapy (16,17). Each culture should ideally be drawn by separate venipuncture or through a separate intravascular device, but not through multiple ports of the same intravascular catheter (18). At least one culture should be drawn from central or longer-term catheters, as differential quantitative bacterial levels may aid in diagnosis of CLABSIs (19,20).

PRINCIPLES OF ANTIBIOTIC THERAPY

Antibiotic Prophylaxis

Widespread application of prophylactic antibiotics, in conjunction with surgical procedures, is common in surgical patients. Nonsurgeons may not be familiar with the appropriate use and goals of prophylactic antibiotics, but it's important that critical care practitioners understand their use. Antibiotics are used "prophylactically" to *prevent* infection(s) that could develop in conjunction with an invasive procedure, most often to prevent infection at the site of the surgical procedure (surgical site infections [SSIs]) (21). The goal of antibiotic prophylaxis is to protect the operative site (incision and operative field) during the procedure, when the site is most vulnerable to microbial inoculation. Prophylactic antibiotics are not a panacea; if not administered properly, antibiotic prophylaxis is ineffective and may even be harmful. Antibiotic prophylaxis does not prevent postoperative *nosocomial* infections, which may occur at an increased rate after prolonged prophylaxis (22), selecting for more resistant pathogens when infection does develop (23).

Surgical wounds can be classified based on the degree to which there is a potential for bacterial contamination (Table 84.4) (21). Antibiotic prophylaxis is indicated for most clean-contaminated and contaminated (or potentially contaminated) operations. Antibiotic prophylaxis of clean surgery is controversial. Where bone is incised (e.g., craniotomy, sternotomy) or a prosthesis is inserted, antibiotic prophylaxis is generally indicated. Some controversy persists with clean surgery of soft tissues (e.g., breast, hernia) (24–27). Lower extremity arterial reconstruction with prosthetic grafts is an example of clean surgery where there is demonstrated benefit of prophylactic antibiotics (28).

Antimicrobial agents for prophylaxis should:

- be a safe agent, as the majority of patients will never develop an infection;
- possess a narrow spectrum of coverage that targets the relevant pathogens that may be present at the surgical site;
- not be an antibiotic relied upon for therapy of established infections; and
- be administered in the optimal manner to prevent infection (29).

The optimal time to give parenteral antibiotic prophylaxis is within 1 hour prior to incision (30). Antibiotics given sooner are ineffective, as are agents given after the incision is closed. The goal is to insure effective concentrations of antibiotic are present in the tissues for the duration of the procedure. Antibiotics with short half-lives (<2 hours, e.g., cefazolin or cefoxitin) should be redosed if the operation is prolonged or bloody (31). Higher doses should be given in obese individuals and patients receiving aggressive resuscitation (e.g., trauma patients). While most guidelines specify a 24-hour *limit* for prophylaxis, single-dose prophylaxis (with intraoperative redosing, if indicated) has shown equivalency to multiple doses for prevention of SSI (32). Antibiotics should not be given to "cover" indwelling drains or catheters, in lavage or irrigation fluid, or as a substitute for poor surgical technique.

It has now been clearly shown that administration of prophylactic antibiotics beyond 24 hours can be harmful. Prolonged prophylaxis increases the risk of nosocomial infections unrelated to the surgical site, and the emergence of multidrug-resistant (MDR) pathogens. Both pneumonia and vascular catheter–related infections have been associated with prolonged prophylaxis (33,34). Continuation of prophylactic antibiotics resulted in a higher proportion of methicillin-resistant *S. aureus* (MRSA) isolates from SSI (23). Disruption of the normal balance of gut flora from longer-duration prophylaxis has been shown to result in overgrowth of the enterotoxin-producing *Clostridium difficile* (35).

TABLE 84.4 Surgical Wound Classification

Class	Status	Description
I	Clean	An uninfected operative wound in which no inflammation is encountered and the respiratory, alimentary, genital, or uninfected urinary tract is not entered.
II	Clean-contaminated	An operative wound in which the respiratory, alimentary, genital, or urinary tracts are entered under controlled conditions and without unusual contamination. (Elective operations involving the biliary tract, bowel, appendix, vagina, and oropharynx are included in this category.)
III	Contaminated	Open, fresh, accidental wounds. In addition, operations with major breaks in sterile technique or gross spillage from the gastrointestinal tract, and incisions in which acute, *nonpurulent* inflammation is encountered.
IV	Dirty-infected	Old traumatic wounds with retained devitalized tissue and those that involve *existing clinical infection* or perforated viscera. The organisms causing postoperative infection were present in the operative field *before* the operation.

Adapted from Mangram AJ, Horan TC, Pearson ML, et al. Guideline for prevention of surgical site infection, 1999. Hospital Infection Control Practices Advisory Committee. *ICHE.* 1999;20(4):250–278.

Therapeutic Antibiotics

When considering antimicrobial therapy for surgical infections, it is critical to remember that surgical infections generally require a "surgical" intervention for resolution, resection, debridement, drainage—operative or percutaneous—removal of foreign body, etc. Further, surgical infections are frequently polymicrobial, especially necrotizing skin and soft tissue infection (SSTI) and IAI. Although antimicrobial therapy is the mainstay of some infections, and required as an adjunct to the surgical therapy of others, the widespread overuse—and misuse—of antibiotics has led to an alarming increase in MDR pathogens. New agents may allow shorter courses of therapy and prophylaxis, which are desirable for cost savings and control of microbial flora, but are not always available.

Empiric Antibiotic Therapy

Empiric antibiotic therapy must be administered carefully. Injudicious therapy could result in undertreatment of established infection, or unnecessary therapy when the patient has only inflammation or bacterial colonization; either may be deleterious. Inappropriate therapy—delay, therapy misdirected against usual pathogens, failure to treat MDR pathogens—leads unequivocally to increased mortality (36–39).

Strategies have been promulgated to optimize antibiotic administration, including reliance upon physician prescribing patterns, computerized decision support (40), administration by protocol (41–47), and formulary restriction programs. Owing to the increasing prevalence of MDR pathogens, it is crucial for initial empiric antibiotic therapy to be targeted appropriately, administered in sufficient dosage to ensure bacterial killing, narrowed in spectrum (*de-escalation*) (48) as soon as possible based on microbiology data and clinical response, and continued only as long as necessary. Appropriate antibiotic prescribing not only optimizes patient care, but also supports infection control practice and preserves microbial ecology (48). Combining these strategies into a unified antibiotic stewardship program has been proven to decrease the incidence of resistant gram-negative health care–associated infections in trauma and surgical ICUs (49).

Choice of Antibiotic

Antibiotic choice is based on several interrelated factors (Table 84.5). Narrow-spectrum coverage is always desired, but the activity of the agent against the identified or likely (for empiric therapy) pathogens is paramount. Estimation of likely pathogens depends on the disease process believed responsible, whether the infection is community-, health care–, or hospital-acquired, and whether MDR organisms are present. Local knowledge of antimicrobial resistance patterns is essential, even at the unit-specific level. Patient-specific factors of importance include age, debility, immunosuppression, intrinsic organ function, prior allergy or other adverse reaction, and recent antibiotic therapy. Institutional factors of importance include guidelines that may specify a particular therapy, formulary availability of specific agents, outbreaks of infections caused by MDR pathogens, and antibiotic control programs.

Numerous agents are available for therapy (Table 84.6) (50–52); these may be chosen based on spectrum, whether broad or targeted (e.g., antipseudomonal, antianaerobic), in addition to the above factors. If a nosocomial gram-positive pathogen is suspected (e.g., wound or SSI, CLABSI, pneumonia) or MRSA is endemic, empiric vancomycin (or linezolid) is appropriate. Some authorities recommend dual-agent therapy for serious *Pseudomonas* infections (i.e., an antipseudomonal β-lactam drug plus an aminoglycoside), but evidence of efficacy is lacking (53). It is important to use at least two antibiotics for empiric therapy of any infection that may be caused by either a gram-positive or gram-negative infection (e.g., nosocomial pneumonia) (54).

TABLE 84.5 Factors Influencing Antibiotic Choice

Activity against known/suspected pathogens
Disease believed responsible
Distinguish infection from colonization
Narrow-spectrum coverage most desirable
Antimicrobial resistance patterns
Patient-specific factors
Severity of illness
Age
Immunosuppression
Organ dysfunction
Allergy
Institutional guidelines/restrictions

TABLE 84.6 Appropriate Antibacterial Agents for Empiric Use

Antipseudomonal
Piperacillin–tazobactam
Cefepime, ceftazidime
Imipenem, meropenem
? Ciprofloxacin, levofloxacin (depending on local susceptibility patterns)
Aminoglycoside
Targeted spectrum
Gram-positive
Glycopeptide
Lipopeptide (not for known/suspected pneumonia)
Oxazolidinone
Gram-negative
Third-generation cephalosporin (not ceftriaxone)
Monobactam
Antianaerobic
Metronidazole
Broad spectrum
Piperacillin–tazobactam
Carbapenems
Fluoroquinolones
Tigecycline (plus an antipseudomonal agent)
Antianaerobic
Metronidazole
Carbapenems
β-Lactam/β-lactamase combination agents
Tigecycline

Role of Antifungal Therapy

The incidence of invasive fungal infections is increasing among critically ill surgical patients. Several conditions are predictors for invasive fungal infection complicating critical illness, including ICU length of stay; altered immune responsiveness; and the number of medical devices placed. Neutropenia, diabetes mellitus, new-onset hemodialysis, total parenteral nutrition, broad-spectrum antibiotic administration, bladder catheterization, azotemia, diarrhea, and corticosteroid therapy are also associated with invasive fungal infection (55,56).

Duration of Antimicrobial Therapy

The endpoint of therapy is largely undefined, in part because quality data are few (41,57,58). If cultures are negative, empiric antibiotic therapy should be stopped in most cases. Unnecessary antibiotic therapy in the absence of infection clearly increases the risk of MDR infection; therefore, therapy beyond 48 to 72 hours with negative cultures usually is unjustifiable. The morbidity of antibiotic therapy includes allergic reactions, development of nosocomial superinfections—fungal, enterococcal, and *C. difficile*–related infections—organ toxicity, promotion of antibiotic resistance, reduced yield from subsequent cultures, and induced vitamin K deficiency with coagulopathy or accentuation of warfarin effect.

If *bona fide* evidence of infection is evident, then treatment is continued as indicated clinically. Some infections can be treated with therapy lasting 5 days or less. Every decision to start antibiotics must be accompanied by a decision regarding the duration of therapy (59); a reason to continue therapy beyond the predetermined endpoint must be compelling. Bacterial killing is rapid in response to effective agents, but the host response may not subside immediately. Therefore, the clinical response of the patient should not be the sole determinant for continuation of therapy. If a patient still has systemic inflammatory response syndrome (SIRS) at the predetermined end of therapy, it is more useful to stop therapy and obtain new cultures to look for persistent or new infection, resistant pathogens, and noninfectious causes of SIRS. Seldom should antibacterial therapy continue for more than 7 to 10 days. This concept was analyzed in the Study to Optimize Peritoneal Infection Therapy (STOP-IT) trial published in the NEJM (60). The two study arms consisted of antibiotic treatment until 2 days after resolution of fever, leukocytosis, and ileus for maximum of 10 days (control group) versus a fixed, short course of antibiotics of 4 ± 1 days (experimental group). The primary outcomes of SSI, recurrent IAI, or death were not different between the experimental group (21.8%) and the control group (22.3%) (95% confidence interval [CI], −7.0 to 8.0; $p = 0.92$). However, there was a significant difference in the median duration of antibiotic therapy of 4.0 days [4.0, 5.0] in the experimental group versus 8.0 days [5.0, 10.0] in the control group (95% CI, −4.7 to −3.3; $P < 0.001$). These results suggest that after an adequate source control procedure, the beneficial effects of systemic antimicrobial therapy are limited to the first few days after intervention. Further, the delay in manifestation of infectious complications in the control group increases the overall time to resolution of all infections. Implementation of this strategy in patients with an IAI who have had adequate source control can effectively cut the duration of antibiotics by half. Keeping this in mind, there are some bacterial infections that require more than 14 days of therapy such as tuberculosis of any site, endocarditis, osteomyelitis, and selected cases of brain abscess, liver abscess, lung abscess, postoperative meningitis, and endophthalmitis.

SPECIFIC CLINICAL SYNDROMES

Surgical Site Infections

According to criteria established by the United States Centers for Disease Control and Prevention (CDC), an SSI is an infection related to an operative procedure that involves only the skin and subcutaneous tissue of the incision. Additionally, the patient must have pain, tenderness, localized swelling, erythema, or heat AND at least one of the following: (1) purulent drainage from the superficial incision; (2) organisms identified from an aseptically obtained specimen from the superficial incision or subcutaneous tissue by a culture or nonculture-based microbiologic testing method which is performed for purposes of clinical diagnosis or treatment; or (3) superficial incision that is deliberately opened by a surgeon and culture or nonculture-based testing is not performed. It is important to remember that a culture- or nonculture-based test that has a negative finding does not meet the criterion for SSI (61). SSIs are classified generally as superficial SSI, deep SSI, and organ space SSI (Fig. 84.1) (21).

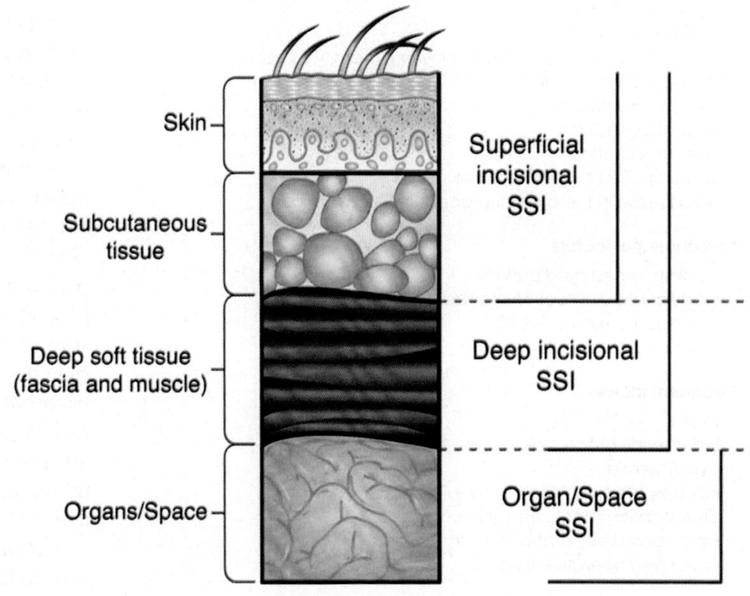

FIGURE 84.1 Classification of surgical site infections by depth of invasion or location. (Redrawn from Horan TC, Gaynes RP, Martone WJ, et al. CDC definitions of nosocomial surgical site infections, 1992: a modification of CDC definitions of surgical wound infections. *Infect Control Hosp Epidemiol.* 1992;13:606–608.)

Pathogenesis of Surgical Site Infection

SSIs are among the most frequently encountered complications in surgical patients, regardless of specialty. Although any patient undergoing an operation is at risk for developing an SSI, rates vary according to the type of operation, with the highest rate seen with abdominal surgery (62). In the 2013 report by the National Healthcare Safety Network (NHSN), coagulase-negative staphylococci and *S. aureus* were the most prevalent SSI pathogens for most types of surgery, whereas SSI occurring from abdominal operations had a predominant gram-negative rod flora (63).

The spectrum of bacterial contamination of the surgical site has been well described (64). The vast majority of SSI arises from the patient's endogenous organisms, typically those present at the site of the procedure. *Clean surgical procedures* affect only integumentary and musculoskeletal soft tissues. *Clean-contaminated procedures* open a hollow viscus (e.g., alimentary, biliary, genitourinary, respiratory tract) under controlled circumstances (e.g., elective colon surgery). *Contaminated procedures* involve extensive introduction of bacteria into a normally sterile body cavity, but too briefly to allow infection to become established during surgery (e.g., penetrating abdominal trauma, enterotomy during adhesiolysis for mechanical bowel obstruction). *Dirty procedures* are performed to control established infection (e.g., colon resection for perforated diverticulitis).

Numerous factors determine whether a patient will develop an SSI, including factors related to the patient, the environment, and the therapy (Table 84.7) (65). As incorporated in the NHSN (66,67), the most recognized factors are the wound category (see Table 84.4), the American Society of Anesthesiologists (ASA) Class ≥ 3 (class 3: chronic active medical illness), and prolonged operative time (procedural time longer than the 75th percentile for each such procedure). According to the NHSN, the risk of SSI increases with an increasing number of risk factors present, irrespective of the type of operation (64). Laparoscopic surgery decreases the incidence of SSI under most circumstances (14) for several reasons, including decreased wound size; limited use of cautery in the abdominal wall; and a diminished stress response to tissue injury.

TABLE 84.7 Risk Factors for Development of Surgical Site Infections

Patient factors
Ascites (for abdominal surgery)
Chronic inflammation
Corticosteroid therapy (controversial)
Obesity
Diabetes
Extremes of age
Hypercholesterolemia
Hypoxemia
Peripheral vascular disease (for lower extremity surgery)
Postoperative anemia
Prior site irradiation
Recent operation
Remote infection
Skin carriage of staphylococci
Skin disease in the area of procedure (e.g., psoriasis)
Environmental factors
Contaminated medications
Inadequate disinfection/sterilization
Inadequate skin antisepsis
Inadequate ventilation
Treatment factors
Drains
Emergency procedure
Hypothermia
Inadequate antibiotic prophylaxis
Oxygenation (controversial)
Prolonged preoperative hospitalization
Prolonged operative time

Host-derived factors contribute importantly to the risk of SSI. Identified risk factors include increased age (14), obesity, malnutrition, diabetes mellitus (4,68), hypocholesterolemia (69), and numerous other factors that are not accounted for specifically by the NHSN system. In one 6-year study of 5,031 patients undergoing noncardiac surgery, the overall incidence of SSI was 3.2% (70). Independent risk factors for the development of SSI included ascites; diabetes mellitus; postoperative anemia; and recent weight loss, but not chronic obstructive pulmonary disorder, tobacco use, or corticosteroid use. In another prospective study of 9,016 patients, 12.5% of patients developed an infection of some type within 28 days after surgery (71). Multivariable analysis showed that decreased serum albumin concentration, increased age, tracheotomy, and amputations were associated with an increased probability of an early infection. Factors associated with readmission due to infection included a dialysis shunt, vascular repair, and an early infection. The 28-day mortality was most influenced by advanced age, low serum albumin concentration, elevated serum creatinine concentration, and early SSI.

In the modern operating room, a lapse in sterile technique has also been shown to increase the rate of SSI. Proper sterilization, ventilation, and skin preparation techniques require continuous vigilance. The operating team must also be attentive to the patient's personal hygiene, as well as their own (e.g., hand scrubbing, hair). Recent data indicate that a brief rinse with soap and water followed by use of an alcohol gel hand rub was equivalent to the prolonged (and ritualized) session at the scrub sink (72). Although this study only yielded Level III evidence, it demonstrated the importance of reviewing the performance of the operating room personnel (including surgeons) and implementing educational strategies if protocol breaches were observed (73).

Broadly speaking, a number of "environmental" factors also have been shown to impact the development of SSI. Hypothermia during surgery is common if patients are not warmed actively, owing to evaporative water losses, administration of room temperature fluids, and other factors (74). Maintenance of normal core body temperature is unequivocally important for decreasing the incidence of SSI. Mild intraoperative hypothermia is associated with an increased rate of SSI following elective colon surgery and diverse operations (75,76). The role of supplemental oxygen in the postoperative period had previously been shown to improve wound healing (77,78), but the role of oxygen on SSI had received much less study. Oxygen has been postulated to have a direct antibacterial effect (78) and it is also important for neutrophil-mediated bacterial killing. However, clinical trials have had conflicting results (79,80). The ischemic milieu of fresh surgical incisions are potentially vulnerable to bacterial invasion. Supplemental oxygenation administration specifically to reduce the incidence of SSI remains plausible, and further studies are needed.

Closure of a contaminated or dirty incision is widely believed to increase the risk of SSI, but few good studies exist to help sort out the multiplicity of wound closure techniques available to surgeons. "Open abdomen" techniques of temporary abdominal closure for management of trauma or severe peritonitis are utilized increasingly. Retrospective studies indicate that antibiotics are not indicated for prophylaxis of the open abdomen, but if infection of the abdominal wall occurs, it is associated with a very high morbidity (81). Inability to achieve primary abdominal closure has been associated with several infectious complications (pneumonia, bloodstream infection, and SSI). Infectious complications, in turn, significantly increased costs from prolonged length of stay, but not mortality (82).

Drains placed in incisions probably cause more infections than they prevent. Drains prevent epithelialization and can become a portal for invasion by pathogens colonizing the skin. Several studies of drains placed into clean or clean-contaminated incisions show that the rate of SSI is not reduced (83,84) and other investigations showed that the incidence of SSI rate was increased (85–88). The preponderance of data supports the concept that drains should be used as little as possible and removed as soon as possible (89). Under no circumstances should prolonged antibiotic "prophylaxis" be administered to "cover" indwelling drains.

Clinicians continue to study modifications of old methods and the utility of new modalities to impact SSI. The use of wound irrigation to reduce the risk of SSI is highly controversial. Routine low-pressure saline irrigation of an incision does not reduce the risk of SSI (90), but lavage with dilute povidone–iodine was reported to reduce the risk of SSI compared with nonantiseptic lavage (91). An increasing body of the literature suggests that intraoperative topical antibiotics can minimize the risk of SSI (92–94), but the use of antiseptics, rather than antibiotics, may minimize the development of resistance. Another recent intervention aimed at reducing SSI is application of negative-pressure wound therapy (NPWT) to closed incisions. Although the evidence for the use of NPWT for the management of open wounds has been described, the data for its use in closed surgical incisions is limited and general recommendations cannot be made at this time, although one meta-analysis did find that closed surgical incision NPWT reduced postoperative wound complications (95).

Diagnosis of Surgical Site Infection

SSI remains largely a clinical diagnosis. Presenting signs and symptoms depends on the depth of infection, typically as early as postoperative day 4 or 5. Clinical signs range from local induration only, to the hallmarks of infection: erythema, edema, tenderness, warm skin, and pain-related immobility. Any or all of these signs may precede wound drainage. In cases of deep incisional SSIs, tenderness may extend beyond the margin of erythema, and crepitus, cutaneous vesicles, or bullae may be present (96). With ongoing infection, the signs of the SIRS herald the development of sepsis. For infections that involve intracavitary space (organ/space), symptoms and signs that are specific to that organ system usually predominate, such as prolonged postoperative ileus, persistent respiratory distress, or altered neurologic status.

Cultures are not mandatory for management of superficial incisional SSIs, particularly if drainage and wound care alone will suffice without antibiotics. In cases of deeper infection or infection that has arisen in the hospital, exudates or drainage specimens should be sent for analysis. Culturing the surgically opened wound (as opposed to the already opened wound, which becomes colonized) by the swab method has been shown to be reliable. Aspiration of a sufficient volume of purulent material using an aseptic technique yields better pathogen identification that swab culturette (21). Computed tomography (CT) and magnetic resonance imaging (MRI) are more sensitive in detecting small amounts of gas in soft tissues than plain radiographs, and CT-guided aspiration or drainage often facilitates treatment, and may serve as definitive source control for an organ/space SSI.

Treatment of Surgical Site Infection

Local surgical control of the infection remains the crucial aspect of therapy, oftentimes by simply opening and draining the incision in cases of superficial incisional SSI. Infections extending below the superficial fascia (deep incisional SSIs) invariably require formal surgical debridement and open wound care to resolve the infection. Vacuum-assisted closure (VAC) and antimicrobial therapy also improved outcomes, but MDR pathogens may complicate resolution of ostensibly simple infections in the postoperative period (97), especially among patients hospitalized for a period before surgery, particularly if they required antimicrobial therapy.

When faced with a potential SSI, the first steps in management are to remove the appropriate sutures/staples, open and examine the suspicious portion of the incision, and decide about further surgical treatment (98). If the infection is not confined to the skin and superficial underlying subcutaneous tissue, urgent surgical exploration and debridement are essential to obtain local control of the infection, remove necrotic tissue, and restore aerobic conditions to prevent further spread of the infection. SSI must also be considered the cause of delayed or failed wound healing and prompt the same decisions as described above (98).

Superficial SSIs (functionally subcutaneous abscesses) rarely lead to systemic infection and usually do not make patients seriously ill. Antibiotic therapy is not indicated for patients who do not have systemic signs of infection. If infection extends to superficial fascia or beneath, or extensive tissue necrosis and liquefaction beyond the obvious limits of the cutaneous signs, there is the possibility of a necrotizing infection and such wounds may necessitate formal exploration in the operating room. Necrotizing soft tissue infections (NSTIs) are true emergencies that need immediate surgical attention. Even modest delays can increase patient mortality substantially. Freischlag et al. (99) showed that mortality increased from 32% to 70% when therapy was delayed more than 24 hours. With an established diagnosis of NSTI, immediate and widespread operative debridement is indicated without waiting for precise determination of the causative pathogen or the identification of a specific clinical symptom. These patients often require planned, sequential, repetitive surgical debridement sessions to control the infection. Broad-spectrum antimicrobial therapy should be given empirically to cover likely pathogens and de-escalated following microbiology speciation.

Organ/space SSIs occur within a body cavity, are directly related to a surgical procedure, and may manifest as intra-abdominal, intrapleural, or intracranial infections. They may remain occult or present with symptoms that mimic incisional SSIs, leading to inadequate initial treatment. Occasionally, organ/space SSI only become apparent when a major complication ensues. The diagnosis of organ/space SSI usually requires some form of imaging (CT, ultrasound, MRI) to confirm the site and extent of infection; adequate source control requires a drainage procedure, whether open or percutaneous.

Experimentally, the value of VAC was first appraised by Morykwas et al. (100) in a swine model in 1997. VAC optimizes blood flow, decreases tissue edema, and removes fluid from the wound bed, thereby facilitating the removal of bacteria from the wound. Mechanical deformation of the wound promotes tissue expansion to cover the defect, and subatmospheric pressure in the milieu may trigger a cascade of intracellular signals that increases the rate of cell division and formation of granulation tissue (101). The clinical value of VAC systems has been described only in small case series and cohort studies, mostly for sternal infections following cardiac surgery, abdominal wall dehiscence, management of complex perineal wounds, or as a method to secure skin grafts (102,103). The absence of well-designed randomized controlled trials precludes more specific recommendations.

SINUSITIS

The paranasal sinuses are normally sterile, but bacterial overgrowth occurs when drainage is impeded. The etiologic agents responsible for most cases of nosocomial sinusitis are those that colonize the naso-oropharynx at high frequency among critically ill patients (104,105). Gram-negative bacilli (particularly *Pseudomonas aeruginosa*) constitute 60% of bacteria isolated from nosocomial sinusitis, whereas gram-positive cocci (typically *S. aureus* and coagulase-negative staphylococci) comprise one-third of isolates, and fungi the remaining 5% to 10% (104,106,107). Sinusitis acquired while in the ICU is most often polymicrobial.

Pathogenesis of Sinusitis

In the ICU, nosocomial sinusitis is an uncommon closed-space infection that is often clinically occult, but that can have serious consequences (108). Although sinusitis should always be part of the differential diagnosis of fever, the incidence is low in comparison to other nosocomial infections in the ICU and the diagnosis can be difficult. The likely pathogenesis of sinusitis is anatomic obstruction of the ostia draining the facial sinuses, especially the maxillary sinuses. Transnasal endotracheal intubation is the leading risk factor, with an incidence of sinusitis estimated to be about 33% after 7 days of intubation. Maxillofacial trauma, with obstruction of drainage by retained blood clots, is another clear risk factor. Nasogastric intubation, nasal packing for epistaxis, and corticosteroid therapy have also been implicated, but the evidence is less convincing.

Diagnosis of Sinusitis

Nosocomial sinusitis is a dangerous, closed-space infection that is increasing in incidence, is difficult to diagnose, and is, therefore, controversial as to its actual incidence and importance (109). Complaints of facial pain or headache may be impossible to elicit and purulent nasal discharge is present in only 25% of proved cases of sinusitis. In the ICU, acute sinusitis is diagnosed most efficiently by CT of the facial bones, followed by sampling using antiseptic technique if mucosal thickening or sinus fluid is documented (110). Microbial analysis of fluid obtained by minimally invasive sinus puncture and aspiration under antiseptic conditions is definitive for the diagnosis. Although less well studied, endoscopic-guided middle meatal tissue culture is a safe alternative for patients who are not candidates for antral puncture (e.g., coagulopathy) (111). Pathogen identification and susceptibility testing permit focused, narrow-spectrum antimicrobial therapy. However, specimen collection is susceptible to contamination by bacteria colonizing the overlying mucosa if rigorous antisepsis is not practiced when obtaining the specimen.

Treatment of Sinusitis

Sinusitis should be suspected in any patient with sepsis, particularly if initial cultures (e.g., blood, sputum, urine, indwelling vascular catheters) are unrevealing. When sinusitis is suspected, the diagnosis is confirmed by maxillary antral tap, lavage, and culture using aseptic technique. Gram-positive cocci, gram-negative bacilli (including *P. aeruginosa*), and fungi (incidence, 8%) are possible pathogens, so initial therapy should be directed at these pathogens, based on local susceptibility patterns. Most antibiotics achieve adequate tissue penetration, so treatment consists of antibiotic therapy, removal of tubes blocking the ostia, and mobilization of the patient (112). The optimal duration of therapy is unknown, so treatment is most often determined by the clinical response. Refractory cases may require repetitive lavage of the sinus, or a more formal drainage procedure.

The role of nasal decongestant agents (NDCA) in the prevention of infectious nosocomial sinusitis has not been convincingly proven. However, one prospective randomized trial in patients at high risk for sinusitis demonstrated a reduction in radiologic sinusitis in those treated with locally applied NDCA and corticosteroids (113). Investigations into prevention should be continued as sinusitis is a predisposing factor for VAP, and may be a source of lower respiratory tract pathogens. There is 85% concordance between pathogens of sinusitis and pneumonia in patients who develop VAP subsequently, lending credence to the hypothesis that purulent sinus drainage inoculates the lower airway.

CENTRAL LINE–ASSOCIATED BLOODSTREAM INFECTION

Critically ill patients often require reliable large-bore central venous access (e.g., femoral, internal jugular, or subclavian vein), but the catheters are highly prone to infection. Strict adherence to infection control and proper insertion technique are crucial for prevention (114), because surgical, and especially trauma, patients are at high risk. When placed under elective (controlled) circumstances, optimal insertion technique includes chlorhexidine skin preparation (not povidone–iodine) (115), draping the entire bed into the sterile field, and donning a cap, a mask, and sterile gown and gloves (116). If there is a break in sterile technique, the risk of infection increases exponentially. Catheters placed emergently without sterile precautions should be removed and replaced (if still needed) at a different site using strict asepsis and antisepsis as soon as the patient's condition permits, but certainly within 24 hours. Infection risk for femoral vein catheters is the highest, whereas catheters placed via the subclavian route have the lowest rates of infection (81). Peripheral vein catheters, peripherally inserted central catheters (PICCs), and tunneled CVCs (e.g., Hickman, Broviac) pose less risk of infection than percutaneous CVCs (117). Information campaigns, educational initiatives (118), and strict adherence to insertion protocols have all been shown to be effective in decreasing the risk of CLABSI. The role of antibiotic- and antiseptic-coated catheters is controversial, but they may help decrease the risk of infection in units that have CLABSI rates exceeding the National Healthcare Safety Network surveillance data targets (119,120).

Pathogenesis of CLABSI

The pathogens isolated in CLABSI are predominantly gram-positive cocci, most commonly methicillin-related *Staphylococcus epidermidis* (MRSE), MRSA, and enterococci. Unfortunately, MRSE is both the most common cause of CLABSI and the most common cause of false-positive blood cultures because of contamination during the collection process. As noted in the section on evaluation of surgical patients with suspected infection, it's critically important to obtain sufficient volume for blood cultures, to obtain samples from multiple sites, and to obtain at least one culture from any central line (11).

Diagnosis of CLABSI

The diagnosis of CLABSI is usually a diagnosis of exclusion. However, in a patient with bacteremia or fungemia with erythema and purulence at the site of central line insertion, the central line can be considered as the source. Another early sign of CLABSI can be the inability to aspirate from the line, as the infected line becomes more thrombogenic. Most authorities consider the isolation of MRSE from a single blood culture to be a contaminant and do not treat, especially if the patient has no indwelling hardware that might become infected secondarily (e.g., prosthetic joint or heart valve). Gram-negative bacillary pathogens are less common (but seldom are contaminants), and fungal CLABSIs are less common in surgical patients than medical patients.

Treatment of CLABSI

The initial treatment for CLABSI involves removal of the suspected catheter (for peripheral or percutaneous CVCs) and parenteral antibiotics. It is not clear whether a positive catheter culture requires therapy beyond catheter removal, absent local signs of infection, or a true-positive blood culture. The historic practice of performing routine guidewire exchange at predefined intervals does *not* decrease the rate of CLABSI and may even increase the incidence. Catheter-related bloodstream infections caused by *S. aureus* requires at least 2 weeks of therapy, although some authorities argue for a longer course (4 to 6 weeks) because of the risk of metastatic infection (e.g., pneumonia, endocarditis). Vancomycin or linezolid is appropriate choice for MRSA (or MRSE when treatment is indicated), with daptomycin as an alternative. Therapy for enterococcal or gram-negative should be dictated by bacterial susceptibility, with no clear consensus as to duration of therapy. Beyond removal of the catheter, treatment of fungal CLABSI is controversial; some authorities recommend at least 2 weeks of systemic antifungal therapy.

C. DIFFICILE–ASSOCIATED DISEASE (CDAD)

C. difficile–associated disease, formerly pseudomembranous colitis, develops because antibiotic therapy disrupts the balance of colonic flora, allowing the overgrowth of *C. difficile*, present in the fecal flora of about 3% of normal hosts. Any antibiotic can induce this selection pressure, even when given appropriately as surgical prophylaxis, although clindamycin, third-generation cephalosporins, and fluoroquinolones have a predilection (121). Paradoxically, even antibiotics used to treat CDAD (e.g., metronidazole) have been associated with CDAD.

Pathogenesis of CDAD

CDAD is unquestionably a nosocomial infection. Spores can persist on inanimate surfaces for prolonged periods, and pathogens can be transmitted from patient to patient by contaminated equipment (e.g., bedpans, rectal thermometers) or on the hands of health care workers. The alcohol gel that is used increasingly for hand disinfection *is not active* against spores of *C. difficile;* therefore, hand washing with soap and water is necessary when caring for an infected patient, or generally during outbreaks.

Diagnosis

The clinical spectrum of CDAD is wide, ranging from asymptomatic (8% of affected patients do not have diarrhea) to life-threatening transmural pancolitis with perforation and septic shock. The typical patient will have fever, abdominal distention, copious diarrhea, and leukocytosis. Colon hemorrhage is rare, and if observed should prompt an alternative diagnosis.

Although there is more than one method for detecting *C. difficile,* the nucleic acid amplification tests (NAAT) for *C. difficile* toxin genes such as PCR are superior to toxins A+B EIA testing as a standard diagnostic test for CDI (122). Most strains of *C. difficile* produce toxin A, but 2% to 3% of stains produce only toxin B, so an assay that detects both toxins A and B is preferred (123). Cultures for *C. difficile* are technically demanding, and are not specific in distinguishing toxin-positive strains, toxin-negative strains, and asymptomatic carriage (121,124). Cultures may be useful in the setting of nosocomial outbreaks to identify isolates for epidemiologic purposes (125). The North American pulse-field gel electrophoresis type 1 (NAP1) strain, now epidemic in many hospitals in the United States, Canada, and Europe, is associated with serious complications (toxic megacolon, leukemoid reactions, septic shock, and death) (126,127). Direct visualization of pseudomembranes is nearly diagnostic of CDAD, but only about 70% of seriously ill patients and 25% of patients with mild disease have pseudomembranes by direct visualization (128), diminishing the role of endoscopy for routine diagnostic use. However, a role for direct visualization may exist if false-negative *C. difficile* toxin assays are suspected (125).

Treatment of CDAD

Treatment of mild cases consists of withdrawal of the putative offending antibiotic. Oral antibiotic therapy is often prescribed, but may or may not be necessary. More severe cases may require parenteral metronidazole or oral or enteral vancomycin (by gavage or enema, if ileus precludes oral therapy); parenteral vancomycin is completely ineffective. Some patients with severe disease may require a colectomy, usually a total abdominal colectomy (127). Colectomy for severe disease has traditionally been the only surgical option for CDAD that is unresponsive to medical therapy. However, more recent reports have shown that minimally invasive surgical techniques coupled with antegrade colonic lavage is associated with improved outcomes (129). In patients with nonfulminant CDAD, a loop ileostomy is formed and the colon is lavaged with warm polyethylene glycol intraoperatively, while postoperative therapy is completed using vancomycin instilled through the colon via the ileostomy. While there are no large trials that demonstrate efficacy, one small trial reported a significant improvement in mortality and colon salvage in the ileostomy and antegrade colonic lavage group compared to historic controls (129). While these early data are promising, questions still remain regarding patient selection and optimal timing of the operation, but is currently not recommended in patients with fulminant or perforated disease (130).

The use of fecal microbiota transplantation (FMT) given to patients with CDAD to repopulate the normal colonic flora is also gaining in popularity as a therapeutic option. Small, retrospective analyses have identified increased cure rates in patients with recurrent CDAD that were treated with FMT and one prospective clinical trial comparing combinations of antibiotics (vancomycin), colonic lavage, and FMT was stopped early because of the superiority of cure rates within the FMT group (131). The delivery of FMT has been a rate-limiting step in its widespread use, but there are currently investigations into delivery via a pill form.

The prevalence of severe disease has increased markedly with the emergence of a new strain of *C. difficile*. This strain has a mutant gene that suppresses toxin production, such that far more toxin is elaborated, resulting in clinically severe disease (126). As this disease continues to evolve, the roles of traditional antibiotic therapy and the role of novel surgical and medical (i.e., FMT) treatments will continue to evolve as well.

PERIANAL ABSCESS AND INFECTION

Perianal abscesses and/or infection, although rare, can occur in the ICU setting. Critical care practitioners should be familiar with perianal infection for several reasons:

- Such infections can easily be missed if clinicians do not have a high index of suspicion and institute a directed examination of the anus and surrounding area.
- Perianal infection is frequently missed by diagnostic modalities employed during workup of sepsis or fever.
- Perianal infections are seen more frequently in immunosuppressed patients.
- These infections can arise in the setting of diarrhea or suboptimal perineal hygiene in immobilized ICU patients.
- Frequently these infections can be treated with relatively simple bedside drainage procedures, although more extensive infections may require formal operative or percutaneous drainage interventions.

Pathogenesis of Perianal Infections

Perianal infections usually arise from the mucosa secondary to obstruction of an anal gland (132,133). In a minority of patients, perianal infections arise from the anoderm or surrounding skin. Immunosuppressed leukemic or bone marrow transplantation patients have been noted to be at increased risk for these infections. In a report of 1,102 patients with leukemia, 6.7% were found to have perianal infection (134); furthermore, perianal abscesses can develop even in the presence of profound granulocytopenia (135).

Overall, the organisms responsible for perianal infection may be changing. Classically, these infections are polymicrobial and arise from endogenous enteric bacteria (132). However, more recent reports show that as many as 37% of ambulatory patients with perianal abscess grew MRSA when the wounds were cultured (136). Perianal infections caused by MRSA were more likely to be associated with extensive induration and erythema on examination, and scant purulence with drainage. The microbiology of perianal infection in immunosuppressed patients also showed a much higher proportion of gram-negative pathogens, including *E. coli, Bacteriodies, Enterococcus,* and *Klebsiella*, than seen in the nonhospitalized population (135).

Diagnosis of Perianal Infections of Perianal Infections

Once identified, the treatment of perianal infections is relatively straightforward. Physical examination is usually sufficient to make the diagnosis, but ultrasound, CT, or MRI may be useful adjuncts in patients with deep-seated infections, ischiorectal infection, or to completely characterize complex fistula (137). Confusion can be avoided when describing the location of an abscess near the rectum by employing standard anatomic terminology, such as right, left, anterior, and posterior—rather than referring to the position of a "clock face" (132).

Treatment of Perianal Infections

Once identified, the treatment of perianal infections is relatively straightforward. Drainage is the mainstay of treatment for perianal abscess (132,133,137). Untreated perianal infections frequently result in development of fistula-in-ano, a complication that may progress to necrotizing perineal infections. Whenever possible, incisions to drain the abscess should be placed as close to the anus as possible, to minimize the impact if an anorectal fistula develops. In the ambulatory population, there's little role for culturing these infections, but cultures should be obtained in ICU setting because of the dramatically altered bacterial flora present in these patients. Antibiotics should also be considered with MRSA infections or if patients have extensive cellulitis (137). Drainage can usually be performed at the bedside under local anesthesia, but some patients may need to be transported to the operating room, or may require more extensive surgical drainage procedures. The role of packing is controversial; practice guidelines from the American Society of Colon and Rectal Surgeons do not recommend routine packing (137). In a small prospective randomized study, no packing of drained perianal abscesses was associated with more rapid resolution of the infection (138).

Key Points

- Surgical patients have multiple sites for potential infection.
- Stresses of surgery plus critical illness often result in significant malnutrition and/or alterations in glucose homeostasis.
- Surgical infections are often polymicrobial, with community organisms during first 72 hours and hospital organisms after 3 days.
- Surgical infections often require an intervention (surgical, procedural, percutaneous), in addition to antibiotics, for resolution.

References

1. De Waele JJ. Early source control in sepsis. *Langenbeck Archives Surg.* 2010;395(5):489–494.
2. Dellinger RP, Levy MM, Rhodes A, et al.; Surviving Sepsis Campaign Guidelines Committee including The Pediatric Subgroup. Surviving sepsis campaign: international guidelines for management of severe sepsis and septic shock, 2012. *Intensive Care Med.* 2013;39(2):165–228.
3. Kobayashi SD, Malachowa N, DeLeo FR. Pathogenesis of *Staphylococcus aureus* abscesses. *Am J Pathol.* 2015;185(6):1518–1527.
4. Latham R, Lancaster AD, Covington JF, et al. The association of diabetes and glucose control with surgical-site infections among cardiothoracic surgery patients. *Infect Contr Hosp Epidemiol.* 2001;22(10):607–612.
5. Ubeda C, Pamer EG. Antibiotics, microbiota, and immune defense. *Trends Immunol.* 2012;33(9):459–466.
6. Shimizu K, Ogura H, Asahara T, et al. Probiotic/synbiotic therapy for treating critically ill patients from a gut microbiota perspective. *Digest Dis Sci.* 2013;58(1):23–32.
7. Minei JP, Nathens AB, West M, et al.; Inflammation and the Host Response to Injury Large Scale Collaborative Research Program Investigators. Inflammation and the host response to injury, a large-scale collaborative project: patient-oriented research core: standard operating procedures for clinical care. II. Guidelines for prevention, diagnosis and treatment of ventilator-associated pneumonia (VAP) in the trauma patient. *J Trauma.* 2006;60(5):1106–1113; discussion 1113.
8. Heyland DK, MacDonald S, Keefe L, Drover JW. Total parenteral nutrition in the critically ill patient: a meta-analysis. *JAMA.* 1998;280(23): 2013–2019.
9. Sinuff T, Muscedere J, Cook DJ, et al.; Canadian Critical Care Trials Group. Implementation of clinical practice guidelines for ventilator-associated pneumonia: a multicenter prospective study. *Crit Care Med.* 2013;41(1):15–23.
10. Barie PS, Hydo LJ, Eachempati SR. Causes and consequences of fever complicating critical surgical illness. *Surg Infect.* 2004;5(2):145–159.
11. O'Grady NP, Barie PS, Bartlett JG, et al.; American College of Critical Care Medicine; Infectious Diseases Society of America. Guidelines for evaluation of new fever in critically ill adult patients: 2008 update from the American College of Critical Care Medicine and the Infectious Diseases Society of America. *Crit Care Med.* 2008;36(4):1330–1349.
12. Bianchi ME. DAMPs, PAMPs and alarmins: all we need to know about danger. *J Leukoc Biol.* 2007;81(1):1–5.
13. Hirsiger S, Simmen HP, Werner CM, et al. Danger signals activating the immune response after trauma. *Mediators Inflamm.* 2012;2012:315941.
14. Garibaldi RA, Cushing D, Lerer T. Risk factors for postoperative infection. *Am J Med.* 1991;91(3B):158S–163S.
15. Trautner BW, Clarridge JE, Darouiche RO. Skin antisepsis kits containing alcohol and chlorhexidine gluconate or tincture of iodine are associated with low rates of blood culture contamination. *Infect Contr Hosp Epidemiol.* 2002;23(7):397–401.
16. Cockerill FR 3rd, Wilson JW, Vetter EA, et al. Optimal testing parameters for blood cultures. *Clin Infect Dis.* 2004;38(12):1724–1730.
17. Mermel LA. Detection of bacteremia in adults: consequences of culturing an inadequate volume of blood. *Ann Intern Med.* 1993;119(4):270.
18. Bates DW. Contaminant blood cultures and resource utilization: the true consequences of false-positive results. *JAMA.* 1991;265(3):365–369.
19. Mermel LA, Allon M, Bouza E, et al. Clinical practice guidelines for the diagnosis and management of intravascular catheter-related infection: 2009 Update by the Infectious Diseases Society of America. *Clin Infect Dis.* 2009;49(1):1–45.
20. Wilson ML, Mitchell M, Morris AJ, et al. *Principles and Procedures for Blood Cultures: Approved Guidelines. CLSI document M47-A,* Clinical and Laboratory Standards Institute (CLSI), Wayne, PA, 2007.
21. Mangram AJ, Horan TC, Pearson ML, et al. Guideline for prevention of surgical site infection, 1999. Hospital Infection Control Practices Advisory Committee. *Infect Control Hosp Epidemiol.* 1999;20(4):250–278; quiz 279–280.
22. Velmahos GC. Severe trauma is not an excuse for prolonged antibiotic prophylaxis. *Arch Surg.* 2002;137(5):537–542.
23. Manian FA, Meyer PL, Setzer J, Senkel D. Surgical site infections associated with methicillin-resistant *Staphylococcus aureus:* do postoperative factors play a role? *Clin Infect Dis.* 2003;36(7):863–868.
24. Tejirian T, DiFronzo LA, Haigh PI. Antibiotic prophylaxis for preventing wound infection after breast surgery: a systematic review and meta-analysis. *J Am Coll Surg.* 2006;203(5):729–734.
25. Cunningham M, Bunn F, Handscomb K. Prophylactic antibiotics to prevent surgical site infection after breast cancer surgery. *Cochrane Database Syst Rev.* 2006(2):CD005360.
26. Aufenacker TJ, Koelemay MJ, Gouma DJ, Simons MP. Systematic review and meta-analysis of the effectiveness of antibiotic prophylaxis in prevention of wound infection after mesh repair of abdominal wall hernia. *Br J Surg.* 2005;93(1):5–10.
27. Sanchez-Manuel FJ, Seco-Gil JL. Antibiotic prophylaxis for hernia repair. In: *Cochrane Database of Systematic Reviews.* New York, NY: Wiley-Blackwell; 2004.
28. Stewart A, Eyers PS, Earnshaw JJ. Prevention of infection in arterial reconstruction. In: *Cochrane Database of Systematic Reviews.* New York, NY: Wiley-Blackwell; 2006.
29. Bratzler DW, Houck PM. Antimicrobial prophylaxis for surgery: an advisory statement from the National Surgical Infection Prevention Project. *Am J Surg.* 2005;189(4):395–404.
30. Classen DC, Evans RS, Pestotnik SL, et al. The timing of prophylactic administration of antibiotics and the risk of surgical-wound infection. *N Engl J Med.* 1992;326(5):281–286.
31. Zanetti G, Giardina R, Platt R. Intraoperative redosing of cefazolin and risk for surgical site infection in cardiac surgery. *Emerg Infect Dis.* 2001;7(5):828–831.
32. McDonald M, Grabsch E, Marshall C, Forbes A. Single-versus multiple–dose antimicrobial prophylaxis for major surgery: a systematic review. *Austr NZ J Surg.* 1998;68(6):388–395.
33. Namias N, Harvill S, Ball S, et al. Cost and morbidity associated with antibiotic prophylaxis in the ICU. *J Am Coll Surg.* 1999;188(3): 225–230.
34. Fukatsu K, Saito H, Matsuda T, et al. Influences of type and duration of antimicrobial prophylaxis on an outbreak of methicillin-resistant *Staphylococcus aureus* and on the incidence of wound infection. *Arch Surg.* 1997;132(12):1320–1325.
35. Morris AM, Jobe BA, Stoney M, et al. *Clostridium difficile* colitis: an increasingly aggressive iatrogenic disease? *Arch Surg.* 2002;137(10):1096–1100.
36. Alvarez-Lerma F. Modification of empiric antibiotic treatment in patients with pneumonia acquired in the intensive care unit. *Intensive Care Med.* 1996;22(5):387–394.
37. Iregui M, Ward S, Sherman G, et al. Clinical importance of delays in the initiation of appropriate antibiotic treatment for ventilator-associated pneumonia. *Chest.* 2002;122(1):262–268.
38. Kollef MH, Ward S, Sherman G, et al. Inadequate treatment of nosocomial infections is associated with certain empiric antibiotic choices. *Crit Care Med.* 2000;28(10):3456–3464.
39. Garnacho-Montero J, Garcia-Garmendia JL, Barrero-Almodovar A, et al. Impact of adequate empirical antibiotic therapy on the outcome of patients admitted to the intensive care unit with sepsis. *Crit Care Med.* 2003; 31(12):2742–2751.
40. Evans RS, Pestotnik SL, Classen DC, et al. A computer-assisted management program for antibiotics and other anti-infective agents. *N Engl J Med.* 1998;338(4):232–238.
41. Niederman MS. Appropriate use of antimicrobial agents: challenges and strategies for improvement. *Crit Care Med.* 2003;31(2):608–616.
42. Kollef MH, Vlasnik J, Sharpless L, et al. Scheduled change of antibiotic classes: a strategy to decrease the incidence of ventilator-associated pneumonia. *Am J Respir Crit Care Med.* 1997;156(4):1040–1048.

43. Gruson D, Hilbert G, Vargas F, et al. Strategy of antibiotic rotation: long-term effect on incidence and susceptibilities of gram-negative bacilli responsible for ventilator-associated pneumonia. *Crit Care Med.* 2003;31(7):1908–1914.
44. Raymond DP, Pelletier SJ, Crabtree TD, et al. Impact of a rotating empiric antibiotic schedule on infectious mortality in an intensive care unit. *Crit Care Med.* 2001;29(6):1101–1108.
45. van Loon HJ, Vriens MR, Fluit AC, et al. Antibiotic rotation and development of gram-negative antibiotic resistance. *Am J Respir Crit Care Med.* 2005;171(5):480–487.
46. Kollef MH. Is antibiotic cycling the answer to preventing the emergence of bacterial resistance in the intensive care unit? *Clin Infect Dis.* 2006;43(Suppl 2):S82–S88.
47. Aarts MA, Granton J, Cook DJ, et al. Empiric antimicrobial therapy in critical illness: results of a Surgical Infection Society survey. *Surg Infect (Larchmt).* 2007;8(3):329–336.
48. Kollef MH, Micek ST. Strategies to prevent antimicrobial resistance in the intensive care unit. *Crit Care Med.* 2005;33(8):1845–1853.
49. Dortch MJ, Fleming SB, Kauffmann RM, et al. Infection reduction strategies including antibiotic stewardship protocols in surgical and trauma intensive care units are associated with reduced resistant gram-negative healthcare-associated infections. *Surg Infect.* 2011;12(1):15–25.
50. Giamarellou H. Treatment options for multidrug-resistant bacteria. *Expert Rev Anti infect Ther.* 2006;4(4):601–618.
51. Bosso JA. The antimicrobial armamentarium: evaluating current and future treatment options. *Pharmacotherapy.* 2005;25(10 Part 2):55S-62S.
52. Padmanabhan RA, LaRosa SP, Tomecki KJ. What's new in antibiotics? *Dermatol Clin.* 2005;23(2):301–312.
53. Kollef MH, Kollef KE. Antibiotic utilization and outcomes for patients with clinically suspected ventilator-associated pneumonia and negative quantitative BAL culture results. *Chest.* 2005;128(4):2706–2713.
54. American Thoracic Society; Infectious Diseases Society of America. Guidelines for the management of adults with hospital-acquired, ventilator-associated, and healthcare-associated pneumonia. *Am J Respir Crit Care Med.* 2005;171(4):388–416.
55. van der Sande FM, Kooman JP, Leunissen KM. Haemodialysis and thermoregulation. *Nephrol Dial Transpl.* 2006;21(5):1450–1451.
56. Torres A, El-Ebiary M. Bronchoscopic BAL in the diagnosis of ventilator-associated pneumonia. *Chest.* 2000;117(4 Suppl 2):198S–202S.
57. Dennesen PJ, van der Ven AJ, Kessels AG, et al. Resolution of infectious parameters after antimicrobial therapy in patients with ventilator-associated pneumonia. *Am J Respir Crit Care Med.* 2001;163(6):1371–1375.
58. Dellinger EP. Duration of antibiotic treatment in surgical infections of the abdomen: undesired effects of antibiotics and future studies. *Eur J Surg Suppl.* 1996(576):29–31; discussion 31–32.
59. Fagon JY, Chastre J, Wolff M, et al. Invasive and noninvasive strategies for management of suspected ventilator-associated pneumonia: a randomized trial. *Ann Intern Med.* 2000;132(8):621–630.
60. Sawyer RG, Claridge JA, Nathens AB, et al. Trial of short-course antimicrobial therapy for intraabdominal infection. *N Engl J Med.* 2015;372(21): 1996–2005.
61. *Surgical site infection event.* CDC website. Available at: http://www.cdc.gov/nhsn/PDFs/pscManual/9pscSSIcurrent.pdf. Published January 2016. Accessed March 27, 2016.
62. Owens PL, Barrett ML, Raetzman S, et al. Surgical site infections following ambulatory surgery procedures. *JAMA.* 2014;311(7):709–716.
63. Sievert DM, Ricks P, Edwards JR, et al.; National Healthcare Safety Network (NHSN) Team and Participating NHSN Facilities. Antimicrobial-resistant pathogens associated with healthcare-associated infections: summary of data reported to the National Healthcare Safety Network at the Centers for Disease Control and Prevention, 2009–2010. *Infect Contr Hosp Epidemiol.* 2013;34(1):1–14.
64. National Nosocomial Infections Surveillance System. National Nosocomial Infections Surveillance (NNIS) System Report, data summary from January 1992 through June 2004, issued October 2004. *Am J Infect Contr.* 2004;32(8):470–485.
65. Barie PS. Surgical site infections: epidemiology and prevention. *Surg Infect.* 2002;3(Suppl 1):S9–21.
66. National Nosocomial Infections Surveillance (NNIS) System Report, Data Summary from January 1992–June 2001, issued August 2001. *Am J Infect Contr.* 2001;29(6):404–421.
67. Mu Y, Edwards JR, Horan TC, et al. Improving risk-adjusted measures of surgical site infection for the national healthcare safety network. *Infect Contr Hosp Epidemiol.* 2011;32(10):970–986.
68. Pomposelli JJ, Baxter JK 3rd, Babineau TJ, et al. Early postoperative glucose control predicts nosocomial infection rate in diabetic patients. *JPEN J Parenter Enteral Nutr.* 1998;22(2):77–81.
69. Delgado-Rodriguez M, Medina-Cuadros M, Martinez-Gallego G, Sillero-Arenas M. Total cholesterol, HDL-cholesterol, and risk of nosocomial infection: a prospective study in surgical patients. *Infect Contr Hosp Epidemiol.* 1997;18(1):9–18.
70. Malone DL, Genuit T, Tracy JK, et al. Surgical site infections: reanalysis of risk factors. *J Surg Res.* 2002;103(1):89–95.
71. Scott JD, Forrest A, Feuerstein S, et al. Factors associated with postoperative infection. *Infect Contr Hosp Epidemiol.* 2001;22(6):347–351.
72. Parienti JJ, Thibon P, Heller R, et al.; Antisepsie Chirurgicale des mains Study Group. Hand-rubbing with an aqueous alcoholic solution vs. traditional surgical hand-scrubbing and 30-day surgical site infection rates: a randomized equivalence study. *JAMA.* 2002;288(6):722–727.
73. Anderson DJ, Podgorny K, Berrios-Torres SI, et al. Strategies to prevent surgical site infections in acute care hospitals: 2014 update. *Infect Contr Hosp Epidemiol.* 2014;35(6):605–627.
74. Hedrick TL, Heckman JA, Smith RL, et al. Efficacy of protocol implementation on incidence of wound infection in colorectal operations. *J Am Coll Surg.* 2007;205(3):432–438.
75. Kurz A, Sessler DI, Lenhardt R. Perioperative normothermia to reduce the incidence of surgical-wound infection and shorten hospitalization: study of Wound Infection and Temperature Group. *N Engl J Med.* 1996;334(19):1209–1212.
76. Flores-Maldonado A, Medina-Escobedo CE, Rios-Rodriguez HM, Fernandez-Dominguez R. Mild perioperative hypothermia and the risk of wound infection. *Arch Med Res.* 2001;32(3):227–231.
77. Gottrup F. Oxygen in wound healing and infection. *World J Surg.* 2004; 28(3):312–315.
78. Knighton DR, Halliday B, Hunt TK. Oxygen as an antibiotic: a comparison of the effects of inspired oxygen concentration and antibiotic administration on in vivo bacterial clearance. *Arch Surg.* 1986;121(2):191–195.
79. Greif R, Akca O, Horn EP, et al.; Outcomes Research Group. Supplemental perioperative oxygen to reduce the incidence of surgical-wound infection. *N Engl J Med.* 2000;342(3):161–167.
80. Pryor KO, Fahey TJ 3rd, Lien CA, Goldstein PA. Surgical site infection and the routine use of perioperative hyperoxia in a general surgical population: a randomized controlled trial. *JAMA.* 2004;291(1):79–87.
81. Miller RS, Morris JA Jr, Diaz JJ Jr, et al. Complications after 344 damage-control open celiotomies. *J Trauma.* 2005;59(6):1365–1371; discussion 1371–1374.
82. Vogel TR, Diaz JJ, Miller RS, et al. The open abdomen in trauma: do infectious complications affect primary abdominal closure? *Surg Infect (Larchmt).* 2006;7(5):433–441.
83. Al-Inany H, Youssef G, Abd ElMaguid A, et al. Value of subcutaneous drainage system in obese females undergoing cesarean section using pfannenstiel incision. *Gynecol Obstet Invest.* 2002;53(2):75–78.
84. Magann EF, Chauhan SP, Rodts-Palenik S, et al. Subcutaneous stitch closure versus subcutaneous drain to prevent wound disruption after cesarean delivery: a randomized clinical trial. *Am J Obstet Gynecol.* 2002;186(6):1119–1123.
85. Siegman-Igra Y, Rozin R, Simchen E. Determinants of wound infection in gastrointestinal operations: the Israeli study of surgical infections. *J Clin Epidemiol.* 1993;46(2):133–140.
86. Noyes LD, Doyle DJ, McSwain NE Jr. Septic complications associated with the use of peritoneal drains in liver trauma. *J Trauma.* 1988;28(3): 337–346.
87. Magee C, Rodeheaver GT, Golden GT, et al. Potentiation of wound infection by surgical drains. *Am J Surg.* 1976;131(5):547–549.
88. Vilar-Compte D, Mohar A, Sandoval S, et al. Surgical site infections at the National Cancer Institute in Mexico: a case-control study. *Am J Infect Contr.* 2000;28(1):14–20.
89. Barie PS. Are we draining the life from our patients? *Surg Infect.* 2002; 3(3):159–160.
90. Platell C, Papadimitriou JM, Hall JC. The influence of lavage on peritonitis. *J Am Coll Surg.* 2000;191(6):672–680.
91. Fournel I, Tiv M, Soulias M, et al. Meta-analysis of intraoperative povidone-iodine application to prevent surgical-site infection. *Br J Surg.* 2010;97(11):1603–1163.
92. Andersen B, Bendtsen A, Holbraad L, Schantz A. Wound infections after appendicectomy. I. A controlled trial on the prophylactic efficacy of topical ampicillin in non-perforated appendicitis. II. A controlled trial on the prophylactic efficacy of delayed primary suture and topical ampicillin in perforated appendicitis. *Acta Chir Scand.* 1972;138(5):531–536.
93. Yoshii S, Hosaka S, Suzuki S, et al. Prevention of surgical site infection by antibiotic spraying in the operative field during cardiac surgery. *Jpn J Thorac Cardiovasc Surg.* 2001;49(5):279–281.
94. O'Connor LT Jr, Goldstein M. Topical perioperative antibiotic prophylaxis for minor clean inguinal surgery. *J Am Coll Surg.* 2002;194(4):407–410.

95. Hyldig N, Birke-Sorensen H, Kruse M, et al. Meta-analysis of negative-pressure wound therapy for closed surgical incisions. *Br J Surg.* 2016;103(5):477–486.
96. Lewis RT. Soft tissue infections. *World J Surg.* 1998;22(2):146–151.
97. Raghavan M, Linden PK. Newer treatment options for skin and soft tissue infections. *Drugs.* 2004;64(15):1621–1642.
98. Turina M, Cheadle WG. Management of established surgical site infections. *Surg Infect.* 2006;7(Suppl 3):s33–41.
99. Freischlag JA, Ajalat G, Busuttill RW. Treatment of necrotizing soft tissue infections. *Am J Surg.* 1985;149(6):751–755.
100. Morykwas MJ, Argenta LC, Shelton-Brown EI, McGuirt W. Vacuum-assisted closure: a new method for wound control and treatment. *Ann Plast Surg.* 1997;38(6):553–562.
101. Venturi ML, Attinger CE, Mesbahi AN, et al. Mechanisms and clinical applications of the vacuum-assisted closure (VAC) device. *Am J Clin Dermatol.* 2005;6(3):185–194.
102. Heller L, Levin SL, Butler CE. Management of abdominal wound dehiscence using vacuum assisted closure in patients with compromised healing. *Am J Surg.* 2006;191(2):165–172.
103. Schaffzin DM, Douglas JM, Stahl TJ, Smith LE. Vacuum-assisted closure of complex perineal wounds. *Dis Colon Rect.* 2004;47(10):1745–1748.
104. Rouby JJ, Laurent P, Gosnach M, et al. Risk factors and clinical relevance of nosocomial maxillary sinusitis in the critically ill. *Am J Respir Crit Care Med.* 1994;150(3):776–783.
105. Westergren V, Forsum U, Lundgren J. Possible errors in diagnosis of bacterial sinusitis in tracheal intubated patients. *Acta Anaesthesiol Scand.* 1994;38(7):699–703.
106. Grindlinger GA, Niehoff J, Hughes SL, et al. Acute paranasal sinusitis related to nasotracheal intubation of head-injured patients. *Crit Care Med.* 1987;15(3):214–217.
107. Aebert H, Hunefeld G, Regel G. Paranasal sinusitis and sepsis in ICU patients with nasotracheal intubation. *Intensive Care Med.* 1988;15(1):27–30.
108. Stein M, Caplan ES. Nosocomial sinusitis: a unique subset of sinusitis. *Curr Opin Infect Dis.* 2005;18(2):147–150.
109. Talmor M, Li P, Barie PS. Acute paranasal sinusitis in critically ill patients: guidelines for prevention, diagnosis, and treatment. *Clin Infect Dis.* 1997;25(6):1441–1446.
110. Vargas F, Bui HN, Boyer A, et al. Transnasal puncture based on echographic sinusitis evidence in mechanically ventilated patients with suspicion of nosocomial maxillary sinusitis. *Intensive Care Med.* 2006;32(6):858–866.
111. Kountakis S. Middle meatal vs antral lavage cultures in intensive care unit patients. *Otolaryngol Head Neck Surg.* 2002;126(4):377–381.
112. Noorbakhsh S, Barati M, Farhadi M, et al. Intensive care unit nosocomial sinusitis at the Rasoul Akram Hospital: Tehran, Iran, 2007–2008. *Iran J Microbiol.* 2012;4(3):146–149.
113. Pneumatikos I, Konstantonis D, Tsagaris I, et al. Prevention of nosocomial maxillary sinusitis in the ICU: the effects of topically applied alpha-adrenergic agonists and corticosteroids. *Intensive Care Med.* 2006;32(4):532–537.
114. Rizzo M. Striving to eliminate catheter-related bloodstream infections: a literature review of evidence-based strategies. *Semin Anesth Periop Med Pain.* 2005;24(4):214–225.
115. Chaiyakunapruk N, Veenstra DL, Lipsky BA, Saint S. Chlorhexidine compared with povidone-iodine solution for vascular catheter-site care: a meta-analysis. *Ann Intern Med.* 2002;136(11):792–801.
116. O'Grady NP, Alexander M, Dellinger EP, et al. Guidelines for the prevention of intravascular catheter-related infections. Centers for Disease Control and Prevention. *MMWR Recomm Rep.* 2002;51(RR-10):1–29.
117. McGee DC, Gould MK. Preventing complications of central venous catheterization. *N Engl J Med.* 2003;348(12):1123–1133.
118. Coopersmith CM, Rebmann TL, Zack JE, et al. Effect of an education program on decreasing catheter-related bloodstream infections in the surgical intensive care unit. *Crit Care Med.* 2002;30(1):59–64.
119. Byrnes MC, Coopersmith CM. Prevention of catheter-related blood stream infection. *Curr Opin Crit Care.* 2007;13(4):411–415.
120. Edwards JR, Peterson KD, Andrus ML, et al.; National Healthcare Safety Network Facilities. National Healthcare Safety Network (NHSN) Report, data summary for 2006 through 2007, issued November 2008. *Am J Infect Contr.* 2008;36(9):609–626.
121. Walker RC, Ruane PJ, Rosenblatt JE, et al. Comparison of culture, cytotoxicity assays, and enzyme-linked immunosorbent assay for toxin A and toxin B in the diagnosis of *Clostridium difficile*-related enteric disease. *Diagn Microbiol Infect Dis.* 1986;5(1):61–69.
122. Surawicz CM, Brandt LJ, Binion DG, et al. Guidelines for diagnosis, treatment, and prevention of Clostridium difficile infections. *Am J Gastroenterol.* 2013;108(4):478–498; quiz 499.
123. Johnson S. Fatal pseudomembranous colitis associated with a variant *Clostridium difficile* strain not detected by toxin a immunoassay. *Ann Intern Med.* 2001;135(6):434.
124. Manabe YC, Vinetz JM, Moore RD, et al. *Clostridium difficile* colitis: an efficient clinical approach to diagnosis. *Ann Intern Med.* 1995;123(11):835–840.
125. DeMaio J, Bartlett JG. Update on diagnosis of *Clostridium difficile*–associated diarrhea. *Curr Clin Top Infect Dis.* 1995;15:97–114.
126. McDonald LC, Killgore GE, Thompson A, et al. An epidemic, toxin gene–variant strain of *Clostridium difficile. N Engl J Med.* 2005;353(23):2433–2441.
127. Lamontagne F, Labbe AC, Haeck O, et al. Impact of emergency colectomy on survival of patients with fulminant *Clostridium difficile* colitis during an epidemic caused by a hypervirulent strain. *Ann Surg.* 2007;245(2):267–272.
128. Talbot RW, Walker RC, Beart RW. Changing epidemiology, diagnosis, and treatment of *Clostridium difficile* toxin-associated colitis. *Br J Surg.* 1986;73(6):457–460.
129. Neal MD, Alverdy JC, Hall DE, et al. Diverting loop ileostomy and colonic lavage: an alternative to total abdominal colectomy for the treatment of severe, complicated *Clostridium difficile* associated disease. *Ann Surg.* 2011;254(3):423–427; discussion 427–429.
130. Luciano JA, Zuckerbraun BS. *Clostridium difficile* infection: prevention, treatment, and surgical management. *Surg Clin North Am.* 2014;94(6):1335–1349.
131. van Nood E, Vrieze A, Nieuwdorp M, et al. Duodenal infusion of donor feces for recurrent *Clostridium difficile. N Engl J Med.* 2013;368(5):407–415.
132. Whiteford MH. Perianal abscess/fistula disease. *Clin Colon Rect Surg.* 2007;20(2):102–109.
133. Klein JW. Common anal problems. *Med Clin North Am.* 2014;98(3):609–623.
134. Chen CY, Cheng A, Huang SY, et al. Clinical and microbiological characteristics of perianal infections in adult patients with acute leukemia. *PloS One.* 2013;8(4):e60624.
135. Cohen JS, Paz IB, O'Donnell MR, Ellenhorn JD. Treatment of perianal infection following bone marrow transplantation. *Dis Colon Rect.* 1996;39(9):981–985.
136. Albright JB, Pidala MJ, Cali JR, et al. MRSA-related perianal abscesses: an underrecognized disease entity. *Dis Colon Rect.* 2007;50(7):996–1003.
137. Steele SR, Kumar R, Feingold DL, et al.; Standards Practice Task Force of the American Society of Colon and Rectal Surgeons. Practice parameters for the management of perianal abscess and fistula-in-ano. *Dis Colon Rect.* 2011;54(12):1465–1474.
138. Perera AP, Howell AM, Sodergren MH, et al. A pilot randomised controlled trial evaluating postoperative packing of the perianal abscess. *Langenbecks Arch Surg.* 2015;400(2):267–271.
139. Schunemann HJ, Oxman AD, Brozek J, et al.; GRADE Working Group. Grading quality of evidence and strength of recommendations for diagnostic tests and strategies. *BMJ.* 2008;336(7653):1106–1110.
140. Dellinger RP, Levy MM, Rhodes A, et al.; Surviving Sepsis Campaign Guidelines Committee including the Pediatric Subgroup. Surviving sepsis campaign: international guidelines for management of severe sepsis and septic shock: 2012. *Crit Care Med.* 2013;41(2):580–637.

CHAPTER

85

Skin Wounds and Musculoskeletal Infection

SHRAVAN KETHIREDDY, MARC J. SHAPIRO, and STEVEN SANDOVAL

INTRODUCTION

Skin and soft tissue infections are common problems in both hospitalized and nonhospitalized patients. For those patients who are hospitalized and, particularly in the intensive care unit (ICU), such infections may cause significant morbidity, even leading to death. In this chapter, we will review the common and important infections occurring on and about the organ system known as the skin, their presentation, diagnosis, classification, and treatment.

TYPES OF WOUNDS ENCOUNTERED

Surgical Site Infections

In the United States alone, the Centers for Disease Control and Prevention (CDC) estimates that 51.4 million inpatient surgical procedures are performed annually (1). Among hospitalized patients who have undergone a surgical procedure, surgical site infections (SSIs) are one of the leading nosocomial infections. Of an estimated 721,800 health care–associated infections (HAIs) occurring during 2011 in US acute care hospitals, 21.8% were attributed to SSIs (2). These infections have significant attributable costs, morbidity, and mortality rates. A study across 129 US Veterans Administration Hospitals (VAH) determined that the average unadjusted difference in cost was $21,040 higher among patients who develop SSIs compared to those who do not (3). Of patients undergoing inpatient surgery, 2% to 5% develop an SSI, and each SSI is associated with approximately 7 to 10 additional postoperative hospital days. SSIs are associated with a 3% mortality rate, and 77% of deaths among these patients are directly attributable to the SSI (4). The effects of SSIs are not only local—such as tissue destruction, pain, scar formation, and septic thrombophlebitis—but also extend systemically to sepsis, shock, organ dysfunction, and death. See Chapter 84 for further discussion of this issue.

Risk Factors

All surgical wounds are at risk for infection. It is important to be aware of the risk factors and, if possible, to take impactful preventative measures. The National Nosocomial Infection Surveillance (NNIS) system, developed in the early 1970s to monitor the incidence of HAIs and their associated risk factors and pathogens, has identified wound infection risk factors as follows:

- Wounds classified as contaminated or dirty
- A patient with an ASA (American Society of Anesthesiologists) physical status score of 3, 4, or 5 prior to operation
- A procedure lasting longer than "T hours," in which T represents the 75th percentile of duration of time expected for that surgery

To identify a patient's risk index category (RIC), each factor, if present, receives a score of 1, with a range between 0 and 3; SSI rates by operative procedure category and risk index is published in NNIS source documents.

The NNIS also publishes recommendations for reducing the risk of SSIs. The weight of these recommendations is based on the scientific evidence used to support the conclusions:

- Category IA: Strongly recommended for implementation and supported by well-designed experimental, clinical, or epidemiologic studies.
- Category IB: Strongly recommended for implementation and supported by some experimental, clinical, or epidemiologic studies and strong theoretical rationale.
- Category II: Suggested for implementation and supported by suggestive clinical or epidemiologic or theoretical rationale.
- No recommendation or unresolved issue: Practice for which insufficient evidence or no consensus regarding efficacy exists.

Category IA recommendations for SSI prevention are as follows:

1. Treat remote infection before performing an elective operation.
2. Do not remove hair from operative sites unless it interferes with surgery and then only use electric clippers just prior to surgery.
3. Select a prophylactic antimicrobial agent with efficacy against the suspected organism, making sure the therapeutic serum levels exist from the beginning of the operation. Mechanical preparation of the colon with enemas and cathartics before elective colorectal operations and the use of nonabsorbable oral antimicrobials the day before operation have been beneficial.

Category IB recommendations for SSI prevention are as follows:

1. Control serum glucose prior to operation.
2. Cease tobacco use 30 days prior to operation.
3. Shower night before surgery using a chlorhexidine product.
4. Prepare the operative site with an antiseptic skin agent.
5. Do not routinely use vancomycin for antimicrobial prophylaxis.
6. The operative team should keep nails short and not wear artificial nails.
7. A 2- to 5-minute preoperative surgical scrub for the surgical team should occur.

Category II recommendations for SSI prevention are as follows:

1. Prepare skin in concentric circles from the incision site outwards.
2. Keep preoperative stay in the hospital as short as possible.
3. Clean underneath each fingernail prior to performing first scrub of the day.

4. Do not wear hand or arm jewelry.
5. Limit the number of personnel entering the operating room.

No recommendation or unresolved issue includes the restriction of scrub suits to the operating suite, or wearing a cover over the scrub suits outside of the operating theater; it is our practice to limit wearing surgical scrubs to the surgical suite.

Pressure or Decubitus Ulcers

From the Latin *decumbere,* "to lie down," the term *decubitus* has been applied to any area that develops an ulcer secondary to prolonged pressure between a bony prominence and an unyielding surface. Thus the term *pressure ulcer* is a more accurate description. Although an issue of long duration, it appears to be first addressed in scientific writing only in the 19th century.

To overcome arterial and capillary hydrostatic pressure and develop subsequent tissue necrosis with ulceration, an individual must be subjected to 32 mmHg pressure at the level of the ischium, sacrum, or heels for a prolonged period of time, usually exceeding 2 hours as reported by Lindan et al. (5). The points of the greatest pressure in the supine patient are seen over the sacrum, heel, and occiput, with pressures at 40 to 60 mmHg (Fig. 85.1).

With the body in a prone position, the chest and knees absorb the greatest pressure, which may be 50 mmHg; when in the sitting position, the ischial tuberosities are under the most pressure, measured at near 100 mmHg (Fig. 85.2). If sensation is intact, ulceration will usually not occur as the incipient pain/discomfort leads to a change in position; this occurs during the sleep cycle as well.

The risk factors associated with pressure ulcer development can be divided into external and internal causes. *Externally,* the patient might be subjected to a constant pressure for a period of time; friction may exist between exposed skin and a surface that remains static; a region may remain moist and may have desquamation, leading to a loss of the epithelial protective mechanism (Fig. 85.3). The placement of splints can also alter a patient's ability to change position in response to pressure-related pain or, in themselves, may cause pressure necrosis. The administration of sedatives or paralytics can also remove the normal feedback pathways that exist to prevent pressure ulcer formation. *Internally,* factors responsible for pressure ulceration include malnutrition (serum albumin levels less than 3.0 g/dL preoperatively), anemia, and/or endothelial dysfunction. Diabetes, peripheral vascular disease, and episodes of hypotension also increase the risk, as do sensory deficits in patients with paralysis (plegia) or weakness (paresis). Patients with dementia may also not be sensitive to the importance of changing position frequently and may also be more prone to pressure ulceration.

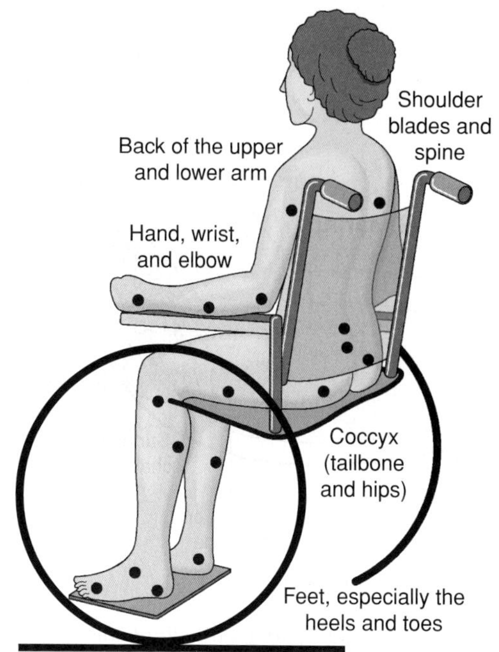

FIGURE 85.2 Pressure points in sitting position.

Most (66%) patients with pressure ulcers are older than 70 years old, with a prevalence rate in nursing homes of 17% to 28%; in contrast, patients admitted with an acute illness have an incidence rate of 3% to 11%. In both subsets of patients, recurrence rates as high as 90% may be seen. The operating room, where patients are immobile, is a high-risk area, and there is a report that up to 25% of all pressure ulcers are initiated there (6).

Anatomic sites affected are primarily the hip and buttocks (67% of the cases involve ischial, trochanteric, and sacral tuberosity); 25% in malleolar, heel, patellar, or pretibial area; with the remainder occurring on the nose, chin, occiput, chest, back, or elbow. In paraplegic patients, pressure ulcers are a leading cause of death, responsible for an 8% mortality rate (7). Overall, an estimated 60,000 people die each year from complications of pressure ulcers. The yearly health care cost in the United States alone is in excess of $1 billion (8).

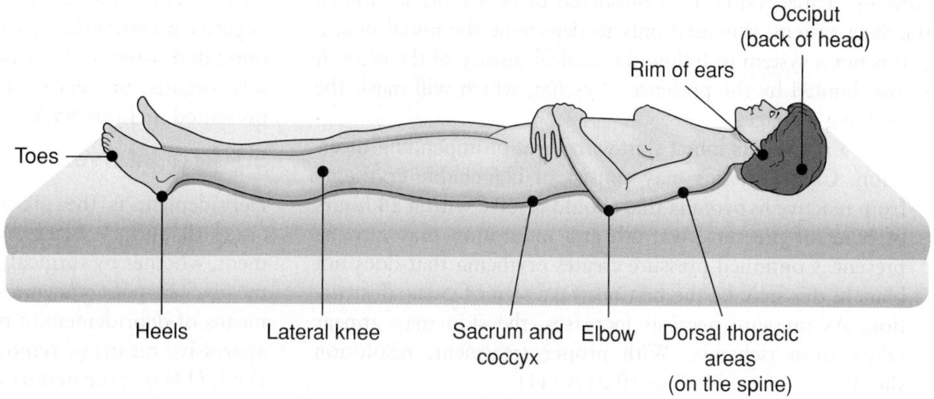

FIGURE 85.1 Pressure points in supine position.

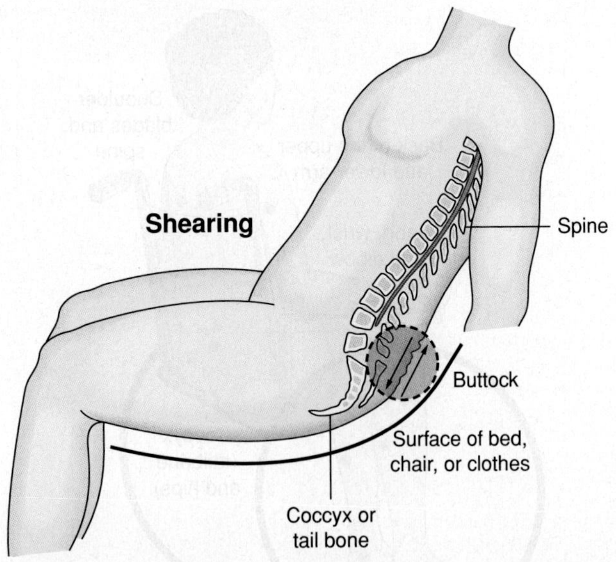

FIGURE 85.3 Shearing effect.

Several scoring systems are used to grade the risk for ulceration. The *Braden scale* is a summation rating scale made up of six subscores, consisting of sensory perception, moisture, activity, mobility, nutrition, and friction/shear, each ranging from 1 to 3 or 4 points, with total scores ranging from 6 to 23. The subscores measure the functional capabilities of the patient that contribute to either higher intensity and duration of pressure or lower tissue tolerance for pressure. A lower Braden score indicates lower levels of functioning with a higher risk for pressure ulcer development.

The *Daniels classification* looks at muscle and subcutaneous tissue breakdown, which occurs before dermal and epidermal changes are observed. Epidermal necrosis occurs later because epidermal cells are able to better withstand prolonged absence of oxygen than cells in the deeper tissues both *in vivo* and *in vitro* (9). Once skin damage is visible, irreversible internal damage may have already occurred (10).

Shea staging describes ulcers that start superficially and progress to deeper structures:

- Grade I: Limited to superficial epidermis and dermis
- Grade II: Involving the epidermis and dermis and extending to the adipose tissue
- Grade III: Extending through the superficial structures and adipose tissue down to muscle
- Grade IV: Complete soft tissue destruction down to bone

Currently, the most widely accepted classification system for pressure ulcers is that produced by the National Pressure Ulcer Advisory Panel (NPUAP). Considered to be a modification of the Shea system, it is used only to determine the initial depth, and is not a system to follow the natural history of the ulcer. It is also limited by the presence of eschar, which will mask the underlying damage.

- *Stage I* represents intact skin with signs of impending ulceration. Clinically, this may consist of blanchable erythema from reactive hyperemia that should resolve within 24 hours of relief of pressure; warmth and induration may also be present. Continued pressure creates erythema that does not blanch; this may be the first outward sign of tissue destruction. As pressure necrosis increases, the skin may appear white from ischemia. With proper treatment, resolution should be expected in 5 to 10 days (11).
- *Stage II* represents a partial-thickness loss of skin involving epidermis and possibly dermis. This lesion may present as an abrasion, blister, or superficial ulceration, with pigmentation changes. These, too, represent a reversible condition.
- *Stage III* represents a full-thickness loss of skin with extension into subcutaneous tissue but not through the underlying fascia. This lesion presents as a crater with or without undermining of adjacent tissue. On examination, this will appear as a necrotic, foul-smelling crater with altered light and dark pigmentation.
- *Stage IV* represents full-thickness loss of skin and subcutaneous tissue and extension into muscle, bone, tendon, or joint capsule. Osteomyelitis with bone destruction, dislocations, or pathologic fractures may be present. Sinus tracts and severe undermining commonly are present.

Treatment

All modalities of care for pressure ulcers fall along four paths.

Pressure Reduction

Frequent—at least every 2 hours—turning and repositioning the patient. Historically, this was adopted because of nursing issues (it took 2 hours for the nurse to rotate all ward patients). Currently, there is debate in the literature as to this being an adequate amount of time. In addition to positioning, mattresses that reduce pressure, such as low-air-loss and air-fluidized beds should be used for patients with stage III and IV ulcers, whereas for stage I and II ulcers, the use of static mattresses such as air, foam, or water overlays are the most beneficial.

Wound Management

Once an ulcer has developed, removal of dead tissue and debris, drainage, and protecting the surrounding healthy tissue are the goals. The pressure needed to clean wounds with no necrotic material is 2 to 5 pounds per square inch (psi). If necrotic debris is present, the pressure required increases by a factor of 2 to 3. The old wound dictum—if it is dry, wet it; if it is wet, dry it—has some validity here. A draining wound needs either a hydrocolloid or alginate, whereas a wound without drainage will respond to simple moist gauze; the surrounding skin of both needs to be kept lubricated, but not wet, to reduce friction. Negative pressure therapy enhances wound healing by reducing edema, increasing the rate of granulation tissue formation, and stimulating circulation. Increased blood flow translates into a reduction in the bacterial load and delivery of infection-fighting leukocytes (12). However, there are significant contraindications for the use of vacuum-assisted or negative pressure therapy including malignancy of the wound, untreated osteomyelitis, nonenteric fistulas, and exposed vessels, organs, or nerves (13). Various dressing categories are presented in Table 85.1.

Surgical Intervention

Debridement is the process of removing devitalized tissue. Stage III and IV ulcers will require some form of debridement, whether by surgical, autolytic, mechanical, or enzymatic means. The patient's wound and overall status will dictate the means of debridement, a more stable patient receiving a more aggressive means of removing the necrotic material. In 1938, Davis (14) was the first to suggest replacing the unstable scar of

TABLE 85.1 Dressing Categories

Category	Properties/Uses
Alginates	Absorption of drainage, dead space obliteration, autolysis of necrotic material
Foams	Absorption of drainage, dead space obliteration, mechanical debridement, moisture retention
Gauzes	Absorption of drainage, dead space obliteration, mechanical debridement, moisture retention
Hydrocolloids	Dead space obliteration, autolysis of necrotic material, moisture retention
Vacuum-assisted closure	Dead space obliteration, induction of granulation
Ostomy appliances	Drainage diversion

a healed pressure sore with a flap of tissue. In 1947, Kostrubala and Greeley recommended excising the bony prominence and adding padding for the exposed bone with local fascia or muscle-fascia flaps. In addition, larger wounds may respond only to the placement of flaps, either fasciocutaneous or musculocutaneous. Flap failure can be seen after insufficient excision of soft tissue and bone, and if systemic factors such as nutritional status are suboptimal.

Nutritional Support

Malnourished patients have a higher susceptibility for ulcer formation. Once formed, these patients also have a diminished ability to heal or to prevent further ulcer formation in other sites. Patients with serum albumin levels less than 3 mg/dL may be candidates for supplemental feedings via enteral or parenteral routes.

PRIMARY BACTERIOLOGIC INFECTIONS

Skin and soft tissue infections are usually easily treated, but have the lethal potential. Any break in the usual protection of the integument, such as occurs with a cut, scrape, insect bite, splinter, or traumatic injury, allows bacteria to enter underlying tissues. Although a scrape or a cut will not usually result in a cellulitis, a tender, firm, painful, and rapidly expanding area of redness on the skin surrounding violation of the skin barrier should be cause for concern. Red streaks between lymph node–bearing areas may be visible, indicative of a potentially spreading infection. Certain areas are more prone in becoming infected depending on the age group, such as facial cellulitis occurring more commonly in adults older than 50 years and in children 6 months to 3 years of age.

The most common causative organisms in skin infections are group A β-hemolytic streptococci and *Staphylococcus aureus.* Depending on the source of contamination and whether the patient is immunocompromised, gram-negative rods and fungus can be seen. If the insult occurs during exposure to fresh water, the causative organism may be *Aeromonas,* a gram-negative rod.

Predisposing states in which a minor break in the skin barrier may lead to a significant infection includes patients with diabetes; immunodeficiency; varicella; venous, arterial or lymphatic insufficiency, such as that seen after lymphatic removal during mastectomy; or vein stripping for varicosities.

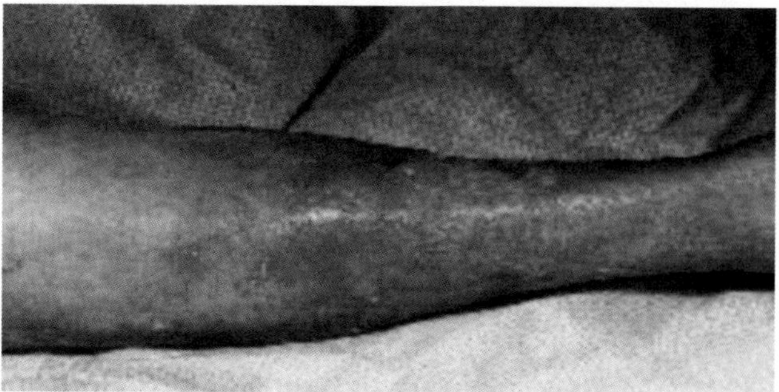

FIGURE 85.4 Erysipelas.

Treatment of uncomplicated cellulitis begins with removing the nidus of infection, cleansing the wound with an antiseptic agent, dressing the wound with an antiseptic ointment if indicated, and considering a course of oral antibiotics, such as dicloxacillin, 500 mg PO (orally) four times a day for 7 days, or cephalexin, 500 mg PO four times a day for 7 days. For patients with a suspected or known penicillin allergy, clindamycin, 400 mg, is given PO four times a day (15).

Erysipelas

Erysipelas (Fig. 85.4) is a form of cellulitis that affects the epidermis primarily, extending into the cutaneous lymphatics. During the Middle Ages, it was referred to as St. Anthony's fire, named after the Egyptian healer who was successful in treating this condition. It shares the same underlying cause as cellulitis with bacterial inoculation into an area of skin violation. It is more commonly seen in children and the elderly. Erysipelas differs from cellulitis in that the inflamed area is distinct from the surrounding skin, being raised and demarcated. Erysipelas is often found on the face; however, it can also develop on the arms and legs. Sometimes the skin will have what is called a *peau d'orange,* or orange peel, look to it. As with cellulitis, *Streptococcus* is the primary organism identified with its toxin responsible for the brisk inflammation associated with this condition.

Treatment consists of elevation of the affected extremity, penicillin, 250 to 500 mg PO or 0.6 to 1.2 million units intramuscularly, given every 4 to 6 hours for a 10- to 20-day course. In cases of penicillin allergy, a macrolide or cephalosporin usually suffices. If the area affected becomes ulcerated, saline dressings changed every 12 hours will assist with wound closure.

Impetigo

Also known as pyoderma, impetigo (Fig. 85.5) is the most common bacterial infection of the skin seen. It is contagious and can happen at any age, but is more common in young children. Patients report skin lesions, often with associated adenopathy, with minimal systemic signs and symptoms. Impetigo may present in two forms: small vesicles with a honey-colored crust known as *impetigo contagiosa,* or purulent-appearing bullae, known as *bullous impetigo* (occurring principally in newborns and young children). While most commonly caused by *S. aureus,* group A β-hemolytic Streptococcus is also

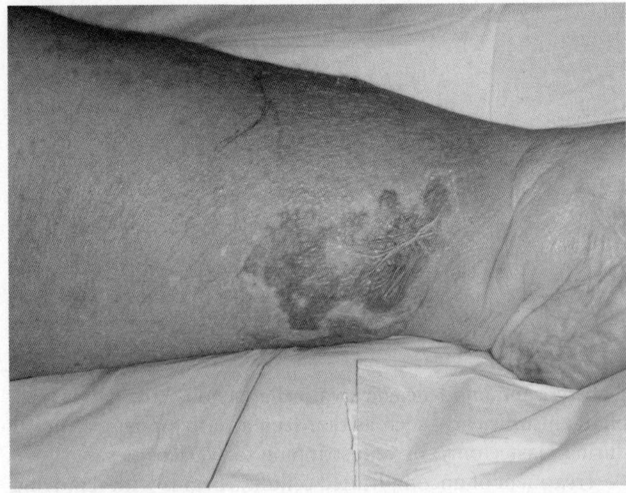

FIGURE 85.5 Impetigo due to *Staphylococcus aureus* in a 68-year-old diabetic who fell onto concrete while walking and developed this lesion after 6 days. This resolved with conservative care and antibiotics.

commonly seen in the over-2-year-old population. Warm temperatures, humidity, poor hygiene, and crowded living conditions can exacerbate the spread of impetigo. When associated with lymphadenitis in deeper infections, the term *ecthyma* is given. While topical mupirocin or retapamulin ointments can be used for treating limited impetigo, systemic therapy is preferred when treating widespread impetigo. Lesions usually resolve completely within 7 to 10 days.

CUTANEOUS FUNGAL INFECTIONS

The most common and important fungal infections that occur in the ICU setting are, for the most part, due to *Candida*, especially *albicans*, *glabrata*, and *tropicalis* (16). In immunocompromised or morbidly obese patients, this usually manifests itself as cutaneous moniliasis and can be treated with topical powders or ointments. Vaginitis, of course, should be treated with suppositories, and funguria is addressed by removing or replacing the urinary catheter, which will be successful in about one-third of patients.

SUBCUTANEOUS TISSUE INFECTIONS AND MYONECROSIS

The clinical distinction between superficial pyodermas and deep subcutaneous infections such as necrotizing fasciitis (NF) is often readily apparent. However, clinically distinguishing between NF and other forms of deep infections is often difficult due to commonalities in clinical presentation, anatomic features, and infecting organisms. Common among all of these types of infections is the variable tendency to form gas as well as the need for surgical exploration to differentiate and treat these processes. For example, clostridial and nonclostridial anerobic cellulitis both result in extensive gas formation, typically present with mild to moderate systemic symptoms, and lack muscle involvement; on the other hand, clostridial myonecrosis presents as a life-threatening infection with significant muscle involvement. The differentiation between these infections is made in the operating room.

The most common gas forming soft tissue infections include clostridial cellulitis, nonclostridial anerobic cellulitis, clostridial myonecrosis (gas gangrene), NF (Types I and II), Fournier gangrene, and synergistic necrotizing cellulitis (Meleney gangrene). Immediate surgical debridement is mandated once the diagnosis of any of these infections is made.

Necrotizing Fasciitis

Synergistic necrotizing cellulitis was first clearly documented in 1926. In their initial report, Brewer and Meleny (17) presented clinical and bacteriologic evidence of symbiotic growth and enhanced invasiveness between anerobic *Streptococcus* and *Staphylococcus aureus*. Their early description of what is now considered a variant of NF defined many of the prominent clinical and anatomic features of this type of infection. An early retrospective case series from the time period between 1958 and 1970 reported 76% mortality among patients with this infection; a mortality rate over twice that reported by contemporary reports, emphasizing that early recognition, surgical debridement, and targeted antimicrobial therapy have dramatically improved survival (18).

The term NF was first coined in 1952 by Wilson (19); the pathology involves the underlying fascia and subcutaneous tissue, but spares muscle. Myositis results in muscle involvement, which becomes exquisitely tender and indurated. The muscle involvement leads to elevation of the creatine phosphokinase (CPK) and can spread over several hours to contiguous muscle groups, thus heightening the need for early diagnosis and treatment. Fournier gangrene is listed here as a separate entity due to its predilection for the perineum.

All of these subgroups have in common pathogenicity with the organisms spreading from subcutaneous tissues to both superficial and deep fascial planes (Fig. 85.6). The local effect is vascular occlusion, ischemia, and necrosis. Prompt recognition is critical due to the rapidity with which this infection progresses. The reported mortality due to NF ranges from 24% to 34%, but decreases to about 12% with prompt recognition and treatment; Fournier gangrene results in a slightly lower mortality rate (15%) (20,21).

NF may be classified as types I and II, Fournier, and gas gangrene; these are discussed in the paragraphs that follows.

Type I (polymicrobial)

Usually occurring after injury or surgery, type I NF can be misdiagnosed as a simple cellulitis; however, as tissue necrosis and hypoxia continue, pain and systemic symptoms of fever, chills, and malaise increase as the underlying tissue liquefies; the overlying skin may show minimal changes. In the later stages, extension into the muscle itself occurs and, over 2 to 3 days, the erythema increases, with occasional bullae formation. Cultures may reveal a combination of aerobic and anaerobic organisms. Deep soft tissue infection of the perineum is termed *Fournier gangrene* (19). Many of these patients have predisposing comorbidities, such as diabetes or the presence of immunosuppressed states. Histologically, thrombosis of blood vessels and abundant bacteria with many polymorphonuclear cells are typically seen.

Type II (group A streptococcal)

Also known, colloquially, as "flesh-eating bacteria" or, by clinicians, as synergistic gangrene of Meleney (Figs. 85.7 and 85.8). As with type I NF, a nearly normal-appearing overlying

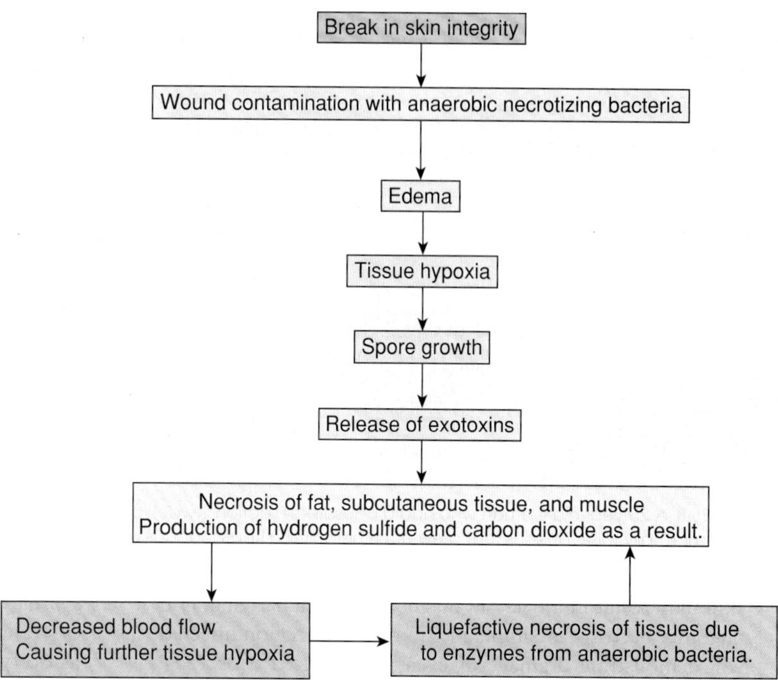

FIGURE 85.6 Pathophysiology of necrotizing fasciitis.

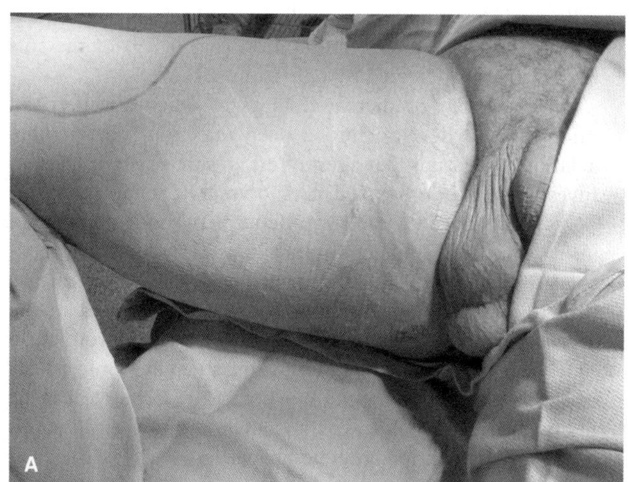

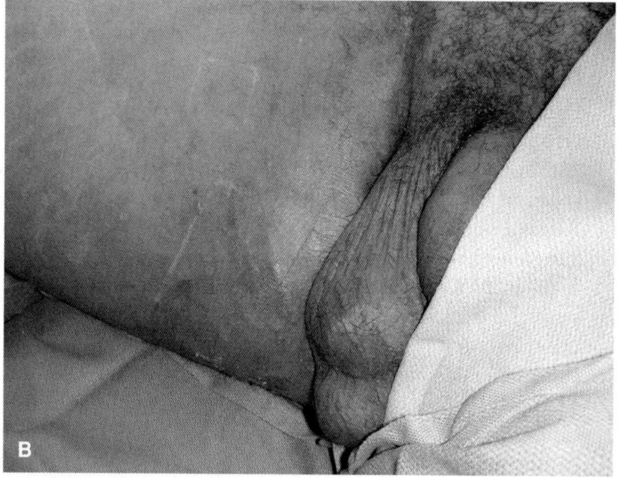

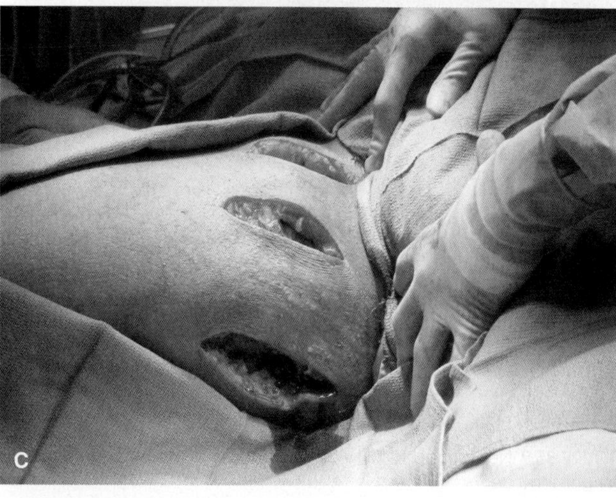

FIGURE 85.7 Meleney synergistic gangrene in a 45-year-old pipe layer who noticed initially a wheal and subsequently required incision and drainage for β-hemolytic streptococcus.

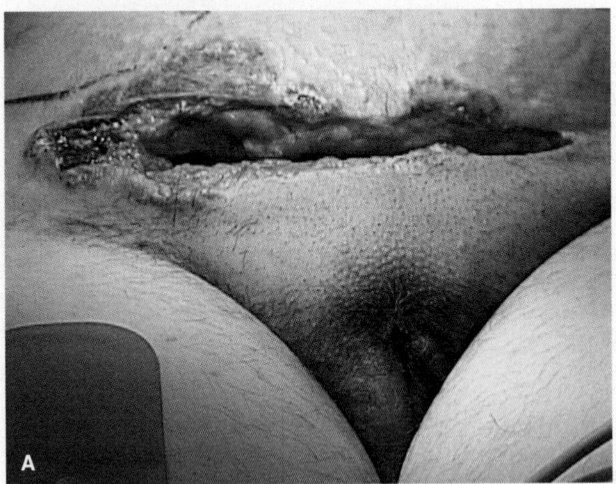

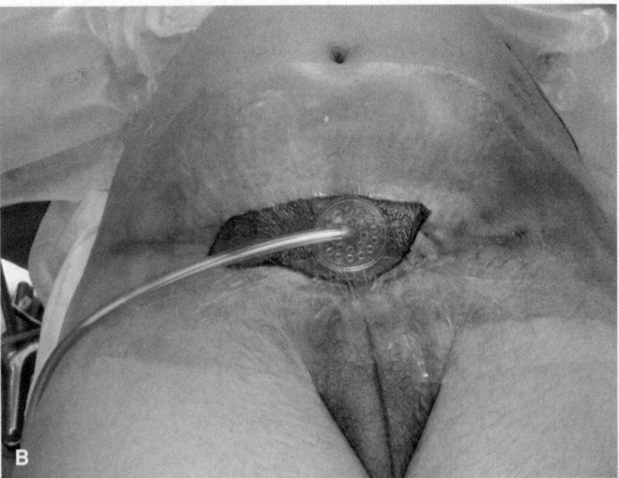

FIGURE 85.8 A 25-year-old woman who had a caesarean section 1 week prior for placenta previa and accreta who, 48 hours later, developed these purplish minimally raised lesions that grew out β-hemolytic streptococcus.

skin may result in a delay in diagnosing the underlying, and ongoing, necrosis. A simple incision into the region affected will demonstrate drainage or even, in advanced cases, gas. Predisposing factors include varicella infection and the use of nonsteroidal anti-inflammatory drugs (NSAIDs) (22). NSAID use is seen as an immunomodulator, which may predispose to this condition. With type II NF, there is an association with the Streptococcal toxic shock syndrome, similar to its Staphylococcal counterpart except for the presence of necrosis as the precipitant event.

Fournier gangrene (idiopathic gangrene of the penis and scrotum)

Although first described in 1764 by Baurienne, this entity received its name from the French venereologist, Jean-Alfred Fournier (23) when, in 1883, he presented a case of gangrene of the perineum in an otherwise healthy young man. In 95% of cases, an identifiable cause can be found, with the disease process originating from the anorectum, the urogenital tract, or the skin of the genitalia: anorectal causes include malignancy, diverticulitis, or appendicitis; urethral injury, urethral stricture, urogenital manipulation, or infection can initiate Fournier's gangrene; finally, cutaneous conditions such as hidradenitis suppurativa or trauma may be precursors. In addition to local predisposing conditions, comorbidities such as leukemia, systemic lupus erythematosus, Crohn disease, HIV, or other conditions of immunodeficiency may be predisposing. Other comorbidities associated with Fournier gangrene include obesity, cirrhosis, vasculitides of the perineum, steroid use, and diabetes.

On examination, the typical Fournier patient will be an elderly male in his sixth or seventh decade of life with one or more of the above comorbidities. Clinically, this patient may have a history of fever and lethargy for approximately 1 week prior to admission. Pain, tenderness, and erythema of the genitalia and overlying skin will progress to a dusky appearance, ultimately with purulent-appearing drainage.

Clostridial myonecrosis (gas gangrene)

A rapidly progressive infection of deep subcutaneous tissue and muscle, gas gangrene is most commonly caused by *Clostridium perfringens* and, less frequently, by *Clostridium septicum*. Most cases arise in the setting of recent surgery or trauma, it does not arise spontaneously as commonly as do types I and II NF. *C. perfringens* (formerly *Clostridium welchii*) is an anaerobic gram-positive spore-forming organism that produces at least 10 distinct exotoxins. The most important exotoxin, leading to human pathogenesis, is the α-toxin, which hemolyzes red blood cells, hydrolyzes cell membranes, and exerts a direct cardiodepressive effect. Within 12 to 24 hours, crepitation (Fig. 85.9) of the soft tissues may be detected by palpation (24,25).

There are no predictive tests as to when a superficial infection will develop into a deep infection, nor is there a laboratory study for identifying a soft tissue infection. Investigation has focused on polymerase chain reaction (PCR) tests specific for streptococcal pyrogenic exotoxin (SPE) genes, variants A, B, and C, along with streptococcal superantigens. These superantigens cause the release of cytokines through binding to a specific segment of the T-cell receptor, resulting in an overwhelming production of TNF-α, IL-1, and IL-6, with subsequent systemic effects of sepsis and septic shock. Work has also centered on the filamentous M-protein, which is anchored to the cell membrane and has antiphagocytic properties (Fig. 85.10).

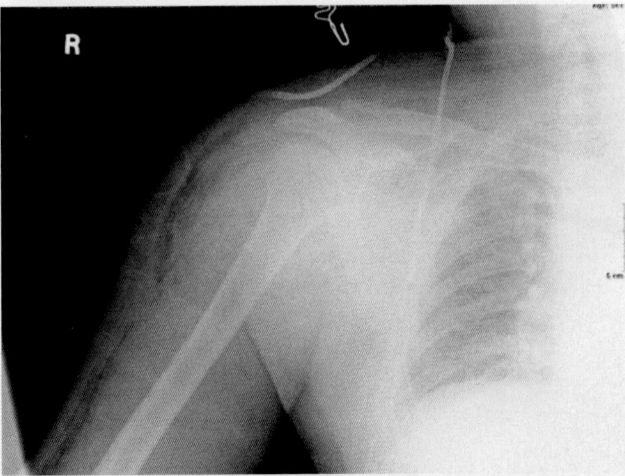

FIGURE 85.9 Necrotizing fasciitis on chest radiograph with soft tissue air in right shoulder.

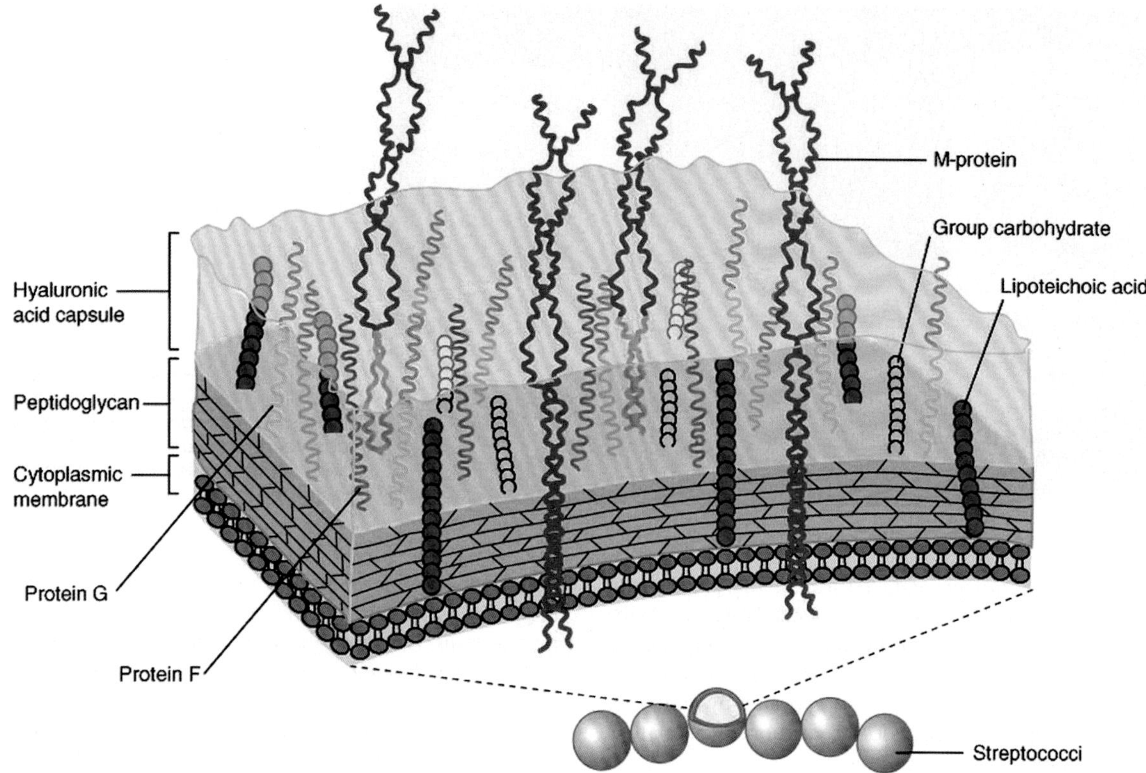

FIGURE 85.10 Action of streptococci.

Imaging Studies for Necrotizing Fasciitis

Imaging studies (Table 85.2), in particular computed tomography (CT), have shown, with great sensitivity, the presence and extent of gas or subcutaneous air. Magnetic resonance imaging (MRI) T2-weighted images (Fig. 85.11) can show well-defined areas of high signal intensity significant for tissue necrosis and, in the absence of gadolinium contrast enhancement on T1 images, reliably detects fascial necrosis in those who might require operative debridement. Ultrasound (US), although able to detect fluid or gas within soft tissues, requires the probe to be applied directly on the involved tissues. Many patients with NF, especially those with Fournier gangrene, may not tolerate this. Additionally, there may be a limitation of visualization related to the anatomic site, causing difficulty in visualizing deep tissues. Yen and colleagues (26) found US to have a sensitivity of 88% and a specificity of 93% (positive predictive value of 83%); their diagnostic criteria included diffuse thickening of the subcutaneous tissue accompanied by fluid accumulation more than 4 mm in depth along the fascial layer.

The diagnosis may also be made with culture and biopsy of the affected tissue; a Gram stain to identify single or multiple organisms is helpful in distinguishing type I from type II NF. Once the diagnosis is made, either on physical examination or through other diagnostic means including culture, biopsy, or excision, multimodality therapy should be used early due to the rapidity of progression.

Therapy

Until the organism is identified, broad-spectrum antibiotics should be administered. For aerobic organisms, one regimen is ampicillin, 8 to 14 g/d intravenously (i.v.) administered in every 6 hours in divided dosages, and gentamicin, 3 mg/kg/d i.v. divided every 8 hours. Penicillin G, 8 to 24 million units/d i.v. given in divided dosages every 4 to 6 hours, in combination with clindamycin, 600 mg i.v. every 6 hours, or metronidazole, not to exceed 4 g/d, provides a two-drug combination for treatment of anerobic organisms. Ampicillin–sulbactam, pipercillin–tazobactam, or carbapenems may also be considered as empiric

TABLE 85.2 Imaging Studies

Type	Role of study	Limitations	Advantages
Ultrasound	Detection of fluid and gas within soft tissues	Requires direct contact, painful	Fast, reproducible, portable to bedside
Magnetic resonance imaging	T2-weighted images. T1-weighted images	Unstable patients unable to tolerate time required for study	High sensitivity for extent of involvement
Plain radiographs	Identification of air in subcutaneous location	Seen in <50% of cases	Fast, reproducible
Computerized tomography	Detection of extent of fluid/gas in soft tissues	Requires transport, dye is nephrotoxic	High sensitivity for extent of involvement

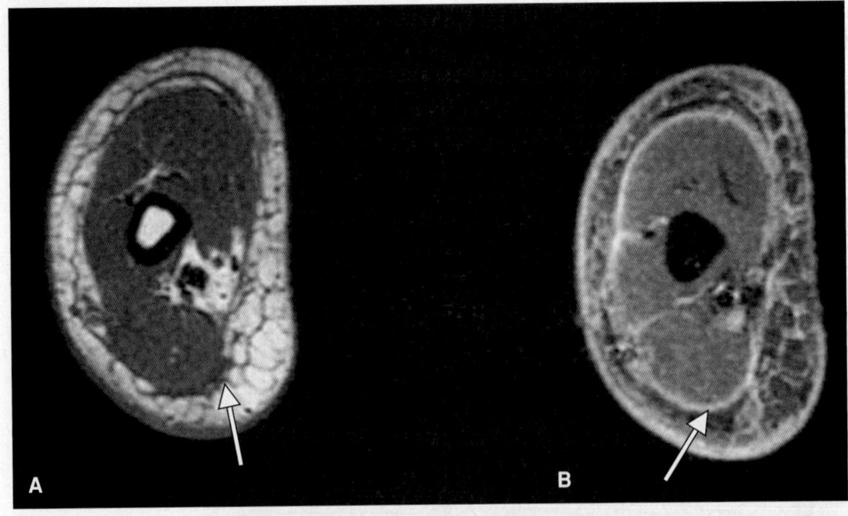

FIGURE 85.11 T1-weighted and T2-weighted MRI of the lower extremity showing fascial thickening and fluid accumulation between the subcutaneous tissues (*arrow*) (A) and fascial layer (*arrow*) (B), respectively, in this patient with necrotizing fasciitis.

treatment until bacteriologic data return. In the presence of group A streptococcal infection, the use of clindamycin may be advantageous as it is not affected by inoculum size or stage of growth. Additionally, clindamycin suppresses toxin production, facilitates phagocytosis of *Streptococcus pyogenes* by inhibiting M-protein synthesis, and suppresses production of regulatory elements controlling cell wall synthesis.

Other nonsurgical modalities include hyperbaric oxygen (HBO), although no prospective study exists to justify its value. HBO can increase the oxygen saturation in infected wounds by a 1000-fold, is bacteriocidal, improves polymorphonuclear leukocytes (PMN) function, and enhances wound healing. There may be better oxygenation and saturation in infected necrotic tissue secondary to HBO-induced vasodilation. HBO has been reported by some to improve patient survival by as much as 50%, and to decrease the number of debridement required to achieve wound control; this is an inconsistent finding (27). A typical treatment protocol involves HBO given aggressively after the first surgical debridement. Three treatment sessions, in a multiplace chamber at 3 atmospheres absolute (ATA) at 100% oxygen for 90 minutes each, can be given in the first 24 hours; in a monoplace chamber (Fig. 85.12), 2.5 to 2.8 ATA, using 100% oxygen for 90 minutes per session may be given. Beginning with the second day, twice-daily treatments are given until granulation tissue is seen, usually requiring a total of 10 to 15 treatments (24). Since clostridial myonecrosis is a monobacterial anaerobic infection, hyperbaric therapy has a greater logistic role in inhibiting clostridial growth and α-toxin production.

Intravenous immunoglobulin (IVIG) has also been used with necrotizing soft tissue infections, although there are no prospective randomized trials to support its use. Case reports indicate that IVIG inhibits activation of T-cells by superantigens and, thereby, decreases the production of TNF-α and IL-6 by T-cells, providing a beneficial effect. The Canadian Streptococcal Study Group, in 1998, compared 21 consecutive patients with group A streptococcal toxic shock syndrome who were administered IVIG, noting a survival benefit rate of 33% (25). Adverse events (AEs) occurred in less than 5% of patients; these AEs may mimic a worsening course of NF. Other AEs include pallor, flushing, fever, muscle aches, hypotension, anaphylaxis, erythema multiforme, and blood-borne pathogen transmission.

Although wide local debridement is the classical therapy for cases of necrotizing soft tissue infections (Table 85.3), initial diagnostic surgical exploration can be limited (28,29). A series of small incisions under local anesthesia can be performed to delineate the extent and presence of muscle or facial necrosis; frozen sections of tissue specimens obtained can establish the diagnosis. However, once the diagnosis is confirmed, *there is no role* for conservative debridement or incision and drainage.

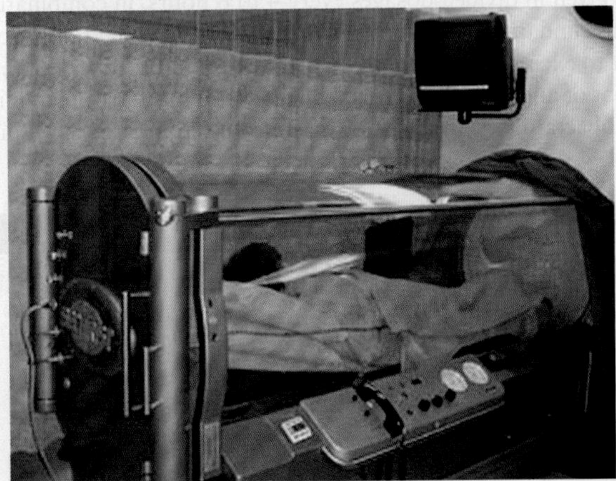

FIGURE 85.12 A monoplace hyperbaric chamber, which may be used to adjunctively treat necrotizing fasciitis.

TABLE 85.3 Clinical Indicators Prompting Wide Surgical Intervention in Necrotizing Fasciitis

Indicator	Remarks
Failure of improvement	After hours of parenteral antibiotics for presumed cellulitis, no decrease in signs and symptoms is detected or if there is progression
Profound toxic effects occurring at the onset of infection	These include malaise, weakness, generalized aching, loss of appetite/concentration
Extensive necrosis	Necrosis or gas is noted in the wound or is evident on radiographs
Compartment syndrome suspected	Edema within muscle group resulting in ischemic injury

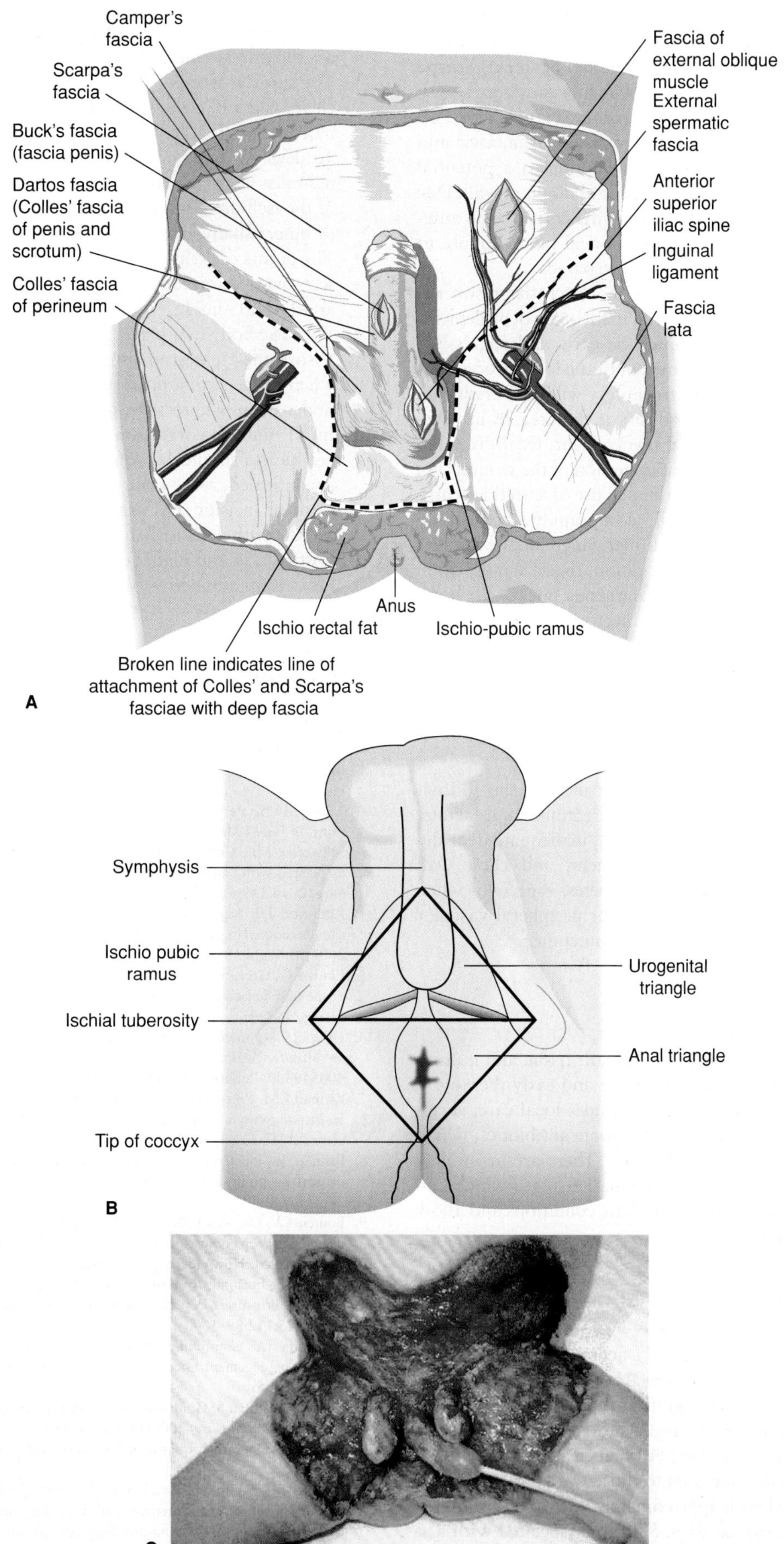

FIGURE 85.13 Fournier gangrene involving the perineum but sparing the penis and testicles; wide debridement has been performed.

In the case of Fournier gangrene, an understanding of the anatomic relationship between the perineum and abdominal wall is important. Below the area of the inguinal ligament, Scarpa fascia blends into the Colles fascia, which is contiguous with the Dartos fascia of the penis and scrotum (Fig. 85.13). This allows a potential space to exist between the Scarpa fascia and abdominal oblique musculature, contributing to a potential spread from the perineum to the anterior abdominal wall. Due to Buck fascia, a deep fascia that covers the corpora and anterior urethra, and due to the retroperitoneal blood supply to the testis, the penis and testicles may be spared.

The two most common pitfalls with a necrotizing soft tissue infection are diagnostic delay and inadequate debridement. Excision of nonviable areas should be early and aggressive, with repeat debridement performed until the local process has been controlled. The use of electrocautery will aid in reducing the considerable operative blood loss if the area of involvement is extensive. With perineal involvement, fecal diversion via colostomy allows for less contamination of the wound site. With urogenital involvement, continued use of a urethral catheter is safe, although occasionally a suprapubic cystostomy will be necessary. In the case of Fournier gangrene, the testicles are usually spared; to prevent desiccation, they are most often placed in a surgically created subcutaneous pocket. If, however, the testes are not viable, an orchiectomy is performed. In all cases of NF, vacuum-assisted closure devices have shown great promise in decreasing time to grafting and closure of the debrided area (see Fig. 85.8B).

Factors Associated with Poor Outcome

Factors associated with poor outcome include the following: older age, female gender, elevated creatinine and lactate, extent of tissue involved (more is worse), inadequate debridement, advanced age, truncal involvement, and chest wall involvement (30). The presence of diabetes, especially when in conjunction with renal dysfunction or peripheral vascular disease (31) is also a marker for a poor outcome.

SUMMARY

The major point to remember with all soft tissue and musculocutaneous infections is that aggressive and early therapy in general yields the best results. This includes local care, surgical debridement, and the use of appropriate antibiotics, which can be guided by the cultures obtained. There are many new topical products coming out on the market place which can further assist in the management of these conditions and allow for improved outcome.

Key Points

- Of HAIs occurring during 2011 acute care hospitals in the United States, 21.8% were attributed to SSIs.
- These infections have significant attributable costs, morbidity, and mortality rates. The average unadjusted difference in cost was $21,040 higher among patients who develop SSIs compared to those who do not. Each SSI is associated with approximately 7 to 10 additional postoperative hospital days. SSIs are associated with a 3% mortality rate; 77% of deaths among these patients are directly attributable to the SSI.
- The surgical wound classification is as follows: Class I, clean; Class II, clean–contaminated; Class III, contaminated; Class IV, dirty.
- To develop tissue necrosis with ulceration, an individual must be subjected to 32 mmHg pressure at the level of the ischium, sacrum, or heels for a prolonged period of time, usually exceeding 2 hours.
- The points of greatest pressure in the supine patient are seen over the sacrum, heel, and occiput, with pressures at 40 to 60 mmHg.
- With the body in a prone position, the chest and knees absorb the greatest pressure, which may be 50 mmHg; when in the sitting position, the ischial tuberosities are under the most pressure, measured at near 100 mmHg.
- In NF, until the organism is identified, broad-spectrum antibiotics should be administered; once the diagnosis is confirmed, *there is no role* for conservative debridement or incision and drainage; the two most common pitfalls with a necrotizing soft tissue infection are diagnostic delay and inadequate debridement.
- HBO is an adjunctive therapy in NF.

References

1. *FastStats: inpatient surgery.* CDC website. Available at: http://www.cdc.gov/nchs/fastats/inpatient-surgery.htm. Updated April 27, 2016; accessed May 1, 2016.
2. Magill SS, Edwards JR, Bamberg W, et al; Emerging Infections Program Healthcare-Associated Infections and Antimicrobial Use Prevalence Survey Team. Multistate point prevalence survey of health care-associated infections. *N Engl J Med.* 2014;370:1198–1208.
3. Schweizer ML, Cullen JJ, Perencevich EN, Vaughan Sarrazin MS. Costs associated with surgical site infections in veterans affairs hospitals. *JAMA Surg.* 2014;149(6):575–581.
4. Anderson DJ, Kaye KS, Classen D, et al. Strategies to prevent surgical site infections in acute care hospitals. *Infect Control Hosp Epidemiol.* 2008;29(Suppl 1):S51–S61.
5. Lindan O, Greenway RM, Piazza JM. Pressure distribution on the surface of the human body: evaluation in lying and sitting positions using a bed of springs and nails. *Arch Phys Med Rehabil.* 1965;46:378.
6. *Up to 25% of bedsores begin in surgery.* Doctor's guide website. Available at: http://www.docguide.com/dg.nsf/printprint/68cbdfa3462eofdd852565c4005496d9. Published March 11, 199;
7. Kirman KM. *Pressure ulcers and wound care.* Medscape website. Available at: http://www.emedicine.com/med/topic2709.htm. Updated April 1, 2015; accessed January 3, 2017.
8. Bennett RG, Bellantoni MF, Ouslander JG. Air-fluidized bed treatment of nursing home patients with pressure sores. *J Am Geriatr Soc.* 1989; 37:235–242.
9. Bouten CV, Oomens CW, Baaijens FP, Bader DL. The etiology of pressure ulcers: skin deep or muscle bound? *Arch Phys Med Rehabil.* 2003;84:616–619.
10. Versluysen M. How elderly patients with femoral fracture develop pressure sores in the hospital. *Br Med J.* 1986;292:1311–1313.
11. Shea JD. Pressure sores: classification and management. *Clin Orthop Rel Res.* 1975;112:89–100.
12. Niezgoda JA. Combining negative pressure wound therapy with other wound management modalities. *Ostomy Wound Manage.* 2005;51(2A Suppl):36–38.
13. Mendez-Eastman S. Guidelines for using negative pressure wound therapy. *Adv Skin Wound Care.* 2001;14(6):314–322.
14. Davis JS. Operative treatment of scars following bed sores. *Surgery.* 1938;3:1.
15. Shapiro MJ, Smith ES, Eachempati SR. Fungal infections and antifungal therapy in the surgical intensive care unit. In: Asensio J, Trunkey D, eds. *Current Therapy of Trauma and Surgical Critical Care.* Philadelphia, PA: Mosby/Elsevier; 2008:702–710.

16. Cruse PJ, Foord R. The epidemiology of wound infections: a 10-year prospective study of 62,939 wounds. *Surg Clin North Am.* 1980;60(1):27–40.
17. Brewer GE, Meleny FL. Progressive gangrenous infection of the skin ad subcutaneous tissues following operation for acute perforative appendicitis: a study in symbiosis. *Ann Surg.* 1926;84:438.
18. Stone HH, Martin JD. Synergistic necrotizing cellulitis. *Ann Surg.* 1972; 175:702–710.
19. Wilson B. Necrotizing fasciitis. *Am Surg.* 1952;18:416–431.
20. Anaya DA, McMahon K, Nathens AB, et al. Predictors of mortality and limb loss in necrotizing soft tissue infections. *Arch Surg.* 2005;140: 151–157; discussion 158.
21. Eke N. Fournier's gangrene: a review of 1726 cases. *Br J Surg.* 2000;87:718–728.
22. Kaul R, McGeer A, Low DE, et al. Population-based surveillance for group A streptococcal necrotizing fasciitis: clinical features, prognostic indicators and microbiologic analysis of 77 cases. Ontario Group A Streptococcal Study. *Am J Med.* 1997;103:18–24.
23. Yanar H, Taviloglu K, Ertekin C, et al. Fournier's gangrene: risk factors and strategies for management. *World J Surg.* 2006;30:1750–1754.
24. Korhonen K, Kuttila K, Niinikoski J. Tissue gas tensions in patients with necrotising fasciitis and healthy controls during treatment with hyperbaric oxygen: a clinical study. *Eur J Surg.* 2000;166(7):530–534.
25. Kaul R, McGeer A, Norrby-Teglund A. Intravenous immunoglobulin therapy for toxic shock syndrome. *Clin Infect Dis.* 1999;28:800–807.
26. Yen ZS, Wang HP, Ma HM, et al. Ultrasonographic screening of clinically suspected necrotizing fasciitis. *Acad Emerg Med.* 2002;9(12):1448–1451.
27. Jallali N, Withey S, Butler PE. Hyperbaric oxygen as adjuvant therapy in the management of necrotizing fasciitis. *Am J Surg.* 2005;189(4):462–468.
28. Yong JM. Rationale for the use of intravenous immunoglobulin in streptococcal necrotizing fasciitis. *Clin Immunother.* 1995;4(1):61–71.
29. Urschel JD. Necrotizing soft tissue infections. *Postgrad Med J.* 1999;75: 645–649.
30. Hammainen P, Kostiainen S. Postoperative necrotizing chest wall infections. *Scand Cardiovasc J.* 1998;32:243–245.
31. Elliot DC, Kufera JA, Myers RA. Necrotizing soft tissue infections: risk factors for mortality and strategies for management. *Ann Surg.* 1996;224: 672–683.

CHAPTER
86
Neurologic Infections

WENDY I. SLIGL and STEPHEN D. SHAFRAN

INTRODUCTION

Infections of the central nervous system (CNS) are often rapidly progressive and can be fatal if left undiagnosed or treatment is delayed. Prompt diagnosis and treatment are, therefore, crucial to decreasing morbidity and mortality. Patients with CNS infections may require intensive care unit (ICU) admission, most commonly for airway protection and mechanical ventilation due to altered mental status. Similarly, patients with undiagnosed CNS infections may be admitted to the ICU, where intensivists can play a role in diagnosis and optimize outcomes with early and effective therapy.

Identification of the presence or absence of focal neurologic findings is important in patients with suspected neurologic infections as this helps to focus the differential diagnosis and identify patients in whom lumbar puncture (LP) may be contraindicated—at least until neuroimaging is completed. The major neurologic infections encountered in the critically ill include acute bacterial meningitis, encephalitis, brain abscess, subdural empyema, epidural abscess, and suppurative intracranial thrombophlebitis. Neurologic findings may also be the result of primary nonneurologic syndromes, such as sepsis, and are covered in other chapters. Neurologic infections in advanced HIV/AIDS are also covered separately.

The CNS is normally protected by various host defenses, the most important of which is the blood–brain barrier. Once microorganisms gain entry, however, they are able to proliferate rapidly due to low concentrations of immunoglobulins and leukocytes in the CNS. Viral, bacterial, mycobacterial, fungal, or parasitic agents can all cause CNS infection. Patient age, underlying host factors, and epidemiologic exposures including travel, animal or vector exposures, and contacts with infectious cases are important risk factors for acquiring specific infections. Prompt physical examination to identify patients in need of urgent interventions—including endotracheal intubation—should be performed, followed by LP and/or imaging studies. New techniques in the areas of molecular diagnostics and neuroimaging have revolutionized the diagnosis of CNS infections. New therapeutic options, as well as improvements in intensive care support, have also enhanced outcomes in these patients.

MENINGITIS

Meningitis—inflammation of the meninges—may be caused by a wide variety of microorganisms (Table 86.1). Infectious agents gain entry to the CSF via hematogenous, transdural, or transparenchymal routes. It is important to consider noninfectious syndromes in the differential diagnosis of meningitis. Such examples include meningeal carcinomatosis, vasculitic syndromes, or drug effect (e.g., nonsteroidal anti-inflammatories, antimicrobials, immunosuppressants, anticonvulsants). Identification of noninfectious conditions is essential, as their therapies differ from those for infectious syndromes; specifically, high-dose corticosteroid therapy may be indicated in some of these cases. Aseptic meningitis refers to inflammation of the meninges not attributed to bacterial infection. Critically ill patients, however, present more commonly with bacterial meningitis by virtue of the more rapid and fulminant presentation.

Acute bacterial meningitis accounts for approximately 1.2 million cases annually worldwide (1). Because untreated bacterial meningitis is universally fatal, early recognition, rapid diagnostic testing, and emergent administration of antimicrobial and adjunctive agents are crucial. The most common meningeal pathogens include *Streptococcus pneumoniae* and *Neisseria meningitidis,* although specific etiologic agents and their frequencies vary with underlying host factors such as age, immune status, and route of acquisition. The case fatality rate for adults with bacterial meningitis is approximately 15% to 30%, and increases with age (2,3). Transient or permanent neurologic sequelae occur in approximately 25% of survivors (4,5). Recent data suggest that survival has improved following recommendations for the adjunctive use of dexamethasone (6).

PATHOPHYSIOLOGY

Bacterial meningitis develops as a result of several mechanisms and involves complex interactions between pathogen virulence and host immune response. Specific microorganisms that colonize the nasopharynx may invade local tissues and subsequently spread to the bloodstream and CNS (7,8). Bacteremia and subsequent CNS invasion may also develop from sources such as pneumonia or urinary tract infection. Last, direct entry from contiguous infection (e.g., sinusitis or mastoiditis), trauma, neurosurgery, or prosthetic devices such as CSF shunts or cochlear implants also occurs. Inflammation and blood–brain barrier injury result from the release of inflammatory cytokines such as interleukin-1 and tumor necrosis factor (9,10). Vasogenic edema and increased intracranial pressure may ensue with subsequent cerebral ischemia, cytotoxic injury, and cellular apoptosis (11). Host factors including functional or anatomic asplenia, complement deficiency, and congenital or acquired immunodeficiency predispose to bacterial meningitis (Table 86.2). Other risk factors for the development of meningitis include recent close contact with a patient with acute bacterial meningitis, recent travel to areas with endemic meningococcal disease, injection drug use, recent neurotrauma or CSF leak, and otorrhea.

The median duration of symptoms prior to hospital admission in bacterial meningitis is short, averaging approximately 24 hours (12). The classic triad of fever, nuchal rigidity, and change in mental status occurs in less than two-thirds of cases; however, almost all patients have at least one of these findings

TABLE 86.1 Causes of Acute Meningitis

	Common	Uncommon
Viruses	Enteroviruses nonpolio Human immunodeficiency virus (HIV) Arboviruses (including West Nile virus, St. Louis encephalitis virus) Herpes simplex virus types 1 and 2 (HSV-1 and HSV-2)	Influenza Parainfluenza Lymphocytic choriomeningitis virus Varicella zoster virus Polio Mumps Cytomegalovirus Epstein–Barr virus Adenovirus
Bacteria	*Streptococcus pneumoniae* *Neisseria meningitidis* *Haemophilus influenzae* *Listeria monocytogenes* Enterobacteriaceae *Staphylococcus aureus* *Mycobacterium tuberculosis* *Borrelia burgdorferi* (Lyme disease) *Streptococcus agalactiae*	*Treponema pallidum* (syphilis) *Rickettsiae* *Mycoplasma* *Brucella* *Chlamydia* *Leptospira*
Fungi	*Cryptococcus neoformans* *Cryptococcus gattii* *Histoplasma capsulatum* *Coccidioides immitis*	*Candida* *Aspergillus* *Blastomyces dermatitidis* *Sporothrix schenckii*
Parasites	None common	*Toxoplasma gondii* *Naegleria fowleri* (free-living amoeba) *Angiostrongylus cantonensis* (eosinophilic meningitis) *Strongyloides stercoralis* (hyperinfection syndrome)
Other infectious syndromes	Parameningeal focus (brain abscess, subdural empyema, epidural abscess) Infective endocarditis	
Noninfectious causes	Medications Intracranial tumor Stroke Lymphoma/leukemia Meningeal carcinomatosis Postprocedure (neurosurgery) Seizure	Autoimmune diseases (SLE, sarcoid, Behçet) Migraine syndromes

SLE, systemic lupus erythematosus.

TABLE 86.2 Predisposing Host Factors to Specific Etiologic Agents of Meningitis

Immunoglobulin deficiency	*Streptococcus pneumoniae*
Asplenia	*S. pneumoniae, Neisseria meningitidis*
Complement deficiency	*N. meningitidis*
Corticosteroid excess	*Listeria monocytogenes, Cryptococcus*
HIV infection	*Cryptococcus, L. monocytogenes, S. pneumoniae*
Bacteremia	*Staphylococcus aureus*, Enterobacteriaceae
Fracture of cribriform plate	*S. pneumoniae*
Basal skull fracture	*S. pneumoniae, Haemophilus influenzae, Streptococcus pyogenes*
Neurotrauma, postneurosurgery	*S. aureus*, coagulase-negative Staphylococci, gram-negative bacilli including *Pseudomonas aeruginosa*

HIV, human immunodeficiency virus.

(3,13). The absence of any of these findings effectively excludes the diagnosis.

Nuchal rigidity can be detected with passive or active flexion of the neck. Tests, such as the Kernig and Brudzinski signs, are well-described physical examination techniques but are neither sensitive nor specific (14). Jolt accentuation (worsening of headache with horizontal rotation of the head two to three times per second) also lacks sensitivity (15). Photophobia, seizures, focal neurologic deficits, and papilledema may be seen on physical examination. Some patients may not manifest the classic signs and symptoms of bacterial meningitis, particularly neonates and those with underlying immunosuppressive conditions including diabetes mellitus, chronic organ failure, neutropenia, chronic corticosteroid use, organ transplantation, and HIV infection. Ten percent to 25% of patients with bacterial meningitis present with septic shock (16,17).

Certain microorganisms may present with specific physical findings. Meningococcal meningitis may present with characteristic skin manifestations consisting of diffuse petechiae and purpura on the distal extremities. Severe cases are described as purpura fulminans. Skin findings occur in approximately one-fourth of bacterial meningitis cases, over 90% of which are due to *N. meningitidis* infection (3).

S. pneumoniae is the most common cause of bacterial meningitis in adults, accounting for 71% of cases in the United States (2). *S. pneumoniae* serotypes causing bacteremic disease are also those commonly responsible for meningitis. Focal infection is common with contiguous or distant sites, including sinusitis, mastoiditis, pneumonia, otitis media, and endocarditis. The major risk factors for pneumococcal meningitis include asplenia, hypogammaglobulinemia, alcoholism, chronic renal or hepatic disease, malignancy, diabetes mellitus, basal skull fracture with CSF leak, and the presence of a cochlear implant.

N. meningitidis commonly causes meningitis in children and young adults. Serogroups B, C, and Y are responsible for most endemic disease in North America (18). Following increasing use of serogroup C and quadrivalent (A, C, Y, W-135) meningococcal vaccines, serogroup B has become the predominant serotype (19). Epidemic disease is most commonly caused by serogroup C, with fewer outbreaks due to serogroup A. In 2000, epidemic W-135 was associated with the Hajj pilgrimage to Mecca in Saudi Arabia (20). Subsequently, meningococcal vaccination has become legally required prior to undertaking this activity. More recent outbreaks have occurred in Gambia and Burkina Faso (21,22). Risk factors for invasive meningococcal disease include nasopharyngeal carriage, terminal complement deficiency, and properdin deficiency (23,24). Although a characteristic rapidly evolving petechial or purpuric rash strongly suggests *N. meningitidis,* a similar rash may be seen in splenectomized patients with overwhelming *S. pneumoniae* or *Haemophilus influenzae* type b infection.

H. influenzae previously accounted for a large proportion of cases of bacterial meningitis; however, widespread vaccination against *H. influenzae* type b has now markedly decreased its incidence. Isolation of *H. influenzae* type b in adults suggests the presence of an underlying condition such as sinusitis, otitis media, pneumonia, diabetes mellitus, alcoholism, CSF leak, asplenia, or immune deficiency.

Listeria monocytogenes meningitis accounts for only 2% of cases of bacterial meningitis in the United States (2) and is associated with similar mortality rates compared to nonlisterial cases. It occurs in neonates, adults older than 50 years of age, and in those with risk factors including alcoholism, malignancy, pregnancy, and immune suppression secondary to corticosteroid therapy or organ transplantation. It is interesting that this infection is seen infrequently in HIV-infected patients; we postulate this may be due to antibiotic prophylaxis—most often with trimethoprim/sulfamethoxazole, which is active against listeria—in HIV patients with low CD4 counts. Pregnant women may be asymptomatic carriers and transmit infection to their infants. *L. monocytogenes* commonly makes up part of the fecal flora of farm animals and can be isolated from soil, water, or contaminated vegetables. Outbreaks have been associated with unpasteurized dairy products such as milk and cheese, as well as vegetables, and processed meats (25–27).

Aerobic gram-negative bacilli can cause meningitis in specific patients. Predisposing risk factors include recent neurosurgery, neonatal status, advanced age, immune suppression, gram-negative bacteremia, and disseminated *Strongyloides stercoralis* hyperinfection syndrome. *Escherichia coli* is a common cause of meningitis in neonates.

Staphylococcus aureus and coagulase-negative staphylococci (CoNS) can both cause meningitis, but are less common. Both Staphylococcal species exist as part of the normal skin flora, predominantly causing infections following neurosurgery or neurotrauma, or when prosthetic material is present, particularly external ventricular drains or ventriculoperitoneal shunts. Some patients with staphylococcal bacterial meningitis have underlying infective endocarditis, paraspinal or epidural infection, sinusitis, osteomyelitis, or pneumonia.

Other less common causes of bacterial meningitis include Enterococci, viridans group Streptococci, β-hemolytic Streptococci, Corynebacterium species (diphtheroids) and *Propionibacterium acnes* (generally only in the setting of prosthetic material), and anaerobic species.

Viruses are the most commonly isolated pathogens in aseptic meningitis. The nonpolio enteroviruses, especially Coxsackie viruses A and B, and echoviruses are common (28), accounting for 85% to 95% of all cases of aseptic meningitis with an identified pathogen (29). Enteroviruses occur worldwide, are transmitted by fecal–oral or respiratory droplet spread, and exhibit summer and fall seasonality in temperate climates. Infants, children, and young adults are commonly affected. Clinical manifestations depend on host age and immune status but generally include abrupt onset of severe headache, fever, nausea, vomiting, photophobia, nuchal rigidity, and malaise. Rash and upper respiratory symptoms are common. Only rarely is illness severe enough to require critical care services.

Arboviruses more commonly cause encephalitis but, rarely, may cause aseptic meningitis. Arboviruses include the flaviviruses (St. Louis encephalitis virus, Colorado tick fever, Japanese encephalitis virus, and West Nile virus), Togaviridae (Eastern equine encephalitis [EEE], Western equine encephalitis [WEE], and Venezuelan equine encephalitis [VEE]), and California serogroup encephalitis viruses, almost all of which are due to La Crosse virus. Arboviruses occur predominantly in the summer and early fall when vector exposure is most likely.

West Nile virus (WNV) came to widespread attention in 1999 when the first North American cases were identified. The virus subsequently spread extensively across North America, and caused three large outbreaks in 2002, 2003, and 2012 (30). WNV infection is asymptomatic in 80% of cases. Symptomatic patients present with West Nile fever (approximately 20%–25%) (31) or neuroinvasive disease (<1%). WNV fever is a self-limited febrile illness characterized by fever, headache, malaise, myalgias, and often a rash (50%). WNV neuroinvasive disease may present as encephalitis, meningitis, or flaccid paralysis. Meningitis, however, is the least common presentation of neuroinvasive disease. Infections occur in late summer or early fall, as nearly all human infections are due to mosquito bites. Rarely, transmission can occur in utero or via donated blood or organ transplantation.

Lymphocytic choriomeningitis (LCM) virus is a zoonotic infection, transmitted by contact with infected rodent (mouse, rat, hamster) secretions or excretions, or rarely via organ transplantation (32–34), which causes aseptic meningitis (35,36). Presenting manifestations include systemic symptoms of fever, myalgias, and malaise, as well as headache and meningismus, with occasional rash, orchitis, arthritis, myopericarditis, and transient alopecia.

Six of the eight recognized human herpesviruses can cause meningitis. Herpes simplex viruses (HSV) are most commonly associated with aseptic meningitis during primary genital infection (37). HSV-2 infection is responsible for most infections, however, HSV-1 genital infection and concomitant meningitis can also occur. Meningitis is much less likely in the setting of genital herpes recurrences. Headache, photophobia, and meningismus are common presenting symptoms. Genital lesions are present in 85% of patients with primary HSV-2 meningitis and generally precede meningeal symptoms by several days.

Herpes zoster aseptic meningitis, with or without typical skin lesions, has also been reported, particularly in older patients. Cytomegalovirus (CMV), Epstein–Barr virus (EBV), and human herpesvirus 6 (HHV-6) are all capable of causing aseptic meningitis but occur very rarely, predominantly in immune-suppressed populations.

HIV-associated aseptic meningitis occurs with primary infection in approximately 5% to 10% of patients (37). Cranial neuropathies may be present along with headache, fever, and meningismus. Symptoms are usually self-limited.

Mumps, now rare as a result of universal vaccination programs, was once a relatively common cause of aseptic meningitis. The clinical manifestations include fever, vomiting, headache, and parotitis in approximately 50% of patients. Meningismus, lethargy, and abdominal pain may also be present. Sporadic outbreaks in susceptible individuals continue to occur worldwide including the United States (38–40).

There are a number of less common causes of aseptic meningitis. Spirochetal meningitis may be caused by *Treponema pallidum* or *Borrelia burgdorferi. T. pallidum,* the etiologic agent of syphilis, is acquired by sexual contact, placental transfer, or direct contact with active lesions; these include *condyloma lata,* mucous patches, or the rash of secondary syphilis. Syphilitic meningitis usually occurs during primary or secondary infection, complicating up to 2% of untreated infections during the first 2 years. *B. burgdorferi* is transmitted by the *Ixodes* tick and causes Lyme disease. It is the most common vector-borne disease in the United States. Meningitis can occur during the first stage of disease, concurrently with *erythema migrans* at the tick bite site. Dissemination of the microorganism in the second stage of disease, 2 to 10 weeks following exposure, may also result in aseptic meningitis. Late or chronic disease may include subacute encephalopathy but not meningitis.

Mycobacterium tuberculosis may cause a subacute or chronic form of meningitis. Infection of the meninges results from rupture of a tuberculous focus into the subarachnoid space. In very young patients, concomitant disseminated systemic infection is common. Epidemiologic risk factors include a known prior history of tuberculosis (TB) exposure, residence in an endemic area, contact with an active case, incarceration, homelessness, and HIV infection. Tuberculin skin testing (TST) is negative in over half of patients with tuberculous meningitis (41,42). A negative skin test, therefore, cannot be used to exclude the diagnosis. Newer tests, such as interferon-gamma release assays (IGRA) and nucleic acid amplification tests (NAT) may be available in some centers.

Fungal meningitis, although uncommon, should be considered particularly given the high mortality associated with untreated infection. *Cryptococcus neoformans* predominantly affects immune-compromised hosts but can also infect the immunocompetent. This encapsulated yeast is distributed worldwide but prefers wet-forested regions with decaying wood and is found in particularly high concentrations in pigeon guano. Risk factors for cryptococcal infection include HIV/AIDS, prolonged corticosteroid therapy, immunosuppression transplantation, malignancy, and sarcoidosis. Clinical presentation is typically indolent, occurring over 1 to 2 weeks, and is characterized by fever, malaise, and headache. Meningismus, photophobia, and vomiting occur in less than one-third of patients. *Cryptococcus gattii,* a serotype usually restricted to tropical climates, emerged on Vancouver Island, British Columbia (BC), Canada in 1999 and has since been responsible for numerous cases of CNS infection in predominantly immunocompetent hosts in BC and the U.S. Pacific Northwest.

Coccidioides immitis, a dimorphic fungus, is found in soil in the dry desert regions of the southwest United States, Mexico, and Central and South America. Infection results after inhalation of arthroconidia, usually following a dust storm or during building construction. Infection is usually confined to the respiratory system in those with competent immune systems. However, extrapulmonary dissemination to the meninges can occur in patients with immune compromise or during pregnancy. Risk factors for the development of disease include travel to or residence in an endemic region and immune deficiency. Coccidioidal meningitis is universally fatal if untreated.

Less common fungal causes of meningitis include *Blastomyces dermatitidis, Histoplasma capsulatum, Sporothrix schenckii,* and rarely, *Candida* species. *B. dermatitidis* and *H. capsulatum* are endemic in the Mississippi and Ohio River Valleys. *S. schenckii* has been reported worldwide, with most cases in the tropical regions of the Americas.

Candida is part of the normal flora of skin and gastrointestinal tract. Candidal CNS infection is most commonly the result of meningeal seeding in candidemic patients. Predisposing risk factors for candidemia include the use of broad-spectrum antibiotics, the presence of indwelling devices such as vascular or urinary catheters, parenteral nutrition, ICU admission, prolonged hospital stay, and immune compromise. Specific risk factors for *Candida* CNS infection include ventricular shunts, trauma, neurosurgery, or lumbar puncture (43,44). *Candida albicans* is the most commonly isolated species; however, non-albicans species are becoming more prevalent, particularly in ICU populations.

Meningitis caused by protozoa or helminths are extremely rare. The free-living amoebas *Acanthamoeba, Balamuthia,* and *Naegleria fowleri* are associated with fresh water exposure. They are usually acquired by individuals diving into contaminated lakes or swimming pools. *N. fowleri* can cause a primary amoebic meningoencephalitis. *Acanthamoeba* and *Balamuthia* rarely cause meningitis; they commonly present as encephalitis. As for helminths, *Angiostrongylus cantonensis* (the rat lungworm) is the classic infectious cause of eosinophilic meningitis (>10% eosinophils in the CSF) (Table 86.3). Humans are incidental hosts and develop neurologic symptoms as a result of larval migration through the CNS. *A. cantonensis* is endemic in Southeast Asia and the Pacific Islands and is acquired by ingesting raw mollusks such as snails or slugs. *Gnathostoma spinigerum,* acquired by ingestion of raw and undercooked fish and poultry, is not primarily neurotropic like *A. cantonensis* but may also cause eosinophilic meningitis as a result of migration of larvae up nerve tracts to the CNS. Gnathostomiasis is endemic in Asia, especially Thailand and Japan, and more recently in Mexico. *Baylisascaris procyonis,* a roundworm infection of raccoons, rarely causes human eosinophilic meningoencephalitis following accidental ingestion of ova from raccoon feces in contaminated water, soil, or foods (45).

TABLE 86.3 Cerebrospinal Fluid Tests in Suspected CNS Infection

Routine Tests	Further Testing
Cell count and differential	Lactate
	Viral studies:
	Enterovirus, HSV, WNV, VZV NAT
	Influenza, EBV, CMV, HHV-6 NAT (selected cases; rare CNS infections)
Protein	AFB stain and Mycobacterial culture
	Mycobacterium tuberculosis NAT
Glucose (preferably with simultaneous serum glucose)	Cryptococcal antigen test (can send serum as well, sensitivity comparable to CSF)
Gram stain	Fungal culture and organism-specific NAT[a]
Bacterial culture and sensitivity	VDRL, FTA-Abs, *Treponema pallidum* NAT[a]
	Cytology
	Cytospin and flow cytometry if available
	Wet mount if PAM suspected
	Lyme-specific Ab and NAT[a]

CNS, central nervous system; NAT, nucleic acid amplification test; HSV, herpes simplex virus; WNV, West Nile virus; VZV, varicella zoster virus; AFB, acid-fast bacillus; CSF, cerebrospinal fluid; VDRL, Venereal Diseases Research Laboratory; FTA-Abs, fluorescent treponemal antibody absorption; PAM, primary amoebic meningoencephalitis.

[a]Experimental, available only in research laboratories.

DIAGNOSIS

Lumbar puncture (LP) should be performed emergently in all patients suspected of having bacterial meningitis unless contraindicated. Unnecessary delays are unfortunately common while neuroimaging is performed to exclude mass lesions. Complications associated with LP are uncommon but may include post-LP headache, infection, bleeding, radicular pain or paresthesias, back pain, and very rarely cerebral herniation (46). A study evaluating the clinical features at baseline associated with abnormal findings on computed tomography (CT) scan, and thus, increased risk of brain herniation, identified: age greater than or equal to 60 years; a history of CNS disease such as a mass lesion, stroke, or focal infection; immune compromise such as HIV or immunosuppressive therapy; a history of seizure within 1 week of presentation; and focal neurologic findings (47). Based on these findings, guidelines for which adult patients should undergo CT prior to LP have been recommended (Table 86.4) (48).

Nosocomial meningitis is rare in nonneurosurgical patients; nevertheless, LP is often performed in hospitalized patients with unexplained fever and/or decreased level of consciousness.

TABLE 86.4 Indications for Imaging Prior to Lumbar Puncture in Adults with Suspected Bacterial Meningitis

Impaired cellular immunity (Advanced HIV infection, immunosuppressive therapy, solid organ or hematopoietic stem cell transplantation)
History of CNS disease (mass lesion, stroke, or focal infection)
New-onset seizure (within 1 wk of presentation)
Papilledema
Abnormal level of consciousness
Focal neurologic deficit (dilated nonreactive pupil, abnormalities of ocular motility, abnormal visual fields, arm or leg drift)

HIV, human immunodeficiency virus; CNS, central nervous system.

The yield of performing an LP in the nonneurosurgical population is extremely low and of questionable utility.

CSF analysis is extremely important in the diagnosis of meningitis. Basic laboratory analyses, including cell count and differential, protein, glucose, Gram stain, and bacterial cultures, are most useful in distinguishing between viral, bacterial, tuberculous, and fungal infection (see Table 86.3).

Bacterial Meningitis

Bacterial meningitis usually presents with an elevated systemic white blood cell (WBC) count due to neutrophilia and left shift (immature forms such as bands and/or myeloids). Leukopenia is occasionally present in severe infection. Thrombocytopenia may be the result of sepsis, disseminated intravascular coagulation, or meningococcemia alone. Renal and hepatic dysfunction may occur as part of multiorgan failure in severe disease. Blood cultures should always be drawn prior to the administration of antimicrobials, particularly if an LP cannot be performed immediately and are positive in 50% to 80% of cases (3,12).

CSF analysis in bacterial meningitis classically reveals a neutrophilic pleocytosis with hundreds to thousands of cells and greater than 80% neutrophils. In fact, a low CSF WBC count is usually a marker of poor prognosis in this setting. The CSF glucose concentration is usually low and should always be compared with a simultaneous serum glucose measurement. An abnormal CSF-to-serum glucose ratio (<0.5) is common in bacterial meningitis—and is often much lower than 0.5. Acute illness in diabetics may increase serum glucose levels markedly, making the CSF-to-serum glucose ratio inaccurate. CSF lactate levels may be useful in distinguishing bacterial from aseptic meningitis (49–51). CSF protein and opening pressure are usually elevated in bacterial meningitis (Table 86.5).

Gram staining permits rapid identification of bacterial species—with a sensitivity of 60% to 90% and specificity of close to 100% in patients with bacterial meningitis (3,51). The

TABLE 86.5 Typical CSF Parameters in Patients with Meningitis

Etiology	WBC Count (cells/microL)	Predominant Cell Type	Protein (mg/dL)	Glucose (mg/dL)	Opening Pressure (cm H_2O)
Normal	0–5	Lymphocyte	15–40	50–75	8–20
Viral	10–500	Lymphocyte[a]	Normal	Normal	9–20
Bacterial	100–5,000	Neutrophil	>100	<40	20–30
Tuberculous	50– 00	Lymphocyte	>100	<40	18–30
Cryptococcal	20–500	Lymphocyte	50–200	<40	18–30

CSF, cerebrospinal fluid.

[a]Neutrophils may predominate in the first 24 hours.

Gram stain is more likely to be positive in patients with high bacterial loads. Gram-positive diplococci suggest *S. pneumoniae* infection, gram-negative diplococci suggest *N. meningitidis* infection, gram-positive rods suggest *L. monocytogenes* infection, and small pleomorphic coccobacilli suggest *H. influenzae* infection.

CSF bacterial cultures are positive in approximately 80% of cases (5,12). The yield decreases significantly in patients treated with antimicrobials prior to CSF collection. Antigen assays (latex agglutination tests) have been used in these cases, but due to their low sensitivity are no longer routinely offered by many laboratories. Broad-based NAT (52) and 16S rDNA-based gene sequencing (53) may be useful for the diagnosis of culture-negative meningitis.

Viral Meningitis

In acute viral meningitis, the CSF cell count is usually in the low hundreds with a lymphocytic predominance. A predominance of neutrophils may be seen in the first 24 hours of disease, occasionally confusing the diagnosis. The CSF glucose concentration is usually within normal range. CSF protein is often mildly elevated, and the opening pressure is usually normal.

Viral cultures and NAT are most commonly used in the diagnosis of viral meningitis, but NAT is more sensitive. Enteroviruses may be cultured from CSF, throat, or rectal swabs, however, CSF NAT testing is both more sensitive and specific. NAT for HSV is also widely available, and in HSV-1 encephalitis, HSV NAT demonstrated a specificity of 99% and sensitivity of 96% when CSF was studied between 48 hours and 10 days from symptom onset (54). False negatives occur mostly within the first 72 hours of infection. The diagnosis of WNV neuroinvasive disease can be made by detection of serum IgM or a fourfold rise in IgG between acute and convalescent titers. WNV NAT of serum and CSF are also available; however, the sensitivity is higher in CSF due to short-lived viremia in humans.

Other Less Common Causes

CSF analysis in syphilitic meningitis is characterized by a mild lymphocytic pleocytosis, decreased glucose, and elevated protein. *T. pallidum* cannot be cultured, so diagnosis must be made using alternate methods, predominantly serology. Direct visualization by darkfield microscopy or direct fluorescent antibody testing may be possible if a primary chancre or skin lesion of secondary syphilis—*condyloma latum* or mucous patch—is present. While *Treponema*-specific enzyme immunoassays (EIA) for IgM and IgG have largely replaced traditional serologic tests, CSF VDRL may be used in the diagnosis of syphilitic meningitis. The specificity is high, but false positives may occur in bloody specimens. The major limitation of CSF VDRL is its low sensitivity, so a negative result should not be used to rule out infection. CSF FTA-Abs is more sensitive; however, false positives are common due to serum antibody leak into the CSF. Last, NAT has been used to detect *T. pallidum* DNA in the CSF but lacks sensitivity and is not available in all centers (55–57).

Lyme meningitis is characterized by a mild lymphocytic pleocytosis, low glucose, and elevated protein. The CSF concentration of *B. burgdorferi* antibody, compared to serum levels, is a sensitive and specific diagnostic method. NAT is currently available only in research laboratories and does not differentiate between infection and remnant DNA from prior cured infection (58). CSF oligoclonal bands and *B. burgdorferi* culture are also available, but neither is sensitive or specific.

The CSF analysis in tuberculosis meningitis demonstrates a lymphocytic pleocytosis, low glucose, and markedly elevated protein and opening pressure. The elevation in protein is particularly marked in the setting of CSF block. Acid-fast bacillus (AFB) smears are generally low yield, but may be optimized by sending large volumes (10–15 mL) of CSF (59). Mycobacterial cultures, although slow growing—taking several weeks—become positive in approximately 70% of cases (59). DNA probes and NAT have recently become available with great improvements in sensitivity and specificity (60). Meningeal biopsy is rarely performed but may show caseating granulomata. Sputum and urine AFB, as well as mycobacterial blood cultures, should also be included as part of the TB workup in these patients. Since CSF AFB microscopy has very low sensitivity and cannot exclude the diagnosis of TB, in most cases the combination of increased WBCs and protein, decreased glucose and negative conventional cultures may be suggestive of TB meningitis, especially in a patient with epidemiologic risk factors for TB (i.e., foreign-born) or positive TST or IGRA, and should prompt consideration of empiric anti-TB therapy.

Cryptococcal meningitis is characterized by a lymphocytic pleocytosis, decreased glucose, and elevated protein. Opening pressures may be markedly elevated. Culture of *C. neoformans* or *C. gattii* from the CSF is diagnostic; however, other simpler tests are now available. Detection of serum or CSF cryptococcal antigen (CrAg) is highly sensitive (>90%) (61). India ink was previously regarded as the standard diagnostic test, but due to its low sensitivity it has been largely replaced by antigen testing. Fungal blood cultures may also be useful, as cryptococcal meningitis occasionally occurs in the setting of disseminated cryptococcal disease, especially in HIV-infected patients.

Other fungal meningitides are similarly characterized by a lymphocytic pleocytosis, low to normal glucose, and an elevated protein. Coccidioidal meningitis may present with an eosinophilic pleocytosis and peripheral eosinophilia. Fungal cultures are diagnostic and are most useful in *Candida* or *Aspergillus* infection. Dimorphic fungal infection may be diagnosed serologically, as isolating these organisms from the CSF is challenging and of low yield (62). Detection of complement-fixing (CF) IgG antibodies or immunodiffusion tests for IgM and IgG in CSF are currently the standard diagnostic tests. Low-titer false positives may occur in the setting of parameningeal foci. As well, false negatives may occur in early disease.

Primary amoebic meningoencephalitis due to *N. fowleri* results in a neutrophilic pleocytosis, increased red blood cells, low glucose, and an elevated protein. Demonstration of motile trophozoites on a wet mount of CSF or biopsy specimens is diagnostic. The diagnosis of *A. cantonensis, G. spinigerum,* or *B. procyonis* requires an appropriate epidemiologic exposure, peripheral blood eosinophilia, and a characteristic eosinophilic pleocytosis. Serologic tests are helpful but performed only in reference laboratories.

TREATMENT

The initial management of the patient with suspected meningitis is primarily guided by epidemiologic risk factors and

TABLE 86.6 Empiric Therapy of Bacterial Meningitis Based on Age and Host Factors

	Most Common Causes	Recommended Therapy
Age: Preterm to less than 1 mo	*Streptococcus agalactiae* *Escherichia coli* *Listeria monocytogenes*	Ampicillin + cefotaxime or ceftriaxone
Age: 1 mo to 50 yrs	*Streptococcus pneumoniae* *Neisseria meningitidis* *Haemophilus influenzae*	Cefotaxime or ceftriaxone + vancomycin + dexamethasone[a]
Age: greater than 50 yrs or alcoholism or other debilitating diseases or impaired cellular immunity	*S. pneumoniae* *L. monocytogenes* Coliform gram-negative bacilli	Ampicillin + cefotaxime or ceftriaxone + vancomycin + dexamethasone[a]
Postneurosurgery, neurotrauma, or cochlear implant	*S. pneumoniae* *Staphylococcus aureus* Coliform gram-negative bacilli *Pseudomonas aeruginosa*	Vancomycin + ceftazidime or cefepime or meropenem
Ventriculitis/meningitis due to infected shunt	Coagulase-negative Staphylococci *S. aureus* Coliform gram-negative bacilli Diphtheroids *Propionibacterium acnes*	Vancomycin + ceftazidime or meropenem

[a]Dexamethasone is efficacious in children with *H. influenzae* and in adults with *S. pneumoniae*. The first dose is to be given 15 to 20 minutes prior to or concomitant with first dose of antibiotic. Dose, 0.15 mg/kg IV every 6 hours for 2 to 4 days; discontinue if microorganism isolated other than listed above.

LP results. The CSF cell count, glucose, and Gram stain are crucial in guiding empiric therapy. If the LP is delayed for any reason, empiric antimicrobial therapy should not be withheld (Table 86.6), as delays in therapy have been associated with adverse clinical outcomes and increased mortality (63–65). The administration of antimicrobials should immediately follow blood culture collection and should not be delayed by neuroimaging or other tests performed prior to LP.

LP should be performed urgently in those with suspected meningitis. A protocol for the management of bacterial meningitis is presented in Figure 86.1. Imaging should be performed prior to LP in specific populations (see Table 86.4) but should not result in delays in antimicrobial therapy. Empiric therapy should be based on age, underlying host factors, and initial CSF Gram stain results, if available (see Table 86.6).

Bacterial Meningitis

The choice of antimicrobial therapy in bacterial meningitis is influenced by blood–CSF barrier penetration, effect of meningeal inflammation on penetration, and bactericidal efficacy. In general, CSF penetration is enhanced in the setting of meningeal inflammation due to increased permeability. Additionally, high lipid solubility, low molecular weight, and low protein binding increase CSF drug levels. Bactericidal efficacy may be decreased in purulent CSF, particularly with aminoglycosides, due to low pH. Penicillins, third-generation cephalosporins, carbapenems, fluoroquinolones, and rifampin achieve high CSF levels and each are bactericidal. While antimicrobials may need to be adjusted based on renal and hepatic function, the doses that follow all assume normal renal function. Therapeutic drug monitoring may be required to ensure adequate levels and prevent toxicity (e.g., vancomycin, aminoglycosides). Antimicrobial therapy should also be adjusted based on culture and susceptibility results as soon as possible (Table 86.7). In suspected meningococcal or *H. influenzae* meningitis, droplet isolation (single room, gowns, gloves, surgical masks, eye protection and dedicated equipment) should be enforced until 24 hours of effective antimicrobial therapy have been completed or an alternate diagnosis is reached. Isolation in other cases of meningitis, including pneumococcal meningitis, is not required.

Streptococcus pneumoniae

Empiric therapy guidelines for pneumococcal meningitis have been recently modified due to increasing penicillin resistance (66–68). *S. pneumoniae* was once uniformly susceptible to penicillin; however, mutations in penicillin-binding proteins have resulted in varying levels of resistance. Empiric therapy therefore consists of a third-generation cephalosporin and vancomycin until susceptibility results become available (48). The recommendation to add vancomycin, however, is based only on a handful of pneumococcal meningitis cases demonstrating third-generation cephalosporin resistance (minimum inhibitory concentration [MIC] ≥2 μg/mL). It should also be noted that vancomycin penetrates the CSF poorly, particularly when dexamethasone is administered concomitantly, so aggressive dosing is required to achieve target trough serum concentrations. Once MICs are available, therapy should be adjusted accordingly. For isolates with penicillin MIC less than 0.06 μg/mL, penicillin G (4 million units IV every 4 hours) or ampicillin (2 g IV every 4 hours) should be used. For isolates with a penicillin MIC of 0.12 μg/mL or higher and ceftriaxone MIC below 1 μg/mL, treatment with a third-generation cephalosporin should be continued; either cefotaxime (2 g IV every 6 hours) or ceftriaxone (2 g IV every 12 hours). For isolates with a ceftriaxone MIC greater than or equal to 1 μg/mL, vancomycin and a third-generation cephalosporin are the recommended therapy; some clinicians administer very high doses of third-generation cephalosporins in these cases. Vancomycin should be dosed 15 to 20 mg/kg/dose (based on actual body weight) every 8 to 12 hours. Subsequent dosing should be adjusted based on serum trough vancomycin concentrations (between 15 and 20 μg/mL). A loading dose of 25 to 30 mg/kg (maximum 2 g) may be used to rapidly achieve target concentrations. Meropenem is a reasonable alternative to the above agents and does not carry the theoretical risk of decreasing seizure threshold as with imipenem. The efficacy of linezolid,

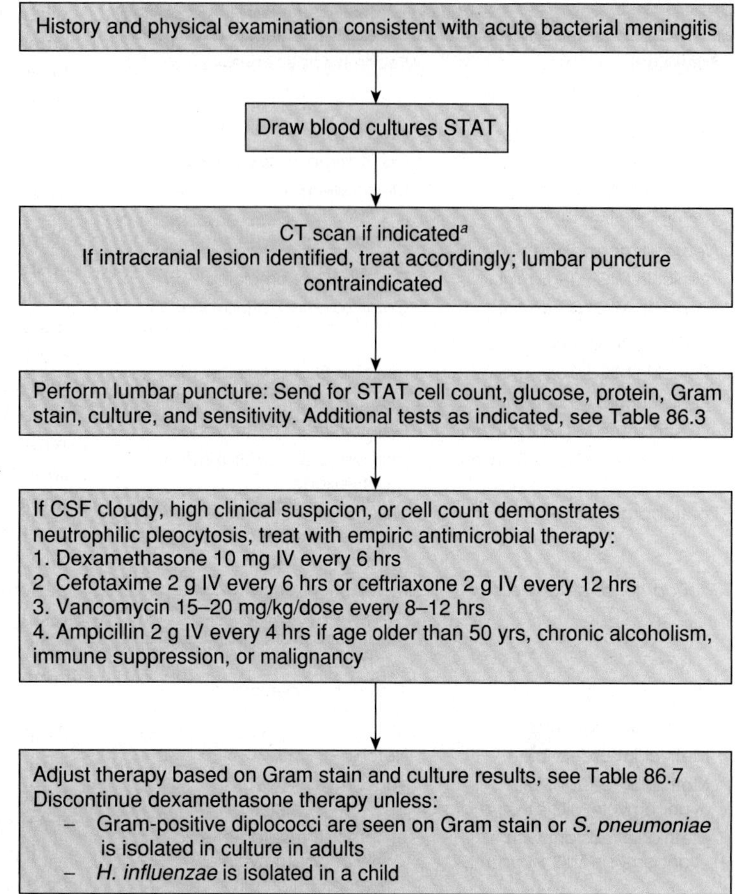

History and physical examination consistent with acute bacterial meningitis
Draw blood cultures STAT
CT scan if indicated[a]
If intracranial lesion identified, treat accordingly; lumbar puncture contraindicated
Perform lumbar puncture: Send for STAT cell count, glucose, protein, Gram stain, culture, and sensitivity. Additional tests as indicated, see Table 86.3
If CSF cloudy, high clinical suspicion, or cell count demonstrates neutrophilic pleocytosis, treat with empiric antimicrobial therapy:
1. Dexamethasone 10 mg IV every 6 hrs
2 Cefotaxime 2 g IV every 6 hrs or ceftriaxone 2 g IV every 12 hrs
3. Vancomycin 15–20 mg/kg/dose every 8–12 hrs
4. Ampicillin 2 g IV every 4 hrs if age older than 50 yrs, chronic alcoholism, immune suppression, or malignancy
Adjust therapy based on Gram stain and culture results, see Table 86.7
Discontinue dexamethasone therapy unless:
– Gram-positive diplococci are seen on Gram stain or S. pneumoniae is isolated in culture in adults
– H. influenzae is isolated in a child
[a]Indications: decreased mental status, focal neurologic deficits, history of CNS disease (mass lesion, stroke, or focal infection), papilledema, new-onset seizure (within 1 week of presentation), impaired cellular immunity.

FIGURE 86.1 Bacterial meningitis protocol.

daptomycin, dalbavancin, and telavancin may be promising for the treatment of highly resistant pneumococcal strains (69,70). Antimicrobial treatment duration is 10 to 14 days. Dexamethasone should be administered prior to or with the first dose of antimicrobial.

Neisseria meningitidis

The empiric treatment of meningococcal meningitis should be a third-generation cephalosporin: cefotaxime (2 g IV every 6 hours) or ceftriaxone (2 g IV every 12 hours); however, therapy should be stepped down to penicillin if susceptibility is confirmed. The duration of treatment is 7 days. Chloramphenicol (25 mg/kg, to a maximum of 1 g IV every 6 hours) is a reasonable alternative in the β-lactam–allergic patient. Meropenem (2 g IV every 8 hours) is another alternative, although there may be cross-reactivity in penicillin-allergic patients. Dexamethasone is not indicated in confirmed meningococcal meningitis.

Haemophilus influenzae

Empiric therapy for *H. influenzae* meningitis is a third-generation cephalosporin. Therapy can be narrowed to ampicillin, 2 g IV every 4 hours if susceptibility is confirmed. A total of 7 days of therapy is recommended. Dexamethasone should be administered as adjunctive therapy in children (71).

Listeria monocytogenes

L. monocytogenes meningitis should be treated with ampicillin 2 g IV every 4 hours. Gentamicin may be added for antimicrobial synergy, but aminoglycosides have poor penetration into CSF and have significant toxicities. When used, gentamicin should be administered as a 2 mg/kg loading dose, followed by 1.7 mg/kg every 8 hours. Trimethoprim/sulfamethoxazole (TMP/SMX), 20 mg/kg/day of the trimethoprim component, divided into 6 to 12 hourly doses, may be used in penicillin-allergic patients. Alternate therapies include meropenem and, potentially, linezolid and rifampin. Third-generation cephalosporins have no activity against *L. monocytogenes*. Treatment duration is 14 to 21 days.

Aerobic Gram-Negative Bacilli

Aerobic gram-negative bacilli should be treated empirically with a third-generation cephalosporin or meropenem. Susceptibility results should guide therapy in consultation with an infectious diseases specialist. For *Pseudomonas aeruginosa* infections, ceftazidime or cefepime, 2 g IV every 8 hours, or meropenem, 2 g IV every 8 hours, with tobramycin 2 mg/kg IV every 8 hours, should be used. Ciprofloxacin or aztreonam are acceptable alternatives if the isolate is susceptible. The duration of therapy is prolonged, generally 21 days.

TABLE 86.7 Specific Therapy of Bacterial Meningitis

Bacterium	Recommended Therapy
Haemophilus influenzae	
β-Lactamase negative	Ampicillin
β-Lactamase positive	Cefotaxime or ceftriaxone
β-Lactamase negative, ampicillin resistant	Meropenem
Neisseria meningitidis	
Penicillin MIC <0.1 μg/mL	Penicillin G or ampicillin
Penicillin MIC ≥0.1 μg/mL	Cefotaxime or ceftriaxone
Streptococcus pneumoniae	
Penicillin MIC ≤0.06 μg/mL	Penicillin G or ampicillin
Penicillin MIC ≥0.12 μg/mL	
Ceftriaxone MIC <0.1 μg/mL	Cefotaxime or ceftriaxone
Ceftriaxone MIC ≥1.0 μg/mL	Vancomycin + cefotaxime or ceftriaxone
Enterobacteriaceae	Cefotaxime or ceftriaxone unless member of SPICEM group[a]
Pseudomonas aeruginosa	Meropenem or ceftazidime or cefepime or aztreonam or ciprofloxacin PLUS tobramycin
Listeria monocytogenes	Ampicillin or penicillin G
Staphylococcus aureus	
Methicillin-susceptible	Nafcillin
Methicillin-resistant with vancomycin MIC ≤1 μg/mL	Vancomycin
Methicillin-resistant with vancomycin MIC >1 μg/mL	Trimethoprim/sulfamethoxazole or daptomycin or linezolid ± rifampin if susceptible
Prosthesis associated	Consider adding rifampin to above choices
Coagulase-negative Staphylococci	Vancomycin
Prosthesis associated	Consider adding rifampin
Streptococcus agalactiae	Ampicillin or penicillin G

MIC, minimum inhibitory concentration.
[a]SPICEM group: includes *Serratia marcescens*, *Providencia*, indole-positive *Proteus* (*P. vulgaris of penneri*), *Citrobacter freundii* group, *Enterobacter* spp, and *Morganella morganii*. These microorganisms carry chromosomal, inducible β-lactamases (ampC), which are capable of inactivating third-generation cephalosporin even if reported to be susceptible. Carbapenems (meropenem has greatest cerebrospinal fluid penetration), fluoroquinolones, or trimethoprim/sulfamethoxazole may be used, if susceptible.

Staphylococcus aureus

Staphylococcal meningitis therapy depends on methicillin susceptibility. Methicillin-susceptible strains should be treated with nafcillin 2 g IV every 4 hours, whereas methicillin-resistant (MRSA) strains should be treated with vancomycin, 15 to 20 mg/kg/dose IV every 8 to 12 hours. Subsequent vancomycin dosing should be adjusted based on serum trough vancomycin concentrations (goal trough 15 to 20 μg/mL). A loading dose of 25 to 30 mg/kg (maximum 2 g) may be used to rapidly achieve target concentrations. Vancomycin is also recommended in patients with serious penicillin allergies. Infected prosthetic material should be removed if possible and antimicrobial therapy continued for 14 days minimum after removal. If removal is not possible, rifampin may be added; however, cure rates are poor with hardware retention. Linezolid, TMP/SMX, daptomycin, telavancin, and dalbavancin may be used as alternate therapies in MRSA meningitis when vancomycin cannot be used or is ineffective (including circumstances of "MIC creep", when vancomycin MIC >1 μg/mL), however further studies are needed to establish efficacy of these agents. Tigecycline should not be used as therapeutic CSF concentrations are not achieved with standard therapy.

Adjunctive Therapies

Adjunctive therapies in bacterial meningitis include corticosteroids, procedures to reduce intracranial pressure, and surgery. Corticosteroid therapy aims to decrease the inflammatory response while allowing antimicrobial therapy to eradicate infection. Although corticosteroid administration may decrease CSF penetration and bactericidal activity of antimicrobials, randomized controlled trials demonstrate benefit with its use (12). In children, the administration of dexamethasone has demonstrated a reduction in the incidence of hearing impairment and severe neurologic complications in *H. influenzae* meningitis (71–73). Adjunctive corticosteroid therapy has also been evaluated in adults, showing a mortality benefit in patients with pneumococcal meningitis (12,72). Based on these results, treatment recommendations suggest dexamethasone, 0.15 mg/kg, be given 10 to 20 minutes before, or at least concomitant with, the first dose of antimicrobial therapy and continued every 6 hours. Dexamethasone should be administered to all patients with suspected bacterial meningitis until Gram stain or culture results are available. Therapy should be continued for 2 to 4 days only if the Gram stain or cultures demonstrate *H. influenzae* in children or *S. pneumoniae* in adults.

Placement of an intracranial pressure monitoring device may be beneficial for patients with bacterial meningitis and elevated intracranial pressure (ICP). Admission to an ICU with expertise in ICP monitoring and management of intracranial hypertension is most appropriate (74). Standard measures—such as CSF drainage, fluid and sodium management, optimization of cerebral perfusion pressure, sedation, temperature control, hyperventilation, and osmotic therapies—should be employed in patients with high ICP (75). Transcranial Doppler ultrasonography and continuous electroencephalography (EEG) monitoring should be applied where possible. Decompressive craniectomy may be considered in patients when maximal medical ICP treatment fails to reduce severe intracranial hypertension. Other surgical interventions may be required, for example, those with basal skull fractures with persistent CSF leaks or dural defects.

Complications

Complications of bacterial meningitis can be divided into neurologic and nonneurologic complications. Neurologic complications include seizures, cerebral edema or infarction, cranial nerve palsies, venous sinus thrombosis, brain abscess, subdural empyema, and coma. Late complications include hearing impairment, obstructive hydrocephalus, learning disabilities, sensory and motor deficits, mental retardation, cortical blindness, and seizures. Nonneurologic complications include septic shock, coagulopathy, and the syndrome of inappropriate antidiuretic hormone secretion (SIADH).

Viral Meningitis

In general, the treatment for viral meningitis is supportive given its benign and self-limited course. Pleconaril has been evaluated for enteroviral meningitis with modest benefit, but remains experimental (76,77). Intravenous immune globulin has been used in agammaglobulinemic patients with chronic enteroviral meningitis. No specific therapy exists for arboviruses, mumps, or LCM. HIV-associated meningitis should be treated with combination antiretroviral therapy.

It is not clear whether antiviral treatment alters the course of HSV meningitis; nevertheless, primary episodes of genital herpes should be treated as per guidelines. Some physicians extend therapy to 14 days with concomitant meningitis. Intravenous acyclovir, dosed 5 mg/kg every 8 hours, has been used in severe disease. Therapy can be stepped down to an oral agent on discharge. Ganciclovir is the treatment of choice for CMV meningitis in immune-compromised hosts.

Other Less Common Etiologies

Syphilitic meningitis does not respond to benzathine penicillin, which is used to treat most forms of syphilis; it requires a 2-week course of high-dose IV penicillin G: 4 million units every 4 hours. Rapid plasma reagin (RPR) titers should be monitored after therapy, and repeat CSF examination should be performed if titers do not decline by fourfold at 6 months after therapy. All HIV patients with syphilitic meningitis should have repeat LP at 6 months following therapy. Patients with penicillin allergy should undergo desensitization, as there are no proven effective alternative therapies for syphilitic meningitis.

The treatment of Lyme meningitis is achieved with ceftriaxone, 2 g daily, or cefotaxime, 2 g IV every 8 hours for 14 to 28 days. Alternate therapy is penicillin, 4 million units every 4 hours, for 14 to 28 days.

The treatment of tuberculous meningitis depends largely on the expected resistance pattern based on country of acquisition and results of susceptibility testing; consultation with an infectious diseases specialist is strongly recommended. In general, standard combination therapy includes isoniazid (INH), rifampin, pyrazinamide, and a fourth drug, either a fluoroquinolone or an injectable aminoglycoside. Ethambutol penetrates CSF poorly and has been largely replaced by fluoroquinolones. If the isolate is fully susceptible, treatment can be narrowed to INH and RIF alone. For drug-resistant TB, therapy should be prescribed by infectious diseases and/or TB services. Treatment should be continued for a minimum of 12 months but may be prolonged for concomitant tuberculoma or in multi–drug-resistant infection. Adjunctive therapy with dexamethasone for the first 2 months has been shown to decrease mortality as well as neurologic deficits and is recommended (78). Pyridoxine, 25 to 50 mg daily, may be administered to prevent INH-related neuropathy.

Therapy for fungal meningitis is complicated by the lack of standardized susceptibility testing and interpretation for many fungi. The area of antifungal therapy, however, is an evolving area with an increasing number of antifungal agents from which to choose.

Cryptococcal meningitis should be treated with a 14-day induction phase of liposomal amphotericin B, 3 to 5 mg/kg/day IV, with or without flucytosine, 100 mg/kg/day PO dosed every 6 hours. Conventional amphotericin B (deoxycholate) may still be used instead of lipid formulations, however, few patients tolerate this therapy. Consolidation therapy with fluconazole, 400 to 800 mg (6 to 12 mg/kg) daily, should be continued for 8 weeks following induction. Maintenance (or suppressive) therapy with fluconazole, 200 mg per day, should be continued in organ transplant recipients for 6 to 12 months or patients with HIV/AIDS until immune reconstitution is achieved. Cryptococcal meningitis may require initial daily therapeutic LPs, an external ventricular drain, or a ventriculoperitoneal shunt to relieve increased intracranial pressure. Echinocandins, such as caspofungin, micafungin, and anidulafungin are not active in cryptococcosis.

The treatment for coccidioidal meningitis is oral fluconazole, 400 mg/day. Some clinicians initiate therapy with a higher dose of 800 mg/day or may add intrathecal amphotericin B. Treatment must be continued lifelong, as relapses are frequently lethal. Newer azoles such as voriconazole or posaconazole may be tried in patients who are refractory to fluconazole, however evidence to support this is limited.

Therapy for *H. capsulatum* meningitis consists of liposomal amphotericin B or amphotericin B deoxycholate. Fluconazole, 800 mg/day, for an additional 9 to 12 months, may be used to prevent relapse. If relapse does occur, long-term therapy with fluconazole or intraventricular amphotericin B is recommended.

For candidal meningitis, the preferred initial therapy is IV liposomal amphotericin B 3 to 5 mg/kg/day, with or without flucytosine, 25 mg/kg dosed every 6 hours and adjusted to maintain serum levels of 40 to 60 μg/mL. Fluconazole therapy, in susceptible species, may be used for follow-up or suppressive therapy. The duration of therapy is at least 4 weeks after resolution of symptoms. All prosthetic material must be removed to achieve cure.

Primary amoebic meningoencephalitis caused by *N. fowleri* is usually fatal. A few cases have had good outcomes with early diagnosis and treatment with high-dose intravenous and intrathecal amphotericin B, rifampicin and steroids to control cerebral edema. Fluconazole, miltefosine, and azithromycin may be additionally prescribed. Eosinophilic meningitis caused by *A. cantonensis* and *G. spinigerum* are treated supportively. Corticosteroids are recommended to decrease the inflammatory response to intracranial larvae. Antihelminthic therapy is relatively contraindicated, as clinical deterioration and death may occur following severe inflammatory reactions to dying larvae.

PREVENTION

Chemoprophylaxis (medications) and immunoprophylaxis (vaccines) are available to prevent infection in close contacts of cases or during outbreaks. Temporary nasopharyngeal carriage with *H. influenzae, N. meningitidis,* and *S. pneumoniae* may occur following exposure to an index case and is a risk factor for the development of invasive disease. Chemoprophylaxis is recommended to eliminate nasopharyngeal carriage in individuals at risk.

Prophylaxis is indicated in selected household/close contacts (those having more than 4 hours < 3 feet from the index case), and child-care or preschool contacts within 5 to 7 days before onset of disease, of cases of *H. influenzae* type b. The recommended therapy is rifampin, 20 mg/kg (usual adult dose of 600 mg daily) for four doses, and should be guided by your local public health department.

Prophylaxis for *N. meningitidis* is also recommended for close contacts of cases. This includes intimate contacts (e.g., kissing) and close contacts with greater than or equal to 4 hours of contact 1 week prior to the onset of illness. Most close contacts include housemates, child-care center contacts, cellmates, and/or military recruits. Medical personnel exposed to oropharyngeal secretions during intubation, nasotracheal suctioning, or mouth-to-mouth resuscitation should also receive chemoprophylaxis. Rifampin, 600 mg orally every 12 hours for a total of four doses, or single doses of ciprofloxacin (500 mg orally) or ceftriaxone (250 mg intramuscularly) are all efficacious. It is recommended that ciprofloxacin be avoided in children younger than 16 years of age and in pregnant women, based on joint cartilage injury demonstrated in animal studies. Chemoprophylaxis is not indicated in *S. pneumoniae* infection.

Vaccination is available for the prevention of *H. influenzae* serogroup b, *N. meningitidis,* and *S. pneumoniae* infections and is part of routine childhood immunization. Unvaccinated children 2 years of age or younger, exposed to an index case, should receive chemoprophylaxis and vaccination.

S. pneumoniae vaccination is available in two preparations: the 23-valent polysaccharide (PPSV23) vaccine and the 13-valent conjugate (PCV13) vaccine. The conjugate vaccine is recommended routinely in all children 23 months of age or less. Adults at high risk of invasive disease—sickle cell disease and other hemoglobinopathies, functional or anatomic asplenia, HIV infection, immune compromise, and chronic medical conditions—and all patients over 65 years of age should receive both PPSV23 and PCV13. Additional specific vaccine recommendations have been published by the United States Advisory Committee on Immunization Practices (79–81). *S. pneumoniae* vaccination is not indicated as postexposure prophylaxis.

Several different meningococcal vaccines are available in the United States, including both conjugate and polysaccharide vaccines. Conjugate vaccines are preferred due to superior immunogenicity. Quadrivalent and monovalent vaccines are available and should be offered to high-risk populations, including those with specific immune deficiencies (see Table 86.2), those traveling to endemic and epidemic regions, laboratory workers routinely exposed to *N. meningitidis,* first-year college students living in dormitories, and military recruits. Vaccination during outbreaks of meningococcal disease due to a serogroup contained in a vaccine should be performed in consultation with public health authorities. A pentavalent meningococcal vaccine is currently under development (82).

ENCEPHALITIS

Encephalitis is defined as inflammation of the brain parenchyma. Although encephalitis and meningitis may present with similar clinical findings, the two syndromes are pathophysiologically distinct. The major distinguishing feature is the presence or absence of normal brain function. Patients with meningitis may be drowsy or lethargic but should have normal cerebral function, whereas those with encephalitis generally have altered mental status. Occasionally patients may present with a combination of findings in an overlap syndrome of meningoencephalitis. It is important to distinguish between the two syndromes, as the etiologic agents and treatments may differ.

Encephalitis is most commonly viral or postinfectious (Table 86.8). Viral encephalitis is caused by direct viral invasion of the CNS whereas postinfectious encephalitis is an immune-mediated process. Unfortunately, it may be difficult to differentiate between the two; however, encephalitis with resolving infectious symptoms suggests a postviral cause. The most common viruses causing postinfectious encephalitis include mumps, measles, varicella zoster virus (VZV), rubella, and influenza.

PATHOPHYSIOLOGY

Access to the CNS is highly virus-specific and occurs via hematogenous or neuronal routes. In hematogenous invasion, viral infection is acquired at an initial site of entry, with primary site replication, transient viremia, and CNS seeding. Retrograde transport within motor and sensory axons to the CNS occurs in the neuronal route of entry. After CNS entry, viruses enter neural cells, causing inflammation and cell dysfunction. Clinical manifestations are the result of specific cell-type invasion. Oligodendroglial cell invasion causes demyelination, whereas cortical invasion results in altered mental status, and neuronal invasion may result in focal or generalized seizures. Thus, focal pathology is the result of specific neural tropism.

Herpes simplex encephalitis (HSE) is the most common cause of sporadic encephalitis in Western countries, accounting for 20% to 40% of cases (83,84). HSE is caused by type 1 virus in greater than 90% of cases, occurs year-round, and affects all age groups. Two-thirds of cases are due to reactivation of the virus in the trigeminal ganglion, with retrograde transport along the olfactory tract to the orbitofrontal and mediotemporal lobes. Untreated HSE has a mortality rate up to 70%, and almost all survivors suffer neurologic sequelae (85,86). Outcomes correlate strongly with the severity of disease at presentation, as well as the time to initiation of antiviral therapy. Other herpes viruses, such as VZV and HHV-6 can rarely cause encephalitis; however they generally affect immune-compromised patients. VZV encephalitis may occur with or without concomitant cutaneous lesions.

Arboviruses are acquired via vector exposure, mainly mosquitoes and ticks. These include EEE, WEE, St. Louis encephalitis, VEE, California encephalitis (caused in most cases by La Crosse virus), Japanese encephalitis, yellow fever, and WNV. Arbovirus-related encephalitides are geographically specific and most prevalent during the summer and early fall months when mosquitoes and ticks are most active.

West Nile virus, first identified in North America in 1999, causes neuroinvasive disease in less than 1% of exposed individuals. It is, however, now the most commonly diagnosed arboviral CNS infection in the United States (87). Neuroinvasive disease most frequently manifests as encephalitis and occurs in those with comorbid disease (88) such as diabetes mellitus, hypertension, renal disease, malignancy, organ transplantation, alcoholism, and advanced age (89–91). Muscle weakness and flaccid paralysis may present concurrently in patients with encephalitis.

Rabies, a zoonotic disease that requires contact with infected animals, should be considered in all cases of encephalitis. Once CNS infection is established, however, the mortality is essentially 100% although survival with aggressive therapy has recently been described (92,93). Rabies can be acquired from many sources including dogs, cats, raccoons, bats, and

TABLE 86.8 Most Common Viral Causes of Encephalitis, Their Vectors or Animal Hosts, and Geographic Distributions

Viral Cause	Vector or Animal Host	Geographic Distribution
Alpha viruses	Mosquitoes	
Eastern equine (EEE)	*Culiseta melanura*	New England
Western equine (WEE)	*Culex tarsalis*	West of Mississippi River
Venezuelan equine (VEE)	*Culex* spp	South and Central America
Flaviviruses	Mosquitoes or ticks	
St. Louis	*Culex* spp	Throughout the United States
West Nile (WNV)	*Culex pipiens* and *tarsalis*	Americas, Africa, Asia, Middle East, Europe
Japanese	*Culex tritaeniorhynchus*	Asia and SE Asia
Murray Valley	*Culex* and *Aedes* spp	Western Australia
Tick-borne Powassan virus Louping ill virus	*Ixodes ricinus* and *persulcatus* ticks	Russia, Central Europe, China, North America, British Isles
Herpes viruses Herpes simplex virus (HSV-1) Varicella zoster virus (VZV) Cytomegalovirus (CMV) Epstein–Barr virus (EBV) Human herpesviruses 6, 7	N/A	Worldwide
Enteroviruses Polioviruses Coxsackieviruses Echoviruses	N/A	Worldwide
Adenoviruses	N/A	Worldwide
Human immunodeficiency virus (HIV)	N/A	Worldwide; particularly high prevalence in sub-Saharan Africa, Central and Southeast Asia, Eastern Europe
Rabies	Dogs, cats, raccoons, wolves, foxes, bats	Worldwide
Colorado tick fever	*Dermacentor andersoni* tick	Western United States and Canada
Mumps	N/A	Unvaccinated populations worldwide
Measles	N/A	Unvaccinated populations worldwide

N/A, not applicable.

foxes. The history of an animal bite, although useful if present, is absent in most cases of rabies.

Nonviral causes of encephalitis include bacterial, rickettsial, fungal, and parasitic infections. Bacterial causes include *Mycoplasma, L. monocytogenes, B. burgdorferi* (Lyme disease), *Leptospira* spp., *Brucella, Legionella, Nocardia, T. pallidum* (syphilis), *Salmonella typhi,* mycobacterial species, *Coxiella burnetii* (Q-fever), and Ehrlichiae. The most common rickettsial species include *Rickettsia rickettsii* (Rocky Mountain spotted fever) and *Rickettsia typhi* (endemic typhus). Fungal causes include *Cryptococcus* spp, *Aspergillus* spp, *Candida, Coccidioides immitis, H. capsulatum,* and *B. dermatitidis.* Finally, *Trypanosoma brucei* complex (African sleeping sickness), malaria, *Toxoplasma gondii, Echinococcus granulosus,* and *Schistosoma* species can cause encephalitis but require epidemiologic exposures or specific risk factors. For example, toxoplasma encephalitis is most common in advanced HIV disease.

DIAGNOSIS

Clinical findings of encephalitis include the classic triad of fever, headache, and altered mental status. The onset of symptoms may be acute, subacute, or chronic; the acuity and severity of symptoms at presentation correlate with prognosis. Encephalitic symptoms may be preceded by a viral prodrome consisting of fever, headache, nausea, vomiting, lethargy, and myalgias.

Disorientation, amnesia, behavioral and speech changes, movement disorders, and focal or diffuse neurologic abnormalities such as hemiparesis, cranial nerve palsies, or seizures are common on presentation; neck stiffness and photophobia may also be noted. VZV, EBV, CMV, measles, and mumps may present with rash, lymphadenopathy, and hepatosplenomegaly. HSE incidence is unrelated to a history of oral or genital lesions.

Laboratory findings may include peripheral leukocytosis or leukopenia. While CSF examination usually reveals a pleocytosis with lymphocytic predominance, neutrophilic predominance may be present early in infection. Red blood cells, in the absence of a traumatic tap, are suggestive of HSV but may be seen in other necrotizing viral encephalitides. Protein levels are usually elevated, and glucose may be normal or slightly decreased. Because viral cultures are rarely positive, molecular methods have become the diagnostic tests of choice. CSF HSV DNA NAT is both sensitive and specific (98% and 94%, respectively) when compared to brain biopsy (94,95), is often positive within the first 24 hours of symptom onset, and remains positive during the first week of antiviral therapy. NAT is available for WNV, VZV, enteroviruses, adenoviruses, rabies, CMV, EBV, and HHV-6 in most reference laboratories. Serology may be diagnostic if IgM is detected or a fourfold rise in acute and convalescent IgG titers is demonstrated. Corneal or neck (posterior, at the hairline) biopsies and saliva NAT can be diagnostic for rabies. Brain biopsy may be considered in patients with encephalitis if all other tests are nondiagnostic.

Other investigations that may aid in diagnosis include EEG, CT, or magnetic resonance imaging (MRI). EEG is particularly helpful in HSE, showing characteristic focal changes (spiked and slow wave patterns) from the temporal regions in greater than 80% of patients. MRI is the most sensitive imaging modality at detecting early viral encephalitis and may show virus-specific changes (e.g., temporal lobe changes in HSE). CT scans are more available on an urgent basis and are useful in ruling out space-occupying lesions; however, they are rarely able to visualize encephalitic changes. Single photon emission computed tomography (SPECT) imaging has also been used in the diagnosis of HSE (96).

TREATMENT

Unfortunately there are few specific therapies for viral encephalitis. Treatment of HSE with acyclovir, 10 mg/kg IV every 8 hours, is the main exception. Treatment should be initiated as soon as possible, as delays in therapy correlate with mortality. Therapy should be started empirically in all patients with encephalitis until confirmatory testing is available, given the dramatic effect on outcome. Acyclovir should also be considered in VZV encephalitis even though data regarding efficacy are only anecdotal. Supportive ICU care, including intubation and mechanical ventilation, may be required. Ganciclovir—or foscarnet for ganciclovir-resistant strains—is used to treat CMV encephalitis. The role of antivirals for EBV and HHV-6 encephalitides is unproven, but ganciclovir or foscarnet should be considered.

Outcomes are related to multiple factors including host age and immune response, organism virulence, and time to effective therapy. Poor outcomes are more common in younger (<1 year of age) and older (>55 years of age) populations. HSE, Japanese encephalitis, and EEE have the highest mortality rates. HSE mortality approaches 70% without therapy but can be reduced to 10% to 30% with early antiviral treatment (86,96–99). Most patients with HSE recover with significant neurologic deficits (paresis, seizures, cognitive and memory deficits).

BRAIN ABSCESS

Brain abscess is an uncommon but potentially life-threatening infection. Characterized by localized intracranial suppurative collections, brain abscesses are usually the result of direct extension of infection (20%–60%) or hematogenous spread. Mortality rates with treatment have decreased dramatically over the past 60 years with advances in imaging, antimicrobials, and neurosurgical therapies (16). Infection begins as a localized area of cerebritis, with subsequent central necrosis, suppuration, and fibrous capsule formation (Table 86.9).

Solitary abscesses are usually the result of contiguous infection including otitis, mastoiditis, frontal or ethmoid sinusitis, or dental infection. Bullet fragments or other foreign bodies may serve as a nidus of infection and develop into abscesses even years after primary injury. Postneurosurgical brain abscesses may also present in a delayed fashion. Multiple abscesses are more commonly the result of hematogenous seeding from chronic pulmonary, endocardial, skin, intra-abdominal, or pelvic infections. A primary site or underlying condition cannot be identified in 20% to 40% of patients with brain abscess.

TABLE 86.9 Risk Factors for Brain Abscess

Otic infection (otitis media, mastoiditis)
Sinusitis (frontal, ethmoid, sphenoid)
Dental infection
Neurosurgical intervention or neurotrauma
Bacterial endocarditis
Neutropenia
Immune compromise (HIV infection, immunosuppressive therapy, solid organ or hematopoietic stem cell transplantation)
Chronic lung infection (abscess, bronchiectasis, empyema)
Congenital heart disease

HIV, human immunodeficiency virus.

The location of brain abscess may be suggestive of the source. Temporal lobe (Fig. 86.2) or cerebellar abscesses commonly result from otic infections, frontal lobe abscesses (Fig. 86.3) from sinusitis or dental infection, and abscesses in the distribution of the middle cerebral artery from hematogenous seeding.

The microbiology of brain abscesses is diverse and depends on the primary site of infection, patient age, and underlying host factors (100). Common aerobic species include streptococci (viridans, anginosus group, and microaerophilic species), which are isolated in up to a third of cases (16,101,102). Aerobic gram-negative bacilli—commonly *Klebsiella pneumoniae, Pseudomonas* spp, *E. coli,* and *Proteus* spp—and *S. aureus*

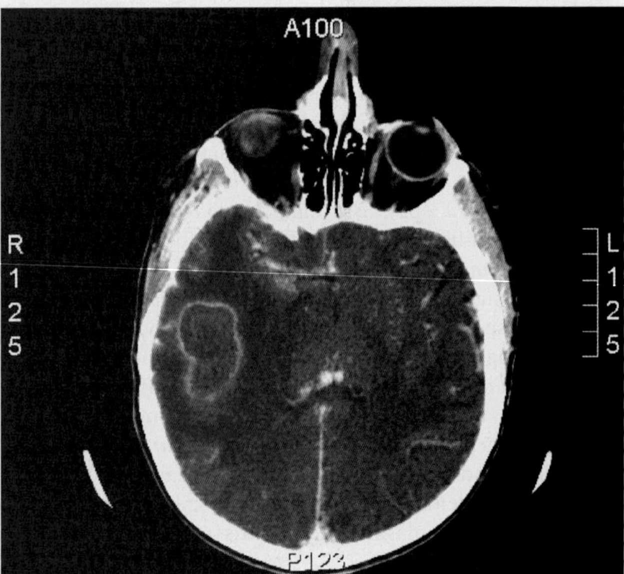

FIGURE 86.2 Axial contrast CT scan of a right temporal lobe abscess. This 36-year-old patient with cyanotic heart disease underwent a previous right craniotomy for subdural hematoma evacuation. Because of the presence of a pacemaker, an MRI could not be performed. The image shows a 3.8- × 2.4-cm abscess in the posterior right temporal lobe underlying the previously noted right craniotomy. Decreased central attenuation of the lesion and surrounding vasogenic edema with uncal and subfalcine herniation are noted. There is no hydrocephalus. Abscess cultures grew *Staphylococcus aureus.*

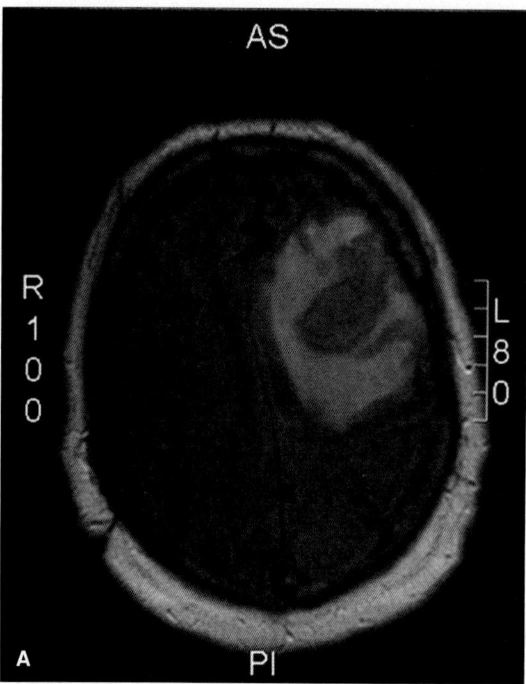

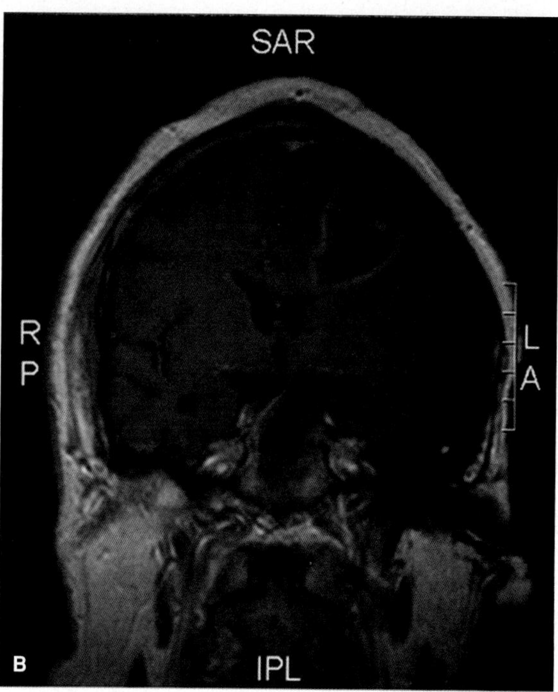

FIGURE 86.3 Axial and coronal MRI images of a frontal brain abscess. This 59-year-old diabetic male presented with a 10-day history of confusion, headache, right upper extremity weakness, as well as a generalized tonic–clonic seizure. Axial T2 FLAIR (**A**) and coronal T1 postgadolinium MRI (**B**) images are shown above demonstrating a 3.4- × 3.4- × 4.3-cm intra-axial frontal lobe abscess with surrounding edema and mass effect. An urgent craniotomy was performed when the patient's level of consciousness decreased abruptly. Approximately 8 mL of pus were drained; cultures grew *Streptococcus anginosus*. Blood cultures were negative and the primary source of abscess was never identified.

are common pathogens with contiguous infection. Less common pathogens, such as *Rhodococcus, Listeria, Nocardia,* mycobacteria, and fungi—including *Candida, Cryptococcus, Aspergillus,* Mucorales (mucormycoses), *Pseudallescheria boydii,* and the dimorphic fungi such as *Histoplasma, Coccidioides,* and *Blastomyces*—cause disease in immune-compromised hosts. Postsurgical and posttraumatic abscesses are usually due to *S. aureus* and aerobic gram-negative bacilli. HIV-infected patients with advanced disease commonly present with *T. gondii* infection.

Anaerobes are present in approximately half of brain abscesses (103), although anaerobic cultures may not be routinely performed in all laboratories and, even if performed, may be falsely negative. Anaerobic species identified may originate from the oropharynx with contiguous head and neck infections, or from the abdomen or pelvis when infection is due to hematogenous seeding. Commonly isolated anaerobes include *Peptostreptococcus, Bacteroides* spp, *Prevotella* spp, *Propionibacterium, Fusobacterium, Eubacterium, Veillonella,* and *Actinomyces.*

Helminths may occasionally cause localized brain infection in immigrant populations. Neurocysticercosis, intracranial infection with the larval cyst of *Taenia solium* (pork tapeworm), is most common and results from the ingestion of *T. solium* ova. *Entamoeba histolytica, Schistosoma japonicum* and *mekongi, Paragonimus,* and *Toxocara* have also been described as causes of brain abscess.

The clinical manifestations of brain abscess are relatively nonspecific, resulting in delays in presentation and diagnosis (Table 86.10). The onset may be acute or chronic, and most of the presenting features are related to the size and location of the abscess; systemic toxicity is uncommon. Headache is the most common presenting symptom and is usually localized to the side of the abscess (16). Sudden worsening of headache may be due to rupture of the abscess into the ventricular space. Fever is present in only half of patients and thus is not a reliable sign. Focal neurologic findings can occur in half of patients and seizures, which can be the first manifestation of disease, develop in 25% of cases. Neck stiffness is most commonly seen with occipital abscesses. Altered mental status and vomiting are late signs, indicating the development of elevated intracranial pressure.

Specific presenting features may correlate with abscess location. Patients with frontal lobe abscesses often present with changes in personality or mental status, hemiparesis, speech difficulties, and seizures. Temporal lobe abscesses may cause visual field defects or dysphasia if located in the dominant hemisphere. Patients with cerebellar abscesses may present with ataxia, nystagmus, and dysmetria. Brainstem abscesses usually extend longitudinally, with minimal compressive effect, and therefore present with few classic features. Papilledema occurs late with increased intracranial pressure.

Imaging of the brain parenchyma is the diagnostic test of choice. LP is contraindicated in patients with focal findings or papilledema and should be avoided in patients with suspected

TABLE 86.10 Common Presenting Features in Brain Abscess

Headache
Mental status changes
Fever
Focal neurologic deficits
Neck stiffness
Papilledema, nausea, or vomiting with increased intracranial pressure
Seizures

brain abscess. CT scanning or MRI should be performed with the choice of test depending on the stability of the patient and availability of the imaging technique (CT is generally more available on an urgent basis or after hours). MRI with gadolinium enhancement is more sensitive than CT in detecting early cerebritis and can more accurately estimate the extent of central necrosis, ring enhancement, and cerebral edema. MRI is also better able to visualize the brainstem, cerebellum, and spinal cord and can detect small lesions, which CT may miss.

Blood cultures should be drawn in all patients with suspected or confirmed brain abscess. Abscess specimens should be obtained by stereotactic CT-guided aspiration or surgery to confirm the diagnosis and guide antimicrobial therapy. Bacterial, mycobacterial, and fungal cultures should be requested. Serology may be helpful for specific causes, such as *T. gondii* and neurocysticercosis. In toxoplasma brain abscess, IgG should be positive, as most infections are due to reactivation, not primary infection. A positive IgG antibody, however, is not specific for *T. gondii* brain abscess. Brain biopsy may establish the diagnosis but is not routinely recommended given the risks involved and availability of less invasive diagnostic methods. Empiric therapy without aspiration for microbiologic samples is not advised except in specific situations where there is a high likelihood of a specific pathogen. For example, empiric treatment for toxoplasma infection may be warranted in a patient with advanced HIV (CD4 count <100 cells/μL) not receiving prophylaxis, with multiple lesions and positive IgG *T. gondii* serology. If clinical and radiologic responses are not evident within 7 to 14 days, a microbiologic specimen should be obtained.

The therapy for brain abscess (Fig. 86.4) requires combination medical and surgical therapy for cure, as antimicrobial therapy alone is rarely effective, with the notable exception of toxoplasmosis. Empiric therapy should be initiated after imaging confirms the presence of an intraparenchymal lesion, pending aspiration for definitive diagnosis. Empiric therapy should be directed by the most likely source and respective pathogens.

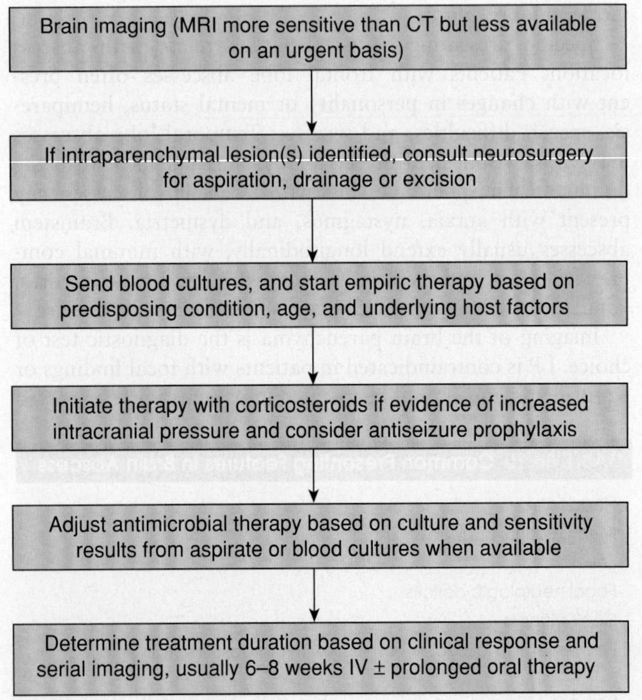

Brain imaging (MRI more sensitive than CT but less available on an urgent basis)
If intraparenchymal lesion(s) identified, consult neurosurgery for aspiration, drainage or excision
Send blood cultures, and start empiric therapy based on predisposing condition, age, and underlying host factors
Initiate therapy with corticosteroids if evidence of increased intracranial pressure and consider antiseizure prophylaxis
Adjust antimicrobial therapy based on culture and sensitivity results from aspirate or blood cultures when available
Determine treatment duration based on clinical response and serial imaging, usually 6–8 weeks IV ± prolonged oral therapy

FIGURE 86.4 Management of brain abscess.

For patients with presumed otic, mastoid, sinus, or dental sources, or temporal or cerebellar abscesses, treatment with a third-generation cephalosporin (cefotaxime, 2 g IV every 4 hours, or ceftriaxone, 2 g IV every 12 hours) and metronidazole (15 mg/kg IV load, followed by 7.5 mg/kg IV every 8 hours) is appropriate.

For patients with suspected hematogenous spread, an antimicrobial with activity against *S. aureus* should be used. Nafcillin 2 g IV every 4 to 6 hours is appropriate in settings with a low prevalence of methicillin resistance. Vancomycin—25 to 30 mg/kg (maximum 2 g) IV load followed by 15 to 20 mg/kg/dose every 8 to 12 hours, with subsequent adjustment based on serum trough vancomycin concentrations (goal trough between 15 and 20 μg/mL)—should be used where methicillin resistance is common or in penicillin-allergic patients. Vancomycin penetrates the CNS poorly and should be used only when indicated. Metronidazole and/or a third-generation cephalosporin may be added, depending on the clinical setting.

For postneurosurgical or posttrauma patients with brain abscess, vancomycin plus meropenem or a cephalosporin with antipseudomonal activity (such as ceftazidime or cefepime), should be used.

Antimicrobial therapy should be adjusted once culture and susceptibility results are available and continued intravenously for 6 to 8 weeks, guided by clinical response and serial imaging. Longer courses of therapy are generally required if the abscess has not been drained. Therapy should be continued until there is complete resolution of symptoms and CT findings. MRI abnormalities may persist for months—serial MRI studies often lead to prolonged and unnecessary antibiotic use and should be avoided (104). Antifungal therapy must be guided by fungal cultures, is generally prolonged, and should be in combination with surgical therapy.

Neurosurgical consultation should be sought at the time of diagnosis. Aspiration through a burr hole with CT or MRI guidance or complete excision following craniotomy are both appropriate treatment options, although aspiration is generally preferred due to reduced neurologic sequelae (105). Surgical excision is indicated in patients with traumatic brain abscesses, fungal abscesses, and large (>2.5 cm) or multiloculated abscesses. If there is no clinical improvement within 1 week of aspiration, mental status declines, or intracranial pressure or abscess size increase despite therapy, surgical excision is indicated. Antibiotic therapy may be shortened to 4 weeks following surgical excision.

Therapy with dexamethasone should be initiated in patients with significant edema and mass effect. Prophylactic antiseizure medications are also frequently administered. Poor prognostic factors in brain abscess include rapid progression, mental status or neurologic impairment on presentation, and rupture into a ventricle (106,107). The most common neurologic sequelae are seizures. With current advances in medical care however, rates of full recovery have substantially improved to 70% (16).

SUBDURAL AND EPIDURAL INFECTIONS

Subdural empyema is an intracranial collection of pus between the dura and arachnoid, while epidural abscesses are located between the dura and overlying skull (intracranial epidural abscess; ICEA) or vertebral column (spinal epidural abscess; SEA). While all are potentially life-threatening infections, with combined medical and surgical therapy, mortality is now well below 10%, and most survivors do so with complete recovery (108–110).

Spread of infection to the subdural and cranial epidural spaces occurs via emissary veins from local or distant sites, by direct extension of cranial osteomyelitis, or due to inoculation during neurosurgical procedures. Common predisposing infections include otic and sinus infections. Other predisposing conditions include traumatic brain injury with skull fracture, infection of a pre-existing hematoma, chronic pulmonary infection, or preceding meningitis.

SEA is nine times more common than ICEA. The epidural space is larger and predominantly posterior in the lumbar area—thus most SEA occurs in this area. SEA originates when the intervertebral disk (diskitis) or vertebral body (osteomyelitis) become infected via hematogenous seeding. Direct compression of the spinal cord or local vascular damage (thrombosis, thrombophlebitis, vasculitis) may ensue. Most abscesses extend approximately three to five vertebral spaces. Risk factors for the development of SEA include bacteremia, infective endocarditis, injection drug use, chronic indwelling catheterization, diabetes mellitus, decubitus ulcers and other chronic skin conditions, back surgery or procedures—such as epidural catheterization, LP, CT-guided needle biopsies—and blunt or penetrating spinal trauma. Secondary hematogenous spread occurs in 25% to 50% of cases.

Subdural empyema and ICEA are invariably polymicrobial, including streptococci, staphylococci, aerobic gram-negative bacilli, and anaerobes. *S. aureus*, Enterobacteriaceae, and *Pseudomonas* are more common following neurosurgical procedures or neurotrauma. In contrast to this, *S. aureus* is the most common pathogen isolated from SEA—approximately two-thirds of cases—with 90% to 95% being monomicrobial (110). *M. tuberculosis* is a common cause of SEA in patients with a previous history of tuberculosis, residence in an endemic region, or other TB risk factors.

Presenting symptoms of subdural empyema or ICEA include fever and headache. Altered mental status progressing to coma, or focal neurologic signs, most commonly hemiparesis or hemiplegia, may be present on admission. Seizures develop in up to 50% of patients. Other focal findings include cranial nerve palsies, homonymous hemianopsia, dysarthria or dysphasia, and ataxia. A fixed, dilated pupil portends imminent cerebral herniation and requires emergent surgical intervention.

SEA presents classically with fever, back pain, and neurologic deficits, however few patients present with all three symptoms (111–112). Back pain is usually the first symptom, with paresthesias, motor weakness, and sensory changes occurring in the affected nerve roots. Bladder and bowel dysfunction, as well as paralysis, are late signs and should prompt urgent surgical consultation.

Routine blood work may demonstrate a peripheral neutrophilia or elevated erythrocyte sedimentation rate (ESR) or C-reactive protein (CRP) (113). Blood cultures should be collected in all patients, especially in SEA as over half of these patients have positive cultures (110).

The diagnostic tests of choice for subdural empyema (Fig. 86.5) or ICEA are contrast CT or MRI—demonstrating typical crescentic or lentiform collections. Imaging of the sinuses, middle ear, and/or mastoids should be performed in the appropriate clinical settings to identify potential sources. For SEA, MRI with gadolinium enhancement is preferred (Fig. 86.6), as CT scanning cannot visualize the spinal cord adequately and is less sensitive at identifying contiguous diskitis or osteomyelitis.

LP is contraindicated in the setting of subdural empyema, ICEA, or SEA; however, studies have shown that CSF analysis is routinely Gram stain–negative and cultures are positive in less than 25% of cases. The highest-yield culture comes from the abscess itself. Ultrasound- or CT-guided drainage should be performed as soon as possible. Bacterial, mycobacterial, and fungal cultures should be requested. Additional studies to diagnose active tuberculosis should be performed (e.g., sputum AFB smears and cultures, and TST or IGRA) in patients with suspected spinal TB.

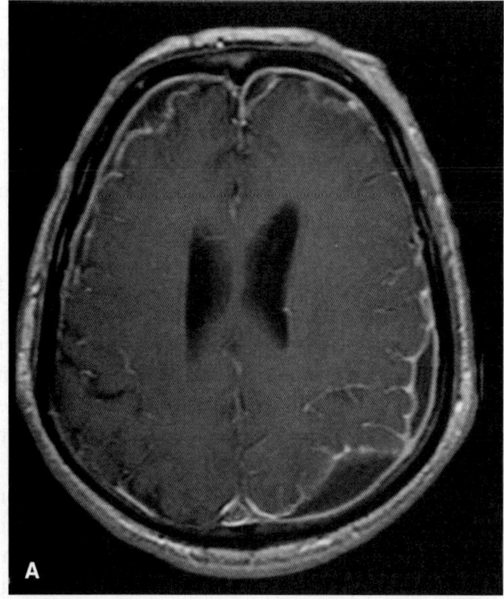

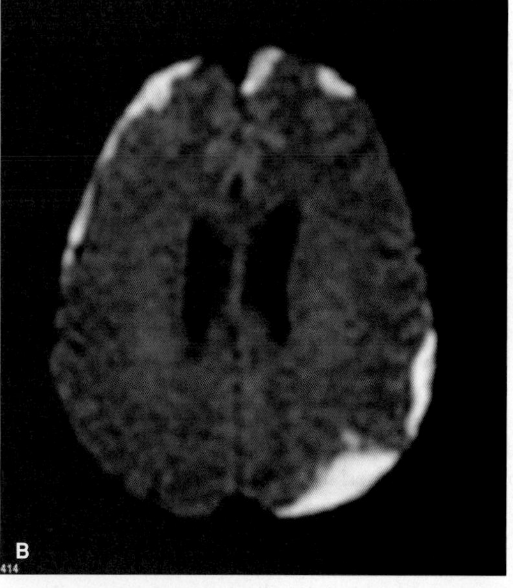

FIGURE 86.5 Axial postgadolinium T1 (**A**) and diffusion (b-1000) MRI (**B**) of subdural empyema. Typical subdural empyemas demonstrating peripheral rim enhancement and central restricted diffusion. There is evidence of leptomeningeal enhancement from meningitis.

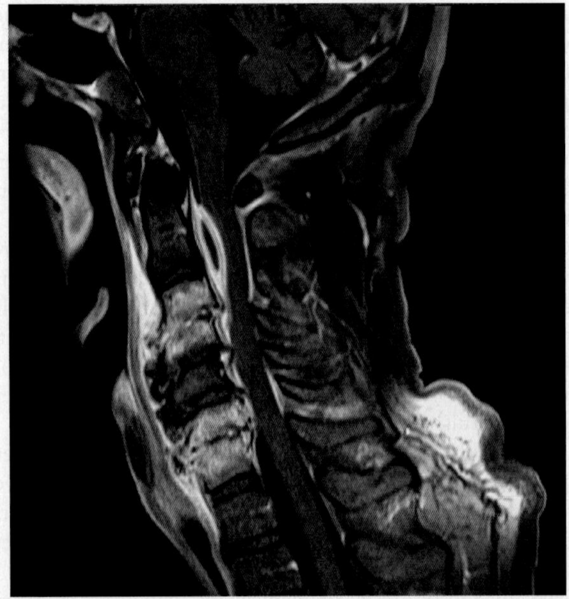

FIGURE 86.6 Sagittal postgadolinium T1 MRI of cervical spinal epidural abscess. This image demonstrates a ventral spinal epidural abscess spanning C2 and C3 levels resulting in compression of the spinal cord. Associated discitis and osteomyelitis can been seen at C3–4 and C6–7.

Treatment of subdural empyema and ICEA requires emergent combined medical and surgical therapy (114). Empiric antimicrobial therapy should be active against staphylococci, streptococci, and gram-negative bacilli (e.g., vancomycin, a third-generation cephalosporin plus metronidazole) and parallels empiric therapies for brain abscess. Surgical drainage is performed via a burr hole or craniotomy. Debridement of necrotic bone and surgical correction of sinus and otic infections are important adjuvant surgical therapies. Antiseizure treatment and/or prophylaxis may be warranted, and standard therapy for increased intracranial pressure should be instituted. Cultures are, of course, required to guide definitive antimicrobial therapy. Intravenous antimicrobial therapy should be administered for 3 to 6 weeks after drainage, depending on clinical response and serial imaging (108). Prolonged therapy (6–8 weeks) may be warranted if contiguous osteomyelitis or mastoiditis is present.

The management of SEA similarly includes empiric antimicrobial therapy with or without surgical decompression, drainage, and/or debridement. Because of the predominance of *S. aureus* infection, empiric therapy is fairly targeted—vancomycin is preferred to ensure coverage of both methicillin-resistant and methicillin-susceptible strains. Medical therapy alone may be successful when blood or abscess aspirate cultures are available to guide therapy and there are no neurologic deficits on presentation (115). Medical therapy is also appropriate in patients with complete paralysis for more than 48 hours—as recovery of neurologic function would be unlikely at this stage (110,116). Surgery should be pursued if neurologic deterioration occurs at any time, or if resolution of the abscess is not evident with medical therapy alone. Definitive antimicrobial therapy is prolonged, usually 6 to 8 weeks, and should be guided by serial imaging to ensure complete resolution of the abscess. Repeat imaging should occur at approximately 4-week intervals or at any time if neurologic deterioration occurs. The most important predictors of neurologic outcome are neurologic status prior to surgery as well as diagnostic delays (110,116).

SUPPURATIVE INTRACRANIAL THROMBOPHLEBITIS

Suppurative intracranial thrombophlebitis is septic venous thrombosis of the cortical veins. It may occur as a complication of sinus, middle ear, mastoid, oropharyngeal, or facial infections. Bacterial meningitis, epidural abscess, or subdural abscess may also result in intracranial suppurative thrombophlebitis.

Anatomically, the location of intracranial infection depends on the original source of infection. In bacterial meningitis, infection is spread via drainage of the meningeal veins into the superior sagittal sinus. The superior sagittal sinus may also be involved following facial, scalp, subdural, and epidural space infections. Otitis media and mastoiditis are the usual causes of lateral sinus and petrosal sinus thromboses. Paranasal sinus, facial, or oropharyngeal infections may result in cavernous sinus thrombosis. Risk factors for cerebral venous stasis include hypercoagulable states—specifically antiphospholipid antibody syndrome—volume depletion, polycythemia, pregnancy, oral contraceptive use, malignancy, sickle cell disease, and traumatic brain injury (117–119).

Bacterial pathogens involved in intracranial suppurative thrombophlebitis depend on the originating source of infection. *S. aureus* is commonly involved following facial infection; otherwise, sinusitis and otitis media pathogens cause most infections; these include staphylococci, streptococci, aerobic gram-negative bacilli, and anaerobes such as *Fusobacterium* and *Bacteroides*. *Aspergillus* and Mucorales rarely cause suppurative intracranial thrombophlebitis and are most often seen in patients with diabetes mellitus or immune compromise.

Clinical manifestations depend on the anatomic sites involved. Septic thrombosis of the superior sagittal sinus presents with fever, headache, confusion, nausea, vomiting, and seizures. Mental status depression and progression to coma may occur rapidly. Upper motor neuron lower extremity weakness or hemiparesis may be present. When septic thrombosis is a complication of bacterial meningitis, nuchal rigidity may also be present.

Cranial nerve palsies may result from compression due to increased pressure in the cavernous sinus. Classic symptoms of septic cavernous sinus thrombosis include fever, headache, diplopia, and retro-orbital pain. Ptosis, proptosis, and chemosis may be present. Venous engorgement of the retinal veins and papilledema are commonly present. Septic transverse sinus thrombosis presents with headache and otitis while sigmoid sinus and internal jugular vein thrombosis may present with neck pain.

MRI demonstrates absence of flow within affected veins and venous sinuses and is the diagnostic test of choice. MR venography can be used to confirm the diagnosis, and sinus imaging should be concomitantly performed. Compared to CT scanning, MRI offers the additional benefits of detecting cerebritis, intracranial abscess, cerebral infarction, hemorrhage, or edema.

The treatment of suppurative intracranial thrombophlebitis includes antimicrobials, surgical therapy, and anticoagulation. The choice of antimicrobial therapy depends on patient risk factors, most probable source of infection, and culture results, if available. In antecedent sinusitis, empiric therapy with cefotaxime or ceftriaxone and metronidazole is a reasonable choice. In cavernous sinus thrombosis, an agent active against *S. aureus* should be included. Antimicrobial therapy should be continued for 6 weeks or until radiographic resolution of thrombosis. Anticoagulation appears to be beneficial in cavernous sinus thrombosis, particularly if used early (119,120).

Key Points

Meningitis

- Untreated acute bacterial meningitis is universally fatal; early recognition, rapid diagnostic testing, and emergent administration of antimicrobials are crucial.
- The absence of fever, nuchal rigidity, and change in mental status effectively excludes the diagnosis of bacterial meningitis.
- *S. pneumoniae* is the most common cause of acute bacterial meningitis in adults. The incidence of *H. influenzae* type b meningitis in the United States has decreased substantially as a result of widespread vaccination.
- LP should be performed urgently in all patients with suspected meningitis. CSF pleocytosis is the hallmark finding. CSF cultures are positive in the majority of patients with bacterial meningitis if obtained prior to antimicrobial therapy.
- Neuroimaging, to rule out mass lesions, should precede LP in patients with abnormal level of consciousness, focal neurologic deficits, papilledema, a history of CNS disease, immune compromise, or seizure within 1 week of presentation.
- Empiric antimicrobial agents should be administered as soon as possible after blood cultures are collected if neuroimaging is to be performed prior to LP or immediately following CSF collection.
- Dexamethasone has been shown to decrease mortality in adults with *S. pneumoniae* and children with *H. influenzae* meningitis, and as such should be administered empirically in all cases of meningitis, before or concomitant with the first dose of antimicrobial.
- Neurologic complications of meningitis include seizure, cerebral edema or infarction, cranial nerve involvement, venous sinus thrombosis, brain abscess, subdural empyema, and coma. Intracranial pressure monitoring and/or other surgical interventions may be required.

Encephalitis

- Encephalitis—inflammation of the brain parenchyma—can most easily be distinguished from meningitis by the finding of altered mental status.
- HSE is the most common cause of sporadic encephalitis in Western countries, accounting for 20% to 40% of cases.
- West Nile virus is the most commonly diagnosed arboviral CNS infection in the United States.
- Clinical findings of encephalitis include the classic triad of fever, headache, and altered mental status.
- Diagnostic tests include CSF analysis and neuroimaging, preferably MRI.
- CSF NAT and/or specific serum tests for plausible etiologies should be pursued.
- Temporal lobe involvement on MRI and EEG are characteristic in HSE.

Brain Abscess

- Brain abscess is characterized by focal intracranial suppurative collection as a result of direct extension or hematogenous spread of infection.
- A solitary abscess is usually the result of contiguous infection from otitis, mastoiditis, sinusitis, or dental infection.
- Multiple abscesses commonly result from hematogenous spread from chronic pulmonary, endocardial, skin, intra-abdominal, or pelvic infections.
- Streptococci are the most common bacteria isolated, often in mixed culture with anaerobes. *S. aureus*, enteric gram negatives, and less common microorganisms (including fungi) are also recognized pathogens.
- Clinical manifestations are nonspecific and depend on the size and location of the abscess. Headache is the most common presenting feature. Systemic toxicity is uncommon.
- MRI is more sensitive than CT scanning and is the neuroimaging test of choice.
- Blood and abscess culture results should be used to tailor antimicrobial therapy, which is generally prolonged—4 to 8 weeks—and guided by serial imaging.
- Surgical excision may be indicated in patients with traumatic brain abscesses, fungal abscesses, and large (>2.5 cm) or multiloculated abscesses.
- Combined medical–surgical therapy results in high cure rates. Poor prognostic factors include rapid progression, mental status or neurologic impairment on presentation, and rupture into a ventricle.

Subdural and Epidural Infections

- Subdural empyema is a collection of pus between the dura and arachnoid.
- Epidural abscesses form between the dura and overlying skull (ICEA) or vertebral column (SEA).
- Presenting symptoms of subdural empyema and ICEA include fever, headache, and a recent history of contiguous otic, mastoid, sinus, or meningeal infection.
- Risk factors for SEA include bacteremia, infective endocarditis, injection drug use, chronic indwelling catheterization, diabetes mellitus, decubitus ulcers and other chronic skin conditions, back surgery or procedures, and trauma.
- *S. aureus* is the most common pathogen in SEA, however tuberculosis should be considered in those at epidemiologic risk.
- Common presenting features of SEA include fever, back pain, and neurologic deficits.
- Contrast CT or MRI is diagnostic in subdural empyema or ICEA.
- MRI is preferred for the diagnosis of SEA.
- Subdural empyema and ICEA require emergent surgical drainage and prolonged antimicrobial therapy, guided, of course, by surgical culture results.

- Management of SEA includes prolonged, 6 to 8 weeks, antimicrobial therapy, serial imaging to ensure resolution of the abscess, and early surgical decompression in selected cases.
- Repeat imaging should occur at approximately 4-week intervals or at any time if neurologic deterioration occurs.

Suppurative Intracranial Thrombophlebitis

- Suppurative intracranial thrombophlebitis—septic venous thrombosis of the cortical veins—is a complication of otic, sinus, mastoid, oropharyngeal, facial, or neurologic (bacterial meningitis, epidural abscess, or subdural abscess) infections.
- Microbiology depends on the source of infection, but staphylococci, streptococci, aerobic gram-negative bacilli, and anaerobic bacteria are the most common pathogens.
- MRI is the diagnostic test of choice as it offers the additional benefits of detecting cerebritis, intracranial abscess, cerebral infarction, hemorrhage, or edema when compared to CT.
- MR venography can be used to confirm the diagnosis.
- Sinus imaging should be concomitantly performed.
- Management includes antimicrobials, surgical therapy, and anticoagulation if not contraindicated.

References

1. Scheld WM, Koedel U, Nathan B, Pfister HW. Pathophysiology of bacterial meningitis: mechanism(s) of neuronal injury. *J Infect Dis.* 2002;186 (Suppl 2):S225–S233.
2. Thigpen MC, Whitney CG, Messonnier NE, et al.; Emerging Infections Programs Network. Bacterial meningitis in the United States, 1998–2007. *N Engl J Med.* 2011;364(21):2016–2025.
3. van de Beek D, de Gans J, Spanjaard L, et al. Clinical features and prognostic factors in adults with bacterial meningitis. *N Engl J Med.* 2004;351 (18):1849–1859.
4. Durand ML, Calderwood SB, Weber DJ, et al. Acute bacterial meningitis in adults: a review of 493 episodes. *N Engl J Med.* 1993;328(1):21–28.
5. Aronin SI, Peduzzi P, Quagliarello VJ. Community-acquired bacterial meningitis: risk stratification for adverse clinical outcome and effect of antibiotic timing. *Ann Intern Med.* 1998;129(11):862–869.
6. Castelblanco RL, Lee M, Hasbun R. Epidemiology of bacterial meningitis in the USA from 1997 to 2010: a population-based observational study. *Lancet Infect Dis.* 2014;14(9):813–819.
7. Stephens DS, Farley MM. Pathogenic events during infection of the human nasopharynx with Neisseria meningitidis and Haemophilus influenzae. *Rev Infect Dis.* 1991;13(1):22–33.
8. Quagliarello V. Dissemination of Neisseria meningitidis. *N Engl J Med.* 2011;364(16):1573–1575.
9. Quagliarello V, Scheld WM. Bacterial meningitis: pathogenesis, pathophysiology, and progress. *N Engl J Med.* 1992;327(12):864–872.
10. Zwijnenburg PJ, van der Poll T, Roord JJ, van Furth AM. Chemotactic factors in cerebrospinal fluid during bacterial meningitis. *Infect Immun.* 2006;74(3):1445–1451.
11. Nudelman Y, Tunkel AR. Bacterial meningitis: epidemiology, pathogenesis and management update. *Drugs.* 2009;69(18):2577–2596.
12. de Gans J, van de Beek D; European Dexamethasone in Adulthood Bacterial Meningitis Study Investigators. Dexamethasone in adults with bacterial meningitis. *N Engl J Med.* 2002;347(20):1549–1556.
13. Attia J, Hatala R, Cook DJ, Wong JG. The rational clinical examination. Does this adult patient have acute meningitis? *JAMA.* 1999;282(2):175–181.
14. Thomas KE, Hasbun R, Jekel J, Quagliarello VJ. The diagnostic accuracy of Kernig's sign, Brudzinski's sign, and nuchal rigidity in adults with suspected meningitis. *Clin Infect Dis.* 2002;35(1):46–52.
15. Nakao JH, Jafri FN, Shah K, Newman DH. Jolt accentuation of headache and other clinical signs: poor predictors of meningitis in adults. *Am J Emerg Med.* 2014;32(1):24–28.
16. Brouwer MC, Coutinho JM, van de Beek D. Clinical characteristics and outcome of brain abscess: systematic review and meta-analysis. *Neurology.* 2014;82(9):806–13.
17. Heckenberg SG, de Gans J, Brouwer MC, et al. Clinical features, outcome, and meningococcal genotype in 258 adults with meningococcal meningitis: a prospective cohort study. *Medicine.* 2008;87(4):185–192.
18. Rosenstein NE, Perkins BA, Stephens DS, et al. The changing epidemiology of meningococcal disease in the United States, 1992–1996. *J Infect Dis.* 1999;180(6):1894–1901.
19. Bijlsma MW, Bekker V, Brouwer MC, et al. Epidemiology of invasive meningococcal disease in the Netherlands, 1960–2012: an analysis of national surveillance data. *Lancet Infect Dis.* 2014;14(9):805–812.
20. Wilder-Smith A, Goh KT, Barkham T, Paton NI. Hajj-associated outbreak strain of Neisseria meningitidis serogroup W135: estimates of the attack rate in a defined population and the risk of invasive disease developing in carriers. *Clin Infect Dis.* 2003;36(6):679–683.
21. Osuorah D, Shah B, Manjang A, et al. Outbreak of serotype W135 Neisseria meningitidis in central river region of the Gambia between February and June 2012: a hospital-based review of paediatric cases. *Nigerian J Clin Prac.* 2015;18(1):41–47.
22. Savadogo M, Kyelem N, Yelbeogo D, et al. [The *Neisseria* meningitidis W135 epidemic in 2012 in Burkina Faso.]. *Bull Soc Pathol Exot.* 2014; 107(1):15–17.
23. Fijen CA, Kuijper EJ, Tjia HG, et al. Complement deficiency predisposes for meningitis due to nongroupable meningococci and *Neisseria*-related bacteria. *Clin Infect Dis.* 1994;18(5):780–784.
24. Sjoholm AG, Kuijper EJ, Tijssen CC, et al. Dysfunctional properdin in a Dutch family with meningococcal disease. *N Engl J Med.* 1988;319(1):33–37.
25. Bula CJ, Bille J, Glauser MP. An epidemic of food-borne listeriosis in western Switzerland: description of 57 cases involving adults. *Clin Infect Dis.* 1995;20(1):66–72.
26. Linnan MJ, Mascola L, Lou XD, et al. Epidemic listeriosis associated with Mexican-style cheese. *N Engl J Med.* 1988;319(13):823–828.
27. Lorber B. Listeriosis. *Clin Infect Dis.* 1997;24(1):1–9.
28. Kupila L, Vuorinen T, Vainionpaa R, et al. Etiology of aseptic meningitis and encephalitis in an adult population. *Neurology.* 2006;66(1):75–80.
29. Connolly KJ, Hammer SM. The acute aseptic meningitis syndrome. *Infect Dis Clin North Am.* 1990;4(4):599–622.
30. Petersen LR, Brault AC, Nasci RS. West Nile virus: review of the literature. *JAMA.* 2013;310(3):308–315.
31. Zou S, Foster GA, Dodd RY, et al. West Nile fever characteristics among viremic persons identified through blood donor screening. *J Infect Dis.* 2010;202(9):1354–1361.
32. Waggoner JJ, Soda EA, Deresinski S. Rare and emerging viral infections in transplant recipients. *Clin Infect Dis.* 2013;57(8):1182–1188.
33. Schafer IJ, Miller R, Stroher U, et al. Notes from the field: a cluster of lymphocytic choriomeningitis virus infections transmitted through organ transplantation-Iowa, 2013. *Am J Transplant.* 2014;14(6):1459.
34. Macneil A, Stroher U, Farnon E, et al. Solid organ transplant-associated lymphocytic choriomeningitis, United States, 2011. *Emerg Infect Dis.* 2012; 18(8):1256–1262.
35. Rousseau MC, Saron MF, Brouqui P, Bourgeade A. Lymphocytic choriomeningitis virus in southern France: four case reports and a review of the literature. *Eur J Epidemiol.* 1997;13(7):817–823.
36. Centers for Disease Control and Prevention (CDC). Notes from the field: lymphocytic choriomeningitis virus infections in employees of a rodent breeding facility—Indiana, May-June 2012. *MMWR Morb Mortal Wkly Rep.* 2012;61(32):622–623.
37. Corey L, Adams HG, Brown ZA, Holmes KK. Genital herpes simplex virus infections: clinical manifestations, course, and complications. *Ann Intern Med.* 1983;98(6):958–972.
38. Centers for Disease Control and Prevention (CDC). Mumps outbreak on a university campus–California, 2011. *MMWR Morb Mortal Wkly Rep.* 2012;61(48):986–989.
39. Barskey AE, Schulte C, Rosen JB, et al. Mumps outbreak in Orthodox Jewish communities in the United States. *N Engl J Med.* 2012;367(18): 1704–1713.
40. Savage E, Ramsay M, White J, et al. Mumps outbreaks across England and Wales in 2004: observational study. *BMJ.* 2005;330(7500):1119–1120.
41. Kent SJ, Crowe SM, Yung A, et al. Tuberculous meningitis: a 30-year review. *Clin Infect Dis.* 1993;17(6):987–994.
42. Klein NC, Damsker B, Hirschman SZ. Mycobacterial meningitis. Retrospective analysis from 1970 to 1983. *Am J Med.* 1985;79(1):29–34.

43. Chow JK, Golan Y, Ruthazer R, et al. Risk factors for albicans and non-albicans candidemia in the intensive care unit. *Crit Care Med.* 2008; 36(7):1993–1998.
44. Blumberg HM, Jarvis WR, Soucie JM, et al.; National Epidemiology of Mycoses Survey(NEMIS) Study Group. Risk factors for candidal bloodstream infections in surgical intensive care unit patients: the NEMIS prospective multicenter study. The National Epidemiology of Mycosis Survey. *Clin Infect Dis.* 2001;33(2):177–186.
45. Gavin PJ, Kazacos KR, Shulman ST. Baylisascariasis. *Clin Microbiol Rev.* 2005;18(4):703–718.
46. Ruff RL, Dougherty JH Jr. Complications of lumbar puncture followed by anticoagulation. *Stroke.* 1981;12(6):879–881.
47. Hasbun R, Abrahams J, Jekel J, Quagliarello VJ. Computed tomography of the head before lumbar puncture in adults with suspected meningitis. *N Engl J Med.* 2001;345(24):1727–1733.
48. Tunkel AR, Hartman BJ, Kaplan SL, et al. Practice guidelines for the management of bacterial meningitis. *Clin Infect Dis.* 2004;39(9):1267–1284.
49. Sakushima K, Hayashino Y, Kawaguchi T, et al. Diagnostic accuracy of cerebrospinal fluid lactate for differentiating bacterial meningitis from aseptic meningitis: a meta-analysis. *J Infect.* 2011;62(4):255–262.
50. Fitch MT, van de Beek D. Emergency diagnosis and treatment of adult meningitis. *Lancet Infect Dis.* 2007;7(3):191–200.
51. Welinder-Olsson C, Dotevall L, Hogevik H, et al. Comparison of broad-range bacterial PCR and culture of cerebrospinal fluid for diagnosis of community-acquired bacterial meningitis. *Clin Micro Infect.* 2007;13(9):879–886.
52. Xu J, Moore JE, Millar BC, et al. Employment of broad range 16S rDNA PCR and sequencing in the detection of aetiological agents of meningitis. *New Microbiol.* 2005;28(2):135–143.
53. Steiner I, Budka H, Chaudhuri A, et al. Viral meningoencephalitis: a review of diagnostic methods and guidelines for management. *Eur J Neurol.* 2010;17(8):999–e57.
54. Fraga D, Muller AL, Czykiel MS, et al. Detection of Treponema pallidum by semi-nested PCR in the cerebrospinal fluid of asymptomatic HIV-infected patients with latent syphilis. *Clin Lab.* 2014;60(12):2051–2054.
55. Dumaresq J, Langevin S, Gagnon S, et al. Clinical prediction and diagnosis of neurosyphilis in HIV-infected patients with early syphilis. *J Clin Microbiol.* 2013;51(12):4060–4066.
56. Garcia P, Grassi B, Fich F, et al. [Laboratory diagnosis of *Treponema pallidum* infection in patients with early syphilis and neurosyphilis through a PCR-based test]. *Rev Chilena Infectol.* 2011;28(4):310–315.
57. Aguero-Rosenfeld ME, Wang G, Schwartz I, Wormser GP. Diagnosis of Lyme borreliosis. *Clin Microbiol Rev.* 2005;18(3):484–509.
58. Thwaites GE, Chau TT, Farrar JJ. Improving the bacteriological diagnosis of tuberculous meningitis. *J Clin Microbiol.* 2004;42(1):378–379.
59. Jayanthi U, Madhavan HN, Therese KL. Nucleic acid amplification tests for diagnosis of tuberculous meningitis. *Lancet Infect Dis.* 2004;4(1):9; discussion 11–12.
60. Tanner DC, Weinstein MP, Fedorciw B, et al. Comparison of commercial kits for detection of cryptococcal antigen. *J Clin Microbiol.* 1994; 32(7):1680–1684.
61. Johnson RH, Einstein HE. Coccidioidal meningitis. *Clin Infect Dis.* 2006; 42(1):103–107.
62. Miner JR, Heegaard W, Mapes A, Biros M. Presentation, time to antibiotics, and mortality of patients with bacterial meningitis at an urban county medical center. *J Emerg Med.* 2001;21(4):387–392.
63. Lu CH, Huang CR, Chang WN, et al. Community-acquired bacterial meningitis in adults: the epidemiology, timing of appropriate antimicrobial therapy, and prognostic factors. *Clin Neurol Neurosurg.* 2002;104(4):352–358.
64. Lepur D, Barsic B. Community-acquired bacterial meningitis in adults: antibiotic timing in disease course and outcome. *Infection.* 2007;35(4):225–231.
65. van de Beek D, de Gans J, Tunkel AR, Wijdicks EF. Community-acquired bacterial meningitis in adults. *N Engl J Med.* 2006;354(1):44–53.
66. Whitney CG, Farley MM, Hadler J, et al.; Active Bacterial Core Surveillance Program of the Emerging Infections Program Network. Increasing prevalence of multidrug-resistant *Streptococcus pneumoniae* in the United States. *N Engl J Med.* 2000;343(26):1917–1924.
67. Centers for Disease Control and Prevention (CDC). Effects of new penicillin susceptibility breakpoints for *Streptococcus pneumoniae*—United States, 2006–2007. *MMWR Morb Mortal Wkly Rep.* 2008;57(50):1353–1355.
68. Mattie H, Stuertz K, Nau R, van Dissel JT. Pharmacodynamics of antibiotics with respect to bacterial killing of and release of lipoteichoic acid by Streptococcus pneumoniae. *J Antimicrob Chemo.* 2005;56(1): 154–159.
69. Mook-Kanamori BB, Rouse MS, Kang CI, et al. Daptomycin in experimental murine pneumococcal meningitis. *BMC Infect Dis.* 2009;9:50.
70. Brouwer MC, McIntyre P, Prasad K, van de Beek D. Corticosteroids for acute bacterial meningitis. *Cochrane Database Syst Rev.* 2013;6:CD004405.
71. van de Beek D, de Gans J, McIntyre P, Prasad K. Corticosteroids for acute bacterial meningitis. *Cochrane Database Syst Rev.* 2007(1):CD004405.
72. McIntyre PB, Berkey CS, King SM, et al. Dexamethasone as adjunctive therapy in bacterial meningitis: a meta-analysis of randomized clinical trials since 1988. *JAMA.* 1997;278(11):925–931.
73. Edberg M, Furebring M, Sjolin J, Enblad P. Neurointensive care of patients with severe community-acquired meningitis. *Acta Anaesthesiol Scand.* 2011;55(6):732–739.
74. Glimaker M, Johansson B, Halldorsdottir H, et al. Neuro-intensive treatment targeting intracranial hypertension improves outcome in severe bacterial meningitis: an intervention-control study. *PloS One.* 2014;9(3):e91976.
75. Desmond RA, Accortt NA, Talley L, et al. Enteroviral meningitis: natural history and outcome of pleconaril therapy. *Antimicrob Agents Chemother.* 2006;50(7):2409–2414.
76. Steiner I, Budka H, Chaudhuri A, et al. Viral encephalitis: a review of diagnostic methods and guidelines for management. *Eur J Neurol.* 2005; 12(5):331–343.
77. Prasad K, Singh MB. Corticosteroids for managing tuberculous meningitis. *Cochrane Database Syst Rev.* 2008(1):CD002244.
78. Tomczyk S, Bennett NM, Stoecker C, et al. Use of 13-valent pneumococcal conjugate vaccine and 23-valent pneumococcal polysaccharide vaccine among adults aged ≥65 years: recommendations of the Advisory Committee on Immunization Practices (ACIP). *MMWR Morb Mortal Wkly Rep.* 2014;63(37):822–825.
79. Centers for Disease Control and Prevention (CDC). Use of 13-valent pneumococcal conjugate vaccine and 23-valent pneumococcal polysaccharide vaccine for adults with immunocompromising conditions: recommendations of the Advisory Committee on Immunization Practices (ACIP). *MMWR Morb Mortal Wkly Rep.* 2012;61(40):816–819.
80. Centers for Disease Control and Prevention (CDC); Advisory Committee on Immunization Practices. Updated recommendations for prevention of invasive pneumococcal disease among adults using the 23-valent pneumococcal polysaccharide vaccine (PPSV23). *MMWR Morb Mortal Wkly Rep.* 2010;59(34):1102–1106.
81. Black SL, Szenborn L, Daly W. A comparative evaluation of two investigational meningococcal ABCWY vaccine formulations: results of a phase 2 randomized, controlled trial. *Vaccine.* 2015;33(21):2500–2510.
82. Mailles A, Stahl JP, Steering Committee and Investigators Group. Infectious encephalitis in France in 2007: a national prospective study. *Clin Infect Dis.* 2009;49(12):1838–1847.
83. Granerod J, Ambrose HE, Davies NW, et al. Causes of encephalitis and differences in their clinical presentations in England: a multicentre, population-based prospective study. *Lancet Infect Dis.* 2010;10(12):835–844.
84. Arciniegas DB, Anderson CA. Viral encephalitis: neuropsychiatric and neurobehavioral aspects. *Curr Psychiatry Rep.* 2004;6(5):372–379.
85. Levitz RE. Herpes simplex encephalitis: a review. *Heart Lung.* 1998; 27(3):209–212.
86. Reimann CA, Hayes EB, DiGuiseppi C, et al. Epidemiology of neuroinvasive arboviral disease in the United States, 1999–2007. *Am J Trop Med Hyg.* 2008;79(6):974–979.
87. Murray K, Baraniuk S, Resnick M, et al. Risk factors for encephalitis and death from West Nile virus infection. *Epidemiol Infect.* 2006;134(6): 1325–1332.
88. Carson PJ, Borchardt SM, Custer B, et al. Neuroinvasive disease and West Nile virus infection, North Dakota, USA, 1999–2008. *Emerg Infect Dis.* 2012;18(4):684–686.
89. Patnaik JL, Harmon H, Vogt RL. Follow-up of 2003 human West Nile virus infections, Denver, Colorado. *Emerg Infect Dis.* 2006;12(7):1129–1131.
90. Nett RJ, Kuehnert MJ, Ison MG, et al. Current practices and evaluation of screening solid organ donors for West Nile virus. *Transpl Infect Dis.* 2012;14(3):268–277.
91. Willoughby RE Jr, Tieves KS, Hoffman GM, et al. Survival after treatment of rabies with induction of coma. *N Engl J Med.* 2005;352(24):2508–2514.
92. Jackson AC. Recovery from rabies. *N Engl J Med.* 2005;352(24):2549–2250.
93. Aurelius E, Johansson B, Skoldenberg B, et al. Rapid diagnosis of herpes simplex encephalitis by nested polymerase chain reaction assay of cerebrospinal fluid. *Lancet.* 1991;337(8735):189–192.
94. Lakeman FD, Whitley RJ. Diagnosis of herpes simplex encephalitis: application of polymerase chain reaction to cerebrospinal fluid from brain-biopsied patients and correlation with disease. National Institute of Allergy and Infectious Diseases Collaborative Antiviral Study Group. *J Infect Dis.* 1995;171(4):857–863.
95. Kataoka H, Inoue M, Shinkai T, Ueno S. Early dynamic SPECT imaging in acute viral encephalitis. *J Neuroimag.* 2007;17(4):304–310.

96. Whitley RJ, Alford CA, Hirsch MS, et al. Vidarabine versus acyclovir therapy in herpes simplex encephalitis. *N Engl J Med.* 1986;314(3):144–149.
97. Skoldenberg B, Forsgren M, Alestig K, et al. Acyclovir versus vidarabine in herpes simplex encephalitis: randomised multicentre study in consecutive Swedish patients. *Lancet.* 1984;2(8405):707–711.
98. Dagsdottir HM, Sigurethardottir B, Gottfreethsson M, et al. Herpes simplex encephalitis in Iceland 1987–2011. *Springerplus.* 2014;3:524.
99. Prasad KN, Mishra AM, Gupta D, et al. Analysis of microbial etiology and mortality in patients with brain abscess. *J Infect.* 2006;53(4):221–227.
100. Felsenstein S, Williams B, Shingadia D, et al. Clinical and microbiologic features guiding treatment recommendations for brain abscesses in children. *Pediatr Infect Dis J.* 2013;32(2):129–135.
101. Lu CH, Chang WN, Lin YC, et al. Bacterial brain abscess: microbiological features, epidemiological trends and therapeutic outcomes. *Q J Med.* 2002;95(8):501–509.
102. Le Moal G, Landron C, Grollier G, et al. Characteristics of brain abscess with isolation of anaerobic bacteria. *Scand J Infect Dis.* 2003;35(5):318–321.
103. Helweg-Larsen J, Astradsson A, Richhall H, et al. Pyogenic brain abscess, a 15 year survey. *BMC Infect Dis.* 2012;12:332.
104. Ratnaike TE, Das S, Gregson BA, Mendelow AD. A review of brain abscess surgical treatment–78 years: aspiration versus excision. *World Neurosurg.* 2011;76(5):431–436.
105. Seydoux C, Francioli P. Bacterial brain abscesses: factors influencing mortality and sequelae. *Clin Infect Dis.* 1992;15(3):394–401.
106. Tseng JH, Tseng MY. Brain abscess in 142 patients: factors influencing outcome and mortality. *Surg Neurol.* 2006;65(6):557–562.
107. Tunkel AR. Subdural empyema, epidural abscess, and suppurative intracranial thrombophlebitis. In: Mandell GL, Bennett JE, Dolin R, eds. *Mandell, Douglas, and Bennett's Principles and Practice of Infectious Diseases.* 8th ed. Philadelphia, PA: Elsevier; 2015:1177–1185.
108. French H, Schaefer N, Keijzers G, Barison D, Olson S. Intracranial subdural empyema: a 10-year case series. *Ochsner J.* 2014;14(2):188–194.
109. Darouiche RO. Spinal epidural abscess. *New Engl J Med.* 2006;355(19):2012–2020.
110. Davis DP, Wold RM, Patel RJ, et al. The clinical presentation and impact of diagnostic delays on emergency department patients with spinal epidural abscess. *J Emerg Med.* 2004;26(3):285–291.
111. Pradilla G, Ardila GP, Hsu W, Rigamonti D. Epidural abscesses of the CNS. *Lancet Neurol.* 2009;8(3):292–300.
112. Reihsaus E, Waldbaur H, Seeling W. Spinal epidural abscess: a meta-analysis of 915 patients. *Neurosurg Rev.* 2000;23(4):175–245.
113. Osborn MK, Steinberg JP. Subdural empyema and other suppurative complications of paranasal sinusitis. *Lancet Infect Dis.* 2007;7(1):62–67.
114. Siddiq F, Chowfin A, Tight R, et al. Medical vs surgical management of spinal epidural abscess. *Arch Intern Med.* 2004;164(22):2409–2412.
115. Sendi P, Bregenzer T, Zimmerli W. Spinal epidural abscess in clinical practice. *Q J Med.* 2008;101(1):1–12.
116. Saposnik G, Barinagarrementeria F, Brown RD Jr, et al.; American Heart Association Stroke Council and the Council on Epidemiology and Prevention. Diagnosis and management of cerebral venous thrombosis: a statement for healthcare professionals from the American Heart Association/American Stroke Association. *Stroke.* 2011;42(4):1158–1192.
117. Ferro JM, Canhao P, Stam J, et al.; ISCVT Investigators. Prognosis of cerebral vein and dural sinus thrombosis: results of the International Study on Cerebral Vein and Dural Sinus Thrombosis (ISCVT). *Stroke.* 2004;35(3):664–670.
118. Southwick FS, Richardson EP Jr, Swartz MN. Septic thrombosis of the dural venous sinuses. *Medicine (Baltimore).* 1986;65(2):82–106.
119. Bhatia K, Jones NS. Septic cavernous sinus thrombosis secondary to sinusitis: Are anticoagulants indicated? A review of the literature. *J Laryngol Otol.* 2002;116(9):667–676.

CHAPTER

87

Infections of the Head and Neck

ANDREW J. REDMANN and ALLEN M. SEIDEN

OTOLOGIC INFECTIONS

Otitis Externa

Acute otitis externa (AOE) is a diffuse inflammation of the external ear canal, which may also involve the pinna or tympanic membrane (1). This condition is also known as "swimmer's ear" or "tropical ear" due to a higher prevalence in individuals with prolonged water exposure during swimming or who live in warm and humid climates. The annual incidence of AOE is about 1:100 to 1:250 within the general population (2).

The external ear is comprised of the auricle and external ear canal. The medial 60% of the external auditory canal is osseous and contains thin skin densely adherent to the underlying periosteum (Fig. 87.1). The lateral 40% of the external auditory canal is cartilaginous and contains a thin layer of subcutaneous tissue between the skin and cartilage. This subcutaneous layer contains hair follicles, sebaceous, and apocrine glands. The skin of the auditory canal migrates from the tympanic membrane outwards, leading to self-cleaning. Cerumen is formed by glandular secretions and sloughed epithelium and provides a chemical and mechanical protective barrier to infection. Cerumen is slightly acidic, maintaining a canal pH of 5 to 6.5, which inhibits bacterial and fungal growth. The lipid content of cerumen prevents maceration and breakdown of the epithelium. Breakdown in this natural defense mechanism allows for opportunistic infections, giving rise to otitis externa (3).

The risk factors for AOE are prolonged exposure to water from swimming; dermatologic conditions such as seborrhea, psoriasis, eczema; trauma from ear cleaning, foreign objects, use of assistive devices such as earplugs or hearing aids, anatomic abnormalities such as exostoses and narrow ear canals, immunocompromising systemic conditions like diabetes, HIV, concomitant ear diseases such as cholesteatoma, suppurative otitis media; and a history of cancer radiotherapy (1).

Presenting symptoms may be otalgia, itching, aural fullness, decreased hearing, and pain with chewing. Patients with AOE will often have disproportionately severe pain and will have significant tenderness when pushed on the tragus, or with manipulation of the posterolateral pinna. Otoscopic examination usually reveals ear canal cellulitis and edema. Depending on the severity of the ear canal swelling the tympanic membrane may or may not be visualized. The ear canal is often filled with purulent discharge and debris. Inflammation may spread to involve the entire auricle and adjacent skin. Regional lymphadenopathy may be present on the examination (1).

Most cases of AOE are bacterial. *Pseudomonas aeruginosa* and *Staphylococcus* species have been found to be the most common pathogens (4,5). Fungal involvement is uncommon in primary AOE. It is more often seen in chronic otitis externa (COE) or as secondary overgrowth following the treatment of bacterial infection.

Initial treatment of otitis externa involves removal of debris from the external ear canal, aggressive pain control, use of topical medications, acidification of the ear canal, and control of predisposing factors. Debridement of the external ear canal allows for removal of infectious material and better penetration of topical medications. In many cases edema of the ear canal will prevent proper penetration of the medicated drop down into the canal. In this situation, placement of a cotton wick directly into the ear canal for several days will facilitate delivery of the medication (1).

Currently, recommended topical preparations consist of antibiotics and steroid combinations. Quinolone antibiotic preparations may have broader microbial coverage and a low risk of contact dermatitis, and are considered first line. Caution should be used when treating with neomycin-containing topical preparations due to a potential for this agent to cause contact sensitivity and in turn lead to worsening of symptoms. Neomycin-containing preparations also have a risk—albeit low—of causing permanent sensorineural hearing loss and should be used with caution in patients with perforated tympanic membranes or tympanostomy tubes. Acetic acid may also be considered as a treatment, but is generally less effective in the long term when compared to antibiotic drops (6). When treating immunocompromised patients, or if otitis externa infection has spread beyond the ear canal, consideration should be given to the use of systemic antibiotics as well, though these are not recommended in otherwise uncomplicated patients. The choice of antibiotics should be based on their antipseudomonal and antistaphylococcal properties (1).

Chronic Otitis Externa

COE is a persistent inflammatory disorder of the ear canal usually caused by repeated mechanical debridement or water exposure. Other potential causes are allergic, contact dermatitis, or dermatologic disorders. Chronic inflammation may lead to development of granulation. The treatment of COE involves debridement, avoidance of ear canal manipulation, elimination of the offending agent, and topical corticosteroids. Tacrolimus has also shown promise in the treatment of refractory COE (7). Regular flushing of the ear canal with a mild acidic solution, such as acetic acid or vinegar and distilled water, can also help to eradicate infection and keep the canal free of debris (7,8).

Otomycosis

Otomycosis is a fungal infection of the external ear canal. It comprises roughly 10% of all cases of otitis externa, and is more common in geographic locations with a warm and humid climate, in patients following long-term topical antibiotic therapy, and in patients with diabetes, HIV, or other immunocompromising conditions (9). The ear canal will often have cellulitis and edema on otoscopic examination. The canal debris may have a cheese-like or grayish appearance with visualized fungal hyphae. *Aspergillus* species and *Candida* species are the

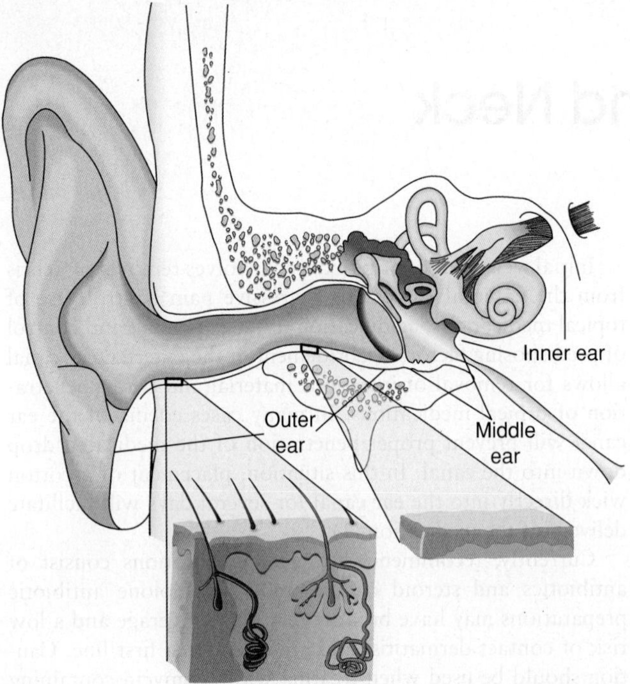

FIGURE 87.1 Anatomic depiction of the external, middle, and inner ear.

most common pathogens (10). Treatment consists of debridement, acidification, and drying of the ear canal. For candidal infections, topical antifungal therapy may also be effective.

Necrotizing Otitis Externa

Malignant or necrotizing otitis externa (MOE) is an aggressive infection that begins as otitis externa but spreads through surrounding tissues toward the skull base. It is seen predominantly in the elderly, diabetic, or immunocompromised patient. *P. aeruginosa* is the most common causative pathogen; however, staphylococcal species are also known to cause the infection (11). Fungal causes of MOE are less common, with *Aspergillus* species the predominating pathogen (12).

MOE initially presents with symptoms and signs of AOE. Subsequently, it may progress to temporal bone osteomyelitis and affect adjacent cranial nerves (VII to XII), blood vessels, and soft tissue. If not treated aggressively, the infection can expand intracranially leading to neurologic symptoms. On otoscopic examination, granulation tissue is classically seen at the bony–cartilaginous junction (11–13). A raised erythrocyte sedimentation rate and abnormal computed tomography (CT) or magnetic resonance imaging (MRI) scan help to confirm the clinical diagnosis. Other imaging techniques that assist in diagnosis include gallium scan, indium-labeled leukocyte scan, technetium bone scan, and single-photon emission tomographs (12,14). Patients will require treatment with systemic antibiotics that cover pseudomonal and staphylococcal infection, including methicillin-resistant *Staphylococcus aureus* (11,12).

Furunculosis (Ear Canal Abscess)

Furunculosis is a localized infection of the ear canal that is usually caused by an infected hair follicle. It may present with otalgia, otorrhea, and localized tenderness. A tender, often fluctuant nodule within the lateral ear canal can be identified on the examination. The most common pathogen is *S. aureus*. The treatment includes application of heat, incision and drainage of the infected area, and systemic antibiotic treatment with staphylococcal coverage (15).

Acute Otitis Media

Acute otitis media is an inflammation of the middle ear, which is generally characterized by the rapid onset of otalgia, aural fullness, and occasionally fever. In the pediatric patient, more common signs are irritability, sleeplessness, and pulling at the affected ear. On pneumatic otoscopy, the tympanic membrane will have a red, opaque, and bulging appearance with decreased mobility due to the accumulation of purulent fluid in the middle ear space. Additionally, the tympanic membrane may rupture, so that patients will present with otorrhea (16,17).

Predominant pathogens in AOM are *Streptococcus pneumoniae, Haemophilus influenzae,* and *Moraxella catarrhalis* (18). Observation for 24 to 48 hours in the case of a nonsevere illness in an otherwise healthy individual greater than 6 months of age is an initial option, with 60% resolving within 24 hours without antibiotic treatment. If symptoms persist, antimicrobial therapy should be initiated. Amoxicillin is recommended for initial treatment of acute otitis media, at a recommended dose of 80 to 90 mg/kg/d. In the case of penicillin allergy, azithromycin, clarithromycin, erythromycin–sulfisoxazole, or trimethoprim–sulfamethoxazole could be used. Due to the increased incidence of β-lactamase–producing organisms, the bacterial coverage should be expanded if there is no improvement within 48 to 72 hours. In very rare cases, if pain or fever is excessive, immediate tympanocentesis or myringotomy may be required, taking care to send purulent fluid for culture in this case (18,19).

Otitis media with effusion is the presence of fluid in the middle ear without signs or symptoms of acute ear infection and should be distinguished from acute otitis media. Otitis media with effusion often occurs as a result of eustachian tube dysfunction, or middle ear inflammation following acute infection. It is most common in the pediatric population between the ages of 6 months and 4 years, although it may occur at any age. On pneumatic otoscopy, the tympanic membrane is often retracted, will have decreased mobility, and an air–fluid level or bubbles are often visualized. Patients often report a decrease in hearing. Otitis media with effusion is often self-limited and is likely to resolve spontaneously within 3 months. If it persists, hearing testing is recommended, particularly in children with language delay, learning problems, or suspicion of significant hearing loss (17,20). In individuals with hearing loss and persistent middle ear effusion for greater than 3 months, myringotomy with tympanostomy tube insertion should be considered (21). Medical treatment, such as decongestants, has not been shown to be effective in the treatment of middle ear effusion. In an adult presenting with a unilateral middle ear effusion, an examination of the nasopharynx should be performed to rule out the possibility of a nasopharyngeal mass causing obstruction of the eustachian tube.

Chronic Otitis Media

Chronic otitis media is diagnosed when infection persists for more than 1 to 3 months. It may present as chronic suppurative otitis media (CSOM), which is characterized by persistent bacterial infection and drainage from the ear, or as chronic otitis media with effusion (COME), which results from unresolving inflammation of the middle ear and persistent middle ear secretions with an intact tympanic membrane. Chronic otitis media may be associated with cholesteatoma, which is a keratin cyst that forms from an accumulation of squamous debris in the middle ear with potential for growth and erosion of surrounding structures (22).

Patients with CSOM will present with hearing loss, painless purulent otorrhea, and a chronic tympanic membrane perforation. Evaluation includes visual examination, bacterial culture, and radiographic imaging. Gram-negative and anaerobic organisms are usually seen on cultures, with *P. aeruginosa* being a predominant organism. Temporal bone CT scan allows evaluation of the extent of disease and reveals potential complications. Medical treatment of CSOM consists of topical debridement, along with topical and systemic antibiotics. Topical drops often consist of antibiotic and steroid combinations (23). Ciprofloxacin is recommended for systemic use; however, it cannot be given to children under 17 years of age. Surgical treatment is performed for eradication of the infection and reconstruction of the middle ear (22).

COME is characterized by persistent hearing loss and a middle ear space filled with thick mucus. Chronic inflammation of the middle ear often begins with obstruction of the eustachian tube. The resulting negative pressure in the middle ear leads to collection of transudate. Secondary to chronic inflammation, the middle ear lining becomes hyperplastic and produces further mucous. On examination, the tympanic membrane is intact and has a thickened, opaque appearance. On pneumatic otoscopy, the tympanic membrane does not move. As the disease progresses the tympanic membrane starts to retract and drape over the ossicles. Nasal obstruction and sinus disease may contribute to Eustachian tube insufficiency and lead to middle ear fluid accumulation. Treatment of COME consists of fluid drainage, which is accomplished by myringotomy with ventilation tube insertion. Treating sinus disease and relieving nasal obstruction may improve eustachian tube function (20).

Acute or chronic forms of otitis media, if left untreated, may lead to extracranial or intracranial complications (Table 87.1). Hearing loss, tympanic membrane perforation, atelectasis of the middle ear, mastoiditis, apical petrositis, facial nerve paralysis, labyrinthitis, and ossicular discontinuity are some of the possible intratemporal sequelae of otitis media. Meningitis, extradural abscess, subdural empyema, encephalitis, brain abscess, sigmoid sinus thrombosis, and hydrocephalus are potential intracranial complications. Intracranial complications should be suspected in individuals presenting with changes in mental status (17,24,25).

TABLE 87.1 Complications of Otitis Media

Intratemporal
- Tympanic membrane perforation
- Mastoiditis
- Petrositis
- Facial nerve paralysis
- Labyrinthitis
- Ossicular discontinuity

Intracranial
- Meningitis
- Extradural abscess
- Subdural empyema
- Encephalitis
- Brain abscess
- Sigmoid sinus thrombosis
- Hydrocephalus

Labyrinthitis

Labyrinthitis is an inflammation or infection of the vestibular apparatus. Patients typically present with vertigo, nausea, vomiting, and malaise. The etiology is most often viral or traumatic, but can be bacterial. Bacterial labyrinthitis most often arises as a spread of infection from meningitis or otitis media. It can be serous or suppurative. Viral infections such as mumps, measles, Lassa fever, varicella-zoster, syphilis, and herpes simplex have been associated with labyrinthitis. Labyrinthitis may or may not be associated with a sensorineural hearing loss, which can be temporary or permanent depending on the etiology, patient's age, and severity of the loss (26).

Idiopathic Facial Paralysis (Bell Palsy)

Idiopathic facial paralysis is an acute unilateral peripheral facial nerve weakness. It is a diagnosis of exclusion, and only made when other causes of paralysis, such as systemic diseases, infection, trauma, central nervous system disorders, and neoplasm, are ruled out. Patients will usually present with abrupt onset of unilateral facial weakness. Other symptoms may include numbness or pain around the ear, decreased taste, and increased sensitivity to sounds (27). Herpes simplex virus is thought to be an etiologic factor for this disease (28). Bell palsy most commonly occurs in individuals between 10 and 40 years of age. Pregnant women and individuals with diabetes mellitus are at a higher risk of developing Bell palsy. Most cases spontaneously improve within 6 months. Residual facial nerve weakness may persist in about 15% of affected individuals (27). In patients older than 16 years of age, the recommended treatment consists of the early administration (first 72 hours) of high-dose prednisone. Antivirals may be added, but have not shown to have benefit apart from steroids (29). Patients should be educated about using artificial tears and protecting the eye during sleep to prevent corneal abrasion and eye infection.

Ramsay Hunt Syndrome

Ramsay Hunt syndrome is caused by reactivation of varicella-zoster virus (VZV) in the geniculate ganglion and is associated with eruption of an auricular or oropharyngeal vesicular rash, facial paralysis, and otalgia (30). In addition, tinnitus, hearing loss, nausea, vomiting, vertigo, and nystagmus can be the accompanying symptoms (31). Patients with Ramsay Hunt syndrome present more severe symptoms and have a worse prognosis for recovery of facial nerve function relative to patients with Bell palsy. The timing between onset of facial paralysis and vesicular eruption may vary. Some patients present with facial paralysis, have a rise in VZV antibody, but never develop cutaneous manifestations. Initiation of early treatment with prednisone and acyclovir is currently recommended (32).

Chondritis/Perichondritis

Chondritis/perichondritis of the ear is an infection of auricular cartilage/perichondrium. It is often caused by penetrating injury to the ear, particularly piercing of the pinna (33). Blunt trauma with auricular hematoma can also lead to infection. Cartilage involvement can also be seen in spreading otitis externa. Because of its relative avascularity, cartilage is more susceptible to infection. Infections are more often reported during warm weather, after exposure to water in pools, lakes, or hot tubs. Patients present with a very tender, erythematous, and indurated auricle. It is generally doughy on palpation and is rarely fluctuant. *P. aeruginosa* has been identified as the most likely cause of the infection, but *S. aureus* must also be considered (33,34). Treatment consists of removing any foreign body, and drainage of any abscess or hematoma. Patients should be treated aggressively with antibiotics that provide coverage for *Pseudomonas*. Cartilage necrosis or subperichondrial fibrosis leading to auricular deformity may be seen following the infectious process. Recurrent auricular chondritis should raise suspicion for the diagnosis of relapsing polychondritis (35).

NASAL INFECTIONS

Septal Abscess

Septal abscesses are collections of pus between the cartilaginous or bony nasal septum and the overlying mucoperichondrium or mucoperiosteum (36). The leading cause is trauma that leads to a septal hematoma, but can also occur after septoplasty. It has also been shown to occur in association with influenza, sinusitis, nasal furuncle, and dental infection. Immunocompromised patients are at a higher risk of dangerous complications. Patients complain of nasal congestion, nasal pain, fever, and headache. On examination, there is evidence of an anterior intranasal mass, as the septum will appear swollen and fluctuant. Most common causative organisms are *S. aureus* and group A β-hemolytic *Streptococcus* (GABHS); however, *Staphylococcus epidermidis, S. pneumoniae, H. influenzae,* and anaerobes are also possible pathogens. Treatment involves antibiotics and surgical drainage. Complications include ischemic necrosis of the septal cartilage, intracranial infections such as meningitis, brain abscess, and subarachnoid empyema (36,37).

Rhinosinusitis

Acute Bacterial Rhinosinusitis

Acute bacterial rhinosinusitis most often develops following a viral upper respiratory infection, and is distinguished by a duration of greater than 10 days (38). Some of the presenting diagnostic symptoms include purulent nasal discharge, nasal congestion, maxillary, tooth or facial pain, and worsening of symptoms following initial improvement, but are not specific for bacterial sinusitis as opposed to viral causes. Predisposing physiologic factors include obstruction of sinus ostia, reduction in number or function of sinus cilia, and a change in the quality of secretions (39). The most common pathogens are *S. pneumoniae, H. influenzae, M. catarrhalis,* and *S. aureus*. In immunocompromised patients, in patients with cystic fibrosis, and in patients with sinusitis of nosocomial origin (on mechanical ventilation, with nasal tubing), *P. aeruginosa* and other aerobic gram-negative rods are common causative pathogens (40). Anaerobic bacteria are usually associated with sinusitis of dental origin (41). It is often difficult to distinguish between viral and bacterial sinusitis. The diagnosis is usually based on

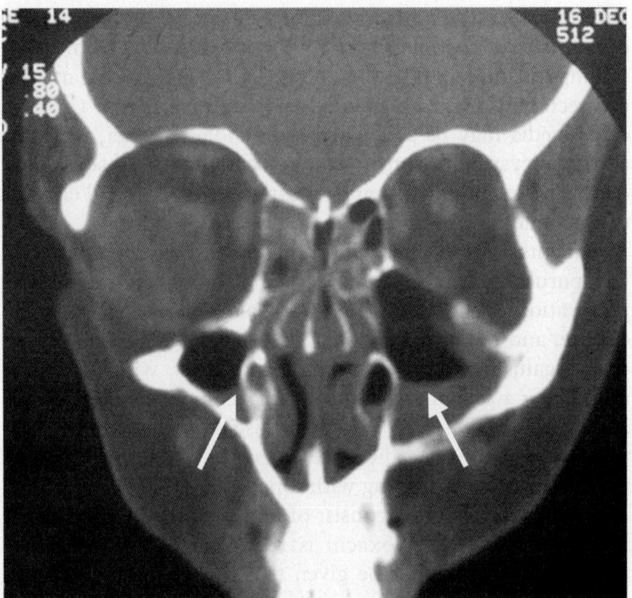

FIGURE 87.2 A coronal computed tomography (CT) image depicting inflammatory sinus disease. A coronal CT without contrast is the preferred radiographic study to evaluate for the presence and extent of sinus infections.

medical history and clinical findings. With bacterial sinusitis, symptoms are usually present for more than 10 days. Sinus puncture with aspiration of sinus contents is the most accurate diagnostic technique; however, since it is invasive it is not commonly used. Radiographic imaging may help confirm the presence of sinus disease. Plain films can be difficult to interpret and should not be ordered. CT findings will include thickened mucosa, sinus opacification, or air–fluid levels, and is the preferred examination although these findings are nonspecific (Fig. 87.2). CT scans are rarely ordered to confirm acute infection unless there is concern about possible complications, such as in the case of frontal or sphenoid sinus infection. Nasal endoscopy will often demonstrate swelling within the middle meatus or sphenoethmoidal recess, with purulent discharge. Antimicrobial treatment of acute sinusitis includes amoxicillin (first line), amoxicillin–clavulanic acid, cephalosporins, trimethoprim–sulfamethoxazole, macrolides, doxycycline, and quinolones (42). Treatment can be supplemented with nasal saline irrigation, antihistamines, decongestants, and intranasal steroids (43). If there is minimal improvement after 2 to 3 days, a change in antibiotics may be indicated. Frontal sinus disease in particular may require early surgical management. If not treated, acute bacterial sinusitis may be complicated by the development of a number of orbital and intracranial complications, particularly when the infection involves the ethmoid, frontal, or sphenoid sinuses, and may require additional surgery to treat the complications (Table 87.2) (44–46).

Chronic Bacterial Rhinosinusitis

Chronic bacterial rhinosinusitis is diagnosed when the symptoms of sinusitis are present for at least 12 weeks. Symptoms include nasal congestion, purulent discharge, facial pressure, and anosmia. Nasal endoscopy may reveal nasal polyps, edema, or purulent discharge. CT findings may reveal mucosal thickening, sinus opacification, polyps, or air–fluid levels (47,48). Predisposing factors include smoking, inhalant allergies, obstruction

TABLE 87.2 Potential Complications of Sinusitis
Acute sinusitis
• Orbital
◦ Periorbital cellulitis
◦ Orbital cellulitis
◦ Subperiosteal abscess
◦ Orbital abscess
◦ Optic neuritis
◦ Cavernous sinus thrombosis
• Intracranial
◦ Meningitis
◦ Epidural abscess
◦ Subdural empyema
◦ Brain abscess
Chronic sinusitis
• Mucocele
• Osteitis/osteomyelitis

of the ostiomeatal complex (Fig. 87.3), immune deficiency, and genetic factors (48). Pathogens are similar to those found in acute infections, with a greater predominance of *Staphylococcus*, *Pseudomonas,* and possibly anaerobes. The most common anaerobic bacteria include *Peptostreptococcus* species, *Fusobacterium* species, *Prevotella,* and *Porphyromonas* species. In cases of *P. aeruginosa,* aminoglycosides, fourth-generation cephalosporins, or fluoroquinolones are used in treatment (40). In chronic bacterial rhinosinusitis (CRS), a prolonged course of antibiotic therapy is often required, ranging from 3 to 6 weeks, with any imaging occurring after the completion of medical therapy. Adjunctive therapy including decongestants, mucolytics, and steroids (both intranasal and oral) may be helpful. In patients with continued symptoms, recent guidelines recommend allergy testing to exclude allergic rhinitis as a contributing factor, as well as considering other immunologic disorders. Testing for cystic fibrosis in younger patients may also be helpful

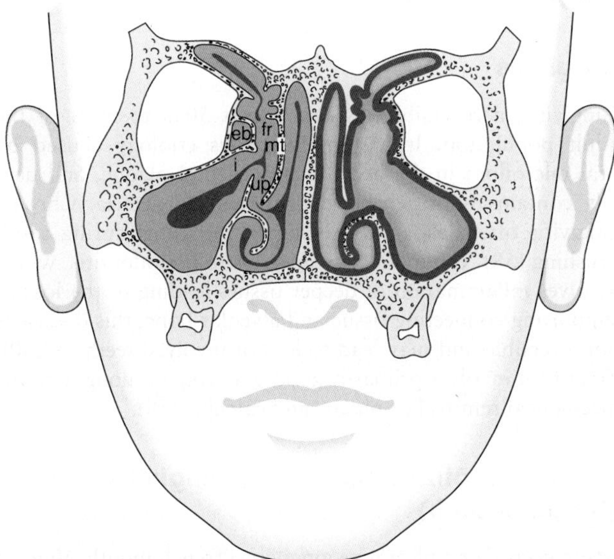

FIGURE 87.3 The ostiomeatal complex, referring to the anterior ethmoid sinus, and the ostia of the maxillary and frontal sinus as they drain into the middle meatus. Most sinus infections begin and persist because of obstruction in this area. The right side depicts these areas swollen; the left demonstrates the postsurgical appearance after the ostiomeatal complex has been opened. Eb, ethmoidal bulla; fr, frontal recess; i, infundibulum; mt, middle turbinate; up, uncinate process.

(43,49). If patients do not respond to medical therapy, functional endoscopic sinus surgery may be indicated (50).

Viral Rhinosinusitis

Viral rhinosinusitis is more common than bacterial. The most common pathogens are rhinovirus, influenza viruses, adenoviruses, parainfluenza viruses, and respiratory syncytial virus (RSV). Inflammatory symptoms of viral rhinosinusitis are thought to be due to the host response to the virus. Patients may present with symptoms of the common cold such as nasal congestion, nasal discharge, sneezing, cough, fever, malaise, and muscle ache. Viral rhinosinusitis is usually self-limited. Antiviral therapy may be used for specific viruses. Nasal saline irrigation and various anti-inflammatory medications may aid with symptomatic relief (51).

Fungal Rhinosinusitis

Acute Necrotizing Fungal Rhinosinusitis. Acute invasive necrotizing fungal rhinosinusitis is a fulminant invasive fungal infection that is often life-threatening. It usually affects immunocompromised patients, such as diabetics, patients with immunodeficiency disorders, and patients undergoing chemotherapy. Patients often present with acute onset of fever, headache, cough, mucosal ulcerations, and epistaxis. On examination, necrotic black turbinates and nasal eschar spreading through mucosa, soft tissue, and bone are seen. Histopathologic evaluation of involved tissue reveals necrosis and inflammatory infiltrate with giant cells, lymphocytes, and neutrophils. Gomori methenamine silver or periodic acid-Schiff histologic fungal stains demonstrate tissue and vascular invasion by fungal hyphae. Most common pathogens are *Aspergillus, Rhizopus,* and *Mucor* species. Treatment involves emergent surgical debridement, intravenous antifungal drugs such as Amphotericin B, and treatment of the underlying immunocompromising disorder. If disease is not treated, it may lead to rapid dissemination and death (52,53).

Chronic Invasive Fungal Rhinosinusitis. Chronic invasive fungal rhinosinusitis is a chronic (greater than 3 months) and slowly invasive fungal infection. It too usually affects immunocompromised patients, particularly diabetics and patients requiring prolonged corticosteroid treatment, but has also been reported in otherwise healthy individuals. Patients may present with orbital apex syndrome due to the extension of the infection into the orbit. This will result in decreased vision, ocular immobility, and proptosis. Erosion may also occur into the infratemporal fossa, the anterior cranial fossa, or the premaxillary region. Histopathology reveals a dense accumulation of hyphae, with a chronic inflammatory infiltrate of lymphocytes, giant cells, and necrotizing granulomas. If left untreated, the disease may invade cerebral blood vessels leading to ischemic injury, or directly invade the brain. Treatment involves repeated surgical debridement and antifungal drugs (52).

Mycetoma

Mycetoma, also described as a fungal ball, is an accumulation of degenerating fungal hyphae within a sinus cavity, most often involving the maxillary sinus. Patients are generally immunocompetent and will present with symptoms of nasal obstruction, postnasal drainage, and localized facial pain. Risk factors include previous sinus surgery, oral–sinus fistula, and chemotherapy treatment. The presence of chronic mucosal

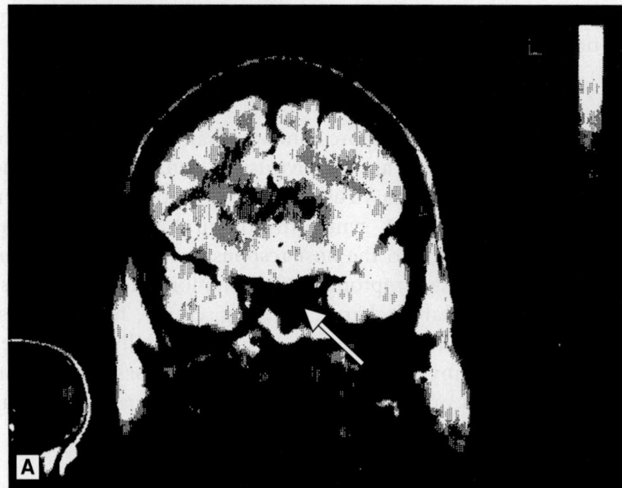

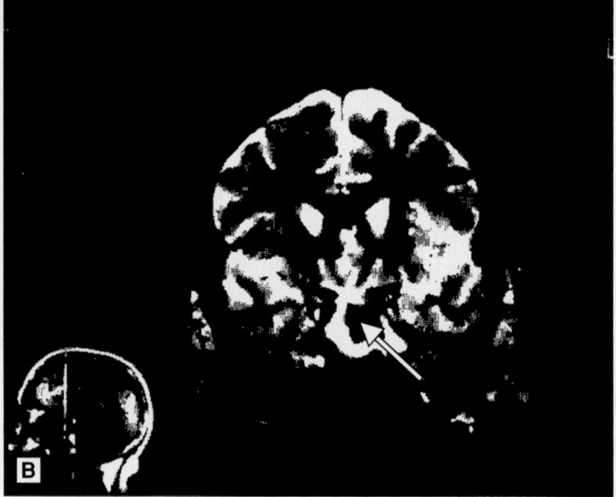

FIGURE 87.4 Magnetic resonance imaging (MRI) of a mycetoma or fungal ball within the sphenoid sinus, demonstrating isodense opacification on T1 images (A), with a ring of enhancement and central attenuation on T2 (B).

inflammation may be noted on nasal endoscopy, along with green–black concretions within the middle meatus. A CT study will reveal sinus opacification, often with areas of calcification. MRI may be definitive, demonstrating isodense opacification on T1 images, with a ring of enhancement and central attenuation on T2 (Fig. 87.4). This result is from ferromagnetic deposits related to the fungal infection. Aspergillus is the most common organism, although fungal cultures are often found to be negative. Treatment involves surgical removal of the fungal ball with adequate drainage of the affected sinus (52,55).

Allergic Fungal Sinusitis

The etiology of allergic fungal sinusitis (AFS) is thought to be in part an allergic response to the presence of noninvasive fungi in the sinus cavity, and has been likened to allergic bronchopulmonary aspergillosis (54,56). Patients will commonly present with hypertrophic sinus disease and nasal polyps. Symptoms of headache, paranasal fullness, and nasal discharge are often reported. Sinus CT often reveals the presence of chronic sinusitis with hyperattenuation present in the opacified sinus, creating an inhomogeneous appearance often with areas of calcification (Fig. 87.5). Serum IgE levels

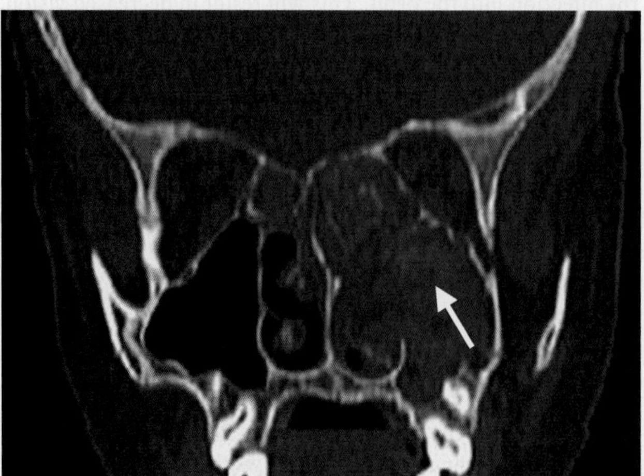

FIGURE 87.5 Computed tomography (CT) of the sinuses in a patient with allergic fungal sinusitis, demonstrating an inhomogeneous appearance with areas of calcification.

are often elevated, and histologic evaluation reveals the presence of allergic mucin, containing fungal hyphae and elevated eosinophils; there is no evidence of mucosal invasion. Intraorbital and intracranial expansion may occur secondary to pressure resorption of surrounding bone. The most common causative agents are *Bipolaris spicifera* and *Curvularia lunata*. Other causative agents are *Exserohilum rostratum, Alternatia* species, and *Aspergillus* species. Treatment consists of sinus surgery to remove the diseased mucosa and allergic mucin, although recurrence is common. Once AFS is diagnosed, if there are no contraindications, treatment with corticosteroids should be initiated. Other treatments include surgical debridement, immunotherapy, antibiotics, and nonsteroidal immunomodulatory medications (57).

ORAL CAVITY

Gingivitis

Gingivitis, a reversible disease, affects 50% to 90% of the adult population. It has an infectious etiology caused by oral microflora in the accumulating dental plaque, and usually contains both aerobic and anaerobic bacteria. Chronic gingivitis often leads to bleeding of the gums during tooth brushing (58). Gingivitis may progress to periodontitis, which involves inflammation of deeper tissues leading to the loss of supporting connecting tissue and alveolar bone; this disease is nonreversible and may lead to loss of involved teeth (59,60). Treatment involves primarily good oral hygiene along with the mechanical removal of plaque and calculus (58).

Acute Necrotizing Ulcerative Gingivitis (Trench Mouth)

Acute necrotizing ulcerative gingivitis (Trench mouth, Vincent stomatitis) is a rare periodontal disease characterized by gingival necrosis, ulceration, pain, and bleeding (61). The disease is most commonly seen in young adults, with patients often presenting with sudden onset of gingival inflammation. Gingival lacerations covered with gray membranes and gingival bleeding are noted on the examination. The causative organisms are

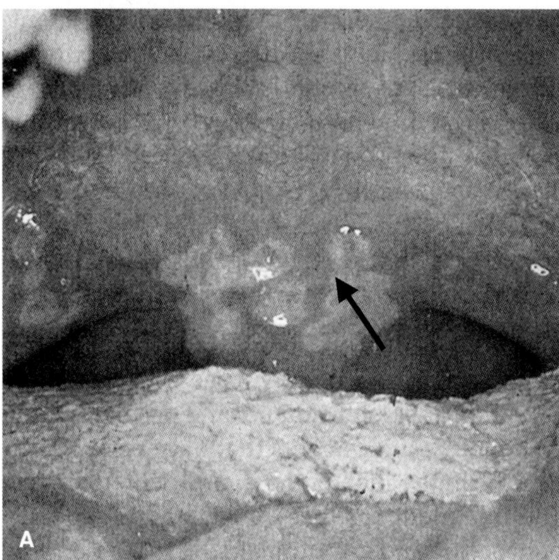

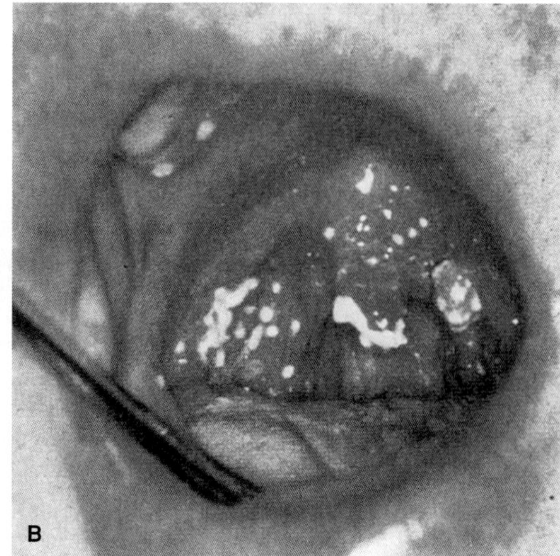

FIGURE 87.6 Oropharyngeal infection by *Candida albicans* (thrush). These photos demonstrate the pseudomembranous form (**A**) associated with yellow–white plaques, and the erythematous form (**B**). (From Walner DL, Shott SR. Infectious and inflammatory disorders. In: Seiden AM, Tami TA, Pensak ML, et al., eds. *Otolaryngology: The Essentials*. New York, NY: Thieme Medical Publishers; 2001:188, with permission.)

fusospirochetal bacteria (*Borrelia vincentii*), which become pathogenic during periods of compromised immune system function. *Bacterioides* and *Selenomonas* species have also been implicated in the disease (61). Diagnosis is based on clinical findings. Risk factors include dental crowding, physical fatigue, increased stress, low socioeconomic status, immunosuppression, smoking, and poor oral hygiene (62). Treatment includes eliminating precipitating factors, treatment of underlying immunosuppression, oral hygiene, mechanical debridement of affected areas, and antibiotics. Penicillin or metronidazole is recommended for antibiotic treatment (62).

Herpetic Gingival Stomatitis

Herpetic gingivostomatitis is an infection due to Herpes simplex virus. Primary infection most commonly manifests in children between the ages of 2 and 5 years. Patients may present with fever and irritability; oropharyngeal pain, mucosal edema, and erythema are often present. Vesicular lesions appear on mobile or nonkeratinized mucosal surfaces (buccal, labial) and attached or keratinized surfaces (gingiva, hard palate); these usually rupture within 24 hours, leaving small ulcers with an elevated margin. Diagnosis is confirmed by viral studies and biopsy. Treatment is usually supportive, although acyclovir may help to shorten the severity and duration of the infection. Once the primary infection resolves, the organism remains dormant, with the reservoir usually being the trigeminal ganglion; periodic reactivation of infection may occur. In most cases, individuals must have an active lesion to be able to transmit the virus (63,64).

Candidiasis

Candidiasis is caused by the overgrowth of *Candida albicans*. Often, the patient is predisposed, with a history of immunosuppression, radiation, or altered microflora following long-term broad-spectrum antibiotic use. In the pseudomembranous form, yellow–white plaques are present that have been likened to milk curds (Fig. 87.6A), whereas in the erythematous form, these plaques have disappeared (Fig. 87.6B). Clinical diagnosis may be confirmed with potassium hydroxide staining revealing fungal hyphae. Initial therapy usually consists of oral hygiene and topical treatment; some of the available agents include oral nystatin preparations, amphotericin lozenges, and clotrimazole troches. Ketoconazole, fluconazole, and itraconazole can be used for systemic treatment if indicated (65).

Odontogenic Infections

Odontogenic infections often originate from infected pulp and may spread to the fascial spaces of the head and neck where an abscess may form (Fig. 87.7). The potential spaces are found around the face (masticator, buccal, canine, and parotid); in the suprahyoid area (submandibular, sublingual, and parapharyngeal); and in the infrahyoid area (retropharyngeal and paratracheal spaces). The most common causative organisms are *S. aureus*, group A streptococci, and anaerobic bacteria. Treatment with broad-spectrum antibiotics is recommended, and surgical drainage is the primary treatment (66,67).

Ludwig Angina

Ludwig angina is an infection that involves the left and right sublingual and submandibular spaces, generally spreading rapidly through fascial planes. It occurs most often in adults with poor dentition, usually from an infection involving the second or third molar. Other sources may include inflammation of the tongue or floor of mouth, and lingual tonsillitis (68,69). Patients will often present with submandibular swelling but not fluctuance, and swelling of the floor of mouth that pushes the tongue upward and backward toward the palate. In the case of advanced disease, patients may present in acute distress with fever, difficulty handling secretions, and dyspnea that favors a seated and head-forward position; infection can be rapidly progressive, leading to airway compromise. Anaerobic organisms and streptococci are the most common cause of Ludwig angina. Treatment requires close airway monitoring, with prophylactic tracheotomy needed for airway protection in most cases, administration of antibiotics, and surgical drainage (68,69).

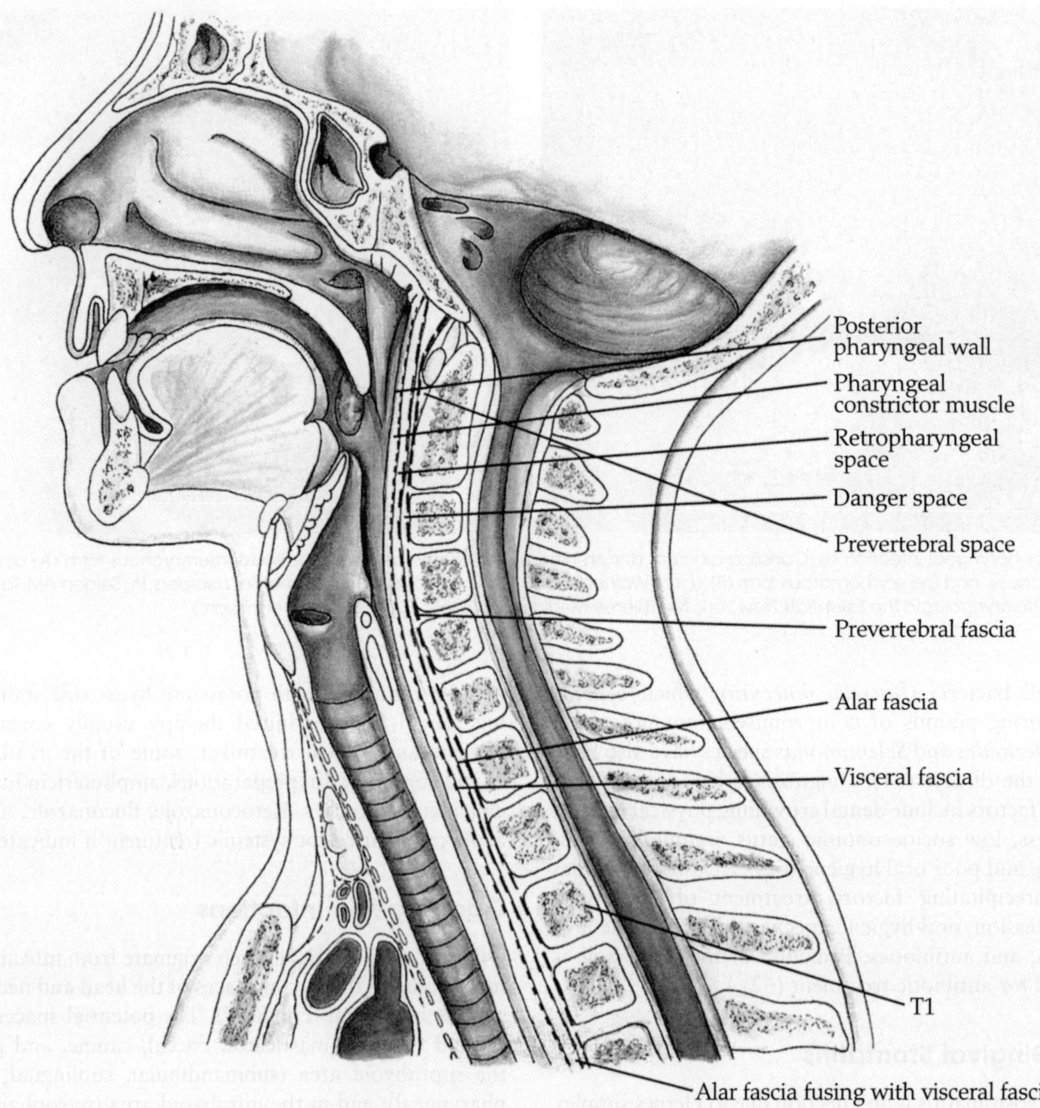

FIGURE 87.7 Schematic representation of the deep fascial spaces of the head and neck. (From Portugal LG, Padhya TA, Gluckman JL. Anatomy and physiology. In: Seiden AM, Tami TA, Pensak ML, et al., eds. *Otolaryngology: The Essentials*. New York, NY: Thieme Medical Publishers; 2001:477, with permission.)

PHARYNX

Tonsillopharyngitis

Tonsillopharyngitis is a common disease characterized by infection of the nasopharynx and oropharynx and its associated lymphoid tissue. Acute tonsillopharyngitis may be caused by viral or bacterial infection, viral being the most common. It is often difficult to distinguish between bacterial and viral causes based on clinical examination. Patients present with fever, malaise, odynophagia, and lymphadenitis. On examination, tonsillar enlargement, erythema, and exudate may be present. Upper respiratory viruses such as rhinovirus, coronavirus, and adenovirus are the most common causes of viral infection (70). The most common cause of bacterial tonsillopharyngitis is a GABHS, which may be diagnosed by performing a group A *Streptococcus* test. Other pathogens have also been associated with the disease such as *M. catarrhalis, H. influenzae, S. aureus*, and *S. pneumoniae* (71). Diphtheria and gonococcal infections should also be considered. If GABHS infection is suspected, antibiotic treatment should be initiated. Penicillin, amoxicillin, erythromycin, and first-generation cephalosporins are the recommended agents; performance of a group A *Streptococcus* test prior to initiation of antibiotic treatment is appropriate (72). If not treated, bacterial tonsillopharyngitis may lead to complications that can be suppurative and nonsuppurative. Nonsuppurative complications include scarlet fever, acute rheumatic fever, and poststreptococcal glomerulonephritis. Suppurative complications include peritonsillar, parapharyngeal, and retropharyngeal cellulites and/or abscess (73,74). In cases of recurrent streptococcal tonsillopharyngitis or infections unresponsive to antimicrobial therapy, tonsillectomy might be indicated (75,76).

Herpangina

Herpangina is a disease that commonly occurs in children (77), with Coxsackie A virus being the most common causative organism (78). Patients will present with fever, malaise, and sore throat. On examination, oropharyngeal erythema is noted, and vesicles and small ulcers are present on the posterior pharynx, often on the uvula and soft palate. The course of herpangina is usually self-limited.

Peritonsillar Abscess

Peritonsillar abscess is the most common deep infection of the head and neck, usually occurring as a complication of bacterial tonsillitis or, less frequently, in cases of infectious mononucleosis, and is most commonly diagnosed in adults or adolescents. Infection may spread through the tonsillar capsule into the space between the tonsil and superior constrictor muscle and sequentially develop into an abscess. Patients will present with increasing pharyngeal pain, dysphagia, trismus, dysarthria, drooling, and a muffled voice. The clinical examination reveals trismus, peritonsillar bulging that displaces the soft palate medially, and uvular deviation toward the opposite side; patients will often have tonsillar exudates and tender cervical lymphadenopathy (79,80). A peritonsillar abscess is usually polymicrobial, with Group A streptococci and anaerobes, the most common pathogens. While the diagnosis is usually made on physical examination, a CT scan of the mid-face and neck may help if there is diagnostic uncertainty, but is usually not necessary. Treatment involves aspiration or incision and drainage of the abscess along with antibiotic therapy, and recent data suggest that steroids may improve outcomes as well (81,82). If the peritonsillar abscess becomes recurrent, a tonsillectomy would be indicated (80). A peritonsillar space infection has the potential for spreading to the parapharyngeal space, the manifestations of which may be delayed.

Lemierre Syndrome

Lemierre syndrome is described as the presence of oropharyngeal infection, sepsis, internal jugular vein thrombosis, and septic emboli caused by *Fusobacterium necrophorum* (83,84). This is a gram-negative anaerobic organism which can be part of the normal human oropharyngeal, gastrointestinal, or genitourinary flora. The disease is currently uncommon due to the availability of antibiotics. Lemiere syndrome most often affects young adults with a recent history of oropharyngeal, tonsillar, or peritonsillar infection. Patients will often present with tenderness and swelling of the lateral neck, secondary to thrombophlebitis of the internal jugular vein. Septic emboli may spread and affect other organs, especially the lungs. Mortality rates approach 5%, and thus the disease requires immediate and aggressive antibiotic treatment with agents such as clindamycin, metronidazole, ampicillin–sulbactam, or ticarcillin–clavulanate for a period of at least 6 weeks (84); in the case of abscess formation, surgical drainage might be required (85). Anticoagulation is controversial, but may be indicated in severe disease (86).

Infectious Mononucleosis

Infectious mononucleosis is a systemic disease caused by Epstein–Barr virus, transmitted via saliva, and most commonly occurring in teenagers and young adults. Patients will present with fever, fatigue, malaise, sore throat, and generalized nontender lymphadenopathy. On examination, one encounters inflamed tonsils with exudate; hepatosplenomegaly may also be present. Diagnosis is confirmed by the presence of atypical lymphocytes on peripheral smear, a positive monospot test, and positive EBV titers; treatment is supportive (87). Corticosteroids are used to decrease inflammation, particularly in cases where airway obstruction is a concern due to marked tonsillar enlargement; in severe cases, where airway obstruction is a concern, establishing a secure airway may be indicated. Patients will develop a rash if treated with amoxicillin for presumed bacterial tonsillitis, thus administration of amoxicillin should be avoided.

LARYNX/AIRWAY

Supraglottitis/Epiglottitis

Epiglottitis is an infectious disease of the epiglottis and supraglottis, most commonly bacterial in origin. It usually has a sudden onset, with patients developing high fever, pain with swallowing, drooling due to difficulty handling secretions, and respiratory distress. On presentation the patient is often found sitting in a hunched forward position with an extended neck and open mouth (sniffing position) (88). On a lateral neck film, edema of the epiglottis and a ballooning of the hypopharynx ("thumb" sign) will be noted (Fig. 87.8). On physical examination, the oral cavity and oropharynx will look remarkably benign. However, on direct visualization, the epiglottis will appear erythematous ("cherry-red") and swollen. Care should be taken with airway manipulation as it may quickly precipitate complete airway obstruction. *H. influenzae* used to be the most common causative agent; however, with the introduction of the vaccine, the incidence of *H. influenza*–related epiglottitis

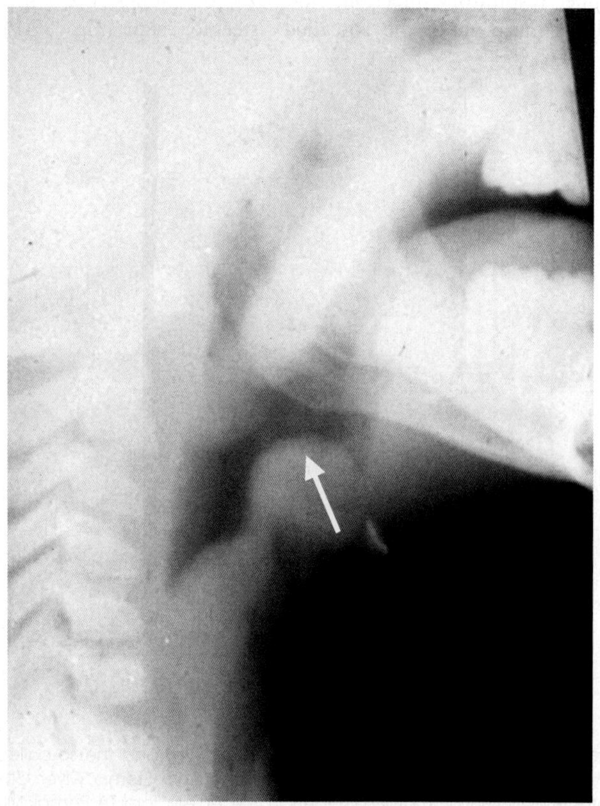

FIGURE 87.8 Lateral plain neck radiograph demonstrating edema (arrow) of the epiglottis associated with epiglottitis.

has significantly decreased (89). Currently, *S. pneumonia* group A and β-hemolytic streptococcus are the most common causative agents (90). Epiglottitis is considered an emergency as it has a potential for rapid complete airway obstruction, particularly in children. When epiglottitis is diagnosed, a secure airway should be established, in most cases, via flexible fiberoptic endotracheal intubation or tracheostomy; the decision to extubate or decannulate the trachea is based upon clinical improvement. Treatment with intravenous antibiotics (ceftriaxone or ampicillin–sublactam) and steroids should be initiated immediately (88,89). Adults may sometimes present with supraglottitis where the epiglottitis is not involved. In these cases, the airway can often be managed more conservatively, although in hospital, observation is required.

Laryngitis

Acute laryngitis most often occurs as part of an upper respiratory infection, and therefore is usually caused by rhinovirus (91). Laryngoscopy reveals diffuse laryngeal erythema and edema, often producing a cough and hoarseness. The treatment is most often supportive, including voice rest, humidification, and occasionally anti-inflammatory medications.

Croup

Croup is an inflammatory disease of the subglottic airway, almost always associated with a viral infection, most commonly parainfluenza and influenza viruses. It is most often seen in children between the ages of 1 and 3 years. Patients usually present with fever, tachypnea, inspiratory stridor, hoarseness, and a barking cough; the history often includes a preceding upper respiratory infection. Radiographic studies reveal subglottic narrowing, the so-called "steeple" sign (Fig. 87.9).

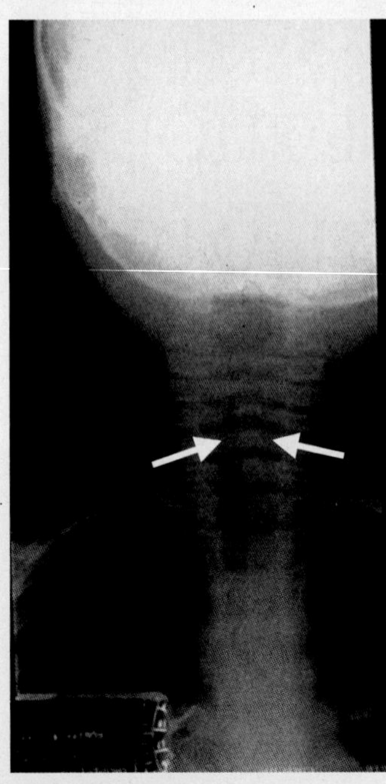

FIGURE 87.9 Subglottic edema causing narrowing and the so-called steeple sign (arrows) associated with croup. (From Stern Y, Myer CM. Infectious and inflammatory disorders. In: Seiden AM, Tami TA, Pensak ML, et al., eds. *Otolaryngology: The Essentials.* New York, NY: Thieme Medical Publisher; 2001:304, with permission.)

Additional diagnostic information can be provided by flexible bedside endoscopy. Depending on the severity of the symptoms, patients might require close observation and establishment of a secure airway. Administration of glucocorticoids is recommended to decrease airway inflammation, and racemic epinephrine treatments are often helpful. In moderate to severe croup, helium–oxygen (heliox) treatment is also of benefit (92). When croup is recurrent, an airway evaluation with laryngoscopy and bronchoscopy is recommended to assess for anatomic abnormalities such as subglottic stenosis (93,94).

Diphtheria

Diphtheria is an infectious disease of the upper airway caused by *Corynebacterium diphtheriae* and is rather rare due to widespread immunization. Patients present with fever and malaise; bloody nasal discharge and pseudomembranes in the nose, oropharynx, and larynx may be noted on examination; the presence of membranes may lead to airway obstruction and respiratory failure. Exotoxins produced by the bacteria may affect the heart, liver, kidney, and brain. Clinical diagnosis is confirmed by bacterial smear and cultures on Löffler or tellurite media. The treatment consists of assuring a secure airway, administration of antitoxin, and antibiotics. Penicillin or erythromycin is recommended for treatment (95).

Bacterial Tracheitis

Bacterial tracheitis is a rare, potentially life-threatening respiratory infection. It is characterized by the presence of thick membranous tracheal secretions that do not readily clear with coughing and may lead to occlusion of the airway. Patients present with fever, cough, stridor, and generalized malaise; there is no response to racemic epinephrine treatment. Radiographic findings often reveal irregular tracheal margins with a normal-appearing epiglottis. Diagnosis is made with direct endoscopic visualization of thick membranous tracheal secretions or the presence of purulent tracheal secretions in the glottis and subglottis (96). The most commonly isolated pathogen is *S. aureus*. Other causative bacterial pathogens include *H. influenzae, S. pneumoniae, Streptococcus pyogenes, M. catarrhalis, Klebsiella,* and *Pseudomonas* species (96–98). If the diagnosis of bacterial tracheitis is made, treatment consists of securing the airway, endoscopically removing tracheal membranes, and administration of antibiotics (97).

NECK

Salivary Gland Infections

Viral Infections

Mumps is a viral infection caused by paramyxovirus and is the most common viral infection that involves the salivary glands. Infected patients display signs of fever and malaise; painful parotid swelling occurs within 24 hours of symptom onset and is often bilateral, with pain upon salivation. Ten percent of patients have submandibular gland involvement; 25% of affected adolescent or adult males will develop orchitis, and 5% of females may present with oophoritis. Pancreatitis and central nervous system involvement may also occur in affected individuals; sensorineural hearing loss may also be seen in mumps. The treatment is usually supportive, although it must be noted that the disease is preventable by vaccination and children have a less severe course than adults (99). Other potential viruses that may infect the salivary glands include Coxsackie A, ECHO, choriomeningitis, parainfluenza types 1 and 3, and cytomegalovirus (99).

Bacterial Infections

Bacterial infections of the salivary glands often develop following salivary stasis, secondary to ductal obstruction by a stone or mass, or a decrease of salivary flow secondary to dehydration. Any sort of intraoral trauma, such as extensive dental work, may also cause an inflammatory obstruction of the duct. The most common causative pathogens are *S. aureus* and *Streptococcus viridans*. The parotid gland is affected more often, likely due to lower bacteriostatic activity of saliva from this gland as compared to the submandibular or sublingual gland. Patients present with pain, swelling, and erythema in the region of the salivary gland, exacerbated by eating; this disorder is most commonly seen in the elderly. Patients may also have fever, malaise, and an elevated white count. Treatment involves hydration to increase salivary flow, massaging of the effected gland, sialogogues, and administration of antistaphyloccocal antibiotics. If there is minimal improvement on conservative treatment, imaging may be considered (CT or ultrasound) to look for abscess. In cases of chronic or recurrent sialadenitis, removal of the obstructing stone via sialoendoscopy or excision of the gland may be indicated (100,101).

Lymphadenitis

Lymphadenitis is an inflammatory process involving lymph nodes, most commonly seen in the pediatric group. Upper respiratory viral infections are the most common cause of cervical lymphadenopathy. This condition is self-limited and usually does not require treatment. Bacterial lymphadenitis most often occurs as a complication of skin or respiratory infection. The commonest causative organisms are *S. aureus* and group A streptococci. Patients may present with tender lymphadenopathy, which may progress to formation of an abscess. If bacterial lymphadenitis is suspected, treatment with β-lactamase-resistant antibiotics is recommended. In case of progression to abscess formation, incision and drainage are indicated (102).

Cat-Scratch Disease

This disease usually presents with subacute solitary or regional lymphadenopathy in patients with a previous contact with a kitten or cat. It is primarily caused by *Bartonella henselae;* however, cases of *Bartonella clarridgeiae* and *Bartonella elizabethae* have been reported. Small red–brown nontender papules may develop at the site of inoculation 3 to 30 days after contact, and lymphadenopathy is seen 1 to 3 weeks after a scratch, bite, or other contact with an infected kitten or cat. The lymph nodes draining the affected site gradually enlarge and are moderately tender, with the overlying skin appearing warm and erythematous. Up to 10% of lesions may require surgical drainage. Histologic examination shows granulomata with multiple microabscesses. The indirect fluorescent antibody test and enzyme immunoassay are used for the detection of specific serum antibody to *B. henselae* (95).

Mycobacterium

Nontuberculous mycobacterial infection is a rare cause of lymphadenitis. It presents as a slowly enlarging, nontender cervical mass. The infection can affect adults; however, it is most commonly found in children less than 5 years of age. It is often diagnosed after the failure to respond to traditional antibiotics. The most common causative pathogen is *Mycobacterium avium–intracellulare;* other reported pathogens are *Mycobacterium scrofulaceum, Mycobacterium kanasasaii, Mycobacterium fortuitum,* and *Mycobacterium cobacterium malmoense* (103,104). Nontuberculous mycobacteria are found ubiquitously in the environment—soil, food, water, animals, etc. The infection is usually acquired from the environment, with no evidence of person-to-person transmission. An intradermal purified protein derivative (PPD) test aids in the diagnosis of nontuberculous lymphadenitis; however, positive cultures will be more definitive (105). Complications include fistula tract formation, and thus complete surgical resection of infected tissues has been the gold standard for the treatment of nontuberculous mycobacterial infections. Treatment with antituberculous medications, such as macrolides (clarithromycin) and rifampin, has also been shown to be effective in some cases. Recent studies have suggested an antibiotic therapeutic trial prior to surgical excision or as an adjunct to surgical excision, though this is controversial, and other data suggest complete excision as the treatment with the lowest likelihood of recurrence (106,107).

Actinomycosis

Actinomycosis is an infection caused by *Actinomyces israelii,* a gram-positive anaerobic bacterium. The disease has multiple presentations and is often misdiagnosed. The majority (>50%) of these infections occur in the head and neck region, most often entering the tissue through an area of prior trauma. As the infection develops, patients will be noted to have a woody induration that eventually leads to central abscess formation. This abscess will generally track to a mucosal surface or externally to the skin, forming a sinus or fistulous tract. The suppurative drainage will contain so-called sulfur granules, yellow flecks containing the bacterial colonies. The diagnosis is best made by culture, but as anaerobic cultures can be unreliable, diagnosis may have to rely on the clinical picture and histology. The organisms stain best with Gram and Gomori methenamine silver stains. Treatment consists of drainage and debridement of the infected area with administration of penicillin (108).

Deep Neck Space Infections

Retropharyngeal Space Abscess

The retropharyngeal space is defined by the prevertebral fascia posteriorly, the posterior layer of the deep cervical fascia anteriorly, the skull base superiorly, and the posterior mediastinum inferiorly (see Fig. 87.7). Infection usually develops from infected retropharyngeal lymph nodes, which receive lymphatic drainage from the paranasal sinuses, nasopharynx, and middle ear, and are more common in children; trauma is another common cause. Patients commonly present with fever, pain upon swallowing, decreased oral intake, drooling, malaise, and torticollis; trismus and neck swelling are often present. The most common causative organisms are *S. pyogenes, S. aureus,* and anaerobic bacteria (109). Lateral radiographic images of the neck in extension reveals thickened prevertebral soft tissue. CT aids in determining the presence of an abscess. Therapy involves the administration of intravenous antibiotics and abscess drainage. Transoral drainage is recommended unless there is extension lateral to the great vessels, i.e., the carotid artery (110). Adjunctive treatments include broad-spectrum antibiotics and steroids postoperatively to decrease swelling. If left untreated, spontaneous rupture of the abscess may lead to aspiration of infectious material; additionally, infection may spread to the parapharyngeal and prevertebral spaces, and lead to mediastinitis or involve the great vessels.

Parapharyngeal Space Abscess

The parapharyngeal space is a potential space that extends from the skull base to the greater cornu of the hyoid bone (see Fig. 87.7). The pharynx and superior constrictor muscle are the medial boundaries; the internal pterygoid muscle, parotid gland, and mandible are lateral structures; the prevertebral fascia lies posteriorly; and the pterygomandibular ligament is an anterior structure that surrounds the parapharyngeal space. The styloid process divides the space into anterior and posterior divisions. Pharyngeal infections, molar tooth infections, gingivitis, and even mastoiditis may spread to the parapharyngeal space. If untreated, infection has the potential to spread to the retropharyngeal space, to the mediastinum, and to involve the great vessels causing internal jugular thrombosis and erosion of the internal carotid artery; airway compromise may also occur. Patients typically present with a prior history of a sore throat or tooth infection. Initial symptoms are fever and pain upon swallowing. Tender, erythematous swelling at the angle of the mandible and parotid is typically found on clinical examination, but it will not appear fluctuant even if an abscess is present. Examination of the pharynx will often reveal medial displacement of the ipsilateral tonsil. Trismus may develop secondary to inflammation of the medial pterygoid muscle. Torticolis toward the opposite side often results from inflammation of lymph nodes under the sternocleidomastoid muscle; patients may also complain of otalgia (111). The most common causative pathogens are *S. aureus*, *S. pyogenes*, and *S. viridans* and anaerobic bacteria (112). CT with contrast aids in the evaluation of the site and the extent of infection, distinguishing between cellulitis and abscess (Fig. 87.10). Parapharyngeal space infections require immediate treatment with intravenous antibiotics and surgical drainage if a large abscess is present (113). This is usually done through an external approach. Transoral drainage is not recommended.

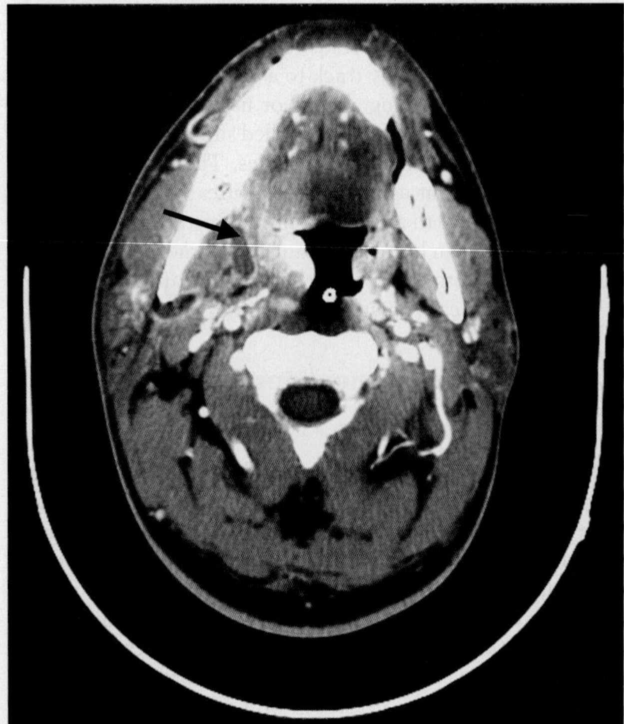

FIGURE 87.10 Computed tomography (CT) of the neck demonstrating a parapharyngeal space abscess.

Key Points

- In a patient presenting with an ear infection, pushing on the tragus will elicit pain if it is an outer or external ear infection, but not if it is a middle ear infection.
- Oral antibiotics are rarely helpful in the treatment of external otitis, a condition that is more effectively treated with topical preparations.
- Otomycosis caused by aspergillus usually presents with grayish black or yellow dots (fungal conidiophores) surrounded by a cotton-like material (fungal hyphae) that is easily visible when examining the ear canal.
- Otitis externa with granulation tissue in a diabetic patient should be considered diagnostic of necrotizing otitis externa and treated aggressively.
- In an adult presenting with a unilateral middle ear effusion, it is essential to evaluate the nasopharynx to rule out the presence of a nasopharyngeal mass obstructing the eustachian tube.
- Auricular perichondritis should be treated early and aggressively to prevent the sequela of auricular deformity. Antibiotics with cartilage penetration, such as fluoroquinolones, are recommended.
- The presence of a nasal septal hematoma or abscess requires immediate drainage to prevent secondary necrosis of the septal cartilage and the subsequent development of a saddle nose deformity.
- A bacterial rather than viral sinus infection should be suspected when symptoms have been present for >7 to 10 days or symptoms are worsening after 5 days. Most sinus infections are of viral etiology
- Ludwig angina can be rapidly progressive and should be considered an airway emergency, with a prophylactic awake tracheotomy recommended in most cases.
- Due to its potential for rapid airway compromise, epiglottitis should be considered an airway emergency.
- Due to its deep location, a parapharyngeal space abscess will cause tender induration of the upper neck, but not fluctuance.

References

1. Rosenfeld RM, Schwartz SR, Cannon CR, et al.; American Academy of Otolaryngology—Head and Neck Surgery Foundation. Clinical practice guideline: acute otitis externa executive summary. *Otolaryngol Head Neck Surg*. 2014;150(2):161–168.

2. Guthrie RM. Diagnosis and treatment of acute otitis externa: an interdisciplinary update. *Ann Otol Rhinol Laryngol.* 1999;17:2–23.
3. Kelly KE, Mohs DC. The external auditory canal: anatomy and physiology. *Otolaryngol Clin North Am.* 1996;29:725–739.
4. Clark WB, Brook I, Bianki D, Thompson DH. Microbiology of otitis exerna. *Otolaryngol Head Neck Surg.* 1997;116:23–52.
5. Schaefer P, Baugh RF. Acute otitis externa: an update. *Am Fam Physician.* 2012;86(11):1055–1061.
6. Kaushik V, Malik T, Saeed SR. Interventions for acute otitis externa. *Cochrane Database Syst Rev.* 2010;(1):CD004740.
7. Kesser BW. Assessment and management of chronic otitis externa. *Curr Opin Otolaryngol Head Neck Surg.* 2011;19(5):341–347.
8. Schapowal A. Otitis externa: a clinical overview. *Ear Nose Throat J.* 2002; 81(8 Suppl 1):21–22.
9. Viswanatha B, Sumatha D, Vijayashree MS. Otomycosis in immunocompetent and immunocompromised patients: comparative study and literature review. *Ear Nose Throat J.* 2012;91(3):114–121.
10. Anwar K, Gohar MS. Otomycosis; clinical features, predisposing factors and treatment implications. *Pak J Med Sci.* 2014;30(3):564–567.
11. Hobson CE, Moy JD, Byers KE, et al. Malignant otitis externa: evolving pathogens and implications for diagnosis and treatment. *Otolaryngol Head Neck Surg.* 2014;151(1):112–116.
12. Kountakis SE, Kemper JV Jr, Chang CY, et al. Osteomyelitis of the base of the skull secondary to Aspergillus. *Am J Otolaryngol.* 1997;18:19–22.
13. Chandler JR. Malignant external otitis. *Laryngoscope.* 1968;78:1257–1294.
14. Okpala NC, Siraj QH, Nilssen E, Pringle M. Radiological and radionuclide investigation of malignant otitis externa. *J Laryngol Otol.* 2005; 119(1):71–75.
15. Bojrab DI, Bruderly T, Abdulrazzak Y. Otitis externa. *Otolaryngol Clin North Am.* 1996;29:761–782.
16. Bluestone CD, Gates GA, Klein JO, et al. Definitions, terminology, and classification of otitis media. *Ann Otol Rhinol Laryngol.* 2002;111:8–18.
17. Lieberthal AS, Carroll AE, Chonmaitree T, et al. Clinical practice guidelines: the diagnosis and management of acute otitis media. *Pediatrics.* 2013;131(3):e964–e999.
18. Hoberman A, Marchant CD, Kaplan SL, Feldman S. Treatment of acute otitis media consensus recommendations. *Clin Pediatr (Phila).* 2002;41:373–390.
19. Rosenfeld RM, Culpepper L, Doyle KJ, et al. American Academy of Pediatrics Subcommittee on Otitis Media with Effusion; American Academy of Family Physicians; American Academy of Otolaryngology—Head and Neck Surgery. Clinical practice guideline: otitis media with effusion. *Otolaryngol Head Neck Surg.* 2004;130(5 Suppl):S95–S118.
20. Jahn AF. Chronic otitis media: diagnosis and treatment. *Med Clin North Am.* 1991;75(6):1277–1291.
21. Rosenfeld RM, Schwartz SR, Pynnonen MA. Clinical practice guideline: tympanostomy tubes in children. *Otolaryngology Head Neck Surg.* 2013;149 (1 Suppl):S1–S35.
22. Kenna MA. Treatment of chronic suppurative otitis media. *Otolaryngol Clin North Am.* 1994;27(3):457–472.
23. van Dongen TM, van der Heijden GJ, Venekamp RP, et al. A trial of treatment for acute otorrhea in children with tympanostomy tubes. *N Engl J Med.* 2014;370(8):723–733.
24. Leskinen K, Jero J. Acute complications of otitis media in adults. *Clin Otolaryngol.* 2005:30(6):511–516.
25. Penido Nde O, Borin A, Iha LC, et al. Intracranial complications of otitis media: 15 years of experience in 33 patients. *Otolaryngol Head Neck Surg.* 2005;132:37–42.
26. Hyden D, Akerlind B, Peebo M. Inner ear and facial nerve complications of acute otitis media with focus on bacteriology and virology. *Acta Otolaryngol.* 2006;126(5):460–466.
27. Ahmed A. When is facial paralysis Bell palsy? Current diagnosis and treatment. *Cleve Clin J Med.* 2005;72(5):398–401, 405.
28. Jackler RK, Furuta Y. Reactiveation of herpes simplex virus type 1 in patients with Bell's palsy. *Am J Otol.* 1998;19:236–245.
29. Baugh RF, Basura GJ, Ishii LE, et al. Clinical practice guideline: Bell's palsy executive summary. *Otolaryngol Head Neck Surg.* 2013;149(5):656–663.
30. Murakiami S, Nakashiro Y, Mizobuchi M, et al. Varicella-zoster virus distribution in Ramsay Hunt syndrome revealed by polymerase chain reaction. *Acta Otolaynqol (Stockholm).* 1998;118:145–149.
31. Kuhweide R, Van de Steene V, Vlaminck S, Casselman JW. Ramsay Hunt syndrome: pathophysiology of cochleovestibular symptoms. *J Laryngol Otol.* 2002;116(10):844–848.
32. Murakami S, Hato N, Horiuch J, et al. Treatment of Ramsay Hunt syndrome with acyclovir–prednisone: significance of early diagnosis and treatment. *Ann Neurol.* 1997;41:353–357.
33. Liu ZW, Chokkalingam P. Piercing associated perichondritis of the pinna: are we treating it correctly? *J Laryngol Otol.* 2013;127(5):505–508.
34. Keene WE, Markum AC, Samadpour M. Outbreak of *Pseudomonas aeruginosa* infections caused by commercial piercing of upper ear cartilage. *JAMA.* 2004;291(8):981–985.
35. Bachor E, Blevins NH, Karmody C, Kühnel T. Otologic manifestations of relapsing polychondritis. Review of literature and report of nine cases. *Auris Nasus Larynx.* 2006;33(2):135–141.
36. Ambrus PS, Eavey RD, Baker AS, et al. Management of nasal septal abscess. *Laryngoscope.* 1981;91:575–582.
37. Canty PA, Berkowitz RG. Hematoma and abscess of the nasal septum in children. *Arch Otolaryngol Head Neck Surg.* 1996;122:1373–1376.
38. van den Broek MF, Gudden C, Kluijfhout WP, et al. No evidence for distinguishing bacterial from viral acute rhinosinusitis using symptom duration and purulent rhinorrhea: a systematic review of the evidence base. *Otolaryngol Head Neck Surg.* 2014;150(4):533–537.
39. Marple BF, Brunton S, Ferguson BJ. Acute bacterial rhinosinusitis: a review of U.S. treatment guidelines. *Otolaryngol Head Neck Surg.* 2006; 135(3):341–348.
40. Brook I. Microbiology and antimicrobial management of sinusitis. *Otolaryngol Clin North Am.* 2004;37(2):253–266, v–vi.
41. Brook I. Sinusitis of odontogenic origin. *Otolaryngol Head Neck Surg.* 2006;135(3):349–355.
42. Chow AW, Benninger MS, Brook I, et al.; Infectious Diseases Society of America. IDSA clinical practice guideline for acute bacterial rhinosinusitis in children and adults. *Clin Infect Dis.* 2012;54(8):e72–e112.
43. Rosenfeld RM, Andes D, Bhattacharyya N. Clinical practice guidelines: adult sinusitis. *Otolaryngol Head Neck Surg.* 2007;137(3 Suppl): S1–S31.
44. Younis RT, Lazar RH, Anand VK. Intracranial complications of sinusitis: a 15-year review of 39 cases. *Ear Nose Throat J.* 2002;81(9):636–638.
45. Jackson LL, Kountakis SE. Classification and management of rhinosinusitis and its complications. *Otolaryngol Clin North Am.* 2005;38(6): 1143–1153.
46. Teinzer F, Stammberger H, Tomazic PV. Transnasal endoscopic treatment of orbital complications of acute sinusitis: the Graz concept. *Ann Otol Rhinol Laryngol.* 2015;124(5):368–373.
47. Benninger MS, Ferguson BJ, Hadley JA, et al. Adult chronic rhinosinusitis: definitions, diagnosis, epidemiology, and pathophysiology. *Otolaryngol Head Neck Surg.* 2003;129(3 Suppl):S1–32.
48. Devaiah AK. Adult chronic rhinosinusitis: diagnosis and dilemmas. *Otolaryngol Clin North Am.* 2004;37(2):243–252.
49. Seidman MD, Gurgel RK, Lin SY, et al.; Guideline Otolaryngology Development Group. AAO-HNSF. Clinical practice guideline: allergic rhinitis. *Otolaryngol Head Neck Surg.* 2015;152(1 Suppl):S1–S43.
50. Smith LF, Brindley PC. Indications, evaluation, complications, and results of functional endoscopic sinus surgery in 200 patients. *Otolaryngol Head Neck Surg.* 1993;108(6):688–696.
51. Winther B, Gwaltney JM Jr, Mygind N, Hendley JO. Viral-induced rhinitis. *Am J Rhinol.* 1998;12(1):17–20.
52. DeShazo RD, Chapin K, Swain RE. Fungal sinusitis. *N Engl J Med.* 1997; 337:254–259.
53. Zuniga MG, Turner JH. Treatment outcomes in acute invasive fungal rhinosinusitis. *Curr Opin Otolaryngol Head Neck Surg.* 2014;22(3): 242–248.
54. Schubert MS. Allergic fungal sinusitis. *Otolaryngol Clin North Am.* 2004; 37(2):301–326.
55. deShazo RD, O'Brien M, Chapin K, et al. Criteria for the diagnosis of sinus mycetoma. *J Allergy Clin Immunol.* 1997;99:475–485.
56. DeShazo RD, Swain RE. Diagnostic criteria for allergic fungal sinusitis. *J Allergy Clin Immunol.* 1995;96:24–35.
57. Plonk DP, Luong A. Current understanding of allergic fungal rhinosinusitis and treatment implications. *Curr Opin Otolaryngol Head Neck Surg.* 2014;22(3):221–226.
58. Pihlstrom BL, Michalowicz BS, Johnson NW. Periodontal diseases. *Lancet.* 2005;306:1809–1820.
59. Preshaw PM, Seymour RA, Heasman PA. Current concepts in periodontal pathogenesis. *Dent Update.* 2004;31:570–578.
60. Tatakis DN, Kumar PS. Etiology and pathogenesis of periodontal diseases. *Dent Clin North Am.* 2005;49:491–516.
61. Johnson BD, Engel D. Acute necrotizing ulcerative gingivitis: a review of diagnosis, etiology and treatment. *J Periodontol.* 1986;57(3):141–150.
62. Rowland RW. Necrotizing ulcerative gingivitis. *Ann Periodontol.* 1999; 4:65–73.
63. Amir J. Clinical aspects and antiviral therapy in primary herpetic gingivostomatitis. *Paediatr Drugs.* 2001;3(8):593–597.

64. Ajar AH, Chauvin PJ. Acute herpetic gingivostomatitis in adults: a review of 13 cases, including diagnosis and management. *J Can Dent Assoc.* 2002;68(4):247–251.
65. Giannini PJ, Shetty KV. Diagnosis and management of oral candidiasis. *Otolaryngol Clin North Am.* 2011;44(1):231–240.
66. Flynn TR. What are the antibiotics of choice for odontogenic infections, and how long should the treatment course last? *Oral Maxillofac Surg Clin North Am.* 2011;23(4):519–536, v–vi.
67. Baker AS, Montgomery WW. Oropharyngeal space infections. *Curr Clin Top Infect Dis.* 1987;8:227–265.
68. Busch RF, Shah D. Ludwig's angina: improved treatment. *Otolaryngol Head Neck Surg.* 1997;117:S172–S175.
69. Baqain ZH, Newman L, Hyde N. How serious are oral infections? *J Laryngol Otol.* 2004;118:561–565.
70. Bastaki JM. Necrotizing tonsillitis caused by group C beta-hemolytic streptococci. *Ear Nose Throat J.* 2015;94(3):E1–E3.
71. Brook I, Gober AE. Increased recovery of *Moraxella catarrhalis* and *Haemophilus influenzae* in association with group A beta-haemolytic streptococci in healthy children and those with pharyngo-tonsillitis. *J Med Microbiol.* 2006;55(Pt 8):989–992.
72. Rufener JB, Yaremchuk KL, Payne SC. Evaluation of culture and antibiotic use in patients with pharyngitis. *Laryngoscope.* 2006;116:1727–1729.
73. Tewfik TL, Al Garni M. Tonsillopharyngitis: clinical highlights. *J Otolaryngol.* 2005;34(Suppl 1):S45–S49.
74. Wessels MR. Clinical practice. Streptococcal Pharyngitis. *N Engl J Med.* 2011;364:648–655.
75. Darrow DH, Siemens C. Indications for tonsillectomy and adenoidectomy. *Laryngoscope.* 2002;112:6–10.
76. Burton MJ, Glasziou PP, Chong LY, Venekamp RP. Tonsillectomy or adenotonsillectomy versus non-surgical treatment for chronic/recurrent acute tonsillitis. *Cochrane Database Syst Rev.* 2014;(11):CD001802.
77. Cherry JD, Jahn CL. Herpangina: the etiologic spectrum. *Pediatrics.* 1965; 36(4):632–634.
78. Zavate O, Avram G, Pavlov E. Coxsackie A virus-associated herpetiform angina. *Virologie.* 1984;35(1):49–53.
79. Johnson RF, Stewart MG, Wright CC. An evidence-based review of the treatment of peritonsillar abscess. *Otolaryngol Head Neck Surg.* 2003; 128(3):332–343.
80. Powell J, Wilson JA. An evidence-based review of peritonsillar abscess. *Clin Otolaryngol.* 2012;37(2):136–145.
81. Hardman JC, McCulloch NA, Nankivell P. Do corticosteroids improve outcomes in peritonsillar abscess? *Laryngoscope.* 2015;125(3):537–538.
82. Shaul C, Koslowsky B, Rodriguez M, et al. Is needle aspiration for peritonsillar abscess still as good as we think? a long-term follow-up. *Ann Otol Rhinol Laryngol.* 2015;124(4):299–304.
83. Moreno S, Garcia Altozano J, Pinilla B, et al. Lemierre's disease: postanginal bacteremia and pulmonary involvement caused by Fusobacterium necrophorum. *Rev Infect Dis.* 1989;11:319–324.
84. Brook I. Microbiology and management of deep facial infections and Lemierre syndrome. *ORL J Otorhinolaryngol Relat Spec.* 2003;65;117–120.
85. Nadkarni MD, Verchick J, O'Neill JC. Lemierre syndrome. *J Emerg Med.* 2005;28;297–299.
86. Ebell MH. Epstein-Barr virus infectious mononucleosis. *Am Fam Physician.* 2004;70(7):1279–1287.
87. Rea TD, Russo JE, Katon W, et al. Prospective study of the natural history of infectious mononucleosis caused by Epstein-Barr virus. *J Am Board Fam Pract.* 2001;14(4):234–242.
88. Carey MJ. Epiglottitis in adults. *Am J Emerg Med.* 1996;14(4):421–424.
89. Shah RK, Roberson DW, Jones DT. Epiglottitis in the Hemophilus influenzae type B vaccine era: changing trends. *Laryngoscope.* 2004;114:557–560.
90. Trollfors B, Nylen O, Carenfelt C, et al. Aetiology of acute epiglottitis in adults. *Scand J Infect Dis.* 1998;30(1):49–51.
91. Monto AS. Epidemiology of viral respiratory infections. *Am J Med.* 2002; 112 (Suppl 6A):4S–12S.
92. Stroud RH, Friedman NR. An update on inflammatory disorders of the pediatric airway: epiglottitis, croup, and tracheitis. *Am J Otolaryngol.* 2001;22(4):268–275.
93. Hadfield TL, McEvoy P, Polotsky Y, et al. The pathology of diphtheria. *J Infect Dis.* 2000;181(Suppl 1):S116–S120.
94. Friedman EM, Jorgensen K, Healy GB, McGill TJ. Bacterial tracheitis: two-year experience. *Laryngoscope.* 1985;95(1):9–11.
95. Mahajan A, Alvear D, Chang C, et al. Bacterial tracheitis, diagnosis and treatment. *Int J Pediatr Otorhinolaryngol.* 1985;10(3):271–277.
96. Salamone FN, Bobbitt DB, Myer CM, et al. Bacterial tracheitis reexamined: is there a less severe manifestation? *Otolaryngol Head Neck Surg.* 2004;131(6):871–876.
97. Johnson A. Inflammatory conditions of the major salivary glands. *Ear Nose Throat J.* 1989;68:94–102.
98. Blitzer A. Inflammatory and obstructive disorders of salivary glands. *J Dent Res.* 1987;66:675–679.
99. Travis LW, Hecht DW. Acute and chronic inflammatory diseases of the salivary glands: diagnosis and management. *Otolaryngol Clin North Am.* 1977;10:329–338.
100. Gosche JR, Vick L. Acute, subacute, and chronic cervical lymphadenitis in children. *Semin Pediatr Surg.* 2006;15(2):99–106.
101. Leung AK, Robson WL. Childhood cervical lymphadenopathy. *J Pediatr Health Care.* 2004;18:3–7.
102. Massei F, Gori L, Macchia P, Maggiore G. The expanded spectrum of Bartonellosis in children. *Infect Dis Clin North Am.* 2005;19:691–711.
103. Flint D, Mahadevan M, Barber C, et al. Cervical lymphadenitis due to non-tuberculous mycobacteria: surgical treatment and review. *Int J Pediatr Otorhinolaryngol.* 2000;53(3):187–194.
104. Danielides V, Patrikakos G, Moerman M, et al. Diagnosis, management and surgical treatment of non-tuberculous mycobacterial head and neck infection in children. *ORL J Otorhinolaryngol Relat Spec.* 2002;64: 284–289.
105. Luong A, McClay JE, Jafri HS, Brown O. Antibiotic therapy for nontuberculous mycobacterial cervicofacial lymphadenitis. *Laryngoscope.* 2005;115:1746–1751.
106. Richtsmeier WJ, Johns ME. Actinomycosis of the head and neck. *CRC Crit Rev Clin Lab Sci.* 1979;11(2):175–202.
107. Kirse DJ, Roberson DW. Surgical management of retropharyngeal space infections in children. *Laryngoscope.* 2001;111:1413–1422.
108. Sethi DS, Stanley RE. Parapharyngeal abscesses. *J Laryngol Otol.* 1991; 105(12):1025–1030.
109. Boscolo-Rizzo P, Marchiori C, Zanetti F, et al. Conservative management of deep neck abscesses in adults: the importance of CECT findings. *Otolaryngol Head Neck Surg.* 2006;135(6):894–899.

CHAPTER

88

Hospital-Acquired Infections

Section I

Catheter-Related Bloodstream Infections

ANDREW DAVIS ASSAF, ELIZABETH WENQIAN WANG, and ISSAM I. RAAD

INTRODUCTION

In 1929, Werner Forssmann (1) inserted the first reported central venous catheter (CVC) in a human being. Sven-Ivar Seldinger, in 1959, described and performed the Seldinger technique, still widely used today in modified form, that facilitated safe access to the central venous system via a catheter (2). Today, the use of CVCs has expanded in the inpatient and outpatient settings, and particularly in the critically ill patients and patients with invasive cancers; a total of more than 13 million CVCs are inserted annually of which 4 million are in cancer patients (3). CVCs serve many purposes including, but not limited to, medication and total parenteral nutrition (TPN) administration, hemodynamic monitoring, and extracorporeal therapies (4). However, these intravascular devices (IVDs) are a conduit for bacterial and fungal invasions, resulting in catheter-related bloodstream infection (CRBSI) (Table 88.1.1) that ultimately can be complicated by septic thrombophlebitis, infective endocarditis (IE), and other metastatic infections, such as lung abscess, brain abscess, and endophthalmitis.

CRBSI is one of the most frequent complications of CVC placement, and certainly the most frequent cause of nosocomial bacteremia (5). More than 400,000 CRBSIs, of which 80,000 occur in the ICU setting, are estimated to occur annually in the United States based on a conservative rate of 0.5 CRBSI per 1,000 catheter days, with an average of 200 catheter days per person and an attributable mortality ranging from 12% to 25% (3,6). Therefore, between 48,000 and 100,000 patients may die from CRBSI annually, of which 9,600 to 20,000 occur in the ICU alone. The average cost of treatment ranges between $33,000 and $75,000 per individual episode of CRBSI in ICU patients, with a gap of more than $26,000 between total cost and reimbursement (7). One study suggested an average of $45,814 per CRBSI with a total annual cost that exceeds $18 billion (8). Non-ICU patients, especially the immunocompromised hosts with CVCs in place, are also at significant risk. These infections are often difficult to diagnose, treat, and prevent; this chapter will concentrate on these aspects of CRBSI.

PATHOGENESIS

Diagnosis, treatment, and prevention of CRBSIs are based on our understanding of the pathogenesis of these infections. For short-term, nontunneled, noncuffed, multilumen catheters—which make up 90% of CRBSIs—the skin insertion site is the source of the colonization; organisms migrate along the external surface of the catheter and through the subcutaneous layers and infect the catheter tip (9,10). For long-term catheters—the cuffed, tunneled, silicone catheters, Hickman or Broviac—or implantable devices, the lumen of the hub or belt of the port is the primary source of entry (11,12). Micro-organisms are introduced via the hands of medical personnel while manipulating the hub during, for example, flushing and drawing of blood (11–13). Of note, colonization is universal after insertion of a CVC, can occur as early as 1 day after insertion, and is quantitatively independent of a catheter-related infection (11).

These sources explain the prevalence of *Staphylococcus aureus*, coagulase-negative *Staphylococcus*, enterococci, nonenteric hospital-acquired gram-negative bacilli (GNB) (*Stenotrophomonas maltophilia, Pseudomonas aeruginosa, Acinetobacter* spp.), mycobacteria, and *Candida* spp. as primary organisms of CRBSI (14). Secondary seeding of the CVC, whereby organisms become blood-borne and colonize the catheter, has been suggested (15,16) to the point of recommending treatment of urinary tract infections prior to CVC insertion to prevent a potential CRBSI (17); however, its role in CRBSI has not been corroborated (17). Contamination of the infusate or additives, such as contaminated heparin flush, is a rare cause of colonization and infection of vascular devices (18–20). The contamination of infusate takes place during the manufacture, solution preparation, or handling by health care worker, and leads to a cluster of bloodstream infections (BSIs) with the same—often unusual—organism. The nationwide outbreaks of *Enterobacter agglomerans* and *Enterobacter cloacae* in 1971 led to widespread changes and surveillance at industry, hospital, and state and federal levels. Even though TPN has been historically associated with CRBSI mainly due to *Candida* spp., there is some evidence suggesting that the etiology is mainly polymicrobial (21). Some studies have suggested that a more acidic TPN solution might suppress bacterial growth and skew the etiology toward *Candida* spp., which is not suppressed by changes in the content pH (22).

The second step in the pathogenesis of CRBSI is the ability of some microbes to form a biofilm of extracellular, polysaccharide-rich slime (23), promoting the adhesiveness of the bacteria to the surface of the CVC. Biofilms form on the external surface of short-term catheters and the internal surface of long-term catheters—that is, those with a dwell time of at least 30 days. This biofilm enables bacteria not only to adhere to the surface of the catheter, but also to resist antibiotics, such that biofilm eradication becomes a difficult task (24). Another factor promoting adherence is the thrombin layer that covers both surfaces of a catheter during its insertion; the rich composition

TABLE 88.1.1 Definitions of Catheter-related Bloodstream Infections (CRBSI)

PROBABLE CRBSI

- Clinical manifestations of infection (fever >38°C, chills/rigors, or hypotension)
- No apparent source of the sepsis/bloodstream infection other than the catheter
- Common skin organisms (e.g., coagulase-negative staphylococci) isolated from two blood cultures from patients with intravascular device or a known pathogen (*Staphylococcus aureus* or *Candida*) isolated from a single blood culture

DEFINITE CRBSI

- Probable CRBSI criteria outlined above with any of the following:
- Differential quantitative blood cultures with 5:1 ratio of the same organism isolated from blood drawn simultaneously from the central venous catheter (CVC) and peripheral vein

or

- Differential positivity time (positive result of culture from a CVC is obtained at least 2 hr earlier than positive result of culture from peripheral blood)

or

- Positive quantitative skin culture whereby the organism isolated from an infected insertion site is identical to that isolated from blood

or

- Isolation of the same organisms from the peripheral blood and from a quantitative or semi-quantitative culture of a catheter segment or tip

of the host's own blood components enables *S. aureus,* for example, to adhere to fibrinogen, coagulase-negative *Staphylococcus* to fibronectin, and *Candida* spp. to fibrin (25–29).

There has been a correlation of catheter site and risk of infection in the past; however, one study has shown that there is no difference in the risk of CRBSI when comparing the femoral and internal jugular sites (30) and that concept has been enforced in the CDC guidelines (31). Avoiding the use of the femoral is for reasons other than infections such as thrombosis (31). In general, the preferential site for nontunneled CVCs is the subclavian vein (31). In terms of catheter site dressings, the CDC recommends using a sterile gauze or sterile transparent dressings to cover the catheter which are to be changed every 2 or 7 days, respectively (31). With the exception of dialysis catheters, the use of antibiotic creams or ointments is not advised as they may promote antimicrobial resistance and fungal growth. In the setting of increasing central line–associated bloodstream infection (CLABSI) rates, the use of chlorhexidine (CHX)-impregnated dressings is acceptable for short-term catheters provided the patient is older than 2 months (31).

CLINICAL MANIFESTATIONS

Clinical manifestations of CRBSIs can be divided into two categories: local and systemic. Local manifestations include erythema, edema, tenderness, and purulent discharge. These signs and symptoms are neither sensitive nor specific, and cannot be relied on to identify catheter colonization or CVC-related BSI. On the one hand, they could be completely absent, especially in immunocompromised and neutropenic patients. On the other hand, peripherally inserted central catheters (PICCs) (inserted in the basilic or cephalic veins) are associated with a 26% rate of sterile local exit site inflammation secondary to irritation of small veins (i.e., cephalic vein) by insertion of a large catheter (32); to this must be added the finding that coagulase-negative staphylococci, the most frequent pathogen involved, incites little local or systemic inflammation (33).

The CDC suggests the following definitions:

1. *Exit-site infection*: Purulent drainage from the catheter exit site, or erythema, tenderness, and swelling within 2 cm of the catheter exit site, and colonization of the catheter, if removed, with or without concomitant BSI.
2. *Port-pocket infection*: Erythema, tenderness, induration, and/or necrosis of the skin or subcutaneous tissues either over or around the reservoir of a totally implanted IVD, and colonization of the device if removed, with or without concomitant BSI.
3. *Tunnel infection:* Erythema, tenderness, and induration of the tissues above the catheter and more than 2 cm from the exit site, along the subcutaneous tract of a tunneled catheter and colonization of the catheter if removed, with or without concomitant BSI.

The systemic features of CRBSIs are generally indistinguishable from those of secondary BSIs arising from other foci of infection, and include fever and chills, which may be accompanied by hypotension, hyperventilation, altered mental status, and nonspecific gastrointestinal manifestations such as nausea, vomiting, abdominal pain, and diarrhea. Deep-seated infections such as endocarditis, osteomyelitis, retinitis, and organ abscess may complicate CRBSIs caused by some virulent organisms such as *S. aureus, P. aeruginosa,* and *Candida albicans.*

DIAGNOSIS

A clinical diagnosis of CRBSI is frequently inaccurate. At this juncture, it is worth noting the difference of *CRBSI* and *CLABSI,* as these terms are often used interchangeably but incorrectly. *CLABSI* is used by CDC's National Healthcare Safety Network (NHSN) to describe any primary BSI in a patient who had a central line within 48 hours of the development of the BSI, and is not related to an infection at another site, such as pyelonephritis or pneumonia. However, other sources of infection, such as mucositis, that are less identifiable, may have led to the BSI, so the diagnosis of CLABSI is nonspecific and overestimates the true incidence of CRBSI. On the other hand, CRBSI is a subcategory of CLABSI for which specific laboratory testing has been done and identifies the catheter as the source of BSI.

Removal of the CVC has been mandatory to prove the CRBSI. Microbiologic methods requiring removal of the CVC were studied with the semi-quantitative roll-plate catheter cultures, developed by Maki et al. (34) in 1977, and considered the gold standard. However, the majority of the catheters were removed unnecessarily, exposing the patient to the complications related to reinsertion of a new CVC and adding to the cost of care. To prevent that, techniques allowing accurate diagnosis without removing the line have been elaborated; these are reviewed (Table 88.1.2).

Catheter-Sparing Diagnostic Methods

Simultaneous Quantitative Blood Cultures

This method consists of obtaining paired quantitative blood cultures (QBCs) simultaneously from the CVC and a peripheral vein. The target is to have both samples drawn less than 10

TABLE 88.1.2 Sensitivity and Specificity of Tests Used in the Diagnosis of CRBSI[a]

Diagnostic Tests	Sensitivity	Specificity
Paired quantitative blood cultures	75–93%	97–100%
Differential time to positivity		
Short-term CVCs	89%	87%
Long-term CVCs	90%	72%
Acridine orange leukocyte cytospin technique	87%	94%
Semi-quantitative culture of catheter tip (roll-plate technique)		
Short-term CVCs	84%	85%
Long-term CVCs	45%	75%
Quantitative catheter culture		
Short-term CVCs	82%	89%
Long-term CVCs	83%	97%

CRBSI, catheter-related bloodstream infection; CVC, central venous catheter.
[a]The data on the sensitivities and specificities are based on a meta-analysis of diagnostic methods by Safdar N, Fine JP, Maki DG. Meta-analysis: methods for diagnosing intravascular device-related bloodstream infection. *Ann Intern Med.* 2005;142(6):451–466.

minutes apart with the same volume of blood. The hypothesis is that the higher load of organisms on the internal lumen of the CVC signifying CRBSI would translate into a colony count from the CVC greater by many folds than the peripheral stick. A CVC/peripheral ratio of CFU/mL of 3:1 has been chosen by the Infectious Diseases Society of America (IDSA) to represent true infection, meaning that the colony count of microbes grown from blood obtained through the catheter hub must be at least threefold greater than the colony count from blood obtained from a peripheral vein (35). However, there are variable reports among the literature which recommend up to a 10:1 ratio (5). A meta-analysis found that QBC is the most accurate, with a pooled sensitivity of 75% to 93% and specificity of 97% to 100% (36). That same study recommended not culturing all catheter tips, but rather culturing *only* if CRBSI is suspected clinically. This method of QBCs is limited by the fact that it is expensive and labor intensive, in addition to the difficulty in obtaining samples through the catheter in some cases (37). The diagnosis of CRBSI should be strongly considered, though not definitively established, when QBCs are drawn from two lumens of the CVC and the colony count for blood from one lumen is at least threefold greater than that from the other lumen.

Differential Time to Positivity

The differential time to positivity (DTP) of qualitative paired CVC and peripheral blood culture has been a more practical test for centers that lack the logistics for QBCs, especially with the introduction of automated radiometric blood culture systems that record the time at which a culture turns positive. The hypothesis suggests that time to positivity of a culture is closely related to the inoculum size of micro-organisms. The technique involves measuring the difference between the time required for culture positivity in simultaneously drawn samples of catheter blood and peripheral blood. In a single-center trial evaluating for CRBSI, a DTP of 120 minutes was associated with 81% sensitivity and 92% specificity for short-term catheters and 93% sensitivity and 75% specificity for long-term catheters (38). A meta-analytic study showed that the DTP of 120 minutes predicts CRBSI, with a pooled sensitivity and specificity of 89% and 87% for short-term catheters and 90% and 72% for long-term catheters, respectively (36). This technique also demands a simultaneous blood draw (within 10 minutes) from the line and the peripheral vein with the *same amount of blood.* One limitation of this study is that its sensitivity could be compromised when antibiotics are given intraluminally at the time of drawing the blood cultures through the catheters (38).

Acridine Orange Cytospin Leukocyte Technique

This test involves 1 mL of ethylenediaminetetraacetic acid (EDTA) blood aspirated through the CVC. The sample is added to 10% formalin saline solution for 2 minutes; the sample is then centrifuged, the supernatant decanted, and the cellular deposit homogenized and cytocentrifuged. A monolayer is stained with 1 in 10,000 acridine orange and viewed under ultraviolet light; a positive test is indicated by the presence of any bacteria (39). This method is expensive but takes only 30 minutes, with a sensitivity of 87% and specificity of 94% (40). This technique has been tested only by a small group of investigators and is not easy to perform correctly in order to reproduce the Kite method (41). One trial showed that this technique anticipated CRBSI earlier than routine measures (42); it is not recommended by the current guidelines of IDSA.

Fluorescence *In Situ* Hybridization on Peptide Nucleic Acid Probes

Fluorescence *in situ* hybridization (FISH) using peptide nucleic acid (PNA) probes is a novel technique in detecting several organisms (43). PNA probes are basically similar in structure to DNA or RNA, but have an uncharged backbone which accounts for its superior stability and improved hybridization when compared to DNA or RNA (43). These characteristics of PNA probes improve binding to certain molecules such as rRNA which makes FISH PNA a superior diagnostic test (43). Interestingly, a study comparing acridine orange cytospin leukocyte technique, FISH PNA and DTP found similar results in terms of sensitivity, specificity, positive predictive value, and negative predictive value (91%, 100%, 100%, and 97%, respectively) (44). In another study, even though FISH PNA was a successful diagnostic tool in patients who experience a BSI, positive results from random CVC sampling did not predict clinical progression to CRBSI as this phenomenon was most likely due to CVC colonization (45).

Diagnostic Methods Requiring Catheter Removal

Semi-Quantitative Roll-Plate Catheter Culture

This method was described by Maki et al. (46) in 1977 and remains the international reference diagnostic method. It consists of rolling a 3- to 5-cm section of the distal tip of the CVC at least four times back and forth over an agar plate surface and incubating overnight. A cutoff of ≥15 CFU defines catheter colonization; if at the same time, a peripheral culture grows the same organism, then a CRBSI is diagnosed. However, this method does not sample the internal lumen of a CVC that is the source of the infection in long-term catheters. Nevertheless, pooled sensitivity and specificity in 14 trials involving short-term catheters were 84% and 85%, respectively (36); this number decreased to 45% and 75%, respectively, with long-term CVCs (i.e., those with more than 30 days of dwell time) (10,47).

Quantitative Catheter Cultures

This type of culture involves flushing or sonicating a catheter segment in broth with the target of retrieving organisms from both surfaces of the line. A threshold of ≥100 CFU (48) correlated best with colonization, although older work (49) used a 1,000 CFU cutoff. CRBSI would be defined by the cutoff of 100 CFU accompanied by a high clinical suspicion and absence of evidence of other sites of infection. As would be expected, the sonication method had a higher sensitivity than the roll-plate method for long-term CVCs (10); however, both sonication and vortexing had the same sensitivity and specificity of the roll-plate method for short-term CVCs (50). Meta-analysis revealed a pooled sensitivity and specificity of 82% and 89% for short-term catheters and 83% and 97% for long-term catheters, respectively (36).

PREVENTIVE STRATEGIES

It should go without saying—but obviously does not—that CVCs should only be used when medically necessary, and should be removed as soon as possible to prevent potential complications. In a large study that included 1,981 ICU months of data, collective antiseptic measures consisting of hand-washing, maximal sterile barriers during insertion, cutaneous antisepsis with CHX, avoidance of femoral site, and removal of CVCs determined to be unnecessary were associated with a significant decrease in CRBSI rate—from 7.7 per 1,000 catheter days to 1.4 per 1,000 catheter days ($p < 0.001$) over 18 months of follow-up (51). In 1992, Cobb et al. (13), in an attempt to reduce catheter-related infection, conducted a controlled study whereby CVCs or pulmonary artery catheters were changed or exchanged over guidewire every 3 days; the former procedure actually resulted in an increase in the risk of mechanical complications, whereas the latter technique increased the risk of BSI. Table 88.1.3 provides a listing of preventive strategies to decrease the risk of CVC colonization. We review below the novel strategies implemented by the Healthcare Infection Control Practices Advisory Committee (HICPAC) and other professional organizations, including the IDSA, Society for Healthcare Epidemiology of America (SHEA), and American Society of Critical Care Anesthesiologists (ASCCA) aiming at controlling all factors that could lead to colonization of the CVC, and hence decreasing the rate of CRBSI.

TABLE 88.1.3 Preventive Measures to Decrease the Risk of Colonization of Central Venous Catheters

- Hand hygiene
- Removing unnecessary catheters
- Avoiding femoral site insertion if possible
- Cutaneous antiseptic agents (2% chlorhexidine-based preparation)
- Maximal sterile barrier (hand-washing, sterile gloves, large drape, and sterile gown, mask, and cap)
- Antimicrobial catheter lock solutions (a combination of an anticoagulant-like heparin or ethylenediaminetetraacetic acid plus an antimicrobial agent, such as vancomycin, minocycline, or ciprofloxacin)
- Antimicrobial coating of catheter (with minocycline/rifampin or chlorhexidine/silver sulfadiazine)

Cutaneous Antiseptics

The HICPAC/CDC guidelines recommend with level 1A evidence—data derived from multiple randomized clinical trials proving general agreement on its effectiveness—the usage of 2% CHX-based preparation (52). Maki et al. (53) prospectively randomized 68 ICU patients to 10% povidone–iodine, 70% alcohol, or 2% aqueous CHX to disinfect the site before insertion of CVCs and for site care every other day thereafter, and demonstrated that 2% aqueous CHX preparation tended to decrease the rate of CRBSI substantially; using lower concentrations of CHX decreased the effectiveness of this method. Tincture of chlorhexidine gluconate 0.5% is no more effective in preventing CRBSI or CVC colonization than 10% povidone–iodine, as demonstrated by a prospective, randomized study in adults (54). A meta-analysis of eight randomized trials found an overall reduction of 49% in catheter-associated BSIs when a disinfectant containing CHX was used (55). A French trial randomly assigned 1,181 ICU patients to CHX-based preparation and 1,168 to povidone–iodine. The CHX preparation was associated with lower incidence of CRBSI, 0.28 versus 1.77 per 1,000 catheter days (95% confidence interval [CI] 0.05 to 0.41, $p = 0.0002$) (56). Finally, the use of a dilute CHX solution for daily baths has been shown to decrease CRBSIs—among other infections—in a variety of settings (57–63).

Maximal Sterile Barrier

This involves wearing a sterile gown, gloves, and a cap, and using a large drape similar to those used in the operating room during the insertion of catheters as opposed to the regular precautions consisting of sterile gloves and a small drape only. The HICPAC/CDC guidelines recommend this technique while inserting CVCs, PICC lines, and pulmonary artery catheters (52) (category 1A) based on a number of studies (64–66). A prospective study conducted by Raad et al. (64) with long-term, nontunneled silicone CVCs and PICC lines in a cancer patient population demonstrated not only a reduction of CRBSIs ($p = 0.03$), but also that this practice was cost effective. Mermel et al. (65), in another prospective study with pulmonary artery catheters, found that less stringent barrier precautions were associated with a significantly increased risk of catheter-related infection (relative risk = 2.1, $p = 0.03$). Of note is that this technique failed to reduce the colonization of CRBSIs associated with arterial catheters (66). It has been shown that dedicated physician education courses can improve compliance with maximal sterile barrier and decrease the incidence of CRBSI (67).

Antimicrobial Catheter-Lock Solutions

Antimicrobial catheter lock involves flushing the catheter lumen and then filling it with 2 to 3 mL of a combination of an anticoagulant plus an antimicrobial agent. The dwell (lock) time varies between clinicians, but 20 to 24 hours is the most preferred. However, this might not be possible if the catheter has to be used (68). This intervention has often been used in long-term CVCs that remain in place longer than 30 days. Henrickson et al. (69) showed that a combination of vancomycin and heparin, with or without ciprofloxacin, was equivalent, but each was superior to heparin alone. Of six studies, four revealed a significant reduction in CRBSI with the above lock solution (70–72), and two demonstrated no benefit (73,74). However, vancomycin–heparin lock solutions may promote the risk of vancomycin resistance and the risk of superinfection with GNB and *Candida* is present since the vancomycin spectrum is limited to gram-positive bacteria. A meta-analysis concluded that the use of a vancomycin lock solution in high-risk patient populations being treated with long-term central IVDs may reduce the risk of BSI with a risk ratio of 0.34 (95% CI, 0.12 to 0.98; $p = 0.04$) (75).

Minocycline and EDTA (M-EDTA), another lock solution, was reported in a prospective randomized trial to significantly reduce the risk of catheter colonization and infection when compared with heparin in long-term hemodialysis CVCs (76). This solution was superior in an *in vitro* biofilm model and in an animal model to vancomycin–heparin lock solution (76–78). A clinical study of pediatric cancer populations showed that M-EDTA significantly reduces the risk of catheter infection and colonization when compared to heparin (79).

In a prospective nonrandomized study of tunneled CVCs in a pediatric cancer population, ethanol as a lock solution reduced the risk of relapse of CRBSI and was well tolerated (80). However, symptoms of fatigue, nausea, dizziness, and headache were reported. The study involved filling the catheter lumen with 2.3 mL of a 74% ethanol solution for 20 to 24 hours. The solution was then flushed through to prevent clotting inside the catheter. Each port was alternately blocked for 3 days, allowing the unblocked port to be used. In a study by Raad et al. (81), M-EDTA in 25% ethanol was found to be highly effective in eradicating organisms embedded in biofilm, even after a short exposure of 15 to 60 minutes. Hence, the addition of a low concentration of ethanol (25%) to M-EDTA could expedite its activity and decrease the necessary dwell time. A prolonged dwell time of more than 8 hours is often required for nonalcohol-based antibiotic lock solutions, which makes their use limited, particularly in critically ill patients or patients requiring TPN.

A meta-analytic study from 2014 (82), which included 23 studies and 2,896 patients, showed that antimicrobial lock solutions led to a 69% reduction in CLABSI compared with heparin, without significantly causing catheter failure due to noninfectious complications. However, one must keep in mind that all of the trials were done in special population patients, such as hemodialysis and oncology patients, patient receiving TPN, and so forth. As there is some concern for the emergence of bacterial resistance associated with utilization of a sole antibiotic agent and not in combination, some have recommended caution when it comes to the widespread indiscriminate prophylactic use of antibiotic-based catheter-lock solutions (82).

Given the fact that heparin, an effective antithrombotic agent, was shown in a study by Shanks et al. (83) to promote the kinetics of biofilm formation by *S. aureus* by enhancing cell–cell interaction and the concern of antibiotic resistance, the future trend will be to move away from heparin and/or antibiotic-based lock solutions. Based on that, several studies have tried to compare heparin with other agents. One study has shown superiority of a combination of ethanol and sodium citrate over heparin in terms of CRBSI prevention and catheter survival (84). Another comparative study has shown superiority of minocycline–EDTA, taurolidine–polyvinylpyrolidine, or ethanol over other current antibiotic-based lock solutions (85). Recently, a novel antimicrobial solution containing 15 μg of nitroglycerin, 4% of citrate, and 22% of ethanol has shown to have *in vitro* activity against all biofilm-producing organisms in as a little at 2 hours (86). However, and while this particular field is very promising, there has yet to be large clinical trials confirming the *in vitro* activity of these novel nonantibiotic, nonheparin-based lock solutions (85).

Antimicrobial Impregnation of Catheters

This technique consists of the impregnation of the external and/or internal surface of the catheter with antiseptic or antibiotics; the slow release of antimicrobials would prevent initial bacterial adherence and biofilm formation, with virtually undetectable serum levels. The HICPAC/CDC, with a category 1B, recommends the use of the coated CVCs described herein. The first-generation catheters were impregnated on the external surface with CHX and silver sulfadiazine (CHX/SSD) (Arrow Gard and Arrow Gard Plus, Arrow International, Inc.). That technique lowered the rate of CRBSI from 7.6 cases per 1,000 catheter days to 1.6 cases per 1,000 catheter days ($p = 0.03$), with a decrease in the rate of colonization (relative risk, 0.56 [95% CI, 0.36 to 0.89]; $p = 0.005$) (9); the estimated cost savings per CVC insertion was $196 (87). However, three subsequent studies failed to show that difference (88–90). This was explained by the fact that short-term catheter infection is due to external colonization, whereas long-term CRBSIs due to internal colonization are not prevented by external coating. Moreover, Mermel (6) showed that these catheters do not protect if the CVC dwell time is more than 3 weeks, secondary to wearing off of the antimicrobial activity. The second-generation CHX/SSD-coated catheters were impregnated on both surfaces. In a multicenter, randomized double-blind prospective study from 14 French ICUs, second-generation catheters failed to decrease the rate of CRBSI (91,92) when compared to noncoated catheters, although they significantly decreased the rate of colonization (11/1,000 catheter days to 3.6/1,000 catheter days, $p = 0.01$).

In 1997, Raad and colleagues (92) developed a catheter impregnated on both surfaces with minocycline–rifampin (M/R). In a prospective randomized, double-blind trial, M/R CVCs showed more efficacy when compared to noncoated catheters. Another prospective trial comparing M/R catheters with first-generation CHX/SSD-impregnated catheters found that the former were three times less likely to be colonized ($p < 0.001$), and CRBSI was 12-fold more likely to occur in the CHX/SSD catheters ($p < 0.002$) (93). The use of antibiotic-impregnated CVCs in medical and surgical units was associated with a significant decrease in nosocomial BSIs, including vancomycin-resistant enterococci (VRE) bacteremia, catheter-related infections, and length of hospital and ICU stay (94). Furthermore, the M/R-coated catheters saved $9,600 per each CRBSI and $81 per each catheter placed when compared to first-generation CHX/SSD (95).

The concern for the emergence of antibiotic-resistant organisms was raised with the catheters coated with M/R. Four prospective studies evaluated the skin at the catheter insertion site before and after the insertion of antibiotic-coated catheters and failed to detect any emergence of resistance (92,93,96,97). A retrospective review of the M/R-coated CVC experience in bone marrow transplant patients also detected no emergence of resistance of staphylococci to either component (98). In a series of prospective randomized studies, the M/R-coated CVCs were shown to bring the risk of CRBSI to a level ≤ 0.3 per 1,000 catheter days in nontunneled, noncuffed CVCs (92,93,97), lower than the 1.4 per 1,000 catheter days achieved with multiple other aseptic measures applied collectively (such as the maximal sterile barrier, CHX cutaneous antisepsis, and hand hygiene).

Two studies by Raad et al. and Jamal and colleagues (99,100) found that minocycline–rifampin impregnated CVCs coated internally and externally with CHX, termed CHX–M/R catheters, were superior to CHX–/SSD (chlorhexidine–silver sulfadiazine) or M/R-coated catheters in preventing biofilm formation and catheter colonization particularly when it comes to *Pseudomonas* and *Candida*. A novel approach using gendine (CHX and gentian violet)-coated CVCs showed promising results in terms of prevention of biofilm formation with no acute systemic exposure of CHX or gentian violet (101); however, clinical trials involving the use of gendine-coated catheters have yet to be initiated.

When all are said and done, CHX/SSD and M/R catheters both reduce CRBSI when compared to noncoated ones. The HICPAC/CDC recommends the use of either if the medical center continues to have higher than national average CRBSI rates despite successful implementation of provider education, maximal sterile barrier and use of CHX preparation with alcohol for skin antisepsis.

Silver-Impregnated Catheters

Other catheters incorporate silver, platinum, and carbon (SPC) into the polyurethane, allowing topical silver ion release (Vantex CVC with oligan, Edwards Life Sciences, Irvine, CA). One prospective randomized study compared these catheters to the M/R-coated type; the latter was more efficacious in reducing, to a significant degree, CVC colonization with gram-positive and gram-negative bacteria ($p = 0.039$); however, the CRBSI rates were low and similar between the two groups (102). In another prospective, randomized, controlled, open-label, multicenter clinical trial, the SPC CVCs failed to show any benefit in reducing CRBSI or colonization (103). A meta-analysis study failed to prove any association between reduced rates of colonization or CRBSI and the use of silver-impregnated catheters (104).

MANAGEMENT

The management of CRBSIs involves confirming the source and cause of infection, determining the choice of antimicrobials, determining the duration of therapy, and deciding whether to remove the invasive device. Confirmation of the infection is dependent on the diagnostic measures outlined above. The duration of therapy depends on whether the infection is complicated (i.e., by a septic phlebitis or endocarditis) or uncomplicated.

Coagulase-Negative Staphylococcus

Coagulase-negative staphylococci are the primary organisms involved in CRBSIs because they are the most common skin organisms; however, and for the same reason, they are the most frequent blood contaminants. One study indicated that QBC collected through CVC, with a cutoff point of 15 CFU/mL, could be a useful laboratory criterion, together with positive clinical findings, for differentiating true bacteremia from false-positive contaminated blood cultures, with a sensitivity of 96%, specificity of 94%, positive predictive value of 86%, and negative predictive value of 98% (105); the IDSA guidelines recommend removing the CVC and treating for 5 to 7 days. Otherwise, if the CVC is to be retained, duration of treatment should be 10 to 14 days, and antibiotic lock therapy should be considered (106). Leaving the CVC in place carries a risk of recurrence of 20% (107). Finally, in the absence of endovascular or orthopedic hardware, and with catheter removal, the patient can be monitored off antibiotics while new blood cultures are drawn to confirm the resolution of bacteremia.

Lock solutions used included vancomycin plus heparin. The limited activity of vancomycin against *Staphylococcus* embedded in biofilms (73,75,108) led investigators to consider other alternatives; minocycline and EDTA, ethanol, or the triple combination (109,110) was used as an alternative. While systemically, vancomycin has been the most frequently used glycopeptide, dalbavancin, a new, long-acting glycopeptide that is dosed weekly, was noted to be superior to vancomycin for adult patients with CRBSIs caused by coagulase-negative *Staphylococcus* and *S. aureus,* including methicillin-resistant *S. aureus* (MRSA) in a phase 2, open-label, randomized, multicenter study; the side effect profile was comparable (111). Linezolid and daptomycin were also used successfully (112,113).

Staphylococcus Aureus

S. aureus CRBSI is associated with high rates of deep-seated infection such as osteomyelitis, septic phlebitis, and endocarditis (114). In addition, Fowler et al. (114) showed that patients whose IVD was not removed were 6.5 times more likely to relapse or die of their infection than were those whose device was removed. IDSA guidelines recommend removing the CVC, as this results in a more rapid response and lower relapse rate but, at the same time, gives the option of keeping it and initiating systemic and lock solutions in the rare and extreme cases of lack of other vascular access, bleeding diathesis, and quality-of-life issues intervene (106). Capdevila et al. (115) used the antibiotic lock technique in addition to standard parenteral therapy for patients with a hemodialysis catheter–related infection. All 40 CRBSIs—including all 12 cases reported to involve *S. aureus*—were cured and the catheter salvaged. The lock solutions most frequently used *in vivo* and *in vitro* are vancomycin plus heparin, or minocycline plus EDTA (71,110). However, the former combination—with or without ceftazidime, depending on the organism—was associated with a 60% failure rate in hemodialysis MRSA catheter infections (116). Another study showed that even though systemic antibiotic therapy was not successful in eradicating most CRBSIs without catheter removal, attempted CVC salvage appeared to have not increased the complication rate even in the setting of *S. aureus* (117). Low-concentration ethanol (25%) is another very appealing component for use in combination lock solutions; Raad and colleagues (81) found that the combination of minocycline–EDTA in 25% ethanol was highly efficacious in eradicating *S. aureus* in biofilm within 60 minutes of dwell time.

For methicillin-sensitive *S. aureus,* nafcillin or first-generation cephalosporins are the first-line agents (100). Vancomycin, linezolid, daptomycin, and dalbavancin (111–113) are all appropriate options for MRSA. Duration of therapy usually consists of 10 to 14 days of intravenous therapy if the CVC is removed, with no deep-seated infection present (106). If fever or bacteremia persists for more than 72 hours after catheter removal, transesophageal echocardiography should be performed to rule out IE, with the intravenous therapy duration expanded to at least 4 weeks (106,118). This is especially important as the frequency of IE in *S. aureus* bacteremia is 25% to 32% (119).

Enterococcus

Enterococcus is the third most common pathogen seen in CRBSI, accounting for about 10% of nosocomial BSIs (120). The IDSA recommends catheter removal and treatment with systemic antibiotics, beginning with ampicillin as the first-line agent of choice; the organism can be treated with vancomycin if ampicillin-resistant. However, 60% of *Enterococcus faecium* and 2% of *Enterococcus faecalis* are now resistant to vancomycin (120); in such cases, linezolid and daptomycin are the agents of choice.

Antibiotics are recommended for 7 to 14 days in the setting of catheter removal, as well as long-term catheter salvage with systemic antibiotics and lock therapy. A transesophageal echocardiogram (TEE) should be pursued to evaluate for IE if the patient has prolonged bacteremia or fever more than 72 hours after the initiation of appropriate antimicrobial therapy, evidence of septic emboli, a new murmur, or embolic phenomena, all of which are also, in the cases of long-term catheters, indications of salvage therapy failure and the need for removal.

There are data regarding combination therapy for enterococcal CRBSI, namely a cell wall–active antimicrobial and an aminoglycoside. Several retrospective cohort studies found no statistically significant difference in outcomes when treated with combination therapy versus monotherapy (121–123).

Gram-Negative Bacilli

GNB bacteremia is rarely due to a CVC; rather, it generally arises from a visceral source of infection such as the genitourinary, pulmonary, or gastrointestinal tracts. However, CRBSIs caused by such organisms as *K. pneumoniae, Enterobacter* spp., *P. aeruginosa* spp., *Acinetobacter* spp., and *Stenotrophomonas maltophilia* have been reported (124,125). Elting and Bodey (124) reported a 15-year experience of 149 episodes of septicemia caused by *Xanthamonas maltophilia* and *Pseudomonas* spp. in cancer patients where the CVC was the most common source. Hanna et al. (125) demonstrated that catheter removal within 72 hours of the onset of the catheter-related GNB was the only independent protective factor against the relapse of infection (OR, 0.13; 95% CI, 0.02 to 0.75; $p = 0.02$). IDSA guidelines (107) recommend removing nontunneled CVCs and treating for 10 to 14 days with systemic antibiotics. Patients at high risk for colonization or infection with multidrug-resistant gram-negative pathogen (i.e., critically ill, neutropenia) should be covered with either two antibiotics of different classes that provide gram-negative activity or a carbapenem as initial therapy. It is considered appropriate to attempt to salvage the CVC in certain situations (see above) using systemic and lock solution therapies. However, lock therapy for GNB CRBSIs is anecdotal; successful cases were salvaged using gentamicin, amikacin, or ceftazidime (106,118).

Candida

Five large prospective studies proved that catheter retention was associated with increased mortality and an increase in the mean duration of candidemia in cases of *Candida* CRBSI (126–130). Hung et al. (128) investigated the predisposing factors and prognostic determinants of candidemia in a Taiwan hospital, and concluded that higher severity scores, nonremoval of the catheter, persistent candidemia, and lack of antifungal therapy adversely affect the outcome. Raad and colleagues (131), in a retrospective study of 404 patients with candidemia and an indwelling CVC, using a multivariate analysis, demonstrated that catheter removal 72 hours or sooner after onset of candidemia improved the response to antifungal therapy exclusively in patients with catheter-related candidemia ($p = 0.04$). IDSA guidelines recommend removing the CVC and treating for 14 days after the last positive blood culture in uncomplicated cases; endophthalmitis merits 6 weeks of therapy (106). Further studies are needed to define the role of antifungal lock solution in these cases. Fluconazole and caspofungin were equivalent to amphotericin B in candidemia, but with a better safety profile (130,131); therefore, fluconazole or caspofungin should be considered in documented cases of catheter-related candidemia. If the rates of fluconazole-resistant *Candida glabrata* and *Candida krusei* in the hospital are high, an echinocandin (caspofungin, micafungin, or anidulafungin) would be the best alternative to amphotericin B.

PERIPHERALLY INSERTED CENTRAL CATHETERS

The use of PICCs is very common in cancer patients, patients receiving TPN, and long-term i.v. antibiotics. Their complication rates, including infection and thrombosis, are low in the outpatient setting (0.4 per 1,000 catheter days) (132,133). There has been speculation that perhaps PICCs are less prone to infection compared to CVCs in the critically ill; this has been proved to be untrue.

In a prospective study in which 115 patients had 251 PICCs placed, Safdar and Maki (127) showed that PICCs used in ICU patients are associated with a rate of CRBSI similar to CVCs placed in internal jugular or subclavian veins (2.1 vs. 2 to 5 per 1,000 catheter days). Nolan et al. (134) performed a retrospective cohort study of 200 PICCs and 200 CVCs placed in the medical ICU adults at Mayo Rochester between 2012 and 2013. Overall, thrombotic and infectious complications were rare following PICC and CVC insertion, with no significant difference in complication rates observed. Finally, the meta-analytic study of Chopra and colleagues (135) identified 23 studies that met eligibility criteria for comparing infection risk of PICC versus CVC. Thirteen studies reported CLABSI rates; PICC-related CLABSI occurred as frequently as CLABSI in CVC. The subcategory where PICC showed a significant infection reduction is in outpatients, *not* in critically ill, hospitalized patients.

Key Points

- CVCs are as much a part of modern ICU practice as are mechanical ventilators and antibiotics.
- When CVCs are placed with the appropriate technique, accessed, and cared for, it is possible to use these devices while approximating a zero incidence of infection.
- PICCs are not lower risk for infectious complication when used in critically ill, hospitalized patients.
- As is typically true in the practice of critical care medicine, it is in the details that the battle is won or lost.

References

1. Smith RN, Nolan JP. Central venous catheters. *BMJ.* 2013;347:f6570.
2. Higgs ZC, Macafee DA, Braithwaite BD, Maxwell-Armstrong CA. The Seldinger technique: 50 years on. *Lancet.* 2005;366(9494):1407–1409.
3. Raad I, Chaftari AM. Advances in prevention and management of central line-associated bloodstream infections in patients with cancer. *Clin Infect Dis.* 2014;59(Suppl 5):S340–S343.
4. American Society of Anesthesiologists Task Force on Central Venous Access, Rupp SM, Apfelbaum JL, Blitt C, et al. Practice guidelines for central venous access: a report by the American Society of Anesthesiologists Task Force on Central Venous Access. *Anesthesiology.* 2012;116(3); 539–573.
5. Gahlot R, Nigam C, Kumar V, et al. Catheter-related bloodstream infections. *Int J Crit Illness Injury Sci.* 2014;4(2):162–167.
6. Mermel LA. Prevention of intravascular catheter-related infections. *Ann Intern Med.* 2000;132(5):391–402.
7. Hollenbeak CS. The cost of catheter-related bloodstream infections: implications for the value of prevention. *J Infus Nurs.* 2011;34(5):309–313.
8. Dimick JB, Pelz RK, Consunji R, et al. Increased resource use associated with catheter-related bloodstream infection in the surgical intensive care unit. *Arch Surg.* 2001;136:229–234.
9. Maki DG, Stolz SM, Wheeler S, Mermel LA. Prevention of central venous catheter-related bloodstream infection by use of an antiseptic impregnated catheter: a randomized controlled trial. *Ann Intern Med.* 1997;127:257–266.
10. Safdar N, Maki DG. The pathogenesis of catheter-related bloodstream infection with noncuffed short-term central venous catheters. *Intensive Care Med.* 2004;30(1):62–67.
11. Raad I, Costerton W, Sabharwal U, et al. Ultrastructural analysis of indwelling vascular catheters: a quantitative relationship between luminal colonization and duration of placement. *J Infect Dis.* 1993;168:400–407.
12. Sitges-Serra A, Puig P, Linares J, et al. Hub colonization as the initial step in an outbreak of catheter-related sepsis due to coagulase negative staphylococci during parenteral nutrition. *J Parenter Enteral Nutr.* 1984;8: 668–672.
13. Cobb DK, High KP, Sawyer RG, et al. A controlled trial of scheduled replacement of central venous and pulmonary artery catheters. *N Engl J Med.* 1991;327:1062–1068.
14. Raad II, Hanna HA. Intravascular catheter-related infections: new horizons and recent advances. *Arch Intern Med.* 2002;162(8):871–878.
15. Kovacevich DS, Faubion WC, Bender JM, et al. Association of parenteral nutrition catheter sepsis with urinary tract infections. *JPEN J Parenter Enteral Nutr.* 1986;10:639–641.
16. Pettigrew RA, Lang SD, Haycock DA, et al. Catheter-related sepsis in patients on intravenous nutrition: a prospective study of quantitative catheter cultures and guideline changes for suspected sepsis. *Br J Surg.* 1985;72:52–55.
17. Anaissie E, Samonis G, Kontoyiannis D, et al. Role of catheter colonization and infrequent hematogeneous seeding in catheter-related-infections. *Eur J Clin Microbiol Infect Dis.* 1995;14(2):134–137.
18. Nosocomial bacteremia associated with intravenous fluid therapy. *MMWR.* 1971;20(Suppl 9):S1–S2.
19. Maki DG, Rhame FS, Mackel DC, Bennett JV. Nationwide epidemic of septicemia caused by contaminated intravenous products. I. Epidemiologic and clinical features. *Am J Med.* 1976;60:471–485.
20. Kimura AC, Calvet H, Higa JI, et al. Outbreak of *Ralstonia pickettii* bacteremia in a neonatal intensive care unit. *Pediatr Infect Dis J.* 2005;24(12): 1099–1103.
21. Marra AR, Opilla M, Edmond MB, Kirby DF. Epidemiology of bloodstream infections in patients receiving long-term total parenteral nutrition. *J Clin Gastroenterol.* 2007;41(1):19–28.
22. Kuwahara T, Kaneda S, Shimono K, Inoue Y. Effects of lipid emulsion and multivitamins on the growth of microorganisms in peripheral parenteral nutrition solutions. *Int J Med Sci.* 2013;10(9):1079–1084.
23. Christensen GD, Simpson WA, Bisno AL, Beachey EH. Adherence of slime producing strains of *Staphylococcus epidermidis* to smooth surfaces. *Infect Immun.* 1982;17:318–326.
24. Anwar H, Strap JL, Chen K, Costerton JW. Dynamic interactions of biofilms of mucoid *Pseudomonas aeruginosa* with tobramycin and piperacillin. *Antimicrob Agents Chemother.* 1992;36(6):1208–1214.
25. Hawiger J, Timmons S, Strong DD, et al. Identification of a region of human fibrinogen interacting with staphylococcal clumping factor. *Biochemistry.* 1982;21:1407–1413.
26. Kuusela P. Fibronectin binds to *Staphylococcus aureus. Nature.* 1978;276: 718–720.
27. Lopes JD, Dos Reis M, Brentani RR. Presence of laminin receptors in *Staphylococcus aureus. Science.* 1985;229:275–277.
28. Vaudaux P, Pittet D, Haeberli A, et al. Host factors selectively increase staphylococcal adherence on inserted catheters: a role for fibronectin and fibrinogen or fibrin. *J Infect Dis.* 1989;160:865–875.
29. Bouali A, Robert R, Tronchin G, Senet JM. Characterization of binding of human fibrinogen to the surface of germ-tubes and mycelium of candida albicans. *J Gen Microbiol.* 1987;133(3):545–551.
30. Marik PE, Flemmer M, Harrison W. The risk of catheter-related bloodstream infection with femoral venous catheters as compared to subclavian and internal jugular venous catheters: a systematic review of the literature and meta-analysis. *Crit Care Med.* 2012;40(8): 2479–2485.
31. O'Grady NP, Alexander M, Burns LA, et al; Healthcare Infection Control Practices Advisory Committee (HICPAC). Guidelines for the prevention of intravascular catheter-related infections. *Clin Infect Dis.* 2011;52(9): e162–e193.
32. Raad I, Davis S, Becker M, et al. Low infection rate and long durability of nontunneled silastic catheters: a safe and cost-effective alternative for long-term venous access. *Arch Intern Med.* 1993;153:1791–1796.
33. Safdar N, Maki DG. Inflammation at the insertion site is not predictive of catheter-related bloodstream infection with short-term, noncuffed central venous catheters. *Crit Care Med.* 2002;30(12):2632–2635.
34. Ryan JA Jr, Abel RM, Abbott WM, et al. Catheter complications in total parenteral nutrition: a prospective study of 200 consecutive patients. *N Engl J Med.* 1974;290(14):757–761.
35. Keutgen X, Ghannam D, Hackett B, et al. Differential quantitative blood cultures (QBC) for the diagnosis of catheter-related bloodstream infection: what is the cutoff ratio? [Abstract D0472]. In: *Programs and Abstracts of the 46th Interscience Conference on Antimicrobial Agents and Chemotherapy.* San Francisco, CA: 2006:27–30.
36. Safdar N, Fine JP, Maki DG. Meta-analysis: methods for diagnosing intravascular device-related bloodstream infection. *Ann Intern Med.* 2005;142(6):451–466.
37. Catton JA, Dobbins BM, Kite P, et al. In situ diagnosis of intravascular catheter-related bloodstream infection: a comparison of quantitative culture, differential time to positivity, and endoluminal brushing. *Crit Care Med.* 2005;33(4):787–791.
38. Raad I, Hanna HA, Alakech B, et al. Differential time to positivity: a useful method for diagnosing catheter-related bloodstream infections. *Ann Intern Med.* 2004;140(1):18–25.
39. Kite P, Dobbins BM, Wilcox MH, McMahon MJ. Rapid diagnosis of central-venous-catheter-related bloodstream infection without catheter removal. *Lancet.* 1999;354:1504–1507.
40. Rushforth JA, Hoy CM, Kite P, Puntis JW. Rapid diagnosis of central venous catheter sepsis. *Lancet.* 1993;342(8868):402–403.
41. Farina C, Bonanomi E, Benetti G, et al. Acridine orange leukocyte cytospin test for central venous catheter-related bloodstream infection: a pediatric experience. *Diagn Microbiol Infect Dis.* 2005;52(4):337–339.
42. Wagner J, Schilcher G, Zollner-Schwetz I, et al. Microbiological screening for earlier detection of central venous catheter-related bloodstream infections. *Eur J Clin Invest.* 2013;43(9):964–969.
43. Stender H. PNA FISH: an intelligent stain for rapid diagnosis of infectious diseases. *Expert Rev Mol Diagn.* 2003;3(5):649–655.
44. Krause R, Salzer HF, Hönigl M, et al. Comparison of fluorescence in situ hybridisation using peptide nucleic acid probes, Gram stain/acridine orange leukocyte cytospin and differential time to positivity methods for detection of catheter-related bloodstream infection in patients after haematopoietic stem cell transplantation. *Clin Microbiol Infect.* 2010;16(10):1591–1593.
45. Rabensteiner J, Theiler G, Duettmann W, et al. Detection of central venous catheter-related bloodstream infections in haematooncological patients. *Eur J Clin Invest.* 2015;45(8):824–832.
46. Maki DG, Weise CE, Sarafin HW. A semiquantitative culture method for identifying intravenous-catheter-related infection. *N Engl J Med.* 1977; 296(23):1305–1309.
47. Rello J, Gatell JM, Almirall J, et al. Evaluation of culture techniques for identification of catheter-related infection in hemodialysis patients. *Eur J Clin Microbiol Infect Dis.* 1989;8(7):620–622.
48. Sherertz RJ, Raad II, Belani A, et al. Three-year experience with sonicated vascular catheter cultures in a clinical microbiology laboratory. *J Clin Microbiol.* 1990;28(1):76–82.
49. Cleri DJ, Corrado ML, Seligman SJ. Quantitative culture of intravenous catheters and other intravascular inserts. *J Infect Dis.* 1980;141(6): 781–786.
50. Bouza E, Alvarado N, Alcala L, et al. A prospective, randomized and comparative study of three different methods for the diagnosis of intravascular catheter colonization. *Clin Infect Dis.* 2005;40(8):1096–1100.

51. Pronovost P, Needham D, Berenholtz S, et al. An intervention to decrease catheter-related bloodstream infections in the ICU. *N Engl J Med.* 2006; 355(26):2725–2732.
52. O'Grady NP, Alexander M, Dellinger EP, et al. Guidelines for the prevention of intravascular catheter-related infections. *MMWR Recomm Rep.* 2002;51(RR-10):1–29.
53. Maki DG, Ringer M, Alvarado CJ. Prospective randomized trial of povidone-iodine, alcohol, and chlorhexidine for prevention of infection associated with central venous and arterial catheters. *Lancet.* 1991; 338(8763):339–343.
54. Humar A, Ostromecki A, Direnfeld J, et al. Prospective randomized trial of 10% povidone–iodine versus 0.5% tincture of chlorhexidine as cutaneous antisepsis for prevention of central venous catheter infection. *Clin Infect Dis.* 2000;31:1001–1007.
55. Chaiyakunapruk N, Veenstra DL, Lipsky BA, Saint S. Chlorhexidine compared with povidone–iodine solution for vascular catheter-site care: a meta-analysis. *Ann Intern Med.* 2002;136:792–801.
56. Mimoz O, Lucet JC, Kerforne T, et al; CLEAN trial investigators. Skin antisepsis with chlorhexidine–alcohol versus povidone iodine–alcohol, with and without skin scrubbing, for prevention of intravascular-catheter-related infection (CLEAN): an open-label, multicentre, randomised, controlled, two-by-two factorial trial. *Lancet.* 2015;386(10008):2069–2077.
57. Popp JA, Layon AJ, Nappo R, et al. Hospital-acquired infections and thermally injured patients: chlorhexidine gluconate baths work. *Am J Infect Control.* 2014;42(2):129–132.
58. Evans HL, Dellit TH, Chan J, et al. Effect of chlorhexidine whole-body bathing on hospital-acquired infections among trauma patients. *Arch Surg.* 2010;145(3):240–246.
59. O'Horo JC, Silva GL, Munoz-Price LS, Safdar N. The efficacy of daily bathing with chlorhexidine for reducing healthcare-associated bloodstream infections: a meta-analysis. *Infect Control Hosp Epidemiol.* 2012;33(3):257–267.
60. Vernon MO, Hayden MK, Trick WE, et al; Chicago Antimicrobial Resistance Project (CARP): Chlorhexidine gluconate to cleanse patients in a medical intensive care unit: the effectiveness of source control to reduce the bioburden of vancomycin-resistant enterococci. *Arch Intern Med.* 2006;166(3):306–312.
61. Bleasdale SC, Trick WE, Gonzalez IM, et al. Effectiveness of chlorhexidine bathing to reduce catheter-associated bloodstream infections in medical intensive care unit patients. *Arch Intern Med.* 2007;167(19):2073–2079.
62. Weber DJ, Rutala WA. Central line-associated bloodstream infections: prevention and management. *Infect Dis Clin North Am.* 2011;25(1): 77–102.
63. Climo MW, Yokoe DS, Warren DK, et al. Effect of daily chlorhexidine bathing on hospital-acquired infection. *N Engl J Med.* 2013;368(6):533–542.
64. Raad II, Hohn DC, Gilbreath B, et al. Prevention of central venous catheter-related infections using maximal sterile barrier precautions during insertion. *Infect Control Hosp Epidemiol.* 1994;15:231–238.
65. Mermel LA, McCormick RD, Springman SR, Maki DG. The pathogenesis and epidemiology of catheter-related infection with pulmonary artery Swan Ganz catheters: a prospective study utilizing molecular subtyping. *Am J Med.* 1991;91(Suppl 3B):197S–205S.
66. Rijnders BJ, Van Wijngaerden E, Wilmer A, Peetermans WE. Use of full sterile barrier precautions during insertion of arterial catheters: a randomized trial. *Clin Infect Dis.* 2003;36(6):743–748.
67. Sherertz RJ, Ely EW, Westbrook DM, et al. Education of physicians-in-training can decrease the risk for vascular catheter infection. *Ann Intern Med.* 2000;132(8):641–648.
68. Segarra-Newnham M, Martin-Cooper EM. Antibiotic lock technique: a review of the literature. *Ann Pharmacother.* 2005;39(2):311–318.
69. Henrickson KJ, Axtell RA, Hoover SM, et al. Prevention of central venous catheter-related infections and thrombotic events in immunocompromised children by the use of vancomycin/ciprofloxacin/heparin flush solution: a randomized, multicenter, double-blind trial. *J Clin Oncol.* 2000;18(6):1269–1278.
70. Schwartz C, Henrickson KJ, Roghmann K, Powell K. Prevention of bacteremia attributed to luminal colonization of tunneled central venous catheters with vancomycin-susceptible organisms. *J Clin Oncol.* 1990;8(9):1591–1597.
71. Carratala J, Niubo J, Fernandez-Sevilla A, et al. Randomized, double-blind trial of an antibiotic-lock technique for prevention of gram-positive central venous catheter-related infection in neutropenic patients with cancer. *Antimicrob Agents Chemother.* 1999;43(9):2200–2204.
72. Garland JS, Henrickson KJ, Maki DG. A prospective randomized trial of vancomycin-heparin lock for prevention of catheter-related bloodstream infection in an NICU (abstract 1734). In: *Program and abstracts of the 2002 Annual Meeting of the Pediatric Academic Societies.* Baltimore, MD: Pediatric Academic Societies; 2002:235.
73. Rackoff WR, Weiman M, Jakobowski D, et al. A randomized, controlled trial of the efficacy of a heparin and vancomycin solution in preventing central venous catheter infections in children. *J Pediatr.* 1995;127(1):147–151.
74. Daghistani D, Horn M, Rodriguez Z, et al. Prevention of indwelling central venous catheter sepsis. *Med Pediatr Oncol.* 1996;26(6):405–408.
75. Safdar N, Maki DG. Use of vancomycin-containing lock or flush solutions for prevention of bloodstream infection associated with central venous access devices: a meta-analysis of prospective, randomized trials. *Clin Infect Dis.* 2006;43(4):474–484.
76. Bleyer AJ, Mason L, Russell G, et al. A randomized, controlled trial of a new vascular catheter flush solution (minocycline-EDTA) in temporary hemodialysis access. *Infect Control Hosp Epidemiol.* 2005;26(6):520–524.
77. Raad I, Chatzinikolaou I, Chaiban G, et al. *In vitro* and *ex vivo* activities of minocycline and EDTA against microorganisms embedded in biofilm on catheter surfaces. *Antimicrob Agents Chemother.* 2003;47(11):3580–3505.
78. Raad I, Hachem R, Tcholakian RK, Sherertz R. Efficacy of minocycline and EDTA lock solution in preventing catheter-related bacteremia, septic phlebitis, and endocarditis in rabbits. *Antimicrob Agents Chemother.* 2002;46(2):327–332.
79. Chatzinikolaou I, Zipf TF, Hanna H, et al. Minocycline-ethylenediamine-tetraacetate lock solution for the prevention of implantable port infections in children with cancer. *Clin Infect Dis.* 2003;36(1):116–119.
80. Dannenberg C, Bierbach U, Rothe A, et al. Ethanol-lock technique in the treatment of bloodstream infections in pediatric oncology patients with Broviac catheter. *J Pediatr Hematol Oncol.* 2003;25(8):616–621.
81. Raad I, Hanna H, Dvorak T, et al. Optimal antimicrobial catheter lock solution, using different combinations of minocycline, EDTA and 25% ethanol: rapid eradication of organisms embedded in biofilm. *Antimicrob Agents Chemother.* 2007;51(1):78–83.
82. Zacharioudakis IM, Zervou FN, Arvanitis M, et al. Antimicrobial lock solutions as a method to prevent central line-associated bloodstream infections: a meta-analysis of randomized controlled trials. *Clin Infect Dis.* 2014; 59(12):1741–1749.
83. Shanks RM, Donegan NP, Graber ML, et al. Heparin stimulates Staphylococcus aureus biofilm formation. *Infect Immun.* 2005;73(8):4596–4606.
84. Vercaigne LM, Allan DR, Armstrong SW, et al. An ethanol/sodium citrate locking solution compared to heparin to prevent hemodialysis catheter-related infections: a randomized pilot study. *J Vasc Access.* 2016; 17(1):55–62.
85. Sherertz RJ, Boger MS, Collins CA, et al. Comparative in vitro efficacies of various catheter lock solutions. *Antimicrob Agents Chemother.* 2006;50(5):1865–1868.
86. Rosenblatt J, Reitzel R, Dvorak T, et al. Glyceryl trinitrate complements citrate and ethanol in a novel antimicrobial catheter lock solution to eradicate biofilm organisms. *Antimicrob Agents Chemother.* 2013; 57(8):3555–3560.
87. Veenstra DL, Saint S, Sullivan SD. Cost-effectiveness of antiseptic impregnated central venous catheters for the prevention of catheter-related bloodstream infection. *JAMA.* 1999;282(6):554–560.
88. Heard SO, Wagle M, Vijayakumar E, et al. Influence of triple-lumen central venous catheters coated with chlorhexidine and silver sulfadiazine on the incidence of catheter-related bacteremia. *Arch Intern Med.* 1998; 158:81–87.
89. Ciresi D, Albrecht RM, Volkers PA, Scholten DJ. Failure of an antiseptic bonding to prevent central venous catheter-related infection and sepsis. *Am Surg.* 1996;62:641–646.
90. Pemberton LB, Ross V, Cuddy P, et al. No difference in catheter sepsis between standard and antiseptic central venous catheters: a prospective randomized trial. *Arch Surg.* 1996;131:986–989.
91. Brun-Buisson C, Doyon F, Sollet JP, et al. Prevention of intravascular catheter-related infection with newer chlorhexidine-silver sulfadiazine-coated catheters: a randomized controlled trial. *Intensive Care Med.* 2004;30(5):837–843.
92. Raad I, Darouiche R, Dupuis J, et al. Central venous catheters coated with minocycline and rifampin for the prevention of catheter-related colonization and bloodstream infections: a randomized, double-blind trial. The Texas Medical Center Catheter Study Group. *Ann Intern Med.* 1997;127:267–274.
93. Darouiche RO, Raad II, Heard SO, et al. Comparison of two anti-microbial impregnated central venous catheters. *N Engl J Med.* 1999;340:1–8.
94. Hanna HA, Raad II, Hackett B, et al. Anderson Catheter Study Group. Antibiotic-impregnated catheters associated with significant decrease in nosocomial and multidrug resistant bacteremias in critically ill patients. *Chest.* 2003;124(3):1030–1038.
95. Shorr AF, Humphreys CW, Helman DL. New choices for central venous catheters: potential financial implications. *Chest.* 2003;124(1):275–284.

96. Chatzinikolaou I, Finkel K, Hanna H, et al. Antibiotic-coated hemodialysis catheters for the prevention of vascular catheter-related infections: a prospective, randomized study. *Am J Med.* 2003;115(5):352–357.
97. Hanna H, Benjamin R, Chatzinikolaou I, et al. Long-term silicone central venous catheters impregnated with minocycline and rifampin decrease rates of catheter-related bloodstream infection in cancer patients: a prospective randomized clinical trial. *J Clin Oncol.* 2004;22(15):3163–3171.
98. Chatzinikolaou I, Hanna H, Graviss L, et al. Clinical experience with minocycline and rifampin-impregnated central venous catheters in bone marrow transplantation recipients: efficacy and low risk of developing staphylococcal resistance. *Infect Control Hosp Epidemiol.* 2003;24(12):961–963.
99. Raad I, Mohamed JA, Reitzel RA, et al. Improved antibiotic-impregnated catheters with extended-spectrum activity against resistant bacteria and fungi. *Antimicrob Agents Chemother.* 2012;56(2):935–941.
100. Jamal MA, Rosenblatt JS, Hachem RY, et al. Prevention of biofilm colonization by gram-negative bacteria on minocycline-rifampin-impregnated catheters sequentially coated with chlorhexidine. *Antimicrob Agents Chemother.* 2014;58(2):1179–1182.
101. Jamal MA, Hachem RY, Rosenblatt J, et al. In vivo biocompatibility and in vitro efficacy of antimicrobial gendine-coated central catheters. *Antimicrob Agents Chemother.* 2015;59(9):5611–5618.
102. Fraenkel D, Rickard C, Thomas P, et al. A prospective, randomized trial of rifampicin-minocycline-coated and silver platinum-carbon-impregnated central venous catheters. *Crit Care Med.* 2006;34(3):668–675.
103. Moretti EW, Ofstead CL, Kristy RM, Wetzler HP. Impact of central venous catheter type and methods on catheter-related colonization and bacteraemia. *J Hosp Infect.* 2005;61(2):139–145.
104. Chen YM, Dai AP, Shi Y, et al. Effectiveness of silver-impregnated central venous catheters for preventing catheter-related blood stream infections: a meta-analysis. *Int J Infect Dis.* 2014;29:279–286.
105. Chatzinikolaou I, Hanna H, Darouiche R, et al. Prospective study of the value of quantitative culture of organisms from blood collected through central venous catheters in differentiating between contamination and bloodstream infection. *J Clin Microbiol.* 2006;44(5):1834–1835.
106. Mermel LA, Allon M, Bouza E, et al. Clinical practice guidelines for the diagnosis and management of intravascular catheter-related infection: 2009 update by the Infectious Diseases Society of America. *Clin Infect Dis.* 2009:49:1–45.
107. Raad I, Davis S, Khan A, et al. Impact of central venous catheter removal on the recurrence of catheter-related coagulase negative staphylococcal bacteremia. *Infect Control Hosp Epidemiol.* 1992;13(4):215–221.
108. Farber BF, Kaplan MH, Clogston AG. *Staphylococcus epidermidis* extracted slime inhibits the antimicrobial action of glycopeptide antibiotics. *J Infect Dis.* 1990;161(1):37–40.
109. Raad I, Buzaid A, Rhyne J, et al. Minocycline and ethylenediaminetetraacetate for the prevention of recurrent vascular catheter infections. *Clin Infect Dis.* 1997;25(1):149–151.
110. Metcalf SC, Chambers ST, Pithie AD. Use of ethanol locks to prevent recurrent central line sepsis. *J Infect.* 2004;49(1):20–22.
111. Raad I, Darouiche R, Vazquez J, et al. Efficacy and safety of weekly dalbavancin therapy for catheter-related bloodstream infection caused by gram-positive pathogens. *Clin Infect Dis.* 2005;40(3):374–380.
112. Birmingham MC, Rayner CR, Meagher AK, et al. Linezolid for the treatment of multidrug-resistant, gram positive infections: experience from a compassionate-use program. *Clin Infect Dis.* 2003;36(2):159–168.
113. Carpenter CF, Chambers HF. Daptomycin: another novel agent for treating infections due to drug-resistant gram-positive pathogens. *Clin Infect Dis.* 2004;38(7):994–1000.
114. Fowler VG Jr, Sanders LL, Sexton DJ, et al. Outcome of *Staphylococcus aureus* bacteremia according to compliance with recommendations of infectious diseases specialists: experience with 244 patients. *Clin Infect Dis.* 1998;27(3):478–486.
115. Capdevila JA, Segarra A, Planes A, et al. Long term follow-up of patients with catheter related sepsis (CRS) treated without catheter removal [abstract J3]. In: *Program and abstracts of the 35th Interscience Conference on Antimicrobial Agents and Chemotherapy (San Francisco).* Washington, DC: American Society for Microbiology; 1995.
116. Poole CV, Carlton D, Bimbo L, Allon M. Treatment of catheter-related bacteraemia with an antibiotic lock protocol: effect of bacterial pathogen. *Nephrol Dial Transplant.* 2004;19(5):1237–1244.
117. Marr KA, Sexton DJ, Conlon PJ, et al. Catheter-related bacteremia and outcome of attempted catheter salvage in patients undergoing hemodialysis. *Ann Intern Med.* 1997;127(4):275–280.
118. Raad II, Sabbagh MF. Optimal duration of therapy for catheter-related *Staphylococcus aureus* bacteremia: a study of 55 cases and review. *Clin Infect Dis.* 1992;14(1):75–82.
119. Abraham J, Mansour C, Veledar E, et al. *Staphylococcus aureus* bacteremia and endocarditis: the Grady Memorial Hospital experience with methicillin-sensitive S aureus and methicillin-resistant S aureus bacteremia. *Am Heart J.* 2004;147(3):536–539.
120. Wisplinghoff H, Bischoff T, Tallent SM, et al. Nosocomial bloodstream infections in US hospitals: analysis of 24,179 cases from a prospective nationwide surveillance study. *Clin Infect Dis.* 2004; 39:309–317.
121. Jones RN, Marshall SA, Pfaller MA, et al. Nosocomial enterococcal blood stream infections in the SCOPE Program: antimicrobial resistance, species occurrence, molecular testing results, and laboratory testing accuracy. SCOPE Hospital Study Group. *Diagn Microbiol Infect Dis.* 1997;29:95–102.
122. Maki DG, Agger WA. *Enterococcal bacteremia:* clinical features, the risk of endocarditis, and management. *Medicine (Baltimore).* 1988;67:248–269.
123. Gray J, Marsh PJ, Stewart D, Pedler SJ. *Enterococcal bacteraemia:* a prospective study of 125 episodes. *J Hosp Infect.* 1994;27:179–186.
124. Elting LS, Bodey GP. Septicemia due to *Xanthomonas* species and non aeruginosa *Pseudomonas* species: increasing incidence of catheter-related infections. *Medicine (Baltimore).* 1990;69(5):296–306.
125. Hanna H, Afif C, Alakech B, et al. Central venous catheter-related bacteremia due to gram-negative bacilli: significance of catheter removal in preventing relapse. *Infect Control Hosp Epidemiol.* 2004;25(8): 646–649.
126. Nguyen MH, Peacock JE Jr, Tanner DC, et al. Therapeutic approaches in patients with candidemia: evaluation in a multicenter, prospective observational study. *Arch Intern Med.* 1995;155:2429–2435.
127. Nucci M, Colombo AL, Silveira F, et al. Risk factors for death in patients with candidemia. *Infect Control Hosp Epidemiol.* 1998;19:846–850.
128. Hung CC, Chen YC, Chang SC, et al. Nosocomial candidemia in a university hospital in Taiwan. *J Formos Med Assoc.* 1996;95:19–28.
129. Rex JH, Bennett JE, Sugar AM, et al. Intravascular catheter-exchange and duration of candidemia. NIAID Mycoses Study Group and the Candidemia Study Group. *Clin Infect Dis.* 1995;21:994–996.
130. Karkowicz MG, Hashimoto LN, Kelly RE Jr, Buescher ES. Should central venous catheters be removed as soon as candidemia is detected in neonates? *Pediatrics.* 2000;106:E63.
131. Raad I, Hanna H, Boktour M, et al. Management of central venous catheters in patients with cancer and candidemia. *Clin Infect Dis.* 2004;38(8): 1119–1127.
132. Morano SG, Latagliata R, Girmenia C, et al. Catheter-associated bloodstream infections and thrombotic risk in hematologic patients with peripherally inserted central catheters (PICC). *Supp Care Cancer.* 2015;23(11): 3289–3295.
133. Safdar N, Maki DG. Risk of catheter-related bloodstream infection with peripherally inserted central venous catheters used in hospitalized patients. *Chest.* 2005;128(2):489–495.
134. Nolan ME, Yadav H, Cawcutt KA, Cartin-Ceba R. Complication rates among peripherally inserted central venous catheters and centrally inserted central catheters in the medical intensive care unit. *J Crit Care.* 2016;31(1):238–242.
135. Chopra V, O'Horo JC, Rogers MA, et al. The risk of bloodstream infection associated with peripherally inserted central catheters compared with central venous catheters in adults: a systematic review and meta-analysis. *Infect Control Hosp Epidemiol.* 2013;34(9):908–918.

Section 2

Respiratory Infections

LISA M. ESOLEN and OLIVIER Y. LEROY

PNEUMONIA

Traditionally, pneumonia has been differentiated as community-acquired or hospital-acquired. For *community-acquired pneumonia* (CAP), the infection either begins while the patient is an outpatient or becomes apparent within the first 48 hours of admission to an acute care hospital. Conversely, a *hospital-acquired pneumonia* (HAP) becomes evident more than 48 hours after admission (1). It has become clear, however, that this simplistic dichotomous classification is not sufficient to characterize all patients suffering from pneumonia. First, among HAPs, those occurring during mechanical ventilation (MV) must be differentiated from others because of epidemiologic, prognostic, and therapeutic factors (2,3). Furthermore, numerous outpatients with frequent health care contact and chronic illnesses that utilize dialysis, chemotherapy, or rehabilitation services cannot be simplistically considered as equivalent to all ambulatory patients. Notably, in most nursing homes and rehabilitation hospitals, patients can receive intensive and/or invasive medical care with exposure to different microbial flora and this places them at an altered risk than otherwise healthy outpatients. We now understand that these situations constitute a separate demographic, now defined as a *health care–associated pneumonia* (HCAP) (3).

Thus, four classes of pneumonia can be distinguished:

1. Community-acquired pneumonia (CAP)
2. Hospital-acquired pneumonia (HAP)
3. Ventilator-associated pneumonia (VAP)
4. Health care–associated pneumonia (HCAP)

We will discuss each of these below, and will also briefly touch on the topics of tracheobronchitis, pleural infections, and pulmonary abscess.

Severe Community-Acquired Pneumonia

Immediate Concerns

CAP is a common infectious disease affecting about 12 per 1,000 adults yearly (4). An intensive care unit (ICU) admission for severe CAP is required for 2% of patients and over 80% of the cases are due to *Streptococcus pneumoniae*. Despite progress in antibiotic therapy and ICU management, the mortality of pneumococcal pneumonia remains high.

Diagnosis

CAP is suspected on the basis of clinical symptoms: cough, dyspnea, sputum production, pleuritic chest pain, and elevated body temperature; these symptoms can be absent or moderated in older patients. However, these signs are not specific of pneumonia; a chest radiograph or computed tomography (CT) scan revealing a new infiltrate is required to document a pneumonia diagnosis, though false-negative results may be seen during early presentations which are complicated by severe dehydration, neutropenia, or with certain pathogens such as *Pneumocystis jirovecci* (4).

The chest radiograph might offer insights into the etiologic diagnosis, with *S. pneumoniae* resulting in a typically lobar pattern, and intracellular pathogens such as mycoplasma typically presenting with an interstitial radiographic pattern. However, these findings are not specific, and caution should be exercised in interpreting radiographs, particularly in critically ill patients. The chest radiograph also allows for staging of severity according to the number of involved lobes, and is helpful to detect complications such as pleural effusions or cavitation. In these situations, CT scan may be advisable for further characterization of the infection, particularly in immunosuppressed patients (e.g., halo or crescent signs in pulmonary aspergillosis of neutropenic patients, cavitation in tuberculosis).

Definition and Decision for ICU Admission

Although there is no gold standard to define severe CAP, criteria do exist that may be used to assess the severity of CAP and define the need for ICU admission.

According to the original American Thoracic Society (ATS) guidelines (5), CAP was considered severe when any one of the following criteria was present:

- Respiratory frequency greater than 30 breaths/min on admission
- Severe respiratory failure ($PaO_2/FiO_2 < 250$ mmHg)
- Requirement for MV
- Bilateral or multilobar or extensive (≥50% within 48 hours of admission) involvement of the chest radiograph
- Shock (systolic blood pressure [SBP] <90 mmHg or diastolic blood pressure <60 mmHg)
- Requirement for vasopressors for more than 4 hours
- Low urine output (<20 mL/hr or <80 mL/4 hr) or acute renal failure requiring dialysis

In 1998, Ewig et al. (6) demonstrated that using any one of these factors as the definition of severe CAP had a high sensitivity but a low specificity; a new definition of severe CAP was proposed, which, in 2001, was adopted by the ATS (7). The diagnosis of CAP was considered severe and requiring ICU admission for patients exhibiting either one of two major criteria (the need for MV and septic shock) or two of three minor criteria (SBP 90 mmHg or below, multilobar involvement on chest radiograph, or PaO_2/FiO_2 less than 250 mmHg) (7). Unfortunately, additional studies suggested that this revised ATS criteria did not discriminate enough to guide decision-making regarding the need for ICU care (8,9).

The British Thoracic Society (BTS) proposed assessing the severity of CAP utilizing three groups of adverse prognostic features: four "core" factors (CURB score: confusion, blood urea nitrogen >19 mg/dL [7 mmol/L], respiratory rate ≥30 breaths/min, and low blood pressure [SBP <90 mmHg and/or diastolic ≤60 mmHg]); two "additional" factors (hypoxemia defined by $SpO_2 < 92\%$ or $PaO_2 < 60$ mmHg [8 kPa] and bilateral or multilobar involvement on chest radiograph); and two "pre-existing" factors (age ≥50 years and the presence of coexisting disease) (10). CAP was considered severe in patients having two or more core adverse prognostic features. In patients exhibiting only one of these core factors, the decision, based on clinical judgment, could be assisted by taking into account pre-existing and additional factors (10).

Finally, in 2007, the ATS and Infectious Disease Society of America (IDSA) drafted a consensus guideline (5) which incorporated much of the CURB score, above, along with the addition of the following elements:

- White blood cell count <4,000 cells/mm^3
- Thrombocytopenia (<100,000 cells/mm^3)
- Nonexposure hypothermia (core temperature <36°C)

Accordingly, ICU admission is now recommended for individuals who meet either major criteria listed below or three of the minor criteria listed as follows:

- Major criteria:
  - Invasive MV
  - Septic shock with the need for vasopressors
- Minor criteria:
  - Respiratory rate ≥30 breaths/min
  - PaO_2/FiO_2 ratio ≤250
  - Multilobar infiltrates
  - Confusion/disorientation (new-onset disorientation to person, place, time)
  - Uremia (BUN level ≥20 mg/dL)
  - Leukopenia (white blood cell count <4,000 cells/mm^3)
  - Thrombocytopenia (<100,000 cells/mm^3)
  - Nonexposure hypothermia (core temperature <36°C)
  - Hypotension requiring aggressive fluid resuscitation.

Diagnostic Studies

Evaluation for the etiologic diagnosis is helpful to confirm the infectious origin of the pulmonary findings and direct appropriate antimicrobial therapy (including secondary de-escalation therapy). Numerous methods are available for the microbiologic diagnosis of pneumonia but, importantly, this analysis is influenced by several factors including the specimen source, the concentration of the organism, the pathogenicity of the organism, and the influence of prior antibiotics.

- Sputum stains and cultures. These require careful interpretation. A sample should only be considered purulent, and valuable for culture and interpretation, if there are more than 25 polymorphonuclear cells (PMNs) and less than 10 squamous epithelial cells per high power field (HPF). A single predominant organism on a Gram stain is suggestive of a specific etiology. But even with this, the yield on culture for certain pathogens can be low, with 30% to 60% of sputum failing to grow the most common pathogen in CAP, *S. pneumoniae,* due to its fastidious growth requirements (11). Other stains can be used according to the particular clinical context and may allow for a positive diagnosis: acid-fast stains for *Mycobacterium tuberculosis,* or various silver stains for cyst wall of *Pneumocystis jirovecii.*
- Alternative specimen collection by more invasive sampling methods (endotracheal aspiration, protected tip bronchoscopic brushings, bronchoalveolar lavage [BAL], and transtracheal aspiration). These methods attempt to bypass the upper airway contamination and are discussed in more detail in the VAP section, but can also be useful in the diagnosis of severe CAP.
- Blood cultures, drawn before antibiotic therapy, are occasionally positive (6% to 20% of cases).
- Urinary antigen assays. The urinary antigen test is about 80% sensitive for the diagnosis of *Legionella pneumophila* type 1 with most of the false negatives being due to *Legionella* species other than *L. pneumophila*. The urinary antigen assay for *S. pneumoniae* shows a high sensitivity (82%) and specificity (97%) in bacteremic pneumonia, but is considerably less sensitive and specific in nonbacteremic pneumococcal pneumonia and in children (12).
- Polymerase chain reaction (PCR) testing. Rapid diagnostic testing by PCR now exists for 12 respiratory pathogens including influenza A (12,13), respiratory syncytial virus, parainfluenza, and coronaviruses. Available tests can detect pathogens in 30 minutes and can often be done at the point of care. The types of specimens acceptable for use (i.e., throat, nasopharyngeal, or nasal; and aspirates, swabs, or washes) vary by test. The specificity and, in particular, the sensitivity of rapid tests are lower than for viral culture and vary by test.
- Serologic testing. The presence of IgM with a titer greater than or equal to 16 generally indicates a recent infection, but this is rarely observed in the initial phase of infection and is rarely useful. A fourfold rise in convalescent antibody titer requires that samples are drawn 2 weeks apart but can be useful for certain pathogens (e.g., *Mycoplasma pneumoniae, Chlamydia pneumoniae, Chlamydophila psittaci, Legionella* spp., *Coxiella burnetii,* adenovirus).

Minimal diagnostic testing for patients admitted to the ICU with CAP can be done via endotracheal aspiration, blood cultures, *L. pneumophila* urinary antigen, and thoracentesis, if pleural effusion is present. Despite the potential for microbiologic testing along with the newer rapid modalities, a definitive diagnosis in CAP is obtained, by some reports, in less than 10% of cases (12). More invasive procedures should be reserved for those patients who are critically ill, immunosuppressed, and those with failure of a first-line treatment (7).

Etiology

Organisms Causing CAP in Hospitalized Patients Requiring ICU Admission. The epidemiology of CAP patients admitted to the ICU does not appear to be different from other hospitalized individuals with CAP. The most frequent pathogen isolated in ICU-hospitalized CAP patients is *S. pneumoniae* (Table 88.2.4) (14–16).

Other pathogens responsible for severe CAP, such as *H. influenzae* or *S. aureus,* occur with less frequency and sometimes as a secondary bacterial superinfection of an underlying influenza infection. Less-frequent pathogens recovered from patients with underlying chronic lung disease include *Pseudomonas aeruginosa* or, in neutropenic patients, *Aspergillus* species.

Drug-resistant Pathogens. A major emerging challenge in the empiric treatment of CAP is the rise of drug-resistant micro-organisms such as community-acquired methicillin-resistant *S. aureus* (CA-MRSA) and penicillin-resistant pneumococci (PRP).

For *S. pneumoniae,* macrolide resistance is above 20% in the United States and greater than 50% in some European and Asian–Pacific countries (17). Decreased susceptibility or resistance to penicillin is observed in 30% to 50% of strains in some studies, and fluoroquinolone resistance has been increasing. While the penicillin resistance is higher for noninvasive

TABLE 88.2.4 Micro-organisms Causing Severe Community-acquired Pneumonia Requiring Admission to the ICU[a]

	Yoshimoto (14)	Leroy (15)	Shorr (16)
Number of patients	72	308	199
Unknown pathogen	55.6%	45–45.9%	43.7%
Streptococcus pneumoniae	13.9%	38.7–41%	44.7%
Haemophilus influenzae	2.8%	15.8–24.5%	10.6%
Legionella pneumophila	2.8%	3.2–3.8%	8.9%
Staphylococcus aureus	2.8%	2.8–7.4%	8.9%
Pseudomonas aeruginosa	8.3%	ND	4.9%
Other gram-positive	2.8%	17–17.9%	ND
Enterobacteriaceae	11.1%	7.5–8.4%	6.5%
Chlamydia spp.	ND	1.9–3.2%	ND
Mycobacterium tuberculosis	2.8%	ND	2.4%
Other	1.4%	3.2–3.8%	13%

ND, no data.
[a]Data presented as number or percentage.

infections, it reached 19% in blood cultures worldwide with risk factors including recent hospitalization, administration of antimicrobials, and immunodeficiency (18,19). The impact of drug resistance on outcome is controversial (20). Some studies have suggested a trend toward higher mortality in patients with pneumococcal pneumonia caused by intermediately resistant strains (21). Fluoroquinolone resistance is increasing, with the prescribing habits of these agents potentially impacting resistance rates (22,23).

Emergence of CA-MRSA with cases of rapidly progressive necrotizing pneumonia, often in previously healthy adults and children, is a new challenge for proper empiric antibiotic choices (24). The further introduction of highly resistant gram-negative pathogens, such as the *Enterobacteriaciae* with extended-spectrum β-lactamases (ESBL) and the emergence of *Klebsiella pneumoniae* with carbapenmase resistance may impact the empiric antimicrobial choices for pneumonia in other clinical settings—ventilator-dependent patients, nosocomially acquired infections—but generally do not impact the etiology of true CAP.

P. aeruginosa are naturally resistant to numerous antibiotics and can elevate to a high-level resistance under treatment. Risk of *P. aeruginosa* is increased in patients presenting with a previous chronic pulmonary disease such as chronic obstructive pulmonary disorder (COPD) or cystic fibrosis, recent antibiotic therapy, or a stay in the hospital, especially the ICU (11,25).

Specific Etiologies in Immunosuppressed Patients

Immunosuppressed patients have an increased risk of severe CAP; these patients have more frequent bacterial pneumonias, with the typical pathogen dependent upon the underlying immune deficiency.

Human immunodeficiency virus (HIV)-infected patients used to have a 25-fold higher risk of developing bacterial pneumonia as compared to the general population (26). This has largely abated due to the use of more active antiretroviral drugs and, in some studies, shows little difference from the general population (27). *P. jirovecii* pneumonia (PJP) remains a frequent acquired immunodeficiency syndrome (AIDS)-defining diagnosis, while less frequent causes include cytomegalovirus (CMV) and mycobacteria.

Patients with chemotherapy-induced neutropenia, particularly when severe (<500 neutrophils/μL) and prolonged (>10 days), have an increased risk of invasive pulmonary aspergillosis as well as severe bacterial pneumonia (28,29). In the proper clinical setting, with cavitary or mass-like lesions, this population may require empiric treatment for *Aspergillus*, usually with a triazole antifungal, such as voriconazole. This risk also exists with targeted monoclonal antibody therapies, which increase the risk of CMV and PJP (30). Patients with solid organ transplant and those receiving antitumor necrosis factor (TNF) monoclonal antibodies both have an increased risk of severe CAP caused by the usual bacterial pathogens, as well as by opportunistic infections such as *P. jirovecii* and *Aspergillus* (31,32).

Treatment

Antibiotic Therapy

Antimicrobial Spectrum. The ideal antibiotic should have a bactericidal activity against the major pathogens responsible for severe CAP. Considerations are given to the severity of clinical presentation, with non-ICU patients being distinguished from ICU patients in terms of empiric therapy. Additionally, special epidemiologic considerations may factor into this decision along with comorbid host conditions that may favor more resistant or unusual pathogens.

Timing of Initial Therapy. The most recent IDSA guideline recommends initial antibiotic administration within 4 hours of admission (25). A reduced mortality (adjusted odds ratio [AOR], 0.85, 95% confidence interval [CI] 0.76 to 0.95) was observed in patients with early therapy in a retrospective study of 18,209 Medicare patients (33). However, other studies contradicted this finding, and suggested that the time to first antibiotic dose was a marker of disease severity rather than an indicator of prognosis (34,35).

Antimicrobial Choices. Drug choice depends on numerous factors, including causative pathogen, pharmacodynamics/pharmacokinetics of the antimicrobial agent, spectrum of activity, adverse events, cost, host factors and, possibly, availability.

The antimicrobial agent must have sufficient diffusion in pulmonary tissues. β-Lactam antibiotics have a good extracellular diffusion, but are ineffective on intracellular organisms; their concentration in the alveolar lining fluid (ALF) reached 10% to 20% of the serum concentration after a single dose. Macrolides, on the other hand, have a variable intracellular distribution—low for erythromycin and elevated for clarithromycin and azithromycin. Fluoroquinolones have an excellent intracellular and extracellular diffusions with levofloxacin having increased activity against *Legionella* species as well as enhanced activity against *S. pneumoniae* (36).

Empiric choices must cover the most common pathogens in severe CAP. While less severe CAP will include *S. pneumoniae*, other atypicals, such as *Mycoplasma*, *Chlamydia*, and respiratory viruses, play a larger role. In severe CAP requiring ICU admission, *S. pneumoniae* remains common, but *S. aureus*,

Legionella, and gram-negative bacilli rise in significance and must be empirically covered. Additionally, there are epidemiologic situations that may contribute to empiric choices. For example, alcoholism raises the concern for oral anaerobes and *Klebsiella,* COPD, and underlying chronic lung disease for *Pseudomonas* and *Moraxella.* Travel history, animal/bird exposures, and intravenous drug abuse may all suggest more unusual pathogens, including *Coccidiodes* species, *Histoplasma,* Hantavirus, or CA-MRSA.

Data suggests that combination regimens which include a macrolide or a quinolone are superior to β-lactam monotherapy for severe CAP (37–39). This is particularly important in cases of bacteremic pneumococcal pneumonia, in which combination therapy was confirmed as superior in an international, multicenter, prospective observational study (38,40,41). Lower mortality was associated with combination therapy for critically ill patients (14-day mortality, 23.4% vs. 55.3%; $p = 0.0015$), but not for all patients receiving combination versus monotherapy (10.4% vs. 11.5%, p = NS). All combinations using a β-lactam had an enhanced response.

The regularly updated guidelines published by North American and European medical societies recommend the utilization of a β-lactam with a macrolide or a respiratory fluoroquinolone. The 2007 IDSA/ATS guidelines concur, and are presented in Table 88.2.5.

Duration of Therapy. Length of treatment may be modified based on the pathogen, response to treatment, comorbid illness, and complications (42). In general, patients with CAP should be treated a minimum of 5 days, but at least until they are afebrile for 72 hours. Longer durations are needed for necrotizing infections caused by *S. aureus*—particularly when bacteremic due to endocarditis and/or metastatic infections—*P. aeruginosa* and *Klebsiella,* which should probably be treated no less than 2 weeks. Similarly, atypical intracellular pathogens are generally treated for a minimum of 2 weeks.

TABLE 88.2.5 Initial Empiric Antibiotic Therapy in Patients Admitted to the ICU for Severe CAP

Clinical Characteristics	Recommended Antibiotics
No *Pseudomonas* or methicillin-resistant *Staphylococcus aureus* (MRSA) or penicillin allergy	β-Lactam (cefotaxime, ceftriaxone, ampicillin/sulbactam) plus azithromycin or a respiratory fluoroquinolone[a]
Patients with penicillin allergy	Respiratory fluoroquinolone, with azithromycin
Suspected *Pseudomonas* infection	Antipseudomonal β-lactam[b] plus Ciprofloxacin or levofloxacin[a] or Aminoglycoside and antipneumococcal fluoroquinolone[a]
Suspected community-acquired MRSA	Addition of vancomycin or linezolid

[a]Dosage of levofloxacin should be 750 mg daily.
Antipseudomonal agents include piperacillin-tazobactam, imipenem, meropenem, or cefepime. Azithromycin can be substituted for penicillin allergy.
Adapted from Mandell LA, Wunderink RG, Anzueto A, et al. Infectious Diseases Society of America/American Thoracic Society consensus guidelines on the management of community-acquired pneumonia in adults. *Clin Infect Dis.* 2007;44(Suppl 2):S27.

Nonantimicrobial Therapy

Besides antimicrobial therapies, most patients admitted to the ICU for severe CAP need additional treatment. End-organ dysfunction, such as respiratory failure, septic shock, or renal failure, require supportive measures. Similarly, the standard care for acutely ill patients (i.e., nutrition, prevention of ICU-related complications, and treatment of underlying diseases) must be utilized.

Activated Protein C. Severe sepsis is associated with a generalized inflammation and a procoagulant response to infection. Activated protein C is an important endogenous modulator of this response; there are reduced levels of activated protein C in most patients with severe sepsis.

Although drotrecogin-α activated, a recombinant form of human activated protein C (r-aPC), exhibits profibrinolytic, antithrombotic, and anti-inflammatory characteristics, and while large studies suggested that treatment with r-aPC significantly decreased 28-day and hospital discharge mortality rates in patients with severe sepsis, although not in lesser ill patients (43–46), this agent was ultimately found to be inefficacious and has been removed from the market.

Corticosteroids. Confalonieri et al. (47) studied hydrocortisone—200 mg i.v. bolus followed by infusion at a rate of 10 mg/hr for 7 days—randomized against placebo in a cohort of 46 patients. Findings included improvements oxygenation, radiographs, shock and multiorgan dysfunction, length of hospital stay, and mortality. While additional randomized trials are needed to recommend routine use for the treatment of severe CAP, use of hydrocortisone is clearly indicated in patients who do not have normal cortisol responses, and screening for occult adrenal insufficiency in patients who remain hypotensive after fluid resuscitation may be warranted. This is at least controversial (see Chapter 46, Sepsis and Septic Shock).

Expected Clinical Course

Evaluation on Day 3. Clinical response to treatment for severe CAP may not be seen in the first 48 hours. Expectations are that fever and oxygenation will, at least, stabilize even though they may not yet begin to improve. Empiric therapy should be continued during this time, allowing for preliminary culture data to return. Upon reassessment with microbiologic data, de-escalation may be supported or therapy modification may be necessary.

Complications and Failure to Improve. A poor clinical response by day 3 may be a sign of treatment failure. However, in the ICU, other diagnoses such as pulmonary embolism or cardiac failure should be considered in this situation. Treatment failure may be due to a non-infectious cause of the pulmonary issue (concomitant cardiac failure, pulmonary embolism), or to an organism not covered by the first-line antimicrobial therapy, thus necessitating a change or addition to the antimicrobial regimen. Other causes of treatment failure can include infectious complications of the pneumonia despite adequate antimicrobial therapy. These include lung abscess, empyema, endocarditis, or other superinfection.

Prognosis

Mortality in patients with severe CAP requiring admission to the ICU remains high, ranging in various series from 18% to

TABLE 88.2.6 Independent Prognostic Factors Associated with Mortality of Patients with Severe CAP

PREADMISSION HEALTH STATUS
- Age >70 yr
- Immunosuppression
- Comorbidities with anticipated death ≤5 yr

INITIAL SEVERITY OF ILLNESS
- Antibiotic administration prior to hospital presentation
- Simplified Acute Physiologic Score (SAPS) I >12 or SAPS II >45
- Septic shock
- Requirement for mechanical ventilation
- Acute renal failure
- Bilateral or multilobar pulmonary involvement
- *K. pneumonia* or *P. aeruginosa* as etiologic agent
- Bacteremia
- Nonaspiration pneumonia

EVOLUTION DURING ICU STAY
- Radiographic spread of pneumonia
- Number of nonpulmonary organs that failed
- Increase in Logistic Organ Dysfunction score from D1 to D3
- Delay in hospital antibiotic administration of more than 4 hr
- Ineffective initial antimicrobial therapy
- Occurrence of nonpneumonia-related complications
- Increase of procalcitonin level in serum from D1 to D3

46% (8,48–54). A meta-analysis of 788 ICU patients found a mean mortality rate of 36.5% (55); in this analysis, Fine and colleagues (55) identified the following 11 factors independently associated with a higher mortality: male gender (OR = 1.3), pleuritic chest pain (OR = 0.5), hypothermia (OR = 5.0), systolic hypotension (OR = 4.8), tachypnea (OR = 2.9), diabetes mellitus (OR = 1.3), neoplastic disease (OR = 2.8), neurologic disease (OR = 4.6), bacteremia (OR = 2.8), leukopenia (OR = 2.5), and multilobar disease (OR = 3.1).

Numerous studies have focused on the prognosis of patients admitted to the ICU for severe CAP (48–50,52–54,56–58). Though inclusion criteria were variable, most independent prognostic factors were similar and demonstrated that, in general, survival in cases of severe CAP depends on the preadmission health status of the patient, the initial severity of illness, and the evolution during the ICU stay (Table 88.2.6). While these findings suggest that there are important nonmodifiable factors which influence mortality, the following points must be underscored:

- The initial empiric antimicrobials must be instituted as soon as possible (<4 hours after hospital admission).
- The empiric antibiotics must be broad enough to cover the most likely pathogens.

Studies have suggested that empiric initial antimicrobial treatment which utilizes a macrolide or a respiratory fluoroquinolone as a second agent to a β-lactam reduces mortality from CAP (37,59,60). Similar results are seen with bacteremic pneumococcal CAP when combination therapy is prescribed (40,41,61). Of note, however, is the fact that in these retrospective analyses, critically ill patients were often excluded. Rello et al. (38) specifically compared multiple antibiotic combinations and the resultant mortality for patients admitted to the ICU with severe CAP. Their major finding was that the addition of empiric aminoglycosides was suboptimal. Wilson and colleagues (62) compared the two regimens which are concordant with the latest IDSA/ATS guideline (β-lactam + macrolide and β-lactam + respiratory quinolone) and found no significant effect on mortality between these two options, though their findings did suggest an increased length of hospital stay when the quinolone was used instead of the macrolide.

Mortality risk can be assessed by the Pneumonia Severity Index (PSI),which stratifies patients into five classes according to the risk of death within 30 days using a two-step approach (63). First, patients with a low risk (class I) are identified by age younger than 50 years and the absence of comorbidities and vital sign abnormalities. For the remaining patients, a score is determined by adding points assigned to age, comorbid conditions, physical findings, laboratory and radiographic abnormalities (Table 88.2.7). According to the value of this score, patients are classified into class II (≤70 points), III (71 to 90 points), IV (91 to 130 points), or V (>130 points). From class I to class V, mortality rates observed were 0.1%, 0.6%, 2.8%, 8.2%, and 29.2%, respectively. Despite major interest in this finding, the indexing of patients in this manner was to identify patients at *low* risk for complications, who might be safely treated as outpatients. Consequently, the implications of the PSI for the medical care of patients exhibiting severe CAP, and requiring admission into an ICU, is unclear.

A specific prediction rule for mortality of patients with severe CAP admitted to an ICU was proposed by Leroy et al. (57), emphasizing both *initial* baseline patient characteristics and the patient's *evolution* during the ICU stay. Upon ICU admission, an initial risk score based on the following six independent variables and their respective point value is established: age 40 years or older (+1 point); anticipated death within 5 years (+1 point); nonaspiration pneumonia (+1 point); chest radiograph involvement greater than one lobe (+1 point); acute respiratory failure requiring MV (+1 point);

TABLE 88.2.7 Criteria and Point Scoring System Used in the Pneumonia Severity Index (Step 2; Classes II–V)

Variables	Points	Variables	Points
Age	Age (yr)	Vital sign abnormality	
Female gender	−10	Altered mental status	+20
Nursing home resident	+10	Respiratory rate >30 breaths/min	+20
		Systolic blood pressure <90 mmHg	+20
		Temperature <35°C or ≥40°C	+15
		Tachycardia >125 beats/min	+10
Comorbidity		Laboratory and radiographic data	
Neoplastic disease	+30		
Liver disease	+20	Arterial pH <7.35	+30
Congestive heart failure	+10	Blood urea nitrogen ≥30 mg/dL	+20
Cerebrovascular disease	+10	Sodium <130 mmol/L	+20
Renal disease	+10	Glucose ≥250 mg/dL	+10
		Hematocrit <30%	+10
		PaO_2 <60 mmHg	+10
		Pleural effusion	+10

Adapted from Fine MJ, Auble TE, Yealy DM, et al. A prediction rule to identify low-risk patients with community-acquired pneumonia. *N Engl J Med.* 1997;336:243.

and septic shock (+3 points). Summation of these points places patients into one of three classes: class I (0 to 2 points; mortality risk is less than 5%), class II (3 to 5 points; mortality risk is 25%), and class III (6 to 8 points, mortality risk is >50%). Step two is to score three independent variables during the ICU stay. These three variables and their point scores are hospital-acquired, lower respiratory tract superinfections (+1 point); nonspecific CAP-related complications (+2 points); and sepsis-related complications (+4 points). This modified risk score most significantly altered the prognosis for patients initially categorized in the moderate range (class II) risk. The adjusted risk score determined subgroups of patients within this class who exhibited significantly different mortality rates ranging from 2% to 86%. Therefore, this score may help clinicians to reassess severe CAP patients during the ICU stay.

Prevention

Immunization remains the most significant method of prevention (25). Two vaccines are available for preventing pneumococcal disease. Pneumococcal polysaccharide vaccine (PPSV23) and pneumococcal conjugate vaccine (PCV13). Currently, the Advisory Committee on Immunization Practices (ACIP) recommends that all adults 65 years of age or older receive one dose of PCV13 followed by PPSV23 one year later. Adults 19 years of age or older who have functional or anatomic asplenia, CSF leaks, cochlear implants, and immunocompromising conditions (HIV, congenital immunodeficiencies, hematologic malignancies, solid organ transplant, chronic renal disease) should receive PCV13, again followed by PPSV23 no sooner than 8 weeks later. PCV13 alone is also recommended for children 2 years of age or greater who have immunocompromising conditions such as asplenia, sickle cell disease, HIV, or other immunocompromising conditions (64–67).

The ACIP recommends that all persons >6 months of age receive influenza vaccination annually. Persons who are between 2 and 49 years of age may receive either the live-attenuated intranasal vaccine or the inactivated intramuscular injection; the inactivated influenza vaccination should be used in persons 50 and older (68).

Ventilator-associated Pneumonia

VAP is defined as a pneumonia occurring in patients undergoing MV. Although usual guidelines suggest a delay of 48 to 72 hours between the beginning of MV and the occurrence of pneumonia to qualify for this diagnosis (69), some data suggest that a pneumonia acquired earlier than the 48th hour of MV could also be considered a VAP (2,70). VAP represents 80% of pneumonia acquired during hospitalization, and is the most frequent hospital-acquired infection in ICUs.

Immediate Concerns

The major considerations regarding VAP are:

- Prevention
- Acceptable "gold standard" for diagnosis
- Increasing rates of nosocomial drug-resistant pathogens

Incidence

The exact incidence of VAP is difficult to assess, as study populations vary widely because the criteria used to define VAP has evolved, especially from organizations such as the United States Centers for Disease Control (CDC). This leads to overlap between VAP and other hospital-acquired lower respiratory tract infections, such as nosocomial tracheobronchitis, nosocomial or community-acquired aspiration, and even non-infectious respiratory illnesses. With no gold standard for diagnosis, studies show very different incidence rates ranging from 5.6% to 82.4% (Table 88.2.8) (70–78). Nevertheless, the CDC reports a decline in the incidence of VAP over the past several years in the United States, with rates up to 6% (79).

While risk for VAP increases the longer the patient is intubated, the daily hazard rate may decrease over time. In a cohort of 1,014 patients ventilated for 48 hours or more, the overall incidence of VAP was 14.8 cases per 1,000 ventilator days. The daily hazard rate for developing VAP was estimated to be 3% per day at day 5 but only 1.3% by day 15 (80). Overall, the risk of infection is the highest during the first 8 to 10 days of MV and increases with the duration of MV (80,81).

Pathogenesis

Pneumonia is essentially the introduction of pathogenic bacteria into the normally sterile lower respiratory tract, where colonization followed by invasive infection may occur (69,82). Bacteria may reach the lower respiratory tract by four different pathogenic mechanisms: (1) contiguous spread; (2) hematogenous spread; (3) inhalation; and (4) aspiration. The first

TABLE 88.2.8 Incidence of Ventilator-associated Pneumonia in the ICU

References	No. of Patients	Characteristics of Patients	Diagnostic Criteria	Incidence of VAP
Torres (71)	322	Medicosurgical patients	Clinical and XR	24%
Chevret (72)	540	Medicosurgical patients	Clinical and XR	12.6%
Baker (73)	514	Trauma patients	Clinical, XR, and Q bacteriologic cultures	5.6%
Chastre (74)	56	Patients with ARDS	Clinical, XR, and Q bacteriologic cultures	55%
Tejada Artigas (75)	103	Trauma patients	Clinical, XR, and Q bacteriologic cultures	22.3%
Ibraham (76)	880	Medicosurgical patients	Clinical and XR	15%
Bouza (77)	356	Heart surgical patients	Clinical, XR, and Q bacteriologic cultures	7.9%
Hilker (78)	17	Patients with acute stroke	Clinical and XR	82.4%

XR, radiologic; ARDS, acute respiratory distress syndrome; Q, quantitative.

two mechanisms of invasion are infrequent (83). Inhalation refers to the direct inoculation of the respiratory tract by way of an aerosol, such as a contaminated ventilator circuit, a nebulized treatment, or even a contaminated bronchoscope; these would all be considered fairly rare events. The major mode of entry for pathogenic bacteria into the lower respiratory tract is by aspiration of oropharyngeal organisms. Colonization of the oropharyngeal airways by pathogenic micro-organisms occurs during the first week of hospitalization and they are more likely to be gram negative and drug-resistant. The endotracheal tube eliminates the protective barriers between the oropharynx and lower respiratory tract, and leakage around the endotracheal tube cuff of secretions, now colonized with more pathogenic bacteria, allows access to the trachea (69,82).

Risk Factors

Patient-related risk factors include male gender, pre-existing pulmonary disease, coma, AIDS, head trauma, age over 60 years, neurosurgical procedures, and multiorgan system failure (84).

The presence of MV alone is associated with a 3- to 21-fold risk of pneumonia (72). The endotracheal tube not only limits the natural elimination of oral secretions contaminated with nosocomial pathogens, but it also impairs ciliary clearance and cough. Furthermore, the MV patient requires other devices, such as nebulizers or humidifiers, which can be an additional, albeit unusual, source of micro-organisms.

Accidental extubation can be distinguished from a more controlled tracheal decannulation as independently elevating the risk for a VAP (85). This may be due to the fact that proper oral care and preparation for the extubation did not occur, and that the patient may be confused or an aspiration risk. GI risk factors include the use of enteral nutrition administered by a nasogastric, rather than a gastrostomy tube, and the use of H_2 blockers and proton pump inhibitors which favor gastric colonization of pathogens due to the elevated pH (80,84).

Other factors that facilitate the inhalation of oropharyngeal secretions include: supine position, patient transportation out of the ICU (86), sedation (87), failed subglottic aspiration of secretions (81), and intracuff pressure less than 20 cm H_2O.

Etiology

VAP may be caused by a wide spectrum of bacteria, and is often polymicrobial (Table 88.2.9) (88–90). *P. aeruginosa, S. aureus,* and gram-negative enteric bacilli are the leading etiologies. However, pathogens may differ according to patient groups, unit types, hospitals, and countries (90). Moreover, the antimicrobial resistance patterns may vary widely with geographic location.

Several studies have tried to identify specific risk factors associated with specific pathogens. The presence of an altered level of consciousness, admission into a medical ICU, and a high Simplified Acute Physiologic Score (SAPS) are independently associated with aspiration of anaerobes (91). In trauma patients, tracheostomy and prior antimicrobial use with cefepime are associated with *Stenotrophomonas maltophilia* (92). Cytotoxic chemotherapy and use of corticosteroids predispose to pneumonia due to *L. pneumophila* (93). Neurosurgery, acute respiratory distress syndrome (ARDS), head trauma, and large-volume pulmonary aspiration have been associated with *Acinetobacter baumannii* (94). COPD, prior use of antibiotics, and duration of MV longer than 8 days are independently associated *P. aeruginosa* (95). Finally, coma is an independent risk factor for VAP caused by *S. aureus* (96). These risk factors are not sufficient to narrow initial empiric therapy, but are considerations when empiric therapy must be broadened in the critical patient for whom microbiologic studies are pending.

TABLE 88.2.9 Micro-organisms Causing Ventilator-associated Pneumonia[a]

	Trouillet (88)	Leroy (89)	Rello (90)
Number of episodes	135	124	290
Number of bacteria identified	245	154	321
Pseudomonas aeruginosa	39 (15.9%)	48 (31.1%)	102 (31.7%)
Acinetobacter baumannii	22 (9%)	9 (5.8%)	38 (11.8%)
Stenotrophomonas maltophilia	6 (2.4%)	8 (5.2%)	8 (2.5%)
Klebsiella species	9 (3.7%)	5 (3.2%)	ND
Escherichia coli	8 (3.3%)	8 (5.2%)	ND
Proteus species	7 (2.9%)	5 (3.2%)	ND
Enterobacter species	5 (2.0%)	7 (4.5%)	ND
Morganella species	4 (1.6%)	—	ND
Serratia species	4 (1.6%)	7 (4.5%)	ND
Haemophilus species	15 (6.1%)	10 (6.5%)	26 (8.1%)
Methicillin-resistant *Staphylococcus aureus*	32 (13.1%)	10 (6.5%)	10 (4.0%)
Methicillin-sensitive *S. aureus*	20 (8.2%)	19 (12.4%)	38 (11.8%)
Streptococcus pneumoniae	3 (1.2%)	9 (5.8%)	25 (7.8%)
Streptococcus species	33 (13.5%)	2 (1.3%)	10 (3.1%)
Enterococcus species	5 (2.0%)	—	ND
Coagulase-negative *Staphylococcus*	4 (1.6%)	1 (0.6%)	ND
Anaerobic pathogens	6 (2.4%)	—	ND

ND, no data.
[a]Data are presented as number and (percentage).

The day of onset of VAP may influence the etiology, making it potentially useful to distinguish early-onset from late-onset VAP. The definitions of early and late-onset VAP may vary, but the IDSA/ATS guidelines define duration of hospitalization fewer than 5 days as early onset, and greater than 5 days as late onset (69,82,97). In early-onset VAP, the main causative pathogens are still community-based and include *S. pneumoniae*, methicillin-susceptible *S. aureus* (MSSA), *H. influenzae,* and susceptible gram-negative enteric bacilli (97). In late-onset VAP, the organisms reflect nosocomial pathogens and include MRSA, *P. aeruginosa, A. baumannii,* and *S. maltophilia.*

Among these potential nosocomial pathogens, the rate of multidrug-resistant (MDR) pathogens has been increasing. Factors associated with the probability of a drug-resistant pathogen are summarized in Table 88.2.10. Duration of hospitalization (and/or MV) and prior exposure to antimicrobial agents are the major risk factors for VAP due to MDR pathogens (88,89,98–101). Finally, VAP due to fungi such as *Candida* species, *Aspergillus* species, or to viruses such as influenza, parainfluenza, and respiratory syncytial virus is uncommon in immunocompetent patients (69).

TABLE 88.2.10 Risk Factors for Multidrug-resistant Pathogens as Causative Organisms in Ventilator-associated Pneumonia

- Admission from a nursing home or an extended-care facility
- History of regular visits to an infusion or dialysis center
- Prior antimicrobial treatment in the preceding 90 d
- Prior use of broad-spectrum antibiotics
- Prior hospitalization in the preceding 90 d
- Current hospitalization for ≥5 d
- Duration of mechanical ventilation ≥7 d
- Immunosuppression
- High level of antibiotic resistance in the community or in local intensive care unit

Diagnostic Strategies and Testing

Pneumonia is suspected when a patient exhibits signs and symptoms suggesting both pulmonary involvement and infection. There remains, however, significant interobserver variation in the interpretation of radiographs and clinical determination of pneumonia such that a clear epidemiologic definition is difficult. The CDC, accordingly, removed radiography altogether as a component of the VAP definition used in the NHSN database and currently uses the following criteria to define ventilator-associated events (VAEs), infection-related ventilator-associated complications (IVAC), and possible ventilator-associated pneumonia (PVAP) (102). For a VAE, the patient must have the following:

- A baseline period of stability or improvement on the ventilator defined by at least 2 calendar days of stable or decreasing daily minimum FiO_2 or PEEP values. The daily minimum FiO_2 or PEEP is the LOWEST value during a calendar day that has been maintained for 1 hour.
- After a period of stability, the patient must have at least one of the following indicators of worsening oxygenation:
  - Increase in daily minimum FiO_s of at least 0.20 (20 points) over the daily minimum FiO_2 from the baseline period, and that increase must be sustained for 2 or more calendar days, or
  - Increase in daily minimum PEEP values of at least 3 cm H_2O over the daily minimum PEEP in the baseline period, sustained for 2 calendar days or longer

In addition to the above criteria, for an IVAC the patient must also have:

- On or after calendar day 3 of MV and within 2 calendar days before or after the onset of worsening oxygenation, the patient meets *both* of the following:
  - Temperature over 38°C or under 36°C, or white blood cell count of at least 12,000 cells/mm^3 or no more than 4,000 cells/mm^3, and
  - A new antimicrobial agent is started and is continued for at least 4 calendar days.

In addition to the above criteria, for a PVAP the patient must also have:

- Positive culture of endotracheal aspirate or BAL or lung tissue or protected tip brush which meet the quantitative or semi-quantitative thresholds defined in the protocol, or
- Purulent respiratory secretions (>25 neutrophils with <10 squamous cells per low powered field, PLUS the organism is identified in one of the following:
  - Sputum, endotracheal aspirate, BAL, lung tissue, protected tip brush, or
- One of the following tests must be positive as defined in the protocol:
  - Pleural culture
  - Lung histopathology is consistent with infection
  - Diagnostic test for *Legionella*
  - Diagnostic test for viral pathogens

The recent ATS/IDSA guidelines propose a "mixed" diagnostic strategy as follows (69):

- The diagnosis of VAP is suspected in the presence of a new or progressive pulmonary infiltrate associated with at least two of the following three infectious signs: fever over 38°C, leukocytosis or leucopenia, and/or purulent secretions. For patients with ARDS, radiographic changes are difficult to analyze, consequently, hemodynamic instability and/or deterioration of blood gases could be considered sufficient to suspect VAP.
- As soon as the diagnosis is suspected, lower respiratory tract samples are obtained for microscopy, and quantitative or semi-quantitative cultures and empiric antimicrobial therapy are started unless there is both a low clinical suspicion for VAP and a negative microscopy of the respiratory sample.
- On days 2 and 3, the results of cultures should be available, and the clinical response is assessed. According to whether the clinical picture is improving or worsening and the results of cultures, antimicrobial therapy will be stopped, de-escalated, or adjusted, and an investigation for other pathogens, other diagnoses, other sites of infection, or complications is performed.

With the ATS/IDSA definition, all acutely ill, MV patients should have a complete daily investigation including physical examination, an anteroposterior portable chest radiograph, measurement of arterial oxygenation saturation, and determination of necessary laboratory values (complete blood count, serum electrolytes, renal function). When VAP is suspected, each patient should have a complete physical examination to search for another source of infection, arterial blood analysis, and blood cultures collected. In cases of large pleural effusions, a diagnostic thoracentesis is indicated unless there is a contraindication. Samples of lower respiratory tract secretions (endotracheal aspirates or bronchoscopic samples) should be quantitatively cultured (69).

Finally, purulent sputum, even when associated with fever and leukocytosis, may be due only to nosocomial tracheobronchitis (103). An additional, more simplistic, definition would add the presence of a new or progressive radiographic infiltrate associated with at least two of three major clinical findings (104).

In addition to the issues with a consistent clinical definition of VAP, numerous techniques have been proposed to identify causative organism(s) of VAP. Blood cultures are rarely positive and a positive result may reflect an extrapulmonary infection (105). Pleural fluid cultures are helpful if positive, but are rarely needed. Analysis of lower respiratory secretions is the most frequently used technique to identify causative organism(s) of VAP. Numerous sampling methods have been described, with the major ones being endotracheal aspiration and bronchoscopic techniques with protected specimen brush (PSB) and/or BAL. These samples may be examined by various stains as described previously under CAP (Gram stains, Giemsa, acid fast stains) and by qualitative, semi-quantitative, and quantitative cultures.

Among all the described microbiologic techniques each have advantages and disadvantages (69,82). Specifically:

- Microscopy and qualitative culture of expectorated sputum or endotracheal aspirates are associated with a high percentage of false-positive results because of colonization of the upper respiratory tract and/or tracheobronchial tree. However, the initial empiric antimicrobial treatment of VAP could be guided by a reliable tracheal aspirate Gram stain.
- Quantitative cultures with a threshold of 10^6 colony-forming units (CFU)/mL to differentiate colonization from lung infection provide a diagnostic accuracy nearly similar to that of quantitative cultures from samples obtained by bronchoscopic techniques (106,107). Moreover, when the culture of endotracheal secretions is sterile in a patient with no recent (<72 hours) change in antimicrobial therapy, the diagnosis of a lower respiratory tract infection can be ruled out with a high probability (the negative predictive value is greater than 90%) (108).
- A PSB allows the collection of uncontaminated specimens from the potentially infected pulmonary area. A threshold set at 10^3 CFU/mL is the most adequate for quantitative cultures (109); false-positive results are infrequent (107). False-negative results may be observed when sampling is performed at an early stage of infection, in a technically incorrect (unaffected pulmonary area) manner, in a patient where a new antimicrobial treatment has been initiated, and/or if the specimens are incorrectly processed.
- BAL explores a larger lung area than PSB. Quantitative cultures of BAL fluid, with a threshold set at 10^4 CFU/mL, provide results similar to those obtained by PSB (109). Microscopic examination of the BAL specimen may add be critical to rule in certain diagnoses (silver staining for *Pneumocytis,* for example) (110,111).

While none of these techniques are without risk of false positives and negatives, an accurate microbiologic diagnosis may reduce VAP mortality (112) and should be attempted.

Antibiotic Treatment

Principles of Initial Empiric Treatment

Prompt initiation of adequate antimicrobials is the cornerstone of treatment for VAP, as studies have shown that inadequate initial coverage is associated with an increased mortality (98,113–115). The excess mortality due to inadequate antimicrobial coverage is not reduced if antibiotics are corrected once bacteriologic data is available (114,115); coverage must be broad initially then de-escalated subsequently. In addition to the proper coverage, Iregui et al. (116) showed that if the antimicrobials were delayed by ≥24 hours, mortality more than doubled (69.7% vs. 28.4%; $p < 0.001$).

Adequate antibiotic therapy could, therefore, be defined as the administration, at an appropriate dose, of at least one antibiotic with good pulmonary penetration, and bactericidal activity against the major causative pathogens, in a timely manner. One of the more common reasons for inadequate initial coverage is the growing pattern of antimicrobial resistant pathogen(s). Consequently, the presence or absence of risk factors for MDR pathogens (see Table 88.2.10) and the local microbiologic patterns must be considered when choosing empiric treatment.

TABLE 88.2.11 Initial Empiric Antibiotic Therapy in Patients with Ventilator-associated Pneumonia

Characteristics of Patient	Recommended Antibiotics and Recommended Dosages[a]
Early-onset VAP and no risk factors for multidrug-resistant pathogens	Ceftriaxone (1–2 g/24 hr) or Levofloxacin (750 mg/24 hr), moxifloxacin (400 mg/24 hr), or ciprofloxacin (400 mg/8 hr) or Ampicillin (1–2 g) plus sulbactam (0.5–1 g)/6 hr or Ertapenem (1 g/24 hr)
Late-onset VAP or risk factors for multidrug-resistant pathogens	Antipseudomonal cephalosporin: cefepime (1–2 g/8–12 hr) or ceftazidime (2 g/8 hr) or Antipseudomonal carbapenem: imipenem (500 mg/6 hr or 1 g/8 hr) or meropenem (1 g/8 hr) or β-Lactam/β-lactamase inhibitor: piperacillin–tazobactam (4.5 g/6 hr) plus Antipseudomonal fluoroquinolone: levofloxacin (750 mg/24 hr) or ciprofloxacin (400 mg/8 hr) or Aminoglycoside[b]: gentamicin (7 mg/kg/24 hr) or tobramycin (7 mg/kg/24 hr) or amikacin (20 mg/kg/24 hr) plus Vancomycin (15 mg/kg/12 hr)[c] or Linezolid (600 mg/12 hr)

[a]Dosages are based on normal hepatic and renal function.
[b]Trough levels for gentamicin and tobramycin should be <1 mg/L and for amikacin should be <4–5 mg/L.
[c]Trough levels for vancomycin should be <15–20 mg/L.
Adapted from American Thoracic Society, Infectious Diseases Society of America. Guidelines for the management of adults with hospital-acquired, ventilator-associated, and health care–associated pneumonia. *Am J Respir Crit Care Med.* 2005;171:388.

Guidelines for Initial Empiric Antibiotic Therapy

The ATS/IDSA guidelines are based on the time of onset of VAP (early vs. late) and the presence of risk factors for MDR pathogens (69). In patients with no risk factors for MDR pathogens and an early-onset VAP (duration of hospitalization <5 days), limited-spectrum monotherapy targeting community-acquired pathogens has been considered appropriate (Table 88.2.11). Conversely, in patients with late-onset VAP (≥5 days) or exhibiting risk factors for MDR pathogens, broad-spectrum combination therapy with antipseudomonal and MRSA coverage is required (Table 88.2.12).

In addition to considering the underlying host factors that may be associated with a specific microbe, recent antibiotic exposure may be important. A patient who develops a VAP while on treatment for an intra-abdominal infection, perhaps with piperacillin–tazobactam, should raise the possibility of MRSA, or an ESBL or carbapenamase-producing gram-negative. In these cases, local epidemiologic patterns have been shown to improve the choice and appropriateness of broader empiric coverage (117,118).

The question of quantitative surveillance cultures of endotracheal aspirates in ventilated patients without evidence

TABLE 88.2.12 Causes of Nonresolution or Deterioration in Patients with Ventilator-associated Pneumonia

Factors	Comments
Wrong initial diagnosis	Many noninfectious processes can mimic VAP: • Pulmonary embolism • Congestive heart failure • Lung contusion • Atelectasis • Chemical pneumonitis from aspiration • ARDS • Pulmonary hemorrhage
Host factors	Despite adequate treatment, many conditions are known to be associated with failure: • Underlying fatal condition • Age >60 yr • Prior pneumonia • Prior antibiotic treatment • Chronic lung diseases
Bacterial factors	Infecting bacteria can be resistant and can acquire resistance during treatment (*Pseudomonas aeruginosa*) Infecting pathogen can be a nonbacterial pathogen: • Mycobacteria • Virus • Fungus Some pathogens, even with effective treatment, are difficult to eradicate (*P. aeruginosa*)
Complications	Complications of initial pneumonia: • Empyema • Lung abscess Other sites of infection: • Urinary tract infection • Catheter-related infection • Sinusitis • Pseudomembranous enterocolitis Drug fever, pulmonary embolism, and sepsis with multiple system organ failure

ARDS, acute respiratory distress syndrome.
Adapted from American Thoracic Society, Infectious Diseases Society of America. Guidelines for the management of adults with hospital-acquired, ventilator-associated, and healthcare-associated pneumonia. *Am J Respir Crit Care Med.* 2005;171:388.

of VAP has been studied to decide whether they may offer important microbial information on patients should they ultimately develop symptoms of a VAP. The issue is whether this knowledge would allow for more immediate proper antibiotic choice. Michel et al. (119) reported 95% concordance between biweekly endotracheal surveillance cultures and a BAL done at the onset of the VAP. Whether this concordance reflects the true etiology of the pneumonic process or simple concordance with colonization, and whether it results in more appropriate antibiotic use and improved survival would require prospective randomized trials.

De-escalation Strategy

Once the results of blood or respiratory tract cultures become available, this strategy recommends the change from a broad-spectrum to a narrow-spectrum antibiotic to which the isolated organism is sensitive (i.e., imipenem to ceftriaxone when the enteric gram-negative bacilli do not exhibit ESBL), as well as removing an antibiotic from an initial combination when the anticipated organism is not recovered (i.e., discontinuation of vancomycin or linezolid when MRSA is not present) (120). Rello and colleagues (121) demonstrated that de-escalation was possible in 31.4% of the 115 patients included in their study.

Duration of Therapy

Until recently, the optimal duration of antibiotic therapy for VAP was unknown; lacking prospective controlled studies, experts empirically recommended a 14 to 21 days of treatment (1). A prospective, multicenter, randomized, double-blind trial was performed to determine whether shorter duration (8 vs. 15 days) therapy was equally effective. Patients receiving appropriate antimicrobial treatment during the shorter course (8 days) had similar survival and relapse rates as compared with patients treated for 15 days. For patients suffering from VAP due to nonlactose fermenting gram-negative bacilli (*P. aeruginosa* and *A. baumannii*), although the outcome was similar in the two groups, there was a trend to greater rates of pulmonary infection recurrences (relapses and/or superinfection) in the short duration of treatment group (122). Consequently, ATS/IDSA guidelines suggest shortening the duration of therapy to 7 days, unless the pathogen is *P. aeruginosa* or *A. baumannii,* as long as the patient exhibits a good clinical response (69). Regardless of the specific treatment duration, if aminoglycosides are used in combination with other agents, they may be stopped after no more than 5 to 7 days (69).

Empiric therapy may safely be discontinued after 72 hours if a noninfectious etiology for the pulmonary infiltrates is discovered, or microbiologic data is negative (123,124).

Specific Antibiotic Regimens

For VAP caused by *P. aeruginosa,* many recommend combination therapy. The purpose of combination therapy is to achieve antibiotic synergy and prevent the emergence of resistant strains during treatment. However, two meta-analyses on treatment of septic patients, showed that the combination β-lactam plus aminoglycoside compared with β-lactam monotherapy provided no clinical benefit (125), nor did it affect the emergence of antimicrobial resistance (126). However, there were a low number of studies evaluated, and the aminoglycoside dosing was outdated. Therefore, these results are probably insufficient to categorically abandon the practice of short-term aminoglycoside–β-lactam combination therapy for pneumonia caused by *P. aeruginosa.*

Vancomycin remains the accepted standard therapy for treatment of serious infections due to MRSA, with linezolid considered an alternative in some circumstances. Two multicenter studies demonstrated equivalence between linezolid and vancomycin for treatment of HAP due to MRSA; when combining these studies there is a suggestion of lower mortality in the linezolid subgroup, though prospective trials are required (127–129). Nevertheless, linezolid may be preferred to vancomycin in patients with or at risk for renal insufficiency (69).

A. baumannii exhibits native resistance to many classes of antimicrobial agents, including carbapenems. Despite the nephrotoxicity of polymyxins, they may be safely used and efficacy has been demonstrated for intravenous colistin in these patients when sensitivity to other antimicrobials is not present (130).

Local Instillation and Aerosolized Antibiotics

Although aminoglycosides and polymyxin B have been used by aerosolization to treat VAP due to pathogens that are resistant to systemic antimicrobials, there is insufficient data to recommend the use of aerosolized antibiotics routinely for treatment of pneumonia (69).

Response to Therapy

Normal Pattern of Resolution

Improvement usually becomes apparent after 48 to 72 hours of adequate antibiotic therapy. Thus, unless there is clinical deterioration, antimicrobial therapy should not be changed during this period (69).

Clinical response is usually first seen with resolution of fever and improvement in oxygenation. Fever typically resolves in about 72 hours and, in patients without ARDS, a PaO_2/FiO_2 ratio >250 should occur within that same timeframe. For patients with ARDS, hypoxemia obviously resolves more slowly and cannot be used to indicate appropriateness of VAP treatment (131).

Radiographic studies do not show rapid resolution when the diagnosis of VAP is accurate; in fact, rapid resolution would suggest an alternative diagnosis. Similarly, while leukocytosis should improve with adequate therapy, the improvement may be confounded by other physiologic stressors and cannot be used as a definitive indicator of successful treatment (131,132).

Reasons for Deterioration or Nonresolution

When a patient fails to improve or exhibits rapid deterioration, several causes may be considered (see Table 88.2.12) (69). In these patients, the following may be considered:

- Antimicrobial choice. The antimicrobial spectrum may need to be broadened to cover more resistant or alternate pathogens. Consideration should be given to repeat culturing of the lower respiratory secretions or use of alternative diagnostic tests (i.e., if not already performed, *Legionella,* rapid viral studies, or search for noninfectious diagnoses).
- Noninfectious process. Consider fever or sepsis due to another site of infection, or occurrence of pulmonary complications such as empyema. If not already done, blood and urine cultures should be performed and a CT scan ought to be considered to evaluate potential thoracic and extrathoracic sites of infection (sinuses, pleural space, abdomen, and pelvis).

Of note, a high percentage of patients may not respond to treatment quickly. Ioanas et al. (133) observed that the rate of nonresponse could be as high as 62%. The main causes were inappropriate initial antimicrobial treatment (23%), superinfections (14%), another site of infection (27%), and a noninfectious process (16%). In 36% of nonresponding patients, no cause could be identified.

Prognosis

Crude mortality rates associated with VAP vary from 24% to 76% (82). The wide range of rates may be due to differences in VAP definitions, diagnostic criteria and, hence, studied populations. It may also in part reflect the pathogenicity of a wide range of causative organisms.

Furthermore, case-control studies comparing attributable mortality of VAP in patients controlled for ICU admission, admitting diagnosis, duration of MV, and severity of underlying comorbid conditions show VAP attributable mortality ranging up to 25% (134–136).

Risk factors associated with death from VAP include (114–116,137–140):

- Underlying comorbidities (malignancy, immunosuppression, anticipated death within 5 years, American Society of Anesthesiology [ASA] score ≥3)
- Age >64 years
- High APACHE II score, simplify Acute Physiology Score <37
- Multilobar disease
- Platelet count <150,000 cells/μL
- Logistic Organ Dysfunction score <4
- Time of onset of VAP <3 days
- Recent surgery
- Hypotension
- Delay in appropriate antibiotic treatment.

Prevention

Basic infection control techniques such as hand washing, glove use, sterile equipment, and adequate staffing help to limit cross-contamination of resistant organisms through health care workers. In addition, there are specific preventative measures that can greatly decrease risk for a VAP (84,141).

First, the primary intervention to reduce any device-associated hospital-acquired infection (HAI) is to minimize the use of the device. Noninvasive positive pressure ventilation should be maximized and is associated with a relative risk reduction for VAP ranging from 0.67 to 0.87. When intubation and MV are necessary, optimizing sedation and weaning protocols may diminish duration of ventilatory support. Continuous aspiration of subglottic secretions by way of a endotracheal tube with a subglottic port that can be attached to continuous suction (about 90 mmHg) to remove oral secretions is associated with a relative risk reduction VAP of 0.45. Raising the head of the bed by a minimum of 30 degrees and up to 45 degrees reduces VAP incidence. Other aspects of a VAP prevention bundle may include stress ulcer prophylaxis, gastrostomy tube feedings as opposed to use of an orogastric or nasogastric tube, proper ventilator circuitry management, and glycemic control (142).

The CDC published 2004 guidelines on the prevention of VAP (143). In that bundled approach to VAP prevention, only four measures were recommended as per Table 88.2.13.

One last, highly controversial, issue is the use of selective digestive decontamination (SDD) (84,141,144). Topical nonabsorbed antimicrobials (usually combining polymyxin, aminoglycoside, and amphotericin B) with or without the addition of a short-duration systemic broad-spectrum antibiotic are ingested. The theory is that these agents will eradicate potential pathogens (gram-negative aerobic intestinal bacteria, *S. aureus,* and fungi) but not the anaerobic flora. Impressive

TABLE 88.2.13 Measures Recommended by the Centers for Disease Control and Prevention to Reduce the Incidence of VAP (143)

- Changing the breathing circuits of ventilators only when they malfunction or are visibly contaminated
- Preferential use of orotracheal rather than nasotracheal tubes
- Use of noninvasive ventilation
- Use of an endotracheal tube with a dorsal lumen to allow drainage of respiratory secretions

TABLE 88.2.14 Micro-organisms That Cause Hospital-acquired Pneumonia[a]

	Valles (146)	Sopena (147)	Kollef (3)
Number of episodes	96	165	835
Number of bacteria identified	75	60	ND
Pseudomonas aeruginosa	18 (24%)	7 (11.7%)	18.4%
Acinetobacter baumannii	1	5 (8.3%)	2.0%
Stenotrophomonas maltophilia	ND	ND	ND
Enterobacteriaceae	7 (9.3%)	8 (13.3%)	16.1%
Haemophilus species	2	2 (3.3%)	5.6%
Legionella pneumophila	9 (12%)	7 (11.7%)	ND
Methicillin-resistant *Staphylococcus aureus*			
Methicillin-sensitive *S. aureus*	9 (12%)	1 (1.6%)	22.9%
Streptococcus pneumoniae	11 (15%)	3 (5%)	26.2%
Streptococcus species	2	16 (26.7%)	3.1%
Enterococcus species	ND	ND	13.9%
Coagulase-negative staphylococcus	ND	ND	ND
Anaerobic pathogens	ND	ND	ND
Aspergillus species	13 (17%)	ND	ND
		7 (11.7%)	ND

ND, no data.
[a]Data are presented as number and/or (percentage).

results have been recently published, though in unblended trials (145). The preventive effects of SDD for VAP are thought to be lower in ICUs with high endemic levels of antibiotic resistance, and, in such cases, SDD may increase the incidence of drug-resistant micro-organisms. Thus, to date, the routine use of SDD in ICUs is not recommended.

Hospital-acquired Pneumonia

HAP can be defined by a number of ways but generally reflects a clinical diagnosis of pneumonia in which symptoms were not incubating on admission or for at least 2 calendar days after admission (3). Data about HAP acquired outside the ICU suggest that most patients have underlying comorbidities (i.e., chronic pulmonary disease, immunosuppression) and develop the pneumonia later in the course of their hospitalization (3,146,147). Microbiologically, the Enterobacteriaceae, *P. aeruginosa,* and MRSA play major causative roles (Table 88.2.14). Mortality rates are variable, similar to VAP, ranging from18% to 50%. ATS/IDSA guidelines suggest that all patients with HAP be managed with antimicrobials as if they were VAP cases (69).

Health Care-associated Pneumonia and Nursing Home Pneumonia

HCAP refers to patients who develop pneumonia in the setting of frequent health care contact. Generally, this includes any patient who was hospitalized in an acute care hospital for >2 days within 90 days of the infection; resides in a nursing home or long-term care facility (LTCF); received recent intravenous antibiotic therapy, chemotherapy, or wound care within 30 days of the current infection; or attends a hospital or hemodialysis clinic.

While HCAP refers to pneumonia in several diverse outpatient populations listed above, it is the second most common infection in LTCFs, with an incidence of 0.3 to 4.7 cases per 1,000 resident days (148). Pneumonia is also an independent risk factor for death in this population with mortality that ranges from 5% to 40% (149,150).

It is important to comment on some differences in the elderly and specifically nursing home (LTCF) population with regard to clinical presentation. Notably, fever and respiratory signs may be minimal, while an altered mental status might be the primary symptom (151). Risk factors for pneumonia include decreased functional status, diminished ability to clear airways, underlying comorbidities (such as COPD and heart disease), swallowing disorders, and use of sedatives. Furthermore, the etiology of HCAP in this population suggests a large proportion of gram-negative bacilli and *S. aureus.* However, when using stricter criteria for sputum interpretation (152), *S. pneumoniae* and *H. influenzae* are major pathogens, while gram-negative bacilli account for 0% to 12% of cases (152,153).

The ATS/IDSA (69) guidelines recommend that, in the hospital, these patients be managed like those with HAP (see Tables 88.2.11 and 88.2.12).

TRACHEOBRONCHITIS

Acute Exacerbations of Chronic Obstructive Pulmonary Disease

Acute exacerbation of COPD (COPD-E) is defined by an alteration in the patient's baseline dyspnea, cough, and/or sputum production (154). The need for ICU or intermediate care unit admission is based on the severity of respiratory failure and/or the presence of associated organ dysfunction (i.e., shock, hemodynamic instability, neurologic disturbances) (154). Therapy in the ICU includes supplemental oxygen, ventilatory support, bronchodilators, corticosteroids, and antibiotics (154); only the latter point will be further discussed here.

The role of bacterial infection in COPD-E remains controversial. As noted by Murphy et al. (155,156), this point is still debated for the following reasons:

- Bacteria routinely colonize the lower respiratory tract of COPD patients.
- Bacteria colonizing the lower respiratory tract vary from one patient to another, as COPD patients are heterogeneous.
- Information provided by sputum culture may not represent conditions in the distal airways.
- Only half of the episodes of acute COPD-E are linked to bacterial causes.
- Animal models are limited by the fact that the most frequently isolated organisms (*S. pneumoniae, H. influenzae, Moraxella catarrhalis*) are exclusively human pathogens.
- Clinical studies on the impact of antibiotic therapy for acute COPD-E suggest that these drugs provide only a small improvement in the most severely ill patients.

Despite this, the ATS/European Respiratory Society Task Force recommends antibiotic treatment in all patients suffering from a severe acute COPD-E requiring ICU admission (154). Two studies support this recommendation. A prospective, randomized, double-blinded, placebo-controlled trial assessing the effects of ofloxacin showed a reduction in mortality, length of hospital stay, and length of MV (157). Similarly, Ferrer et al. (158) observed that inadequate initial antibiotic treatment increased hospital mortality and was associated with failure of noninvasive ventilation. Inadequacy of initial empiric treatment mainly occurred when colonizing pathogens were not the usual community-acquired pathogens (*S. pneumoniae, H. influenzae, M. catarrhalis*), but were instead nonfermenting (*P. aeruginosa*) or enteric gram-negative bacilli.

Current recommendations include treatment with amoxicillin/clavulanate or respiratory fluoroquinolones (gatifloxacin, levofloxacin, moxifloxacin) (154). If *Pseudomonas* spp. or *Enterobacteriaceae* spp. are suspected, combination therapy should be considered with a β-lactam antibiotic and an antipseudomonal fluoroquinolone or an aminoglycoside (154,159).

Nosocomial Tracheobronchitis

Few studies have addressed nosocomial tracheobronchitis acquired during MV (160). In a retrospective analysis of 2,128 patients mechanically ventilated more than 48 hours, the incidence of nosocomial tracheobronchitis was 10.6%, without any significant difference between medical (9.9%; 165 of 1,655) and surgical patients (15.3%; 36 of 234) (103). In patients without underlying chronic pulmonary disease, the incidence was similarly 8% (161). The interval between initiation of MV and occurrence of tracheobronchitis averaged approximately10 days. In medical patients, nosocomial tracheobronchitis was significantly associated with age under 60 years (OR = 1.8), COPD (OR = 1.57), and receiving prior antibiotics within the 2 weeks of ICU admission (OR = 1.52). Major pathogens identified in tracheal aspirate cultures were *P. aeruginosa, A. baumannii,* and MRSA.

The impact of nosocomial tracheobronchitis on patient outcome is unclear. Two case-control studies compared patients with and without nosocomial tracheobronchitis. In both COPD patients and in those without chronic pulmonary disease, nosocomial tracheobronchitis was associated with longer durations of MV and ICU stay, but no increased mortality (161,162).

Indications for antibiotic treatment in these patients remain unclear. There is, however, increasing evidence that antimicrobial therapy, when targeted against a purulent endotracheal aspirate culture, may reduce duration of MV and the rate of VAP (162–164).

LUNG ABSCESS

Lung abscesses may be associated with aspiration pneumonia, poor dental hygiene, alcohol consumption, or chronic lung disease (165). It is relatively uncommon in developed countries, where it occurs mostly in immunosuppressed patients or as a postobstructive complication. Risk factors and underlying diseases are listed in Table 88.2.15 (165,166).

TABLE 88.2.15 Risk Factors and Underlying Diseases of Adult Patients with Community-acquired Lung Abscess[a]

	Hammond (165)	Wang (166)
Number of patients	34	90
Smoking	ND	57%
Chronic lung disease	29%	37%
Diabetes mellitus	ND	31%
Previous aspiration pneumonia	29%	32%
Malignancy	3%	19%
Alcohol abuse	38%	14%
Dental caries	26%	ND
CNS disease	9%	11%
Chronic liver disease	ND	11%
Steroid use/SLE	9%	6%
None	12%	18%

ND, no data; CNS, central nervous system; SLE, systemic lupus erythematosus.
[a]Data are presented as number or percentage.

Bacteriology

Anaerobes play a more dominant role in cases of parenchymal abscess as compared with pneumonia. Some studies note anaerobes to be the cause in 60% to 80% of cases (167), usually in a polymicrobial setting. Hammond et al. (165) in a study of 34 patients with community-acquired lung abscess, identified 2.3 bacterial species per episode; anaerobes were identified in 75% of cases. Contrary to those findings, a study of 90 patients with lung abscesses in Taiwan observed polymicrobial infection in only 20% of cases, while gram-negative bacilli, notably *K. pneumoniae*, were identified 47% of the time and anaerobes were isolated in 31% (Table 88.2.16) (166).

Diagnosis

Blood cultures and sputum examination are rarely positive (165,166). Methods to obtain a specimen uncontaminated by upper airway bacteria include percutaneous aspiration, transtracheal aspiration, or thoracentesis from empyema fluid. With the exception of thoracentesis when appropriate, the other invasive measures are rarely performed.

Antimicrobial Therapy

Lung abscesses are generally treated successfully with prolonged systemic antibiotic therapy. The preferred choice, based on the high frequency of anaerobes, is clindamycin or

TABLE 88.2.16 Pathogens Isolated from Adult Patients with Community-acquired Lung Abscess[a]

	Hammond (165)	Wang (166)
Number of patients	34	90
Number of bacteria identified	79	118
Anaerobes	59 (75%)	40 (34%)
Microaerophilic streptococci	7 (20%)	11 (12%)
Prevotella	17 (50%)	8 (9%)
Bacteroides	4 (12%)	6 (7%)
Fusobacterium	4 (12%)	3 (3%)
Porphyromonas	7 (20%)	1 (1%)
Gram-negative bacilli	3 (9%)	42 (47%)
Klebsiella pneumoniae	2 (6%)	30 (33%)
Gram-positive cocci	12 (35%)	30 (33%)
Streptococcus milleri	ND	19 (21%)
Staphylococcus aureus	5 (15%)	2 (2%)
Viridans streptococci	7 (20%)	5 (5%)
Other	5 (15%)	5 (5%)

ND, no data.
[a]Data are presented as number and (percentage).

a β-lactamase inhibitor/aminopenicillin (167,168). Both regimens obtain cure rates between 60% and 70% with a 3-week course of therapy. Surgical resection or an invasive drainage procedures of the diseased lung and abscess are sometimes necessary (169,170).

EMPYEMA (PLEURAL INFECTION)

Pathophysiology

The pleural space is normally sterile. Pleural effusion is favored by an increase in the hydrostatic pressure, a decrease of oncotic pressure, or alterations of pleural permeability. Infection follows contamination of pleural fluid. The formation of an empyema is arbitrarily divided into three phases: (1) an exudative phase with accumulation of pus; (2) a fibropurulent phase with fibrin deposition and loculation of pleural exudate; and (3) an organization phase with fibroblast proliferation leading to scar formation and lung entrapment (171).

In up to 50% of cases, empyema is a complication of pneumonia; approximately one-fourth of empyemas are due to a traumatic or iatrogenic injury (surgery, thoracentesis, chest tube placement). In the remaining cases, pleural infection is due to a contiguous infection (i.e., mediastinum, esophagus, subdiaphragmatic areas) extending to the pleura (171).

Bacteriology

The bacterial etiology of empyema depends on the underlying mechanism leading to pleural colonization. With 75% of empyemas developing as a complication of pneumonia or traumatic or iatrogenic injury, most isolated aerobic organisms are *Streptococcus* species, *S. pneumoniae,* and *S. aureus.* The main isolated aerobic gram-negative organisms are *Klebsiella* species, *P. aeruginosa, H. influenzae,* and *Escherichia coli.* These organisms are commonly part of a mixed growth with anaerobes; anaerobic isolates are identified in 12% to 34% of cultures. They can cause empyema without aerobic copathogens in about 15% of cases (171,172).

Treatment

Identification of Pleural Effusion

In patients suffering from empyema, clinical symptoms may include fever, chills, chest pain—particularly with inspiration—and night sweats. Physical examination tends to show diminished breath sounds and, possibly, a friction rub. In patients on MV, these signs may be more difficult to ascertain (171). Chest radiography shows blunting of the costo-diaphragmatic angle when the volume of pleural fluid exceeds 200 mL. The presence of a concomitant pulmonary infiltrate suggests a parapneumonic effusion which may or may not have evolved to an empyema (172). Ultrasonography is useful in unstable or critically ill patients, since it allows for a guided diagnostic aspiration and may yield characteristics more suggestive of an empyema (loculations or septations) as opposed to a simple effusion (171).

Indication for Pleural Fluid Sampling

In most cases, diagnostic pleural fluid sampling (thoracentesis) is recommended in patients with pleural effusion and an associated pneumonia or recent chest surgery or trauma (172). Once obtained, the pleural fluid should be sent pH, lactic dehydrogenase (LDH), glucose levels, and a white blood cell count; Gram stain and cultures should be ordered. Empyema usually has a pH value of less than 7.0, an LDH level greater than 1,000 IU/L, a glucose level less than 40 mg/dL, and positive Gram stain and/or culture (171).

Characteristics of the fluid should differentiate between empyema and simple or complicated para-pneumonic effusions (172). In a simple para-pneumonic effusion, the fluid should appear clear, the pH is >7.2, LDH is <1,000 IU/L, glucose level is >40 mg/dL, and no organism is identified on Gram stain or culture. In a complicated para-pneumonic effusion, the studies may be mixed with pleural fluid appearing clear to somewhat cloudy, pH <7.2 (but not <7.0); LDH level >1,000 IU/L; glucose level <40 mg/dL; and the Gram stain and/or culture are positive.

Antibiotics

Treatment of empyema requires adequate antimicrobial therapy, drainage of pus, and re-expansion of the lung.

Both penicillins and cephalosporins exhibit good penetration into the pleural space. They are the drugs of choice for treating empyemas due to *Streptococcus* species and *S. pneumoniae*. Nafcillin is the drug of choice for MSSA infection. Third-generation cephalosporins and carbapenems are preferred choices in case of empyema due to gram-negative aerobic bacilli. Infections due to MRSA and penicillin- and cephalosporin-resistant *S. pneumoniae* should be treated with vancomycin. Aminoglycosides do not penetrate into the pleural space well and have poor activity in acidic pleural fluid. When anaerobic organisms are causative pathogens, a β-lactam combined with a β-lactamase inhibitor, imipenem, metronidazole, and clindamycin are the drugs of choice (171,172).

When cultures are negative, antibiotics must be chosen empirically according to the likely pathogens and the clinical setting. Guidelines from the BTS suggest the following (172):

- Community-acquired empyema: Second- and third-generation cephalosporins, amoxicillin, β-lactam–β-lactamase inhibitor combination, meropenem, clindamycin, or benzyl penicillin combined with quinolone
- Hospital-acquired infection, such as empyema following a HAP or VAP, or after recent chest surgery: Antipseudomonal penicillins (piperacillin–tazobactam, ticarcillin–clavulanic acid), carbapenems, or third-generation cephalosporins combined with vancomycin.
- BTS guidelines suggest that a duration of 3 weeks is likely needed.

Chest Tube Drainage

Prompt chest tube drainage is indicated in patients with frankly purulent or turbid/cloudy pleural fluid. Similarly, patients with a pleural fluid pH less than 7.2 and the presence of pathogens identified by Gram stain or culture should receive chest tube drainage (172). Furthermore, when there is not clinical improvement with antimicrobials alone or when the pleural fluid becomes loculated, drainage should be considered.

The use of intrapleural fibrinolytic drugs have not shown consistent benefit. In a randomized, double-blind trial comparing intrapleural streptokinase (250,000 IU twice daily for 3 days) to placebo among 427 studied patients, streptokinase did not reduce mortality, need for drainage surgery, duration of hospital stay, and it did not improve radiographic and spirometric outcomes (173). The routine use of fibrinolytic treatment for patients requiring chest tube drainage for empyema or complicated para-pneumonic effusion is not recommended based on a meta-analysis of available data (174).

Surgical Treatment

Surgical treatment must be considered in all patients who do not resolve the infection despite antibiotics and chest tube drainage. Different surgical approaches have been described. The choice between video-assisted thoracoscopic surgery (VATS), open thoracic drainage, or thoracotomy with decortication depends on the patient status (age, comorbidity), surgeon preferences, and anatomy of pleural effusion assessed by recent thoracic CT scanning (172).

SUMMARY

Pneumonia remains a common and morbid infection in the community in hospitalized and in ventilated patients. Management of severe pneumonia in the ICU may be challenging as the diagnosis can be difficult, and no gold standard exists for the definition of VAP. Preventive strategies for CAP are limited to influenza and pneumococcal vaccinations. However, in the hospitalized critically ill, mechanically ventilated patient, more opportunity exists for aggressive preventative measures focused on oral care and management of oral secretions.

Despite adequate treatment, the death rate remains elevated, ranging from 18% to 46% in CAP, and 24% to 76% in VAP. Adequate antimicrobial therapy is paramount for successful treatment but is increasingly complex. Drug choice depends on numerous factors: pharmacodynamics/pharmacokinetics, spectrum, hospital or health care exposure, dosing schedule, adverse events, costs, and availability. The rise of antimicrobial resistance complicates therapeutic guidelines and empiric therapy needs to be regularly adapted to local resistance patterns.

Key Points

- Lower respiratory tract infections in the critical care population are common and include pneumonia, tracheobronchitis, and pleural space infections. Pneumonia carries significant morbidity and mortality depending upon certain host factors, presenting signs and symptoms, and the timing of initial and appropriate antimicrobial therapy.
- Traditionally, pneumonia was simply categorized as either community- or hospital-acquired, but the complexity of interactions between patients and the health care environment has led to further subdivisions which are now: CAP, HCAP, HAP, or VAP.
- The diagnosis of pneumonia depends on various clinical elements including signs of a systemic inflammatory response syndrome, impaired oxygenation, radiographic infiltrates, and microbial testing but, importantly, there is no one simple gold standard for diagnosis.
- Of the major categories of pneumonia, prevention strategies are most clearly defined for VAP, where certain "bundled" interventions are associated with dramatic decreases in incidence.
- Bacterial pathogens that predominate as causes of lower respiratory infections have evolved more resistant antimicrobial patterns, particularly in the hospital environment, making choices of empiric therapy more difficult and reliant on local resistance patterns.

ACKNOWLEDGMENT
The authors thank Serge Alfandari, MD, MSc, for his contribution to this topic in the previous edition.

References

1. Hospital-acquired pneumonia in adults: diagnosis, assessment of severity, initial antimicrobial therapy, and preventive strategies: a consensus statement, American Thoracic Society, November 1995. *Am J Respir Crit Care Med.* 1996;153:1711–1725.
2. Ewig S, Bauer T, Torres A. The pulmonary physician in critical care: nosocomial pneumonia. *Thorax.* 2002;57:366–371.
3. Kollef MH, Shorr A, Tabak YP, et al. Epidemiology and outcomes of health-care–associated pneumonia: results from a large US database of culture-positive pneumonia. *Chest.* 2005;128:3854.
4. Bartlett JG, Mundy LM. Community-acquired pneumonia. *N Engl J Med.* 1995;333:1618–1624.
5. Niederman MS, Bass JB Jr, Campbell GD, et al. Guidelines for the initial management of adults with community-acquired pneumonia: diagnosis, assessment of severity, and initial antimicrobial therapy. *Am Rev Respir Dis.* 1993;148:1418–1426.
6. Ewig S, Ruiz M, Mensa J, et al. Severe community-acquired pneumonia: assessment of severity criteria. *Am J Respir Crit Care Med.* 1998;158:1102–1108.
7. Niederman MS, Mandell LA, Anzueto A, et al.; American Thoracic Society. Guidelines for the management of adults with community-acquired pneumonia: diagnosis, assessment of severity, antimicrobial therapy, and prevention. *Am J Respir Crit Care Med.* 2001;163:1730–1754.
8. Angus DC, Marrie TJ, Obrosky DS, et al. Severe community-acquired pneumonia: use of intensive care services and evaluation of American and British Thoracic Society Diagnostic criteria. *Am J Respir Crit Care Med.* 2002;166:717–723.
9. Riley PD, Aronsky D, Dean NC. Validation of the 2001 American Thoracic Society criteria for severe community-acquired pneumonia. *Crit Care Med.* 2004;32:2398–2402.
10. British Thoracic Society Standards of Care Committee. BTS guidelines for the management of community acquired pneumonia in adults. *Thorax.* 2001;56(Suppl 4):IV1–64.
11. Rello J, Rodriguez A, Torres A, et al. Implications of COPD in patients admitted to the intensive care unit by community-acquired pneumonia. *Eur Respir J.* 2006;27:1210–1216.
12. Bartlett JG. Diagnostic tests for agents of community-acquired pnueumonia. *Clin Infect Dis.* 2011:52(Suppl 4):S296–S304.
13. Cox NJ, Subbarao K. Influenza. *Lancet.* 1999;354:1277–1282.
14. Yoshimoto A, Nakamura H, Fujimura M, Nakao S. Severe community-acquired pneumonia in an intensive care unit: risk factors for mortality. *Intern Med.* 2005;44:710–716.
15. Leroy O, Saux P, Bedos JP, Caulin E. Comparison of levofloxacin and cefotaxime combined with ofloxacin for ICU patients with community-acquired pneumonia who do not require vasopressors. *Chest.* 2005;128:172–183.
16. Shorr AF, Bodi M, Rodriguez A, et al.; CAPUCI Study Investigators. Impact of antibiotic guideline compliance on duration of mechanical ventilation in critically ill patients with community-acquired pneumonia. *Chest.* 2006;130:93–100.
17. Hyde TB, Gay K, Stephens DS, et al.; Active Bacterial Core Surveillance/Emerging Infections Program Network. Macrolide resistance among invasive *Streptococcus pneumoniae* isolates. *JAMA.* 2001;286:1857–1862.
18. Hoban DJ, Doern GV, Fluit AC, et al. Worldwide prevalence of antimicrobial resistance in *Streptococcus pneumoniae, Haemophilus influenzae,* and *Moraxella catarrhalis* in the SENTRY Antimicrobial Surveillance Program, 1997–1999. *Clin Infect Dis.* 2001;32(Suppl 2):S81–S93.

19. Hoban D, Baquero F, Reed V, Felmingham D. Demographic analysis of antimicrobial resistance among *Streptococcus pneumoniae:* worldwide results from PROTEKT 1999–2000. *Int J Infect Dis.* 2005;9:262–273.
20. Metlay JP, Hofmann J, Cetron MS, et al. Impact of penicillin susceptibility on medical outcomes for adult patients with bacteremic pneumococcal pneumonia. *Clin Infect Dis.* 2000;30:520–528.
21. Falco V, Almirante B, Jordano Q, et al. Influence of penicillin resistance on outcome in adult patients with invasive pneumococcal pneumonia: is penicillin useful against intermediately resistant strains? *J Antimicrob Chemother.* 2004;54:481–488.
22. Low DE. Quinolone resistance among pneumococci: therapeutic and diagnostic implications. *Clin Infect Dis.* 2004;38(Suppl 4):S357–S362.
23. Deshpande LM, Sader HS, Debbia E, et al. Emergence and epidemiology of fluoroquinolone-resistant *Streptococcus pneumoniae* strains from Italy: report from the SENTRY Antimicrobial Surveillance Program (2001–2004). *Diagn Microbiol Infect Dis.* 2006;54:157–164.
24. Francis JS, Doherty MC, Lopatin U, et al. Severe community-onset pneumonia in healthy adults caused by methicillin-resistant *Staphylococcus aureus* carrying the Panton-Valentine leukocidin genes. *Clin Infect Dis.* 2005;40:100–107.
25. Mandell LA, Wunderink RG, Anzueto A, et al. Infectious Diseases Society of America/American Thoracic Society consensus guidelines on the management of community-acquired pneumonia in adults. *Clin Infect Dis.* 2007;44(Suppl 2):S27–S72.
26. Feikin DR, Feldman C, Schuchat A, Janoff EN. Global strategies to prevent bacterial pneumonia in adults with HIV disease. *Lancet Infect Dis.* 2004;4:445–455.
27. Le Moing V, Rabaud C, Journot V, et al.; APROCO Study Group. Incidence and risk factors of bacterial pneumonia requiring hospitalization in HIV-infected patients started on a protease inhibitor-containing regimen. *HIV Med.* 2006;7:261–267.
28. Pagano L, Caira M, Fianchi L. Pulmonary fungal infection with yeasts and pneumocystis in patients with hematological malignancy. *Ann Med.* 2005;37:259–269.
29. Rano A, Agusti C, Benito N, et al. Prognostic factors of non-HIV immunocompromised patients with pulmonary infiltrates. *Chest.* 2002;122:253–261.
30. Martin SI, Marty FM, Fiumara K, et al. Infectious complications associated with alemtuzumab use for lymphoproliferative disorders. *Clin Infect Dis.* 2006;43:16–24.
31. Cervera C, Agusti C, Angeles Marcos M, et al. Microbiologic features and outcome of pneumonia in transplanted patients. *Diagn Microbiol Infect Dis.* 2006;55:47–54.
32. Colombel JF, Loftus EV Jr, Tremaine WJ, et al. The safety profile of infliximab in patients with Crohn's disease: the Mayo clinic experience in 500 patients. *Gastroenterology.* 2004;126:19–31.
33. Houck PM, Bratzler DW, Nsa W, et al. Timing of antibiotic administration and outcomes for Medicare patients hospitalized with community-acquired pneumonia. *Arch Intern Med.* 2004;164:637–644.
34. Waterer GW, Kessler LA, Wunderink RG. Delayed administration of antibiotics and atypical presentation in community-acquired pneumonia. *Chest.* 2006;130:11–15.
35. Metersky ML, Sweeney TA, Getzow MB, et al. Antibiotic timing and diagnostic uncertainty in Medicare patients with pneumonia: is it reasonable to expect all patients to receive antibiotics within 4 hours? *Chest.* 2006;130:16–21.
36. Pedro-Botet L, Yu VL. Legionella: macrolides or quinolones? *Clin Microbiol Infect.* 2006;12(Suppl 3):25–30.
37. Gleason PP, Meehan TP, Fine JM, et al. Associations between initial antimicrobial therapy and medical outcomes for hospitalized elderly patients with pneumonia. *Arch Intern Med.* 1999;159:2562–2572.
38. Rello J, Catalan M, Diaz E, et al. Associations between empirical antimicrobial therapy at the hospital and mortality in patients with severe community-acquired pneumonia. *Intensive Care Med.* 2002;28:1030–1035.
39. Mortensen EM, Restrepo MI, Anzueto A, Pugh J. The impact of empiric antimicrobial therapy with a β-lactam and fluoroquinolone on mortality for patients hospitalized with severe pneumonia. *Crit Care.* 2006;10:R8.
40. Waterer GW, Somes GW, Wunderink RG. Monotherapy may be suboptimal for severe bacteremic pneumococcal pneumonia. *Arch Intern Med.* 2001;161:1837–1842.
41. Martinez JA, Horcajada JP, Almela M, et al. Addition of a macrolide to a beta-lactam-based empirical antibiotic regimen is associated with lower in-hospital mortality for patients with bacteremic pneumococcal pneumonia. *Clin Infect Dis.* 2003;36:389–395.
42. Bartlett JG, Dowell SF, Mandell LA, et al. Practice guidelines for the management of community-acquired pneumonia in adults. Infectious Diseases Society of America. *Clin Infect Dis.* 2000;31:347–382.
43. Bernard GR, Vincent JL, Laterre PF, et al. Recombinant human protein C Worldwide Evaluation in Severe Sepsis (PROWESS) study group. Efficacy and safety of recombinant human activated protein C for severe sepsis. *N Engl J Med.* 2001;344:699–709.
44. Angus DC, Laterre PF, Helterbrand J, et al.; PROWESS Investigators. The effect of drotrecogin alfa (activated) on long-term survival after severe sepsis. *Crit Care Med.* 2004;32:2199–2206.
45. Laterre PF, Garber G, Levy H, et al.; PROWESS Clinical Evaluation Committee. Severe community-acquired pneumonia as a cause of severe sepsis: data from the PROWESS study. *Crit Care Med.* 2005;33:952–961.
46. Abraham E, Laterre PF, Garg R, et al.; Administration of Drotrecogin Alfa (Activated) in Early Stage Severe Sepsis (ADDRESS) Study Group. Drotrecogin alfa (activated) for adults with severe sepsis and a low risk of death. *N Engl J Med.* 2005;353:1332–1341.
47. Confalonieri M, Urbino R, Potena A, et al. Hydrocortisone infusion for severe community-acquired pneumonia: a preliminary randomized study. *Am J Respir Crit Care Med.* 2005;171:242–248.
48. Pachon J, Prados MD, Capote F, et al. Severe community-acquired pneumonia: etiology, prognosis, and treatment. *Am Rev Respir Dis.* 1990;142:369–373.
49. Almirall J, Mesalles E, Klamburg J, et al. Prognostic factors of pneumonia requiring admission to the intensive care unit. *Chest.* 1995;107:511–516.
50. Leroy O, Santré C, Beuscart C, et al. A five-year study of severe community-acquired pneumonia with emphasis on prognosis in patients admitted to an intensive care unit. *Intensive Care Med.* 1995;21:24–31.
51. Pascual FE, Matthay MA, Bacchetti P, Wachter RM. Assessment of prognosis in patients with community-acquired pneumonia who require mechanical ventilation. *Chest.* 2000;117:503–512.
52. Paganin F, Lilienthal F, Bourdin A, et al. Severe community-acquired pneumonia: assessment of microbial aetiology as mortality factor. *Eur Respir J.* 2004;24:779–785.
53. Tejerina E, Frutos-Vivar F, Restrepo MI, et al.; International Mechanical Ventilation Study Group. Prognosis factors and outcome of community-acquired pneumonia needing mechanical ventilation. *J Crit Care.* 2005;20:230–238.
54. Boussekey N, Leroy O, Alfandari S, et al. Procalcitonin kinetics in the prognosis of severe community-acquired pneumonia. *Intensive Care Med.* 2006;32:469–472.
55. Fine MJ, Smith MA, Carson CA, et al. Prognosis and outcomes of patients with community-acquired pneumonia: a meta-analysis. *JAMA.* 1996;275:134–141.
56. Torres A, Serra-Batlles J, Ferrer A, et al. Severe community-acquired pneumonia: epidemiology and prognostic factors. *Am Rev Respir Dis.* 1991;144:312–318.
57. Leroy O, Devos P, Guery B, et al. Simplified prediction rule for prognosis of patients with severe community-acquired pneumonia in ICUs. *Chest.* 1999;116:157–165.
58. Wilson PA, Ferguson J. Severe community-acquired pneumonia: an Australian perspective. *Intern Med J.* 2005;35:699–705.
59. Houck PM, MacLehose RF, Niederman MS, Lowery JK. Empiric antibiotic therapy and mortality among medicare pneumonia inpatients in 10 western states: 1993, 1995, and 1997. *Chest.* 2001;119:1420–1426.
60. Brown RB, Iannini P, Gross P, Kunkel M. Impact of initial antibiotic choice on clinical outcomes in community-acquired pneumonia: analysis of a hospital claims-made database. *Chest.* 2003;123:1503–1511.
61. Baddour LM, Yu VL, Klugman KP; International Pneumococcal Study Group. Combination antibiotic therapy lowers mortality among severely ill patients with pneumococcal bacteremia. *Am J Respir Crit Care Med.* 2004;170:440–444.
62. Wilson BZ, Anzueto A, Restrepo MI, et al. Comparison of two guideline-concordant antimicrobial combinations in elderly patients hospitalized with severe community-acquired pneumonia. *Crit Care Med.* 2012;40(8):2310–2314.
63. Fine MJ, Auble TE, Yealy DM, et al. A prediction rule to identify low-risk patients with community-acquired pneumonia. *N Engl J Med.* 1997;336:243–250.
64. Kobayashi M, Bennett NM, Gierke R, et al. Intervals between PCV13 and PPSV23 vaccines: recommendations of the Advisory Committee on Immunization Practices (ACIP). *MMWR Morb Mortal Wkly Rep.* 2015;64(34):944–947.
65. Prevention of pneumococcal disease among infants and children – use of 13-valent pneumococcal conjugate vaccine and 23-valent pneumococcal polysaccharide vaccine – recommendations of the Advisory Committee on Immunization Practices (ACIP). *MMWR Recomm Rep.* 2010;59(RR11):1–18.

66. Whitney CG, Farley MM, Hadler J, et al.; Active Bacterial Core Surveillance of the Emerging Infections Program Network. Decline in invasive pneumococcal disease after the introduction of protein-polysaccharide conjugate vaccine. *N Engl J Med.* 2003;348:1737–1746.
67. Kyaw MH, Lynfield R, Schaffner W, et al.; Active Bacterial Core Surveillance of the Emerging Infections Program Network. Effect of introduction of the pneumococcal conjugate vaccine on drug-resistant *Streptococcus pneumoniae*. *N Engl J Med.* 2006;354:1455–1463.
68. Advisory Committee on Immunization Practices, Smith NM, Bresee JS, et al. Prevention and control of influenza Recommendations of the Advisory Committee on Immunization Practices (ACIP). *MMWR Recomm Rep.* 2006;55 (RR10):1–42.
69. American Thoracic Society, Infectious Diseases Society of America. Guidelines for the management of adults with hospital-acquired, ventilator-associated, and healthcare-associated pneumonia. *Am J Respir Crit Care Med.* 2005;171:388–416.
70. Rello J, Ollendorf DA, Oster G, et al.; VAP Outcomes Scientific Advisory Group. Epidemiology and outcomes of ventilator-associated pneumonia in a large US database. *Chest.* 2002;122:2115–2121.
71. Torres A, Aznar R, Gatell JM, et al. Incidence, risk, and prognosis factors of nosocomial pneumonia in mechanically ventilated patients. *Am Rev Respir Dis.* 1990;142:523–528.
72. Chevret S, Hemmer M, Carlet J, Langer M. Incidence and risk factors of pneumonia acquired in intensive care units: results from a multicenter prospective study on 996 patients. European Cooperative Group on Nosocomial Pneumonia. *Intensive Care Med.* 1993;19:256–264.
73. Baker AM, Meredith JW, Haponik EF. Pneumonia in intubated trauma patients: microbiology and outcomes. *Am J Respir Crit Care Med.* 1996; 153:343–349.
74. Chastre J, Trouillet JL, Vuagnat A, et al. Nosocomial pneumonia in patients with acute respiratory distress syndrome. *Am J Respir Crit Care Med.* 1998;157:1165–1172.
75. Tejada Artigas A, Bello Dronda S, Chacon Valles E, et al. Risk factors for nosocomial pneumonia in critically ill trauma patients. *Crit Care Med.* 2001;29:304–309.
76. Ibrahim EH, Tracy L, Hill C, et al. The occurrence of ventilator-associated pneumonia in a community hospital: risk factors and clinical outcomes. *Chest.* 2001;120:555–561.
77. Bouza E, Perez A, Munoz P, et al. Ventilator-associated pneumonia after heart surgery: a prospective analysis and the value of surveillance. *Crit Care Med.* 2003;31:1964–1970.
78. Hilker R, Poetter C, Findeisen N, et al. Nosocomial pneumonia after acute stroke: implications for neurological intensive care medicine. *Stroke.* 2003;34:975–981.
79. Dudek MA, Horan TC, Pererson KD, et al. National Healthcare Safety Nework (NHSN) report, data summary for 2009, device-associated module. *Am J Infect Control.* 2011;39:349–367.
80. Cook DJ, Walter SD, Cook RJ, et al. Incidence of and risk factors for ventilator-associated pneumonia in critically ill patients. *Ann Intern Med.* 1998;129:433–440.
81. Rello J, Sonora R, Jubert P, et al. Pneumonia in intubated patients: role of respiratory airway care. *Am J Respir Crit Care Med.* 1996;154: 111–115.
82. Chastre J, Fagon JY. Ventilator-associated pneumonia. *Am J Respir Crit Care Med.* 2002;165:867–903.
83. Rello J, Diaz E, Rodriguez A. Advances in the management of pneumonia in the intensive care unit: review of current thinking. *Clin Microbiol Infect.* 2005;11(Suppl 5):30–38.
84. Bonten MJ, Kollef MH, Hall JB. Risk factors for ventilator-associated pneumonia: from epidemiology to patient management. *Clin Infect Dis.* 2004;38:1141–1149.
85. de Lassence A, Alberti C, Azoulay E, et al.; OUTCOMEREA Study Group. Impact of unplanned extubation and reintubation after weaning on nosocomial pneumonia risk in the intensive care unit: a prospective multicenter study. *Anesthesiology.* 2002;97:148–156.
86. Kollef MH, von Harz B, Prentice D, et al. Patient transport from intensive care increases the risk of developing ventilator-associated pneumonia. *Chest.* 1997;112:765–773.
87. Kollef MH. Ventilator-associated pneumonia: a multivariate analysis. *JAMA.* 1993;270:1965–1970.
88. Trouillet JL, Chastre J, Vuagnat A, et al. Ventilator-associated pneumonia caused by potentially drug-resistant bacteria. *Am J Respir Crit Care Med.* 1998;157:531–539.
89. Leroy O, Girardie P, Yazdanpanah Y, et al. Hospital-acquired pneumonia: microbiological data and potential adequacy of antimicrobial regimens. *Eur Respir J.* 2002;20:432–439.
90. Rello J, Sa-Borges M, Correa H, et al. Variations in etiology of ventilator-associated pneumonia across four treatment sites: implications for antimicrobial prescribing practices. *Am J Respir Crit Care Med.* 1999;160:608–613.
91. Dore P, Robert R, Grollier G, et al. Incidence of anaerobes in ventilator-associated pneumonia with use of a protected specimen brush. *Am J Respir Crit Care Med.* 1996;153:1292–1298.
92. Hanes SD, Demirkan K, Tolley E, et al. Risk factors for late-onset nosocomial pneumonia caused by *Stenotrophomonas maltophilia* in critically ill trauma patients. *Clin Infect Dis.* 2002;35:228–235.
93. Carratala J, Gudiol F, Pallares, et al. Risk factors for nosocomial *Legionella pneumophila* pneumonia. *Am J Respir Crit Care Med.* 1994;149:625–629.
94. Baraibar J, Correa H, Mariscal D, et al. Risk factors for infection by *Acinetobacter baumannii* in intubated patients with nosocomial pneumonia. *Chest.* 1997;112:1050–1054.
95. Rello J, Ausina V, Ricart M, et al. Risk factors for infection by *Pseudomonas aeruginosa* in patients with ventilator-associated pneumonia. *Intensive Care Med.* 1994;20:193–198.
96. Rello J, Quintana E, Ausina V, et al. Risk factors for *Staphylococcus aureus* nosocomial pneumonia in critically ill patients. *Am Rev Respir Dis.* 1990;142:1320–1324.
97. Torres A, Carlet J. Ventilator-associated pneumonia. European Task Force on ventilator-associated pneumonia. *Eur Respir J.* 2001;17:1034–1045.
98. Porzecanski I, Bowton DL. Diagnosis and treatment of ventilator-associated pneumonia. *Chest.* 2006;130:597–604.
99. Rello J, Torres A, Ricart M, et al. Ventilator-associated pneumonia by *Staphylococcus aureus:* comparison of methicillin-resistant and methicillin-sensitive episodes. *Am J Respir Crit Care Med.* 1994;150:1545–1549.
100. Trouillet JL, Vuagnat A, Combes A, et al. *Pseudomonas aeruginosa* ventilator-associated pneumonia: comparison of episodes due to piperacillin-resistant versus piperacillin-susceptible organisms. *Clin Infect Dis.* 2002;34:1047–1054.
101. Leroy O, Jaffre S, D'Escrivan, et al. Hospital-acquired pneumonia: risk factors for antimicrobial-resistant causative pathogens in critically ill patients. *Chest.* 2003;123:2034–2042.
102. Raoof S, Baumann MH. Ventilator-associated events: the new definition. *Am J Crit Care.* 2014;23(1):7–9.
103. Nseir S, Di Pompeo C, Pronnier P, et al. Nosocomial tracheobronchitis in mechanically ventilated patients: incidence, aetiology and outcome. *Eur Respir J.* 2002;20:1483–1489.
104. Fabregas N, Ewig S, Torres A, et al. Clinical diagnosis of ventilator associated pneumonia revisited: comparative validation using immediate post-mortem lung biopsies. *Thorax.* 1999;54:867–873.
105. Luna CM, Videla A, Mattera J, et al. Blood cultures have limited value in predicting severity of illness and as a diagnostic tool in ventilator-associated pneumonia. *Chest.* 1999;116:1075–1084.
106. Marquette CH, Copin MC, Wallet F, et al. Diagnostic tests for pneumonia in ventilated patients: prospective evaluation of diagnostic accuracy using histology as a diagnostic gold standard. *Am J Respir Crit Care Med.* 1995;151:1878–1888.
107. Torres A, Martos A, Puig de la Bellacasa J, et al. Specificity of endotracheal aspiration, protected specimen brush, and bronchoalveolar lavage in mechanically ventilated patients. *Am Rev Respir Dis.* 1993;147:952–957.
108. Blot F, Raynard B, Chachaty E, et al. Value of Gram stain examination of lower respiratory tract secretions for early diagnosis of nosocomial pneumonia. *Am J Respir Crit Care Med.* 2000;162:1731–1737.
109. Baselski VS, el-Torky M, Coalson JJ, et al. The standardization of criteria for processing and interpreting laboratory specimens in patients with suspected ventilator-associated pneumonia. *Chest.* 1992;102(Suppl 1):571.
110. Timsit JF, Cheval C, Gachot B, et al. Usefulness of a strategy based on bronchoscopy with direct examination of bronchoalveolar lavage fluid in the initial antibiotic therapy of suspected ventilator-associated pneumonia. *Intensive Care Med.* 2001;27:640–647.
111. Chastre J, Fagon JY, Bornet-Lecso M, et al. Evaluation of bronchoscopic techniques for the diagnosis of nosocomial pneumonia. *Am J Respir Crit Care Med.* 1995;152:231–240.
112. Fagon JY, Chastre J, Wolff M, et al. Invasive and noninvasive strategies for management of suspected ventilator-associated pneumonia: a randomized trial. *Ann Intern Med.* 2000;132:621–630.
113. Alvarez-Lerma F. Modification of empiric antibiotic treatment in patients with pneumonia acquired in the intensive care unit. ICU-Acquired Pneumonia Study Group. *Intensive Care Med.* 1996;22:387–394.
114. Kollef MH, Ward S. The influence of mini-BAL cultures on patient outcomes: implications for the antibiotic management of ventilator-associated pneumonia. *Chest.* 1998;113:412–420.
115. Luna CM, Vujacich P, Niederman MS, et al. Impact of BAL data on the therapy and outcome of ventilator-associated pneumonia. *Chest.* 1997;111:676–685.

116. Iregui M, Ward S, Sherman G, et al. Clinical importance of delays in the initiation of appropriate antibiotic treatment for ventilator-associated pneumonia. *Chest.* 2002;122:262–268.
117. Ioanas M, Cavalcanti M, Ferrer M, et al. Hospital-acquired pneumonia: coverage and treatment adequacy of current guidelines. *Eur Respir J.* 2003;22:876–882.
118. Ibrahim EH, Ward S, Sherman G, et al. Experience with a clinical guideline for the treatment of ventilator-associated pneumonia. *Crit Care Med.* 2001;29:1109–1115.
119. Michel F, Franceschini B, Berger P, et al. Early antibiotic treatment for BAL-confirmed ventilator-associated pneumonia: a role for routine endotracheal aspirate cultures. *Chest.* 2005;127:589–597.
120. Hoffken G, Niederman MS. Nosocomial pneumonia: the importance of a de-escalating strategy for antibiotic treatment of pneumonia in the ICU. *Chest.* 2002;122:2183–2196.
121. Rello J, Vidaur L, Sandiumenge A, et al. De-escalation therapy in ventilator-associated pneumonia. *Crit Care Med.* 2004;32:2183–2190.
122. Chastre J, Wolff M, Fagon JY, et al.; PneumA Trial Group. Comparison of 8 vs 15 days of antibiotic therapy for ventilator-associated pneumonia in adults: a randomized trial. *JAMA.* 2003;290:2588–2598.
123. Micek ST, Ward S, Fraser VJ, Kollef MH. A randomized controlled trial of an antibiotic discontinuation policy for clinically suspected ventilator-associated pneumonia. *Chest.* 2004;125:1791–1799.
124. Kollef MH, Kollef KE. Antibiotic utilization and outcomes for patients with clinically suspected ventilator-associated pneumonia and negative quantitative BAL culture results. *Chest.* 2005;128:2706–2713.
125. Paul M, Benuri-Silbiger I, Soares-Weiser K, Leibovici L. Beta lactam monotherapy versus beta lactam-aminoglycoside combination therapy for sepsis in immunocompetent patients: systematic review and meta-analysis of randomised trials. *BMJ.* 2004;328:668.
126. Bliziotis IA, Samonis G, Vardakas KZ, et al. Effect of aminoglycoside and beta-lactam combination therapy versus beta-lactam monotherapy on the emergence of antimicrobial resistance: a meta-analysis of randomized, controlled trials. *Clin Infect Dis.* 2005;41:149–158.
127. Rubinstein E, Cammarata S, Oliphant T, Wunderink R; Linezolid Nosocomial Pneumonia Study Group. Linezolid (PNU-100766) versus vancomycin in the treatment of hospitalized patients with nosocomial pneumonia: a randomized, double-blind, multicenter study. *Clin Infect Dis.* 2001;32:402–412.
128. Wunderink RG, Cammarata SK, Oliphant TH, Kollef MH; Linezolid Nosocomial Pneumonia Study Group. Continuation of a randomized, double-blind, multicenter study of linezolid versus vancomycin in the treatment of patients with nosocomial pneumonia. *Clin Ther.* 2003;25:980–992.
129. Wunderink RG, Rello J, Cammarata SK, et al. Linezolid vs vancomycin: analysis of two double-blind studies of patients with methicillin-resistant *Staphylococcus aureus* nosocomial pneumonia. *Chest.* 2003; 124:1789–1797.
130. Garnacho-Montero J, Ortiz-Leyba C, Jimenez-Jimenez FJ, et al. Treatment of multidrug-resistant *Acinetobacter baumannii* ventilator-associated pneumonia (VAP) with intravenous colistin: a comparison with imipenem-susceptible VAP. *Clin Infect Dis.* 2003;36:1111–1118.
131. Vidaur L, Gualis B, Rodriguez A, et al. Clinical resolution in patients with suspicion of ventilator-associated pneumonia: a cohort study comparing patients with and without acute respiratory distress syndrome. *Crit Care Med.* 2005;33:1248–1253.
132. Luna CM, Blanzaco D, Niederman MS, et al. Resolution of ventilator-associated pneumonia: prospective evaluation of the clinical pulmonary infection score as an early clinical predictor of outcome. *Crit Care Med.* 2003;31:676–682.
133. Ioanas M, Ferrer M, Cavalcanti M, et al. Causes and predictors of nonresponse to treatment of intensive care unit-acquired pneumonia. *Crit Care Med.* 2004;32:938–945.
134. Nseir S, Di Pompeo C, Soubrier S, et al. Impact of ventilator-associated pneumonia on outcome in patients with COPD. *Chest.* 2005;128:1650–1656.
135. Bercault N, Boulain T. Mortality rate attributable to ventilator-associated nosocomial pneumonia in an adult intensive care unit: a prospective case-control study. *Crit Care Med.* 2001;29:2303–2309.
136. Fagon JY, Chastre J, Hance AJ, et al. Nosocomial pneumonia in ventilated patients: a cohort study evaluating attributable mortality and hospital stay. *Am J Med.* 1993;94:281–288.
137. Moine P, Timsit JF, De Lassence A, et al.; OUTCOMEREA study group. Mortality associated with late-onset pneumonia in the intensive care unit: results of a multi-center cohort study. *Intensive Care Med.* 2002;28:154–163.
138. Dupont H, Montravers P, Gauzit R, et al.; Club d'Infectiologie en Anesthésie-Réanimation. Outcome of postoperative pneumonia in the Eole study. *Intensive Care Med.* 2003;29:179–188.
139. Leroy O, Meybeck A, d'Escrivan T, et al. Impact of adequacy of initial antimicrobial therapy on the prognosis of patients with ventilator-associated pneumonia. *Intensive Care Med.* 2003;9:2170–2173.
140. Clec'h C, Timsit JF, De Lassence A, et al. Efficacy of adequate early antibiotic therapy in ventilator-associated pneumonia: influence of disease severity. *Intensive Care Med.* 2004;30:1327–1333.
141. Alp E, Voss A. Ventilator associated pneumonia and infection control. *Ann Clin Microbiol Antimicrob.* 2006;5:7.
142. Isakow W, Kollef MH. Preventing ventilator-associated pneumonia: an evidence-based approach of modifiable risk factors. *Semin Respir Crit Care Med.* 2006;27:5–17.
143. Tablan OC, Anderson LJ, Besser R, et al.; Healthcare Infection Control Practices Advisory Committee, Centers for Disease Control and Prevention. Guidelines for preventing health-care–associated pneumonia, 2003: recommendations of the CDC and the Healthcare Infection Control Practices Advisory Committee. *MMWR Recomm Rep.* 2004;53(RR-3):1–36.
144. van Nieuwenhoven CA, Buskens E, van Tiel FH, Bonten MJ. Relationship between methodological trial quality and the effects of selective digestive decontamination on pneumonia and mortality in critically ill patients. *JAMA.* 2001;286:335–340.
145. de Jonge E, Schultz M, Spanjaard L, et al. Effects of selective decontamination of the digestive tract on mortality and acquisition of resistant bacteria in intensive care: a randomized controlled trial. *Lancet.* 2003;362:1011–1016.
146. Valles J, Mesalles E, Mariscal D, et al. A 7-year study of severe hospital-acquired pneumonia requiring ICU admission. *Intensive Care Med.* 2003;29:1981–1988.
147. Sopena N, Sabria M; Neunos 2000 Study Group. Multicenter study of hospital-acquired pneumonia in non-ICU patients. *Chest.* 2005;127:213–219.
148. Capitano B, Nicolau DP. Evolving epidemiology and cost of resistance to antimicrobial agents in long-term care facilities. *J Am Med Dir Assoc.* 2003;4(3Suppl):S90–S99.
149. Mylotte JM, Goodnough S, Tayara A. Antibiotic-resistant organisms among long-term care facility residents on admission to an inpatient geriatrics unit: retrospective and prospective surveillance. *Am J Infect Control.* 2001;29:139–144.
150. Dosa D. Should I hospitalize my resident with nursing home-acquired pneumonia? *J Am Med Dir Assoc.* 2006;7(Suppl 3):S74–S80, 73.
151. Crossley KB, Peterson PK. Infections in the elderly. *Clin Infect Dis.* 1996;22:209–215.
152. Muder RR. Pneumonia in residents of long-term care facilities: epidemiology, etiology, management, and prevention. *Am J Med.* 1998;105:319–330.
153. Mylotte JM. Nursing home-acquired pneumonia: update on treatment options. *Drugs Aging.* 2006;23(5):377–390.
154. Celli BR, MacNee W; ATS/ERS Task Force. Standards for the diagnosis and treatment of patients with COPD: a summary of the ATS/ERS position paper. *Eur Respir J.* 2004;23:932–946.
155. Murphy TF, Sethi S, Niederman MS. The role of bacteria in exacerbations of COPD: a constructive view. *Chest.* 2000;118:204–209.
156. Saint S, Bent S, Vittinghoff E, Grady D. Antibiotics in chronic obstructive pulmonary disease exacerbations: a meta-analysis. *JAMA.* 1995;273:957–960.
157. Nouira S, Marghli S, Belghith M, et al. Once daily oral ofloxacin in chronic obstructive pulmonary disease exacerbation requiring mechanical ventilation: a randomised placebo-controlled trial. *Lancet.* 2001;358:2020–2025.
158. Ferrer M, Ioanas M, Arancibia F, et al. Microbial airway colonization is associated with noninvasive ventilation failure in exacerbation of chronic obstructive pulmonary disease. *Crit Care Med.* 2005;33:2003–2009.
159. Ewig S, Soler N, Gonzalez J, et al. Evaluation of antimicrobial treatment in mechanically ventilated patients with severe chronic obstructive pulmonary disease exacerbations. *Crit Care Med.* 2000;28:692–697.
160. Cavalcanti M, Valencia M, Torres A. Respiratory nosocomial infections in the medical intensive care unit. *Microbes Infect.* 2005;7:292–301.
161. Nseir S, Di Pompeo C, Soubrier S, et al. Effect of ventilator-associated tracheobronchitis on outcome in patients without chronic respiratory failure: a case-control study. *Crit Care.* 2005;9:R238–R245.
162. Nseir S, Di Pompeo C, Soubrier S, et al. Outcomes of ventilated COPD patients with nosocomial tracheobronchitis: a case-control study. *Infection.* 2004;32:210–216.
163. Nseir S, Ader F, Marquette CH. Nosocomial tracheobronchitis. *Curr Opin Infect Dis.* 2009;22:148–153.
164. Craven DE, Chroneou A, Zias N, Hjalmarson KI. Ventilator-associated tracheobronchitis: the impact of targeted antibiotic therapy on patient outcomes. *Chest.* 2009;135:521–528.
165. Hammond JM, Potgieter PD, Hanslo D, et al. Etiology and antimicrobial susceptibility patterns of micro organisms in acute community-acquired lung abscess. *Chest.* 1995;108:937–941.

166. Wang JL, Chen KY, Fang CT, et al. Changing bacteriology of adult community-acquired lung abscess in Taiwan: *Klebsiella pneumoniae* versus anaerobes. *Clin Infect Dis.* 2005;40:915–922.
167. Bartlett JG. The role of anaerobic bacteria in lung abscess. *Clin Infect Dis.* 2005;40:923–925.
168. Allewelt M, Schuler P, Bolcskei PL, et al. Study group on aspiration pneumonia. Ampicillin + sulbactam vs clindamycin +/- cephalosporin for the treatment of aspiration pneumonia and primary lung abscess. *Clin Microbiol Infect.* 2004;10:163–170.
169. Podbielski FJ, Rodriguez HE, Wiesman IM, et al. Pulmonary parenchymal abscess: VATS approach to diagnosis and treatment. *Asian Cardiovasc Thorac Ann.* 2001;9:339–341.
170. Herth F, Ernst A, Becker HD. Endoscopic drainage of lung abscesses: technique and outcome. *Chest.* 2005;127:1378–1381.
171. Bryant RE, Salmon CJ. Pleural empyema. *Clin Infect Dis.* 1996;22:747–762; quiz 763–764.
172. Davies CW, Gleeson FV, Davies RJ; Pleural Diseases Group, Standards of Care Committee, British Thoracic Society. BTS guidelines for the management of pleural infection. *Thorax.* 2003;58(Suppl 2):ii18–ii28.
173. Maskell NA, Davies CW, Nunn AJ, et al.; First Multicenter Intrapleural Sepsis Trial (MIST1) Group. U.K. Controlled trial of intrapleural streptokinase for pleural infection. *N Engl J Med.* 2005;352:865–874.
174. Tokuda Y, Matsushima D, Stein GH, Miyagi S. Intrapleural fibrinolytic agents for empyema and complicated parapneumonic effusions: a meta-analysis. *Chest.* 2006;129:783–790.

Section 3

Urinary Tract Infections

MARC LEONE, GARY DUCLOS, and CLAUDE MARTIN

INTRODUCTION

The intensive care units (ICUs) represent a meeting point between the most seriously ill patients receiving aggressive therapy and the most resistant pathogens, which are selected by the use of broad-spectrum antimicrobial therapy. ICU patients require indwelling devices associated with an increased risk of infection. Most patients who are hospitalized in ICUs receive an indwelling urinary catheter to monitor diuresis; urinary tract infection (UTI) remains a leading cause of nosocomial infections with significant morbidity, mortality, and additional hospital costs (1,2).

Although UTI represents 30% to 40% of nosocomial infections (3), its prevalence in patients admitted to ICU is about 10%, depending on ICU patient's type (1). In a large European survey, UTI is the third most common cause of infections in ICU (4). Another study suggests that the incidence of urosepsis, which is defined as an inflammation of the upper urinary tract that causes sepsis and bacteremia occurs in approximately 18% of the ICU patient population (5). The aim of this review is to focus on the prevention and management of UTI in patients hospitalized in ICU.

DEFINITIONS

In ICU, UTI is the consequence of the presence of an indwelling catheter (Table 88.3.17). This results in the concept of catheter-associated UTI (CAUTI) (Table 88.3.18), which is defined by Center of Disease Control and prevention (CDC) by the presence of three criteria: presence of an indwelling urinary bladder catheter (IUBC) for more than 2 days; bacteria in the bladder of a patient; and at least one of the following signs of symptoms: fever (>38°C), suprapubic tenderness or costovertebral angle pain. Bacteriuria was defined as the detection of ≥10^5 organisms/mL of urine with no more than two species of organisms (6). In the ICU, the clinical symptoms can be missing due to the patient's lack of awareness.

TABLE 88.3.17 Symptomatic Urinary Tract Infection: Patient Must Meet Criteria 1, 2, and 3

Criterion 1
Patient has at least one of the following signs or symptoms: • Fever (>38°C) in a patient that is ≤65 yr of age • Suprapubic tenderness* • Costovertebral angle pain or tenderness* • Urinary frequency* • Urinary urgency* • Dysuria*
Criterion 2
Patient has a urine culture with no more than two species of organisms, at least one of which is a bacteria of ≥10^5 CFU/mL
Criterion 3
• Patient has/had an indwelling urinary catheter but it has/had not been in place >2 calendar days on the date of event or • Patient did not have a urinary catheter in place on the date of event nor the day before the date of event

*Only for interactive patients.
From Catheter-associated urinary tract infections (CAUTI). CDC website. Available at: http://www.cdc.gov/HAI/ca_uti/uti.html. Updated October 16, 2015; accessed October 31, 2015.

Pathophysiology

With the exception of distal urethra, the urinary tract is normally sterile. The resistance to UTI is influenced by exposure to uropathogenic bacteria, age, hormonal status, and urine flow (7,8). The insertion of an IUBC allows organisms to gain access to the bladder; the device induces an inflammation of the urethra, allowing bacteria to ascend into the bladder in the space between the urethral mucosa and the catheter. CAUTI usually follows formation of biofilm, which consists of adherent micro-organisms, their extracellular products, and host components deposited on both the internal and external catheter surface. The biofilm protects organisms from both antimicrobials and the host immune response

TABLE 88.3.18 Catheter-associated Urinary Tract Infection (CAUTI): Patient Must Meet Criteria 1, 2, and 3

Criterion 1 Patient had an indwelling urinary catheter that had been in place for >2 d on the date of event (day of device placement = day 1) *and* was either: • Still present on the date of event, or • Removed the day before the date of event
Criterion 2 Patient has at least one of the following signs or symptoms: • Fever (>38.0°C) • Suprapubic tenderness • Costovertebral angle pain or tenderness • Urinary urgency • Urinary frequency • Dysuria
Criterion 3 Patient has a urine culture with no more than two species of organisms, at least one of which is a bacteria of ≥10⁵ CFU/mL ***Notes*** • An indwelling urinary catheter in place would constitute "other recognized cause" for patient complaints of "frequency" "urgency" or "dysuria" and therefore these cannot be used as symptoms when catheter is in place. • Fever and hypothermia are nonspecific symptoms of infection and cannot be excluded from UTI determination because they are clinically deemed due to another recognized cause.

From Catheter-associated urinary tract infections (CAUTI). CDC website. Available at: http://www.cdc.gov/HAI/ca_uti/uti.html. Updated October 16, 2015; accessed October 31, 2015.

(7,9). The ascending route of infection is predominant in women because of the short urethra and contamination with the anal flora. Intraluminal contamination is less frequent, and is related to reflux of pathogens from the drainage system into the bladder. This contamination occurs in case of failure of closed drainage or contamination of urine in the collection bag.

Microbiology

The isolated pathogens among ICU patients with bacteriuria are essentially *Escherichia coli, Pseudomonas aeruginosa,* and *Enterococcus* species (1,10,11); polymicrobial infections represent only 5% to 12% (3,10) of cases. In the largest report investigating nosocomial infections in ICU patients, gram-negative bacteria are responsible for 70% of CAUTIs (1). During this period, resistance to antimicrobials increased, especially the rates of resistance to third-generation cephalosporins for *E. coli* (up to 60%) and for *Klebsiella pneumoniae* (68%) (Table 88.3.19) (1).

Risk Factors

In ICU patients, UTIs are associated with the presence of an IUBC. Among 10,755 patients in a trauma center, risk factors were female gender (59%) and age (>57 years old) (12). Accordingly to prior studies, female gender, length of ICU stay, prior use of antibiotics, severity score at admission, and duration of catheterization were independently associated with an increased risk of catheter-associated bacteriuria (13–15). These results emphasize that preventing or reducing the duration of catheterization is the most important intervention. In a tertiary care hospital, the initial indication for the placement of a urinary catheter was unjustified in 15% of patients and unclear in 28% of patients (14); as a result, the length of stay and cost of care were increased (15). In the medical ICU, an excessively prolonged use of urinary catheter for monitoring urine output resulted in 64% of the total unjustified patient days (16).

Impact of CAUTIs in ICU

Although adverse consequences of asymptomatic UTIs are described during pregnancy or in nursing home (17,18), the real impact of ICU-acquired CAUTIs on outcome remains unclear. In a general hospital population, Platt et al. (19)

TABLE 88.3.19 Percentage of Pathogens Associated with Nosocomial Urinary Tract Infections

	Study			
Pathogen	**Leone (10) (*N* = 53)**	**Laupland (23) (*N* = 290)**	**Gaynes (11) (*N* = 4,109)**	**Rosenthal (1) (*N* = 3,225)**
Gram-negative				
Escherichia coli	39	23	26	47
Pseudomonas aeruginosa	22	10	16.3	26.5
Enterobacter species	15	3	6.9	–
Acinetobacter acinus	11	–	1.6	3.9
Proteus species	11	5	–	–
Klebsiella species	11	5	9.8	19
Citrobacter species	2	1	–	–
Gram-positive				
Enterococcus species	4	15	17.4	2.8
Staphylococcus aureus	2	1	3.6	0.3
Coagulase-negative *Staphylococcus*	2	5	4.9	–
Yeast				
Candida albicans	2	20	–	–
Candida non-*albicans*		8	–	–

TABLE 88.3.20 Rates of Sepsis According to Each Site

	Study		
Site	Vincent (4) (*N* = 7,087)	Vincent (21) (*N* = 1,177)	Angus (22) (*N* = 192,980)
Lung	63.5%	68%	44%
Abdomen	19.6%	22%	8.6%
Blood	15.1%	20%	17.3%
Urine	14.3%	14%	9.1%

showed that nosocomial UTIs were associated with a significant attributable mortality; the picture is probably different in a specific ICU population. Indeed, even after controlling for many risk factors, UTIs have a higher incidence in ICUs than on conventional wards (20), although urinary tract is the source of sepsis in only 10% to 14% of cases, far from that seen in the lung (Table 88.3.20) (1,4,21,22). The development of an ICU-acquired UTIs is associated with a prolonged ICU stay and crude rate of mortality (2,10); however, adequately powered studies demonstrate that UTIs are not dependent factors for mortality (2,23).

Urosepsis is defined as an inflammation of the upper urinary tract that causes seeding of the blood with bacteria, resulting in local and distant destruction of tissues. In a retrospective study, urinary tract was responsible for 21% of the health care–acquired bloodstream infection. The incidence was 1.4 urinary bloodstream per 10,000 patients days of IUBC, with an associated mortality rate at 15% (24). These results are similar in ICU population. In another retrospective study, a total of 105 CAUTIs were identified; only 6% resulted in positive bloodstream infections. The mortality rates of the patients were not influenced by the presence of CAUTI (5). Accordingly, in a prospective randomized study, 6 out of 60 patients with an IUBC and asymptomatic bacteriuria developed urosepsis (25). Risk factors of developing an urinary tract–related bloodstream infection were neutropenia, renal disease, male gender, insulin, and immunosuppressant therapy (26).

Finally, the CAUTIs result in a significant increase in cost. An episode of symptomatic nosocomial CAUTI in hospitalized patients was associated with an additional cost of US$749—1,007/admission (24,25). Among the nosocomial infections, UTIs had the lowest daily antibiotic cost per infected patient (27).

DIAGNOSTIC TOOLS IN THE ICU

The diagnosis of urosepsis should be entertained each time a patient has a febrile episode. Because of the prevalence of bacteriuria in patients with urinary catheters, some have advocated daily monitoring of urine in catheterized patients; however, routine daily bacteriologic monitoring of the urine from all catheterized patients is not an effective way to decrease the incidence of symptomatic, catheter-associated UTI and is not recommended (28)

Some clinical trials assess the effectiveness of urinary dipsticks (leukocyte esterase and nitrite) for screening patients instead of quantitative urine culture in ICU (Table 88.3.21) (29,30). Leukocyte esterase activity is an indicator of pyuria and urinary nitrite production an indicator of bacteriuria. In an older medical ICU study, it had been demonstrated that

TABLE 88.3.21 Assessing Urinary Reagent Strips in the ICU

	Study		
Parameter	Tissot (29)	Mimoz (32)	Legras (31)
Prevalence	31%	38%	42%
Sensitivity	87%	84%	90%
Specificity	61%	41%	65%
Positive predictive value	31%	46%	61%
Negative predictive value	96%	81%	91%

the urinary dipstick strategy was a rapid and cost-effective test with which to screen asymptomatic catheterized patients (29;31,32). This effectiveness was observed only for a positive quantitative urine culture level of 10^5 organisms/mL; in these cases, the urinary dipstick strategy decreased the cost of nosocomial infection diagnosis and the daily workload in the microbiology laboratory. The authors concluded that the urinary dipsticks were a cost-effective test for screening asymptomatic catheterized patients in a medical ICU (29). During a 2-year period, however, Coman et al. (30) did not show an impact of urinary dipstick on symptomatic CAUTI with fever or hypothermia. The Cochrane review concluded that the effectiveness of urinary dipstick remains unresolved due to the lack of good quality studies (33). The use of dipsticks instead of quantitative urine culture cannot be recommended for symptomatic CAUTIs in ICU patients. Guidelines recommend that asymptomatic bacteriuria or funguria should not be screened for in patients with IUBCs (34). Hence, in symptomatic patients, quantitative urine culture with Gram stain examination is recommended to obtain rapid identification of the pathogen.

PREVENTION OF UTI IN THE ICU

Most measures, described below, are useful only in units with a restrictive policy of catheterization (Table 88.3.22).

Urinary Drainage System

For preventing infection, the maintenance of a closed, sterile drainage system is recommended (35); this was described for the first time in 1928 (36), and its benefit has been subsequently re-enforced. In a randomized study, a subgroup analysis, which considered patients not receiving an antibiotic treatment, showed a reduction in mortality in the group using the closed system (37). Historically, "open systems" were large, uncapped glass bottles. The drainage catheters were inserted into the glass bottles, often below the level of urine; urine was stagnant, and bacteria could easily grow and ascend through the drainage catheter. The introduction of closed drainage systems was an improvement, dramatically reducing the rate of bacteriuria. However, in the modern era, several studies failed to confirm the benefit of complex closed system compared with simple devices (38,39).

Two studies focused specifically on ICU patients (40,41), comparing a two-chamber drainage system with a complex closed drainage system. In a randomized and prospective trial, 311 patients requiring an IUBC for longer than 48 hours

TABLE 88.3.22 Comparative Studies Performed in the ICU on the Prevention of Catheter-associated Urinary Tract Infection

	Study			
Parameter	Leone (34) ($N = 311$)	Leone (35) ($N = 224$)	Thibon (40) ($N = 199$)	Bologna (41) ($N = 108$)
Method	Prospective, not randomized	Prospective, randomized	Prospective, Randomized, multicenter	Prospective, not randomized, multicenter
Rate of bacteriuria (%)	8	12	11	8.1 vs 4.9
Study group	Two-chamber simple closed drainage system	Two-chamber simple closed drainage system	Catheter coated with hydrogel and silver salts	Hydrogel latex Foley catheter with silver metal
Control group	Complex closed system	Complex closed system	Standard catheter	Standard catheter
Conclusion	No difference	No difference	No difference	No difference

were assigned to the two-chamber drainage system group or to a complex closed drainage system group to compare the rates of bacteriuria. Rates of UTIs were 12.1 and 12.8 episodes/1,000 catheter days, respectively ($p > 0.05$) (40). The data extracted from the literature do not support the use of complex closed drainage systems in ICU patients in view of the increased cost (42).

For the management of drainage systems, owing to the lack of specific studies in ICU, guidelines may be viewed as recommendations at best. The following are reasonable suggestions: only persons who know the correct technique of aseptic insertion and maintenance of the catheter should handle catheters; hospital personnel should be given periodic in-service training stressing the correct techniques and potential complications of urinary catheterization; hand-washing should be done immediately before and after any manipulation of the catheter site or apparatus; if small volumes of fresh urine are needed for examination, the distal end of the catheter, or preferably the sampling port if present, should be cleansed with a disinfectant, and urine then aspirated with a sterile needle and syringe; larger volumes of urine for special analyses should be obtained aseptically from the drainage bag; unobstructed flow should be maintained; to achieve free flow of urine, (1) the catheter and the collecting tube should be kept from kinking; (2) the collecting bag should be emptied regularly using a separate collecting container for each patient (the draining spigot and nonsterile collecting container should never come in contact); (3) poorly functioning or obstructed catheters should not be irrigated in routine but replaced after reconsidering indication of urinary catheter; (4) collecting bags should always be kept below the level of the bladder; and (5) IUBCs should not be changed at arbitrary fixed intervals (34,43,44).

Type of Urethral Catheters

There is a vast literature stressing the efficacy of antiseptic impregnated catheters, including silver oxide or silver alloy, and antibiotic-impregnated catheters in hospitalized patients (45–47). In the largest RCT, Pickard et al. showed a nonclinically relevant benefit of using nitrofural-impregnated catheters to reduce CAUTI versus silver-coated or standard catheters (47). Diagnosis of CAUTI was supported by microbiologic culture and use of antibiotic, but the difference is probably not clinically relevant (48). A recent Cochrane meta-analysis compared the effectiveness of different indwelling urethral catheters in reducing risk of CAUTI for short-term catheterization (<14 days) (42); silver oxide and silvery alloy catheters were not associated with a reduction of CAUTI in short-term catheterized hospitalized adults. Catheters coated with a combination of minocycline and rifampin or nitrofurazone may be beneficial in reducing bacteriuria and symptomatic CAUTI in hospitalized males catheterized less than 2 weeks, but this requires further assessment (42). Comparison of nitrofurazone-coated and silver alloy–coated catheters results in a superiority of antibiotic-coated in reducing bacteriuria and symptomatic CAUTI, but the magnitude of reduction was low and hence may not be clinically relevant (42). However, those catheters are more expensive and are more likely to cause discomfort than standard catheters (42).

In ICU patients, a randomized, prospective, double-blind multicenter trial compared catheters coated with hydrogel and silver salts with classical urinary tract catheters (49). The cumulative incidence of UTIs associated with catheterization was 11.1% overall, 11.9% for the control group, and 10% for the coated catheter group. The odds ratio was 0.82 (95% confidence interval [CI]: 0.30 to 2.20) (49). In a prior blind prospective trial, standard latex IUBCs were switched for a hydrogel latex IUBC with a monolayer of silver metal applied to the inner and outer surfaces of the catheter. The adjusted CAUTI rates during the baseline and intervention periods were 8.1 and 4.9 infections/1,000 device days, respectively ($p = 0.13$) (47). With respect to long-term bladder drainage, a Cochrane meta-analysis showed that no eligible trials compared alternative routes of catheter insertion or catheter types (48).

Meatal Care

Twice daily cleansing with povidone–iodine solution and daily cleansing with soap and water have failed to reduce CAUTIs; thus, at this time, daily meatal care with either of these two regimens cannot be endorsed (34). A randomized, controlled, prospective clinical trial involving 696 hospitalized medical and surgical patients was undertaken to determine the effectiveness of 1% silver sulfadiazine cream applied twice daily to the urethral meatus in preventing transurethral catheter-associated bacteriuria. The overall incidence of bacteriuria was similar in both groups ($p = 0.56$) (42). In the absence of study performed in a specific ICU patient population, the expert opinion may be followed and daily soap cleansing seems to be an appropriated care (44).

There are no data available on the level of sterility required to insert the urinary catheter. Experts recommend that catheters should be inserted using aseptic technique and sterile equipment; gloves, drape, and sponges should be used for insertion. However, in a prospective study conducted in the operating room, 156 patients underwent preoperative urethral catheterization, randomly allocated to "sterile" or "clean/nonsterile" technique groups. There was no statistical difference between the two groups with respect to the incidence of UTI, but the cost differs considerably between the two groups (43). A Cochrane meta-analysis of 31 trials showed no evidence that the incidence of CAUTI is affected by the use of aseptic or clean technique for intermittent catheterization in long-term bladder management (50).

Bladder Irrigation and Antiseptic in the Drainage System

The objective of antibiotic irrigation is to clear the bacteria from the urinary tract. A randomized study compared 89 patients receiving a neomycin–polymyxin irrigant administered through closed urinary catheters to 98 patients not given irrigation. Eighteen of 98 (18%) of the patients not given irrigation became infected, as compared with 14 of 89 (16%) of those given irrigation, and the organisms from patients with irrigation were more resistant (51). Another study was conducted in urology patients, evaluating the effect of povidone–iodine bladder irrigation prior to catheter removal on subsequent bacteriuria. Of 264 patients, 138 received irrigation and 126 were controls. Urine cultures were positive in 22% in the control group and 18% in the study group (52). Thus, irrigation methods failed to demonstrate an efficacy in surgical patients and meta-analysis does not shows any benefit for long-term catheterization management (53). Experts do not recommend its use in ICU patients (34,44).

In ICU, the addition of antimicrobial agents in the drainage device has not been studied. The largest study investigating the effect of H_2O_2 insertion in the drainage device of 353 patients compared to 315 control patients failed to show a benefit in treated patients. It is noteworthy that 68% of these patients required an IUBC for hemodynamic monitoring, with antimicrobial therapy prescribed in 75% of patients, suggesting these results can apply to ICU patients (54). Experts recommend not using any kind of irrigation unless obstruction is anticipated, as might occur with bleeding after prostatic or bladder surgery (34,44).

Alternatives to the Urinary Catheter

For selected patients, other methods of urinary drainage such as condom catheter drainage, suprapubic catheterization, and intermittent urethral catheterization should be used as alternatives to an IUBC. While there are few data available in ICU to assess these alternative devices, there is evidence that suprapubic catheterization have advantages over indwelling catheters with respect to bacteriuria, recatheterization, and discomfort after abdominal or pelvic surgery (55–57). The use of condom linked to a collection bag has been evaluated in a study comparing two periods of 6 months, in which 167 patients were included. The occurrence of bacteriuria was significantly decreased for the period using the condoms (26.7% vs. 2.4%) (58). A recent study comparing microbiology reports from cultures collected from external versus indwelling catheters shows no difference in species that colonize, but did not analyze UTI incidence (59). A randomized trial of 75 males older than 40 years compared condom and indwelling catheters. Morbidity risk (bacteriuria, symptomatic UTI, or death) was higher in the catheterized group (hazard ratio = 4.84, 95% CI = 1.46 to 16.02; $p = 0.02$). Patients reported that condom catheters were more comfortable ($p = 0.02$) and less painful ($p = 0.02$) than indwelling catheters (60). The use of intermittent catheterization was also associated with a lower risk of bacteriuria than indwelling urethral catheter; such a procedure has not been systematically investigated in ICU patients (42,61,62).

Miscellaneous Measures

While there is a low risk of bacteremia during the urinary catheterization (63), the administration of prophylactic antimicrobial therapy at the time of catheterization leads to a reduction in bacteriuria and pyuria (64). The efficacy of antibiotic treatment has been assessed as optimal for catheterization lasting less than 14 days in perioperative and nonsurgical patients (64). However, the prophylactic use of antibiotic in ICU can be detrimental for the ecology in increasing the resistance of bacteria. This practice must, therefore, be discouraged in ICU. It is noteworthy that in most ICU studies 75% of patients with an indwelling catheter required antibiotics for different reasons (10).

Care bundles seem efficient to reduce CAUTI in conventional wards. A large survey compared American hospitals applying the "Keystone bladder bundle initiative" (65) with those not applying it (64). The compliant hospitals had better prevention of CAUTI related to improved assessment of initial indication, use of bladder scanner, removal reminder, and/or systematic stop orders (66,67). In the ICU, use of a daily checklist to systematically review invasive devices may increase compliance with recommendations for preventing nosocomial infection, but as of this writing, there is no reduction of CAUTI (68). Emerging work aiming at removing biofilm in order to prevent CAUTI by using low-energy ultrasound (69) or lytic bacteriophages (70) are underway; to date, they are not applicable to the bedside.

In conclusion, few preventive measures have demonstrated efficacy in reducing the rate of UTIs in the ICU. Additionally, the clinical significance of bacteriuria remains uncertain. Consequently, general measures with good adherence to hygiene procedures are more relevant than expensive devices to fight infections.

TREATMENT OF CAUTIS IN THE ICU

The management of CAUTI has not been evaluated in ICU patients. Several nonspecific measures, including hydration, have been advocated in the therapy of UTI. Adequate hydration would appear to be important although there is no evidence that it improves the effectiveness of an appropriate antimicrobial therapy (71). The management of complicated UTIs in the ICU may include mechanical intervention. Consequently, appropriate diagnostic tests and urologic consultation should be included in the algorithm of the management of these patients (Fig. 88.3.1).

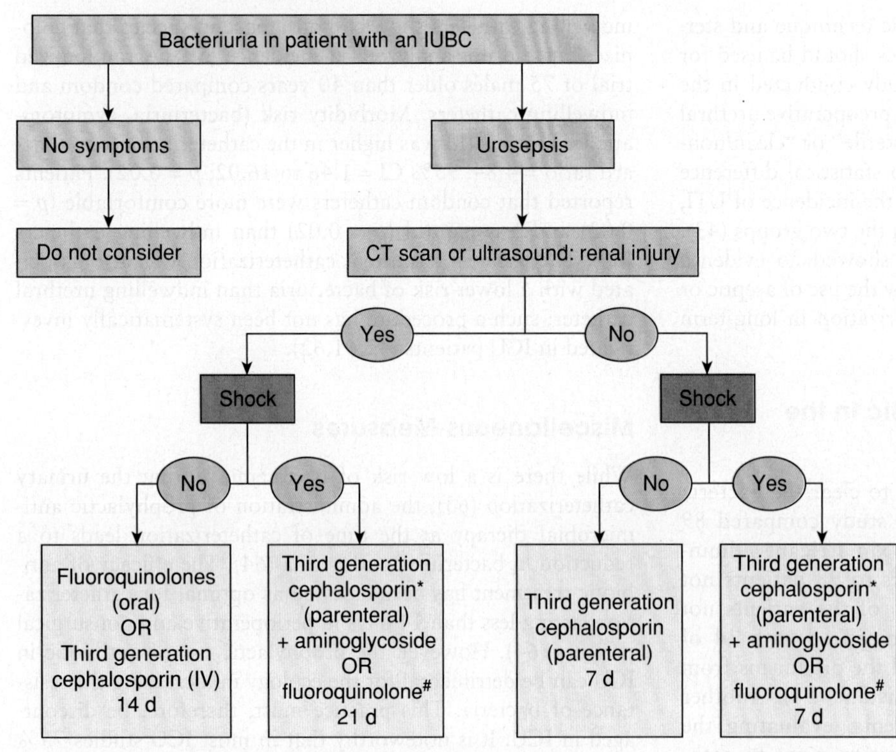

FIGURE 88.3.1 Suggested algorithm for the management of urinary tract infections related to an indwelling catheter in the ICU. *Discuss the need for antipseudomonal coverage according to the duration of hospitalization, prior medical history, and local ecology. #Discuss if renal failure.

Management of Asymptomatic Bacteriuria

Expert opinion holds that asymptomatic catheter-associated bacteriuria does not require treatment or screening in the ICU (34,72). However, antimicrobial treatment may be considered for asymptomatic women with a CAUTI that persists 48 hours after catheter removal (73). In a specific ICU population, 60 patients with an IUBC for longer than 48 hours who developed an asymptomatic positive urine culture were randomized to receive either a 3-day course of antibiotics associated with the replacement of the indwelling urethral catheter 4 hours after first antibiotic administration or no antibiotics and no catheter replacement; six patients, equally distributed in the two groups, developed urosepsis and the profile of bacterial resistance was similar in the two groups. Hence, treating a positive urine culture in an asymptomatic patient with an indwelling urethral catheter does not reduce the occurrence of urosepsis (25).

Management of Symptomatic Urinary Tract Infections

Choice of Antimicrobial Agents

The optimal characteristics of agents to treat UTIs must include activity against the major pathogens involved in these infections, good tissue penetration, and minimal side effects. High urinary levels should be present for an adequate period to eliminate the organisms, since disappearance of bacteriuria is correlated to the sensitivity of the pathogen and to the urine concentration of the antimicrobial agent (74). Inhibitory urinary concentrations are achieved after administration of essentially all commonly used antibiotics. However, an antibiotic achieving active concentrations in the renal tissue is required for infection of the renal tissue; the antibiotic concentration in the serum or plasma can be used as surrogate markers for the antibiotic concentrations in the renal tissue (75). For drugs with concentration-dependent time-kill activity such as the aminoglycosides or the fluoroquinolones, the peak antibiotic concentration is the most important parameter for the *in vivo* effect. Experimentally, gentamicin and fluoroquinolone treatment are both more effective than β-lactam antibiotics in rapid bacterial killing (Table 88.3.23) (75).

Clinical studies have shown that the renal concentrations of cephalosporins remain higher than the minimal inhibitory concentration for the most common bacteria during the time interval between the administrations of two doses (76–78). In contrast, β-lactam antibiotics with a low pKa and poor lipid solubility penetrate poorly into the prostate, except for some cephalosporins. Good to excellent penetration into the prostatic tissue has been demonstrated with many antimicrobial agents, such as aminoglycosides, fluoroquinolones, sulfonamides, and nitrofurantoin (79).

In ICU patients, the pharmacokinetics of β-lactam and aminoglycosides antibiotics may be profoundly altered due the dynamic and unpredictable pathophysiologic changes that occur in critical illness (80). Consequently, therapeutic drug monitoring may optimize antibiotic therapy (81) especially in septic shock and when continuous renal replacement therapy (CRRT) is used, to individualize dosing and to ensure optimal antibiotic exposure (82). The side effects of treatment should be minimized at both the individual and the community levels. Many patients develop renal failure, associated with inability to concentrate antimicrobial agents in the urine.

Otherwise, antimicrobial treatment should produce a minimal effect on the bacterial flora of the community (83). From this standpoint, there is significant literature demonstrating that the use of fluoroquinolone is associated with the emergence of resistant pathogens (84–87). This implies that an indication for antibacterial therapy should be weighed thoroughly and fluoroquinolones should be used in accordance with sensitivity testing (88). Hence, it is of importance to stress that UTI should not be treated before the results of sensitivity testing, except in patients with pyelonephritis and those with

TABLE 88.3.23 Antimicrobial Treatment of Urinary Tract Infections. Each Empirical Treatment Must Be Adapted to the Susceptibility Testing Results

Source of infection	Pathogens	Treatment	Duration
Acute prostatitis (without bacteremia)	*E. coli, Proteus* sp., *Klebsiella* sp., *Enterococcus* sp., *S. aureus, N. gonorrhoeae, C. trachomatis*	Ofloxacin 200 mg × 2 (oral)	28 d
Acute prostatitis (with bacteremia)	*E. coli, Proteus* sp., *Klebsiella* sp., *Enterococcus* sp., *S. aureus, N. gonorrhoeae, C. trachomatis*	Ofloxacin 200 mg × 2 (oral) or Ceftriaxone 2 g/d and Gentamicin 3 to 8 mg/kg/d i.v.	28 d 3 d
Chronic bacterial prostatitis	*E. coli, Proteus* sp., *Klebsiella* sp., *Enterococcus* sp., *S. aureus, N. gonorrhoeae, C. trachomatis*	Ofloxacin 200 mg × 2 (oral) or Trimethoprim 160 mg/sulfamethoxazole 800 mg × 2/d (oral)	28 d
Acute pyelonephritis (uncomplicated)	Enterobacteriaceiae, *E. coli, Proteus* sp., *Enterococcus* sp.	Ciprofloxacin 500 mg × 2/d (oral) *If oral route not possible:* Ceftriaxone 2 g/day i.v.	14 d
Acute pyelonephritis (complicated)	Enterobacteriaceiae, *E. coli, Proteus* sp., *Enterococcus* sp.	Ciprofloxacin 500 mg × 2/d (oral) or Ceftriaxone 2 g/d i.v. and Gentamicin 3–8 mg/kg/d	14–21 d 3 d

severe sepsis or septic shock who require empirical antimicrobial therapy.

Cystitis

As acute uncomplicated cystitis is infrequent in ICU patients, most recommendations focus on the treatment of nonhospitalized women, which makes their relevance in the ICU patients questionable; *E. coli* is the evident target pathogen. The 2010 IDSA guidelines recommend treatment with trimethoprim–sulfamethoxazole for 3 days, nitrofurantoin monohydrate for 3 days, or fosfomycin–trometamol in single dose as standard therapy for acute uncomplicated cystitis (89). Single-dose therapy is less effective in eradicating initial bacteriuria than longer durations, but considering the minimal resistance and low propensity for collateral damage, it is still an appropriate choice (89,90). In contrast, a meta-analysis determined that 3 days of antibiotic therapy is similar to 5 to 10 days in achieving symptomatic cure during uncomplicated UTIs, while the longer treatment is more effective in obtaining bacteriologic cure. Consequently, such durations should be considered for the treatment of women in whom eradication is critical (91). Among fluoroquinolones, ofloxacin, ciprofloxacin, and levofloxacin are highly efficient in 3-day regimens but have a propensity for collateral damage and should be reserved for important uses other than acute cystitis and thus should be considered alternative antimicrobials for acute cystitis (89). The rate of adverse events causing antimicrobial withdrawal tends to be lower with norfloxacin and ciprofloxacin than with other quinolones (92).

Antibiotic treatment of UTI depends on the antibiotic being able to inhibit the growth of, or to kill, the bacteria present in the urinary tract; this is related to the concentration of antibiotics at the site of infection. Very high concentrations of antibiotics with renal clearance are obtained in urine. Consequently, even in the presence of pathogens exhibiting *in vitro* resistance, the high concentrations of antibiotics in urine inhibit the growth of pathogens, rending them effective to treat UTI.

Prostatitis

For outpatients, bacterial prostatitis is a common diagnosis and a frequent indication for antibiotics. Although urethral instrumentation and prostatic surgery are known causes of prostatitis, the incidence of prostatitis among ICU patients has never been assessed, and there is only a weak relation between acute and chronic prostatitis.

Acute prostatitis is an acute infection producing local heat, tenderness, and fever, with the presence of IgA and IgG bacteria-specific immunoglobulins in the prostatic secretions. Most patients with chronic prostatitis have no history of positive urine or urethral cultures (93).

In ICU patients, the rate of acute bacterial prostatitis remains unknown; the patient presents septic, but without an evident source of infection. There may be a history of urine retention due to bladder outlet obstruction. Rectal examination, a crucial step in the diagnosis, reveals a warm, swollen, and tender prostate; the prostatic fluid contains leukocytes and the pathogen responsible for the infection. However, massage of the prostate is proscribed to avoid bacteremia. Acute bacterial prostatitis is a serious infection with fever, intense local pain, and general symptoms. Parenteral administration of high doses of bactericidal antibiotics, such as a broad-spectrum penicillin, a third-generation cephalosporin or fluoroquinolone, should be administered (94). For initial therapy, any of these antibiotics may be combined with an aminoglycoside. Oral therapy can be substituted and continued for a total of 2 to 4 weeks after apyrexia is obtained (94). Fluoroquinolones are the drugs of choice to treat acute prostatitis because of their excellent penetration in the tissue and secretions (95,96). The targeted pathogens are *E. coli, Proteus* sp., *Klebsiella* sp., *Enterococcus* sp., *Staphylococcus aureus, Neisseria gonorrhoeae,* and *Chlamydia trachomatis* (97). For acute prostatitis occurring without bacteremia, antimicrobial treatment consists of oral ofloxacin 200 mg twice per day for 28 days (98); ceftriaxone 2 g/d has good prostatic tissue penetration and represents an alternative to ofloxacin (99). Gentamicin 3 mg/kg/d is added in the presence of positive blood cultures. French guidelines suggest that, if possible, bacterial identification be secured before starting a treatment (100). Of importance, urethral instrumentation should be discouraged and if acute retention occurs, suprapubic drainage of urine is required. Treatment of chronic prostatitis is based on the oral administration of ofloxacin 200 mg twice per day, or trimethroprim 160 mg–sulfamethazole 800 mg twice per day for at least 28 days (94). The indications for this treatment should be discussed with specialists.

Acute Pyelonephritis

The urine of patients with suspicion of complicated pyelonephritis should be cultured and a Gram stain of the spun urine performed. Blood cultures, which are positive in 36% of women not admitted to ICU, are also required (101). There is poor specific data available in the literature on the management of acute pyelonephritis requiring ICU admission. A case series of 68 patients with severe acute pyelonephritis showed 57% had renal dysfunction, 47% shock status, and 56% required ICU admission; additionally, 75% of the patients had radiologic evidence of urinary tract obstruction requiring drainage. Rate of bacteremia was higher than in cases of uncomplicated pyelonephritis, with 57% positive bloodstream cultures (102). All patients with acute pyelonephritis should have an ultrasound examination or a renal computed tomography scan to evaluate for obstruction and stones.

For uncomplicated acute pyelonephritis, the 2010 IDSA guidelines suggest the following: First, oral ciprofloxacin (500 mg twice daily) for 7 days, with or without an initial 400 mg dose of intravenous ciprofloxacin, is an appropriate choice for therapy in patients not requiring hospitalization where the prevalence of resistance of community uropathogens to fluoroquinolones is known not to exceed 10%. In addition, oral trimethoprim–sulfamethoxazole (160/800 mg twice daily for 14 days) is an appropriate choice for therapy if the uropathogen is known to be susceptible. In a comparative study, 255 outpatients were randomized to oral ciprofloxacin, 500 mg twice per day for 7 days followed by placebo for 7 days versus trimethoprim–sulfamethoxazole, 160/800 mg twice per day for 14 days. A 7-day ciprofloxacin regimen was associated with better bacteriologic and clinical cure rates than a 14-day trimethoprim–sulfamethoxazole regimen (103). The second conclusion is that oral β-lactam agents are less effective than other available agents for the treatment of pyelonephritis. Indeed, there is a relatively high prevalence of organisms causing acute pyelonephritis that are resistant to ampicillin, and even for susceptible organisms, there is a significantly increased recurrence rate in patients given ampicillin compared with those given trimethroprim–sulfamethazole. If an oral β-lactam agent is used, an initial intravenous dose of a long-acting parenteral antimicrobial, such as 1 g of ceftriaxone or a consolidated 24-hour dose of an aminoglycoside, is recommended. In any event, 10 to 14 days of therapy with β-lactam appears to be adequate for the majority of women (89).

Patients with pyelonephritis requiring hospitalization should be initially treated with an i.v. antimicrobial regimen, such as a fluoroquinolone, an aminoglycoside, with or without ampicillin, an extended-spectrum cephalosporin or extended-spectrum penicillin, with or without an aminoglycoside, or a carbapenem. The choice between these agents should be based on local resistance data, and the regimen should be tailored on the basis of susceptibility results (89). The targeted bacteria are *Enterobacter* sp., *E. coli, Proteus* sp., and *Enterococcus* sp. Ciprofloxacin, 500 mg twice daily, is administered orally for 14 to 21 days as soon as fever decreases; gentamicin, 3 to 8 mg/kg/day intravenously, is added during the first 3 days.

In all cases, plasma peak concentration (30 minutes after end of perfusion) of gentamicin must reach six to eight times the minimal inhibitory concentration (MIC) of treated bacteria to guarantee efficient treatment. Interestingly, oral ciprofloxacin is as effective as the i.v. regimen in the initial empirical management of complicated pyelonephritis (104), and gatifloxacin is as effective as ciprofloxacin (105). If needed, ceftriaxone (2 g/d i.v.) is an alternative choice to ciprofloxacin. Further, the success rates are similar in patients given ceftriaxone or ertapenem (106).

The drainage of urine must be urgently performed using bladder catheterization, percutaneous nephrostomy drainage, or definitive surgery. Antimicrobial treatment is administered after urine and blood specimen collection. The antibiotic selection is based on the result of the Gram stain of the urine and the knowledge of the local ecology. Antimicrobial treatment should be adapted to the susceptibility testing results as soon as possible, and de-escalation be performed in favor of a narrow-spectrum antibiotic.

Specificities of Complicated UTIs in the ICU

Although there is little in the literature on the treatment of UTIs in the ICU, one presumes the need for i.v. antibiotics for these patients because of the possibility of bacteremia or sepsis. The guidelines from the Surviving Sepsis Campaign state that (i) antibiotic therapy should be started within the first hour of recognition of severe sepsis, after appropriate cultures have been obtained; (ii) initial empirical anti-infective therapy should include one or more drugs that have activity against the likely pathogens and that penetrate the presumed source of sepsis; (iii) monotherapy is as effective as combination therapy with a β-lactam and an aminoglycoside as empiric therapy of patients with severe sepsis or septic shock (107). Hence, empirical antimicrobial therapy should include drugs with good penetration in the urinary tract, and the choice is guided by the susceptibility patterns of micro-organisms in the hospital. For the septic shock patients whose presumed source is urine, we recommend, empirically, a combination of a β-lactam antibiotic with antipseudomonal activity and an aminoglycoside. This broad-spectrum treatment is narrowed as soon as the results of the susceptibility testing are known. The durations of treatment should be tailored to the source of infection.

Management of Candiduria

Candiduria represents from 3% to 15% of catheter-associated UTI in the ICU (10, 23,108). *Candida albicans* and *C. (Torulopsis) glabrata* are found in 46% to 60%, and 31% of cases, respectively (108,109). According to the international guidelines, colonized patients without evidence of infection do not require treatment (110,111). But the contributing cause should be addressed such as changing or removing the IUBC and discontinuing inappropriate antibiotic therapy (34). Fluconazole may be the best option for treating candiduria, in case of urologic surgery, for example, but only if the species is *C. albicans* (110); voriconazole or amphotericin B may be more effective against non-*albicans* species (111).

Clinician reaction to isolating *Candida* organisms in urine was assessed in a retrospective review of 133 consecutive patients. The average patient age was 68.8 years old, most (78%) had an IUBC, and many (35%) were in the ICU. In response to culture results, clinicians initiated antifungal therapy in 80 instances (60%); treatment was often based on a single culture result without evidence of infection (66%) and in the absence of risk of invasive disease. Removal of the IUBC was never attempted and antibiotics were rarely discontinued or modified (1.3%). Fluconazole was the most frequently utilized (52%) agent, followed by amphotericin-B bladder irrigation (32%), and combined fluconazole/amphotericin-B bladder irrigation (15%). Therapy was more frequently initiated in ICU cases (77% vs. 56%; $p = 0.02$) (112). These results show a worrisome lack of adherence to established guidelines.

A prospective, randomized trial compared fungal eradication rates among 316 hospitalized patients with candiduria treated with fluconazole (200 mg) or placebo daily for 14 days. Candiduria cleared by day 14 in 50% of the patients receiving fluconazole and 29% of those receiving placebo, with higher eradication rates among patients completing 14 days of therapy. While fluconazole initially produced high eradication rates, cultures at 2 weeks revealed similar candiduria rates among treated and untreated patients. In 41% of the catheterized subjects, candiduria was resolved as the result of catheter removal only. The outcomes of patients were not provided in the results (113).

Bladder irrigation using amphotericin B has been proposed as an alternative technique to clear *Candida* from the urine. A comparative and randomized study of 109 elderly patients showed that fungiuria was eradicated in 96% of the patients treated with amphotericin B, and 73% of those treated with fluconazole ($p < 0.05$). One month after study enrollment, the mortality rate associated with all causes was greater among patients who were treated with amphotericin B bladder irrigation than among those who received oral fluconazole therapy (41% vs. 22%, respectively; $p < 0.05$); this finding suggests that irrigation therapy could be associated with poorer survival (114). Reviews suggest that amphotericin B bladder irrigation is as effective as oral fluconazole to treat asymptomatic candiduria. The best method is to use continuous irrigation for more than 5 days. The level of the literature cannot allow drawing definitive conclusions (115).

There has only been one study performed in ICU patients developing candiduria, which reached the same conclusions; unfortunately, methodologic issues restrict the interest of this study. The authors retrospectively compared three means to manage candiduria in ICU patients: successful bladder irrigation with amphotericin B (10/27 patients), failure of bladder irrigation requiring the use of parenteral amphotericin B (n = 17/27), and patients treated with parenteral fluconazole (n = 20). Severity score on the day of admission was significantly lower in the first group than in the two others. However, the mortality rate was 53% and 5% in patients who failed bladder irrigation and in patients receiving fluconazole, respectively (116). These results must be considered with caution because of serious methodologic limitations. However, these data indicate that bladder irrigation of critically ill patients has a negative survival advantage.

Key Points

- Preventing or reducing the duration of catheterization is the most important intervention in preventing CAUTIs.
- The initial indication for the placement of an IUBC was unjustified in 15% of patients and unclear in 28% of patients.
- Pathogens among ICU patients with bacteriuria are *E. coli, P. aeruginosa, Enterococcus* species, 70% of cases.
- Polymicrobial infections represent only 5% to 12% of cases.
- Comparison of nitrofurazone-coated and silver alloy–coated catheters results in a superiority of antibiotic-coated in reducing bacteriuria and symptomatic CAUTI, but the magnitude of reduction is low and hence may not be clinically relevant.
- Bacteria in the bladder constitute a reservoir for the development of multiresistant bacterial strains.
- The rate of bacteriuria may be used as a marker of the level of care in the ICU.
- Prevention of UTIs in the ICU is not improved by the use of expensive devices, but can reflect the level of general unit hygiene.
- While management of UTIs in the ICU is poorly described in the literature, it is reasonably clear that there is no need to treat asymptomatic bacteriuria.
- Although infrequent, severe sepsis whose source is urine requires empirical broad-spectrum antimicrobial treatment based upon the local bacterial ecology. Treatment is de-escalated after identification of the pathogen and reporting of the susceptibility testing.

References

1. Rosenthal VD, Maki DG, Mehta Y, et al. International Nosocomial Infection Control Consortium (INICC) report, data summary of 43 countries for 2007–2012: device-associated module. *Am J Infect Control.* 2014;42:942–956.
2. Chant C, Smith OM, Marshall JC, et al. Relationship of catheter-associated urinary tract infection to mortality and length of stay in critically ill patients: a systematic review and meta-analysis of observational studies. *Crit Care Med.* 2011;39:1167–1173.
3. Wagenlehner FM, Cek M, Naber KG, et al. Epidemiology, treatment and prevention of healthcare-associated urinary tract infections. *World J Urol.* 2012;30:59–67.
4. Vincent JL, Rello J, Marshall J, et al.; EPIC II Group of Investigators. International study of the prevalence and outcomes of infection in intensive care units. *JAMA.* 2009;302:2323–2329.
5. Tedja R, Wentink J, O'Horo JC, et al. Catheter-associated urinary tract infections in intensive care unit patients. *Infect Control Hosp Epidemiol.* 2015;36:1330–1334.
6. *Catheter-associated urinary tract infections (CAUTI).* CDC website. Available at: http://www.cdc.gov/HAI/ca_uti/uti.html. Updated October 16, 2015; accessed October 31, 2015.
7. Flores-Mireles AL, Walker JN, Caparon M, et al. Urinary tract infections: epidemiology, mechanisms of infection and treatment options. *Nat Rev Microbiol.* 2015;13:269–284.
8. Stapleton AE. Urinary tract infection pathogenesis: host factors. *Infect Dis Clin North Am.* 2014;28:149–159.
9. Jacobsen SM, Shirtliff ME. Proteus mirabilis biofilms and catheter-associated urinary tract infections. *Virulence.* 2011;2:460–465.
10. Leone M, Albanèse J, Garnier F, et al. Risk factors of nosocomial catheter-associated urinary tract infection in a polyvalent intensive care unit. *Intensive Care Med.* 2003;29:1077–1080.
11. Gaynes R, Edwards JR. National Nosocomial Infections Surveillance System. Overview of nosocomial infections caused by gram-negative bacilli. *Clin Infect Dis Off Publ Infect Dis Soc Am.* 2005;41:848–854.
12. Bottiggi AJ, White KD, Bernard AC, Davenport DL. Impact of device-associated infection on trauma patient outcomes at a major trauma center. *Surg Infect.* 2015;16:276–280.
13. Tissot E, Limat S, Cornette C, Capellier G. Risk factors for catheter-associated bacteriuria in a medical intensive care unit. *Eur J Clin Microbiol Infect Dis Off Publ Eur Soc Clin Microbiol.* 2001;20:260–262.
14. Burton DC, Edwards JR, Srinivasan A, et al. Trends in catheter-associated urinary tract infections in adult intensive care units-United States, 1990–2007. *Infect Control Hosp Epidemiol.* 2011;32:748–756.

15. Apisarnthanarak A, Rutjanawech S, Wichansawakun S, et al. Initial inappropriate urinary catheters use in a tertiary-care center: incidence, risk factors, and outcomes. *Am J Infect Control.* 2007;35:594–599.
16. Jain P, Parada JP, David A, Smith LG. Overuse of the indwelling urinary tract catheter in hospitalized medical patients. *Arch Intern Med.* 1995; 155:1425–1429.
17. Schnarr J, Smaill F: Asymptomatic bacteriuria and symptomatic urinary tract infections in pregnancy. *Eur J Clin Invest.* 2008;38 Suppl 2:50–57.
18. Platt R. Adverse consequences of asymptomatic urinary tract infections in adults. *Am J Med.* 1987;82:47–52.
19. Platt R, Polk BF, Murdock B, et al. Mortality associated with nosocomial urinary-tract infection. *N Engl J Med.* 1982;307:637–642.
20. Mnatzaganian G, Galai N, Sprung CL, et al. Increased risk of bloodstream and urinary infections in intensive care unit (ICU) patients compared with patients fitting ICU admission criteria treated in regular wards. *J Hosp Infect.* 2005;59:331–342.
21. Vincent J-L, Sakr Y, Sprung CL, et al. Sepsis in European intensive care units: results of the SOAP study. *Crit Care Med.* 2006;34:344–353.
22. Angus DC, Linde-Zwirble WT, Lidicker J, et al. Epidemiology of severe sepsis in the United States: analysis of incidence, outcome, and associated costs of care. *Crit Care Med.* 2001;29:1303–1310.
23. Laupland KB, Bagshaw SM, Gregson DB, et al. Intensive care unit-acquired urinary tract infections in a regional critical care system. *Crit Care Lond Engl.* 2005;9:R60–R65.
24. Fortin E, Rocher I, Frenette C, et al. Healthcare-associated bloodstream infections secondary to a urinary focus: the Québec provincial surveillance results. *Infect Control Hosp Epidemiol.* 2012;33:456–462.
25. Leone M, Perrin AS, Granier I, et al. A randomized trial of catheter change and short course of antibiotics for asymptomatic bacteriuria in catheterized ICU patients. *Intensive Care Med.* 2007;33:726–729.
26. Greene MT, Chang R, Kuhn L, et al. Predictors of hospital-acquired urinary tract-related bloodstream infection. *Infect Control Hosp Epidemiol.* 2012;33:1001–1007.
27. Inan D, Saba R, Gunseren F, et al. Daily antibiotic cost of nosocomial infections in a Turkish university hospital. *BMC Infect Dis.* 2005;5:5.
28. Garibaldi RA, Mooney BR, Epstein BJ, et al. An evaluation of daily bacteriologic monitoring to identify preventable episodes of catheter-associated urinary tract infection. *Infect Control IC.* 1982;3:466–470.
29. Tissot E, Woronoff-Lemsi MC, Cornette C, et al. Cost-effectiveness of urinary dipsticks to screen asymptomatic catheter-associated urinary infections in an intensive care unit. *Intensive Care Med.* 2001;27:1842–1847.
30. Coman T, Troché G, Semoun O, et al. Diagnostic accuracy of urinary dipstick to exclude catheter-associated urinary tract infection in ICU patients: a reappraisal. *Infection.* 2014;42:661–668.
31. Legras A, Cattier B, Perrotin D. Dépistage des infections urinaires dans un service de réanimation: intérêt des badelettes réactives. *Med Mal Infect.* 1993;23:34–36.
32. Mimoz O, Bouchet E, Edouard A, et al. Limited usefulness of urinary dipsticks to screen out catheter-associated bacteriuria in ICU patients. *Anaesth Intensive Care.* 1995;23:706–707.
33. Krogsbøll LT, Jørgensen KJ, Gøtzsche PC: Screening with urinary dipsticks for reducing morbidity and mortality. *Cochrane Database Syst Rev.* 2015;1:CD010007.
34. Hooton TM, Bradley SF, Cardenas DD, et al. Diagnosis, prevention, and treatment of catheter-associated urinary tract infection in adults. 2009 International Clinical Practice Guidelines from the Infectious Diseases Society of America. *Clin Infect Dis Off Publ Infect Dis Soc Am.* 2010;50:625–663.
35. Warren JW. Catheter-associated urinary tract infections. *Int J Antimicrob Agents.* 2001;17:299–303.
36. Kunin CM, McCormack RC. Prevention of catheter-induced urinary-tract infections by a new sterile closed drainage system. *Antimicrob Agents Chemother.* 1965;5:631–638.
37. Platt R, Polk BF, Murdock B, et al. Reduction of mortality associated with nosocomial urinary tract infection. *Lancet Lond Engl.* 1983;1:893–897.
38. Huth TS, Burke JP, Larsen RA, et al. Clinical trial of junction seals for the prevention of urinary catheter-associated bacteriuria. *Arch Intern Med.* 1992;152:807–812.
39. DeGroot-Kosolcharoen J, Guse R, Jones JM. Evaluation of a urinary catheter with a preconnected closed drainage bag. *Infect Control Hosp Epidemiol.* 1988;9:72–76.
40. Leone M, Garnier F, Antonini F, et al. Comparison of effectiveness of two urinary drainage systems in intensive care unit: a prospective, randomized clinical trial. *Intensive Care Med.* 2003;29:410–413.
41. Leone M, Garnier F, Dubuc M, et al. Prevention of nosocomial urinary tract infection in ICU patients: comparison of effectiveness of two urinary drainage systems. *Chest.* 2001;120:220–224.
42. Lam TB, Omar MI, Fisher E, et al. Types of indwelling urethral catheters for short-term catheterisation in hospitalised adults. *Cochrane Database Syst Rev.* 2014;9:CD004013.
43. Umscheid CA, Agarwal RK, Brennan PJ, et al. Updating the guideline development methodology of the Healthcare Infection Control Practices Advisory Committee (HICPAC). *Am J Infect Control.* 2010;38:264–273.
44. National Clinical Guideline Centre (UK). Infection: prevention and control of healthcare-associated infections in primary and community care: partial update of NICE clinical guideline. Avaialable at: http://www.ncbi.nlm.nih.gov/books/NBK115271./ Published 2012; accessed November 11, 2015.
45. Stensballe J, Tvede M, Looms D, et al. Infection risk with nitrofurazone-impregnated urinary catheters in trauma patients: a randomized trial. *Ann Intern Med.* 2007;147:285–293.
46. Schumm K, Lam TB. Types of urethral catheters for management of short-term voiding problems in hospitalised adults. *Cochrane Database Syst Rev.* 2008;CD004013.
47. Pickard R, Lam T, MacLennan G, et al. Antimicrobial catheters for reduction of symptomatic urinary tract infection in adults requiring short-term catheterisation in hospital: a multicentre randomised controlled trial. *Lancet Lond Engl.* 2012;380:1927–1935.
48. Leone M. Prevention of CAUTI: simple is beautiful. *Lancet Lond Engl.* 2012;380:1891–1892.
49. Thibon P, Le Coutour X, Leroyer R, Fabry J. Randomized multi-centre trial of the effects of a catheter coated with hydrogel and silver salts on the incidence of hospital-acquired urinary tract infections. *J Hosp Infect.* 2000;45:117–124.
50. Prieto J, Murphy CL, Moore KN, et al. Intermittent catheterisation for long-term bladder management. *Cochrane Database Syst Rev.* 2014;9:CD006008.
51. Warren JW, Platt R, Thomas RJ, et al. Antibiotic irrigation and catheter-associated urinary-tract infections. *N Engl J Med.* 1978;299:570–573.
52. Schneeberger PM, Vreede RW, Bogdanowicz JF, et al. A randomized study on the effect of bladder irrigation with povidone-iodine before removal of an indwelling catheter. *J Hosp Infect.* 1992;21:223–229.
53. Hagen S, Sinclair L, Cross S. Washout policies in long-term indwelling urinary catheterisation in adults. *Cochrane Database Syst Rev.* 2010; CD004012.
54. Thompson RL, Haley CE, Searcy MA, et al. Catheter-associated bacteriuria: failure to reduce attack rates using periodic instillations of a disinfectant into urinary drainage systems. *JAMA.* 1984;251:747–751.
55. Vandoni RE, Lironi A, Tschantz P. Bacteriuria during urinary tract catheterization: suprapubic versus urethral route: a prospective randomized trial. *Acta Chir Belg.* 1994;94:12–16.
56. McPhail MJ, Abu-Hilal M, Johnson CD. A meta-analysis comparing suprapubic and transurethral catheterization for bladder drainage after abdominal surgery. *Br J Surg.* 2006;93:1038–1044.
57. Healy DA, Walsh CA, Walsh SR. Suprapubic versus transurethral bladder catheterization following pelvic surgery. *Curr Opin Obstet Gynecol.* 2013;25:410–413.
58. Harti A, Bouaggad A, Barrou H, et al. [Prevention of nosocomial urinary tract infection: vesical catheter versus Penilex]. *Cah Anesth.* 1994;42: 31–34.
59. Grigoryan L, Abers MS, Kizilbash QF, et al. A comparison of the microbiologic profile of indwelling versus external urinary catheters. *Am J Infect Control.* 2014;42:682–684.
60. Saint S, Kaufman SR, Rogers MA, et al. Condom versus indwelling urinary catheters: a randomized trial. *J Am Geriatr Soc.* 2006;54:1055–1061.
61. Tang MW, Kwok TC, Hui E, Woo J. Intermittent versus indwelling urinary catheterization in older female patients. *Maturitas.* 2006;53:274–281.
62. Ghalayini IF, Al-Ghazo MA, Pickard RS. A prospective randomized trial comparing transurethral prostatic resection and clean intermittent self-catheterization in men with chronic urinary retention. *BJU Int.* 2005;96: 93–97.
63. Bregenzer T, Frei R, Widmer AF, et al. Low risk of bacteremia during catheter replacement in patients with long-term urinary catheters. *Arch Intern Med.* 1997;157:521–525.
64. Lusardi G, Lipp A, Shaw C. Antibiotic prophylaxis for short-term catheter bladder drainage in adults. *Cochrane Database Syst Rev.* 2013;7: CD005428.
65. Saint S, Olmsted RN, Fakih MG, et al. Translating health care-associated urinary tract infection prevention research into practice via the bladder bundle. *Jt Comm J Qual Patient Saf Jt Comm Resour.* 2009;35:449–455.
66. Saint S, Greene MT, Kowalski CP, et al. Preventing catheter-associated urinary tract infection in the United States: a national comparative study. *JAMA Intern Med.* 2013;173:874–879.
67. Meddings J, Rogers MA, Krein SL, et al. Reducing unnecessary urinary catheter use and other strategies to prevent catheter-associated urinary tract infection: an integrative review. *BMJ Qual Saf.* 2014;23:277–289.

68. Byrnes MC, Schuerer DJ, Schallom ME, et al. Implementation of a mandatory checklist of protocols and objectives improves compliance with a wide range of evidence-based intensive care unit practices. *Crit Care Med.* 2009;37:2775–2781.
69. Hazan Z, Zumeris J, Jacob H, et al. Effective prevention of microbial biofilm formation on medical devices by low-energy surface acoustic waves. *Antimicrob Agents Chemother.* 2006;50:4144–4152.
70. Carson L, Gorman SP, Gilmore BF. The use of lytic bacteriophages in the prevention and eradication of biofilms of *Proteus mirabilis* and *Escherichia coli. FEMS Immunol Med Microbiol.* 2010;59:447–455.
71. Beetz R. Mild dehydration: a risk factor of urinary tract infection? *Eur J Clin Nutr.* 2003;57(Suppl. 2):S52–S58.
72. Nicolle LE, Bradley S, Colgan R, et al. Infectious Diseases Society of America guidelines for the diagnosis and treatment of asymptomatic bacteriuria in adults. *Clin Infect Dis Off Publ Infect Dis Soc Am.* 2005;40:643–654.
73. Harding GK, Nicolle LE, Ronald AR, et al. How long should catheter-acquired urinary tract infection in women be treated? A randomized controlled study. *Ann Intern Med.* 1991;114:713–719.
74. Stamey TA, Fair WR, Timothy MM, et al. Serum versus urinary antimicrobial concentrations in cure of urinary-tract infections. *N Engl J Med.* 1974;291:1159–1163.
75. Frimodt-Møller N. Correlation between pharmacokinetic/pharmacodynamic parameters and efficacy for antibiotics in the treatment of urinary tract infection. *Int J Antimicrob Agents.* 2002;19:546–553.
76. Leone M, Albanèse J, Tod M, et al. Ceftriaxone (1 g intravenously) penetration into abdominal tissues when administered as antibiotic prophylaxis during nephrectomy. *J Chemother Florence Italy.* 2003;15:139–142.
77. Leroy A, Oser B, Grise P, et al. Cefixime penetration in human renal parenchyma. *Antimicrob Agents Chemother.* 1995;39:1240–1242.
78. Saito I, Saiko Y, Tahara T, et al. Penetration of cefpirome into renal and prostatic tissue. *Int J Clin Pharmacol Res.* 1993;13:317–324.
79. Charalabopoulos K, Karachalios G, Baltogiannis D, et al. Penetration of antimicrobial agents into the prostate. *Chemotherapy.* 2003;49:269–279.
80. Udy AA, Roberts JA, Lipman J. Clinical implications of antibiotic pharmacokinetic principles in the critically ill. *Intensive Care Med.* 2013; 39:2070–2082.
81. Sime FB, Roberts MS, Peake SL, et al. Does β-lactam pharmacokinetic variability in critically ill patients justify therapeutic drug monitoring? A systematic review. *Ann Intensive Care.* 2012;2:35.
82. Ulldemolins M, Vaquer S, Llauradó-Serra M, et al. Beta-lactam dosing in critically ill patients with septic shock and continuous renal replacement therapy. *Crit Care Lond Engl.* 2014;18:227.
83. Neu HC. Optimal characteristics of agents to treat uncomplicated urinary tract infections. *Infection.* 1992;20 Suppl 4:S266–S271.
84. Ray GT, Baxter R, DeLorenze GN. Hospital-level rates of fluoroquinolone use and the risk of hospital-acquired infection with ciprofloxacin-nonsusceptible *Pseudomonas aeruginosa. Clin Infect Dis Off Publ Infect Dis Soc Am.* 2005;41:441–449.
85. Pakyz AL, Lee JA, Ababneh MA, et al. Fluoroquinolone use and fluoroquinolone-resistant *Pseudomonas aeruginosa* is declining in US academic medical centre hospitals. *J Antimicrob Chemother.* 2012;67:1562–1564.
86. Lafaurie M, Porcher R, Donay J-L, et al. Reduction of fluoroquinolone use is associated with a decrease in methicillin-resistant *Staphylococcus aureus* and fluoroquinolone-resistant *Pseudomonas aeruginosa* isolation rates: a 10 year study. *J Antimicrob Chemother.* 2012;67:1010–1015.
87. Gallini A, Degris E, Desplas M, et al. Influence of fluoroquinolone consumption in inpatients and outpatients on ciprofloxacin-resistant *Escherichia coli* in a university hospital. *J Antimicrob Chemother.* 2010;65: 2650–2657.
88. Naber KG, Witte W, Bauernfeind A, et al. Clinical significance and spread of fluoroquinolone resistant uropathogens in hospitalised urological patients. *Infection.* 1994;22(Suppl. 2):S122–S127.
89. Gupta K, Hooton TM, Naber KG, et al. International clinical practice guidelines for the treatment of acute uncomplicated cystitis and pyelonephritis in women: A. 2010 update by the Infectious Diseases Society of America and the European Society for Microbiology and Infectious Diseases. *Clin Infect Dis Off Publ Infect Dis Soc Am.* 2011;52:e103–120.
90. Matsumoto T, Muratani T, Nakahama C, Tomono K. Clinical effects of 2 days of treatment by fosfomycin calcium for acute uncomplicated cystitis in women. *J Infect Chemother.* 2011;17(1):80–86.
91. Milo G, Katchman EA, Paul M, et al. Duration of antibacterial treatment for uncomplicated urinary tract infection in women. *Cochrane Database Syst Rev.* 2005;(2):CD004682.
92. Rafalsky V, Andreeva I, Rjabkova E. Quinolones for uncomplicated acute cystitis in women. *Cochrane Database Syst Rev.* 2006;(3):CD003597.
93. Krieger JN, Riley DE. Prostatitis: what is the role of infection. *Int J Antimicrob Agents.* 2002;19:475–479.
94. *Urological infections.* European Association of Urology website. https://uroweb.org/guideline/urological-infections/. Accessed November 14, 2015.
95. Hurtado FK, Weber B, Derendorf H, et al. Population pharmacokinetic modeling of the unbound levofloxacin concentrations in rat plasma and prostate tissue measured by microdialysis. *Antimicrob Agents Chemother.* 2014;58:678–686.
96. Wagenlehner FM, Naber KG. Current challenges in the treatment of complicated urinary tract infections and prostatitis. *Clin Microbiol Infect Off Publ Eur Soc Clin Microbiol Infect Dis.* 2006;12(Suppl 3):67–80.
97. Schneider H, Ludwig M, Hossain HM, et al. The 2001 Giessen Cohort Study on patients with prostatitis syndrome: an evaluation of inflammatory status and search for microorganisms. 10 years after a first analysis. *Andrologia.* 2003;35:258–262.
98. Ulleryd P, Sandberg T. Ciprofloxacin for 2 or 4 weeks in the treatment of febrile urinary tract infection in men: a randomized trial with a 1 year follow-up. *Scand J Infect Dis.* 2003;35:34–39.
99. Martin C, Viviand X, Cottin A, et al. Concentrations of ceftriaxone (1,000 milligrams intravenously) in abdominal tissues during open prostatectomy. *Antimicrob Agents Chemother.* 1996;40:1311–1313.
100. Caron F. [Diagnosis and treatment of community-acquired urinary tract infections in adults: what has changed: comments on the 2008 guidelines of the French Health Products Safety Agency (AFSSAPS)]. *Presse Médicale Paris Fr 1983.* 2010;39:42–48.
101. Smith WR, McClish DK, Poses RM, et al. Bacteremia in young urban women admitted with pyelonephritis. *Am J Med Sci.* 1997;313:50–57.
102. Chung VY, Tai CK, Fan CW, et al. Severe acute pyelonephritis: a review of clinical outcome and risk factors for mortality. *Hong Kong Med J Xianggang Yi Xue Za Zhi Hong Kong Acad Med.* 2014;20:285–289.
103. Talan DA, Stamm WE, Hooton TM, et al. Comparison of ciprofloxacin (7 days) and trimethoprim-sulfamethoxazole (14 days) for acute uncomplicated pyelonephritis pyelonephritis in women: a randomized trial. *JAMA.* 2000;283:1583–1590.
104. Mombelli G, Pezzoli R, Pinoja-Lutz G, et al. Oral vs intravenous ciprofloxacin in the initial empirical management of severe pyelonephritis or complicated urinary tract infections: a prospective randomized clinical trial. *Arch Intern Med.* 1999;159:53–58.
105. Naber KG, Bartnicki A, Bischoff W, et al. Gatifloxacin 200 mg or 400 mg once daily is as effective as ciprofloxacin 500 mg twice daily for the treatment of patients with acute pyelonephritis or complicated urinary tract infections. *Int J Antimicrob Agents.* 2004;23(Suppl 1):S41–53.
106. Wells WG, Woods GL, Jiang Q, et al. Treatment of complicated urinary tract infection in adults: combined analysis of two randomized, double-blind, multicentre trials comparing ertapenem and ceftriaxone followed by appropriate oral therapy. *J Antimicrob Chemother.* 2004;53(Suppl 2):ii67–74.
107. Dellinger RP, Levy MM, Rhodes A, et al. Surviving sepsis campaign: international guidelines for management of severe sepsis and septic shock: 2012. *Crit Care Med.* 2013;41:580–637.
108. Padawer D, Pastukh N, Nitzan O, et al. Catheter-associated candiduria: risk factors, medical interventions, and antifungal susceptibility. *Am J Infect Control.* 2015;43:e19–22.
109. Leone M, Albanèse J, Antonini F, et al. Long-term epidemiological survey of *Candida* species: comparison of isolates found in an intensive care unit and in conventional wards. *J Hosp Infect.* 2003;55:169–174.
110. Behzadi P, Behzadi E, Ranjbar R. Urinary tract infections and *Candida albicans. Cent Eur J Urol.* 2015;68:96–101.
111. Kauffman CA. Diagnosis and management of fungal urinary tract infection. *Infect Dis Clin North Am.* 2014;28:61–74.
112. Ayeni O, Riederer KM, Wilson FM, et al. Clinicians' reaction to positive urine culture for Candida organisms. *Mycoses.* 1999;42:285–289.
113. Sobel JD, Kauffman CA, McKinsey D, et al. Candiduria: a randomized, double-blind study of treatment with fluconazole and placebo. The National Institute of Allergy and Infectious Diseases (NIAID) Mycoses Study Group. *Clin Infect Dis Off Publ Infect Dis Soc Am.* 2000;30:19–24.
114. Jacobs LG, Skidmore EA, Freeman K, et al. Oral fluconazole compared with bladder irrigation with amphotericin B for treatment of fungal urinary tract infections in elderly patients. *Clin Infect Dis Off Publ Infect Dis Soc Am.* 1996;22:30–35.
115. Tuon FF, Amato VS, Penteado Filho SR. Bladder irrigation with amphotericin B and fungal urinary tract infection–systematic review with meta-analysis. *Int J Infect Dis IJID Off Publ Int Soc Infect Dis.* 2009;13:701–706.
116. Nassoura Z, Ivatury RR, Simon RJ, et al. Candiduria as an early marker of disseminated infection in critically ill surgical patients: the role of fluconazole therapy. *J Trauma.* 1993;35:290–294.

Section 4

Adult Gastrointestinal Infections

LAYTH AL-JASHAAMI and HERBERT L. DUPONT

INTRODUCTION

Acute diarrhea and acute gastroenteritis with vomiting occurring outside the hospital are most often secondary to viral infection. Most cases of health care–associated diarrhea are not etiologically defined, with *Clostridium difficile* being the most important definable cause of illness, identified in 10% to 20% of cases. In the United States, approximately 179 million cases of acute diarrhea occur each year, amounting to 0.6 episodes/person/yr, with approximately 11,255 deaths yearly, of which 83% occur in adults 65 years of age or older (1). The most communicable enteric pathogens are noroviruses and *Shigella* spp. due to their low inoculum requirements, stability in the environment, and because children often harbor the pathogens (2).

Diarrhea is commonly defined as passage of three or more loose stools/d or passage a total stool weight/volume of 250 g/mL of unformed stool/d. The following definitions have been suggested taking into account diarrheal duration:

- *Acute*—up to 14 days
- *Persistent*—14 days or more
- *Chronic*—30 days or more

The cause of the diarrheal illness is divided into three groups: viruses, bacteria, and bacterial toxins and protozoal parasites. Noninfectious causes of diarrhea are characteristically associated with chronic diarrhea.

The severity of diarrhea can be determined functionally:

- Mild—requires no change in activities
- Moderate—requires a change in activities but does not disable
- Severe—disables, usually confining the affected person to bed. It is the severe forms of diarrhea that usually lead to hospitalization

ETIOLOGY OF ACUTE DIARRHEA IN THE UNITED STATES

Diarrhea can be divided into community-acquired, health care–acquired, and traveler's diarrhea (TD). Community-acquired acute infectious diarrhea is caused by various micro-organisms including bacteria, viruses, and parasites. With widespread use of rotavirus vaccine in the United States, the major viral pathogens seen are a number of noroviruses of which genogroup II, genotype 4 is the most important (3). Noroviruses cause approximately half of all diarrhea for which a cause of illness can be found; noroviruses are usually intense but persist for no more than 60 hours, and do not usually require therapy. For the elderly and infirm, especially after organ and stem cell transplantation, the noroviruses can cause severe and chronic illness and may be fatal (3). Most cases of diarrhea in the community have undefinable causes of illness using currently available diagnostic tests.

The etiology of diarrheal cases presenting to a hospital and hospital-acquired diarrhea is different from the community-based diarrhea. Diarrhea acquired in the hospital is generally not associated with a definable pathogen, although the most important definable pathogen in hospital-acquired diarrhea is *C. difficile*.

EVALUATION OF THE PATIENT WITH SEVERE DIARRHEA

Emergency Department

The first priority in the ED is to evaluate the stability and hydration status of the patient by examining vital signs, mucous membranes, sensorium, and looking for postural hypotension. Rehydration is the mainstay of treatment of gastrointestinal infection; many cases can be treated and maintained using oral rehydration therapy (ORT), although in the United States, most patients with any degree of dehydration are treated with i.v. fluids. Secondly, electrolyte disturbances need to be sought and corrected; electrolyte imbalances may vary depending on the cause and also on other comorbid conditions. The primary concern is to immediately reverse circulatory or organ failure resulting from loss of fluid and salt.

Diagnostic investigations for identifying the causative agent should be done either simultaneously or after stabilization of the patient. Most of the cases requiring hospitalization are due to bacterial causes rather than viral, which tend to be mild. Epidemiologic history and clinical features may provide clues to the diagnosis, for example, prior travel to an economically developing country suggests a bacterial cause of diarrhea. Diarrhea in a person receiving antibacterial or chemotherapeutic drugs suggests *C. difficile* as the etiologic agent. Proctitis in a male with a history of having unprotected receptive anal intercourse suggests sexually transmitted pathogens including *Neisseria gonorrhoeae*, *Chlamydia trachomatis*, herpes simplex, or *Treponema pallidum*. A diagnostic algorithm is provided to help identify important steps in the workup of patients with acute diarrhea (Fig. 88.4.2).

If the patient with diarrhea is taking a proton pump inhibitor (PPI), they are susceptible to a large number of enteric pathogens (4) as acidic pH of the stomach is one of the important barriers to prevent enteric infection.

The laboratory will help establish the diagnosis. Finding many fecal leukocytes in stool indicates the patient has diffuse colonic inflammation; occult blood in the stool supports an inflammatory type of diarrhea. Other tests for colonic inflammation include studies for the presence of lactoferrin or calprotectin, constituents of polymorphonuclear

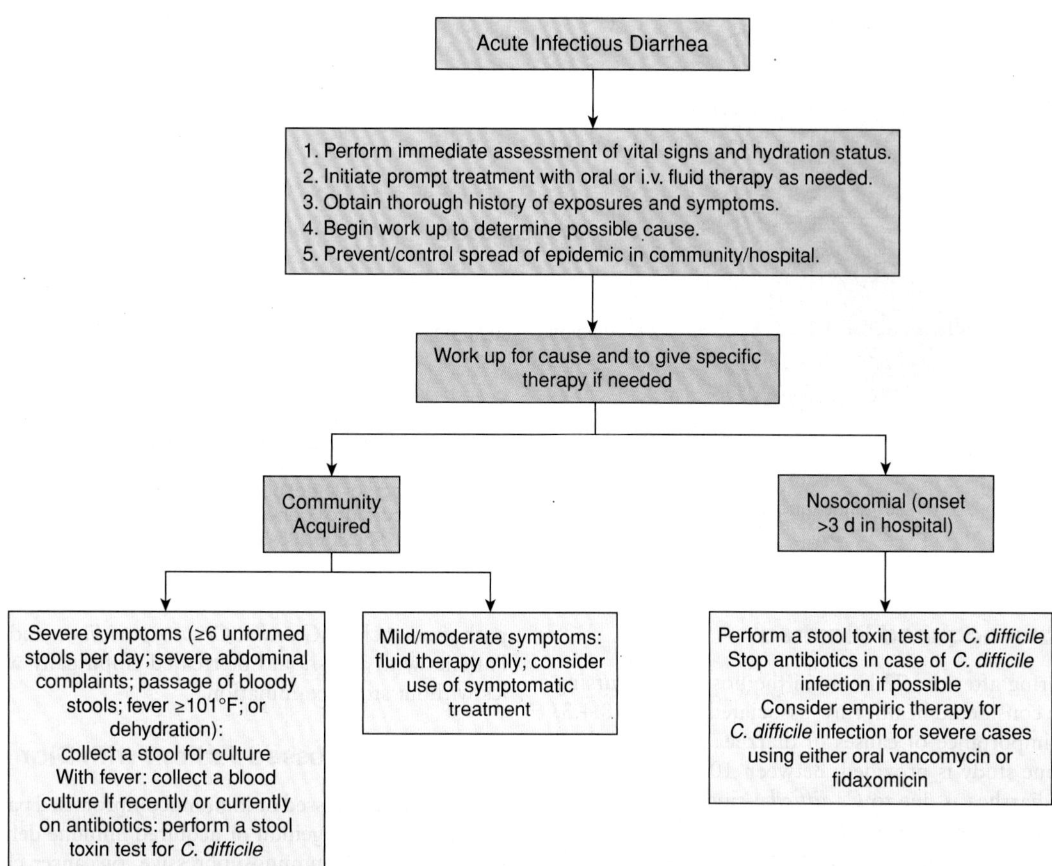

FIGURE 88.4.2 Flow chart showing approach to the evaluation of a patient with acute infectious diarrhea.

leukocytes (5). Gross blood in the stool with mucus may indicate a dysenteric pathogen, such as *Shigella, Campylobacter, Salmonella,* Shigatoxin-producing *Escherichia coli* (often *E. coli* O157:H7) or *C. difficile.* Stool cultures, parasite examination, or stool toxin test for *C. difficile* may help define the cause of the illness. Some characteristics, when present, requiring aggressive and thorough laboratory workup are fever over 102°F (38.9°C), severe diarrhea, presence of dehydration, presence of dysentery, and coexistence of important immunosuppressive disorder. Physical examination is important and should focus on vital signs—fever, heart rate, and blood pressure including postural hypotension—volume status, abdominal tenderness, and systemic complications. Rectal examination should be performed to assess stool for gross and occult blood; painful hemorrhoids from frequent defecation may be detected. A white blood count may reveal leukocytosis or a shift to the left in neutrophils suggesting a severe inflammatory process of the gut; this finding warrants stool studies, culture if the diarrhea is community acquired and *C. difficile* fecal toxin test if health care–associated. Eosinophilia may be seen in parasitic infection (e.g., strongyloidiasis).

Once disease onset, presentation, and progression of associated symptoms are evaluated, and immediate laboratory work has been performed, it may be useful to categorize the diarrhea into one of two physiologic classifications: noninflammatory and inflammatory (Table 88.4.24). A subcategory of inflammatory is hemorrhagic or dysenteric diarrhea; distinction of the specific type of diarrhea is helpful to focus on appropriate empiric management options.

TABLE 88.4.24 Classification of Acute Diarrhea Based on Findings of Fecal Markers of Inflammation (Leukocytes or Lactoferrin) or Presence of Gross Fecal Blood

Types of Diarrhea	Possible Causes	Measures to Be Taken
Noninflammatory (negative for fecal inflammatory markers or dysentery)	Toxin-mediated, viral, noninvasive pathogens like *Vibrio cholerae,* ETEC, EAEC, enteric viruses, protozoal parasites like *Giardia* or *Cryptosporidium*	Oral/i.v. fluid replacement and empiric therapy if required
Inflammatory (clinical colitis or presence of fecal inflammatory markers (e.g., leukocytes, calprotectin, lactoferrin) or presence of dysentery)	*Shigella, Salmonella,* STEC, *Entamoeba histolytica, Campylobacter, Clostridium difficile*	Oral/i.v. fluid therapy based on hydration status and thorough laboratory investigations with specific antibiotic therapy if indicated[a]

ETEC, enterotoxigenic *E. coli;* EAEC, enteroaggregative *E. coli;* STEC, Shiga toxin–producing *E. coli.*
[a]Specific therapies are listed in Table 27.

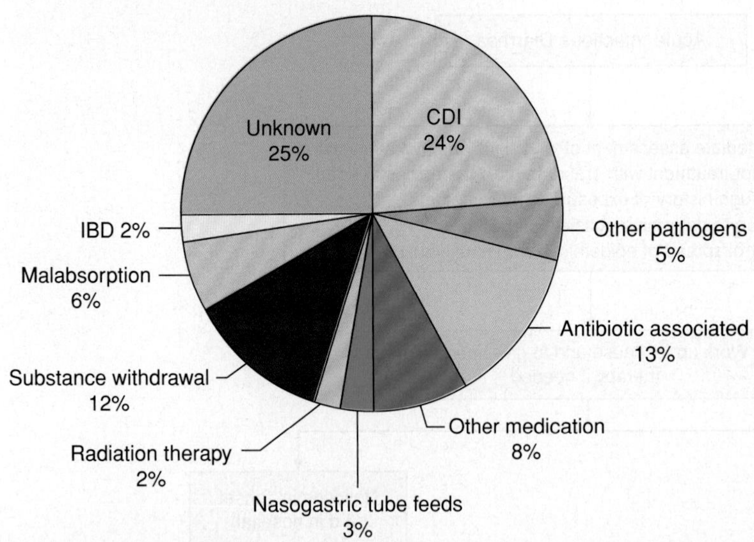

FIGURE 88.4.3 Relative importance of etiologic agents in hospital-acquired diarrhea. This figure shows the percentage of incidence of each of the common diarrhea-causing bacteria. CDI, *Clostridium difficile* infection; IBD, inflammatory bowel disease. (Adapted from McFarland LV. Epidemiology of infectious and iatrogenic nosocomial diarrhea in a cohort of general medicine patients. *Am J Infect Control.* 1995;23(5):295–305.)

Health Care–acquired Diarrhea

Illness occurring after the 72 hours in the hospital or nursing home can be considered health care–associated. In Fig. 88.4.3, the relative importance of causes of diarrhea in hospitalized patients in one study is provided. Between 10% and 30% of nosocomial diarrhea is due to *C. difficile;* since 10% to 20% of institutionalized patients are colonized with this organism during hospitalization and because most acute diarrhea developing in the hospital is not caused by *C. difficile* the PCR test for fecal toxin often gives a false-positive result (6).

The other important causes of nosocomial diarrhea include antibiotics, chemotherapeutic agents, PPIs, tube feedings, laxatives, other drugs, and various iatrogenic and idiopathic conditions (see Fig. 88.4.3).

It is appropriate, in all hospital-associated diarrheas when a patient is receiving antibacterial treatment, to consider *C. difficile* as the causative agent, and empiric treatment is advisable only in the more severe cases while laboratory tests are pending. Rarely, other pathogens can be found in hospital- and nursing home–associated diarrhea, including rotaviruses.

The International Traveler Returning with Diarrhea

TD may occur when persons travel from industrialized to developing tropical and semitropical areas with reduced levels of personal and food hygiene. TD is the most common travel-related infectious illness, occurring in up to 40% of travelers to regions of Asia, Africa, and Latin America. Among US travelers, the majority of cases of TD occur in individuals returning from Latin America and the Caribbean, but the greatest risk is noted after travel to the Indian subcontinent (7); bacterial enteropathogens cause as much as 80% of TD cases.

The world has been classified into three different risk groups: low, intermediate, and high risk, based on the frequency of TD in the traveling public. The important causes of TD are Enterotoxigenic *E. coli* (ETEC), enteroaggregative *E. coli* (EAEC), noroviruses, *Campylobacter, Shigella,* and *Salmonella.* Less commonly, parasitic agents cause TD and should be suspected in persistent illness; important parasitic pathogens include *Giardia, Cryptosporidium,* and *Cyclospora.* Patients with TD should be treated empirically with antibiotics without stool examination.

Immunosuppressed Patient with Diarrhea

An immunosuppressed or immunocompromised patient, including those with congenital or acquired immune deficiency, HIV/AIDS, receipt of immunosuppressive, or cancer chemotherapy drugs, will have increased susceptibility to diarrhea. The etiology of diarrheal diseases in immunocompromised hosts is different from that of other populations in that they are at risk of developing infections from various opportunistic organisms in addition to the routine diarrheal pathogens. The use of various chemotherapy drugs or immunomodulators, such as cyclosporine, mycophenolate mofetil, tacrolimus, or sirolimus may result in drug-induced diarrhea (8); diarrhea in transplant recipients can also be due to graft versus host disease (GVHD). The most commonly identified organisms to consider as causes of diarrhea in this group of patients are *C. difficile* and noroviruses; other causes are *Salmonella, Cryptosporidium, Isospora, Cyclospora,* cytomegalovirus, and *Mycobacterium avium–intracellulare* complex. A thorough and quick evaluation for identifying the causative organism is the key in treating and controlling diarrhea in this patient population. Appropriate rapid diagnostic tests may include direct stool examination for ova, cysts, and parasites; stool test for *C. difficile* toxin; polymerase chain reaction (PCR) for cytomegalovirus or herpesvirus; stool cultures; and blood cultures. If the above tests do not provide a specific diagnosis, endoscopy and mucosal biopsy should be pursued to establish an etiologic diagnosis (9). Abdominal computed tomography (CT) may detect mucosal thickening or other changes of ischemic, hemorrhagic, or inflammatory colitis, and it is the preferred diagnostic study when both intra-abdominal disease and intestinal disease are expected (10).

Patient with Extraintestinal Disease and Diarrhea

Diagnostic evaluation of patients with diarrhea and systemic symptoms and signs will often take the clinician's focus

TABLE 88.4.25 Classification of Dehydration in a Patient with Acute Diarrhea (11)

Dehydration		Symptoms	Suggested Management
Mild dehydration	3–5% loss in body weight	Increased thirst and slightly dry mucous membranes	Oral rehydration solution (ORS) 50 mL/kg over first 2–4 hr
Moderate dehydration	6–9% loss in body weight	Loss of skin turgor, dry mucous membranes, tenting of skin	ORS 100 mL/kg over first 2–4 hr
Severe dehydration	≥10% loss in body weight	Lethargy, altered consciousness, prolonged skin retraction time, cool extremities, decreased capillary refill	Immediate i.v. fluid replacement with 20 mL/kg of lactated Ringer solution to restore perfusion and mental status. Continue with 100 mL/kg ORS or i.v. 5% dextrose and 1/2 normal saline at two times the maintenance rate.

Adapted from Duggan C, Santosham M, Glass RI. The management of acute diarrhea in children: oral rehydration, maintenance, and nutritional therapy. *MMWR*. 1992; 41(RR-16):1–20.

away from the gut for the diagnosis. Blood cultures, CT of the abdomen, and serology (for *Entamoeba histolytica*) may help determine the primary cause of the disease. In cases of sepsis, blood cultures and stool studies may provide the diagnosis; systemic complications are often seen with invasive bacterial and parasitic infections. Systemic complications of enteric infection include hemolytic uremic syndrome (HUS) or thrombotic thrombocytopenic purpura (TTP), Guillain–Barré syndrome, reactive arthritis, iritis, postinfectious irritable bowel syndrome, sepsis, infective endocarditis, and abdominal abscesses or localized abscess elsewhere, or pyogenic arthritis. In immunocompromised patients with diarrhea, systemic complications can occur with any of the etiologic agents. Antimotility drugs should not be used in dysenteric and febrile diarrhea without effective concomitant antibiotics as they can prolong or complicate the disease. Amoebiasis, which is uncommon in the United States, shows an extended spectrum of extraintestinal complications including liver abscess and disseminated infection.

MANAGEMENT OF ACUTE DIARRHEA

Dehydration

Dehydration is defined as excess loss of body fluids resulting in fluid and electrolyte abnormalities; classifications of dehydration are provided (Table 88.4.25).

Dry skin and dry mucous membranes, sunken eyes, decreased urine output, loss of skin turgor, dizziness/lightheadedness are all manifestations of moderate to severe dehydration. Dehydration is the most common serious complication of diarrhea and should be promptly recognized and managed in all patients. Patients in an ICU, with other comorbid conditions and extremes of age, need to be vigorously treated to avoid life-threatening complications of dehydration. Routine testing of electrolytes in patients with severe diarrhea offers some value in guiding fluid management in the ICU setting (12).

Rehydration can be done depending on severity of the dehydration either by oral or i.v. routes. Where available, oral rehydration salt (ORS) solution can be used in mild or moderate dehydration and for maintenance of hydration after i.v. fluid administration in severe dehydration. Standard or reduced osmolarity (low salt) ORS formulations are preferable where available. In dehydration due to cholera-like profuse watery diarrhea with massive fluid loses, reduced-osmolarity ORS may lead to subclinical reduction of body electrolytes, making standard ORS preferable in this dehydrating form of diarrhea for outpatients (13). In the United States, ORS is not readily available, but Pedialyte or Ricelyte can be used to maintain hydration and treat minor degrees of dehydration for outpatients. For inpatients with cholera-like diarrhea in the United States, i.v. fluids are preferentially used; specific fluid replacement strategies based on severity are presented in Table 88.4.25.

Dysentery

Dysentery is defined as passage of bloody stools suggesting bacterial colitis (14). The four major causes of bloody diarrhea in the United States, in descending order of frequency of occurrence, are *Shigella, Campylobacter,* nontyphoid *Salmonella,* and Shiga toxin–producing *E. coli* (15). Single cases of dysentery with high fever should be treated with azithromycin empirically. For nonfebrile or low-grade fever with dysentery in an outbreak with multiple cases, stools studies should be performed to look for the etiology, including Shiga toxin–producing *E. coli,* before considering therapy. Empiric and specific antibiotic treatments are provided in Tables 88.4.26 and 88.4.27.

TABLE 88.4.26 Empiric Antimicrobial Therapy of Acute Diarrhea (16–19,20)

Indication	Recommended Therapy
Febrile dysentery: fever (temperature > 100.2°F (>38°C)) plus dysentery (passage of grossly bloody stools)	Azithromycin 500 mg PO daily for 3 d
Moderate to severe traveler's diarrhea with fever and dysentery	Azithromycin 1,000 mg PO single dose
Moderate to severe traveler's diarrhea without fever and dysentery	Rifaximin, 200 mg tid for 3 d; or ciprofloxacin, 500 mg bid for 3 d
Severe hospital-acquired diarrhea in a patient with comorbidity and prior receipt of antibacterial therapy	Vancomycin, 125 mg every 6 hr orally; or fidaxomicin 200 mg bid for 10–14 d (preferred) i.v. metronidazole 500 mg every 8 hr if cannot take oral medications.

bid, twice a day; PO, orally; tid, three times a day.

TABLE 88.4.27 Specific Therapy for Pathogen-Specific Diarrhea, Once Etiologic Diagnosis Is Established (1,20,21)

Identified Pathogen	Suggested Antimicrobial Therapy
Clostridium difficile First or second bout	Vancomycin 125 mg qid for 10–14 d; or fidaxomicin 200 mg bid for 10–14 d Fulminant cases: oral vancomycin 500 mg every 6 hr for 10–14 d
Recurrent (≥3 bouts)	Tapered or pulsed doses of vancomycin for 3–5 wk or fecal microbial transplantation, if available
Salmonella sp. (treat only for suspected sepsis based on presence of high-risk host*)	For high-risk host[a]: Fluoroquinolones: ciprofloxacin 500 mg bid; or levofloxacin 500 mg once a day for 7–10 d; or slow i.v. infusion of ceftriaxone, 1–2 g once daily for 7–10 d (14 d in patients with immunosuppression)
Shigella	Fluoroquinolones, dosed as in *Salmonella* above, given for 3 d; or azithromycin 500 mg once daily for 3 d
Campylobacter	Azithromycin 500 mg once a day for 3 d; or erythromycin 500 mg bid for 5 d
Shigatoxin-producing *E. coli* (STEC)	No antimotility drugs, antibiotic treatment not usually given as they may increase the risk of occurrence of hemolytic uremic syndrome
Enterotoxigenic *E. coli* (ETEC)	Rifaximin 200 mg tid for 3 d; or fluoroquinolone in above dose for 1–3 d; or azithromycin 1,000 mg in single dose
Enteroaggregative *E. coli* (EAEC)	Same as ETEC
Enteropathogenic *E. coli* (EPEC)	Same as *Shigella*, plus perform susceptibility testing to refine treatment
Enteroinvasive *E. coli* (EIEC)	Same as *Shigella*
Vibrio cholerae infection (cholera)	Doxycycline single 300 mg dose
Noncholeraic Vibrio diarrhea	Ciprofloxacin 750 mg once daily for 3 d, or azithromycin 500 mg once daily for 3 d
Aeromonas/Plesiomonas shigelloides	Same as *Shigella*
Yersinia	Same as *Shigella*
Entamoeba histolytica	Metronidazole 750 mg tid for 5 d, plus either diloxanide furoate 500 mg tid for 10 d or paromomycin 25–35 mg/kg/d divided in 3 daily doses for 7 d
Giardia	Tinidazole 2 g orally in single dose, nitazoxanide 500 mg twice daily for 3 da, or metronidazole 250 mg tid for 5–7 d
Cryptosporidium	Nitazoxanide 500 mg bid for 3 to 14 d
Cyclospora	TMP-SMZ 160 and 800 mg, respectively, bid for 7 d; in immunosuppressed patients, TMP-SMZ treatment is given for ≥14 d followed by 3 times weekly for up to 10 wk
Cystoisospora	TMP-SMZ 160 and 800 mg, respectively, qid for 10 d
Microsporidium	Albendazole 400 mg bid for 14–28 d or fumagillin, 20 mg bid for 14 d
Cytomegalovirus	Ganciclovir 5 mg/kg i.v. every 12 hr for 14 d, or valganciclovir 900 mg twice daily orally for 21 d; maintenance dose of either agent may then be needed
Strongyloides	Ivermectin 200 μg/d orally for 2 d, or albendazole 400 mg twice daily for 7 d
Norovirus	Fluid and electrolyte therapy, consider bismuth subsalicylate symptomatic therapy
Rotavirus	Fluid and electrolyte therapy

bid, twice a day; ETEC, enterotoxigenic *E. coli*; qid, four times a day; tid, three times a day; TMP-SMZ, trimethoprim-sulfamethoxazole.

[a]High-risk patients for *Salmonella* enterica species (nontyphoid *Salmonella*): Any subject who is toxic with fever >102°F (39°C), with age <3 months or ≥65 years, and or with malignancy or AIDS, on steroids, with inflammatory bowel disease or renal failure, or undergoing hemodialysis, with hemoglobinopathy such as sickle cell disease. Patients with simple gastroenteritis are best not given antibacterial drugs.

Clostridium difficile Infection and Colitis

C. difficile infection (CDI) was first identified as a causative agent of antibiotic-associated diarrhea in the early 1970s, associated with clindamycin use. The organism is a gram-positive, spore-forming anaerobic bacteria that produces an enterotoxin known as toxin A and a cytotoxin called toxin B; there is a third type of toxin produced, called binary toxin, which is an actin-specific ADP ribosylating toxin that is associated with more severe disease. Toxin A causes necrosis, increased intestinal permeability, and inhibition of protein synthesis. Toxin B is thought to become effective once the gut wall has been damaged. Over the past two decades, an increased virulence of CD strains has evolved, making the disease more severe. The virulence relates to higher levels of toxin production and greater rates of sporulation, which relates to recurrences. The North American PFGE type 1 strain (NAP1) or PCR ribotype 027 strain has been particularly virulent, with higher death and recurrence rates. The incidence of CDI has been rising for the past 20 years; recent surveys in 183 hospitals among 11,282 patients noted 452 patients with one or more health care–associated infection, with gastrointestinal infections seen in 17.1%, and CDI being the most important diagnosis identified in 12.1% of health care–associated infections (22). Since a higher number of hospital associated diarrhea cases do not have CDI plus the fact that *C. difficile* PCR-based diagnostic tests will be positive in colonized patients without diarrhea, *only unformed stool should be tested for C. difficile,* unless the patient has ileus.

Major risk factors for CDI include antimicrobial use, age older than 65 years, severity of existing health condition, use of other drugs such as chemotherapeutic agents and PPIs, renal insufficiency, and gastrointestinal surgery. In CDI, advanced age and comorbidity, plus severity of underlying impairment, predict frequency of infection and outcome (23). Host conditions may influence susceptibility to CDI, such as inflammatory bowel disease (24), IBS (25), and failure to develop serum antibodies to toxin A of *C. difficile.*

When assessing institutionalized individuals, such as nursing home patients with diarrhea, associated risk factors for CDAD should be considered. Some of the risk factors other than antibiotic use and comorbidity are low albumin level (<2.5 g/dL), recent admission to a health care institution, and use of PPIs (26). In nonhospitalized patients with other predisposing conditions such as cancer, prolonged antibiotic usage—especially with first-generation cephalosporins, fluoroquinolones, or clindamycin—is a recognized risk factor for CDI. The risk is greatest with clindamycin, followed by fluoroquinolones and β-lactam drugs (cephalosporins and penicillins); all antibiotics show a risk for causing CDI except for vancomycin, the major therapeutic drug when given orally.

CDI caused by a spore-forming organism resists curative therapy and recurs in approximately 25% of properly treated cases, often within 7 to 14 days, but occasionally as long as 60 days after completion of therapy. Risk factors for early recurrence of CDI are renal failure; white blood cell counts greater than 15,000 cells/μL with the initial episode, and first episode of community-acquired CDI. Failure to mount a serum antibody response to toxin A during an initial episode of CDI is associated with CD recurrence (27).

Despite the growing incidence of CD and the increased knowledge about CDI, there is no gold standard diagnostic test to diagnose CDI. Diagnosis of CDI is based on both clinical and laboratory findings. The customary way to make the diagnosis is to recover a toxigenic strain of CD through detection one or both of the known CD toxins, A and B, in stool samples by commercial tissue culture cytotoxin assay for toxin B, enzyme immunoassay (EIA) for one or both of the toxins or RT-PCR. Toxigenic culture is a sensitive method of diagnosing CDI, but this test as well as the tissue culture cytotoxin assay takes 3 days to complete, making them impractical for deciding about therapy needs. The EIA is specific testing for toxin but it lacks sensitivity and the PCR while the most sensitive test lacks specificity for CDI as it fails to determine carriers from infected patients. Many groups are going to a two-step diagnostic approach, using very sensitive glutamine dehydrogenase (GDH) screening followed by rejection of patients with negative tests as not having CDI and testing the positive reactions by EIA (28). GDH is an enzyme found in all strains of *C. difficile* but because it is found in other bacteria, it is not a standalone test.

In a highly probable clinical case with severe disease or fragile clinical picture, it is often advisable to initiate prompt empiric treatment before stool test results are back, or even in the face of negative laboratory tests for the toxins. In these cases, colonoscopy, abdominal CT, or measurement of fecal inflammatory markers could be considered to provide additional evidence of CDI.

Treatment of Acute Diarrhea

Prompt diagnosis and treatment are important to successful management of CDI (see Tables 88.4.26 and 88.4.27). CDI can be classified into mild, moderate, and severe. Cessation of causative antibiotic use if possible is important and, in very mild cases, it may be enough to result in cure without further treatment. While previous recommendations were made to use oral metronidazole for mild CDI, the drug has serious flaws because it is nearly 100% absorbed, resulting in very low fecal levels (29). Most experts in the field now reserve metronidazole use for i.v. administration when no oral therapy is possible because of ileus or other condition. For therapy of mild to severe cases, oral vancomycin or fidaxomicin is recommended. For first recurrence of CDI, the same drug, oral vancomycin or fidaxomicin, can be used again since resistance development is not a reason for recurrence in infection caused by this spore-forming organism. When two or more recurrences occur, the primary problem is intestinal dysbiosis (decrease in number of species/phyla and evenness of counts of the various pathotypes) limiting colonization resistance (30). Fecal microbiota transplantation (FMT) is the most effective treatment in these cases (31). Other approaches, since FMT is not available everywhere, including longer-term oral vancomycin given intermittently or in pulse therapy (20).

Diarrhea Epidemics in the Hospital

Early identification and controlling the spread of rare hospital epidemics of enteric disease are the keys to successful management. Universal protocols of isolation and personal hygiene measures play an important role. Cohorting subjects by putting infected persons in contiguous areas away from uninfected persons and using dedicated hospital personnel for their care is an important strategy. Judicious use of antibiotics in the hospital and prompt discontinuation of possible inciting drugs also can be helpful. Agents showing potential for epidemics in hospitals are *C. difficile, Salmonella* spp., *Shigella, Campylobacter, Vibrio, Aeromonas, Yersinia,* noroviruses, and rotavirus. Early therapy of treatable enteric pathogens should occur (see Table 88.4.27). Health care worker and patient education regarding various personal hygiene and isolation procedures could help in stopping the spread within the institution.

Prevention of Diarrhea in the Hospital

Appropriate use of antibiotics in hospitalized patients, along with the use of the narrowest-spectrum antibiotics possible to treat their infection will preserve gut flora helpful in the prevention of CDI. Additionally, at least in a research setting, *Saccharomyces* has been used to prevent CDI (32). Other drugs in future study may be effective and reasonable to use to prevent CDI in hospitalized patients (33). Enteric isolation practices for patients with known enteric infection in the hospital will help prevent the spread of diarrhea and lower its incidence, as will effective and widespread hand washing with soap and water. A systematic review and meta-analysis of studies from the developing world and from US and Australian childcare settings estimated that hand-washing with soap reduces the risk for diarrheal diseases in hospitals by 42% to 47% (34); alcohol-based hand cleaners are not effective against strains of *C. difficile*. Patients with CDI and the health care workers caring for them must use under regular effective hand washing with soap and water, use disposable thermometers for recording temperature, and employ meticulous environmental cleaning with chlorine-based bleach products in clinical settings to prevent spread of infections in the hospital.

Live, oral, human-bovine (Pentavalent/RV5) rotavirus vaccine (RotaTeq) recommended for routine use in infants in the United States since 2006 has had a great impact on the morbidity associated with rotavirus infection in children in the United States (35) in addition to decreasing rates of rotavirus-associated gastroenteritis among adults, since rotavirus vaccine is being used in children (36).

Key Points

- Noroviruses cause approximately half of all diarrhea for which a cause of illness can be found.
- Noroviruses are usually intense but persist for no more than 60 hours, and do not usually require therapy.
- For the elderly and infirm, especially after organ and stem cell transplantation. the noroviruses can cause severe and chronic illness and may be fatal.
- Between 10% and 30% of nosocomial diarrhea is due to *C. difficile*.
- Since 10% to 20% of institutionalized patients are colonized with this organism during hospitalization and because most acute diarrhea developing in the hospital is not caused by *C. difficile, the PCR test for fecal toxin often gives a false-positive result.*
- Since a very significant number of hospital associated diarrhea cases do not have CDI plus the fact that *C. difficile* PCR-based diagnostic tests will be positive in colonized patients without diarrhea, *only unformed stool should be tested for CD,* unless the patient has ileus.
- Immunosuppressed or immunocompromised patients will have increased susceptibility to diarrhea.
- Antimotility drugs should not be used in dysenteric and febrile diarrhea without effective concomitant antibiotics as they can prolong or complicate the disease.
- Patients with CDI and the health care workers caring for them must employ effective hand-washing with soap and water, disposable thermometers for recording temperature, and meticulous environmental cleaning with chlorine-based bleach products in clinical settings to prevent spread of infections in the hospital.

References

1. DuPont HL. Acute infectious diarrhea in immunocompetent adults. *N Engl J Med.* 2014;370(16):1532–1540.
2. Wikswo ME, Hall AJ, Centers for Disease C, Prevention. Outbreaks of acute gastroenteritis transmitted by person-to-person contact—United States, 2009–2010. *MMWR Surveill Summ.* 2012;61(9):1–12.
3. Centers for Disease C, Prevention. Emergence of new norovirus strain GII.4 Sydney–United States, 2012. *MMWR Morb Mortal Wkly Rep.* 2013; 62(3):55.
4. Bavishi C, DuPont HL. Systematic review: the use of proton pump inhibitors and increased susceptibility to enteric infection. *Aliment Pharmacol Ther.* 2011;34(11–12):1269–1281.
5. Darkoh C, Turnwald BP, Koo HL, et al. Colonic immunopathogenesis of *Clostridium difficile* infections. *Clin Vaccine Immunol.* 2014;21(4):509–517.
6. Koo HL, Van JN, Zhao M, et al. Real-time polymerase chain reaction detection of asymptomatic *Clostridium difficile* colonization and rising *C. difficile*-associated disease rates. *Infect Control Hosp Epidemiol.* 2014; 35(6):667–673.
7. Steffen R, Hill DR, DuPont HL. Traveler's diarrhea: a clinical review. *JAMA.* 2015;313(1):71–80.
8. Ginsburg PM, Thuluvath PJ. Diarrhea in liver transplant recipients: etiology and management. *Liver Transpl.* 2005;11(8):881–890.
9. Donowitz M, Kokke FT, Saidi R. Evaluation of patients with chronic diarrhea. *N Engl J Med.* 1995;332(11):725–729.
10. Horton KM, Corl FM, Fishman EK. CT evaluation of the colon: inflammatory disease. *Radiographics.* 2000;20(2):399–418.
11. Duggan C, Santosham M, Glass RI. The management of acute diarrhea in children: oral rehydration, maintenance, and nutritional therapy. *MMWR.* 1992;41(RR-16):1–20.
12. Wathen JE, MacKenzie T, Bothner JP. Usefulness of the serum electrolyte panel in the management of pediatric dehydration treated with intravenously administered fluids. *Pediatrics.* 2004;114(5):1227–1234.
13. Murphy C, Hahn S, Volmink J. Reduced osmolarity oral rehydration solution for treating cholera. *Cochrane Database Syst Rev.* 2004(4):CD003754.
14. Pfeiffer ML, DuPont HL, Ochoa TJ. The patient presenting with acute dysentery—a systematic review. *J Infect.* 2012;64(4):374–386.
15. Talan D, Moran GJ, Newdow M, et al. Etiology of bloody diarrhea among patients presenting to United States emergency departments: prevalence of *Escherichia coli* O157:H7 and other enteropathogens. *Clin Infect Dis.* 2001;32(4):573–580.
16. Tribble DR, Sanders JW, Pang LW, et al. Traveler's diarrhea in Thailand: randomized, double-blind trial comparing single-dose and 3-day azithromycin-based regimens with a 3-day levofloxacin regimen. *Clin Infect Dis.* 2007;44(3):338–346.
17. DuPont HL. Azithromycin for the self-treatment of traveler's diarrhea. *Clin Infect Dis.* 2007;44(3):347–349.
18. DuPont HL, Ericsson CD. Prevention and treatment of traveler's diarrhea. *N Engl J Med.* 1993;328(25):1821–1827.
19. DuPont HL, Ericsson CD, Farthing MJ, et al. Expert review of the evidence base for self-therapy of travelers' diarrhea. *J Travel Med.* 2009;16(3):161–171.
20. DuPont HL. Diagnosis and management of *Clostridium difficile* infection. *Clin Gastroenterol Hepatol.* 2013;11(10):1216–1223.
21. DuPont HL. Clinical practice: bacterial diarrhea. *N Engl J Med.* 2009; 361(16):1560–1569.
22. Magill SS, Edwards JR, Bamberg W, et al. Multistate point-prevalence survey of health care-associated infections. *N Engl J Med.* 2014;370(13):1198–1208.
23. Andrews CN, Raboud J, Kassen BO, Enns R. *Clostridium difficile*-associated diarrhea: predictors of severity in patients presenting to the emergency department. *Can J Gastroenterol.* 2003;17(6):369–373.
24. Ananthakrishnan AN, McGinley EL, Saeian K, Binion DG. Temporal trends in disease outcomes related to *Clostridium difficile* infection in patients with inflammatory bowel disease. *Inflamm Bowel Dis.* 2011;17(4):976–983.
25. Dial S, Kezouh A, Dascal A, et al. Patterns of antibiotic use and risk of hospital admission because of *Clostridium difficile* infection. *Can Med Assoc J.* 2008;179(8):767–772.
26. Al-Tureihi FI, Hassoun A, Wolf-Klein G, Isenberg H. Albumin, length of stay, and proton pump inhibitors: key factors in *Clostridium difficile*-associated disease in nursing home patients. *J Am Med Direct Assoc.* 2005;6(2):105–1058.
27. Kyne L, Warny M, Qamar A, Kelly CP. Association between antibody response to toxin A and protection against recurrent *Clostridium difficile* diarrhoea. *Lancet.* 2001;357(9251):189–193.
28. Goldenberg SD, Cliff PR, Smith S, et al. Two-step glutamate dehydrogenase antigen real-time polymerase chain reaction assay for detection of toxigenic *Clostridium difficile. J Hosp Infect.* 2010;74(1):48–54.
29. Bolton RP, Culshaw MA. Faecal metronidazole concentrations during oral and intravenous therapy for antibiotic associated colitis due to Clostridium difficile. *Gut.* 1986;27(10):1169–1172.
30. Reeves AE, Theriot CM, Bergin IL, et al. The interplay between microbiome dynamics and pathogen dynamics in a murine model of *Clostridium difficile* infection. *Gut Microbes.* 2011;2(3):145–158.
31. Sha S, Liang J, Chen M, et al. Systematic review: faecal microbiota transplantation therapy for digestive and nondigestive disorders in adults and children. *Aliment Pharmacol Ther.* 2014;39(10):1003–1032.
32. McFarland LV. Meta-analysis of probiotics for the prevention of antibiotic associated diarrhea and the treatment of *Clostridium difficile* disease. *Am J Gastroenterol.* 2006;101(4):812–822.
33. DuPont HL. Chemoprophylaxis of *Clostridium difficile* infections in high risk hospitalized patients. *Clin Gastroenterol Hepatol.* 2014;12:1862–1864.
34. Curtis V, Cairncross S. Effect of washing hands with soap on diarrhoea risk in the community: a systematic review. *Lancet Infect Dis.* 2003;3(5):275–281.
35. Cortes JE, Curns AT, Tate JE, et al. Rotavirus vaccine and health care utilization for diarrhea in U.S. children. *N Engl J Med.* 2011;365(12):1108–1117.
36. Anderson EJ, Shippee DB, Weinrobe MH, et al. Indirect protection of adults from rotavirus by pediatric rotavirus vaccination. *Clin Infect Dis.* 2013;56(6):755–760.

CHAPTER

89

Fungal and Viral Infections

PALASH SAMANTA, GHADY HAIDAR, MINH LY NGUYEN, CORNELIUS J. CLANCY, and M. HONG NGUYEN

FUNGAL INFECTIONS

Fungal Pathogens

Medically relevant fungi are classically considered as one of three types of organism: yeasts, molds, or dimorphic agents. The yeasts grow as smooth colonies on culture plates. Microscopically, they are oval or spherical, and they reproduce by budding. The two most common human yeast pathogens are *Candida* and *Cryptococcus* spp. The molds appear as fuzzy colonies on agar plates. Histopathologically, they have hyphae, which are tubular or filamentous morphologies that grow by branching and longitudinal extension. Hyphae can be septated (i.e., with cross walls perpendicular to hyphal cell wall) or aseptated (no cross walls). The most common human pathogens are *Aspergillus* and *Rhizopus* spp. The term *dimorphic fungi* is used to describe the endemic fungi, which are found in distinct geographic locations. These fungi grow as filaments in the environment at ambient temperatures and as yeasts at higher body temperatures. The three most common pathogens are *Histoplasma capsulatum*, *Coccidioides immitis*, and *Blastomyces dermatitidis*. Clinicians should recognize that the term dimorphic fungi, as commonly used in the medical literature, is misleading. *Candida albicans*, although not grouped with the endemic dimorphic fungi, frequently assumes filamentous morphologies in tissue (pseudohyphae and hyphae).

Most fungal pathogens, except for *Candida* spp., are widespread in nature and are acquired by inhalation into the lungs. In immunocompetent hosts, inhaled fungi are generally arrested in the lungs by the host immune system. *Candida* spp, with the exception of *Candida parapsilosis*, are part of the human gastrointestinal flora, and infections with these organisms are usually endogenous in origin.

Due to the widespread environmental distribution of many fungal pathogens and the presence of *Candida* as human commensals, the diagnosis of infection (i.e., fungal disease) is often difficult to distinguish from colonization. As such, definitive diagnoses generally require either the presence of the organism at sterile sites or histopathology demonstrating tissue-invasive disease. Since many fungi show morphologies that are indistinguishable by histopathology (e.g., *Aspergillus* spp vs. *Fusarium* spp and other acute-angle branching, septated molds), identification of the organism from culture is the only means to ascertain the etiologic agent.

In intensive care unit (ICU) settings, *Candida* spp and, to a much lesser extent, *Aspergillus* are the major fungal pathogens. This chapter will concentrate on these fungi.

Infections Caused by *Candida* Species (Candidiasis)

Candida spp cause a wide range of clinical syndromes, from benign cutaneous to fatal deep-seated infections (Table 89.1). *Candida* spp can affect otherwise healthy patients, as well as those with defective immune systems. In the ICU setting, the most common and serious form of disease is invasive candidiasis, which will be the focus of the rest of this section. Other types of candidiasis are alluded to in Table 89.1.

Invasive candidiasis comprises candidemia and deep-seated candidiasis. In general, about 50% of the primary candidemia seeds deep-seated organs causing secondary deep-seated candidiasis. On the other hand, less than 20% of primary deep-seated candidiasis is associated with secondary candidemia. Invasive candidiasis therefore encompasses three different entities: candidemia in the absence of deep-seated candidiasis, candidemia associated with deep-seated candidiasis, and deep-seated candidiasis (1). Although candidemia is the most common type of invasive candidiasis studied clinically, recent data suggested that deep-seated candidiasis, such as intra-abdominal candidiasis (IAC), might be much more common than recognized (1,2).

Most epidemiologic surveys of invasive candidiasis are based on candidemia, which accounts for 5 to 10 episodes per 1,000 ICU admissions, and represents 5% to 10% of all ICU-acquired infections (3). Candidemia is the second most common cause of mortality from blood stream infection in the ICUs in the United States (4), and is associated with excess ICU and hospital stays and increased costs of care (5–7); crude mortality rates range from 35% to 67% (4,8,9). IAC is the most common form of deep-seated candidiasis, and the second most common cause of ICU admissions for invasive candidiasis (10–13). IAC includes peritonitis, pancreatitis, biliary tract infections, and intra-abdominal abscesses.

Pathophysiology

Invasive candidiasis may stem from endogenous or exogenous sources, although the former are predominant. Derangement of the host immune system, overgrowth of *Candida* on mucosal surfaces, and breaches of host mucosa predispose patients to invasive candidiasis. Exogenous acquisitions, from hands of health care workers, via use of vascular catheters, contaminated solutions, cardiac valves, and so forth, have been associated with invasive candidiasis, especially candidemia. Indeed, up to one-third of candidemia may be attributable to nosocomial clusters, and the highest risk is in the ICUs (14).

The leading predisposing factors for invasive candidiasis include prolonged ICU stay, previous surgery (especially solid organ transplant [SOT] and gastrointestinal surgery), acute renal failure, receipt of antibacterial agents or hyperalimentation, and the presence of a central venous catheter (CVC). In these settings, *Candida* colonization of different body sites and immunosuppression are major risk factors. SOT recipients are at highest risk among the surgical patients, particularly small bowel, liver, and pancreas recipients, in whom the prevalence ranges from 9% to 59%; the types of surgical procedure and posttransplant immunosuppression confer additional risk.

TABLE 89.1 Major Clinical *Candida* Syndromes

Type of Candidiasis	Specific Clinical Syndromes	Frequency	Risk Factors	Types of Hosts	Treatment
Cutaneous: skin, nails		Most common form of candidiasis; Self-limited	Prolonged exposure of skin to moisture	Immunocompetent Immunocompromised	Topical antifungals
Mucocutaneous: Mucous membranes of the mouth, esophagus, vagina	Oropharyngeal	About 25% in patients with solid tumors and 60% in patients with hematologic malignancies and/or following bone marrow transplantation; up to 90% in AIDS	Extremes of age, broad-spectrum antibiotics, inhaled or systemic steroids, radiation to the head and neck	Immunocompetent Immunocompromised, especially patients receiving cytotoxic chemotherapy or systemic immunosuppressive therapy, those with AIDS, malignancy, or chronic mucocutaneous candidiasis	Topical or systemic azole agents
	Esophagitis	15–20% in AIDS	Broad-spectrum antibiotics, acid-suppressive therapy, prior gastric surgery, mucosal barrier injury, inhaled or systemic steroids, esophageal motility disorders	Mostly immunocompromised, especially patients receiving cytotoxic chemotherapy or systemic immunosuppressive therapy, those with AIDS or malignancy	Systemic antifungal agents: oral azole (preferred treatment), parenteral echinocandin or AmB
	Vaginitis	70–75% of healthy adult women	Pregnancy, diabetes mellitus, and broad-spectrum antibiotics	Immunocompetent Immunocompromised	Topical or systemic azole agents
Disseminated candidiasis			Colonization with *Candida*, broad-spectrum antibiotics, end-stage renal disease, central venous catheters, critically ill patients, hyperalimentation, GI surgery, burn patients, neonates	Immunocompetent Immunocompromised, especially granulocytopenia, bone marrow or solid organ transplant, chemotherapy, mucositis	Systemic antifungal agents

AIDS, acquired immunodeficiency syndrome; AmB, amphotericin B; GI, gastrointestinal.

Although risk factors are well defined, the diversity of factors and underlying diseases associated with invasive candidiasis make it difficult to reliably identify large subgroups of patients within the ICU who might merit particular attention or targeted interventions.

C. albicans is the most common *Candida* species involved in invasive candidiasis, followed by *C. glabrata*, *C. tropicalis*, and *C. parapsilosis*. Other species are less common and often associated with underlying malignancy or chemotherapy. Whereas *C. tropicalis* and *C. glabrata* are found largely in adults, *C. parapsilosis* is the leading pathogen in the neonatal population. In many tertiary care centers, *C. glabrata* has surpassed *C. albicans* to become the most common *Candida* sp in invasive candidiasis, accounting for up to 35% of all candidemias (15,16). Among non-*albicans Candida* species, *C. krusei* and *C. glabrata* are particularly important because of their resistance and decreased susceptibility to fluconazole, respectively (17).

Diagnosis

Clinical manifestations of invasive candidiasis are often nonspecific, and fever is frequently the first and only sign. Signs that should raise concern for candidemia are papulopustular or macronodular skin lesions or ocular involvement such as chorioretinitis or endophthalmitis. Symptoms of sepsis, severe sepsis, or septic shock can be presenting symptoms in critically ill patients. Deep-seated infections often present with findings localized to the particular tissue site.

The diagnosis of invasive candidiasis is a challenge due to nonspecific clinical manifestations and the low sensitivity of microbiologic culture techniques. Furthermore, *Candida* spp are common colonizers of humans, which often makes it difficult to differentiate between colonization and true infections when organisms are isolated from the urine and other nonsterile sites.

Cultures. Blood culture is the gold standard and should be routinely obtained among patients who have suggestive signs and symptoms or those at high risk for invasive candidiasis. However, it is positive in less than 50% of patients (1). Overall, the sensitivity of blood culture is impacted by the mechanisms of pathogenesis: it is highly sensitive in the setting of CVC-associated candidemia (1), but is much less sensitive when candidemia stems from extracellular sources (deep-seated sites) or from translocation across the gastrointestinal mucosa. Blood culture is further limited by time to positivity, with the median time of 2 to 3 days, ranging from 1 to more than 7 days (1,18). For deep-seated candidiasis, the gold standard of diagnosis is culture of sterilely collected samples, a procedure that can be challenging. In this setting, blood culture sensitivity is only 25%, and blood culture may take up to 4 weeks longer than nonculture tests to turn positive. The poor sensitivity and slow time to positivity of culture are important considerations because delays in antifungal therapy are associated with poor outcomes (19,20).

Given the potential for antifungal resistance among the non-*albicans Candida* spp, isolates recovered from blood or sterile sites should be identified to the species level. The availability of special fungal media (such as CHROMagar), rapid in situ hybridization techniques, DNA sequencing, and other molecular methods such as MALDI TOF have shown promising results (21,22).

Studies have demonstrated that azole minimum inhibitory concentrations (MICs) correlate with the likelihood of success in treating patients. Nevertheless, antifungal susceptibility testing of *Candida* is not routinely performed in most clinical laboratories, and it is not considered the standard of care, unlike antibacterial susceptibility testing. In fact, antifungal susceptibility patterns are predictable in most cases based on species and prior exposure to antifungal agents (23). For this reason, it has generally been believed that identification of isolates to the species level is more important than MIC data in the management of individual patients. However, triazole resistance among *C. glabrata* has risen to a degree that it is difficult to select these agents as therapy in the absence of susceptibility testing. Similarly, resistance among *C. albicans, C. tropicalis,* and *C. parapsilosis* has also been increasingly reported, especially at tertiary care institutions where azole agents are extensively used. Cross-resistance to other azoles is often seen, which limits the utility of this class against fluconazole-resistant isolates. For these reason, antifungal susceptibility testing should be incorporated in the clinical microbiology laboratory workflow to guide the management of patients with invasive candidiasis.

Resistance among *Candida* spp to the echinocandin class of antifungals is uncommon, except for *C. glabrata*, where the rate of resistance can be as high as 13% at certain institutions (24,25). The most important risk factors for echinocandin resistance among *C. glabrata* are prior prolonged exposure to this agent, especially in the setting of breakthrough infection. In one study, 36% of echinocandin-resistant *C. glabrata* were associated with cross-resistance to the triazoles, yielding multi–drug-resistant phenotypes and limiting therapeutic options (26). Amphotericin B resistance is difficult to document using current testing methods. Resistance among *C. lusitaniae* and *C. guilliermondii* isolates is well described but not seen with all isolates. Clinicians should probably avoid amphotericin B if elevated MICs are documented. At centers where candidiasis is a particular problem and antifungal use is widespread, it is useful to conduct periodic susceptibility testing to generate an institutional antibiogram. Clinicians should be aware if such reports exist at their institution, as susceptibility patterns against different species can be used to guide empiric antifungal therapy.

Nonculture Diagnostics. Efforts have been devoted to develop non–culture-based diagnostic tests for invasive candidiasis. *β D-glucan assay* (Fungitell; Associates of Cape Cod, Massachusetts) is a pan-fungal diagnostic assay that detects a nonantigenic cell wall component of most pathogenic fungi, including *Aspergillus*, *Candida*, and *Pneumocystis*, but not *Mucorales* and *Cryptococcus* (27). In the United States, the Fungitell assay (BDG) has been approved by the Food and Drug Administration for the diagnosis of invasive fungal infections, with positive and negative tests defined as at least 80 pg/mL and below 60 pg/mL, respectively. Levels of 60 to 79 pg/mL are considered indeterminate. BDG becomes positive earlier than blood culture, and is a relatively sensitive, but nonspecific, test. In meta-analyses, the pooled BDG sensitivity and specificity for diagnosing invasive candidiasis were 75% to 80% and 80%, respectively (28,29). In a few studies evaluating nonneutropenic critically ill patients with candidemia or IAC, the sensitivity and specificity of BDG ranged from 52% to 100% and 58% to 94%, respectively (30). A major drawback of BDG is its low specificity and positive predictive value for invasive candidiasis. Indeed, BDG is not specific for *Candida*, as it also detects other fungi such as *Aspergillus*, *Fusarium*, and *Trichosporon*. Furthermore, numerous factors might cause false-positive BDG tests, including fungal colonization, disruption of GI mucosa, bacteremia, hemodialysis with cellulose membranes, glucan-contaminated blood collection tubes and surgical gauze, administration of human blood products, and use of certain broad-spectrum antibiotics (1,31). In general, false-positive BDG results are rare in healthy controls, but common in patients with bacteremia and ICU residents (32).

Detection of *Candida* DNA using polymerase chain reaction (PCR) is a potentially useful diagnostic test that enables early detection of invasive candidiasis. A meta-analysis of 54 studies with 4,694 patients demonstrated that PCR in whole blood had pooled sensitivity and specificity for suspected invasive candidiasis of 95% and 92%, respectively (33). In probable invasive candidiasis, the sensitivity of PCR was 85%, higher than that of the blood culture (38%). To date, PCR data for patients colonized with *Candida* are limited, but overall, there was trend toward lower specificity (30). Major limitations of PCR are the lack of standardized methodologies and multicenter validation of assay performance (33,34). In 2015, U.S. Food and Drug Administration approved the T2Candida assay (T2 Biosystems, Massachusetts), which amplifies and detects *Candida* DNA within whole blood by PCR and T2 magnetic resonance (T2MR), respectively. The test is able to detect five most common *Candida* spp (*C. albicans, C. glabrata, C. parapsilosis, C. tropicalis,* and *C. krusei*). Published clinical study on the T2Candida assay is limited to a report of 250 contrived blood specimens spiked with five Candida spp and 1,501 control patients with *Candida*-negative blood culture (35). In this setting, the sensitivity and specificity were 91% and 99%, respectively. A potential advantage of T2Candida assay is time to test positivity (mean time of 4.4 hours) compared with automated blood culture (2–5 days). A potential advantage of T2Candida over BDG is its ability to speciate *Candida* and to identify poly-*Candida* fungemia. Nevertheless, studies are required to evaluate the performance of T2Candida assay in real time among patients with invasive candidiasis.

The overwhelming majority of studies of nonculture diagnostics have focused on candidemia. Nonculture tests are unlikely to be more sensitive than blood cultures for diagnosing primary candidemia, but may shorten turn-around times. A potential role of nonculture tests is in the diagnosis of blood culture–negative, deep-seated candidiasis (34,36). Assays may accomplish this goal by detecting *Candida* antigens or DNA that are released from deep tissue sites or that persist in blood after viable cells are eliminated (37). Indeed, two recent studies assessed the role of BDG among prospectively enrolled patients with deep-seated candidiasis (34,38), in both studies, the sensitivities of BDG (65% and 67%, respectively) were higher than blood culture (21% and 7%, respectively). Along the same line, PCR has also been shown to be superior to BDG in diagnosing deep-seated candidiasis. In a prospective study of 24 patients with deep-seated candidiasis in whom samples were collected at the same time for testing, the sensitivities were 88% with PCR, 62% with BDG, and 17% with blood culture (34). These studies suggest that nonculture diagnostics may be useful adjuncts to blood cultures, and identify some patients who are currently undiagnosed.

Treatment

Invasive Candidiasis. The major antifungal agents and the current guidelines for management of invasive candidiasis are summarized in Tables 89.2 and 89.3, respectively (39). In general, the selection of an antifungal agent for the treatment of invasive candidiasis should take into account the severity of illness of patients, the target organ involved, history of recent azole or echinocandin use, previous episodes of candidiasis, and antifungal drug intolerance. Echinocandin should be the first-line treatment for critically ill patients with invasive candidiasis. This class of antifungal exhibits potent candidacidal activity and is highly efficacious in the treatment of invasive candidiasis in randomized comparative trials (40). It also has favorable tolerance and safety profile. The only limitation is the need for intravenous administration. The three echinocandins—anidulafungin, caspofungin, and micafungin—are considered therapeutically equivalent. Fluconazole can be considered an acceptable alternative to echinocandin for noncritically ill patients with no recent azole exposures and who are considered unlikely to be infected with azole-resistant *Candida* isolates. Transition from an echinocandin to fluconazole can be safely done for patients who are clinically stable and who are infected with fluconazole-susceptible *Candida* isolates. Voriconazole offers little advantage over fluconazole during initial therapy for invasive candidiasis, but has a role as step-down oral therapy for selected cases of invasive candidiasis due to *C. krusei*. Amphotericin B formulations can be considered an acceptable alternative for patients not able to tolerate an echinocandin or azole agents, or who are infected with multi–drug-resistant *Candida* species. Lipid formulations of amphotericin B are better tolerated than amphotericin deoxycholate and have less nephrotoxicity.

All patients with candidemia should have an ophthalmologic examination to rule out retinal involvement. In addition, all vascular catheters should be removed if possible. *Candida* spp tend to form biofilms on catheters, which can render otherwise susceptible isolates resistant to antifungal agents.

Candida Recovered from Urine or Sputum/Bronchoalveolar Lavage. As mentioned above, *Candida* spp are part of endogenous flora and frequent colonizers of mucosal surfaces. In the ICU setting, urine and sputum are the two most common sites of colonization.

***Candida* in the Urine.** *Candida* spp are now the most common organisms recovered from the urine of surgical ICU patients. The risk factors include urinary catheters, old age, and receipt of antibacterial agents. Unlike the assessment of bacteriuria, colony counts and urine analysis are not helpful in deciding whether candiduria is of clinical importance (41,42). Many studies have demonstrated that asymptomatic candiduria in the low-risk patient is of little clinical relevance and should not be treated. In a small subset of patients, candiduria is a marker for invasive candidiasis. Treatment is indicated for symptomatic patients and those who are neutropenic, have undergone a urologic manipulation, or received a kidney transplant. Treatment entails removal of the urinary catheter and therapy with a systemic antifungal agent (fluconazole or amphotericin B) for 7 to 14 days. Echinocandins do not penetrate well, and voriconazole and isavuconazole do not accumulate in active forms in the urine, thus should not be used for renal candidiasis. In the event that catheter removal is not possible, changing the catheter might be of benefit and should be performed. For cystitis due to fluconazole-resistant *Candida* spp, an alternative treatment is amphotericin deoxycholate (50 mg/mL) bladder irrigation for 5 days.

***Candida* in the Sputum.** Specimens from the airways—sputum, tracheal aspirates, and BAL—are frequently contaminated with oropharyngeal flora, including *Candida* spp. Despite the frequency with which *Candida* spp are isolated from the respiratory tree of ICU patients, primary *Candida* pneumonia is extremely rare; cases are generally encountered among neutropenic hosts. The diagnosis of *Candida* pneumonia requires evidence of parenchymal invasion by hyphae on a biopsy specimen. Antifungal therapy should not be instituted in response to *Candida* isolates recovered from respiratory samples. In fact, strategies of not identifying or reporting *Candida* spp in respiratory samples decrease length of stay, hospital costs, and unnecessary antifungal therapy, without any negative effects on the accurate diagnosis of *Candida* pneumonia or patient outcome (43).

Controversies

Given the nonspecific clinical manifestations, low yield of blood cultures, and high mortality rates of invasive candidiasis, investigators have studied three treatment strategies in the absence of a definitive diagnosis:

- Prophylactic strategy: Administration of an antifungal agent at a period of high risk to prevent candidiasis.
- Preemptive strategy: Administration of an antifungal agent to treat suspected invasive candidiasis based on particular warning signs.
- Empiric therapy: Administration of an antifungal agent in persistently febrile patients without a known source or with no response to appropriate antibacterial agents.

Prophylactic Strategy. The role of prophylactic antifungal therapy is controversial, as results from several clinical trials are contradictory. The most popular antifungal agent used for prophylaxis is fluconazole, given its benign side effect profile and good absorption. Five meta-analyses showed that antifungal prophylaxis (mostly fluconazole) reduced invasive candidiasis (44–47), but only one analysis showed reduction in mortality (47). It should be pointed out that only a small subset of patients is at sufficient risk for invasive candidiasis to justify this strategy. Thus, universal prophylaxis to all ICU patients is not warranted. To date, the specific patient populations that would benefit most are not clearly defined. However, populations in which antifungal prophylaxis may be useful include patients with gastric perforation, gastrointestinal dehiscence and/or leakage, status-post multiple abdominal procedures, surgical treatment for pancreatic infection, and liver transplant recipients with significant risk factors for invasive candidiasis (choledochojejunostomy, prolonged operative time, receipt of substantial amount of blood products, *Candida* infection within the preceding 3 months, and living donor transplant).

TABLE 89.2 Available Systemic Antifungal Agents

Class of Antifungal	Mechanisms of Actions of Specific Drugs	Routes of Administration and Daily Doses	Spectrum of Activity	Side Effects and Toxicity
Polyene	Potent antifungal agents that act by binding to ergosterol in the fungal cell membrane, leading to leakage and cell death Amphotericin B (AmB), available in three formulations: • AmB deoxycholate (dAmB; often called conventional AmB) • AmB lipid complex (ABLC) • Liposomal AmB (L-AmB)	IV for invasive candidiasis Usual daily dosages: dAmB, 0.5–1.5 mg/kg ABLC, 5 mg/kg L-AmB, 3–5 mg/kg	AmB is active (fungicidal) against most pathogenic fungi, except the following: *Trichosporon beigelii, Aspergillus terreus, Pseudallescheria boydii, Malassezia furfur, Fusarium* spp. Some *Candida lusitaniae* and *C. guilliermondii* isolates are resistant.	Infusion-related (fever, chills, and myalgia). Nephrotoxicity: Azotemia, electrolyte wasting (potassium, magnesium), renal tubular acidosis. Overall, the lipid-based formulations of AmB are less nephrotoxic.
Azoles	Inhibition of cytochrome P450 14α-demethylase, an enzyme involved in the sterol biosynthesis pathway Fluconazole	PO and IV Usual daily dosage: 6 mg/kg. Doses of 12 mg/kg are increasingly used to overcome intermediately susceptible (i.e., dose-dependent) organisms.	Fungistatic agent, active against *Candida* spp, *Cryptococcus* spp, and *Coccidioides immitis. Candida krusei* is intrinsically resistant, and resistance has been reported among isolates of several other *Candida* spp, especially *C. glabrata*. No activity against molds. Limited activity against *Histoplasma capsulatum, Blastomyces dermatitidis*, and *Sporothrix schenckii*.	In general, well-tolerated. Hepatotoxicity is rare.
	Itraconazole	PO (solution preferred) Daily dosage: PO: 200 mg bid	Active against yeasts, molds, and dimorphic fungi. Limited activity against *Fusarium* and Zygomycetes. Resistance has been reported among *Candida* and *Aspergillus* spp.	Generally benign. Hepatotoxicity is rare.
	Voriconazole	PO and IV Daily dosage: IV: load with 6 mg/kg every 12 hrs X1 day, then 4 mg/kg bid. PO: 200–300 mg bid	Active against yeasts, molds and dimorphic fungi. Variable activity against *Fusarium*. Limited activity against Zygomycetes. Resistance has been reported among *Candida* and *Aspergillus* spp.	Dose-related, transient visual disturbances, skin rash, and elevated hepatic enzyme levels have been reported.
	Posaconazole	PO, suspension Daily dosage: 200 mg/day QID	Active against yeasts, molds (including Zygomycetes) and dimorphic fungi. Variable activity against *Fusarium*.	Nausea and headache. Rash, dry skin, nausea, taste disturbance, abdominal pain, dizziness, and flushing can occur. Posaconazole can cause abnormalities in liver function.
	Isavuconazole	PO (delayed release), IV Daily dosage: 300 mg BID × 1 day, then 300 mg daily PO (delayed release), IV Daily dosage: 200 mg q8 hrs × 6 doses, then 200 mg daily	Active against yeasts, molds (including Zygomycetes) and dimorphic fungi.	GI side effect, elevated liver enzymes
Glucan synthesis inhibitors (echinocandins)	Block the synthesis of a major fungal cell wall component, 1-3-β-D-glucan Caspofungin Anidulafungin Micafungin	IV Caspofungin: 70 mg load, then 50 mg daily Anidulafungin: 200 mg, then 100 mg/day Micafungin: 100 mg/kg	Activity is mainly against *Candida* spp and *Aspergillus* spp. No activity against *Cryptococcus* or Zygomycetes.	Side effects are limited Liver toxicity

TABLE 89.3 Recommended Antifungal Agents against Invasive Candidiasis

Host	Primary Therapy	Alternative Therapy	Comments
Nonneutropenic	*Recommended:* Caspofungin, 70 mg IV once, then 50 mg/day IV *or* Anidulafungin, 200 mg IV for 1 dose, then 100 mg/day IV *or* Micafungin, 100 mg/day IV *Acceptable alternatives:* Fluconazole,[a] 800 mg load then 400–800 mg/day IV or PO *or* AmB, 0.6–1 mg/kg/day IV *or* lipid formulation of AmB (3–5 mg/kg/day) *Others:* Voriconazole, 400 mg (6 mg/kg) IV every 12 hrs for 2 doses, then 200–300 mg (3–4 mg/kg/day) IV every 12 hrs (can be switched to 200–300 mg bid PO after 3 days)	AmB, 0.7 mg/kg IV plus fluconazole, 800 mg IV or PO for 4 to 7 days, then fluconazole, 800 mg/day	Transition from an echinocandin to fluconazole can be safely done for patients who are clinically stable, infected with fluconazole-susceptible *Candida* isolate, in whom blood cultures have sterilized. Duration: 14 days after the documented blood culture clearance and resolution of signs and symptoms Removal of all vascular catheters
Neutropenic	*Recommended:* Caspofungin, 70 mg IV once, then 50 mg/day IV *or* Anidulafungin, 200 mg IV for 1 dose, then 100 mg/day IV *or* Micafungin, 100 mg/day IV *Alternatives:* AmB, 0.7–1 mg/kg/day IV *or* lipid formulations of AmB, 3–5 mg/kg/day IV *or* Fluconazole,[a] 800 mg load, then 400–800 mg/day IV or PO Voriconazole, 400 mg (6 mg/kg) IV every 12 hrs for 2 doses, then 200–300 mg (3–4 mg/kg/day) IV every 12 hrs (can be switched to 200–300 mg bid PO after 3 days)		Duration: 14 days after the last positive blood culture, resolution of signs and symptoms, and of neutropenia Removal of vascular catheters if possible (controversial issue)

[a]Fluconazole is an acceptable alternative for treatment of invasive candidiasis in selected patients who are not critically ill, considered not infected with fluconazole-resistant *Candida*, or have not received previous azole agents.

Preemptive Strategy. There have been two randomized trials evaluating preemptive echinocandin antifungal approaches among ICU patients. The first trial utilized a clinical prediction rule to identify medical–surgical ICU patients with invasive candidiasis (48). There was a trend toward a reduction in proven or probable invasive candidiasis in the caspofungin arm of the trial (9.8%, 10/102) versus the control arm (16.7%, 14/84; $p = 0.14$); however, there was no difference in mortality between the two groups. The second trial targeted high-risk surgical ICU patients with intra-abdominal infection for randomization to micafungin or placebo (49). Although patients in the micafungin arm had significantly reduced *Candida* colonization indices, there were no differences in the rates of invasive candidiasis, mortality, or organ failure between the 2 arms. Taken together, these studies demonstrate that precise ICU subgroups that may benefit from preemptive antifungal therapy against invasive candidiasis are not yet identified.

Empiric Strategy. Empiric administration of antifungal agents, although widely employed by some practitioners, has not been validated in clinical trials. A randomized controlled trial evaluating empiric fluconazole among medical–surgical ICU patients with persistent fevers despite broad-spectrum antibiotics failed to show significantly reduced rates of invasive candidiasis (5% in the fluconazole arm and 9% in the placebo arm) or improved outcomes. This trial suggests that empiric antifungal therapy solely based on nonspecific clinical features is unlikely to be of benefit.

In summary, optimal approaches for incorporating clinical prediction rules and/or nonculture diagnostics into management strategies remain undefined. An important step moving forward is the identification of a biomarker with substantial negative predictive value to safely discontinue empiric antifungal therapy among patients at low-to-moderate risk of IC (pretest likelihood of 3%–10%) and positive predictive value to trigger preemptive therapy among patients at moderate-to-high risk of IC (pretest likelihood about 10%–35%) (36). In clinical settings where pretest likelihood for IC is high (>25%–35%), the optimal strategy might be universal prophylaxis. On the other hand, in clinical settings where pretest likelihood is very low (<3%), routine nonculture testing or prophylactic or preemptive therapy might not be necessary (36).

Infections Caused by *Aspergillus* Species (Aspergillosis)

Aspergillus spp are less common human pathogens in the ICU than *Candida* spp but cause greater morbidity and mortality. These molds are ubiquitous in the environment; in normal hosts, they are generally saprophytes that colonize the bronchopulmonary tree. Most infections caused by *Aspergillus* spp originate from the inhalation of fungal spores into the lungs. Cases of direct skin inoculation of *Aspergillus* have been described in association with the insertion of intravenous devices or the taping of arm boards to the extremities.

Patients with severe burns can also develop local burn wound infections. Regardless of the portal of entry, any local form of aspergillosis can disseminate to various sites if host immune function is impaired.

Almost any organ may be involved in disseminated aspergillosis, including integument (onychomycosis, cutaneous aspergillosis), ear (otomycosis), respiratory tract (sinusitis, pneumonia, empyema), heart (endocarditis, myocarditis), gastrointestinal tract (GI, hepatosplenic aspergillosis), central nervous system (CNS) (cerebral aspergillosis, meningitis), eye (endophthalmitis), bone (osteomyelitis, mediastinitis), and so forth. The lungs and sinuses are the two most common primary sites of aspergillosis; the CNS is the most common secondary site.

The four classical clinical syndromes of pulmonary aspergillosis are presented in Table 89.4. This section will focus

TABLE 89.4 Clinical Spectrum of Aspergillosis

Clinical Syndromes	Description and Epidemiology	Predisposing Factors	Clinical Characteristics	Outcome
Aspergilloma	Fungus ball (a mass of fungal mycelia, inflammatory cells, tissue debris) within a pre-existing lung cavity Usually, the fungus does not invade the surrounding lung parenchyma or blood vessels 17% of patients with pre-existing lung cavity have aspergilloma	Pre-existing lung cavity	Often asymptomatic. Some develop hemoptysis. Chest radiograph shows a mobile intracavitary mass with an air crescent in the periphery.	Asymptomatic patients: No treatment. Symptomatic patients: Intracavitary AmB or antimold azole agents. Surgical resection: Reserved for patients with massive hemoptysis; carries significant morbidity and mortality.
Allergic bronchopulmonary aspergillosis (ABPA)	Hypersensitivity reaction to *Aspergillus* colonization of the tracheobronchial tree. This can occur by itself or in conjunction with *Aspergillus* sinusitis 7–10% of patients with steroid-dependent asthma and 7% of patients with cystic fibrosis have ABPA. The incidence is much less among all patients with asthma (<1%)	Patients with asthma or cystic fibrosis	Typical presentations: fever and pulmonary infiltrates unresponsive to antibacterial therapy; cough with mucous plugs. Suggestive findings: asthma, eosinophilia, a positive skin test result for *Aspergillus fumigatus*, serum IgE level >1,000 IU/dL, fleeting pulmonary infiltrates, central bronchiectasis, mucoid impaction, and positive test results for *Aspergillus* precipitins.	Systemic corticosteroids (inhaled steroids have no effect). For recurrent ABPA, itraconazole in conjunction with systemic steroids speeds the resolution of symptoms and facilitates steroid taper.
Chronic necrotizing aspergillosis	Chronic, indolent destructive process of the lung due to invasion by *Aspergillus* The rate of disease is not known	Underlying lung disease. Patients with mild immunosuppression, diabetes, poor nutrition, chronic lung diseases (such as COPD, inactive tuberculosis, previous radiation therapy, pneumoconiosis, cystic fibrosis), lung infarction, sarcoidosis. This syndrome can also follow aspergilloma	Typical presentations: fever, cough, sputum production, and weight loss for several months. Chest radiographs show an infiltrative process with or without a fungal ball. The diagnosis requires confirmation by demonstration of fungal tissue invasion and the growth of *Aspergillus* species on culture.	Systemic antifungal therapy with voriconazole (or itraconazole) or lipid formulations of AmB. Caspofungin might also be considered. Surgical resection is considered if the disease is focal and refractory to antifungal therapy.
Invasive aspergillosis	Rapidly progressive, often fatal infection Characterized by fungal invasion of blood vessels. Infection can disseminate to various organs Epidemiology: refer to discussion in text	Patients with profound immunosuppression: prolonged neutropenia; recipients of bone marrow transplant or solid organ transplant; advanced AIDS or chronic granulomatous disease; severe burn	Typical presentations: fever refractory to antibacterial agents, cough, pleuritic chest pain, or hemoptysis. Suggestive chest radiograph findings: pulmonary nodules with or without surrounding halo sign, crescent sign (indicative of cavitation), wedge-shaped or pleural-based nodules or infiltrates.	Systemic antifungal therapy with voriconazole. Itraconazole, lipid formulations of amphotericin B, and caspofungin are alternative treatments.

COPD, chronic obstructive pulmonary disease; AIDS, acquired immunodeficiency syndrome.

on the two syndromes most commonly encountered in ICU settings: chronic necrotizing pulmonary aspergillosis (CNPA) and invasive pulmonary aspergillosis (IPA). In both of these diseases, *Aspergillus* spp invades tissue and blood vessels, causing necrosis and possibly disseminating to the brain and elsewhere. Of note, entities similar to allergic aspergillosis and invasive aspergillosis (IA) are also found in the sinuses.

Pathophysiology

The major risk factors for IA include neutropenia and other defects of the immune system (Table 89.5). IA is estimated to occur in 5% to 13% of patients who have undergone hematopoietic stem cell transplant (HSCT), 5% to 25% of patients who have received SOT, and 10% to 20% of patients receiving intensive chemotherapy for leukemia. Other well-recognized risk factors for IA are chronic granulomatous disease and other immunodeficiencies, cystic fibrosis, the use of high-dose corticosteroids, and other conditions associated with cell-mediated immune defects such as acquired immunodeficiency syndrome (AIDS) and the use of TNF-α-inhibitors to treat rheumatologic and other autoimmune diseases. The disease is not as common in patients with less profound immunosuppression and exceedingly uncommon in immunocompetent hosts. Nevertheless, *Aspergillus* has been increasingly recognized as a pathogen of critically ill patients without the classical risk factors that are summarized in Table 89.5 (50). Indeed, fatal IA has been reported among patients with no known immunosuppression who develop sepsis and multiorgan dysfunction syndrome (MODS). It is speculated that sepsis displays a biphasic immunologic pattern: an early hyperinflammatory phase followed by a compensatory anti-inflammatory response syndrome/immunoparalysis state (51). Patients colonized with *Aspergillus* might develop IA during sepsis-induced immunoparalysis state. IPA can also complicate influenza (52–54), and has a predilection for patients with underlying comorbid conditions. Corticosteroid therapy during hospitalization has been linked to worse outcomes in influenza-associated IPA (54). Influenza A causes necrosis of columnar ciliated epithelium, rendering the airways susceptible to secondary opportunistic pathogens; it also suppresses phagocytosis and killing of organisms by alveolar macrophages. With worsening pneumonia following influenza A, *Aspergillus* should be added to the list of potential secondary pathogens such as *Staphylococcus aureus* and *Streptococcus pneumoniae*, particularly if there is no evidence of secondary bacterial pneumonia.

Critically ill patients with Child C liver cirrhosis and those with chronic obstructive pulmonary disease (COPD) treated with systemic and/or inhaled corticosteroids are recognized to be at risk for IA (50,55–61). Low doses of steroids and brief courses of high-dose steroids have been shown to cause an accelerated course of IPA in patients with underlying lung disease such as COPD, asthma, sarcoidosis, and berylliosis (62). IPA complicating COPD has also been rarely described outside the setting of steroid use (61,63). Finally, diabetes, end-stage heart failure, malnutrition, alcohol abuse, severe burns, prolonged ICU stays, and near drowning have all been described as host factors for IA (50,57,64).

Although there are over 100 species of *Aspergillus*, only a few cause diseases in humans. The most common species causing invasive infection is *Aspergillus fumigatus*; *A. flavus, A. terreus, A. nidulans, A. lentulus,* and *A. niger* are less common causes of invasive disease. *Avicularia versicolor* is usually considered an environmental contaminant. However, with the expansion of the immunosuppressed population, the list of esoteric species implicated in clinical infection continues to increase; thus, even previously "nonpathogenic" species can cause true disease in the right clinical setting.

Diagnosis

Culture and Histopathology. The diagnosis of IA is problematic. Since *Aspergillus* spores are ubiquitous, they are common colonizers of the bronchopulmonary tree. A definitive diagnosis, therefore, requires histologic evidence of tissue invasion by hyphal elements, as well as culture of the organism. It should be noted that the sensitivity of tissue culture and biopsy in diagnosing IA is low (e.g., 50% and 30% for

TABLE 89.5 Common Predisposing Factors to Invasive Aspergillosis

Underlying Conditions	Notes	Predisposing Factors
Allogeneic HSCT	Risk highest for transplantation from an unrelated donor > HLA-mismatched related donor > HLA-matched related donor	Early after BMT: receipt of T-cell–depleted or CD34-selected stem cell products; neutropenia; use of steroids; CMV disease; respiratory viral infections
		1–6 mo: defective cellular immunity; use of steroids
		>6 mo: use of steroids for GVHD; CMV disease
Cord blood transplant	Higher risk of fungal infections than other allograft recipients during the early and late transplant period	Early: slower myeloid engraftment >6 mo: use of steroids for GVHD
Autologous HSCT	Lowest risk of infections among the bone marrow transplants	Use of CD34-enriched autografts Use of previous potent immunosuppression for treatment of refractory malignancy
Solid organ transplant	Lung transplant has the highest risk	Immunosuppression to treat allograft rejection
Neutropenia	Highest risk among patients treated with chemotherapy for acute leukemia or aplastic anemia	Intensity (absolute neutrophil count <200 cells/μL) and duration of neutropenia (more than 10 days)
Receipt of immunosuppressive therapy	Therapy for autoimmune diseases	Receipt of high-dose steroids (dose equivalent to prednisone >20 mg for >3 wks), antilymphocyte immunoglobulin, anti-TNF-α agents, and other immunosuppressive drugs
AIDS	Advanced HIV infection with CD4+ <100 cells/μL	

CMV, cytomegalovirus; GVHD, graft versus host disease; TNF, tumor necrosis factor.

bronchoalveolar lavage fluid [BALF] culture and lung biopsies, respectively). Moreover, recovery of *Aspergillus* from the blood is extremely rare, with a sensitivity of approximately 5% in cases of IA. In immunocompromised hosts, a positive culture from a respiratory sample (sputum or BAL) is highly associated with invasive pulmonary disease.

The Clinical and Laboratory Standards Institute (CLSI) has developed standardized methods for performing susceptibility testing on filamentous fungi. However, MICs should be interpreted with caution, as interpretive breakpoints that correlate with clinical outcomes do not currently exist. Susceptibility testing of *Aspergillus* spp and other molds should therefore not be routinely performed, but reserved for cases where there is clinical failure despite optimal antifungal therapy, or for epidemiologic purposes.

Nonculture Diagnostics. Nonculture diagnostic markers, if sufficiently sensitive and specific, should theoretically allow for the early, rapid diagnosis of fungal infections, thus resulting in the earlier initiation of antifungal therapy. Several markers exist for the diagnosis of IA. We will focus on galactomannan (GM), BDG, and PCR.

GM, a heteropolysaccharide cell wall component of *Aspergillus*, can be detected in the blood and BALF. A double-sandwich enzyme-linked immunosorbent assay (ELISA) (Platelia *Aspergillus* enzyme immunoassay, Bio-Rad Laboratories, Hercules, CA, USA) has been approved by the FDA for the diagnosis of IA. The cut-off value for positivity recommended by the manufacturer and FDA is an optical density index of 0.5. However, the best cut-off for defining and positive result continues to spark debate (65,66). The performance of serum and BALF GM varies widely across different clinical settings, and has been most extensively studied in neutropenic patients with hematologic malignancy and HSCT recipients. In two large meta-analyses, the pooled sensitivity and specificity of serum GM for patients with proven or probable IA were 71% and 82% to 89%, respectively (67,68). However, these values showed marked variability across patient populations, study designs, and definitions of IA. The serum GM test is clearly superior in neutropenic patients with hematologic malignancy and HSCT recipients in whom the sensitivity was 70% and 82%, respectively, while the specificity was 92% and 86%, respectively (67). It performs poorly in SOT recipients with IA, in whom the sensitivity and specific are 22% and 84%, respectively (67).

GM testing in BALF is more sensitive than in serum (67–69). The increased sensitivity may come at the price of decreased specificity, particularly in lung transplant recipients, in whom positive GM tests cannot differentiate between invasive disease and airway colonization (70,71). There are limited data investigating the use of GM in nonclassic hosts, including the critically ill and patients with COPD. In general, the serum test performs poorly in these patients (sensitivity of 42%–51%) (72), whereas GM within BALF is more sensitive (88%) (59).

False-positive GM results have been reported with the use of antibiotics such as amoxicillin–clavulanate, colonization with other molds (*Penicillium, Fusarium, Paecilomyces, Histoplasma, Blastomyces*), and the use of Plasmalyte in BAL. Notably, current formulations of the antibiotic piperacillin/tazobactam, which was historically linked to false-positive GM assays, no longer contain GM and are thus unlikely to lead to false-positive results (73). Both serum and BAL GM can be rendered falsely negative with the receipt of mold-active antifungal therapy.

There is limited information on the diagnostic performance of BDG specifically for IA, but a retrospective study of patients with malignancy demonstrated a sensitivity and specificity of 88% and 90%, respectively. Sensitivity among ICU patients and SOT recipients is lower (66%). As mentioned above, BGD is limited by low specificity (about 44%) and positive predictive value (10%–12%); combining both BG and GM assays or higher BDG cut-off values may result in greater accuracy in the diagnosis of IA.

Although *PCR assays* are promising diagnostic tests for IA, their use in clinics remains limited because few assays have been standardized and validated, and the role of PCR testing in patient management is not established. Overall, *Aspergillus* PCR is more sensitive than culture in blood and respiratory fluids. In a meta-analysis, the sensitivity and specificity of serum or whole-blood PCR assays for IA were 84% and 76%, respectively (74). The sensitivity of *Aspergillus* PCR on BAL fluid was higher than within blood, but in many instances its specificity was lower. The lower specificity in BAL might be due to the fact that lungs are often colonized by *Aspergillus*, and that PCR is not able to differentiate colonization from disease or to distinguish different *Aspergillus* spp. The high negative predictive value of BAL PCR (usually ≥95%) suggests a role in ruling out IPA.

Radiology. In neutropenic patients and bone marrow transplant recipients, high-resolution CT scan of the chest has become an important adjunct to the diagnosis of IPA. One or more nodules surrounded by halo signs (ground glass opacity or haziness) are early findings of angioinvasive mold infections; cavitation with air-crescent sign is a late finding (75). Although these lesions are highly suggestive of IPA in high-risk patients, it should be emphasized that other infections (other fungi, *Nocardia*, and so forth) can also present with halo signs. In one study, classic CT scan findings led to the earlier diagnosis of IPA, more timely administration of antifungal therapy, and improved outcome.

Of note, halo signs have not been validated outside patients with hematologic malignancies and HSCT recipients. In SOT recipients, for instance, ground glass opacification, peribronchial consolidation, macronodules, and mass-like consolidations are commonly seen in IPA, and the halo and air-crescent signs rarely occur (76). Similar findings have been observed in COPD patients, or those who are critically ill but otherwise immunocompetent, with IPA, who develop nonspecific consolidations, nodules, and cavities but almost never have halo or air-crescent signs (55,60,72).

Treatment

Voriconazole is the first-line therapy against IA, as it has been proven superior to conventional amphotericin B. Isavuconazole might be an alternative therapeutic agent as it was shown to be noninferior to voriconazole for the primary treatment of suspected invasive IA in a randomized comparative study (77). In that study, isavuconazole was better tolerated than voriconazole, with fewer study drug–related adverse events. To date, there have not been head-to-head comparisons of voriconazole versus lipid formulations of amphotericin B. Therapy is generally prolonged for at least 6 to 12 weeks or until the primary infection is resolved. The role of other systemic antifungal

TABLE 89.6 Recommended Antifungal Agents against Aspergillosis

Antifungal Agents	Primary Therapy	Notes
Monotherapy		
Voriconazole	More effective and yields better outcome than conventional AmB. There have not been head-to-head comparisons between voriconazole and lipid formulations of AmB.	
Isavuconazole	Noninferior to voriconazole against IA (77)	Better tolerated than voriconazole
Posaconazole	Has not been evaluated as initial monotherapy for invasive aspergillosis.	Yields favorable response (42%) when used as salvage therapy (78)
Caspofungin	Has not been evaluated as initial monotherapy for invasive aspergillosis.	Yields favorable response (45%) when used as salvage therapy. To date only caspofungin has been evaluated for invasive aspergillosis among echinocandins (80)
Lipid formulations of AmB	Have not been evaluated in controlled trials.	Anecdotal reports demonstrating efficacy as salvage therapy
Combination therapy		
Liposomal formulations of AmB and caspofungin	Have not been evaluated in controlled trials.	Yield favorable outcome in 40–60% of patients (83)
Voriconazole and echinocandin	Combination therapy with voriconazole and anidulafungin led to higher survival in subgroups of patients with IA.	Superior to voriconazole alone in salvage therapy of invasive aspergillosis (82,84)

agents is summarized in Table 89.6 (78,79). Alternative therapies include lipid formulations of AmB. Echinocandins are effective in salvage therapy (either alone or in combination) against IA, but we do not recommend their routine use as monotherapy for the primary treatment of IA (80,81). The combination of an echinocandin and voriconazole for primary therapy should be considered in the setting of severe disease, especially in patients with hematologic malignancy and those with profound and persistent neutropenia (82).

Therapeutic drug monitoring (TDM) should be performed once the steady state has been reached to enhance therapeutic efficacy and minimize toxicities potentially attributable to the azoles (itraconazole, voriconazole, and solution formulation of posaconazole). Whether TDM is helpful or necessary with the extended release or intravenous formulations of posaconazole or for isavuconazole is not known at the current time.

Debridement of the involved sinuses or primary cutaneous aspergillosis should be performed in conjunction with systemic antifungal therapy. Recent data show that combined antifungal therapy and surgical resection of single lesions from the lungs or CNS might clear the infection faster than antifungal therapy alone, improve outcome, and prevent reactivation during consecutive chemotherapy courses (85–89). The procedures are generally well tolerated and associated with low rates of complications and mortality.

VIRAL INFECTIONS

Recent years have seen the emergence of unexpected viral diseases with high case fatality rates, including Hantavirus pulmonary syndrome (HPS), West Nile virus (WNV) encephalitis, severe adult respiratory syndrome, Middle East respiratory syndrome coronaviruses (MERS-CoV), and avian influenza. There are several reasons for critical care physicians to be familiar with a range of viral infections and to consider these in their differential diagnoses (90). First, there is a small window of time to effectively intervene with antiviral agents in many of these diseases. Second, the timely identification of persons with potentially infectious viral diseases has significant public health implications and may reduce the risk of transmission to other persons. Third, in the era of long-distance travel, clinicians must recognize previously unfamiliar diseases. Finally, viruses such as those causing hemorrhagic fevers are possible agents of bioterrorism.

In general, viral infections can be diagnosed by several means:

- Serologic tests: The antibody response to viral antigens can be detected in the serum of patients with viral infections. An IgM response usually indicates recent exposure to a virus, whereas the presence of IgG reflects past exposure. Serologic testing, in general, does not provide real-time results to guide clinical management.
- Culture: Several types of cells are available for growing viruses, and no single cell line is appropriate for all of them. Therefore, it is helpful for the laboratory to know which virus the clinician suspects.
- Pathology: Histologic examination of biopsy and autopsy tissues may demonstrate changes that are typical of certain viruses (e.g., DNA viruses usually produce inclusions in the cytoplasm).
- Detection of viral antigens: Viral antigens can be detected in tissues by direct or indirect immunofluorescence using appropriate antibodies.
- Amplification of viral nucleic acids: Small copy numbers of viral DNA and RNA can be detected by PCR and reverse transcription-PCR (RT-PCR), respectively. Real-time amplification methods permit simultaneous detection and quantification of viral nucleic acids.

Table 89.7 lists the leading viruses that might be encountered in the ICU, as of the writing of this chapter. We will review major viral illnesses encountered in critically ill patients, their diagnosis, and treatment. A review of human immunodeficiency virus (HIV) medicine is covered in Chapter 91.

TABLE 89.7 Viral Pathogens Most Likely to Be Encountered in the ICU

Family	Viruses	Acute Critical Illness
DNA viruses		
Adenoviridae	Adenovirus	Myocarditis
Hepadnaviridae	Hepatitis B	Fulminant liver failure, myocarditis
	Hepatitis delta virus	Fulminant liver failure
Herpesviridae	Herpes simplex	Myocarditis, meningoencephalitis
	Varicella zoster	Pneumonitis, encephalitis
	Cytomegalovirus	Opportunistic infection in immunosuppressed hosts
	EBV	Fulminant liver failure
	HHV8 (Kaposi sarcoma virus)	Pulmonary or GI bleeding in HIV
Papovaviridae	JC, BK, other polyomavirus	Renal failure, encephalitis
Parvoviridae	Parvovirus B19	Myocarditis
Poxviridae	Vaccinia	Postvaccinia vaccine complication
RNA viruses		
Arenaviridae	Lymphocytic choriomeningitis virus	Encephalitis
	South American hemorrhagic fever	Hemorrhagic fever
Bunyaviridae	California encephalitis	Encephalitis
	Hantavirus pulmonary syndrome	Pneumonitis
	Bunyavirid hemorrhagic fever	Hemorrhagic fever
Coronaviridae	Coronavirus (including SARS associated)	Pneumonitis
Filoviridae	Marburg	Hemorrhagic fever
	Ebola	Hemorrhagic fever
Flaviviruses	Yellow fever	Encephalitis
	Dengue, dengue hemorrhagic fever	Hemorrhagic fever
	Japanese encephalitis	Encephalitis
	West Nile encephalitis	Encephalitis
	St. Louis encephalitis	Encephalitis
	Tick-borne encephalitis	Encephalitis
	Hepatitis C	Myocarditis
Orthomyxoviridae	Influenza virus	Pneumonitis, myocarditis
	Avian influenza	Pneumonitis
Paramyxoviridae	Parainfluenza	Pneumonitis
	Mumps	Myocarditis
	Respiratory syncytial virus	Pneumonitis in children, IC
	Human metapneumovirus	Encephalitis, myocarditis
	Measles virus (rubeola)	
Picornaviridae	Enterovirus	Myocarditis
	Hepatitis A	Fulminant hepatic failure
	Poliovirus	Myocarditis
	Coxsackievirus, echovirus, and newer enteroviruses	Myocarditis
	Rhinovirus	
Retroviridae	Human T-cell lymphotropic virus I and II	Acute adult T-cell leukemia
	Human immunodeficiency virus	Refer to Chapter 91
Rhabdoviridae	Vesicular stomatitis virus and related virus	Encephalitis
	Rhabdovirus	
Togaviridae	Rubella virus (German measles)	Myocarditis

EBV, Epstein–Barr virus; HHV-8, human herpes virus 8; GI, gastrointestinal; SARS, severe acute respiratory syndrome; IC, intensive care.

Viral Infections on Admission to the ICU

Viral Pneumonitis

The two major sites of viral infections that require ICU admission are the respiratory tract and CNS. However, other organs such as heart, liver, gastrointestinal tract, pancreas, and muscle may also be involved in severe infections. Viruses have been increasingly recognized as causes of community-acquired pneumonia, and account for approximately 3% to 10% of the cases. In a French ICU, bronchoscopy of 41 patients with severe pneumonia revealed that 30% of all BALs and 63% of bacteria-negative BALs were positive for a respiratory virus (91). Influenza A and B are the most common causes of viral pneumonia in immunocompetent adults, followed by other respiratory viruses such as parainfluenza, adenovirus, respiratory syncytial virus (RSV), HSV, varicella zoster, coronavirus, and human metapneumovirus. These viruses can cause severe pneumonia with acute respiratory distress syndrome requiring mechanical ventilation. A major challenge in caring for patients with community-acquired pneumonia is that viruses often co-exist with bacteria. Furthermore, viruses might worsen bacterial pneumonia.

It is difficult to differentiate bacterial from viral pneumonia, but patients who have viral pneumonia often have a less severe illness and may complain of a dry hacking cough. Cultures are often necessary to make a definitive diagnosis. The radiographic findings of viral pneumonia are generally nonspecific, ranging from minimal changes on chest radiograph to hyperinflation or bilateral reticular opacities that are diffuse in distribution. Uncommonly, viral pneumonias can be associated with thickened interlobular septae that result in Kerley B lines. Viral pneumonias are rarely associated with pleural effusions, unless complicated by secondary bacterial pneumonia (92). CT scan of the chest may show poorly defined air space nodules, patchy areas of peribronchial ground glass opacity, and consolidation.

Influenza Virus

In the United States, epidemics of influenza typically occur during the winter. Approximately 66% of patients hospitalized with influenza are older than 64 years of age. Morbidity and mortality are highest among the elderly, children younger than 2 years of age, and persons of any age who have comorbid illnesses such as cardiac, pulmonary, or renal diseases, diabetes mellitus, and/or immunosuppression.

Human infections are caused by influenza A, B, or C viruses. Wild birds are the natural host for influenza A, and the virus infects humans, birds, pigs, and other animals. Influenza B and C viruses are usually found only in humans. Influenza A and B can cause severe disease and occur in epidemics. Influenza A can also be responsible for pandemics. Influenza C, on the other hand, causes only mild illness in humans and does not result in epidemics or pandemics.

Influenza A viruses are divided into subtypes on the basis of the two main surface glycoproteins, hemagglutinin (HA) and neuraminidase (NA). There are 18 known HA and 11 known NA subtypes of influenza A. New influenza virus variants result from frequent antigenic change, termed *antigenic drift*, resulting from point mutations that occur during viral replication. Influenza B viruses undergo antigenic drift less rapidly than influenza A viruses. The 2009–2010 influenza A pandemic, caused by a novel H1N1 human-swine-avian reassortant virus, was associated with high morbidity and mortality, especially among children and young adults (93). Most deaths were related to respiratory failure resulting from severe pneumonia and acute respiratory distress syndrome.

Immunity to surface antigens, particularly HA, reduces the likelihood of infection and severity of disease. Antibody against one influenza virus type or subtype confers limited or no protection against another type or subtype of influenza. Furthermore, antibody to one antigenic variant of influenza virus might not completely protect against a new antigenic variant of the same type or subtype. Antigenic drift is the basis for seasonal epidemics and the reason for the incorporation of one or more new strains in each year's influenza vaccine. More dramatic antigenic changes, or shifts, occur less frequently and can result in the emergence of a novel influenza virus with the potential to cause a pandemic.

Transmission. Influenza is transmitted from person-to-person through close contact or inhalation of droplets following sneezing, coughing, talking, or by contact with infected fomites. Infected people might transmit viral particles to others beginning one day before and 5 to 7 days after the first onset of symptoms.

Diagnosis. The classic influenza symptoms in healthy adults include abrupt fever, myalgia, headaches, and upper respiratory symptoms. In elderly or immunocompromised hosts, these classic symptoms might be absent, and patients might present only with fever and altered mental status.

Influenza-associated lower respiratory tract infections can be classified into four general forms (94):

- Influenza without radiographic evidence of pneumonia: Up to 30% of hospitalized patients with influenza have no evidence of pulmonary infiltrates (95).
- Viral pneumonia followed by bacterial pneumonia: The true incidence is unknown. The most common bacteria are *S. aureus* and *S. pneumoniae.*
- Rapidly progressive diffuse viral pneumonia: This entity may be decreasing due to the increased rate of influenza vaccination in the elderly.
- Concomitant viral and bacterial pneumonia: In addition to *S. aureus* and *S. pneumoniae*, the most common bacterium is *Haemophilus influenzae.* These patients are generally more ill than the other groups, with a higher rate of ICU admission and greater morbidity. Poor outcomes result from worsening of underlying heart or lung conditions, secondary bacterial pneumonia, toxic shock syndrome, endotoxemia, myopericarditis, cytokine-induced shock syndrome, encephalitis, and transverse myelitis.

Several tests can be performed to diagnose influenza. Nasopharyngeal swabs, nasal washes, and aspirates obtained within the first 4 days of illness are preferred respiratory samples.

- *Rapid influenza tests* can provide results within 30 minutes, and some distinguish between influenza A and B. The overall sensitivity is 50% to 70%, with a specificity of 90% to 95%. These tests are useful in the diagnosis of individual patients and in detecting outbreaks.
- *Direct immunofluorescent antibody (DFA) staining* requires 2 to 4 hours for results. It distinguishes influenza A and B and is often performed in a panel that also detects parainfluenza and RSVs.
- *RT-PCR* is more sensitive and specific than other influenza tests, and distinguishes both influenza A and B. Some tests can distinguish specific influenza subtypes. A disadvantage of RT-PCR is that results may not be available in a clinically relevant time frame to direct clinical management decisions.
- Multiplex PCR respiratory virus panel (RVP) allows the simultaneous detection of a wide range of pathogens, mostly viruses but also atypical bacteria such as *Mycoplasma pneumoniae*, *Chlamydophila pneumoniae*, *Legionella pneumophila*, and *Bordetella pertussis.*
- *Viral culture* might take up to 10 days. Culture is essential for determining influenza A subtypes and distinguishing influenza A or B strains, information that can be incorporated into the following year's vaccine.
- *Serology* is used mainly for research or public health investigations, as results are not helpful for clinical decision making.

Treatment. Two classes of antiviral drugs are available for the prevention and treatment of influenza (Table 89.8):

- *Amantadine* and *rimantadine* target the M2 protein of influenza A and are not effective against other influenza viruses. These agents have not been recommended since 2006 due to the emergence of a high level of resistance. Both amantadine and rimantadine are generally well tolerated, but CNS side effects are more common in the elderly. Dosing modification is based on renal function.
- *Oral oseltamivir, inhaled zanamivir,* and *intravenous peramivir* are NA inhibitors that are active for prevention and therapy against both influenza A and influenza B. They

TABLE 89.8 Antiviral Agents (Excluding Anti-HIV, Anti-HBV, and Anti-HCV Drugs)

Drugs	Description	Viral Agents	Infection and Sites	Dose in Patients with Normal Renal Function	Toxicities	Viral Resistance	Mechanism of Resistance
Acyclovir	Acyclic guanosine nucleoside analogue	HSV-1, HSV-2, and VZV	Mucocutaneous HSV infection HSV or VZV encephalitis or VZV pneumonitis	400 mg tid PO or 5 mg/kg q8h IV (also available as topical agent) 10 mg/kg q8h IV	Headache, nausea Renal, neurologic toxicities	<1% in immunocompetent hosts 6–8% in immunocompromised hosts 11–17% in patients with AIDS and transplant recipients	Most common: no or low production of viral thymidine kinase (TK) → cross-resistant to penciclovir and ganciclovir Altered TK substrate specificity Altered viral DNA polymerase
Valacyclovir	L-valine ester prodrug of acyclovir	HSV-1, HSV-2, and VZV	Mucocutaneous HSV Cutaneous HZV	1 g bid PO 1 g tid PO	Similar to acyclovir		Same as acyclovir
Famciclovir	Ester prodrug of penciclovir	HSV-1, HSV-2, and VZV	Mucocutaneous HSV Cutaneous VZV	125–500 mg bid PO 500–750 mg bid to tid PO	Headache, nausea, and diarrhea		Inactive against TK-deficient strains of HSV and VZV
Ganciclovir	Acyclic guanosine nucleoside analogue	HSV-1, HSV-2, VZV, CMV, EBV	CMV retinitis, pneumonitis, or other organ disease	5 mg/kg q12h IV	Hematologic	About 8% of isolates in AIDS patients are resistant to ganciclovir after a course of therapy; resistance also documented among transplant recipients	Mutation of UL97 gene or of viral DNA polymerase Some ganciclovir-resistant strains with DNA polymerase mutations are cross-resistant to foscarnet and cidofovir
Valganciclovir	Ester prodrug of ganciclovir	CMV	CMV retinitis	900 mg bid po	Hematologic	Same as ganciclovir	Same as ganciclovir
Foscarnet	Pyrophosphate analogue	HSV-1, HSV-2, VZV, CMV, HIV	CMV HSV VZV	60 mg/kg q8h IV or 90 mg/kg IV q12h IV 40 mg/kg q8h or 60 mg/kg q12h IV 60–90 mg/kg q12h IV	Renal (azotemia, acute tubular necrosis)	<5% of patients on foscarnet therapy Metabolic and electrolyte imbalance Neurotoxicity (tremor, headache)	Point mutations in DNA polymerase of HSV and CMV, and reverse transcriptase of HIV. In general, no cross-resistance with ganciclovir or cidofovir, although some ganciclovir-resistant strains with DNA polymerase mutations are cross-resistant to foscarnet and cidofovir
Cidofovir	Nucleotide analogue	HSV-1, HSV-2, VZV, HHV-6, HHV-8, CMV, EBV, DNA viruses (papilloma, poyloma, pox viruses)	CMV retinitis	5 mg/kg once a week IV	Renal (proximal tubular dysfunction), Ocular (anterior uveitis or ocular hypotony)	Uncommon	Ganciclovir-resistant CMV (due to DNA polymerase mutations plus UL97 mutations) and some foscarnet-resistant CMV strains are cross-resistant to cidofovir

(Continued)

TABLE 89.8 Antiviral Agents (Excluding Anti-HIV, Anti-HBV, and Anti-HCV Drugs) (*Continued*)

Drugs	Description	Viral Agents	Infection and Sites	Dose in Patients with Normal Renal Function	Toxicities	Viral Resistance	Mechanism of Resistance
Amantadine Rimantadine	Tricyclic amine	Influenza A	Influenza A within 48 hrs of symptoms	100 mg bid po	Gastrointestinal complaints and neurologic toxicities (rimantadine has lower neuro effects)	Up to 30% of patients treated shed-resistant viruses by the fifth day	Cross-resistance between amantadine and rimantadine Resistant viruses remain susceptible to neuraminidase inhibitors
Zanamivir	Neuraminidase inhibitor	Influenza A, B	Influenza within 48 hrs of symptoms	10 mg bid via inhalation	Bronchospasm		
Oseltamivir	Neuraminidase inhibitor	Influenza A, B	Influenza within 48 hrs of symptoms	75 mg bid po 600 mg IV	Neuropsych, nausea		Diarrhea, constipation, insomnia, and high blood pressure.
Peramivir	Neuraminidase inhibitor	Influenza A, B	Influenza within 48 hrs of symptoms				
Ribavirin	Nucleoside analogue	RSV	RSV in infants	6 g/300 mL over 12–18 hr/day via aerosol	Teratogenic, embryotoxic Anemia	No viral resistance has been detected (except for Sindbis virus)	
		Hepatitis C	Hepatitis C	500–600 bid po (together with IFN)	Reversible hyperbilirubinemia		
		Lassa fever or Hantavirus		IV, may be obtained from CDC			

work best if initiated within 48 hours of clinical symptoms. Although all antiviral medications lessen symptoms and shorten the duration of illness, only oseltamivir has been shown to reduce lower respiratory tract complications requiring antibiotics. Patients with asthma or COPD are advised to have a fast-acting inhaled bronchodilator available when inhaling zanamivir. Zanamivir should be stopped if patients develop difficulty breathing.

Prevention. Yearly vaccination is the best means to prevent influenza. Vaccination is particularly important in people who are at high risk of having serious complications, such as those 65 years of age or older, and those with cardiac or pulmonary diseases, diabetes or other metabolic diseases, renal dysfunction, hemoglobinopathies, or immunosuppression, or people (physicians, nurses) caring for those at high risk for serious complications. During influenza outbreaks within an institution or community, public health practice is to combine influenza vaccine and antiviral medications. The vaccine is given to the exposed patients and staff, and the antiviral agent is also given for about 2 weeks until the vaccine takes effect.

Respiratory Syncytial Virus

RSV causes acute respiratory illness in persons of all ages. The annual frequency of RSV infection in the elderly and high-risk adults is about 5.5% (96). Among patients admitted to a hospital for community-acquired pneumonia, RSV is second to influenza among viral causes. RSV and influenza A result in comparable lengths of stay, admissions to ICUs, and mortality (8% and 7%, respectively). There are subtypes of RSV (A and B), with subtype A causing more severe disease.

Transmission. RSV is transmitted person-to-person through close contact or inhalation of large droplets following sneezing or coughing, or by contact with infected fomites. In the United States, RSV outbreaks occur in the winter. In tropical regions, outbreaks occur usually in the rainy season.

Diagnosis. The clinical presentation varies depending on the patient's age and health status. Older children and young adults typically present with upper respiratory symptoms or tracheobronchitis. The elderly and immunocompromised may develop pneumonia. Wheezing occurs in 35% of elderly patients with RSV infection. The presentations can be difficult to differentiate from other causes of viral illnesses, including influenza. In general, however, the upper respiratory infection (URI) symptoms tend to last longer than those caused by other respiratory viruses, and are associated with a bronchitic cough and wheezing (96). Findings on chest radiograph range from focal interstitial or lobar consolidations to diffuse alveolar interstitial infiltrates. Infections are particularly severe in compromised hosts, with a mortality of 30% to 100% in bone marrow transplant recipients (97).

The diagnosis is made by viral detection (by culture or immunofluorescence) or by detection of viral antigens, RNA, or serology. Cultures are performed on respiratory secretions and require 4 to 14 days for results. Rapid assays using *antigen capture technology* can be performed in less than 30 minutes, and sensitivity and specificity approach 90%. Multiplex PCR RVP enables simultaneous diagnosis of multiple respiratory pathogens. In general, the diagnosis is more difficult to establish in adults than in children due to the low titers of viral shedding.

Treatment. Therapy is mainly supportive. Bronchodilators may help to relieve bronchospasm in some patients. Early use of inhaled ribavirin has been shown to reduce morbidity and mortality in adult bone marrow transplant patients who develop RSV infections (97). More aggressive therapy with combined ribavirin, intravenous immunoglobulin with high titers of neutralizing RSV antibody, and/or steroids can be considered in immunosuppressed patients with severe RSV pneumonia (96–98).

Varicella Zoster Virus

Varicella zoster virus (VZV) causes chickenpox or shingles. Primary infection usually occurs in childhood and is generally a benign self-limited illness in immunocompetent hosts. Although pneumonia is an uncommon complication of varicella in healthy children, it is the most frequent complication in healthy adults. The reported incidence rate is about 2.3 in 400 cases in the United States, and the overall mortality is between 10% and 30% (99,100). In patients with respiratory failure due to varicella pneumonia who require mechanical ventilation, mortality rates approach 50% despite institution of aggressive therapy and supportive measures. Cigarette smoking, pregnancy, immunosuppression, and male sex are risk factors for varicella pneumonia (99,100).

Diagnosis. Varicella pneumonia develops insidiously 1 to 6 days after the onset of the vesicular rash, with symptoms of cough, shortness of breath, fever, and occasionally pleuritic chest pain or hemoptysis. Examination of the chest may reveal rhonchi or wheezes. Chest radiograph typically reveals diffuse or patchy nodular infiltrates with a prominent peribronchial distribution. Reticular markings, pleural effusions, and hilar adenopathy may be seen as well (101).

Treatment. Prompt treatment with intravenous acyclovir at a dose of 10 mg/kg every 8 hours has been associated with clinical improvement and resolution of pneumonia. The addition of steroids for the treatment of life-threatening varicella pneumonia is controversial, and has not been well studied. In one study, patients who received steroids as adjunctive therapy had shorter hospitalizations and ICU stays and no mortality (102,103). Rapid institution of extracorporeal life support has been reported to improve outcome in patients with severe life-threatening varicella pneumonia (104).

Prevention. Two doses of chickenpox vaccine are about 98% effective at preventing chickenpox, and are recommended for children, adolescents, and adults.

Hantavirus Pulmonary Syndrome

Among the agents causing HPS, the *Sin Nombre* (Spanish for "nameless" or "without a name") virus that caused the 1993 Four Corners outbreak in the southwestern United States is the most severe. Many Hantaviruses are shed in the urine, feces, or saliva of infected rodents, and transmission to humans occurs via aerosols (105). The deer mouse *Peromyscus maniculatus* is the predominant reservoir. A total of 690 cases of HPS have been reported in the United States through January 6, 2016 (http://www.cdc.gov/hantavirus/surveillance/).

Diagnosis. The incubation period is 1 to 3 weeks, after which patients experience fever, muscle pain, and fatigue; some patients also experience headache, dizziness, vomiting, or diarrhea. Four to 10 days later, patients develop cough and respiratory distress. In general, there are no defined sets of symptoms and signs that reliably distinguish HPS from other forms of noncardiogenic pulmonary edema or adult respiratory distress syndrome (ARDS). Features associated with HPS are thrombocytopenia, hemoconcentration, leukocytosis with increased band forms on differential, hypoalbuminemia, and lactic acidosis. The classic diagnostic triad includes thrombocytopenia, neutrophilia, and an immunoblast count of greater than 10% of the total lymphocytes. Shock and lactic acidosis are associated with poor prognosis; the case fatality ratio is 30% to 40%.

Clinicians should consider HPS in the differential diagnosis of previously healthy patients from endemic areas who present with fever greater than 101°F and develop bilateral diffuse interstitial edema of the lungs within 72 hours of hospitalization. The edema can resemble ARDS on chest radiograph.

Laboratory tests for confirmation of HPS include serology, immunohistochemistry of infected tissue, and RT-PCR in tissue and blood. Serology, an ELISA of IgG test in conjunction with the IgM-capture test, is available in some state health laboratories and the CDC. Immunohistochemistry of tissues using specific monoclonal and polyclonal antibodies is a sensitive method for laboratory confirmation of hantaviral infections. RT-PCR is very prone to cross-contamination and should be considered an experimental technique (http://www.cdc.gov/hantavirus/technical/hps/diagnostics.html).

Treatment. There is no specific antiviral therapy for HPS, and treatment is mainly supportive, with early initiation of mechanical ventilation to treat respiratory failure. In specialized centers, the use of extracorporeal membrane oxygenation (ECMO) should be considered in patients with a cardiac index of less than 2.5 L/min/m^2 despite inotropes (106). A placebo-controlled double-blind trial of intravenous ribavirin for the treatment of Hantavirus cardiopulmonary syndrome in North America was terminated early due to the drug's probable ineffectiveness (107).

Severe Acute Respiratory Syndrome

Severe acute respiratory syndrome (SARS) is a serious pulmonary illness caused by a coronavirus that jumped species from semidomesticated animals to humans and spread from China to Hong Kong in late 2002 (http://www.cdc.gov/sars/) (108,109). The infection is spread by close person-to-person contact via respiratory droplets; incubation period is 2 to 10 days. The patients first experience a high fever associated with chills, headache, and myalgia. Diarrhea is seen in approximately 10% to 20% of patients. Two to 7 days later, patients develop a dry nonproductive cough and hypoxia that progresses to ARDS and multiple organ dysfunction. Ten percent to 20% of patients require mechanical ventilation. RT-PCR, serology, and cultures of blood, stool, and nasal secretions are possible diagnostic tools but have shortcomings that make routine clinical use difficult. There is no specific treatment against the SARS-associated coronavirus, and supportive care remains the principal therapeutic alternative. Ribavirin and corticosteroids have been used, but their efficacy has not been established. Mortality approximates 11%. Infection control practices are extremely important in halting the progression of an outbreak.

Middle East Respiratory Syndrome Coronavirus. Middle East respiratory syndrome (MERS) is a severe viral respiratory illness caused by a novel coronavirus (MERS-CoV). It was first reported in Saudi Arabia in 2012 and has since spread to several other countries; dromedary camels are thought to be the primary animal host for MERS-CoV. Case clusters suggest that human-to-human transmission occurs. Indeed, secondary cases have occurred in health care and household settings. The incubation period ranges from 2 to 14 days. Most people develop severe acute respiratory illness, including fever, cough, and shortness of breath; diarrhea, nausea, and vomiting can also occur. Severe complications, such as pneumonia and kidney failure, develop, and most of the patients died. Virus can be found in lower respiratory tract samples and this shedding may persist for several weeks. Virus can be detected by real-time reverse-transcriptase PCR (RT-PCR). Several serology assays are available for the detection of MERS-CoV antibodies. The CDC has developed a two-stage approach, which uses an ELISA for screening followed by an indirect immunofluorescence test or microneutralization test for confirmation. Management involves mainly supportive care.

Other Viruses

Although uncommon in adults, adenovirus pneumonia outbreaks have been described among military recruits and among adults in chronic care facilities (110). Diagnosis is established by culture of a nasopharyngeal aspirate or swab, throat swab, or sputum. Other viruses associated with acute pneumonias in adults include measles, parainfluenza, human metapneumovirus, and rarely, parvovirus.

Viral Meningitis and Encephalitis

The terms, *viral meningitis* and *encephalitis*, refer to infections of the leptomeninges and brain parenchyma, respectively. The important feature that differentiates viral meningitis and encephalitis is the presence or absence of altered sensorium. Patients with viral meningitis may be lethargic and have severe headache, but their cerebral function remains normal. In encephalitis, cerebral functions are abnormal, including altered mental status, altered behavior and personality changes, speech or movement disorder, and focal neurologic deficits. Viral meningitis and encephalitis are common, with the reported incidence of 11 and 7 per 100,000 person-years, respectively. Some patients may have both a parenchymal and meningeal process that is called *meningoencephalitis*.

Viral (Aseptic) Meningitis

The common causes of viral meningitis are summarized in Table 89.9 (111,112). Other viruses such as Epstein–Barr virus (EBV), cytomegalovirus (CMV), human herpes virus 6 (HHV-6), and herpes zoster (reactivation of VZV infection) are less common causes of aseptic meningitis. Arboviruses such as St. Louis encephalitis and California encephalitis (SLE and CE, respectively) more commonly cause encephalitis or meningoencephalitis but can also cause aseptic meningitis.

The clinical presentations of viral meningitis are nonspecific with fever, headache, photophobia, and nuchal rigidity as common symptoms. Helpful clues to the diagnosis include travel to arbovirus endemic areas, exposure history (rodents, ticks), sexual activity (herpes simplex virus type 2 [HSV-2]), and contact with other people with similar symptoms (enteroviruses). Clinicians should look for pharyngitis and pleurodynia (enteroviruses), rash (zosteriform rash of VZV, vesicular rash

TABLE 89.9 Common Causes of Viral Meningitis and Encephalitis

Types of Infection	Viral Pathogen	Comments
Viral meningitis	Enterovirus	Most common cause of viral meningitis >50 serotypes of enteroviruses Can cause meningitis or meningoencephalitis
	Herpes simplex type 2	Associated with genital herpes infection
	HIV	Generally develops at the time of HIV seroconversion
	Lymphocytic choriomeningitis	Sporadic cause of meningitis Can cause meningitis or meningoencephalitis
	Adenovirus	Rare cause of viral meningitis Can cause severe meningoencephalitis in children
Encephalitis	Japanese encephalitis	Most common cause worldwide
	Herpes simplex type 1	Most common cause of sporadic viral encephalitis Associated with focal symptoms
	Arboviruses	Transmitted by mosquitoes or ticks.
	CMV, VZV	Causes disease in immunocompromised patients only
Guillain–Barré syndrome	Influenza Herpes virus (EBV, CMV, HSV, CMV) HIV HBV (acute and chronic) Zika virus (113)	 Transmitted by *Aedes aegypti* mosquitoes in specific geographic areas

HIV, human immunodeficiency virus; CMV, cytomegalovirus; VZV, varicella zoster virus.

of HSV, maculopapular rash of measles or enteroviruses), and adenopathy (primary HIV or EBV). Cerebrospinal fluid (CSF) findings include white blood cells (WBCs) less than 500/μL, of which greater than 50% are lymphocytes; protein less than 80 mg/dL; normal glucose; and negative Gram stain. CSF should be sent for bacterial and viral cultures, HSV PCR, and HIV viral load. Other tests that can be sent if indicated include enterovirus PCR and acute/convalescent serologic testing for specific viruses.

If the patient is neither immunocompromised nor toxic appearing, one can observe without giving antibiotic therapy. Treatment for enteroviral meningitis is mostly supportive (pain management and hydration). Pleconaril, which inhibits viral attachment to host cells and viral uncoating, has shown disappointing results in the treatment of enteroviral meningitis. If the patient is immunosuppressed, elderly, or toxic appearing, or has received antibiotics before presentation, one may consider empiric antibiotics for 48 hours while waiting for culture results.

Viral Encephalitis

In the United States, the most common cause of sporadic encephalitis is Herpes simplex type 1 (HSV-1). Arboviruses account for approximately 5% of viral encephalitis, with SLE virus being the most common. Clues to arboviral infection include the season (arboviruses cause disease when mosquitoes are active, whereas HSV-1 can occur at any time), location (woody or marshy areas would suggest viruses such as the cause of Colorado tick fever or nonviral illness such as Lyme disease or Rocky Mountain spotted fever), geographic region (SLE occurs in the midwest and southern United States, whereas WNV occurs in multiple continents), or a history of animal exposure (rabies). Clues on physical examination include parotitis (mumps); flaccid paralysis (WNV); tremors of the eyelids, tongue, lips, and extremities (SLE); or findings of hydrophobia, aerophobia, and hyperactivity (rabies).

The CSF findings can be similar to those of viral meningitis. Depending on clinical suspicion, the CSF can also be sent for PCR for enteroviruses, HSV, or CMV. Acute and convalescent sera against specific viral pathogens such as arboviruses, and lymphocytic choriomeningitis virus (LCMV) might also be useful in determining a cause. CT scan with IV contrast or magnetic resonance imaging (MRI) should be obtained to exclude an intracranial process (cerebritis, abscess, subdural empyema, mass occupying lesions) or to detect findings suggestive of a viral cause. Temporal and basal frontal lobe involvement suggests HSV encephalitis, whereas basal ganglia and thalamic involvement suggest Eastern equine encephalitis.

Until HSV encephalitis is ruled out, acyclovir at 10 mg/dL IV every 8 hours should be considered in patients with suspected viral encephalitis.

HSV Encephalitis. HSV encephalitis is a fulminant hemorrhagic and necrotizing meningoencephalitis that involves primarily the temporal and basal frontal cortices and the limbic system (114). HSV-1 accounts for most fatal cases of sporadic encephalitis in adults. HSV-1 encephalitis can arise either from primary infections or reactivation of a latent infection; there is no difference in outcomes among patients suffering encephalitis from a primary or reactivation HSV infection. HSV-2 accounts for herpes encephalitis in 80% to 90% of neonates and children.

Clinical Manifestations

The most common early symptoms are fever and headache. Additional symptoms include meningeal irritation, nausea, vomiting, altered consciousness, and generalized seizures. Other changes are referable to the involved areas of the brain and include anosmia, memory loss, abnormal behavior, speech defects, olfactory and gustatory hallucinations, and focal seizures. There can be rapid progression of the disease in some patients with the development of focal paralysis, hemiparesis, and coma.

Diagnosis

The diagnosis of HSV encephalitis can be strongly suggested if the typical clinical presentations are associated with specific findings on electroencephalogram (EEG) and MRI. The typical EEG findings are focal temporal abnormalities, which are found in about 80% of patients; periodic lateralized epileptiform discharges also suggest HSV encephalitis, although they are not as specific. In HSV encephalitis, a normal EEG essentially excludes the diagnosis. The typical MRI appearance is medial temporal abnormalities that do not respect hippocampal borders. CSF findings are similar to other cases of viral meningoencephalitis. Isolation of HSV from the CSF is rare, occurring in less than 5% of cases. A definitive diagnosis is made by detection of HSV DNA in CSF by PCR, which is very sensitive and specific. The availability of PCR has largely obviated the need for brain biopsy, which was the previous gold standard diagnostic test.

Treatment

Morbidity and mortality are reduced by early antiviral therapy. Intravenous acyclovir, 10 mg/kg every 8 hours, is continued for 14 to 21 days. There is a 5% relapse rate after the discontinuation of antiviral therapy.

Rabies. Rabies is caused by neurotropic RNA viruses. In addition to the classic rabies virus, at least 10 other rabies-related viruses can cause clinically indistinguishable fatal encephalitis (115). Rabies has a worldwide distribution and is found throughout the United States except Hawaii. In developing countries, dogs are the major reservoir. Wild animals remain the most important reservoir in the United States; most reported cases occur in carnivores (raccoons in the northeast, skunks in the south and southwest, and foxes in the southwest and Alaska) or insectivorous bats. In the United States, there has been an average of three fatal human cases per year since 1980 (112).

Acquisition of rabies usually occurs after a bite from an infected animal or scratching and licking by a rabid animal. Cases have also been reported after solid organ, cornea, or vascular tissue transplantation from unsuspected rabies-infected individuals.

Clinical Manifestations

Human rabies assumes two forms: furious (encephalitic) and paralytic (dumb). The furious form (observed in 80% of patients) manifests as hyperactivity, hydrophobia, pharyngeal spasms, and aerophobia. The paralytic presentation can mimic Guillain–Barré syndrome with quadriparesis, sphincter involvement, and late cerebral involvement. Some bat-associated rabies may present atypically with neuropathic pain, sensory or motor deficits, choreiform movements of the bitten limb, focal brainstem signs, myoclonus, and seizures. Regardless of presentation, the disease is almost always fatal.

Diagnosis

The diagnosis can be confirmed in several ways: (a) detection of viral RNA in saliva by RT-PCR; (b) biopsy of the nape of the neck for detection of RNA or viral antigen within hair follicles by RT-PCR or immunofluorescence staining, respectively; (c) antibodies in serum and CSF; (d) the presence of pathognomonic Negri bodies (eosinophilic neuronal cytoplasmic inclusions) in brain biopsy.

Treatment

There is no proven effective treatment for rabies after the onset of illness. Only six survivors have been reported, five of whom received postexposure vaccination. The sixth patient survived after induction of coma and treatment with ribavirin and amantadine (116). Rabies vaccination after the onset of illness is not recommended and may be detrimental. After definitive diagnosis, the primary focus is comfort care.

Management of patients with rabies poses no greater risk to health care providers than caring for patients with more common infections. Adherence to standard precautions should be maintained, including gloves, gowns, masks, eye protection, and face shield (particularly during intubation or suctioning). Because of the lack of effective treatment, postexposure prophylaxis should be initiated as soon as possible after exposure to rabid or unknown animals. This includes the administration of human rabies immune globulin and rabies vaccination (Human diploid cell vaccine or purified chick embryo cell vaccine).

West Nile Virus. WNV is a single-stranded RNA virus that can infect humans, mosquitoes, and animals such as birds and horses. In temperate climates, WNV is transmitted primarily in the summer or early fall, whereas transmission can occur year round in warmer climates. Most human WNV infections result from mosquito bites. Infection can also be transmitted via transfusion of WNV-infected blood products, transplacental fetal infection, and transplantation of infected organs.

Clinical Manifestations

Patients infected with WNV can be asymptomatic (80%), develop West Nile fever (WNF, 20%) or West Nile neuroinvasive disease (WNND, less than 1%). WNND includes meningitis, encephalitis, and acute flaccid paralysis. WNV encephalitis is more common in the elderly or immunocompromised patients. The incubation period ranges from 3 to 14 days, and symptoms generally last 3 to 6 days. Patients with WNF or WNND present with an abrupt onset of fever, headache, fatigue, anorexia, gastrointestinal complaints, myalgia, lymphadenopathy, and generalized nonpruritic maculopapular rash. Patients with WNND also present with altered mental status (46%–74%), tremor (12%–80% of patients), extrapyramidal features such as rigidity or bradykinesia (67%), and cerebellar abnormalities (11%–57%). Myoclonus, which is present in 33% of cases, is a clue to WN infection since it is rare in other causes of viral encephalitis. Seizures are unusual (1%–16%).

Diagnosis

Diagnosis of WNV infection is based on a high index of suspicion and obtaining specific laboratory tests. An IgM antibody capture ELISA (MAC-ELISA) can detect WNV in nearly all CSF and serum specimens from WNV-infected patients. Because IgM antibody does not cross the blood–brain barrier, IgM antibody in the CSF strongly suggests acute CNS infection. WNV testing of patients with encephalitis, meningitis, or other serious CNS infections can be obtained through local or state health departments.

Treatment

Treatment is supportive, with hospitalization, IV fluids, respiratory support, and prevention of secondary infections for patients with severe disease. Although ribavirin and interferon α-2b were found to have some activity against WNV in vitro, no controlled studies have been completed. The role of corticosteroids has not been assessed.

Viral Infections Acquired during Intensive Care Unit Stay

Herpes family viruses have been recognized as pathogens in immunosuppressed transplant patients and HIV/AIDS patients. Recently, they have been increasingly reported as pathogens in the nonimmunosuppressed critically ill. A retrospective review demonstrated that at least 14% of chronic critically ill surgical patients had occult CMV or HSV infection/reactivation (117).

CMV Infection

CMV infects about 60% to 70% of people during their lifetimes. Like other members of the herpes family, CMV becomes latent or persistent after primary infection. The infection can reactivate at a later time, especially in the settings of immunodeficiency or significant stress from operations or injuries.

Transmission. CMV can be found in body secretions (e.g., urine, saliva, sputum, breast milk, semen, and cervical fluid) or in circulating mononuclear and polymorphonuclear cells, vascular endothelium, and renal epithelium. CMV spreads from person-to-person by contact with body fluids. Transmission is particularly high among toddlers in day care. Day care employees are also at significant risk for CMV exposure and/or infection, as are health care personnel with direct patient contact. Congenital transmission from a mother with acute infection during pregnancy is a significant cause of neurologic abnormalities and deafness in newborns. CMV can also be transmitted by breastfeeding, blood transfusion, or receipt of an organ transplant. The major risk factors for CMV disease in SOT recipients are CMV mismatch (i.e., transplantation of a CMV-positive organ into a CMV-seronegative recipient) and the degree of immunosuppression.

Clinical Manifestations. Most immunocompetent children and adults who are infected with CMV do not develop symptoms. Some may experience an illness resembling infectious mononucleosis with fever, swollen glands, and mild hepatitis. Rare complications of primary CMV infection include hepatitis, interstitial pneumonia, Guillain–Barré syndrome, meningoencephalitis, pericarditis, myocarditis, thrombocytopenia, and hemolytic anemia. In patients who are immunocompromised, primary CMV infection can be life threatening; myelosuppression, encephalitis, hepatitis, pneumonitis, retinitis, and GI infection are the most common manifestations. Moreover, reactivation of latent CMV also causes disease in immunocompromised hosts, although typically milder than primary infection. In general, the severity of CMV disease is related to the degree of immunosuppression. CMV appears to target allografts in particular. Hepatitis, for example, is common in liver transplant recipients, pancreatitis in pancreatic transplant, and pneumonitis in lung and heart–lung transplant. CMV pneumonia is highest among bone marrow transplant recipients.

In SOT recipients, CMV infections predispose to other opportunistic infections, especially fungal or *Pneumocystis* infections. CMV infection can also affect graft survival, causing early allograft rejection in renal transplant recipients, chronic allograft rejection in cardiac transplant recipients (allograft atherosclerosis), and vanishing bile duct syndrome in liver transplant recipients.

In CMV serology-positive immunocompetent patients admitted to an ICU, CMV viremia can be detected in almost a third of patients after 2 weeks in the ICU (118). The presence of viremia was associated with increased in hospitalization stay, duration of mechanical ventilation, severe sepsis, and death.

Diagnosis. Since CMV can be shed in biologic fluids from patients with no evidence of CMV disease, the gold standard for diagnosis remains finding intranuclear inclusion bodies in histologically examined tissue. CMV infection may be confirmed by in situ hybridization or direct or indirect staining of intranuclear inclusions using specific antibodies linked to an indicator system; histopathology is limited by poor sensitivity.

CMV excretion in the saliva and urine is common in patients who are immunocompromised and is generally of little consequence. In contrast, viremia in organ transplant patients identifies CMV infection, which encompasses a spectrum ranging from asymptomatic viremia to CMV syndrome to CMV disease with tissue-invasive disease.

In bone marrow transplant recipients, the sensitivity of viremia as a marker for CMV pneumonia is 60% to 70%; lack of viremia also has a high negative predictive value. In general, detection of CMV or its products in the blood of transplant recipients is a basis for starting antiviral therapy. The value of positive CMV tests in the nontransplant ICU patient is less clear. Further studies are needed to elucidate the impact of CMV infection/reactivation in critically ill patients and to clarify the effects of CMV treatment on morbidity and mortality.

Management. Ganciclovir, foscarnet, and cidofovir are IV antiviral agents active against CMV. Valganciclovir, an oral prodrug of ganciclovir, has a 10-fold greater bioavailability than oral ganciclovir. To date, the efficacy of anti-CMV therapy has been evaluated primarily in immunocompromised hosts (transplant recipients and AIDS patients). CMV disease in transplant recipients is typically treated with a 3-week course of ganciclovir. Foscarnet is an alternative for patients who cannot tolerate, or fail to respond to, ganciclovir; but experience is more limited, and foscarnet is associated with high rates of nephrotoxicity. CMV retinitis requires a longer course of systemic therapy; intravitreal administration of ganciclovir or fomivirsen, an antisense inhibitor of CMV, is frequently used in addition to systemic therapy. Although long-term maintenance therapy is required for AIDS patients who do not undergo immune reconstitution, this strategy is generally not required for transplant recipients. Recurrence of CMV disease, which can occur in up to 25% of transplant recipients, appears to respond to ganciclovir as well as the initial episode.

CMV resistance to antivirals is a major problem among transplant recipients and in patients with AIDS. The overall incidence of ganciclovir-resistant CMV infection is about 2%, but the range varies widely. Resistance to cidofovir and foscarnet has also been reported, but it is less common. Among organ transplant recipients, risk factors for ganciclovir resistance include CMV serology mismatch (donor-positive, recipient-negative), T-cell depletion, prolonged antiviral exposure, very high viral loads, multiple episodes of CMV disease, more intensive immunosuppression, and suboptimal antiviral drug concentrations due to reduced absorption or poor compliance (119). CMV resistance results primarily from mutations in the phosphotransferase gene UL97, which do not generally confer cross-resistance to cidofovir or foscarnet. Mutations in the DNA polymerase gene UL54 may also lead to high-level resistance to ganciclovir and may confer cross-resistance to cidofovir and/or foscarnet. Drug-resistant CMV within blood or body fluid can be genetically detected by sequencing UL97 and UL54. This test is commercially available, but expensive and does not furnish a quantitative result (119). Moreover, interpretation of results requires knowledge of specific mutations proven by resistance transfer. Phenotypic assay using plaque reduction provides a quantitative result, but requires recovery of virus. The assay may take at least 4 weeks to complete, thus might not be practical for clinical use (119).

HSV Infection

HSV-1 and HSV-2 are closely related, but the epidemiology of infections by the viruses is distinct. HSV-1 is transmitted mainly by contact with infected saliva, and HSV-2 by contact with genital tract lesions. HSV-1 is acquired more commonly and at an earlier age than HSV-2. By the age of 50 years, over 90% of people have antibodies against HSV-1. Consistent with this, HSV-1 is also more common among ICU patients.

Clinical Manifestations. HSV encephalitis and meningitis are discussed above. HSV-1 can infect virtually any mucocutaneous or visceral site. Typically, primary infections are associated with systemic signs and symptoms, mucosal and extramucosal involvement, longer duration of symptoms and viral shedding, and higher complication rates. Gingivostomatitis and pharyngitis are the most common clinical syndromes of HSV-1 infection. Lesions are ulcerative with or without exudates, and can be difficult to differentiate from bacterial pharyngitis. HSV-1 also has a predilection for regenerating epithelium. Therefore, healing partial-thickness skin burns, skin donor sites, skin diseases (e.g., eczema, pemphigus, Darier disease), and areas of cutaneous trauma are common sites of infection. HSV-1 keratitis is the most frequent cause of corneal blindness. HSV-1 can also cause chorioretinitis—a sign of disseminated infection—and acute necrotizing retinitis, affecting both immunocompetent and immunocompromised hosts.

In immunocompromised hosts and patients with atopic eczema or burns, severe orofacial HSV lesions can rapidly spread and disseminate infection. Bone marrow and SOT recipients are at highest risk for HSV reactivation during the preengraftment period or within the first month after transplant. Complications include pneumonitis, tracheobronchitis, esophagitis, hepatitis, and disseminated viral infection.

HSV-1 shedding is observed in immunocompetent but critically ill patients. In one study, HSV-1 was recovered from the mouth swabs or respiratory secretions of 27% of patients requiring mechanical ventilation (120). Although the presence of HSV was associated with a higher APACHE II score and increased mortality (121), it is not clear whether HSV was the cause of the excess deaths or simply a marker for impaired immune function. HSV-1 may predispose to subsequent bacterial or fungal infection (120).

Diagnosis. The diagnosis of HSV-1 infection can be made using a direct immunofluorescence test or by culture of tissue or aspirated fluid. Serology is helpful in diagnosing primary HSV infection. Improved testing methods have led to increased detection of HSV-1 in ICU patients. As with CMV, however, it is often unclear whether HIV-1 is an active pathogen or merely a marker of immune dysfunction. Large randomized trials are needed to determine the impact of CMV and HSV isolation from respiratory specimens of patients in the ICU and the effect of treatment on morbidity and mortality of critically ill patients.

Management. For mucocutaneous and visceral infections, acyclovir or related agents (famciclovir and valacyclovir) are the standard therapy. For disseminated disease or encephalitis due to HSV-1, intravenous acyclovir is recommended. For HSV keratitis, debridement along with topical therapy with idoxuridine or vidarabine is the treatment of choice. Other ophthalmologic disease such as chorioretinitis or retinal necrosis requires systemic antiviral therapy.

Key Points

- Early and appropriate antifungal treatment improves outcomes of patients with invasive fungal infections.
- Diagnosis of invasive candidiasis is difficult due to nonspecific clinical manifestations, low sensitivity of blood culture, and time to culture positivity.
- Deep-seated candidiasis is diagnosed by culture of sterilely collected samples. Nonculture diagnostics, such as β-D-glucan and PCR, might improve the diagnosis of invasive candidiasis. Blood culture sensitivity is only 50%, and may take up to 4 weeks longer than nonculture tests to turn positive.
- Emergence of resistance against both triazoles and echinocandins merits vigilance. An important risk factor for antifungal resistance among *Candida* spp is prior drug exposure, especially in the setting of breakthrough infection.
- Antifungal susceptibility testing should be available to guide the management of patients with invasive candidiasis.
- Echinocandins are first-line treatment for critically ill patients with invasive candidiasis. Therapy can be safely changed to an azole once clinical improvement is achieved.
- IA occurs most commonly in immunocompromised patients, especially those with hematologic malignancies, prolonged neutropenia, HSCT or organ transplant, and receipt of prolonged and high-dose corticosteroids. However, there has been an increase in recognition of IA in the ICU setting, among hosts without well-recognized host factors. These include patients with end-stage lung disease (especially those with COPD on inhaled steroids), advanced AIDS, decompensated liver cirrhosis, and status-post recent influenza infection.
- Voriconazole is the first-line treatment for patients with IA. There might be a role for adjunctive echinocandin therapy, at least until therapeutic voriconazole levels are achieved.
- Respiratory viruses account for up to 10% of community-acquired pneumonia, and can cause severe pneumonia leading to respiratory failure and acute

respiratory distress syndrome. In the ICU, influenza virus is the most common viral cause of severe community-acquired pneumonia.
- Clinicians need to maintain high clinical suspicion for viral illness since the window of opportunity for treatment is often very narrow.
- Latent viruses, such as CMV or HSV, can reactivate in critically ill (immunocompromised or immunocompetent) patients in the ICU. Although latent viruses can cause pneumonia (or other diseases) in the immunocompromised patients, the significance of viral reactivation in the immunocompetent patients is not known.
- There is a critical need for new antiviral therapies that expand the rather limited present armamentarium. Until that time, vaccination, strict infection control, and other preventive strategies are the best hope for the control of viral infections.

References

1. Clancy CJ, Nguyen MH. Finding the "missing 50%" of invasive candidiasis: how nonculture diagnostics will improve understanding of disease spectrum and transform patient care. *Clin Infect Dis*. 2013;56:1284–1292.
2. Kullberg BJ, Arendrup MC. Invasive candidiasis. *N Engl J Med*. 2016; 374:794–795.
3. Eggimann P, Bille J, Marchetti O. Diagnosis of invasive candidiasis in the ICU. *Ann Intensive Care*. 2011;1:37.
4. Wisplinghoff H, Bischoff T, Tallent SM, et al. Nosocomial bloodstream infections in US hospitals: analysis of 24,179 cases from a prospective nationwide surveillance study. *Clin Infect Dis*. 2004;39:309–317.
5. Moran C, Grussemeyer CA, Spalding JR, et al. Comparison of costs, length of stay, and mortality associated with *Candida glabrata* and *Candida albicans* bloodstream infections. *Am J Infect Control*. 2010;38:78–80.
6. Wilson LS, Reyes CM, Stolpman M, et al. The direct cost and incidence of systemic fungal infections. *Value Health*. 2002;5:26–34.
7. Hassan I, Powell G, Sidhu M, et al. Excess mortality, length of stay and cost attributable to candidaemia. *J Infect*. 2009;59:360–365.
8. Marriott DJ, Playford EG, Chen S, et al. Determinants of mortality in non-neutropenic ICU patients with candidaemia. *Crit Care*. 2009;13:R115.
9. Bassetti M, Righi E, Ansaldi F, et al. A multicenter study of septic shock due to candidemia: outcomes and predictors of mortality. *Intensive Care Med*. 2014;40:839–845.
10. Blot SI, Vandewoude KH, De Waele JJ. Candida peritonitis. *Curr Opin Crit Care*. 2007;13:195–199.
11. Carneiro HA, Mavrakis A, Mylonakis E. *Candida* peritonitis: an update on the latest research and treatments. *World J Surg*. 2011;35:2650–2659.
12. Montravers P, Dupont H, Gauzit R, et al. Candida as a risk factor for mortality in peritonitis. *Crit Care Med*. 2006;34:646–652.
13. Sandven P, Qvist H, Skovlund E, et al.; theNorwegian Yeast Study Group. Significance of *Candida* recovered from intraoperative specimens in patients with intra-abdominal perforations. *Crit Care Med*. 2002;30: 541–547.
14. Asmundsdottir LR, Erlendsdottir H, Haraldsson G, et al. Molecular epidemiology of candidemia: evidence of clusters of smoldering nosocomial infections. *Clin Infect Dis*. 2008;47:e17–e24.
15. Pfaller MA, Diekema DJ, Jones RN, et al. International surveillance of bloodstream infections due to *Candida* species: frequency of occurrence and in vitro susceptibilities to fluconazole, ravuconazole, and voriconazole of isolates collected from 1997 through 1999 in the SENTRY antimicrobial surveillance program. *J Clin Microbiol*. 2001;39:3254–3259.
16. Bodey GP, Mardani M, Hanna HA, et al. The epidemiology of *Candida glabrata* and *Candida albicans* fungemia in immunocompromised patients with cancer. *Am J Med*. 2002;112:380–385.
17. Cleveland AA, Harrison LH, Farley MM, et al. Declining incidence of candidemia and the shifting epidemiology of *Candida* resistance in two US metropolitan areas, 2008–2013: results from population-based surveillance. *PloS One*. 2015;10:e0120452.
18. Pfeiffer CD, Samsa GP, Schell WA, et al. Quantitation of *Candida* CFU in initial positive blood cultures. *J Clin Microbiol*. 2011;49:2879–2883.
19. Morrell M, Fraser VJ, Kollef MH. Delaying the empiric treatment of candida bloodstream infection until positive blood culture results are obtained: a potential risk factor for hospital mortality. *Antimicrob Agents Chemother*. 2005;49:3640–3645.
20. Garey KW, Rege M, Pai MP, et al. Time to initiation of fluconazole therapy impacts mortality in patients with candidemia: a multi-institutional study. *Clin Infect Dis*. 2006;43:25–31.
21. Halliday CL, Kidd SE, Sorrell TC, Chen SC. Molecular diagnostic methods for invasive fungal disease: the horizon draws nearer? *Pathology*. 2015;47:257–269.
22. Arvanitis M, Anagnostou T, Fuchs BB, et al. Molecular and nonmolecular diagnostic methods for invasive fungal infections. *Clin Microbiol Rev*. 2014;27:490–526.
23. Rex JH, Pfaller MA. Has antifungal susceptibility testing come of age? *Clin Infect Dis*. 2002;35:982–989.
24. Shields RK, Nguyen MH, Clancy CJ. Clinical perspectives on echinocandin resistance among *Candida* species. *Curr Opin Infect Dis*. 2015; 28:514–522.
25. Alexander BD, Johnson MD, Pfeiffer CD, et al. Increasing echinocandin resistance in *Candida glabrata*: clinical failure correlates with presence of FKS mutations and elevated minimum inhibitory concentrations. *Clin Infect Dis*. 2013;56:1724–1732.
26. Perlin DS. Echinocandin resistance in Candida. *Clin Infect Dis*. 2015;61 (Suppl 6):S612–S667.
27. Haidar GF, Nguyen MH. Diagnostic modalities for invasive mould infections among hematopoietic stem cell transplant and solid organ recipients: performance characteristics and practical roles in the clinic. *J Fungi*. 2015;1:252–276.
28. Karageorgopoulos DE, Vouloumanou EK, Ntziora F, et al. Beta-D-glucan assay for the diagnosis of invasive fungal infections: a meta-analysis. *Clin Infect Dis*. 2011;52:750–770.
29. Lu Y, Chen YQ, Guo YL, et al. Diagnosis of invasive fungal disease using serum (1–>3)-beta-D-glucan: a bivariate meta-analysis. *Intern Med*. 2011; 50:2783–2791.
30. Leon C, Ostrosky-Zeichner L, Schuster M. What's new in the clinical and diagnostic management of invasive candidiasis in critically ill patients. *Intensive Care Med*. 2014;40:808–819.
31. Martin-Mazuelos E, Loza A, Castro C, et al. beta-D-Glucan and *Candida albicans* germ tube antibody in ICU patients with invasive candidiasis. *Intensive Care Med*. 2015;41:1424–1432.
32. Wheat LJ. Approach to the diagnosis of invasive aspergillosis and candidiasis. *Clin Chest Med*. 2009;30:367–377.
33. Avni T, Leibovici L, Paul M. PCR diagnosis of invasive candidiasis: systematic review and meta-analysis. *J Clin Microbiol*. 2011;49:665–670.
34. Nguyen MH, Wissel MC, Shields RK, et al. Performance of *Candida* real-time polymerase chain reaction, beta-D-glucan assay, and blood cultures in the diagnosis of invasive candidiasis. *Clin Infect Dis*. 2012;54:1240–1248.
35. Mylonakis E, Clancy CJ, Ostrosky-Zeichner L, et al. T2 magnetic resonance assay for the rapid diagnosis of candidemia in whole blood: a clinical trial. *Clin Infect Dis*. 2015;60:892–899.
36. Clancy CJ, Nguyen MH. Undiagnosed invasive candidiasis: incorporating non-culture diagnostics into rational prophylactic and preemptive antifungal strategies. *Exp Rev Anti-infect Ther*. 2014;12:731–734.
37. Kasai M, Francesconi A, Petraitiene R, et al. Use of quantitative real-time PCR to study the kinetics of extracellular DNA released from *Candida albicans*, with implications for diagnosis of invasive candidiasis. *J Clin Microbiol*. 2006;44:143–150.
38. Tissot F, Lamoth F, Hauser PM, et al. Beta-glucan antigenemia anticipates diagnosis of blood culture-negative intraabdominal candidiasis. *Am J Resp Crit Care Med*. 2013;188:1100–1109.
39. Pappas PG, Kauffman CA, Andes DR, et al. Executive summary: clinical practice guideline for the management of candidiasis: 2016 update by the Infectious Diseases Society of America. *Clin Infect Dis*. 2016;62:409–417.
40. Andes DR, Safdar N, Baddley JW, et al. Impact of treatment strategy on outcomes in patients with candidemia and other forms of invasive candidiasis: a patient-level quantitative review of randomized trials. *Clin Infect Dis*. 2012;54:1110–1122.
41. Kauffman CA. Candiduria. *Clin Infect Dis*. 2005;41(Suppl 6):S371–S376.
42. Kauffman CA. Diagnosis and management of fungal urinary tract infection. *Infect Dis Clin North Am*. 2014;28:61–74.
43. Barenfanger J, Arakere P, Cruz RD, et al. Improved outcomes associated with limiting identification of *Candida* spp. in respiratory secretions. *J Clin Microbiol*. 2003;41:5645–5649.
44. Playford EG, Webster AC, Sorrell TC, Craig JC. Antifungal agents for preventing fungal infections in non-neutropenic critically ill patients. *Cochrane Database System Rev*. 2006:CD004920.

45. Shorr AF, Chung K, Jackson WL, et al. Fluconazole prophylaxis in critically ill surgical patients: a meta-analysis. *Crit Care Med.* 2005;33:1928–1935.
46. Vardakas KZ, Samonis G, Michalopoulos A, et al. Antifungal prophylaxis with azoles in high-risk, surgical intensive care unit patients: a meta-analysis of randomized, placebo-controlled trials. *Crit Care Med.* 2006;34:1216–1224.
47. Cruciani M, de Lalla F, Mengoli C. Prophylaxis of *Candida* infections in adult trauma and surgical intensive care patients: a systematic review and meta-analysis. *Intensive Care Med.* 2005;31:1479–1487.
48. Ostrosky-Zeichner L, Shoham S, Vazquez J, et al. MSG-01: a randomized, double-blind, placebo-controlled trial of caspofungin prophylaxis followed by preemptive therapy for invasive candidiasis in high-risk adults in the critical care setting. *Clin Infect Dis.* 2014;58:1219–1226.
49. Knitsch W, Vincent JL, Utzolino S, et al. A randomized, placebo-controlled trial of preemptive antifungal therapy for the prevention of invasive candidiasis following gastrointestinal surgery for intra-abdominal infections. *Clin Infect Dis.* 2015;61:1671–1678.
50. Vandewoude KH, Blot SI, Depuydt P, et al. Clinical relevance of *Aspergillus* isolation from respiratory tract samples in critically ill patients. *Crit Care.* 2006;10:R31.
51. Hartemink KJ, Paul MA, Spijkstra JJ, et al. Immunoparalysis as a cause for invasive aspergillosis? *Intensive Care Med.* 2003;29:2068–2071.
52. Clancy CJ, Nguyen MH. Acute community-acquired pneumonia due to *Aspergillus* in presumably immunocompetent hosts: clues for recognition of a rare but fatal disease. *Chest.* 1998;114:629–634.
53. Adalja AA, Sappington PL, Harris SP, et al. Isolation of *Aspergillus* in three 2009 H1N1 influenza patients. *Influenza Other Resp Viruses.* 2011;5:225–229.
54. Alshabani K, Haq A, Miyakawa R, et al. Invasive pulmonary aspergillosis in patients with influenza infection: report of two cases and systematic review of the literature. *Exp Rev Resp Med.* 2015;9:89–96.
55. Meersseman W, Vandecasteele SJ, Wilmer A, et al. Invasive aspergillosis in critically ill patients without malignancy. *Am J Resp Crit Care Med.* 2004;170:621–625.
56. Dimopoulos G, Piagnerelli M, Berre J, et al. Disseminated aspergillosis in intensive care unit patients: an autopsy study. *J Chemother.* 2003;15:71–75.
57. Garnacho-Montero J, Amaya-Villar R, Ortiz-Leyba C, et al. Isolation of *Aspergillus* spp. from the respiratory tract in critically ill patients: risk factors, clinical presentation and outcome. *Crit Care.* 2005;9:R191–R199.
58. Rello J, Esandi ME, Diaz E, et al. The role of *Candida* sp isolated from bronchoscopic samples in nonneutropenic patients. *Chest.* 1998;114:146–149.
59. Meersseman W, Lagrou K, Maertens J, Van Wijngaerden E. Invasive aspergillosis in the intensive care unit. *Clin Infect Dis.* 2007;45:205–216.
60. Bulpa P, Dive A, Sibille Y. Invasive pulmonary aspergillosis in patients with chronic obstructive pulmonary disease. *Eur Resp J.* 2007;30:782–800.
61. Vadnerkar A, Clancy CJ, Celik U, et al. Impact of mold infections in explanted lungs on outcomes of lung transplantation. *Transplantation.* 2010;89:253–260.
62. Palmer LB, Greenberg HE, Schiff MJ. Corticosteroid treatment as a risk factor for invasive aspergillosis in patients with lung disease. *Thorax.* 1991;46:15–20.
63. Ali ZA, Ali AA, Tempest ME, Wiselka MJ. Invasive pulmonary aspergillosis complicating chronic obstructive pulmonary disease in an immunocompetent patient. *J Postgrad Med.* 2003;49:78–80.
64. Dimopoulos G, Frantzeskaki F, Poulakou G, Armaganidis A. Invasive aspergillosis in the intensive care unit. *Ann NY Acad Sci.* 2012;1272:31–39.
65. Lamoth F, Alexander BD. Nonmolecular methods for the diagnosis of respiratory fungal infections. *Clin Lab Med.* 2014;34:315–336.
66. Zou M, Tang L, Zhao S, et al. Systematic review and meta-analysis of detecting galactomannan in bronchoalveolar lavage fluid for diagnosing invasive aspergillosis. *PloS One.* 2012;7:e43347.
67. Pfeiffer CD, Fine JP, Safdar N. Diagnosis of invasive aspergillosis using a galactomannan assay: a meta-analysis. *Clin Infect Dis.* 2006;42:1417–1427.
68. Leeflang MM, Debets-Ossenkopp YJ, Visser CE, et al. Galactomannan detection for invasive aspergillosis in immunocompromized patients. *Cochrane Database System Rev.* 2008:CD007394.
69. Guo YL, Chen YQ, Wang K, et al. Accuracy of BAL galactomannan in diagnosing invasive aspergillosis: a bivariate metaanalysis and systematic review. *Chest.* 2010;138:817–824.
70. Luong ML, Clancy CJ, Vadnerkar A, et al. Comparison of an *Aspergillus* real-time polymerase chain reaction assay with galactomannan testing of bronchoalveolar lavage fluid for the diagnosis of invasive pulmonary aspergillosis in lung transplant recipients. *Clin Infect Dis.* 2011;52:1218–1226.
71. Pasqualotto AC, Xavier MO, Sanchez LB, et al. Diagnosis of invasive aspergillosis in lung transplant recipients by detection of galactomannan in the bronchoalveolar lavage fluid. *Transplantation.* 2010;90:306–311.
72. Guinea J, Torres-Narbona M, Gijon P, et al. Pulmonary aspergillosis in patients with chronic obstructive pulmonary disease: incidence, risk factors, and outcome. *Clin Microbiol Infect.* 2010;16:870–877.
73. Vergidis P, Razonable RR, Wheat LJ, et al. Reduction in false-positive *Aspergillus* serum galactomannan enzyme immunoassay results associated with use of piperacillin-tazobactam in the United States. *J Clin Microbiol.* 2014;52:2199–2201.
74. Arvanitis M, Ziakas PD, Zacharioudakis IM, et al. PCR in diagnosis of invasive aspergillosis: a meta-analysis of diagnostic performance. *J Clin Microbiol.* 2014;52:3731–3742.
75. Greene RE, Schlamm HT, Oestmann JW, et al. Imaging findings in acute invasive pulmonary aspergillosis: clinical significance of the halo sign. *Clin Infect Dis.* 2007;44:373–379.
76. Park YS, Seo JB, Lee YK, et al. Radiological and clinical findings of pulmonary aspergillosis following solid organ transplant. *Clin Radiol.* 2008;63:673–680.
77. Maertens JA, Raad II, Marr KA, et al. Isavuconazole versus voriconazole for primary treatment of invasive mould disease caused by *Aspergillus* and other filamentous fungi (SECURE): a phase 3, randomised-controlled, non-inferiority trial. *Lancet.* 2016;387:760–769.
78. Walsh TJ, Raad I, Patterson TF, et al. Treatment of invasive aspergillosis with posaconazole in patients who are refractory to or intolerant of conventional therapy: an externally controlled trial. *Clin Infect Dis.* 2007;44:2–12.
79. Herbrecht R, Denning DW, Patterson TF, et al. Voriconazole versus amphotericin B for primary therapy of invasive aspergillosis. *N Engl J Med.* 2002;347:408–415.
80. Kartsonis NA, Saah AJ, Joy Lipka C, et al. Salvage therapy with caspofungin for invasive aspergillosis: results from the caspofungin compassionate use study. *J Infect.* 2005;50:196–205.
81. Aliff TB, Maslak PG, Jurcic JG, et al. Refractory *Aspergillus* pneumonia in patients with acute leukemia: successful therapy with combination caspofungin and liposomal amphotericin. *Cancer.* 2003;97:1025–1032.
82. Marr KA, Schlamm HT, Herbrecht R, et al. Combination antifungal therapy for invasive aspergillosis: a randomized trial. *Ann Intern Med.* 2015;162:81–89.
83. Kontoyiannis DP, Hachem R, Lewis RE, et al. Efficacy and toxicity of caspofungin in combination with liposomal amphotericin B as primary or salvage treatment of invasive aspergillosis in patients with hematologic malignancies. *Cancer.* 2003;98:292–299.
84. Marr KA, Boeckh M, Carter RA, Kim HW, Corey L. Combination antifungal therapy for invasive aspergillosis. *Clin Infect Dis.* 2004;39:797–802.
85. Matt P, Bernet F, Habicht J, et al. Predicting outcome after lung resection for invasive pulmonary aspergillosis in patients with neutropenia. *Chest.* 2004;126:1783–1788.
86. Matt P, Bernet F, Habicht J, et al. Short- and long-term outcome after lung resection for invasive pulmonary aspergillosis. *Thorac Cardiovasc Surg.* 2003;51:221-225.
87. Ali R, Ozkalemkas F, Ozcelik T, et al. Invasive pulmonary aspergillosis: role of early diagnosis and surgical treatment in patients with acute leukemia. *Ann Clin Microbiol Antimicrob.* 2006;5:17.
88. Cesaro S, Cecchetto G, De Corti F, et al. Results of a multicenter retrospective study of a combined medical and surgical approach to pulmonary aspergillosis in pediatric neutropenic patients. *Pediatr Blood Cancer.* 2007;49:909–913.
89. Middelhof CA, Loudon WG, Muhonen MD, et al. Improved survival in central nervous system aspergillosis: a series of immunocompromised children with leukemia undergoing stereotactic resection of aspergillomas: report of four cases. *J Neurosurg.* 2005;103:374–378.
90. Kelesidis T, Mastoris I, Metsini A, Tsiodras S. How to approach and treat viral infections in ICU patients. *BMC Infect Dis.* 2014;14:321.
91. Legoff J, Guerot E, Ndjoyi-Mbiguino A, et al. High prevalence of respiratory viral infections in patients hospitalized in an intensive care unit for acute respiratory infections as detected by nucleic acid-based assays. *J Clin Microbiol.* 2005;43:455–457.
92. Kim EA, Lee KS, Primack SL, et al. Viral pneumonias in adults: radiologic and pathologic findings. *Radiographics.* 2002;22(Spec No):S137–S149.
93. Writing Committee of the WHO Consultation on Clinical Aspects of Pandemic (H1N1) 2009 Influenza, Bautista E, Chotpitayasunondh T, et al. Clinical aspects of pandemic 2009 influenza A (H1N1) virus infection. *N Engl J Med.* 2010;362:1708–1719.
94. Louria DB, Blumenfeld HL, Ellis JT, et al. Studies on influenza in the pandemic of 1957-1958. II. Pulmonary complications of influenza. *J Clin Invest.* 1959;38:213–265.
95. Oliveira EC, Marik PE, Colice G. Influenza pneumonia: a descriptive study. *Chest.* 2001;119:1717–1723.

96. Falsey AR, McElhaney JE, Beran J, et al. Respiratory syncytial virus and other respiratory viral infections in older adults with moderate to severe influenza-like illness. *J Infect Dis.* 2014;209:1873–1881.
97. McColl MD, Corser RB, Bremner J, Chopra R. Respiratory syncytial virus infection in adult BMT recipients: effective therapy with short duration nebulised ribavirin. *Bone Marrow Transplant.* 1998;21:423–425.
98. Neemann K, Freifeld A. Respiratory syncytial virus in hematopoietic stem cell transplantation and solid-organ transplantation. *Curr Infect Dis Rep.* 2015;17:490.
99. Feldman S. Varicella-zoster virus pneumonitis. *Chest.* 1994;106:22S–27S.
100. Gogos CA, Bassaris HP, Vagenakis AG. Varicella pneumonia in adults: a review of pulmonary manifestations, risk factors and treatment. *Respir Int Rev Thorac Dis.* 1992;59:339–343.
101. Schlossberg D, Littman M. Varicella pneumonia. *Arch Intern Med.* 1988; 148:1630–1632.
102. Mer M, Richards GA. Corticosteroids in life-threatening varicella pneumonia. *Chest.* 1998;114:426–431.
103. Adhami N, Arabi Y, Raees A, et al. Effect of corticosteroids on adult varicella pneumonia: cohort study and literature review. *Respirology.* 2006;11:437–441.
104. Lee WA, Kolla S, Schreiner RJ Jr, et al. Prolonged extracorporeal life support (ECLS) for varicella pneumonia. *Crit Care Med.* 1997;25:977–982.
105. Hartline J, Mierek C, Knutson T, Kang C. Hantavirus infection in North America: a clinical review. *Am J Emerg Med.* 2013;31:978–982.
106. Serna D, Brenner M, Chen JC. Severe Hantavirus pulmonary syndrome: a new indication for extracorporeal life support? *Crit Care Med.* 1998; 26:217–218.
107. Mertz GJ, Miedzinski L, Goade D, et al. Placebo-controlled, double-blind trial of intravenous ribavirin for the treatment of hantavirus cardiopulmonary syndrome in North America. *Clin Infect Dis.* 2004;39:1307–1313.
108. Holmes KV. SARS-associated coronavirus. *N Engl J Med.* 2003;348: 1948–1951.
109. Booth CM, Stewart TE. Severe acute respiratory syndrome and critical care medicine: the Toronto experience. *Crit Care Med.* 2005;33:S53-60.
110. Klinger JR, Sanchez MP, Curtin LA, et al. Multiple cases of life-threatening adenovirus pneumonia in a mental health care center. *Am J Resp Crit Care Med.* 1998;157:645–649.
111. Swanson PA 2nd, McGavern DB. Viral diseases of the central nervous system. *Curr Opin Virol.* 2015;11:44–54.
112. Desmond RA, Accortt NA, Talley L, et al. Enteroviral meningitis: natural history and outcome of pleconaril therapy. *Antimicrob Agents Chemother.* 2006;50:2409–2414.
113. Broutet N, Krauer F, Riesen M, et al. Zika virus as a cause of neurologic disorders. *N Engl J Med.* 2016;374(16):1506–1509.
114. Whitley RJ. Herpes simplex encephalitis: adolescents and adults. *Antiviral Res.* 2006;71:141–148.
115. Hemachudha T, Wacharapluesadee S, Laothamatas J, Wilde H. Rabies. *Curr Neurol Neurosci Rep.* 2006;6:460–468.
116. Centers for Disease C, Prevention. Recovery of a patient from clinical rabies—Wisconsin, 2004. *MMWR.* 2004;53:1171–1173.
117. Davis LE, DeBiasi R, Goade DE, et al. West Nile virus neuroinvasive disease. *Ann Neurol.* 2006;60:286–300.
118. Limaye AP, Kirby KA, Rubenfeld GD, et al. Cytomegalovirus reactivation in critically ill immunocompetent patients. *JAMA.* 2008;300:413–422.
119. Drew WL. Cytomegalovirus resistance testing: pitfalls and problems for the clinician. *Clin Infect Dis.* 2010;50:733-736.
120. Bruynseels P, Jorens PG, Demey HE, et al. Herpes simplex virus in the respiratory tract of critical care patients: a prospective study. *Lancet.* 2003; 362:1536–1541.
121. Ong GM, Lowry K, Mahajan S, et al. Herpes simplex type 1 shedding is associated with reduced hospital survival in patients receiving assisted ventilation in a tertiary referral intensive care unit. *J Med Virol.* 2004;72:121–125.

CHAPTER

90

Infections in the Immunocompromised Host

KAREN DOUCETTE and JAY A. FISHMAN

INTRODUCTION

The population of immunocompromised patients has expanded greatly due to broader application of immunosuppressive therapies combined with improved survival following organ and stem cell transplantation, cancer chemotherapy, and other chronic diseases requiring immunosuppressive therapy. In addition, monoclonal antibody therapies have revolutionized the treatment of rheumatologic as well as other systemic inflammatory and autoimmune conditions; use of such "biologic" agents results in selected immune deficits and the associated infectious complications. Despite advances in prophylactic and antimicrobial therapies, infectious complications remain a leading complication of immunosuppressive and immunomodulatory therapies.

Familiarity with the clinical presentation, differential diagnosis, and management of infectious complications in immunocompromised patients is essential in critical care medicine. An understanding of the nature of the patient's underlying immune deficits, both innate (e.g., neutropenia) or adaptive (B- or T-cell) immune deficits, and an assessment of the timing, intensity and virulence of epidemiologic exposures, will generally define the most likely pathogens responsible for infectious syndromes.

PATHOPHYSIOLOGY

The risk of infection and spectrum of likely pathogens in the immunocompromised host is determined by the interaction of two factors:

- The epidemiologic exposures of the patient including the timing, intensity, and virulence of the organisms to which the individual is exposed.
- The patient's "net state of immunosuppression," a conceptual measure of all host factors potentially contributing to the risk for infection (Table 90.1) including anatomic defects and exogenous immunosuppression. Specific immunosuppressive therapies and deficits predispose to specific types of infection (Table 90.2).

Consideration of these factors for each patient allows the development of a differential diagnosis for "infectious syndromes." Additional clues to possible etiologies of infection can be obtained from a careful epidemiologic exposure history including travel, occupation, hobbies, animal contact, exposure to ill contacts, and recent hospitalizations.

In critical care units, the most commonly encountered immunocompromised hosts are those with neutropenia, on systemic corticosteroids, following solid organ or stem cell transplantation and, increasingly, those on immunomodulatory therapies.

The Neutropenic Patient

Neutropenic patients, generally as a result of cytotoxic chemotherapy for hematologic or solid tumors, are among the most commonly encountered immunocompromised hosts. The relationship between the absolute neutrophil count (ANC) and risk of infection was described by Bodey et al., who correlated the risk for infection with the degree (usually neutrophil counts <500 cells/μL) and duration of neutropenia, notably in leukemic patients (1,2). A reduction in ANC impairs the innate host immune responses of inflammation, phagocytosis, and antigen presentation, making clinical diagnosis more difficult—via the absence of erythema or pulmonary infiltrates—and predisposing the neutropenic patient to bacterial and fungal infections, usually from endogenous colonization.

Historically, gram-negative organisms such as *Escherichia coli, Klebsiella* species, and *Pseudomonas aeruginosa* accounted for most bloodstream infections (2); gram-positive organisms, particularly *Streptococcus* species and coagulase-negative *Staphylococcus*, are now isolated in almost two-thirds of bloodstream infections (3). This shift from gram-negative to gram-positive infections (recalling a prior shift from gram-positive to gram-negative with the early deployment of cephalosporins) is related to the near universal placement of central venous catheters (CVCs) in patients undergoing chemotherapy, as well as the impact of fluoroquinolone prophylaxis on the risk of gram-negative infections (4).

The risk of opportunistic fungal infection increases with the duration and severity of neutropenia (5). Up to one-third of febrile neutropenic patients who fail to respond to a 1-week course of empiric antibacterial therapy have systemic fungal infections, most commonly (over 80%) due to *Candida* or *Aspergillus* species (6,7). The epidemiology of invasive fungal infections has evolved with the growing "at-risk" population and increased use of azole prophylaxis. Over half of the bloodstream isolates at most centers are due to non-*albicans Candida* species with increasing intrinsic (e.g., seen with *Candida krusei*) or acquired (e.g., seen with *Candida glabrata*) fluconazole resistance (8). Similarly, neutropenic patients have been found to become infected with highly resistant non-*Aspergillus* molds in addition to *Aspergillus* species (9,10).

The Corticosteroid-Treated Patient

Corticosteroids have been used for the treatment of inflammatory, autoimmune, and lymphoproliferative diseases and for prevention of allograft rejection since the 1950s, and remain an integral part of management of many of these conditions today. Corticosteroids have a broad range of effects on the immune system (11). Treatment with corticosteroids results in reduced proliferation of B and T lymphocytes, reduced release of tumor necrosis factor (TNF) and fever, inhibition of neutrophil adhesion to endothelial cells, inhibition of macrophage differentiation, and reduced recruitment of mononuclear cells, including monocytes, to sites of immune inflammation (11,12). In addition, these agents suppress cellular (Th1) immunity and promote humoral (Th2) immunity (11).

TABLE 90.1 Factors Contributing to the Net State of Immunosuppression

Immunosuppressive therapy
- Type
- Temporal sequence
- Intensity
- Cumulative dose

Prior therapies
- Chemotherapy or antimicrobials

Mucocutaneous barrier integrity
- Surgery
- Catheters
- Lines
- Drains
- Fluid collections

Neutropenia, lymphopenia
- Often drug induced

Underlying immune deficiency
- Hypogammaglobulinemia (e.g., from proteinuria)
- Complement deficiencies
- Autoimmune diseases (e.g., systemic lupus erythematosus)
- Other disease states
  - Human immunodeficiency virus
  - Lymphoma/leukemia

Metabolic conditions
- Uremia
- Malnutrition
- Diabetes mellitus
- Cirrhosis

Immunomodulatory viral infections
- Cytomegalovirus
- Hepatitis B and C
- Respiratory viruses

The risk of infection in corticosteroid-treated patients is related to the dose and duration of therapy (13,14). Those treated with more than 10 to 20 mg/day of prednisone for more than 3 to 4 weeks are at risk for infectious complications. Corticosteroids place the host at risk for fungal, viral, protozoal, and intracellular bacterial infections. Common pathogens to be considered in corticosteroid-treated patients presenting with a suspected infectious complication include *Pneumocystis jirovecii, Listeria monocytogenes, Legionella,* and *Nocardia* species. Bolus treatments with corticosteroids (e.g., for graft-vs.-host or autoimmune disease) may convert colonization (e.g., Aspergillus) to invasive infection.

The Solid Organ Transplant Patient

With improvements in surgical techniques and immunosuppressive therapy, a growing number of people are living with solid organ transplants. Intensified immunosuppression has decreased the incidence of graft rejection, while infectious complications are an important cause of morbidity and mortality. Interestingly, both a recent case-controlled and retrospective cohort study suggest that in hospital mortality in abdominal organ transplant patients with bacteremia and/or sepsis is lower than in the general population (15,16). Further confirmation of these results as well as additional research to understand the mechanism of this finding are needed.

Although all transplant recipients are at increased risk of infection compared to the general population, the risk of infection in an individual recipient is determined largely by the degree of exposure to potential pathogens and the overall or "net state of immunosuppression" (see Table 90.1) (17). These patients are differentiated from other immunocompromised hosts by the technical aspects (complex surgery) and the need for lifelong immune suppression to maintain graft function.

In an individual, the net state of immunosuppression is determined by the immunosuppressive agents selected as well as the dose, duration, and sequence of use. In addition,

TABLE 90.2 Infections Associated with Specific Immune Defects

Defect	Common Causes	Associated Infections
Granulocytopenia	Leukemia, cytotoxic chemotherapy, acquired immunodeficiency syndrome (AIDS), drug toxicity, Felty syndrome	Enteric gram negatives, *Pseudomonas, Staphylococcus aureus, Staphylococcus epidermidis,* streptococci, *Aspergillus, Candida,* and other fungi
Neutrophil chemotaxis	Diabetes, alcoholism, uremia, Hodgkin disease, trauma (burns), Lazy leukocyte syndrome, connective tissue disease	*S. aureus, Candida,* streptococci
Neutrophil killing	Chronic granulomatous disease, myeloperoxidase deficiency	*S. aureus, Escherichia coli, Candida, Aspergillus, Torulopsis*
T-cell defects	AIDS, congenital lymphoma, sarcoidosis, viral infection, connective tissue disease, organ transplants, steroids	Intracellular bacteria (*Legionella, Listeria, Mycobacteria*), herpes simplex virus, varicella zoster virus, cytomegalovirus, Epstein–Barr virus, parasites (*Strongyloides, Toxoplasma*), fungi (*Candida, Cryptococcus*) *Pneumocystis jirovecii*
B-cell defects	Congenital/acquired agammaglobulinemia, burns, enteropathies, splenic dysfunction, myeloma, acute lymphocytic leukemia	*Streptococcus pneumoniae, Haemophilus influenzae, Salmonella* and *Campylobacter* spp, *Giardia lamblia*
Splenectomy	Surgery, sickle cell, cirrhosis	*S. pneumoniae, H. influenzae, Salmonella* spp, *Capnocytophaga*
Complement	Congenital/acquired defects	*S. aureus, Neisseria* spp, *H. influenzae, S. pneumoniae*
Anatomic	Vascular/Foley catheters, incisions, anastomotic leaks, mucosal ulceration, vascular insufficiency	Colonizing organisms, resistant nosocomial organisms

factors such as underlying immune deficiencies, metabolic derangements, the presence of foreign bodies (e.g., surgical drains, CVCs) or fluid collections, and infection with immune-modulating viruses such as cytomegalovirus (CMV), Epstein–Barr virus (EBV) or human immunodeficiency virus (HIV) contribute to the risk of infection (17,18).

With standardized immunosuppressive regimens, specific infections vary in a predictable pattern depending on the time elapsed since transplantation (Fig. 90.1) (17). This is a reflection of the changing risk factors over time including surgery/hospitalization, immune suppression, acute and chronic rejection, emergence of latent infections, and exposures to novel community infections. The pattern of infection changes with the immunosuppressive regimen–for example, use of pulse dose steroids or T-cell depletion for graft rejection—intercurrent viral infections, neutropenia, or significant epidemiologic exposures, such as travel or food. The timeline remains a useful starting point, although it has been altered by the introduction of newer immunosuppressive agents (e.g., sirolimus) and patterns of use including reduced use of corticosteroids and increased use of antibody-based induction therapies. Routine antimicrobial prophylaxis, improved molecular assays, antimicrobial resistance, transplantation in HIV- and hepatitis C virus (HCV)-infected individuals have also impacted the timeline (18). Figure 90.1 demonstrates three overlapping periods of risk for infection after transplantation, each most often associated with unique groups of pathogens.

- The perioperative period to *approximately 4 weeks after transplantation*, reflecting surgical and technical complications. Most infections are related to the surgery, similar to those occurring in the complex general surgical population, such as pneumonia, surgical site, urinary tract, and CVC-associated infections caused by typical bacterial and fungal pathogens such as *Candida*. Nosocomial pathogens including methicillin-resistant *Staphylococcus aureus* (MRSA), vancomycin-resistant enterococcus (VRE), fluconazole-resistant *Candida* species, *Clostridium difficile, P. aeruginosa,* and carbapenem-resistant *Enterobacteriaceae* are increasingly common. Uncommonly, infections may be transmitted from a bacteremic or fungemic donor with potentially serious complications, including seeding of the vascular suture line. The use of prophylactic antibiotics in the recipient, directed by donor culture results, may allow organs from infected donors to be safely used without compromising transplant outcomes (19–21).
- The risk for infections in the period from *1 to 6 to 12 months after transplantation* are driven largely by the rapidity of tapering of immunosuppression, the use of antilymphocyte "induction" therapy, the use of antiviral (anti-CMV) and anti-*Pneumocystis* prophylaxis, and the reactivation of latent viral infections. Opportunistic infections include viral (CMV, varicella zoster virus [VZV], EBV, HCV), bacterial (*Nocardia*, *Listeria*, and tuberculosis), fungal (*Aspergillus, Pneumocystis,* and *Cryptococcus*), or parasitic (*Toxoplasma* and *Strongyloides*) infections.
- The period *beyond 6 to 12 months after transplantation* reflect community-acquired exposures and some unusual pathogens based on the level of maintenance immunosuppression. Commonly, these include viral respiratory infections, pneumococcal pneumonia, and gastroenteritis. Herpes simplex, CMV, and shingles infections may emerge. Intense exposure to an opportunistic pathogen may result in disease; transplant recipients should be counseled to avoid high-risk exposures such as unpasteurized milk products (22). Recipients requiring augmentation of immunosuppression for management of graft rejection, as well as those with chronic or recurrent CMV or HCV infections, remain at risk for other opportunistic infections, particularly *P. jirovecii*, invasive fungal infection, and EBV-associated, posttransplant lymphoproliferative disease (PTLD) (19–25).

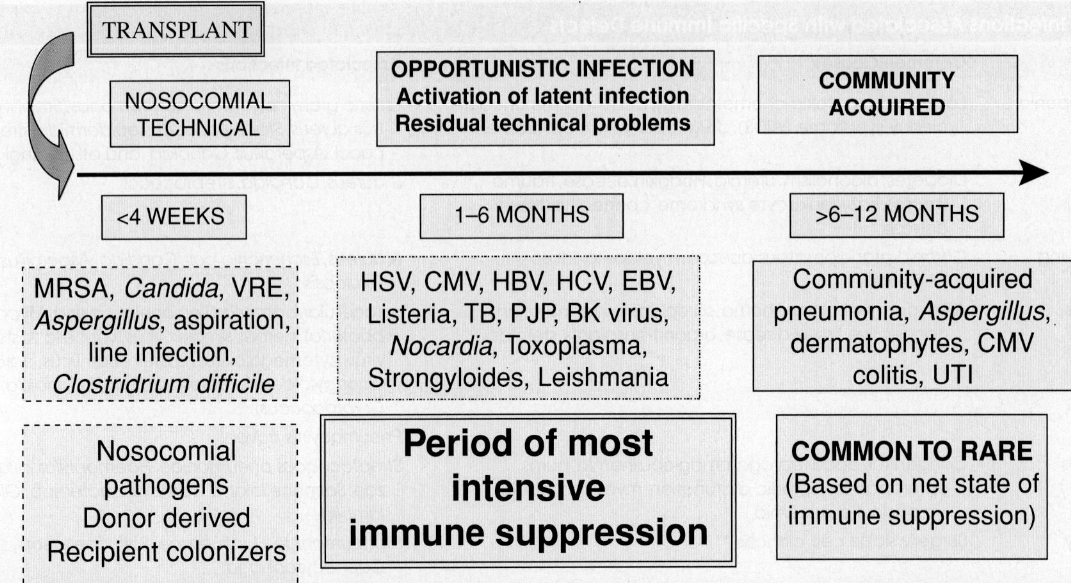

FIGURE 90.1 The timeline of infection after transplantation. MRSA, methicillin-resistant *Staphylococcus aureus;* VRE, vancomycin-resistant enterococcus; HSV, herpes simplex virus; CMV, cytomegalovirus; HBV, hepatitis B virus; EBV, Epstein–Barr virus; TB, tuberculosis; PJP, *Pneumocystic jirovecii;* UTI, urinary tract infection. (Adapted from Fishman JA, Rubin RH. Infection in organ-transplant recipients. *N Engl J Med.* 1998;338(24):1741.)

Hematopoietic Stem Cell Transplant Recipients

A growing number of patients undergo allogeneic and autologous hematopoietic stem cell transplantation (HSCT) procedures for both malignant and nonmalignant conditions (26). Despite advances, severe infectious complications are common, with up to 40% of HSCT recipients requiring intensive care unit (ICU) admission, and 60% of these needing mechanical ventilation, which is associated with a high mortality rate (27,28). Although traditionally poor, the outcomes of HSCT recipients admitted to the ICU are improving with advances in infection prevention, diagnosis and management, and ICU care (29); the combination of allogeneic transplantation, mechanical ventilation, and vasopressor use is predictive of mortality (30).

Advances in stem cell source and nonmyeloablative conditioning have resulted in shorter periods of neutropenia and less severe mucositis and hepatic venoocclusive disease; the risk of early bacterial infections is decreased while the risks of late viral, fungal, and bacterial infections persist (31,32). In part this reflects increased use of positively selected CD34+ progenitor cells for transplant which results in significant T-lymphocyte and monocyte depletion of the graft and therefore increases the risk of opportunistic infection while reducing malignant cells and reducing graft-versus-host disease (GVHD) (32). Reduced-intensity or nonmyeloablative-conditioning regimens have been developed in attempt to extend these therapies to older and more medically complex patients (34) and although the period of neutropenia is shorter, and potent antitumor effects result from these transplants, patients remain at high risk for GVHD necessitating significant immunosuppression for GVHD prophylaxis (31,33–35). As a result of pretransplant chemotherapy, with or without total-body irradiation, both humoral- and cell-mediated immunity are diminished. Natural host barrier defenses are also impaired by mucositis and the use of vascular access catheters.

The timeline of infectious complications in the HSCT recipient is generally divided into three phases.

- **The pre-engraftment phase**—the period from conditioning therapy to engraftment when patients are neutropenic. Prolonged neutropenia carries the risk for bacterial and fungal infections. Similar to other neutropenic hosts, there has been a shift from predominantly gram-negative to gram-positive—coagulase-negative *Staphylococci*, *Streptococci*, *Enterococci*—bacterial infections with the use of fluoroquinolone prophylaxis, to which the streptococci are generally resistant (4). Many centers use azole prophylaxis to reduce the incidence of candidemia; however, azole-resistant fungemia remains common (36,37). Herpes simplex virus may also reactivate during this phase but can be prevented with prophylactic acyclovir in seropositive HSCT recipients.
- The second phase, from **engraftment to day 100** or for the duration of treatment for acute GVHD, is characterized by deficits in cellular immunity. The most important pathogens in this period are viral, particularly CMV and adenovirus, and invasive mold infections. The most common manifestations of CMV disease in HSCT recipients are pneumonia and gastrointestinal disease (38). Despite treatment with intravenous ganciclovir and CMV-hyperimmune globulin or intravenous immunoglobulin, the mortality from CMV pneumonitis remains high at 50% or greater (38). The use of ganciclovir or valganciclovir for prophylaxis or preemptive therapy has resulted in a decreased risk of CMV infection during this period, with most infections now occurring after discontinuation (39). Adenovirus may produce severe hepatitis.

  Interstitial pneumonitis is an important clinical syndrome presenting during the postengraftment phase; etiologies include CMV, respiratory viruses, or idiopathic pneumonia syndrome (IPS, which is overdiagnosed). *P. jirovecii* can be eliminated as a cause of pneumonitis with TMP-SMX prophylaxis. Respiratory viral infections, such as influenza, respiratory syncytial virus (RSV), parainfluenza virus, and human metapneumovirus are commonly recognized as etiologies of pneumonia in HSCT (40). A number of noninfectious etiologies must also be considered in the differential diagnosis, including IPS and diffuse alveolar hemorrhage.

  Most invasive mold infections occur during the postengraftment phase, and are associated with treatment of acute GVHD (37). Although *Aspergillus* continues to be the predominant pathogen, non-*Aspergillus* molds, including Zygomycetes, *Fusarium*, and *Scedosporium* species are important pathogens in this population (41,42). Invasive mold infections generally present as pulmonary nodules or pneumonia, but invasive fungemia with septic emboli, sinus disease, and disseminated disease including central nervous system (CNS) involvement are other common presentations.
- In the **late phase, beyond day 100 following engraftment** and with chronic GVHD, the incidence of infection is determined by the level of immunosuppression required for the GVHD. Beyond 100 days post transplant, there is gradual recovery of humoral and cellular immune function, but immune reconstitution is often incomplete and antimicrobial prophylaxis may simply shift risk to later periods (43). Up to 40% of HSCT recipients develop VZV infection, generally as a result of reactivation of latent infection, with most cases occurring during the first year. Late CMV disease may occur and is associated with a history of early CMV disease and GVHD (44). Late invasive mold infections may occur, particularly in those with GVHD and preceding viral (CMV) infection. About one-third of patients with chronic GVHD may develop recurrent infection with encapsulated bacteria (sinopulmonary, bacteremia) (45). The predominant pathogen is *Streptococcus pneumoniae* (often with antimicrobial resistance) as well as *Haemophilus influenzae* and *S. aureus*. This risk is related to a deficit in opsonizing antibody (4,36,40,44–52).

The Patient Treated with Immunomodulatory Agents

There are a growing number of immunomodulatory agents, generally targeting specific cell populations and cytokines, commonly used in clinical practice (53). As more patients are treated with these therapies and with longer-term follow-up, understanding of the risk of infection associated with these biologic compounds will be refined.

Tumor necrosis factor-α (TNF-α) antagonists are effective in the treatment of rheumatoid arthritis, active inflammatory bowel disease, psoriasis, and ankylosing spondylitis, and are amongst the best characterized in terms of infectious risk. There are currently five marketed in the United States: Infliximab (Remicade, Centocor Inc.), etanercept (Enbrel, Amgen and Wyeth Pharmaceuticals), adalimumab (Humira, Abbott), certolizumab pegol (Cimzia, UCB Inc.), and golimumab (Simponi, Janssen). Blockade of TNF-α, a proinflammatory cytokine, results in improvement in systemic inflammatory conditions; however, TNF-α, along with interferon-γ and other cytokines, is an important component in maintaining cellular immunity and, in animal studies, preventing bacterial deep tissue infections.

Tuberculosis has been associated with use of TNF-α antagonists due to cell-mediated immune deficits (54,55). Rates are three- to fourfold higher with adalimumab and infliximab compared to etanercept (56,57). In general, cases have occurred in those with risk factors for latent tuberculosis infection. As a result, tuberculosis skin testing (TST) or interferon-gamma-release assay (IGRA) and chest radiography are recommended in patients prior to the initiation of a TNF-α antagonist as well as the newer biologic agents. Regardless of TST or IGRA data, tuberculosis (and nontuberculous mycobacterial infections) should be considered in the differential diagnosis in a patient presenting with compatible symptoms and after a TNF-α antagonist. Infections with fungi (histoplasmosis, aspergillosis, coccidiomycosis, and candidiasis), bacteria (listeriosis, nocardiosis), parasites (leishmaniasis), and viruses (herpes zoster, hepatitis B and C reactivation) have also been associated with the use of TNF-α antagonists. In 2008 the FDA issued a black box warning regarding endemic mycoses and TNF-α antagonists, although the exact degree of risk appears to vary based on intensity of exposure (55).

Rituximab (Rituxan, Genentech Inc. and Biogen Idec) is a chimeric murine/human monoclonal antibody to the CD20 epitope expressed on B lymphocytes but not plasma cells. Treatment with rituximab results in rapid depletion of circulating CD20+ B cells. This agent is approved for the treatment of CD20+ B-cell lymphoma, as well as in combination with methotrexate in rheumatoid arthritis. Rituximab has also been used for the treatment of PTLD, immune thrombocytopenic purpura, autoimmune hemolytic anemia, systemic lupus erythematosus, multiple sclerosis, GVHD, and treatment of antibody-mediated graft rejection (58). Following rituximab therapy, antibody production is maintained by plasma cells. Peripheral B-cell recovery takes 3 to 12 months (59). Approximately 5% of people can develop persistent hypogammaglobulinemia after rituximab treatment, increasing infectious risk (60–62). Fatal hepatitis B reactivation (63,64) and progressive multifocal leukoencephalopathy (PML), a demyelinating disease of the CNS caused by human JC polyomavirus, have been associated with rituximab (65).

Numerous other biologic agents are currently approved or undergoing study (53). Table 90.3 summarizes selected approved agents, mechanism of action, associated infectious risks, and approved indications.

DIAGNOSIS

The signs and symptoms of infection are often muted in immunocompromised hosts with infectious syndromes (66). Minor complaints may be the only clues to localize infections. A physical examination should be completed, with particular focus on organ systems commonly involved with infectious complications including the skin, respiratory tract including sinuses, CNS, and urinary tract. Cutaneous lesions may be the earliest manifestation of disseminated infection. Examination of the skin should include the perirectal area, looking for evidence of erythema or tenderness; this is a common site of infection and source of fever notably in neutropenic patients.

In neutropenic patients, fever, defined as a single oral temperature of 38.3°C (101°F) or higher or a temperature of

TABLE 90.3 Selected Biologic Agents, Mechanisms of Action, Food and Drug Administration (FDA)-Approved Indications and Associated Infections

Biologic Agent	Mechanism of Action	FDA-Approved Indications	Associated Infectious Risk
Natalizumab (Tysabri)	Integrin receptor antagonist	Relapsing multiple sclerosis moderately to severely active Crohn disease with failure or intolerance to conventional therapies including TNF inhibitors	Progressive multifocal leukoencephalopathy/JC virus herpes encephalitis and meningitis
Abatacept (Orencia)	Selective costimulation modulator; inhibits T cell (T lymphocyte) activation by binding to CD80 and CD86, thereby blocking interaction with CD28	Adult rheumatoid arthritis Juvenile idiopathic arthritis	Sepsis Pneumonia Blunted response to immunizations; live vaccines contraindicated
Ustekinumab (Stelara)	IgG1 k_1 monoclonal antibody that binds with specificity to the p40 protein subunit used by both the IL-12 and IL-23 cytokines	Moderate to severe plaque psoriasis and active psoriatic arthritis	Serious bacterial, fungal, and viral infections including disseminated mycobacterial disease, *Salmonella* and reactivation of hepatitis B
Tocilizumab (Actemra)	Binds specifically to both soluble and membrane-bound IL-6 receptors and inhibits signaling	Adult rheumatoid arthritis Polyarticular juvenile idiopathic arthritis Systemic juvenile idiopathic arthritis	Serious infections leading to hospitalization or death including tuberculosis, bacterial (pneumonia, UTI), invasive fungal (*Aspergillus*), and viral (herpes zoster) infections as well as pneumocystis pneumonia
Tofacitinib (Xeljanz)	Janus kinase (JAK) inhibitor	Adult rheumatoid arthritis with inadequate response to methotrexate	Serious and sometimes fatal infections. The most common serious infections reported include pneumonia, cellulitis, herpes zoster, and urinary tract infection; tuberculosis and other mycobacterial infections, esophageal candidiasis, pneumocystosis, CMV, and BK virus have been reported

38°C (100.4°F) or higher for an hour or more, may be the only indication of infection (6). About 50% of neutropenic patients with fever have a documented infection, and about 20% of those with neutrophil counts less than 100 cells/μL have bacteremia (2–7,9,10,67,68). Up to 50% of neutropenic patients with a normal chest radiograph and fever lasting 2 days, despite empiric antibiotic therapy, will have findings on chest CT suggestive of pneumonia that were not appreciated on plain radiograph (69). A daily search for subtle signs and symptoms of infection should be undertaken if unexplained fever persists.

Basic investigations include a CBC with differential, serum creatinine, liver enzymes, and liver function tests in addition to *cultures of blood, urine, and sputum prior to antimicrobial therapy*. A chest radiograph should be performed and, if normal, a CT scan should be obtained in the patient with pulmonary symptoms. Collection of additional specimens is guided by the clinical presentation and preliminary investigations (e.g., stool cultures and examination for parasites and *C. difficile* toxin, blood for CMV nucleic acid testing [NAT], respiratory viral studies, viral swabs for HSV, and VZV from skin lesions).

Delays in appropriate therapy may compromise outcome necessitating an aggressive approach to making a specific microbiologic diagnosis. Based upon the clinical stability of the patient, the severity of immune deficits, and the most likely cause of infection, the physician may initiate empiric therapy while awaiting the results of investigations, or therapy may be deferred until clinical data become available. Increasingly, infections in compromised hosts are due to organisms with antimicrobial resistance patterns that make selection of empiric therapy more difficult. Compromised hosts have an increased susceptibility to community-acquired organisms (MRSA, extended-spectrum beta lactamase (ESBL) producing gram negatives and multi–drug-resistant *Pneumococcus*) and nosocomial pathogens (VRE, fluconazole-resistant *Candida* species and carbapenem-resistant *Enterobacteriaceae*). All microbiologic isolates require susceptibility testing in immunocompromised patients. Consultation with an infectious diseases specialist may be useful to assist in decisions regarding empiric therapy and for guidance regarding appropriate investigations, specimen collection, and transport.

Whenever tissue or body fluids are collected, appropriate histologic and microbiologic investigations should be performed, and consultation with the pathologist and/or microbiologist is recommended to ensure appropriate testing. Diagnosis of many pathogens that cause disease in immunocompromised hosts requires special stains (e.g., modified acid-fast stain for *Nocardia,* silver or immunofluorescent stains for *P. jirovecii*) or culture media (e.g., for *Mycobacteria* species). In addition, given that noninfectious etiologies such as organ rejection, drug toxicity, and GVHD are often in the differential diagnosis, histology is integral to making a definitive diagnosis and invasive diagnosis should be considered early in the patient's course. The diagnosis of virally mediated diseases such as tissue-invasive CMV (70) and EBV-associated PTLD (71) may require histology for diagnosis.

TREATMENT

The Neutropenic Patient

After appropriate microbiologic studies, empiric antimicrobial therapy is indicated in neutropenic patients at the onset of fever or, in the case of suspected infection, without fever (6). In critically ill neutropenic patients, there is no single empiric regimen appropriate for all patients (6,72–74). The selection of an initial empiric antibiotic regimen should take into consideration the general trend of increasing gram-positive infections, the local hospital epidemiology, including the susceptibility patterns of isolates from neutropenic patients, in addition to the clinical presentation, epidemiologic exposures, and prior antimicrobial use.

Options include monotherapy with (a) a third- or fourth-generation cephalosporin (e.g., ceftazidime or cefepime), (b) an antipseudomonal carbapenem such as imipenem or meropenem, or (c) piperacillin–tazobactam. Dual therapy, such as an antipseudomonal β-lactam plus an aminoglycoside or fluoroquinolone may be used or, for inpatients with recent surgery or vascular access catheters, a glycopeptide such as vancomycin can be combined with one- or two-drug therapy.

The initial empiric addition of vancomycin therapy in febrile neutropenia has not been shown to alter outcomes in patients without pulmonary infiltrates, septic shock, clinically documented infections likely due to gram-positive organisms such as CVC or skin and soft tissue infections, or documented gram-positive infections resistant to the primary empiric therapy (75). Vancomycin use has also been associated with the emergence of vancomycin-resistant enterococci; its use in febrile neutropenic patients should be limited as indicated above.

For those with an identified source of infection, usually less than half of patients, antimicrobial therapy can be tailored based on culture results. Those who defervesce on empiric antibacterial therapy should have the antimicrobials continued to complete a therapeutic course appropriate for the defined infection and until neutrophil recovery.

Controversy persists regarding the optimal timing of adding antifungal therapy. In patients who have been in the ICU for more than 5 to 7 days and have been hypotensive or otherwise critically ill, anti-*Candida* therapy may be added after cultures are obtained (76,77). In others who have failed to defervesce on empiric antibiotic therapy after 5 to 7 days, and in whom no source of infection is identified, there is a high risk of systemic fungal infection, and empiric antifungal therapy should be added (5–7,72). Amphotericin B is the historical gold standard for empiric therapy in this setting; however, lipid products of amphotericin B (e.g., liposomal amphotericin B [AmBisome, Astellas] and amphotericin B lipid complex [Abelcet, Elan]) have similar efficacy with less toxicity (78). In the United States, liposomal amphotericin or echinocandins (caspofungin (79)) are approved for empiric therapy of fever in neutropenia. Other agents may have efficacy such as voriconazole (80), other echinocandins (e.g., anidulafungin and micafungin), and posaconazole (81). Renal and hepatic function, potential drug interactions, cost, and suspected source of fungal infection are all considerations when choosing an initial empiric antifungal agent. In those with confirmed invasive aspergillosis, voriconazole is the drug of choice although no direct clinical trial comparison with liposomal amphotericin has been performed. Limited data suggest that combination therapy with these agents with an echinocandin may improve outcomes in highly selected patients (52,82,83).

Although the use of hematopoietic growth factors such as granulocyte colony-stimulating factor (G-CSF) increase the neutrophil count, they have not been shown to have benefit in the management of febrile neutropenia and routine use is not recommended (84,85).

TABLE 90.4 Treatment Modalities for Common Opportunistic Infections

Infectious Agent	Primary Therapy	Secondary Therapy	Other Considerations
Pneumocystis jirovecii (PCP)	TMP-SMX, dosed as 15–20 mg/kg/day of TMP component, divided every 6–8 hrs × 21 days	• Atovaquone 750–1,500 mg orally bid • Dapsone 100 mg orally plus TMP as above • Clindamycin 600 mg IV every 6 hrs plus primaquine 15–30 mg/day (as base)	Adjunctive use of corticosteroids common but not evidence based in non-HIV patients
Listeria monocytogenes	***Empiric or confirmed:*** Ampicillin 2 g IV every 4 hrs × 21 days or more ***For synergy:*** Ampicillin plus TMP-SMX 20 mg/kg/day divided every 6 hrs	Ampicillin plus gentamicin 2 mg/kg IV load, then 1.7 mg/kg IV every 8 hrs	
Legionella pneumophila and other species	Levofloxacin 250–750 mg IV every 24 hrs × 7–14 days	Azithromycin 500 mg daily for 7–14 days	
Nocardia spp	TMP-SMX, dosed as 15 mg/kg/day of TMP component, divided every 6–12 hrs, PO or IV	• Imipenem 500 mg IV every 6 hrs plus amikacin 7.5 mg/kg IV every 12 hrs (with normal renal function) both × 3–4 wks, then switch to PO regimen • Linezolid 300–600 mg orally bid • Ceftriaxone 2 g bid	• Based on antimicrobial susceptibility pattern • Surgical resection of necrotic material often necessary • Therapy duration is 6–12 mo; for central nervous system infection 9–12 mo

The Corticosteroid-Treated Patient

Common pathogens to be considered in corticosteroid-treated patients presenting with suspected infection include bacterial sepsis, *P. jirovecii* (PCP), *L. monocytogenes*, *Legionella*, and *Nocardia* species. Those requiring prolonged steroid therapy are appropriate candidates for prophylaxis with TMP-SMX which has broad antibacterial as well as anti-*Pneumocystis* and anti-*Toxoplasma* activity (86); in the absence of prophylaxis, PCP remains common. Overly rapid tapering of corticosteroids may provoke adrenal insufficiency including nausea, abdominal pain, hypotension, and confusion, and may be precipitated by simultaneous infections. Table 90.4 summarizes the antimicrobial treatment of these common opportunistic infections (86–104).

The Solid Organ Transplant Patient

Treatment of infections in transplant recipients may be complicated by rapid progression, precipitation of rejection, and antimicrobial toxicity related to drug interactions or nephrotoxicity; whenever possible, prevention of infections is therefore a principal goal. Approaches to prevention include donor and recipient history and serologic screening, TST or IGRA screening, and pretransplant immunization of recipients.

All potential organ donors and recipients should undergo a thorough history and physical examination to identify risk factors for infection and potential latent infections. This includes information regarding travel/residence, occupational, and risk behavior (e.g., injection drug use) and exposure histories (e.g., tuberculosis). Commonly utilized serologic tests for screening donors and recipients include HIV-1 and -2; HCV antibodies; hepatitis B surface antigen (HBsAg); hepatitis B core antibody (anti-HBc total ± IgM); hepatitis B surface antibody (anti-HBs) (some centers); CMV-IgG antibodies; EBV antibody panel; syphilis screen (rapid plasma reagin [RPR] or syphilis enzyme immune assay); *Toxoplasma* antibody; HSV IgG (some centers); and VZV IgG in recipients.

Optimally, immunization against vaccine-preventable diseases should be completed prior to transplantation and as early in the course of the disease as possible. This is based on three principal factors (a) the response to vaccine declines with progressive end-organ failure; (b) despite this, the response to vaccination may be better before transplantation than after; and (c) live viral vaccines (e.g., mumps, measles, rubella [MMR], varicella/herpes zoster) are generally contraindicated post transplant. Attention to the appropriate and timely administration of as many immunizations as possible is of particular importance in pediatric transplant candidates. National immunization guidelines should be followed by consultation with an infectious diseases specialist. In addition to routine vaccinations, all transplant candidates should receive a pneumococcal vaccine, yearly influenza vaccine, and hepatitis B vaccine. Hepatitis B vaccination, with a documented serologic response, allows for the safe use of anti–HBc-positive nonhepatic donors, thus expanding the donor pool (105). Susceptible individuals should receive varicella vaccine (live vaccine) a minimum of 4 weeks prior to transplantation. The optimal treatment of HCV (pre- or posttransplant) is under investigation.

Transplant candidates should undergo TB screening with TST/IGRA and risk factor assessment prior to transplantation. There is a 50- to 100-fold increased risk of tuberculosis (TB) following organ transplantation, with an increased risk of dissemination compared to the general population (106,107). Management of TB post transplant is also associated with significant morbidity and mortality, and its therapy is complicated by the multiple drug interactions between antituberculous and antirejection medications (107,108).

Disease-Specific Prevention and Management

Cytomegalovirus. CMV remains a significant cause of morbidity in organ transplant recipients; strategies for prevention have decreased the morbidity of CMV. The risk of CMV disease depends on a number of factors, including the donor and recipient serostatus, as well as the immunosuppression, particularly the use of antilymphocyte antibody (ALA) preparations for induction or treatment of rejection.

The American Society of Transplantation Guidelines on CMV prevention and management (109) should be used to guide institutional approaches to CMV prevention in conjunction with local CMV epidemiology, available laboratory support, and infrastructure. If both the donor and recipient are CMV-negative, antiherpes virus prophylaxis (for HSV and VZV) is generally used for the first 3 to 12 months post transplantation. However, 5% to 10% of such patients may develop community-acquired CMV at some time post transplant. Those who are CMV-seronegative and receive a seropositive organ are at greater risk of a primary CMV infection. Such patients should receive prophylaxis with valganciclovir (900 mg/day corrected for renal function) for 100 days; 200 days in kidney recipients and 12 months in lung recipients (109–112). In CMV-seropositive recipients, either prophylaxis with valganciclovir or preemptive therapy based on routine monitoring via a sensitive assay (e.g., quantitative CMV NAT) have been used. Given the high risk of CMV infection and disease in seropositive lung and heart–lung recipients, prophylaxis is generally preferred. All patients at risk for CMV who receive lymphocyte-depleting agents for induction or treatment of rejection should receive antiviral prophylaxis.

CMV disease refers to the presence of symptoms attributable to CMV in the face of viral replication, and can be further divided into (a) "CMV syndrome" and (b) tissue-invasive disease. "CMV syndrome" is defined by the constellation of fever greater than 38°C, neutropenia or thrombocytopenia, and the detection of CMV in the blood by antigenemia, PCR, or shell viral culture. Tissue-invasive disease requires a biopsy for confirmation, except in the case of retinitis, and is defined by the presence of signs or symptoms of organ dysfunction in association with histologic evidence of CMV in the affected tissue (113). Established CMV syndrome or tissue-invasive disease should be treated with intravenous ganciclovir, 5 mg/kg every 12 hours or valganciclovir 900 mg orally twice daily (114). Therapy should be continued for a minimum of 14 days and until symptoms have resolved and viremia has cleared (i.e., until the CMV PCR/antigenemia is undetectable) in order to minimize the risk of relapse (115,116). Gastrointestinal disease may present with diarrhea and with negative NAT testing of blood samples.

Ganciclovir-resistant CMV is an emerging problem; risk factors include donor–recipient mismatch, in which the donor is seropositive and the recipient seronegative; prolonged use of ganciclovir/valganciclovir; suboptimal ganciclovir levels; intense immunosuppression; and high CMV viral load. If ganciclovir resistance is suspected, infectious diseases/microbiology should be consulted for consideration of molecular resistance testing and either alternative (e.g., foscarnet, cidofovir) or adjunctive (CMV-Ig) therapies (117).

Epstein–Barr Virus and Posttransplant Lymphoproliferative Disease. Primary EBV infection after transplantation has been identified as the most important risk factor for PTLD, a complication with mortality reported to range as high as 40% to 60%. This risk is exacerbated by the occurrence of CMV disease and treatment with polyclonal or monoclonal ALA. Use of belatacept immunosuppression has been associated with increased risk of PTLD in the EBV D+/R- transplant population, notably involving the central nervous system (118,119). Studies comparing transplant recipients having received antiviral prophylaxis with either acyclovir or ganciclovir to historical controls suggest some benefit of antiviral prophylaxis (120). More recently, quantitative EBV viral load monitoring has also been shown to decrease the risk of PTLD (121). In those at high risk for PTLD (i.e., EBV donor seropositive/recipient seronegative), preventative strategies with antiviral prophylaxis and/or EBV viral load monitoring may be considered. If EBV viremia is detected, immunosuppression reduction should be considered.

PTLD represents a highly diverse spectrum of disease with variable clinical presentation, from benign B-cell proliferation (mononucleosis) to true monoclonal malignancy. It may be nodal or extranodal, localized or disseminated, and commonly involves the allograft. The diagnosis of PTLD requires histologic confirmation and staging of the disease (122).

Options for the treatment of PTLD depend on the histology and stage of the disease; however, in all cases, attempts should be made to reduce or withdraw immunosuppression. Additional considerations for treatment will depend on the clinical presentation, histology, and stage of disease (122). A multidisciplinary approach to management is generally indicated with collaboration of the transplant physician with hematology/oncology, infectious diseases, and surgery specialists, depending on the clinical setting. In addition to immunosuppression reduction or withdrawal, potential options for therapy include antiviral agents, intravenous immunoglobulin, surgical resection, and local radiation. The use of rituximab, the anti-CD20 monoclonal antibody, is an attractive second-line option if reduction in immunosuppression alone fails, given its low toxicity and response rates, which range from 61% to 76% (123). Cytotoxic chemotherapy is generally considered a third-line option due to a high incidence of toxicity in this population.

***Pneumocystis jirovecii* (formerly *P. carinii*).** In the absence of prophylaxis, Pneumocystis pneumonia occurs in 5% to 15% of solid organ transplant recipients. Prophylaxis with TMP-SMX, one single-strength tablet daily, essentially eliminates this risk and is indicated in all nonallergic transplant recipients for a minimum of 6 months following transplantation. This also acts as prophylaxis for a number of other infections such as *Nocardia*, *Listeria,* and community-acquired pneumonia. In sulfa-allergic patients, dapsone 100 mg daily or atovaquone 1,500 mg daily are alternatives (124).

Toxoplasmosis. Toxoplasmosis is of particular concern among cardiac transplant recipients given that the site of latency is the cardiac muscle. Seronegative recipients of a seropositive heart are at risk due to donor transmission and primary infection, and therefore require prophylaxis. TMP-SMX has been used effectively for prophylaxis as one double-strength tablet daily; lifelong prophylaxis is recommended (125).

Treatment of Infectious Syndromes in Immunocompromised Hosts

The management of infectious complications in immunocompromised hosts can be complex, and thus, consultation with local infectious diseases specialists is recommended.

Fever and Pulmonary Infiltrate

Immunocompromised hosts are susceptible to both common and unusual respiratory pathogens. In those presenting with fever and a pulmonary infiltrate, the differential diagnosis is broad and includes both infectious and noninfectious

TABLE 90.5 Differential Diagnosis of Fever and Pulmonary Infiltrate in Organ Transplant Recipients

Chest Radiograph Finding	Acute Onset	Subacute/Chronic Onset
Consolidation	Bacteria	Fungal
	Pulmonary embolism	*Nocardia*
	Hemorrhage	Tuberculosis
	Pulmonary edema	Viral (adenovirus)
Reticulonodular	Pulmonary edema	*Pneumocystis carinii (jirovecii)*
	Viral	Drug reaction (including sirolimus)
	P. carinii (jirovecii)	
	Bacterial	Viral
Nodular	Bacterial	Fungal
		Nocardia
		Tuberculosis
		Tumor (including PTLD)

PTLD, posttransplant lymphoproliferative disease.

etiologies. Infection is ultimately identified in 75% to 90% of such cases in organ transplant patients, and dual processes or sequential infections are common. Because pneumonia may rapidly progress in immunocompromised hosts with a resultant high mortality, initial empiric therapy directed at the most likely pathogens should be considered *following* the collection of blood and sputum cultures, viral respiratory studies, a complete blood count, and serum creatinine; consultation with pulmonary and infectious diseases specialists is recommended. Identification of the pathogen is key to directing appropriate therapy, and thus, early invasive diagnostic tests (e.g., bronchoscopy, lung biopsy) should be considered, particularly in those who are critically ill or fail to respond to initial empiric therapy.

Findings on chest radiograph combined with the clinical presentation, rate of progression, exposure history, and assessment of the net state of immunosuppression can help narrow the differential diagnosis. Table 90.5 summarizes the differential diagnosis based on chest radiographic findings and clinical presentation. Chest CT may be useful to delineate the extent of pulmonary disease and guide invasive diagnostic tests.

Central Nervous System Infections

Similar to pulmonary infections, the presentation of CNS infection in compromised hosts may differ from the general population due to immunosuppression. Fever may or may not be present, and the presentation can be subtle, with headache or minor changes in mental status. The differential diagnosis in those presenting with neurologic symptoms—with or without fever—is broad, including both infectious and noninfectious etiologies. Clinical presentations include meningitis—acute or subacute/chronic—encephalitis, seizures, focal neurologic deficits, and progressive cognitive impairment. Among the common causes of infection are *L. monocytogenes* and *Cryptococcus neoformans*, as well as the common community-acquired bacteria pathogens. Metastatic infection due to *Aspergillus*, *Mucormycoses,* and *Nocardia* species are observed. In those with underlying solid tumor or hematologic malignancy, metastatic disease including meningeal involvement must also be considered. Table 90.6 lists the most common causes of these symptoms. Consultation with infectious diseases/microbiology should be considered to assist in diagnosis and to ensure that appropriate samples are collected for diagnostic testing. Cerebral spinal fluid analysis after neuroimaging with CT and/or magnetic resonance imaging (MRI) should be obtained in all such individuals.

TABLE 90.6 Common Central Nervous System Infections in Transplant Recipients

Community-acquired pathogens
- Pneumococcus
- Meningococcus
- *Listeria monocytogenes*
- Herpes simplex virus
- *Cryptococcus neoformans*
- Lyme disease

Metastatic infection
- Bacteremia (endocarditis)
- *Mycobacterium tuberculosis*
- *Aspergillus*
- *Nocardia* species
- *Strongyloides stercoralis* (gram-negative meningitis)
- Mucoraceae (sinuses)
- Dematiaceae—cerebral phaeohyphomycosis (skin)
- *Histoplasma* and *Pseudallescheria/Scedosporium, Fusarium*

Other central nervous system processes
- Cytomegalovirus (nodular angiitis)
- Varicella zoster virus
- Human herpesvirus 6
- *Toxoplasma gondii*
- JC virus (progressive multifocal leukoencephalopathy)
- West Nile virus, lymphocytic choriomeningitis virus
- Lymphoma (PTLD)
- *Naegleria/Acanthamoeba*

Key Points

- Because of the impaired inflammatory response, the classic signs and symptoms of infection may be absent in immunocompromised patients. For example, an organ transplant recipient with a perforated viscus may present with fever but without clinical evidence of peritonitis; a neutropenic patient with pneumonia may have cough but absence of a pulmonary infiltrate on chest radiograph. A thorough, repeated history and physical examination is vital, and is the basis upon which investigations and management are directed in order to achieve a rapid diagnosis and early appropriate therapy.
- Assessment of the immune deficits based on the underlying condition, immunosuppressive/immunomodulatory therapies, and other risk factors—surgery, surgical drains, vascular access, antimicrobial therapies, mucositis, epidemiology—will suggest the most probable pathogens.

- An aggressive initial approach to diagnosis is generally warranted given the broad spectrum of pathogens potentially causing disease in this population. Routine noninvasive investigations—for example, cultures of blood, urine, and sputum; chest radiograph—should be performed, and invasive procedures such as biopsy and bronchoscopy/endoscopy considered early. Delay in diagnosis due to reluctance to perform invasive diagnostic tests often results in delays of appropriate therapy and/or exposure to toxicities of unneeded therapies and compromises treatment outcomes.
- Initial empiric antimicrobial therapy is often warranted due to the severity of initial presentation and/or potential for rapid clinical deterioration. Microbiologic specimens obtained prior to antimicrobial therapy will facilitate microbiologic diagnosis and directed therapy that will limit toxicities and improve patient outcome.

References

1. Bodey GP, Buckley M, Sathe YS, Freireich EJ. Quantitative relationships between circulating leukocytes and infection in patients with acute leukemia. *Ann Intern Med.* 1966;64(2):328–340.
2. Bodey GP, Rodriguez V, Chang HY, Narboni. Fever and infection in leukemic patients: a study of 494 consecutive patients. *Cancer.* 1978;41(4):1610–1622.
3. Peacock JE, Herrington DA, Wade JC, et al. Ciprofloxacin plus piperacillin compared with tobramycin plus piperacillin as empirical therapy in febrile neutropenic patients: a randomized, double-blind trial. *Ann Intern Med.* 2002;137(2):77–87.
4. Leibovici L, Paul M, Cullen M, et al. Antibiotic prophylaxis in neutropenic patients: new evidence, practical decisions. *Cancer.* 2006;107(8): 1743–1751.
5. Gerson SL, Talbot GH, Hurwitz S, et al. Prolonged granulocytopenia: the major risk factor for invasive pulmonary aspergillosis in patients with acute leukemia. *Ann Intern Med.* 1984;100(3):345–351.
6. Freifeld AG, Bow EJ, Sepkowitz KA, et al. Clinical practice guideline for the use of antimicrobial agents in neutropenic patients with cancer: 2010 update by the infectious diseases society of America. *Clin Infect Dis.* 2011;52(4):e56–e93.
7. Pizzo PA, Robichaud KJ, Gill FA, Witebsky FG. Empiric antibiotic and antifungal therapy for cancer patients with prolonged fever and granulocytopenia. *Am J Med.* 1982;72(1):101–111.
8. Wisplinghoff H, Ebbers J, Geurtz L, et al. Nosocomial bloodstream infections due to *Candida* spp. in the USA: species distribution, clinical features and antifungal susceptibilities. *Int J Antimicrob Agents.* 2014;43(1):78–81.
9. Pagano L, Girmenia C, Mele L, et al. Infections caused by filamentous fungi in patients with hematologic malignancies: a report of 391 cases by GIMEMA Infection Program. *Haematologica.* 2001;86(8):862–870.
10. Richardson MD. Changing patterns and trends in systemic fungal infections. *J Antimicrob Chemother.* 2005;56(Suppl 1):i5–i11.
11. Franchimont D. Overview of the actions of glucocorticoids on the immune response: a good model to characterize new pathways of immunosuppression for new treatment strategies. *Ann N Y Acad Sci.* 2004;1024:124–137.
12. Boumpas DT, Chrousos GP, Wilder RL, et al. Glucocorticoid therapy for immune-mediated diseases: basic and clinical correlates. *Ann Intern Med.* 1993;119(12):1198–1208.
13. Dale DC, Petersdorf RG. Corticosteroids and infectious diseases. *Med Clin North Am.* 1973;57(5):1277–1287.
14. Stuck AE, Minder CE, Frey FJ. Risk of infectious complications in patients taking glucocorticosteroids. *Rev Infect Dis.* 1989;11(6):954–963.
15. Kalil AC, Syed A, Rupp ME, et al. Is bacteremic sepsis associated with higher mortality in transplant recipients than in nontransplant patients? A matched case-control propensity-adjusted study. *Clin Infect Dis.* 2015;60(2):216–222.
16. Donnelly JP, Locke JE, MacLennan PA, et al. Inpatient mortality among solid organ transplant recipients hospitalized for sepsis and severe sepsis. *Clin Infect Dis.* 2016;63(2):186–194.
17. Fishman JA, Rubin RH. Infection in organ-transplant recipients. *N Engl J Med.* 1998;338(24):1741–1751.
18. Fishman JA, Issa NC. Infection in organ transplantation: risk factors and evolving patterns of infection. *Infect Dis Clin North Am.* 2010; 24(2):273–283.
19. Lopez-Navidad A, Domingo P, Caballero F, et al. Successful transplantation of organs retrieved from donors with bacterial meningitis. *Transplantation.* 1997;64(2):365–368.
20. Lumbreras C, Sanz F, Gonzalez A, et al. Clinical significance of donor-unrecognized bacteremia in the outcome of solid-organ transplant recipients. *Clin Infect Dis.* 2001;33(5):722–726.
21. Freeman RB, Giatras I, Falagas ME, et al. Outcome of transplantation of organs procured from bacteremic donors. *Transplantation.* 1999; 68(8):1107–1111.
22. Avery RK, Michaels MG, AST Infectious Diseases Community of Practice. Strategies for safe living after solid organ transplantation. *Am J Transplant.* 2013;13(Suppl 4):304–310.
23. Wilck MB, Zuckerman RA, AST Infectious Diseases Community of Practice. Herpes simplex virus in solid organ transplantation. *Am J Transplant.* 2013;13(Suppl 4):121–127.
24. Le J, Gantt S, AST Infectious Diseases Community of Practice. Human herpesvirus 6, 7 and 8 in solid organ transplantation. *Am J Transplant.* 2013;13(Suppl 4):128–137.
25. Pergam SA, Limaye AP, AST Infectious Diseases Community of Practice. Varicella zoster virus in solid organ transplantation. *Am J Transplant.* 2013;13(Suppl 4):138–146.
26. Ljungman P, Bregni M, Brune M, et al. Allogeneic and autologous transplantation for haematological diseases, solid tumours and immune disorders: current practice in Europe 2009. *Bone Marrow Transplant.* 2010;45(2):219–234.
27. Soubani AO, Kseibi E, Bander JJ, et al. Outcome and prognostic factors of hematopoietic stem cell transplantation recipients admitted to a medical ICU. *Chest.* 2004;126(5):1604–1611.
28. Afessa B, Tefferi A, Hoagland HC, et al. Outcome of recipients of bone marrow transplants who require intensive-care unit support. *Mayo Clin Proc.* 1992;67(2):117–122.
29. Huynh TN, Weigt SS, Belperio JA, et al. Outcome and prognostic indicators of patients with hematopoietic stem cell transplants admitted to the intensive care unit. *J Transplant.* 2009;2009:917294.
30. Soubani AO. Critical care considerations of hematopoietic stem cell transplantation. *Crit Care Med.* 2006;34(9 Suppl):S251–S267.
31. Junghanss C, Marr KA. Infectious risks and outcomes after stem cell transplantation: Are nonmyeloablative transplants changing the picture? *Curr Opin Infect Dis.* 2002;15(4):347–353.
32. Ramaprasad C, Pursell KJ. Infectious complications of stem cell transplantation. *Cancer Treat Res.* 2014;161:351–370.
33. Kawabata Y, Hirokawa M, Komatsuda A, Sawada K. Clinical applications of CD34+ cell-selected peripheral blood stem cells. *Ther Apher Dial.* 2003;7(3):298–304.
34. Baron F, Storb R. Allogeneic hematopoietic cell transplantation following nonmyeloablative conditioning as treatment for hematologic malignancies and inherited blood disorders. *Mol Ther.* 2006;13(1):26–41.
35. Sandmaier BM, McSweeney P, Yu C, Storb R. Nonmyeloablative transplants: preclinical and clinical results. *Semin Oncol.* 2000;27(2 Suppl 5): 78–81.
36. Marr KA, Seidel K, White TC, Bowden RA. Candidemia in allogeneic blood and marrow transplant recipients: evolution of risk factors after the adoption of prophylactic fluconazole. *J Infect Dis.* 2000;181(1):309–316.
37. Pagano L, Caira M, Nosari A, et al. Fungal infections in recipients of hematopoietic stem cell transplants: results of the SEIFEM B-2004 study—Sorveglianza Epidemiologica Infezioni Fungine Nelle Emopatie Maligne. *Clin Infect Dis.* 2007;45(9):1161–1170.
38. Ljungman P, Hakki M, Boeckh M. Cytomegalovirus in hematopoietic stem cell transplant recipients. *Infect Dis Clin North Am.* 2010;24(2):319–337.
39. Boeckh M, Nichols WG, Chemaly RF, et al. Valganciclovir for the prevention of complications of late cytomegalovirus infection after allogeneic hematopoietic cell transplantation: a randomized trial. *Ann Intern Med.* 2015;162(1):1–10.
40. Martino R, Porras RP, Rabella N, et al. Prospective study of the incidence, clinical features, and outcome of symptomatic upper and lower respiratory tract infections by respiratory viruses in adult recipients of hematopoietic stem cell transplants for hematologic malignancies. *Biol Blood Marrow Transplant.* 2005;11(10):781–796.
41. Walsh TJ, Groll A, Hiemenz J, et al. Infections due to emerging and uncommon medically important fungal pathogens. *Clin Microbiol Infect.* 2004;10(Suppl 1):48–66.
42. Richardson M, Lass-Florl C. Changing epidemiology of systemic fungal infections. *Clin Microbiol Infect.* 2008;14(Suppl 4):5–24.

43. Marr KA. Delayed opportunistic infections in hematopoietic stem cell transplantation patients: a surmountable challenge. *Hematology Am Soc Hematol Educ Program*. 2012;2012:265–270.
44. Boeckh M, Leisenring W, Riddell SR, et al. Late cytomegalovirus disease and mortality in recipients of allogeneic hematopoietic stem cell transplants: importance of viral load and T-cell immunity. *Blood*. 2003; 101(2):407–414.
45. Atkinson K, Storb R, Prentice RL, et al. Analysis of late infections in 89 long-term survivors of bone marrow transplantation. *Blood*. 1979; 53(4):720–731.
46. Winston DJ, Schiffman G, Wang DC, et al. Pneumococcal infections after human bone-marrow transplantation. *Ann Intern Med*. 1979;91(6):835–841.
47. Boeckh M, Bowden R. Cytomegalovirus infection in marrow transplantation. *Cancer Treat Res*. 1995;76:97–136.
48. Meyers JD, Flournoy N, Thomas ED. Risk factors for cytomegalovirus infection after human marrow transplantation. *J Infect Dis*. 1986; 153(3):478–488.
49. Boeckh M. Current antiviral strategies for controlling cytomegalovirus in hematopoietic stem cell transplant recipients: prevention and therapy. *Transpl Infect Dis*. 1999;1(3):165–178.
50. Jantunen E, Ruutu P, Niskanen L, et al. Incidence and risk factors for invasive fungal infections in allogeneic BMT recipients. *Bone Marrow Transplant*. 1997;19(8):801–808.
51. Walsh TJ, Groll AH. Emerging fungal pathogens: evolving challenges to immunocompromised patients for the twenty-first century. *Transpl Infect Dis*. 1999;1(4):247–261.
52. Herbrecht R, Denning DW, Patterson TF, et al. Voriconazole versus amphotericin B for primary therapy of invasive aspergillosis. *N Engl J Med*. 2002;347(6):408-415.
53. Novosad SA, Winthrop KL. Beyond tumor necrosis factor inhibition: the expanding pipeline of biologic therapies for inflammatory diseases and their associated infectious sequelae. *Clin Infect Dis*. 2014;58(11):1587–1598.
54. Keane J, Gershon S, Wise RP, et al. Tuberculosis associated with infliximab, a tumor necrosis factor alpha-neutralizing agent. *N Engl J Med*. 2001;345(15):1098–1104.
55. Rychly DJ, DiPiro JT. Infections associated with tumor necrosis factor-alpha antagonists. *Pharmacotherapy*. 2005;25(9):1181–1192.
56. Dixon WG, Hyrich KL, Watson KD, et al. Drug-specific risk of tuberculosis in patients with rheumatoid arthritis treated with anti-TNF therapy: results from the British Society for Rheumatology Biologics Register (BSRBR). *Ann Rheum Dis*. 2010;69(3):522–528.
57. Winthrop KL, Weinblatt ME, Daley CL. You can't always get what you want, but if you try sometimes (with two tests—TST and IGRA—for tuberculosis) you get what you need. *Ann Rheum Dis*. 2012;71(11):1757–1760.
58. Rastetter W, Molina A, White CA. Rituximab: expanding role in therapy for lymphomas and autoimmune diseases. *Annu Rev Med*. 2004; 55:477–503.
59. Maloney DG, Grillo-Lopez AJ, White CA, et al. IDEC-C2B8 (Rituximab) anti-CD20 monoclonal antibody therapy in patients with relapsed low-grade non-Hodgkin's lymphoma. *Blood*. 1997;90(6):2188–2195.
60. Casulo C, Maragulia J, Zelenetz AD. Incidence of hypogammaglobulinemia in patients receiving rituximab and the use of intravenous immunoglobulin for recurrent infections. *Clin Lymphoma Myeloma Leuk*. 2013;13(2):106–111.
61. Gottenberg JE, Ravaud P, Bardin T, et al. Risk factors for severe infections in patients with rheumatoid arthritis treated with rituximab in the autoimmunity and rituximab registry. *Arthritis Rheum*. 2010;62(9):2625–2632.
62. Diwakar L, Gorrie S, Richter A, et al. Does rituximab aggravate pre-existing hypogammaglobulinaemia? *J Clin Pathol*. 2010;63(3):275–277.
63. Tsutsumi Y, Ogasawara R, Kamihara Y, et al. Rituximab administration and reactivation of HBV. *Hepat Res Treat*. 2010;2010:182067.
64. Evens AM, Jovanovic BD, Su YC, et al. Rituximab-associated hepatitis B virus (HBV) reactivation in lymphoproliferative diseases: meta-analysis and examination of FDA safety reports. *Ann Oncol*. 2011;22(5):1170–1180.
65. Bharat A, Xie F, Baddley JW, et al. Incidence and risk factors for progressive multifocal leukoencephalopathy among patients with selected rheumatic diseases. *Arthritis Care Res (Hoboken)*. 2012;64(4):612–615.
66. Sickles EA, Greene WH, Wiernik PH. Clinical presentation of infection in granulocytopenic patients. *Arch Intern Med*. 1975;135(5):715–719.
67. Empiric antifungal therapy in febrile granulocytopenic patients. EORTC International Antimicrobial Therapy Cooperative Group. *Am J Med*. 1989; 86(6 Pt 1):668–672.
68. Wisplinghoff H, Bischoff T, Tallent SM, et al. Nosocomial bloodstream infections in US hospitals: analysis of 24,179 cases from a prospective nationwide surveillance study. *Clin Infect Dis*. 2004;39(3):309–317.
69. Heussel CP, Kauczor HU, Heussel G, et al. Early detection of pneumonia in febrile neutropenic patients: use of thin-section CT. *AJR Am J Roentgenol*. 1997;169(5):1347–1353.
70. Ljungman P, Griffiths P, Paya C. Definitions of cytomegalovirus infection and disease in transplant recipients. *Clin Infect Dis*. 2002;34 (8):1094–1097.
71. Preiksaitis JK, Keay S. Diagnosis and management of posttransplant lymphoproliferative disorder in solid-organ transplant recipients. *Clin Infect Dis*. 2001;33(Suppl 1):S38–S46.
72. Hughes WT, Armstrong D, Bodey GP, et al. 2002 guidelines for the use of antimicrobial agents in neutropenic patients with cancer. *Clin Infect Dis*. 2002;34(6):730–751.
73. Viscoli C, Cometta A, Kern WV, et al. Piperacillin-tazobactam monotherapy in high-risk febrile and neutropenic cancer patients. *Clin Microbiol Infect*. 2006;12(3):212–216.
74. Bow EJ, Rotstein C, Noskin GA, et al. A randomized, open-label, multicenter comparative study of the efficacy and safety of piperacillin-tazobactam and cefepime for the empirical treatment of febrile neutropenic episodes in patients with hematologic malignancies. *Clin Infect Dis*. 2006;43(4):447–459.
75. Cometta A, Kern WV, De Bock R, et al. Vancomycin versus placebo for treating persistent fever in patients with neutropenic cancer receiving piperacillin-tazobactam monotherapy. *Clin Infect Dis*. 2003;37(3):382–389.
76. Rex JH, Sobel JD. Prophylactic antifungal therapy in the intensive care unit. *Clin Infect Dis*. 2001;32(8):1191–1200.
77. Ostrosky-Zeichner L, Pappas PG. Invasive candidiasis in the intensive care unit. *Crit Care Med*. 2006;34(3):857–863.
78. Wingard JR, White MH, Anaissie E, et al. A randomized, double-blind comparative trial evaluating the safety of liposomal amphotericin B versus amphotericin B lipid complex in the empirical treatment of febrile neutropenia. L Amph/ABLC Collaborative Study Group. *Clin Infect Dis*. 2000;31(5):1155–1163.
79. Walsh TJ, Teppler H, Donowitz GR, et al. Caspofungin versus liposomal amphotericin B for empirical antifungal therapy in patients with persistent fever and neutropenia. *N Engl J Med*. 2004;351(14):1391–1402.
80. Walsh TJ, Pappas P, Winston DJ, et al. Voriconazole compared with liposomal amphotericin B for empirical antifungal therapy in patients with neutropenia and persistent fever. *N Engl J Med*. 2002;346 (4):225–234.
81. Ullmann AJ, Cornely OA. Antifungal prophylaxis for invasive mycoses in high risk patients. *Curr Opin Infect Dis*. 2006;19(6):571–576.
82. Marr KA, Schlamm HT, Herbrecht R, et al. Combination antifungal therapy for invasive aspergillosis: a randomized trial. *Ann Intern Med*. 2015;162 (2):81–89.
83. Schiffer CA. Granulocyte transfusion therapy. *Curr Opin Hematol*. 1999; 6(1):3–7.
84. American Society of Clinical Oncology. Update of recommendations for the use of hematopoietic colony-stimulating factors: evidence-based clinical practice guidelines. *J Clin Oncol*. 1996;14(6):1957–1960.
85. Berghmans T, Paesmans M, Lafitte JJ, et al. Therapeutic use of granulocyte and granulocyte-macrophage colony-stimulating factors in febrile neutropenic cancer patients: a systematic review of the literature with meta-analysis. *Support Care Cancer*. 2002;10(3):181–188.
86. Fishman JA. Prevention of infection due to *Pneumocystis carinii*. *Antimicrob Agents Chemother*. 1998;42(5):995–1004.
87. Hughes WT. *Pneumocystis carinii* versus *Pneumocystis jirovecii (jiroveci)* Frenkel. *Clin Infect Dis*. 2006;42(8):1211–1212.
88. LaRocque RC, Katz JT, Perruzzi P, Baden LR. The utility of sputum induction for diagnosis of Pneumocystis pneumonia in immunocompromised patients without human immunodeficiency virus. *Clin Infect Dis*. 2003;37(10):1380–1383.
89. Stover DE, Zaman MB, Hajdu SI, et al. Bronchoalveolar lavage in the diagnosis of diffuse pulmonary infiltrates in the immunosuppressed host. *Ann Intern Med*. 1984;101(1):1–7.
90. Kovacs JA, Ng VL, Masur H, et al. Diagnosis of *Pneumocystis carinii* pneumonia: improved detection in sputum with use of monoclonal antibodies. *N Engl J Med*. 1988;318(10):589–593.
91. Fishman JA. Treatment of infection due to *Pneumocystis carinii*. *Antimicrob Agents Chemother*. 1998;42(6):1309–1314.
92. Freitag NE, Jacobs KE. Examination of Listeria monocytogenes intracellular gene expression by using the green fluorescent protein of *Aequorea victoria*. *Infect Immun*. 1999;67(4):1844–1852.
93. Lorber B. Listeriosis. *Clin Infect Dis*. 1997;24(1):1–9; quiz 10–11.
94. Taege AJ. Listeriosis: recognizing it, treating it, preventing it. *Cleve Clin J Med*. 1999;66(6):375–380.
95. Gellin BG, Broome CV. Listeriosis. *JAMA*. 1989;261(9):1313–1320.

96. MacGowan AP, Holt HA, Bywater MJ, Reeves DS. In vitro antimicrobial susceptibility of Listeria monocytogenes isolated in the UK and other *Listeria* species. *Eur J Clin Microbiol Infect Dis.* 1990;9(10):767–770.
97. Merle-Melet M, Dossou-Gbete L, Maurer P, et al. Is amoxicillin-cotrimoxazole the most appropriate antibiotic regimen for listeria meningoencephalitis? Review of 22 cases and the literature. *J Infect.* 1996;33(2):79–85.
98. Roig J, Sabria M, Pedro-Botet ML. *Legionella* spp.: community acquired and nosocomial infections. *Curr Opin Infect Dis.* 2003;16(2):145–151.
99. Saravolatz LD, Burch KH, Fisher E, et al. The compromised host and Legionnaires' disease. *Ann Intern Med.* 1979;90(4):533–537.
100. Den Boer JW, Yzerman EP. Diagnosis of *Legionella* infection in Legionnaires' disease. *Eur J Clin Microbiol Infect Dis.* 2004;23(12):871–878.
101. Pedro-Botet L, Yu VL. Legionella: macrolides or quinolones? *Clin Microbiol Infect.* 2006;12 Suppl 3:25–30.
102. McNeil MM, Brown JM. The medically important aerobic actinomycetes: epidemiology and microbiology. *Clin Microbiol Rev.* 1994;7(3): 357–417.
103. Lerner PI. Nocardiosis. *Clin Infect Dis.* 1996;22(6):891–903.
104. Smego RA Jr., Moeller MB, Gallis HA. Trimethoprim-sulfamethoxazole therapy for *Nocardia* infections. *Arch Intern Med.* 1983;143(4): 711–718.
105. Chung RT, Feng S, Delmonico FL. Approach to the management of allograft recipients following the detection of hepatitis B virus in the prospective organ donor. *Am J Transplant.* 2001;1(2):185–191.
106. Kotloff RM, Ahya VN, Crawford SW. Pulmonary complications of solid organ and hematopoietic stem cell transplantation. *Am J Respir Crit Care Med.* 2004;170(1):22–48.
107. Subramanian AK, Morris MI, Practice AIDC. *Mycobacterium tuberculosis* infections in solid organ transplantation. *Am J Transplant.* 2013;13:68–76.
108. Singh N, Paterson DL. Mycobacterium tuberculosis infection in solid-organ transplant recipients: impact and implications for management. *Clin Infect Dis.* 1998;27(5):1266–1277.
109. Razonable RR, Hayden RT. Clinical utility of viral load in management of cytomegalovirus infection after solid organ transplantation. *Clin Microbiol Rev.* 2013;26(4):703–727.
110. Paya C, Humar A, Dominguez E, et al. Efficacy and safety of valganciclovir vs. oral ganciclovir for prevention of cytomegalovirus disease in solid organ transplant recipients. *Am J Transplant.* 2004;4(4):611–620.
111. Humar A, Lebranchu Y, Vincenti F, et al. The efficacy and safety of 200 days valganciclovir cytomegalovirus prophylaxis in high-risk kidney transplant recipients. *Am J Transplant.* 2010;10(5):1228–1237.
112. Finlen Copeland CA, Davis WA, et al. Long-term efficacy and safety of 12 months of valganciclovir prophylaxis compared with 3 months after lung transplantation: a single-center, long-term follow-up analysis from a randomized, controlled cytomegalovirus prevention trial. *J Heart Lung Transplant.* 2011;30(9):990–996.
113. Razonable RR, Humar A, Practice AIDC. Cytomegalovirus in solid organ transplantation. *Am J Transplant.* 2013;13:93–106.
114. Asberg A, Humar A, Rollag H, et al. Oral valganciclovir is noninferior to intravenous ganciclovir for the treatment of cytomegalovirus disease in solid organ transplant recipients. *Am J Transplant.* 2007;7(9): 2106–2113.
115. Sia IG, Wilson JA, Groettum CM, et al. Cytomegalovirus (CMV) DNA load predicts relapsing CMV infection after solid organ transplantation. *J Infect Dis.* 2000;181(2):717–720.
116. Humar A, Kumar D, Boivin G, Caliendo AM. Cytomegalovirus (CMV) virus load kinetics to predict recurrent disease in solid-organ transplant patients with CMV disease. *J Infect Dis.* 2002;186(6):829–833.
117. Kotton CN, Kumar D, Caliendo AM, et al. Updated international consensus guidelines on the management of cytomegalovirus in solid-organ transplantation. *Transplantation.* 2013;96(4):3333–3360.
118. Larsen CP, Grinyo J, Medina-Pestana J, et al. Belatacept-based regimens versus a cyclosporine A-based regimen in kidney transplant recipients: 2-year results from the BENEFIT and BENEFIT-EXT studies. *Transplantation.* 2010;90(12):1528–1535.
119. Vincenti F, Charpentier B, Vanrenterghem Y, Rostaing L, Bresnahan B, Darji P, et al. A phase III study of belatacept-based immunosuppression regimens versus cyclosporine in renal transplant recipients (BENEFIT study). *Am J Transplant.* 2010;10(3):535–546.
120. Green M, Reyes J, Webber S, Rowe D. The role of antiviral and immunoglobulin therapy in the prevention of Epstein-Barr virus infection and post-transplant lymphoproliferative disease following solid organ transplantation. *Transpl Infect Dis.* 2001;3(2):97–103.
121. Lee TC, Savoldo B, Rooney CM, et al. Quantitative EBV viral loads and immunosuppression alterations can decrease PTLD incidence in pediatric liver transplant recipients. *Am J Transplant.* 2005;5(9):2222–2228.
122. Allen UD, Preiksaitis JK. Epstein-Barr virus and posttransplant lymphoproliferative disorder in solid organ transplantation. *Am J Transplant.* 2013;13(Suppl 4):107–120.
123. Milpied N, Vasseur B, Parquet N, et al. Humanized anti-CD20 monoclonal antibody (Rituximab) in post transplant B-lymphoproliferative disorder: a retrospective analysis on 32 patients. *Ann Oncol.* 2000;11(Suppl 1):113–116.
124. Martin SI, Fishman JA, AST Infectious Diseases Community of Practice. *Pneumocystis* pneumonia in solid organ transplantation. *Am J Transplant.* 2013;13(Suppl 4):272–279.
125. Schwartz BS, Mawhorter SD, AST Infectious Diseases Community of Practice. Parasitic infections in solid organ transplantation. *Am J Transplant.* 2013;13:280–303.

CHAPTER

91

Human Immunodeficiency Virus in the Intensive Care Unit

KATHLEEN M. AKGÜN, KRISTINA CROTHERS, and LAURENCE HUANG

INTRODUCTION

Human immunodeficiency virus (HIV)-infected patients require critical care for various reasons that may or may not be related to their underlying immunodeficiency. The evaluation of HIV-infected persons admitted to the intensive care unit (ICU) requires consideration of all processes that can occur in HIV-*un*infected persons, as well as those particular to HIV infection, namely opportunistic infections (OIs), neoplasms, and HIV-associated comorbidities or toxicities associated with antiretroviral therapy (ART). Management of acute, life-threatening conditions requires institution of similar therapies in HIV-infected persons as in HIV-uninfected persons, with awareness of potential drug toxicities and drug interactions that can occur in those on ART.

This chapter reviews the critical care of HIV-infected patients, including causes of ICU admission and patient outcomes. Special emphasis is placed on the etiology and management of respiratory failure, particularly that due to *Pneumocystis jirovecii* pneumonia (PCP), which carries an especially high mortality risk. Other major indications for ICU admission and the potential impact of combination ART on the critical care of HIV-infected patients are summarized.

EPIDEMIOLOGY OF HIV-INFECTED PATIENTS IN THE ICU

ICU Admission Rates and Outcomes

The first cases of HIV/AIDS were reported in 1981. Since that time, there have been many developments in the treatment of HIV and its associated diseases, most notably the introduction of highly active, combination ART in 1996. Rates of ICU admission and mortality related to ICU admission for HIV-infected patients have shifted multiple times during the AIDS epidemic.

Overall, there has been a steady decline in ICU mortality after the introduction of ART, mirroring a general improvement in survival in critically ill HIV-uninfected populations. In studies from San Francisco General Hospital, ICU mortality decreased significantly from 37% in 1992–1995 to 29% in 1996–1999 and 31% in 2000–2004 (1–3 Is it possible to include the Nickas and Wachter reference here (Currently reference number 6)? Please advise if this would require too many changes to keep the references in order of their first appearance.). More contemporary multicenter cohorts from the Veterans Health Administration in the United States (U.S.) and from France have reported further improvements in ICU outcomes. Thirty-day mortality among HIV-infected patients from the Veterans Aging Cohort Study (VACS) admitted to the ICU between 2002 and 2010 was 19% (4). Similarly, the French Collège des Utilisateurs de Base de données en Réanimation (CUB-Réa) network, including ICU admissions between 1999 and 2010, reported ICU mortality of 17.6% (5). In recent studies, the average reported in-hospital mortality for HIV-infected patients admitted to the ICU ranged between 19% and 40%, with a median ICU length of stay of 2 to 11 days (2,4–13) (Table 91.1).

In HIV-infected patients on ART, overall survival has improved, resulting in an increase in the number of persons living and aging with HIV. Patients aging with HIV are developing non–AIDS-related medical comorbidities that account for a growing proportion of hospitalizations and ICU admissions (4,5,14,15). Improved survival and increasing prevalence of non–AIDS-related comorbidities likely influence medical decision making by patients and providers, contributing to pursuit of more aggressive life-supporting measures in the ICU for patients living with HIV (8,16).

Despite decreasing hospitalization rates for HIV-infected patients, ICU admission rates have not changed substantially in the ART era (2,7–9,16,17). Approximately 5% to 18% of hospital admissions for HIV-infected patients involve ICU care (8,12,15). While a significant proportion (range 17%–40%) of HIV-infected patients continue to be admitted to the ICU without prior known HIV infection (8,9,17), this may be less frequent in more contemporary cohorts with access to HIV testing and ART. In addition, approximately 30% to 50% of patients are not on ART at the time of admission (8,9,12,15), attributable to new diagnoses among patients not yet in care and barriers to treatment or compliance among patients with known HIV infection.

Indications for ICU Admission

Studies of critically ill HIV-infected patients indicate that the spectrum of diseases requiring ICU admission is changing in the setting of ART. Early in the epidemic, most patients were admitted with an AIDS-associated condition, most often PCP. Increasingly, patients with HIV infection are admitted with a non–AIDS-associated condition. Data from San Francisco General Hospital found a high proportion of patients (79%) admitted with non–AIDS-related conditions from 2000 through 2004 (3). Similarly, in VACS, approximately 80% of ICU admissions were for non–HIV-associated conditions (4). Likewise, in CUB-Réa, the proportion of admissions for main diagnosis of non–AIDS-defining conditions increased significantly from 74% to 83% between 1999–2001 and 2008–2010, respectively (5).

Acute respiratory failure is the most common indication for ICU care, accounting for approximately 21% to 59% of ICU admissions in HIV-infected patients (2–6,9–12,17–20); *Pneumocystis jirovecii* was the responsible pathogen in approximately 25% to 50% of these patients in earlier investigations (6,10,21). Although decreased in some studies (5,7,15), it remains a significant cause of respiratory failure in recent studies, accounting for 14% to nearly 50% of cases of respiratory

TABLE 91.1 Mortality Associated with ICU Admission among HIV-Infected Patients in the Combination ART Era

Setting (reference)	ICU Patients (*N*)	Time Period	HIV Unknown at Admission	ART at Admission	HIV or AIDS-Related Illness	Overall ICU Mortality	Independent Predictors of ICU or In-Hospital Mortality[a]
University hospital, Jacksonville, FL (11)	141	1995–1999	—	—	—	30%[b]	Transfer from another hospital ward, APACHE II score
University hospital, Paris, France (9)	230	1997–1999	40%	28%	37%	20%	SAPS II score, mechanical ventilation, Omega score
University hospital, Paris, France (8)	236	1998–2000	28%	50%	50%	25%	PCP with pneumothorax; mechanical ventilation; Kaposi sarcoma; inotropic support; CD4+ count <50 cells; SAPS II score
Urban hospital, New York, NY (12)	259	1997–1999	—	48%	60%	30%	Mechanical ventilation; admission with HIV-related illness
Urban hospital, New York, NY (7)	53	2001	—	52%	33%	29%[b]	No multivariate analysis provided; low albumin associated with increased mortality on univariate analysis
Urban hospital, San Francisco, CA (2)	295	1996–1999	7%	25%	37%	29%[b]	Mechanical ventilation; PCP; APACHE II scores >13; albumin <2.6 g/dL; AIDS-associated diagnosis
Hospital Virgen de la Victoria, Malaga, Spain (22)	49	1997–2003	31%	31%	61%	57%	Not reported
Urban hospital, San Francisco, CA (3)	281 (311 admissions)	2000–2004	Not reported	33%	21%	31%	Mechanical ventilation Albumin, per 1 g/dL decrease
University hospital, The Netherlands (13)	117 (127 admissions)	1990–2008	13%	23%	52%	37%	1-yr mortality: mechanical ventilation, APACHE II >20, older age
VACS: 8 Department of Veterans Affairs medical ICUs (4)	539	2002–2010	Not reported	71%	15%	18% (30 days)	VACS Risk Index Infection, respiratory, noncardiovascular admission diagnoses (vs. cardiovascular)
CUB-Réa, Paris, France (5)	6,373	1999–2010	Not reported	Not reported	21.9% (main diagnosis)	17.6%	Malignancy, liver disease

[a]In order of descending magnitude of association.
[b]Data given as in-hospital rather than ICU mortality.
ICU, intensive care unit; HIV, human immunodeficiency virus; ART, antiretroviral therapy; AIDS, acquired immunodeficiency syndrome; APACHE, Acute Physiology and Chronic Health Evaluation; SAPS, Simplified Acute Physiology Score; PCP, *Pneumocystis* pneumonia. VACS, Veterans Aging Cohort Study

failure, particularly in HIV-infected patients who are not on ART (2,3,5,7,12,22). Bacterial pneumonia (BP) is also a frequent cause of acute respiratory failure and in some studies is now as common (2) or more common (5,7,17,23) than PCP.

Sepsis is an increasingly frequent indication for ICU admission, accounting for 10% to 57% of all admissions for HIV-infected patients during recent years (3–5,9,24). Other commonly reported causes of ICU admission include CNS dysfunction (11%–27%), gastrointestinal (GI) and liver diagnoses (4%–15%), and cardiovascular disease (8%–18%) (2–6,9,10,19,21). Other reasons for ICU admission unrelated to immunodeficiency include trauma, routine postoperative care, noninfectious pulmonary diseases such as asthma and pulmonary embolism, renal failure, metabolic disturbances, and drug overdose. Given the frequent coinfection with hepatitis C among patients with HIV, liver disease may be increasing as a cause of death (4,24–26), and complications related to cirrhosis often require ICU admission. In addition, solid organ transplantation (liver, kidney) is currently being studied in HIV-infected patients; thus, these patients may also be encountered in the ICU setting.

Predictors of Mortality during ICU Admission

Mortality in the ICU has improved for HIV-infected patients but remains substantially higher than uninfected comparators, even after adjusting for ICU admission diagnosis (4,24,27). The highest mortality rates for HIV-infected patients requiring ICU admission are associated with sepsis, respiratory failure, chronic liver disease, and malignancy (3–5,17). Mortality rates of approximately 50% (6,19) and as high as 68% have been reported for sepsis (27,28). Among HIV-infected patients coinfected with hepatitis C admitted for severe sepsis, 30-day mortality can be as high as 82% (24). If respiratory failure is due to PCP, mortality remains nearly 50% (2,3,12) and is increased if complicated by PCP-associated pneumothorax (2,8). For AIDS patients admitted to the ICU for other HIV-related reasons, the reported mortality is generally lower. For example, the reported mortality for CNS dysfunction is 20% to 48% (6,10,11,19,29), whereas the mortality for GI disease is approximately 30% to 35% (6,10,11).

As ART use increases and HIV-infected patients are living longer, the impact of HIV-related versus non–HIV-related conditions on ICU mortality is changing. Although HIV-related conditions remain important predictors for mortality, they are becoming less common in areas with access to ART (5). Comorbidities such as chronic liver disease and cancer are increasingly important predictors of ICU mortality in HIV-infected patients (4,5,27).

Mortality during hospitalization is also related to the severity of the acute illness (Table 91.1). Predictors of increased hospital mortality include the need for mechanical ventilation and disease severity (as assessed by scoring systems such as the Simplified Acute Physiology Score II [SAPS II], the Acute Physiology and Chronic Health Evaluation II [APACHE II] score, and the VACS Index, a mortality prediction tool including biomarkers for HIV-specific and general organ dysfunction) (2,4–6,9,12,19,30). ICU mortality has also been related to the preadmission health status of the patient. Patients with a decreased serum albumin level or a history of weight loss may also have a higher mortality (2,3,6,19). The CD4+ T-cell count and the plasma HIV RNA level have generally not been independent predictors of short-term mortality during the ICU stay (2,6,7,11,12,21,30). However, long-term mortality after ICU admission has been related to the underlying severity of HIV disease in most studies (6,19,21). Long-term survival following ICU discharge is improved compared with the pre-ART era (8,9,13).

Impact of Antiretroviral Therapy on ICU Mortality

The full impact of ART on outcomes of HIV patients in the ICU remains unclear, as prospective, randomized trials assessing the initiation of ART on outcomes in critically ill patients have not been completed. Two retrospective studies conducted at San Francisco General Hospital suggest that ART may improve outcomes in critically ill HIV patients. In a review of all HIV-infected patients admitted to the ICU between 1996 and 1999, patients receiving combination ART at the time of ICU admission were less likely to present with two conditions associated with decreased survival, an AIDS-associated diagnosis and decreased serum albumin, but ART itself was not independently associated with survival (2). In a study of all HIV-infected patients with PCP who were admitted to the ICU at San Francisco General Hospital between 1996 and mid-2001, patients who were on ART at the time of ICU admission or started ART during hospitalization had an improved survival compared to patients not receiving ART (31). However, in another study from New York City, ICU mortality was not different in patients admitted between 1997 and 1999 when comparing patients receiving ART versus those not on ART (12). Furthermore, the prior use of ART was not associated with differences in overall hospital mortality or length of stay (12). Another study found that although ICU mortality had improved in recent years, this improvement could not be attributed to ART because none of the patients received this therapy (32). Conclusions regarding the impact of ART on outcomes are limited by the nonrandomized nature of these retrospective studies and by the inability to measure potential bias in the selection of patients received ART. In addition, these studies do not address treatment failure, drug resistance, or medication nonadherence prior to or after ICU admission, all of which influence long-term outcome (12).

IMMEDIATE CONCERNS IN MANAGING CRITICALLY ILL HIV-INFECTED PATIENTS

The initial management of critically ill HIV-infected patients includes all the immediate concerns in HIV-uninfected patients such as securing a stable airway and ensuring adequate respiration and circulation. The immediate management of patients with respiratory failure depends on the underlying reason for respiratory compromise, but consideration of OIs is warranted early in the course of care to ensure prompt diagnostic evaluation and initiation of appropriate antibiotic therapy. Management of patients in shock consists of similar strategies as in HIV-uninfected patients and depends on the cause of shock, with use of volume resuscitation, vasopressors, and/or inotropic agents as appropriate to maintain adequate mean arterial pressures and systemic perfusion. For patients with septic shock, guideline-based therapy focusing on early identification, fluid resuscitation, appropriate antimicrobials, and other ICU support should be instituted (33,34). Given the increased association of HIV with cardiovascular disease, cardiomyopathy (35), and adrenal insufficiency (36), providers should be alert to the possibility that these conditions may also cause shock in HIV-infected patients.

Certain aspects of the patient's history are important for initiating early appropriate management. The degree of immunosuppression related to HIV infection, reflected by the CD4+ cell count, is a critical determinant of risk for OIs. In addition, use of and adherence to ART and prophylactic antibiotics, as well as intravenous drug use and exposures to endemic fungi and mycobacteria, are key components of the patient's history. The evaluation and management of the most common indications for ICU admission among HIV-infected patients are discussed in detail below.

PULMONARY MANIFESTATIONS OF HIV

Spectrum of Respiratory Diseases and Approach to Diagnosis

Although the spectrum of diseases leading to respiratory failure has changed during the ART era, acute respiratory failure is still the most common cause of ICU admission for HIV-infected patients in studies throughout the world (2,4–6,9,11,12,20,37). Respiratory failure can occur from a multitude of causes including infections, neoplasms, drug overdose, and cardiac and neurologic conditions that may be both HIV- and non–HIV-related. Rapid diagnosis and initiation of appropriate therapy is crucial, particularly in patients with HIV-associated infections. Although these conditions have typical signs and symptoms, many of the presentations can overlap and patients may occasionally present with more than one etiology for their respiratory failure. Therefore, definitive diagnosis should be pursued whenever possible. It is important to remember that all the conditions leading to respiratory failure in the HIV-uninfected patient also occur in those with HIV infection. Diagnoses such as pulmonary embolism, asthma, chronic obstructive pulmonary disease, and cardiogenic pulmonary edema also present with respiratory failure, and appropriate testing should be performed.

Pneumocystis Pneumonia (PCP)

PCP has historically been the most common cause of respiratory failure in AIDS patients, but its frequency has declined (6,10,21,38). PCP is caused by the organism *P. jirovecii*, formerly *Pneumocystis carinii*. The number of patients admitted to the ICU with PCP has decreased since the introduction of ART, but it remains an important cause of morbidity and mortality in the HIV-infected ICU patient. In the 1980s, patients with PCP who were admitted to the ICU had a mortality rate as high as 81%, with mortality for those individuals requiring mechanical ventilation approaching 90% (39). The introduction of adjunctive corticosteroids for moderate to severe PCP in the mid-1980s led to an improvement in mortality to approximately 60% (40–42). Since that time, there has been little change in outcomes from severe PCP, with later studies still reporting a hospital mortality of approximately 60% (2,6). The primary critical care factors that determine mortality in patients with PCP are the need for mechanical ventilation and the development of a pneumothorax. Either of these factors portends a poor prognosis, and the occurrence of both concurrently is almost uniformly fatal (2,43). Other factors that have been reported to be associated with mortality in some studies include low serum albumin, admission to the ICU after 3 to 5 days of hospitalization, increased age, and elevated serum lactate dehydrogenase (LDH) (2,32,43–45).

Clinical Presentation. PCP is most frequent in patients with a CD4+ cell count below 200 cells/μL, with the risk of PCP increasing as the CD4+ count decreases below that level (46,47). Although use of PCP prophylaxis decreases the incidence of PCP, patients receiving prophylaxis may still develop PCP, especially if severely immunocompromised (48). However, many patients with PCP do not know that they are HIV-infected, and therefore never receive PCP prophylaxis. Published studies have reported that 28% to 57% of patients admitted to the ICU are diagnosed with PCP as their first manifestation of HIV; thus clinicians need to consider PCP in *any* patient with a consistent clinical picture if the patient's HIV status is unknown (31,43). Additional risk factors for PCP other than a low CD4+ cell count include the presence of oropharyngeal candidiasis and prior PCP.

The symptoms of PCP can be nonspecific but include fever, tachypnea, dyspnea, and cough. The cough associated with PCP is most often nonproductive or productive of clear sputum. Patients with purulent sputum are more likely to have BP. The pace and duration of symptoms is also important in distinguishing PCP from BP. Unlike in the HIV-uninfected immunosuppressed population, HIV-infected patients with PCP generally report the subacute onset of symptoms progressing over several weeks, with the median duration of symptoms in one study being 28 days (49).

Many patients with PCP have an unremarkable lung examination, with inspiratory crackles being the most frequent abnormal finding. They will often manifest hypoxemia and an increased alveolar–arterial oxygen gradient. Laboratory tests can suggest the diagnosis but are often nonspecific. The white blood cell count can be normal, decreased, or increased. Serum LDH is often elevated in patients with PCP but a normal serum LDH does not rule out the diagnosis (50–52). Also, multiple pulmonary and nonpulmonary conditions can result in an elevated LDH, so an elevated LDH does not rule in the diagnosis. In general, the LDH is more useful as a prognostic rather than a diagnostic test. The degree of elevation correlates with outcome and response to therapy, and patients with a rising serum LDH in the face of treatment have a worse prognosis (52). The arterial blood gas in PCP demonstrates hypoxemia and a widened alveolar–arterial gradient ($P_{A-a}O_2$), which can be seen in any pulmonary disease but is useful in determining the need for adjunctive corticosteroids and ICU care. Finally, 1,3 β-D-Glucan, which is a component of fungal cell walls, is often elevated in PCP and other fungal infections.

The classic chest radiographic appearance of PCP is a diffuse interstitial, reticular, or granular infiltrate (Fig. 91.1); PCP can also result in focal airspace consolidation, although this presentation is less common. Infiltrates are occasionally unilateral or asymmetric and, in patients receiving aerosolized pentamidine for prophylaxis, there may be an upper lobe predominance. In general, the pattern (reticular or granular) is more suggestive of the diagnosis than the distribution. Severe PCP is similar to the acute respiratory distress syndrome (ARDS) in causing widespread capillary leak that results in

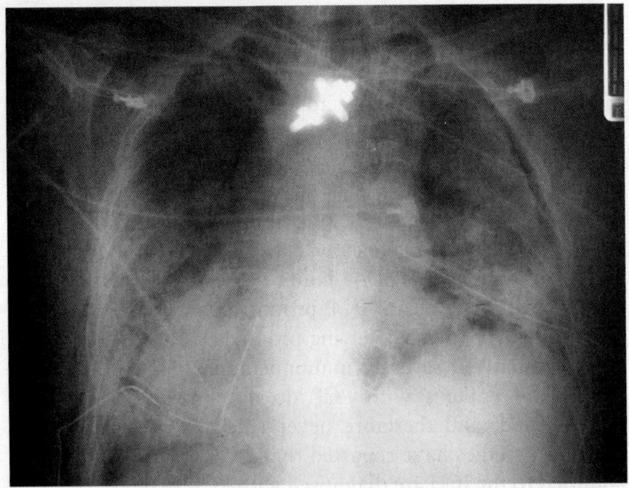

FIGURE 91.1 Portable chest radiograph from a patient with *Pneumocystis* pneumonia demonstrating diffuse bilateral infiltrates and pneumothoraces.

bilateral radiographic infiltrates, and these two entities may be indistinguishable radiographically. Single or multiple cysts or pneumatoceles occur in about 10% to 20% of patients, and these changes can be seen before, during, or after PCP treatment (53,54). Patients with PCP are at risk for developing spontaneous pneumothoraces, and PCP should be high in the differential for any HIV-infected patient presenting with a pneumothorax. Radiographic findings such as pleural effusions or lymphadenopathy are uncommon in PCP, and their presence should lead the clinician to consider alternate or concurrent diagnoses. High-resolution CT scans can be helpful in demonstrating diffuse ground glass opacities typical of PCP, but these findings are nonspecific.

Diagnosis. Although patients may present with typical signs and symptoms of PCP, a definitive diagnosis is preferred, particularly in patients in the ICU. Many HIV-associated respiratory diseases have overlapping or nonspecific presentations, which makes it difficult for even experienced clinicians to diagnose empirically. Definitive diagnosis allows for the timely administration of appropriate antibiotics and avoids exposure to unnecessary medications. We are currently unable to culture *Pneumocystis* and, thus, the diagnosis relies on microscopic visualization of the organism in a respiratory sample from a patient with a compatible clinical presentation.

PCP can be diagnosed either through examination of induced sputum or from samples obtained at bronchoscopy. Spontaneous sputum is generally not acceptable for diagnosis of PCP (55). In the ICU, bronchoscopy with bronchoalveolar lavage (BAL) is generally the primary means of diagnosis although endotracheal aspirates have also been used. For patients with HIV infection, BAL has a sensitivity of well over 90% for diagnosis of PCP and should be performed as early as possible in undiagnosed patients (56). Transbronchial biopsy does not add significantly to the yield for PCP in an HIV-infected individual and is technically challenging in an intubated patient on mechanical ventilation; however, it may be useful in diagnosing other pulmonary infections that are also in the differential (57). It is reasonable to perform transbronchial biopsy as part of the initial procedure when the probability of PCP is low or as a follow-up test when the initial BAL is nondiagnostic.

Traditional staining methods for PCP include Gomori methenamine silver, toluidine blue O stain, or a modified Wright–Giemsa stain. Immunofluorescent antibody staining can also be used to examine induced sputum or BAL and has a high sensitivity (58,59). Newer polymerase chain reaction (PCR)-based methods have been reported; PCR can also detect *Pneumocystis* DNA in persons without microscopic PCP who are considered to be colonized with the organism.

Treatment and Corticosteroids. The duration of PCP treatment is 21 days. First-line therapy for moderate to severe PCP is intravenous trimethoprim/sulfamethoxazole (TMP/SMX) (Table 91.2). TMP/SMX is curative in 60% to 86% of patients (60,61). The dosage of TMP/SMX is 15 to 20 mg/kg of trimethoprim and 75 to 100 mg/kg of sulfamethoxazole daily, divided every 6 to 8 hours. TMP/SMX is associated with a high rate of adverse reactions, particularly in those with HIV infection. Approximately one-fourth to one-half of patients will develop therapy-limiting toxicity (49,60,62–64). Adverse reactions to TMP/SMX include nausea, vomiting, integumentary rash, elevation of transaminases, hyponatremia, hyperkalemia, renal insufficiency, and bone marrow suppression.

Intravenous pentamidine isethionate is the preferred alternative treatment for patients who cannot tolerate TMP/SMX or who have failed treatment. Patients should receive 3 to 4 mg/kg/day of pentamidine. Some studies have found that the efficacy of pentamidine is similar to TMP/SMX, but others have reported a lower survival rate with pentamidine (61% vs. 86% for TMP/SMX) (60,61,65). Pentamidine has several serious adverse effects that can limit therapy and may be seen in as many as 50% of patients. Toxicity from pentamidine includes nausea, vomiting, hypotension, bone marrow suppression, hepatic transaminitis, and nephrotoxicity. Glucose levels should be monitored in patients receiving pentamidine because it is toxic to pancreatic islet cells and can result in initial hypoglycemia from a surge of insulin release, followed by hyperglycemia from inadequate insulin. Some patients can even progress to chronic diabetes mellitus. Pancreatitis also occurs with pentamidine and may be fatal (66,67). Other side effects that have been reported include myoglobinuria,

TABLE 91.2 Summary of Treatment Regimens for PCP in the ICU in Decreasing Order of Preference[a]

Agent	Dose
Trimethoprim–sulfamethoxazole	15–20 mg/kg/day trimethoprim with 75–100 mg/kg/day sulfamethoxazole IV, divided every 6–8 hrs Can switch to PO if substantial clinical improvement (e.g., transfer out of ICU)
Pentamidine isethionate	3–4 mg/kg/day IV, infused over >60 min Start at 4 mg/kg but can reduce to 3 mg/kg if substantial clinical improvement (e.g., transfer out of ICU) or toxicity
Clindamycin/primaquine	600 mg IV every 6 hrs or 900 mg IV every 8 hrs (clindamycin) 30 mg (base) PO daily (primaquine)
Adjunctive therapy: Prednisone if PaO_2 <70 mmHg or A-a gradient ≥35 mmHg	40 mg PO every 12 hrs for 5 days, 40 mg PO daily for 5 days, 20 mg PO daily for 11 days

[a]Duration of PCP treatment is 21 days.
PCP, *Pneumocystis* pneumonia; ICU, intensive care unit; IV, intravenously; PO, by mouth; PaO_2, arterial oxygen tension; A-a, alveolar–arterial.

hyperkalemia, and increases in creatinine kinase. Pentamidine also has cardiac side effects, leading to bradycardia, prolonged Q-T intervals, and ventricular arrhythmias (68,69).

When TMP/SMX and pentamidine are either ineffective or toxic, it is possible to use clindamycin and primaquine as another salvage regimen option, but this use may be limited in the ICU because primaquine is administered orally and its absorption may be impaired. Clindamycin should be dosed from 600 to 900 mg every 6 to 8 hours intravenously, with primaquine given 15 to 30 mg orally daily. Patients should be tested for glucose-6-phosphate dehydrogenase (G6PD) deficiency before starting primaquine; side effects include rash, diarrhea, and methemoglobinemia.

Adjunctive corticosteroids have been shown to decrease mortality in those patients with moderate to severe PCP (41,42,70,71). A meta-analysis of all randomized trials of corticosteroids found that the administration of corticosteroids was associated with a risk ratio of 0.56 for mortality and 0.38 for requiring mechanical ventilation (72,73). Patients with a room air arterial oxygen pressure less than 70 mmHg or with an alveolar–arterial gradient 35 mmHg or greater should receive corticosteroids. Corticosteroid therapy should be started within 24 to 72 hours of initiation of PCP treatment, regardless of whether the diagnosis is confirmed or only suspected. Corticosteroids act to reduce the inflammatory response seen during the first few days of treatment, thereby lessening the occurrence of respiratory deterioration. The recommended regimen is 40 mg of oral prednisone given twice daily for 5 days, then 40 mg once daily for 5 days, and 20 mg daily for 11 days. If patients are unable to tolerate oral medications, intravenous methylprednisolone or dexamethasone can be substituted.

Treatment Failure. Due to the increased inflammatory response during the initial phase of treatment, clinical deterioration can frequently be seen in the first 3 to 5 days of PCP treatment. Patients may experience worsening hypoxemia and increasing respiratory distress, and radiographic infiltrates may progress. This worsening is likely due to an inflammatory response to dead or dying organisms that results in increased capillary permeability and formation of pulmonary edema. Assessment of treatment failure is challenging given this potential for initial worsening combined with the inability to culture *Pneumocystis* or to determine antibiotic sensitivities. In general, treatment should be continued for at least 5 to 7 days before diagnosing treatment failure and switching to another agent. It is important to remember that other processes present at baseline or processes that have developed since admission can explain the patient's lack of improvement, and these diagnoses must be excluded before concluding that treatment failure is solely to blame. Other frequent diagnoses to consider include nosocomial, community-acquired, or other opportunistic pneumonia and cardiogenic or noncardiogenic pulmonary edema. Patients who worsen or fail to improve while receiving PCP treatment should undergo diagnostic procedures such as chest CT, sputum cultures, or echocardiography as clinically indicated. Repeat bronchoscopy is useful to identify pathogens other than PCP but is not useful to evaluate treatment failure because *Pneumocystis* can persist in the BAL, even in patients who are successfully treated (74).

It is unknown if treatment failure is more likely in patients with previous exposure to anti-*Pneumocystis* prophylaxis. *Pneumocystis* develops mutations at the dihydropteroate synthase (DHPS) locus with exposure to sulfa- or sulfone-containing medications such as TMP/SMX and dapsone (75–77). In other microorganisms, mutations at this locus have been shown to produce resistance to TMP/SMX, but the evidence for clinically important resistance in *Pneumocystis* is not clear-cut. Some authors have found an increased mortality and rate of treatment failure in patients with DHPS mutations (78–81), but others have not observed this association (76,82). In general, most patients with previous exposure to TMP/SMX or dapsone respond to treatment with TMP/SMX, and it should still be regarded as first-line therapy for these patients.

Ventilatory Support. Because the physiology of PCP is very similar to that of ARDS, principles of ventilatory management should be the same. Barotrauma (or volutrauma) is of particular concern in ventilated patients with PCP, as the development of a pneumothorax heralds a poor prognosis. Although patients with PCP were not included in the ARDSnet study published in 2000, these patients should probably be ventilated in a similar fashion—with tidal volumes of 6 mL/kg of ideal body weight and levels of positive end-expiratory pressure (PEEP) as needed to maintain oxygenation according to the ARDSnet guidelines (83). Noninvasive positive pressure ventilation (NIPPV) with continuous positive airway pressure (CPAP) or bilevel positive airway pressure (BiPAP) may be useful in patients with PCP. One study found that use of noninvasive ventilation decreased the rate of intubation, lowered the number of pneumothoraces, and improved survival (84). Thus, NIPPV may be tried as a first-line ventilation mode in patients with PCP who are awake, cooperative, and able to protect their airway. High-flow oxygen delivered through nasal cannula may improve outcome for patients with hypoxemic respiratory failure, although its role in HIV-infected patients with PCP and other pulmonary conditions has not specifically been studied (85).

Bacterial Pneumonia

BP is significantly more frequent in HIV-infected compared to uninfected individuals, despite an overall decline in incidence (86,87). Earlier initiation and more widespread use of ART, as well as TMP/SMX for PCP prophylaxis in eligible individuals, have contributed to an overall decline in the numbers of cases of HIV-associated BP (29,88,89). Although absolute numbers of cases of BP have declined since the introduction of ART, BP now accounts for a greater percentage of ICU admissions for respiratory failure since the number of PCP cases has also declined (2,11). Similarly, nosocomial or hospital-acquired pneumonia (HAP) has also declined since the introduction of ART but remains common in mechanically ventilated patients (90). Risk factors for BP include injection drug use, cigarette smoking, older age, and lower CD4+ cell count, although BP can occur in patients at any CD4+ cell count and with increasing frequency as the CD4+ cell count declines (89,91–93).

BP can be associated with significant morbidity and with increased short- and long-term mortality in HIV-infected patients (94). CD4+ cell count below 100 cells/μL, shock, and radiographic progression have been associated with mortality from BP in HIV-infected patients (95). ICU mortality in HIV-infected patients admitted with BP has been reported between 17% and 24% (5,7).

Clinical Presentation. Clinical presentation of BP in the HIV-infected patient is similar to that in the HIV-uninfected population. Patients typically present with an acute onset of fever, cough, shortness of breath, and purulent sputum. Chest radiographs frequently reveal lobar infiltrates that may progress to an ARDS-like picture in severe cases. The most common causes of BP in HIV include *Streptococcus pneumoniae* and *Haemophilus influenzae. Pseudomonas aeruginosa* and *Staphylococcus aureus* are also frequent causes of BP, particularly hospital-acquired cases, but can be community-acquired as well. Drug-resistant *S. pneumoniae* and *S. aureus* are common in HIV-infected patients, particularly in those on macrolide prophylaxis for *Mycobacterium avium* complex (MAC) and in injection drug users (96–98). Atypical pneumonia with *Mycoplasma pneumoniae* is reported in approximately 20% to 30% of HIV-infected patients with community-acquired pneumonia (CAP) but is less commonly a cause of ICU admission (99). HIV-infected patients are more likely to be bacteremic, particularly those with *S. pneumoniae* infection (100). Additionally, the incidence of bacteremia increases as the CD4+ lymphocyte count declines.

Diagnosis and Treatment. Diagnosis and treatment for both CAP and HAP should generally follow published guidelines, although these guidelines do not specifically address pneumonia in HIV-infected patients (101,102). Blood cultures should be obtained, and sputum should be sent for Gram stain and culture. Bronchoscopy should be considered, particularly in cases of ventilator-associated pneumonia or when the diagnosis is uncertain to assess for other OIs. Additional diagnostic evaluation such as pneumococcal and legionella urinary antigen testing may be useful. Treatment should include empiric coverage for the organisms above. Because of the higher incidence of pseudomonal and staphylococcal pneumonia in HIV-infected patients with severe pneumonia, it is important to initiate coverage for these organisms. As methicillin-resistant *Staphylococcus aureus* (MRSA) is common in HIV infection and is associated with decreased survival (90), empiric antibiotics effective against this pathogen are warranted particularly in injection drug users and in patients with other risk factors for multi–drug-resistant organisms pending results of cultures and antimicrobial sensitivities. Empirical monotherapy with a macrolide is not advised in HIV-infected patients, particularly if they are critically ill and are already on macrolide prophylaxis for MAC because of increasing pneumococcal resistance rates (103). Patients on TMP/SMX prophylaxis may be more likely to have penicillin- and TMP/SMX-resistant *S. pneumoniae.* For patients with CD4+ lymphocyte counts less than 100 cells/μL, consideration should be given to including coverage against *P. aeruginosa.*

Other Respiratory Diseases

Other respiratory diseases that occur in HIV-infected ICU patients include *Mycobacteria tuberculosis* pneumonia; fungal pneumonias such as *Cryptococcus neoformans*, *Histoplasma capsulatum*, *Coccidioides immitis*, and *Aspergillus fumigatus*; cytomegalovirus (CMV) pneumonia; and *Toxoplasma gondii* pneumonitis. Malignancies such as Kaposi sarcoma and non-Hodgkin lymphoma can also lead to respiratory failure, but they are far less common than infections.

IMMUNE RECONSTITUTION INFLAMMATORY SYNDROME

Immune reconstitution inflammatory syndrome (IRIS) encompasses a paradoxical worsening of clinical status in the setting of recovery of the immune system following immunosuppression, typically after the initiation of ART in HIV-infected patients. IRIS is thought to result from immune activation and dysregulated host inflammatory responses to previously recognized or subclinical infections, or in response to cancer or self-antigens (104–106). Immunopathogenesis of IRIS may be different depending upon the pathogen (105).

Clinical Presentation

IRIS can occur days to months after ART is started, with the majority of cases occurring within the first 1 to 3 months (106). Immune reconstitution is most often seen in infection with *Mycobacterium tuberculosis*, *Cryptococcus*, CMV, *Pneumocystis*, MAC, and endemic fungi (106–108). Cancers such as Kaposi sarcoma can also cause IRIS. Manifestations of IRIS that can result in the need for ICU care include meningitis, pneumonitis, hepatitis, and pericarditis. Cryptococcal meningitis has been associated with increased mortality. Respiratory failure secondary to IRIS is most common in tuberculosis and PCP (109,110). Paradoxical worsening in these cases presents with fever, hypoxemia, and new or increased radiographic infiltrates.

Diagnosis and Treatment

The diagnosis of IRIS is one of exclusion, as IRIS can be difficult to distinguish from acute OIs or other etiologies on the basis of clinical features alone. It is thus imperative that other causes of clinical deterioration, such as a new infection, drug resistance, or inadequate drug levels against a known infection, are sought and ruled out before assigning a diagnosis of IRIS.

Treatment is generally supportive, and ART should be continued whenever possible. Nonsteroidal anti-inflammatory agents can be used to decrease inflammation. Steroids are not routinely given, but may be indicated if the excessive inflammatory response is particularly harmful, such as in the setting of life-threatening complications including meningitis, central nervous system lesions, or airway involvement. In these cases, prednisone or methylprednisolone at approximately 1.5 mg/kg of body weight per day for 2 weeks followed by 0.75 mg/kg/day for an additional 2 weeks are recommended while monitoring clinical response (103).

SEPSIS

Sepsis is increasingly common among HIV-infected patients admitted to the ICU. In the ART era, more deaths in the HIV population have been attributed to sepsis and bacteremia (111–113). Amongst ICU patients, severe sepsis is associated with higher mortality compared to other indications for ICU admission (24,113). Furthermore, severe sepsis may be associated with greater mortality in HIV-infected patients compared to HIV-uninfected patients (24,27,112).

In-hospital mortality has been reported to be between 40% and 60% (9,28,30,112,114), with worse outcomes associated with higher severity of illness scores (30,113). Longer-term outcomes are also poor, with 6-month mortality reported at 60% (113). However, in published studies of HIV-infected critically ill patients, the majority of patients admitted with sepsis in these studies were severely immunocompromised with CD4+ cell counts below 200 cells/μL, and many were not on ART (112,113). Prognosis and outcomes, particularly following hospitalization, should be considered in this context.

Clinical Presentation

Clinical presentation of sepsis, severe sepsis, and septic shock are the same in HIV-infected as in non–HIV-infected persons. Providers should consider a broad differential diagnosis, including bacterial as well as nonbacterial causes for infection, and ensure adequate source control in the case of invasive infections. Pneumonia is generally reported as the leading cause of sepsis in HIV-infected persons, with bloodstream and intra-abdominal infections common sources as well (24,27,112,113). Nosocomial infections are frequent in HIV-infected persons in studies from the United States and Europe, with gram negatives such as *P. aeruginosa*, *Klebsiella pneumoniae*, *Enterobacter* species, and gram-positive organisms such as *S. aureus* and *S. pneumoniae*. By way of contrast, in other parts of the world, such as in studies from Uganda, sepsis is frequently due to bacteremia from *M. tuberculosis* (115,116).

Diagnosis and Treatment

Care of the HIV-infected patient with sepsis should follow current guidelines (34). Broad-spectrum antibiotics should be based on the patient's CD4+ cell count, the presumed source as noted above, and previous use of prophylactic antibiotics that might predispose to resistant bacteria. Clinicians should consider empiric coverage and diagnostic evaluation for bacterial infections, PCP, mycobacterial diseases, endemic fungi, and other OIs as suggested by the patient's presentation. Because HIV-infected patients may have an increased risk for adrenal insufficiency, steroids should be considered in patients who are persistently hypotensive despite adequate fluid resuscitation and vasopressors.

NEUROLOGIC MANIFESTATIONS OF HIV

The spectrum of neurologic disorders requiring critical care for patients with HIV infection includes all the causes commonly seen in the HIV-uninfected population in addition to particular OIs, neoplasms, and sequelae of HIV. As many as 80% of these conditions required mechanical ventilation among HIV-infected patients in an earlier series (117). Nonetheless, neurologic causes of ICU admission may be decreasing. Coma as the ICU admission diagnosis decreased from 29% in 1999–2001 to 15% in 2008–2010 in CUB-Réa (5). In the most recent reports from San Francisco General Hospital, neurologic diagnoses accounted for 16% of ICU admissions and delirium diagnosis was associated with approximately 75% survival (2,3). Another study found that CNS toxoplasmosis and progressive multifocal leukoencephalopathy (PML) had decreased, but the incidence of ischemic stroke, hemorrhagic stroke, and primary CNS lymphoma had increased (118).

CNS toxoplasmosis is one of the most frequent CNS infections seen, although the number of cases has fallen dramatically with the introduction of ART (119,120). Patients typically present with fever, headache, focal neurologic deficits, and a decreased level of consciousness; seizures can also occur. CT scan reveals characteristic ring-enhancing lesions

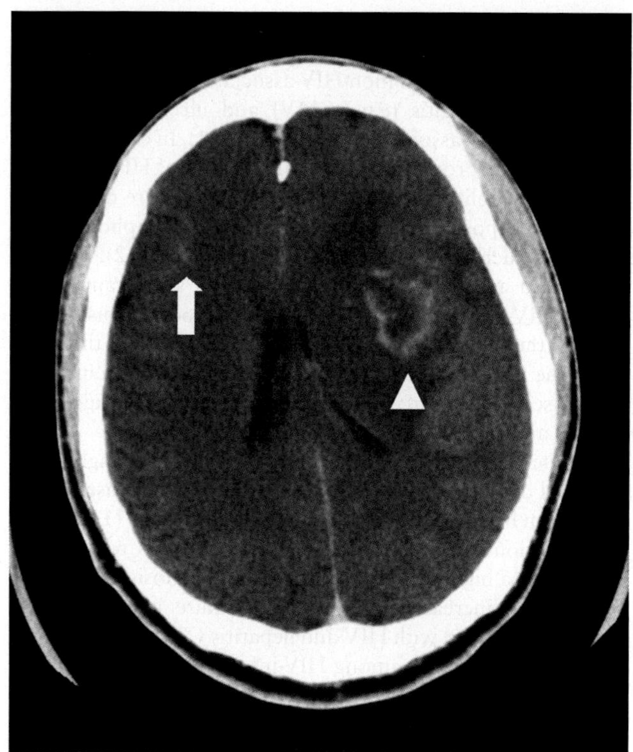

FIGURE 91.2 Contrast-enhanced head computed tomography scan from an AIDS patient with headache, word-finding difficulty, and several seizures showing a left frontoparietal ring-enhancing lesion (*arrowhead*) with mass effect on the lateral ventricle and a subtler focus of enhancement on the right at the gray–white junction (*arrow*). (Courtesy of Cheryl Jay, M.D., Associate Clinical Professor of Neurology, University of California, San Francisco.)

(Fig. 91.2). Similar findings can also be seen with CNS lymphoma. Treatment for CNS toxoplasmosis is pyrimethamine given as a 200-mg loading dose, followed by 50 to 75 mg orally every 24 hours, with sulfadiazine at a dose of 1 to 1.5 g every 6 hours orally. Patients should also receive 10 to 20 mg of folic acid daily while receiving pyrimethamine. Other CNS infections that are seen in HIV infection include bacterial and *C. neoformans* meningitis. Diagnosis of *C. neoformans* is confirmed by visualization of encapsulated yeast on cerebrospinal fluid (CSF), a positive CSF culture, or a positive CSF cryptococcal antigen. Treatment should be initiated with liposomal amphotericin B (3–4 mg/kg/day intravenously) and flucytosine (100 mg/kg/day orally, divided into four doses). Repeated lumbar puncture is often required to normalize CSF pressure. Other CSF infections that occur in HIV include PML, which is a progressive demyelinating disease, CMV, and herpes simplex virus. Any of these diseases can worsen and present with a neurologic IRIS in the setting of introduction of ART (118).

GASTROINTESTINAL MANIFESTATIONS OF HIV

GI diseases, in particular liver diseases, have increased as a cause of death in HIV-infected patients (111). These diseases are either the primary cause or a complicating factor in the ICU admission of many HIV-infected patients. As in the HIV-uninfected population, significant GI bleeding often results in ICU admission. Upper GI bleeding is more common than lower GI bleeding, and approximately half of the cases are HIV-related (121). Common HIV-associated diagnoses include infectious esophagitis (e.g., CMV) and ulcers, Kaposi sarcoma, and AIDS-associated lymphoma (121). In cases of lower GI bleeding, approximately 70% are a result of HIV infection (121). CMV colitis and idiopathic colon ulcers are most common, but Kaposi sarcoma, AIDS-associated lymphoma, and infections such as MAC may also contribute (122). Hemorrhoids and anal fissures can also result in significant bleeding in HIV-infected patients with thrombocytopenia (123). Care of the HIV-infected patient with a GI bleed is the same as for the HIV-uninfected patient and should include immediate resuscitation, source identification, reversal of coagulation defects, and achievement of hemostasis.

Coinfection with HIV and hepatitis C is increasingly common and complicates the management of both diseases. Mortality from hepatitis C has increased in recent years (124–127), and infection in HIV-infected individuals seems to be more severe with a higher mortality and risk of cirrhosis (128–132). There is an increased risk of renal failure in hospitalized patients coinfected with HIV and hepatitis C (133,134). Hepatitis B is also common among HIV-infected patients.

Other GI conditions that are common in HIV-infected patients include peritonitis and bowel perforation. The most common cause of life-threatening abdominal pain is small bowel or colon peritonitis from CMV (135). Kaposi sarcoma, AIDS-associated lymphoma, and mycobacterial infection have also been associated with bowel perforation (122). Pancreatitis can also be seen, particularly with exposure to certain antiretroviral medications or pentamidine. AIDS cholangiopathy can result from various infectious and neoplastic processes and can be asymptomatic or present with fulminant biliary sepsis (122). In addition to the usual care of cholangitis with intravenous fluids and broad-spectrum antibiotics, endoscopic retrograde cholangiopancreatography (ERCP) with sphincterotomy may be helpful in patients with common bile duct dilatation (135).

OTHER HIV-ASSOCIATED CONDITIONS

Cardiac Disease

Since the introduction of ART, there has been growing evidence that HIV-infected patients are developing premature atherosclerosis, and cardiovascular disease is a primary cause of non–HIV-related deaths in these patients (111,136). Although the literature has been conflicting, HIV-infected patients have an elevated risk of cardiovascular disease compared to uninfected patients in recent studies when controlling for other risk factors and confounders (137,138). Thus, HIV-infected patients may be commonly admitted to the ICU with acute coronary syndromes.

The increased risk for cardiovascular disease in HIV-infected patients is in part explained by a high prevalence of metabolic abnormalities, chronic inflammation, and other cardiac risk factors such as cigarette smoking. The development of metabolic abnormalities that contribute to atherosclerosis has been associated with the use of nonnucleoside reverse transcriptase inhibitors (NNRTIs) and/or protease inhibitors (PIs). Elevated triglycerides, hypercholesterolemia, decreased high-density lipoproteins, glucose intolerance, and frank diabetes have all been associated with various antiretrovirals (139–142). There may also be direct endothelial effects of PIs or HIV itself that play a role in the development of vascular complications. Chronic inflammation and immune activation associated with HIV infection have also been associated with risk for cardiovascular events (143).

Congestive heart failure may also be an indication for ICU admission. In the precombination ART era, HIV was associated with dilated cardiomyopathy that was often severe. In the ART era, however, systolic heart failure has decreased in prevalence, while diastolic dysfunction has increased, often in association with traditional cardiac risk factors (144).

There are few data on treatment or outcomes of cardiac disease specifically in the HIV-infected population. In the absence of specific data, treatment of acute coronary syndromes should be the same as in the HIV-uninfected population. HIV-infected patients should be referred for cardiac surgery and coronary artery bypass grafting when appropriate. Heart failure should also be managed similarly as in HIV-uninfected patients.

Renal Disease

HIV-infected patients are at risk of acute and chronic renal failure that can either lead to ICU admission or complicate care in the ICU. Baseline renal function is abnormal in approximately 30% of HIV-infected patients. HIV-associated nephropathy has decreased with the use of ART but is still a common cause of end-stage renal disease (145–147). Renal dysfunction can occur from use of certain antiretroviral medications and other therapies such as pentamidine, TMP/SMX, and amphotericin B. HIV-infected patients who are coinfected with hepatitis C also have an increased risk of renal failure (133,148). Other common comorbidities including hypertension and diabetes are emerging as major risk factors for end-stage renal disease in HIV-infected patients who achieve viral suppression (148).

Acute kidney injury is likely more common in HIV-infected patients, occurring in 66% of all HIV-infected patients admitted to the ICU with nearly one-third requiring renal replacement therapy (149). The diagnostic workup and treatment of renal dysfunction in HIV-infected patients is similar to that for the HIV-uninfected patient and should include renal ultrasound to rule out obstruction, examination of the urine, discontinuation of nephrotoxic medications, and renal biopsy if indicated. Dialysis should be offered to appropriate patients.

Metabolic Abnormalities

Metabolic abnormalities are common in the HIV-infected ICU patient. As described above, lipid and glucose abnormalities are often seen. Hyperglycemia secondary to drugs such as pentamidine also occurs in this population. It has been noted that hospitalized patients with HIV have high rates of hyponatremia (150–152). Causes of hyponatremia include hypovolemia, adrenal insufficiency, drugs, and the syndrome of inappropriate antidiuretic hormone (SIADH). A high incidence of adrenal abnormalities has been noted on autopsy of HIV-infected patients (153–155). Causes of adrenal pathology include infections such as CMV, tumors such as Kaposi sarcoma, and drugs such as ketoconazole and pentamidine (156). The clinical significance of the adrenal abnormalities is uncertain, but it seems that HIV-infected patients have a higher likelihood of adrenal dysfunction (36,157). Adrenal insufficiency can present with hyperkalemia, hyponatremia, and hypotension, and patients with these symptoms should be evaluated and treated appropriately. As with HIV-uninfected patients, adrenal insufficiency may be common in sepsis.

Lactic acidosis is another metabolic abnormality that can occur in HIV-infected patients receiving ART. This syndrome was first described in the 1990s and can occur with any nucleoside/nucleotide reverse transcriptase inhibitor (NRTI) but is most commonly seen with didanosine and stavudine (158,159). Mitochondrial toxicity secondary to impaired synthesis of adenosine triphosphate (ATP)-generating enzymes is believed to be the cause of lactic acidosis (160–162). Patients particularly at risk of developing lactic acidosis from these drugs include those with a creatinine clearance less than 70 mL/min and a nadir CD4+ cell count below 250 cells/μL (163). Although some patients may have only an asymptomatic lactic acidosis, others present with life-threatening acidemia. These patients also commonly complain of abdominal pain, nausea, and vomiting. Hepatic steatosis and transaminitis also occur, and patients can progress to respiratory failure and shock.

In any patient presenting with these symptoms, an arterial lactate level should be checked and all antiretroviral medications discontinued if the level is greater than 5 mmol/L. Supportive care should be administered with bicarbonate therapy and hemodialysis if necessary. Based on anecdotal data, riboflavin, thiamine, and L-carnitine may reverse toxicity (164–167). Riboflavin is administered at a dose of 50 mg daily with 50 mg/kg of L-carnitine, and 100 mg of thiamine. Although the exact length of treatment is unknown, it should be continued at least until acidosis resolves.

Fever of Unknown Origin

Fever is common in all ICU patients. The differential for fever is broad in the HIV-infected patient and includes infections, neoplasms, medications, and collagen vascular diseases. Several studies have examined the etiology of fevers of unknown origin in those with HIV infection. Most studies have found that infectious causes are responsible for most prolonged fevers in the HIV-infected patient, with mycobacterial diseases diagnosed most commonly. PCP, cryptococcus, histoplasma, CMV, and bacterial infections are also seen (168,169). The most common neoplastic cause of prolonged fever is lymphoma. Patients receiving ART are less likely to present with a fever of unknown origin than those not receiving ART (170).

Recurrent fever in an HIV-infected ICU patient should also prompt evaluation of those conditions commonly seen in HIV-uninfected ICU patients. Common infectious causes of fever in the ICU include HAP, catheter-related infections, sinusitis, and pseudomembranous colitis. Noninfectious causes include drug reactions, pancreatitis, venous thromboembolism, acalculous cholecystitis, adrenal insufficiency, and thyroid storm. A thorough physical examination and imaging studies should be obtained, often including CT scan of the chest, abdomen, and pelvis. Diagnostic workup should include standard evaluation for infections such as blood, sputum, and urine cultures. Bronchoscopy with BAL should be performed in patients who demonstrate a new infiltrate on chest radiograph or have a worsening respiratory status. Testing should be performed for mycobacterial and fungal pathogens. Other diagnostic options include fluorodeoxyglucose (FDG)/positron emission tomography (PET), bone marrow biopsy and culture, and lymph node biopsy (171–174). Generally, workup should be performed as would be done in the HIV-uninfected population.

ANTIRETROVIRAL THERAPY IN THE ICU

Treatment Strategies

HIV-infected patients may be receiving ART at the time of ICU admission or may have ART initiated in the ICU. The use of ART in critically ill patients presents distinct issues related to patient involvement, drug delivery, drug dosing, drug interactions, and antiretroviral-associated toxicities. The success of ART in decreasing HIV-associated morbidity and mortality has raised questions regarding the ability of ART to improve outcomes in critically ill HIV-infected patients, the HIV patients with the highest short-term mortality, and it is important for the critical care physician to consider ART in every HIV-infected patient.

There are several factors related to using ART in the ICU that are important to consider. ART improves immune function. In chronic HIV infection, improving immune function with ART significantly reduces the risk of OIs and neoplasms. This could contribute to reductions in morbidity and mortality in critically ill HIV-infected patients by decreasing the risk of subsequent HIV-associated diseases. ART is also important in treating conditions such as PML that otherwise lack effective therapy. For patients already receiving ART, discontinuing therapy could result in the selection of drug-resistant virus that could limit future therapy. This is especially true if patients are receiving efavirenz or nevirapine, as these antiretrovirals have longer half-lives than other antiretroviral medications. As a result, levels of these medications may persist as the levels of the other antiretroviral medications decrease, resulting in functional monotherapy.

ART is also associated with several risks. Current ART guidelines recommend implementing a series of patient-based strategies and patient involvement to optimize adherence to ART, strategies that are often impossible in a critically ill ICU patient (175). Drug interactions and ART-associated toxicities can also complicate management. Pharmacokinetic interactions can occur during drug absorption, metabolism, and elimination of the antiretroviral(s) as well as the interacting drug. In addition, there are uncertainties surrounding dosing in acute and multiple organ system failures. These uncertainties could place patients at risk for subtherapeutic drug levels and drug resistance or, conversely, supratherapeutic levels and toxicity. IRIS could result in significant clinical worsening of an already critical disease. The potential threat of this syndrome may make physicians reluctant to initiate ART in the ICU.

There are now several randomized clinical trials to support the initiation of ART in acutely ill HIV-infected patients with OIs but no randomized clinical trials and no consensus guidelines to assist in decisions regarding ART use in the ICU, particularly amongst mechanically ventilated patients with respiratory failure, as these patients have not been represented in prior clinical trials. Only a few retrospective studies address some of the clinical issues that critical care clinicians face. Although decisions regarding ART use in the ICU require a

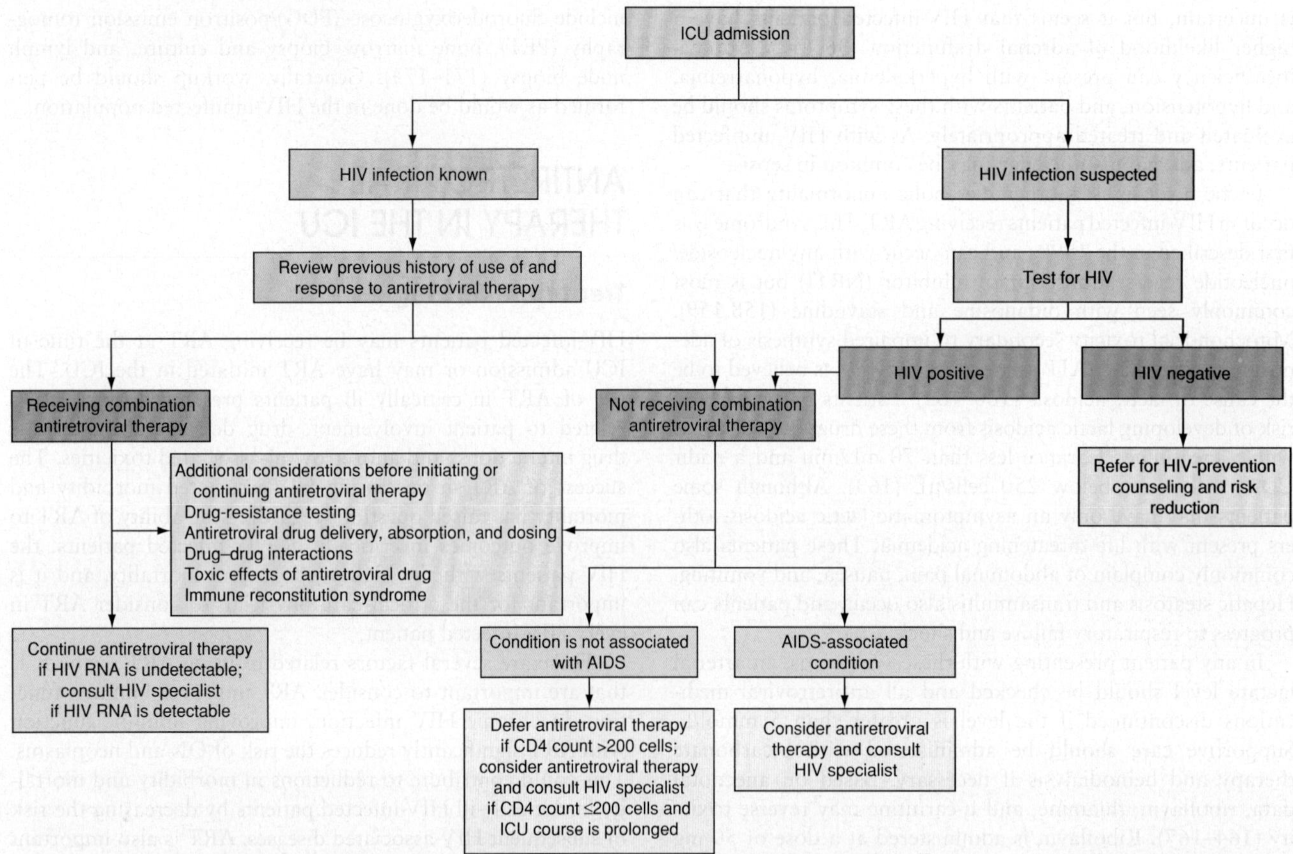

FIGURE 91.3 Treatment strategies for patients with HIV in the ICU. This algorithm provides a framework for making decisions regarding the use of antiretroviral therapy in the ICU. (Adapted from Huang L, Quartin A, Jones D, et al. Intensive care of patients with HIV infection. *N Engl J Med.* 2006;355:179. Copyright © 2006 Massachusetts Medical Society. Reprinted with permission.)

case-by-case basis review, Huang et al. (176) suggested the following general framework (Fig. 91.3). Patients receiving ART prior to ICU admission who have evidence of virologic suppression (plasma HIV RNA below the limit of detection) should continue ART, if possible. These patients should have no contraindications to continuing ART such as drug interactions or ART-associated toxicities. Prompt placement of a feeding tube is especially critical in these patients. In patients whose plasma HIV RNA is detectable despite ART, the risks of continuing ART may outweigh the benefits of incomplete HIV viral suppression, especially if the CD4+ cell count response has been poor. In these individuals, switching to a new ART regimen may be preferable to continuing a potentially failing regimen. However, consultation with an expert in HIV medicine should be obtained prior to any decision to continue, switch, or discontinue ART.

Patients not receiving ART prior to ICU admission represent the largest proportion of HIV-infected patients admitted to the ICU in most published studies (2,7–9). Two studies from the ART era suggest that patients admitted with an AIDS-defining diagnosis, especially PCP, have the poorest prognosis and, thus, the greatest theoretical benefit from ART (2,31). Although one study found that patients receiving or started on ART during ICU admission for PCP had decreased mortality (25% vs. 63%), this study was retrospective and based on a limited number of patients.

Based on the limited available data, ART initiation should be deferred in HIV-infected patients admitted to the ICU with a non–AIDS-associated condition (see Fig. 91.3) (176). The immediate prognosis in these patients is generally better than for an AIDS-associated diagnosis, and the short-term outcome is most likely related to successful treatment of the underlying non-AIDS condition (2). As a result, the risks of ART initiation in the ICU outweigh the short-term benefits of this therapy. If, however, patients remain in the ICU for a prolonged period, ART (and OI prophylaxis) should be considered if the patients have a CD4+ cell count less than 200 cells/μL since the risk of OIs is increased below this CD4+ count.

In contrast, ART should be considered for HIV-infected patients admitted to the ICU with an AIDS-associated diagnosis. This is especially true for patients whose condition is worsening despite optimal ICU management and treatment for the AIDS-associated condition. In these individuals, the prognosis is dire, and aggressive measures are warranted. Patients who receive ART should be followed for development of IRIS, and consultation with an expert in HIV medicine should be obtained.

Drug Delivery, Dosing, and Interactions

All of the currently approved antiretroviral medications are dispensed orally, either as tablets or capsules, with the sole exception of enfuvirtide, a fusion inhibitor that is delivered subcutaneously. Several antiretrovirals are available in an oral solution, oral suspension, or in an oral powder, but only zidovudine has an intravenous formulation. If the medications

TABLE 91.3 Examples of Common ICU Medications and Potentially Serious Life-Threatening Interactions with Antiretrovirals

Drug	Antiretroviral	Interaction
Sedatives/analgesics		
Midazolam	All PIs, Efavirenz (EFV) Elvitegravir/cobicistat/tenofovir disoproxil fumarate/emtricitabine (EVG/c/TDF/FTC)	Increased midazolam expected Do not coadminister oral midazolam and these ARVs Parenteral midazolam can be used with caution as a single dose and given in a monitored situation for procedural sedation
Fentanyl	All PIs	Increased fentanyl possible
Methadone	Ritonavir-boosted PIs Most NNRTIs	Decreased methadone AUC Opioid withdrawal may occur
Methadone	Zidovudine (ZDV)	Increased ZDV AUC Monitor for ZDV-related adverse effects
Oxycodone	Ritonavir-boosted lopinavir (LPV/r)	Increased oxycodone AUC Monitor for opioid-related adverse effects
Gastrointestinal agents		
Antacids	Atazanavir (ATV) (unboosted and boosted), fosamprenavir, and tipranavir (boosted)	Decreased PI AUC Administer PI >2 hrs before or >1–2 hrs after antacid administration
Antacids	Rilpivirine (RPV)	Decreased RPV Administer antacid >2 hrs before or >4 hrs after RPV
Antacids (Aluminum, Magnesium ± Calcium containing)	Dolutegravir (DTG), elvitegravir/cobicistat/tenofovir disoproxil fumarate/emtricitabine (EVG/c/TDF/FTC)	Administer integrase strand transfer inhibitor >2 hrs before or >2–6 hrs after antacid administration
Antacids (aluminum–magnesium containing)	Raltegravir (RAL)	Do not coadminister Al-Mg hydroxide antacids and RAL
H_2 receptor antagonists	Atazanavir (ATV) (unboosted and boosted), fosamprenavir (unboosted)	Decreased PI AUC Administer PI >2 hrs before H_2 receptor antagonist administration
H_2 receptor antagonists	Rilpivirine (RPV)	Decreased RPV Administer H_2 receptor antagonist >12 hrs before or >4 hrs after RPV
Proton pump inhibitors (PPIs)	Atazanavir (ATV) (unboosted and boosted) Delavirdine	Decreased ATV levels PPIs are not recommended in patients receiving unboosted ATV
Proton pump inhibitors (omeprazole)	Tipranavir (boosted)	Decreased omeprazole levels May need to increase omeprazole dose
Proton pump inhibitors (omeprazole)	Rilpivirine (RPV)	Contraindicated. Do not coadminister

Note: There are also important drug interactions between antiretroviral medications and a wide spectrum of medications that may be used in critically ill patients, including anticoagulants and antiplatelets, anticonvulsants, antidepressants and antipsychotics, antimicrobials, cardiac medications, corticosteroids, HMG-CoA reductase inhibitors, and phosphodiesterase Type 5 (PDE5) inhibitors. Please refer to https://aidsinfo.nih.gov/guidelines for the latest information.

ICU, intensive care unit; ARV, antiretroviral; AUC, area under the curve; NRTI, nucleoside reverse transcriptase inhibitor; NNRTI, nonnucleoside reverse transcriptase inhibitor; PI, protease inhibitor; PPI, proton pump inhibitor.

that are only available as tablets or capsules are to be continued or initiated in the ICU, then these medications need to be crushed and reconstituted for delivery via feeding tube. As an additional consideration, the administration of many antiretrovirals requires the interruption of enteral feedings that are usually delivered continuously, while other antiretrovirals should be taken with food to minimize adverse effects.

Critical illness may complicate the absorption of antiretroviral medications. Decreased gastric motility (177,178), continuous feeding (179), nasogastric suctioning, and gastric alkalinization recommended for stress ulcer prophylaxis (34) may contribute to variations in the absorption of enterally administered drugs. H_2 blockers and proton pump inhibitors, used for stress ulcer prophylaxis, are contraindicated with certain antiretroviral medications, necessitating the use of alternative prophylaxis agents or antiretroviral medications (Table 91.3) (175). Absorption of subcutaneously injected medications may also be altered (180,181). Furthermore, atypical drug volumes of distribution and compromise of elimination pathways due to acute organ failures may confound the achievement of appropriate drug levels (182).

The impact of acute and multiple organ system failures on the pharmacokinetics of antiretroviral medications, particularly when used in combination, have been largely unstudied. The presence of renal insufficiency or hepatic impairment will affect antiretroviral dosing. Renal insufficiency will reduce the clearance of all NRTIs except abacavir and will require dose adjustment of these NRTIs. Patients with renal insufficiency cannot use the fixed-dose NRTI combinations if each component has a different dose adjustment. Instead, each antiretroviral must be used individually and dosed accordingly. Liver impairment will reduce the hepatic metabolism of abacavir, nevirapine (an NNRTI), and many PIs and integrase strand transfer inhibitors (INSTIs), and will require dose adjustment of these medications. Finally, as the patient's renal and hepatic functions change, the dose of these medications must be readjusted accordingly.

Antiretroviral medications, especially NNRTIs and ritonavir-boosted PI regimens, have several important drug interactions with other medications (Table 91.3). These interactions involve other HIV-associated medications, including those for OI treatment or prevention, and common ICU medications, especially benzodiazepines. Midazolam, a benzodiazepine of choice in the ICU, should be avoided in nonventilated patients who are receiving efavirenz (an NNRTI) or PIs, as benzodiazepine drug levels may be markedly increased (175). For mechanically ventilated patients, any resulting increased sedation may be a relative, rather than an absolute, contraindication. However, excess sedation is a significant factor in patients weaning from a ventilator and nearing extubation. Other drug–drug interactions may require close monitoring, dose adjustment (increase or decrease), or avoidance of a specific antiretroviral medication and/or the other drug.

Drug Toxicity

In general, the newer antiretroviral medications possess better safety profiles compared to their predecessors. Nevertheless, several antiretrovirals are associated with potentially life-threatening and serious adverse effects (Table 91.4).

TABLE 91.4 Potentially Life-Threatening and Serious Adverse Effects of Antiretroviral Agents

Life-threatening and Adverse Effect	Principal Antiretroviral Agent	Onset	Prevention/Monitoring and Management
Dermatologic			
Hypersensitivity reaction (HSR)—fever, diffuse rash; may progress to hypotension, respiratory distress, and vascular collapse	Abacavir (ABC) Check HLA-B*5701 status; patients who are HLA-B*5701-positive are at highest risk; ABC is contraindicated if HLA-B*5701-positive	Onset, 9 days (median); approximately 90% occur within first 6 wks; symptoms worsen with continuation of ABC	• Discontinue ABC and other ARVs • Rule out other causes of symptoms • Discontinue other potential agent(s) • Do not rechallenge patients with ABC after suspected HSR regardless of HLA-B*5701 status
Stevens–Johnson syndrome (SJS), toxic epidermal necrolysis (TEN)	Chiefly NNRTIs Nevirapine (NVP) more than other NNRTIs Reported cases with NRTIs, PIs, and raltegravir (RAL)	Onset within first few days to weeks	• NVP: 2-wk lead in period with 200 mg QD dosing, then increase to 200 mg BID or 400 mg QD (XR tablet) • Repeat 2-wk lead in period if therapy is discontinued for >7 days • Discontinue NNRTI and other ARVs • Rule out other causes of symptoms • Discontinue other potential agent(s) • Do not rechallenge patients with NNRTI
Neurologic			
CNS effects including somnolence, insomnia, abnormal dreams, hallucination, psychosis, depression, and suicidal ideation	Efavirenz (EFV)	Approximately 50% may have some symptoms Onset within first few days; most symptoms subside or diminish after 2–4 wks but symptoms may necessitate discontinuation in some	• Administer at bedtime or 2–3 hrs before bedtime for nonintubated, nonsedated patients • Take on an empty stomach to reduce CNS effects • Consider discontinuing EFV if symptoms persist and cause significant impairment or exacerbation of psychiatric illness
Gastrointestinal			
Hepatotoxicity	All ARVs; nevirapine (NVP) > other NNRTIs, tipranavir (TPV)/ritonavir (RTV) > other PIs Tipranavir (TPV)/Ritonavir (RTV) is contraindicated in hepatic insufficiency (Child-Pugh B or C)	Frequency varies with ARV Onset (NRTIs), months to years; PIs generally weeks to months Risk of severe hepatotoxicity from NVP is increased in ARV-naive	• Monitor liver enzymes • For symptomatic patients, discontinue all ARVs • Rule out other causes of hepatotoxicity • Discontinue other potential agent(s)
Pancreatitis	Didanosine (ddI), also stavudine (d4T)	Onset usually weeks to months	• Avoid in patients with a history of pancreatitis • Monitoring of serum amylase/lipase in asymptomatic patients is generally not recommended • Discontinue offending ARV • Rule out other causes of pancreatitis • Discontinue other potential agent(s)
Hematologic			
Bone marrow suppression (macrocytic anemia and neutropenia)	Zidovudine (AZT, ZDV)	Onset, weeks to months	• Avoid use in patients at risk • Avoid other bone marrow suppressants if possible • Monitor CBC with differential • Switch to another NRTI if there is an alternative • Discontinue concomitant bone marrow suppressants if there are alternatives • Blood transfusion and other therapies as indicated

TABLE 91.4 Potentially Life-Threatening and Serious Adverse Effects of Antiretroviral Agents (*Continued*)

Life-threatening and Adverse Effect	Principal Antiretroviral Agent	Onset	Prevention/Monitoring and Management
Lactic acidosis, hepatic steatosis ± pancreatitis (severe mitochondrial toxicities)	NRTIs, especially stavudine (d4T), didanosine (ddI), and zidovudine (AZT, ZDV)	Rare, but mortality up to 50% in some case series; mortality high if serum lactate >10 mmol/L Insidious onset, months; GI prodrome	• Routine monitoring of lactic acid is generally not recommended • Discontinue ARV if this syndrome is highly suspected • May require IV bicarbonate infusion, hemodialysis, or hemofiltration
Renal			
Nephrolithiasis, urolithiasis, crystalluria	Indinavir (IDV) and Atazanavir (ATV)	Onset is any time after beginning of therapy, especially at times of decreased fluid intake	• Maintain hydration, increase hydration at first sign of darkened urine • Monitor serum creatinine, urinalysis • Consider switching to alternative agent • Stent placement may be required
Nephrotoxicity	Tenofovir disoproxil fumarate (TDF): increased serum creatinine, proteinuria, hypophosphatemia, hypokalemia Indinavir (IDV), potentially tenofovir (TDF): increased serum creatinine, hydronephrosis	Frequency unknown Onset: IDV, months; TDV, weeks to months	• Avoid use of other nephrotoxic medications • Maintain hydration, increase hydration at first sign of darkened urine • Monitor serum creatinine, urinalysis, serum potassium and phosphorus • Stop offending agent (generally reversible)

This table only lists potential life-threatening and serious adverse effects with an onset starting from initial dose up to months after initiation of therapy. However, there are several important adverse effects including cardiovascular effects, hyperlipidemia, insulin resistance or diabetes mellitus, and osteonecrosis that may result from antiretroviral therapy.

ARV, antiretroviral; NNRTI, nonnucleoside reverse transcriptase inhibitor; QD, daily; BID, twice a day; NRTI, nucleoside reverse transcriptase inhibitor; PI, protease inhibitor; CBC, complete blood count.

Adapted from Guidelines for the Use of Antiretroviral Agents in HIV-1-Infected Adults and Adolescents. These guidelines are updated frequently, and the most recent information is available on the AIDS*info* Web site: http://AIDSinfo.nih.gov. Accessed June 3, 2015.

Abacavir is associated with a hypersensitivity syndrome that, in rare cases, can lead to death if the patient is rechallenged. The rash associated with nevirapine can be severe, presenting with systemic symptoms and, in rare cases, progressing to Stevens–Johnson syndrome and toxic epidermal necrosis. Efavirenz is associated with mental status alterations that may be attributed erroneously to analgesics, sedatives, or the sleep-disrupted schedule in the ICU. These complications may be difficult to recognize as secondary to ART. If toxicities to antiretroviral agents are suspected, the offending agent should be discontinued promptly. Since antiretroviral drug resistance can develop within days of a partially suppressive regimen, all antiretroviral medications should be discontinued or a replacement drug should be substituted for the suspected agent. Consultation with an expert in HIV medicine is recommended for patients with suspected antiretroviral-associated toxicities.

HIV TESTING IN THE ICU

In the current era, 13% to 40% of patients are unaware of their HIV infection at the time of their ICU admission (2,7–9). For these patients, the first opportunity for HIV testing and diagnosis occurs in an ICU setting. Thus, critical care physicians need to consider evaluation for HIV risk factors and HIV testing in the ICU.

In general, HIV testing should be performed whenever HIV infection is suspected. Most states, per the Centers for Disease Control and Prevention (CDC) recommendations, do not require separate written consent for HIV testing, and instead, general informed consent for medical care includes HIV testing unless the patient declines screening. However, laws are not uniform across all states and local institutional policies may vary. HIV testing and disclosure requirements can present challenges to critical care physicians. If local requirements for testing cannot be obtained or HIV testing is refused, physicians must weigh the risks and benefits of diagnostic procedures and empiric therapy without a confirmed diagnosis; these decisions may harm patients with and without HIV infection.

CONTROL OF HIV INFECTION IN THE ICU

Blood-borne Pathogen Precautions

Risks for occupational transmission of HIV depend on the type and severity of exposure. Potentially infectious fluids include blood, any visibly bloody body fluid, semen, vaginal secretions, and cerebrospinal, synovial, pleural, peritoneal, pericardial, and amniotic fluid. Transmission may occur via percutaneous injury or via contact with mucous membranes or nonintact skin with infectious material. The average risk for transmission of HIV following a percutaneous exposure to HIV-infected blood is estimated to be approximately 0.3%; transmission after mucous membrane exposure is estimated to be approximately 0.09% (183).

Primary preventive measures should be used to decrease the risk of exposure to HIV, as well as other infections including hepatitis B and C. Health care workers should use universal precautions for handling blood and body fluids for all patients, regardless of known HIV status. These precautions include the routine use of personal protective equipment such as gloves, face protection, and gown, depending on the nature of the procedure, anticipated contact with blood or bodily fluids, and the potential for splashing or splattering of fluids. Additional components of a primary prevention strategy include work practice controls—for example, not recapping needles, announcing all sharps introduced onto or removed from the field, not leaving sharps on the field—and engineering controls—for example, self-retracting needles, needleless systems, and sharps disposal containers.

Management of Needle Sticks

In health care workers exposed to potentially infectious body fluids, secondary prevention measures should be used promptly. The first step in postexposure management is the immediate provision of first aid in the event of broken skin or other wound. Exposures should be reported promptly to the appropriate contact at each facility. If the HIV status of the source patient is unknown, evaluation of the risk factors and HIV testing following proper consent procedures should be performed.

In workers with a potential exposure to HIV, postexposure prophylaxis (PEP) should be offered urgently. PEP should begin within hours of exposure, as data suggest that PEP is likely to be more effective if started shortly after exposure (183,184). If a source patient's HIV status is unknown, PEP should be started immediately rather than delayed, particularly if ascertainment of HIV status will be delayed by hours to days.

Preferred PEP regimens should consist of three (or more) antiretroviral drugs for 4 weeks (183,184). A recommended regimen by the US Public Health Service is a backbone of emtricitabine plus tenofovir (often dispensed as Truvada, a fixed-dose combination tablet) with raltegravir as the third drug (183). This regimen has the advantage of being potent, tolerable, conveniently administered, and has minimal drug interactions. Alternative recommendations are also available, depending upon HIV resistance patterns of the source patient and any comorbidities or use of concurrent medications in the health care worker. If three antiretroviral drugs cannot be used, two are acceptable (184). Expert consultation should be considered early, particularly in cases with exposure to documented HIV drug resistance. Substantial side effects are associated with PEP. Because of toxicity, PEP is not justified in exposures that have a negligible risk for transmission of HIV.

Health care workers with potential exposure to HIV should undergo serial HIV antibody testing. The CDC-recommended schedule is initial testing at the time of exposure, with repeat testing at 6 weeks, 12 weeks, and 6 months after exposure. HIV testing should be extended to 12 months in those who become infected with hepatitis C virus after dual exposure to HIV and hepatitis C. Health care workers should also receive counseling to discuss ways to decrease risk of exposures in the future, measures to decrease the risk of secondary transmission, and side effects of any treatments, as well as medical evaluation. Reevaluation should occur within 72 hours after exposure. PEP should be discontinued if HIV testing of the source patient is negative.

Respiratory Isolation

As with HIV-uninfected patients, HIV-infected patients with suspected airborne-spread infections should be placed in respiratory isolation. Airborne precautions in the hospital setting consist of the use of personal protective equipment in the form of respirators and engineering controls such as the use of negative pressure rooms (185). Diseases requiring airborne isolation precautions include tuberculosis, varicella (chickenpox and herpes zoster), measles, and the severe acute respiratory syndrome (SARS) (185). Because tuberculosis is common in the HIV-infected population and is often difficult to distinguish from other types of pneumonia, most HIV-infected patients with respiratory symptoms and chest radiographic abnormalities should be considered for respiratory isolation. The immune status of staff caring for the patient should also be considered, and limiting the number of staff exposed to the patient may be warranted. Patients with suspected airborne-transmitted diseases should wear a surgical mask during transport. Criteria for removing patients from respiratory isolation vary by disease. For example, patients with tuberculosis can be removed from respiratory isolation when the patient is on effective therapy, is clinically improving, and has three consecutive negative sputum smears for acid-fast bacilli on different days, or tuberculosis has been ruled out.

SUMMARY

The outcome for HIV-infected ICU patients has improved dramatically since the beginning of the AIDS epidemic. The spectrum of admitting diagnoses in the ICU has shifted to include more non–HIV-related conditions and diagnoses related to side effects of ART. Because many patients are admitted to the ICU as their first manifestation of HIV, clinicians also need to consider a diagnosis of HIV in any patient with a compatible clinical history. Issues regarding continuing or starting HIV therapy are complex, and although ART seems to have had some impact on the outcomes of critically ill HIV-infected patients, much remains to be discovered about its role in the ICU. Unfortunately, few data exist to guide clinicians in this difficult decision, and until future randomized, controlled studies examine this question, physicians must balance the risks and benefits for individual patients.

Key Points

- Intensive care survival of HIV-infected patients has improved over the course of the AIDS epidemic with survival rates that justify ICU care for most patients.
- Diagnoses such as BP, sepsis, and non–AIDS-related conditions have increased in frequency since the introduction of highly active ART.
- Definitive diagnosis of pneumonia is highly recommended in patients with HIV. Early bronchoscopy with BAL should be performed in patients with pneumonia who do not have an established microbiologic diagnosis.
- Despite decreasing numbers of cases of *Pneumocystis* pneumonia (PCP), PCP is still common in HIV-infected patients. It is associated with a high mortality, particularly in those patients with a pneumothorax while on mechanical ventilation. Many patients admitted with PCP are not aware of their HIV status.
- First-line treatment for PCP is intravenous trimethoprim/sulfamethoxazole, although many patients develop side effects. Corticosteroids should be given to those meeting oxygenation criteria.

- IRIS can result in pneumonitis, meningitis, hepatitis, and pericarditis. Respiratory failure is most often from tuberculosis and PCP. The syndrome occurs after starting ART and needs to be distinguished from acute OIs.
- Patients can develop fatal lactic acidosis as a result of antiretroviral medications. Treatment consists of drug discontinuation. Administration of riboflavin, thiamine, and L-carnitine might be helpful but is unproven.
- Coinfection with HIV and hepatitis C is increasingly common and can complicate ICU care.
- Administration of ART in the ICU is challenging because of the multiple side effects and drug interactions, difficulty with administration of oral medications, and the possibility of inducing viral resistance; however, use of these medications may be beneficial in certain patients.

References

1. Morris A, Masur H, Huang L. Current issues in critical care of the human immunodeficiency virus-infected patient. *Crit Care Med.* 2006;34(1):42–49.
2. Morris A, Creasman J, Turner J, et al. Intensive care of human immunodeficiency virus-infected patients during the era of highly active antiretroviral therapy. *Am J Respir Crit Care Med.* 2002;166(3):262–267.
3. Powell K, Davis JL, Morris AM, et al. Survival for patients with HIV admitted to the ICU continues to improve in the current era of combination antiretroviral therapy. *Chest.* 2009;135(1):11–17.
4. Akgun KM, Tate JP, Pisani M, et al. Medical ICU admission diagnoses and outcomes in human immunodeficiency virus-infected and virus-uninfected veterans in the combination antiretroviral era. *Crit Care Med.* 2013;41(6):1458–1467.
5. Barbier F, Roux A, Canet E, et al. Temporal trends in critical events complicating HIV infection: 1999–2010 multicentre cohort study in France. *Intensive Care Med.* 2014;40(12):1906–1915.
6. Nickas G, Wachter RM. Outcomes of intensive care for patients with human immunodeficiency virus infection. *Arch Intern Med.* 2000;160(4): 541–547.
7. Narasimhan M, Posner AJ, DePalo VA, et al. Intensive care in patients with HIV infection in the era of highly active antiretroviral therapy. *Chest.* 2004;125(5):1800–1804.
8. Vincent B, Timsit JF, Auburtin M, et al. Characteristics and outcomes of HIV-infected patients in the ICU: impact of the highly active antiretroviral treatment era. *Intensive Care Med.* 2004;30(5):859–866.
9. Casalino E, Wolff M, Ravaud P, et al. Impact of HAART advent on admission patterns and survival in HIV-infected patients admitted to an intensive care unit. *AIDS.* 2004;18(10):1429–1433.
10. Rosen MJ, Clayton K, Schneider RF, et al. Intensive care of patients with HIV infection: utilization, critical illnesses, and outcomes. Pulmonary Complications of HIV Infection Study Group. *Am J Respir Crit Care Med.* 1997;155(1):67–71.
11. Afessa B, Green B. Clinical course, prognostic factors, and outcome prediction for HIV patients in the ICU: the PIP (pulmonary complications, ICU support, and prognostic factors in hospitalized patients with HIV) study. *Chest.* 2000;118(1):138–145.
12. Khouli H, Afrasiabi A, Shibli M, et al. Outcome of critically ill human immunodeficiency virus-infected patients in the era of highly active antiretroviral therapy. *J Intensive Care Med.* 2005;20(6):327–333.
13. van Lelyveld SF, Wind CM, Mudrikova T, et al. Short- and long-term outcome of HIV-infected patients admitted to the intensive care unit. *Eur J Clin Microbiol Infect Dis.* 2011;30(9):1085–1093.
14. Rentsch C, Tate JP, Akgun KM, et al. Alcohol-related diagnoses and all-cause hospitalization among HIV-infected and uninfected patients: a longitudinal analysis of United States veterans from 1997 to 2011. *AIDS Behav.* 2016;20(3):555–645.
15. Akgun KM, Gordon K, Pisani M, et al. Risk factors for hospitalization and medical intensive care unit (MICU) admission among HIV-infected veterans. *J Acquir Immune Defic Syndr.* 2013;62(1):52–59.
16. Nuesch R, Geigy N, Schaedler E, Battegay M. Effect of highly active antiretroviral therapy on hospitalization characteristics of HIV-infected patients. *Eur J Clin Microbiol Infect Dis.* 2002;21(9):684–687.
17. Coquet I, Pavie J, Palmer P, et al. Survival trends in critically ill HIV-infected patients in the highly active antiretroviral therapy era. *Crit Care.* 2010;14(3):R107.
18. Gill JK, Greene L, Miller R, et al. ICU admission in patients infected with the human immunodeficiency virus: a multicentre survey. *Anaesthesia.* 1999;54(8):727–732.
19. Lazard T, Retel O, Guidet B, et al. AIDS in a medical intensive care unit: immediate prognosis and long-term survival. *JAMA.* 1996;276(15): 1240–1245.
20. Chiang HH, Hung CC, Lee CM, et al. Admissions to intensive care unit of HIV-infected patients in the era of highly active antiretroviral therapy: etiology and prognostic factors. *Crit Care.* 2011;15(4):R202.
21. Casalino E, Mendoza-Sassi G, Wolff M, et al. Predictors of short- and long-term survival in HIV-infected patients admitted to the ICU. *Chest.* 1998;113(2):421–429.
22. Palacios R, Hidalgo A, Reina C, et al. Effect of antiretroviral therapy on admissions of HIV-infected patients to an intensive care unit. *HIV Med.* 2006;7(3):193–196.
23. Barbier F, Coquet I, Legriel S, et al. Etiologies and outcome of acute respiratory failure in HIV-infected patients. *Intensive Care Med.* 2009;35(10): 1678–1686.
24. Medrano J, Alvaro-Meca A, Boyer A, et al. Mortality of patients infected with HIV in the intensive care unit (2005-2010): significant role of chronic hepatitis C and severe sepsis. *Crit Care.* 2014;18(4):475.
25. Mocroft A, Brettle R, Kirk O, et al. Changes in the cause of death among HIV positive subjects across Europe: results from the EuroSIDA study. *AIDS.* 2002;16(12):1663–1671.
26. Smit C, Geskus R, Walker S, et al. Effective therapy has altered the spectrum of cause-specific mortality following HIV seroconversion. *AIDS.* 2006;20(5):741–749.
27. Silva JM Jr., dos Santos Sde S. Sepsis in AIDS patients: clinical, etiological and inflammatory characteristics. *J Int AIDS Soc.* 2013;16:17344.
28. Rosenberg AL, Seneff MG, Atiyeh L, et al. The importance of bacterial sepsis in intensive care unit patients with acquired immunodeficiency syndrome: implications for future care in the age of increasing antiretroviral resistance. *Crit Care Med.* 2001;29(3):548–556.
29. Kohli R, Lo Y, Homel P, et al. Bacterial pneumonia, HIV therapy, and disease progression among HIV-infected women in the HIV epidemiologic research (HER) study. *Clin Infect Dis.* 2006;43(1):90–98.
30. Greenberg JA, Lennox JL, Martin GS. Outcomes for critically ill patients with HIV and severe sepsis in the era of highly active antiretroviral therapy. *J Crit Care.* 2012;27(1):51–57.
31. Morris A, Wachter RM, Luce J, et al. Improved survival with highly active antiretroviral therapy in HIV-infected patients with severe *Pneumocystis carinii* pneumonia. *AIDS.* 2003;17(1):73–80.
32. Miller RF, Allen E, Copas A, et al. Improved survival for HIV infected patients with severe *Pneumocystis jirovecii* pneumonia is independent of highly active antiretroviral therapy. *Thorax.* 2006;61(8):716–721.
33. Rivers E, Nguyen B, Havstad S, et al. Early goal-directed therapy in the treatment of severe sepsis and septic shock. *N Engl J Med.* 2001;345(19): 1368–1377.
34. Dellinger RP, Levy MM, Rhodes A, et al. Surviving sepsis campaign: international guidelines for management of severe sepsis and septic shock: 2012. *Crit Care Med.* 2013;41(2):580–637.
35. Hsue PY, Waters DD. What a cardiologist needs to know about patients with human immunodeficiency virus infection. *Circulation.* 2005;112(25): 3947–3957.
36. Marik PE, Kiminyo K, Zaloga GP. Adrenal insufficiency in critically ill patients with human immunodeficiency virus. *Crit Care Med.* 2002;30(6): 1267–1273.
37. Sarkar P, Rasheed HF. Clinical review: respiratory failure in HIV-infected patients—a changing picture. *Crit Care.* 2013;17(3):228.
38. Akgun KM, Huang L, Morris A, et al. Critical illness in HIV-infected patients in the era of combination antiretroviral therapy. *Proc Am Thorac Soc.* 2011;8(3):301–307.
39. Wachter RM, Luce JM, Turner J, et al. Intensive care of patients with the acquired immunodeficiency syndrome: outcome and changing patterns of utilization. *Am Rev Respir Dis.* 1986;134(5):891–896.
40. Wachter RM, Russi MB, Bloch DA, et al. *Pneumocystis carinii* pneumonia and respiratory failure in AIDS: improved outcomes and increased use of intensive care units. *Am Rev Respir Dis.* 1991;143(2):251–256.
41. Bozzette SA, Sattler FR, Chiu J, et al. A controlled trial of early adjunctive treatment with corticosteroids for *Pneumocystis carinii* pneumonia in the acquired immunodeficiency syndrome. California Collaborative Treatment Group. *N Engl J Med.* 1990;323(21):1451–1457.

42. el-Sadr W, Sidhu G, Diamond G, et al. High-dose corticosteroids as adjunct therapy in severe *Pneumocystis carinii* pneumonia. *AIDS Res.* 1986;2(4):349–355.
43. Bedos JP, Dumoulin JL, Gachot B, et al. *Pneumocystis carinii* pneumonia requiring intensive care management: survival and prognostic study in 110 patients with human immunodeficiency virus. *Crit Care Med.* 1999;27(6):1109–1115.
44. Antinori A, Maiuro G, Pallavicini F, et al. Prognostic factors of early fatal outcome and long-term survival in patients with *Pneumocystis carinii* pneumonia and acquired immunodeficiency syndrome. *Eur J Epidemiol.* 1993;9(2):183–189.
45. Forrest DM, Zala C, Djurdjev O, et al. Determinants of short- and long-term outcome in patients with respiratory failure caused by AIDS-related *Pneumocystis carinii* pneumonia. *Arch Intern Med.* 1999;159(7):741–747.
46. Phair J, Munoz A, Detels R, et al. The risk of *Pneumocystis carinii* pneumonia among men infected with human immunodeficiency virus type 1. Multicenter AIDS Cohort Study Group. *N Engl J Med.* 1990;322(3):161–165.
47. Stansell JD, Osmond DH, Charlebois E, et al. Predictors of *Pneumocystis carinii* pneumonia in HIV-infected persons. Pulmonary complications of HIV infection Study Group. *Am J Respir Crit Care Med.* 1997;155(1): 60–66.
48. Saah AJ, Hoover DR, Peng Y, et al. Predictors for failure of *Pneumocystis carinii* pneumonia prophylaxis. Multicenter AIDS Cohort Study. *JAMA.* 1995;273(15):1197–1202.
49. Kovacs JA, Hiemenz JW, Macher AM, et al. *Pneumocystis carinii* pneumonia: a comparison between patients with the acquired immunodeficiency syndrome and patients with other immunodeficiencies. *Ann Intern Med.* 1984;100(5):663–671.
50. Kales CP, Murren JR, Torres RA, Crocco JA. Early predictors of in-hospital mortality for *Pneumocystis carinii* pneumonia in the acquired immunodeficiency syndrome. *Arch Intern Med.* 1987;147(8):1413–1417.
51. Zaman MK, White DA. Serum lactate dehydrogenase levels and *Pneumocystis carinii* pneumonia: diagnostic and prognostic significance. *Am Rev Respir Dis.* 1988;137(4):796–800.
52. Garay SM, Greene J. Prognostic indicators in the initial presentation of *Pneumocystis carinii* pneumonia. *Chest.* 1989;95(4):769–772.
53. Sandhu JS, Goodman PC. Pulmonary cysts associated with *Pneumocystis carinii* pneumonia in patients with AIDS. *Radiology.* 1989;173(1):33–35.
54. Kennedy CA, Goetz MB. Atypical roentgenographic manifestations of *Pneumocystis carinii* pneumonia. *Arch Intern Med.* 1992;152(7):1390–1398.
55. Metersky ML, Aslenzadeh J, Stelmach P. A comparison of induced and expectorated sputum for the diagnosis of *Pneumocystis carinii* pneumonia. *Chest.* 1998;113(6):1555–1559.
56. Golden JA, Hollander H, Stulbarg MS, Gamsu G. Bronchoalveolar lavage as the exclusive diagnostic modality for *Pneumocystis carinii* pneumonia: a prospective study among patients with acquired immunodeficiency syndrome. *Chest.* 1986;90(1):18–22.
57. Cadranel J, Gillet-Juvin K, Antoine M, et al. Site-directed bronchoalveolar lavage and transbronchial biopsy in HIV-infected patients with pneumonia. *Am J Respir Crit Care Med.* 1995;152(3):1103–1106.
58. Kovacs JA, Ng VL, Masur H, et al. Diagnosis of *Pneumocystis carinii* pneumonia: improved detection in sputum with use of monoclonal antibodies. *N Engl J Med.* 1988;318(10):589–593.
59. Ng VL, Yajko DM, McPhaul LW, et al. Evaluation of an indirect fluorescent-antibody stain for detection of *Pneumocystis carinii* in respiratory specimens. *J Clin Microbiol.* 1990;28(5):975–979.
60. Sattler FR, Cowan R, Nielsen DM, Ruskin J. Trimethoprim-sulfamethoxazole compared with pentamidine for treatment of *Pneumocystis carinii* pneumonia in the acquired immunodeficiency syndrome: a prospective, noncrossover study. *Ann Intern Med.* 1988;109(4):280–287.
61. Klein NC, Duncanson FP, Lenox TH, et al. Trimethoprim-sulfamethoxazole versus pentamidine for *Pneumocystis carinii* pneumonia in AIDS patients: results of a large prospective randomized treatment trial. *AIDS.* 1992;6(3): 301–305.
62. Gordin FM, Simon GL, Wofsy CB, Mills J. Adverse reactions to trimethoprim-sulfamethoxazole in patients with the acquired immunodeficiency syndrome. *Ann Intern Med.* 1984;100(4):495–499.
63. Wofsy CB. Use of trimethoprim-sulfamethoxazole in the treatment of *Pneumocystis carinii* pneumonitis in patients with acquired immunodeficiency syndrome. *Rev Infect Dis.* 1987;9(Suppl 2):S184–S194.
64. Hardy WD, Feinberg J, Finkelstein DM, et al. A controlled trial of trimethoprim-sulfamethoxazole or aerosolized pentamidine for secondary prophylaxis of *Pneumocystis carinii* pneumonia in patients with the acquired immunodeficiency syndrome. AIDS Clinical Trials Group Protocol 021. *N Engl J Med.* 1992;327(26):1842–1848.
65. Masur H. Prevention and treatment of pneumocystis pneumonia. *N Engl J Med.* 1992;327(26):1853–1860.
66. Salmeron S, Petitpretz P, Katlama C, et al. Pentamidine and pancreatitis. *Ann Intern Med.* 1986;105(1):140–141.
67. Zuger A, Wolf BZ, el-Sadr W, Simberkoff MS, Rahal JJ. Pentamidine-associated fatal acute pancreatitis. *JAMA.* 1986;256(17):2383–2385.
68. Gonzalez A, Sager PT, Akil B, et al. Pentamidine-induced torsade de pointes. *Am Heart J.* 1991;122(5):1489–1492.
69. Quadrel MA, Atkin SH, Jaker MA. Delayed cardiotoxicity during treatment with intravenous pentamidine: two case reports and a review of the literature. *Am Heart J.* 1992;123(5):1377–1379.
70. MacFadden DK, Edelson JD, Hyland RH, et al. Corticosteroids as adjunctive therapy in treatment of *Pneumocystis carinii* pneumonia in patients with acquired immunodeficiency syndrome. *Lancet.* 1987;1(8548):1477–1479.
71. Walmsley S, Salit IE, Brunton J. The possible role of corticosteroid therapy for pneumocystis pneumonia in the acquired immune deficiency syndrome (AIDS). *J Acquir Immune Defic Syndr.* 1988;1(4):354–360.
72. Briel M, Boscacci R, Furrer H, Bucher HC. Adjunctive corticosteroids for *Pneumocystis jiroveci* pneumonia in patients with HIV infection: a meta-analysis of randomised controlled trials. *BMC Infect Dis.* 2005;5:101.
73. Briel M, Bucher HC, Boscacci R, Furrer H. Adjunctive corticosteroids for *Pneumocystis jiroveci* pneumonia in patients with HIV-infection. *Cochrane Database Syst Rev.* 2006(3):CD006150.
74. Shelhamer JH, Ognibene FP, Macher AM, et al. Persistence of *Pneumocystis carinii* in lung tissue of acquired immunodeficiency syndrome patients treated for pneumocystis pneumonia. *Am Rev Respir Dis.* 1984;130(6): 1161–1165.
75. Lane BR, Ast JC, Hossler PA, et al. Dihydropteroate synthase polymorphisms in *Pneumocystis carinii. J Infect Dis.* 1997;175(2):482–485.
76. Ma L, Borio L, Masur H, Kovacs JA. *Pneumocystis carinii* dihydropteroate synthase but not dihydrofolate reductase gene mutations correlate with prior trimethoprim-sulfamethoxazole or dapsone use. *J Infect Dis.* 1999;180(6):1969–1978.
77. Huang L, Crothers K, Atzori C, et al. Dihydropteroate synthase gene mutations in *Pneumocystis* and sulfa resistance. *Emerg Infect Dis.* 2004;10(10):1721–1728.
78. Helweg-Larsen J, Benfield TL, et al. Effects of mutations in *Pneumocystis carinii* dihydropteroate synthase gene on outcome of AIDS-associated *P. carinii* pneumonia. *Lancet.* 1999;354(9187):1347–1351.
79. Kazanjian P, Armstrong W, Hossler PA, et al. *Pneumocystis carinii* mutations are associated with duration of sulfa or sulfone prophylaxis exposure in AIDS patients. *J Infect Dis.* 2000;182(2):551–557.
80. Takahashi T, Hosoya N, Endo T, et al. Relationship between mutations in dihydropteroate synthase of *Pneumocystis carinii* f. sp. hominis isolates in Japan and resistance to sulfonamide therapy. *J Clin Microbiol.* 2000;38(9):3161–3164.
81. Crothers K, Beard CB, Turner J, et al. Severity and outcome of HIV-associated *Pneumocystis pneumonia* containing *Pneumocystis jirovecii* dihydropteroate synthase gene mutations. *AIDS.* 2005;19(8):801–805.
82. Navin TR, Beard CB, Huang L, et al. Effect of mutations in *Pneumocystis carinii* dihydropteroate synthase gene on outcome of P carinii pneumonia in patients with HIV-1: a prospective study. *Lancet.* 2001; 358(9281):545–549.
83. Ventilation with lower tidal volumes as compared with traditional tidal volumes for acute lung injury and the acute respiratory distress syndrome. The Acute Respiratory Distress Syndrome Network. *N Engl J Med.* 2000; 342(18):1301–1308.
84. Confalonieri M, Calderini E, Terraciano S, et al. Noninvasive ventilation for treating acute respiratory failure in AIDS patients with *Pneumocystis carinii* pneumonia. *Intensive Care Med.* 2002;28(9):1233–1238.
85. Frat JP, Thille AW, Mercat A, et al. High-flow oxygen through nasal cannula in acute hypoxemic respiratory failure. *N Engl J Med.* 2015;372(23): 2185–2196.
86. Sogaard OS, Lohse N, Gerstoft J, et al. Hospitalization for pneumonia among individuals with and without HIV infection, 1995–2007: a Danish population-based, nationwide cohort study. *Clin Infect Dis.* 2008;47(10):1345–1353.
87. Segal LN, Methe BA, Nolan A, et al. HIV-1 and bacterial pneumonia in the era of antiretroviral therapy. *Proc Am Thorac Soc.* 2011;8(3):282–287.
88. Alves C, Nicolas JM, Miro JM, et al. Reappraisal of the aetiology and prognostic factors of severe acute respiratory failure in HIV patients. *Eur Respir J.* 2001;17(1):87–93.
89. Puro V, Serraino D, Piselli P, et al. The epidemiology of recurrent bacterial pneumonia in people with AIDS in Europe. *Epidemiol Infect.* 2005; 133(2):237–243.

90. Franzetti F, Grassini A, Piazza M, et al. Nosocomial bacterial pneumonia in HIV-infected patients: risk factors for adverse outcome and implications for rational empiric antibiotic therapy. *Infection*. 2006;34(1):9–16.
91. Hirschtick RE, Glassroth J, Jordan MC, et al. Bacterial pneumonia in persons infected with the human immunodeficiency virus: pulmonary complications of HIV Infection Study Group. *N Engl J Med*. 1995;333(13):845–851.
92. Crothers K, Griffith TA, McGinnis KA, et al. The impact of cigarette smoking on mortality, quality of life, and comorbid illness among HIV-positive veterans. *J Gen Intern Med*. 2005;20(12):1142–1145.
93. Le Moing V, Rabaud C, Journot V, et al. Incidence and risk factors of bacterial pneumonia requiring hospitalization in HIV-infected patients started on a protease inhibitor-containing regimen. *HIV Med*. 2006;7(4):261–267.
94. Sogaard OS, Lohse N, Gerstoft J, et al. Mortality after hospitalization for pneumonia among individuals with HIV, 1995–2008: a Danish cohort study. *PLoS One*. 2009;4(9):e7022.
95. Cordero E, Pachon J, Rivero A, et al. Community-acquired bacterial pneumonia in human immunodeficiency virus-infected patients: validation of severity criteria. The Grupo Andaluz para el Estudio de las Enfermedades Infecciosas. *Am J Respir Crit Care Med*. 2000;162(6):2063–2068.
96. Bedos JP, Chevret S, Chastang C, et al. Epidemiological features of and risk factors for infection by *Streptococcus pneumoniae* strains with diminished susceptibility to penicillin: findings of a French survey. *Clin Infect Dis*. 1996;22(1):63–72.
97. Meynard JL, Barbut F, Blum L, et al. Risk factors for isolation of *Streptococcus pneumoniae* with decreased susceptibility to penicillin G from patients infected with human immunodeficiency virus. *Clin Infect Dis*. 1996;22(3):437–440.
98. Madhi SA, Petersen K, Madhi A, et al. Increased disease burden and antibiotic resistance of bacteria causing severe community-acquired lower respiratory tract infections in human immunodeficiency virus type 1-infected children. *Clin Infect Dis*. 2000;31(1):170–176.
99. Shankar EM, Kumarasamy N, Balakrishnan P, et al. Detection of pulmonary *Mycoplasma pneumoniae* infections in HIV-infected subjects using culture and serology. *Int J Infect Dis*. 2007;11(3):232–238.
100. Afessa B, Green B. Bacterial pneumonia in hospitalized patients with HIV infection: the Pulmonary Complications, ICU Support, and Prognostic Factors of Hospitalized Patients with HIV (PIP) Study. *Chest*. 2000;117(4):1017–1022.
101. American Thoracic Society; Infectious Diseases Society of America. Guidelines for the management of adults with hospital-acquired, ventilator-associated, and healthcare-associated pneumonia. *Am J Respir Crit Care Med*. 2005;171(4):388–416.
102. Mandell LA, Wunderink RG, Anzueto A, et al. Infectious Diseases Society of America/American Thoracic Society consensus guidelines on the management of community-acquired pneumonia in adults. *Clin Infect Dis*. 2007;44(Suppl 2):S27–S72.
103. Guidelines for the prevention and treatment of opportunistic infections in HIV-infected adults and adolescents. Recommendations from the Centers for Disease Control and Prevention, the National Institutes of Health, and the HIV Medicine Association of the Infectious Diseases Society of America. AIDSinfo website. http://aidsinfo.nih.gov/contentfiles/lvguidelines/adult_oi.pdf. Accessed June 26, 2013.
104. Crothers K, Huang L. Pulmonary complications of immune reconstitution inflammatory syndromes in HIV-infected patients. *Respirology*. 2009;14(4):486–494.
105. Chang CC, Sheikh V, Sereti I, French MA. Immune reconstitution disorders in patients with HIV infection: from pathogenesis to prevention and treatment. *Curr HIV/AIDS Rep*. 2014;11(3):223–232.
106. Manzardo C, Guardo AC, Letang E, et al. Opportunistic infections and immune reconstitution inflammatory syndrome in HIV-1-infected adults in the combined antiretroviral therapy era: a comprehensive review. *Expert Rev Anti Infect Ther*. 2015;13(6):751–767.
107. Shelburne SA III, Hamill RJ, Rodriguez-Barradas MC, et al. Immune reconstitution inflammatory syndrome: emergence of a unique syndrome during highly active antiretroviral therapy. *Medicine (Baltimore)*. 2002;81(3):213–227.
108. Muller M, Wandel S, Colebunders R, et al. Immune reconstitution inflammatory syndrome in patients starting antiretroviral therapy for HIV infection: a systematic review and meta-analysis. *Lancet Infect Dis*. 2010;10(4):251–261.
109. Wislez M, Bergot E, Antoine M, et al. Acute respiratory failure following HAART introduction in patients treated for *Pneumocystis carinii* pneumonia. *Am J Respir Crit Care Med*. 2001;164(5):847–851.
110. Dean GL, Williams DI, Churchill DR, Fisher MJ. Transient clinical deterioration in HIV patients with *Pneumocystis carinii* pneumonia after starting highly active antiretroviral therapy: another case of immune restoration inflammatory syndrome. *Am J Respir Crit Care Med*. 2002;165(12):1670; author reply.
111. Palella F Jr Baker RK, Moorman AC, et al. Mortality in the highly active antiretroviral therapy era: changing causes of death and disease in the HIV outpatient study. *J Acquir Immune Defic Syndr*. 2006;43(1):27–34.
112. Cribbs SK, Tse C, Andrews J, et al. Characteristics and outcomes of HIV-infected patients with severe sepsis: continued risk in the post-highly active antiretroviral therapy era. *Crit Care Med*. 2015;43(8):1638–1645.
113. Japiassu AM, Amancio RT, Mesquita EC, et al. Sepsis is a major determinant of outcome in critically ill HIV/AIDS patients. *Crit Care*. 2010;14(4):R152.
114. Rosen MJ, Narasimhan M. Critical care of immunocompromised patients: human immunodeficiency virus. *Crit Care Med*. 2006;34(9 Suppl):S245–S250.
115. Jacob ST, Moore CC, Banura P, et al. Severe sepsis in two Ugandan hospitals: a prospective observational study of management and outcomes in a predominantly HIV-1 infected population. *PLoS One*. 2009;4(11):e7782.
116. Jacob ST, Pavlinac PB, Nakiyingi L, et al. *Mycobacterium tuberculosis* bacteremia in a cohort of HIV-infected patients hospitalized with severe sepsis in Uganda–high frequency, low clinical suspicion [corrected] and derivation of a clinical prediction score. *PLoS One*. 2013;8(8):e70305.
117. Bedos JP, Chastang C, Lucet JC, et al. Early predictors of outcome for HIV patients with neurological failure. *JAMA*. 1995;273(1):35–40.
118. Subsai K, Kanoksri S, Siwaporn C, et al. Neurological complications in AIDS patients receiving HAART: a 2-year retrospective study. *Eur J Neurol*. 2006;13(3):233–239.
119. Sonneville R, Ferrand H, Tubach F, et al. Neurological complications of HIV infection in critically ill patients: clinical features and outcomes. *J Infect*. 2011;62(4):301–308.
120. George BP, Schneider EB, Venkatesan A. Encephalitis hospitalization rates and inpatient mortality in the United States, 2000–2010. *PLoS One*. 2014;9(9):e104169.
121. Chalasani N, Wilcox CM. Gastrointestinal hemorrhage in patients with AIDS. *AIDS Patient Care STDS*. 1999;13(6):343–346.
122. Lew E, Dieterich D, Poles M, Scholes J. Gastrointestinal emergencies in the patient with AIDS. *Crit Care Clin*. 1995;11(2):531–560.
123. Betz ME, Gebo KA, Barber E, et al. Patterns of diagnoses in hospital admissions in a multistate cohort of HIV-positive adults in 2001. *Med Care*. 2005;43(9 Suppl):III3–14.
124. Bica I, McGovern B, Dhar R, et al. Increasing mortality due to end-stage liver disease in patients with human immunodeficiency virus infection. *Clin Infect Dis*. 2001;32(3):492–497.
125. Monga HK, Rodriguez-Barradas MC, Breaux K, et al. Hepatitis C virus infection-related morbidity and mortality among patients with human immunodeficiency virus infection. *Clin Infect Dis*. 2001;33(2):240–247.
126. Sulkowski MS, Thomas DL. Hepatitis C in the HIV-infected patient. *Clin Liver Dis*. 2003;7(1):179–194.
127. Antiretroviral Therapy Cohort Collaboration. Causes of death in HIV-1–infected patients treated with antiretroviral therapy, 1996–2006: collaborative analysis of 13 HIV cohort studies. *Clin Infect Dis*. 2010;50(10):1387–1396.
128. Greub G, Ledergerber B, Battegay M, et al. Clinical progression, survival, and immune recovery during antiretroviral therapy in patients with HIV-1 and hepatitis C virus coinfection. The Swiss HIV Cohort Study. *Lancet*. 2000;356(9244):1800–1805.
129. Sansone GR, Frengley JD. Impact of HAART on causes of death of persons with late-stage AIDS. *J Urban Health*. 2000;77(2):166–175.
130. Dodig M, Tavill AS. Hepatitis C and human immunodeficiency virus coinfections. *J Clin Gastroenterol*. 2001;33(5):367–374.
131. Chen TY, Ding EL, Seage GR III, Kim AY. Meta-analysis: increased mortality associated with hepatitis C in HIV-infected persons is unrelated to HIV disease progression. *Clin Infect Dis*. 2009;49(10):1605–1615.
132. Hernando V, Perez-Cachafeiro S, Lewden C, et al. All-cause and liver-related mortality in HIV positive subjects compared to the general population: differences by HCV co-infection. *J Hepatol*. 2012;57(4):743–751.
133. Wyatt CM, Arons RR, Klotman PE, Klotman ME. Acute renal failure in hospitalized patients with HIV: risk factors and impact on in-hospital mortality. *AIDS*. 2006;20(4):561–565.
134. Wyatt CM, Malvestutto C, Coca SG, et al. The impact of hepatitis C virus coinfection on HIV-related kidney disease: a systematic review and meta-analysis. *AIDS*. 2008;22(14):1799 1–807.
135. Wilcox CM. Serious gastrointestinal disorders associated with human immunodeficiency virus infection. *Crit Care Clin*. 1993;9(1):73–88.
136. Sackoff JE, Hanna DB, Pfeiffer MR, Torian LV. Causes of death among persons with AIDS in the era of highly active antiretroviral therapy: New York City. *Ann Intern Med*. 2006;145(6):397–406.

137. Freiberg MS, Chang CC, Kuller LH, et al. HIV infection and the risk of acute myocardial infarction. *JAMA Intern Med.* 2013;173(8):614–622.
138. Islam FM, Wu J, Jansson J, Wilson DP. Relative risk of cardiovascular disease among people living with HIV: a systematic review and meta-analysis. *HIV Med.* 2012;13(8):453–468.
139. Grunfeld C, Kotler DP, Hamadeh R, et al. Hypertriglyceridemia in the acquired immunodeficiency syndrome. *Am J Med.* 1989;86(1):27–31.
140. Hommes MJ, Romijn JA, Endert E, et al. Insulin sensitivity and insulin clearance in human immunodeficiency virus-infected men. *Metabolism.* 1991;40(6):651–656.
141. Carr A, Samaras K, Burton S, et al. A syndrome of peripheral lipodystrophy, hyperlipidaemia and insulin resistance in patients receiving HIV protease inhibitors. *AIDS.* 1998;12(7):F51–F58.
142. Friis-Moller N, Sabin CA, Weber R, et al. Combination antiretroviral therapy and the risk of myocardial infarction. *N Engl J Med.* 2003; 349(21):1993–2003.
143. Deeks SG, Tracy R, Douek DC. Systemic effects of inflammation on health during chronic HIV infection. *Immunity.* 2013;39(4):633–645.
144. Remick J, Georgiopoulou V, Marti C, et al. Heart failure in patients with human immunodeficiency virus infection: epidemiology, pathophysiology, treatment, and future research. *Circulation.* 2014;129(17):1781–1789.
145. Gupta SK, Eustace JA, Winston JA, et al. Guidelines for the management of chronic kidney disease in HIV-infected patients: recommendations of the HIV Medicine Association of the Infectious Diseases Society of America. *Clin Infect Dis.* 2005;40(11):1559–1585.
146. Berliner AR, Fine DM, Lucas GM, et al. Observations on a cohort of HIV-infected patients undergoing native renal biopsy. *Am J Nephrol.* 2008; 28(3):478–486.
147. Wyatt CM. The kidney in HIV infection: beyond HIV-associated nephropathy. *Top Antivir Med.* 2012;20(3):106–110.
148. Abraham AG, Althoff KN, Jing Y, et al. End-stage renal disease among HIV-infected adults in North America. *Clin Infect Dis.* 2015;60(6):941–949.
149. Randall D, Brima N, Walker D, et al. Acute kidney injury among HIV-infected patients admitted to the intensive care unit. *Int J STD AIDS.* 2015;26(13):915–921.
150. Agarwal A, Soni A, Ciechanowsky M, et al. Hyponatremia in patients with the acquired immunodeficiency syndrome. *Nephron.* 1989;53(4):317–321.
151. Cusano AJ, Thies HL, Siegal FP, et al. Hyponatremia in patients with acquired immune deficiency syndrome. *J Acquir Immune Defic Syndr.* 1990;3(10):949–953.
152. Vitting KE, Gardenswartz MH, Zabetakis PM, et al. Frequency of hyponatremia and nonosmolar vasopressin release in the acquired immunodeficiency syndrome. *JAMA.* 1990;263(7):973–978.
153. Guarda LA, Luna MA, Smith JL Jr, et al. Acquired immune deficiency syndrome: postmortem findings. *Am J Clin Pathol.* 1984;81(5):549–557.
154. Klatt EC, Shibata D. Cytomegalovirus infection in the acquired immunodeficiency syndrome: clinical and autopsy findings. *Arch Pathol Lab Med.* 1988;112(5):540–544.
155. Lo J, Grinspoon SK. Adrenal function in HIV infection. *Curr Opin Endocrinol Diabetes Obes.* 2010;17(3):205–209.
156. Kibirige D, Ssekitoleko R. Endocrine and metabolic abnormalities among HIV-infected patients: a current review. *Int J STD AIDS.* 2013;24(8):603–611.
157. Grinspoon SK, Bilezikian JP. HIV disease and the endocrine system. *N Engl J Med.* 1992;327(19):1360–1365.
158. Chattha G, Arieff AI, Cummings C, Tierney LM Jr. Lactic acidosis complicating the acquired immunodeficiency syndrome. *Ann Intern Med.* 1993;118(1):37–39.
159. Freiman JP, Helfert KE, Hamrell MR, Stein DS. Hepatomegaly with severe steatosis in HIV-seropositive patients. *AIDS.* 1993;7(3):379–385.
160. Lonergan JT, Behling C, Pfander H, et al. Hyperlactatemia and hepatic abnormalities in 10 human immunodeficiency virus-infected patients receiving nucleoside analogue combination regimens. *Clin Infect Dis.* 2000;31(1):162–166.
161. Margolis AM, Heverling H, Pham PA, Stolbach A. A review of the toxicity of HIV medications. *J Med Toxicol.* 2014;10(1):26–39.
162. Tan DH, Walmsley SL. Management of persons infected with human immunodeficiency virus requiring admission to the intensive care unit. *Crit Care Clin.* 2013;29(3):603–620.
163. Bonnet F, Bonarek M, Morlat P, et al. Risk factors for lactic acidosis in HIV-infected patients treated with nucleoside reverse-transcriptase inhibitors: a case-control study. *Clin Infect Dis.* 2003;36(10):1324–1328.
164. Fouty B, Frerman F, Reves R. Riboflavin to treat nucleoside analogue-induced lactic acidosis. *Lancet.* 1998;352(9124):291–292.
165. Luzzati R, Del Bravo P, Di Perri G, et al. Riboflavin and severe lactic acidosis. *Lancet.* 1999;353(9156):901–902.
166. Brinkman K, Vrouenraets S, Kauffmann R, et al. Treatment of nucleoside reverse transcriptase inhibitor-induced lactic acidosis. *AIDS.* 2000;14(17): 2801–2802.
167. Claessens YE, Cariou A, Monchi M, et al. Detecting life-threatening lactic acidosis related to nucleoside-analog treatment of human immunodeficiency virus-infected patients, and treatment with L-carnitine. *Crit Care Med.* 2003;31(4):1042–1047.
168. Hot A, Schmulewitz L, Viard JP, Lortholary O. Fever of unknown origin in HIV/AIDS patients. *Infect Dis Clin North Am.* 2007;21(4):1013–1032.
169. Babu C, McQuillan O, Kingston M. Management of pyrexia of unknown origin in HIV-positive patients. *Int J STD AIDS.* 2009;20(6):369–372.
170. Lozano F, Torre-Cisneros J, Santos J, et al. Impact of highly active antiretroviral therapy on fever of unknown origin in HIV-infected patients. *Eur J Clin Microbiol Infect Dis.* 2002;21(2):137–139.
171. Davison JM, Subramaniam RM, Surasi DS, et al. FDG PET/CT in patients with HIV. *AJR Am J Roentgenol.* 2011;197(2):284–294.
172. Hayakawa K, Ramasamy B, Chandrasekar PH. Fever of unknown origin: an evidence-based review. *Am J Med Sci.* 2012;344(4):307–316.
173. Martin C, Castaigne C, Tondeur M, et al. Role and interpretation of fluorodeoxyglucose-positron emission tomography/computed tomography in HIV-infected patients with fever of unknown origin: a prospective study. *HIV Med.* 2013;14(8):455–462.
174. Quesada AE, Tholpady A, Wanger A, et al. Utility of bone marrow examination for workup of fever of unknown origin in patients with HIV/AIDS. *J Clin Pathol.* 2015;68(3):241–245.
175. Guidelines for the use of antiretroviral agents in HIV-1-infected adults and adolescents. AIDSinfo website. https://aidsinfo.nih.gov/contentfiles/lvguidelines/adultandadolescentgl.pdf. Accessed June 15, 2015.
176. Huang L, Quartin A, Jones D, Havlir DV. Intensive care of patients with HIV infection. *N Engl J Med.* 2006;355(2):173–181.
177. Heyland DK, Tougas G, King D, Cook DJ. Impaired gastric emptying in mechanically ventilated, critically ill patients. *Intensive Care Med.* 1996; 22(12):1339–1344.
178. Tarling MM, Toner CC, Withington PS, et al. A model of gastric emptying using paracetamol absorption in intensive care patients. *Intensive Care Med.* 1997;23(3):256–260.
179. Mimoz O, Binter V, Jacolot A, et al. Pharmacokinetics and absolute bioavailability of ciprofloxacin administered through a nasogastric tube with continuous enteral feeding to critically ill patients. *Intensive Care Med.* 1998;24(10):1047–1051.
180. Dorffler-Melly J, de Jonge E, Pont AC, et al. Bioavailability of subcutaneous low-molecular-weight heparin to patients on vasopressors. *Lancet.* 2002;359(9309):849–850.
181. Priglinger U, Delle Karth G, Geppert A, et al. Prophylactic anticoagulation with enoxaparin: Is the subcutaneous route appropriate in the critically ill? *Crit Care Med.* 2003;31(5):1405–1409.
182. Townsend PL, Fink MP, Stein KL, Murphy SG. Aminoglycoside pharmacokinetics: dosage requirements and nephrotoxicity in trauma patients. *Crit Care Med.* 1989;17(2):154–157.
183. Kuhar DT, Henderson DK, Struble KA, et al. Updated US Public Health Service guidelines for the management of occupational exposures to human immunodeficiency virus and recommendations for postexposure prophylaxis. *Infect Control Hosp Epidemiol.* 2013;34(9):875–892.
184. Kaplan JE, Dominguez K, Jobarteh K, Spira TJ. Postexposure prophylaxis against human immunodeficiency virus (HIV): new guidelines from the WHO: a perspective. *Clin Infect Dis.* 2015;60(Suppl 3):S196–S199.
185. Rebmann T. Management of patients infected with airborne-spread diseases: an algorithm for infection control professionals. *Am J Infect Control.* 2005;33(10):571–579.

CHAPTER

92

Unusual Infections

SANKAR SWAMINATHAN

INTRODUCTION

This chapter describes the epidemiology, clinical presentation, diagnosis, therapy, and prevention of several relatively unusual infections. Although the incidence of these infections in the United States is low, they have the potential to cause rapidly progressive disease, and to present unique problems in management and infection control in the critical care setting. Since rapid treatment is essential in many of these infections, prompt diagnosis is also important. Additionally, many of the organisms causing these infectious diseases have gained new relevance as potential biologic warfare agents. The epidemiology, clinical presentation, and management of infections resulting from an intentional release of micro-organisms may differ significantly from disease resulting from traditional modes of spread. In addition to an intentional bioterrorist attack, large social disruptions that affect housing, public hygiene, and mass migration have the potential to allow epidemic transmission of some of these agents. Outbreaks of diseases previously thought to be under control have occurred as a result of natural disasters and human activities, both in the United States and abroad. Climate change has led to changes in disease prevalence in many parts of the globe due to changing habitats of disease vectors. Finally, globalization, leading to increasing travel of humans, transport of animals and plant materials, increases the likelihood that hitherto unusual infections will become more prevalent in the United States. Recognition of such unusual infections will require familiarity with their epidemiology and clinical presentation and will allow diagnosis and treatment in a timely fashion.

TULAREMIA

Tularemia is a multisystem zoonotic infection caused by a gram-negative coccobacillus, *Francisella tularensis*. Tularemia, named after Tulare County, California, where the disease was first characterized in ground squirrels (1), has been recognized since the 1800s and is primarily transmitted through contact with infected animals, contaminated food and water, or arthropod bites (2). Tularemia has been listed as a Tier 1 agent (3). The Department of Health and Human Services/Centers for Disease Control and Prevention (HHS/CDC) has designated those select agents and toxins that present the greatest risk of deliberate misuse with the most significant potential for mass casualties or devastating effects to the economy, critical infrastructure; or public confidence as Tier 1 agents. High-priority agents include organisms that pose a risk to national security because they can be easily disseminated or transmitted from person to person, result in high mortality rates and have the potential for major public health impact, might cause public panic and social disruption and require special action for public health preparedness (4).

Epidemiology

The incidence of tularemia in the United States has declined since the 1950s, and is currently less than 200 cases per year (5–7). Cases occur throughout the continental United States and Alaska in small sporadic clusters. Most cases are centered around Missouri, Kansas, Oklahoma, and Arkansas. Incidence is also high in other Western states such as South Dakota and Wyoming. Tularemia primarily occurs during the summer months, most likely due to the increased exposure to biting arthropods. Cases also occur during the fall and winter and are linked to hunting and handling infected animals. Perhaps because of a greater likelihood of exposure to animals and arthropods, there is a 3 to 1 preponderance of male to female cases. Most recent cases in the United States have been in young adults, although a significant percentage of cases occurs among children below the age of 14 (8). Inhalational exposures have occurred in Martha's Vineyard in Massachusetts and were associated with mowing grass and cutting brush (9).

In the United States, ticks and biting flies are the most important arthropod vectors. Major animal reservoirs are lagomorphs (rabbits and hares), and rodents including prairie dogs, squirrels, and rats. Mosquitoes were implicated as a primary vector in Scandinavia in one large outbreak (10). Direct contact with infected animals is another significant mode of transmission (11). Hunting, trapping, butchering animal carcasses, and handling meat are all risk factors for tularemia. Contamination of food and water by rodents and other carriers has also been linked to human infection. The organism survives well in cold, moist conditions and can withstand freezing. Finally, cats and other carnivores may transiently carry organisms in their mouths or claws and thereby transmit infection to humans (12). Pets may also increase the likelihood of tick-borne transmission to humans. Inhalational exposure may occur in the laboratory or as the consequence of a deliberate release of weaponized *Francisella* cultures. Human-to-human transmission of tularemia is not known to occur.

Clinical Presentation

Tularemia has been classically described as presenting in one of six syndromes: ulceroglandular, oculoglandular, glandular, pharyngeal, typhoidal, and pneumonic (13). However, it is clear that individual patients may have symptoms of several of these types simultaneously. After initial entry into the host, either through cutaneous inoculation, ingestion, or inhalation, *Francisella* organisms multiply at the site of infection (14); a vigorous inflammatory response ensues, leading to subsequent necrosis. The organism multiplies within macrophages and travels to regional lymph nodes, kidney, liver, lung, and spleen (15). The meninges and pericardium are occasionally involved secondarily in untreated tularemia. Inhalation or cutaneous inoculation of 10 to 50 organisms is sufficient for infection

(16,17). Symptoms usually begin 3 to 5 days after infection, although longer incubation periods are possible (18).

Differences in clinical presentation may be partly attributable to the type and route of infection. Thus tick-borne infection is more likely to result in skin lesions on the head and neck, trunk, and perineum, whereas animal-associated infections more commonly result in upper extremity lesions (19). Ingestion of contaminated water or food is more likely to cause pharyngeal infection. Inoculation into mucous membranes of the eye results in the oculoglandular syndrome, an ocular lesion with local lymphadenopathy. Inhalation of the organism leads to the pneumonic form of tularemia, although other forms of tularemia can also cause prominent pulmonary involvement through hematogenous dissemination. A typhoidal form of tularemia occurs in less than 30% of cases, in which there are no characteristic localized mucocutaneous or glandular signs or symptoms. The distinction between typhoidal and nontyphoidal infections appears to reflect differences in the host response. In nontyphoidal forms, there is a vigorous inflammatory reaction and the prognosis is good in comparison to typhoidal infection, which has a higher mortality and in which pneumonia is more common (19). Certain strains of *F. tularensis* may be associated with higher mortality, up to 24%, but it is 2% overall (20).

In general, the onset of systemic symptoms in tularemia is abrupt, and includes fever, headache, myalgia, coryza, cough, malaise, and chest pain or tightness. In mucocutaneous infection, the presenting complaint is usually painful lymphadenopathy, which may precede or follow the skin lesion; in the purely glandular form, there is no apparent skin lesion. Skin lesions usually begin as erythematous, painful papules which progress to necrotic ulcers that are slow to heal. Enlarged lymph nodes are also slow to resolve and may suppurate. In ocular infection, a painful conjunctivitis occurs. Pharyngeal tularemia presents as an exudative pharyngitis with adenopathy that is unresponsive to standard therapy. Tularemic pneumonia is characterized by fever, cough, and pleuritic pain, but sputum production and hemoptysis are unusual. A relative bradycardia, with a normal pulse despite an elevated temperature is common (40%) in tularemia, and may be a useful diagnostic finding (19). Chest x-ray findings include hilar adenopathy, patchy or less commonly, lobar infiltrates, and pleural effusions.

Although there has not been a documented biologic attack with weaponized tularemia, several probable aspects of such an occurrence are worth noting to allow early recognition and management. If there were an aerosolized release of organisms, cases are likely to be pneumonic, although aerosolized tularemia would also be likely to result in ocular and cutaneous forms (2). Occurrence of tularemia in urban settings and among healthy individuals should also prompt suspicion of a biologic attack. Onset of symptoms is expected to be rapid, and as described above, closely resemble the acute onset of influenza. The differential diagnosis of pneumonia due to an aerosolized biologic weapon attack would include anthrax, plague, and Q fever. Important distinguishing characteristics between these etiologies would include a more rapid and fulminant course in both anthrax and plague. In addition, pneumonic anthrax would not be expected to cause bronchopneumonia, but would result in mediastinal widening. Pneumonic plague results in frankly purulent sputum with hemoptysis and rapid progression. Laboratory testing is important in distinguishing between these various entities (see below), but initial empiric treatment will, by necessity, require diagnosis based primarily on clinical and epidemiologic data.

Diagnosis

Cultures for *F. tularensis* require incubation on special supportive media. The laboratory must be notified in advance if tularemia is suspected, both to perform appropriate testing as well as to institute protective measures to prevent infection of laboratory workers. Cultures of pharyngeal washings, sputum, and fasting gastric aspirates are most likely to yield positive results whereas blood samples are usually negative (21). Direct fluorescent staining of specimens or PCR can be performed by specialized laboratories for relatively rapid diagnosis. Serology is positive approximately 10 days after infection. While serology is not helpful for diagnosis of acute infection, it is useful for confirmation of suspected cases. It is important to promptly contact the hospital epidemiologist or infection control practitioner, and the local health department in cases of tularemia to aid in management and diagnosis of suspected outbreaks. It is also imperative to notify the microbiology laboratory if tularemia is suspected to prevent exposure and infection of laboratory personnel.

Treatment

The first-line treatment for tularemia is streptomycin, with gentamicin as an acceptable alternative, although experience with gentamicin is relatively sparse. Quinolone therapy has been reported to be successful although failures have also been reported. Relapse despite appropriate therapy has been noted in 38.6% of patients (22). Treatment regimens for most of the select agents have been devised for either a contained casualty setting or a mass casualty setting (Table 92.1). The recommendations for the latter situation take into account the likelihood that services may be limited and parenteral or inpatient therapy may not be possible. The first-line treatment of tularemia in a contained casualty setting is an aminoglycoside, either streptomycin or gentamicin (2,23). Alternatives are doxycycline, chloramphenicol, or ciprofloxacin, given intravenously. Treatment with aminoglycosides or ciprofloxacin should be given for a minimum of 10 days, and with doxycycline or chloramphenicol for 14 to 21 days. In a mass casualty setting or for postexposure prophylaxis, oral doxycycline or ciprofloxacin for 14 days is recommended. As is the case with other organisms described later in this chapter, several potentially toxic antibiotics that are not routinely given to children or pregnant women are included in the recommended treatment regimens. For example, the use of tetracyclines and quinolones carries the risk of potential side effects in pregnant women and children. Nevertheless, given the high mortality of tularemia, these agents are recommended as acceptable alternatives if aminoglycosides cannot be administered or are not available. The CDC website should be consulted for the most current details regarding the CDC recommendations for treatment as well as more detailed information regarding usage in renal failure and in special situations (23).

PLAGUE

Plague, caused by the gram-negative bacillus *Yersinia pestis*, is one of the oldest and most feared illnesses known to man.

TABLE 92.1 Treatment Recommendations for Tularemia

Contained Casualty Setting
Adults
Preferred choices
Streptomycin, 1 g IM twice daily
Gentamicin, 5 mg/kg IM or IV once daily
Alternative choices
Doxycycline, 100 mg IV twice daily
Chloramphenicol, 15 mg/kg IV 4 times daily
Ciprofloxacin, 400 mg IV twice daily
Children
Preferred choices
Streptomycin, 15 mg/kg IM twice daily (not to exceed 2 g/d)
Gentamicin, 2.5 mg/kg IM or IV 3 times daily
Alternative choices
Doxycycline
If weight 45 kg or more, 100 mg IV
If weight less than 45 kg, 2.2 mg/kg IV twice daily
Chloramphenicol, 15 mg/kg IV 4 times daily.
Ciprofloxacin, 15 mg/kg IV twice daily
Pregnant Women
Same as adults above except chloramphenicol is not recommended
Mass Casualty Setting
Adults, including pregnant women
Doxycycline, 100 mg orally twice daily
Ciprofloxacin, 500 mg orally twice daily
Children
Doxycycline
If weight 45 kg or more, 100 mg IV
If weight less than 45 kg, 2.2 mg/kg IV twice daily
Ciprofloxacin, 15 mg/kg IV twice daily[a]
For full details and most current treatment recommendations, the reader is referred to the CDC website (23).

[a]Ciprofloxacin dosage should not exceed 1 g/d in children.

Millions of people were killed by three pandemics occurring in AD 540, the Middle Ages, and in the late 19th century (24,25). Plague has been developed by various groups and nations as a biologic weapon since the 1950s, and has been listed as an important potential agent of bioterrorism (4).

Epidemiology

Plague is primarily a rural disease that occurs in all continents except Australia (24). Although most common in rural settings in developing nations, sporadic clusters occur regularly in the United States. For example, 107 cases were reported in the United States between 1990 and 2005, with a median number of seven cases per year (8). However, in 2006, 13 cases were reported in the first 10 months of the year (8). Most cases occur between spring and autumn in the Western states where the disease in enzootic in wild rodents. Humans are infected by being bitten by infected rodent fleas, or handling infected animals, either domestic pets or wild animals. Worldwide, the most important reservoir is the domestic rat, but as in the United States, sylvatic foci (in wild animals) also exist (26). Human-to-human transmission can occur in pneumonic plague, but requires close contact. The last known case acquired in this manner in the United States was reported in 1925 (27).

Clinical Manifestations

The three main types of plague are bubonic, septicemic, and pneumonic. Although there is no current experience with pneumonic plague acquired from a biologic attack, the clinical presentation is expected to differ from that of natural infection and is discussed below.

Bubonic Plague

This is the most common type of plague, occurring in 76% of the cases reported in the United States between 1990 and 2005 (8). Large numbers of bacteria are inoculated at the site of the flea bite and multiply locally, followed by rapid replication in nearby lymph nodes (26). The incubation period is between 2 and 7 days. There is abrupt onset of fever, chills, and headache. The characteristic bubo typically develops as a smooth, firm oval mass which is extremely tender. The overlying skin is warm and erythematous, but suppuration is rare. The primary lesion is often inapparent, but can develop into an ulcer. The most common site of the buboes is in the femoral lymph nodes, but they are also seen in inguinal, cervical, and axillary locations depending on the location of the inoculation. Bacteremia occurs in about 25% of cases and, in untreated cases, the mortality approximates 50% (8,26). In untreated cases, deterioration is usually rapid, with progression of typical signs of shock and death occurring as early as 2 to 3 days.

Septicemic Plague

This is defined as plague in the absence of an apparent bubo. As with other systemic infections without clear localization, diagnosis of septicemic plague is often delayed and the prognosis is thus poorer. In the United States from 1990 to 2005, 18% of reported plague cases were defined as septicemic, although 38% of the cases in 2006 were of this variety (8). A useful clue to the diagnosis of septicemic plague is that gastrointestinal symptoms of nausea and vomiting, diarrhea, and abdominal pain were prominent in several recent cases (8). Disseminated intravascular coagulation may develop rapidly with cutaneous and visceral hemorrhage. Rapidly progressive gangrene may also develop in this setting. Both septicemic plague and pneumonic plague are fatal if untreated. Even with treatment, mortality rates of 33% in septicemic plague were reported from New Mexico in the 1980s (28).

Pneumonic Plague

This presentation may develop secondary to either bubonic or septicemic plague. The incidence of secondary pulmonary involvement approximates 12% (24). Recent cases of primary pneumonic plague in the United States have either occurred from laboratory accidents or from exposure to cats (29). Pneumonic plague is similar to other acute pneumonia with abrupt onset of fever and dyspnea. Watery or purulent, and bloody sputum is produced and is highly infectious. Transmission is by respiratory droplets, and therefore, simple respiratory isolation with droplet precautions is sufficient. The CXR usually reveals bronchopneumonia, and multilobar consolidation or cavitation may be seen (30). Primary pneumonic plague is a rapidly progressive condition with a mortality rate of approximately 50% (27).

Clues to plague arising as the result of a biologic attack include cases outside areas of known enzootic infection; occurrences in an area without associated rodent die-offs, and numerous cases of pneumonia in otherwise healthy patients (30). In general, routine laboratory tests are not markedly different from those seen in other causes of fulminant pneumonia and sepsis. The white blood cell count is often markedly elevated and fibrin degradation products are detectable in cases where disseminated intravascular coagulation is present (31).

Diagnosis

The peripheral white blood cell count is invariably elevated and blood cultures are often positive. High-grade bacteremia may permit direct visualization of bacteria in the blood smear (31). Specialized laboratory tests to definitively and rapidly identify *Y. pestis* are not widely available. When plague is suspected, coordination with state public health officials and the CDC will allow more specialized tests and susceptibility testing to be performed. Blood, sputum, lymph node aspirates, and lesion swabs should be examined by Gram or Wright–Giemsa stain for the presence of bipolar-staining gram-negative bacilli, which appear to have the appearance of safety pins. The laboratory should be alerted to the possibility of plague so that appropriate biosafety procedures can be followed.

Treatment

The recommendations for therapy of plague provided here are derived from the recommendations of the Working Group on Civilian Biodefense and the CDC (30). Treatment recommendations for plague are complicated by the lack of clinical efficacy trials, lack of experience with widespread pneumonic plague, and potentially unpredictable clinical responses in infections due to a biologic attack. While some recommendations are not FDA-approved uses of the antibiotics, they are the consensus recommendations for the best alternatives for therapy in various situations and clinical scenarios.

The historically proven effective antibiotic therapy for plague has been streptomycin. Because of the limited availability of streptomycin, gentamicin—used successfully to treat plague—is the recommended alternative (32). Doxycycline and quinolones are effective against plague and are recommended alternatives. While ciprofloxacin is the officially recommended quinolone, levofloxacin has also been FDA-approved for treatment of plague. For pregnant women and children, the use of tetracyclines and quinolones carry the risk of potential side effects. Nevertheless, given the high mortality of plague, these agents are recommended as acceptable alternatives if aminoglycosides cannot be administered or are not available. In the setting of a mass casualty, oral regimens are recommended as these allow treatment of large numbers of people and they are also useful in settings where parenteral therapy may not be possible.

The recommended duration of therapy for plague (Table 92.2) is 10 days and oral therapy should be substituted when the patient's condition improves. Duration of postexposure prophylaxis to prevent plague infection is 7 days. For full details regarding usage in pregnant women and children as well as in special settings including renal failure, please consult the CDC website where the most current recommendations may be found (32,33).

TABLE 92.2 Recommendations for Treatment of Patients with Pneumonic Plague in Contained and Mass Casualty Settings and for Postexposure Prophylaxis

Contained Casualty Setting
Adults
Preferred choices
Streptomycin, 1g IM twice daily
Gentamicin, 5 mg/kg IM or IV once daily or 2 mg/kg loading dose followed by 1.7 mg/kg IM or IV three times daily
Alternative choice:
Doxycycline:
100 mg IV twice daily or
200 mg IV once daily
Ciprofloxacin, 400 mg IV twice daily
Chloramphenicol, 25 mg/kg IV 4 times daily
Children
Preferred choices
Streptomycin, 15 mg/kg IM twice daily (maximum daily dose 2 g)
Gentamicin, 2.5 mg/kg IM or IV 3 times daily[†]
Alternative choices:
Doxycycline:
If 45 kg or more, give adult dosage
If less than 45 kg, give 2.2 mg/kg IV twice daily (maximum 200 mg/d)
Ciprofloxacin, 15 mg/kg IV twice daily
Chloramphenicol, 25 mg/kg IV 4 times daily
In children, ciprofloxacin dose should not exceed 1 g/d, and chloramphenicol should not exceed 4 g/d. Children younger than 2 yr should not receive chloramphenicol.
Pregnant women
Same as adults above except chloramphenicol is not recommended.
Mass Casualty Setting and Postexposure Prophylaxis
Adults, including pregnant women
Preferred choices
Doxycycline, 100 mg orally twice daily
Ciprofloxacin, 500 mg orally twice daily
Alternative choices
Chloramphenicol, 25 mg/kg orally 4 times daily
Children
Preferred choices
Doxycycline:
If 45 kg or more give adult dosage
If less than 45 kg then give 2.2 mg/kg orally twice daily
Ciprofloxacin, 20 mg/kg orally twice daily
Alternative choices
Chloramphenicol, 25 mg/kg orally 4 times daily (maximum 200 mg/dL)

ANTHRAX

An extremely rare disease in the United States until the bioterrorism attacks of 2001, anthrax is caused by a gram-positive spore-forming bacillus, *Bacillus anthracis*. However, anthrax was tested as a biologic weapon by the United States in the 1960s and by several other countries until at least the 1970s. The technology to produce highly infectious anthrax spores and disseminate them widely as an aerosol exists and is known to have been developed for use as a biological warfare agent (34). It is therefore important for all physicians to be aware of the manifestations of anthrax and especially of the expected characteristics of an outbreak due to a biological attack.

Epidemiology

There are three major modes of infection with anthrax: inhalational, cutaneous, and gastrointestinal. *Cutaneous anthrax* is the most common type of anthrax. However, it is still extremely rare in the United States with 224 cases having been reported in the 50 years from 1944 to 1994 (35). Barring exposure to intentionally produced anthrax, *inhalational anthrax* is even less common and occurs primarily in those with occupational or laboratory exposure. Prior to 2001, there were only 18 cases of inhalational anthrax reported from 1900 to 1978 (36). *Gastrointestinal anthrax* is most commonly reported where improperly cooked meat contaminated with large numbers of anthrax bacilli has been consumed (37).

Clinical Manifestations

The presentation of anthrax due to a biologic attack is still incompletely characterized. Most of the information relevant to inhalational anthrax from anthrax manufactured as a biologic weapon is from the 2001 US attacks and an unintentional release in Sverdlosk, Russia, in 1979 (38). There were 11 cases of inhalational anthrax resulting from the exposures in 2001. Several aspects of the pathophysiology of inhalational anthrax are highly relevant to the clinician. Infection occurs after spores are inhaled and deposited in the alveoli. The spores are phagocytosed by macrophages and transported to regional lymph nodes where they germinate and replicate vegetatively (39). There may be a period of extended latency in the lymph node because of spores that remain dormant. Therefore, although the usual period of incubation is 2 to 6 days, cases have occurred as late as 6 weeks after exposure to aerosolized anthrax (38). When replication does occur, toxin production leads to edema, necrosis, and hemorrhage.

Typical symptoms are fever and chills, chest discomfort and dyspnea, severe fatigue, and vomiting. Two stages may occur with an initial period of improvement followed by rapid deterioration. The initial finding on chest x-ray is a widened mediastinum due to mediastinal lymph node involvement (40). A hemorrhagic mediastinal lymphadenitis ensues, often accompanied by bloody pleural effusions. Eight of 11 patients in 2001 developed bloody pleural effusions, and 10 of 11 had radiologic evidence of mediastinal adenopathy (41). Although anthrax does not cause a typical bronchopneumonia, pulmonary infiltrates, or consolidation were observed in 8 of 11 cases. In addition, in an autopsy series from the Sverdlosk outbreak, primary focal hemorrhagic necrotizing pneumonia was described in 11 of 42 cases (42).

An important point emphasized by Lucey is that while there are three known modes of exposure—inhalational, cutaneous, and gastrointestinal—anthrax may actually present as meningitis, which was the initial presentation of the index case in 2001 (34). Further, as many as 50% of inhalational anthrax cases may develop meningitis (42). Anthrax causes a rapidly progressive hemorrhagic meningitis with characteristic large gram-positive bacilli in the CSF. Similarly, although the portal of infection is the lung, hemorrhagic submucosal lesions may develop in the gastrointestinal tract along with mesenteric infection; such lesions were seen in 39 of 42 of the autopsy cases reported in the Sverdlosk outbreak and in one 2001 case (42,43). Importantly, this patient presented with primarily gastrointestinal symptoms (43).

The diagnosis of inhalational anthrax may be difficult, especially in the early stages. In addition to the signs and symptoms listed above, tachycardia and severe diaphoresis may be present. Rhinorrhea or sore throat is common in viral respiratory infections, but were uncommon in inhalational anthrax (44). A high index of clinical suspicion should be maintained especially as the risk of exposure may be unknown in the early stages of a biologic attack. Blood cultures are invariably positive if obtained prior to antibiotics.

Cutaneous anthrax is also expected to occur as a result of a biologic anthrax attack. Cutaneous cases occurred up to 12 days after the exposure in the Sverdlovsk outbreak (38). The initial lesion is a papule or macule leading to ulceration at the site of inoculation within 2 days, followed by vesiculation. The lesion is painless although it may be highly pruritic, and the vesicular fluid contains large amounts of bacteria. The characteristic depressed, black eschar that subsequently develops is painless. Surrounding edema is often a prominent feature of cutaneous anthrax lesions. In the one case of cutaneous anthrax that developed in a 7-month-old infant in 2001, microangiopathic hemolytic anemia and renal insufficiency occurred (45).

Diagnosis

Blood cultures should be obtained promptly if anthrax is suspected; blood smears should be examined for the presence of organisms. Chest x-ray and chest CT scans should be obtained to look for evidence of mediastinal widening, pleural effusions, and parenchymal abnormalities. Thoracentesis of any pleural effusions should be performed and lumbar puncture should be done as indicated. The clinical microbiology laboratory and the state public health department should both be notified of the possibility of anthrax. If indicated, specimens can be sent to specialized laboratories participating in the Laboratory Response Network for specific testing such as immunohistochemical staining or PCR. Cutaneous lesions, especially vesicle fluid, should be swabbed for stain and culture. Punch biopsy of the periphery of lesions may also be performed and analyzed by immunohistochemistry or PCR if the Gram stain is negative. Nasal swabs are not sensitive indicators of exposure or infection and should not be used to diagnose or rule out infection in individual patients (46). Sputum culture is generally negative in inhalational anthrax.

Treatment

The current recommendations for therapy of anthrax provided here are derived from the recommendations of the CDC expert panel on anthrax treatment and prevention (Tables 92.3 to 92.5) (47). As with recommendations for plague, the recommendations are based on expert opinion and a risk–benefit calculation that takes into account the extremely high mortality of inhalational anthrax. As such, the recommendations include therapy with drugs that are not specifically FDA-approved for anthrax and drugs that may have potential side effects in pregnant women and children. Adjunctive measures that may be helpful are discussed after antibiotic therapy.

TABLE 92.3 Intravenous Treatment for Systemic Anthrax with Possible/Confirmed Meningitis[a]

Bactericidal Agent (Fluoroquinolone)
Ciprofloxacin, 400 mg every 8 hr
or
Levofloxacin, 750 mg every 24 hr
or
Moxifloxacin, 400 mg every 24 hr
PLUS
Bactericidal agent (β-lactam)
For all strains, regardless of penicillin susceptibility or if susceptibility is unknown
Meropenem, 2 g every 8 hr
or
Imipenem, 1 g every 6 hr[b]
or
Doripenem, 500 mg every 8 hr
or
Alternatives for penicillin-susceptible strains
Penicillin G, 4 million units every 4 h
or
Ampicillin, 3 g every 6 hr
PLUS
Protein synthesis inhibitor
Linezolid, 600 mg every 12 hr[c]
or
Clindamycin, 900 mg every 8 hr
or
Rifampin, 600 mg every 12 hr[d]
or
Chloramphenicol, 1 g every 6–8 hr[e]

[a]Duration of treatment: 2–3 wk or more until clinical criteria for stability are met (see text). Patients exposed to aerosolized spores will require prophylaxis to complete an antimicrobial drug course of 60 d from onset of illness (see Technical Appendix Table 2 (postexposure prophylaxis)). Systemic anthrax includes anthrax meningitis; inhalation, injection, and gastrointestinal anthrax; and cutaneous anthrax with systemic involvement, extensive edema, or lesions of the head or neck. Preferred drugs are indicated in boldface. Alternative drugs are listed in order of preference for treatment for patients who cannot take first-line treatment, or if first-line treatment is unavailable.
[b]Increased risk for seizures associated with imipenem/cilastatin treatment.
[c]Linezolid should be used with caution in patients with thrombocytopenia because it might exacerbate it. Linezolid use for more than 14 d has additional hematopoietic toxicity.
[d]Rifampin is not a protein synthesis inhibitor. However, it may be used in combination with other antimicrobial drugs on the basis of its in vitro synergy.
[e]Should only be used if other options are not available because of toxicity concerns.
From CDC technical appendix available through http://www.ncbi.nlm.nih.gov/pmc/articles/PMC3901462/.

Antibiotic Regimens

Several factors are important in choosing an empiric regimen for inhalational anthrax and other systemic forms of anthrax. The 60% survival rate in the 2001 cases, which were treated with multidrug regimens, was superior to historical experience. Partly because of these data, the CDC has recommended the use of a quinolone and at least one other bactericidal agent capable of achieving therapeutic levels in the CNS, plus a third drug, for the initial treatment of systemic anthrax with confirmed or possible meningitis. Other factors considered were the possibility of engineered or primary drug resistance. Although penicillin is FDA-approved for anthrax, the presence of inducible β-lactamases dictate against the use of penicillin alone. Parenteral therapy is recommended initially. Once meningitis has been ruled out, the regimen may be simplified, and these recommendations are summarized in Table 92.4. Recommendations for cutaneous anthrax consist of treatment with a single drug, preferably a quinolone or a tetracycline (see Table 92.5).

TABLE 92.4 Intravenous Therapy for Systemic Anthrax When Meningitis Has Been Excluded[a]

Bactericidal Drug
For all strains, regardless of penicillin susceptibility or if susceptibility is unknown
Ciprofloxacin, 400 mg every 8 hr
or
Levofloxacin, 750 mg every 24 hr
or
Moxifloxacin, 400 mg every 24 hr
or
Meropenem, 2 g every 8 hr
or
Imipenem, 1 g every 6 hr[b]
or
Doripenem, 500 mg every 8 hr
or
Vancomycin, 60 mg/kg/d intravenous divided every 8 h (maintain serum trough concentrations of 15–20 μg/mL)
or
Alternatives for penicillin-susceptible strains
Penicillin G, 4 million units every 4 hr
or
Ampicillin, 3 g every 6 hr
PLUS
Protein synthesis inhibitor
Clindamycin, 900 mg every 8 hr
or
Linezolid, 600 mg every 12 hr[c]
or
Doxycycline, 200 mg initially, then 100 mg every 12 hr[d]
or
Rifampin, 600 mg every 12 hr[e]

[a]Duration of treatment: for 2 wk until clinical criteria for stability are met (see text). Patients exposed to aerosolized spores will require prophylaxis to complete an antimicrobial drug course of 60 d from onset of illness (see Technical Appendix Table 2 (postexposure prophylaxis)). Systemic anthrax includes anthrax meningitis; inhalation, injection, and gastrointestinal anthrax; and cutaneous anthrax with systemic involvement, extensive edema, or lesions of the head or neck. Preferred drugs are indicated in boldface. Alternative drugs are listed in order of preference for treatment for patients who cannot take first-line treatment, or if first-line treatment is unavailable.
[b]Increased risk for seizures associated with imipenem/cilastatin treatment.
[c]Linezolid should be used with caution in patients with thrombocytopenia because it might exacerbate it. Linezolid use for more than 14 d has additional hematopoietic toxicity.
[d]A single 10–14 d course of doxycycline is not routinely associated with tooth staining.
[e]Rifampin is not a protein synthesis inhibitor. However, it may be used in combination with other antimicrobials drugs on the basis of its in vitro synergy.
From CDC technical appendix available through http://www.ncbi.nlm.nih.gov/pmc/articles/PMC3901462/.

The duration of therapy is an important consideration both in treatment and in postexposure prophylaxis. Although the longest period of latency in the Sverdlovsk episode was reported to be 43 days, viable spores have been demonstrated in the mediastinal lymph nodes of monkeys as late as 100 days after exposure, and disease has occurred 98 days after exposure (48,49). In addition, antibiotic treatment may prevent disease, but it also prevents the development of an effective immune

TABLE 92.5 Oral Treatment for Cutaneous Anthrax Without Systemic Involvement[a]

For All Strains, Regardless of Penicillin Susceptibility or if Susceptibility is Unknown
Ciprofloxacin, 500 mg every 12 hr
or
Doxycycline, 100 mg every 12 hr
or
Levofloxacin, 750 mg every 24 hr
or
Moxifloxacin, 400 mg every 24 hr
or
Clindamycin, 600 mg every 8 hr[b]
or
Alternatives for penicillin-susceptible strains
Amoxicillin, 1 g every 8 hr
or
Penicillin VK, 500 mg every 6 hr

[a]Preferred drugs are indicated in **boldface**. Alternative drugs are listed in order of preference for treatment for patients who cannot take first-line treatment, or if first-line treatment is unavailable. Duration of treatment is 60 d for bioterrorism-related cases and 7–10 d for naturally acquired cases.
[b]Based on in vitro susceptibility data, rather than studies of clinical efficacy.

response. Therefore, treatment regimens are recommended for 60 days with close follow-up after discontinuation of antibiotics. Postexposure prophylaxis recommendations are given in Table 92.6, and consist of a single oral drug, similar to the recommendations for the treatment of cutaneous anthrax.

Corticosteroids

Although data are lacking, corticosteroids may be helpful in cutaneous anthrax with edema and in bacterial meningitis (50–52). Therefore, the consensus recommendations are to use corticosteroids in patients on prior steroid therapy, cases with edema, especially of the head and neck, meningitis, and vasopressor-resistant shock (47).

TABLE 92.6 Recommendations for Postexposure Prophylaxis of Anthrax

For All Strains, Regardless of Penicillin Susceptibility or if Susceptibility is Unknown
Ciprofloxacin, 500 mg every 12 hr
or
Doxycycline, 100 mg every 12 hr
or
Levofloxacin, 750 mg every 24 hr
or
Moxifloxacin, 400 mg every 24 hr
or
Clindamycin, 600 mg every 8 hr[b]
or
Alternatives for penicillin-susceptible strains
Amoxicillin, 1 g every 8 hr
or
Penicillin VK, 500 mg every 6 hr

[a]Preferred drugs are indicated in **boldface**. Alternative drugs are listed in order of preference for treatment for patients who cannot take first-line treatment or if first-line treatment is unavailable.
[b]Based on in vitro susceptibility data rather than studies of clinical efficacy.
From CDC technical appendix available through http://www.ncbi.nlm.nih.gov/pmc/articles/PMC3901462/.

Procedures and Surgical Interventions

Aggressive thoracostomy tube placement and drainage of pleural effusions are recommended to maximize pulmonary function and to remove the potentially deleterious effects of toxin-containing effusions. Surgery, while generally not indicated, may be required in cases of gastrointestinal anthrax or in cases of deep soft tissue infection.

Antibody Treatment

There are two antibody preparations which could potentially be used for anthrax. The first, raxibacumab, is a recombinant, humanized monoclonal antibody directed against protective antigen (PA) of the anthrax bacillus. It has proven efficacy in rabbits and monkeys and was well tolerated in a Phase I human trial (53,54). Raxibacumab has been approved by the FDA for treatment and postexposure prophylaxis. The second antibody preparation consists of anthrax immune globulin from pooled human sera from patients immunized with anthrax vaccine. Like raxibacumab, it is also effective in animal studies and was well tolerated in humans (47,55). This anthrax immune globulin preparation is not FDA-approved but could be used under an Investigational New Drug (IND) protocol or an Emergency Use Authorization during a declared emergency.

Prevention

Postexposure prophylaxis with antibiotics should be administered to all exposed patients as soon as possible after exposure and continued for 60 days (see Table 92.6). A three-dose series of Adsorbed Vaccine Anthrax may be administered combined with antibiotic prophylaxis (56).

VIRAL HEMORRHAGIC FEVER

The major diseases that will be considered in this section are Marburg, Ebola, and Lassa fevers. Marburg and Ebola viruses are filoviruses, whereas Lassa virus is an arenavirus with different clinical characteristics. Nevertheless, they have the potential to create similar problems in hospital management because of the sometimes dramatic nature of the illness and the potential for human-to-human transmission. The largest outbreak of Ebola to occur to date began in Western Africa in 2014 and is ongoing at the time of publication. There is now an extensive body of guidelines and practice recommendations regarding evaluation, diagnosis, and treatment of Ebola virus disease (EVD) from various nongovernmental organizations, the World Health Organization (WHO), and the CDC. A summary of the most pertinent recommendations is provided here, but due to the complex and evolving nature of the ongoing outbreak, the reader is advised to consult the CDC website for the most recent recommendations.

Epidemiology and Virology

Ebola (EBOV) and Marburg (MARV) viruses are related, but serologically noncross-reactive. There are five species of EBOV: Bundibugyo ebolavirus (BEBOV), Côte d'Ivoire ebolavirus (CIEBOV), Reston ebolavirus (REBOV), Sudan ebolavirus (SEBOV), and Zaire ebolavirus (ZEBOV). Since 1976, there have been approximately a dozen outbreaks of Ebola in Africa, with mortality generally ranging from 53% to 88% (57). Most cases have been due to ZEBOV, although an outbreak of 425 cases in Uganda due to SEBOV occurred in 2000 and 2001 (58). Mortality with ZEBOV is higher than with SEBOV, with the lowest mortalities reported for BEBOV (59–61). The natural reservoir is thought to include fruit bats with transmission to nonhuman primates, but the details of the enzootic cycle remain to be fully resolved (62).

Ebola transmission has ranged from 3% to 17% in household contacts (63). Transmission is related to contact with sicker patients in later stages of disease, when viremia may reach very high titers in bodily fluid and in skin (58,63–65). Nosocomial transmission is associated with percutaneous exposure and mucous membrane or cutaneous exposure to infected body fluids. The skin of patients is also infected and may serve as a source of secondary transmission (66).

Initial infection of humans has been associated with contact with wild game, particularly "bush meat" from nonhuman primates and with bats. Secondary transmission is linked to contact with blood and other bodily fluids during provision of health care, by reuse of contaminated needles and syringes, and to preparation of the bodies of victims for burial during traditional rites which involve bathing and touching the bodies of the deceased. Droplet and, possibly, small-particle aerosol transmission is thought to have occurred in the Reston outbreak but has not been documented in human-to-human transmission (66). Pigs may also be a reservoir for REBOV, although there are no documented human cases of disease associated with transmission from swine (67).

During the latest outbreak in Africa, the countries of Guinea, Sierra Leone, and Liberia have been most severely affected. As of March 2015, there have been almost 25,000 cases with approximately 10,000 deaths (Table 92.7). In addition, there was limited transmission to Nigeria, Mali, and Senegal, with 20, 9, and 1 cases, respectively. There is currently no ongoing transmission in those countries and they have been declared free of EVD. There have been several imported cases of EVD diagnosed in the United States. The first case diagnosed in the United States was a traveler from Liberia who arrived while incubating EVD and the second was a physician who was also asymptomatic on arrival but was incubating an infection acquired while providing medical services in Guinea prior to returning to the United States. Two health care workers were infected in the United States while caring for the patient from Liberia. One nurse was infected while caring for an EVD patient in Spain. There have also been several health care workers transferred to the United States for further medical treatment. All of these patients survived with the exception of the Liberian patient. There have been eight cases of documented human infection with REBOV in the United States from contact with imported monkeys from the

TABLE 92.7 Incidence of EVD in Africa 2014 to 2015

Country	Total Cases		
(Suspected, Probable, and Confirmed)	Laboratory-Confirmed Cases	Total Deaths	
Guinea	3,331	2,911	2,192
Liberia	9,482	3,150	4,241
Sierra Leone	11,696	8,469	3,663
Total	24,509	14,530	10,096

Adapted from the CDC: http://www.cdc.gov/vhf/ebola/outbreaks/2014-west-africa/case-counts.html.

Philippines. Infections with this Reston strain of Ebola virus have been subclinical.

Marburg virus has been associated with six outbreaks since the disease was recognized in 1976 in German and Yugoslav laboratory workers infected by African green monkeys of Ugandan origin (68). Since then, there have been six other clusters of infection in Africa, the most recent in Angola and the Democratic Republic of Congo. Involving more than 400 people, the mortality was 83% and 90%, respectively, in these last two outbreaks. MARV infections are transmitted by exposure to infected primate blood or cell culture or probably by direct exposure to virus from fruit bats (66,69–71). Secondary transmission occurs from exposure to blood and body fluids, as well as by intimate contact.

Lassa virus causes a chronic infection of rodents, and is endemic throughout West Africa (72). Transmission to humans is through exposure to infected rodents, primarily through contact with urine from chronically and asymptomatically animals (73). Person-to-person transmission is thought to be primarily via contact with infected bodily fluids, although aerosol transmission may also occur. Incubation is between 7 and 21 days. Other arenaviruses are present worldwide in rodent reservoirs and are a potential source of new clinical syndromes (72).

Clinical Manifestations

The clinical picture of Ebola and Marburg infections is similar (66). The incubation period is usually between 8 and 10 days with an overall range of 2 to 21 days. Abrupt onset of fever, weakness, myalgias, and headache is typical. A characteristic maculopapular rash is described by day 5 of the illness. Nausea and vomiting, abdominal pain, diarrhea, and hypotension may occur by 4 to 7 days, followed by confusion, bleeding, and shock. Bleeding is usually not profuse although a bleeding diathesis is seen in at least 50% of patients; chest pain and pharyngitis are also common. Photophobia, lymph node enlargement, jaundice, and pancreatitis are all manifestations of widespread organ involvement. CNS involvement may manifest as obtundation or coma. By the second week, there is either a period of defervescence and improvement, or further deterioration with multiorgan system failure. Disseminated intravascular coagulation, as well as hepatic and renal failure may ensue; convalescence is often protracted. As described above, Ebola–Reston has not led to any known human deaths. There is viremia with infection of all organs, leading to necrosis in areas of viral replication (74). Pathogenesis is thought to be also due to cytokine release leading to increased vascular permeability and hemodynamic instability (75).

Lassa fever presents with relatively nonspecific signs and symptoms, making recognition of cases in the initial stages difficult (72,76). A combination of fever, retrosternal pain, pharyngitis, and proteinuria has been suggested to be indicative of Lassa fever (76). A diffuse capillary leak syndrome in the second week of illness is a cardinal manifestation of this disorder. Mortality of hospitalized cases ranges from 15% to 25%. Seventh cranial nerve deafness is a common sequela of Lassa infection, occurring in approximately one-third of cases (77); persistent vertigo is another reported side effect (78). The pathogenic mechanism of Lassa fever is not well understood, but there is variable necrosis in affected organs and the systemic manifestations of vascular dysfunction may be due to soluble macrophage-derived factors.

Diagnosis

A history of travel to endemic areas and a clinical syndrome compatible with viral hemorrhagic fever (VHF) are key elements of making a diagnosis. Nevertheless, a cluster of cases with signs and symptoms indicative of VHF may the first clue of a biologic attack. Specialized testing for Marburg and Ebola, including PCR and direct antigen visualization in clinical samples, is available through reference laboratories and the CDC. Contact with local public health authorities and the CDC will allow testing according to approved protocols. An extensive series of protocols has been established for handling of clinical samples to prevent exposure of clinicians and laboratory personnel and is available on the CDC website at http://www.cdc.gov/vhf/ebola/healthcare-us/laboratories/specimens.html. Lassa virus is easily cultured as the levels of viremia are usually high; RT-PCR may also be used to identify Lassa virus.

Treatment

Treatment of Marburg and EVD is primarily supportive. There is no proven effective specific antiviral therapy. Ribavirin and interferon have been previously ineffective. Several recent patients who have survived were treated with a combination of four monoclonal antibodies directed against Ebola virus antigens and open trials with this product are underway. Whether administration of serum from convalescent patients is useful in the treatment of EVD is unknown. Unnecessary movement or manipulation of the patient should be avoided. Contact and respiratory isolation of the patient is necessary including use of goggles and face shields to prevent exposure to body fluids (79). Prevention of nosocomial exposure and infection is of paramount importance. The complexities of protocols for the use of appropriate personal protective equipment and infection control are beyond the scope of this chapter and CDC guidelines should be followed in all cases of suspected or proven viral hemorrhagic fever. Transfer to specialized treatment centers may also be appropriate. Vaccines that have shown promise in primate models are currently under evaluation but are not available for routine clinical use.

In cases of Lassa fever, where the aspartate transaminase levels exceed 150 IU/L, early treatment with intravenous ribavirin has been reported to be beneficial in tapering doses over 12 days (80).

SMALLPOX

Smallpox is caused by infection with variola, a double-stranded DNA orthopoxvirus. Smallpox, one of the most feared and lethal diseases known to man, was virtually eliminated as a natural threat by vaccination (81). By 1980, WHO declared it to be eradicated worldwide, with the last case known to have occurred naturally in 1977. In the United States, universal childhood vaccination ended in 1972. Thus, most people in the United States today are susceptible to smallpox infection. The anthrax attacks in 2001 again raised the possibility of smallpox being used as a biologic weapon. Smallpox is classified as a Tier 1 bioterrorism agent, a high-priority organism that poses a risk to national security (3,4) and should be considered one of the most dangerous agents because of its high infectiousness, capability for rapid spread, the lack of effective treatment, and the capacity to induce mass social disruption and overburden the public health system.

Epidemiology

Smallpox is spread by direct close contact via large droplet inhalation (82); there are no known animal reservoirs. Spread can also occur by contact with lesions or infected fomites. Household spread has been reported to range from 30% to 80% (83). Smallpox outbreaks were most common during the winter and early spring (84). All ages are susceptible although, historically, vaccination rates and prior infection modulated the attack rates among different groups. Patients are most contagious when they have a rash although they may be infectious during the symptomatic prodrome prior to the development of skin lesions (see below). Incubation is from 7 to 17 days, during which period the patient is not infectious.

Clinical Manifestations

During the prodromal phase, the patient experiences high fever with back pain and prostration (81). The rash follows within a day or two, with more lesions on the face, oral mucosa, and extremities than on the trunk—termed a centrifugal pattern. The lesions begin as macules, progress to vesicles, and then finally pustules over the first week. Fever is usually persistent throughout the period of rash development. The lesions are deep seated, firm, painful, and—importantly for the diagnosis—all lesions are at the same stage of development at each phase. All of these characteristics of the rash serve to differentiate it from the rash of chickenpox, which is superficial, lesions appear in crops, are centripetal in distribution, and are associated with a relatively mild prodrome. The extent of the smallpox rash correlates with mortality, which may range from 10% to 75%; in fatal cases, death usually occurs by the second week. The lesions begin to crust over after 7 to 9 days, and the patient is noninfectious only after all scabs have fallen off. Scarring and pitting result in the characteristic pock-marked appearance of survivors. The pathologic damage in smallpox is generally confined to the skin and mucous membranes, although virus is present throughout the internal organs (81). The systemic manifestations and fatalities are attributed to toxinemia and antigenemia.

Vaccine-modified smallpox presents as a milder illness with fewer lesions and mortality less than 10% (81). A hemorrhagic form of smallpox may occur in which there is diffuse erythema, followed by petechial hemorrhages; it is reported to have mortality approaching 100% (85). In malignant or "flat" smallpox, discrete lesions do not develop, but confluent rubbery lesions are present (86). A form of smallpox known as variola minor, with much milder symptoms and mortality less than 10%, is now known to be due to a genetically distinct strain of the virus (87).

Diagnosis

Specimens of vesicular or pustular fluid should be obtained for culture and electron microscopic examination; these are transported in double-sealed leak-proof containers designed for transport of body fluids. Specimens should be handled only in BSL-4 laboratories and public health authorities should be notified if a case of smallpox is suspected to assist with specimen handling. The diagnosis of orthopoxvirus infection can be made by electron microscopic examination and speciation can be performed by molecular techniques such as PCR and DNA sequencing.

Treatment and Prevention

While a full discussion of infection control and vaccination protocols is beyond the scope of this text, the following principles should be followed (88). The patient should be isolated, and contact and airborne precautions should be instituted when a case of smallpox is suspected. All personnel who had face-to-face contact with the patient should be vaccinated, as should all personnel who had contact with the patient while the latter was febrile. Local health authorities should be contacted immediately and the CDC will provide assistance with prioritizing contacts for vaccination and monitoring. It should also be noted that contraindications to vaccinations do not apply to high-risk exposures. Treatment is primarily supportive, and is aimed at maintaining hemodynamic stability and treating secondary infections. Vaccination is most effective when administered within 72 of exposure, but may mitigate symptoms and severity of disease if administered after 72 hours. A vaccinia immune globulin product may be available from the CDC to manage vaccine adverse effects.

MONKEYPOX

Monkeypox is a disease clinically similar to smallpox that has been sporadically reported in Africa since 1960. Pronounced lymphadenopathy is an additional sign of monkeypox that may help differentiate it from smallpox (89,90). Monkeypox is thought to be endemic in rodents and transmitted to humans via direct animal contact, with occasional human-to-human transmission. In 2003, there was a large cluster of human cases in the United States associated with prairie dogs that had become infected by imported African rodents (91). Although there were no fatalities, several patients required hospitalization. Vaccination against smallpox is thought to ameliorate symptoms and lessen the likelihood of infection. Cidofovir, an antiviral agent, has activity against monkeypox in vitro, and may be used in severe infection, although there are no clinical data regarding its effectiveness (92).

MALARIA

Malaria, the fourth largest killer of children under five, causes over 350 million clinical episodes and one million deaths per year. While a comprehensive discussion of the management of malaria will not be possible here, we will cover the recognition and treatment of severe malaria, which may be encountered in the critical care setting in a nonendemic setting. As such, this chapter will focus on infection with *Plasmodium falciparum*, the strain of the parasite which is most likely to cause high-level parasitemia and severe, life-threatening malaria.

Epidemiology

Malaria is endemic throughout much of the world, with the greatest number of cases in Africa and Asia (93). Malaria has been officially eradicated in the United States since 1970, but approximately 1,200 cases are reported annually (94), mostly in travelers from endemic areas. Other cases are due to local transmission from infected mosquitoes (so-called "airport malaria"), congenital malaria, and malaria acquired from blood transfusion. Local transmission of malaria in the United States has occurred at least 11 times since 1970, with 20 probable cases (95). In a recent outbreak in Florida, seven cases were verified as being caused by the same strain of *P. vivax* (95). Thus, domestic transmission of malaria is possible especially in warmer regions of the United States.

In endemic areas, many adults are partially immune to malaria and, although infected, may even be asymptomatic. Children are particularly prone to infection and to developing severe disease. Other high-risk groups include pregnant women, asplenic individuals, and other immunocompromised hosts.

Clinical Manifestations

Malaria typically has an incubation period of 1 to 3 weeks. However, this may be extended by partial immunity or chemoprophylaxis. Therefore, it has been suggested that any traveler returning from an endemic area should be considered at risk for development of malaria for as long as 3 months (96). The clinical presentation is usually nonspecific: fever and headache are universally present, and myalgia, sweats, and weakness are common. Paroxysmal and cyclical fever, while classically associated with malaria, are not consistently present. Especially in the case of falciparum malaria, the fever is often continuous. While other infections are common in malaria-endemic areas, malaria should be considered as one of the most likely diagnoses in any patient with a consistent clinical picture and travel history. If malaria is suspected, prompt infectious disease consultation is indicated, to help with management and assess the likelihood of alternate diagnoses.

The pathogenesis of malaria is complex and related to both direct effects of the parasite on erythrocytes and the vasculature, and indirect effects on cytokine production, tissue oxygen consumption, and other systemic effects (96). Several aspects of the biology of *P. falciparum* are relevant to the development of severe malaria. *P. falciparum* sequesters itself in the venous microcirculation of virtually all tissues, including the brain. Hypoglycemia is common during *P. falciparum* infection and is thought to be due to oxygen consumption by replicating parasites as well as due to increased tissue metabolism. Severe anemia may occur and is due to lysis of infected erythrocytes as well as to clearance of uninfected erythrocytes, and decreased erythrocyte production. Thus the anemia in severe malaria is often normochromic and normocytic. This combination of factors aggravates tissue hypoxia and leads to metabolic acidosis. A capillary leak syndrome due to parasite sequestration and cytokine production may lead to pulmonary edema. Renal failure in malaria is multifactorial and is more common in adults than children. Hemoglobinuria may be severe enough to cause dark urine, termed, when present, blackwater fever.

Diagnosis

The gold standard for diagnosis of malaria remains microscopic identification of parasites on the blood smear. However, rapid diagnostic tests (RDTs) based on antigen detection are becoming widely available and facilitate diagnosis within minutes. These tests allow the identification of the infection as falciparum or non-falciparum, and are highly sensitive and specific, although sensitivity and specificity decline with lower levels of parasitemia. Examination of thick and thin blood smears should be performed immediately by trained personnel. If the initial examination is negative, smears should be repeated every 12 to 24 hours for a total of 48 to 72 hours (94). When parasites are detected, the percentage of parasitemia can be calculated by counting the number of infected and noninfected RBCs. The number of WBCs in the microscopic field can also be used as an internal standard to aid in estimated parasite density and percentage when thick smears are examined. Malaria is a nationally notifiable disease and the state health authorities should be notified when a diagnosis of malaria is made. The Centers for Disease Control and Prevention maintains a 24-hour malaria hotline to assist clinicians with the management of suspected and confirmed malaria cases (97).

Treatment

It should be emphasized that patients, particularly those who are nonimmune, may deteriorate rapidly. Thus hospitalization of patients during the initial phase of treatment is prudent. Furthermore, nonimmune patients may have severe illness before manifesting high degrees of parasitemia. Therefore, patients who manifest any of the symptoms or signs of severe malaria and have any degree of parasitemia on blood smear should be treated as a case of severe malaria. The WHO has promulgated criteria for the diagnosis of severe malaria (Table 92.4 and footnote to Table 92.8) (98). Cases that meet these criteria should be treated with intravenous therapy. Intravenous quinidine gluconate and artesunate are currently the only available parenteral drugs recommended for severe malaria in the United States. Artesunate is recommended by the WHO in preference to quinidine for the treatment of severe malaria and has now been used for many years in other countries. Artesunate may be obtained under an IND protocol from the CDC if patients have severe disease, a high level of parasitemia, an

TABLE 92.8 Recommendations for Treatment of Severe Malaria from All Regions

Adult Dosage
Quinidine gluconate[a] plus one of the following: doxycycline, tetracycline, or clindamycin
Quinidine gluconate: 6.25 mg base/kg (= 10 mg salt/kg) loading dose IV over 1–2 hr, then 0.0125 mg base/kg/min (= 0.02 mg salt/kg/min) continuous infusion for at least 24 hr. An alternative regimen is 15 mg base/kg (= 24 mg salt/kg) loading dose IV infused over 4 hr, followed by 7.5 mg base/kg (= 12 mg salt/kg) infused over 4 hr every 8 hr, starting 8 hr after the loading dose (see package insert). Once parasite density is less than 1% and patient can take oral medication, complete treatment with oral quinine. Quinidine/quinine course = 7 d in Southeast Asia, 3 d in Africa or South America.
Doxycycline: If patient not able to take oral medication, give 100 mg IV every 12 hr and then switch to oral doxycycline (as soon as patient can take oral medication (100 mg po bid). For IV use, avoid rapid administration. Treatment course = 7 d.
Tetracycline: 250 mg po 4 times daily.
Clindamycin: 20 mg base/kg/d po divided 3 times daily. If patient not able to take oral medication, give 10 mg base/kg loading dose IV followed by 5 mg base/kg IV every 8 hr. Switch to oral clindamycin (oral dose as above) as soon as patient can take oral medication. For IV use, avoid rapid administration. Treatment course = 7 d.
Investigational New Drug (contact CDC for information):
Artesunate followed by one of the following: Atovaquone/proguanil (Malarone™), Doxycycline (Clindamycin in pregnant women), or Mefloquine
Pediatric Dosage
Quinidine gluconate[a] plus one of the following:
Doxycycline,[b] tetracycline,[b] or clindamycin
Quinidine gluconate: Same mg/kg dosing and recommendations as for adults.
Doxycycline: 2.2 mg/kg po every 12 hr.
If patient not able to take oral medication, may give IV. For children 45 kg, use same dosing as for adults. For IV use, avoid rapid administration. Treatment course = 7 d.
Tetracycline: 25 mg/kg/day po divided 4 times daily.
Clindamycin: 20 mg base/kg/day po divided 3 times daily. If patient not able to take oral medication, give 10 mg base/kg loading dose IV followed by 5 mg base/kg IV every 8 hr. Switch to oral clindamycin (oral dose as above) as soon as patient can take oral medication. For IV use, avoid rapid administration. Treatment course = 7 d.
Investigational new drug (contact CDC for information): Artesunate followed by one of the following: Atovaquone-proguanil (Malarone), Clindamycin, or Mefloquine

[a]Persons with a positive blood smear OR history of recent possible exposure and no other recognized pathology who have one or more of the following clinical criteria **(impaired consciousness/coma, severe normocytic anemia, renal failure, pulmonary edema, ARDS, circulatory shock, disseminated intravascular coagulation, spontaneous bleeding, acidosis, hemoglobinuria, jaundice, repeated generalized convulsions, and/or parasitemia of more than 5%)** are considered to have manifestations of more severe disease. Severe malaria is most often caused by *P. falciparum*. Patients diagnosed with severe malaria should be treated aggressively with parenteral antimalarial therapy. Treatment with IV quinidine should be initiated as soon as possible after the diagnosis has been made. Patients with severe malaria should be given an intravenous loading dose of quinidine unless they have received more than 40 mg/kg of quinine in the preceding 48 hr or if they have received mefloquine within the preceding 12 hr. Consultation with a cardiologist and a physician with experience treating malaria is advised when treating malaria patients with quinidine. During administration of quinidine, blood pressure monitoring (for hypotension) and cardiac monitoring (for widening of the QRS complex and/or lengthening of the Q–Tc interval) should be monitored continuously and blood glucose (for hypoglycemia) should be monitored periodically. Cardiac complications, if severe, may warrant temporary discontinuation of the drug or slowing of the intravenous infusion. Pregnant women diagnosed with severe malaria should be treated aggressively with parenteral antimalarial therapy. Doxycycline and tetracycline are not indicated for use in children less than 8 years old. For children less than 8 yr old with chloroquine-resistant *P. falciparum*, atovaquone–proguanil and artemether–lumefantrine are recommended treatment options; mefloquine can be considered if no other options are available.

inability to take oral medications, a lack of timely access to intravenous quinidine, quinidine intolerance, or contraindications or quinidine failure. Postartemisinin delayed hemolysis (PADH) can occur 1 to 3 weeks after therapy with artesunate. Two aspects of quinidine therapy in this setting are important to remember. The first is the possibility of ventricular dysrhythmias; prolongation of the Q–T_C interval is commonly seen during quinidine therapy and careful monitoring of the electrocardiogram and electrolytes are mandatory. Combination with other drugs that may prolong the Q–T_C interval should be avoided. The second is the propensity of quinidine and quinine to cause hypoglycemia. Given the likelihood of hypoglycemia in severe malaria due to the disease itself, serum glucose must be carefully monitored and supplemented as necessary. Given these considerations, quinidine should be administered in an intensive care unit, with the assistance of a cardiologist as needed.

It is recommended by the CDC that exchange transfusion be considered in cases where parasitemia exceeds 10% or when severe complications are present (99,100). Although the benefits have not been proven in a randomized trial, exchange transfusion has the potential benefit of both reducing parasite burden and circulating cytokines and toxins. Exchange transfusion is recommended until parasitemia is below 1%. The CDC may also be contacted for advice at the Malaria Hotline.

ROCKY MOUNTAIN SPOTTED FEVER

Rocky Mountain spotted fever (RMSF) is a disease that presents with nonspecific signs and symptoms, for which there is not a specific RDT. Unless treated appropriately, RMSF has a high mortality. It is therefore important for the practicing clinician to have a high index of suspicion for RMSF and to be familiar with its epidemiology, clinical manifestations, and treatment.

Epidemiology

RMSF is caused by *Rickettsia rickettsii*, an intracellular bacterium that is transmitted in the United States primarily by the dog tick, *Dermacentor variabilis*, in the Eastern states, and the wood tick, *Dermacentor andersonii*, in the Rocky Mountain States, as well as by the brown dog tick, *Rhipicephalus sanguineus*, throughout the United States. Ticks are also the primary reservoir for *R. rickettsii*. Despite the name, most cases of RMSF occur in the Southeastern United States, and over 60% of reported cases are from North Carolina, Missouri, Tennessee, Oklahoma, and Arkansas (101). However, cases have been reported in all 48 continental states except Vermont and Maine (102). The incidence of RMSF has risen sharply over the past decade, and is now over 6 cases per million, with approximately 2,000 cases reported per year in the United States. Most cases occur between April and September with a peak in June and July. Although children have been reported to be at highest risk of RMSF, the peak incidence currently is in those aged 55 to 64 (101,102). Although males are reported to be at higher risk, a recent study of children with RMSF found more cases among girls than boys (103). Most bites are unnoticed and the tick must be attached for 6 to 10 hours for feeding and infection to take place.

Clinical Manifestations and Pathogenesis

The rickettsial organisms primarily target and infect endothelial cells (104). The primary pathology consists of diffuse cell injury and increased vascular permeability caused by cell-to-cell spread of the organisms after initial hematogenous and lymphatic seeding. Infection occurs in virtually all internal organs and vascular injury occurs in lung, heart, brain, gastrointestinal tract, and skin, as well as other sites.

Symptoms typically begin 2 to 14 days after the tick bite. Virtually all patients experience the classical triad of fever, headache, and rash (103,105,106). However, it should be emphasized that the rash is only present in about 50% of cases within the first 3 days. Rash usually appears by the 2nd to 5th day, but is absent in about 10% of patients. The rash is often faint in the initial stages and may be more difficult to detect in patients with dark skin (106). It begins as a blanching, pink maculopapular exanthem, most commonly beginning at the wrists and ankles, and develops into palpable lesions that spread centrally. The rash subsequently becomes petechial and may involve the palms and soles. Progression to petechiae is a sign of progressive disease. Commonly associated symptoms occurring in more than 50% of patients are myalgias, nausea, vomiting, and abdominal pain. The serum AST is often elevated and thrombocytopenia and hyponatremia occur in up to 50% of cases (106). Atypical symptoms such as cough, diarrhea, or sore throat may predominate in children, complicating diagnosis.

CNS abnormalities occur in about 25% and carry a poor prognosis. CSF abnormalities are observed in one-third of patients and consist of pleocytosis and elevated protein levels, although the CSF glucose is usually normal. A fulminant form of the disease, with death occurring in the first five days, has been described; glucose-6-phosphate dehydrogenase deficiency has been linked to this form of the disease (107). Neurologic deficits and limb loss are the most serious sequelae observed in survivors of RMSF (108).

Diagnosis

Delay in diagnosis and delay in seeking medical attention are associated with poor outcome in RMSF. Therefore, empiric therapy should not await the result of laboratory testing. Factors that are likely to lead to delay in diagnosis include absence of rash or delayed appearance of the rash, no history of tick bite, and presentation early in the course of disease (106,109,110). *R. rickettsii* can be isolated in culture or demonstrated by immunohistochemistry in tissue specimens. Blood culture or PCR is insensitive due to the low number of circulating organisms. Serology is useful for confirmation of diagnosis. Diagnosis should, therefore, be made on the basis of epidemiologic and clinical findings described above.

Treatment

The recommended therapy for RMSF in both adults and children is doxycycline, administered at a dose of 100 mg twice daily for adults and 2.2 mg/kg body weight twice daily for children under 45 kg (111). Treatment of suspected RMSF should be instituted promptly with doxycycline either intravenously or orally. Doxycycline for RMSF is not contraindicated in children (111). Outcome is superior with doxycycline compared to other antibiotic regimens. Therapy is continued for 7 to 14 days and a minimum of 3 days after the patient has defervesced.

Key Points

- The epidemiology, clinical presentation, and management of infections resulting from an intentional release of microorganisms may differ significantly from disease resulting from traditional modes of spread.
- The HHS/CDC has designated those select agents and toxins that present the greatest risk of deliberate misuse with the most significant potential for mass casualties or devastating effects to the economy, critical infrastructure or public confidence as Tier 1 agents.
- Recommendations for a mass casualty setting take into account the likelihood that services may be limited and parenteral or inpatient therapy may not be possible. Therefore, several potentially toxic antibiotics that are not routinely given to children or pregnant women are included in the recommended treatment regimens.
- While there are three known modes of exposure—inhalational, cutaneous, and gastrointestinal—anthrax may present as meningitis, and as many as 50% of inhalational anthrax cases may develop meningitis.
- A prolonged latency period may occur after anthrax exposure. Postexposure antibiotic prophylaxis is therefore continued for 60 days with subsequent monitoring of the patient.
- Nonimmune malaria patients may have severe illness before manifesting high degrees of parasitemia. Therefore, those who meet criteria for severe malaria and have any degree of parasitemia should be hospitalized and treated with intravenous therapy.
- Close cooperation with the CDC and local public health authorities should be initiated in all cases of suspected viral hemorrhagic fever and transfer to specialized care facilities should be considered.
- The rash of RMSF may not be present initially or may never develop. Delay in diagnosis and delay in seeking medical attention are associated with poor outcome in RMSF. Therefore, empiric therapy should not await the result of laboratory testing.
- Smallpox is highly infectious. The patient should be isolated, and contact and airborne precautions should be instituted when a case of smallpox is suspected. Specimens should be handled only in BSL-4 laboratories and public health authorities should be notified to assist with specimen handling.

References

1. McCoy G. A plague-like illness of rodents. *Public Health Bull.* 1911;43: 53–71.
2. Dennis DT, Inglesby TV, Henderson DA, et al. Tularemia as a biological weapon: medical and public health management. *JAMA.* 2001;285:2763–2773.
3. Centers for Disease Control and Prevention (CDC), Department of Health and Human Services (HHS). Possession, use, and transfer of select agents and toxins: biennial review. Final rule. *Fed Reg.* 2012;77:61083–61115.
4. Emergency preparedness and response, bioterrorism agents/diseases. CDC website. Available at: http://www.bt.cdc.gov/agent/agentlist-category.asp. Accessed March 13, 2015.
5. Boyce JM. Recent trends in the epidemiology of tularemia in the United States. *J Infect Dis.* 1975;131:197–199.
6. Dennis DT. Tularemia. In: Wallace R, Doebbeling BN, eds. *Public Health and Preventive Medicine.* 14th ed. Stamford, CO: Appleton & Lange; 1998;354–357.
7. Reported tularemia cases by year—United States, 1950–2013. CDC website. Available at: http://www.cdc.gov/tularemia/statistics/year.html. Accessed March 15, 2015.
8. Centers for Disease Control and Prevention (CDC). Human plague—four states, 2006. *MMWR Morb Mortal Wkly Rep.* 2006;55:940–943.
9. Feldman KA, Enscore RE, Lathrop SL, et al. An outbreak of primary pneumonic tularemia on Martha's Vineyard. *N Engl J Med.* 2001;345:1601–1606.
10. Christenson B. An outbreak of tularemia in the northern part of central Sweden. *Scand J Infect Dis.* 1984;16:285–290.
11. Young LS, Bickness DS, Archer BG, et al. Tularemia epidemia: Vermont, 1968. Forty-seven cases linked to contact with muskrats. *N Engl J Med.* 1969;280:1253–1260.
12. Capellan J, Fong IW. Tularemia from a cat bite: case report and review of feline-associated tularemia. *Clin Infect Dis.* 1993;16:472–475.
13. Penn RL. Francisella tularensis (tularemia). In: Bennett JE, Dolin R, Blaser MJ, ed. *Mandell, Douglas, and Bennett's Principles and Practice of Infectious Diseases.* 8th ed. Vol. 2. Philadelphia, PA: Churchill Livingstone/Elsevier; 2015:2590–2602.
14. Penn RL. Tularemia. In: Mandell GL, Bennett JE, Dolin R, eds. *Principles and Practice of Infectious Diseases.* 6th ed. Vol. 2. New York, NY: Churchill Livingstone; 2004:2674–2683.
15. Fortier AH, Green SJ, Polsinelli T, et al. Life and death of an intracellular pathogen: *Francisella tularensis* and the macrophage. *Immunol Ser.* 1994;60:349–361.
16. Saslaw S, Eigelsbach HT, Wilson HE, et al. Tularemia vaccine study. I. Intracutaneous challenge. *Arch Intern Med.* 1961;107:689–701.
17. Saslaw S, Eigelsbach HT, Prior JA, et al. Tularemia vaccine study. II. Respiratory challenge. *Arch Intern Med.* 1961;107:702–714.
18. Sanders CV, Hahn R. Analysis of 106 cases of tularemia. *J LA State Med Soc.* 1968;120:391–393.
19. Evans ME, Gregory DW, Schaffner W, et al. Tularemia: a 30-year experience with 88 cases. *Medicine (Baltimore).* 1985;64:251–269.
20. Kugeler KJ, Mead PS, Janusz AM, et al. Molecular epidemiology of *Francisella tularensis* in the United States. *Clin Infect Dis.* 2009;48:863–870.
21. Overhol EL, Tigert WD, Kadul PJ, et al. An analysis of forty-two cases of laboratory-acquired tularemia: treatment with broad spectrum antibiotics. *Am J Med.* 1961;30:785–806.
22. Maurin M, Pelloux I, Brion JP, et al. Human tularemia in France, 2006–2010. *Clin Infect Dis.* 2011;53:e133–e141.
23. Consensus statement: tularemia as a biological weapon: medical and public health management. CDC website. Available at: http://www.bt.cdc.gov/agent/tularemia/tularemia-biological-weapon-abstract.asp#4. Accessed March 13, 2015.
24. Perry RD, Fetherston JD. *Yersinia pestis*: etiologic agent of plague. *Clin Microbiol Rev.* 1997;10:35–66.
25. Slack P. The black death past and present. 2. Some historical problems. *Trans R Soc Trop Med Hyg.* 1989;83:461–463.
26. Butler T, Dennis DT. Plague. In: Mandell GL, Bennett JE, Dolin R, eds. *Principles and Practice of Infectious Diseases.* 6th ed. vol. 2. New York, NY: Churchill Livingstone; 2004:2691–2701.
27. Meyer KF. Pneumonic plague. *Microbiol Mol Biol Rev.* 1961;25:249–261.
28. Hull HF, Montes JM, Mann JM. Septicemic plague in New Mexico. *J Infect Dis.* 1987;155:113–118.
29. Gage KL, Dennis, DT, Orloski KA, et al. Cases of cat-associated human plague in the Western US, 1977–1998. *Clin Infect Dis.* 2000;30:893–900.
30. Inglesby TV, Dennis DT, Henderson DA, et al. Plague as a biological weapon: medical and public health management. *JAMA.* 2000;283:2281–2290.
31. Butler T. A clinical study of bubonic plague: observations of the 1970 Vietnam epidemic with emphasis on coagulation studies, skin histology and electrocardiograms. *Am J Med.* 1972;53:268–276.
32. Plague: resources for clinicians. CDC website. Available at: http://www.cdc.gov/plague/healthcare/clinicians.html. Accessed November 13, 2016.
33. Plague as a biological weapon: medical and public health management. CDC website. Available at: http://www.bt.cdc.gov/Agent/Plague/plague-biological-weapon-abstract.asp#therapy. Accessed March 14, 2015.
34. Lucey D. Anthrax. In: Mandell GL, Bennett JE, Dolin R, eds. *Principles and Practice of Infectious Diseases.* 6th ed. Vol. 2. New York, NY: Churchill Livingstone; 2004:3618–3624.
35. Centers for Disease Control and Prevention. Summary of notifiable diseases, 1945–1994. *MMWR Morb Mortal Wkly Rep.* 1994;43:70–78.
36. Brachman PS. Inhalation anthrax. *Ann N Y Acad Sci.* 1980;353:83–93.

37. Sirisanthana T, Brown AE. Anthrax of the gastrointestinal tract. *Emerg Infect Dis*. 2003;8:649–651.
38. Meselson M, Guillemin J, Hugh-Jones M, et al. The Sverdlovsk anthrax outbreak of 1979. *Science*. 1994;266:1202–1208.
39. Hanna PC, Ireland JA. Understanding *Bacillus anthracis* pathogenesis. *Trends Microbiol*. 1999;7:180–182.
40. Jernigan JA, Stephens DS, Ashford DA, et al. Bioterrorism-related inhalational anthrax: the first 10 cases reported in the United States. *Emerg Infect Dis*. 2001;7:933–944.
41. Bartlett JG, Inglesby TV Jr, Borio L. Management of anthrax. *Clin Infect Dis*. 2002;35:851–858.
42. Abramova FA, Grinberg LM, Yampolskaya OV, et al. Pathology of inhalational anthrax in 42 cases from the Sverdlovsk outbreak of 1979. *Proc Natl Acad Sci U S A*. 1993;90:2291–2294.
43. Borio L, Frank D, Mani V, et al. Death due to bioterrorism-related inhalational anthrax: report of 2 patients. *JAMA*. 2001;286:2554–2559.
44. Hupert N, Bearman GM, Mushlin AI, et al. Accuracy of screening for inhalational anthrax after a bioterrorist attack. *Ann Intern Med*. 2003; 139:337–345.
45. Freedman A, Afonja O, Chang MW, et al. Cutaneous anthrax associated with microangiopathic hemolytic anemia and coagulopathy in a 7-month-old infant. *JAMA*. 2002;287:869–874.
46. Kiratisin P, Fukuda CD, Wong A, et al. Large-scale screening of nasal swabs for Bacillus anthracis: descriptive summary and discussion of the National Institutes of Health's experience. *J Clin Microbiol*. 2002;40:3012–3016.
47. Hendricks KA, Wright ME, Shadomy SV, et al. Centers for Disease Control and Prevention expert panel meetings on prevention and treatment of anthrax in adults. *Emerg Infec Dis*. 2014;20:e130687.
48. Henderson DW, Peacock S, Belton FC. Observations on the prophylaxis of experimental pulmonary anthrax in the monkey. *J Hyg (Lond)*. 1956;54:28–36.
49. Glassman HN. Industrial inhalation anthrax. *Microbiol Mol Biol Rev*. 1966;30:657–659.
50. Sejvar JJ, Tenover FC, Stephens DS. Management of anthrax meningitis. *Lancet Infect Dis*. 2005;5:287–295.
51. de Gans J, van de Beek D; European Dexamethasone in Adulthood Bacterial Meningitis Study Investigators. Dexamethasone in adults with bacterial meningitis. *N Engl J Med*. 2002;347(20):1549–1556.
52. Demirdag K, Ozden M, Saral Y, et al. Cutaneous anthrax in adults: a review of 25 cases in the eastern Anatolian region of Turkey. *Infection*. 2003;31(5):327–330.
53. Migone T-S, Subramanian GM, Zhong J, et al. Raxibacumab for the treatment of inhalational anthrax. *N Engl J Med*. 2009;361:135–144.
54. Subramanian GM, Cronin PW, Poley G, et al. A phase 1 study of PAmAb, a fully human monoclonal antibody against *Bacillus anthracis* protective antigen, in healthy volunteers. *Clin Infect Dis*. 2005;41(1):12–20.
55. Walsh JJ, Pesik N, Quinn CP, et al. A case of naturally acquired inhalation anthrax: clinical care and analyses of anti-protective antigen immunoglobulin G and lethal factor. *Clin Infect Dis*. 2007;44(7):968–971.
56. Wright JG, Quinn CP, Shadomy S, et al. Use of anthrax vaccine in the United States: recommendations of the Advisory Committee on Immunization Practices (ACIP), 2009. *MMWR Recomm Rep*. 2010;59(RR-6): 1–30.
57. Ebola hemorrhagic fever. CDC website. Available at: http://www.cdc.gov/ncidod/dvrd/spb/mnpages/dispages/ebotabl.htm. Accessed February 1, 2007.
58. Towner JS, Rollin PE, Bausch DG, et al. Rapid diagnosis of Ebola hemorrhagic fever by reverse transcription-PCR in an outbreak setting and assessment of patient viral load as a predictor of outcome. *J Virol*. 2004;78:4330–4341.
59. MacNeil A, Farnon EC, Wamala J, et al. Proportion of deaths and clinical features in Bundibugyo Ebola virus infection, Uganda. *Emerg Infect Dis*. 2010;16:1969–1972.
60. World Health Organization. Ebola haemorrhagic fever in Sudan, 1976: report of a WHO/International Study Team. *Bull World Health Organ*. 1978;56:247–270.
61. World Health Organization. Ebola haemorrhagic fever in Zaire, 1976. *Bull World Health Organ*. 1978;56:271–293.
62. Leroy EM, Kumulungui B, Pourrut X, et al. Fruit bats as reservoirs of Ebola virus. *Nature*. 2005;438:575–576.
63. Baron RC, McCormick JB, Zubeir OA. Ebola virus disease in southern Sudan: hospital dissemination and intrafamilial spread. *Bull World Health Organ*. 1983;61:997–1003.
64. Bausch DG, Towner JS, Dowell SF, et al. Assessment of the risk of Ebola virus transmission from bodily fluids and fomites. *J Infect Dis*. 2007; 196(Suppl 20):S142–S147.
65. Dowell SF, Mukunu R, Ksiazek TG, et al. Transmission of Ebola hemorrhagic fever: a study of risk factors in family members, Kikwit, Democratic Republic of the Congo, 1995. Commission de Lutte contre les Epidemies a Kikwit. *J Infect Dis*. 1999;179(Suppl 1):S87–S91.
66. Geisbert TW. Marburg and Ebola hemorrhagic viruses (filoviruses). In: Bennett JE, Dolin R, Blaser MJ, ed. *Mandell, Douglas, and Bennett's Principles and Practice of Infectious Diseases*. 8th ed, Vol 2. Philadelphia, PA: Churchill Livingstone/Elsevier; 2015:1995–1999.
67. Barrette RW, Metwally SA, Rowland JM, et al. Discovery of swine as a host for the Reston ebolavirus. *Science*. 2009;325:204–206.
68. Centers for Disease Control and Prevention. Chronology of Marburg hemorrhagic fever outbreaks. CDC website. Available at: https://www.cdc.gov/vhf/marburg/resources/outbreak-table.html. Updated October 9, 2014; accessed November 13, 2016.
69. Bausch DG, Nichol ST, Muyembe-Tamfum JJ, et al. Marburg hemorrhagic fever associated with multiple genetic lineages of virus. *N Engl J Med*. 2006;355:909–919.
70. Towner JS, Khristova ML, Sealy TK, et al. Marburg virus genomics and association with a large hemorrhagic fever outbreak in Angola. *J Virol*. 2006;80:6497–6516.
71. Towner JS, Pourrut X, Albarino CG, et al. Marburg virus infection detected in a common African bat. *PLoS One*. 2007;2:e764.
72. Peters C. Lymphocytic choriomeningitis virus, Lassa virus, and the South American hemorrhagic fevers. In: Mandell GL, Bennett JE, Dolin R, eds. *Principles and Practice of Infectious Diseases*. 6th ed, Vol 2. New York, NY: Churchill Livingstone; 2004:2090–2098.
73. Keenlyside RA, McCormick JB, Webb PA, et al. Case-control study of *Mastomys natalensis* and humans in Lassa virus-infected households in Sierra Leone. *Am J Trop Med Hyg*. 1983;32:829–837.
74. Zaki SR, Goldsmith CS. Pathologic features of filovirus infections in humans. *Curr Top Microbiol Immunol*. 1999;235:97–116.
75. Geisbert TW, Young HA, Jahrling PB, et al. Pathogenesis of Ebola hemorrhagic fever in primate models: evidence that hemorrhage is not a direct effect of virus-induced cytolysis of endothelial cells. *Am J Pathol*. 2003;163:2371–2382.
76. McCormick JB, King IJ, Webb PA, et al. A case-control study of the clinical diagnosis and course of Lassa fever. *J Infect Dis*. 1987;155: 445–455.
77. Cummins D, McCormick JB, Bennett D, et al. Acute sensorineural deafness in Lassa fever. *JAMA*. 1990;264:2093–2096.
78. Rose JR. An outbreak of encephalomyelitis in Sierra Leone. *Lancet*. 1957; 273:914–916.
79. Ebola virus disease. U.S. healthcare workers and settings. CDC website. Available at: http://www.cdc.gov/vhf/ebola/healthcare-us/index.html. Accessed 3/15/2015.
80. McCormick JB, King IJ, Webb PA, et al. Lassa fever: effective therapy with ribavirin. *N Engl J Med*. 1986;314:20–26.
81. Fenner F, Henderson DA, Arita I, et al. Smallpox and its eradication. Available at: http://whqlibdoc.who.int/smallpox/9241561106.pdf. Accessed March 15, 2015.
82. Wehrle PF, Posch J, Richter KH, et al. An airborne outbreak of smallpox in a German hospital and its significance with respect to other recent outbreaks in Europe. *Bull World Health Organ*. 1970;43:669–679.
83. Damon I. Orthopoxviruses: vaccinia (smallpox vaccine), variola (smallpox), monkeypox, and cowpox. In: Mandell GL, Bennett JE, Dolin R, eds. *Principles and Practice of Infectious Diseases*. 6th ed, vol 2. New York, NY: Churchill Livingstone; 2004:1742–1751.
84. Joarder A, Tarantola D, Tulloch J. *The Eradication of Smallpox from Bangladesh*. New Delhi: World Health Organization South-East Asia Regional Office; 1980.
85. Downie AW, Fedson DS, Saint Vincent L, et al. Haemorrhagic smallpox. *J Hyg (Lond)*. 1969;67:619–629.
86. Rao A. *Smallpox*. Bombay: Kothari Book Depot; 1972.
87. Esposito JJ, Knight JC. 1985. Orthopoxvirus DNA: a comparison of restriction profiles and maps. *Virology*. 1985;143:230–251.
88. The CDC smallpox response plan and guidelines. CDC website. Available at: http://www.bt.cdc.gov/agent/smallpox/response-plan/index.asp#annex. Accessed 03/13/2015.
89. Nalca A, Rimoin AW, Bavari S, et al. Reemergence of monkeypox: prevalence, diagnostics, and countermeasures. *Clin Infect Dis*. 2005;41:1765–1771.
90. Huhn GD, Bauer AM, Yorita K, et al. Clinical characteristics of human monkeypox, and risk factors for severe disease. *Clin Infect Dis*. 2005;41:1742–1751.
91. Reed KD, Melski JW, Graham MB, et al. The detection of monkeypox in humans in the Western hemisphere. *N Engl J Med*. 2004;350:342–350.

92. Updated Interim CDC guidance for use of smallpox vaccine, cidofovir, and vaccinia immune globulin (VIG) for prevention and treatment in the setting of an outbreak of monkeypox infections. CDC website. Available at: http://www.cdc.gov/ncidod/monkeypox/treatmentguidelines.htm. Accessed 1/25/2007.
93. World malaria report 2005. WHO website. Available at: http://rbm.who.int/wmr2005/. Accessed 01/27/2005.
94. Treatment of malaria. Part 1. Reporting and epidemiology: evaluation and diagnosis. CDC website. Available at: http://www.cdc.gov/malaria/diagnosis_treatment/clinicians1.htm. Accessed March 15, 2015.
95. Local transmission of Plasmodium vivax Malaria—Palm Beach County, Florida, 2003. CDC website. Available at: http://www.cdc.gov/mmwr/preview/mmwrhtml/mm5238a3.htm. Accessed 01/25/2007.
96. Fairhurst R, Wellems T. Plasmodium species (malaria). In: Bennett JE, Dolin R, Blaser MJ, eds. *Mandell, Douglas, and Bennett's Principles and Practice of Infectious Diseases*. 8th ed, vol 2. Philadelphia, PA: Churchill Livingstone/Elsevier; 2015:3070–3090.
97. Malaria diagnosis and treatment in the United States. CDC website. Available at: http://www.cdc.gov/malaria/diagnosis_treatment/index.html. Accessed March 15, 2015.
98. Severe falciparum malaria. World Health Organization, Communicable Diseases Cluster. *Trans R Soc Trop Med Hyg*. 2000;94(Suppl 1):S1–S90.
99. Zucker JR, Campbell CC. Malaria: principles of prevention and treatment. *Infect Dis Clin North Am*. 1993;7:547–567.
100. Powell VI, Grima K. Exchange transfusion for malaria and Babesia infection. *Transfus Med Rev*. 2002;16:239–250.
101. Rocky Mountain spotted fever (RMSF). CDC website. Available at: http://www.cdc.gov/rmsf/stats/index.html. Accessed March 15, 2015.
102. Dalton MJ, Clarke MJ, Holman RC, et al. National surveillance for Rocky Mountain spotted fever, 1981–1992: epidemiologic summary and evaluation of risk factors for fatal outcome. *Am J Trop Med Hyg*. 1995;52:405–413.
103. Buckingham SC, Marshall GS, Schutze GE, et al. Clinical and laboratory features, hospital course, and outcome of Rocky Mountain spotted fever in children. *J Pediatr*. 2007;150:180–184.
104. Walker DH, Valbuena GA, Olano JP. Pathogenic mechanisms of diseases caused by Rickettsia. *Ann NY Acad Sci*. 2003;990:1–11.
105. Kirk JL, Fine DP, Sexton DJ, et al. Rocky Mountain spotted fever: a clinical review based on 48 confirmed cases, 1943–1986. *Medicine (Baltimore)*. 1990;69:35–45.
106. Helmick CG, Bernard KW, D'Angelo LJ. Rocky Mountain spotted fever: clinical, laboratory, and epidemiological features of 262 cases. *J Infect Dis*. 1984;150:480–488.
107. Walker DH, Hawkins HK, Hudson P. Fulminant Rocky Mountain spotted fever. Its pathologic characteristics associated with glucose-6-phosphate dehydrogenase deficiency. *Arch Pathol Lab Med*. 1983;107:121–125.
108. Archibald LK, Sexton DJ. Long-term sequelae of Rocky Mountain spotted fever. *Clin Infect Dis*. 1995;20:1122–1125.
109. Kirkland KB, Wilkinson WE, Sexton DJ. Therapeutic delay and mortality in cases of Rocky Mountain spotted fever. *Clin Infect Dis*. 1995;20:1118–1121.
110. Hattwick MA, Retailliau H, O'Brie, RJ, et al. Fatal Rocky Mountain spotted fever. *JAMA*. 1978;240:1499–1503.
111. Centers for Disease Control and Prevention. Diagnosis and management of tick-borne rickettsial diseases in the United States—Rocky Mountain spotted fever, ehrlichioses, and anaplasmosis: a practical guide for physicians and other health care and public health professionals. *MMWR*. 2006;55(RR-4):1–28.

CHAPTER

93

Emergent Pandemic Infections

LENNOX K. ARCHIBALD and GAUTAM SUBBAIAH KALYATANDA

INTRODUCTION

An epidemic of communicable infection that becomes very widespread, affects a whole region or continent, or spreads over several countries and affects many people is termed a pandemic. Three key factors set the conditions for a pandemic: the emergence of a new strain of microorganism; the ability of that strain to infect humans and cause serious illness: that is, the capacity of the organism to cause disease in an infected host (pathogenicity) and the severity of the disease produced (virulence); and the ability of the microorganism to spread easily among humans. Within intensive care units (ICUs) in tertiary care hospitals, factors that decrease transmission of communicable infection between individuals (e.g., reducing the likelihood of contact through isolation), adherence to infection control guidelines, immunization, herd immunity, increasing levels of natural immunity following infection, or depression of agent reservoirs and viability by control programs or seasonal climatic change are offset by the ICU environment, where patients generally have relatively high severity of illness scores and in situ medical devices (e.g., intravascular and urinary catheters), and antimicrobial prescribing remains uncurbed. Compounding the problem are fluctuations in staffing levels, varying degrees of immunization or vaccination among patients, and exposure of patients to health care personnel who move freely among other patients and health care personnel within the institution.

The relevance and importance of pandemic preparedness in critical care medicine is underscored by the reality that while there has been a general decrease in the total number of beds in US hospitals during the 1990s, the number of ICU beds has increased during the same period (1). This increase in the numbers of ICU beds suggest larger numbers of critically ill patients are being admitted to the inpatient services with the expected parallel increases in medical device usage and antimicrobial prescribing. The increases in device use and severity of illness scores increase the susceptibility of ICU patients to health care–associated infections—a problem compounded by the crowding that one would expect with the increased patient census in the event of a pandemic. In the wake of a pandemic, tertiary care hospitals with large numbers of beds will, by default, have to provide critical care management for greater numbers of patients in the first instance. The implications of this scenario are serious and complex, and include the increased human and material resources that would be required to manage very sick patients during a pandemic; limited availability of designated areas for cohorting patients who need to be isolated; the logistics of implementing and maintaining adherence to infection control practices and procedures during a pandemic; and the ever present risk of transmission of the pandemic agent among patients and personnel who may be called upon to "float" in other areas of the hospital.

This chapter addresses the following true or potentially emergent pandemic infections:

- Severe acute respiratory syndrome (SARS)—a true pandemic caused by a previously unrecognized corona virus
- Avian influenza—not yet a true pandemic but one which infectious diseases experts believe is imminent and long overdue
- Dengue fever and Dengue hemorrhagic fever—a mosquito-borne infection that has insidiously spread across the globe and considered a pandemic by many experts
- Tuberculosis—a pandemic caused by *Mycobacterium tuberculosis* and largely attributable directly to the nearly almost four-decade-long human immunodeficiency virus (HIV) pandemic
- Infections caused by *Staphylococcus aureus* resistant to methicillin group penicillins (methicillin-resistant *S. aureus* [MRSA])—perhaps the only bacterial microorganism that to reach pandemic proportions in health care settings around the world during the space of three decades
- Cholera

The importance of being able to address illnesses like Dengue has implications for the management of the newly recognized emerging infections caused by the Middle East respiratory syndrome coronavirus (MERS-CoV) and the Zika virus, which will be discussed briefly at the conclusion of the chapter.

The SARS pandemic in 2002 emerged suddenly and unexpectedly, affected health care workers, but was successfully controlled through the application of basic infection control principles and guidelines that had already been established, ratified, and validated. The expected, but not-as-yet seen, emergence of the impending avian influenza pandemic has underscored the importance of preparedness for an event that is so oftentimes decried as "crying wolf" by some and at the same time characterized as "a matter of when rather than if" by others. The fact remains that should an influenza pandemic occur, substantial numbers of persons with the infection will certainly require critical care management, underscoring the need for preparedness from diagnostic, management, control, and preventive perspectives. Although the epidemiology of the respective infections and public health preparedness will be alluded to, this chapter focuses more on the diagnosis and management of the infections, the relevant infection prevention and control interventions for the respective infections, and the obstacles that might be faced by ICU care givers during a pandemic.

SEVERE ACUTE RESPIRATORY SYNDROME

In November 2002, the Centers for Disease Control and Prevention (CDC) and the World Health Organization (WHO) reported an investigation of a multicountry outbreak of unexplained pneumonia referred to as SARS—officially, the first pandemic of the 21st century (2–5). SARS began as an outbreak of atypical pneumonia among patients in the Guangdon province, China. A Chinese physician, who had taken care of patients with SARS, subsequently traveled to Hong Kong and transmitted the infection to guests at the Metropole Hotel. These guests, in turn, unwittingly became the index cases for SARS outbreaks in Canada, Hong Kong, Singapore, Vietnam, and Taiwan (6–9). Subsequently, the condition was reported in more than 8,400 people globally and resulted in over 800 deaths (6,8,10). The case-fatality rate was estimated at 13% for patients under 60 years and 43% for those over 60 years (11).

SARS is caused by a novel strain of coronavirus (SARS-CoV) that was first identified in Canada in early March 2003 (12). Because genetic changes occur frequently in these viruses, it is thought that the outbreak might have been facilitated by cross species transmission of the virus; exotic animals from a Guangdong marketplace are likely to have been the immediate origin of the SARS-CoV that infected humans in the winters of 2002–2003 and 2003–2004 (13). Before the SARS pandemic, coronaviruses already were known to be ubiquitous and were recognized as the underlying cause of illness in various animals, including pigs, cattle, dogs, cats, and chickens, and had been found to be associated with upper respiratory infections and sometimes pneumonia in humans (14). Although the natural reservoir of SARS-CoV remains uncharacterized, the virus has been isolated from all of the above animals as well as civet cats, a delicacy in the Far East (15,16).

The primary mode of transmission of SARS-CoV is direct or indirect contact of mucous membranes (eyes, nose, or mouth) with large infectious respiratory droplets (17–19). This mode of transmission suggests that the major risk factor for infection in susceptible persons is intimate direct contact with one or more individuals who are already infected or colonized. However, the unusually rapid transmission of SARS-CoV suggests that airborne transmission through droplet nuclei (i.e., droplets <10 μm in diameter) might by playing a significant role in transmission. Droplet nuclei (the mode of transmission of influenza, measles, and tuberculosis), enable SARS-CoV to reach the lung alveoli in at-risk contacts (20). This would explain why aerosol-producing procedures, such as bronchoscopy or nebulized medication, have been implicated as independent risk factors in SARS-CoV transmission and outbreaks (21–23). The hospital environment provides an efficient site for transmission of SARS-CoV infection and, because the virus survives for many days in feces and when dried on environmental surfaces, fomites can play a role in transmission (24). The problem is compounded by the difficulty in differentiating SARS from other clinical syndromes (25).

The phenomenon of "superspreading events" plays an important role in the transmission of SARS-CoV in health care settings (19,22,26–28). The mechanism of "superspreading events" involves SARS-CoV transmission from one individual to several secondary cases (22,23,25,26,29,30). Risk factors associated with "superspreading events" include high severity of illness scores, higher age, and increased numbers of secondary contacts (25). Superspreading has played major roles in the transmission of SARS-CoV within health care settings in Singapore and Toronto (12,25,26,31,32).

SARS is characterized by rapid onset of high fever, malaise, myalgia, chills, rigors, and sore throat, followed by shortness of breath, cough, and radiographic evidence of pneumonia (10,12,26,29,33). The median incubation period ranged is generally between 4 and 7 days (range 2 to 10) (21). Some patients develop profuse watery diarrhea, though, as stated above, the role of feco-oral transmission remains uncharacterized (33). After 1 week (34,35) of illness, patients with SARS frequently develop respiratory failure, which often requires critical care management for respiratory support and mechanical ventilation (10,33). Chest radiographs frequently show nonspecific patchy opacification, but may be normal during the early stages of the infection (34). Because of the nonspecific clinical manifestations at presentation, all cases of community-acquired pneumonia are suspect during a SARS pandemic, and a history of exposure to a patient with probable SARS or travel to SARS-affected geographic areas should heighten clinical suspicion and increase the likelihood of the diagnosis (36). In patients with suspected SARS or patients who develop respiratory symptoms during a SARS pandemic, the workup for known causes of community-acquired pneumonia should certainly be performed, and appropriate specimens should be sent to the designated State Health Department or CDC for viral identification and serologic analysis.

Laboratory features include lymphopenia, thrombocytopenia, and elevated levels of lactate dehydrogenase, aspartate aminotransferase, and creatinine kinase (12). SARS-CoV can be detected by the polymerase chain reaction (PCR) in respiratory secretions and other body fluids; however, PCR is not sensitive during the early stages of the illness. Specific SARS-CoV antibodies are detectable, but play little or no role in making a diagnosis during the acute stages of the pneumonia, especially during a pandemic. However, detection of antibodies provides a retrospective diagnosis as part of clinical confirmation or surveillance activities. In virologically or serologically documented infections caused by SARS-CoV, viral RNA may persist for some time in patients who seroconvert, and some patients may lack an antibody response to SARS-CoV more than 21 days after illness onset. An upsurge of antibody response is associated with the aggravation of respiratory failure that requires ventilator support (37). The presence of underlying disease, high initial C-reactive protein levels, and positive SARS-CoV in nasopharyngeal aspirate samples are associated with a higher risk of respiratory failure and mortality (36).

Prevention and Control of SARS

In Canada, transmission of the SARS-CoV occurred predominantly among health care workers, presumably through close contact with symptomatic persons (12,38). Health care workers made up a large proportion of cases, accounting for 37% to 63% of suspected SARS cases in highly affected countries (17,39–41). Thus, the basic tenets of prevention and control include institution and implementation of traditional infection control practices and procedures, early detection and prompt isolation of infected patients, contact tracing, and quarantine of contact persons (27,42). Because SARS-CoV is likely not going to be identified before recommended infection control precautions are implemented, the primary strategy to reduce transmission is early recognition and isolation of patients who might have the syndrome. In Vietnam and Canada, the pandemic was brought under control through the institution of a constellation of interventions that included the following: (i) early detection, and prompt isolation of case-patients;

(ii) implementation of traditional infection control practices (i.e., scrupulous handwashing, and environmental decontamination; (iii) use of personal protective equipment, where deemed necessary; (iv) initiation of surveillance activities for patients with SARS; and (v) education and training of patients, relatives, and care givers (43,44).

Transmission of SARS-CoV may occur on an aircraft when infected persons fly during the asymptomatic phase of illness (45). Moreover, because asymptomatic persons (i.e., unrecognized cases) remain a significant source of transmission, a detailed travel history for patients during a pandemic is essential—more specifically, travel to or from SARS-endemic regions. In a retrospective cohort study of nurses in Toronto, assisting during intubation, suctioning before intubation, and manipulation of oxygen masks were found to be significant risk factors for acquiring SARS (27). This study also found that consistently wearing a mask, regardless of type (i.e., whether surgical or particulate respirator N-95 type) was protective for nurses and resulted in an 80% reduction in risk of infection (27). Of note, the risk of SARS-CoV transmission and infection among nurses who consistently wore N-95 masks was approximately half that for the surgical mask; however, this difference was not statistically different (27). These data concur with the findings of Seto et al., who established that both surgical and N-95 masks were protective against SARS for health care workers in Hong Kong (19), and with anecdotal reports from Bach Mai hospital in Hanoi, Vietnam, where SARS was controlled and contained largely through adherence to basic infection control principles, use of surgical masks, and quarantine of close contacts (unpublished communication, Bach Mai Hospital, Hanoi, Vietnam). Finally, Loeb et al. established unequivocally that use of personal protective equipment (N-95 masks, gowns, gloves, and goggles) were important preventive measures when caring for SARS patients (27). Ultimately, improvement in the outcomes of patients with SARS is dependent on heightened levels of clinical suspicion, rapid case detection and isolation, strict attention and adherence to infection control policies and guidelines, and development of reliable diagnostic tests and effective antiviral and immunomodulatory agents, and vaccines (36,37).

INFLUENZA

Influenza is an acute febrile illness that is caused by a group of respiratory viruses that primarily infect the columnar cells of the upper respiratory tract. Humans are the major hosts of these viruses, which are the most important cause of wintertime respiratory morbidity throughout the world. Despite vaccines and antiviral therapies, influenza epidemics still occur every year. The occurrence of three major influenza pandemics during the 20th century was not an aberration but rather a manifestation of the continuing emergence of virulent strains of a virus that has adapted for efficient human transmission and which continues to undergo point mutations and genetic exchange or reassortment (46,47). The magnitude of influenza outbreaks during the winter is dictated by the trilateral interaction between the influenza virus, susceptible persons, and the environment in which this interaction takes place. Intrinsic viral factors that determine the size of an outbreak for a particular year include the degree of molecular change in the virus compared with the previous year, and the pathogenicity and virulence of the new winter strain. Patient factors that determine the size of the outbreak for a particular year include the numbers of susceptible individuals and the proportion of individuals who received that year's influenza vaccine. Important environmental factors that facilitate transmission include crowding, the ever-present issue with hospital ICUs.

Influenza viruses belong to the orthomyxovirus family; these viruses are enveloped, pleomorphic, and contain negative, single-stranded RNA, which are organized into eight gene segments that code for ten proteins. They are classified into three major serotypes—influenza A, B, and C—based on differences in a stable, internal ribonucleoprotein antigen. Two surface glycoproteins—hemagglutinin and neuraminidase—constitute the major antigens and are therefore the prime targets of the protective host immune response and vaccine prophylaxis.

Influenza A is the most extensively studied of the three types; influenza B is more antigenically stable and usually occurs in more localized outbreaks; influenza C appears to be a relatively minor cause of disease and differs considerably from A and B types, possessing only seven RNA segments and no neuraminidase. Only influenza A and B cause epidemic infections and disease in humans.

Hemagglutinin is so named because of its ability to agglutinate red blood cells from chickens or guinea pigs in vitro, and facilitates viral attachment to the host respiratory epithelial cells via sialic acid-containing receptors. Once bound, hemagglutinin facilitates the entry of the viral genome into the target cells by causing the fusion of host endosomal membrane with the viral membrane; antibody to hemagglutinin is protective. The neuraminidase glycoprotein is involved in viral entry into the host cell by helping release virions from cells, and is important in the process of the viral envelope fusion with the host cell membrane as a prerequisite to viral entry into the human cell. Antibodies to neuraminidase appear to modify disease severity by inhibiting the spread of virus in the infected host and limiting the amount of virus released from host cells.

Among the 18 known hemagglutinins subtypes (H1 through H18) and eleven neuraminidase glycoprotein subtypes (N1 through N11) of influenza A viruses, three major subtypes of hemagglutinins (H1, H2, and H3) and two subtypes of neuraminidases (N1 and N2) are currently in general circulation among people (H1N1, H1N2, H3N2). The three 20th century pandemics were caused by strains of avian influenza A viruses classified as H1N1 for 1918, H2N2 for 1957, and H3N2 for the 1968 pandemic virus. The 1968 H3N2 strain had the same neuraminidase glycoprotein as the 1957 H2N2 strain. Influenza viruses are named on the basis of the following nomenclature: type/geographic source/strain number/year isolated (specific H and N subtypes). Thus, for the 2015/2016 influenza season, the vaccine includes A/California/7/2009 (H1N1) 09-like virus, A/Switzerland/9715293/2013 (H3N2)-like virus, B/Phuket/3073/2013-like virus, and B/Brisbane/60/2008-like antigens (CDC, Atlanta, GA). These viruses were used because they are representative of influenza viruses that are anticipated to circulate in the United States during the 2015–2016 influenza season and have favorable growth properties in eggs (CDC, Atlanta, GA).

A key feature of influenza A viruses is their ability to undergo periodic antigenic change, more commonly and to a much greater degree than other respiratory viruses. These antigenic changes occur through two completely different mechanisms: antigenic "drift" and antigenic "shift." In antigenic drift, point mutations in the hemagglutinin or neuraminidase genes cause minor antigenic changes to the main surface glycoproteins resulting in strain variants. Antigenic drift within major subtypes can involve either the hemagglutinin or neuraminidase antigen or the genes encoding nonstructural proteins, and can result from a single mutation on the viral RNA. *Antigenic drift* is a continuous process that leads to emergence of strain variants, most of which form evolutionary dead ends. Eventually, however, a strain becomes predominant worldwide for 1 to 3 years on average. Immunity against one strain might be limited and antibodies formed to older viruses gradually lose their ability to protect against newer strains. As a result, people recurrently become susceptible to influenza and vaccine strains must be updated annually. Only antigenic drifts in the hemagglutinin have been described for influenza B viruses.

Antigenic shift is the emergence of a novel human influenza virus subtype through genetic reassortment between human and animal viruses or through direct animal- or poultry-to-human transmission resulting in a virus bearing new hemagglutinin or neuraminidase antigens. Basically, reassortment occurs when an avian virus and human-adapted virus "swap genes" in a coinfected cell of an animal or human, and a third virus results that can be readily transmitted by and between humans. Antigenic shift is relatively infrequent and, because there is little or no immunity to a novel virus, it remains the initiating event for pandemics, which occur if there is efficient and sustained virus transmission among humans. Compared with regular seasonal epidemics, the emergence of a novel influenza virus through antigenic shift will result in greater numbers of infections and more serious illness among infected persons. Antigenic shifts are associated with epidemics and pandemics of influenza A (c.f., antigenic drifts which are associated with more localized outbreaks).

The incubation period of the influenza A virus is about 2 days. Symptoms characteristically begin with the abrupt onset of fever (>37.8°C), chills, headache, myalgia, and malaise, anorexia, sore throat, coughing, sneezing, and shortness of breath. Fever peaks within 24 hours of onset and lasts 1 to 5 days. Within 6 to 12 hours, the illness reaches maximum severity and a dry nonproductive cough develops. Symptoms may range from afebrile respiratory illnesses, similar to the common cold, to systemic involvement with relatively little involvement of the respiratory system. In uncomplicated influenza, physical findings are generally few or nonspecific and may improve over 2 to 5 days, followed by gradual improvement although the illness may last for 1 week or more. Some patients develop persistent weakness or easy fatigability that may last for several weeks. The clinical outcome is directly dependent on the viral load, which peaks at about 48 hours after exposure. The larger the infecting dose of virus, the more severe the course of illness. Viral shedding begins 24 to 48 hours before the onset of symptoms and continues for about a week after the onset of the illness.

Complications Associated with Influenza A

Influenza can result in significant pulmonary (involving the tracheobronchial tree and lungs) and extrapulmonary complications. Pulmonary complications include acute viral or secondary bacterial pneumonia. Persons at high risk for influenza complications include the following: children under 2 years; adults over 65 years; pregnant and postpartum women (within 2 weeks after delivery); American Indians and Alaska Natives; persons who are morbidly obese (BMI >40); residents of long-term care facilities; persons with immunosuppression; persons under 19 years who are receiving long-term aspirin therapy; persons with chronic medical conditions, such as chronic obstructive pulmonary disease, chronic cardiovascular disease, cirrhosis of the liver, chronic renal failure, diabetes, long-standing rheumatoid arthritis; immunocompromised patients; or neurologic and neurodevelopmental conditions; the elderly are particularly susceptible.

The respiratory epithelium becomes damaged within 24 hours of infection, rendering the patient susceptible to secondary bacterial pneumonia. At-risk patients usually develop secondary bacterial pneumonia 4 to 14 days after the onset of influenza symptoms. Bacterial pathogens that commonly cause superinfection include *Streptococcus pneumoniae*, *S. aureus*, *Haemophilus influenzae*, or group A *Streptococcus*. Bacterial superinfection can develop at any time in the acute or convalescent phase of the infection and is often characterized by an abrupt worsening of the patient's condition after initial stabilization. Although acute viral pneumonia is relatively uncommon, patients with significant underlying cardiovascular disease appear to be most susceptible and commonly affected. Mortality rates among patients with bacterial pneumonia and acute viral pneumonia are relatively high in the elderly.

The clinician must be alert because patients with viral pneumonia usually present with the typical features of influenza but then develop an exacerbation of respiratory symptoms, hemoptysis, and respiratory failure. Chest radiographs in patients with viral pneumonia generally have a reticular interstitial pattern rather than radiologic characteristics of consolidation; blood gases reflect severe hypoxemia; and cultures of the blood and respiratory tract are generally negative for bacterial growth.

Extrapulmonary complications include musculoskeletal abnormalities, such as myositis and rhabdomyolysis; neurologic sequelae—encephalopathy, encephalitis, transverse myelitis, or Guillain–Barré syndrome; myocarditis; and rarely, Reye syndrome (48). The latter is almost never seen nowadays with the decreased use of aspirin as an antipyretic and analgesic in children. Mortality rates attributable to influenza in patients with underlying chronic medical conditions are probably underestimated because many of these patients die ostensibly through exacerbation of the underlying chronic respiratory or cardiovascular condition, which in fact rendered them susceptible to the influenza virus in the first place.

Avian Influenza A

Influenza A viruses naturally infect avian and mammalian species; wild aquatic birds are considered the prime reservoir. Through antigenic shift, influenza A viruses that are naturally resident in wild waterfowl (e.g., aquatic ducks, geese, and swans) acquire the potential for transmission to humans. Viruses are shed in respiratory secretions and feces of birds and can survive at low temperatures and low humidity for days to weeks. Avian influenza A viruses are classified in one of the following two categories: low pathogenic or highly pathogenic forms. The criteria for high pathogenicity include one or more of the following: (i) any avian influenza A virus that is lethal for 4-week-old chickens in the laboratory; (ii) any H5 or H7 virus that has a multibasic amino acid sequence at the hemagglutinin cleavage site; or (iii) any non-H5 or non-H7 that kills one to five of eight inoculated chickens and grows in cell culture without trypsin (49); low pathogenic infections are generally much milder in all avian species. With rare exceptions, highly pathogenic avian influenza viruses are usually H5 or H7 subtypes.

Risk factors for H5N1 infection include the presence in the household and the handling of dead or sick poultry in an H5N1-affected area, and lack of access to an indoor water source (50). Human-to-human transmission, though limited, has been documented and is particularly relevant for health care personnel—a retrospective case-control study has presented epidemiologic evidence that H5N1 viruses were transmitted from patients to health care workers (51). Some studies suggest that exposure alone to persons who might be a source of H5N1 infection might not necessarily be the only risk factor for this mode of transmission (50,52,53). These data suggest two possible mechanisms for transmission: inhalation or conjunctival deposition of large infectious droplets that could travel short distances, or presence or consumption of infected poultry in the home (54).

The incubation period for human avian influenza A (H5N1) infection is 2 to 8 days but may be as long as 17 days (48). The clinical course in humans is characterized by rapid deterioration and high mortality rates. Patients tend to develop high viremic levels and intense inflammatory responses—a finding that had been established previously for seasonal influenza A virus strains (55). Early symptoms of influenza A H5N1 include a high fever, diarrhea, vomiting, abdominal pain, chest pain, and bleeding from the nose and gums (48). Pneumonia that did not respond to antimicrobials is a common complication, suggesting that the process is likely a viral pneumonia, usually without bacterial superinfection at the time of hospitalization (48). Data from Vietnam suggest that multifocal consolidation involving at least two zones is the most common radiographic abnormality at the time of admission (48). In severe cases, respiratory failure occurs within 3 to 5 days after the onset of symptoms and may progress to the acute respiratory distress syndrome (ARDS) within a week from the time of onset of illness (56). Other documented complications include the reactive hemophagocytic syndrome, extensive hepatic central lobular necrosis, acute renal tubular necrosis, rhabdomyolysis, pancytopenia, cardiac dilatation, and dysrhythmias, ventilator-associated pneumonia (VAP), pulmonary hemorrhage, pneumothorax, or the systemic inflammatory response syndrome (SIRS) without documented bacteremia (48,56–60).

The mortality rate among patients who acquire influenza A (H5N1) infection is high. Since 2003, over 50% of persons who have been treated for avian H5N1 infection have died, with the highest death rates among persons younger than 15 years in Thailand (48). The most common cause of death is progressive respiratory failure.

Laboratory Diagnostic Tests

Common laboratory findings include leucopenia (especially lymphopenia), thrombocytopenia, raised aminotransferase levels, and elevated creatinine levels (48). Diagnosis of influenza requires collection of appropriate clinical specimens. For example, respiratory viruses grow in the epithelial lining of the nasal mucosa. Thus, a nasal wash is the optimal specimen for recovering respiratory viruses. Because the influenza virus is enveloped, it is less stable and may become nonviable during specimen collection and processing. The specimen, ideally, should be transported immediately to the laboratory in a sterile container; specimens that cannot be delivered immediately to the laboratory should be refrigerated until transported. Dry nasal swabs, throat swabs, or calcium alginate swabs are not appropriate for recovering respiratory viruses and should be discouraged. Unlike human influenza A infection, avian influenza (H5N1) is more commonly detected in, and has higher viral RNA levels in, pharyngeal versus nasal specimens (48).

Rapid enzyme immunoassay (EIA) testing of nasal washes for influenza A and B are available and are useful in the outpatient clinic or the emergency room. In these settings, physicians may use the EIA test results to discharge patients or to initiate prompt therapy and infection control measures. The EIA test is approved for nasopharyngeal swabs, though nasal washes afford the best sensitivity. Rapid antigen tests are less sensitive in detecting influenza A (H5N1) infections compared with real-time PCR assays (56).

Rapid inpatient diagnosis is achievable through use of fluorescent antibody to directly detect the influenza antigen. This immunofluorescence testing of properly taken specimens for influenza A and B is usually performed with a respiratory viral battery that includes adenovirus; influenza A and B; parainfluenza 1, 2, and 3; and respiratory syncytial virus. The fluorescent antibody test has a relatively high sensitivity and specificity and turnaround time is approximately 2 hours. Fluorescent antibody-negative specimens should be cultured for the above respiratory viruses (influenza cell cultures take about 5 to 7 days to grow). As with respiratory syncytial virus, viral culture is the gold standard for laboratory diagnosis of influenza A.

Serologic testing requires testing of paired serum specimens: the first taken during the acute phase; the second taken 2 to 4 weeks later; the diagnosis is made by demonstrating a fourfold or greater increase in complement-fixing or hemagglutination inhibition antibody titers in the paired serum specimens. However, serologic testing for influenza A and B has a low sensitivity. For these reasons, serologic testing is not useful for diagnosis in the acute phase of influenza; it may, however, be used for establishing a retrospective diagnosis and for surveillance activities and epidemiologic studies.

Rapid influenza antigen diagnostic test (RIDT) platforms are now used by the majority of hospitals in the United States and generally yield results within 30 minutes. In areas of low prevalence, false-negatives are frequent and specificity is reduced (61). A negative RIDT does not exclude a diagnosis of influenza. Thus, all hospitalized and all high-risk patients with suspected or confirmed influenza should be treated as soon as possible without waiting for confirmatory testing (62). The CDC has published a comprehensive guidance for clinicians on the use of RIDTs at http://www.cdc.gov/flu/professionals/diagnosis/clinician_guidance_ridt.htm#figure 1.

Therapy

Medical management of influenza A infection comprises three essential components: (i) symptomatic, supportive therapy—rest, fluid replacement (oral or intravenous as deemed appropriate), and cautious use of analgesics, keeping in mind the association between salicylate use and Reye syndrome in children; (ii) initiation of antiviral therapy; and (iii) timely anticipation of complications, such as bacterial superinfection. Antimicrobial prophylaxis has not been shown to increase or reduce the risks for developing bacterial superinfection. However, there is always a risk that empirical antimicrobial therapy could increase the emergence of antimicrobial resistance among microorganisms in the respiratory tract.

Antiviral treatment is recommended as soon as possible for all persons with suspected or confirmed influenza requiring hospitalization or who have progressive, severe, or complicated illness regardless of previous health or vaccination status. Treatment should not be delayed while the results of diagnostic testing are pending.

Neuraminidase inhibitors, such as Oseltamivir and Zanamivir are the mainstay antiviral agents currently prescribed. They act by inhibiting the cleavage of the virus from sialic acid, which blocks the release of new virus thereby preventing the propagation of infection. Oseltamivir is FDA approved for patients ages one and older and therapy should be started within 24 to 48 hours of symptoms. Neuraminidase inhibitors are active against both influenza A and B; for hospitalized patients, treatment with oral or enterically administered Oseltamivir is recommended. Limited data suggest that Oseltamivir administered by oro/nasogastric tube is well absorbed in critically ill patients with influenza, including those persons on continuous renal replacement therapy (CRRT), or patients on extracorporeal membrane oxygenation (ECMO). In patients with severe influenza disease, inhaled Zanamivir is not recommended because of lack of data for use in this patient population. Finally, for patients who remain severely ill after 5 days of treatment, longer treatment courses may be considered.

At the present time, there are insufficient data to support *routine* IV Peramivir in hospitalized patients. However, for critically ill patients who cannot tolerate or absorb oral Oseltamivir because of suspected or known gastric stasis, malabsorption, or gastrointestinal bleeding, the use of intravenous Peramivir or investigational intravenous Zanamivir may be considered. If Peramivir is used in severely ill patients, single dose treatment should not be given. For severely ill patients, adult dose of 600 mg IV once daily for 5 days is recommended (dose for children >6 years: 10 mg/kg once daily [≤600 mg] for 5 days); minimum of 5 days duration (63).

Adamantanes, such as amantadine and rimantadine, are M2 protein blockers that used to be active against influenza A. These M2 protein blockers work by causing a loss in ion channel function, inhibition of ribonucleoprotein release, and of the uncoating process. However, the occurrence of adamantane resistance among circulating influenza A viruses increased rapidly worldwide beginning during 2003–2004. The percentage of influenza A virus isolates submitted from throughout the world to the World Health Organization Collaborating Center for Surveillance, Epidemiology, and Control of Influenza at CDC that were adamantane-resistant increased from 0.4% during 1994–1995 to 12.3% during 2003–2004 (64). High levels of resistance to the adamantanes (amantadine and rimantadine) persist among the influenza A viruses currently circulating (65–68). Moreover, the adamantanes are not effective against influenza B viruses (65). For this reason, amantadine and rimantadine are not recommended for antiviral treatment or chemoprophylaxis of currently circulating influenza A virus strains at the present time.

Current recommendations for treating influenza A are summarized as follows:

- Oral oseltamivir (Tamiflu)—recommended for treatment of all ages and chemoprophylaxis for age over 3 months
- Inhaled zanamivir (Relenza): effective against influenza A and B. Used when predominant circulating strain is resistant to Tamiflu and recommended for treatment in persons aged over 7 years and chemoprophylaxis for age over 5 years
- Intravenous peramivir (Rapivab): approved on December 19, 2014, for the treatment of acute *uncomplicated* influenza in persons over 18 years (600-mg dose infused over 15 to 30 minutes).

Patients with suspected influenza A (H5N1) should promptly receive a neuraminidase inhibitor pending the results of diagnostic laboratory testing (48); early treatment provides the greatest clinical benefit (56). Any patient with suspected or confirmed influenza in the following categories should be treated with a neuraminidase inhibitor:

- All hospitalized patients
- Has severe, complicated, or progressive illness, including individuals in the outpatient setting, who have severe or prolonged progressive symptoms or who develop complications such as pneumonia
- Individuals who are at higher risk for influenza complications (hospitalized or outpatient). Patients in this group include the following:
  - Children younger than 2 years (although all children younger than 5 years are considered at higher risk for complications from influenza, the highest risk is for those younger than 2 years)
  - Adults aged 65 years and older
  - Persons with chronic pulmonary (including asthma), cardiovascular (except hypertension alone), renal, hepatic, hematologic (including sickle cell disease), and metabolic disorders (including diabetes mellitus), or neurologic and neurodevelopment conditions (including disorders of the brain, spinal cord, peripheral nerve, and muscle such as cerebral palsy, epilepsy [seizure disorders], stroke, intellectual disability [mental retardation], moderate to severe developmental delay, muscular dystrophy, or spinal cord injury)
  - Persons with immunosuppression, including that caused by medications or by HIV infection
  - Women who are pregnant or postpartum (within 2 weeks after delivery)
  - Persons aged younger than 19 years who are receiving long-term aspirin therapy
  - American Indians/Alaska Natives
  - Persons who are morbidly obese (i.e., body mass index is equal to or >40)
  - Residents of nursing homes and other chronic-care facilities.

Antiviral treatment may be prescribed on the basis of clinical judgment for any previously healthy (non-high risk) patient with suspected or confirmed influenza. When indicated, antiviral treatment should be started as soon as possible after illness onset. Ideally, treatment should be initiated within 48 hours of symptom onset and should not be delayed even for a few hours to wait for the results of testing; a negative RIDT does not rule out a diagnosis of influenza.

Of note, antiviral therapy initiated after 48 hours can still be beneficial in some patients. Some observational studies of hospitalized patients suggest that treatment might still be beneficial when initiated 4 or 5 days after symptom onset. Observational data in pregnant women have shown antiviral treatment to provide benefit when started 3 or 4 days after onset and a randomized placebo-controlled study suggested clinical benefit when Oseltamivir was initiated 72 hours after illness onset among febrile children with uncomplicated influenza (66,69–72).

Resistance to oseltamivir has been recognized and documented; in addition, some influenza viruses may become resistant to oseltamivir and peramivir during antiviral treatment with one of these agents and remain susceptible to zanamivir. For this reason, investigational use of intravenous zanamivir should be considered for treatment of severely ill patients with Oseltamivir-resistant influenza virus infection.

Adverse events associated with neuraminidase inhibitors have been recognized and documented: oral Oseltamivir is associated with a slightly increased risk of nausea and vomiting over placebo. However, these symptoms are mild and transient and improve when taken with food. Inhaled zanamivir can cause bronchospasm and is not recommended for persons with underlying airways disease such as asthma, COPD. Intravenous peramivir is associated with a slightly increased risk of diarrhea and neutropenia over placebo.

The utility of antiviral therapy in noncomplicated influenza infection remains a highly debatable issue. Some studies have shown that oseltamivir therapy is associated with modest reduction in the duration of symptoms and virus shedding in people with uncomplicated influenza infections, even when treatment was started 48 hours or longer after illness onset (69). Overall, though, there is a paucity of data on the utility of antiviral agents in patients who have already developed complications, such as viral pneumonia or bacterial superinfection. Neuraminidase inhibitors are efficacious in preventing febrile illness though systemic infection can still occur; they also provide a degree of protection against the next wave of the pandemic virus (73). The role of corticosteroids and immunomodulators, such as interferon alpha, remains uncharacterized.

Infection Control within the Health Care Setting

Transmission of influenza in health care settings is well documented, and can occur between patients and health care personnel or health care workers can transmit the virus to patients or other health care workers. During a pandemic, control and prevention of influenza A (H5N1) transmission in the inpatient setting requires institution of current guidelines for the prevention of transmission in health care settings (74); scrupulous attention to infection control practices and procedures, including strict attention to handwashing and hygienic practices in conjunction with established guidelines for the prevention of hospital-acquired pneumonia (42,48,74). As recommended for the control of SARS, use of N-95 masks has been shown to be effective in reducing person-to-person transmission. However, surgical masks are acceptable if N-95 masks are not available (19,27,75).

The best prevention for influenza is to avoid the illness, though this is largely unavoidable during a pandemic. Annual influenza vaccination is recommended for all high-risk patients (e.g., those with chronic lung or cardiac disease) and their close contacts, including medical personnel and household members and universal vaccination of all children is recommended (76). However, it is widely appreciated that should an avian influenza A pandemic occur, a vaccine against the pandemic strain will not be immediately available. Moreover, because the major determinant of protection afforded by the influenza vaccine recipient is the generation of hemagglutinin antibodies that provide protection approximately 2 weeks after administration, immediate benefit will not be rendered to vaccine recipients. Chemoprophylaxis with Oseltamivir once daily for 7 to 10 days has been suggested for persons who might have had an unprotected exposure to avian influenza H5N1 (48,77,78). Other data suggest that preexposure prophylaxis might warrant consideration if there is evidence that the influenza A (H5N1) strain is being transmitted person-to-person with increased efficiency or if there is a likelihood of a high-risk exposure (48).

DENGUE

Dengue fever is a mosquito-borne disease caused by a Flavivirus, and is currently the most common arthropod-borne viral disease in the world. Though most cases have been reported in Asia, the number of countries with endemic Dengue activity has increased dramatically in recent decades (79–82). The Dengue fever virus is now endemic in over 100 tropical and subtropical countries in Southeast Asia, Africa, the Western Pacific, Africa, the Americas, the Caribbean, and the Eastern Mediterranean (83). The annual occurrences of Dengue fever and its serious sequelae—Dengue hemorrhagic fever—are estimated at about 100 million and 500,000 cases, respectively, with an estimated mortality rate of 25,000 per year (79,81,83). Because many of the countries where the virus is endemic remain popular tourist areas and international travelers can both acquire and spread Dengue virus infection, the public and clinical implications of this infection remain pertinent to critical care specialists in both developed and economically less-developed countries (79–81,83–85).

The Dengue fever virus is a small mosquito-borne virus from the viral family *Flaviviridae*, genus *Flavivirus*, and contains a single strand of nonsegmented, positive sense RNA enclosed in a tight envelope. Disease is caused by four closely related but antigenically distinct serotypes—DENV types 1 to 4. Worldwide, the virus is transmitted person-to-person primarily by the female *Aedes aegypti* mosquito (79–81,83–86); in the continental United States, two major Dengue vectors, *Ae. aegypti* and *Ae. albopictus* mosquitoes, are widely distributed and are likely to play important roles in transmission of the virus in North America during a Dengue fever pandemic (81,87). These are day-biting species well adapted to urban settings and found inside and around houses, particularly in places where clean stagnant water has collected in receptacles, such as tires, domicile house rainwater tanks, empty oil drums, discarded plastic containers and soft drink cans, or plant pots. Humans are the principal reservoir for the Dengue virus and are able to sustain a viremia for up to 10 days after acquiring the infection; there is no known natural animal reservoir of infection. After it takes a blood meal from an infected human, the mosquito vector transmits the virus to new hosts during subsequent blood feeds. Transmission of Dengue virus infection in patient care settings and among laboratory personnel has been described and attributed largely to mucocutaneous contact with infected blood from travelers, needle stick injury, or blood transfusion (88–94).

The incubation period of Dengue fever ranges from 3 to 14 days during which the virus multiplies in lymph nodes. Infection with any of the four serotypes can cause disease ranging from mild infection (Dengue fever) with complete recovery to severe disease (i.e., Dengue hemorrhagic fever and Dengue shock syndrome) that may result in substantial morbidity and mortality. "Typical" Dengue fever has an abrupt onset and is characterized by high fever, headache, retro-orbital pain worsened by moving the eyes, pain in the joints, limbs, and muscles ("breakbone fever"), and a rash that resembles sunburn. Other symptoms include abdominal pain and vomiting, and cough is particularly common in children. On examination, the face is usually flushed, the eyes congested, and cervical lymph nodes enlarged. The fever lasts for about a week, but after 2 to 4 days often falls to normal, returning after another 24 hours, giving rise to the so-called saddle-back fever curve. During the second fever phase, the patient often develops a characteristic maculopapular rash over the entire body except the face, and the pulse tends to be disproportionately slow. Uncomplicated Dengue fever is a mild form of the condition with the characteristic clinical features of fever, joint ache, severe headaches, weakness, and skin rashes. This form of Dengue fever is not fatal, rarely affects children, and usually lasts just 3 to 4 days.

Through a mechanism known as antibody-dependent enhancement (or *immune enhancement*), previous or sequential infection with the Dengue virus increases the risk for progression to Dengue hemorrhagic fever and Dengue shock syndrome in subsequent infections, which are also more likely on reinfection with a different serotype (95,96). The immunologic response is an anamnestic reaction with IgG antibodies persisting from the previous infection. Dengue hemorrhagic fever is characterized by high fever, alteration in microvascular permeability leading to plasma leakage, hepatomegaly, and circulatory failure—the key feature of *Dengue shock syndrome* (85,95,97). The patient's face is pale or mottled and cyanosed, skin clammy and cold, and pulse thready. In addition, the palms and soles become red and edematous, and the patient may develop petechiae and purpuric lesions. Bleeding varies from these skin lesions to epistaxis, bleeding from the gums or gastrointestinal tract, or hematuria. Unless urgently treated, death ensues from profound shock, severe bleeding, or both within a few hours of presentation.

Plasma leakage is a result of damage to endothelial cells during the course of Dengue infection; this damage is attributable to cytokine release rather than a cytopathic effect of the virus itself on the endothelium (87,95). Progression to the Dengue hemorrhagic syndrome is not uniform among persons infected with the Dengue virus. Several factors determine whether or not an infected person will develop the syndrome:

- HLA gene linkage or ethnicity has been shown to make a person susceptible or resistant to the virus; for example, persons of African ethnicity harbor a gene that proffers resistance, and Dengue hemorrhagic fever appears to occur rarely in European travelers (87,98–100).
- Vascular permeability is age related with very young children and the elderly most susceptible (81,101,102).
- Differences in intrinsic virulence of various virus strains explain the ability of some strains, more than others, to cause progression of Dengue fever to Dengue hemorrhagic fever and the Dengue shock syndrome (87,95).

Vascular permeability is the key feature in Dengue hemorrhagic fever; however, as Halstead pointed out, at its onset, vascular permeability exhibits only subtle changes, which can make early diagnosis difficult (87,95,103). The sphygmomanometer cuff tourniquet test has been widely used to screen children for vascular permeability, and though a positive test is an early correlate of Dengue hemorrhagic fever (87), the test itself has a sensitivity of only 42% and a specificity of 94% (104–107). The tourniquet test is carried out by inflating a blood pressure cuff to midway between the systolic and diastolic BP for 15 minutes. The number of petechiae that form within a 2.5-cm diameter circle are counted; greater than 20 petechiae is suggestive of capillary fragility. It should be borne in mind that a negative tourniquet test alone does not exclude an ongoing Dengue infection.

A better screening test for incipient Dengue hemorrhagic fever and early evidence of vascular permeability is detection of protein or heparin sulfate in acute-phase urine (87,107,108). The diagnosis is made principally on epidemiologic and clinical grounds, but may be confirmed by serologic testing. Dengue hemorrhagic fever should be suspected in children with WHO-defined clinical criteria: that is, sudden fever that stays high for 2 to 7 days, hemorrhagic manifestations, and hepatomegaly. Hemorrhagic manifestations include at least a positive tourniquet test and petechiae, purpura, ecchymoses, bleeding gums, hematemesis, or melena.

There are no specific therapies for Dengue fever, Dengue hemorrhagic fever, or Dengue shock syndrome, which must be differentiated from the toxic shock syndrome. Treatment is directed against the shock and hemorrhage rather than against the infection. Clinical outcomes are largely dependent on careful history and physical examination, and a low threshold of suspicion among physicians for the diagnosis, especially among travelers who present with symptoms (83). Dengue fever, Dengue hemorrhagic fever, and Dengue shock syndrome cause substantial morbidity; death rates can be as high as 30% if these complications are not managed properly (84,87,95,102,109–111). Although vaccines for flaviviruses, such as yellow fever and Japanese encephalitis, are available, Dengue vaccine is still under development, made complicated by the need to incorporate all four virus serotypes into a single preparation (81,82,84,110–112). Thus, until a safe and effective tetravalent vaccine becomes available, prevention will be attained only through vector control programs and avoidance of mosquito bites through protective gear and insect repellent.

Summary

In summary, Dengue fever and Dengue hemorrhagic fever have reached pandemic proportions in countries across the globe and Dengue has become one of the most important tropical diseases in the first decade of the 21st century (79). The resurgence has been linked to population growth, urbanization, air travel, and changes in the environment that have all favored extension of the ranges of the mosquito vector or its ability to thrive. Unfortunately, lack of or inadequate existing surveillance activities have resulted in reduced ascertainment of the early stages of epidemic transmission, with gross underreporting of cases until the epidemic is recognized as Dengue (79,113). Travelers returning from endemic regions are at particular risk of acquiring Dengue fever. Persons who travel repeatedly to countries with high Dengue endemicity put themselves at risk of becoming reinfected with a different serotype of the Dengue virus thereby predisposing themselves to Dengue hemorrhagic fever. In the characterization of fever in the tropics or among returning travelers, clinicians need to have a high degree of suspicion and maintain Dengue high on their list of differential diagnoses following a thorough history and physical examination.

TUBERCULOSIS: FALLOUT OF THE HUMAN IMMUNODEFICIENCY VIRUS PANDEMIC

Before the HIV pandemic, *M. tuberculosis* infection and disease were already endemic in many economically less-developed countries, though not at pandemic proportions. With the onset of the HIV pandemic, there has been a dramatic, parallel increase in rates of tuberculosis among HIV-infected patients, especially those in sub-Saharan Africa, Southeast Asia, and increasingly, the Indian subcontinent; over 80% of all patients with tuberculosis live in sub-Saharan Africa and Asia (114). Tuberculosis now ranks alongside HIV as a leading cause of death worldwide: the death toll attributed to HIV in 2014 was estimated at 1.2 million, which included almost one-half million deaths attributed to tuberculosis among HIV-positive people (114); worldwide, 9.6 million people are estimated to have fallen ill with *M. tuberculosis* infection in 2014—12% of the 9.6 million new TB cases in 2014 were HIV-positive (114).

The WHO generally considers *M. tuberculosis* infections a true pandemic that is linked primarily with immunosuppression resulting from HIV infection, though the problem has certainly been compounded by other factors associated with poverty, such as overcrowding, malnutrition, lack of access to health care, and poor sanitation, made particularly worse in refugee camps resulting from natural and man-made disasters and war (114). The fact remains that at the middle of the second decade of the 21st century, tuberculosis remains a leading cause of death worldwide.

The major issues relevant to the management of tuberculosis within the critical care setting include the following:

- The ability of clinicians to recognize active or disseminated tuberculosis
- The need to have a low threshold of suspicion for active tuberculosis when interpreting sputum smear results and abnormal chest radiographs, especially for at-risk patients or individuals who resided in HIV-endemic regions
- The importance of collecting appropriate sputum specimens for screening smears and cultures, and rational interpretation of results
- The utility and interpretation of tuberculin skin tests and interferon gamma assays
- The timely institution of infection control measures for the prevention of transmission of the tubercle bacillus from infected patients or health care personnel to other individuals in the unit through isolation of patients with active disease or positive smears in properly designed rooms maintained at negative pressure differentials
- Collection of appropriate sputum specimens for follow-up smears and cultures per CDC's recommendations (115,116)
- Involvement of infection control and occupational health personnel in the preventive decision making for patients and staff who might have been exposed inadvertently to persons with active tuberculosis (74,115,116)
- Awareness by all health care personnel of the basic tenets of guidelines published by CDC for the prevention of tuberculosis in health care settings (74,115,116)

Perhaps the most insidious occurrence resulting from the tuberculosis pandemic is the emergence of strains of *M. tuberculosis* resistant to standard antituberculous agents. During the 1990s, multidrug-resistant (MDR) tuberculosis, defined as resistance to at least both isoniazid and rifampin, emerged as a threat to therapy, control, and prevention of tuberculosis, both in the United States and worldwide (117–120). MDR tuberculosis is associated with the ready availability and over-prescribing of antituberculous agents. The treatment of MDR tuberculosis has clinical and public health implications largely related to the fact that therapy requires the use of alternative second-line drugs that are more expensive, toxic, and less effective than first-line isoniazid- and rifampin-based regimens (118,119).

There have now been numerous reports of tuberculosis caused by extensively drug-resistant (XDR) strains of *M. tuberculosis* (i.e., strains resistant to practically all second-line agents) (114,121–124). To assess the frequency and distribution of XDR tuberculosis, CDC and WHO carried out a survey of an international network of tuberculosis laboratories during 1993 through 2004 (127). Of 17,690 *M. tuberculosis* isolates characterized, 20% were MDR and 2% were found to be XDR. In addition, the study found that 4% of MDR tuberculosis cases in the United States were in fact caused by XDR *M. tuberculosis* (122). In October 2006, the WHO Global Task Force on XDR tuberculosis met in Geneva, Switzerland, to review available information on the emergence of XDR tuberculosis and to recommend measures to prevent and control this serious international public health threat (125). The Task Force approved the following revised laboratory case definition for XDR tuberculosis: "XDR tuberculosis is tuberculosis showing resistance to at least rifampin and isoniazid, which is the definition of MDR tuberculosis, in addition to any fluoroquinolone, and to at least one of the three following injectable drugs used in antituberculosis treatment: capreomycin, kanamycin, and amikacin" (125).

CDC and WHO have deemed XDR tuberculosis a serious emerging public health threat, raising the specter of a pandemic of untreatable tuberculosis (120,122). Patients with XDR tuberculosis generally have poor outcomes, prolonged infectious periods and limited treatment options. Thus, rapid detection of drug-resistant strains, enhanced infection control and the development of new therapeutics remain the basis of management in the inpatient setting (126). The current management of patients with MDR/XDR tuberculosis is difficult and complex. There is an increasing, but still as yet limited, body of literature that provides evidence for the use of carbapenems (ertapenem, imipenem, meropenem) in treating MDR and XDR tuberculosis (127,128). The therapeutic difficulty is underscored by the lack of comprehensive four-drug protocols to treat XDR-tuberculosis. Moreover, despite recent scientific advances in MDR/XDR tuberculosis care, decisions for the management of patients with MDR/XDR tuberculosis often rely on expert opinions, rather than on clinical evidence (129,130). Ultimately, strategies for treating cases of difficult MDR-/XDR-tuberculosis will rely on harnessing existing drugs (e.g., newer generation fluoroquinolones, high-dose isoniazid, linezolid, and pyrazinamide) in the best combinations and dosing schedules, together with adjunctive surgery in carefully selected cases (131).

Compounding the problem is the emergence of totally drug-resistant (TDR) tuberculosis (124,132). The first cases of TDR tuberculosis were reported in Italy in 2007 (133). These strains show in vitro resistance to all first- and second-line antituberculosis drugs (isoniazid, rifampicin, streptomycin, ethambutol, pyrazinamide, ethionamide, paraaminosalicylic acid, cycloserine, ofloxacin, amikacin, ciprofloxacin, capreomycin, kanamycin). Subsequently, cases were reported in Iran, India, and South Africa. The treatment of TDR tuberculosis includes agents with disputed or minimal effectiveness against *M. tuberculosis* and the fatality rate is high (132). MDR tuberculosis is difficult to cure and requires 18 to 24 months of treatment after sputum culture conversion with a regimen that consists of four to six medications with toxic side effects. Moreover, the attributable mortality is significantly greater than that associated with susceptible strains of *M. tuberculosis*. Following clinical trials, FDA has approved use of bedaquiline (an oral diarylquinoline) under the provisions of the accelerated approval regulations for "serious or life-threatening illnesses" (132,134,135).

METHICILLIN-RESISTANT *STAPHYLOCOCCUS AUREUS*

S. aureus is an important cause of infections of the skin, soft tissue, wounds, respiratory tract, urinary tract, central nervous system, and the bloodstream, and can be rapidly fatal if not treated effectively. Soon after the introduction of antimicrobials, *S. aureus* resistance to penicillin became widespread, quickly followed by resistance to semisynthetic penicillinase-resistant antimicrobials, such as methicillin, oxacillin, and nafcillin (i.e., MRSA)—first detected in the United Kingdom in 1960 (136). By the 1980s, MRSA had spread throughout health care institutions worldwide and in the United States, thereby compromising the effectiveness of therapy for staphylococcal infections, and dramatically increasing the empiric use of vancomycin, with its own attendant risks.

By 2006, MRSA was recognized as the most commonly identified antimicrobial-resistant pathogen in many parts of the world, including Europe, the Americas, North Africa, the Middle East, and East Asia (137). Grundmann et al. have pointed out that the increases in MRSA rates in these regions should be taken seriously because it is possible that the threshold for losing control might actually be low, albeit not well defined (137).

It is estimated that some 2 billion individuals are carrying *S. aureus* worldwide and between 2 and 53 million people carry MRSA across the globe (138). Despite more awareness among health care professionals of the adverse implications associated with MRSA colonization and infection, and despite more attention being paid to implementation of infection control guidelines, the prevalence of health care–associated MRSA infections in US acute care hospitals remains significant—the myriad of MRSA publications in the medical literature attests to the fact that MRSA is beating current prevention and control efforts.

In recent years, epidemics of hospital-acquired MRSA infections have highlighted attributable risk factors both intrinsic to the patient (e.g., age, underlying chronic heart or pulmonary disease, connective tissue disorders, high severity of illness scores, diabetes mellitus, immunosuppression, dialysis) and extrinsic (invasive medical devices and foreign bodies, surgical wounds, contact with other patients or health care personnel who are carriers). The clinical and diagnostic issues that must be addressed in ICUs and some of the tenets of infection control and hospital epidemiology that are necessary for the prevention of MRSA infection among unaffected patients, medical personnel, and other ancillary health care personnel have been made more complicated by the relatively recent emergence of community-associated MRSA.

Antimicrobial resistance among MRSA isolates is linked to a large mobile genetic element known as the staphylococcal cassette chromosome *mec* (SSC*mec*) gene that has been introduced into methicillin-susceptible *S. aureus* strains (the origin of this *mec* element remains unknown). The SCC*mec* element carries a methicillin-resistance determinant—*mecA*—that encodes for an additional penicillin-binding protein (PBP2A) with reduced affinity for beta-lactam antimicrobials, in addition to the regulatory genes (*mec I* and *mecRI*) of *mec A* (137,139). Five types of SCC*mec* (SCC*mec* I–V) have been described; most health care–associated strains carry either type I, II, or III, whereas community-acquired MRSA tend to be predominantly type IV and less commonly type V.

Individuals colonized with MRSA in their anterior nares can function as reservoirs for the organism over long periods (140). Recognition of colonized individuals is important because such persons may become infected; in the critical care setting, these persons may be a source of infection or colonization to other patients or health care personnel. Various epidemiologic studies have shown that the risk factors for MRSA carriage are similar to those for MRSA infection and include hospitalization (particularly in ICUs, surgery wards, other nursing units with documented high prevalence rates), invasive medical device use, the elderly, open wounds, underlying debilitation, proximity to other patients infected or colonized with MRSA, prior detection of MRSA, diabetes mellitus, treatments by injection, prior antimicrobial therapy, long inpatient stays, prior nursing home stays, visits at home by a nurse, or long periods of antimicrobial therapy (140–143). Health care personnel caring for MRSA-infected or MRSA-colonized patients with risk factors may themselves become colonized with MRSA and subsequently transmit the organism to noncolonized at-risk patients. Work carried out by Huang et al. have established that approximately 29% of newly detected MRSA carriers develop invasive disease within 18 months (144–146). There is now ample evidence that MRSA does not simply replace methicillin-susceptible *S. aureus* as a cause of health care–associated infection, but rather adds to the burden of infections caused by *S. aureus*.

In 2006, population-based estimates of nasal carriage of *S. aureus*, MRSA and identification of risk factors for carriage were carried out by two groups that independently analyzed the 2001–2002 National Health and Nutrition Examination Survey (NHANES) data for the noninstitutionalized US population, including children and adults (138,147,148). The findings of both groups were similar: close to 90 million persons (i.e., 32% of the US population) were colonized with *S. aureus*; and the prevalence of MRSA among *S. aureus* isolates was 2.6%, for an estimated population carriage of MRSA of 0.8% or 2.2 million persons adults. One of the studies also found that while *S. aureus* colonization prevalence was highest in participants 6 to 11 years old, MRSA colonization was associated with age 60 years of age or greater, and not necessarily with recent health care exposure (138).

Standard approaches to preventing MRSA transmission include implementing CDC guidelines that recommend isolation of patients colonized or infected with MRSA in a private or dedicated room, and use of gowns, gloves, and masks when appropriate, by all personnel entering the room (i.e., contact isolation). Many hospitals actively screen all patients when they are admitted to high-risk hospital areas (i.e., ICUs, transplant units, or surgical wards), and implement appropriate contact isolation for those identified as carriers. This approach, referred to as "active screening and isolation," minimizes the possibility of transmitting MRSA between patients via the hands or clothes of health care workers, and has been effective in some centers (149–152). The major criticism of "active screening and isolation" programs is that it takes about 3 days on average from the time a nasal screening swab is obtained from a patient and is logged in the microbiology laboratory specimen receiving station, to the time the information that a patient is indeed an MRSA carrier gets reported back to those who need to know in the inpatient service. Person-to-person MRSA transmission may occur during those 3 days. Therefore, decreasing the time it takes to identify a patient as an MRSA carrier will eliminate this delay and may provide a rational strategy for reducing the transmission of MRSA in the inpatient setting. There has been an increasing body of literature regarding new methods for rapid identification of MRSA from clinical specimens (150,152–154). Few studies, however, have established the utility of rapid MRSA identification in reducing MRSA transmission and infection in the critical care setting (150,153,155–160).

In 1993, new strains of MRSA were identified among people in Western Australia who had not been in contact with the health care system (161). Since then, there has been a worldwide recognition of the emergence of community-associated MRSA strains. Previously healthy young adults are particularly affected and numerous reports of community-associated MRSA have been reported involving children, prison inmates, Alaskan Natives, Native Americans, Pacific Islanders, intravenous drug abusers, the homeless, children in daycare, athletes who participate in contact sports, and military personnel, though infections are by no means restricted to these populations. A single toxin, Panton-Valentine leukocidin (PVL), has been linked by epidemiologic studies to community-associated MRSA infection. Subsequent studies, however, have established that MRSA strains lacking PVL are just as likely to be virulent and to cause severe infection as PVL-positive strains, suggesting that PVL is not the major virulence determinant of community-associated MRSA.

Approximately 85% of community-associated MRSA infections involve the skin and subcutaneous tissues, with the most common presentations being an abscess or folliculitis in otherwise healthy individuals who do not have MRSA-associated risk factors. A predominant clone of community-associated MRSA, the US 300 clone, appears to be the predominant cause of community-onset *S. aureus* skin and soft-tissue infection. Also, the presence of unique virulence factors may be responsible for potentially lethal necrotizing pneumonia and other invasive infections in both immunocompetent and immunosuppressed individuals. Community-associated MRSA isolates are generally susceptible to multiple classes of antimicrobials other than beta-lactams, and infections can be treated with trimethoprim—sulfamethoxazole, doxycycline, or clindamycin; for severe infections, vancomycin, daptomycin, quinupristin/dalfopristin, or linezolid can be used, though delay in initiating appropriate antimicrobial therapy for severe infections can cause substantial morbidity or even be life-threatening (162–164).

The diversity of strain types involved in epidemiologically clear outbreaks of MRSA suggests the spread of genetic information among different strains that have strong predispositions for causing infections in hospital patients. Alternatively, the association could be due merely to the fact that resistance provides a dramatic marker that increases the likelihood that an epidemic will be recognized and investigated. If so, as infection control personnel in hospitals initiate surveillance activities and develop more sensitive means for recognizing outbreaks and clusters of infections, and more effectively share surveillance data with their counterparts in other local hospitals (e.g., through area-wide surveillance systems supported by local health departments), interhospital transmission of infection will likely be more readily recognized and controlled. The main obstacle to endeavors that properly and comprehensively address the clinical and public health challenges of MRSA infections both in hospitals and the community remains the changing face of health care in the United States. Adding to the complexity of the issue are the uncharacterized confounding variables of long-term care facilities, free-standing medical clinics and surgery centers, and home care, where substantial amounts of patient care are now provided or delivered. Admission of these varied populations to ICUs adds to the complexity of inter- and intrahospital transmission of MRSA, and continues to render control of MRSA transmission in critical care units a perennial problem notwithstanding prevention and control efforts.

Control and Prevention

That endemic and epidemic health care–associated infections are preventable have periodically been reaffirmed by the myriad of single-center studies published over the past three decades dealing with the unequivocal effect of handwashing with soap and water, proper care of urinary catheters, respirators, intravascular catheters, and surgical wounds, numerous evidence-based infection control guidelines published by CDC, and position papers issued by the Society of Healthcare Epidemiology of America, the Association of Practitioners of Infection Control, and the Infectious Diseases Society of America (82,176–178). However, according to CDC data, although overall rates of health care–associated infections at the main anatomic sites (i.e., bloodstream, respiratory tract, wounds, urine) have been falling, infections caused by MRSA have been increasing in hospitals across the United States.

There is little doubt that we would not be where we are today had more attention been paid to the published evidence-based data regarding which interventions have been effective in controlling the transmission of health care–associated, antimicrobial-resistant pathogens. After decades of discussing control of antimicrobial-resistant health care–associated pathogens in the medical literature, there is actually very little evidence of success either in the control of the infections caused by these pathogens or in halting the increasing incidence of resistance among isolates. The myriad articles published have in effect helped explain this failure because much of the published data on health care–associated infections have been carried out in hospitals that had implemented untried control programs or had substantially ineffective programs. Moreover, despite all the resources put into surveillance activities and "quality programs" for health care–associated infections in facilities across the country, there remains substantial variation in surveillance activities from one medical center to another, inconsistent use of effective control measures—for example, surveillance cultures not being performed as recommended, or failure of hospitals to use effective measures due to lack of commitment by health care companies and administrators alike to initiate and sustain these measures. In addition, there appears to be moderate compliance with goals to optimize antimicrobial use, and to detect, report, and control the spread of antimicrobial-resistant pathogens.

In the Netherlands and Nordic countries, rates of health care–associated MRSA infections have been held to less than 3% through programs that include screening of patients and exposed health care workers in aggressive "search and destroy" MRSA prevention programs (165–175). There are some differences in the choice of measures and target groups in the search and destroy strategy toward MRSA in some countries. For example, in the draft of a new Norwegian MRSA guideline it is suggested to have a search and destroy strategy in hospitals, while the measures outside health care institutions are targeted toward people with the highest risk of transmitting the bacteria to hospitals or nursing homes (165). American guidelines advocate an approach similar to the search and destroy paradigm (176); the value of obtaining screening cultures in areas with high MRSA endemicity, however, remains controversial (137).

Numerous reports presented at various Annual Meetings of the Society for Healthcare Epidemiology of America have repeatedly shown control of endemic or epidemic MRSA infections through implementation of the SHEA guidelines with more emphasis on contact precautions and less on standard precautions. In fact, CDC has never been able to provide any evidence-based data showing that standard precautions and passive surveillance have led to the control of MRSA in health care settings.

The tenets of the SHEA guidelines are based on identification and containment of spread through the following (176):

- Active surveillance cultures to identify the reservoir for spread
- Routine hand hygiene
- Barrier precautions for patients known or suspected to be colonized or infected with MRSA
- Implementation of an antimicrobial stewardship program
- Decolonization or suppression of colonized patients

There is increasing evidence that screening of high-risk patients combined with a comprehensive prevention program consisting of contact precautions and scrupulous hand hygiene program can reduce transmission of MRSA (136,142,143,149–152,168,170,175,177–184). Grundmann et al. have pointed out that virtually all published analyses comparing the costs of screening patients on admission and using contact precautions when dealing with colonized patients with the cost savings made by preventing health care–associated MRSA infections have concluded that the combination of surveillance cultures and barrier precautions results in substantial cost savings for health care facilities (137).

In summary, active surveillance cultures for MRSA in the ICU setting with isolation of colonized persons is a highly effective strategy for control of MRSA. Isolation purely on the basis of history of previous detection, at least for MRSA, appears to be of little benefit. Standard precautions and isolation of the occasional patient recognized to be colonized through routine clinical cultures are minimally effective. The onus is now on health care professionals and health care administrators to invest intelligently in prevention programs, to enhance existing surveillance activities in targeted areas, and to avoid regarding death and morbidity attributable to MRSA as inevitable. However, it must be equally understood and appreciated by relatives, the patients themselves, lawyers, administrators, and health care personnel alike that the following types of patients are particularly susceptible to or likely to acquire health care–associated MRSA infections: those born very prematurely; the elderly; those who are debilitated or have severe congenital abnormalities; patients with diabetes mellitus, connective tissue disorders, or end-stage respiratory, liver, renal, or cardiac disease; patients with solid organ or hematologic malignancies; transplant patients; patients on steroids or immunosuppressive agents; and patients with numerous invasive medical devices or who have undergone one or more major surgical procedures or other invasive procedures.

The challenge that faces us now is controlling transmission of strains of community-associated MRSA that become endemic within the inpatient setting, especially in ICUs. New MRSA clones have emerged in the community that combine antimicrobial resistance with easy transmissibility and virulence (137,183). The worry is that these could take hold in hospitals, where patients are particularly vulnerable.

CHOLERA

Cholera is a secretory gastroenteritis caused by *Vibrio cholerae*, a small, comma-shaped gram-negative microorganism. The natural reservoir is aquatic invertebrates in brackish or marine environments. The spread of cholera is primarily through ingestion of fecally contaminated water or food. Cholera is endemic in Asia, Africa, the Middle East and parts of Oceania and there are an estimated 3 to 5 million cases, and over 100,000 deaths each year around the world. In endemic areas, the disease is most common in children. However, nonimmune adults traveling to an endemic region is susceptible and at risk of acquiring the infection. Since 1817, there have been seven recorded cholera pandemics that affected populations across the entire globe, resulting in hundreds of thousands of deaths (184–186); the seventh pandemic began in 1961 and affects 3 to 5 million people each year, killing 120,000. CDC and WHO surveillance data indicate that there has been an ongoing global pandemic in Asia, Africa, and Latin America for the last four decades. Resource-poor areas continue to report the vast majority of cases with the African continent having the worst case fatality rates. There are 139 serotypes of *V. cholerae*, defined by the O surface antigen; the continuing pandemics are caused by two serogroups: O1 or O139.

V. cholerae is sensitive to gastric acid. Thus, the infectious inoculum in healthy hosts is relative large (about 10^{10} organisms). In persons who have achlorhydria, are taking antacids, or have had gastrectomy, the infectious inoculum is much lower ($\leq 10^6$). The organism tends to colonize the small intestine and secretes one major (cholera toxin) and two minor enterotoxins. The cholera toxin binds to the ganglioside on the small bowel epithelium and activates adenylate cyclase, which in turn leads to accumulation of cycle adenosine monophosphate (cAMP). The increased levels of cAMP inhibit sodium absorption and increase chloride secretion, leading to the characteristic, profuse, watery diarrhea.

The incubation period is 1 to 5 days. Profuse watery diarrhea containing flecks of mucus (the so-called "rice-water stools") is the hallmark of cholera. This is followed by vomiting without retching, rapid heart rate, loss of skin elasticity due to dehydration, dry mucous membranes, low blood pressure, thirst, muscle cramps as a result of electrolyte shifts, restlessness or irritability. Patients characteristically do not have fever, abdominal pain, or tenesmus.

Isolation and identification of *V. cholerae* serogroup O1 or O139 by culture of a stool specimen remains the gold standard for the laboratory diagnosis of cholera. Cary Blair media is ideal for transport, and the selective thiosulfate–citrate–bile salts agar (TCBS) is ideal for isolation and identification. Laboratory test results usually reveal an elevated hematocrit, elevated blood urea nitrogen and creatinine, an elevated anion gap with significantly reduced bicarbonate levels and a metabolic acidosis.

Management of patients with cholera involves prompt aggressive fluid and electrolyte replacement–effective therapy can decrease mortality from greater than 50% to less than 0.2% (184). Replacement fluid and electrolytes should be administered intravenously in patients with severe dehydration, patients with moderate dehydration who are unable to take fluids orally, and patients who are purging copious amounts (>10 mL/kg/hr). The treatment and rehydration of cholera, based on the degree of dehydration, is summarized in a useful document published by the WHO (187). Antimicrobial therapy is merely adjunct to rehydration therapy and should be reserved for patients with severe dehydration only. In patients with severe disease, antibiotics can ameliorate the duration of symptoms and fluid requirements:

- For adults, doxycycline is given as a single dose 300 mg or tetracycline 12.5 mg/kg, four times a day for 3 days
- For young children: erythromycin 12.5 mg/kg, four times a day for 3 days
- For children under 6 months of age: 10 mg daily for 10 days
- For children 6 months to 5 years of age: 20 mg daily for 10 days

Of note, normal feeding should continue during treatment, if at all possible.

Infection control is of paramount importance. Chemoprophylaxis with antibiotics is not indicated for health care providers. One needs to protect oneself from contamination: the basic tenets of prevention in the inpatient setting are as follows:

1. Scrupulous hand hygiene with soap and clean water before and after taking care of a patient. If no water and soap are available, use an alcohol-based hand cleaner (with at least 60% alcohol).
2. Cut fingernails.
3. Isolate cholera patients:
   a. Stool, vomit, and soiled clothes of patients are highly contagious.
   b. Patients' utensils need to be washed and disinfected with chlorine.
   c. Cholera patients have to be in a special ward, isolated from other patients.

At present, two oral cholera vaccines are available: Dukoral (manufactured by SBL Vaccines) and ShanChol (manufactured by Shantha Biotec in India), which are WHO prequalified. These are two-dose vaccines; thus, multiple weeks can elapse before people receiving the vaccines are protected. Further, vaccines offer incomplete protection; therefore, vaccination should not replace standard prevention and control measures. In the United States, cholera vaccines are not yet available, and the disease is a reportable infection.

POTENTIAL PANDEMIC INFECTIONS: IMPLICATIONS FOR ICUs

Over the past 5 years, two viruses with the potential for pandemic spread have emerged: the Middle East respiratory syndrome coronavirus (MERS-CoV) and the Zika virus. One bacteria—*V. cholera*—has been associated with infections of Pandemic proportions over the past 100 years.

MERS-CoV

Most people infected with MERS-CoV develop severe acute respiratory illness. MERS-CoV infection was first reported in Saudi Arabia in 2012 and has since spread to several other countries. As of September 30, 2015, a total of 1,589 laboratory-confirmed cases of infection with MERS-CoV have been reported to the WHO. Although most cases of MERS-CoV have occurred in Saudi Arabia and the United Arab Emirates, cases have been reported in Europe, the United States, and Asia in people who travelled from the Middle East or their contacts (188). Epidemiologic and genomic studies show zoonotic transmission to humans from camels and possibly bats. In contrast to the SARS-CoV pandemic, very limited global spread of fatal MERS-CoV has occurred outside the Arabian Peninsula (189,190). Both community-acquired and hospital-acquired cases of MERS-CoV infection have been reported with little human-to-human transmission reported in the community. Clinical features of MERS-CoV range from asymptomatic or mild disease to ARDS and multiorgan failure resulting in death, especially in individuals with underlying comorbidities. Zumla has underscored the fact that although MERS-CoV continues to be an endemic, low-level public health threat, there is always a risk that the virus could mutate, leading to increased person-to-person transmissibility, thereby increasing its pandemic potential (188). No specific drug treatment exists for MERS-CoV and there is no vaccination available at the present time. Supportive care is the mainstay of therapy; the use of convalescent plasma has been suggested as a potential therapy based on existing evidence from other viral infections (190). Corticosteroids used empirically have showed no survival benefit. Various trial therapies have included interferon alpha and ribavirin; these were tested in severely ill patients and showed an improvement in survival at 14 days but not at 28 days. Other investigational agents have included cyclophilin inhibitors, inhibitors of MERS-CoV cell receptors (CD26), and MERS neutralizing antibodies. None of these agents have been shown to be effective. CDC and ECDC recommend airborne isolation for patients at health care facilities. The WHO recommends airborne precautions during aerosol-generating procedures. Eye protection should be used when heath care workers care for probable or confirmed patients. Since it is not known how long the virus is present in respiratory secretions, patients should remain on contact and airborne precautions until discharge. Exposed individuals should be monitored for any symptoms, for 14 days, from date of exposure. Health care workers in contact or taking care of MERS patients are a high risk for acquiring the infection. Prolonged shedding occurs since the virus was found to be excreted even after 1 month of illness (96,188).

Zika Virus

The emergence of the Zika virus is more recent phenomenon: it is a flavivirus that emerged in Brazil in 2015 and then rapidly spread throughout the tropical and subtropical Americas, and the Caribbean. It is transmitted largely by the *Aedes* mosquito (191). Based on clinical criteria alone, Zika virus infection cannot be reliably distinguished from infections caused by two other common arboviruses transmitted by Dengue virus and Chikungunya virus. One or more of the following symptoms can be associated with Dengue or Zika: fever, rash, conjunctivitis, arthralgia, myalgia, or headache; unlike Dengue, hemorrhage and shock are not characteristic of Zika virus infection. Since specific diagnosis would be difficult at the time of presentation, the key factor for prevention of intrahospital transmission is obtaining a detailed travel history and implementation of contact and airborne precautions until a diagnosis is made.

Key Points

- We have highlighted infections that have caused pandemics or, in the case of avian influenza, Dengue, MERS-CoV, or cholera, has a high potential to do so.
- Patients with any of these infections may require management in an ICU. Knowledge of these infections is important for ICU personnel if appropriate management, as well as infection control and preventive measures, is to be instituted in a timely manner.
- The common threads running through all of these pandemic infections include the need for physicians to have high indices of clinical suspicion and, early on, consider these diagnoses and the importance of infection control, surveillance, and education for staff and patients alike.
- Apart from infections caused by MRSA and tuberculosis, critical care management of SARS, influenza, Dengue, MERS-CoV, and cholera are largely supportive.
- SARS was controlled largely through early detection and implementation of traditional infection control practices, environmental decontamination, use of personal protective equipment, surveillance activities, and education and training of patients, relatives, and caregivers.
- Avian influenza, where there have been outbreaks, has largely been controlled through early recognition, scrupulous attention to infection control practices and procedures, appropriate use of surgical masks, institution of established guidelines for the prevention of hospital-acquired pneumonia, and annual influenza vaccination for all high-risk patients and their close contacts—including medical personnel as well as household members.
- Dengue and Zika virus infection must be considered in the characterization and workup of fever among returning international travelers, especially persons returning from Central and South America, Puerto Rico, and the Eastern Caribbean islands. Clinicians in critical care medicine need to have a high degree of suspicion for the associated clinical syndromes.
- Preventing the transmission of tuberculosis in the inpatient setting is made all the more imperative because of the limited therapeutic options available once a patient has acquired infection caused by MDR, XDR, and totally resistant strains. Compounding the risk of tuberculosis in the in-patient setting is the looming possibility of transmission of untreatable XDR strains to previously healthy humans, including health care personnel.
- Control and prevention of MRSA infections, too, have been made especially difficult since the emergence of community-associated strains that have insidiously crept into the in-patient setting, raising the possibility of transmission of MRSA to healthy personnel with no obvious risk factors. Antimicrobial therapeutic options for MRSA infection are also limited largely to vancomycin, daptomycin, and ceftaroline; idiosyncratic reactions or renal dysfunction reduces these choices even further.

References

1. Archibald L, Phillips L, Monnet D, et al. Antimicrobial resistance in isolates from inpatients and outpatients in the United States: increasing importance of the intensive care unit. *Clin Infect Dis.* 1997;24(2):211–215.
2. Centers for Disease Control and Prevention. Revised U.S. surveillance case definition for severe acute respiratory syndrome (SARS) and update on SARS cases—United States and worldwide, December 2003. *MMWR Morb Mortal Wkly Rep.* 2003;52(49):1202–1206.
3. Centers for Disease Control and Prevention. Update: severe acute respiratory syndrome—United States, May 14, 2003. *MMWR Morb Mortal Wkly Rep.* 2003;52(19):436–438.
4. Centers for Disease Control and Prevention. Update: outbreak of severe acute respiratory syndrome—worldwide, 2003. *MMWR Morb Mortal Wkly Rep.* 2003;52(13):269–272.
5. Centers for Disease Control and Prevention. Outbreak of severe acute respiratory syndrome—worldwide, 2003. *MMWR Morb Mortal Wkly Rep.* 2003;52(11):226–228.
6. Ksiazek TG, Erdman D, Goldsmith CS, et al. A novel coronavirus associated with severe acute respiratory syndrome. *N Engl J Med.* 2003; 348(20):1953–1966.
7. Berger A, Drosten C, Doerr HW, et al. Severe acute respiratory syndrome (SARS): paradigm of an emerging viral infection. *J Clin Virol.* 2004; 29(1):13–22.
8. Drosten C, Gunther S, Preiser W, et al. Identification of a novel coronavirus in patients with severe acute respiratory syndrome. *N Engl J Med.* 2003;348(20):1967–1976.
9. Kuiken T, Fouchier RA, Schutten M, et al. Newly discovered coronavirus as the primary cause of severe acute respiratory syndrome. *Lancet.* 2003;362(9380):263–270.
10. Peiris JS, Guan Y, Yuen KY. Severe acute respiratory syndrome. *Nature Med.* 2004;10(12 Suppl):S88–S97.
11. Donnelly CA, Ghani AC, Leung GM, et al. Epidemiological determinants of spread of causal agent of severe acute respiratory syndrome in Hong Kong. *Lancet.* 2003;361(9371):1761–1766.
12. Poutanen SM, Low DE, Henry B, et al. Identification of severe acute respiratory syndrome in Canada. *N Engl J Med.* 2003;348(20):1995–2005.

13. Li W, Wong SK, Li F, et al. Animal origins of the severe acute respiratory syndrome coronavirus: insight from ACE2-S-protein interactions. *J Virol.* 2006;80(9):4211–4219.
14. Weiss SR, Navas-Martin S. Coronavirus pathogenesis and the emerging pathogen severe acute respiratory syndrome coronavirus. *Microbiol Molec Biol Rev. MMBR*. 2005;69(4):635–664.
15. Fouchier RA, Kuiken T, Schutten M, et al. Aetiology: Koch's postulates fulfilled for SARS virus. *Nature*. 2003;423(6937):240.
16. Martina BE, Haagmans BL, Kuiken T, et al. Virology: SARS virus infection of cats and ferrets. *Nature*. 2003;425(6961):915.
17. Varia M, Wilson S, Sarwal S, et al. Investigation of a nosocomial outbreak of severe acute respiratory syndrome (SARS) in Toronto, Canada. *CMAJ*. 2003;169(4):285–292.
18. Yu IT, Sung JJ. The epidemiology of the outbreak of severe acute respiratory syndrome (SARS) in Hong Kong: what we do know and what we don't. *Epidemiol Infect*. 2004;132(5):781–786.
19. Seto WH, Tsang D, Yung RW, et al. Effectiveness of precautions against droplets and contact in prevention of nosocomial transmission of severe acute respiratory syndrome (SARS). *Lancet*. 2003;361(9368):1519–1520.
20. Tang JW, Li Y, Eames I, et al. Factors involved in the aerosol transmission of infection and control of ventilation in healthcare premises. *J Hosp Infect*. 2006;64(2):100–114.
21. Centers for Disease Control and Prevention. Revised U.S. surveillance case definition for severe acute respiratory syndrome (SARS) and update on SARS cases—United States and worldwide, December 2003. *MMWR Morbid Mortal Wkly Rep*. 2003;52(49):1202–1206.
22. Christian MD, Loutfy M, McDonald LC, et al. Possible SARS coronavirus transmission during cardiopulmonary resuscitation. *Emerg Infect Dis*. 2004;10(2):287–293.
23. Wong TW, Lee CK, Tam W, et al. Cluster of SARS among medical students exposed to single patient, Hong Kong. *Emerg Infect Dis*. 2004; 10(2):269–276.
24. Dowell SF, Simmerman JM, Erdman DD, et al. Severe acute respiratory syndrome coronavirus on hospital surfaces. *Clin Infect Dis*. 2004;39(5): 652–657.
25. Shen Z, Ning F, Zhou W, et al. Superspreading SARS events, Beijing, 2003. *Emerg Infect Dis*. 2004;10(2):256–260.
26. Centers for Disease Control and Prevention. Update: Severe respiratory illness associated with Middle East Respiratory Syndrome Coronavirus (MERS-CoV)—worldwide, 2012–2013. *MMWR Morbid Mortal Wkly Rep*. 2013;62(23):480–483.
27. Loeb M, McGeer A, Henry B, et al. SARS among critical care nurses, Toronto. *Emerg Infect Dis*. 2004;10(2):251–255.
28. Ofner M, Lem M, Sarwal S, et al. Cluster of severe acute respiratory syndrome cases among protected health care workers—Toronto, April 2003. *Canada Communicable Dis Rep*. 2003;29(11):93–97.
29. Tsang KW, Ho PL, Ooi GC, et al. A cluster of cases of severe acute respiratory syndrome in Hong Kong. *N Engl J Med*. 2003;348(20):1977–1985.
30. Wong RS, Hui DS. Index patient and SARS outbreak in Hong Kong. *Emerg Infect Dis*. 2004;10(2):339–341.
31. Centers for Disease Control and Prevention. Cluster of severe acute respiratory syndrome cases among protected health-care workers—Toronto, Canada, April 2003. *MMWR Morbid Mortal Wkly Rep*. 2003;52(19): 433–436.
32. Centers for Disease Control and Prevention. Severe acute respiratory syndrome—Singapore, 2003. *MMWR Morbid Mortal Wkly Rep*. 2003; 52(18):405–411.
33. Peiris JS, Yuen KY, Osterhaus AD, Stohr K. The severe acute respiratory syndrome. *N Engl J med*. 2003;349(25):2431–241.
34. Lapinsky SE, Hawryluck L. ICU management of severe acute respiratory syndrome. *Intensive Care Med*. 2003;29(6):870–875.
35. Raboud J, Shigayeva A, McGeer A, et al. Risk factors for SARS transmission from patients requiring intubation: a multicentre investigation in Toronto, Canada. *PloS One*. 2010;5(5):e10717.
36. Hsueh PR, Yang PC. Severe acute respiratory syndrome (SARS): an emerging infection of the 21st century. *J Formosan Med Assoc Taiwan*. 2003;102(12):825–839.
37. Hsueh PR, Hsiao CH, Yeh SH, et al. Microbiologic characteristics, serologic responses, and clinical manifestations in severe acute respiratory syndrome, Taiwan. *Emerg Infect Dis*. 2003;9(9):1163–1167.
38. Poutanen SM, McGeer AJ. Transmission and control of SARS. *Curr Infect Dis Rep*. 2004;6(3):220–227.
39. Chen KT, Twu SJ, Chang HL, et al. SARS in Taiwan: an overview and lessons learned. *Int J Infect Dis*. 2005;9(2):77–85.
40. Twu SJ, Chen TJ, Chen CJ, et al. Control measures for severe acute respiratory syndrome (SARS) in Taiwan. *Emerg Infect Dis*. 2003;9(6):718–720.
41. Masur H, Emanuel E, Lane HC. Severe acute respiratory syndrome: providing care in the face of uncertainty. *JAMA*. 2003;289(21):2861–2863.
42. Tablan OC, Anderson LJ, Besser R, et al. Guidelines for preventing health-care–associated pneumonia, 2003: recommendations of CDC and the Healthcare Infection Control Practices Advisory Committee. *MMWR Recommend Rep*. 2004;53(RR-3):1–36.
43. Shaw K. The 2003 SARS outbreak and its impact on infection control practices. *Public Health*. 2006;120(1):8–14.
44. McDonald LC, Simor AE, Su IJ, et al. SARS in healthcare facilities, Toronto and Taiwan. *Emerg Infect Dis*. 2004;10(5):777–781.
45. Olsen SJ, Chang HL, Cheung TY, et al. Transmission of the severe acute respiratory syndrome on aircraft. *N Engl J Med*. 2003;349(25):2416–2422.
46. Taubenberger JK, Morens DM. 1918 Influenza: the mother of all pandemics. *Emerg Infect Dis*. 2006;12(1):15–22.
47. Kilbourne ED. Influenza pandemics of the 20th century. *Emerg Infect Dis*. 2006;12(1):9–14.
48. Beigel JH, Farrar J, Han AM, et al. Avian influenza A (H5N1) infection in humans. *N Engl J Med*. 2005;353(13):1374–1385.
49. Pearson JE. International standards for the control of avian influenza. *Avian Dis*. 2003;47(3 Suppl):972–975.
50. Dinh PN, Long HT, Tien NT, et al. Risk factors for human infection with avian influenza A H5N1, Vietnam, 2004. *Emerg Infect Dis*. 2006; 12(12):1841–1847.
51. Buxton Bridges C, Katz JM, Seto WH, et al. Risk of influenza A (H5N1) infection among health care workers exposed to patients with influenza A (H5N1), Hong Kong. *J Infect Dis*. 2000;181(1):344–348.
52. Areechokchai D, Jiraphongsa C, Laosiritaworn Y, et al. Investigation of avian influenza (H5N1) outbreak in humans—Thailand, 2004. *MMWR Suppl*. 2006;55(1):3–6.
53. Ungchusak K, Auewarakul P, Dowell SF, et al. Probable person-to-person transmission of avian influenza A (H5N1). *N Engl J Med*. 2005;352(4): 333–340.
54. Bridges CB, Kuehnert MJ, Hall CB. Transmission of influenza: implications for control in health care settings. *Clin Infect Dis*. 2003;37(8): 1094–1101.
55. de Jong MD, Simmons CP, Thanh TT, et al. Fatal outcome of human influenza A (H5N1) is associated with high viral load and hypercytokinemia. *Nature Med*. 2006;12(10):1203–1207.
56. Chotpitayasunondh T, Ungchusak K, Hanshaoworakul W, et al. Human disease from influenza A (H5N1), Thailand, 2004. *Emerg Infect Dis*. 2005;11(2):201–209.
57. Chan PK. Outbreak of avian influenza A(H5N1) virus infection in Hong Kong in 1997. *Clin Infect Dis*. 2002;34(Suppl 2):S58–S64.
58. To KF, Chan PK, Chan KF, et al. Pathology of fatal human infection associated with avian influenza A H5N1 virus. *J Med Virol*. 2001;63(3):242–246.
59. To KK, Ng KH, Que TL, et al. Avian influenza A H5N1 virus: a continuous threat to humans. *Emerg Microbes Infect*. 2012;1(9):e25.
60. Yuen KY, Chan PK, Peiris M, et al. Clinical features and rapid viral diagnosis of human disease associated with avian influenza A H5N1 virus. *Lancet*. 1998;351(9101):467–471.
61. Centers for Disease Control and Prevention. Evaluation of 11 commercially available rapid influenza diagnostic tests—United States, 2011–2012. *MMWR Morbid Mortal Wkly Rep*. 2012;61(43):873–876.
62. Centers for Disease Control and Prevention. Evaluation of rapid influenza diagnostic tests for detection of novel influenza A (H1N1) virus—United States, 2009. *MMWR Morbid Mortal Wkly Rep*. 2009;58(30):826–829.
63. de Jong MD, Ison MG, Monto AS, et al. Evaluation of intravenous peramivir for treatment of influenza in hospitalized patients. *Clin Infect Dis*. 2014;59(12):e172–e185.
64. Bright RA, Medina MJ, Xu X, et al. Incidence of adamantane resistance among influenza A (H3N2) viruses isolated worldwide from 1994 to 2005: a cause for concern. *Lancet*. 2005;366(9492):1175–1181.
65. Fiore AE, Fry A, Shay D, Gubareva L, et al. Antiviral agents for the treatment and chemoprophylaxis of influenza: recommendations of the Advisory Committee on Immunization Practices (ACIP). *MMWR Recomm Rep*. 2011;60(1):1–24.
66. Prevention of influenza: recommendations for influenza immunization of children, 2007–2008. *Pediatrics*. 2008;121(4):e1016–e1031.
67. Update: influenza activity—United States, August 30–October 31, 2009. *MMWR Morbid Mortal Wkly Rep*. 2009;58(44):1236–1241.
68. Li F, Ma C, Wang J. Inhibitors targeting the influenza virus hemagglutinin. *Curr Med Chem*. 2015;22(11):1361–1382.
69. Fry AM, Goswami D, Nahar K, et al. Efficacy of oseltamivir treatment started within 5 days of symptom onset to reduce influenza illness duration and virus shedding in an urban setting in Bangladesh: a randomised placebo-controlled trial. *Lancet Infect Dis*. 2014;14(2):109–118.

70. Louie JK, Yang S, Acosta M, et al. Treatment with neuraminidase inhibitors for critically ill patients with influenza A (H1N1)pdm09. *Clin Infect Dis*. 2012;55(9):1198–1204.
71. Siston AM, Rasmussen SA, Honein MA, et al. Pandemic 2009 influenza A(H1N1) virus illness among pregnant women in the United States. *JAMA*. 2010;303(15):1517–1525.
72. Yu H, Feng Z, Uyeki TM, et al. Risk factors for severe illness with 2009 pandemic influenza A (H1N1) virus infection in China. *Clin Infect Dis*. 2011;52(4):457–465.
73. Monto AS. Vaccines and antiviral drugs in pandemic preparedness. *Emerg Infect Dis*. 2006;12(1):55–60.
74. Sehulster L, Chinn RY. Guidelines for environmental infection control in health-care facilities: recommendations of CDC and the Healthcare Infection Control Practices Advisory Committee (HICPAC). *MMWR Recomm Rep*. 2003;52(RR-10):1–42.
75. Aiello AE, Murray GF, Perez V, et al. Mask use, hand hygiene, and seasonal influenza-like illness among young adults: a randomized intervention trial. *J Infect Dis*. 2010;201(4):491–498.
76. Centers for Disease Control P. Prevention and control of influenza with vaccines: recommendations of the Advisory Committee on Immunization Practices (ACIP), 2011. *MMWR Morbid Mortal Wkly Rep*. 2011;60(33):1128–1132.
77. Welliver R, Monto AS, Carewicz O, et al. Effectiveness of oseltamivir in preventing influenza in household contacts: a randomized controlled trial. *JAMA*. 2001;285(6):748–754.
78. Hayden FG, Belshe R, Villanueva C, et al. Management of influenza in households: a prospective, randomized comparison of oseltamivir treatment with or without postexposure prophylaxis. *J Infect Dis*. 2004;189(3):440–449.
79. Gubler DJ. Epidemic Dengue/Dengue hemorrhagic fever as a public health, social and economic problem in the 21st century. *Trends Microbiol*. 2002;10(2):100–103.
80. Gubler DJ, Meltzer M. Impact of Dengue/Dengue hemorrhagic fever on the developing world. *Adv Virus Res*. 1999;53:35–70.
81. Guzman MG, Halstead SB, Artsob H, et al. Dengue: a continuing global threat. *Nature Rev Microbiol*. 2010;8(12 Suppl):S7–S16.
82. Shepard DS, Undurraga EA, Betancourt-Cravioto M, et al. Approaches to refining estimates of global burden and economics of Dengue. *PLoS Negl Trop Dis*. 2014;8(11):e3306.
83. Wilder-Smith A, Schwartz E. Dengue in travelers. *N Engl J Med*. 2005; 353(9):924–932.
84. Achee NL, Gould F, Perkins TA, et al. A critical assessment of vector control for Dengue prevention. *PLoS Neglect Trop Dis*. 2015;9(5):e0003655.
85. Isturiz RE, Gubler DJ, Brea del Castillo J. Dengue and Dengue hemorrhagic fever in Latin America and the Caribbean. *Infect Dis Clin North Am*. 2000;14(1):121–140.
86. Lambrechts L, Scott TW, Gubler DJ. Consequences of the expanding global distribution of *Aedes albopictus* for Dengue virus transmission. *PLoS Negl Trop Dis*. 2010;4(5):e646.
87. Halstead SB. More Dengue, more questions. *Emerg Infect Dis*. 2005;11(5): 740–741.
88. Chen LH, Wilson ME. Nosocomial Dengue by mucocutaneous transmission. *Emerg Infect Dis*. 2005;11(5):775.
89. Chen LH, Wilson ME. Transmission of Dengue virus without a mosquito vector: nosocomial mucocutaneous transmission and other routes of transmission. *Clin Infect Dis*. 2004;39(6):e56–e60.
90. de Wazieres B, Gil H, Vuitton DA, Dupond JL. Nosocomial transmission of Dengue from a needlestick injury. *Lancet*. 1998;351(9101):498.
91. Gupta V, Bhoi S, Goel A, Admane S. Nosocomial Dengue in health-care workers. *Lancet*. 2008;371(9609):299.
92. Morgan C, Paraskevopoulou SM, Ashley EA, Probst F, Muir D. Nosocomial transmission of Dengue fever via needlestick: an occupational risk. *Trav Med Infect Dis*. 2015;13(3):271–273.
93. Nemes Z, Kiss G, Madarassi EP, et al. Nosocomial transmission of Dengue. *Emerg Infect Dis*. 2004;10(10):1880–1881.
94. Wagner D, de With K, Huzly D, et al. Nosocomial acquisition of Dengue. *Emerg Infect Dis*. 2004;10(10):1872–1873.
95. Halstead SB. Pathogenesis of Dengue: dawn of a new era. *F1000Res*. 2015;4.
96. Halstead SB, O'Rourke EJ. Dengue viruses and mononuclear phagocytes. I. Infection enhancement by non-neutralizing antibody. *J Exp Med*. 1977;146(1):201–217.
97. Halstead SB, O'Rourke EJ. Resuscitation of patients with Dengue hemorrhagic fever/Dengue shock syndrome [editorial response]. *Clin Infect Dis*. 1999;29(4):795–796.
98. Alagarasu K, Mulay AP, Singh R, et al. Association of HLA-DRB1 and TNF genotypes with Dengue hemorrhagic fever. *Hum Immunol*. 2013; 74(5):610–617.
99. Cardozo DM, Moliterno RA, Sell AM, et al. Evidence of HLA-DQB1 contribution to susceptibility of Dengue serotype 3 in Dengue patients in southern Brazil. *J Trop Med*. 2014;2014:968262.
100. Loeb M. Genetic susceptibility to West Nile virus and Dengue. *Publ Health Genom*. 2013;16(1–2):4–8.
101. Guzman MG, Alvarez M, Halstead SB. Secondary infection as a risk factor for Dengue hemorrhagic fever/Dengue shock syndrome: an historical perspective and role of antibody-dependent enhancement of infection. *Arch Virol*. 2013;158(7):1445–1459.
102. Guzman MG, Kouri G. Dengue and Dengue hemorrhagic fever in the Americas: lessons and challenges. *J Clin Virol*. 2003;27(1):1–13.
103. Pang T, Cardosa MJ, Guzman MG. Of cascades and perfect storms: the immunopathogenesis of Dengue haemorrhagic fever–Dengue shock syndrome (DHF/DSS). *Immunol Cell Biol*. 2007;85(1):43–45.
104. Antunes AC, Oliveira GL, Nunes LI, et al. Evaluation of the diagnostic value of the tourniquet test in predicting severe Dengue cases in a population from Belo Horizonte, State of Minas Gerais, Brazil. *Rev Soc Brasil Med Trop*. 2013;46(5):542–546.
105. Cao XT, Ngo TN, Wills B, et al. Evaluation of the World Health Organization standard tourniquet test and a modified tourniquet test in the diagnosis of Dengue infection in Viet Nam. *Trop Med Int Health*. 2002;7(2):125–132.
106. Mayxay M, Phetsouvanh R, Moore CE, et al. Predictive diagnostic value of the tourniquet test for the diagnosis of Dengue infection in adults. *Trop Med Int Health*. 2011;16(1):127–133.
107. Norlijah O, Khamisah AN, Kamarul A, et al. Repeated tourniquet testing as a diagnostic tool in Dengue infection. *Med J Malaysia*. 2006;61(1):22–27.
108. Wills BA, Oragui EE, Dung NM, et al. Size and charge characteristics of the protein leak in Dengue shock syndrome. *J Infect Dis*. 2004;190(4):810–818.
109. Diaz-Quijano FA, Villar-Centeno LA, Martinez-Vega RA. Predictors of spontaneous bleeding in patients with acute febrile syndrome from a Dengue endemic area. *J Clin Voirol*. 2010;49(1):11–15.
110. Zhang H, Zhou YP, Peng HJ, et al. Predictive symptoms and signs of severe Dengue disease for patients with Dengue fever: a meta-analysis. *BioMed Res Int*. 2014;2014:359308.
111. Martin J, Hermida L. Dengue vaccine: an update on recombinant subunit strategies. *Acta virologica* 2016;60(1):3–14.
112. Thisyakorn U, Thisyakorn C. Latest developments and future directions in Dengue vaccines. *Ther Adv Vacc*. 2014;2(1):3–9.
113. Gubler DJ. *Aedes aegypti* and *Aedes aegypti*-borne disease control in the 1990s: top down or bottom up. Charles Franklin Craig Lecture. *Am J Trop Med Hygiene*. 1989;40(6):571–578.
114. World Health Organization. *Global Tuberculosis Report 2015*. Geneva: World Health Organization; 2015.
115. Jensen PA, Lambert LA, Iademarco MF, Ridzon R. Guidelines for preventing the transmission of *Mycobacterium tuberculosis* in health-care settings, 2005. *MMWR Recomm Rep*. 2005;54(RR-17):1–141.
116. Taylor Z, Nolan CM, Blumberg HM. Controlling tuberculosis in the United States: recommendations from the American Thoracic Society, CDC, and the Infectious Diseases Society of America. *MMWR Morb Mortal Week Rep*. 2005;54(RR-12):1–81.
117. Babu GR, Laxminarayan R. The unsurprising story of MDR-TB resistance in India. *Tuberculosis*. 2012;92(4):301–306.
118. Daley CL, Caminero JA. Management of multidrug resistant tuberculosis. *Semin Resp Crit Care Med*. 2013;34(1):44–59.
119. Prasad R, Gupta N, Singh M. Multidrug resistant tuberculosis: trends and control. *Ind J Chest Dis Allied Sci*. 2014;56(4):237–246.
120. Streicher EM, Muller B, Chihota V, et al. Emergence and treatment of multidrug resistant (MDR) and extensively drug-resistant (XDR) tuberculosis in South Africa. *Infect Genet Evol*. 2012;12(4):686–694.
121. Amaral L, Kristiansen JE. Phenothiazines: an alternative to conventional therapy for the initial management of suspected multidrug resistant tuberculosis: a call for studies. *Int J Antimicrob Agents*. 2000;14(3):173–176.
122. Centers for Disease Control and Prevention. Emergence of *Mycobacterium tuberculosis* with extensive resistance to second-line drugs—worldwide, 2000-2004. *MMWR Morb Mortal Week Rep*. 2006;55(11):301–305.
123. Dheda K, Gumbo T, Gandhi NR, et al. Global control of tuberculosis: from extensively drug-resistant to untreatable tuberculosis. *Lancet Resp Med*. 2014;2(4):321–338.
124. Klopper M, Warren RM, Hayes C, et al. Emergence and spread of extensively and totally drug-resistant tuberculosis, South Africa. *Emerg Infect Dis*. 2013;19(3):449–455.
125. Extensively drug-resistant tuberculosis (XDR-TB): recommendations for prevention and control. *Rel Epidemiol*. 2006;81(45):430–432.
126. Banerjee R, Schecter GF, Flood J, Porco TC. Extensively drug-resistant tuberculosis: new strains, new challenges. *Exp Review Anti-infect Ther*. 2008;6(5):713–724.

127. Sotgiu G, D'Ambrosio L, Centis R, et al. Carbapenems to treat multidrug and extensively drug-resistant tuberculosis: a systematic review. *Int J Mol Sci*. 2016;17(3):373.
128. Wilson JW, Tsukayama DT. Extensively drug-resistant tuberculosis: principles of resistance, diagnosis, and management. *Mayo Clin Proc*. 2016;91(4):482–495.
129. Jakab Z, Acosta CD, Kluge HH, Dara M. Consolidated action plan to prevent and combat multidrug- and extensively drug-resistant tuberculosis in the WHO European region 2011-2015: cost-effectiveness analysis. *Tuberculosis*. 2015;95(Suppl 1):S212–S216.
130. Lange C, Abubakar I, Alffenaar JW, et al. Management of patients with multidrug-resistant/extensively drug-resistant tuberculosis in Europe: a TBNET consensus statement. *Eur Resp J*. 2014;44(1):23–63.
131. Chang KC, Yew WW. Management of difficult multidrug-resistant tuberculosis and extensively drug-resistant tuberculosis: update 2012. *Respirology*. 2013;18(1):8–21.
132. Parida SK, Axelsson-Robertson R, Rao MV, et al. Totally drug-resistant tuberculosis and adjunct therapies. *J Intern Med*. 2015;277(4):388–405.
133. Migliori GB, De Iaco G, Besozzi G, et al. First tuberculosis cases in Italy resistant to all tested drugs. *Euro Surveill*. 2007;12(5):E0705171.
134. Provisional CDC guidelines for the use and safety monitoring of bedaquiline fumarate (Sirturo) for the treatment of multidrug-resistant tuberculosis. *MMWR Recomm Rep*. 2013;62(RR-09):1–12.
135. Calligaro GL, Moodley L, Symons G, Dheda K. The medical and surgical treatment of drug-resistant tuberculosis. *J Thorac Dis*. 2014;6(3):186–195.
136. Jevons MP, Coe AW, Parker MT. Methicillin resistance in staphylococci. *Lancet*. 1963;1(7287):904–907.
137. Grundmann H, Aires-de-Sousa M, Boyce J, Tiemersma E. Emergence and resurgence of meticillin-resistant *Staphylococcus aureus* as a public-health threat. *Lancet*. 2006;368(9538):874–885.
138. Kuehnert MJ, Kruszon-Moran D, Hill HA, et al. Prevalence of *Staphylococcus aureus* nasal colonization in the United States, 2001-2002. *J Infect Dis*. 2006;193(2):172–179.
139. Hartman B, Tomasz A. Altered penicillin-binding proteins in methicillin-resistant strains of *Staphylococcus aureus*. *Antimicrob Agents Chemother*. 1981;19(5):726–735.
140. Marschall J, Muhlemann K. Duration of methicillin-resistant *Staphylococcus aureus* carriage, according to risk factors for acquisition. *Infect Control Hosp Epidemiol*. 2006;27(11):1206–1212.
141. Hidron AI, Kourbatova EV, Halvosa JS, et al. Risk factors for colonization with methicillin-resistant Staphyl*ococcus aureus* (MRSA) in patients admitted to an urban hospital: emergence of community-associated MRSA nasal carriage. *Clin Infect Dis*. 2005;41(2):159–166.
142. Lucet JC, Chevret S, Durand-Zaleski I, et al. Prevalence and risk factors for carriage of methicillin-resistant *Staphylococcus aureus* at admission to the intensive care unit: results of a multicenter study. *Arch Intern Med*. 2003;163(2):181–188.
143. Troillet N, Carmeli Y, Samore MH, et al. Carriage of methicillin-resistant *Staphylococcus aureus* at hospital admission. *Infect Control Hosp Epidemiol*. 1998;19(3):181–185.
144. Calfee DP, Salgado CD, Milstone AM, et al. Strategies to prevent methicillin-resistant *Staphylococcus aureus* transmission and infection in acute care hospitals: 2014 update. *Infect Control Hosp Epidemiol*. 2014;35(Suppl 2):S108–S132.
145. Huang SS, Platt R. Risk of methicillin-resistant *Staphylococcus aureus* infection after previous infection or colonization. *Clin Infect Dis*. 2003; 36(3):281–285.
146. Huang SS, Yokoe DS, Hinrichsen VL, et al. Impact of routine intensive care unit surveillance cultures and resultant barrier precautions on hospital-wide methicillin-resistant *Staphylococcus aureus* bacteremia. *Clin Infect Dis*. 2006;43(8):971–978.
147. Datta R, Platt R, Yokoe DS, Huang SS. Environmental cleaning intervention and risk of acquiring multidrug-resistant organisms from prior room occupants. *Arch Internal Med*. 2011;171(6):491–494.
148. Mainous AG III, Hueston WJ, Everett CJ, Diaz VA. Nasal carriage of *Staphylococcus aureus* and methicillin-resistant *S aureus* in the United States, 2001-2002. *Ann Fam Med*. 2006;4(2):132–137.
149. Glick SB, Samson DJ, Huang ES, et al. Screening for methicillin-resistant *Staphylococcus aureus*: a comparative effectiveness review. *Am J Infect Control*. 2014;42(2):148–155.
150. Noorani HZ, Adams E, Glick S, et al. Screening for Methicillin-Resistant Staphylococcus aureus (MRSA): Future Research Needs: Identification of Future Research Needs from Comparative Effectiveness Review no. 102. Rockville, MD; 2013.
151. Clancy M, Graepler A, Wilson M, et al. Active screening in high-risk units is an effective and cost-avoidant method to reduce the rate of methicillin-resistant *Staphylococcus aureus* infection in the hospital. *Infect Control Hosp Epidemiol*. 2006;27(10):1009–1017.
152. Khoury J, Jones M, Grim A, et al. Eradication of methicillin-resistant *Staphylococcus aureus* from a neonatal intensive care unit by active surveillance and aggressive infection control measures. *Infect Control Hosp Epidemiol*. 2005; 26(7):616–621.
153. Hubner C, Hubner NO, Wegner C, Flessa S. Impact of different diagnostic technologies for MRSA admission screening in hospitals: a decision tree analysis. *Antimicrob Resist Infect Control*. 2015;4:50.
154. Tenover FC. Rapid detection and identification of bacterial pathogens using novel molecular technologies: infection control and beyond. *Clin Infect Dis*. 2007;44(3):418–423.
155. Carroll KC. Rapid diagnostics for methicillin-resistant Staphylococcus aureus: current status. *Mole Diagn Ther*. 2008;12(1):15–24.
156. Hirvonen JJ. The use of molecular methods for the detection and identification of methicillin-resistant Staphylococcus aureus. *Biomark Med*. 2014;8(9):1115–1125.
157. Palavecino EL. Rapid methods for detection of MRSA in clinical specimens. *Methods Mol Biol (Clifton, NJ)*. 2014;1085:71–83.
158. Tacconelli E, De Angelis G, de Waure C, et al. Rapid screening tests for meticillin-resistant *Staphylococcus aureus* at hospital admission: systematic review and meta-analysis. *Lancet Infect Dis*. 2009;9(9):546–554.
159. Harbarth S, Masuet-Aumatell C, Schrenzel J, et al. Evaluation of rapid screening and pre-emptive contact isolation for detecting and controlling methicillin-resistant *Staphylococcus aureus* in critical care: an interventional cohort study. *Crit Care*. 2006;10(1):R25.
160. Roisin S, Laurent C, Denis O, et al. Impact of rapid molecular screening at hospital admission on nosocomial transmission of methicillin-resistant *Staphylococcus aureus*: cluster randomised trial. *PloS One*. 2014;9(5):e96310.
161. Turnidge JD, Bell JM. Methicillin-resistant *Staphylococcal aureus* evolution in Australia over 35 years. *Microb Drug Resist*. 2000;6(3):223–229.
162. Lessa FC, Mu Y, Ray SM, et al. Impact of USA300 methicillin-resistant *Staphylococcus aureus* on clinical outcomes of patients with pneumonia or central line-associated bloodstream infections. *Clin Infect Dis*. 2012;55(2):232–241.
163. Nair N, Kourbatova E, Poole K, et al. Molecular epidemiology of methicillin-resistant *Staphylococcus aureus* (MRSA) among patients admitted to adult intensive care units: the STAR*ICU trial. *Infect Control Hosp Epidemiol*. 2011;32(11):1057–1063.
164. Wang JT, Liao CH, Fang CT, et al. Incidence of and risk factors for community-associated methicillin-resistant *Staphylococcus aureus* acquired infection or colonization in intensive-care-unit patients. *J Clin Microbiol*. 2010;48(12):4439–4444.
165. Elstrom P, Aavitsland P. [Meticillin resistant *Staphylococcus aureus* in Norway]. *Tidsskr Nor Laegeforen*. 2008;128(23):2730–2733.
166. Daniels-Haardt I, Verhoeven F, Mellmann A, et al. [EUREGIO-projekt MRSA-net Twente/Munsterland. Creation of a regional network to combat MRSA]. *Gesundheitswesen*. 2006;68(11):674–678.
167. Higgins A, Lynch M, Gethin G. Can "search and destroy" reduce nosocomial methicillin-resistant *Staphylococcus aureus* in an Irish hospital? *J Hosp Infect*. 2010;75(2):120–123.
168. Holzknecht BJ, Hardardottir H, Haraldsson G, et al. Changing epidemiology of methicillin-resistant *Staphylococcus aureus* in Iceland from 2000 to 2008: a challenge to current guidelines. *J Clin Microbiol*. 2010;48(11):4221–4227.
169. Souverein D, Houtman P, Euser SM, et al. Costs and benefits associated with the MRSA search and destroy policy in a hospital in the Region Kennemerland, The Netherlands. *PloS One*. 2016;11(2):e0148175.
170. Sturenburg E. Rapid detection of methicillin-resistant *Staphylococcus aureus* directly from clinical samples: methods, effectiveness and cost considerations. *Germ Med Sci*. 2009;7:Doc06.
171. Traa MX, Barboza L, Doron S, et al. Horizontal infection control strategy decreases methicillin-resistant *Staphylococcus aureus* infection and eliminates bacteremia in a surgical ICU without active surveillance. *Crit Care Med*. 2014;42(10):2151–2157.
172. van der Zee A, Hendriks WD, Roorda L, et al. Review of a major epidemic of methicillin-resistant *Staphylococcus aureus*: the costs of screening and consequences of outbreak management. *Am J Infect Control*. 2013;41(3):204–209.
173. Wagener J, Seybold U. [MRSA—hygiene management, diagnostics and treatment]. *Dtsch Med Wochenschr*. 2014;139(13):643–651.
174. Wassenberg MW, Bonten MJ. [The Dutch MRSA policy can and should be different]. *Ned Tijdschr Geneeskd*. 2010;154(45):A2575.
175. Widner A, Nobles DL, Faulk C, et al. The impact of a "search and destroy" strategy for the prevention of methicillin-resistant *Staphylococcus aureus* infections in an inpatient rehabilitation facility. *PM R*. 2014;6(2):121–126.
176. Muto CA, Jernigan JA, Ostrowsky BE, et al. SHEA guideline for preventing nosocomial transmission of multidrug-resistant strains of *Staphylococcus aureus* and Enterococcus. *Infect Control Hosp Epidemiol*. 2003;24(5):362–386.

177. Byrne FM, Wilcox MH. MRSA prevention strategies and current guidelines. *Injury*. 2011;42(Suppl 5):S3–S6.
178. Harbarth S. Control of endemic methicillin-resistant *Staphylococcus aureus*: recent advances and future challenges. *Clin Microbiol Infect*. 2006;12(12):1154–1162.
179. Kjonegaard R, Fields W, Peddecord KM. Universal rapid screening for methicillin-resistant Staphylococcus aureus in the intensive care units in a large community hospital. *Am J Infect Control*. 2013;41(1):45–50.
180. Kock R, Becker K, Cookson B, et al. Systematic literature analysis and review of targeted preventive measures to limit healthcare-associated infections by meticillin-resistant *Staphylococcus aureus*. *Euro Surveill*. 2014;19(29):pii: 20860.
181. McKinnell JA, Miller LG, Eells SJ, et al. A systematic literature review and meta-analysis of factors associated with methicillin-resistant *Staphylococcus aureus* colonization at time of hospital or intensive care unit admission. *Infect Control Hosp Epidemiol*. 2013;34(10):1077–1086.
182. Polisena J, Chen S, Cimon K, et al. Clinical effectiveness of rapid tests for methicillin resistant *Staphylococcus aureus* (MRSA) in hospitalized patients: a systematic review. *BMC Infect Dis*. 2011;11:336.
183. Robinson DA, Kearns AM, Holmes A, et al. Re-emergence of early pandemic *Staphylococcus aureus* as a community-acquired meticillin-resistant clone. *Lancet*. 2005;365(9466):1256–1258.
184. Harris JB, LaRocque RC, Qadri F, et al. Cholera. *Lancet*. 2012;379(9835):2466–2476.
185. Mukhopadhyay AK, Takeda Y, Balakrish Nair G. Cholera outbreaks in the El Tor biotype era and the impact of the new El Tor variants. *Curr Top Microbiol Immunol*. 2014;379:17–47.
186. Siddique AK, Cash R. Cholera outbreaks in the classical biotype era. *Curr Top Microbiol Immunol*. 2014;79:1–16.
187. First steps for managing an outbreak of acute diarrhoea. WHO Global Task Force on Cholera Control, 2010. Available at http://www.who.int/cholera/publications/firststeps/en/. Accessed March 28, 2016.
188. Zumla A, Hui DS, Perlman S. Middle East respiratory syndrome. *Lancet*. 2015;386(9997):995–1007.
189. Al-Tawfiq JA, Zumla A, Memish ZA. Coronaviruses: severe acute respiratory syndrome coronavirus and Middle East respiratory syndrome coronavirus in travelers. *Curr Opin Infect Dis*. 2014;27(5):411–417.
190. Arabi Y, Balkhy H, Hajeer AH, et al. Feasibility, safety, clinical, and laboratory effects of convalescent plasma therapy for patients with Middle East respiratory syndrome coronavirus infection: a study protocol. *SpringerPlus*. 2015;4:709.
191. Waggoner JJ, Pinsky BA. Zika virus: diagnostics for an emerging pandemic threat. *J Clin Microbiol*. 2016;54(4):860–867.

CHAPTER 94

Chest Pain and Acute Coronary Syndrome: Non–ST-Elevation Acute Coronary Syndrome and ST-Elevation Myocardial Infarction

ACHILLE GASPARDONE and GREGORY A. SGUEGLIA

INTRODUCTION

Chest pain represents an important symptom deserving immediate evaluation in the intensive care unit (ICU). Moreover, the differential diagnosis of chest pain is extensive, ranging from benign musculoskeletal etiologies to life-threatening cardiac diseases. Acute coronary syndrome (ACS), including myocardial infarction (MI) with or without ST-segment elevation, represents one of the most ominous causes of chest pain since it significantly increases both morbidity and mortality of critically ill patients. Observational studies highlighted the higher complexity of MI patients originally hospitalized for another reason (1,2). Yet, the availability of effective treatments for ACS to minimize permanent myocardial damage requires an understanding of this condition to provide appropriate and immediate care.

Owing to its significance and frequency, MI will be the main focus of this chapter with special emphasis on specific issues that may arise in the ICU. The general approach to the patient with chest pain and differential diagnosis of chest pain in the ICU will be described in the Diagnosis section.

PATHOPHYSIOLOGY

Acute Myocardial Infarction

Sudden conversion of a stable atherosclerotic plaque to an unstable atherothrombotic lesion is the initiating event of acute myocardial infarction (AMI). Coronary plaque activation, including fissuring, rupture, or erosion exposes the subendothelial matrix to circulating blood, leading to platelets adhesion and activation, thrombin generation, and thrombus formation. This is a dynamic process involving cyclic transitions including total vessel occlusion, partial vessel occlusion, and intermittent or permanent reperfusion (3). Plaques that rupture, often termed vulnerable plaques, tend to have a thin fibrous cap over a central core of foam cells, lipids, and necrotic debris (Fig. 94.1). Inflammation is considered to play a critical role in plaque rupture by driving the release by activated macrophages of proteolytic enzymes that progressively weaken the fibrous cap, eventually leading to plaque rupture, typically near its junction with normal endothelium (3). Acute hemodynamic stress synergistically associated with increased adrenergic tone is considered another important trigger of plaque rupture.

The extent of the thrombotic reaction within coronary lumen determines the severity of coronary arterial obstruction, and the volume of affected myocardium determines the clinical course of the patient. Total occlusion of an artery supplying a substantial volume of myocardium typically drives ST-segment elevation myocardial infarction (STEMI) while a persistent injury causing partial occlusion of the vessel determines non–ST-segment elevation myocardial infarction (NSTEMI).

Coronary artery narrowing caused by thrombus causes a rapid reduction of myocardial perfusion, resulting in an acute mismatch between oxygen supply and demand. Distal microembolization of thrombus and disrupted plaque components may further reduce perfusion of the distal microvasculature. Additionally, a variety of vasoactive mediators are released from the cells interplaying in thrombus formation and can cause vessel constriction and further worsening of the picture (4). Furthermore, in critically ill patients, acute myocardial ischemia may also be caused by an increase of myocardial oxygen demand in the presence of a fixed (not activated) epicardial coronary artery stenosis. Oxygen supply is dependent on the available oxygen, that is, the oxygen-carrying capacity of the blood, the perfusion pressure, and resistance to coronary blood flow. Indeed, any fixed stenosis in an epicardial coronary artery may limit the increase of myocardial blood flow, upsetting the normal supply–demand balance and precipitating ischemia in circumstances of increased myocardial oxygen demand, which is dependent on heart rate, blood pressure, contractility, and wall stress. In the critically ill patient, fever, pain, and endogenous and exogenous catecholamines promote tachycardia, increased myocardial contractility, and the generation of higher wall tension, all of which increase myocardial oxygen demand. On the other hand, oxygen supply may be diminished as a result of blood loss, anemia, iatrogenic hypotension, or respiratory disease. Like critical illness, recovery from major trauma or surgical interventions places extra demands on the myocardium by increasing oxygen consumption.

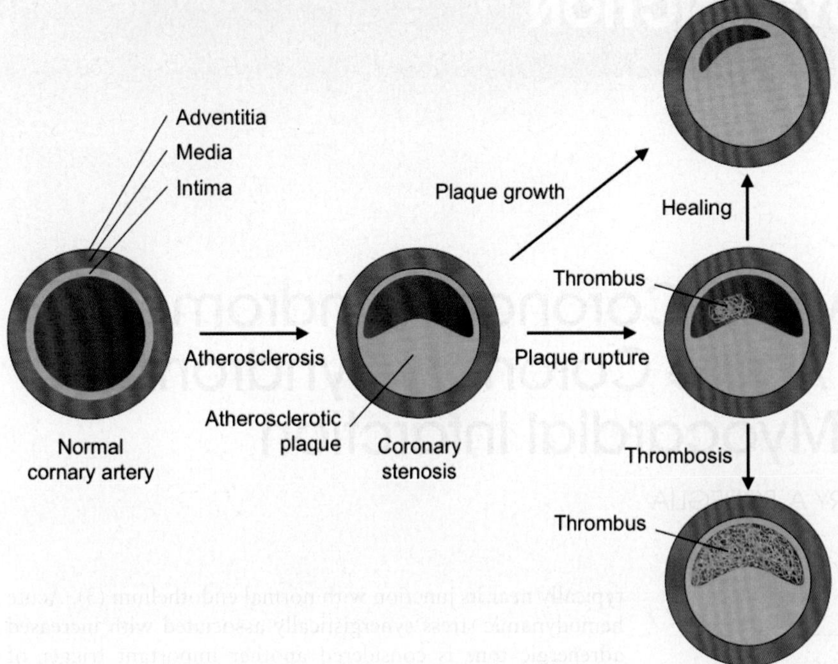

FIGURE 94.1 Initiation, progression, and complication of human coronary atherosclerotic plaque.

Coronary artery spasm, which is a sudden, intense vasoconstriction of an epicardial coronary artery causing vessel occlusion or near occlusion, represents a less frequent cause of myocardial ischemia. Coronary artery spasm typically represents the cause of Prinzmetal variant angina; functional vessel occlusion is usually transient although when being prolonged it may cause AMI (5). Another cause of epicardial coronary spasm is cocaine use that can cause prolonged interruption of coronary blood flow leading to myocardial infarction and life-threatening arrhythmias.

Complications

After an AMI, mechanical problems that result from dysfunction or disruption of critical myocardial structures may occur portending a significantly worse outcome. Cardiogenic shock usually results from extensive loss of left ventricle contractile function, but may occur with other mechanical complications of AMI. Indeed, right ventricle infarction may lead to decreased compliance and decreased systolic function thus causing venous congestion and low cardiac output. Severe ischemia or infarction can lead to papillary muscle dysfunction or rupture, resulting in mitral valve regurgitation of varying severity. The posterior medial papillary muscle, in association with inferior wall infarction is most commonly affected as it has a single blood supply; the anterior medial papillary muscle with its dual blood supply is less affected. Ventricular septal defects may occur with extensive anterior and inferior wall infarction. The size of the defect and extent of the left-to-right shunt determine the clinical features, usually dominated by shock. Acute free wall rupture is a catastrophic event presenting with severe hypotension with relatively unchanged electrocardiogram (ECG) although it is occasionally subacute. Of note, shock may also occur in patients with relative or absolute hypovolemia, especially in those with increased vagal tone due to the Bezold–Jarisch reflex.

In the long term, the left ventricle will undergo a transformation of its size and shape through a process known as negative remodeling. This enlargement which is proportional to the scar extension has a detrimental effect on left ventricular function eventually leading to chronic heart failure.

Additionally, potentially life-threatening cardiac dysrhythmias may result from electrical instability due to ischemia, conduction disturbances, and excessive sympathetic stimulation. Sinus tachycardia, resulting from pain, anxiety, or heart failure is the most common supraventricular arrhythmia in patients with AMI. Sinus bradycardia is usually seen in the setting of inferior ischemia as a result of the high concentration of vagal efferent nerves in the inferior-posterior wall and sinus node. Atrial fibrillation, seen less frequently, has as its underlying causes atrial ischemia, excess catecholamines, and heart failure–induced increased left atrial pressure. Tachycardia increases myocardial oxygen consumption and may increase infarct size. Moreover, ventricular tachycardias are of high life-threatening potential. The most common ventricular dysrhythmias are polymorphic ventricular tachycardia and ventricular fibrillation originating from area of active ischemia that determines electrical instability.

Conduction blocks may represent another manifestation of AMI. Atrioventricular block is most often evident in case of inferior ischemia or infarction because of excessive vagal tone or hypoperfusion through the atrioventricular nodal branches. Right bundle branch block or left posterior fascicular block may also occur in this setting because branches from the posterior descending artery perfuse both the proximal third of the right bundle and the left posterior fascicle.

In case of anterior ischemia, hypoperfusion involves the distal right bundle, the main left bundle, and the left anterior fascicle that are usually supplied by the left anterior descending artery. Under these circumstances atrioventricular block is more typically infranodal causing junctional or ventricular rhythm.

TABLE 94.1 Causes of Chest Pain in the ICU

Cardiovascular
Angina
Myocardial infarction
Aortic valve stenosis
Aortic dissection or aortic ulcer
Congestive heart failure
Pericarditis
Pulmonary
Pulmonary embolism
Pneumothorax
Pneumonia
Pleurisy
Tracheobronchitis
Chest tubes
Gastrointestinal
Esophageal reflux or spasm
Peptic ulcer disease
Cholecystitis
Pancreatitis
Hepatic capsule distention
Subdiaphragmatic abscess
Musculoskeletal
Costochondritis or Tietze syndrome
Arthritis
Postcardiopulmonary resuscitation trauma
Postoperative pain
Neurologic
Herpes zoster
Compression neuropathy
Psychological
Anxiety
Panic disorder
Depression
Hysteria

TABLE 94.2 Differentiating Cardiac Ischemic from Noncardiac Chest Pain

Favoring Ischemic Origin	Against Ischemic Origin
Character of pain	
Constricting	Sharp
Squeezing	Knifelike
Burning	Stabbing
Heaviness	
Location of pain	
Substernal	Left submammary area
Across midthorax	Left hemithorax
Radiation of pain	
Arms, forearms	
Shoulders	
Interscapular region	
Neck	
Teeth	
Duration of pain	
Minutes	Seconds
	Hours (no evidence of myocardial damage)

DIAGNOSIS

Diagnosis of chest pain in the ICU is compelling, and particularly challenging, due to numerous cardiac and noncardiac potentially life-threatening causes and comorbidities (Table 94.1). Every patient with chest pain should rapidly have a comprehensive evaluation including assessment of symptoms at presentation, clinical history and examination of the cardiovascular system, standard 12-lead ECG, and evaluation of serum markers of myocardial injury. When AMI is diagnosed, risk stratification based on the data obtained during the initial workup is a next step to predict the risk of adverse events and guide optimal treatment.

Clinical Assessment

Initial patient assessment is directed to accurately characterize the patient's discomfort and identify its location, duration, aggravating, and relieving factors. Classic presentation of myocardial ischemia is substernal chest pain described as pressure, squeezing, or a sensation of suffocation (Table 94.2). Some patients may however describe aching, burning, or tightness. The pain frequently radiates to the left arm, and less frequently, to the right arm, the neck, and the jaw. Epigastric or interscapular pain is seldom reported. The discomfort of AMI is similar to that of myocardial ischemia but is more severe, longer in duration, and is not usually relieved with nitroglycerin. Typically, peak intensity is not instantaneous but is reached in a crescendo pattern.

Dyspnea is frequently associated to chest pain and may be the major symptom in a number of patients with ACS. Also, in some patients, especially women and the elderly, other atypical symptoms including diaphoresis, palpitation, dizziness, nausea, and vomiting may be prevalent or associated to more typical ischemic chest pain. In some cases, myocardial infarction may occur without any symptoms. A review of patient's medical history should aim at identifying cardiovascular risk factors, previous cardiovascular disease, and other conditions affecting the oxygen supply–demand ratio or acting as ischemia precipitants.

Physical Examination

The examination should include assessment of hemodynamic status and a screening neurologic evaluation. Physical signs of myocardial ischemia are frequently limited and nonspecific, especially in the critically ill patient; vital signs abnormalities can suggest a perturbation in cardiac function. Indeed, bradycardia may reflect conduction tissue ischemia whereas tachycardia and hypotension may be due to impaired left ventricle contractility and low cardiac output. Jugular venous distention usually reflects right ventricle failure, whereas diaphoresis and cyanosis are due to peripheral vasoconstriction and poor cardiac output, respectively.

Auscultation of the heart may reveal a newly appearing third or fourth heart sound indicating acute ventricular dysfunction. A new systolic murmur suggests mitral valve regurgitation due to papillary muscle ischemia. Auscultation of the lungs may reveal different degrees of pulmonary edema caused

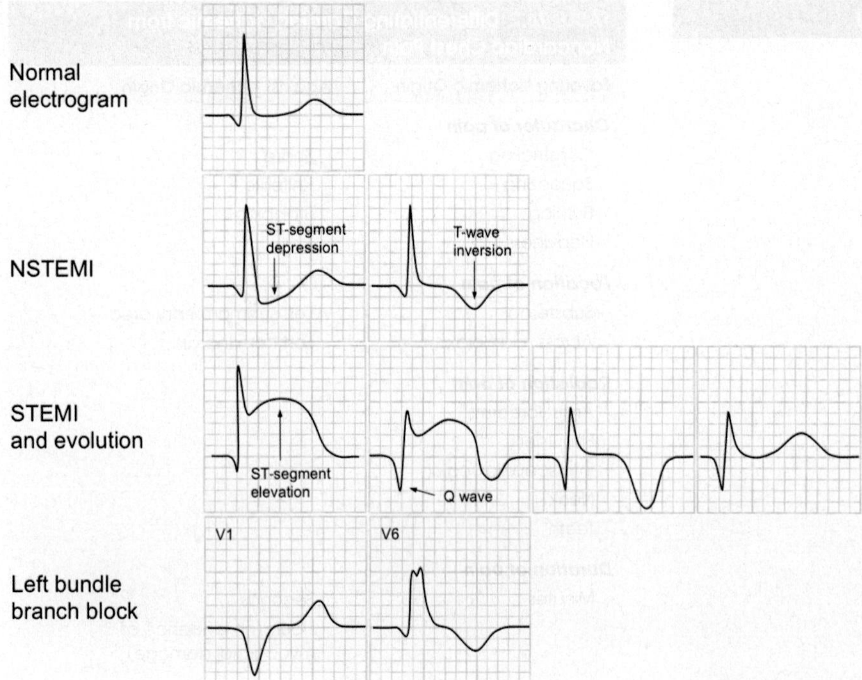

FIGURE 94.2 Main electrocardiographic patterns in acute myocardial infarction.

by left ventricle impairment. Importantly, peripheral pulses palpation and blood pressure measurement in both arms complete physical examination.

Electrocardiogram

Every patient complaining of new onset chest pain should have an ECG immediately. Moreover, critically ill ICU patients should have routine ECGs, especially in case of a significant change in vital or physical signs. Most frequently, myocardial ischemia causes repolarization abnormalities including T-wave inversion and ST-segment depression while ST-segment elevation is consistent with transmural myocardial infarction and is generally followed by appearance of Q waves and T-wave inversion (Fig. 94.2). A new occurring left bundle branch block is considered equivalent of an anterior wall STEMI. However, previous left bundle branch block and pacing can interfere with the electrocardiographic diagnosis of coronary ischemia. Isolated T-wave abnormalities are more difficult to interpret due to their poor specificity, especially in ICU where multiple conditions including chronic hypertension, pulmonary embolism, hyperventilation, neurologic events, anxiety, extracardiac diseases, and several drugs may produce T-wave changes very similar to those generally caused by myocardial ischemia.

Specific ECG leads explore different coronary arteries. Indeed, leads II, III, and aVF typically explore the right coronary artery; leads I, aVL, V5, and V6 explore the left circumflex artery; and precordial leads V1 to V4 explore left anterior descending artery. Occasionally, ST-segment elevation in V1–V2 may reflect a posterior wall ischemia and conversely, ST-segment depression in V1–V2 may reflect a posterior wall MI. Accordingly, reciprocal ST-segment depression in mirror-image leads is frequently observed in STEMI. Of note, positive inflection and ST elevation in lead aVR, usually negative, may be indicative of left main occlusion and deserves maximal attention (Table 94.3).

Additionally, the ECG is useful to document possible complications of myocardial ischemia or myocardial infarction, such dysrhythmias or conduction blocks that require specific and urgent management.

Biomarkers of Myocardial Injury

When myocardial injury occurs a variety of biochemical compounds are released into the blood. Assessment of myocardial injury most commonly relies on the measurement of the enzyme creatine kinase (CK), its dimeric isoform CK-MB (muscle and brain subunits) and the structural proteins cardiac troponin T or I. After an AMI, CK and CK-MB start increasing within 4 to 6 hours, peak within 18 to 24 hours, and remain elevated for 48 to 72 hours. Troponins appear at 2 to 6 hours after symptom onset, peak at 15 to 20 hours, and remain elevated for 5 to 7 days (Fig. 94.3).

Increase of CK and CK-MB are very sensitive to diagnose AMI, but trace amounts are generally present in blood and, as these enzymes are also present in other tissues, their rising values may reflect other conditions such as trauma or surgery. Troponins are very specific to myocardial tissue and are gener-

TABLE 94.3 ECG Definition of Coronary Territory

ECG Abnormality	Coronary Territory
Leads II, III, and aVF	Typically the RCA
Leads I, aVL, V5, and V6	Typically the left circumflex artery
Precordial leads V1 to V4	Typically the LAD artery
ST-segment elevation in V1–V2	Occasionally reflects posterior wall (PW) ischemia
ST-segment depression in V1–V2	May reflect PWMI
Positive inflection and ST elevation, lead aVR	May indicate left main occlusion

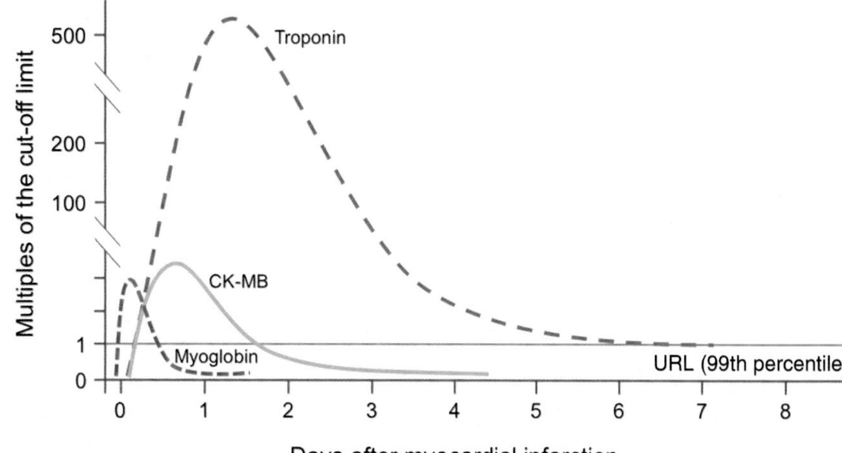

FIGURE 94.3 Release curves of main markers of myocardial injury.

ally not detectable in blood, although their elevation can result from causes of myocardial injury other than ACSs (Table 94.4). Furthermore, troponins are cleared by the kidney and may show persisting mild elevation in patients with advanced renal failure. Therefore, the value of these markers must always be interpreted critically in the clinical context and according to their timetable of release. Recently a new high sensitivity test for troponin assessment have been introduced in routine practice; by using this test it is possible to design a release curve within 3 to 6 hours from the onset of chest pain that, in uncertain cases, is extremely useful to rule out an acute myocardial ischemia.

Other Blood Tests and Imaging

Blood chemistry is essential to acquire important information about main organs and whole body function to guide diagnosis and implementation of the best treatment. Arterial blood gas analysis provides useful data on pulmonary gas exchange and acid/base balance, and has a specific role in differential diagnosis. Cardiac natriuretic peptides are useful diagnostic and prognostic markers for patients with heart failure. D-dimer is a fibrin degradation product being measured to rule out the presence of an inappropriate blood clot such as occurring in pulmonary embolism. Chest radiography is particularly useful to assess for pulmonary edema and other conditions involving lungs and pleurae. It also provides some potentially useful insight on heart and great vessels. Echocardiography is very helpful tool for a bedside assessment of global and regional left ventricular function. Regional function analysis includes evaluation of both wall thickening and wall motion toward the left ventricular center. Myocardial segments with abnormal contractility coexisting with areas of normal contractile myocardium are highly suggestive ischemic heart disease. On the other hand, areas of thinned and akinetic myocardium suggest scarred or chronically hypoperfused myocardium. Echocardiography can also reveal heart valve abnormalities, pericardial disease, and some aortic disorders.

Although computed tomography has the ability to identify epicardial coronary stenosis, its role in the assessment of chest pain is mainly limited to the imaging of pulmonary structures and great vessels in a differential diagnostic workup. Triple rule out computed tomography aiming at excluding the three most important causes of chest pain in a single examination is appealing although its role appears still uncertain (6).

TABLE 94.4 Nonischemic Causes of Cardiac Troponin Elevation

Tachydysrhythmias or bradydysrhythmias
Severe aortic stenosis
Aortic dissection
Hypertrophic cardiomyopathy
Myocarditis
Shock
Severe anemia
Hypertension with and without left ventricle hypertrophy
Cardiac contusion
Surgery
Defibrillator shock
Rhabdomyolysis with cardiac involvement
Cardiotoxicity
Mental stress and Takotsubo cardiomyopathy
Pulmonary embolism
Sepsis
Critical illness
Severe kidney disease
Severe acute neurologic disease
Infiltrative disease (amyloidosis, sarcoidosis)
Strenuous exercise

Differential Diagnosis

Acute Myocardial Infarction

The diagnosis of AMI relies on criteria established by a committee grouping the European Society of Cardiology (ESC), the American College of Cardiology (ACC), the American Heart Association (AHA), and the World Heart Federation (WHF). Indeed, according to the Third Universal Definition, AMI is a clinical event consequent to the death of cardiac myocytes (myocardial necrosis) that is caused by ischemia (as opposed to other etiologies) (7). According to this definition, spontaneous myocardial infarction—also known as type 1—occurs in cases of detection of a rise and/or fall of cardiac biomarker values (preferably cardiac troponin) with at least one value above the 99th percentile upper reference limit (URL) and with at least one of the following: symptoms of ischemia, ischemic ECG changes, identification of an intracoronary thrombus by angiography, or imaging evidence of new loss of viable myocardium or a new regional wall motion abnormality.

ECG findings consistent with STEMI are: new ST elevation at the J point in two anatomically contiguous leads using the following diagnostic thresholds: 0.1 mV (1 mm) or more in all leads other than V2–V3. In V2-V3 leads the following diagnostic thresholds apply: 0.2 mV (2 mm) or more in men 40 years or older; 0.25 mV (2.5 mm) or more in men under 40 years; or 0.15 mV (1.5 mm) or more in women.

Findings consistent with NSTEMI are: new horizontal or down-sloping ST depression 0.05 mV (0.5 mm) or more in two anatomically contiguous leads and/or T inversion 0.1 mV (1 mm) or more in two anatomically contiguous leads with prominent R wave or R/S ratio greater than 1.

The other types of myocardial infarction identified according to the Third Universal Definition are as follows: type 2, myocardial infarction due to ischemic blood supply/demand imbalance; type 3, cardiac death presumed to be caused by myocardial infarction when markers of myocardial injury are unavailable; type 4a, myocardial infarction associated with percutaneous coronary intervention (arbitrary defined by elevation of biomarker values higher than five times 99th percentile URL in patients with normal baseline values or a rise of values over 20% if the baseline values are elevated but stable or falling); type 4b, myocardial infarction related to stent thrombosis; and type 5, myocardial infarction associated to coronary artery bypass grafting (arbitrary defined by elevation of biomarker values over 10 times the 99th percentile URL in patients with normal baseline values) (7).

Takotsubo Cardiomyopathy

Takotsubo cardiomyopathy starts abruptly and unpredictably, with symptoms of chest pain and, often, shortness of breath, usually triggered by an emotionally or physically stressful event (stress cardiomyopathy), especially in postmenopausal women. Typically, ECG changes mimic an anterior wall myocardial infarction whereas coronary arteries lack significant obstructions. During the evaluation of the patient, generally a bulging out of the left ventricular apex is found associated with preserved function of the bases. This apical ballooning is the hallmark of the syndrome that has been termed Takotsubo after a resemblance with the traditional Japanese octopus pot (8). For the final diagnosis, coronary angiography is needed.

Pericarditis

Typically, in this disorder, chest pain changes with the person's position. The physical examination may reveal a pericardial friction rub, and ECG abnormalities include diffuse ST-segment elevation, PR depression, and peaked T waves. Generally, ECG signs are out of proportion to the clinical scenario; an ECG clue of the diagnosis of pericarditis is that ST-segment elevation is often concave whereas it is typically convex in STEMI. Also, reciprocal ST depression does not occur in pericarditis. Markers of myocardial injury may be elevated when the inflammatory process spreads toward the contiguous myocardium (epimyocarditis). Echocardiography is useful to evaluate pericardial effusion—which can, however, occur in AMI—and in assessing left ventricle wall motion, which is typically normal in pericarditis despite persisting ongoing pain and electrocardiographic abnormalities.

Myocarditis

Symptoms and ECG findings, frequently, are similar to those of AMI. Physical examination and echocardiography may point toward left ventricle dysfunction. Clinical history will generally reveal insidious onset and recent viral syndrome. Frequently coronary angiography is needed to rule out coronary artery disease.

Acute Aortic Dissection

Sharp, tearing chest pain radiating through the chest to the back is the typical presentation of aortic dissection. Typically, the maximal intensity of pain is reached immediately. Pulse and/or blood pressure often generally diminished in the left arm and/or in the legs. Proximal extension of the dissection to the coronary arteries can result in compression of the proximal coronary arteries and AMI. Chest radiography may reveal an enlarged mediastinum and echocardiography may show a dissection flap in the proximal ascending aorta; definitive diagnosis is obtained by computed tomography.

Pulmonary Embolism

Tachycardia and tachypnea associated with diffuse chest pain but without evidence of pulmonary edema suggests pulmonary embolism. Cough may be present. Echocardiography helps to rule out left ventricle wall motion abnormalities and identify right ventricular strain (enlargement, wall motion abnormalities, tricuspid regurgitation). The most frequent ECG finding is sinus tachycardia with nonspecific ST-segment and T-wave changes; the $S_1Q_3T_3$ pattern (a large S wave in lead I, a Q wave in lead III, and an inverted T wave in lead III) is classic, although rarely seen. Final diagnosis is achieved with ventilation–perfusion lung scan, pulmonary angiogram, or with the computed tomographic angiography.

Pneumothorax

Pain is usually sharp, sudden, and accompanied by dyspnea. Pneumothorax can also have a significant impact on oxygenation and hemodynamics. Auscultation and percussion of the chest often reveal decreased breath sounds and hyperresonance of the affected side. Tracheal deviation, jugular venous distention, hypotension, and shock are indicators of an immediate life-threatening process (tension pneumothorax). Chest radiographs are usually diagnostic when the lung parenchyma is normal, whereas in patients with severe underlying pulmonary disease, a computed tomography scan of the chest often is necessary to make the diagnosis.

Esophageal Disorders

Gastroesophageal reflux disease (GERD), esophageal motility disorders, and esophageal hyperalgesia can cause chest pain very similar to cardiac ischemic pain. Notably, esophageal pain is frequently relieved with nitroglycerin, which is also frequently administered to relieve myocardial ischemic pain. Moreover, both disorders can coexist, thus complicating the diagnosis. Workup for coronary artery disease should always be completed before attributing the pain to GERD. Characteristics suggestive of an esophageal origin of chest pain are postprandial symptoms, relief with antacids or with standing, and lack of pain radiation.

Less obvious causes of chest pain related to esophageal injury include mucosal damage by ingested pills. Occasionally, nasogastric tubes have been found to be the culprit of significant esophageal trauma with resultant chest pain. Moreover, acute increases in intra-abdominal pressure have been associated with esophageal wall rents and rupture. The presence of subcutaneous emphysema, pleural effusion, or mediastinal air on chest radiograph is suggestive of esophageal perforation.

Acute Cholecystitis

This disorder can sometimes mimic the symptoms and ECG findings of inferior wall myocardial infarction. Tenderness in the right upper abdominal quadrant, fever, and elevated leukocyte count favor cholecystitis.

Costochondritis

Inflammation of the costochondral joints frequently results in chest wall pain. This pain is exacerbated by applying pressure over the affected area, by deep breathing, or by coughing. Often, patients can point to the exact area of inflammation.

Tietze syndrome is similar to costochondritis but is differentiated by notable swelling of the costal cartilage that is commonly palpable on examination.

Risk Assessment

Risk stratification using clinical and laboratory markers allows for rapid estimation of the risk of an adverse outcome and provides optimal guidance of treatment to prevent both ischemic and bleeding events. Evolving risk assessment can similarly be used to determine the most appropriate level of care and monitoring.

Killip Classification. This is not a rigorous risk score, but a very rapid and effective system of risk assessment of patients with myocardial infarction. Class I includes individual with no clinical signs of heart failure, Class II includes those with rales or crackles in the lungs, a third heart sound, and elevated jugular venous pressure, Class III are patients with frank, acute pulmonary edema, and Class IV are those with cardiogenic shock or severe hypotension.

Thrombolysis in Myocardial Infarction Risk Scores. The thrombolysis in myocardial infarction (TIMI) risk score is a well-validated scoring system used to predict the 14-day risk of death, myocardial infarction, or urgent revascularization in patients with NSTEMI (9). It is composed of seven independent predictors: age, cardiovascular risk factors, previous coronary artery disease, aspirin use within the prior week, two or more angina episodes in the prior 24 hours, ST-segment deviation greater than 0.5 mm, and elevation of markers of myocardial injury.

A TIMI risk score predicting 30-day adverse events in patients with STEMI has been developed as well, and includes different variables: Killip class, age, cardiovascular risk factors, low systolic blood pressure, high heart rate, low weight, anterior ST elevation or left bundle branch block, time to treatment longer than 4 hours (10). In both cases, the probability of an adverse event proportionally rises with the TIMI risk score.

Global Registry of Acute Coronary Events Score. The Global Registry of Acute Coronary Events (GRACE) score was developed from an international registry with a population of patients across the entire spectrum of ACS (11). It is composed of the following items: age, heart rate, systolic blood pressure, serum creatinine, Killip class, cardiac arrest at admission, elevation of markers of myocardial injury, ST-segment deviation. Patients with GRACE score over 140 have high risk of in-hospital mortality, whereas values between 109 and 140 identify those with an intermediate risk.

Can Rapid Risk Stratification of Unstable Angina Patients Suppress Adverse Outcomes with Early Implementation of the ACC/AHA Guidelines (CRUSADE) Bleeding Score. The CRUSADE score has relatively high accuracy for estimating bleeding risk by incorporating admission and treatment variables: baseline hematocrit, creatinine clearance, heart rate, gender, signs of heart failure at presentation, prior vascular disease, diabetes mellitus, systolic blood pressure (12). The risk of bleeding increases progressively with the CRUSADE score.

TREATMENT

The main objective of treatment for suspected myocardial ischemia is to restore the oxygen supply–demand balance. Hence, the early management of the patients simultaneously involves relief of ischemic pain, reperfusion therapy, and antithrombotic treatment. At this stage, it is also very important to initiate the prevention of myocardial infarction complications.

Anti-Ischemic Drugs

Oxygen

Supplemental oxygen should be administered to all patients whose saturation is over 90% or in respiratory distress. In patients with normal oxygen saturation, supplemental oxygen may be harmful and is not recommended (13).

Analgesics

Effective analgesia is important to reduce sympathetic stimulation caused by pain and anxiety, thereby decreasing cardiac workload and risks associated with excess catecholamines. Opioids are particularly helpful: Morphine sulfate (2–5 mg IV, every 10–30 minutes) is a very effective analgesic and has additional venodilatory effects that may reduce preload, lower the end-diastolic pressure, and improve hemodynamics. Moreover, morphine has been suggested to help with reducing reperfusion injury and myocardial preconditioning (an increased capacity of myocardium to resist to the ischemic insult) (14). Fentanyl (25–50 µg IV, every 5–30 minutes) is another effective analgesic drug. Care must be taken to avoid respiratory depression with cumulative doses of opioid. Moreover, a retrospective study showed that morphine use is associated with a slight increase of death in patients with NSTEMI (15), probably because of an interference with the antiplatelet effect of $P2Y_{12}$ receptors blockers (16).

Nitroglycerin

Nitroglycerin acts by reducing preload through venodilation and afterload by arteriolar dilation, promoting coronary vasodilation, relieving coronary vasospasm or vasoconstriction, and by putative effects upon platelet aggregability. These effects act synergically to improve myocardial blood flow and relieve ischemia. Nitroglycerin may be administered sublingually with close monitoring of hemodynamics, and additional doses may be given as long as they are tolerated hemodynamically. For more accurate control, IV nitroglycerin may be initiated and titrated until symptoms are controlled. Extreme care should also be taken before giving nitrates to patients with profound hemodynamic compromise such as those with right ventricle infarction and those with severe aortic stenosis. In this setting, patients are dependent upon preload to maintain cardiac output, and nitrates can cause severe hypotension. In addition, nitroglycerin is contraindicated in patients who have taken a phosphodiesterase inhibitor (sildenafil, vardenafil, tadalafil) for erectile dysfunction or pulmonary hypertension within the previous 24 hours (or perhaps as long as 36 hours with tadalafil).

β-Blockers

β-Blockers act by reducing heart rate, blood pressure, and left ventricle contractility, thereby reducing myocardial oxygen demand. Additionally the reduction of heart rate increases diastolic time resulting in improved coronary blood flow and oxygen supply. The main contraindications include low output state, high risk for cardiogenic shock, bradycardia, atrioventricular conduction defects, and reactive airway disease. Some β-blockers have β_1-selective properties that minimize the risk of bronchospasm (e.g., metoprolol) and/or membrane-stabilizing activity, a kind of type I antidysrhythmic effect, which is valuable for the prevention of ischemia-induced ventricular dysrhythmias (e.g., propranolol). In a polled analysis on 2,537 patients enrolled in primary angioplasty trials, those who received β-blocker therapy before primary angioplasty, compared to those who did not, had lower adjusted in-hospital mortality (OR 0.41, 95% CI 0.20–0.84) and nonsignificantly lower 1-year mortality (OR 0.72, 95% CI 0.47–1.08). Moreover, in a recent study on 270 patients with anterior STEMI undergoing primary percutaneous coronary intervention, early intravenous metoprolol (5 mg IV, every 2 minutes up to three times) before reperfusion reduced infarct size and increased left ventricular ejection fraction with no excess of adverse events during the first 24 hours (17).

Calcium Channel Antagonists

These agents are effective antianginal drugs but, given their adverse effects and the mortality benefit of β-blockers, they should be considered for only second-line therapy, with the notable exception of ACS in the setting of variant angina where they represent the mainstay of therapy.

Antiplatelet Drugs

Aspirin

Aspirin acts by irreversibly inhibiting cyclooxygenase-1, thus reducing the generation of thromboxane A_2, a potent vasoconstrictor and mediator of platelet aggregation. In an analysis of pooled data from nearly 200,000 patients, aspirin produced a 30% reduction of the combined end point of subsequent nonfatal myocardial infarction, nonfatal stroke, or vascular death in patients with AMI (18). The study also outlined that there was no significant difference in efficacy between lower and higher daily doses and that the addition of a second antiplatelet agent significantly improved the combined end point. Unless there are specific contraindications, such as intolerance or allergy, active bleeding or high hemorrhagic risk, aspirin should be given to all patients with ACS as soon as possible and continued indefinitely. Low-dose aspirin (75–100 mg daily) should be preferred due to increased risk of gastrointestinal bleeding in patients on higher dose (300–325 mg daily) (19).

Clopidogrel

Clopidogrel blocks the binding of adenosine diphosphate (ADP) to the platelet receptor $P2Y_{12}$, thereby inhibiting activation of the glycoprotein (GP) IIb/IIIa complex and platelet aggregation. In the CURE trial, the addition of clopidogrel to aspirin in patients with NSTEMI has shown to significantly reduce the risk of myocardial infarction, stroke, or cardiovascular death both in patients treated medically and in those undergoing percutaneous coronary intervention (20,21), thus establishing a sound basis for dual antiplatelet therapy in ACS.

Clopidogrel should be administered as an initial loading dose of 300 or 600 mg followed by 75 mg daily. A 600-mg loading dose is indicated in patients undergoing urgent percutaneous coronary intervention as it achieves platelet inhibition more rapidly (22). Contraindications to clopidogrel are the same as for aspirin. Clopidogrel is a prodrug and has to be converted to its active form by the CYP2C19 isoform of the hepatic cytochrome P450. Genetic polymorphisms may be present, with certain patients having reduced CYP2C19 function and consequently lower plasma levels of the active metabolite. In addition, several drugs may interfere with CYP2C19 function. Tests for genetic polymorphisms and clinical assays for assessment of platelet inhibition are currently available although their role in clinical practice is uncertain (23).

Prasugrel

Prasugrel has a more rapid onset of action and is able to achieve higher degrees of platelet inhibition than clopidogrel. Furthermore, prasugrel does not require conversion by CYP2C19 and effectively suppresses platelet activity in a larger numbers of patients than clopidogrel. Prasugrel was compared to clopidogrel in the TRITON-TIMI 38 trial of 13,608 moderate- to high-risk ACS patients undergoing percutaneous coronary intervention, including 3,534 with STEMI (24). Prasugrel was given with a loading dose of 60 mg and maintenance dose of 10 mg/day, while clopidogrel was given with a 300-mg loading dose and a 75-mg/day maintenance dose. For patients with NSTEMI, the coronary anatomy had to be known before randomization (clopidogrel and prasugrel were given after coronary angiography). At 15-month follow-up, the primary efficacy end point (cardiovascular death, nonfatal myocardial infarction, or nonfatal stroke) occurred significantly less often in patients treated with prasugrel (HR 0.81, 95% CI 0.73–0.90). The safety end point of a major bleeding event not associated with coronary artery bypass graft surgery occurred significantly more often in patients treated with prasugrel (HR 1.32, 95% CI 1.03–1.68). Post hoc analysis identified three predictors of bleeding with prasugrel: a history of stroke or transient ischemic attack, at least 75 years of age, and body weight no more than 60 kg.

In the TRILOGY ACS trial, prasugrel was compared to clopidogrel in 9,326 patients treated with aspirin with ACS in whom percutaneous coronary intervention was not performed (25). Prasugrel was given with a loading dose of 30 mg and a maintenance dose of 10 mg/day in patients under 75 years or 5 mg/day for those at least 75 years or weighed no more than 60 kg; clopidogrel was given with a 300-mg loading dose and a 75-mg/day maintenance dose. There was no statistically significant difference in the rate of the primary end point in the 7,243 patients under 75 years between those who received prasugrel and those who received clopidogrel (HR 0.91, 95% CI 0.79–1.05). The rates of severe and intracranial bleeding were not statistically significantly different. In a separate analysis of the 2,083 individuals at least 75 years of age, the risks of the primary end point and TIMI major bleeding increased progressively with age (26).

Ticagrelor

Ticagrelor differs from the thienopyridines (clopidogrel and prasugrel) in that it binds reversibly rather than irreversibly to $P2Y_{12}$ platelet receptor, is a direct drug and has a more rapid onset of action than clopidogrel. It belongs to a new chemical class of antiplatelet agents, the cyclopentyltriazolopyrimidines. Similar to prasugrel, treatment with ticagrelor leads to more intense platelet inhibition than clopidogrel. The efficacy and safety of ticagrelor were evaluated in the PLATO trial in which 18,624 patients with ACS were randomly assigned to either ticagrelor (180-mg loading dose followed by 90 mg twice daily) or clopidogrel (300–600 mg loading dose followed by 75 mg daily). In this trial, 38% of patients had STEMI with intended percutaneous coronary intervention. Treatment was started as soon as possible after hospital admission (27,28). At 12 months, the composite primary end point (first event of death from vascular causes, myocardial infarction, or stroke) occurred significantly less often in patients receiving ticagrelor (HR 0.84, 95% CI 0.77–0.92). There was no significant difference in the rates of major bleeding between the ticagrelor and clopidogrel groups (11.6% vs. 11.2%). The primary outcome was similar to the entire study population in three prespecified subgroups: patients with chronic kidney disease (HR 0.77, 95% CI 0.65–0.90) (29), patients who underwent coronary artery bypass graft surgery and were receiving study drug treatment less than 7 days before surgery (HR 0.84, 95% CI 0.60–1.16) (30), and patients with planned noninvasive management (12.0% vs. 14.3%; HR 0.85, 95% CI 0.73–1.00) (31). Of note, another prespecified subgroup analysis found a potentially clinically important interaction between treatment and region: the composite primary end point occurred more often with ticagrelor for patients enrolled in the United States (32). Among 37 baseline and postrandomization factors, only aspirin dose explained a substantial fraction (80%–100%) of the interaction (p = 0.00006). Therefore, aspirin should be administered only at a daily dose of no more than 100 mg when used in conjunction with ticagrelor.

Glycoprotein IIb/IIIa Inhibitors

GP IIb/IIIa inhibitors—abciximab, eptifibatide, and tirofiban—act on the final common pathway of platelet aggregation by preventing fibrinogen-mediated platelet cross-linking via GP IIb/IIIa receptors. Conclusions from early trials are of limited applicability to patients treated today with the routine use of $P2Y_{12}$ receptor blockers and percutaneous coronary intervention, however these agents may still be considered in high-risk patients (especially high troponin increase) as adjunctive antiplatelet therapy (33). Two large trials of similar but not identical design did not demonstrate a significant benefit of early compared with delayed use of GP IIb/IIIa inhibitor, even in high-risk patients with NSTEMI who are scheduled to undergo early percutaneous coronary intervention (34,35). Moreover, the early use of GP IIb/IIIa use was associated with a significantly increased risk of bleeding. In the ISAR-REACT 4 trial, which compared bivalirudin to heparin plus GP IIb/IIIa inhibitor in STEMI patients receiving aspirin and clopidogrel, the rate of death, recurrent MI, or urgent target-vessel revascularization was similar between the two groups, but bleeding occurred significantly more often in those receiving heparin plus GP IIb/IIIa inhibitor (36). In STEMI patients, the HEAT-PPCI trial called into question the need for the routine use of GP IIb/IIIa inhibitor in patients receiving heparin plus a potent oral antiplatelet agent such as prasugrel or ticagrelor (37).

Gp IIb/IIIa inhibitors can be associated with thrombocytopenia, which is sudden and severe. Therefore, the platelet count should be monitored frequently in patients receiving GP IIb/IIIa inhibitors. If the platelet count falls below 100,000 cells/μL, or to less than 25% of its pretreatment level, the possibility of pseudothrombocytopenia, a laboratory artifact of no clinical concern, should be eliminated by examination of a blood smear for the presence of platelet clumping. The platelet count should be repeated using a tube containing sodium citrate and heparin rather than EDTA as a preservative, if platelet clumping is observed. If pseudothrombocytopenia is ruled out by the above procedures, the GP IIb/IIIa inhibitor should be discontinued.

Anticoagulant Drugs

Thrombin activity at the site of plaque rupture may result in delayed or incomplete reperfusion of occluded vessels and contributes to reocclusion. Thrombin is a central mediator of clot formation through its activation of platelets, conversion of fibrinogen to fibrin, and activation of factor XIII, leading to fibrin cross-linking and clot stabilization. The heparins, including unfractionated heparin and the low–molecular-weight heparins, are indirect thrombin inhibitors that complex with antithrombin and convert antithrombin from a slow to a rapid inactivator of thrombin, and factor Xa. The direct thrombin inhibitors bind to and inactivate one or more of the active sites on the thrombin molecule (Fig. 94.4).

Heparins

In combination with aspirin, either unfractioned heparin or low–molecular-weight heparin has been shown to reduce the risk of death or myocardial infarction as compared to aspirin alone (38). Trials comparing a low–molecular-weight heparin, usually enoxaparin, to unfractionated heparin in ACS found that enoxaparin leads to better outcomes in patients managed with a conservative strategy (39,40). On the other hand, for patients undergoing an early invasive strategy, unfractioned heparin may be preferable in patients at high bleeding risk due to the increased risk of bleeding seen with enoxaparin (41). There is no evidence to support the use of other low–molecular-weight heparin in preference to enoxaparin. Indeed, these drugs appear to have equivalent efficacy to unfractioned heparin, may be less effective than enoxaparin, and may be associated with higher rates of major bleeding.

Intravenous unfractioned heparin is best administered on a weight basis starting with a bolus of 60 units/kg followed by continuous infusion at a rate of 12 units/kg/hr. Heparin requirement are however variables and optimal therapeutic benefit with minimization of bleeding is best accomplished with activated partial thromboplastin time (aPTT) maintenance at 50 to 70 seconds.

Like unfractioned heparin, enoxaparin inactivates factor Xa, but has a lesser effect on thrombin. Enoxaparin has several advantages over unfractioned heparin, including a more predictable anticoagulant effect, a reduced likelihood of inducing immune-mediated thrombocytopenia, subcutaneous administration, and does not require laboratory monitoring. On the other hand, reversal with protamine sulfate is possible

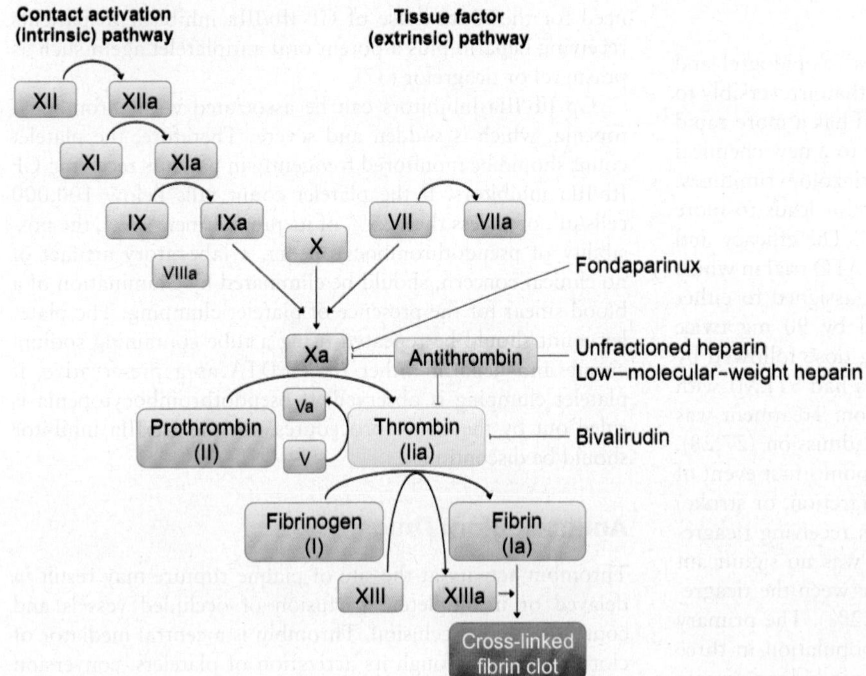

FIGURE 94.4 Interaction between anticoagulant drugs and the coagulation cascade.

for unfractioned heparin but not for enoxaparin. All heparins require dose adjustment in patients with renal insufficiency.

Therapy with heparin may be complicated by immune-mediated heparin-induced thrombocytopenia. Its incidence is approximately 2.5% in patients exposed to unfractioned heparin for more than 4 days, but is much lower in patients treated with unfractioned heparin for 4 days or less (0.2%), and in those treated with low–molecular-weight heparin (0.2%) (42). In patients with a history of heparin-induced thrombocytopenia, or in whom heparin-induced thrombocytopenia develops or is suspected while on unfractioned heparin therapy, the preferred anticoagulant is bivalirudin.

Direct Thrombin Inhibitors

Bivalirudin is the most studied and used of this category of drugs that have been developed to overcome intrinsic limitations to unfractioned heparin therapy in patients with acute MI such as heparin-induced thrombocytopenia or ineffective inactivation of thrombin bound within a clot. The efficacy and safety of bivalirudin (alone or with a GP IIb/IIIa inhibitor) compared to unfractioned heparin or enoxaparin (both with a GP IIb/IIIa inhibitor) was evaluated in the ACUITY trial of almost 14,000 patients with moderate- to high-risk ACS undergoing percutaneous revascularization (43). Bivalirudin alone was noninferior to unfractioned heparin or enoxaparin for the rate of ischemic complications (RR 1.08, 95% CI 0.93–1.24), while the rate of major bleeding was significantly lower with bivalirudin monotherapy (RR 0.53, 95% CI 0.43–0.65). Similar findings were reported by the ISAR-REACT 4 trial (36). Of note, a substudy of the ACUITY trial showed that patients who were switched from unfractioned heparin or enoxaparin had similar outcomes compared to those not switched (44).

In STEMI, bivalirudin was assessed in three main trials: HORIZONS AMI (45), BRIGHT (46), and HEAT PPCI (37). Overall, these studies found similar or worse rates of a composite primary outcome with bivalirudin compared to heparin, comparable rates of bleeding when heparin is given without a GP IIb/IIIa inhibitor, and increase in the risk of acute stent thrombosis with bivalirudin.

Fondaparinux

Fondaparinux is a synthetic pentasaccharide that is a highly selective inhibitor of factor Xa. It selectively binds antithrombin, inducing a conformational change resulting in a dose-dependent inhibition of factor Xa. In the OASIS-5 trial comparing fondaparinux (2.5 mg/day) to enoxaparin (1 mg/kg twice daily) in ACS, the two groups of patients had similar rates of the primary end point, defined as death, myocardial infarction, or refractory ischemia at 9 days, while a reduction in the primary end point was found with fondaparinux at 30 days and 6 months due to a significant reduction of death (47). Notably, the rate of major bleeding was significantly reduced with fondaparinux (HR 0.52, 95% CI 0.44–0.61). However, fondaparinux was associated with a small but significant increase in catheter-related thrombi (in patients undergoing percutaneous coronary intervention) compared to enoxaparin.

The OASIS-6 trial results showed a trend toward worse outcomes with fondaparinux compared to heparin in patients treated with primary PCI, thus advising against fondaparinux use in STEMI (48).

Statins

Beside well-known lipid-lowering effects, statins appear to have a vascular protective pleiotropic action already effective in the acute phase of myocardial infarction. Based on the significant reduction of death, stroke, and myocardial infarction observed in the MIRACL and PROVE IT-TIMI 22 trials, intensive statin therapy with atorvastatin 80 mg/day should be initiated as early as possible in all patients with ACS (49,50). This treatment should be continued for at least 30 days after which dose can be adjusted on patient's lipid levels.

Myocardial Revascularization

Prompt restoration of myocardial blood flow is essential to optimize myocardial salvage and to reduce mortality in patients with STEMI. Multiple randomized trials have shown enhanced survival and a lower rate of intracranial hemorrhage and recurrent myocardial infarction with primary percutaneous coronary intervention compared to fibrinolysis (51). As a result, primary percutaneous coronary intervention is recommended for any patient with STEMI who can undergo the procedure in a timely manner by persons skilled in the procedure (52,53). Timely is defined as an ideal first medical contact to revascularization time of 90 minutes or less for patients in a percutaneous coronary intervention center or 120 minutes or less for patients who are in a nonpercutaneous coronary intervention capable hospital and are then taken to a percutaneous coronary intervention center. If the diagnosis of STEMI is made 12 to 24 hours after symptom onset, the performance of primary percutaneous coronary intervention is reasonable if the patient has severe heart failure, hemodynamic or electrical instability, or persistent ischemic symptoms. Randomized trials of routine late percutaneous coronary intervention have shown an improvement in left ventricular function but not in hard clinical end points (54,55).

If primary percutaneous coronary intervention is not available on site, rapid transfer to a percutaneous coronary intervention center can produce better outcomes than fibrinolysis, as long as the door-to-balloon time, including interhospital transport time, is less than 90 minutes.

Fibrinolytic therapy is recommended in qualifying patients (Table 94.5) with symptom onset within 12 hours who cannot receive primary percutaneous coronary intervention within 120 minutes of diagnosis. A number of different fibrinolytic regimens have been evaluated and each agent has its own preferred dosing regimen (Table 94.6).

In patients with NSTEMI, prospective trials have demonstrated that fibrinolytic therapy is not beneficial (56). On the other hand, NSTEMI patients at very high risk of adverse outcomes because of hemodynamic instability, severe left ventricular dysfunction, recurrent or persistent angina despite intensive medical therapy, new or worsening mitral regurgitation, or sustained ventricular tachycardia must be referred for urgent coronary angiography and revascularization. For patients lacking these very high-risk characteristics, randomized trials have shown benefit of an early invasive approach essentially in higher-risk NSTEMI. While the optimal timing is uncertain, the majority of patients undergo coronary revascularization early (within 24 hours). A widely used strategy to guide invasive versus conservative strategy is based on risk score calculation. The choice of revascularization procedure after angiography depends upon the location and extent of disease. Among patients with an appropriate lesion, percutaneous coronary intervention is most often performed, but coronary artery bypass surgery is usually preferred for the treatment of patients with left main or left main equivalent disease, or three- or two-vessel disease involving the left anterior descending artery with left ventricular dysfunction or diabetes (57). Yet, coronary artery bypass grafting is infrequently performed in patients with STEMI. The main indications are limited to emergent or urgent surgical revascularization related to failure of fibrinolysis or percutaneous coronary intervention, or hemodynamically important mechanical complications.

TABLE 94.5 Contraindications to the Use of Thrombolytic Therapy in Patients with STEMI

Absolute contraindications
History of any intracranial hemorrhage
History of ischemic stroke within the previous 3 mo, with the important exception of acute ischemic stroke seen within 3 hrs, which may be treated with thrombolytic therapy
Presence of a cerebral vascular malformation or a primary or metastatic intracranial malignancy
Symptoms or signs suggestive of an aortic dissection
A bleeding diathesis or active bleeding, with the exception of menses thrombolytic therapy may increase the risk of moderate bleeding, which is offset by the benefits of thrombolysis
Significant closed-head or facial trauma within the preceding 3 mo
Relative contraindications
History of chronic, severe, poorly controlled hypertension or uncontrolled hypertension at presentation (blood pressure >180 mmHg systolic and/or >110 mmHg diastolic severe hypertension at presentation can be an absolute contraindication in patients at low risk)
History of ischemic stroke more than 3 mo previously
Dementia
Any known intracranial disease that is not an absolute contraindication
Traumatic or prolonged (>10 min) cardiopulmonary resuscitation
Major surgery within the preceding 3 wks
Internal bleeding within the preceding 2 to 4 wks or an active peptic ulcer
Noncompressible vascular punctures
Pregnancy
Current warfarin therapy—the risk of bleeding increases as the INR increases
For streptokinase: a prior exposure (>5 days previously) or allergic reaction to these drugs

TABLE 94.6 Thrombolytic Regimens for Acute ST-Elevation Myocardial Infarction

Drug	Recommended IV Regimen[a]
Alteplase (accelerated regimen)	15 mg bolus
	then
	0.75 mg/kg (maximum 50 mg) over 30 min
	then
	0.5 mg/kg (maximum 35 mg) over the next 60 min
Tenecteplase	Single bolus over 5 to 10 sec based on body weight:
	<60 kg: 30 mg
	60–69 kg: 35 mg
	70–79 kg: 40 mg
	80–89 kg: 45 mg
	≥90 kg: 50 mg
Reteplase	10 units over 2 min then repeat 10 unit bolus at 30 min
Streptokinase[b]	1.5 million units over 30–60 min

[a]All patients are also given aspirin 162 to 325 mg and, with alteplase, reteplase, and tenecteplase, unfractionated heparin as a 60 units/kg bolus (maximum 4,000 units) followed by an intravenous infusion of 12 units/kg per hour (maximum 1,000 units per hour) adjusted to target aPTT of 50 to 70 seconds. Heparin has not been definitively shown to improve outcomes with non–fibrin-specific agents such as streptokinase. However, heparin is recommended with streptokinase in patients who are at high risk for systemic thromboembolism (large or anterior myocardial infarction, atrial fibrillation, previous embolus, or known left ventricular thrombus).

[b]Elevated risk of hypersensitivity reaction with repeated doses.

The benefit of revascularization must be weighed against the increase in mortality associated with coronary artery bypass grafting in the first 3 to 7 days after STEMI. Thus, if the patient has stabilized, surgery should be delayed to allow myocardial recovery.

Management of Complications

Given their multiple potential causes, acute heart failure and cardiogenic shock represent the most frequent complication of acute MI. In these patients, hemodynamic monitoring is often necessary to optimize volume status, cardiac output, and peripheral oxygen delivery. Moreover, a number of invasive approaches and support may help managing cardiogenic shock. The intra-aortic balloon pump (IABP) provides a beneficial hemodynamic effect by increasing coronary perfusion in diastole and augmenting cardiac output by creating reduced afterload during systole. In contrast, inotropic agents augment cardiac output at the expense of increased myocardial oxygen consumption. These agents also have an undesirable prodysrhythmic effect. However, the IABP has not been shown to reduce mortality in patients with cardiogenic shock complicating AMI (58), and the role of newer circulatory support devices is still poorly defined (59). The IABP is, however, essential to assist stabilization allowing for urgent surgery in patients with mitral valve regurgitation because of papillary muscle dysfunction or rupture and in those with ventricular septal defects. Alternatively, percutaneous closure of postinfarction ventricular septal defect is a reasonably effective treatment for these extremely high-risk patients. Mortality remains high, but patients who survive to discharge do well in the longer term (60). In patients with decreased ejection fraction following myocardial infarction, angiotensin-converting enzyme inhibitors positively affects ventricular remodeling and significantly improve prognosis (61).

When low cardiac output is due to ischemia-induced right ventricle dysfunction, treatment is, in several ways, opposed to the management of left ventricle dysfunction. It includes early maintenance of right ventricle preload and reduction of its afterload. Because of their influence on right ventricle preload, drugs routinely used in management of acute MI, such as nitrates and diuretics, may reduce cardiac output and produce severe hypotension in case of right ventricle ischemia. Indeed, a common clinical presentation is profound hypotension after administration of sublingual nitroglycerin, with the degree of hypotension often out of proportion to the ECG severity of the infarction. The primary treatment is vigorous volume expansion to raise the right ventricular filling pressure and eventually restore the left ventricular stroke volume. Although this is a critical step, inotropic support (especially dobutamine) should be initiated promptly if cardiac output fails to improve after 0.5 to 1 L of fluid has been administered (62). Indeed, excessive volume loading may further complicate the right side filling pressure increase and cause right ventricular dilatation, resulting in decreased left ventricle output secondary to a shift of the interventricular septum toward the left ventricle.

Attempt to suppress ventricular premature complexes and nonsustained ventricular tachycardia in patients with AMI has been shown not to improve outcome and, with some drugs, to actually increase mortality (63). β-Blockers and correction of electrolyte disturbances are general preventive measures. However, when nonsustained ventricular tachycardic episodes are frequent and/or causes hemodynamic compromise, treatment with additional β-blockade or, if necessary, intravenous amiodarone or—if amiodarone is not available—lidocaine may be useful.

Sustained monomorphic ventricular tachycardia, even when hemodynamically tolerated, must be treated urgently because of its deleterious effect on cardiac output, possible exacerbation of myocardial ischemia, and the risk of deterioration into ventricular fibrillation. After an initial attempt with amiodarone 150 mg IV, synchronized electrical cardioversion using an initial energy of 100 joules, with brief anesthesia, should be administered. If ventricular tachycardia persists, subsequent shocks at increasing energy can be given as necessary.

Polymorphic ventricular tachycardia is a poorly tolerated dysrhythmia representing a life-threatening emergency that should be treated with unsynchronized electrical shocks (defibrillation). A biphasic waveform defibrillator is preferable since the success rate for defibrillation is higher than with monophasic waveforms. For biphasic defibrillators, the initial shock should be at 120 to 200 joules, with subsequent shocks at the highest available biphasic energy level (200 joules for most devices); for monophasic defibrillators, shocks at 360 joules should be used.

In case of conduction blocks developing in the setting of inferior ischemia, transvenous pacing allows management of a patient developing hemodynamic instability, becoming symptomatic, or presenting bradycardia-dependent ventricular arrhythmias until effective reperfusion is achieved, which generally restores normal atrioventricular conduction. When a conduction block manifests during anterior ischemia or infarction, prognosis is generally poorer and higher-degree atrioventricular block are more frequent.

CONTROVERSIES

Despite the fact that treatment of ACS is a top priority in the health systems of industrialized countries, significant improvements are needed in the organization of care, in available therapeutic options, and in effective preventive strategies.

Higher-risk patients, such as those with STEMI, have a better prognosis if treated by primary percutaneous coronary intervention rather than thrombolysis. However, this advantage is time-dependent and much effort is directed at reducing the delay time to transcatheter revascularization. On the other hand, thrombolysis could be anticipated in such a way that is impossible to achieve with primary percutaneous intervention, especially in patients who are already hospitalized but require very complex management, as occurs in ICU patients. This and other strategies potentially useful for improving access of critically ill patients to myocardial revascularization have been substantially neglected so far.

Antithrombotic therapy plays a major role in the treatment of ACS. Recent trials on new antithrombotic agents for the treatment of patients with ACS have shown that improvement in effectiveness is almost consistently associated with lower safety. Yet, a significant amount of data suggests that individual response to antithrombotic drugs may have an important genetic basis. Genotype-guided antithrombotic represents a first step toward individualized medicine but has still not provided convincing evidence of efficacy.

When looking at complications of myocardial infarction, available treatments are extremely scarce, which is somewhat surprising in the light of the multiplicity of interplaying factors. Especially, medical therapy is almost entirely limited to boost residual myocardial function rather than attempting to avoid its overall impairment. On the other hand, there is much excitement with newer approaches allowing several kinds of left ventricular percutaneous repair such as staminal therapy.

But an ounce of prevention is worth a pound of cure. Indeed, improved understanding of the intimate mechanisms driving atherothrombosis is probably the best pathway to early identification of people who will suffer ACS and who are at risk of a major mechanical complication; this is certainly the future of coronary artery medicine.

Key Points

Presentation

- Typically constricting substernal pain radiating to left arm
- Atypical presentation frequent in hospitalized patients
- Dyspnea and congestive heart failure frequent

Diagnosis

- Ischemic changes on 12-lead ECG
- Elevation of markers of myocardial injury
- Risk stratification

Treatment

- Anti-ischemic therapy (oxygen, analgesia, nitroglycerin, β-blockers)
- Antiplatelet therapy (aspirin, clopidogrel or prasugrel or ticagrelor) and anticoagulant therapy (unfractioned heparin or low–molecular-weight heparin or direct thrombin inhibitors or fondaparinux)
- Myocardial revascularization (percutaneous coronary intervention, thrombolysis if percutaneous revascularization not possible)

References

1. Dai X, Bumgarner J, Spangler A, et al. Acute ST-elevation myocardial infarction in patients hospitalized for noncardiac conditions. *J Am Heart Assoc*. 2013;2:e000004.
2. Garberich RF, Traverse JH, Claussen MT, et al. ST-elevation myocardial infarction diagnosed after hospital admission. *Circulation*. 2014;129: 1225–1232.
3. Fuster V, Kovacic JC. Acute coronary syndromes: pathology, diagnosis, genetics, prevention, and treatment. *Circ Res*. 2014;114:1847–1851.
4. Hirsh PD, Hillis LD, Campbell WB, et al. Release of prostaglandins and thromboxane into the coronary circulation in patients with ischemic heart disease. *N Engl J Med*. 1981;304:685–691.
5. Romagnoli E, Lanza GA. Acute myocardial infarction with normal coronary arteries: role of coronary artery spasm and arrhythmic complications. *Int J Cardiol*. 2007;117:3–5.
6. Ayaram D, Bellolio MF, Murad MH, et al. Triple rule-out computed tomographic angiography for chest pain: a diagnostic systematic review and meta-analysis. *Acad Emerg Med*. 2013;20:861–871.
7. Thygesen K, Alpert JS, Jaffe AS, et al. Third universal definition of myocardial infarction. *J Am Coll Cardiol*. 2012;60:1581–1598.
8. Pelliccia F, Greco C, Vitale C, et al. Takotsubo syndrome (stress cardiomyopathy): an intriguing clinical condition in search of its identity. *Am J Med*. 2014;127:699–704.
9. Antman EM, Cohen M, Bernink PJ, et al. The TIMI risk score for unstable angina/non-ST elevation MI: a method for prognostication and therapeutic decision making. *JAMA*. 2000;284:835–842.
10. Morrow DA, Antman EM, Charlesworth A, et al. TIMI risk score for ST-elevation myocardial infarction: a convenient, bedside, clinical score for risk assessment at presentation. An intravenous nPA for treatment of infarcting myocardium early II trial substudy. *Circulation*. 2000;102:2031–2037.
11. Granger CB, Goldberg RJ, Dabbous O, et al. Predictors of hospital mortality in the global registry of acute coronary events. *Arch Intern Med*. 2003;163:2345–2353.
12. Subherwal S, Bach RG, Chen AY, et al. Baseline risk of major bleeding in non-ST-segment-elevation myocardial infarction: the CRUSADE (Can Rapid risk stratification of Unstable angina patients Suppress ADverse outcomes with Early implementation of the ACC/AHA Guidelines) Bleeding Score. *Circulation*. 2009;119:1873–1882.
13. Stub D, Smith K, Bernard S, et al. Air versus oxygen in ST-segment elevation myocardial infarction. *Circulation*. 2015;131:2143–2150.
14. Rentoukas I, Giannopoulos G, Kaoukis A, et al. Cardioprotective role of remote ischemic periconditioning in primary percutaneous coronary intervention: enhancement by opioid action. *JACC Cardiovasc Interv*. 2010;3:49–55.
15. Meine TJ, Roe MT, Chen AY, et al. Association of intravenous morphine use and outcomes in acute coronary syndromes: results from the CRUSADE Quality Improvement Initiative. *Am Heart J*. 2005;149:1043–1049.
16. Parodi G, Valenti R, Bellandi B, et al. Comparison of prasugrel and ticagrelor loading doses in ST-segment elevation myocardial infarction patients: RAPID (Rapid Activity of Platelet Inhibitor Drugs) primary PCI study. *J Am Coll Cardiol*. 2013;61:1601–1606.
17. Ibanez B, Macaya C, Sanchez-Brunete V, et al. Effect of early metoprolol on infarct size in ST-segment-elevation myocardial infarction patients undergoing primary percutaneous coronary intervention: the Effect of Metoprolol in Cardioprotection During an Acute Myocardial Infarction (METOCARD-CNIC) trial. *Circulation*. 2013;128:1495–1503.
18. Collaborative meta-analysis of randomised trials of antiplatelet therapy for prevention of death, myocardial infarction, and stroke in high risk patients. *BMJ*. 2002;324:71–86.
19. Mehta SR, Bassand JP, Chrolavicius S, et al. Dose comparisons of clopidogrel and aspirin in acute coronary syndromes. *N Engl J Med*. 2010; 363:930–942.
20. Yusuf S, Zhao F, Mehta SR, et al. Effects of clopidogrel in addition to aspirin in patients with acute coronary syndromes without ST-segment elevation. *N Engl J Med*. 2001;345:494–502.
21. Mehta SR, Yusuf S, Peters RJ, et al. Effects of pretreatment with clopidogrel and aspirin followed by long-term therapy in patients undergoing percutaneous coronary intervention: the PCI-CURE study. *Lancet*. 2001;358:527–533.
22. Cuisset T, Frere C, Quilici J, et al. Benefit of a 600-mg loading dose of clopidogrel on platelet reactivity and clinical outcomes in patients with non-ST-segment elevation acute coronary syndrome undergoing coronary stenting. *J Am Coll Cardiol*. 2006;48:1339–1345.
23. Bonello L, Tantry US, Marcucci R, et al. Consensus and future directions on the definition of high on-treatment platelet reactivity to adenosine diphosphate. *J Am Coll Cardiol*. 2010;56:919–933.
24. Wiviott SD, Braunwald E, McCabe CH, et al. Prasugrel versus clopidogrel in patients with acute coronary syndromes. *N Engl J Med*. 2007; 357:2001–2015.
25. Roe MT, Armstrong PW, Fox KA, et al. Prasugrel versus clopidogrel for acute coronary syndromes without revascularization. *N Engl J Med*. 2012; 367:1297–1309.
26. Roe MT, Goodman SG, Ohman EM, et al. Elderly patients with acute coronary syndromes managed without revascularization: insights into the safety of long-term dual antiplatelet therapy with reduced-dose prasugrel versus standard-dose clopidogrel. *Circulation*. 2013;128:823–833.
27. Wallentin L, Becker RC, Budaj A, et al. Ticagrelor versus clopidogrel in patients with acute coronary syndromes. *N Engl J Med*. 2009;361: 1045–1057.
28. Sgueglia GA, Tarantini G, Niccoli G. Ticagrelor in ST-elevation myocardial infarction. *Curr Vasc Pharmacol*. 2012;10:458–462.
29. James S, Budaj A, Aylward P, et al. Ticagrelor versus clopidogrel in acute coronary syndromes in relation to renal function: results from the Platelet Inhibition and Patient Outcomes (PLATO) trial. *Circulation*. 2010; 122:1056–1067.
30. Held C, Asenblad N, Bassand JP, et al. Ticagrelor versus clopidogrel in patients with acute coronary syndromes undergoing coronary artery bypass surgery: results from the PLATO (Platelet Inhibition and Patient Outcomes) trial. *J Am Coll Cardiol*. 2011;57:672–684.

31. James SK, Roe MT, Cannon CP, et al. Ticagrelor versus clopidogrel in patients with acute coronary syndromes intended for non-invasive management: substudy from prospective randomised platelet inhibition and patient outcomes (PLATO) trial. *BMJ*. 2011;342:d3527.
32. Mahaffey KW, Wojdyla DM, Carroll K, et al. Ticagrelor compared with clopidogrel by geographic region in the Platelet Inhibition and Patient Outcomes (PLATO) trial. *Circulation*. 2011;124:544–554.
33. Kastrati A, Mehilli J, Neumann FJ, et al. Abciximab in patients with acute coronary syndromes undergoing percutaneous coronary intervention after clopidogrel pretreatment: the ISAR-REACT 2 randomized trial. *JAMA*. 2006;295:1531–1538.
34. Stone GW, Bertrand ME, Moses JW, et al. Routine upstream initiation vs deferred selective use of glycoprotein IIb/IIIa inhibitors in acute coronary syndromes: the ACUITY Timing trial. *JAMA*. 2007;297:591–602.
35. Giugliano RP, White JA, Bode C, et al. Early versus delayed, provisional eptifibatide in acute coronary syndromes. *N Engl J Med*. 2009;360:2176–2190.
36. Kastrati A, Neumann FJ, Schulz S, et al. Abciximab and heparin versus bivalirudin for non-ST-elevation myocardial infarction. *N Engl J Med*. 2011; 365:1980–1989.
37. Shahzad A, Kemp I, Mars C, et al. Unfractionated heparin versus bivalirudin in primary percutaneous coronary intervention (HEAT-PPCI): an open-label, single centre, randomised controlled trial. *Lancet*. 2014;384:1849–1858.
38. Eikelboom JW, Anand SS, Malmberg K, et al. Unfractionated heparin and low-molecular-weight heparin in acute coronary syndrome without ST elevation: a meta-analysis. *Lancet*. 2000;355:1936–1942.
39. Cohen M, Demers C, Gurfinkel EP, et al. A comparison of low-molecular-weight heparin with unfractionated heparin for unstable coronary artery disease: Efficacy and Safety of Subcutaneous Enoxaparin in Non-Q-Wave Coronary Events Study Group. *N Engl J Med*. 1997;337:447–452.
40. Gurfinkel E, Duronto E, Colorio C, et al. Thrombotic reactant markers in non-ST segment elevation acute coronary syndromes treated with either enoxaparin (low molecular weight heparin) or unfractionated heparin. *J Thromb Thrombolysis*. 1999;8:227–232.
41. Ferguson JJ, Califf RM, Antman EM, et al. Enoxaparin vs unfractionated heparin in high-risk patients with non–ST-segment elevation acute coronary syndromes managed with an intended early invasive strategy: primary results of the SYNERGY randomized trial. *JAMA*. 2004;292:45–54.
42. Martel N, Lee J, Wells PS. Risk for heparin-induced thrombocytopenia with unfractionated and low-molecular-weight heparin thromboprophylaxis: a meta-analysis. *Blood*. 2005;106:2710–2715.
43. Stone GW, McLaurin BT, Cox DA, et al. Bivalirudin for patients with acute coronary syndromes. *N Engl J Med*. 2006;355:2203–2216.
44. White HD, Chew DP, Hoekstra JW, et al. Safety and efficacy of switching from either unfractionated heparin or enoxaparin to bivalirudin in patients with non-ST-segment elevation acute coronary syndromes managed with an invasive strategy: results from the ACUITY (Acute Catheterization and Urgent Intervention Triage Strategy) trial. *J Am Coll Cardiol*. 2008;51:1734–1741.
45. Stone GW, Witzenbichler B, Guagliumi G, et al. Bivalirudin during primary PCI in acute myocardial infarction. *N Engl J Med*. 2008;358:2218–2230.
46. Han Y, Guo J, Zheng Y, et al. Bivalirudin vs heparin with or without tirofiban during primary percutaneous coronary intervention in acute myocardial infarction: the BRIGHT randomized clinical trial. *JAMA*. 2015;313: 1336–1346.
47. Yusuf S, Mehta SR, Chrolavicius S, et al. Comparison of fondaparinux and enoxaparin in acute coronary syndromes. *N Engl J Med*. 2006;354:1464–1476.
48. Yusuf S, Mehta SR, Chrolavicius S, et al. Effects of fondaparinux on mortality and reinfarction in patients with acute ST-segment elevation myocardial infarction: the OASIS-6 randomized trial. *JAMA*. 2006;295:1519–1530.
49. Schwartz GG, Olsson AG, Ezekowitz MD, et al. Effects of atorvastatin on early recurrent ischemic events in acute coronary syndromes: the MIRACL study: a randomized controlled trial. *JAMA*. 2001;285:1711–1718.
50. Cannon CP, Braunwald E, McCabe CH, et al. Intensive versus moderate lipid lowering with statins after acute coronary syndromes. *N Engl J Med*. 2004;350:1495–1504.
51. Keeley EC, Boura JA, Grines CL. Primary angioplasty versus intravenous thrombolytic therapy for acute myocardial infarction: a quantitative review of 23 randomised trials. *Lancet*. 2003;361:13–20.
52. Steg PG, James SK, Atar D, et al. ESC Guidelines for the management of acute myocardial infarction in patients presenting with ST-segment elevation. *Eur Heart J*. 2012;33:2569–2619.
53. O'Gara PT, Kushner FG, Ascheim DD, et al. 2013 ACCF/AHA guideline for the management of ST-elevation myocardial infarction: a report of the American College of Cardiology Foundation/American Heart Association Task Force on Practice Guidelines. *J Am Coll Cardiol*. 2013;61:e78–e140.
54. Schomig A, Mehilli J, Antoniucci D, et al. Mechanical reperfusion in patients with acute myocardial infarction presenting more than 12 hours from symptom onset: a randomized controlled trial. *JAMA*. 2005;293:2865–2872.
55. Hochman JS, Lamas GA, Buller CE, et al. Coronary intervention for persistent occlusion after myocardial infarction. *N Engl J Med*. 2006;355: 2395–2407.
56. Anderson HV, Cannon CP, Stone PH, et al. One-year results of the Thrombolysis in Myocardial Infarction (TIMI) IIIB clinical trial: a randomized comparison of tissue-type plasminogen activator versus placebo and early invasive versus early conservative strategies in unstable angina and non-Q wave myocardial infarction. *J Am Coll Cardiol*. 1995;26:1643–1650.
57. Windecker S, Kolh P, Alfonso F, et al. 2014 ESC/EACTS Guidelines on myocardial revascularization: the Task Force on Myocardial Revascularization of the European Society of Cardiology (ESC) and the European Association for Cardio-Thoracic Surgery (EACTS) Developed with the special contribution of the European Association of Percutaneous Cardiovascular Interventions (EAPCI). *Eur Heart J*. 2014;35:2541-2619.
58. Thiele H, Zeymer U, Neumann FJ, et al. Intraaortic balloon support for myocardial infarction with cardiogenic shock. *N Engl J Med*. 2012;367:1287–1296.
59. Werdan K, Gielen S, Ebelt H, Hochman JS. Mechanical circulatory support in cardiogenic shock. *Eur Heart J*. 2014;35:156–167.
60. Calvert PA, Cockburn J, Wynne D, et al. Percutaneous closure of postinfarction ventricular septal defect: in-hospital outcomes and long-term follow-up of UK experience. *Circulation*. 2014;129:2395–2402.
61. ACE Inhibitor Myocardial Infarction Collaborative Group. Indications for ACE inhibitors in the early treatment of acute myocardial infarction: systematic overview of individual data from 100,000 patients in randomized trials. *Circulation*. 1998;97:2202–2212.
62. Kinch JW, Ryan TJ. Right ventricular infarction. *N Engl J Med*. 1994;330: 1211–1217.
63. Echt DS, Liebson PR, Mitchell LB, et al. Mortality and morbidity in patients receiving encainide, flecainide, or placebo: the Cardiac Arrhythmia Suppression Trial. *N Engl J Med*. 1991;324:781–788.

CHAPTER
95

Evaluation and Management of Heart Failure

MUSTAFA AHMED, ANITA SZADY, JUAN VILARO, and JUAN M. ARANDA, JR.

INTRODUCTION

Despite advances in the prevention, diagnosis, and management of cardiovascular disease, heart failure (HF) continues to be a major burden on morbidity, mortality, and cost to our community (1). Systolic HF is a complex syndrome of structural, functional, and biologic alterations characterized by abnormalities in cardiac function that cause inadequate blood supply to tissues. The issues of poor perfusion or lack of "forward flow" are complicated by "backward flow" which produce congestion in the lungs, liver dysfunction, and renal venous hypertension (cardiorenal syndrome) (2). No matter the etiology, damage to the heart muscle starts a cascade of events that lead to neurohormonal abnormalities such as the sympathetic nervous system, the renin–angiotensin–aldosterone system (RAAS), and vasopressin activation (3). The end result is a symptomatic patient with decrease exercise tolerance with an underlying systemic neurohormonal activation associated with poor prognosis (4).

HF is now a serious public health concern. It is estimated that 6 million Americans have HF, with an associated 3 million hospital discharges per year. Half of these discharges are related to diastolic HF or impaired relaxation of the heart (5). Although patients with diastolic HF have better prognosis, they have the same number of hospitalization as those with systolic HF (6). Despite evidence-based medicine, mortality at 5 years is 50% for HF with 30-day mortality after hospital discharge at 10% to 12%. (1) In-hospital mortality if admitted with a systolic blood pressure less than 100 mmHg and a serum creatinine 2.0 mg/dL is estimated to be approximately 16% (7). Additionally, 30-day readmission rates continue to be problematic, presently 30% of all HF patients will be readmitted to a hospital within that time frame. As our medical community struggles to keep HF patients out of the hospital, estimated costs related to HF issues have risen to 29 billion dollars a year (1). The purpose of this chapter is to review the pathophysiology, diagnosis, treatment options, and controversies in HF as it pertains to the critical care patient.

PATHOPHYSIOLOGY

Determinants of Contractility

Myocardial contraction is regulated by the interaction of contractile proteins, calcium (Ca^{2+}), and cyclic adenosine monophosphate (cAMP). The contractile proteins include actin, myosin, and the troponin complex. Actin and myosin engage when cytosolic Ca^{2+} concentrations increase in the presence of adequate levels of adenosine triphosphate (ATP). This influx of Ca^{2+} is regulated by the troponin complex. Troponin T has a Ca^{2+} binding site, whose affinity for Ca^{2+} is further regulated by Troponin I. When Ca^{2+} is bound, tropomyosin undergoes a conformational change which allows for the actin–myosin interaction and contraction (8). Subsequent removal of Ca^{2+} from the cytosol results in dissociation from the troponin complex, with subsequent cessation of actin–myosin cross-linkage. This event signals the end of contractile activity and the start of relaxation—a process known as *inactivation* (9).

Delivery and removal of Ca^{2+}, and alterations in its cytosolic concentrations, are the basis of normal contractility and relaxation of the myocardium. Therefore, alterations in this mechanism result in abnormalities. Ca^{2+} can enter the cell via gated, voltage-dependent channels, or via a sodium-calcium exchange. This can be augmented with elevations in cAMP which, in turn, results in an increase in Ca^{2+} influx by recruitment of additional voltage-dependent channels. The process of recruiting previously dormant Ca^{2+} channels occurs via cAMP-mediated transfer of phosphates to phospholamban, a protein linked to the voltage-gated channels. The Ca^{2+} that enters through this mechanism causes a release of additional Ca^{2+} from the sarcoplasmic reticulum, a phenomenon termed Ca^{2+}-dependent Ca^{2+} release (10). The Ca^{2+} released from the sarcoplasmic reticulum binds to troponin with subsequent contractile activity.

While enhanced Ca^{2+} kinetics have been demonstrated to result in hypercontractile states, regardless of the underlying cause, the failing ventricle is known to have abnormalities in Ca^{2+} handling.

Determinants of Relaxation

Ca^{2+}-dependent mechanisms are also responsible for normal and abnormal ventricular relaxation. Cessation of the inward Ca^{2+} current—or inactivation—by closure of voltage-limited channels of the sarcolemma begins the period of relaxation, with the rate and extent of Ca^{2+} removal affecting the rate and extent of relaxation. Impairment of LV relaxation occurs secondary to increased levels of Ca^{2+} within the myocyte in diastole (11), owing to diminished function of the SR uptake pump, decreased expression at the genetic level for this pump, decreased phospholamban activity (12), as well as the downregulation and inhibition of β-receptors (13,14).

Mediators of Contractility

The contractile state of the myocardium is altered by a number of mediators which act independently. Chief among these are G proteins and their interactions with β-receptors and nitric oxide (NO).

β-Receptors

Adrenergic stimulation of the myocyte results increased production of cAMP, resulting in more Ca^{2+} influx via β-receptor operated

Ca^{2+} channels (15,16) specifically, stimulation of β-receptors on the cell surface results in activation of adenylate cyclase (AC) and subsequent increases in cAMP levels. This results in increased Ca^{2+} influx, with resultant increases in contractile force. The coupling between β-receptors and AC occurs through guanine cyclic nucleotides, also known as G proteins (17).

Alterations in β-receptor production also lead to various disease states. As an example, in dilated cardiomyopathies, both β_1-receptor mRNA and absolute receptor levels were found to be depressed (13). This is likely the mechanism for the catecholamine insensitivity observed in failing hearts (18).

Nitric Oxide

NO also affects cardiac contractility. It has been found in many tissue types, including ventricular myocytes, where its physiologic effects are mediated via cGMP. NO inhibition has been demonstrated to augment the positive inotropic effects of β-agonists as well as limit the negative inotropic effects of cholinergic agents. NO also plays a role in excitation, LV relaxation, and modulation of heart rate; its activity is altered in HF (19).

Calcium, Contractile Protein, and Collagen in Heart Failure

HF, either acute or chronic, results from loss of myocytes or loss of intrinsic contractility within individual myocytes. As previously mentioned, Ca^{2+} handling is essential in the regulation of myocardial contraction. Numerous abnormalities in the above discussed mechanisms and pathways are found in the failing heart, including a prolonged intracellular Ca^{2+} elevation, impaired reuptake into the sarcoplasmic reticulum, and increased activity in the Na-Ca^{2+} exchanger (20,21).

The troponin complex, as well as myosin, have altered gene expression in the failing myocardium (22). In addition to abnormalities of the contractile proteins, the collagen scaffolding of the myocytes is altered, due to a respond to pressure overload as well as up regulation of metalloproteinase which are responsible for the degradation of collagen within the extracellular matrix (23).

Compensatory Adaptations in the Failing Heart

In the face of myocardial injury, a number of compensatory mechanisms exist to help maintain cardiac output. This includes increases in preload, myocardial remodeling with dilatation and increase of myocardial mass, catecholamine surge, and the activation of the RAAS (24,25). These changes lead to increases in effective circulating blood volume, blood pressures, and peripheral vascular resistance, at the expense of an ever increasing ventricular dilatation.

Remodeling has two distinct patterns in response to volume overload or pressure overload. The former results in an eccentric hypertrophy, while the latter results in a concentric hypertrophy (26). The eccentric hypertrophy of volume overload leads to a series of replication of sarcomeres, elongation of myocytes, and ventricular dilatation, thereby resulting in increased mass and chamber enlargement. The concentric hypertrophy of pressure overload is characterized by the parallel replication of myofibrils and thickening of individual contractile units, resulting in increased mass without chamber enlargement. As HF continues to progress, these compensatory mechanisms are no longer able to maintain cardiac output, and decompensated HF ensues.

Neurohormonal Derangements in Heart Failure

Multiple neurohormonal pathways are activated in patients with HF as further compensatory mechanisms in reaction to the effects of decreased cardiac output. The pathways involved include the sympathetic nervous system, RAAS, natriuretic peptide (NP) release, and the nonosmotic release of vasopressin. Derangements of these pathways contribute to fluid retention and symptoms of volume overload seen in patients with HF. These neurohormonal pathways are intricately intertwined and each is a key component in the pathogenesis of HF (27–29).

A decrease in cardiac output leads to decreased effective arterial filling pressure, which is sensed by receptors in the carotid sinus, aortic arch, left ventricle, and afferent arteriole of the kidney. This sensed decrease in filling pressure triggers activation of the sympathetic nervous system and the release of norepinephrine (noradrenalin), as well as the nonosmotic release of vasopressin from the supraoptic and paraventricular nuclei in the brain. Norepinephrine binds to β-adrenergic receptors in the heart in an effort to increase heart rate and thereby cardiac output, and to α_1-adrenergic receptors on blood vessels causing arterial and venous constriction in order to increase arterial filling pressure. The increase in afterload caused by norepinephrine stimulating α_1-adrenergic receptors on blood vessels causes further left ventricular dysfunction and further stimulation of the sympathetic nervous system. Stimulation of cardiac β-adrenergic receptors leads to the tachycardia often seen in decompensated HF patients. Norepinephrine also activates the RAAS via activation of juxtaglomerular cells in the kidney (27,29). Stimulation of the juxtaglomerular cells in the afferent arteriole of the kidney causes the release of renin, which converts angiotensinogen to angiotensin I, which is converted to angiotensin II by angiotensin-converting enzyme (ACE). Angiotensin II acts as a powerful peripheral vasoconstrictor, stimulates the release of aldosterone from the adrenal cortex, and stimulates sodium and water reabsorption by binding to angiotensin AT1-receptors in the proximal tubule and collecting duct of the kidney (29,30). It also directly stimulates the thirst center in the brain, causing the release of vasopressin, which leads to increased fluid intake.

Aldosterone increases sodium and water reabsorption in the distal tubule and collecting duct of the kidney; vasopressin acts in the collecting duct of the kidney to stimulate water reabsorption as well (27,30,31). The combined effects of these neurohormonal pathways ultimately lead to sodium and water retention, and the symptoms of volume overload.

Although these compensatory mechanisms are designed to counteract the effects of decreased arterial filling pressure, they also have deleterious effects that contribute to the pathogenesis of HF. Both angiotensin II and aldosterone have been shown to cause myocyte necrosis, fibroblast proliferation, and myocardial fibrosis, collectively known as cardiac remodeling (32–34). Blockade of angiotensin II and aldosterone has been shown to prevent the ventricular remodeling that occurs in HF and improve survival (35–37). It is important to note the cyclical nature of the stimulation of both the sympathetic nervous system and the RAAS in HF. The sympathetic release of norepinephrine not only worsens left ventricular function by increasing afterload on the already failing ventricle, thus propagating further stimulation of the sympathetic nervous system, it also ultimately leads to the release of both angiotensin II and aldosterone, both of which further contribute to left ventricular dysfunction through the stimulation of cardiac remodeling, and the reabsorption of sodium and water.

Another group of neurohormones produced in response to the failing heart has been determined to be beneficial. These include the NPs made in response to left ventricular dilatation. These hormones have natriuretic and vasodilatory properties that are beneficial in patients with HF; their function being an attempt to counteract the deleterious effects of aldosterone and angiotensin II. Levels of NPs are elevated in patients with HF (38), this can be of utility when making a diagnosis of HF, and to differentiate causes of dyspnea (39), as well as a prognostic tool for HF outcomes and discharge readiness (40). Despite elevated circulating NPs, patients may continue to deteriorate, as their beneficial effects are rapidly overwhelmed by more potent vasoconstrictor substances.

Another substance with vasodilatory properties is bradykinin. One mechanism for vasodilatation with ACE inhibitors (ACEIs) is that degradation of bradykinin is inhibited by this class of drugs, since kininase, the enzyme that degrades bradykinin, is also known as ACE. Additionally, cytokines are produced in abnormal amounts in the HF patient, including interleukins and TNF-α. Once left ventricular dysfunction is present, the overexpression of these compounds contributes to the progression of HF, promoting left ventricular dilatation and remodeling (41); this contributes to the proinflammatory state of HF.

The Case of Heart Failure with Preserved Ejection Fraction

Diastolic dysfunction, now commonly referred to as the clinical syndrome of HF with preserved ejection fraction (HFpEF) remains an area of active research to refine our understanding of its etiologies and treatment. Recent advances along these lines have been made, in large part, due to evaluation of myocardial tissue. This has resulted in a new model of HFpEF based on structural alterations in the cardiomyocyte and fibrosis resulting in incomplete relaxation and increased ventricular stiffness, as well as abnormal intramyocardial signaling, and increased oxidative stress (42). This new paradigm suggests that HFpEF is the end result of a cascade of events initially triggered by the presence of comorbid conditions, most importantly obesity, diabetes, and hypertension, which create a systemic proinflammatory state. This leads to increased production of reactive oxygen species (ROS) which limits NO availability and leads to endothelial dysfunction, which in turn decreases G protein activity which results in cardiomyocyte hypertrophy and concentric LV remodeling and a stiffening of the cardiomyocyte. This, in addition to collagen deposition, causes the abnormalities of LV relaxation.

The Proinflammatory State and Endothelial Dysfunction

The chronic diseases which often accompany HFpEF are critical to creating the proinflammatory state which allows for the conditions to evolve to create this entity of HF. TNF-α, IL-1β, IL-4, and IL-8 are all increased in obesity (43) while hypertension leads to systemic oxidative stress (44). Chronic obstructive lung disease, iron deficiency, diabetes, and renal disease have also been studied with similar derangements noted in the secretion of cytokines (42). This systemic inflammatory state, as marked by elevations in TNF-α and IL-6, has been demonstrated to be predictive of incident HFpEF (45) while these and other markers of inflammation have been noted to be elevated in cross-sectional, observational studies in patients with HFpEF (46).

The proinflammatory cytokine release leads to endothelial production of ROS as well as endothelial mitochondrial dysfunction (47). This results in a blunted vasodilator response at the level of the coronary microcirculation, indicating impaired endothelium-mediated NO bioavailability and has been linked to prognosis in patients with HFpEF (48,49).

Hypertrophy, Relaxation, and Stiffness

The demonstrated lower NO bioavailability in HFpEF results in lower protein kinase G (PKG) activity. PKG functions as a stop to myocardial hypertrophy, and therefore, results in cardiomyocyte hypertrophy (50,51). This same pathway affects relaxation and stiffness demonstrated in numerous small and large animal model of HFpEF. This, along with collagen deposition, leads to fibrosis via proliferation of fibroblasts and profibrotic growth hormones (52,53).

Taken together, the above mechanisms suggest a different pathogenesis for HFpEF when compared to HF with reduced ejection fraction (HFrEF, systolic dysfunction), which may have important diagnostic and therapeutic implications.

DIAGNOSIS

In the critical care setting, new-onset acute HF and/or acute exacerbations of chronic HF are both encountered frequently. Early recognition of any developing HF syndrome and rapid characterization of the patient's hemodynamic profile are essential to providing optimal management.

Clinical symptoms of HF traditionally include new or progressively worsening dyspnea, fatigue, abdominal and lower extremity swelling, weight gain, orthopnea, and paroxysmal nocturnal dyspnea, all direct manifestation of hypervolemia and increased vascular congestion. Chest discomfort with anginal features is not uncommon, even in the absence of obstructive coronary disease, due to increased myocardial oxygen demand from high ventricular filling pressures and pulmonary hypertension. In addition, symptoms of severe low output such as abdominal pain, lightheadedness, and confusion are all less specific but many times indicators of the most ominous outcomes in HF patients, particularly in the ICU setting.

On examination, signs of an active clinical HF syndrome may include visible respiratory distress, increased jugular venous pressure, resting tachycardia, an s3 or s4 gallop on cardiac auscultation, newly heard, or increasing intensity of, mitral or tricuspid regurgitation murmurs, peripheral edema, ascites, diminished breath sounds, and crackles on pulmonary auscultation, particularly in dependent lung zones. Occasionally pulmonary edema will manifest as wheezing rather than crackles. In the setting of severe low output states, profound hypotension, cool extremities, tachypnea, and lethargy, many times without any signs of hypervolemia, are all manifestations of impaired end-organ perfusion and impending shock.

The diagnosis of any clinically suspected HF is strongly supported by increased serum levels of NPs, namely, BNP and, NT-pro-BNP (N-terminal-pro-Brain Natriuretic Peptide). These peptides are released from myocardial tissue in response to increased myocardial stretch, a circumstance common to all HF patients due to congestion and elevated intracardiac filling pressures (54).

The normal serum values for NPs seem to increase with age, making absolute cutoff values for diagnosing HF difficult to define; however, values that optimize sensitivity and specificity have been proposed: NT-pro-BNP values of 450, 900, and 1,800 pg/mL in patients aged under 50, 50 to 75, and over 75 years, respectively, can readily identify patients who symptoms of dyspnea are related to underlying HF (55). It is important to note that NPs have a particularly high sensitivity and negative predictive value for the diagnosis of acute HF, hence normal levels can be quite helpful in "ruling out" HF as the primary cause of any new or worsening symptoms. However, due to the breakdown of NPs occurring largely in adipose tissue, obese patients may have overt HF syndromes with normal or near normal NP levels, making the false-negative rate in these patients notably higher (56). Acute or chronic renal insufficiency, sepsis, pulmonary embolism, and stroke can all be associated with increased NP levels, even in the absence of clinically evident HF, and should be considered in the setting of an abnormally elevated BNP or NT-pro-BNP (54,57).

In patients with acute HF syndromes, worsening of renal function is very common, mainly due to reductions in effective renal perfusion that lead to decreased GFR. However, there are additional, less understood, cardiorenal interactions and pathways that seem to perpetuate further dysfunction in both organ systems independent of alterations in renal blood flow (58). The traditionally taught "prerenal" pattern of azotemia with an elevated BUN/creatinine ratio rarely reflects true hypovolemia in HF patients, but is rather a marker of more advanced HF, decreased cardiac output, and increased hospital mortality (59). Renal venous hypertension secondary to severe central venous congestion also contributes to worsening azotemia and may confound volume management (2).

If there is significant elevation in right heart pressures, liver enzyme abnormalities are frequently present. In chronic HF, decreased albumin and modest elevation in alkaline phosphatase levels predominate, largely a result of passive hepatic congestion (60). In acute HF, impaired perfusion from decreased cardiac output may be associated with acute hepatocellular necrosis and marked elevations in serum aminotransferases. Cardiogenic ischemic hepatitis ("shock liver") may ensue following an episode of profound hypotension in patients with acute HF (61).

A transthoracic echocardiogram should be obtained on any patient with clinically suspected HF. In addition to providing detailed assessment of cardiac chamber size, structure, and function, including left ventricular ejection fraction (LVEF), it frequently allows estimation of intracardiac and pulmonary pressures, all of which can be severely abnormal even in the setting of normal LVEF. The most definitive way of confirming the diagnosis of acute decompensated HF is demonstrating the typical derangements in hemodynamics that characterize the disease process. This can be accomplished noninvasively with echo, as noted above, or by invasive heart catheterization, with or without continuous hemodynamic monitoring with a balloon-tipped pulmonary artery (Swan–Ganz) catheter. The hallmark of decompensated HF is a significantly increased left ventricular filling pressure, typically estimated from the pulmonary artery postcapillary wedge pressure (PCWP), also called the pulmonary artery occlusion pressure (PAOP), with a depressed cardiac output and cardiac index. Pulmonary hypertension, at least to a mild degree, is typically present, but when severe, should raise suspicion for more chronic or advanced HF, or additional noncardiac causes. Invasive heart catheterization allows for calculation of numerous additional hemodynamic parameters such as systemic and pulmonary vascular resistance, and right ventricular stroke work index, all of which can be used to tailor management strategies for each individual patient and define prognosis. Table 95.1 shows

TABLE 95.1 Hemodynamic Parameters: Normal Adult Ranges

Parameter	Equation	Normal Range
Arterial oxygen saturation (SAO_2)		95–100%
Mixed venous saturation (MVO_2)		60–80%
Arterial blood pressure (BP)	Systolic (SBP), Diastolic (DBP)	100–140 mmHg, 60–90 mmHg
Mean arterial pressure (MAP)	(SBP + 2(DBP))/3	70–105 mmHg
Right atrial pressure/central venous pressure (RAP/CVP)		2–6 mmHg
Right ventricular pressure (RVP)	Systolic (RVSP), Diastolic (RVDP)	15–30 mmHg, 2–8 mmHg
Pulmonary artery pressure (PAP)	Systolic (PASP), Diastolic (PADP)	15–30 mmHg, 8–15 mmHg
Mean pulmonary artery pressure (MPAP)	(PASP + 2(PADP))/3	9–18 mmHg
Pulmonary artery occlusion pressure (PAOP)		6–12 mmHg
Left atrial pressure (LAP)		4–12 mmHg
Cardiac output (CO)	HR × SV/1,000	4.0–8.0 L/min
Cardiac index (CI)	CO/BSA	2.5–4.0 L/min/m^2
Stroke volume (SV)	CO/HR × 1,000	60–100 mL/beat
Stroke volume index (SVI)	CI/HR × 1,000 or SV/BSA	33–47 mL/m^2/beat
Systemic vascular resistance (SVR)	80 × (MAP–RAP)/CO	800–1200 dynes • sec/cm^5
Transpulmonic gradient (TPG)	MPAP–PAOP	<10 mmHg
Pulmonary vascular resistance	(MPAP–RAP)/CO	<250 dynes • sec/cm^5
Left ventricular stroke work index (LVSWI)	SVI × (MAP–PAOP) × 0.0136	50–62 g/m^2/beat
Right ventricular stroke work index (RVSWI)	SVI × (MPAP–RAP) × 0.0136	5–10 g/m^2/beat

normal adult ranges for hemodynamic parameters measurable with invasive catheterization.

MANAGEMENT

The optimal treatment strategy for patients with HF depends on numerous clinical factors, particularly the presence or absence of active decompensation. In the critical care setting, management strategies for *acute* HF syndromes are much more relevant and will be the focus of this chapter.

Once acute decompensated HF has been confirmed or become the leading diagnosis, initial treatment should focus on decongestion and maximizing end-organ perfusion. The specific treatment regimen needed to accomplish these goals depends largely on the hemodynamic profile, which typically will fall into one of four main categories, depending on the adequacy of end-organ perfusion and degree of hypervolemia (Fig. 95.1). Early hemodynamic characterization, and therefore initial treatment strategy, can be accomplished in many patients at the bedside simply by measuring systemic blood pressure and central venous pressure (62).

The most common profile is "warm and wet," which characterizes patients who are not overtly hypotensive and have evidence of hypervolemia, with preserved overall end-organ perfusion. In these patients, afterload reduction and volume management are the main goals of care, accomplished mostly with vasodilator and diuretic therapy. Common vasodilators with proven efficacy in the management of HF patients include nitrates, ACEIs, angiotensin receptor blockers (ARBs), and hydralazine.

Loop diuretics should be used first line for treatment of congestion related to hypervolemia. Intravenous administration, rather than oral, increases bioavailability, onset of action, and peak effect, and is therefore the preferred method in the critical care setting. Bolus dosing or continuous infusions appear to be equally safe and effective with regard to net volume loss over a given time period (63). However, in our experience continuous infusions are sometimes better tolerated in patients with marginal blood pressure, possibly due to less abrupt redistributions of intra- and extravascular volume compared to bolus dosing.

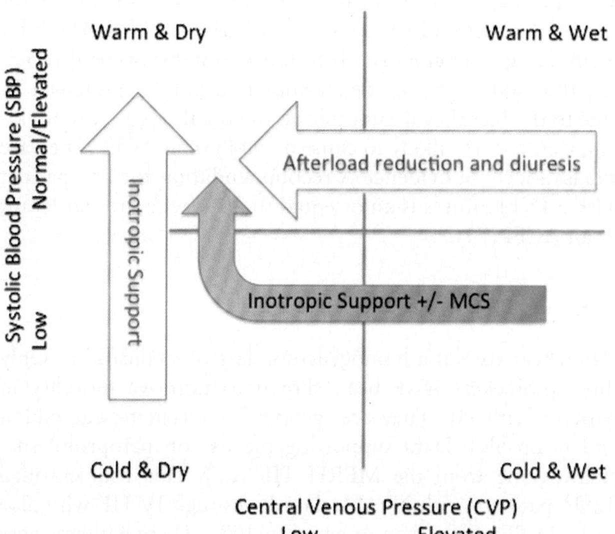

FIGURE 95.1 Rapid hemodynamic assessment.

Resistance to loop diuretics, also called diuretic "braking," can be encountered, particularly in patients who are receiving loop diuretics chronically or have impaired renal function. If patients cannot be brought to euvolemia with a loop diuretic–based strategy, several ways of intensifying the regimen for volume management exist. Providing a dose of thiazide diuretic, given orally or intravenously 30 minutes prior to loop diuretic dosing, potentiates the diuretic effect and can result in large increases in urine output (64). Frequent electrolyte monitoring and replacement is crucial in this setting as the diuretic combination can quickly cause severe deficiencies, namely hypokalemia and hypomagnesemia, which in turn precipitate atrial and ventricular dysrhythmias.

Nesiritide, a synthetic form of B-type NP, can be highly effective in patients with severe congestion and suboptimal response to diuretics. It has natriuretic, diuretic, and vasodilator effects, and reduces neurohormonal activation. It is administered by continuous infusion with an initial bolus typically not recommended due to risk of causing profound hypotension. Although no clear benefits in HF outcomes have been demonstrated with nesiritide compared to traditional loop diuretic regimens, it remains a valuable option for volume management, especially in the setting of loop diuretic resistance (65,66).

In many HF patients, the predominant hemodynamic alteration is a markedly reduced cardiac output, characterized by severe symptomatic hypotension that essentially contraindicates the use of vasodilators or diuretics by themselves, the so-called "cold and wet" profile. In these patients several inotropes and vasopressors can be used to maximize end-organ perfusion, facilitate volume management, and provide symptom relief. It is crucial to understand that the predominant hemodynamic effect of these agents varies depending on the dose. Table 95.2 outlines the mechanism of action, dose range, and special considerations for vasopressors and inotropes used in HF.

For catecholaminergic agents at low to moderate doses, positive inotropic effects will generally predominate. At high doses, all can be potentially detrimental to cardiac function due to increased afterload from excessive vasoconstrictive effect and extreme tachycardia (67). Multiple markers of cardiac output and end-organ perfusion, rather than systemic blood pressure alone, should guide titration of inotropes and vasopressors to optimal doses for HF treatment. Both dobutamine and milrinone, the most commonly utilized inotropic agents, can worsen hypotension due to vasodilation from peripheral β_2-receptor stimulation. If poorly tolerated, it is reasonable to delay initiation of inotropes until risk of precipitating overt shock is lower. Low-dose dopamine or norepinephrine, used alone or started preemptively/simultaneously with low-dose inotropes, can readily offset this risk of worsening hypotension. Used at the right doses, they facilitate initial hemodynamic stabilization of severely decompensated HF patients. This is particularly true for patients with any degree of acidosis or worsening end-organ function, where rescuing them from overt shock is critical.

Mental status, urine output, capillary refill, mixed venous oxygen saturation (drawn from the PA catheter or central venous access), and lactic acid levels can all be assessed, serially over time if needed, to determine if cardiac output is

TABLE 95.2 Vasoactive Medications in Heart Failure

Agent	Mechanism of Action	Considerations in HF
Dopamine	Activates dopaminergic and adrenergic receptors. At 0.5–3 μg/kg/min may increase blood flow to the renal vasculature. At 3–10 μg/kg/min, binds to β_1-receptors, promotes norepinephrine release and increase contractility and chronotropy. At more than 10 μg/kg/min, α_1-effects dominate and result in vasoconstriction.	May cause arrhythmias, tachycardia At higher doses will increase SVR and potentially decrease CO
Dobutamine	Strongly stimulates β_1- and β_2-receptors, potent inotrope with weaker chronotropic effects. At doses less than 5 μg/kg/min, may cause mild vasodilatation due to β_2-, α_1-, and smooth muscle effects. Vasoconstriction predominates at higher doses.	May cause arrhythmias, tachycardia. Increases myocardial oxygen demand and may worsen ischemia.
Epinephrine	Endogenous catecholamine with high affinity for β_1-, β_2-, and α_1-receptors in cardiac and smooth muscle. β effects more pronounced at low dose, α-effects at higher doses.	May cause arrhythmias, tachycardia. Prolonged use at high dose can stimulate myocyte death and myocardial necrosis.
Milrinone	Phosphodiesterase 3 inhibitor, which increases cAMP levels leading to increased contractility. Potent inotrope and vasodilator.	May cause arrhythmias. Caution initiation as single agent with hypotension as decreases in preload, afterload, and SVR may cause severe hypotension.
Norepinephrine	Potent α_1-agonist with modest β_1-activity. Powerful vasoconstrictor with less potent inotropic effects. Minimal chronotropic effects.	Can be useful when trying to avoid increases in heart rate. Prolonged use can be toxic to the myocyte by inducing apoptosis.
Phenylephrine	Essentially pure α_1-adrenergic activity with no effect on heart rate.	Severe vasoconstriction for rapid correction of hypotension, useful for patients with severe hypotension and critical aortic stenosis. Caution prolonged use with LV dysfunction as CO will decrease
Vasopressin	Stimulates V1 and V2 receptors, resulting in vascular smooth muscle constriction and enhanced renal water reabsorption	Dose-dependent increase in SVR will decrease CO. Effects are preserved in hypoxic and acidotic states

HF, heart failure; SVR, systemic vascular resistance; CO, cardiac output.

adequate, worsening, or improving. In refractory cases, temporary mechanical support, in the form of an intra-aortic balloon pump or percutaneous left ventricular assist device, should be considered.

Evidence-Based Therapy for Chronic Systolic Heart Failure

The mainstays of treatment for HF are medications that modulate the neurohormonal cascade. These medications include ACEIs, ARBs, β-blockers, and mineralocorticoid antagonists. It is important to use evidence-based medications approved for HF and to titrate them to evidence-based doses as much as possible to achieve maximum benefit.

ACE Inhibitors and Angiotensin Receptor Blockers

ACEIs inhibit the enzyme ACE that converts angiotensin I to angiotensin II, a potent vasoconstrictor, simulator of the release of aldosterone, and contributor to left ventricular remodeling. Bradykinin, which induces NO-mediated vasodilatation, is degraded by ACE. Angiotensin I is converted to angiotensin II by tissue chymases as well, but the main pathway is via ACE. Data supporting the use of these medications come from three landmark trials: Consensus I, VHEFT II, and the SOLVED Treatment Trial. Consensus I enrolled 253 patients with NYHA class IV HF and randomized them to either enalapril 40 mg daily versus placebo. The result was a 27% reduction in mortality in the enalapril group. The mortality benefit in the enalapril group was found to be mainly due to a reduction in death from progressive HF (68). The VHEFT II study enrolled 804 patients with NYHA class II and III HF. These patients were randomized to either enalapril 20 mg daily versus hydralazine 300 mg daily plus isosorbide dinitrate 160 mg daily. The result was a 28% reduction in mortality in the enalapril group (69). The SOLVED Treatment Trial enrolled 2,569 patients with NYHA class II and III HF. Patients were randomized to enalapril 20 mg daily versus placebo. The result was a 16% reduction in morality in the enalapril group. Analysis showed that the mortality benefit in the enalapril group was mainly due to a reduction in death from progressive HF (70). Due to these overwhelming data, use of an ACEI is a class I level of evidence A for any patient with a LVEF of 40% or lower (71). ARBs inhibit the binding of angiotensin II to the angiotensin type II receptor, thus inhibiting the deleterious effects of angiotensin II. Due to the fact they do not inhibit the breakdown of bradykinin, they are less likely to cause a cough than ACEI. They are a class I level of evidence A recommendation for any patient with a LVEF of less than or equal to 40% who are intolerant of an ACEI (71).

β-Blockers

β-Blockers are not a homogeneous class of medications. Only three β-blockers have been shown to improve morality in patients with HF. They are metoprolol succinate, carvedilol, and bisoprolol. Data supporting the use of metoprolol succinate came from the MERIT HF trial. This trial enrolled 3,991 patients with NYHA class II through IV HF who also had a LVEF of less than or equal to 40%. These patients were randomized to metoprolol succinate 200 mg daily versus placebo. It is important to note that 95% of patients enrolled were either on an ACEI or an ARB. The results were a 41% risk reduction in sudden cardiac death, a 49% risk reduction in death from HF, a 30% risk reduction in the number of HF hospitalizations, and a 36% risk reduction in the number of days hospitalized for HF in the metoprolol succinate group (72). A substudy of the MERIT-HF trial looked at left ventricular volumes by MRI. Patients in the metoprolol succinate group had statistically significant decreases in left ventricular volumes and mass compared to placebo (73).

The CIBIS II study evaluated the efficacy of bisoprolol. This trial enrolled 2,647 patients with NYHA class III and IV HF who had a LVEF less than or equal to 35% and randomized them to bisoprolol 10 mg daily versus placebo; 96% of enrolled patients were either on an ACEI or an ARB. The results were a 42% reduction in sudden cardiac death and a 32% reduction in the combined end point of morality and admission for HF (74).

Carvedilol was evaluated in the COPERNICUS trial. This trial evaluated 2,289 patients with NYHA class III and IV HF with a LVEF of 25% or less; 97% of patients in this trial were on an ACEI or an ARB. Patients were randomized to carvedilol 25 mg twice daily versus placebo. Patients in the carvedilol group had a 35% risk reduction in mortality when compared to placebo (75). Use of a β-blocker is a class I level of evidence A recommendation for any patient with a LVEF of 40% or less (71).

Mineralocorticoid Antagonists

Mineralocorticoid antagonists block the binding of aldosterone to the mineralocorticoid receptor. Aldosterone is known to cause ventricular remodeling and fibrosis in HF. There are three landmark trials supporting the use of mineralocorticoid antagonists in the HF population. The RALES study evaluated 1,663 patients with NYHA class III and IV HF and a LVEF of 35% or less. They were randomized to spironolactone 25 mg daily, with a target of 50 mg daily, added to optimal medical therapy versus optimal medical therapy alone. In this trial, 95% of patients were on an ACEI or an ARB, and 10% were on a β-blocker. The trial has been criticized due to the low number of patients receiving a β-blocker. The results showed a 30% reduction in all-cause death, a 31% reduction in death from cardiovascular causes, and a 30% reduction in HF hospitalizations in the spironolactone group. Patients in the spironolactone group also had statistically significant improvement in NYHA functional class when compared to the optimal medical therapy group (76). It is important to note that the exclusion criteria for this trial included a creatinine of 2.5 mg/dL or higher. The addition of a mineralocorticoid antagonist to an ACEI or an ARB can cause life-threatening hyperkalemia, and the patients creatinine and serum potassium levels much be watched carefully during initiation of this class of medications.

The use of a mineralocorticoid receptor antagonist post myocardial infarction was evaluated in the EPHESUS trial. This trial enrolled 6,642 patients who were post acute myocardial infarction and had a LVEF of 40% or less and either clinical symptoms of HF or the diagnosis of diabetes mellitus. Patients were randomized to eplerenone 25 mg daily, with a target of 50 mg daily, in addition to optimal medical therapy versus optimal medical therapy alone. It is important to note 87% of these patients were on an ACEI or an ARB and 75% were on a β-blocker. The results noted a 15% reduction in mortality in the Eplerenone group (77).

The EMPHASIS HF trial evaluated the use of the mineralocorticoid receptor antagonist Eplerenone in patients with NYHA class II HF and a LVEF no greater than 30%. Enrollees also had to have been hospitalized for HF within the previous 6 months of enrollment or had to have had a BNP of 250 pg/mL or more at the time of enrollment. Patients were randomized to Eplerenone 50 mg daily added to optimal medical therapy versus optimal medical therapy alone. In this trial, 97% of patients were on an ACEI or an ARB and 86% were on a β-blocker. The results were a 24% decrease in cardiovascular death, a 42% decrease in HF hospitalizations, and a 37% decrease in the combined end point of death from cardiovascular causes or HF hospitalizations in the Eplerenone group (78). Addition of a mineralocorticoid receptor antagonist to optimal medical therapy with a β-blocker and ACEI or ARB is a class I level of evidence A for any patient with a LVEF of 35% or less, and NYHA symptom class II through IV. Patients with NYHA class II HF should have a recent history of HF hospitalization or elevated BNP (71). Mineralocorticoid receptor antagonists are also a class I level of evidence B recommendation for patients who are post acute myocardial infarction who have a LVEF of 40% or less and have HF symptoms or who are diabetic (71).

Controversies in Heart Failure

Some of the most difficult decisions affecting practitioners who care for patients with advanced HF are hemodynamic monitoring in the critically ill patient and when to refer patients for advanced HF therapies (cardiac transplantation or ventricular assist device). The utility of continuous hemodynamic monitoring in the advanced HF patient was evaluated in the ESCAPE trial (79). ESCAPE enrolled 433 patients with decompensated HF and randomized them to treatment guided by a pulmonary artery catheter versus clinically guided therapy. The trials primary end point was days alive out of the hospital 6 months after randomization. The trial showed no benefit in the primary end point in patients who underwent continuous hemodynamic monitoring with a pulmonary artery catheter as compared to those who were treated based on clinical assessment, and there were more adverse events noted in the pulmonary artery catheter cohort. The ESCAPE trial was specifically designed to determine if the routine use of continuous hemodynamic monitoring was useful in decompensated HF patients. Any patient who may have benefited from or needed acute hemodynamic monitoring was not included in the trial by design. Given this, there are certain patients with acute decompensated HF who should undergo temporary continuous hemodynamic monitoring with a pulmonary artery catheter in order to guide therapy. According to the ACC/AHA guidelines (2), patients who would benefit from monitoring are those patients whose volume status is difficult to determine clinically and have either evidence of hypoperfusion, such as worsening renal function or rising serum lactic acid, or respiratory distress despite treatment. Other patients who should be considered for hemodynamic monitoring are those whose systolic blood pressure remains low, or who remain symptomatic despite initial therapy; those whose volume status, perfusion status, or systemic or pulmonary vascular resistance are uncertain; or those who require vasoactive agents (71). Ideally, hemodynamic assessment should occur prior to initiation of vasoactive agents. Assessment of hemodynamics should also be performed on any patient being considered for temporary mechanical circulatory support (71). Hemodynamic monitoring in these patients should be short term, and should be discontinued once the patient's clinical status begins to improve, or further monitoring is not needed to guide therapy.

With respect to when to evaluate a patient for advanced HF therapies, a timely referral to a center which specializes in advanced HF therapies is critical to the outcome of the patient. Advanced HF therapies are generally reserved for patients with stage D HF. The Heart Failure Society of America's definition of stage D HF is "the presence of progressive and/or persistent severe signs and symptoms of heart failure despite optimized medical, surgical, and device therapy. It is generally accompanied by frequent hospitalization, severely limited exertional tolerance and poor quality of life, and is associated with high morbidity and mortality. Importantly, the progressive decline should be primarily driven by the heart failure syndrome" (80). Defining stage D HF in the individual patient is often difficult. Multiple guidelines are available to aid in the diagnosis (Table 95.3), but often no one set of guidelines is adequate. Indicators that a patient is declining and should be referred for advanced HF therapies include frequent hospitalizations

TABLE 95.3 Definitions of Stage D Heart Failure

American College of Cardiology/American Heart Association (71)

- Repeated (≥2) hospitalizations or ED visits for HF in the past year
- Progressive deterioration in renal function (e.g., rise in BUN and creatinine)
- Weight loss without other cause (e.g., cardiac cachexia)
- Intolerance to ACEIs due to hypotension and/or worsening renal function
- Intolerance to β-blockers due to worsening HF or hypotension
- Frequent systolic blood pressure <90 mmHg
- Persistent dyspnea with dressing or bathing requiring rest
- Inability to walk one block on the level ground due to dyspnea or fatigue
- Recent need to escalate diuretics to maintain volume status, often reaching daily furosemide equivalent dose >160 mg/day and/or use of supplemental metolazone therapy
- Progressive decline in serum sodium, usually to <133 mEq/L
- Frequent ICD shocks

Interagency Registry for Mechanically Assisted Circulatory Support (INTERMACS)(81)

- Profile 1: Critical cardiogenic shock. Patients with life-threatening hypotension despite rapidly escalating inotropic support, critical organ hypoperfusion, often confirmed by worsening acidosis and/or lactate levels. "Crash and burn." Definitive intervention needed within hours.
- Profile 2: Progressive decline. Patient with declining function despite intravenous inotropic support may be manifest by worsening renal function, nutritional depletion, and inability to restore volume balance. "Sliding on inotropes." Also describes declining status in patients unable to tolerate inotropic therapy. Definitive intervention needed within few days.
- Profile 3: Stable but inotrope dependent. Patient with stable blood pressure, organ function, nutrition, and symptoms on continuous intravenous inotropic support (or a temporary circulatory support device or both), but demonstrating repeated failure to wean from support due to recurrent symptomatic hypotension or renal dysfunction "Dependent stability."
- Profile 4: Resting symptoms. Patient can be stabilized close to normal volume status but experiences daily symptoms of congestion at rest or during ADL. Doses of diuretics generally fluctuate at very high levels. More intensive management and surveillance strategies should be considered, which may in some cases reveal poor compliance that would compromise outcomes with any therapy. Some patients may shuttle between 4 and 5. Definitive intervention elective over period of weeks to few months.
- Profile 5: Exertion intolerant. Comfortable at rest and with ADL but unable to engage in any other activity, living predominantly within the house. Patients are comfortable at rest without congestive symptoms, but may have underlying refractory elevated volume status, often with renal dysfunction. If underlying nutritional status and organ function are marginal, patient may be more at risk than INTERMACS 4, and require definitive intervention. Variable urgency depends on maintenance of nutrition, organ function, and activity.
- Profile 6: Exertion limited. Patient without evidence of fluid overload is comfortable at rest, and with activities of daily living and minor activities outside the home but fatigues after the first few minutes of any meaningful activity. Attribution to cardiac limitation requires careful measurement of peak oxygen consumption, in some cases with hemodynamic monitoring to confirm severity of cardiac impairment. "Walking wounded."
- Profile 7: Advanced NYHA III. A placeholder for more precise specification in future, this level includes patients who are without current or recent episodes of unstable fluid balance, living comfortably with meaningful activity limited to mild physical exertion.

European Society of Cardiology(82)

- Episodes of fluid retention (pulmonary and/or systemic congestion, peripheral edema) and/or of reduced cardiac output at rest (peripheral hypoperfusion)
- Objective evidence of severe cardiac dysfunction, shown by at least one of the following:
  - A low LVEF (<30%)
  - A severe abnormality of cardiac function on Doppler echocardiography with a pseudonormal or restrictive mitral inflow pattern
- High LV filling pressures (mean PCWP >16 mmHg, and/or mean RAP >12 mmHg by pulmonary artery catheterization)
- High BNP or NT-ProBNP plasma levels, in the absence of noncardiac causes
- Severe impairment of functional capacity shown by one of the following:
  - Inability to exercise
  - 6-MWT distance 300 m
  - Peak VO_2 less than 12 to 14 mL/kg/min
- History of 1 or more HF hospitalization in the past 6 mo

for HF despite optimal medical therapy; inability to tolerate evidence-based medical therapies due to hypotension or renal dysfunction; functional decline; escalation of diuretics; refractory arrhythmias; ICD firing; and cardiac cachexia (81,82). Objective measurements that indicate a patient may have progressed to stage D HF include a 6-minute walk distance of less than 300 m and peak oxygen consumption on cardiopulmonary exercise stress test of less than 12 to 14 mL/kg/min. Unfortunately, referrals are often made too late to advanced HF centers. Patient acuity and frailty are often issues with late referrals. Data from INTERMACS (Interagency Registry for Mechanically Assisted Circulatory Support) (83) show that patients with an INTERMACS scores of 1 or 2 have a higher mortality compared with patients who have lower INTERMACS scores. Implant trends have mirrored this data, with less INTERMACS 1 and 2 patients receiving durable devices due to their increased mortality. Patients should be referred for evaluation for advanced HF therapies before they reach INTERMACS 1 or 2 scores. Ideally, they should be referred for initial evaluation when they are INTERMACS score 5 or 6. Frailty is a known predictor of death, HF hospitalization, and quality of life in patients with HF and those undergoing cardiac surgery. Multiple definitions of frailty exist, but most include measurements of unintentional weight loss and malnutrition (usually <10 lb in the past year, serum albumin <3.3 mg/dL, respectively), weakness as measured by hand grip strength (<30 kg for men, <20 kg for women), gait speed (5 m gait speed <0.5 m/sec), level of physical activity, and level of exhaustion. Satisfying more than 3 of 5 of the preceding criteria qualify for the diagnosis of frailty (84). Muscle wasting (sarcopenia) and cachexia are related to frailty and are also predictive of morbidity and mortality. Sarcopenia is defined as a muscle mass more than 2 standard deviations below the mean measured in young adults of the same sex and ethnic background (85). Cachexia is defined as a metabolic syndrome that is associated with an underlying illness such as HF that is characterized by loss of muscle with or without loss of fat. The prominent clinical feature is weight loss (86). Frailty has been associated with worse outcomes after destination LVAD placement. In a study evaluating frailty in destination therapy LVAD patients, frailty was associated with a hazard ratio of 1.7 for death in patients determined to be intermediately frail, and 3.08 for those who were determined to be frail (10). Rehospitalizations were also found to be increased in the intermediately frail (hazard ratio 1.7), and frail patients (hazard ratio 1.42) (87). Referral to an advanced HF center should occur prior to a patient reaching a state of frailty that would preclude intervention.

SUMMARY

HF is a pervasive and progressive condition affecting an increasing number of patients. Therefore, familiarity with its pathophysiology and treatment are essential to effective patient care in the modern critical care unit. Despite a large repository of data and guidelines to direct therapy, one must be sure to provide patient-specific care, while keeping in mind appropriate goals of care. A multidisciplinary approach to these patients is of great utility in determining timely and effective interventions, ranging from pharmacologic remedies, mechanical circulatory support, and palliative care.

Key Points

- Understanding the mechanisms and pathophysiology of the failing heart can aid in management.
- Early diagnosis of an HF syndrome and recognition of its severity is critical to providing a good outcome.
- The basis of HF therapy is neurohormonal blockade.
- Therapy should be step-wise and escalated to maximal tolerated doses.
- Failure of response to routine medical therapy may suggest the need for vasoactive infusions, and invasive hemodynamic monitoring can be beneficial in this setting.
- Patients with advanced HF syndromes should be managed in a multidisciplinary fashion with consideration of early referral to a VAD/transplant center.

References

1. Braunwald E. Heart failure. *JACC Heart Fail.* 2013;1:1–20.
2. Ross E. Congestive renal failure: the pathophysiology and treatment of renal venous hypertension. *J Cardiac Fail.* 2012;12:930–938.
3. Tavares M, Rezlan E, Vostroknoutova I, et al. New pharmacologic therapies for acute heart failure. *Crit Care Med.* 2008;36(1 Suppl):S112–S120.
4. Cohn JN, Johnson GR, Shabetai R, et al. Ejection fraction, peak exercise oxygen consumption, cardiothoracic ratio, ventricular arrhythmias, and plasma norepinephrine as determinants of prognosis in heart failure. The V-HeFT VA Cooperative Studies Group. *Circulation.* 1993;87(6 Suppl):V15–V16.
5. Adams KF, Fonarow GC, Emerman CL, et al; ADHERE Scientific Advisory Committee and Investigators. Characteristics and outcomes of patients hospitalized for heart failure in the United States: rationale, design, and preliminary observations from the first 100,000 cases in the Acute Decompensated Heart Failure National Registry (ADHERE). *Am Heart J.* 2005;149: 209–216.
6. Dauterman KW, Go AS, Rowell R, et al. Congestive heart failure with preserved systolic function in a statewide sample of community hospitals. *J Card Fail.* 2001;7:221–228.
7. Abraham WT, Fonarow GC, Albert NM, et al; OPTIMIZE-HF Investigators and Coordinators. Predictors of in-hospital mortality in patients hospitalized for heart failure: Insights from the Organized Program to Initiate Lifesaving Treatment in Hospitalized Patients with Heart Failure (OPTIMIZE-HF). *J Am Coll Cardiol.* 2008;52:347–356.
8. Housmans PR, Lee NK, Blinks JR. Active shortening retards the decline of the intracellular calcium transient in mammalian heart muscle. *Science.* 1983;221:159–161.
9. Brustsaert DL, Rademakers FE, Sys SU. Triple control of relaxation: implications in cardiac disease. *Circulation.* 1984;69:190–196.
10. Kohmoto O, Spitzer KW, Movsesian MA, Barry WH. Effects of intracellular acidosis on [Ca^{2+}]i transients, transsarcolemmal Ca^{2+} fluxes, and contraction in ventricular myocytes. *Circ Res.* 1990;66:622–632.
11. Gwatheny JK, Slawsky MT, Hajjar RJ, et al. Role of intracellular calcium handling in force-interval relationships of human ventricular myocardium. *J Clin Invest.* 1990;85:1599–1613.
12. Feldman MD, Copelas L, Gwathmey JK, et al. Deficient production of cyclic AMP: pharmacologic evidence of an important cause of contractile dysfunction in patients with end-stage heart failure. *Circulation.* 1987;75:331–339.
13. Ungerer M, Böhm M, Elce JS, et al. Altered expression of beta-adrenergic receptor kinase and beta 1-adrenergic receptors in the failing human heart. *Circulation.* 1993;87:454–463.
14. Feldman MD, Alderman JD, Aroesty JM. Depression of systolic and diastolic myocardial reserve during atrial pacing tachycardia in patients with dilated cardiomyopathy. *J Clin Invest.* 1988;82:1661–1669.
15. Katz AM. Cyclic adenosine monophosphate effects on the myocardium: a man who blows hot and cold with one breath. *J Am Coll Cardiol.* 1983;2: 143–149.
16. Homey CJ, Graham RM. Molecular characterization of adrenergic receptors. *Circ Res.* 1985;56:635–650.
17. Neer EJ, Clapham DE. Roles of G protein subunits in transmembrane signaling. *Nature.* 1988;333:129–134.

18. Schranz D, Droege A, Broede A, et al. Uncoupling of human cardiac beta-adrenoceptors during cardiopulmonary bypass with cardioplegic cardiac arrest. *Circulation.* 1993;87:422–426.
19. Cotton JM, Kearney MT, Shah AM. Nitric oxide and myocardial function in heart failure: friend or foe? *Heart.* 2002;88:564–566.
20. Piacentino V 3rd, Weber CR, Chen X, et al. Cellular basis of abnormal calcium transients of failing human ventricular myocytes. *Circ Res.* 2003;92:651–658.
21. Flesch M, Schwinger RH, Schnabel P, et al. Sarcoplasmic reticulum Ca^{2+} ATPase and phospholamban mRNA and protein levels in end-stage heart failure due to ischemic or dilated cardiomyopathy. *J Mol Med (Berl).* 1996;74:321–332.
22. Abraham WT, Gilbert EM, Lowes BD, et al. Coordinate changes in myosin heavy chain isoform gene expression are selectively associated with alterations in dilated cardiomyopathy phenotype. *Mol Med.* 2002;8:750–760.
23. Thomas CV, Coker ML, Zellner JL, et al. Increased matrix metalloproteinase activity and selective upregulation in LV myocardium from patients with end-stage dilated cardiomyopathy. *Circulation.* 1998;97:1708–1715.
24. Meerson FZ. The myocardium in hyperfunction, hypertrophy, and heart failure. *Circ Res.* 1998;25(Suppl 2):1–163.
25. Cohn JN, Ferrari R, Sharpe N. Cardiac remodeling—concepts and clinical implications: a consensus paper from an international forum on cardiac remodeling. Behalf of an International Forum on Cardiac Remodeling. *J Am Coll Cardiol.* 2000;35:569–582.
26. Calderone A, Takahashi N, Izzo NJ Jr, et al. Pressure- and volume-induced left ventricular hypertrophies are associated with distinct myocyte phenotypes and differential induction of peptide growth factor mRNAs. *Circulation.* 1995;92:2385–2390.
27. Sica DA. Sodium and water retention in heart failure and diuretic therapy: basic mechanics. *Cleve Clin J Med.* 2006;73(Suppl 2):S2–S7; discussion S30–S33.
28. Francis GS, Benedict C, Johnstone DE, et al. Comparison of neuroendocrine activation in patients with left ventricular dysfunction with and without congestive heart failure: a substudy of the Studies of Left Ventricular Dysfunction (SOLVD). *Circulation.* 1990;82:1724–1729.
29. Schrier RW, Abraham WT. Hormones and hemodynamics in heart failure. *N Engl J Med.* 1999;341:577–585.
30. Johnson LR, Byrne JH. *Essential Medical Physiology.* 2nd ed. Philadelphia, PA: Lippincott-Raven; 1998.
31. Brunton L. *Goodman & Gillman's The Pharmacological Basis of Therapeutics.* 11th ed. Boston, MA: McGraw-Hill; 2006.
32. Tan LB, Jalil JE, Pick R, et al. Cardiac myocyte necrosis induced by angiotensin II. *Circ Res.* 1991;69:1185–1195.
33. Thohan V, Torre-Amione G, Koerner MM. Aldosterone antagonism and congestive heart failure; a new look at an old therapy. *Curr Opin Cardiol.* 2004;19:301–308.
34. Weber KT, Brilla CG. Pathological hypertrophy and cardiac interstitium: fibrosis and renin-angiotensin-aldosterone system. *Circulation.* 1991; 83:1849–1865.
35. Konstam MA, Kronenberg MW, Rousseau MF, et al. Effects of the angiotensin converting enzyme inhibitor enalapril on the long term progression of left ventricular dilatation in patients with asymptomatic systolic dysfunction. SOLVD (Studies of Left Ventricular Dysfunction) Investigators. *Circulation.* 1993;88:2277–2283.
36. Swedberg K, Eneroth P, Kjekshus J, Wilhelmsen L. Hormones regulating cardiovascular function in patients with severe congestive heart failure and their relation to mortality. The CONSENSUS Trial Study Group. *Circulation.* 1990;82:1730–1736.
37. Pitt B, Zannad F, Remme WJ, et al. The effect of spironolactone on morbidity and mortality in patients with severe heart failure. *N Engl J Med.* 1999;341:709–717.
38. Worster A, Balion CM, Hill SA, et al. Diagnostic accuracy of BNP and NT-proBNP in patients presenting to acute care settings with dyspnea: a systematic review. *Clin Biochem.* 2008;41:250–259.
39. Januzzi JL Jr, Camargo CA, Anwaruddin S, et al. The N-terminal proBNP investigation of dyspnea in the emergency department (PRIDE) study. *Am J Cardiol.* 2005;95:948–954.
40. Maisel A, Mueller C, Adams K Jr, et al. State of the art: using natriuretic peptide levels in clinical practice. *Eur J Heart Fail.* 2008;10:824–839.
41. Effect of enalapril on mortality and the development of heart failure in asymptomatic patients with reduced left ventricular ejection fractions. The SOLVD Investigators. *N Engl J Med.* 1992;327:685–691.
42. Paulus WJ, Tschöpe C. A novel paradigm for heart failure with preserved ejection fraction: comorbidities drive myocardial dysfunction and remodeling through coronary microvascular endothelial inflammation. *J Am Coll Cardiol.* 2013;62:263–271.
43. Taube A, Schlich R, Sell H, et al. Inflammation and metabolic dysfunction: links to cardiovascular disease. *Am J Physiol Heart Circ Physiol.* 2012; 302:H2148–H2165.
44. Hummel SL, Seymour EM, Brook RD, et al. Low-sodium dietary approaches to stop hypertension diet reduces blood pressure, arterial stiffness, and oxidative stress in hypertensive heart failure with preserved ejection fraction. *Hypertension.* 2012;60:1200–1206.
45. Kalogeropoulos A, Georgiopoulou V, Psaty BM, et al; Health ABC Study Investigators. Inflammatory markers and incident heart failure risk in older adults: the Health ABC (Health, Aging, and Body Composition) study. *J Am Coll Cardiol.* 2010;55:2129–2137.
46. Collier P, Watson CJ, Voon V, et al. Can emerging biomarkers of myocardial remodelling identify asymptomatic hypertensive patients at risk for diastolic dysfunction and diastolic heart failure? *Eur J Heart Fail.* 2011; 13:1087–1095.
47. Griendling KK, Sorescu D, Ushio-Fukai M. NAD(P)H oxidase: role in cardiovascular biology and disease. *Circ Res.* 2000;86:494–501.
48. Akiyama E, Sugiyama S, Matsuzawa Y, et al. Incremental prognostic significance of peripheral endothelial dysfunction in patients with heart failure with normal left ventricular ejection fraction. *J Am Coll Cardiol.* 2012;60:1778–1786.
49. Lam CS, Brutsaert DL. Endothelial dysfunction: a pathophysiologic factor in heart failure with preserved ejection fraction. *J Am Coll Cardiol.* 2012;60:1787–1789.
50. Calderone A, Thaik CM, Takahashi N, et al. Nitric oxide, atrial natriuretic peptide, and cyclic GMP inhibit the growth-promoting effects of norepinephrine in cardiac myocytes and fibroblasts. *J Clin Invest.* 1998; 101:812–818.
51. Falcão-Pires I, Hamdani N, Borbély A, et al. Diabetes mellitus worsens diastolic left ventricular dysfunction in aortic stenosis through altered myocardial structure and cardiomyocyte stiffness. *Circulation.* 2011; 124:1151–1159.
52. Kasner M, Westermann D, Lopez B, et al. Diastolic tissue Doppler indexes correlate with the degree of collagen expression and cross-linking in heart failure and normal ejection fraction. *J Am Coll Cardiol.* 2011;57:977–985.
53. Zannad F, Radauceanu A. Effect of MR blockade on collagen formation and cardiovascular disease with a specific emphasis on heart failure. *Heart Fail Rev.* 2005;10:71–78.
54. McCullough PA, Duc P, Omland T, et al. B-type natriuretic peptide and renal function in the diagnosis of heart failure: an analysis from the Breathing Not Properly Multinational Study. *Am J Kidney Dis.* 2003;41:571–579.
55. Januzzi JL Jr, Chen-Tournoux AA, Moe G. Amino-terminal pro-B-type natriuretic peptide testing for the diagnosis or exclusion of heart failure in patients with acute symptoms. *Am J Cardiol.* 2008;101:29–38.
56. Krauser DG, Lloyd-Jones DM, Chae CU, et al. Effect of body mass index on natriuretic peptide levels in patients with acute congestive heart failure: a ProBNP Investigation of Dyspnea in the Emergency Department (PRIDE) substudy. *Am Heart J.* 2005;149:744–750.
57. Rudiger A, Gasser S, Fischler M, et al. Comparable increase of B-type natriuretic peptide and amino-terminal pro-B-type natriuretic peptide levels in patients with severe sepsis, septic shock, and acute heart failure. *Crit Care Med.* 2006;34:2140–2144.
58. Ronco C, McCullough P, Anker SD, et al; Acute Dialysis Quality Initiative (ADQI) consensus group. Cardio-renal syndromes: report from the consensus conference of the acute dialysis quality initiative. *Eur Heart J.* 2010;31:703–711.
59. Fonarow GC, Adams KF Jr, Abraham WT, et al. Risk stratification for in-hospital mortality in acutely decompensated heart failure: classification and regression tree analysis. *JAMA.* 2005;293:572–580.
60. Poelzl G, Ess M, Mussner-Seeber C, et al. Liver dysfunction in chronic heart failure: prevalence, characteristics and prognostic significance. *Eur J Clin Invest.* 2012;42:153–163.
61. Vyskocilova K, Spinarova L, Spinar J, et al. Prevalence and clinical significance of liver function abnormalities in patients with acute heart failure. *Biomed Pap Med Fac Univ Palacky Olomouc Czech Repub.* 2014.
62. Nohria A, Lewis E, Stevenson LW. Medical management of advanced heart failure. *JAMA.* 2002;287:628–640.
63. Felker GM, Lee KL, Bull DA, et al; NHLBI Heart Failure Clinical Research Network. Diuretic strategies in patients with acute decompensated heart failure. *N Engl J Med.* 2011;364:797–805.
64. Ellison DH. The physiologic basis of diuretic synergism: its role in treating diuretic resistance. *Ann Intern Med.* 1991;114:886–894.
65. Chen HH, Anstrom KJ, Givertz MM, et al; NHLBI Heart Failure Clinical Research Network. Low-dose dopamine or low-dose nesiritide in acute heart failure with renal dysfunction: the ROSE acute heart failure randomized trial. *JAMA.* 2013;310:2533–2543.

66. O'Connor CM, Starling RC, Hernandez AF, et al. Effect of nesiritide in patients with acute decompensated heart failure. *N Engl J Med.* 2011;365: 32–43.
67. Overgaard CB, Dzavik V. Inotropes and vasopressors: review of physiology and clinical use in cardiovascular disease. *Circulation.* 2008;118:1047–1056.
68. Effects of enalapril on mortality in severe congestive heart failure: results of the Cooperative North Scandinavian Enalapril Survival Study (CONSENSUS). The CONSENSUS Trial Study Group. *N Eng J Med.* 1987;316:1429–1435.
69. Cohn JN, Johnson G, Ziesche S, et al. A comparison of enalapril with hydralazine-isosorbide dinitrate in the treatment of chronic congestive heart failure. *N Eng J Med.* 1991;325:303–310.
70. Effect of enalapril on survival in patients with reduced left ventricular ejection fractions and congestive heart failure. The SOLVD Investigators. *N Engl J Med.* 1991;325:293–302.
71. Yancy CW, Jessup M, Bozkurt B, et al; American College of Cardiology Foundation; American Heart Association Task Force on Practice Guidelines. 2013 ACCF/AHA Guideline for the Management of Heart Failure: a report of the American College of Cardiology Foundation/American Heart Association Task Force on Practice Guidelines. *J Am Coll Cardiol.* 2013;62:e147–e239.
72. Effect of metoprolol CR/XL in chronic heart failure: Metoprolol CR/XL Randomised Intervention Trial in Congestive Heart Failure (MERIT-HF). *Lancet.* 1999;353:2001–2007.
73. Groenning BA, Nilsson JC, Sondergaard L, et al. Antiremodeling effects on the left ventricle during beta-blockade with metoprolol in the treatment of chronic heart failure. *J Am Coll Cardiol.* 2000;36:2072–2080.
74. The Cardiac Insufficiency Bisoprolol Study II (CIBIS-II): a randomised trial. *Lancet.* 1999;353:9–13.
75. Packer M, Coats AJ, Fowler MB, et al; Carvedilol Prospective Randomized Cumulative Survival Study Group. Effect of carvedilol on survival in severe chronic heart failure. *N Eng J Med.* 2001;344:1651–1658.
76. Pitt B, Zannad F, Remme WJ, et al. The effect of spironolactone on morbidity and mortality in patients with severe heart failure. *N Engl J Med.* 1999;341:709–717.
77. Pitt B, Remme W, Zannad F, et al; Eplerenone Post-Acute Myocardial Infarction Heart Failure Efficacy and Survival Study Investigators. Eplerenone, a selective aldosterone blocker, in patients with left ventricular dysfunction after myocardial infarction. *N Engl J Med.* 2003;348:1309–1321.
78. Zannad F, McMurray JJ, Krum H, et al; EMPHASIS-HF Study Group. Eplerenone in patients with systolic heart failure and mild symptoms. *N Engl J Med.* 2011;364:11–21.
79. Binanay C, Califf RM, Hasselblad V, et al; Escape Investigators and ESCAPE Study Coordinators. Evaluation study of congestive heart failure and pulmonary artery catheterization effectiveness: the ESCAPE trial. *JAMA.* 2005;294:1625–1633.
80. Fang JC, Ewald G, Allen L, et al; Heart Failure Society of America Guidelines Committee. Advanced (stage D) heart failure: a statement from the Heart Failure Society of America Guidelines Committee. *J Card Fail.* 2015; 21:519–534.
81. Stevenson LW, Pagani FD, Young JB, et al. INTERMACS profiles of advanced heart failure: the current picture. *J Heart Lung Transplant.* 2009;28:535–541.
82. Metra M, Ponikowski P, Dickstein K, et al. Advanced chronic heart failure: a position statement from the Study Group on Advanced Heart Failure of the Heart Failure Association of the European Society of Cardiology. *Eur J Heart Fail.* 2007;9:684–694.
83. Kirklin JK, Naftel DC, Pagani FD, et al. Sixth INTERMACS annual report: a 10,000-patient database. *J Heart Lung Transplant.* 2014;33:555–564.
84. Afilalo J, Alexander KP, Mack MJ, et al. Frailty assessment in the cardiovascular care of older adults. *J Am Coll Cardiol.* 2014;63:747–762.
85. Muscaritoli M, Anker SD, Argilés J, et al. Consensus definition of sarcopenia, cachexia and pre-cachexia: Joint document elaborated by Special Interest Groups (SIG) "cachexia-anorexia in chronic wasting diseases" and "nutrition in geriatrics". *Clin Nutr.* 2010;29:154–159.
86. Evans WJ, Morley JE, Argilés J, et al. Cachexia: a new definition. *Clin Nutr.* 2008;27:793–799.
87. Dunlay SM, Park SJ, Joyce LD, et al. Frailty and outcomes after implantation of left ventricular assist device as destination therapy. *J Heart Lung Transplant.* 2014;33:359–365.

CHAPTER

96

Cardiac Mechanical Assist Devices

EROL V. BELLI and CHARLES T. KLODELL, JR.

IMMEDIATE GOALS AND PURPOSE OF USE

Cardiac mechanical assist devices are used during periods of hemodynamic instability and persistent low cardiac output in an attempt to restore normal hemodynamic parameters. The primary goal of their use is to normalize inflow and drainage of vital organs so that kidney and liver function return to normal with improved hemostatic potential. The deleterious effects of elevated atrial pressure on many of the major organs are well known, with the lungs being most adversely affected. Increased central venous pressure is also particularly detrimental to the liver and kidneys, causing outflow disorders that compromise organ function. Elevated atrial and central venous pressures, secondary to ventricular dysfunction, are often rapidly normalized by the use of cardiac mechanical assist devices.

There is a stepwise progression of therapy that is followed in the intensive care unit (ICU) with respect to cardiac assist interventions. Therapy begins with inotropic and vasodilator drugs and, if the sought-after end point is not achieved, typically progresses to the use of an intra-aortic balloon pump. Ultimately, mechanical ventricular assist device (VAD) placement may be necessary, and often may occur without intervening use of a balloon pump. In this chapter, we will briefly discuss these devices with special emphasis on the indications, contraindications, placement, complications, and potential pitfalls.

INTRA-AORTIC BALLOON PUMP

Indications

- Acute myocardial infarction and shock: 10% to 15% of acute myocardial infarctions may require hemodynamic support with the temporary use of an intra-aortic balloon pump (Fig. 96.1). This may translate into as many as 1.5 million patients annually
- Unstable angina
- Prophylaxis for high-risk surgery or percutaneous coronary intervention
- Acute mitral insufficiency
- Ventricular septal rupture following an ischemic event (usually several days after ischemic insult)
- Postcardiotomy failure: Inability to separate patient from cardiopulmonary bypass following cardiac surgical procedure
- Traumatic myocardial contusion with low cardiac output

Contraindications

- *Aortic insufficiency (AI):* Leaking of the aortic valve makes the use of an intra-aortic balloon pump potentially detrimental. During periods of diastolic augmentation, enhanced reversal of flow actually exacerbates the AI.
- *Atheromatous aorta:* Patients who are known to have severe atheromatous disease of the aorta are poor candidates for balloon pump therapy. There is the risk of atheroembolization, either distally or retrograde into the cerebral vasculature, during pump use or manipulation.
- *Severe peripheral vascular disease or aortic dissection:* The balloon pump is typically inserted in a retrograde fashion from the groin. This relative contraindication of peripheral vascular disease can be overcome by the use of alternate insertion techniques.

Techniques of Insertion

The most commonly used method of intra-aortic balloon pump insertion is via the retrograde Seldinger technique in the femoral artery (Fig. 96.2). This can be performed with or without a vascular sheath, depending on size of the femoral artery. The balloon pump is then carefully inserted over the wire into the descending aorta to a point immediately distal to the left subclavian artery. When there has already been an incision made to the groin related to coronary artery bypass cannulation or some other intervention, it is possible to insert the balloon pump via direct arterial access.

In special circumstances, there are alternate sites for insertion. This is especially true in patients who either have their balloon pump for an extended period of time or have a need for ambulation during balloon pump use. In these circumstances, a balloon pump may also be placed directly through the axillary artery (1). When placed via the axillary artery, a sheath is not routinely used for placement. In more extreme circumstances, placement may require an antegrade approach either directly into the arch or through a small graft sewn onto the ascending aorta or arch and tunneled to the chest wall (2,3). This method may be necessary for patients with coexisting peripheral vascular disease and postcardiotomy failure to wean during cardiopulmonary bypass.

Verification of Location

It is important that the appropriate location of the balloon pump be confirmed after insertion. It should be positioned just distal to the left subclavian artery in the descending thoracic aorta (Fig. 96.3). A more proximal placement risks an increased incidence of cerebral atheroembolization or of thromboembolization from microthrombi forming on the balloon pump itself. A more distal placement may cause the pump to impede the visceral arteries. The location of the balloon pump may be verified either by fluoroscopy, transesophageal echocardiography, or a chest roentgenogram. The tip

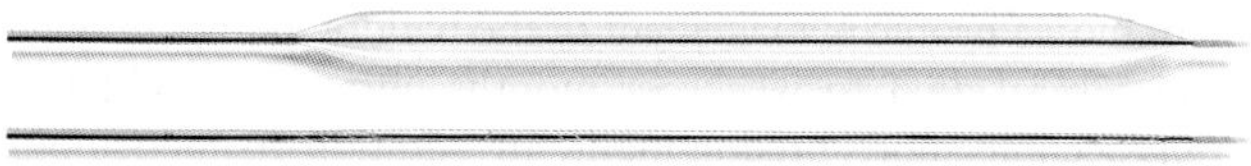

FIGURE 96.1 Example of standard 7.5-French 40-mL intra-aortic balloon pulsation.

should be high in the left chest in appropriate relation to the aortic arch and distal to the left subclavian artery.

It is also important to select the appropriate-sized balloon pump for the patient. Balloon pumps are manufactured in various sizes, ranging from those appropriate for a small infant to those used in large adults (Fig. 96.4); the standard adult size is 40 mL. The manufacturer's labeling and recommendations and the patient's habitus should be considered in size selection.

Mechanism of Action

There are two complimentary effects of an intra-aortic balloon pump. The first is the diastolic augmentation of coronary blood flow. The balloon pump is carefully timed to the cardiac cycle so that the pump inflates during aortic valve closure and thus enhances the diastolic pressure in the proximal aorta. This allows increased coronary blood flow and enhanced myocardial oxygen delivery. The second action involves the afterload reduction at the time of cardiac systole, thereby allowing enhanced runoff for the failing ventricle. The balloon should be properly timed to deflate during aortic valve opening, thereby creating a pocket of reduced afterload and thus enhancing the ability of the heart to eject the blood during systole. This action serves to lower the left ventricular

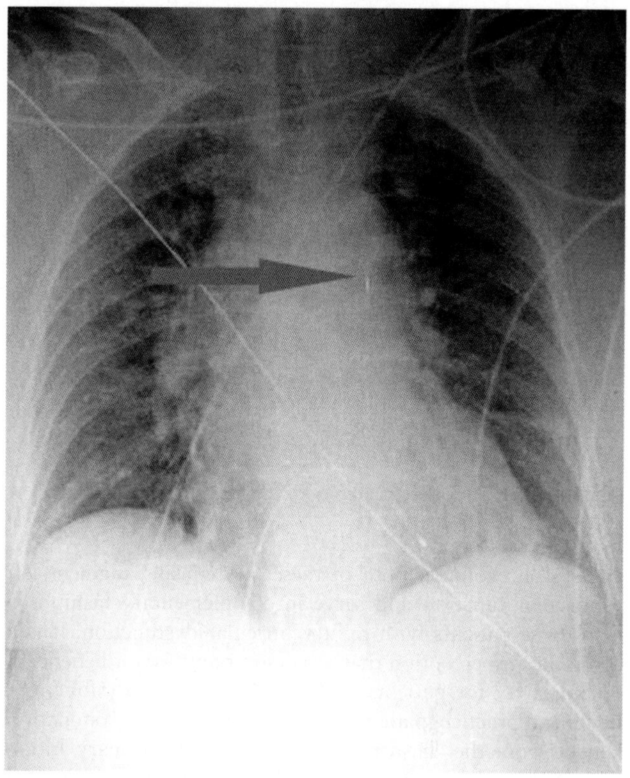

FIGURE 96.3 Chest radiograph showing intra-aortic balloon pulsation in place. Distal tip is marked.

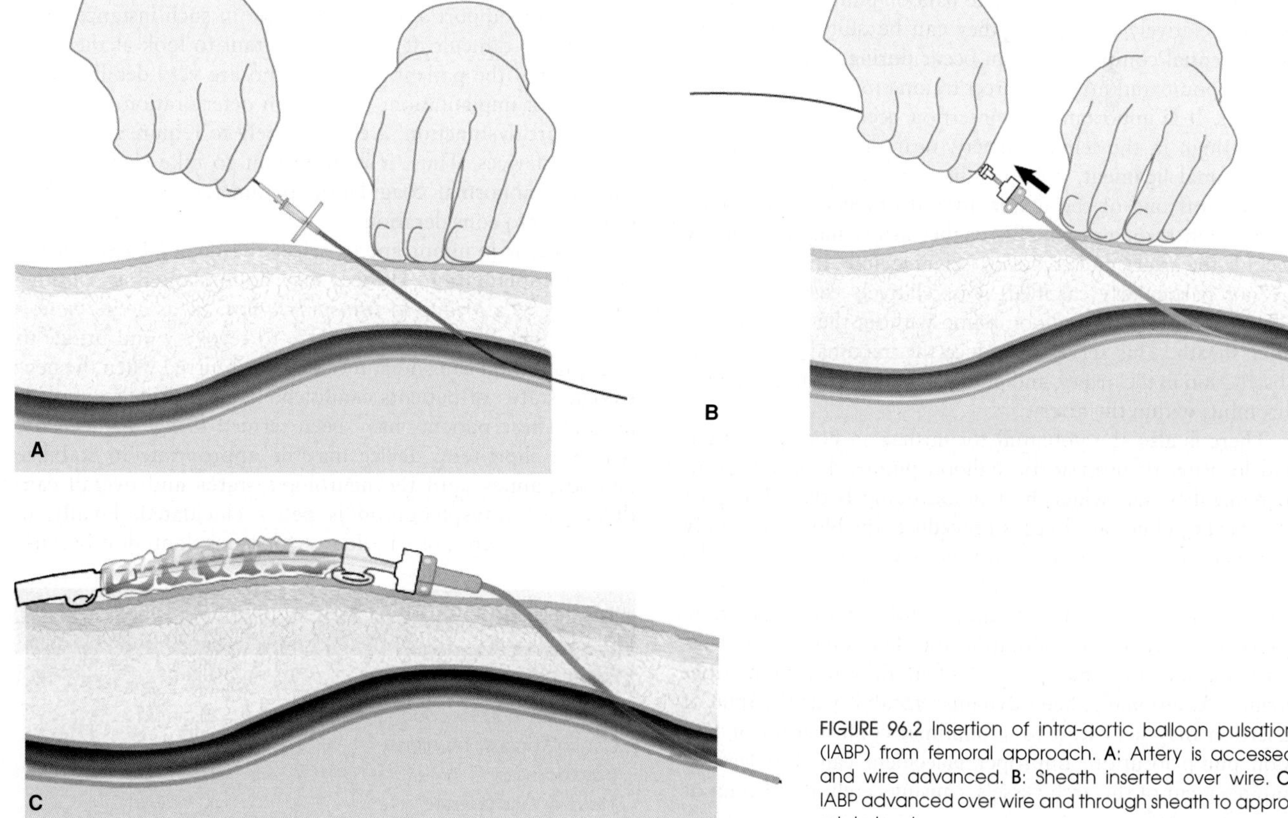

FIGURE 96.2 Insertion of intra-aortic balloon pulsation (IABP) from femoral approach. **A**: Artery is accessed and wire advanced. **B**: Sheath inserted over wire. **C**: IABP advanced over wire and through sheath to appropriate level.

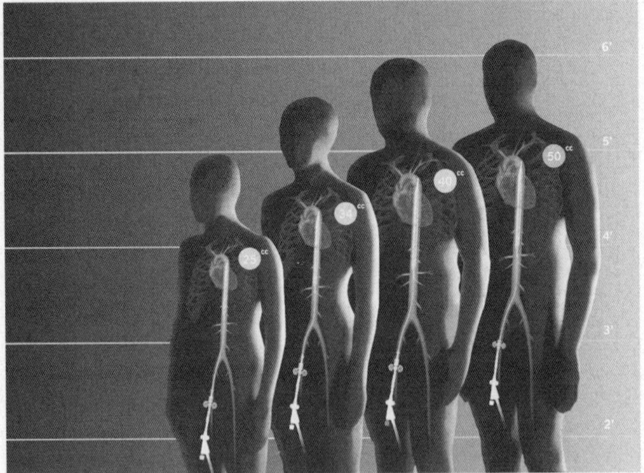

FIGURE 96.4 Different sizes of intra-aortic balloon pulsation devices.

end-systolic volume. Both of these mechanisms augment left ventricular function and serve in complementary fashion to help those patients with right ventricular dysfunction. It is a common misperception that a balloon pump is not beneficial, or indicated, for patients with right ventricular dysfunction. In clinical practice, patients with right ventricular dysfunction benefit from the diastolic augmentation of coronary blood flow in the right coronary artery. Additional benefit is derived from the reduced left ventricular end-diastolic pressure and left atrial pressure, thereby allowing increased forward flow and decreased afterload for the failing right ventricle.

Complications

Although complications related to balloon pump insertion and use are relatively infrequent, they can be quite serious. The first potential complication can occur during insertion of the balloon pump and involves direct trauma to the arterial insertion site. It is important that insertion occurs relatively high in the thigh in the femoral artery, near the inferior edge of the inguinal ligament. It is possible for a misplaced balloon to shear off one of the major arterial branches. Misplacing the balloon through a smaller-caliber artery may completely occlude the artery and create an ischemic limb. In arteries that are not particularly calcified, it is relatively easy to use the dilator and place the balloon pump without the use of a vascular sheath. This serves to reduce the maximal diameter of obstruction in the artery, and perhaps reduces the potential for thrombus within the artery.

There is also the potential for mishap in both placement and location of intra-aortic balloon pumps. It is important to remember that when the balloon pump is placed as part of a cardiopulmonary bypass procedure, the blood is equally oxygenated in the arterial and venous vessels because of the bypass oxygenator. Additionally, there is zero pulsatile flow at the time of insertion, making it difficult to differentiate artery from vein. This situation has led some to inadvertently place balloon pumps via the femoral vein into the right atrium. Additionally, hemodynamic instability at the time of insertion may also lead to suboptimal confirmation of balloon pump location. Improper placement can thus lead to impingement of the arch vessels, causing cerebral ischemia or thromboembolism.

In more chronic management of the balloon pump, ranging from several days to weeks or months, infectious complications become more predominant. In addition to meticulous sterile insertion techniques, balloon pumps also require daily attention from the nursing staff. Like any other percutaneously inserted central catheter, they have the potential to become a source of infection. Attention to the insertion site for signs of erythema or purulence and close monitoring of the patient's temperature is mandatory in all patients using a balloon pump. When a patient's hemodynamic status fails to stabilize with balloon pump therapy, a VAD is the next course of progressive therapy.

VENTRICULAR ASSIST DEVICES

Preoperative Considerations

Indications for VADs include unstable hemodynamic measurements and failure to stabilize measurements with other less invasive therapies previously discussed. Common hemodynamic parameters that are indications for a VAD placement are listed in Table 96.1.

In the preoperative assessment, it is important to determine the likelihood that right ventricular support will be needed as a course of therapy. There are several scoring systems that are commonly used (4–6). Most of these scoring systems center on the calculation of right ventricular stroke work index and other hemodynamic indices such as transpulmonary gradient, right atrial pressure, and tricuspid annular plane excursion (7,8). Generally, practitioners should use caution if the central venous pressure is greater than the pulmonary capillary wedge pressure, or if the patient's central venous pressure is greater than 20 mmHg after optimization. Dependence on the right ventricle to support a left-sided device in such instances may prove to be difficult. It is also important to look at the overall illness of the patient. Patients who are very debilitated at the time of implantation, with organ deterioration caused by right heart dysfunction, are more likely to require right-sided support devices. Thus, it is important to take elevated liver enzymes, abnormal coagulation parameters, and renal dysfunction into consideration.

Finally, it is important to select the device based on the goal of implantation. Devices may be implanted as a *bridge to recovery*, a *bridge to transplantation*, or as a *destination therapy*. The lines between bridge to recovery and bridge to transplantation can sometimes become blurred when the neurologic status of patients cannot be defined prior to implantation. These patients have been termed *bridge to decision*, where a short-term device may be appropriate to stabilize hemodynamics until the neurologic status and overall candidacy for transplantation is better elucidated. Finally, in patients who are not candidates for transplantation because

TABLE 96.1 Hemodynamic Parameters Suggesting Need for Mechanical Support

Parameter	Values
Pulmonary capillary wedge pressure	>20 mmHg
Central venous pressure	>20 mmHg
Cardiac index	<2.0 L/m^2
Mean arterial pressure	<60 mmHg

of age or end-organ dysfunction, consideration of destination therapy may be appropriate. Destination therapy refers to permanent device implantation, intended to remain in use for the duration of the patient's lifetime. Patients may migrate between these defined groups based on a center's transplant protocols.

Preparation of the Patient

Before the operative implantation of the VAD, it is often useful to have a period of volume optimization, or a preoperative "tune up." This is done to ensure that right ventricular function is as well preserved as possible for placement of a left VAD, and may include diuretic and inotropic therapy. In some cases, where the decision for biventricular support is difficult, a 24- to 48-hour period of intra-aortic balloon pumping may be a useful prognostic indicator. This helps to demonstrate the response of the right ventricular function to a reduced left ventricular end-diastolic pressure (9). During this period of optimization, it is ideal to use an arterial pressure monitor and a pulmonary artery catheter to allow fine tuning of medications and volume status.

It is essential that attention be given to antimicrobial prophylaxis during the period of preoperative optimization. This usually involves selective skin decontamination with Hibiclens scrub (Regent Medical, London, UK). Additionally, Bactroban (mupirocin) is often used to reduce the number of pathogens in the nasal passages of the patient. It may also be useful to use red cell augmentation in patients who are having semielective implants, as frequently there may be a 5- to 7-day delay before implantation, during which time erythropoiesis-stimulating drugs, such as erythropoietin, can be combined with iron supplementation to achieve a significant increase of hematocrit.

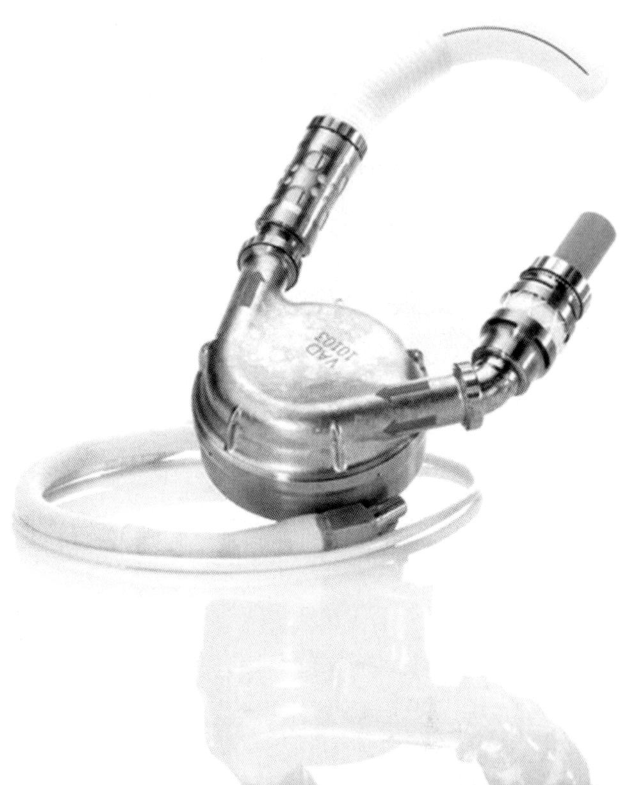

FIGURE 96.5 HeartMate XVE. An example of a pulsatile pusher plate device. (Courtesy of Thoratec Corp, Pleasanton, CA.)

Classification of Ventricular Assist Devices

Flow Type

The devices may be classified by the type of flow:

- **Pulsatile:** In these devices, the intermittent relocation of a pusher plate or blood sack emits a pulsatile wave similar to that of the natural heart (Fig. 96.5).
- **Axial flow:** The term *nonpulsatile* is frequently applied to these devices, although this is a misnomer. These pumps actually have a central blade that rotates at a rapid rate, similar to a jet engine in an airplane (Fig. 96.6). The native function of the left ventricle does intermittently augment the inflow to the pump, which generates a pulsatile output at appropriate speeds.
- **Centripetal flow:** These pumps have a continuous spinning impeller that generates a flow similar to axial pumps. However, the more advanced pumps may be magnetically levitated to function without bearings (Figs. 96.7 and 96.8).

Mechanism

- **Pneumatic:** These pumps are operated by air, where intermittent external application of compressed gas through a tube to a blood sac emits the pulse of the pump.
- **Electric:** Electric pumps are driven by batteries or AC current via an adapter. They may have the axial flow motor or the pusher plate-driven motor (see Figs. 96.5 and 96.6).

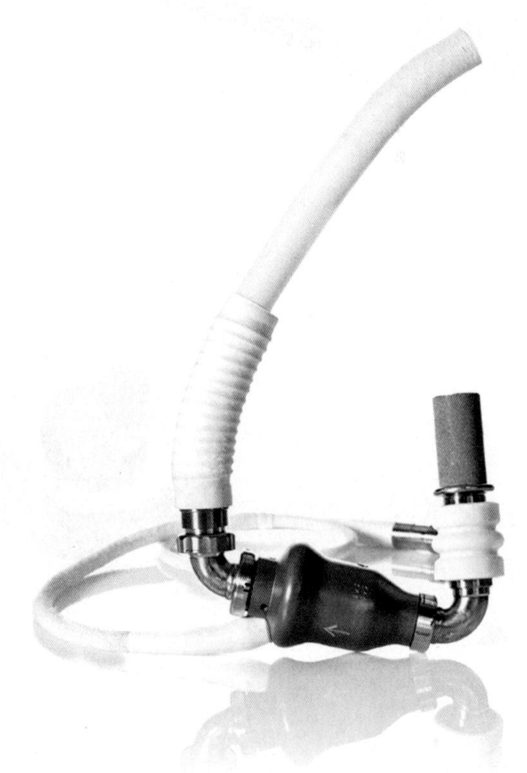

FIGURE 96.6 HeartMate II. An example of an axial flow device. (Courtesy of Thoratec Corp, Pleasanton, CA.)

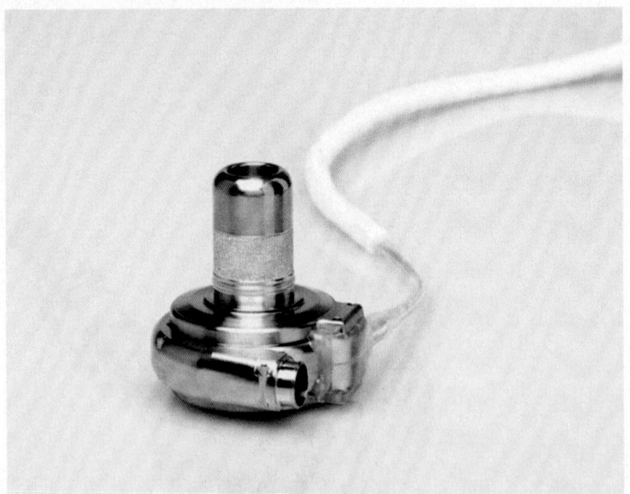

FIGURE 96.7 HVAD, Magnetically levitated, centripetal pump. (Courtesy of Heartware, Framingham, MA.)

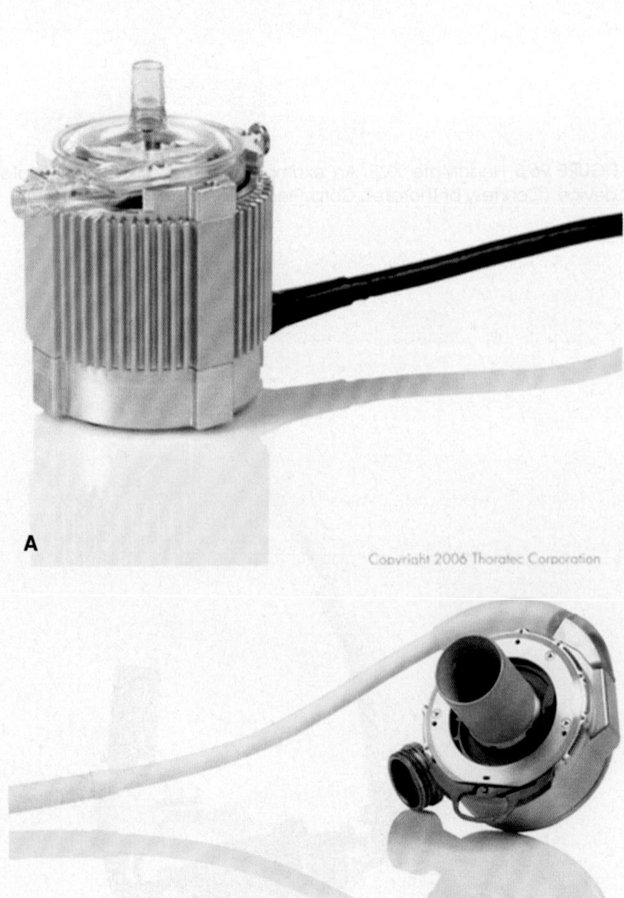

B

FIGURE 96.8 Thoratec CentriMag (A) and HeartMate III (B, in development). Examples of magnetically levitated ventricular assist devices. (Courtesy of Thoratec Corp, Pleasanton, CA.)

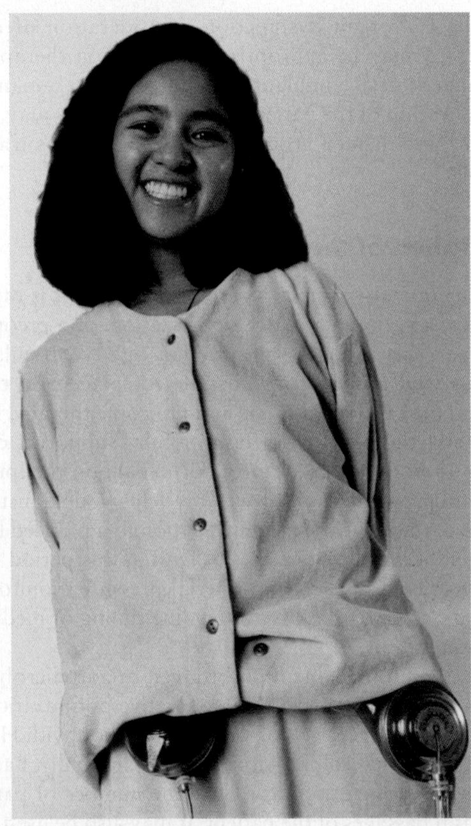

FIGURE 96.9 Picture diagram of HeartMate XVE implanted, an intracorporeal LVAD. (Courtesy of Thoratec Corp, Pleasanton, CA.)

Location

- **Paracorporeal:** These pumps are placed outside of, but in continuity with, the body, usually connected via transcutaneous cannulas that are surgically implanted into the heart.
- **Intracorporeal:** This term typically refers to those pumps that are placed completely within the body with only a drive line exiting the skin (Fig. 96.9). The main pumping mechanism is within the body, rather than external to it.
- **Percutaneous:** *Percutaneous* refers to a small group of pumps that are indicated for extremely short-term use and are inserted transcutaneously, either via the femoral vein and then transseptally into the left atrium, or retrograde across the aortic valve (Figs. 96.10 and 96.11).

Potential Duration of Support Based on Device Type

- **Short term:** These devices are placed to resolve immediate hemodynamic instability as either a bridge to recovery, a bridge to decision, or for use during a short-term procedure. Their use is intended for hours to weeks.
- **Medium term:** These devices are inserted with the intention of being used to allow recovery of the native heart function, or as a short-term bridge to transplantation. They are indicated for weeks to months.
- **Long term:** These devices are intended to be used for either long-term bridge patients who will require an extended period of time to acquire donor hearts or for those patients who may potentially have the device as destination therapy.

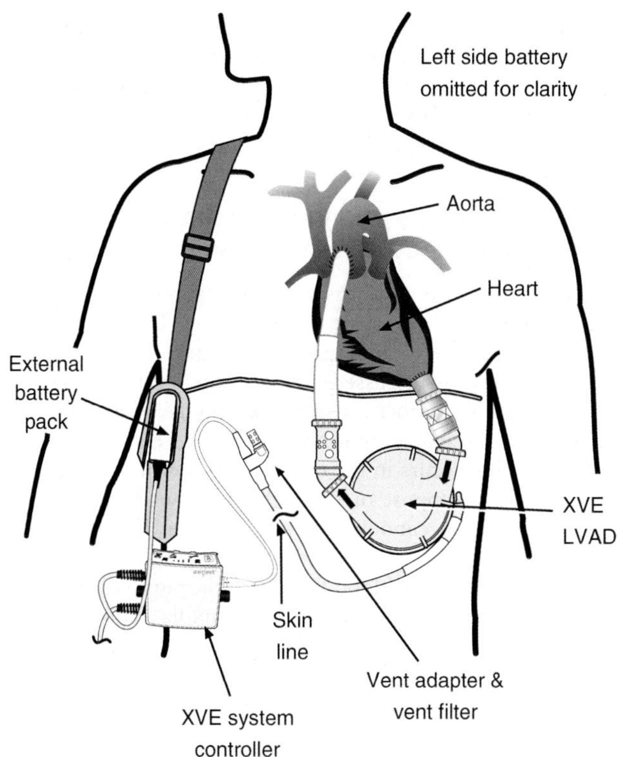

FIGURE 96.10 Impella (Abiomed). Temporary percutaneous ventricular assist device. (Courtesy of Abiomed, Danvers, MA.)

Important Implications for Potential Emergency Situations While the Patient Is Supported by Ventricular Assist Devices

It is important to understand the physiologic implications of each VAD, not only while they are in use, but also during periods of unintended pump arrest. One of the critical differentiations between the various types of pumps is the presence or absence of valves, and the potential for retrograde flow during periods of pump stoppage. In the devices with valves, a pump arrest merely means that the augmented flow no longer exists, and the presence of valves should prevent retrograde flow. This is a key point to consider during emergency management. The pumps with no valves, such as the axial flow devices, will allow volumes in excess of 1.5 L per minute of retrograde flow during periods of pump arrest. This degree of acute AI will frequently lead to ventricular arrhythmias and cardiovascular collapse. Knowledge of these internal components and working mechanisms leads to proper decision-making during emergencies. Health care providers must know whether the pump can be temporally actuated via an external mechanism (blood sac pumps) by an individual (as opposed to the driver), and whether or not the pump electronics are defibrillation-compatible.

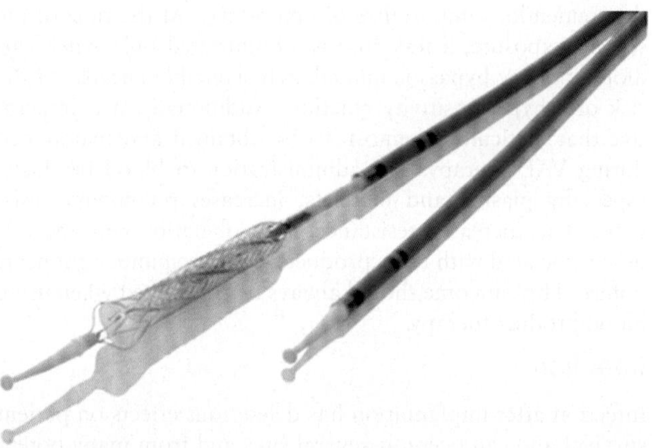

FIGURE 96.11 Thoratec PHP. Another example of a percutaneous device in development. (Courtesy of Thoratec Corp, Pleasanton, CA.)

Management of the Post-Left Ventricular Assist Device Patient

Most VAD centers strive to support patients with left-sided devices only and limit the number of patients who require right VADs whenever possible. Patients on single ventricular support are more mobile and more rapidly rehabilitated. Thus, a major focus of post–left VAD management is the stabilization of right heart function and prevention of right heart failure. To accomplish this goal, the most important factor is the selection of patients who have sustainable right ventricular hemodynamic parameters preoperatively. The previously discussed period of optimization often allows patients with marginal right ventricular function to have significant improvement. This is crucial and ranks just under the requirement that the right heart can support the function of the left VAD. Additionally, right heart function is frequently supported for some period of time with inotropic therapy. The most commonly used drugs are dobutamine or a phosphodiesterase inhibitor such as milrinone (9). Aggressive attempts are made to lower the pulmonary artery resistance by using nitrosodilators, such as sodium nitroprusside, nitroglycerin, and inhaled NO. There is some enthusiasm for the use of inhaled prostacyclin as a less expensive alternative to inhaled NO (10,11). Other more novel options in evolution include the use of orally available, direct-acting drugs on the pulmonary vasculature, such as the use of sildenafil, a phosphodiesterase type 5 inhibitor (12,13).

After placement of a left VAD, meticulous care of the drive-line site is important to reduce the risk of ascending infection. This typically involves diligent immobilization of the drive line and the use of topical treatments, initially several times a day. In cases where infection is noted at the drive-line site despite all efforts, topical treatments can be used with success (14).

Dysfunction and Complications of Left Vads

Cannula Kinking

In the paracorporeal devices, this is particularly problematic. Shifting of patient position or rolling in the bed can lead to either dislodgement or, more frequently, kinking of the transcutaneous cannula. This will lead to flow alarms and sudden dysfunction of the device, and can usually be addressed by simply removing the kink in the cannula. Often, centers have found it beneficial to keep a folded towel under the device to keep it off the patient's skin and to keep the cannulas straight. With the intracorporeal devices, this problem is usually secondary to device migration, either from chest closure in the operating room, postoperative ambulation, or postoperative weight fluctuations. With intracorporeal devices, this frequently requires reoperation for adjustment of the device.

Thrombosis and Embolism

The Achilles heel of all device therapy remains the poorly understood human coagulation system and the effects of foreign bodies in the bloodstream. Depending on the specific device selected, the type of valves within the device, and predicted presence of pseudointimal formation in the pump, variable amounts of anticoagulation are recommended by the manufacturer (4). Regardless of the anticoagulation therapy used, thrombosis, embolism, and bleeding events are a concern with all devices. It is important to treat patients with any new symptom, such as abdominal pain or a cold leg, as if it were a thromboembolic event. With appropriate management of anticoagulation and diligent patient care, these events are relatively infrequent. The risk of cerebrovascular accident increases with longer VAD support time and the presence of infection (15).

Mechanical Device Issues

The devices themselves may have mechanical issues related to valve dysfunction or problems with either bearings or motor wear. These are addressed in the materials supplied by the manufacturers. All of the devices require some type of ongoing surveillance and assessment for wear and potential mechanical failure, which may require pump exchange.

Patent Foramen Ovale and Hypoxemia Following Left Ventricular Assist Placement

Patients need to be carefully screened in the operating room with TEE and provocation maneuvers during a bubble test to identify a patent foramen ovale. With the altered hemodynamics following left VAD placement, the left atrial pressure is suddenly dramatically lower than the right atrial pressure. This allows even the smallest patent foramen ovale to become clinically significant, with right-to-left shunting occurring and resultant hypoxemia. A recent report described partial digital occlusion of the main pulmonary artery as a provocative maneuver to be used during the bubble study (16). Such a maneuver enhances the intraoperative detection of patent foramen ovale during device placement. A patent foramen ovale discovered in the operating room prior to placement of the VAD and those discovered after the device is activated in the operating room should be closed at that time. There are some reports of patients being treated with percutaneous closure, when discovered as a cause of persistent hypoxemia several hours or days following device placement (17).

Tricuspid and Aortic Regurgitation

After successful implantation of VADs and weaning of inotropic support, significant improvement may be seen in a patient's hemodynamics. Postoperative echocardiography may reveal unloading of the left ventricle with improvement in right ventricular function and mitral regurgitation (18). Preoperative AI and tricuspid regurgitation (TR) being the exceptions. Moderate to severe TR has been shown not to improve immediately after VAD implantation and is associated with longer length of hospital stay, need for longer inotropic support, and a trend toward decreased survival (19). It is therefore recommended the tricuspid valve be repaired at the time of implantation. AI does not improve and actually progresses over the duration of support; this can affect device performance and end-organ function (18,20). What to do with AI at the time of implantation is surgeon and center dependent, with some choosing to replace the valve with a bioprosthetic device and others sewing the aortic valve shut which makes the patient completely VAD dependent for any outflow from the left ventricle.

Right Heart Failure and the Potential Need for a Right Ventricular Assist Device

One of the greatest concerns when implanting a left VAD is the potential need for right VAD therapy. This risk can be minimized by careful adherence to the post–left VAD management protocols discussed earlier in the chapter. However, despite one's best efforts, a small percentage of patients will still develop refractory right heart failure necessitating device therapy. If this occurs in the operating room, it is possible to use temporary support of the right heart while the cardiopulmonary bypass cannulae are still in place. This is done by using a "Y" off the arterial line and clamping the line to the aorta, thus redirecting blood flow from the pump directly into the pulmonary artery via a separate cannula. This sets up a circuit in which the blood is drawn from the right atrium, oxygenated by the cardiopulmonary bypass circuit, and then returned to the pulmonary artery. The effect of superoxygenated blood on the pulmonary artery may result in a reduction in pulmonary resistance over several minutes and obviate the need for a right VAD. This is often referred to as a *Berlin bridge* and may be a beneficial intermediate step before placing a right VAD when right ventricular dysfunction is apparent in the operating room. When right heart dysfunction and failure develop several days after a left VAD placement, some type of short-term device support may be required if the heart remains refractory to initial interventions. These interventions include the multiple levels of pharmacotherapy previously discussed.

Bleeding

One of the most common complications related to VAD therapy is bleeding. This is most common during the perioperative period, but can also occur with anticoagulation during device use. Individual institutions must make the decision regarding the appropriateness of aprotinin therapy. It has been our standard practice to use a full dose of aprotinin (full Hammersmith protocol, see package insert) at the time of device implantation and with subsequent transplantation because of the tremendous importance of hemostasis. At the time of the second exposure, a test dose is administered only when cardiopulmonary bypass is immediately available because of the risk of a hypersensitivity reaction. Additionally, it is imperative that meticulous hemostasis be obtained and maintained during VAD therapy. The administration of blood products, especially plasma and platelets, increases pulmonary resistance. This increased resistance, in combination with the volume associated with these products, can precipitate right heart failure. This outcome should always be considered when using blood product therapy.

Infection

Infection after implantation has deleterious effects on patient survival and can occur at several sites and from many potential sources (21). Almost every patient has had several hospital stays prior to implantation and exposure to several nosocomial sources, such as indwelling urinary catheters or invasive line monitoring. Strict sterile technique is needed intraoperatively as well as prophylactic broad-spectrum antibiotics preoperatively that are continued postoperatively to decrease infection incidence. Infections of the drive line and pocket may not require complete device removal, but if the patient is experiencing sepsis, consideration must be given to removal.

Ventricular Dysrhythmias

Ventricular dysrhythmias occur in up to 22% of patients after implantation. They are defined as early (<1 week) or late (>1 week) (22). Those occurring early are associated with a significant increase in mortality as compared to late. Antidysrhythmics may be of use for prevention, but the cause is often unknown and may be related to subendocardial ischemia, postoperative inotropic support, or myocyte remodeling.

Patient Factors

These include the patient factors related to the devices such as accidental disconnects, where a patient, in spite of optimal education from physicians and VAD staff, simultaneously disconnects all power sources to their device, resulting in pump stoppage. Additionally, traction injuries are common. Particular attention should be given to entering and exiting vehicles and traversing through narrow doorways, as these seem to be particularly problematic for the drive lines of VADs.

TRANSITION FROM ICU TO THE FLOOR AND OUTPATIENT MANAGEMENT

It is beyond the scope of this chapter to discuss personnel management. However, dedicated staff members are essential and must be thoroughly trained to deal with outpatient management of VADs. Communication and current knowledge of the device is paramount to the success of the VAD program. This requires the establishment of community resources and alternate caregiver training so that there is redundancy at every level of the system. Although minor problems with these patients and their devices are not uncommon, most are easily handled if the support staff are prepared and adequately trained. Mechanical assist devices can enhance not only the quantity, but also the quality of life for these patients.

Key Points

- There are many options for mechanical support to help restore persistent low cardiac output.
- The preoperative evaluation of right heart function is imperative prior to insertion of mechanical assist devices. This helps to maximize patient benefit and prevent the need for a secondary device.
- There are several classification systems available for VADs; knowing your institutions selected devices and their mechanism of action is of utmost importance.
- There are many reported complications of mechanical assist devices, but infection and thrombosis remain throughout the device lifespan.
- Multidisciplinary management is needed during preoperative evaluation, intraoperative implantation, and postoperative care for mechanical assist device patients.

References

1. Marcu CB, Donohue TJ, et al. Intraaortic balloon pump insertion through the subclavian artery. Subclavian artery insertion of IABP. *Heart Lung Circ.* 2006;15(2):148–150.
2. Kaplan LJ, Weiman DS, Langan N, et al. Safe intraaortic balloon pump placement through the ascending aorta using transesophageal ultrasound. *Ann Thorac Surg.* 1992;54(2):374–375.
3. Meldrum-Hanna WG, Deal CW, et al. Complications of ascending aortic intraaortic balloon pump cannulation. *Ann Thorac Surg.* 1985;40(3):241–244.
4. Fukamachi K, McCarthy PM, Smedira NG, et al. Preoperative risk factors for right ventricular failure after implantable left ventricular assist device insertion. *Ann Thorac Surg.* 1999;68(6):2181–2184.
5. Kavarana MN, Pessin-Minsley MS, Urtecho J, et al. Right ventricular dysfunction and organ failure in left ventricular assist device recipients: a continuing problem. *Ann Thorac Surg.* 2002;73(3):745–750.
6. Ochiai Y, McCarthy PM, Smedira NG, et al. Predictors of severe right ventricular failure after implantable left ventricular assist device insertion: analysis of 245 patients. *Circulation.* 2002;106(12 Suppl 1):I198–I202.
7. Puwanant S, Hamilton KK, Klodell CT, et al. Tricuspid annular motion as a predictor of severe right ventricular failure after left ventricular assist device implantation. *J Heart Lung Transplant.* 2008;27(10):1102–1107.
8. Wang Y, Simon MA, Bonde P, et al. Decision tree for adjuvant right ventricular support in patients receiving a left ventricular assist device. *J Heart Lung Transplant.* 2012;31(2):140–149.
9. Klodell CT, Staples ED, Aranda JM Jr., et al. Managing the post-left ventricular assist device patient. *Congest Heart Fail.* 2006;12(1):41–45.
10. Fattouch K, Sbraga F, Bianco G, et al. Inhaled prostacyclin, nitric oxide, and nitroprusside in pulmonary hypertension after mitral valve replacement. *J Card Surg.* 2005;20(2):171–176.
11. Muzaffar S, Shukla N, Angelini GD, et al. Inhaled prostacyclin is safe, effective, and affordable in patients with pulmonary hypertension, right-heart dysfunction, and refractory hypoxemia after cardiothoracic surgery. *J Thorac Cardiovasc Surg.* 2004;128(6):949–950.
12. Lobato EB, Beaver T, Muehlschlegel J, et al. Treatment with phosphodiesterase inhibitors type III and V: milrinone and sildenafil is an effective combination during thromboxane-induced acute pulmonary hypertension. *Br J Anaesth.* 2006;96(3):317–322.
13. Trachte AL, Lobato EB, Urdaneta F, et al. Oral sildenafil reduces pulmonary hypertension after cardiac surgery. *Ann Thorac Surg.* 2005;79(1):194–197.
14. Baradarian S, Stahovich M, Krause S, et al. Case series: clinical management of persistent mechanical assist device driveline drainage using vacuum-assisted closure therapy. *ASAIO J.* 2006;52(3):354–356.
15. Tsukui H, Abla A, Teuteberg JJ, et al. Cerebrovascular accidents in patients with a ventricular assist device. *J Thorac Cardiovasc Surg.* 2007;134(1):114–123.
16. Majd RE, Kavarana MN, Bouvette M, et al. Improved technique to diagnose a patent foramen ovale during left ventricular assist device insertion. *Ann Thorac Surg.* 2006;82(5):1917–1918.
17. Kavarana MN, Rahman FA, Recto MR, et al. Transcatheter closure of patent foramen ovale after left ventricular assist device implantation: intraoperative decision making. *J Heart Lung Transplant.* 2005;24(9):1445.
18. Topilsky Y, Oh JK, Atchison FW, et al. Echocardiographic findings in stable outpatients with properly functioning HeartMate II left ventricular assist devices. *J Am Soc Echocardiogr.* 2011;24(2):1571–1569.
19. Piacentino V III, Williams ML, Depp T, et al. Impact of tricuspid valve regurgitation in patients treated with implantable left ventricular assist devices. *Ann Thorac Surg.* 2011;91(5):1342–1346.
20. Aggarwal A, Raghuvir R, Eryazici P, et al. The development of aortic insufficiency in continuous-flow left ventricular assist device-supported patients. *Ann Thorac Surg.* 2013;95(2):493–498.
21. Topkara VK, Kondareddy S, Malik F, et al. Infectious complications in patients with left ventricular assist device: etiology and outcomes in the continuous-flow era. *Ann Thorac Surg.* 2010;90(4):1270–1277.
22. Bedi M, Kormos R, Winowich S, et al. Ventricular arrhythmias during left ventricular assist device support. *Am J Cardiol.* 2007;99(8):1151–1153.

CHAPTER

97

Valvular Heart Disease

KATHIRVEL SUBRAMANIAM and JEAN-PIERRE YARED

INTRODUCTION

Critically ill patients with valvular heart disease (VHD) presenting to the intensive care unit (ICU) fall into three primary categories: patients who are critically ill as a result of acute-onset, newly acquired VHD; patients with exacerbation or complications of pre-existing VHD; or patients with concomitant VHD who are critically ill from other causes.

Diseases of the mitral or aortic valve are the most common. Patients usually present with instability secondary to dysfunction of the left atrium (LA) and left ventricle (LV), which, if severe, causes pulmonary hypertension and right ventricular failure. Decompensated left-sided valvular lesions often present with diminished cardiac output (CO), tissue hypoperfusion, and pulmonary venous hypertension with pulmonary edema. Isolated right-sided valvular lesions present with reduced CO and systemic venous congestion. Management is determined by the type of lesion and its severity, and is modified by coexisting derangements. The patient's history, physical examination, chest radiography, and echocardiography help in determining the need for invasive measurements such as arterial blood pressure, cardiac filling pressures, CO, mixed venous oxygen saturation, and derived variables such as systemic vascular and pulmonary vascular resistances. Invasive monitoring is particularly useful for guiding and assessing the response to treatment. However, invasive monitoring of these critically ill patients presents several technical challenges and limitations: The risk of vascular injury and bleeding increases when patients are receiving anticoagulants for mechanical valves or atrial fibrillation; proper positioning of a flow-directed pulmonary artery balloon catheter (pulmonary artery catheter [PAC]) may be very difficult in presence of an enlarged right atrium, right ventricle, or tricuspid regurgitation (TR). Advancement of the catheter may precipitate malignant dysrhythmias that are poorly tolerated, especially in presence of severe aortic stenosis (AS). Interpretation of hemodynamic data are often more difficult in presence of valvular disease. However, although absolute values of pulmonary capillary wedge pressure (PCWP) do not reflect ventricular volume because of decreased ventricular compliance, the PAC can provide useful information about trends in left ventricular filling pressures, CO, and mixed venous oxygenation. Continuous echocardiographic monitoring can provide useful information both with regard to LV diastolic volume and wall motion abnormalities indicative of ischemia. ECG monitoring is essential for detection and treatment of rhythm disturbances and ischemia. However, detection of ischemia is often difficult because of left ventricular hypertrophy and conduction blocks.

Critically ill patients with VHD generally present with circulatory and respiratory compromise, and frequently with acute kidney injury, hepatic, and other organ dysfunction. Initial interventions aim at controlling circulatory shock and respiratory failure, treating the cause of critical illness, and preventing or reversing associated organ dysfunction. The type and severity of VHD as well as acute precipitating events must be determined. Acute cardiac events include valve thrombosis, endocarditis, myocardial infarction, ruptured chordae tendineae, or new cardiac dysrhythmias. Noncardiac factors exacerbating VHD include pulmonary embolism, uncontrolled hypertension, infection, endocrine abnormalities—particularly diabetic ketoacidosis or hyperthyroid crisis—and acute renal failure. Finally, critical illness unrelated to VHD further impairs cardiac function and increases the complexity of management.

DIAGNOSIS

A thorough history taking and physical examination are essential for the overall assessment of severity of illness. However, the relative impact of VHD on the patient's status often requires more advanced diagnostic tools. Electrocardiography may reveal concomitant ischemic heart disease, left ventricular hypertrophy, atrial abnormalities, arrhythmias, or right ventricular hypertrophy. Chest radiography helps in assessing the presence or severity of pulmonary edema, pleural effusions, or lung parenchymal abnormalities. Transthoracic echocardiography (TTE) is essential to characterize the valvular lesions, atrial size, and ventricular systolic and diastolic function, as well as identify abnormal masses, pericardial pathology, and pulmonary artery pressure. If the quality of the TTE is not optimal, transesophageal echocardiography (TEE) should be performed.

CRITICAL ILLNESS IN PATIENTS WITH UNDERLYING VALVULAR HEART DISEASE

Several common therapeutic interventions must be addressed irrespective of the type and severity of the valve lesions. Antibiotic prophylaxis for endocarditis is important since community-acquired, as well as nosocomial, infections are common in critically ill patients, particularly when invasive procedures are undertaken or indwelling catheters are inserted.

Fever and increased work of breathing may increase oxygen demand and CO to a degree not well tolerated, and should be treated vigorously. Sinus tachycardia and atrial fibrillation with rapid ventricular response are poorly tolerated by patients with stenotic lesions because of the decrease in left ventricular filling time, decreased CO, and hypotension. Treatment of dysrhythmias includes correction of electrolyte abnormalities, judicious use of digoxin, and administration of β-adrenergic blockers, calcium channel blockers, amiodarone, or other antidysrhythmic drugs. Hemodynamically compromised patients who do not promptly respond to the above measures may need urgent cardioversion.

CRITICAL ILLNESSES CAUSED BY SPECIFIC VALVULAR ABNORMALITIES

Aortic Stenosis

AS is the most common isolated primary VHD and is usually caused by a fibrocalcific process. In areas where rheumatic heart disease is prevalent, it is often associated with mitral valve disease. Patients with AS may require ICU admission because of acute cardiogenic shock, pulmonary edema, severe angina, ventricular dysrhythmias, or, less commonly, atrial fibrillation and systemic embolization.

Pathophysiology

Chronic obstruction to forward blood flow causes compensatory concentric hypertrophy of the LV. Hypertrophy decreases LV compliance, increases oxygen demand and dependence of ventricular filling on left atrial contractions. As diastolic dysfunction progresses, the risk of pulmonary edema, subendocardial ischemia, and ventricular dysrhythmias increases. The inability to increase forward flow during exercise and associated peripheral vasodilatation can cause hypotension, syncope, and sudden death. The triad of symptoms—syncope, angina, and dyspnea—indicates severe AS and requires surgical intervention. Clinical signs of common valve lesions are noted in Table 97.1.

Diagnosis

Common features on ECG include left ventricular hypertrophy with strain pattern, left bundle branch block, and left atrial hypertrophy (biphasic P waves in precordial lead V_1). Chest radiography may reveal a boot-shaped heart, calcification of the aortic valve, poststenotic dilatation of the aorta, and pulmonary venous congestion. Echocardiography is the principal modality for confirming the diagnosis of AS (Fig. 97.1); the severity of AS is determined by mean gradient and peak velocity across the aortic valve and calculation of valve area (Table 97.2; Fig. 97.2). It is important to recognize that the gradients will be lower with severe AS if the flow across the valve is reduced by hypovolemia or by poor left ventricular function. Dobutamine stress testing can be used to evaluate the contractile reserve and true gradients in patients with low-flow, low-gradient AS (1). Coronary angiography is indicated in patients with AS before surgery to rule out associated coronary artery disease (CAD).

Treatment

Stabilization of the patient with AS presenting with myocardial ischemia, dysrhythmias, and/or pulmonary edema requires maintenance or restoration of atrioventricular synchrony, coronary perfusion pressure, LV contractility, and preload as well as avoidance of tachycardia. Drugs commonly used to treat ischemia, dysrhythmias, or pulmonary edema (vasodilators, antidysrhythmics, diuretics) carry significant risks in patients with AS because they often cause myocardial depression, vasodilation, or a decrease in preload that result in hypotension. Sedative drugs such as propofol and dexmedetomidine can cause significant vasodilatation and hypotension in patients with AS and fixed CO, and therefore should be avoided when possible. Narcotics can relieve pain and discomfort without significant myocardial depression and are usually well tolerated.

Fluids may be necessary to restore adequate LV filling and CO. However, excessive fluid administration may cause pulmonary edema because it increases end-diastolic pressure in the noncompliant LV. LV hypertrophy renders the atrial contraction—and thus sinus rhythm and preload—more crucial for diastolic filling of the LV. Atrial fibrillation should be reversed with prompt cardioversion and initiation of antidysrhythmic therapy with amiodarone and/or β-blocking drugs. If cardioversion is unsuccessful, pharmacologic control of the ventricular rate is essential. It is important to avoid tachycardia, which will decrease the diastolic ventricular filling time, coronary perfusion, and increase the risk of ischemia. Severe bradycardia also should be avoided because severe AS results in a fixed stroke volume, therefore potentially reducing CO. Afterload reduction is indicated only in patients with significant systemic hypertension; otherwise, because of the fixed CO, it often leads to severe hypotension and compromise of coronary perfusion pressure. Vasopressors such as phenylephrine may be necessary in patients with optimized volume and myocardial contractile status. Inotropes may be needed if myocardial dysfunction and hypotension occur. In severe cases, patients may benefit from insertion of an intra-aortic balloon counterpulsation pump (IABP) to improve coronary perfusion pressure and decrease LV afterload.

Definitive Therapy

Considering the unfavorable natural history of AS, any ICU patient with severe AS who continues to deteriorate despite medical therapy should be assessed for possible balloon valvotomy, percutaneous or transthoracic aortic valve replacement (AVR), or open valve replacement. Balloon valvotomy affords temporary improvement in transvalvular gradient—usually with restenosis in about 6 months—and may serve as a bridge to definitive surgery. Balloon valvotomy is often very effective for young adults and adolescents with bicuspid valves, although it carries a mortality of 10% in patients with calcific AS (2). Transcatheter aortic valve implantation (TAVI) has become an acceptable method of treatment in high-risk patients with AS. Cao et al., in their meta-analysis, have shown comparable outcomes for both open surgical treatment and TAVI (3). Acutely decompensated AS presenting as cardiogenic shock has also been treated by TAVI; while mortality is higher compared to elective TAVI, it can be considered as a reasonable rescue therapy (4).

Aortic Regurgitation

The most common causes of acute aortic regurgitation (AR) are infective endocarditis and diseases involving the aortic root. Infective endocarditis results in leaflet perforation, vegetations, or perivalvular fistula. Acute aortic dissection from pre-existing aortic aneurysm or from trauma may cause avulsions of the annulus and tears of the cusps. Severe, acute hypertension may also cause sudden onset of AR that often reverses after control of hypertension. The causes of chronic

TABLE 97.1 Clinical Signs in Valvular Heart Disease

	Aortic Stenosis	Aortic Regurgitation	Acute Mitral Regurgitation	Chronic Mitral Regurgitation	Mitral Stenosis
General signs	Nothing remarkable	Look for Marfan syndrome, ankylosing spondylitis, or seronegative arthropathies	Tachypnea, circulatory shock	Tachypnea	Mitral facies (malar flush), tachypnea, peripheral cyanosis
Pulse	Small volume (parvus) and late peaking (tardus)	Water-hammer pulse, wide pulse pressure	Sinus tachycardia	Irregularly irregular in AF	Reduced or normal volume, irregularly irregular in AF
Neck and JVP	Prominent a wave	Prominent carotid pulsations (Corrigan sign)	Prominent a wave	Absent a wave in AF	Prominent a wave in PHT, absent a wave in AF
Precordium	Sustained, nondisplaced or slightly displaced apical impulse, palpable S_4, systolic thrill at the base and at carotids	Diffuse, hyperdynamic and displaced apical impulse	Nondisplaced hyperdynamic apical impulse, systolic thrill	Hyperdynamic, inferolateral displaced apical impulse, parasternal heave (LAE)	Tapping apical impulse (palpable S_1), palpable P_2 and parasternal heave in PHT, diastolic thrill rarely
AUSCULTATION					
S_1	Soft	Soft in acute AR	Normal/soft	Soft	Loud
S_2	Narrow split or reverse split S_2, absent A_2 in severe AS	P_2 loud in acute AR	Accentuated P_2/wide paradoxical split	Normal P_2/wide paradoxical split	P_2 loud in PHT
S_3/S_4	Prominent S_4	S_3 heard	Present/present	Present/absent	
Clicks and added sounds	Systolic ejection click indicates mobile valve			Midsystolic click in MVP	Opening snap
Murmur	Systolic soft musical murmur, decreasing intensity in advanced disease	High-pitched, long diastolic murmur in chronic versus low-pitched short diastolic murmur in acute AR along left sternal border, diastolic murmur of early mitral diastolic closure	Early systolic loud radiating toward base (anterior directed jet) or axilla (posterior directed jet)	Holosystolic, soft or harsh and radiating toward axilla/back, late systolic murmur in MVP	Middiastolic murmur with late diastolic accentuation best heard at apex

AF, Atrial fibrillation; PHT, pulmonary hypertension; LAE, left atrial enlargement; MVP, mitral valve prolapse; AR, aortic regurgitation; AS, aortic stenosis.

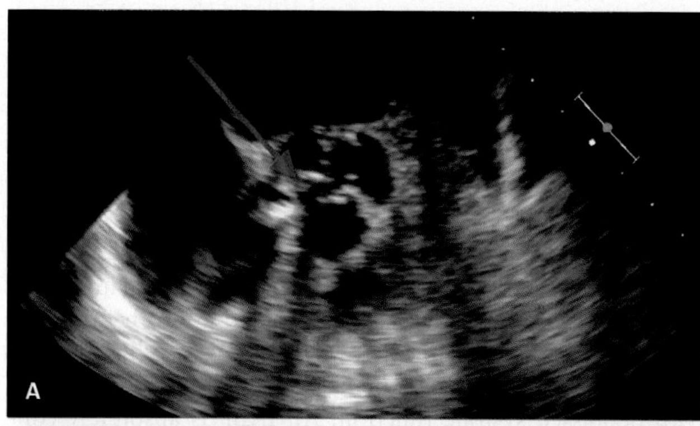

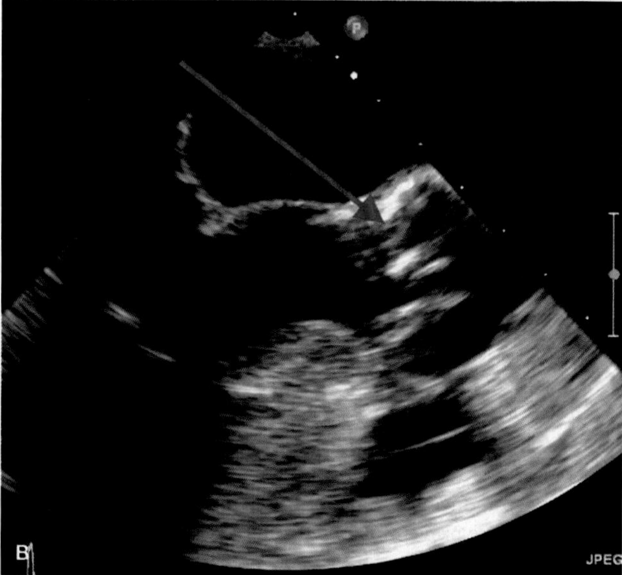

FIGURE 97.1 Mid esophageal aortic valve short axis (A) and long axis (B). TEE views showing calcified aortic valve leaflets with valve stenosis.

AR are diverse involving the valve or the aortic root. Primary valvular diseases include congenital bicuspid valve, prolapse of aortic cusp, rheumatic heart disease, calcific degenerative disease, connective tissue diseases, and subacute bacterial endocarditis. Diseases associated with aortic root dilatation include systemic hypertension, Marfan disease (Fig. 97.2), Ehlers–Danlos disease, granulomatous diseases of the aorta, senile and cystic medial degeneration, annuloaortic ectasia, and syphilis. Patients with AR may present to the critical care physician either because of acute decompensation of chronic AR or due to acute onset of severe regurgitation.

Pathophysiology

In chronic AR, the LV dilates and hypertrophies due to volume overload. This keeps wall stress in check and maintains normal forward stroke volume. As the disease progresses and the compensatory limit is reached, the wall stress begins to rise and systolic function deteriorates, with decreasing forward stroke volume as well as increasing LV end-diastolic volume (LVEDV) and LVEDP, resulting in heart failure. During the relatively asymptomatic phase, the patient develops symptoms at a rate of 3.7% per year. The presence of symptoms, systolic dysfunction, and an increase in end-systolic dimensions indicate severe and decompensated AR.

In acute AR, the LV is subject to a sudden increase in volume, with no opportunity for a compensatory increase in compliance and eccentric hypertrophy to occur. Therefore, AR of a lesser severity may markedly increase end-diastolic pressures, causing acute pulmonary venous congestion and pulmonary edema. Symptoms become more severe as the regurgitant orifice size increases, and with bradycardia as the duration of diastole increases.

TABLE 97.2 Echocardiographic Assessment of Aortic Stenosis (AS)

	Mild AS	Moderate AS	Severe AS
Valve area (cm^2)	>1.5	1–1.5	<1
Mean transvalvular gradient (mmHg)	<25	25–40	>40
Jet velocity of blood flow across the valve (m/s)	<3	3–4	>4

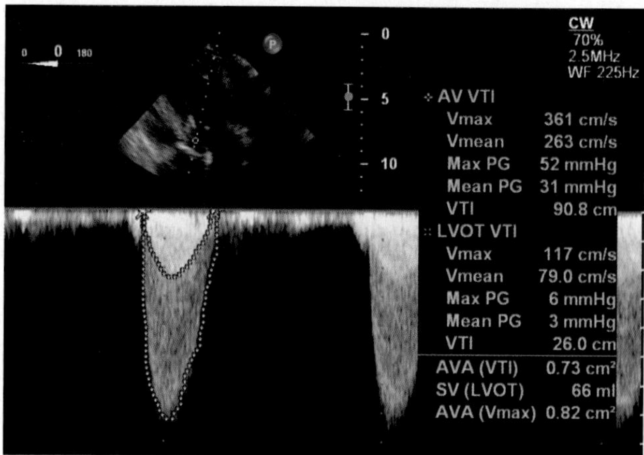

FIGURE 97.2 Spectral Doppler through the aortic valve showing aortic valve gradients and calculated aortic valve area.

Diagnosis

An ECG is performed to rule out ischemic heart disease in situations of acute AR. The chest radiograph may reveal cardiomegaly in chronic AR or pulmonary congestion with a normal-sized heart in acute AR. Echocardiography is essential to determine the mechanism and severity of AR, and identifies perivalvular pathology (e.g., an abscess) or associated aortic pathology such as acute aortic dissection. In the presence of normal leaflets, the aortic valve can be preserved surgically (AV repair). Diseased valve with vegetations, calcifications, and restrictions usually end up in AVR. Other techniques such as computerized tomographic (CT) scanning, magnetic resonance imaging (MRI), and aortography have been used. Each modality has its own advantages and disadvantages (5). TEE is clearly superior to MRI and CT scanning to characterize the valve pathology in cases of acute dissection, and obviates the need for aortography (Fig. 97.3). TEE is also readily available, can be done at the bedside and will avoid transport of hemodynamically unstable acute AR patients to radiology suite. TEE can also identify the dissection flaps causing coronary artery occlusion. Analysis of wall motion abnormalities may also help in ruling out coronary artery involvement in dissections. Coronary angiography may be necessary to rule out ischemic heart disease before surgery, in patients with chronic AR.

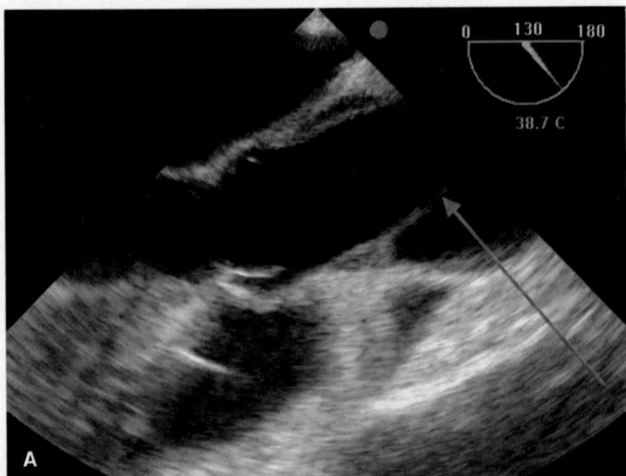

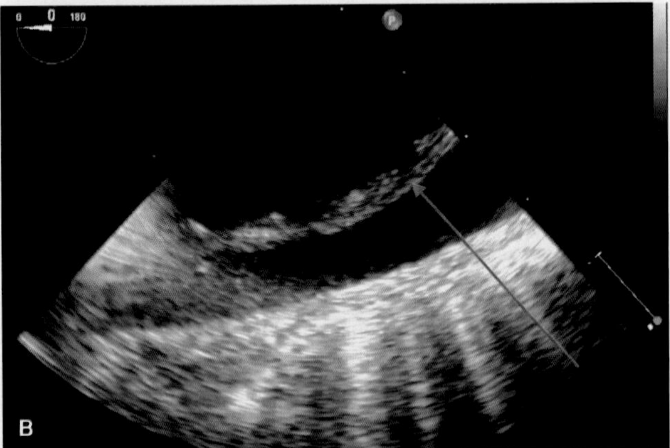

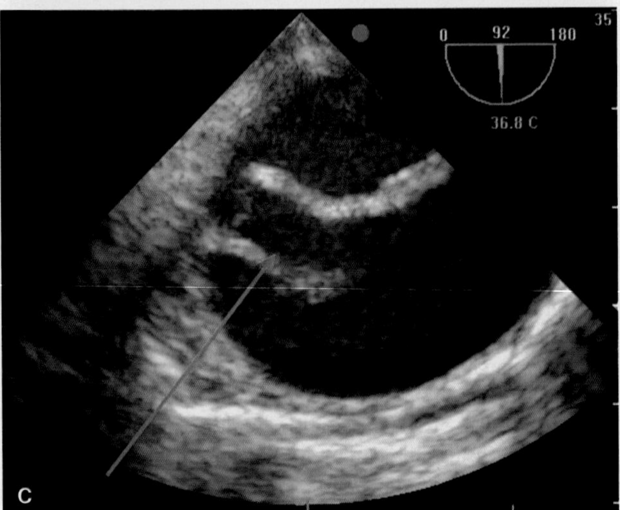

FIGURE 97.3 A: TEE images showing type A aortic dissection in the ascending aorta. B: Dissection flap in the aortic arch, with *arrows* showing the intimal flap. C: Type B aortic dissection in the descending aorta.

Treatment

While medical therapy may allow patients with mild acute AR to reach a chronic compensated state, patients with acute AR are generally ill enough to require ICU admission and/or emergency AVR. Patients with ascending aortic dissections and acute-onset AR will require immediate surgical management. In the absence of aortic dissection, the medical management of acute AR aims at optimizing CO and systemic perfusion, reduce pulmonary venous congestion, and treat any associated disorder. Invasive monitoring is initiated and intravascular volume is optimized. Moderate tachycardia is beneficial in maintaining CO, and decreases the regurgitant fraction by decreasing the duration of diastole. β-Blockers should be administered with careful hemodynamic monitoring because they depress cardiac function, increase the duration of diastole, and can precipitate circulatory failure. Hypertension and increased afterload are to be avoided; afterload reduction is indicated with arterial vasodilators such as nitroprusside. Inotropic therapy is advised only in patients with depressed systolic function. An IABP is absolutely contraindicated in patients with AR, as it will increase the regurgitant fraction.

In patients with chronic AR who present with an acute decompensation, a search should be made for the precipitating cause, with particular attention to possible infectious endocarditis. Most patients stabilize with medical therapy, but early elective surgery should be considered, as the outlook for medically treated symptomatic patients is poor. Decompensated patients who do not improve with aggressive medical therapy should undergo emergency valve replacement. Mortality with medical therapy alone in this group approaches 100%, while many moribund patients will survive with surgery.

In contrast to other causes of AR, inotropic therapy is avoided in patients with aortic dissection, as it occurs as a result of long-standing, poorly controlled hypertension or trauma. Left ventricular contractility is preserved and inotropes are not indicated. Moreover, β-adrenergic blockade is often necessary to reduce the velocity of LV ejection and aortic wall stress, therefore preventing extension of the aortic dissection or aortic rupture.

Mitral Stenosis

Mitral stenosis (MS) is mostly related to rheumatic heart disease. Degenerative calcific stenosis, congenital stenosis, and connective tissue disorders such as systemic lupus erythematosus and Lutembacher syndrome (atrial septal defect with MS) are other causes for MS. Atrial myxomas and left atrial ball-valve thrombus can present with intermittent obstruction to mitral inflow and mimic MS.

Pathophysiology

In rheumatic MS, inflammation of the connective tissue leads to leaflet thickening and calcification, and commissural and chordal fusion. Ultimately, many patients are left with a funnel-shaped mitral apparatus. As the condition progresses, left atrial pressure and the transmitral gradient increase, thus maintaining flow. However, the subsequent increase in pulmonary venous pressure leads to hydrostatic pulmonary edema. Pulmonary vasoconstriction increases pulmonary arterial pressure and right ventricular afterload. Over the course of rheumatic heart disease, persistently elevated pulmonary arterial pressure leads to intimal hyperplasia and medial hypertrophy. These structural changes are permanent and result in fixed pulmonary hypertension. Right ventricular dilatation and failure result in tricuspid insufficiency and systemic venous congestion, respectively. The impact of MS on CO is initially determined by the limitation to flow across the narrowed mitral orifice. However, as pulmonary hypertension

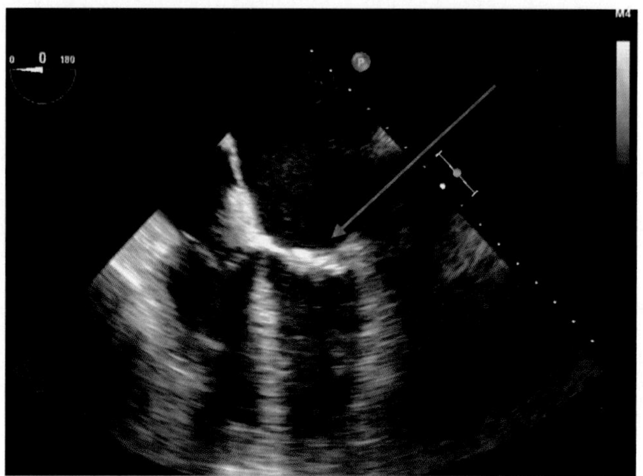

FIGURE 97.4 Midesophageal four chamber TEE view showing severe calcified and fused rheumatic mitral leaflets (*arrow*).

progresses, right ventricular failure may become severe enough to limit CO. Similarly, progression of rheumatic disease with its associated inflammation, fibrosis, and calcium deposition may impair left ventricular function. Although this effect is not a major determinant of CO in patients with MS, it may become important to consider in some patients after surgical repair. In such situations, the increase in transmitral flow may expose the LV to a sudden increase in preload, causing failure.

Diagnosis

The ECG may show left atrial enlargement, right ventricular hypertrophy, and atrial fibrillation. Chest radiography shows straightening of the left heart border, indicating left atrial and pulmonary artery enlargement. Echocardiographic findings include doming of the anterior leaflet, decreased leaflet mobility, increased leaflet calcification and thickness (Fig. 97.4), commissural fusion, calcification of the subvalvular apparatus, increased LA size, and the presence of an LA thrombus (Fig. 97.5). Color flow may show associated mitral regurgitation (MR). Doppler echocardiography allows quantification of severity of MS by calculation of pressure gradients and mitral valve area (Table 97.3; Fig. 97.6). Pressure half-time method is most commonly used to calculate mitral valve area. Evaluation of severity of associated TR and estimation of pulmonary artery systolic pressure can also be done using echocardiography. Cardiac MRI is increasingly being used in the evaluation of stenotic valvular lesions; it measures valve area by planimetry. Its advantage over echocardiography is the lack of dependence upon good echocardiographic windows. Patients with MS often present to the ICU with acute cardiogenic pulmonary edema. Precipitating factors such as infective endocarditis, fever, anxiety, pain, atrial fibrillation, and pregnancy should be identified. Occlusion from an enlarging atrial myxoma should be ruled out. Right-sided heart failure with hepatic dysfunction, acute hemoptysis, systemic embolism, and hoarseness of voice may also be present.

TABLE 97.3 Echocardiographic Evaluation of Severity of Mitral Stenosis

Method	Normal	Mild	Moderate	Severe
Valve area (cm^2)	4–6	1.5–2.5	1.0–1.5	<1.0
Mean pressure gradient (mmHg)		<5	6–10	>10
Pressure half-time (msec)	40–70	70–150	150–200	>220

Treatment

New-onset atrial fibrillation with hemodynamic instability should be treated with cardioversion. Cardioversion of a patient with atrial fibrillation of unknown duration or that is known to have persisted for more than 48 hours must be preceded by 3 weeks of anticoagulation or by a TEE to exclude the presence of left atrial thrombus. Anticoagulation should be continued for 4 weeks following cardioversion because the enlarged LA remains "stunned" and does not recover a normal contractile state immediately following cardioversion (6).

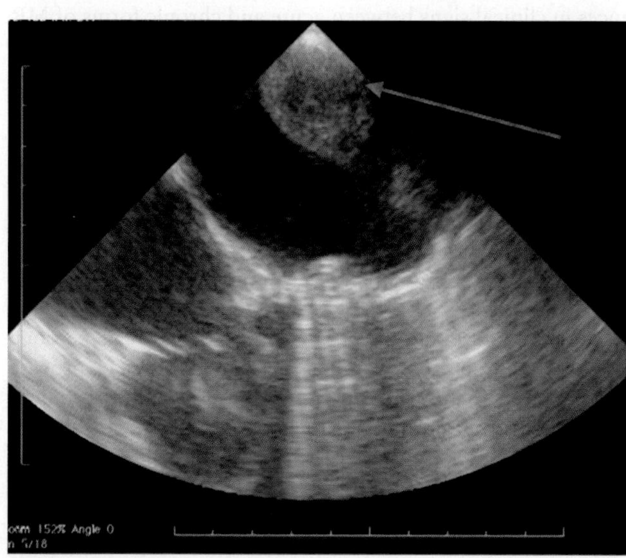

FIGURE 97.5 Prosthetic mitral stenosis with stasis in the left atrium leading to thrombus formation (*arrow*).

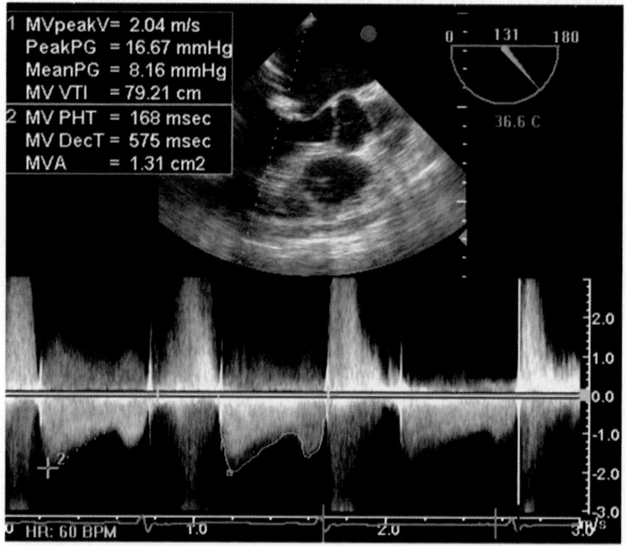

FIGURE 97.6 Spectral Doppler through mitral valve showing higher mean gradient and reduced valve area indicating moderate mitral stenosis (compare the values in Table 97.3).

Anticoagulants should also be used in patients with a prior embolic event and left atrial diameter greater than 55 mm by echocardiography (7). Antidysrhythmics, such as amiodarone, may be used to maintain sinus rhythm but should not be expected to provide indefinite success.

Patients admitted with pulmonary edema benefit from oxygen, diuretics, morphine, anxiolytics, and digoxin; the latter is especially useful in patients with atrial dysrhythmias and congestive heart failure. Sympathetic nervous system activity is increased in patients with MS, worsening the symptom complex; β-blockers are very useful in this situation. Intravenous nesiritide, a synthetic human natriuretic peptide, is also used in the critically ill patients with acute decompensated cardiac failure and pulmonary hypertension (8,9). If the patient is hypotensive, inotropes to improve left ventricular function may not be useful, but may worsen tachycardia and pulmonary edema. Inodilators however may be useful in improving right ventricular dysfunction and reducing pulmonary hypertension. Systemic blood pressure may need to be supported with vasopressors, with the caveat that they may adversely impact pulmonary vascular resistance. The most effective way to support RV function is to decrease pulmonary vascular resistance by administering inhaled vasodilators such as nitric oxide (NO) and epoprostenol. Although inhaled NO decreases PVR and improves right heart function, it may increase left-sided filling pressures in patients with LV dysfunction by increasing blood flow to the pulmonary venous system (10,11). Careful titration and monitoring is required while administering NO to patients with MS as pulmonary edema has been reported in patients with heart failure after treatment with inhaled NO (12). As the LV is usually underfilled, assessment of volume status should focus on the RV. Observation of trends in CVP is useful, especially when a sudden increase occurs, reflecting worsening TR and RV failure.

Emergency invasive intervention is rarely required to relieve MS. If the precipitating events are controlled, elective surgery or balloon valvotomy may be indicated. Balloon valvotomy is possible in patients with pliable leaflets, no commissural fusion, and minimal subvalvular calcification. Because of extensive calcifications and marked anatomic distortion, mitral valve repair may not be possible in rheumatic mitral disease, and valve replacement is necessary in those patients.

Mitral Regurgitation

The mitral valve apparatus is composed of the valve leaflets, mitral annulus, chordae tendineae, and papillary muscles. Any disruption in its integrity may result in MR. One of the major breakthroughs in the management of MR was the functional classification of MR by Carpentier in early 1980s (13) (Table 97.4).

Acute onset of severe MR can lead to acute pulmonary edema and cardiogenic shock. Acute MR may be caused by infection (infective endocarditis with leaflet perforations, vegetations, or periprosthetic valvular leaks); connective tissue or myxomatous disorders (chordal rupture; Fig. 97.7); or ischemic heart disease (infarction and rupture of papillary muscles (Fig. 97.8), or papillary muscle dysfunction due to ischemia). Acute rheumatic mitral valvulitis as the cause of MR is less common today. Patients with MR present to the critical care physician either because of decompensated chronic MR or due to acute onset of severe regurgitation.

TABLE 97.4 Functional Classification of Mitral Regurgitation (MR)

Type of MR	Pathology	Disease
I	Normal motion of leaflets	Endocarditis (leaflet perforation) or various etiologies causing LV dysfunction (annular dilatation)
II	Increased leaflet motion with free edge of the leaflet traveling above the plane of the annulus; this is due to chordal elongation or rupture, papillary muscle rupture	Degenerative myxomatous valve disease
IIIA	Restricted leaflet motion during diastole and systole	Rheumatic heart disease
IIIB	Restricted leaflet motion during systole, papillary muscle displacement	Ischemic or dilated cardiomyopathy

Pathophysiology

Chronic MR leads to adaptation of the LV by dilatation and eccentric hypertrophy. Over many years of increasing regurgitant volume, systolic function may fail, resulting in decreased LVEF, increased LVEDP, and pulmonary hypertension. Left atrial (LA) dilatation leads to atrial fibrillation. While chronic MR is rarely the direct cause of critical illness, chronic MR often renders the management of a critically ill patient more complex. In acute MR, on the other hand, the regurgitant volume is ejected into the normal, noncompliant left atrium, causing an acute increase in left atrial pressure, which is transmitted to the pulmonary venous system, resulting in pulmonary edema, acute pulmonary hypertension, and RV strain or failure. Sudden volume overload causes further distension of the LV and MV apparatus that increases the regurgitant fraction and decreases forward stroke volume and CO. Systemic vascular resistance rises, further increasing the regurgitant fraction, ultimately leading to cardiogenic shock. The differences in clinical signs between acute and chronic forms of MR are given in Table 97.1.

Diagnosis

The ECG may show atrial fibrillation, left ventricular hypertrophy, right ventricular strain, or myocardial ischemia or infarction. Chest radiograph may show cardiomegaly indicating pre-existing heart disease. Pulmonary venous congestion and/or edema with a normal-sized heart indicate acute MR.

Echocardiography remains the standard for the diagnosis of MR. Bedside TTE often reveals the mechanism of MR. Qualitative and quantitative assessment of MR can be done by color and spectral Doppler methods. TEE may provide better detail because of superior resolution and better definition of anatomic details of the mitral valve apparatus and mechanism and severity of MR. Three-dimensional echocardiography is a revolution in the management of MR by providing accurate diagnosis and precise location of the lesions (Fig. 97.9). Indices of left ventricular function such as LVEF are unreliable in the presence of severe MR. Ejection fraction in MR is increased when contractility is normal. Normal LVEF

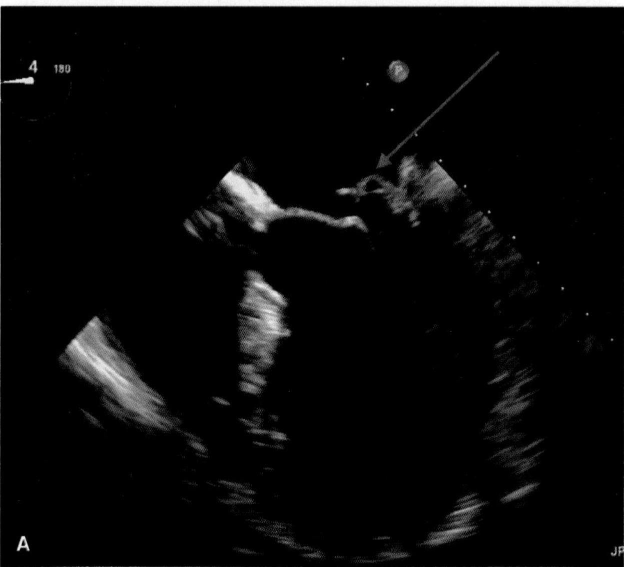

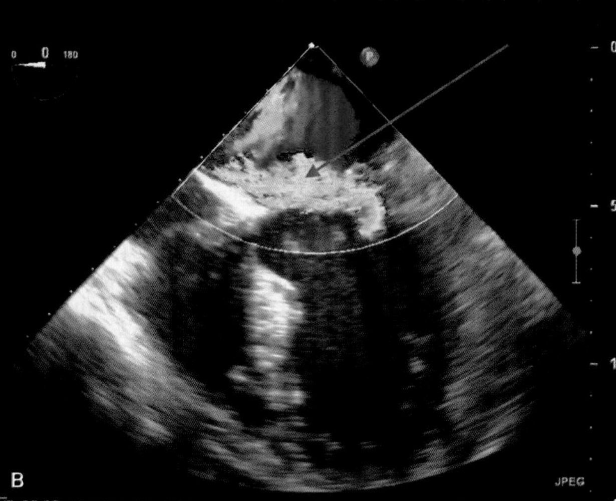

FIGURE 97.7 Two-dimensional echocardiography showing the posterior leaflet prolapse and ruptured chordae (A) leading to severe anteriorly directed eccentric mitral regurgitation (B).

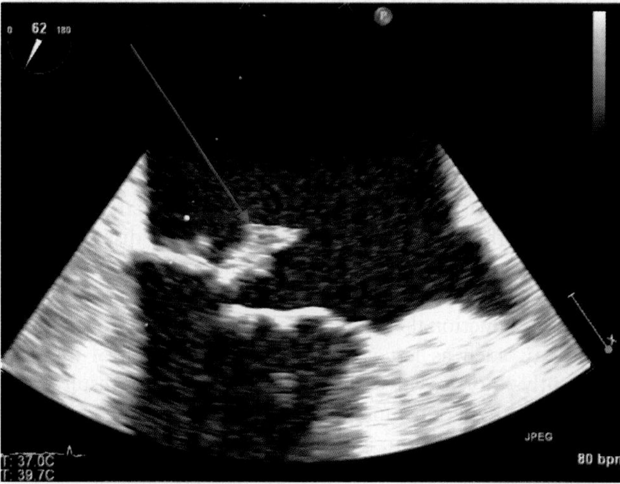

FIGURE 97.8 Papillary muscle rupture and prolapse into left atrium (*arrow*).

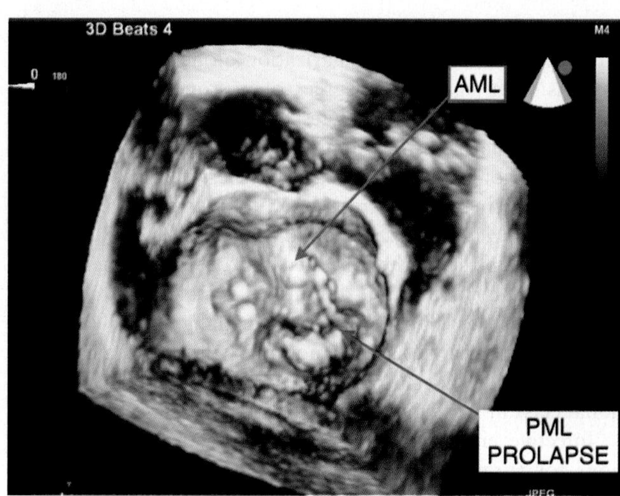

FIGURE 97.9 Three-dimensional echocardiography of mitral valve surgeon's view showing anterior mitral leaflet (AML) and prolapsed posterior mitral leaflet (PML) in the same patient as that in Figure 97.7.

indicates a significant loss of myocardial function; when LVEF is reduced to 50% or less, advanced myocardial dysfunction is generally present (14). The American Heart Association/American College of Cardiology (AHA/ACC) guidelines recommend medical treatment when EF is less than 30% and surgical treatment, even in asymptomatic patients, with EF less than 60% to prevent progression of disease (7). Urgent coronary angiography is indicated in presence of myocardial ischemia or infarction since the culprit lesion may be amenable to catheter-based or open surgical interventions. In the case of chordal rupture or infective endocarditis without risk factors for CAD, angiography may be deferred.

Treatment

In acute, severe MR, medical therapy has a limited role and is aimed at controlling circulatory shock and preserving organ function in preparation for surgical intervention; early valve surgery is lifesaving. When ischemic heart disease is present, therapy should aim at maintaining coronary perfusion pressure and reducing myocardial oxygen consumption. A moderate degree of sinus tachycardia is desirable as it helps maintain forward flow and limits diastolic distension of the LV. Hypertension and elevation of SVR are undesirable as they increase the regurgitant fraction and exacerbate heart failure and pulmonary edema. In the normotensive patient, arterial vasodilators—such as nitroprusside—can increase forward flow and decrease the regurgitant fraction. The initial treatment of arterial hypotension should aim at restoring an acceptable CO. Inotropic agents are often useful, but vasoconstrictors are rarely necessary. Diuretics may be needed to reduce pulmonary venous congestion. When patients fail to respond adequately to medical management, IABP may be lifesaving, as it increases forward flow and systemic pressure while decreasing preload and afterload. It is effective in increasing coronary perfusion pressure, reducing oxygen consumption, and maintaining a favorable balance between myocardial oxygen supply and demand.

The surgical intervention is determined by the nature of the lesion. Chordal rupture or prolapse of the posterior leaflet can be repaired. Catheter-based or surgical revascularization alone may improve ischemic MR in selected patients with reversible, ischemia-related papillary muscle dysfunction without rupture (15). However, revascularization alone may leave these patients with significant degrees of postoperative MR (16). Current lines of evidence suggest that a combination of complete revascularization with mitral valve repair or replacement with posterior chordal sparing is the best surgical treatment for acute ischemic MR refractory to medical management and nonsurgical revascularization techniques (17). Mitral valve annuloplasty is the preferred approach for ischemic MR due to annular dilatation, diminished systolic contraction of the annulus, or papillary muscle malalignment. Papillary muscle rupture carries a high mortality without surgical intervention; surgery does improve the long-term outcome in functional class in these patients.

Infective endocarditis is treated with antibiotics. Indications for surgery include congestive heart failure refractory to medical treatment, uncontrolled infection despite antibiotics, recurrent systemic embolism, perivalvular or pericardial extension of infection, fungal endocarditis, and prosthetic valve endocarditis. If urgent surgery is indicated, it should not be delayed for microbiologic clearance (7).

Mitral valve prolapse (MVP) is the most prevalent VHD and the most common cause of MR. Patients with this condition may present to the ICU because of severe MR, atrial fibrillation with transient ischemic attacks, prolonged QT syndrome and tachydysrhythmias, pulmonary hypertension, cerebral embolism from MVP-related fibrin, infective endocarditis, or even sudden death (18). Medical stabilization and elective surgical repair of the mitral valve are recommended therapies.

Mitraclip is a percutaneous catheter-based system, which can be used to treat severe MR in patients who will not tolerate open surgical repair. Mitraclip decreases severity of MR, improves the functional NYHA classification and quality of life. Mitraclip procedure can be used for symptomatic patients with functional or degenerative MR. Short-term outcomes such as duration of hospital stay, transfusion rate, duration of mechanical ventilation, and ICU stay are improved compared with open surgical treatment. Long-term efficacy of this procedure is yet to be established (19,20).

Tricuspid Stenosis

Tricuspid stenosis (TS) is usually related to rheumatic heart disease; involvement of the mitral valve is common. Other causes include carcinoid syndrome, infective endocarditis, congenital stenosis or atresia, and methysergide toxicity. Functional obstruction can be caused by right atrial tumors and thrombi.

Pathophysiology

Obstruction to right ventricular inflow results in systemic venous congestion: elevated jugular venous pulse (JVP), congestive hepatomegaly, and peripheral edema. Diastole is shortened by increasing heart rate, thus causing dramatic increases in transvalvular gradients. Most patients are symptomatic from coexisting MS. The presence of systemic venous congestion out of proportion to pulmonary venous congestion should raise the suspicion for involvement of the tricuspid valve.

Diagnosis

The ECG may show evidence of RA enlargement—a P wave exceeding 2.5 mm in lead II and 1.5 mm in V_1. RA enlargement may increase the distance from sinus node to atrioventricular node, causing first-degree heart block; atrial fibrillation may occur in advanced disease. The chest radiograph may show cardiomegaly and RA enlargement, and calcification of the valve may be evident. Typically, echocardiographic visualization shows thickened leaflets, limited mobility, and a dome-shaped structure in diastole. Right ventricular function and the presence of tumor, thrombus, and vegetations can also be assessed. Spectral and color Doppler methods allow calculation of pressure gradients to grade the stenosis—that is, mild less than 5 mmHg, moderate 5 to 10 mmHg, and severe greater than 10 mmHg—and valve area.

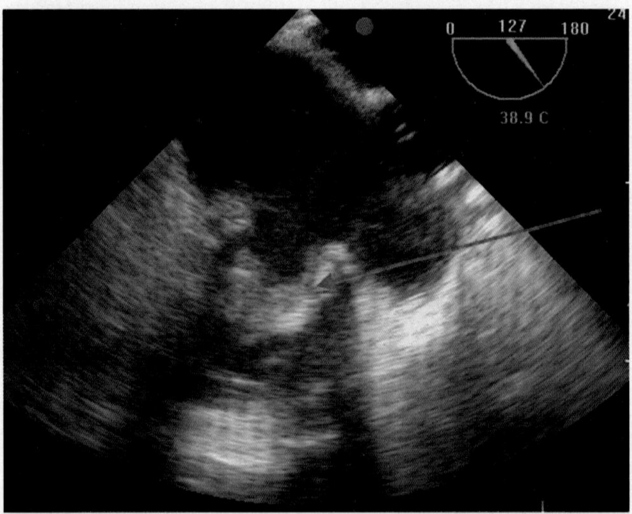

FIGURE 97.10 Midesophageal bicaval view showing complete obstruction of tricuspid valve (*arrow*) by infected vegetation in a patient with IV drug use.

Treatment

Complete obstruction of the tricuspid valve by vegetations, thrombus, and/or tumors is an indication for emergency valve surgery (Fig. 97.10). As seen in other valvular lesions the disease progresses slowly becoming symptomatic as obstruction to flow increases. Sodium restriction, careful diuresis, rate control, and anticoagulation are helpful, but surgical correction is required when the transvalvular gradient exceeds 5 mmHg and the valve area falls below 2 cm^2. Percutaneous valvotomy or, more often, a bioprosthetic valve replacement is necessary. Mechanical valves are avoided when possible because of the very high risk of thromboembolism in this position.

Tricuspid Regurgitation

TR can be classified as structural or functional. Structural diseases of the valve are caused by rheumatic disease, infective endocarditis, carcinoid syndrome, radiation therapy, Marfan syndrome, congenital heart disease, or tricuspid valve prolapse. Functional TR is usually secondary to left-sided pathology, such as left ventricular failure or mitral or—less frequently—aortic valve disease, but may also result from pulmonary hypertension, pulmonic stenosis (PS), right ventricular (RV) infarction, and dilated cardiomyopathy; a small number of cases may not have an etiology identified. While most cases of TR are chronic, an acute presentation may occur following penetrating trauma, RV infarction, infective endocarditis, and repeated endomyocardial biopsies following heart transplantation.

Pathophysiology

Acute TR increases RA pressure and systemic venous congestion. Over time, the RA dilates, with the possible sequelae of atrial fibrillation and thrombus formation. Formation of an RA thrombus may lead to pulmonary and systemic emboli, the latter in patients with patent foramen ovale. RV volume overload leads to eccentric hypertrophy and dilatation. RV systolic dysfunction develops, leading to further decompensation and dilatation, which in turn causes annular dilatation and an increase in the severity of TR. The left heart also suffers from low CO because the RV fails to deliver enough blood to the LV. Ventricular interdependence and paradoxical septal motion also decrease left ventricular output in patients with RV volume overload.

Diagnosis

Symptoms of low CO and venous congestion are present in these patients. Shock and hypotension may develop following acute TR after RV infarction or papillary muscle rupture. Other patients maintain blood pressure but demonstrate signs of right-sided failure. Distended neck veins with a prominent c-v wave, pulsatile hepatomegaly, a precordial bulge, and parasternal heave from RV hypertrophy; soft S_1, prominent P_2, and right-sided S_3 from RV dilatation; pansystolic thrill; and a murmur heard at the left lower sternal border are associated signs. Cases of isolated tricuspid valve endocarditis may disseminate emboli to the lungs, resulting in multiple septic emboli and abscess formation. Peripheral stigmata of infective emboli are usually absent, but may indicate paradoxical embolism or left-sided lesions if present.

The ECG may show atrial fibrillation, right axis deviation, RV hypertrophy, and a right bundle branch block. Right-sided leads will show ST elevation in RV infarction and may be associated with LV inferior wall infarction. Enlarged RV and cardiomegaly are seen on chest radiography. Echocardiography can yield details about the structural issues with the tricuspid valve—prolapse, vegetations, annular diameter, and rheumatic disease—and helps to rule out thrombus and patent foramen ovale. The diagnosis of a patent foramen ovale is important, since the elevated right atrial pressure frequently exceeds left atrial pressure, causing a right-to-left shunt that may cause refractory hypoxemia (Fig. 97.11). Severity of TR can be assessed by hepatic venous systolic flow reversal using spectral pulse wave Doppler and estimation of regurgitant orifice area (>40 mm^2 is severe). Also, right ventricular systolic pressure can be estimated by continuous wave Doppler signal of TR (Fig. 97.12). Augmenting ultrasound signal with 10% air, 10% patient's blood, and 80% saline will improve the accuracy of estimated pulmonary artery systolic pressures by echocardiography (21). RV systolic pressure is usually greater than 60 mmHg in functional TR while it is less than 40 mmHg in structural TR, when measured directly by right heart catheterization.

Treatment

In general, the hemodynamic impact of acute TR is less severe and can be effectively managed by improving LV function, reducing PVR, or with diuresis. In rare instances, acute severe TR may require valvular surgery when the process is refractory to medical therapy. Once stabilized, these patients' long-term prognosis depends on the etiology and severity of the TR. Patients tolerate mild and moderate degrees of chronic TR in the presence of normal LV function. Correction of left-sided heart lesions and treatment of left-sided failure and pulmonary hypertension take priority. If functional TR is significant with annular enlargement (Fig. 97.13), surgical intervention may be needed. Ring annuloplasty can improve TR and survival in these patients (22). Cardiac resynchronization therapy with biventricular pacemakers and the Dor procedure (endoventricular circular patch plasty) help patients with functional TR due to systolic heart failure (23).

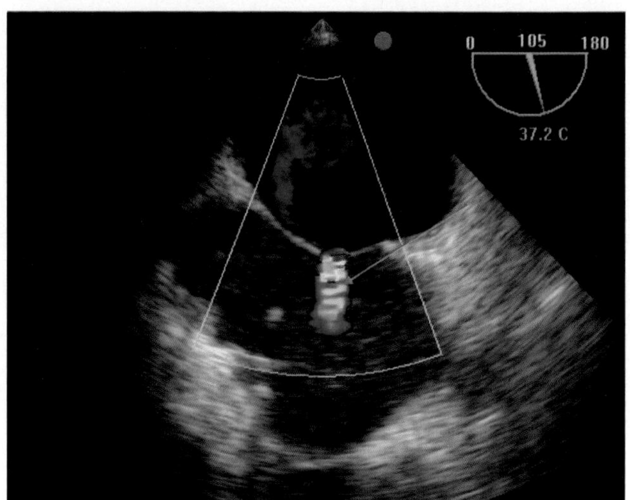

FIGURE 97.11 Midesophageal bicaval view showing color flow through patent foramen ovale (*arrow*).

Rheumatic TR may be treated with open valvotomy or valve replacement. Valves compromised by infective endocarditis can simply be removed after an aggressive course of antibiotics. Valve replacement can be performed later if there is no recurrence of drug abuse in these patients. When acute TR is the result of RV infarction, the usual management of acute coronary insufficiency must be observed, including β-blockers, aspirin, fluids, thrombolysis, coronary angiography, angioplasty, and stenting and, in suitable patients, coronary artery bypass grafting.

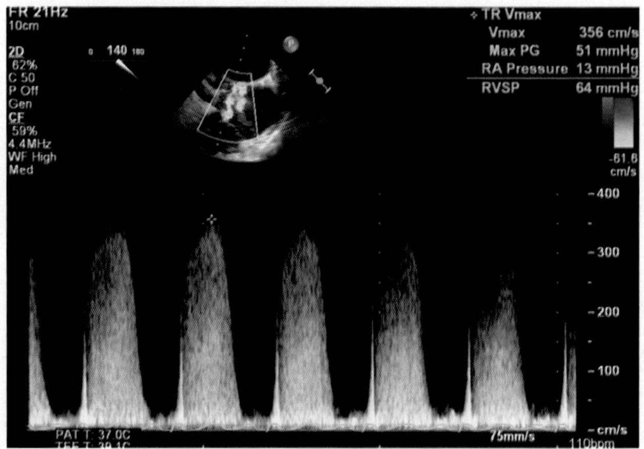

FIGURE 97.12 Estimation of right ventricular systolic pressure using continuous wave Doppler through tricuspid regurgitation jet. Calculation is given in the right upper corner.

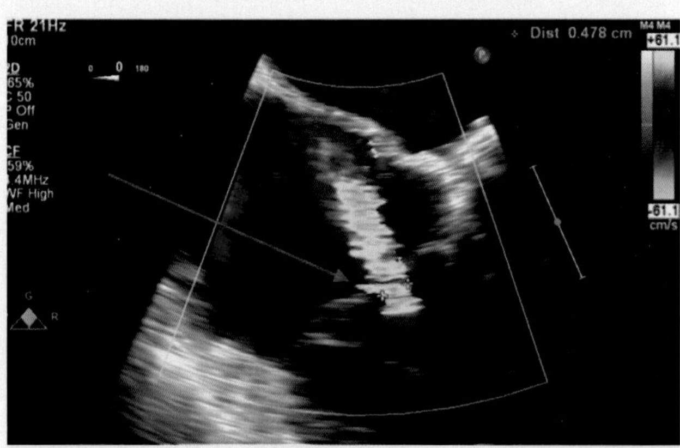

FIGURE 97.13 Functional tricuspid regurgitation (*arrow*) with enlarged annulus'.

Pulmonic Stenosis

PS is usually congenital. While valvular PS does occur in isolation, subvalvular and supravalvular stenosis usually comprise part of a larger syndrome. Severe forms, or those associated with other cardiac anomalies, are generally identified and treated in childhood. Acquired forms of pulmonary stenosis include rheumatic, carcinoid disease; infundibular stenosis from pulmonary hypertension; extrinsic compression from aneurysm of the sinus of Valsalva; tumors; and scarring from previous surgery.

Pathophysiology

PS causes obstruction to right ventricular outflow and right ventricular hypertrophy. If right ventricular failure or TR develops, systemic venous hypertension can result. The degree of stenosis, once established, tends to be stable; if decompensation does not occur in childhood, subsequent deterioration is unlikely. Occasionally, patients manifest increasing right ventricular outflow obstruction, perhaps caused by secondary infundibular hypertrophy.

Mild PS is often asymptomatic. Patients with more severe stenosis commonly develop fatigue, atypical chest pain, and syncope. When right ventricular failure or TR occurs, systemic venous hypertension may be present. Elevated right atrial pressures in the presence of a patent foramen ovale or atrial septal defect can result in a right-to-left shunt at the atrial level.

Diagnosis

Physical examination typically reveals a large jugular venous a wave. In the absence of right ventricular failure or TR, jugular venous pressure remains normal. A left parasternal systolic lift is common with significant PS. The murmur is best heard at the left upper sternal border and typically radiates to the left clavicle. A palpable thrill may be present. The intensity of the murmur does not correlate well with severity, but increasing duration and late systolic peaking are indicators of significant stenosis. An ejection click is usually present. As severity increases, P_2 is increasingly delayed; thus, wide splitting of the second sound indicates more severe stenosis.

The ECG is normal in mild PS. With increasing severity, right ventricular hypertrophy and right atrial enlargement are common. The chest radiograph may reveal poststenotic dilatation of the main and left pulmonary arteries. Echocardiography is particularly useful in assessing the valve morphology, calculating pressure gradients across the pulmonic valve, grading the severity of stenosis, and evaluating right ventricular function. The presence of other congenital abnormalities, TR, and right atrial enlargement can also be ruled out by echocardiography. Cardiac catheterization provides confirmation of pressure gradients, full hemodynamic assessment, and identification of associated pulmonary artery branch stenosis. Pulmonary stenosis is graded based on the peak pressure gradient: mild, with a gradient of 25 to 49 mmHg; moderate, 50 to 75 mmHg; and severe, greater than 75 mmHg.

Treatment

Currently, balloon valvuloplasty is recommended for symptomatic patients and those with a peak gradient greater than 50 mmHg. Surgical valvuloplasty is reserved for severe calcification, dysplasia, endocarditis, and previous valvuloplasty failure. Medical management includes infective endocarditis prophylaxis, treatment of right heart failure and atrial fibrillation, and anticoagulation to prevent thromboembolic complications.

Pulmonic Insufficiency

Pulmonic insufficiency (PI) generally has a benign course as an isolated abnormality. The natural history is that of the associated lesions. PI may be secondary to pulmonary hypertension or, rarely, to leaflet damage caused by infectious endocarditis, rheumatic fever, or carcinoid syndrome. Occasionally, PI is congenital.

Pathophysiology

In the absence of pulmonary hypertension, volume overload of the right ventricle is well tolerated. Decompensation with resulting right ventricular failure can occur when pulmonary hypertension develops from other causes. PI is usually an incidental auscultatory finding in patients admitted to the ICU for other reasons. Physical findings include the typical decrescendo diastolic murmur along the upper left sternal border. The intensity of the murmur does not correlate well with the severity of regurgitation.

Diagnosis

The ECG is usually normal. The presence of right ventricular hypertrophy suggests pulmonary hypertension. The chest radiograph is normal in mild insufficiency. The pulmonary trunk may be prominent when the insufficiency is moderate to severe. Pulmonary hypertension may be present. Echocardiography with Doppler study can be useful for differentiating pulmonic from aortic insufficiency and for establishing right heart chamber sizes and associated abnormalities.

Treatment

Specific treatment is rarely required. However, therapy should be directed toward control of pulmonary hypertension when present. When the right heart fails, diuretics and sodium restriction are useful, and some clinicians suggest that cardiac glycosides are helpful. Surgical treatment (bioprosthetic valve replacement) is reserved for advanced right heart failure. In patients with a remote repair of tetralogy of Fallot and chronic PI, RV dilatation has been linked to sudden death. This has led some clinician investigators to pursue valve replacement in early stages of RV dilatation.

Mixed Valve Lesions

Mitral Stenosis with Regurgitation

The combination of pressure and volume overload on LA favors early development of symptoms, atrial fibrillation, and congestive heart failure. Because transvalvular gradients may overestimate the degree of stenosis, Doppler measurement of valve area should be considered. Three-dimensional measurement of valve area by planimetric method is useful in these situations. Decision making is complex, and intervention is often required before either of the lesions reaches a severe degree. Moderate MR is a contraindication for balloon valvotomy.

Aortic Stenosis and Regurgitation

This combination causes both pressure and volume overload on the LV. The predominant lesion is indicated by the size of the LV: a normal-sized, but hypertrophied, LV signifies predominant AS; a dilated LV suggests dominant AR. As with combined MS and MR, transvalvular gradients may overestimate AS, so planimetry or the continuity equation method should be considered. The threshold for surgery is lowered as compared to single valve–defect patients. Those with severe AS with accompanying AR should be operated on in higher calculated valve areas or in the presence of mild symptoms. Surgery in patients with predominant AR with accompanying AS can be delayed until symptoms develop or asymptomatic LV dysfunction becomes apparent on echocardiography (enlarged ventricular dimensions).

Mitral Stenosis and Aortic Stenosis

This combination causes serial obstructions resulting in reduced CO and early development of pulmonary venous congestion and hypertension. Low transvalvular gradients characterize this AS because of low CO. Mitral valvotomy is done first, followed by AVR as indicated. Double valve replacement is recommended in patients with significant stenosis in both valves.

Mitral Stenosis and Aortic Regurgitation

This combination creates a challenge for the physician attempting to make a diagnosis. MS decreases the volume overload of AR, and AR attenuates antegrade mitral valve flow by increasing LV diastolic pressure, thereby decreasing transmitral gradients. Balloon mitral valvotomy followed by AVR, as indicated, is a reasonable approach. Double valve replacement is recommended in patients with significant lesions in both valves.

Mitral Regurgitation and Aortic Stenosis

AS aggravates MR by increasing the afterload. MR, by its pressure release effect, obscures even severe AS. Systolic function remains normal with low transaortic gradients. If both lesions are severe, AVR with mitral valve repair or replacement is necessary. Moderate or mild MR may improve after AVR for AS, especially if there is no anatomic lesion in the mitral valve. Intraoperative TEE plays an important role in this decision.

Mitral Regurgitation and Aortic Regurgitation

These lesions create additive volume loads on the LV; consequently, the sequelae of dyspnea and LV dysfunction appear sooner. Mitral valve annuloplasty is done along with AVR if MR is severe with no anatomic lesions in the MV.

Prosthetic Valve Dysfunction

Prosthetic valves in common use are broadly divided into mechanical, bioprosthetic, and homograft valves. Mechanical valves need lifelong anticoagulation, while bioprosthetic valves do not require long-term anticoagulation. However, bioprosthetic valves have a shorter life span and are prone to degenerative changes and failure. Acute valvular complications may result from infective endocarditis, paravalvular leak, valve ring abscess, thrombosis, pannus formation, degenerative calcification, lipid infiltration, dehiscence of the valve, and strut fracture. Acute, complete valvular obstruction may lead to sudden death in the absence of surgical intervention.

Progressive congestive cardiac failure is a common presentation with stenosis and regurgitation. Embolic phenomenon, hemolytic anemia—indicating a paravalvular leak, and a new atrioventricular block—indicating a valve ring abscess may be other presenting symptoms. Prosthetic valve thrombosis may present with nonspecific cardiac symptoms. Normally functioning prosthetic valves are associated with clicks and murmurs; hence, disappearance of clicks or a new or changing murmur is important in making the diagnosis.

Echocardiography is essential to make a diagnosis in these patients. As previously noted, TEE is more sensitive and specific in the evaluation of prosthetic valve pathologies than TTE; echocardiography has replaced cardiac catheterization in these cases. Excessive rocking motion of the valve ring with perivalvular leak may indicate valve dehiscence (Fig. 97.14) or underlying infective process. Limited motion of the valve components could be due to thrombus, pannus formation, or because of degenerative changes with thickening and calcification. Presence of a vegetation (Fig. 97.15), leaflet perforation, and periannular thickening (abscess formation; Fig. 97.16) confirms the diagnosis of infective endocarditis. Other complications of prosthetic endocarditis include pseudoaneurysm and fistula formation with adjacent cardiac chambers, which can be readily identified with two-dimensional echocardiography and color Doppler. Calculation of transvalvular gradients help in the diagnosis of prosthetic valve obstruction. Gradients depend on the type and size of the valve and dynamic conditions such as CO, blood volume, heart rate, and contractility. Therefore, it is recommended that the measurements be compared to the control values obtained immediately after valve replacement. It has also been suggested that it may be more appropriate to calculate the prosthetic valve area using the continuity equation:

$$\text{Area}_1 \times \text{velocity time integral}_1 = \text{area}_2 \times \text{velocity time integral}_2$$

Fluoroscopy may be needed in some cases to identify the nature of the disease and assess the effects of thrombolysis.

Medical therapy is directed toward treatment of congestive heart failure—diuretics, vasodilators, and inotropes; initiation of antibiotics for infective endocarditis after obtaining blood cultures; and thrombolysis for certain cases of prosthetic valve thrombosis. Staphylococcal organisms predominate in early (<60 days post placement) prosthetic valve endocarditis, whereas in late (>60 days post placement) endocarditis, there are equal percentages of infection caused by streptococcal and staphylococcal organisms (24); empiric antibiotics are started until culture results and sensitivities are available. Virtually all early cases of prosthetic valve endocarditis require surgery. Systemic embolism, periannular extension, persistent sepsis,

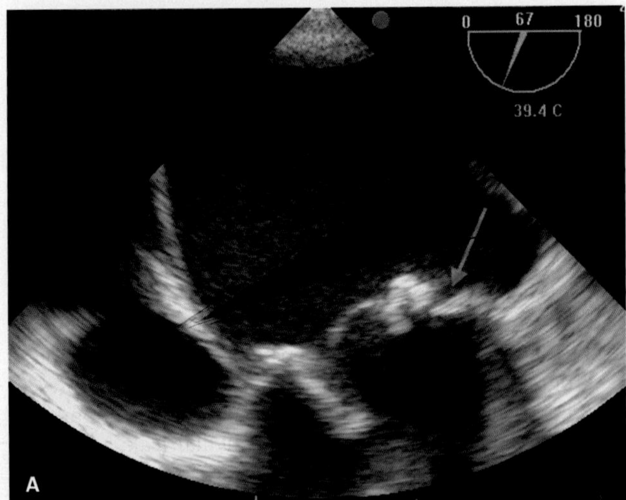

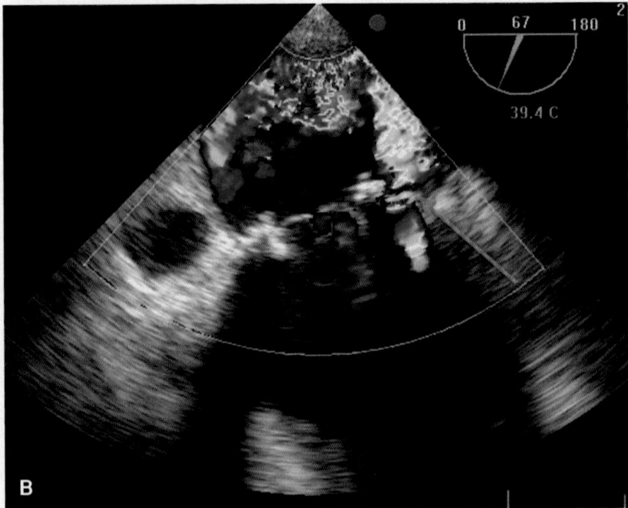

FIGURE 97.14 Two dimensional TEE image. A: Showing dehiscence (*arrow*) and color flow Doppler. B: Showing associated paravalvular leak (*arrow*) in the bio prosthetic mitral valve.

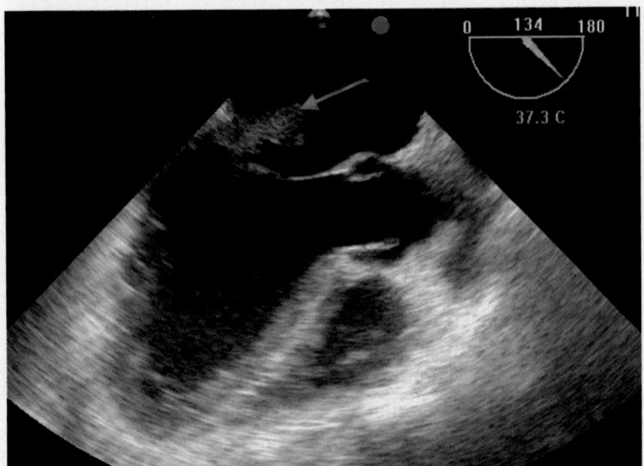

FIGURE 97.15 TEE image showing infective vegetation attached to AML (*arrow*).

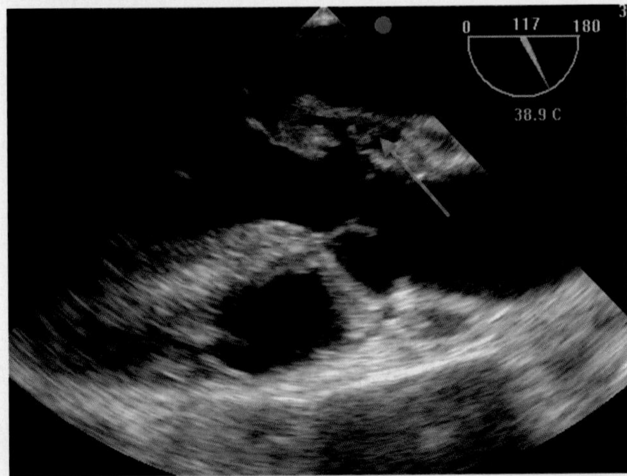

FIGURE 97.16 TEE image, midesophageal long axis showing periannular aortic abscess with cavitation (*arrow*).

difficult organisms, and congestive heart failure are some other indications for surgery in native valve or prosthetic valve endocarditis (25).

Surgery is indicated in prosthetic valve thrombosis if the patient is in advanced heart failure and unstable. ECMO can be used to stabilize the patient perioperatively. Surgery is also indicated if thrombus burden as detected by TEE is high (more than 0.8 cm^2 thrombus area). Fibrinolytic therapy is recommended for right-sided thrombosis with a large clot burden or New York Heart Association class III to IV symptoms. Fibrinolysis for left-sided lesions is reserved for patients in whom emergency surgery is high risk or contraindicated because this is associated with a 12% to 15% risk of cerebral embolism (26). Ultimately, all prosthetic valve lesions require valve replacement surgery. Reoperative mortality is high in this patient population.

IMPORTANT CONSIDERATIONS IN THE TREATMENT OF RIGHT VENTRICULAR FAILURE SECONDARY TO VALVULAR HEART DISEASE

Chronic pulmonary hypertension and RV failure secondary to VHD presents major therapeutic challenges to the intensive care physician. These patients are usually debilitated with low CO and pulmonary, hepatic, and renal dysfunction. Patients develop hepatic failure secondary to congestive hepatic cirrhosis. Ascites, malnutrition, reduced systemic vascular resistance, jaundice, coagulopathy, and the hepatorenal syndrome are the manifestations of hepatic dysfunction. The management of hepatorenal syndrome is challenging and will require invasive monitoring and, often, renal replacement therapy.

Treatment of pulmonary hypertension in the critically ill patient should be directed toward the treatment of the volume overload related to the underlying VHD such as MS. Decreasing afterload in MR or AR may increase the forward flow and decrease the pulmonary arterial pressures; inotropes may be added in some situations to improve CO. In general, medical treatment of underlying VHD takes the priority and urgent surgical treatment is indicated in patients with acute valvular obstruction and resultant RV failure. This approach, combined with maintenance of adequate coronary perfusion pressure, forms the mainstay of treatment of acute RV failure. Exacerbating factors of pulmonary hypertension, such as hypoxemia, hypercarbia, acidosis, hypothermia, hypervolemia, and increased intrathoracic pressure, should be corrected aggressively (27,28).

Pulmonary vasodilators should be used with caution in patients with left ventricular dysfunction as they increase the blood flow through the pulmonary circulation and can precipitate acute pulmonary edema. Recent advances in pharmacology provide intensivists with a wide variety of options for selective pulmonary vasodilatation, with studies favoring the use of inhaled prostaglandins and NO (29). Inhaled pulmonary vasodilators are preferred over intravenous agents because they do not decrease systemic blood pressure and also do not increase shunt fraction. Many newer drugs—including NO donors and inhaled phosphodiesterase inhibitors or prostacyclins or prostaglandins—are promising and may decrease pulmonary vascular resistance and promote CO; their impact on patient outcome is yet unclear.

References

1. Bermejo J, Yotti R. Low-gradient aortic valve stenosis: value and limitations of dobutamine stress testing. *Heart*. 2007;93(3):298–302.
2. Lieberman EB, Bashore TM, Hermiller JB, et al. Balloon aortic valvuloplasty in adults: failure of procedure to improve long-term survival. *J Am Coll Cardiol*. 1995;26:1522–1528.
3. Cao C, Ang SC, Indraratna P, et al. Systematic review and meta-analysis of transcatheter aortic valve implantation versus surgical aortic valve replacement for severe aortic stenosis. *Ann Cardiothorac Surg*. 2013;2:10–23.
4. Frerker C, Schewel J, Schlüter M, et al. Emergency transcatheter aortic valve replacement in patients with cardiogenic shock due to acutely decompensated aortic stenosis. *EuroIntervention*. 2016;11:1530–1536.
5. Shiga T, Wajima Z, Apfel CC, et al. Diagnostic accuracy of transesophageal echocardiography, helical computed tomography, and magnetic resonance imaging for suspected thoracic aortic dissection: systematic review and meta-analysis. *Arch Intern Med*. 2006;166:1350–1356.
6. Dabek J, Gasior Z, Monastyrska-Cup B, et al. Cardioversion and atrial stunning. *Pol Merkur Lekarski*. 2007;22:224–228.
7. Bonow RO, Carabello BA, Chatterjee K, et al. American College of Cardiology/American Heart Association Task Force on Practice Guidelines. 2008 focused update incorporated into the ACC/AHA 2006 guidelines for the management of patients with valvular heart disease: A report of the American College of Cardiology/American Heart Association Task Force on Practice Guidelines (Writing Committee to revise the 1998 guidelines for the management of patients with valvular heart disease). Endorsed by the Society of Cardiovascular Anesthesiologists, Society for Cardiovascular Angiography and Interventions, and Society of Thoracic Surgeons. *J Am Coll Cardiol*. 2008;52(13):e1–e142.
8. Maisel AS. Nesiritide: a new therapy for the treatment of heart failure. *Cardiovasc Toxicol*. 2003;3:37–42.
9. Keating GM, Goa KL. Nesiritide: a review of its use in acute decompensated heart failure. *Drugs*. 2003;63:47–70.
10. Loh E, Stamler JS, Hare JM, Loscalzo J, Colucci WS. Cardiovascular effects of inhaled nitric oxide in patients with left ventricular dysfunction. *Circulation*.1994;90:2780–2785.
11. Semigran MJ, Cockrill BA, Kacmarek R, et al. Hemodynamic effects of inhaled nitric oxide in heart failure. *J Am Coll Cardiol*. 1994;24: 982–988.
12. Bocchi EA, Bacal F, Auler JO Jr, et al. Inhaled nitric oxide leading to pulmonary edema in stable severe heart failure. *Am J Cardiol*. 1994; 74: 70–72.
13. Carpentier A. Cardiac valve surgery: the "French correction." *J Thorac Cardiovasc Surg*. 1983;86:323–337.
14. Gillam LD, Ford-Mukkamala L. Assessment of ventricular systolic function. In: Mathew JP, Ayoub CM, eds. *Clinical Manual and Review of Transesophageal Echocardiography*. New York: McGraw-Hill; 2005:74–90.
15. Durate IG, Shen Y, McDonald MJ, et al. Treatment of mitral regurgitation and coronary disease by coronary bypass alone: late results. *Ann Thorac Surg*. 1999;68:426–430.
16. Prifti E, Bonacchi M, Frati G, et al. Ischemic mitral valve regurgitation grade II-III–Correction in patients with impaired left ventricular function undergoing simultaneous coronary revascularization. *J Heart Valve Dis*. 2001;10:754–762.
17. Edmunds LH Jr. Ischemic mitral regurgitation. In: *Cardiac Surgery in the Adult*. New York: McGraw-Hill; 1997:657.
18. Fontana ME, Sparks EA, Boudoulas H, et al. Mitral valve prolapse and the mitral valve prolapse syndrome. *Curr Probl Cardiol*. 1991;16:309–375.
19. Vakil K, Roukoz H, Sarraf M, et al. Safety and efficacy of the MitraClip® system for severe mitral regurgitation: a systematic review. *Catheter Cardiovasc Interv*. 2014;84(1):129–136.
20. Kothandan H, Vui KH, Khung KY, Nian CH. Anesthesia management for MitraClip device implantation. *Ann Card Anaesth*. 2014;17(1):17–22.
21. Jeon D, Luo H, Iwami T, et al. The usefulness of a 10% air–10% blood–80% saline mixture for contrast echocardiography—Doppler measurement of pulmonary artery systolic pressure. *J Am Coll Cardiol*. 2002;39: 124–129.
22. Onoda K, Yasuda F, Takao M, et al. Long-term follow-up after Carpentier-Edwards ring annuloplasty for tricuspid regurgitation. *Ann Thorac Surg*. 2000;70:796–799.
23. Trichon BH, O'Connor CM. Secondary mitral and tricuspid regurgitation accompanying left ventricular systolic dysfunction: Is it important and how is it treated? *Am Heart J*. 2002;144:373–376.
24. Karchmer AW. Infective endocarditis. In: Braunwald E, Zipes DP, Lippy P, eds. *Heart Disease: A Textbook of Cardiovascular Medicine*. 6th ed. Philadelphia, PA: WB Saunders; 2001:1723.
25. Prendergast BD, Tornos P. Valvular heart disease: changing concepts in disease management. Surgery for infective endocarditis: who and when? *Circulation*. 2010;121:1141–1152.
26. Roudaut R, Labbe T, Lorient-Roudaut MF, et al. Mechanical cardiac valve thrombosis: Is fibrinolysis justified? *Circulation*. 1992;86(Suppl5): II8–II15.
27. Minai OA, Yared JP, Kaw R, et al. Perioperative risk and management in patients with pulmonary hypertension. *Chest*. 2013;144:329–340.
28. Subramaniam K, Yared JP. Management of pulmonary hypertension in the operating room. *Semin Cardiothorac Vasc Anesth*. 2007;11:119–136.
29. Blaise G, Langleben D, Hubert B. Pulmonary arterial hypertension: pathophysiology and anesthetic approach. *Anesthesiology*. 2003;99:1415–1432.

CHAPTER

98

Cardiac Dysrhythmias

MATTHEW S. MCKILLOP, WILLIAM M. MILES, and JAMIE B. CONTI

BRADYARRHYTHMIAS

Bradycardia is a common finding in hospitalized patients, especially during sleep. An increase in vagal tone or a decrease in sympathetic outflow may result in sinus bradycardia, sinus pauses, or atrioventricular (AV) nodal block—all physiologic findings that may have no clinical significance. Bradyarrhythmias can generally be categorized as either sinoatrial (SA) or AV conduction abnormalities.

Sinoatrial Abnormalities

Sinus pauses may be caused by either SA conduction block or sinus arrest. SA conduction block occurs when impulses generated by the sinus node are not transmitted to the surrounding atrial myocardium due to peri-SA nodal tissue slowing or conduction block. The three categories are first-, second-, and third-degree SA block. First-degree SA block is not manifested on electrocardiogram (ECG) as it is merely the delay between the sinus impulse formation and atrial activation. Second-degree SA block can be type I or type II. Type I (Wenckebach) is manifest by group beating with progressive shortening of PP intervals until a P wave is absent. The subsequent PP interval is usually less than twice the shortest previous PP cycle. Type II SA block has fixed PP intervals followed by a pause without a P wave. This pause is twice the previous PP interval (Fig. 98.1). Third-degree SA block is also not apparent on the surface ECG as no sinus impulse can escape the SA node. This disorder cannot be differentiated from sinus arrest.

Sinus arrest is the failure of automaticity in which no impulses are generated by the sinus node (Fig. 98.2). *Sick sinus syndrome* is dysfunction of the sinus node or SA conduction in which no adequate escape mechanism is present resulting in symptomatic bradycardia. There are intrinsic and extrinsic causes of SA abnormalities. The most prevalent intrinsic cause of sinus node dysfunction is aging with replacement of sinus nodal tissue and the surrounding atrium by fibrotic degeneration. Extrinsic causes of sinus node dysfunction include drugs (Table 98.1), electrolyte abnormalities (hyperkalemia), endocrine disorders (hypothyroidism), neurally mediated conditions (vasovagal syncope), and intracranial hypertension.

Diagnosis and Treatment

1. Record a 12-lead ECG.
2. If hypotension or significant symptoms (i.e., dizziness or presyncope) are absent, no immediate treatment is required. Symptoms dictate the treatment plan. Asymptomatic bradycardia due to sinus node dysfunction is not usually an emergency.
3. Evaluate the ECG for the following:
   - Evidence of acute myocardial infarction (MI)
   - Mechanism of bradycardia
   - P-wave regularity (sinus or an ectopic atrial rhythm)
   - Abrupt pauses or group beating in the sinus rhythm (suggests SA block)
   - P waves without QRS complexes (suggests AV block)
   - QRS axis and width for coexistent bundle branch block
4. In cases of sinus bradycardia, give no treatment unless hypotension or symptoms are present. If there are symptoms, then consider giving intravenous (IV) atropine, 0.04 mg/kg of body weight.
5. In cases of SA block or sinus arrest, give no treatment unless hypotension or symptoms are present or the rhythm is drug induced (*stop drug*).
6. If sick sinus syndrome is present, then treatment depends on first excluding and/or reversing identified reversible causes. If bradycardia persists, especially in the context of symptoms (dizziness, presyncope, or congestive heart failure), further intervention is usually required.

Atrioventricular Conduction Abnormalities

AV conduction abnormalities can be categorized as first-, second-, or third-degree AV block. In first-degree AV block, every P wave is conducted to the ventricles but with a prolonged PR interval (usually defined as >200 msec). Second-degree AV block is characterized by intermittent P waves not conducted to the ventricles and is further broken down into type I (Wenckebach), type II, and two-to-one conduction. Third-degree AV block demonstrates no conduction between the atrium and ventricles. To establish the diagnosis of complete or third-degree AV block, the sinus rate is faster than the ventricular rate, and there must be no observed consistent relationship between the P waves and QRS complexes.

Noninvasive Methods for Determining Site of Block

In AV block, the conduction abnormality may be located within the AV node, the His bundle, or the bundle branches (1,2). Determining the location of block is important as this will affect immediate and long-term treatment. A 12-lead ECG and diagnostic maneuvers are helpful in establishing the level of block. Baseline intervals on the ECG, including PR interval, QRS duration, and axis, are important. Responses to noninvasive interventions, including IV atropine administration, exercise, or vagal maneuvers may also help differentiate between AV nodal and infranodal (below the AV node) block (Table 98.2). Specifically, interventions that slow AV nodal conduction, such as carotid sinus massage or other vagal maneuvers, will worsen AV nodal block. However, because of sinus slowing and the decreased rate of His–Purkinje stimulation in these situations, infranodal AV block may actually improve. Conversely, interventions that improve AV nodal conduction, such as exercise and atropine, can worsen infranodal AV block

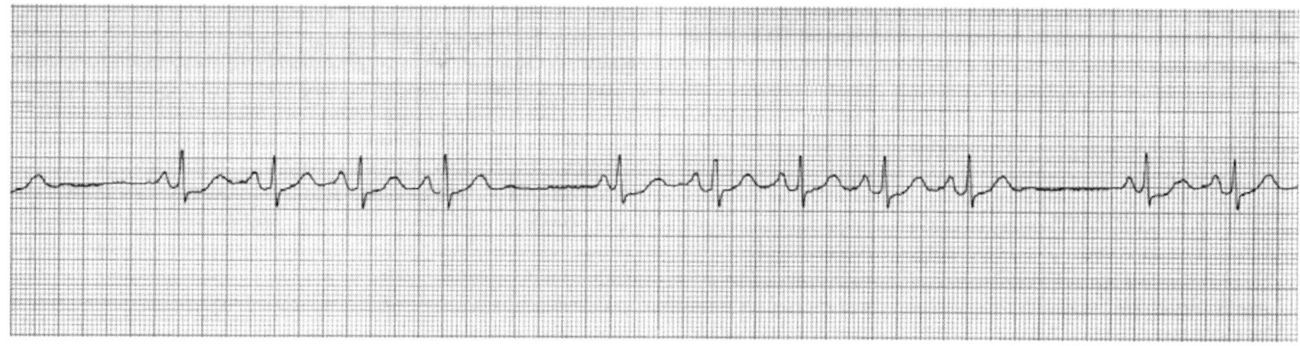

FIGURE 98.1 Lead II rhythm strip. Second-degree type II sinoatrial block. The P–P interval is initially 720 msec and appears to prolong to 1,440 msec (exactly twice the prior P–P interval).

because the acceleration of electrical stimulation into the His–Purkinje system worsens conduction if this tissue is diseased whereas healthy tissue will allow accelerating conduction without interruption.

First-Degree AV Block or Prolonged PR Interval

The PR interval is a reflection of intra-atrial and AV conduction time and is measured from the onset of the P wave to the beginning of the QRS complex. Conduction delay in the atrium, AV node, bundle of His, or bundle branches all may result in a prolonged PR interval. The longer the PR interval becomes, the more likely the delay resides in the AV node.

Second-Degree Type I AV Block (AV Wenckebach)

In second-degree AV block, type I (AV Wenckebach), there is progressive lengthening of the PR interval culminating in a blocked P wave (Fig. 98.3). The QRS duration may be narrow or wide, depending on the presence of bundle branch block. When the QRS is narrow, it suggests the block is at the level of the AV node and will improve with atropine or exercise and worsen with carotid sinus massage. It can be seen in young healthy individuals with increased vagal tone, especially nocturnally. It is commonly due to reversible causes such as AV nodal slowing drugs.

Second-Degree Type II AV Block

In second-degree AV block, type II the PR intervals are normal or slightly prolonged and are exactly the same length before and after the nonconducted P waves (Fig. 98.4). As opposed to second-degree, type I block, AV conduction may worsen with sinus acceleration due to atropine or exercise and may improve with carotid massage. Type II second-degree AV block is most likely located below the AV node, residing in the His bundle if there is a narrow QRS duration (rare) or in the bundle branches if there is wide QRS duration (common). These patients are often symptomatic with dyspnea, fatigue, and syncope, and can progress to complete AV block.

Two-to-One AV Block

In a two-to-one AV block, every other P wave conducts to the ventricle, and the conducted PR interval may be either normal or prolonged (Fig. 98.5). The level of block—AV nodal versus infranodal—cannot be determined with certainty without an electrophysiology study. A narrow QRS duration suggests that the block is in the AV node or rarely the His bundle, whereas a wide QRS suggests block in the bundle branches.

Third-Degree AV Block or Complete AV Block

In complete AV block there is no P wave to QRS relationship. The sinus rate (P-to-P intervals) is faster than the escape rate. The ventricular escape rate is usually less than 50 beats per minute (bpm), with the exception of a congenital AV block (Fig. 98.6). If the escape rhythm has a narrow QRS complex, then it originates in the AV junction and the site of block is either AV nodal or, less likely, the His bundle. If the QRS is wide, the site of block is likely within the bundle branches. If occasional P waves are observed to capture the ventricle but most do not, then the term high-grade or advanced AV block may be used.

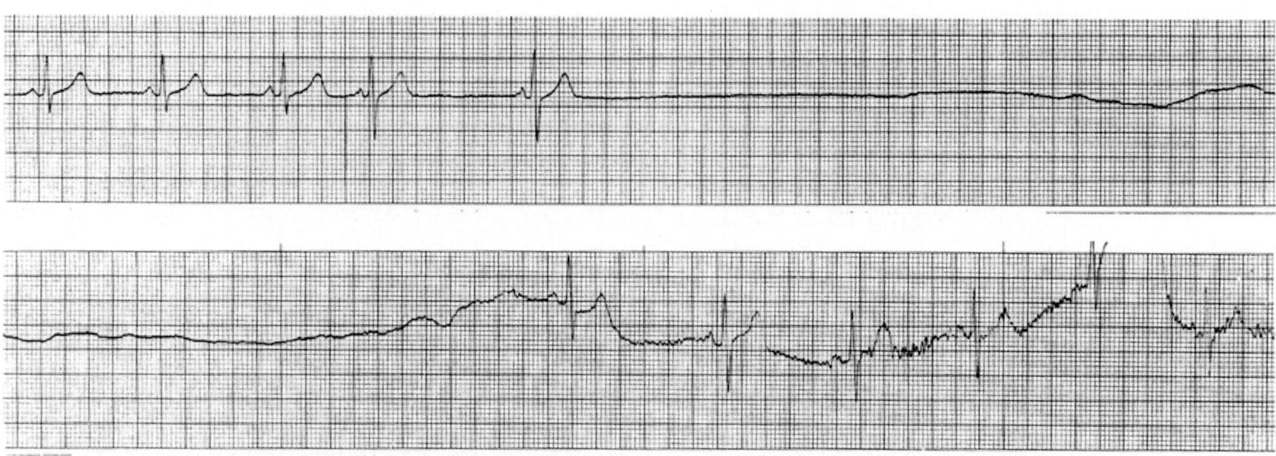

FIGURE 98.2 Lead II rhythm strip. Sinus arrest with no ventricular escape.

TABLE 98.1 Drugs Affecting Sinus Node Function

Antiarrhythmics
Class IA (quinidine, procainamide, disopyramide)
Class IC (flecainide, propafenone)
Class III (sotalol, amiodarone)
β-Blocking agents
Calcium channel blockers
Verapamil
Diltiazem
Cardiac glycosides
Miscellaneous
Lithium
Cimetidine
Diphenylhydantoin
Clonidine and dexmedetomidine

TABLE 98.2 Noninvasive Interventions to Determine Site of Atrioventricular (AV) Block

Intervention	AV Nodal Site of Block	Infranodal Site of Block
Atropine	AV block improves	AV block worsens
Exercise	AV block improves	AV block worsens
Carotid sinus massage	AV block worsens	AV block improves

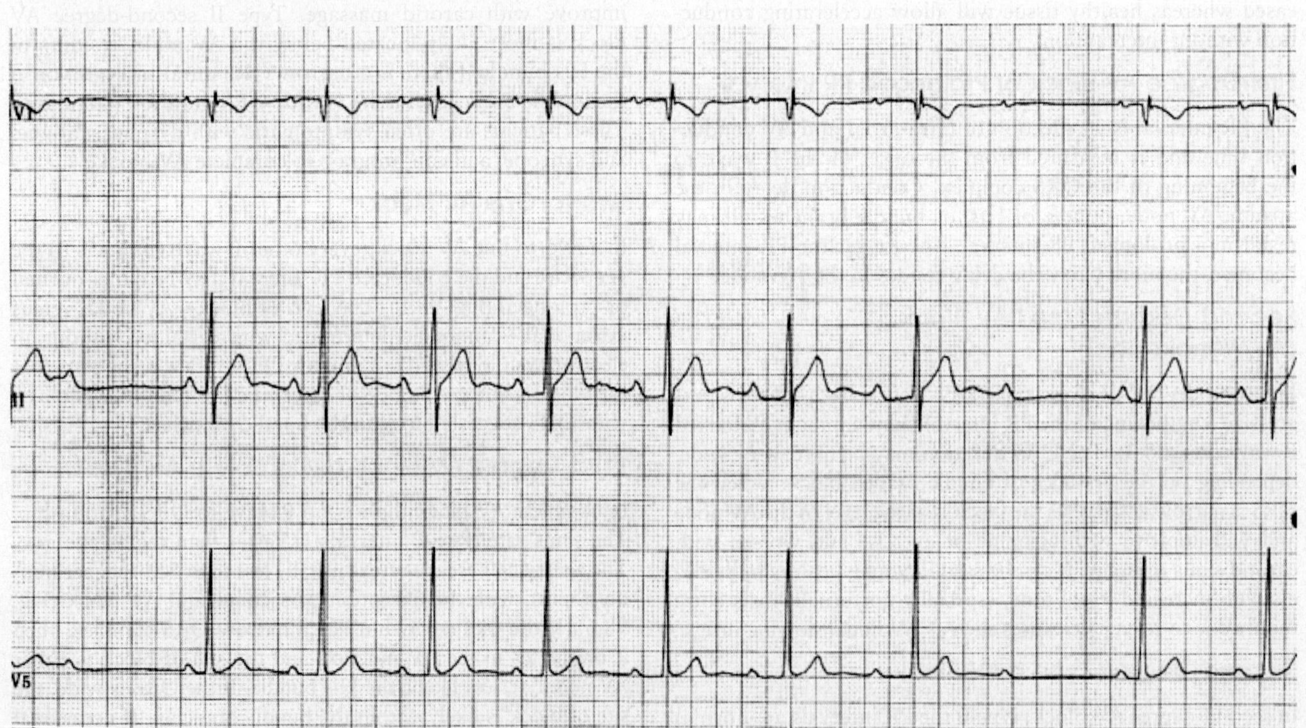

FIGURE 98.3 Simultaneous leads V1, II, and V5. Sinus rhythm with type I second-degree atrioventricular conduction block.

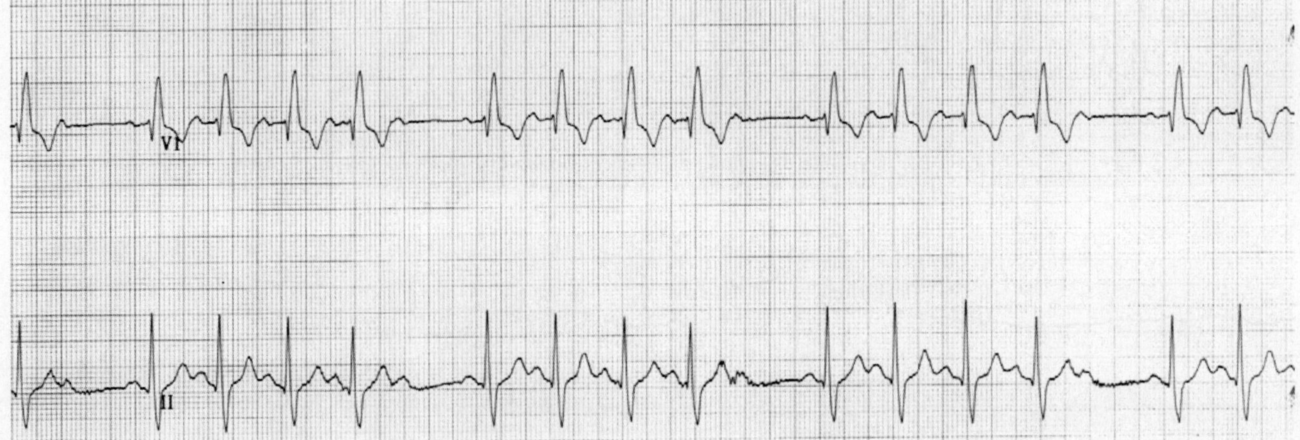

FIGURE 98.4 Simultaneous leads V1, II, and V5. Sinus rhythm with second-degree type II atrioventricular conduction block.

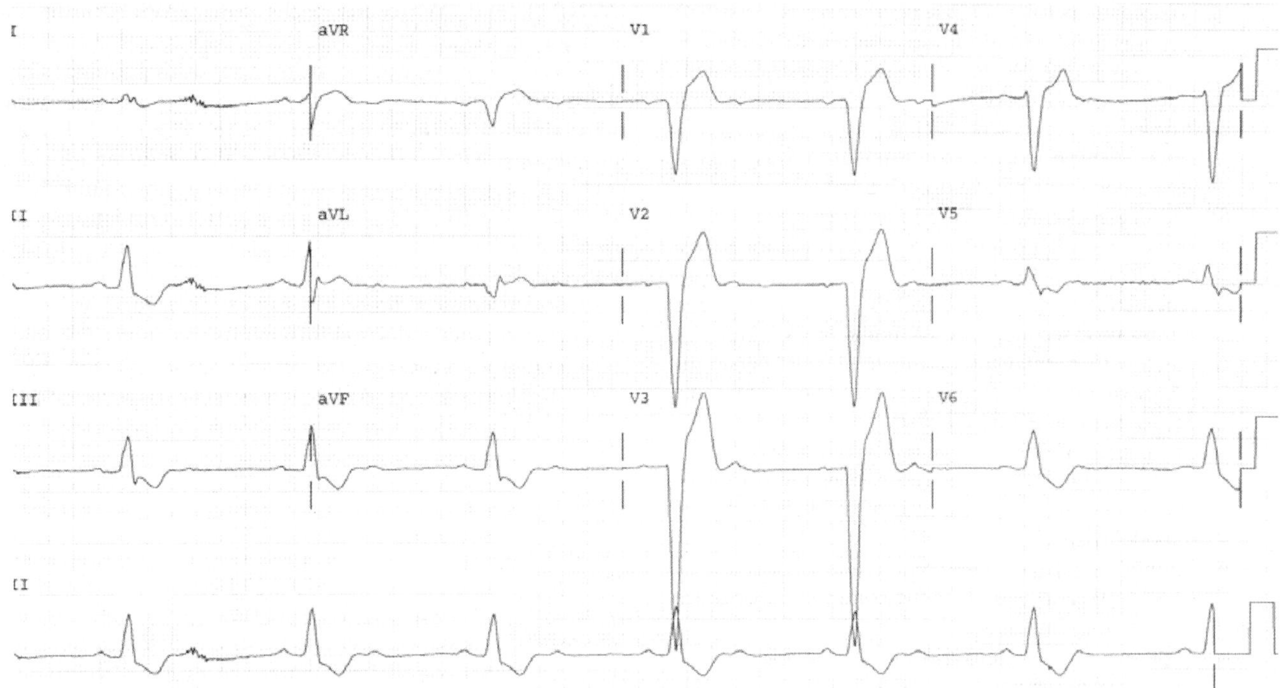

FIGURE 98.5 A 12-lead electrocardiogram. Sinus rhythm with 2:1 atrioventricular conduction block. The normal PR interval when conducted and the left bundle branch block suggest block below the His bundle.

General Pacing Considerations for AV Conduction Abnormalities

1. Record a 12-lead ECG and try to determine site of block by noninvasive methods.
2. In the setting of an acute inferior wall MI, the site of block is usually the AV node and is usually transient with successful reperfusion.
   a. Insert a temporary pacemaker if there is hemodynamic compromise secondary to heart block.
   b. Proceed to permanent pacing if there is persistent hemodynamic compromise, continued symptoms due to ongoing AV nodal block, or persistent high-grade or complete AV block.
3. In the setting of an acute anterior MI, the site of block is considered likely to be infranodal especially in the context of a wide QRS.
   a. Insert a temporary pacemaker if there is hemodynamic compromise secondary to heart block.

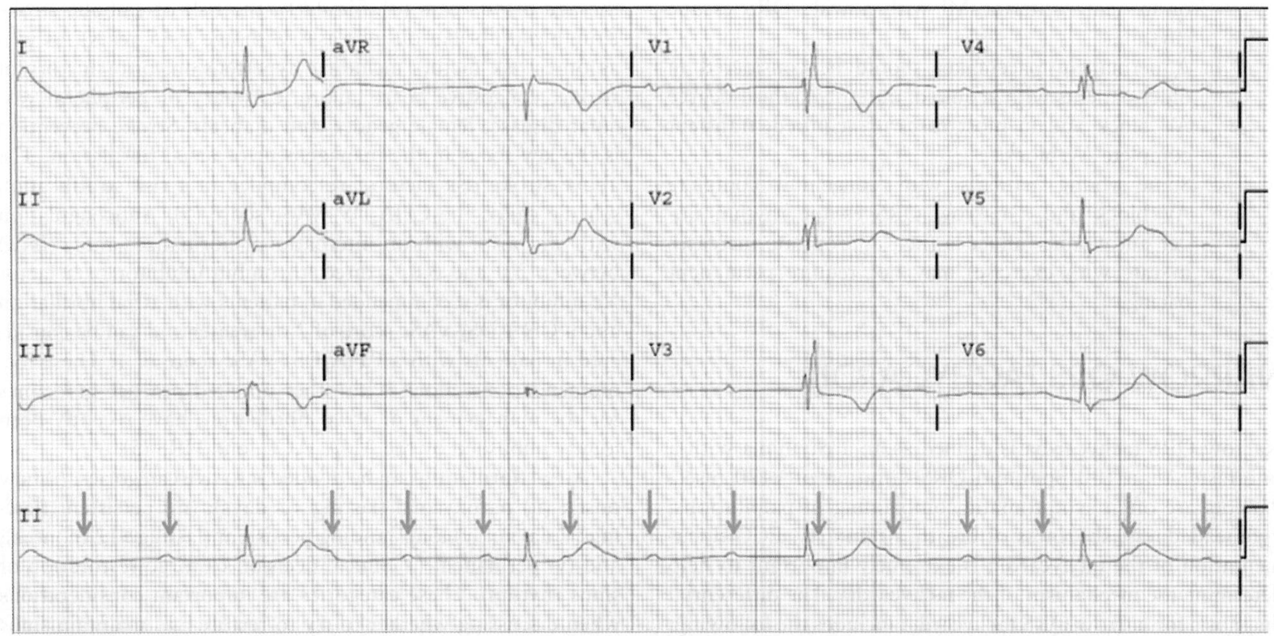

FIGURE 98.6 A 12-lead electrocardiogram. Sinus rhythm with third-degree AV conduction block and a ventricular escape rhythm. The *arrows* indicate P waves.

   b. Proceed to permanent pacing if there is persistent hemodynamic compromise, continued symptoms due to ongoing AV nodal block, or persistent high-grade or complete AV block.
   c. Proceed to permanent pacing, if the transient AV block is suspected to be infranodal and associated with a persistent bundle branch block.
4. Second-degree AV block, Type I
   a. Progressive PR prolongation is present prior to AV conduction block.
   b. Proceed to temporary pacing if there is hemodynamic compromise secondary to AV nodal block (rare).
   c. Proceed to permanent pacing if there is persistent hemodynamic compromise or continued symptoms due to ongoing AV nodal block.
5. Second-degree AV block, Type II
   a. If there is no PR progressive prolongation prior to block, then the site of block is most likely in the infranodal tissue.
   b. Temporary pacemaker is required when associated with significant hemodynamic compromise or unrelenting symptoms.
   c. A permanent pacemaker should be considered in most cases of infranodal AV block.
6. Two-to-one AV block
   a. A relatively short PR interval (≤160 msec) with a wide QRS suggests infranodal block.
   b. A temporary pacemaker is indicated in patients with significant hemodynamic compromise, unrelenting symptoms, or with a wide QRS following an acute anterior MI.
   c. Observe other periods on telemetry or rhythm strips for evidence of 3:2 (Wenckebach) second-degree AV block, type I or second-degree AV block, type II to help define the level of block.
7. Third-degree AV block
   a. A temporary pacemaker is indicated in patients with hemodynamic compromise, unrelenting symptoms, or in acute anterior MI with a wide QRS escape rhythm.
   b. A permanent pacemaker should be considered in older patients with acquired, unresolved third-degree AV block and in most cases of acquired, transient complete AV block.
   c. Some young patients with congenital complete AV block and a narrow QRS escape rhythm under autonomic influence (i.e., appropriate increases in rate with exercise) may not require permanent pacing.

NARROW QRS TACHYCARDIA

Narrow QRS tachycardia is defined as an arrhythmia with a rate faster than 100 bpm and QRS duration of <120 msec. Patients are often symptomatic complaining of palpitations, lightheadedness, shortness of breath, or anxiety. ECG documentation of the tachycardia is extremely important to help determine the mechanism of the tachycardia. The differential diagnosis for narrow QRS tachycardia includes the following: sinus tachycardia, atrial tachycardia, atrial flutter, atrial fibrillation, junctional tachycardia, AV nodal reentry tachycardia (AVNRT), and AV reentry tachycardia (AVRT) using an accessory pathway.

A 12-lead ECG can be helpful in distinguishing sinus tachycardia from other narrow QRS tachycardias by allowing the evaluation of the morphology of the P wave. A P-wave morphology that is distinctly different than sinus or a P wave that is notably absent suggests the mechanism is unlikely to be originating from the sinus node. Atrial fibrillation is an irregular tachycardia due to a rapid, irregular atrial rhythm with variable AV conduction. The ventricular response to the more organized atrial flutter rhythm can be regular or irregular depending on conduction through the AV node. The three most common causes of regular paroxysmal narrow QRS tachycardia are AVNRT, AVRT, and atrial tachycardia, respectively (3,4).

Atrial Flutter

Atrial flutter typically has an atrial rate of 250 to 350 bpm. The most common form of atrial flutter uses a right atrial macroreentrant circuit that includes the cavotricuspid isthmus (the region of tissue between the tricuspid valve and the inferior vena cava). Typical atrial flutter has a classic "sawtooth" pattern of atrial activation in the inferior leads of the ECG (Fig. 98.7). Flutter waves can be better appreciated during rapid tachycardia upon slowing of the ventricular response by carotid sinus massage.

Atrial Fibrillation

Atrial fibrillation is the most common supraventricular tachyarrhythmia in the United States (3,4). The atrial rhythm is irregular with an atrial rate of 350 to 500 bpm (Fig. 98.8). It is a major cause of cardiovascular morbidity and mortality, with an increased risk of death, congestive heart failure, and stroke. The incidence of atrial fibrillation increases with age, with a lifetime risk of one in four men and women older than the age of 40 years (4). Similarly, the risk of embolic stroke from atrial fibrillation increases with age (>65 years), as well as other risk factors including hypertension, prior history of stroke, congestive heart failure, coronary or peripheral vascular disease, female gender, and diabetes. Stroke prevention is the key focus in the management of atrial fibrillation. The above stroke risk factors are compiled in a risk stratification scheme called the CHA_2DS_2-VASc score (5). Anticoagulation with warfarin, with an international normalized ratio (INR) between 2.0 and 3.0, a direct thrombin inhibitor or a factor Xa inhibitor is recommended in patients with atrial fibrillation and a CHA_2DS_2-VASc score of 2 or greater and can be considered in patients with a CHA_2DS_2-VASc score of 1. These recommendations, along with other updated practice guidelines for the management of atrial fibrillation, have recently been jointly published by the AHA, ACC, and HRS (5).

Atrial fibrillation can be divided into five categories: (i) new onset; (ii) paroxysmal (lasting <7 days); (iii) persistent (lasting >7 days); (iv) longstanding persistent (lasting >12 months); and (v) permanent (a clinical decision to forgo restoration of sinus rhythm). These categories are important considerations when discussing whether to try to restore and maintain sinus rhythm as the longer atrial fibrillation persists, the harder it becomes to achieve that goal.

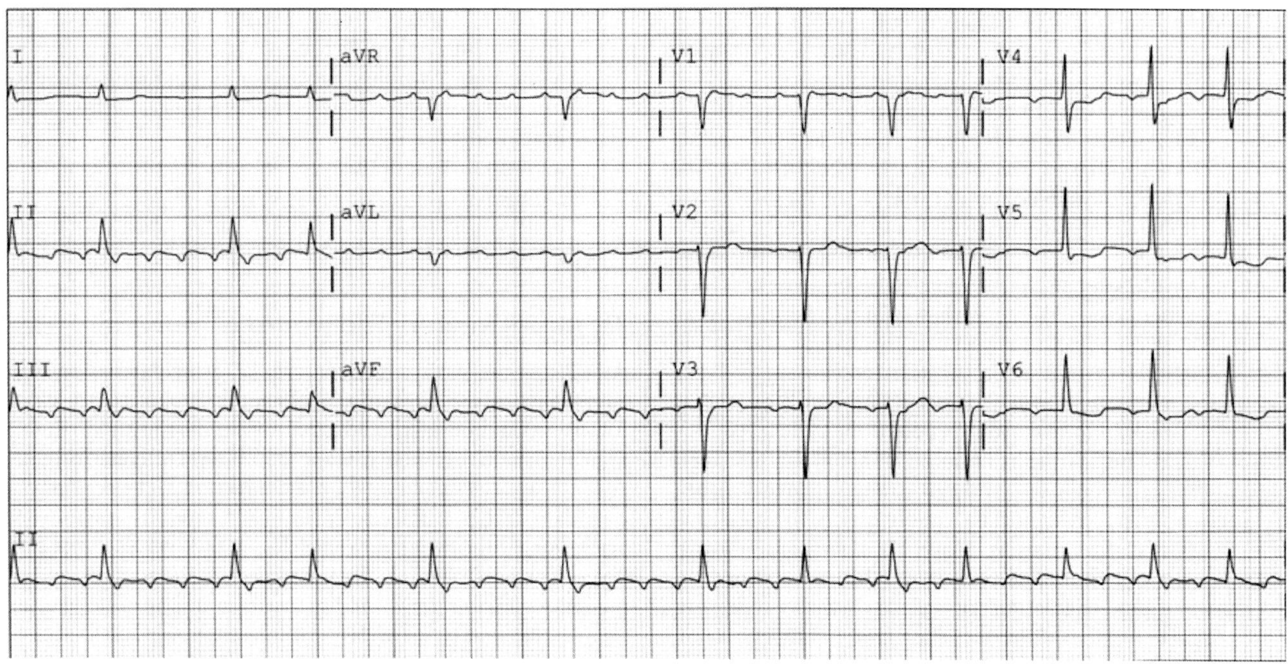

FIGURE 98.7 A 12-lead electrocardiogram. Atrial flutter with variable atrioventricular conduction.

Acute Treatment

1. Recent onset (<48 hours, preferably with documentation of onset) without significant heart disease and stable:
   a. Pharmacologic cardioversion with flecainide (300 mg per mouth once), propafenone (600 mg per mouth once), procainamide (5–10 mg/kg IV over 20 minutes), ibutilide (1 mg IV over 10 minutes), then repeat (after 10 minutes), or amiodarone (1,000 mg IV over first 24 hours)
   b. Electrical cardioversion with sedation
2. Recent onset (<48 hours) and unstable: Proceed with immediate cardioversion

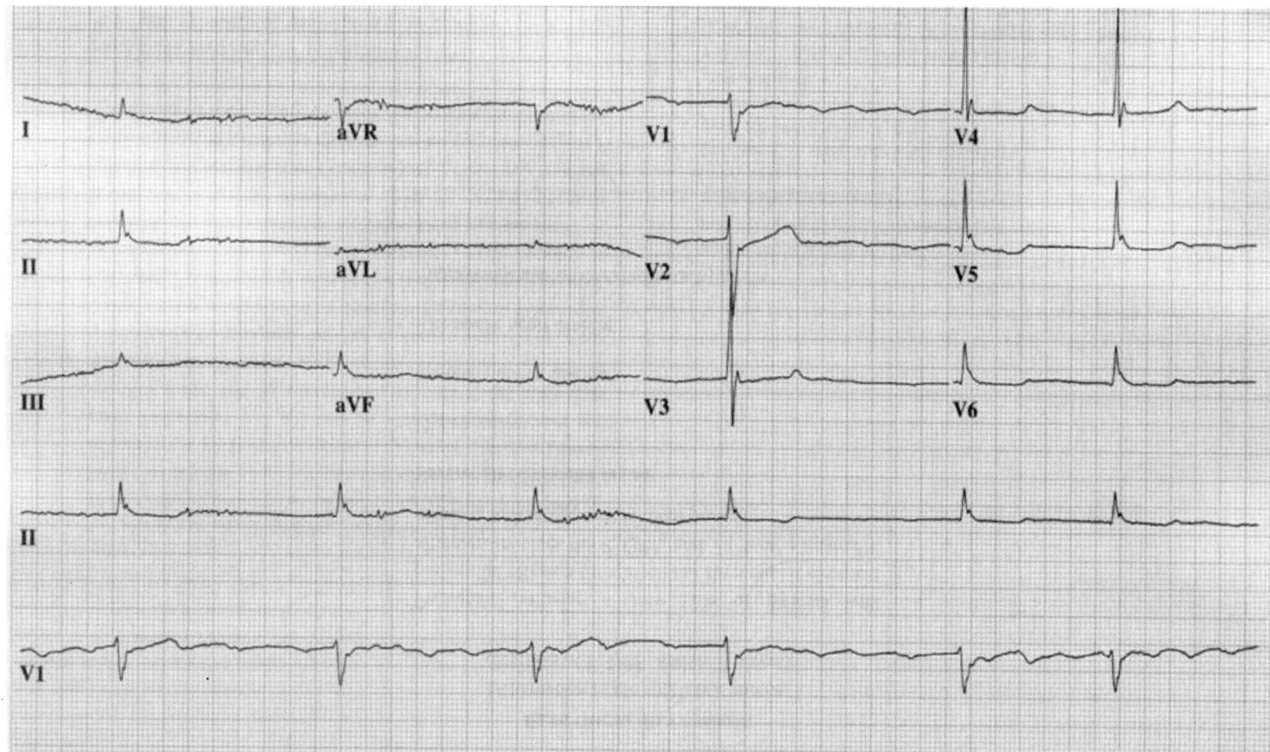

FIGURE 98.8 A 12-lead electrocardiogram. Atrial fibrillation with slow ventricular response. Note that there are no discernible P waves and that the rhythm is irregular.

3. More than 48 hours (or unsure of duration) and stable:
   a. Control ventricular rate with β-blockers or non-dihydropyridine calcium channel blockers
   b. Patients with two or more risk factors on the CHA_2DS_2-VASc score should receive oral anticoagulation with warfarin, with a goal of INR of 2.0 to 3.0, a direct thrombin inhibitor or a factor Xa inhibitor.
   c. If there is a plan to restore sinus rhythm with cardioversion or antiarrhythmic medications and the atrial fibrillation has been present for over 48 hours, then either anticoagulate with warfarin (maintaining at least 3 consecutive weeks of therapeutic INR levels prior to cardioversion) or start and continue a direct thrombin inhibitor or factor Xa inhibitor for at least 3 weeks prior to cardioversion. If the patient requires or desires earlier restoration of sinus rhythm, then the patient may undergo transesophageal echocardiography prior to cardioversion. If no intracardiac thrombus is identified, then proceed with cardioversion. The patient should be continued on oral anticoagulation for at least 4 weeks following cardioversion regardless of the CHA_2DS_2-VASc score. Anticoagulation beyond those 4 weeks is dependent on the $CHADS_2$-VASc score. (5).
4. More than 48 hours and difficulty obtaining adequate rate control: Proceed with transesophageal echocardiogram and cardioversion.
   a. If no thrombus, then cardiovert and anticoagulate as above.
   b. If thrombus is present, then anticoagulate and control rate until thrombus has resolved.

AV Nodal Reentry Tachycardia

AVNRT is the most common form of a regular paroxysmal supraventricular tachycardia (SVT) and is due to reentry utilizing AV nodal and perinodal atrial tissue. The heart rhythm is regular, usually between 130 and 250 bpm. Different forms of AVNRT are classified based on the direction and electrophysiologic properties of the circuit. Typically, there is simultaneous activation of the atria and ventricles, with P waves either hidden or partially visible at the end of the QRS (Fig. 98.9A), producing a pseudo-r′ in V1 and pseudo-s in inferior leads during tachycardia that is not present in sinus rhythm (Fig. 98.9B,C).

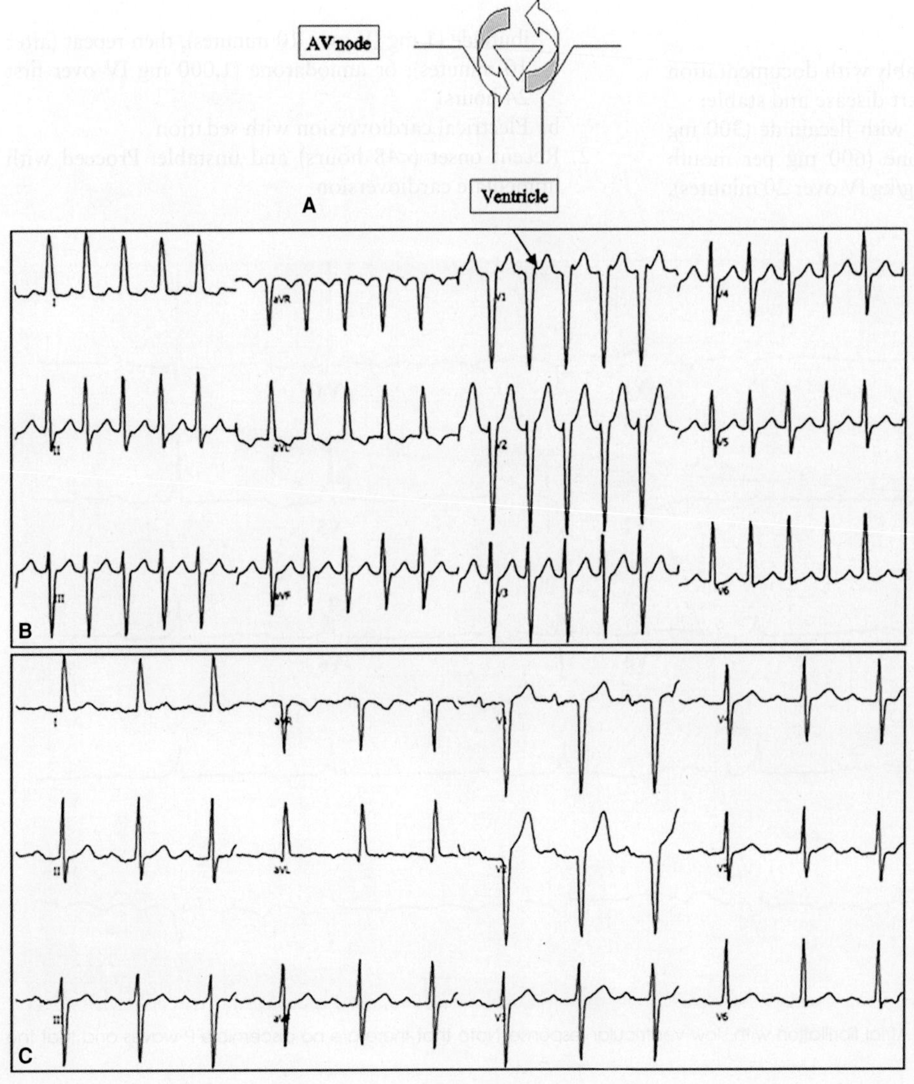

FIGURE 98.9 A: Schematic of atrioventricular (AV) nodal reentry tachycardia where the ventricle is passively activated. B: The most common form is anterograde conduction down a slow AV nodal pathway and retrograde atrial activation via a fast AV nodal pathway showing AVNRT with a pseudo-r′ in lead V1 denoted by the *arrow*. C: A 12-lead electrocardiogram showing sinus rhythm of the same patient in (B). Note that there is no r′ in lead V1.

AV Reentry Tachycardia

AVRT is due to reentry involving an accessory pathway, an abnormal electrical connection between the atria and ventricle (6). During sinus rhythm, if the accessory pathway conducts anterograde, then a short PR interval, broad QRS, and a slurring of the upstroke of the QRS (i.e., a delta wave with ventricular pre-excitation typical of the Wolff–Parkinson–White pattern), may be present on surface 12-lead ECG (Fig. 98.10A). The tachycardia that typically results has a narrow QRS due to anterograde conduction down the AV node followed by retrograde atrial activation via the accessory pathway. This circuit is termed orthodromic AVRT (Fig. 98.10B). Antidromic AV reentry (the reverse of this circuit) will be discussed below in the section on pre-excited tachycardias. Both the atria and ventricles are essential parts of these tachycardia circuits. Orthodromic AV reentry is a regular paroxysmal tachycardia, usually with the RP interval less than the PR interval (Fig. 98.10C).

If atrial fibrillation occurs in a patient with an anterograde-conducting accessory pathway, the fibrillatory impulses can conduct rapidly to the ventricle via the accessory pathway resulting in variable QRS morphologies due to differing amounts of fusion in ventricular activation via the accessory pathway versus the AV node (Fig. 98.10D). Rarely, this rapid ventricular activation can degenerate into ventricular fibrillation causing sudden cardiac death. If pre-excited atrial fibrillation is hemodynamically unstable, then it should be electrically cardioverted. However, if the patient is hemodynamically stable, then one can consider the use of IV ibutilide or procainamide as first-line medical therapy to slow AP conduction

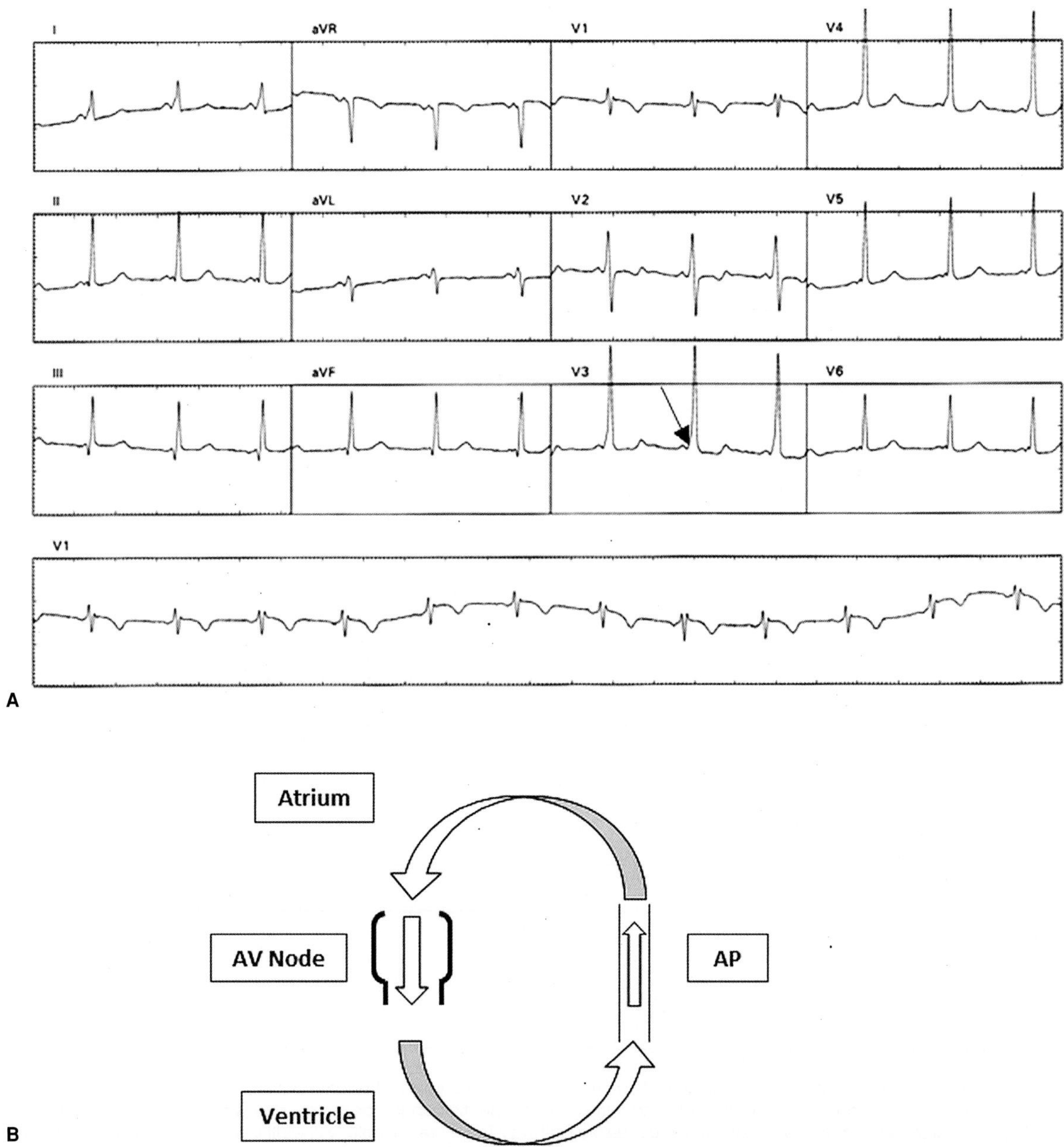

FIGURE 98.10 A: A 12-lead electrocardiogram. Sinus rhythm with ventricular pre-excitation manifested as a delta wave (*arrow*), consistent with Wolff–Parkinson–White syndrome. B: Schematic of orthodromic atrioventricular (AV) reentrant tachycardia with anterograde ventricular activation from the AV node and retrograde activation via an accessory pathway (AP). (*Continued*)

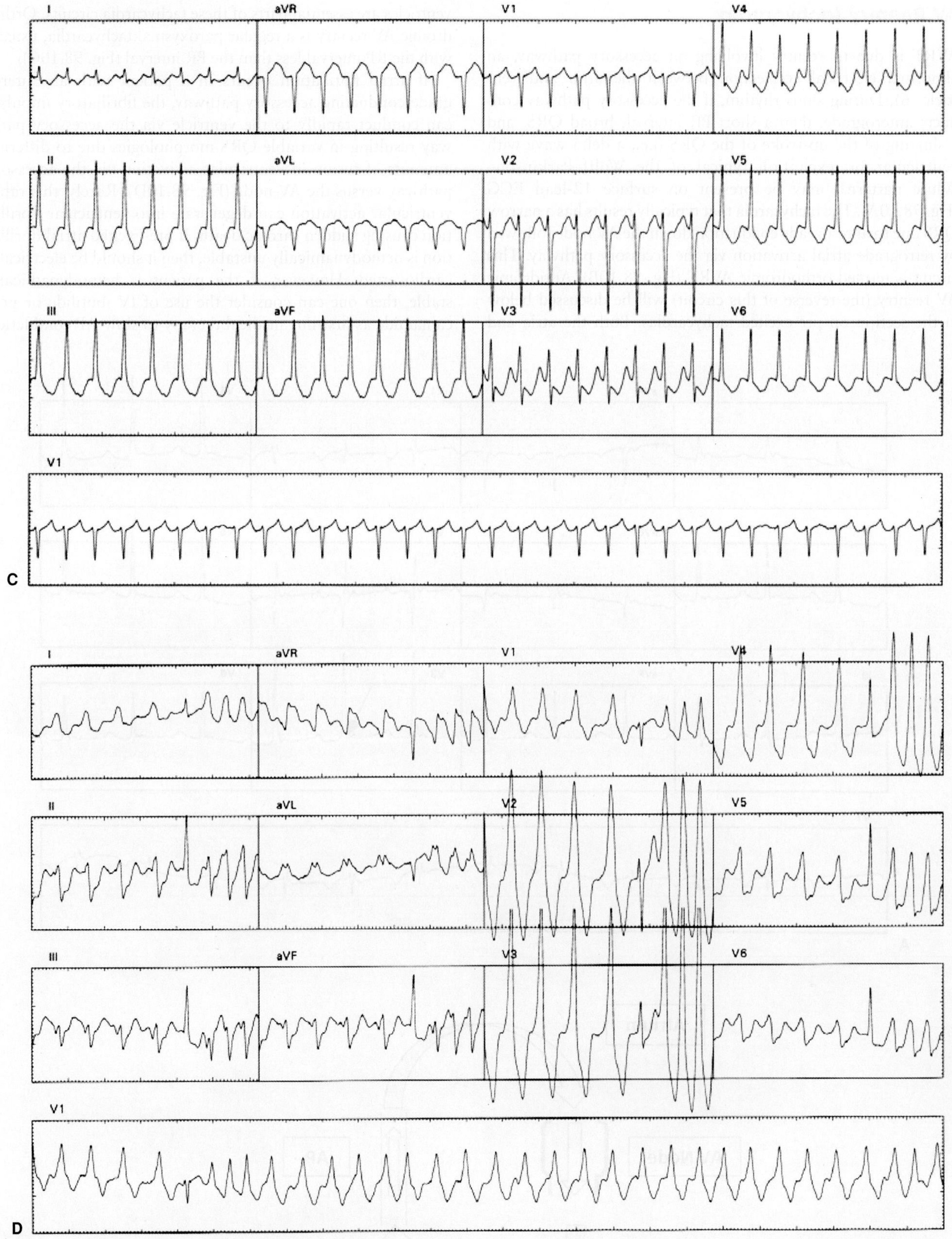

FIGURE 98.10 (*Continued*) C: A 12-lead electrocardiogram. Narrow-complex tachycardia in the same patient was found to be AV reentrant tachycardia with anterograde conduction down the AV node and retrograde conduction up the accessory pathway. D: A 12-lead electrocardiogram. Atrial fibrillation in a patient with anterograde conducting accessory pathway. There are variable QRS widths, as there is conduction simultaneously down both the AV node and the accessory pathway. This patient is at risk for ventricular fibrillation and sudden cardiac death.

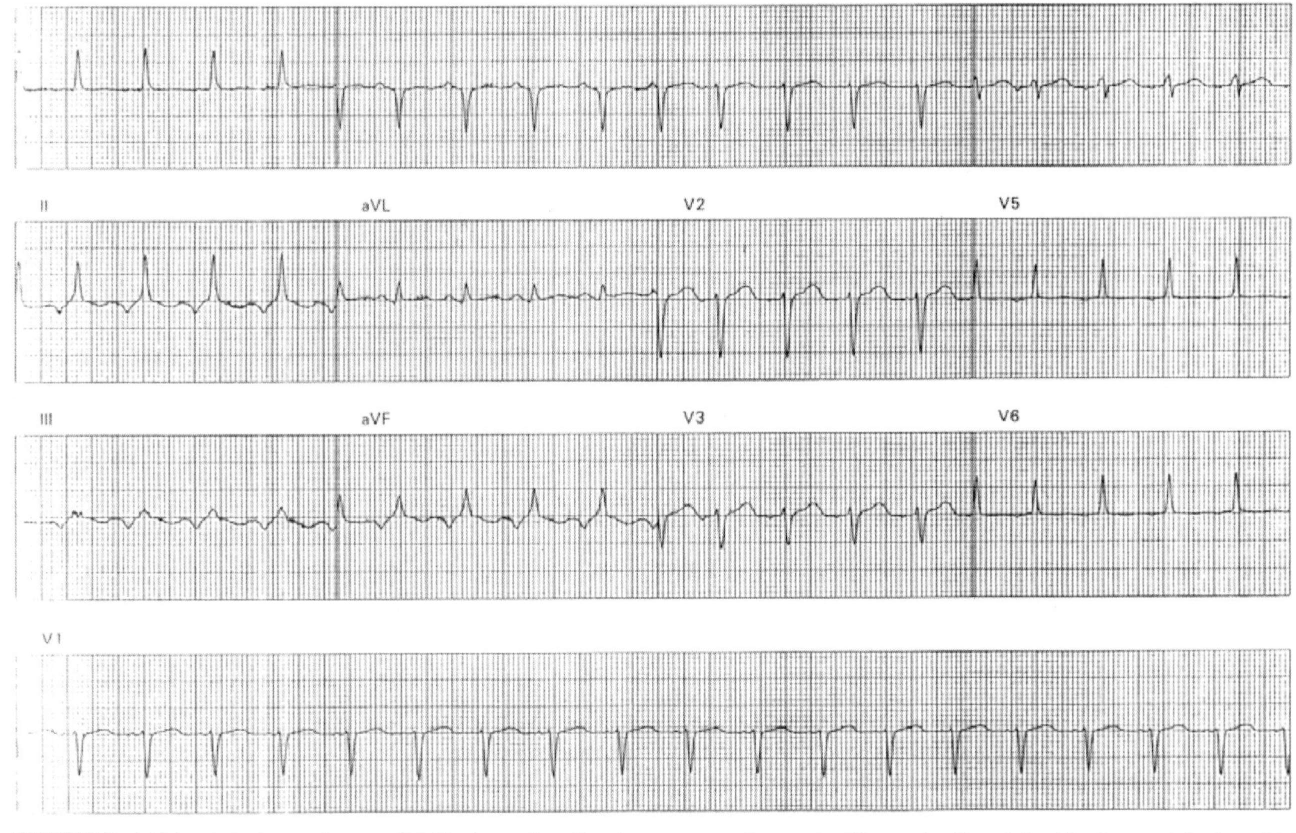

FIGURE 98.11 A 12-lead electrocardiogram. Atrial tachycardia with a P wave preceding each QRS complex. The origin of the P wave is the low atrial septum.

and/or terminate atrial fibrillation, as other drug therapies can cause hypotension and further hemodynamic compromise without affecting the properties of the accessory pathway or converting to sinus rhythm.

Acute Treatment of Regular Narrow-Complex Tachycardia

1. Record 12-lead ECG during tachycardia and in sinus rhythm; record the termination of the tachycardia.
2. Vagal maneuver; if no termination, then 6 mg of rapid IV adenosine bolus injection. If no effect, then repeat with 12 mg of IV adenosine preferably through central IV access.
3. If tachycardia continues, then consider β-blockers or non-dihydropyridine calcium channel blockers (if normal left ventricular function) for attempted slowing and/or block of AV nodal conduction and resultant rate control or interruption of the reentrant circuit.
4. If tachycardia persists and/or the patient at any point becomes hemodynamically unstable, then proceed to cardioversion with adequate sedation.

Atrial Tachycardia

During episodes of atrial tachycardia, an ectopic (nonsinus) P wave precedes the QRS complex. These tachycardias tend to stop and start abruptly, and AV block can occur during tachycardia. The atrial rate is regular, with P-to-P intervals ranging between 120 and 250 bpm. The site of origin of the tachycardia within the atria can often be localized using the ECG morphology of the P wave (Fig. 98.11). Atrial tachycardias may be paroxysmal, persistent, or incessant (i.e., recurs almost immediately despite attempts at termination). Paroxysmal tachycardias can originate from a focal area of the myocardium or may be due to a larger reentrant circuit. Incessant atrial tachycardia is rare but important to recognize; patients who are in tachycardia a majority of the time may develop tachycardia-induced dilated cardiomyopathy.

WIDE QRS TACHYCARDIA

There are three causes of wide-complex tachycardia: ventricular tachycardia (VT), pre-excited tachycardia, and SVT with baseline bundle branch block (fixed) or aberrant conduction (functional/intermittent bundle branch block). A correct and rapid diagnosis is essential as incorrect treatment may result in hemodynamic decompensation and death (7,8).

Ventricular Tachycardia

Independent atrial and ventricular activity (AV dissociation) is an important electrocardiographic finding when present but is visible on surface 12-lead ECG in only about 10% to 25% of patients (Fig. 98.12). Physical examination findings of an irregular jugular pulse, known as cannon "A" waves, varying intensity of the first heart sound, and beat-to-beat changes in systolic blood pressure all are consistent with AV dissociation.

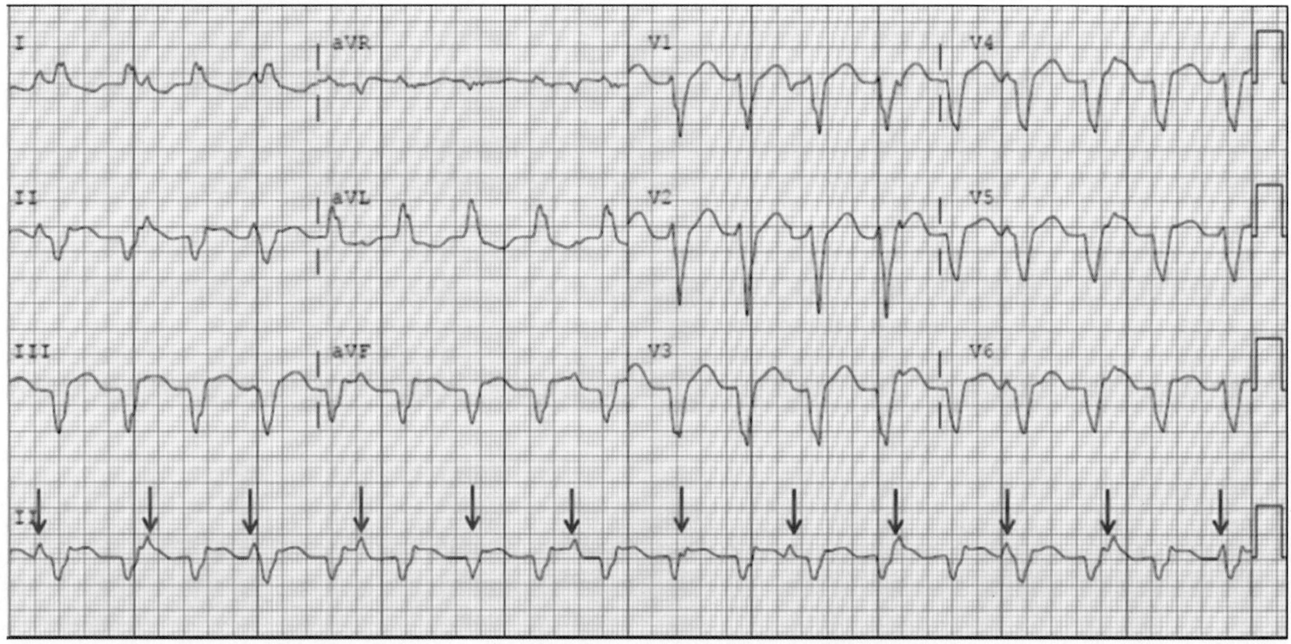

FIGURE 98.12 A 12-lead electrocardiogram. Ventricular tachycardia with atrioventricular dissociation (*arrows* indicate sinus P waves) and negative QRS concordance.

In addition, the presence of supraventricular capture beats (sinus beats that are conducted to the ventricle with a narrow QRS during a wide-complex tachycardia) or fusion beats (sinus beats that fuse with the wide-complex beat, resulting in a QRS that is narrower than the tachycardia) are diagnostic of VT (Fig. 98.13). The wide QRS of VT does not usually mimic the morphology of a true bundle branch block; therefore, careful examination of the QRS morphology can sometimes differentiate VT from right or left bundle branch aberrant conduction. In addition, if all the QRS complexes in the precordial leads V1 to V6 are going in the same direction (concordance), this is suggestive of the diagnosis of VT (see Fig. 98.12). Furthermore, the wider the QRS, the more likely that tachycardia is ventricular in origin. Hemodynamic stability, age of the patient, and ventricular rate or regularity should be used with caution to distinguish between supraventricular and VT, as they can be misleading.

Supraventricular Tachycardia with Aberrancy

SVT with a wide QRS can result from either functional or intermittent bundle branch aberrancy or a fixed bundle branch block. The pattern of aberrancy is usually in the form of a typical left or right bundle branch block, and a prior sinus rhythm 12-lead ECG can help determine the presence of an underlying or fixed bundle branch block (Fig. 98.14).

Pre-Excited Tachycardia

Patients with anterograde conducting AV accessory pathways can have wide-complex tachycardias referred to as pre-excited tachycardias, where the activation of the ventricles is largely or exclusively through the accessory pathway. In the antidromic AV reentry variety, the atrial impulse travels to the

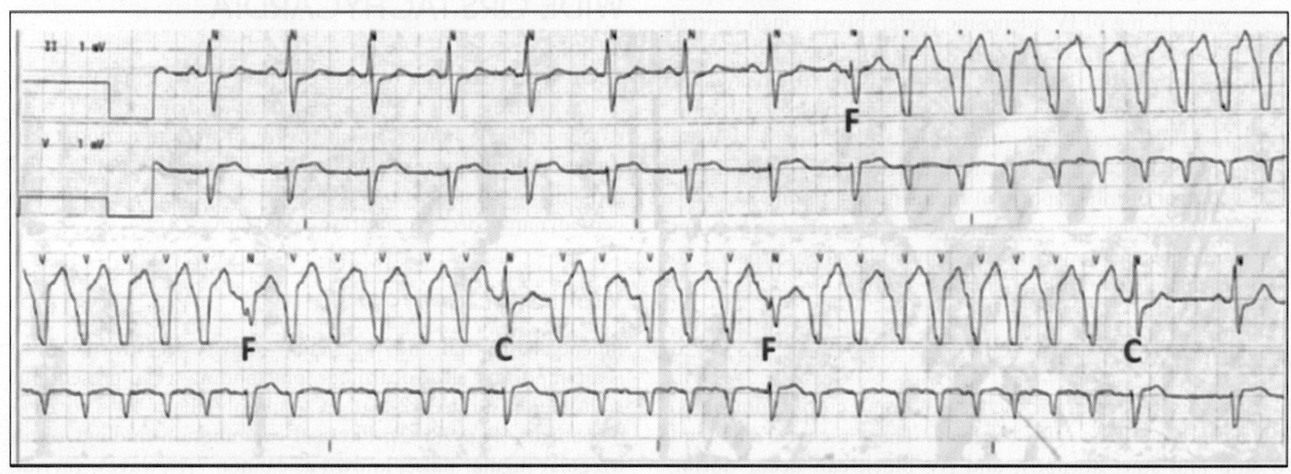

FIGURE 98.13 A 12-lead electrocardiogram. Sinus rhythm with the onset of ventricular tachycardia. AV dissociation is evidenced by capture (C) and fusion beats (F).

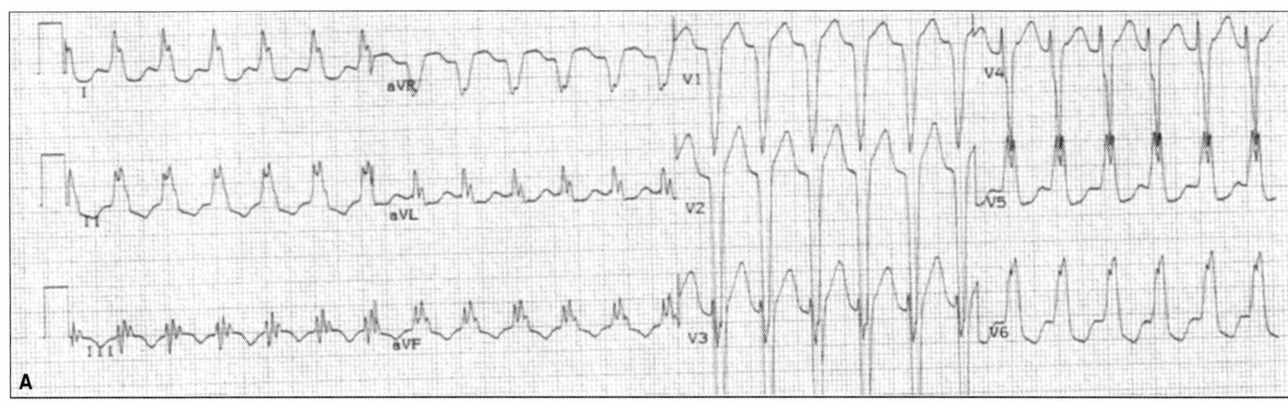

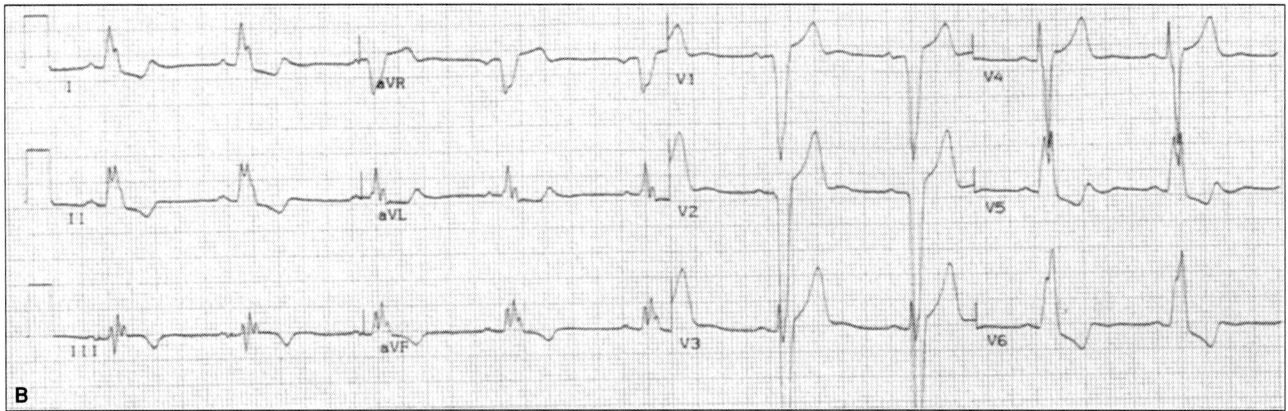

FIGURE 98.14 **A**: A 12-lead electrocardiogram. Supraventricular tachycardia having a wide QRS with a typical-appearing left bundle branch block pattern. **B**: A 12-lead electrocardiogram of the same patient with the typical left bundle branch block present in sinus rhythm, establishing a fixed conduction defect.

ventricle anterograde via the accessory pathway and returns to the atrium retrograde via the AV node (Fig. 98.15). A more rare variety of pre-excited wide-complex tachycardia involves anterograde conduction through one accessory pathway and retrograde conduction via a second accessory pathway or pathway–pathway tachycardia. Atrial tachycardias, atrial fibrillation, or atrial flutter can also conduct via accessory pathways to produce pre-excited tachycardias.

Treatment of Wide QRS Tachycardia

Monomorphic wide-complex tachycardia that is thought to be ventricular in origin in a stable patient can be treated with IV amiodarone (150 mg IV over 10 minutes; repeat as needed to a maximum dose of 2.2 g IV per 24 hours). If amiodarone is not successful or the patient develops hemodynamic instability or symptoms, then electrical cardioversion with adequate sedation is appropriate (9).

If the wide-complex tachycardia is thought to be SVT with aberrant conduction, then adenosine administration is recommended (6 mg rapid IV push followed by 12 mL of saline, if no effect, 12 mg IV push of adenosine can be tried). Adenosine may be therapeutic (terminating the tachycardia by blocking the AV node) if the patient has a reentrant SVT involving the AV node, or diagnostic (causing transient increase in AV block) if the patient has atrial fibrillation, atrial flutter, or atrial tachycardia. In the latter cases, if the patient remains stable, then rate-controlling IV drugs with longer-lasting effects, such as β-blockers or diltiazem, may be administered. Avoid the administration of IV verapamil if the patient has left ventricular dysfunction, heart failure, and/or if there is a possibility that the rhythm could be ventricular in origin, as verapamil has been shown to cause hemodynamic deterioration and death (7). If the patient is hemodynamically unstable, then synchronized cardioversion is appropriate (9).

In a patient with ventricular pre-excitation who is in atrial fibrillation with evidence of anterograde conduction down the accessory pathway, first-line medical therapy should be IV procainamide (25 to 50 mg/min up to 17 mg/kg maximum if normal renal function) or IV ibutilide, 1 mg over 10 minutes (may be repeated once). These drugs block the rapid conduction over the accessory pathway and may also terminate the atrial fibrillation. If there is no effect, then proceed with cardioversion with adequate sedation. If the patient is unstable, then perform immediate cardioversion (9).

Torsade de Pointes

Many antiarrhythmic agents, noncardiac drugs, and nonprescription medications can cause QT prolongation (Fig. 98.16) resulting in polymorphic VT also known as torsade de pointes (10). The mechanism is thought to be related to different repolarization times within the layers of ventricular myocardium leading to a dispersion of refractoriness. This dispersion of refractoriness when combined with early after depolarization events (triggered early ventricular ectopic impulses also induced by these drugs) leads to ventricular arrhythmia (11,12).

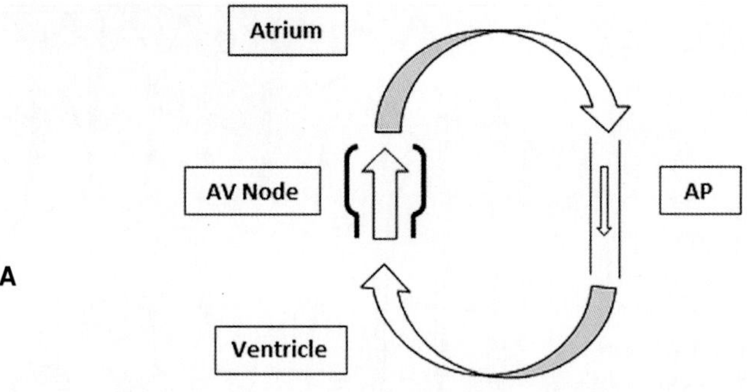

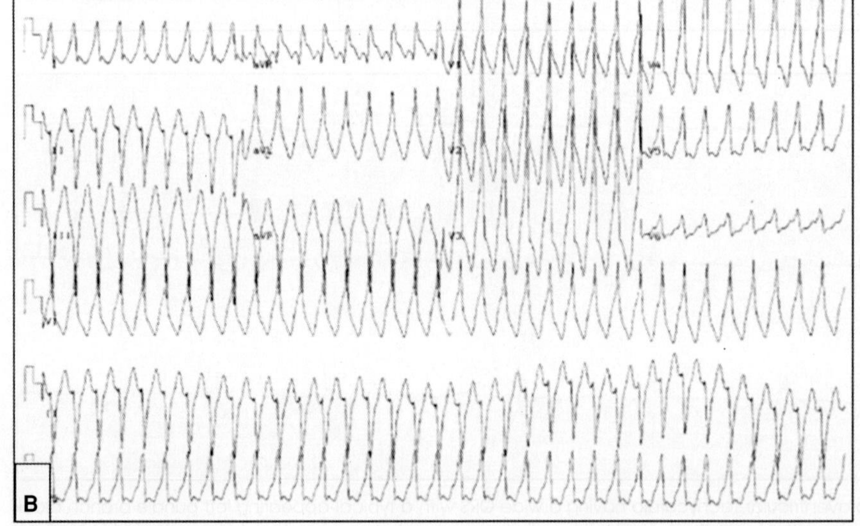

FIGURE 98.15 A: Schematic of antidromic AV reentry tachycardia, a pre-excited tachycardia with anterograde conduction down the accessory pathway and retrograde conduction up the AV node. B: A 12-lead electrocardiogram. Wide-complex tachycardia found to be antidromic AV reentry tachycardia.

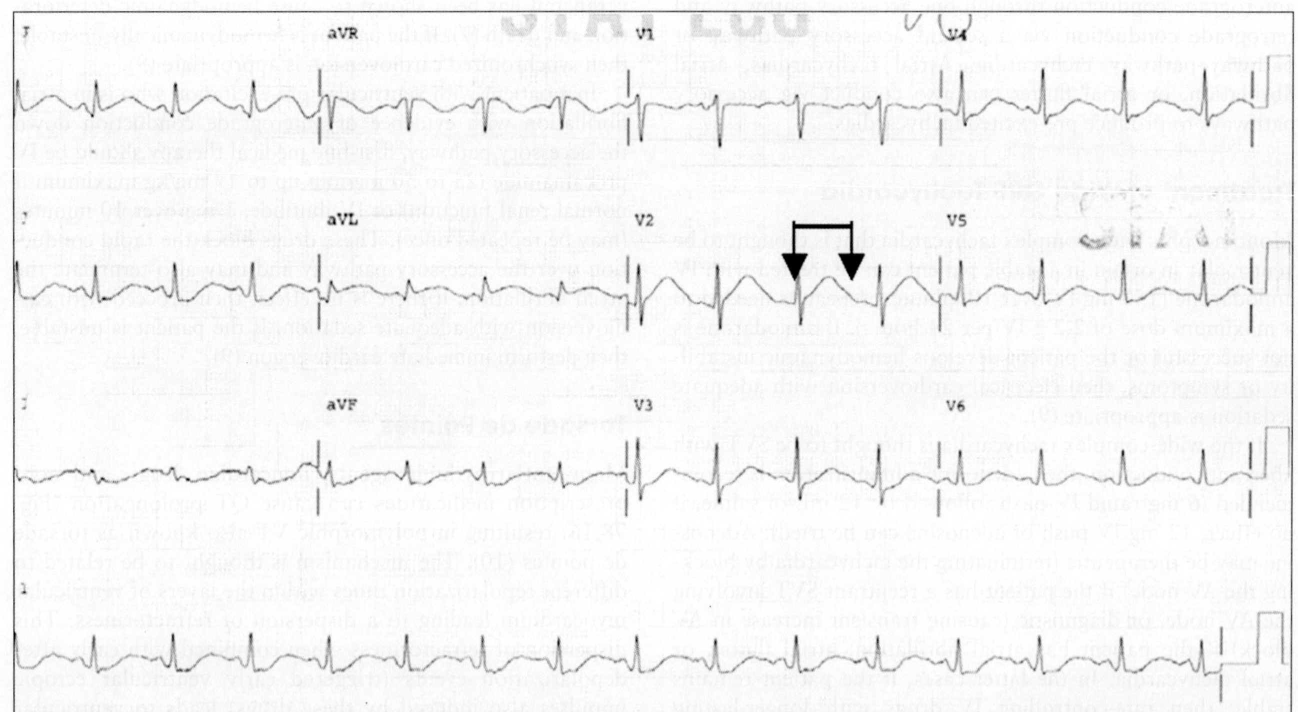

FIGURE 98.16 A 12-lead electrocardiogram. Sinus rhythm with a long QT interval (*arrows* indicate QT measured at approximately 520 msec).

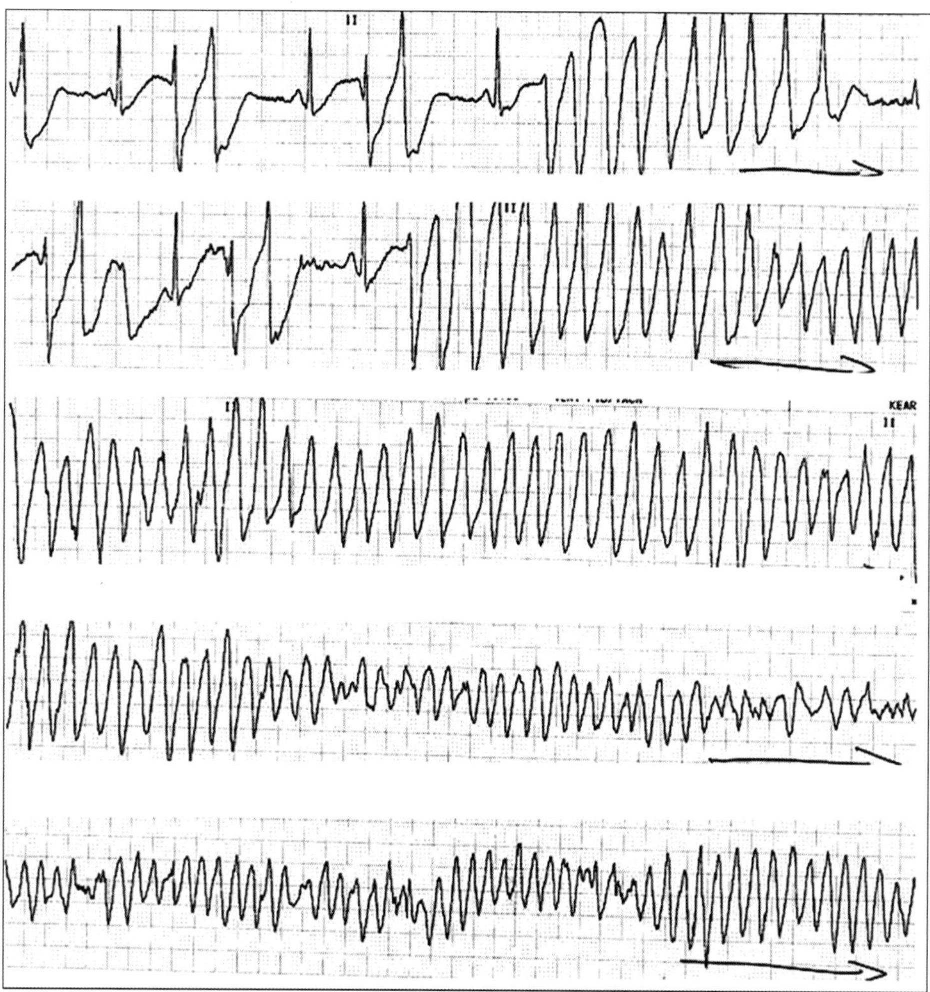

FIGURE 98.17 Lead II rhythm strip. Long QT interval with torsade de pointes.

Torsade de pointes is a polymorphic VT with beat-to-beat changes in the QRS axis (Fig. 98.17). There is QT prolongation, often with a pause or bradycardia-dependent initiation of the arrhythmia. If a drug is responsible for prolonging the QT duration, then it should be discontinued. The administration of 1 to 2 g of IV magnesium can be effective for the treatment of torsade de pointes, even when serum magnesium is normal. Hypokalemia should also be corrected. Close monitoring is essential, and if bradycardia persists and is contributing to induction of the polymorphic VT, then give atropine or institute temporary pacing. Isoproterenol infusion, between 1 and 4 μg/min, can also be used transiently to increase the heart rate while temporary pacing is being established.

Digitalis

Digitalis is used both for heart failure and atrial fibrillation management. It is a positive inotrope. It also slows the ventricular rate during atrial fibrillation, increases vagal tone, causes diuresis, and vasodilates. Digitalis has a narrow therapeutic window, with women requiring lower doses than men (12). Unrecognized digitalis intoxication is a problem often missed by clinicians (13,14) because the symptoms of digitalis intoxication are nonspecific (gastrointestinal symptoms, visual changes, neuropsychiatric problems, and weakness), and serum drug levels do not necessarily correlate well with toxicity. It is important for any health care professional caring for patients who take digitalis to be familiar with ECG findings consistent with digitalis toxicity (14).

Arrhythmias due to digitalis toxicity include atrial tachycardia, junctional tachycardia, VT, and bradyarrhythmias, including AV block. Many other comorbidities and conditions can potentiate digitalis toxicity, including sympathetic stimulation, hypokalemia, hypercalcemia, hypomagnesemia, diuretics, ischemia and reperfusion, and heart failure. Digitalis toxicity results in a combination of increased cardiac automaticity and conduction slowing. This can manifest itself as: (i) bradycardia when the heart rate was previously normal or fast; (ii) atrial tachyarrhythmia with dissociated, regular ventricular activity secondary to complete AV block; (iii) VT with variable exit block leading to regular or irregular R-to-R intervals and bidirectional QRS morphologies (10).

The treatment of digitalis toxicity depends on the clinical condition and not the drug level. The first step when suspecting digitalis toxicity is to discontinue the medication. Patient rest, continuous ECG monitoring, and correction of electrolyte abnormalities will often help. If the arrhythmia is life threatening, administering digitalis antibodies or phenytoin may be indicated (10). The patient's kidney function must be determined to estimate the severity of the suspected intoxication.

Key Points

- If no symptoms or hemodynamic changes are present during sinus bradycardia, then treatment is rarely necessary.
- If sinus bradycardia is present, then exclude and/or reverse any identified reversible causes.
- Intervention in patients with asymptomatic sinus rhythm with first-degree AV block or second-degree AV block, type 1 is rarely necessary.
- Intervention in asymptomatic patients with sinus rhythm with second-degree AV block, type 2 may be needed as they are at risk to progress to high-grade AV block.
- A temporary pacemaker is indicated in any bradycardic rhythm with significant symptoms and/or hemodynamic collapse.
- A permanent pacemaker should be considered in older patients with acquired, unresolved third-degree AV block and in most cases of acquired, transient complete AV block.
- The three most common causes of regular paroxysmal narrow QRS tachycardia are AVNRT, AVRT, and atrial tachycardia, respectively.
- AV nodal reentry and AVRTs involve the AV node as a part of their circuit, and therefore, AV nodal blocking vagal maneuvers and IV adenosine can abruptly terminate these rhythms.
- Vagal maneuvers and IV adenosine administration during atrial tachycardia or atrial flutter does not typically terminate these rhythms, but instead can lead to transient AV block "unmasking" the P waves leading to a diagnosis.
- There are three causes of wide-complex tachycardia: VT, pre-excited tachycardia, and SVT with baseline bundle branch block (fixed) or aberrant conduction (functional/intermittent bundle branch block).

References

1. OS N. *Cardiac Arrhythmias: Electrophysiology, Diagnosis, and Management*. Baltimore, MD: Lippincott Williams & Wilkins; 1979.
2. Bar FW, Brugada P, Dassen WR, et al. Differential diagnosis of tachycardia with narrow QRS complex (shorter than 0.12 second). *Am J Cardiol*. 1984;54:555–560.
3. Wolf PA, Abbott RD, Kannel WB. Atrial fibrillation: a major contributor to stroke in the elderly: the Framingham study. *Arch Intern Med*. 1987; 147:1561–1564.
4. Lloyd-Jones DM, Wang TJ, Leip EP, et al. Lifetime risk for development of atrial fibrillation: the Framingham study. *Circulation*. 2004;110: 142–146.
5. January C, Wann L, Alpert J, et al. AHA/ACC/HRS 2014 guidelines for the management of patients with atrial fibrillation: executive summary. *J Am Coll Cardiol*. 2014;64:2246–2280.
6. Wellens HJJ, Brugada P, Penn OC. The management of pre-excitation syndromes. *JAMA*. 1987;257(17):2325–2333.
7. Buxton AE, Marchlinski FE, Doherty JU, et al. Hazards of intravenous verapamil for sustained ventricular tachycardia. *Am J Cardiol*. 1987; 59:1107–1110.
8. Stewart RB, Bardy GH, Greene HL. Wide complex tachycardia: misdiagnosis and outcome after emergent therapy. *Ann Intern Med*. 1986;104: 766–771.
9. Okin PM, Devereux RB, Nieminen MS, et al. Management of symptomatic bradycardia and tachycardia. *Circulation*. 2005;112;67–77.
10. Conover HW. *The ECG in Emergency Decision Making*. Vol 1. St. Louis, MO: Saunders Elsevier; 2006.
11. Zipes DP, Jalife J. *Cardiac Electrophysiology From Cell to Bedside*. 5th ed. Philadelphia, PA: Saunders Elsevier; 2009.
12. Adams KF Jr, Gheorghiade M, Uretsky BF, et al. Clinical benefits of low serum digoxin concentrations in heart failure. *J Am Coll Cardiol*. 2002;39: 946–953.
13. Gandhi AJ, Vlasses PH, Morton DJ, et al. Economic impact of digoxin toxicity. *Pharmacoeconomics*. 1997;12:175–181.
14. Williamson KM, Thrasher KA, Fulton KB, et al. Digoxin toxicity: an evaluation in current clinical practice. *Arch Intern Med*. 1998;158: 2444–2449.

CHAPTER

99

Pericardial Disease

CARSTEN M. SCHMALFUSS

INTRODUCTION

The normal pericardium forms a sac around the heart and proximal large arteries and veins. It has a thin visceral mesothelial layer that closely adheres to the epicardial surface of the heart. The parietal layer consists of the same thin mesothelium and a thicker (up to 2 mm), fairly nonelastic fibrous layer on the outside. Physiologically, the space between both mesothelial layers contains 20 to 30 mL of fluid.

The fibrous part of the pericardium is attached to the surrounding mediastinal structures and holds the heart in its position within the chest. It limits cardiac dilatation, contributes to the interventricular interaction, and primarily affects diastolic function. The smooth mesothelial surfaces and the pericardial fluid between them reduce friction and act as a barrier to inflammation from surrounding structures. The pericardium is well innervated, and pathologic processes can cause severe episodic or continuous pain.

The intrapericardial pressure is usually negative; it is approximately equal to and varies with the pleural pressure at the same hydrostatic level. Pericardial pressure affects myocardial transmural pressure by the following relationship:

Transmural pressure
= cavitary pressure − adjacent intrapericardial pressure

Because the intrapericardial pressure is normally negative, this usually adds to the normal transmural pressure gradient (1).

The relationship between intrapericardial and pleural pressures causes a simultaneous fall of pressures in both spaces during inspiration and leads to an increased venous return into the right chambers (increased preload), with a subsequent increase in cardiac output. Inspiration influences filling and cardiac output of the left heart only indirectly and very little. The parietal pericardium is very resistant to acute stretching but adapts and expands to great dimension when subjected to a chronic stretching process. The pericardial pressure–volume curve is generally flat as pericardial volume increases, and when further distention is impossible, a sharp rise in the intrapericardial pressure occurs. This exponential curve accounts for the rapid clinical response when even small amounts of fluid are removed in cardiac tamponade (2).

This chapter deals with the most common clinical pericardial problems encountered in critical care medicine. They include acute pericarditis, pericardial effusion, cardiac tamponade, and pericardial constriction.

ACUTE PERICARDITIS

Pathophysiology

Inflammation of the pericardial sac results in acute pericarditis and is either an isolated problem or part of a systemic process. Exudation of inflammatory fluid into the pericardial space can result in pericardial effusion. Depending on the frequency and time course, pericarditis can be acute, recurrent, or chronic. Common causes of acute pericarditis are shown in Table 99.1. Most often, clinically recognizable pericarditis in the adult is idiopathic. In these cases, various viruses are often the suspected causes; an etiologic agent is infrequently demonstrated. The most commonly demonstrated virus is the Coxsackie B group, which causes myopericarditis in children and pleuropericarditis in adults—also called Bornholm disease (3). ECHO, influenza, Epstein–Barr, varicella, hepatitis, mumps, and human immunodeficiency viruses can also cause pericarditis.

Up to one-third of patients with end-stage renal disease will develop uremic pericarditis. Most of them have not started dialysis when they present with pericarditis, and the symptoms usually disappear after beginning or increasing the frequency of dialysis (4). There is no direct association with serum blood urea nitrogen level or serum creatinine and the acute illness. However, it is suspected that increased toxin levels from declining renal function cause the inflammatory process. It is important to remember that the uremic patient is susceptible to infections and that the pericarditis may be infectious. Last but not least, the underlying disease process leading to the renal insufficiency (i.e., lupus erythematosus) may also be the cause for the pericardial inflammation.

Acute pericarditis after myocardial injury is thought to be due to direct irritation of the visceral mesothelium. In the past, pericarditis occurred in up to 20% of patients after transmural myocardial infarction; recently, the frequency has decreased due to the increased use of reperfusion therapy—that is, thrombolytic therapy or angioplasty (5). Typically, symptoms occur 1 to 3 days after the myocardial damage and can mimic recurrent angina pectoris. If the patient is receiving anticoagulants, the inflammation can lead to hemorrhagic intrapericardial effusion and possibly cardiac tamponade. Acute pericardial inflammation is also found after open-heart surgery, implantation of cardiac pacemakers, percutaneous coronary interventions, or external cardiac trauma, and the presentation is similar to that after transmural infarction.

The postpericardiotomy syndrome was originally described as postmyocardial infarction pericarditis. Later, Engle and Ito (6) noted the same clinical syndrome in children and adults who experienced an opening of the pericardium. The syndrome occurs in 10% to 30% of patients who have undergone pericardiotomy and is thought to be an immune complex reaction to the patient's own pericardium (7). In contrast to pericarditis caused by myocardial injury, these patients usually have symptoms of chest pain and fever beginning several weeks to months after cardiac surgery or other myocardial injury.

Neoplastic pericarditis is most often caused by cancer of the lung, breast, or esophagus as well as lymphoma and melanoma (8). The tumor directly invades the pericardial space or metastasizes through lymphatics or blood vessels; primary

TABLE 99.1 Common Causes of Pericarditis

Idiopathic
Viral
Uremic
Neoplastic
Metastatic
Contiguous spread
Primary
Autoimmune
Systemic lupus erythematosus
Postpericardiotomy syndrome (Dressler)
Rheumatoid arthritis
Scleroderma
Postmyocardial infarction
Bacterial
Parasitic
Mycotic
Trauma with contusion of the heart
Aortic dissection or ventricular rupture
Radiation-induced
Myxedema
Drug-induced
Procainamide
Hydralazine
Quinidine
Isoniazid
Methysergide
Daunorubicin
Penicillin
Streptomycin
Phenylbutazone
Minoxidil
Sarcoid
Amyloidosis
Acute pancreatitis
Chylopericardium

pericardial tumors like mesothelioma are rare. The likelihood of finding previously undiagnosed cancer in a patient presenting with pericarditis is about 6% to 7% (9). In patients with known malignancy pericarditis is caused by cancer in only 50% to 60%; idiopathic pericarditis and radiation-induced pericarditis are the most common benign causes (10,11). The prognosis of neoplastic pericarditis and effusion is poor.

Pericarditis is also seen in patients with systemic lupus erythematosus, rheumatoid arthritis, and scleroderma. Inflammation of the pericardium is often the first manifestation of lupus in female patients; this diagnosis should be ruled out during the workup for a first episode of idiopathic pericarditis. Radiation pericarditis often follows a mediastinal dose of 4,000 rad or more and can lead to pericardial effusion and acute cardiac tamponade. The long-term effects of radiation also can lead to constrictive pericarditis.

Pericarditis caused by infectious organisms other than viruses is less frequent now than it was in the preantibiotic era. Pneumonia is still the most common cause; others include sepsis from peritonitis and urinary tract infection, or direct spread of the infectious process from mediastinitis or necrotizing fasciitis of the head or neck. Immunocompromised and elderly patients are more prone to infectious pericarditis than the general population. In adults, *Staphylococcus aureus* is still the most common organism, and there is an apparent decline in infections with *Streptococcus* spp, *Pneumococcus* spp, and *Haemophilus influenzae*.

Tuberculous pericarditis was once a common cause of acute and constrictive pericarditis, but with the overall decline of tuberculosis, it has become a rare entity in the United States (12). More recently, states with a high percentage of immigrants have again reported rising numbers of tuberculous pericarditis (13). One to two percent of patients with pulmonary tuberculosis will develop tuberculous pericarditis (14). Mycobacterial infection must be ruled out in any case of suspected purulent pericarditis.

The most common fungal organism to cause pericarditis is *Histoplasma capsulatum*. Histoplasmosis in the United States is most common in the Mississippi and Ohio River Valleys (15). Diagnosis is usually delayed and made by positive fungal culture of the pericardial fluid and/or a significant rise of serologic antibody titers (>1:32) against *H. capsulatum*.

Diagnosis

The typical patient presenting with pericarditis is young and was previously healthy. Symptoms of acute pericarditis include sharp and, usually, persistent chest pain that is generally increased with respiration and motion. It is worse in the supine position and usually improves sitting up and/or with shallow breathing. The pain can radiate to the neck, and dyspnea may also be present. Other common findings preceding or accompanying pericarditis are fever, myalgia, malaise, and tachycardia. The characteristic and pathognomonic three-component friction rub is best described as coarse, leathery, and superficial—like "pulling Velcro." The rub is only intermittently heard during the episode of pericarditis, and therefore, it is important to auscultate frequently. The patient is ideally examined in a quiet setting in an upright position leaning forward; the rub is best heard at the left sternal border or the cardiac apex.

An electrocardiogram (ECG) should be obtained in every patient presenting with chest pain. Four ECG stages, evolving over hours to days and weeks, have been described:

- Stage I includes classic and diffuse ST elevations with a concave ST segment and significant PR-segment depression (Fig. 99.1)
- Stage II is normalization of the ECG
- Stage III is the development of diffuse T-wave inversion that may persist or normalize
- Stage IV is final normalization of the ECG (16)

The ECG may show all, several, or none of the stages during an episode of acute pericarditis. Atrial arrhythmias are rare but do occur in acute pericarditis (17) and can be the first manifestation of acute pericarditis. However, sustained atrial or ventricular arrhythmias are suggestive of concomitant myocarditis.

The key to an ECG diagnosis of pericarditis is the diffuse nature of the ECG changes, the absence of localization to a particular ECG anatomic area, PR-segment depression, and the absence of ST depression except in lead aVR.

Every patient suspected to have pericarditis should have a chest radiograph taken. It will be normal in most cases of pericarditis; a new finding of an enlarged cardiac silhouette is, however, suggestive of a pericardial effusion (>200 mL) and should be further evaluated.

The laboratory may report positive acute-phase reactants (especially the erythrocyte sedimentation rate [ESR]) and an

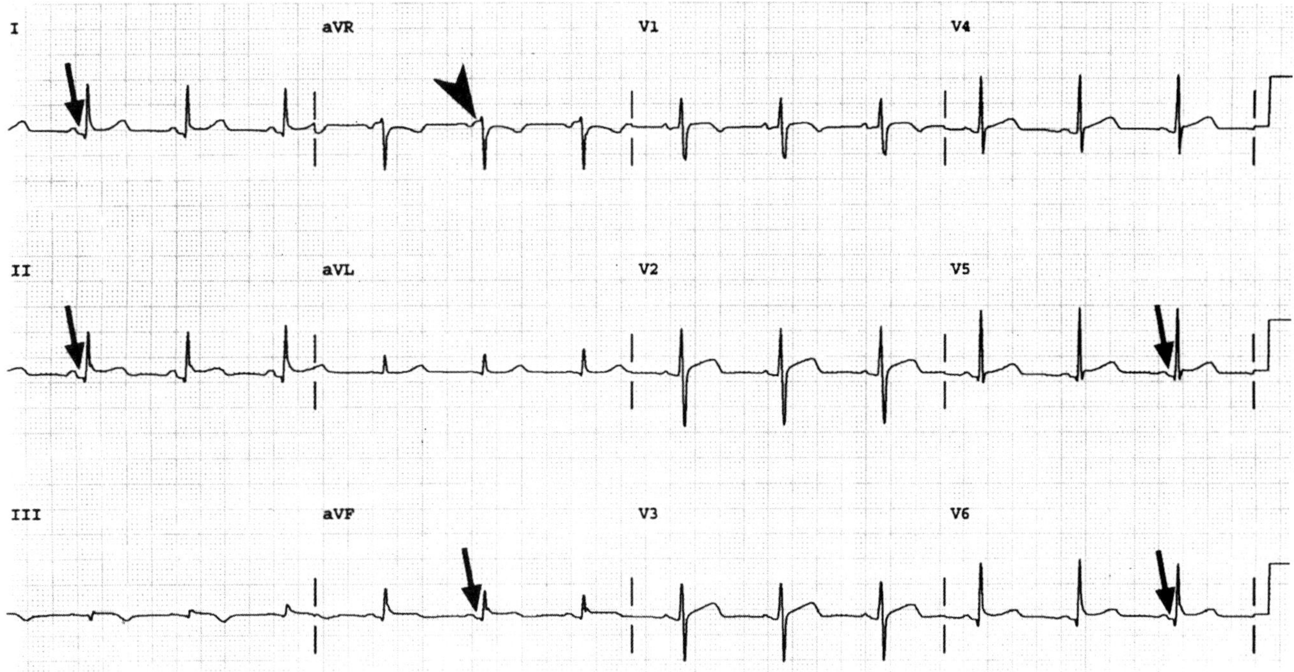

FIGURE 99.1 Electrocardiogram of a patient with acute pericarditis. Note the PR-segment depressions (*arrows*) and convex ST-segment elevations in the inferolateral leads and PR-segment elevation (*arrowhead*) and ST-segment depression in lead aVR consistent with stage I of electrocardiogram findings in acute pericarditis.

elevated white blood cell count; however, these are nonspecific findings. Cardiac troponin T or I and CK-MB isoenzymes are cardiac—but not pericardium—specific and are often found minimally elevated in acute pericarditis. Viral studies may confirm a viral cause of the pericarditis; however, their yield is low, and the result does not change management. In cases of suspected infectious etiology, cultures from blood and pericardial fluid, if available, should be examined for bacterial and mycobacterial pathogens.

Echocardiography should be performed in every patient with the suspected diagnosis of pericarditis to evaluate for and follow pericardial effusion (Fig. 99.2) and to help diagnose cardiac tamponade.

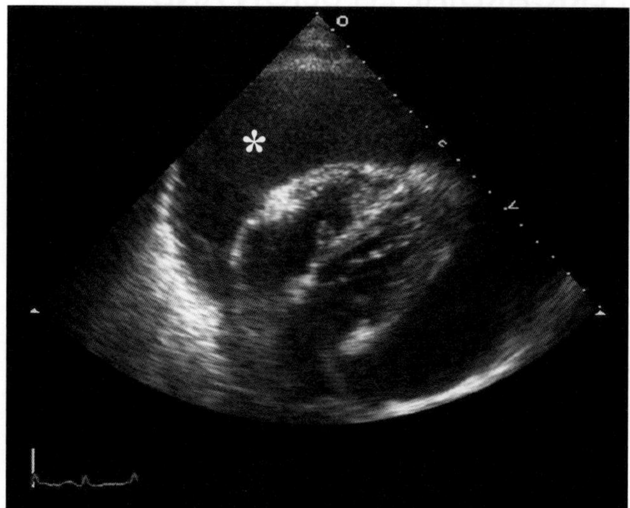

FIGURE 99.2 Subcostal echocardiogram showing a giant pericardial effusion (*asterisk*) in a patient with neoplastic pericarditis.

The triad of typical chest pain, pericardial friction rub, and the aforementioned ECG changes confirms the diagnosis of acute pericarditis. However, this diagnosis should be made only after life-threatening conditions with similar presentation (acute coronary syndrome, pulmonary embolism, aortic dissection, and cardiac tamponade) have been ruled out. Electrocardiographic differential diagnosis also includes variant angina, hypertrophic cardiomyopathy, and the benign finding of early repolarization—all of which can mimic the ECG changes described earlier (Table 99.2).

Aside from history and physical examination, ECG, chest radiographs, blood work, and echocardiogram, it may be necessary to evaluate the patient with computed tomography (CT) of the chest to rule out pulmonary embolism or aortic dissection (Fig. 99.3).

Treatment

Patients with acute pericarditis have a high likelihood of uncomplicated recovery and can be treated outside the hospital. However, several factors are described as being associated with a complicated course (Table 99.3) and patients with any of these factors should be hospitalized for their initial treatment (18).

TABLE 99.2 Differential Diagnosis of Pericardial Effusion

- Acute coronary syndrome
- Pulmonary embolism
- Aortic dissection
- Cardiac tamponade
- ECG diagnosis
  - Variant angina
  - Hypertrophic cardiomyopathy
  - Benign finding of early repolarization

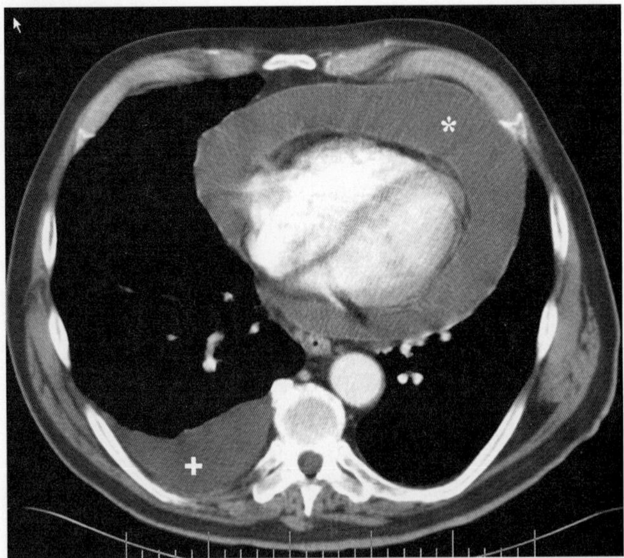

FIGURE 99.3 Computed tomography (CT) of the chest with large pericardial effusion (*asterisk*) and small right-sided pleural effusion (*plus sign*). The dark rim between the pericardial effusion and the right heart represents epicardial fat.

Acute idiopathic or viral pericarditis usually responds to nonsteroidal anti-inflammatory drugs (NSAIDs). The drug regimen consists of high-dose aspirin (325–975 mg three to four times daily for 4 weeks); with the addition of a proton pump inhibitor to lessen gastrointestinal effects. Alternatively, indomethacin (25–50 mg four times daily) or ibuprofen (400–600 mg four times daily) can be given. Recently, Imazio et al. (19) found that routine use of colchicine (0.5 mg twice daily for 3 months) in addition to aspirin or ibuprofen—compared to aspirin or ibuprofen alone—in patients with a first episode of acute pericarditis significantly reduced incessant or recurrent pericarditis. Colchicine added to NSAID treatment (0.5 mg twice daily for 6 months) has also been shown to be effective for patients who have had multiple recurrences of their acute pericarditis (20). Diarrhea is a known side effect of colchicine and may cause discontinuation of drug therapy in about 10% of patients.

Symptoms of acute pericarditis respond rapidly to systemic steroids, but there seems to be an increase in relapse after tapering (21). Therefore, corticosteroid therapy should be reserved only for patients with recurrent pericarditis not responding to NSAIDs and colchicine. The recommended daily regimen is 0.2 to 0.5 mg/kg of prednisone for at least 1 month before slowly tapering the dose by 2.5 to 5 mg/wk until the drug is withdrawn (22). The possible side effects of corticosteroid treatment include peptic ulcer disease, sodium retention, hypokalemia, hyperglycemia, osteoporosis, Cushing syndrome, and suppression of the adrenal axis. Treatment with corticosteroids also requires the exclusion of infection or an appropriate antibiotic regimen before initiation of therapy.

TABLE 99.3 Presenting Factors Predicting Complicated Course

- Fever >8°C
- Symptoms developing over weeks in immunocompromised patient
- Traumatic pericarditis
- Patient on oral anticoagulants
- Large effusion (>20 mm) or tamponade
- Failure to respond to nonsteroidal anti-inflammatory drugs

The treatment of choice for uremic pericarditis consists of intensive, initially daily dialysis therapy. Heparin should be used sparingly during dialysis to reduce the risk of intrapericardial hemorrhage and possible tamponade. The presence of acute pericarditis in acute myocardial infarction also requires caution with the use of intravenous anticoagulants. These drugs are not, however, absolutely contraindicated. Thrombolytic agents have been reported to lead to cardiac tamponade and should be used with caution in the patient with acute myocardial infarction and acute pericarditis.

The postpericardiotomy syndrome is usually self-limited if left untreated; however, the disease may increase the risk of early coronary artery bypass graft closure. Therefore, aggressive treatment has been recommended; NSAIDs often decrease symptoms and speed up recovery (23). Colchicine compared to placebo given perioperatively (0.5 mg twice daily 72 hours before and for 1 month after cardiac surgery) significantly reduced the incidence of postpericardiotomy syndrome and showed nonsignificant reduction of postoperative atrial fibrillation (24). Refractory cases may occur but usually respond rapidly to systemic corticosteroids as outlined above. Advocates of corticosteroid therapy claim that this treatment reduces the incidence of late constrictive pericarditis.

Nonviral infectious etiology of pericarditis requires prompt evacuation of purulence from the pericardium, usually by operative intervention, because of the need to establish a definitive diagnosis, eradicate the infection, and prevent constrictive pericarditis.

Recurrence of acute pericarditis is quite common and often requires long-term drug therapy as noted above. In a few selected cases refractory to medical therapy, radical pericardiectomy may need to be considered (21).

In general, acute pericarditis symptoms subside within several days to weeks. The major immediate complication is cardiac tamponade, which occurs in less than 5% of patients. For diagnostic and treatment approach in patients with suspected acute uncomplicated or complicated pericarditis, see Figure 99.4.

PERICARDIAL EFFUSION AND CARDIAC TAMPONADE

Pathophysiology

Pericardial effusion often develops with acute pericarditis. It is caused by an inflammatory exudation and an occlusion of the normal drainage through epicardial venous and lymphatic systems by the inflammatory process. The most common causes of tamponade include idiopathic pericarditis, cancer of the lung and breast, lymphoma, renal failure, and tuberculosis (25). Pericardial effusion may also occur in the absence of pericardial inflammation—for example, as a hemorrhagic effusion from internal sources such as a pacemaker, angioplasty, coronary artery bypass grafting (CABG) surgery, aortic dissection, ventricular rupture—or external cardiac trauma. Regardless of their size, pericardial effusions can either be clinically silent or cause hemodynamic compromise. The latter situation is called *cardiac tamponade. The most important factor contributing to the development of cardiac tamponade is not the*

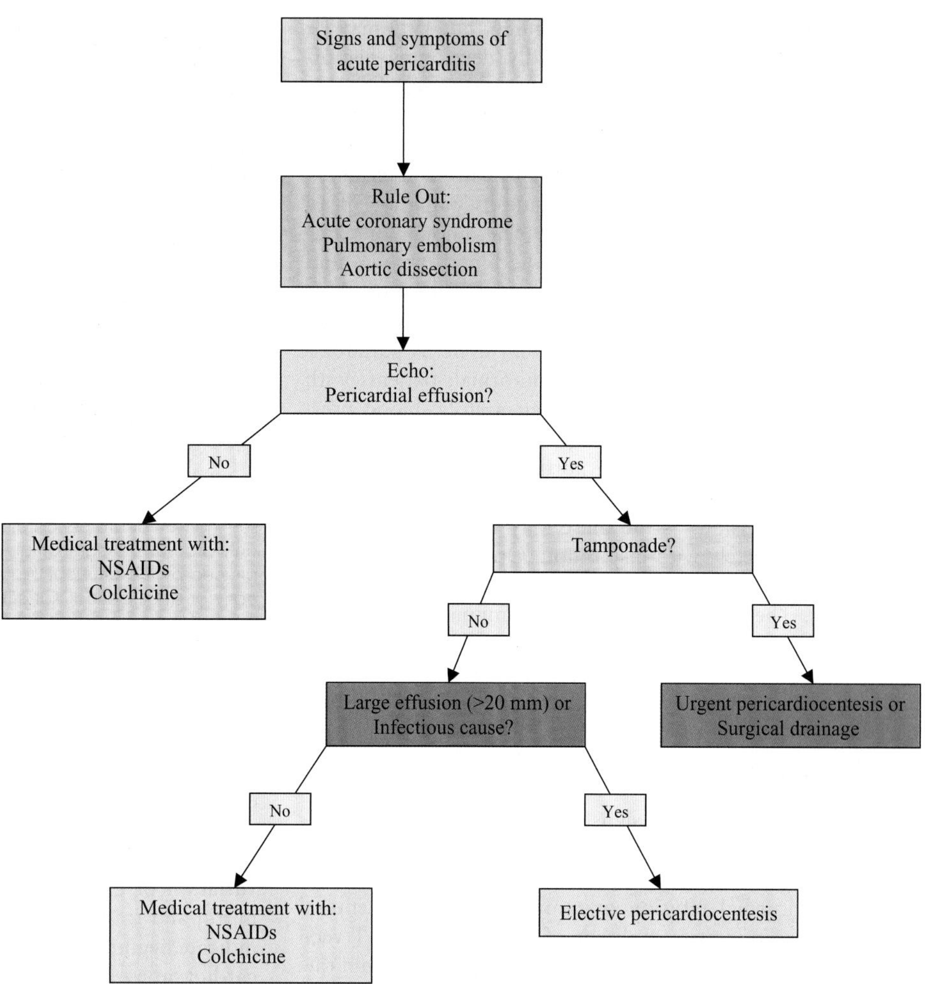

FIGURE 99.4 Diagnostic and treatment algorithm for patients presenting with signs and symptoms of acute pericarditis.

total amount of pericardial fluid but the rate at which it accumulates. The pericardium resists sudden stretching but can gradually expand in response to a chronic distending force. A small but rapidly developing effusion—less than 200 mL—in a trauma patient can cause tamponade, because the fibrous pericardial membrane does not have enough time to stretch and accommodate the increased volume. Conversely, a patient with a very large pericardial effusion—1,000 mL—developing over weeks or months may be completely asymptomatic, given that the parietal pericardium has had time to adjust to the increased volume.

It is also important to note that the pressure–volume curve for the stretchable pericardium is curvilinear; a large amount of fluid accumulating over a long time raises the intrapericardial pressure very little. However, at some point, the ability of the pericardium to stretch further is exceeded, and the addition of a very small volume raises the intrapericardial pressure significantly. Once the intrapericardial pressure exceeds the filling pressures of the right atrium and/or the right ventricle, central venous pressure rises, cardiac output drops, and cardiac tamponade—and consequently cardiogenic shock—occur (26,27). Physiologically, the total cardiac volume is limited, and volume in one chamber can increase only if volume in another chamber decreases. This physiologic interdependence of the ventricles is accentuated in cardiac tamponade when right ventricular (RV) filling during inspiration causes a significant decrease in left ventricular (LV) filling and a significant decrease in stroke volume. This inspiratory drop in systolic blood pressure of greater than 10 mmHg, termed *pulsus paradoxus*, is very suggestive of cardiac tamponade in a patient presenting with hypotension and tachycardia, but it is not specific and can also present in other conditions such as chronic obstructive pulmonary disease (COPD), pulmonary embolism, pneumothorax, acute asthma, and hypovolemic shock (28).

Cardiac tamponade is a serious problem that, if not treated aggressively and rapidly, may be fatal. Treatment may be successful if diagnosed in a timely fashion, and thus cardiac tamponade needs to be included in the initial differential diagnosis of cardiogenic shock or pulseless electrical activity.

Diagnosis

The patient with early pericardial tamponade is often confused, agitated, pale, and diaphoretic and complains of chest pain and dyspnea. Initially, compensatory catecholamine release, caused by a decreased cardiac output, leads to sinus tachycardia and often to peripheral vasoconstriction. Later in the course, bradycardia occurs, indicating imminent pulseless electrical activity and cardiorespiratory arrest unless the effusion is immediately decompressed.

Classic clinical signs include jugular venous distention (JVD), demonstrating a rapid x-descent but no y-descent because of right atrial and ventricular compression throughout the entire diastolic cycle. In this situation, the central venous pressure is usually greater than 15 mmHg, but JVD may be missing in trauma patients with rapidly developing hemorrhagic tamponade or in patients with uremic pericarditis due to volume depletion from blood loss or dialysis, respectively (*low-pressure tamponade*).

Pulsus paradoxus is often present and can be ascertained through invasive arterial pressure tracing by palpation of an artery or with a sphygmomanometer. The amount of paradox is gauged by measuring the systolic blood pressure and observing the difference in the level at which the Korotkoff sounds are heard only during expiration and the level at which they are heard throughout the respiratory cycle. A paradoxical pulse greater than 10 mmHg is abnormal; patients with tamponade physiology often drop their systolic blood pressure more than 20 mmHg with inspiration. Paradoxical pulse is absent in patients with severe aortic insufficiency or atrial septal defect and is difficult to assess in acute cardiac tamponade with hypotension, as the pulse may be unobtainable or disappear completely with inspiration. Other clinical signs of cardiac tamponade are distant and muffled heart sounds and clear lungs. The patient with chronic tamponade may present with a low-output state, right upper quadrant pain caused by swelling of the hepatic capsule, or even ascites and lower extremity edema. The two main differential diagnoses for cardiac tamponade are tension pneumothorax and pulmonary edema; both conditions can present with tachycardia, hypotension, and JVD.

The ECG usually shows signs of acute pericarditis, including sinus tachycardia, PR depression, and abnormal T-wave changes. Electrical alternans of the ECG is pathognomonic of large pericardial effusion or tamponade; it represents a change of direction and amplitude of the P, QRS, and T vectors with every other heartbeat, and probably results from the "swinging" movement of the heart in a large volume of fluid. A change of the QRS vector alone is the most common finding (29). As mentioned above, the finding is highly specific for large effusion or tamponade, but its absence does not rule out large effusion or tamponade, particularly if they develop rapidly.

The chest radiograph may show a globular heart hanging down in the mediastinum—*the water bottle heart.* It is also helpful to rule out diagnoses presenting similarly to tamponade, such as tension pneumothorax and pulmonary edema.

Cardiac tamponade is a clinical diagnosis based on the previously described symptoms and findings. However, the best adjunctive test to assess for pericardial effusion and cardiac tamponade is the echocardiogram (30). Pericardial effusion is seen as an echo-free space surrounding the heart. An echocardiogram can detect even very small amounts of pericardial effusion (<20 mL), helps to estimate amount and distribution of the effusion, and visualizes clot or tumor in the fluid if present. Small effusions (<1 cm) are seen only inferolaterally and around the right atrium (Fig. 99.5). Effusions causing tamponade are mostly large (>2 cm) and circumferential. Effusions seen with acute tamponade are usually smaller than those seen with chronic tamponade. An echocardiogram can distinguish pericardial from pleural effusion; pericardial effusion tracks between the inferolateral wall and the descending thoracic aorta in the parasternal long axis view and separates both structures (Fig. 99.6), whereas pleural effusion is found only posterior to the aorta in this view.

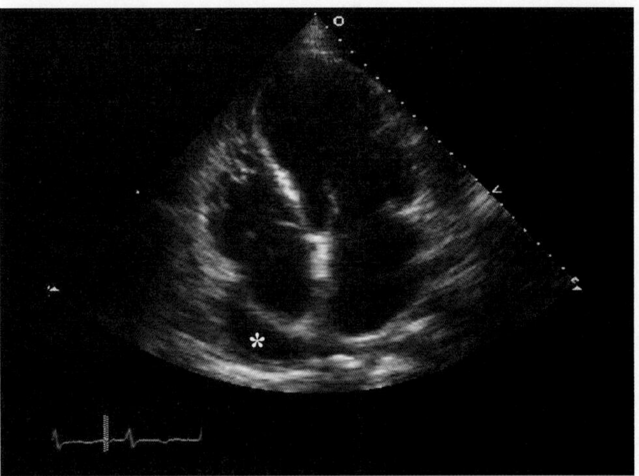

FIGURE 99.5 Apical four-chamber view echocardiogram in patient presenting with acute pericarditis. The very small pericardial effusion is seen only around the right atrial wall (*asterisk*). The right atrium is not compressed by the effusion. This location may be the only one in which an early or small pericardial effusion can be seen in a patient with poor subcostal windows.

Once a pericardial effusion begins to compromise the hemodynamics, there are several characteristic echocardiographic findings. There is diastolic collapse, first of the right atrium, and then right ventricle, both of which worsen during expiration when right-sided filling is reduced (31,32). Diastolic collapse lasting more than one-third of diastole is considered indicative for tamponade (Fig. 99.7). Reciprocal respiratory variation of greater than 20% and 30% of the peak transmitral and transtricuspid Doppler velocities respectively does indicate beginning of tamponade physiology (Fig. 99.8). Echocardiography is a very useful tool to assess pericardial effusion and determine its hemodynamic significance. However, life-saving treatments for an unstable or deteriorating patient

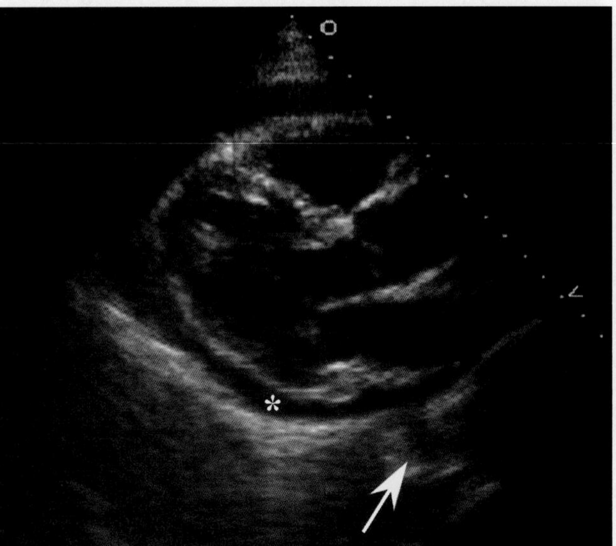

FIGURE 99.6 Parasternal long-axis echocardiographic view in a patient presenting with clinical symptoms of acute pericarditis. There is a small- to moderate-sized concentric effusion (*asterisk*). It tracks between the inferolateral wall and the descending thoracic aorta (*arrow*) and thereby confirms the diagnosis of pericardial effusion. A pleural effusion may be seen in the same inferolateral location but would not separate the heart from the aorta.

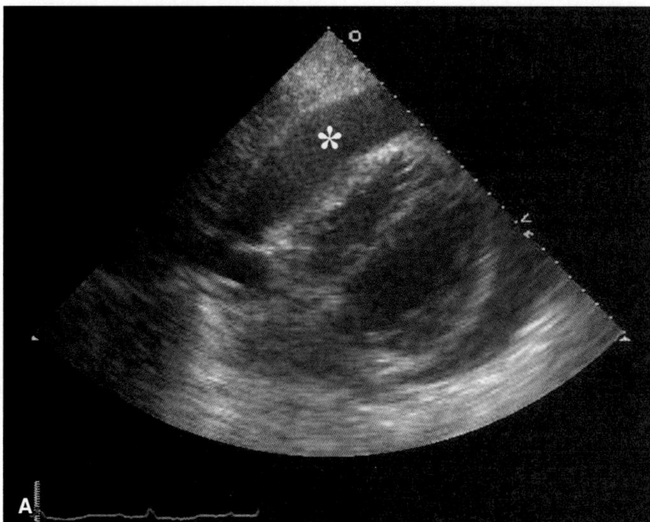

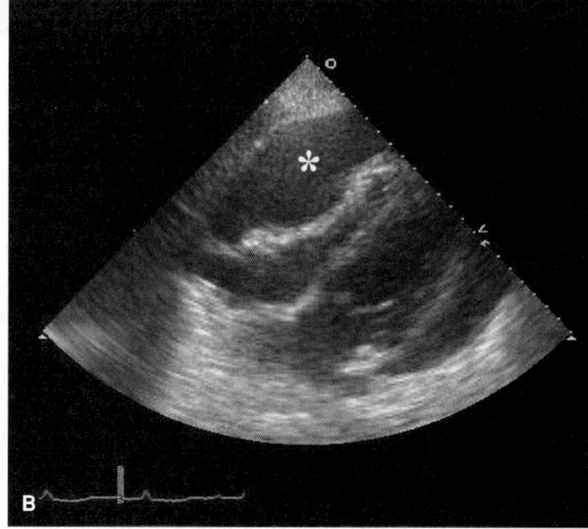

FIGURE 99.7 Subcostal echocardiogram in a patient with cardiogenic shock. Compared to early systole **(A)**, there is significant collapse of the right ventricular free wall until very late into the diastolic filling phase **(B)**, consistent with pericardial tamponade. The treatment of choice is immediate decompression of the effusion (*asterisk*) by percutaneous or surgical drainage.

suffering from cardiac tamponade should not be delayed by waiting for an echocardiogram to be performed.

The invasive hemodynamic profile of acute cardiac tamponade is characteristic and can be assessed by placement of a pulmonary artery catheter. The right-sided cardiac pressures are elevated, and the diastolic pressures equilibrate. The mean right atrial pressure, RV diastolic pressure, pulmonary artery diastolic pressure, and the pulmonary capillary wedge pressure are elevated and are measured within 2 to 3 mmHg of each other. The pressure contour does not show a dip and plateau sign as seen in constrictive pericarditis. The pressures in chronic congestive heart failure are elevated but do not equilibrate in diastole. These measurements made in the intensive care unit (ICU) setting can confirm the diagnosis of cardiac tamponade.

Treatment

Patients with newly diagnosed pericardial effusion, without tamponade physiology, should be monitored in the hospital for 24 to 48 hours, with at least one repeat echocardiogram prior to discharge. A repeat echocardiogram should be performed in patients with large pericardial effusions 4 to 6 weeks after the initial presentation or with change in symptoms suggestive of beginning hemodynamic significance of the pericardial effusion.

Patients diagnosed with cardiac tamponade, defined as systolic blood pressure less than 110 mmHg or pulsus paradoxus greater than 10 mmHg, should receive immediate aggressive fluid resuscitation with normal saline to increase right-sided filling pressures to at least temporarily stabilize hemodynamics. Additionally, inotropic support with dobutamine, dopamine, isoproterenol, or norepinephrine may be needed to further stabilize the blood pressure. More definitive treatment with percutaneous pericardiocentesis or surgically created pericardial window should follow promptly. Any patient presenting with traumatic hemopericardium should be treated surgically (33).

Pericardiocentesis should be performed in any patient with acute tamponade and hemodynamic compromise, or when an infectious or malignant cause of the pericardial effusion is suspected. The procedure is usually performed in the cardiac

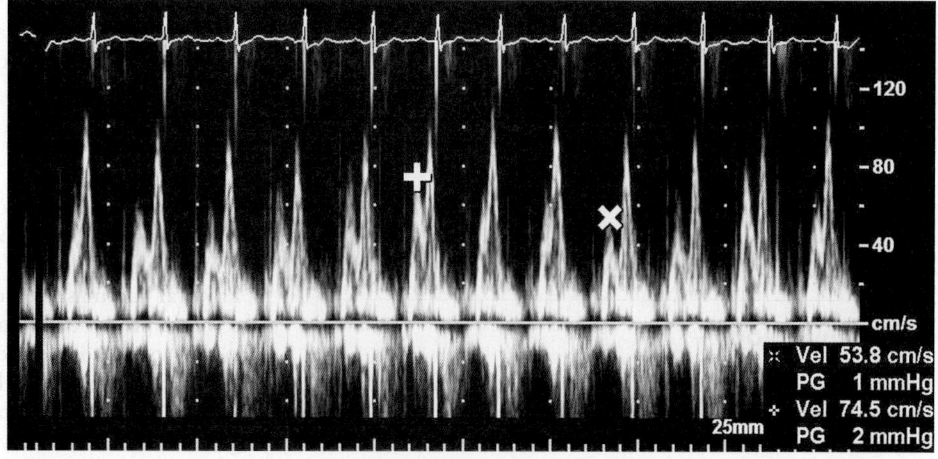

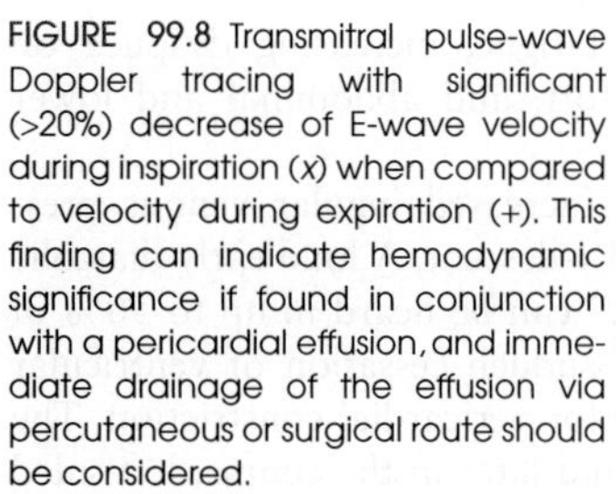

FIGURE 99.8 Transmitral pulse-wave Doppler tracing with significant (>20%) decrease of E-wave velocity during inspiration (*x*) when compared to velocity during expiration (+). This finding can indicate hemodynamic significance if found in conjunction with a pericardial effusion, and immediate drainage of the effusion via percutaneous or surgical route should be considered.

TABLE 99.4 Diagnostic Tests on Pericardial Fluid

- Complete blood count and differential
- Microbiology (Gram stain, culture, acid-fast bacillus smear)
- Chemistry (glucose, protein, albumin, lactate dehydrogenase, amylase)
- Cytology

catheterization laboratory, but in an emergency, may be done at the bedside if clinically necessary (33).

The patient should be placed in a supine position at a 45-degree angle. The area between the xiphoid and the left costal arch should be sterilely prepped using a tinted (so clinicians can see where they have prepped) chlorhexidine–alcohol solution and draped in the usual fashion, and anesthetized with a 1% or 2% lidocaine solution. A 7.6-cm (3-in) aspiratory needle (16–18 gauge) with a short bevel should be directly attached to a three-way stop cock and a 50-mL syringe, and the needle advanced with negative pressure at an angle of 30 to 45 degrees to the abdominal wall and oriented in a posterocephalad direction toward the left shoulder (34). Once it enters the pericardial space, fluid can be easily removed. Removal of a small amount of fluid may provide significant clinical improvement. A temporary catheter is then placed into the pericardial space via Seldinger technique and connected to a bag draining to gravity for several days. This approach provides more complete drainage and reduces the risk for reaccumulation of the effusion. The first sample of fluid retrieved should be sent for microbiologic studies and several other diagnostic tests (Table 99.4).

Echocardiography can be used to locate the ideal spot for percutaneous puncture (35). It is helpful to determine the distance from the surface to the effusion and demonstrates liver or lung tissue that may be in the projected path of the needle. After the puncture, an echocardiogram confirms the correct position when bubbles generated with sterile, agitated saline injected through the needle are demonstrated within the pericardial effusion. Complications of this procedure include pneumothorax, myocardial and coronary artery laceration, dysrhythmias, and death. If the patient with acute cardiac tamponade can be stabilized by volume expansion and vasopressor support, a safer and equally effective drainage of pericardial fluid can be accomplished by surgical subxiphoid pericardial resection and drainage (33). Subxiphoid resection can be performed in a sterile environment under local anesthesia; pericardial fluid can be removed and pericardial tissue obtained for biopsy and culture (36).

Malignant recurrent pericardial effusions often require surgical creation of a pericardial window to allow fluid to drain into the adjacent pleural space. More recently, percutaneous balloon pericardiotomy has been developed as a nonsurgical approach to create such a window and to drain large pericardial effusions (37).

CONSTRICTIVE PERICARDITIS

Pathophysiology

Constrictive pericarditis occurs when chronic inflammation leads to scarring and, in some cases, calcification of the pericardium. Tuberculosis is the most common cause of constrictive pericarditis worldwide; the leading causes in the United States are idiopathic pericarditis, previous mediastinal radiation, or cardiac surgery (33). The thickened (>2–3 mm) and shrunken pericardium leads to compromise of diastolic filling and elevation and equalization of end-diastolic pressures in all four cardiac chambers (38). Of note is that up to 20% of patients with surgically proven constriction may present without any pericardial thickening (39) (Fig. 99.9). Contrary to pericardial tamponade, the initial diastolic ventricular filling is not inhibited and is very rapid (dip on central pressure tracing). However, once the ventricular volume has reached the limits allowed by the constricted pericardium, filling abruptly ceases (plateau on central pressure tracing). Together, these two findings compose the dip and plateau or square root sign of constrictive pericarditis seen during pulmonary artery catheterization (Fig. 99.10). The signs and symptoms of constrictive pericarditis generally develop over a prolonged period and are similar to those of biventricular congestive heart failure, restrictive cardiomyopathy, cor pulmonale, cirrhosis, and pericardial tamponade. Features of cardiac tamponade and constrictive pericarditis can occur simultaneously, referred to as *effusive-constrictive pericarditis*. This likely represents a transitional state from effusive to constrictive pericarditis, and is commonly seen in patients with thoracic neoplasm who present with malignant pericardial effusion and constrictive pericarditis after radiation to the chest.

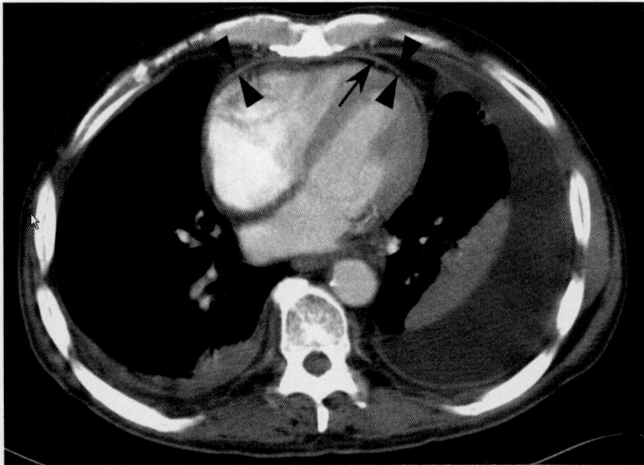

FIGURE 99.9 Axial slice of chest computed tomography in a patient with clinical findings of severe right heart failure. The pericardium is well seen (*arrowheads*) due to the separation from the myocardium by a very small pericardial effusion (*arrow*). Of note is that the pericardium is neither thickened (maximally 3 mm in thickness) nor calcified; however, preoperative cardiac catheterization results and the intraoperative findings during surgical pericardial stripping confirmed the diagnosis of constrictive pericarditis.

Diagnosis

Patients often complain of fatigue, increasing dyspnea on exertion, abdominal discomfort, and abdominal and lower extremity swelling.

Physical findings include increased jugular venous pressure with a prominent *x*- and *y*-descent. A loud early diastolic sound, a “pericardial knock,” can be heard in up to 50% of patients. It is caused by the sudden cessation of ventricular filling and is pathognomonic for pericardial constriction. The lungs remain clear initially, and later in the course, left-sided

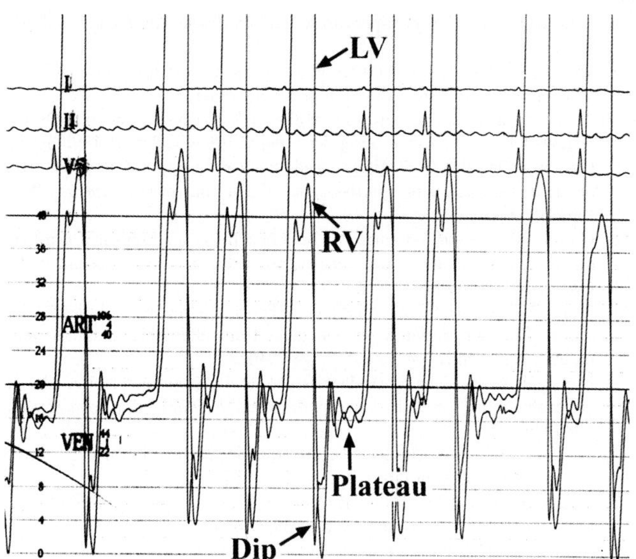

FIGURE 99.10 Right (RV) and left ventricular (LV) pressure tracings in a patient with clinical findings consistent with constrictive pericarditis. The early diastolic dip is followed by plateau, with elevation and equalization of right and left ventricular pressures. Note that contrary to ventricular discordance, the dip and plateau sign is classic but not specific for constrictive pericarditis and can be found in several other medical conditions (see text for details). The ECG tracing shows atrial fibrillation seen often in constrictive pericarditis.

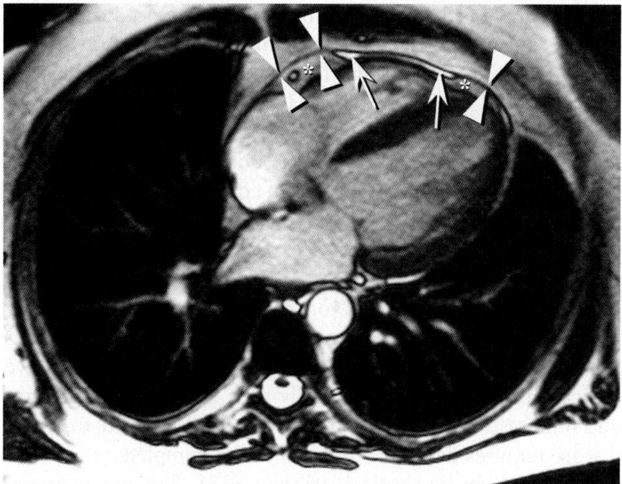

FIGURE 99.11 Four-chamber view of electrocardiogram (ECG)-gated cardiac magnetic resonance imaging (MRI) in a patient with suspected pericardial constriction. The normal-appearing pericardium (*arrowheads*) is very precisely visualized in areas with pericardial effusion (*arrows*) and with pericardial fat (*asterisk*) only. The outstanding soft tissue imaging capabilities of MRI make it preferable over cardiac computed tomography (CT) to evaluate the pericardium in patients with no or very little pericardial effusion.

or bilateral pleural effusions develop. The liver is enlarged secondary to congestion; ascites, splenomegaly, and significant lower extremity edema are also present. Unlike in cardiac tamponade, blood pressure is maintained, and less than 20% of patients have a significant pulsus paradoxus. A lateral chest radiograph may show pericardial calcium in up to 50%.

The ECG findings are nonspecific and include T-wave inversions, low voltage, and atrial fibrillation. Echocardiography is helpful to distinguish right heart failure from pericardial constriction; however echocardiographic findings are not specific for the diagnosis of pericardial constriction. They include paradoxical septal motion, rapid deceleration of the early diastolic mitral inflow velocity (E wave), significant respiratory variation of mitral inflow velocity (>20%), and normal mitral valve annular tissue Doppler velocity. In the absence of a pericardial effusion, a thickened pericardium is often hard to distinguish from the myocardium. On the other hand, cardiac CT and cardiac magnetic resonance imaging (MRI) are very useful imaging modalities to precisely determine the pericardial thickness. Cardiac MRI is better suited to image soft tissues and can, in contrast to CT, show normal pericardium, even in the absence of pericardial effusion (Fig. 99.11). Furthermore, tagged cine MRI is able to demonstrate adhesions between the pericardium and myocardium (40) and contrast-enhanced cardiac MRI is able to identify patients with active inflammation and transient constrictive pericarditis which may resolve with anti-inflammatory therapy (41,42).

Cardiac catheterization pressure tracings are still the gold standard to diagnose constrictive pericarditis and to differentiate it from restrictive cardiomyopathy. The hemodynamic findings of elevated and equalized diastolic pressures in all four chambers and the dip and plateau sign are classic, although not very specific for constriction. In contrast, respiratory variation of ventricular pressures (RV pressure rises and

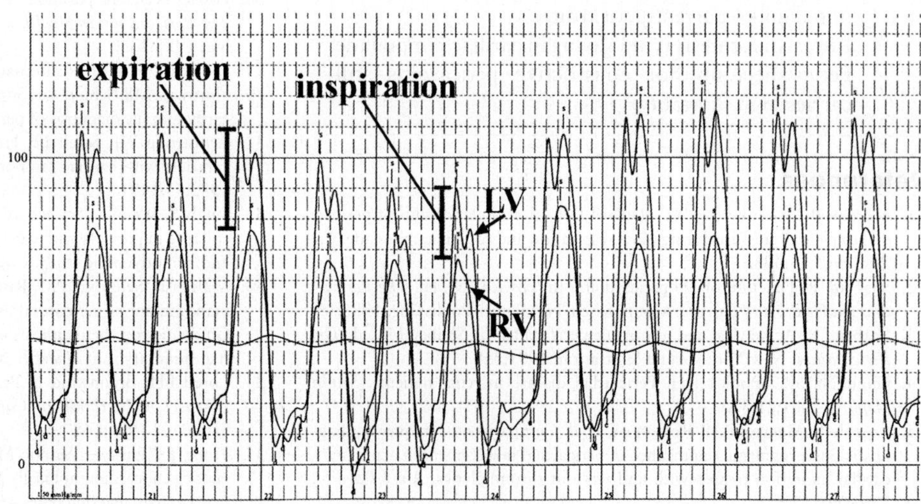

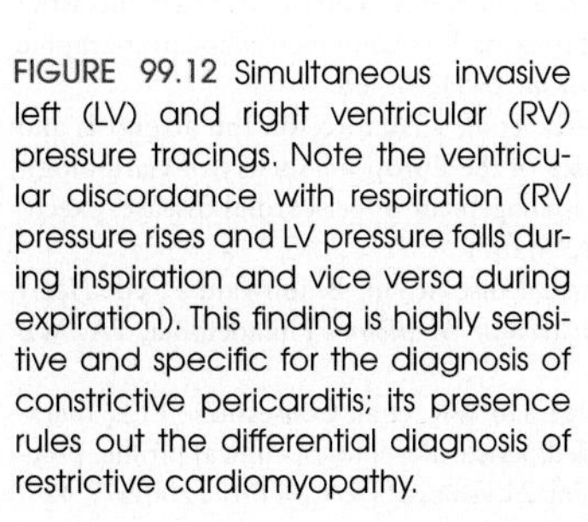

FIGURE 99.12 Simultaneous invasive left (LV) and right ventricular (RV) pressure tracings. Note the ventricular discordance with respiration (RV pressure rises and LV pressure falls during inspiration and vice versa during expiration). This finding is highly sensitive and specific for the diagnosis of constrictive pericarditis; its presence rules out the differential diagnosis of restrictive cardiomyopathy.

LV pressure falls during inspiration and vice versa during expiration, causing ventricular discordance) has been shown to be highly sensitive and specific for the diagnosis of constrictive pericarditis (43) (Fig. 99.12). Hemodynamically silent constrictive pericarditis can be evaluated by performing volume loading during catheterization; the initially normal right and left heart pressures may elevate and equilibrate in diastole.

Treatment

Patients with acute onset of constrictive symptoms may improve significantly with medical treatment that includes NSAIDs, colchicine, and steroids (44). Chronic constrictive pericarditis can be treated initially with diuretics, and sodium and fluid restriction, if symptoms are mild. Moderate to severe disease requires definitive treatment with complete removal of the pericardium by surgical stripping (33). This major procedure is still associated with a perioperative mortality of 8% to 14% (45,46), it can be life-saving and improves symptoms drastically in most patients; however, poor outcome is likely if the constriction is radiation-induced.

ACKNOWLEDGMENTS

I would like to thank Dr. Ilona Schmalfuss, Radiology and the Medical Media Service, particularly Mr. John Richardson, both at the Malcom Randall VA Medical Center, for their assistance with the figures for this chapter.

Key Points

- Presentation
  - Pericardial diseases are relatively rare
  - Acute pericarditis can relapse
  - Pericardial constriction develops over time
  - Cardiac tamponade presents acutely and is life threatening
- Diagnosis
  - Diagnose pericarditis after exclusion of life-threatening other causes for symptoms
  - Always include ECG and echocardiogram early in the work-up
  - Consider cardiac CT and MRI if initial work-up is inconclusive
- Treatment and outcome
  - NSAIDs and colchicine are first-line therapy for initial and recurrent pericarditis
  - Pericardiocentesis is life-saving in cardiac tamponade
  - Pericardiectomy for constrictive pericarditis still carries high mortality

References

1. Morgan BC, Guntheroth WG, Dillard DH, et al. Relationship of pericardial to pleural pressure during quiet respiration and cardiac tamponade. *Cir Res.* 1965;16:493.
2. Shabetai R. Function of the pericardium. In: Fowler NO, ed. *The Pericardium in Health and Disease.* Mount Kisco, NY: Futura Publishing; 1985:19.
3. Shabetai R. Acute viral and idiopathic pericarditis. In: Shabetai R, ed. *The Pericardium.* New York: Grune & Stratton; 1981:348.
4. Gunukula SR, Spodick DH. Pericardial disease in renal patients. *Semin Nephro.* 2001;21:52.
5. Coreale E, Maggioni AP, Romano S, et al. Comparison of frequency, diagnostic and prognostic significance of pericardial involvement in acute myocardial infarction treated with and without thrombolytics. *Am J Cardiol.* 1993;71:1377.
6. Engle MA, Ito T. The post-pericardiotomy syndrome. *Am J Cardiol.* 1961; 7:73.
7. Engle MA, McCabe JC, Ebert PA, et al. The post-pericardiotomy syndrome and antiheart antibodies. *Circulation.* 1974;49:401.
8. Abraham KP, Reddy V, Gattuso P, et al. Neoplasms metastatic to the heart: review of 3314 consecutive autopsies. *Am J Cardiovasc Pathol.* 1990;3:195.
9. Permanyer-Miralda G, Sagrista-Sauleda J, Soler-Soler J, et al. Primary acute pericardial disease: a prospective series of 231 consecutive patients. *Am J Cardiol.* 1985;56:623.
10. Gornik HL, Gerhard-Herman M, Beckman JA, et al. Abnormal cytology predicts poor prognosis in cancer patients with pericardial effusion. *J Clin Oncol.* 2005;23:5211.
11. Posner MR, Cohen GI, Skarin AT, et al. Pericardial disease in patients with cancer. The differentiation of malignant from idiopathic and radiation-induced pericarditis. *Am J Med.* 1981;71:407.
12. McCaughan BC, Schaff HV, Piehler JM, et al. Early and late results of pericardiectomy for constrictive pericarditis. *J Thorac Cardiovasc Surg.* 1985;89:340.
13. Trautner BW, Darouiche RO. Tuberculous pericarditis: optimal diagnosis and management. *Clin Infect Dis.* 2001;33:954.
14. Larrieu AJ, Tyers GFO, Williams EH, et al. Recent experience with tuberculous pericarditis. *Ann Thorac Surg.* 1980;29:464.
15. Hammerman KJ, Powell KE, Tosh FE, et al. The incidence of hospitalized cases of systemic mycotic infections. *Sabouraudia.* 1974;12:33.
16. Spodick DH. Diagnostic electrocardiographic sequences in acute pericarditis. *Circulation.* 1973;48:575.
17. Spodick DH. Arrhythmias during acute pericarditis (100 cases). *JAMA.* 1976;235:39.
18. Imazio M, Demichellis B, Parrini I, et al. Day-hospital treatment of acute pericarditis: a management program for outpatient therapy. *J Am Coll Cardiol.* 2004;43:1042.
19. Imazio M, Brucato A, Cemin R, et al. A randomized trial of colchicine for acute pericarditis. *N Engl J Med.* 2013;369:1522–1528.
20. Imazio M, Belli R, Brucato A, et al. Efficacy and safety of colchicine for treatment of multiple recurrences of pericarditis (CORP-2): a multicenter, double-blind, placebo controlled, randomized trial. *Lancet.* 2014; 383: 2232–2237
21. Shabetai R. Recurrent pericarditis: recent advances and remaining questions. *Circulation.* 2005;112:1921.
22. Imazio M, Brucato A, Cumetti D, et al. Corticosteroids for recurrent pericarditis: high versus low doses: a nonrandomized observation. *Circulation.* 2008;118:667–671.
23. Urschel HC, Razzuk MA, Gardner M, et al. Coronary artery bypass occlusion secondary to postpericardiotomy syndrome. *Ann Thorac Surg.* 1976;22:528.
24. Imazio M, Brucato A, Ferrazzi P, et al. Colchicine for prevention of post-pericardiotomy syndrome and postoperative atrial fibrillation: the COPPS-2 randomized clinical trial. *JAMA.* 2014;312:1016–1023.
25. Guberman BA, Fowler NO, Engel PJ, et al. Cardiac tamponade in medical patients. *Circulation.* 1981;64:633.
26. Fowler NO. Physiology of cardiac tamponade and pulsus paradoxus. *Mod Concept Cardiovasc Dis.* 1978;48:115.
27. Shabetai R. Cardiac tamponade. In: Shabetai R, ed. *The Pericardium.* New York: Grune & Stratton; 1981:224.
28. Fowler NO. The paradoxical pulse (pulses paradoxus). In: Fowler NO, ed. *The Pericardium in Health and Disease.* Mount Kisco, NY: Futura Publishing; 1985:235.
29. Spodick DH. Electric alternation of the heart. *Am J Cardiol.* 1962;10:155.
30. Horowitz MS, Schultz CS, Stinson EB, et al. Sensitivity and specificity of echocardiographic diagnosis of pericardial effusion. *Circulation.* 1974;50:239.
31. Armstrong WF, Schilt BF, Helper DJ, et al. Diastolic collapse of the right ventricle with cardiac tamponade: an echocardiographic study. *Circulation.* 1982;65:1491.
32. Singh S, Wann S, Schuchard GH, et al. Right ventricular and right atrial collapse in patients with cardiac tamponade: a combined echocardiographic and hemodynamic study. *Circulation.* 1984;70:966.
33. Maisch B, Seferovic PM, Ristic AD, et al. Task force on the diagnosis and management of pericardial diseases of the European Society of Cardiology. Guidelines on the diagnosis and management of pericardial disease: executive summary. *Eur Heart J.* 2004;25:587.
34. Lorell BH, Braunwald E. Pericardial disease. In: Braunwald E, ed. *Heart Disease: A Textbook of Cardiovascular Medicine.* Philadelphia, PA: WB Saunders; 1984:1487.
35. Tsang TS, Enriquez-Sarano M, Freeman WK, et al. Consecutive 1127 therapeutic echocardiographically guided pericardiocenteses: clinical profile, practice patterns, and outcomes spanning 21 years. *Mayo Clin Proc.* 2002;77:429.

36. Santos GH, Frater RW. The subxiphoid approach in the treatment of pericardial effusion. *Ann Thorac Surg*. 1977;23:468.
37. Wang HJ, Hsu KL, Chiang FT, et al. Technical and prognostic outcomes of double-balloon pericardiotomy for large malignancy-related pericardial effusions. *Chest*. 2002;122:893.
38. Shabetai R. Constrictive pericarditis. In: Shabetai R, ed. *The Pericardium*. New York: Grune & Stratton; 1981:154.
39. Talreja DR, Edwards DW, Danielson GK, et al. Constrictive pericarditis in 26 patients with histologically normal pericardial thickness. *Circulation*. 2003;108:1852.
40. Kojima S, Yamada N, Goto Y, et al. Diagnosis of constrictive pericarditis by tagged cine magnetic resonance imaging. *N Engl J Med*. 1999;341:373.
41. Aquaro GD, Barison A, Cagnolo A, et al. Role of tissue characterization by Cardiac Magnetic Resonance in the diagnosis of constrictive pericarditis. *Int J Cardiovasc Imaging*. 2015;31:1021–1031.
42. Welch TD, Oh JK Constrictive pericarditis: old disease, new approaches. *Curr Cardiol Rep*. 2015;17:20.
43. Hurrell DG, Nishimura RA, Higano ST, et al. Value of dynamic respiratory changes in left and right ventricular pressures for the diagnosis of constrictive pericarditis. *Circulation*. 1996;93:2007.
44. Haley JH, Tajik J, Danielson GK, et al. Transient constrictive pericarditis: causes and natural history. *J Am Coll Cardiol*. 2004;43:271.
45. Mutyaba AK, Balkaran S, Cloete R, et al. Constrictive pericarditis requiring pericardiectomy at Groote Schuur Hospital, Cape Town, South Africa: causes and perioperative outcomes in the HIV era (1990–2012). *J Thorac Cardiovasc Surg*. 2014;148:3058–3065.
46. Vistarini N, Chen C, Mazine A, et al. Pericardiectomy for constrictive pericarditis: 20 years of experience at the Montreal Heart Institute. *Ann Thorac Surg*. 2015;100(1):107–113.

CHAPTER

100

Acute Hypertension Management in the ICU

ELIZABETH MAHANNA GABRIELLI, VIVEK SABHARWAL, and THOMAS P. BLECK

INTRODUCTION

Hypertension is extraordinarily common, with over 1 billion individuals affected worldwide in 2000, 26% of the worldwide population in 2010, and projections of 29% of the population by 2025 (1,2). Between 1% and 2% of persons with chronic hypertension have hospital admissions related to cardiovascular disease (3,4). Because hypertension is so common, and because such a wide variety of conditions can be categorized as hypertensive emergencies, acutely elevated blood pressure is still a factor in a substantial number of medical visits to emergency departments and a frequent problem in the intensive care unit (ICU) (Table 100.1) (5,6).

Hypertensive crisis (Table 100.2) is defined as a systolic blood pressure greater than 180 mmHg or a diastolic blood pressure greater than 120 mmHg (7). Hypertensive crises may then be divided into two categories: hypertensive emergency and hypertensive urgency. *Hypertensive emergency* is now defined by the above elevated blood pressure measurements along with impending or continued organ dysfunction (7). This means the blood pressure elevation itself does not need to be directly responsible for causing end-organ damage, as it was previously defined. For example, acute hypertension is usually the result of, rather than the immediate cause of, an acute ischemic stroke. If the patient is to be treated with thrombolytics, it becomes imperative to maintain the blood pressure within certain narrow limits to minimize the risk of hemorrhagic transformation while at the same time not compromising cerebral blood flow. Thus, in this chapter, we define a hypertensive emergency as being associated with impending or continued organ dysfunction. Although the term *malignant hypertension* has been discouraged by some, it is still widely used in the literature to describe the syndrome where organ dysfunction is a direct *consequence* of the elevated blood pressure, rather than an epiphenomenon. The presence of papilledema is not necessarily required for the diagnosis of malignant hypertension to be made (3,8).

In contrast, a *hypertensive urgency* is defined as a condition with severe blood pressure elevation and no target-organ damage, such that the blood pressure can be decreased more gradually over the course of several hours, often with oral medications. It is therefore the presence or absence of organ dysfunction, rather than the absolute degree of blood pressure elevation, which determines whether a patient is classified as having a hypertensive emergency or urgency. It is not always clear how clinicians distinguish between hypertensive urgencies and the situation where a patient simply has severe, poorly controlled, chronic hypertension.

We will discuss the pathophysiology, diagnosis, and treatment of acute hypertension in the ICU both in a general manner and when pertaining to specific end-organ disease state.

PATHOPHYSIOLOGY OF HYPERTENSION-INDUCED END-ORGAN DYSFUNCTION

Blood flow to organs is kept relatively constant despite variations in blood pressure. This process is called *autoregulation*, and its limits are usually between mean arterial pressure (MAP) values of about 50 and 150 mmHg. Increases in blood pressure induce arteriolar smooth muscle contraction and vasoconstriction, while reductions lead to vasodilatation. Extreme hypertension exceeding the upper range of autoregulation causes edema, hemorrhage, and organ dysfunction, while reductions in blood pressure beyond the lower limits of autoregulation result in tissue hypoperfusion and ischemia (Fig. 100.1). In addition to a widespread, systemic myogenic response, there are also more organ-specific vascular regulatory mechanisms to protect against the effects of acute hypertension. The likelihood of end-organ damage increases not only with the absolute degree of blood pressure elevation, but also with the rate at which this occurs (8). With chronic hypertension, there is hypertrophy in the walls of small arteries and arterioles, and the autoregulatory curve is shifted to the right, such that blood flow can be maintained constant, even at unusually high blood pressures. Conversely, ischemia may occur when blood pressure falls to levels that would otherwise be well tolerated. In the setting of neurologic injury, autoregulation is often impaired, and cerebral blood flow becomes directly dependent on blood pressure (Fig. 100.1).

Normal endothelial function is necessary for the regulation of vascular tone, blood pressure, and regional blood flow (Fig. 100.2). The endothelium is involved in maintaining a delicate balance between vasodilating substances (e.g., nitric oxide, bradykinin, prostacyclin) and vasoconstrictors (e.g., endothelin), as well as between coagulation and fibrinolysis. Elevations in humoral vasoconstrictors leads to acute elevation in systemic vascular resistance and could trigger a hypertensive crisis (9–11). Thrombotic microangiopathy (TMA), endothelial dysfunction, elevated thrombin generation, and platelet activation, with enhanced fibrinolysis, have been associated with hypertensive crisis and ischemic complications (12). Platelet activation in particular has been found in both hypertensive emergency and urgency, and may be an early finding of hypertensive crisis (12). When blood pressure is elevated, natriuretic peptides are released from the endothelium, which in turn induce sodium and water loss, with decreased intravascular volume (8). Excessive activation of the renin–angiotensin system causes vasoconstriction and inflammation, and has been demonstrated to cause hypertensive emergencies in animal models, an effect that can be inhibited with the use of angiotensin-converting enzyme (ACE) inhibitors (13,14). Angiotensin II levels are elevated in most cases of malignant hypertension, particularly when the

TABLE 100.1 Types of Hypertensive Emergencies

Malignant hypertension
- Posterior reversible encephalopathy syndrome (PRES)/ hypertensive encephalopathy
- Retinopathy and papilledema
- Acute heart failure
- Myocardial ischemia
- Malignant nephrosclerosis and acute renal failure
- Microangiopathy

Neurocritical care emergencies
- Acute ischemic stroke requiring thrombolysis
- Acute intracerebral hemorrhage
- Subarachnoid hemorrhage
- Severe hypertension following craniotomy
- Cerebral hyperperfusion syndrome (postendarterectomy or stenting)
- Normal perfusion pressure breakthrough (postarteriovenous malformation resection)

Cardiovascular emergencies
- Acute myocardial infarction
- Acute heart failure
- Aortic dissection
- Severe hypertension following cardiovascular surgery

Preeclampsia/eclampsia

TABLE 100.2 Definitions

- **Hypertensive emergency:** Any condition where hypertension is causing or potentially exacerbating organ dysfunction and should be lowered emergently.
- **Hypertensive urgency:** Severe hypertension that is not associated with acute organ dysfunction and requires gradual reduction in blood pressure over several hours.
- **Malignant hypertension:** A syndrome in which uncontrolled hypertension directly causes organ dysfunction (note that this is a subtype of hypertensive emergency). Although previous definitions have sometimes mandated the presence of retinopathy with papilledema, this is only one of several possible clinical manifestations, and is not necessarily be required.

etiology is a renal condition (15). Increased risk of hypertensive emergency has been associated with the presence of the DD genotype of the ACE gene (16). As the blood pressure rises dramatically, endothelial compensatory mechanisms fail, and injury ensues with subsequent fibrinoid necrosis, increased permeability, and inflammation. Therefore, paradoxically, both hyperemia and TMA and ischemia develop during a hypertensive crisis (12) (Fig. 100.2).

DIAGNOSIS, ETIOLOGY, AND MANIFESTATION

Malignant Hypertension

The peak incidence of malignant hypertension occurs between the ages of 40 and 50, with risk factors including poor long-term blood pressure control, lack of a primary care physician, noncompliance with antihypertensive medications, male gender, African-American ethnicity, illicit drug use, and lower socioeconomic status (17–20). Prior to the availability of effective antihypertensive therapy, the mortality of malignant hypertension was very high, with approximately 80% of patients dying within a year; hence, the term *malignant* (21).

At least 90% to 95% of patients with chronically elevated blood pressure can be classified as having "essential" hypertension, meaning that the underlying cause is multifactorial and not specifically known. A small proportion of patients have "secondary" hypertension, where there is an identifiable and sometimes treatable condition that is responsible for raising blood pressure (22). In contrast, among patients who present with malignant hypertension, as many as 50% to 80% may have a secondary etiology (23). Other clues that should alert clinicians to the possibility of secondary hypertension include a history of blood pressure that is resistant to medical therapy, sudden worsening in a previously well-controlled patient, and the onset of hypertension at an unusually young or old age (24).

Renovascular disease, the most common cause of secondary hypertension, may be present in as many as 45% of patients

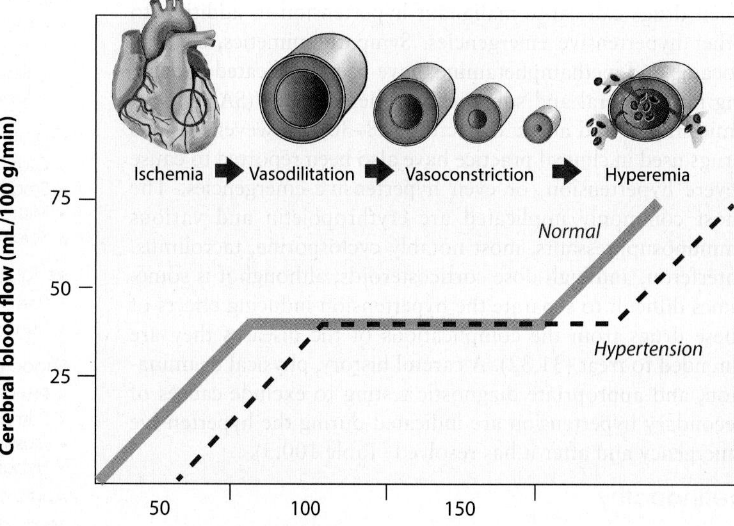

FIGURE 100.1 Cerebral blood flow autoregulation. Effect of changes in cerebral perfusion pressure on cerebral blood flow and vascular caliber in normal and hypertensive patients (*dashed line*).

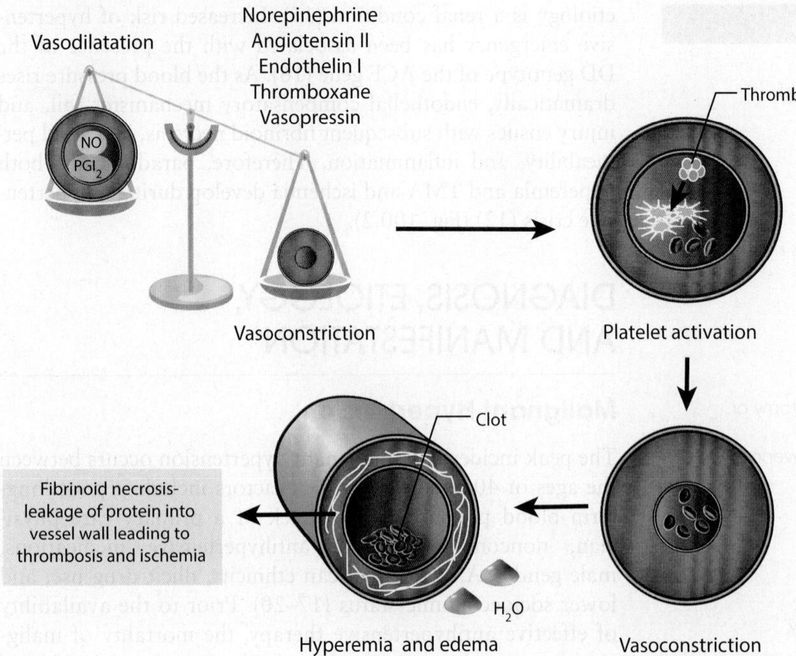

FIGURE 100.2 Simplified pathophysiology of acute hypertension-induced organ dysfunction. Endothelial system balances between vasodilatation and vasoconstriction. In hypertensive crisis the scales dip to vasoconstriction due to the following mediators: norepinephrine, angiotensin II, endothelin I, thromboxane, vasopressin. Thrombin leads to platelet activation, which leads to further vasoconstriction. Clot forms inside of vessel, which leads to both fibrinoid necrosis and results in thrombosis and ischemia, as well as destruction of endothelial cells leading to hyperemia, edema, and leakage of fluid and red blood cells.

with severe or malignant hypertension, although the proportion is higher in Caucasians than African Americans (25). Features that suggest renovascular hypertension include atherosclerotic vascular disease in other organ systems, systolic–diastolic abdominal bruits, a history of deterioration in renal function with exposure to ACE inhibitors or angiotensin II receptor blockers (ARBs), recurrent flash pulmonary edema, and small kidneys (determined by ultrasound or other imaging).

Hypertension is almost universally present in patients with acute or chronic kidney disease, especially when the etiology is a glomerulonephropathy (26). Hypertension is a common manifestation of obstructive sleep apnea, and can be improved by the administration of noninvasive positive airway pressure (27). Various and rare endocrinologic causes, including primary aldosteronism, Cushing syndrome, hypercalcemia, hyperthyroidism or hypothyroidism, and pheochromocytoma, are also responsible for a small proportion of cases. Several illicit drugs can cause malignant hypertension in addition to other hypertensive emergencies. Sympathomimetics, such as cocaine and methamphetamine, have been implicated in causing intracerebral and subarachnoid hemorrhage (SAH), ischemic stroke, and aortic dissection (28–30). However, various drugs used in clinical practice have also been reported to cause severe hypertension, or even hypertensive emergencies. The most commonly implicated are erythropoietin and various immunosuppressants, most notably cyclosporine, tacrolimus, interferon, and high-dose corticosteroids, although it is sometimes difficult to separate the hypertension-inducing effects of these drugs from the complications of the diseases they are intended to treat (31,32). A careful history, physical examination, and appropriate diagnostic testing to exclude causes of secondary hypertension are indicated during the hypertensive emergency and after it has resolved (Table 100.3).

Retinopathy

Endothelial damage and leakage of plasma proteins into the retina lead to edema and the formation of hard exudates. Focal areas of ischemia and infarction within the nerve fiber layer cause white areas, called *cotton wool spots,* to appear. Breakdown of the blood–retinal barrier results in the emergence of flame-shaped hemorrhages within the retina. The development of papilledema has historically been used to differentiate "accelerated" from "malignant" hypertension. However, the presence or absence of papilledema has little impact on the natural history and prognosis of hypertensive emergencies, nor should it significantly alter management (33). The mechanism of papilledema may include elevated intracranial pressure (ICP), which is known to be present in some patients with hypertensive encephalopathy, as well as ischemia of the optic

TABLE 100.3 Etiologies of Malignant Hypertension

Essential hypertension
Secondary hypertension
• Renovascular disease
• Atherosclerosis, thrombosis
• Fibromuscular dysplasia
• Medium and large vessel vasculitis
Glomerular disease
• Glomerulonephritis
• Small vessel vasculitis
• Microangiopathies
• Scleroderma
Renal parenchymal disease
• Polycystic kidney disease (and others)
• Renin-producing tumors
Endocrine causes
• Pheochromocytoma
• Primary hyperaldosteronism
• Cushing syndrome
• Hypercalcemia
Aortic coarctation
Medications (e.g., cyclosporine, tacrolimus, erythropoietin)
Sympathomimetic drugs (e.g., cocaine, amphetamines)

nerve head (34). It should be noted that ophthalmoscopic examination for hypertensive retinopathy has relatively high rates of inter- and intraobserver variability, particularly among nonophthalmologists (35).

Nephropathy and Microangiopathy

Certain conditions causing acute renal failure may cause hypertensive emergencies, but severely elevated blood pressure can also cause renal dysfunction, a condition called *malignant nephrosclerosis*. Renal biopsies reveal fibrinoid necrosis, hyperplastic arteriolitis, neutrophilic infiltration, and thrombosis of glomerular capillaries (12). The histologic appearance can be difficult to distinguish from other microangiopathies, such as hemolytic-uremic syndrome (HUS) and thrombotic thrombocytopenic purpura (TTP) (36). It is therefore not surprising that more than a quarter of patients with malignant hypertension, especially those with acute renal failure, have typical clinical features of microangiopathy, including thrombocytopenia, elevated lactate dehydrogenase, and schistocytes on blood smear (12,37). Impaired renal perfusion leads to greater activation of the renin–angiotensin system, which further augments vasoconstriction, fluid retention, and blood pressure elevation. The earliest evidence of renal involvement is the presence of abnormal urine sediment, with proteinuria, hematuria, and the appearance of red and white blood cell casts. This is followed by the development of acute renal failure, which is sometimes severe enough for patients to require dialysis, and occasionally results in end-stage renal disease.

Neurologic Hypertensive Emergencies

Stroke

Acute stroke is one of the most common indications for which emergent blood pressure control may be necessary, and often the most frequent form of end-organ damage in a consecutive series of patients with hypertensive emergencies (5). Stroke is the second leading cause of death worldwide, and is also a major reason for long-term disability. Cerebral ischemia is responsible for 70% to 80% of strokes, while intracerebral hemorrhage (ICH) and SAH account for 5% to 20%, and 1% to 7%, respectively (38,39).

Hypertensive ICH is thought to be due to long-standing hypertension. The shear forces at the point of acute angles from large vessels to smaller perforating vessels and chronic hypertension cause atherosclerosis, fibroblast proliferation, lipid deposits in the vessel wall, and collagen replacing smooth muscle cells over prolonged periods of time. All of this weakens the vessels and decreases their compliance, thereby putting them at risk for rupture (Fig. 100.3) (40–43). In 1868, Charcot and Bouchard described microaneurysms as the cause of bleeding; these microaneurysms have since been found to be subadventitial hemorrhages and extravascular clots (42,43). Most often ruptures occur in the lenticulostriate vessels, causing hemorrhage into the basal ganglia; the thalamostriate vessels, causing hemorrhage into the thalamus; the pontine perforators, causing pontine hemorrhage; cerebellar vessels and, less often, the small vessels in the cortex causing hemorrhage in the parenchyma. ICH can also be due to hemorrhage in an intraparenchymal lesion such as in tumor, either primary or metastatic, or amyloid angiopathy (39).

Overall, more than 80% of patients with ischemic or hemorrhagic strokes are initially hypertensive to some degree (39,44). Even without treatment, the blood pressure usually declines gradually over the first several hours or days in-hospital; however, most patients with acute ICH are treated for acute hypertension (45). For instance, in the recent INTERACT 2 trial, 42.9% of 1,430 patients in the conservative arm were treated to keep SBP less than 180 mmHg, and 90.1% of 1,399 patients were treated in the aggressive arm to keep SBP less than 140 mmHg (46). In addition, in the well-known National Institute of Neurological Disorders and Stroke (NINDS) trial

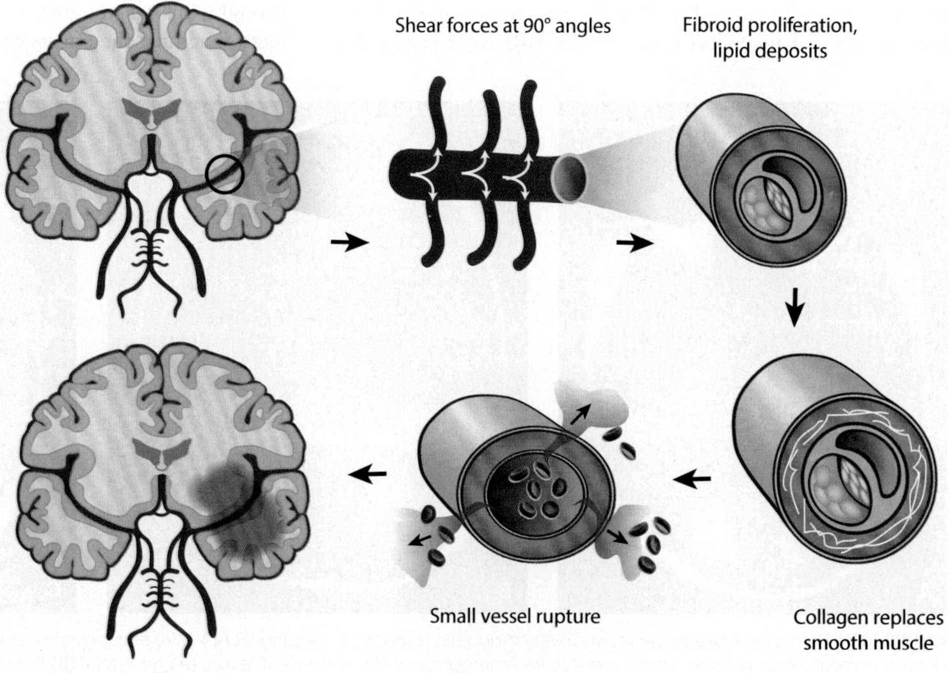

FIGURE 100.3 Simplified pathophysiology of hypertensive intracerebral hemorrhage. The cerebral arterial system with the small lenticulostriate vessels, thalamostriate, pontine perforators join at sharp angles. Close-up of the lenticulostriate vessels off of the middle cerebral artery with shear forces. Over time these shear forces lead to changes in the endothelium including fibroblast proliferation and lipid deposits. Eventually collagen replaces smooth muscle cells which leads to decreased compliance of the small vessels. These compromised vessels eventually rupture.

evaluating recombinant tissue plasminogen activator (rt-PA) for the management of acute ischemic stroke, 19% of patients had an initial blood pressure of more than 185/110 mmHg, and 60% had a blood pressure of more than 180/105 mmHg during the first 24 hours in-hospital (47). Whether or not it is appropriate (see Treatment section), more than half of these patients receive antihypertensive medications during the first few days of hospitalization (48). The incidence of hypertension with SAH is somewhat lower, but aggressive treatment is often advocated in order to minimize the initial risk of rebleeding from the aneurysm (49,50).

Posterior Reversible Encephalopathy Syndrome

The clinical manifestations of posterior reversible encephalopathy syndrome (PRES) in the setting of acute blood pressure elevation are collectively described by the term "hypertensive encephalopathy" characterized by the subacute development of neurologic signs and symptoms and may include headache, altered mental status, seizures, and visual disturbances (51). Headaches are usually generalized, severe, and poorly responsive to analgesics and improve rapidly with treatment of hypertension (52). Altered mental status can range from lethargy and confusion to stupor and coma, although the latter is unusual. The posterior predominance of PRES is reflected by the frequent occurrence of unilateral or bilateral visual disturbances, including hemianopsia, visual neglect, cortical blindness, Anton syndrome (patient is not aware of blindness), and visual hallucinations. Focal seizures originating in the occipital regions have also been described, although they most often generalize, and may be recurrent (53).

The characteristic clinical features and magnetic resonance imaging (MRI) findings of vasogenic edema in posterior white matter led to the description of a clinical radiologic syndrome, now most commonly termed *posterior reversible encephalopathy syndrome* (PRES), but previously known as *reversible posterior leukoencephalopathy syndrome* (RPLS) and *hypertensive encephalopathy syndrome* (HTE) (51,54). Although cerebral edema can sometimes be seen on computed tomography (CT) scans, PRES is best visualized using T2 and fluid-attenuated inversion recovery (FLAIR) MRI sequences. Diffusion-weighted image (DWI) MRI has confirmed that vasogenic edema is much more prominent than cytotoxic edema and, although PRES is usually "reversible," some patients do develop ischemic strokes (55). Interestingly, lesions with increased diffusion-weighted and decreased apparent diffusion coefficient (ADC) values, which normally correspond to ischemic stroke, later have completely reversed on MRI (51). Many patients do not adhere perfectly to the typical patterns of PRES: gray matter involvement of the cerebral cortex and basal ganglia, as well as edema occurring in the frontal lobes, posterior fossa, and brainstem are found in 10% to 30% of cases (51); it is rare for only one vascular territory to be involved (Fig. 100.4A–C).

The pathophysiology of PRES is both not completely understood and controversial. The older hypothesis is hypertension can lead to vasoconstriction by autoregulation and subsequent hypoperfusion, ischemia, and cerebral edema (51). The newer hypothesis is severe elevations in blood pressure eventually cause a breakdown of the blood–brain barrier, with subsequent development of vasogenic cerebral edema. White matter is less tightly packed than the overlying cerebral cortex thereby making it more vulnerable to the spread of edema. Although occurring most commonly in association with severe hypertension, there are other conditions that may at least predispose to, if not directly cause, the development of PRES, perhaps because they induce endothelial toxicity. PRES has been described in association with certain medications—most notably cyclosporine (32,51)—and other immunosuppressive agents, as well as in the setting of microangiopathies, connective tissue diseases, vasculitis, and preeclampsia (56). Endothelial injury, therefore, seems to be a common link between these conditions (51). Because of the importance of endothelium in autoregulation, injury may lead to an inability to vasodilate, leading to hypoperfusion, thereby arguing for the older hypothesis of pathogenesis. As to why PRES most often occurs posteriorly is up to some debate. Based on a histofluorescence study from the 1970s, showing a greater concentration of sympathetic fibers around arterioles in the anterior brain, it is thought this allows greater vasoconstriction and relative protection against the effects of severe hypertension (57). A more

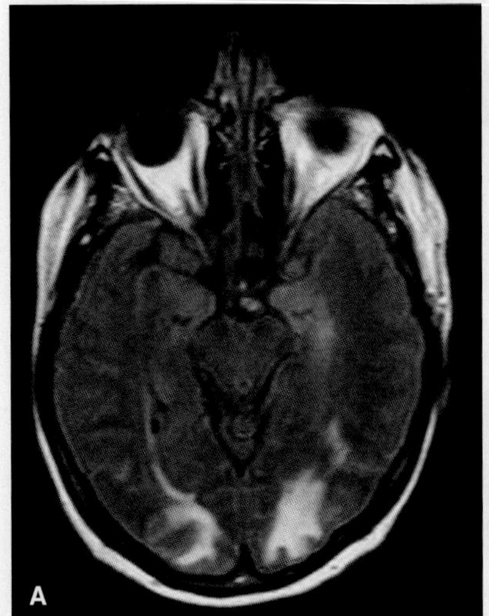

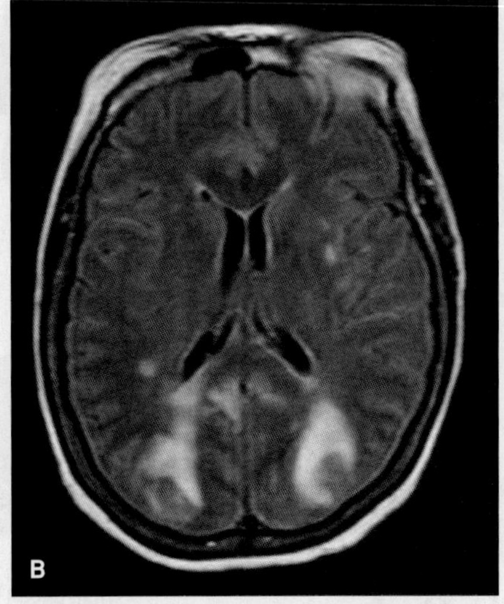

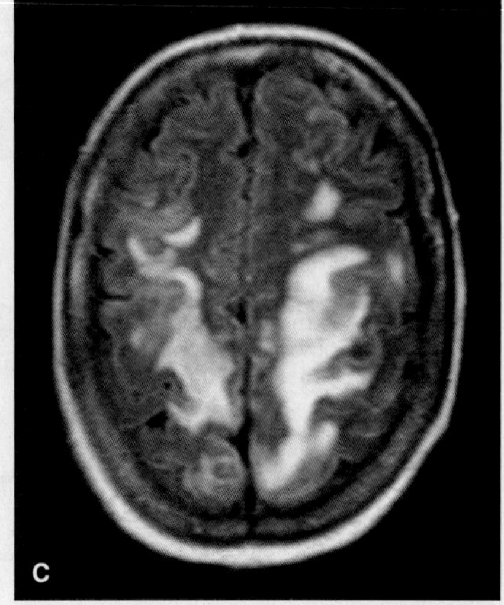

FIGURE 100.4 Fluid-attenuated inversion recovery magnetic resonance imaging (FLAIR–MRI) sequences of a 58-year-old woman who presented with altered mental status, seizures, and hypertensive emergency at three different levels, **(A)** midbrain, **(B)** basal ganglia, and **(C)** more superiorly. The findings are consistent with posterior reversible encephalopathy syndrome.

recent study looking into quantifying perivascular nerve fibers in human cerebral arteries has shown a greater concentration of sympathetic fibers around the posterior cerebral arteries and posterior communicating arteries. This then lends itself to the hypothesis that greater sympathetic innervation leads to vasoconstriction and possibly hypoperfusion, endothelial injury, and cerebral edema (51,58). This further leads to controversy and questions into the exact pathophysiology of PRES.

Cardiovascular Hypertensive Emergencies

Approximately 20% of patients with malignant hypertension present with cardiac complications, which may include myocardial ischemia or pulmonary edema (59). Many patients have a pre-existing history of chronic hypertension with already existing left ventricular hypertrophy and diastolic dysfunction, while a smaller subset also has impaired systolic function. Left ventricular hypertrophy increases myocardial oxygen requirements while also outstripping vascular supply and compressing coronary arterioles. The increased afterload associated with severe hypertension further increases myocardial wall stress and oxygen demand, such that ischemia occurs, especially if there is also concomitant coronary artery disease. Increased wall thickness and changes to the extramyocardial collagen network impair myocardial relaxation, and cause pressure within the left ventricle to rise at relatively lower volumes during diastole. As a result, even small increases in intravascular volume and afterload can produce pulmonary edema (60).

Acute Heart Failure

Acute heart failure is responsible for 5% to 10% of hospital admissions, with hospital mortality of about 4%, increasing to more than 50% at 1 year. In a large American registry, 73% of patients had a history of chronic hypertension, and 50% were hypertensive at admission (61). In patients presenting with flash pulmonary edema, acute hypertension is particularly common, and is likely to be both a consequence *and* contributing cause. Patients suspected of having acute heart failure should have a chest x-ray, echocardiogram, electrocardiogram, oxygen saturation, blood chemistry, full blood counts, and natriuretic peptide measurements (62). If the measured NT-pro-BNP or BNP level is less than the cut-off points of, respectively, 300 pg/mL and 100 pg /mL, acute heart failure can be ruled out (62). These tests have the goal of determining if ventilation and oxygenation are adequate, if the patient is hypotensive or in shock, has life-threatening tachy- or brady-dysrhythmias, acute valvular disease, or acute coronary syndrome (ACS). The patient may need noninvasive or invasive ventilation, cardioversion, pacing, inotrope infusion, mechanical circulatory support, or coronary reperfusion (62). A history of chronic hypertension exists in 40% to 70% of patients with ACSs, and about 30% have an elevated blood pressure when initially assessed (63,64). Severe uncontrolled hypertension at admission (>180/110 mmHg) is a relative contraindication to thrombolysis for ST-elevation myocardial infarction (STEMI) (65). ACS is diagnosed by clinical symptoms of chest pain and ST changes on electrocardiogram, but troponin biomarkers have the most utility, approaching 100% sensitivity (66,67). In fact, chest pain syndromes without troponin biomarker elevation are excluded from the definition of ACS and, instead, are classified as a subtype of severe stable coronary artery disease (66).

Aortic Dissection

Aortic dissection is a relatively rare condition, with an annual incidence of between 3 and 6 cases/100,000 persons/year, with about two-thirds being Stanford type A (involving the ascending aorta or the arch) and one-third being type B (involving the descending aorta) (68,69). With modern medical and surgical therapy, the mortality has decreased from as high as 90% to approximately 47% for type A who survive to admission, and 13% for type B (69). About 65% to 70% of patients have a history of chronic hypertension and, in one study, 46% of patents had documented systolic blood pressure of greater than 180 mmHg in the prior 5 years before dissection. Most patients (70%) with type B dissection have an admission systolic pressure of more than 150 mmHg, compared with just over a third of those with type A dissections, of whom approximately 25% actually present with hypertension or in frank shock (68). The pathophysiology and mechanism by which hypertension predisposes to aortic dissection is still under investigation. Current postulates stem from decreased flow in the vasa vasorum; when this flow is decreased, there is inadequate oxygen delivery to the entire thickness of the aortic wall. This leads to ischemic outer media, decreased smooth muscle cells, and changes in the elastic laminae, leading to stiffness of the outer media. Interlaminar shear forces occur between the healthy inner layer and stiff outer layer, which eventually lead to aortic dissection (70,71).

Perioperative Hypertension

Preoperative hypertension is thought to be a perioperative risk factor for mortality, major morbidity, prolonged length of stay, and readmission (72), although this is questioned. Classically, operative cases have been canceled for hypertension greater than 180/110 mmHg. However, a study of 989 hypertensive patients who had a diastolic pressure of greater than 100 mmHg just prior to surgery were either treated with intranasal nifedipine and immediate surgery, or surgery was delayed with slower lowering of the blood pressure over a course of days; delaying surgery did not improve outcomes (73). Increased pulse pressure—the systolic pressure minus diastolic pressure–has been shown to yield increased risk for perioperative cerebral events and mortality in patients having cardiac surgery (74). The American Heart Association now recommends weighing the risk of delaying nonemergent surgery to control severely elevated blood pressure—greater than 180/100 mmHg—versus proceeding (75).

Intraoperative blood pressure elevations of greater than 20% of baseline blood pressures are considered to be a hypertensive emergency (76). Intraoperative hypertension has the highest incidence during carotid, abdominal aortic, peripheral vascular, abdominal, and intrathoracic operations. Depending upon the patient population, type of surgery, and how hypertension is defined, 3% to 34% of operative interventions are complicated by postoperative hypertension in the recovery room or ICU, with the most important risk factors being inadequately controlled pain and a pre-existing history of hypertension, especially if antihypertensives were withdrawn in the preoperative period (77,78). Elevations in blood pressure occur most often during the initial 30 to 60 minutes after surgery, may last for several hours, and have been associated with higher rates of postoperative hemorrhage and myocardial ischemia in certain patient populations (77). Hypertension is particularly frequent following neurosurgical and cardiovascular procedures, occurring in, respectively, 54% to 91% and 30% to 80% of patients undergoing craniotomy and coronary artery bypass grafting (79–81). The elevation in blood pressure is postulated to be due to increases in sympathetic tone and vascular resistance (77,82).

Pregnancy-Induced Hypertension

Hypertension complicates approximately 6% to 8% of pregnancies, and is responsible for 18% of maternal deaths in the United States, 26% of maternal deaths in Latin America and the Caribbean, and 9% of the deaths in Africa and Asia (83). Pregnancy-induced hypertension (PIH) encompasses gestational hypertension, preeclampsia, and eclampsia. *Gestational hypertension* is defined as blood pressure elevation, greater than 140/90 mmHg beginning after 20 weeks gestation and resolving by 12 weeks postpartum. *Eclampsia* is defined as gestational hypertension with proteinuria, greater than or equal to 300 mg in 24 hours, or as proteinuria in women with known hypertension but who previously did not have proteinuria prior to 20 weeks gestation. Preeclampsia is associated with vasoconstriction, endothelial dysfunction, platelet aggregation, and increased coagulation (83). Preeclampsia occurs in 2% to 8% of pregnancies with important risk factors including nulliparity, antiphospholipid antibodies, diabetes mellitus, obesity, family history, multiple (twin) pregnancies, maternal age over 40, and a previous history during other pregnancies. Maternal complications can include progression to eclampsia, pulmonary edema, microangiopathy, renal failure, and placental abruption. The most common neonatal complications are prematurity and intrauterine growth restriction. Most cases of PIH do not present until after 36 weeks of gestation. Recently, a multicenter, randomized control trial looked at the induction of labor versus expectant monitoring for gestational hypertension or mild preeclampsia after 36 weeks' gestation (HYPITAT) (84). This study found induction of labor resulted in a lower incidence of poor maternal outcome and therefore recommend for inducing labor (84). Eclampsia is defined as the development of severe neurologic manifestations, including seizures and a depressed level of consciousness, in women with preeclampsia, which is not attributed to another cause. It complicates 1% to 2% of severe preeclampsia and 79% of cases have signs and symptoms in the week prior to the event: headache in 56%, hypertension in 48%, proteinuria in 46%, visual disturbances in 23%, and epigastric pain in 17% (83).

TREATMENT

Pharmacologic Agents

An ideal pharmacologic agent (Table 100.4) for treatment of hypertensive emergencies should have a rapid onset in order to immediately reduce the progression of organ failure, but should also be short acting and easy to titrate to avoid excessively lowering the blood pressure below the range of autoregulation of cerebral, coronary, and renal arterial systems. Because of this, intravenous agents should be used, rather than ones requiring the sublingual or intramuscular routes (85). The following agents are the most commonly used.

β-Blockers

Labetalol is the most commonly used intravenous β-blocker (and α-blocker) for the management of hypertensive emergencies. One of its unique properties is that when given intravenously, it blocks both α- and β-receptors, although the nonselective β-blocking effect is more prominent at a ratio of 1:7 (85). Labetalol is usually administered as 10- to 20-mg boluses, which can be repeated every 15 minutes until the desired effect is achieved. Blood pressure lowering begins within 2 to 5 minutes, with maximal effect after about 5 to 15 minutes and elimination half-life of around 5.5 hours (85). Labetalol can also be delivered as an infusion, beginning at a dose of 1 to 2 mg/min. It has been demonstrated to be safe and effective in the management of severe hypertension, with advantages that it does not cause reflex tachycardia, has little effect on cerebral blood flow or ICP, and does not decrease cardiac output (85,86). Because of its lipophilic nature, labetalol does not cross the placenta well, and there is extensive

TABLE 100.4 Intravenous Pharmacologic Agents for Management of Hypertensive Emergencies

Drug	Dose	Onset	Duration	Precautions
Labetalol	10–20 mg boluses 1–4 mg/min infusion	5–15 min	2–4 hrs	Bradycardia, heart block; LV dysfunction; asthma
Esmolol	0.5 mg/kg load, 50–200 μg/kg/min	5 min	10–30 min	Bradycardia, heart block; LV dysfunction; asthma
Nicardipine	3–15 mg/min	5–15 min	30–60 min	Rebound tachycardia
Clevidipine	2–32 mg/hrs	2–6 min	2–10 min	Reflexive tachycardia; rebound hypertension; each 100 mL vial has 20 g of soya bean oil
Fenoldopam	0.1–1.6 μg/kg/min	5–15 min	20–60 min	Glaucoma
Nitroprusside	0.25–10 μg/kg/min (ideally less than 2 μg/kg/min)	Immediate	1–10 min	Cyanide toxicity with prolonged infusions; coronary steal; ↑ ICP
Nitroglycerin	10–200 μg/min	Immediate	3–10 min	Severe hypotension in hypovolemic patients; ↑ ICP; contraindicated if on PDE-5 inhibitors
Enalaprilat	0.625–2.5-mg bolus, every 6 hrs	15 min	4–6 hrs	Renal failure; hyperkalemia
Hydralazine	10–20 mg every 4–6 hrs	5–20 min	2–6 hrs	Reflex tachycardia; ischemic heart disease

ICP, intracranial pressure; LV, left ventricular; PDE-5, phosphodiesterase-5.

experience using it in pregnancy, making it one of the preferred agents in the management of preeclampsia and eclampsia (83).

Esmolol is an extremely short-acting, relatively cardioselective β-blocker, with onset within less than a minute, and a unique metabolism by red blood cell esterases such that its duration of action is only 10 to 20 minutes; in anemic patients the half-life can be increased. A loading dose of 0.5 mg/kg is administered over 1 minute, followed by an infusion of 50 μg/kg/min, which can be adjusted as often as every 5 minutes to a maximum dose of 200 μg/kg/min. This maximum dose is due to the toxicities of the solvent, propylene glycol: renal toxicity, elevated osmolar gap, metabolic acidosis, cardiac arrhythmias, seizures, and hemolysis (87). Esmolol is a useful agent when blood pressure is elevated and cardiac output is preserved, especially when there are concerns about myocardial ischemia. Because it decreases heart rate as well as myocardial contractility, cardiac output is lowered. It may also cause bronchospasm and, therefore, should be used in caution in patients with low cardiac output or chronic obstructive pulmonary disease (85).

Nicardipine

Nicardipine is a second-generation dihydropyridine calcium channel blocker (CCB) that inhibits calcium influx through L-type channels, thereby preventing smooth muscle contraction, particularly in vascular smooth muscle, rather than cardiac myocytes. Thus, nicardipine causes arterial vasodilatation, with minimal venodilatation or change in cardiac output. It increases stroke volume and coronary blood flow leading to a favorable oxygen consumption versus supply ratio (85). It is most often administered as an intravenous infusion, beginning at 3 to 5 mg/hr, to a maximum of 15 mg/hr, but it can also be given as 0.5- to 3-mg boluses, and dosing has been reported up to 30 to 45 mg/hr. Because of a distribution half-life of less than 3 minutes and an intermediate elimination half-life of less than 45 minutes, nicardipine has a relatively rapid onset and offset (88). It has compared favorably with sodium nitroprusside (NTP) in clinical trials, with therapeutic targets achieved in a similar amount of time, fewer episodes of severe hypotension, and less frequent dose adjustment (88,89). Nicardipine has been used in a variety of settings, including malignant hypertension, perioperative hypertension, hemorrhagic stroke, preeclampsia, and acute heart failure. It is generally well tolerated, with few adverse effects when used with caution. Given that nicardipine may increase cerebral blood flow, one might expect that it would raise ICP. Although this has been reported, it does not appear to be a major concern in most studies (85,90).

Clevidipine

Clevidipine is a third-generation, intravenous, dihydropyridine calcium channel antagonist. It selectively inhibits L-type channels, which inhibits the influx of calcium leading to smooth muscle relaxation. This equates to potent arterial vasodilatory properties with little effect on myocardial inotropy and venous capacitance. It has been shown to significantly increase stroke volume and cardiac output (91). Clevidipine has a rapid onset of about 2 minutes, with goal blood pressure being reached within 6 minutes and steady state reached in 15 minutes. It is metabolized by red blood cell esterases and has a half-life of around 2 minutes. It also has numerous antioxidative properties, increases NO concentrations, and decreases intracellular calcium concentration (85,91). Initial infusion rate is recommended at 2 mg/hr and may be doubled every 90 seconds to reach target blood pressure. The US guidelines recommend using a lower dose increase and at 5- to 10-minute intervals as the target blood pressure is neared. The maximum dose is 32 mg/hr, with a maximum of 1,000 mL/24-hour period and maximum infusion period of 72 hours (91). Clevidipine has been shown to be safe in treatment of acute ICH, acute ischemic stroke, SAH, perioperative hypertension, acute heart failure, and patients with renal dysfunction and severe hypertension. It is available in many European countries for blood pressure control in the perioperative setting and in the United States when oral therapy is not feasible (91).

Fenoldopam

Fenoldopam is a selective dopamine-1 (DA-1)-receptor agonist, which produces peripheral, renal, splanchnic, and, to a lesser degree, coronary vasodilatation. Stimulation of DA-1 receptors also promotes natriuresis. Unlike dopamine, fenoldopam does not have any effect on DA-2 receptors, nor does it act at the α- or β-adrenergic receptor level. It does not cross the blood–brain barrier, and therefore has no effect on intraparenchymal dopamine receptors. There are cranial endothelial DA-1 receptors and, therefore, fenoldopam causes some cerebral vasodilation. It is typically administered in doses of 0.025 to 1 μg/kg/min, and begins to lower blood pressure after as little as 2 minutes, although the maximal effect is not seen for at least 20 to 30 minutes or more; with discontinuation of an infusion, the elimination half-life is less than 10 minutes. Reflex tachycardia, related to activation of the baroreflex, may occur and can be attenuated with concomitant use of a β-blocker (92). A theoretical advantage of fenoldopam is improved renal blood flow, but clinical trials have shown conflicting results in decreases in renal replacement therapy or death (93–96). Fenoldopam has been demonstrated to be effective at controlling blood pressure in hypertensive emergencies, with efficacy similar to nitroprusside, but has shown no clear improvement in outcomes; it has also been considerably more expensive than NTP (97), although this may be changing with the upheaval of the US generic drug market. Overall, fenoldopam seems to have few adverse effects. It does raise intraocular pressure, and should therefore probably be avoided in patients with a known history of glaucoma (98,99).

Sodium Nitroprusside

NTP has been used in the management of hypertensive emergencies for over 40 years, and continues to be used, largely because of its rapid onset, short duration of action, affordability—although the upheavals in the US generic drug market may be changing this—familiarity, and efficacy (8,100). Sodium nitroprusside is a potent arterial and venous vasodilator, which has an onset within less than 30 seconds and a duration of action of only 2 to 3 minutes, such that cessation of the infusion allows blood pressure to rise back to previous levels within 1 to 10 minutes. Cardiac output is either preserved or increased, and cardiac filling pressures decrease (85). The mechanism of action involves the release of NO into the bloodstream, activation of guanylate cyclase, and subsequent conversion of guanosine triphosphate (GTP) to cyclic guanosine monophosphate (cGMP) in vascular smooth muscle, which in turn inhibits the intracellular movement of calcium. The usual starting dose of sodium nitroprusside is 0.25 to 0.5 μg/kg/min, and it is increased in increments of 0.5 μg/kg/min every 5 to 10 minutes until the goal blood pressure is achieved.

Sodium nitroprusside has the potential for several serious, life-threatening complications. First, despite lowering preload and afterload, sodium nitroprusside may induce coronary steal, whereby excessive vasodilatation of coronary arterioles shunts blood away from ischemic regions (85). This effect may help explain the findings of a large clinical trial in which patients with acute myocardial infarction and high left ventricular filling pressures had worse outcomes when treated with nitroprusside within the first 8 hours, but improved outcomes thereafter (101).

Second, NTP is often avoided in neurologic emergencies because of the observation that it vasodilates cerebral vasculature, increases cerebral blood volume, and therefore raises ICP (85,102). The demonstration of this phenomenon is not entirely consistent in the literature, and it may be avoidable with a somewhat slower administration (103).

Third, each nitroprusside molecule has five cyanide moieties, such that cyanide makes up 44% of the drug's molecular weight (85). Cyanide is metabolized by transulfuration in the liver to thiocyanate, which is 100 times less toxic than cyanide, and is cleared in the urine and stool; when this pathway is overwhelmed, cyanide accumulates and causes toxicity. Patients receiving sodium nitroprusside are particularly vulnerable when treated with prolonged, high-dose infusions, especially if hepatic and renal function are impaired, or if sulfur stores are depleted because of malnutrition (100). Cyanide blocks oxidative phosphorylation and essentially causes tissue anoxia and lactic acidosis despite adequate oxygen delivery, leading to high venous oxygen saturation levels. Manifestations of cyanide poisoning include depressed mental status, seizures, and, eventually, bradycardia and hemodynamic collapse. Cyanide levels are not easily monitored, and the development of lactic acidosis is a late finding. The development of tachyphylaxis to nitroprusside, with consequent increasing dose requirements, may be a harbinger of toxicity (100).

Treatment of cyanide poisoning consists of discontinuation of sodium nitroprusside, supportive care with the delivery of 100% oxygen, and the administration of sodium nitrite (300 mg IV), followed by sodium thiosulfate (12.5 gm IV). The use of sodium nitrite is controversial, as it actually causes the production of methemoglobin, which, although also potentially toxic, binds avidly to cyanide. Sodium thiosulfate acts as a sulfur donor to promote the formation of thiocyanate, and has been used effectively as monotherapy. Hydroxycobalamin combines with cyanide to form cyanocobalamin, and may provide synergy with sodium thiosulfate. Both agents have been used prophylactically with infusions of nitroprusside to prevent cyanide accumulation. Accumulation of thiocyanate, although far less toxic than cyanide, may also cause complications (104). The coadministration of thiosulfate infusions in patients receiving nitroprusside infusions, in the 4 to 10 μg/kg/min range, has been advocated.

Because of these concerns, and despite sodium nitroprusside's extensive track record, it should be administered at as low a dose as possible, and for as short a duration as possible. It has been argued sodium nitroprusside should only be used in patients with normal renal and hepatic function and only after newer, alternative agents have failed (85).

Nitroglycerin

Because nitroglycerin produces more venous, than arterial, dilatation, it is usually not used as first-line therapy for hypertensive emergencies, unless there is concurrent pulmonary edema or myocardial ischemia. When either of these are the case, it is usually started at 5 to 10 μg/min, and can be titrated up every 5 to 10 minutes to doses as high as 200 to 300 μg/min. Particular caution must be exercised in the setting of hypovolemia (85). Patients using drugs for erectile dysfunction should not be given nitroglycerin or nitroprusside, as this may induce profound hypotension (80). As with nitroprusside, there are case reports of nitroglycerin increasing ICP, such that it should be used with caution in brain-injured patients (105).

Enalaprilat

Enalaprilat is an ACE inhibitor in intravenous form. Its effect is not seen for about 15 minutes, takes an hour to reach peak effect, and lasts for up to 6 hours. As with all ACE inhibitors, patients who have decreased renal perfusion are at risk for acute renal injury and hyperkalemia if given this drug (85).

TREATMENT FOR SPECIFIC HYPERTENSIVE EMERGENCIES

Malignant Hypertension

Because of the shift in the autoregulatory curve that occurs with prolonged hypertension, rapid reductions in blood pressure may cause organ ischemia (106). With hypertensive urgencies, the blood pressure should therefore be reduced carefully and gradually with oral medications over the course of several days. It is not precisely known how long it takes for the autoregulatory curve to recover and shift back toward the left, thus, the initial goal should never be normal blood pressure.

With hypertensive emergencies, the blood pressure must be reduced immediately, with an initial goal of no more than a 15% reduction. Specific treatment goals should be individualized to ensure that the pressure is reduced sufficiently for organ failure to resolve without compromising perfusion. To facilitate keeping blood pressure within a narrow range, placement of an arterial catheter and careful observation in the ICU are recommended.

Neurologic

Acute Ischemic Stroke

Although acute hypertension is common in patients with ischemic stroke, optimal treatment remains uncertain. The greatest priority in these patients is to preserve as much of the ischemic penumbra as possible and to avoid hemorrhagic conversion and malignant cerebral edema. Because autoregulation is usually impaired within the penumbra, pressure reductions may cause blood flow to fall, which in turn may increase infarct size (107). However, several older observational studies have inconsistent results, demonstrating lowering blood pressure may cause worsened, better, or no change in clinical outcome (108–111). Preliminary pilot studies have suggested that transcranial Doppler middle cerebral artery (MCA) flow velocities, cerebral perfusion as determined by MRI, and neurologic examination may improve with supranormal augmentation of blood pressure using a vasopressor (112). The International Stroke Trial of more than 17,000 patients found a U-shaped relationship, where the best outcomes occurred in patients with a presenting systolic blood pressure of about 150 mmHg (113). The 2013 American Stroke Association guidelines currently recommend not treating hypertension unless the systolic pressure exceeds 220 mmHg, the diastolic pressure exceeds 120 mmHg, or there is another medical condition which would benefit from lowering the blood pressure (111). Finally, in a large, multicenter, randomized and controlled study in which patients were randomized to reduction of blood pressure by 25% within 24 hours and to less than 140/90 mmHg within 7 days versus discontinuing all antihypertensive medications, there was no difference in death or major disability at 14 days, at hospital discharge, or at 3-month follow-up (114).

The exception to this rule is if the patient is a candidate for intravenous or, possibly, intra-arterial thrombolysis. Of patients who receive intravenous rt-PA for treatment of acute ischemic stroke, 5% to 6% will develop ICH (115). Whether lowering blood pressure helps to limit this risk is not certain. However, patients in whom systolic and diastolic pressure could not easily be lowered to, respectively, less than 185 mmHg and 110 mmHg, were excluded from the definitive clinical trial (116). Patients who did receive thrombolysis had a goal blood pressure of less than 180/105 mmHg. Approximately 10% of patients require intravenous antihypertensive therapy prior to receiving thrombolysis, while 25% to 30% require treatment in the 24 hours after thrombolysis (47).

Intracerebral Hemorrhage

Good neurologic recovery is very uncommon if the volume of ICH exceeds 30 to 60 mL. Hematoma growth is a dynamic process that occurs over several hours, with a significant proportion of patients having detectable expansion even within the first few hours after presentation to the ED or ICU (117). Patients with early hematoma enlargement have substantially worse outcomes, and it is likely that therapy that can limit this early growth will improve outcomes. Numerous studies have suggested that patients with higher blood pressure at presentation are more likely to develop hematoma expansion and have a higher mortality (118,119). The main reason for previous concern for lowering the blood pressure has been the observation that there is reduced blood flow around areas of ICH and the belief that this represents an ischemic penumbra that could be compromised with lower blood pressure. However, studies using positive emission tomography and MRI have suggested that decreased flow surrounding ICH is appropriate for the corresponding reduction in cerebral metabolic rate (120). Furthermore, cerebral blood flow autoregulation in this region appears to be preserved, such that lowering blood pressure does not adversely impact regional blood flow (121).

Based on these data, the INTensive Blood Pressure Reduction in Acute Cerebral Hemorrhage Trial (INTERACT) 1 and 2, and Antihypertensive Treatment of Acute Cerebral Hemorrhage (ATACH) I and II were undertaken (46,122). The INTERACT 2 trial reported results in the Spring of 2013, demonstrating that intensive lowering of systolic blood pressure to less than 140 mmHg within 6 hours of onset did not result in a change in rate of death or severe disability. However, ordinal analysis of modified Rankin scores did show improvement in functional outcomes with intensive blood pressure control (46). ATACH II is an ongoing, multicenter, 5-year, randomized, controlled, phase-III trial to determine if intensive blood pressure lowering within 3 hours of onset and for 24 hours by intravenous nicardipine decreases the likelihood of death or disability by 10% at 3 months, compared to conservative treatment (122). The current American Heart Association guidelines from 2010 were promulgated prior to completion of these studies, and state that for patients with systolic blood pressure of 150 to 220 mmHg, its acute lowering to 140 mmHg is probably safe (39).

Subarachnoid Hemorrhage

Nontraumatic SAH results from a ruptured intracranial aneurysm in more than 80% of cases (49). The risk of recurrent hemorrhage from the aneurysm is 4% to 13.6% within the first 24 hours (50). Risk factors associated with rebleeding include longer time to securing of the aneurysm, worse admission neurologic examination, previous sentinel headaches, larger aneurysm size, and systolic blood pressure greater than 160 mmHg. Many centers attempt to decrease the risk of recurrent hemorrhage by reducing blood pressure prior to securing the aneurysm, with review articles often citing goal systolic pressures of less than 140 to 180 mmHg (49). However, the efficacy of this practice remains uncertain, with conflicting results from observational studies. Particular caution should be exercised when treating patients with high-grade SAH who are stuporous or comatose, because these patients may have a raised ICP, and excessive reduction in blood pressure may compromise cerebral perfusion and promote ischemia. Current American Heart Association guidelines recognize the lack of evidence on how intensely to control the blood pressure, but state that decreasing the systolic blood pressure to less than 160 mmHg is reasonable (50).

After the aneurysm has been treated, the most concerning complication is the development of cerebral vasospasm and delayed ischemic neurologic deficits (DINDs), which occur in approximately 20% to 40% of patients, with maximum risk between days 7 and 10 after the event, resolving by post bleed day 21 (50). Hypertension should not routinely be treated during this time, even at relatively high levels, since this practice increases the risk of DIND. If clinical vasospasm develops, first-line therapy actually involves hemodynamic augmentation, using vasopressors to raise blood pressure in order to increase cerebral blood flow and improve cerebral perfusion in conjunction with endovascular treatments such as intra-arterial vasodilator infusions and balloon angioplasty (50).

CARDIOVASCULAR HYPERTENSIVE EMERGENCIES

Acute Heart Failure and Pulmonary Edema

Acute hypertension exists in the majority of patients presenting with flash pulmonary edema, and is likely to be both a consequence and contributing cause (61,123). The venodilating properties of nitroglycerin make it an excellent initial choice as an antihypertensive in both normotensive and hypertensive patients, especially if there is failure to improve after administration of a loop diuretic. In titrating the dose of intravenous nitroglycerin, clinicians should be aware that relatively large doses, often in excess of 100 μg/min, may be required to significantly lower cardiac filling pressures and improve symptoms (124). Patients who benefit from aggressive afterload reduction, such as those with acute aortic or mitral regurgitation (if not hypotensive), may require a more potent arterial vasodilator than nitroglycerin, such as nitroprusside or nicardipine.

Although ACE inhibitors are standard care for chronic heart failure, there is little evidence of benefit for acute decompensated heart failure. The only intravenous preparation, enalaprilat, was potentially harmful when routinely administered to patients within the first 24 hours following STEMI, and is therefore not recommended (125). Considerable caution must be exercised when intubating hypertensive patients with acute pulmonary edema, since it is very common for blood pressure to drop precipitously with sedation and positive pressure ventilation. Noninvasive ventilation should be considered in dyspneic patients with pulmonary edema but, again, may reduce blood pressure with initiation and should be used in caution in patients in shock (62). Another agent that has been proposed for use in acute heart failure is nesiritide (recombinant human brain natriuretic peptide). However, it has not been demonstrated to improve clinically important outcomes when compared with standard therapy (126), may worsen renal function (127), and has been linked to a possible increased risk of short-term death (128). In a trial comparing low-dose dopamine or low-dose nesiritide in addition to diuretic therapy in patients in acute heart failure with renal dysfunction, neither drug improved congestion or renal function (129). In a recent international, multicenter, randomized controlled trial, clevidipine was demonstrated to be faster and more effective in reducing blood pressure into the target range, and in reducing dyspnea symptoms when compared to standard of care intravenous blood pressure lowering agents (130).

Acute Coronary Syndromes

Although definitive therapy for ACSs involves antithrombotic agents and revascularization, other steps can be taken to decrease oxygen consumption. Oxygen consumption is increased by increases in heart rate, contractility, and wall stress. Wall stress is estimated by Laplace's equation:

$$\text{Stress} = \text{pressure} \times \text{radius}/(2 \times \text{wall thickness}).$$

β-Blockers decrease heart rate, contractility, and blood pressure, and are recommended for all ACS patients without a contraindication. β-blockers have been shown to decrease mortality by 28% to 34%, decrease the reinfarction rate by 18%, and cardiac arrest by 15% (131). Intravenous β-blockers must be used with caution in patients with reduced left ventricular systolic function and in those in whom there is concern about impaired cardiac conduction (e.g., inferior myocardial infarction). A large clinical trial of early intravenous, followed by oral, β-blockade in patients with STEMI demonstrated an increased risk of cardiogenic shock, mostly in high-risk patients: age greater than 70, systolic blood pressure less than 120 mmHg, and heart rate greater than 110 beats/min (131). ACE inhibitors decrease afterload and oxygen consumption; captopril, ramipril, and trandolapril have all been shown to reduce mortality in patients with heart failure and after myocardial infarction (131). ACE inhibitors should be given within 24 hours of myocardial infarction in patients with a left ventricular ejection fraction of less than 40% or heart failure (131). If the blood pressure remains significantly elevated, especially with ongoing chest pain or pulmonary edema, then nitroglycerin should be used. In addition to reducing oxygen consumption by decreasing preload and left ventricular end-diastolic volume, nitrates also vasodilate coronary arteries, especially at the site of plaque disruption. If three sublingual tablets (0.4 mg over 5 minutes) are ineffective, then an intravenous infusion should be started and adjusted to alleviate chest pain and reduce blood pressure (10% reduction in normotensive patients, 30% reduction in hypertensive patients) (65). Use of nitroglycerin in combination with phosphodiesterase inhibitors can cause profound hypotension and, therefore, nitrates should be avoided in patients who have taken sildenafil and tadalafil. The aldosterone receptor antagonist, eplerenone, has been shown to further reduce mortality in patients with acute myocardial infarction with heart failure who have already been treated with a β-blocker or ACE inhibitor. CCBs should only be used in patients for augmented hemodynamic control, not as routine primary agents. Caution must be taken with dihydropyridine CCBs, nifedipine and amlodipine, as they can cause reflex tachycardia, and caution must be taken with nondihydropyridine CCBs, verapamil and diltiazem, in patients with heart failure and pulmonary edema due to their negative inotropic effects (131). Preconditioning strategies such as remote upper limb transient ischemia by suprainflation of blood pressure cuff have been shown to reduce all-cause mortality in comparison to standard care. Cyclosporine administration for postconditioning to prevent reperfusion injury is currently being studied in Europe in the larger Cyclosporine and Prognosis in Acute MI Patients (CIRCUS; NCT01502774) trial.

Aortic Dissection

The purpose of emergently lowering blood pressure in aortic dissection is to decrease shear stress on the aorta and limit propagation of the intimal tear and false lumen. In order to concomitantly reduce both blood pressure and the force of left ventricular contraction, first-line therapy consists of a β-blocker or, if contraindicated, a CCB with negative inotropic and chronotropic properties (e.g., diltiazem or verapamil). Pure vasodilators should not be used in isolation. If possible, the heart rate should be lowered to less than 60 beats/min, and the blood pressure reduced as much as can be tolerated, ideally below a systolic pressure of 120 mmHg. Because patients often have substantial chest discomfort, the use of opiates to ameliorate pain may greatly reduce antihypertensive requirements. If the blood pressure remains elevated despite adequate β-blockade, a vasodilator can be added. There is extensive experience with nitroprusside in this setting, although other agents have also been used (88,132).

Perioperative Hypertension

Perioperative hypertension is a common phenomenon, as previously mentioned, especially after vascular surgery, neurosurgery, intrathoracic surgery, and abdominal surgery. Almost all of the agents previously mentioned have been studied and the choice of agent should depend upon the patient's specific comorbidities and operation.

Hypertension occurs in the setting of craniotomy more often than with any other type of surgery (79). Neurosurgery results in the release of large amounts of vasoactive substances that raise blood pressure, including catecholamines, endothelin, and renin (133). Importantly, severe hypertension occurring intraoperatively or during the first 12 postoperative hours has been associated with a higher risk of intracranial hemorrhage complicated craniotomy (79). Recently a clinical trial found nicardipine to be superior to esmolol in the treatment of emergence hypertension after intracranial tumor resection (81).

Mild intraoperative hypotension is sometimes used for vascular neurosurgical procedures, such as microsurgical excision or endovascular obliteration of arteriovenous malformations (AVMs) in order to reduce the risk of hemorrhage. With AVM, the sudden "repressurization" of previously hypotensive arterioles may contribute to the development of regional hyperemia, edema, and bleeding, a condition sometimes referred to as "normal perfusion pressure breakthrough." Consequently, hypertension should be avoided in the immediate postoperative period; indeed, systolic blood pressure is frequently kept between 90 and 110 mmHg in the immediate postoperative period. Conversely, the sacrifice of vascular branches during the procedure, or vasospasm from surgical manipulation and retraction, may also create areas of relative underperfusion, such that hypotension would also be deleterious (134).

There are certain neurosurgical procedures where tight postoperative blood pressure control is particularly important. In most patients undergoing carotid stenting or endarterectomy, the sudden resolution of carotid stenosis results in a sudden, asymptomatic, 20% to 40% increase in ipsilateral cerebral blood flow. However, in some patients, the increase can be much more profound, to the degree that it overcomes the autoregulatory capacity of the corresponding, previously hypoperfused territory. The resulting cerebral hyperperfusion syndrome (CHS) is characterized by the presence of vasogenic edema, which resembles PRES in that there is a posterior predilection. Patients who are most vulnerable are those with relatively severe carotid stenosis and poor collateral circulation, but postoperative hypertension is also an important risk factor. CHS is treated with tight blood pressure control, but agents that cause cerebral vasodilatation, including nitroprusside ideally should be avoided (135).

Preeclampsia and Eclampsia

Although hypertensive encephalopathy and eclampsia have largely been considered separate entities, they have a similar pathophysiology and essentially the same MRI findings, PRES (136). Definitive treatment for severe preeclampsia and eclampsia is delivery, but careful intravenous blood pressure control is frequently also necessary.

Treatment of hypertension in severe preeclampsia has not been shown to improve perinatal outcomes, and may actually contribute to a decrease in neonatal birth weight (137). Thus, pharmacologic therapy is not recommended unless the degree of blood pressure elevation is severe (defined as SBP exceeding 160 mmHg or DBP exceeding 105 to 110 mmHg) or there are end-organ complications. Oral medications, with a systolic goal pressure of 140 to 155 mmHg and a diastolic goal of 90 to 105 mmHg, may be sufficient in the absence of organ dysfunction, but more rapid and tighter control is necessary for severe preeclampsia and eclampsia. Although there has been extensive experience with intravenous hydralazine (5 to 10 mg every 15–20 minutes to a maximum dose of 30 mg), this agent has a relatively slow onset, has not commonly been used as an infusion, may overshoot blood pressure goals, and has recently been linked to worse outcomes, including more placental abruption, adverse effects on fetal heart rate, lower Apgar scores, and a greater need for cesarean section (138). Other intravenous agents that have been successfully and safely used include labetalol and nicardipine (88,139). In addition, magnesium sulfate should be given to prevent the development of seizures in patients with severe preeclampsia, and should be used to prevent further seizures should eclampsia occurs (140).

SUMMARY

Treatment of acute hypertension and hypertensive crisis is common in the ICU. Determining the underlying cause, and how it is affecting end organs, is paramount in selecting the best treatment options. Manifestations in the course of a hypertensive emergency may impact all organs, but especially the cardiovascular system and brain, and this greatly affects therapeutic options and goals. With few exceptions from the rule (aortic dissection or severe pulmonary edema), the patient's blood pressure should be reduced in a stepwise approach, and with precision, by intravenous medications rapidly delivered, while monitoring the cardiovascular and central nervous systems. The selection of the ideal antihypertensive agent depends on both the cause and the end-organ dysfunction as detailed in this chapter.

Key Points

- Extreme hypertension exceeding the upper range of autoregulation causes edema, hemorrhage, and organ dysfunction, while reductions in blood pressure beyond the lower limits of autoregulation result in tissue hypoperfusion and ischemia.
- Normal endothelial function is necessary for the regulation of vascular tone, blood pressure, and regional blood flow.
- Ideal pharmacologic agents for treatment of hypertensive emergencies have a rapid onset, are short-acting and are easy to titrate.

References

1. Hajjar I, Kotchen TA. Trends in prevalence, awareness, treatment, and control of hypertension in the United States, 1988–2000. *JAMA.* 2003;290(2):199–206.
2. Kearney PM, Whelton M, Reynolds K, et al. Global burden of hypertension: analysis of worldwide data. *Lancet.* 2005;365(9455):217–223.
3. Calhoun D, Oparil S. Treatment of hypertensive crisis. *N Engl J Med.* 1990;323(17):1177–1183.
4. Wu PH, Yang CY, Yao ZL, et al. Relationship of blood pressure control and hospitalization risk to medication adherence among patients with hypertension in Taiwan. *Am J Hypertens.* 2010;23(2):155–160.
5. Zampaglione B, Pascale C, Marchisio M, Cavallo-Perin P. Hypertensive urgencies and emergencies. Prevalence and clinical presentation. *Hypertension.* 1996;27(1):144–147.
6. Karras DJ, Ufberg JW, Heilpern KL, et al. Elevated blood pressure in urban emergency department patients. *Acad Emerg Med.* 2005;12(9):835–843.

7. ESH/ESC Task Force for the Management of Arterial Hypertension. 2013 Practice guidelines for the management of arterial hypertension of the European Society of Hypertension (ESH) and the European Society of Cardiology (ESC): ESH/ESC Task Force for the Management of Arterial Hypertension. *J Hypertens.* 2013;31(10):1925–1938.
8. Vaughan CJ, Delanty N. Hypertensive emergencies. *Lancet.* 2000;356 (9227):411–417.
9. Marik PE, Rivera R. Hypertensive emergencies: an update. *Curr Opin Crit Care.* 2011;17(6):569–580.
10. Ault MJ, Ellrodt AG. Pathophysiological events leading to the end-organ effects of acute hypertension. *Anm J Emerg Med.* 1985;3(6 Suppl):10–15.
11. Wallach R, Karp RB, Reves JG, et al. Pathogenesis of paroxysmal hypertension developing during and after coronary bypass surgery: a study of hemodynamic and humoral factors. *Am J Cardiol.* 1980;46(4):559–565.
12. van den Born BJ, Lowenberg EC, van der Hoeven NV, et al. Endothelial dysfunction, platelet activation, thrombogenesis and fibrinolysis in patients with hypertensive crisis. *J Hypertens.* 2011;29(5):922–927.
13. Montgomery HE, Kiernan LA, Whitworth CE, et al. Inhibition of tissue angiotensin converting enzyme activity prevents malignant hypertension in TGR (mREN2) 27. *J Hypertens.* 1998;16(5):635–643.
14. Han Y, Runge MS, Brasier AR. Angiotensin II induces interleukin-6 transcription in vascular smooth muscle cells through pleiotropic activation of nuclear factor-kappa B transcription factors. *Circ Res.* 1999;84(6):695–703.
15. Davies D, Beevers D, Briggs J, et al. Abnormal relation between exchangeable sodium and the renin-angiotensin system in malignant hypertension and in hypertension with chronic renal failure. *Lancet.* 1973;301(7805): 683–686.
16. Espinel E, Tovar JL, Borrellas J, et al. Angiotensin-converting enzyme i/d polymorphism in patients with malignant hypertension. *J Clin Hypertens.* 2005;7(1):11–15.
17. Bennett NM, Shea S. Hypertensive emergency: case criteria, sociodemographic profile, and previous care of 100 cases. *Am J Public Health.* 1988;78(6):636–640.
18. Shea S, Misra D, Ehrlich MH, et al. Predisposing factors for severe, uncontrolled hypertension in an inner-city minority population. *N Engl J Med.* 1992;327(11):776–781.
19. Bender SR, Fong MW, Heitz S, Bisognano JD. Characteristics and management of patients presenting to the emergency department with hypertensive urgency. *J Clin Hypertens.* 2006;8(1):12–18.
20. Tisdale JE, Huang MB, Borzak S. Risk factors for hypertensive crisis: importance of out-patient blood pressure control. *Fam Practice.* 2004; 21(4):420–424.
21. Keith NM, Wagener HP, Kernohan JW. The syndrome of malignant hypertension. *Arch Intern Med.* 1928;41(2):141–188.
22. Chobanian AV, Bakris GL, Black HR, et al. The seventh report of the joint national committee on prevention, detection, evaluation, and treatment of high blood pressure: the JNC 7 report. *JAMA.* 2003;289(19):2560–2571.
23. Scarpelli PT, Livi R, Caselli G-M, et al. Accelerated (malignant) hypertension: a study of 121 cases between 1974 and 1996. *J Nephrol.* 1997;10(4):207–215.
24. Hemmelgarn BR, Zarnke KB, Campbell N, et al. The 2004 Canadian Hypertension Education Program recommendations for the management of hypertension: Part I—Blood pressure measurement, diagnosis and assessment of risk. *Can J Cardiol.* 2004;20(1):31–40.
25. Mann SJ, Pickering TG. Detection of renovascular hypertension: state of the art: 1992. *Ann Intern Med.* 1992;117(10):845–853.
26. Buckalew VM Jr, Berg RL, Wang S-R, et al. Prevalence of hypertension in 1,795 subjects with chronic renal disease: the modification of diet in renal disease study baseline cohort. *Am J Kidney Dis.* 1996;28(6):811–821.
27. Becker HF, Jerrentrup A, Ploch T, et al. Effect of nasal continuous positive airway pressure treatment on blood pressure in patients with obstructive sleep apnea. *Circulation.* 2003;107(1):68–73.
28. Levine SR, Brust JC, Futrell N, et al. Cerebrovascular complications of the use of the crack form of alkaloidal cocaine. *N Engl J Med.* 1990;323 (11):699–704.
29. Green RM, Kelly KM, Gabrielsen T, et al. Multiple intracerebral hemorrhages after smoking "crack" cocaine. *Stroke.* 1990;21(6):957–962.
30. Hsue PY, Salinas CL, Bolger AF, et al. Acute aortic dissection related to crack cocaine. *Circulation.* 2002;105(13):1592–1595.
31. Delanty N, Vaughan C, Frucht S, Stubgen P. Erythropoietin-associated hypertensive posterior leukoencephalopathy. *Neurology.* 1997;49(3):686–689.
32. Schwartz R, Bravo S, Klufas R, et al. Cyclosporine neurotoxicity and its relationship to hypertensive encephalopathy: CT and MR findings in 16 cases. *AJR Am J Roentgenol.* 1995;165(3):627–631.
33. Ahmed M, Walker J, Beevers DG, Beevers M. Lack of difference between malignant and accelerated hypertension. *Br Med J (Clin Res Ed).* 1986;292 (6515):235–237.
34. Hammond S, Wells JR, Marcus DM, Prisant LM. Ophthalmoscopic findings in malignant hypertension. *J Clin Hypertens.* 2006;8(3):221–223.
35. Dimmitt S, Eames S, Gosling P, et al. Usefulness of ophthalmoscopy in mild to moderate hypertension. *Lancet.* 1989;333(8647):1103–1106.
36. Alpers CE. The kidney. In: *Robbins and Cotran: Pathological Basis of Disease.* 7th ed. Philadelphia, PA: Saunders; 2005:955–1022.
37. van den Born BJ, Honnebier UP, Koopmans RP, van Montfrans GA. Microangiopathic hemolysis and renal failure in malignant hypertension. *Hypertension.* 2005;45(2):246–251.
38. Feigin VL, Lawes CM, Bennett DA, Anderson CS. Stroke epidemiology: a review of population-based studies of incidence, prevalence, and case-fatality in the late 20th century. *Lancet Neurol.* 2003;2(1):43–53.
39. Morgenstern LB, Hemphill JC 3rd, Anderson C, et al. Guidelines for the management of spontaneous intracerebral hemorrhage: a guideline for healthcare professionals from the American Heart Association/American Stroke Association. *Stroke.* 2010;41(9):2108–2129.
40. Manno EM. Update on intracerebral hemorrhage. *Continuum (Minneap, Minn).* 2012;18(3):598–610.
41. Manno EM, Atkinson JL, Fulgham JR, Wijdicks EF. Emerging medical and surgical management strategies in the evaluation and treatment of intracerebral hemorrhage. *Mayo Clin Proc.* 2005;80(3):420–433.
42. Ferro JM, Canhao P, Peralta R. Update on subarachnoid haemorrhage. *J Neurol.* 2008;255(4):465–479.
43. Qureshi AI, Tuhrim S, Broderick JP, et al. Spontaneous intracerebral hemorrhage. *N Engl J Med.* 2001;344(19):1450–1460.
44. Wallace J, Levy L. Blood pressure after stroke. *JAMA.* 1981;246(19): 2177–2180.
45. Jauch EC, Lindsell CJ, Adeoye O, et al. Lack of evidence for an association between hemodynamic variables and hematoma growth in spontaneous intracerebral hemorrhage. *Stroke.* 2006;37(8):2061–2065.
46. Anderson CS, Heeley E, Huang Y, et al. Rapid blood-pressure lowering in patients with acute intracerebral hemorrhage. *N Engl J Med.* 2013; 368(25):2355–2365.
47. Brott T, Lu M, Kothari R, et al. Hypertension and its treatment in the NINDS rt-PA stroke trial. *Stroke.* 1998;29(8):1504–1509.
48. Lindenauer P, Mathew M, Ntuli T, et al. Use of antihypertensive agents in the management of patients with acute ischemic stroke. *Neurology.* 2004;63(2):318–323.
49. Suarez JI, Tarr RW, Selman WR. Aneurysmal subarachnoid hemorrhage. *N Engl J Med.* 2006;354(4):387–396.
50. Connolly ES Jr, Rabinstein AA, Carhuapoma JR, et al. Guidelines for the management of aneurysmal subarachnoid hemorrhage: a guideline for healthcare professionals from the American Heart Association/American Stroke Association. *Stroke.* 2012;43(6):1711–1737.
51. Staykov D, Schwab S. Posterior reversible encephalopathy syndrome. *J Intensive Care Med.* 2012;27(1):11–24.
52. Stott V, Hurrell M, Anderson T. Reversible posterior leukoencephalopathy syndrome: a misnomer reviewed. *Intern Med J.* 2005;35(2):83–90.
53. Bakshi R, Bates VE, Mechtler LL, et al. Occipital lobe seizures as the major clinical manifestation of reversible posterior leukoencephalopathy syndrome: magnetic resonance imaging findings. *Epilepsia.* 1998;39(3): 295–299.
54. Hinchey J, Chaves C, Appignani B, et al. A reversible posterior leukoencephalopathy syndrome. *N Engl J Med.* 1996;334(8):494–500.
55. Covarrubias DJ, Luetmer PH, Campeau NG. Posterior reversible encephalopathy syndrome: prognostic utility of quantitative diffusion-weighted MR images. *Am J Neuroradiol.* 2002;23(6):1038–1048.
56. Schwartz RB, Feske SK, Polak JF, et al. Preeclampsia-eclampsia: clinical and neuroradiographic correlates and insights into the pathogenesis of hypertensive encephalopathy 1. *Radiology.* 2000;217(2):371–376.
57. Beausang-Linder M, Bill A. Cerebral circulation in acute arterial hypertension; protective effects of sympathetic nervous activity. *Acta Physiol Scand.* 1981;111(2):193–199.
58. Bleys RL, Cowen T, Groen GJ, et al. Perivascular nerves of the human basal cerebral arteries: I. Topographical distribution. *J Cereb Blood Flow Metab.* 1996;16(5):1034–1047.
59. Lip GY, Beevers M, Beevers G. The failure of malignant hypertension to decline: a survey of 24 years' experience in a multiracial population in England. *J Hypertens.* 1994;12(11):1297–1305.
60. Aurigemma GP, Gaasch WH. Clinical practice. Diastolic heart failure. *N Engl J Med.* 2004;351(11):1097–1105.
61. Adams KF, Fonarow GC, Emerman CL, et al. Characteristics and outcomes of patients hospitalized for heart failure in the United States: rationale, design, and preliminary observations from the first 100,000 cases in the Acute Decompensated Heart Failure National Registry (ADHERE). *Am Heart J.* 2005;149(2):209–216.

62. McMurray JJ, Adamopoulos S, Anker SD, et al. ESC guidelines for the diagnosis and treatment of acute and chronic heart failure 2012: The Task Force for the Diagnosis and Treatment of Acute and Chronic Heart Failure 2012 of the European Society of Cardiology. Developed in collaboration with the Heart Failure Association (HFA) of the ESC. *Eur J Heart Fail.* 2012;14(8):803–869.
63. Yusuf S, Mehta SR, Chrolavicius S, et al. Comparison of fondaparinux and enoxaparin in acute coronary syndromes. *N Engl J Med.* 2006;354 (14):1464–1476.
64. Chen Z, Pan H, Chen Y, et al. Early intravenous then oral metoprolol in 45,852 patients with acute myocardial infarction: randomised placebo-controlled trial. *Lancet.* 2005;366(9497):1622–1632.
65. Antman EM, Anbe DT, Armstrong PW, et al. ACC/AHA guidelines for the management of patients with ST-elevation myocardial infarction—executive summary: a report of the American College of Cardiology/American Heart Association Task Force on Practice Guidelines (Writing Committee to Revise the 1999 Guidelines for the Management of Patients With Acute Myocardial Infarction). *J Am Coll Cardiol.* 2004;44(3):671–719.
66. Fuster V, Kovacic JC. Acute coronary syndromes: pathology, diagnosis, genetics, prevention, and treatment. *Circ Res.* 2014;114(12):1847–1851.
67. Weber M, Bazzino O, Navarro Estrada JL, et al. Improved diagnostic and prognostic performance of a new high-sensitive troponin T assay in patients with acute coronary syndrome. *Am Heart J.* 2011;162(1): 81–88.
68. Hagan PG, Nienaber CA, Isselbacher EM, et al. The International Registry of Acute Aortic Dissection (IRAD): new insights into an old disease. *JAMA.* 2000;283(7):897–903.
69. Howard DP, Banerjee A, Fairhead JF, et al. Population-based study of incidence and outcome of acute aortic dissection and premorbid risk factor control: 10-year results from the Oxford Vascular Study. *Circulation.* 2013;127(20):2031–2037.
70. Osada H, Kyogoku M, Ishidou M, et al. Aortic dissection in the outer third of the media: What is the role of the vasa vasorum in the triggering process? *Eur J Cardiothorac Surg.* 2013;43(3):e82–e88.
71. Angouras D, Sokolis DP, Dosios T, et al. Effect of impaired vasa vasorum flow on the structure and mechanics of the thoracic aorta: implications for the pathogenesis of aortic dissection. *Eur J Cardiothorac Surg.* 2000;17(4):468–473.
72. Sanders RD. How important is perioperative hypertension? *Anaesthesia.* 2014;69(9):948–953.
73. Weksler N, Klein M, Szendro G, et al. The dilemma of immediate preoperative hypertension: to treat and operate, or to postpone surgery? *J Clin Anesth.* 2003;15(3):179–183.
74. Vaccarino V, Berger AK, Abramson J, et al. Pulse pressure and risk of cardiovascular events in the systolic hypertension in the elderly program. *Am J Cardiol.* 2001;88(9):980–986.
75. Fleisher LA, Beckman JA, Brown KA, et al. ACC/AHA 2007 guidelines on perioperative cardiovascular evaluation and care for noncardiac surgery: executive summary: a report of the American College of Cardiology/American Heart Association Task Force on Practice Guidelines (Writing Committee to Revise the 2002 Guidelines on Perioperative Cardiovascular Evaluation for Noncardiac Surgery). *Anesth Analg.* 2008;106(3):685–712.
76. Goldberg ME, Larijani GE. Perioperative hypertension. *Pharmacotherapy.* 1998;18(5):911–914.
77. Marik PE, Varon J. Perioperative hypertension: a review of current and emerging therapeutic agents. *J Clin Anesth.* 2009;21(3):220–229.
78. Gal TJ, Cooperman LH. Hypertension in the immediate postoperative period. *Br J Anaesth.* 1975;47(1):70–74.
79. Basali A, Mascha EJ, Kalfas I, Schubert A. Relation between perioperative hypertension and intracranial hemorrhage after craniotomy. *Anesthesiology.* 2000;93(1):48–54.
80. Leslie J. Incidence and aetiology of perioperative hypertension. *Acta Anaesthesiol Scand Suppl.* 1993;99:5–9.
81. Bebawy JF, Houston CC, Kosky JL, et al. Nicardipine is superior to esmolol for the management of postcraniotomy emergence hypertension: a randomized open-label study. *Anesth Analg.* 2015;120(1):186–192.
82. Varon J, Marik PE. Perioperative hypertension management. *Vasc Health Risk Manag.* 2008;4(3):615–627.
83. Steegers EA, von Dadelszen P, Duvekot JJ, Pijnenborg R. Pre-eclampsia. *Lancet.* 2010;376(9741):631–644.
84. Koopmans CM, Bijlenga D, Groen H, et al. Induction of labour versus expectant monitoring for gestational hypertension or mild pre-eclampsia after 36 weeks' gestation (HYPITAT): a multicentre, open-label randomised controlled trial. *Lancet.* 2009;374(9694):979–988.
85. Varon J. Treatment of acute severe hypertension: current and newer agents. *Drugs.* 2008;68(3):283–297.
86. Orlowski JP, Shiesley D, Vidt DG, et al. Labetalol to control blood pressure after cerebrovascular surgery. *Crit Care Med.* 1988;16(8):765–768.
87. Arroliga AC, Shehab N, McCarthy K, Gonzales JP. Relationship of continuous infusion lorazepam to serum propylene glycol concentration in critically ill adults. *Crit Care Med.* 2004;32(8):1709–1714.
88. Curran MP, Robinson DM, Keating GM. Intravenous nicardipine: its use in the short-term treatment of hypertension and various other indications. *Drugs.* 2006;66(13):1755–1782.
89. Neutel JM, Smith DH, Wallin D, et al. A comparison of intravenous nicardipine and sodium nitroprusside in the immediate treatment of severe hypertension. *Am J Hypertens.* 1994;7(7 Pt 1):623–628.
90. Nishiyama T, Yokoyama T, Matsukawa T, Hanaoka K. Continuous nicardipine infusion to control blood pressure after evacuation of acute cerebral hemorrhage. *Can J Anaesth.* 2000;47(12):1196–1201.
91. Keating GM. Clevidipine: a review of its use for managing blood pressure in perioperative and intensive care settings. *Drugs.* 2014;74(16):1947–1960.
92. Murphy MB, Murray C, Shorten GD. Fenoldopam: a selective peripheral dopamine-receptor agonist for the treatment of severe hypertension. *N Engl J Med.* 2001;345(21):1548–1557.
93. Tumlin JA, Finkel KW, Murray PT, et al. Fenoldopam mesylate in early acute tubular necrosis: a randomized, double-blind, placebo-controlled clinical trial. *Am J Kidney Dis.* 2005;46(1):26–34.
94. Elliott WJ, Weber RR, Nelson KS, et al. Renal and hemodynamic effects of intravenous fenoldopam versus nitroprusside in severe hypertension. *Circulation.* 1990;81(3):970–977.
95. Bove T, Zangrillo A, Guarracino F, et al. Effect of fenoldopam on use of renal replacement therapy among patients with acute kidney injury after cardiac surgery: a randomized clinical trial. *JAMA.* 2014;312(21):2244–2253.
96. Biancofiore G, Bindi ML, Miccoli M, et al. Intravenous fenoldopam for early acute kidney injury after liver transplantation. *J Anesth.* 2015;29(3):426–432.
97. Devlin JW, Seta ML, Kanji S, Somerville AL. Fenoldopam versus nitroprusside for the treatment of hypertensive emergency. *Ann Pharmacother.* 2004;38(5):755–759.
98. Elliott WJ, Karnezis TA, Silverman RA, et al. Intraocular pressure increases with fenoldopam, but not nitroprusside, in hypertensive humans. *Clin Pharmacol Ther.* 1991;49(3):285–293.
99. Everitt DE, Boike SC, Piltz-Seymour JR, et al. Effect of intravenous fenoldopam on intraocular pressure in ocular hypertension. *J Clin Pharmacol.* 1997;37(4):312–320.
100. Friederich JA, Butterworth JF 4th. Sodium nitroprusside: twenty years and counting. *Anesth Analg.* 1995;81(1):152–162.
101. Cohn JN, Franciosa JA, Francis GS, et al. Effect of short-term infusion of sodium nitroprusside on mortality rate in acute myocardial infarction complicated by left ventricular failure: results of a Veterans Administration cooperative study. *N Engl J Med.* 1982;306(19):1129–1135.
102. Davis RF, Douglas ME, Heenan TJ, Downs JB. Brain tissue pressure measurement during sodium nitroprusside infusion. *Crit Care Med.* 1981;9(1):17–21.
103. Marsh ML, Aidinis SJ, Naughton KV, et al. The technique of nitroprusside administration modifies the intracranial pressure response. *Anesthesiology.* 1979;51(6):538–541.
104. Hall VA, Guest JM. Sodium nitroprusside-induced cyanide intoxication and prevention with sodium thiosulfate prophylaxis. *Am J Crit Care.* 1992;1(2):19–25.
105. Ghani GA, Sung YF, Weinstein MS, et al. Effects of intravenous nitroglycerin on the intracranial pressure and volume pressure response. *J Neurosurg.* 1983;58(4):562–565.
106. Reed WG, Anderson RJ. Effects of rapid blood pressure reduction on cerebral blood flow. *Am Heart J.* 1986;111(1):226–228.
107. Powers WJ. Acute hypertension after stroke: the scientific basis for treatment decisions. *Neurology.* 1993;43(3 Pt 1):461–467.
108. Castillo J, Leira R, Garcia MM, et al. Blood pressure decrease during the acute phase of ischemic stroke is associated with brain injury and poor stroke outcome. *Stroke.* 2004;35(2):520–526.
109. Chamorro A, Vila N, Ascaso C, et al. Blood pressure and functional recovery in acute ischemic stroke. *Stroke.* 1998;29(9):1850–1853.
110. Zhang Y, Reilly KH, Tong W, et al. Blood pressure and clinical outcome among patients with acute stroke in Inner Mongolia, China. *J Hypertens.* 2008;26(7):1446–1452.
111. Jauch EC, Saver JL, Adams HP Jr, et al. Guidelines for the early management of patients with acute ischemic stroke: a guideline for healthcare professionals from the American Heart Association/American Stroke Association. *Stroke.* 2013;44(3):870–947.
112. Rordorf G, Koroshetz WJ, Ezzeddine MA, et al. A pilot study of drug-induced hypertension for treatment of acute stroke. *Neurology.* 2001;56(9): 1210–1213.

113. Leonardi-Bee J, Bath PM, Phillips SJ, Sandercock PA. Blood pressure and clinical outcomes in the International Stroke Trial. *Stroke.* 2002;33(5):1315–1320.
114. He J, Zhang Y, Xu T, et al. Effects of immediate blood pressure reduction on death and major disability in patients with acute ischemic stroke: the CATIS randomized clinical trial. *JAMA.* 2014;311(5):479–489.
115. Hill MD, Buchan AM, Canadian Alteplase for Stroke Effectiveness Study (CASES) Investigators. Thrombolysis for acute ischemic stroke: results of the Canadian Alteplase for Stroke Effectiveness Study. *CMAJ.* 2005;172(10):1307–1312.
116. Tissue plasminogen activator for acute ischemic stroke. The National Institute of Neurological Disorders and Stroke rt-PA Stroke Study Group. *N Engl J Med.* 1995;333(24):1581–1587.
117. Brott T, Broderick J, Kothari R, et al. Early hemorrhage growth in patients with intracerebral hemorrhage. *Stroke.* 1997;28(1):1–5.
118. Willmot M, Leonardi-Bee J, Bath PM. High blood pressure in acute stroke and subsequent outcome: a systematic review. *Hypertension.* 2004;43(1):18–24.
119. Leira R, Davalos A, Silva Y, et al. Early neurologic deterioration in intracerebral hemorrhage: predictors and associated factors. *Neurology.* 2004;63(3):461–467.
120. Zazulia AR, Diringer MN, Videen TO, et al. Hypoperfusion without ischemia surrounding acute intracerebral hemorrhage. *J Cereb Blood Flow Metab.* 2001;21(7):804–810.
121. Powers WJ, Zazulia AR, Videen TO, et al. Autoregulation of cerebral blood flow surrounding acute (6 to 22 hours) intracerebral hemorrhage. *Neurology.* 2001;57(1):18–24.
122. Qureshi AI, Palesch YY. Antihypertensive Treatment of Acute Cerebral Hemorrhage (ATACH) II: design, methods, and rationale. *Neurocrit Care.* 2011;15(3):559–576.
123. Kramer K, Kirkman P, Kitzman D, Little WC. Flash pulmonary edema: association with hypertension and reoccurrence despite coronary revascularization. *Am Heart J.* 2000;140(3):451–455.
124. Elkayam U, Akhter MW, Singh H, et al. Comparison of effects on left ventricular filling pressure of intravenous nesiritide and high-dose nitroglycerin in patients with decompensated heart failure. *Am J Cardiol.* 2004;93(2):237–240.
125. Sigurdsson A, Swedberg K. Left ventricular remodelling, neurohormonal activation and early treatment with enalapril (CONSENSUS II) following myocardial infarction. *Eur Heart J.* 1994;15(Suppl B):14–19.
126. O'Connor CM, Starling RC, Hernandez AF, et al. Effect of nesiritide in patients with acute decompensated heart failure. *N Engl J Med.* 2011;365(1):32–43.
127. Sackner-Bernstein JD, Skopicki HA, Aaronson KD. Risk of worsening renal function with nesiritide in patients with acutely decompensated heart failure. *Circulation.* 2005;111(12):1487–1491.
128. Sackner-Bernstein JD, Kowalski M, Fox M, Aaronson K. Short-term risk of death after treatment with nesiritide for decompensated heart failure: a pooled analysis of randomized controlled trials. *JAMA.* 2005;293(15):1900–1905.
129. Chen HH, Anstrom KJ, Givertz MM, et al. Low-dose dopamine or low-dose nesiritide in acute heart failure with renal dysfunction: the ROSE acute heart failure randomized trial. *JAMA.* 2013;310(23):2533–2543.
130. Peacock WF, Chandra A, Char D, et al. Clevidipine in acute heart failure: results of the A Study of Blood Pressure Control in Acute Heart Failure—a pilot study (PRONTO). *Am Heart J.* 2014;167(4):529–536.
131. Soukoulis V, Boden WE, Smith SC Jr, O'Gara PT. Nonantithrombotic medical options in acute coronary syndromes: old agents and new lines on the horizon. *Circ Res.* 2014;114(12):1944–1958.
132. Tsai TT, Nienaber CA, Eagle KA. Acute aortic syndromes. *Circulation.* 2005;112(24):3802–3813.
133. Olsen KS, Pedersen CB, Madsen JB, et al. Vasoactive modulators during and after craniotomy: relation to postoperative hypertension. *J Neurosurg Anesthesiol.* 2002;14(3):171–179.
134. Hashimoto T, Young WL. Anesthesia-related considerations for cerebral arteriovenous malformations. *Neurosurg Focus.* 2001;11(5):e5.
135. van Mook WN, Rennenberg RJ, Schurink GW, et al. Cerebral hyperperfusion syndrome. *Lancet Neurol.* 2005;4(12):877–888.
136. Zeeman GG, Hatab MR, Twickler DM. Increased cerebral blood flow in preeclampsia with magnetic resonance imaging. *Am J Obstet Gynecol.* 2004;191(4):1425–1429.
137. von Dadelszen P, Magee LA. Fall in mean arterial pressure and fetal growth restriction in pregnancy hypertension: an updated metaregression analysis. *J Obstet Gynecol Can.* 2002;24(12):941–945.
138. Magee LA, Cham C, Waterman EJ, et al. Hydralazine for treatment of severe hypertension in pregnancy: meta-analysis. *BMJ.* 2003;327(7421):955–960.
139. Mabie WC, Gonzalez AR, Sibai BM, Amon E. A comparative trial of labetalol and hydralazine in the acute management of severe hypertension complicating pregnancy. *Obstet Gynecol.* 1987;70(3 Pt 1):328–333.
140. Altman D, Carroli G, Duley L, et al. Do women with pre-eclampsia, and their babies, benefit from magnesium sulphate? The Magpie trial: a randomised placebo-controlled trial. *Lancet.* 2002;359(9321):1877–1890.

CHAPTER

101

Heart–Lung Interactions

MICHAEL R. PINSKY

INTRODUCTION

Perhaps the most obvious and least understood aspect of cardiopulmonary disease is the profound and intimate relation between cardiac and pulmonary dysfunction. Heart–lung interactions go in both directions: they include the effect of the circulation on ventilation wherein acute ventricular failure causes hypoxemia and ischemic respiratory failure; and the effect of ventilation on circulation where hyperinflation can induce tamponade and spontaneous inspiration acute heart failure. Although, most references to heart–lung interactions usually refer to the effect of ventilation on the circulation, the opposite interactions also exist and are relevant to the bedside clinician. Since the initial publication of this chapter in the 4th edition of this textbook in 2009 few new advances in our understanding of heart–lung interactions have evolved, but several new applications of those principles have entered into clinical practice. Those changes are reflected in this version of the chapter.

Heart–lung interactions can be grouped into interactions that involve three basic concepts that usually coexist (1,2). First, spontaneous ventilation is exercise, requiring O_2 and blood flow, thus placing demands on cardiac output, and producing CO_2, adding additional ventilatory stress on CO_2 excretion. Second, inspiration increases lung volume above resting end-expiratory volume. Thus, some of the hemodynamic effects of ventilation are due to changes in lung volume and chest wall expansion. Third, spontaneous inspiration decreases intrathoracic pressure (ITP); whereas positive-pressure ventilation increases ITP. Thus the differences between spontaneous ventilation and positive-pressure ventilation primarily reflect the differences in ITP swings and the energy necessary to produce them.

THE EFFECTS OF CARDIOVASCULAR DYSFUNCTION ON VENTILATION

Cardiogenic shock can induce hydrostatic pulmonary edema, causing, or worsening if extant, acute hypoxic respiratory failure. Furthermore, circulatory shock, by limiting blood flow to the respiratory muscles, can induce respiratory muscle failure and respiratory arrest. These points underscore a fundamental aspect of ventilation, namely that it is exercise, and like any form of exercise, it must place a certain metabolic demand on the cardiovascular system (3). If cardiovascular reserve is limited, this metabolic demand may exceed the heart's ability to deliver O_2 to meet the increased metabolic activity associated with spontaneous ventilation. Thus, ventilator-dependent patients with cardiovascular insufficiency may not be able to wean from mechanical ventilation because the metabolic demand is too great. Failure to wean from mechanical ventilation often reflects cardiovascular insufficiency. Becuase the increased stress only occurs during the weaning trial, such insufficiency may not be apparent prior to weaning attempts.

Under conditions of normal cardiovascular conditions, respiratory muscle blood flow is not the limiting factor determining maximal ventilatory effort even with marked respiratory efforts. Although ventilation normally requires less than 5% of total O_2 consumption (3), if the work of breathing is increased, such as in pulmonary edema, pulmonary fibrosis, or bronchospasm, the work cost of breathing can increase to 25% of total O_2 consumption (3–6). If cardiac output (CO) is limited, then blood flow to all organs—including the respiratory muscles—may be compromised, inducing both tissue hypoperfusion and lactic acidosis (7–10). Under these severe heart failure conditions, respiratory muscle failure may develop despite high central neuronal drive (11). Supporting spontaneous ventilation by the use of mechanical ventilation will reduce O_2 consumption, resulting in an increased SvO_2 for a constant CO and arterial O_2 content (CaO_2). Thus, intubation and mechanical ventilation in patients in severe heart failure will not only decrease the work of breathing, but increased the available O_2 delivery to other vital organs, decreasing serum lactate levels. These cardiovascular benefits are not limited to intubated patients but can also be seen with noninvasive ventilation mask continuous positive airway pressure (CPAP) (12).

Ventilator-dependent patients who fail to wean during spontaneous breathing trials often have impaired baseline cardiovascular performance that may be apparent (13). More commonly, however, the patients develop overt signs of heart failure only during spontaneous breathing trials. The heart failure presentation can be dramatic, with the acute development of pulmonary edema (13,14), myocardial ischemia (15–18), tachycardia, and gut ischemia (19). Because breathing is exercise, all subjects will increase their CO in response to a spontaneous breathing trial. However, those that subsequently fail to wean demonstrate a reduction in mixed venous O_2, consistent with a failing cardiovascular response to an increased metabolic demand (20). Importantly, the increased work of breathing may come from the endotracheal tube flow resistance (21). Thus, some subjects who fail a spontaneous breathing trial may actually be able to breathe on their own if extubated. Clearly, weaning from mechanical ventilatory support is a cardiovascular stress test. Numerous studies have documented weaning-associated ischemic ECG changes and thallium cardiac blood flow scan-related signs of ischemia in both subjects with known coronary artery disease (15) and those with normal coronaries (17,18). Using this same logic in reverse, placing patients with severe heart failure and/or ischemia on mechanical ventilatory support by either intubation and ventilation (22) or noninvasive CPAP (23) often reverses myocardial ischemia.

Since weaning from artificial ventilatory support is cardiovascular stress, if a subject has reduced cardiovascular reserve, then their ability to wean may be impaired. Several recent studies have documented that they could predict which patients would fail a spontaneous breathing trial by indirect measures of their baseline cardiovascular reserve. Gruartmoner et al. (24) used the microvascular reoxygenation rate measured by noninvasive near infrared spectroscopy on the thenar eminence following a total blood pressure cuff hand vascular occlusion as a measure of cardiovascular reserve: a delayed reoxygenation rate reflecting impaired reserve. They showed that those patients with a delayed reoxygenation rate failed to wean from mechanical ventilation significantly more often than those with a normal reoxygenation rate. Similarly, Dres et al. (25) measured the ability of a ventilated patient to increase their CO by at least 10% in response to a passive leg-raising maneuver, as a measure of cardiovascular reserve. They showed that patients who could not increase their blood flow were more likely to not successfully wean from mechanical ventilation.

HEMODYNAMIC EFFECTS OF VENTILATION AND VENTILATORY MANEUVERS

Ventilation can profoundly alter cardiovascular function. The specific response seen will be dependent on myocardial reserve, circulating blood volume, blood flow distribution, autonomic tone, endocrinologic responses, lung volume, ITP, and the surrounding pressures for the remainder of the circulation (26,27). Relevant to this issue is the relation between airway pressure (Paw) and ITP: the transpulmonary pressure. Paw is relatively easy to measure (28,29), whereas ITP is not.

Positive-pressure ventilation-induced increases in Paw do not necessarily equate to proportional increases in ITP. The primary determinants of the hemodynamic responses to ventilation are due to changes in ITP and lung volume (30), not Paw. The relation between Paw, ITP, pericardial pressure (Ppc) and lung volume varies with spontaneous ventilatory effort, lung and chest wall compliance. Lung expansion during positive-pressure inspiration pushes on the surrounding structures distorting them and causing their surface pressures to increase, increasing lateral wall, diaphragmatic, juxtacardiac pleural pressure (Ppl) and Ppc (31). Only lung and thoracic compliance determine the relation between end-expiratory Paw and lung volume in the sedated and paralyzed patient. However, if a ventilated patient actively resist lung inflation or sustains expiratory muscle activity at end-inspiration, then end-inspiratory Paw will exceed resting Paw for that lung volume. Similarly, if the patient activity prevents full exhalation by expiratory breaking, then for the same end-expiratory Paw, lung volume may be higher than predicted from end-expiratory Paw values. At end-expiration, if the respiratory system is at rest, Paw equals alveolar pressure and lung volume is at functional residual capacity (FRC). If incomplete exhalation occurs, then alveolar pressure will exceed Paw. The difference between measured Paw and alveolar pressure is called intrinsic PEEP. Finally, if chest wall compliance decreases, as may occur with increased abdominal pressure, both Paw and ITP will increase for the same tidal breath.

Since the heart is fixed within a cardiac fossa and cannot displace in any direction, juxtacardiac Ppl will increase more than lateral chest wall or diaphragmatic Ppl during inspiration. Ppc is the outside pressure to LV intraluminal ventricular pressure determining LV filling. Ppc and ITP may not be similar, nor increase by similar amounts with the application of positive Paw, if the pericardium acts as a limiting membrane (32,33). With pericardial restraint, as in tamponade, Ppc exceeds juxtacardiac Ppl (34). With progressive increases in PEEP, juxtacardiac Ppl will increase toward Ppc levels, whereas Ppc will initially remain constant. Once these two pressures equalize, further increases in PEEP by increasing lung volume will increase both juxtacardiac Ppl and Ppc in parallel. Thus, if pericardial volume restraint exists, as may occur with acute cor pulmonale or tamponade, then juxtacardiac Ppl will underestimate Ppc.

The presence of lung parenchymal disease, airflow obstruction, and extra-pulmonary processes that directly alter chest wall–diaphragmatic contraction or intra-abdominal pressure may also alter these interactions. Static lung expansion occurs as Paw increases because the transpulmonary pressure (Paw relative to ITP) increases. If lung injury induces alveolar flooding or increased pulmonary parenchyma stiffness, then greater increases in Paw will be required to distend the lungs to a constant end-inspiratory volume (9,31,35). Thus, the primary determinants of the increase in Ppl and Ppc during positive-pressure ventilation are lung volume change and chest wall compliance, not Paw change (36). Since acute lung injury (ALI) is often nonhomogeneous, with aerated areas of the lung displaying normal specific compliance, increases in Paw above approximately 30 cm H_2O will overdistend these aerated lung units (37). Vascular structures that are distended will have a greater increase in their surrounding pressure than collapsible structures that do not distend (38). Despite this nonhomogeneous alveolar distention, if tidal volume is kept constant, then Ppl increases equally, independent of the mechanical properties of the lung (35,39,40). Thus, under constant tidal volume conditions, changes in peak and mean Paw will reflect changes in the mechanical properties of the lungs and patient coordination, but may not reflect changes in ITP. Thus, one cannot predict the amount of change in ITP or Ppc that will occur in a given patient as PEEP is varied. Accordingly, assuming some constant fraction of Paw transmission to the pleural surface as a means of calculating the effect of increasing Paw on ITP is inaccurate and potentially dangerous if used to assess transmural intrathoracic vascular pressures. However, if the patient has a pulmonary artery catheter in situ, then one can estimate end-expiratory ITP. The ability to measure "on-PEEP" intrathoracic vascular pressures by calculating the airway pressure transmission index to the pleural space (41) or by briefly removing PEEP while these pressures are directly measured (40) has been shown to be accurate under a variety of clinical conditions. The ratio of end-inspiratory to end-expiratory pulmonary artery diastolic pressure (reflecting ITP changes) to Paw (reflecting alveolar pressure changes) defines the pulmonary transmission index. If one assumes that lung compliance is linear over the given tidal volume, then the product of this transmission index and PEEP represents the end-expiratory ITP.

HEMODYNAMIC EFFECTS OF CHANGES IN LUNG VOLUME

Changing lung volume alters autonomic tone, pulmonary vascular resistance and, at high lung volumes, compresses the heart in the cardiac fossa, limiting absolute cardiac volumes analogous to cardiac tamponade. However, unlike tamponade where Ppc selectively increases in excess of Ppl, with hyperinflation both juxtacardiac Ppl and Ppc increase together.

Autonomic Tone

Cyclic changes in lung volume induce cyclic changes in autonomic inflow. The lungs are richly enervated with integrated somatic and autonomic fibers that originate, traverse through, and end in the thorax. These neuronal pathways mediate many homeostatic processes through the autonomic nervous system that alter both instantaneous cardiovascular function and steady-state cardiovascular status (42,43). Lung inflation to normal tidal volumes (<8 mL/kg) induces parasympathetic withdrawal, increasing heart rate. This inspiration-induced cardioacceleration is referred to as respiratory sinus arrhythmia (44). The presence of respiratory sinus arrhythmia connotes normal autonomic control (45), and is used in diabetics with peripheral neuropathy to assess peripheral dysautonomia (46). Inflation to larger tidal volumes (>15 mL/kg) decreases heart rate by a combination of both increased vagal tone (47) and sympathetic withdrawal. The sympathetic withdrawal also creates arterial vasodilation (42,48–52). This inflation–vasodilatation response induces expiration-associated reductions in LV contractility in healthy volunteers (53), and in ventilator-dependent patients with the initiation of high-frequency ventilation (42) or hyperinflation (50). Humeral factors, including compounds blocked by cyclooxygenase inhibition (54), released from pulmonary endothelial cells during lung inflation may also induce this depressor response (55–57). However, these interactions do not appear to grossly alter cardiovascular status (58). Although overdistention of aerated lung units in patients with ALI may induce such cardiovascular depression, unilateral lung hyperinflation (unilateral PEEP) does not appear to influence systemic hemodynamics (59). Thus, these cardiovascular effects are of uncertain clinical significance.

Ventilation also compresses the right atrium and, through this mechanical effect, alters control of intravascular fluid balance. Both positive-pressure ventilation and sustained hyperinflation decrease right atrial stretch, stimulating endocrinologic responses that induce fluid retention. Plasma norepinephrine, plasma rennin activity (60,61), and atrial natriuretic peptide (62) increase during positive-pressure ventilation owing to right atrial collapse. Potentially, one of the benefits of the use of nasal CPAP in patients with CHF is to decrease plasma atrial natriuretic peptide activity in parallel with improvements in blood flow (63,64). Thus, some of the observed benefit of CPAP therapy in heart failure patients may be mediated through humoral mechanisms.

Pulmonary Vascular Resistance

Right ventricular (RV) ejection performance is much more limited by changes in ejection pressure than is LV ejection performance, because the right ventricle has thin walls that cannot distribute increased wall stress. Sudden increases in pulmonary vascular resistance, if associated with increases in pulmonary arterial pressure, can induce cardiovascular collapse. In this context, changing lung volume changes pulmonary vascular resistance. The mechanisms inducing these changes are often complex, often conflicting, and include both humoral and mechanical interactions. Increasing lung volume occurs because transpulmonary pressure increases. For example, although obstructive inspiratory efforts, as occur during obstructive sleep apnea, are usually associated with increased RV afterload, the increased afterload is due primarily to either increased vasomotor tone (hypoxic pulmonary vasoconstriction) or backward LV failure, and not lung volume–induced changes in pulmonary vascular resistance (65,66). However, RV afterload increases with obstructive sleep apnea; since RV afterload can be defined as the maximal RV systolic wall stress during contraction (67), it is a function of the maximal product of the RV free wall radius of curvature (a function of end-diastolic volume) and transmural pressure (a function of systolic RV pressure) during ejection (68). Systolic RV pressure equals transmural pulmonary artery pressure (Ppa). Increases in transmural Ppa impede RV ejection (69), decreasing RV stroke volume (70), and inducing RV dilation and passive impedance to venous return (54,56). If not relieved quickly, acute cor pulmonale rapidly develops (71). Furthermore, if RV dilation and RV pressure overload persist, RV free wall ischemia and infarction can develop (72). Importantly, rapid fluid challenges in the setting of acute cor pulmonale can precipitate profound cardiovascular collapse due to excessive RV dilation, RV ischemia, and compromised LV filling.

The pulmonary vasculature constricts if alveolar PO_2 (P_AO_2) decreases below 60 mmHg (73). This process of hypoxic pulmonary vasoconstriction is mediated, in part, by variations in the synthesis and release of nitric oxide by endothelial nitric oxide synthase localized on pulmonary vascular endothelial cells and in part by an NAD/NADH voltage-dependent calcium channel in the pulmonary vasculature. Hypoxic pulmonary vasoconstriction, by reducing pulmonary blood flow to hypoxic lung regions, minimizes shunt blood flow. However, if generalized alveolar hypoxia occurs then pulmonary vasomotor tone increases, increasing pulmonary vascular resistance and impeding RV ejection (67). Importantly, at low lung volumes, alveoli spontaneously collapse as a result of loss of interstitial traction and closure of the terminal airways. This collapse causes both absorption atelectasis and alveolar hypoxia. Patients with acute hypoxemic respiratory failure have small lung volumes and are prone to spontaneous alveolar collapse (74,75). Therefore, pulmonary vascular resistance is often increased in patients with acute hypoxemic respiratory failure due to small lung volumes and atelectasis (e.g., ALI).

Mechanical ventilation may reduce pulmonary vasomotor tone and pulmonary artery pressure, decreasing RV afterload by many related processes. First, hypoxic pulmonary vasoconstriction can be inhibited if O_2-enriched inspired gas increases P_AO_2 (76–79) or if the mechanical breaths and PEEP, by recruiting collapsed alveolar units, increases P_AO_2 in those local alveoli (30,80–82). Second, mechanical ventilation often reverses respiratory acidosis by increasing alveolar ventilation, which itself stimulates pulmonary vasoconstriction (79). Finally, decreasing central sympathetic output by sedation during mechanical ventilation will also reduce vasomotor tone (59,83,84).

Increases in lung volume directly increase pulmonary vascular resistance by compressing the alveolar vessels (74,81,82). The actual mechanisms by which this occurs have not been completely resolved, but appear to reflect differential extraluminal pressure gradient–induced vascular compression. The pulmonary circulation can be conceptually viewed as existing in two distinct compartments based on the pressure outside, either alveolar pressure (alveolar vessels) or extra-alveolar or ITP (extra-alveolar vessels) (81). The small pulmonary arterioles, venules, and alveolar capillaries sense alveolar pressure as their surrounding pressure, whereas the large pulmonary arteries and veins, as well as the heart and intrathoracic great vessels of the systemic circulation, sense interstitial pressure or ITP as their surrounding pressure. Since alveolar pressure minus ITP is the transpulmonary pressure, and increasing lung volume requires transpulmonary pressure to increase, such increases in lung volume must increase the extraluminal pressure gradient from extra-alveolar vessels to alveolar vessels. Increases in lung volume progressively increase alveolar vessel resistance, becoming measurable above FRC (Fig. 101.1) (77,85). Since the intraluminal pressure in the pulmonary arteries is generated by RV ejection relative to ITP, but the outside pressure of the alveolar vessels is alveolar pressure, if transpulmonary pressure exceeds intraluminal pulmonary arterial pressure, then the pulmonary vasculature will collapse where extra-alveolar vessels pass into alveolar loci, reducing the vasculature cross-sectional area and increasing pulmonary vascular resistance. Hyperinflation can create significant pulmonary hypertension and may precipitate acute RV failure (acute cor pulmonale) (86) and RV ischemia (72) especially in patients prone to hyperinflation (e.g., COPD). Thus, PEEP may increase pulmonary vascular resistance if it induces lung overdistention (87). Similarly, if lung volumes are reduced, increasing lung volume back to baseline levels by the use of PEEP decreases pulmonary vascular resistance by reversing hypoxic pulmonary vasoconstriction (88). Relevant to these findings, Vieillard-Baron et al. (89) reviewed their echocardiographic studies for all patients with acute respiratory distress syndrome (ARDS) on mechanical ventilation with PEEP before and after the era of protective lung ventilation, and found the incidence of acute right heart syndrome to be approximately 40% before protective lung ventilation, decreasing to approximately 25% afterward. Thus, protective lung ventilation by minimizing overdistention may limit acute cor pulmonale but does not eliminate it in ARDS patients.

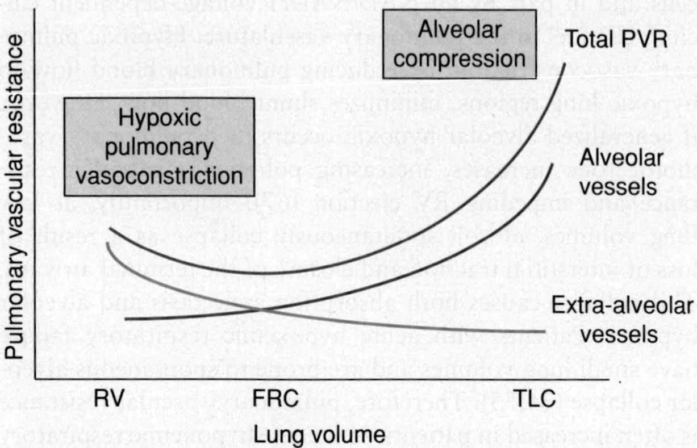

FIGURE 101.1 Schematic diagram of the relation between changes in lung volume and pulmonary vascular resistance, where the extra-alveolar and alveolar vascular components are separated. Note that pulmonary vascular resistance is minimal at resting lung volume or functional residual capacity (FRC). As lung volume increases toward total lung capacity (TLC) or decreases toward residual volume (RV), pulmonary vascular resistance also increases. However, the increase in resistance with hyperinflation is due to increased alveolar vascular resistance, whereas the increase in resistance with lung collapse is due to increased extra-alveolar vessel tone.

Ventricular Interdependence

Although LV preload must eventually be altered by changes in RV output, because the two ventricles are in series, changes in RV end-diastolic volume can also alter LV preload by altering LV diastolic compliance by the mechanism of ventricular interdependence (90). Ventricular interdependence functions through two separate processes. First, increasing RV end-diastolic volume will induce an intraventricular septal shift into the LV, decreasing LV diastolic compliance (91). Thus, for the same LV filling pressure, RV dilation will decrease LV end-diastolic volume and, therefore, CO. Second, if pericardial restraint limits absolute biventricular filling, then RV dilation will increase Ppc without septal shift (2,92). This ventricular interaction is believed to be the major determinant of the phasic changes in arterial pulse pressure and stroke volume seen in tamponade, and is referred to as pulsus paradoxus. Pulsus paradoxus can be demonstrated during loaded spontaneous inspiration in normal subjects as an inspiration-associated decrease is pulse pressure. Maintaining a constant rate of venous return, either by volume resuscitation (93) or vasopressor infusion (29) will minimize hyperinflation-induced cardiac compression.

Hyperinflation-Induced Cardiac Compression

As lung volume increases, the heart is compressed between the expanding lungs (94), increasing juxtacardiac ITP. This compressive effect of the inflated lungs can be seen with either spontaneous (95) or positive-pressure–induced hyperinflation (5,40,96–98). As described above, both Ppc and ITP are increased and no pericardial restraint exists. This decrease in apparent LV diastolic compliance (93) was previously misinterpreted as impaired LV contractility, because LV stroke work for a given LV end-diastolic pressure or pulmonary artery occlusion pressure is decreased (99,100). However, when such patients are fluid resuscitated to return LV end-diastolic volume to its original level, both LV stroke work and CO also returned to their original levels (93,101) despite the continued application of PEEP (102).

HEMODYNAMIC EFFECTS OF CHANGES IN INTRATHORACIC PRESSURE

The heart within the thorax is a pressure chamber within a pressure chamber. Therefore, changes in ITP will affect the pressure gradients for both systemic venous return to the RV and systemic outflow from the LV, independent of the heart itself. Increases in ITP, by increasing right atrial pressure and decreasing transmural LV systolic pressure, will reduce the pressure gradients for venous return and LV ejection, decreasing intrathoracic blood volume. Using the same argument, decreases in ITP will augment venous return and impede LV ejection and increase intrathoracic blood volume; everything else follows from these simple truths.

Venous Return

Blood flows back from the systemic venous reservoirs into the right atrium through low pressure–low resistance venous conduits (103). Right atrial pressure is the backpressure for venous return; ventilation alters both right atrial pressure and venous reservoir pressure. It is these changes in right atrial and venous capacitance vessel pressure that induce most of the observed cardiovascular effects of ventilation. Pressure in the upstream venous reservoirs is called mean systemic pressure and is, itself, a function of blood volume, peripheral vasomotor tone, and the distribution of blood within the vasculature (104). Usually mean systemic pressure does not change rapidly during positive-pressure ventilation, whereas right atrial pressure does owing to concomitant changes in ITP. Thus, variations in right atrial pressure represent the major factor determining the fluctuation in pressure gradient for systemic venous return during ventilation (105,106). The positive-pressure inspiration increases in right atrial pressure, decreases the pressure gradient for venous return, decreasing RV filling (70) and RV stroke volume (70,105,107–115). During normal spontaneous inspiration, the opposite occurs (2,29,70,71,109,112,116,117). The detrimental effect of positive-pressure ventilation on CO can be minimized by either fluid resuscitation to increase mean systemic pressure (29,107,118,119) or by keeping both mean ITP and swings in lung volume as low as possible. Accordingly, prolonging expiratory time, decreasing tidal volume, and avoiding PEEP all minimize this decrease in systemic venous return to the RV (4,26,105,109–113,120).

However, if positive-pressure ventilation-induced increases in right atrial pressure always proportionally decreased venous return, then most patients would display profound cardiovascular insufficiency when placed on mechanical ventilator support and especially so when given increased levels of PEEP. Fortunately, when lung volumes increase, the diaphragm descends, compressing the abdominal compartment and increasing intra-abdominal pressure (121,122). Since a large proportion of venous blood exists in intra-abdominal vasculature, it is pressurized as well, increasing mean systemic pressure. Accordingly, the pressure gradient for venous return is often not reduced by PEEP (118). Inspiration-induced abdominal pressurization by diaphragmatic descent is probably the primary mechanism by which the decrease in venous return is minimized during positive-pressure ventilation (123–128). However, laparotomy, by abolishing the inspiration-associated increases in intra-abdominal pressure, makes surgery patients especially sensitive to mechanical ventilation and is one of the reasons why abdominal surgery patients often leave the operating room many liters positive.

Spontaneous inspiratory efforts usually increase venous return because of the combined decrease in right atrial pressure (2,28,110–112) and increase in intra-abdominal pressure (121,122), described above. However, this augmentation of venous return is limited (129,130) because as ITP decreases below atmospheric pressure, central venous pressure also becomes subatmospheric, collapsing the great veins as they enter the thorax and creating a flow-limiting segment (103).

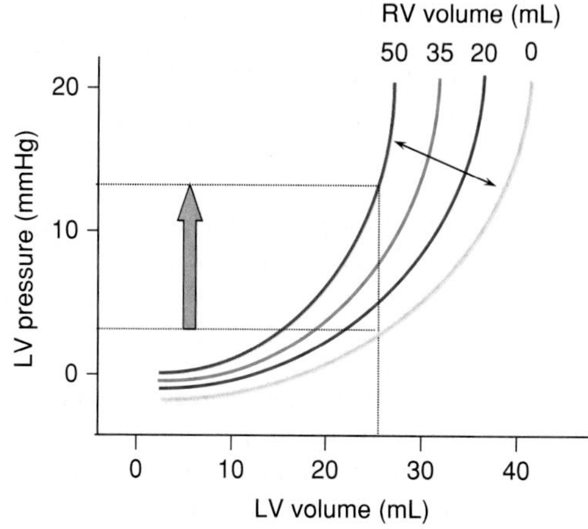

FIGURE 101.2 Schematic diagram of the effect of increasing right ventricular (RV) volumes on the left ventricular (LV) diastolic pressure–volume (filling) relationship. Note that increasing RV volumes decrease LV diastolic compliance, such that a higher filling pressure is required to generate a constant end-diastolic volume. (Adapted from Taylor RR, Covell JW, Sonnenblick EH, Ross J Jr. Dependence of ventricular distensibility on filling the opposite ventricle. *Am J Physiol.* 1967;213:711–718.)

Ventricular Interdependence

Since spontaneous inspiration increases RV filling, it will also directly alter LV diastolic compliance by the process of ventricular interdependence. Increasing RV volume decreases LV diastolic compliance, while decreasing RV volume increases LV diastolic compliance, although the positive-pressure ventilation effect of increased LV diastolic compliance is usually minimal (Fig. 101.2) (90,131–134).

However, the spontaneous inspiration-induced RV volume increase reduces the LV diastolic compliance and is the primary cause for the inspiration-associated decrease in LV stroke volume and pulse pressure (89,91,134,135). If the pulse pressure change is greater than 10 mmHg, or 10% of the mean pulse pressure, then it is referred to as pulsus paradoxus (2). Since spontaneous inspiratory efforts can also occur during positive-pressure ventilation, the use of ventilation-associated pulse pressure variation (PPV) during positive-pressure ventilation can reflect ventricular interdependence. Presently, positive-pressure–induced changes in pulse pressure and LV stroke volume have been advocated to be a useful parameter of preload-responsiveness (136). However, in order to assess volume responsiveness using PPV, it is essential that no spontaneous inspiratory efforts be present. These points are discussed in greater detail in the next section.

Changes in ITP can directly and indirectly alter LV afterload by altering both LV end-diastolic volume and ejection pressure. LV ejection pressure can be estimated as arterial pressure relative to ITP. Since baroreceptor mechanisms located in the extrathoracic carotid body maintain arterial pressure constant relative to atmosphere, if arterial pressure were to remain constant as ITP increased, then transmural LV pressure and thus

LV afterload would decrease. Similarly, if transmural arterial pressure were to remain constant as ITP decreased then LV wall tension would increase (137). Thus, under steady-state conditions, increases in ITP decrease LV afterload and decreases in ITP increase LV afterload (138,139). The spontaneous inspiration-associated decrease in ITP-induced increase in LV afterload is one of the major mechanisms thought to be operative in the wean-induced LV ischemia described in the first part of this chapter, since increased LV afterload must increase myocardial O_2 consumption (MVO_2). Thus, spontaneous ventilation not only increases global O_2 demand by its exercise component (3–5), but also increases MVO_2.

Profoundly negative swings in ITP commonly occur during forced spontaneous inspiratory efforts in patients with bronchospasm and obstructive breathing. This condition may rapidly deteriorate into acute heart failure and pulmonary edema (65), as has been described for airway obstruction (asthma, upper airway obstruction, vocal cord paralysis) or stiff lungs (interstitial lung disease, pulmonary edema, and ALI), as these swings may selectively increase LV afterload and may be the cause of the LV failure and pulmonary edema (1,51,65,66) seen, especially if LV systolic function is already compromised (13,140). Clearly, weaning from mechanical ventilation is a selective LV stress test (137,141,142). Similarly, improved LV systolic function is observed in patients with severe LV failure placed on mechanical ventilation (142).

The improvement in LV functional seen with positive-pressure ventilation in subjects with severe heart failure is self-limited, because venous return also decreases, limiting total blood flow. However, the effect of removing large negative swings of ITP on LV performance will also act to reduce LV afterload, but will not be associated with a change in venous return because, until ITP becomes positive, venous return remains constant. Thus, removing negative ITP swings on LV afterload will selectively reduce LV afterload in a fashion analogous to increasing ITP, but without the effect on CO (23,29,103,143–145). This concept has been validated to be a very important clinical approach for patients with obstructive sleep apnea. For example, the cardiovascular benefits of positive airway pressure in nonintubated patients can be seen with CPAP therapy for heart failure patients (146,147). Even low levels of CPAP, if they inhibit airway obstruction, will be beneficial (148,149). Prolonged nighttime nasal CPAP can selectively improve respiratory muscle strength, as well as LV contractile function if the patients have pre-existent heart failure (150,151); these benefits are associated with reductions of serum catecholamine levels (152). Furthermore, CPAP therapy now forms the fundamental first step in the management of acute cardiogenic pulmonary edema, because it both abolishes the negative swings in ITP during inspiration while sustaining alveolar oxygenation, and it does this from the very first breath it delivers (153,154).

USING HEART–LUNG INTERACTIONS TO DIAGNOSE CARDIOVASCULAR INSUFFICIENCY

Since the cardiovascular response to positive-pressure breathing is determined by the baseline cardiovascular state, ventilation-associated changes in arterial pulse pressure and stroke volume should be inferential for dynamic changes in venous return and the responsiveness of the heart to these transient and cyclic changes in preload (155). Both arterial pulse pressure (diastole to systole) and systolic pressure variations during positive-pressure ventilation nicely describe preload-responsiveness, with threshold values of greater than 10% variability compared to mean values in a patient on 8 mL/kg or more, adapted to the ventilation and without dysrhythmias (136). This technique can be modified to assess stroke volume variation (SVV) (156) and has profound clinical potential as newer monitoring devices allow for the bedside display of both PPV and SVV. In subjects on controlled mechanical ventilation, a PPV of more than 13% or an SVV of more than 10% accurately predict preload-responsiveness. Since a primary cardiovascular management decision in shock is whether or not to give intravascular fluids to increase blood flow (157), knowing if a patient is volume responsive before giving fluids will both prevent overhydration of nonresponsive patients and aid in monitoring the response to fluid resuscitation in responsive ones. This approach has been termed functional hemodynamic monitoring because it uses a repetitive known physiologic perturbation to drive a readout physiologic signal defining cardiovascular reserve. This application of heart–lung interactions has been validated in many prospective clinical trials, reviewed in a meta-analysis (158). This practical application of heart–lung interactions is now commonplace. Importantly, a basic understanding of the principles described in this chapter is an essential part of the training of acute care physicians. For example, the ITP-induced PPV and SVV, caused by the positive pressure breath, would be inaccurate if tidal volume were to vary from breath to breath. Similarly, if chest wall compliance were to decrease, owing to increased intra-abdominal pressure limiting diaphragmatic descent, then the accuracy of these measures would also decline.

Many functional hemodynamic monitoring approaches take advantage of these dynamic transients to measure either the capacity of the ventricles to fill as the pressure gradient for ventricular filling changes, or for the ventricles to proportionally eject this varying amount of volume (159). As described above, both spontaneous and positive-pressure breathing, by altering the pressure gradients for venous return to the right ventricle, can be used to assess both right and left ventricular preload reserve (160). For dynamic changes in venous return to alter LV stroke volume or arterial pulse pressure, then both RV and LV preload reserve need to be present. Dynamic venous flow changes during spontaneous and positive-pressure ventilation identify RV preload reserve, and can be measured indirectly by the dynamic changes in inferior vena caval (161), superior vena caval (162), and internal jugular venous diameters (163). Threshold values above 10% to 15% change in diameter define volume-responsiveness.

Because both SVV and PPV sensitivity degrade during spontaneous ventilation, low tidal volume ventilation, severe cor pulmonale and other extremes of physiology (164), alterative tests have been proposed. Specifically, performing passive leg-raising maneuvers to transiently increase venous return while concomitantly monitoring transient changes in left-sided CO is very sensitive and specific predictor of volume responsiveness under most conditions (165). It also becomes inaccurate when intra-abdominal hypertension exists because the pressure gradient for venous return is altered less (166).

Key Points

- Spontaneous ventilation is exercise.
  - Failure to wean may connote cardiovascular insufficiency.
  - Weaning is a cardiovascular stress test.
  - Breathing loads both the heart and lungs.
- Changes in lung volume alter autonomic tone, pulmonary vascular resistance, and at high lung volumes compress the heart in the cardiac fossa in a fashion analogous to cardiac tamponade.
  - Low lung volumes increase pulmonary vasomotor tone by stimulating hypoxic pulmonary vasoconstriction.
  - High lung volumes increase pulmonary vascular resistance by increasing transpulmonary pressure.
- Spontaneous inspiration and spontaneous inspiratory efforts decrease intrathoracic pressure.
  - Increasing venous return.
  - Increasing LV afterload.
- Positive-pressure ventilation increases intrathoracic pressure.
  - Decreasing venous return.
  - The decrease in venous return is mitigated by the associated increase in intra-abdominal pressure.
  - Decreasing LV afterload.
  - Abolishing negative swings in ITP selectively reduces LV afterload without reducing venous return.

ACKNOWLEDGMENTS

Supported in part by the NIH grants HL074316, HL120877 HL07820, and NR013912.

References

1. Bromberger-Barnea B. Mechanical effects of inspiration on heart functions: a review. *Fed Proc.* 1981;40:2172–2177.
2. Wise RA, Robotham JL, Summer WR. Effects of spontaneous ventilation on the circulation. *Lung.* 1981;159:175–192.
3. Roussos C, Macklem PT. The respiratory muscles. *N Engl J Med.* 1982; 307:786–797.
4. Grenvik A. Respiratory, circulatory and metabolic effects of respiratory treatment. *Acta Anaesthesiol.* 1966. (19 Suppl):1–122.
5. Shuey CB, Pierce AK, Johnson RL. An evaluation of exercise tests in chronic obstructive lung disease. *J Appl Physiol.* 1969;27:256–261.
6. Stock MC, David DW, Manning JW, Ryan ML. Lung mechanics and oxygen consumption during spontaneous ventilation and severe heart failure. *Chest.* 1992;102:279–283.
7. Kawagoe Y, Permutt S, Fessler HE. Hyperinflation with intrinsic PEEP and respiratory muscle blood flow. *J Appl Physiol (1985).* 1994;77:2440–2448.
8. Aubier M, Vires N, Sillye G, et al. Respiratory muscle contribution to lactic acidosis in low cardiac output. *Am Rev Respir Dis.* 1982;126:648–652.
9. Frazier SK, Stone KS, Schertel ER, et al. A comparison of hemodynamic changes during the transition from mechanical ventilation to T-piece, pressure support, and continuous positive airway pressure in canines. *Biol Res Nurs.* 2000;1:253–264.
10. Magder S, Erian R, Roussos C. Respiratory muscle blood flow in oleic acid-induced pulmonary edema. *J Appl Physiol.* 1986;60:1849–1856.
11. Vires N, Sillye G, Rassidakis A, et al. Effect of mechanical ventilation on respiratory muscle blood flow during shock. *Physiologist.* 1980;23:1–8.
12. Baratz DM, Westbrook PR, Shah K, Mohsenifar Z. Effects of nasal continuous positive airway pressure on cardiac output and oxygen delivery in patients with congestive heart failure. *Chest.* 1992;102:1397–1401.
13. Lemaire F, Teboul JL, Cinoti J, et al. Acute left ventricular dysfunction during unsuccessful weaning from mechanical ventilation. *Anesthesiology.* 1988;69:171–179.
14. Richard C, Teboul JL, Archambaud F, et al. Left ventricular dysfunction during weaning in patients with chronic obstructive pulmonary disease. *Intensive Care Med.* 1994;20:171–172.
15. Hurford WE, Lynch KE, Strauss HW, et al. Myocardial perfusion as assessed by thallium-201 scintigraphy during the discontinuation of mechanical ventilation in ventilator-dependent patients. *Anesthesiology.* 1991;74:1007–1016.
16. Abalos A. Leibowitz AB, Distefano D, et al. Myocardial ischemia during the weaning period. *Am J Crit Care.* 1992;1:32–36.
17. Chatila W, Ani S, Guaglianone D, et al. Cardiac ischemia during weaning from mechanical ventilation. *Chest.* 1996;109:1421–1422.
18. Srivastava S, Chatila W, Amoateng-Adjepong Y, et al. Myocardial ischemia and weaning failure in patients with coronary disease: an update. *Crit Care Med.* 1999;27:2109–2112.
19. Mohsenifar Z, Hay A, Hay J, et al. Gastric intramural pH as a predictor of success or failure in weaning patients from mechanical ventilation. *Ann Intern Med.* 1993;119:794–798.
20. Jabran A, Mathru M, Dries D, Tobin MJ. Continuous recordings of mixed venous oxygen saturation during weaning from mechanical ventilation and the ramifications thereof. *Am J Respir Crit Care Med.* 1998; 158:1763–1769.
21. Straus C, Lewis B, Isebey D, et al. Contribution of the endotracheal tube and the upper airway to breathing workload. *Am J Respir Crit Care Med.* 1998;157:23–30.
22. Rasanen J, Nikki P, Heikkila J. Acute myocardial infarction complicated by respiratory failure: the effects of mechanical ventilation. *Chest.* 1984;85:21–28.
23. Rasanen J, Vaisanen IT, Heikkila J, et al. Acute myocardial infarction complicated by left ventricular dysfunction and respiratory failure: the effects of continuous positive airway pressure. *Chest.* 1985;87:156–162.
24. Gruartmoner G, Mesquida J, Masip J, et al. Tissue oxygen saturation (StO_2) during weaning from mechanical ventilation: an observational study. *Eur Respir J.* 2014;43:143–150.
25. Dres M, Teboul JL, Anguel N, et al. Passive leg raising performed before a spontaneous breathing trial predicts weaning-induced cardiac dysfunction. *Intensive Care Med.* 2015;41:487–494.
26. Cournaud A, Motley HL, Werko L, et al. Physiologic studies of the effect of intermittent positive pressure breathing on cardiac output in man. *Am J Physiol.* 1948;152:162–174.
27. Tyberg JV, Grant DA, Kingma I, et al. Effects of positive intrathoracic pressure on pulmonary and systemic hemodynamics. *Respir Physiol.* 2000;119:171–179.
28. Milic-Emili J, Mead J, Turner JM, Glauser EM. Improved method for assessing the validity of the esophageal balloon technique. *J Appl Physiol.* 1964;19: 207–211.
29. Braunwald E, Binion JT, Morgan WL Jr, Sarnoff SJ. Alterations in central blood volume and cardiac output induced by positive pressure breathing and counteracted by metraminol (Aramine). *Circ Res.* 1957;5:670–675.
30. Whittenberger JL, McGregor M, Berglund E, Borst HG. Influence of state of inflation of the lung on pulmonary vascular resistance. *J Appl Physiol.* 1960;15:878–882.
31. Novak RA, Matuschak GM, Pinsky MR. Effect of ventilatory frequency on regional pleural pressure. *J Appl Physiol.* 1988;65:1314–1323.
32. Kingma I, Smiseth OA, Frais MA, et al. Left ventricular external constraint: relationship between pericardial, pleural and esophageal pressures during positive end-expiratory pressure and volume loading in dogs. *Ann Biomed Eng.* 1987;15:331–346.
33. Tsitlik JE, Halperin HR, Guerci AD, et al. Augmentation of pressure in a vessel indenting the surface of the lung. *Ann Biomed Eng.* 1987; 15:259–284.
34. Pinsky MR, Guimond JG. The effects of positive end- expiratory pressure on heart-lung interactions. *J Crit Care.* 1991;6:1–11.
35. Romand JA, Shi W, Pinsky MR. Cardiopulmonary effects of positive pressure ventilation during acute lung injury. *Chest.* 1995;108:1041–1048.
36. O'Quinn RJ, Marini JJ, Culver BH, et al. Transmission of airway pressure to pleural pressure during lung edema and chest wall restriction. *J Appl Physiol.* 1985;59:1171–1177.
37. Gattinoni L, Mascheroni D, Torresin A, et al. Morphological response to positive end-expiratory pressure in acute respiratory failure. *Intensive Care Med.* 1986;12:137–142.
38. Globits S, Burghuber OC, Koller J, et al. Effect of lung transplantation on right and left ventricular volumes and function measured by magnetic resonance imaging. *Am J Respir Crit Care Med.* 1994;149:1000–1004.
39. Scharf SM, Ingram RH Jr. Effects of decreasing lung compliance with oleic acid on the cardiovascular response to PEEP. *Am J Physiol.* 1977; 233:H635–H641.
40. Pinsky MR, Vincent JL, DeSmet JM. Estimating left ventricular filling pressure during positive end-expiratory pressure in humans. *Am Rev Respir Dis.* 1991;143:25–31.

41. Teboul JL, Pinsky MR, Mercat A, et al. Estimating cardiac filling pressure in mechanically ventilated patients with hyperinflation. *Crit Care Med.* 2000;28:3631–3636.
42. Glick G, Wechsler AS, Epstein DE. Reflex cardiovascular depression produced by stimulation of pulmonary stretch receptors in the dog. *J Clin Invest.* 1969;48:467–472.
43. Painal AS. Vagal sensory receptors and their reflex effects. *Physiol Rev.* 1973;53:59–88.
44. Anrep GV, Pascual W, Rossler R. Respiratory variations in the heart rate. I. The reflex mechanism of the respiratory arrhythmia. *Proc R Soc Lond B Biol Sci.* 1936;119:191–217.
45. Taha BH, Simon PM, Dempsey JA, et al. Respiratory sinus arrhythmia in humans: an obligatory role for Vagal feedback from the lungs. *J Appl Physiol (1985).* 1995;78:638–645.
46. Bernardi L, Calciati A, Gratarola A, et al. Heart rate-respiration relationship: computerized method for early detection of cardiac autonomic damage in diabetic patients. *Acta Cardiol.* 1986;41:197–206.
47. Persson MG, Lonnqvist PA, Gustafsson LE. Positive end-expiratory pressure ventilation elicits increases in endogenously formed nitric oxide as detected in air exhaled by rabbits. *Anesthesiology.* 1995;82:969–974.
48. Cassidy SS, Eschenbacher WI, Johnson RL Jr. Reflex cardiovascular depression during unilateral lung hyperinflation in the dog. *J Clin Invest.* 1979;64:620–626.
49. Daly MB, Hazzledine JL, Ungar A. The reflex effects of alterations in lung volume on systemic vascular resistance in the dog. *J Physiol.* 1967; 188:331–351.
50. Shepherd JT. The lungs as receptor sites for cardiovascular regulation. *Circulation.* 1981;63:1–10.
51. Stalcup SA, Mellins RB. Mechanical forces producing pulmonary edema in acute asthma. *N Engl J Med.* 1977;297:592–596.
52. Vatner SF, Rutherford JD. Control of the myocardial contractile state by carotid chemo- and baroreceptor and pulmonary inflation reflexes in conscious dogs. *J Clin Invest.* 1978;63:1593–1601.
53. Karlocai K, Jokkel G, Kollai M. Changes in left ventricular contractility with the phase of respiration. *J Auton Nerv Syst.* 1998;73:86–92.
54. Said SI, Kitamura S, Vreim C. Prostaglandins: release from the lung during mechanical ventilation at large tidal ventilation. *J Clin Invest.* 1972; 51:83a.
55. Bedetti C, Del Basso P, Argiolas C, Carpi A. Arachidonic acid and pulmonary function in a heart-lung preparation of guinea-pig: modulation by PCO_2. *Arch Int Pharmacodyn Ther.* 1987;285:98–116.
56. Berend N, Christopher KL, Voelkel NF. Effect of positive end- expiratory pressure on functional residual capacity: role of prostaglandin production. *Am Rev Respir Dis.* 1982;126:641–647.
57. Pattern MY, Liebman PR, Hetchman HG. Humorally mediated decreases in cardiac output associated with positive end-expiratory pressure. *Microvasc Res.* 1977;13:137–144.
58. Berglund JE, Halden E, Jakobson S, Svensson J. PEEP ventilation does not cause humorally mediated cardiac output depression in pigs. *Intensive Care Med.* 1994;20:360–364.
59. Fuhrman BP, Everitt J, Lock JE. Cardiopulmonary effects of unilateral airway pressure changes in intact infant lambs. *J Appl Physiol Respir Environ Exerc Physiol.* 1984;56:1439–1448.
60. Payen DM, Brun-Buisson CJ, Carli PA, et al. Hemodynamic, gas exchange, and hormonal consequences of LBPP during PEEP ventilation. *J Appl Physiol.* 1987;62:61–70.
61. Frage D, de la Coussaye JE, Beloucif S, et al. Interactions between hormonal modifications during PEEP-induced antidiuresis and antinatriuresis. *Chest.* 1995;107:1095–1100.
62. Frass M, Watschinger B, Traindl O, et al. Atrial natriuretic peptide release in response to different positive end-expiratory pressure levels. *Crit Care Med.* 1993;21:343–347.
63. Wilkins MA, Su XL, Palayew MD, et al. The effects of posture change and continuous positive airway pressure on cardiac natriuretic peptides in congestive heart failure. *Chest.* 1995;107:909–915.
64. Shirakami G, Magaribuchi T, Shingu K, et al. Positive end-expiratory pressure ventilation decreases plasma atrial and brain natriuretic peptide levels in humans. *Anesth Analg.* 1993;77:1116–1121.
65. Fletcher EC, Proctor M, Yu J, et al. Pulmonary edema develops after recurrent obstructive apneas. *Am J Respir Crit Care Med.* 1999;160:1688–1696.
66. Chen L, Shi Q, Scharf SM. Hemodynamic effects of periodic obstructive apneas in sedated pigs with congestive heart failure. *J Appl Physiol.* 2000;88:1051–1060.
67. Maughan WL, Shoukas AA, Sagawa K, Weisfeldt ML. Instantaneous pressure-volume relationships of the canine right ventricle. *Circ Res.* 1979; 44:309–315.
68. Sibbald WJ, Driedger AA. Right ventricular function in disease states: pathophysiologic considerations. *Crit Care Med.* 1983;11:339–345.
69. Piene H, Sund T. Does pulmonary impedance constitute the optimal load for the right ventricle? *Am J Physiol.* 1982;242:H154–H160.
70. Pinsky MR. Determinants of pulmonary arterial flow variation during respiration. *J Appl Physiol.* 1984;56:1237–1245.
71. Theres H, Binkau J, Laule M, et al. Phase-related changes in right ventricular cardiac output under volume-controlled mechanical ventilation with positive end-expiratory pressure. *Crit Care Med.* 1999;27:953–958.
72. Johnston WE, Vinten-Johansen J, Shugart HE, Santamore WP. Positive end-expiratory pressure potentates the severity of canine right ventricular ischemia-reperfusion injury. *Am J Physiol.* 1992;262:H168–H176.
73. Madden JA, Dawson CA, Harder DR. Hypoxia-induced activation in small isolated pulmonary arteries from the cat. *J Appl Physiol.* 1985;59: 113–118.
74. Hakim TS, Michel RP, Chang HK. Effect of lung inflation on pulmonary vascular resistance by arterial and venous occlusion. *J Appl Physiol.* 1982;53:1110–1115.
75. Quebbeman EJ, Dawson CA. Influence of inflation and atelectasis on the hypoxic pressure response in isolated dog lung lobes. *Cardiovas Res.* 1976;10:672–677.
76. Brower RG, Gottlieb J, Wise RA, et al. Locus of hypoxic vasoconstriction in isolated ferret lungs. *J Appl Physiol.* 1987;63:58–65.
77. Hakim TS, Michel RP, Minami H, Chang K. Site of pulmonary hypoxic vasoconstriction studied with arterial and venous occlusion. *J Appl Physiol.* 1983;54:1298–1302.
78. Marshall BE, Marshall C. A model for hypoxic constriction of the pulmonary circulation. *J Appl Physiol.* 1988;64:68–77.
79. Marshall BE, Marshall C. Continuity of response to hypoxic pulmonary vasoconstriction. *J Appl Physiol.* 1980;49:189–196.
80. Dawson CA, Grimm DJ, Linehan JH. Lung inflation and longitudinal distribution of pulmonary vascular resistance during hypoxia. *J Appl Physiol Respir Environ Exerc Physiol.* 1979;47:532–536.
81. Howell JB, Permutt S, Proctor DF, et al. Effect of inflation of the lung on different parts of the pulmonary vascular bed. *J Appl Physiol.* 1961; 16:71–76.
82. West JB, Dollery CT, Naimark A. Distribution of blood flow in isolated lung: relation to vascular and alveolar pressures. *J Appl Physiol.* 1964;19:713–724.
83. Fuhrman BP, Smith-Wright DL, Kulik TJ, Lock JE. Effects of static and fluctuating airway pressure on the intact, immature pulmonary circulation. *J Appl Physiol.* 1986;60:114–122.
84. Thorvalson J, Ilebekk A, Kiil F. Determinants of pulmonary blood volume: effects of acute changes in airway pressure. *Acta Physiol Scand.* 1985;125:471–479.
85. Lopez-Muniz R, Stephens NL, Bromberger-Barnea B, et al. Critical closure of pulmonary vessels analyzed in terms of Starling resistor model. *J Appl Physiol.* 1968;24:625–635.
86. Block AJ, Boyson PG, Wynne JW. The origins of cor pulmonale, a hypothesis. *Chest.* 1979;75:109–114.
87. Vieillard-Baron A, Loubieres Y, Schmitt JM, et al. Cyclic changes in right ventricular output impedance during mechanical ventilation. *J Appl Physiol.* 1999;87:1644–1650.
88. Canada E, Benumnof JL, Tousdale FR. Pulmonary vascular resistance correlated in intact normal and abnormal canine lungs. *Crit Care Med.* 1982;10:719–723.
89. Vieillard-Baron A, Schmitt JM, et al. Acute cor pulmonale in acute respiratory distress syndrome submitted to protective ventilation: incidence, clinical implications, and prognosis. *Crit Care Med.* 2001;29:1551–1555.
90. Taylor RR, Corell JW, Sonnenblick EH, Ross J Jr. Dependence of ventricular distensibility on filling the opposite ventricle. *Am J Physiol.* 1967;213:711–718.
91. Brinker JA, Weiss I, Lappe DL, et al. Leftward septal displacement during right ventricular loading in man. *Circulation.* 1980;61:626–633.
92. Takata M, Harasawa Y, Beloucif S, Robotham JL. Coupled vs. uncoupled pericardial restraint: effects on cardiac chamber interactions. *J Appl Physiol.* 1997;83:1799–1813.
93. Marini JJ, Culver BN, Butler J. Mechanical effect of lung distention with positive pressure on cardiac function. *Am Rev Respir Dis.* 1980; 124:382–386.
94. Butler J. The heart is in good hands. *Circulation.* 1983;67:1163–1168.
95. Cassidy SS, Wead WB, Seibert GB, Ramanathan M. Changes in left ventricular geometry during spontaneous breathing. *J Appl Physiol.* 1987;63: 803–811.
96. Hoffman EA, Ritman EL. Heart–lung interaction: effect on regional lung air content and total heart volume. *Ann Biomed Eng.* 1987;15:241–257.

97. Olson LE, Hoffman EA. Heart–lung interactions determined by electron beam x-ray CT in laterally recumbent rabbits. *J Appl Physiol.* 1995;78:417–427.
98. Jayaweera AR, Ehrlich W. Changes of phasic pleural pressure in awake dogs during exercise: potential effects on cardiac output. *Ann Biomed Eng.* 1987;15:311–318.
99. Cassidy SS, Robertson CH Jr, Pierce AK, et al. Cardiovascular effects of positive end-expiratory pressure in dogs. *J Appl Physiol.* 1978;4:743–749.
100. Conway CM. Hemodynamic effects of pulmonary ventilation. *Br J Anaesth.* 1975;47:761–766.
101. Jardin F, Farcot JC, Boisante L. Influence of positive end-expiratory pressure on left ventricular performance. *N Engl J Med.* 1981;304:387–392.
102. Berglund JE, Halden E, Jakobson S, Landelius J. Echocardiographic analysis of cardiac function during high PEEP ventilation. *Intensive Care Med.* 1994;20:174–180.
103. Guyton AC, Lindsey AW, Abernathy B, et al. Venous return at various right atrial pressures and the normal venous return curve. *Am J Physiol.* 1957;189:609–615.
104. Goldberg HS, Rabson J. Control of cardiac output by systemic vessels: circulatory adjustments of acute and chronic respiratory failure and the effects of therapeutic interventions. *Am J Cardiol.* 1981;47:696–702.
105. Pinsky MR. Instantaneous venous return curves in an intact canine preparation. *J Appl Physiol Respir Environ Exerc Physiol.* 1984;56:765–771.
106. Kilburn KH. Cardiorespiratory effects of large pneumothorax in conscious and anesthetized dogs. *J Appl Physiol.* 1963;18:279–283.
107. Chevalier PA, Weber KC, Engle JC, et al. Direct measurement of right and left heart outputs in Valsalva-like maneuver in dogs. *Proc Soc Exper Biol Med.* 1972;139:1429–1437.
108. Guntheroth WC, Gould R, Butler J, et al. Pulsatile flow in pulmonary artery, capillary and vein in the dog. *Cardiovasc Res.* 1974;8:330–337.
109. Guntheroth WG, Morgan BC, Mullins GL. Effect of respiration on venous return and stroke volume in cardiac tamponade: mechanism of pulsus paradoxus. *Circ Res.* 1967;20:381–390.
110. Guyton AC. Effect of cardiac output by respiration, opening the chest, and cardiac tamponade. In: *Circulatory Physiology: Cardiac Output and Its Regulation.* Philadelphia, PA: Saunders; 1963:378–386.
111. Holt JP. The effect of positive and negative intrathoracic pressure on cardiac output and venous return in the dog. *Am J Physiol.* 1944;142:594–603.
112. Morgan BC, Abel FL, Mullins GL, et al. Flow patterns in cavae, pulmonary artery, pulmonary vein and aorta in intact dogs. *Am J Physiol.* 1966;210:903–909.
113. Morgan BC, Martin WE, Hornbein TF, et al. Hemodynamic effects of intermittent positive pressure respiration. *Anesthesiology.* 1960;27:584–590.
114. Scharf SM, Brown R, Saunders N, Green LH. Hemodynamic effects of positive pressure inflation. *J Appl Physiol.* 1980;49:124–131.
115. Jardin F, Vieillard-Baron A. Right ventricular function and positive-pressure ventilation in clinical practice: from hemodynamic subsets to respirator settings. *Intensive Care Med.* 2003;29:1426–1434.
116. Scharf SM, Brown R, Saunders N, et al. Effects of normal and loaded spontaneous inspiration on cardiovascular function. *J Appl Physiol.* 1979;47:582–590.
117. Groeneveld AB, Berendsen RR, Schneider AJ, et al. Effect of the mechanical ventilatory cycle on thermodilution right ventricular volumes and cardiac output. *J Appl Physiol (1985).* 2000;89:89–96.
118. Van den Berg P, Jansen JR, Pinsky MR. The effect of positive-pressure inspiration on venous return in volume loaded post-operative cardiac surgical patients. *J Appl Physiol (1985).* 2002;92:1223–1231.
119. Magder S, Georgiadis G, Cheong T. Respiratory variation in right atrial pressure predict the response to fluid challenge. *J Crit Care.* 1992;7:76–85.
120. Harken AH, Brennan MF, Smith N, Barsamian EM. The hemodynamic response to positive end-expiratory ventilation in hypovolemic patients. *Surgery.* 1974;76:786–793.
121. Fessler HE, Brower RG, Wise RA, Permutt S. Effects of positive end-expiratory pressure on the canine venous return curve. *Am Rev Respir Dis.* 1992;146:4–10.
122. Takata M, Robotham JL. Effects of inspiratory diaphragmatic descent on inferior vena caval venous return. *J Appl Physiol (1985).* 1992;72:597–607.
123. Matuschak GM, Pinsky MR, Rogers RM. Effects of positive end-expiratory pressure on hepatic blood flow and hepatic performance. *J Appl Physiol (1985).* 1987;62:1377–1383.
124. Chihara E, Hasimoto S, Kinoshita T, et al. Elevated mean systemic filling pressure due to intermittent positive-pressure ventilation. *Am J Physiol.* 1992;262:H1116–H1121.
125. Takata M, Wise RA, Robotham JL. Effects of abdominal pressure on venous return: abdominal vascular zone conditions. *J Appl Physiol (1985).* 1990;69:1961–1972.
126. Barnes GE, Laine GA, Giam PY, et al. Cardiovascular responses to elevation of intra-abdominal hydrostatic pressure. *Am J Physiol.* 1985;248:R208–R213.
127. Lichtwarck-Aschoff M, Zeravik J, Pfeiffer UJ. Intrathoracic blood volume accurately reflects circulatory volume status in critically ill patients with mechanical ventilation. *Intensive Care Med.* 1992;18:142–145.
128. Brecher GA, Hubay CA. Pulmonary blood flow and venous return during spontaneous respiration. *Circ Res.* 1955;3:40–214.
129. Terada N, Takeuchi T. Postural changes in venous pressure gradients in anesthetized monkeys. *Am J Physiol.* 1993;264:H21–H25.
130. Scharf S, Tow DE, Miller MJ, et al. Influence of posture and abdominal pressure on the hemodynamic effects of Mueller's maneuver. *J Crit Care.* 1989;4:26–34.
131. Rankin JS, Olsen CO, Arentzen CE, et al. The effects of airway pressure on cardiac function in intact dogs and man. *Circulation.* 1982;66:108–120.
132. Robotham JL, Rabson J, Permutt S, Bromberger-Barnea B. Left ventricular hemodynamics during respiration. *J Appl Physiol.* 1979;47:1295–1303.
133. Ruskin J, Bache RJ, Rembert JC, Greenfield JC Jr. Pressure-flow studies in man: effect of respiration on left ventricular stroke volume. *Circulation.* 1973;48:79–85.
134. Olsen CO, Tyson GS, Maier GW, et al. Dynamic ventricular interaction in the conscious dog. *Circ Res.* 1983;52:85–104.
135. Janicki JS, Weber KT. The pericardium and ventricular interaction, distensibility and function. *Am J Physiol.* 1980;238:H494–H503.
136. Michard F, Boussat S, Chemla D, et al. Relation between respiratory changes in arterial pulse pressure and fluid responsiveness in septic patients with acute circulatory failure. *Am J Respir Crit Care Med.* 2000;162:134–138.
137. Beyar R, Goldstein Y. Model studies of the effects of the thoracic pressure on the circulation. *Ann Biomed Eng.* 1987;15:373–383.
138. Buda AJ, Pinsky MR, Ingels NB, et al. Effect of intrathoracic pressure on left ventricular performance. *N Engl J Med.* 1979;301:453–459.
139. Pinsky MR, Summer WR, Wise RA, et al. Augmentation of cardiac function by elevation of intrathoracic pressure. *J Appl Physiol.* 1983;54: 950–955.
140. Beach T, Millen E, Grenvik A. Hemodynamic response to discontinuance of mechanical ventilation. *Crit Care Med.* 1973;1:85–90.
141. Cassidy SA, Wead WB, Seibert GB, Ramanathan M. Geometric left-ventricular responses to interactions between the lung and left ventricle: positive pressure breathing. *Ann Biomed Eng.* 1987;15:285–295.
142. Scharf SM, Brown R, Warner KG, Khuri S. Intrathoracic pressure and left ventricular configuration with respiratory maneuvers. *J Appl Physiol.* 1989;66:481–491.
143. Sharpey-Schaffer EP. Effects of Valsalva maneuver on the normal and failing circulation. *Br Med J.* 1955;1:693–699.
144. Khilnani S, Graver LM, Balaban K, Scharf SM. Effects of inspiratory loading on left ventricular myocardial blood flow and metabolism. *J Appl Physiol.* 1992;72:1488–1492.
145. Sibbald WH, Calvin J, Driedger AA. Right and left ventricular preload, and diastolic ventricular compliance: implications of therapy in critically ill patients. *Critical Care State of the Art.* Vol 3. Fullerton, CA: Society of Critical Care; 1982.
146. DeHoyos A, Liu PP, Benard DC, Bradley TD. Haemodynamic effects of continuous positive airway pressure in humans with normal and impaired left ventricular function. *Clin Sci Colch.* 1995;88:173–178.
147. Naughton MT, Rahman MA, Hara K, et al. Effect of continuous positive airway pressure on intrathoracic and left ventricular transmural pressures in patients with congestive heart failure. *Circulation.* 1995;91:1725–1731.
148. Philip-Joet FF, Paganelli FF, Dutau HL, Saadjian AY. Hemodynamic effects of bi-level nasal positive airway pressure ventilation in patients with heart failure. *Respiration.* 1999;66:136–143.
149. Buckle P, Millar T, Kryger M. The effect of short-term nasal CPAP on Cheyne-Stokes respiration in congestive heart failure. *Chest.* 1992;102:31–35.
150. Granton JT, Naughton MT, Benard DC, et al. CPAP improves inspiratory muscle strength in patients with heart failure and central sleep apnea. *Am J Respir Crit Care Med.* 1996;153:277–282.
151. Kaneko Y, Floras JS, Usui K, et al. Cardiovascular effects of continuous positive airway pressure in patients with heart failure and obstructive sleep apnea. *N Engl J Med.* 2003;348:1233–1241.
152. Naughton MT, Benard DC, Liu PP, et al. Effects of nasal CPAP on sympathetic activity in patients with heart failure and central sleep apnea. *Am J Respir Crit Care Med.* 1995;152:473–479.
153. Lin M, Yang YF, Chiang HT, et al. Reappraisal of continuous positive airway pressure therapy in acute cardiogenic pulmonary edema. Short-term results and long-term follow-up. *Chest.* 1995;107:1379–1386.
154. Bersten AD, Holt AW, Vedig AE, et al. Treatment of severe cardiogenic pulmonary edema with continuous positive airway pressure delivered by face mask. *N Engl J Med.* 1991;325(26);1825–1830.

155. Denault AY, Gasior TA, Gorcsan J 3rd, et al. Determinants of aortic pressure variation during positive-pressure ventilation in man. *Chest.* 1999;116:176–186.
156. Monnet X, Rienzo M, Osman D, et al. Esophageal Doppler monitoring predicts fluid responsiveness in critically ill ventilated patients. *Intensive Care Med.* 2005;31(9):1195–1201.
157. Cecconi M, De Backer D, Antonelli M, et al. Consensus on Circulatory Shock and Hemodynamic Monitoring, Task Force of the European Society of Intensive Care Medicine. *Intensive Care Med.* 2014;49:1795–1815.
158. Benes J, Giglio M, Brienza N, Michard F. The effects of goal-directed fluid therapy based on dynamic parameters on post-surgical outcome: a meta-analysis of randomized controlled trials. *Crit Care.* 2014;18:584.
159. Perner A, De Backer D. Understanding hypovolaemia. *Intensive Care Med.* 2014;40:613–615.
160. Pinsky MR. The hemodynamic consequences of mechanical ventilation: an evolving story. *Intensive Care Med.* 1997;23:493–503.
161. Feissel M, Michard F, Faller J, Teboul JL. The respiratory variation in inferior vena cava diameter as a guide to fluid therapy. *Intensive Care Med.* 2004;30:1834–1837.
162. Vieillard-Baron A, Chergui K, Rabiller A, et al. Superior vena cava collapsibility as a gauge of volume status in ventilated septic patients. *Intensive Care Med.* 2004;30:1734–1739.
163. Guarracino F, Ferro B, Forfori F, et al. Jugular vein distensibility predicts fluid responsiveness in septic patients. *Crit Care.* 2014;18:647.
164. De Backer D, Heenen S, Piagnerelli M, et al. Pulse pressure variations to predict fluid responsiveness: influence of tidal volume. *Intensive Care Med.* 2005;31:517–523.
165. Monnet X, Rienzo M, Osman D, et al. Passive leg raising predicts fluid responsiveness in the critically ill. *Crit Care Med.* 2006;34:1402–1407.
166. Mahjoub Y, Touzeau J, Airapetian N, et al. The passive leg-raising maneuver cannot accurately predict fluid responsiveness in patients with intra-abdominal hypertension. *Crit Care Med.* 2010;38:1824–1829.

CHAPTER

102

Mechanical Ventilation

PAUL B. BLANCH

IMMEDIATE CONCERNS

Ventilation/Perfusion (V_A/Q) in the Normal Lung

The lung's primary function is to add oxygen (O_2) to, and remove carbon dioxide (CO_2) from, blood passing through the pulmonary capillary beds. For this to occur, the gas we breathe must be "matched" to the blood flowing through our lungs. Average minute alveolar ventilation (V_A), for a healthy adult, is 4.0 liters (L) per minute (min), while resting cardiac output (Q) is 5.0 L/min; it follows that optimal ventilation–perfusion matching (V_A/Q ratio) is 4 L/min divided by 5 L/min or 0.8. Perfect V_A/Q matching is unlikely because the distribution of gas and blood flow vary across the lungs fields for several reasons. Both gases and blood have mass and are therefore gravity dependent (Fig. 102.1); as a result, both increase as we progress from apex to the base of the lung. Gravity's effect on blood flow is however, predominant; it has been estimated that in an upright subject, 6 times as much blood passes through each lung's base, compared to its apex, whereas only 2½ times as much air reaches each lung's base. These different gradients dictate that V_A/Q ratio rises progressively, from the bottom to the top of the lungs.

Furthermore, the lungs are comprised of millions of alveoli, connected to each other and eventually to the trachea by a labyrinth of pathways, and interconnections (pores of Kohn). Few connections are consistent in either length or diameter; this effect conspires to further disrupt the distribution of inhaled gases. Even the healthiest athletes exhibit areas of shunt and dead space (Fig. 102.2). About 30% of the air a healthy adult breathes each minute is wasted as dead space ventilation (V_D) and 3% to 5% of their cardiac output passes through the lungs without undergoing gas exchange (shunt). Any pathophysiologic stimulus that acutely increases or decreases ventilation or cardiac output is likely to have a pronounced impact upon V_A/Q ratios and in turn, upon oxygenation and CO_2 removal.

Positive Pressure Breathing

Positive pressure mechanical ventilation, unlike normal breathing, increases transpulmonary pressure, reduces venous return. The balance of these two forces affect cardiac output. Positive pressure breathing also preferentially forces gas into areas of the lung with the lowest airway resistance (R_{aw}) and highest compliance (C_{RS}). It is not uncommon for ventilated patients to require airway pressures (P_{aw}) of 30 cm H_2O or more; yet, normal systolic pulmonary arterial pressures seldom exceed 20 to 25 mmHg (27 to 34 cm H_2O). It follows that during positive pressure inflations, if intraluminal alveolar pressure exceeds the hydrostatic pressure, blood flow and gas exchange cease—until alveolar pressure falls below hydrostatic levels again during exhalation. Given these factors, it is easy to understand how mechanical ventilation often disrupts V_A/Q, and why up to 60% or more of each positive pressure breath is wasted as V_D. Allowing patients to breathe spontaneously, between mechanical breaths, significantly reduces mean transpulmonary and transluminal pressures, improves venous return and often cardiac output, which in turn, improves V_A/Q.

V_A/Inequalities in Respiratory Failure

It is not necessary that alveoli be completely deprived of V_A or Q for life-threatening symptoms to exist. When significant areas of a patient's lungs receive too much or too little V_A or Q, these regions exhibit abnormally high or low V_A/Q ratios, referred to as *relative shunt* and *relative dead space* (Fig. 102.3). Relative shunt and V_D are extremely common in the intensive care unit (ICU) setting and disrupt CO_2 removal and oxygenation just as quickly as, comparable, but smaller areas of absolute V_D or shunt.

Conditions Affecting Lung Structure

Along with conditions that effect only V_A or Q, there are a number of disorders that actually damage lung structure. Furthermore, failure to properly manage the ventilator, in some situations, may play a role in determining the ultimate severity of, and progression of the lung disease (1–7). Critical care personnel called upon to manage ventilators for these patients, whether in a primary or consulting role, must possess a thorough understanding of the pathophysiology and treatment of acute respiratory failure.

Reductions in the arterial partial pressure of oxygen (PaO_2) and carbon dioxide ($PaCO_2$) are characteristic of the early stages of acute respiratory distress syndrome (ARDS). Widespread, but not uniform, alveolar destabilization and collapse (atelectasis) are hallmarks of ARDS. If ARDS is not aggressively managed in its early stages, pulmonary consolidation (secondary to atelectasis) develops and may lead to a fibroprolific phase; the chances for recovery are significantly reduced if the disease progresses to this point (8). Hypoxemia results from both relative and absolute shunting caused by complete or partial alveolar collapse and the continued perfusion of these lung regions.

Ventilator Support

With respect to therapy, a shifting emphasis in the role of mechanical ventilation has occurred. Positive-pressure ventilation was clearly responsible for the decrease in mortality following the poliomyelitis epidemic. Yet, a similar reduction in mortality has been slow to respond following the widespread application of mechanical ventilatory support to ARDS, or to acute exacerbations of chronic obstructive pulmonary disease (COPD). Although this is in part due to the multisystem

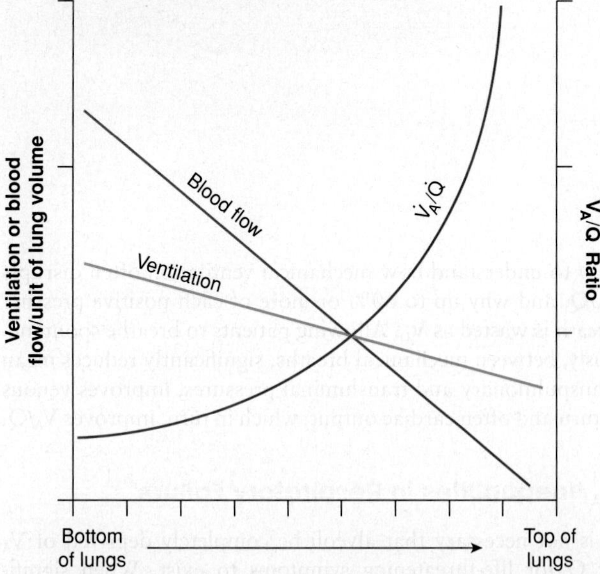

FIGURE 102.1 The effects of gravity on ventilation–perfusion ratio (V_A/Q). In the upright subject, gravity affects V_A, Q, and concomitantly, the V_A/Q ratio. Gravitational forces pull on both the gases we breathe and pulmonary blood flow; as a result, V_A and Q increase from a lung's apex to its base. Because of blood's greater mass, gravity's effect upon Q predominates; it is estimated that Q at a lung's base is six times as great as at its apex, compared to only 2½ times as much V_A at the lung's base versus its apex. The resultant V_A/Q ratio is therefore greater at the lung apices than the bases.

dysfunction that frequently accompanies such problems, it now appears that the inappropriate use of mechanical ventilation has played a significant role.

Poliomyelitis, Guillain–Barré syndrome, and other neuromuscular disease states produce respiratory insufficiency because of mechanical and neural failure to control diaphragmatic-driven ventilation. In the absence of complications such as aspiration of gastric contents, pulmonary parenchymal function remains intact. By contrast, ARDS represents a failure of gas exchange that is related almost entirely to parenchymal involvement. Furthermore, neuromuscular and musculoskeletal function generally remains unimpaired during ARDS, although there are exceptions, such as flail chest associated with underlying pulmonary contusion after trauma. Even in this situation however, the musculoskeletal abnormality is of secondary importance compared with the underlying lung contusion.

Even the simplest ventilator provides a satisfactory means for sustaining V_A when neuromuscular and musculoskeletal problems predominate. Yet, it would be very surprising if a simple ventilator performed equally well in the therapy of ARDS, in which an entirely different spectrum of pathophysiologic changes occurs. Thus, when a decrease in residual alveolar volume is present—whether caused by surfactant depletion, partial airway obstruction, interstitial and alveolar pulmonary edema, or a combination of these factors—a simple mechanical ventilator can have salutary effects only while it restores alveolar volume and improves oxygen exchange during the inhalation phase provided, of course, that ventilatory pressures do not approach or exceed pulmonary hydrostatic pressures. During exhalation, the beneficial effects of inflation quickly dissipate, especially if alveolar volume is allowed to return to its starting point.

In fact, opening alveoli during inhalation, and allowing them to close again during exhalation, may exacerbate the problem. It seems that when alveoli collapse, surfactant activity is lost; there are two putative theories to explain this: (a) surfactant molecules are forced into close proximity during collapse; ultimately they collide and clump together (9,10); and/or (b) surfactant is forced up, into the airways, during alveolar collapse (11)—once in the airways, surfactant is either damaged, or removed by ciliary action.

Positive End-Expiratory Pressure

Reduced levels of surfactant, such as occur during ARDS, lead to widespread atelectasis and hypoxemia; these conditions respond poorly to mechanical ventilation alone. The law of Laplace states that pressure inside a spherical structure is directly proportional to tension in that structure's wall and inversely proportional to its radius. Normally, alveolar surface forces, at alveolar-capillary membranes, are essentially identical. Laplace's law dictates that a loss of surfactant means a greater pressure is required to keep smaller alveoli open (Fig. 102.4). When this occurs, smaller alveoli empty into larger ones, eventually collapsing. A plot of the lung's pressure–volume relationship, during ARDS, helps to better visualize this phenomenon (Fig. 102.5). Without adequate surfactant, significant portions of the lungs collapse at end-exhalation. During inhalation, as pressure is applied to the airways (*x*-axis), nothing initially happens. However, when the applied pressure reaches sufficient magnitude, in this instance 14 cm H_2O, some

A. Absolute shunt—low $\dot{V}_A/\dot{Q}$ ratio

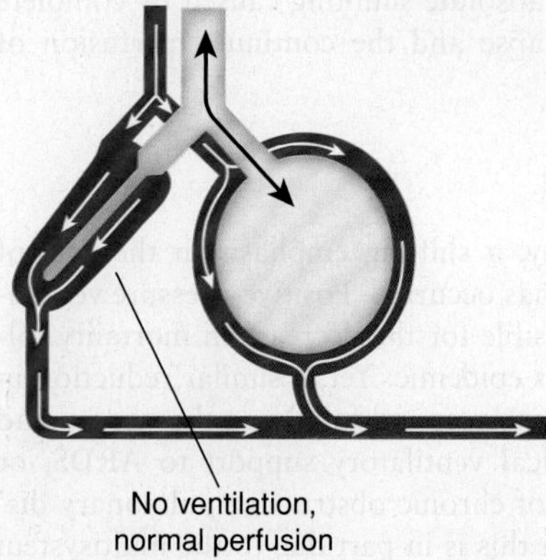

B. Alveolar dead space—high $\dot{V}_A/\dot{Q}$ ratio

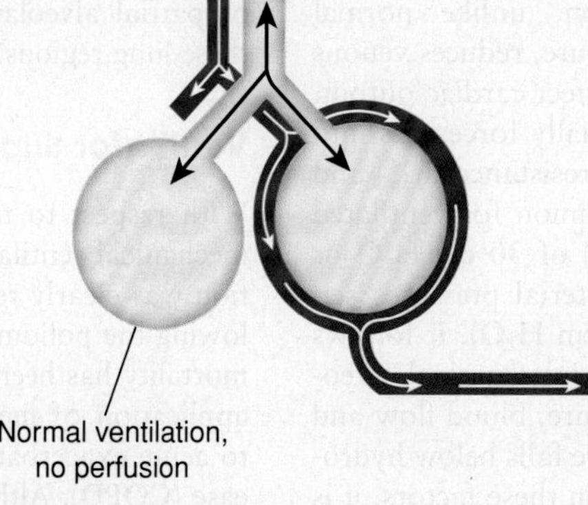

FIGURE 102.2 Ventilation–perfusion (V_A/Q) abnormalities. A: Absolute shunt—low V_A/Q ratio. An intrapulmonary, or absolute, shunt occurs when blood continues to perfuse collapsed, or otherwise unventilated alveoli–blood literally shunts past, or bypasses the lung, without participating in gas exchange. B: Alveolar dead space—high V_A/Q ratio. Dead space or wasted ventilation exists when alveoli receive ventilation but no blood flow.

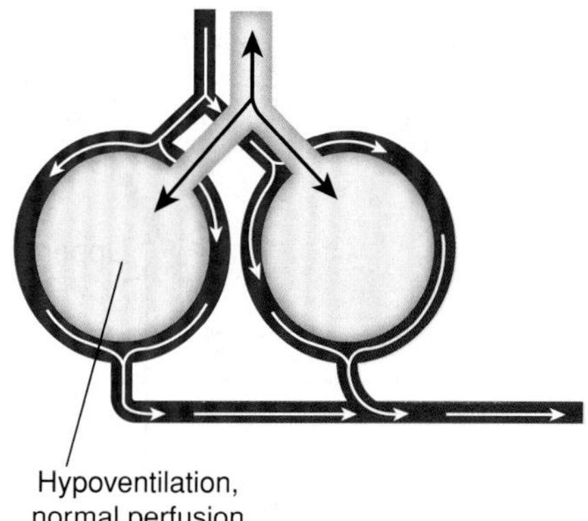

FIGURE 102.3 Relative ventilation–perfusion (V_A/Q) abnormalities. **A:** Relative shunt—low V_A/Q ratio. A relative shunt occurs when an alveolus receives too much Q in relation to V_A. **B:** Relative dead space—high V_A/Q ratio. Relative dead space exists when an alveolus receives too much V_A relative to its Q.

of the collapsed alveoli start to open and gas begins entering the lungs. This "opening" pressure is commonly referred to as the *lower inflection point*, and provides the theoretical underpinnings for the use of positive end-expiratory pressure (PEEP). That is, an ARDS-related surfactant deficiency predisposes to alveolar collapse, unless counteracted by force. Clinically, the easiest way to accomplish this goal is by maintaining PEEP, preferably somewhat above the lower inflection point (12). Because the therapeutic objective is to prevent alveolar collapse—that is to say, keep the alveoli open—the approach is often referred to as the *open lung* approach (13,14).

Combining mechanical ventilation and PEEP usually decreases shunt and improves oxygenation (15–18), often significantly; nevertheless, ARDS mortality rates have failed to improve. The reasons for this are complex, but theories for these failures are starting to emerge (19). It now appears that, to reduce ARDS-associated morbidity and mortality, we must avoid the risks associated with both low-volume (4–7) and high-volume (1–3) lung injury. To accomplish this, all tidal ventilation must occur between the lower and upper inflection points (19). This sounds easy; but bedside determination of inflection points is difficult; nevertheless, it's worth the effort.

To date, a universally agreed upon ventilatory approach, or mode, for managing critically ill patients has failed to emerge. Considering the wide variety of conditions ameliorated by mechanical ventilation, and the extreme range of severity between patients with the same problem, a single, always best, approach may not exist. Clinicians, therefore, must understand and recognize the potential and limitations of their favored approaches.

VENTILATOR CLASSIFICATION

Positive versus Negative Pressure

Today, virtually all ventilators function by providing some variant of positive pressure. Yet, during the polio epidemic, "iron lungs" or negative pressure ventilators were in common use. Negative pressure devices require that the patient's body be tightly enclosed within a tube or box, while the head remained outside. Once the patient is sealed inside, a pump or bellows evacuates gas, from inside the box; this creates a negative pressure around the patient's thorax, making atmospheric pressure positive in relation to alveolar pressure. As a result, gas flows from the mouth to alveoli, trying to equalize the pressure difference. Because this process is nearly identical to normal breathing, negative pressure ventilators tend to provide better V_A/Q ratios (20) and produce less interference with cardiac output (21) than positive pressure counterparts. Nevertheless, these devices quickly lost favor for a number of compelling reasons: (a) iron lungs are very large

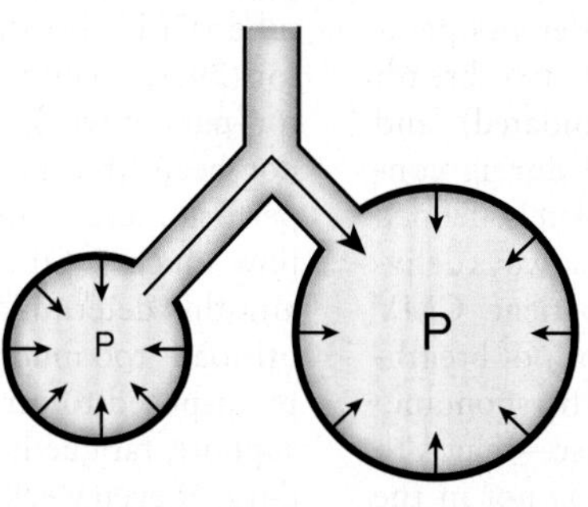

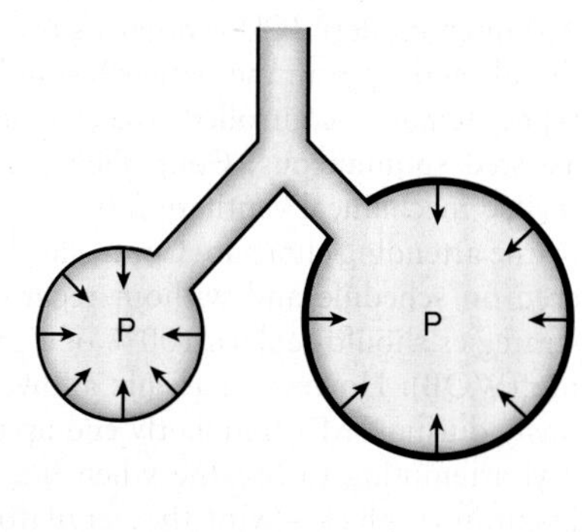

$$P = \frac{2T}{r}$$

FIGURE 102.4 Laplace's law and its effect on alveoli. Laplace's law states pressure (P), inside a sphere, is directly proportional the tension in the walls (T) and inversely proportional to the sphere's radius. **A:** Without surfactant. Wall or surface tension in both large and small alveoli is about the same. As a result, a greater pressure develops in the smaller alveolus, which then proceeds to empty into adjacent, larger alveoli. **B:** With surfactant. The surface tension reducing properties of surfactant increase as individual surfactant molecules get closer together. This property counteracts Laplace's law, and reduces the tendency for small alveoli to empty into nearby larger alveoli.

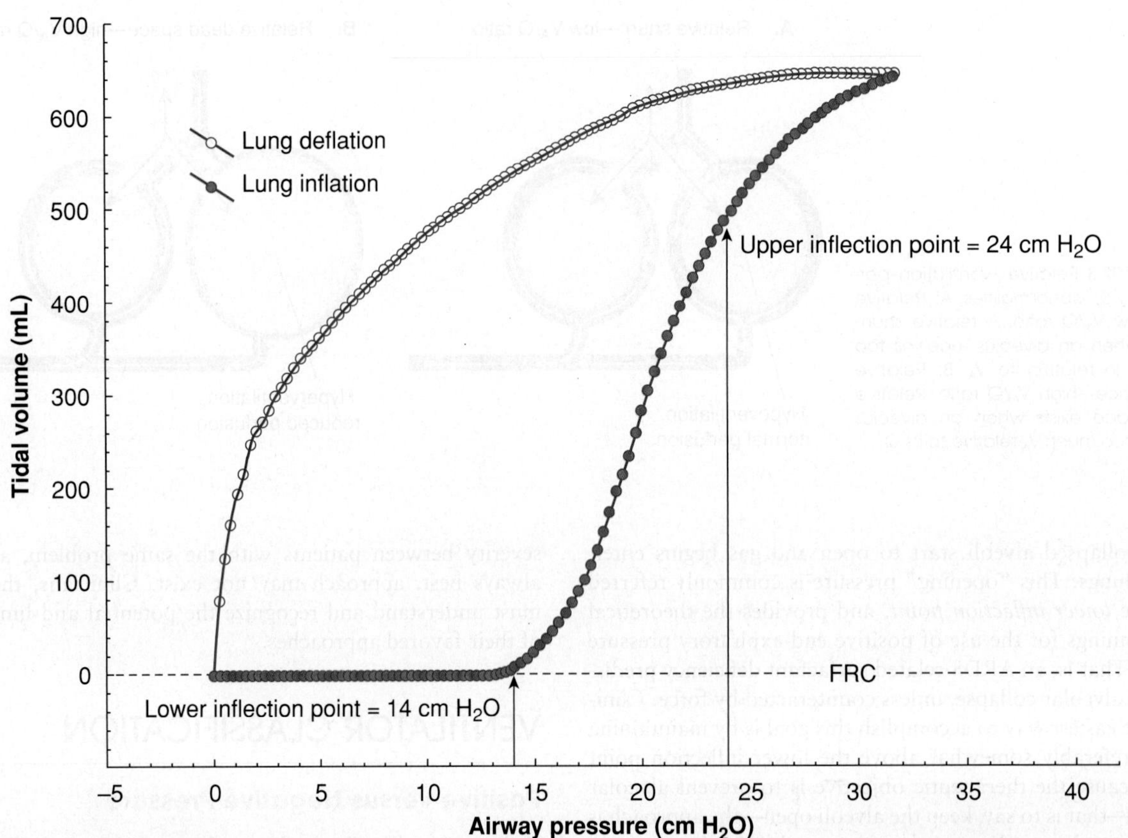

FIGURE 102.5 Inflation and deflation characteristics in the surfactant-deficient lung. Surfactant deficient alveoli generally remain open throughout exhalation (*open circles*); at end-exhalation, unstable alveoli empty into adjacent, larger alveoli and collapse. This phenomenon reduces functional residual capacity (FRC), often significantly. Furthermore, once collapsed, alveoli tend to stay collapsed until a relatively high pressure is applied. In this idealized example, airway pressure is steadily increased to inflate the lungs (*solid circles*). Note airway pressure reaches 14 cm H_2O, before any measurable volume enters the lungs; at this point (*lower inflection point*), collapsed alveoli begin to open, the lungs begin to accept volume, and the pressure–volume curve changes slope upward. Alveoli continue to open, those already open expand, and airway pressure continues to rise until the average patent alveoli begin to approach their maximum volume. At this point, the pressure–volume curve flattens—in other words, from this point on, larger changes in pressure will be required to produce a complimentary change in volume. This slope change is referred as the *upper inflection point*. Although the pressure–volume curve may be difficult to measure at the bedside, avoiding ventilator-induced lung injury requires that all mechanical ventilation occur between the upper and lower inflection points; that is, patient airway pressure should not be allowed above the upper inflection point, or below the lower inflection point.

and difficult to move; (b) maintaining an air-tight seal around the patient's neck, *without irritation*, is nearly impossible; (c) personnel responsible for providing patient monitoring and routine care could not easily access important areas of their patient's body.

Controlled versus Assisted Breaths

Although modern ICU ventilators offer many different operational modes, from the patient's standpoint, only two breath types remain: controlled (mechanical or mandated) and assisted spontaneous. Controlled breaths, used during controlled mechanical ventilation (CMV), are completely defined by the attending clinician. Controlled breaths are always delivered on schedule and without regard for the patient. CMV strategies should replace 100% of a patient's work of breathing (WOB). However, patients allowed to breathe spontaneously during CMV frequently end up out of phase—that is to say, attempting to breathe when the ventilator is not in the inspiratory phase—with the ventilator. Also known as *dyssynchrony*, out of phase breathing during CMV produces very high patient WOB (22). Assisted-spontaneous breathing strategies involve a work-sharing approach between the patient and ventilator (23). Theoretically speaking, a work-sharing approach makes perfect sense; ideally, the ventilator functions to "unload" WOB the patient cannot tolerate. Critically ill patients face an above normal workload, primarily from their pulmonary disease process and, secondarily from their artificial breathing apparatus, including the endotracheal tube (ETT), breathing circuits, humidifiers, and the ventilator (24,25). Unfortunately, there is a fatal flaw in the ventilator–patient work sharing concept: until recently (26) we have not been able to find a reliable, readily available, easy-to-perform, and noninvasive methodology for determining just how much WOB our patients can actually tolerate (27–29), and this determination is absolutely crucial. If the ventilator off-loads too much work, the patient's respiratory muscles are predisposed to atrophy. If the ventilator provides insufficient support, fatigue is likely. Either scenario can add unnecessary days, or even weeks, to the period time patients require ventilatory support. Fatigued or weak patients make poor candidates for weaning and attempts at liberation from the ventilator;

moreover, the risk for developing ventilator-associated pneumonia (VAP) correlates directly to the time spent receiving ventilatory support (30). Research suggests that the diaphragm, which evolved to contract without interruption from birth until death, begins to loose contractility shortly after initiating CMV (31); the loss of contractility is time-dependent and continues to worsen as mechanical ventilation is prolonged (31).

Ventilator Breaths: Defining Characteristics

The idea of trying to classify each ventilator type—to better understand how specific ventilators interacts with and affect physiology—remains as common today as ever. Yet, today's ventilators include so many modes and options that they are near impossible to classify. For a time, some tried to classify ventilator modes (32), but even this strategy is no longer reliable because many ventilators now incorporate dual-mode capabilities—the ability to switch modes *within* an individual ventilator breath.

Instead of trying to classify ventilators, modes, or even submodes, it may be easier to develop and use a standardized set of terms, and describe the breath types in use. This is possible because, regardless of ventilator or breath type, all ventilator breaths are delivered in four distinct phases or variables (Fig. 102.6).

Phase or Control Variables

Each ventilator breath must begin, for some reason and at some specific moment in time. The physical change that initiates a breath is known as the *trigger variable* (labeled A in Fig. 102.6). Once a breath is triggered "on," the ventilator must somehow, precisely manage how gas is forced into the patient's lungs; the physical characteristic managed during lung inflation is the *control variable* (labeled B in Fig. 102.6). After delivering the prescribed volume or pressure, inflation must end. This physical change responsible for ending inflation is called the *cycle variable* or cycling (labeled C in Fig. 102.6). Immediately following inhalation is exhalation, or the *exhalation variable* (labeled D in Fig. 102.6). Unlike the previous three variables, use of an exhalation variable is optional.

In early attempts at ventilator classification, author(s) often used the term *cycling* for both breath initiation and termination. Do *not* confuse the breath initiation, triggering, with breath termination, cycling; the ambiguous use of the term "cycling" continues to produce confusion.

All ventilators systematically, change the pressure, flow, and volume with respect to time. It follows that, when characterizing any of the four phase variables, pressure, flow, volume, or time are the only possible physical characteristics a ventilator could change or control, during any phase of respiratory cycle (Table 102.1). It is also important to note that

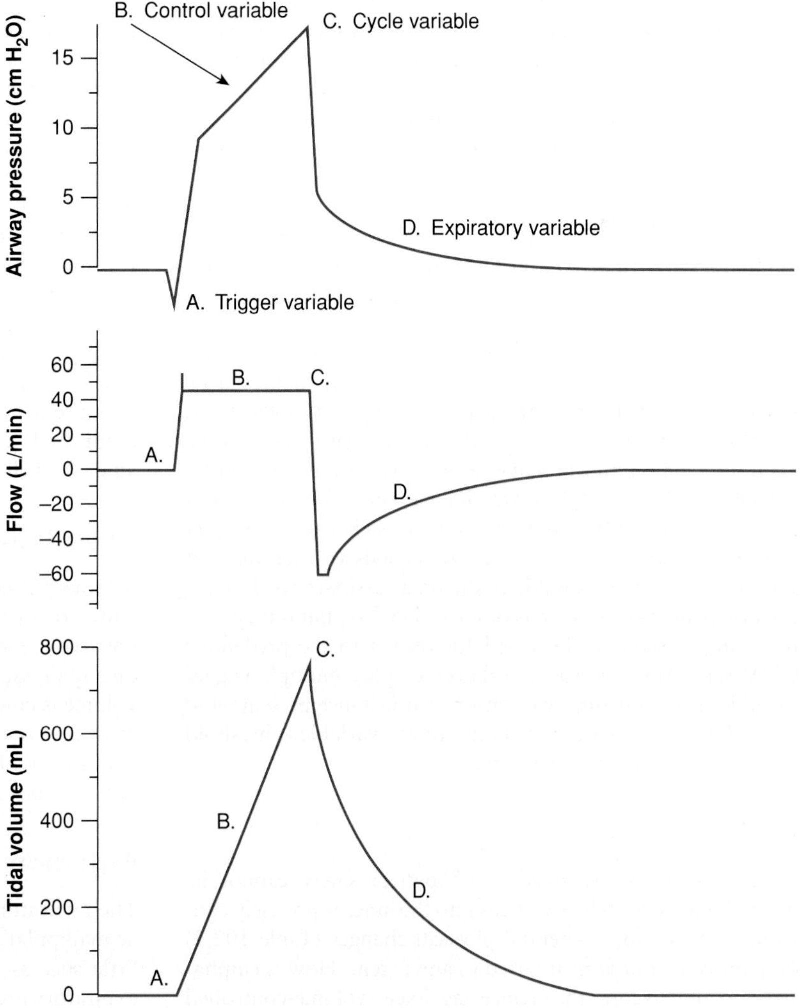

FIGURE 102.6 Pressure, flow, and volume curves for a mechanical ventilator breath. **A**: The trigger variable. The trigger variable is the physical characteristic used, by the ventilator, to initiate a mechanical inflation of the lungs. In this case, pressure falls before the breath starts; the represented ventilator breath is likely pressure-triggered. **B**: Control variable. For patient safety, the ventilator must precisely control an important aspect involved with inflating the patient's lungs. For this breath, flow is held constant; the ventilator is described as flow-controlled. **C**: Cycle variable. Each mechanical breath must end such that the lungs are properly filled and then allow the patient to exhale. The physical characteristic that determines appropriate lung filling, is the cycle variable. This example shows the breath ending after the control variable (flow) has continued for a specific interval of time; this ventilator is time-cycled. **D**: Expiratory variable. Modern ventilators either control pressure during exhalation or they do not. In this example, pressure returns to ambient (0 cm H_2O), so this ventilator has no operative expiratory variable.

TABLE 102.1 Ventilator Breath Classification

Breath Variable	Variable Characteristics	Frequency of Use and Example
Trigger	Time	Common, IMV, CMV, PCV, APRV
	Pressure	Common, SIMV, AC, PSV, CPAP
	Flow	Common, SIMV, AC, PSV, CPAP
	Volume	Infrequent, SIMV (some neonatal ventilators)
Inspiratory control	Time	Never
	Pressure	Common, all pressure-based breaths
	Flow	Common, most volume-based breaths
	Volume	Infrequent, some piston ventilators
Cycle	Time	Common, PCV, APRV
	Pressure	Common, IPPB
	Flow	Common, PSV
	Volume	Common, all volume-targeted modes
Expiratory	Time	Never
	Pressure	Common, CPAP, PEEP, NEEP
	Flow	Infrequent, retard
	Volume	Never

while some of these characteristics correlate and may change together, in direction and magnitude, they do not always do so. The practical side of this translates into an important tenet: ventilators can only control one characteristic at a time. This does not however, preclude using multiple characteristics, provided they are used in a logical sequence, and one at a time.

Trigger Variable

Ventilators are triggered "on" by time, pressure, flow, or volume. Today's ventilators however, often depend upon multiple trigger variables, used sequentially. For example, with a trigger sensitivity set for 2 (actually, –2 cm H_2O), breath rate set to 10 breaths per minute (bpm), and in the CMV mode, this ventilator has, at least, two trigger variables. First, breaths may be pressure-triggered when the ventilator is in the expiratory phase and baseline airway pressure is reduced by 2 cm H_2O, or more. If, however, the patient makes no attempt to breathe; the CMV rate timer counts reaches 0 and a time-triggered breath results—exactly 6 seconds(s) after the last ventilator breath. This mode is known as assist-control (A/C), because patients can assist as often as they like, but if they stop breathing (assisting), the ventilator reverts to the predefined CMV rate. Another way ventilators employ multiple trigger variables is by utilizing two sensors, for instance pressure and flow; triggering occurs in response to the variable's threshold (pressure or flow), breached first.

Control Variable

Once a breath is triggered "on," patient safety cannot be assured unless the delivery of gas into the lungs is precisely controlled. Of the four potential physical changes (Table 102.1) only pressure and *flow* are used to any extent. Flow is emphasized to underscore an engineering issue: volume-controlled ventilators are actually flow-controlled. There are several reasons for this. First, the integral of flow, with respect to time, is volume. It follows that by precisely controlling inspiratory flow (V_I), for a preset inspiratory time (T_I), produces an exact tidal volume (V_T), based on the following equation:

$$V_T = V_I \times T_I \quad (1)$$

Algebraically speaking, the operator can preset only two of these variables, in this case V_I and T_I; the third variable (V_T) cannot be preset; it is a consequence of V_I and T_I. Given a choice however, most clinicians prefer to preset the V_I and V_T; in this situation, T_I becomes the consequential or resultant variable. In an effort to obviate this preference, most of today's ventilators use an algebraic variant of equation 1:

$$V_T/V_I = T_I \quad (2)$$

This design allows operators to preset V_T and V_I. Furthermore, because the operator actually predefines V_T—referring to the ventilator as a volume-controller, or as volume-controlled ventilation (VCV)—this is perfectly acceptable; this nomenclature will be used henceforth.

Volume-controlled strategies differ markedly from pressure-controlled ventilation (PCV). When we opt for VCV, our priorities are clear: we wish to prescribe (preset) V_T, V_I, and flow pattern. If we wish these parameters reliably delivered, then airway pressure (P_{aw}) must not be restricted. When P_{aw} is allowed to vary, V_T, V_I, and flow pattern are delivered, regardless of the patient's pulmonary mechanics (Fig. 102.7). High peak inflation pressures (PIP) are a concern; so, ventilators allow clinicians to preset a maximum, safe level of P_{aw}; this setting, referred to as a *high pressure limit*, which functions as a cycle variable—that is, ending inspiration (or diverting gas flow), the moment P_{aw} violates the established threshold. Keep in mind though, cycling via high pressure limit truncates breath delivery, negates volume-control, and reduces V_T.

Pressure-controlled strategies allow us to preset a desired P_{aw} and T_I; conversely, V_T, V_I, and flow waveform cannot be predetermined. Pressure-controlled breaths always generate an exponentially decelerating flow pattern; the individual's C_{RS} and R_{aw} determine the magnitude of V_I and V_T (Fig. 102.8) (33,34). Inasmuch as PCV does not control V_T, and preset pressure never varies, clinicians must insure PCV is carefully monitored; always carefully set low/high V_T alarms (if available), as well as low/high minute ventilation alarms.

Cycle Variable

All four physical changes are commonly used for cycling ventilator breaths. Pressure-cycling is common during intermittent positive pressure breathing (IPPB); flow-cycling predominates during pressure support ventilation (PSV) and, either time or volume is common during VCV. Without question, time is the most commonly used cycle variable, particularly if one remembers that with today's VCVs, cycling occurs when T_I lapses, not in response to delivered volume.

Expiratory Variable

The expiratory phase is the least varied of the four; attempts at manipulating the expiratory phase variable have met with little success. Varying flow resistance (retard), negative end-expiratory pressure (NEEP) and PEEP have all been thoroughly

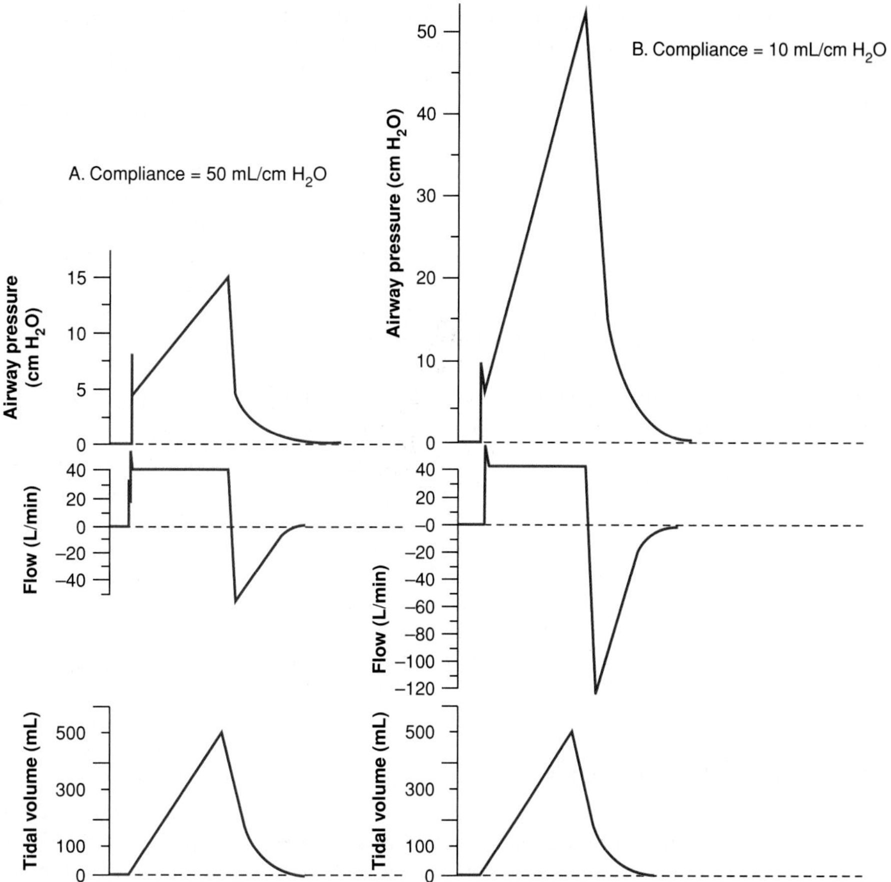

FIGURE 102.7 Response of volume-controlled ventilation (VCV) to a sudden change in respiratory system compliance (C_{RS}). **A:** Compliance = 50 mL/cm H_2O. An airway pressure, flow, and tidal volume curve for a patient with this C_{RS} and receiving VCV. **B:** Compliance = 10 mL/cm H_2O. An airway pressure, flow, and tidal volume curve, for the same patient as shown in panel A except, the patient's C_{RS} is acutely reduced. Note volume and flow are essentially unaffected, but, airway pressure is dramatically elevated as the ventilator required far more pressure to provide the same flow and volume into the much stiffer lungs.

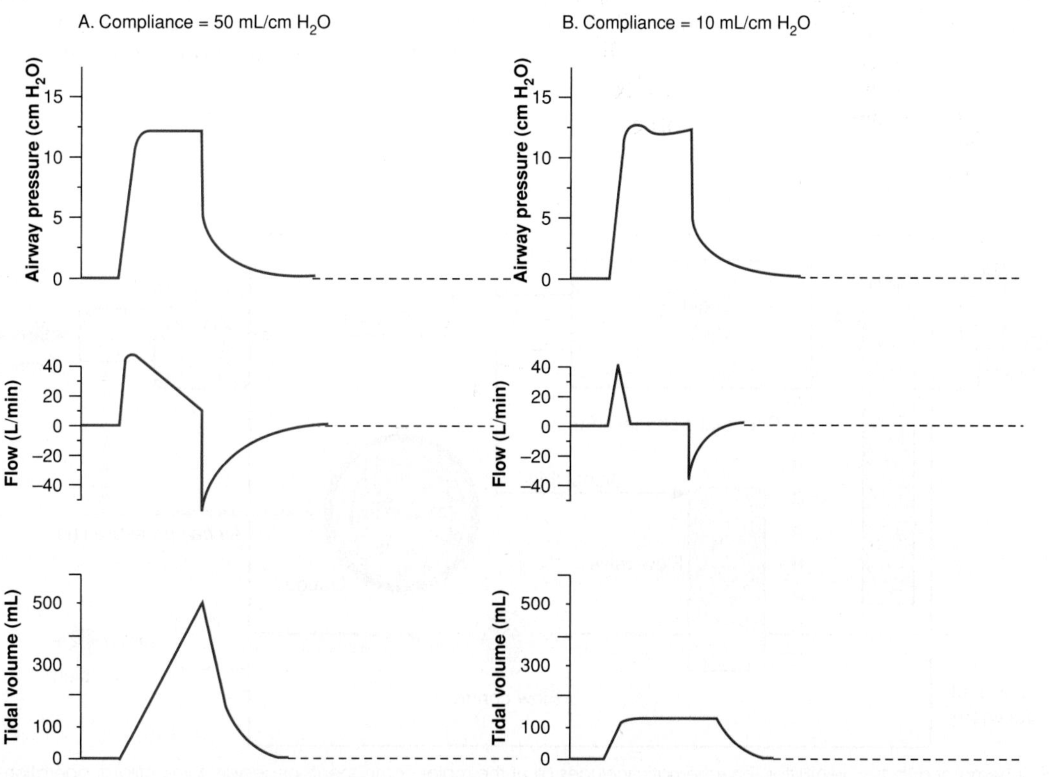

FIGURE 102.8 Response of pressure-controlled ventilation (PCV) to a sudden change in respiratory system compliance (C_{RS}). **A:** Compliance = 50 mL/cm H_2O. An airway pressure, flow, and tidal volume curve for a patient with this C_{RS} and receiving PCV. **B:** Compliance = 10 mL/cm H_2O. An airway pressure, flow, and tidal volume curve, for the same patient as shown in panel A except, the patient's C_{RS} is acutely reduced. Note pressure is essentially unaffected, but, flow and volume are dramatically reduced as the far stiffer lungs accept much less flow and volume at the same airway pressure.

tried and discarded. Compelling evidence however, substantiates using continuous positive airway pressure (CPAP) and PEEP to restore or increase functional residual capacity (FRC) (35–37), reduce shunt and improve oxygenation (15–18), and reduce WOB (38).

Classifying Breaths

The four phase variables (trigger, control, cycle, expiratory) provide us with an easy-to-use and understand method for classifying ventilator breaths. It makes sense classifying by breath behavior because today's ventilators offer so many breath types. For instance, the breath depicted in Figure 102.6 is pressure-triggered, volume-controlled, and time- or volume-cycled; there is no exhalation phase variable. In Figures 102.7 and 102.8, the breaths are time-triggered, volume-controlled and time- or volume-cycled and, time-triggered, pressure-controlled, and time-cycled, respectively. Some ventilator modes like intermittent mandatory ventilation (IMV) or synchronized IMV (SIMV) allow two different breath types. Mandated breaths might be time-triggered, volume-controlled and time-cycled; while in-between scheduled breaths, spontaneous breaths might be pressure-triggered, pressure-controlled and pressure-cycled.

VENTILATOR DESIGN

Modern ICU ventilators are expensive and seemingly complex; yet, while the electronics may be complicated, basic ventilator component configuration is simple and has changed very little over the past 20 years. In simplest form, a mechanical ventilator requires only a few essential components (Fig. 102.9).

Power Sources

Pneumatics

Ventilators must have power. Most patients require, at least, some oxygen; this makes the energy stored within compressed oxygen a reliable and convenient power source. Gas-powered ventilators are called *pneumatic*. The powering gas source can be oxygen or compressed air, as long as the gas source is free of contaminants, debris, and is dry. Hospital oxygen supplies virtually never pose contamination or water concerns; whether in bulk form or in cylinders, oxygen is certified clean and pure (99.99%). Compressed air sources are however, a completely different matter. Compressors aspirate air from the environment; if aspirated air is contaminated, so too will be the compressed air. There have been instances of hospitals locating compressor intakes too close to parking lots and, on occasion, compressing exhaust gases along with air. Also, environmental air contains water vapor, some of which condenses and becomes liquid during the compression process; any and all water must be removed or it can cause serious damage to ventilators and other pneumatic equipment. Finally, most compressors use rapidly moving pistons or rotors to compress the air; operating at such high speed requires lubrication. Compressed air, for human consumption, should never involve using an oil-lubricated device. Small oil particles are compressed along with the air and can cause serious lung injury, if inhaled.

Despite potential drawbacks associated with using compressed air sources, pneumatic ventilators offer several advantages, particularly when used for transport. For instance, a pneumatic ventilator is always ready to go; they never require time-consuming recharging as battery-powered units do. Moreover, pneumatic ventilators use no expensive batteries, power supplies, or electric cables that can fail or must be periodically replaced. Furthermore, batteries often contain

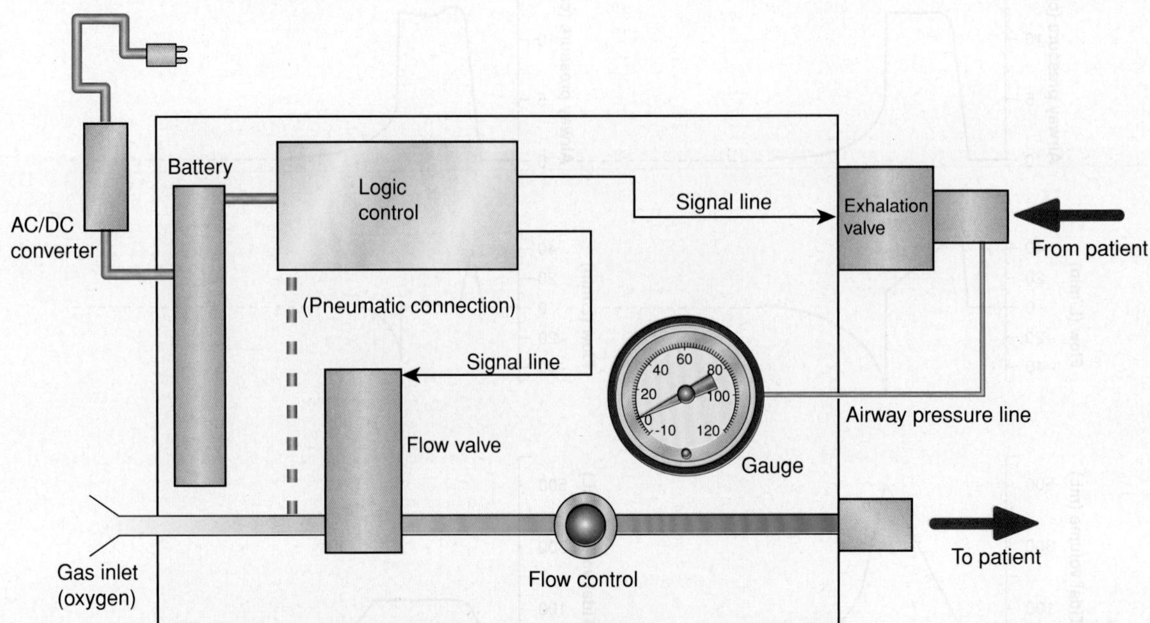

FIGURE 102.9 Schema of a "basic" ventilator. This schematic includes all of the major components necessary for ventilator operation. The logic component provides timing signals responsible for the inspiratory and expiratory phases. Ventilator logic must also synchronize the onset of each breath by the closing of the exhalation valve. Ventilator logic may be provided by fluidics, analog electronics, digital electronics (microprocessors), or pneumatics. All ventilators, regardless of simplicity, are either electrically powered with or without battery back-up, or pneumatically powered. None so far are powered by both.

extremely toxic components—lead, cadmium, lithium, and so forth—and must be properly disposed or recycled, often at hospital expense. Pneumatic ventilators are also exceptionally robust; many pneumatic components will operate through many millions of actuations without failure. They are also reasonably priced and easy to maintain.

Electric Power

Electricity is cheap, reliable, and, in most countries, virtually ubiquitous. As a result, electricity powers most ventilators. Electrically powered units utilize alternating current (AC), AC converted to direct current (DC), battery, or some combination (see Fig. 102.9). Unfortunately, ventilators are either pneumatically or electrically powered, never both. As a result, if power outages are likely, clinicians must consider their alternatives carefully; ventilators with battery back-up are great, but will only operate for, at best, a few hours. Few, if any of us have considered how ventilator-dependent patients would be ventilated in the event of an extended loss of electricity. This point is not simply a theoretical one, as just such a scenario occurred following hurricane Katrina (39).

Conventional Ventilator Logic

All ventilators require some sort of logic to coordinate the timing of inhalation (I) and exhalation (E), as well as actuating the flow/volume delivery mechanism and the exhalation valve (see Fig 102.9).

Traditionally, ventilator logic involved pneumatics, standard electronics, fluidics, or some combination of these. To initiate and maintain inhalation, logic signals simultaneously activate both the flow/volume delivery system and the exhalation valve. At the same time, ventilator logic is responsible for timing or controlling inhalation and, for monitoring breath delivery; the ventilator's logic must be prepared to cycle the breath "off" if the high P_{aw} limit is breached, or when cycling criteria is met.

Microprocessor-Controlled Logic

The first microprocessor-controlled ventilator was introduced in the early 1980s. Today, microprocessor-controlled logic dominates virtually every category of mechanical ventilation. Given that a microprocessor, or central processing unit (CPU), has virtually no influence on ventilator performance per se; it's not unreasonable to wonder why microprocessor ventilators are so popular. The answer is, in a nutshell, that they are far more flexible and vastly safer than any other type of ventilator. Some of the many advantages offered by today's CPU-controlled ventilators are listed in Table 102.2.

TABLE 102.2 Advantages of Microprocessor-Controlled Ventilators

General versatility
- Capable of providing virtually any desired mode of positive-pressure ventilation
- Ability to provide a wide variety of inspiratory flow waveforms
- Choice of cycling or trigger variable in many modes pressure ventilation or proportional assist ventilation (PAV)

Monitoring
- Real-time monitoring and alarms for a variety of ventilatory parameters
- Ability to measure and display lung-thorax compliance (C_{LT}), airway resistance (R_{aw}), plateau pressure, minute exhaled ventilation, auto-PEEP
- On-board computer memory saves, for later retrieval, ventilation data for trend analysis

Computer correction and safety
- Capable of automatically correcting for many internal variations that might affect prescribed tidal volume (V_T) or target pressure
- Able to automatically maintain the set inspiratory flow rate, waveform, and V_T, even when the patient's impedance (C_{LT}, R_{aw}) decreases or increases
- Measured and displayed tidal and minute volumes corrected to BTPS
- Measures compliance/compression of the specific breathing circuit and humidifier in use compensates for the "lost" volume on a breath-by-breath basis
- Monitors all critical computer and patient parameters declares an inoperative condition, terminates ventilation, opens the safety valve (to allow spontaneous breathing from the room), or begins a backup mode of ventilation any time a dangerous situation is detected
- Saves and stores, for later retrieval and analysis, any and all errors, including patient alarms or other important issues detected during operation

Display and communications capability
- Ability to process and display any and all monitored data, and important patient ventilation parameters
- Ability to communicate and interface with remote monitors
- Ability to communicate with separate microcomputers (personal computers) for monitoring and storage of data

Repairs and maintenance
- Provide troubleshooting programs or extensive testing programs that pinpoint problems, facilitate repairs, and minimize down-time
- Contain few moving parts maintenance may involve only routine filters changes
- Modular design and easily removable printed circuit boards facilitate repair

Relational Logic

An advantage offered only by a CPU is an ability to answer relational questions. A CPU can easily evaluate the "truth" of simple relational expressions such as: is $x < y$?, $x = y$?, or is $x > y$? A relational question can either be *true* or *false*. For instance, x might be the patient's P_{aw} and y the operator-selected high pressure limit. During each breath, the CPU could be instructed to evaluate, every few milliseconds, the relational expression is $x > y$? If the answer is *false*, then the ventilator breath continues; if the answer is *true*, then the breath would cycled "off" and the over-pressure alarms sounded and/or illuminated. Modern CPUs evaluate simple expressions with blinding speed. In fact, microprocessor-controlled ventilators evaluate dozens of relational expressions, in a specific sequence, continuously, until each mechanical breath is safely delivered.

Logical Expressions

Microprocessors can also evaluate logical expressions or operate on the results of a relational question; logical operations follow the rules of Boolean algebra. For example, NOT true is false and NOT false is true. The AND function operates on two relational questions and requires that they both be true for the result to be true. That is, true AND true is true, but true AND false is false. The OR function also operates on two relational questions but only requires one of the questions to be true for the result to be true; true OR false is true and false OR false is false.

As an example, a CPU might evaluate the following two questions: Is exhaled V_T less than inhaled V_T, divided by 2? AND is the operator setting for V_T unchanged? If answered true AND true, then the ventilator might be instructed to warn clinicians of low exhaled V_T; from there the patient's breathing circuit and ET cuff could then be quickly checked for leaks. With these simple building blocks, powerful algorithms can be devised that monitor all aspects of ventilator operations and make today's mechanical ventilators safer than ever before.

Computer Memory

A CPU, no matter how powerful or fast, cannot function without memory. How could a CPU answer the relational question: "Is x (P_{aw}) greater than y (airway pressure limit)," if it couldn't remember the value of x or y? Additionally, how would a CPU know when, or how often, to answer relational questions?

In our example, the value for x (P_{aw}) varies continuously as a function of time, while the value for y (airway pressure limit) may remain constant; on the other hand, y will most likely vary from one patient to the next. Somehow, the CPU must be able to update the values for x and y as often as they change. This requires, easily erasable memory, known as *random access memory* (RAM). There is a caveat, however: easily erased means volatile, and volatile means easily lost. For instance, valuable data might be lost the instant power is lost. As a result, ventilator CPUs cannot operate safely without battery backup to maintain critical data stored in RAM; without a patient's *exact* data safely stored, the ventilator could malfunction, even if power was lost for an instant. Data stored in RAM is bidirectional; this means the CPU can store (write) information into RAM and read it later. Memory is limited, so the CPU must use its memory over and over again. Suppose the area used for storing a patient's pressure limit (y) is already "occupied" and the operator changes the pressure limit; the CPU simply "writes over"—thereby erasing—the pre-existing pressure limit value.

Instructions for how to use data stored in RAM, and the sequence and timing of all functions carried out by the CPU, reside is a different type of memory known as *read only memory* (ROM). This form of memory is nonvolatile and not easily altered. It is this memory that queues the CPU as to how often and when to evaluate the relational and logical operations. In fact, the entire sequence, or code, responsible for every conceivable ventilator function is stored in ROM. The use of ROM comes with a caveat too: ROM is nonvolatile; but it is not impervious. Even the slightest change in a critical instruction could harm a patient. As a result, ventilator CPUs *must* have powerful "watchdog" systems that constantly evaluate every aspect of their behavior. Watchdogs always err on the side of safety—should they detect anything out of the ordinary they immediately terminate CPU operation, protect the patient, and alert the operator of the malfunction, often referred to as a *vent-inop*. Once a "bizarre" or unusual behavior has been detected, manufacturers insure that CPU integrity be verified *before* the ventilator will function again. Unfortunately, too often, vent-inop conditions require technical assistance from a biomedical engineer or factory representative. To obviate such problems, engineers have tried two, or even three, CPUs, which are programmed to constantly evaluate each other. This strategy eliminates the need for watchdogs; but, in the case of only two CPUs, does not eliminate the problem: when one CPU detects a "problem," who decides which CPU is still functioning properly? With a three CPU design, there is always a "referee"; the aberrant CPU, once detected can be shut off leaving two CPUs to continue safely operating the ventilator until it can be safely replaced.

Ventilator Control Systems

Open-Loop Control

Open-loop ventilator designs (Fig. 102.10) are economical and straightforward, but functionally limited. Ventilators employing open-loops offer VCV or PCV; they seldom provide both. Open-loop systems are also not fault-tolerant. For instance, suppose over time and with prolonged usage, a ventilator's flow valve gradually drifts out of calibration. Now, the signal designed to produce 0.75 L/s, yields only 0.60 L/s and V_T is preset to 0.75 L. This patient will receive a V_T no greater than 0.6 L, and the ventilator, even if CPU controlled, would have no way of detecting this problem.

Closed-Loop Control

Closed-loop or feedback designs (Fig 102.11) are far more complex and expensive than open-loop designs. In return, they deliver exceptional accuracy and automatically correct for many common failures and variances. Using the same preset V_T of 0.75 L and V_I of 0.75 L/s, a closed-loop ventilator delivers the requested V_T even if the flow-valve is no longer calibrated—thereby protecting the patient. Given the example above, ventilator logic opens the flow valve, expecting 0.75 L/s; yet, a flow sensor, located just downstream from the flow valve, measures the actual flow (0.6 L/s) and sends an electric signal, proportional to measured flow, to the comparator (see Fig. 102.11). The comparator functions to analyze (electrically) the difference between the measured flow and actuating signals; if the signals are identical nothing happens, if the signals vary, the comparator provides an output signal, proportional in magnitude to the difference. The comparator's output adds to, or removes from, the existing signal actuating the valve–in this case, the combined signals open the valve to produce a higher flow. Comparators function nearly instantaneously; so, the flow valve's output can be corrected repeatedly, as often as the valve's response time and the programmed T_I allow. A response time of 10 ms, allows a 100 corrections in a T_I of one second, if necessary.

Closed-loop feedback also corrects the ventilator outputs when affected by changing pulmonary impedance, different breathing circuits, and high resistance humidifiers. Closed-loop designs that incorporate flow and pressure sensors do not require separate valves for VCV and PCV. In this instance, a flow valve is either opened and a prescribed V_T delivered, or the valve is opened to provide an initial high flow and a closed-loop pressure algorithm maintains any desired target pressure by manipulating the valve's output flow based upon the target pressure.

Closed-loop designs require accurate, onboard flow and pressure sensors as well as sophisticated control algorithms, these are relatively costly and can be damaged by rough handling. For these reasons, transport ventilators often incorporate open-loop designs.

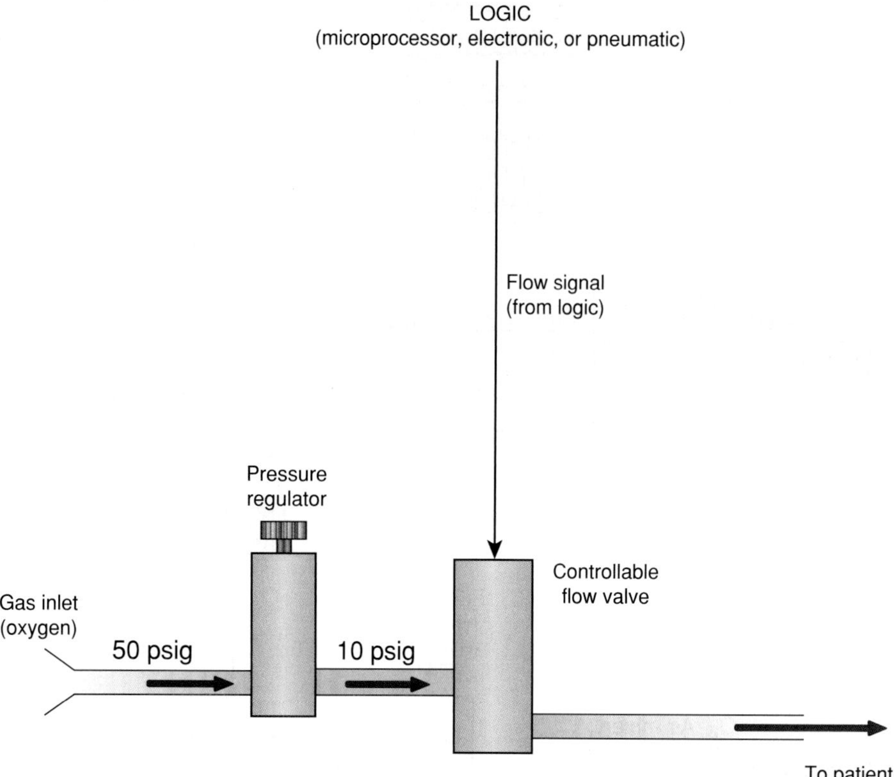

FIGURE 102.10 Schema of open-loop ventilator control. Virtually all positive-pressure ventilators control flow (shown) or pressure during each mechanical breath. The simplest control system involves a properly synchronized signal, from the logic element, that produces the output (flow); the ventilator does not verify accuracy so the operator must do so.

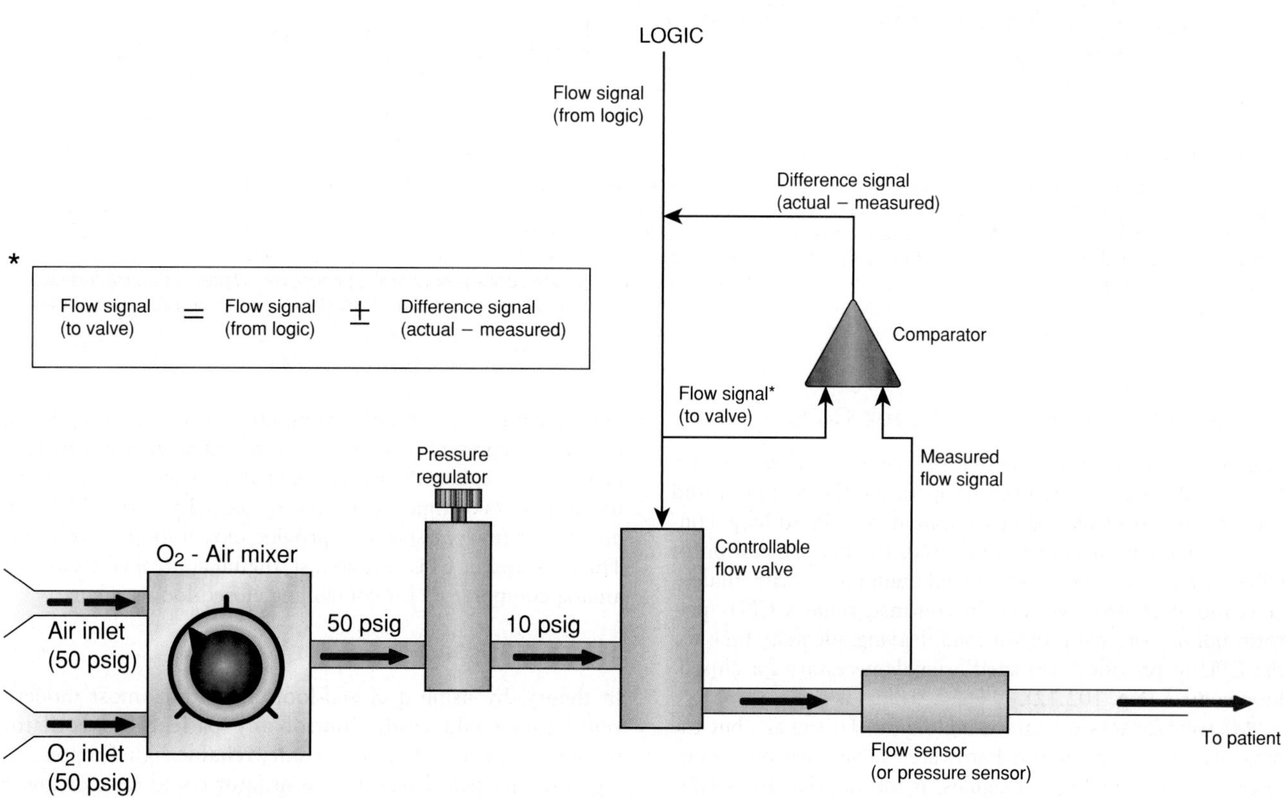

FIGURE 102.11 Schema of closed-loop ventilator control. Ventilator reliability and accuracy is vastly improved by measuring the actual output (flow), comparing the measured to desired, and correcting the actuating signal by the difference. At the onset of each breath, a signal from the ventilator's logic actuates (opens) the output valve. The resultant output (flow) is measured immediately by a flow sensor positioned downstream. The flow sensor converts measured gas flow into an analog electric signal, which is routed to one side of an electronic comparator. The actuating signal (actual) from the logic element is fed into the other side of the comparator, where it is compared to the measured signal. If the two signals differ, the comparator adds (or subtracts) an amount of electricity, proportional to the signal difference, to (or from) the actuating signal. The entire loop requires only about 10 milliseconds to complete; that means the actual signal could theoretically be "corrected" as many as 100 times in a typical mechanical breath lasting just 1 second. Normally however, it only requires a few iterations before the measured and desired signals are identical.

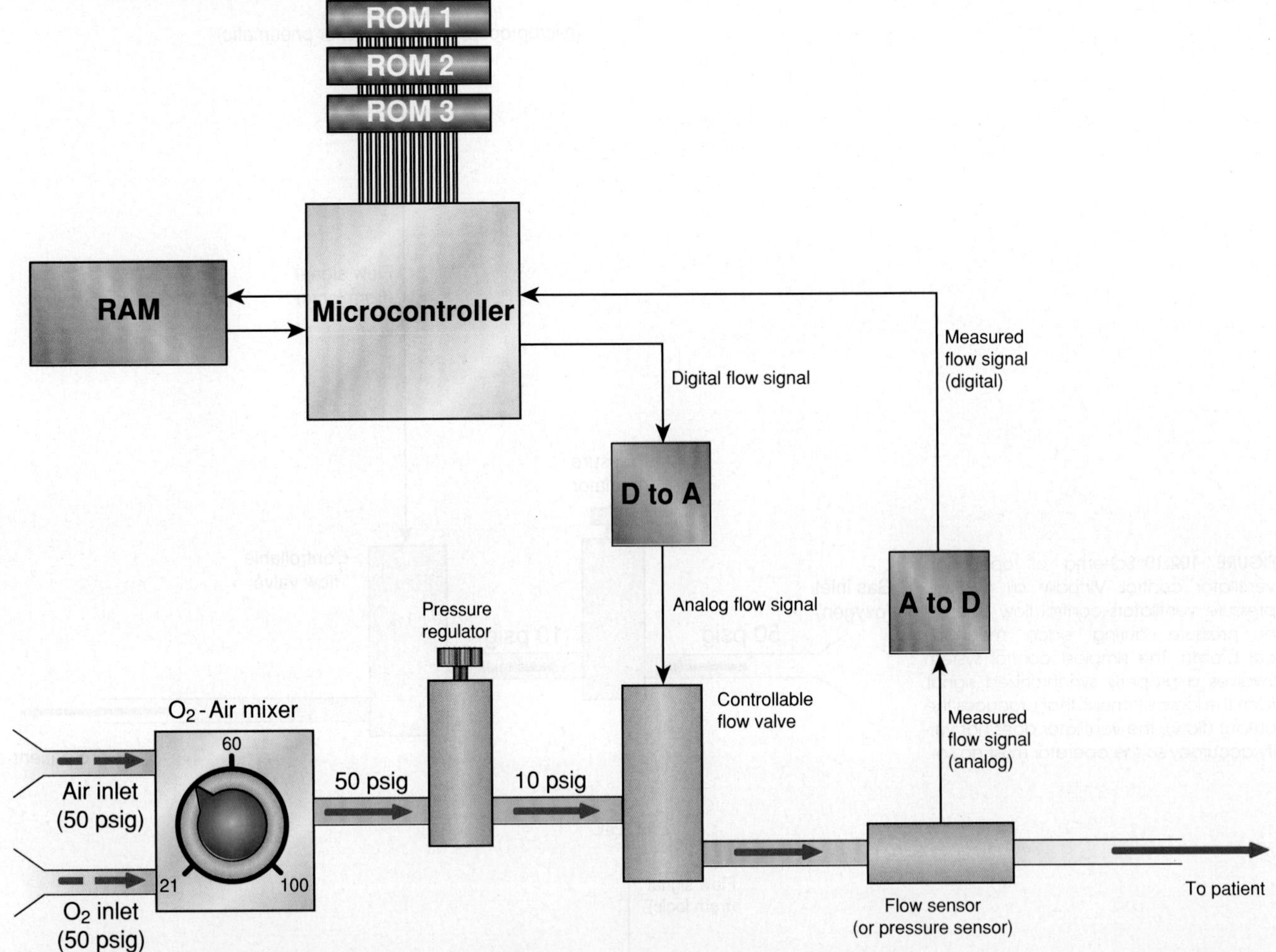

FIGURE 102.12 Schema of a microprocessor-controlled, closed-loop control system. First-generation microprocessor-controlled ventilators combined digital (D) signals converted to analog (A), with an analog closed-loop system. This approach was necessary because digital control of closed-loop feedback added several time-consuming steps: corrected signals had to be converted D to A before they could operate ventilator valves; the measured signal had to be converted A to D before the microprocessor could compare it to desired and determine an appropriate correction. Unfortunately, microprocessors available at the time were simply not fast enough to adequately monitor lung inflation *and* provide corrected closed-loop signals. Today's microprocessors easily perform billions of operation/second, and most second- or third-generation microprocessor-controlled ventilators provide closed-loop control using only digital signal processing.

Microprocessors and Closed-Loop Control

The first CPU-powered ventilators were too slow to perform all of the tasks involved in operating the ventilator and provide the corrected signals required for closed-loop control. To maintain accuracy and speed, the first generation of CPU-powered ventilators combined digital logic with analog, closed-loop control systems. In contrast, today's CPUs perform billions of operations/second, leaving adequate time for the CPU to provide "corrected" signals necessary for closed-loop control (Fig. 102.12).

Microprocessors operate using digital (D) signals, but the majority of our real-world hardware (valves, sensors, transducers) require analog (A) signals. It follows that for a CPU to actuate a valve, a digital signal, from the CPU, must first be converted to analog; this takes place in a D to A signal processing chip (see Fig. 102.12). Analog information, such as a measured flow signals, must be similarly converted, A to D, before the CPU can use them. During closed-loop control, once a measured signal is converted, A to D, and reaches the CPU, it is compared to the current actuating signal; based upon the difference the CPU computes a new actuating signal; its digital representation is sent to the D to A; from there it proceeds to replace the existing signal. As each of these transformations take time, it is easy to see why early CPUs did not have sufficient speed to provide closed-loop corrections. The most recent CPUs are so fast, digital control rivals that of analog comparators for controlling closed-loop systems.

Future of Closed-Loop Control

In theory, by using a closed-loop algorithm, most modern ventilators could easily control any patient or ventilator parameter, provided there is a safe, reliable signal representing that parameter. That is, a ventilator could raise or lower the breathing rate, or V_T, in order to maintain a target CO_2 level; or, the ventilator might raise or lower the fractional inspired oxygen (F_iO_2), or CPAP level, to achieve a specified, target oxygen level. These possibilities still remain on the horizon, as the FDA ponders whether or not closed-loop control of such critical patient parameters will ultimately be as safe as the current generation of ventilators. Although some argue that the FDA is being overly cautious, it's easy to imagine the potential for harm should a future ventilator fail to properly manage a life-sustaining parameter such as CO_2 or O_2. Nevertheless, the topic of whether future ventilators should be managed by computers or by experienced clinicians has become very popular at many of today's respiratory therapy meetings. There are strong emotions and arguments from both sides: yet, it seems almost inevitable that computers will ultimately be allowed to control most or all of a patient's vital parameters. Primarily, this is because educating, training, and providing the necessary experience to provide for sufficient numbers of respiratory therapists is an expensive and daunting task.

CONVENTIONAL MECHANICAL VENTILATORY TECHNIQUES

Compliance and Resistance—The End-Inspiratory Plateau

Operational Principles

The terms *postinflation hold*, *end-inspiratory pause*, and *end-inspiratory plateau* (EIP) all refer to the same ventilator routine; instead of allowing the patient to exhale the instant V_T delivery is complete, the ventilator stops gas flow but does not allow the patient to exhale until a pre-specified period time, the EIP, elapses (Fig. 102.13). The EIP is considered part of T_I because the V_T volume remains in the lungs and the patient does not exhale until the EIP is complete; ventilators often allow EIP to persist as long as 2 seconds. Although this may not seem excessive, when combined with the existing T_I, EIPs are often long enough to adversely impact hemodynamics and are poorly tolerated by spontaneously breathing patients.

Clinical Applications

An EIP has been advocated as a method to improve the distribution of inhaled gases, thereby decreasing V_D/V_T and $PaCO_2$ (40). Theoretically, this makes sense; if inhalation was long enough, gas redistribution into slow-filling spaces would improve overall distribution (41). Gas redistribution during EIP, is thought to result secondary to collateral ventilation and Pendelluft flow.

Collateral ventilation occurs when gas enters alveoli from adjacent alveoli through channels in the alveolar walls (Pores of Kohn) or through cross-communications between bronchioles (Lambert canals). *Pendelluft flow* occurs when, during EIP, volume from fast-filling spaces redistributes into slow-filling

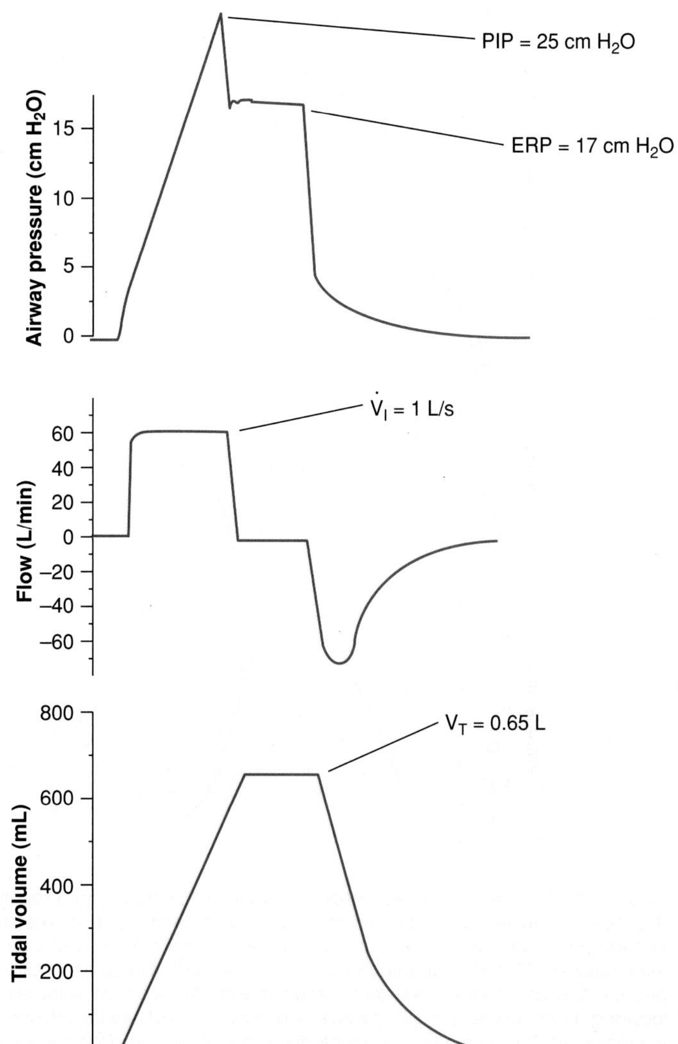

FIGURE 102.13 Compliance and resistance determination in the ventilator patient. Respiratory system compliance (C_{RS}) and airway resistance (R_{aw}) determination, by end-inspiratory plateau (EIP), requires volume-controlled mode, square flow pattern, inspiratory flow rate (V_I) of exactly 1 Liter (L)/second (s) (or, 60 L/min), and an EIP of 0.25 second or more. In this example, the peak inflation pressure (PIP) reaches 25 cm H_2O, the instant flow ceases. After the preset tidal volume (V_T) is delivered, the EIP begins, that is, gas flow from the ventilator ceases and the patient is not permitted to exhale. During the EIP, pressure equilibrates between the lungs and breathing circuit and elastic recoil pressure (ERP) of the lungs can be measured at the airway opening. The greater the difference between a patient's PIP and ERP, the greater the R_{aw}. Compliance is computed by dividing V_T (0.65 L) by measured ERP minus the baseline pressure (0 cm H_2O), and is given in units of L/cm H_2O or mL/cm H_2O. Resistance is computed as PIP minus ERP divided by V_I (must be 1 L/s) and is stated in units of cm H_2O/L/s. In this example, C_{RS} is 0.038 L/cm H_2O and R_{aw} is 8 cm H_2O/L/s.

spaces. Such gas flow is caused by regional pressure gradients that arise as a consequence of maldistribution secondary to positive pressure inflation.

The EIP is seldom used to improve distribution, but rather to determine C_{RS} and R_{aw}. During the plateau time, as gas flow ceases, the flow resistive component of PIP disappears. The remaining pressure, the plateau pressure, also reflects the static elastic recoil pressure (ERP) of the lungs. Exhaled V_T, PIP, and ERP are used in determining the patient's C_{RS} and R_{aw} (Table 102.3). These measurements are often performed routinely to assess the patient's progress or gauge the response to bronchodilators.

Inspiratory Flow Waveforms

Before the advent of microprocessor-powered ventilators, different ventilator brands delivered gas flow using a wide variety of methodologies: pistons, injectors, bellows, solenoids, and so forth. Each flow generating technique produced a different inspiratory flow patterns: square or constant (Fig. 102.14A), sinusoidal, decelerating (Fig. 102.14B), or accelerating. Clinicians immediately began to wonder which waveform was best, or, could matching specific waveforms with specific pulmonary conditions make a difference? To this day, these questions

TABLE 102.3 Measurement of Compliance and Airway Resistance

Definition: End-inspiratory pause (EIP) may be used to differentiate dynamic (C_{RS}) (L/cm H_2O) from static lung-thorax compliance (C_{RS}) (L/cm H_2O) and to determine airway resistance (R_{aw}) (cm H_2O/L/s).

1. Dynamic $C_{RS} = V_T$/(PIP – baseline airway pressure)
   Where: V_T = exhaled tidal volume (L);
   PIP = peak inflation pressure (cm H_2O);
   Baseline airway pressure = atmospheric pressure, continuous positive airway pressure (CPAP) (cm H_2O), or positive end-expiratory pressure (PEEP) (cm H_2O).
   e.g., C_{RS} = 0.65 L/(25 cm H_2O–0 cm H_2O) = 0.026 L/cm H_2O
2. Static $C_{RS} = V_T$/(ERP–baseline airway pressure)
   Where: ERP = static elastic recoil pressure of the respiratory system (cm H_2O);
   e.g., C_{RS} = 0.65 L/(17 cm H_2O–0 cm H_2O) = 0.038 L/cm H_2O
3. R_{aw} = (PIP–ERP) × V_I
   Where: V_I = inspiratory flow rate[a] (L/s)
   e.g., R_{aw} = (25 cm H_2O–17 cm H_2O) × 1 L/s = 8 cm H_2O/L/s

[a]The selected inspiratory flow pattern must be constant (square).

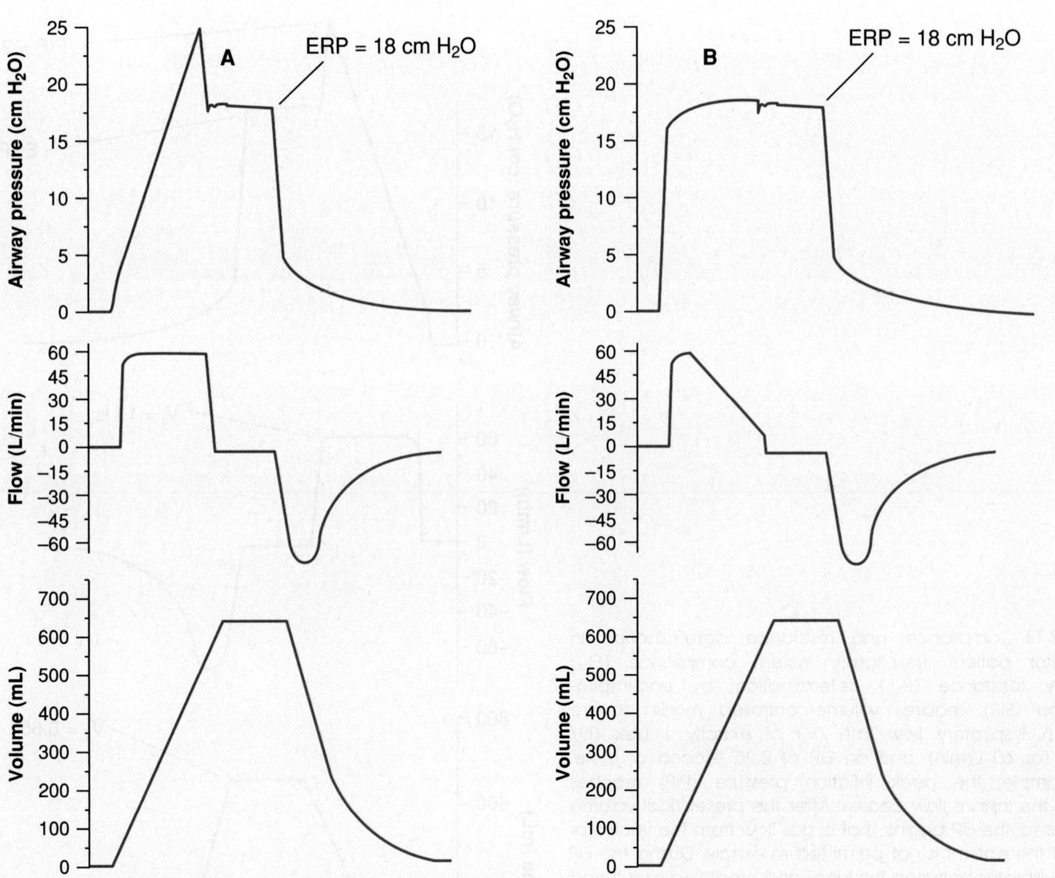

FIGURE 102.14 Differences in peak inflation pressure (PIP) when using a square or decelerating inspiratory flow (V_I) waveform. **A:** An airway pressure (P_{aw}), flow, and volume curve for a typical volume-controlled breath delivered using a square V_I waveform. Following breath delivery, an end-inspiratory plateau (EIP) terminates gas flow and allows pressure to equilibrate between the lungs and airway opening; at equilibration, P_{aw} reflects the elastic recoil pressure (ERP) of the respiratory system—that is, of the lungs and thorax combined. Note the PIP of this breath is nearly 25 cm H_2O. **B:** An airway pressure, flow, and volume curve for the same breath, delivered to the same patient, except using a decelerating V_I waveform in this instance. Again, following breath delivery, an EIP allows determination of ERP. Note the PIP of this breath is 8 cm H_2O lower than for the square waveform; nevertheless, the measured ERP (18 cm H_2O), is exactly the same as that using the square flow pattern; this occurs because a decelerating flow pattern reduces gas flow, to near zero (as during an EIP), *before* the breath cycles "off" and the EIP begins.

remain essentially unresolved. Some tried various waveforms and found little or no difference in the distribution of ventilation (42). Other studies, modeling multiple lung compartments with different R_{aw}, showed improved distribution with the decelerating waveform compared to others (43,44). Clinical reports confirmed the utility of a decelerating pattern (45–47). In one investigation, V_T, T_I, I:E ratio, and ventilator rate were held constant. Compared to the constant flow pattern, the decelerating waveform significantly reduced patient PIP, $PaCO_2$, V_D/V_T ratio, and alveolar-to-arterial oxygen pressure gradient $P_{(A\text{-}a)}O_2$ (46). However, mean P_{aw} was significantly greater, predisposing to adverse hemodynamic effects.

In addition to the potential to improve distribution, decelerating waveforms significantly reduce PIP, especially when contrasted to square (see Fig. 102.14) or accelerating patterns. Some clinicians opt for a decelerating pattern believing the lower PIPs may help protect their patients from ventilator-induced lung injury (VILI). This logic is flawed; the pulmonary edema and lung injury, often seen during mechanical ventilation, are now believed the consequence of excessive volume (volutrauma), rather than excessive pressure (barotrauma) (48,49). Furthermore, the main determinant of volutrauma appears to be end-inspiratory lung volume (the overall lung distension), rather than the FRC (which depends upon PEEP) (19,37). Based on this information, reducing PIP by waveform selection offers no advantage; patients supported using VCV receive the same V_T, and therefore overall lung expansion, regardless of waveform.

Inspiratory flow waveforms impact yet another aspect of mechanical ventilation, patient-ventilator synchrony. During any form of patient-triggered mechanical ventilation, the spontaneous inspiratory effort may extend well into mechanical inflation. If at any point spontaneous flow-demand exceeds the preset V_I, flow starvation results. Flow starvation distorts pressure patterns and exaggerates WOB. Decelerating flow patterns often provide initial V_I sufficient to meet patient demand; however, as the breath proceeds and V_I decelerates patient demand may suddenly exceed the available flow and dyssynchrony and flow starvation follow. Management of flow starvation of this nature can, on occasion, be as simple as switching from a decelerating to a constant waveform using a V_I set to a value equal to, or greater than, the peak flow used with the decelerating waveform (Fig. 102.15).

Controlled Ventilation

Operational Principles

Mechanical ventilation is indicated when spontaneous ventilation is inadequate or absent. Physiologically, this means the

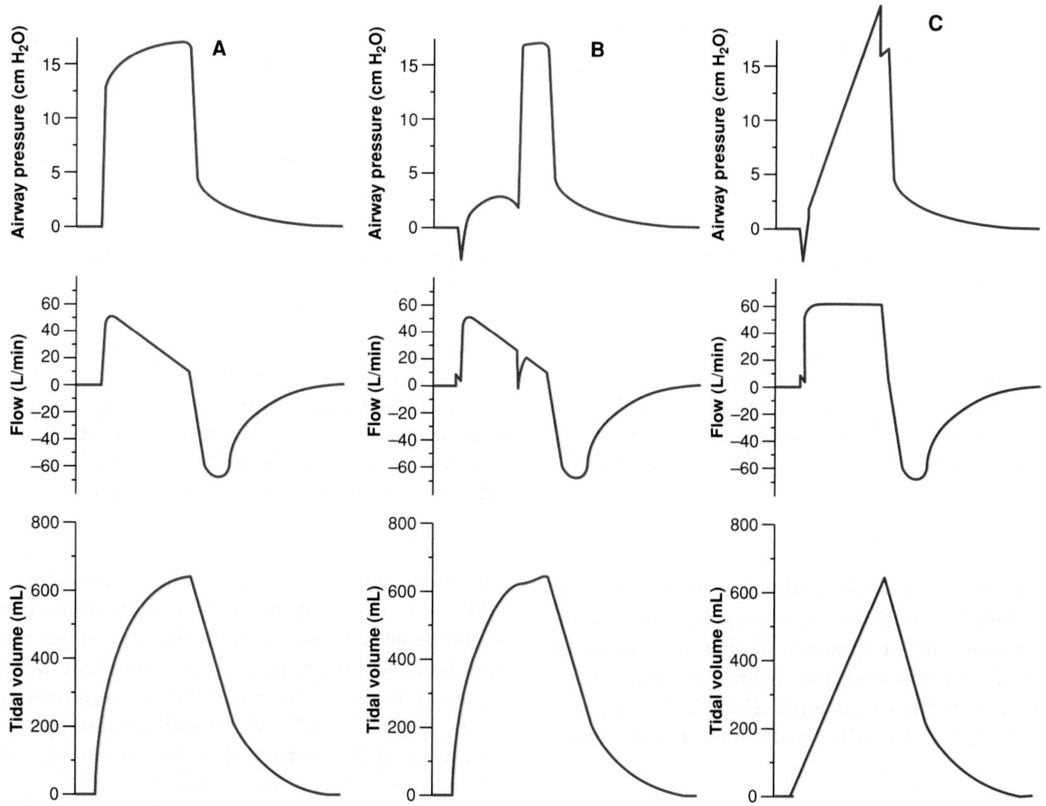

FIGURE 102.15 Improving patient-ventilator synchrony using a square instead of decelerating flow waveform, during volume-controlled ventilation (VCV). **A:** An airway pressure (P_{aw}), flow, and tidal volume (V_T) curve for a heavily sedated or very relaxed patient, receiving VCV. **B:** An airway pressure, flow, and V_T curve for the same patient, except the patient is awake, alert, and "fighting the ventilator"; that is, attempting to breathe spontaneously during a machine-delivered breath. Note that both the P_{aw} pressure pattern and V_I pattern are distorted by the patient's effort. Distortions are often exacerbated by the selected flow pattern, particularly the decelerating pattern, which progressively reduces V_I, while patient flow demands may remain high. In situations where the patient flow demand exceeds V_I from the ventilator, a tremendous additional workload is imposed upon the patient; this predisposes to fatigue and makes managing the patient difficult. **C:** An airway pressure, flow, and V_T curve for the same patient, making the same effort to breathe spontaneously, except the selected V_I pattern is switched from decelerating to square. Note that peak V_I is nearly identical in each case; yet, by maintaining a high flow longer, a square flow pattern better meets the patient flow demand.

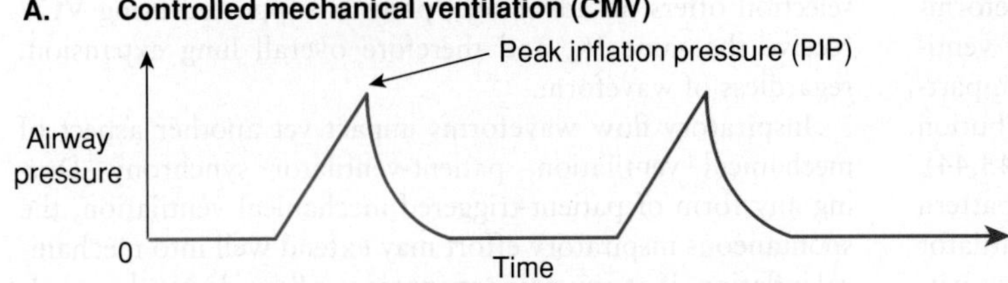

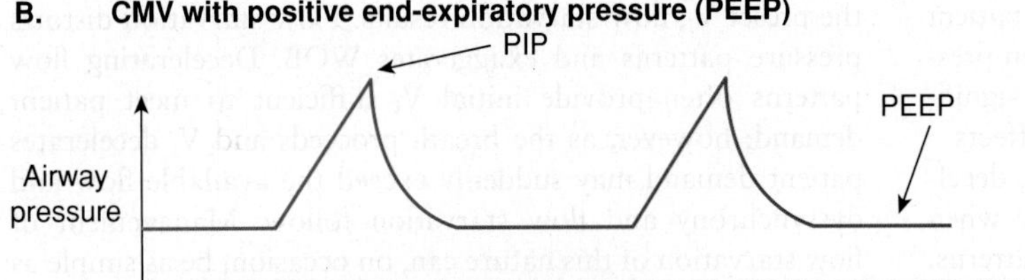

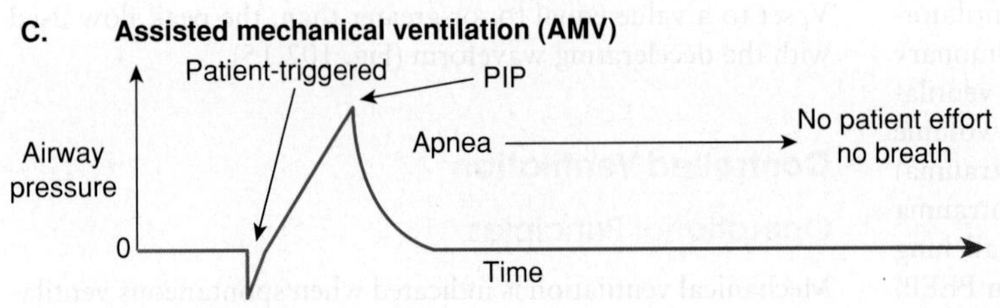

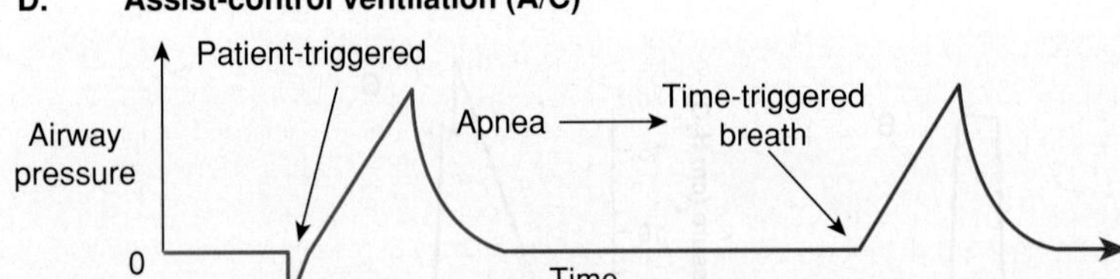

FIGURE 102.16 Conventional mechanical ventilatory airway pressure patterns. A: Controlled mechanical ventilation (CMV). Mechanical breath rate, tidal volume (V_T), and inspiratory flow rate (V_I) and pattern are all selected and set by the operator and cannot be altered appreciably by patient efforts to breathe. B: CMV with positive end-expiratory pressure (PEEP). Exhalation stops at a predetermined pressure above ambient (PEEP level). If the PEEP is adequate, it mechanically stabilizes and prevents alveolar collapse secondary to ARDS. C: *Assisted mechanical ventilation (AMV).* Tidal volume and V_I are prescribed and set by the operator and cannot be altered, regardless of patient effort; the patient is, however, completely responsible determining breathing rate, by physically triggering the ventilator. D: *Assist-control ventilation (A/C).* This mode combines AMV with a CMV back-up. This is accomplished using two trigger variables, for instance pressure and time, and initiating a breath to whichever occurs first. The operator sets V_T, V_I and pattern, CMV rate, and trigger sensitivity. After each breath, regardless of which variable triggered the breath, the CMV rate timing clock is restarted. Following this, if a spontaneous effort triggers a breath, before the CMV timer lapses, the breath is pressure-triggered and the CMV clock restarted. If the patient fails to breathe or cannot spontaneously trigger, the CMV clock will run down and the next breath will be time-triggered. Using the A/C strategy, patients may breathe as rapidly as they desire, but never at rate lower than CMV mechanical rate setting.

patient is incapable of maintaining acceptable $PaCO_2$ and arterial pH levels. CMV delivers an operator-selected breathing rate, V_T, peak V_I, and flow pattern; CMV operates completely independent of patient efforts to breathe (Fig. 102.16A). When patients attempt to breathe during CMV, the result can be violent patient-ventilator dyssynchrony. Consequently, patients supported by CMV often require hyperventilation—to blunt the normal stimulus to breathe—heavy sedation, or even pharmacologic paralysis.

Clinical Applications

Indications for CMV and CMV with PEEP (Fig. 102.16B) include apnea, ARDS, central nervous system depression, drug overdose, or neuromuscular dysfunction. For this subset of patients, an accidental disconnection from the ventilator, or a ventilator failure, is life-threatening. Thus, CMV requires vigilant monitoring and carefully set disconnect and failure-to-cycle alarms.

Patient-Triggered Ventilation

Operational Principles

There are two basic forms of patient-triggered breaths: mechanical and spontaneous. Patient-triggered mechanical breaths (Fig. 102.16C) are nearly identical to CMV breaths in that the V_T, peak V_I, and flow pattern are all operator-selected; the only difference is assisted mechanical ventilation (AMV) requires the patient trigger each and every breath. It follows that when supported by AMV, a patient must not experience an acute apneic episode; if they do, all ventilation ceases. Concern for this possibility, explains why so few physicians opted to use AMV, before ventilators came equipped with back-up ventilator modes. For AMV, a back-up mode might allow the operator to select desired CMV settings that the ventilator defaults to and uses in the event of apnea.

Clinical Applications

Patient-triggered ventilation is considered a vital link between CMV and extubation. In theory, it allows the patient to breathe spontaneously, in preparation for removal of the ventilator. Spontaneous breathing is never consistent however, meaning AMV is extraordinarily difficult to optimize to a patient's efforts. If the preset V_I, V_T, or both are too high, patient WOB falls to essentially zero; if they are insufficient, or the patient becomes dyssynchronous WOB skyrockets.

CMV Backup

The use of dual trigger variables allowed clinicians to safely use AMV well before the incorporation of back-up modes. Patient-triggered support, with a time-triggered CMV backup was coined *assist/controlled ventilation* (A/C) (Fig. 102.16D). When using A/C, the operator sets a minimum acceptable breathing rate, using the CMV rate control, and adjusts trigger sensitivity (usually pressure). As with AMV, the patient triggers breaths, as often as desired, by breaching the trigger threshold. If the patient stops breathing however, or the spontaneous breathing rate drops below the preset minimum, time-triggered CMV intercedes until a clinician investigates, or adequate breathing activity resumes.

Potential Problems

AMV and CMV, used alone or in conjunction, predispose to hyperventilation, ventilator-induced V_A/Q abnormalities, and excessive WOB. These untoward effects are related to anxiety driven ventilator-patient dyssynchrony, and maldistribution of ventilation, respectively. A disproportionate amount of the V_T is delivered anteriorly to nondependent lung regions with decreased perfusion when patients are in the supine position (50). Conversely, spontaneous breathing tends to promote better V_A/Q distribution. Some studies have demonstrated that V_D increases during CMV and AMV, with or without PEEP (51,52). Downs and Mitchell (51) reported increases in V_D were related to the rate of mechanical breathing, regardless of the ventilatory pattern, mode, and whether or not PEEP was used.

As mentioned, ventilator-patient dyssynchrony is very common during CMV, AMV, and A/C modes of ventilation. These modes all require preset V_T, V_I, and flow waveforms while patient breathing patterns frequently vary. When patient flow demand exceeds that provided by the ventilator, the WOB imposed on the patient may become excessive (22). Recent trends requiring the use of smaller mechanical tidal volumes has exacerbated the issue (53). Patients allowed to breathe spontaneously, while receiving low V_T, lung-protective ventilation, will likely suffer from both flow and volume starvation (Fig. 102.17); the additional WOB can be enormous. Clinicians facing this situation are left with few palatable options; increasing V_T and V_I predispose to ventilator-induced lung injury; yet, continued sedation or paralysis will undoubtedly complicate or prolong the weaning process.

Intermittent Mandatory Ventilation

Operational Principles

With spontaneous breathing rates often exceeding 100 bpm, infants with hyaline membrane disease confounded even the best early efforts at patient-ventilator synchronization. The simple concept of providing a continuous flow, from which these babies could breathe spontaneously between mandated mechanical breaths (54–56), resulted in a new ventilatory mode referred to as IMV. After proving its utility on neonates, IMV was later advocated for adults, especially those difficult to wean from mechanical ventilation (57). Neonatal IMV systems provided a continuous flow of gas, throughout the respiratory cycle; tidal ventilation was accomplished by simply closing the exhalation valve and diverting flow into the lungs (54,55).

When applying IMV, the operator pre-selects the desired ventilator rate, V_T, V_I, and flow pattern; in this aspect, it does

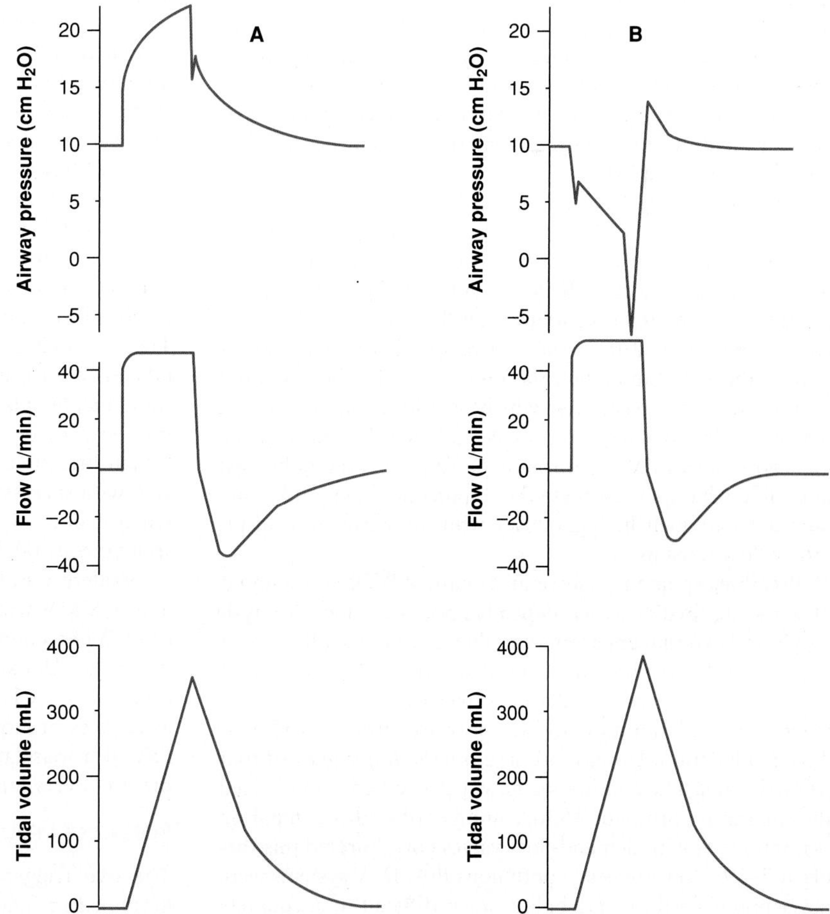

FIGURE 102.17 Flow and volume starvation during low tidal volume (V_T) ventilation. **A**: An airway pressure (P_{aw}), flow, and tidal volume (V_T) curve for a heavily sedated or very relaxed patient receiving, lung-protective, low V_T ventilation. **B**: An airway pressure, flow, and V_T curve for the same patient who is now, awake, alert, and "fighting the ventilator." Note that because both flow and V_T are insufficient, P_{aw} remains below baseline pressure throughout the entire inspiratory phase of the mechanical breath; distortions of this magnitude are frequently encountered if patients are allowed to breathe spontaneously when using lung-protective, low V_T ventilation.

not differ from CMV. With IMV however, the patient breathes spontaneously, as often as desired, between sequential positive pressure breaths. In theory, a designed and adjusted IMV system provides an unrestricted gas flow equal to, or greater than, the patient's peak, spontaneous V_I demand; these conditions minimize WOB. Early IMV systems were "homemade" (58,59), leading some to opine that reported failures resulted due to poor system design, not due to IMV per se (60).

Clinical Applications

Most clinicians select an IMV mandated breathing rate sufficient to compliment the patient's own spontaneous breathing and still maintain an acceptable alveolar ventilation, meaning P_aCO_2, and pH. Mandated breathing rates of 4 to 6 were popular because they provided an adequate V_A, in the event of apnea. When patients with pre-existing COPD were managed using IMV and compared to others managed using patient-triggered ventilation, IMV offered better control of P_aCO_2 and pH (61,62). When IMV is combined with CPAP, the cardiopulmonary effects are improved when compared to CMV or A/C modes of ventilation; as a result, IMV makes it possible to maintain higher mean expiratory positive pressures with fewer deleterious effects on venous return and cardiac output (63,64).

Potential Problems

IMV and CMV share many similarities, such as preset V_T, V_I, and flow waveform. Furthermore, with both modes, all mandated breaths are time-triggered, unresponsive to any patient effort. During IMV however, the patient may breathe spontaneously, as desired. It follows that, occasionally, a time-triggered breath might be delivered at or near end-inhalation for a spontaneous breath, a phenomenon referred to as breath-stacking; if the stacked volumes were large enough, they would predispose to elevated PIP and mean P_{aw}, leading to subsequent cardiovascular embarrassment; without any compelling evidence validating this hypothesis, many clinician nevertheless completely avoided IMV.

The concept of providing an unimpeded, continuous gas flow equal to, or exceeding, the patient's peak spontaneous V_I demand, introduced an unexpected consequence into developing safe and effective IMV systems: finding a humidifier capable handling the potentially high flow rates. Poulton and Downs (65) studied the issue and reported that with exception of the Bird humidifier, the others tested either imposed significant flow resistance—which would certainly impact patient WOB—or failed to provide sufficient humidity at the high flow rates IMV often required. Today's commonly used humidifiers have solved these developmental issues and easily humidify extremely high gas flows, while imparting little inspiratory flow resistance.

Breathing spontaneously requires patient WOB; the amount of work required however, depends upon a number of physiologic and external apparatus variables such as C_{RS}, R_{aw}, effort required to trigger breaths (if needed), available flow to that demanded, ETT size, exhalation valve performance, and the magnitude and duration of the pressure drop experienced during inhalation. Downs (60) and others (66) suggested that properly adjusted continuous-flow IMV systems minimized the apparatus portion of WOB; a number of studies comparing continuous-flow to demand-flow valves corroborated this theory (67–69). Nevertheless, continuous-flow IMV systems were never popular—they were bulky, noisy, difficult to adequately humidify, required frequent readjustment, and wasted massive amounts of gas. Clinicians therefore prevailed upon manufacturers to refine and improve their demand valves or demand flow systems. Gradually, demand-flow system performance improved; by 1985, Katz et al. (70) reported comparing seven demand-flow CPAP systems against a continuous-flow system (at 60 L/min) and reported some demand-flow systems performed as well or better than the continuous-flow system.

Synchronized Intermittent Mandatory Ventilation

Operational Principles

Clinical concerns about potential for breath-stacking stimulated the development of SIMV, which allows patient-triggered mandated breaths. That is, like the A/C mode of ventilation, SIMV employed two trigger variables, usually pressure and time; if the patient failed to trigger, an IMV breath was time triggered when the rate clock reached zero. Operators established SIMV by setting patient rate, V_T, V_I, flow waveform, and trigger sensitivity. Otherwise, like IMV, the patient was free to breathe spontaneously as desired.

Clinical Applications

Proponents believed SIMV would eliminate breath-stacking, promote patient-ventilator synchrony, and minimize cardiovascular effects. These benefits were not easily substantiated. Shapiro et al. (71) reported mean intrapleural pressure was substantially lower with SIMV than IMV in normal volunteers. Hasten et al. (72) compared SIMV and IMV in 25 critically ill patients, finding that, although PIP was higher, blood pressure, cardiac output, stroke index, central venous pressure, and pulmonary artery pressure did not differ significantly. In a similar study, Heenan et al. (73) studied anesthetized, near-drowned dogs ventilated with IMV or SIMV. Again, no differences were noted with respect to cardiac output, stroke volume, intrapleural pressure, and intrapulmonary shunt. Mean airway pressure and PIP were significantly elevated with IMV, and some breath-stacking occurred, but the authors noted no adverse effects from these differences. Based on these data, SIMV seems to offer little clinical advantage compared to IMV with CPAP. There is a logical explanation for these findings, however: spontaneously breathing, critically ill patients seldom inspire large spontaneous tidal volumes from CPAP systems. In fact, a high rate, low V_T breathing pattern is extremely common; indeed, a high breathing frequency (f) to V_T or f/V_T ratios correlates well with successful extubation (74). So, IMV breath-stacking, when it does occur, is unlikely to result in dangerously high spontaneous tidal volumes, PIP, or cardiovascular interference.

Modern ventilators all incorporate SIMV and, in the United States, SIMV with PSV is now the preferred ventilatory mode (75). When combined with PSV, synchronization is an absolute must. Unlike assisted or unassisted spontaneous breaths taken from a CPAP system, PSV breaths are frequently large—as large as or larger than the mandated V_T; during SIMV with PSV, if a mandatory breath stacks on a relatively large PSV breath, a very large and dangerous V_T *would* result.

Potential Problems

The two trigger variables used with SIMV cannot be programmed to function as flawlessly as during A/C ventilation.

For instance, if the SIMV rate is 8 bpm, but the patient is breathing spontaneously at a rate varying between 30 and 40 bpm, exactly which of the 30 to 40 breaths should be selected for synchronization? If every fifth breath is selected, and the breath rate is 40 bpm, the patient gets exactly 8 mandated bpm; but what happens if the spontaneous rate suddenly drops to 30 bpm? To overcome this dilemma, ventilator logic divides 60 seconds by the preset SIMV rate—in this case 60/8 = 7.5 seconds—so the ventilator opens a new timing window every 7.5 seconds. The ventilator is programmed to synchronize to the *first patient effort in each timing window*, if the patient makes no effort during the window, the breath is delivered at the end of our example 7.5-second interval; this results in the desired SIMV rate, at least most of the time. Problems still occur, however. During apnea, a bizarre pattern often results. Because the patient fails to make an effort, a mandated breath occurs at the very end of a timing window; but, the next successive time window opens immediately, even before the just delivered mandated breath can be exhaled. Exhalation therefore proceeds well into the next timing window. If, at the end of this exhalation, P_{aw} falls a few cm H_2O below baseline pressure, as often happens, the ventilator often mistakes this pressure drop for the first patient effort in the timing window and delivers a second successive SIMV breath—a phenomenon often referred to as *auto-triggering*. But the strange behavior doesn't end there. Because the ventilator has already "synchronized" to the first breath in the present timing window, and because the patient is apneic, it will not trigger again until the next successive timing window expires. A breathing pattern consisting of two consecutive mandated breaths, followed by 15 seconds without a mandated breath, followed by two consecutive mandated breaths repeats, over and over (Fig. 102.18). Despite the bizarre appearance, the patient actually receives the 8 mandated bpm requested, just not in the pattern expected. Auto-triggering is easily rectified by increasing trigger sensitivity—to a point just below the pressure drop noted at end-exhalation. There is a caveat to this solution however. Increasing trigger sensitivity makes triggering more difficult. Therefore, the operator must be sure to readjust the sensitivity as soon as spontaneous breathing activity resumes.

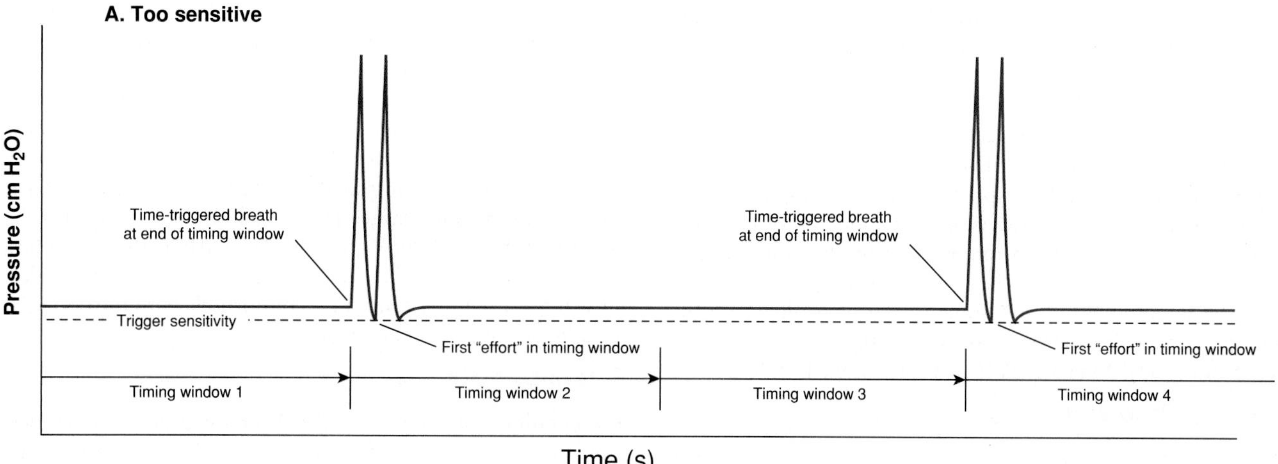

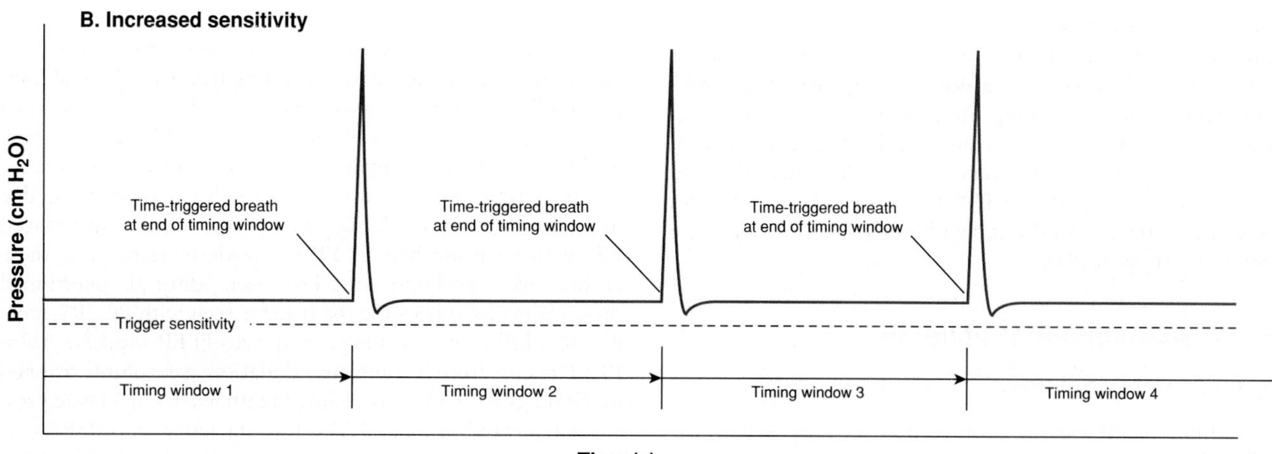

FIGURE 102.18 Synchronized intermittent mandatory ventilation (SIMV) and autotriggering during apnea. **A:** Too sensitive. An airway pressure curve demonstrating how trigger sensitivity set for normal breathing may be too sensitive during apnea. SIMV modes are programmed to synchronize to the first patient effort in each timing window. When no effort occurs, as during apnea, the ventilator must time trigger at the end of the timing window. If sensitivity is set too low (1 to 2 cm H_2O), exhalation from the previous breath may appear as the first effort in the next timing window and auto-trigger a breath. This scenario results in a bizarre breathing pattern: two breaths in succession, followed by a very long pause and two breaths in succession, the pattern then repeats. Interestingly, this pattern delivers the preset breathing rate, just not in the sequence expected. **B:** Increased sensitivity. An airway pressure curve of the same apneic patient except, trigger sensitivity is increased to a pressure lower than that occurring during exhalation; this eliminates autotriggering and results in a more uniform pattern of ventilation.

Pressure Support Ventilation

Operational Principles

PSV likely developed as a method to counteract the additional WOB imposed by early, poorly designed demand valves and demand-flow systems (28). As demand systems improved, the WOB imposed by the breathing apparatus approached zero; still, patients often struggled to overcome the WOB imposed by the ETT (29,30). Furthermore, increased R_{aw} and/or reduced C_{RS} increased patient physiologic WOB, often significantly (76). There were plenty of reasons to continue using PSV.

Pressure support is an assisted spontaneous breathing mode; it can be used alone, or in conjunction with SIMV. It is patient-triggered, pressure-controlled, and is generally flow-cycled (at 25% to 50% of peak V_I). Patients receiving PSV control their own breathing rate, and exert some control over V_T, peak V_I and T_I. Originally, operators preset only the desired PSV level, in cm H_2O above the baseline pressure. PSV however, generates very high initial V_I; on occasion, the flow was too high for patient comfort (77). This shortcoming was corrected in the latest generation of ventilators by adding a "rise time" control. Clinicians use this control to adjust peak V_I during PSV, up or down, to meet patient needs.

Clinical Application

Pressure support has replaced CPAP as the spontaneous breathing mode used during SIMV. PSV helps to reduce WOB by partially unloading the respiratory muscles. Approaches to the use of PSV vary; some advocate just enough PSV to counteract any additional WOB imposed by the breathing apparatus, and ETT (25,27,29,78), while others try to neutralize both the imposed WOB and some of the physiologic WOB, enough to provide comfort and avoid fatigue. With back-up modes for safety, some use PSV as a standalone (79,80).

Potential Problems

Despite its promise, PSV may have created more problems than it solved. If set too low, the patient continues to struggle and may fatigue; set too high, the patient does essentially no work and is predisposed to disuse atrophy of the respiratory muscles. Confounding matters are two unresolved problems: first, no one has developed a noninvasive, easy-to-use, reliable method for determining the proper PSV level; and second, patient demands vary considerably, and a single PSV level cannot possibly meet every conceivable patient demand level. Studies suggest that if PSV levels are managed around the clock, patients spend less significantly less time receiving ventilatory support (81).

Pressure-Controlled Ventilation

Operational Principles

As outlined in the classification section, in today's ICU virtually all mechanical breaths are either volume- or pressure-controlled. Pressure-controlled breaths can be used for CMV, A/C, mandated SIMV breaths, as well as for pressure-controlled inverse-ratio ventilation (PC-IRV). Operators set the desired ventilator rate, T_I, target pressure (above baseline) and, for A/C or SIMV, trigger sensitivity. After a PCV breath is triggered, flow and pressure rise rapidly to the preset pressure; upon reaching the preset pressure, flow decelerates as needed to maintain that pressure until the preset T_I elapses. For patient-triggered modes, the same rise time control used for PSV adjusts the initial rate flow rate and pressure rise in PCV; on occasion, an appropriate adjustment of the rise time control significantly enhances patient comfort. For those acutely ill with ARDS, PC-IRV is sometimes applied. Using PC-IRV however, requires sedation and, sometimes, neuromuscular blockade; awake and alert patients seldom tolerate the extended T_I intervals—with I:E ratios up to 4:1—used during PC-IRV without "fighting" the ventilator.

Clinical Applications

Clinicians opt for PCV instead of VCV for three reasons, or some combination thereof: (a) to provide higher initial and average V_I for patients breathing spontaneously during mechanical breaths; (b) to control PIP and limit the possibility of VILI; and/or (c) to use PC-IRV. Although several studies report improvements in oxygenation at lower PIP using PC-IRV with infants (82,83), its use in adults (84,85) remains limited. Clearly, PC-IRV elevates mean P_{aw}, which in turn raises FRC. Proponents of PC-IRV, however, claimed similar improvements in oxygenation those seen using VCV, but at much lower CPAP or PEEP levels. Using PCV as a method to control PIP, and minimize the risk of VILI, is an interesting approach. However, if the culprit in VILI is the end-inspiratory lung volume, not the PIP, then the approach is terribly flawed. That is, during PCV the patient is free to interact with the ventilator. If the patient inhales deeply during any pressure-controlled breath, the resultant spontaneous V_T may be quite large. Thus, while PCV may control P_{aw} precisely, it fails to limit V_T to a safe level. Along the same lines, using PCV, to provide higher peak and average V_I, only makes sense if the attending clinician is comfortable with the potential for a large range in spontaneous V_T.

Potential Problems

The defining characteristics of PCV are high peak V_I, decelerating flow waveform, and no control over V_T. At one extreme, PCV continues to control pressure even if the ETT occludes and V_T drops to zero; at the other extreme, a vigorous patient effort often produces very large spontaneous V_T, especially when compared to the V_T delivered with no patient effort. Clinicians using PCV must carefully set high and low V_T and minute ventilation alarms to avoid these problems, as well as keep a close eye on ventilator graphics, if available. Often, these problems are visually apparent well before adverse responses.

For a time, PC-IRV was popular; this was, in part, due to claims that the mode increased oxygenation and reduced PIP, without using high PEEP or CPAP. In retrospect, these authors were probably mistaken. Two editorials questioned these claims by suggesting the benefits seen with PC-IRV *were* due to PEEP—that is, undetected auto-PEEP (86,87). *Auto-PEEP* results from incomplete exhalation; gas volume trapped in the lungs from the proceeding breath, exerts an elastic pressure similar to PEEP or CPAP—thus the name auto-PEEP. Gas trapping results for two primary reasons: incomplete time for exhalation, or premature airway collapse. Inverse ratios, as used in PC-IRV, reduce exhalation time, often significantly; hence PC-IRV predisposes to air trapping or auto-PEEP. Furthermore, during normal exhalation, auto-PEEP exists only in the lungs, not in the breathing circuit, making it difficult to detect; for this reason, some have even called it *occult-PEEP* (88). Auto-PEEP can, however, be estimated at the bedside, if one suspects its existence (88). A patient's total PEEP must take into consideration auto-PEEP:

$$\text{Total PEEP} = \text{applied PEEP} + \text{auto-PEEP} \quad (3)$$

Once this concept was understood, clinicians began routinely monitoring for auto-PEEP. Interestingly, interest in PC-IRV waned almost concomitantly providing strong circumstantial evidence that auto-PEEP was indeed responsible, in part, for PC-IRV's initial success in adults. Today's mechanical ventilators measure auto-PEEP "on request," presuming the patient makes no effort to breathe during the measurement.

SPONTANEOUS BREATHING

CPAP and Spontaneous PEEP

Operational Principles

Given the improvements in oxygenation, V_A/Q, C_{RS}, and WOB attributed to using PEEP or CPAP during mechanical ventilation (14–16,68,69) it seems logical to use them as stand-alone modes. With CPAP, both inspiratory and expiratory pressures remain positive. As a practical matter, the inspiratory pressures are lower than expiratory, during CPAP. This occurs for three reasons: (a) during inspiration, the removal of gas from the continuous flow by the patient causes pressure to fall; (b) triggering a demand CPAP system generally requires that pressure fall; (c) the CPAP system cannot meet the patient's inspiratory flow demands. By definition, spontaneous PEEP requires that the patient reduce P_{aw} to zero or less during the inspiratory phase; P_{aw} returns to the PEEP level during exhalation. Spontaneous PEEP differs from CPAP in that the large pressure fluctuations during inspiration impose a significantly greater WOB on the patient (89) (Fig. 102.19). When tolerated however, the same large pressure swings improve venous return and cardiac output (90). Conversely, CPAP reduces patient WOB, but at the expense of decreased venous return.

Years ago, most CPAP and PEEP devices were "homemade"—there were no commercially available systems. Modern ventilators easily provide either spontaneous PEEP or CPAP, and have obviated the need for homemade systems, particularly in the ICU setting. Using a ventilator to provide

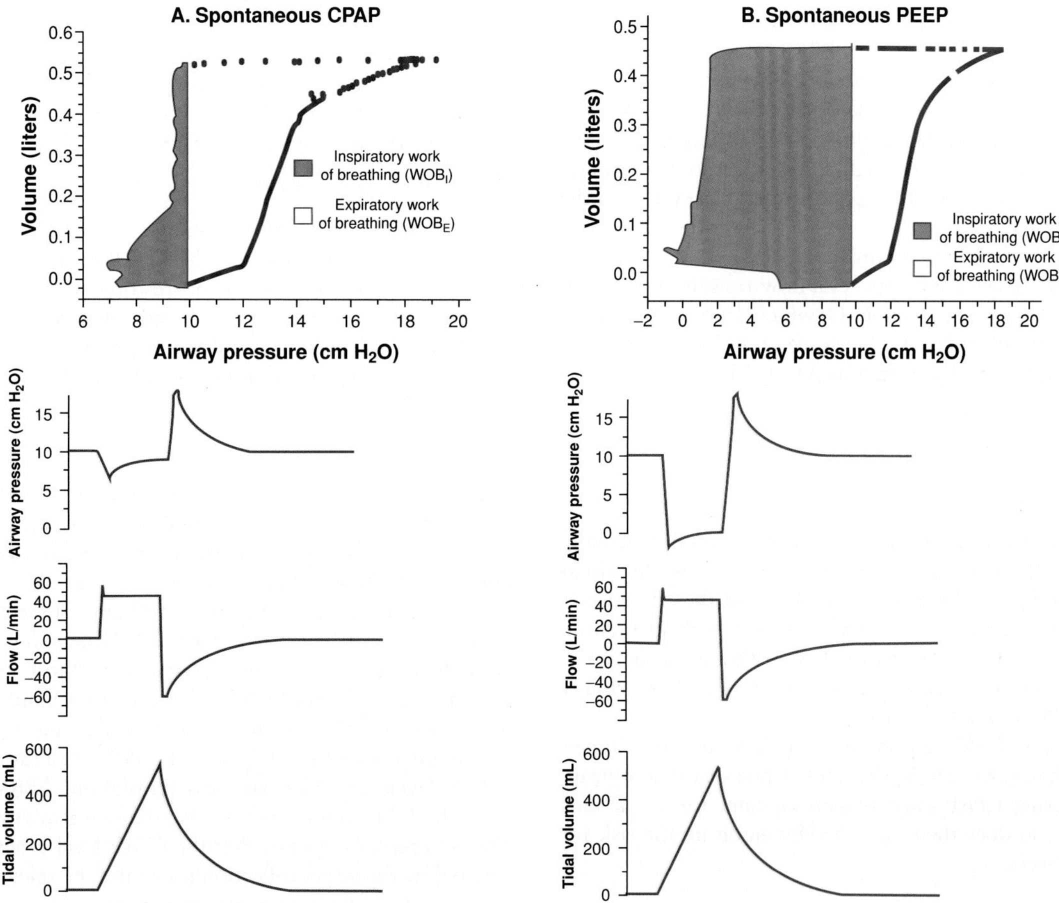

FIGURE 102.19 Work imposed by spontaneous continuous positive airway pressure (CPAP) or positive end-expiratory pressure (PEEP) breathing systems. The inspiratory work of breathing (WOB_I), encountered by patients breathing spontaneously, is impacted by the type of breathing system. Additional workloads, imposed upon spontaneously breathing patients, are determined by measuring the area under the curve obtained by plotting airway pressure (P_{aw}) versus volume (V_T) loops taken at the proximal airway (i.e., at the endotracheal tube opening). End-expiratory pressure is 10 cm H_2O, while the simulated patient effort is identical for both systems. The additional WOB_I (*solid areas*) is computed from the area within the P_{aw}–V_T loop while P_{aw} remains below the starting point (10 cm H_2O). With the CPAP system, P_{aw} initially falls to 7 cm H_2O (during triggering), but quickly returns to 9 cm H_2O for the remainder of inspiration; with the spontaneous PEEP system, the same patient effort initially reduces P_{aw} to –2 cm H_2O, but it quickly returns to 0 cm H_2O. The computed WOB_I, for the CPAP system, is approximately 0.1 Joules (J) and for PEEP system 0.48 J, an increase of 480%. The expiratory work of breathing (WOB_E) is generally a nonfactor; the energy required to exhale is provided by the energy released as patients' highly elastic lungs, which were stretched during inflation, recoil to their resting position (like releasing a just-inflated party balloon).

spontaneous PEEP or CPAP has distinct advantages; if the patient deteriorates, the ventilator is already on hand. Furthermore, modern ventilators often incorporate back-up modes that automatically begin ventilating patients when predefined criteria are met. For example, mechanical ventilation may begin in response to a 15- to 60-second period of apnea.

The optimum level PEEP or CPAP can be difficult to determine. For this reason, clinicians often start with a conservative level and then titrate up using quantitative criteria such as: serial blood gases (91,92), oximetry (93), computers (94), or even conjunctival oximetry (95).

Clinical Applications

The rationale for applying spontaneous PEEP or CPAP is the same, whether they are used with or without mechanical ventilation; both techniques improve oxygenation, V_A/Q, C_{RS}, FRC, and WOB. Furthermore, CPAP/PEEP prevents airway collapse during exhalation and reduces the potential for low-volume lung injury.

Potential Problems

Both spontaneous PEEP and CPAP impose an additional workload on the patient's respiratory muscles. Of the two, there is no argument that spontaneous PEEP imposes a far greater workload. However, even a "perfect" CPAP system—one that allows little, or no pressure deflection during inhalation—still does not eliminate the additional WOB imposed by the patient's ET. If an ET is too small, kinks, or becomes partially occluded, the patient's WOB may be intolerable, even with the best CPAP system.

Consider the following example:

Suppose a patient's ET imposes a flow resistance of 10 cm H_2O/L/s, CPAP is set at 10 cm H_2O, which drops to 8 cm H_2O at mid-inspiration, and peak V_I measures 60 L/min; pressure at the carinal end of the ET at mid-inspiration is:

$$\begin{aligned}&\text{Pressure (at the carina)}\\&= \text{CPAP} - (\text{resistance at } V_I + \text{pressure drop})\\&= 10 - (10 + 2)\\&= -2 \text{ cm } H_2O\end{aligned}$$

What *appears* as CPAP in the breathing circuit is actually spontaneous PEEP at the carinal end of the ET. In this situation, maintaining CPAP at the carinal end of the ET requires an airway pressure of 20 cm H_2O or more; in this situation, a PSV setting of 10 cm H_2O would neutralize most the WOB imposed by the ET. It also demonstrates why PSV has virtually replaced CPAP in the ICU setting.

Spontaneous CPAP, especially at high levels, may hyperinflate the lungs, elevate V_D/V_T, and depress cardiac output. Clinicians using CPAP must remain vigilant, for as patients improve so too does their C_{RS}, thereby elevating the risk for these side effects.

Airway Pressure Release Ventilation

Operational Principles

Unlike conventional mechanical ventilation, APRV establishes an elevated baseline pressure—or CPAP level—ostensibly to restore FRC; tidal ventilation occurs by decreasing, or releasing, the CPAP. APRV allows unrestricted spontaneous breathing at all times, even during releases. Interestingly, with conventional ventilation, a higher breathing rate means a higher mean P_{aw}, which, in turn, reduces venous return and cardiac output; with APRV however, a higher breathing rate actually lowers the mean P_{aw}. As a result, APRV has far less influence on cardiovascular parameters than a comparable level of CPAP.

During the process of initiating APRV, the operator presets the desired CPAP level, number of releases/minute (or breath rate), release time, and release pressure. Although it is possible to set V_T during APRV, it is a difficult trial-and-error process. V_T is limited by the CPAP level, release pressure, release time, and patient C_{RS}. For example, suppose a patient's CPAP level is set at 10 cm H_2O, C_{RS} is 50 mL/cm H_2O, and the release pressure set to 0 cm H_2O. The maximum V_T for this patient is (assuming complete exhalation) as follows:

$$\begin{aligned}V_T &= \text{change in pressure} \times C_{RS}\\&= (10 - 0) \text{ cm } H_2O \times 50 \text{ mL/cm } H_2O = 500 \text{ mL}\end{aligned} \quad (4)$$

Release volume or V_T also varies with release time; we only get the maximum V_T only if release time is long enough for the lungs to completely empty. On many occasions, however, oxygenation deteriorates when using a release pressure of zero. When this happens, raising the release pressure will restore oxygenation (96); but unless the CPAP level is raised concomitantly, V_T will fall. When switching from conventional mechanical ventilation to APRV, some suggest and adequate V_T results by setting CPAP at 1.5 to 2 times that required during conventional ventilation (97,98).

Clinical Applications

Proponents believe APRV should minimize barotrauma because PIP never surpasses the CPAP level and maximum lung volume never exceeds the restored FRC. In addition, APRV lowers physiologic V_D and improves oxygenation (96,99,100). If these assertions are proven accurate, APRV might be used in place of conventional ventilation, for virtually any and all patients.

Potential Problems

There is a potential flaw in the potential for APRV to minimize barotrauma. That is, APRV as described and studied does not, necessarily, eliminate the risk for low-volume lung injury (4–7). If avoiding VILI requires that all tidal ventilation take place between the lower and upper inflection points, as some now believe (19), then APRV may fail to protect patients; especially if release pressures of 0 to 6 cm H_2O are used as reported (96,99,100). On the other hand, given that the volumetric distance between the lower and upper inflection point is often small and that APRV maintains the same $PaCO_2$ levels as CMV with less ventilation, APRV may well offer the best lung-protective, ventilatory strategy available. This assumes, of course, that the CPAP level is set to a pressure below the upper inflection point and the release level to a pressure above the lower inflection point (19).

Apneustic Anesthesia Ventilation

Operational Principles

AAV is a variant of APRV often referred to as *intermittent CPAP*. AAV differs from APRV in that it is only applied to patients with normal lung compliance. As a result, the selected CPAP level does not restore FRC; rather, AAV produces a higher than normal FRC, but in all other aspects is identical to APRV. The concept was patented by John B. Downs and later described by Bratzke et al. (101). They studied surgical patients exposing them to alternating trials of AAV and to CMV, the standard form of ventilation used in the operating room. During AAV, many statistically significant differences were found: patients required lower minute ventilation to achieve the same P_aCO_2, lower V_D, lower $P_{(a\text{-}et)}$ CO_2 (arterial–end tidal CO_2 measurement), lower peak P_{aw}, and a higher mean P_{aw}. Clearly, when compared to CMV, AAV provides a more efficient form of ventilation at lower peak P_{aw}.

Clinical Applications

Perioperative and postoperative pulmonary dysfunction is a common phenomenon (101–103). The use of CPAP as a target pressure during AAV maintains an open lung, thereby preventing atelectasis and minimizing the need for supplemental oxygen (104). Furthermore, like APRV, AAV allows the patient to breathe at any time during the breathing cycle. This facet makes AAV useful for all types of anesthetic procedures including conscious sedation. Unfortunately, although it appears that AAV could potentially alleviate many perioperative and postoperative pulmonary complications and offers a more efficient form of ventilation, it is seldom used.

Potential Problems

As a rule, AAV will generate a slightly higher mean P_{aw} than conventional mechanical ventilation; as a result AAV might result in a reduced venous return. If a reduced venous return could in anyway comprise the patient, the clinician might consider using CMV. Otherwise, AAV is as safe as any other mode of mechanical ventilation.

SPECIAL TECHNIQUES

Pressure-Targeted Volume Ventilation

Operational Principles

For years, the Food and Drug Administration (FDA) resisted approving any sort of "smart" ventilator setting. Pressure-targeted, volume ventilation, pressure-regulated volume control (PRVC), or volume ventilation plus represent a distinct departure from that stance; this mode is far more automated than any before it. To initiate the mode, the operator presets a ventilator rate, V_T, T_I, and trigger sensitivity (if patient-triggering is desired). Upon connecting the patient, the ventilator performs up to three test breaths. Test breaths are, as a rule, square flow pattern, volume-controlled breaths with a short end-inspiratory pause. Assuming one of the test breaths is not disturbed by patient attempts to breathe, the ventilator determines the patient's C_{RS} (see Fig. 102.13, and Table 102.3). Once V_T and C_{RS} are known, the ventilator rearranges and solves equation 4:

$$\text{Pressure change (target)} = V_T/C_{RS}$$

Having determined the target pressure, the ventilator switches, from the test breath protocol, into what amounts to a smart PCV. For safety reasons, the ventilator begins PRVC, using a pressure, substantially below that calculated (above). The ventilator "watches" the exhaled V_T and gradually, over the next 5 to 10 mechanical breaths, ramps up its pressure until the exhaled V_T equals that requested. At this point, the operator must thoughtfully set the ventilator's high P_{aw} limit, based upon the current target pressure and the maximum P_{aw} deemed safe for the patient. This setting is crucial because PRVC is not limited to the initial or starting target pressure. In fact, PRVC changes target pressure quite often, within limits, in order to maintain an exhaled V_T equal to that requested. If for instance, patient C_{RS} suddenly deteriorates, V_T also falls in direct proportion, and concomitantly. The ventilator immediately detects the reduced exhaled V_T and increases target pressure at a rate of 2 or 3 cm H_2O per breath. Target pressure continues to increase, with each breath, until either exhaled V_T is restored, or target pressure reaches a value no greater than high P_{aw} limit minus 2 to 3 cm H_2O. The same but opposite response occurs should C_{RS} improve and V_T increase; that is, target pressure is reduced by 2 or 3 cm H_2O, until the exhaled V_T is re-established; but, target pressure can go no lower than baseline pressure (PEEP or CPAP level, if applicable) plus 3 cm H_2O.

Clinical Applications

In theory, PRVC combines the best aspects of both VCV and PCV—consistent V_T, delivered at lower PIP with high initial peak V_I. Some clinicians will consider using this mode for its ability to deliver the same V_T at lower PIP. There is no doubt this strategy works to lower PIP, but the same V_T produces the same ERP, regardless of how that volume is forced into the lungs (see Fig. 102.14). This explains why, in two carefully controlled studies comparing PRVC to VCV found significantly lower PIPs, but were unable to detect any difference in outcome (104,105).

Others might consider using PRVC for its ability to provide high initial peak V_I, reduce WOB, and better synchronize with spontaneously active patients. Kallet et al. (53) looked at this issue during lung-protective ventilation and concluded PCV and PRVC offer no advantage in reducing WOB, when compared to VCV with a high preset V_I.

Potential Problems

Conceptually, PRVC appears inherently safer than traditional PCV because it automatically maintains the preset V_T. Nevertheless, if the operator does not carefully set the high P_{aw} limit, PRVC may produce unexpected and dangerous changes. For instance, imagine a patient supported by PRVC with a V_T of 500 mL and a target pressure of 25 cm H_2O; the operator sets a high P_{aw} limit of 50 cm H_2O. Suppose this patient develops an acute tension pneumothorax and the effected lung collapses. The patient's apparent C_{RS} would suddenly be reduced by one-half, or more. If the mode were traditional PCV, V_T would be reduced to the same extent, thereby leaving the contralateral lung inflated by essentially the same V_T as prior to the pneumothorax. In contrast, V_T would also be initially reduced with PRVC but, almost immediately, PRVC would begin increasing the target pressure at 3 cm H_2O per breath in an effort to re-establish the preset exhaled volume. If the desired V_T was re-established by 47 cm H_2O (high P_{aw} limit minus 3 cm H_2O), then the entire initial V_T, for both lungs, is forced into the remaining good lung, risking hyperinflation and damage to this lung as well.

PROPORTIONAL ASSIST VENTILATION

Operational Principles

As explained, PSV unloads potentially fatiguing workloads from spontaneously breathing patients. Unfortunately, it is difficult to determine the needed level of PSV, and PCV does not accommodate changes in patient breathing pattern. As a consequence, PSV either over supports or under supports the patient most of the time. Ideally, we need a variable support mode that automatically raises or lowers its response to maintain the same level of support, regardless of patient effort. Younes proposed such a mode, which he named proportional assist ventilation (PAV) (106,107). This mode relies upon what is referred to as the equation of motion of the respiratory system, which states:

$$P_{aw} = V_T/C_{RS} + V_I \times R_{aw} \quad (5)$$

If C_{RS} and R_{aw} are known and the ventilator measures V_T and V_I instantaneously, as it provides them, the work required—measured as pressure—is easily computed, regardless of effort level; recall that work is defined as the integral of P_{aw} with respect to time. If the ventilator also knows the ETT size and flow resistance, which is stored in ROM, the ventilator can compute nearly the total WOB, although this approach cannot determine the work to inflate chest wall. Estimating patient WOB, in real-time, throughout each and every breath, allows the ventilator to unload any quantifiable amount, or percentage, of that WOB; in fact, most PAV systems are preset to unload a specific percentage of the total WOB provided by the ventilator. For instance, if PAV was preset for 50%, the ventilator would measure the work being performed and provide exactly half of it. By measuring V_I and V_T, many times within each breath, PAV provides 50% of the work generated, regardless of how much or little effort the patient expends.

Assuming PAV works as theorized, it should meet a patient's varying needs by proportionally varying its response, a feature PSV cannot match. Nevertheless, PAV brings us no closer to a quantifiable and reliable method for determining an appropriate level of support; that is, we do not know what percentage of the total WOB the patient can tolerate. Manufacturers recommend starting PAV at a high percentage and gradually tapering down as the patient improves; the statement simply states the obvious, and applies equally well to PSV.

Clinical Applications

If PAV proves effective, clinicians should use it in any instance when they'd previously used PSV. So far, PAV remains unproven and controversial. Giannouli et al. (108) compared different levels of PSV and PAV; they reported that PAV seemed more synchronous, but the differences had no effect on gas exchange or spontaneous breathing rate. Hart et al. (109) compared PAV to PSV, in patients with neuromuscular and chest wall deformity, and concluded both modes produced similar improvements. Finally, Passam et al. (110) compared different levels of PSV and PAV on breathing pattern, WOB, and gas exchange in mechanically ventilated, hypercapnic COPD patients. They concluded that in COPD, although both PAV and PSV produced similar improvements in blood gases, higher levels of PSV often resulted in efforts that failed to trigger breaths, whereas under similar circumstances PAV developed the "runaway" phenomenon. Runaway occurs when, during PAV, the ventilator begins to trigger on and cycle off at rates much higher than the patient's actual spontaneous breathing frequency. Finally, another group reported PAV was not superior to PSV in unloading the respiratory muscles following artificially increased ventilatory demand (111). These failures have some to questioning whether PAV represents any improvement over PSV (112,113).

Potential Problems

Based upon existing research, patients respond very differently to PAV than to PSV; yet the end results so far, appear similar. To date, we have over 20 years of clinical experience using PSV. It makes little sense switching to PAV, without a compelling reason to do so, especially if PAV is going to affect patients differently, and in ways we may not yet understand. One of those differences involves the previously mentioned runaway, which results when the pressure provided by PAV exceeds the patient's elastance (inverse of C_{RS}) and R_{aw}, and persists into the exhalation phase. The physiologic problems that might result during runaway PAV remain to be thoroughly understood and unexplained.

ARDS NETWORK PROTOCOL

Operational Principles

ARDS is a syndrome of inflammation and increased permeability associated with an acute onset of hypoxemia (arterial partial pressure of oxygen/fractional inspired oxygen [P_aO_2/F_iO_2] < 200 mmHg) accompanied by infiltrates on x-ray that cannot be explained by left atrial or pulmonary capillary hypertension (pulmonary artery occlusion pressure >18 mmHg) (115). Acute lung injury (ALI) refers to a milder form of ARDS that is defined by a somewhat better P_aO_2/F_iO_2 *less than* 300 mmHg (114).

For many years, despite vast improvements in overall care, the mortality associated with ARDS remained unacceptably high. Gattinoni et al. (115–117) proposed that patients with ARDS had areas of essentially normal lung coexisting with the consolidated areas so often seen on x-ray, even when the lungs appeared completely consolidated. Furthermore, because the normal areas of the lung were small compared to the infiltrated and consolidated areas, they described the ARDS affected patient as having *baby lungs* (116,117). They also proposed that, because the collapsed and congested areas could not be easily ventilated, if at all, most of a patient's mechanical ventilation was directed into the normal areas of lung. This caused hyperinflation, damage, and ultimately inflammation and infiltration (115–117). This sequence became known as VILI and formed the basis of the operative hypothesis of the ARDS Network. That is, mechanical ventilation itself can further injure the ARDS, or ALI damaged lung (118). The basic goal of the protocol is aimed at minimizing any additional lung damage while maintaining adequate gas exchange. To validate the hypothesis, the ARDS network randomized patients to a lower V_T (6–8 mL/kg) ventilation strategy and compared that to patients receiving a 12 mL/kg ventilation strategy (118). Patients in the lower V_T group demonstrated a 22% relative reduction in mortality and formed the cornerstone for the ARDS Network Protocol (118).

Clinical Applications

The ARDS Network believes that low V_T ventilation (LTVV) reduces the damaging, excessive stretch of lung tissue and alveoli (the so-called volutauma) caused by high V_T mechanical ventilation, and recommend their protocol as the standard of care for patients with ALI and ARDS (119). They suggest implementation begin by using CMV with a V_T of 8 mL/kg of body weight and a breathing rate of up to 35 breaths/min to achieve a minute ventilation of 7 to 9 L/min. PEEP is set to at least 5 cm H_2O to achieve an oxygen saturation (SpO_2) of 88% to 95%; the F_iO_2 is then titrated down, maintaining an acceptable SpO_2, with an F_iO_2 less than or equal to 0.7. Subsequently, while maintaining adequate ventilation and oxygenation, V_T is reduced to 7 mL/kg and finally 6 mL/kg; ideally V_T should reach 6 mL/kg in 4 hours or less. The use of higher PEEP levels is associated with increased survival for those with severe ARDS, but tended to produce more damage in those with milder forms of ALI (119–121). During care, ventilator adjustments are made with the primary goal of sustaining an EIP (or plateau pressure) at less than 30 cm H_2O, while providing adequate ventilation and oxygenation. Prone positioning of the patient is also recommended.

Potential Problems

Patients with severe ARDS are not easily managed, especially when trying to employ such low tidal volumes. Frequently, patients continue to deteriorate, and maintaining an EIP *less than* 30 cm H_2O may be impossible. In such circumstances recommended approaches include the following: (a) reduce the V_T to 4 mL/kg; (b) sedate heavily to reduce asynchrony; (c) consider permissive hypercapnia or even extracorporeal membrane oxygenation (ECMO). In addition, using the EIP obtained using only the mechanical ventilator can be misleading; that is, the ventilator produced EIP is the static pressure produced by the entire respiratory system (lungs and chest wall combined). Obese and other postsurgical patients may exhibit significantly reduced chest wall compliance (C_{CW}), which in turn acts to elevate the ventilator measured EIP. Therefore, to accurately measure the maximum pressure exerted on the lungs requires esophageal manometry. Using this technique, the pressure exerted by the chest wall can be separated from that exerted by the lungs themselves.

Clearly, LTVV improves mortality, yet too many patients still succumb to this devastating complex. It follows that LTVV is, at best, a partial answer; many questions remain unanswered. For example, why is CMV the only ventilator mode recommended by the ARDS Network? What about ventilator techniques like APRV, with its increased efficiency of ventilation, PRVC, or even PCIRV? Also, does breathing frequency play a role in lung damage? There is evidence suggesting that lower breathing rates, even with somewhat higher V_T and high PEEP can reduce barotrauma when compared to CMV (122). Limiting the ventilator technique to CMV seems unscientific, without compelling evidence that suggests using CMV is demonstrably superior to other approaches. Nevertheless, the ARDS Network Protocol or using some form of LTVV provides an effective approach as we await further research.

Neurally Adjusted Ventilatory Assist

Operational Principles

The optimal method for synchronizing a ventilator to an aggressively breathing patient remains an unsolved problem. Patient–ventilator asynchrony may predispose to any of a number of problems: flow starvation; delayed triggering, erratic cycling, and other forms of asynchrony; intrinsic PEEP; muscle dysfunction or dystrophy; inability to adapt to altered metabolic situations; and inability to respond adequately to the tiny signals produced by neonatal and pediatric patients. Understanding the reason most ventilators do not consistently synchronize begins by reviewing the neuroventilatory coupling mechanism (Fig. 102.20).

Most modern ventilators use either a drop in airway pressure or an onset of flow to trigger a breath, and because these occur at the very end of the neuroventilatory pathway, synchronization often fails; especially when the patient is a rapidly breathing neonate, pediatric patient, or very

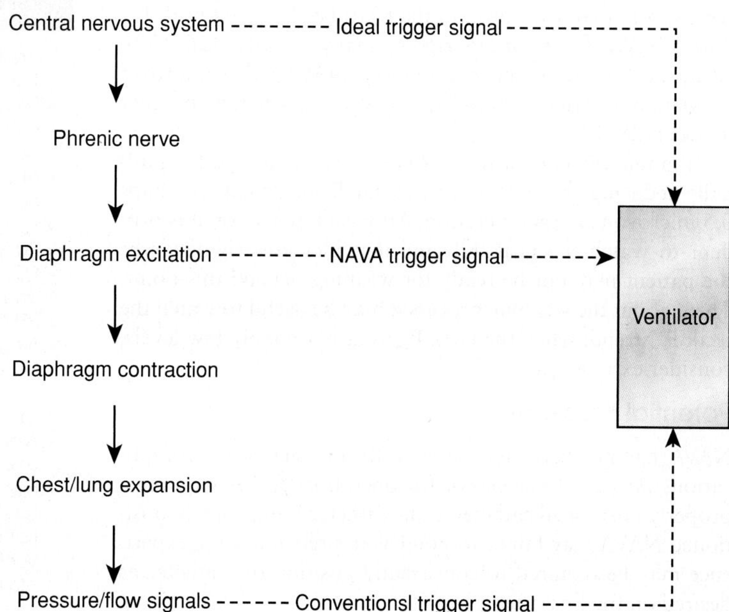

FIGURE 102.20 The neuroventilatory pathway showing the propagation of a spontaneous breath starting at the central nervous system and ending with chest movement and the movement of gas into the lungs. Also shown are: the ideal point for detecting a breath triggering signal, the point at which NAVA triggers a breath, and the point at which conventional ventilators trigger a breath. While NAVA is not ideal it is a vast improvement over conventional trigger signals. For this reason, NAVA synchronizes to patient efforts more efficiently than conventional approaches.

tachypneic adult. Beck et al. (123) showed that during SIMV the synchronized portion of the breathing cycle is actually 53% asynchronous versus only 47% synchronous as measured by neural timing. Thille et al. (124) demonstrated that 25% of patients exhibit a high incidence of inspiratory asynchrony during assisted ventilation. They also showed that a high incidence of asynchrony predisposes to a prolongation of mechanical ventilation and that patients with frequent, ineffective triggering may receive excess levels of ventilatory support. Finally, patient–ventilator asynchrony during assisted ventilation is associated with higher auto-PEEP levels, higher peak P_{aw}, and hypoxemia (124).

Neurally adjusted ventilatory assist (NAVA) provides for inspiratory pressure controlled by diaphragmatic EMG, called the Edi signal. The Edi is measured in microvolts using a properly positioned special nasogastric catheter. The Edi signals rises and falls with inspiration and expiration. During inspiration peak Edi is in the range of 11 ± 5 microvolts and 3 ± 2 microvolts during exhalation. Ventilatory assistance during NAVA is proportional to patient effort as measured by the Edi signal:

Inspiratory pressure (cm H_2O above PEEP) = NAVA level (cm H_2O/microvolt) × Edi (above minimum Edi)

Technical capabilities of the mode may include the following: all breaths can be spontaneous, trigger/cycle variables based on chest/diaphragm movement, automatic coordination of mandatory and spontaneous breaths, reduction of auto-PEEP, unrestricted V_T, and automatic adjustment of support (flow and pressure) to meet demand. At this time, NAVA is only available on the Maquet Servo-i ventilator.

Clinical Applications

For those with access to the Servo-i, NAVA is often the mode of choice for neonatal and pediatric populations. It is also suitable for use in adults who, for one reason or another, fail to synchronize adequately to more conventional approaches. Many papers are appearing in the literature documenting measurable improvements during NAVA compared to other approaches, especially in neonates or pediatric patients. Brodessoule et al. (125) demonstrated improved synchrony. Beck et al. (126) showed that NAVA improves synchrony even with substantial leaks around the ET tube. Lowered peak P_{aw} during NAVA has been reported by many authors (126–130). Also, several authors have noted that NAVA either improves or maintains arterial blood gases when compared to other modes (128–130).

Weaning the patient from NAVA is accomplished by gradually reducing the NAVA level in small increments, perhaps 0.5 microvolts at each iteration. After each reduction it is prudent to watch the peak Edi and if it increases significantly, the patient may not be ready for weaning beyond this point. Throughout the weaning process it may be useful to watch the peak P_{aw} trend; when the peak P_{aw} is at reasonably low levels, consider extubation.

Potential Problems

NAVA has not been associated with any significant complications *per se*. Nevertheless, for operation NAVA requires a properly positioned catheter. If the catheter is improperly positioned NAVA may fail to respond as desired and some experience may be required to consistently position the catheter as desired on the first attempt.

TRANSPORT VENTILATION

Automatic or Manual Ventilation

Ventilation during transport is still often supported using a self-inflating bag (e.g., the Ambu device), a flow-inflating (Mapleson) system, or oxygen-powered breathing devices (Elder demand valve or a similar device). This is, indeed, surprising, in an era dominated by evidence-based medicine. The use of bags and valves, even in the most skilled hands, results in significant breath-to-breath differences in V_T, respiratory rate, minute ventilation, PIP and, in some cases, inspired fraction of oxygen (F_iO_2). These differences, acting alone or in combination, may disrupt arterial blood gases by the end of even a short intrahospital transport (131–134). Furthermore, bags and valves may not deliver an effective level of PEEP/CPAP, and can make spontaneous breathing difficult. A portable ventilator, with the proper capabilities, is clearly a better choice.

Important Features for Transport Ventilation

Typical ICU mechanical ventilators are too large, cumbersome, and fragile to use for routine transports. Repairing a $40,000 ICU ventilator, unintentionally tipped over or dropped during a rushed transport, could easily cost as much or more than the purchase price of a new transport ventilator. Ruggedness is one of the more important, but often overlooked, characteristics desired in a transport ventilator (Table 102.4). Most practitioners opt for units that are electrically powered, with battery backup; nevertheless, an ideal unit would also work when powered only by compressed air or oxygen. Several hospitals in hurricane Katrina's wake lost electric power for days following the storm. Absolutely nothing electric worked and batteries were all dead in a few hours; yet, they had plenty of oxygen. Left without properly equipped, pneumatically powered ventilators, however, these physicians and nurses simply could not adequately ventilate their sickest patients (39).

TABLE 102.4 Desirable Characteristics for Transport Ventilators

- Adult/pediatric use (>5 kg or 11 lb)
- Transportable, rugged (<15 lb), and easily stored
- Power source (pneumatic/electric with battery backup)
- Battery life a minimum of 3 hr
- Nonproprietary, single use, universal breathing circuit
- NBC filter compliant (for use in nuclear, biologic, or chemically hazardous environments)
- V_T (50–3,000 mL)
- Rate (spontaneous: 100 breaths/min)
- F_iO_2 (at least 0.6 and 1.0, preferably adjustable between 0.21 and 1.0)
- PEEP/CPAP (0–20 cm H_2O)
- Trigger sensitivity (<5 cm H_2O, regardless of CPAP level)
- Inspiratory time (adjustable to 3.0 s)
- Breath types: Volume control (VC) and/or pressure control (PC), spontaneous continuous positive airway pressure (CPAP)
- Alarms (audible and visual) should include:
  Low pressure/disconnect
  High pressure (3–75 cm H_2O)
  Loss of power (pneumatic or electric)
  Battery low (if applicable)
  Vent-inop
  Alarm silence (at least 60 s)

Unfortunately, there are no currently manufactured, transport or emergency ventilators that can be powered either electrically or pneumatically. It seems only reasonable that disaster preparedness teams consider having at least a few pneumatic transport ventilators available; at present, with certain exceptions, this does not seem to be the case.

Spontaneous Breathing during Transport

Disaster preparedness, for possible mass casualty scenarios or avian flu outbreaks, has taken the country by storm. To meet the demand, many companies are either modifying existing ventilators for emergency use, or are bringing new products to market. Currently, dozens of brands of transport and emergency ventilators are available; this makes the selection process truly difficult, at best.

Perhaps however, a transport ventilator's spontaneous breathing capabilities provide us with a useful metric. Clearly, the act of spontaneous breathing reduces V_D (51,52,135,136). True spontaneous breathing however, dramatically improves virtually every parameter associated with V_A/Q matching. Putensen et al. (135) compared APRV, which allows unrestricted spontaneous breathing, to PSV, which provides pressure-assistance during each spontaneous breath. The APRV group demonstrated improved V_A/Q matching, venous return, right ventricular end-diastolic filling, stroke index, PaO_2, O_2 delivery, and mixed venous oxygen content, when compared to PSV (134). In addition, APRV reduced V_D, intrapulmonary shunting, pulmonary vascular resistance, and O_2 extraction when compared to PSV (134). Given the compelling strength of the data, it's surprising so few clinicians consider idea of spontaneous breathing during transport. Perhaps this oversight developed because so few transport ventilators allow effortless spontaneous breathing. Some might argue that patients do not really need to breathe spontaneously during a 10-minute transport. On the other hand, heavy sedation, paralysis, and CMV really do not appear to be in the best interest of potential avian flu victims.

Most true emergency or transport ventilators simply do not facilitate spontaneous breathing. Making matters worse, many use optional PEEP valves, which attach to the exhalation valve, and demand valves that trigger at subambient pressure; these greatly magnify patient WOB as compared to CPAP, often requiring a herculean effort to trigger and maintain flow during spontaneous breaths (see Fig. 102.19). To circumvent these issues, clinicians take one of several approaches: heavily sedate or even paralyze patients they plan to transport, thus allowing the use of CMV; or moderately sedate patients, allowing them to use the A/C mode of ventilation with minimal patient interaction.

For those wishing to avoid sedatives and paralytic agents, the transport ventilator needed is one that allows unimpeded, extremely low WOB spontaneous breathing. The pNeuton ventilator (Airon Corporation) is pneumatic and claims spontaneous WOB comparable to that of an ICU ventilator; unfortunately, this claim has not been scientifically validated. Without scientific data, testing ventilators by actually breathing on them will often expose a system's strengths and weaknesses, in terms of its spontaneous breathing claims. Considering the potential benefit to patients allowed to spontaneously breathe during transport, it is surprising there are so few scientific studies thoroughly examining WOB, as it applies to transport ventilators. Furthermore, the studies done so far are now dated; that is, they do not include many of today's newer and more popular models. For example, one study found the LTV 1000 (Pulmonetics) consistently produced WOB values comparable to those of critical care ventilators (135).

The LTV 1000 has two distinct drawbacks as a transport ventilator. First, it will not tolerate the many "crash landings" most transport ventilators must endure. Second, the LTV 1000 uses a very precise, high-speed turbine compressor. When used in a dehumidified, heated and air-conditioned environment, like a hospital, the LTV 1000 will likely work for many hours without incident. On the other hand, if the LTV 1000 is even briefly exposed to the heat and humidity, often found outdoors, and is then moved back indoors, a potential exists for condensation to develop on the turbine's bearings. If this occurs, the lifespan of the turbine can be dramatically shortened.

SIDE EFFECTS AND COMPLICATIONS

Spontaneous Breathing

An understanding of the effects of any form of positive airway pressure requires a working knowledge of the physiology that drives spontaneous breathing. Normal, spontaneous inspiration, at ambient pressure, involves contraction of the diaphragm. As the diaphragm contracts, a pressure gradient develops between the pleural space and the mouth; in response air rushes from the mouth into the lungs. During expiration, the diaphragm relaxes, the gradient reverses, and the gas leaves the lungs.

Hemodynamics

Return of venous blood to the heart is dependent upon the pressure gradient between the peripheral vasculature and the right atrium. If mean pressure rises or right atrial pressure (RAP) falls, venous return increases. Conversely, a fall in mean pressure or a rise in RAP decreases venous return. Because output of the right ventricle depends on the venous return to it, factors that alter mean pressure and RAP also affect cardiac output (136).

Intrapleural Pressure Changes

A decrease in intrapleural pressure during inhalation is associated with a similar decrease in RAP, and this enhances venous return. During exhalation, intrapleural pressure increases and venous return falls; these fluctuations are familiar to anyone who has viewed a recording of central venous pressure (CVP) in a spontaneously breathing patient.

Ventricular Interdependence

Because the right and left ventricles are surrounded by the pericardium, volume changes in one chamber affect the other. An increase in right ventricular volume during inspiration pushes the interventricular septum toward the left (posteriorly), thereby increasing left ventricular pressure; thereby increasing left ventricular pressure; this in turn reduces left ventricular filling and changes the spatial configuration and compliance of the left ventricle.

Left Ventricular Afterload

The decrease in intrapleural pressure is also transmitted to the left ventricle. At the peak of spontaneous inspiration (lowest intrapleural pressure), the left ventricular end-diastolic pressure is reduced correspondingly. In contrast, the pressure that must be developed by the ventricle to perfuse the systemic vessels outside the thoracic cavity remains the same. Because the ventricle is initiating contraction from a lower baseline pressure, however, the gradient of pressure that must be generated is increased.

The increment in necessary wall tension represents an increase of the left ventricular afterload, and may be tolerated poorly by patients with ischemia heart disease and compromised ventricular function. Spontaneous breathing with PEEP, which requires greater decrements in airway pressure and pleural pressures for gas to flow, predisposes to this chain of events. Conversely, a properly functioning CPAP system, which requires minimal deflections in airway and intrapleural pressures, minimizes such changes.

Pulmonary Vascular Changes

Expansion of the lungs also affects hemodynamic function. Alveolar vessels are compressed and elongated while pressure and alveolar volume increase. Extra-alveolar vessels, however, are opened by traction of lung inflation, with a consequent decrease in their resistance. When the alveolar vessels are engorged, inspiration decreases net pulmonary blood volume, and pulmonary venous return to the left ventricle may rise. Conversely, when alveolar vessels contain less blood, spontaneous inspiration changes alveolar blood volume very little, but a net increase in pulmonary blood volume and a concomitant decrease in pulmonary venous flow to the left ventricle occurs.

Spontaneous PEEP and CPAP

Common hemodynamic alterations seen during spontaneous PEEP or CPAP involve five major areas:

1. *Decreased venous return*: Most studies confirm increased intrapleural pressures, secondary to the increased mean airway pressures used by these modalities. This reduces the mean pressure/RAP gradient, which in turn reduces venous return. The heart has less blood to pump and output falls.
2. *Decreased right ventricular function*: Acute respiratory failure and PEEP/CPAP may, in some circumstances, increase pulmonary vascular resistance. Conceivably, the right ventricle might fail under these conditions; yet, this is probably not a major direct cause positive-pressure–induced cardiovascular insufficiency.
3. *Decreased left ventricular function*: Left ventricular dysfunction can result from increased mean airway pressures, but the changes are most likely the result of right ventricular dilatation and encroachment. Some investigators question this hypothesis, however. Prewitt and Wood (137) suggest that, in selected instances (e.g., high PEEP), 50% of the reduction in cardiac output results from left ventricular failure (138).
4. *Neural and humoral depression*: In canine cross-circulation studies, PEEP applied to one dog's lungs resulted in a reduction in cardiac output in both animals (140). The nature and composition of the depressant substance or substances is unknown.
5. *Reduction of endocardial blood flow*: It has been suggested that an increased mean airway pressure may act to impede coronary arterial blood flow (140). Such a decrease has been demonstrated, experimentally, during the use of PEEP.

Most studies show that spontaneous PEEP does not affect circulatory function adversely, as long as patients are not hypovolemic. These observations oddly, are diametrically opposed to those expected during normal breathing. This phenomenon is best explained by the fact that PEEP is not generally used on *normal* lungs; when it is, FRC is raised above normal, often significantly. With more volume in the lungs, even during exhalation, venous return may be compromised. When either PEEP or CPAP are used therapeutically, however, patients invariably have reduced compliance and a significantly reduced FRC. Collapsed and underventilated alveoli produce hypoxic vasoconstriction in the affected areas; this often markedly increases pulmonary vascular resistance and abnormal loading of the right ventricle. As end-expiratory pressure is raised, FRC increases back toward normal and underventilated alveoli re-expand; this releases some of the hypoxic vasoconstriction and unloading of the right ventricle may occur.

Sturgeon et al. (90) reported the effects of 15 cm H_2O spontaneous CPAP, 15 cm H_2O spontaneous PEEP, and zero pressure on a group of patients following coronary artery bypass grafting. When receiving spontaneous PEEP, this groups cardiac output was 1 L/min more when compared to spontaneous CPAP or zero pressure. The authors suggested that the very large intrapleural pressure drops of greater than 15 cm H_2O, required to breathe from 15 cm H_2O PEEP, resulted in a substantially greater venous return. Also, as pleural pressure increased back to the 15 cm H_2O baseline during exhalation, the associated and likely pericardial compression may have aided ventricular ejection.

Large intrapleural pressure fluctuations are not always beneficial and could easily overfill the right ventricle, resulting in an elevated left ventricular afterload. It is quite possible a "worst case scenario" might involve a patient with severe coronary artery disease and left ventricular failure, managed using a high level of spontaneous PEEP. The resultant increase in the left ventricular afterload, on an already failing myocardium, would predispose to a dramatic and potentially dangerous fall in systemic cardiac output as well as acute pulmonary edema. Substituting a properly functioning spontaneous CPAP system with a minimal trigger sensitivity would, all other things being equal, unload the left ventricle by decreasing the preloading of the right ventricle.

MECHANICAL VENTILATION

Hemodynamics

Falling Pressures

As a rule, any form of positive pressure breathing will reduce venous return and decrease right ventricular preload; with normal lungs the effect is pronounced. Even modest increases in airway pressure will elevate the FRC well above normal; an increased intrapleural pressure from the over-expanded lungs presses the pericardium and compresses the heart. These conditions make interpreting filling pressures a challenge, as the CVP and pulmonary artery occlusion pressure may be elevated while ventricular stroke volumes are actually decreased.

Ventricular Function

As stated, the elevated airway pressures associated with positive pressure breathing increase the right ventricular afterload and in turn, decrease venous inflow to the right heart. At the same time, transmural aortic pressure, left ventricular afterload, and end-systolic left ventricular volume fall. The reduced output volume is easily restored by intravascular volume expansion—enough to counteract some or all of airway pressure on venous return. If, after re-expansion of intravascular volume, the source of elevated airway pressure (i.e., ventilator or PEEP/CPAP system) is suddenly removed, a venous return surge which may be well beyond the initial baseline predisposes the patient to acute pulmonary edema (141,142); this complication is especially likely if the patient's left ventricle is compromised.

Robotham et al. (143) summarized the known and postulated effects of positive pressure inflation of the lungs on cardiopulmonary function—most of these have already been reviewed. They concluded that mechanical ventilation may act as a (relatively) noninvasive cardiac assist device and deserves further evaluation as such.

The hemodynamic effects of spontaneous breathing, with or without CPAP, and those secondary to positive pressure ventilation become complicated when combined as during IMV/SIMV with CPAP. The cumulative effect likely depends upon the relative contributions of spontaneous versus mandated breaths, as well as the absolute values of the inspiratory and expiratory pressures, V_T, baseline cardiovascular status, intravascular volume, and so forth. Ventilator performance also plays an important role, especially during spontaneous breathing.

A difficult to trigger CPAP system, or a poorly designed and slow to respond demand-flow valve, often require major inspiratory efforts by the patient. These factors were the primary reason many early trials of IMV failed; that is, patients were simply fatigued to the point of failure by work imposed by the system—not by the technique.

Barotrauma and Ventilator-Induced Lung Injury

For many years, the concept of pulmonary barotrauma was limited to extra-alveolar air leaks. It is now abundantly clear that human lungs can be damaged, internally, by the ventilator with or without air leaks; this type of damage is known as ventilator-associated lung injury (VALI).

Extra-Alveolar Air Leaks

All forms of mechanical ventilation, whether by virtue of positive or negative pressure, rhythmically drive air in and out of the lungs. As outlined, mechanical ventilation disrupts normal hemodynamics, alters V_A/Q ratios, and occasionally damages the lungs. Pulmonary barotrauma (PBT) represents the "classic" form of VALI. Pulmonary barotrauma includes pneumothorax, pneumomediastinum, pneumopericardium, pneumoperitoneum, pneumoretroperitoneum, subcutaneous air, and air embolization—either venous or arterial. Interestingly, none of these conditions actually describe *lung injury*. Rather, each of these represents a form of extra-alveolar air—each occurs after the lung fabric is torn and an air leak follows. Air leaks occur following a tear in the fabric of lung parenchyma. If the tear involves the visceral pleura, a pneumothorax often results as the air quickly moves into the pleural space, whose pressure is negative, relative to alveolar pressure, most of the time. Tension pneumothorax is the most threatening variety of this problem, and can obliterate cardiac output if not immediately decompressed. When an air leak occurs away from the pleura, the repeated stretching associated with positive pressure ventilation, facilitates the dissection of air along the perivascular sheaths that parallel the airways. Eventually, the dissecting air reaches the pulmonary hilum, where it may invade the subcutaneous tissues of the neck, or enter the mediastinum and beyond. Rarely, the rent exposes a vessel large enough for air to enter; and, with sufficient air pressure changes (positive or negative), air may enter the circulation. Scuba divers that ascend too rapidly, or hold their breath while surfacing, can easily rupture their lungs. Because divers normally surface with their head up, the air bubbles rise and may reach the brain. Cerebral air emboli can be fatal, particularly when the diver cannot be quickly recompressed in a hyperbaric chamber.

A common misconception, that PEEP and CPAP increase the incidence of barotrauma, persists even today. Yet, no increase in the incidence of barotrauma occurs when positive pressure ventilation and CPAP are compared with positive pressure alone (144).

CONCLUSION

Mechanical ventilators continue to evolve rapidly, in complexity, design, and function. It is quite likely this brisk pace will persist for many years to come. As outlined, it also seems likely that controversies regarding how and when to use ventilators safely and effectively, will not be conclusively resolved any time soon. This set of circumstances means those of us responsible for prescribing, operating, monitoring, or repairing ventilators must rise to the challenge of maintaining an up-to-date knowledge base. This is no easy task, but one that will result in significant benefits for all parties involved.

Key Points

- Consider ventilation/perfusion in the healthy lung and how it changes during respiratory failure.
- How are PEEP/CPAP or positive pressure breathing useful when managing respiratory failure?
- Define the four phases of any mechanical ventilator breath.
- What is the difference between triggering and cycling as it pertains to a ventilator breath and why does it matter?
- What is an EIP and compliance, how are they measured and used?

- What is RAM and ROM and how are they used in a mechanical ventilator?
- What is the difference between open-loop and closed-loop ventilator designs?
- Define "flow starvation" during mechanical inflation and how it is best managed?
- Describe "occult PEEP" and how it is measured at the bedside?
- How does AAV differ from APRV?
- Explain why managing work of breathing is so important to patients undergoing mechanical ventilation.
- How does proportional assist ventilation (PAV) differ from pressure support ventilation (PSV) and why neither completely solves the problem of managing a patient's work of breathing?

References

1. Kolobow T, Moretti MP, Famagalli R, et al. Severe impairment of lung function induced by high peak airway pressure during mechanical ventilation. *Am Rev Respir Dis*. 1987;135:312.
2. Tsuno K, Prato P, Kolobow T. Acute lung injury from mechanical ventilation at moderately high airway pressures. *J Appl Physiol*. 1990;69:956.
3. Bowton DL, Kong DL. High tidal volume ventilation increases lung water in oleic acid-injured rabbit lungs. *Crit Care Med*. 1989;17:908.
4. Hernandez LA, Cohen PJ, May AL, et al. Mechanical ventilation increases microvascular permeability in oleic injured lungs. *J Appl Physiol*. 1990;69:2057.
5. Taskar V, Evander JJE, Robertson B, et al. Surfactant dysfunction makes lungs vulnerable to repetitive collapse and reexpansion. *Am J Respir Crit Care Med*. 1997;155:313.
6. Argiras EP, Blakeley CR, Dunnill MS, et al. High PEEP decreases hyaline membrane formation in surfactant deficient lungs. *Br J Anaesth*. 1987; 59:1278.
7. Muscedere JG, Mullen JBM, Gan K, et al. Tidal ventilation at low airway pressures can augment lung injury. *Am J Respir Crit Care Med*. 1994;149:1327.
8. Martin C, Papazian L, Payan MJ, et al. Pulmonary fibrosis correlates with adult respiratory distress syndrome: a study in mechanically ventilated patients. *Chest*. 1995;107:196.
9. Fariday EE, Permutt S, Riley RL. Effect of ventilation on surface forces in excised dogs' lungs. *J Appl Physiol*. 1966;21:1453.
10. Brown ES, Johnson RP, Clements JA. Pulmonary surface tension. *J Appl Physiol*. 1959;14:717.
11. Fariday EE. Effect of ventilation on movement of surfactant in the airways. *Respir Physiol*. 1976;27:323 .
12. Dreyfuss D, Saumon G. Should the lungs be rested or recruited? The Charybdis and Scylla of ventilator management. *Am J Respir Crit Care Med*. 1994; 149:1066.
13. Lachmann B. Open up the lung and keep the lung open. *Intensive Care Med*. 1992;18:319.
14. va Kaam AH, Haitsma JJ, De Jaegere A, et al. Open lung ventilation improves gas exchange and attenuates secondary lung injury in a piglet model of meconium aspiration. *Crit Care Med*. 2004;32(2):443.
15. Falke KJ, Pontoppidan H, Kumar A, et al. Ventilation with end-expiratory pressure in acute lung disease. *J Clin Invest*. 1972;51:2315.
16. Suter PM, Fairley HB, Isenberg MD. Optimum end-expiratory pressure in patients with acute pulmonary failure. *N Engl J Med*. 1975;292:284.
17. Matamis D, Lemaire F, Harf A, et al. Total respiratory pressure-volume curves in the adult respiratory distress syndrome. *Chest*. 1984;86:58.
18. Benito S, Lemaire F. Pulmonary pressure-volume relationship in acute respiratory distress syndrome in adults: role of positive end-expiratory pressure. *J Crit Care*. 1990;5:27.
19. Dreyfuss D, Saumon G. Ventilator-induced lung injury: lessons from experimental studies. *Am J Resp Crit Care Med*. 1998;157:294.
20. Fernandez E, Weiner P, Meltzer E, et al. Sustained improvement in gas exchange after negative pressure ventilation for 8 hours per day on 2 successive days in chronic airflow limitation. *Am Rev Respir Dis*. 1991;144(2):390.
21. Skarburkis M, Rivero A, Fitchett D, et al. Hemodynamic effects of continuous negative chest pressure ventilation in heart failure. *Am Rev Respir Dis*. 1990;141:938.
22. Marini JJ, Capps JS, Culver BH. The inspiratory work of breathing during assisted mechanical ventilation. *Chest*. 1985;87(5):612.
23. Banner MJ, Kirby RR, Gabrielli A, et al. Partially and totally unloading the respiratory muscles based upon real-time measurements of work of breathing: a clinical approach. *Chest*. 1994;106(6):1835.
24. French CJ, Bellomo R, Buckmaster J. Effect of ventilation equipment on imposed work of breathing. *Crit Care Resus*. 2001;3(3):148.
25. Bersten AD, Rutten AJ, Verdig AE, et al. Additional work of breathing imposed by endotracheal tubes, breathing circuits, and intensive care ventilators. *Crit Care Med*. 1989;17(7):671.
26. Banner MJ, Euliano NR, Brennan V, et al. Power of breathing determined non-invasively using an artificial neural network in patients with respiratory failure. *Crit Care Med*. 2006;34:1052.
27. Banner MJ, Kirby RR, Blanch PB, et al. Decreasing imposed work of breathing apparatus to zero using pressure support ventilation. *Crit Care Med*. 1993;21(9):1338.
28. Kacmarek RM. The role of pressure support ventilation in reducing work of breathing. *Respir Care*. 1988;33(2):99.
29. Fiastro JF, Habib MP, Quan SF. Pressure support compensation for inspiratory work due to endotracheal tubes and demand continuous positive airway pressure. *Chest*. 1988;93(3):499.
30. Myny D, Depuydt P, Colardyn F, et al. Ventilator-associated pneumonia in a tertiary care ICU: analysis of risk factors for acquisition and mortality. *Acta Clin Belg*. 2005;60(3):114.
31. Jubran A. Critical illness and mechanical ventilation: effects on the diaphragm. *Respir Care*. 2006;51(9):1054.
32. Branson RD, Chatburn RL. Technical description and classification of modes of ventilator operation. *Respir Care*. 1992;37(9):1026.
33. Blanch PB, Jones MR, Layon AJ, et al. Pressure-preset ventilation. Part I. Physiologic and mechanical considerations. *Chest*. 1993;104(2):590.
34. Blanch PB, Jones MR, Layon AJ, et al. Pressure-preset ventilation. Part II. Mechanics and safety. *Chest*. 1993;104(3):904.
35. Hopewell PC, Murray JF. Effects of continuous positive pressure ventilation in experimental pulmonary edema. *J Appl Physiol*. 1976;40:568.
36. Luce JM, Huang TW, Robertson HT, et al. The effects of prophylactic expiratory positive airway pressure on the resolution of oleic acid-induced injury in dogs. *Ann Surg*. 1983;197:327.
37. Dreyfuss D, Saumon G. The role of tidal volume, FRC and end-inspiratory volume in the development of pulmonary edema following mechanical ventilation. *Am Rev Respir Dis*. 1993;148:1194.
38. Smith TC, Marini JJ. Impact of PEEP on lung mechanics and work of breathing in severe airflow obstruction. *J Appl Physiol*. 1988;65(4):1488.
39. de Boisblanc BP. Blackhawk, please come down: reflections on a hospital's struggle to survive in the wake of hurricane Katrina. *Am Rev Respir Crit Care Med*. 2005;172(10):1239.
40. Fuleihan SF, Wilson RS, Pontoppidan H. Effect of mechanical ventilation with end-expiratory pause on blood gas exchange. *Anesth Analg*. 1976;55:122.
41. Banner MJ, Lampotang S. Clinical use of inspiratory and expiratory waveforms. In: Kacmarek RM, Stoller JK, eds. *Current Respiratory Care*. Philadelphia, PA: BC Decker; 1988:139.
42. Dammann JF, McAslan TC. Optimal flow pattern for mechanical ventilation of the lungs. *Crit Care Med*. 1977;5:128.
43. Hedenstierna G, Johansson H. Different flow patterns and their effect on gas distribution in a lung model. *Acta Anaesthesiol Scand*. 1973;17: 190.
44. Jansson L, Jonson B. A theoretical study of flow patterns of ventilators. *Scand J Respir Dis*. 1972;55:237.
45. Al-Saady N, Bennett ED. Decelerating inspiratory flow waveform improves lung mechanics and gas exchange in patients on intermittent positive-pressure ventilation. *Intensive Care Med*. 1985;11:68.
46. Baker AB, Colliss JE, Cowie RW. Effects of varying inspiratory flow waveforms and time in intermittent positive-pressure ventilation. II. Various physiologic variables. *Br J Anaesth*. 1977;49:1221.
47. Johansson H, Lofstrom JB. Effects on breathing mechanics and gas exchange of different inspiratory gas flow patterns during anesthesia. *Acta Anaesthesiol Scand*. 1975;19:8.
48. Dreyfuss D, Soler G, Basset C, et al. High inflation pressure pulmonary edema: respective effects of high airway pressure, high tidal volume, and positive end-expiratory pressure. *Am Rev Respir Dis*. 1988;137:1159.
49. Dreyfuss D, Saumon G. Barotrauma is volutrauma, but which volume is the one responsible? *Intensive Care Med*. 1992;18:139.
50. Froese AB, Bryan AC. Effects of anesthesia and paralysis on diaphragmatic mechanics in man. *Anesthesiology*. 1974;41:242.
51. Downs JB, Mitchell LA. Pulmonary effects of ventilatory pattern following cardiopulmonary bypass. *Crit Care Med*. 1976;4:295.

52. Murphy EJ, Downs JB. Ventilator induced ventilation-perfusion mismatching. *Anesthesiology*. 1976;45:A345.
53. Kallet RH, Campbell AR, Dicker RA, et al. Work of breathing during lung-protective ventilation in patients with acute lung injury and acute respiratory distress syndrome: a comparison between volume and pressure-regulated breathing modes. *Respir Care*. 2005;50(12):1623.
54. Kirby RR, Robison E, Schultz J. Continuous flow ventilation as an alternative to assisted or controlled ventilation in infants. *Anesth Analg*. 1972;51:871.
55. Kirby RR, Robison E, Shultz J. A new pediatric volume ventilator. *Anesth Analg*. 1971;50:533.
56. Munson ES, Eger EI II. Controlled ventilation in the newborn. *Anesthesiology*. 1963;24:871.
57. Downs JB, Klein EF, Desautels D. Intermittent mandatory ventilation: a new approach to weaning patients from mechanical ventilators. *Chest*. 1973; 64:331.
58. Desautels DA. PEEP and open IMV systems. *Respir Care*. 1977;22(11):1230.
59. Bruining HA. Two simple assemblies for the application of intermittent mandatory ventilation with positive end expiratory pressure. *Intensive Care Med*. 1984;10(1):33.
60. Downs JB. Inappropriate applications of IMV. *Chest*. 1980;78(6):897.
61. Groeger JS, Levinson MR, Carlon GC. Assist control versus synchronized intermittent mandatory ventilation during acute respiratory failure. *Crit Care Med*. 1989;17:607.
62. Kirby RR. Synchronized intermittent mandatory ventilation versus assist control: just the facts ma'am. *Crit Care Med*. 1989;17:706.
63. Kirby RR, Perry JC, Calderwood HW. Cardiorespiratory effects of high end-expiratory pressure. *Anesthesiology*. 1975;43:533.
64. Kirby RR, Downs JB, Civetta JM. High level positive end-expiratory pressure (PEEP) in acute respiratory insufficiency. *Chest*. 1975;67:156.
65. Poulton TJ, Downs JB. Humidification of rapidly flowing gas. *Crit Care Med*. 1981;9:59.
66. Op't Holt TB. Work of breathing and other aspects of patient interaction with PEEP devices and systems. *Respir Care*. 1988;33(6):444.
67. Op't Holt TB, Hall MW, Bass JB, et al. Comparisons of changes in airway pressure during continuous positive airway pressure (CPAP) between demand valve and continuous flow devices. *Respir Care*. 1982;27(10):1200.
68. Gibney NR, Wison RS, Pontoppidan H. Comparison of work of breathing on high gas flow and demand valve continuous positive airway pressure systems. *Chest*. 1982;82(6):692.
69. Henry WC, West GA, Wilson RA. A comparison of the oxygen cost of breathing between a continuous-flow CPAP system and a demand-flow system. *Respir Care*. 1983;28(10):1273.
70. Katz JA, Kraemer RW, Gjerde GE. Inspiratory work and airway pressure with continuous positive airway pressure delivery systems. *Chest*. 1985;88(4):519.
71. Shapiro BA, Harrison RA, Walton JR. Intermittent demand ventilation (IDV): a new technique for supporting ventilation in critically ill patients. *Respir Care*. 1976;21:521.
72. Hasten RW, Downs JB, Heenan TJ. A comparison of synchronized and nonsynchronized intermittent mandatory ventilation. *Respir Care*. 1980;25:554.
73. Heenan TJ, Downs JB, Douglas ME. Intermittent mandatory ventilation: is synchronization important? *Chest*. 1980;77:598.
74. Yang KL, Tobin MJ. A prospective study of indexes predicting the outcome of trials of weaning from mechanical ventilation. *N Engl J Med*. 1991;324(21):1445.
75. Esteban A, Anzueto A, Alia I, et al. How is mechanical ventilation employed in the intensive care unit? An international utilization review. *Am J Respir Crit Care Med*. 2000;161:1450.
76. Brochard L, Harf A, Lorino H, et al. Inspiratory pressure support prevents diaphragmatic fatigue during weaning from mechanical ventilation. *Am Rev Resp Dis*. 1989;33:99.
77. MacIntyre NR, Ho LI. Effects of initial flow rate and breath termination criteria on pressure support ventilation. *Chest*. 1991;99:134.
78. Bolder PM, Healy EJ, Bolder AR, et al. The extra work of breathing through adult endotracheal tubes. *Anesth Analg*. 1986;65:853.
79. MacIntyre NR. Weaning from mechanical ventilatory support: volume-assisting intermittent breaths versus pressure-assisting every breath. *Respir Care*. 1988;33:121.
80. MacIntyre NR. Pressure support ventilation. *Prob Crit Care*. 1990;4:225.
81. Kirton OC, DeHaven B, Hudson-Civetta J, et al. Re-engineering ventilatory support to decrease days and improve resource utilization. *Ann Surg*. 1996;224(3):396.
82. Reynolds EOR. Effect of alterations in mechanical ventilator settings on pulmonary gas exchange in hyaline membrane disease. *Arch Dis Child*. 1971;46:159.
83. Spahr RC, Klein AM, Brown DR, et al. Hyaline membrane disease: a controlled study of inspiratory to expiratory ratio and its management by ventilator. *Am J Dis Child*. 1980;134:373.
84. Tharatt RS, Allen RP, Albertson TE. Pressure controlled inverse ratio ventilation in severe adult respiratory failure. *Chest*. 1988;94:755.
85. Gurevitch MJ, Van Dyke J, Young ES, et al. Improved oxygenation and lower peak airway pressure in severe adult respiratory syndrome: treatment with inverse ratio ventilation. *Chest*. 1986;89:211.
86. Duncan SR, Rizk NW, Raffin TA. Inverse ratio ventilation: PEEP in disguise? (editorial). *Chest*. 1989;92:390.
87. Kacmarek RM, Hess D. Pressure-controlled inverse-ratio ventilation: panacea or auto-PEEP? (editorial). *Respir Care*. 1990;35(10):945.
88. Pepe P, Marini JJ. Occult positive end-expiratory pressure in mechanically ventilated patients with airflow obstruction: the auto-PEEP effect. *Am Rev Respir Dis*. 1982;126(1):166.
89. Gherini S, Peters RM, Virgilio RW. Mechanical work on the lung and work of breathing with positive end expiratory pressure and continuous positive airway pressure. *Chest*. 1979;76:251.
90. Sturgeon CL, Douglas ME, Downs JB, et al. PEEP and CPAP: cardiopulmonary effects during spontaneous ventilation. *Anesth Analg*. 1977;56:633.
91. Kirby RR, Downs JB, Civetta JM, et al. High level positive end-expiratory pressure (PEEP) in acute respiratory failure. *Chest*. 1975;67(2):156.
92. Civetta JM, Kirby RR. Criteria for optimum PEEP. *Respir Care*. 1977;22 (11):1171.
93. Rasanen J, Downs JB, DeHaven B. Titration of continuous positive airway pressure by real-time oximetry. *Chest*. 1987;92(5):853.
94. Mrochen H. Optimum PEEP using a desk top computer. *Int J Biomed Comput*. 1982;13(4):303.
95. Kram HB, Appel PL, Fleming AW, et al. Determination of optimum positive end-expiratory pressure by means of conjunctival oximetry. *Surgery*. 1987;101(3):329.
96. Rasanen J, Cane R, Downs JB, et al. Airway pressure release ventilation in severe acute respiratory failure. *Crit Care Med*. 1989;17:S32.
97. Banner MJ, Kirby RR, Banner TE. Airway pressure release ventilation in patients with acute respiratory failure. *Crit Care Med*. 1989;17(4):S32.
98. Florete O, Banner MJ, Banner TE, et al. Airway pressure release ventilation in a patient with acute pulmonary injury. *Chest*. 1989;96:679.
99. Stock MC, Downs JB, Frolicher DA. Airway pressure release ventilation. *Crit Care Med*. 1987;15:462.
100. Garner W, Downs JB, Stock MC, et al. Airway pressure release ventilation: a human trial. *Chest*. 1988;94:779.
101. Bratzke E, Downs JB, Smith RA. Intermittent CPAP: a new mode of ventilation during general anesthesia. *Anesthesiology*. 1998;89:334.
102. Strandberg A, Tokics L, Brismar B, et al. Atelectasis during anesthesia and in the postoperative period. *Acta Anaesthesiol Scand*. 1986:30(2):154.
103. Badenes R, Lozano A, Belda FJ. Postoperative pulmonary dysfunction and mechanical ventilation in cardiac surgery. *Crit Care Res Pract*. 2015;2015:420513.
104. D'Angio CT, Chess PR, Kovacs SJ, et al. Pressure-regulated volume control vs synchronized intermittent mandatory ventilation for very low birth weight infants: a randomized controlled trial. *Acrh Pediatr Adolesc Med*. 2005;159(9):868.
105. Gulager H, Nielsen SL, Carl P, et al. A comparison of volume control and pressure-regulated volume control in acute respiratory failure. *Crit Care*. 1997;1(2):75.
106. Younes M. Proportional assist ventilation, a new approach to ventilatory support. Theory. *Am Rev Respir Dis*. 1992;145(1):114.
107. Younes M, Puddy A, Roberts D, et al. Proportional assist ventilation: results of an initial clinical trial. *Am Rev Respir Dis*. 1992;145(1):121.
108. Giannouli E, Webster K, Roberts D, et al. Response of ventilator-dependent patients to different levels of pressure support and proportional assist. *Am J Respir Crit Care Med*. 1999;159(6):1716.
109. Hart N, Hunt A, Polkey MI, et al. Comparison of proportional assist ventilation and pressure support ventilation in chronic respiratory failure due to neuromuscular and chest wall deformity. *Thorax*. 2002;57(11):979.
110. Passam F, Hoing S, Prinianakis G, et al. Effect of different levels of pressure support and proportional assist ventilation on breathing pattern, work of breathing, and gas exchange in mechanically ventilated hypercapnic COPD patients with acute respiratory failure. *Respiration*. 2003;70(4):355.
111. Varelmann D, Wrigge H, Zinserling J, et al. Proportional assist versus pressure support ventilation in patients with acute respiratory failure: cardiorespiratory responses to artificially increased ventilatory demand. *Crit Care Med*. 2005;33(9):2125.
112. Vitacca M. New things are not always better: proportional assist ventilation vs pressure support ventilation. *Intensive Care Med*. 2003;29(7):1038.

113. Appendini L. Proportional assist ventilation: back to the future? *Respiration*. 2003;70(4):345.
114. Bernard GR, Artigas A, Brigham KL, et al. American-European Consensus Conference on ARDS: definitions, mechanisms, relevant outcomes and clinical trial coordination. *Am J Resp Care Med*. 1994;149(3):818.
115. Gattinoni L, Pesenti A, Torresin A, et al. Adult respiratory distress syndrome profiles by computed tomography. *J Thorac Image*. 1986;3:25.
116. Gattinoni L, Pesenti A, et al. ARDS: the non-homogeneous lung; facts and hypothesis. *Intesive Crit Care Dig*. 1987;6:1.
117. Gattinoni L, Pesenti A. The concept of 'baby lung. *Intensive Care Med*. 2005;31(6):776.
118. Ventilation with lower tidal volumes as compared with traditional tidal volume for acute lung injury and acute respiratory distress syndrome. The Acute Respiratory Distress Syndrome Network. *N Engl J Med*. 2000; 342:1301.
119. Briel M, Meade M, Mercal A, et al. Higher vs lower positive end-expiratory pressure in patients with acute lung injury and acute respiratory distress syndrome: systemic review and meta-analysis. *JAMA*. 2010;303(9):865.
120. Brower R, Lanker P, MacIntyre N, et al. Higher versus lower positive end-expiratory pressure in patients with acute respiratory distress syndrome. National Heart, Lung, and Blood Institute ARDS Clinical Trial Network. *N Engl J Med*. 2004;351(4):327.
121. Meade M, Cook D, Guyatt G, et al. Ventilation strategy using low tidal volumes, recruitment maneuvers, and high positive end-expiratory pressure for acute lung injury and acute respiratory distress syndrome: a randomized controlled trial. *JAMA*. 2008;229(6):637.
122. Mathru M, Rao T, Venus B. Ventilator-induced barotauma in controlled mechanical ventilation versus intermittent mandatory ventilation. *Crit Care Med*. 1983;11(5):359.
123. Beck J, Tucci M, Emeriaud G, et al. Prolonged neural expiratory time induced by mechanical ventilation in infants. *Pediatr Res*. 2004;55:747.
124. Thille A, Rodriguez P, Cabello B, et al. Patient-ventilator asynchrony during assisted mechanical ventilation. *Intensive Care Med*. 2006;32:1515.
125. Brodssoule A, Emeriaud G, Morneau S, et al. Neurally adjusted ventilatory assist improves patient-ventilator interaction in infants as compared with conventional ventilation. *Pediatr Res*. 2012;72(2):194.
126. Beck J, Reilly M, Grasselli G, et al. Patient-ventilator interaction during neutrally adjusted ventilatory assist in low birth weight infants. *Pediatr Res*. 2009;65(6):663.
127. Stein H, Alosh H, Ethington P, et al. Prospective crossover comparison between NAVA and pressure control ventilation on premature neonates. *J Perinatol*. 2013;33:452.
128. Breatnach C, Conlon N, Stack M, et al. A prospective crossover comparison of neutrally adjusted ventilatory assist and pressure support ventilation in a pediatric intensive care unit population. *Pediatr Crit Care Med*. 2010;11(1):7.
129. Alander M, Petoniemi T, Kontiokar T. Comparison of pressure-, flow-, and NAVA-triggering in pediatric and neonatal ventilatory care. *Pediatr Pulmonol*. 2012;47(1):76.
130. Stein H, Howard D. Neurally adjusted ventilatory assist in neonates weighing <1500 grams: a retrospective analysis. *J Pediatr*. 2012;160(5):786.
131. Gervais HW, Eberle B, Konietzke D, et al. Comparison of blood gases of ventilated patients during transport. *Crit Care Med*. 1987;15(8):761.
132. Braman SS, Dunn SM, Amico CA, et al. Complications of intrahospital transport in critically ill patients. *Ann Intern Med*. 1987;107(4):469.
133. Hurst JM, Davis JR, Branson RD, et al. Comparison of blood gases during transport using two methods of ventilatory support. *J Trauma*. 1989;29(12):1637.
134. Nakamura T, Fujino Y, Uchiyama A, et al. Intrahospital transport of critically ill patients using ventilator with patient-triggering function. *Chest*. 2003;123(1):159.
135. Putensen C, Mutz NJ, Putensen-Himmer G, et al. Spontaneous breathing during ventilatory support improves ventilation–perfusion distribution in patients with acute respiratory distress syndrome. *Am J Respir Crit Care Med*. 1999;159(4):1241.
136. Austin PN, Campbell RS, Johannigman JA, et al. Work of breathing of seven portable ventilators. *Resuscitation*. 2001;49(2):159.
137. Prewitt RM, Wood LH. Effects of positive end-expiratory pressure on ventricular function in dogs. *Am J Physiol*. 1972;236:H534.
138. Pinsky MR. Cardiovascular effects of ventilatory support and withdrawl. *Anesth Analg*. 1994;79:567.
139. Patten MT, Liebman PR, Hechtman HB. Humorally medicated decrease in cardiac output associated with positive end-expiratory pressure. *J Microvasc Res*. 1977;13:137.
140. Laver MB. The pulmonary response to trauma and mechanical ventilation: its consequences on hemodynamic function. *World J Surg*. 1983;7:31.
141. Beach T, Millen E, Grenvik A. Hemodynamic response to discontinuation of mechanical ventilation. *Crit Care Med*. 1973;1:85.
142. Robotham JL, Cherry D, Mitzner W, et al. A reevaluation of the hemodynamic consequences of intermittent positive pressure ventilation. *Crit Care Med*. 1983;11:783.
143. Kumar A, Pontoppidan H, Falke KJ, et al. Pulmonary barotrauma during mechanical ventilation. *Crit Care Med*. 1973:1:181.
144. Kirby RR. Best PEEP: issues and choices in the selection and monitoring of PEEP levels. *Respir Care*. 1988;33:569.

CHAPTER
103
Noninvasive Ventilatory Support Modes

MASSIMO ANTONELLI, GENNARO DE PASCALE, and GIUSEPPE BELLO

INTRODUCTION

Noninvasive ventilation (NIV) refers to the provision of ventilatory assistance using techniques that do not bypass the upper airway. The theoretical advantages of NIV include avoiding the complications associated with endotracheal intubation, improving patient comfort, and preserving airway defense mechanisms. NIV may be delivered through various devices including negative and positive-pressure ventilators. During the first half of the 20th century, negative-pressure ventilation was the main means of providing mechanical ventilatory assistance outside the anesthesia suite. Because of several disadvantages relative to negative-pressure ventilation, including patient discomfort, restrictions on positioning, lack of airway protection, problems with correct fitting, time-consuming application, and lack of portability, negative-pressure ventilators have seen diminishing use in favor of positive-pressure assistance modes since the early 1960s. Therefore, only positive-pressure support modes are discussed here.

The following sections deal with the history and epidemiology of NIV, as well as currently available equipment and techniques, practical applications, appropriate indications, and possible adverse effects. In this chapter, continuous positive airway pressure (CPAP) delivered noninvasively is referred to as CPAP. The use of intermittent positive-pressure ventilation (IPPV) with or without positive end-expiratory pressure (PEEP) is referred to as NIV.

BACKGROUND

The first report of noninvasive positive-pressure dates to 1912, when Bunnell (1) used a face mask to maintain lung expansion during thoracic surgery. In 1936, Poulton and Oxon (2) used a vacuum cleaner to generate gas flow and a spring-loaded valve to oppose expiration to treat a patient with cardiogenic pulmonary edema (CPE). A number of studies conducted by Barach et al. (3–5) over the 1930s showed that CPAP delivered through a face mask could be useful in the treatment of CPE and other forms of respiratory failure. Noninvasive IPPV administered through a mouthpiece was first described by Motley (6) in the 1940s and was used widely until the early 1980s, either for aerosol delivery in patients with chronic obstructive pulmonary disease (COPD) and asthma, or as a means of ventilatory assistance. The use of noninvasive IPPV declined sharply after the demonstration of lack of benefit in comparison to simple nebulizing treatments (7).

The proliferation of NIV occurred during the 1980s, after the introduction of nasal mask ventilation in the management of obstructive sleep apnea (8). Despite a lack of randomized controlled trials, NIV became the ventilatory mode of first choice for patients with neuromuscular diseases and chest wall deformities (9–12). In the early 1990s, the encouraging results obtained in the treatment of acute respiratory failure (ARF) by using NIV (13–15) stimulated investigation on various applications in the acute care setting. The desire of avoiding complications of endotracheal intubation (16–19), potentially lowering morbidity and mortality rates in selected patients with ARF (20–23), has been the major driving force of the increasing use of NIV in the acute care setting over the past decades.

In their 28-day international study on patients admitted to 361 ICUs who received mechanical ventilation for more than 12 hours, Esteban et al. (24) found that NIV through a facial mask was used in 4.9% of overall patients and in 16.9% of patients ventilated because of an exacerbation of COPD. Similarly, in a prospective 3-week survey of 70 French ICUs performed in 2002, Demoule et al. (25) showed that 23% of patients requiring ventilatory assistance received NIV as a first-line treatment; a significant increase compared to 1997 (16%) (26). Also the incidence of NIV for patients admitted to the ICU without tracheal intubation was strongly implemented.

Interestingly, NIV-implementing programs outside the ICU coordinated by a medical emergency team (MET) may also be introduced in clinical practice, with a high success rate and few complications (27). The estimated utilization rate in the clinical setting remains markedly varied, mainly due to differences in physician knowledge and adequate equipment (28).

EQUIPMENT AND TECHNIQUES

The following paragraphs will discuss various interfaces and ventilatory modes available for administration of NIV; cough-enhancing techniques will also be described.

Interfaces

Interfaces are devices that connect ventilator tubing to the face, allowing the delivery of pressurized gas into the airway during NIV. Currently available interfaces include nasal and oronasal masks, helmets, and mouthpieces. Selection of a comfortable interface that fits properly is a key issue for the success of NIV.

Nasal Masks

The standard nasal mask is a triangular or cone-shaped clear plastic device that fits over the nose and uses a soft cushion or flange to seal over the skin (Fig. 103.1). Because of the pressure exerted over the bridge of the nose, the mask may cause skin irritation and redness, and occasionally ulceration (Fig. 103.2). For the occasional patient who cannot tolerate commercially available masks, custom-molded, individualized masks that conform to facial contours of the patient can be constructed. Several types of strap systems have been used to hold the mask in place. Depending on the interface, straps

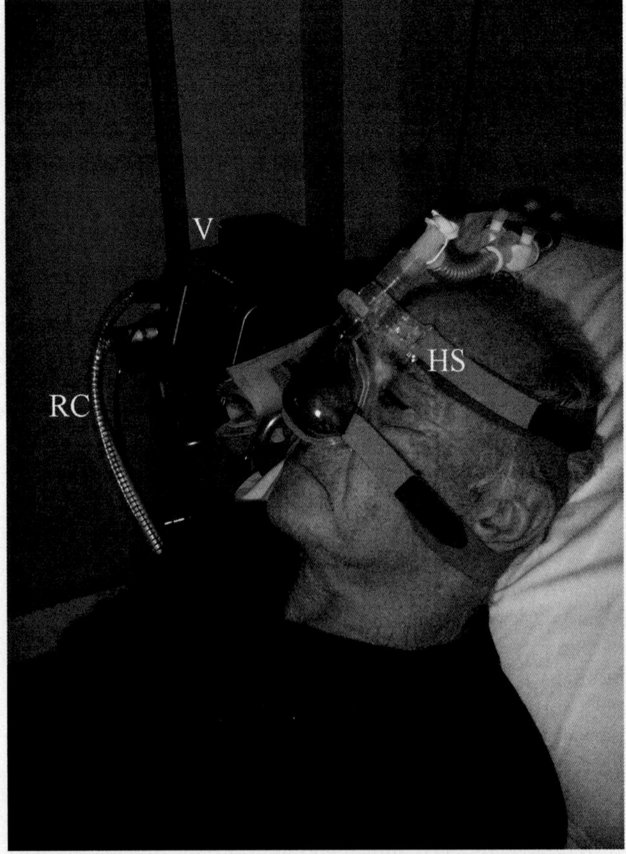

FIGURE 103.1 Noninvasive ventilation delivered through a nasal mask. HS, head straps; RC, respiratory circuit; V, ventilator. (Photograph printed with the permission of the patient.)

attach at two or as many as five points on the mask and may be provided with Velcro fasteners. The nasal mask is generally preferred for chronic administration of NIV. In patients with a nasogastric tube, a seal connector in the dome of the mask may be used to avoid air leakage.

Nasal Pillows

Nasal pillows or seals consist of soft rubber or silicone plugs that are inserted directly into the nostrils (Fig. 103.3). As they exert no pressure over the bridge of the nose, nasal pillows

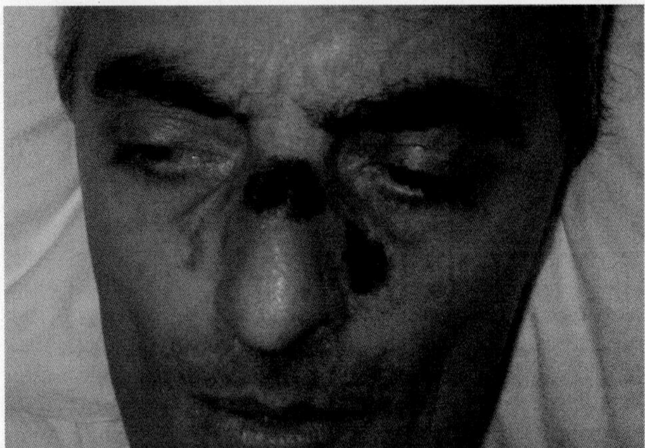

FIGURE 103.2 Skin lesions caused by a mask. Please note that the point at major risk to develop a skin necrosis is the bridge of the nose. (Photograph printed with the permission of the patient.)

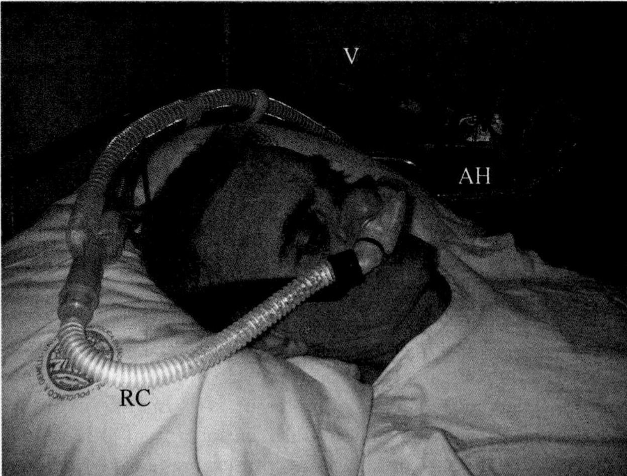

FIGURE 103.3 Noninvasive ventilation delivered through nasal pillows. AH, active humidifier; RC, respiratory circuit; V, ventilator. (Photograph printed with the permission of the patient.)

may be useful in patients who develop irritation or ulceration on the nasal bridge while using nasal or oronasal masks.

Oronasal Masks

Oronasal or face masks cover both the nose and the mouth (Fig. 103.4). The oronasal mask is largely used in patients with copious air leaking through the mouth during nasal

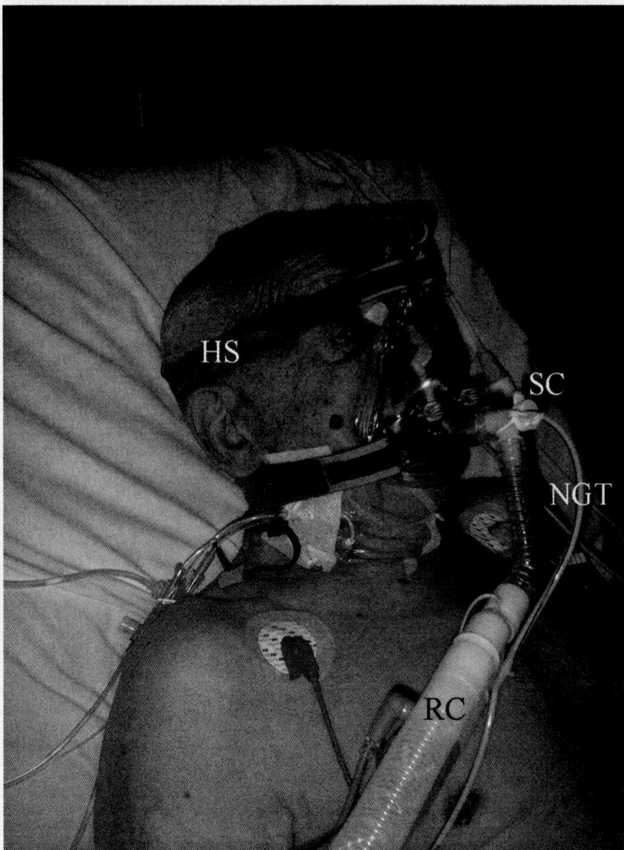

FIGURE 103.4 Noninvasive ventilation delivered through an oronasal mask. HS, head straps; NGT, nasogastric tube; RC, respiratory circuit; SC, seal connection. (Photograph printed with the permission of the patient.)

mask ventilation. Interference with speech, eating, and expectoration, and the likelihood of claustrophobic reactions, are greater with oronasal than with nasal masks. In the acute setting, however, oronasal masks are preferable to nasal masks because dyspneic patients are mouth breathers, predisposing to greater air leakage during nasal mask ventilation. The oronasal masks, like the nasal mask, may cause skin necrosis over the nasal bridge (29). When the opening pressure of the upper esophageal sphincter (25 to 30 cm H_2O) is overcome, the positioning of a nasogastric tube may protect from gastric distension, even though this is not a common event.

A type of oronasal mask is the "full" face mask, which is made of clear plastic and uses a soft silicone flange that seals around the perimeter of the face avoiding direct pressure on facial structures. Over last years, new face mask models have been diffused with the aim at improving patient comfort and interface performance. Characteristics of recent models of full face mask include a lightweight design, a seal connector specifically dedicated to the passage of the feeding tube, a soft and thin membrane of the mask contour, and a mask holder that incorporates more than four points of attachment to secure the head straps.

Helmet

The standard helmet (Fig. 103.5) is made of transparent latex-free polyvinyl chloride, and is secured by two armpit braces at the plastic ring that joins the helmet with a seal connection soft collar adherent to the neck (30,31). The pressure increase during ventilation makes the soft collar sealing comfortable to the neck and shoulders, avoiding air leakage (30). The whole apparatus is connected to an ICU ventilator by a standard respiratory circuit. The two ports of the helmet act as inlet and outlet for inspiratory and expiratory gas flows. The inspiratory and expiratory valves are those of the mechanical ventilator. A specific connector placed in the plastic ring can be used to allow the passage of a nasogastric tube, thus reducing air leaks. A security valve is used to reduce the risk of asphyxia. The patient is allowed to drink through a straw or to be fed a liquid diet. Two inner inflatable cushions may be used to increase comfort and reduce the internal volume. The main

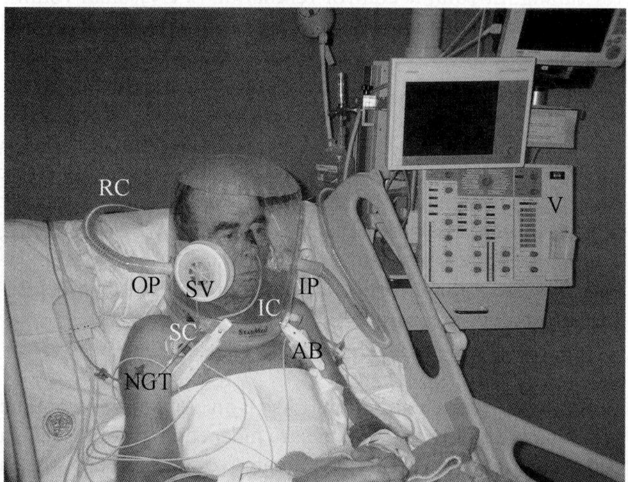

FIGURE 103.5 Noninvasive ventilation delivered through a helmet. AB, armpit braces; IC, inflated cushion; IP, inlet port; NGT, nasogastric tube; OP, outlet port; RC, respiratory circuit; SC, seal connection; SV, security valve. (Photograph printed with the permission of the patient.)

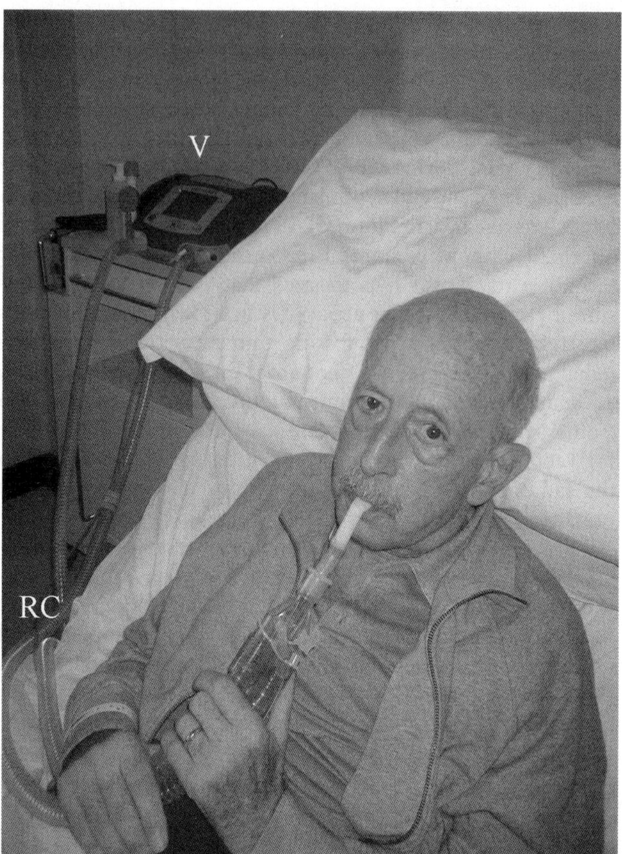

FIGURE 103.6 Noninvasive ventilation delivered through a mouthpiece. RC, respiratory circuit; V, ventilator. (Photograph printed with the permission of the patient.)

advantages of the helmet include a good tolerability in both adult and pediatric populations (32), with a satisfactory interaction of the patients with the environment; a lower risk of dermal lesions; and, compared with the mask, easier applicability to any patient regardless of the face contour. In a recent model of helmet, a zip opening ensures patient accessibility without the need to remove the interface, and alternative fastening systems on the top of the helmet cab avoid skin damage along the braces of the armpits.

Mouthpieces

Mouthpieces are simple and inexpensive devices used to provide NIV for as long as 24 hours a day to patients with chronic respiratory failure (Fig. 103.6). If nasal air leaking reduces efficacy, ventilator tidal volume may be increased or cotton plugs or nose clips may be used for occluding the nostrils. NIV via mouthpieces has proved to be a valid alternative to tracheostomy in some patients with chronic respiratory muscle insufficiency (33).

CPAP and Ventilatory Modes

Continuous Positive Airway Pressure

CPAP delivers a constant pressure throughout spontaneous inspiration and exhalation without assisting inspiration. Because spontaneous breathing is not assisted, this technique requires an intact respiratory drive and adequate alveolar ventilation. CPAP increases functional residual capacity and opens underventilated alveoli, thus decreasing right-to-left intrapulmonary shunt and improving oxygenation and lung mechanics (34). Moreover, CPAP may reduce the work of breathing and dyspnea in COPD patients by counterbalancing the inspiratory threshold load imposed by intrinsic PEEP (35). Effects on hemodynamics during CPAP have been widely described. By lowering left ventricular transmural pressure in patients with left congestive heart failure, CPAP may reduce left ventricular afterload without compromising cardiac index (36,37). For several years, it was hypothesized that positive airway pressure, by increasing right atrial pressure (38), reduced venous return by decreasing the pressure gradient between mean systemic filling pressure and right atrial pressure (39). However, as demonstrated in experimental (40,41) and human (42) studies, positive airway pressure does not affect the gradient for venous return, because pleural pressure is transmitted to the same extent to both the mean systemic and right atrial pressures. CPAP can be applied by various devices including low-flow generators with an inspiratory reservoir, high-flow jet venturi circuits (Fig. 103.7)—both of them with an expiratory mechanical or water valve—and bilevel and critical care ventilators. Continuous positive pressure may be administered using the demand flow (DF) or the gold standard continuous flow (CF) system. With DF CPAP, the patient has to trigger a preset pressure to open the demand valve, whereas with CF CPAP, no valves are present. The work of breathing is significantly greater with the DF system than with the CF system (43–45). It is crucial to provide an adequate airflow rate for maintaining a continuous positive pressure, especially in dyspneic patients who breathe at high-flow rates. A low CPAP level may be obtained by delivering oxygenation through high-flow nasal cannula (HFNC). During HFNC at a flow rate of 35 L/min in patients with the mouth closed, a mean nasopharyngeal airway pressure of 2.7 cm H_2O has been measured (46).

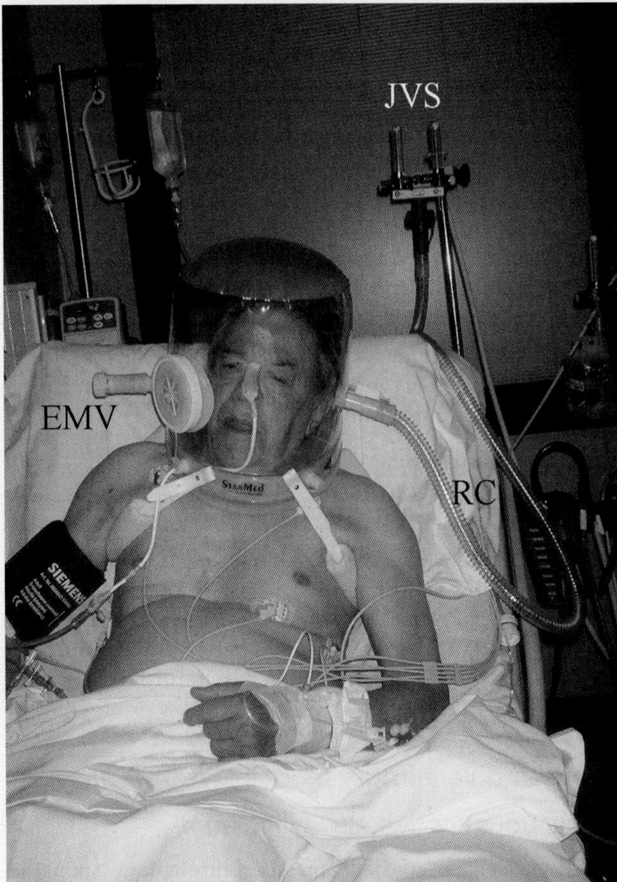

FIGURE 103.7 Helmet continuous positive airway pressure (CPAP) delivered by a high-flow jet venturi system. EMV, expiratory mechanical valve; JVS, jet venturi system; RC, respiratory circuit. (Photograph printed with the permission of the patient.)

Pressure Support Ventilation

Pressure support ventilation (PSV) is a pressure-triggered, pressure-targeted, flow-cycled mode of ventilation. It delivers a preset inspiratory pressure to assist spontaneous breathing, augmenting spontaneous breaths and offsetting the work imposed by the breathing apparatus. A sensitive patient-initiated trigger causes the delivery of inspiratory pressure support that is maintained throughout inspiration, and a reduction in inspiratory flow drives the ventilator to cycle into expiration. Therefore, the patient can control either inspiratory duration or breathing rate.

Bilevel Positive Airway Ventilation

In bilevel positive airway pressure (BiPAP), a valve sets two pressure levels, the expiratory positive airway pressure (EPAP) level, and the inspiratory positive airway pressure (IPAP) level, even in the presence of rapidly changing flows. With this technique, ventilation is produced by the cyclic delta pressure between the IPAP and EPAP. EPAP also recruits underventilated lung and offsets eventual intrinsic PEEP.

Controlled Mechanical Ventilation

In the mandatory controlled mechanical ventilation (CMV) mode, no patient effort is required, as full ventilatory support is provided. In this mode, ventilator settings include inflation pressure or tidal volume, frequency, and the timing of each breath. Pressure control ventilation (PCV) delivers time-cycled preset inspiratory and expiratory pressures with adjustable inspiratory-to-expiratory ratios at a controlled rate. The resulting tidal volume is determined by the compliance of the lungs and chest wall, and the resistance to flow of ventilator tubing. In volume control ventilation (VCV), tidal volume is set and the resulting pressure depends on the thoracic and circuit compliance.

Assist/Control Ventilation

In assist/control (A/C) ventilation, the ventilator delivers a breath either when triggered by the patient's inspiratory effort (assist) or independently, if such an effort does not occur within a preselected time period (control). When triggering occurs, the ventilator delivers an identical breath to mandatory breaths; volume-cycled and pressure-limited or pressure-targeted modes are available.

Proportional Assist Ventilation

Proportional assist ventilation (PAV) is an alternative technique in which both flow and volume are independently adjusted. In this technique, the ventilator generates volume and pressure in proportion to the patient's effort, increasing comfort and so improving success and compliance with NIV (47). Despite the promising concept, there is a substantial lack of large clinical studies (48).

Techniques to Assist Cough

The cough mechanism may be severely impaired in neuromuscular diseases when weak expiratory muscles are combined with a markedly reduced vital capacity. An effective cough depends on the ability to generate adequate expiratory airflow, estimated at more than 160 L/min (49), which is determined by lung and chest wall elasticity, airway conductance, and expiratory muscle force. Additionally, intact glottic function is needed for yielding high peak expiratory cough flows. Manually assisted coughing consists of quick thrusts applied to the abdomen using the palms of the hands, timed to coincide with the patient's cough effort. The maneuver should be applied cautiously after meals and with the patient positioned semi-upright to reduce the risk of aspiration of gastric contents.

Manually assisted coughing may enhance expiratory force, but it does not increase inspired volume, so that patients with severely restricted volumes may still achieve insufficient cough flows. Such a limitation may be overcome by using the mechanical insufflator–exsufflator (MI-E) (Fig. 103.8), which delivers a positive inspiratory pressure of 30 to 40 cm H_2O via a face mask and then rapidly switches to an equal negative pressure (50). The positive pressure produces an adequate tidal volume, whereas the negative pressure stimulates the high peak expiratory cough flows. An MI-E may be combined with manually assisted coughing to further augment cough effectiveness. In a randomized trial, patients who were extubated and allocated to three daily sessions of MI-E experienced a lower rate of reintubations and postextubation ICU length of stay (51). In any event, all the techniques used to assist cough can be performed effectively and frequently by skilled caregivers, with minimal discomfort to the patient.

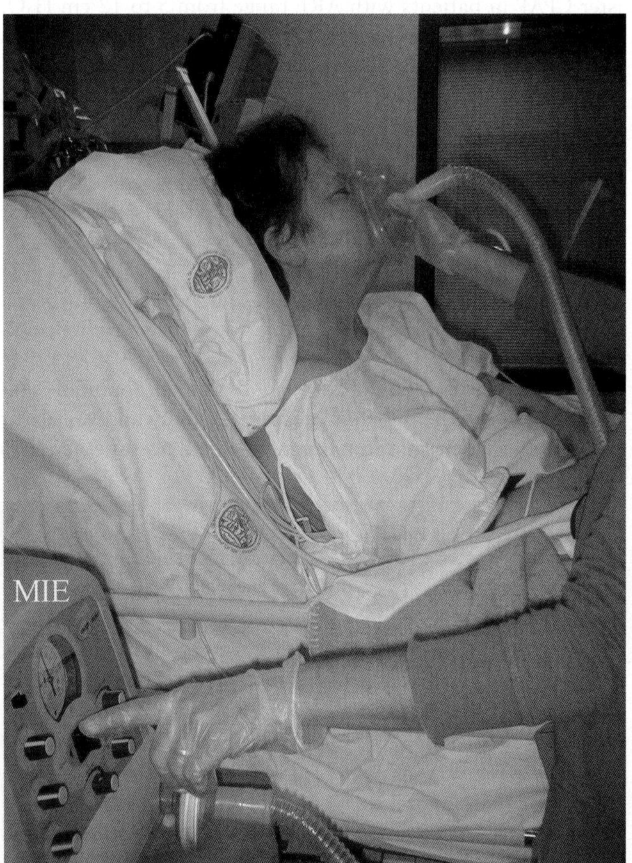

FIGURE 103.8 Mechanical insufflator–exsufflator (MIE). (Photograph printed with the permission of the patient.)

TABLE 103.1 Criteria for Noninvasive Ventilation Discontinuation and Endotracheal Intubation

- Technique intolerance (pain, discomfort, or claustrophobia)
- Inability to improve gas exchanges and/or dyspnea
- Hemodynamic instability or evidence of shock, cardiac ischemia, or ventricular dysrhythmia
- Inability to improve mental status within 30 min after the application of NIV in hypercapnic, lethargic COPD patients or agitated hypoxemic patients

PRACTICAL APPLICATION

NIV should be considered early when patients first develop signs of incipient respiratory failure needing ventilatory assistance. It is crucial that caregivers can identify patients who are likely to benefit from NIV and exclude those for whom NIV would be unsafe. Once the decision to institute NIV has been taken, an interface and ventilatory mode must be chosen, and a close monitoring in an appropriate hospital location must be provided. The initial approach should consist in fitting the interface and familiarizing the patient with the apparatus, explaining the purpose of each piece of equipment. Patients should be motivated and reassured by the clinician, instructed to coordinate their breathing with the ventilator, and encouraged to communicate any discomfort or fears. Collaboration among medical practitioners including physicians, respiratory therapists, and nurses is critical to the success of NIV. Aggressive physiotherapy is crucial during the periods of NIV discontinuation. Endotracheal intubation must be rapidly accessible, when indicated (Table 103.1).

Patient Selection

The criteria for selecting appropriate patients to receive NIV for ARF include clinical indicators of acute respiratory distress, such as moderate-to-severe dyspnea, tachypnea, accessory muscle use and paradoxical abdominal breathing, and gas exchange deterioration. Blood gas parameters aid in identifying patients with acute or acute superimposed on chronic CO_2 retention. A conscious and cooperative patient is crucial for initiating NIV (Table 103.2), although hypercapnic patients with narcosis who are otherwise good candidates for NIV may be an exception (52,53).

TABLE 103.2 Contraindications to Noninvasive Ventilation

- Coma, seizures, or severe central neurologic disturbances
- Inability to protect the airway or clear respiratory secretions
- Unstable hemodynamic conditions (blood pressure or rhythm instability)
- Upper airway obstruction
- Severe upper gastrointestinal bleeding
- Recent facial surgery, trauma, burns, deformity, or inability to fit the interface (unless a helmet is used)

During NIV, patients can achieve a level of control and independence totally different from when intubated, and sedation is infrequently required. If benzodiazepines or opiates are administered, caution is advised to prevent undue hypoventilation. NIV should be avoided in patients with hemodynamic instability and in those who are unable to protect the airways (i.e., coma, impaired swallowing) (see Table 103.2). Patients with severe hypoxemia (PaO_2/FiO_2 <100) or morbid obesity (>200% of ideal body weight) should be closely managed only by experienced personnel and with a low threshold for endotracheal intubation (20,21,54). In the presence of a pneumothorax, NIV can be initiated provided an intercostal drain is inserted. Criteria for NIV discontinuation and endotracheal intubation must be thoroughly considered to avoid dangerous delays (see Table 103.1).

Identification of predictors of success or failure may help in recognizing patients who are appropriate candidates for NIV and those in whom NIV is not likely to be effective, thereby avoiding its application and unnecessary delays before invasive ventilation is given.

Predictors of NIV failure observed in COPD patients with ARF are the following:

- Lower arterial pH at baseline (55,56)
- Greater severity of illness, as indicated by Acute Physiology and Chronic Health Evaluation (APACHE) II score (57)
- Inability to coordinate with the ventilator (57)
- Inability to minimize the amount of mouth leak with nasal mask ventilation (57)
- Less efficient or less rapid correction of hypercapnia, pH, or tachypnea in the early hours (57)
- Functional limitations caused by COPD before ICU admission, evaluated using a score correlated to home activities of daily living (ADL) (56)

Predictors of NIV failure observed in hypoxemic patients with ARF are the following:

- Higher severity score (Simplified Acute Physiology Score [SAPS] II ≥35 (58), SAPS II >34 (59), higher SAPS II (60))
- Older age (>40 years) (58)
- Presence of acute respiratory distress syndrome (ARDS) or community-acquired pneumonia (58,60,61)
- Failure to improve oxygenation after 1 hour of treatment (PaO_2/FiO_2 ≥146 (58), PaO_2/FiO_2 ≥175 (59))
- Higher respiratory rate under NIV (61)
- Need for vasopressors (61)
- Need for renal replacement therapy (61)

Ventilation Mode Selection

The choice of the correct ventilatory mode is crucial for achieving physiologic and clinical benefit during NIV. However, each ventilation mode has theoretical advantages and limitations.

Work of breathing during ARF may be significantly reduced if the selection is made properly. In a physiologic study (62) performed in hypoxemic patients with ARF, noninvasive PSV combined with PEEP improved dyspnea and gas exchange, and lowered neuromuscular drive and inspiratory muscle effort; in these patients, CPAP used alone improved oxygenation but failed to unload the respiratory muscles.

The application of external PEEP is a valid strategy to counterbalance the effects of dynamic hyperinflation in patients with acute hypercapnic exacerbations of COPD. In this setting, NIV delivered through different ventilator modes can provide respiratory muscle rest and improve respiratory physiologic parameters. No difference in clinical outcome or arterial blood gases between patients ventilated in ACV and PSV modes has been found, even though PSV is in general better accepted by the patients and associated with fewer side effects in comparison with ACV mode (63). However, in patients with severe chest wall deformity or obesity, who typically need higher inflation pressures, VCV may be preferred.

Triggering systems are critical to the success of NIV in both assist and control modes. During assisted ventilation, flow triggering reduces breathing effort more effectively as compared with pressure triggering, obtaining a better patient–ventilator interaction (64). Similarly, in COPD patients, the increase of expiratory trigger (10% to 70% of peak expiratory flow) may reduce the magnitude of delayed cycling, intrinsic PEEP and nontriggering breaths (65).

There are no clear recommendations or specific requirements from bench studies on the performance of NIV ventilators and interfaces (66). Personal experience, clinical setting, etiology, and severity of the pathologic process responsible for ARF should lead physicians' decisions; however assisted modes, particularly PSV, are more often used. As regards pressure-targeted ventilation, it is thought that starting at low pressures to facilitate patient tolerance (appropriate initial pressures are a CPAP of 3 to 5 cm H_2O and an inspiratory pressure of 8 to 12 cm H_2O above CPAP) is appropriate and then, if necessary, to gradually increase pressures, as tolerated, to obtain alleviation of dyspnea, decreased respiratory rate, adequate exhaled tidal volume, and good patient–ventilator interaction (Table 103.3). Pressures commonly used to administer CPAP in patients with ARF range from 5 to 12 cm H_2O. In patients with hypoxemic ARF and bilateral pulmonary infiltrates, undergoing 10 cm H_2O CPAP delivered via a helmet, adding a 25 cm H_2O sigh for 8 seconds, once a minute, improved oxygenation (67). Oxygen supplementation should be targeted to achieve an oxygen saturation above 92% or between 85% and 90% in patients at risk of worsening hypercapnia. A modality that provides a backup rate is necessary for patients with inadequate ventilatory drive.

Patient-Ventilator interaction and Carbon Dioxide Rebreathing

NIV tolerance is strictly correlated with an optimal synchrony between the patient's breathing activity and ventilator parameters. When an optimal patient–ventilator interaction is

TABLE 103.3 Proposed Ventilator Settings for Pressure Support Ventilation Mode

	Initial Setting	Treatment Setting
PEEP	3–5 cm H_2O	Slowly increased to up to 8–12 cm H_2O in hypoxemic patients
PSV	8–12 cm H_2O	Increased as tolerated to 20 cm H_2O to obtain an exhaled tidal volume of about 7 mL/kg and respiratory rate <25 breaths/min
FiO_2	Titrated to achieve an arterial saturation >90% or 85–90% in patients at risk of worsening hypercapnia	Titrated to achieve an arterial saturation >90% or 85–90% in patients at risk of worsening hypercapnia

lacking, increase in the work of breathing and patient discomfort may be remarkable (68). Patient–ventilator asynchrony may be determined by a number of events including ineffective triggering, double-triggering, auto-triggering, premature cycling, and delayed cycling.

During NIV in PS modality, several forms of patient–ventilator asynchrony may occur, causing breathing discomfort. In a multicenter French study, the level of pressure support and the magnitude of leaks were identified as independent predictors of increased patient–ventilator asynchrony (number of ineffective breaths and delayed cycling) (69). In addition, ineffective triggering due to excessive levels of PS (17.5 cm H_2O vs. 15 cm H_2O) and less sensitive inspiratory triggers has been shown contributing to longer duration of mechanical ventilation (17.5 vs. 7.5 days) (70). Eventual air leaks during noninvasive PSV may impede the inspiratory flow decay required to open the expiratory valve, thereby prolonging inspiratory flow. In these circumstances, air leaks should be minimized by optimizing the fitting or size of the interface, or even switching to another type of interface. To reduce leaks, it may also be helpful to decrease ventilator pressure settings as much as allowed by clinical parameters. In older machines, when an air leak occurs, an option to obtain a better patient–ventilator interaction is to select pressure-limited, time-cycled ventilation modes, or even PSV mode with a maximal inspiratory time. With ventilators that allow changing the cycling off criteria (expiratory trigger), raising the cycling off airflow threshold (i.e., the percentage of peak inspiratory flow at which transition from inspiration to expiration occurs) can activate an earlier switchover to expiration, thus avoiding prolonged insufflations and patient–ventilator asynchrony.

Pressurization rate is another parameter that can be modified during PS NIV in order to reduce patient–ventilator asynchrony. In COPD patients, faster values are able to reduce the diaphragmatic metabolic consumption (expressed as pressure time product) but may determine significant air leaks and poor tolerance (71). Similarly, in hypoxemic subjects, a "fast" pressure ramp significantly decreased the work of breathing even though either the lowest or the highest pressurization rates were associated with patient discomfort (72). In the presence of significant air leaks, pressure-targeted modes are preferred to deliver NIV as they can maintain delivered tidal volume better than volume-targeted modes (73). In new ventilators, an NIV algorithm, usually referred to as "NIV mode," measures and compensates leaks in order to minimize their detrimental impact on patient–machine synchrony (74,75). Neurally adjusted ventilatory assist (NAVA) seems to a very promising mode to help improve adaptation during NIV (76–78).

An optimal ventilator setting should also take into account the type of interface used to deliver NIV. It has been advised that the highest PEEP and PS levels clinically indicated and tolerated by the patient should be applied when NIV is administered with the helmet, in order to increase the elastance of the system, enhancing the trigger sensitivity (79). Vargas et al. (80) suggested that increasing both PEEP and PS levels and using the highest pressurization rate may be suitable when providing NIV through this interface. In their study, the helmet with the same settings as the face mask was associated with less inspiratory-muscle unloading and with worse patient–ventilator asynchrony. In contrast, specific settings with a fast ramp and higher pressures provided results similar to the mask, ameliorating the inspiratory trigger delay, without discomfort. In addition, as observed in a helmet NIV bench study, a double tube circuit (with one inspiratory and one expiratory line) seems to improve patient–ventilator interaction and reduce the rate of wasted efforts, compared with a standard circuit (a Y-piece connected only to one port of the helmet) (81).

Humidification

Prolonged exposure of tracheobronchial epithelium to cool and dry gases may be a clinical issue during NIV. So, both humidification and warming may be required to prevent upper airways irritation. Two humidifying devices are commonly used with ICU ventilators: heated humidifiers (HHs), and heat and moisture exchangers (HMEs). The latter are the most commonly used due to their simplicity and cost-effectiveness. However, because the HMEs are placed between the Y-piece and the patient, they add a substantial amount of dead space, compared to an HH, which is placed in the inspiratory circuit. In addition, compared to HHs, HMEs may increase resistance to flow (82).

Heated humidification during NIV in patients with ARF can minimize work of breathing and improve CO_2 clearance. In a physiologic study on nine COPD patients with hypercapnic ARF requiring NIV, Lellouche et al. (83) showed that the use of HMEs, compared with HHs, greatly increased work of breathing. Nonetheless, despite significantly higher minute ventilation during the HME study phase, arterial partial pressure of CO_2 ($PaCO_2$) was not different. By way of contrast, in another study on 24 patients with ARF undergoing face mask NIV with HME or HH, Jaber et al. (84) found that HME was associated with a significantly higher $PaCO_2$.

Given the above-mentioned physiologic implications, in a recent randomized clinical trial, a multicenter French study group tested the hypothesis that HH use during NIV, compared with HME, could reduce the rate of intubation in patients with ARF (both hypoxemic and hypercapnic). Surprisingly, no differences in terms of intubation rate, ICU or hospital length of stay and ICU mortality were observed between the two groups, even in the subgroup of hypercapnic patients (85). In addition, no difference in the patients' mucosal dryness was reported with HH in comparison with HME. The authors concluded that HHs during NIV cannot be recommended as a first-line treatment in all patients with ARF but they may be considered in the presence of persistent high $PaCO_2$ levels associated with threatening encephalopathy. Additionally, in COPD patients under long-term NIV, no firm conclusion can be drawn on the type of humidification system to be used. A randomized crossover 1-year study on 16 COPD patients receiving long-term NIV with either HH or HME, showed that compliance with treatment and occurrence of infections were similar with HH and HME, albeit patients with HH showed less dryness of the throat (86). Of note, at the end of this study, a higher number of patients decided to continue NIV with HH.

Monitoring

In the acute setting, patients can initiate NIV anywhere, at the onset of the acute respiratory distress, but after initiation, they should be transferred to an ICU or a step-down unit for continuous monitoring until they are sufficiently stable to be moved to a medical ward. During transfers, NIV and monitoring should not be discontinued. The early use of NIV for less acutely ill patients with COPD on a medical ward seems to be effective,

TABLE 103.4 Monitoring of Patients Receiving Noninvasive Ventilation in the Acute Care Setting

- Level of consciousness
- Comfort
- Chest wall motion
- Accessory muscle recruitment
- Patient–ventilator synchrony
- Respiratory rate
- Exhaled tidal volume
- Flow and pressure waveforms
- Heart rate
- Blood pressure
- Continuous electrocardiography
- Continuous oximetry
- Arterial blood gas at baseline, after 1–2 hr, and as clinically indicated
- Level of consciousness

but if pH is lower than 7.30, admission to an environment with intensive care monitoring is highly recommended (87).

Monitoring of patients undergoing NIV is aimed at determining whether the initial goals are being achieved, including relief of symptoms, reduced work of breathing, improved or stable gas exchange, good patient–ventilator synchrony, and patient comfort (Table 103.4). Gas exchange is monitored by continuous oximetry and arterial blood gases at baseline, after 30 to 60 minutes, and as clinically indicated; physiologic responses are evaluated by continuous electrocardiography, respiratory rate, blood pressure, and heart rates. Finally, dyspnea, as well as tolerance of the technique, symptoms of impaired sleep, patient–ventilator asynchrony, and air leaking can be easily assessed through patient queries, bedside observation, and flow, volume, and pressure waveform analysis. If a poor response to NIV occurs and the specific measures used to correct the situation fail to address an adequate improvement, NIV should be considered a failure, and invasive ventilation should be promptly considered.

INDICATIONS

Acute Exacerbations of Chronic Obstructive Pulmonary Disease (COPD-E)

In patients with ARF resulting from acute COPD-E, the use of NIV has been proven to be effective in ameliorating dyspnea, improving vital signs and gas exchange (87–91), preventing endotracheal intubation (88–91), and improving hospital survival (87,88,90). Consequently, there is a general agreement concerning the early use of NIV in such patients (92,93). In a 10 years (from 1998 to 2008) prevalence study on more than 7 million patients with acute COPD-E, a 462% increase in NIV use and a 42% decline in invasive mechanical ventilation use were observed. Surprisingly, the study documented a rising mortality rate in the subgroup of patients who needed endotracheal intubation after failing NIV (94). Such findings were explained by patients' severity, the time before NIV failure and possible difficulties with the interface tolerance (95).

In COPD patients with acute respiratory decompensations, the increased flow resistance and the impossibility to complete the expiration before inspiration determine high levels of dynamic hyperinflation, and substantial shortening of the diaphragm and the inspiratory intercostals and accessory muscles, thereby reducing their mechanical efficiency and endurance. The need to overcome the inspiratory threshold load due to auto-PEEP and to drive the tidal volume against airway resistances increases the respiratory muscle fatigue. During NIV, the combination of external PEEP and PSV offsets the auto-PEEP level and reduces the work of breathing that the inspiratory muscles must generate to produce the tidal volume (96).

In an early study on the use of face mask NIV in patients with ARF, Meduri et al. (13) obtained improvements of gas exchanges and avoided endotracheal intubation in a group of COPD patients. Soon thereafter, Brochard et al. (14) described the short-term (45 minutes) physiologic effects of inspiratory assistance with a face mask on gas exchange and respiratory-muscle work in 11 patients with COPD and evaluated the therapeutic use of the technique in 13 patients with COPD-E, comparing the results in the latter group with the results of conventional treatment in 13 matched historical-control patients. In the physiologic study, arterial pH rose from 7.31 to 7.38 ($p < 0.01$), $PaCO_2$ fell from 68 to 55 mmHg ($p < 0.01$), PaO_2 rose from 52 to 69 mmHg ($p < 0.05$), and respiratory rate reduced from 31 to 21 breaths per minute ($p < 0.01$) (14). Only 1 of 13 patients treated with NIV needed intubation, as compared with 11 of the 13 historical controls ($p < 0.001$). In addition, the NIV-treated patients were weaned from the ventilator faster and spent less time in the ICU than did the control subjects (14). Subsequently, numerous randomized controlled trials using NIV in ARF caused by COPD have been published (Table 103.5).

In the first randomized, prospective study on 60 COPD patients, Bott et al. (89) compared NIV delivered through nasal mask with conventional therapy as a treatment of ARF. Patients receiving NIV had a significant reduction of $PaCO_2$, dyspnea score, and 30-day mortality (10% vs. 30%). A multicenter European trial (88) on the efficacy of NIV in acute COPD-E randomized 85 COPD patients to receive face mask PSV or conventional treatment (oxygen therapy plus drugs). After 1 hour of NIV, respiratory rate, but not $PaCO_2$, showed a significant decrease. The group of patients treated with NIV had a significantly lower intubation rate, a lower complication rate (14% vs. 45%), length of hospital stay, and mortality rate. In another randomized study on 23 COPD patients that compared NIV with conventional treatment, the investigators reported a reduction of intubation rate, with a significant improvement in PaO_2, heart rate, and respiratory rate in the NIV group, even though $PaCO_2$ did not significantly decrease (90). A randomized study on 30 COPD patients with ARF (91) confirmed that early application of NIV facilitates gas exchange improvement, reduces the need for invasive mechanical ventilation, and decreases the duration of hospitalization. In a randomized trial on 50 acute COPD-E patients, NIV reduced weaning time, shortened the length of stay in the ICU, decreased the incidence of nosocomial pneumonia, and improved 60-day survival rates (99). Other and more recent prospective randomized controlled studies on patients with ARF due to COPD-E (103,104) have confirmed the benefit of applying NIV in improving clinical status and blood gases.

A randomized prospective study by Conti et al. (102) compared the short- and long-term response to face mask NIV

TABLE 103.5 Main Randomized Controlled Studies Using Noninvasive Ventilation in Chronic Obstructive Pulmonary Disease

Reference	Population	Site	Intervention (NIV/control)	Sample Size (NIV/control)	Need for ETI (NIV/control, %)	ICU LOS (NIV/control, days)	Hospital LOS (NIV/control, days)	Survival (NIV/control, %)
Bott et al., 1993 (89)	COPD	Ward	ACV/UMC	30/30	0.0/6.6	NA/NA	9/9	90[a]/70
Brochard et al., 1995 (88)	COPD	ICU	PSV/UMC	43/42	25.6[a]/73.8	7 ± 3[a]/19 ± 13	23 ± 17[a]/35 ± 33	90.7[a]/71.4
Kramer et al., 1995 (90)	Varied	ICU	BiPAP/UMC	11/8[b]	9.1[a]/66.6[b]	NA/NA	14.9 ± 3.3/17.3 ± 3.0[b]	NA/NA
Barbé et al., 1996 (97)	COPD	Ward	BiPAP/UMC	10/10	0/0	NA/NA	10.6 ± 0.9/11.3 ± 1.3	100/100
Angus et al., 1996 (98)	COPD	IRCU	PSV/UMC	9/8	NA/NA	NA/NA	NA/NA	100/62.5
Celikel et al., 1998 (91)	COPD	ICU	PSV/UMC	15/15	6.7[a]/40.0	NA/NA	11.7 ± 3.5[a]/14.6 ± 4.7	100/93.3
Nava et al., 1998 (99)	Weaning	ICU	PSV/PSV (invasive)	25/25	NA/NA	15.1 ± 5.4[a]/24 ± 13.7	NA/NA	92[a]/72
Confalonieri et al., 1999 (100)	CAP	IRCU	PSV/UMC	12/11[b]	0.0[a]/54.6[b]	0.25 ± 2.1[a]/7.6 ± 2.2[b]	14.9 ± 3.4/22.5 ± 3.5[b]	91.7/81.8[b]
Plant et al., 2000 (87)	COPD	Ward	BiPAP/UMC	118/118	15[a]/27	NA/NA	NA/NA	90[a]/80
Martin et al., 2000 (101)	Varied	ICU	BiPAP/UMC	12/11[b]	25/45[b]	NA/NA	NA/NA	92/91[b]
Conti et al., 2002 (102)	COPD	ED	PSV/ACV, PSV (invasive)	23/26	52/NA	22 ± 1/21 ± 20	NA/NA	74/54

NIV, noninvasive ventilation; ETI, endotracheal intubation; ICU; intensive care unit; LOS, length of stay; COPD, chronic obstructive pulmonary disease; ACV, assist control ventilation; UMC, usual medical care; NA, not applicable; BiPAP, bilevel positive airway pressure; IRCU, intermediate respiratory care unit; PSV, pressure support ventilation; Weaning, patients in whom NIV was used to facilitate weaning from mechanical ventilation; CAP, community-acquired pneumonia.

[a]Significant difference.

[b]Subset analysis.

versus invasive conventional ventilation in COPD patients with ARF failing to sustain the initial improvement with conventional medical therapy in the emergency department and needing ventilatory assistance. In this study, the intubation rate of 52% in the NIV group was higher than in other randomized controlled trials, which is not surprising given the higher severity of illness of these patients, as evidenced by the mean pH of 7.2, compared with 7.27 in the study of Brochard et al. (88) and 7.32 in the study of Plant et al. (87). Although the patients who received NIV were sicker than those reported in previous studies, they showed a trend toward a lower incidence of nosocomial pneumonia during the ICU stay and a better outcome at a 1-year follow-up, as well as no significant differences in ICU and hospital mortality, overall complications, duration of mechanical ventilation and ICU. These findings support early use of NIV during the course of acute exacerbation of COPD patients. However, if NIV is started later, after the failure of medical treatment, it is comparable to invasive mechanical ventilation in terms of survival.

In a matched case-control study conducted in ICU, 64 COPD patients with advanced ARF (pH ≤7.25, $PaCO_2$ ≥70 torr, and respiratory rate ≥35 breaths/min) prospectively received NIV, and their outcomes were compared with those of a control group of 64 COPD patients (105). NIV had a high rate of failure (40/64), although mortality rate, duration of mechanical ventilation, and lengths of ICU and post-ICU stay were not different between the two groups, and the NIV group had fewer complications. In this study, patients who failed NIV were not harmed by the delayed institution of invasive ventilation, and those who avoided endotracheal intubation had a clear-cut benefit. Based on these results, the authors suggested that in COPD patients with advanced ARF, it might be worthwhile to attempt a trial of NIV prior to a shift to invasive ventilation with endotracheal intubation.

In summary, NIV should be considered the first-line therapeutic option to prevent endotracheal intubation and improve outcome in patients with exacerbations of COPD who have no contraindication to NIV (see Table 103.3).

Asthma

NIV is considered an option in asthmatic patients at risk for endotracheal intubation. However, mechanical ventilation may be dangerous in patients with asthma, first, by worsening lung hyperinflation with the risk of causing barotrauma, and second, by inducing hemodynamic deterioration by increased intrathoracic pressure. To date, guidelines for NIV in severe asthma are not supported by strong data. In one study (106), only 2 of 17 severe asthmatic patients (average initial pH of 7.25 and $PaCO_2$ of 65 mmHg) required intubation after starting therapy with face mask PSV, and the use of NIV was associated with a rapid correction of gas exchange abnormalities and improvement in dyspnea. A retrospective analysis of 33 asthmatic patients treated with NIV or invasive mechanical ventilation (107) found that, although the NIV patients were less hypercapnic than the other group, gas exchange and vital signs improved rapidly in the NIV group, and only three patients eventually required endotracheal intubation. A prospective, randomized, placebo-controlled study compared 15 patients with acute asthma who received NIV plus conventional therapy versus conventional therapy alone, and found an improvement in lung function and decreased hospital admission rate in the NIV group (108). In contrast, another randomized trial found no significant advantages of NIV in patients with acute asthma (109), and medical therapy alone can be highly effective in the management of asthmatic patients (110). Therefore, in the absence of clear evidence, no conclusions can be drawn regarding the relative effectiveness of NIV versus conventional therapy in acute exacerbations of asthma.

Hypoxemic Respiratory Failure

Trials of NIV in patients with hypoxemic respiratory failure, defined as those with ARF not related to COPD, have yielded conflicting results. In hypoxemic ARF patients, NIV has been adopted to decrease the amount of work of breathing, correct the rapid shallow breathing, and prevent respiratory muscle fatigue and endotracheal intubation. The studies reviewed in these sections have been conducted on heterogeneous groups of patients with hypoxemic respiratory failure, whereas the analyses of homogeneous patient populations are discussed under each specific topic. Randomized controlled trials using NIV in hypoxemic ARF patients are shown in Table 103.6.

Meduri et al. (13) in 1989 reported one of the first clinical applications of NIV in patients with hypoxemic respiratory failure. Subsequently, Pennock et al. (116) reported a 50% success in a large group of patients with ARF of different causes, and similar good results were achieved using NIV with nasal mask in a second study (117). Wysocki et al. (111) randomized 41 non-COPD patients with ARF to NIV delivered by face mask versus conventional medical therapy. NIV reduced the need of endotracheal intubation, the duration of ICU stay, and mortality rate only in those patients with hypercapnia ($PaCO_2$ >45 mmHg), while having no significant advantages in the hypoxemic group without concomitant hypercarbia. On the basis of these results, the investigators concluded that NIV may not be beneficial in all forms of ARF not related to COPD. In a study conducted by Meduri et al. (118) on the use of NIV to treat respiratory failure of varied origins, 41 of 158 patients were hypoxemic. These patients required endotracheal intubation in only 34% of cases and showed a mortality rate of 22% compared with a predicted mortality (using the APACHE II score) of 40%. In a pilot study on patients with hematologic malignancies complicated by ARF (119), 15 of 16 individuals showed a significant improvement in blood gases and respiratory rate within the first 24 hours of nasal mask NIV treatment.

Antonelli et al. (20) conducted a prospective, randomized study comparing NIV via a face mask to endotracheal intubation with conventional mechanical ventilation in 64 patients with hypoxemic ARF who required ventilatory assistance after failure to improve with aggressive medical therapy. After 1 hour of mechanical ventilation, both groups had a significant improvement in oxygenation. Ten (31%) patients treated with NIV required endotracheal intubation. Patients randomized to conventional ventilation developed significantly more frequent septic complications such as pneumonia or sinusitis (31% vs. 3%). Among survivors, NIV patients had a lower duration of mechanical ventilation ($p = 0.006$) and a shorter ICU stay ($p = 0.002$). On the basis of these results, this trial suggested that NIV may lead to more favorable outcomes than conventional ventilation in the management of patients with hypoxemic respiratory failure. Conversely, Wood et al.

TABLE 103.6 Main Randomized Controlled Studies Using Noninvasive Ventilation I\In Nonchronic Obstructive Pulmonary Disease

Reference	Population	Site	Intervention (NIV/control)	Sample size (NIV/control)	Need for ETI (NIV/control, %)	ICU LOS (NIV/control, days)	Hospital LOS (NIV/control, days)	Survival (NIV/control, %)
Wysocki et al., 1993 (111)	Varied	ICU	PSV + PEEP/UMC	21/20	62/70	17 ± 19/25 ± 23	NA/NA	65/70
Antonelli et al., 1998 (20)	AHRF	ICU	PSV + PEEP/ACV, SIMV	32/32	31.3/NA	9 ± 7[a]/16 ± 17	NA/NA	68.8/50.0
Wood et al., 1998 (112)	Varied	ED	Bi PAP/UMC	16/11	45.5/43.8	5.8 ± 5.5/4.9 ± 3.2	17.4 ± 34.3/9.1 ± 5.7	75/100
Girault et al., 1999 (113)	Weaning	ICU	PSV, ACV/PSV	17/16	NA/NA	12.4 ± 6.8/14.1 ± 7.5	27.7 ± 13.1/27.1 ± 14.3	100/87.5
Confalonieri et al., 1999 (100)	CAP	IRCU	PSV/UMC	16/17[b]	37.5/47.1[b]	2.9 ± 1.8/4.8 ± 1.7[b]	17.9 ± 2.9/15.1 ± 2.8[b]	62.5[a,c]/76.5[b]
Antonelli et al., 2000 (21)	IC	ICU	PSV + PEEP/UMC	20/20	20/70[a]	5.5 ± 3/9 ± 4[a]	NA/NA	65/45
Martin et al., 2000 (101)	Varied	ICU	BiPAP/UMC	16/13[b]	37.5[a]/77.0[b]	NA/NA	NA/NA	75/46[b]
Hilbert et al., 2001 (114)	IC	ICU	PSV + PEEP/UMC	26/26	46/77[a]	7 ± 3/10 ± 4	NA/NA	50/81[a]
Ferrer et al., 2003 (115)	AHRF	ICU	BiPAP/UMC	51/54	25[a]/52	9.6 ± 12.6/11.3 ± 12.6	20.7 ± 16.6/26.8 ± 19.8	82[a]/61

NIV, noninvasive ventilation; ETI, endotracheal intubation; ICU, intensive care unit; LOS, length of stay; PSV, pressure support ventilation; PEEP, positive end-expiratory pressure; UMC, usual medical care; NA, not applicable; AHRF, acute hypoxemic respiratory failure; ACV, assist control ventilation; SIMV, synchronous mandatory ventilation; ED, emergency department; BiPAP, bilevel positive airway pressure; Weaning, patients in whom NIV was used to facilitate weaning from mechanical ventilation; CAP, community-acquired pneumonia; IRCU, intermediate respiratory care unit; IC, immunocompromised.

[a]Significant difference.

[b]Subset analysis.

[c]Hospital survival (no difference noted in 2-month mortality).

(112) had a substantially negative evaluation of the use of NIV when applied to patients with hypoxemic ARF. These investigators randomized 27 patients in the emergency department to receive conventional medical therapy or NIV for the treatment of hypoxemic respiratory failure. The 16 patients who were randomized to the NIV group had an intubation rate and duration of ICU stay similar to the 11 patients who received medical treatment alone, but there was a trend toward a greater rate of hospital mortality among the patients in the NIV group compared to patients in the conventional medical therapy group. Several factors may have influenced these negative results of this study. Among patients requiring endotracheal intubation, those of the NIV group had a longer delay to intubation (26 vs. 4.8 hours, $p = 0.055$). In addition, it cannot be excluded that a sicker patient population was randomized to NIV. Indeed, the NIV population had a lower PaO_2 (60 vs. 71), fewer patients with COPD (12% vs. 36%), and more patients with pneumonia (44% vs. 18%), ARDS, and interstitial lung disease (1 vs. 0). Furthermore, the NIV group had a higher APACHE II score (18 vs. 16), and more required admission to an ICU (81% vs. 64%).

In a study on 10 hemodynamically stable patients with severe acute lung injury or ARDS (120), NIV had a high success rate (66%) and high hospital survival (70%). Three of the six patients who received NIV as initial mode of ventilatory assistance were discharged from the ICU within 48 hours. Survival for the 10 patients was 70%, and duration of successful NIV ranged from 23 to 80 hours. Ferrer et al. (121) have prospectively randomized 105 patients with severe hypoxemic ARF to receive NIV or high-concentration oxygen. Compared with oxygen therapy, NIV decreased the need for intubation (13 [25%] vs. 28 [52%]), the incidence of septic shock (6 [12%] vs. 17 [31%]), and ICU mortality (9 [18%] vs. 21 [39%]), and increased the cumulative 90-day survival (all, $p < 0.05$). Additionally, the improvement of tachypnea and arterial hypoxemia was higher in the NIV group. In a physiologic study performed by L'Her et al. (122) in patients with acute lung injury, noninvasive PSV combined with PEEP improved dyspnea and gas exchange and lowered neuromuscular drive and inspiratory muscle effort.

In ARDS, transient loss of positive pressure during mechanical ventilation may seriously compromise lung recruitment and gas exchange. For this reason, most NIV studies have excluded patients with ARDS, and limited data are currently available in the literature. The first application of NIV (via face mask CPAP) in patients with increased permeability pulmonary edema ARDS was reported by Barach et al. in 1938 (4). In 1982, Covelli et al. (123) applied face mask CPAP in 35 patients with ARDS of varied causes, with all patients improving their oxygenation within the first hour of therapy. Only five patients were ultimately intubated, two from mask discomfort and three from a change in mental status and lack of cooperation. In two randomized studies, Antonelli et al. (20,21) reported that among patients with ARDS ($n = 31$), NIV avoided intubation in 60%, whereas in their trial including a small number of ARDS patients ($n = 7$), Ferrer et al. (121) reported an 86% intubation rate. Two NIV observational studies involving 98 ARDS patients reported an intubation rate of 50% (58,120), which was similar in patients with ARDS of pulmonary or extrapulmonary origin (58). Antonelli et al. (59) prospectively investigated, under close ICU observation, the application of NIV as first-line intervention in 147 patients with early ARDS. NIV improved gas exchange and avoided intubation in 54% of treated patients. Avoidance of intubation was associated with less ventilator-associated pneumonia (2% vs. 20%, $p < 0.001$) and a lower ICU mortality rate (6% vs. 53%, $p < 0.001$). SAPS II more than 34 and a PaO_2/FIO_2 less than 175 after 1 hour of NIV were independently associated with NIV failure and need for endotracheal intubation. Caution is, however, required when NIV is used in hypoxemic patients. In a large prospective French survey (524 patients), NIV failure was found to be independently associated with ICU mortality in patients with "de novo" ARF rather than in those ones affected by CPE or COPD-E (124). In 2012, a new ARDS definition was promulgated (125). Therefore, further studies in such setting could be useful in order to better identify patients who can benefit from early NIV application. A decisional flow chart may be adopted in applying NIV to patients with ARDS (Fig. 103.9).

The above findings are, for the most part, supportive of the use of NIV to treat hypoxemic patients without hypercapnia. However, an extremely prudent approach is needed, limiting the application of NIV to hemodynamically stable patients who can be closely monitored in the ICU where endotracheal intubation is promptly available.

Cardiogenic Pulmonary Edema

Applying positive air pressure has been shown to decrease the work of breathing (34) and left ventricular afterload while maintaining cardiac index (37), thereby benefiting patients with cardiac dysfunction and ARF. The use of mask CPAP in patients with CPE was first described in the 1930s by Poulton and Oxon (2) and Barach et al. (3,4). More recently, several studies have examined responses to NIV of patients with CPE (126–137). In a large randomized controlled trial (138), the use of both NIV and CPAP in patients with acute CPE resulted in faster improvement of respiratory distress and metabolic disturbance, compared with standard oxygen therapy; early mortality, within first 7 days, did not significantly differ.

A systematic review and meta-analysis performed by Collins et al. (139) suggested that early application of NIV in the emergency department can decrease the relative risk of mortality by 39% and the necessity of endotracheal intubation by 57% when compared with standard medical therapy alone. However, in patients with CPE, NIV should not be viewed as the exclusive therapy, but should be accompanied by the aggressive conventional medical treatment.

In the comparison of NIV modalities, BiPAP has the potential advantage over CPAP of assisting the respiratory muscles during inspiration, which would result in faster alleviation of dyspnea and exhaustion (140). Nevertheless, according to all available data, there is no evidence to suggest superiority of either CPAP or BiPAP in terms of intubation or mortality, even in patients with CPE and hypercapnia (139,141,142). A recent meta-analysis on randomized trials comparing CPAP and BiPAP with standard therapy has showed that CPAP is able to reduce mortality and the need for intubation (especially in the presence of CPE of ischemic origin) but does not reduce the incidence of new myocardial infarction episodes compared with standard therapy (143). Differently, the BiPAP modality seems to reduce the need for intubation without improving the rate of mortality

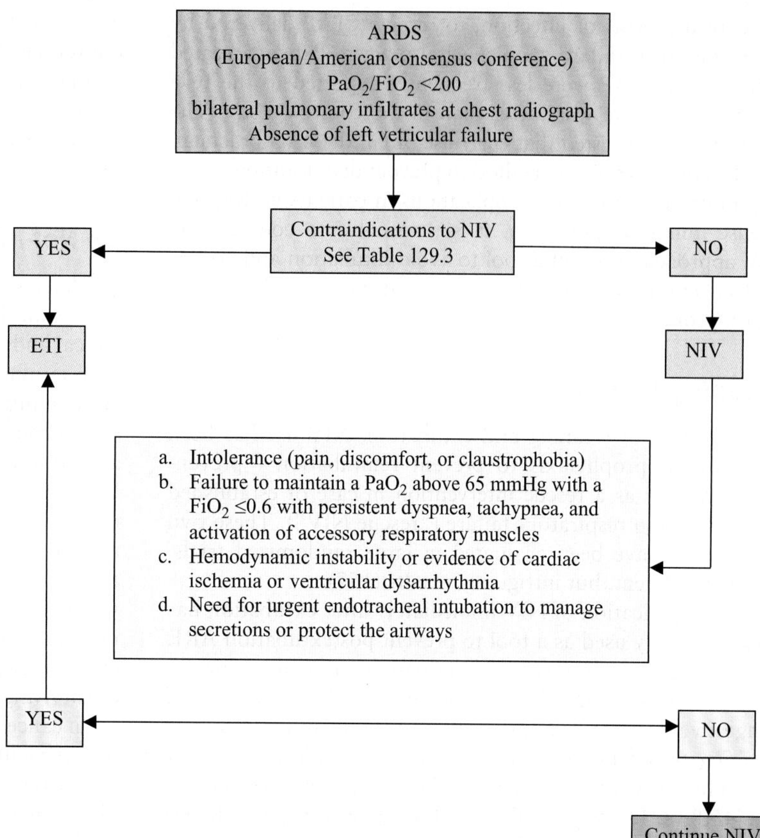

FIGURE 103.9 Decisional flow chart for the application of noninvasive ventilation to acute respiratory distress syndrome (ARDS). CPAP, continuous positive airway pressure; ETI, endotracheal intubation; FiO_2, fraction of inspired oxygen; NIV, noninvasive ventilation; PaO_2, partial pressure of arterial oxygen; PEEP, positive end-expiratory pressure.

or new myocardial infarction. In the management of suspected acute CPE in the prehospital setting, helmet CPAP has been used as first-line treatment, allowing prompt improvement in respiratory and hemodynamic parameters. This new approach was shown to be feasible, safe, and clinically effective (144).

In conclusion, NIV should be strongly considered as a first-line treatment in patients with CPE.

Immunocompromised Patients

Immunocompromised patients in whom respiratory failure develops often require mechanical ventilatory assistance. Endotracheal intubation is associated with numerous complications (16–19) and, in immunosuppressed patients, invasive mechanical ventilation is associated with a significant risk of death (145–147). The benefit of NIV in immunocompromised patients with ARF has been evaluated in two interventional trials (21,114), as well as in a substantial number of observational studies (61,119,148–155); a large part of the research has been conducted in oncohematologic patients. Antonelli et al. (21) included 40 recipients of solid-organ transplantation with hypoxemic ARF who were randomized to receive NIV versus standard oxygen therapy; patients treated with NIV more often achieved a better oxygenation with lower ETI and ICU mortality rates. Similarly, Hilbert et al. (114) randomized 52 hypoxemic ARF patients with pneumonia and immunosuppression to therapy with NIV or supportive oxygen only, showing a reduction in the need for ETI and hospital mortality rate in NIV-treated patients compared with conventionally treated controls. Unlike these interventional trials, observational studies of NIV in cancer patients with ARF have yielded conflicting results. Indeed, although most of these observational studies reported improved outcomes for these patients after NIV treatment as compared with invasive mechanical ventilation, some studies failed to show any beneficial effect of NIV (152,155). In a retrospective analysis of 137 hematologic patients admitted to the ICU with severe hypoxic ARF, Depuydt et al. (155) found that the use of NIV within 24 hours after ICU admission was not associated with better outcome as compared with invasive ventilation or supplemental oxygen only; in multivariate regression analysis, higher cancer-specific severity of illness score upon admission and more organ failure after 24 hours of ICU admission were significantly associated with increased ICU or in-hospital mortality, but the initial type of respiratory support was not. The disagreement between these findings and those of most other studies may be explained by differences in study design or patient selection, as not all forms of ARF are appropriate to be treated with NIV. As pointed out by the authors, the patients of their study might have been too ill to benefit from a trial of NIV, because as many as 74% of them met the criteria for ARDS, which has been shown to be significantly associated with NIV failure in hematologic patients (61). A large observational multicenter Italian survey investigated the clinical impact of NIV use in 1,302 hematologic patients admitted to ICU with ARF (60). The authors, after a propensity score analysis, confirmed the role of NIV treatment ab initio (from the beginning) as an independent predictor of survival. On the other hand, CPAP has been also used to treat cancer patients with ARF in order to prevent ICU admission. Squadrone et al. (156) randomized 40 patients with hematologic malignancy, recruited in the hematologic ward during the early phases of ARF, with PaO_2/FiO_2 levels between 200 and 300, and without a secure diagnosis of infection, to receive CPAP delivered by the helmet or standard supplemental oxygen. Patients treated with helmet CPAP were less frequently admitted to the ICU and their ETI rate was lower than in the control group. The investigators suggested that early use of CPAP was a practical, simple, and inexpensive method to prevent deterioration of the respiratory function and complications in patients undergoing intense immunosuppression. It is reasonable to consider the NIV approach as a useful tool to avoid intubation and associated infectious complications in selected patients with immunocompromised states.

Weaning Process

In the setting of weaning and extubation, NIV use has been proposed as prophylaxis to prevent reintubation ("preventive NIV") or as a rescue intervention in case of established postextubation respiratory failure ("rescue NIV"). These two approaches have been evaluated in large randomized trials, yielding different, but intriguing, results (157).

Early application of NIV immediately after extubation has been efficiently used as a tool to prevent postextubation ARF. Nava et al., in a multicenter randomized trial involving 97 patients with specific risk factors for postextubation ARF (i.e., congestive heart failure, excessive secretions, more than one weaning trial failure), observed that NIV application for at least 8 hours significantly decreased the rate of extubation failure (4/48 vs. 12/49; $p = 0.027$) and was associated with lower ICU mortality (10%; $p < 0.01$) (158).

Similarly, Ferrer et al. (159) randomized 162 mechanically ventilated patients who tolerated a spontaneous breathing trial but had increased risk for ARF after extubation (i.e., age more than 65 years, cardiac failure as the cause of intubation, APACHE II severity of illness score more than 12) to receive NIV for 24 hours versus conventional management with oxygen therapy. In the NIV group, ARF after extubation was less frequent ($p = 0.029$) and the ICU mortality was lower ($p = 0.015$), whereas 90-day survival did not change significantly between groups. Interestingly, in patients with hypercapnia ($PaCO_2$ >45 mmHg) during the spontaneous breathing trial, NIV use could significantly improve ICU mortality and 90-day survival.

The other potential application of NIV (i.e., as rescue strategy for postextubation ARF) has been investigated in multicenter randomized controlled trials. Keenan et al. (160) studied the effectiveness of NIV compared with standard medical therapy in preventing the need for endotracheal intubation in 81 patients who developed ARF during the first 48 hours after extubation. Comparing the two groups, no significant difference was found in rates of reintubation or duration of mechanical ventilation, in hospital mortality or ICU or hospital length of stay. Similarly, in a study conducted by Esteban et al. (161), no benefits from NIV were found in avoiding reintubation in patients who had developed ARF after extubation, and NIV was even associated with higher mortality rates as compared with patients treated according to standard treatment. In this study, the time from extubation to reintubation was longer in patients who received NIV.

In a more recent clinical trial, Girault et al. compared three early weaning/extubation techniques (conventional invasive weaning group; NIV group; standard oxygen therapy group) in 208 patients with chronic hypercapnic respiratory failure (162). Although, no differences were observed in the reintubation rate within the first 7 days, NIV was able to shorten the intubation duration and the risk of postextubation ARF.

In summary, NIV approach has to be considered to reduce the risk of postextubation ARF. However, further studies are needed to better define which patient categories are most likely to benefit from its application during weaning process.

Do-Not-Intubate Orders

To date, some confusion does remain on applying NIV in do-not-intubate patients, with some warning of the potential ethical and economic cost of delaying the inevitable in patients with terminal respiratory failure (163). This has stimulated a large number of research studies on the usefulness of NIV in such a context (164). In one study of 30 patients, most elderly and suffering from COPD, in whom invasive ventilation was "contraindicated or postponed," 18 patients (60%) were able to be successfully weaned from nasal mask NIV (165). In a trial conducted on 114 patients who declined intubation but accepted NIV to treat their ARF (166), 49 patients (43%) survived to discharge. Those patients who were awake, suffering from congestive heart failure or COPD, and those with a more efficient cough mechanism had an increased probability of survival.

In cancer patients at the end of life who have a stated desire to receive life-prolonging treatment, NIV may be of benefit as it may relieve dyspnea while preserving the ability to communicate, as well as decrease the need for sedatives, and prolong life for a period of time sufficient to accomplish personal tasks or realize possible end-of-life desires.

In those patients with the do-not-intubate order in whom the technique is unlikely to provide any survival or qualitative benefits, NIV should be avoided, whereas it might be considered when the acute process responsible for ARF is known to respond well to the technique, such as CPE or COPD exacerbation. Prior to initiation of NIV in these terminally ill patients, it is critical that the patient, family, and clinicians have a clear understanding of the possible outcomes of NIV. The caring clinician should inform the dying patients and their loved ones about the potential use of NIV, including the risks, benefits, and alternatives, and assure them that NIV can be withdrawn at any time if it fails to achieve the previously defined goals or the patient cannot tolerate the technique. In those cancer patients who cannot communicate, NIV should be discouraged as one of the theoretical advantages of palliative NIV is maintenance of the patient's ability to communicate. Throughout the management of any terminal patient with ARF, the caregiver must remember that not guaranteeing a quality death is a serious and irretrievable error. Finally, controversy remains about which is the most appropriate setting to deliver palliative NIV in end-of-life care.

Postoperative Patients

Thoracic and upper abdominal surgery are associated with a prolonged deterioration in postoperative gas exchange, as well as reduction in functional residual capacity, PaO_2, and forced vital capacity (167,168). Mask CPAP was initially used by Bunnell (1) in 1912 to maintain lung expansion in patients undergoing thoracic surgery, and by Boothby et al. (169) in 1940 for treating postoperative hypoxemic ARF. Applying mask CPAP or NIV improves oxygenation and pulmonary function following upper abdominal surgery (167,170–172) or coronary artery bypass graft (173–175). Squadrone et al. (171) randomized 209 patients who developed severe hypoxemia after major elective abdominal surgery to receive oxygen or oxygen plus CPAP. CPAP-treated patients had a lower intubation rate (1% vs. 10%) and a lower occurrence rate of pneumonia (2% vs. 10%), infection (3% vs. 10%), and sepsis (2% vs. 9%) (all $p < 0.05$) than patients treated with oxygen alone. NIV improves gas exchange and reduces the need for intubation after lung resection (176,177) or bilateral lung transplantation (178).

A recent systematic-review summarized the results of 29 articles where the use of preventive and therapeutic NIV was investigated in postsurgical patients (179). Thoracoabdominal/bariatric surgical interventions and solid-organ transplants were included. Arterial blood gases improvement and intubation rate reduction were the main benefits associated with the use of NIV. Thus, despite the limitations of available data and the need of new randomized trials, accumulating evidence supports the use of NIV/CPAP to reduce respiratory postoperative complications in selected patients.

Obstructive Sleep Apnea

CPAP is recognized to be effective in correcting the respiratory and arousal abnormalities and improving sleep quality in OSA syndrome (180,181). CPAP is believed to act by pneumatically "splinting" the pharyngeal airway, thus preventing its collapse during sleep (182,183). Additionally, nasal NIV has been used in patients with ARF following obstructive sleep apnea syndrome, with improvements in clinical status and arterial blood gas values (184).

Trauma

ARF in trauma patients is generally associated with reduced pulmonary compliance and functional residual capacity, and subsequent restrictive defects (185). In a study of 33 trauma patients with ARF who received face mask CPAP, Hurst et al. (185) found rapid improvements in gas exchange, avoiding intubation in 94% of the cases. In a retrospective survey of 46 trauma patients with ARF who had been given mask NIV, 33 patients (72%) were successfully weaned to spontaneous breathing (186). In another study (187), NIV used as first-line treatment in 22 patients with ARF due to blunt chest trauma resulted in rapid improvement in blood gases and respiratory rate, and avoided intubation in 18 patients (82%). In a study of patients with acute hypoxemic respiratory failure needing ventilatory assistance, Antonelli et al. (20) reported that 7 of the 32 patients (22%) randomized to receive NIV had trauma with pulmonary contusion or atelectasis. NIV was associated with a rapid improvement in oxygenation, and all seven patients avoided intubation and survived. Interestingly, Chiumello et al. performed a meta-analysis of ten studies addressing the use of NIV in patients with chest trauma who developed mild-to-severe respiratory failure (188). There was no difference between CPAP and PS NIV in terms of mortality, but the latter could significantly increase arterial oxygenation, leading to a reduction in the intubation rate and infectious complications incidence. However, despite the favorable results obtained, large randomized studies are still needed before definitive recommendations on the use of NIV in posttraumatic ARF can be made.

Restrictive Diseases

NIV has a role in the treatment of respiratory failure caused by some types of restrictive thoracic diseases. Bach et al. (189) demonstrated that NIV can prolong survival while decreasing the respiratory morbidity and hospitalization rates in patients with Duchenne muscular dystrophy. Using NIV prevented intubation in 7 of 11 episodes of ARF in a group of 9 patients with myasthenic crises (190). In ARF due to pulmonary fibrosis, prognosis is poor even when invasive mechanical ventilation is used (191). Aggressive respiratory physiotherapy is crucial in all patients with thoracic restriction.

Bronchoscopy

In nonintubated patients, severe hypoxemia is an accepted contraindication to fiberoptic bronchoscopy (FB). Since PaO_2 routinely decreases after uncomplicated FB, these patients are at high risk for developing ARF or serious cardiac arrhythmias. Performing bronchoscopy during NIV has been described either in at-risk patients who were initially breathing spontaneously and who started NIV to assist bronchoscopy, or in patients who were already receiving NIV and were scheduled to perform bronchoscopy (192–195). Antonelli et al. (192,193) proposed a technique to perform FB with bronchoalveolar lavage in hypoxemic, nonintubated patients by means of facial mask NIV (Fig. 103.10). The fiberoptic bronchoscope was passed through a T adapter and then advanced transnasally. The technique was safe and effective in avoiding gas exchange worsening during FB, allowing early and accurate diagnosis of pneumonia, and preventing undesired intubation in spontaneously breathing, hypoxemic patients. Alternately, if a helmet is adopted, the bronchoscope is passed through the specific seal connector placed in the plastic ring of the helmet. The internal adjustable diaphragm of the seal connection can prevent loss of the respiratory gases, maintaining ventilation throughout bronchoscopy (194).

Conscious sedation using propofol target-controlled infusion (TCI) techniques seems to be a promising approach to assist bronchoscopy in hypoxemic patients under NIV (196). Similarly bronchoscopy under sedation with remifentanil TCI

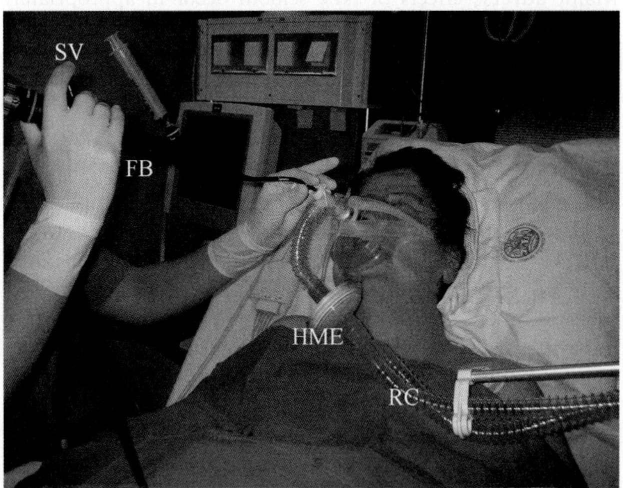

FIGURE 103.10 Fiberoptic bronchoscopy performed during noninvasive ventilation delivered through an oronasal mask. FB, fiberoptic bronchoscope; HME, heat and moisture exchanger; RC, respiratory circuit; SC, seal connection; SV, suction valve. (Photograph printed with the permission of the patient.)

has been safely and effectively used in critically ill patients undergoing spontaneous ventilation (197). During the last several years, dexmedetomidine use has been widely implementing in the clinical practice as a sedative agent, although few data are available in patients undergoing NIV (198). Due to its favorable pharmacologic profile, dexmedetomidine might be suitable as an adjuvant agent during bronchoscopy in spontaneous breathing critically ill patient with respiratory failure.

Pediatric Population

A growing body of evidence supports the use of NIV in children with ARF. Early case reports showed the safety and efficacy of the technique in the setting of cystic fibrosis, non-CPE and aspiration lung injury. One of the largest observational survey was reported by Essouri et al. (199) who described the application of NIV in 114 consecutive pediatric patients during a 5-year period. Even though only 22% of subjects with ARDS avoided endotracheal intubation, the authors reported an overall clinical success rate of 77%. More recently, a randomized controlled trial compared NIV treatment to standard therapy in 50 children with ARF, mainly due to bronchiolitis (200). The authors observed that patients undergoing NIV in PS modality had a sudden improvement in respiratory parameters and a significantly lower intubation rate (28% vs. 60%). Usually, facial masks have been considered the first choice to deliver CPAP/NIV. However, due to several possible disadvantages associated with its application in the pediatric population, helmet use is progressively increasing in this setting. Better tolerance of the interface may contribute to the reduction of sedatives used during spontaneous breathing (201). New assisted ventilatory modalities (e.g., NAVA) have been recently promoted in the pediatric setting in order to optimize child–ventilator interaction (202).

ADVERSE EFFECTS AND COMPLICATIONS

Major adverse effects of NIV seldom occur in appropriately selected patients and are minimized when the technique is applied by experienced caregivers (203). The most frequently encountered complications are related to the interface, ventilator airflow or pressure, or patient–ventilator interaction.

The pressure of the mask over the bridge of the nose may induce discomfort, erythema, or ulceration (see Fig. 103.2). There are various remedies to ameliorate this complication such as application of a hydrocolloid sheet over the nasal bridge or switching to alternative interfaces. Air leakage under the mask into the eyes may cause conjunctival irritation, and excessive pressure may be responsible for sinus or ear pain. To minimize these problems, refitting the mask or lowering inspiratory pressure may be useful. Patient–ventilator asynchrony is a common cause of NIV failure and is often related to patient agitation or inability of the ventilator to sense the onset of patient expiration because of excessive air leaking. Judicious use of sedatives may be safe and effective in the treatment of NIV failure due to low tolerance (204), and minimizing air leaks (73,205) may improve patient–ventilator synchrony.

Presumably because of the low inflation pressure used compared with invasive ventilation, NIV is well tolerated hemodynamically, but it should be avoided in patients with an unstable hemodynamic status, dysrhythmias, or uncontrolled ischemia until these problems are stabilized. Gastric insufflation occurs commonly, but is usually well tolerated. Aspiration pneumonia has been reported in as many as 5% of patients (106); the risk for aspiration is minimized by excluding patients with compromised upper airway function or problems clearing secretions and positioning a nasogastric tube in those with excessive gastric distention, an ileus, or nausea or vomiting. Although pneumothoraces occur very infrequently, inspiratory pressures should be kept at the minimum effective level in patients with bullous lung disease.

SUMMARY

To date, the best-established indication for NIV in the acute care setting is ARF related to COPD-E. However, evidence has been rapidly accumulating to support application of NIV to treat many other types of ARF in selected patients. Further research should better define indications and patient selection criteria, as well as establish optimal techniques of administration.

Key Points

- NIV has the potential of avoiding the complications associated with endotracheal intubation, improving patient comfort, and preserving speech and airway defense mechanisms.
- Advances in patient–ventilator interfaces and ventilatory modes have fostered the increasing use of NIV in the acute care setting.
- The choice of ventilatory mode should be dictated by personal experience, as well as the patient's respiratory drive and etiologic factors and severity of the underlying disease causing respiratory failure.
- It is crucial to identify patients who are likely to benefit from NIV and exclude those for whom NIV would be unsafe.
- Several factors are critical to the success of NIV: properly timed initiation, comfortable and well-fitting interface, patient preparation, careful ventilatory mode selection, and respiratory physiotherapy.
- Patients should receive NIV in an intensive care unit or a step-down unit for continuous monitoring until sufficient stabilization.
- NIV can be used to avoid intubation, *but not to replace it*. Invasive ventilation remains the method of choice for patients with respiratory failure who have contraindications to NIV.
- NIV is indicated as the ventilator mode of first choice in selected patients with COPD-E.
- In acute hypoxemic respiratory failure without hypercapnia, NIV can be used as long as patients are hemodynamically stable and are closely monitored in the intensive care unit to avoid dangerous delays if intubation becomes necessary.
- NIV has a central role in the management of ARF of varied causes, improving patient outcome and efficiency of care in the acute setting.

References

1. Bunnel S. The use of nitrous oxide and oxygen to maintain anesthesia and positive pressure for thoracic surgery. *JAMA*. 1912;58:835.
2. Poulton EP, Oxon DM. Left-sided heart failure with pulmonary edema: its treatment with the "pulmonary plus pressure machine." *Lancet*. 1936; 231:981.
3. Barach AL, Martin J, Eckman M. Positive-pressure respiration and its application for the treatment of acute pulmonary edema and respiratory obstruction. *Proc Am Soc Clin Invest*. 1937;16:664.
4. Barach AL, Martin J, Eckman M. Positive-pressure respiration and its application to the treatment of acute pulmonary edema. *Ann Intern Med*. 1938;12:754.
5. Barach AL, Swenson P. Effect of breathing gases under positive pressure on lumens of small and medium sized bronchi. *Arch Intern Med*. 1939; 63:946.
6. Motley HL, Lang LP, Gordon B. Use of intermittent positive pressure breathing combined with nebulization in pulmonary disease. *Am J Med*. 1948;5:853.
7. The Intermittent Positive Pressure Breathing Trial Group. Intermittent positive pressure breathing therapy of chronic obstructive pulmonary disease. *Ann Intern Med*. 1983;99:612.
8. Sullivan CE, Issa FG, Berthon-Jones M, et al. Reversal of obstructive sleep apnea by continuous positive airway pressure applied through the nares. *Lancet*. 1981;1:862.
9. Rideau Y, Gatin G, Bach J, et al. Prolongation of life in Duchenne's muscular dystrophy. *Acta Neurol Belg*. 1983;5:118.
10. Kerby GR, Mayer LS, Pingleton SK. Nocturnal positive pressure ventilation via nasal mask. *Am Rev Respir Dis*. 1987;135:738.
11. Ellis ER, Bye PT, Bruderer JW, et al. Treatment of respiratory failure during sleep in patients with neuromuscular disease: positive-pressure ventilation through a nose mask. *Am Rev Respir Dis*. 1987;135:148.
12. Bach JR, Alba AS. Management of chronic alveolar hypoventilation by nasal ventilation. *Chest*. 1990;97:52.
13. Meduri GU, Conoscenti CC, Menashe P, et al. Noninvasive face mask ventilation in patients with acute respiratory failure. *Chest*. 1989;95:865.
14. Brochard L, Isabey D, Piquet J, et al. Reversal of acute exacerbations of chronic obstructive lung disease by inspiratory assistance with a face mask. *N Engl J Med*. 1990;95:865.
15. Elliott MW, Steven MH, Phillips GD, et al. Noninvasive mechanical ventilation for acute respiratory failure. *BMJ*. 1990;300:358.
16. Zwillich CW, Pirson DJ, Creagh CE, et al. Complications of assisted ventilation. *Am J Med*. 1974;57:161.
17. Stauffer JL, Olson DE, Petty TL. Complications and consequences of endotracheal intubation. *Am J Med*. 1981;70:65.
18. Craven DE, Kunches LM, Kilinsky V, et al. Risk factors for pneumonia and fatality in patients receiving continuous mechanical ventilation. *Am Rev Respir Dis*. 1986;113:792.
19. Pingleton SK. Complications of acute respiratory failure. *Am Rev Respir Dis*. 1988;137:1463.
20. Antonelli M, Conti G, Rocco M, et al. A comparison of noninvasive positive-pressure ventilation and conventional mechanical ventilation in patients with acute respiratory failure. *N Engl J Med*. 1998;339:429.
21. Antonelli M, Conti C, Bufi M, et al. Noninvasive ventilation for treatment of acute respiratory failure in patients undergoing solid organ transplantation. *JAMA*. 2000;283:235.
22. Nourdine K, Combes P, Carton MJ, et al. Does noninvasive ventilation reduce the ICU nosocomial infection risk? A prospective clinical survey. *Intensive Care Med*. 1999;25:567.
23. Girou E, Schortgen F, Delclaux C, et al. Association of noninvasive ventilation with nosocomial infections and survival in critically ill patients. *JAMA*. 2000;284:2361.
24. Esteban A, Anzueto A, Frutos F, et al. Characteristics and outcomes in adult patients receiving mechanical ventilation: a 28-day international study. *JAMA*. 2002;287:345.
25. Demoule A, Girou E, Richard JC, et al. Increased use of noninvasive ventilation in French intensive care units. *Intensive Care Med*. 2006; 32:1747.
26. Carlucci A, Richard JC, Wysocki M, et al. Noninvasive versus conventional mechanical ventilation. An epidemiologic survey. *Am J Respir Crit Care Med*. 2001;163:874.
27. Cabrini L, Idone C, Colombo S, et al. Medical emergency team and noninvasive ventilation outside ICU for acute respiratory failure. *Intensive Care Med*. 2009;35:339.
28. Maheshwari V, Paioli D, Rothaar R, Hill NS. Utilization of noninvasive ventilation in acute care hospitals: a regional survey. *Chest*. 2006;129:1226.
29. Antonelli M, Conti G. Noninvasive ventilation in intensive care unit patients. *Curr Opin Crit Care*. 2000;6:11.
30. Antonelli M, Conti G, Pelosi P, et al. New treatment of acute hypoxemic respiratory failure: noninvasive pressure support ventilation delivered by helmet: a pilot controlled trial. *Crit Care Med*. 2002;30:602.
31. Antonelli M, Pennisi MA, Pelosi P, et al. Noninvasive positive pressure ventilation using a helmet in patients with acute exacerbation of chronic obstructive pulmonary disease: a feasibility study. *Anesthesiology*. 2004;100:16.
32. Piastra M, Antonelli M, Chiaretti M, et al. Treatment of acute respiratory failure by helmet-delivered non-invasive ventilation in children with acute leukemia: a pilot study. *Intensive Care Med*. 2004;30:472.
33. Bach JR, Alba AS, Saporito LR. Intermittent positive pressure ventilation via the mouth as an alternative to tracheostomy for 257 ventilator users. *Chest*. 1993;103:174.
34. Katz JA, Marks JD. Inspiratory work with and without continuous positive airway pressure in patients with acute respiratory failure. *Anesthesiology*. 1985;63:598.
35. Petrof BJ, Legere M, Goldberg P, et al. Continuous positive airway pressure reduced work of breathing and dyspnea during weaning from mechanical ventilation in severe chronic obstructive pulmonary disease. *Am Rev Respir Dis*. 1990;141:281.
36. Rasanen J, Heikkila J, Downs J, et al. Continuous positive airway pressure by face mask in acute cardiogenic pulmonary edema. *Am J Cardiol*. 1985;55:296.
37. Naughton MT, Rahman MA, Hara K, et al. Effect of continuous positive airway pressure on intrathoracic and left ventricular transmural pressures in patients with congestive heart failure. *Circulation*. 1995;91:1725.
38. Scharf SM, Caldini P, Ingram RH. Cardiovascular effects of increasing airway pressure in the dog. *Am J Physiol*. 1977;232:H35.
39. Braunwald E, Binion JT, WL Morgan, et al. Alterations in central blood volume and cardiac output induced by positive pressure breathing counteracted by metaraminol (Aramine). *Circ Res*. 1957;5:670.
40. Fessler H, Brower R, Wise R, et al. Effects of positive end-expiratory pressure on the gradient for venous return. *Am Rev Respir Dis*. 1991;143:19.
41. Nanas S, Magder S. Adaptation of the peripheral circulation to PEEP. *Am Rev Respir Dis*. 1992;146:688.
42. Jellinek H, Krenn H, Oczenski W, et al. Influence of positive airway pressure on the pressure gradient for venous return in humans. *J Appl Physiol*. 2000;88:926.
43. Gibney RT, Wilson RS, Pontoppidan H. Comparison of work of breathing on high gas flow and demand valve continuous positive airway pressure systems. *Chest*. 1982;82:692.
44. Beydon L, Chasse M, Harf A, et al. Inspiratory work of breathing during spontaneous ventilation using demand valves and continuous flow systems. *Am Rev Respir Dis*. 1988;138:300.
45. Sassoon CSH, Lodia R, Rheeman CH, et al. Inspiratory muscle work of breathing during flow-by, demand-flow and continuous-flow systems in patients with chronic obstructive pulmonary disease. *Am Rev Respir Dis*. 1992;145:1219.
46. Parke R, McGuinness S, Eccleston M. Nasal high-flow therapy delivers low level positive airway pressure. *Br J Anaesth*. 2009;103:886.
47. Younes M, Puddy A, Roberts D, et al. Proportional assist ventilation: results of an initial clinical trial. *Am Rev Respir Dis*. 1992;145:121.
48. Conti G, Costa R. Technological development in mechanical ventilation. *Curr Opin Crit Care*. 2010;16:26.
49. Bach JR, Saporito LR. Criteria for extubation and tracheostomy tube removal for patients with ventilatory failure: a different approach to weaning. *Chest*. 1996;110:1566.
50. Bach JR. Mechanical insufflation-exsufflation: comparison of peak expiratory flows and manually assisted and unassisted coughing techniques. *Chest*. 1993;104:1553.
51. Gonçalves MR, Honrado T, Winck JC, Paiva JA. Effects of mechanical insufflation-exsufflation in preventing respiratory failure after extubation: a randomized controlled trial. *Crit Care*. 2012;16(2):R48.
52. Diaz GG, Alcaraz AC, Talavera JC, et al. Noninvasive positive-pressure ventilation to treat hypercapnic coma secondary to respiratory failure. *Chest*. 2005;127:952.
53. Scala R, Naldi M, Archinucci I, et al. Noninvasive positive pressure ventilation in patients with acute exacerbations of COPD and varying levels of consciousness. *Chest*. 2005;128:1657.
54. Pankow W, Hijjeh N, Schuttler F, et al. Influence of noninvasive positive pressure ventilation on inspiratory muscle activity in obese subjects. *Eur Respir J*. 1997;10:2847.
55. Ambrosino N, Foglio K, Rubini F, et al. Noninvasive mechanical ventilation in acute respiratory failure due to chronic obstructive pulmonary disease: correlates for success. *Thorax*. 1995;50:755.

56. Moretti M, Cilione C, Tampieri A, et al. Incidence and causes of non-invasive mechanical ventilation failure after initial success. *Thorax*. 2000;55:819.
57. Soo Hoo GW, Santiago S, Williams AJ. Nasal mechanical ventilation for hypercapnic respiratory failure in chronic obstructive pulmonary disease: determinants of success and failure. *Crit Care Med*. 1994;22:1253.
58. Antonelli M, Conti G, Moro ML, et al. Predictors of failure of noninvasive positive pressure ventilation in patients with acute hypoxemic respiratory failure: a multicenter study. *Intensive Care Med*. 2001;27:1718.
59. Antonelli M, Conti G, Esquinas A, et al. A multiple-center survey on the use in clinical practice of noninvasive ventilation as a first-line intervention for acute respiratory distress syndrome. *Crit Care Med*. 2007;35:18.
60. Gristina GR, Antonelli M, Conti G, et al. Noninvasive versus invasive ventilation for acute respiratory failure in patients with hematologic malignancies: a 5-year multicenter observational survey. *Crit Care Med*. 2011;39:2232.
61. Adda M, Coquet I, Darmon M, et al. Predictors of noninvasive ventilation failure in patients with hematologic malignancy and acute respiratory failure. *Crit Care Med*. 2008;36:2766.
62. L'Her E, Deye N, Lellouche F, et al. Physiologic effects of noninvasive ventilation during acute lung injury. *Am J Respir Crit Care Med*. 2005; 172:1112.
63. Vitacca M, Rubini F, Foglio K, et al. Noninvasive modalities of positive pressure ventilation improve the outcome of acute exacerbations in COLD patients. *Intensive Care Med*. 1993;19:450.
64. Nava S, Ambrosino N, Bruschi C, et al. Physiological effects of flow and pressure triggering during non invasive mechanical ventilation in patients with chronic obstructive pulmonary disease. *Thorax*. 1997;52:249.
65. Tassaux D, Gainnier M, Battisti A, Jolliet P. Impact of expiratory trigger setting on delayed cycling and inspiratory muscle workload. *Am J Respir Crit Care Med*. 2005;172:1283.
66. Olivieri C, Costa R, Conti G, et al. Bench studies evaluating devices for noninvasive ventilation: critical analysis and future perspectives. *Intensive Care Med*. 2012;38:160.
67. Cammarota G, Vaschetto R, Turucz E, et al. Influence of lung collapse distribution on the physiologic response to recruitment maneuvers during noninvasive continuous positive airway pressure. *Intensive Care Med*. 2011;37:1095–1102.
68. Kondili E, Prinianakis G, Georgopoulos D. Patient-ventilator interaction. *Br J Anaesth*. 2003;91:106.
69. Vignaux L, Vargas F, Roeseler J, et al. Patient-ventilator asynchrony during non-invasive ventilation for acute respiratory failure: a multicenter study. *Intensive Care Med*. 2009;35:840.
70. Thille AW, Rodriguez P, Cabello B, et al. Patient-ventilator asynchrony during assisted mechanical ventilation. *Intensive Care Med*. 2006;32:1515.
71. Prinianakis G, Delmastro M, Carlucci A, et al. Effect of varying the pressurisation rate during noninvasive pressure support ventilation. *Eur Respir J*. 2004;23:314.
72. Chiumello D, Pelosi P, Croci M, et al. The effects of pressurization rate on breathing pattern, work of breathing, gas exchange and patient comfort in pressure support ventilation. *Eur Respir J*. 2001;18:107.
73. Mehta S, McCool FD, Hill NS. Leak compensation in positive pressure ventilators: a lung model study. *Eur Respir J*. 2001;17:259.
74. Vignaux L, Tassaux D, Carteaux G, et al. Performance of noninvasive ventilation algorithms on ICU ventilators during pressure support: a clinical study. *Intensive Care Med*. 2010;36:2053–2059.
75. Carteaux G, Lyazidi A, Cordoba-Izquierdo A, et al. Patient-ventilator asynchrony during noninvasive ventilation: a bench and clinical study. *Chest*. 2012;142:367–376.
76. Schmidt M, Dres M, Raux M, et al. Neurally adjusted ventilatory assist improves patient-ventilator interaction during postextubation prophylactic noninvasive ventilation. *Crit Care Med*. 2012; 40:1738.
77. Bertrand PM, Futier E, Coisel Y, et al. Neurally adjusted ventilator assist versus pressure support ventilation for noninvasive ventilation during acute respiratory failure: a cross-over physiological study. *Chest*. 2013;143:30.
78. Cammarota G, Olivieri C, Costa R, et al. Noninvasive ventilation through a helmet in postextubation hypoxemic patients: physiologic comparison between neurally adjusted ventilatory assist and pressure support ventilation. *Intensive Care Med*. 2011;37:1943.
79. Moerer O, Fischer S, Hartelt M, et al. Influence of two different interfaces for noninvasive ventilation compared to invasive ventilation on the mechanical properties and performance of a respiratory system: a lung model study. *Chest*. 2006;129:1424.
80. Vargas F, Thille A, Lyazidi A, et al. Helmet with specific settings versus facemask for noninvasive ventilation. *Crit Care Med*. 2009;37:1921.
81. Ferrone G, Cipriani F, Spinazzola G, et al. A bench study of 2 ventilator circuits during helmet noninvasive ventilation. *Respir Care*. 2013; 58:1474–1481.
82. Iotti GA, Olivei MC, Palo A, et al. Unfavorable mechanical effects of heat and moisture exchangers in ventilated patients. *Intensive Care Med*. 1997;23:399.
83. Lellouche F, Maggiore SM, Deye N, et al. Effect of the humidification device on the work of breathing during noninvasive ventilation. *Intensive Care Med*. 2002;28:1582.
84. Jaber S, Chanques G, Matecki S, et al. Comparison of the effects of heat and moisture exchangers and heated humidifiers on ventilation and gas exchange during noninvasive ventilation. *Intensive Care Med*. 2002; 28:1590.
85. Lellouche F, L'Her E, Abroug F, et al. Impact of the humidification device on intubation rate during noninvasive ventilation with ICU ventilators: results of a multicenter randomized controlled trial. *Intensive Care Med*. 2014;40:211.
86. Nava S, Cirio S, Fanfulla F, et al. Comparison of two humidification systems for long-term noninvasive mechanical ventilation. *Eur Respir J*. 2008;32:460.
87. Plant PK, Owen JL, Elliott MW. Early use of noninvasive ventilation for acute exacerbations of chronic obstructive pulmonary disease on general respiratory wards: a multicenter randomized controlled trial. *Lancet*. 2000;355:1931.
88. Brochard L, Mancebo J, Wysocki M, et al. Noninvasive ventilation for acute exacerbations of chronic obstructive pulmonary disease. *N Engl J Med*. 1995;333:817.
89. Bott J, Carroll MP, Conway JH, et al. Randomized controlled trial of nasal ventilation in acute ventilatory failure due to chronic obstructive airways disease. *Lancet*. 1993;341:1555.
90. Kramer N, Meyer TJ, Meharg J, et al. Randomized, prospective trial of noninvasive positive pressure ventilation in acute respiratory failure. *Am J Respir Crit Care Med*. 1995;151:1799.
91. Celikel T, Sungur M, Ceyhan B, et al. Comparison of noninvasive positive pressure ventilation with standard medical therapy in hypercapnic acute respiratory failure. *Chest*. 1998;114:1636.
92. Organized jointly by the American Thoracic Society, the European Respiratory Society, the European Society of Intensive Care Medicine, and the Societe de Reanimation de Langue Francaise, and approved by ATS Board of Directors, December 2000. International Consensus Conferences in Intensive Care Medicine: noninvasive positive pressure ventilation in acute respiratory failure. *Am J Respir Crit Care Med*. 2001;163:283.
93. Mehta S, Hill NS. Noninvasive ventilation. *Am J Respir Crit Care Med*. 2001;163:540.
94. Chandra D, Stamm JA, Taylor B, et al. Outcomes of noninvasive ventilation for acute exacerbations of chronic obstructive pulmonary disease in the United States, 1998–2008. *Am J Respir Crit Care Med*. 2012;185: 152–159.
95. Elliott MW, Nava S. Noninvasive ventilation for acute exacerbations of chronic obstructive pulmonary disease: "Don't think twice, it's alright!" *Am J Respir Crit Care Med*. 2012;185:121–123.
96. Appendini L, Palessio A, Zanaboni S, et al. Physiologic effects of positive end-expiratory pressure and mask pressure support during exacerbations of chronic obstructive pulmonary disease. *Am J Respir Crit Care Med*. 1994;149:1069.
97. Barbé F, Togores B, Rubi M, et al. Noninvasive ventilatory support does not facilitate recovery from acute respiratory failure in chronic obstructive pulmonary disease. *Eur Respir J*. 1996;9:1240.
98. Angus RM, Ahmed AA, Fenwick LJ, et al. Comparison of the acute effects on gas exchange of nasal ventilation and doxapram in exacerbations of chronic obstructive pulmonary disease. *Thorax*. 1996;51:1048.
99. Nava S, Ambrosino N, Clini E, et al. Noninvasive mechanical ventilation in the weaning of patients with respiratory failure due to chronic obstructive pulmonary disease: a randomized, controlled trial. *Ann Intern Med*. 1998;128:721.
100. Confalonieri M, Potena A, Carbone G, et al. Acute respiratory failure in patients with severe community-acquired pneumonia: a prospective randomized evaluation of noninvasive ventilation. *Am J Respir Crit Care Med*. 1999;160:1585.
101. Martin TJ, Hovis JD, Constantino JP, et al. A randomized prospective evaluation of noninvasive ventilation for acute respiratory failure. *Am J Respir Crit Care Med*. 2000;161:807.
102. Conti G, Antonelli M, Navalesi P, et al. Noninvasive vs. conventional mechanical ventilation in patients with chronic obstructive pulmonary disease after failure of medical treatment in the ward: a randomized trial. *Intensive Care Med*. 2002;28:1701.

103. Thys F, Roeseler J, Reynaert M, et al. Noninvasive ventilation for acute respiratory failure: a prospective randomised placebo-controlled trial. *Eur Respir J*. 2002;20:545.
104. Dikensoy O, Ikidag B, Filiz A, et al. Comparison of non-invasive ventilation and standard medical therapy in acute hypercapnic respiratory failure: a randomised controlled study at a tertiary health centre in SE Turkey. *Int J Clin Pract*. 2002;56:85.
105. Squadrone E, Frigerio P, Fogliati C, et al. Noninvasive vs. invasive ventilation in COPD patients with severe acute respiratory failure deemed to require ventilatory assistance. *Intensive Care Med*. 2004;30:1303.
106. Meduri GU, Cook TR, Turner RE, et al. Noninvasive positive pressure ventilation in status asthmaticus. *Chest*. 1996;110:767.
107. Fernandez MM, Villagra A, Blanch L, et al. Non-invasive mechanical ventilation in status asthmaticus. *Intensive Care Med*. 2001;27:486.
108. Soroksky A, Stav D, Shpirer I. A pilot prospective, randomized, placebo-controlled trial of bilevel positive airway pressure in acute asthmatic attack. *Chest*. 2003;123:1018.
109. Holley MT, Morrissey TK, Seaberg DC, et al. Ethical dilemmas in a randomized trial of asthma treatment: can Bayesian statistical analysis explain the results? *Acad Emerg Med*. 2001;8:1128.
110. Levy BD, Kitch B, Fanta CH. Medical and ventilatory management of status asthmaticus. *Intensive Care Med*. 1998;24:105.
111. Wysocki M, Tric L, Wolff MA, et al. Noninvasive pressure support ventilation in patients with acute respiratory failure. *Chest*. 1993;103:907.
112. Wood KA, Lewis L, Von Harz B, et al. The use of noninvasive positive pressure ventilation in the emergency department. *Chest*. 1998;113:1339.
113. Girault C, Daudenthun I, Chevron V, et al. Noninvasive ventilation as a systematic extubation and weaning technique in acute-on-chronic respiratory failure: a prospective, randomized controlled study. *Am J Respir Crit Care Med*. 1999;160:86.
114. Hilbert G, Gruson D, Vargas F, et al. Noninvasive ventilation in immunosuppressed patients with pulmonary infiltrates, fever, and acute respiratory failure. *N Engl J Med*. 2001;344:481.
115. Ferrer M, Esquinas A, Leon M, et al. Noninvasive ventilation in severe hypoxemic respiratory failure: a randomized clinical trial. *Am J Respir Crit Care Med*. 2003;168:1438.
116. Pennock BE, Crawshaw L, Kaplan PD. Noninvasive nasal mask ventilation for acute respiratory failure. *Chest*. 1994;105:441.
117. Lapinsky SE, Mount DNB, Mackey D, et al. Management of acute respiratory failure due to pulmonary edema with nasal positive pressure support. *Chest*. 1994;105:229.
118. Meduri GU, Turner RE, Abou-Shala N, et al. Noninvasive positive pressure ventilation via face mask. *Chest*. 1996;109:179.
119. Conti G, Marino P, Cogliati A, et al. Noninvasive ventilation for the treatment of acute respiratory failure in patients with hematologic malignancies: a pilot study. *Intensive Care Med*. 1998;24:1283.
120. Rocker GM, Mackensie M-G, Willilams B, et al. Noninvasive positive pressure ventilation: successful outcome in patients with acute lung injury/ARDS. *Chest*. 1999;115:173.
121. Ferrer M, Esquinas A, Leon M, et al. Noninvasive ventilation in severe hypoxemic respiratory failure: a randomized clinical trial. *Am J Respir Crit Care Med*. 2003;168:1438.
122. L'Her E, Deye N, Lellouche F, et al. Physiologic effects of noninvasive ventilation during acute lung injury. *Am J Respir Crit Care Med*. 2005; 172:1112.
123. Covelli HD, Weled BJ, Beekman JF. Efficacy of continuous positive airway pressure administered by face mask. *Chest*. 1982;81:147.
124. Demoule A, Girou E, Richard JC, et al. Benefits and risks of success or failure of noninvasive ventilation. *Intensive Care Med*. 2006;32:1756.
125. Ranieri VM, Rubenfeld GD, Thompson BT, et al.; ARDS Definition Task Force. Acute respiratory distress syndrome: the Berlin Definition. *JAMA*. 2012;307:2526.
126. Bersten AD, Holt AW, Vedig AE, et al. Treatment of severe cardiogenic pulmonary edema with continuous positive airway pressure delivered by face mask. *N Engl J Med*. 1991;325:1825.
127. Mehta S, Jay GD, Woolard RH, et al. Randomized prospective trial of bilevel versus continuous positive airway pressure in acute pulmonary edema. *Crit Care Med*. 1997;25:620.
128. Bellone A, Monari A, Cortellaro F, et al. Myocardial infarction rate in acute pulmonary edema. *Crit Care Med*. 2004;32:1860.
129. Masip J, Betbese AJ, Paez J, et al. Non-invasive pressure support ventilation versus conventional oxygen therapy in acute cardiogenic pulmonary edema: a randomized study. *Lancet*. 2000;356:2126.
130. Levitt MA. A prospective, randomized trial of BIPAP in severe acute congestive heart failure. *J Emerg Med*. 2001;21:363.
131. Kelly CA, Newby DE, McDonagh TA, et al. Randomised controlled trial of continuous positive airway pressure and standard oxygen therapy in acute pulmonary oedema. *Eur Heart J*. 2002;23:1379.
132. Nava S, Carbone G, Dibatista N, et al. Noninvasive ventilation in cardiogenic pulmonary edema. *Am J Respir Crit Care Med*. 2003;168:1432.
133. Cross AM, Cameron P, Kierce M, et al. Non-invasive ventilation in acute respiratory failure. *Emerg Med J*. 2003;20:531.
134. L'Her E, Duquesne F, Girou E, et al. Noninvasive continuous positive airway pressure in elderly cardiogenic pulmonary edema patients. *Intensive Care Med*. 2004;30:882.
135. Park M, Sangean MC, Volpe MC, et al. Randomized, prospective trial of oxygen, continuous positive airway pressure, and bilevel positive airway pressure by face mask in acute cardiogenic pulmonary edema. *Crit Care Med*. 2004;32:2407.
136. Crane SD, Elliott MW, Gilligan P, et al. Randomised controlled comparison of continuous positive airways pressure, bilevel non-invasive ventilation, and standard treatment in emergency department in patients with acute cardiogenic pulmonary oedema. *Emerg Med J*. 2004;21:155.
137. Bellone A, Vettorello M, Monari A, et al. Noninvasive pressure support ventilation vs. continuous positive airway pressure in acute hypercapnic pulmonary edema. *Intensive Care Med*. 2005;31:807.
138. Gray A, Goodacre S, Newby DE, et al.; 3CPO Trialists. Noninvasive ventilation in acute cardiogenic pulmonary edema. *N Engl J Med*. 2008; 359(2):142.
139. Collins SP, Mielniczuk LM, Whittingham HA, et al. The use of noninvasive ventilation in emergency department patients with acute cardiogenic pulmonary edema: a systematic review. *Ann Emerg Med*. 2006;48:260.
140. Wysocki M. Noninvasive ventilation in acute cardiogenic pulmonary edema: better than continuous positive airway pressure? *Intensive Care Med*. 1999;25:1.
141. Masip J, Roque M, Sanchez B, et al. Noninvasive ventilation in acute cardiogenic pulmonary edema: systematic review and meta-analysis. *JAMA*. 2005;294:3124.
142. Ho KM, Wong K. A comparison of continuous and bi-level positive airway pressure non-invasive ventilation in patients with acute cardiogenic pulmonary oedema: a meta-analysis. *Crit Care*. 2006;10:R49.
143. Weng CL, Zhao YT, Liu QH, et al. Meta-analysis: Noninvasive ventilation in acute cardiogenic pulmonary edema. *Ann Intern Med*. 2010;152: 590–600.
144. Foti G, Sangalli F, Berra L, et al. Is helmet CPAP first line pre-hospital treatment of presumed severe acute pulmonary edema? *Intensive Care Med*. 2009;35:656–662.
145. Estopa R, Torres-Marti A, Kastanos N, et al. Acute respiratory failure in severe hematologic disorders. *Crit Care Med*. 1984;12:26.
146. Blot F, Guignet M, Nitenberg G, et al. Prognostic factors for neutropenic patients in an intensive care unit: respective roles of underlying malignancies and acute organ failures. *Eur J Cancer*. 1997;33:1031.
147. Ewig S, Torres A, Riquelme R, et al. Pulmonary complications in patients with haematological malignancies treated at a respiratory ICU. *Eur Respir J*. 1998;12:116.
148. Tognet E, Mercatello A, Polo P, et al. Treatment of acute respiratory failure with non-invasive intermittent positive pressure ventilation in haematological patients. *Clin Intensive Care*. 1994; 5:282.
149. Varon J, Walsh GL, Fromm RE Jr. Feasibility of noninvasive mechanical ventilation in the treatment of acute respiratory failure in postoperative cancer patients. *J Crit Care*. 1998;13:55.
150. Azoulay E, Alberti C, Bornstain C, et al. Improved survival in cancer patients requiring mechanical ventilatory support: impact of noninvasive mechanical ventilatory support. *Crit Care Med*. 2001;29:519.
151. Azoulay E, Thiéry G, Chevret S, et al. The prognosis of acute respiratory failure in critically ill cancer patients. *Medicine (Baltimore)*. 2004;83:360.
152. Depuydt PO, Benoit DD, Vandewoude KH, et al. Outcome in noninvasively and invasively ventilated hematologic patients with acute respiratory failure. *Chest*. 2004;126:1299.
153. Rabbat A, Chaoui D, Montani D, et al. Prognosis of patients with acute myeloid leukaemia admitted to intensive care. *Br J Haematol*. 2005;129:350.
154. Rabitsch W, Staudinger T, Locker GJ, et al. Respiratory failure after stem cell transplantation: improved outcome with non-invasive ventilation. *Leuk Lymphoma*. 2005;46:1151.
155. Depuydt PO, Benoit DD, Roosens CD, et al. The impact of the initial ventilatory strategy on survival in hematological patients with acute hypoxemic respiratory failure. *J Crit Care*. 2010;25:30.
156. Squadrone V, Massaia M, Bruno B, et al. Early CPAP prevents evolution of acute lung injury in patients with hematologic malignancy. *Intensive Care Med*. 2010;36:1666.

157. Agarwal R, Aggarwal AN, et al. Role of noninvasive positive-pressure ventilation in postextubation respiratory failure: a meta-analysis. *Respir Care.* 2007;52:1472.
158. Nava S, Gregoretti C, Fanfulla F, et al. Noninvasive ventilation to prevent respiratory failure after extubation in high-risk patients. *Crit Care Med.* 2005;33:2465–2470.
159. Ferrer M, Valencia M, Nicolas JM, et al. Early noninvasive ventilation averts extubation failure in patients at risk: a randomized trial. *Am J Respir Crit Care Med.* 2006;173:164.
160. Keenan SP, Powers C, McCormack DG, et al. Noninvasive positive-pressure ventilation for postextubation respiratory distress: a randomized controlled trial. *JAMA.* 2002;287:3238.
161. Esteban A, Frutos-Vivar F, Ferguson ND, et al. Noninvasive positive-pressure ventilation for respiratory failure after extubation. *N Engl J Med.* 2004;350:2452.
162. Girault C, Bubenheim M, Abroug F, et al.; VENISE Trial Group. Noninvasive ventilation and weaning in patients with chronic hypercapnic respiratory failure: a randomized multicenter trial. *Am J Respir Crit Care Med.* 2011;184:672.
163. Clarke DE, Vaughan L, Raffin TA. Noninvasive positive pressure ventilation for patients with terminal respiratory failure: the ethical and economic costs of delaying the inevitable are too great. *Am J Crit Care.* 1994;3:4.
164. Azoulay E, Kouatchet A, Jaber S, et al. Noninvasive mechanical ventilation in patients having declined tracheal intubation. *Intensive Care Med.* 2013;39:292.
165. Benhamou D, Girault C, Faure C, et al. Nasal mask ventilation in acute respiratory failure. Experience in elderly patients. *Chest.* 1992;102:912.
166. Levy M, Tanios MA, Nelson D, et al. Outcomes of patients with do-not-intubate orders treated with noninvasive ventilation. *Crit Care Med.* 2004;32:2002.
167. Craig DB. Postoperative recovery of pulmonary function. *Anesth Analg.* 1981;60:46.
168. Linder KH, Lotz P, Ahnefeld FW. Continuous positive airway pressure effect on functional residual capacity, vital capacity and its subdivisions. *Chest.* 1987;92:66.
169. Boothby WM, Mayo Cw, Lovelace WR II. The use of oxygen and oxygen-helium, with special reference to surgery. *Surg Clin North Am.* 1940;20:1107.
170. Joris JL, Sottiaux TM, Chiche JD, et al. Effect of bi-level positive airway pressure (BiPAP) nasal ventilation on the postoperative pulmonary restrictive syndrome in obese patients undergoing gastroplasty. *Chest.* 1997; 111:665.
171. Squadrone V, Coha M, Cerutti E, et al. Continuous positive airway pressure for treatment of postoperative hypoxemia: a randomized controlled trial. *JAMA.* 2005;293:589.
172. Jaber S, Chanques G, Sebbane M et al. Non-invasive positive pressure ventilation in patients with respiratory failure due to severe acute pancreatitis. *Respiration.* 2006;73:166.
173. Pinilla J, Oleniuk FH, Tan L, et al. Use of a nasal continuous positive airway pressure mask in the treatment of postoperative atelectasis in aortocoronary bypass surgery. *Crit Care Med.* 1990;18:836.
174. Pennock BE, Kaplan PD, Carlin BW, et al. Pressure support ventilation with a simplified ventilatory support system administered with a nasal mask in patients with respiratory failure. *Chest.* 1991;100:1371.
175. Matte P, Jacquet L, Van Dyck M, et al. Effects of conventional physiotherapy, continuous positive airway pressure and non-invasive ventilatory support with bilevel positive airway pressure after coronary artery bypass grafting. *Acta Anaesthesiol Scand.* 2000;44:75.
176. Aguilo R, Togores B, Pons S, et al. Noninvasive ventilatory support after lung resectional surgery. *Chest.* 1997;112:117.
177. Auriant I, Jallot A, Hervè O, et al. Non-invasive ventilation reduces mortality in acute respiratory failure following lung resection. *Am J Respir Crit Care Med.* 2001;164:1231.
178. Rocco M, Conti G, Antonelli M, et al. Non-invasive pressure support ventilation in patients with acute respiratory failure after bilateral lung transplantation. *Intensive Care Med.* 2001;27:1622.
179. Chiumello D, Chevallard G, Gregoretti C. Non-invasive ventilation in postoperative patients: a systematic review. *Intensive Care Med.* 2011; 37:918.
180. Jenkinson C, Davies RJ, Mullins R, et al. Comparison of therapeutic and subtherapeutic nasal continuous positive airway pressure for obstructive sleep apnoea: a randomised prospective parallel trial. *Lancet.* 1999; 353:2100.
181. Loredo JS, Ancoli-Israel S, Kim EJ, et al. Effect of continuous positive airway pressure versus supplemental oxygen on sleep quality in obstructive sleep apnea: a placebo-CPAP-controlled study. *Sleep.* 2006;29:564.
182. Abbey NC, Block AJ, Green D, et al. Measurement of pharyngeal volume by digitized magnetic resonance imaging. Effect of nasal continuous positive airway pressure. *Am Rev Respir Dis.* 1989;140:717.
183. Schwab RJ, Pack AI, Gupta KB, et al. Upper airway and soft tissue structural changes induced by CPAP in normal subjects. *Am J Respir Crit Care Med.* 1996;154:1106.
184. Sturani C, Galavotti V, Scarduelli C, et al. Acute respiratory failure, due to severe obstructive sleep apnoea syndrome, managed with nasal positive pressure ventilation. *Monaldi Arch Chest Dis.* 1994;49:558.
185. Hurst JM, DeHaven CB, Branson RD. Use of CPAP mask as the sole mode of ventilatory support in trauma patients with mild to moderate respiratory insufficiency. *J Trauma.* 1985;25:1065.
186. Beltrame F, Lucangelo U, Gregori D, et al. Noninvasive positive pressure ventilation in trauma patients with acute respiratory failure. *Monaldi Arch Chest Dis.* 1999;54:109.
187. Xirouchaki N, Kondoudaki E, Anastasaki M, et al. Noninvasive bilevel positive pressure ventilation in patients with blunt thoracic trauma. *Respiration.* 2005;72:517.
188. Chiumello D, Coppola S, Froio S, et al. Noninvasive ventilation in chest trauma: systematic review and meta-analysis. *Intensive Care Med.* 2013;39:1171.
189. Bach JR, Ishikawa Y, Kim H. Prevention of pulmonary morbidity for patients with Duchenne muscular dystrophy. *Chest.* 1997;112:1024.
190. Rabinstein A, Wijdicks EF. BiPAP in acute respiratory failure due to myasthenic crisis may prevent intubation. *Neurology.* 2002;59:1647.
191. Fumeaux T, Rothmeier C, Jolliet P. Outcome of mechanical ventilation for acute respiratory failure in patients with pulmonary fibrosis. *Intensive Care Med.* 2001;27:1868.
192. Antonelli M, Conti G, Riccioni L, et al. Noninvasive positive-pressure ventilation via face mask during bronchoscopy with BAL in high-risk hypoxemic patients. *Chest.* 1996;110:724.
193. Antonelli M, Conti G, Rocco M, et al. Noninvasive positive-pressure ventilation vs. conventional oxygen supplementation in hypoxemic patients undergoing diagnostic bronchoscopy. *Chest.* 2002;121:1149.
194. Antonelli M, Pennisi MA, Conti G, et al. Fiberoptic bronchoscopy during noninvasive positive pressure ventilation delivered by helmet. *Intensive Care Med.* 2003;29:126.
195. Baumann HJ, Klose H, Simon M, et al. Fiber optic bronchoscopy in patients with acute hypoxemic respiratory failure requiring noninvasive ventilation: a feasibility study. *Crit Care.* 2011;15:R179.
196. Clouzeau B, Bui HN, Guilhon E, et al. Fiberoptic bronchoscopy under noninvasive ventilation and propofol target-controlled infusion in hypoxemic patients. *Intensive Care Med.* 2011;37:1969.
197. Chalumeau-Lemoine L, Stoclin A, Billard V, et al. Flexible fiberoptic bronchoscopy and remifentanil target-controlled infusion in ICU: a preliminary study. *Intensive Care Med.* 2013;39:53.
198. Devlin JW, Al-Qadheeb NS, Chi A, et al. Efficacy and safety of early dexmedetomidine during noninvasive ventilation for patients with acute respiratory failure: a randomized, double-blind, placebo-controlled pilot study. *Chest.* 2014;145:1204.
199. Essouri S, Chevret L, Durand P, et al. Noninvasive positive pressure ventilation: five years of experience in a pediatric intensive care unit. *Pediatr Crit Care Med.* 2006;7:329.
200. Yañez LJ, Yunge M, Emilfork M, et al. A prospective, randomized, controlled trial of noninvasive ventilation in pediatric acute respiratory failure. *Pediatr Crit Care Med.* 2008;9:484.
201. Chidini G, Piastra M, Marchesi T, et al. Continuous positive airway pressure with helmet versus mask in infants with bronchiolitis: an RCT. *Pediatrics.* 2015;135:e868.
202. Piastra M, De Luca D, Costa R, et al. Neurally adjusted ventilatory assist vs pressure support ventilation in infants recovering from severe acute respiratory distress syndrome: nested study. *J Crit Care.* 2014;29:312.e1.
203. Hill NS. Complications of noninvasive positive pressure ventilation. *Respir Care.* 1997;42:432.
204. Constantin JM, Schneider E, Cayot-Constantin S, et al. Remifentanil-based sedation to treat noninvasive ventilation failure: a preliminary study. *Intensive Care Med.* 2006;33(1):82.
205. Calderini E, Confalonieri M, Puccio PG, et al. Patient–ventilator asynchrony during noninvasive ventilation: the role of expiratory trigger. *Intensive Care Med.* 1999;25:662.

CHAPTER
104

Invasive Ventilatory Support Modes

CLAUDIA CRIMI, RAIMIS MATULIONIS, DEAN R. HESS, and LUCA M. BIGATELLO

INTRODUCTION

Mechanical ventilation (MV) facilitates gas exchange by substituting, in full or in part, for the action of the respiratory muscles. MV can be provided by applying positive pressure to the proximal airway (positive pressure ventilation [PPV]) or negative pressure ventilation (NPV) to the chest wall. PPV is by far the most commonly used for acute respiratory failure, and is delivered either through an endotracheal or a tracheostomy tube (invasive ventilation), or through a face mask or similar interface applied to the upper airway (noninvasive ventilation, see Chapter 103). This chapter focuses on invasive ventilator modes; many of the principles herein illustrated can be applied to noninvasive MV as well.

PHYSICS OF VENTILATION

During spontaneous breathing, air flows into the lungs as the result of negative intrathoracic pressure generated by the respiratory muscles (P_{MUS}). Exhalation occurs passively due to the elastic recoil pressure accrued during inspiration. P_{MUS} is opposed by the resistance to gas flow imposed by the airways (R_{AW}) and by the static elastance (E, stiffness) of the lungs and chest wall (1):

$$P_{MUS} = P_R + P_E \quad (1)$$

where P_R is the pressure required to overcome R_{AW} and P_E the pressure required to overcome E. During PPV, the driving pressure for air to flow is applied by the ventilator (P_{VENT}) and, in certain modes, by the patient (P_{MUS}) as well:

$$P_{APPL} = P_{MUS} + P_{VENT} = P_R + P_E \quad (2)$$

where P_{APPL} is the total pressure applied, either by the respiratory muscles (P_{MUS}), the ventilator (P_{VENT}), or both. P_E is determined by the elastance of the respiratory system (E) and the size of the tidal volume (V_T):

$$P_E = E \times V_T \quad (3)$$

Using the more familiar entity of compliance (C, the reciprocal of E)

$$P_E = V_T/C \quad (4)$$

P_R is determined by the flow rate of gas ($\dot{V}$) and the R_{AW}

$$P_R = \dot{V} \times R_{AW} \quad (5)$$

The full interaction between patient and ventilator is described by the *equation of motion of the respiratory system* (1).

$$P_{APPL} = P_{MUS} + P_{VENT} = \dot{V} \times R_{AW} + V_T/C \quad (6)$$

This relatively simple mathematical model has two valuable practical implications: (a) it allows measurement of the patient's respiratory mechanics at the bedside; and (b) it can be used to predict the independent variable, for example, airway pressure (P_{AW}), for a given value of the set variable ("control"), for example, the V_T (2). The first function is widely implemented in modern ventilators: we know the set variable, for example, V_T, and the ventilator measures the resulting variable, that is, P_{AW}:

$$C = V_T/P_{AW} \quad (7)$$

$$R_{AW} = P_{AW}/\dot{V} \quad (8)$$

This is accurate if the patient is passively ventilated (P_{MUS} = 0). If the respiratory muscles are contributing to the V_T, measuring mechanics as described may not be accurate, because P_{APPL} is now the result of P_{VENT} and P_{MUS}, but P_{MUS} is unknown. In clinical practice, P_{MUS} can be estimated by measuring the change in intrathoracic pressure in the esophagus (P_{ESO}) by means of an esophageal balloon.

The second function forms the basis of the ventilator-control model used in the modern classifications of ventilatory modes (2). The equation shows that for any mode of ventilation only one variable (P_{AW} or $\dot{V}$) can be controlled at one time, that is, on volume-control ventilation (VCV) $\dot{V}$ is fixed, so we cannot fix the pressure. V_T and $\dot{V}$ are very closely related functions: $\dot{V}$ is the time derivative of V_T, and volume is the time-integral of $\dot{V}$, such that we only need to speak about *pressure control* and *volume control.*

DESCRIPTION OF A VENTILATOR BREATH

There are three principal components of a ventilator breath: how inspiration begins (trigger), what limits the size of the breath (limit), and how inspiration ends (cycle).

The Trigger

Breaths are triggered either by the patient or by the ventilator (3). If the ventilator initiates the breath, the trigger is time, that is, the operator sets a respiratory rate, and the ventilator will deliver the breath at time intervals to achieve that rate. If the breath is initiated by the patient, inspiration starts when the ventilator detects a pressure or flow change at the airway (pressure trigger and flow trigger), or an electrical signal from diaphragmatic activity in neurally adjusted ventilatory assist (NAVA, later in this chapter).

With *pressure trigger* (Fig. 104.1) the ventilator senses a decrease of P_{AW} relative to end-expiration, that is, 0 cm H_2O or positive end-expiratory pressure (PEEP). A preset decrease of $P_{AW,}$ generally 0.5 to 2 cm H_2O, will result in closure of the expiratory valve, opening of the inspiratory valve, and delivery of gas to the airway. With *flow trigger,* the ventilator

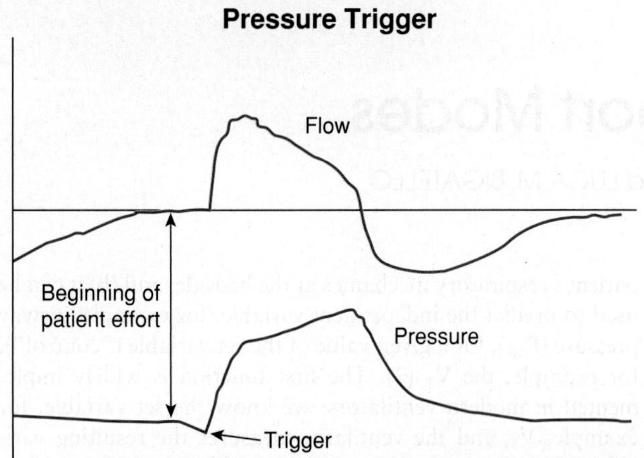

FIGURE 104.1 Pressure triggering and flow triggering. With flow triggering, the negative deflection in airway pressure is deeper than flow triggering. This indicates that, if properly set, flow triggering may require less patient work.

senses a change in flow relative to a baseline continuous low flow (bias flow) of gas through the ventilator circuit that most ventilators use in conjunction with flow triggering. A decrease in this bias flow, generally 1 to 3 L/min, will result in initiation of the inspiratory phase. In the special case of NAVA, an electrode array mounted on a special nasogastric feeding tube senses the change in electrical activity of the diaphragm. The change in P_{AW}, $\dot{V}$, or electrical signal that triggers inspiration is usually caused by the contraction of the respiratory muscles, but can result from artifacts such as transmission of cardiac oscillations (4), air leaks in the system, or movement of the circuit from water condensate.

In modern ventilators, both flow and pressure triggers are very sensitive (5), and if the trigger sensitivity is set correctly, both modalities are clinically effective (6). If trigger sensitivity is diminished by incorrect setting, failure to trigger spontaneous breaths may increase effort and tax the patient's reserve. Failure to trigger is often generated by a physiologic problem such as auto-PEEP (7) or respiratory muscle weakness, and requires attention by the clinician to be detected and corrected.

The Limit

The limit variable determines the size of the breath. This is the independent or control variable—that is, the variable set and controlled by the ventilator. Within limits set by alarms and safety mechanisms, this variable is applied independently of the patient's respiratory mechanics or inspiratory effort. When volume is the preset variable (VCV), the $\dot{V}$ and V_T are set and the P_{AW} can vary. When pressure is the preset limit variable (pressure-control ventilation [PCV] and pressure support ventilation [PSV]), the P_{AW} is set, and $\dot{V}$ and V_T are variable.

The Cycle

The cycle variable is what ends the breath. This can be V_T, $\dot{V}$, P_{AW}, or time. In older ventilators, inspiration was volume-cycled when the volume was delivered from a bellows (Puritan-Bennett MA-1) or piston (Emerson Post-Operative). In modern ventilators, time is the cycle criteria with both VCV and PCV. With PSV, the cycle is usually flow: inspiration ends when the flow rate reaches a fraction of the peak flow. During VCV or PCV, pressure cycle is an alarm condition that avoids application of unsafe high pressure to the airway.

MODES OF VENTILATION

Organization

A mode of ventilation describes the pattern of breathing delivered with a ventilator. Unfortunately, a disproportionate number of proprietary designations exist for a relatively simple structure that is best explained by the *equation of motion of the respiratory system* Eqs. (6 through 8). That is, (a) for any mode of ventilation only one variable is controlled at one time; even in dual modes, where both pressure and volume may be targeted, this occurs in separate phases of the mechanical breath; and, (b) the result of what is set on the ventilator dependent on the setting itself and the patient's mechanics, that is, compliance, resistance, and spontaneous effort. The updated classification of ventilator modes describes three basic components: the control variable, the breath sequence, and the targeting scheme (Fig. 104.2). The control variable is what *limits* the breath, and is discussed in the previous section. Hence, with VCV the P_{AW} varies, and with PCV, the V_T varies.

The possible breath sequences are continuous mandatory ventilation (CMV), continuous spontaneous ventilation (CSV), and intermittent mandatory ventilation (IMV). With CMV (also assist/control ventilation [ACV]), every breath is a mandatory breath type, whether *initiated* from the ventilator or from the patient. With CSV, every breath is a spontaneous breath type. With IMV, spontaneous breathing is allowed between mandatory breaths, so that there will be a mix of mandatory and spontaneous breaths. With CMV or IMV, a minimum rate is set on the ventilator, and the patient can trigger at a more rapid rate. With CSV, there is no set rate other than the alarm parameter (for minute volume or breaths per minute or both) set on the ventilator.

The targeting schemes represent the predetermined goals of ventilator output. The *set-point* scheme includes most of the traditional modes such as VCV, PCV, and PSV. More complex schemes such as *servo* and *adaptive* include proportional assist ventilation (PAV) and volume support (VS) respectively.

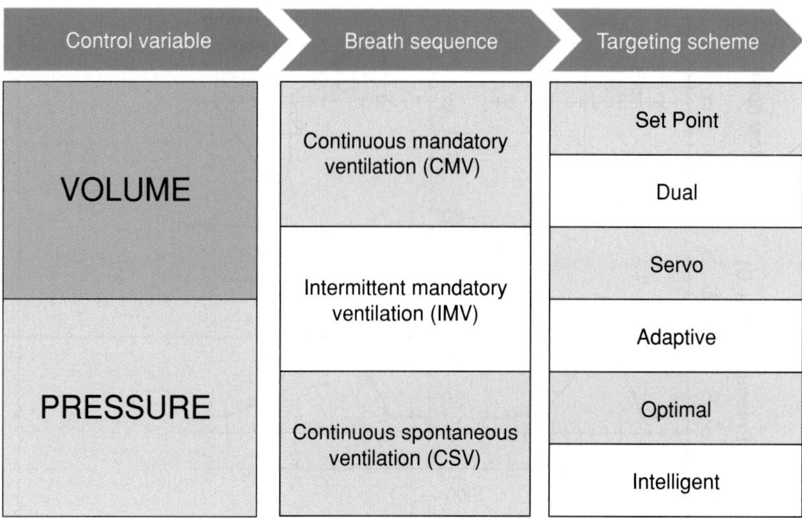

FIGURE 104.2 The taxonomy of ventilator modes: a new classification scheme to describe ventilation modes. (Adapted from Chatburn R. Classification of ventilator modes: update and proposal for implementation. *Respir Care.* 2007;53(3):323.)

A complete description of the targeting schemes is available in Table 104.1.

Continuous Mandatory Ventilation

With CMV (also called Assist/Control, A/C) the ventilator supplies full support of the patient's effort. Disadvantages are the possibilities of hyperventilation and of asynchrony. Hyperventilation (the patient always receives the full breath, even when triggering at a high frequency) is uncommon, because the minute ventilation (V_E) is rapidly blunted by the decrease in $PaCO_2$ that follows hyperventilation (8). Asynchrony occurs more frequently, particularly when the level of support is insufficient (see Chapter 105). CMV A/C can be delivered in both volume- and pressure-control modes.

Volume-Control Ventilation

With VCV, the ventilator controls the inspiratory flow and time to deliver the resultant V_T. In some cases (e.g., Draeger ventilators) V_T, $\dot{V}$, and T_i (inspiratory time) are each set. In this case, an inspiratory breath hold occurs if the set inspiratory time is greater than that required to deliver the V_T at the selected $\dot{V}$. For example, for a V_T of 0.5 L, inspiratory flow of 60 L/min, and inspiratory time 1 second, a 0.5 second breath hold will result. On other ventilators (e.g., Puritan-Bennett 840) an inspiratory hold is set separately.

For VCV, V_T, and Ti are the independent variables, and P_{AW} is the dependent variable, as dictated by the *equation of motion of the respiratory system* Eq. (6), (9,10). Hence, during VCV, the inspiratory pressure applied by the ventilator will increase with a higher V_T, higher $\dot{V}$, lower C, and higher R_{AW}. Because $\dot{V}$ is fixed, a vigorous inspiratory effort will lower the inspiratory pressure, creating asynchrony (9). This can be observed by inspecting the airway pressure waveform (see Chapter 105). In patients with acute respiratory failure, who may have a high respiratory drive, $\dot{V}$ should be carefully set to meet the patient's demand in order to avoid asynchrony and increased (WOB) (11).

Volume-control breaths are generally delivered with a constant inspiratory flow waveform, or square wave. On most ventilators, the inspiratory flow can also be set to a descending ramp waveform. With such a flow pattern, the preset peak inspiratory flow is reached early during the breath, after which flow decreases in a linear fashion, reaching a low level at end inspiration (Fig. 104.3). Given the low inspiratory flow at end inspiration, the peak inspiratory pressure (PIP) is lower and approaches the plateau pressure (P_{PLAT}). Note that, in order to accommodate the lower flow and deliver the same V_T, the inspiratory time will be longer for a descending ramp than

TABLE 104.1 Targeting Schemes Used in Current Mechanical Ventilators

Targeting Scheme	Characteristics	Example Mode Names
Set point	The ventilator will provide an output that matches a target parameter (e.g., pressure limit, V_T, inspiratory flow) set by the operator.	ACV, VCV, SIMV, PCV, BiLevel, PSV
Dual	The ventilator can switch between pressure and volume signal to control the breath size in an attempt to guarantee minute ventilation.	Volume assured PSV CMV with pressure limited
Servo	The ventilator output automatically follows a varying input (e.g., lung mechanics, diaphragmatic activity, airway resistance).	ATC, PAV, NAVA
Adaptive	One target of the ventilator is automatically adjusted to achieve another target as the patient's condition changes.	Autoflow; PRVC, VS
Optimal	One target of the ventilator is automatically adjusted to optimize another target (using ventilatory mechanics measurements) to minimize the work of breathing.	ASV
Intelligent	Ventilator's targets are automatically adjusted according to an artificial rule-based expert system.	SmartCare®

ACV, assisted control ventilation; VCV, volume-controlled ventilation; SIMV, synchronized intermittent mandatory ventilation; PCV, pressure-controlled ventilation; PSV, pressure support ventilation; CMV, continuous mandatory ventilation; ATC, automatic tube compensation; PAV, proportionally assist ventilation; NAVA, neurally adjusted ventilatory assist; PRVC, pressure-regulated volume control; VS, volume support; ASV, adaptive support ventilation. (Adapted from Chatburn R. Classification of ventilator modes: update and proposal for implementation. *Respir Care.* 2007;53(3):323.)

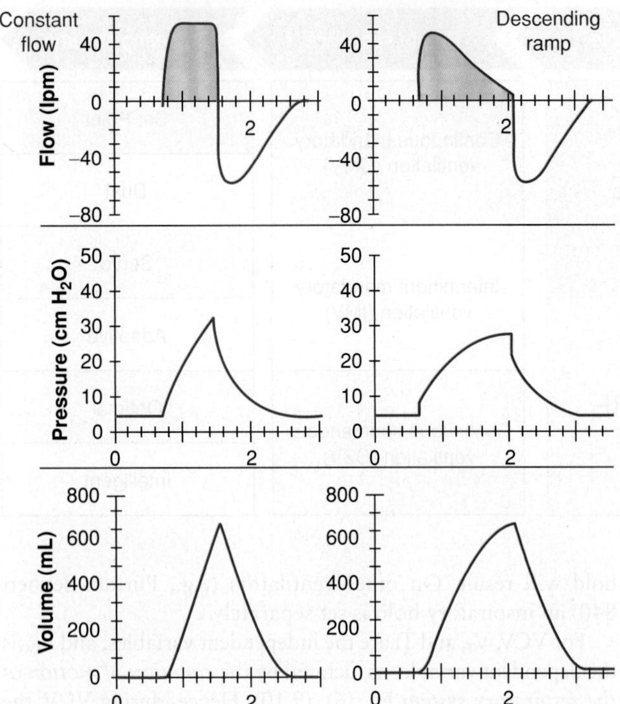

FIGURE 104.3 Flow, pressure, and volume waveforms during volume-control ventilation with constant flow (**left**), and descending ramp (**right**) obtained in a lung model. Note that with the descending ramp flow the peak pressure is lower, the inspiratory time is longer, and, given the low inspiratory flow at end inspiration, the peak inspiratory pressure (PIP) is lower and approaches the plateau pressure (P_{PLAT}). By definition the tidal volume (area under the curve of the flow trace) is unchanged.

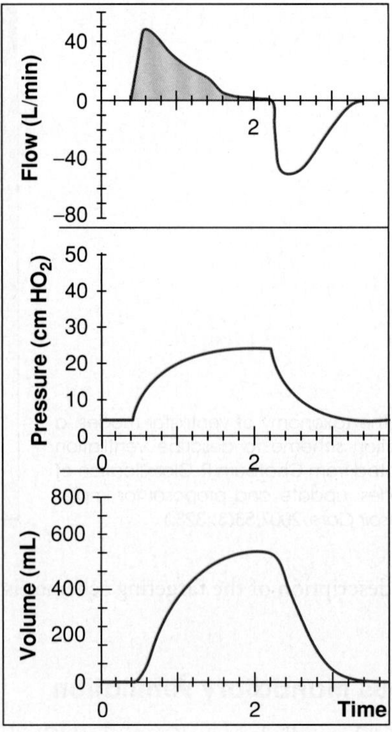

FIGURE 104.4 Flow, pressure, and volume waveforms during pressure-control ventilation. In this instance the inspiratory flow rate reaches 0 before the end of inspiration (*blue area*). Hence, the airway pressure at end inspiration is a true plateau pressure (P_{PLAT}).

for a constant flow waveform. The longer inspiratory time may result in better oxygenation, but the effect is modest. The longer inspiratory time may also increase the risk or air trapping (auto-PEEP) and hemodynamic compromise.

The main advantage of VCV is the ability to control the V_T. This may be important when the $PaCO_2$ must be closely controlled, such as in patients with traumatic brain injury, or when a low V_T is desired as part of a lung-protective ventilation strategy (12,13). Limitations of VCV are related to the fixed V_T and inspiratory flow pattern. This can result in asynchrony in actively breathing patients if efforts are not made to set the inspiratory flow appropriately or to provide adequate sedation (14). With VCV, a high PIP may occur with changes in lung mechanics. However, this only increases the risk of lung injury if the high PIP is associated with an increase in plateau pressure (P_{PLAT}). Accordingly, it is important to monitor P_{PLAT} regularly when VCV is used.

Pressure-Control Ventilation

With PCV, inspiratory pressure and time are set on the ventilator. In some cases (e.g., Draeger ventilators), the set pressure is the total inspiratory pressure, but more commonly it is the pressure above PEEP. For PCV, inspiratory pressure and time are the independent variables. The dependent variables are inspiratory $\dot{V}$ and V_T, as dictated by the *equation of motion of the respiratory system* Eq. (6). Hence, during PCV, inspiratory $\dot{V}$ and V_T will increase with a higher set inspiratory pressure, higher C, and lower R_{AW}. Also, $\dot{V}$ and V_T will increase if the patient generates a vigorous inspiratory effort (i.e., high P_{MUS}). Compared to VCV, this may improve patient-ventilator synchrony (15) but with an increased risk of overdistention lung injury (ventilator-induced lung injury, VILI).

During PCV, the inspiratory flow waveform is a descending ramp (Fig. 104.4). After triggering, the ventilator delivers gas to the airway at a rate dependent on the capability of the ventilator, respiratory mechanics, and patient effort. The set pressure is applied to the airway until the set time is reached. The slope of the descending portion of the inspiratory flow waveform will also depend on the lung mechanics (Fig. 104.5). The initial flow is high, flow descent rapid, and the resulting V_T small when C is low, for example, ARDS, pulmonary fibrosis, and large pleural effusions. The initial flow is low, flow descent slow, and V_T large when R_{AW} is high, for example, chronic obstructive pulmonary disease (COPD) and asthma.

Many current ventilators allow for the adjustment of the rise time (or pressurization rate), which is the time required to reach the set pressure at the onset of inspiration. A fast rise time (the ventilator reaches the target pressure quickly) is associated with a high flow at the onset of inspiration. A slow rise time (the ventilator reaches the target pressure slowly) is associated with a low flow at the onset of inspiration (Fig 104.6). Patients with a high respiratory drive benefit from a fast rise time; patients with a lower respiratory drive might benefit from a slow rise time (16).

A potential advantage of PCV is that it limits the pressure applied to the alveoli (P_{ALV}, clinically estimated by the P_{PLAT}) and the risk of VILI. However, it is important to note that this benefit occurs only if the patient is making no inspiratory effort, because any inspiratory efforts of the patient will increase the transpulmonary distending pressure during PCV. This theoretical advantage of PCV has not been confirmed by appropriately designed clinical trials. The variable inspiratory

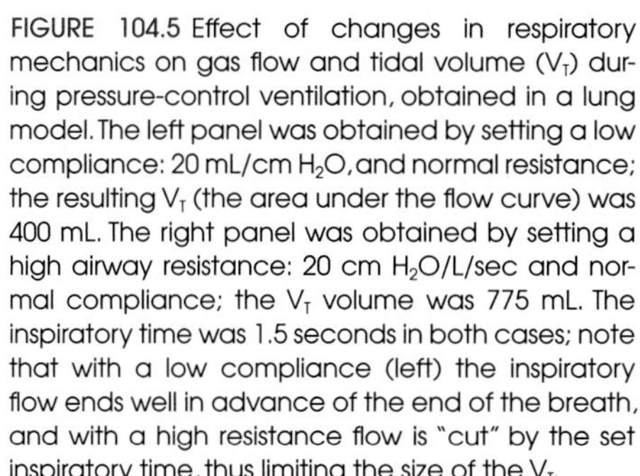

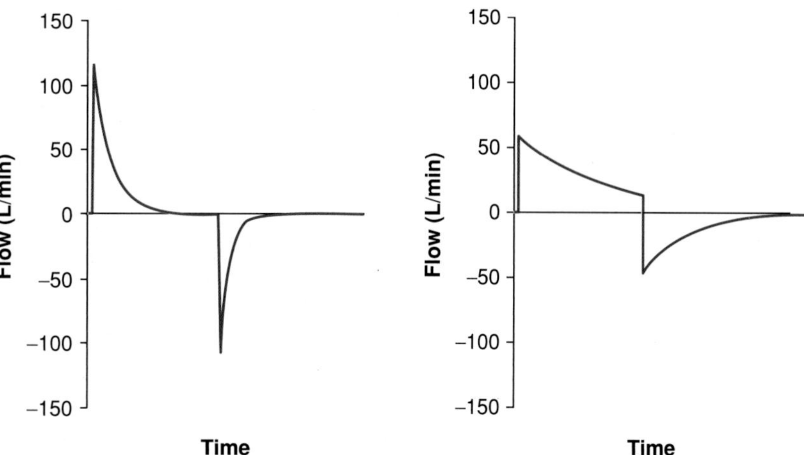

FIGURE 104.5 Effect of changes in respiratory mechanics on gas flow and tidal volume (V_T) during pressure-control ventilation, obtained in a lung model. The left panel was obtained by setting a low compliance: 20 mL/cm H_2O, and normal resistance; the resulting V_T (the area under the flow curve) was 400 mL. The right panel was obtained by setting a high airway resistance: 20 cm H_2O/L/sec and normal compliance; the V_T volume was 775 mL. The inspiratory time was 1.5 seconds in both cases; note that with a low compliance (left) the inspiratory flow ends well in advance of the end of the breath, and with a high resistance flow is "cut" by the set inspiratory time, thus limiting the size of the V_T.

flow pattern may improve patient–ventilator synchrony during active breathing efforts (15). It seems that in patients receiving small V_T during lung-protective strategy, a variable-flow, pressure-targeted breath improves breathing effort compared to a fixed, volume-targeted breath (17).

The square pressure waveform of PCV (and of VCV with a descending ramp flow waveform) produces a higher mean airway pressure than constant flow VCV because the target pressure is reached rapidly and remains at that level through the breath (see Figs. 104.3 and 104.4); this may produce better alveolar recruitment for the same end-inspiratory airway pressure (18). Also, the low end-inspiratory flow with PCV may improve the distribution of ventilation, which may increase PaO_2 and decrease PCO_2, but the effect is usually modest (19).

A limitation of PCV is the inability to guarantee a V_T and a stable $PaCO_2$. With PCV, changes in respiratory mechanics can result in hypoventilation. In particular, PCV can cause hypoventilation in the presence of dynamic hyperinflation and auto-PEEP. For example, if the inspiratory pressure is set at 15 cm H_2O and the PEEP is zero, the driving pressure is 15 cm H_2O. If the patient develops dynamic hyperinflation and auto-PEEP of 10 cm H_2O, the driving pressure is 5 cm H_2O, with consequent hypoventilation. With VCV, this will not occur because the set V_T is delivered regardless of the level of auto-PEEP, albeit with a higher PIP and P_{PLAT}.

The selection of PCV or VCV is based chiefly on individual preference. If V_T, P_{PLAT}, and transpulmonary distending pressure (see Chapter 105) are carefully monitored, either PCV or VCV can be used safely and effectively. Moreover current data from RCTs are insufficient to confirm or refute whether PCV or VCV offers any advantage for patients with acute respiratory failure due to ARDS (20).

Adaptive Pressure Control. Adaptive pressure control allows the ventilator to control pressure based on a volume feedback loop. Because the ventilator controls either pressure or volume, but not both at the same time, there is no divergence from the *law of motion of the respiratory system* Eq. (6). With adaptive pressure control, the ventilator delivers PCV and adjusts the pressure control in the attempt to keep V_T constant.

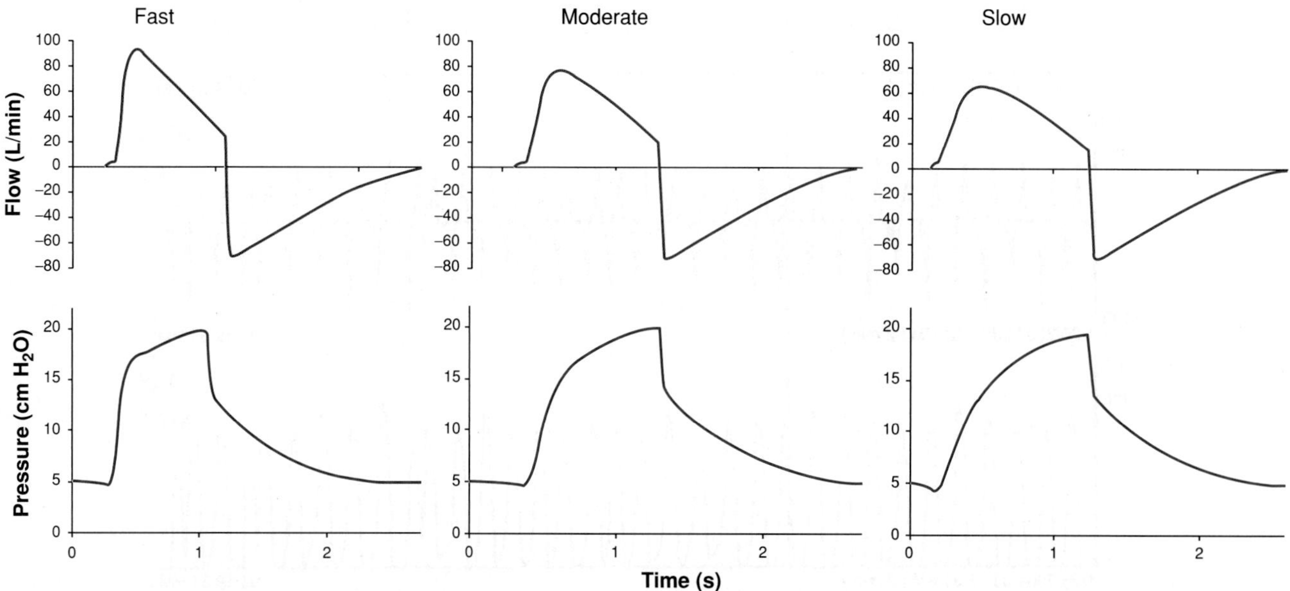

FIGURE 104.6 Flow and pressure waveforms obtained at increasing rise times of inspiratory flow at a pressure support of 20 cm H_2O. The fastest flow delivery (**left**) results in a rapid reach of the set pressure, thus favoring synchrony for high demand breaths. The slowest delivery (**right**) may be more comfortable during quiet, unstressed breathing. (Adapted from Gibbons FK, Hess DR. Mechanical ventilation. In: Bigatello LM, ed. *Critical Care Handbook of the Massachusetts General Hospital.* 4th ed. Philadelphia, PA: Lippincott Williams & Wilkins; 2006.)

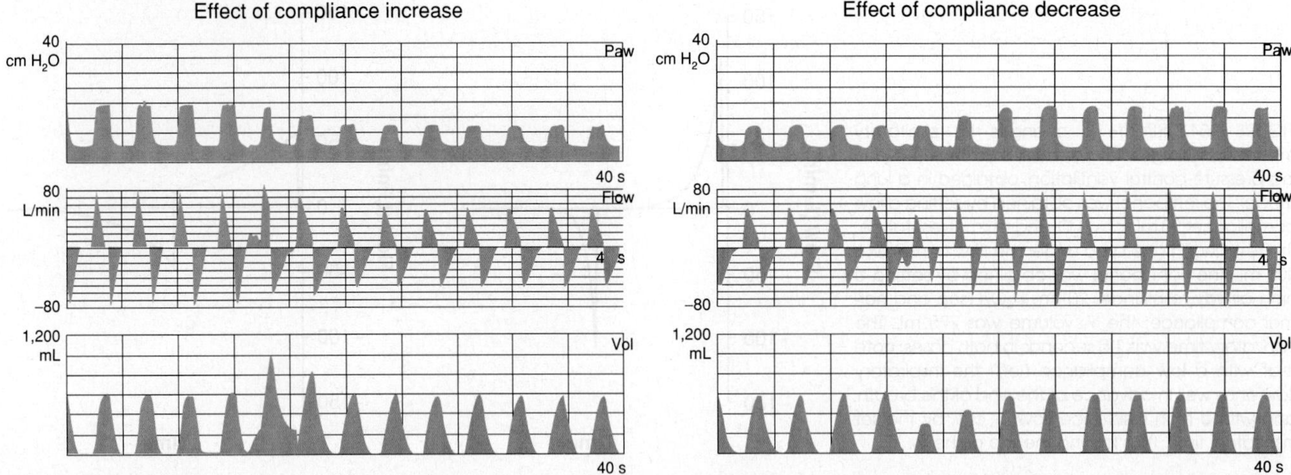

FIGURE 104.7 Adaptive pressure control with a set tidal volume of 600 mL. Left: effects of an increase in lung compliance. The first four breaths are at steady state; with the fifth and sixth breaths the tidal volume (V_T) is higher due to an increase in compliance as indicated by the steady airway pressure (P_{AW}). From the sixth breath, P_{AW} starts decreasing, and the original V_T is restored. Right panel: effects of a decrease in lung compliance. The first four breaths are at steady state; with the fifth breath the V_T is lower due to a decrease in compliance as indicated by a steady P_{AW}. From the sixth breath the P_{AW} is increasing, and the original V_T is restored. (Adapted from Branson RD, Johannigman JA. The role of ventilator graphics when setting dual-control modes. *Respir Care.* 2005;50:187, with permission.)

Pressure-regulated volume control (PRVC) (21–27) (Maquet, CareFusion), AutoFlow (Draeger), VC+ (Puritan-Bennett), PCV-Volume Guaranteed (PCV-VG, GE), Adaptive pressure ventilation (Hamilton, Galileo) are trade names of gas delivery that function in a similar manner. Each mode increases or decreases the pressure breath-to-breath by no more than 3 cm H_2O per breath to deliver the desired V_T. The pressure limit fluctuates between PEEP and 5 cm H_2O below the upper pressure alarm setting, as illustrated by the example in Figure 104.7. An alarm occurs if the V_T and maximum pressure settings are incompatible. The proposed advantage of dual control is the ability of the ventilator to meet patient demand (an advantage of PCV) while maintaining a constant V_E (an advantage of VCV). However, the V_T and transpulmonary distending pressure during PRVC can potentially exceed safe limits, as illustrated by the example in Figure 104.8 (24). This is of particular concern if these modes are utilized to limit the size of the V_T to avoid VILI, suggesting that these modes

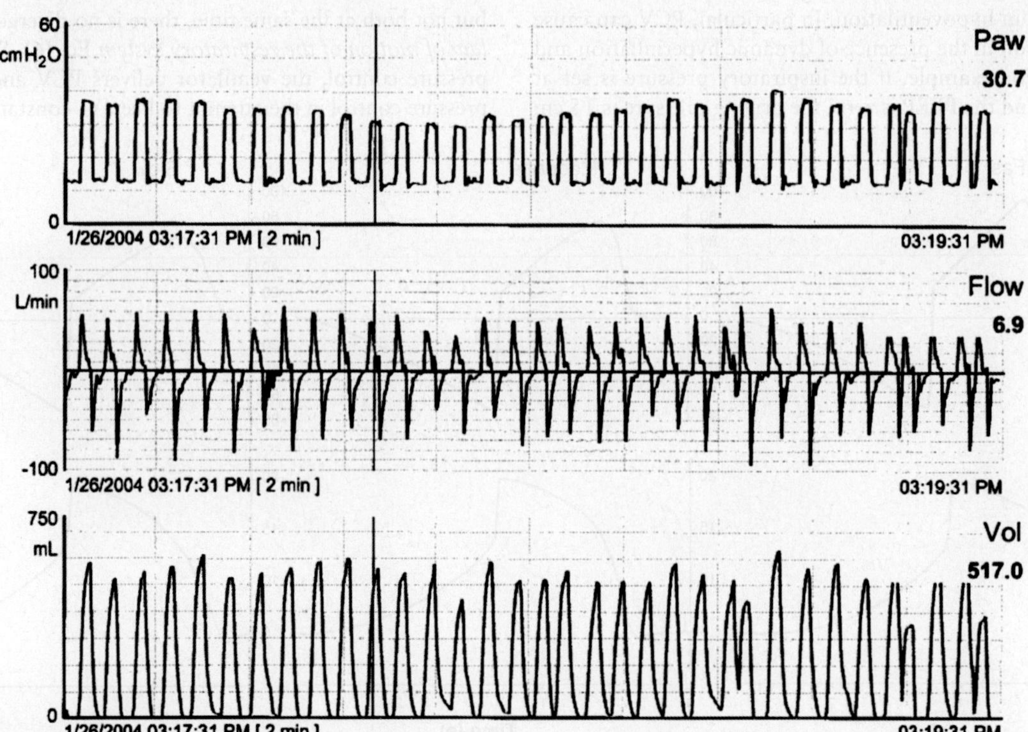

FIGURE 104.8 Airway pressure (P_{AW}), flow, and volume waveforms demonstrating the response of a dual-control algorithm over a 2-minute period with varying patient effort. The tidal volume varies above and below the target (500 mL) by as much as 150 mL. (From Branson RD, Johannigman JA. The role of ventilator graphics when setting dual-control modes. *Respir Care.* 2005;50:187, with permission.)

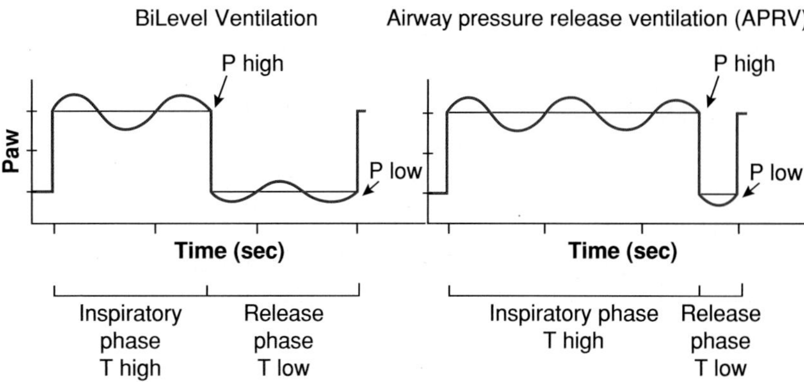

FIGURE 104.9 Airway pressure (P_{AW}) waveform during BiLevel (**left**) and airway pressure release ventilation (APRV, **right**). Superimposed changes of P_{AW} due to spontaneous breathing activity are shown at both P_{AW} levels: P-high and P-low. With BiLevel, P-high and P-low are set of the same duration; without spontaneous breathing the BiLevel trace would be undistinguishable from pressure-control ventilation (PCV). With APRV, P-high is much longer than P-low, with the purpose to enhance alveolar recruitment; without spontaneous breathing, this would be again PCV, with an extreme I:E ratio. (Adapted with permission from Seymour C, Frazer M, Reilly PM, Fuchs BD. Airway pressure release and biphasic intermittent positive airway pressure ventilation: Are they ready for prime time? *J Trauma.* 2007;62:1298–1309.)

may not be as safe as traditional VCV when used as part of a lung-protective ventilation strategy. Moreover, if patient effort increases, the level of support decreases, which could result in asynchrony and discomfort (28). Additionally, as the pressure level is reduced, mean airway pressure will fall, potentially resulting in a fall in PaO_2. Because this mode depends on the measured V_T, any errors in measurement will also result in decision errors.

Pressure Control Inverse Ratio Ventilation. With PCIRV the T_i is set longer than the expiratory time T_e. The result is a higher mean airway pressure (see Chapter 105) and enhanced lung recruitment, but also a higher potential for air trapping and hemodynamic compromise. In the past, this ventilatory strategy was used with the rationale that it improves lung recruitment (e.g., ARDS) (29,30). However, this approach likely results in little additional alveolar recruitment unless auto-PEEP results from the short expiratory time.

Bilevel Positive Airway Pressure (BiLevel) Ventilation and Airway Pressure Release Ventilation. Current-generation expiratory valves that are used with PCV allow the delivery of additional inspiratory flow if the P_{AW} decreases below the set value, thereby permitting spontaneous breathing during the inspiratory phase of the ventilator. This happens with modes of ventilation such as BiLevel and APRV (31,32). Ambiguity exists in the nomenclature of these modes (7), in part because of proprietary technology used by different manufacturers. For example, BiLevel (Covidien), Biphasic (CareFusion), BiVent (Maquet), and BiPAP and APRV by Draeger and GE. For clarity, in this section we will use the terms BiLevel and APRV.

During fully controlled ventilation, BiLevel is identical to PCV, and APRV is Bi-Level with extreme inverse I:E ratio. The patient can breathe spontaneously at the two set levels of pressure (P-high and P-low; Fig. 104.9). P-high is equivalent to a continuous positive airway pressure (CPAP) level that is held for a set time (T-high). The CPAP phase is intermittently released to a set P-low level (CPAP at a lower pressure) generally of brief duration (T-low), and the high CPAP is then reestablished. Spontaneous breathing may be superimposed at both pressure levels, and is independent of time cycling. Spontaneous breathing can be supported with PSV. With APRV, the set duration of P-high is extreme, and the short time at P-low is intended to deliver a mandatory breath in reverse from a traditional positive pressure breath. The minute ventilation during both these modes results from the amount of spontaneous breathing, the difference between the two pressure levels, and the frequency at which the pressure is released to the lower level. The P-high level is the main determinant of arterial oxygenation, but the additional spontaneous breaths may further improve gas exchange by preferentially recruiting the dependent lung regions (33,34). The duration of T-low is set sufficiently short to interrupt expiratory flow and maintain alveolar recruitment due to air trapping.

The potential advantage of these modes is lung recruitment and improved oxygenation at a relatively low airway pressure (the P-high) and possibly higher mean airway pressure. In addition, maintaining spontaneous breathing provides further recruitment to lung segments adjacent to the diaphragm and may decrease the need for sedation. On the other hand, a long inspiratory time may prove uncomfortable in some patients. A concern with APRV is the high transpulmonary pressure that can be generated during spontaneous breathing at P-high, as this could potentially results in injurious distending pressures. The use of these modes in clinical practice is limited by the lack of evidence for improved outcomes. APRV improves oxygenation through lung recruitment (35) while maintaining spontaneous breathing, attractive features in diseases like ARDS. However, it may also increase ventilator days and ICU length of stay (36), possibly due to the complexity of implementation.

Synchronized Intermittent Mandatory Ventilation

With SIMV, the ventilator provides a mandatory breath rate. If the patient breathes at a higher rate, the additional breaths are unsupported (Fig. 104.10). If the patient has no spontaneous breathing efforts, SIMV, CMV, and A/CV are synonymous. The mandatory breaths are synchronized to patient trigger effort, and can be volume control, pressure control, or adaptive pressure control. It has been traditionally taught that during SIMV the ventilator does the work for the mandatory breaths, and the patient does the work for the spontaneous breaths, thus integrating effort and support. As such, weaning from the ventilator would occur by progressively decreasing the mandatory breath rate. However, this has not been confirmed by either physiologic or outcome studies (37,38). Inspiratory effort may be as great during mandatory breaths as during spontaneous breaths, as shown in Figure 104.10, thus denying the purpose of unloading the work of breathing with the mandatory breath. The combination of mandatory and spontaneous breaths can also lead to asynchrony (39).

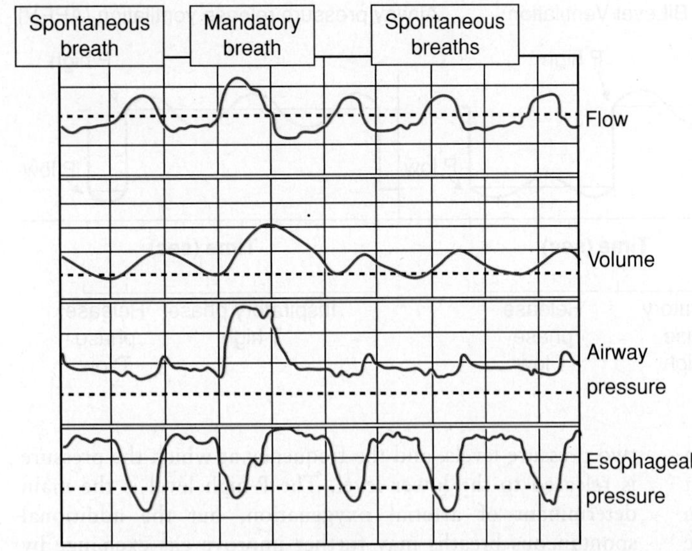

FIGURE 104.10 Synchronized intermittent mandatory ventilation (SIMV). Flow, volume, airway pressure, and esophageal pressure waveforms are shown. Note the persistence of the patient's own negative intrathoracic pressure during the mandatory breath. (Adapted from Hess D, Branson RD. Ventilators and weaning modes. *Respir Care Clin North Am.* 2000;6(9):407, with permission.)

Part of the SIMV shortcomings can be resolved by supporting spontaneous breathing with PSV (Fig. 104.11); this has become a routine addition when SIMV is used. A particular way to accomplish this goal of supporting the spontaneous breaths with SIMV is with BiLevel (Covidien) (PCV+ in the Draeger). This mode allows delivering PSV as the primary mode with a low number (typically 1–4) of BiLevel mandatory breaths that can be thought of as sighs (40). The mandatory breaths are set at relative high P_{AW} to provide recruitment, for example, 25 to 30 cm H_2O, and a relatively long inspiratory time, for example, 3 to 4 seconds (Fig. 104.12). With the PCV+ mode, these mandatory breaths are BiLevel breaths that allow spontaneous breathing during the sigh, thus further enhancing recruitment (40).

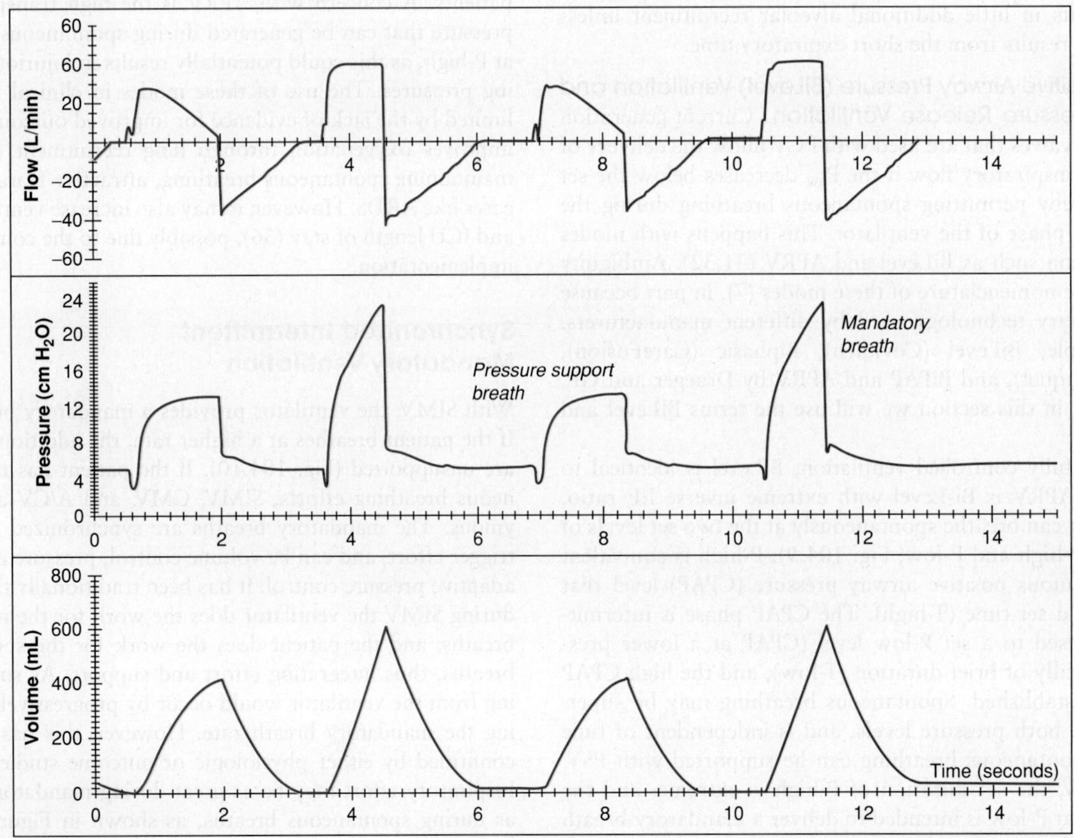

FIGURE 104.11 Synchronized intermittent mandatory ventilation (SIMV). Flow, airway pressure, and volume waveforms obtained in a lung model. The mandatory breaths are constant flow, volume-controlled ventilation, and the spontaneous breaths are pressure support ventilation.

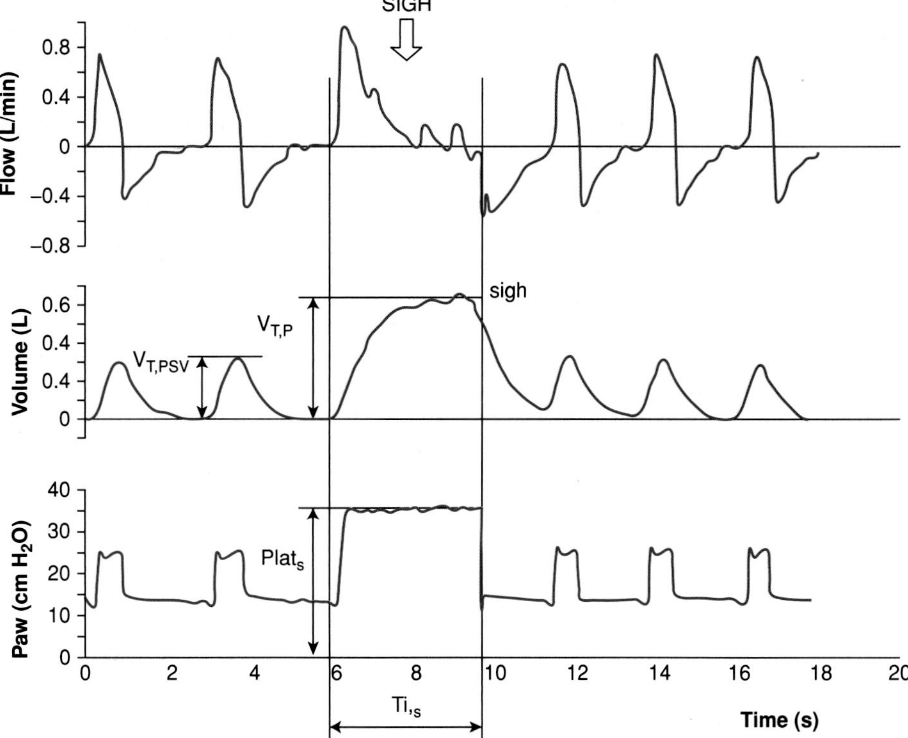

FIGURE 104.12 Using a sigh breath in conjunction with pressure support ventilation. The patient is ventilated with a Draeger Evita 4 in PCV+ mode. Paw is airway pressure. (Adapted from Patroniti N, Foti G, Cortinovis B, et al. Sigh improves gas exchange and lung volume in patients with acute respiratory distress syndrome undergoing pressure support ventilation. *Anesthesiology.* 2002;96:788, with permission.)

Continuous Spontaneous Ventilation

Continuous Positive Airway Pressure

CPAP provides positive P_{AW} throughout the respiratory cycle, promoting recruitment and possibly decreasing work of breathing (41). This is traditionally accomplished by maintaining $\dot{V}$ at the airway higher than the patient's inspiratory $\dot{V}$. Such a system is still occasionally employed without the support of a ventilator, with the high gas flow coming directly from a regulator at the gas source (42). When delivered by a mechanical ventilator, the need to supply very high $\dot{V}$ is generally circumvented by substituting CPAP with PSV, for example, 2 cm H_2O (Fig. 104.13). This is possible in modern ventilators by virtue of very

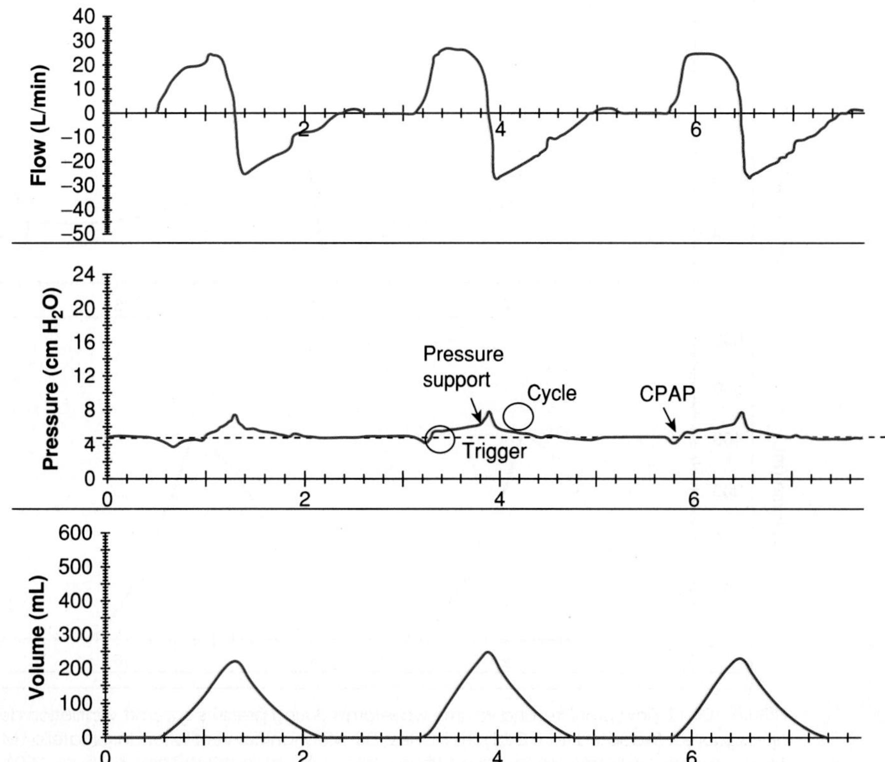

FIGURE 104.13 Flow, pressure, and volume waveforms during continuous positive airway pressure (CPAP) by a ventilator. The airway pressure fluctuates above and below the set CPAP level of 5 cm H_2O (see text for explanation).

low-resistance exhalation valves and minimal time delay for triggering and cycling.

CPAP is used to treat hypoxemia by maintaining alveolar recruitment throughout the respiratory cycle, to treat acute cardiogenic pulmonary edema by raising intrathoracic pressure, and to counterbalance auto-PEEP in patients with obstructive lung disease.

Pressure Support Ventilation

With PSV, the ventilator applies a set inspiratory pressure to assist each patient-initiated breath (Fig. 104.14) (43). The early part of inspiration is similar to PCV. Once the patient triggers the ventilator, inspiratory $\dot{V}$ is delivered at a variable rate, and the rise time can be adjusted (44,45). When the set inspiratory pressure is reached, $\dot{V}$ decreases with a variable decay (see above: PCV). The size of the V_T is the result of the set inspiratory pressure, the patient's mechanics, and the patient's inspiratory effort (see Chapter 105). Differently from PCV, where inspiration ends by time, with PSV inspiration ends when the inspiratory flow falls to a ventilator-preset value, such as 25% of the peak flow. Most current ventilators allow the clinician to adjust the fraction of the inspiratory flow at which inspiration ends—the expiratory sensitivity (Fig. 104.15) (46–50). Setting a high expiratory sensitivity (e.g., 50% of the peak rate) will shorten the duration of the breath, which may be desirable in situation of expiratory flow limitation and slow flow decay such as COPD. A low expiratory sensitivity (e.g., 5% of the peak rate) will prolong the duration of the breath, which may be desirable in situation of a low compliance such as ARDS.

SmartCare® (Draeger) is a closed-loop application (using ventilator output as a feedback signal to adjust the system toward the desired output) of PSV designed for ventilator weaning (51). It adapts the level of PSV to the patient's ventilatory needs, with the goal to keep the patient within a comfort zone. Comfort is defined primarily as a respiratory

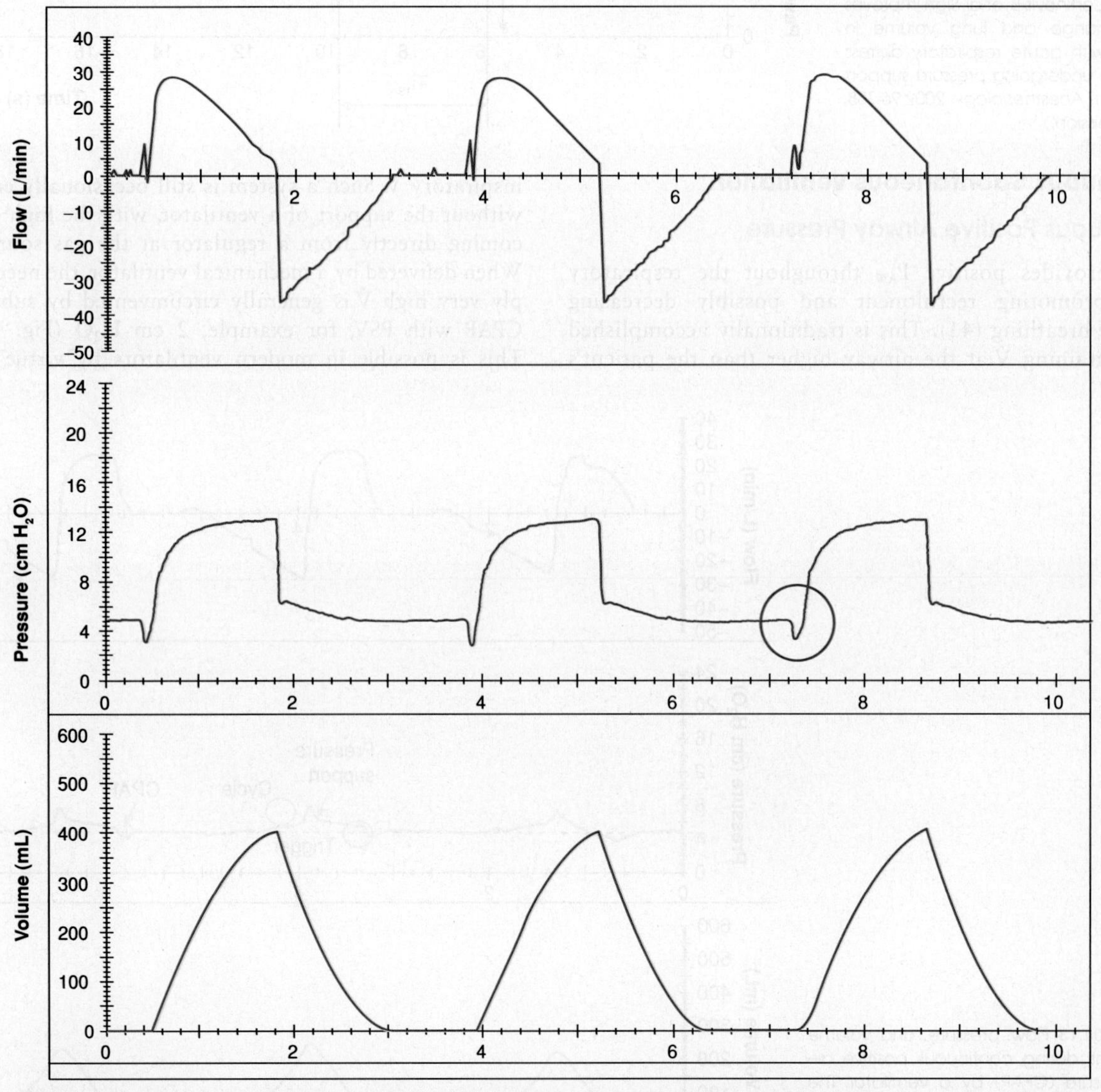

FIGURE 104.14 Flow, pressure, and volume waveforms during pressure support ventilation delivered by a lung model. All breaths are triggered. (Adapted from Gibbons FK, Hess DR. Mechanical ventilation. In: Bigatello LM, ed. *Critical Care Handbook of the Massachusetts General Hospital.* 4th ed. Philadelphia, PA: Lippincott Williams & Wilkins; 2006.)

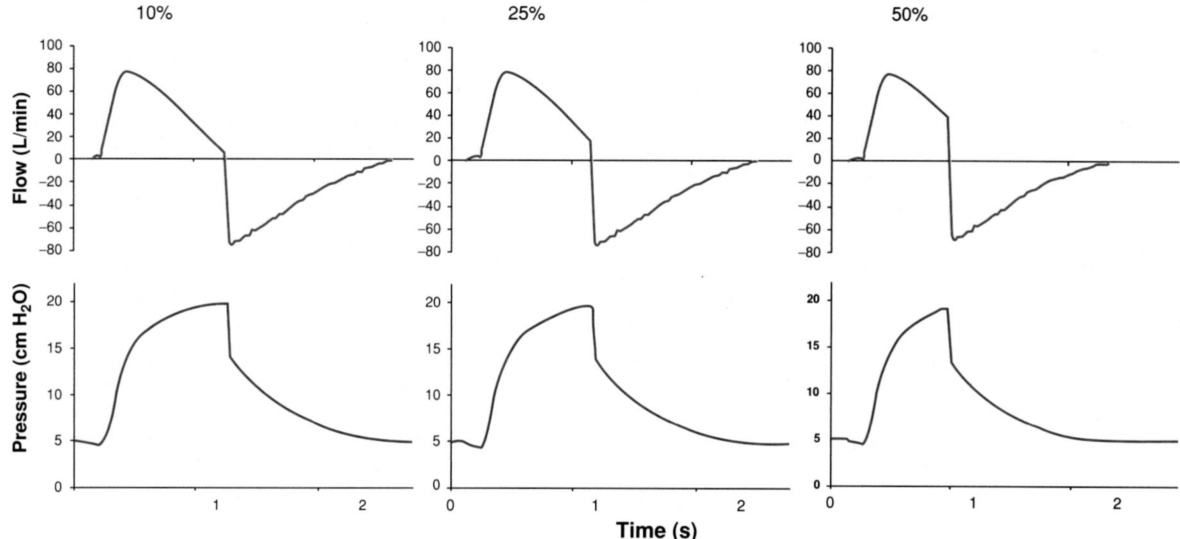

FIGURE 104.15 Examples of flow termination criteria of 10%, 25%, and 50% using a Puritan-Bennett 840 ventilator with pressure support of 15 cm H_2O and PEEP 5 cm H_2O. (Adapted from Gibbons FK, Hess DR. Mechanical ventilation. In: Bigatello LM, ed. *Critical Care Handbook of the Massachusetts General Hospital*. 4th ed. Philadelphia, PA: Lippincott Williams & Wilkins; 2006.)

rate that can vary in the range of 15 to 30 breaths/min, a V_T above a minimum threshold (>300 mL), and an end-tidal CO_2 ($PetCO_2$) below a maximum threshold (usually <55 mmHg). The level of support is periodically adapted by the system in increments or decrements of 2 to 4 cm H_2O. The system automatically tries to reduce the pressure level to a minimum value. At this value, a spontaneous breathing trial is performed. If successful, a message on the screen recommends removal from the ventilator (i.e., extubation). This mode was shown to reduce the duration of MV as compared with physician-controlled weaning (52), but these data were not confirmed by subsequent studies (53,54). A recent Cochrane review (55) suggested that, SmartCare may result in reduced duration of weaning time, days on MV, and length of stay in ICU with no increase in adverse events, but due to a substantial heterogeneity in trials reporting weaning duration, further randomized controlled trials need to better evaluate its clinical role on patients' outcome (56).

Volume support uses PSV in a manner analogous to the use by PRVC of PCV (21–27). In other words, the ventilator adjusts the inspiratory pressure according to a set minimum V_T. If the patient's effort increases (higher V_T for the set level of PSV), the ventilator decreases the support of the next breath. If the compliance or patient effort decreases, the ventilator increases the support to maintain the set V_T. This combines the attributes of PSV with the guaranteed minimum V_T. A concern with this mode is that the ventilator takes away support if the patient's respiratory demand increases and V_T exceeds what was set. This results in increased WOB (28).

AutoMode is a dual-controlled mode available on the Maquet ventilators (21,22). It provides automated weaning from PCV to PSV, and automated escalation of support if patient effort diminishes. The ventilator provides PRVC if the patient is making no breathing efforts. If the patient triggers two consecutive breaths, the ventilator switches to VS. If the patient becomes apneic, the ventilator switches back to PRVC. AutoMode can also switch between PCV and PSV or VCV and VS.

Adaptive Support Ventilation

ASV is based on the *minimal work-of-breathing* concept. The patient will breathe at a V_T and respiratory frequency that minimizes the elastic and resistive loads while maintaining oxygenation and acid-base balance (57). The ventilator attempts to deliver 100 mL/kg V_E (expired minute volume) for an adult and 200 mL/kg for a child. This can be adjusted by setting the % V_E control from 20% to 350%, which allows the clinician to provide full ventilatory support or encourage spontaneous breathing and facilitate weaning. When first connected to the patient, the ventilator delivers a series of test breaths and measures C, R_{AW}, and auto-PEEP. The input of body weight allows the ventilator's algorithm to choose a required V_E. Lung mechanics are measured on a breath-to-breath basis, and ventilator settings are altered to meet the desired targets. If the patient breathes spontaneously, the ventilator will support breaths. Spontaneous and mandatory breaths can be combined to meet the minute ventilation target. The pressure limit of both the mandatory and spontaneous breaths is adjusted continuously. This means that ASV is continuously using adaptive pressure control for mandatory and spontaneous breaths.

The ventilator adjusts the I:E ratio and inspiratory time of mandatory breaths by calculation of the expiratory time constant (compliance × resistance) and maintains sufficient expiratory time to prevent auto-PEEP. If the patient is triggering, the number of mandatory breaths decreases and the ventilator chooses a pressure support that maintains a tidal volume sufficient to ensure alveolar ventilation based on a dead space calculation of 2.2 mL/kg. ASV can provide pressure-limited, time-cycled ventilation, add adaptive pressure control, allow for mandatory breaths and spontaneous breaths (SIMV + PSV), and eventually switch to pressure support (adaptive pressure control with PSV).

Tube Compensation

Tube compensation (TC) is designed to overcome the flow-resistive work of breathing imposed by the endotracheal or tracheostomy tube (58,59). It uses the known resistive coefficients of the artificial airway (tracheostomy or endotracheal tube) and measurement of instantaneous flow to apply a pressure proportional to resistance throughout the total respiratory cycle. With TC, the ventilator targets the tracheal pressure, rather than proximal airway pressure, increasing the proximal airway pressure necessary to overcome the flow-resistive properties of the artificial airway (Fig. 104.16). The clinician can set the fraction of tube resistance for which compensation is desired (e.g., 50% compensation rather than full compensation). On some ventilators, TC can be used with any mode, whereas on others, it can be used only with CPAP. Because in vivo tracheal tube resistance tends to be greater than in vitro resistance, incomplete compensation for endotracheal tube resistance may occur. Additionally, kinks or bends in the tube as it traverses the upper airway and accumulation of secretions in the inner lumen will change the tube's resistive coefficient and result in incomplete compensation. Available evidence suggests that TC can effectively compensate for resistance through the artificial airway but has not shown improved outcomes with this mode (60,61). At present there is no convincing evidence that TC is a superior mode for SBT except for patients with a resistive work of breathing imposed by the tracheal tube (62).

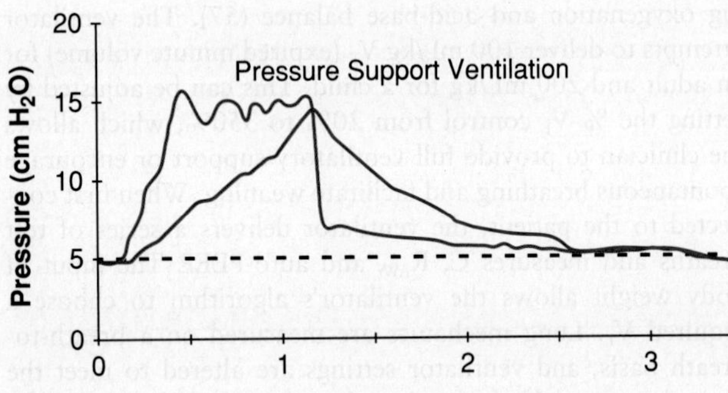

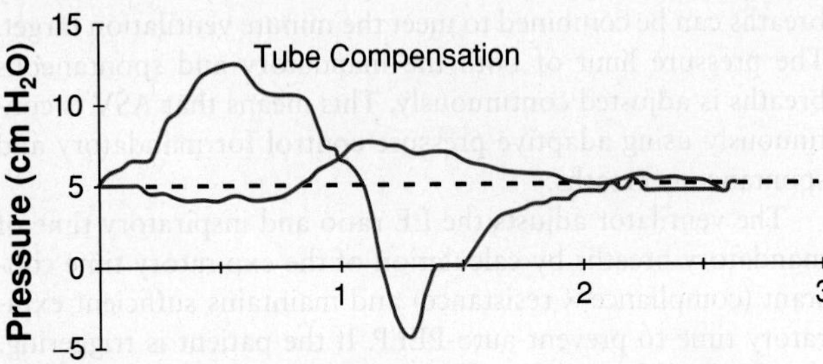

FIGURE 104.16 Tube compensation. Pressure waveforms from the trachea (*blue lines*) and the proximal airway (*red lines*) during pressure support ventilation and automatic tube compensation. Note that the tracheal pressure fluctuates very little during automatic tube compensation. (Adapted from Fabry B, Haberthur C, Zappe D, et al. Breathing pattern and additional work of breathing in spontaneously breathing patients with different ventilatory demands during inspiratory pressure support and automatic tube compensation. *Intensive Care Med.* 1997;23:545, with permission.)

Proportional Assist Ventilation

With PAV (63–65), the ventilator applies inspiratory pressure as a positive feedback controller, where respiratory E and R are the feedback signal gains, defined as K_1 (cm H_2O/L) and K_2 (cm H_2O/L/sec), respectively, following the *equation of motion of the respiratory system* Eq. (6).

$$P_{APPL} = K_1 \times V + K_2 \times \dot{V} \qquad (9)$$

where K_1 and K_2 substitute E and R_{AW}, respectively. K_1 and K_2 are the preset values of volume and flow gains of the proportional assist ventilator. The ventilator measures the patient's instantaneous inspiratory flow rate and provides the set support through a rapid positive feedback loop (Fig. 104.17).

PAV should provide optimal patient–ventilator synchrony by following and amplifying the patient's inspiratory flow on a breath-by-breath basis. This differs from PSV, in which the level of support is constant regardless of demand, and VCV, in which the level of support decreases when demand increases. It is important to note that, like other continuous spontaneous breathing modes, PAV requires the presence of an intact ventilatory drive. A dangerous runaway,

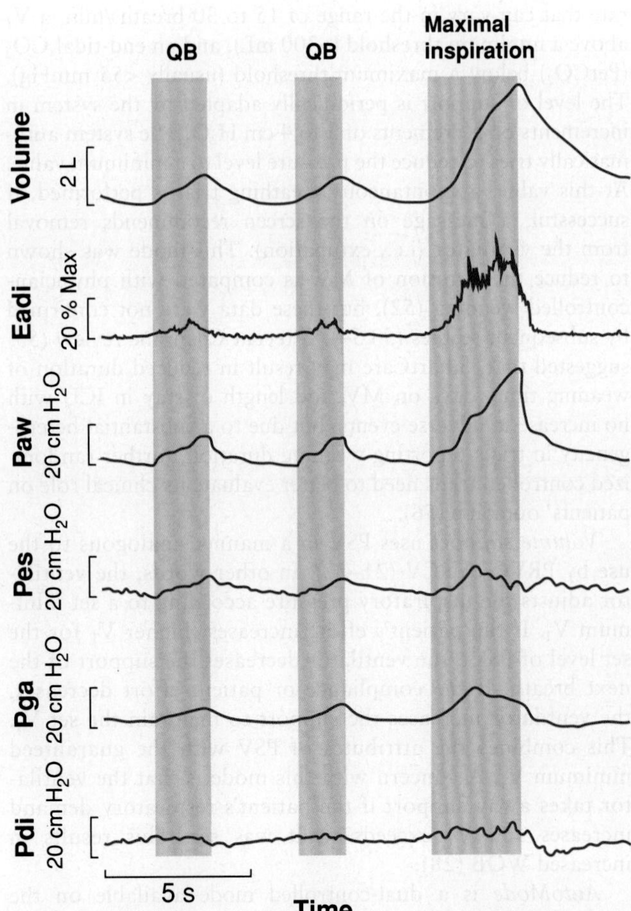

FIGURE 104.17 Airway pressure (P_{AW}), flow, and volume waveforms during proportional assist ventilation. Note that the P_{AW} varies with the inspiratory flow and volume demands of the patient. (Adapted from Marantz S, Patrick W, Webster K, et al. Response of ventilator-dependent patients to different levels of proportional assist. *J Appl Physiol.* 1996;80:397, with permission.)

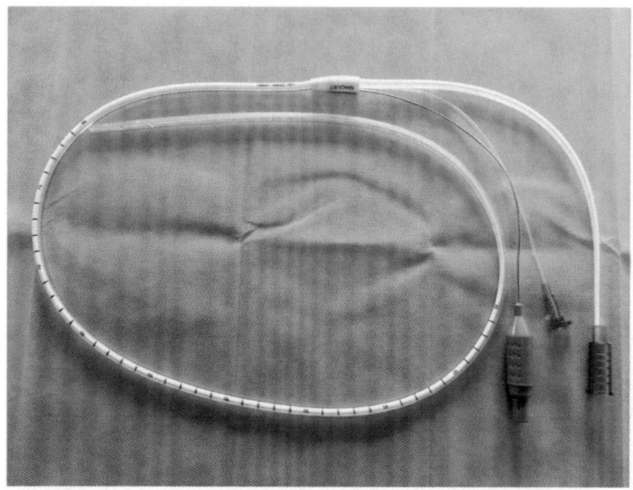

FIGURE 104.18 The NAVA catheter. It is a special catheter (called the Edi Catheter), fitted with an array of 10 electrodes (nine measuring and one reference electrode); it comes in different sizes ranging from 6 to 16 Fr. and are chosen according to the patient's height. A Nose-Ear-Xiphoid (NEX) measurement protocol distance is used for each patient to determine insertion length. Like an ordinary feeding tube, the Edi Catheter is placed in the esophagus and captures the electrical activity of the diaphragm (Edi). (Courtesy of Alberto Noto MD, Department of Anesthesia and Critical Care, Policlinico G. Martino, Messina, Italy.)

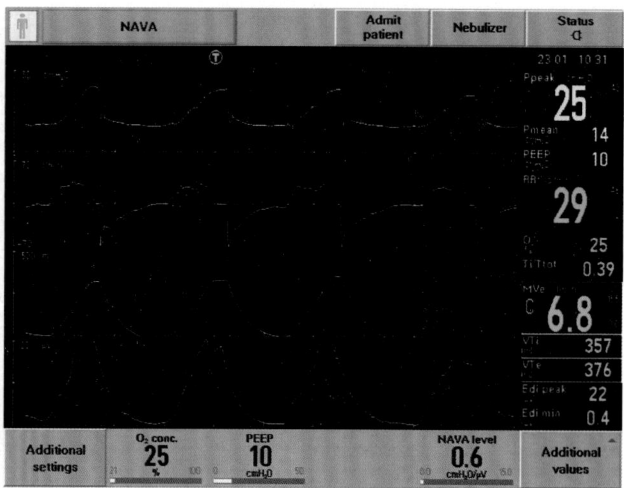

FIGURE 104.19 A screenshot showing a patient ventilating in the neurally adjusted ventilatory assist (NAVA) mode. Due to the continuous adjustments of airway pressure (at the top, reflecting ventilatory assist) with changes in diaphragmatic electrical activity (at the bottom, reflecting neural drive) during changes in tidal and end-expiratory lung volumes there is a perfect match between the neural demand and delivered support. (Adapted from Hopkins P, Hadfield D. The use of neurally adjusted ventilatory assist to unmask and overcome critical dyssynchrony in flow–triggered pressure support. Cure & Care website. http://www.cureandcareportal.com/use-neurally-adjusted-ventilatory-assist-unmask-overcome-critical-dyssynchrony-flow-triggered-pressure-support/. Accessed May 23, 2017.)

that is, a continuous increase in respiratory support, may occur in situation like a large air leak, where the ventilator does not record an end to the inspiratory flow and continues to amplify the support. This is a similar situation to the prolonged inspiratory time that can occur with an air leak during PSV.

A concern with PAV is its dependence on measures of R_{AW} and E. These can be difficult to measure during spontaneous breathing, and they change frequently over the course of MV. In its initial application, the clinician measured (or estimated) compliance and resistance and set the proportion of inspiratory support that the ventilator would provide, generally as a percentage of elastic and resistive work, respectively. In a newer algorithm of PAV (PAV+, Puritan-Bennett 840/980), the ventilator applies a 300-msec end-inspiratory and end-expiratory pause every 8 to 15 breaths to measure R_{AW}, E, and auto-PEEP. The clinician sets the trigger, the cycle (3 L/min default), and the % support. For example, for 50% support, half of the work of breathing is performed by the patient and half by the ventilator.

As with PSV, PAV is able to unload the respiratory muscles (66,67) to optimize patient–ventilator synchrony, and to diminish sleep disruptions (68–71). Just like PSV, PAV can also be delivered through noninvasive ventilation.

Neurally Adjusted Ventilatory Assist

NAVA delivers a variable support in proportion to the patient's effort by measuring the electrical activity of the diaphragm (EAdi) and applying a gain selected on the ventilator (72,73). The ventilator is triggered and cycled based on the EAdi value, which directly reflects the activity of the neural respiratory output, provided that motor neuron disease is not present. EAdi is measured by an electromyography electrode array located on a special nasogastric tube at the position of the diaphragm (Fig. 104.18). Correct position of the catheter is mandatory to obtain a representative EAdi signal from the diaphragm (74).

The inspiratory pressure applied by the ventilator is determined by the following equation:

$$P_{AW} = \text{NAVA level} \times \text{EAdi} \quad (10)$$

The NAVA level reflects the amount of WOB reduced by the ventilator. The level is usually set between 1 and 4 cm $H_2O/\mu V$ and it can be adjusted over time in small increments. Is it possible to set any value between 0 and 15 cm $H_2O/\mu V$ (75)? Because NAVA's trigger is based on diaphragmatic activity rather than pressure or flow measured at the proximal airway, triggering is not adversely affected in patients with flow limitation and auto-PEEP, but at the same time it is not useful in patients with weak respiratory drive or motor neuron disease. NAVA is effective in optimizing patient–ventilator synchrony compared to conventional ventilatory modes (76–79). However, there is still a paucity of data regarding its effect on clinical outcomes (80). Like PAV, NAVA can be used in both invasive and noninvasive ventilation (81). A representative trace of NAVA is shown in Figure 104.19.

SUMMARY

The plethora of settings available for the various modes on modern ventilators can be overwhelming. New modes are often based on technical and engineering capability rather than a clear clinical superiority over previously available modes. There is little evidence that any mode improves patient outcome. Patient outcomes are affected more by how the mode is used than by the mode per se.

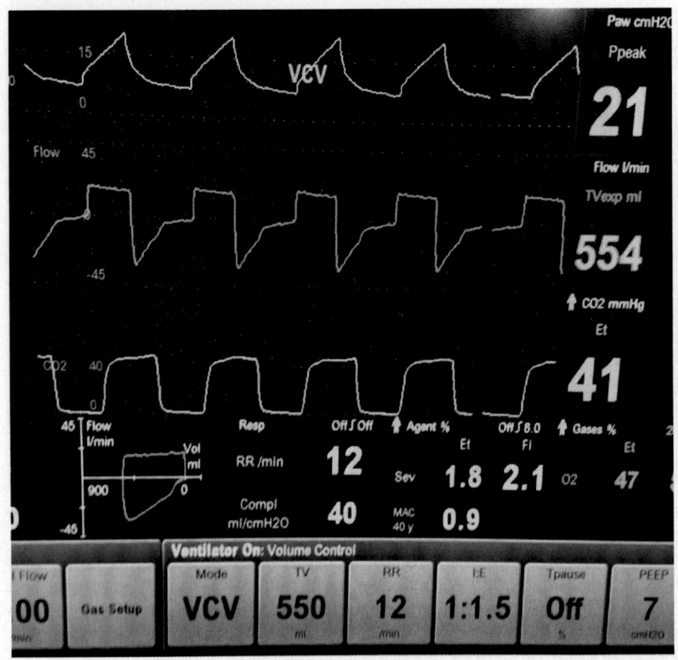

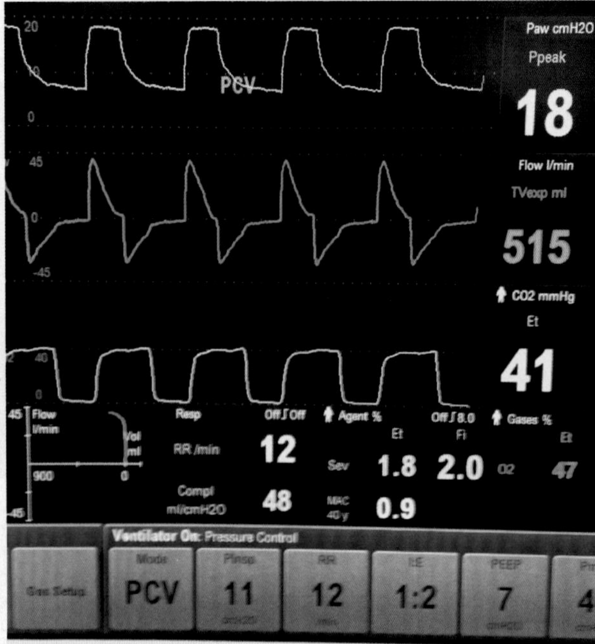

FIGURE 104.20 Ventilator screens showing waveforms for volume-control ventilation (VCV) and pressure-control ventilation (PCV) obtained in the same patient, achieving comparable tidal volume (V_T) and minute ventilation (VE). Airway pressure is at the top, flow in the middle, and exhaled CO_2 at the bottom. Note the same V_T on VCV (set) and PCV (result of the set P_{AW}), and the same end-tidal CO_2.

Key Points

- The *equation of motion of the respiratory system* Eq. (6) provides the structure for understanding MV. The result of any variable set on the ventilator (the *control* variable) depends on the setting itself, the patient's mechanics and any active inspiratory effort.
- Pressure control (PCV) and volume control (VCV) differ not only in what is set on the ventilator (the *control* variable) and what is variable, but also in how the breath is delivered in each mode (Fig. 104.20). With VCV, the inspiratory flow is fixed and set by the operator, while with PCV it is variable, and it is the result of the set pressure and the patient's mechanics and effort. Hence, with PCV the inspired gas may distribute more evenly through an inhomogeneous lung, and the spontaneous breathing activity may synchronize more easily with the ventilator.
- When setting a lung-protective strategy of low tidal volume (V_T) and low driving pressure, the desired V_T can be obtained in either volume- (VCV) or pressure (PCV)-control ventilation. However, VCV assures the size of the V_T, whereas PCV may allow it to increase beyond the desired limit due to changes in respiratory mechanics or an increased patient effort.
- BiLevel ventilation in the absence of spontaneous breathing is indistinguishable from PCV. With spontaneous breathing activity, breaths occur at both high and low pressure levels. As such, BiLevel is a form of synchronized intermittent mandatory ventilation (SIMV) and, as with SIMV, the spontaneous breaths can be supported with PSV. However, unlike SIMV, spontaneous breathing can occur also at the high pressure level, which can be applied for longer periods of time to enhance alveolar recruitment.
- Both assist-control ventilation (ACV) and synchronized intermittent mandatory ventilation (SIMV) can be delivered in the volume-control and the pressure-control modes even though not all ventilators provide all four combinations. During both volume- and pressure-control SIMV the spontaneous breaths can be supported by PSV.
- During PSV, a fast time constant (i.e., low compliance and normal resistance) as is seen in acute respiratory distress syndrome (ARDS), may result in a low mean airway pressure and low tidal volume; a slow time constant (i.e., normal or high compliance and high resistance) as is seen in asthma/COPD, may result in a high mean airway pressure, large tidal volumes, and auto-PEEP.

References

1. Otis AB, Fenn WO, Rahn H. Mechanics of breathing in man. *J Appl Physiol.* 1950;2:592–607.
2. Chatburn RL. Classification of ventilator modes: update and proposal for implementation. *Resp Care.* 2007;52:301–323.
3. Racca F, Squadrone V, Ranieri VM. Patient–ventilator interaction during the triggering phase. *Respir Care Clin North Am.* 2005;11:225.
4. Imanaka H, Nishimura M, Takeuchi M, et al. Autotriggering caused by cardiogenic oscillation during flow-triggered mechanical ventilation. *Crit Care Med.* 2000;28:402.
5. Richard JC, Carlucci A, Breton L, et al. Bench testing of pressure support ventilation with three different generations of ventilators. *Intensive Care Med.* 2002;28:1049.
6. Goulet R, Hess D, Kacmarek RM. Pressure vs. flow triggering during pressure support ventilation. *Chest.* 1997;111:1649.
7. Ranieri VM, Grasso S, Fiore T, et al. Auto-positive end-expiratory pressure and dynamic hyperinflation. *Clin Chest Med.* 1996;17:379.
8. Hudson LD, Hurlow RS, Craig KC, et al. Does intermittent mandatory ventilation correct respiratory alkalosis in patients receiving assisted mechanical ventilation? *Am Rev Respir Dis.* 1985;130:1071.

9. Nilsestuen JO, Hargett KD. Using ventilator graphics to identify patient–ventilator asynchrony. *Respir Care*. 2005;50:202.
10. Hess DR, Medoff BD, Fessler MB. Pulmonary mechanics and graphics during positive pressure ventilation. *Int Anesthesiol Clin*. 1999;37:15.
11. Marini JJ, Rodriguez RM, Lamb V. The inspiratory workload of patient-initiated mechanical ventilation. *Am Rev Respir Dis*. 1986;134:902.
12. The Acute Respiratory Distress Syndrome Network. Ventilation with lower tidal volumes as compared with traditional tidal volumes for acute lung injury and the acute respiratory distress syndrome. *N Engl J Med*. 2000; 342:1301.
13. Amato MB, Meade MO, Slutsky AS, et al. Driving pressure and survival in the acute respiratory distress syndrome. *N Engl J Med*. 2015;372:745.
14. Hess DR, Thompson BT. Patient–ventilator dyssynchrony during lung protective ventilation: what's a clinician to do? *Crit Care Med*. 2006;34:231.
15. MacIntyre NR, McConnell R, Cheng KC, et al. Patient–ventilator flow dyssynchrony: flow-limited versus pressure-limited breaths. *Crit Care Med*. 1997;25:1671.
16. Uchiyama A, Imanaka H, Taenaka N. Relationship between work of breathing provided by a ventilator and patients' inspiratory drive during pressure support ventilation; effects of inspiratory rise time. *Anaesth Intensive Care*. 2001;29:349.
17. Yang LY, Huang YC, Macintyre NR. Patient-ventilator synchrony during pressure-targeted versus flow-targeted small tidal volume assisted ventilation. *J Crit Care*. 2007;22:252–257.
18. Davis K Jr, Branson RD, Campbell RS, et al. Comparison of volume control and pressure control ventilation: Is flow waveform the difference? *J Trauma*. 1996;41:808.
19. Abraham E, Yoshihara G. Cardiorespiratory effects of pressure controlled ventilation in severe respiratory failure. *Chest*. 1990;98:1445–1449.
20. Chacko B, Peter JV, Tharyan P, et al. Pressure-controlled versus volume-controlled ventilation for acute respiratory failure due to acute lung injury (ALI) or acute respiratory distress syndrome (ARDS). *Cochrane Database Syst Rev*. 2015;1.
21. Branson RD, Davis K Jr. Dual control modes: combining volume and pressure breaths. *Respir Care Clin North Am*. 2001;7:397.
22. Branson RD, Campbell RS, Davis K Jr. New modes of ventilatory support. *Int Anesthesiol Clin*. 1999;37:103.
23. Branson RD, Johannigman JA. What is the evidence base for the newer ventilation modes? *Respir Care*. 2004;49:742.
24. Branson RD, Johannigman JA. The role of ventilator graphics when setting dual-control modes. *Respir Care*. 2005;50:187.
25. Branson RD, Johannigman JA, Campbell RS, et al. Closed-loop mechanical ventilation. *Respir Care*. 2002;47:427.
26. Hess D, Branson RD. Ventilators and weaning modes. *Respir Care Clin North Am*. 2000;6:407.
27. D'Angio CT, Chess PR, Kovacs SJ, et al. Pressure-regulated volume control ventilation vs. synchronized intermittent mandatory ventilation for very low-birth-weight infants: a randomized controlled trial. *Arch Pediatr Adolesc Med*. 2005;159:868.
28. Jaber S, Delay JM, Matecki S, et al. Volume-guaranteed pressure-support ventilation facing acute changes in ventilatory demand. *Intensive Care Med*. 2005;31:1181.
29. Mercat A, Titiriga M, Anguel N, et al. Inverse ratio ventilation (I/E = 2/1) in acute respiratory distress syndrome: a six-hour controlled study. *Am J Respir Crit Care Med*. 1997;155:1637.
30. Kacmarek RM, Hess D. Pressure-controlled inverse-ratio ventilation: panacea or auto-PEEP? *Respir Care*. 1990;35:945.
31. Habashi NM. Other approaches to open-lung ventilation: airway pressure release ventilation. *Crit Care Med*. 2005;33:S228.
32. McCunn M, Habashi NM. Airway pressure release ventilation in the acute respiratory distress syndrome following traumatic injury. *Int Anesthesiol Clin*. 2002;40(3):89.
33. Putensen C, Mutz NJ, Putensen-Himmer G, et al. Spontaneous breathing during ventilatory support improves ventilation-perfusion distributions in patients with acute respiratory distress syndrome. *Am J Respir Crit Care Med*. 1999;159:1241.
34. Putensen C, Zech S, Wrigge H, et al. Long-term effects of spontaneous breathing during ventilatory support in patients with acute lung injury. *Am J Respir Crit Care Med*. 2001;164:43.
35. Dart BW 4th, Maxwell RA, Richart CM, et al. Preliminary experience with airway pressure release ventilation in a trauma/surgical intensive care unit. *J Trauma*. 2005;59:71–76.
36. Maxwell RA, Green JM, Waldrop J, et al. A randomized prospective trial of airway pressure release ventilation and low tidal volume ventilation in adult trauma patients with acute respiratory failure. *J Trauma*. 2010;69:501–510.
37. Marini JJ, Smith TC, Lamb VJ. External work output and force generation during synchronized intermittent mechanical ventilation: effect of machine assistance on breathing effort. *Am Rev Respir Dis*. 1988;138:1169.
38. Imsand C, Feihl F, Perret C, et al. Regulation of inspiratory neuromuscular output during synchronized intermittent mandatory ventilation. *Anesthesiology*. 1994;80:13.
39. Robinson BR, Blakeman TC, Toth P, et al. Patient-ventilator asynchrony in a traumatically injured population. *Respir Care*. 2013;58:1847–1855.
40. Patroniti N, Foti G, Cortinovis B, et al. Sigh improves gas exchange and lung volume in patients with acute respiratory distress syndrome undergoing pressure support ventilation. *Anesthesiology*. 2002;96:788.
41. Lenique F, Habis M, Lofaso F, et al. Ventilatory and hemodynamic effects of continuous positive airway pressure in left heart failure. *Am J Respir Crit Care Med*. 1997;155(2):500–505.
42. Mistraletti G, Giacomini M, Sabbatini G, et al. Noninvasive CPAP with facemask: comparison among new air-entrainment masks and the Boussignac valve. *Resp Care*. 2015;305–312.43.
43. Hess DR. Ventilator waveforms and the physiology of pressure support ventilation. *Respir Care*. 2005;50:166.
44. Chiumello D, Pelosi P, Croci M, et al. The effects of pressurization rate on breathing pattern, work of breathing, gas exchange and patient comfort in pressure support ventilation. *Eur Respir J*. 2001;18(1):107.
45. Chiumello D, Pelosi P, Taccone P, et al. Effect of different inspiratory rise time and cycling off criteria during pressure support ventilation in patients recovering from acute lung injury. *Crit Care Med*. 2003;31:2604.
46. Du HL, Yamada Y. Expiratory asynchrony. *Respir Care Clin North Am*. 2005;11:265.
47. Du HL, Amato MB, Yamada Y. Automation of expiratory trigger sensitivity in pressure support ventilation. *Respir Care Clin North Am*. 2001;7:503.
48. Yamada Y, Du HL. Analysis of the mechanisms of expiratory asynchrony in pressure support ventilation: a mathematical approach. *J Appl Physiol*. 2000;88:2143.
49. Tassaux D, Gainnier M, Battisti A, et al. Impact of expiratory trigger setting on delayed cycling and inspiratory muscle workload. *Am J Respir Crit Care Med*. 2005;172:1283.
50. Tokioka H, Tanaka T, Ishizu T, et al. The effect of breath termination criterion on breathing patterns and the work of breathing during pressure support ventilation. *Anesth Analg*. 2001;92:161.
51. Dojat M, Brochard L. Knowledge-based systems for automatic ventilatory management. *Respir Care Clin North Am*. 2001;7:379.
52. Lellouche F, Mancebo J, Jolliet P, et al. A multicenter randomized trial of computer-driven protocolized weaning from mechanical ventilation. *Am J Respir Crit Care Med*. 2006;174:894.
53. Rose L, Presneill J, Johnston L, et al. A randomised, controlled trial of conventional versus automated weaning from mechanical ventilation using SmartCare/PS. *Intensive Care Med*. 2008:1788–1795.
54. Schädler D, Engel C, Elke G, et al. Automatic control of pressure support for ventilator weaning in surgical intensive care patients. *Am J Respir Crit Care Med*. 2012:637–644.
55. Burns KE, Lellouche F, Nisenbaum R, et al. Automated weaning and SBT systems versus non-automated weaning strategies for weaning time in invasively ventilated critically ill adults. *Cochrane Database Syst Rev*. 2014;(9):CD008638.
56. Rose L, Schultz MJ, Cardwell CR, et al. Automated versus non-automated weaning for reducing the duration of mechanical ventilation for critically ill adults and children: a Cochrane systematic review and meta-analysis. *Critical Care*. 2015:19:48
57. Campbell RS, Branson RD, Johannigman JA. Adaptive support ventilation. *Respir Care Clin North Am*. 2001;7:425.
58. Guttmann J, Haberthur C, Mols G, et al. Automatic tube compensation (ATC). *Minerva Anestesiol*. 2002;68:369.
59. Guttmann J, Haberthur C, Mols G. Automatic tube compensation. *Respir Care Clin North Am*. 2001;7:475.
60. Haberthur C, Mols G, Elsasser S, et al. Extubation after breathing trials with automatic tube compensation, T-tube, or pressure support ventilation. *Acta Anaesthesiol Scand*. 2002;46:973.
61. Cohen JD, Shapiro M, Grozovski E, et al. Extubation outcome following a spontaneous breathing trial with automatic tube compensation versus continuous positive airway pressure. *Crit Care Med*. 2006;34:682.
62. Tanios MA, Epstein SK. Spontaneous breathing trials: Should we use automatic tube compensation? *Respir Care*. 2010;55(5):640–642.
63. Grasso S, Ranieri VM. Proportional assist ventilation. *Respir Care Clin North Am*. 2001;7:465.
64. Navalesi P, Costa R. New modes of mechanical ventilation: proportional assist ventilation, neurally adjusted ventilatory assist, and fractal ventilation. *Curr Opin Crit Care*. 2003;9:51.

65. Sinderby C, Navalesi P, Beck J, et al. Neural control of mechanical ventilation in respiratory failure. *Nat Med.* 1999;5:1433.
66. Delaere S, Roeseler J, D'hoore W, et al. Respiratory muscle workload in intubated, spontaneously breathing patients without COPD: pressure support vs. proportional assist ventilation. *Intensive Care Med.* 2003;29:949–954.
67. Ranieri VM, Giuliani R, Mascia L, et al. Patient-ventilator interaction during acute hypercapnia: pressure-support vs proportional-assist ventilation. *J Appl Physiol.* 1996:426-436.
68. Kondili E, Prinianakis G, Alexopoulou C, et al. Respiratory load compensation during mechanical ventilation-proportional assist ventilation with load-adjustable gain factors versus pressure support. *Intensive Care Med.* 2006:692–699.
69. Xirouchaki N, Kondili E, Vaporidi K, et al. Proportional-assist ventilation with load-adjustable gain factors in critically ill patients: comparison with pressure support. *Intensive Care Med.* 2008;34:2026–2034.
70. Costa R, Spinazzola G, Cipriani F, et al. A physiologic comparison of proportional assist ventilation with load-adjustable gain factors (PAV+) versus pressure support ventilation (PSV). *Intensive Care Med.* 2011:1494–1500.
71. Bosma K, Ferreyra G, Ambrogio C, et al. Patient-ventilator interaction and sleep in mechanically ventilated patients: pressure support versus proportional assist ventilation. *Crit Care Med.* 2007;35:1048–1054.
72. Navalesi P, Costa R. New modes of mechanical ventilation: proportional assist ventilation, neurally adjusted ventilatory assist, and fractal ventilation. *Curr Opin Crit Care.* 2003;9:51.
73. Sinderby C, Navalesi P, Beck J, et al. Neural control of mechanical ventilation in respiratory failure. *Nat Med.* 1999;5:1433.
74. Barwing J, Ambold M, Linden N, et al. Evaluation of the catheter positioning for neurally adjusted ventilatory assist. *Intensive Care Med.* 2009;35: 1809–1814.
75. Patroniti N, Bellani G, Saccavino E, et al. Respiratory pattern during neurally adjusted ventilatory assist in acute respiratory failure patients. *Intensive Care Med.* 2012;38:230–239.
76. Colombo D, Cammarota G, Bergamaschi V, et al. Physiologic response to varying levels of pressure support and neurally adjusted ventilatory assist in patients with acute respiratory failure. *Intensive Care Med.* 2008;34:2010–2018.
77. Spahija J, de Marchie M, Albert M, et al. Patient-ventilator interaction during pressure support ventilation and neurally adjusted ventilatory assist. *Crit Care Med.* 2010;38:518–526.
78. Passath C, Takala J, Tuchscherer D, et al. Physiologic response to changing positive end-expiratory pressure during neurally adjusted ventilatory assist in sedated, critically ill adults. *Chest.* 2010;138:578–587.
79. Brander L, Leong-Poi H, Beck J, et al. Titration and implementation of neurally adjusted ventilatory assist in critically ill patients. *Chest.* 2009;135:695–703.
80. Navalesi P, Longhini F. Neurally adjusted ventilatory assist. *Curr Opin Crit Care.* 2015;21:58–64.
81. Piquilloud L, Tassaux D, Bialais E, et al. Neurally adjusted ventilatory assist (NAVA) improves patient-ventilator interaction during noninvasive ventilation delivered by face mask. *Intensive Care Med.* 2012;38:1624–1631.

CHAPTER

105

Bedside Interpretation of Ventilatory Waveforms

ETTORE CRIMI, MASSIMILIANO PIRRONE, DEAN R. HESS, and LUCA M. BIGATELLO

INTRODUCTION

Modern ventilators provide a continuous graphic display of the basic physiologic determinants of ventilation: pressure (P), flow ($\dot{V}$), and volume (V). They also have the capability of performing diagnostic maneuvers measuring important physiologic variables such as airway plateau pressure (P_{PLAT}) and auto-positive end-expiratory pressure (or intrinsic PEEP, $PEEP_i$) at the bedside. In addition, recognition of abnormal ventilator waveforms allows detection of conditions such as missed triggering and patient–ventilator asynchrony. This chapter focuses on the use of ventilator waveforms to facilitate bedside management of mechanical ventilation for patients with acute respiratory failure.

MEASUREMENT OF PRESSURE (P), FLOW ($\dot{V}$), AND VOLUME (V)

The ability of modern ventilators to display graphics and numeric data of P, $\dot{V}$, and V has become possible due to the availability of cost-effective sensor-transducer devices and the proliferation of microelectronic and digital technology. What used to be limited to delicate instruments in the physiology laboratory is now compacted at relatively low cost in critical care ventilators. Airway pressure (P_{AW}) is measured in most ventilators by solid-state transducers, such as piezoresistive or strain gauge transducers. Although P_{AW} is best measured distal to the endotracheal tube (tracheal pressure) or at the proximal airway, these locations interfere to different degrees with patient care, and are not practical for continuous clinical monitoring. Hence, pressure transducers are now located inside the ventilator at the inspiratory and expiratory valves, alternating measurements at the expiratory limb during inspiration and inspiratory limb during exhalation.

Gas flow to and from the patient may be measured by screen or orifice pneumotachographs (1,2) that record the pressure drop across a known resistance and derive the flow according to Ohm's law (2):

$$\text{Resistance (R)} = \Delta P/\dot{V} \qquad (1)$$

where R will be the resistance imposed by the airways: R_{AW}. Thermal cooling (or hot wire) pneumotachographs estimate $\dot{V}$ from the amount of heat loss as gas flows across the device, applying the principle of thermal convection. As is the case of P_{AW} measurements, most ventilators measure $\dot{V}$ at the inspiratory and expiratory valves rather than at the airway. Flow sensors are calibrated for air/oxygen mixtures; thus, inaccuracies can occur in the presence of other gases, such as helium–oxygen mixtures (Heliox) (3), unless the ventilator is designed to make appropriate corrections.

Tidal volume (V_T) is measured by time integration of the flow signal. When gas flow is not measured at the proximal airway, there is a difference between volume output from the ventilator and the volume delivered to the patient due to the *compressible volume* of the ventilator circuit. This is the volume of gas that is lost in the compliant structures of the system (circuit tubing) and through gas compression. Current ventilators compensate for this lost volume by measuring the compliance of the breathing circuit at the time of the initial automatic setup, and calculate a factor (generally 3–4 mL/cm H_2O), which is automatically added to the set V_T (4). Additional potential sources of error in volume measurements include gas conditioning by heating and humidification, which increase gas volume after the inspiratory flow sensor, and differences between the inspired and expired flow/volume due to oxygen consumption. Generally, these are small inaccuracies that fall within the margin of error of the flow sensors (± 0%).

Monitoring Functions

Common functions present in microprocessor-driven ventilators include the ability to perform diagnostic maneuvers that can be used to assess physiologic variables at the bedside. The most common of these functions are the end-inspiratory and end-expiratory pauses (Fig. 105.1).

- An *end-inspiratory pause* is used to estimate alveolar pressure, respiratory compliance (C), and airways resistance (R_{AW}). During volume-control ventilation (VCV) with constant inspiratory flow, a manual or programmed end-inspiratory pause generates a characteristic pattern where the peak inspiratory pressure (PIP) is followed by a rapid descent to a plateau, which constitutes the plateau pressure (P_{PLAT}). When the inspiratory pause is of sufficient duration (0.8–2 seconds), it ensures cessation of gas flow and equilibration between the pressure at the proximal airway (the P_{PLAT}) and in the alveoli (P_{ALV}). Measurement of P_{PLAT} requires full patient relaxation because any spontaneous breathing effort would cause changes due to the decrease in pleural pressure. The presence of a leak in the system (within either the patient or the ventilator) will also prevent reaching a stable P_{PLAT}. The end-inspiratory pause maneuver is limited to a single breath at the time to avoid asynchrony.
- An *end-expiratory pause* is used to estimate auto-PEEP when the lungs fail to empty to functional residual capacity (FRC) at end expiration (dynamic hyperinflation). An end-expiratory pause of sufficient duration allows equilibration between P_{ALV} and P_{AW}. Just as for the P_{PLAT}, the measurement of auto-PEEP is invalidated by the presence of spontaneous breathing efforts and air leaks (5).
- *Airway occlusion pressure* is the value of negative airway pressure generated in the first 100 msec ($P_{0.1}$) of an occluded

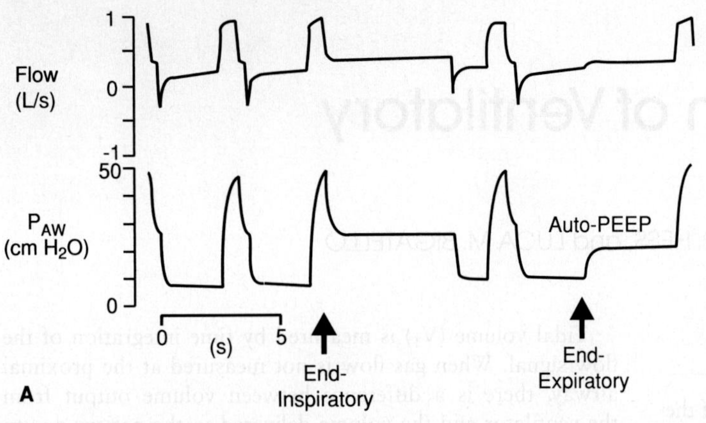

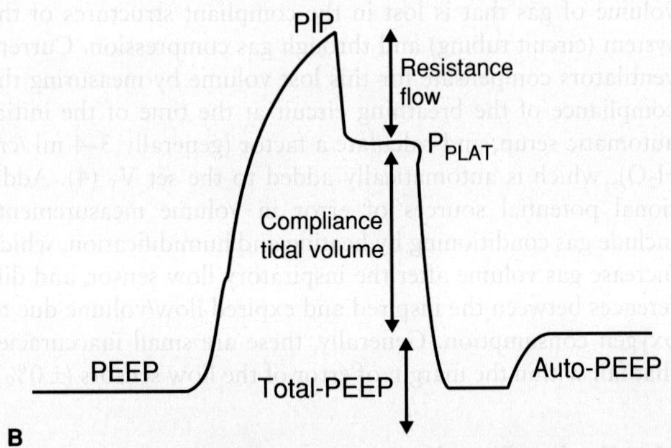

FIGURE 105.1 A: Flow and airway pressure (P_{AW}) waveforms in a mechanically ventilated patient with chronic obstructive pulmonary disease, showing an end-inspiratory and an end-expiratory pause. B: Diagram of a typical airway pressure waveform during mechanical ventilation. The difference between peak inspiratory pressure (PIP) and plateau pressure (P_{PLAT}) is determined by airways resistance and end-inspiratory flow. The difference between P_{PLAT} and PEEP is determined by compliance and tidal volume. (A: Modified from Putensen C, Mutz NJ, Putensen-Himmer G, et al. Spontaneous breathing during ventilatory support improves ventilation-perfusion distributions in patients with acute respiratory distress syndrome. *Am J Respir Crit Care Med.* 1999;159:1241, with permission. B: From Fisher D, Hess D. Respiratory monitoring. In: Bigatello LM, ed. *Critical Care Handbook of the Massachusetts General Hospital.* 4th ed. Philadelphia, PA: Lippincott Williams & Wilkins; 2006:33–52.)

inspiratory effort. Since the early part of inspiration is largely independent of voluntary effort, $P_{0.1}$ is used as an index of ventilatory drive (6). Some ventilators can perform this measurement automatically, with seemingly equal accuracy as the manual measurement (7).

- *Maximum inspiratory pressure (PI_{max})* is the most negative pressure generated during a maximal inspiratory effort against an occluded airway. It is an index of the strength of the inspiratory muscles and has been used in the assessment of readiness for ventilator weaning. The off-ventilator measurement technique uses a one-way valve, allowing exhalation but not inspiration for about 15 to 20 seconds, provided the maneuver is safely tolerated (8). Some ventilators perform this measurement electronically by occluding both inspiratory and expiratory valves for a set time. The manual and ventilator method differ in the starting lung volume, which is residual volume (the subject is coached to exhale fully) in the manual method, and FRC in the automatic method.
- *The Rapid Shallow Breathing Index (RSBI)* is the ratio of respiratory frequency to V_T in liters, commonly used as a screening criterion for readiness to wean/extubate in the setting of a spontaneous breathing trial (SBT) (9). Ventilator-derived measures of RSBI provide equivalent values to those obtained manually with a Wright respirometer (10), except that the ventilator count may fail to detect untriggered breaths (see Patient–Ventilator Asynchrony, below), which occur in patients with chronic obstructive pulmonary disease (COPD) and with severe muscle weakness. The use of pressure support ventilation (PSV) or continuous positive airway pressure (CPAP) during SBT can decrease work of breathing by as much as 40% (11) and significantly affect RSBI values (12,13). Therefore, unless a patient is breathing through an unusually narrow airway, such as endotracheal tube of less than 7.0 mm internal diameter, we recommend avoiding additional support during an SBT of standard duration, that is, 20 to 30 minutes (14). Finally, overreliance on RSBI as the main or only weaning predictor may result in prolonged weaning time (15).

SPECIFIC USES

Breath Delivery

Delivery of a ventilator breath is determined by the interaction between the machine's operation and the patient's physiology, which is described by the *equation of motion of the respiratory system* (Chapter 104):

$$P_{APPL} = P_{VENT} + P_{MUS} = V_T/C + \dot{V} \times R \quad (2)$$

where P_{APPL} is the pressure applied to generate the breath, P_{VENT} is the pressure applied by the ventilator, and P_{MUS} is the pressure generated by the respiratory muscles. Understanding the interaction between ventilator (P, V_T, and $\dot{V}$) and patient (C and R) greatly aids the understanding of the principles of ventilation. In the previous chapter we used this approach to describe how the ventilator delivers different types of breaths. Here, we will use the same basic approach to describe how these breaths can be affected by changes in ventilatory settings, changes in physiologic variables, and specific disease states.

Pressure, Flow, and Volume Waveforms

Most ventilators allow multiple graphic and numeric display options including continuous measurements, ventilator settings, alarm limits, and operational information. Graphic options may include adjusting scales, sweep speed, color coding of various ventilatory modes and breathing cycle phases, freezing of a desired screen, and performing precise measurements with a cursor. By convention, inspiratory events are displayed as positive and expiratory events as negative.

Loops

In addition to the time-based graphics of P, V, and $\dot{V}$, ventilators can display these variables as pressure over volume (P-V loop) and flow over volume ($\dot{V}$-V loop). These graphics may be used to visualize and diagnose specific clinical situations.

- Dynamic P-V loops provide useful information regarding the state of lung inflation at end inspiration when $\dot{V}$ has reached minimal or zero value. Caution must be paid in identifying the contribution of lung C to the state of lung inflation in the early part of inspiration, when $\dot{V}$ is high and hence R_{AW} is high (Fig. 105.2).
- $\dot{V}$-V loops are commonly used in the diagnosis and treatment of *expiratory flow limitation* in ambulatory patients with asthma and COPD, and they can provide useful clinical information in intubated patients as well. Expiratory flow limitation occurs because of increased resistance to airflow from excessive secretions and bronchospasm. In this situation, expiratory flow decays rapidly at the beginning of exhalation and subsequently tapers off to a prolonged low flow phase, which may not reach 0 flow before the next breath starts. Figure 105.3 shows a severely limited expiratory flow with an early rapid drop and subsequent long and slow expiratory phase. Figure 105.4 shows both a normal and an abnormal expiratory flow pattern, where the flow decays slowly in the last part of expiration and does not reach 0 flow before the end of the breath. The inability to reach 0 flow indicates that exhalation ends at a lung volume higher than FRC, which exerts an abnormal pressure, or auto-PEEP ($PEEP_i$) (16–18). The next breath will start only after auto-PEEP is overcome, thus increasing work of breathing.
- $\dot{V}$-V loops are useful in the detection of *air leaks* that cause a loss of volume with each breath, as well as a difference between the delivered and the exhaled tidal volume. Air leaks can occur within the ventilator system, for example, at the ventilator circuit, between the ventilator and the patient, for example, at connections between a thoracostomy tube and a drainage device, and within the patient when a bronchopleural fistula is present. Regardless of their location, air leaks cause a characteristic failure of the $\dot{V}$-V loop to close at the end of expiration, because a portion of the inspired tidal volume does not return to the site of measurement on the expiration side (Fig. 105.5).

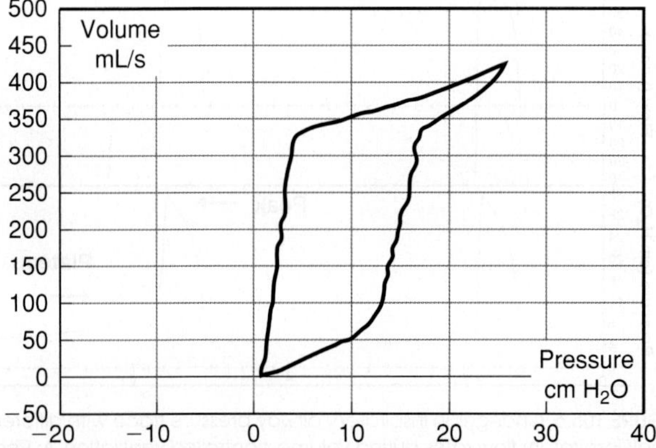

FIGURE 105.2 Pressure–volume loop showing hyperinflation as abrupt increase of pressure at the end of inspiration. (From Nilsestuen JO, Hargett KD. Using ventilator graphics to identify patient–ventilator asynchrony. *Respir Care*. 2005;50:202–234, with permission.)

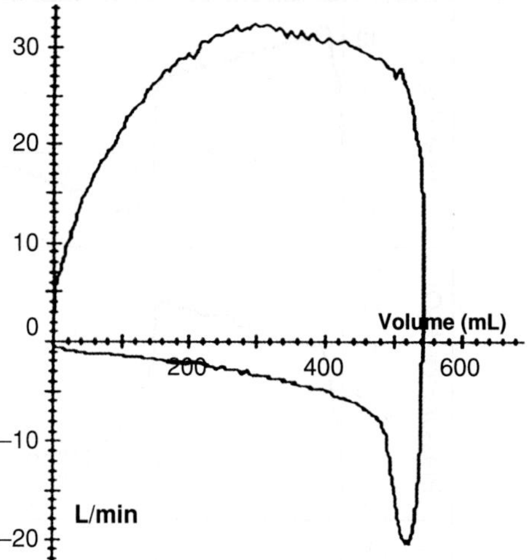

FIGURE 105.3 Flow–volume loop during mechanical ventilation. Severe expiratory flow limitation, like in asthma and COPD: flow falls rapidly immediately after the onset of expiration, then remains at a very slow rate without ever reaching the 0-flow line.

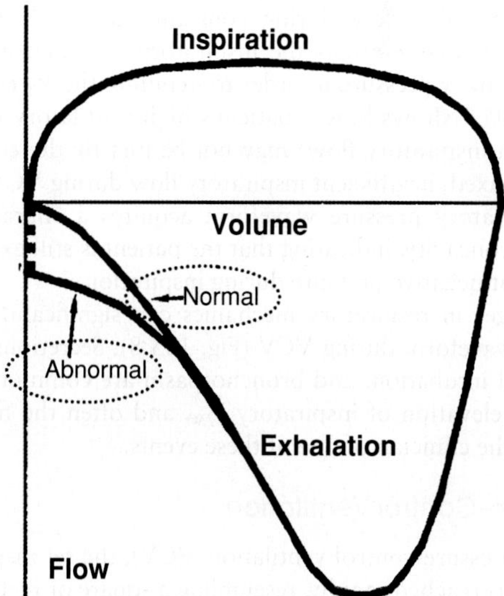

FIGURE 105.4 Flow–volume loop during mechanical ventilation, showing normal and abnormal expiratory patterns. Normally, expiratory flow "closes the loop"—that is, reaches 0 flow before the next inspiration starts. With expiratory flow limitation, like in asthma and COPD, flow may not reach baseline (0 flow) before the next inspiration starts, thus failing to close the loop, which remains truncated. (Modified from Dhand R. Ventilator graphics and respiratory mechanics in the patient with obstructive lung disease. *Respir Care*. 2005;50:246–261, with permission.)

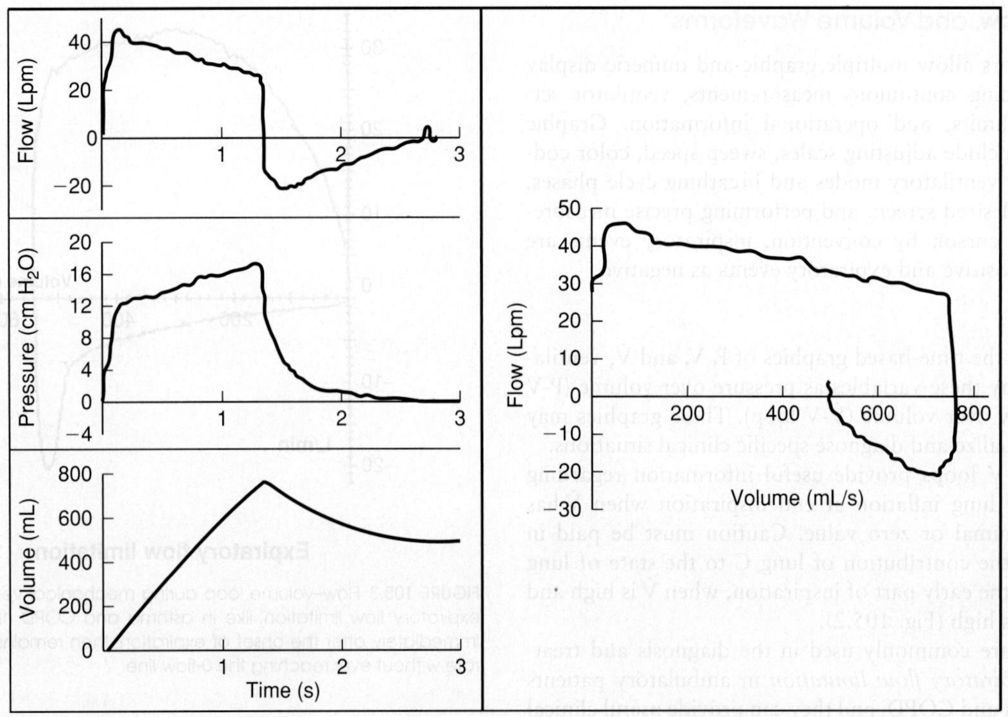

FIGURE 105.5 Detection of an air leak by ventilator waveform analysis. On the **left**, traces of flow, pressure, and volume. The flow trace shows a smaller area (= volume) in expiration than in inhalation, indicating a loss of volume. The volume trace that does not reach baseline, also indicating a loss of volume. On the **right**, the flow–volume loop fails to close at end exhalation. (Modified from Lucangelo U, Bernabe F, Blanch L. Respiratory mechanics derived from signals in the ventilator circuit. *Respir Care.* 2005;50:55–65, with permission.)

Variations in Ventilatory Waveforms

Volume-Control Ventilation

During VCV, airway pressure waveforms can be affected by changes in ventilator settings and in the patient's respiratory mechanics. Figure 105.6 shows the result of setting a higher peak inspiratory flow during constant flow VCV (19,20). The higher flow shortens the inspiratory time and increases the inspiratory pressure in order to maintain the V_T constant. Figure 105.7 shows how a patient's high ventilatory demand (i.e., high inspiratory flow) may not be met by the combination of a fixed, insufficient inspiratory flow during VCV. Here, the inspiratory pressure waveform acquires a characteristic upward concavity, indicating that the patient is still exerting a significant negative pressure during inspiration.

Changes in respiratory mechanics can significantly affect the P_{AW} waveform during VCV (Fig. 105.8). Secretions, endobronchial intubation, and bronchospasm are common causes of acute elevation of inspiratory P_{AW}, and often the first sign alerting the clinician of one of these events.

Pressure-Control Ventilation

During pressure-control ventilation (PCV), the set inspiratory pressure is reached rapidly, resembling a square or rectangular wave. This is due to the unique way the inspiratory flow is delivered. With PCV, the flow is variable and is affected by the combination of the capability of each ventilator to generate high flows, the patient's respiratory mechanics, and the patient's own effort (21). Once the set inspiratory pressure is reached, the flow decreases exponentially to maintain the pressure for the desired time, with the decay of the flow

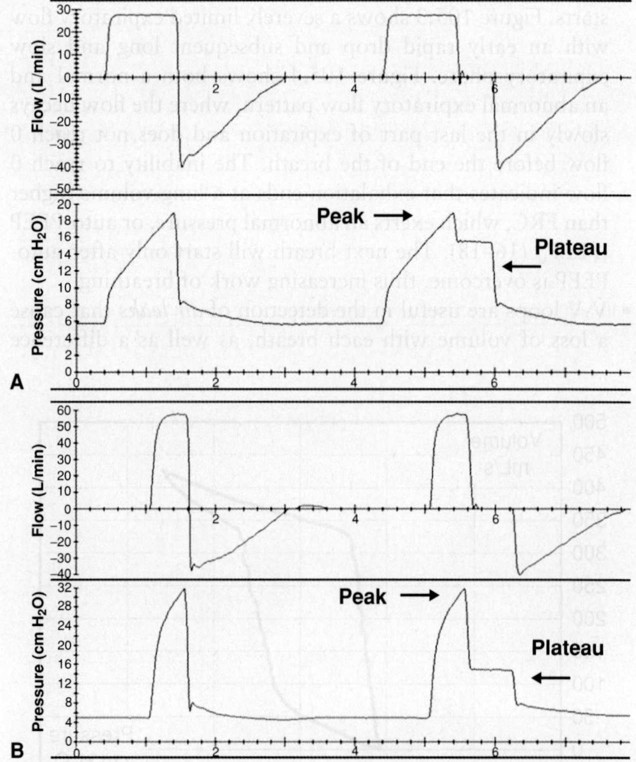

FIGURE 105.6 Changes in inspiratory airway pressure trace with different peak inspiratory flow rates during volume-controlled ventilation. A: Peak inspiratory flow rate = 30 L/min, tidal volume 500 mL. B: Peak inspiratory flow rate = 60 L/min, tidal volume 500 mL. The higher flow rate is associated with higher peak—but not plateau—inspiratory airway pressure and a shorter inspiratory time; the tidal volume is the same by default.

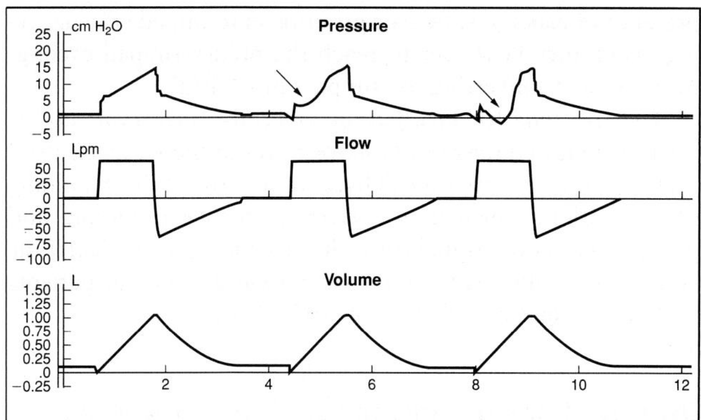

FIGURE 105.7 Examples of inadequate peak inspiratory flow rate during volume-controlled ventilation. The *arrows* point to the scooped appearance of the airway pressure waveform that is due to the patient's own vigorous inspiratory effort. (Modified from Nilsestuen JO, Hargett KD. Using ventilator graphics to identify patient-ventilator asynchrony. *Respir Care.* 2005;50:202–234, with permission.)

rate largely dependent on the *time constant* (τ) of the respiratory system:

$$\tau = R_{AW} \times C_{RS} \quad (3)$$

Tau (τ) is a measure of the time required to achieve a new steady state in a mechanical system (22). One τ is the time necessary to inhale or exhale 63% of the final lung volume. A slow τ is characteristic of a respiratory system with high airway resistance (R_{AW}) and normal or increased respiratory system compliance (C_{RS}). Such a set of mechanics is present in asthma and COPD where the decay of the inspiratory flow is slow and the duration of inspiration may cut into the ongoing flow and limit V_T. Conversely, a fast τ occurs in a system with normal R_{AW} and low C_{RS}, such as ARDS, where the decay of the inspiratory flow is steep and the V_T will be low for a set value of inspiratory pressure. Of note, this reasoning does not apply to the descending ramp waveform of VCV, where the flow is fixed. Figure 105.9 shows how the duration of the PCV breath and the time-decay of the inspiratory flow may affect the size of V_T for a given set inspiratory pressure. When the breath ends before the inspiratory flow has reached zero, the V_T can be increased by a longer inspiratory time. In addition, a stable plateau in the P_{AW} trace occurs at end inspiration (P_{PLAT}) because there is no flow at that time.

Pressure Support Ventilation

With PSV, the P_{AW} waveform approximates a square wave, similarly to PCV. However, differently from PCV, with PSV the breath is not cycled by time, but by flow, which is when the down sloping inspiratory flow reaches a fraction of the peak inspiratory flow, generally 25%. Most ventilators allow adjustments of this 25% cycling-off criterion (*expiratory sensitivity*). Ending the breath at a higher percentage of the peak inspiratory flow shortens the inspiratory time, potentially improving synchrony in patients with long respiratory time constants (above). A lower percentage setting may increase the V_T if a sufficient inspiratory flow is still present at that point during inspiration, and improve synchrony in patients with short respiratory time constants (Fig. 105.10) (23).

PSV also provides backup cycling criteria designed to minimize patient–ventilator asynchrony. For example, inspiration terminates early when the inspiratory pressure plateau rises 2 to 3 cm H_2O above the set pressure (Fig. 105.11) (24). This phenomenon is characteristic of COPD, where a long

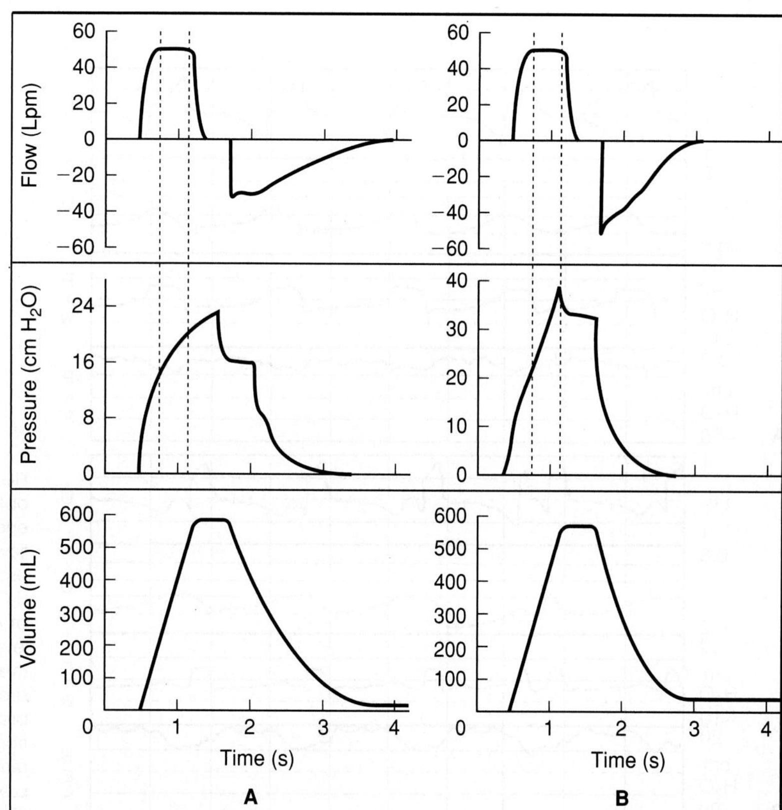

FIGURE 105.8 Airway pressure, flow, and volume waveforms during volume-controlled ventilation with normal (A) and decreased (B) compliance. As the compliance lowers, the peak inspiratory pressure and plateau pressure increase. Tidal volume stays the same. (Modified from Lucangelo U, Bernabe F, Blanch L. Respiratory mechanics derived from signals in the ventilator circuit. *Respir Care.* 2005;50:55–65, with permission.)

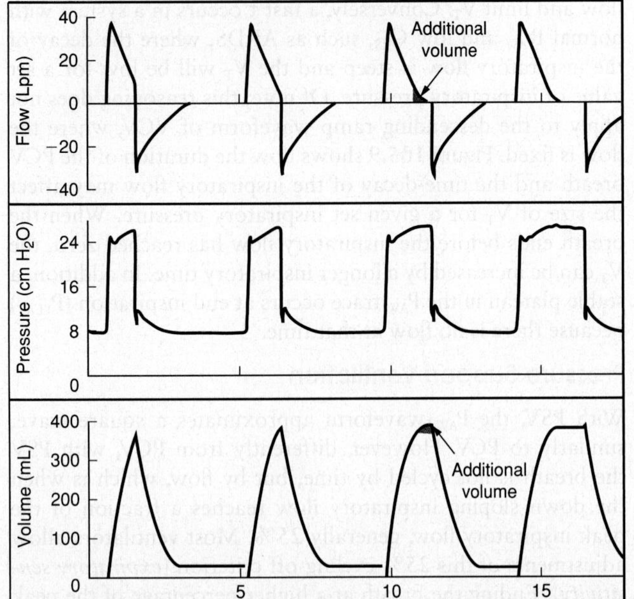

FIGURE 105.9 Effects of changes in inspiratory time during pressure-controlled ventilation. As the duration of inspiration progressively increases from left to right, the tidal volume also increases (*arrows*). Once the inspiratory time is sufficiently long that the inspiratory flow reaches baseline before the end of inspiration (last breath), no further volume is gained. (Modified from Lucangelo U, Bernabe F, Blanch L. Respiratory mechanics derived from signals in the ventilator circuit. *Respir Care.* 2005;50:55–65, with permission.)

time-constant may prolong inspiration beyond the neural inspiratory time, causing the patient to actively exhale thus increasing P_{AW}. A second backup criterion consists of setting a maximum inspiratory time. This feature is helpful in the presence of leaks of sufficient proportion to impede the decaying inspiratory flow ever to reach the predetermined cycling-off level thus converting the support in a CPAP.

The *rise time* (or *insufflation time, pressurization rate*) is the time required for the ventilator to reach the set inspiratory pressure. A faster rise time delivers more flow at the beginning of inspiration, which may correct ineffective triggering and patient–ventilator asynchrony due to long mechanical time constants (COPD) (25), and may relieve dyspnea in patients with high respiratory drive (Fig. 105.12) (26).

Bedside Uses of Physiologic Measurements and Graphic Display

Assessment of Respiratory Mechanics

The electronic performance of *end-inspiratory* and *end-expiratory pauses* allows the measurement of respiratory compliance (C) and resistance (R) at the bedside. The ventilator is set in the VCV mode with a constant inspiratory flow pattern. Care must be paid to minimize the patient's own respiratory efforts, which would invalidate the measurements. This may be accomplished by overriding the patient's own drive by transiently hyperventilating, administering a short-acting sedative-hypnotic, or even inducing pharmacologic neuromuscular blockade. A thorough risk–benefit evaluation has to be made before resorting to these interventions.

Compliance of the Respiratory System (C_{RS}). C_{RS} (mL/cm H_2O) comprises the individual compliances of lung (C_L) and chest wall (C_{CW}). It is acutely reduced in ARDS, atelectasis, pulmonary edema, pneumonia, pleural effusions, abdominal distention, and pneumothorax, and is increased in asthma and

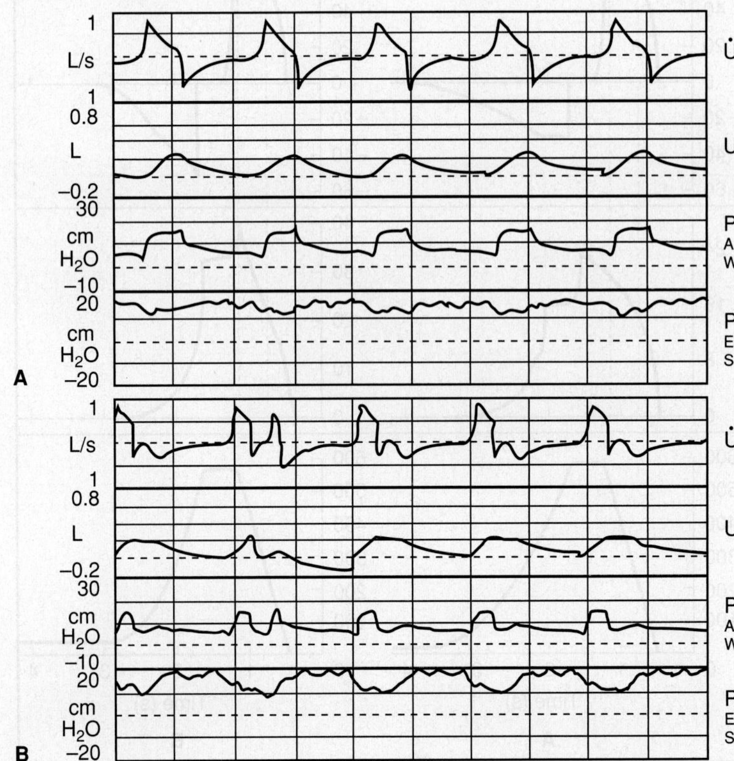

FIGURE 105.10 Two pressure support ventilation traces obtained with different expiratory sensitivity. In **A**, the breath ends when the inspiratory flow (V̇) reaches 5% of the peak flow (low sensitivity): tidal volume (V) is approximately 300 mL, esophageal pressure (PES) change approximately 5 cm H_2O, and all breaths are synchronous. In **B**, the breath ends at 45% of the peak flow rate (high sensitivity): At the same level of inspiratory pressure (P_{AW}) and a similar tidal volume, there is significant patient–ventilator asynchrony, demonstrated by an attempted (all breaths) or successful (second breath) triggering effort during early exhalation. (Modified from Tokioka H, Tanaka T, Ishizu T, et al. The effect of breath termination criterion on breathing patterns and the work of breathing during pressure support ventilation. *Anesth Analg.* 2001;92:161–165, with permission.)

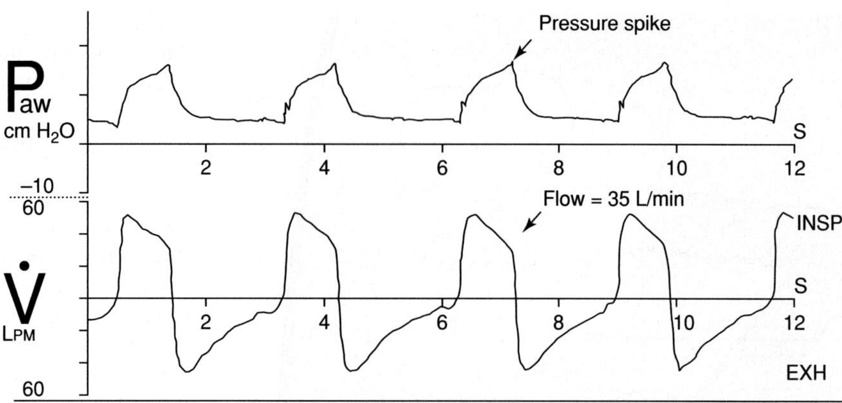

FIGURE 105.11 Termination of pressure support ventilation breaths by a pressure criterion, rather than the default flow criterion. Once the set inspiratory pressure (P_{AW}) is reached and maintained to begin a plateau, a further increase in pressure cycles the ventilator off. This backup setting is intended to decrease patient–ventilator asynchrony when a patient generates a positive P_{AW} to end inspiration. This occurs typically in patients with long time constants, such as in COPD and asthma. (From Branson RD, Campbell RS. Pressure support ventilation, patient-ventilator synchrony, and ventilator algorithms. *Respir Care.* 1998;43:1045–1047, with permission.)

emphysema. C_{RS} is measured by applying an *end-inspiratory pause*, separating PIP and P_{PLAT} (see Fig. 105.1). The P_{PLAT}, not the PIP, is the pressure of reference in measuring C_{RS}, because it is measured at 0 flow, hence not affected by resistance of flow through the airways (R_{AW}). The pressure difference between P_{PLAT} and PEEP is due to the size of the V_T and the value of C_{RS} (27):

$$C_{RS} = V_T/(P_{PLAT} - PEEP) \tag{4}$$

This measurement of C_{RS}, also called *static compliance* (28), is relatively simple and more than valid for routine clinical use, but it also has limitations:

- It is measured at just one lung volume, the current V_T. Although under normal circumstances, the relationship between P and V in the respiratory system is linear within a physiologic range of lung volumes, pathologies such as ARDS may alter this relationship so that C may vary significantly within a relatively narrow range of lung volumes. In these cases, more complex methods to evaluate respiratory C at different lung volumes are indicated (29).
- It assumes the respiratory system as a single compartment, which may underestimate the complexity of regional compliances. This occurs frequently in ARDS, pneumonia, obesity, or pneumothorax, invalidating—to a variable degree—our standard assessment of C. The coexistence of lung regions with different mechanical properties leads to unbalanced regional lung inflation where the well-aerated areas (higher C) receive most of the V_T, and the poorly aerated areas (lower C) see only minimal changes in volume (Fig. 105.13).

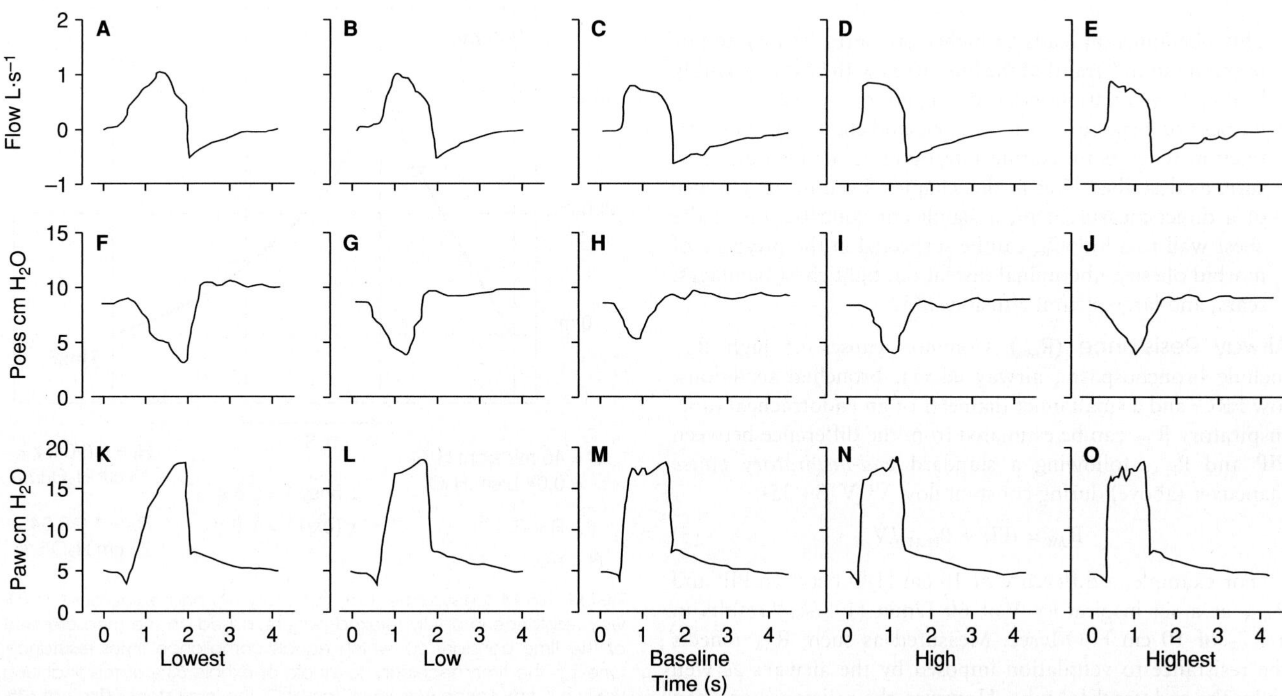

FIGURE 105.12 Effects of a progressive increase of the inspiratory pressurization rate during pressure support ventilation, from breath A to breath E. Note the different shapes of the flow and airway pressure (P_{AW}) traces, and the variable esophageal pressure gradient (Poes), which suggests that the optimal support (i.e., lowest inspiratory effort) was obtained at the intermediate setting (breath C). (From Chiumello D, Pelosi P, Croci M, et al. The effects of pressurization rate on breathing pattern, work of breathing, gas exchange and patient comfort in pressure support ventilation. *Eur Respir J.* 2001;18:107–114, with permission.)

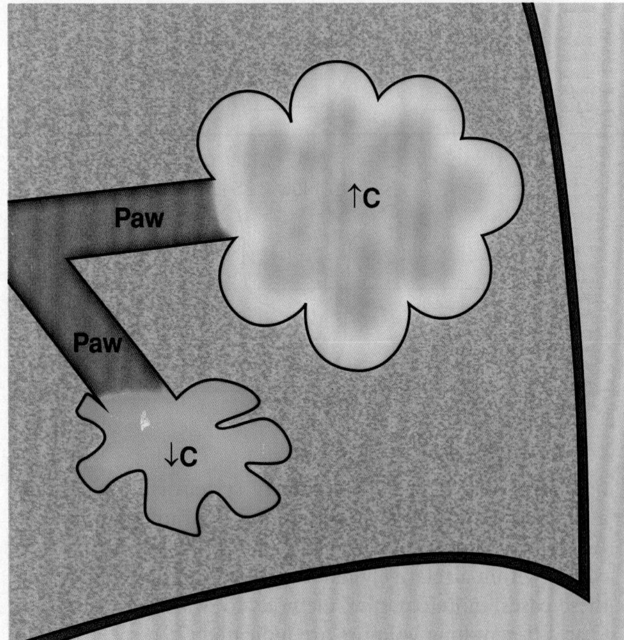

FIGURE 105.13 Effects of PEEP and recruitment maneuvers on a heterogeneous lung. When the lung is recruited at end expiration by PEEP, collapsed alveoli are reopened and end-expiratory lung volume increases. However, the change in alveolar volume will be greater in alveoli with normal C (healthy alveolus, in *blue*) than in alveoli with low C (collapsed/consolidated alveolus, in *green*), generating overdistention and possibly injury to healthy alveoli. When the lung is recruited at end inspiration by a recruitment maneuver the same principle applies, with further chance of recruiting the low compliance alveoli and further risk of overdistending the compliant alveoli. Note that the same alveolar pressure that may injure healthy alveoli may or may not be sufficient to recruit the collapsed/consolidated alveoli.

This phenomenon leads to higher pressures (stress) and/or overdistention (strain) of the lung areas with best C, possibly leading to ventilation-induced lung injury (30–32).

- It does not distinguish between lung and chest wall. This distinction requires measuring intrathoracic (or pleural) pressure, as described later in this chapter. Even in the absence of a direct measurement, a significant contribution of the chest wall to a low C_{RS} can be suspected in the presence of morbid obesity, abdominal distention, tight chest bandages, scars, and large pleural effusions (33).

Airway Resistance (R_{AW}). Common causes of high R_{AW} include bronchospasm, airway edema, bronchial secretions, low FRC, and a small inner diameter of an endotracheal tube. Inspiratory R_{AW} can be estimated from the difference between PIP and P_{PLAT} following a standard *end-inspiratory pause* maneuver (above) during constant flow VCV (34,35):

$$R_{AW} = (PIP - P_{PLAT})/\dot{V} \quad (5)$$

For example, a difference of 10 cm H_2O between PIP and P_{PLAT} at a set inspiratory $\dot{V}$ of 60 L/min (1 L/sec) results in a R_{AW} of 10 cm H_2O/L/sec. Measured as such, R_{AW} reflects the resistance to ventilation imposed by the airways as well as by the endotracheal tube. However, the resistance of clean endotracheal tubes is known, and one can use this knowledge (36,37) and clinical judgment (presence of secretions within the tube) in estimating the airway-versus-equipment contribution to R_{AW} (38). The resistance imposed by the ventilator circuit (generally minimal) is not part of this measurement. This is because modern ventilators measure pressure during inhalation through the expiratory line and during exhalation through the inspiratory line, which becomes identical to placing the pressure transducer directly on the proximal airway.

R_{AW} is affected by flow, lung volume, and phase of respiration. Inspiratory R_{AW} is typically lower than expiratory R_{AW} due to the increased diameter of the airways during inspiration, particularly in patients with COPD and dynamic hyperinflation (39). This phenomenon is evident in obese patients with severely reduced FRC, where lung collapse causes local airway closure and regionally different R, leading to heterogeneous lung inflation (40). R_{AW} can also be estimated from the time constant ($\tau = R \times C$) of the respiratory system Eq. (3). This method permits to calculate both inspiratory and expiratory R_{AW} (Fig. 105.14).

Auto-PEEP ($PEEP_i$). Auto-PEEP (cm H_2O) is the result of incomplete emptying of the lung at end expiration, causing an increase in end-expiratory lung volume and pressure (39,41–43). This is due to *expiratory flow limitation* characteristic of asthma and COPD. Figures 105.15B and 105.16 show representative traces of expiratory flow limitation. Auto-PEEP can be quantified by means of a standard *end-expiratory pause* maneuver shown in Figures 105.1 and 105.16.

Mean P_{AW}. Many desired as well as adverse effects of mechanical ventilation can be traced through the measurement of the mean P_{AW}. Mean P_{AW} is the average pressure value measured throughout one respiratory cycle. Hence, mean P_{AW} is determined by PIP, PEEP, the inspiratory-to-expiratory (I:E) time

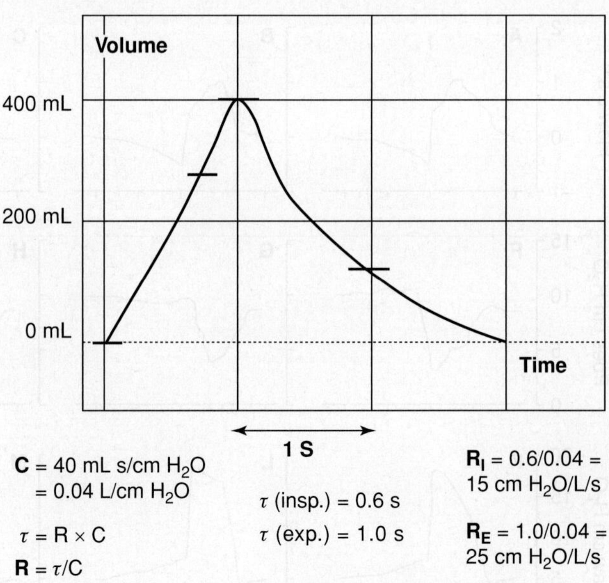

FIGURE 105.14 Measurement of inspiratory (R_I) and expiratory (R_E) airway resistance in a fully relaxed patient, based on the measurement of the time constant (τ), which equals compliance times resistance. One τ is the time necessary to inhale or exhale 63% of the final lung volume. Compliance was 40 mL/cm H_2O; the inspiratory τ (time at 63% of inspiratory volume, *horizontal line*) was 0.6 second, and the expiratory τ (time at 63% of inspiratory volume, *horizontal line*) was 1 second. Values of R_I and R_E are shown. (From Nims RG, Conner EH, Comroe JH Jr. The compliance of the human thorax in anesthetized patients. *J Clin Invest.* 1955;34:744–750, with permission.)

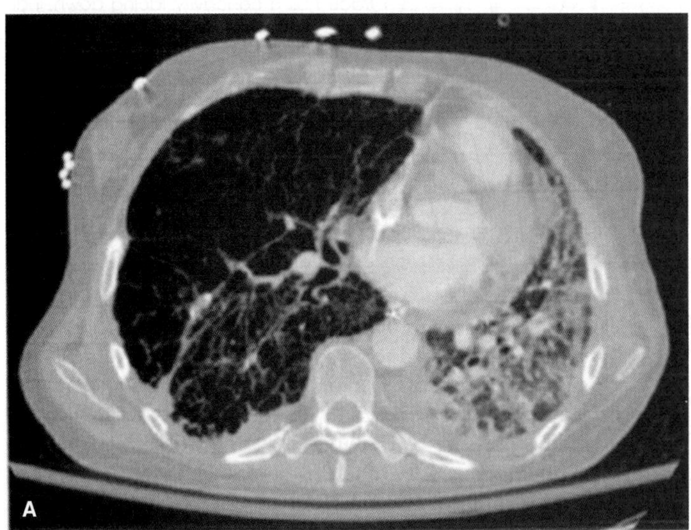

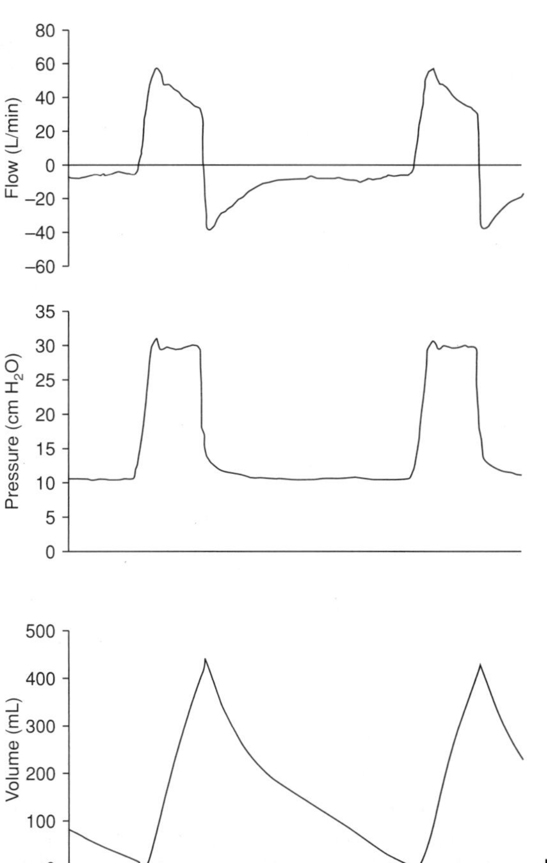

FIGURE 105.15 Acute lung injury in a transplanted lung. **A:** Computed tomogram showing severe emphysema of the right (native) lung and diffuse edema and consolidation of the left (transplanted) lung. **B:** Ventilator waveforms, compatible with a two-compartment model. The initial part of the breath, coming from the transplanted lung (seen best in the expiratory flow trace) has a fast time constant; the second part of the breath has a very slow time constant, because of the high resistance and high compliance of the emphysematous native lung.

ratio, and the inspiratory pressure waveform. During PCV, the inspiratory pressure waveform is rectangular and mean P_{AW} is estimated as:

$$\text{Mean } P_{AW} = (\text{PIP} - \text{PEEP}) \times (\text{Ti/Ttot}) + \text{PEEP} \quad (6)$$

where Ti is inspiratory time and Ttot is total cycle time. For example, with a PIP of 40 cm H_2O, PEEP of 10 cm H_2O, Ti of 1 second, and respiratory rate (f) 20/min (Ti/Ttot = 0.33), mean P_{AW} is 20 cm H_2O. During constant flow VCV, the inspiratory pressure waveform is triangular and mean P_{AW} can be estimated as:

$$\text{Mean } P_{AW} = 0.5 \times (\text{PIP} - \text{PEEP}) \times (\text{Ti/Ttot}) + \text{PEEP} \quad (7)$$

For example, with a PIP of 25 cm H_2O, PEEP 5 cm H_2O, Ti 1.5 seconds, f 20/min (Ti/Ttot = 0.5), mean P_{AW} is 10 cm H_2O. Many current microprocessor ventilators display mean P_{AW} from integration of the P_{AW} waveform. Typical mean P_{AW} values for fully ventilated patients are 5 to 10 cm H_2O (normal), 10 to 20 cm H_2O (airflow obstruction), and 15 to 30 cm H_2O (ARDS).

Pressure–Time Waveforms. Measuring the overall pressure changes of the respiratory system throughout a mechanical breath (*dynamic compliance*) may be a useful indicator of the behavior of the respiratory system during mechanical ventilation (44–47). For example, pressure changes measured over time under conditions of constant flow can provide information on alveolar recruitment and overdistention (stress index). A constant slope of the airway pressure suggests that there is no change in compliance during tidal ventilation; a downward concavity indicates an increase in compliance (i.e., lung

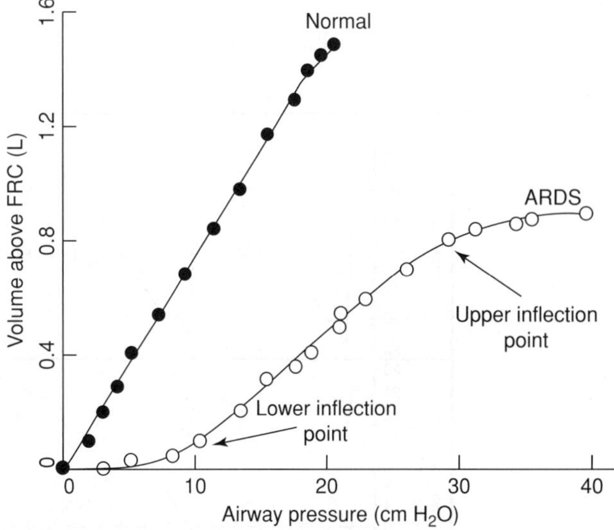

FIGURE 105.16 Flow and pressure traces in a patient with expiratory flow limitation from emphysema. The expiratory flow (**top** trace, down) has an immediate sharp decrease in rate, then a very slow plateau throughout expiration, never reaching baseline (0 flow). In the second-to-last breath, after a failed attempt to trigger a breath, an end-expiratory pause set on the ventilator shows the presence of auto-PEEP.

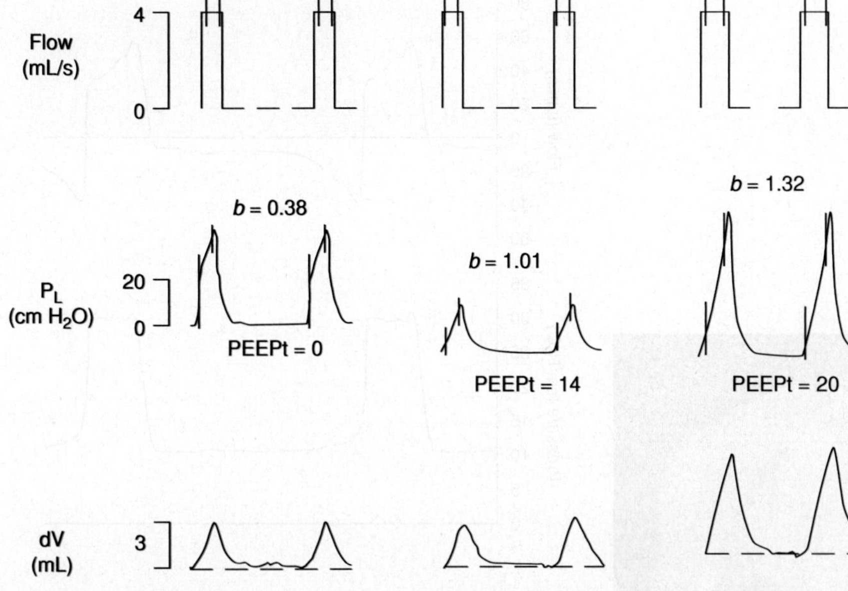

FIGURE 105.17 Analysis of the pressure over time (P-t) curve during constant inspiratory flow. The coefficient *b* describes the shape of the P-t curve. When *b* is less than 1 (**left**), the P-t trace has a concavity facing up, indicating an increasing compliance throughout inflation, related to ongoing alveolar recruitment. When *b* is greater than 1 (**right**), the P-t trace has a concavity facing down, indicating a decreasing compliance, related to alveolar overdistention. When *b* = 1 (**middle**), the P-t curve is linear, indicating a constant compliance throughout inflation and hence minimal alveolar recruitment/stress. (Modified from Ranieri VM, Zhang H, Mascia L, et al. Pressure–time curve predicts minimally injurious ventilatory strategy in an isolated rat lung model. *Anesthesiology.* 2000;93:1320–1328, with permission.)

recruitment); and an upward concavity suggests a decrease in compliance (i.e., overdistention) (46,47) (Fig. 105.17).

Intrathoracic or Pleural Pressure (P_{PL}). P_{PL} is estimated by measuring the pressure in the lower third of the esophagus with an esophageal balloon catheter (48–50). Esophageal pressure (P_{ESO}) is used as a surrogate of pleural pressure to estimate lung and chest wall compliance (C_L and C_{CW}), to quantify auto-PEEP and work of breathing during assisted modes of ventilation, and to evaluate the degree of diaphragmatic dysfunction (28). The measurement of P_{PL} is of great value in the assessment of respiratory mechanics and can be used by experienced clinicians at the bedside as well (Fig. 105.18) (48).

Transpulmonary Pressure (P_{TP}). P_{TP} is the difference between the pressure inside the alveoli (P_{ALV}) and the pressure surrounding the lung (pleural pressure, P_{PL}) (Fig. 105.19):

$$P_{TP} = P_{ALV} - P_{PL} \quad (8)$$

As in vivo measurements of P_{ALV} and P_{PL} are not feasible, P_{ALV} is usually assumed to be approximately equal to the static pressure at the airway opening (P_{PLAT}, PEEP) and P_{PL} equal to the esophageal pressure (P_{ESO}). P_{TP} is usually described as the distending pressure of the lungs, as it best describes the sum of the interactions of P_{PL} and P_{ALV} across the lungs. As P_{ESO} can be elevated in the setting of ARDS, obesity, or increased intra-abdominal pressure, the use of P_{TP} allows the titration of positive pressure according to the actual pressure applied to the lung. To allow optimal recruitment, PEEP could be increased until P_{TP} becomes positive at end expiration, to keep airways and alveoli open during the tidal cycle (51). End-inspiratory P_{TP} is evaluated by calculating the $P_{PLAT} - P_{ESO}$ difference during an inspiratory hold. It is useful in the assessment of safety pressure thresholds: an end-inspiratory P_{TP} lower than 20 cm H_2O is generally considered safe (52).

Compliance of Lungs and Chest Wall (C_L, C_{CW}). Measurement of end-inspiratory P_{ESO} ($P_{ESO,i}$) and end-expiratory

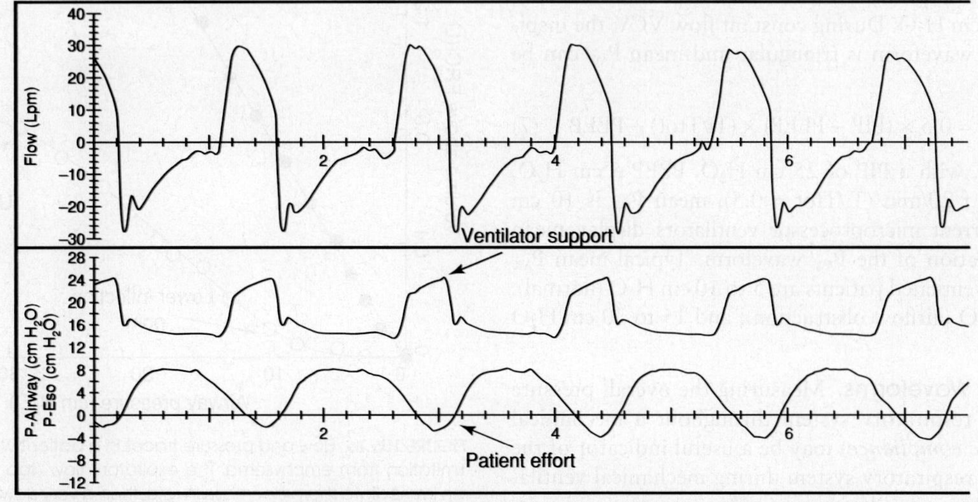

FIGURE 105.18 Flow, airway pressure, and esophageal pressure traces during pressure-controlled ventilation. At each breath, the esophageal pressure shows negative swings of approximately 10 cm H_2O, indicating active inspiratory efforts.

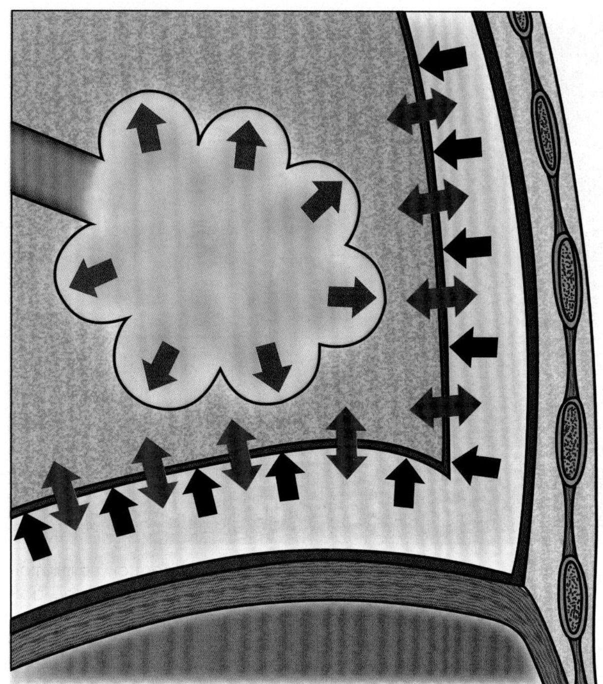

FIGURE 105.19 The transpulmonary pressure (P_{TP} *blue arrows*) describes the interaction between the forces acting inside the lung (alveolar pressure, P_{ALV}, *red arrows*) and the forces acting outside of the lung (P_{PL}, *black arrows*). During positive-pressure ventilation, P_{PL} acts as a force directed against the lung; in static conditions (end expiration or end inspiration) this pressure is sensed by the alveoli—P_{ALV}. When P_{ALV} is higher than P_{PL}, P_{TP} is positive and it represents a pressure vector oriented outside of the lung (lung-expanding force). If P_{ALV} is lower than P_{PL}, P_{TP} represents a pressure vector oriented inside the lung (collapsing force).

P_{ESO} ($P_{ESO,e}$) allows to distinguish the two components of C_{RS}: C_{CW} and C_L:

$$1/C_{RS} = 1/C_{CW} + 1/C_L \tag{9}$$

$$C_{CW} = V_T/(P_{ESO,i} - P_{ESO,e}) \tag{10}$$

$$C_L = V_T/[(P_{PLAT} - P_{ESO,i}) - (PEEP - P_{ESO,e})] \tag{11}$$

or

$$C_L = V_T/(P_{TP,i} - P_{TP,e}) \tag{12}$$

The partitioning of the elastic properties of the respiratory system is useful to understand whether a low C_{RS} as a whole might be due to low C_L, low C_{CW}, or both. Impairment of the elastic properties of the chest wall, as in morbid obesity, pneumoperitoneum, or increased intra-abdominal pressure, gives us an indication that additional pressure needs to be applied to the lung and transmitted to pleural space in order to achieve adequate thoracic inflation (53). As the chest wall becomes stiffer, the proportion of P_{AW} that is spent for lung distention becomes smaller. The degree of stiffness of the chest wall (low C_{CW}) must be taken into account when titrating P_{AW} to recruit the lung of ARDS, because higher P_{AW} levels might be needed to achieve the desired recruitment, without the same risk of injuring the lung. Using P_{TP} rather than P_{PLAT} as a target of P_{AW} titration has been shown to be safe and effective (54).

Patient-Ventilator Asynchrony

Asynchronous interactions between the patient's own effort and the machine's support may occur at any time in the course of mechanical ventilation. Asynchrony may worsen gas exchange, cause hemodynamic instability, and generate additional mechanical load that hinders ventilator weaning (55–58).

- *Insufficient gas flow support* can occur when the patient's ventilatory demand is higher than the inspiratory flow rate supplied by the ventilator. Increased inspiratory work during VCV can be detected by looking at the inspiratory pressure waveform (see Fig. 105.7), which acquires a characteristic upward concavity, indicating that the patient is exerting a significant negative (additional work of breathing) during inspiration (20).
- *Missed triggering* due to dynamic hyperinflation and auto-PEEP can occur with any mode of ventilation (59). Common to this phenomenon is a characteristic notching of the expiratory flow trace aiming toward the 0-flow line, as if to start a breath, but not going over it (see Fig. 105.16). This indicates an attempt to trigger breaths that do not generate sufficient pressure to overcome auto-PEEP (e.g., 10 cm H_2O) and reach the needed negative pressure threshold (e.g., 2 cm H_2O) to trigger the new breath. The significance of this phenomenon is twofold. First, it constitutes wasted respiratory

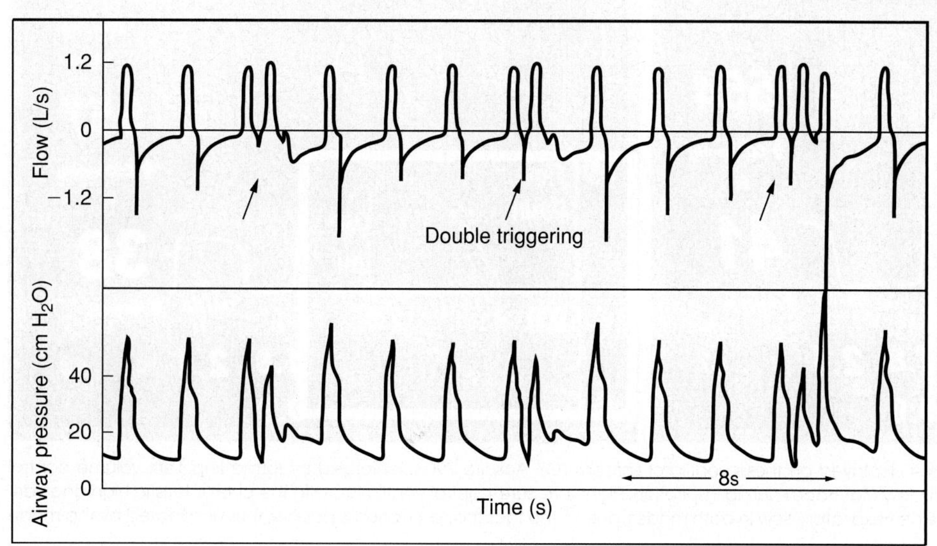

FIGURE 105.20 Double triggering during volume-controlled ventilation. Several breaths (*arrows*) start immediately after the previous breath, without allowing full exhalation. This phenomenon is characteristic of situations where the ventilator provides insufficient inspiratory flow, time, or volume to satisfy the patient's demand. (From Thille AW, Rodriguez P, Cabello B, et al. Patient-ventilator asynchrony during assisted mechanical ventilation. *Intensive Care Med.* 2006;32:1515–1522, with permission.)

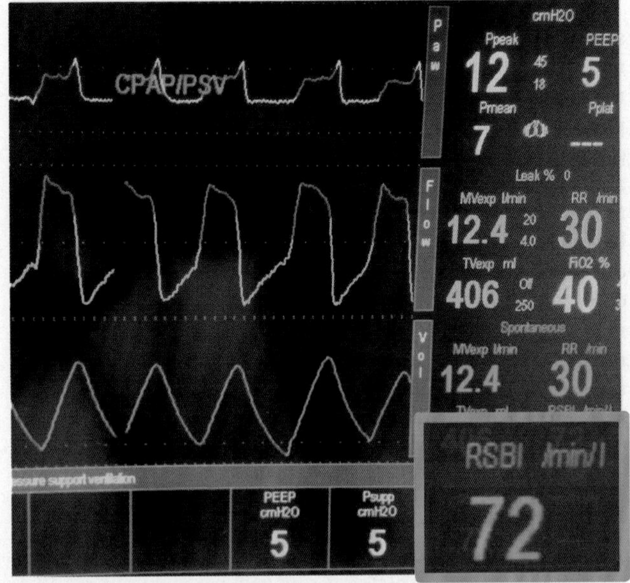

FIGURE 105.21 The Rapid Shallow Breathing Index (RSBI) is displayed on this ventilator screen (GE Engstrom Carestation), enlarged by formatting, in the "spontaneous breathing trial" function. Patient is on pressure support ventilation with set inspiratory pressure of 5 cm H_2O and PEEP of 5 cm H_2O. Patient is breathing 30 bpm with a tidal volume of 406 mL, which gives a RSBI of 72, a value normally associated with successful weaning.

work, that is, no volume is generated. Second, it may mislead the clinician reading the ventilator display to underestimate the true respiratory rate that the patient is trying to develop.

- *Missed triggering* can also occur with severe neuromuscular disease such as Guillain–Barré syndrome, where even a routine triggering threshold of −2 cm H_2O may at times constitute an overwhelming elastic load to work against.

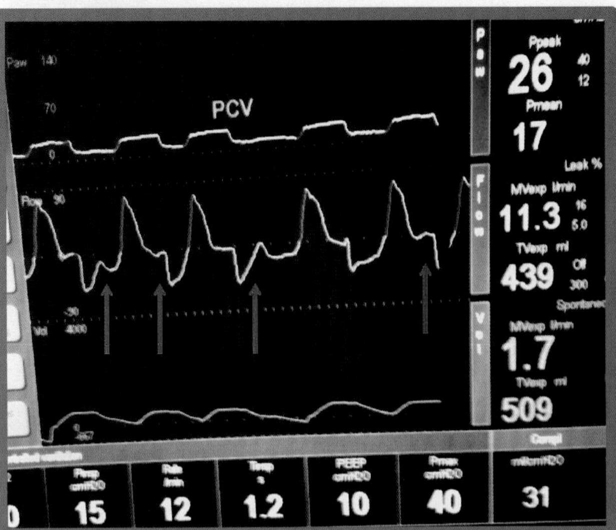

FIGURE 105.23 Missed triggering during pressure-control ventilation (PCV). Airway pressure (P_{AW}) on top, set at 15 mmHg (tabs at the bottom). Flow ($\dot{V}$) at the bottom, not set (PCV), reaching 30 L/min. The four *arrows* indicate multiple attempts to trigger the ventilator, where the expiratory flow rapidly ascends toward the 0 line, but does not cross it, hence does not generate a breath. This is likely due to expiratory flow limitation and auto-PEEP ($PEEP_i$).

- *Inadequate inspiratory time* can cause a discrepancy between the patient's own ventilatory pattern and the one set on the ventilator. This phenomenon can occur during PSV and can be aided by changing the expiratory sensitivity parameter, as shown in Figure 105.10. It can also occur during VCV or PCV (28,60) when an insufficient inspiratory time or low set V_T may result in a new breathing effort starting during or immediately after the ongoing cycle (*double triggering*) (Fig. 105.20). The patient's high demand is sufficient to close the expiratory

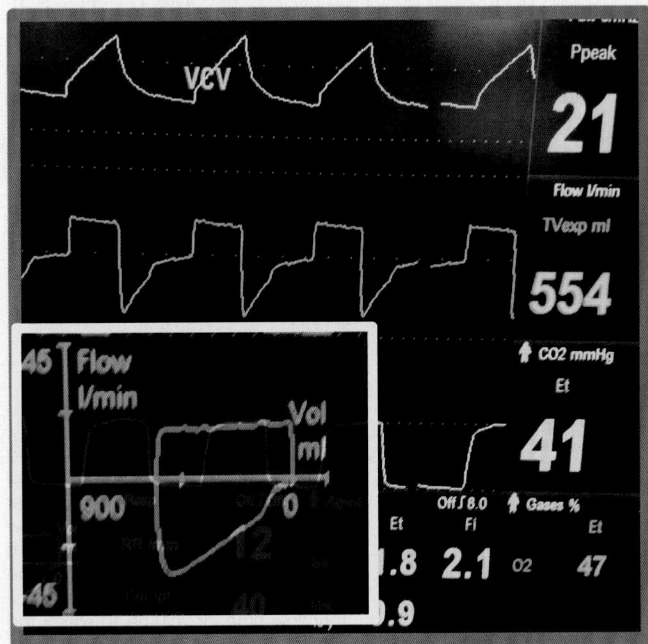

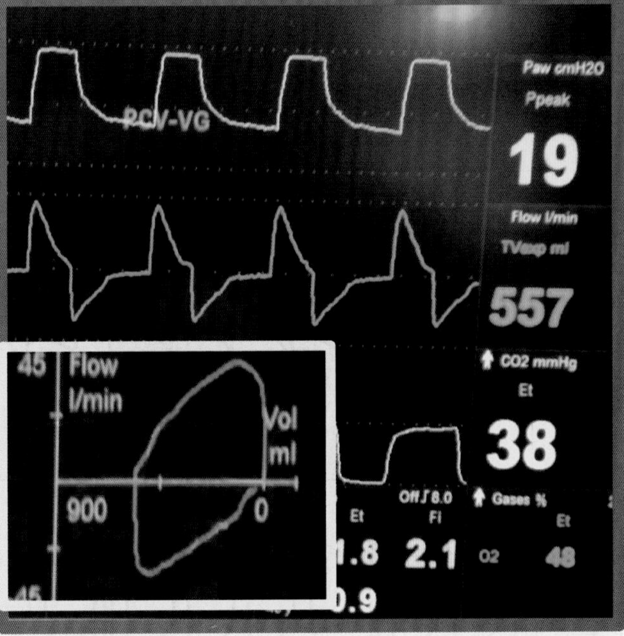

FIGURE 105.22 Flow–volume ($\dot{V}$-V) loops are displayed on these ventilator screens (GE Aespire 7900), enlarged by formatting. **Left**: volume control ventilation with the characteristic constant flow (flat trace) during inspiration. **Right**: pressure-control ventilation with the characteristic high and variable inspiratory flow. Note the similar pattern of expiratory flow in both modes, due to the fact that expiration is passive, thus unaffected by the mode of ventilation.

valve early in exhalation and trigger a second inspiration before exhalation is completed. The occurrence of double triggering in ARDS patients ventilated in assist control volume can result in higher V_T than recommended and increase the risk of ventilator-induced lung injury; this asynchrony may be prevented by increasing the inspiratory time (61).

- *Reverse triggering* describes the occurrence of diaphragmatic muscle contractions elicited by the ventilator, potentially affecting P_{TP} and V_T, and promoting muscle and lung damage (62).

SUMMARY

Modern ventilators measure and display physiologic information during mechanical ventilation. The observation of the pressure, volume, and flow traces may help clinicians to evaluate respiratory mechanics in real time, adjust ventilator settings, and detect equipment abnormalities. In addition, it offers the opportunity to learn and teach applied respiratory physiology at the bedside.

Key Points

- The end-inspiratory and end-expiratory pause functions on the ventilator provide measurement and display of basic respiratory mechanics in intubated patients (see Fig. 105.1).
- The Rapid Shallow Breathing Index (RSBI: respiratory rate/tidal volume in liters) is commonly used as a screening tool in the weaning process. Many ventilators display it on the screen when in the appropriate function, for example, "SBT" or "weaning" (Fig. 105.21).
- Flow–volume ($\dot{V}$-V) loops can be displayed during mechanical ventilation to complement the standard airway pressure (P_{AW}) and $\dot{V}$ over time traces (Fig. 105.22).
- Analysis of pressure and flow waveforms during mechanical ventilation can reveal the presence of expiratory flow limitation, auto-PEEP, and missed triggering (Fig. 105.23).
- The respiratory rate displayed on a ventilator screen may be deceiving. With missed triggering (Tip 4) the displayed rate is slower than the actual rate, possibly misleading the clinician evaluating readiness for extubation. With double triggering (see Fig. 105.20) the ventilator may or may not count the extra attempts to breathe, depending upon the resulting flow and pressure recorded.
- Calculating a single value of compliance or resistance to describe the respiratory system mechanics in the setting of lung heterogeneity (e.g., ARDS or asthma; see Figs. 105.13 and 105.15) may be too simplistic to guide effective ventilator management.
- Measuring esophageal pressure changes during mechanical ventilation aids in the titration of positive pressure (e.g., PEEP) in patients with altered mechanics, such as in ARDS, morbid obesity, and abdominal distention.

References

1. Sanborn WG. Monitoring respiratory mechanics during mechanical ventilation: Where do the signals come from? *Respir Care*. 2005;50:28–52.
2. Sullivan WJ, Peters GM, Enright PL. Pneumotachographs: theory and clinical application. *Respir Care*. 1984;29:736–749.
3. Hess DR. Heliox and noninvasive positive-pressure ventilation: a role for heliox in exacerbations of chronic obstructive pulmonary disease? *Respir Care*. 2006;51:640–650.
4. Hess D, McCurdy S, Simmons M. Compression volume in adult ventilator circuits: a comparison of five disposable circuits and a non-disposable circuit. *Respir Care*. 1991;36:1113–1118.
5. Gottfried SB, Reissman H, Ranieri VM. A simple method for the measurement of intrinsic positive end-expiratory pressure during controlled and assisted modes of mechanical ventilation. *Crit Care Med*. 1992;20:621–629.
6. Brenner M, Mukai DS, Russell JE, et al. A new method for measurement of airway occlusion pressure. *Chest*. 1990;98:421–427.
7. Kuhlen R, Hausmann S, Pappert D, et al. A new method for P0.1 measurement using standard respiratory equipment. *Intensive Care Med*. 1995;21:554–560.
8. Marini JJ, Smith TC, Lamb V. Estimation of inspiratory muscle strength in mechanically ventilated patients: the measurements of maximal inspiratory pressure. *J Crit Care*. 1986;1:32–38.
9. Tobin MJ, Jubran A. Variable performance of weaning-predictor tests: role of Bayes' theorem and spectrum and test-referral bias. *Intensive Care Med*. 2006;32:2002–2012.
10. Patel KN, Ganatra KD, Bates HJ, et al. Variation in the rapid shallow breathing index associated with common measurement techniques and conditions. *Resp Care*. 2009;54:1462–1466.
11. Tobin MJ. Extubation and the myth of "minimal ventilator settings." *Am J Respir Crit Care Med*. 2012;185:349–350.
12. Kheir F, Myers L, Desai NR, et al. The effect of flow trigger on rapid shallow breathing index measured through the ventilator. *J Intensive Care Med*. 2015;30:103–106.
13. Desai NR, Myers L, Simeone F. Comparison of 3 different methods used to measure the rapid shallow breathing index. *J Crit Care*. 2012;4:418.e1–e6.
14. Purro A, Appendini L, De Gaetano A, et al. Physiologic determinants of ventilator dependence in long-term mechanically ventilated patients. *Am J Respir Crit Care Med*. 2000;161:1115–1123.
15. Tanios MA, Nevins ML, Hendra KP, et al. A randomized, controlled trial of the role of weaning predictors in clinical decision making. *Crit Care Med*. 2006;34:2530–2535.
16. Jubran A, Tobin MJ. Use of flow-volume curves in detecting secretions in ventilator-dependent patients. *Am J Respir Crit Care Med*. 1994;150:766–769.
17. Brown K, Sly PD, Milic-Emili J, et al. Evaluation of the flow-volume loop as an intra-operative monitor of respiratory mechanics in infants. *Pediatr Pulmonol*. 1989;6:8–13.
18. Dhand R. Ventilator graphics and respiratory mechanics in the patient with obstructive lung disease. *Respir Care*. 2005;50:246–261.
19. Kondili E, Prinianakis G, Georgopoulos D. Patient–ventilator interaction. *Br J Anaesth*. 2003;91:106–119.
20. Marini JJ, Rodriguez RM, Lamb V. The inspiratory workload of patient-initiated mechanical ventilation. *Am Rev Respir Dis*. 1986;134:902–909.
21. Bernasconi M, Ploysongsang Y, Gottfried SB, et al. Respiratory compliance and resistance in mechanically ventilated patients with acute respiratory failure. *Intensive Care Med*. 1988;14:547–553.
22. Brunner JX, Laubscher TP, Banner MJ, et al. A simple method to measure total expiratory time constant based on the passive expiratory flow-volume curve. *Crit Care Med*. 1995;23:1117–1122.
23. Tokioka H, Tanaka T, Ishizu T, et al. The effect of breath termination criterion on breathing patterns and the work of breathing during pressure support ventilation. *Anesth Analg*. 2001;92:161–165.
24. Branson RD, Campbell RS. Pressure support ventilation, patient–ventilator synchrony, and ventilator algorithms. *Respir Care*. 1998;43:1045–1047.
25. Thille AW, Cabello B, Galia F, et al. Reduction of patient-ventilator asynchrony by reducing tidal volume during pressure-support ventilation. *Intensive Care Med*. 2008;34:1477–1486.
26. Chiumello D, Pelosi P, Croci M, et al. The effects of pressurization rate on breathing pattern, work of breathing, gas exchange and patient comfort in pressure support ventilation. *Eur Respir J*. 2001;18:107–114.
27. D'Angelo E, Calderini E, Torri G, et al. Respiratory mechanics in anesthetized paralyzed humans: effects of flow, volume, and time. *J Appl Physiol*. 1989;67:2556–2564.
28. Truwit JD, Marini JJ. Evaluation of the thoracic mechanics in the ventilated patients, I: primary measurements. *J Crit Care*. 1988;3:133–150.
29. Harris RS. Pressure-volume curves of the respiratory system. *Respir Care*. 2005;50:78–98.
30. Grasso S, Stripoli T, Sacchi M, et al. Inhomogeneity of lung parenchyma during the open lung strategy. *Am J Respir Crit Care Med*. 2009;180:415–423.

31. Terragni PP, Rosboch G, Tealdi A, et al. Tidal hyperinflation during low tidal volume ventilation in acute respiratory distress syndrome. *Am J Respir Crit Care Med.* 2007;175:160–166.
32. Gattinoni L, Protti A, Caironi P, et al. Ventilator-induced lung injury: the anatomical and physiological framework. *Crit Care Med.* 2010;38:S539–S548.
33. Ranieri VM, Giuliani R, Mascia L, et al. Chest wall and lung contribution to the elastic properties of the respiratory system in patients with chronic obstructive pulmonary disease. *Eur Respir J.* 1996;9:1232–1239.
34. Lucangelo U, Bernabe F, Blanch L. Respiratory mechanics derived from signals in the ventilator circuit. *Respir Care.* 2005;50:55–65.
35. Hess D, Tabor T. Comparison of six methods to calculate airway resistance during mechanical ventilation in adults. *J Clin Monit.* 1993;9:275–282.
36. Rossi A, Gottfried SB, Higgs BD, et al. Respiratory mechanics in mechanically ventilated patients with respiratory failure. *J Appl Physiol.* 1985;58:1849–1858.
37. Polese G, Lubli P, Poggi R, et al. Effects of inspiratory flow waveforms on arterial blood gases and respiratory mechanics after open heart surgery. *Eur Respir J.* 1997;10:2820–2824.
38. Mietto C, Pinciroli R, Piriyapatsom A, et al. Tracheal tube obstruction in mechanically ventilated patients assessed by high-resolution computed tomography. *Anesthesiology.* 2014;121:1226–1235.
39. Smith TC, Marini JJ. Impact of PEEP on lung mechanics and work of breathing in severe airflow obstruction. *J Appl Physiol.* 1988;65:1488–1499.
40. Pellegrino R, Gobbi A, Antonelli A, et al. Ventilation heterogeneity in obesity. *J Appl Phys.* 2014;116:1175–1181.
41. Marini JJ, Culver BH, Kirk W. Flow resistance of exhalation valves and positive end-expiratory pressure devices used in mechanical ventilation. *Am Rev Respir Dis.* 1985;131:850–854.
42. Ranieri VM, Grasso S, Fiore T, et al. Auto-positive end-expiratory pressure and dynamic hyperinflation. *Clin Chest Med.* 1996;17:379–394.
43. Blanch L, Bernabe F, Lucangelo U. Measurement of air trapping, intrinsic positive end-expiratory pressure, and dynamic hyperinflation in mechanically ventilated patients. *Respir Care.* 2005;50:110–123.
44. Bates JH, Rossi A, Milic-Emili J. Analysis of the behavior of the respiratory system with constant inspiratory flow. *J Appl Physiol.* 1985;58:1840–1848.
45. Lichtwarck-Aschoff M, Kessler V, Sjostrand UH, et al. Static versus dynamic respiratory mechanics for setting the ventilator. *Br J Anaesth.* 2000;85:577–586.
46. Ranieri VM, Zhang H, Mascia L, et al. Pressure–time curve predicts minimally injurious ventilatory strategy in an isolated rat lung model. *Anesthesiology.* 2000;93:1320–1328.
47. Grasso S, Terragni P, Mascia L, et al. Airway pressure–time curve profile (stress index) detects tidal recruitment/hyperinflation in experimental acute lung injury. *Crit Care Med.* 2004;32:1018–1027.
48. Benditt JO. Esophageal and gastric pressure measurements. *Respir Care.* 2005;50:68–75.
49. Petit JM, Milic-Emili G. Measurement of endoesophageal pressure. *J Appl Physiol.* 1958;13:481–485.
50. Walterspacher S, Isaak L, Guttmann J, et al. Assessing respiratory function depends on mechanical characteristics of balloon catheters. *Respir Care.* 2014;59:1345–1352.
51. Talmor D, Sarge T, Malhotra A, et al. Mechanical ventilation guided by esophageal pressure in acute lung injury. *N Engl J Med.* 2008;359:2095–2104.
52. Gattinoni L, Carlesso E, Cadringher P, et al. Physical and biological triggers of ventilator-induced lung injury and its prevention. *Eur Resp J Suppl.* 2003;47:15s–25s.
53. Gattinoni L, Chiumello D, Carlesso E, Valenza F. Bench-to-bedside review: chest wall elastance in acute lung injury/acute respiratory distress syndrome. *Crit Care.* 2004;8:350–355.
54. Sarge T, Talmor D. Targeting transpulmonary pressure to prevent ventilator induced lung injury. *Minerva Anestesiol.* 2009;75:293–299.
55. Nilsestuen JO, Hargett KD. Using ventilator graphics to identify patient–ventilator asynchrony. *Respir Care.* 2005;50:202–234.
56. Georgopoulos D, Prinianakis G, Kondili E. Bedside waveforms interpretation as a tool to identify patient–ventilator asynchronies. *Intensive Care Med.* 2006;32:34–47.
57. Younes M, Riddle W. Relation between respiratory neural output and tidal volume. *J Appl Physiol.* 1984;56:1110–1119.
58. Younes M. Patient–ventilator interaction with pressure-assisted modalities of ventilator support. *Semin Respir Med.* 1993;14:299–322.
59. Leung P, Jubran A, Tobin MJ. Comparison of assisted ventilator modes on triggering, patient effort, and dyspnea. *Am J Respir Crit Care Med.* 1997; 155:1940–1948.
60. Hess DR, Medoff BD, Fessler MB. Pulmonary mechanics and graphics during positive pressure ventilation. *Int Anesthesiol Clin.* 1999;37:15–34.
61. Chanques G, Kress JP, Pohlman A, et al. Impact of ventilator adjustment and sedation-analgesia practices on severe asynchrony in patients ventilated in assist-control mode. *Crit Care Med.* 2013;41:2177–2187.
62. Akoumianaki E, Lyazidi A, Rey N, et al. Mechanical ventilation-induced reverse-triggered breaths: a frequently unrecognized form of neuromechanical coupling. *Chest.* 2013;143:927–938.

CHAPTER

106

Weaning from Mechanical Ventilation

FRANCO LAGHI, HAMEEDA SHAIKH, and DEJAN RADOVANOVIC

INTRODUCTION

The process of discontinuing mechanical ventilation is known as *weaning*. Although often lifesaving, mechanical ventilation can be associated with life-threatening complications (1). Therefore, it is essential to safely discontinue mechanical ventilation at the earliest possible time. Unfortunately, both investigators and clinicians alike assign different meanings to this term. For some, most common definitions of weaning include gradual reduction in ventilator support when patients are recovering from respiratory failure, the act of removing patients from the ventilator with extubation of the endotracheal tube, or disconnection of the tracheotomy tube.

To overcome these differences, a framework of seven stages of weaning has been proposed (Fig. 106.1) (2). Stage 1 is preweaning, when patients are too ill to be considered ready for weaning (e.g., patients requiring high levels of oxygen (O_2) and positive end-expiratory pressure (PEEP)). All ventilated patients begin at stage 1. In some large series, 13% to 26% of patients never go beyond stage 1 (3–5). During stage 1, measurement of weaning predictors is inappropriate and potentially dangerous.

Stage 2 is the period of diagnostic triggering. This is the time when a physician begins to think that the patient *might* be ready to come off the ventilator. Failure to engage in this period of diagnostic triggering may be the greatest impediment to prompt weaning (2). Most patients that have been ventilated for a week or longer and are recruited in randomized controlled trials (RCTs) of different weaning techniques can often be successfully discontinued on the first day of active weaning (6). This observation raises the possibility that, in many patients, discontinuation of mechanical ventilation could have been performed a day or so earlier if physicians had considered earlier that the patient *might have been* ready to come off the ventilator.

Stage 3 is the time to obtain physiologic measurements that serve as predictors (*weaning predictors*) and to interpret them in the context of each patient's unique clinical condition. During stage 4 (*weaning trial*), ventilatory support is either gradually decreased over hours or days (e.g., gradual reduction in pressure support), or it is removed abruptly and completely (T-tube trial). Approximately 20% to 30% of patients deemed ready for a weaning trial will develop severe distress during the first trial of spontaneous breathing, requiring the resumption of mechanical ventilation (7). This highlights the importance of the weaning trial within the framework of the weaning process. In stage 5, patients who succeeded the weaning trial are extubated. Patients who did not succeed the weaning trial are returned to ventilator support. Stages 6 and 7 apply to patients who do poorly after extubation. Stage 6 is continuation of ventilator support with noninvasive positive pressure ventilation (NIPPV). Stage 7 is reintubation, accompanied by the reinstitution of mechanical ventilation (2).

This chapter will review the pathophysiology of weaning failure, and the clinical use of predictors of weaning outcome and techniques of weaning. Finally, extubation failure will be discussed. Areas of active research and controversial topics will be highlighted throughout the chapter.

PATHOPHYSIOLOGY OF WEANING FAILURE

Various disease states, alone or in combination, may cause weaning failure. From a pathophysiologic standpoint, it is useful to consider these disease states in terms of those characterized by a failure of the lungs as a gas exchange unit, and those characterized by a failure of the ventilatory pump. In a third group of patients, psychological factors may contribute to weaning failure.

Impaired Gas Exchange

Conditions characterized by failure of the lungs as a gas exchange unit include those associated with ventilation–perfusion mismatching and (less often) conditions associated with increased shunt (7). The typical consequence of impaired gas exchange is development of hypoxemia (7). Impaired gas exchange is a common finding among patients considered for a trial of weaning. For example, the mean arterial-to-inspired oxygen ratio (PaO_2/FiO_2) in more than 600 patients enrolled in weaning studies of the Spanish Lung Failure Collaborative Group ranged from 200 to 335 mmHg (8,9).

The ratio of dead space to tidal volume (V_D/V_T)—an approximation of impaired gas exchange due to lung units with abnormally high ventilation–perfusion ratios—is normally about 0.30 at rest (10). In patients requiring prolonged mechanical ventilation, the ratio can reach or even exceed 0.74 (11). Patients can compensate for the increase in dead space by increasing minute ventilation by as much as 2.5 times. Such an increase in minute ventilation poses a minor challenge when respiratory mechanics and respiratory muscles are normal; for example, the development of hypercapnia is uncommon with pulmonary vascular disease (12). Likewise, in the presence of large shunts, increases in minute ventilation can be sufficient to prevent hypercapnia (13). Accordingly, an increase in dead-space ventilation or shunt should not be considered the primary mechanisms responsible for weaning failure, unless there is a concurrent abnormality in the mechanical load of the respiratory muscles or in their contractile performance (12), or there are concurrent abnormalities in the control of breathing. For example, increases in dead-space ventilation may develop during weaning trials as the result of rapid shallow breathing and dynamic hyperinflation (14). Finally, an increased production in carbon dioxide (CO_2) can probably only be a contributory factor and not the sole cause of weaning failure (15).

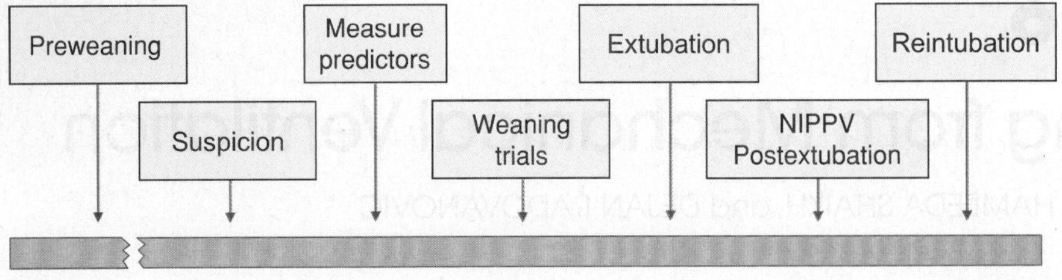

FIGURE 106.1 Seven stages of weaning. Stage 1 is preweaning, a stage that many patients never get beyond. Stage 2 is the period of diagnostic triggering, the time when a physician begins to think that the patient might be ready come off the ventilator. Stage 3 is the time of measuring and interpreting weaning predictors. Stage 4 is the time of decreasing ventilator support (abruptly or gradually). Stage 5 is either extubation (of a weaning success patient) or reinstitution of mechanical ventilation (in a weaning failure patient). Stage 6 is use of noninvasive positive pressure ventilation (NIPPV) after extubation. Stage 7 is reintubation. Failure to appreciate stage 2 probably leads to the greatest delays in weaning. (From Tobin MJ, Jubran A. Weaning from mechanical ventilation. In: Tobin MJ, ed. *Principles and Practice of Mechanical Ventilation.* 3rd ed. New York, NY: McGraw-Hill; 2013:1308.)

Impaired Ventilatory Pump

Impairment of the ventilatory pump can occur in conditions characterized by impaired control of breathing, abnormal respiratory mechanics (increased mechanical load), diminished respiratory muscle performance, impaired cardiovascular performance, and psychological factors.

Impaired Control of Breathing

Many weaning-failure patients develop hypercapnia (7). Specific conditions such as central alveolar hypoventilation secondary to neurologic lesions (trauma, infections, stroke) can contribute to, or cause, weaning failure. In most weaning failure patients, however, estimations of respiratory drive indicate that drive is increased, and not decreased (7,16). In these patients with high respiratory drive, hypercapnia is often accompanied by a marked shortening of inspiratory time coupled with shortening of expiratory time (Fig. 106.2). The shortening of both inspiratory time and expiratory time results in an elevation in the respiratory frequency and a marked decrease of tidal volume (17). The combined elevation in respiratory frequency and decrease in tidal volume is referred to as rapid shallow breathing and has been recognized as the physiologic hallmark of weaning failure (7). It has been suggested that, by stimulating pulmonary or bronchial receptors (stretch or irritant), an increased mechanical load on the respiratory muscles may trigger such a rapid and shallow breathing pattern (7). An elevated neuromuscular inspiratory drive in weaning failure patients does not necessarily translate into full respiratory muscle recruitment (Fig. 106.3) (18).

In some patients, a decrease in drive relative to the ventilatory demands may still contribute to weaning failure (14). Whether sleep deprivation decreases respiratory drive remains controversial (19,20).

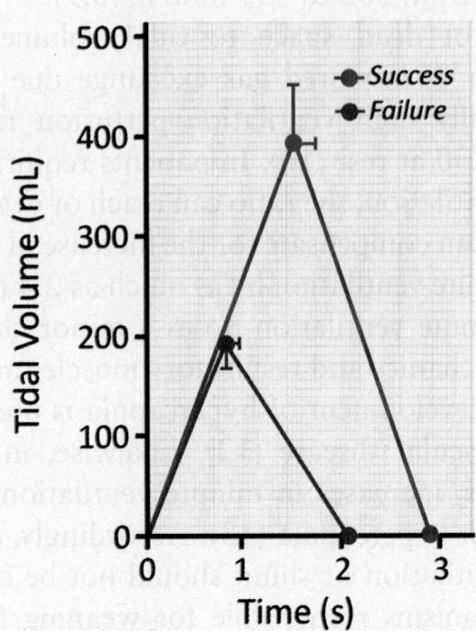

FIGURE 106.2 The mean respiratory cycle during spontaneous breathing in seven weaning-failure patients and ten weaning-success patients. The early termination of inspiratory time in the weaning-failure patients lead to a decrease in tidal volume (V_T). The decrease in inspiratory time, coupled with a decrease in expiratory time, resulted in a faster respiratory frequency (bars represent one standard error). (Adapted from Tobin MJ, Perez W, Guenther SM, et al. The pattern of breathing during successful and unsuccessful trials of weaning from mechanical ventilation. *Am Rev Respir Dis.* 1986;134(6):1111–1118.)

Increased Mechanical Load

Patients who fail a weaning trial usually experience an increased mechanical load on the respiratory muscles (Fig. 106.4) (14,16,21–24). Of interest, before the onset of a trial of spontaneous respiration (i.e., T-tube trial), Jubran and Tobin (25) reported that lung resistance, static elastance, and intrinsic PEEP during passive ventilation are equivalent in weaning failure and

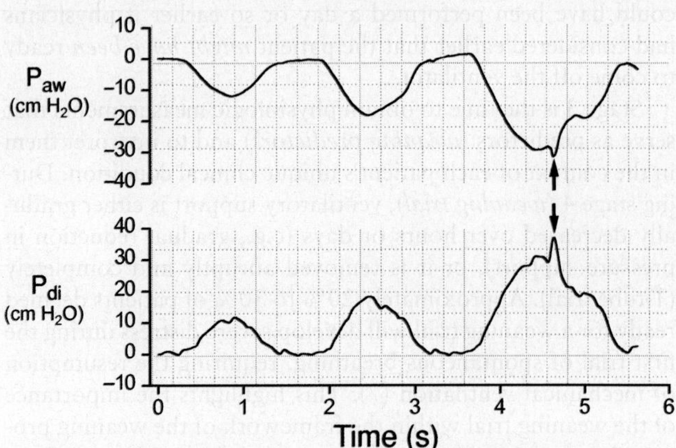

FIGURE 106.3 Continuous recordings of airway pressure (P_{aw}) and transdiaphragmatic pressure (P_{di}) during airway occlusion in a patient with COPD after an unsuccessful trial of spontaneous breathing. Phrenic nerve stimulation (*arrows*) during the maximal inspiratory effort resulted in a detectable superimposed twitch. That a twitch could be superimposed during the maximal effort indicates that diaphragmatic activation was incomplete.

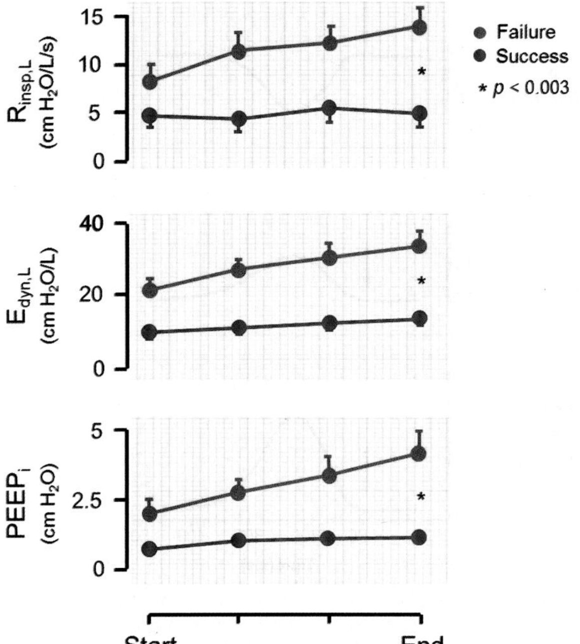

FIGURE 106.4 Inspiratory resistance of the lung ($R_{insp,L}$), dynamic lung elastance ($E_{dyn,L}$), and intrinsic positive end-expiratory pressure ($PEEP_i$) in 17 weaning-failure patients and 14 weaning-success patients. Data displayed were obtained during the second and last minute of a T-tube trial, and at one-third and two-thirds of the trial duration. Between the onset and end of the trial, the failure group developed increases in $R_{insp,L}$ ($p < 0.009$), $E_{dyn,L}$($p < 0.0001$), and $PEEP_i$ ($p < 0.0001$) and the success group developed increases in $E_{dyn,L}$ ($p < 0.006$) and $PEEP_i$ ($p < 0.02$). Over the course of the trial, the failure group had higher values of $R_{insp,L}$ ($p < 0.003$), $E_{dyn,L}$ ($p < 0.006$), and $PEEP_i$ ($p < 0.009$) than the success group. (From Jubran A, Tobin MJ. Pathophysiologic basis of acute respiratory distress in patients who fail a trial of weaning from mechanical ventilation. *Am J Respir Crit Care Med.* 1997;155(3):906–915.)

weaning success patients. This difference indicates that one or more factors associated with the act of spontaneous breathing are responsible for the marked difference between failure and success patients during a weaning trial (2).

Several circumstances can be responsible for an abnormal mechanical load, such as bronchoconstriction, bronchial edema, pulmonary edema (14), and lung inflammation (21,22). Rapid shallow breathing can aggravate the abnormalities in lung elastance, intrinsic PEEP, and carbon dioxide clearance (14). Expiratory muscle recruitment can also increase intrinsic PEEP (26) and breathing effort (24,27,28).

Several lines of evidence support the likelihood that increased mechanical load contributes to weaning failure. First, during spontaneous respiration, mechanical load is greater in weaning failure patients than in weaning success patients (14,16). Second, in patients who required mechanical ventilation for 6 to 70 days, progression to successful weaning was associated with an improvement in work of breathing per liter of minute ventilation (29); work of breathing per liter of minute ventilation is a function of compliance, resistance, tidal volume, and minute ventilation (29). Third, in weaning failure patients, neuromuscular drive is higher than in patients who are successfully weaned (16). Despite a greater neuromuscular drive, the mean inspiratory flow in weaning failures is similar to the mean inspiratory flow in weaning successes (16), indicating that for any given change in drive, the flow resistance and compliance characteristics of the respiratory system in weaning failure patients limit the capacity of neuromuscular drive to produce the otherwise expected changes in ventilation.

Inadequate Performance of the Respiratory Muscles

Respiratory muscle weakness and respiratory muscle fatigue can decrease the capacity of these muscles to generate and sustain tension. Direct quantification of respiratory muscle tension is clinically impossible. Therefore, measurements of pressure produced by respiratory muscle contractions are used as an indirect means to determine whether inadequate performance of the respiratory muscles is responsible for weaning failure.

Respiratory Muscle Weakness. (1) *Detection of respiratory muscle weakness in critically ill patients.* Measurements of airway pressure during maximal voluntary inspiratory efforts are used to evaluate global inspiratory muscle strength (30). In healthy subjects, maximum inspiratory airway pressure is usually more negative than −80 cm H_2O (30). In mechanically ventilated patients recovering from an episode of acute respiratory failure, maximum inspiratory airway pressure can range from less negative than −20 cm H_2O to about −100 cm H_2O (5,14,16). Values of maximal airway pressure during voluntary maneuvers depend greatly on level of motivation and comprehension of the maneuver, and are therefore often not obtainable in critically ill patients (see Fig. 106.3). Thus, it is not surprising that, in patients requiring short-term mechanical ventilation, measurements of maximum inspiratory airway pressure commonly do not differentiate between weaning successes and weaning failure patients (5,24,29,31,32).

In contrast, transdiaphragmatic pressures elicited by single stimulations of the phrenic nerves—or twitch pressure—are independent of patients' motivation and eliminate the influence of the central nervous system (33). Activation can be achieved with either an electrical stimulator or a magnetic stimulator (33), though the latter is easier to use in mechanically ventilated patients (Fig. 106.5) (24,34,35).

In healthy volunteers, magnetic stimulation elicits twitch pressures which average 31 to 39 cm H_2O (30). In ambulatory patients with severe chronic obstructive pulmonary disease (COPD), twitch pressures average 19 to 20 cm H_2O (36,37). The value of transdiaphragmatic twitch pressure in patients recovering from an episode of acute respiratory failure is about half of that recorded in ambulatory patients with severe COPD (Fig. 106.6) (24,34,35,38). This marked reduction in twitch pressure indicates the presence of respiratory muscle weakness in most of these patients. Moreover, it has been suggested that the severity of diaphragm weakness may correlate with poor patient outcomes (38). In a study of 60 critically ill patients, a transdiaphragmatic twitch pressure of less than 10 cm H_2O was associated with increased mortality and a longer duration of mechanical ventilation (38).

Respiratory muscle weakness in critically ill patients can result from pre-existing conditions or from new onset conditions.

(1) Weakness due to pre-existing conditions: Pre-existing conditions that can cause respiratory muscle weakness include disorders such as neuromuscular diseases, malnutrition, and endocrine disturbances. Pre-existing conditions can be recognized before instituting mechanical ventilation, when ventilator support is being delivered or when the patient fails a weaning trial.

Neuromuscular Disorders. According to the level of anatomical involvement, neuromuscular disorders can be grouped

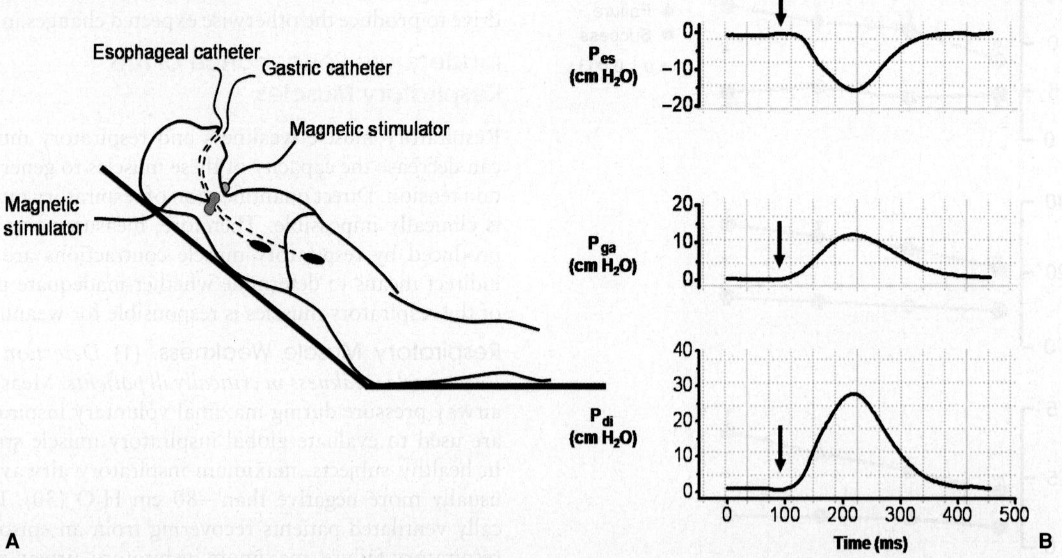

FIGURE 106.5 Twitch pressure recordings following magnetic stimulation of the phrenic nerves. A: An esophageal and a gastric balloon catheter are passed through the nares. Magnetic stimulation of the phrenic nerves elicits diaphragmatic contraction. B: Continuous recordings of esophageal (P_{es}) and gastric pressures (P_{ga}) and transdiaphragmatic pressure (P_{di})—calculated by subtracting P_{es} from P_{ga}. Phrenic nerve stimulation (*arrows*) results in contraction of the diaphragm with consequent fall in intrathoracic pressure (negative deflection of P_{es}) and rise in intra-abdominal pressure (positive deflection of P_{ga}). These swings in pressure are responsible for transdiaphragmatic twitch pressure. The smaller the transdiaphragmatic twitch pressure, the smaller the force generation capacity of the diaphragm. (Adapted from Laghi F. Hypoventilation and respiratory muscle dysfunction. In: Parrillo JE, Dellinger RP, eds. *Critical Care Medicine: Principles of Diagnosis and Management in the Adult*. 4th ed. St Louis, MO: Mosby; 2014: 674–691.)

in those involving the central nervous system (e.g., multiple sclerosis, amyotrophic lateral sclerosis), motor neuron (e.g., spinal cord compression, postpolio syndrome, amyotrophic lateral sclerosis), peripheral nerves (e.g., Guillain–Barré syndrome), neuromuscular junction (e.g., botulism, myasthenia gravis), and peripheral muscles (e.g., inflammatory myopathies, myotonic dystrophy, Duchenne's muscular dystrophy) (18).

Hypercapnic respiratory failure usually occurs when respiratory muscle strength falls to 39% of the predicted normal value (39). Gibson et al. (40), however, have described several patients with neuromuscular disease who had a normal partial pressure of CO_2 despite decreases in respiratory muscle strength to less than 20% of predicted. Conversely, some patients with only moderate respiratory muscle weakness displayed hypercapnia (Fig. 106.7) (40). In other words,

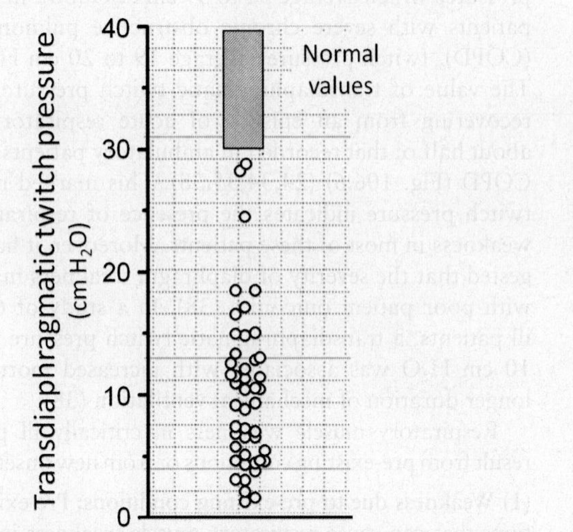

FIGURE 106.6 Transdiaphragmatic pressure in response to single stimulations (twitch stimulation) of the phrenic nerves recorded in ventilated patients recovering from acute respiratory failure. The boxed area represents the 95% confidence interval of values obtained in healthy subjects. The decreased transdiaphragmatic twitch pressure in patients indicates presence of diaphragmatic weakness. (From Laghi F. Ventilator-induced diaphragmatic dysfunction: is there a dim light at the end of the tunnel? *Crit Care Med.* 2011;39:903.)

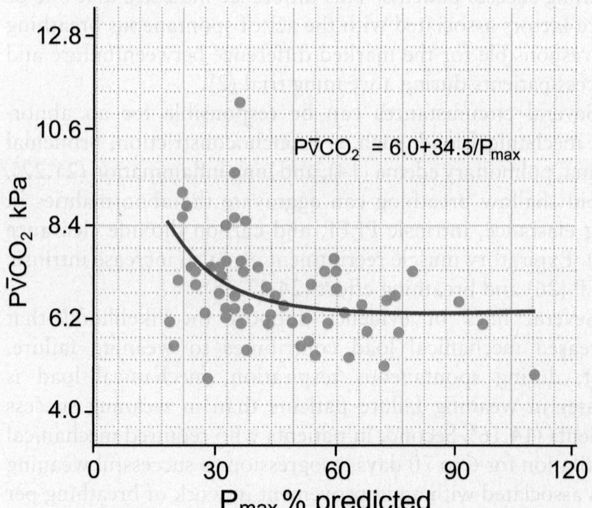

FIGURE 106.7 Relationship between muscle strength and mixed venous partial pressure of CO_2 ($P\bar{V}CO_2$) in patients with respiratory muscle weakness. Respiratory muscle strength is the arithmetic sum of maximum static inspiratory and expiratory mouth pressures ($P_{max} = PI_{max} + PE_{max}$). As respiratory muscle weakness became more severe, $P\bar{V}CO_2$ increased, although considerable variability was observed among patients. (Adapted from Gibson GJ, Gilmartin JJ, Veale D, et al. Respiratory muscle function in neuromuscular disease. In: Jones NL, Killian KJ, eds. Breathlessness. *The Campbell Symposium*. Hamilton, ON: Boehringer-Ingelheim; 1992.)

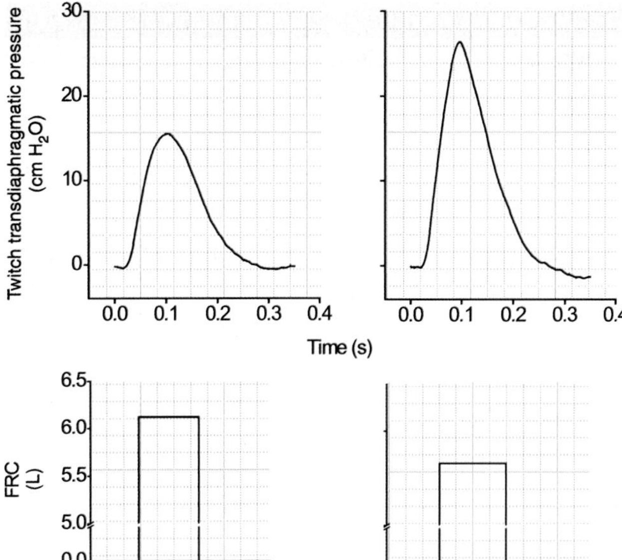

FIGURE 106.8 Twitch transdiaphragmatic pressure elicited by phrenic nerve stimulation (**top**) and functional residual capacity (FRC) (**bottom**) in a patient with severe emphysema before (**left**) and after (**right**) lung volume reduction surgery. The increase in transdiaphragmatic pressure after surgery was in part due to a decrease in the operating lung volume as demonstrated by the decrease in functional residual capacity. (Based on data from Laghi F, Jubran A, Topeli A, et al. Effect of lung volume reduction surgery on neuromechanical coupling of the diaphragm. *Am J Respir Crit Care Med.* 1998;157(2):475–483.)

reductions in muscle strength do not consistently predict the degree of alveolar hypoventilation in this setting.

Hyperinflation. Hyperinflation is a common pre-existing problem in patients with obstructive lung diseases (41,42), but can also occur *de novo* in patients with pneumonia, acute respiratory distress syndrome, and chest trauma (15). Hyperinflation forces inspiratory muscles to operate at an unfavorable position of the length-tension relationship (Fig. 106.8) (43). Gross hyperinflation resulting in flattening of the diaphragm decreases the size of the zone of apposition leading to less effective rib cage expansion during diaphragmatic contraction (18). An increase in lung elastance secondary to hyperinflation also worsens the workload of inspiratory muscles as they are forced to operate against both the elastic recoil of the lungs and the chest wall (18). The functional consequences of dynamic hyperinflation contribute to weaning failure (44). In patients with acute respiratory distress syndrome, the impairment of inspiratory muscle function as a consequence of hyperinflation, however, is less likely because these patients breathe at a low lung volume despite dynamic hyperinflation (45,46).

Malnutrition. Malnutrition is highly prevalent among critically ill patients requiring mechanical ventilation, and is associated with poor prognosis (47). Malnutrition decreases muscle mass and respiratory muscle strength both in humans and laboratory animals (18).

In malnourished patients, inspiratory weakness (48–50), fatigability (49), and dyspnea (49) are partially reversible with nutritional support. The process is slow and, in laboratory animals, can take months of refeeding for muscle mass to return to normal values (51). To date, it remains unclear whether malnutrition by itself can cause sufficient respiratory muscle weakness to produce weaning failure. It is more likely for malnutrition to be a contributory factor rather than the sole cause of weaning failure.

Endocrine Disturbances. Endocrine disturbances, including acromegaly, hypothyroidism, and hyperthyroidism can adversely affect respiratory muscle function (52). Proteolysis of myofibrillar proteins by the ubiquitin–proteasome proteolytic system is probably responsible for respiratory muscle catabolism and weakness of hyperthyroidism (52). This mechanism is implicated in the muscle wasting associated with acidosis, renal failure, denervation, cancer, diabetes, AIDS, trauma, and burns (18).

(2) **Weakness due to new onset conditions**: New-onset respiratory muscle weakness may result from conditions which are unique to critically ill patients or from conditions common in other settings. The former include ventilator-associated respiratory muscle dysfunction, sepsis-associated myopathy, and intensive care unit (ICU)-acquired paresis. All these conditions are often associated with alterations in respiratory muscle structure and recovery, if it occurs at all, is slow. In contrast, respiratory muscle weakness due to acid–base disorders, electrolyte disturbances, decreased oxygen delivery, or medications are not necessarily associated with alterations in respiratory muscle structure and the recovery is usually rapid once the underlying triggering factor has been corrected.

Ventilator-associated Respiratory Muscle Dysfunction. In laboratory animals, controlled mechanical ventilation delivered for 1 to 11 days can decrease diaphragmatic force generation by 20% to more than 50% (Fig. 106.9) and it can cause similar decreases in diaphragmatic endurance (15,53).

Several mechanisms, including structural injury, oxidative stress, muscle fiber remodeling, muscle atrophy—with attendant reduction in myofibril synthesis and increased myofibril proteolysis—appear to be responsible for ventilator-associated respiratory muscle dysfunction (54). In two RCTs (55,56), investigators reported that administration of antioxidants was associated with a reduction in the duration of mechanical ventilation both medical and surgical critically ill patients. Whether this decrease in duration of mechanical ventilation was due in part to the potential positive effects of antioxidants on the respiratory muscles remains to be determined.

Atrophy of respiratory muscle fibers appears to be mechanistically linked in the development of ventilator-induced

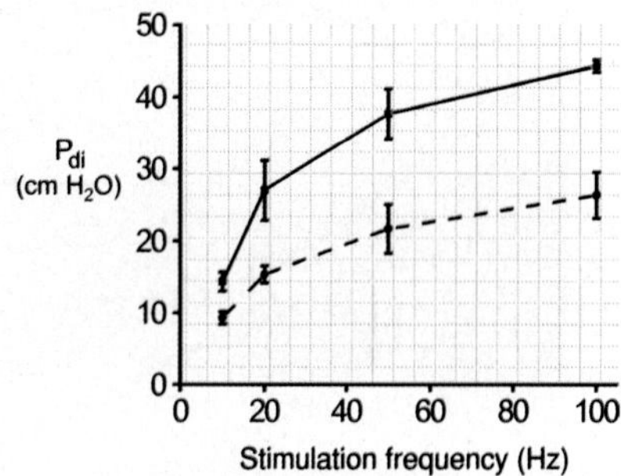

FIGURE 106.9 Transdiaphragmatic pressure (P_{di}) response to phrenic nerve stimulation before (*solid line*) and after 11 days (*dashed line*) of mechanical ventilation. That the transdiaphragmatic pressure recorded after 11 days of mechanical ventilation shows a decrease response to all stimulation frequencies is suggestive of ventilator-associated diaphragmatic dysfunction. (Adapted from Anzueto A, Peters JI, Tobin MJ, et al. Effects of prolonged controlled mechanical ventilation on diaphragmatic function in healthy adult baboons. *Crit Care Med.* 1997;25:1187.)

TABLE 106.1 Characteristics of Types of Muscle Fibers

	Type I	Type IIa	Type IIx	Type IIb
Contractile properties				
Velocity of shortening	+	++	+++	++++
Tetanic Force	+	+	++	++
Endurance	++++	+++	++	+
Work efficiency[a]	+++	++	++	+
Histochemistry				
Mitochondrial volume density	+++	+++	++	+
ATP consumption rate	+	++	+++	++++
Oxidative enzymes	+++	+++	++	+
Glycolytic enzymes	+	++	+++	++++
Glycogen	+	++	++	+++
Capillary supply	+++	+++	++	+
Diameter	+	++	++	+++

[a]Amount of work performed per unit of adenosine triphosphate consumed.

A single myosin heavy chain isoform is typically expressed within an adult skeletal muscle fiber. Fibers classified as Type I, IIa, IIx, and IIb express myosin heavy chain isoform I (or slow), IIa, IIx, and IIb, respectively. Type IIx fibers have been reported in peripheral muscles of humans and animals and in the diaphragm of animals. Type IIx fibers have not been reported in the human diaphragm. More than one myosin heavy chain isoform is expressed in a few fibers (about 14% of adult rat diaphragm co-expresses myosin heavy chain isoforms IIb and IIx, and less than 1% co-expresses myosin heavy chain isoforms I and IIa). While the velocity of muscle contraction depends primarily on the myosin heavy chain isoform, the velocity of muscle relaxation is mainly determined by troponin C calcium binding and release, and by calcium reuptake by the sarco-endoplasmic reticulum calcium-adenosine triphosphatase (SERCA). Several SERCA isoenzymes have been identified: SERCA 1 is expressed in Type II fibers (fast calcium reuptake); and SERCA 2a is expressed in Type I (slow calcium reuptake). The density of pumping sites largely accounts for different rates of calcium uptake in fast- and slow-twitch muscle fibers. Despite this separation of tasks, velocity of contraction and velocity of relaxation tend to parallel each other; Type II fibers contract and relax with a greater velocity than Type I fibers. Slower velocity of relaxation allows fusion of repetitive twitches at lower frequencies of stimulation as compared with fast relaxations. Impairment of SERCA activity has been implicated in the development of fatigue and in disease states including heart failure and corticosteroid myopathy.

From Laghi F, Tobin MJ. Disorders of the respiratory muscles. *Am J Respir Crit Care Med.* 2003; 168:10.

muscle dysfunction. This possibility is supported by the study of Levine et al. (57), who compared costal diaphragm biopsies of 14 brain-dead organ donors maintained on controlled mechanical ventilation for 18 to 72 hours with those of eight patients ventilated for less than 2 hours during surgery to remove solitary pulmonary nodules. In this study, prolonged controlled mechanical ventilation was associated with 57% atrophy of slow fibers and 53% atrophy of fast fibers (Table 106.1) (57). Muscle fiber atrophy has also been linked to increased ubiquitin–proteasome proteolysis (58).

Considering that decreases in protein synthesis seem to contribute to ventilator-associated respiratory muscle dysfunction (58), it would seem biologically plausible that administration of anabolic factors—such as growth hormone—might be of benefit in ventilated patients. Unfortunately, when growth hormone has been administered to patients requiring prolonged mechanical ventilation, duration of mechanical ventilation was not decreased nor was muscle strength increased (59). Of concern was the report that recombinant growth hormone can increase mortality of critically ill patients (60).

Sepsis-associated Myopathy. Sepsis, a common occurrence in critically ill patients (61,62), can produce ventilatory failure by causing respiratory muscle dysfunction and increased metabolic demands (18). Septic animals develop failure of neuromuscular transmission due to increased sarcolemmal electric potential, and failure of excitation–contraction coupling (18). Mechanisms responsible for failure of excitation–contraction coupling include the cytotoxic effect of free radicals (62), ubiquitin–proteasome proteolysis, the cytotoxic

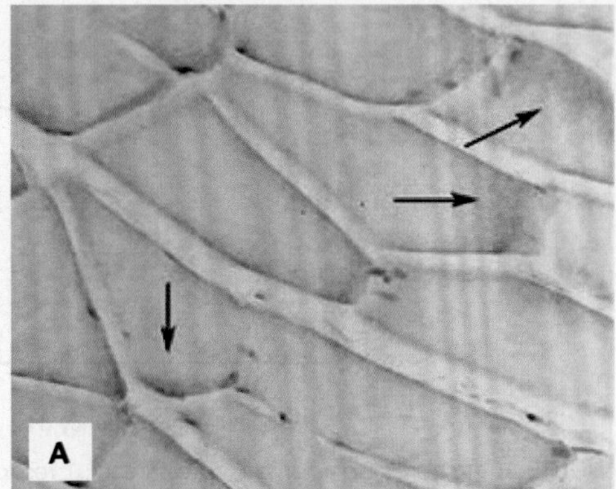

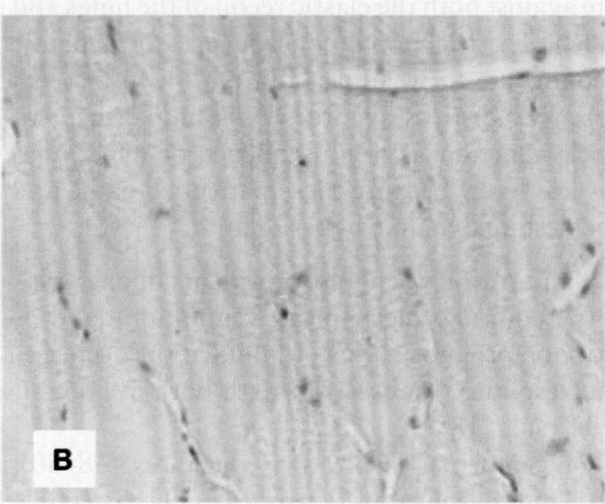

FIGURE 106.10 (A) A sample of gastrocnemius muscle obtained from an adult Sprague–Dawley rat injected 12 hours earlier with *E. coli* endotoxin (20 mg/kg). The section was stained with an antibody to inducible nitric oxide synthase. Positive staining (*brown coloration, arrows*) is evident inside the fibers. (B) A sample of gastrocnemius muscle obtained from a rat injected 12 hours earlier with normal saline. No positive staining is evident. (From Laghi F, Tobin MJ. Disorders of the respiratory muscles. *Am J Respir Crit Care Med.* 2003;168:10. Photomicrographs provided by Dr. Sabah N. Hussain, Royal Victoria Hospital, Montreal, Canada.)

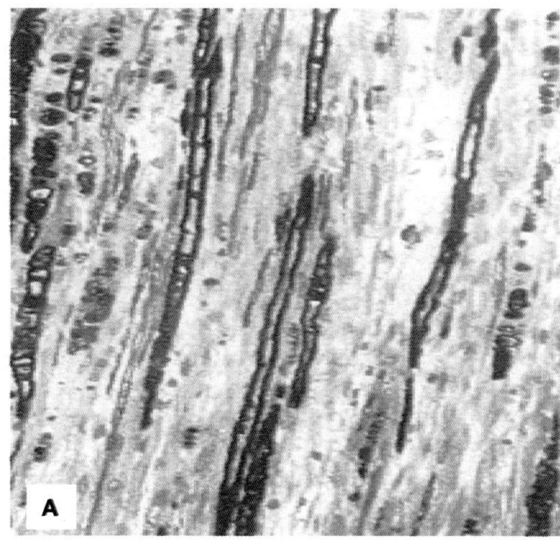
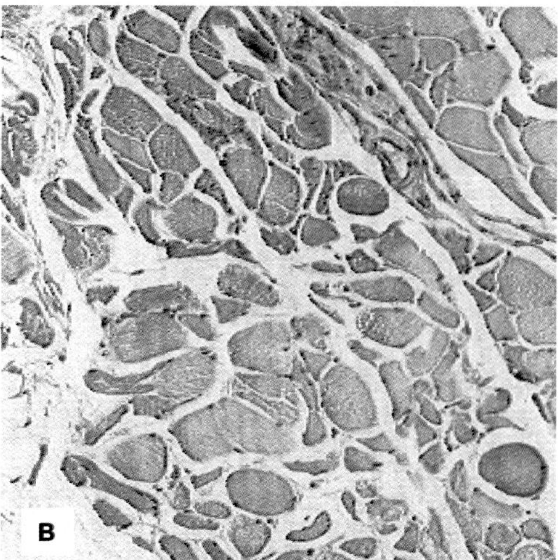

FIGURE 106.11 Transverse section of a peripheral motor nerve (deep peroneal nerve, **A**) and of a skeletal muscle (intercostal, **B**) in patients who developed profound weakness following a prolonged hospital course characterized by sepsis, multiple organ failure syndrome, and inability to wean from mechanical ventilation. **A**: The long, thin dark structures seen in the left panel are myelin sheaths that contain axons. The axons are degenerating and dying; following death, they disintegrate. The myelin surrounding the disintegrating axons collapses around the axonal debris to form *ovoids of myelin*, seen better on the lateral portions. **B**: Amid muscle fibers that are normal in size and shape there are atrophic ones that appear small and that have developed contours with acute angles. These findings are consistent with denervation atrophy secondary to axonal degeneration, so called critical illness polyneuropathy. (From Zochodne DW, Bolton CF, Wells GA, et al. Critical illness polyneuropathy: a complication of sepsis and multiple organ failure. *Brain.* 1987;110:819.)

effect of nitric oxide (Fig. 106.10) and its metabolites, and a decrease in mitochondrial content with associated reduction in energy-rich phosphates (62,63).

ICU-acquired Paresis. While cared for in the ICU, critically ill patients can develop muscle weakness and, occasionally, paralysis. Some of these patients have evidence of axonal degeneration and denervation atrophy (Fig. 106.11) (18). This constellation of findings is known as critical illness polyneuropathy (Table 106.2). Sensory involvement is usually more limited than motor involvement. Critical illness polyneuropathy has been considered one of the manifestations of multiple organ failure syndrome. Sepsis and multiple organ failure, though, are not essential prerequisites for the development of critical illness polyneuropathy (18). Tight control of hyperglycemia may reduce the risk of polyneuropathy and the duration of mechanical ventilation (64). It has been speculated that the known neurotoxic effects of hyperglycemia play a role in the development of critical illness polyneuropathy, and that the anti-inflammatory and neuroprotective effects of insulin contribute to the protective effects of tight hyperglycemic control (65). The administration of corticosteroids has not been linked with an increased risk of developing critical illness polyneuropathy (66,67).

In some ICU patients with muscle weakness or paralysis, there is evidence of isolated myopathy (critical illness myopathy) rather than axonopathy (18). Patients developing isolated myopathy often have been treated with steroids

TABLE 106.2 Electromyographic Findings

	Axonal Injury	Myelin Injury	Neuromuscular Conduction Defect	Myopathy
Compound muscle action potential (amplitude)[a]	Reduced	Normal to slightly reduced	Normal[b]	Normal
Sensory nerve action potential (amplitude)[c]	Reduced	Normal to reduced	Normal	Normal
Conduction velocity	Normal to slightly reduced	Reduced	Normal	Normal
Spontaneous muscle depolarization[d]	Present	Absent	Absent	None to present
Amplitude of compound muscle action potential with stimulation at 3 Hz[e]	Unchanged	Unchanged	Decreased	Unchanged
Motor unit activation	Decreased	Decreased	Normal	Increased

Although features of myopathy can be recorded by electromyographic studies, electromyography cannot always distinguish critical illness myopathy from critical illness polyneuropathy, and muscle biopsies may be needed.

Examples of injuries and deficits: axonal injury, critical illness myopathy; myelin injury, Guillain-Barré; neuromuscular conduction defect, myasthenia, prolonged neuromuscular blockade; myopathy, critical illness myopathy.

[a]Elicited by motor nerve stimulation.

[b]Decreased in the Lambert–Eaton syndrome.

[c]Elicited by sensory nerve stimulation.

[d]Spontaneous muscle depolarization (caused by denervation) is detected by presence of fibrillation potentials and positive sharp waves.

[e]Repetitive nerve stimulation is performed to exclude neuromuscular transmission defects such as prolonged neuromuscular paralysis.

From Laghi F, Tobin MJ. Disorders of the respiratory muscles. *Am J Respir Crit Care Med.* 2003;168:10.

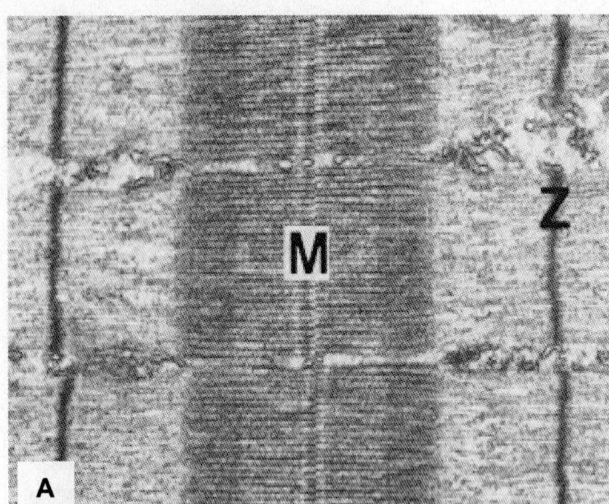

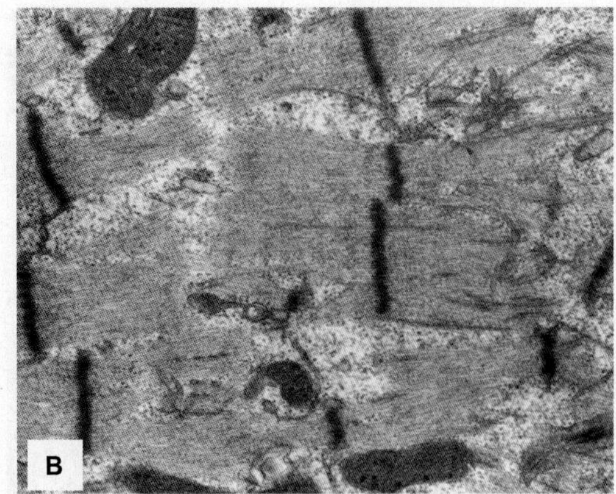

FIGURE 106.12 Electron micrographs of normal skeletal muscle (A) and skeletal muscle from a patient who received steroids and the neuromuscular blocking agent vecuronium during a hospitalization with status asthmaticus followed by flaccid quadriplegia (B). Compared with the normal structure, the patient developed extensive loss of thick (myosin) myofilaments and relative preservation of thin (actin) filaments. Muscle strength returned to normal 2 months after discontinuation of vecuronium. M, M-line formed by myosin filaments and M-line proteins; Z, Z-disk formed by a lattice of filaments that join the actin filaments of one sarcomere with the actin filaments of the adjacent sarcomere. (A: From Eisenberg BR. In: Bradley WG, Gardner-Medwin D, Walton JN, eds. *Recent Advances in Myology.* Amsterdam: Excerpta Medica; 1975; B: From Danon MJ, Carpenter S. Myopathy with thick filament (myosin) loss following prolonged paralysis with vecuronium during steroid treatment. *Muscle Nerve.* 1991;14:1131.)

and neuromuscular blocking agents (e.g., patients with status asthmaticus) (18). Muscle biopsies demonstrate a general decrease in myofibrillar protein content and a selective loss of thick filaments (myosin) within Type I and Type II fibers (Fig. 106.12). Subtypes of critical illness myopathy, including rhabdomyolysis and frank myonecrosis, have been occasionally reported (Fig. 106.13) (65,68). Experimental data in laboratory animals (69) and in critically ill patients suggest that critical illness myopathy may result from several coexisting processes including a decrease in mRNA substrates for actin and myosin due to pretranslational defects (69), decrease in myosin mRNA (70), induction of myofiber-specific ubiquitin/proteasome pathways (71), and local immune activation (72).

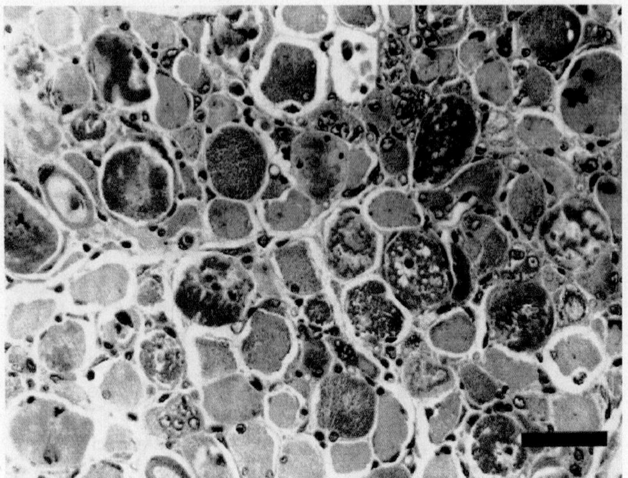

FIGURE 106.13 Transverse section of a peripheral skeletal muscle (rectus femoris) in a patient with necrotizing myopathy of the critically ill. Several muscle fibers demonstrate an obvious panfascicular destructive process. The destructive process is associated with myophagocytosis and small, regenerating muscle fibers that contain groups of vesicular nuclei and prominent nucleoli. Bar, 50 µm. (From Ramsay DA, Zochodne DW, Robertson DM, et al. A syndrome of acute severe muscle necrosis in intensive care unit patients. *J Neuropathol Exp Neurol.* 1993;52:387.)

In recent years, it has become increasingly apparent that critical illness neuropathy and myopathy often coexist (66,73–75). It has become common to refer to patients who become weak while in the ICU, as a result of acquired neuropathy and/or myopathy, as simply having critical illness neuromyopathy or, more simply, ICU-acquired paresis (73–75). ICU-acquired paresis has been reported to be an independent risk factor of prolonged weaning (75,76) and to be associated with respiratory muscle weakness (77,78).

Acid–Base Disorders. Alkalosis, either metabolic or respiratory, does not affect skeletal muscle strength (79) and may improve endurance (80). Whether acidosis, either metabolic or respiratory, impairs respiratory muscle function remains controversial (15).

Electrolyte Disturbances. Respiratory muscle function may be impaired by decreased levels of phosphate, calcium, magnesium, and potassium (18).

Medications. Weakness can result from medications that have a direct myotoxic effect, such as blockade of myocyte glycoprotein synthesis and electron transport caused by statins (inhibitors of the hydroxy-methylglutaryl coenzyme A reductase) used in patients with hyperlipidemia or nucleoside analogues used in patients with human immunodeficiency virus (18). Weakness can also result with neuromuscular blocking agents and aminoglycosides, which interfere with neuromuscular transmission (18).

In acutely ventilated patients, paralysis (including the respiratory muscles) can persist after discontinuation of neuromuscular blocking agents (81–83). Recovery from prolonged neuromuscular blockade is usually reported to begin within 2 days of the last dose of neuromuscular blocking agents (81,82). This contrasts with the prolonged course of critical illness myopathy or neuropathy (70,84). It is thus unlikely, if not impossible, for prolonged neuromuscular blockade to cause long-term ventilator dependence (85). Dose adjustment of neuromuscular blocking agents based on frequent monitoring of peripheral muscle responsiveness (Table 106.2) may permit faster recovery of neuromuscular function and spontaneous respiration (83). Treatment consists primarily of waiting for clearance of the neuromuscular blocking agents or their metabolites (65). Reversal of neuromuscular blockade with a cholinesterase has been used to establish a diagnosis. However, in the presence of high concentrations of neuromuscular blocking agents—or their metabolites—recovery is usually incomplete or transitory (65).

Limitations in the Current Classification of Respiratory Muscle Weakness

When studying respiratory muscle weakness leading to weaning failure, it is necessary to bear in mind the current limited understanding of these conditions. First, the distinction between pre-existing conditions and new-onset conditions can be arbitrary. Second, conditions which are pre-existing—such as malnutrition and hyperinflation—can worsen during the course of an unrelated critical illness. Third, the nosology is often unsatisfactory—consider the nebulous distinction between ICU-acquired paresis and sepsis-associated myopathy, or between ICU-acquired paresis and ventilator-associated respiratory muscle dysfunction. Fourth, conditions in which respiratory muscle weakness is associated with muscle damage can also display some degree of muscle atrophy—consider diaphragmatic atrophy in cases of ventilator-associated respiratory muscle dysfunction. Fifth, there is limited laboratory specificity to differentiate the various conditions causing weakness in the ICU. Sixth, in any given patient, more than one mechanism may be responsible for respiratory muscle weakness. Lastly, respiratory muscle weakness can be combined with a depressed drive—for example, in the setting of hypercapnia-induced hypoventilation (18).

Respiratory Muscle Fatigue

Contractile fatigue occurs when a sufficiently large respiratory load is applied over a sufficiently long period (86–88). Contractile fatigue can be short-lasting or long-lasting (Fig. 106.14). Short-lasting fatigue results from accumulation of inorganic phosphate, failure of the membrane electrical potential to propagate beyond T-tubules and, to a much lesser extent, intramuscular acidosis (18). Short-lasting fatigue appears to have a protective function because it can prevent injury to the sarcolemma caused by forceful muscle contractions (18). Long-lasting fatigue is consistent with the development of, and recovery from, muscle injury (Fig. 106.15) (18). Several mechanisms may contribute to muscle injury. These include activation of calpain (a calcium-dependent nonlysosomal protease), increased muscle temperature, and excessive production of reactive oxygen species (18). Muscle injury can also be caused by eccentric contractions, in other words, contraction of a muscle, while it is stretched by external forces (18). Eccentric contractions can occur during ineffective inspiratory

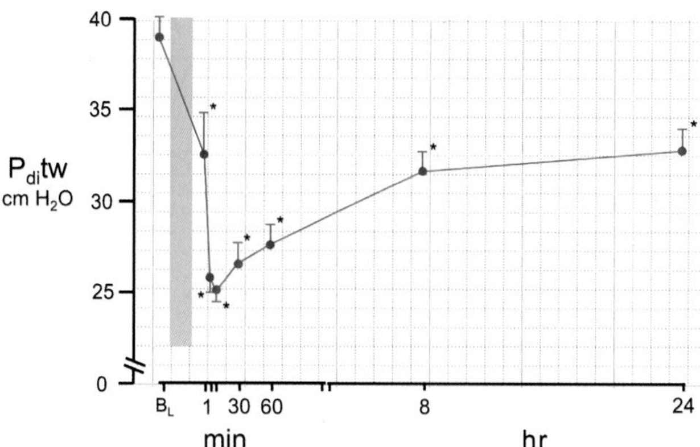

FIGURE 106.14 Induction of diaphragmatic fatigue (*stippled bar*) produced a significant fall in transdiaphragmatic pressure elicited by twitch stimulation of phrenic nerves ($P_{di}tw$). Significant recovery of twitch pressure was noted in the first 8 hours after completion of the fatigue protocol; no further change was observed between 8 and 24 hours, and the 24-hour value was significantly lower than baseline. The delay in reaching the nadir of twitch transdiaphragmatic pressure probably results from twitch potentiation, induced by repeated contractions, which was present at the end of the protocol. Values are mean ± SE. *Significant difference compared with baseline value, $p <$ 0.01. (Adapted from Laghi F, D'Alfonso N, Tobin MJ. Pattern of recovery from diaphragmatic fatigue over 24 hours. *J Appl Physiol.* 1995;79:539.)

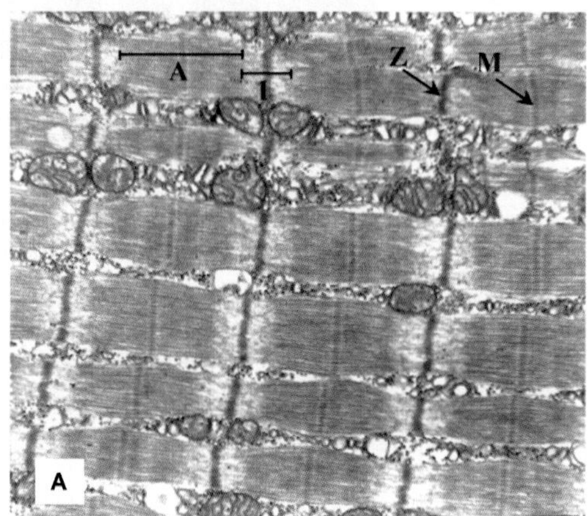

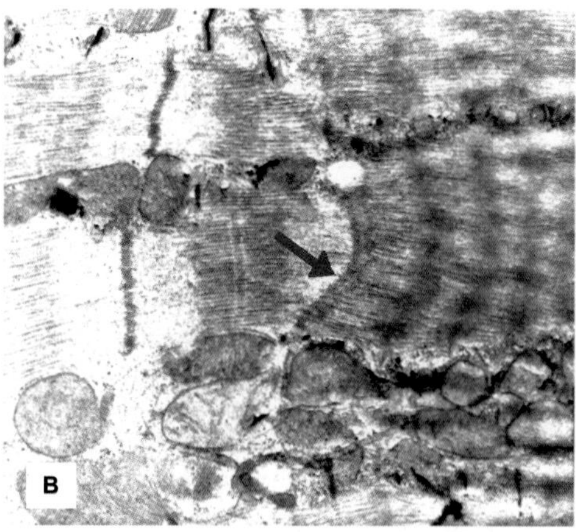

FIGURE 106.15 Electron micrographs of longitudinal sections from the costal diaphragm of a healthy control hamster (A) and a hamster exposed to 6 days of resistive loading (B). **A**: Normal sarcomeres with distinct A-bands, I-bands, Z-bands, and M-lines that are aligned between adjacent myofibrils. **B**: Load-induced damage recognizable by Z-band streaming (*arrow*) and disruption of sarcomeric structure (**right section**) with loss of distinct A-bands and I-bands. Z-band streaming is attributed to a loss of cytoskeletal protein elements such as desmin, alpha-actinin, and vimentin (magnification 16,500x for both micrographs). (From Laghi F, Tobin MJ. Disorders of the respiratory muscles. *Am J Respir Crit Care Med.* 2003;168:10. Electron micrographs provided by Drs. David C. Walker and Darlene W. Reid, University of British Columbia, Vancouver, Canada.)

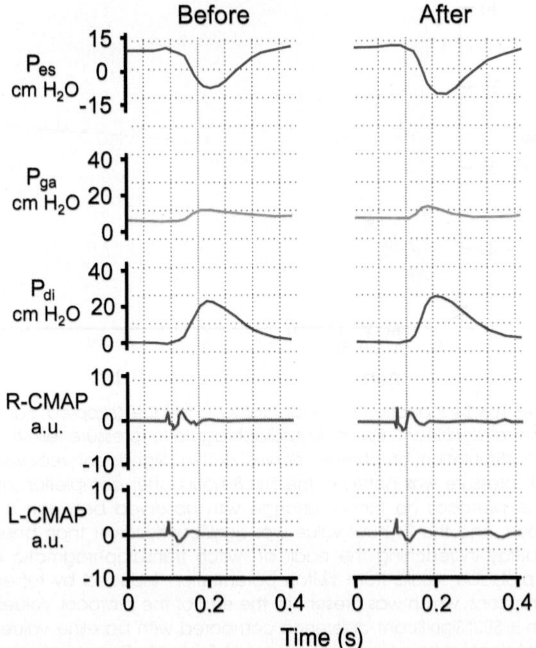

FIGURE 106.16 Esophageal pressure (P_{es}), gastric pressure (P_{ga}), transdiaphragmatic pressure (P_{di}), and compound motor action potentials (CAMP) of the right and left hemidiaphragms after phrenic nerve stimulation before and after a failed trial of weaning. The end-expiratory value of P_{es} and the amplitude of the right and left CAMPs were the same before and after the trial, indicating that the stimulations were delivered at the same lung volume and that the stimulations achieved the same extent of diaphragmatic recruitment. The amplitude of twitch P_{di} elicited by phrenic nerve stimulation was the same before and after weaning. (From Laghi F, Cattapan SE, Jubran A, et al. Is weaning failure caused by low-frequency fatigue of the diaphragm? *Am J Respir Crit Care Med.* 2003;167:120.)

efforts, which have been associated with worse weaning outcome both in the acute (89) and chronic settings (90), and with ventilator dependence (16,90).

Whether critically ill patients develop short-lasting or long-lasting contractile fatigue of the respiratory muscles has long been debated. Patients who fail a trial of weaning from mechanical ventilation are at particular risk of developing fatigue because they experience marked increases in respiratory load (14,16,24). The addition of a new injury to the respiratory muscles secondary to the development of contractile fatigue might be the ultimate determinant of whether or not some patients are ever successfully weaned.

Laghi et al. (24) measured the contractile response of the diaphragm to phrenic nerve stimulation in nine patients who failed a weaning trial; seven patients who were successfully weaned served as control subjects. The weaning failure patients experienced a greater respiratory load. Moreover, the *tension-time index*[1] of the diaphragm—an index of the ability of the diaphragm to sustain a given inspiratory load—was greater in the failure group than in the success group ($p = 0.01$). Nevertheless, not a single patient developed a decrease in transdiaphragmatic twitch pressure elicited by phrenic nerve stimulation (Fig. 106.16). The failure to develop fatigue is surprising because seven of the nine weaning failure patients had a tension-time index above 0.15, the putative threshold for task failure and fatigue.

The increase in tension-time index over the course of the weaning trial and predicted time to task failure are shown in Figure 106.17. At the point that the physician reinstituted mechanical ventilation, patients were predicted to be an average of 13 minutes away from task failure. In other words, patients display clinical manifestations of severe respiratory distress for a substantial time before they develop fatigue. In an intensive care setting, these clinical signs will lead attendants to reinstitute mechanical ventilation before fatigue has time to develop.

Impaired Cardiovascular Performance

Spontaneous respiratory efforts decrease intrathoracic pressure, and thus increase the pressure gradient for systemic venous return (91). In addition, decreases in intrathoracic pressure raise the left ventricular afterload, causing additional stress on the left ventricle (91). In patients with coronary artery disease, the increased stress can alter myocardial perfusion and cause transient left ventricular dilation (92).

The occurrence of myocardial ischemia during periods of spontaneous respiration has been associated with a greater risk of weaning failure (93) and greater risk of ventilator dependence (94). A proximal mechanism likely responsible for ventilator dependence in patients with myocardial ischemia

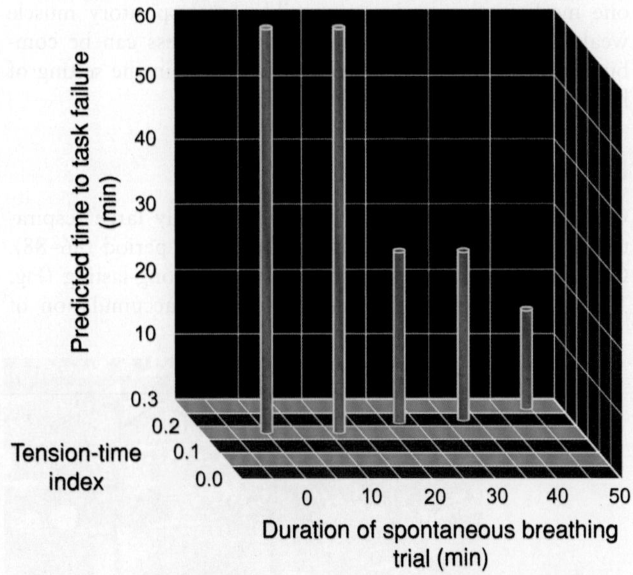

FIGURE 106.17 The interrelationship between the duration of a spontaneous breathing trial, tension-time index of the diaphragm, and predicted time to task failure in nine patients who failed a trial of weaning from mechanical ventilation. The patients breathed spontaneously for an average of 44 minutes before a physician terminated the trial. At the start of the trial, tension-time index was 0.17, and the formula of Bellemare and Grassino (285) predicted that patients could sustain spontaneous breathing for another 59 minutes before developing task failure. As the trial progressed, tension-time index increased and predicted time to the development of task failure decreased. At the end of the trial, tension-time index reached 0.26; that patients were predicted to sustain spontaneous breathing for another 13 minutes before developing task failure clarifies why patients did not develop a decrease in diaphragmatic twitch pressure. In other words, physicians interrupted the trial based on clinical manifestations of respiratory distress before patients had sufficient time to develop contractile fatigue. (From Laghi F, Tobin MJ. Disorders of the respiratory muscles. *Am J Respir Crit Care Med.* 2003;168:10.)

[1] The tension-time index of the diaphragm (TT_{di}) is calculated by multiplying two ratios: the respiratory duty cycle (T_i/T_{tot}), i.e., inspiratory time divided by the time of a total respiratory cycle, and the mean transdiaphragmatic inspiratory pressure per breath divided by the maximum transdiaphragmatic inspiratory pressure (P_{di}/P_{dimax}).

(94) and in patients with impaired left ventricular function (95) is the increase in transmural pulmonary artery occlusion pressure during spontaneous respiration (96). Mechanisms by which increases in transmural pulmonary artery occlusion pressure could contribute to weaning failure include worsening pulmonary mechanics and decreased gas exchange (91).

In the acute setting, oxygen consumption at the completion of a weaning trial is equivalent in weaning-success and weaning-failure patients (97). The manner in which the cardiovascular system meets oxygen demands, however, differs between the two groups. In weaning successes, oxygen transport increases, mainly resulting from an increase in cardiac index; in weaning failures, the increase in demand is met by an increase in oxygen extraction, resulting in a decrease in mixed venous oxygen saturation (Fig. 106.18). A decrease in mixed venous oxygen saturation is consistent with a failing cardiovascular response to an increased metabolic demand (91).

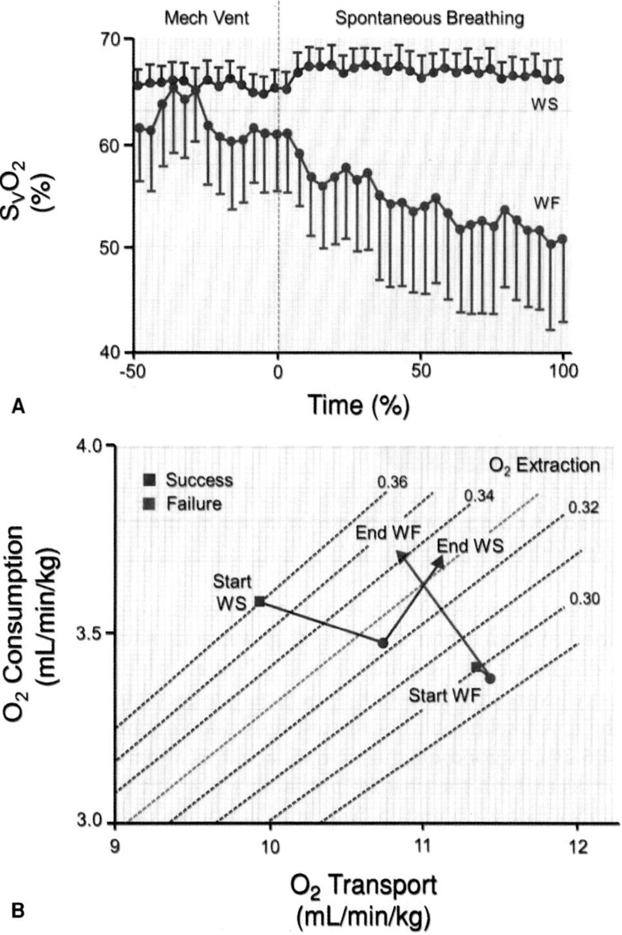

FIGURE 106.18 A: Mixed venous oxygen saturation (SvO_2) during mechanical ventilation and a trial of spontaneous breathing in eleven weaning success patients (WS, *blue symbols*) and in eight weaning failure patients (WF, *red symbols*). During mechanical ventilation, SvO_2 was similar in the two groups ($p = 0.28$). Between the onset (*dashed line*) and the end of the trial, SvO_2 decreased in the failure group ($p < 0.01$) whereas it remained unchanged in the success group ($p = 0.48$). Over the course of the trial, SvO_2 was lower in the failure group than in the success group ($p < 0.02$). Bars = SE. **B**: Oxygen transport, oxygen consumption, and isopleths of oxygen extraction ratio in the success (WS, *blue symbols*) and failure (WF, *red symbols*) groups during mechanical ventilation (*squares*) and at the onset (*circles*) and end (*triangles*) of a spontaneous breathing trial. See text for details. (Adapted from Jubran A, Mathru M, Dries D, et al. Continuous recordings of mixed venous oxygen saturation during weaning from mechanical ventilation and the ramifications thereof. *Am J Respir Crit Care Med.* 1998;158:1763.)

High variability in hemodynamic response during failure to wean has been reported by Zakynthinos et al. (31). It is unclear whether the absent interaction between weaning failure and oxygen consumption in some of the patients studied by Zakynthinos et al. (31) was due to depression of the respiratory centers, limited capacity to extract oxygen, or limited cardiac reserve (98), including diastolic dysfunction (99).

Psychological Factors

Patients who require mechanical ventilation are commonly affected by psychological problems such as anxiety, agitation, delirium, depression, apathy, and posttraumatic stress disorder (PTSD) (100). Overall 50% to 80% of patients receiving mechanical ventilation in adult ICUs develop delirium at some point during the ICU stay (101–103). In these patients, delirium has been associated with greater likelihood of discharge to a nursing home or long-term care facility and with increased mortality at 1 year (103). As with the high prevalence of delirium, PTSD has also been reported to be very common in acutely and chronically ventilated patients (104,105). Duration of mechanical ventilation, use of sedative agents, and presence and severity of PTSD appear causally linked, and may influence duration of mechanical ventilation and psychological function after discharge (106). Finally, in patients with prolonged respiratory failure, the rate of weaning failure and death is higher in patients with anxiety or depression than in those without such disorders (107).

Possible mechanisms for psychological dysfunction in mechanically ventilated patients include respiratory discomfort, severity of illness, medication side effects, sleep deprivation, and sensory deprivation (Fig. 106.19) (104,108–111). The delivery of mechanical ventilation itself can cause psychological dysfunction (106,109). Mechanical ventilation limits mobility, fosters isolation, impairs communication, and interferes with or blocks patient control over the act of breathing. Anxiety and depression can decrease motivation, interfere with performing simple tasks, and decrease self-esteem (106).

PREDICTION OF WEANING OUTCOME

Research on prediction of weaning outcome employs the tools of medical decision analysis (2). Therefore, before discussing weaning-predictor tests, it is useful to review the principles of medical decision analysis.

Medical Decision Analysis

Diagnostic tests are designed to screen for a condition and to confirm the condition. The characteristics of screening tests and confirmatory tests differ, and only rarely will a single diagnostic test fulfill both functions (112).

The primary goal of weaning-predictor tests is screening (2). A good weaning-predictor test, like any good screening test, should miss no patient who has the condition under consideration—i.e., to be ready for a weaning trial. This means that a good weaning-predictor test must have a low

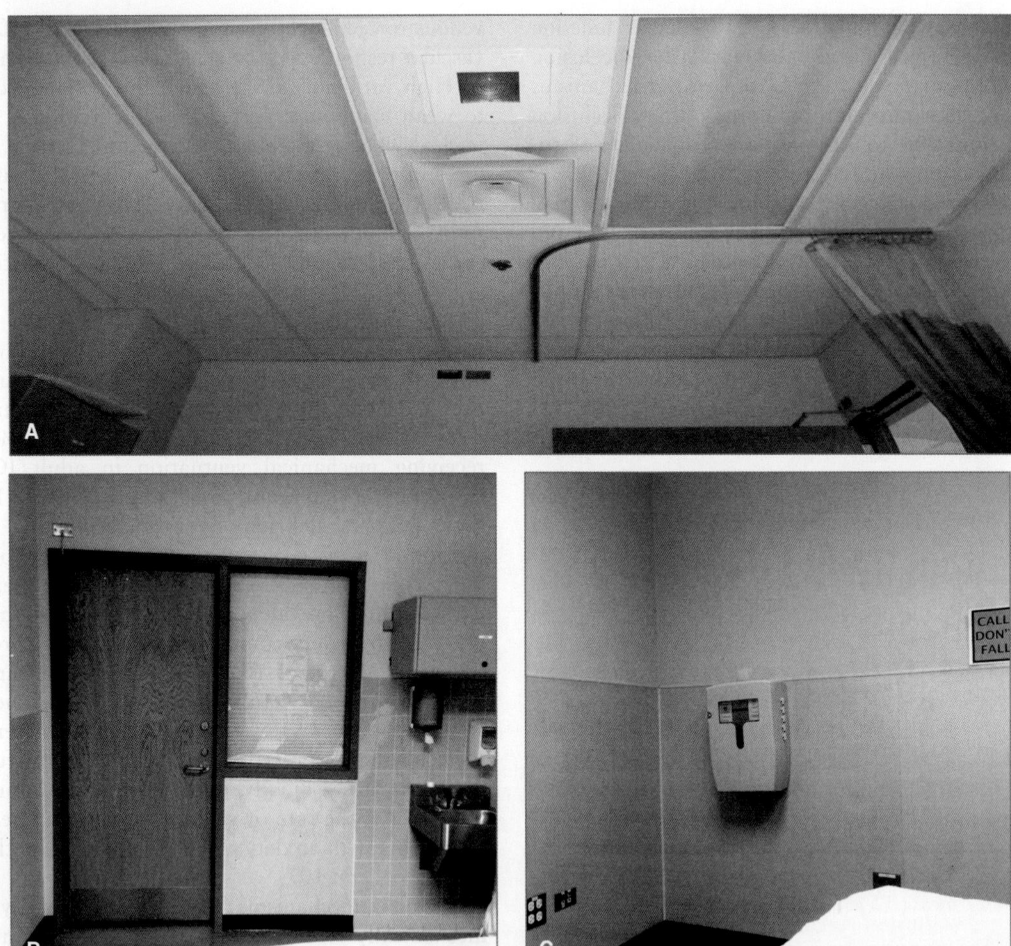

FIGURE 106.19 The environment where ventilated patients are being cared for can promote sensory deprivation through the lack of windows with a view (B), bare walls (C), and tedious ceiling (A). (From Shaikh H, Morales D, Laghi F. Weaning from mechanical ventilation. *Semin Respir Crit Care Med.* 2014;35(4):451–468.)

rate of false-negative results—high sensitivity (Fig. 106.20) (112,113). A high rate of false-positive results (low specificity) is acceptable (112,113).

The process of weaning entails measurement of weaning predictors, a trial of weaning, and a trial of extubation (see Fig. 106.1) (2). Each step in this sequence is a diagnostic test. Measurements of weaning predictors (screening tests) are used to diagnose readiness for a weaning trial. The trial of weaning (confirmatory test of the screening tests) itself is used to screen for readiness to extubate. Extubation (confirmatory test of the weaning trial) is used to diagnose/screen for readiness to maintain spontaneous respiration. To apply diagnostic tests (screening or confirmatory) in sequence introduces critical confounders in the interpretation of studies designed to assess the reliability of a pre-existing predictor test. These confounders are spectrum bias, test-referral bias, and base-rate fallacy (114). In the case of weaning, *spectrum bias* arises when the study population in a new investigation contains more (or fewer) sick patients than the population in which the diagnostic test was first developed (112). *Test-referral bias* arises when the results of the weaning-predictor test being assessed are used to choose patients for a reference-standard test—i.e., passing a weaning trial that leads to extubation (114). *Base-rate fallacy* occurs when physicians fail to take into account the pretest probability of the disorder (114).

Pre-test probability is a physician's estimate of the likelihood of a particular condition (e.g. weaning outcome) before a diagnostic test is undertaken (2). Posttest probability, typically expressed as positive- or negative-predictive value, is the new likelihood after the test results are obtained (see Fig. 106.20). A good diagnostic tests achieves a marked increase or decrease in the posttest probability over the pretest probability. For every test in every medical subspecialty, the magnitude of change between pre-test probability and posttest probability is determined by Bayes' theorem (114). Three factors alone determine the magnitude of the pre- to posttest change: sensitivity, specificity, and pre-test probability. It is commonly assumed that sensitivity and specificity remain constant for a test. In truth, test-referral bias, a common occurrence in studies of weaning tests, leads to major changes in sensitivity and specificity (112). Likewise, major changes in pretest probability arise as a consequence of spectrum bias (112). All of these factors need to be carefully considered when reading a study that evaluates the reliability of a weaning-predictor test.

Weaning-Predictor Tests

Several weaning-predictor tests have been proposed and studied over the years. These tests include measurements

		Gold Standard Success	Gold Standard Fail
Test (f/V_T)	Positive (≤100)	TP	FP
	Negative (>100)	FN	TN

TP = Test predicts weaning success and patient actually succeeds
TN = Test predicts weaning failure and patient actually fails
FP = Test predicts weaning success and patient actually fails
FN = Test predicts weaning failure and patient actually succeeds

$$\text{Sensitivity} = \frac{TP}{TP + FN} = TPR = [1 - FNR]$$

$$\text{Specificity} = \frac{TN}{TN + FP} = TNR = [1 - FPR]$$

$$PPV = \frac{TP}{TP + FP}$$

$$NPV = \frac{TN}{TN + FN}$$

FN Rate = 1 - Sensitivity

FP Rate = 1 - Specificity

Likelihood ratio for a positive test = TPR / FPR = sensitivity / (1 - specificity)

Likelihood ratio for a negative test = FNR / TNR = (1 – sensitivity) / specificity

Prevalence = TP + FN / (TP + TN + FP + FN)

Diagnostic accuracy = [TP + TN] / [TP + TN + FP + FN]

FIGURE 106.20 A 2 × 2 tabular display of the characteristics of diagnostic tests. The vertical columns represent the results of the gold standard test. The horizontal rows represent the results of the index test. Readings of $f/V_t \leq 100$ are classified as positive test results and readings >100 are classified as negative test results. The relationship of these binary results to the outcome of a T-tube weaning trial forms a decision matrix that has four possible combinations. (From Tobin MJ, Jubran A. Weaning from mechanical ventilation. In: Tobin MJ, ed. *Principles and Practice of Mechanical Ventilation.* New York, NY: McGraw-Hill; 2006:1185.)

of breathing pattern, pulmonary gas exchange, and muscle strength. To this list we must add new approaches such as echocardiography, measurements of B-type natriuretic peptide levels, diaphragm ultrasonography, and esophageal pressure monitoring. The goal of any weaning-predictor test is to safely speed up the weaning process (2).

Respiratory Frequency-to-Tidal Volume Ratio (f/V_t)

The ratio of respiratory frequency to tidal volume (f/V_t)[2] is measured during 1 minute of spontaneous breathing (5). The higher the f/V_t ratio, the more severe the rapid shallow breathing and the greater the likelihood of unsuccessful weaning. An f/V_t ratio of 100 best discriminates between successful and unsuccessful attempts at weaning (Fig. 106.21) (5).

The f/V_t can be recorded with a handheld spirometer after disconnecting the patient's endotracheal tube from the ventilator circuit (Fig. 106.22) (5). The f/V_t can be also recorded with the use of the pneumotachograph within the ventilator as long as the patient is in the "flow-by" mode and PEEP, pressure

[2]For example, for a spontaneous respiratory rate of 24 breaths/min, and a spontaneous tidal volume of 600 mL (0.6 L), the $f/V_t = 24/0.6 = 40$.

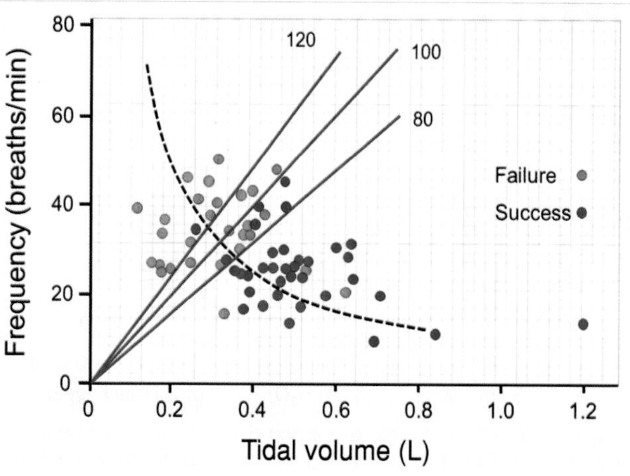

FIGURE 106.21 Isopleths for the ratio of respiratory frequency to tidal volume (f/V_t) recorded reported by Yang and Tobin in clinically stable patients considered ready to undergo a weaning trial by their primary physicians. The isopleths represent different degrees of rapid shallow breathing. For the patients indicated by the points to the left of the isopleth representing 100 breath/min/L, the likelihood that a weaning trial would fail was 95%, whereas for the patients indicated by the points to the right of this isopleth, the likelihood of a successful weaning outcome was 80%. The hyperbola represents a minute ventilation of 10 L/min, a criterion commonly used to predict weaning outcome; this criterion was of little value in discriminating between the successfully weaned patients (*blue circles*) and the patients in whom weaning failed (*red circles*). (Adapted from Yang KL, Tobin MJ. A prospective study of indexes predicting the outcome of trials of weaning from mechanical ventilation. *N Engl J Med.* 1991;324:1445–1450.)

support and continuous positive airway pressure (CPAP) are all set at zero (115). If present, tube compensation must be set at the lowest possible compensatory parameter or, if possible, it should be turned off. These steps are necessary to avoid the inaccurate prediction of weaning outcome. For instance,

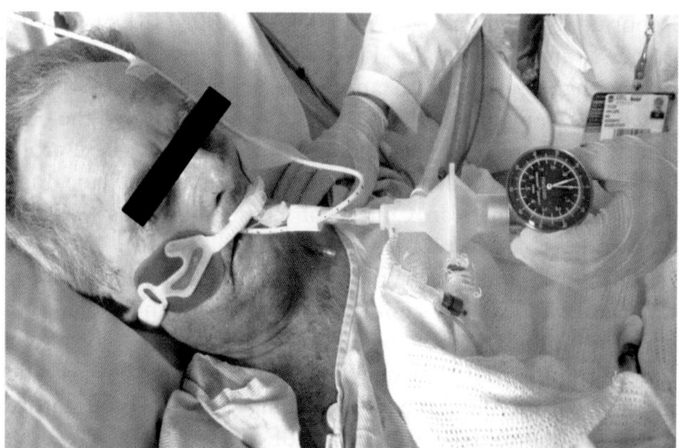

FIGURE 106.22 Technique to record of frequency over tidal volume ratio (f/V_t) with a handheld spirometer. The endotracheal tube is disconnected from the ventilator. A handheld spirometer connected to a filter is attached to the end of the endotracheal tube. When recording f/V_t it is important that the patient's breathing pattern achieves equilibrium before starting the measurement as mechanical ventilation can depress respiratory motor output and, thus, apneic pauses and shallow breaths can occur during the first minute after disconnecting a patient from the ventilator. To avoid this pitfall the clinician must wait until the patient has established a regular respiratory rhythm, a process that can take about one minute. When regular respiratory rhythm has been established the clinician will be able to measure f/V_t over the subsequent minute. (From Shaikh H, Morales D, Laghi F. Weaning from mechanical ventilation. *Semin Respir Crit Care Med.* 2014;35(4):451–468.)

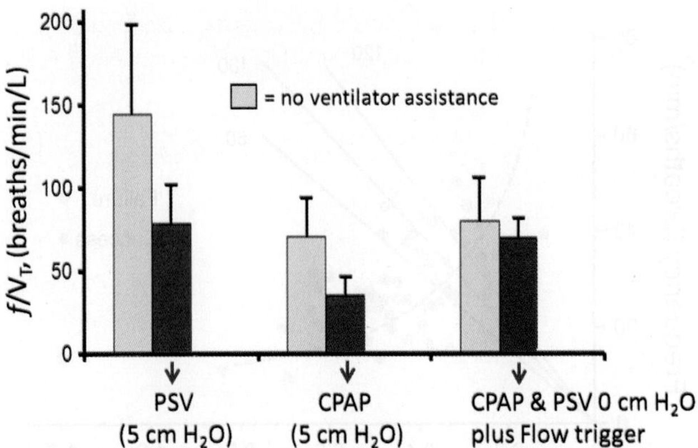

FIGURE 106.23 Effect of pressure support (PSV), continuous positive airway pressure (CPAP), and flow trigger on frequency-to-tidal volume ratio (f/V_t). **Left**: In 21 patients with COPD, f/V_t recorded with a handheld spirometer while patients received no ventilator assistance was 145 ± 121 (standard deviation (SD)); the addition of pressure support 5 cm H_2O caused f/V_t to decrease to 79 ± 53 (45% decrease) (280–282). **Center**: In 33 postoperative patients, the f/V_t recorded with a handheld spirometer while patients received no ventilator assistance was 71 ± 23 (SD); the addition of CPAP 5 cm H_2O caused f/V_t to decrease to 36 ± 14 (49% decrease) (283). **Right**: In 80 patients cared for in a medical ICU, f/V_t recorded with a handheld spirometer while patients received no ventilator assistance was 80 ± 30 (SD). The corresponding value of f/V_t recorded while patients were connected to the ventilator with CPAP and PSV both set at 0 cm H_2O plus flow trigger decreased to 70 ± 26 (12% decrease) (284). (From Shaikh H, Morales D, Laghi F. Weaning from mechanical ventilation. *Semin Respir Crit Care Med.* 2014;35(4):451–468.)

the use of pressure-support ventilation of 5 or 10 cm H_2O decreased f/V_t by 20% to 80% as compared to unassisted breathing (Fig. 106.23) (17). The use of CPAP of 5 cm H_2O decreases the f/V_t by 20% to 50% as compared to unassisted breathing (17).

The initial evaluation of f/V_t was reported in 1991 (5). Since then, this test has been evaluated in more than 25 studies. Reported sensitivity ranges from 0.35 to 1.00 (114). Specificity ranges from 0.00 to 0.89 (114). At the first glance, this wide scatter suggests that f/V_t is an unreliable predictor of weaning outcome. Many of the investigators, however, ignored the possibility of test-referral bias and spectrum bias (2). These problems were compounded by an Evidence-Based Medicine Task Force of the American College of Chest Physicians (ACCP), who undertook a meta-analysis of the studies (116).

The Task Force calculated pooled likelihood ratios for f/V_t, and judged the summated values to signify that f/V_t was not a reliable predictor of weaning success. Accordingly, they recommended that clinicians should start the weaning process with a spontaneous breathing trial (a confirmatory test), and the initial few minutes of the trial as a screening test (116,117). This recommendation, however, is untenable because the studies included in the meta-analysis exhibited significant heterogeneity in pretest probability of successful outcome (114). Such marked heterogeneity prohibits the undertaking of a reliable meta-analysis (118,119). When data from the studies included in the meta-analysis were entered into a Bayesian model with pretest probability as the operating point, the reported positive-predictive and negative-predictive values were significantly correlated with the values predicted by the original report (5) of f/V_t—i.e., $r = 0.86$ ($p < 0.0001$) and, $r = -0.82$ ($p < 0.0001$), respectively (Figs. 106.24 and 106.25) (114).

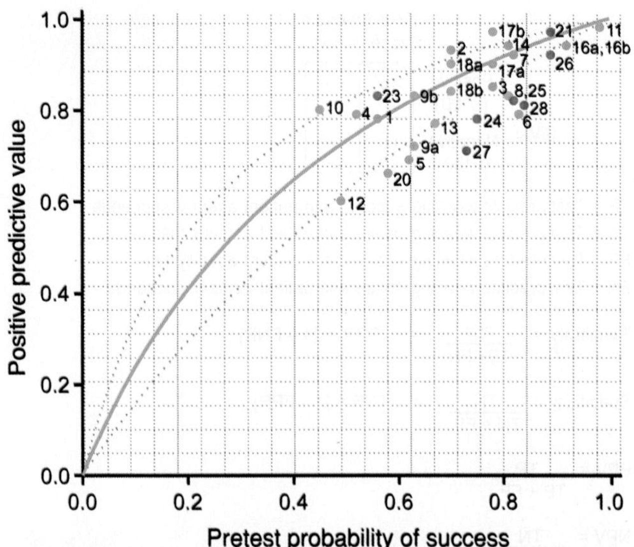

FIGURE 106.24 Positive predictive value (posttest probability of successful outcome) for f/V_t plotted against pretest probability of successful outcome. Studies included in the ACCP Task Force's meta-analysis (116) are indicated by *blue symbols*; studies undertaken after publication of the Task Force's report are indicated by *red symbols*. The curve is based on the sensitivity, specificity originally reported by Yang and Tobin (5) and Bayes' formula for 0.01-unit increments in pretest probability between 0.00 and 1.00. The *lines* represent the upper and lower 95% confidence intervals for the predicted relationship of the positive-predictive values against pretest probability. The observed positive predictive value in a study is plotted against the pre-test probability of weaning success (prevalence of successful outcome). Studies 5, 6, 11, 18a, 18b, and 24 include measurements of f/V_t obtained during pressure support. Studies 14 and 1 include measurements obtained in pediatric patients. Studies 7, 18a, 18b, and 28 used f/V_t threshold values below 65. (From Tobin MJ, Jubran A. Variable performance of weaning-predictor tests: role of Bayes' theorem and spectrum and test-referral bias. *Intensive Care Med.* 2006;32:2002.)

The primary task of a weaning-predictor test is screening, which requires a high sensitivity (112,113). The average sensitivity in all of the studies on f/V_t was 0.89, and 85% of the studies reveal sensitivities above 0.90 (114). This sensitivity compares well with commonly used diagnostic tests: creatinine phosphokinase and troponin T for the diagnosis of acute myocardial infarction, sensitivity of 0.94 and 0.98, respectively; chest x-ray for lung cancer, 0.60; stress EKG for myocardial ischemia, 0.61 for women and 0.72 for men, and sensitivity to diagnose endocarditis of less than 0.60 to 0.70 with transthoracic echocardiography and between 0.75 and 0.95 with transesophageal echocardiography (2). The sensitivity of a spontaneous breathing trial is unknown.

Since screening is the primary purpose of a weaning-predictor test, it is important that the test be performed early in a patient's ventilator course. Figures 106.24 and 106.25, however, reveal that pretest probability of weaning success was 75% or higher in more than half the studies of weaning-predictor tests, a percentage that far exceeds what one would expect from a screening test. In other words, most physicians inappropriately delayed the undertaking of weaning-predictor tests, increasing the likelihood of weaning success. A simple way for a physician to assess his or her own timeliness in initiating weaning is to estimate the number of times he/she obtained positive results on weaning-predictor tests over the preceding 6 months. If a physician working in a typical

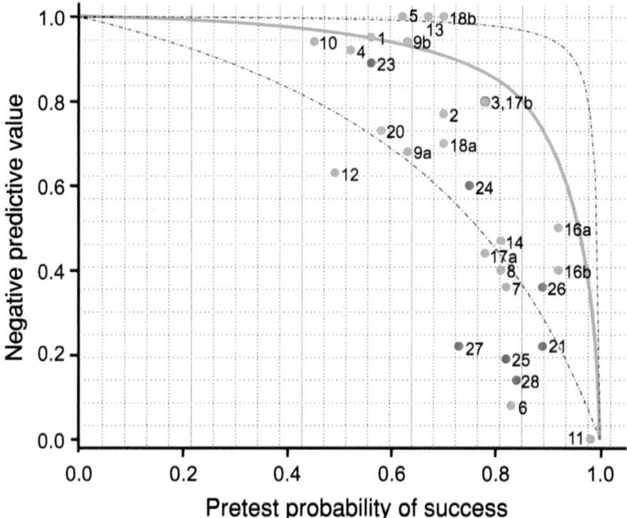

FIGURE 106.25 Negative predictive value (posttest probability of unsuccessful outcome) for f/V_T. Studies included in the ACCP Task Force's meta-analysis (116) are indicated by *blue symbols;* studies undertaken after publication of the Task Force's report are indicated by red symbols. The curve, its 95% confidence intervals, and placement of a study on the plot are described in the legend of Figure 106.24. The observed negative predictive value in a study is plotted against the pretest probability of weaning success (prevalence of successful outcome). Note study 11, which has a negative-predictive value of 0.00 and specificity of 0.00. These values suggest that f/V_T is an unreliable test (and this will also be the natural conclusion reached by a meta-analysis of likelihood ratio). Instead, a negative predictive value of 0.00 and specificity of 0.00 are the values predicted for the pretest probability of weaning success of 98.2% reported in study 11. (From Tobin MJ, Jubran A. Variable performance of weaning-predictor tests: role of Bayes' theorem and spectrum and test-referral bias. *Intensive Care Med.* 2006;32:2002.)

medical ICU estimates that he/she obtained positive results 70% or more of the time, they should consider that they are being too slow in initiating weaning (2).

Pulmonary Gas Exchange

Mechanical ventilation is virtually never discontinued in a patient who has severe hypoxemia, such as arterial oxygen tension (PaO_2) less than 55 mmHg with inspired oxygen fraction (FiO_2) greater than 0.40. Arterial-to-inspired oxygen ratio (PaO_2/FiO_2), alveolar–arterial oxygen tension gradient, and arterial/alveolar oxygen tension ratio (PaO_2/PaO_2) are indices derived from arterial blood gas measurements proposed as predictors of weaning outcome. Of these indices only PaO_2/PaO_2 has been prospectively evaluated, and it has performed poorly as predictor of weaning outcome (5). The study (5) was marred by test-referral bias—i.e., patients with severe hypoxia were excluded from the study population. Therefore, it is not possible to conclude that the poor performance of PaO_2/PaO_2 means that indices derived from arterial blood gas measurements are of no value in predicting weaning outcome. While threshold values of the efficiency of indices derived from arterial blood gas measurements cannot be recommended for weaning prediction, weaning attempts are not recommended in patients with borderline hypoxemia.

Minute Ventilation

A minute ventilation of less than 10 L/min was a classic index used to predict a successful weaning outcome (120). When prospectively assessed, however, minute ventilation has a high rate of false-negative and false-positive results and cannot be recommended as a predictor of weaning outcome (2).

Maximum Inspiratory Pressure

The use of maximum inspiratory pressure as a weaning predictor stems from a study by Sahn and Lakshminarayan (120). They found that all patients with a maximum inspiratory pressure value more negative than −30 cm H_2O were successfully weaned, whereas all patients with a maximum inspiratory pressure less negative than −20 cm H_2O failed a weaning trial. In most successive investigations, these threshold values have shown poor sensitivity and specificity (5,24,29,31,32).

VITAL CAPACITY

The normal vital capacity is usually between 65 and 75 mL/kg, and a value of 10 mL/kg or more has been suggested to predict a successful weaning outcome (2). In a study of 10 patients with Guillain–Barré syndrome, Chevrolet and Deleamont (121) reported that vital capacity was helpful in guiding the weaning process. Patients with a vital capacity of less than 7 mL/kg were unable to tolerate as few as 15 minutes of spontaneous breathing. As vital capacity increased to more than 15 mL/kg with recovery from the illness, patients were safely extubated. Apart from unique circumstances, such as patients with Guillain–Barré syndrome, vital capacity is rarely used as a weaning predictor, and it is often unreliable (2).

B-Type Natriuretic Peptide

The mechanical stretch of atrial or ventricular cardiomyocytes caused by pressure overload, volume overload or both, triggers the release of pro-brain natriuretic peptide (pro-BNP), a prohormone. Pro-BNP is rapidly cleaved into a biologically active peptide (BNP) and its inactive N-terminal fragment (NT-proBNP) (122). Several investigators have evaluated the accuracy of BNP and NT-proBNP in identifying the likelihood and presence of cardiac causes of weaning failure. To date, however, there is substantial discrepancy in the results of the studies assessing the capacity of natriuretic peptides to predict weaning outcome. For some investigators, the change in peptide concentration over the course of a weaning trial has the greatest predictive power (123); others suggest utilizing baseline values (124). Some report that BNP is more dependable than NT-proBNP (125) while others report the opposite (123). The threshold values that differentiate between weaning-success and weaning-failure patients diverge greatly among the investigations.

Echocardiography

During a spontaneous breathing trial, an increase in left ventricular afterload may impair ventricular compliance, while myocardial ischemia and right ventricular dysfunction may cause an increase in left ventricular filling pressures, resulting in pulmonary edema (126). These findings are especially prominent in patients with known cardiac disorders and can lead to task failure of cardiac origin. Pulmonary edema can be detected by an increase in the pulmonary artery occlusion pressure (i.e., pressure >18 mmHg) (96,127) measured by pulmonary artery catheterization (98). Lamia et al. (127) reported that weaning-induced increases in pulmonary artery occlusion pressure can be predicted noninvasively through the computation of indices such as the E/A ratio and the E/E' ratio.[3] These indices are obtained using transthoracic echocardiography (128). Investigation into the relationship between transthoracic echocardiography and weaning outcomes, however, has yielded contrasting results. In three such studies, cardiac indices failed to predict weaning outcome (129–131). In contrast, two additional studies describe a good sensitivity and specificity for E/E' in predicting weaning failure (99,126). When compared to patients who were successfully weaned from the ventilator, patients with weaning failure demonstrated a significant increase in the E/E' ratio during the weaning trial (99,126).

Differences in the inclusion and exclusion criteria among the studies are responsible for large spectrum biases and do not allow for the generalization of the results. Some investigators excluded patients with known cardiac disorders (126,129) or compared patients with different diuretic treatments prior to the weaning trial (129,130). Moreover, technical issues often forced the investigators to perform the assessments in a group of patients that does not reflect a typical critical care setting, excluding patients with poor acoustic windows (99,130,131), arrhythmias (126,130,131), mitral stenosis (131), and a pacemaker (130). Although transthoracic echocardiography can be a useful bedside tool for an intensivist (132), its utility as a predictor of weaning outcome is limited at present.

Diaphragm Ultrasonography

Diaphragmatic ultrasonography is a promising noninvasive technique to identify diaphragmatic dysfunction in ventilated patients (133,134). Recently, Kim et al. (135) used ultrasonography to assess the impact of diaphragmatic dysfunction in 88 patients deemed ready for a trial of spontaneous respiration, and with no history of diaphragmatic disease. Diaphragmatic dysfunction was defined as either a vertical excursion of the muscle of less than 10 mm or as paradoxical movements. Twenty-four patients (29%) had evidence of diaphragmatic dysfunction. Compared with patients without dysfunction, those with dysfunction had longer weaning time (17 vs. 4 days, $p < 0.01$) and total ventilation time (24 vs. 9 days $p < 0.01$). Future studies are necessary to assess the role of diaphragm ultrasonography in identifying patients at high risk of difficulty weaning.

Esophageal Pressure Measurement

Esophageal pressure can be measured using a water-filled esophageal catheter or, more often, using an air-filled system consisting of a catheter provided with a distal thin-walled balloon (136). These catheters, which are inserted nasally or orally, provide an estimation of pleural pressure and, thus, they are used in a variety of computations including the estimation of the respiratory effort and the calculation of work of breathing (Fig. 106.26) (137). In 1995, Gluck et al. (138) evaluated a commercial system that calculated work of breathing, based in part on esophageal pressure measurement, to expedite the weaning process. The use of esophageal pressure measurements shortened the need for mechanical ventilation by setting a more aggressive pace of weaning when compared with conventional care. More recently, Jubran et al. (139) have shown that monitoring the *change* in esophageal pressure—the esophageal pressure trend index—during the course of a weaning trial, can be used to predict weaning outcome. Although the application of esophageal pressure measurement in the management of weaning from mechanical ventilation has shown promising results, it remains a relatively unused technology given the technical requirements of correct esophageal balloon placement (140).

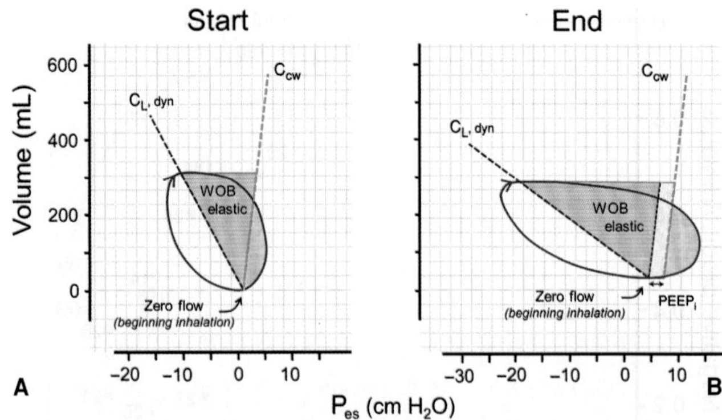

FIGURE 106.26 Representative esophageal pressure–volume loops in a patient with moderate COPD at the start (A) and end of a failed weaning trial (B). *Blue dashed line* represents dynamic lung compliance ($C_{L,dyn}$); *green dashed line* represents the chest wall compliance (C_{cw}). The resistive work is represented as the area to the left of dynamic lung compliance line, the elastic work is represented as the area between the dynamic lung compliance line and the chest wall compliance line (*dark blue area*), and inspiratory effort to overcome intrinsic positive end-expiratory pressure ($PEEP_i$) is the pressure required to start inspiratory flow (*light blue area* in B). Total inspiratory work of breathing is the sum of elastic and resistive work. The area to the right of the chest wall compliance line represents expiratory work (*orange area*). Over the course of the trial, the patient developed $PEEP_i$ and an increase in total inspiratory work of breathing. When partitioned, the increase in inspiratory work was mostly due to an increase in the elastic component. The increase in elastic work made the clinician suspicious for subclinical pulmonary edema. Accordingly, the patient had a coronary angiography that showed critical obstructions involving the left anterior descending coronary artery and the left obtuse marginal artery. Next, he underwent a balloon angioplasty and stent placement. Few days later, the patient was successfully weaned from the ventilator.

WEANING TRIALS

When a screening test is positive—for example, a low f/V_t—the clinician proceeds to a confirmatory test (112)—for example, pressure support of 6 to 8 cm H_2O or spontaneous respiration through a T-Tube (Fig. 106.27). The goal of a positive result on a confirmatory test-no respiratory distress at the conclusion of the pressure-support trial or T-tube trial-is to rule in a condition, in this case, a high likelihood that a patient will tolerate a trial of extubation (112). An ideal confirmatory

[3]Transthoracic echocardiography employs conventional pulsed-wave Doppler techniques and tissue Doppler imaging (TDI) to perform hemodynamic and myocardial motion measurements. These instruments allow the estimation of the flow velocity during early passive diastolic filling of the left ventricle (identified with E mitral annular inflow wave) and the early diastolic myocardial relaxation velocity below the baseline as the annulus ascends from the apex (identified with E_a or E'). An increase of the E/E' ratio (usual cutoff = 8) reveals increased left ventricular filling pressures and correlates to pulmonary capillary wedge pressure (128).

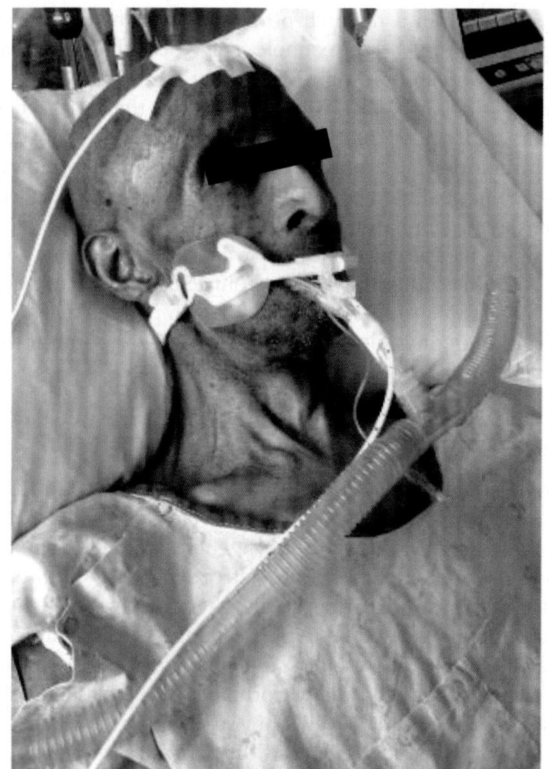

FIGURE 106.27 Unassisted breathing through a T-tube circuit. During a weaning trial of unassisted breathing the patient is disconnected from the ventilator and breathes through a T-tube circuit without continuous positive airway pressure. The T-tube is connected to an oxygen source with an FiO_2 usually set at 0.40. During the trial, we monitor transcutaneous oxygen saturation, cardiac activity, and blood pressure. Concurrently, we observe the patient for development of respiratory distress. Patients who tolerate the T-tube trial for at least 30 minutes are considered for a trial of extubation. Only in selected patients do we perform arterial blood gas analysis before extubation. Patients who do not tolerate the trial are reconnected to the ventilator and are usually reassessed the following day. (From Shaikh H, Morales D, Laghi F. Weaning from mechanical ventilation. *Semin Respir Crit Care Med.* 2014;35(4):451–468.)

test has a very low rate of false-positive results; that is, a high specificity (112). Unfortunately, the specificity of a spontaneous breathing trial is not known. Indeed, its specificity will never be known, because its determination would require an unethical experiment: extubating all patients who fail a weaning trial and counting how many require reintubation (2).

The major weaning techniques used include intermittent mandatory ventilation (IMV), pressure support, T-tube trials, or some combination of these three. Recently, NIPPV has been used to facilitate extubation in selected patients.

Intermittent Mandatory Ventilation (IMV)

For many years, IMV was the most popular method of weaning from mechanical ventilation (141). With IMV weaning, the ventilator's mandatory rate is reduced in steps of 1 to 3 breaths per minute, and an arterial blood gas is obtained about 30 minutes after each rate change (142). Unfortunately, titrating the ventilator's mandatory rate according with the results of arterial blood gases can produce a false sense of security. As little as 2 to 3 IMV breaths per minute can achieve acceptable blood gases, but these values provide no information regarding the patient's work of breathing (2). At IMV rates of 14 breaths per minute or less, the patient's work of breathing may be excessive (143,144) both during the ventilator-assisted breaths and the intervening spontaneous breaths. The fact that, as the IMV rate is decreased, inspiratory work increases progressively not only for the spontaneous breaths, but also for the assisted breaths, is largely due to the inability of the respiratory center to adapt its output rapidly to intermittent support (144). By providing inadequate respiratory muscle rest, IMV is likely to delay, rather than facilitate, discontinuation of mechanical ventilation in difficult-to-wean patients (8).

Pressure Support

When pressure support is used for weaning, the level of pressure is reduced gradually and titrated on the basis of the patient's respiratory frequency (145). When the patient tolerates a pressure support of approximately 6 to 8 cm H_2O with a PEEP 5 cm H_2O, he or she is extubated (146). This strategy is based on the belief that such "minimal levels" of support are solely overcoming the resistance produced by the endotracheal tube and ventilator circuit (145,146). This belief, however, disregards the edema and the inflammation that develop in the upper airways after an endotracheal tube has been in place for a day or more (147). Upon removal of the tube, the work produced by breathing through the swollen airway is about the same as that caused by breathing through an endotracheal tube (147)—this should hold true as long as the internal diameter of the endotracheal tube is not too small and there is no accumulation of dense secretions within it (148). The addition of a small amount of pressure support produces surprisingly large reductions in inspiratory work in ventilated patients: 5 cm H_2O decreases inspiratory work by 31 to 38%, and 10 cm H_2O decreases work by 46 to 60% (146). Independently, the addition of 5 cm H_2O of PEEP can decrease the work of breathing by as much as 40% in ventilated patients (146). In conclusion, in most cases, any level of pressure support would overcompensate and may give misleading information (149).

T-Tube Trials

The use of repeated T-tube trials several times a day is the oldest method for conducting a weaning trial (141). The patient receives an enriched supply of oxygen through a T-tube circuit. Initially 5 to 10 minutes in duration, T-tube trials were extended and repeated several times a day until the patient could sustain spontaneous ventilation for several hours. This approach has become unpopular because it requires considerable time on the part of the ICU staff.

Today, it is usual to limit a T-tube trial to once a day (Fig. 106.27). Performing single, daily T-tube trials is as effective as performing such trials several times a day (8), but is much simpler. If the trial is successful, the patient is extubated. If the trial is unsuccessful, the patient is given at least 24 hours of respiratory muscle rest with full ventilator support before another trial is performed (2).

Patients are judged to have failed a T-tube trial when they develop severe tachypnea, increased accessory muscle activity, diaphoresis, facial signs of respiratory distress, oxygen desaturation, tachycardia, arrhythmias, or hypotension. The degree of change in these variables, however, varies from report to report. A standardized approach to patient monitoring during a T-tube trial does not exist. Indeed, there is no agreement as to whether the monitoring of any specific variable helps in deciding whether to continue a T-tube trial for an initially planned duration, prolong it, or curtail it (2).

Comparison of Weaning Methods

In patients undergoing their first weaning trial who have both a high pretest probability of weaning success (e.g., uncomplicated postoperative patients), and who have required short-term mechanical ventilation, weaning with IMV is probably as effective as weaning with T-tube trials (150). Moreover, in patients with good weaning parameters undergoing their first trial of weaning, investigators reported that pressure support and the T-tube trials are "appropriate approaches for spontaneous breathing trials before extubation" (151,152).

In difficult-to-wean patients who have failed at least one weaning trial, however, weaning methods are not equally effective (141). For example, the period of weaning is as much as three times as long with IMV compared to T-tube trials (8) or pressure-support trials (153). In contrast, in a study involving patients with respiratory difficulties upon weaning, the weaning time with pressure-support and T-tube trials was similar (153). In another study, T-tube trials halved the weaning time compared to pressure support (8). Accordingly, our approach is to use T-tube trials rather than pressure-support trials.

Weaning by Protocol versus Usual Care

The use of human-driven protocols for weaning versus usual care has been compared in several trials (154), six of which are particularly relevant (3,155–159). The reports of Namen et al. (155), Randolph et al. (156), and Krishnan et al. (157) show no advantage for a protocol approach. The reports of Kollef et al. (3), Marelich et al. (158), and and Ely et al. (159) are viewed as evidence for the superiority of a protocol approach to weaning.

In the trial of Kollef et al. (3), however, no advantage for weaning by protocol was observed in three of the four study ICUs. In the fourth unit, where an advantage for a protocol approach to weaning was observed, patients assigned to usual care were sicker than those assigned to protocol management; this confounding factor markedly weakens (if not destroys) any assertion that protocol weaning was superior (2).

Although Marelich et al. (158) suggest the superiority of the weaning-by-protocol approach, they found no advantage over usual care in one of the two study ICUs. The study of Ely et al. (159) does not consist of a straightforward comparison of protocol versus nonprotocol care. All of the patients in the intervention arm were weaned by T-tube or flow-by trials, whereas 76% of the patients in the nonintervention arm were managed by SIMV alone or in combination with pressure support. Physiologic studies and randomized trials have repeatedly shown that SIMV is the least effective weaning modality (8,145). With this fundamental difference in techniques, it is impossible to use data from this study to form a judgment about the efficacy of a protocol *per se*. Instead the report of Ely et al. (159) can be viewed primarily as another study of SIMV, confirming the reports of Brochard et al. (145) and Esteban et al. (8), that SIMV slows weaning.

That the use of a protocol does not improve weaning outcome should not be surprising (113,160). One needs to make a distinction between the use of algorithms in research protocols and their subsequent application in everyday practice. The algorithm in a research protocol is specified with exacting precision (161). For example, if f/V_t less than or equal to 100 is the nodal point for advancement to a T-tube trial, then patients with an f/V_t of 100 will undergo the trial, whereas patients with an f/V_t of 101 will return to mechanical ventilation for another 24 hours. An experienced clinician, however, would think it silly to comply with a protocol that decided an entire day of ventilator management on a one-unit difference in a single measurement of f/V_t or any other weaning predictor (160). Instead, physicians customize the knowledge generated by research to the particulars of each patient. The careful application of physiologic principles is likely to outperform an inflexible application of a protocol.

Computerized Approaches to Weaning

A novel strategy of weaning entails the use of modified ventilators equipped with computer-driven closed-loop knowledge-based algorithms (162–164). These modified ventilators continuously monitor respiratory frequency (f), V_T, and end-tidal CO_2 tension, and repeatedly alter the level of delivered pressure support based on iterative changes in these three variables (162). The pace of pressure-support reduction is tailored according to the needs and performance of the patient. Once a predesignated minimal level of pressure support is reached, the ventilator automatically subjects the patient to a weaning trial, conducted at a low level of pressure support. If the patient develops no distress, a message is displayed on the screen recommending the removal of the ventilator.

Lellouche et al. (165) were the first to perform a large RCT in Europe comparing the computerized ventilator (SmartCare, Lubeck, Germany) against standardized written instructions. They concluded that, compared with usual care, the computerized system decreased weaning duration from a median of 5 to 3 days ($p = 0.01$) and decreased total duration of mechanical ventilation from 12 to 7.5 days ($p = 0.003$) (Fig. 106.28A). These positive results have been recently confirmed by Burns et al. (166) that showed how patients randomized in the computerized system had shorter median times to first successful spontaneous breathing trial (1.0 vs. 4.0 days; $p < 0.0001$), extubation (3.0 vs. 4.0 days; $p = 0.02$), and successful extubation (4.0 vs. 5.0 days; $p = 0.01$).

An Australian RCT (167), using the same ventilator employed by Lellouche et al. (165) and Burns et al. (166), found no difference in the median time to successful extubation. At least two factors contributed to this negative result. First, most patients enrolled in the studies of Lellouche et al. (165) and Burns et al. (166) were medical patients, whereas 78% of enrollees in the study of Rose et al. (167) were surgical patients, which are typically less challenging to wean (150). In this regard, it is worth noting that computerized weaning in a bench model performed poorly in the presence of Cheyne–Stokes respiration (164), a pattern of breathing that is likely more common among medical than among surgical patients. Second, the nurse-to-patient ratio in the study of Rose et al. (167) was 1:1, increasing the likelihood that frequent clinical assessment of the patients in the usual care arm added to the equivalency of the results.

A fourth RCT of computerized weaning versus usual care was undertaken in Brazil by Taniguchi et al. (163). These Brazilian researchers, employing a slightly different computerized system from the previous investigators, found no difference in

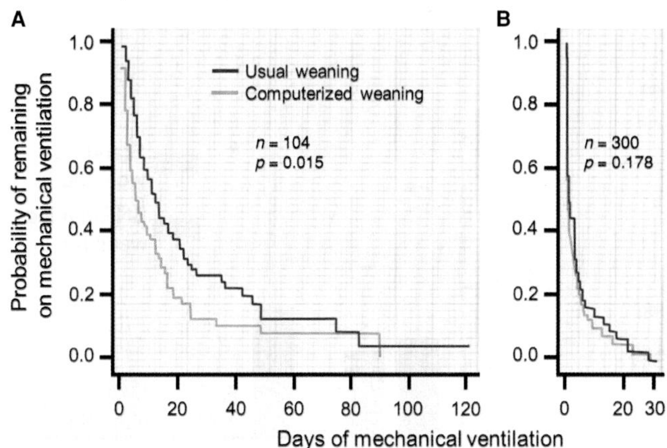

FIGURE 106.28 Computerized approaches to weaning. **A:** Kaplan–Meier analysis of weaning time until successful extubation or death in 70 patients randomized to usual weaning (*purple line*) and 74 patients randomized to computerized weaning (*blue line*). The probability of remaining on mechanical ventilation in this study in which medical patients accounted for more than two-thirds of randomized subjects was significantly reduced with the computer-driven weaning (log-rank test, $p = 0.015$). **B:** Kaplan–Meier curves for overall ventilation time in 150 patients randomized to usual weaning (*purple line*) and 150 patients randomized to computerized weaning (*blue line*). The probability of remaining on mechanical ventilation in this study that enrolled only surgical patients was not reduced by computer-driven weaning (log-rank test, $p = 0.178$). (**A:** Adapted from Lellouche F, Mancebo J, Jolliet P, et al. A multicenter randomized trial of computer-driven protocolized weaning from mechanical ventilation. *Am J Respir Crit Care Med*, 2006;174:894–900; **B:** Adapted from Schädler D, Engel C, Elke G, et al. Automatic control of pressure support for ventilator weaning in surgical intensive care patients. *Am J Respir Crit Care Med*. 2012;185:637–644.)

weaning duration with the two approaches. Patients enrolled by Taniguchi et al. (163) consisted solely of postoperative patients. The lack of benefit from computerized weaning in surgical patients is further supported by a recent report (168) that found no difference between weaning using the computerized approach and weaning based on standardized written instructions in 300 surgical patients (Fig. 106.28B).

MANAGEMENT OF WEANING FAILURE PATIENT

Weaning attempts that are repeatedly unsuccessful usually signify either incomplete resolution of the illness that precipitated mechanical ventilation or the development of new problems. A thorough diagnostic evaluation with correction of reversible pathologies is mandatory. Important aspects in the care of these patients include the optimization of ventilator settings and optimization of cardiovascular function. In addition, selected patients may benefit from NIPPV, respiratory muscle training, physical and occupational therapy, and psychological interventions (17).

Optimization of Ventilator Settings

Careful adjustment of the ventilator settings is necessary to minimize work of breathing. It is important to spot the presence of intrinsic PEEP, as this will interfere with ventilator triggering (41). A careful interpretation of flow, volume, and airway pressure waveform at the bedside is essential to monitor patient–ventilator interaction (7). Considering the purported association between asynchronies and duration of mechanical ventilation (89), intensivists should actively adjust ventilator settings in patients who experience asynchronies (7,42). Alternatively, they may consider the use of novel modes of mechanical ventilation such as neurally adjusted ventilatory assist (169,170). Of note, whether reducing the number of asynchronies decreases the duration of mechanical ventilation in the problem patient remains to be determined.

Noninvasive Pressure-Support Ventilation to Expedite Weaning and Extubation

In selected patients (i.e., patients with COPD) who fail weaning trials, investigators have evaluated the possibility to extubate them to NIPPV. This strategy stems from the work of Nava et al. (171) published in 1998. In that study, duration of ventilator support, ICU length of stay, incidence of nosocomial pneumonia, and 60-day survival were better with early extubation plus application of NIPPV than with gradual weaning of invasive ventilation. These results have been replicated by some (172,173) but not all investigators (174). In the latest and largest study thus far, Girault et al. (174) reported that, compared to conventional weaning from invasive mechanical ventilation, NIPPV instituted when patients had just failed a trial of spontaneous breathing decreased the duration of intubation. NIPPV, however, did not reduce reintubation rate within 7 days of extubation. Moreover, NIPPV did not reduce morbidity and 28-day mortality. In this study, rescue NIPPV was successfully used in patients randomized to the control group who developed respiratory distress following extubation. It is thus possible that one of the contributing factors to the negative results of Girault et al. (174) was this liberal use of rescue NIPPV in the control group. Accordingly, the use of NIPPV to expedite weaning and extubation in COPD remains controversial.

Optimization of Cardiovascular Function

Cardiac dysfunction can be assessed using bedside transthoracic echocardiography as it can provide information regarding the status of the right and left ventricles and ischemia-induced ventricular dysfunction during weaning (99,148). Volume overload should be treated before carrying out a weaning trial as volume overload has been associated with worse weaning outcome (96,175).

In an RCT of 304 patients allocated to either a BNP-driven or physician-driven strategy of fluid management during ventilator weaning using a computer-driven weaning system, Mekontso et al. (124) reported a shorter time to successful extubation in the intervention group as compared with the control group: median (interquartile range [IQR]) of 42 (21–108) hours versus 59 (23–140) hours, respectively ($p = 0.034$) (Fig. 106.29). These effects were especially pronounced in patients with left ventricular systolic dysfunction. Whether intravenous inotropic agents such as dobutamine should be used in difficult-to-wean patients remains controversial (91).

Respiratory Muscle Training

The growing recognition that many weaning-failure patients have severe respiratory muscle weakness has been the springboard of an RCT designed to determine whether inspiratory

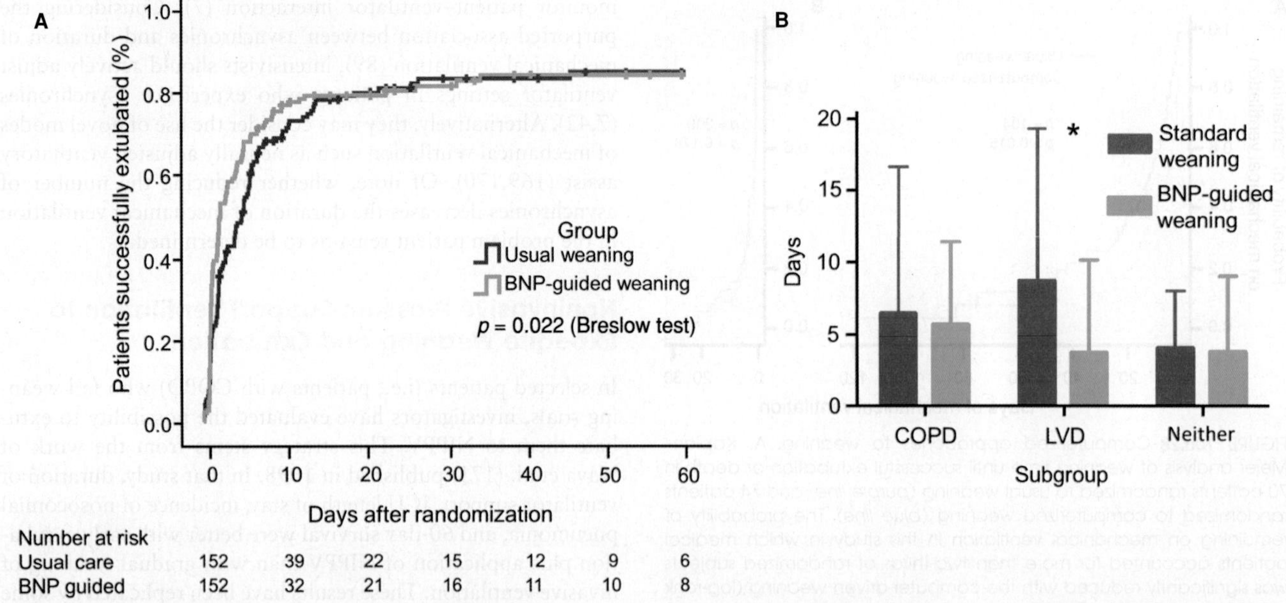

FIGURE 106.29 Natriuretic peptide–driven fluid management during ventilator weaning. A: Kaplan–Meier analysis of probability of successful extubation in 152 patients randomized to usual care (*red line*) and 152 patients randomized to weaning guided by B-type natriuretic peptide (BNP) (*green line*). The probability of successful extubation was increased with the BNP-guided strategy ($P = 0.022$, Breslow test). Compared with the control group, the BNP-guided group had a higher proportion of patients receiving diuretics, resulting in a significantly more negative fluid balance during the weaning period. There was no difference in length of stay, ICU mortality, or hospital mortality. B: Mean (SD) time to successful weaning from invasive and noninvasive ventilation in patients with COPD, left ventricular systolic dysfunction (LVD), or neither. The differences between the two strategies in time to successful weaning were significant only in patients with LVD, suggesting a stronger effect of BNP-guided fluid management in this subgroup than in the other two subgroups (*$P < 0.05$ between the usual care and BNP-guided groups; Mann–Whitney test). (From Mekontso DA, Roche-Campo F, Kouatchet A, et al. Natriuretic peptide-driven fluid management during ventilator weaning: a randomized controlled trial. *Am J Respir Crit Care Med.* 2012;186(12):1256–1263.)

muscle-strength training would improve the weaning outcome of patients who had received mechanical ventilation for about 1 to 2 months (176). Strength training was achieved with the use of a commercial threshold inspiratory muscle training device equipped with an adjustable spring-loaded valve (Fig. 106.30). Five days a week, patients in the intervention group were

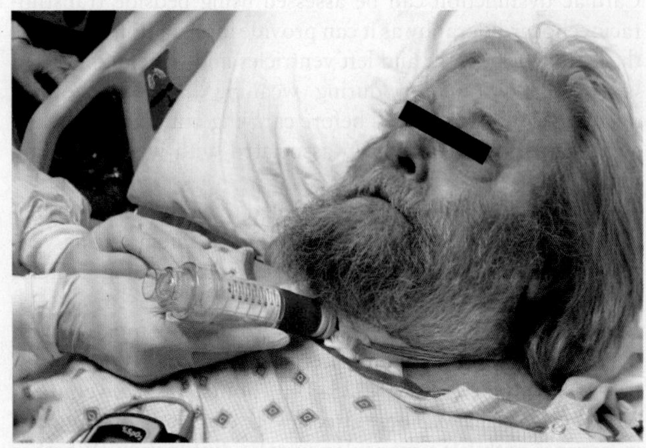

FIGURE 106.30 Inspiratory threshold device used for inspiratory muscle training. This device contains an adjustable, spring-loaded, mushroom valve. To inhale through the device, the patient must generate an inspiratory pressure that is sufficient to compress the spring of the mushroom valve. To keep the valve open throughout inhalation, the inspiratory pressure must be maintained above the threshold pressure. The patient exhales through the training device via a low-resistance, one-way, silicone rubber diaphragm (see text for details). (From Shaikh H, Morales D, Laghi F. Weaning from mechanical ventilation. *Semin Respir Crit Care Med.* 2014;35(4):451–468.)

required to perform four sets of 6 to 10 threshold-loaded inspirations; between each set, patients were returned to the ventilator for 2 minutes. During these sessions, the spring-loaded valve in the threshold device was adjusted to the highest pressure setting that the patient could consistently open during each inspiration. In contrast, patients in the sham arm inhaled through an inspiratory muscle training device that contained a large hole, with the result that little pressure was required to generate airflow. Upon completion of the study, 71% patients in the strength-training arm were weaned as compared with 47% patients in the sham arm ($p = 0.039$). In addition, over the course of the trial, patients in the strength-training arm exhibited an increase in maximal inspiratory pressure from 44 ± 18 to 54 ± 18 cm H_2O ($p < 0.0001$); corresponding values of maximal inspiratory pressure in the sham arm were 44 ± 18 and 45 ± 20 cm H_2O.

The results of this study suggest that the use of a simple device (a threshold loader) can markedly increase the weanability of patients requiring long-term mechanical ventilation. The challenges now are to reproduce these findings, determine whether further adjustments to the training regimen might achieve an even greater level of success, and investigate whether the use of a threshold loading device may increase the weanability of patients in the acute care setting.

Physical and Occupational Therapy to Aid Weaning

In 1974, Petty (177) hypothesized that ambulation in mechanical ventilation patients could be a useful strategy to improve strength and coordination during weaning. This hypothesis was tested 35 years later by Schweickert et al. (77). At two university hospitals, the investigators enrolled patients who had received less than 72 hours of mechanical ventilation and who had exhibited functional independence 2 weeks before admission. From an initial screening of 1,161 patients, 104 were enrolled. Of these, 49 were randomized to early exercise and mobilization (physical and occupational therapy), starting on the day of enrollment, and 55 to usual care that did not include routine physical therapy. The primary end point, the number of patients returning to independent functional status at hospital discharge, was reached by 29 (59%) patients in the intervention group and 19 (35%) in the control group (p = 0.02). Duration of mechanical ventilation was also shorter in the intervention group, 3.4 days (IQR: 2.3 to 7.3) versus 6.1 days (IQR: 4.0 to 9.6; p = 0.02).

More recently, in a single-center study, Denehy et al. (178) compared usual care against an exercise rehabilitation program that commenced during the ICU admission and continued into the outpatient setting. At the conclusion of the study, the investigators reported no difference in the duration of mechanical ventilation in the two groups of patients. Moreover, there was no difference in ICU length of stay, mortality, and 6-minute walking distance 12 months after ICU discharge. Of note, the *a priori* enrollment goal of 200 patients was not reached.

The studies of Schweickert et al. (77) and Denehy et al. (178) raise several important questions. Can physical and occupational therapy shorten the duration of mechanical ventilation in the type of patients excluded from the studies such as patients with significant baseline-dependent functional status or who have been ventilated for more than 72 hours? Can alternative strategies, such as transcutaneous neuromuscular electrical stimulation (179–181) alone or in combination with anabolic agents (182), be of benefit in selected patients who are not candidates or who do not tolerate physical and occupational therapy? Finally, is it more cost-effective to combine a limited number of physical and occupational therapy sessions with transcutaneous neuromuscular electrical stimulation than it is to perform an intensive program of physical and occupational therapy alone (77)?

Psychological Interventions

The negative impact of psychological factors on weaning underscores the need for active screening for delirium, depression, anxiety, and PTSD (100,105,107). Aggressive treatment of depression may increase the likelihood of weaning (183,184). Biofeedback therapy (185,186), weaning in specialized centers (187), and improving the patients' environment, communication, and mobility (106,188) have been used to decrease psychological problems in ventilated patients (100). Whether novel adjuncts such as music therapy may benefit anxious patients who repeatedly fail weaning remains to be determined (189).

Role of Sedation in Weaning

Pharmacologic agents that produce sedation are almost invariably used in patients receiving mechanical ventilation. The goal is to decrease anxiety and agitation, enhance patient–ventilator synchronization, and facilitate patient care (17). More than 15 years ago, Kress et al. (190) undertook an RCT in 128 adult patients receiving mechanical ventilation in a medical ICU and concluded that daily interruption of sedation resulted in a shorter duration of mechanical ventilation and a shorter ICU stay. Girard et al. (191) extended these findings by combining daily interruption of sedation with spontaneous breathing trials. The paired intervention resulted in more days breathing without ventilator assistance, and earlier discharge from both the ICU and the hospital. In an accompanying editorial, Brochard (192) pointed out several problems with the design of the study including the absence of a requirement to stop sedatives in the control group before a spontaneous breathing trial, the timing of weaning onset, and markedly increased rate of failed weaning trials in the control arm that render the interpretation of this study highly problematic.

More recently, Mehta et al. (193) reported that among 430 mechanically ventilated adults, the addition of daily sedation interruption to protocolized sedation designed to maintain a comfortable yet arousable state equivalent did not shorten the duration of mechanical ventilation or ICU stay. In a third study, Shehabi et al. (102) noted that a daily interruption of sedation increased the overall need for benzodiazepines and the workload of the nurses. Strøm et al. (194) went even further and, in a single-blinded study of 140 mechanically ventilated patients, sought to determine if complete withholding of sedation would be superior to daily interruption of sedation. Withholding all sedations was associated with significantly more days without ventilator assistance (mean: 4.2 days, 95% CI 0.3 to 8.1 days), and earlier discharge from both the ICU and hospital. Agitated delirium was more frequent in the intervention group than in the control group (20% vs. 7%; p = 0.04) (194). Two years later, a neuropsychologist interviewed 13 patients from each group and concluded that there were no differences in terms of quality of life, depression and anxiety (195). The investigators concluded that "a protocol of no sedation applied to critically ill patients undergoing mechanical ventilation does not increase the risk of long-term psychological sequelae" (195). Two interdependent observations, however, limit the strength of this conclusion. First, only a minority of patients enrolled in the original study were available for the follow-up neuropsychologist's interview (195). Second, it is likely that the incidence of psychological problems would have been higher among patients who declined the interview than among those who agree to it (196).

In view of the above findings, we use sedation in most of our patients requiring invasive mechanical ventilation—particularly early in the ICU course. Our goal is to maintain a comfortable yet arousable state whenever possible. If this goal is impractical, we try daily interruptions of sedation. Only later in the ICU course, do we administer sedation on an as-needed basis and, in selected patients, we withhold sedation altogether.

EXTUBATION

Decisions about weaning and extubation are commonly merged. Merging these two decisions, however, can cause patient mismanagement (197). When a patient tolerates a weaning trial without distress, a clinician feels reasonably confident that the patient will be able to sustain spontaneous ventilation after extubation. However, passing a weaning trial without distress is not the only consideration. The clinician also must consider whether the patient will be able to maintain a patent upper airway after extubation.

Removal of an endotracheal tube is typically performed under controlled conditions after the patient has satisfactorily tolerated a weaning trial (197). Enteral feeding is temporally withheld for about 4 hours. When possible, the head of the bed should be at 30 to 90 degrees from the horizontal (198). The endotracheal tube, mouth, and upper airway are suctioned, paying attention to the collection of secretions above an inflated cuff, as inadequate clearing of secretions can result in postextubation laryngospasm (198). Some clinicians recommend keeping a suction catheter in place, aiming for the catheter to barely protrude from the distal end of the endotracheal tube as the cuff is deflated; this step is taken in an attempt to capture any secretions sitting on the top of an inflated cuff that may fall into the airway after deflating the cuff. Some clinicians inflate the lungs with an Ambubag immediately before pulling out the endotracheal tube, hoping that the larger-than-usual ensuing exhalation will push secretions upward and outward (199). The cuff is then deflated, and the endotracheal tube is withdrawn (Fig. 106.31). After the removal of the endotracheal tube, the patient is given supplemental oxygen titrated to oxygen saturation, being particularly cautious with a patient who is at risk of carbon dioxide retention. Patients may have impaired airway protection reflexes immediately after extubation (200,201), and aspiration can be silent—that is, aspiration can occur without coughing (202). If speech is impaired for more than 24 hours, indirect laryngoscopy should be undertaken to assess vocal cord function. Oral intake should be delayed in patients who have been intubated for a prolonged period (200,201).

In the hours following extubation, patients are carefully monitored for their ability to protect the upper airway and sustain ventilation. Most patients will display progressive improvement, allowing the discontinuation of supplemental

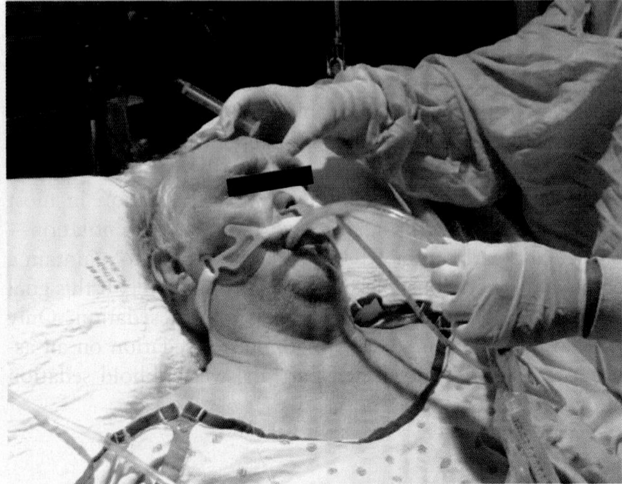

FIGURE 106.31 Extubation. In terms of medical decision analysis, extubation is a confirmatory test of the weaning trial. That is, extubation is used to diagnose/screen for readiness to maintain spontaneous respiration. Extubation is typically performed under controlled conditions. Enteral feeding is temporally withheld for about four hours. Following extubation, the patient is given supplemental oxygen. The development of severe respiratory distress after extubation, if sufficient to require reintubation, is associated with a high mortality rate. (From Shaikh H, Morales D, Laghi F. Weaning from mechanical ventilation. *Semin Respir Crit Care Med.* 2014;35(4):451–468.)

oxygen and ultimate discharge from the ICU. Between 2% and 30% (165,203–209) of patients, however, experience respiratory distress in the postextubation period. Many, but not all, require reinsertion of the endotracheal tube and mechanical ventilation (174). These patients are commonly classified as *extubation failures*. In contrast to the relatively short time required to recognize that a patient is failing a weaning trial, the time course for the development of postextubation distress extends over a longer span. In the study of Epstein et al. (210), for example, 33% of reintubations occurred within the first 12 hours after extubation, and 42% occurred after 24 hours.

The mortality rate among patients who require reintubation is more than six times as high as the mortality rate among patients who tolerate extubation (9). The reason for the higher mortality rate is unknown. It might be related to the development of new problems after extubation or to complications associated with reinsertion of a new tube or that the need for reintubation reflects greater severity of the underlying illness (197). Recent data suggest that reintubation following a planned extubation may affect survival independently of the underlying illness severity (211,212).

Causes of Postextubation Distress

The listed indications for reintubation vary considerably from study to study. Of these, postextubation upper airway obstruction has attracted the most attention.

Postextubation Upper Airway Obstruction

Upper airway obstruction is one of the most urgent and potentially lethal medical emergencies. Complete airway obstruction lasting for as little as 4 to 6 minutes can cause irreversible brain damage (13). The upper airway, which encompasses the passage between the nares and carina, can be obstructed by functional or anatomic causes. Among the former are vocal cord paralysis, paradoxical vocal cord motion, and laryngospasm. Among the latter are trauma (including arytenoid dislocation), burn, granulomas, infections, foreign bodies, tumors, tracheomalacia, compression by a hematoma in close proximity to the airway, and supraglottic, retroarytenoidal, or subglottic edema (13). Edema can develop after only 6 hours of intubation (15). A thinner mucosa covering the cartilage of the vocal processes, less resistance to trauma, and smaller laryngeal diameter are probably responsible for the greater prevalence of laryngeal edema in female than male patients (15). Other risk factors associated with the development of laryngeal edema include traumatic intubation, excessively large tube size, excessive tube mobility secondary to insufficient fixation, patient fighting against the tube or trying to speak, excessive pressure in the cuff, too frequent or too aggressive tracheal suctioning, occurrence of infections or hypotension, and the presence of a nasogastric tube-because these tubes predispose to gastroesophageal reflux (13). It is also possible that a biochemical reaction between the tube material and the airway mucosa may cause laryngeal edema (15). Life-threatening obstruction-either functional and anatomic-can occur postoperatively in patients with redundant pharyngeal soft tissue-such as in sleep apnea-and loss of muscle tone related to the postanesthetic state (13).

A number of investigators have reported that upper airway obstruction accounts for about 15% of patients requiring reintubation (9,210,213). When upper airway obstruction occurs, it typically becomes manifest within 3 to 12 hours after extubation (214–216). In the case of postextubation laryngeal edema, symptoms occur within 5 minutes postextubation in 47% of patients, within 6 to 30 minutes postextubation in 33% of patients, and after more than 30 minutes postextubation in 20% of patients (217). Symptoms rarely occur until 75% of the upper airway lumen has been obliterated (218,219). Occasionally, symptoms may not occur until the diameter of the airway is reduced to 5 mm (220).

Upper airway obstruction causes stridor only if the patient is capable of generating sufficient airflow; if airflow is insufficient, obstruction may cause hypercapnia, hypoxemia, or paradoxical breathing, but not stridor. Women are more susceptible to postextubation stridor than men (214,221,222). Among patients who develop stridor, 1% to 69% require reintubation (214,215,221,223). Many (214,215,222,223), but not all (217,221), investigators have noted that the rate of postextubation stridor increases in proportion to the duration of mechanical ventilation. Stridor usually occurs during inhalation in the presence of upper airway obstruction and during exhalation in the presence of lower airway obstruction, and it can be biphasic with midtracheal stenosis (224).

The first warning of airway obstruction in an unconscious patient may be failure of a jaw–thrust maneuver to open the airway or the inability to ventilate with a bag-valve. Wheezing may be present or absent. Thoracoabdominal paradox may be prominent. Sympathetic discharge is high, and patients are diaphoretic, tachycardic, and hypertensive. As asphyxia progresses, bradycardia, hypotension, and death ensue (13). Arterial blood gases are not particularly helpful, because they are not specific to airway patency and they may show little change until a patient is *in extremis* (15).

TABLE 106.3 Indications and Contraindications for Noninvasive Ventilation in Patients with COPD Who Fail Extubation

Indications
Clinical observations
Moderate-to-severe dyspnea
Tachypnea
Accessory muscle use, abdominal paradox
Impaired gas exchange
Acute or acute-on-chronic hypercapnic respiratory failure ($PaCO_2$> 45 mmHg, pH < 7.35)
Hypoxemia ($PaO_2/FiO_2 \le 200$)[a]
Contraindications
Absolute
Bradypnea, respiratory arrest, immediate need for intubation
Life-threatening hypoxemia
Unable to fit mask
Upper airway obstruction
Undrained pneumothorax
Vomiting/severe upper gastrointestinal bleed
Relative
Agitated, uncooperative
Severe hypercapnic encephalopathy (Glasgow Coma Scale score < 10)
Inability to protect the airway
Impaired swallowing or cough
Excessive secretions
Recent upper airway or upper gastrointestinal surgery
Multiple organ failure
Medically unstable
Uncontrolled cardiac ischemia or arrhythmia
Hypotensive shock

[a]Noninvasive ventilation should be used with caution in exacerbations of COPD accompanied with hypoxemia.

From Shaikh H, Morales D, Laghi F. Weaning from mechanical ventilation. *Semin Respir Crit Care Med.* 2014;35(4):451–468.

Other Causes of Postextubation Distress

Conditions other than upper airway obstruction that cause postextubation distress include bronchopulmonary disorders including aspiration or excessive secretions, congestive heart failure, encephalopathy, and other conditions (210). The frequency of a particular cause differs among studies. For example, cardiac failure accounted for 23% of the cases of Epstein et al. (210), 7% of the cases of Esteban et al. (9), but none of the cases of Smina et al. (213) or De Bast et al. (216).

Predictors of Postextubation Distress

Because reintubation causes serious complications in some patients, attempts are made to predict its likely occurrence. A number of physiologic variables have been evaluated for their ability to predict this likelihood. For some patients, the likelihood of reintubation is considered so high that a clinician may proceed to tracheotomy without first attempting extubation (197) (Table 106.4).

Ability to Sustain Spontaneous Respiration

A true-positive result of a T-tube trial is defined as a patient who tolerates the trial without distress, is then extubated, and does not require reintubation (197). The usual rate of reintubation is 15% to 20%—sometimes lower—but reintubation rates of 24% up to 29% (205–207,216) have been reported by some investigators. These percentages represent all the false-positive test results—that is, patients who tolerate the T-tube trial but require reintubation after extubation—and mean that the positive predictive value and specificity of passing a T-tube trial in predicting that a patient will not require reintubation is less than 100%. To measure the false-negative rate (see Fig. 106.21) would require extubation of patients who fail a T-tube trial and counting how many do *not* require reintubation. For obvious ethical reasons, this number is not known. Given the natural caution of physicians, it can be confidently assumed that it is higher than 0% (197).

Weaning-Predictor Tests

Several investigators have examined the ability of weaning-predictor tests to predict the development of distress after extubation. The question posed is along these lines, "Does f/V_t or some other predictor test, measured before a T-tube trial, predict the likelihood of reintubation?" To answer this question with scientific validity, it is imperative to avoid test-referral bias. This can be avoided if the investigators take steps to ensure that clinicians do *not* perform a T-tube trial or are *not* taking the results of the T-tube trial into account when deciding whether to extubate the study patients. In other words, a decision to extubate the patient must be taken before the T-tube trial, and must proceed even if the patient exhibits significant distress during the trial—a strategy which raises ethical concerns.

Zeggwagh et al. (225) are the only group of investigators who assessed the ability of weaning-predictor tests to forecast development of distress after extubation without performing a weaning trial after the weaning predictors had been recorded. The investigators prospectively studied 101 patients at the point that their ICU physicians contemplated weaning. They measured a series of physiologic measurements during 2 minutes of spontaneous breathing; the results of these measurements were not communicated to the primary team. The team then extubated the patients without first undertaking any form of weaning trial.

Reintubation was necessary in 37% of the patients. Several variables predicted the need for reintubation with a reasonable degree of accuracy. For example, f/V_t had sensitivity of 0.77 and specificity of 0.79, with an area under a receiver operating curve (ROC) curve of 0.81 ± 0.06; maximum expiratory pressure had a sensitivity of 0.52 and specificity 0.92, with an area under an ROC curve of 0.73 ± 0.07. The investigators developed a model based on three variables: f/V_t, maximum expiratory pressure, and vital capacity. The area under the ROC curve for the model was 0.91 ± 0.04 for a development data series and 0.86 ± 0.06 for a validation data series. The accuracy of weaning predictors to predict the development of distress after extubation in this study (225) contrasts sharply with their limited accuracy in studies where the investigators permitted a weaning trial (which altered clinician's extubation decisions) between measurement of the predictors and extubation (197). This difference in diagnostic accuracy is likely due to test-referral bias (2). An important aspect of this study (225) is that the results suggest that undertaking a weaning trial before extubation is useful; the rate of reintubation in the study of Zeggwagh et al. (225) was about double that reported in studies in which weaning trials precede extubation (197).

Cuff-Leak Test

The presence of an endotracheal tube makes it extremely difficult to evaluate the structure and function of the airway before extubation. The amount of air leaking around the outside of an endotracheal tube on deflating the balloon cuff has been used by a number of investigators to predict upper airway obstruction after extubation (Fig. 106.32) (197). For several

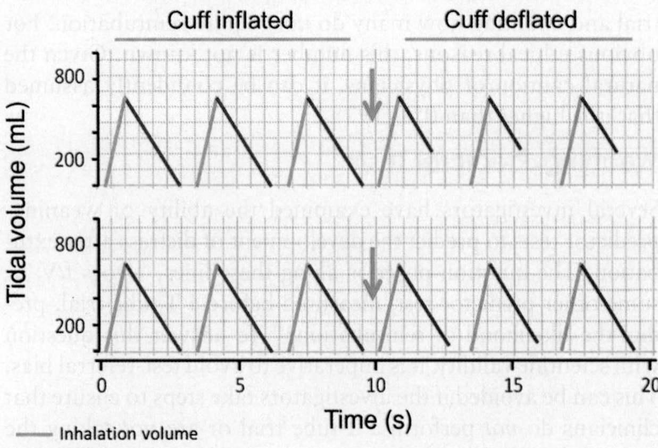

FIGURE 106.32 Cuff-leak test. Schematic representation of tidal volume recorded by the ventilators' inspiratory pneumotach (*blue line*) and by the ventilators' expiratory pneumotach (*red line*) during inhalation and exhalation in two patients before and after deflation of the cuff on the endotracheal tube (*arrow*). **Top**: The patient develops a large leak after cuff deflation (positive test result), as signified by the expired tidal volume being markedly smaller than the inspired tidal volume. **Bottom**: The patient develops a small leak after cuff deflation (negative test result), as signified by the expired tidal volume being only about 40 to 75 mL or 6% to 12% less than the inspired tidal volume. (From Shaikh H, Morales D, Laghi F. Weaning from mechanical ventilation. *Semin Respir Crit Care Med.* 2014;35(4):451–468.)

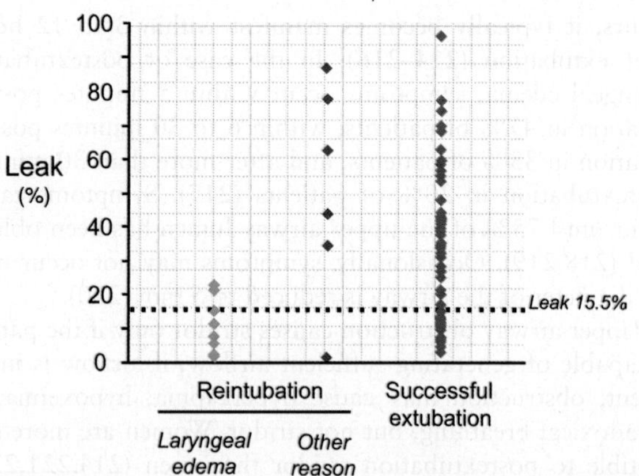

FIGURE 106.33 Cuff leak calculated as the percentage difference between exhaled tidal volume when the cuff of the endotracheal tube was inflated and then deflated. Eight of 76 patients (11%) required reintubation for laryngeal edema. In this study, patients requiring reintubation for laryngeal edema had a smaller leak than the other patients. The best cutoff value for air leak was 15.5%. Small or absent cuff leaks, however, did not necessarily translate in reintubation. The positive predictive value of a leak less than 15.5% was only 25%—i.e., a patient with a small cuff leak still had 75% chance of being extubated without requiring reintubation for laryngeal edema. (Adapted from De Bast Y, De Backer D, Moraine JJ, et al. The cuff leak test to predict failure of tracheal extubation for laryngeal edema. *Intensive Care Med.* 2002;28:1267.)

reasons, however, it is difficult to provide general recommendations on how to perform and interpret a cuff-leak test (197).

First, the method for performing the test has not been standardized. In particular, none of the investigators addressed the setting of inspired tidal volume, which may influence the size of the leak; the method for quantifying the leak varies between absolute units (milliliters) and percentage of inspired tidal volume. Second, the outcome criterion is not always clearly stated: rate of reintubation for any reason, occurrence of stridor of any severity, or occurrence of stridor that requires reintubation. The rates of stridor vary considerably among studies, suggesting that investigators used different criteria; admittedly, it is not obvious that severity of stridor can be graded in any reproducible manner. Third, in some studies, it is not clear whether the investigators carefully excluded reasons for reintubation other than stridor. If a patient is reintubated because of left ventricular failure, it is not logic to expect the cuff-leak test to predict such an event. Fourth, the thresholds for defining a significant leak vary. Fifth, all calculations of test performance are inevitably overestimates, because none of the investigators split their data-set into training and validation subsets. Finally, in adult patients, small or absent cuff leaks do not necessarily translate in the development of stridor or the need for reintubation, and vice versa (Fig. 106.33) (216,222,226–228). In view of all the above observations, some investigators reason that in adult patients, failing a cuff-leak test should not be used as an indication for either delaying extubation or initiating other specific therapy (222,226,229) but, possibly, as an indicator of increasing vigilance at the time of extubation (229). Factors which may contribute to small or absent cuff leaks in patients who do not develop postextubation distress include:secretions located around the endotracheal tube; head and neck position; presence or absence of sedation; and large endotracheal tube relative to the size of the patient's larynx (222,230). When upper airway obstruction due to laryngeal edema is of concern, intensivists may opt to administer systemic corticosteroids before extubation (217).

Laryngeal Ultrasound

In intubated patients, laryngeal ultrasonography can delineate the anatomical structures of the larynx, and it can record the shape and width of the column of air—both within and around the endotracheal tube—which passes through the vocal cords (230). The difference between the air column width before and during a cuff leak test is measured and has been studied as a possible predictor of postextubation laryngeal stridor due to laryngeal edema (Fig. 106.34). So far, five prospective studies show contrasting results. Three of them found a positive relation between the air column width and the likelihood of postextubation stridor—the smaller the air column width, the higher the occurrence of stridor (230–232). In contrast, the remaining two found a very low sensitivity and positive predictive value of the air column width in predicting postextubation stridor (227,228), even when combined with indirect laryngoscopic examination (232). Moreover, with the exception of few patients in one study (228), no investigator has specifically addressed the reliability of air column width measurements in obese patients, or in patients with endotracheal tubes with an inner diameter smaller than 7.5 mm. Finally, no study has addressed the use of laryngeal ultrasonography in difficult-to-wean patients. Accordingly, it is premature to use laryngeal ultrasonography as a screening tool to predict postextubation stridor.

Secretions and Cough

A proportion of patients fail either a weaning attempt or an extubation attempt because of excessive airway secretions. Investigators have evaluated measurements of secretions as predictors of postextubation distress (213,233–236). Salam et al. (234) tested cough strength by means of cough peak flow in 88 patients deemed ready for extubation. Cough peak flow was lower in extubation failures than extubation successes: 58 ± 5 (SE) versus 80 ± 4 L/min. A threshold peak flow of

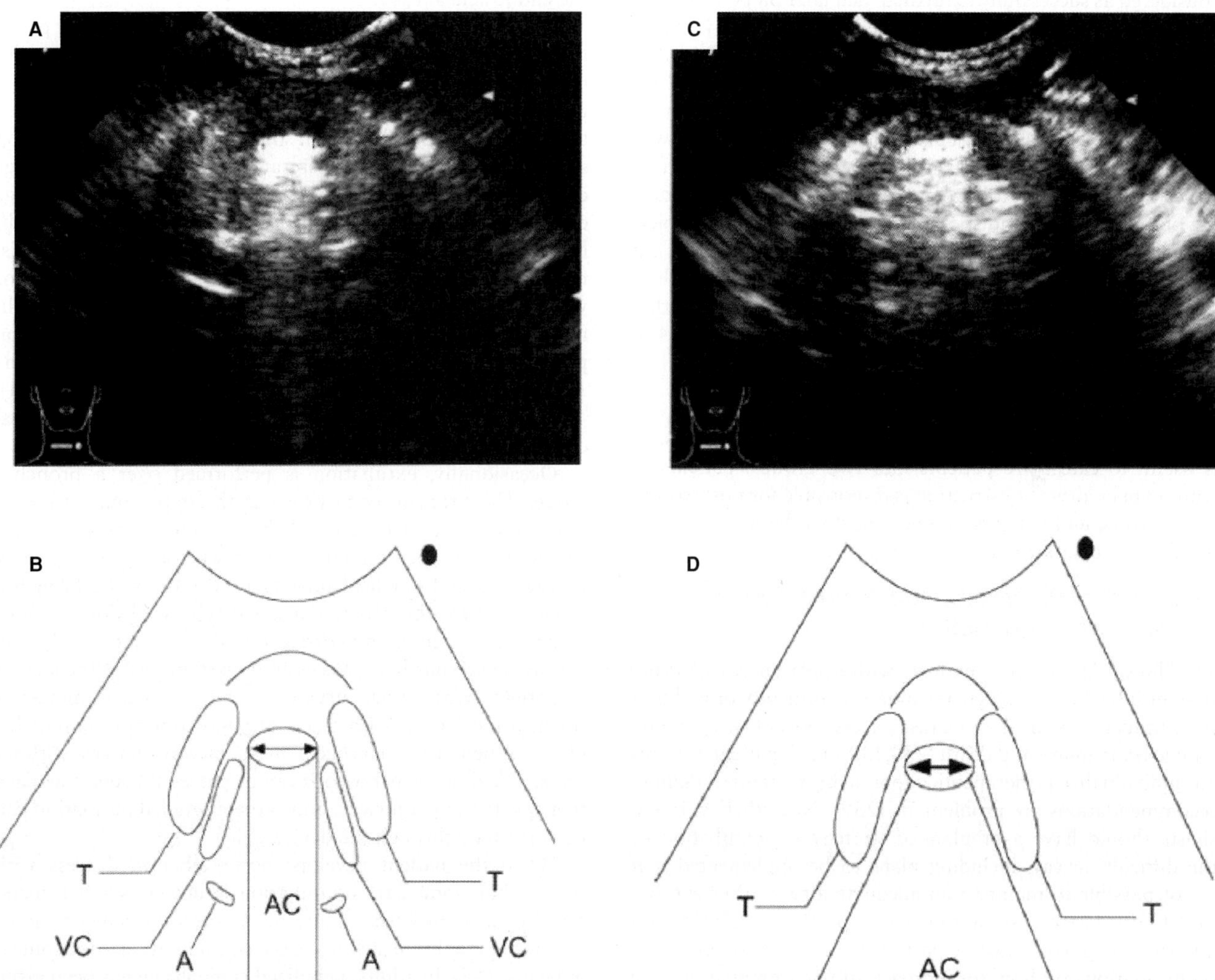

FIGURE 106.34 Laryngeal ultrasound in an intubated patient who did not develop postextubation stridor. When the cuff on the endotracheal tube is inflated—ultrasound (A) and schematic illustration (B)—the column of air (AC) passing through the true vocal cords (VC) is square-shaped. The hypoechoic true vocal cords can be seen on both sides of the air-column. The hyperechoic arytenoid cartilages (A) are located behind the true vocal cords and next to the air-column. When the cuff is deflated—ultrasound (C) and schematic illustration (D)—the column of air passing through the true vocal cords becomes trapezoid and the air-column width increases. In addition, the acoustic shadow of the laryngeal air-column masks the arytenoid cartilages and part of the true vocal cords. T, thyroid cartilage. *Arrows*, width of the air column. (From Ding LW, Wang HC, Wu HD, et al. Laryngeal ultrasound: a useful method in predicting post-extubation stridor. A pilot study. *Eur Respir J*. 2006;27:384.)

less than or equal to 60 L/min had a sensitivity of 0.77, and a specificity 0.66, likelihood ratio 2.3, and risk ratio 4.8.

Neurologic Assessment

Some ventilated patients demonstrate good respiratory function and tolerate a T-tube trial without distress, yet their physicians are reluctant to extubate them because they fear that the patients will not be able to protect their airway after extubation (197). Concern about protecting the airway most often arises in a patient with evidence of brain injury. Three groups of investigators—Coplin et al. (235), Namen et al. (155), and Salam et al. (235)—have studied the role of brain function in patients being considered for extubation. The careful study by Coplin et al. (235) demonstrated that a depressed level of consciousness—quantified with the Glasgow Coma Scale score—and absence of a gag reflex should not be used as the sole indication for prolonged intubation.

Conversely, a Glasgow Coma Scale score ≥8 was considered by Namen et al. (155) helpful in predicting successful extubation in brain-injury patients. The fact that half of the patients considered as successfully extubated died later on because they were part of the withdrawal of life-support therapy makes these data impossible to interpret. While the previous studies were conducted in patients with brain injury, Salam et al. (234) evaluated neurologic function as a predictor of reintubation in medical–cardiac ICU patients. Neurologic performance was quantified by requesting patients to perform four simple tasks (237): open their eyes, follow an observer with their eyes, grasp the observer's hand, and stick out their tongue. Patients tolerating extubation performed a higher number of tasks than did the reintubated patients: 3.8 ± 0.1 versus 2.9 ± 0.5. The failure to perform any of the four tasks predicted reintubation with a sensitivity of 0.42, a specificity of 0.91, and a risk ratio of 4.3.

Treatment of Postextubation Distress

When considering therapies for postextubation distress, it is useful to categorize patients into two groups: patients in whom upper airway obstruction is responsible for postextubation distress, and patients in whom postextubation distress is not due to upper airway obstruction.

Treatment of Postextubation Distress due to Upper Airway Obstruction

The clinical approach to patients with upper airway obstruction must be dictated by great caution, as difficulty or inability to reintubate a patient can cause excess morbidity, including anoxic brain injury and death (238,239). Each patient requires an individualized therapeutic approach; therefore, definite recommendations are problematic (239). Nevertheless, intensivists should have a preplanned strategy for extubation of the difficult airway, including plans to be implemented if it is not possible to maintain an adequate airway after extubation (239). Close consultation with an anesthesiologist and an otolaryngologist must be part of this strategy. Because recommendations on how to approach difficult extubations are essentially based on small clinical series or case reports, the appropriate weighting of each recommendation is a matter of judgment and may be influenced by specific expertise at particular institutions. Upper airway obstruction may worsen suddenly because resistance varies with the fourth power of the radius. A slight change in airway anatomy may dramatically increase resistive load (240). For example, manipulation of the upper airway by an inexperienced clinician may induce edema, which can markedly increase airway resistance and induce asphyxia. In general, pharmacotherapy cannot reverse mechanical obstruction (13). To ensure adequate oxygen stores before extubation, patients should be preoxygenated with an FiO_2 of 1.0 for 3 or more minutes (239,241).

Steps for the care of patients with no cuff leak and no identified complicating factors and those for patients with identified complicating factors with or without cuff leak will be discussed separately.

Approach to Patients with No Cuff Leak and No Identified Complicating Factors. When upper airway obstruction is suspected because the patient has failed a cuff-leak test, one possibility is to proceed with extubation while having an anesthesiologist at the bedside. Intubation equipment has to be readily accessible (242). If the patient develops postextubation distress, and reintubation is deemed necessary, the anesthesiologist is immediately available to proceed with reinsertion of the endotracheal tube.

Before extubation, the anesthesiologist may consider placement of an airway exchange catheter (AEC) through the endotracheal tube (Fig. 106.35) (243–246). Following extubation, the AEC is secured, and humidified oxygen can be insufflated through its central lumen. If the patient does not develop stridor or other signs of respiratory difficulty, the exchange catheter is removed after a variable period of time; exchange catheters have been left in place for up 72 hours (243). If, however, the patient develops postextubation respiratory distress, and reintubation is deemed necessary, the AEC (with or without the help of laryngoscope) (198) can be used to facilitate reintubation (243–245). Should tracheal reintubation prove complicated, jet ventilation can be delivered through the AEC as a bridge to more definitive treatment (199,241,244). To avoid the risk of aspiration, patients should not be fed enterally while the AEC is in place (244).

Occasionally, extubation is performed over a bronchoscope. The bronchoscope provides the opportunity to visually assess the upper airway. When significant abnormalities are noted, the operator must decide whether to immediately reinsert the endotracheal tube or to withdraw the bronchoscope and treat the patient conservatively (see below, racemic epinephrine, heliox, and corticosteroids). The laryngeal mask airway device has been successfully used to rescue the airway in patients with upper airway obstruction when emergency tracheal intubation with direct laryngoscopy was impossible (247). When using laryngeal mask airway devices without grills, a flexible bronchoscope can be passed through the mask to assess the upper airway, and catheter-guided intubation can be performed through the device (247).

When the patient develops postextubation distress with stridor, but immediate reintubation is not considered necessary, some intensivists administer aerosolized epinephrine or racemic epinephrine as long as the compounds are not contraindicated (15). In adults, nebulized epinephrine has been given at a dose of 0.5 mg/kg of 1:1,000 solution, and aerosolized racemic epinephrine has been given at doses ranging from 0.25 to 0.75 mL of a 2.25% solution in 2.0 to 3.5 mL of normal saline (15). In patients with laryngeal edema the response to aerosolized epinephrine or racemic epinephrine can be dramatic but short-lived (15). Therefore, if there is a positive

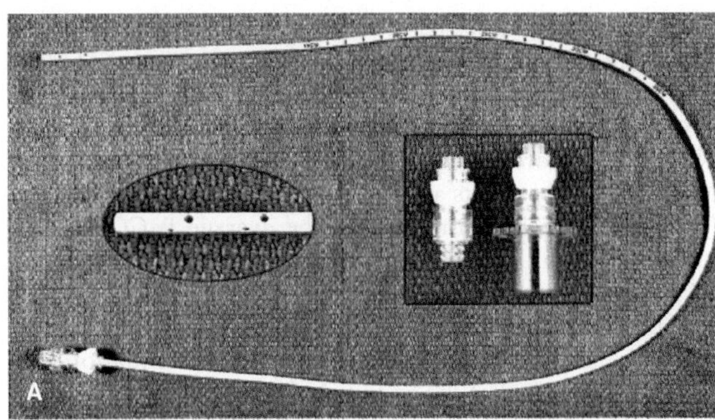

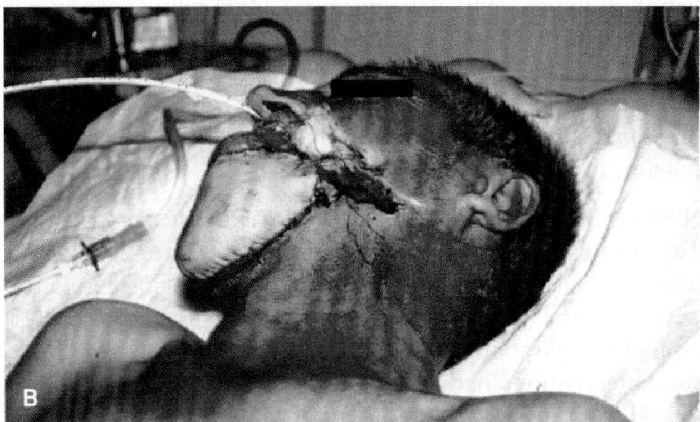

FIGURE 106.35 **A**: The airway exchange catheter is a semi-rigid catheter designed to maintain airway access following tracheal extubation. **Left inset**: In the distal 3 cm, several side holes are built into the catheter to allow delivery of gas if needed. **Right inset**: In the proximal end, a 15-mm connector for attachment to oxygen tubing (**right**) and a Luer lock connector (**left**) for attachment to jet ventilator circuit. **B**: A representative patient following maxillofacial reconstructive surgery. The airway exchange catheter is emerging from the right nostril and is connected to an oxygen source. At the time of surgery the endotracheal tube—through which the airway exchange catheter had been introduced at the time of extubation—was placed nasally. Airway exchange catheters have been used as stylet to facilitate reintubation of medical and surgical patients through the oral and nasal routes (see text for details). (**A**: From Loudermilk EP, Hartmannsgruber M, Stoltzfus DP, et al. A prospective study of the safety of tracheal extubation using a pediatric airway exchange catheter for patients with a known difficult airway. *Chest.* 1997;111:1660; **B**: From Dosemeci L, Yilmaz M, Yegin A, et al. The routine use of pediatric airway exchange catheter after extubation of adult patients who have undergone maxillofacial or major neck surgery: a clinical observational study. *Crit Care.* 2004;8:R385.)

response and patients do not develop side effects, nebulization of epinephrine or racemic epinephrine can be repeated every 1 to 4 hours; repeated doses of racemic epinephrine every 30 to 60 minutes have also been used (15). The employment of the racemic form of epinephrine rather than the homologous levo-isomer is based on the supposition that the former produces epinephrine's vasoconstrictor action without rebound vasodilation, and with fewer side effects such as tachycardia, hypertension, and tremor. The stated different actions, however, may have arisen from comparisons of inappropriate dosages (197). In children with postextubation stridor, levo-epinephrine is as effective as the more expensive racemic epinephrine (15).

High-dose corticosteroids—for example, dexamethasone 4 to 8 mg intravenously every 8 to 12 hours (248,249), tapered based on symptoms—may be administered alone or together with aerosolized racemic epinephrine. Whether corticosteroids should be administered before extubation in children or in adults remains controversial. The timing of administration seems to contribute to the therapeutic effect (15). All positive trials started corticosteroids 6 to 24 hours before planned extubation (217,250,251), and more recently, François et al. (217) reported that, compared to placebo, intravenous methylprednisolone started 12 hours before a planned extubation in patients being intubated for more than 36 hours, reduced the incidence of postextubation laryngeal edema from 22% to 3% ($p < 0.0001$) and reduced the incidence of reintubation from 8% to 4% ($p = 0.02$). On the other hand, all negative trials started corticosteroids 30 minutes to 6 hours before extubation (214,221,252). In contrast to common practice in weaning, directed to the prevention of iatrogenic complications, the approach of François et al. (217) may systematically delay the extubation time by 12 hours in patients deemed ready for extubation. Therefore, the administration of corticosteroids in every patient intubated for more than 36 hours seems premature, while it may be justifiable in patients with a high suspicion of laryngeal edema and no contraindications to steroids.

For patients who do not require high FiO_2, helium–oxygen mixture (heliox)[4] may be tried (249,253–258). The goal of this low-density gas mixture is to reduce work of breathing by decreasing the pressure drop associated with turbulent flow across the obstruction. In most cases of airway obstruction, the response to heliox can be seen in minutes (254). If heliox is ineffective, it is likely that turbulent flow is not playing an important role in the patient's stridor. Even when effective, the use of helium–oxygen mixtures should not engender a false sense of security (240).

Finally, some authors also use noninvasive ventilation—CPAP (259) or bi-level positive airway pressure (BIPAP) (231,254,259)—alone or in combination with heliox (255). Neither heliox nor noninvasive ventilation has curative properties on their own. Yet, they may be able to "buy time" until the underlying cause of upper airway obstruction has resolved (e.g., laryngeal edema treated with high-dose corticosteroids). None of these pharmacologic and nonpharmacologic strategies have been studied systematically. If stridor does not respond to initial measures or recurs while patients are being treated with noninvasive ventilation, reintubation is usually necessary.

Racemic epinephrine, systemic corticosteroids, heliox, and noninvasive ventilation should be used only in carefully selected patients. Occasionally, the decision to defer intubation may give time to the obstruction of the upper airway to progress to a point at which intubation becomes more difficult, if not impossible (253). Similarly, pharmacologic strategies and noninvasive ventilation should not supplant endotracheal intubation when the upper airway obstruction is critical and expected to progress—e.g., upper airway infection, upper airway tumor awaiting surgery, or radiation therapy (253).

Approach to Patients with Identified Complicating Factors with or without Cuff Leak. It may be prudent to have both an anesthesiologist and an otolaryngologist—the latter with an available tracheostomy tray open and ready to use—at the bedside during extubation of patients who fail a cuff-leak test and are known to be at high risk for complications. This is

[4]Mixtures of heliox and oxygen containing less than 70% helium are probably of little or no mechanical benefit (254).

the case for patients that had stridor during the original intubation, in patients with a history of self-extubation, those who experienced a traumatic intubation, patient who needed for multiple attempts at direct tracheal intubation, unsuccessful direct laryngoscopy followed by intubation using an alternate method such as fibreoptic intubation or nasal intubation, in patients with abnormal anatomy,[5] or in patients with cervical immobility or instability (244). If the patient develops postextubation distress, and the anesthesiologist is unable to reinsert the endotracheal tube, the surgeon will be immediately available to perform a cricothyrotomy or tracheostomy. If time permits, and the patient is conscious and moving sufficient air to speak, some clinicians consider best to transport the patient to the operating room (260); otherwise, the procedure should be performed at the bedside. Although percutaneous tracheostomy is gaining in popularity, it is best performed in an already intubated patient and not as an emergency procedure (260).

Unless upper airway tumor is considered as a possible cause of upper airway obstruction, endoscopic visualization of the upper airway before extubation has limited value (261), and it is usually not performed. In some high-risk patients, clinicians may decide to perform an elective tracheostomy (244). A patient with an obstructed airway should not be sedated until the airway has been secured, as minimal sedation may precipitate acute respiratory failure (13).

Treatment of Postextubation Distress Not due to Upper Airway Obstruction

As with patients developing postextubation distress due to upper airway obstruction, patients developing postextubation distress due to other causes require individualized therapy—e.g., chest tube for pneumothorax, bronchodilators for bronchoconstriction, and diuretics for volume overload or negative pressure pulmonary edema (13). In addition to specific therapies, investigators have studied the usefulness of NIPPV as a means of preventing the occurrence of respiratory failure after successful extubation (262,263) and as rescue therapy to treat new-onset respiratory failure after extubation (208,264).

NIPPV to Prevent Respiratory Failure after Successful Extubation. Older age, severity of illness, cardiac failure, longer duration of ventilation, and development of hypercapnia ($PaCO_2 > 45$ mmHg) during a spontaneous breathing trial are some of the factors associated with postextubation respiratory failure and need for reintubation (262,263). In a prospective study of 106 patients with a chronic pulmonary disorder, mainly COPD, who were hypercapnic during a successful spontaneous breathing trial, Ferrer et al. (263) assessed the efficacy of NIPPV to avert postextubation respiratory failure. Inspiratory pressure was set between 12 and 20 cm H_2O. Expiratory pressure was set between 5 and 6 cm H_2O. As compared to conventional medical management, continuous use of NIPPV delivered during the first 24 hours after extubation reduced the frequency of respiratory failure from 48% to 15% ($p < 0.0001$). The mean time from extubation to respiratory failure was 29 ± 13 (SD) hours in the NIPPV group and 17 ± 18 hours in the conventional management group ($p = 0.098$).

By study design (263), NIPPV was used as rescue therapy in all patients who developed postextubation respiratory failure independent of original allocation. This is the likely reason why reintubation rate was similar in both groups of patients. Ninety-day mortality was lower in patients assigned to NIPPV than in patients assigned to conventional management ($p = 0.015$). In this study (263), the average $PaCO_2$ during mechanical ventilation of patients randomized to NIPPV was 48 ± 6 mmHg, and at the end of the breathing trial, it was 55 ± 6 mmHg. In patients randomized to conventional management, the average $PaCO_2$ during mechanical ventilation was 48 ± 7 mmHg, and at the end of the breathing trial, it was 53 ± 5 mmHg. These observations raise two points. First, NIPPV should be considered in the first 24 hours after successful extubation in hypercapnic patients with COPD who experience a worsening in $PaCO_2$ during the trial of spontaneous breathing. Second, whether hypercapnic patients with COPD who do not experience an increase in $PaCO_2$ during a trial of spontaneous breathing should receive prophylactic NIPPV after extubation remains to be determined.

NIPPV as a Rescue of Postextubation Respiratory Failure. Two groups of investigators have reported that rescue NIPPV was not beneficial in a mixed population of postextubated patients who had developed respiratory distress during the 48 hours from extubation (208,264). In the first study (264), the two interventions had similar rates of reintubation (72% in the NIPPV group, 69% in the usual care group) and hospital mortality (31% for both groups). In the second study (208), the rates of reintubation were identical (48% vs. 48%), but there was a significantly higher time to reintubation (12 vs. 2.5 hours) and ICU mortality (25% and 14%) for the group treated with NIPPV when compared to the arm treated with usual care. In these two studies, the level of ventilator assistance—pressure support of 5 cm H_2O (264) or delivered V_T of as little as 5 mL/kg (208)—may have been inadequate to truly test the efficacy of NIPPV in this circumstance. This possibility is supported by two recent studies conducted in patients with chronic pulmonary disorders, most of whom had COPD (174,263). The first study demonstrated rescue NIPPV prevented reintubation in 75% of patients with postextubation respiratory failure (263). The mean inspiratory pressure used was 17 ± 3 (SD) cm H_2O (263). In the second study (174), rescue NIPPV prevented reintubation in 45% of patients. Here the inspiratory pressure was titrated to achieve an expiratory V_T greater than 7 mL/kg (174).

NIPPV Postextubation: Putting All Together. In summary, we favor the use of NIPPV after a planned extubation (i.e., patients who have passed a T-tube trial) as long as the following caveats are borne in mind (265): (a) NIPPV for weaning and extubation must be reserved mainly for patients with COPD—particularly those who are hypercapnic; (b) patients must be good candidates for NIPPV (Table 106.4); (c) patients should have been easy to intubate; (d) before extubation, patients must be comfortable and well oxygenated on levels of pressure support and FiO_2 that can be safely delivered via mask after extubation, for example, pressure support <15 to 20 cm H_2O and FiO_2 <0.4 to 0.5. In regard to the role of NIPPV in weaning from hypoxemic respiratory failure, so far insufficient data are available. Finally, very seldom do we use either sedation or analgesia during NIPPV, and when we do use such medications, we do not use them together (266).

[5]Patients who had undergone maxillofacial or major neck surgery, morbidly obese patients, soft tissue swelling due to trauma or allergic reactions, goiter or other masses.

TABLE 106.4 Possible Predictors of Postextubation Distress

Ability to sustain spontaneous ventilation
Weaning-predictor tests
Cuff-leak test
Laryngeal ultrasound
Secretions and cough
Neurologic assessment

High-Flow Nasal Oxygen for Postextubation Distress. Supplemental oxygen represents first-line treatment in patients with acute hypoxemic respiratory failure (267). Oxygen therapy can be delivered by means of standard, low-flow devices, or by higher-flow devices, such as the Venturi mask, that utilize the Bernoulli effect to provide a more consistent flow rate and a higher FiO_2 when compared to conventional low-flow systems (268). The FiO_2 delivered by these devices, however, depend greatly on a patient's respiratory effort—i.e., the higher the peak inspiratory flow, the greater the entrainment of *room air*, in turn lowering the delivered FiO_2 (269). High-flow oxygen via nasal cannula (HFNC) is a newer oxygen delivery system with potentially important physiologic and clinical effects. HFNC can generate flow rates of up to 60 L/min; by exceeding a patient's peak inspiratory flow, it minimizes the entrainment of room air and can thereby deliver an FiO_2 much more closely matched to the set concentration (270). In addition, the high-operative gas flow creates both a small amount of flow-dependent nasopharyngeal PEEP, and produces a washout effect on the upper airways dead space by creating an oxygen reservoir (268,271). A reduction in inspiratory effort, along with a decreased respiratory rate (272,273), may be the mechanism by which HFNC improves patient comfort (272,274,275). Given its physiologic effects, Maggiore et al. (275) recently evaluated the role of HFNC in the management of patients immediately after extubation. In a series of 105 patients with a PaO_2/FiO_2 ratio of less than 300 prior to extubation, patients were randomized to receive either HFNC or Venturi mask for 48 hours after extubation. Patients in the HFNC group demonstrated superior oxygenation, less discomfort, and better tolerance of the delivery device. Moreover, the need for NIPPV postextubation and the rate of reintubation were less in the HFNC group than in the Venturi mask group. Unfortunately, the study was not powered to provide definitive conclusions in regards to weaning outcome. A trial specifically designed to test whether HFNC is superior to Venturi mask in reducing the reintubation rates in patients with moderate hypoxemia is currently ongoing (ClinicalTrials.gov:NCT02107183).

TRACHEOSTOMY AND LONG-TERM ACUTE CARE HOSPITALS

Patients who receive mechanical ventilation and cannot be extubated often undergo tracheostomy. A tracheostomy is considered more comfortable and thus may allow for a lowering of sedative and narcotic doses. In a recent meta-analysis that included 14 trials enrolling 2,406 patients, Szakmany et al. (276) reported that early tracheostomy (within 10 days of intubation) leads to more procedures and a shorter duration of sedation. Early tracheostomy, however, did not reduce mortality, duration of mechanical ventilation, ICU stay, or ventilator-associated pneumonia (276).

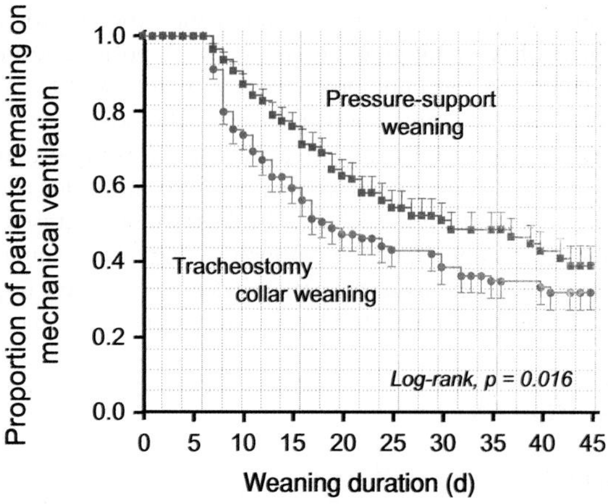

FIGURE 106.36 Weaning in patients requiring prolonged mechanical ventilation (>21 days) and cared for at long-term acute care hospital (LTACH). Kaplan–Meier plot of proportion of patients remaining on mechanical ventilation in the pressure support arm (*blue line*, *n* = 152) and the tracheostomy collar arm (*orange line*, *n* = 160). Weaning time was greater with pressure support than with tracheostomy collar (log rank, *p* = 0.016). After adjusting for baseline covariates (chosen *a priori*) that can influence weaning duration in a Cox proportional hazards model, rate of successful weaning was 1.43 times higher with trach-collar than with pressure support. Mortality was equivalent in the pressure-support and tracheostomy collar groups at 6 months and at 12 months. (Adapted from Jubran A, Grant BJ, Duffner LA, et al. Effect of pressure support vs unassisted breathing through a tracheostomy collar on weaning duration in patients requiring prolonged mechanical ventilation: a randomized trial. *JAMA*. 2013;309(7):671–677.)

Tracheostomized patients requiring prolonged mechanical ventilation (>21 days) are commonly weaned in long-term acute care hospitals (LTACHs). In these centers, weaning is started as soon as possible, as about 20% of patients succeed weaning at their first trial of unsupported respiration. The best time window for successful weaning seems to be within the initial 3 weeks from transfer to an LTACH (148,277,278).

In a recent study of more than 300 tracheostomized patients cared for in an LTACH, Jubran et al. (279) compared the effect of unassisted breathing through a tracheostomy collar versus pressure support on weaning duration. In that study, weaning by unassisted breathing through a tracheostomy resulted in shorter median weaning time (15 days with tracheostomy collar vs. 19 days with pressure support) (Fig. 106.36). Weaning mode had no effect on survival at 6 months (51% with tracheostomy collar vs. 56% with pressure support) and 12 months (60% with tracheostomy collar vs. 66% with pressure support) (279). When liberation from mechanical ventilation ultimately becomes improbable (more than 1 month of a structured, multidisciplinary weaning approach), home ventilation has to be considered (277,278).

CONCLUSION

In conclusion, to reduce the possibility of delayed weaning or premature extubation, clinicians should contemplate a two-step diagnostic strategy: irst, measurement of weaning predictors, and second, a weaning trial. Each step constitutes a diagnostic test, and therefore, clinicians must be aware of the scientific principles of diagnostic testing when they interpret the information produced by each step (2). The key point is for physicians to consider the possibility that a patient *just may* be able to tolerate weaning. Such diagnostic triggering is facilitated through use of a screening test and is the rationale for measurement of weaning-predictor tests (2). A positive result on a screening test (weaning-predictor test) is followed by a confirmatory test (weaning trial) to increase the possibility that a patient will successfully tolerate extubation. It is important not to postpone the use of a screening test by waiting for a more complex diagnostic test, such as a T-tube trial. In contrast to our greater understanding of the pathophysiology of weaning failure, our understanding of the pathophysiology of severe respiratory distress in the postextubation period remains rudimentary.

Key Points

Pathophysiology of Weaning

- Most patients who fail a trial of weaning from mechanical ventilation demonstrate progressive impairment of pulmonary mechanics.
- Weakness of respiratory muscles that predates the episode of critical illness, or that which develops during the course of it, may be an important contributing factor to failure to wean from mechanical ventilation.

Screening Tests for Weaning from Mechanical Ventilation

- To avoid iatrogenic complications related to mechanical ventilation, physicians must maintain a high index of suspicion that a patient *may* be ready for a weaning trial. Accordingly, clinicians must employ screening tests with the highest possible sensitivity to identify patients appropriate for a weaning trial.
- The ratio of respiratory frequency to tidal volume (f/V_t) has been extensively evaluated and is the most reliable screening test with regards to weaning, carrying a sensitivity of 0.89.
- Evaluating shifts in cardiorespiratory parameters, such as left ventricular filling pressure and esophageal pressure, may have a complimentary role in testing for readiness to wean from mechanical ventilation.

Weaning Trial and Extubation

- Among the weaning techniques, T-tube trials and pressure-support trials perform better than IMV trials.
- The role of computerized approaches to weaning, particularly in medical–ICU patients, appears promising.
- Postextubation distress is difficult to predict and often leads to reintubation, an event that carries a six-fold increase in mortality when compared to successful extubation.
- One of the main causes of postextubation distress is upper airway obstruction; respiratory failure, congestive heart failure, and excessive secretions are less commonly involved.
- NIPPV can be a valuable option to prevent and treat postextubation respiratory distress in selected hypercapnic patients with COPD without upper airway obstruction.

ACKNOWLEDGMENTS

The authors are grateful to Dr. Martin Tobin for his comments on the specific content of this chapter.

References

1. Provost KA, El Solh A. Complications associated with mechanical ventilation. In: Tobin MJ, ed. *Principles and Practice of Mechanical Ventilation.* 3rd ed. New York, NY: McGraw-Hill; 2013:973–993.
2. Tobin MJ, Jubran A. Weaning from mechanical ventilation. In: Tobin MJ, ed. *Principles and Practice of Mechanical Ventilation.* 3rd ed. New York, NY: McGraw-Hill; 2013:1307–1351.
3. Kollef MH, Shapiro SD, Silver P, et al. A randomized, controlled trial of protocol-directed versus physician-directed weaning from mechanical ventilation. *Crit Care Med.* 1997;25(4):567–574.
4. Epstein SK. Etiology of extubation failure and the predictive value of the rapid shallow breathing index. *Am J Respir Crit Care Med.* 1995;152(2):545–549.
5. Yang KL, Tobin MJ. A prospective study of indexes predicting the outcome of trials of weaning from mechanical ventilation. *N Engl J Med.* 1991;324(21):1445–1450.
6. Laghi F, Morales D. Predictors of weaning from mechanical ventilation. *Eur Respir Mon.* 2012;55:169–190.
7. Tobin MJ, Laghi F, Jubran A. Ventilatory failure, ventilator support, and ventilator weaning. *Compr Physiol.* 2012;2(4):2871–2921.
8. Esteban A, Frutos F, Tobin MJ, et al. A comparison of four methods of weaning patients from mechanical ventilation. Spanish Lung Failure Collaborative Group. *N Engl J Med.* 1995;332(6):345–350.
9. Esteban A, Alia I, Tobin MJ, et al. Effect of spontaneous breathing trial duration on outcome of attempts to discontinue mechanical ventilation. Spanish Lung Failure Collaborative Group. *Am J Respir Crit Care Med.* 1999;159(2):512–518.
10. West JB. *Pulmonary Pathophysiology: The Essentials.* 8th ed. Philadelphia, PA: Lippincott Williams & Wilkins; 2012.
11. Gluck EH. Predicting eventual success or failure to wean in patients receiving long-term mechanical ventilation. *Chest.* 1996;110(4):1018–1024.
12. Younes M. Mechanisms of ventilatory failure. *Curr Pulmonol.* 1993;14:243–292.
13. Laghi F, Tobin MJ. Indications for mechanical ventilation. In: Tobin MJ, ed. *Principles and Practice of Mechanical Ventilation.* 3rd ed. New York, NY: McGraw-Hill; 2013:101–138.
14. Jubran A, Tobin MJ. Pathophysiologic basis of acute respiratory distress in patients who fail a trial of weaning from mechanical ventilation. *Am J Respir Crit Care Med.* 1997;155(3):906–915.
15. Laghi F. Weaning from mechanical ventilation. In: Gabrielli A, Layon AJ, Yu M, eds. *Civetta, Taylor, and Kirby's Handbook of Critical Care.* 4th ed. Philadelphia, PA: Lippincott Williams & Wilkins; 2009:1991–2028.
16. Purro A, Appendini L, De Gaetano A, et al. Physiologic determinants of ventilator dependence in long-term mechanically ventilated patients. *Am J Respir Crit Care Med.* 2000;161(4 Pt 1):1115–1123.
17. Shaikh H, Morales D, Laghi F. Weaning from mechanical ventilation. *Semin Respir Crit Care Med.* 2014;35(4):451–468.
18. Laghi F, Tobin MJ. Disorders of the respiratory muscles. *Am J Respir Crit Care Med.* 2003;168(1):10–48.
19. Cooper KR, Phillips BA. Effect of short-term sleep loss on breathing. *J Appl Physiol.* 1982;53(4):855–858.
20. Spengler CM, Shea SA. Sleep deprivation per se does not decrease the hypercapnic ventilatory response in humans. *Am J Respir Crit Care Med.* 2000;161(4 Pt 1):1124–1128.
21. Zakynthinos SG, Vassilakopoulos T, Roussos C. The load of inspiratory muscles in patients needing mechanical ventilation. *Am J Respir Crit Care Med.* 1995;152(4 Pt 1):1248–1255.
22. D'Angelo E, Calderini E, Robatto FM, et al. Lung and chest wall mechanics in patients with acquired immunodeficiency syndrome and severe *Pneumocystis carinii* pneumonia. *Eur Respir J.* 1997;10(10):2343–2350.
23. Appendini L, Purro A, Patessio A, et al. Partitioning of inspiratory muscle workload and pressure assistance in ventilator-dependent COPD patients. *Am J Respir Crit Care Med.* 1996;154(5):1301–1309.
24. Laghi F, Cattapan SE, Jubran A, et al. Is weaning failure caused by low-frequency fatigue of the diaphragm? *Am J Respir Crit Care Med.* 2003;167(2):120–127.
25. Jubran A, Laghi F, Mazur M, et al. Partitioning of lung and chest-wall mechanics before and after lung volume reduction surgery. *Am J Respir Crit Care Med.* 1998;158(1):306–310.
26. Parthasarathy S, Jubran A, Laghi F, Tobin MJ. Sternomastoid, rib-cage and expiratory muscle activity during weaning failure. *J Appl Physiol.* 2007;103(1):140–147. doi: 10.1152/japplphysiol.00904.2006.
27. Zakynthinos SG, Vassilakopoulos T, Zakynthinos E, et al. Contribution of expiratory muscle pressure to dynamic intrinsic positive end-expiratory pressure: validation using the Campbell diagram. *Am J Respir Crit Care Med.* 2000;162(5):1633–1640.

28. Parthasarathy S, Jubran A, Tobin MJ. Cycling of inspiratory and expiratory muscle groups with the ventilator in airflow limitation. *Am J Respir Crit Care Med.* 1998;158(5 Pt 1):1471–1478.
29. Fiastro JF, Habib MP, Shon BY, Campbell SC. Comparison of standard weaning parameters and the mechanical work of breathing in mechanically ventilated patients. *Chest.* 1988;94(2):232–238.
30. Tobin MJ, Laghi F. Monitoring respiratory muscle function. In: Tobin MJ, ed. *Principles and Practice of Intensive Care Monitoring.* New York, NY: McGraw-Hill; 1998:497–544.
31. Zakynthinos S, Routsi C, Vassilakopoulos T, et al. Differential cardiovascular responses during weaning failure: effects on tissue oxygenation and lactate. *Intensive Care Med.* 2005;31(12):1634–1642.
32. Sassoon CS, Mahutte CK. Airway occlusion pressure and breathing pattern as predictors of weaning outcome. *Am Rev Respir Dis.* 1993;148(4 Pt 1): 860–866.
33. Laghi F, D'Alfonso N, Tobin MJ. A paper on the pace of recovery from diaphragmatic fatigue and its unexpected dividends. *Intensive Care Med.* 2014;40(9):1220–1226.
34. Cattapan SE, Laghi F, Tobin MJ. Can diaphragmatic contractility be assessed by airway twitch pressure in mechanically ventilated patients? *Thorax.* 2003;58(1):58–62.
35. Watson AC, Hughes PD, Louise HM, et al. Measurement of twitch transdiaphragmatic, esophageal, and endotracheal tube pressure with bilateral anterolateral magnetic phrenic nerve stimulation in patients in the intensive care unit. *Crit Care Med.* 2001;29(7):1325–1331.
36. Polkey MI, Kyroussis D, Hamnegard CH, et al. Diaphragm strength in chronic obstructive pulmonary disease. *Am J Respir Crit Care Med.* 1996;154(5):1310–1317.
37. Laghi F, Jubran A, Topeli A, et al. Effect of lung volume reduction surgery on diaphragmatic neuromechanical coupling at 2 years. *Chest.* 2004; 125(6):2188–2195.
38. Supinski GS, Callahan LA. Diaphragm weakness in mechanically ventilated critically ill patients. *Crit Care.* 2013;17(3):R120.
39. Braun NM, Arora NS, Rochester DF. Respiratory muscle and pulmonary function in polymyositis and other proximal myopathies. *Thorax.* 1983;38(8):616–623.
40. Gibson GJ, Gilmartin JJ, Veale D, et al. Respiratory muscle function in neuromuscular disease. In: Jones NL, Killian KJ, eds. *Breathlessness: The Campbell Symposium.* Hamilton: Boehringer-Ingelheim; 1992:66–73.
41. Laghi F, Goyal A. Auto-PEEP in respiratory failure. *Minerva Anestesiol.* 2012;78(2):201–221.
42. Laghi F. Mechanical ventilation in chronic obstructive pulmonary disease. In: Tobin MJ, ed. *Principles and Practice of Mechanical Ventilation.* 3rd ed. New York, NY: McGraw-Hill; 2013:741–759.
43. Laghi F, Jubran A, Topeli A, et al. Effect of lung volume reduction surgery on neuromechanical coupling of the diaphragm. *Am J Respir Crit Care Med.* 1998;157(2):475–483.
44. Tobin MJ, Laghi F, Brochard L. Role of the respiratory muscles in acute respiratory failure of COPD: lessons from weaning failure. *J Appl Physiol.* 2009;107(3):962–970.
45. Koutsoukou A, Armaganidis A, Stavrakaki-Kallergi C, et al. Expiratory flow limitation and intrinsic positive end-expiratory pressure at zero positive end-expiratory pressure in patients with adult respiratory distress syndrome. *Am J Respir Crit Care Med.* 2000;161(5):1590–1596.
46. Pelosi P, Cereda M, Foti G, et al. Alterations of lung and chest wall mechanics in patients with acute lung injury: effects of positive end-expiratory pressure. *Am J Respir Crit Care Med.* 1995;152(2):531–537.
47. Faisy C, Rabbat A, Kouchakji B, Laaban JP. Bioelectrical impedance analysis in estimating nutritional status and outcome of patients with chronic obstructive pulmonary disease and acute respiratory failure. *Intensive Care Med.* 2000;26(5):518–525.
48. Murciano D, Rigaud D, Pingleton S, et al. Diaphragmatic function in severely malnourished patients with anorexia nervosa: effects of renutrition. *Am J Respir Crit Care Med.* 1994;150(6 Pt 1):1569–1574.
49. Schols AM, Soeters PB, Mostert R, et al. Physiologic effects of nutritional support and anabolic steroids in patients with chronic obstructive pulmonary disease: a placebo- controlled randomized trial. *Am J Respir Crit Care Med.* 1995;152(4 Pt 1):1268–1274.
50. Ryan CF, Whittaker JS, Road JD. Ventilatory dysfunction in severe anorexia nervosa. *Chest.* 1992;102(4):1286–1288.
51. Lanz JK Jr, Donahoe M, Rogers RM, Ontell M. Effects of growth hormone on diaphragmatic recovery from malnutrition. *J Appl Physiol.* 1992; 73(3):801–805.
52. Laghi F, Adiguzel N, Tobin MJ. Endocrinological derangements in COPD. *Eur Respir J.* 2009;34(4):975–996.
53. Anzueto A, Peters JI, Tobin MJ, et al. Effects of prolonged controlled mechanical ventilation on diaphragmatic function in healthy adult baboons. *Crit Care Med.* 1997;25(7):1187–1190.
54. Petrof BJ, Hussain SN. Ventilator-induced diaphragmatic dysfunction: what have we learned? *Curr Opin Crit Care.* 2016;22(1):67–72.
55. Crimi E, Liguori A, Condorelli M, et al. The beneficial effects of antioxidant supplementation in enteral feeding in critically ill patients: a prospective, randomized, double-blind, placebo-controlled trial. *Anesth Analg.* 2004;99(3):857–863.
56. Nathens AB, Neff MJ, Jurkovich GJ, et al. Randomized, prospective trial of antioxidant supplementation in critically ill surgical patients. *Ann Surg.* 2002;236(6):814–822.
57. Levine S, Nguyen T, Taylor N, et al. Rapid disuse atrophy of diaphragm fibers in mechanically ventilated humans. *N Engl J Med.* 2008;358(13): 1327–1335.
58. Levine S, Biswas C, Dierov J, et al. Increased proteolysis, myosin depletion, and atrophic AKT-FOXO signaling in human diaphragm disuse. *Am J Respir Crit Care Med.* 2011;183(4):483–490.
59. Pichard C, Kyle U, Chevrolet JC, et al. Lack of effects of recombinant growth hormone on muscle function in patients requiring prolonged mechanical ventilation: a prospective, randomized, controlled study. *Crit Care Med.* 1996;24(3):403–413.
60. Takala J, Ruokonen E, Webster NR, et al. Increased mortality associated with growth hormone treatment in critically ill adults. *N Engl J Med.* 1999;341(11):785–792.
61. Fredriksson K, Tjader I, Keller P, et al. Dysregulation of mitochondrial dynamics and the muscle transcriptome in ICU patients suffering from sepsis induced multiple organ failure. *PLoS One.* 2008;3(11):e3686.
62. Callahan LA, Supinski GS. Sepsis-induced myopathy. *Crit Care Med.* 2009;37(10 Suppl):S354–S367.
63. Fredriksson K, Hammarqvist F, Strigard K, et al. Derangements in mitochondrial metabolism in intercostal and leg muscle of critically ill patients with sepsis-induced multiple organ failure. *Am J Physiol Endocrinol Metab.* 2006;291(5):E1044–E1050.
64. Hermans G, Wilmer A, Meersseman W, et al. Impact of intensive insulin therapy on neuromuscular complications and ventilator dependency in the medical intensive care unit. *Am J Respir Crit Care Med.* 2007;175(5): 480–489.
65. Deem S, Lee CM, Curtis JR. Acquired neuromuscular disorders in the intensive care unit. *Am J Respir Crit Care Med.* 2003;168(7):735–739.
66. Khan J, Harrison TB, Rich MM, Moss M. Early development of critical illness myopathy and neuropathy in patients with severe sepsis. *Neurology.* 2006;67(8):1421–1425.
67. Bednarik J, Vondracek P, Dusek L, et al. Risk factors for critical illness polyneuromyopathy. *J Neurol.* 2005;252(3):343–351.
68. Bolton CF. Neuromuscular manifestations of critical illness. *Muscle Nerve.* 2005;32(2):140–163.
69. Mozaffar T, Haddad F, Zeng M, et al. Molecular and cellular defects of skeletal muscle in an animal model of acute quadriplegic myopathy. *Muscle Nerve.* 2007;35(1):55–65.
70. Larsson L, Li X, Edstrom L, et al. Acute quadriplegia and loss of muscle myosin in patients treated with nondepolarizing neuromuscular blocking agents and corticosteroids: mechanisms at the cellular and molecular levels. *Crit Care Med.* 2000;28(1):34–45.
71. Di Giovanni S, Molon A, Broccolini A, et al. Constitutive activation of MAPK cascade in acute quadriplegic myopathy. *Ann Neurol.* 2004;55(2): 195–206.
72. de Letter MA, van Doorn PA, Savelkoul HF, et al. Critical illness polyneuropathy and myopathy (CIPNM): evidence for local immune activation by cytokine-expression in the muscle tissue. *J Neuroimmunol.* 2000; 106(1–2):206–213.
73. De Jonghe B, Sharshar T, Lefaucheur JP, et al. Paresis acquired in the intensive care unit: a prospective multicenter study. *JAMA.* 2002;288(22): 2859–2867.
74. Lefaucheur JP, Nordine T, Rodriguez P, Brochard L. Origin of ICU acquired paresis determined by direct muscle stimulation. *J Neurol Neurosurg Psychiatry.* 2006;77(4):500–506.
75. De Jonghe B, Bastuji-Garin S, Sharshar T, et al. Does ICU-acquired paresis lengthen weaning from mechanical ventilation? *Intensive Care Med.* 2004;30(6):1117–1121.
76. Latronico N, Shehu I, Seghelini E. Neuromuscular sequelae of critical illness. *Curr Opin Crit Care.* 2005;11(4):381–390.
77. Schweickert WD, Pohlman MC, Pohlman AS, et al. Early physical and occupational therapy in mechanically ventilated, critically ill patients: a randomised controlled trial. *Lancet.* 2009;373(9678):1874–1882.

78. De JB, Bastuji-Garin S, Durand MC, et al. Respiratory weakness is associated with limb weakness and delayed weaning in critical illness. *Crit Care Med.* 2007;35(9):2007–2015.
79. Juan G, Calverley P, Talamo C, et al. Effect of carbon dioxide on diaphragmatic function in human beings. *N Engl J Med.* 1984;310(14):874–879.
80. Roberts PA, Loxham SJ, Poucher SM, et al. Bicarbonate-induced alkalosis augments cellular acetyl group availability and isometric force during the rest-to-work transition in canine skeletal muscle. *Exp Physiol.* 2002;87(4):489–498.
81. de Lemos JM, Carr RR, Shalansky KF, et al. Paralysis in the critically ill: intermittent bolus pancuronium compared with continuous infusion. *Crit Care Med.* 1999;27(12):2648–2655.
82. Segredo V, Caldwell JE, Matthay MA, et al. Persistent paralysis in critically ill patients after long-term administration of vecuronium. *N Engl J Med.* 1992;327(8):524–528.
83. Rudis MI, Sikora CA, Angus E, et al. A prospective, randomized, controlled evaluation of peripheral nerve stimulation versus standard clinical dosing of neuromuscular blocking agents in critically ill patients. *Crit Care Med.* 1997;25(4):575–583.
84. de Seze M, Petit H, Wiart L, et al. Critical illness polyneuropathy: a 2-year follow-up study in 19 severe cases. *Eur Neurol.* 2000;43(2):61–69.
85. Whetstone Foster JG, Clark AP. Functional recovery after neuromuscular blockade in mechanically ventilated critically ill patients. *Heart Lung.* 2006;35(3):178–189.
86. Laghi F, Topeli A, Tobin MJ. Does resistive loading decrease diaphragmatic contractility before task failure? *J Appl Physiol.* 1998;85(3):1103–1112.
87. Laghi F, Harrison MJ, Tobin MJ. Comparison of magnetic and electrical phrenic nerve stimulation in assessment of diaphragmatic contractility. *J Appl Physiol.* 1996;80(5):1731–1742.
88. Laghi F, D'Alfonso N, Tobin MJ. Pattern of recovery from diaphragmatic fatigue over 24 hours. *J Appl Physiol.* 1995;79(2):539–546.
89. Thille AW, Rodriguez P, Cabello B, et al. Patient-ventilator asynchrony during assisted mechanical ventilation. *Intensive Care Med.* 2006;32(10):1515–1522.
90. Chao DC, Scheinhorn DJ, Stearn-Hassenpflug M. Patient-ventilator trigger asynchrony in prolonged mechanical ventilation. *Chest.* 1997;112(6):1592–1599.
91. Gomez H, Pinsky MR. Effect of mechanical ventilation on heart-lung interactions. In: Tobin MJ, ed. *Principles and Practice of Mechanical Ventilation.* 3rd ed. New York, NY: McGraw-Hill; 2013:821–850.
92. Hurford WE, Lynch KE, Strauss HW, et al. Myocardial perfusion as assessed by thallium-201 scintigraphy during the discontinuation of mechanical ventilation in ventilator-dependent patients. *Anesthesiology.* 1991;74(6):1007–1016.
93. Srivastava S, Chatila W, Amoateng-Adjepong Y, et al. Myocardial ischemia and weaning failure in patients with coronary artery disease: an update. *Crit Care Med.* 1999;27(10):2109–2112.
94. Hurford WE, Favorito F. Association of myocardial ischemia with failure to wean from mechanical ventilation. *Crit Care Med.* 1995;23(9):1475–1480.
95. Nozawa E, Azeka E, Ignez ZM, et al. Factors associated with failure of weaning from long-term mechanical ventilation after cardiac surgery. *Int Heart J.* 2005;46(5):819–831.
96. Lemaire F, Teboul JL, Cinotti L, et al. Acute left ventricular dysfunction during unsuccessful weaning from mechanical ventilation. *Anesthesiology.* 1988;69(2):171–179.
97. Jubran A, Mathru M, Dries D, Tobin MJ. Continuous recordings of mixed venous oxygen saturation during weaning from mechanical ventilation and the ramifications thereof. *Am J Respir Crit Care Med.* 1998;158(6):1763–1769.
98. Richard C, Teboul JL. Weaning failure from cardiovascular origin. *Intensive Care Med.* 2005;31(12):1605–1607.
99. Moschietto S, Doyen D, Grech L, et al. Transthoracic echocardiography with Doppler tissue imaging predicts weaning failure from mechanical ventilation: evolution of the left ventricle relaxation rate during a spontaneous breathing trial is the key factor in weaning outcome. *Crit Care.* 2012;16(3):R81.
100. Skrobik Y. Psychological problems in the ventilated patient. In: Tobin MJ, ed. *Principles and Practice of Mechanical Ventilation.* 3rd ed. New York, NY: McGraw-Hill; 2013:1259–1266.
101. Ely EW, Shintani A, Truman B, et al. Delirium as a predictor of mortality in mechanically ventilated patients in the intensive care unit. *JAMA.* 2004;291(14):1753–1762.
102. Shehabi Y, Bellomo R, Reade MC, et al. Early intensive care sedation predicts long-term mortality in ventilated critically ill patients. *Am J Respir Crit Care Med.* 2012;186(8):724–731.
103. Repetz N, Ciccolella DE, Criner GJ. Long-term outcome of patients with delirium on admission to a multidisciplinary ventilator rehabilitation unit (VRU). *Am Respir Crit Care Med.* 2001;163:A889.
104. Kress JP, Gehlbach B, Lacy M, et al. The long-term psychological effects of daily sedative interruption on critically ill patients. *Am J Respir Crit Care Med.* 2003;168(12):1457–1461.
105. Jubran A, Lawm G, Duffner LA, et al. Post-traumatic stress disorder after weaning from prolonged mechanical ventilation. *Intensive Care Med.* 2010;36(12):2030–2037.
106. Martin UJ, Criner GJ. Psychological problems in the ventilated patient. In: Tobin MJ, ed. *Principles and Practice of Mechanical Ventilation.* 2nd ed. New York, NY: McGraw-Hill; 2006:1137–1151.
107. Jubran A, Lawm G, Kelly J, et al. Depressive disorders during weaning from prolonged mechanical ventilation. *Intensive Care Med.* 2010;36(5):828–835.
108. Hanly PJ. Sleep in the ventilated patient. In: Tobin MJ, ed. *Principles and Practice of Mechanical Ventilation.* 2nd ed. New York, NY: McGraw-Hill; 2006:1173–1183.
109. Banzett RB, Brown R. Addressing respiratory discomfort in the ventilated patient. In: Tobin MJ, ed. *Principles and Practice of Mechanical Ventilation.* 2nd ed. New York, NY: McGraw-Hill; 2006:1153–1162.
110. Dubois MJ, Bergeron N, Dumont M, et al. Delirium in an intensive care unit: a study of risk factors. *Intensive Care Med.* 2001;27(8):1297–1304.
111. Ely EW, Gautam S, Margolin R, et al. The impact of delirium in the intensive care unit on hospital length of stay. *Intensive Care Med.* 2001;27(12):1892–1900.
112. Feinstein AR. *Clinical Epidemiology: The Architecture of Clinical Research.* Philadelphia, PA: WB Saunders; 1985.
113. Tobin MJ, Jubran A. Weaning from mechanical ventilation. In: Tobin MJ, ed. *Principles and Practice of Mechanical Ventilation.* 3rd ed. New York, NY: McGraw-Hill; 2006:1307–1351.
114. Tobin MJ, Jubran A. Variable performance of weaning-predictor tests: role of Bayes' theorem and spectrum and test-referral bias. *Intensive Care Med.* 2006;32(12):2002–2012.
115. Patel KN, Ganatra KD, Bates JH, Young MP. Variation in the rapid shallow breathing index associated with common measurement techniques and conditions. *Respir Care.* 2009;54(11):1462–1466.
116. Meade M, Guyatt G, Cook D, et al. Predicting success in weaning from mechanical ventilation. *Chest.* 2001;120(6 Suppl):400S–424S.
117. MacIntyre NR, Cook DJ, Ely EW Jr, et al. Evidence-based guidelines for weaning and discontinuing ventilatory support: a collective task force facilitated by the American College of Chest Physicians; the American Association for Respiratory Care; and the American College of Critical Care Medicine. *Chest.* 2001;120(6 Suppl):375S–395S.
118. Brand R, Kragt H. Importance of trends in the interpretation of an overall odds ratio in the meta-analysis of clinical trials. *Stat Med.* 1992;11(16):2077–2082.
119. Schmid CH, Lau J, McIntosh MW, Cappelleri JC. An empirical study of the effect of the control rate as a predictor of treatment efficacy in meta-analysis of clinical trials. *Stat Med.* 1998;17(17):1923–1942.
120. Sahn SA, Lakshminarayan S. Bedside criteria for discontinuation of mechanical ventilation. *Chest.* 1973;63(6):1002–1005.
121. Chevrolet JC, Deleamont P. Repeated vital capacity measurements as predictive parameters for mechanical ventilation need and weaning success in the Guillain-Barre syndrome. *Am Rev Respir Dis.* 1991;144(4):814–818.
122. Vanderheyden M, Bartunek J, Goethals M. Brain and other natriuretic peptides: molecular aspects. *Eur J Heart Fail.* 2004;6(3):261–268.
123. Grasso S, Leone A, De Michele M, et al. Use of N-terminal pro-brain natriuretic peptide to detect acute cardiac dysfunction during weaning failure in difficult-to-wean patients with chronic obstructive pulmonary disease. *Crit Care Med.* 2007;35(1):96–105.
124. Mekontso DA, Roche-Campo F, Kouatchet A, et al. Natriuretic peptide-driven fluid management during ventilator weaning: a randomized controlled trial. *Am J Respir Crit Care Med.* 2012;186(12):1256–1263.
125. Zapata L, Vera P, Roglan A, et al. B-type natriuretic peptides for prediction and diagnosis of weaning failure from cardiac origin. *Intensive Care Med.* 2011;37(3):477–485.
126. Papanikolaou J, Makris D, Saranteas T, et al. New insights into weaning from mechanical ventilation: left ventricular diastolic dysfunction is a key player. *Intensive Care Med.* 2011;37:1976–1985.
127. Lamia B, Maizel J, Ochagavia A, et al. Echocardiographic diagnosis of pulmonary artery occlusion pressure elevation during weaning from mechanical ventilation. *Crit Care Med.* 2009;37(5):1696–1701.
128. Nagueh SF, Middleton KJ, Kopelen HA, et al. Doppler tissue imaging: a noninvasive technique for evaluation of left ventricular relaxation and estimation of filling pressures. *J Am Coll Cardiol.* 1997;30(6):1527–1533.
129. Schifelbain LM, Vieira SR, Brauner JS, et al. Echocardiographic evaluation during weaning from mechanical ventilation. *Clinics (Sao Paulo).* 2011;66(1):107–111.
130. Caille V, Amiel JB, Charron C, et al. Echocardiography: a help in the weaning process. *Crit Care.* 2010;14(3):R120.

131. Gerbaud E, Erickson M, Grenouillet-Delacre M, et al. Echocardiographic evaluation and N-terminal pro-brain natriuretic peptide measurement of patients hospitalized for heart failure during weaning from mechanical ventilation. *Minerva Anestesiol.* 2012;78(4):415–425.
132. Zieleskiewicz L, Muller L, Lakhal K, et al. Point-of-care ultrasound in intensive care units: assessment of 1073 procedures in a multicentric, prospective, observational study. *Intensive Care Med.* 2015;41(9):1638–1647.
133. Goligher EC, Laghi F, Detsky ME, et al. Measuring diaphragm thickness with ultrasound in mechanically ventilated patients: feasibility, reproducibility and validity. *Intensive Care Med.* 2015;41(4):642–649.
134. Matamis D, Soilemezi E, Tsagourias M, et al. Sonographic evaluation of the diaphragm in critically ill patients: technique and clinical applications. *Intensive Care Med.* 2013;39(5):801–810.
135. Kim WY, Suh HJ, Hong SB, et al. Diaphragm dysfunction assessed by ultrasonography: influence on weaning from mechanical ventilation. *Crit Care Med.* 2011;39(12):2627–2630.
136. Zin WA, Milic-Emili J. Esophageal pressure monitoring. In: Tobin MJ, ed. *Principles and Practice of Intensive Care Monitoring.* New York, NY: McGraw-Hill; 1998:545–552.
137. Akoumianaki E, Maggiore SM, Valenza F, et al. The application of esophageal pressure measurement in patients with respiratory failure. *Am J Respir Crit Care Med.* 2014;189(5):520–531.
138. Gluck EH, Barkoviak MJ, Balk RA, et al. Medical effectiveness of esophageal balloon pressure manometry in weaning patients from mechanical ventilation. *Crit Care Med.* 1995;23(3):504–509.
139. Jubran A, Grant BJ, Laghi F, Parthasarathy S, Tobin MJ. Weaning prediction: esophageal pressure monitoring complements readiness testing. *Am J Respir Crit Care Med.* 2005;171(11):1252–1259.
140. Mauri T, Yoshida T, Bellani G, et al. Esophageal and transpulmonary pressure in the clinical setting: meaning, usefulness and perspectives. *Intensive Care Med.* 2016;42(9):1360–1373. doi: 10.1007/s00134-016-4400-x. Epub 2016 Jun 22.
141. Tobin MJ. Remembrance of weaning past: the seminal papers. *Intensive Care Med.* 2006;32(10):1485–1493.
142. Sassoon CS. Intermittent mechanical ventilation. In: Tobin MJ, ed. *Principles and Practice of Mechanical Ventilation.* 2nd ed. New York, NY: McGraw-Hill; 2006:201–220.
143. Marini JJ, Smith TC, Lamb VJ. External work output and force generation during synchronized intermittent mechanical ventilation: effect of machine assistance on breathing effort. *Am Rev Respir Dis.* 1988;138(5):1169–1179.
144. Imsand C, Feihl F, Perret C, Fitting JW. Regulation of inspiratory neuromuscular output during synchronized intermittent mechanical ventilation. *Anesthesiology.* 1994;80(1):13–22.
145. Brochard L, Lellouche F. Pressure-support ventilation. In: Tobin MJ, ed. *Principles and Practice of Mechanical Ventilation.* 3rd ed. New York, NY: McGraw-Hill; 2013:199–226.
146. Tobin MJ. Extubation and the myth of "minimal ventilator settings." *Am J Respir Crit Care Med.* 2012;185(4):349–350.
147. Straus C, Louis B, Isabey D, et al. Contribution of the endotracheal tube and the upper airway to breathing workload. *Am J Respir Crit Care Med.* 1998;157(1):23–30.
148. Perren A, Brochard L. Managing the apparent and hidden difficulties of weaning from mechanical ventilation. *Intensive Care Med.* 2013;39(11): 1885–1895.
149. Cabello B, Thille AW, Roche-Campo F, et al. Physiological comparison of three spontaneous breathing trials in difficult-to-wean patients. *Intensive Care Med.* 2010;36(7):1171–1179.
150. Tomlinson JR, Miller KS, Lorch DG, et al. A prospective comparison of IMV and T-piece weaning from mechanical ventilation. *Chest.* 1989; 96(2):348–352.
151. Esteban A, Alia I, Gordo F, et al. Extubation outcome after spontaneous breathing trials with T-tube or pressure support ventilation. The Spanish Lung Failure Collaborative Group. *Am J Respir Crit Care Med.* 1997;156(2 Pt 1):459–465.
152. Haberthur C, Mols G, Elsasser S, et al. Extubation after breathing trials with automatic tube compensation, T-tube, or pressure support ventilation. *Acta Anaesthesiol Scand.* 2002;46(8):973–979.
153. Brochard L, Rauss A, Benito S, et al. Comparison of three methods of gradual withdrawal from ventilatory support during weaning from mechanical ventilation. *Am J Respir Crit Care Med.* 1994;150(4):896–903.
154. Blackwood B, Burns KE, Cardwell CR, O'Halloran P. Protocolized versus non-protocolized weaning for reducing the duration of mechanical ventilation in critically ill adult patients. *Cochrane Database Syst Rev.* 2014;11:CD006904.
155. Namen AM, Ely EW, Tatter SB, et al. Predictors of successful extubation in neurosurgical patients. *Am J Respir Crit Care Med.* 2001;163(3 Pt 1):658–664.
156. Randolph AG, Wypij D, Venkataraman ST, et al. Effect of mechanical ventilator weaning protocols on respiratory outcomes in infants and children: a randomized controlled trial. *JAMA.* 2002;288(20):2561–2568.
157. Krishnan JA, Moore D, Robeson C, Rand CS, Fessler HE. A prospective, controlled trial of a protocol-based strategy to discontinue mechanical ventilation. *Am J Respir Crit Care Med.* 2004;169(6):673–678.
158. Marelich GP, Murin S, Battistella F, et al. Protocol weaning of mechanical ventilation in medical and surgical patients by respiratory care practitioners and nurses: effect on weaning time and incidence of ventilator-associated pneumonia. *Chest.* 2000;118(2):459–467.
159. Ely EW, Baker AM, Evans GW, Haponik EF. The prognostic significance of passing a daily screen of weaning parameters. *Intensive Care Med.* 1999;25(6):581–587.
160. Tobin MJ. Of principles and protocols and weaning. *Am J Respir Crit Care Med.* 2004;169(6):661–662.
161. Morris AH. Algorithm-based decision making. In: Tobin MJ, ed. *Principles and Practice of Intensive Care Monitoring.* New York, NY: McGraw-Hill; 1998:1355–1381.
162. Laghi F. Weaning: can the computer help? *Intensive Care Med.* 2008; 34(10):1746–1748.
163. Taniguchi C, Eid RC, Saghabi C, et al. Automatic versus manual pressure support reduction in the weaning of post-operative patients: a randomised controlled trial. *Crit Care.* 2009;13(1):R6.
164. Morato JB, Sakuma MT, Ferreira JC, Caruso P. Comparison of 3 modes of automated weaning from mechanical ventilation: a bench study. *J Crit Care.* 2012;27(6):741–748.
165. Lellouche F, Mancebo J, Jolliet P, et al. A multicenter randomized trial of computer-driven protocolized weaning from mechanical ventilation. *Am J Respir Crit Care Med.* 2006;174(8):894–900.
166. Burns KE, Meade MO, Lessard MR, et al. Wean earlier and automatically with new technology (the WEAN study): a multicenter, pilot randomized controlled trial. *Am J Respir Crit Care Med.* 2013;187(11):1203–1211.
167. Rose L, Presneill JJ, Johnston L, Cade JF. A randomised, controlled trial of conventional versus automated weaning from mechanical ventilation using SmartCare/PS. *Intensive Care Med.* 2008;34(10):1788–1795.
168. Schadler D, Engel C, Elke G, et al. Automatic control of pressure support for ventilator weaning in surgical intensive care patients. *Am J Respir Crit Care Med.* 2012;185(6):637–644.
169. Spahija J, de MM, Albert M, et al. Patient-ventilator interaction during pressure support ventilation and neurally adjusted ventilatory assist. *Crit Care Med.* 2010;38(2):518–526.
170. Piquilloud L, Vignaux L, Bialais E, et al. Neurally adjusted ventilatory assist improves patient-ventilator interaction. *Intensive Care Med.* 2011; 37(2):263–271.
171. Nava S, Ambrosino N, Clini E, et al. Noninvasive mechanical ventilation in the weaning of patients with respiratory failure due to chronic obstructive pulmonary disease: a randomized, controlled trial. *Ann Intern Med.* 1998;128(9):721–728.
172. Girault C, Daudenthun I, Chevron V, et al. Noninvasive ventilation as a systematic extubation and weaning technique in acute-on-chronic respiratory failure: a prospective, randomized controlled study. *Am J Respir Crit Care Med.* 1999;160(1):86–92.
173. Ferrer M, Esquinas A, Arancibia F, et al. Noninvasive ventilation during persistent weaning failure: a randomized controlled trial. *Am J Respir Crit Care Med.* 2003;168(1):70–76.
174. Girault C, Bubenheim M, Abroug F, et al. Noninvasive ventilation and weaning in patients with chronic hypercapnic respiratory failure: a randomized multicenter trial. *Am J Respir Crit Care Med.* 2011;184(6):672–679.
175. Wiedemann HP, Wheeler AP, Bernard GR, et al. Comparison of two fluid-management strategies in acute lung injury. *N Engl J Med.* 2006; 354(24):2564–2575.
176. Martin AD, Smith BK, Davenport PD, et al. Inspiratory muscle strength training improves weaning outcome in failure to wean patients: a randomized trial. *Crit Care.* 2011;15(2):R84.
177. Petty TL. Chronic airway obstruction. In: Petty TL, ed. *Intensive and Rehabilitative Respiratory Care.* Philadelphia, PA: Lea & Febiger; 1974: 115–135.
178. Denehy L, Skinner EH, Edbrooke L, et al. Exercise rehabilitation for patients with critical illness: a randomized controlled trial with 12 months of follow-up. *Crit Care.* 2013;17(4):R156.
179. Zanotti E, Felicetti G, Maini M, Fracchia C. Peripheral muscle strength training in bed-bound patients with COPD receiving mechanical ventilation: effect of electrical stimulation. *Chest.* 2003;124(1):292–296.
180. Routsi C, Gerovasili V, Vasileiadis I, et al. Electrical muscle stimulation prevents critical illness polyneuromyopathy: a randomized parallel intervention trial. *Crit Care.* 2010;14(2):R74.

181. Laghi F, Jubran A. Treating the septic muscle with electrical stimulations. *Crit Care Med*. 2011;39(3):585–586.
182. Hsieh LC, Chien SL, Huang MS, et al. Anti-inflammatory and anticatabolic effects of short-term beta-hydroxy-beta-methylbutyrate supplementation on chronic obstructive pulmonary disease patients in intensive care unit. *Asia Pac J Clin Nutr*. 2006;15(4):544–550.
183. Johnson CJ, Auger WR, Fedullo PF, Dimsdale JE. Methylphenidate in the 'hard to wean' patient. *J Psychosom Res*. 1995;39(1):63–68.
184. Rothenhausler HB, Ehrentraut S, von Degenfeld G, et al. Treatment of depression with methylphenidate in patients difficult to wean from mechanical ventilation in the intensive care unit. *J Clin Psychiatry*. 2000;61(10):750–755.
185. Holliday JE, Hyers TM. The reduction of weaning time from mechanical ventilation using tidal volume and relaxation biofeedback. *Am Rev Respir Dis*. 1990;141(5 Pt 1):1214–1220.
186. Acosta F. Biofeedback and progressive relaxation in weaning the anxious patient from the ventilator: a brief report. *Heart Lung*. 1988;17(3): 299–301.
187. Elpern EH, Silver MR, Rosen RL, Bone RC. The noninvasive respiratory care unit: patterns of use and financial implications. *Chest*. 1991;99(1): 205–208.
188. Martin UJ, Hincapie L, Nimchuk M, et al. Impact of whole-body rehabilitation in patients receiving chronic mechanical ventilation. *Crit Care Med*. 2005;33(10):2259–2265.
189. Hunter BC, Oliva R, Sahler OJ, et al. Music therapy as an adjunctive treatment in the management of stress for patients being weaned from mechanical ventilation. *J Music Ther*. 2010;47(3):198–219.
190. Kress JP, Pohlman AS, O'Connor MF, Hall JB. Daily interruption of sedative infusions in critically ill patients undergoing mechanical ventilation. *N Engl J Med*. 2000;342(20):1471–1477.
191. Girard TD, Kress JP, Fuchs BD, et al. Efficacy and safety of a paired sedation and ventilator weaning protocol for mechanically ventilated patients in intensive care (Awakening and Breathing Controlled trial): a randomised controlled trial. *Lancet*. 2008;371(9607):126–134.
192. Brochard L. Sedation in the intensive-care unit: good and bad? *Lancet*. 2008;371(9607):95–97.
193. Mehta S, Burry L, Cook D, et al. Daily sedation interruption in mechanically ventilated critically ill patients cared for with a sedation protocol: a randomized controlled trial. *JAMA*. 2012;308(19):1985–1992.
194. Strom T, Martinussen T, Toft P. A protocol of no sedation for critically ill patients receiving mechanical ventilation: a randomised trial. *Lancet*. 2010;375(9713):475–480.
195. Strom T, Stylsvig M, Toft P. Long-term psychological effects of a no-sedation protocol in critically ill patients. *Crit Care*. 2011;15(6):R293.
196. Griffiths RD. Sedation, delirium and psychological distress: let's not be deluded. *Crit Care*. 2012;16(1):109.
197. Tobin MJ, Laghi F. Extubation. In: Tobin MJ, ed. *Principles and Practice of Mechanical Ventilation*. 3rd ed. New York, NY: McGraw-Hill; 2013:1353–1374.
198. de la Linde Valverde CM. [Extubation of the difficult airway]. *Rev Esp Anestesiol Reanim*. 2005;52(9):557–570.
199. Gal TG. Airway management. In: Miller RD, ed. *Miller's Anesthesia*. 6th ed. Philadelphia, PA: Elsevier, Churchill Livingstone; 2005:1617–1652.
200. Leder SB, Cohn SM, Moller BA. Fiberoptic endoscopic documentation of the high incidence of aspiration following extubation in critically ill trauma patients. *Dysphagia*. 1998;13(4):208–212.
201. El Solh A, Okada M, Bhat A, Pietrantoni C. Swallowing disorders post orotracheal intubation in the elderly. *Intensive Care Med*. 2003;29(9): 1451–1455.
202. Barquist E, Brown M, Cohn S, et al. Postextubation fiberoptic endoscopic evaluation of swallowing after prolonged endotracheal intubation: a randomized, prospective trial. *Crit Care Med*. 2001;29(9):1710–1713.
203. Leitch EA, Moran JL, Grealy B. Weaning and extubation in the intensive care unit: clinical or index-driven approach? *Intensive Care Med*. 1996;22(8):752–759.
204. Conti G, Montini L, Pennisi MA, et al. A prospective, blinded evaluation of indexes proposed to predict weaning from mechanical ventilation. *Intensive Care Med*. 2004;30(5):830–836.
205. Dojat M, Harf A, Touchard D, et al. Evaluation of a knowledge-based system providing ventilatory management and decision for extubation. *Am J Respir Crit Care Med*. 1996;153(3):997–1004.
206. Cohen JD, Shapiro M, Grozovski E, Singer P. Automatic tube compensation-assisted respiratory rate to tidal volume ratio improves the prediction of weaning outcome. *Chest*. 2002;122(3):980–984.
207. Maldonado A, Bauer TT, Ferrer M, et al. Capnometric recirculation gas tonometry and weaning from mechanical ventilation. *Am J Respir Crit Care Med*. 2000;161(1):171–176.
208. Esteban A, Frutos-Vivar F, Ferguson ND, et al. Noninvasive positive-pressure ventilation for respiratory failure after extubation. *N Engl J Med*. 2004;350(24):2452–2460.
209. Thille AW, Richard JC, Brochard L. The decision to extubate in the intensive care unit. *Am J Respir Crit Care Med*. 2013;187(12):1294–1302.
210. Epstein SK, Ciubotaru RL. Independent effects of etiology of failure and time to reintubation on outcome for patients failing extubation. *Am J Respir Crit Care Med*. 1998;158(2):489–493.
211. Thille AW, Harrois A, Schortgen F, et al. Outcomes of extubation failure in medical intensive care unit patients. *Crit Care Med*. 2011;39(12):2612–2618.
212. Frutos-Vivar F, Esteban A, Apezteguia C, et al. Outcome of reintubated patients after scheduled extubation. *J Crit Care*. 2011;26(5):502–509.
213. Smina M, Salam A, Khamiees M, et al. Cough peak flows and extubation outcomes. *Chest*. 2003;124(1):262–268.
214. Darmon JY, Rauss A, Dreyfuss D, et al. Evaluation of risk factors for laryngeal edema after tracheal extubation in adults and its prevention by dexamethasone: a placebo-controlled, double-blind, multicenter study. *Anesthesiology*. 1992;77(2):245–251.
215. Jaber S, Chanques G, Matecki S, et al. Post-extubation stridor in intensive care unit patients: risk factors evaluation and importance of the cuff-leak test. *Intensive Care Med*. 2003;29(1):69–74.
216. De Bast Y, De Backer D, Moraine JJ, et al. The cuff leak test to predict failure of tracheal extubation for laryngeal edema. *Intensive Care Med*. 2002;28(9):1267–1272.
217. Francois B, Bellissant E, Gissot V, et al. 12–h pretreatment with methylprednisolone versus placebo for prevention of postextubation laryngeal oedema: a randomised double-blind trial. *Lancet*. 2007;369(9567):1083–1089.
218. Dane TE, King EG. A prospective study of complications after tracheostomy for assisted ventilation. *Chest*. 1975;67(4):398–404.
219. Pearson FG, Goldberg M, da Silva AJ. Tracheal stenosis complicating tracheostomy with cuffed tubes. Clinical experience and observations from a prospective study. *Arch Surg*. 1968;97(3):380–394.
220. Stauffer JL, Olson DE, Petty TL. Complications and consequences of endotracheal intubation and tracheotomy: a prospective study of 150 critically ill adult patients. *Am J Med*. 1981;70(1):65–76.
221. Ho LI, Harn HJ, Lien TC, et al. Postextubation laryngeal edema in adults. Risk factor evaluation and prevention by hydrocortisone. *Intensive Care Med*. 1996;22(9):933–936.
222. Kriner EJ, Shafazand S, Colice GL. The endotracheal tube cuff-leak test as a predictor for postextubation stridor. *Respir Care*. 2005;50(12):1632–1638.
223. Sandhu RS, Pasquale MD, Miller K, Wasser TE. Measurement of endotracheal tube cuff leak to predict postextubation stridor and need for reintubation. *J Am Coll Surg*. 2000;190(6):682–687.
224. Ferrari LR, Gotta AW. Anesthesia for otolaringologic surgery. In: Barash PG, Cullen BF, Stoelting RK, eds. *Clinical Anesthesia*. 5th ed. Philadelphia, PA: Lippincott Williams & Wilkins; 2006:997–1012.
225. Zeggwagh AA, Abouqal R, Madani N, et al. Weaning from mechanical ventilation: a model for extubation. *Intensive Care Med*. 1999;25(10): 1077–1083.
226. Engoren M. Evaluation of the cuff-leak test in a cardiac surgery population. *Chest*. 1999;116(4):1029–1031.
227. Mikaeili H, Yazdchi M, Tarzamni MK, et al. Laryngeal ultrasonography versus cuff leak test in predicting postextubation stridor. *J Cardiovasc Thorac Res*. 2014;6(1):25–28.
228. Patel AB, Ani C, Feeney C. Cuff leak test and laryngeal survey for predicting post-extubation stridor. *Indian J Anaesth*. 2015;59(2):96–102.
229. Deem S. Limited value of the cuff-leak test. *Respir Care*. 2005;50(12): 1617–1618.
230. Ding LW, Wang HC, Wu HD, et al. Laryngeal ultrasound: a useful method in predicting post-extubation stridor: a pilot study. *Eur Respir J*. 2006;27(2):384–389.
231. Venkategowda PM, Mahendrakar K, Rao SM, et al. Laryngeal air column width ratio in predicting post extubation stridor. *Indian J Crit Care Med*. 2015;19(3):170–173.
232. Sutherasan Y, Theerawit P, Hongphanut T, et al. Predicting laryngeal edema in intubated patients by portable intensive care unit ultrasound. *J Crit Care*. 2013;28(5):675–680.
233. Khamiees M, Raju P, DeGirolamo A, et al. Predictors of extubation outcome in patients who have successfully completed a spontaneous breathing trial. *Chest*. 2001;120(4):1262–1270.
234. Salam A, Tilluckdharry L, Amoateng-Adjepong Y, Manthous CA. Neurologic status, cough, secretions and extubation outcomes. *Intensive Care Med*. 2004;30(7):1334–1339.
235. Coplin WM, Pierson DJ, Cooley KD, et al. Implications of extubation delay in brain-injured patients meeting standard weaning criteria. *Am J Respir Crit Care Med*. 2000;161(5):1530–1536.

236. Vallverdu I, Calaf N, Subirana M, et al. Clinical characteristics, respiratory functional parameters, and outcome of a two-hour T-piece trial in patients weaning from mechanical ventilation. *Am J Respir Crit Care Med.* 1998;158(6):1855–1862.
237. Kress JP, O'Connor MF, Pohlman AS, et al. Sedation of critically ill patients during mechanical ventilation: a comparison of propofol and midazolam. *Am J Respir Crit Care Med.* 1996;153(3):1012–1018.
238. Cheney FW, Posner KL, Lee LA, et al. Trends in anesthesia-related death and brain damage: a closed claims analysis. *Anesthesiology.* 2006; 105(6):1081–1086.
239. Practice guidelines for management of the difficult airway: an updated report by the American Society of Anesthesiologists Task Force on Management of the Difficult Airway. *Anesthesiology.* 2003;98(5):1269–1277.
240. King EG, Sheehan GJ, McDonnell TJ. Upper airway obstruction. In: Hall JB, Schmidt GA, Wood LD, eds. *Principles of Critical Care.* New York, NY: McGraw-Hill; 1992:1710–1718.
241. Cooper SD, Benumof JL. Airway algorithm: safety considerations. In: Murell RC, Eichhorn JH, eds. *Patient Safety in Anesthetic Practice.* New York, NY: Churchill Livingstone; 1997:221–262.
242. Practice guidelines for management of the difficult airway: a report by the American Society of Anesthesiologists Task Force on Management of the Difficult Airway. *Anesthesiology.* 1993;78(3):597–602.
243. Cooper RM. The use of an endotracheal ventilation catheter in the management of difficult extubations. *Can J Anaesth.* 1996;43(1):90–93.
244. Loudermilk EP, Hartmannsgruber M, Stoltzfus DP, Langevin PB. A prospective study of the safety of tracheal extubation using a pediatric airway exchange catheter for patients with a known difficult airway. *Chest.* 1997;111(6):1660–1665.
245. Dosemeci L, Yilmaz M, Yegin A, et al. The routine use of pediatric airway exchange catheter after extubation of adult patients who have undergone maxillofacial or major neck surgery: a clinical observational study. *Crit Care.* 2004;8(6):R385–R390.
246. Walz JM, Zayaruzny M, Heard SO. Airway management in critical illness. *Chest.* 2007;131(2):608–620.
247. Cook TM, Silsby J, Simpson TP. Airway rescue in acute upper airway obstruction using a ProSeal Laryngeal mask airway and an Aintree catheter: a review of the ProSeal Laryngeal mask airway in the management of the difficult airway. *Anaesthesia.* 2005;60(11):1129–1136.
248. Schmidt GA, Hall JB. Management of the ventilated patient. In: Hall JB, Schmidt GA, Wood LD, eds. *Principles of Critical Care Medicine.* 3rd ed. New York, NY: McGraw-Hill; 2005:481–468.
249. Donlon JV, Doyle DJ, Feldman MA. Anesthesia for eye, ear, nose and throat surgery. In: Miller RD, ed. *Miller's Anesthesia.* 6th ed. Philadelphia, PA: Elsevier, Churchill Livingstone; 2005:2527–2555.
250. Anene O, Meert KL, Uy H, et al. Dexamethasone for the prevention of postextubation airway obstruction: a prospective, randomized, double-blind, placebo-controlled trial. *Crit Care Med.* 1996;24(10):1666–1669.
251. Cheng KC, Hou CC, Huang HC, et al. Intravenous injection of methylprednisolone reduces the incidence of postextubation stridor in intensive care unit patients. *Crit Care Med.* 2006;34(5):1345–1350.
252. Tellez DW, Galvis AG, Storgion SA, et al. Dexamethasone in the prevention of postextubation stridor in children. *J Pediatr.* 1991;118(2):289–294.
253. Gehlbach B, Kress JP. Upper airway obstruction. In: Hall JB, Schmidt GA, Wood LD, eds. *Principles of Critical Care Medicine.* 3rd ed. New York, NY: McGraw-Hill; 2005:455–464.
254. Orr JB. Helium-oxygen gas mixtures in the management of patients with airway obstruction. *Ear Nose Throat J.* 1988;67(12):866–869.
255. Jaber S, Carlucci A, Boussarsar M, et al. Helium-oxygen in the postextubation period decreases inspiratory effort. *Am J Respir Crit Care Med.* 2001;164(4):633–637.
256. Skrinskas GJ, Hyland RH, Hutcheon MA. Using helium-oxygen mixtures in the management of acute upper airway obstruction. *Can Med Assoc J.* 1983;128(5):555–558.
257. Boorstein JM, Boorstein SM, Humphries GN, Johnston CC. Using helium-oxygen mixtures in the emergency management of acute upper airway obstruction. *Ann Emerg Med.* 1989;18(6):688–690.
258. Berkenbosch JW, Grueber RE, Graff GR, Tobias JD. Patterns of helium-oxygen (heliox) usage in the critical care environment. *J Intensive Care Med.* 2004;19(6):335–344.
259. Sundaram RK, Nikolic G. Successful treatment of post-extubation stridor by continuous positive airway pressure. *Anaesth Intensive Care.* 1996;24(3): 392–393.
260. Khosh MM, Lebovics RS. Upper airway obstruction. In: Parrillo JE, Dellinger PR, eds. *Critical Care Medicine. Principles of Diagnosis and Management in the Adult.* 2nd ed. St Louis, MO: Mosby; 2001:808–825.
261. Benjamin B. Prolonged intubation injuries of the larynx: endoscopic diagnosis, classification, and treatment. *Ann Otol Rhinol Laryngol Suppl.* 1993; 160:1–15.
262. Ferrer M, Valencia M, Nicolas JM, et al. Early noninvasive ventilation averts extubation failure in patients at risk: a randomized trial. *Am J Respir Crit Care Med.* 2006;173(2):164–170.
263. Ferrer M, Sellares J, Valencia M, et al. Non-invasive ventilation after extubation in hypercapnic patients with chronic respiratory disorders: randomised controlled trial. *Lancet.* 2009;374(9695):1082–1088.
264. Keenan SP, Powers C, McCormack DG, Block G. Noninvasive positive-pressure ventilation for postextubation respiratory distress: a randomized controlled trial. *JAMA.* 2002;287(24):3238–3244.
265. Hill NS. Noninvasive positive-pressure ventilation. In: Tobin MJ, ed. *Principles and Practices of Mechanical Ventilation.* 3rd ed. New York, NY: McGraw-Hill; 2013:447–494.
266. Muriel A, Penuelas O, Frutos-Vivar F, et al. Impact of sedation and analgesia during noninvasive positive pressure ventilation on outcome: a marginal structural model causal analysis. *Intensive Care Med.* 2015; 41(9):1586–1600.
267. Kallstrom TJ. AARC Clinical Practice Guideline: oxygen therapy for adults in the acute care facility—2002 revision & update. *Respir Care.* 2002; 47(6):717–720.
268. Spoletini G, Alotaibi M, Blasi F, Hill NS. Heated humidified high-flow nasal oxygen in adults: mechanisms of action and clinical implications. *Chest.* 2015;148(1):253–261.
269. Bazuaye EA, Stone TN, Corris PA, Gibson GJ. Variability of inspired oxygen concentration with nasal cannulas. *Thorax.* 1992;47(8):609–611.
270. Chanques G, Riboulet F, Molinari N, et al. Comparison of three high flow oxygen therapy delivery devices: a clinical physiological cross-over study. *Minerva Anestesiol.* 2013;79(12):1344–1355.
271. Saslow JG, Aghai ZH, Nakhla TA, et al. Work of breathing using high-flow nasal cannula in preterm infants. *J Perinatol.* 2006;26(8):476–480.
272. Frat JP, Thille AW, Mercat A, et al. High-flow oxygen through nasal cannula in acute hypoxemic respiratory failure. *N Engl J Med.* 2015; 372(23):2185–2196.
273. Corley A, Caruana LR, Barnett AG,et al. Oxygen delivery through high-flow nasal cannulae increase end-expiratory lung volume and reduce respiratory rate in post-cardiac surgical patients. *Br J Anaesth.* 2011;107(6):998–1004.
274. Cuquemelle E, Pham T, Papon JF, et al. Heated and humidified high-flow oxygen therapy reduces discomfort during hypoxemic respiratory failure. *Respir Care.* 2012;57(10):1571–1577.
275. Maggiore SM, Idone FA, Vaschetto R, et al. Nasal high-flow versus Venturi mask oxygen therapy after extubation: effects on oxygenation, comfort, and clinical outcome. *Am J Respir Crit Care Med.* 2014;190(3):282–288.
276. Szakmany T, Russell P, Wilkes AR, Hall JE. Effect of early tracheostomy on resource utilization and clinical outcomes in critically ill patients: meta-analysis of randomized controlled trials. *Br J Anaesth.* 2015; 114(3):396–405.
277. Scheinhorn DJ, Hassenpflug MS, Votto JJ, et al. Post-ICU mechanical ventilation at 23 long-term care hospitals: a multicenter outcomes study. *Chest.* 2007;131(1):85–93.
278. Polverino E, Nava S, Ferrer M, et al. Patients' characterization, hospital course and clinical outcomes in five Italian respiratory intensive care units. *Intensive Care Med.* 2010;36(1):137–142.
279. Jubran A, Grant BJ, Duffner LA, et al. Effect of pressure support vs unassisted breathing through a tracheostomy collar on weaning duration in patients requiring prolonged mechanical ventilation: a randomized trial. *JAMA.* 2013;309(7):671–677.
280. Brochard L, Harf A, Lorino H, Lemaire F. Inspiratory pressure support prevents diaphragmatic fatigue during weaning from mechanical ventilation. *Am Rev Respir Dis.* 1989;139(2):513–521.
281. Jubran A, Van de Graaff WB, Tobin MJ. Variability of patient-ventilator interaction with pressure support ventilation in patients with chronic obstructive pulmonary disease. *Am J Respir Crit Care Med.* 1995;152(1): 129–136.
282. MacIntyre NR. Respiratory function during pressure support ventilation. *Chest.* 1986;89(5):677–683.
283. El-Khatib MF, Jamaleddine GW, Khoury AR, Obeid MY. Effect of continuous positive airway pressure on the rapid shallow breathing index in patients following cardiac surgery. *Chest.* 2002;121(2):475–479.
284. Kheir F, Myers L, Desai NR, Simeone F. The effect of flow trigger on rapid shallow breathing index measured through the ventilator. *J Intensive Care Med.* 2015;30(2):103–106.
285. Bellemare F, Grassino A. Effect of pressure and timing of contraction on human diaphragm fatigue. *J Appl Physiol.* 1982;53:1190.

CHAPTER

107

High-Frequency Ventilation

ALYAA EL HAZAMI and NIALL D. FERGUSON

INTRODUCTION

Acute respiratory distress syndrome (ARDS) is responsible for significant morbidity and mortality in the critically ill population (1–5). The use of mechanical ventilation in this population is important to sustain life but the goal has shifted dramatically over the last few decades, from aiming to achieve normal blood gases to instead minimizing ventilator-induced lung injury (VILI). The recognition of the critical role that VILI plays in the outcome of adults with ARDS has driven significant interest in alternative modes of ventilation that might be more lung protective. High-frequency ventilation (HFV) is a family of ventilatory modes that falls into this category. High-frequency oscillatory ventilation (HFOV) is the most extensively studied mode, and this chapter focuses on its use in the adult population.

DEFINITIONS, TERMINOLOGY, AND SUBTYPES

HFV is a collection of ventilatory modes, grouped together by their common property of employing high respiratory rates, all greater than 60 breaths/min (6,7). In addition to HFOV, other modes in this group include high-frequency jet ventilation (HFJV), high-frequency percussive ventilation (HFPV), and high-frequency positive-pressure ventilation (HFPPV).

High-Frequency Jet Ventilation

HFJV is a mode of ventilation in which gas is delivered through a small-bore catheter into the lungs at rates of 100 to 150 breaths/min (8). Delivered tidal volume is still small, but higher than just the volume exiting the jet, as the jets entrain an additional flow of gas by the *Choanda effect*. Exhalation is passive during HFJV; therefore, gas trapping or dynamic hyperinflation can be an issue. In practice, a conventional ventilator is set up as a "slave" to the jet to provide positive end-expiratory pressure (PEEP), along with basic monitoring and alarms.

HFJV is a very efficient mode for removing CO_2. Additionally, because of HFJV's very high flow rates and the differing pulmonary time constants in the clinical setting of bronchopleural fistulae (9), this mode of ventilation is implied to have beneficial effects in the presence of this disorder; however, these benefits have not been verified during objective testing (10,11). Concerns with HFJV relate to the delivery of high pressures (10–15 pounds per square inch, equivalent to 700 to 1,000 cm of water), unpredictable tidal volumes, and the development of dynamic hyperinflation (12), all of which may worsen VILI rather than minimize it. In addition, problems with adequate humidification of inspired gas and the subsequent risks of tracheobronchitis have been noted and documented. On the other hand, the greatest asset of HFJV is its ability to provide adequate ventilation while minimizing the chest motion normally associated with the respiratory cycle. This has led to the restricted use of HFJV in the operating room during procedures involving the airways as well as those requiring limited movements related to the respiratory cycle, such as ablation atrial arrhythmogenic foci and hepatic lesions with radiofrequency ablation (13,14), or renal stones treated with extracorporeal shock-wave lithotripsy (15,16).

High-Frequency Percussive Ventilation

HFPV is the newest and least well-studied of the HFV modes. It combines a high-frequency rate of 200 to 900 breaths/min superimposed on a conventional pressure mode of ventilation (17). HFPV is reported to enhance the clearance of respiratory secretions and has been successfully used in this regard in patients with burns and inhalational injury (17,18).

High-Frequency Oscillatory Ventilation

High-frequency oscillation (HFO) is a mode of mechanical ventilation with very high respiratory rates of 3 to 15 Hz (equivalent to 180 to 900 breaths/min), generating very small tidal volumes around a set mean airway pressure (mP_{aw}). Tidal volumes are small with HFO, often smaller than the anatomic dead space, in the range of 1 to 2 mL/kg (19). HFO has been widely and effectively used in neonates and children for close to 30 years (20–24). Only in the late 1990s did this device became available in the adult ICU; previous versions of this ventilator were only capable in oscillating patients under 35 kg. In contrast to other HFV modes, humidification is less of an issue during HFO, as a continuous bias flow of humidified gas is passed in front of an oscillating membrane (Fig. 107.1). Another advantage of HFO over other HFV is its active expiration, which may account for more control of ventilation and CO_2 elimination, and the lack of important gas trapping and hyperinflation (25,26). A resistance valve at the end of the bias flow circuit regulates the mean airway pressure. The elegance of HFO is that it allows for "decoupling" of oxygenation and ventilation. In general, alveolar ventilation, and thus carbon dioxide elimination, is dependent on the frequency and tidal volume but are relatively independent of lung volume (26,27). In contrast, oxygenation is typically proportional to the fraction of inspired oxygen and the mean airway pressure and lung volume (27,28).

PHYSIOLOGY

Mechanisms of Gas Transport during High-Frequency Oscillation

In addition to relying on bulk flow, adequate CO_2 removal during HFO is achieved through a number of alternative

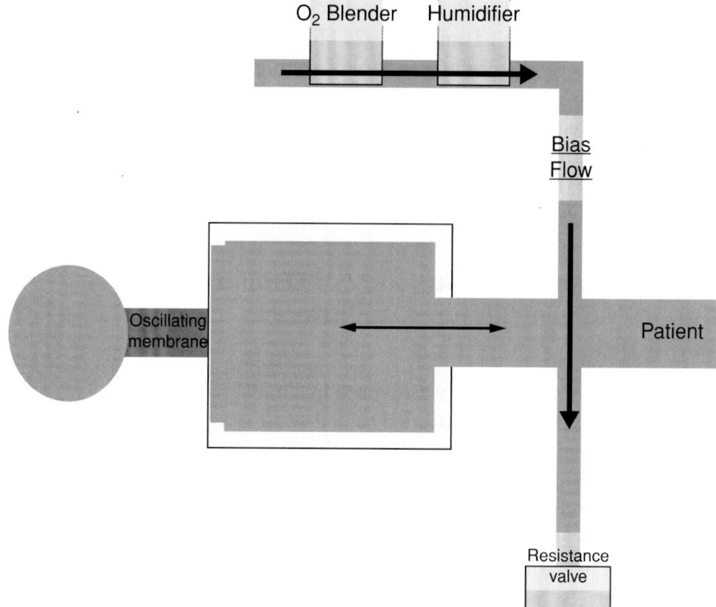

FIGURE 107.1 Schematic overview of the high-frequency oscillation (HFO) circuit. (Adapted from Ferguson ND, Stewart TE. New therapies for adults with acute lung injury: high-frequency oscillatory ventilation. *Crit Care Clin.* 2002;18:91–106, with permission.)

mechanisms including convective streaming due to asymmetric velocity profiles, Pendelluft, cardiogenic mixing, and diffusion (Fig. 107.2). A full explanation of these physiologic principles can be found in a number of papers reviewing this physiology in detail (7,19,29–36). During HFOV, alveolar ventilation is influenced by the frequency of oscillations, the inspiratory/expiratory (I/E) ratio, and the peak-to-peak pressure gradient (delta P) which is generated by the force of the diaphragm movement. The major message from these theoretical and experimental studies is that CO_2 elimination—which is

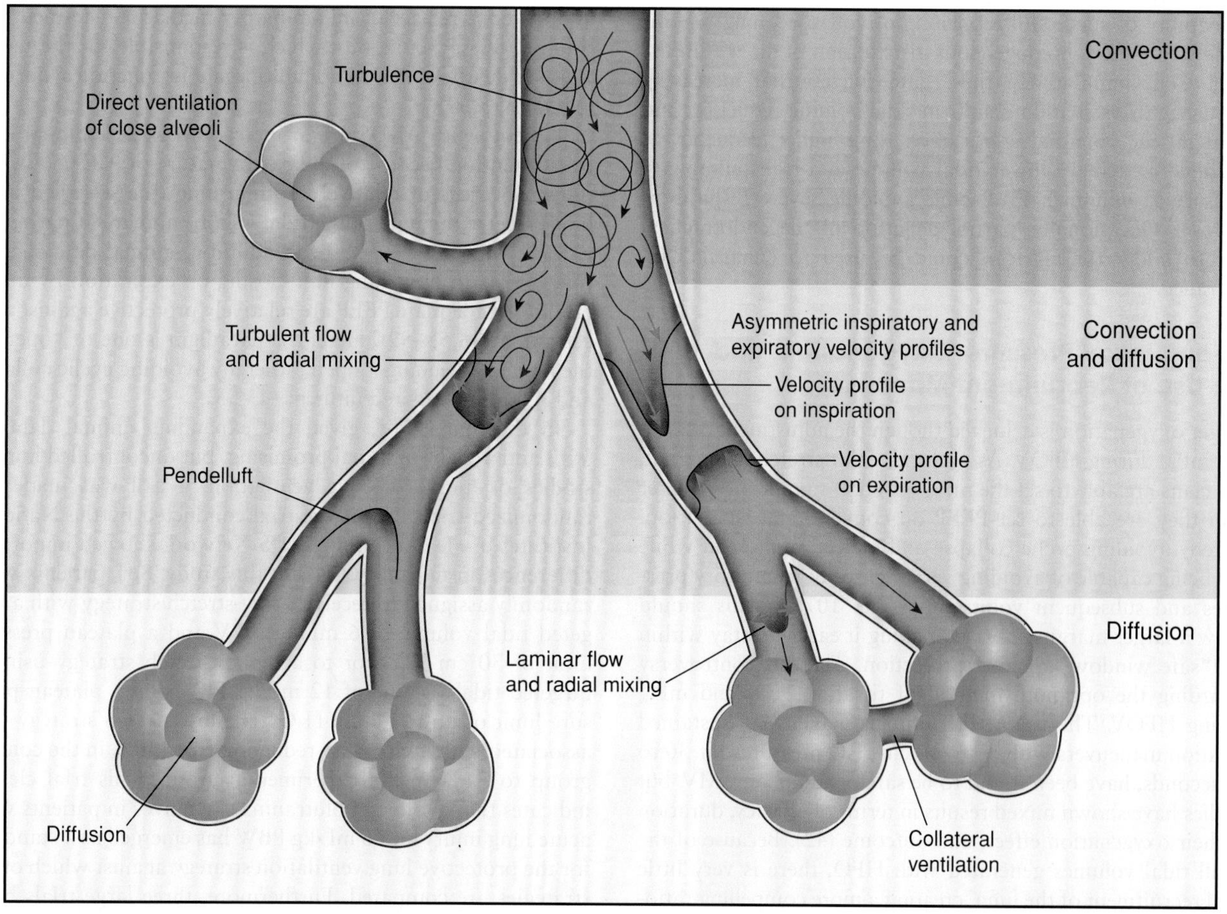

FIGURE 107.2 Mechanisms of gas transport during HFOV. (Adapted from Slutsky AS, Drazen JM. Ventilation with small tidal volumes. *N Engl J Med.* 2002;347:630–631, with permission.)

inversely proportional to $PaCO_2$—is described by the relationship: $f^aV_T{}^b$, where $a = -1$ and $b = -2$. However, this relationship is not as straightforward as it may seem, as tidal volume is inversely proportional to frequency with most HFO ventilators. In contrast to conventional ventilation, where increasing the respiratory rate will usually augment elimination of CO_2, during HFOV one decreases frequency to increase of elimination CO_2.

Tidal Volume and Frequency of Oscillation during High-Frequency Oscillatory Ventilation

Tidal volume is not routinely measured in clinical practice during the use of HFOV but assumed to be low. It is known to be inversely related to frequency due to the decrease in inspiratory time with increasing frequency (26). Many investigators have explored this issue reporting tidal volumes in adults with ARDS during HFOV usually range from 1 to 2.5 cc/kg predicted body weight (PBW) (19,37). Changes in delta P have a comparatively smaller effect on tidal volume in adults with ARDS (38,39). The relationship between the frequency of oscillation and the tidal volume generated during HFOV was clearly demonstrated in a recent animal ARDS model when HFOV at frequencies of 3, 6, and 9 Hz generated tidal volumes of 4.8, 2.7, and 1.8 mL/kg, respectively (40). This study also showed that despite application of the same mP_{aw}, higher frequencies were associated with lower transpulmonary pressure. Moreover, higher frequencies of oscillation enhanced the probability of successful reopening of collapsed lung regions leading to a more homogeneous distribution of air within the lung (41). Cumulatively, these data suggest that increasing frequency of oscillation results in tidal volume reduction and highlight the potential importance using higher frequency as tolerated to achieve lower tidal volume and transpulmonary pressure to minimize VILI while avoiding severe respiratory acidosis. Occasionally, partial deflation of the endotracheal cuff to allow for air leak could be used to enhance CO_2 clearance.

Mean Airway Pressure, Oxygenation, and the Use of Recruitment Maneuver

Target oxygenation is achieved though the adjustment of FiO_2 and mP_{aw} during HFOV. As cyclic alveolar stretch is minimal, clinicians are able to set the mP_{aw} on HFO significantly higher than they are able to set PEEP on conventional ventilation, thereby avoiding cyclic collapse and atelectrauma, and while still being capable of avoiding very high-peak inspiratory pressures and subsequent volutrauma (Fig. 107.3). This should allow a larger margin of error, making it easier to stay within the "safe window" of lung protection. There is controversy regarding the optimum method of titration FiO_2 and mP_{aw} during HFOV. The use of recruitment maneuvers, sustained inflation maneuvers with 30 to 40 cm H_2O pressures for 30 to 40 seconds, have been found to be safe in adults on CMV, but studies have shown mixed results in terms of efficacy, duration of their oxygenation effect, and outcome (42). Because of the small tidal volumes generated with HFO, there is very little tidal recruitment of the lung, creating a more compelling rationale for recruitment maneuvers (RMs) during HFO compared with conventional ventilation (28,43–45).

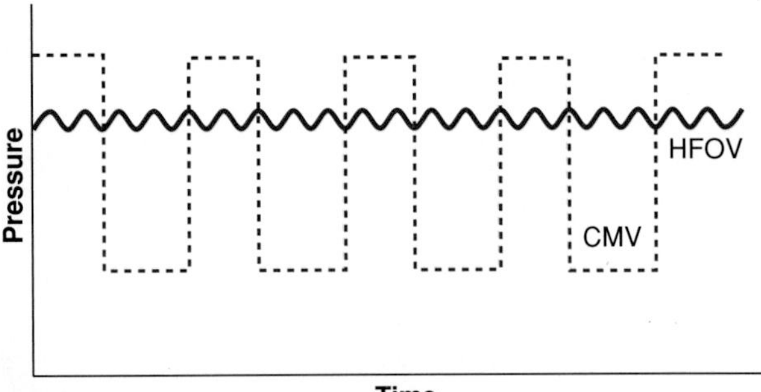

FIGURE 107.3 Pressure–time curve contrasts tidal variations in airway pressure associated with conventional ventilation (*dashed line*) and high-frequency oscillation (*solid line*). HFOV, high-frequency oscillation ventilation; CMV, conventional mechanical ventilation. (Adapted from Ferguson ND, Stewart TE. New therapies for adults with acute lung injury: high-frequency oscillatory ventilation. *Crit Care Clin.* 2002;18:91–106, with permission.)

RATIONALE FOR USE

Mechanical ventilation, although necessary to preserve life, can itself aggravate or cause lung damage, referred to as VILI. The pathophysiologic principles of VILI are complex and overlapping. These include high tidal volumes causing overdistention (volutrauma) (46–54); recruitment and derecruitment of unstable lung units (atelectrauma) (46,55–59); and oxygen toxicity (60,61). All of these mechanisms can lead to the local and systemic release of inflammatory mediators—termed biotrauma (38,55,56,62–68), which is responsible for the major cause of death in ARDS and multiorgan dysfunction syndrome (MODS) (5,69).

Patients with ARDS are at increased risk of regional lung overdistention because of the patchy nature of ARDS (70,71); the small areas of relatively normal lung (the so-called baby lung) receive the bulk of the tidal volume and are at particular risk of volutrauma (72,73). In addition, animal data suggest that efforts to limit lung unit closing on expiration by maintaining an adequate PEEP are relatively protective against atelectrauma (46,55–59). Here, the paradigm is one of "opening the lung and keeping it open," thereby avoiding cyclic collapse and recruitment/derecruitment (43,55).

In the mid-1990s, given the expanding animal data on VILI and in light of initial promising, but uncontrolled human studies of lung-protective ventilation, a call was made for randomized trials. The large trial conducted by the National Institutes of Health (NIH) ARDS Network showed important differences in mortality (74). In this study, 861 patients were randomly assigned to receive a low-stretch strategy with a targeted tidal volume of 6 mL/kg PBW and a plateau pressure limit of 30 cm H_2O, or to a higher-stretch strategy using a targeted tidal volume of 12 mL/kg PBW and a plateau pressure limit of up to 50 cm H_2O. The low-stretch strategy was associated with a mortality reduction from 40% in the control group to 31% in the experimental group. This trial clearly indicates that avoiding volutrauma saves lives in patients with acute lung injury and 6 mL/kg PBW has emerged as a standard for the protective lung ventilation strategy against which other strategies are compared. Furthermore, three large trials have subsequently been conducted comparing higher versus lower levels of PEEP while controlling tidal volumes in all patients

(75–77). When combined in an individual patient data meta-analysis (78), these trials demonstrate a mortality benefit for patients with moderate-to-severe ARDS when they receive higher levels of PEEP.

Therefore, a strategy that minimizes overdistention, by delivering small tidal volumes, and keeps the lung open, via the facilitation of alveolar recruitment and prevention of cyclical opening and closing of the alveolar units through the application of a higher mean airway pressure, should be the ideal mode in patients with ARDS. HFOV would appear an ideal mode for achieving these goals.

IMPLEMENTATION

Neonatal Studies

The longest clinical experience and the most rigorous evaluation of HFO have both been in the neonatal population. Multiple RCTs of HFO in neonates using an open-lung approach have demonstrated HFO to be safe and effective in improving oxygenation (79), with possible trends toward reduction of chronic lung disease in adolescence (80). However, meta-analyses comparing HFOV with CMV showed no effect on mortality at 28 to 30 days of age or at term equivalent age, and inconsistent effects but a possible reduction of chronic lung disease at term equivalent age (22,23,79). Interpreting the neonatal HFO literature is challenging due to differences in study populations (preterm vs. term), interventions (degree of lung recruitment targeted), the timing of HFO (immediately after birth vs. later), and by the introduction of exogenous surfactant as a standard therapy in the 1990s. In addition, it is important to realize that the baseline mortality rate in infant respiratory distress syndrome is an order of magnitude less than that seen in adults with severe ARDS. All of these factors mean that results from neonatal studies cannot be directly extrapolated to adult populations.

Observational Studies in Adults

Almost all of these studies evaluated HFOV as rescue therapy for patients with severe disease who "failed" conventional ventilation. Despite being limited by their uncontrolled nature and by selection bias, consistent messages arise that HFO is usually effective in improving oxygenation, with no obvious increased rates of complications. These studies of HFOV as rescue therapy in adults are summarized in Table 107.1.

Randomized Controlled Trials in Adults

A summary of randomized control trials (RCT) comparing HFOV to controlled mechanical ventilation in adults with ARDS is included in Table 107.2. We divide them into two groups; before and after 2013, as 2013 was the year when two landmark RCTs comparing HFOV with conventional mechanical ventilation were published.

Randomized Control Trials Published Prior to 2013

A few randomized controlled trials evaluated HFOV use in ARDS in comparison to conventional ventilation prior to 2013. Two of these trials (92,93) were planned and started prior to the completion of the first ARDS Network study that showed benefit from strict control of tidal volumes (74). None of the RCTs demonstrated safety concerns. The Multicenter Oscillatory Ventilation for Acute Respiratory Distress Syndrome (MOAT) Trial by Derdak et al. (92) was the first RCT that compared HFOV with CMV in adults with moderate to severe ARDS. It included 148 patients from 13 university-affiliated medical centers. There were significant improvements in oxygenation with HFOV and an impressive trend toward a mortality benefit with HFOV (RR 0.72; 95% CI 0.50 to 1.04) despite more than 10% of the control group crossing over to HFOV. It is important to recognize that the parameters of the CMV arms of the studies by Derdak et al. (92) and Bollen et al. (93) may have been relatively injurious, having been designed and initiated in the 1990s. The mean tidal volumes applied were high (10.6 mL/kg PBW and 8.1 ± 1.6 mL/kg PBW at 48 hours, respectively). HFOV was considered well tolerated and safe in moderate-to-severe ARDS and warranted the need of larger studies to demonstrate outcome benefit of HFOV.

Multiple meta-analyses of the use of HFOV in adults with ARDS have been published. A 2010 systematic review and meta-analysis (96) included eight trials of HFO as an initial ventilation strategy for early ARDS with total enrollment of 419 patients with ARDS (PaO_2/FiO_2 ratio of 112) in seven trials. The analysis showed that there was improvement in oxygenation with an increase in PO_2/FiO_2 ratio by 16% to 24% and mortality reduction at hospital discharge or 30 days (risk ratio 0.77, 95% CI 0.61 to 0.98, $P = 0.03$). However, many limitations to these data are implied by the quality of the studies included including the high mortality and injurious higher tidal volumes (>8 mL/kg PBW) in the control group. Although the subgroup *post hoc* analysis showed a similar benefit in trials that implemented lower tidal volumes (≤8 mL/kg) in the control group, the number of patients was considerably low ($n = 98$) such that solid conclusions could not be generated. These data in conjunction with those derived from the animal studies and theoretical principles, called for the conduction of the larger RCTs.

Randomized Control Trials Published in 2013

The two most recent and largest multicenter RCTs of HFOV in adults with ARDS were published in early 2013. Both the Oscillation for Acute Respiratory Distress Syndrome Treated Early (OSCILLATE) Trial ($N = 548$) (94) and the Oscillation in ARDS (OSCAR) trial ($N = 795$) (95) were designed to compare HFOV to a conventional mechanical ventilation strategy in adults with early moderate-to-severe ARDS and revealed interesting results. The two study protocols are compared and contrasted in Table 107.3. The OSCILLATE trial was designed to test the early application of an HFOV strategy targeting lung recruitment with higher mean airway pressures compared with conventional lung-protective mechanical ventilation also targeting lung recruitment with higher PEEP. This trial was stopped early because of increased in-hospital mortality in the HFOV group (47% vs. 35%; relative risk of death with HFOV 1.33; 95% CI 1.09 to 1.64; $P = 0.005$). Meanwhile, the OSCAR trial compared a different HFOV strategy versus usual care conventional ventilation found no difference between HFOV and CMV in all-cause 30-day mortality (41.7% vs. 41.1%; $P = 0.85$) and in in-hospital mortality (50.1% vs. 48.4%).

TABLE 107.1 Observational Studies of HFOV in ARDS

Study	*N*	Baseline Characteristics	Design	Mean Time of CMV Prior to HFOV	Complications	Main Findings	Mortality	Comment
Fort (81)	17	PaO_2/FiO_2: 68.6 ± 21.6 OI: 49 APACHE II: 23	Prospective	5.12 ± 4.3 d	Barotrauma 6% ETT obstruction 6%	Improved oxygenation	53%	Baseline OI and duration of CMV associated with ↑ mortality
Mehta (82)	24	PaO_2/FiO_2: 99 ± 39 OI: 33 APACHE II: 22	Prospective	5.7 ± 5.6 d	Barotrauma 8% ETT obstruction 4%	Improved oxygenation	67%	HFO appears safe and improves O_2 in rescue setting
Andersen (83)	16	PaO_2/FiO_2: 92 OI: 28 APACHE II: 27	Retrospective	7.2 d	Barotrauma 6%	Improved oxygenation	31%	HFO appears safe and improves O_2 in rescue setting
David (84)	42	OI: 23 APACHE II: 28	Prospective	3 d	Barotrauma 2%	Improved oxygenation	43%	HFO appears safe and improves O_2 in rescue setting Subset analysis showed higher 30-d mortality rate in patients without oxygenation improvement after 24 hr on HFOV (71%)
Cartotto (85)	25	Burn patients with ARDS (28% inhalation injury) PaO_2/FiO_2: 98 ± 26 OI: 27 APACHE II: 16	Retrospective	4.8 ± 4.4 d	Barotrauma 0%	Improved oxygenation	28%	HFO appears safe and improves O_2 in rescue setting
Mehta (86)	156	PaO_2/FiO_2: 91 ± 48 OI: 31 APACHE II: 24	Retrospective	5.6 ± 7.6 d	Barotrauma 21%	Improved oxygenation	62%	Baseline OI and duration of CMV associated with ↑ mortality
Ferguson (87) (TOOLS)	25	IO: 23 APACHE II: 24	Prospective, multiple-center, single-intervention pilot study	5.8–50.5 hr	Barotrauma 8–20%	Rapidly improved oxygenation		
Finkielman (88)	14	PaO_2/FIO_2: 73 ± 20 OI: 35 APACHE II: 35	Retrospective	1.8 ± 1.1 d	Barotrauma 0%	Improved oxygenation	57%	HFO appears safe and improves O_2 in rescue setting
Fessler (89)	30	APACHE II: 25 PaO_2/FiO_2: 78	Retrospective	3.1 ± 3 d	Barotrauma 20%	Improved oxygenation	63%	Used high frequency >6 Hz (median is 9 Hz)
Adhikari (90)	190	APACHE II: 28	Retrospective	2 d		62.5% had a positive oxygenation response after 2 hr of HFOV	128 of 189 patients died in hospital	No independent predictors of positive oxygenation response to HFOV Reasons for HFOV discontinuation included death or withdrawal of life support (39.1%), significant improvement in respiratory failure (37.6%), and inadequate improvement (23.3%)
Camporota (91)	102	APACHE II: 24.1 PaO_2/FiO_2: 93.8 ± 38	Retrospective	45 hr	Barotrauma 2%	Changes in PaO_2/FiO_2 of HFOV helped identify patients that are more likely to survive	30-d mortality (56%)	Improvement of >38% in PaO_2/FiO_2 occurring at any time within the first 72 hr, was the best predictor of survival at 30 d

HFO, high-frequency oscillation; ARDS, acute respiratory distress syndrome; OI, oxygen index; ETT, endotracheal tube; CMV, conventional mechanical ventilation.

TABLE 107.2 Randomized Controlled Trials of HFOV in ARDS

Study	*N*	Baseline Characteristics	Mean Days of CMV Prior to HFOV	Complications	Main Findings	Comment
Derek (92)	148	APACHE II: 22 PaO_2/FiO_2: <115 OI: 25	2.8	No significant difference between CMV and HFOV regarding hemodynamic variables, barotraumas, and mucus plugging	Improved oxygenation with HFOV for the first 24 hr	Mortality: HFOV: 37% CV 52%
Bollen (93)	61	OI: HFOV: 25 CV: 18 APACHE II: 21	2.1	HFOV: hypotension (10.8%), air leak (2.7%) CV: hypotension (4.2%), air leak (4.2%)	Significant improvement in oxygenation initially compared with CMV	No difference in mortality The study was stopped early
Ferguson (94) (OSCILLATE trial)	548	APACHE II: 29 (both groups) PaO_2/FiO_2: HFOV: 121 ± 46 CMV: 114 ± 38	HFOV: 2.5 ± 3.3 CMV: 1.9 ± 2.3	HFOV group required more vasopressors (91 vs. 84%), higher doses of midazolam (199 vs. 141 mg/d), and had more paralysis (83 vs. 68%) than CMV group	Mortality was higher in the HFOV group as compared to CMV (47 vs. 35%)	
Young (95) (OSCAR)	795	APACHE II: 21.7 (both groups) PaO_2/FiO_2: 113 ± 38 (both groups)	HFOV: 2.2 ± 2.3 CMV: 2.2 ± 2.3	No significant difference in the number of days on which patients received inotropic agents or pressor infusions (2.8 ± 5.6 d in conventional ventilation group vs. 2.9 ± 4.5 d in HFOV group)	41.7% in the HFOV group and in 163 of 397 patients (41.1%) in the conventional-ventilation group ($P = 0.18$)	

TABLE 107.3 Characteristics of OSCAR and OSCILLATE Trials Study Design and Methodology

	OSCAR	OSCILLATE	Comments
Study design	Multicenter randomized control trial 29 ICUs all in the UK 795 patients (HFOV: 398, CMV: 397)	Multicenter randomized control trial 39 ICUs in several countries, mainly North America 548 patients (HFOV: 275, CMV: 273)	The OSCILLATE trial planned to recruit 1200 patients but was terminated early. Most of OSCILLATE trial centers are experienced with HFOV use in OSCAR trial; only 9 centers had previous experience with HFOV.
Patient characteristics	APACHE II: 21.8 (at ICU admission) Age: 55.9 ± 16.2 yr Duration of mechanical ventilation before randomization (days): HFOV: 2.1 ± 2.1 CMV: 2.2 ± 2.3 PaO_2/FiO_2 ratio (mmHg): HFOV and CMV: 113 ± 38	APACHE II: 29 (at randomization) Age: 55 ± 16 yr Duration of mechanical ventilation before randomization (d): HFOV: 2.5 ± 3.3 CMV: 1.9 ± 2.3 PaO_2/FiO_2 ratio (mmHg): HFOV: 121 ± 46 CMV: 114 ± 38	Baseline characteristics were similar in both studies except for APACHE II score and time of calculation
Ventilatory strategy			
HFOV arm	The initial settings were a ventilation frequency of 10 Hz, an mP_{aw} of 5 cm H_2O above the P_{plat} of CMV at enrollment. Hypoxemia was treated by increasing the mP_{aw} and then by increasing the FiO_2 level. Titration of FiO_2 as first step before reducing mP_{aw} in the weaning process	Initial mP_{aw} value was 30 cm H_2O (highest value allowed 38 cm H_2O). Further titration is based on a strict protocol.	The result is lower mP_{aw} in the OSCAR trial than OSCILLATE trial on day 1 (26.9 ± 6.2 cm H_2O vs. 31 ± 2.6 cm H_2O) Ventilatory frequencies of oscillation used in OSCAR trial was higher than those in OSCILLATE trial Differences in I:E ratio between trials (1:1 in OSCAR and 1:2 in OSCILLATE) may diminish the effective difference in intrathoracic mean airway pressures
CMV arm	According to local practice in the participating ICUs. However, encouraged to use pressure-controlled ventilation targeting a tidal volume of 6 to 8 mL/kg of PBW, and to use the combinations of PEEP and FiO_2 values that were used in the ARDS Network study.	Adhered to a strict protocol of target V_T of 6 mL/kg PBW or less and P_{plat} of 35 cm H_2O or less. PEEP levels were high, based on modified previously published PEEP/FiO_2 tables.	The result is higher tidal volumes (8.3 ± 2.9 mL/kg PBW vs. 6.1 ± 1.3 mL/kg PBW) and lower PEEP levels (11.4 ± 3.6 cm H_2O vs. 18 ± 3.0 cm H_2O) in the OSCAR trial than OSCILLATE trial.
Recruitment maneuver	Recruitment maneuvers were not mandated in either arm	Recruitment maneuvers (sustained inflation of 40 cm H_2O for 40 s) were performed repeatedly.	

Ppalt, plateau pressure; mP_{aw}, mean airway pressure; CMV, controlled mechanical ventilation; HFOV, high-frequency oscillatory ventilation; PEEP, positive end-inspiratory pressure; PBW, predicted body weight.

The difference in the outcomes of the two studies can be attributed to multiple factors. The most significant is the ventilatory management of both arms. The adherence to the low-tidal volume strategy in OSCILLATE trial could contribute to the lower mortality rate in the control group in comparison to the OSCAR trial (35% vs. 48%). In addition, the early termination of the OSCILLATE trial might have exaggerated the harm of HFOV. As to why neither trial was able to show a beneficial effect of HFOV despite much theoretical promise, this is also likely multifactorial. These factors include that the incremental increase in lung protective ventilation with HFOV may have been smaller than anticipated, and that adverse effects related to HFOV (e.g. need for more sedation, increased vasopressor requirements, effects of higher mean airway pressures on the right heart) outweighed any potential benefit.

With the inclusion of the OSCILLATE and OSCAR trials result, a meta-analysis (97) analyzed six RCTs comparing HFOV to CMV in early moderate-to-severe ARDS. The majority of patients (84%) were from OSCAR and OSCILATE trials. Compared with conventional mechanical ventilation, HFOV did not significantly reduce the mortality at 28 or 30 days (pooled relative risk was 1.051 (95% CI: 0.813 to 1.358). This study concluded that HFOV should not be utilized as a mode of mechanical ventilation in patients with early moderate-to-severe ARDS due to lack of mortality benefit in comparison to low tidal volume, high PEEP mechanical ventilation, and a possible trend toward higher mortality. These results should not necessarily be extended to the use of HFOV as a rescue therapy in patients with refractory hypoxemia as none of the included studies evaluated that indication.

COMPLICATIONS

In comparison to controlled mechanical ventilation, patients ventilated with HFOV require more vasoactive medications. This hemodynamic effect could be attributed to high mean airway pressures increasing right ventricular afterload or reducing venous return and the negative effect on left ventricle performance at the presence of low filling pressures (98–100). It also could be attributed to the higher doses of sedatives used for HFOV patients (94,95,101). Adequate sedation and analgesia during HFOV in necessary to ensure patient–ventilator synchrony. The incidence of barotrauma in patients ventilated by HFOV did not differ from those ventilated with controlled mechanical ventilation (92,93,97,102).

FUTURE DIRECTIONS

Research in the field of the ventilatory care of ARDS patients and the prevention of VILI has been the focus of many investigators in critical care. Despite the physiologic rationale and encouraging initial data, the outcome of the use of HFOV has been disappointing. Patients with mild disease and nonrecruitable lung are likely not good candidates for HFO as increasing mean airway pressure that may lead to overdistention of some lung regions without increased aeration of collapsed or flooded alveoli worsened alveolar stress and strain (103).

We believe that HFOV should not be used routinely in adults with ARDS. Future clinical use and studies should be tailored to include targeted patient populations. ARDS patients who might benefit from what HFOV has to offer include those with severe ARDS and important hypoxemia despite lung-protective lung ventilation utilizing high PEEP and other evidence-based adjunct therapies such as prone positioning and paralysis (78,104,105) as a "rescue" therapy. In addition, dynamic assessment of a patient's response to HFOV may be useful. In a retrospective study, patients with improved oxygenation following HFOV, which is a surrogate of recruitability, seemed to benefit more from HFOV (91).

CONCLUSION

In summary, HFOV should not be recommended for routine use in adults with ARDS because of a lack of survival benefit with the application of HFOV and possibly trend toward harm. HFOV might be considered as a "rescue therapy" in patients who have failed lung-protective low tidal volume conventional mechanical ventilation after the utilization of more supported therapeutic intervention, such as higher PEEP (78), neuromuscular blockade (104), and prone positioning (105).

Key Points

- HFV modes are characterized by generation of very low tidal volumes at high frequencies and HFOV is the most commonly used mode.
- Ventilator-induced lung injury may worsen lung injury in patients with ARDS and induce multiple organ dysfunction through multiple mechanisms. Ventilator strategies should avoid volutrauma by using low tidal volumes, and avoid atelectrauma and oxygen toxicity through lung recruitment.
- HVOC does not reduce mortality in comparison to low tidal volume conventional mechanical ventilation utilizing high PEEP in patients with early moderate-to-severe ARDS, and therefore should not be used routinely in this population.
- HFOV might be used as a rescue mode of ventilation in patients with severe respiratory failure when oxygenation is not achievable by optimal low tidal volume and high PEEP-controlled mechanical ventilation and the application of evidence-based adjuvant therapy such as prone positioning.

References

1. Rubenfeld GD, Caldwell E, Peabody E, et al. Incidence and outcomes of acute lung injury. *N Engl J Med.* 2005;353:1685–1693.
2. Bersten AD, Edibam C, Hunt T, Moran J. Incidence and mortality of acute lung injury and the acute respiratory distress syndrome in three Australian states. *Am J Respir Crit Care Med.* 2002;165:443–448.
3. Villar J, Sulemanji D, Kacmarek RM. The acute respiratory distress syndrome: incidence and mortality, has it changed? *Curr Opin Crit Care.* 2014;20:3–9.
4. Wang CY, Calfee CS, Paul DW, et al. One-year mortality and predictors of death among hospital survivors of acute respiratory distress syndrome. *Intensive Care Med.* 2014;40:388–396.
5. Estenssoro E, Dubin A, Laffaire E, et al. Incidence, clinical course, and outcome in 217 patients with acute respiratory distress syndrome. *Crit Care Med.* 2002;30:2450–2456.
6. Froese AB, Bryan AC. High frequency ventilation. *Am Rev Respir Dis.* 1987;135:1363–1674.

7. Drazen JM, Kamm RD, Slutsky AS. High-frequency ventilation. *Physiol Rev.* 1984;64:505–543.
8. Klain M, Smith RB. High frequency percutaneous transtracheal jet ventilation. *Crit Care Med.* 1977;5:280–287.
9. Wood MJ, Lin ES, Thompson JP. Flow dynamics using high-frequency jet ventilation in a model of bronchopleural fistula. *Br J Anaesth.* 2014;112:355–366.
10. Roth MD, Wright JW, Bellamy PE. Gas flow through a bronchopleural fistula. Measuring the effects of high-frequency jet ventilation and chest-tube suction. *Chest.* 1988;93:210–213.
11. Ritz R, Benson M, Bishop MJ. Measuring gas leakage from bronchopleural fistulas during high-frequency jet ventilation. *Crit Care Med.* 1984;12:836–837.
12. Spackman DR, Kellow N, White SA, et al. High frequency jet ventilation and gas trapping. *Br J Anaesth.* 1999;83:708–714.
13. Goode JS Jr, Taylor RL, Buffington CW, et al. High-frequency jet ventilation: utility in posterior left atrial catheter ablation. *Heart Rhythm.* 2006;3:13–19.
14. Biro P, Spahn DR, Pfammatter T. High-frequency jet ventilation for minimizing breathing-related liver motion during percutaneous radiofrequency ablation of multiple hepatic tumours. *Br J Anaesth.* 2009;102:650–653.
15. Warner MA, Warner ME, Buck CF, Segura JW. Clinical efficacy of high frequency jet ventilation during extracorporeal shock wave lithotripsy of renal and ureteral calculi: a comparison with conventional mechanical ventilation. *J Urol.* 1988;139:486–487.
16. Mucksavage P, Mayer WA, Mandel JE, Van Arsdalen KN. High-frequency jet ventilation is beneficial during shock wave lithotripsy utilizing a newer unit with a narrower focal zone. *Can Urol Assoc J.* 2010;4:333–335.
17. Salim A, Martin M. High-frequency percussive ventilation. *Crit Care Med.* 2005;33:S241–S245.
18. Reper P, Heijmans W. High-frequency percussive ventilation and initial biomarker levels of lung injury in patients with minor burns after smoke inhalation injury. *Burns.* 2015;41:65–70.
19. Hager DN, Fessler HE, Kaczka DW, et al. Tidal volume delivery during high-frequency oscillatory ventilation in adults with acute respiratory distress syndrome. *Crit Care Med.* 2007;35:1522–1529.
20. Froese AB, Butler PO, Fletcher WA, Byford LJ. High-frequency oscillatory ventilation in premature infants with respiratory failure: a preliminary report. *Anesth Analg.* 1987;66:814–824.
21. Bryan AC. The oscillations of HFO. *Am J Respir Crit Care Med.* 2001;163:816–817.
22. Cools F, Offringa M, Askie LM. Elective high frequency oscillatory ventilation versus conventional ventilation for acute pulmonary dysfunction in preterm infants. *Cochrane Database Syst Rev.* 2015;3:CD000104.
23. Elective high-frequency oscillatory ventilation versus conventional ventilation for acute pulmonary dysfunction in preterm infants. *Neonatology.* 2013;103:7–8.
24. Arnold JH, Truog RD, Thompson JE, Fackler JC. High-frequency oscillatory ventilation in pediatric respiratory failure. *Crit Care Med.* 1993;21:272–278.
25. Bryan AC, Slutsky AS. Long volume during high frequency oscillation. *Am Rev Respir Dis.* 1986;133:928–930.
26. Slutsky AS, Kamm RD, Rossing TH, et al. Effects of frequency, tidal volume, and lung volume on CO_2 elimination in dogs by high frequency (2–30 Hz), low tidal volume ventilation. *J Clin Invest.* 1981;68:1475–1484.
27. Suzuki H, Papazoglou K, Bryan AC. Relationship between PaO_2 and lung volume during high frequency oscillatory ventilation. *Acta Paediatr Jpn.* 1992;34:494–500.
28. Kolton M, Cattran CB, Kent G, et al. Oxygenation during high-frequency ventilation compared with conventional mechanical ventilation in two models of lung injury. *Anesth Analg.* 1982;61:323–332.
29. Alzahrany M, Banerjee A, Salzman G. Flow transport and gas mixing during invasive high frequency oscillatory ventilation. *Med Eng Phys.* 2014;36:647–658.
30. Chang HK. Mechanisms of gas transport during ventilation by high-frequency oscillation. *J Appl Physiol Respir Environ Exerc Physiol.* 1984;56:553–563.
31. Schmid ER, Knopp TJ, Rehder K. Intrapulmonary gas transport and perfusion during high-frequency oscillation. *J Appl Physiol Respir Environ Exerc Physiol.* 1981;51:1507–1514.
32. Slutsky AS. Gas mixing by cardiogenic oscillations: a theoretical quantitative analysis. *J Appl Physiol Respir Environ Exerc Physiol.* 1981;51:1287–1293.
33. Slutsky AS, Brown R. Cardiogenic oscillations: a potential mechanism enhancing oxygenation during apneic respiration. *Med Hypotheses.* 1982;8:393–400.
34. Cybulsky IJ, Abel JG, Menon AS, et al. Contribution of cardiogenic oscillations to gas exchange in constant-flow ventilation. *J Appl Physiol (1985).* 1987;63:564–570.
35. Slutsky AS, Drazen JM. Ventilation with small tidal volumes. *N Engl J Med.* 2002;347:630–631.
36. Slutsky AS, Drazen FM, Ingram RH Jr., et al. Effective pulmonary ventilation with small-volume oscillations at high frequency. *Science.* 1980;209:609–671.
37. Hager DN, Fuld M, Kaczka DW, et al. Four methods of measuring tidal volume during high-frequency oscillatory ventilation. *Crit Care Med.* 2006;34:751–757.
38. Slutsky AS, Tremblay LN. Multiple system organ failure: is mechanical ventilation a contributing factor? *Am J Respir Crit Care Med.* 1998;157:1721–1725.
39. Chiumello D, Pristine G, Slutsky AS. Mechanical ventilation affects local and systemic cytokines in an animal model of acute respiratory distress syndrome. *Am J Respir Crit Care Med.* 1999;160:109–116.
40. Liu S, Yi Y, Wang M, et al. Higher frequency ventilation attenuates lung injury during high-frequency oscillatory ventilation in sheep models of acute respiratory distress syndrome. *Anesthesiology.* 2013;119:398–411.
41. Bauer K, Brucker C. The role of ventilation frequency in airway reopening. *J Biomech.* 2009;42:1108–1113.
42. Fan E, Wilcox ME, Brower RG, et al. Recruitment maneuvers for acute lung injury: a systematic review. *Am J Respir Crit Care Med.* 2008;178:1156–1163.
43. Lachmann B. Open up the lung and keep the lung open. *Intensive Care Med.* 1992;18:319–321.
44. Froese AB. The incremental application of lung-protective high-frequency oscillatory ventilation. *Am J Respir Crit Care Med.* 2002;166:786–787.
45. Froese AB. Role of lung volume in lung injury: HFO in the atelectasis-prone lung. *Acta Anaesthesiol Scand Suppl.* 1989;90:126–130.
46. Webb HH, Tierney DF. Experimental pulmonary edema due to intermittent positive pressure ventilation with high inflation pressures: protection by positive end-expiratory pressure. *Am Rev Respir Dis.* 1974;110:556–565.
47. Dreyfuss D, Soler P, Basset G, Saumon G. High inflation pressure pulmonary edema. Respective effects of high airway pressure, high tidal volume, and positive end-expiratory pressure. *Am Rev Respir Dis.* 1988;137:1159–1164.
48. Parker JC, Hernandez LA, Longenecker GL, Peevy K, Johnson W. Lung edema caused by high peak inspiratory pressures in dogs: role of increased microvascular filtration pressure and permeability. *Am Rev Respir Dis.* 1990;142:321–328.
49. Dreyfuss D, Basset G, Soler P, Saumon G. Intermittent positive-pressure hyperventilation with high inflation pressures produces pulmonary microvascular injury in rats. *Am Rev Respir Dis.* 1985;132:880–884.
50. Kolobow T, Moretti MP, Fumagalli R, et al. Severe impairment in lung function induced by high peak airway pressure during mechanical ventilation: an experimental study. *Am Rev Respir Dis.* 1987;135:312–315.
51. Tsuno K, Miura K, Takeya M, et al. Histopathologic pulmonary changes from mechanical ventilation at high peak airway pressures. *Am Rev Respir Dis.* 1991;143:1115–1120.
52. Dreyfuss D, Saumon G. Ventilator-induced lung injury: lessons from experimental studies. *Am J Respir Crit Care Med.* 1998;157:294–323.
53. Hernandez LA, Peevy KJ, Moise AA, Parker JC. Chest wall restriction limits high airway pressure-induced lung injury in young rabbits. *J Appl Physiol (1985).* 1989;66:2364–2368.
54. Steinberg J, Schiller HJ, Halter JM, et al. Tidal volume increases do not affect alveolar mechanics in normal lung but cause alveolar overdistension and exacerbate alveolar instability after surfactant deactivation. *Crit Care Med.* 2002;30:2675–2683.
55. Tremblay LN, Slutsky AS. Ventilator-induced lung injury: from the bench to the bedside. *Intensive Care Med.* 2006;32:24–33.
56. Tremblay L, Valenza F, Ribeiro SP, et al. Injurious ventilatory strategies increase cytokines and c-fos m-RNA expression in an isolated rat lung model. *J Clin Invest.* 1997;99:944–952.
57. Steinberg JM, Schiller HJ, Halter JM, et al. Alveolar instability causes early ventilator-induced lung injury independent of neutrophils. *Am J Respir Crit Care Med.* 2004;169:57–63.
58. Muscedere JG, Mullen JB, Gan K, Slutsky AS. Tidal ventilation at low airway pressures can augment lung injury. *Am J Respir Crit Care Med.* 1994;149:1327–1334.
59. Dos Santos CC, Slutsky AS. Invited review: mechanisms of ventilator-induced lung injury: a perspective. *J Appl Physiol (1985).* 2000;89:1645–1655.
60. Bryan CL, Jenkinson SG. Oxygen toxicity. *Clin Chest Med.* 1988;9:141–152.

61. Davis WB, Rennard SI, Bitterman PB, Crystal RG. Pulmonary oxygen toxicity: early reversible changes in human alveolar structures induced by hyperoxia. *N Engl J Med*. 1983;309:878–883.
62. Tremblay LN, Miatto D, Hamid Q, et al. Injurious ventilation induces widespread pulmonary epithelial expression of tumor necrosis factor-alpha and interleukin-6 messenger RNA. *Crit Care Med*. 2002;30:1693–1700.
63. Tremblay LN, Slutsky AS. Ventilator-induced injury: from barotrauma to biotrauma. *Proc Assoc Am Phys*. 1998;110:482–488.
64. Guery BP, Welsh DA, Viget NB, et al. Ventilation-induced lung injury is associated with an increase in gut permeability. *Shock*. 2003;19:559–563.
65. Choi WI, Quinn DA, Park KM, et al. Systemic microvascular leak in an in vivo rat model of ventilator-induced lung injury. *Am J Respir Crit Care Med*. 2003;167:1627–1632.
66. Imai Y, Parodo J, Kajikawa O, et al. Injurious mechanical ventilation and end-organ epithelial cell apoptosis and organ dysfunction in an experimental model of acute respiratory distress syndrome. *JAMA*. 2003;289:2104–2112.
67. Ranieri VM, Suter PM, Tortorella C, et al. Effect of mechanical ventilation on inflammatory mediators in patients with acute respiratory distress syndrome: a randomized controlled trial. *JAMA*. 1999;282:54–61.
68. dos Santos CC, Slutsky AS. The contribution of biophysical lung injury to the development of biotrauma. *Annu Rev Physiol*. 2006;68:585–618.
69. Montgomery AB, Stager MA, Carrico CJ, Hudson LD. Causes of mortality in patients with the adult respiratory distress syndrome. *Am Rev Respir Dis*. 1985;132:485–489.
70. Gattinoni L, Pelosi P, Vitale G, et al. Body position changes redistribute lung computed-tomographic density in patients with acute respiratory failure. *Anesthesiology*. 1991;74:15–23.
71. Gattinoni L, Caironi P, Pelosi P, Goodman LR. What has computed tomography taught us about the acute respiratory distress syndrome? *Am J Respir Crit Care Med*. 2001;164:1701–1711.
72. Roupie E, Dambrosio M, Servillo G, et al. Titration of tidal volume and induced hypercapnia in acute respiratory distress syndrome. *Am J Respir Crit Care Med*. 1995;152:121–128.
73. Gattinoni L, Pesenti A. The concept of "baby lung." *Intensive Care Med*. 2005;31:776–784.
74. Network TARDS. Ventilation with lower tidal volumes as compared with traditional tidal volumes for acute lung injury and the acute respiratory distress syndrome. The Acute Respiratory Distress Syndrome Network. *N Engl J Med*. 2000;342:1301–1308.
75. Meade M, Cook D, Guyatt G, et al. Ventilation strategy using low tidal volumes, recruitment maneuvers, and high positive end-expiratory pressure for acute lung injury and acute respiratory distress syndrome: a randomized controlled trial. *JAMA*. 2008;299:637–645.
76. Mercat A, Richard JC, Vielle B, et al. Positive end-expiratory pressure setting in adults with acute lung injury and acute respiratory distress syndrome: a randomized controlled trial. *JAMA*. 2008;299:646–655.
77. Brower RG, Lanken PN, MacIntyre N, et al. Higher versus lower positive end-expiratory pressures in patients with the acute respiratory distress syndrome. *N Engl J Med*. 2004;351:327–336.
78. Briel M, Meade M, Mercat A, et al. Higher vs lower positive end-expiratory pressure in patients with acute lung injury and acute respiratory distress syndrome: systematic review and meta-analysis. *JAMA*. 2010;303:865–873.
79. Duyndam A, Ista E, Houmes RJ, et al. Invasive ventilation modes in children: a systematic review and meta-analysis. *Crit Care*. 2011;15:R24.
80. Zivanovic S, Peacock J, Alcazar-Paris M, et al. Late outcomes of a randomized trial of high-frequency oscillation in neonates. *N Engl J Med*. 2014;370:1121–1130.
81. Fort P, Farmer C, Westerman J, et al. High-frequency oscillatory ventilation for adult respiratory distress syndrome: a pilot study. *Crit Care Med*. 1997;25:937–947.
82. Mehta S, Lapinsky S, Hallett D, et al. Prospective trial of high-frequency oscillation in adults with acute respiratory distress syndrome. *Crit Care Med*. 2001;29:1360–1369.
83. Andersen FA, Guttormsen AB, Flaatten HK. High frequency oscillatory ventilation in adult patients with acute respiratory distress syndrome: a retrospective study. *Acta Anaesthesiol Scand*. 2002;46:1082–1088.
84. David M, Weiler N, Heinrichs W, et al. High-frequency oscillatory ventilation in adult acute respiratory distress syndrome. *Intensive Care Med*. 2003;29:1656–1665.
85. Cartotto R, Ellis S, Gomez M, et al. High frequency oscillatory ventilation in burn patients with the acute respiratory distress syndrome. *Burns*. 2004;30:453–463.
86. Mehta S, Granton J, MacDonald RJ, et al. High-frequency oscillatory ventilation in adults: the Toronto experience. *Chest*. 2004;126:518–527.
87. Ferguson ND, Chiche JD, Kacmarek RM, et al. Combining high-frequency oscillatory ventilation and recruitment maneuvers in adults with early acute respiratory distress syndrome: the Treatment with Oscillation and an Open Lung Strategy (TOOLS) Trial pilot study. *Crit Care Med*. 2005; 33:479–486.
88. Finkielman JD, Gajic O, Farmer JC, et al. The initial Mayo Clinic experience using high-frequency oscillatory ventilation for adult patients: a retrospective study. *BMC Emerg Med*. 2006;6:2.
89. Fessler HE, Hager DN, Brower RG. Feasibility of very high-frequency ventilation in adults with acute respiratory distress syndrome. *Crit Care Med*. 2008;36:1043–1048.
90. Adhikari NK, Bashir A, Lamontagne F, et al. High-frequency oscillation in adults: a utilization review. *Crit Care Med*. 2011;39:2631–2644.
91. Camporota L, Sherry T, Smith J, et al. Physiological predictors of survival during high-frequency oscillatory ventilation in adults with acute respiratory distress syndrome. *Crit Care*. 2013;17:R40.
92. Derdak S, Mehta S, Stewart TE, et al. High-frequency oscillatory ventilation for acute respiratory distress syndrome in adults: a randomized, controlled trial. *Am J Respir Crit Care Med*. 2002;166:801–808.
93. Bollen C, van Well G, Sherry T, et al. High frequency oscillatory ventilation compared with conventional mechanical ventilation in adult respiratory distress syndrome: a randomized controlled trial [ISRCTN24242669]. *Crit Care*. 2005;9:R430–R439.
94. Ferguson N, Cook D, Guyatt G, et al. High-frequency oscillation in early acute respiratory distress syndrome. *N Engl J Med*. 2013;368:795–805.
95. Young D, Lamb SE, Shah S, et al. High-frequency oscillation for acute respiratory distress syndrome. *N Engl J Med*. 2013;368:806–813.
96. Sud S, Sud M, Friedrich JO, et al. High frequency oscillation in patients with acute lung injury and acute respiratory distress syndrome (ARDS): systematic review and meta-analysis. *BMJ*. 2010;340:c2327.
97. Gu XL, Wu GN, Yao YW, et al. Is high-frequency oscillatory ventilation more effective and safer than conventional protective ventilation in adult acute respiratory distress syndrome patients? A meta-analysis of randomized controlled trials. *Crit Care*. 2014;18:R111.
98. Smailys A, Mitchell JR, Doig CJ, et al. High-frequency oscillatory ventilation versus conventional ventilation: hemodynamic effects on lung and heart. *Physiol Rep*. 2014;2:e00259.
99. David M, von Bardeleben RS, Weiler N, et al. Cardiac function and haemodynamics during transition to high-frequency oscillatory ventilation. *Eur J Anaesthesiol*. 2004;21:944–952.
100. Nakagawa R, Koizumi T, Ono K, et al. Cardiovascular responses to high-frequency oscillatory ventilation during acute lung injury in sheep. *J Anesth*. 2007;21:340–347.
101. Burry LD, Seto K, Rose L, et al. Use of sedation and neuromuscular blockers in critically ill adults receiving high-frequency oscillatory ventilation. *Ann Pharmacother*. 2013;47:1122–1129.
102. Ferguson ND, Cook DJ, Guyatt GH, et al. High-frequency oscillation in early acute respiratory distress syndrome. *N Engl J Med*. 2013;368: 795–805.
103. Gattinoni L, Caironi P, Cressoni M, et al. Lung recruitment in patients with the acute respiratory distress syndrome. *N Engl J Med*. 2006;354: 1775–1786.
104. Papazian L, Forel J-M, Gacouin A, et al. Neuromuscular blockers in early acute respiratory distress syndrome. *N Engl J Med*. 2010;363:1107–1116.
105. Guerin C, Reignier J, Richard JC, et al. Prone positioning in severe acute respiratory distress syndrome. *N Engl J Med*. 2013;368:2159–2168.

CHAPTER

108

Oxygen Therapy, Respiratory Care, and Monitoring

VITTORIA COMELLINI, LARA PISANI, and STEFANO NAVA

INTRODUCTION

Supplemental oxygen is one of the most widely used therapies for people admitted to the hospital and it is used across the whole range of specialties. Although oxygen therapy is used as a medical treatment in both acute and chronic setting, it is often administered improperly. The major problems consist in the fact that about this topic there are strongly held beliefs, but very few randomized controlled trials and frequently health care professionals receive conflicting advice about oxygen use from different "experts" during their clinical training and during their careers, and many are confused about the oxygen's prescription and use. This chapter will give a comprehensive and practical overview of oxygen pathophysiologic effects, current modalities for its delivery, and monitoring in the critical care setting. In order to give a more complete view about the management of patients with acute respiratory failure (ARF), we will also discuss the other respiratory monitoring techniques in the intensive care unit (ICU) and in specific circumstances like during noninvasive ventilation (NIV).

OXYGEN THERAPY

Oxygen makes up 21% of the atmosphere we breathe; in the air it exists in a diatomic molecular form (O_2, molecular weight [MW] 16 g/mol) that is the state in which we administer oxygen to our patients as a respiratory gas, either pure oxygen or in mixtures with air or helium (Heliox). While the gaseous state is most clinically relevant, oxygen can be found in liquid and solid states as well, under appropriate conditions.

Oxygen was not discovered as a separate gas until the late 18th century, when the Swedish apothecary, Karl W. Scheele in 1772, made a series of experiments with mercuric oxide and potassium nitrate and, heating these two elements, obtained a gas that caused candles to burn more brightly; he did not, however, rush to publication. In the same years, the English amateur chemist Joseph Priestley liberated oxygen by intensely heating mercurius calcinatus (mercuric oxide) placed over liquid mercury in a closed vessel; he called this new gas "dephlogisticated air" (1).

The first notice about the use of oxygen as a remedy in disease dates back to 1870 (2). Although oxygen life-supporting role was understood, it took about 150 years for the gas to be used in a proper way: during the first 150 years after this discovery, the therapeutic use of oxygen was sporadic, erratic, and controversial.

Currently, oxygen is administered for three main indications, but only one is evidence-based. First, oxygen is given to correct hypoxemia as there is good evidence that severe hypoxemia is harmful. Second, oxygen is administered to ill patients in case they might become hypoxemic. Recent evidence suggests that this practice may actually place patients at increased risk of developing the toxic effects mediated by reactive oxygen species (ROS) (3), leading to tissue damage and absorption atelectasis. Third, a very high proportion of medical oxygen is administered because most clinicians believe that oxygen can alleviate breathlessness. However, there is no evidence that oxygen holds this beneficial effect in nonhypoxemic patients and there is evidence of lack of effectiveness in nonhypoxemic breathless patients with chronic obstructive pulmonary disease (COPD) and advanced cancer (4,5).

PATHOPHYSIOLOGY

Respiration is the process that involves the exchange of oxygen and carbon dioxide (CO_2) between the environment and a living organism. Oxygen is indispensable for the aerobic metabolism of cells, so it is essential for humans to maintain a safe level of this gas in the bloodstream. Several mechanisms exist to regulate breathing in such a way that it is maintained within quite a narrow range. Inside the lungs, oxygen passes from inspired air into the bloodstream, and its diffusion depends on alveolar oxygen pressure. Most of the oxygen in the blood is bound to a carrying protein contained in red blood cells and called hemoglobin, whereas, normally, only a small amount is dissolved in the blood itself. Under normal conditions, almost all of the oxygen-carrying capacity of hemoglobin in the blood is used when the oxygen saturation (SaO_2) is in the normal range, 95% to 98%. Therefore, giving supplementary oxygen to a healthy young person will increase the saturation level only slightly from about 97% to 99% or a maximum of 100%, producing only a very small increase in amount of oxygen made available to the tissues.

Hypoxemia is the result of respiratory failure, a condition that leads to inadequate oxygen delivery (DO_2) to the tissues (partial respiratory failure) and/or to inadequate removal of carbon dioxide (global respiratory failure). The most common form of hypoxemia occurs when there is sufficient oxygen-carrying capacity—in patients with a normal level of hemoglobin—but insufficient oxygen uptake in the lungs. This can be the result of poor ventilation of areas of lung or abnormalities of gas exchange during illnesses such as pneumonia. This form of hypoxemia is the easiest to treat with oxygen therapy; on the contrary oxygen therapy is less effective in other situations, including anemia where there is a low carrying capacity or intoxications where the carrying capacity of hemoglobin has been reduced by a toxic substance. For example, carbon monoxide (CO), by combining with hemoglobin to form carboxyhemoglobin (HbCO), blocks oxygen binding to hemoglobin despite having a normal level of oxygen in the lungs and in the blood.

Oxygen therapy increases alveolar oxygen (PAO_2) and is, therefore, effective only when alveolar capillary units have some functional ventilation. In turn, it is ineffective if there is a pure shunt, such as pulmonary arteriovenous malformations, where mixed venous blood does not pass through an alveolar capillary unit. There will be, in this situation, a small overall increase in PaO_2 due to an increase in dissolved oxygen in the pulmonary venous blood from ventilated alveolar capillary units, which is minor compared with the oxygen carried by hemoglobin. Despite this, there is good evidence that breath-hold times can be increased by breathing oxygen (6,7). The same principles are used to preoxygenate, actually denitrogenate, patients before intubation during anesthesia; it is thought that the additional breath-hold time is produced not by the marginal increase in blood oxygen levels but by the increased reservoir of oxygen in the lungs after breathing oxygen-enriched air. In poorly ventilated alveoli (i.e., low ventilation/perfusion ratio [V/Q]), PAO_2 will be low and increasing FiO_2 will increase PAO_2 and therefore PaO_2 (7). When there is a diffusion barrier due to increased alveolar capillary membrane thickness, such as in fibrotic lung disease (6), increasing PAO_2 will augment the rate of diffusion across the alveolar capillary membrane by increasing the concentration gradient.

TREATMENT

Oxygen represents the first line of treatment for hypoxemia in those patients who are not breathless, aiming to achieve normal or near-normal oxygen saturation. For critically ill patients with an oxygen saturation below the target, after having ascertained that the airway is clear, oxygen should be administered as soon as possible and the flow rates should be adjusted to keep the oxygen saturation (SpO_2) in the target range, or at least above 90% (8,9). Indeed when prescribing oxygen therapy, the health care professional should indicate the target SpO_2 range rather than prescribing a fixed dose of oxygen or FiO_2. The clinician may indicate a starting dose, the device and the flow rate, but there needs to be an agreed-on system for adjusting the oxygen dose upward or downward according to the patient's needs. It is important to consider that every requirement for an increased dose of oxygen is an indication for urgent clinical reassessment of the patient, repeating arterial blood gas (ABG) measurements in most instances. The SpO_2 should be monitored continuously until the patient is stable and, as soon as ABG measurements are available, the patient's further treatment should be guided by the results of this test.

Some subjects, especially those older than 70 years, may have SpO_2 measurements below 94% and yet do not require oxygen therapy if clinically stable. Despite this, a reduction of more than 3% in a patient's usual SpO_2, even if it remains within the target range, may be the first evidence of an acute illness. It is known that oxygenation is reduced in the supine position, so fully conscious hypoxemic patients should ideally be allowed to maintain the most upright posture possible, or the most comfortable posture for the patient, unless there are contraindications (e.g., skeletal or spinal trauma, severe hypotension). A wide variation in SpO_2 characterizes sleep: all healthy subjects in all age groups routinely have transient dips overnight with a mean saturation nadir of 90.4% (10). These decrements should be interpreted with caution, monitoring the subject for few minutes in order to determine whether the hypoxemia is sustained or just a transient, normal nocturnal dip.

There are several medical emergencies in which patients are likely to suffer from hypoxemia, including cardiac arrest, major trauma, shock, major sepsis, anaphylaxis, major pulmonary hemorrhage, massive hemoptysis, major head injury, and near-drowning. In all these conditions initial treatment should involve high-concentration oxygen, aiming at an SpO_2 of 94% to 98% pending availability of satisfactory ABG measurements or until the airway is secured by endotracheal intubation. High-concentration oxygen is additionally recommended during resuscitation and in case of CO poisoning, taking into account that in this condition patients have a normal level of PaO_2 but a greatly reduced level of oxygen bound to hemoglobin because this has been displaced by the CO (11). Pulse oximetry cannot screen for CO exposure, as it does not differentiate carboxyhemoglobin from oxyhemoglobin and ABG analysis will show an apparently normal SaO_2. The blood carboxyhemoglobin level must be measured to assess the degree of CO poisoning. The half-life of carboxyhemoglobin in a patient breathing room air is approximately 300 minutes; this decreases to 90 minutes with high-concentration oxygen via a reservoir mask. The most important treatment for a patient with CO poisoning is, therefore, to give high-dose oxygen via a reservoir mask. Comatose patients or those with severe mental impairment should be endotracheally intubated and ventilated with 100% oxygen. The role of hyperbaric oxygen remains controversial (12,13).

Patients who present serious illness but are not critical or greatly hypoxic—pneumonia, acute asthma, lung cancer, interstitial lung disease, pneumothorax, pleural effusion, pulmonary embolism, acute heart failure with hypoxemia, stroke with hypoxemia, labor with hypoxemia, postoperative breathlessness or hypoxemia, or severe anemia with breathlessness—can be treated with medium-dose oxygen therapy with a target SpO_2 range of 94% to 98%. Generally, breathless and hypoxemic patients do not have a firm diagnosis at the time of presentation to the hospital. For most acutely hypoxemic patients whose medical problem is not yet diagnosed, an SpO_2 range of 94% to 98% will avoid the potential risks associated with hypoxemia or hyperoxia. Aiming for an SpO_2 in the normal range will also have the effect of using the lowest effective FiO_2, avoiding risks such as absorption atelectasis and V/Q mismatch. The priority for such patients is to make a specific diagnosis as early as possible and to institute specific treatment for the underlying condition. Early ABG measurement is mandatory in the management of patients with sudden unexplained hypoxemia.

Patients with chronic lung disease may tolerate a low SpO_2 chronically when clinically stable; however, these resting oxygen levels may not be adequate for tissue oxygenation during acute illness or in those conditions where oxygen demand increases. For those patients with COPD (14–22) or other known risk factors that can predispose to hypercapnic respiratory failure with acidosis—morbid obesity, chest wall deformities, or neuromuscular disorders, cystic fibrosis, severe lung scarring from old tuberculosis, overdose of respiratory depressant drugs—a target SpO_2 range of 88% to 92% is suggested pending the availability of ABG results. For this subgroup of patients, it is recommended that treatment is carefully titrated with ABG measurements in order to prevent episodes of hypercapnic respiratory failure, using, if necessary, noninvasive or invasive mechanical ventilation. Noninvasive ventilation is recommended for patients with COPD with hypercapnia and a pH less than 7.35 despite 1 hour of standard medical treatment (23,24).

On the contrary, there are no published trials supporting the use of oxygen to relieve breathlessness in nonhypoxemic patients, and there is evidence from randomized studies that oxygen does not relieve breathlessness compared with air in nonhypoxemic patients with COPD who are breathless following exertion (25).

Oxygen Delivery Devices

Oxygen can be delivered to spontaneously breathing patients through a very wide range of devices that are described in the following. But first we note the main method of storage and provision of oxygen. Compressed gas can be contained at a very high pressure into cylinders that come in an array of sizes and, hence, capacity ranging from small portable cylinders for individual use to large ones suitable for hospital use. Additionally, oxygen exists in a liquid form, which is obtained from atmospheric oxygen by fractional distillation and is stored in pressure tanks; it has to be evaporated into gas before use. Finally, oxygen can be obtained from the concentrators.

Returning to delivery devices for oxygen therapy, they are typically classified into two groups: variable flow or fixed-flow equipment. The term variable flow relates to the fact that as the patient's respiratory pattern changes, delivered oxygen is diluted with room air. This results in a widely inconsistent and fluctuating FiO_2. In fact, despite some commonly published figures for delivered FiO_2 at given flow rates, the actual FiO_2 delivered to the patient by various devices is neither precise nor predictable. Variable flow devices include nasal catheter, nasal cannulae, transtracheal oxygen catheter, and various oxygen masks. Fixed-flow equipment, on the other hand, provides the entire patient's inspired gas with a precisely controlled FiO_2; when applied appropriately, the FiO_2 delivered to the patient is therefore constant, regardless of ventilatory pattern. Fixed-flow devices include air-entrainment masks, large-volume aerosol systems, and large-volume humidifier systems.

The choice of a specific system will depend upon the clinical status of the patients, the dose of oxygen required, and the tolerance of the patient for the device. Oxygen should be humidified, whenever possible, in order to prevent dried secretions to obstructing smaller airways. A nasal cannula provides oxygen through oxygen supply tubing with two soft prongs that are inserted into the nares. It can deliver low and medium-dose oxygen concentrations—respectively with low- and high-flow devices—that, flowing into the nasopharynx, mixes with room air; consequently, the FiO_2 varies depending upon factors such as respiratory rate, tidal volume, oxygen flow rate, and extent of mouth breathing. Although one might expect mouth breathing to reduce the efficiency of nasal cannulae, the majority of studies have shown that mouth breathing results in either the same inspired oxygen concentration or a higher concentration, especially when the respiratory rate is increased. This is important because patients with acute breathlessness are likely to breathe quickly and via the mouth rather than the nose. As there is marked individual variation in breathing pattern, the flow rate must be adjusted based on SpO_2 and, where necessary, ABG measurements. The formula to calculate the FiO_2 delivered with nasal cannula is:

$$FiO_2 = 20\% + (4 \times \text{oxygen liter flow})$$

Low-flow nasal cannulae typically deliver rates between 1 and 4 L/min with an FiO_2 that varies from 25% to 40% (26). Generally, low-flow nasal cannulae are used to deliver oxygen to an adult with a low oxygen requirement; this system is lightweight and inexpensive. In addition, the patient can talk and feed without interruption of oxygen delivery. On the other hand, they are of limited use during the stabilization of acutely ill patients, since they cannot reliably deliver high concentrations of oxygen. Moreover, some patients may experience discomfort, nasal dryness, and epistaxis at flows above 4 L/min, especially if it is maintained for many hours, even when a bubble humidifier is used. Therefore, if higher oxygen flow rates and FiO_2 are needed, it is better to use a mask.

Masks are the most frequently used oxygen delivery system; they are indicated in patients who breathe spontaneously, especially if they are strictly mouth breathers, and who require FiO_2 that cannot be delivered using nasal cannulae. The device should be placed over the patient's nose and mouth and secured with an elastic strap fitted around the head. There exist several different types of masks, characterized by the range of oxygen concentration that can be delivered and the possibility to avoid carbon dioxide rebreathing. However, the masks have some disadvantages, such as the risk for aspiration if the patient vomits, and limitations in communication, coughing, and eating. Moreover, masks are not suitable for patients with hypercapnic respiratory failure, because of the risk of rebreathing associated with their use.

The simple face mask delivers moderate amounts of oxygen with a higher concentration than nasal cannula; it receives the oxygen through a tube connected at the base of the mask, delivering oxygen flows between 6 and 10 L/min. The mask itself, with its volume of 100 to 300 mL, serves as a reservoir. Room air enters through the holes on each side of the mask and mixes with pure oxygen, thereby decreasing the percentage of oxygen inspired by the patient; the final concentration generally varies between 35% and 50%, depending on the patient's respiratory rate and the mask fit (27–29). Thus, precise concentration of oxygen cannot be reliably delivered. Using this mask, an oxygen flow rate greater than 5 L/min is recommended to prevent rebreathing of carbon dioxide (28,30).

A specific type of simple mask is the Venturi mask, the operation of which is based upon the Venturi principle: pure oxygen flows into the mask and is diluted with air entrained via ports on the Venturi valve. The amount of air entrained into the mask is related to the thickness of the ports and to the flow of oxygen into the system. The proportion of air entrained remains essentially the same through a range of oxygen flow rates and, therefore, the Venturi mask delivers the same oxygen concentration as the flow rate is increased (the minimum suggested flow rate is written on each Venturi device). Because this high-flow mask provides an accurate concentration of oxygen to the patient, regardless of the flow rate, it is suitable for patients needing a known concentration of oxygen. For patients with a high respiratory rate, the flow rate is set above the minimum indicated on the valve so as to exceed the inspiratory flow rate of the patient.

A simple mask connected to a reservoir is defined a partial rebreathing mask. This kind of mask needs oxygen flow rates of between 10 and 12 L/min and delivers an oxygen concentration ranging between 50% and 60% (28,31). During inspiration, air is drawn predominantly from the fresh oxygen contained in the reservoir. Despite the fact that this compartment contains some exhaled gases as well, gases in the reservoir are oxygen rich because the early exhaled air that flows into the reservoir from respiratory dead space is oxygen rich and contains little carbon dioxide (31,32). To avoid this commingling of pure oxygen flow with exhaled gas, and to avoid the risk of rebreathing, it can be used a nonrebreathing face mask with reservoir and one-way valves. This system is composed of one-way valves over the exhalation ports that allow the egress of expired gases during exhalation and prevent room air from entering the mask during inspiration (33). Another one-way valve is located between the mask and the reservoir in order to prevent flow of exhaled gases into the reservoir. With this mask, oxygen should flow into the reservoir at 8 to 15 L/min and, in any case, the flow should be adjusted to prevent the collapse of reservoir. Notwithstanding the fact that, with this aid, an FiO_2 of up to 95% can be achieved (34), the real oxygen concentration inhaled by the patient is variable and not accurately predictable, depending on the flow rate and the breathing pattern.

High-Flow Nasal Cannulae (HFNC)

All the conventional high-flow oxygen delivery systems discussed above are not well tolerated by the patients due to discomfort, obtrusiveness, and insufficient heating and humidification of the inspired gases (35–37). To obviate these disadvantages, effort has been spent over the past two decades to develop and validate an alternative oxygen delivery system: the high-flow nasal cannulae (HFNC). This device provides a gas mixture, with an FiO_2 ranging from 0.21 to nearly 1.0 to nares via nasal prolongs. The presence of an oxygen blender allows the desired FiO_2 to be set and delivered, adjusting it independently from the flow rate, which can reach a maximum of 60 L/min. In addition, the gas mixture can be warmed to body temperature and saturated with water via an inline humidifier. Several studies showed that the use of HFNC was associated with a greater comfort and tolerance, lower dyspnea, lower dryness of upper airways, and lower desiccation of secretions, compared to conventional face masks (38–40). One of the consequences of inhaling a warmed and fully humidified gas mixture is the maintenance of the integrity of mucociliary function, consequently rendering secretions easier to mobilize. This produces a decrease in the work imposed on muscles for expectoration. Another beneficial effect of this device consists in its ability of generate a flow rate that exceeds the patient's peak inspiratory flow rate, in most cases, guaranteeing that there is less room air mixed with the inspired gas, and the desired FiO_2 is more reliably delivered to the patient (41,42). This is particularly useful for patients in respiratory distress, who often have inspiratory flow rates that exceed those that can be delivered by standard systems (33). Patients with respiratory distress can also benefit from the continuous wash out of carbon dioxide from the anatomic dead space (43,44), occurring with HFNC, especially at higher flow rates (45). Over the last 10 years, multiple studies have shown that HFNC generate a positive pressure inside the nasopharynx and esophagus during both inspiration and expiration (46,47). Perhaps as a consequence, HFNC may reduce the work of breathing by providing inspiratory assistance, which increases the tidal volume, reduces respiratory rate, and counterbalances autoPEEP, especially in COPD patients (48–50). Although HFNC has been proposed as a management tool for various conditions, including hypoxemic respiratory failure, cardiogenic pulmonary edema, as well as to prevent respiratory failure in postoperative and postextubation patients, the data available for adult applications of HFNC are limited (51).

For patients who have a tracheostomy or a transtracheal fistula, oxygen can be delivered through a tracheostomy mask or a transtracheal catheter. These devices deliver high-flow oxygen directly into trachea, promoting gas exchange; indeed they can reduce the work of breathing and augment carbon dioxide removal. When oxygen is given in this way for a prolonged period, humidification and suctions to remove the mucus from the airways are indicated.

RESPIRATORY CARE AND MONITORING IN THE ICU

Respiratory monitoring in critically ill patients is mandatory to detect inadequate oxygenation, acid–base imbalance and tissue hypoperfusion at an early stage. The correct use and interpretation of data from bedside assessment can improve patient outcomes. We describe here the potential clinical value of advanced respiratory monitoring technologies, according with a recent published consensus (52).

Monitoring Systems

Gas Exchange

The diagnosis of hypoxemia is essentially based on two parameters: oxygen saturation and arterial oxygen tension. The amount of oxygen carried in the blood is often expressed in terms of oxygen saturation of circulating hemoglobin. This is what is meant by "oxygen saturation level" (SpO_2, SaO_2), defined as one of the five vital signs. If the measurement is checked using pulse oximeter, rather than via an ABG measurement (SaO_2), it is called the SpO_2: for adults aged less than 70 years, the normal range is approximately 95% to 98% at sea level, and it declines gradually within this age range (53). The mean SpO_2 may be lower in older people; however, it is difficult to dissociate the effects of advancing age from the effects of the disease which are common in old age (54,55). If the oxygen saturation is measured directly from an arterial blood sample, it is called the SaO_2 (56–58).

Alternatively, it is possible to measure the oxygen tension of the blood (PaO_2), known as the "partial pressure of oxygen." This measurement can be expressed in kilopascals (kPa, normal range 12.0 to 14.6 kPa) or in millimeters of mercury (normal range 90 to 110 mmHg for young adults) and it is usually obtained from an arterial specimen. More rarely, it is obtained from arteriolized earlobe blood. In both cases, it is preferable to use local anesthesia to obtain these specimens, except in emergencies or if the patient is unconscious or anesthetized. The presence of a normal saturation measured by SpO_2 does not exclude the need for performing ABG analysis, especially among critically ill patients. Indeed SpO_2 can be normal in a patient with an alteration of pH or arterial carbon dioxide tension ($PaCO_2$) or with anemia. Therefore, ABG analysis should be evaluated early in all critically ill patients, in all subjects having an unexpected or inappropriate SpO_2, in any case of increasing breathlessness in a patient with previously stable hypoxemia, in a stable patient who deteriorates and requires a significantly increased FiO_2 to maintain a constant SpO_2, in any patient with risk factors for hypercapnic respiratory failure who develops acute breathlessness, deteriorating oxygen saturation or drowsiness, or other symptoms of CO_2 retention. Additionally, ABG analysis should be performed in breathless patients who are thought to be at risk of metabolic conditions such as diabetic ketoacidosis or metabolic acidosis due to renal failure, in acutely breathless or critically ill patients with poor peripheral circulation in whom a reliable oximetry signal cannot be obtained, or in the presence of any other evidence that would indicate that ABG blood gas results would be useful in the patient's management, for example, an unexpected change in "track and trigger" systems such as a sudden rise of several units in the medical early warning score (MEWS) or an unexpected fall in SpO_2 of 3% or more, even if within the target range (59).

Before evaluating the oxygenation of a patient, it's important to record the FiO_2 and the PaO_2/FiO_2 ratio; the latter is a quick and simple parameter that refers to the ratio of arterial oxygen partial pressure to fractional inspired oxygen. According to the Berlin definition of acute respiratory distress syndrome (ARDS; see Chapter 109), patients are categorized into three different categories (mild, moderate, or severe), based on the PaO_2/FIO_2 ratio (60). Although it has limitations, the PaO_2/FIO_2 ratio is a very useful clinical parameter used for predicting outcome and response to therapy in patients with ARDS (61).

As mentioned above, when assessing the level of oxygenation of critically ill patients with respiratory failure, PaO_2 and SaO_2 (or SpO_2) are the main determinants and are most frequently used; however, there are many conditions where they may not provide sufficient information about the adequacy of oxygen delivery (DO_2). Indeed this parameter relies on many determinants, such as passive oxygen diffusion into the arterial blood, but also on oxygen-carrying capacity of blood, adequate cardiac output, and local control of blood flow to the organs. Global DO_2 is the product of cardiac output (CO) and arterial oxygen content (CaO_2); CaO_2 is, in turn, the product of SaO_2, hemoglobin concentration and a constant reflecting hemoglobin–oxygen binding capacity (6). In the case of V/Q abnormalities, anemia, or low CO, the $PA–aO_2$ gradient or the PaO_2/FiO_2 ratio may be more sensitive indicators and correlate better with the adequacy of DO_2.

Devices for Titration of Oxygen Flow

Over the past several years, devices have been developed that automatically adjust—in a closed-loop manner—oxygen flow to spontaneously breathing patients, maintaining a set oxygenation target, such as the O_2 flow regulator (62) and the free O_2 (63). It is recognized that the oxygen flow administered to the patient is not always optimal; patient's needs vary during the day, and even in healthy people, episodes of oxygen desaturation may occur during daily activities or during sleep. These drops in saturation occur more frequently in the critically ill patient and in those affected by COPD (64), inducing complications such as reduction in exercise tolerance (65), pulmonary hypertension, right heart failure, polycythemia, and increased mortality (66). Some studies have found that oxygen therapy is not optimally prescribed in COPD patients; that the commonly prescribed, fixed dose, usually titrated at rest, may not meet the patient's needs during an exacerbation, inducing both hypoxemia and hyperoxia, with their attendant complications (67–70). It would be preferable, therefore, to tailor the oxygen flow to the actual changing need of the patient, and to titrate the flow rate based upon an SpO_2 signal to maintain a target saturation, for example, a target of 93% or more (71). This adjustment in oxygen flow minimizes episodes of desaturation, avoids excessive administration that may produce respiratory acidosis, and maintains stable SpO_2 at all activity levels.

Transcutaneous Arterial Carbon Dioxide Pressure

Transcutaneous carbon dioxide monitoring ($PtcCO_2$) is a noninvasive method used to estimate the $PaCO_2$. It is able to give an electrochemical measurement of $PaCO_2$ by warming the skin and inducing hyperperfusion (72). Although there is a good concordance between arterial and transcutaneous $PaCO_2$ values (73), the role of $PtcCO_2$ in the adult intensive care setting remains unclear. Major issues include the need for frequent recalibration and the mismatch in presence of hyperoxia, hypoperfusion, improper electrode placement, and tissue edema. Additionally, skin breakdown and tissue loss can occur, especially if the probe is left in place for long time (74).

Volumetric Capnography

Volumetric capnography is a noninvasive technique that examines the CO_2 concentration in exhaled air as a function of expired volume by using infrared light. As described for the first time by Aitken and Clarke–Kennedy (75), the capnogram curve represents one respiratory cycle and has several components: the first part of the waveform (phase I) represents the CO_2 from the airway (dead space), the second part (phase II) is a sharp rise (beginning of exhalation) that coincides with the transition between airway and alveolar gas. The highest portion of this segment is called the end-tidal CO_2 and represents the maximum pressure of CO_2 at the end of breath; normally it is between 35 and 40 mmHg. The phase III corresponds to the CO_2 eliminated from the alveoli (plateau line). The homogeneity of the gas distribution and alveolar ventilation are the major determinants of the capnogram's shape.

In addition, dead space can be deduced noninvasively using volumetric capnography (76–78). It has, thus, been useful in the monitoring of various diseases, particularly when V/Q mismatch is present, such as in pulmonary thromboembolism (79), interstitial lung disease, and acute lung injury, as well as in patients undergoing mechanical ventilation (52,80). However, this technique needs a complex equipment which represents a limitation of its use in clinical practice (52).

Respiratory System Mechanics

The respiratory system includes both passive (lung and the chest wall) and active structures (respiratory muscles); these components have both elastic and resistive properties. The elasticity is defined as a driving pressure variation (ΔP) over a change in volume (ΔV). Resistance is expressed as the ratio between the pressure change and the gas flow ($\dot{V}$) variation ($\Delta P/\Delta \dot{V}$). It is not possible to separate the chest wall and the lung from the respiratory muscles, and so the respiratory mechanics properties can be evaluated only when the respiratory muscle activity is quiescent (patient deeply sedated or paralyzed). During passive mechanical ventilation, compliance is calculated as the ratio between V_T and plateau pressure (P_{plat}) minus positive end-expiratory pressure (PEEP). On the other hand, the difference between peak or maximal pressure (P_{MAX}) and plateau pressure (P_{plat}) over a constant $\dot{V}$ define the resistance (81,82).

During volume-controlled ventilation, with a constant flow, it is possible to calculate both the resistive forces and the compliance of the respiratory system by performing easily bedside end-inspiratory and end-expiratory occlusion maneuvers. Briefly, after the end-inspiratory occlusion technique, the rapid pressure drop from P_{MAX} to P_{plat} represents the pressure required to move the flow through the airways and the endotracheal tube (ETT). The following slow drop until a plateau depends mainly on the elastic properties of the system. With the end-expiratory occlusion, clinicians can evaluate the values for intrinsic (auto) PEEP and total PEEP. Thus, compliance and resistance measurements provided by ventilators performing end-inspiratory and end-expiratory pauses, as well as the interpretation of P/V curves with the identification of the lower (LIP) and upper (UIP) inflection points, furnish useful information to optimize mechanical ventilation management according with the underlying diseases.

Esophageal and Transpulmonary Pressure

The esophageal pressure (P_{es}) is an acceptable surrogate of pleural pressure and can be measured by using an esophageal balloon catheter. Thanks to this correlation, it is possible to estimate the transpulmonary pressure (P_{TP}), the pressure needed to distend the lungs, as the difference between the airway pressure (P_{aw}) and the pleural pressure (P_{pl}); it is also possible to measure the gastric pressure (P_{ga}) and, consequently, the transdiaphragmatic pressure (P_{di}), which results from the difference between P_{ga} and P_{es}, by adding a gastric balloon.

Recently, a Pleural Pressure Working Group (PLUG) reviewed the newest information on esophageal pressure monitoring in patients with respiratory failure (83). Currently, the measurement of P_{es} in mechanically ventilated patients is often performed in an attempt to detect and treat patient/ventilator asynchrony, to measure work of breathing and to guide weaning, and to optimize mechanical ventilation in patients with ARDS. ARDS is characterized by a decrease in respiratory system compliance due to the presence of alveolar and interstitial fluid, and the loss of surfactant. The standard of care for mechanically ventilated patients with ARDS includes low tidal volume (V_t = 6 mL/kg of predicted body weight) and low plateau pressure ($P_{plat} \leq 30$ cm H_2O) (84). PEEP is also applied in order to maintain open air spaces and to prevent the cyclic opening and closing of alveoli that produces the ventilator-induced lung injury (85,86). As previously mentioned, clinicians optimize ventilator support by monitoring the airway pressure, assuming that the P_{aw} reflects the P_{TP}. On the other hand, because the P_{aw} represents the sum of pressure across the lung and the chest wall, in case of chest compliance reduction, as one would see with obese patients, as well as in patients with edema or with abdominal distension, it does not always correspond to the pressure seen by the lung (87).

Therefore, the P_{es} has been proposed to calculate the end-expiratory P_{TP} and to set PEEP so as to prevent the cyclic lung recruitment and derecruitment that are present when P_{pl} is greater than P_{aw} at the end of expiration (88). As shown by the EPVent study (89), the strategy that uses P_{es} to adjust PEEP in order to achieve end-expiratory P_{TP} between 0 and 10 cm H_2O (the esophageal pressure–guided group) significantly improves oxygenation and compliance compared with the control group in which PEEP was set according to the patient's PaO_2 and FiO_2 (gas exchange–based PEEP group). Based upon these considerations, the use of the P_{es} to optimize ventilator setting in ARDS patients seems more useful to avoid both under- and over-lung distension compared to the use of airway pressure as guide.

The Procedure

Although advances in electronic and computer technology over the last decades have generated several ventilators with additional pressure transducers that provide P_{es} measurement at the patient's bedside, the most commonly used procedure is performed via esophageal and gastric balloons that are now commercially available. The passage of the catheters through the nasal cavity may cause pain, irritation, cough, and sometimes vomiting. Thus, initial preparation of the awake patient includes the local nebulization of lidocaine and a mild dose of sedative, if the patient is particularly anxious. Placing the patient into the semi-recumbent position is the best approach to the insertion of the balloon (90). Usually two operators are required for the operation, the first one dedicated to extend the neck of the patient, with the second one very slowly introducing the catheter into the nares, preferably the one appearing to be unoccluded or less occluded.

The esophageal balloon should be first pushed into the stomach and moved backward step by step until it passes through the esophageal sphincter where the waveform during inspiration will begin to become negative. The balloon is then positioned roughly in the middle third of the esophagus where the "occlusion test" is performed (91). The gastric catheter's position is checked by pushing over the patient's abdomen to see a clear positive pressure swing. Once the catheter is in place, it needs to be fixed with tape at the nostril, and 1 mL of air is then inserted with a syringe and then slowly removed until about 0.3 to 0.4 mL remain (92–96).

Despite being relatively well standardized, the technique for measuring respiratory mechanics requires special attention to avoid errors and complications. Patient should be fasting to reduce the risk of vomiting. Additionally, disorders of the mouth, pharynx—tumors, cervical spine disease, or pharyngoesophageal diverticulum—and esophageal pathologies—tumor, strictures secondary to radiation or chemical burns, medications or ulcers, Schatzki's ring, or foreign bodies—may represent relative and absolute contraindications to the examination (92). Clinicians must pay careful attention to patients with pre-existing cardiac dysrhythmias, as catheter placement may increase the risk of complication, as well as of a vagal reflex syndrome. Finally, neuromuscular problems—stroke, Parkinson's disease, Huntington's disease, multiple sclerosis, myasthenia gravis, muscular dystrophy, polymyositis, amyotrophic lateral sclerosis or scleroderma—may also make balloon passage difficult (92).

Lungs Volumes

Direct Measurement of End-Expiratory Lung Volume

The lung volume at the end of passive expiration is defined functional residual capacity (FRC). The term end-expiratory lung volume (EELV) is the more precise term to describe the lung volume when PEEP is applied during mechanical ventilation. The measurement of FRC and EELV is useful for the management of patients with ARDS that present a reduction in lung volume. To calculate the EELV we can use several methods. The closed dilution technique requires the calculation of a known soluble gas volume (helium or methane) in expired breath. Recently, bedside EELV measurement using nitrogen or O_2 and CO_2 sensors in ICU ventilators—so-called washout/wash-in techniques—have been proposed in clinical practice (52). EELV estimation may help to set PEEP and monitor alveolar recruitment maneuver responses in patients with ARDS when combined with compliance measures (97).

Lung Ultrasound

Over the past decade, the use of lung ultrasound (LUS), supported by emerging data, has increased in different clinical settings. The International Consensus Conference provided recommendations and indications for LUS in order to standardize this technique (98). Actually, LUS is considered an accurate tool for bedside respiratory monitoring in the ICUs. In fact, LUS allows detection of pleural effusion, differentiation of consolidation potentially secondary to pulmonary embolism, pneumonia, or atelectasis, and as a tool to rule out pneumothorax and diaphragmatic dysfunction. Moreover, thoracic ultrasound is used as a tool to guide thoracentesis and for placement of thoracostomy tubes or central venous lines. LUS is also able to monitor the effects of therapy in various acute lung diseases, including acute pulmonary edema, ARDS, community-acquired pneumonia, and ventilator-associated pneumonia (98,99). Thoracic ultrasound has some advantages compared to the chest radiography and CT scan, including portability and the ability to perform real-time imaging. In addition, LUS does not expose the patient to ionizing radiation. The major limitations include the need for staff training and the inability to give precise information in case of deep lesions without consolidation/effusion and/or paravertebral lesions, along with technical challenges in obese or edematous patients (100).

Respiratory Monitoring During Noninvasive Ventilation

NIV is a useful therapeutic modality for many patients and its use in the ICU has increased in the last two decades. As success with NIV depends on several factors, monitoring during NIV should be directed to identify and, if possible, resolving the issues that are associated with failure of this mode of ventilation, in order to improve patient's outcomes. As noted by Olzyman et al. (101), the possible causes of immediate NIV failure—that is, failure within minutes to less than 1 hour of initiation of NIV—are a weak cough reflex and/or excessive secretions, severe neurologic impairment, patient–ventilator asynchrony, and intolerance and agitation. Thus, an accurate evaluation of vital signs, respiratory muscle function, cough effectiveness, and degree of consciousness is mandatory prior to initiation if NIV. In addition, unstable patients with ARF should be closely monitored with ABG analysis, both to establish the baseline severity and to avoid delay in endotracheal intubation in case of worsening gas exchange.

Patient–ventilator interaction is an important issue that ICU staff should take into account when using NIV. In fact, high inspiratory ventilator pressures and the presence of air leaks are major determinants of NIV asynchronies (52,102). Although recent technologic advances—for instance, new NIV algorithms and modes such as neurally adjusted ventilator assistance (NAVA)—have been designed to reduce the occurrence of patient–ventilator asynchrony (103–105), bedside methods, including evaluation of spontaneous versus ventilator-delivered breaths and accessory muscle use should be always considered initially. Additionally, air leaks can be identified by following the inspired and expired tidal volume values, and the presence of autoPEEP can be expected when the flow does not reach zero at the end of expiration. These simple measures, in association with flow and pressure waveform observations on the ventilator screen, should be used by physicians to detect "gross" patient–ventilator mismatching. In patients receiving NIV for acute COPD exacerbation, optimization of the ventilator settings by analyzing flow and pressure waveforms on the screen ("optimized ventilation") is a more efficient manner to set the ventilator than by considering only numerical data ("standard ventilation") in terms of gas exchange and NIV success (106).

Finally, NIV interface intolerance is another important reason of failure when attempting to utilize NIV for an acute episode. Consequently, sedation should be considered part of the strategy aimed at improving NIV acceptance, mainly related to minimizing interface discomfort (101,107).

In conclusion, it is advisable for every clinician prescribing NIV to have an experience in clinical, pharmacologic, and technologic competences as well as in monitoring skills in order to improve patient outcomes and to avoid delays in endotracheal intubation, especially in patient with *de novo* hypoxemic respiratory failure (108).

Key Points

- Oxygen therapy should be handled carefully in critically ill patients according to the underline cause of respiratory failure.
- Oxygen therapy can be delivered via different devices. The choice of the most appropriate system should be made based upon patient's clinical status, level of required oxygen supply, and patient's tolerance and comfort. The use of HFNC is associated with a greater comfort and tolerance, lower dyspnea, lower dryness of upper airways, compared to standard oxygen. However, the data available for adult applications of HFNC are limited.
- Critically ill patients should be closely monitored in order to detect the early onset of acute respiratory distress and failure to maintaining adequate saturation, to avoid oxygen toxicity and its side effects. On the other hand, respiratory monitoring is essential to identify the causes of the disease involved and the effects of treatment.

References

1. Priestley J. *Experiments and Observations on Different Kinds of Air*. London, J. Johnson. 1775; revised 1790.
2. Smith AH. *Oxygen Gas as a Remedy in Disease*. New York, NY: D. Appleton & Company; 1870.
3. Bryan CL, Jenkinson SG. Oxygen toxicity. *Clin Chest Med*. 1988;9:141–152.
4. O'Neill B, Mahon JM, Bradley J. Short-burst oxygen therapy in chronic obstructive pulmonary disease. *Respir Med*. 2006;100:1129–1138.
5. Clemens KE, Klaschik E. Symptomatic therapy of dyspnea with strong opioids and its effect on ventilation in palliative care patients. *J Pain Symptom Manag*. 2007;33:473–481.
6. Marks B, Mitchell DG, Simelaro JP. Breath-holding in healthy and pulmonary compromised patients: effects of hyperventilation and oxygen inspiration. *J Magn Reson Imaging*. 1997;7:595–597.
7. McCarthy RM, Shea S, Deshpande VS, et al. Coronary MR angiography: true FISP imaging improved by prolonging breath holds with preoxygenation in healthy volunteers. *Radiology*. 2003;227:283–288.
8. Bowton DL, Scuderi PE, Haponik EF. The incidence and effect on outcome of hypoxemia in hospitalised medical patients. *Am J Med*. 1994;97:38–46.
9. Slutsky AS. Consensus conference on mechanical ventilation. Part I. European Society of Intensive Care Medicine, the ACCP and the SCCM. *Intensive Care Med*. 1994;20:64–79.
10. Gries RE, Brooks LJ. Normal oxyhemoglobin saturation during sleep: how low does it go? *Chest*. 1996;110:1489–1492.
11. Kao LW, Nanagas KA. Toxicity associated with carbon monoxide. *Clin Lab Med*. 2006;26:99–125.
12. Juurlink DN, Buckley NA, Stanbrook MB, et al. Hyperbaric oxygen for carbon monoxide poisoning. *Cochrane Database Syst Rev*. 2005;(1):CD002041.
13. Weaver LK, Valentine KJ, Hopkins RO. Carbon monoxide poisoning: risk factors for cognitive sequelae and the role of hyperbaric oxygen. *Am J Respir Crit Care Med*. 2007;176:491–497.
14. Plant PK, Owen JL, Elliott MW. One year period prevalence study of respiratory acidosis in acute exacerbations of COPD: implications for the provision of noninvasive ventilation and oxygen administration. *Thorax*. 2000;55:550–554.
15. Warrel DA, Edwards RHT, Godfrey S, et al. Effect of controlled oxygen therapy on arterial blood gases in acute respiratory failure. *BMJ*. 1970;2:452–455.
16. Campbell EJM. The management of acute respiratory failure in chronic bronchitis and emphysema. *Am Rev Respir Dis*. 1967;96:26–39.
17. Lopez-Majano V, Dutton RE. Regulation of respiration during oxygen breathing in COLD. *Am Rev Respir Dis*. 1973;108:232–240.
18. Aubier M, Murciano D, Milic Emili J, et al. Effects of the administration of O2 on ventilation and blood gases in patients with chronic obstructive pulmonary disease during acute respiratory failure. *Am Rev Respir Dis*. 1980;122:747–754.
19. Johnson JE, Peacock MD, Hayes JA, et al. Forced expiratory flow is reduced by 100% oxygen in patients with chronic obstructive pulmonary disease. *South Med J*. 1995;88:443–449.
20. Refsum HE. Relationship between state of consciousness and arterial hypoxaemia and hypercapnia in patients with pulmonary insufficiency, breathing air. *Clin Sci*. 1963;25:361–367.
21. Joosten SA, Koh MS, Bu X, et al. The effects of oxygen therapy in patients presenting to an emergency department with exacerbation of chronic obstructive pulmonary disease. *Med J Aust*. 2007;186:235–238.
22. Campbell EJ. A method of controlled oxygen administration which reduces the risk of carbon-dioxide retention. *Lancet*. 1960;2:12–24.
23. National Institute for Clinical Excellence (NICE). Chronic obstructive pulmonary disease. NICE Guideline CG12. Available at: http://www.nice.org.uk/guidance/CG12/niceguidance/pdf/English. 2004.
24. British Thoracic Society Standards of Care Committee. Non-invasive ventilation in acute respiratory failure. *Thorax*. 2002;57:192–211.
25. Abernethy AP, McDonald CF, Frith PA, et al. Effect of palliative oxygen versus room air in relief of breathlessness in patients with refractory dyspnoea: a double-blind, randomised controlled trial. *Lancet*. 2010;376(9743):784–793.
26. Wettstein RB, Shelledy DC, Peters JI. Delivered oxygen concentrations using low-flow and high-flow nasal cannulas. *Respir Care*. 2005;50:604–609.
27. Bateman NT, Leach RM. ABC of oxygen: acute oxygen therapy. *BMJ*. 1998;317:798–801
28. Myers TR, American Association for Respiratory Care (AARC). AARC Clinical Practice Guideline: selection of an oxygen delivery device for neonatal and pediatric patients—2002 revision & update. *Respir Care*. 2002;47:707–716.
29. Milross J, Young IH, Donnelly P. The oxygen delivery characteristics of the Hudson Oxy-one face mask. *Anaesth Intensive Care*. 1989;17:180–184.
30. Jensen AG, Johnson A, Sandstedt S. Rebreathing during oxygen treatment with face mask: the effect of oxygen flow rates on ventilation. *Acta Anaesthesiol Scand*. 1991;35:289–292.
31. King BR, King C, Coates WC. Critical procedures. In: Gausche-Hill M, Fuchs S, Yamamoto L, eds. *APLS: The Pediatric Emergency Medicine Resource*. 4th ed. Sudbury, MA: Jones and Bartlett; 2004:686.
32. Ludwig S. Resuscitation: pediatric basic and advanced life support. In: Fleisher GR, Ludwig S, eds. *Textbook of Pediatric Emergency Medicine*. Baltimore, MD: Williams & Wilkins; 1993:3.
33. Scarfone RJ. Airway adjuncts, oxygen delivery, and suctioning of the upper airway. In: Henretig FM, King C, eds. *Textbook of Pediatric Emergency Medicine Procedures*. Philadelphia, PA: Lippincott Williams & Wilkins, 1997:101.
34. Boumphrey SM, Morris EA, Kinsella SM. 100% inspired oxygen from a Hudson mask-a realistic goal? *Resuscitation*. 2003;57:69–72.
35. Kallstrom TJ. AARC Clinical Practice Guideline: oxygen therapy for adults in the acute care facility—2002 revision & update. *Respir Care*. 2002:47:717–720.
36. Shapiro BA, Kacmarek RM, Cane RD, et al. *Clinical Application of Respiratory Care*. 4th ed. St. Louis, MA: Mosby-Year Book; 1991.
37. Chanques G, Constantin JM, Sauter M, et al. Discomfort associated with underhumidified high-flow oxygen therapy in critically ill patients. *Intensive Care Med*. 2009:35:996–1003.
38. Roca O, Riera J, Torres F, et al. High-flow oxygen therapy in acute respiratory failure. *Respir Care*. 2010:55(4):408–413.
39. Tiruvoipati R, Lewis D, Haji K, et al. High-flow nasal oxygen vs. high-flow face mask: a randomized crossover trial in extubated patients. *J Crit Care*. 2010:25:463–468.
40. Rittayamai N, Tscheikuna J, Rujiwit P. High-flow nasal oxygen versus conventional oxygen therapy after endotracheal extubation: a randomized crossover physiologic study. *Respir Care*. 2014; 59(4):485–490.
41. Sim MAB, Dean P, Kinsella J, et al. Performance of oxygen delivery devices when the breathing pattern of respiratory failure is simulated. *Anaesthesia*. 2008:63:938–940.
42. Wagstaff TA, Soni N. Performance of six types of oxygen delivery devices at varying respiratory rates. *Anaesthesia*. 2007:62:492–503.
43. Sztrymf B, Messika J, Bertrans F, et al. Beneficial effects of humidified high flow oxygen in critical care patients: a prospective pilot study. *Intensive Care Med*. 2011:37:1780–1786.
44. Lenglet H, Sztrymf B, Leroy C, et al. Humidified high flow nasal oxygen during respiratory failure in the emergency department: feasibility and efficacy. *Respir Care*. 2012:57(11):1873–1878.
45. Frizzola M, Miller TL, Rodriguez ME, et al. High-flow nasal cannula: impact on oxygenation and ventilation in an acute lung injury model. *Pediatr Pulmonol*. 2011:46(1):67–74.
46. Hasan RA, Habib RH. Effects of flow-rate and airleak at the nares and mouth opening on positive distending pressure delivery using commercially available high-flow nasal cannula systems: a lung model study. *Pediatr Crit Care Med*. 2011:12(1):e29–e33.
47. Parke RL, Ecclestone ML, McGuinness SP. The effects of flow on airway pressure during nasal high-flow oxygen therapy. *Respir Care*. 2011:56(8):1151–1155.
48. Braunlich J, Beyer D, Mai D, et al. Effects of nasal high flow on ventilation in volunteers, COPD and idiopathic pulmonary fibrosis patients. *Respiration*. 2013;85(4):319–325.
49. Mundel T, Feng S, Tatkov S, et al. Mechanisms of nasal high-flow on ventilation during wakefulness and sleep. *J Appl Physiol*. 2013:114:1058–1065.
50. Corley A, Caruana LR, Barnett AG, et al. Oxygen delivery through high-flow nasal cannulae increase end-expiratory lung volume and reduce respiratory rate in post-cardiac surgical patients. *Br J Anaesth*. 2011:107(6):998–1004.
51. Spoletini G, Alotaibi M, Blasi F, et al. Heated humidified high-flow nasal oxygen in adults: mechanism of action and clinical implications. *Chest*. 2015;148(1):253–261.
52. Brochard L, Martin GS, Blanch L, et al. Clinical review: respiratory monitoring in the ICU—a consensus of 16. *Crit Care*. 2012;16(2):219.
53. Crapo RO, Jensen RL, Hegewald M, et al. Arterial blood gas reference values for sea level and an altitude of 1,400 meters. *Am J Respir Crit Care Med*. 1999;160(5 Pt 1):1525–1531.
54. Hardie JA, Vollmer WM, Buist AS, et al. Reference values for arterial blood gases in the elderly. *Chest*. 2004;125:2053–2060.
55. Blom H, Mulder M, Verweij W. Arterial oxygen tension and saturation in hospital patients: effect of age and activity. *BMJ*. 1988;297:720–721.

56. Wilson AT, Channer KS. Hypoxaemia and supplemental oxygen therapy in the first 24 hours after myocardial infarction: the role of pulse oximetry. *J R Coll Physicians Lond.* 1997;31:657–661.
57. Levin KP, Hanusa BH, Rotondi A, et al. Arterial blood gas and pulse oximetry in initial management of patients with community-acquired pneumonia. *J Gen Intern Med.* 2001;16:590–598.
58. Moed BR, Boyd DW, Andring RE. Clinically inapparent hypoxemia after skeletal injury: the use of the pulse oximeter as a screening method. *Clin Orthop.* 1993;293:269–273.
59. O'Driscoll BR, Howard LS, Davison AG. BTS, guidelines for emergency oxygen use in adult patients. *Thorax.* 2008;63:vi1–vi68.
60. Ferguson ND, Fan E, Camporota L, et al. The Berlin definition of ARDS: an expanded rationale, justification, and supplementary material. *Intensive Care Med.* 2012;38:1573–1582.
61. Villar J, Fernández RL, Ambrós A, et al. Acute Lung Injury Epidemiology and Natural History Network: a clinical classification of the acute respiratory distress syndrome for predicting outcome and guiding medical therapy. *Crit Care Med.* 2015;43(2):346–353.
62. Cirio S, Nava S. Pilot study of a new device to titrate oxygen flow in hypoxic patients on long-term oxygen therapy. *Respir Care.* 2011;56(4):429–434.
63. Lellouche F, L'her E. Automated oxygen flow titration to maintain constant oxygenation. *Respir Care.* 2012;57(8):1254–1262.
64. Kim V, Benditt JO, Wise RA, et al. Oxygen therapy in chronic obstructive pulmonary disease. *Proc Am Thorac Soc.* 2008; 5(4):513–518.
65. O'Donnell DE, Bain DJ, Webb KA. Factors contributing to relief of exertional breathlessness during hyperoxia in chronic airflow limitation. *Am J Respir Crit Care Med.* 1997;155(2):530–535.
66. Boushy SF, Thompson HK Jr, North LB, et al. Prognosis in chronic obstructive pulmonary disease. *Am Rev Respir Dis.* 1973;108(6):1373–1383.
67. Aubier M, Murciano D, Milic-Emili J, et al. Effects of the administration of O_2 on ventilation and blood gases in patients with chronic obstructive pulmonary disease during acute respiratory failure. *Am Rev Respir Dis.* 1980;122(5):747–754.
68. Sassoon CS, Hassell KT, Mahutte CK. Hyperoxic-induced hypercapnia in stable chronic obstructive pulmonary disease. *Am Rev Respir Dis.* 1987; 135(4):907–911.
69. Plant PK, Owen JL, Elliott MW. One year period prevalence study of respiratory acidosis in acute exacerbations of COPD: implications for the provision of non-invasive ventilation and oxygen administration. *Thorax.* 2000;55(7):550–554.
70. Hale KE, Gavin C, O'Driscoll BR. Audit of oxygen use in emergency ambulances and in a hospital emergency department. *Emerg Med J.* 2008; 25(11):773–776.
71. Carone M, Patessio A, Appendini L, et al. Comparison of invasive and non-invasive saturation monitoring in prescribing oxygen during exercise in COPD patients. *Eur Respir J.* 1997;10(2):446–451.
72. Monaco F, Nickerson BG, McQuitty JC. Continuous transcutaneous oxygenand carbon dioxide monitoring in the pediatric ICU. *Crit Care Med.* 1982;10:765–766.
73. Rodriguez P, Lellouche F, Aboab J, et al. Transcutaneous arterial carbon dioxide pressure monitoring in critically ill adult patients. *Intensive Care Med.* 2006;32(2):309–312
74. Coates BM, Chaize R, Goodman DM, et al. Performance of capnometry in non-intubated infants in the pediatric intensive care unit. *BMC Pediatr.* 2014;14:163.
75. Aitken RS, Clark-Kennedy AE. On the fluctuation in the composition of the alveolar air during the respiratory cycle in muscular exercise. *J Physiol.* 1928;65(4):389–411.
76. Wolff G, Brunner JX. Series dead space volume assessed as the mean value of a distribution function. *Int J Clin Monit Comput.* 1984;1(3): 177–181.
77. Tusman G, Sipmann FS, Borges JB, et al. Validation of Bohr dead space measured by volumetric capnography. *Intensive Care Med.* 2011;37(5): 870–874.
78. Fletcher R, Jonson B, Cumming G, et al. The concept of deadspace with special reference to the single breath test for carbon dioxide. *Br J Anaesth.* 1981;53(1):77–88.
79. Verschuren F, Heinonen E, Clause D, et al: Volumetric capnography as a bedside monitoring of thrombolysis in major pulmonary embolism. *Intensive Care Med.* 2004;30:2129–2132.
80. Kelly AM, Klim S. Agreement between arterial and transcutaneous PCO_2 in patients undergoing non-invasive ventilation. *Respir Med.* 2011;105: 226–229.
81. Lu Q, Rouby JJ. Measurement of pressure-volume curves in patients on mechanical ventilation: methods and significance. *Crit Care.* 2000;4(2): 91–100.
82. Harris RS. Pressure-volume curves of the respiratory system. *Respir Care.* 2005;50(1):78–98.
83. Akoumianaki E, Maggiore SM, Valenza F, et al. The application of esophageal pressure measurement in patients with respiratory failure. *Am J Respir Crit Care Med.* 2014;189(5):520–531.
84. The Acute Respiratory Distress Syndrome Network. Ventilation with lower tidal volumes as compared with traditional tidal volumes for acute lung injury and the acute respiratory distress syndrome. *N Engl J Med.* 2000;342(18):1301–1308.
85. Gattinoni L, Carlesso E, Cressoni M. Selecting the 'right' positive end-expiratory pressure level. *Curr Opin Crit Care.* 2015;21(1):50–57
86. Chiumello D, Guerin C. Understanding the setting of PEEP from esophageal pressure in patients with ARDS. *Intensive Care Med.* 2015;41(8):1465–1467.
87. Chiumello D, Guerin C. Understanding the setting of PEEP from esophageal pressure in patients with ARDS. *Intensive Care Med.* 2015;41(8):1465–1467.
88. Brochard L. Measurement of esophageal pressure at bedside: pros and cons. *Curr Opin Crit Care.* 2014;20(1):39–46.
89. Talmor D, Sarge T, Malhotra A, et al. Mechanical ventilation guided by esophageal pressure in acute lung injury. *N Engl J Med.* 2008;359:2095–2104.
90. Baydur A, Cha EJ, Sassoon CS. Validation of esophageal balloon technique at different lung volumes and postures. *J Appl Physiol.* 1987;62:315–321.
91. Benditt JO. Esophageal and gastric pressure measurements. *Respir Care.* 2005;50(1):68–75.
92. Zin WA, Milic-Emili J. Esophageal pressure measurement. In: Hamid Q, Shannon J, Martin J, eds. *Physiologic Basis of Respiratory Disease.* New York, NY: BC Decker Inc; 2005:639–647.
93. Polese G, Serra A, Rossi A. Respiratory mechanics in the intensive care unit. *Eur Respir Mon.* 2005;31:195–206.
94. Gappa M, Colin AA, Goetz I, et al. ERS/ATS Task Force on Standards for Infant Respiratory Function Testing. Passive respiratory mechanics: the occlusion techniques. *Eur Respir J.* 2001;17(1):141–148.
95. Benditt JO. Esophageal and gastric pressure measurements. *Respir Care.* 2005;50(1):68–75.
96. Hedenstierna G. Esophageal pressure: benefit and limitations. *Minerva Anestesiol.* 2012;78(8):959–966.
97. Dellamonica J, Lerolle N, Sargentini C, et al. PEEP-induced changes in lung volume in acute respiratory distress syndrome: two methods to estimate alveolar recruitment. *Intensive Care Med.* 2011;37:1595–1604.
98. Volpicelli G, Elbarbary M, Blaivas M, et al. International evidence based recommendations for point-of-care lung ultrasound. *Intensive Care Med.* 2012;38:577–591.
99. Bouhemad B, Zhang M, Lu Q, et al. Clinical review: bedside lung ultrasound in critical care practice. *Crit Care.* 2007;11:205.
100. Via G, Storti E, Gulati G, et al. Lung ultrasound in the ICU: from diagnostic instrument to respiratory monitoring tool. *Minerva Anestesiol.* 2012;78:1282–1296.
101. Ozyilmaz E, Ugurlu AO, Nava S. Timing of noninvasive ventilation failure: causes, risk factors, and potential remedies. *BMC Pulm Med.* 2014;14:19.
102. Vignaux L, Vargas F, Roeseler J, et al. Patient-ventilator asynchrony during non-invasive ventilation for acute respiratory failure: a multicenter study. *Intensive Care Med.* 2009;35:840–846.
103. Schmidt M, Dres M, Raux M, et al. Neurally adjusted ventilatory assist improves patient-ventilator interaction during postextubation prophylactic noninvasive ventilation. *Crit Care Med.* 2012;40(6):1738–1744.
104. Cammarota G, Olivieri C, Costa R, et al. Noninvasive ventilation through a helmet in postextubation hypoxemic patients: physiologic comparison between neurally adjusted ventilatory assist and pressure support ventilation. *Intensive Care Med.* 2011;37(12):1943–1950.
105. Doorduin J, Sinderby CA, Beck J, et al. Automated patient-ventilator interaction analysis during neurally adjusted non-invasive ventilation and pressure support ventilation in chronic obstructive pulmonary disease. *Crit Care.* 2014;18(5):550.
106. Di Marco F, Centanni S, Bellone A, et al. Optimization of ventilator setting by flow and pressure waveforms analysis during noninvasive ventilation for acute exacerbations of COPD: a multicentric randomized controlled trial. *Crit Care.* 2011;15:R283.
107. Longrois D, Conti G, Mantz J, et al. Sedation in non-invasive ventilation: do we know what to do (and why)? *Multidisc Respir Med.* 2014;9:56.
108. Demoule A, Girou E, Richard JC, et al. Benefits and risks of success or failure of noninvasive ventilation. *Intensive Care Med.* 2006;32(11):1756–1765.

CHAPTER
109

Acute Lung Injury and Acute Respiratory Distress Syndrome

ETTORE CRIMI, CARL W. PETERS, MIHAE YU, ROBERT N. SLADEN, ANDREA GABRIELLI, and A. JOSEPH LAYON

OVERVIEW

The acute respiratory distress syndrome (ARDS) is a devastating injury to the lungs, characterized by diffuse pulmonary inflammation, hypoxemia, and respiratory distress (1). In 1994, the American–European Consensus Committee (AECC) on ARDS defined diagnostic criteria to include acute onset; bilateral radiographic infiltrates; pulmonary artery occlusion pressure (PAOP) 18 mmHg or less, or no evidence of left atrial hypertension; and PaO_2/FiO_2 ratio of 300 mmHg or less for ALI and 200 mmHg or less for ARDS (2).

Most of the clinical investigation done on ARDS in the past decade is based upon this far from perfect definition. Respiratory distress is common to many pulmonary processes. Bilateral radiographic infiltrates may be seen with cardiogenic pulmonary edema, pneumonitis, and several other entities. The PaO_2/FiO_2 ratio may be influenced by therapy, especially positive end-expiratory pressure (PEEP) and the FiO_2 itself. It seems specious to separate "acute lung injury" (ALI) from ARDS when the two terms reflect only a different severity of the—apparently—same processes. Heart failure may be present at a PAOP less than 18 mmHg and may coexist with ARDS, but heart failure may not be present with a PAOP of 18 mmHg or higher.

The new consensus Berlin definition addresses the limits of the AECC definition, by excluding the ALI term, removing the PAOP criteria, introducing PEEP level criteria and including the use of computed tomography (CT) images and bedside echocardiography for the assessment of the pulmonary edema (3). The new criteria include (a) onset within 1 week of a known clinical insult or new or worsening respiratory system; (b) bilateral opacities secondary to pulmonary edema and not explained by effusions, lobar and lung collapse or pulmonary nodules, present on chest radiograph or CT scan; (c) respiratory failure not explained by cardiac failure or fluid overload; echocardiography can be used as objective assessment to exclude hydrostatic pulmonary edema; (d) severity of hypoxemia defined as mild ($PaO_2/FiO_2 > 200$ but <300 mmHg with PEEP or continuous positive airway pressure (CPAP) ≥ 5 cm H_2O); moderate ($PaO_2/FiO_2 > 100$ but <200 mmHg with PEEP ≥ 5 cm H_2O); and severe ($PaO_2/FiO_2 \leq 100$ mmHg with PEEP ≥ 5 cm H_2O).

To better define the range of lung injury, Murray et al. (4) in 1988 described the Lung Injury Score (LIS) based on chest radiographic findings, degree of hypoxemia (using PaO_2/FiO_2 values), compliance of the pulmonary system (if ventilated), and PEEP levels (Table 109.1). A patient was considered to have ARDS if the score was more than 2.5. Whether this scoring system contributes additional descriptive value is debatable, since the mortality rate is impacted more by the comorbidities, such as sepsis or cirrhosis (5,6), than by the LIS value, and the LIS does not add accuracy either to the AECC (7) or Berlin definitions (8).

Multiple risk factors for ARDS have been identified, with sepsis syndrome having the highest prevalence (30% to 50%) (9–12). The pathogenesis for pulmonary and extrapulmonary causes for ALI may be different (13); the Consensus Committee categorized ARDS into direct versus indirect causes (Tables 109.2 and 109.3) (2). Secondary predisposing factors described in the literature are alcohol abuse, chronic lung disease, and a low systemic pH (10).

ARDS should be considered the final common pathway of a very heterogeneous group of insults. Although the pulmonary injury is widespread, it does not uniformly affect lung tissue; this nonuniformity has important therapeutic consequences. There are also two broad etiologies of ARDS (13): In *pulmonary ARDS* (generally corresponding to "direct" disease), there is primary lung injury (e.g., pneumonia) that involves the alveolar epithelium, and may be confined to single organ failure. In *extrapulmonary ARDS* (generally corresponding to "indirect" disease), the inflammatory effect of a remote insult—usually sepsis—reaches the capillary endothelium via a SIRS phenomenon, and lung failure becomes one more component of multiple organ dysfunction syndrome (MODS). Although there are important differences in pathophysiology, the outcome between ARDS of pulmonary and extrapulmonary origin does not appear to differ greatly. While the vast majority of studies reviewed here consider ARDS to be a single entity, questions remain as to whether this is true.

The reported incidence of ARDS is variable. In 1972, the National Heart and Lung Institute Task Force on Respiratory Disease estimated the incidence to be 150,000 cases per year, or 71 patients per 100,000 people. Although the "true" incidence of ARDS as defined by the LIS may be lower—1.5 to 8 cases per 100,000 people—the incidence of ALI was found to be 89 cases per 100,000, which approximates the previous value (11,14). A more recent study reported the incidence of ALI to be 78.8 cases per 100,000 and for ARDS to be 58.7 cases per 100,000 (12).

OUTCOME

The cause of death in ARDS patients is more often associated with MODS than deficient oxygenation. The overall mortality rate has declined from 68% in the 1980s to 36% in 1993 (14), and presently ranges widely from 30% to 58% (4–19), depending on the specific patient group—based on age and etiology of lung injury—being studied. A recent observational study showed that, even with the use of lung-protective strategy, overall ICU and hospital mortality can be still higher

TABLE 109.1 Lung Injury Score

Chest roentgenogram score	
0	No alveolar consolidation
1	Alveolar consolidation in one quadrant
2	Alveolar consolidation in two quadrants
3	Alveolar consolidation in three quadrants
4	Alveolar consolidation in four quadrants
Hypoxemia (PaO_2/FiO_2) score	
0	≥300
1	225–299
2	175–224
3	100–174
4	<100
Respiratory system compliance score (mL/cm H_2O)	
0	≥80
1	60–79
2	40–59
3	20–39
4	≤19
PEEP score (cm H_2O)	
0	≤5
1	6–8
2	9–11
3	12–14
4	≥15
Final value	
0	No lung injury
1–2.5	Acute lung injury
>2.5	Severe lung injury (acute respiratory distress syndrome)

than 40% (20). ARDS patients who leave the hospital seem to have no increased risk of subsequent death when matched for comorbidities (21).

Families and intensive care unit (ICU) patients frequently ask about the long-term outcomes and quality of life after ARDS. As with all heterogeneous diseases, outcome varies. Lung mechanics in ARDS survivors may return to normal in the year after hospital discharge, but pulmonary gas exchange abnormalities may persist (22). Spirometry is likely to be normal at 6 months, but the Short Form General Health Survey (SF-36) score was low in one study (23). Mild-to-moderate deterioration in health-related quality of life (QOL), as measured by the Sickness Impact Profile, has been reported (24). Thus, ARDS appears to add a functional burden of reduced

TABLE 109.2 Major Categories of Acute Respiratory Distress Syndrome Risk

Direct
- Pneumonia
- Aspiration
- Pulmonary contusion
- Fat emboli
- Near-drowning
- Inhalational injury
- Reperfusion after lung transplant or pulmonary embolectomy

Indirect
- Sepsis
- Severe trauma with shock
- Multiple transfusions
- Cardiopulmonary bypass
- Drug overdose
- Acute pancreatitis
- Multiple transfusions

ARDS, acute respiratory distress syndrome.
From Bernard GR, Artigas A, Brigham KL, et al. The American-European Consensus Conference on ARDS. *Am J Respir Crit Care Med.* 1994;149:818.

TABLE 109.3 Conditions Associated with Acute Respiratory Distress Syndrome

Shock
- Hemorrhagic
- Septic
- Cardiogenic
- Anaphylactic

Trauma
- Burns
- Fat emboli
- Lung contusion
- Nonthoracic trauma (especially head trauma)
- Near-drowning

Infection
- Viral pneumonia
- Bacterial pneumonia
- Fungal pneumonia
- Gram-negative sepsis
- Tuberculosis

Inhalation of toxic gases
- Oxygen
- Smoke
- NO_2, NH_3, Cl_2
- Cadmium
- Phosgene

Drug ingestion
- Cocaine
- Heroin
- Methadone
- Barbiturates
- Ethchlorvynol
- Thiazides
- Fluorescein
- Propoxyphene
- Salicylates
- Chlordiazepoxide
- Colchicine
- Dextran 40

Metabolic
- Uremia
- Diabetic ketoacidosis

Miscellaneous
- Pancreatitis
- Postcardiopulmonary bypass
- Postcardioversion
- Multiple transfusions
- DIC
- Leukoagglutinin reaction
- Eclampsia
- Air or amniotic fluid emboli
- Bowel infarction
- Carcinomatosis
- Aspiration of gastric contents (especially with pH < 2.5)

ARDS, acute respiratory distress syndrome; NO_2, nitrogen dioxide; NH_3, ammonia; Cl_2, chlorine; DIC, disseminated intravascular coagulation.
From Taylor RW, Duncan CA. The adult respiratory distress syndrome. *Res Med.* 1983;1:17.

QOL to survivors compared to non-ARDS patients who survived a major illness (25,26); nonetheless, as many as 78% of patients return to work (23). Cognitive dysfunction, depression, anxiety, and post-traumatic stress disorder can commonly occur in ARDS survivors (27,28). Determining whether the quality of life is "good" after a devastating illness is likely a personal decision.

Patients with ARDS who die within the first several days do so because of the underlying condition and respiratory failure. Many of those who survive the original insult succumb to sepsis or MODS. Of those who survive ARDS, most return to their premorbid state of respiratory function by about 6 months after extubation (24). Long-term outcomes are quite good even among patients who developed life-threatening hypoxemia, if they survived their hospitalization (29). This relatively optimistic view of post-ARDS outcome has been seriously challenged and is likely a gross oversimplification (see Chapter 12).

PATHOPHYSIOLOGY

The inciting process in ALI is the pathologic loss of integrity of the alveolar–capillary membrane complex associated with exuberant inflammation, with increased endothelial and epithelial permeability and leakage of proteinaceous edema and cellular components into the interstitial and alveolar spaces. This occurs in response to some provocative stimulus, which may arise from various disease processes or physical or chemical insults, including primary pulmonary or extrapulmonary events (see Tables 109.2 and 109.3). While the details of lung injury may differ between primary and secondary causes (30), the differences in overt clinical consequences are difficult to identify when comparing patients from either general category.

The initial acute event that induces disruption of the alveolar epithelial or capillary endothelial cells in the exudative phase of ARDS yields denuded alveolar basement membrane and dysfunctional or destroyed surfactant and types 1 and 2 pneumocytes (Table 109.4). Demarginated "activated" neutrophils within the pulmonary circulation release inflammatory mediators, degrading the integrity of capillary endothelial cell junctions and allowing the influx of proteinaceous plasma fluid, erythrocytes, and inflammatory cells into the interstitium (31,32). Interstitial fluid volume eventually exceeds lymphatic clearance capabilities, flooding the alveoli with hemorrhagic plasma. Thickened interstitium is "stiffer" and worsens pulmonary compliance, yielding a scenario of restrictive physiology. Loss and dysfunction of surfactant (33) increases alveolar surface tension, thus producing alveolar collapse. Ongoing inflammation initiates the coagulation cascade within the microcapillaries, with platelet deposition (34) obliterating the capillary luminal cross-sectional area, disrupting blood flow, and raising pulmonary artery pressure. Further recruitment of activated neutrophils into the interstitium (31,32) augments the inflammatory cycle of capillary permeability, interstitial edema, and continuous alveolar macrophage activation (Fig. 109.1) (35).

Accumulation of proinflammatory mediators such as tumor necrosis factor-α (TNF-α), interleukin-1β (IL-1β), and IL-8 in the alveolar fluid of ARDS patients (36) portends the amplified production of cytokine and toxic reactive oxygen and nitrogen radical species (37,38) (Table 109.5). The highly complex network mediating inflammation in ARDS also includes signaling pathways activated by Toll-like receptor, mitochondrial derived products, and posttranslational modification (i.e., ubiquitination), all potential therapeutic targets (39).

Activated complement components accumulate with fibrin and immunoglobulins to form alveolar hyaline membranes, further worsening compliance. Fibroproliferation and accelerated collagen deposition may begin early in the inflammatory sequence and continue into the proliferative phase (7 to 21 days) (40,41), with thickening of the alveolar walls already denuded of type 1 pneumocytes (35,42).

While the original inciting event may resolve, judicious correction of persistent metabolic and infectious issues, and meticulous attention to appropriate ventilatory techniques, must continue in order to minimize iatrogenic contributions to self-sustaining inflammation (see Ventilator-Induced Lung Injury below). Evolution into the *fibrotic phase* occurs, generally, after 3 to 4 weeks. Variable degrees of fibrosis and parenchymal tissue loss (40) yield "diffuse alveolar damage," the histologic correlate of advanced ARDS, characterized by widespread and severe damage to the alveolar–capillary unit (40). Microcystic and macrocystic areas abut dilated ectatic bronchi, with fibrotic noncompliant septa and collapsed alveoli—no longer tethered open by healthy surrounding tissue—and interwoven with thrombosed capillaries that provide no capacity for gas exchange (i.e., dead-space ventilation) (40). Hypoxemia from tenaciously collapsed, fibrotic, shunt-producing alveoli accompanies the hypercarbia and

TABLE 109.4 Histopathologic Changes in Acute Respiratory Distress Syndrome

	Exudative Phase	Proliferative Phase	Fibrotic Phase
Macroscopic	Heavy, rigid, dark	Heavy, gray	Cobblestoned
Microscopic	Hyaline membranes	Barrier disruption	Fibrosis
	Edema	Edema	Macrophages
	Neutrophils	Alveolar type II cell proliferation	Lymphocytes
	Epithelial > endothelial damage	Myofibroblast infiltration	Matrix organization
		Neutrophils	Deranged acinar architecture
		Alveolar collapse	Patchy emphysematous change
		Alveoli filled with cells and organizing matrix	
		Epithelial apoptosis	
		Fibroproliferation	
Vasculature	Local thrombus	Loss of capillaries	Myointimal thickening
		Pulmonary hypertension	Tortuous vessels

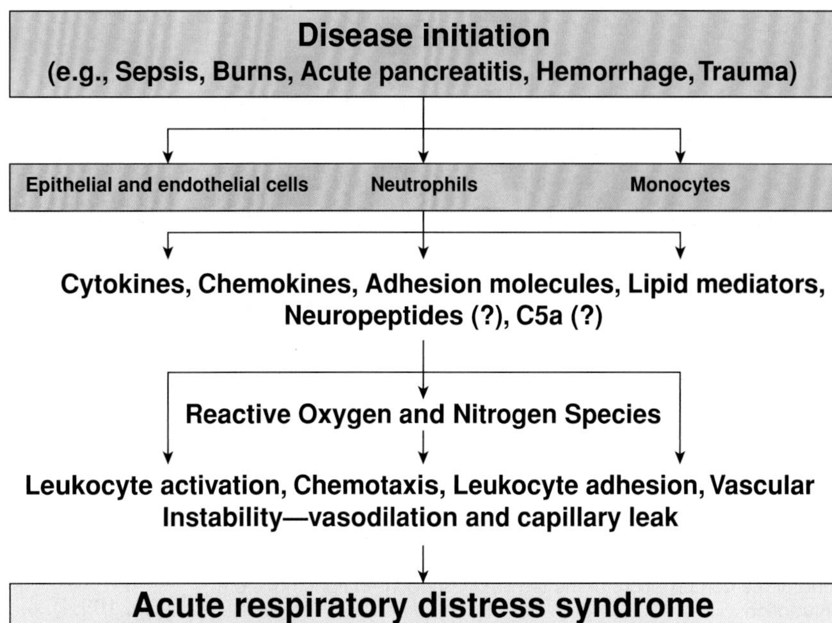

FIGURE 109.1 Pathogenesis of acute respiratory distress syndrome. (Data from Bhatia M, Moochhala S. Role of inflammatory mediators in the pathophysiology of acute respiratory distress syndrome. *J Pathol.* 2004;202(2):145–156.)

respiratory acidosis of large dead-space fractions from nongas exchanging overdistended alveoli, dilated cystic areas, and thrombosed non–CO_2-excreting pulmonary capillaries.

Clinical Presentation Physical Examination

After the inciting event, several hours to a day may pass before clinically apparent respiratory failure ensues. Based on work by Gomez (43), the clinical findings in ARDS may be roughly grouped into four phases (Table 109.6). Tachypnea and tachycardia usually develop during the first 12 to 24 hours. The skin may appear moist and cyanotic; intercostal and accessory respiratory muscles become actively involved in supporting ventilation. A dramatic increase in work of breathing can be appreciated at a glance from the bedside. High-pitched end-expiratory crackles are heard throughout all lung fields. Increasing agitation, lethargy, and obtundation may occur as the syndrome progresses. Because these clinical findings may become apparent long after hypoxemia develops, careful attention to arterial blood gas analysis is warranted in patients at risk for ARDS.

TABLE 109.5 Inflammatory Mediators in Acute Respiratory Distress Syndrome

Inflammatory Mediator	Function
TNF-α	Proinflammatory; neutrophil activation
IL-1β	Proinflammatory; neutrophil activation
IL-6	Leukocyte growth/activation; proliferation of myeloid progenitor cells; acute-phase response; pyrexia
IL-10	Anti-inflammatory; inhibits release of proinflammatory cytokines
TGF-β	Resolution of tissue injury; proinflammatory
GM-CSF	Host defense; hematologic growth factor
PAF	Platelet activation; neutrophil activation and chemotaxis
ICAM-I	Neutrophil adhesion
C5a	Leukocyte chemoattractant; dual pro- and anti-inflammatory role
Substance P	Proinflammatory
Chemokines	Leukocyte activation and chemotaxis
VEGF	Endothelial cytokine; plays a role in angiogenesis and vascular permeability
IGF-I	Alveolar macrophage–derived growth factor; profibrotic
KGF	Epithelial-specific growth factor; important for lung development repair
Reactive oxygen and nitrogen species	Regulation of vascular tone, antimicrobial action

TABLE 109.6 Progression of Clinical Findings in Acute Respiratory Distress Syndrome

Phase 1: Acute injury
- Normal physical examination and chest radiograph
- Tachycardia, tachypnea, and respiratory alkalosis develop

Phase 2: Latent period
- Lasts approximately 6–48 hr after injury
- Patient appears clinically stable
- Hyperventilation and hypocapnia persist
- Mild increase in work of breathing
- Widening of the alveolar-arterial oxygen gradient
- Minor abnormalities on physical examination and chest radiograph

Phase 3: Acute respiratory failure
- Marked tachypnea and dyspnea
- Decreased lung compliance
- Diffuse infiltrates on chest radiograph
- High-pitched crackles heard throughout all lung fields

Phase 4: Severe abnormalities
- Severe hypoxemia unresponsive to therapy
- Increased intrapulmonary shunting
- Metabolic and respiratory acidosis

From Taylor RW. The adult respiratory distress syndrome. In: Kirby RR, Taylor RW, eds. *Respiratory Failure.* Chicago, IL: Year Book Medical Publishers; 1986:208.

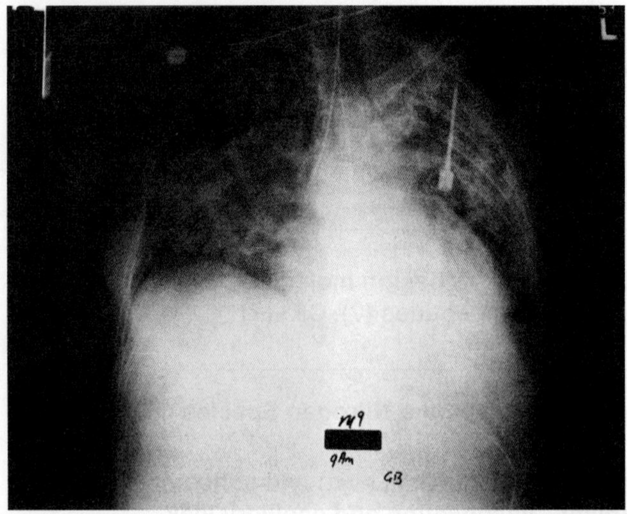

FIGURE 109.2 Diffuse interstitial and panacinar infiltrates are seen in a 36-year-old patient with acute respiratory distress syndrome. Also notice one of the complications of the respiratory support—a right mainstem intubation.

Lung Imaging

The changes seen on the chest radiograph in ARDS are characteristic but nonspecific, rarely revealing the etiology of the syndrome. Acutely, pulmonary edema is seen; interstitial infiltrates progress to a diffuse, fluffy, panacinar pattern (Fig. 109.2). Although it may be difficult to differentiate from cardiogenic pulmonary edema, there is generally an absence of pulmonary vascular redistribution, pleural effusion, or cardiomegaly. The panacinar infiltrates may consolidate and, with time, take on a patchy or nodular pattern. If the patient improves, radiographic results may revert to normal. If the disorder progresses, a pattern of diffuse interstitial fibrosis may ensue (Fig. 109.3). Therapeutic interventions may alter the radiographic findings. Pulmonary infiltrates may increase with injudicious fluid administration. Positive pressure ventilation and PEEP may lead to hyperinflation, and subcutaneous, mediastinal, retroperitoneal, and intraperitoneal emphysema, or pneumothorax. Mainstem bronchus intubation may lead to ipsilateral pneumothorax or contralateral lung collapse (Fig. 109.4).

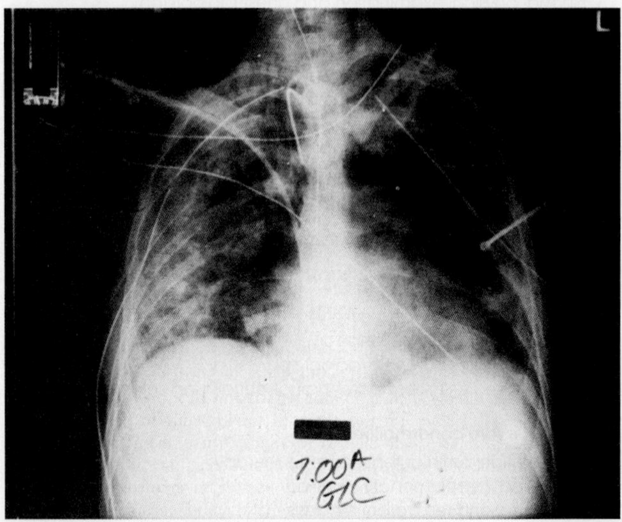

FIGURE 109.3 A pattern of diffuse interstitial fibrosis can be seen in this 52-year-old patient with acute respiratory distress syndrome.

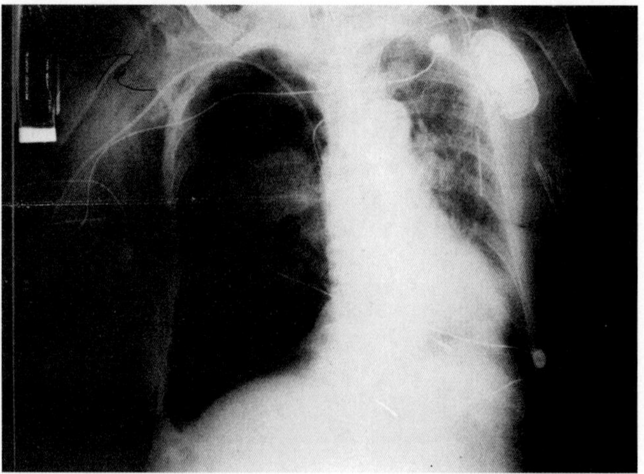

FIGURE 109.4 This 70-year-old patient with acute respiratory distress syndrome has a right tension pneumothorax and right mainstem intubation.

Whereas a two-dimensional chest radiograph may suggest diffuse homogeneous infiltrates, the chest CT scan usually demonstrates remarkably inhomogeneous lung involvement. Dependent regions of the lung appear to be much more involved than nondependent regions. Although chest CT scanning is not always practical in the day-to-day management of patients with ARDS, in investigational trials, it has provided a vivid image of dramatically reduced lung volumes. The chest CT also may be useful in demonstrating the presence and magnitude of pneumothoraces and pleural effusions not well visualized on the standard chest radiograph. It is also useful for the positioning of thoracostomy tubes in patients with loculated pneumothoraces.

TREATMENT

General Therapeutic Measures

Nutritional Support

The gut serves a critical function beyond the absorption and transport of nutrients. Enteral nutrition seems to have an advantage over parenteral nutrition in preventing gastrointestinal atrophy, maintaining normal gut flora, and preserving immune function in surgical patients (44). Enteral nutrition should be started within 24 to 48 hours. The ARDS Network EDEN multicenter trial showed no difference in the short-term functional outcome measures, including mortality and days without mechanical ventilation, for the initial 6 days of either full feeding (about 80% of caloric goals achieved) or trophic feeding (about 20% of caloric goals achieved) (45). Longer-term outcomes were subsequently assessed and there were no differences at either 6- or 12-month follow-up in physical parameters (anthropometrics, muscle strength, pulmonary function, and 6-minute walking distance) or cognitive assessment (46). Chapter 150 details the importance of nutrition in the critically ill.

Fluid Management

Fluid management in ARDS has been controversial. As the permeability of the alveolar–capillary membrane increases, pulmonary edema develops at lower pulmonary capillary pressures. When a strategy of fluid restriction and diuresis is undertaken, extravascular lung water (EVLW) is decreased, as is the duration of mechanical ventilation. While mortality in ARDS seems to be associated with net fluid gain, adequate intravascular volume must be maintained to avoid tissue hypoperfusion; we recommend that the minimal amount of fluid be given, and that judicious attempts at diuresis be undertaken in the hemodynamically stable patient (47). A large study conducted by the National Heart, Lung, and Blood Institute (NHLBI) Acute Respiratory Distress Syndrome Clinical Trials Network (48) found no difference in 60-day mortality when comparing liberal and conservative fluid management strategies. Although the time allowed to enrollment was long (48 hours) and may not have captured the initial resuscitation, in light of the shorter ventilator and ICU days with conservative fluid management and associated improvement in pulmonary function when compared to liberal use of fluid, our routine practice is a conservative fluid strategy. There is some recent evidence that a fluid-conservative approach increases the risk of long-term dysfunction (27).

Bronchodilators

Multiple factors may lead to airflow obstruction in patients with ARDS, including mucosal and interstitial edema, airway secretions, and atelectasis. Airway hyperreactivity also contributes to increased airflow resistance in many patients with ARDS, in both the acute and chronic phases. Aerosolized β-agonists can decrease airway resistance, even in patients without underlying chronic obstructive pulmonary disease or asthma. By reducing airway resistance, the work of breathing can be decreased. Aerosolized β-agonists might have anti-inflammatory activity and promote alveolar fluid absorption, but have not shown clinical benefit in prevention and treatment of ARDS (49–51). We recommend a therapeutic trial of inhaled bronchodilators in patients with wheezing, in those with increased resistance as measured directly, or in patients with high peak airway pressures (52).

Steroids

The use of corticosteroids in the treatment of the various phases of ARDS is the basis of controversy and ongoing investigation. The cytokine-mediated inflammatory response to an inciting event in ARDS intuitively suggests that suppression of that response would be therapeutic, but studies are equivocal in reporting benefit. Steroid use in different phases of ARDS has been meticulously investigated, but the dynamic nature of the inflammatory process has made the findings in individual studies difficult to extrapolate to varying illnesses at varying times. Furthermore, infectious risks of corticosteroid use aside, their prolonged use risks profoundly detrimental neuromuscular effects, even further compounded when employed with nondepolarizing neuromuscular blocking agents—often used in ARDS patients to facilitate efficient mechanical ventilation (53). Thus, routine use of corticosteroids is not advocated, especially in the acute phase of ARDS. During the late phase, fibroproliferation often occurs in response to tissue injury and is associated with persistent inflammation. In this setting, fever and SIRS are present in the absence of infection. A small uncontrolled trial suggested that improvement in "late" ARDS patients—those mechanically ventilated for approximately 15 days—with progressive fibroproliferation may be seen when corticosteroid treatment begins during that period (54). Proponents of this therapy recommend that a trial of corticosteroids be instituted in such patients *after* infection has been excluded. The NHLBI ARDS Clinical Trials Network (55) conducted a randomized multicenter controlled trial of steroid use in 180 patients with ARDS of at least 7 days' duration. While there was no difference overall in mortality at 60 and 180 days, steroids imparted a higher number of ventilator-free days and earlier departure from the ICU in the first 28 days. Those given methylprednisolone after day 13 of ARDS, however, had a higher mortality than controls. Meduri et al (56) found reductions in length of mechanical ventilation, and ICU stay and in mortality in early septic/ARDS patients receiving "low-dose" methylprednisolone infusions. While there have been several recent reviews and meta-analyses addressing corticosteroid use in ARDS (52–61), varying population groups and treatment regimens and differing end points and definitions of "success" in the studies make broadly inclusive recommendations difficult to formulate. Even the impact of steroids on mortality varies positively or negatively with different groups of patients. In general, corticosteroids are not effective in ameliorating cytokine-induced inflammation in ARDS in a clinically significant way and routine use of corticosteroids is, therefore, not advocated, especially in the acute phase. There are, however, some subgroups of patients in whom corticosteroids may have a positive effect. One example may be the late phase, during which fibroproliferation often occurs in response to tissue injury. This response is damaging to the lung and is associated with persistent cytokine-mediated inflammation (62). Lung injury is characterized by endothelial and epithelial damage, as well as augmented fibroblast proliferation, which may be lessened by steroid treatment. Proponents of this therapy recommend that a trial of corticosteroids be instituted in patients with severe ARDS *after* infection has been excluded (54).

Neuromuscular Blockade

The use of neuromuscular blockade in ARDS patients has been controversial. A recent trial showed that early administration of short term (48 hours) infusion of cisatracurium besylate in patients with severe ARDS (e.g., $PaO_2/FiO_2 \leq 120$ mmHg) reduces in-hospital mortality without increasing muscle weakness (63). The use of neuromuscular blockade in the early phase of severe ARDS can minimize patient–ventilator dyssynchrony, the implementation of a lung-protective strategy and ultimately limit the VILI (64,65).

Monitoring

Monitoring the patient with ARDS is similar to that performed on other critically ill patients (Table 109.7). Detailed descriptions of monitoring techniques that are essential to reduce or prevent the occurrence of significant complications are found in earlier chapters. Careful titration of therapy is best guided by monitoring clinical, laboratory, and cardiorespiratory variables. Our practice is to use, minimally an arterial line, pulse oximetry, and capnography in patients with ARDS. More invasive devices—central venous pressure (CVP), pulmonary artery catheter—may be required based on the clinical situation.

Standard Management

Progress has been made in the management of ARDS, as suggested by the number of large studies and meta-analyses

TABLE 109.7 Monitoring the Patient with Acute Respiratory Distress Syndrome[a]

Level I

Temperature, heart rate, respiratory rate, arterial blood pressure, pulse oximetry, capnography
Weight
Intake and output
Caloric intake
Physical examination, with special emphasis on:
- Skin (texture, turgor, perspiration, emphysema)
- Respiratory (breathing pattern, lung examination)
- Cardiovascular (heart examination, peripheral pulses)
- Abdominal
- Neurologic (mental status)

Continuous ECG monitoring
Chest radiography
Laboratory (CBC, electrolytes)
Arterial pressure monitoring/blood gases
Vital capacity
Negative inspiratory pressure
Dead space/tidal volume ratio (VDb/bVT)
Tracheal tube cuff pressures
Ventilator settings
Pressure–volume relationship: lung and chest wall compliance and airways resistance

Level II

Minimally invasive CO/CI with pulse waveform variability evaluation of preload
Pulmonary artery catheter: pulmonary artery pressures, PAOP waveforms, CI, mixed venous blood gases, stroke volume index, ventricular stroke work indices, systemic and pulmonary vascular resistance, arterial and mixed venous oxygen content, oxygen transport, arteriovenous content difference, oxygen consumption, oxygen extraction, venous admixture.

ECG, electrocardiographic; CBC, complete blood cell count; CO/CI, cardiac output/cardiac index; PAOP, pulmonary artery occlusion pressure.
[a]Various monitoring techniques have been divided into three arbitrary levels. The levels are roughly ordered in terms of increasing invasiveness and sophistication. The exact monitoring modalities selected and the frequency with which measurements are made must be individualized.
From Taylor RW. The adult respiratory distress syndrome. In: Kirby RR, Taylor RW, eds. *Respiratory Failure*. Chicago, IL: Year Book Medical Publishers; 1986:208.

published in the last decade. Over this time, data have been gathered addressing modes of therapy and ancillary support techniques previously initiated and practiced empirically. Despite considerable progress, however, many questions await definitive resolution, as will become apparent in the discussion that follows. Due to the complex metabolic and pulmonary aberrations that characterize ARDS, treatment strategies can be divided into those directed toward respiratory support and all other therapeutic measures.

Respiratory Support

Mechanical ventilatory support, most often via an endotracheal tube, is fundamental to the management of ARDS, as perturbations of gas exchange and respiratory mechanics associated with this syndrome exceed the limits of compensation that most individuals are able to muster without mechanical assistance; it is as fundamental and integral to the management of the patient with ARDS as is exogenous insulin to the diabetic or antibiotics to the treatment of infections. The indications for respiratory support include hemodynamic instability, protection and maintenance of the airway, inability to maintain PaO_2 above 55 mmHg on an FiO_2 of 0.6 or less, the need for positive airway pressure, and progressive ventilatory insufficiency with rising respiratory rate and hypercarbia. The presence of several or all of these features in most individuals with ARDS mandates endotracheal intubation and mechanical ventilation to optimize gas exchange and minimize work of breathing. Noninvasive positive pressure ventilation (NIPPV) has been employed in some instances for those with less severe pulmonary impairment and preserved mental status (66), although studies are few, with fairly high rates of eventual endotracheal intubation (67,68). Broad recommendations regarding the use of NIPPV in ARDS are difficult to make in the absence of large prospective studies due to the heterogeneity of patient populations, comorbidities, and diversity of the inciting pathophysiology (66).

Lung CT studies have demonstrated the distribution of areas of alveolar collapse and distension characteristic of ARDS to be regional rather than diffuse. Alveolar collapse predominates in dependent areas, producing venous admixture and hypoxemia, while nondependent areas manifest airway destruction with hyperinflation, often to the point of exclusion of pulmonary capillary blood flow (dead space) (69,70). These alveolar morphologies, however, are not strictly related to dependency within the chest cavity, as is clearly visible in Figure 109.5. Areas of atelectasis, producing shunt and airway/alveolar destruction, and areas of overdistension, producing dead space, may be randomly distributed and interspersed with areas of spared pulmonary tissue, thereby generating profound ventilation/perfusion mismatch.

The use of mechanical ventilation in ARDS has evolved dramatically over the last 30 years. Techniques of mechanical ventilation commonly employed through the decade of the 1980s led to use of what would now be described by most practitioners and investigators as "high" tidal volumes (V_t), with FiO_2 supplemented well above ambient. Subsequently, the observation was made (71,72) that ventilation of healthy laboratory animals with high V_t induced profound clinical and histologic deterioration that was difficult to distinguish from those of ARDS. In a retrospective study in 1990, Hickling et al. observed an apparent improved mortality in

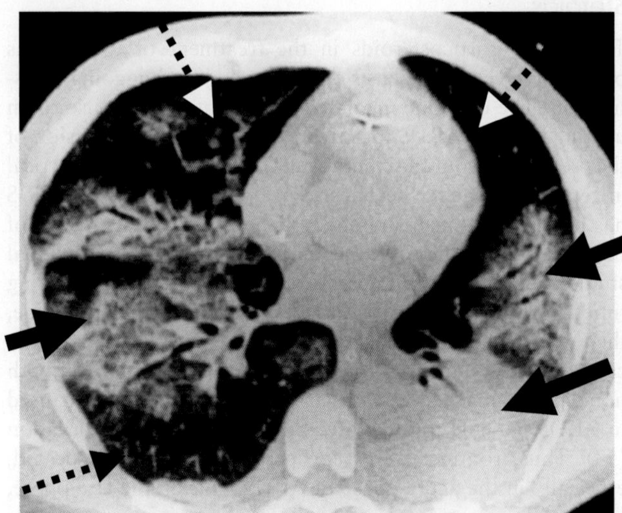

FIGURE 109.5 Computed tomography scan of the chest of a patient with acute respiratory distress syndrome. *Solid arrows* show dense parenchymal opacification resulting in shunt. The *broken lines* show relatively "normal"-appearing lung but that can suffer from overdistension, resulting in dead space. (From Desai SR. Acute respiratory distress syndrome: imaging of the injured lung. *Clin Radiol.* 2002;57(1):8–17; with permission.)

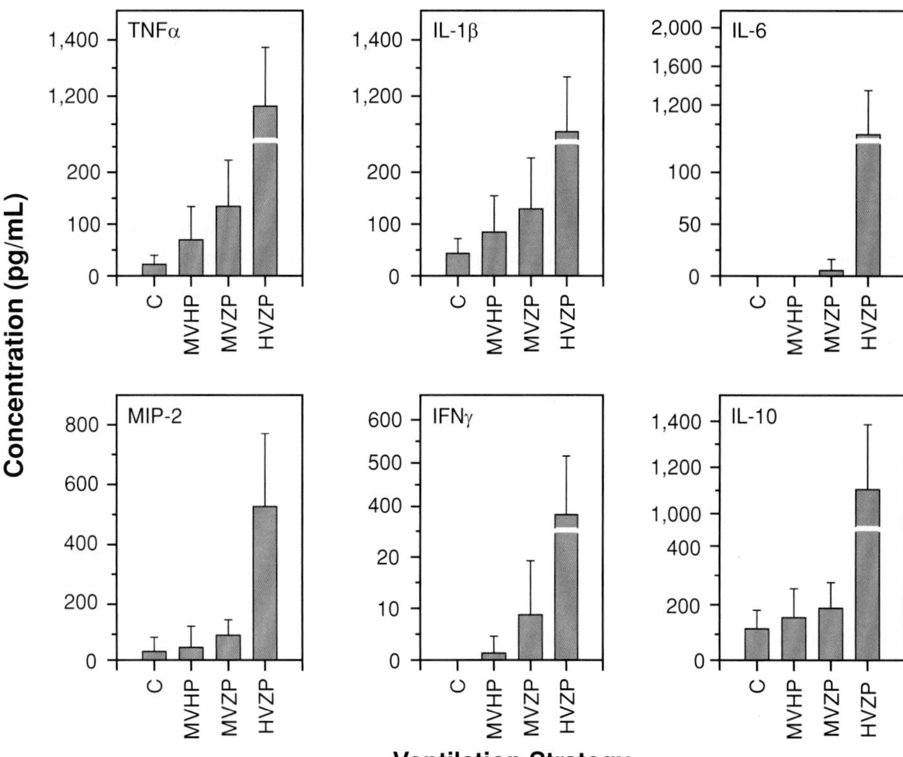

FIGURE 109.6 The effect of ventilation strategy on inflammatory mediator concentration. High tidal volume strategy resulted in higher levels. C, control: V_t = 7 mL/kg, PEEP = 3 cm H_2O; MVHP, moderate-volume, high PEEP: V_t = 15 mL/kg, PEEP = 10 cm H_2O; HVZP, high-volume, zero PEEP: V_t = 40 mL/kg; MVZP, moderate-volume, zero PEEP: V_t = 15 mL/kg. TNF-α, tumor necrosis factor-α; IL-1β, interleukin-1β; IL-6, interleukin-6; MIP-2, macrophage inflammatory protein 2; IFNγ, interferon-γ. (Adapted from Tremblay L, Valenza F, Ribeiro SP, et al. Injurious ventilatory strategies increase cytokines and c-fos m-RNA expression in an isolated rat lung model. *J Clin Invest.* 1997;99(5):944–952.)

ARDS patients with lower than "traditional" V_t (73). Subsequent investigations yielding conflicting results mandated the ARMA (acute respiratory distress syndrome network low tidal volume) trial of mechanical ventilation, with limited V_t and plateau pressures compared to the higher values in common use at the time (74). The result was a reduction in mortality from 40% to 31% with the experimental protocol parameters. While the ARMA study has been criticized from a number of standpoints (75), none is sufficiently compelling to negate the persuasiveness of its results. In our practice, low V_t ventilation (V_t = 6–8 mL/kg ideal body weight) is considered standard, maintaining a plateau pressure—as a surrogate of transpulmonary pressure—30 cm H_2O or less. Tidal volumes exceeding these parameters have been implicated in generating lung injury caused by mechanical ventilation itself. This phenomenon, termed *ventilator-induced lung injury* (VILI), is a by-product of the interaction of mechanical ventilation and the cytokine proliferation that is a fundamental pathophysiologic feature of ARDS (76,77). As described below, components of VILI include (a) *barotrauma*, the appearance of air outside the airways and alveoli, attributed to airway pressures that exceed certain thresholds; (b) *volutrauma*, increased alveolar and capillary permeability due to alveolar overdistension and leading to pulmonary edema; and (c) *atelectrauma*, the destructive repetitive opening and closing of stiff, collapsed, surfactant-depleted, fibrotic alveoli with thickened interstitium that are associated with cyclic positive pressure ventilation. Excessive alveolar stretch is associated with inflammatory cytokine proliferation, in particular during excursions into ranges of tidal volume that induce VILI (78,79) (Fig. 109.6). Of note, this cytokine proliferation can be limited by using a lung-protective ventilation strategy (79).

The importance of V_t limitation as a guide to appropriate mechanical ventilation in the acutely injured lung may be more easily understood when viewed within a conceptual framework of patchy, unevenly distributed alveolar injury. When such an injured lung receives a positive pressure breath, the gas distribution is impacted by the variability of compliance and resistance in the injured and healthy areas. Flow preferentially enters unaffected (i.e., low resistance, relatively high compliance) pulmonary tissue, risking unintentional overdistension and injury of these normal areas (80) despite inflation with an "appropriate" V_t based on body weight. This is often termed *the baby lung phenomenon* (81), since the volume of unaffected lung parenchyma within the ARDS patient's thorax more closely approximates that of a child than an adult. Delivered V_t, therefore, must more closely approximate those appropriate for a smaller lung, usually on the order of 6 to 8 mL/kg; exceeding these volumes risks iatrogenic perpetuation of lung injury, since a positive pressure breath inflates a smaller volume of lung tissue than would be predicted by ideal body weight.

The importance of PEEP and recruitment maneuvers in providing efficient ventilator management of ARDS patients warrants further discussion. While the traditional approach of oxygen supplementation may improve the PaO_2 within the limits of a marginal FRC, such supplementation should be looked upon only as a temporizing measure. Prolonged high FiO_2 use risks toxicity and absorption atelectasis, while leaving the underlying cause of hypoxemia neither identified nor corrected. Recovery of FRC by reinflation of atelectatic areas using recruitment maneuvers and PEEP will restore gas flow to previously nonaerated areas of lung (82–86). These modalities of treatment are commonly utilized in the modern strategy of ARDS treatment (87,88). Areas of particularly tenacious atelectasis will often require an inspiratory time (T_i) equal to several inspiratory time constants (one "time constant" equals product of compliance and resistance, both easily measurable by current ventilators) to achieve inflation. Insufficient T_i may leave such areas persistently collapsed, worsening shunt fraction and compromising FRC and oxygenation. Despite the most heroic efforts, a substantial percentage of ARDS patients harbor lung tissue that is only variably "PEEP recruitable" (85). The benefit of recruitment maneuvers and PEEP can be understood within the context of the *Law of LaPlace* (actually the Young–LaPlace equation), which states that the pressure difference across a fluid interface is equal to the surface tension times the mean curvature of the surface. In pulmonary physiology and ARDS, this means that the pressure difference between alveolar gas and alveolar epithelium contracts the alveolus inward unless counteracted by surfactant. Furthermore, the relationship between surface tension and alveolar radius is inverse. Thus, the smaller the alveolar radius, the greater the force contracting it even further inward (i.e., toward collapse). Since surfactant decreases surface tension, the inward force within a collapsed alveolus is greater than that within its surfactant-replete, healthy, "noncollapsed" neighbor with lower surface tension, resulting in a temporary high-pressure requirement to open a collapsed alveolus. The alveolus may then be maintained open, with PEEP exceeding the alveolar closing pressure. Because low Vt (6 mL/kg) followed by PEEP in itself is generally ineffective in expanding collapsed alveoli, a "recruitment maneuver," the temporary application of airway pressure far above any possible alveolar retractive force, may be warranted to open and stabilize collapsed alveoli (89–91), preventing exposure to repetitive cyclic collapse and associated destructive shear forces by maintaining an "open lung" (Fig. 109.7); while there are several ways to perform this maneuver, our preferred method is to utilize esophageal pressure as an inference of pleural pressure, and push the transpulmonary pressure to 20 to 25 cm H_2O.

The benefit of PEEP was recently addressed and showed, surprisingly, that no difference was achieved in discharge or survival between ICU patients receiving high- or low-PEEP regimens (87). Flaws in the study may have contributed to this result, as the table defining PEEP levels was altered after the study had begun. More recently, no significant improvement in all-cause mortality rates was noted in two studies of ARDS patients managed with an "open-lung" approach, involving the addition of modestly higher levels of PEEP and recruitment maneuvers compared to a regimen utilizing a tidal volume of 6 mL/kg and approximately 10 cm H_2O PEEP (88). There are still controversies on the best method to select the adequate level of PEEP that guarantees lung recruitment without overdistension (92). The use of a PEEP/FiO_2 table approach achieves more effective lung recruitment than methods based on lung mechanics (93,94). Nonetheless, in the patient with a noncompliant abdominal or chest wall, use of the PEEP table may be dramatically inadequate. In these cases, in which there is significant difficulty with oxygenation—and these comprise about 20% of our ARDS population—the measurement of transpulmonary pressure using esophageal pressure as inferential of pleural pressure is mandatory. Patients who would have been placed prone or started on extracorporeal membrane oxygenation were kept from these procedures using this technique to measure transpulmonary pressure and optimize pulmonary mechanics.

The selection of V_t is intimately linked to the pressure–volume curve. Optimal gas exchange with minimal alveolar injury is achieved when the lung is positioned on the vertical portion of the pressure–volume curve (Fig. 109.8). This minimizes collapse in areas of high time constants and overdistension in normal areas. Once alveolar re-expansion is optimized, which may take several hours of vigilance to titrate V_t and mean airway pressure, optimal inflation is maintained with PEEP as ventilation is then conducted along the expiratory limb of the curve, lowering mean pressures overall (see Fig. 109.8). There is wide acceptance of the use of low V_t/limited plateau pressure ventilation techniques, directed toward gas exchange along the expiratory curve once inflation has been achieved, with the goal of preserving the integrity of pulmonary parenchyma not yet affected by inflammation and to allow healing of diseased areas. Since compliance varies between individual alveoli, a given inspiratory pressure may hold some in overdistension while others are minimally opened; the curve depicted in Figure 109.8 actually represents an averaged compliance. A not uncommon observation when monitoring gas exchange in ARDS is hypercarbia with mild acidemia, often more uncomfortable for the clinician to observe than the patient to experience. However, "permissive hypercapnia" is safe and acceptable (95) when not contraindicated by underlying medical condition (e.g., elevated intracranial pressure), though it

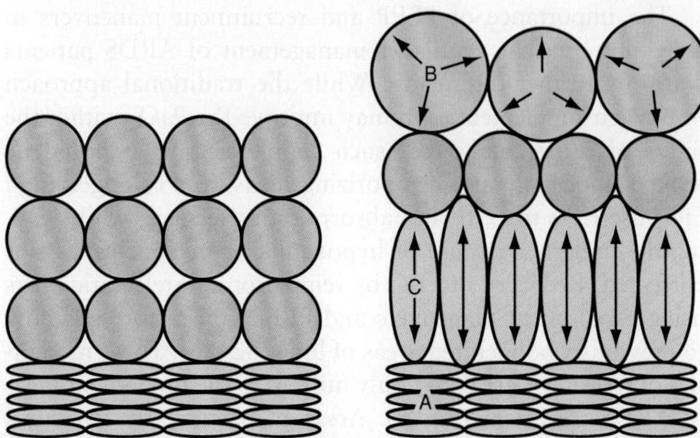

FIGURE 109.7 Atelectrauma and the interdependence of lung units. (Adapted from Moloney ED, Griffiths MJ. Protective ventilation of patients with acute respiratory distress syndrome. *Br J Anaesth.* 2004;92(2):261–270.)

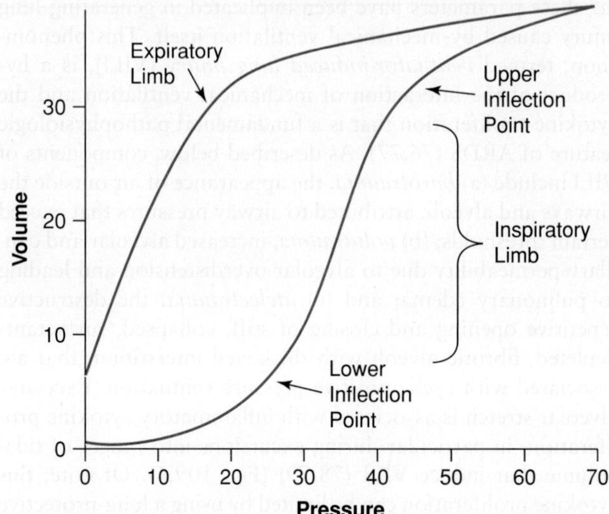

FIGURE 109.8 Pressure–volume curve of an idealized lung, showing both the inspiratory and expiratory limbs as well as the upper and lower inflection points.

often warrants protocol-delivered sedation. This may be understood by visualizing a variety of pressure–volume curves depicting compliance curves for variously distensible alveoli. The pressure to aerate sufficient numbers of tenaciously collapsed alveoli may overdistend more compliant areas such that the increased dead space precludes adequate ventilation.

The mode of mechanical ventilation used in ARDS is likely more dependent on the comfort level of the practitioner than on "best evidence." *Pressure control ventilation* (PCV) offers the theoretical advantages of limiting peak airway pressure, a component that may be associated with VILI (77). PCV may decrease work of breathing, possibly due to the variable flow rate (96). PCV is a ventilatory mode that is time initiated, pressure limited, and time cycled. PCV delivers a square pressure wave that provides tight control of the inflation pressure equal to the applied pressure plus PEEP. This mode also allows precise adjustment of inspiratory time at the expense of expiratory time—that is, increased inspiratory to expiratory (I:E) ratio, or "inverse ratio ventilation" (IRV). Mean airway pressure is substantially increased without an increase in peak airway pressure, promoting alveolar recruitment while—again, theoretically—attenuating barotrauma and volutrauma. With PC–IRV, mean airway pressures are typically increased from less than 10 to between 20 and 30 cm H_2O; inspiratory time—if the ventilator is set, for example, at 10 breaths/min—between 3 and 5 seconds; and I:E ratio between 1:1 and 3:1. Indeed, IRV may be considered an alternative (or adjunct) to PEEP in providing airway pressure therapy during inspiration instead of expiration, and with limited peak airway pressure.

To date, the hypothesis that PC–IRV results in a better outcome than standard volume–limited ventilation has not been rigorously tested (97,98). Moreover, IRV may result in inadequate exhalation time, air trapping, and the generation of intrinsic PEEP ("auto-PEEP"), leading to barotrauma and CO_2 retention. Paradoxically, hypercarbia occurring during PC–IRV may be improved by decreasing the ventilator rate to allow additional time for CO_2 elimination. Nonetheless, high time-constant, low-compliance lung segments may benefit from the ability to control the inspiratory time and the prolonged, but controlled, plateau pressures that PCV allows (99).

Airway pressure release ventilation (APRV), also known as invasive bi-level ventilation, combines the advantages of improved alveolar recruitment, lung protection, and spontaneous ventilation. In this mode, a sustained 3- to 4-second high airway pressure—the upper PEEP level—of 20 to 30 cm H_2O is intermittently released for one-half to one second to the lower level of PEEP (5 to 10 cm H_2O), while allowing spontaneous breathing to occur throughout the cycle (100). This technique optimizes alveolar recruitment by increasing mean airway pressure while restricting the peak airway pressure to the upper PEEP level, and can maintain oxygenation and ventilation at lower airway pressures than conventional ventilation (100). This mode is useful in the transition from PC–IRV to ventilatory weaning with intermittent mandatory ventilation (IMV) or pressure support, but it has not been subjected to randomized outcome trials (101,102).

Advantageous aspects of both volume- and pressure-controlled ventilation can be combined in advanced circuitry ventilators in a mode termed *pressure-regulated volume control* (VC+). This mode allows the practitioner to select the mechanical rate, V_t, inspiratory time, pressure support level (if desired), FiO_2, PEEP level, and maximal values for PIP and V_t. When VC+ is selected, the ventilator adjusts the pressure to deliver the desired V_t, changing the pressure by about 3 cm H_2O every third breath or so. As compliance worsens, V_t is maintained up to the maximal set PIP, which will not be exceeded. When compliance improves, the ventilator automatically decreases the inspiratory pressure to keep the V_t within the set range. A single V_t delivered above the set maximal value generates a ventilator alarm. Thus, the potential problems one might see with standard volume ventilation (excessive peak pressure to deliver the target V_t) or PC ventilation (improving compliance, producing a dangerously high V_t) are obviated with this mode of ventilation.

Prone Positioning

A progressive decrease in transpulmonary pressure—the force distending the alveoli, defined as the difference between alveolar pressure (P_A) and pleural pressure (P_{pl})—with dependency manifests itself as airway collapse in the dependent portions of the inflamed lung. When proceeding from ventral to dorsal areas in the supine position, transpulmonary pressure—the outward traction force keeping the airways "tethered" open—no longer exceeds alveolar surface tension, and collapse occurs in dependent areas. In the absence of adequate PEEP, inflation of dependent alveoli, once achieved, cannot be maintained, and inspiratory volume is preferentially directed into nondependent areas of the lung (103). Preferential distribution of perfusion to dependent areas with collapsed alveoli contributes to ventilation/perfusion mismatch and intrapulmonary shunt (104). A logical step to realign distribution of inflated alveoli with pulmonary perfusion is to turn the patient prone, alleviating many factors contributing to airway collapse. These factors include the position of cardiac mass that no longer impinges on the retrocardiac lung parenchyma, patterns of diaphragm movement, gravitational redistribution of perfusion, and chest wall mechanics (103). Prone positioning at high PEEP levels in ARDS patients decreases hyperinflation, alveolar instability, and increases alveolar recruitment (105). It also shows beneficial hemodynamic effects, reducing right ventricular afterload and increasing cardiac preload (106).

Although few large studies have documented improvements in oxygenation without significant improvement in outcomes (107–109), a recent multicenter study clearly showed that early application of prolonged prone position (more than 16 hours per day) in patients with severe ARDS significantly reduces mortality (16% prone group vs. 32.8% nonprone group) (110). Considerable skill and experience are needed to pronate to prevent potential pressure-bearing ventral body structures—face, eyes, chest, and knees—and accidental device removal.

High-Frequency Ventilation

High-frequency ventilation (HFV) is a technique that minimizes the risk of ventilator associated lung injury (VALI) and atelectrauma by avoiding both excessive inspiratory volumes and repetitive airway collapse produced by conventional cyclic ventilation in the noncompliant ARDS lung, while maintaining higher mean airway pressures (Fig. 109.9). Subcategories of HFV include high-frequency positive pressure ventilation, high-frequency oscillatory ventilation, and high-frequency jet ventilation. Respiratory rates range from 50 to 2,400 breaths/min, the latter rate produced in oscillatory ventilation.

High-frequency oscillation (HFO) potentially provides lung protection in ARDS by avoiding alveolar distension

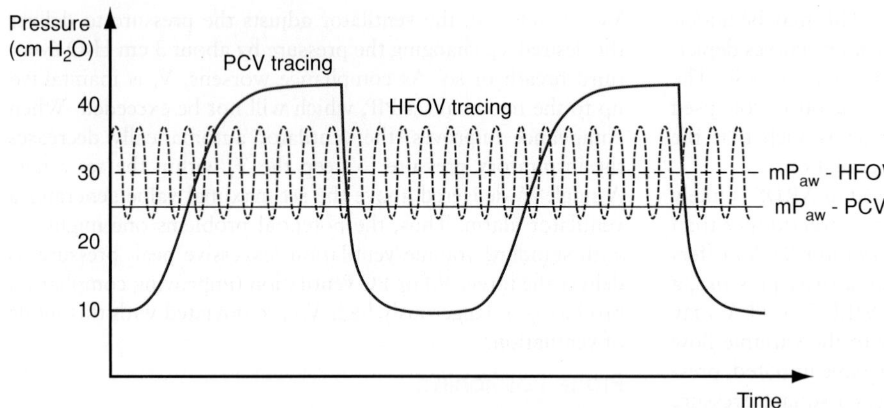

FIGURE 109.9 Depiction of airway pressures—peak and mean—in high-frequency oscillatory ventilation (HFOV) as compared to pressure control ventilation (PCV). (Adapted from Chan KP, Stewart TE, Mehta S. High-frequency oscillatory ventilation for adult patients with ARDS. *Chest.* 2007;131(6):1907–1916.)

and collapse (111). Oscillation is provided at rates of 180 to 900 cycles/min—or 3 to 15 Hz, where 1 Hz = 60 cycles/min or 1 cycle/s—with below dead-space V_t (0.1 to 0.3 mL/kg), high gas flow, and an active expiratory phase. High levels of PEEP are necessary to support the mean airway pressure and maintain alveolar recruitment. HFO provides a number of management challenges, including the necessity for deep sedation, muscle paralysis, a firm bed surface, with increased risk of pressure injury, and difficulty with humidification of inspired gas.

Despite its theoretical benefits and some initial favorable data from small clinical trials (112–114), two recent large multicenter trials showed no benefits of early application of HFO in patients with moderate-to-severe ARDS (115,116), with one study stopped early due to an increased in-hospital mortality in the HFO group when compared to a lung-protective ventilation strategy with low V_t and higher levels of PEEP (115). There may still be some utility for HVO as a salvage technique.

Extracorporeal Life Support

ARDS-related respiratory failure particularly refractory to the most aggressive support measures may warrant the temporary use of mechanical gas exchange devices for pulmonary support while native lung tissue recovers. The process, known as *extracorporeal life support* (ECLS) or ECMO (extracorporeal membrane oxygenation), employs a membrane oxygenator, a blood warmer, and pump systems in parallel with components of the central circulation, depending on the intensity of support required. Blood is withdrawn from the venous system—typically via the internal jugular vein—anticoagulated, oxygenated, decarbonated, adjusted to appropriate temperature, and then returned via the femoral vein (venovenous ECLS) or the right carotid or femoral artery (venoarterial ECLS), depending on the physiologic system(s) requiring support. Either function can be supported alone or together. ECLS is supportive only, bridging the patient's vital cardiopulmonary functions until definitive therapy is instituted. ECLS should not be used as a salvage procedure once irreversible loss of organ function is thought to have occurred (117). During the actual functioning of the bypass circuit, ventilator settings are turned to minimal, thereby avoiding the additional pulmonary insult that VALI would impart.

Initial studies, such as the U.S. ECMO trial (1974 to 1977), used ECMO with complete lung collapse; the unfortunate result was dismal survival (9%). Over the next 10 years, Gattinoni et al. (118) demonstrated the effectiveness of maintaining low levels of lung ventilation (pressure limit 35 cm H_2O, rate 3 to 5 breaths/min) by utilizing low-flow venovenous ECMO for CO_2 removal. In Gattinoni's hands, this approach, termed *low-frequency positive pressure ventilation with extracorporeal CO_2 removal* (LFPPV-$ECCO_2R$), was associated with a 49% survival in very severe ARDS patients (118). In survivors, lung function improved within 48 hours. In a subsequent randomized study carried out in the United States, Morris et al. (119) compared LFPPV–$ECCO_2R$ with PC–IRV using computerized protocols in 40 patients. There was no statistical significance in 30-day survival—33% versus 42% ($p = 0.8$)—but the study size was small.

At present, ECLS is well established in neonatology and pediatrics (120,121), but use in the adult population is less widespread. In the most experienced center, the University of Michigan at Ann Arbor (http//www.med.umich.edu/ecmo/intro.htm), consideration is given to use of ECLS when all maximally supportive measures yield an arterial–alveolar O_2 difference of more than 600 with hypercarbia and persistently reduced compliance (117). Survival may exceed 50%, despite several potential complications, including coagulopathy with bleeding, stroke, pulmonary thromboembolism, ischemic bowel, sepsis, and MODS. Considerable experience and expertise in this complex, expensive, and resource-intensive procedure is required to maximize outcome. Venovenous ECMO may be a lifesaving intervention in selected patients with primary ARDS, especially ischemic–perfusion injury after double lung transplantation. A salutary outcome is predicated on good cardiovascular function, the absence of MODS, and relatively rapid (less than 72 hours) improvement in lung function.

Inhaled Vasodilators

Fundamental to the pathophysiology of ARDS is the phenomenon of ventilation/perfusion mismatch–induced shunt-related hypoxemia. The phenomenon of hypoxic pulmonary vasoconstriction (HPV), which may be viewed evolutionarily as a mechanism to "isolate and exclude" the pathologic hypoxic collapsed alveoli, carries a price of right heart pressure elevation. The influence of HPV extends beyond the collapsed areas; well-aerated alveoli may abut remotely constricted vessels, increasing dead-space ventilation and further straining the right ventricle. When airway inflation and stabilization via optimization of mechanical ventilation do not suffice to alleviate collapse, vasodilators may be employed. Intravenous agents, such as sodium nitroprusside, affect all vessels, frequently worsening hypoxemia by dilating and perfusing

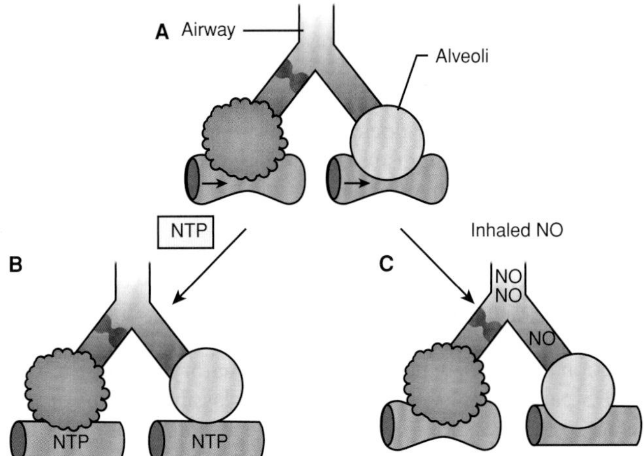

FIGURE 109.10 Intravenous versus inhaled vasodilator effects on pulmonary circulation. A: Shows two idealized alveoli, one occluded (left) and the other normal; both have hypoxic pulmonary vasoconstriction (HPV)-induced decreased pulmonary blood flow. B: Shows the result of using an intravenous vasodilator: HPV is removed to both the occluded and nonoccluded alveoli, resulting in significant shunt. C: Shows the result of utilization of inhaled nitric oxide (NO): HPV is reversed in the area of the ventilated alveolus, but not the obstructed one. NTP, nitroprusside. (Adapted from Lunn RJ. Inhaled nitric oxide therapy. *Mayo Clin Proc.* 1995;70(3):247–255.)

collapsed areas. Aerosolized vasoactive medications, such as nitric oxide or prostaglandin-I, diffuse from ventilated alveoli and result in relaxation of endothelial smooth muscle within remotely constricted vascular beds, thus improving ventilation/perfusion matching while vessels adjacent to collapsed alveoli remain unaffected. Selective vasodilation in ventilated areas decreases shunt fraction and contributes to alleviation of pulmonary hypertension (Fig. 109.10) (122,123).

Nitric oxide (NO) was discovered to be an endogenous compound with vasoactive properties in the late 1980s (124,125); its mechanism of action is through the generation of cyclic guanosine monophosphate (cGMP) (125). NO's rapid absorption and inactivation by hemoglobin restrict its effects to the pulmonary circulation (126). While clinical trials have repeatedly documented improvement in pulmonary artery pressures and oxygenation with NO in ALI/ARDS, there is no evidence that overall mortality is reduced (127,128). Haphazard use of NO is inadvisable in that substantial potential toxicities exist, including free radical formation, production of nitrogen dioxide (NO_2) (129), and generation of methemoglobin. The rate of formation of NO_2 from oxygen and NO depends on the concentration of oxygen and the square of the NO concentrations. The Occupational Safety and Health Administration has set safety limits of 5 ppm for NO_2, as it can cause pathologic changes to the lungs at doses of 25 ppm. At extremely high doses, pulmonary edema, hemorrhage, and death have been seen in animal models. NO_2 levels should be monitored as closely as possible to the endotracheal tube (130). In clinical trials using NO at 5 to 40 ppm, NO_2 has not been a significant problem.

Methemoglobinemia is another potential, but rare, complication of NO administration. About 80% to 90% of inhaled NO is absorbed within the bloodstream, where it reacts with hemoglobin within the red blood cell to form nitrosyl–hemoglobin and methemoglobin. The primary factor determining the development of methemoglobinemia is the dose of NO, although the hemoglobin level, oxygen saturation, and methemoglobin reductase also play a role. In the United States, Native Americans more frequently have methemoglobin reductase deficiency—either partial or complete—and therefore are more susceptible to methemoglobinemia. Closer monitoring of such patients is warranted. In clinical trials using NO at 5 to 40 ppm, methemoglobinemia has not been a significant problem. Finally, the cost of inhaled NO is surprisingly steep (131), warranting the closest scrutiny of its use in "marginal" situations.

Surfactant Replacement

Surfactant is a phospholipid, a protein material produced by type II epithelial pneumocytes, secreted along the alveolar surface and acting to decrease surface tension to prevent alveolar collapse. Hydrophilic surfactant proteins A and D contribute to the immune response (132), while hydrophobic types B and C facilitate monolayer formation within the alveolus (133). Pulmonary epithelial injury and surfactant dysfunction from direct or indirect injury destabilize alveoli, leading to the collapse, venous admixture, hypoxemia, and a decreased lung compliance characteristic of ARDS.

Surfactant replacement therapy in adults has been, thus far, unsuccessful. After an encouraging phase I/II trial of recombinant surfactant protein C–based surfactant supplement (134), a phase III trial of the same material improved oxygenation without lowering mortality or the number of ventilator days in adult patients with ARDS (135).

COMPLICATIONS

Significant morbidity or mortality may occur during supportive therapy for ARDS. Most aspects of supportive care transcend the specifics of ARDS, and the clinician should be aware of these potential complications, many of which are outlined by Pingleton (Table 109.8) (136). Attention to detail decreases complications and may improve outcome in ARDS. As suggested earlier, the ARDS patient is so exquisitely sensitive to the smallest subtleties of mechanical ventilation that discussion of the main potential sequelae of suboptimal mechanical ventilation, namely VILI, is provided in detail below.

Ventilator-Induced Lung Injury

To date, the only mode of management with which outcome in ARDS patients can predictably be improved is the optimal use of mechanical ventilation, using low V_t with PEEP (137). As in all things medical, specific techniques of ventilator management carry risks and benefits. While mechanical assistance with gas exchange may be lifesaving, mechanical ventilation may contribute simultaneously to worsening the overall inflammatory process and the eventual triumph of MODS leading to death. In fact, the very process of mechanical ventilatory support can, if conducted suboptimally, provoke edematous morphologic and microscopic pulmonary changes indistinguishable from those associated with commonly recognized ARDS-inducing processes (77). Again, in ARDS, nonhomogeneous distribution of areas of consolidated, noncompliant lung, featuring thickened interstitium and fluid- and debris-filled alveoli residing adjacent to unaffected areas, causes maldistribution of positive pressure ventilation, exceeding injurious pressure and volume thresholds in healthy areas, while not affecting inflamed tissues. The additional inflammatory insult induced by suboptimal mechanical

TABLE 109.8 Complications Associated with Acute Respiratory Distress Syndrome

Pulmonary
- Pulmonary emboli
- Pulmonary barotrauma
- Pulmonary fibrosis
- Oxygen toxicity

Gastrointestinal
- Gastrointestinal hemorrhage
- Ileus
- Gastric distension
- Pneumoperitoneum

Renal
- Renal failure
- Fluid retention

Cardiovascular
- Invasive catheters
- Arrhythmia
- Hypotension
- Low cardiac output

Infection
- Sepsis
- Nosocomial pneumonia

Hematologic
- Anemia
- Thrombocytopenia
- Disseminated intravascular coagulation

Other
- Hepatic
- Endocrine
- Neurologic
- Psychiatric
- Malnutrition

Complications attributable to intubation and extubation
- Prolonged attempt at intubation
- Intubation of a mainstem bronchus
- Premature extubation
- Self-extubation

Complications associated with endotracheal/tracheostomy tubes
- Tube malfunction
- Nasal necrosis
- Paranasal sinus infection
- Tracheal stenosis
- Tracheomalacia
- Polyps
- Erosion
- Fistulae
- Airway obstruction
- Hoarseness

Complications attributable to operation of the ventilator
- Machine failure
- Alarm failure
- Alarms silenced
- Inadequate nebulization or humidification

Complications occurring during positive airway pressure therapy
- Alveolar hypoventilation
- Alveolar hyperventilation
- Massive gastric distension
- Barotrauma
- Atelectasis
- Pneumonia
- Hypotension

From Taylor RW. The adult respiratory distress syndrome. In: Kirby RR, Taylor RW, eds. *Respiratory Failure.* Chicago, IL: Year Book Medical Publishers; 1986:208.

ventilation technique is termed *ventilator-associated lung injury.* The ARMA study (74) revealed the importance of low-volume ventilation in ARDS, with substantial improvement in several indices using 6 mL/kg rather than 12 mL/kg V_t. While criticized, the findings document the importance of avoiding several putative mechanisms of pathologic effect:

- Excess alveolar hyperinflation with associated increased permeability and cytokine release
- Escape of alveolar air outside the confines of alveoli
- Destructive sheer-stress influence of repetitive inflation/collapse of unstable alveoli.

Each of these phenomena contributes to pulmonary dysfunction and perpetuation of the inflammatory response in the ARDS patient, and thus each has been classified. *Barotrauma* refers to the presence of air outside the alveoli when receiving positive pressure ventilation. Air leaks track along the perivascular sheath to the mediastinum and pleural cavities, or along fascial planes to extrathoracic areas (138). It seems intuitive that such occurrences are related to pressures exceeding the limits of tissue structural integrity, but the issue is clearly more complicated, since musicians are repeatedly able to generate 150 cm H_2O airway pressure with no sequelae (139). It is speculated that barotrauma represents regional overinflation in areas of diseased lung, such areas thereby being particularly at risk for structural failure and air leak (139). *Volutrauma* occurs when excessive inspiratory volumes induce microvascular edema (140); the offending agent appears to be excessive *volume*, rather than the excessive *pressure* required to supply that volume. Resultant mechanical stretch triggers changes in the alveolar–capillary barrier (79), and in proliferation of inflammatory cytokines (75), resulting in interstitial and alveolar proteinaceous edema, decreased compliance, and hyaline membrane formation. Compromised surfactant production and function leads to increased surface tension, provoking alveolar collapse with increased venous admixture and subjecting alveolar epithelium to the tissue-destructive shear stresses of recruitment/derecruitment in the process known as *atelectrauma.* While the use of PEEP to maintain diseased distal alveoli splinted "open" has not definitively been demonstrated to improve outcome (79, and earlier discussion, above), improvements in oxygenation and pulmonary compliance with PEEP mandate its routine use in ARDS. Of note is the complex relationship between mechanical ventilation and patchy maldistribution throughout the lung in areas of varying ratios of ventilation and perfusion, with atelectatic areas abutting hyperinflated bullous and cystic areas. While collapsed noncompliant airways require high initial opening pressures consistent with the Law of LaPlace (within the context of pulmonary physiology, the following formula is appropriate: $P = 2t/R$, where P = pressure, t = tension, and R = radius), such high pressure is transmitted throughout the lung, overdistending more compliant airways both through direct influence and by an unequally distributed traction force upon the adjacent airways, as depicted in Figure 109.7. Implicit in such heterogeneous patterns of gas distribution is the initiation of the destructive sequelae associated with inflation of each subregion of lung, as delineated above.

Furthermore, over the last few years, there has been recognition of the inflammatory cytokine release, as well as alveolar and interstitial neutrophil infiltration associated with ventilator-related pulmonary disruption, leading to MODS (76,141). While it is indisputable that "excessive" V_t

ventilation augments systemic cytokine levels (79), the specific causal relationship with worse outcome has yet to be validated. The ALVEOLI study (87), which examined the variation of short-term indices—28-day mortality and number of ventilator-free days—with modulation of PEEP, was discontinued early based on lack of improvement in outcome with high PEEP levels. Thus, the optimal inspiratory pressure, or level of PEEP for a given ARDS patient's pressure–volume curve, can be exceedingly difficult to identify despite the potentially severe consequences of failure to do so. While dependent areas of tenaciously collapsed, high time-constant alveoli may require the equivalent of repeated and prolonged high-pressure recruitment maneuvers to achieve inflation and avoid atelectrauma, simultaneous transmission of such pressure to compliant alveoli incurs the risk of inducing volutrauma and inciting inflammation. Clearly, in those with advanced lung injury, the "optimal" inspiratory pressure, in reality, reflects a statistical bell curve of widely variable individual alveolar compliances. The clinician must vary inspiratory time, plateau pressure, PEEP, and tidal volume to inflate stiff alveoli while not persistently overdistending the normal ones. Such important actions are required because of the dynamic and changing compliance profiles of the inflamed lung.

Key Points

- ARDS is commonly seen with the systemic inflammatory response syndrome (SIRS) and the MODS.
- Risk factors for developing ARDS include SIRS, sepsis, pulmonary contusion, aspiration, inhalation of toxic substances, near-drowning, long-bone fractures, pancreatitis, diffuse pneumonia, and multiple blood transfusions.
- Most patients with ARDS demonstrate similar clinical and pathologic features, irrespective of the cause of the ALI.
- The lung's response to injury can be divided into an exudative phase, a proliferative phase, and a fibrotic phase.
- A variety of inflammatory mediators have been implicated in the pathogenesis of ALI.
- The neutrophil plays a central role in ALI.
- The severe hypoxemia associated with this syndrome is caused by intrapulmonary shunting that occurs with interstitial edema, and alveolar flooding and collapse.
- A reduction in functional residual capacity (FRC) and lung compliance are the hallmarks of ARDS.
- Radiographic changes seen in patients with ARDS are characteristic but nonspecific, and rarely reveal the etiology of the syndrome.

Essential Diagnostic Tests and Procedures

- History and physical examination
- Chest radiograph
- Arterial blood gas measurements
- Further diagnostic tests based on the clinical circumstances

Initial Therapy

- Most patients require early endotracheal intubation and positive pressure ventilation.
- The goal of mechanical ventilation is to provide adequate oxygenation and carbon dioxide elimination while keeping complications, such as oxygen toxicity, ventilator-associated lung injury, and hemodynamic compromise, to a minimum.

References

1. Kollef MH, Schuster D. The acute respiratory distress syndrome. *N Engl J Med.* 1995;332:27.
2. Bernard GR, Artigas A, Brigham KL, et al. The American-European Consensus Conference on ARDS. *Am J Respir Crit Care Med.* 1994;149:818.
3. Ranieri VM, Rubenfeld GD, Thompson BT, et al. Acute respiratory distress syndrome: the Berlin definition. *JAMA.* 2012;307:2526–2533.
4. Murray JF, Matthay MA, Luce JM, et al. An expanded definition of the adult respiratory distress syndrome. *Am Rev Respir Dis.* 1988;138:720.
5. Matthay MA. Conference summary—acute lung injury. *Chest.* 1999;116: 119S–126S.
6. Zilberberg MD, Epstein SK. Acute lung injury in the medical ICU: comorbid conditions, age, etiology, and hospital outcome. *Am J Respir Crit Care Med.* 1998;157(Pt 1):1159–1164.
7. Moss M, Goodman PL, Heinig M, et al. Establishing the relative accuracy of three new definitions of the adult respiratory distress syndrome. *Crit Care Med.* 1995;23:1629.
8. Kangelaris KN, Calfee CS, May AK, et al. Is there still a role for the lung injury score in the era of the Berlin definition ARDS? *Ann Intensive Care.* 2014;4:4.
9. Hudson LD, Milberg JA, Anardi D, et al. Clinical risks of the development of the acute respiratory distress syndrome. *Am J Respir Care.* 1995; 151:293.
10. Hudson LD, Steinberg KP. Epidemiology of acute lung injury and ARDS. *Chest.* 1999;116:74S.
11. Ware LB, Matthay MA. The acute respiratory distress syndrome. *N Engl J Med.* 2000;342:1334.
12. Rubenfield GD, Caldwell E, Peabody E, et al. Incidence and outcomes of acute lung injury. *N Engl J Med.* 2005;353:1685.
13. Rocco PRM, Zin WA. Pulmonary and extrapulmonary acute respiratory distress syndrome: are they different? *Curr Opin Crit Care.* 2005;11:10.
14. Milberg JA, Davis DR, Steinberg KP, et al. Improved survival of patients with acute respiratory distress syndrome (ARDS): 1983–1993. *JAMA.* 1995; 273(4):306–309.
15. Abel SJC, Finney SJ, Brett SJ, et al. Reduced mortality in association with acute respiratory distress syndrome (ARDS). *Thorax.* 1998;53:292.
16. Taylor RW, Duncan CA. The adult respiratory distress syndrome. *Res Med.* 1983;1:17.
17. Brun-Buisson C, Minelli C, Bertolini G, et al. Epidemiology and outcome of acute lung injury in European intensive care units: results from the ALIVE study. *Intensive Care Med.* 2004;30:51–61.
18. Luhr OR, Antonsen K, Karlsson M, et al. Incidence and mortality after acute respiratory failure and acute respiratory distress syndrome in Sweden, Denmark, and Iceland: the ARF Study Group. *Am J Respir Crit Care Med.* 1999;159:1849–1861.
19. Bersten AD, Edibam C, Hunt T, et al. Incidence and mortality of acute lung injury and the acute respiratory distress syndrome in three Australian states. *Am J Respir Crit Care Med.* 2002;165:443–448.
20. Villar J, Blanco J, Añón JM, et al. The ALIEN study: incidence and outcome of acute respiratory distress syndrome in the era of lung protective ventilation. *Intensive Care Med.* 2011;37:1932–1941.
21. Davidson TA, Rubenfeld GD, Caldwell ES, et al. The effect of acute respiratory distress syndrome on long-term survival. *Am J Respir Crit Care Med.* 1999;160:1838.
22. Luce JM. Acute lung injury and the acute respiratory distress syndrome. *Crit Care Med.* 1998;26:369–376.
23. Herridge MS, Cheung AM, Tansey CM, et al. One-year outcomes in survivors of the acute respiratory distress syndrome. *N Engl J Med.* 2003; 348:683.
24. McHugh LG, Milberg JA, Whitecomb ME, et al. Recovery of function in survivors of the acute respiratory distress syndrome. *Am J Respir Crit Care Med.* 1994;150:90.
25. Davidson TA, Caldwell ES, Curtis JR, et al. Reduced quality of life in survivors of acute respiratory distress syndrome compared with critically ill control patients. *JAMA.* 1999;281:354.

26. Weinert CR, Gross CR, Kangas JR, et al. Health-related quality of life after acute lung injury. *Am J Respir Crit Care Med.* 1997;156:1120.
27. Mikkelsen ME, Christie JD, Lanken PN, et al. The adult respiratory distress syndrome cognitive outcomes study: long-term neuropsychological function in survivors of acute lung injury. *Am J Respir Crit Care Med.* 2012;185:1307–1315.
28. Bienvenu OJ, Colantuoni E, Mendez-Tellez PA, et al. Cooccurrence of and remission from general anxiety, depression, and posttraumatic stress disorder symptoms after acute lung injury: a 2-year longitudinal study. *Crit Care Med.* 2015;43:642–653.
29. Khandelwal N, Hough CL, Bansal A, et al. Long-term survival in patients with severe acute respiratory distress syndrome and rescue therapies for refractory hypoxemia. *Crit Care Med.* 2014;42:1610–1618.
30. Pelosi P, D'Onofrio D, Chiumello D, et al. Pulmonary and extrapulmonary acute respiratory distress syndrome are different. *Eur Respir J (Suppl).* 2003;42:48s–56s.
31. Lee WL, Downey GP. Neutrophil activation and acute lung injury. *Curr Opin Crit Care.* 2001;7(1):1–7.
32. Abraham E. Neutrophils and acute lung injury. *Crit Care Med.* 2003;31 (4 Suppl):S195–199.
33. Frerking I, Günther A, Seeger W, et al. Pulmonary surfactant: functions, abnormalities and therapeutic options. *Intensive Care Med.* 2001;27(11): 1699–1717.
34. Idell S. Coagulation, fibrinolysis, and fibrin deposition in acute lung injury. *Crit Care Med.* 2003;31(4 Suppl):S213–S220.
35. Pittet JF, Mackersie RC, Martin TR, et al. Biological markers of acute lung injury: prognostic and pathogenetic significance. *Am J Respir Crit Care Med.* 1997;155(4):1187–1205.
36. Park WY, Goodman RB, Steinberg KP, et al. Cytokine balance in the lungs of patients with acute respiratory distress syndrome. *Am J Respir Crit Care Med.* 2001;164:1896–1903.
37. Fink MP. Role of reactive oxygen and nitrogen species in acute respiratory distress syndrome. *Curr Opin Crit Care.* 2002;8:6–11.
38. Bhatia M, Moochhala S. Role of inflammatory mediators in the pathophysiology of acute respiratory distress syndrome. *J Pathol.* 2004;202:145–156.
39. Han S, Mallampalli RK. The acute respiratory distress syndrome: from mechanism to translation. *J Immunol.* 2015;194:855–860.
40. Tomashefski JF Jr. Pulmonary pathology of acute respiratory distress syndrome. *Clin Chest Med.* 2000;21:435–466.
41. Bellingan GJ. The pulmonary physician in critical care: the pathogenesis of ALI/ARDS. *Thorax.* 2002;57:540–546.
42. Marshall RP, Bellingan G, Webb S, et al. Fibroproliferation occurs early in the acute respiratory distress syndrome and impacts on outcome. *Am J Respir Crit Care Med.* 2000;162:1783–1788.
43. Gomez AC: Pulmonary insufficiency in non-thoracic trauma. *J Trauma.* 1968;8:666.
44. Moore FA, Feliciano DV, Andrassy RJ, et al. Early enteral feeding, compared with parenteral, reduces postoperative septic complications. *Ann Surg.* 1992;216:172.
45. Rice TW, Wheeler AP, Thompson BT, et al. Initial trophic vs full enteral feeding in patients with acute lung injury: the EDEN randomized trial. *JAMA.* 2012; 307:795–803.
46. Needham DM, Dinglas VD, Bienvenu OJ, et al. One year outcomes in patients with acute lung injury randomised to initial trophic or full enteral feeding: prospective follow-up of EDEN randomised trial. *Br Med J.* 2013; 346:f1532
47. Schuster D. Fluid management in ARDS: "keep them dry" or does it matter? *Intensive Care Med.* 1995;21:101.
48. National Heart, Lung, and Blood Institute Acute Respiratory Distress Syndrome (ARDS) Clinical Trials Network. Comparison of two fluid-management strategies in acute lung injury. *N Engl J Med.* 2006;354(24):2564–2575.
49. Matthay MA, Brower RG, Carson S, et al. National Heart, Lung, and Blood Institute Acute Respiratory Distress Syndrome (ARDS) Clinical Trials Network. Randomized, placebo-controlled clinical trial of an aerosolized b2-agonist for treatment of acute lung injury. *Am J Respir Crit Care Med.* 2011;184:561–568.
50. Gao Smith F, Perkins GD, Gates S, et al.; BALTI-2 study investigators. Effect of intravenous b-2 agonist treatment on clinical outcomes in acute respiratory distress syndrome (BALTI-2): a multicentre, randomised controlled trial. *Lancet.* 2012;379:229–235.
51. Perkins GD, Gates S, Park D et al. The beta agonist lung injury trial prevention. A randomized controlled trial. *Am J Respir Crit Care Med.* 2014;189:674–683.
52. Wright P, Carmichael L, Bernard G. Effect of bronchodilators on lung mechanics in the acute respiratory distress syndrome (ARDS). *Chest.* 1994;106:157.
53. Stoelting RK. *Pharmacology and Physiology in Anesthetic Practice.* 3rd ed. Philadelphia, PA: Lippincott–Raven; 1999:196.
54. Meduri GU, Chinn AJ, Leeper KV, et al. Corticosteroid rescue treatment of progressive fibroproliferation in late ARDS. Patterns of response and predictors of outcome. *Chest.* 1994;105:1516–1527.
55. Steinberg KP, Hudson LD, Goodman RB, et al.; The National Heart, Lung, and Blood Institute Acute Respiratory Distress Syndrome (ARDS) Clinical Trials Network. Efficacy and safety of corticosteroids for persistent acute respiratory distress syndrome. *N Engl J Med.* 2006;354:1671–1684.
56. Meduri GU, Golden E, Freire AX, et al. Methylprednisolone infusion in early severe ARDS: results of a randomized controlled trial. *Chest.* 2007; 131:954–963.
57. Meduri GU, Marik PE, Chrousos GP, et al. Steroid treatment in ARDS: a critical appraisal of the ARDS network trial and the recent literature. *Intensive Care Med.* 2008;34:61–69.
58. Peter JV, John P, Graham PL, et al. Corticosteroids in the prevention and treatment of acute respiratory distress syndrome (ARDS) in adults: meta-analysis. *BMJ.* 2008;336:1006–1009.
59. Calfee CS, Matthay MA. Nonventilatory treatments for acute lung injury and ARDS. *Chest.* 2007;131:913–920.
60. Hudson LD, Hough CL. Therapy for late-phase acute respiratory distress syndrome. *Clin Chest Med.* 2006;27:671–677.
61. Bream-Rouwenhorst HR, Beltz EA, Ross MB, et al. Recent developments in the management of acute respiratory distress syndrome in adults. *Am J Health Syst Pharm.* 2008;65:29–36.
62. Meduri GU, Headley S, Tolley E, et al. Plasma and BAL cytokine response to corticosteroid rescue treatment in late ARDS. *Chest.* 1995;103:1315.
63. Papazian L, Forel JM, Gacouin A, et al. Neuromuscular blockers in early acute respiratory distress syndrome. *N Engl J Med.* 2010;363:1107–1116.
64. Alhazzani W, Alshahrani M, Jaeschke R, et al. Neuromuscular blocking agents in acute respiratory distress syndrome: a systematic review and meta-analysis of randomized controlled trials. *Crit Care.* 2013;17:R43.
65. Hraiech S, Dizier S, Papazian L. The use of paralytics in patients with acute respiratory distress syndrome. *Clin Chest Med.* 2014;35:753–763.
66. Antonelli M, Conti G, Esquinas A, et al. A multiple-center survey on the use in clinical practice of noninvasive ventilation as a first-line intervention for acute respiratory distress syndrome. *Crit Care Med.* 2007;35:18–25.
67. Ferrer M, Esquinas A, Leon M, et al. Noninvasive ventilation in severe hypoxemic respiratory failure: a randomized clinical trial. *Am J Respir Crit Care Med.* 2003;168:1438–1444.
68. Keenan SP, Sinuff T, Cook DJ, et al. Does noninvasive positive pressure ventilation improve outcome in acute hypoxemic respiratory failure? A systematic review. *Crit Care Med.* 2004;32:2516–2523.
69. Rouby JJ, Puybasset L, Cluzel P, et al. Regional distribution of gas and tissue in acute respiratory distress syndrome. II. Physiological correlations and definition of an ARDS Severity Score. CT Scan ARDS Study Group. *Intensive Care Med.* 2000;26:1046–1056.
70. Puybasset L, Gusman P, Muller JC, et al. Regional distribution of gas and tissue in acute respiratory distress syndrome. III. Consequences for the effects of positive end-expiratory pressure. CT Scan ARDS Study Group. *Intensive Care Med.* 2000;26:1215–1227.
71. Kolobow T, Moretti MP, Fumagalli R, et al. Severe impairment in lung function induced by high peak airway pressure during mechanical ventilation: an experimental study. *Am Rev Respir Dis.* 1987;135:312–315.
72. Tsuno K, Prato P, Kolobow T. Acute lung injury from mechanical ventilation at moderately high airway pressures. *J Appl Physiol.* 1990;69:956–961.
73. Hickling KG, Henderson SJ, Jackson R. Low mortality associated with low volume pressure limited ventilation with permissive hypercapnia in severe adult respiratory distress syndrome. *Intensive Care Med.* 1990;16:372–377.
74. Acute Respiratory Distress Syndrome Network. Ventilation with lower tidal volumes as compared with traditional tidal volumes for acute lung injury and the acute respiratory distress syndrome. *N Engl J Med.* 2000; 342:1301–1308.
75. Tremblay LN, Slutsky AS. Ventilator-induced lung injury: from the bench to the bedside. *Intensive Care Med.* 2006;32:24–33.
76. Tremblay L, Valenza F, Ribeiro SP, et al. Injurious ventilatory strategies increase cytokines and c-fos m-RNA expression in an isolated rat lung model. *J Clin Invest.* 1997;99:944–952.
77. Slutsky AS, Ranieri VM. Ventilator-induced lung injury. *N Engl J Med.* 2013;369:2126–2136.
78. Belperio JA, Keane MP, Lynch JP III, et al. The role of cytokines during the pathogenesis of ventilator-associated and ventilator-induced lung injury. *Semin Respir Crit Care Med.* 2006;27:350–364.
79. Ranieri VM, Suter PM, Tortorella C, et al. Effect of mechanical ventilation on inflammatory mediators in patients with acute respiratory distress syndrome: a randomized controlled trial. *JAMA.* 1999;282:54–61.

80. Terragni PP, Rosboch G, Tealdi A, et al. Tidal hyperinflation during low tidal volume ventilation in acute respiratory distress syndrome. *Am J Respir Crit Care Med.* 2007;175:160–166.
81. Gattinoni L, Pesenti A. The concept of "baby lung." *Intensive Care Med.* 2005;31:776–784.
82. Barbas CS, de Matos GF, Pincelli MP, et al. Mechanical ventilation in acute respiratory failure: recruitment and high positive end-expiratory pressure are necessary. *Curr Opin Crit Care.* 2005;11:18–28.
83. Amato MB, Barbas CS, Medeiros DM, et al. Effect of a protective-ventilation strategy on mortality in the acute respiratory distress syndrome. *N Engl J Med.* 1998;338:347–354.
84. Lachmann B. Open up the lung and keep the lung open. *Intensive Care Med.* 1992;18:319–321.
85. Gattinoni L, Caironi P, Cressoni M, et al. Lung recruitment in patients with the acute respiratory distress syndrome. *N Engl J Med.* 2006;354: 1775–1786.
86. Dueck R. Alveolar recruitment versus hyperinflation: a balancing act. *Curr Opin Anaesthesiol.* 2006;19:650–654.
87. Brower RG, Lanken PN, MacIntyre N, et al.; National Heart, Lung, and Blood Institute ARDS Clinical Trials Network. Higher versus lower positive end-expiratory pressures in patients with the acute respiratory distress syndrome. *N Engl J Med.* 2004;351:327–336.
88. Meade MO, Cook DJ, Guyatt GH, et al.; Lung Open Ventilation Study Investigators. Ventilation strategy using low tidal volumes, recruitment maneuvers, and high positive end-expiratory pressure for acute lung injury and acute respiratory distress syndrome: a randomized controlled trial. *JAMA.* 2008;299:637–645.
89. Borges JB, Okamoto VN, Matos GF, et al. Reversibility of lung collapse and hypoxemia in early acute respiratory distress syndrome. *Am J Respir Crit Care Med.* 2006;174(3):268–278.
90. Lapinsky SE, Mehta S. Bench-to-bedside review: recruitment and recruiting maneuvers. *Crit Care.* 2005;9:60–65.
91. Medoff BD, Harris RS, Kesselman H, et al. Use of recruitment maneuvers and high-positive end-expiratory pressure in a patient with acute respiratory distress syndrome. *Crit Care Med.* 2000;28:1210–1216.
92. Gattinoni L, Carlesso E, Cressoni M. Selecting the 'right' positive end-expiratory pressure level. *Curr Opin Crit Care.* 2015;21:50–57.
93. Chiumello D, Cressoni M, Carlesso E, et al. Bedside selection of positive end-expiratory pressure in mild, moderate, and severe acute respiratory distress syndrome. *Crit Care Med.* 2014;42:252–264.
94. Gulati G, Novero A, Loring SH, et al. Pleural pressure and optimal positive end-expiratory pressure based on esophageal pressure versus chest wall elastance: incompatible results. *Crit Care Med.* 2013;41:1951–1957.
95. Laffey JG, O'Croinin D, McLoughlin P, et al. Permissive hypercapnia: role in protective lung ventilatory strategies. *Intensive Care Med.* 2004; 30:347–356.
96. Kallet RH, Campbell AR, Alonso JA, et al. The effects of pressure control versus volume control assisted ventilation on patient work of breathing in acute lung injury and acute respiratory distress syndrome. *Respir Care.* 2000;45:1085–1096.
97. Shanholtz C, Brower R. Should inverse ratio ventilation be used in adult respiratory distress syndrome. *Am J Respir Crit Care Med.* 1994;149: 1354–1358.
98. Mercat A, Graïni L, Teboul JL, et al. Cardiorespiratory effects of pressure-controlled ventilation with and without inverse ratio in the adult respiratory distress syndrome. *Chest.* 1993;104:871–875.
99. Esteban A, Alía I, Gordo F, et al. Prospective randomized trial comparing pressure-controlled ventilation and volume-controlled ventilation in ARDS. For the Spanish Lung Failure Collaborative Group. *Chest.* 2000;117: 1690–1696.
100. Habashi NM. Other approaches to open-lung ventilation: airway pressure release ventilation. *Crit Care Med.* 2005;33:S228–S240.
101. Kaplan LJ, Bailey H, Formosa V. Airway pressure release ventilation increases cardiac performance in patients with acute lung injury/adult respiratory distress syndrome. *Crit Care.* 2001;5:221–226.
102. Putensen C, Zech S, Wrigge H, et al. Long-term effects of spontaneous breathing during ventilatory support in patients with acute lung injury. *Am J Respir Crit Care Med.* 2001;164:43–49.
103. Pelosi P, Brazzi L, Gattinoni L. Prone position in acute respiratory distress syndrome. *Eur Respir J.* 2002;20:1017–1028.
104. West JB, Dollery CT, Naimark A. Distribution of blood flow in isolated lung; relation to vascular and alveolar pressures. *J Appl Physiol.* 1964; 19:713–724.
105. Cornejo RA, Díaz JC, Tobar EA, et al. Effects of prone positioning on lung protection in patients with acute respiratory distress syndrome. *Am J Respir Crit Care Med.* 2013;188:440–448.
106. Jozwiak M, Teboul JL, Anguel N, et al. Beneficial hemodynamic effects of prone positioning in patients with acute respiratory distress syndrome. *Am J Respir Crit Care Med.* 2013;188:1428–1433.
107. Gattinoni L, Tognoni G, Pesenti A, et al.; Prone-Supine Study Group. Effect of prone positioning on the survival of patients with acute respiratory failure. *N Engl J Med.* 2001;345:568–573.
108. Guerin C, Gaillard S, Lemasson S, et al. Effects of systematic prone positioning in hypoxemic acute respiratory failure: a randomized controlled trial. *JAMA.* 2004;292:2379–2387.
109. Mancebo J, Fernández R, Blanch L, et al. A multicenter trial of prolonged prone ventilation in severe acute respiratory distress syndrome. *Am J Respir Crit Care Med.* 2006;173:1233–1239.
110. Guérin C, Reignier J, Richard JC, et al Prone positioning in severe acute respiratory distress syndrome. *N Engl J Med.* 2013;368:2159–2168.
111. Derdak S. High-frequency oscillatory ventilation for acute respiratory distress syndrome in adult patients. *Crit Care Med.* 2003;31(4 Suppl): S317–S323.
112. Derdak S, Mehta S, Stewart TE, et al.; Multicenter Oscillatory Ventilation For Acute Respiratory Distress Syndrome Trial (MOAT) Study Investigators. High-frequency oscillatory ventilation for acute respiratory distress syndrome in adults: a randomized, controlled trial. *Am J Respir Crit Care Med.* 2002;166:801–808.
113. Bollen CW, van Well GT, Sherry T, et al. High frequency oscillatory ventilation compared with conventional mechanical ventilation in adult respiratory distress syndrome: a randomized controlled trial. *Crit Care.* 2005;9:R430–R439.
114. Sud S, Sud M, Friedrich JO, et al. High frequency oscillation in patients with acute lung injury and acute respiratory distress syndrome (ARDS): systematic review and meta-analysis. *BMJ.* 2010;340:c2327.
115. Ferguson ND, Cook DJ, Guyatt GH, et al. High-frequency oscillation in early acute respiratory distress syndrome. *N Engl J Med.* 2013;368: 795–805.
116. Young D, Lamb SE, Shah S, et al. High-frequency oscillation for acute respiratory distress syndrome. *N Engl J Med.* 2013;368:806–813.
117. Brown JK, Haft JW, Bartlett RH, et al. Acute lung injury and acute respiratory distress syndrome: extracorporeal life support and liquid ventilation for severe acute respiratory distress syndrome in adults. *Semin Respir Crit Care Med.* 2006;27:416–425.
118. Gattinoni L, Pesenti A, Mascheroni D, et al. Low-frequency positive-pressure ventilation with extracorporeal CO_2 removal in severe acute respiratory failure. *JAMA.* 1986;256:881–886.
119. Morris AH, Wallace CJ, Menlove RL, et al. Randomized clinical trial of pressure-controlled inverse ratio ventilation and extracorporeal CO_2 removal for adult respiratory distress syndrome. *Am J Respir Crit Care Med.* 1994;149:295–305.
120. Lequier L. Extracorporeal life support in pediatric and neonatal critical care: a review. *J Intensive Care Med.* 2004;19:243–258.
121. Skinner SC, Hirschl RB, Bartlett RH. Extracorporeal life support. *Semin Pediatr Surg.* 2006;15:242–250.
122. Pison U, López FA, Heidelmeyer CF, et al. Inhaled nitric oxide reverses hypoxic pulmonary vasoconstriction without impairing gas exchange. *J Appl Physiol.* 1993;74:1287–1292.
123. Rossaint R, Falke KJ, López F, et al. Inhaled nitric oxide for the adult respiratory distress syndrome. *N Engl J Med.* 1993;328:399–405.
124. Palmer RM, Ferrige AG, Moncada S. Nitric oxide release accounts for the biological activity of endothelium-derived relaxing factor. *Nature.* 1987; 327:524–526.
125. Moncada S, Palmer RM, Higgs EA. Nitric oxide: physiology, pathophysiology, and pharmacology. *Pharmacol Rev.* 1991;43:109–142.
126. Cooper CE. Nitric oxide and iron proteins. *Biochim Biophys Acta.* 1999; 1411:290–309.
127. Taylor RW, Zimmerman JL, Dellinger RP, et al.; Inhaled Nitric Oxide in ARDS Study Group. Low-dose inhaled nitric oxide in patients with acute lung injury: a randomized controlled trial. *JAMA.* 2004;291(13):1603–1609.
128. Adhikari NK, Burns KE, Friedrich JO, et al. Effect of nitric oxide on oxygenation and mortality in acute lung injury: systematic review and meta-analysis. *BMJ.* 2007;334:779.
129. Lowson SM. Inhaled alternatives to nitric oxide. *Crit Care Med.* 2005; 33:S188–S195.
130. Puybasset L, Rouby JJ, Mourgeon E, et al. Factors influencing cardiopulmonary effects of inhaled nitric oxide in acute respiratory failure. *Am J Respir Crit Care Med.* 1995;152(1):318–328.
131. Pierce CM, Peters MJ, Cohen G, et al. Cost of nitric oxide is exorbitant [Letter to the Editor]. *BMJ.* 2002;325:336.
132. Wright JR. Immunoregulatory functions of surfactant proteins. *Nat Rev Immunol.* 2005;5:58–68.

133. Stevens TP, Sinkin RA. Surfactant replacement therapy. *Chest*. 2007; 131:1577–1582.
134. Spragg RG, Lewis JF, Wurst W, et al. Treatment of acute respiratory distress syndrome with recombinant surfactant protein C surfactant. *Am J Respir Crit Care Med*. 2003;167:1562–1566.
135. Spragg RG, Lewis JF, Walmrath HD, et al. Effect of recombinant surfactant protein C-based surfactant on the acute respiratory distress syndrome. *N Engl J Med*. 2004;351:884–892.
136. Pingleton SK. Complications associated with the adult respiratory distress syndrome. *Clin Chest Med*. 1982;5:143.
137. Villar J, Kacmarek RM, Pérez-Méndez L, et al. A high positive end-expiratory pressure, low tidal volume ventilatory strategy improves outcome in persistent acute respiratory distress syndrome: a randomized, controlled trial. *Crit Care Med*. 2006;34(5):1311–1318.
138. Gammon RB, Shin MS, Buchalter SE. Pulmonary barotrauma in mechanical ventilation: patterns and risk factors. *Chest*. 1992;102:568–572.
139. Bouhuys A. Physiology and musical instruments. *Nature*. 1969;221: 1199–2004.
140. Dreyfuss D, Soler P, Saumon G. Mechanical ventilation-induced pulmonary edema. Interaction with previous lung alterations. *Am J Respir Crit Care Med*. 1995;151:1568–1575.
141. Kawano T, Mori S, Cybulsky M, et al. Effect of granulocyte depletion in a ventilated surfactant-depleted lung. *J Appl Physiol*. 1987;62:27–33.

CHAPTER
110

Extracorporeal Circulation for Respiratory or Cardiac Failure

ROBERT H. BARTLETT, JONATHAN W. HAFT, and WILLIAM R. LYNCH

INTRODUCTION

You probably turned to this chapter because you are caring for a patient with acute heart or lung failure, and the patient is failing despite your best treatment. The risk of death for your patient is over 80%, any way you measure it. The patient might be a woman with pneumonia, a child who cannot come off cardiopulmonary bypass, a man with acute respiratory distress syndrome (ARDS), or an emergency department (ED) patient undergoing cardiopulmonary resuscitation (CPR). Your only option to improve survival is extracorporeal life support (ECLS) with mechanical artificial organs.

ECLS is the use of an artificial heart (pump) and lung (membrane oxygenator) to replace organ function for days, weeks, or months to allow time for diagnosis, treatment, organ recovery, or organ replacement. The indications for ECLS are acute, severe heart or lung failure, not improving with conventional management. In a patient with an 80% to 100% risk of dying, the healthy survival results with ECLS ranges from 40% in cardiac arrest with CPR to 95% in neonatal meconium aspiration. ECLS is routine treatment in every major neonatal intensive care unit (ICU) and pediatric cardiac surgery program. Why is ECLS not used routinely in every adult ICU and emergency room? The reasons have been complexity, expense, the need for special equipment and experienced personnel, and education. Improvements in the technology for ECLS are changing this landscape.

BACKGROUND

The heart–lung machine was developed by John Gibbon, culminating in the first successful heart operation using a heart–lung machine in 1954 (1). Dr. Gibbon's motivation was to develop a technique to treat massive pulmonary embolism, but what resulted instead was the entire field of intracardiac surgery. The artificial heart was simply a blood pump, and the artificial lung was direct exposure of the flowing blood to gaseous oxygen. For cardiac surgery, all the venous return is diverted into the machine and pumped into the systemic circulation, leaving the heart empty long enough to complete the operative procedure. The opportunity to operate directly on the heart was miraculous, but the heart–lung machine itself caused damage to the blood, resulting in fatal complications when used for more than 4 hours. The major cause of blood damage was the direct exposure of blood to gas (2,3). Interposing a gas exchange membrane of plastic (4) or cellulose (5) between the flowing blood and the gas solved most of the blood-damage problems. Silicone membranes became available in the 1960's and artificial lungs with clinical application were designed and studied (4–10). By eliminating the gas interface it was possible to use a modified heart–lung machine for days at a time, and the physiology and pathophysiology of prolonged extracorporeal circulation were worked out in the laboratory (11–13).

The first successful use of prolonged life support with a heart–lung machine was conducted by J. Donald Hill and colleagues in 1971 (14). The patient was a young man suffering from ARDS, a newly recognized entity at that time; at the same time, the discipline we call critical care was evolving. After Hill's case, several other successful cases were reported in children and adults with severe pulmonary and cardiac failure (15), and extracorporeal support looked like it might be the answer to the epidemic of ARDS. A multicenter clinical trial of prolonged extracorporeal circulation for adults with ARDS was commissioned by the National Institutes of Health in 1975. This was the first prospective randomized trial of a life support technique in acute fatal illness in which the endpoint was death. There were many problems with the design and execution of that clinical trial, but from it we learned that the mortality for all patients with ARDS was 66%, and the mortality for severe ARDS was 90%, with or without ECLS. We learned that extracorporeal support attempted by inexperienced teams, in venoarterial (VA) mode for 1 week without protecting the lung from ventilator injury, did not improve the ultimate survival in severe ARDS. We learned (the hard way) the mistakes to avoid when conducting a prospective trial in acute fatal illness. And finally, we developed a name for the technology: extracorporeal membrane oxygenation (ECMO). The results of that study were published in 1979 (16). Laboratory and clinical research on ECLS in adults essentially stopped for a decade because of those results. However, the results in neonatal respiratory failure were very encouraging.

We reported the first successful case of ECLS for respiratory failure in a newborn infant in 1976 (17). Our laboratory had been studying membrane oxygenator development and prolonged extracorporeal circulation in animals for 10 years. We, and others, had used extracorporeal support for postoperative cardiopulmonary failure in children with the first successful pediatric cardiac case in 1972 (18), and we treated 40 newborn patients over the next 5 years with 50% survival (21). Neonatologists and surgeons from other institutions joined us to learn the technology; by 1986, 18 neonatal centers had successful ECMO teams (22).

Our group conducted the first prospective randomized trial of ECMO in neonatal respiratory failure, using an adaptive design to correct some of the mistakes we had made in the earlier adult trial (23). Another prospective randomized trial was carried out by O'Rourke et al. (24) at the Boston Children's Hospital. ECMO became standard treatment for severe neonatal respiratory failure by 1986, and standard treatment for severe cardiac failure in children by 1990.

Kolobow (25) showed that high ventilator inspiratory pressure (lung stretch) and high FiO_2 caused severe lung injury. Gattinoni et al. (26) and Kolobow (25) separated respiration from oxygenation by removing CO_2 by extracorporeal circulation (making ventilation unnecessary) and oxygenating by insufflation. Using extracorporeal CO_2 removal, they prevented stretch injury, and reported 56% survival in severe ARDS. These observations led to renewed interest in ECLS for adult respiratory failure. By the 1990s, several groups reported similar results (27–29). The value of avoiding lung stretch injury has been verified in many studies (30–32), decreasing the incidence of iatrogenic lung injury (and decreasing the need for ECLS). Even with these and other improvements, the mortality for ARDS in otherwise healthy patients was still 30% (32) and ECLS use related to ARDS remained limited to few expert centers.

ECLS technology continued to evolve with the most significant developments occurring in pumps, oxygenators, and cannulae. Centrifugal pump design addressed heat generation and blood stasis, resulting in minimal pump-related hemolysis. Oxygenator design shifted toward polymethylpentene (PMP) membranes which allowed for decreased blood path resistance, improved gas exchange characteristics, and prolonged reliable use. New, dual lumen cannulae came to the market place making practical single-site cannulation for adult venovenous (VV) bypass. These technological advancements also began to change the bedside model of care. Historically, the complexity of the technology obligated the bedside presence of a technology "specialist"; the modern ECLS technology is simpler to operate and more reliable. In essence, the technology has an improved "safety profile." This has made practical ECLS bedside care by the experienced critical care nurse with support from the technology "specialist" (33).

While interest in adult ECLS was reinvigorated by these technological advancements, real excitement was generated by two events in 2009: The publication of the CESAR Trial (34) results and the coincidental H1N1 Influenza A pandemic. The CESAR Trial (Conventional Ventilatory Support versus Extracorporeal Membrane Oxygenation for Severe Adult Respiratory Failure) was conducted in the UK from 2001 to 2006 and evaluated a strategy of adult ARDS management that compared transfer to a single center (Glenfield Hospital, Leicester) with ECMO capabilities to a control group of patients managed locally with conventional means. Primary endpoints were mortality and disability at 6 months; 90 patients were randomized to each group. The Glenfield group had 63% (57/90) alive without disability at 6 months compared with the control group that had 47% (41/87) without disability at 6 months. ECMO was used for 68 (75%) of the Glenfield patients, while 16 were managed with conventional means; 5 died prior to arrival. The control group was managed at multiple participating centers without an agreed-upon protocol for conventional care. Glenfield, as the expert center, had access to ECMO *but also had a fixed protocol of care.* Detractors argued that the intent-to-treat analysis and lack of protocols for critical care and ventilator management in the control centers weakened the conclusions (35).

Early in 2009, there was the emergence of a new H1N1 virus causing an influenza pandemic and the World Health Organization estimated that there were over 200 million cases (36). Early reports described a severe form of hypoxic–hypercarbic respiratory failure, predominately in young patients, also seen in the obese and pregnant women. Patients were refractory to conventional management with mechanical ventilation, so ECMO was offered as "rescue therapy." As the pandemic circled the globe, from the southern to the northern hemisphere, reports began to emerge. Australia and New Zealand reported 68 patients supported with ECMO with 75% survival (37). Italy reported the collective of 14 ECMO centers with 68% survival to discharge in H1N1 ARDS patients supported with ECMO (38). Similar reports came out of England, France, and the United States (39–42). CESAR and ECMO use in H1N1 adult ARDS, coupled with modern ECLS technology, changed the landscape of ECMO practice across the world.

The use of ECMO allows study of patients who would otherwise have died, unveiling many aspects of respiratory pathophysiology and treatment. As the technology developed, it was standardized, disseminated, studied, and improved in an organized fashion by the actual users of the technology. This group of investigators and clinicians organized as the Extracorporeal Life Support Organization (ELSO) in 1989. For the last 27 years, this group has developed guidelines, published the standard textbook in the field (43), and maintained a registry of ECLS cases.

ECLS TECHNIQUE AND PHYSIOLOGY

ECLS is simply the use of a modified heart–lung machine to provide gas exchange (and systemic perfusion if necessary) to prolong the life of a patient when native heart and lung function is not adequate to sustain life. The technique, indications, methods, and results are described in detail in the book *ECMO: Extracorporeal Cardiopulmonary Support in Critical Care* published by the ELSO (https://www.elso.org) (43). The heart–lung machine used for cardiac surgery is modified, both in devices and technology, to be used for days, weeks, or even months in the ICU. The technique is invasive and complex. A large (23 to 31 French catheter) is inserted into the inferior vena cava or right atrium; venous blood is drained, passed through an artificial lung, and pumped back into the patient, either into the aorta (VA bypass) or into the right atrium (VV bypass). VA bypass puts the artificial lung in parallel with the native lungs and substitutes for both heart and lung function. In VV bypass, the artificial lung is in series with the native lungs and the patient is reliant on his own hemodynamics for pulmonary and systemic perfusion. ECLS allows decreasing the ventilator to nondamaging "rest" settings (typically FiO_2 0.3, pressure 20/10, rate 4), decreasing vasoactive drugs, and optimizing other aspects of treatment.

Because the surfaces of the extracorporeal devices are plastic, it is necessary to anticoagulate the blood; this is most commonly done with a continuous infusion of heparin. Heparin is titrated to a low, but constant, level of anticoagulation and can be measured by whole blood activated clotting time (ACT) with the goal being 1.5 times normal. While this level of heparinization prevents thrombosis in the circuit, platelets still adhere to the plastic surfaces, becoming activated. The platelets then aggregate, break free into the circulation, and are removed by the reticuloendothelial system. Because heparinization and thrombocytopenia are necessary components of ECLS, the major risk of this mode of therapy is bleeding.

Significant bleeding is rarely a serious problem, but it does require a protocolized strategy of measuring coagulation profiles and platelet count, titrating heparin dose and platelet infusions accordingly. Properly managed, ECLS can be used for weeks without hemolysis, device failure, clotting, or bleeding. The technology must be learned and practiced by the ICU team and also endorsed by the entire hospital. Management of the patient during ECLS requires attending to the technology while addressing the critical care issues of the patient.

In *respiratory failure*, VV access is preferred. Gas exchange across the native lungs is usually minimal during the first several days of ECLS; therefore, the patient is totally dependent on the technology. As lung function returns, systemic blood oxygenation and CO_2 clearance improve, and the extracorporeal blood flow rate is gradually decreased, allowing the native lungs to assume a larger percentage of gas exchange. It is practical and safe to allow these patients to be awake and active, with extubation and ambulation as possibilities. When native lung function is sufficient, ECLS is weaned off and the patient is supported with non-damaging ventilator settings; cannulae are removed and recovery continues. Patients successfully weaned off ECLS have a 90% likelihood of complete recovery.

In *cardiac failure*, VA access is required. Arterial access is typically via the femoral artery, with distal limb perfusion assured by placing a small reperfusion line in the distal femoral artery or in the posterior tibial artery (46). Inotropes and pressors are weaned off, and systemic perfusion is maintained by extracorporeal flow. Lung function usually returns to normal in a day or two, and the patient can be awakened and extubated. When the patient is stable, and the function of other organs can be determined, a decision can be made about bridging to recovery or to ventricular assist device (VAD) and transplantation. When ECLS is used for cardiac support, the pulmonary and left ventricular blood flow is minimal; this can result in two problems. First, if the heart stops altogether, the left atrium and ventricle will gradually distend with bronchial venous blood, leading to high left atrial pressure and pulmonary edema. This is recognized by the lack of systemic arterial pulsatility. If this is the case, the left side of the heart must be decompressed, either by direct catheterization of the left atrium or by creation of an atrial septal defect. The second problem with VA bypass in the totally failing heart is thrombosis in the left atrium or left ventricle; this will occur even in the presence of systemic heparinization. Thrombosis is diagnosed by echocardiography; if a patient has left atrial or left ventricular thrombus, it is important to avoid spontaneous left ventricular function and the clot can be extracted at the time of VAD placement.

CLINICAL RESULTS

The most recent data from the ELSO registry are shown in Table 110.1. Participation in the ELSO is voluntary, but almost all cases treated with ECLS in established centers are included in the registry. There are currently over 65,000 patients listed in this Registry and the volume has doubled in the last decade. ECLS use in neonates has remained stable while the significant growth noted has been realized in pediatric and adult populations. Much data is collected, but the most important statistic is hospital discharge survival. ECLS is a life-support technique, applied only to patients with a high risk (80% to 100%) of dying who are not expected to survive with conventional treatment. The mortality risk is measured differently in different age groups.

TABLE 110.1 Overall Patient Outcomes with ECLS for Cardiac and Respiratory Failure[a]

	Total	Survival with ECLS	Survival to Discharge
Neonatal			
Respiratory	27,728	23,358 (84%)	20,592 (74%)
Cardiac	5,810	3,600 (62%)	2,389 (41%)
ECPR	1,112	712 (64%)	449 (40%)
Pediatric			
Respiratory	6,569	4,327 (66%)	3,760 (57%)
Cardiac	7,314	4,825 (66%)	3,679 (50%)
ECPR	2,370	1,313 (55%)	976 (41%)
Adult			
Respiratory	7,008	4,587 (65%)	4,026 (57%)
Cardiac	5,603	3,129 (56%)	2,294 (41%)
ECPR	1,657	639 (39%)	471 (28%)
Total	65,171	46,490 (71%)	38,636 (59%)

[a]Extracorporeal Life Support Organization registry data, January 2015. The data for 2014 are incomplete.

ECLS, extracorporeal life support; ECPR, extracorporeal cardiopulmonary resuscitation.

Neonatal Respiratory Failure

The largest group of patients treated with ECLS is newborn infants with respiratory failure, of which there are only a few causes. ECLS survival for meconium aspiration, infant respiratory distress syndrome (IRDS), primary pulmonary hypertension of the newborn (PPHN), and neonatal sepsis is 80% to 95%, but only 60% for congenital diaphragmatic hernia. Excluding diaphragmatic hernias, these excellent results exist because respiratory failure in neonates does not destroy lung tissue. The pathophysiology is pulmonary hypertension with right-to-left shunting through the ductus arteriosus (persistent fetal circulation). During ECLS, the pulmonary vasculature relaxes, the ductus closes, and lung recovery occurs promptly. The problem in congenital diaphragmatic hernia is that the hernia compresses the lungs and causes bilateral lung hypoplasia *in utero* in addition to pulmonary vasospasm. The hypoplastic lungs may be too small to support the infant to recovery.

About 10% of surviving patients have some neurologic disability, with the most common being some degree of hearing loss. This is lower than the incidence of complications in critically ill infants not treated with ECLS, indicating that these are the complications of profound illness in the newborn. While the use of ECLS in neonatal respiratory failure has decreased since the introduction of nitric oxide, there are still approximately 1,000 new cases per year entered into the ELSO registry.

Pediatric Respiratory Failure

Severe respiratory failure in older children is relatively rare, compared to the incidence in newborn infants and adults, with the most common causes being viral or bacterial pneumonia.

Survival rate approximates 66%, varying based on the primary condition. The effectiveness of ECLS in pediatric respiratory failure was demonstrated in a contemporary matched-pairs study by Green et al. (47). Most children with respiratory failure can be managed successfully with VV access. The most common cause of death is progressive lung destruction from the primary infection, or brain damage from the period of hypoxia and ischemia that preceded ECLS. These children are all essentially normal in follow-up. Once the lung recovers, pulmonary function and exercise tolerance return to normal.

Adult Respiratory Failure

The cause of ARDS is a primary lung event in about half the cases (viral or bacterial pneumonia, aspiration, pulmonary vasculitis, etc.), and secondary to extrapulmonary causes in the others (shock, trauma, pancreatitis, sepsis). The overall mortality for ARDS approximates 30%, even with excellent management. ECLS is indicated for those patients who have a high mortality risk within the first week after intubation. These patients are relatively easy to identify; they have an alveolar–arterial (A-a) gradient for oxygen greater than 600 on day 2, 3, or 4 following initial intubation. The mortality risk for those patients is approximately 80%, and the recovery rate with ECLS in these same patients approximates 70% (48–51). Patients on the ventilator more than 5 days pre-ECLS have a lesser chance of recovery; hence the overall survival rate for ECLS treatment of ARDS is approximately 57%. The University of Michigan has reported the largest experience with ECLS for ARDS; in that series, the overall survival rate was 52% (48). More recently, they reported their experience with 2,000 ECLS patients, of which 353 were adult respiratory patients, with survival to discharge of 50% (52). These series are large enough to characterize the patient population and identify the likelihood of recovery based on age and days on mechanical ventilation.

Adult respiratory ECLS requires VV bypass, with high blood flow adequate to sustain oxygenation and CO_2 removal. Lung rest, diuresis, and prone positioning have led to the 50% to 60% survival, discussed above. The dual lumen cannulae make single-site cannulation possible for VV bypass. The cannulae are designed to be placed in the right internal jugular vein, using fluoroscopy to confirm safe placement. It is practical to minimize sedation, extubate and help patients out of bed so they can ambulate and participate in physical therapy (53,54). Severe ARDS treated without ECLS requires uncomfortable modes of ventilation. With this discomfort comes the dependency on heavy sedation or even paralytics. The critical care literature has well-described survival and quality-of-life risks related to sedation (55–57) and these risks can be minimized with ECLS.

Cardiac Failure in Children

VA ECLS is currently the only mechanical support system available for children in the United States. Most of the children treated with ECLS have cardiac failure following a cardiac operative intervention, usually for congenital heart disease. These patients cannot be weaned from cardiopulmonary bypass in the operating room, or are weaned but remain in profound cardiac failure despite full inotropic support following surgical intervention. Patients who cannot be weaned from cardiopulmonary bypass are attached to ECLS using the same cannulae used for cardiopulmonary bypass, typically in the right atrium and aorta. If the patient has been weaned off bypass and the chest is closed, vascular access is gained by cannulation of the right internal jugular vein and right common carotid artery, as in newborn respiratory failure. This same vascular access is used for children with myocarditis or cardiomyopathy. Because ECLS is commonly used directly after cardiopulmonary bypass, bleeding is a more common occurrence in cardiac patients than in respiratory patients. This is best managed by maintaining the chest open with a sterile plastic sheet over the open wound and blood drainage tubes placed in the chest. In this way, the amount of bleeding can be observed directly, and it is easy to re-explore the chest, which is often required every 8 to 12 hours for the first day on ECLS. Bleeding is managed by maintaining the heparinization at very low levels (1.25 times the upper limit of normal ACT), maintaining platelet count over 100,000 cells/μL, and adding epsilon-aminocaproic acid (Amicar) to minimize fibrinolysis. In larger patients (adolescents/adults), if high ECLS flows (more than 3 L/min) can be maintained through a modern polymethylpentene membrane oxygenator, it can be practical to run without anticoagulation for days. While this strategy can be used to control patient bleeding, it places the extracorporeal circuit at risk for thrombus formation and failure. In these cases, it is important to keep a primed extracorporeal circuit available so that the circuit can be changed if clotting occurs.

Generalized fluid overload is a common problem associated with cardiac failure in children. Diuresis is begun immediately with ECLS; if satisfactory negative fluid balance cannot be achieved with continuous infusion of diuretics, continuous hemofiltration may be instituted. Survival with ECLS in pediatric cardiac failure is 40% to 50% (58).

Cardiac Failure in Adults

The experience with ECLS for cardiac failure in adults is shown in Table 110.1. The most common indication for ECLS for cardiac support in adults is acute myocardial failure following myocardial infarction or heart failure following cardiac operation. Vascular access is usually achieved by cannulation of the right atrium via the right internal jugular or femoral vein, with arterial return retrograde via the femoral artery. Intra-aortic balloon pumping is possible in adults and will support approximately 40% of the cardiac output. Most patients treated with ECLS have failed balloon pumping, as well as full inotropic support. If a balloon pump is in place through one of the femoral arteries, it is best left in place because of the risk of bleeding once the device has been removed. The opposite femoral artery is used for arterial access; distal limb perfusion is assured as previously described.

Adult patients in acute cardiac failure are candidates for left ventricular assist device (LVAD) placement as a bridge to recovery or a bridge to transplantation. However, in the acute failure situation it is best to institute ECLS first, stabilize the circulation and gas exchange, and determine if other organs are functioning, most importantly the brain. If severe brain injury has occurred, ECLS is discontinued, avoiding the futile and expensive LVAD placement. The survival for ECLS in adult cardiac failure is 40% to 50% (59–62).

EXTRACORPOREAL LIFE SUPPORT FOR CARDIOPULMONARY RESUSCITATION

ECLS can be used in association with resuscitation to support cardiac and pulmonary function in cardiac arrest or profound shock. In this application, the ECLS circuit must be primed and available within minutes. Therefore, ECLS for cardiopulmonary resuscitation (ECPR) cases are done primarily in established ECLS centers, which have both the equipment and the team to institute ECLS on a moment's notice. The limiting factor in establishing ECLS in these cases is vascular access. It is difficult to get rapid arterial and venous access in a patient in full cardiac arrest. Most successful ECPR cases have been in patients who arrested, then briefly resuscitated, with simple vascular access gained following initial resuscitation. Then, ECLS cannulae can be placed over a wire through smaller catheters if, and when, the patient arrests again or proceeds to cardiogenic shock or intractable dysrhythmias. In our institution, we consider ECPR for patients who have been in cardiac arrest for less than 5 minutes. A few patients who have been arrested with full and well-documented resuscitation for over an hour have been treated successfully, but if the arrest has been prolonged, and if profound metabolic acidosis exists, then establishing ECLS is often futile. The overall results for successful, healthy survival after ECPR is approximately 40%, much better than the 5% successful results of external message only (63–67).

OTHER APPLICATIONS OF ECLS

The ability to totally control perfusion and gas exchange with an extracorporeal system offers unique opportunities in other aspects of acute medical care. Profound hypothermia can be treated by extracorporeal support; this is particularly important because patients who are hypothermic may develop ventricular fibrillation during external warming. Hypothermia associated with exsanguinating hemorrhage in the operating room can be treated successfully with ECLS. Perfusion is maintained during the period of bleeding, and hypothermia can be maintained to protect organ function. After bleeding is controlled, blood is returned to the patient associated with warming to avoid the coagulopathy caused by low temperature. Hyperthermic perfusion can be established, either for total body warming or for regional warming, as an adjunct to cancer chemotherapy.

ECLS can be used to specifically resolve hypercarbia, requiring flows equivalent to about 10% to 20% of the cardiac output. This is being used to support hypercarbic COPD patients and patients with status asthmaticus (68–70).

Septic shock was once considered a contraindication to ECLS. However, sepsis often clears during ECLS, and this has become a standard indication in our institution. It is common for patients in septic shock to regain normal vascular tone and to come off all vasopressors within a day or two of instituting ECLS (71). This is partly related to establishing healthy perfusion and gas exchange, and partly related to adsorption of inflammatory mediators by the plastic in the circuit.

ECLS has also been used to support perfusion in potential organ donors, particularly in situations in which death prior to organ donation occurs because of cardiac arrest following elective withdrawal of ventilator support (72).

SUMMARY

A decade ago, you might have turned to this chapter as a last resort for a patient dying in your ICU. You would have likely been an intensivist doing your best with unconventional ventilation modes, an oscillator or NO; ECLS was not available in your hospital. Today, you may be a pulmonologist who has been learning about ECMO at your national meetings. Perhaps you are an ED physician just returning from an ELSO Course on Adult ECMO and you are interested to learn more. Maybe you are a cardiothoracic surgeon who has been asked to help start an ECMO program by your ICU or ED. Maybe you are a hospital administrator charged with understanding the finances related to ECLS. ECLS has evolved in the past 10 years because of modern affordable technology and evidence that ECLS is cost effective and life sustaining. Patients are walking the critical care unit while on ECLS. Unheard of when the previous edition was written.

ECLS sustains cardiac and pulmonary function by mechanical means for patients with profound cardiac or respiratory failure. The technology includes extracorporeal vascular access, perfusion devices, and management of anticoagulation. ECLS does not treat cardiac or pulmonary failure, but offers hours or days of time to establish a diagnosis and allow time for organ recovery or replacement. Overall success is measured as survival because ECLS is used only in patients at a high risk of dying from acute heart or lung failure. Healthy survival ranges from 95% in some cases of newborn respiratory failure to 40% when ECLS is used as adjunct to cardiac resuscitation.

Key Points

- ECMO (ECLS) provides cardiopulmonary support in severe heart or lung failure.
- For support of circulation, ECLS is used in the VA mode. For respiratory failure, ECLS is used in the VV mode.
- The extracorporeal circuit includes a blood pump, membrane oxygenator, and heat exchanger.
- During ECLS, blood is anticoagulated with continuous infusion of heparin or a direct thrombin inhibitor.
- The major risk is clotting in the circuit or bleeding in the patient.
- The success (healthy hospital discharge) rate is 50% for cardiac support, 65% for respiratory support.

References

1. Gibbon JH. Application of a mechanical heart and lung apparatus to cardiac surgery. *Minn Med*. 1954;37:171.
2. Lee WH Jr, Krumhar D, Fonkalsrud EW, et al. Denaturation of plasma proteins as a cause of morbidity and death after intracardiac operations. *Surgery*. 1961;50:29–39.
3. Dobell ARC, Mitri M, Galva R, et al. Biological evaluation of blood after prolonged recirculation through film and membrane oxygenators. *Ann Surg*. 1965; 161:617–622.

4. Clowes GH Jr, Hopkins AL, Neville WE. An artificial lung dependent upon diffusion of oxygen and carbon dioxide through plastic membranes. *J Thorac Surg*. 1956;32:630–637.
5. Kolff WJ, Effler DB. Disposable membrane oxygenator (heart lung machine) and its use in experimental and clinical surgery while the heart is arrested with potassium citrate according to the Melrose technique. *Trans Am Soc Artif Intern Organs*. 1956;2:13–21.
6. Pierce EC II. Modification of the Clowes membrane lung. *J Thorac Cardiovasc Surg*. 1960;39:438.
7. Kolobow T, Bowman RL. Construction and evaluation of an alveolar membrane artificial heart-lung. *Trans Am Soc Artif Intern Organs*. 1963;9:238.
8. Bramson ML, Osborn JJ, Main FB, et al. A new disposable membrane oxygenator with integral heat exchanger. *J Thorac Cardiovasc Surg*. 1965; 50:391.
9. Landé AJ, Dos SJ, Carlson RG, et al. A new membrane oxygenator-dialyzer. *Surg Clin North Am*. 1967;47:1461.
10. Bartlett RH, Isherwood J, Moss RA, et al. A toroidal flow membrane oxygenator: four day partial bypass in dogs. *Surg Forum*. 1969;20:152–153.
11. Kolobow T, Zapol W, Pierce J. High survival and minimal blood damage in lambs exposed to long term (1 week) veno-venous pumping with a polyurethane chamber roller pump with and without a membrane blood oxygenator. *Trans Am Soc Artif Intern Organs*. 1969;15:172–177.
12. Bartlett RH, Fong SW, Burns NE, et al. Prolonged partial venoarterial bypass: physiologic, biochemical and hematologic responses. *Ann Surg*. 1974;180:850–856.
13. Fong SW, Burns NE, Williams G, et al. Changes in coagulation and platelet function during prolonged extracorporeal circulation (ECC) in sheep and man. *Trans Am Soc Artif Intern Organs*. 1974;20:239–246.
14. Hill JD, O'Brien TG, Murray JJ, et al. Extracorporeal oxygenation for acute post-traumatic respiratory failure (shock-lung syndrome): use of the Bramson membrane lung. *N Engl J Med*. 1972;286:629–634.
15. Bartlett RH. Extracorporeal life support for cardiopulmonary failure. *Curr Probl Surg*. 1990;27(10):621–705.
16. Zapol WM, Snider MT, Hill JD, et al. Extracorporeal membrane oxygenation in severe acute respiratory failure: a randomized prospective study. *JAMA*. 1979;242:2193–2196.
17. Bartlett RH, Gazzaniga AB, Jefferies R, et al. Extracorporeal membrane oxygenation (ECMO) cardiopulmonary support in infancy. *Trans Am Soc Artif Intern Organs*. 1976;22:80–88.
18. Bartlett RH, Gazzaniga AB, Fong SW, et al. Prolonged extracorporeal cardiopulmonary support in man. *J Thorac Cardiovasc Surg*. 1974;68:918–932.
19. White JJ, Andrews HG, Risemberg H, et al. Prolonged respiratory support in newborn infants with a membrane oxygenator. *Surgery*. 1971;70:288–296.
20. Dorson WJ, Baker E, Cohen ML, et al. A perfusion system for infants. *Trans Am Soc Artif Intern Organs*. 1969;15:155.
21. Bartlett RH, Andrews AF, Toomasian JM, et al. Extracorporeal membrane oxygenation (ECMO) for newborn respiratory failure: 45 cases. *Surgery*. 1982;92:425–433.
22. Toomasian JM, Snedecor SM, Cornell R, et al. National experience with extracorporeal membrane oxygenation (ECMO) for newborn respiratory failure: data from 715 cases. *Trans Am Soc Artif Intern Organs*. 1988;34: 140–147.
23. Bartlett RH, Roloff DW, Cornell RG, et al. Extracorporeal circulation in neonatal respiratory failure: a prospective randomized study. *Pediatrics*. 1985; 4:479–487.
24. O'Rourke PP, Crone R, Vacanti J, et al. Extracorporeal membrane oxygenation and conventional medical therapy in neonates with persistent pulmonary hypertension of the newborn: a prospective randomized study. *Pediatrics*. 1989;84:957–963.
25. Kolobow T. On how to injure healthy lungs (and prevent sick lungs from recovering). *Trans Am Soc Artif Intern Organs*. 1988;34:31–34.
26. Gattinoni L, Pesenti A, Mascheroni D, et al. Low frequency positive pressure ventilation with extracorporeal CO_2 removal in severe acute respiratory failure. *JAMA*. 1986;256:881–886.
27. Lewandowski K, Rossaint R, Pappert D, et al. High survival rate in 122 ARDS patients managed according to a clinical algorithm including extracorporeal membrane oxygenation. *Intensive Care Med*. 1997;23:819–835.
28. Ullrich R, Larber C, Roder G, et al. Controlled airway pressure therapy, nitric oxide inhalation, prime position, and ECMO as components of an integrated approach to ARDS. *Anesthesiology*. 1999;91:1577–1586.
29. Kolla S, Awad SA, Rich PB, et al. Extracorporeal life support for 100 adult patients with severe respiratory failure. *Ann Surg*. 1997;226:544–566.
30. Hickling K, Walsh J, Henderson S, et al. Low mortality in adult respiratory distress syndrome using low-volume, pressure-limited ventilation with permissive hypercapnia: a prospective study. *Crit Care Med*. 1994;22(10): 1568.
31. Amato MB, Barbas CSV, Mederos DM, et al. Effect of a protective ventilator strategy on mortality in the acute respiratory distress syndrome. *N Engl J Med*. 1998;338(6):347–354.
32. The Acute Respiratory Distress Syndrome network. Ventilation with lower tidal volumes as compared with traditional volumes for ARDS. *N Engl J Med*. 2000;342:1301–1308.
33. Freeman R, Nault C, Mowry J, Baldridge P. Expanded resources through utilization of a primary care giver extracorporeal membrane oxygenation model. *Crit Care Nurse Q*. 2012;35:39–49.
34. Peek GJ, Mugford M, Tiruvoipati R, et al. Efficacy and economic assessment of conventional ventilator support versus extracorporeal membrane oxygenation for severe adult respiratory failure (CESAR): a multicenter randomized controlled trial. *Lancet*. 2009;374:1351-63.35.
35. Zwischenberger JB, Lynch JE. Will CESAR answer the adult ECMO debate? *Lancet*. 2009;374:1307–1308.
36. Pandemic influenza A(H1N1) 2009: report of the Review Committee on the Functioning of the International Health Regulations (2005) in relation to pandemic (H1N1) 2009. 64thWorld Health Assembly, May 5, 2011, pp 49–65.
37. The Australia and New Zealand Extracorporeal Membrane Oxygenation (ANZ ECMO) Influenza Investigators. Extracorporeal membrane oxygenation for 2009 influenza A(H1N1) acute respiratory distress syndrome. *JAMA*. 2009;302:1888–1895.
38. Patroniti N, Zangrillo A, Pappalardo F, et al. The Italian ECMO network experience during the 2009 influenza A(H1N1) pandemic: preparation for severe respiratory emergency outbreaks. *Intensive Care Med*. 2011;37:1447–1457.
39. Noah MA, Peek GJ, Finney SJ, et al. Referral to an extracorporeal membrane oxygenation center and mortality among patients with severe 2009 influenza A(H1N1). *JAMA*. 2011;306:1659–1668.
40. Pham T, Combes A, Roze H, Richard JC. Extra-corporal membrane oxygenation (ECMO) for influenza A(H1N1) induced acute respiratory distress: preliminary results of a pairwise-matched propensity based analysis. *Am J Respir Crit Care Med*. 2012;185:A6013.
41. Pham T, Combes A, Roze H, Richard JC. Extra-corporal membrane oxygenation (ECMO) for influenza A(H1N1) induced acute respiratory distress syndrome (ARDS): analysis of the factors associated with death in 122 French patients. *Am J Respir Crit Care Med*. 2012;185:A6019.
42. Luyt CE, Combes A, Becquemin MH, et al. Long-term outcomes of pandemic 2009 influenza A (H1N1)-associated severe acute respiratory distress syndrome. *Chest*. 2012;142(3):583–592.
43. Annich GM, Lynch WR, MacLaren G, et al. *ECMO in Extracorporeal Cardiopulmonary Support in Critical Care*. 4th ed. Ann Arbor, MI: ELSO.
44. Young G. New anticoagulants in children. *Hematology*. 2008:245-250.
45. Bates SM, Weitz JI. The mechanism of action of thrombin inhibitors. *J Invasive Cardiol*. 2000;12:1–12.
46. Spurlock D, Toomasian JM, Romano MA, et al. A simple technique to prevent limb ischemia during veno-arterial ECMO using the femoral artery: the posterior tibial approach. *Perfusion*. 2011;27:141–145.
47. Green TP, Timmons OD, Fackler JC, et al. The impact of extracorporeal membrane oxygenation on survival in pediatric patients with acute respiratory failure: Pediatric Critical Care Study. *Crit Care Med*. 1996;24:323–329.
48. Hemmila MR, Rowe SA, Boules TN, et al. Extracorporeal life support for severe acute respiratory syndrome in adults. *Ann Surg*. 2004;240(4):595–605.
49. Peek GJ, Moore HM, Sosnowski AW, et al. Extracorporeal membrane oxygenation for adult respiratory failure. *Chest*. 1997;112:759–764.
50. Ullrich R, Lorber C, Roder G, et al. Controlled airway pressure therapy, nitric oxide inhalation, prone position, and extracorporeal membrane oxygenation (ECMO) as components of an integrated approach to ARDS. *Anesthesiology*. 1999;91:1577–1586.
51. Linden V, Palmer K, Reinhard J, et al. High survival in adult patients with acute respiratory distress syndrome treated by extracorporeal membrane oxygenation, minimal sedation, and pressure supported ventilation. *Intensive Care Med*. 2000;26:1630–1637.
52. Gray BW, Haft JW, Hirsch JC, Annich GM, Hirschl RB, Bartlett RH. Extracoporeal life support: experience with 2,000 patients. *ASAIO J*. 2015;61:2–7.
53. Schweickert WD, Pohlman MC, Pohlman AS, et al. Early physical and occupational therapy in mechanically ventilated, critically ill patients: a randomized controlled trial. *Lancet*. 2009;373:1874–1882.
54. Needham DM, Korupolu R, Zanni JM, et al. Early physical medicine and rehabilitation for patients with acute respiratory failure: a quality improvement project. *Arch Phys Med Rehabil*. 2010;91:536–542.
55. Kress JP, Vinayak AG, Levitt J, et al. Daily sedative interruption in mechanically ventilated patients at risk for coronary artery disease. *Crit Care Med*. 2007;35:365–371.
56. Kress JP, Gehlbach B, Lacy M, et al. The long-term psychological effects of daily sedative interruption on critically ill patients. *Am J Respir Crit Care Med*. 2003;168:1457–1461.

57. Girard TD, Kress JP, Fuchs BD, et al. Efficacy and safety of a paired sedation and ventilator weaning protocol for mechanically ventilated patients in intensive care (Awakening and Breathing Controlled trial): a randomized controlled trial. *Lancet*. 2008;371:126–134.
58. Thourani VH, Kirshbom PM, Kanter KR, et al. Venoarterial ECMO in pediatric cardiac support. *Ann Thorac Surg*. 2006;82:138–194.
59. Pagani FD, Aaronson KD, Dyke DB, et al. Assessment of an extracorporeal life support LVAD bridge to heart transplant strategy. *Ann Thorac Surg*. 2000; 70(6):1977–1984.
60. Muehreke DD, McCarthy PM, Stewart RW, et al. Extracorporeal membrane oxygenation for postcardiotomy cardiogenic shock. *Ann Thorac Surg*. 1996; 61:684–691.
61. Magovern GJ, Simpson KA. Extracorporeal membrane oxygenation for adult cardiac support: the Allegheny experience. *Ann Thorac Surg*. 1999;68: 655–661.
62. Diddle JW, Almodovar MC, Rajagopal ST, et al. Extracoporeal membrane oxygenation for the support of adults with myocarditis. *Crit Care Med*. 2015;43:1016–1025.
63. Younger JG, Schreiner RJ, Swaniker F, et al. Extracorporeal resuscitation of cardiac arrest. *Acad Emerg Med*. 1999;6(7):700–707.
64. Massetti M, Tasle M, Le Page O, et al. Back from irreversibility: extracorporeal life support for prolonged cardiac arrest. *Ann Thorac Surg*. 2005;79: 178–183.
65. de Mos N, van Listenburg RR, McCrindle B, et al. Pediatric intensive care unit cardiac arrest: incidence, survival and predictive factors. *Crit Care Med*. 2006;34:1209–1215.
66. Morris MC, Wernovsky G, Nadkarni VM. Survival outcomes after extracorporeal cardiopulmonary resuscitation instituted during active chest compressions following refractory in-hospital pediatric cardiac arrest. *Pediatr Crit Care Med*. 2004;5:440–446.
67. Barrett CS, Bratton SL, Salvin JW, et al. Neurological injury after extracorporeal memebrane oxygenation use to aid pediatric cardiopulmonary resuscitation. *Pediatric Crit Care Med*. 2009;10:445-51.
68. Hermann A, Staudinger T, Bojic A, et al. First experience with a new miniaturized pump-driven venovenous extracorporeal CO_2 removal system (iLA Activve): a retrospective data analysis. *ASAIO J*. 2014;60:342–347.
69. Agerstrand CL, Bacchetta MD, Brodie D. ECMO for adult respiratory failure: current use and evolving applications. *ASAIO J*. 2014;60:255–262.
70. Shapiro MB, Kleaveland AC, Bartlett RH. Extracoporeal life support for status asthmaticus. *Chest*. 1993;103:1651–1654.
71. MacLaren G, Butt W, Best D, et al. Extracorporeal membrane oxygenation for refractory septic shock in children: one institution's experience. *Pediatr Crit Care Med*. 2007;8(5):447–451.
72. Magliocca JF, Magee JC, Rowe SA, et al. Extracorporeal support for organ donation after cardiac death safely expands the donor pool. *J Trauma*. 2005;58(6):1095–1101.

CHAPTER

111

Drowning

ELIZABETH MAHANNA GABRIELLI, ANDREA GABRIELLI, PEGGY WHITE, A. JOSEPH LAYON, and JEROME H. MODELL

DEFINITIONS AND DESCRIPTIONS

Several definitions and multiple terminologies have appeared during the past half-century regarding the description of victims who suffer a fatal or near-fatal event from being submerged in water and other liquids. Some of the descriptors have had modifications placed on them and, furthermore, their meaning was somewhat lost when translated into some languages other than English. Because drowning is a global problem, in association with the World Congress on Drowning in Amsterdam, The Netherlands, on June 26 to 28, 2002, a group of experts was convened from multiple countries to develop a definition of "drowning" that would be applicable in multiple languages worldwide (1). Although unanimity may not have been present on every term discussed, there clearly was a consensus to simplify the terminology for international application. What follows is the consensus of that group with comment and, in some cases, slight modification representing the bias of the authors of this chapter.

THE DROWNING PROCESS

Drowning is the process resulting from primary respiratory impairment from submersion or immersion in a liquid medium. Implicit in this definition is that a liquid-to-air interface must be present at the entrance to the victim's airway, thus precluding the possibility of the victim to breathe air. Although it is possible to suffer a drowning episode in multiple types of liquid, this chapter will be confined to the most common use of the terminology, namely drowning in water.

The drowning process is a continuum that begins when the victim's airway is initially below the surface of the water. At this time, the victim first will voluntarily hold his or her breath. Some victims will swallow significant quantities of water during this time. This period of voluntary breath-holding, which has been found in human volunteers to last an average of 87 seconds at rest and shorter with exercise (2), is followed by an involuntary period of laryngospasm secondary to water in the oropharynx or at the level of the larynx acting as a foreign body (3). During this period of breath-holding and laryngospasm, the patient cannot breathe; therefore, oxygen is depleted and carbon dioxide is not eliminated. This results in the patient becoming hypercarbic, hypoxic, and acidotic (4).

As the levels of carbon dioxide increase in the blood and levels of oxygen decrease, respiratory efforts become very active but no exchange of air occurs because of the obstruction at the larynx. Victims who subsequently recover and recall this period frequently describe it as being quite terrifying and painful as they struggle, creating intense negative intrapleural pressure breathing against a closed glottis (5). As the patient's arterial oxygen tension drops further, laryngospasm abates, and the patient then actively breathes water. Further evidence of the magnitude of negative pressure created during laryngospasm is the fact that the lungs of drowning victims frequently demonstrate significant hyperinflation at autopsy (6).

The amount of liquid a drowning victim inhales varies considerably (4). Studies comparing the biochemical changes occurring in humans after a drowning episode with those in experimental animals suggest that, while the volume of liquid actually inhaled varies, only 15% of persons who die in the water aspirate in excess of 22 mL/kg of water (7), and the percentage is considerably less in those who survive (4). Changes occur in the lung, body fluids, and electrolyte concentrations, which are dependent on both the composition and volume of the liquid aspirated (8–10).

RESUSCITATION

A victim can be rescued at any time during the drowning process and given the appropriate resuscitation measures, in which case the process is interrupted. The victim may recover with the initial resuscitation efforts or after subsequent therapy aimed at eliminating hypoxia, hypercarbia, and acidosis and restoring normal organ function. If the patient is not removed from the water, then circulatory arrest will occur, and, in the absence of effective resuscitative efforts, multiple organ dysfunction and death will result, primarily from tissue hypoxia.

Although the tolerance to hypoxia of various tissues is different, it should be noted that the brain is the organ most at risk for permanent detrimental changes from relative brief periods of hypoxia. Frequently, the question is asked, "How long can a person be submerged and still be rescued and resuscitated back to a normal life?" While, obviously, there are no controlled human studies on this subject, the limiting time factor is likely the duration that cerebral hypoxia can be tolerated before irreversible changes occur. Irreversible damage to brain tissue is reported to begin approximately 3 minutes after the PaO_2 falls below 30 mmHg under normothermic conditions in otherwise normal people (11). Such data suggest that if the victim is rescued and effective resuscitation efforts are applied within 3 minutes of the cessation of respiration (i.e., submersion in water), the vast majority of such victims should be able to be resuscitated and suffer no permanent brain damage. Further, because the period of voluntary breath-holding and laryngospasm is thought to last for approximately 1½ to 2 minutes (2,12), persons who are retrieved within that time frame will likely not suffer lung damage secondary to the aspiration of liquid. Once the 3-minute time frame has been exceeded, although some normal survivors are reported, it becomes less likely that normal survival will result from resuscitation efforts. This time frame may be prolonged if hypothermia occurs rapidly because it decreases the cerebral requirement for oxygen (13,14).

Trained divers have been shown to be able to voluntarily hold their breath for much longer periods of time, approaching 4 to 5 minutes without complication (15). Persons who become hypothermic due to immersion or submersion in extremely cold water will rapidly develop hypothermia, which protects the brain by decreasing its oxygen requirement, and prolongs survival (13,16). In the latter case, seemingly miraculous recoveries of patients who have been submerged for over 20 minutes have been reported (17). It should be noted, however, that hypothermia is a two-edged sword; although it can protect the brain from oxygen deprivation, it also can cause death in the water secondary to its effect on the conduction system of the heart, resulting in circulatory arrest either by asystole or ventricular fibrillation (18,19).

The drowning process can be altered by the initiating event, such as if the victim suffers trauma, develops syncope, or unconsciousness, has a circulatory arrest either by asystole or ventricular fibrillation as the precipitating event, hyperventilates prior to breath-holding under water, or has a convulsive disorder that leads him or her to become incapacitated, thereby becoming submerged, or if the victim's judgment and/or motor function is impaired by significant parenteral levels of depressant drugs, including alcohol. For example, in the victim who suffers a concussion from a blow to the head, subsequent recollection of the events is unlikely. If trauma results in a cervical fracture, disastrous damage to the spinal cord may occur acutely and, thus, motor function may be lost below that level. If the victim has a circulatory arrest either by asystole or ventricular fibrillation as a precipitating event, respiration will cease, and it is highly unlikely that significant amounts of water will be breathed into the lung given that active respiration is necessary for this to occur. If the victim hyperventilates prior to breath-holding under water, it has been shown that the breath-holding breaking point can be extended until the level of hypoxia is so severe that consciousness is lost, and thus the victim actively breathes in water (2,12). The effect of drug usage is variable, depending on the level of depression and the patient's response. There is considerable variation in tolerance to depressant drugs and alcohol and their effects on performance and orientation. To better understand what to expect in each victim, the initiating event should be reported in every case if it is known.

Drowning episodes can lead to many possible outcomes. On the most basic level there are two outcomes: death or survival. Of the survivors there are, however, many outcomes: no residual damage, to minor neurologic difficulty to severe disability, bedridden and requiring continual nursing care.

CLASSIFICATIONS

Numerous terms have been used to describe the episode of submersion and its sequelae. Many of these have fallen out of favor due to the confusion in meaning (Table 111.1). The terms *drowning* and *near-drowning* have been used for decades in an attempt to separate these outcomes (20). At the World Congress on Drowning, however, it became apparent that their meaning was not felt to be clear when translated into some languages (1). Furthermore, a victim could have no signs of spontaneous physiologic function and, therefore, be "drowned"; however, once resuscitative efforts were applied, they would respond positively and survive to varying degrees and, thus, the term applied to them would have to be changed to "near-drowned" (21). In addition, there is another group who do not die acutely, but die later of complications from their drowning episode. In this case, the question is, were they "near-drowned" or were they "drowned?"

TABLE 111.1 Description of Meaning of Current Terms and Former Terms Used to Describe the Submersion Episode and Its Sequelae

Term	Meaning	Still in Use
Drowning	Death secondary to undergoing the drowning episode either acutely in the water or later of consequences directly resulting from the submersion episode	Yes
Near-drowning	Survival from a submersion episode, now replaced by "the victim survived the drowning episode"	No
Witnessed drowning	The act of submersion is witnessed by bystanders; formally "active drowning"	Yes
Unwitnessed drowning	The act of submersion is not witnessed by bystanders; formally "passive or silent drowning"	Yes
Secondary drowning	Another medical condition caused the victim to submerge (i.e., syncope or while a victim is recovering from a drowning episode), another medical condition arises due to the submersion episode (i.e., ARDS)	No
Dry drowning	Liquid has not been aspirated in a submersion episode	No

The definition of "drowned" we believe to be fairly clear—namely, death secondary to undergoing the drowning episode. "Near-drowned" presents a significantly greater problem of understanding. We believe that the term "drowned" should be retained for both those who die acutely in the water and those who die later of consequences directly resulting from the submersion episode. However, we agree with the consensus of the World Congress members that "near-drowned" may lead to unnecessary confusion and, therefore, should be replaced by terminology such as "the victim survived the drowning episode" and then describe the ultimate condition of the victim.

Other terms that have appeared in the literature over the past few decades that we believe are confusing and should be abandoned are as follows.

Dry versus Wet Drowning

Because all drowning occurs in liquid, by definition, they are all wet. This terminology has been used by some to categorize drowning victims into those who aspirate liquid into the lungs and those who do not. Frequently, it is not possible to determine at the scene of the accident whether the victim actually did aspirate water. This is particularly true when the quantity of water aspirated is small. Further, if evidence of fluid aspiration is not detected in the victim who dies or is discovered dead in the water, the diagnosis may be suspect (22,23). In these cases, one should look for other explanations such as acute mechanical standstill of the heart, from asystole or ventricular fibrillation, or, for that matter, whether the victim was actually alive when he or she first became submerged.

Active versus Passive versus Silent Drowning

This terminology has been used by some to separate those victims who are observed to be struggling at the surface of the water from those who are first discovered when they are actually submerged and motionless. It has been shown with underwater cameras that even victims who were not seen to be in difficulty on the surface of the water by observers may have had unrecognized active motion while submerged. We believe, therefore, that these terms should be abandoned in favor of the terms "witnessed," when the episode is witnessed from the onset of submersion/immersion to the time of rescue, or "unwitnessed," when a body is found in the water without direct knowledge of how long ago the incident occurred.

Secondary Drowning

This terminology has been used by some to describe a situation when a precipitating event from another origin (e.g., syncope) causes a victim to be below the surface of the water, and then he/she drowns. On the other hand, some use this terminology to describe a victim who appears to be recovering from a drowning episode in the hospital and then develops adult respiratory distress syndrome. Not only is this terminology confusing but also, in the latter instance, a patient does not experience a second submersion or drowning episode, and therefore, this terminology should be abandoned.

PATHOPHYSIOLOGY

There have been extensive studies both in animals (7–9,16, 20,24–35) and in humans (4,6,22,36–41) over the past century in an attempt to quantify the changes that occur as a result of a drowning episode. What has consistently been shown is that, acutely, drowning produces asphyxia (i.e., hypoxia, hypercarbia, and acidosis). The hypercarbia is due to absent or ineffective ventilation, and is readily correctable when aggressive mechanical ventilation is instituted. The hypoxia that occurs initially is not as readily correctable and may be persistent for long periods of time (8–10). This hypoxia is first due to apnea, and then primarily to intrapulmonary shunting from alveoli that are perfused but not being ventilated, or not being ventilated adequately (33). The acidosis is mixed, and the respiratory component rapidly disappears with effective ventilation. The patient is, however, frequently left with significant metabolic acidosis due to anaerobic metabolism during the period of time that profound tissue hypoxia secondary to absent or ineffective respiration and cardiac output was present. The hallmark of this high anion gap metabolic acidosis is an increased level of serum lactic acid.

Pulmonary

While intrapulmonary shunting occurs after both freshwater and seawater aspiration, the etiology is different (Table 111.2) (13,34,42). In the case of freshwater, the aspirated water alters the surface tension properties of pulmonary surfactant. Thus, the alveoli become unstable and do not maintain their normal shape or patency, resulting in an increase in both absolute and relative intrapulmonary shunt (33,34). Seawater does not change the surface tension properties of pulmonary surfactant but, because it is hypertonic, it pulls fluid from the circulation into the alveoli, disrupts the capillary–alveolar membrane, which leads to further permeability and thus producing obstruction to gas exchange at the alveolar level (42); bronchoconstriction also has been reported after aspiration of even small quantities of water (29).

Freshwater, being hypotonic, is absorbed very rapidly into the circulation and, because of the transient hypervolemia that occurs and the change in the surface tension properties of pulmonary surfactant, pulmonary edema results. The pulmonary edema is most commonly described as frothy or foamy and blood-tinged. This coloring is secondary to the presence of free plasma hemoglobin from the rupture of some red blood cells due to the absorption of hypotonic fluid into the circulation in the face of hypoxia (43). Pulmonary edema also occurs when sea water is aspirated, secondary to a semipermeable membrane effect because the seawater is hypertonic compared to plasma. Even though the etiology of the hypoxia is different between freshwater and seawater aspiration, the result of both is to increase intrapulmonary shunt, decreased compliance, and bronchospasm all of which requires aggressive therapy (13,33,42,44,45).

Extensive studies of serum electrolyte concentrations after drowning have shown that only 15% of victims who die in the water aspirate more than 22 mL/kg of water. In patients who survive, the percentage is much less and, thus, significant changes in serum electrolyte concentrations that require treatment are rarely observed (7), with the only exception being, perhaps, victims of drowning in the Dead Sea (46).

The treatment of the respiratory lesion requires providing mechanical ventilatory support in a fashion that will restore an adequate functional residual capacity and keep the alveoli open during all phases of the respiratory cycle, thus

TABLE 111.2 Freshwater versus Seawater Effects on Pulmonary Physiology during Aspiration

	Freshwater Aspiration	Seawater Aspiration
Intrapulmonary shunting	Present	Present
Surface tension	Altered	Not altered
Fluid movement	Into circulation	Into alveoli
Capillary-alveolar membrane	Disrupted due to altered surface tension	Disrupted due to increased intra-alveolar fluid
Pulmonary edema	Present, due to increased pulmonary circulatory volume	Present, due to increased intra-alveolar fluid
Bronchoconstriction	Present	Present
Compliance	Decreased	Decreased

decreasing the intrapulmonary shunt. Obviously, if foreign material such as sand, silt, or plant life is aspirated into the lung, it may produce obstruction, and it should be removed via bronchoscopy.

Cardiovascular

The cardiovascular changes that occur during a drowning episode can best be ascribed to inadequate oxygenation. Although fatal dysrhythmia, such as ventricular fibrillation, is rarely documented in human drowning victims, ventricular fibrillation can occur with profound hypoxia, especially if very significant changes in serum potassium and serum sodium result from the movement of fluid and rupture of red blood cells. Usually the sequence of cardiac dysrhythmias progresses from tachycardia to bradycardia, then pulseless electrical activity and finally asystole (42,47). Although a wide variety of cardiac dysrhythmias have been reported (20), particularly in animal models, rarely do they require specific therapy other than improving oxygenation, correcting severe metabolic acidosis, fluid resuscitation, and correcting temperature (13,42). More common problems are profound hypoxia and the leak of fluid into the lung as pulmonary edema, resulting in a relative hypovolemia in the patient. It has been shown by multiple investigators that to treat this hypovolemia, it may be necessary to infuse significant amounts of intravenous fluid to maintain an adequate effective circulating blood volume, even in the face of pulmonary edema (27,45). Without such therapy, even though the arterial oxygen tension might have improved with mechanical ventilatory support, the delivery of oxygen to the tissues remains compromised and incompatible with supplying adequate tissue oxygenation (45).

Neurologic

The neurologic injury that occurs during drowning, like cardiovascular complications, can also be attributed to hypoxia and its risk is similar to patients who require cardiopulmonary resuscitation (CPR) from other etiologies (13). When cerebral flood flow drops to less than 20 mL/100g/min, cerebral metabolic oxygen demands exceed oxygen supply, and neuronal ischemia will begin to occur and permanent injury can occur within 4 to 10 minutes to the hippocampus, basal ganglia, and cerebral cortex (48,49). As previously discussed, hypothermia commonly occurs with the drowning incident and, if this is the case, it may have neuroprotective qualities and decrease the amount of neurologic injury expected to occur for the length of period with decreased oxygen delivery; this occurs due to the decrease in cerebral metabolic rate at lower temperatures as, for each degree of Celsius below 37°, the cerebral metabolic rate decreases by 5% to 7%.

In addition to the primary injury at the time of the event, there is also secondary injury and delayed neuronal cell death (49). There are complex cellular signals and responses to both hypoxia and to reperfusion, which may lead to subsequent pro-death signaling (49).

Renal

Detrimental changes in renal function are rarely seen in persons recovering from near-drowning. However, when present, they likely are the result of inadequate perfusion and oxygenation rather than anything specifically related to the drowning episode *per se*. Some have emphasized the need for the kidneys to clear free plasma hemoglobin after freshwater drowning; however, significant levels of free plasma hemoglobin have rarely been reported in such patients. This is likely due to the fact that for red blood cells to rupture and release enough hemoglobin into the plasma during a drowning episode to require specific therapy for its clearance, it requires transfer of substantial volumes of free water into the circulation in the face of hypoxia (43); as stated above, this rarely occurs.

INITIAL RESCUE AND RESUSCITATION

To ensure survival after a drowning episode, it is imperative that one never lose sight of the fact that time is of the essence. The longer a person is without the ability to breathe air, the more profound are the hypoxia and permanent damage to vital tissues. Thus, those who are entrusted with guarding swimming facilities must never lose sight of the fact that continual vigilance is required to recognize a victim in distress, and that the victim must be removed from the water and resuscitative measures begun in a timely fashion. Frequently, bodies are discovered motionless in a pool, without anyone in attendance being able to pinpoint the length of time that the victim was submerged. If an individual is not noted to be making purposeful movements for more than 10 seconds, rescue attempts should be initiated. The individual responsible for safety at the pool should always be in proper attire and in position to initiate such a rescue and complete it within 20 seconds of the recognition of the problem.

While removing the victim from the water, care should be taken to avoid complicating neck injuries when they are suspected. Routine stabilization of the neck is unnecessary unless the circumstances leading to the drowning episode suggest that trauma was likely (50). These circumstances include a history of diving, use of a water slide, signs of injury, or evidence of alcohol intoxication. If neck injury is suspected, gentle immobilization of the head should be accomplished, securing it in a neutral position. However, if the neck appears to be obviously deformed and the patient has pain with neck movement, the neck should be immobilized in the existing position.

If the victim is apneic, the airway should rapidly be cleared of foreign material, a patent airway secured, and mouth-to-mouth resuscitation started immediately. It is preferable to begin artificial ventilation in the water if it can be accomplished without jeopardizing the safety of the rescuer. Starting resuscitation efforts while in water increases the chances of a good outcome by threefold compared to waiting until a victim is brought to land (51). In-water resuscitation efforts are, therefore, ventilation alone due to the inability to perform chest compressions (50). It should be remembered that not all victims are in a state of cardiac arrest when the rescue attempt begins. They may be in a state of vasoconstriction or have a significant bradycardia, in which case, if effective ventilation is started, the myocardium will be re-oxygenated, and increased cardiac activity will result in improved tissue perfusion.

Upon removing the victim from the water, he or she should rapidly be assessed for the presence of both spontaneous respiration and cardiac activity. In the absence of these, the airway should be inspected rapidly to ensure that there is no mechanical obstruction, and artificial respiration and cardiac compression should be instituted without delay. Although, chest compression alone—without artificial respiration—is an alternate resuscitation method that has been proposed for victims of dysrhythmic cardiac arrest, it must be emphasized that these recommendations do not apply to the drowning victim because the pathophysiologic lesion in the lungs requires active attempts at reinflation and stabilization of the alveoli. Therefore, cardiac arrest following drowning is more likely due to asphyxia, and thus, immediate provision of ventilation is recommended (50). Resuscitation efforts should follow the traditional airway-breathing-circulation (ABC) sequence, which starts with 5 initial rescue breaths, then 30 chest compressions, then 2 rescue breaths, then 30 chest compressions, and repeated until return of spontaneous circulation occurs. Five initial breaths are recommended instead of two due to water in the airways in difficulty performing the initial breaths (50,52,53).

PATIENT TRANSPORT AND EMERGENCY MEDICAL SERVICES

Neither equipment nor properly trained personnel are usually available at the site to provide advanced cardiac life support, including endotracheal intubation, intravenous access, drug therapy, and electrical defibrillation. However, these measures should be instituted when indicated and when the proper equipment and properly trained personnel are available. It is crucial that someone other than the individual rescuing and resuscitating the patient contact emergency medical services (EMS) as rapidly as possible so that they can respond in a timely fashion and perform advanced cardiac life-support treatment on the victim.

Whenever a drowning victim has to be transported to a location or facility such as a hospital emergency room, it is important that a call be made promptly to inform the emergency room personnel of the exact circumstances, type of treatment instituted, and condition of the patient en route so that they will be prepared to accept the patient and render appropriate therapy immediately upon arrival.

When moving a critically ill drowning victim, it is imperative to remember the fragility of such patients because they can decompensate in a matter of a few seconds or minutes if appropriate therapy is withdrawn. Examples of such situations are movement (a) from the scene to the EMS vehicle, (b) from the EMS vehicle to the hospital emergency department, or (c) from the hospital emergency department to other hospital locations for testing, such as radiology, or for treatment, such as the intensive care unit (ICU). Thus, every attempt should be made to continue essential therapy at all times.

Treatment in the Emergency Department

In the emergency department, a thorough evaluation of the patient should be performed, keeping in mind that the most serious problems that require immediate therapy are pulmonary insufficiency and cardiovascular instability, which result in inadequate delivery of oxygen to vital tissues. If the victim is responding fully, does not require respiratory or cardiovascular support, and has a normal oxyhemoglobin saturation while breathing room air, it is unlikely that the victim has aspirated a significant amount of water, and observation may be all that is necessary. At the other extreme is the patient who is still unconscious and requires extensive pulmonary and cardiovascular support in an attempt to normalize vital signs and produce adequate cardiac output and tissue oxygenation. Thus, a cookbook-type treatment that would apply to *every* victim cannot be prescribed. However, the treating physician should keep in mind that increased intrapulmonary shunt and poorly matched ventilation-to-perfusion ratios are the rule rather than the exception for the victim who has aspirated a significant quantity of water.

Therapy must be aimed at improving ventilation-to-perfusion ratios and restoring adequate residual lung volume to optimally oxygenate the blood. A relative hypovolemia frequently is present due to fluid shifts between the lung and the circulation. These can be accentuated by the increase in mean intrathoracic pressure that occurs with mechanical ventilatory support. Thus, evaluation of effective circulating blood volume and replenishment of intravascular fluid volume to physiologic levels is important as a primary concern.

If the patient is a victim of seawater drowning and has aspirated sufficient water to produce hypernatremia, we might be better advised to use an agent such as *tris*-(hydroxymethyl) aminomethane (*Tris*) buffer; 2-amino-2-hydroxyl-1,3-propandiol (THAM) to avoid compounding the hypernatremia. However, once again, it should be noted that the quantity of water aspirated is seldom sufficient to produce such significant changes in serum electrolyte concentrations, except perhaps when the drowning occurs in water of extreme hypersalinity such as the Dead Sea (46).

Changes in serum electrolyte concentrations and hemoglobin and hematocrit of sufficient magnitude to justify specific therapy are rare, as are alterations in renal function other than those that might be expected in the hypovolemic, hypoxic, or markedly acidotic patient.

The patient's level of consciousness on admission to the emergency room has been shown to markedly influence outcome (54,55). The most important consideration here is to provide adequate oxygenation and perfusion and to avoid producing increased intracranial pressure if possible. Treatments aimed specifically at preservation of cerebral function have not been shown to be particularly beneficial to date (49,55,56).

If the patient requires diagnostic testing in a distant location such as the radiology department, it is imperative that adequate personnel and equipment accompany the patient to ensure that optimum therapy is not interrupted at any time during transport or when performing the procedure. Likewise, transportation to the ICU should be done with a "full team approach." Should optimum therapy be interrupted during any of these time periods, adverse consequences should be anticipated.

Drowning episodes in cold water may produce significant hypothermia. There are several methods of rewarming that have been recommended including, but not necessarily limited to, heating blankets, warmed intravenous fluids, warmed humidification of breathing circuits, gastric lavage, and cardiopulmonary bypass. The method used should be tailored to the resources available and the condition of the patient. It must be remembered, however, that rewarming peripheral tissues before the patient's circulation is capable of supplying adequate amounts of oxygenated blood can compound the situation and increase the degree of metabolic acidosis.

IN-HOSPITAL THERAPY: POSTRESUSCITATION CARE

Expert intensive care is vital to survival once optimal prehospital and emergency department management have been performed. Hemodynamic instability after cardiac arrest, respiratory insufficiency, and severe neurologic impairment are all criteria for admission to the ICU. The administrative structure of the hospital's critical care service dictates the setting to which the patient is admitted. A recent attempt to classify survivors of drowning based on the severity of symptoms on a scale of 1 to 6 recommends ICU admission for all pediatric patients requiring high concentrations of oxygen, with or without the need for invasive ventilation (57).

Respiratory Support

Although the degree of intrapulmonary shunting after drowning is variable from one patient to the next, if the patient is breathing adequately to clear carbon dioxide, the single most important method of treatment in reversing hypoxemia is the application of continuous positive airway pressure (CPAP). The amount of CPAP applied must be individualized because the degree of atelectasis, the amount of pulmonary edema, and the magnitude of the intrapulmonary shunt varies between patients. In great measure, this will depend on the type and quantity of the water aspirated. Although the mechanism for producing the intrapulmonary shunt is different between freshwater and seawater (34), Lee (58) found no statistically significant difference between the PaO_2/FiO_2 ratio in patients after the two types of aspiration.

The pathophysiologic mechanism involved in freshwater drowning is lowering of the sodium concentration in the alveolus, thus changing the surface tension characteristics of pulmonary surfactant (34). The alteration in the surface tension properties of pulmonary surfactant increases alveolar surface tension upon compression of the surfactant layer and results in alveolar volume loss. Also, pulmonary capillaries become more permeable, resulting in an increase in interstitial lung water that eventually compresses alveoli and promotes volume loss and causes pulmonary edema. Based on the severity of the acute respiratory derangement, this "abnormal surfactant state" has been termed mild, moderate or severe acute respiratory distress syndrome (ARDS) (59).

ARDS represent a final common pathway that accompanies a number of physiologic insults that may occur after drowning, including respiratory obstruction, aspiration of water or gastric contents, and global hypoxemia from cardiovascular insufficiency or cardiac arrest. Unfortunately, ARDS often can be clinically and radiologically confused with acute pulmonary edema from left ventricular dysfunction or fluid overload of different etiologies.

Both CPAP and positive end-expiratory pressure (PEEP) have the capability to restore lung volume and improve oxygenation in many patients with decreased lung volume, especially functional residual capacity. However, there are some differences in their function. By definition, CPAP means that airway pressure remains positive during all phases of the respiratory cycle. With PEEP, during the inspiratory phase of a spontaneous breath, circuit pressures drop to zero or become negative as a result of a vigorous inspiratory effort by the patient. Because PEEP with spontaneous ventilation increases the work of breathing, it may increase pressure gradients between the pulmonary vasculature and the alveoli, thereby leading to more pulmonary edema. Also, it does not forcibly inflate alveoli with abnormal surfactant after freshwater drowning (33). Thus, CPAP is more beneficial than PEEP for spontaneously breathing drowning victims (44,60).

Both CPAP and PEEP increase expiratory pressure; thus, air is trapped within the lungs during the expiratory phase of respiration. This results in an increase in residual lung volume in many patients with ARDS. As alveolar units re-expand, intrapulmonary shunt decreases, and improvement is seen in oxygenation and compliance. The increase in compliance decreases the work of breathing (61). The degree of lung volume restoration roughly correlates with the improvement in oxygenation. As lung volume increases toward normal, gas exchange continues to improve. It has been shown, however, that while the above beneficial effect is found with CPAP in many victims of both freshwater and seawater drowning (60,62), unless mechanical breaths are added, PEEP does not improve the ventilation-to-perfusion ratio after freshwater drowning (33,44,60). Additionally, in some freshwater drowning victims, CPAP alone does not produce an adequate response, and hence, mechanical breaths should be added (44).

When ARDS develops and oxygen desaturation occurs, an FiO_2 of 1.0 is initially recommended to attempt to restore adequate oxygenation. Increased work of breathing, severe hypoxemia, and hypercarbia are all indications for instituting mechanical ventilation. Ordinarily, CPAP is titrated to achieve an oxygen saturation greater than 95%, with the lowest possible inspired oxygen (FiO_2) levels down to an FiO_2 of 0.4 or less. We routinely increase CPAP at the bedside in increments of 3 to 5 cm H_2O in an attempt to achieve an oxygen saturation of 95%, and subsequently, the FiO_2 is gradually decreased to reach a PaO_2/FiO_2 of greater than 300 mmHg. Increased dead-space ventilation and decreased preload are the two most important adverse effects that can limit the use of CPAP. Once adequate PaO_2/FiO_2 has been achieved, CPAP can slowly be weaned based on improvement of patient lung compliance and general clinical conditions.

Mechanical Ventilation

CPAP therapy alone is not sufficient in the case of the patient who is apneic, hypoventilating, or hypercarbic, or shows little to no improvement in ventilation-to-perfusion matching while breathing spontaneously. In these patients, mechanical ventilatory breaths must also be provided. In general, mechanical ventilation in patients with ALI or ARDS can be applied either noninvasively or invasively (i.e., face mask vs. endotracheal tube, respectively). Noninvasive ventilation is reserved for milder cases of ARDS or pulmonary edema when the patient is awake, cooperative, triggering spontaneous ventilation, and has his/her swallowing and protective laryngeal reflexes intact. Although successful experience with noninvasive positive pressure ventilation (NPPV) for patients with respiratory failure other than from chronic obstructive pulmonary disease (COPD) is growing (63), potential complications include gastric distention, nasal congestion, regurgitation and aspiration of stomach contents, nasal bridge ulceration, and eye irritation (64). Several modes of mechanical ventilation and adjunct therapies are available; while not specifically used in drowning, their use has proven valuable in the ventilatory support of any patient with ARDS. A list of the most commonly used forms in drowning victims follows. Invasive mechanical ventilation modes for patients with ARDS have been discussed in Chapters 104 and 109. The same principles apply to patients whose cause for ARDS is drowning.

Nitric Oxide

Inhaled nitric oxide (NO) appears to act selectively on the pulmonary vascular bed and only in those areas associated with adequate ventilation, locally reversing hypoxic pulmonary vasoconstriction and increasing oxygenation. However, outcome in terms of mortality or number of days alive and off mechanical ventilation between patients treated with NO and those not treated has not changed when the effect of NO is studied in a prospective randomized fashion (65). Nevertheless, reducing the level of mechanical ventilatory support or FiO_2 needed to achieve adequate oxygenation is a potential benefit that could reduce barotrauma and the side effects of treatment. There are two case reports published in which NO was used in drowning victims: one in a 16-year-old boy in which both oxygenation and pulmonary hypertension improved with no untoward cardiovascular events (66), and the second a 21-year-old man in which both NO and prone positioning were used which lead to improvement in oxygenation and extubation within 5 days (67).

Prone Positioning

Rotation of patients from supine to prone may cause rapid improvement in oxygenation that may last for up to 12 hours (68). With this maneuver, there is a relatively high risk of inadvertent extubation and removal of invasive monitors; nonetheless, oxygenation improves mainly because the nondependent dorsal portion of the lung has a higher air-to-tissue ratio (69). Obviously, the risks and benefits need to be considered before using this technique in any specific patient.

Bronchodilator Therapy

Small airway closure has been shown to occur even with aspiration of relatively small amounts of water (26). Thus, bronchodilator therapy should be considered in patients when bronchospasm is thought to be present.

Surfactant

ARDS from drowning involves both quantitative (seawater) and qualitative (freshwater) alterations in lung surfactant (34,70). Although the use of exogenous surfactant has been shown to lower mortality in neonates with respiratory distress syndrome (71) and a few successful case reports in drowned children have been reported (72–74), this effect in adults has been disappointing, and its prohibitive cost makes its use infrequent.

Prophylactic Antibiotics

Prophylactic antibiotics are not needed in most drowning victims, and the use of broad-spectrum antibiotics may enhance the emergence of resistant organisms, as well as the potential for *Clostridium difficile* infection. Pneumonia is often misdiagnosed due to the consolidation which appears on radiographs due to water in the alveoli (13). It has been shown only about 12% of patients rescued from a drowning episode developed pneumonia and required antibiotic treatment (75). An exception represents survival from drowning in heavily contaminated water such as stagnant ponds or public spas, where *Pseudomonas* species are endemic. Our initial choice in this situation is usually a fourth-generation cephalosporin with broad gram-negative coverage. In other patients, antibiotics are not recommended unless the patient develops evidence of infection, in which case cultures and sensitivities will guide the choice of antibiotics to be given.

Cardiovascular Support

By the time a drowning victim reaches the ICU, cardiac dysrhythmias are rarely a problem. If witnessed in the emergency department or the ICU, the most common cause of arrhythmias is severe hypoxia, and providing adequate ventilation and oxygenation will usually restore a normal rhythm. If not, drug therapy or, in the case of severe ventricular arrhythmias, electrical intervention is appropriate. Hypotension may require initial pharmacologic support, but it should be remembered that the hypotension seen in drowning victims is predominantly due to fluid shifts resulting in hypovolemia (27,45). This hypovolemia may be accentuated when mechanical ventilatory techniques that increase mean intrathoracic pressure are used (45).

Experimental studies have shown that, whereas mechanical ventilation and CPAP will decrease intrapulmonary shunt and increase PaO_2, because of the detrimental effect on cardiac output, tissue perfusion is compromised. In one study, attempting to increase oxygen delivery by use of vasopressors and inotropes was not productive, but fluid administration to increase blood volume resulted in an increased cardiac output and oxygen delivery (45).

Precise fluid replacement is dependent on an accurate assessment of effective circulating blood volume. To this end, monitoring the patient with a pulmonary artery catheter or transesophageal echocardiography is extremely helpful.

Temperature Management

As previously mentioned, many drowning victims are hypothermic upon rescue and upon presentation to the hospital. Deciding to keep a patient hypothermic or induce hypothermia is largely based on extrapolation of studies of therapeutic hypothermia in cardiac arrest and asphyxia (49). In cardiac arrest there have been multiple studies showing improvement in neurologic outcome with therapeutic hypothermia. In two landmark, randomized controlled trials, moderate hypothermia, 32° to 34°C, was induced in patients after return of spontaneous circulation after ventricular fibrillation arrest for 12 to 24 hours and was compared to standard temperature care and showed improvement in neurologic outcome in the mild hypothermia arm (76,77). International guidelines began recommending therapeutic hypothermia in comatose patients after cardiac arrest in 2003 and this then extended to patients with in-hospital arrest and arrest from initially nonshockable rhythms. In 2013, another landmark multicenter, randomized study compared targeted temperature therapy of 33°C versus normothermia at 36°C in patients suffering out-of-hospital arrest presumed of cardiac etiology, not finding a difference in outcomes between the two arms, and both had improved neurologic outcomes compared to previous studies (78,79).

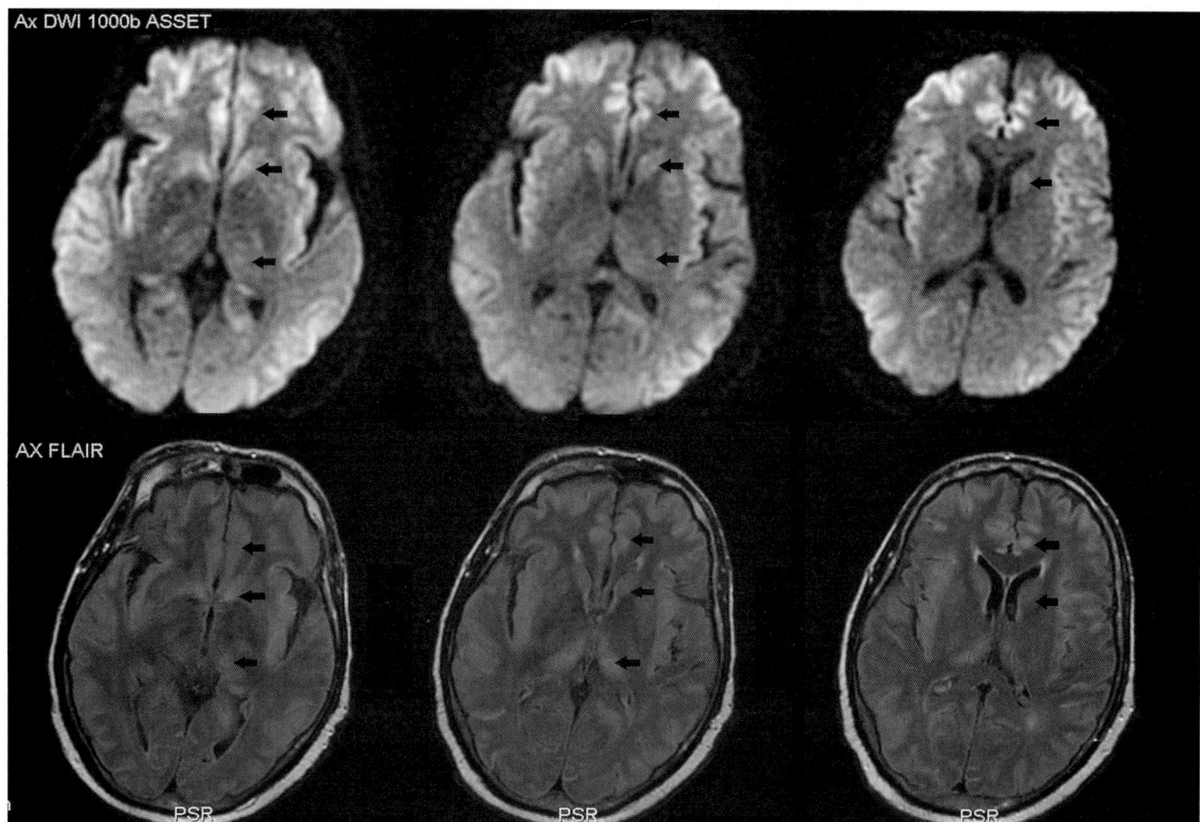

FIGURE 111.1 MRI of anoxic brain injury showing confluent T2/FLAIR signal hyperintensity with diffusion hyperintensity involving the cerebral cortex bilaterally, the bilateral thalami, and to a lesser degree the caudate heads.

This has since raised the question if the therapeutic benefits of targeted temperature therapy are in avoiding fever rather than in hypothermia itself, but clearly establishes temperature should be controlled (79).

Therapeutic hypothermia in asphyxia has been studied almost primarily in neonates but also in children. A Cochrane review of eight randomized controlled trials and two other subsequent meta-analyses of neonates with intrapartum asphyxia and moderate-to-severe encephalopathy found hypothermia had a beneficial effect on mortality and major neurodevelopmental disability at 18 months (80–82).

Therapeutic hypothermia has only been sparsely studied in drowning itself. More than two decades ago, two small retrospective studies examined deep, prolonged hypothermia with and without barbiturate therapy and found only an increase in survival of patients in persistent vegetative state (49,56,83). Two cases of drowning associated with cardiopulmonary arrest and requirement of extracorporeal membrane oxygenation were reported in which a hypothermic state was maintained for 6 days; both survived without neurologic sequelae (84). In contrast to the previous studies of deep hypothermia, mild hypothermia and targeted temperature therapy, as have been studied in cardiac arrest, should be a point for future investigation in drowning victims.

Central Nervous System Support

The two most important factors influencing morbidity and mortality in victims surviving drowning are severe respiratory insufficiency and permanent neurologic impairment secondary to cerebral hypoxia (Fig. 111.1). Despite improvement in emergency and intensive pulmonary and cardiovascular care, neurologic outcome in drowning patients is directly related to the initial duration of hypoxia from the onset of submersion until effective CPR is provided. The Glasgow coma scale (GCS) score mirrors this relationship during the first few hours after submersion. As in other neurologic injury, care is often separated into neuromonitoring and neuroprotective strategies; we discuss both below.

NEUROPROTECTION STRATEGIES

Unfortunately, there is a lack of evidence to guide any neuroprotective strategies specifically for the drowning victim (49). Much of the research regarding drowning victims has focused more on the pulmonary and cardiovascular systems. Attempting to study different neuroprotective strategies in drowning victims is difficult, if not impossible, given the rarity and heterogeneity of the events (49). It is also unknown if there are any differences in cerebral injury from saltwater versus freshwater drowning (49). Temperature management and therapeutic hypothermia, previously discussed, have possible benefits if extrapolated to the drowned patient. Barbiturates have been studied and were specifically part of the HYPER (hypothermia, hyperventilation, steroids, dehydration, barbiturate coma, and neuromuscular blockade) therapy, introduced in the late 1970s to control intracranial pressure postdrowning; barbiturates had mixed results in outcomes (85–87). Barbiturates then were specifically studied in the pediatric population, which showed no improvement in outcome and the drugs have since fallen out of favor (88). Magnesium therapy, allopurinol, and erythropoietin have all been studied in neonatal asphyxia and hypoxic–ischemic encephalopathy (49). A recent review and meta-analysis of magnesium for neuroprotection in hypoxic–ischemic encephalopathy reviewed five studies, finding improvement in short-term outcomes and only a trend toward improved mortality (89). Allopurinol has been extensively studied in hypoxic–ischemic encephalopathy due to its inhibition of xanthine oxidase, which may reduce delayed cell death (90). A recent Cochrane review did not show a statistically significant difference in the risk of death or severe neurodevelopmental disability (90). A large ongoing multicenter trial, the ALLO-trial, is studying antenatal allopurinol during fetal hypoxia (91). Erythropoietin has been shown to have neuroprotective qualities by modulating antioxidant enzyme activity and the genetic expression of apoptosis; numerous trials show promise in hypoxic–ischemic encephalopathy in newborns (49).

NEUROMONITORING

No single neuromonitoring modality is considered the gold standard, and the use of multimodality monitoring is recommended in this population. Severity of illness can be estimated by the quality of resuscitative efforts on the scene, patient age, submersion time, temperature, initial pH, hyperglycemia, and presenting neurologic examination (92). The following discussion includes evidence from patients suffering from anoxia secondary to drowning or near-drowning or cardiac arrest; studies reviewed include the adult and pediatric population. It is important to consider the use of hypothermia after anoxic event and patient age, both of which may impact neuroprognostication (93).

The pediatric population is of considerable concern because the increased neuroplasticity of their immature neurologic system makes recovery more difficult to predict. This can be extrapolated to an extent to young adults, making prognostication difficult in this population. Nonetheless, it is important to keep in mind that no one modality is the gold standard, and multiple modalities should be utilized to provide a clearer picture of the damage, prognostication, and to guide resuscitation.

NEUROLOGIC EXAMINATION

The neurologic examination is an important monitor for secondary injury, and has less of an impact with prognostication in hypoxic–ischemic encephalopathy (92). However, it is important to realize that the neurologic examination can be clouded by the use of neuromuscular blockade, sedatives, and narcotics; in these circumstances, the physical examination can be unreliable. We recommend allowing more than five-drug half-lives (depending on the patient's ability to metabolize the medications) prior to predicting neurologic outcomes via neurologic examination.

Several grading scales can be used to classify patients, the most frequently being the GCS, pupillary response, corneal reflex, and motor responses (92–94). Patients who present awake have better prognosis than those who present comatose. A GCS score of less than 5 combined with no pupillary response at presentation, 24 and 48 hours is associated with poor outcome (92). The American Academy of Neurology states clinical findings that predict poor outcome in anoxia after cardiac arrest include myoclonus, status epilepticus (SE) within the first 24 hours, absence of pupillary responses on days 1 to 3, absent corneal reflexes within 1 to 3 days, and absent or extensor motor responses after 3 days (94,95). One study evaluating pediatric patients with hypoxic–ischemia found a GCS score of less than 5 after 24 hours was always associated with poor outcome (96). These results are further echoed in patients treated with hypothermia after arrest (97). It should be emphasized that the neurologic examination, especially motor response, is an unreliable predictor of neurologic outcome when used alone and should be correlated with clinical circumstance and other neuromonitoring modalities (97).

INTRACRANIAL PRESSURE MONITORING

Hypoxic injury leading to cell death and subsequent cerebral edema makes ICP monitoring a logical choice for monitoring and prognostication in this population. Poor outcomes have been associated with sustained ICPs above 20 mmHg and CPP below 50 mmHg (98). Regardless of the pathophysiology of elevated ICP with cerebral anoxia, the risks of invasive ICP monitoring may outweigh the benefits, and currently is not in the mainstream of monitoring modalities. Earlier studies on ICP monitoring in this population showed mixed results and unreliable prediction of outcome with CPP just below normal (99).

SOMATOSENSORY EVOKED POTENTIALS

The use of somatosensory evoked potentials (SSEPs) has been validated as an alternative method of confirming brain death in the United States. SSEPs can also be used for prognostication in patients with anoxic encephalopathy, with the absence of bilateral cortical responses at 24 hours after injury closely correlating with poor prognosis (95). More definitively, absent cortical responses with SSEPs at 1 week have been shown to have 100% positive predictive value for poor outcome after cardiac arrest (95,100). These results are more predictive when combined with serum levels of neuron-specific enolase greater than or equal to 33 μg/L (95). A systematic review comparing SSEPs to clinical examination, including pupil and motor responses, to predict poor and favorable outcomes in pediatric TBI showed that SSEPs provided better reliability in predicting favorable and poor outcomes. In addition, SSEPs showed good reliability with the use of NMB and sedation when compared to the clinical examination (100). Similar findings are reported in a study of anoxic encephalopathy after cardiac arrest in adults (101). Absent bilateral median nerve SSEPs along with pupillary response, corneal reflexes, and motor response after 72 hours after arrest correlated to poor outcome (101). In another study of adults after cardiac arrest, bilateral absence of SSEPs was always predictive of an unfavorable prognosis, defined as death or persistent vegetative state (96).

ELECTROENCEPHALOGRAPHY

In patients with hypoxic encephalopathy due to cardiac arrest, EEG findings of SE or suppression correlated with nonsurvivability, and nonreactive EEG correlated highly with in-hospital mortality (93). EEG may thus have both prognostic and therapeutic utility. While evidence of SE increases mortality and morbidity, its recognition and management may improve outcome (97).

Renal Support

Albuminuria, hemoglobinuria, oliguria, and anuria, while rare, have all been described in drowning victims secondary to acute tubular necrosis from hypoxemia, rhabdomyolysis, or both. Hypothermia leads to reduced blood flow to the skin and muscle, preserving core temperature and central organ perfusion. The pathophysiology of acute rhabdomyolysis is probably secondary to tissue hypoxia from acute vessel constriction, due to the competitive need for heat conservation; skeletal myolysis and increased circulating myoglobin will result. Acute renal failure may be aggravated by acute tubular necrosis secondary to hemodynamic instability.

Acute tubular necrosis and rhabdomyolysis require early and vigorous treatment directed at correcting hypovolemia, improving oxygenation, and enhancing heme protein elimination. Volume replacement therapy aims to restore normal blood flow and enhance renal oxygen supply; the medullary ascending limb of Henle loop is most vulnerable to hypoxic injury. Invasive monitoring may be necessary to provide adequate intravascular volume. The window of opportunity for restoration of intravascular volume and volume expansion is likely within 6 hours or less of the acute event.

If rhabdomyolysis is present, enhancing the elimination of heme protein helps to limit tubular damage. Intravenous fluids should be increased to 400 mL/hr and may need to be as high at 1,000 mL/hr with a goal of 3 mL/kg/hr of urine output (102). Systemic alkalinization of the urine with sodium bicarbonate increases the solubility and, therefore, the elimination of heme protein (102,103). A urine pH between 6.5 and 8 produces a myoglobin solubility of around 80% and is a reasonable goal. Caution should be taken with administration of sodium bicarbonate as it may worsen hypocalcemia associated with rhabdoymyolysis (102). However, in a patient with low urine output, massive doses of sodium bicarbonate may be associated with volume overload secondary to an acute increase in intravascular osmolarity (102,104). In these cases, when the hemodynamic goal is mild hypervolemia, the weak diuretic acetazolamide may be a valid alternative. Acetazolamide increases the excretion of bicarbonate in urine as a result of the inhibition of the enzyme carbonic anhydrase. However, diuretics, particularly in patients on significant ventilatory support, may adversely affect venous filling and cardiac output. Mannitol, an osmotic diuretic, has also been used in rhabdomyolysis due to the increased urinary flow, excretion of nephrotoxins, its ability to pull fluid from the injured muscles due to its osmotic properties, and its free-radical scavenging properties (102).

Manipulating the renal output by means of significantly altering the effective circulating blood volume in drowning victims frequently has a detrimental effect on pulmonary and cardiovascular function. Therefore, a fine-tuned balancing act is frequently required to not adversely affect one organ system while treating another.

Other Concerns

Severe metabolic acidosis from low systemic oxygen delivery and resulting anaerobic metabolism should be corrected. We recommend correction of the base deficit with bicarbonate or acetate solutions to maintain a pH no lower than 7.20. Mechanical ventilation is adjusted frequently with the help of arterial blood gas determinations to maintain a $PaCO_2$ between 35 and 40 mmHg. Lactic acid levels are checked frequently for a few hours after resuscitation. In fact, while base deficit and single absolute levels of lactic acidosis do not necessarily correlate with the development of multiple organ failure and survival, the rate of lactic acid clearance does (105). Because significant electrolyte abnormalities requiring specific therapy are rarely observed in the drowning victim, normal saline is used as replacement fluid. Isotonic solution also provides less chance of aggravating cerebral edema.

PREVENTION

An awareness of the hidden dangers of recreational activities in and around water, and close supervision of infants, children, and adolescents are the secrets to preventing a significant number of drowning incidents. Swimming pools should be enclosed by security fences to prevent small children from entering the water inadvertently or unsupervised. By identifying age-related drowning risks, communities can reduce drowning rates. Effective CPR and water safety skills should be encouraged in the community, particularly for parents with small children who own home pools. Furthermore, children who can swim should never do so alone or without adult supervision. Everyone participating in water sports should wear an approved personal flotation device. Adolescents need to be taught to swim and informed about the dangers of alcohol and other drug consumption during water sport activities. Between 13 and 19 years of age, risk-taking behavior increases significantly in boys; therefore, extra counseling is warranted. Alcohol should never be consumed, regardless of age, while swimming or engaging in water sports. Swimming with a partner is particularly important for individuals with medical conditions that may abruptly alter their level of consciousness, such as seizure disorders, cardiac disease, and several metabolic diseases. Emergency gear for rescuing and resuscitating drowning victims should be readily available at the poolside. The specific gear required may vary with the size, access, and ownership of the facility.

The community expects the government to enforce safety rules, promote health education through medical and nonmedical personnel, and punish individuals who transgress basic safety rules and regulations. Despite recent advances in CPR and more sophisticated intensive care medicine, drowning victims with poor GCS scores have a high likelihood of living in a vegetative state as a result of the initial injury. When this occurs, making life or death decisions regarding withdrawal of life support by relatives and health professionals represents a significant stressful event. At the time of this writing, prevention is still the most fundamental way to limit neurologic disasters from drowning.

Key Points

- Because cardiac arrest following drowning is more likely due to asphyxia, immediate provision of ventilation is recommended and not chest compressions alone.
- Drowning in both freshwater and seawater produces intrapulmonary shunting, although from differing mechanisms.
- The single most important method of treatment in reversing hypoxemia is the application of CPAP.
- Prophylactic antibiotics are not needed in most cases.
- Targeted temperature management and hypothermia have been shown to improve neurologic outcomes in anoxic injury due to cardiac arrest and may be helpful in drowning victims.

References

1. Idris A, Berg R, Bierens J, et al. Recommended guidelines for uniform reporting of data from drowning: the "Utstein style." *Circulation.* 2003;108(20):2565–2574.
2. Albert B, Craig J. Causes of loss of consciousness during underwater swimming. *J Appl Physiol.* 1961;16(4):583–586.
3. Swann H. Resuscitation in semi-drowning. *Artificial Respiration: Theory and Application.* New York, NY: Harper & Row; 1962:202-24.
4. Modell JH, Graves SA, Ketover A. Clinical course of 91 consecutive near-drowning victims. *Chest J.* 1976;70(2):231–238.
5. Lowson JA. Sensations in drowning. *Edinb Med J.* 1903;13:41–45.
6. Fuller R. The 1962 Wellcome prize essay. Drowning and the postimmersion syndrome: a clinicopathologic study. *Military Med.* 1963;128:22–36.
7. Modell JH, Davis J. Electrolyte changes in human drowning victims. *Anesthesiology.* 1969;30(4):414.
8. Modell JH, Moya F, Newby EJ, et al. The effects of fluid volume in seawater drowning. *Ann Intern Med.* 1967;67(1):68–80.
9. Modell JH, Moya F. Effects of volume of aspirated fluid during chlorinated fresh water drowning. *Anesthesiology.* 1966;27(5):662.
10. Modell JH, Gaub M, Moya F, et al. Physiologic effects of near drowning with chlorinated fresh water, distilled water and isotonic saline. *Anesthesiology.* 1966;27(1):33–41.
11. Leach R, Treacher D. ABC of oxygen: oxygen transport—2. Tissue hypoxia. *BMJ.* 1998;317(7169):1370.
12. Craig AB. Underwater swimming and loss of consciousness. *JAMA.* 1961;176(4):255–258.
13. Szpilman D, Bierens JJ, Handley AJ, Orlowski JP. Drowning. *N Engl J Med.* 2012;366(22):2102–2110.
14. Polderman KH. Application of therapeutic hypothermia in the ICU: opportunities and pitfalls of a promising treatment modality. Part 1: indications and evidence. *Intensive Care Med.* 2004;30(4):556–575.
15. Ferretti G, Costa M, Ferrigno M, et al. Alveolar gas composition and exchange during deep breath-hold diving and dry breath holds in elite divers. *J Appl Physiol.* 1991;70(2):794–802.
16. Gray SW. Respiratory movements of rat during drowning and influence of water temperature upon survival after submersion. *Am J Physiol.* 1951;167(1):95–102.
17. Kvittingen TD, Naess A. Recovery from drowning in fresh water. *BMJ.* 1963;1(5341):1310.3.
18. Modell JH, Gabrielli A. Cardiopulmonary resuscitation following drowning. In: *Cardiopulmonary Resuscitation.* New York, NY: Springer; 2005:407–424.
19. Mouritzen C, Andersen M. Myocardial temperature gradients and ventricular fibrillation during hypothermia. *J Thorac Cardiovasc Surg.* 1965;49:937–944.
20. Modell JH. *The Pathophysiology and Treatment of Drowning and Near-Drowning.* New York, NY: Charles C Thomas Publisher; 1971.
21. Modell J. Drown versus near-drown: a discussion of definitions. *Crit Care Med.* 1981;9(4):351.
22. Modell JH, Bellefleur M, Davis JH. Drowning without aspiration: is this an appropriate diagnosis? *J Forens Sci.* 1999;44(6):1119–1123.
23. Lunetta P, Modell JH, Sajantila A. What is the incidence and significance of "dry-lungs" in bodies found in water? *Am J Forens Med Pathol.* 2004;25(4):291–301.
24. Lougheed D, Janes J, Hall G. Physiological studies in experimental asphyxia and drowning. *Can Med Assoc J.* 1939;40(5):423.
25. Halmagyi DF, Colebatch H. Ventilation and circulation after fluid aspiration. *J Appl Physiol.* 1961;16(1):35–40.
26. Colebatch H, Halmagyi D. Lung mechanics and resuscitation after fluid aspiration. *J Appl Physiol.* 1961;16(4):684–696.
27. Redding JS, Voigt GC, Safar P. Treatment of sea-water aspiration. *J Appl Physiol.* 1960;15(6):1113–1136.
28. Colebatch H, Halmagyi D. Reflex pulmonary hypertension of fresh-water aspiration. *J Appl Physiol.* 1963;18(1):179–185.
29. Colebatch H, Halmagyi D. Reflex airway reaction to fluid aspiration. *J Appl Physiol.* 1962;17(5):787–794.
30. Fainer DC, Martin CG, Ivy A. Resuscitation of dogs from fresh water drowning. *J Appl Physiol.* 1951;3(7):417–426.
31. Redding JS, Cozine RA. Restoration of circulation after fresh water drowning. *J Appl Physiol.* 1961;16(6):1071–1074.
32. Redding J, Voigt GC, Safar P. Drowning treated with intermittent positive pressure breathing. *J Appl Physiol.* 1960;15(5):849–854.
33. Modell JH, Moya F, Williams H, Weibley T. Changes in blood gases and A-aDO_2 during near-drowning. *Anesthesiology.* 1968;29(3):456–465.
34. Giammona ST, Modell JH. Drowning by total immersion: effects on pulmonary surfactant of distilled water, isotonic saline, and sea water. *Am J Dis Child.* 1967;114(6):612–616.
35. Spitz W, Blanke R. Mechanism of death in fresh-water drowning: 1. an experimental approach. *Arch Pathol.* 1961;71(1):661.
36. Modell JH, Davis JH, Giammona ST, et al. Blood gas and electrolyte changes in human near-drowning victims. *JAMA.* 1968;203(5):337–343.
37. Hasan S, Avery WG, Fabian C, Sackner MA. Near drowning in humans: a report of 36 patients. *Chest J.* 1971;59(2):191–197.
38. Fainer DC. Near drowning in sea water and fresh water. *Ann Intern Med.* 1963;59(4):537–541.
39. Fuller RH. The clinical pathology of human near-drowning. *Proc R Soc Med.* 1963;56(1):33.
40. Moritz AR. Chemical methods for the determination of death by drowning. *Physiol Rev.* 1944;24(1):70–88.
41. Butt M, Jalowayski A, Modell J, Giammona S. Pulmonary function after resuscitation from near-drowning. *Anesthesiology.* 1970;32(3):275.
42. Orlowski JP, Abulleil MM, Phillips JM. The hemodynamic and cardiovascular effects of near-drowning in hypotonic, isotonic, or hypertonic solutions. *Ann Emerg Med.* 1989;18(10):1044–1049.
43. Modell J, Kuck E, Ruiz B, Heinitsh H. Effect of intravenous vs. aspirated distilled water on serum electrolytes and blood gas tensions. *J Appl Physiol.* 1972;32(5):579–584.
44. Bergquist R, Vogelhut M, Modell J, et al. Comparison of ventilatory patterns in the treatment of freshwater near-drowning in dogs. *Anesthesiology.* 1980;52(2):142–148.
45. Tabeling BB, Modell JH. Fluid administration increases oxygen delivery during continuous positive pressure ventilation after freshwater near-drowning. *Crit Care Med.* 1983;11(9):693–696.
46. Yagil Y, Stalnikowicz R, Michaeli J, Mogle P. Near drowning in the Dead Sea: electrolyte imbalances and therapeutic implications. *Arch Intern Med.* 1985;145(1):50–53.
47. Grmec Š, Strnad M, Podgoršek D. Comparison of the characteristics and outcome among patients suffering from out-of-hospital primary cardiac arrest and drowning victims in cardiac arrest. *Int J Emerg Med.* 2009;2(1):7–12.
48. Smith M-L, Auer R, Siesjö B. The density and distribution of ischemic brain injury in the rat following 2–10 min of forebrain ischemia. *Acta Neuropathol.* 1984;64(4):319–332.
49. Topjian AA, Berg RA, Bierens JJ, et al. Brain resuscitation in the drowning victim. *Neurocrit Care.* 2012;17(3):441–467.
50. Hoek TLV, Morrison LJ, Shuster M, et al. Part 12: cardiac arrest in special situations 2010 American Heart Association guidelines for cardiopulmonary resuscitation and emergency cardiovascular care. *Circulation.* 2010;122(18 Suppl 3):S829–S861.
51. Szpilman D, Soares M. In-water resuscitation—is it worthwhile? *Resuscitation.* 2004;63(1):25–31.
52. Soar J, Perkins GD, Abbas G, et al. European Resuscitation Council Guidelines for Resuscitation 2010 Section 8. Cardiac arrest in special circumstances: electrolyte abnormalities, poisoning, drowning, accidental hypothermia, hyperthermia, asthma, anaphylaxis, cardiac surgery, trauma, pregnancy, electrocution. *Resuscitation.* 2010;81(10):1400–1433.

53. Rosen P, Stoto M, Harley J. The use of the Heimlich maneuver in near drowning: Institute of Medicine report. *J Emerg Med.* 1995;13(3): 397–405.
54. Conn AW, Montes JE, Barker GA, Edmonds JF. Cerebral salvage in near-drowning following neurological classification by triage. *Can Anaesth Soc J.* 1980;27(3):201–210.
55. Modell JH, Graves SA, Kuck EJ. Near-drowning: correlation of level of consciousness and survival. *Can Anaesth Soc J.* 1980;27(3):211–215.
56. Bohn DJ, Biggar WD, Smith CR, et al. Influence of hypothermia, barbiturate therapy, and intracranial pressure monitoring on morbidity and mortality after near-drowning. *Crit Care Med.* 1986;14(6):529–534.
57. Orlowski JP, Szpilman D. Drowning: rescue, resuscitation, and reanimation. *Pediatr Clin North Am.* 2001;48(3):627–646.
58. Lee KH. A retrospective study of near-drowning victims admitted to the intensive care unit. *Ann Acad Med Singapore.* 1998;27(3):344–346.
59. ARDS Definition Task Force; Ranieri VM, Rubenfeld GD, Thompson BT, et al. Acute respiratory distress syndrome: the Berlin Definition. *JAMA.* 2012;307(23):2526–2533.
60. Ruiz BC, Calderwood HW, Modell JH, Brogdon JE. Effect of ventilatory patterns on arterial oxygenation after near-drowning with fresh water: a comparative study in dogs. *Anesth Analg.* 1973;52(4):570–576.
61. Suter PM, Fairley B, Isenberg MD. Optimum end-expiratory airway pressure in patients with acute pulmonary failure. *N Engl J Med.* 1975; 292(6):284–289.
62. Modell JH, Calderwood HW, Ruiz BC, et al. Effects of ventilatory patterns on arterial oxygenation after near-drowning in sea water. *Anesthesiology.* 1974;40(4):376–384.
63. Antonelli M, Conti G, Rocco M, et al. A comparison of noninvasive positive-pressure ventilation and conventional mechanical ventilation in patients with acute respiratory failure. *N Engl J Med.* 1998;339(7):429–435.
64. Rabatin JT, Gay PC. Noninvasive ventilation. *Mayo Clin Proc.* 1999;74(8): 817–820.
65. Dellinger RP, Zimmerman JL, Taylor RW, et al. Effects of inhaled nitric oxide in patients with acute respiratory distress syndrome: results of a randomized phase II trial. Inhaled Nitric Oxide in ARDS Study Group. *Crit Care Med.* 1998;26(1):15–23.
66. Takano Y, Hirosako S, Yamaguchi T, et al. [Nitric oxide inhalation as an effective therapy for acute respiratory distress syndrome due to near-drowning: a case report.] *Nihon Kokyuki Gakkai Zasshi.* 1999;37(12): 997–1002.
67. Lee JM, Lee JH, Lee C-T, Cho Y-J. Successful recovery after drowning by early prone ventilatory positioning and use of nitric oxide gas: a case report. *Korean J Crit Care Med.* 2011;26(3):196–199.
68. Jolliet P, Bulpa P, Chevrolet JC. Effects of the prone position on gas exchange and hemodynamics in severe acute respiratory distress syndrome. *Crit Care Med.* 1998;26(12):1977–1985.
69. Pelosi P, Tubiolo D, Mascheroni D, et al. Effects of the prone position on respiratory mechanics and gas exchange during acute lung injury. *Am J Respir Crit Care Med.* 1998;157(2):387–393.
70. Petty TL, Reiss OK, Paul GW, et al. Characteristics of pulmonary surfactant in adult respiratory distress syndrome associated with trauma and shock. *Am Rev Respir Dis.* 1977;115(3):531–536.
71. Corbet A, Bucciarelli R, Goldman S, et al. Decreased mortality rate among small premature infants treated at birth with a single dose of synthetic surfactant: a multicenter controlled trial. American Exosurf Pediatric Study Group 1. *J Pediatr.* 1991;118(2):277–284.
72. Cubattoli L, Franchi F, Coratti G. Surfactant therapy for acute respiratory failure after drowning: two children victim of cardiac arrest. *Resuscitation.* 2009;80(9):1088–1089.
73. Suzuki H, Ohta T, Iwata K, et al. Surfactant therapy for respiratory failure due to near-drowning. *Eur J Pediatr.* 1996;155(5):383–384.
74. Onarheim H, Vik V. Porcine surfactant (Curosurf) for acute respiratory failure after neardrowning in 12 year old. *Acta Anaesthesiol Scand.* 2004;48(6):778–781.
75. Van Berkel M, Bierens J, Lie R, et al. Pulmonary oedema, pneumonia and mortality in submersion victims: a retrospective study in 125 patients. *Intensive Care Med.* 1996;22(2):101–107.
76. Bernard SA, Gray TW, Buist MD, et al. Treatment of comatose survivors of out-of-hospital cardiac arrest with induced hypothermia. *N Engl J Med.* 2002;346(8):557–563.
77. Mild therapeutic hypothermia to improve the neurologic outcome after cardiac arrest. *N Engl J Med.* 2002;346(8):549–556.
78. Nielsen N, Wetterslev J, Cronberg T, et al. Targeted temperature management at 33 C versus 36 C after cardiac arrest. *N Engl J Med.* 2013;369(23): 2197–2206.
79. Rittenberger JC, Callaway CW. Temperature management and modern post-cardiac arrest care. *N Engl J Med.* 2013;369(23):2262–2263.
80. Jacobs SE, Hunt R, Tarnow-Mordi WO, et al. Cooling for newborns with hypoxic ischaemic encephalopathy. *Evidence-Based Child Health Cochrane Rev J.* 2008;3(4):1049–1115.
81. Shah PS. Hypothermia: a systematic review and meta-analysis of clinical trials. *Semin Fetal Neonatal Med.* 2010;15(5):238–246.
82. Tagin MA, Woolcott CG, Vincer MJ, et al. Hypothermia for neonatal hypoxic ischemic encephalopathy: an updated systematic review and meta-analysis. *Arch Pediatr Adolesc Med.* 2012;166(6):558–566.
83. Biggart MJ, Boh DJ. Effect of hypothermia and cardiac arrest on outcome of near-drowning accidents in children. *J Pediatr.* 1990;117(2):179–183.
84. Guenther U, Varelmann D, Putensen C, Wrigge H. Extended therapeutic hypothermia for several days during extracorporeal membrane-oxygenation after drowning and cardiac arrest: two cases of survival with no neurological sequelae. *Resuscitation.* 2009;80(3):379–381.
85. Conn A, Edmonds J, Barker G. Near-drowning in cold fresh water: current treatment regimen. *Can Anaesth Soc J.* 1978;25(4):259–265.
86. Bohn DJ, Biggar WD, Smith CR, et al. Influence of hypothermia, barbiturate therapy, and intracranial pressure monitoring on morbidity and mortality after near-drowning. *Crit Care Med.* 1986;14(6):529–534.
87. Conn A, Modell J. Current neurological considerations in near-drowning (editorial). *Can Anaesth Soc J.* 1980;27:197.
88. Nussbaum E, Maggi JC. Pentobarbital therapy does not improve neurologic outcome in nearly drowned, flaccid-comatose children. *Pediatrics.* 1988;81(5):630–634.
89. Tagin M, Shah P, Lee K. Magnesium for newborns with hypoxic-ischemic encephalopathy: a systematic review and meta-analysis. *J Perinatol.* 2013;33(9):663–669.
90. Chaudhari T, McGuire W. Allopurinol for preventing mortality and morbidity in newborn infants with hypoxic-ischaemic encephalopathy. *Cochrane Database Syst Rev.* 2012;7:Cd006817.
91. Kaandorp JJ, Benders MJ, Rademaker CM, et al. Antenatal allopurinol for reduction of birth asphyxia induced brain damage (ALLO-Trial): a randomized double blind placebo controlled multicenter study. *BMC Pregn Childb.* 2010;10:8.
92. Ballesteros MA, Gutierrez-Cuadra M, Munoz P, Minambres E. Prognostic factors and outcome after drowning in an adult population. *Acta Anaesthesiol Scand.* 2009;53(7):935–940.
93. Fugate JE, Wijdicks EF, Mandrekar J, et al. Predictors of neurologic outcome in hypothermia after cardiac arrest. *Ann Neurol.* 2010;68(6):907–914.
94. Wijdicks EF, Hijdra A, Young GB, et al. Practice parameter: prediction of outcome in comatose survivors after cardiopulmonary resuscitation (an evidence-based review): report of the Quality Standards Subcommittee of the American Academy of Neurology. *Neurology.* 2006;67(2):203–210.
95. Zandbergen EG, Hijdra A, Koelman JH, et al. Prediction of poor outcome within the first 3 days of postanoxic coma. *Neurology.* 2006;66(1):62–68.
96. Mandel R, Martinot A, Delepoulle F, et al. Prediction of outcome after hypoxic–ischemic encephalopathy: a prospective clinical and electrophysiologic study. *J Pediatr.* 2002;141(1):45–50.
97. Rossetti AO, Oddo M, Logroscino G, Kaplan PW. Prognostication after cardiac arrest and hypothermia: a prospective study. *Ann Neurol.* 2010;67(3):301–307.
98. Nussbaum E, Galant SP. Intracranial pressure monitoring as a guide to prognosis in the nearly drowned, severely comatose child. *J Pediatr.* 1983; 102(2):215–218.
99. Tasker RC, Matthew DJ, Helms P, et al. Monitoring in non-traumatic coma. Part I: invasive intracranial measurements. *Arch Dis Child.* 1988; 63(8):888–894.
100. Carter BG, Butt W. A prospective study of outcome predictors after severe brain injury in children. *Intensive Care Med.* 2005 31(6):840–845.
101. Bouwes A, Binnekade JM, Verbaan BW, et al. Predictive value of neurological examination for early cortical responses to somatosensory evoked potentials in patients with postanoxic coma. *J Neurol.* 2012;259:537–541
102. Bosch X, Poch E, Grau JM. Rhabdomyolysis and acute kidney injury. *N Engl J Med.* 2009;361(1):62–72.
103. Better OS, Stein JH. Early management of shock and prophylaxis of acute renal failure in traumatic rhabdomyolysis. *N Engl J Med.* 1990;322(12): 825–829.
104. Eneas JF, Schoenfeld PY, Humphreys MH. The effect of infusion of mannitol-sodium bicarbonate on the clinical course of myoglobinuria. *Arch Intern Med.* 1979;139(7):801–805.
105. Bakker J, Gris P, Coffernils M, et al. Serial blood lactate levels can predict the development of multiple organ failure following septic shock. *Am J Surg.* 1996;171(2):221–226.

CHAPTER

112

Severe Asthma Exacerbation

PARASKEVI A. KATSAOUNOU, IOANNA SIGALA, and THEODOROS VASSILAKOPOULOS

DEFINITION AND CHARACTERISTICS OF SEVERE ASTHMA

Different Phenotypes

Asthma is a heterogeneous disease, usually characterized by chronic airway inflammation. It is defined by the history of respiratory symptoms such as wheezing, shortness of breath, chest tightness, and cough that vary over time and in intensity, together with variable expiratory airflow limitation (1). The prevalence of severe asthma is 5% to 10% (1–3) or lower (4); despite this low prevalence, it is responsible for 50% of asthma costs and some of the near-fatal asthma episodes.

It is imperative to use a recognized common definition of severe asthma to distinguish other terms and definitions that are usually included in its definition or used as synonyms (Table 112.1). Because of the complexity of asthma as a disease—which is mostly a collection of different phenotypes, rather than a single, specific disease with a unifying pathogenic mechanism—various clinical definitions have been proposed through national and international guidelines, working groups, and workshops, which incorporate symptoms, lung function, exacerbations, and treatment (1,2,5–7). In the original European Network description, patients with severe asthma were defined as those who were difficult to control after evaluation and treatment by an asthma specialist for a year or more (5,6).

The definition of severe asthma has been recently updated for patients aged more than 6 years old by the European Respiratory Society/American Thoracic Society Task Force on Severe Asthma (2). Asthma severity can be assessed retrospectively after an asthmatic patient has been on regular controller treatment for several months, from the level of treatment required to control his/her symptoms and exacerbations (1,2,5,6). Therefore, severe asthma is defined as disease requiring medications according to GINA steps 4 and 5 of asthma treatment (Table 112.2) in order to be "controlled" or which remains "uncontrolled" (Table 112.3) (1,2) despite this therapy. Although asthma is usually controllable if guidelines for asthma management are strictly followed, a minority of asthma patients remain difficult to control even with maximal therapy. Therefore, before establishing the definition of severe asthma, it is mandatory to distinguish it from uncontrolled disease (Table 112.4) (1,2). To do so, comorbidities, alternative diagnosis, and adherence and exposure to triggers should be assessed. Then, severe asthma is reserved for patients with refractory disease and those in whom response to treatment of comorbidities is incomplete. Asthma control has two domains (Table 112.5): symptom control and future risk of adverse outcomes.

The previously used term "current clinical control" has been renamed "symptom control" in order to emphasize that these measures are not sufficient for assessment of disease control, since future risk assessment for adverse outcomes is also needed. "Independent" risk factors are those that are significant after adjustment for the level of symptom control. Poor symptom control and exacerbation risk should not be simply combined numerically, as they may have different causes and may need different treatment strategies (1,2). To conclude, severe asthma treatment consists of high-dose inhaled corticosteroids (ICS) (Table 112.6), plus a second controller (LABA [long-acting beta agonist] or leukotriene modifier/theophylline) and/or systemic corticosteroids (CS) (1,2).

Since severe asthma is a heterogenic disease with a variety of clinical presentations, physiologic characteristics, and outcomes, asthma phenotyping has emerged. A phenotype is defined as the integration of different characteristics that are the product of the interaction of the patient's genes with the environment. At least four to six phenotypes of severe asthma have been identified (Fig. 112.1). The value of phenotyping is to increase understanding of the pathophysiology and natural history of the disease and link specific phenotypes to genotypes in order to develop targeted treatments. The phenotyping can be done from very different perspectives. Numerous attempts at classifying potential phenotypes of severe asthma have been proposed. Although these phenotypes may overlap, there is reasonable supporting evidence for the presence of at least six—and likely more—severe asthma phenotypes (Table 112.7; Fig. 112.1), as defined by clinical parameters (natural history, clinical presentation, atopy, airflow obstruction), type of inflammation, and treatment-related parameters (1,8–13).

Therefore, some patients with severe asthma may use phenotype-guided add-on treatment (1,2). Patients with severe allergic asthma, in which there are elevated IgE levels, may benefit from anti-IgE therapy (Evidence A), and leukotriene receptor antagonists (LRTAs) may be helpful for patients found to be aspirin sensitive (Evidence B). Other potential phenotype-targeted therapies in severe asthma are shown in Table 112.8.

From a clinical point of view, three categories of patients with severe asthma seem to be of particular importance:

- those with frequent severe asthma exacerbations
- those with fixed airway obstruction
- those with oral steroid dependency

Together, these three categories cover most of the patients classified with difficult-to-control asthma.

PATHOPHYSIOLOGY

Respiratory Mechanics

The main pathophysiologic mechanism of acute severe asthma is pulmonary hyperinflation (14) caused by a combination of factors (Fig. 112.2). The driving force for expiratory flow is reduced because of an abnormally low pulmonary elastic recoil, the etiology of which is uncertain (15,16). Persistent activation of the inspiratory muscles during expiration causes

TABLE 112.1 Terms and Definitions in Severe Asthma

Term	Definition
Severe asthma (ERS/ATS, 2014)	• Asthma that requires treatment with high-dose ICS and LABA (or leukotriene modifier/theophylline) for the previous year or systemic CS for ≥50% of the previous year to prevent it from becoming "uncontrolled" or which remains "uncontrolled" despite this therapy • Controlled asthma that worsens on tapering of these high doses of ICS or systemic CS (or additional biologics)
Severe persistent asthma (NHLBI/GINA, 2006)	Continual symptoms, frequent nocturnal symptoms, limited activity, frequent exacerbations, FEV_1 or PEV < 60% predicted, PEF variability > 30%
Severe/refractory asthma (ATS workshop consensus, 2000)	Definition requires at least one major criterion and two minor criteria are met, other disorders have been excluded, exacerbating factors have been treated, and patient is generally compliant. Major: • Treatment requires continuous or near continuous (≥50% of year) oral corticosteroids • Treatment requires high dose (>880 μg/d fluticasone or equivalent) inhaled corticosteroids Minor: • Asthma symptoms needing short-acting β-agonist use on a daily or near-daily basis • Need for additional daily treatment with a controller medication (e.g., long-acting β-agonist, theophylline, or leukotriene antagonist) • Persistent airway obstruction (FEV_1 < 80% predicted, diurnal peak expiratory flow variability >20%) • One or more urgent care visits for asthma per year • Three or more oral steroid bursts per year • Prompt clinical deterioration with ≤25% reduction in oral or intravenous corticosteroid dose • Near-fatal asthma event in the past
Severe asthma (ENFUMOSA, 1999)	Diagnosis requires at least three of the following: • Seen by a consultant in asthma >2 per year • Has persistent symptoms and decreased symptoms quality of life • Has received maximal asthma therapy (high dose ICS) with documented adherence • History of respiratory failure/intubation • Has repeated low FEV_1 (<70% predicted)
Status asthmaticus	Severe airway obstruction and asthmatic symptoms persist despite the administration of standard acute asthma therapy
Difficult to treat asthma	Failure to achieve asthma control when maximally recommended doses of inhaled therapy are prescribed for at least 6–12 mo. Ongoing factors such as comorbidities, poor adherence, and allergen exposure interfere with achieving good asthma control.
Refractory asthma	Asthmatic patients with confirmed asthma diagnosis whose symptoms or exacerbations remain poorly controlled despite high dose ICS plus a second controller and/or systemic corticosteroids and management of comorbidities or whose asthma control deteriorates when this treatment is stepped down.
Steroid-resistant asthma (1993)	Failure of FEV_1 or PEF to improve >15% after 14-d course of, at least, 40 mg/d of prednisone.
Steroid-dependent asthma	Asthma that can be controlled only with oral corticosteroids, but in contrast to corticosteroid-resistant there is a response to corticosteroids, although only when high doses are given.
Irreversible asthma (1998)	Persistent airflow obstruction despite maximum controller therapy: presumably related to airway and parenchymal structural alterations.
Near-fatal asthma (1991)	Attack associated with respiratory failure, intubation, and/or hemodynamic and metabolic compromise.
Fixed airway obstruction	Persistent airflow obstruction despite maximal controller therapy; presumably related to airway and parenchymal structural alterations.
Brittle asthma (1971)	Unstable, unpredictable asthmatics with wide variability in PEF Type I: persistent PEF variability (>40%) despite controller therapy Type II: prone to sudden, dramatic falls in PEF
Asthma related to specific triggers or circumstances	Premenstrual asthma: Worsening of asthma 7 d premenstrually Aspirin-induced asthma Exercise-induced asthma

TABLE 112.2 Asthma Treatment for Severe Asthma

	Step 4	Step 5
Controller		
Preferred controller choice	Medium/high ICS/LABA	High ICS/LABA Refer for add-on treatment (e.g., IgE)
Other controller options	Low dose ICS + LTRA (or theophylline) Tiotropium	Low-dose OCS Tiotropium Refer for add-on treatment (e.g., IgE)
Reliever	As needed SABA or low-dose ICS/formoterol	

Adapted from Global Initiative for Asthma. Global strategy for asthma management and prevention 2015. Available: http://ginasthma.org/

outward recoil of the chest wall, further reducing the driving force for expiration (17). At the same time, resistance to airflow is greatly augmented because of severely reduced airway caliber and, perhaps, also narrowing of the glottic aperture during expiration (18). Expiration is prolonged, so that the following inspiration starts before static equilibrium is reached. Consequently, the end-expiratory alveolar pressure remains positive, a phenomenon known as auto-PEEP or intrinsic PEEP ($PEEP_i$) (19,20).

It should be noted that the lung is extremely inhomogeneous during an episode of acute severe asthma. The distribution of bronchial obstruction is uneven because of both anatomical reasons—variable amounts of secretions, edema,

TABLE 112.3 Uncontrolled Asthma

Defined as at least one of the below:

Poor symptom control

- Asthma Control Questionnaire consistently >1.5
- Asthma Control Test <20
- Or "not well controlled" by NAEPP/GINA guidelines

Frequent severe exacerbations

- ≥2 bursts of systemic corticosteroids (>3 d each) in the previous year

Serious exacerbations

- ≥1 hospitalization, ICU stay, or mechanical ventilation in the previous year

Airflow limitation

- FEV_1 < 80% predicted (in the face of reduced FEV_1/FVC defined as less than the lower limit of normal)

Controlled asthma that worsens on tapering of high doses of inhaled corticosteroids (see Table 112.6) or systemic corticosteroids or additional biologics

bronchospasm—and variable external compression exerted on the distal airways by intrathoracic positive pressure during expiration (21). Thus, illustratively, four parallel compartments can be recognized (Fig. 112.3): compartment A represents the portion of the lung with neither bronchial obstruction nor hyperinflation; compartment B is the part of the lung where the airways are entirely obstructed during the whole respiratory cycle (mucous plugging); in compartment C obstruction appears only during expiration, inducing alveolar hyperinflation and high $PEEP_i$; in compartment D partial obstruction of the airways is present throughout the respiratory cycle causing a lesser extent of alveolar hyperinflation and $PEEP_i$ than in compartment C.

Hyperinflation has several detrimental consequences (22). Firstly, the load the inspiratory muscles are facing is increased for a variety of reasons. As already noted, expiration ends before the respiratory system reaches elastic equilibrium at functional residual capacity (FRC), and thus a positive elastic

TABLE 112.4 Distinguishing between Severe and Uncontrolled Asthma

Confirm asthma diagnosis
• The asthma diagnosis should have been confirmed, evaluated and managed from an asthma specialist for more than 3 mo.
• If evidence of variable airflow limitation on spirometry or other testing consider halving ICS dose and repeating lung function after 2–3 wk.
• Check if patient has action plan.
• Consider referring for challenge test.
	Check for:
	• Recurrent respiratory infections
	• Upper airway dysfunction
	• Concurrent COPD
	• Diseases that mimic asthma
	  • Bronchiectasis
	  • Constrictive bronchiolitis
	  • COD
	  • CHF
	  • ABPA
	  • Churg–Strauss syndrome
	  • Eosinophilic pneumonia
	  • Thyrotoxicosis

Investigate for comorbidities	• Chronic sinusitis/ nasal polyps • Obesity • Gastroesophageal reflux disease • Obstructive sleep apnea • Psychological/psychiatric disorders (personality trait, symptom perception, anxiety, depression) • Vocal cord dysfunction • Hyperventilation syndrome • Hormonal influences (premenstrual, menarche, menopause, thyroid disorders)
Check for incorrect inhaler use and adherence • Dry powder inhalers may be used to deliver short-acting β_2-agonist as an alternative to pressurized metered dose inhaler and spacer during worsening asthma or exacerbations. • Watch patients use their inhaler; check again inhaler checklist. • Show correct method and recheck up to 3 times. Recheck each time. • Have empathic discussion to identify poor adherence. • Ask about beliefs, cost of medications and refill frequency. Check if the patient has a written asthma action plan. • Ask about the patient's attitudes and goals for their asthma and medication.	Medication/regimen factors: • Difficulties using inhaler device (e.g., arthritis) • Burdensome regimen (e.g., multiple times per day) • Multiple different inhalers Unintentional poor adherence: • Misunderstanding about instructions • Forgetfulness • Absence of a daily routine • Cost Intentional poor adherence: • Perception that treatment is not necessary • Denial or anger about asthma or its treatment • Inappropriate expectations • Concerns about side effects (real or perceived) • Dissatisfaction with health care providers • Stigmatization • Cultural or religious issues • Cost
Check persistent exposure to triggers • Triggers at home or workplace should be removed wherever possible.	• Exposure to tobacco smoke • Occupational sensitizers • Dietary factors • Drugs (NSAIDs, β-blockers, aspirin, ACE inhibitors) • Unidentified allergens (fungal infections, molds)

ACE, angiotensin converting enzyme; NSAIDs, nonsteroidal anti-inflammatory drugs.

Adapted from Global Initiative for Asthma. Global strategy for asthma management and prevention 2015. Available: http://ginasthma.org/; and Chung KF, Wenzel SE, Brozek JL, et al. International ERS/ATS guidelines on definition, evaluation and treatment of severe asthma. *Eur Respir J.* 2014;43:343–373.

TABLE 112.5 Assessment of Asthma Control in Adults, Adolescents, and Children 6–11 Years Old

	Asthma Symptom Control			Level of Asthma Symptom Control		
Current Clinical Control	**In the past 4 wk, has the patient had:**	**Yes**	**No**	**Well controlled**	**Partly controlled**	**Uncontrolled**
	Daytime asthma symptoms more than twice/week?			None of these	1–2 of these	3–4 of these
	Any night waking due to asthma?					
	Reliever needed for symptoms* more than twice/week?					
	Any activity limitation due to asthma?					
Risk Factors for Poor Asthma Outcomes						
Future risk of adverse outcomes	**Potentially modifiable independent risk factors for flare-ups (exacerbations)**					
	Uncontrolled asthma symptoms				Having ≥1 increases the risk of exacerbations even if symptoms are well controlled	
	High SABA use (with increased mortality if >1 × 200-dose canister/mo)					
	Inadequate ICS					
	Poor adherence					
	Incorrect inhaler technique					
	Exposures: smoking; allergen exposure if sensitized					
	Comorbidities:					
	Obesity, rhinosinusitis, confirmed food allergy					
	Sputum or blood eosinophilia					
	Pregnancy					
	Low FEV_1, especially if <60% predicted					
	Major psychological or socioeconomic problems					
	Other major independent risk factors for flare-ups (exacerbations)					
	Ever intubated or in intensive care unit for asthma				Having ≥1 increases the risk of exacerbations even if symptoms are well controlled	
	≥1 severe exacerbation in last 12 mo					
	Risk factors for developing fixed airflow limitation					
	Lack of ICS treatment					
	Exposures: tobacco smoke, noxious chemicals, occupational exposures					
	Low initial FEV_1, chronic mucus hypersecretion, sputum or blood eosinophilia					
	Risk factors for medication side effects					
	Systemic: frequent OCS, long-term, high-dose and/or potent ICS; also taking P450 inhibitors					
	Local: high-dose or potent ICS, poor inhaler technique					

FEV_1, forced expiratory volume in 1 s; ICS, inhaled corticosteroid; OCS, oral corticosteroid; P450 inhibitors, cytochrome P450 inhibitors such as ritonavir, ketoconazole, itraconazole; SABA, short-acting β_2-agonist.
*Excludes reliever taken before exercise.
Adapted from Global Initiative for Asthma. Global strategy for asthma management and prevention 2015. Available: http://ginasthma.org/.

TABLE 112.6 Definition of High Daily Dose of Various ICSs in Relation to Patient Age

	Threshold Daily Dose in Mg Considered as High	
Inhaled Corticosteroid	**Age 6–12 yr**	**Age >12 yr**
Beclomethasone dipropionate	≥800 (DPI or CFC MDI) ≥320 (HFA MDI)	≥2,000 (DPI or CFC MDI) ≥1,000 (HFA MDI)
Budesonide	≥800 (MDI or DPI)	≥1,600 (MDI or DPI)
Ciclesonide	≥160 (HFA MDI)	≥320 (HFA MDI)
Fluticasone propionate	≥500 (HFA MDI or DPI)	≥000 (HFA MDI or DPI)
Mometasone furoate	≥500 (DPI)	≥800 (DPI)
Triamcinolone acetonide	≥1,200	≥2,000

CFC, chlorofluorocarbon; DPI, dry powder inhaler; HFA, hydrofluoroalkane; MDI, metered-dose inhaler.
As CFC preparations are being taken from the market, medication inserts for HFA preparations should be carefully reviewed by the clinician for the equivalent correct dosage.
Adapted from Global Initiative for Asthma. Global strategy for asthma management and prevention 2015. Available: http://ginasthma.org/; and Chung KF, Wenzel SE, Brozek JL, et al. International ERS/ATS guidelines on definition, evaluation and treatment of severe asthma. *Eur Respir J.* 2014;43:343–373.

recoil pressure ($PEEP_i$) remains. During the next inspiration, the inspiratory muscles have to develop an equal amount of pressure before the airway pressure becomes negative (subatmospheric), with subsequent initiation of airflow. Secondly, due to hyperinflation tidal breathing occurs at a steeper portion of the pressure–volume curve of the lung, further increasing the load. Thirdly, as FRC increases, tidal breathing may take place at that portion of the chest wall static pressure–volume curve where either positive recoil pressure exists, i.e., the chest wall tends to move inwards, or its expanding tendency is reduced. This is contrasted with the tendency of the chest wall to expand when tidal breathing begins from normal FRC. Furthermore, with severe hyperinflation, the marked flattening of the diaphragm causes its costal and crural fibers to be arranged in series and perpendicularly to the chest wall. Contraction of these perpendicularly oriented fibers results in paradoxical inward movement of the lower rib cage. This distortion of the chest wall during inspiration elevates the elastic load. In summary, hyperinflation imposes a threshold load to initiate breathing and greatly augments the elastic load once breathing has started. Of course, acute severe asthma also increases the resistive load to breathe due to the obstruction of the

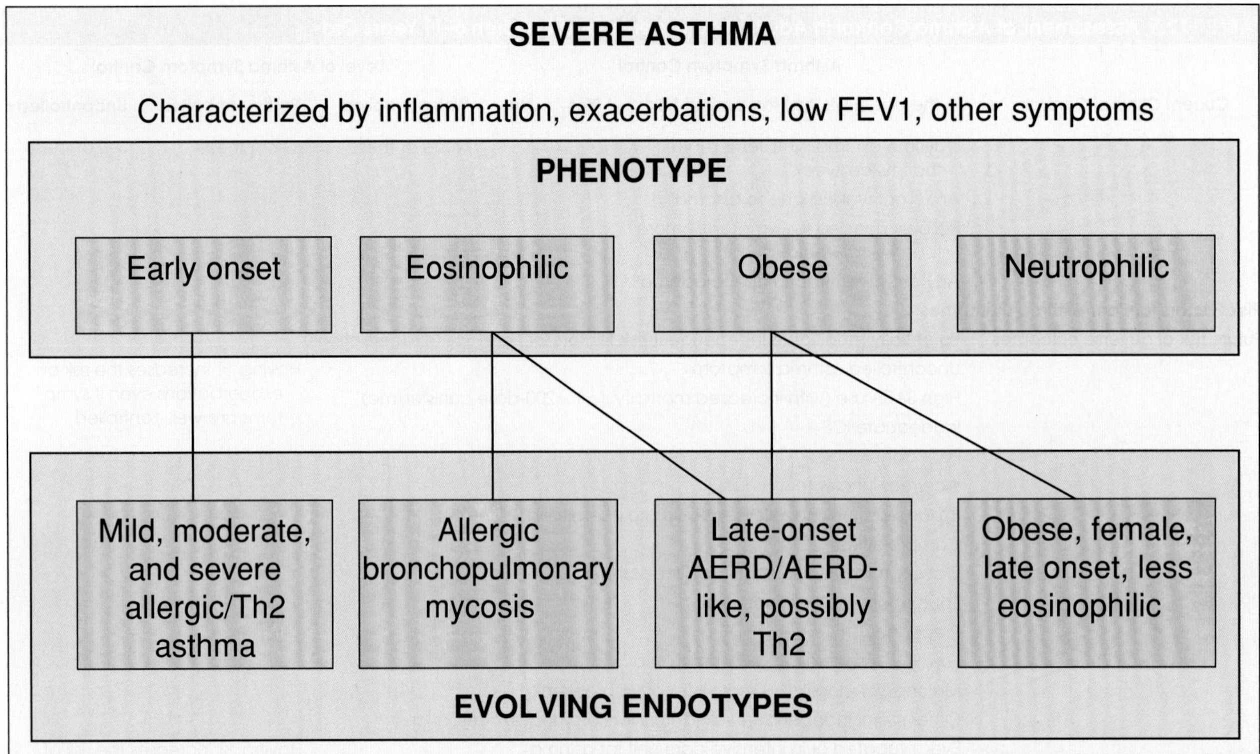

FIGURE 112.1 Severe asthma phenotypes. (Adapted from Wenzel S. Severe asthma: from characteristics to phenotypes to endotypes. *Clin Exp Allergy.* 2012;42:650–658.)

airways caused by bronchoconstriction, copious secretions, and mucous plugging.

At the same time that the load is severely increased, hyperinflation compromises the force generating capacity of the diaphragm for a variety of reasons (Fig. 112.4) (22,23). First, the respiratory muscles, like other skeletal muscles, obey the length–tension relationship (Fig. 112.5). At any given level of activation, changes in muscle fiber length alter tension development. This is because the force-tension developed by a muscle depends on the interaction between actin and myosin fibrils, i.e., the number of myosin heads attaching and thus pulling the actin fibrils closer within each sarcomere. The optimal fiber length (L_o) where tension is maximal is the length at which all myosin heads attach and pull the actin fibrils. Below this length (as with hyperinflation which shortens the diaphragm) actin–myosin interaction becomes suboptimal and tension development declines. Second, as lung volume increases, the zone of apposition of the diaphragm decreases in size, and a larger fraction of the rib cage becomes exposed to pleural pressure

TABLE 112.7 Phenotypes of Asthma

Natural history
- Early-onset (childhood-onset)
- Late-onset (adult-onset)

Type of airway inflammation
- Predominantly eosinophilic
- Predominantly neutrophilic
- Pauci-inflammatory phenotype

Response to treatment
- Steroid dependent
- Steroid resistant
- Steroid-sensitive

Severity
- Mild
- Moderate
- Severe
- Near-fatal asthma
- Fatal asthma

Pattern of bronchoconstriction
- Brittle
- Stable
- Fixed obstruction

Presence or absence of atopy
- Atopic
- Nonatopic

Major trigger factor
- Gastric asthma
- Aspirin-sensitive asthma
- Hormonal asthma

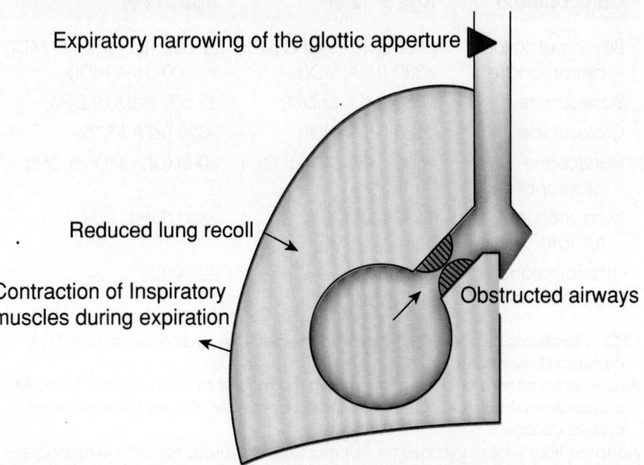

FIGURE 112.2 Mechanisms responsible for dynamic hyperinflation in asthma.

TABLE 112.8 Potential Phenotype-Targeted Therapies in Severe Asthma

Characteristic	Associations	Specifically Targeted Treatments
Severe allergic asthma	Blood and sputum eosinophils High serum IgE high FeNO	Anti-IgE (adults and children) Anti-IL-4/IL-13 Anti-IL-4 receptor
Eosinophilic asthma	Blood and sputum eosinophils Recurrent exacerbations High FeNO	Anti-IL-5 Anti-IL-4/IL-13 Anti-IL-4 receptor
Neutrophilic asthma (rare in children)	Corticosteroid insensitivity Bacterial infections	Anti-IL-8 CXCR2 antagonists Anti-LTB4 (adults and children) Macrolides (adults and children)
Chronic airflow obstruction	Airway wall remodeling as increased airway wall thickness	Anti-IL-13 Bronchial thermoplasty
Recurrent exacerbations	Sputum eosinophils in sputum Reduced response to ICS and/or OCS	Anti-IL5 Anti-IgE (adults and children)
Corticosteroid insensitivity	Increased neutrophils in sputum	p38 MAPK inhibitors Theophylline (adults and children) Macrolides (adults and children)

FeNO, exhaled nitric oxide fraction; IL, interleukin; LTB4, leukotriene B4; ICS, inhaled corticosteroid; OCS, oral corticosteroid; MAPK, mitogenactivated protein kinase.
Unless otherwise stated, these potential treatments apply to adults.
Adapted from Chung KF, Wenzel SE, Brozek JL, et al. International ERS/ATS guidelines on definition, evaluation and treatment of severe asthma. *Eur Respir J.* 2014;43:343–373.

(see Fig. 112.3). Hence, the diaphragm's inspiratory action on the rib cage diminishes. When lung volume approaches total lung capacity, the zone of apposition all but disappears (see Fig. 112.4), and the diaphragmatic muscle fibers become oriented horizontally internally. The insertional force of the diaphragm is then expiratory, rather than inspiratory, in direction. Third, the resulting flattening of the diaphragm increases its radius of curvature (R_{di}) and, thus, diminishes its pressure-generating capacity (P_{di}) for the same tension development (T_{di}). This is because when a muscle contracts it generates tension, not pressure. Because of the geometry of the diaphragm, tension (T_{di}) is transformed into pressure (P_{di}), obeying the law of Laplace which states:

$$P_{di} = 2T_{di}/R_{di}$$

where R_{di} is the radius of the curvature of the diaphragm (see Fig. 112.4).

The imbalance between the load faced by the respiratory muscles and their capacity to develop force (22) results in dyspnea (22–25) and predisposes the respiratory muscle to the development of fatigue (22,23), which is a terminal event,

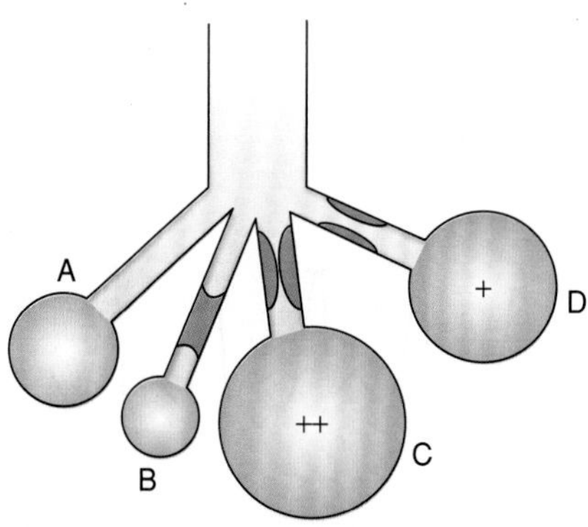

FIGURE 112.3 Effect of varying amounts of airway obstruction on end-expiratory alveolar volumes and pressures. (Adapted from Oddo M, Feihl F, Schaller MD, et al. Heliox improves pulsus paradoxus and peak expiratory flow in nonintubated patients with severe asthma. *Intensive Care Med.* 2006;32:501–510.)

likely to be present in asthmatic crisis necessitating intubation and mechanical ventilation (MV).

Gas Exchange

Widespread occlusion of the airways leads to development of extensive areas of alveolar units in which ventilation (V) is severely reduced but perfusion (Q) is maintained, i.e., areas with very low V/Q ratios, frequently lower than 0.1. Intrapulmonary shunt appears to be rare in the majority of patients because of the collateral ventilation and the effectiveness of the hypoxic pulmonary vasoconstriction (26,27). Hypoxemia is, therefore, common in every asthmatic crisis of some severity; mild hypoxia is easily corrected with the administration of relatively low concentrations of supplemental oxygen. More severe hypoxemia and the need for higher concentrations of supplemental oxygen may relate to some contribution of shunt physiology.

Dead space increases substantially in most severe cases, due to alveolar overdistention, i.e., areas with very high V/Q ratios (27,28). This is accompanied by increased CO_2 production due to the increased work performed by the respiratory muscles. The respiratory muscles are unable to further increase minute ventilation and thus hypercapnia ensues. However, even if minute ventilation were increased, it might not correct hypercapnia because it would lead to a vicious cycle of worsening hyperinflation with more alveolar overdistention and thus increased dead space (27,28). It should be noted, nevertheless, that in milder attacks reflex hyperventilation may lead to hypocapnia; however, as the severity of asthma attack increases, PCO_2 builds up first toward normal levels, and then, as respiratory failure impends, to supra-normal values.

Cardiovascular System Effects

Acute, severe asthma may also compromise hemodynamics. During expiration, due to the presence of dynamic hyperinflation, increased intrathoracic pressure impedes venous return. During the ensuing inspiration, forceful inspiratory muscle contraction renders intrathoracic pressure negative again,

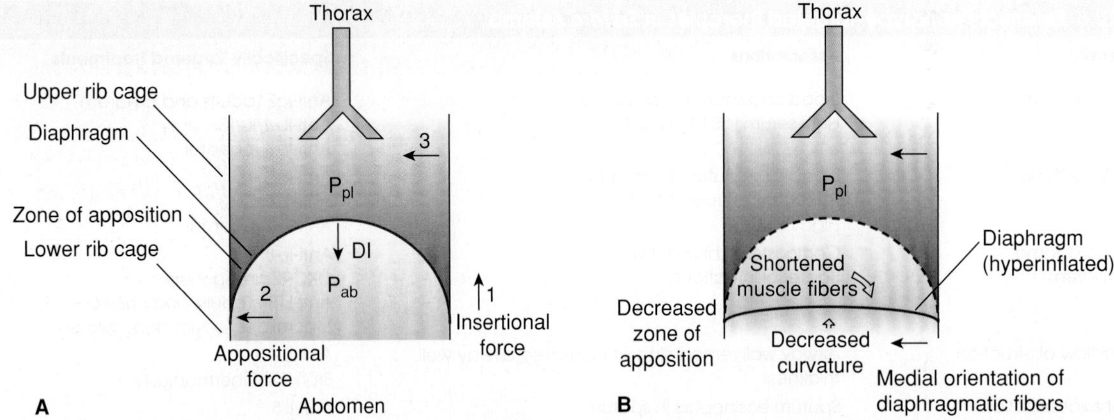

FIGURE 112.4 A: Actions of the diaphragm: When the diaphragm contracts, a caudally oriented force is being applied on the central tendon and the dome of the diaphragm descends (DI). Furthermore, the costal diaphragmatic fibers apply a cranially oriented force to the upper margins of the lower six ribs that has the effect of lifting and rotating them outward (insertional force, *arrow 1*). The zone of apposition makes the lower rib cage part of the abdomen and the changes in pressure in the pleural recess between the apposed diaphragm and the rib cage are almost equal to the changes in abdominal pressure. Pressure in this pleural recess rises rather than falls during inspiration because of diaphragmatic descent, and the rise in abdominal pressure is transmitted through the apposed diaphragm to expand the lower rib cage (*arrow 2*). All these effects result in expansion of the lower rib cage. On the upper rib cage, isolated contraction of the diaphragm causes a decrease in the anteroposterior diameter and this expiratory action is primarily due to the fall in pleural pressure (*arrow 3*). B: Deleterious effects of hyperinflation on the diaphragm.

rapidly increasing venous return. Rapid right ventricular filling during inspiration shifts the interventricular septum toward the left ventricle, leading to its incomplete filling during diastole, and thus, to left ventricular diastolic dysfunction. The large negative intrathoracic pressure generated during inspiration increases left ventricular afterload and impairs systolic emptying (22). Pulmonary artery pressure may also be increased due to lung hyperinflation, thereby resulting in increased right ventricular afterload (22). These events in acute, severe asthma may accentuate the normal inspiratory reduction in left ventricular stroke volume and systolic pressure, leading to the appearance of *pulsus paradoxus*, defined as a reduction of greater than 10 mmHg of the arterial systolic pressure during inspiration (Fig. 112.6) (29,30). A variation greater than 12 mmHg in systolic blood pressure between inspiration and expiration represents a sign of severity in asthmatic crisis. In advanced stages, when ventilatory muscle fatigue ensues, pulsus paradoxus (31) will decrease or disappear as force generation declines. This finding is a harbinger of impeding respiratory arrest.

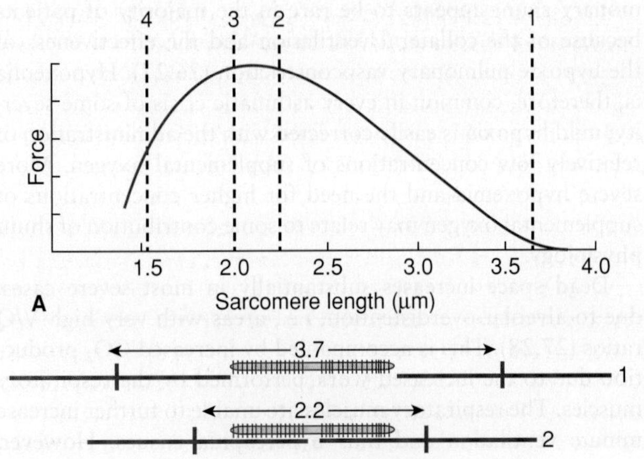

FIGURE 112.5 Isometric force at different sarcomere lengths. A: Force generated. B: Arrangements of actin-myosin filaments at different sarcomere lengths. The optimal length is where all myosin heads belonging to each myosin fibril come into contact (and thus exert attracting force) with actin filaments. At lengths less than 2.0 μm, actin filaments begin to overlap, and at still shorter lengths, the myosin filaments come into contact. At lengths greater than 2 μm, increasing numbers of myosin heads do not come into contact with actin filaments. Values are for frog muscle. Mammalian actin (thin) filaments are slightly longer so the corresponding sarcomere lengths are 1, 4.0 μm; 2, 2.5 μm; 3, 2.4 μm; and 4, 1.6 μm. (Adapted from Gordon AM, Huxley AF, Julian FJ. The variation in isometric tension with sarcomere length in vertebrate muscle fibres. *J Physiol.* 1966;184:170–192.)

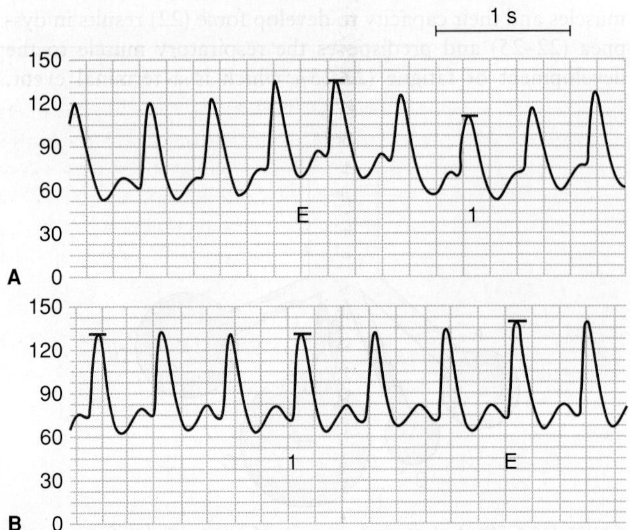

FIGURE 112.6 Arterial pressure of an asthmatic patient when breathing air (A) and heliox (B). Pulsus paradoxus was lower when the patient was breathing heliox. E, expiration; I, inspiration. (Adapted from Manthous CA, Hall JB, Caputo MA, et al. *Am J Respir Crit Care Med.* 1995;151:310–314.)

Clinicopathologic Patterns of Asthmatic Attacks

Exacerbations

Asthma exacerbations represent an acute or subacute worsening in symptoms and lung function from the patient's usual status, or in some cases, the initial presentation of asthma (1). The precise definition of a severe asthmatic exacerbation is an issue that presents difficulties. The terms *episodes*, *attacks*, and *acute severe asthma* are also often used, but they have variable meanings. The term *flare-up* is preferred for use in asthmatic patients (1).

Acute asthma exacerbations may have different levels of severity, as shown in Table 112.9.

Critical asthma syndrome represents the most severe subset of asthma exacerbations, and the critical asthma syndrome is an umbrella term for *life-threatening asthma*, status asthmaticus, and *near-fatal asthma*. The term *status asthmaticus* relates severity to outcome and has been used to define a severe asthmatic exacerbation that does not respond—the quantification of responsiveness has limitations—to and/or responds in a delayed manner to repetitive or continuous administration of short-acting inhaled β_2-adrenergic receptor agonists (SABA) in the emergency setting.

The term *acute severe asthma* is widely used, and relates to the severe presenting signs, symptoms, and cardio respiratory abnormalities observed. However, the presentation does not foretell outcome.

TABLE 112.9 Levels of Severity of Acute Asthma Exacerbations

Near-fatal asthma	Raised $PaCO_2$ and/or requiring mechanical ventilation with elevated inflation pressures
Life-threatening asthma	Any one of the following in a patient with severe asthma: • PEF < 33% best or predicted • SpO_2 < 92% • PaO_2 < 8 kPa • Normal $PaCO_2$ • Exhaustion • Silent chest • Bradycardia • Arrhythmia • Coma • Feeble respiratory effort • Cyanosis • Confusion • Hypotension
Acute severe asthma	Any one of: • PEF 33–50% best or predicted • Respiratory rate ≥5 breaths/min • Heart rate ≥110 beats/min • Inability to complete sentences in one breath
Moderate asthma exacerbation	Increasing symptoms • PEF >50–75% best or predicted • No features of acute severe asthma
Status asthmaticus	Severe asthmatic exacerbation that does not respond to SABA
Brittle asthma	**Type 1:** wide PEF variability (>40% diurnal variation for > 0% of the time over a period >150 d) despite intense therapy **Type 2:** sudden severe attacks on a background of apparently well-controlled asthma

Near-fatal asthma (NFA) defines mainly the resolution of a severe asthmatic exacerbation in a patient previously admitted into the ICU and/or mechanically supported. Although, most often, severe asthmatic exacerbation results from asthmatic patients with severe or uncontrolled asthma, any patient with asthma may experience a severe asthmatic exacerbation during his/her life. Occasionally, acute severe asthma may present as a new problem in a patient who is unaware of having asthma and the diagnosis has to be established at the emergency department (ED).

The time course of the asthmatic crisis, as well as the severity of airway obstruction, may vary broadly. Exacerbations usually occur in response to exposure to common allergens and external agents (viral upper respiratory tract infection, pollen or pollution, nonsteroidal anti-inflammatory agents, food allergens) and/or poor adherence with controller medication; however, a subset of patients present more acutely and without exposure to known risk factors. The group of asthmatic patients that fall into the category of fatal asthma are usually those with difficult to treat asthma, although theoretically all asthmatics may experience a severe exacerbation. Severe exacerbations can occur even in patients with mild or well-controlled asthma. Patients who are at increased risk of asthma-related death should be identified, and flagged for more frequent review. These patients include those with/who:

- Have a history of near-fatal asthma requiring intubation and MV
- Have had a hospitalization or emergency care visit for asthma in the last year
- Are currently using or have recently stopped using oral glucocorticosteroids
- Are not currently using inhaled glucocorticosteroids
- Are overdependent on rapid-acting inhaled β_2-agonists, especially those who use more than one canister of salbutamol (or equivalent) monthly
- Have repeated presentation to the ED for asthma care, especially if in the last year
- Have brittle asthma
- Have a history of noncompliance with an asthma medication plan
- Have home exposure to air conditioning and dusty conditions
- Male gendered
- Have atopy and sensitivity to *Altenaria* spp.
- Have a difference in perception of dyspnea
- Are more than 40 years of age
- Have a smoking history
- Have hyperinflation on chest radiograph
- Receive suboptimal medical advice
- Failure to attend appointments
- Have had self-discharge from hospital
- Have a history of psychiatric disease (psychosis, depression, other psychiatric illness, or deliberate self-harm) or psychosocial problems (denial, employment problems, income problems, social isolation, childhood abuse, severe domestic, marital or legal stress) including the use of sedatives (current or recent major tranquillizer use)
- Have a history of alcohol or drug abuse
- Are obese
- Have learning difficulties

In summary, health care professionals must be aware that patients with severe asthma and one or more adverse psychosocial factors are at risk of death. Without prompt and appropriate

TABLE 112.10 Different Patterns of Fatal Asthma

	Scenario of Asthma Death	
Variable	Type 1: Slow-onset–late arrival	Type 2: Sudden-onset fatal asphyxic asthma
Time course	Subacute worsening (d)	Acute deterioration (hr)
Frequency	~80–85%	~15–20%
Airways	Extensive mucous plugging	More or less "empty" bronchi
Inflammation	Eosinophils	Neutrophils
Response to treatment	Slow	Faster
Prevention	Possible	(?)

treatment, status asthmaticus may result in ventilatory failure and death. Annual worldwide deaths of asthma have been estimated at 25,000 and occur mostly outside the hospital and in the older age groups (32). Most deaths from asthma (80% to 85%) occur in patients with severe and poorly controlled disease who gradually deteriorate over days or weeks. Mortality in asthma ranges from 0.4% to 12%; asthma patients usually die of respiratory failure outside the hospital, and of barotrauma and/or sepsis after ICU admission. No serious dysrhythmias are encountered. Lung morphology in fatal asthma is mainly characterized by overinflation, atelectasis, bronchospasm, luminal narrowing, and microscopic pathology that shows:

- Inflammation of bronchioles
- Patchy necrosis of the epithelium
- Increase of basement membrane collagen
- Submucosal glandular hyperplasia
- Hypertrophy and hyperplasia of bronchial smooth muscle
- Mucus plugging of bronchi, casts

Two different patterns of fatal asthma have been described (Table 112.10).

Type I Scenario of Asthma Death: Slow-Onset–Late Arrival

Slow-onset asthma exacerbations are mainly related to faults in management (inadequate treatment, noncompliance to therapy, inappropriate control, psychological factors) that should be investigated and corrected in every patient in advance. An inappropriate response to dyspnea may be an important factor. Repeated peak expiratory flow (PEF) measurements, when available, may document subacute worsening of expiratory flow over several days before the appearance of severe symptoms. This pattern of asthma death is generally considered preventable.

A variation of this pattern is a history of unstable disease, which is partially responsive to treatment, on which a major attack is superimposed. In both situations, hypercapnic respiratory failure and mixed acidosis ensue and the patient succumbs to asphyxia, or if MV is applied, to complications such as barotrauma and ventilator-associated pneumonia. Pathologic examination in such cases shows extensive plugging of the airways by dense and tenacious mucus mixed with inflammatory and epithelial cells ("endobronchial mucus suffocation"), epithelial denudation, mucosal edema, and an intense eosinophilic infiltration of the submucosa.

Type II Scenario of Asthma Death: Sudden-Onset Asphyctic Fatal Asthma Exacerbation

In a small proportion of patients, lung function may deteriorate severely in under an hour, leading to sudden and unexpected death from asthma, termed *sudden*, without obvious antecedent long-term deterioration of asthma control. Affected individuals rapidly develop severe hypercapnic respiratory failure with combined metabolic and respiratory acidosis, and succumb to asphyxia. If treated medically and/or with MV, however, they present a faster rate of improvement than patients with slow-onset asthmatic crisis. Pathologic examination in such cases shows "empty" airways (no mucus plugs) in some patients and in almost all patients there is a greater proportion of neutrophils than eosinophils infiltrating the submucosa. It is unclear whether the presence of neutrophils is an epiphenomenon or it directly contributes to the fatal attacks.

A significant volume of research is currently dedicated to unraveling the characteristics of airway remodeling in patients with severe asthma, showing that smooth muscle alteration is the key structural alteration that distinguishes severe from moderate asthma. Phenotypic change in airway smooth muscle might contribute to the difficulty in obtaining adequate control in some patients with severe asthma. Sudden asphyxic asthma death is associated with inflammatory infiltrates both of proximal and distal lung tissues, with the outer wall of small membranous bronchioles being the main site of inflammatory changes.

DIAGNOSIS

There are four parameters that should be investigated before the diagnosis of severe asthma is made for the first time (see Table 112.4):

1. Asthma diagnosis (1,2,33). Confirmation of the diagnosis is important, because in 12% to 50% of people assumed to have severe asthma, asthma is not found to be the correct diagnosis.
2. Unrecognized aggravating comorbidities (1,2,33,34) such as chronic rhinosinusitis, recurrent respiratory tract infections, gastroesophageal reflux, obstructive sleep apnea, psychiatric problems, and obesity; these factors, if found, should be treated.
3. Noncompliance with therapy, either incorrect inhaler use or nonadherence.
4. Continuing exposure to sensitizing agents. Numerous factors such as ongoing (low-dose) allergen exposure at home or at work can aggravate the inflammatory process in the airways and contribute to lack of control of the disease. Once the relationship with the sensitizing agent has been established, the patient must be encouraged to take avoidance measures. Smoking is another important factor that may contribute to the lack of adequate response, and therefore, it is imperative that smoking cessation be suggested.

If these four factors are excluded and the diagnosis remains consistent with severe asthma, a therapeutic trial of systemic

CS therapy—preferably intravenously or intramuscularly—should be performed. If the cause was noncompliance, the best attainable lung function may be seen.

CLINICAL PRESENTATION

Clinical Assessment of Exacerbations Severity

Exacerbations represent a change in symptoms and lung function from the patient's usual status. The signs of exacerbation severity should be immediately assessed (Table 112.11), and include:

- Dyspnea
- Alteration in the level of consciousness
- Temperature
- Pulse rate
- Respiratory rate
- Blood pressure
- Ability to complete sentences without taking a breath
- Use of accessory muscles.

Simultaneously, complicating factors (e.g., anaphylaxis, pneumonia, atelectasis, pneumothorax, or pneumomediastinum) and signs of alternative conditions that could explain acute breathlessness, such as cardiac failure, upper airway dysfunction, inhaled foreign body, or pulmonary embolism should be assessed for.

Functional Assessment of Exacerbation Severity

PEF/FEV_1

It is strongly recommended that PEF or forced expiratory volume in 1 second (FEV_1) be recorded and quantified in the context of the patient's previous lung function or predicted values, before treatment is initiated and without unduly delaying treatment. Their decrease reflects decrease in expiratory airflow. In the acute setting, these measurements are more reliable indicators of the severity of the exacerbation than symptoms. The frequency of symptoms may, however, be a more sensitive measure of the onset of an exacerbation than PEF. A minority of patients may perceive symptoms poorly and experience a significant decline in lung function without a perceptible change in symptoms. This situation especially affects patients with a history of near-fatal asthma and also appears to be more common in males.

The measurement of lung function should be monitored at one hour intervals until a clear response to treatment has occurred or a plateau is reached.

Oxygen Saturation ($SatO_2$)

Oxygen saturation should also be closely monitored, preferably by pulse oximetry. This is especially useful in children if they are unable to perform PEF. In children, oxygen saturation is normally above 95%, and a value below 92% is a predictor of the need for hospitalization. Saturation levels less than 90% in children or adults signal the need for aggressive therapy. Subject to clinical urgency, saturation should be assessed before oxygen is commenced, or 5 minutes after oxygen is removed or when saturation stabilizes.

Arterial Blood Gas Analysis

These measurements are not routinely required. They should be considered for patients with a PEF or FEV_1 below 50% of predicted, or for those who do not respond to initial treatment or are deteriorating. Analysis of arterial blood gases (ABGs) is important in the management of patients with acute severe asthma and useful for decisions regarding hospital admission or tracheal intubation, but is not predictive of outcome. In the early stages of acute severe asthma, analysis of

TABLE 112.11 Clinical and Functional Assessment of Severe Asthma Exacerbations

Variable	Severe Exacerbation	Imminent Respiratory Arrest
Symptoms		
Dyspnea	At rest Hunched forward	
Speech	Single words, not sentences or phrases	
Alertness	Usually agitated	Drowsy or confused
Signs		
Respiratory rate	Often >30 breaths/min	
Heart rate	>120 beats/min	Bradycardia
Pulsus paradoxus*	Often present >25 mmHg	Absence suggests respiratory muscle fatigue
Use of accessory muscles and suprasternal reactions	Usually evident	Abdominal paradox (paradoxical thoracoabdominal movement)
Wheeze	Usually loud	Absence of wheeze "Silent chest"
Functional assessment		
PEF (after initial bronchodilator, % predicted or % personal best)	<40% (50%) of predicted or personal best (<100 L/min adults), *or* Response lasts <2 hr	<25% of predicted or personal best
PaO_2	<60 mmHg Possible cyanosis	
$PaCO_2$	>42 mmHg Possible respiratory failure	
$SatO_2$	<90%	

*Significant reduction of the arterial systolic pressure in inspiration, variation > 12 mmHg between inspiration and expiration

The presence of several parameters, but not necessarily all, indicates the general classification of the exacerbation.

Adapted from Global Initiative for Asthma. Global strategy for asthma management and prevention 2015. Available: http://ginasthma.org/; and Papiris SA, Manali ED, Kolilekas L, et al. Acute severe asthma: new approaches to assessment and treatment. *Drugs.* 2009;69:2363–2391.

TABLE 112.12 Staging of Severe Asthma Crisis by Arterial Blood Gases

Stage 1	Stage 2	Stage 3	Stage 4	Stage 5
Normal $PaCO_2$	↑ $PaCO_2$	↑ $PaCO_2$	Normal	↑ $PaCO_2$ Respiratory failure
Normal PaO_2	Normal PaO_2 Hyperventilation has led to normalization of PaO_2.	↓ PaO_2 Hyperventilation is now unable to compensate totally for a widened $P(A\text{-}a)O_2$.	↓↓↓ PaO_2 Inspiratory fatigue is now prominent.	↓↓↓PaO_2 These findings indicate an impending respiratory arrest.

ABGs usually reveals mild hypoxemia, hypocapnia and respiratory alkalosis; if the deterioration in the patient's clinical status lasts for a few days there may be some compensatory renal bicarbonate loss. As the severity of airflow obstruction increases, $PaCO_2$ first normalizes (Table 112.12) and then, subsequently, increases because of the patient's exhaustion, inadequate alveolar ventilation, and/or an increase in physiologic dead space. Hypercapnia is not usually observed for FEV_1 values higher than 25% of predicted normal, but in general there is no correlation between airflow rates and gas exchange markers. Furthermore, paradoxical deterioration of gas exchange while flow rates improve after the administration of β-adrenergic agonists is not uncommon. Respiratory acidosis is always present in hypercapnic patients who rapidly deteriorate, and in severe, advanced stage disease, metabolic (lactic) acidosis may coexist. The pathogenesis of lactic acidosis in the acutely severe asthmatic patient remains to be fully elucidated. There are several mechanisms that are probably involved: the use of high-dose, parenteral β-adrenergic agonists, the increased work of breathing resulting in anaerobic metabolism of the ventilatory muscles and overproduction of lactic acid, the eventually coexisting tissue hypoxia, and the decreased lactate clearance by the liver because of hypoperfusion. A normal $PaCO_2$ in a distressed asthmatic patient should alert the physician to respiratory fatigue and the danger of respiratory arrest. This classification system is best applied after initial aggressive treatment of asthmatic patients and may be inappropriate if applied before initial therapy.

Supplemental controlled oxygen should be continued while ABGs are obtained. A PaO_2 below 60 mmHg and normal or increased $PaCO_2$ (especially >45 mmHg) indicates respiratory failure. Fatigue and somnolence suggest that $PaCO_2$ may be increasing and airway intervention may be needed.

Laboratory and Radiographic Data

Severe asthma exacerbation may show right ventricular strain on electrocardiogram that resolves with clinical improvement. Chest x-ray (CXR) is not routinely recommended; in adults, CXR should be considered if a complicating or alternative cardiopulmonary process is suspected (especially in older patients), or for patients who are not responding to treatment where a pneumothorax may be difficult to diagnose clinically. Similarly, in children, routine CXR is not recommended unless there are physical signs suggestive of pneumothorax, parenchyma disease, or an inhaled foreign body. Features associated with positive CXR findings in children include fever, no family history of asthma, and localized lung examination; Table 112.13 presents further details (1,2).

THERAPEUTIC APPROACHES: MANAGEMENT OF ACUTE SEVERE ASTHMA

Most of the following management is recommended from GINA guidelines 2015 and British Thoracic Society guidelines (1,32,35). Early diagnosis and treatment of asthma exacerbations are the best strategy for management. Severe exacerbations are potentially life-threatening; patients at high risk of asthma-related death require special attention, particularly intensive education, monitoring, and care, and should be encouraged to seek urgent care early in the course of their exacerbation, meaning they should seek their physician promptly or, depending on the organization of local health services, proceed to the nearest clinic or hospital that provides emergency access for patients with acute asthma. Early home management of asthma exacerbations is of paramount importance as it avoids treatment delay and prevents clinical deterioration. The effectiveness of care depends on the abilities of the patients and/or their families, and on the availability

TABLE 112.13 Laboratory Investigations and Diagnostic Tests for Patients with Difficult to Control Asthma

Diagnostic tests
- Peripheral blood
  - Erythrocyte sedimentation rate
  - Full blood count (eosinophils)
  - Total serum IgE
  - Specific IgE to common and less common allergens
  - Free-T4, thyroid-stimulating hormone

Lung function
- Spirometry (pre- and post-bronchodilator)
- Lung volumes
- Arterial blood gases
- Histamine challenge test

Radiology
- Chest x-ray
- Sinus computed tomography

Additional tests for comorbidities and alternative diagnoses
- Nasal endoscopy
- 24-hr esophageal pH monitoring or trial with proton pump inhibitors
- Polysomnography
- Bronchoscopy
- High-resolution computed tomography scan of the thorax
- D-dimer
- Antineutrophilic cytoplasmic antibody
- IgG against *Aspergillus fumigatus*

of emergency care equipment (peak flow meter, appropriate medications, nebulizer, supplemental oxygen).

Thus, prompt management of acute asthma exacerbation in adults should include the following steps:

1. Recognition of acute asthma (see Table 112.9).
2. Self-treatment. Many patients with asthma, and all patients with severe asthma, should have an agreed written action plan and their own peak flow meter, with regular checks of inhaler technique and compliance. They should know how to recognize early signs of worsening of their asthma, when and how to increase their medication, and when to seek medical assistance. Asthma action plans can decrease hospitalization and deaths from this disorder. Prompt communication between the patient and clinician about any serious deterioration of asthma control should be encouraged. A respiratory specialist should follow up patients admitted with severe asthma for at least 1 year after the admission. However, patients, their families, and their physicians frequently underestimate the severity of asthma.
3. Initial assessment. All possible initial contact personnel (practice receptionists, ambulance call takers) should be aware that asthma patients complaining of respiratory symptoms may be at risk and should have immediate access to a doctor or trained asthma nurse. The assessments required to determine whether the patient is suffering from an acute attack of asthma, the severity of the attack, and the nature of treatment required are detailed in Tables 112.10 and 112.11.
4. Prevention of acute deterioration. A register of patients at risk may help primary care health professionals to identify patients who are more likely to die from their asthma. A system should be in place to ensure that these patients are contacted if they fail to attend for follow-up.
5. Criteria for referral. Refer to hospital any patients with features of acute severe or life-threatening asthma. Other factors, such as failure to respond to treatment, social circumstances, or concomitant disease, may warrant hospital referral.
6. Criteria for admission. Criteria for determining whether a patient should be discharged from the ED or admitted to the hospital have been succinctly reviewed and stratified based on consensus opinion (1,2,32,35).

Asthmatics that require hospitalization are those with any feature of a life-threatening or near-fatal attack; those with any feature of a severe attack persisting after initial treatment; those with a pretreatment FEV_1 or PEF below 25% of predicted or of personal best, or those with a post-treatment FEV_1 or PEF below 40% of predicted or personal best.

Those patients whose peak flow is greater than 75% best or predicted 1 hour after initial treatment may usually be discharged from ED unless they meet any of the following criteria: still have significant symptoms, concerns about compliance, living alone/socially isolated, psychological problems, physical disability or learning difficulties, previous near-fatal or brittle asthma, exacerbation despite adequate dose steroid tablets prepresentation, presentation at night, pregnancy. Asthmatics that *could be discharged* are those with post-treatment FEV_1 or PEF of 40% to 60% of predicted, provided that adequate follow-up is available in the community and that compliance is assured; those with post-treatment FEV_1 or PEF over 60% of predicted can be discharged with significantly less immediate concern.

For patients discharged from the ED, at a minimum, a 7-day course of oral glucocorticosteroids for adults and a shorter course (3 to 5 days) for children should be prescribed, along with continuation of bronchodilator therapy. For most patients, regular controller therapy should be prescribed and increased controller doses should be used for at least 2 to 4 weeks after discharge. The bronchodilator can be used on an as-needed basis, based on both symptomatic and objective improvement, until the patient returns to his or her pre-exacerbation use of rapid acting inhaled β_2-agonists. Ipratropium bromide is unlikely to provide additional benefit beyond the acute phase and may be quickly discontinued. In adult patients with moderate-to-severe asthma, not controlled with high-dose ICSs, tiotropium bromide (a long-acting muscarinic antagonist) can be prescribed as it improves lung function and symptoms (1,2), and modestly reduces the risk of severe exacerbation. One must check the patient's inhaler technique, their use of a peak flow meter to monitor therapy at home, and adherence. Patients discharged from the ED with a peak flow meter and an action plan have a better response than those discharged without these resources; the action plan should be reviewed and written guidance provided.

Other issues that should be addressed are identification of factors that precipitated the exacerbation and implementation of strategies for their future avoidance; evaluation of the asthmatic's response to the exacerbation; ensuring early follow-up after any exacerbation; reviewing the patient's symptom control and risk factors for further exacerbations; and informing the patient's primary care practice within 24 hours of ED or hospital discharge following an asthma exacerbation. Ideally this communication should be directly with a named individual responsible for asthma care within the practice, by means of fax or email.

Pharmacologic Treatment

The aims of treatment are to relieve airflow obstruction and hypoxemia as quickly as possible, and to prevent future relapses (Table 112.14). Response to treatment may take time, and patients should be closely monitored using clinical as well as objective measurements. The increased treatment should continue until measurements of lung function (PEF or FEV_1) return to their previous best (ideally) or plateau, at which time a decision to admit or discharge can be made based on these values. Patients who can be safely discharged will have responded within the first 2 hours, at which time decisions regarding patient disposition can be made.

Schematically, management plan of acute severe asthma in adults is shown in Figure 112.7. In the ED, a brief history regarding time of onset, cause of exacerbation, severity of symptoms (especially in comparison to previous attacks), prior hospitalizations and/or ED visits for asthma, prior intubation or ICU admission, and complicating illness may be useful for treatment decisions. The primary therapies and the intensity of pharmacologic treatment and patient's surveillance should correspond to the severity of the exacerbation and, for severe acute asthma, will include the therapies discussed in the following sections.

Oxygen

High-flow oxygen should be given to all patients with severe acute asthma as these individuals are hypoxemic. This may be

TABLE 112.14 Pharmacologic Management of Patients with Acute Severe Asthma in the ED

Drug	Comments
Salbutamol (albuterol) solution for inhalation: single-dose 2.5 mg (2.5 mL)	2.5 mg (2.5 mL) by nebulization continuously for 1 hr, then reassess Thereafter, clinical response or occurrence of serious adverse effects influences the frequency of administration
Ipratropiun bromide	Nebulized ipratropium bromide (0.5 mg/2.5 mL, 4–6 hr) combined with salbutamol May mix in the same nebulizer with salbutamol
Corticosteroids	Methylprednisolone 40 mg IV or hydrocortisone 200 mg IV or prednisone 50 mg PO Consider high-dose inhaled corticosteroids
Magnesium sulfate	A single 1.2–2.0 g infusion over 20 min in adults
Methylxanthines	Avoid; poor evidence and serious adverse effects
Leukotriene receptor antagonists	A single 7–14 mg infusion of montelukast over 5 min
Epinephrine (adrenaline): 1:1,000 (1 mg/mL)	0.3–0.4 mL of a 1:1,000 (1 mg/mL) solution subcutaneously every 20 min for three doses in case of no response (last chance to avoid intubation)
Terbutaline (1 mg/mL)	0.25 mg subcutaneously every 20 min for 3 doses. Preferable to epinephrine in pregnancy
Heliox	Helium/oxygen mixture in a ratio of 80:20 or 70:30

Adapted from Global Initiative for Asthma. Global strategy for asthma management and prevention 2015. Available: http://ginasthma.org/; and Papiris SA, Manali ED, Kolilekas L, et al. Acute severe asthma: new approaches to assessment and treatment. *Drugs*. 2009;69:2363-2391.

corrected urgently using high concentrations of inspired oxygen by either nasal cannulae or mask. Unlike patients with chronic obstructive pulmonary disease (COPD), there is little danger of precipitating hypercapnia with high-flow oxygen. Hypercapnia indicates the development of near-fatal asthma and the need for emergency specialist/anesthetic intervention. An SpO_2 of at least 92% must be achieved, and an SpO_2 over 95% is desired in pregnant women, children, and in patients with coexistent cardiac disease. In severe exacerbations, controlled low-flow oxygen therapy using SpO_2 to maintain saturation at 93% to 95% is associated with better physiologic outcomes than with high-flow 100% oxygen therapy. However, oxygen therapy should not be withheld if SpO_2 is not available. Once the patient has stabilized, consider weaning them off oxygen using SpO_2 to guide the need for ongoing oxygen therapy (1,2,32,35).

β_2-Agonist Bronchodilators

Inhaled β_2-agonists are the cornerstone of asthma treatment and are administered in the form of *short-acting β_2-agonists* (SABA). Continuous or repetitive nebulization of rapid-acting β_2-agonists is the safest and most effective means of reversing airflow obstruction, and should be administered as early as possible (1,32,35). In most cases of acute asthma, inhaled β_2-agonists given in high doses act quickly to relieve bronchospasm and have few side effects. There is no evidence for any difference in efficacy between salbutamol and terbutaline. In acute asthma without life-threatening features, β_2-agonists can be administered by repeated activations of a metered-dose inhaler via an appropriate large-volume spacer, or by wet nebulization. The most cost-effective and efficient delivery is by pMDI with a spacer (Evidence level A); evidence is less robust in severe and near-fatal asthma. In view of the theoretical risk of oxygen desaturation while using air-driven compressors to nebulize β_2-agonist bronchodilators, oxygen-driven nebulizers are preferred. Systematic reviews of intermittent versus continuous nebulized SABA in acute asthma provide conflicting results. One found no significant differences in lung function or hospital admissions, but a later review with additional studies found reduced hospitalizations and better lung function with continuous compared with intermittent nebulization, particularly in patients with worse lung function. An earlier study in hospitalized patients found that intermittent, on-demand therapy led to a significantly shorter hospital stay, fewer nebulizations, and fewer palpitations when compared with 4-hourly intermittent therapy. A reasonable approach to inhaled SABA in exacerbations, therefore, would be to initially use continuous therapy, followed by intermittent on-demand therapy for hospitalized patients. There is no evidence to support the routine use of intravenous (IV) β_2-agonists in patients with severe asthma exacerbations (Evidence level A). In severe asthma, with PEF below 50% of personal best or FEV_1 less than 50% predicted, and asthma that is poorly responsive to an initial bolus dose of β_2-agonist, continuous nebulization should be considered. Continuous nebulization of β_2-agonists may also be more effective in children. Larger doses and more frequent dosing intervals for inhaled β-agonist therapy are needed in acute severe asthma because of decreased deposition at site of action, itself resultant from low tidal volumes and narrowed airways, alteration in dose–response curve, and altered duration of activity. *Repeated doses* of β_2-agonists should be given at 15- to 30-minute intervals, or continuous nebulization of salbutamol at 5 to 10 mg/hr used if there is an inadequate response to initial treatment. Higher bolus doses (e.g., 10 mg of salbutamol) are unlikely to be more effective.

Continuous or repetitive nebulization of salbutamol is preferred because of its potency, 4- to 6-hour duration of action, and β_2-selectivity. The usual dose is 2.5 mg of salbutamol (0.5 mL) in 2.5 mL of normal saline for each nebulization (see Table 112.14). Nebulized β_2-agonists should be continued until a significant clinical response is achieved or serious side effects, such as severe tachycardia or dysrhythmias, appear. Prior ineffective use of β_2-agonists does not preclude their use and does not limit their efficacy. Inhaled therapy with β_2-agonists appears to be equal to, or even better than, IV infusion in treating airway obstruction in adults with severe asthma (meta-analysis has excluded subcutaneous trials). IV β_2-agonists should be reserved for those patients in whom inhaled therapy cannot be used reliably. Although most rapid-acting β_2-agonists have a short duration of effect, the long-acting bronchodilator formoterol, which has both a rapid onset of action and a long duration of effect, has been shown to be equally effective without increasing side effects,

INITIAL ASSESSMENT

- **Brief history:** Exclude other diagnoses than asthma, time of onset, cause of exacerbation, severity of symptoms especially in comparison to previous attacks, prior hospitalizations and/or ED visits for asthma, prior intubation or intensive care admission, complicating illness
- **Focused physical examination:** Auscultation, use of accessory muscles, heart rate, respiratory rate, color, alertness, vital signs
- **Objective testing:** PEF or FEV_1, SpO_2, arterial blood gas analyses if patient in extremis

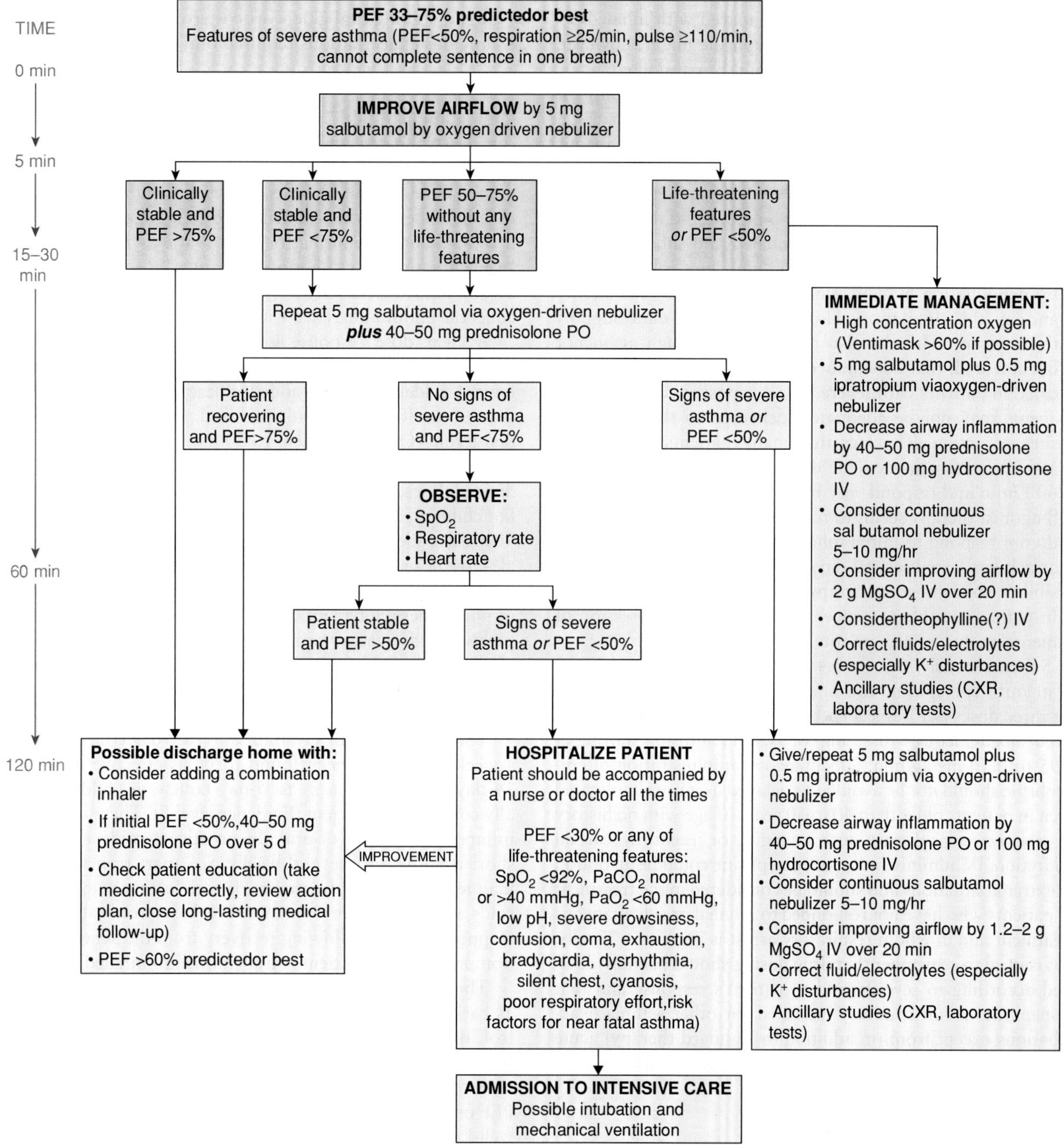

FIGURE 112.7 Management of acute severe asthma in adults in the emergency department. PEF, peak expiratory flow; FEV_1, forced expiratory volume in 1 second; CXR, chest x-ray.

although it is considerably more expensive. The importance of this feature of formoterol is that it provides support and reassurance regarding the use of a combination of formoterol and budesonide early in asthma exacerbations.

Two types of nebulizer systems are available for inhalation therapy: the face mask and the hand-held nebulizer with a mouthpiece. The mouthpiece is preferred because it delivers more drug, but it requires more patient cooperation because a good seal must be maintained around the mouthpiece. In the severely ill asthmatic patient, the face mask system may be necessary. When β_2-selective agents are delivered parenterally or orally, they lose much of their β_2-selectivity, so terbutaline loses its β-selectivity and offers no advantages over epinephrine. When subcutaneous terbutaline is compared with subcutaneous epinephrine, equal cardiac side effects are seen. Oral β_2-selective agents should not be used as primary treatment for patients with acute asthma because the therapeutic-to-toxicity ratio is less than that with inhaled agents. Subcutaneous β-agonist therapy (epinephrine) also has a disadvantageous therapeutic-to-toxicity ratio when compared with inhaled β_2-selective agonists. Subcutaneous epinephrine might, however, be useful in several situations and should be considered:

- In children in whom inhaled agents are often difficult to administer. In addition, the pediatric population has a reduced susceptibility to β_1-toxicity, making subcutaneous administration a useful route of drug delivery.
- In seriously ill asthmatic patients with impending respiratory arrest in whom rapid delivery of β-agonists to the airway is desirable. The combination of inhaled and subcutaneously administered β-agonists in this circumstance could enhance bronchodilation by delivering the drug both by the airway and by the circulation. However, no clear data support this concept. There is also a concern, although again not documented, that subcutaneous adrenergic therapy is indicated in patients with severe bronchospasm because inhaled agents may not be adequately delivered to the peripheral sites of action. The fact that many patients with severe asthma present in extreme distress with a PEF rate below 60 L/min and respond very briskly to continuous nebulized β-agonist therapy seems to refute this contention. If patients do not respond to initial inhaled therapy, particularly if the attack has lasted several days and mucus plugging is a possibility, subcutaneous therapy could be attempted.
- In patients unable to cooperate secondary to depression of mental status, apnea, or coma.

Subcutaneously, 0.3 to 0.4 mL of a solution of 1:1,000 (1 mg/mL) epinephrine can be administered every 20 minutes for three doses (see Table 112.14). Terbutaline can be administered subcutaneously (0.25 mg) or as an IV infusion starting at 0.05 to 0.10 mg/kg/min. Subcutaneous administration of epinephrine should *not* be avoided or delayed as it is well tolerated even in patients older than 40 to 50 years of age with no history of cardiovascular disease, such as angina or recent myocardial infarction. IV administration of epinephrine could be an option in extreme situations and should be considered in the treatment of patients who have not responded to inhaled or subcutaneous treatment and in whom respiratory arrest is imminent. Finally, it is critical to remember that drug dosing should be individualized according to severity and to patient's response and that epinephrine is not routinely indicated for other asthma exacerbations except from (in addition to standard therapy) acute asthma associated with anaphylaxis and angioedema.

Steroids

Systemic CS speed resolution (1,32,35) of exacerbations and prevent relapse, and should be utilized in all but the mildest exacerbations in adults, adolescents, and children aged 6 to 11 years (Evidence level A). Where possible, systemic CSs should be administered to the patient within 1 hour of presentation, as they lower hospitalization rates and improve pulmonary function. They also reduce the risk of relapses, rehospitalization, requirement for β_2-agonist therapy, all-cause mortality in elderly asthmatics, and more generally reduce mortality from asthma. The earlier they are given in the acute attack the better the outcome.

Systemic CSs in adequate doses should be administered in all cases of acute asthma, especially if:

- The initial rapid-acting inhaled β_2-agonist therapy fails to achieve lasting improvement
- The exacerbation develops even though the patient was already taking oral glucocorticosteroids
- Previous exacerbations required oral glucocorticosteroids

Route of Delivery

Oral administration is as effective as IV, provided tablets can be swallowed and retained. The oral route is preferred because it is quicker, less invasive, and less expensive; for children, a liquid formulation is preferred to tablets. IV CSs can be administered when patients are too dyspneic to swallow, if the patient is vomiting, or when patients require noninvasive ventilation or intubation. In patients discharged from the ED, an intramuscular CS may be helpful, especially if there are concerns about adherence with oral therapy.

A clear dose response is usually seen at dosages below 40 mg/d of methylprednisone or equivalent; however, there is limited evidence of any added efficacy when dosages higher than 60 to 80 mg/d are administered. Daily doses of oral corticosteroid (OCS) equivalent to 50 mg prednisolone as a single morning dose (see Table 112.14), or 200 mg hydrocortisone in divided doses, are adequate for most patients (Evidence level B). For children, an OCS dose of 1 to 2 mg/kg up to a maximum of 40 mg/d is adequate. Minimal or no side effects occur with a single large dose of IV steroid. The benefit derived by the asthmatic is probably from a combination of enhancement of β_2-receptor responsiveness, interruption of arachidonic acid inflammatory pathways, decrease in capillary basement membrane permeability, decreased leukocyte attachment, modulation of calcium migration intracellularly, reduction in airway mucus production, and suppression of immunoglobulin E receptor binding.

The OCS is usually given for a 5- to 7-day course in adults; a-week course has been found to be as effective as a 10- to 14-day course, and a 3- to 5-day course in children is usually considered sufficient (Evidence level B). There is no benefit in tapering the dose of oral glucocorticosteroids, either in the short term or over several weeks. So, apart from patients on maintenance steroid treatment or rare instances in which steroids are required for 3 or more weeks, steroid tablets can be stopped abruptly following recovery from the acute exacerbation provided the patient is transitioned to inhaled steroids.

The intensification of a patient's CS therapy should begin as early as possible, at the first sign of loss of asthma control. Because benefits from CS treatment are not usually seen before 6 to 12 hours, early administration is necessary. Their onset of action may be seen in 2 hours in studies measuring PEF or 6 hours in studies measuring FEV_1 (32). In addition to well-known side effects of CS administration (hyperglycemia, hypertension, hypokalemia, psychosis, susceptibility to infections), myopathy should be considered in the intubated and mechanically ventilated patient (see below).

Inhaled Corticosteroids

High-dose ICSs given within the first hour after presentation reduces the need for hospitalization in patients not receiving systemic CSs (Evidence level A), but there is no firm evidence to suggest that inhaled steroids can substitute for steroid tablets in treating patients with acute severe or life-threatening asthma, despite some promising results. When given in addition to systemic CSs, evidence is conflicting (Evidence level B). Overall, ICSs are well tolerated; however, the agent, dose, and duration of treatment with ICSs in the management of asthma in the ED remain unclear.

If the patient is discharged, they should be prescribed regular ongoing ICS treatment since the occurrence of a severe exacerbation is a risk factor for future exacerbations (Evidence level B) and ICS-containing medications significantly reduce the risk of asthma-related death or hospitalization (Evidence level A). For short-term outcomes, such as relapse requiring admission, symptoms, and quality of life, a systematic review found no significant differences when ICSs were added to systemic CSs after discharge. There was some evidence, however, that post-discharge ICS were as effective as systemic CSs for milder exacerbations, but the confidence limits were wide (Evidence level B). ICSs should be started as soon as possible, or continued, at the beginning of the chronic asthma management plan as they can be as effective as oral steroids at preventing relapses, although cost may be a problem.

Anticholinergics

Ipratropium Bromide

Ipratropium bromide is a short-acting anticholinergic, although producing less bronchodilation at peak effect than a β_2-agonist, is supported from the literature as adjunctive therapy in patients with severe acute asthma (1,2,32,35). Treatment in the ED with both SABA and ipratropium was associated with fewer hospitalizations and greater improvement in PEF and FEV_1 compared with SABA alone for adults and children with moderate–severe exacerbations.

Ipratropium bromide appears to reliably augment the bronchodilating effect of β-agonists in acute asthma and is particularly useful in the presence of β-blockade. Combining nebulized ipratropium bromide with a nebulized β_2-agonist has been shown to produce significantly greater bronchodilation than a β_2-agonist alone, leading to a faster recovery, a shorter duration of admission, lower hospitalization rates, greater improvement in PEF and FEV_1, and should be administered before methylxanthines are considered. The recommended dose is 0.25 to 0.5 mg by nebulizer; this can be combined with an albuterol dose. Without any doubt, nebulized ipratropium bromide in a dose of 0.5 mg every 4 to 6 hours should be added to β_2-agonist treatment for patients with severe acute or life-threatening asthma, or in those with a poor initial response to β_2-agonist therapy (see Table 112.14).

The hand-held mouthpiece nebulizer system should be used if anticholinergic medication is being administered. Contamination of the ocular area with precipitation of narrow-angle glaucoma may occur in susceptible individuals if a face mask is used for delivery of an anticholinergic agent.

Magnesium

IV magnesium sulfate, usually given as a single 1.2 to 2 g infusion over 20 minutes, can help reduce hospital admission rates in certain patients (1,2,32,35). A single dose of IV magnesium sulfate should be considered for patients with:

- Acute severe asthma, with FEV_1 25% to 30% predicted at presentation
- Adults and children who fail to respond to initial treatment
- Life-threatening or near-fatal asthma

Magnesium's potential to reverse bronchoconstriction is multifactorial, based upon characteristics of inhibition of the calcium channel and decreased acetylcholine release. Considerable controversy exists as to the potential benefit of magnesium as adjunctive therapy in acute asthma. A single dose of IV magnesium is safe and sometimes effective in severe acute asthma, although the responsive patients cannot be predicted. The safety and efficacy of repeated doses have not been assessed in asthmatic patients; repeated doses could give rise to hypermagnesemia with muscle weakness and respiratory failure. More studies are needed to determine the optimal frequency and dose of IV magnesium sulfate therapy (1,2,72). Although it has been tried, it is unclear if nebulized salbutamol administered in isotonic magnesium sulfate solution provides greater benefit than if it is delivered in normal saline.

Agents Not Recommended (And Why)

Methylxanthines: Aminophylline and Theophylline

In the ED, methylxanthines are of debated efficacy and not generally recommended (1,2,32,35). Theophylline, when compared with a placebo, is clearly an effective bronchodilator in the patient with acute bronchospasm but, in view of the effectiveness and relative safety of rapid-acting β_2-agonists, has a minimal role in the management of acute asthma. The question, however, is whether theophylline plus adequate dosing of an inhaled β-agonist produces greater bronchodilation than adequate dosing of β-agonist alone in the patient with acute asthma. The majority of studies have demonstrated no significant additional improvement in physiologic or outcome variables when theophylline is added to full doses of inhaled β-agonist therapy.

Theophylline has also been demonstrated *in vitro* and *in vivo* to have nonbronchodilator effects of potential clinical benefit. It increases diaphragmatic endurance, is a respiratory muscle inotrope, and a nonspecific respiratory stimulant. It is doubtful, however, that any of these effects exert a significant clinical impact. Lastly, theophylline has been shown to have anti-inflammatory properties, but at very low (<10 μg/mL) concentrations. All patients evaluated for acute bronchospasm who have been receiving a theophylline preparation should have a theophylline level determined, the results of which are useful in later dosing decisions.

In addition to its questionable efficacy, theophylline toxicity is a concern. Its use is associated with severe and potentially fatal side effects, particularly in those on long-term therapy with sustained-release theophylline; a therapeutic range of serum theophylline at 8 to 12 μg/mL minimizes risk for toxicity. The theophylline levels correlate, however, only roughly with toxicity. The longer acting the oral theophylline compound, the more likely it is to be associated with a higher initial level. If aminophylline is to be used, a decreased loading dose (2 mg/kg) is recommended in the severely bronchospastic asthmatic patient who admits to poor or partial compliance in taking medications. Without any doubt, some patients with near-fatal or life-threatening asthma, as well as patients admitted to the ICU, with a poor response to initial therapy, may gain additional benefit from IV aminophylline. The drug is loaded at

5 mg/kg over 20 minutes (unless on maintenance oral therapy), followed by an infusion of 0.5 to 0.7 mg/kg/hr, and is added to full-dose inhaled β-agonist; higher doses may be used in children. A 1 mg/kg IV aminophylline dose increases the serum level roughly by 2 µg/mL, with considerable scatter. A 5 mg/kg dose is, therefore, estimated to give a level of approximately 10 µg/mL. This relationship of loading dose to incremental increase in blood level can also be used for additional dosing considerations after theophylline level is known. The rate of metabolism is highly variable and may be affected by many factors. Factors that decrease aminophylline clearance and necessitate lowering of infusion rates include use of cimetidine, erythromycin, upper respiratory tract infections, pneumonia, and so forth. If IV aminophylline is given to patients receiving oral aminophylline or theophylline, blood levels should be checked on admission; levels should be checked daily for all patients receiving aminophylline infusions.

To conclude, IV aminophylline and theophylline IV should not be used in the management of asthma exacerbations in view of their poor efficacy and safety profile, and the greater effectiveness and relative safety of SABA. In adults with severe asthma exacerbations, add-on treatment with aminophylline does not improve outcomes compared with SABA alone.

Leukotriene Modifiers

There are little data to suggest a role for leukotriene modifiers in acute asthma and, therefore, these agents are not recommended (1,2,32,35).

ICS/LABA Combinations

The role of these medications in the ED or hospital is unclear. One study showed that high-dose budesonide/formoterol in patients in the ED, all of whom received prednisolone, had a similar efficacy and safety profile to SABA. The data on salmeterol added to OCS for hospitalized patients were not adequately powered to support a recommendation.

Antibiotics

Evidence does not support a role of antibiotics in asthma exacerbations unless there is strong evidence of lung or sinus infection: fever or purulent sputum, radiographic evidence of pneumonia, purulent sinus drainage; hence, routine administration of antibiotics is not recommended. Aggressive treatment with CSs should be implemented before antibiotics are considered. When an infection precipitates an exacerbation of asthma, it is likely to be viral in nature.

Helium–Oxygen Therapy

A blended mixture of helium and oxygen (heliox) is available in mixtures of 60:40, 70:30, and 80:20. Heliox is less dense than air and can be delivered through a tight-fitting nonrebreathing mask or, in the intubated patient, through the ventilator circuit. This less dense gas mixture results in decreased airway resistance. Studies have shown the ability of heliox to decrease *pulsus paradoxus* and improve both inspiratory and expiratory flows. Heliox may have potential benefit in delaying need for intubation while bronchodilators exert their effect, as well as decreasing peak airway pressures in the mechanically ventilated patient. In the latter case, its potential to decrease auto-PEEP, may be particularly useful. A mixture of 60:40 of heliox can be used as initial therapy with carefully monitoring oxygenation status. Recalibration of gas blenders and flow meters is required to obtain accurate measurement of oxygen concentration and tidal volumes when this mixture is used in the mechanically ventilated patient. It must be remembered that, despite reported anecdotal success, no controlled trials have demonstrated an alteration of outcome variables and, therefore, the use of heliox in adults with acute asthma cannot be recommended as *standard* therapy on the basis of present evidence. The mixture might be considered for patients who do not respond to standard therapy (see Table 112.14).

Intravenous Fluids

There are no controlled trials, or even observational or cohort studies, of differing fluid regimens in acute asthma. Some patients with acute asthma require rehydration and correction of electrolyte imbalance. Hypokalemia can be caused or exacerbated by β_2-agonist and/or steroid treatment and must be corrected. Aggressive hydration is not recommended for adults or older children but may be indicated for infants and young children.

Chest Physiotherapy and Mucolytics

These treatment modalities are mentioned only to note that they have no role in the treatment of severe, acute asthma.

Sedatives

Sedation should be strictly avoided during exacerbations of asthma because of the respiratory depressant effect of anxiolytic and hypnotic drugs. An association between the use of these drugs and avoidable asthma deaths has been demonstrated.

REFERRAL TO THE INTENSIVE CARE UNIT

All patients transferred to the ICU should be accompanied by a physician suitably equipped and skilled to perform endotracheal intubation, if necessary. Indications for admission to the ICU or a high-dependency unit include patients requiring ventilatory support and those with severe acute or life-threatening asthma who are failing to respond to therapy, as evidenced by:

- Deteriorating PEF
- Persisting or worsening hypoxia
- Hypercapnia
- Worsening acidosis
- Exhaustion, feeble respiration
- Drowsiness, confusion
- Coma or respiratory arrest

Indications for Endotracheal Intubation

Careful and repeat assessment of patients with severe asthmatic exacerbations is mandatory. Not all patients admitted to the ICU need invasive MV. The exact time to intubate is based mainly on clinical judgment (36–39):

- Patients presenting with apnea or coma should be intubated immediately.
- Progressive exhaustion, patient fatigue, and worsening hypercapnia despite maximal therapy together with altered level of consciousness are indications for intubation.
- Maintaining adequate oxygenation (and oxygen transport) with supplemental oxygen is seldom a problem even in very

severe asthma and is a relatively uncommon reason for intubation.
- If the patient is cooperative, hypercapnia and fatigue do not necessarily mandate intubation because noninvasive ventilation may be an option (see below).

Intubation

Intubation may be performed by either the nasal or the oral route, the latter allowing for the insertion of a larger tube that facilitates suctioning, important for removing tenacious mucus plugs mobilized during recovery, and offers less resistance to flow. A larger endotracheal tube reduces flow-resistive pressure during inspiration, of significance during weaning, but not important during controlled MV. Given the extraordinary high resistance of the patient's airways, the effect of the larger bore tube on expiratory flow is also trivial (28,39).

Intubation should be performed by the most skilled operator available to avoid repeated airway manipulation which may induce laryngospasm and worsened bronchoconstriction. Satisfactory local anesthesia of the oropharynx, nasopharynx, and larynx is essential. Table 112.15 summarizes drugs used to facilitate intubation of patients with severe asthma (28,40). It should be stressed that many of these drugs reduce vascular tone and combined with decreased venous return due to hyperinflation, may cause profound hypotension. This may require rapid infusion of IV fluids and manual ventilation via a bag-valve-mask device at a slow rate or even temporary apnea to decrease hyperinflation; lack of response suggests the presence of tension pneumothorax.

Mechanical Ventilation

Noninvasive Positive Pressure Ventilation

Although of proven benefit in the treatment of COPD exacerbation, noninvasive positive pressure ventilation (NIPPV) is still considered controversial in the treatment of acute severe asthma attack (1), related to the lack of large scale randomized studies showing its worth. However, NIPPV has a strong physiologic basis in favor of its use (41) and, due to this, it has gained acceptance in centers experienced in NIPPV.

NIPPV can be considered for asthmatic patients at risk for endotracheal intubation from progressive exhaustion (42). There are a few extant prospective randomized controlled trials: Soroksky et al. (43) in normocapnic asthmatic patients showed that a short trial of NIPPV in the ED decreased hospitalization rate, respiratory frequency, and improved spirometric indices of pulmonary function; Gupta et al. (44) found significantly shorter ICU and hospital stay in the group treated with NIPPV. Although a mortality benefit was not demonstrated (43–45) with the use of NIPPV in severe asthma patients, there are some data showing improved physiologic parameters (43,46–48), and reduced intubation rates (49) without worsened patient prognosis, that is, there was no subsequent complications in NIPPV failure patients requiring escalation of treatment to intubation and MV (49). Pallin et al. (50), in a retrospective study, showed that NIPPV use in severe acute asthma patients, not in cardiorespiratory arrest, was safe in the ED and ICU, with no hemodynamic or barotraumatic complications, no need for escalation of therapy—that is, endotracheal intubation and MV—and no deaths. All these studies (44,49,50) support the use of NIPPV in carefully selected and monitored patients, if performed by team with significant experience in the use of NIPPV, always keeping in mind that an NIPPV trial should not unnecessarily delay endotracheal intubation, if it becomes necessary.

Suggested criteria for an NIV trial include (51) (1) respiratory rate greater than 25 breaths/min; (2) heart rate greater than 110 beats/min; (3) use of accessory respiratory muscles; (4) hypoxemia, but with a PaO_2/FIO_2 greater than 200 mmHg; (5) hypercapnia, but with $PaCO_2$ less than 60 mmHg; and (6) FEV_1 less than 50% predicted.

Absolute contraindications for the use of NIPPV in asthma are emergency intubation for cardiorespiratory resuscitation, hemodynamic and/or electrocardiographic instability, life-threatening hypoxemia, and an altered level of consciousness. The presence of severe hypercapnia on hospital admission should alert the clinician to the high risk of endotracheal intubation, despite not being a contraindication to NIPPV *per se* (52). Interestingly, among severe asthmatics admitted to the ICU, patients successfully treated with NIPPV had less hypercapnia (mean $PaCO_2$ 53 ± 13 mmHg; mean pH 7.28 ± 0.008) than those who eventually underwent endotracheal intubation (mean $PaCO_2$ 89 ± 29 mmHg; mean pH 7.05 ± 0.21) (36). An NIPPV "trial" is also best avoided in the presence of severe patient agitation, poor patient cooperation, or a lack of trained/experienced staff.

When used, NIPPV should be started with low levels of inspiratory pressure support (5 to 10 cm H_2O) and PEEP (3 to 5 cm H_2O). Pressure support should be progressively increased by 2 cm H_2O every 15 minutes, the goal being to reduce

TABLE 112.15 Drugs Used for Intubation in Acute Severe Asthma

Agent	Dose	Advantages	Side Effects	Contraindications
Midazolam	1 mg IV slowly, every 2–3 min until the patient allows positioning and airways inspection	Amnesia Muscle relaxation	Hypotension Respiratory depression	
Ketamine	1–2 mg/kg IV at a rate of 0.5 mg/kg/min	No respiratory depression No hypotension Short-lasting bronchodilation	Increased laryngeal reflexes Increased laryngeal secretions Sympathomimetic effects (hypertension, tachycardia) Increased intracranial pressure Delirium Hallucinations (prevented by midazolam coadministration)	Atherosclerosis Hypertension Increased intracranial pressure
Propofol	60–80 mg/min initial intravenous infusion up to 2.0 mg/kg	Rapid onset and resolution of sedation Bronchodilation	Hypotension Respiratory depression	Hemodynamic instability

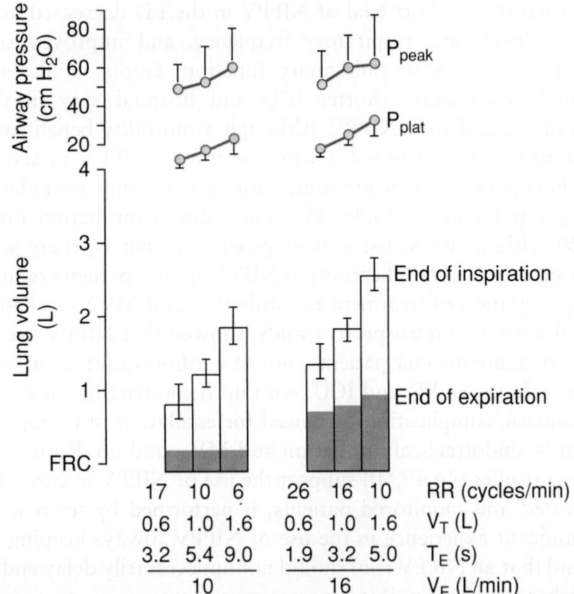

FIGURE 112.8 Effect of respiratory rate and tidal volume variations on airway pressures and lung volumes during mechanical ventilation of acute severe asthma. FRC, functional residual capacity; P_{peak}, peak inspiratory pressure; P_{plat}, end-inspiratory plateau pressure; RR, respiratory rate; V_T, tidal volume; T_E, expiratory time; V_E, minute ventilation. All conditions are for a square inspiratory flow of 100 L/min. (Adapted from Tuxen D, Lane S. The effects of ventilatory pattern on hyperinflation, airway pressures, and circulation in mechanical ventilation of patients with severe air-flow obstruction. *Am Rev Respir Dis.* 1987;136:872–879.)

respiratory rate below 25 breaths/min, monitoring ABG analysis and patient comfort, while keeping peak inspiratory pressure below 25 cm H_2O. Future prospective, randomized, controlled trials are required to definitely establish the role of NIPPV in severe acute asthma.

Invasive Mechanical Ventilation

The goal of MV is to buy time until pharmacotherapy can reverse the underlying pathophysiologic features of airway inflammation, mucus plugging, and bronchoconstriction. The main strategy of ventilatory support is to minimize hyperinflation and avoid excessive airway pressure (overdistention) (21,28); thus, controlled hypoventilation or permissive hypercapnia is often required (53,54). Controlled ventilation is often used because of the need for deep sedation—with or without muscle paralysis to avoid patient–ventilator asynchrony and to achieve controlled hypoventilation (21,28). Volume-controlled ventilation is usually preferable to pressure control as the latter carries the risk of delivering variable tidal volume with sometimes unacceptably low alveolar ventilation in conditions of fluctuating high airway resistance and hyperinflation (21,28).

The most important parameter to achieve the goal of reducing end-expiratory lung volume (i.e., hyperinflation) is a reduction in the administered minute ventilation (i.e., <10 L/min) (Figs. 112.8 and 112.9) (55). For a given level of minute ventilation, the end-expiratory lung volume will be similar regardless of the combination of tidal volume and respiratory rate. However, for any level of minute ventilation and with constant (square wave) inspiratory flow rate, end-inspiratory lung distention is minimized by a combination of low tidal volume (V_t) and high respiratory rate (see Fig. 112.8). This is because in the inhomogeneous asthmatic lung, most of the V_t delivered by positive pressure ventilation goes to the parts of lung parenchyma with almost normal mechanical characteristics (compartment A; see Fig. 112.3). Because such "mechanically normal" areas represent only a small fraction of the total asthmatic lung, they become overdistended. Thus, the lower V_t would cause less end-inspiratory lung overdistention. When keeping minute ventilation, V_t, and respiratory rate constant, increasing inspiratory flow allows inspiratory time (T_i) to be reduced and, thus, expiratory time (T_e) to be increased. When minute ventilation is high (>10 L/min), increasing inspiratory flow and, thus, reducing T_i allows a decrease in lung hyperinflation (see Fig. 112.9). It should be stressed, however, that prolonging T_e is not very effective in decreasing dynamic hyperinflation when minute ventilation is below 10 L/min (56). This is because flow progressively

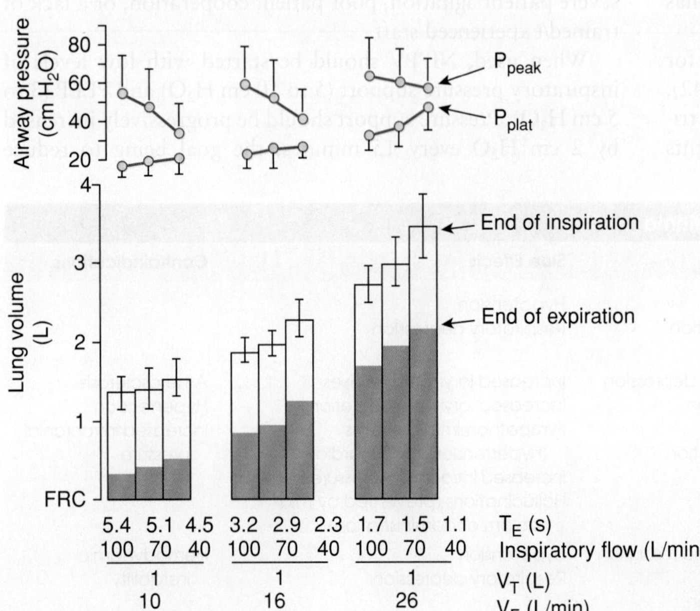

FIGURE 112.9 Effect of inspiratory flow variations on airway pressures and lung volumes during mechanical ventilation in acute severe asthma. FRC, functional residual capacity; P_{peak}, peak inspiratory pressure; P_{plat}, end-inspiratory plateau pressure; RR, respiratory rate; V_T, tidal volume; T_E, expiratory time; V_E, minute ventilation. (Adapted from Tuxen D, Lane S. The effects of ventilatory pattern on hyperinflation, airway pressures, and circulation in mechanical ventilation of patients with severe airflow obstruction. *Am Rev Respir Dis.* 1987;136:872–879.)

TABLE 112.16 Initial Ventilatory Settings in Status Asthmaticus

Setting	Recommendation
Mode	Volume control ventilation
Minute ventilation	<10 L/min
Tidal volume	6–8 mL/kg ideal body weight
Respiratory rate	10–15 breaths/min
PEEP	Titration trial (increments of 2 cm H_2O)
Expiratory time	> 4 s
Inspiratory flow	60–80 L/min
Inspiratory to expiratory ratio	>1:3
FiO_2	Maintain SpO_2 93–95%
P_{plat}	<30 cm H_2O

FIO_2, fraction of inspired oxygen; PEEP, positive end-expiratory pressure; P_{plat}, end-inspiratory plateau pressure; SaO_2, oxygen saturation.

decreases during expiration, so prolonging expiration will allow additional time for expiration at a point at which expiratory flows are low, and thus the additional volume that could be exhaled (the integral of flow over time) is modest; this decrease in dynamic hyperinflation is even less when respiratory rate is low. Thus, at any given minute ventilation, inspiratory flow should be 60 to 80 L/min (Table 112.16), as further prolonging T_e by greater inspiratory flow will not significantly reduce hyperinflation.

The optimal inspiratory flow waveform with volume-controlled ventilation is not entirely clear. For a given tidal volume, T_i will be shorter and, thus, T_e longer when constant flow (square wave) rather than decelerating flow is used. However, the effect of this on reducing hyperinflation is clinically insignificant (see previous discussion). At identical levels of V_t, T_i, and P_{plat}, a square wave results in a higher peak inspiratory pressure (P_{peak}) than does a decelerating wave. This consideration has limited clinical relevance because P_{peak} is highly dependent on inspiratory flow-resistive properties; therefore, P_{peak} does not reflect alveolar distention pressure in most of the (57) (i.e., increased airway resistance combined with high inspiratory flow rate may result in P_{peak} above 50 cm H_2O but without increased risk of barotraumas). Nevertheless, a lower P_{peak} may mean less overdistension of alveoli distal to the least obstructed airways, as these are the most exposed to high pressure in the central airways. Another reason to minimize P_{peak} and, thus, to prefer the decelerating over the square waveform, is that delivery of the full V_t is less easily interrupted by opening of the pop-off safety valve of the ventilator, securing a steadier minute ventilation (40).

Monitoring of Hyperinflation and Overdistension

Dynamic hyperinflation can be monitored in two different ways:

1. By measuring the volume passively exhaled from end inspiration to the static functional residual capacity in the course of a prolonged apnea and subtracting the delivered tidal volume (V_{EI}) (55). Although this is the most accurate way of measuring dynamic hyperinflation and estimating the attendant risks of hypotension and barotrauma, the need for complete muscle relaxation, with its potential complications (see below), and practical aspects of the measurement reduce its clinical applicability (21). Furthermore, it cannot measure the volume of air trapped behind collapsed airways.
2. By measuring the average pressure developed in the airways at the end of expiration ($PEEP_i$) after occluding the airways and allowing sufficient time for equilibration (the end-expiratory occlusion technique) (20,42). This pressure represents the average recoil pressure of the respiratory system at the end of expiration, and is an indirect measure of the end-expiratory lung volume and thus of hyperinflation. However, it should be kept in mind that, in acute asthmatic crisis, the measurement of $PEEP_i$ sometimes yields unexpectedly low values, presumably reflecting airway closure (42). This is because the pressure developed behind noncommunicating airways, which might be quite high because of regional hyperinflation, does not contribute to the static $PEEP_i$ measurement by the end-expiratory occlusion technique (Fig. 112.10). Thus, the average airway pressure at the end of expiration might underestimate the pressure that corresponds to the end-expiratory lung volume. Absence of respiratory muscle activity is required for a valid measurement, because expiratory efforts can artifactually increase the measured end-expiratory occlusion pressure (59). In such cases, insertion of a gastric balloon is required to measure the increase in the gastric pressure during expiratory efforts and subtract it from the measured end-expiratory occlusion pressure to obtain the actual $PEEP_{i,st}$ (Fig. 112.11) (59).

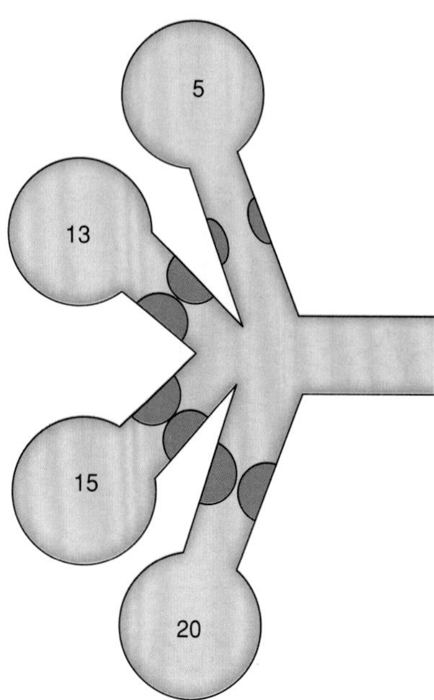

FIGURE 112.10 Hypothetical model suggesting a mechanism whereby measured auto-PEEP (positive end-expiratory pressure) by the end-expiratory occlusion technique may underestimate the severity of hyperinflation because of widespread airway closure at end-expiration. Measured auto-PEEP reflects only the end-expiratory alveolar pressure in lung units that are in communication with the proximal airway at end expiration. (Adapted from Leatherman JW, Ravenscraft SA. Low measured auto-positive end-expiratory pressure during mechanical ventilation of patients with severe asthma: hidden auto-positive end-expiratory pressure. *Crit Care Med.* 1996;24:541–546.)

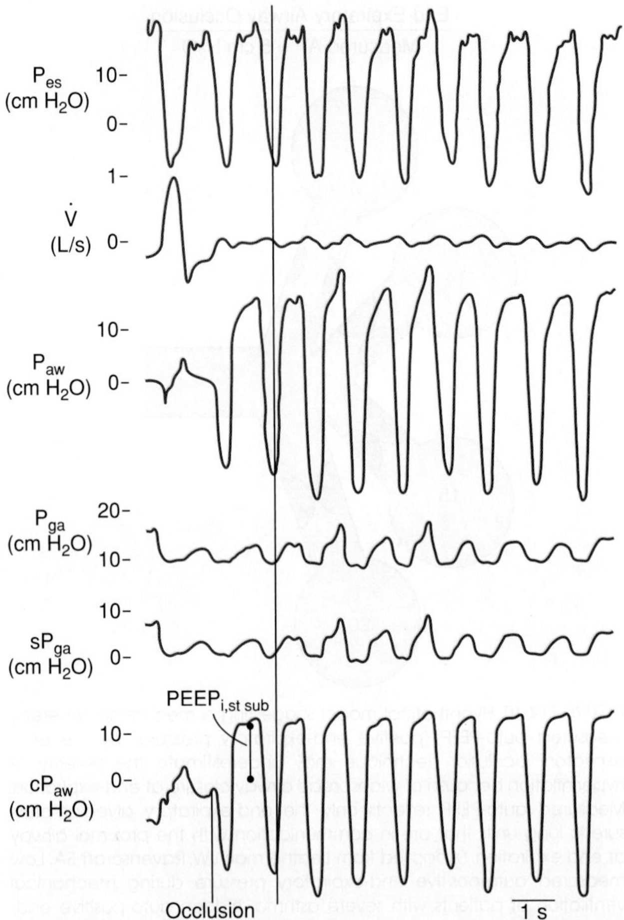

FIGURE 112.11 Correction of $PEEP_{i,st}$ measurement for expiratory muscle contraction with the use of a gastric balloon. Recordings of esophageal (P_{es}), airway (P_{aw}), gastric (P_{ga}), "suppressed" gastric pressure (sP_{ga}), and online "corrected" airway pressure (cP_{aw}) in a representative actively expiring patient during airway occlusion. sP_{ga} is the P_{ga} tracing suppressed to zero at its lowest value at the end-inspiratory level (*vertical line*) where expiratory muscle activity is nil, that is, at this level it was given the value of zero irrespective of its true value relative to atmospheric pressure. cP_{aw} is obtained by subtracting sP_{ga} from Paw. Note a consistent end-expiratory plateau in cP_{aw} despite marked variability in P_{ga} swings. From this plateau $PEEP_{i,st\ sub}$ was measured. (Adapted from Zakynthinos SG, Vassilakopoulos T, Zakynthinos E, et al. Correcting static intrinsic positive end-expiratory pressure for expiratory muscle contraction: validation of a new method. *Am J Respir Crit Care Med.* 1999;160:785–790.)

Combined Estimation of Hyperinflation and Overdistention

This can be achieved by measuring the average pressure developed in the airways at the end of inspiration after occluding the airways (end-inspiratory occlusion) and allowing sufficient time for equilibration (plateau pressure [P_{plat}]). This P_{plat} represents the recoil pressure of the respiratory system at end inspiration and, compared with the $PEEP_{i,st}$ value, is usually less prone to underestimation artifacts due to airway closure, as the delivered V_t may open airways that collapse during expiration. Furthermore, P_{plat} is increased both by increases in the end-expiratory lung volume (hyperinflation) and by overdistension (large V_t for the lung compliance). Thus, P_{plat} is the recommended variable for monitoring lung hyperinflation and overdistention during MV in asthmatic patients (56,60). An end-inspiratory pause of several seconds is required for an accurate measurement of P_{plat} because of the prolonged equilibration time of the extremely heterogeneous asthmatic lung (21,56); P_{plat} should not exceed 30 cm H_2O (58). P_{peak}, in contrast to P_{plat}, is not useful for assessing lung hyperinflation in asthmatic patients because it depends strongly on airway resistance and inspiratory flow.

The Role of Extrinsic PEEP

Controlled Mechanical Ventilation

The addition of PEEP during controlled MV in asthma patients results in a variable and unpredictable response (56,58–60). In some patients, external PEEP ($PEEP_e$) causes overinflation (56,61,62); in others, FRC and $PEEP_i$ (61–63) are decreased, and in still others no response to PEEP is observed until $PEEP_e$ exceeds baseline $PEEP_i$ (61,62). This might be because there is great heterogeneity of the asthmatic lung with various combinations of the previously described compartments in each patient.

- If the predominant site of increased resistance to airflow is located in the central, noncollapsible airways, and the transmural pressure of peripheral, collapsible bronchi and bronchioles remain positive throughout expiration, passive exhalation is not flow-limited (62–64), and the applied $PEEP_e$ extends all the way up to the alveoli, increasing end-expiratory lung volume (21,62,65).
- If the prevailing pathophysiology is flow limitation of peripheral, collapsible bronchi, and bronchioles, the addition of PEEP will not affect end-expiratory lung volume until $PEEP_e$ exceeds baseline $PEEP_i$. This is explained by the classic waterfall theory of flow limitation, which suggests that expiratory flow is determined by pressure gradients up to the choke point (point of flow limitation) and that conditions downstream from the choke point have no influence on expiratory flow (66–68). By analogy, the level of the lake downstream from a waterfall is said to have no influence on the water flow falling into it (provided that the lake level does not exceed the waterfall's edge). The water flow would be determined basically by the difference in level between the headspring and the edge of the waterfall. Because $PEEP_e$ represents the level of the downstream lake in such an analogy, it follows that $PEEP_e$ application either should have no influence on expiratory flow or should only impair it when $PEEP_i$ is approached (59).
- If the prevailing pathophysiology is sticky airway closure during exhalation, trapping some highly pressurized air, application of $PEEP_e$ (associated with transiently high end-inspiratory pressures) might reopen such a disconnected lung unit and then, because of airway hysteresis, this $PEEP_e$ might be enough to prevent expiratory airway recollapse in the next breath, promoting appropriate progressive deflation of overinflated lung (a recruiting effect analogous to that described in acute respiratory distress syndrome) (61,69).

Thus, a $PEEP_e$ trial—a stepwise application of PEEP in increments of 2 cm H_2O every 5 minutes—with measurement of the P_{plat} at each step might be a useful bedside approach. If P_{plat} decreases, application of $PEEP_e$ is deflating the lung and is beneficial (61); if P_{plat} increases, $PEEP_e$ should be withdrawn.

Assisted Mechanical Ventilation

At the resolution phase, when inspiratory muscle activity resumes and the patient triggers the ventilator, low levels of

$PEEP_e$ may be useful. This is because $PEEP_e$ may decrease muscle effort required to trigger the ventilator by providing part of the threshold pressure that $PEEP_i$ represents, which the inspiratory muscles have to overcome before airway pressure becomes negative and the ventilator is triggered (70). Keeping in mind that the existence of the waterfall effect is not guaranteed, and also that flow-limited and flow-unlimited pathways may coexist in these conditions, a prudent trial of $PEEP_e$ to a level lower than $PEEP_i$ is worth pursuing, with titration for patient comfort under close monitoring of airway and blood pressures (65). Frequent reassessment is essential because the adequate level of $PEEP_e$ is subject to change as lung mechanics and ventilatory requirements evolve.

Permissive Hypercapnia

The ventilatory strategy described is accompanied by variable levels of hypercapnia, with values averaging between 60 and 70 mmHg, but sometimes exceeding 100 mmHg (28,32,65). At times hypercapnia is unavoidable, rather than permissive (see Pathophysiology: Gas Exchange). The physiologic and untoward effects of hypercapnia are related to acute reduction of intracellular pH, due to high CO_2 diffusability, and the interested reader should consult excellent detailed reviews (54). However, effective compensatory mechanisms return intracellular pH to nearly normal within 1 to 3 hours, which explains why even extreme degrees of normoxic hypercapnia are well tolerated. Except in patients with raised intracranial pressure or severe myocardial depression, the respiratory acidosis induced by permissive hypercapnia does not need to be treated (28,53,65). In ventilated asthmatic patients CO_2 production should be reduced by the use of sedation, analgesia, and antipyretics to reduce hypercapnia (21). If these measures are insufficient, muscle relaxants may be considered (21). In acute asthma, hypercapnia usually improves within the first 12 hours of MV (probably as a result of the time-dependent effect of CSs).

Hypercapnia depresses myocardial contractility, relaxes systemic arterioles, and increases the tone in venous capacitance vessels. In the absence of β-blockade, reflex sympathetic stimulation offsets the depressed contractility (54). The integrated hemodynamic response to acute hypercapnia in patients with normal cardiac function is an increase in cardiac output (CO) accompanied by decreased systemic vascular resistance (54). In patients with underlying left ventricular dysfunction, adverse hemodynamic effects may ensue including severe hypotension and dysrhythmias, so cautious use of permissive hypercapnia is suggested in this situation (28).

Hypercapnia reversibly increases cerebral blood flow and intracranial pressure (54), which may prove disastrous in patients with intracranial pathology (53,71). A clinical challenge is presented by patients who have experienced profound cerebral anoxia secondary to respiratory arrest before intubation, in which clinicians face the therapeutic dilemma of brain protection *versus* controlled hypoventilation for addressing the asthmatic crisis. Although not supported by strong clinical data, blood alkalinization may be considered in this context. A slow infusion of sodium bicarbonate should be used, as rapid bicarbonate administration in the context of suppressed ventilatory drive may transiently raise the $PaCO_2$, thus worsening intracellular and cerebrospinal acidosis. Other buffers such as *tris*-hydroxymethyl aminomethane (tromethamine, Tham) or Carbicarb (a mixture of sodium carbonate and bicarbonate) do not have these disadvantages, but clinical experience with these agents is quite limited (72).

Sedation

Hypercapnia stimulates the respiratory center, increasing the drive to the respiratory muscles (54). Thus, controlled hypoventilation requires deep sedation to suppress respiratory muscle activity. Benzodiazepines can be safely used (73,74), as can propofol, with its rapid onset of action and—with short term use—lack of accumulation, and bronchodilating action (75,76); there is a risk of hypotension with propofol, particularly in hypovolemic patients (77). Ketamine has anesthetic, sedative, analgesic, and bronchodilating effects. In anesthetic (77,78) or subanesthetic (79) doses, ketamine reduced bronchospasm and was associated with favorable outcome in refractory cases of asthma. However, ketamine increases tracheobronchial secretions and intracranial pressure. Thus, ketamine should not be used in established or suspected anoxic encephalopathy. The addition of opioids to either benzodiazepines or propofol may help suppress the ventilatory drive, at times allowing paralysis to be avoided. The natural opioid morphine can cause allergic reactions and, because of histamine release, bronchoconstriction (80); it should thus be avoided. The synthetic opioids fentanyl or remifentanil should be used instead; remifentanil potently suppresses the ventilatory drive (81) and has a rapid onset and offset of action.

Despite the use of deep sedation, patient–ventilator asynchrony can be a problem that requires muscle paralysis, particularly in the presence of acute hypercapnia. Neuromuscular blocking agents (NMBAs) should be given as intermittent IV boluses rather than as a continuous infusion (82) to reduce the dose and duration of administration (83). Repeat boluses of NMBA should only be administered when patient–ventilator asynchrony reappears that cannot be suppressed by increasing the dose of opioid. With this strategy of NMBA, neuromuscular monitoring with "train of four," nerve stimulation becomes less obligatory.

Administration of Bronchodilators

β_2-agonists are preferably given as repeated inhaled doses rather than as continuous IV infusion because of faster onset of action and lesser incidence of adverse side effects with the former mode of administration (84,85). Aerosolized salbutamol (albuterol in North America) can be delivered via metered dose inhalers or nebulizers. Metered-dose inhalers—if possible, with the use of a spacer device—are preferred to nebulizers because of less cost and inconvenience of use, lower risk of bacterial contamination, better reproducibility of dosing, and faster maximal bronchodilation (86,87).

Humidification

Heated wire humidifiers are preferable to heat and moisture exchangers. The latter add to expiratory airway resistance and increase dead space—being inserted between the endotracheal tube and the Y-piece of ventilator tubing—and therefore contribute to hypercapnia (21).

Weaning

Once dynamic hyperinflation has abated sufficiently, as assessed by a substantial resolution of wheezing on chest auscultation and decrease of P_{plat} and $PEEP_i$, weaning should be initiated using standard procedures (88). Suppression of respiratory muscle activity with controlled hypoventilation should be maintained for as short a time as possible to prevent ventilator-induced diaphragmatic dysfunction (89). Weaning is normally rapidly achieved in patients with severe acute asthma (90). Weaning difficulty in the absence of persistent severe airway obstruction must raise the suspicion of myopathy induced by previous administration of NMBAs and CSs (see below).

COMPLICATIONS AND MORTALITY

Controlled hypoventilation for severe acute asthma has significantly reduced complications and mortality compared with conventional MV aiming at normalizing blood gases (73,74,76,91–93). The mortality of patients mechanically ventilated for severe acute asthma has been under 10% in all studies, except two, after 1990 (91,92); a frequently reported cause of death is cerebral anoxia secondary to prehospital cardiac arrest (21,28).

Hypotension

The most frequent complication of MV in asthmatic patients is hemodynamic instability manifested as hypotension (21,28,74,92,94), usually occurring at the initiation of ventilation (see above), which can occasionally be life-threatening (92). This mechanism is easily verified by temporarily disconnecting the patient from the ventilator (1 minute, under close monitoring of SpO_2) and documenting an immediate increase in blood pressure. Ventilation should be resumed with lower V_t and respiratory rate, and adequate volume expansion should rapidly follow (94). When hypotension is unresponsive to ventilator disconnection, tension pneumothorax must be suspected (21,28).

Pneumothorax

Barotrauma is the second most frequently reported complication. Controlled hypoventilation does not confer complete protection against pneumothorax, but decreases its incidence from 30% to less than 10% (74,93). Although usually not reported as a direct cause of mortality when rapidly diagnosed and adequately treated, barotrauma can still be life-threatening (91).

Myopathy

Diffuse paresis of voluntary muscles (frequently termed acute quadriplegic myopathy) has been observed on cessation of NMBA administration in asthmatic patients, lasting from a few hours to months, sometimes involving the respiratory muscles and, thus, delaying ventilator weaning (95–98). A deleterious interaction of combined treatment with NMBAs and CSs has been implicated in the pathogenesis of this complication (99). The duration of muscle relaxation (91) and the cumulative dose of NMBAs increase the risk (100). Electromyography typically shows acute myopathy usually confirmed by mildly elevated levels of creatine–phosphokinase and thick filament necrosis on muscle biopsy, which is often seen on light microscopy but found more definitely on electron microscopy (98–100). There is no specific treatment; the best approach is to avoid NMBAs and steroids, or to use these medications as sparingly as possible.

Key Points

- Although, most often, severe asthmatic exacerbation results from asthmatic patients with severe or uncontrolled asthma, any patient with asthma may experience a severe asthmatic exacerbation during his/her life.
- The group of asthmatic patients that is mainly responsible for fatal asthma are usually those with difficult to treat asthma.
- Early home management of asthma exacerbations is of paramount importance as it avoids treatment delay and prevents clinical deterioration.
- Asthma is a disease that should be diagnosed, treated, and controlled; if uncontrolled, it needs be closely followed so that asthmatics do not end up in the ICU.
- Lessons learned from asthmatic deaths include the following:
  - Most deaths can be avoided, because severe asthma crisis requiring hospitalization usually progresses over more than 6 hours.
  - Factors that lead to death are nonreferral to a specialist and inadequate steroid dosage and monitoring of disease.
  - Patients with severe asthma and psychiatric disease or psychosocial problems may experience near-fatal asthma.
  - Patients with a history of near-fatal asthma or unstable asthma should be treated only by specialists who should closely follow these patients for at least 1 year after admission.
- Early identification and treatment of asthma are essential.
- After establishing the diagnosis of severe asthma, all exacerbating factors should be identified and treated.
- Aggressive use of inhaled bronchodilator therapy plus systemic anti-inflammatory therapy (although not immediately effective) is a fundamental element of therapy of acute asthma exacerbation.
- The primary cause of respiratory demise in the patient with severe asthma is acute respiratory acidosis and ventilator insufficiency. Acute respiratory acidosis may lead to depressed level of consciousness and loss of airway protection.
- Patients with status asthmaticus may be unresponsive to initial therapeutic intervention and may require prolonged and aggressive therapy.
- Patients failing drug therapy should be considered early for intubation and MV.
- Intubation and MV increase morbidity and mortality in patients with status asthmaticus.
- The role of NIPPV in the treatment of the failing patient is not clearly established. However, in an experienced environment, a trial of NIPPV can be considered in carefully selected patients with hypercapnia and excessive work of breathing with no obvious contraindication for NIV. In face of failing treatment, early intubation should be considered.
- Controlled hypoventilation (permissive hypercapnia) in order to avoid hyperdistention and hyperinflation is the cornerstone of MV in status asthmaticus.

References

1. Global Initiative for Asthma. Global strategy for asthma management and prevention 2015. Available: http://ginasthma.org. Accessed June 23, 2017.
2. Chung KF, Wenzel SE, Brozek JL, et al. International ERS/ATS guidelines on definition, evaluation and treatment of severe asthma. *Eur Respir J*. 2014;43:343–373.
3. European Lung Foundation. Asthma. In: Gibson G, Loddenkemper R, Sibille Y, Lundback B, eds. *European Lung White Book*. European Respiratory Society; 2013.
4. Hekking PP, Wener RR, Amelink M, et al. The prevalence of severe refractory asthma. *J Allergy Clin Immunol*. 2015;135:896–902.
5. American Thoracic Society. Proceedings of the ATS workshop on refractory asthma: current understanding, recommendations, and unanswered questions. *Am J Respir Crit Care Med*. 2000;162:2341–2351.
6. European Network for Understanding Mechanisms of Severe Asthma. The ENFUMOSA cross-sectional European multicentre study of the clinical phenotype of chronic severe asthma. *Eur Respir J*. 2003;22:470–477.
7. Wenzel S. Severe asthma in adults. *Am J Respir Crit Care Med*. 2005; 172:149–160.
8. Moore WC, Peters SP. Severe asthma: an overview. *J Allergy Clin Immunol*. 2006;117:487–494.
9. Moore WC, Meyers DA, Wenzel SE, et al. Identification of asthma phenotypes using cluster analysis in the Severe Asthma Research Program. *Am J Respir Crit Care Med*. 2010;181:315–323.
10. Wenzel S. Severe asthma: from characteristics to phenotypes to endotypes. *Clin Exp Allergy*. 2012;42:650–658.
11. Wenzel SE. Asthma: defining of the persistent adult phenotypes. *Lancet*. 2006;368:804–813.
12. Wenzel SE. Asthma phenotypes: the evolution from clinical to molecular approaches. *Nat Med*. 2012;18:716–725.
13. Wenzel SE. Complex phenotypes in asthma: current definitions. *Pulm Pharmacol Ther*. 2013;26:710–715.
14. McFadden ER Jr, Kiser R, DeGroot WJ. Acute bronchial asthma: relations between clinical and physiologic manifestations. *N Engl J Med*. 1973; 288:221–225.
15. Colebatch HJ, Finucane KE, Smith MM. Pulmonary conductance and elastic recoil relationships in asthma and emphysema. *J Appl Physiol*. 1973;34:143–153.
16. McCarthy DS, Sigurdson M. Lung elastic recoil and reduced airflow in clinically stable asthma. *Thorax*. 1980;35:298-302.
17. Martin J, Powell E, Shore S, et al. The role of respiratory muscles in the hyperinflation of bronchial asthma. *Am Rev Respir Dis*. 1980;121: 441–447.
18. Collett PW, Brancatisano T, Engel LA. Changes in the glottic aperture during bronchial asthma. *Am Rev Respir Dis*. 1983;128: 719–723.
19. Briscoe WA, McLemorE GA Jr. Ventilatory function in bronchial asthma. *Thorax*. 1952;7:66–77.
20. Pepe PE, Marini JJ. Occult positive end-expiratory pressure in mechanically ventilated patients with airflow obstruction: the auto-PEEP effect. *Am Rev Respir Dis*. 1982;126:166–170.
21. Oddo M, Feihl F, Schaller MD, Perret C. Management of mechanical ventilation in acute severe asthma: practical aspects. *Intensive Care Med*. 2006;32: 501–510.
22. Vassilakopoulos T, Zakynthinos S, Roussos C. Respiratory muscles and weaning failure. *Eur Respir J*. 1996;9:2383–2400.
23. Vassilakopoulos T, Zakynthinos S, Roussos C. Muscle function: basic concepts. In: Marini JJ, Slutsky AS, eds. *Physiologic Basis of Ventilator Support*. New York: Marcel Dekker; 1998:103–152.
24. Lougheed MD, Lam M, Forkert L, et al. Breathlessness during acute bronchoconstriction in asthma: pathophysiologic mechanisms. *Am Rev Respir Dis*. 1993;148:1452–1459.
25. Lougheed DM, Webb KA, O'Donnell DE. Breathlessness during induced lung hyperinflation in asthma: the role of the inspiratory threshold load. *Am J Respir Crit Care Med*. 1995;152:911–920.
26. Rodriguez-Roisin R, Ballester E, Roca J, et al. Mechanisms of hypoxemia in patients with status asthmaticus requiring mechanical ventilation. *Am Rev Respir Dis*. 1989;139:732–739.
27. Rodriguez-Roisin R. Acute severe asthma: pathophysiology and pathobiology of gas exchange abnormalities. *Eur Respir J*. 1997;10:1359–1371.
28. Leatherman J. Mechanical ventilation for severe asthma. *Chest*. 2015;147: 1671–1680.
29. Martin J, Jardim J, Sampson M, Engel LE. Factors influencing pulsus paradoxus in asthma. *Chest*. 1981;80:543–549.
30. Shim C, Williams MH Jr. Pulsus paradoxus in asthma. *Lancet*. 1978;1: 530–531.
31. Manthous CA, Hall JB, Caputo MA, et al. Heliox improves pulsus paradoxus and peak expiratory flow in nonintubated patients with severe asthma. *Am J Respir Crit Care Med*. 1995;151:310–314.
32. Papiris SA, Manali ED, Kolilekas L, et al. Acute severe asthma: new approaches to assessment and treatment. *Drugs*. 2009;69:2363–2391.
33. Bel EH. Clinical phenotypes of asthma. *Curr Opin Pulm Med*. 2004;10: 44–50.
34. Holgate ST, Polosa R. The mechanisms, diagnosis, and management of severe asthma in adults. *Lancet*. 2006;368:780–793.
35. British Thoracic Society; Scottish Intercollegiate Guidelines network. British guideline on the management of asthma: a national clinical guideline. Available: https://www.brit-thoracic.org.uk/document-library/clinical-information/asthma/btssign-asthma-guideline-2016. Last accessed July 29, 2017.
36. Fernandez MM, Villagra A, Blanch L, Fernandez R. Non-invasive mechanical ventilation in status asthmaticus. *Intensive Care Med*. 2001;27: 486–492.
37. Ram FS, Wellington S, Rowe B, Wedzicha JA. Non-invasive positive pressure ventilation for treatment of respiratory failure due to severe acute exacerbations of asthma. *Cochrane Database Syst Rev*. 2005;CD004360.
38. Tuxen DV, Williams TJ, Scheinkestel CD, et al. Use of a measurement of pulmonary hyperinflation to control the level of mechanical ventilation in patients with acute severe asthma. *Am Rev Respir Dis*. 1992;146: 1136–1142.
39. Brenner B, Corbridge T, Kazzi A. Intubation and mechanical ventilation of the asthmatic patient in respiratory failure. *Proc Am Thorac Soc*. 2009; 6:371–379.
40. Corbridge TC, Hall JB. The assessment and management of adults with status asthmaticus. *Am J Respir Crit Care Med*. 1995;151:1296–1316.
41. Pallin M, Naughton MT. Noninvasive ventilation in acute asthma. *J Crit Care*. 2014;29:586–593.
42. Leatherman JW, Ravenscraft SA. Low measured auto-positive end-expiratory pressure during mechanical ventilation of patients with severe asthma: hidden auto-positive end-expiratory pressure. *Crit Care Med*. 1996;24:541–546.
43. Soroksky A, Stav D, Shpirer I. A pilot prospective, randomized, placebo-controlled trial of bilevel positive airway pressure in acute asthmatic attack. *Chest*. 2003;123:1018–1025.
44. Gupta D, Nath A, Agarwal R, Behera D. A prospective randomized controlled trial on the efficacy of noninvasive ventilation in severe acute asthma. *Respir Care*. 2010;55:536–543.
45. Lim WJ, Mohammed AR, Carson KV, et al. Non-invasive positive pressure ventilation for treatment of respiratory failure due to severe acute exacerbations of asthma. *Cochrane Database Syst Rev*. 2012;12:CD004360.
46. Brandao DC, Lima VM, Filho VG, et al. Reversal of bronchial obstruction with bi-level positive airway pressure and nebulization in patients with acute asthma. *J Asthma*. 2009;46:356–361.
47. Galindo-Filho VC, Brandao DC, Ferreira RC, et al. Noninvasive ventilation coupled with nebulization during asthma crises: a randomized controlled trial. *Respir Care*. 2013;58:241–249.
48. Soma T, Hino M, Kida K, Kudoh S. A prospective and randomized study for improvement of acute asthma by non-invasive positive pressure ventilation (NPPV). *Intern Med*. 2008;47:493–501.
49. Murase K, Tomii K, Chin K, et al. The use of non-invasive ventilation for life-threatening asthma attacks: changes in the need for intubation. *Respirology*. 2010;15:714–720.
50. Pallin M, Hew M, Naughton MT. Is non-invasive ventilation safe in acute severe asthma? *Respirology*. 2015;20:251–257.
51. Soroksky A, Klinowski E, Ilgyev E, et al. Noninvasive positive pressure ventilation in acute asthmatic attack. *Eur Respir Rev*. 2010;19:39–45.
52. Cappiello JL, Hocker MB. Noninvasive ventilation in severe acute asthma. *Respir Care*. 2014;59: e149–e152.
53. Darioli R, Perret C. Mechanical controlled hypoventilation in status asthmaticus. *Am Rev Respir Dis*. 1984;129:385–387.
54. Feihl F, Perret C. Permissive hypercapnia: how permissive should we be? *Am J Respir Crit Care Med*. 1994;150:1722–1737.
55. Tuxen DV, Lane S. The effects of ventilatory pattern on hyperinflation, airway pressures, and circulation in mechanical ventilation of patients with severe air-flow obstruction. *Am Rev Respir Dis*. 1987;136:872–879.
56. Leatherman JW, McArthur C, Shapiro RS. Effect of prolongation of expiratory time on dynamic hyperinflation in mechanically ventilated patients with severe asthma. *Crit Care Med*. 2004;32:1542–1545.
57. McFadden ER Jr. Acute severe asthma. *Am J Respir Crit Care Med*. 2003; 168:740–759.

58. Ninane V, Yernault JC, de TA. Intrinsic PEEP in patients with chronic obstructive pulmonary disease: role of expiratory muscles. *Am Rev Respir Dis*. 1993;148: 1037–1042.
59. Zakynthinos SG, Vassilakopoulos T, Zakynthinos E, et al. Correcting static intrinsic positive end-expiratory pressure for expiratory muscle contraction: validation of a new method. *Am J Respir Crit Care Med*. 1999;160:785–790.
60. Slutsky AS. Consensus conference on mechanical ventilation—January 28–30, 1993 at Northbrook, Illinois, USA. Part 2. *Intensive Care Med*. 1994;20:150–162.
61. Caramez MP, Borges JB, Tucci MR, et al. Paradoxical responses to positive end-expiratory pressure in patients with airway obstruction during controlled ventilation. *Crit Care Med*. 2005;33:1519–1528.
62. Tuxen DV. Detrimental effects of positive end-expiratory pressure during controlled mechanical ventilation of patients with severe airflow obstruction. *Am Rev Respir Dis*. 1989;140:5–9.
63. Qvist J, Andersen JB, Pemberton M, Bennike KA. High-level PEEP in severe asthma. *N Engl J Med*. 1982;307:1347–1348.
64. McFadden ER Jr, Ingram RH Jr, Haynes RL, Wellman JJ. Predominant site of flow limitation and mechanisms of postexertional asthma. *J Appl Physiol Respir Environ Exerc Physiol*. 1977;42:746–752.
65. Marini JJ. Should PEEP be used in airflow obstruction? *Am Rev Respir Dis*. 1989;140:1–3.
66. Dawson SV, Elliott EA. Wave-speed limitation on expiratory flow-a unifying concept. *J Appl Physiol Respir Environ Exerc Physiol*. 1977;43: 498–515.
67. Pride NB, Permutt S, Riley RL, Bromberger-Barnea B. Determinants of maximal expiratory flow from the lungs. *J Appl Physiol*. 1967;23:646–662.
68. Tobin MJ, Lodato RF. PEEP, auto-PEEP, and waterfalls. *Chest*. 1989;96: 449–451.
69. Marini JJ. Positive end-expiratory pressure in severe airflow obstruction: more than a "one-trick pony"? *Crit Care Med*. 2005;33:1652–1653.
70. Smith TC, Marini JJ. Impact of PEEP on lung mechanics and work of breathing in severe airflow obstruction. *J Appl Physiol (1985)*. 1988;65: 1488–1499.
71. Meduri GU, Cook TR, Turner RE, et al. Noninvasive positive pressure ventilation in status asthmaticus. *Chest*. 1996;110:767–774.
72. Levraut J, Grimaud D. Treatment of metabolic acidosis. *Curr Opin Crit Care*. 2003;9:260–265.
73. Bellomo R, McLaughlin P, Tai E, Parkin G. Asthma requiring mechanical ventilation: a low morbidity approach. *Chest*. 1994;105:891–896.
74. Williams TJ, Tuxen DV, Scheinkestel CD, et al. Risk factors for morbidity in mechanically ventilated patients with acute severe asthma. *Am Rev Respir Dis*. 1992;146:607–615.
75. Conti G, Ferretti A, Tellan G, et al. Propofol induces bronchodilation in a patient mechanically ventilated for status asthmaticus. *Intensive Care Med*. 1993;19:305.
76. Kearney SE, Graham D, Atherton ST. Acute severe asthma treated by mechanical ventilation: a comparison of the changing characteristics over a 17 year period. *Respir Med*. 1998;92:716–721.
77. Mirenda J, Broyles G. Propofol as used for sedation in the ICU. *Chest*. 1995;108:539–548.
78. Hemming A, MacKenzie I, Finfer S. Response to ketamine in status asthmaticus resistant to maximal medical treatment. *Thorax*. 1994;49:90–91.
79. Sarma VJ. Use of ketamine in acute severe asthma. *Acta Anaesthesiol Scand*. 1992;36:106–107.
80. Golembiewski JA. Allergic reactions to drugs: implications for perioperative care. *J Perianesth Nurs*. 2002;17:393–398.
81. Bouillon T, Bruhn J, Radu-Radulescu L, et al. A model of the ventilatory depressant potency of remifentanil in the non-steady state. *Anesthesiology*. 2003;99:779–787.
82. Shapiro BA, Warren J, Egol AB, et al. Practice parameters for sustained neuromuscular blockade in the adult critically ill patient: an executive summary. Society of Critical Care Medicine. *Crit Care Med*. 1995;23: 1601–1605.
83. de Lemos JM, Carr RR, Shalansky KF, et al. Paralysis in the critically ill: intermittent bolus pancuronium compared with continuous infusion. *Crit Care Med*. 1999;27:2648–2655.
84. Rodrigo GJ. Inhaled therapy for acute adult asthma. *Curr Opin Allergy Clin Immunol*. 2003;3:169–175.
85. Travers AH, Rowe BH, Barker S, et al. The effectiveness of IV beta-agonists in treating patients with acute asthma in the emergency department: a meta-analysis. *Chest*. 2002;122:1200–1207.
86. Duarte AG, Momii K, Bidani A. Bronchodilator therapy with metered-dose inhaler and spacer versus nebulizer in mechanically ventilated patients: comparison of magnitude and duration of response. *Respir Care*. 2000;45: 817–823.
87. Duarte AG. Inhaled bronchodilator administration during mechanical ventilation. *Respir Care*. 2004;49:623–634.
88. Vassilakopoulos T, Roussos C, Zakynthinos S. Weaning from mechanical ventilation. *J Crit Care*. 1999;14:39–62.
89. Vassilakopoulos T. Ventilator-induced diaphragm dysfunction: the clinical relevance of animal models. *Intensive Care Med*. 2008;34:7–16.
90. Mansel JK, Stogner SW, Petrini MF, Norman JR. Mechanical ventilation in patients with acute severe asthma. *Am J Med*. 1990;89:42–48.
91. Afessa B, Morales I, Cury JD. Clinical course and outcome of patients admitted to an ICU for status asthmaticus. *Chest*. 2001;120:1616–1621.
92. Rosengarten PL, Tuxen DV, Dziukas L, et al. Circulatory arrest induced by intermittent positive pressure ventilation in a patient with severe asthma. *Anaesth Intensive Care*. 1991;19:118–121.
93. Peters JI, Stupka JE, Singh H, et al. Status asthmaticus in the medical intensive care unit: a 30-year experience. *Respir Med*. 2012;106:344–348.
94. Berlin D. Hemodynamic consequences of auto-PEEP. *J Intensive Care Med*. 2014;29:81–86.
95. Danon MJ, Carpenter S. Myopathy with thick filament (myosin) loss following prolonged paralysis with vecuronium during steroid treatment. *Muscle Nerve*. 1991;14:1131–1139.
96. David WS, Roehr CL, Leatherman JW. EMG findings in acute myopathy with status asthmaticus, steroids and paralytics: clinical and electrophysiologic correlation. *Electromyogr Clin Neurophysiol*. 1998;38:371–376.
97. Griffin D, Fairman N, Coursin D, et al. Acute myopathy during treatment of status asthmaticus with corticosteroids and steroidal muscle relaxants. *Chest*. 1992;102:510–514.
98. Leatherman JW, Fluegel WL, David WS, et al. Muscle weakness in mechanically ventilated patients with severe asthma. *Am J Respir Crit Care Med*. 1996;153:1686–1690.
99. Behbehani NA, Al-Mane F, D'yachkova Y, et al. Myopathy following mechanical ventilation for acute severe asthma: the role of muscle relaxants and corticosteroids. *Chest*. 1999;115:1627–1631.
100. Douglass JA, Tuxen DV, Horne M, et al. Myopathy in severe asthma. *Am Rev Respir Dis*. 1992;146:517–519.

CHAPTER

113

Acute Respiratory Failure in Chronic Obstructive Pulmonary Disease

MARCELO BRITTO PASSOS AMATO, MARCELO PARK, and EDUARDO LEITE VIEIRA COSTA

INTRODUCTION

Chronic obstructive pulmonary diseases (COPDs) are a group of disorders characterized by airflow limitation that is not fully reversible (1). Being the fourth leading cause of death worldwide (and projected to be the first in 2030), COPD is responsible for a remarkable public health burden. There are several diseases under this designation (Table 113.1), the most common of which are chronic bronchitis and emphysema. These two disorders represent the extremes of the COPD spectrum and usually coexist in COPD patients. Bronchitis is predominantly a disease of the airways and presents as a chronic productive cough for at least 3 months during 2 consecutive years, while emphysema is a disease of the parenchyma and consists of permanent airspace enlargement associated with rupture of the alveolar septa.

The common final pathway leading to COPD is an increased inflammatory response to inhaled particles or gases, of which the most common is cigarette smoke. Occupational exposure to fumes and dusts and use of indoor biomass cooking also account for a significant proportion of cases, especially among nonsmokers in whom they represent roughly a third of cases. The inflammatory process involves the airways and the lung parenchyma, leading to mucosal gland hypertrophy and disruption of alveolar septa with loss of elastic recoil. These alterations ultimately lead to the obstructive ventilatory defect that defines COPD (2,3). Some patients develop pulmonary hyperinflation caused by the loss of elastic recoil and increased airway resistance. During exacerbations, there might be a secondary dynamic pulmonary hyperinflation (2,4) caused by the increased ventilatory requirement and shortened expiratory time (5). The capacity of the respiratory muscles to generate inspiratory pressure is limited by their shortened operating length and impaired geometric arrangement (6). Long-term steroid use and/or malnutrition also contribute to strength impairment in many patients with severe chronic disease (7).

Only about 15% of all smokers will develop the full-blown syndrome with overt clinical symptoms, although a half of elderly smokers fulfill the criteria for COPD (8). The degree of obstruction correlates best with the smoking load, traditionally measured in pack-years. Rarely, the disease results from an inborn imbalance between the proteases and antiproteases present in the lung, as occurs in the autosomal recessive α_1-antitrypsin deficiency (9).

CLINICAL FINDINGS

The clinical manifestations of COPD appear late in the course of the disease. There is initially a slow decline in lung function that goes unnoticed over the years (10). Cough is the first finding, usually after the patient has been a smoker for many years. After about 20 years of smoking, some patients begin to notice shortness of breath on exertion, reflecting the progressive airflow limitation that is characteristic of the disease. The dyspnea worsens slowly over time, although sometimes patients deny the deterioration of lung function because they slowly adapt their level of activity to their exercise capacity. The decrease in lung function might become steeper during exacerbations, with a slow recovery to baseline levels (at most) after resolution of the decompensation. It can be useful to assess COPD-related symptoms in a systematic manner. One widely used scale to gauge breathlessness is the modified British Medical Research Council Questionnaire or mMRC (Table 113.2). For a more comprehensive assessment of the health status, the COPD assessment test (CAT; Table 113.3) can be used. Either the mMRC or the CAT can be used in the combined COPD assessment (see Spirometry section below).

Spirometry

Spirometry is the most important functional test for the diagnosis and the classification of severity of the disease. It consists of a forced exhalation after a deep inspiration while the patient is connected to a pneumotachograph. The ratio of the forced expiratory volume in the first second of the exhalation (FEV_1) to the forced vital capacity is diagnostic of an obstructive ventilatory defect if below 0.7 (1). The FEV_1 is a useful marker of the disease severity (Table 113.4) and is well suited as a longitudinal monitor of lung function (10). The degree of airflow limitation is also associated with the prevalence of exacerbations. However, because of the weak correlation between the patients' health status and the severity of airflow obstruction, we recommend a combined assessment, which considers not only the severity of the airflow limitation but also symptoms (CAT; see Table 113.3) or the degree of breathlessness (mMRC; see Table 113.2). In this combined assessment, the history of previous exacerbations can substitute the degree of airflow limitation (Table 113.5).

TABLE 113.1 Diseases Associated with Chronic Obstructive Pulmonary Disease
Chronic bronchitis
Emphysema
Bronchiolitis
Bronchiectasis
Tuberculosis
α_1-Trypsin deficiency

TABLE 113.2 Severity of Breathlessness Assessment According to the Modified British Medical Research Council (mMRC)

Grade 0	I only get breathless with strenuous exercise
Grade 1	I get short of breath when hurrying on the level or walking up a slight hill
Grade 2	I walk slower than people of the same age on the level because of breathlessness, or I have to stop for breath when walking on my own pace on the level
Grade 3	I stop for breath after walking about 100 m or after a few minutes on the level
Grade 4	I am too breathless to leave the house or I am breathless when dressing or undressing

TABLE 113.4 Classification of Severity of Airflow Limitation According to GOLD

In patients with FEV_1/FVC <0.7 (postbronchodilator):	
1: Mild COPD	FEV_1 = 80% predicted
2: Moderate COPD	50% = FEV_1 <80% predicted
3: Severe COPD	30% = FEV_1 <50% predicted
4: Very severe COPD	FEV_1 <30% predicted

GOLD, Global Initiative for Chronic Obstructive Lung Disease; COPD, chronic obstructive pulmonary disease; FEV_1, forced expiratory volume in the first second of the exhalation; FVC, forced vital capacity. (From the Global Strategy for the Diagnosis, Management and Prevention of COPD, Global Initiative for Chronic Obstructive Lung Disease (GOLD) 2016. Available from: http://www.goldcopd.org/.)

Lung Volume and Diffusing Capacity

Lung volumes can be measured using whole-body plethysmography or gas dilution (helium or nitrogen washout) techniques. In emphysema, both total lung capacity and residual volume may be increased because of loss of lung elastic recoil. The carbon monoxide diffusing capacity may be diminished with the progression of the disease, reflecting the impaired gas exchange due to loss of the functional parenchyma. Although not required for the diagnosis of COPD, both lung volumes and diffusing capacity can be used to characterize its severity. Both measurements are part of the COPD workup especially when techniques such as volume reduction surgery or placement of endobronchial valves are being considered.

Chest Radiographic Findings

Chest radiographic alterations usually occur late in the course of the disease, and there is no alteration pathognomonic of COPD. The radiograph is usually normal in mild disease; changes reflecting airway disease and hyperinflation may appear with disease progression. Sometimes it is possible to see enlarged bronchial walls reflected as an increase in bronchovascular markings. Emphysema is manifested by an increased lucency of the lungs. In smokers, these changes are more prominent in the upper lobes, while in α_1-antitrypsin deficiency, they are more likely in basal zones. With hyperinflation, the chest becomes vertically elongated with low, flattened diaphragmatic domes. The heart shadow is also vertical and narrow. The retrosternal airspace is increased on the lateral view, and the sternal-diaphragmatic angle exceeds 90 degrees. Radiographic computerized tomography is more sensitive and specific for the presence of emphysema, but it is rarely required. It is most useful in the preoperative evaluation for lung volume reduction surgery or to plan the placement of endobronchial valves (11,12).

Arterial Blood Gases

Both pulse oximetry and arterial blood gases can be used to determine the need of home oxygen therapy. If oxygen saturation is below 92% on pulse oximetry while breathing room air, an arterial blood sample should be obtained. If PaO_2 is below 55 mmHg, long-term oxygen therapy is indicated. When between 55 and 59 mmHg, home oxygen is recommended only if there is polycythemia or signs of right heart failure.

EXACERBATION

COPD exacerbation can be defined as an acute event characterized by an increase in dyspnea, cough, or sputum production that requires therapy (13). The two most commonly identified precipitating factors are infection—viral, such as *Rhinovirus* spp or influenza, and bacterial, such as *Haemophilus influenzae*, *Streptococcus pneumoniae*, *Moraxella catarrhalis*, *Enterobacteriaceae* spp, or *Pseudomonas* spp—as well as environmental exposure to air pollutants. However, in about one-third of cases, no underlying cause is identified. Infectious agents can also be recovered from some patients with stable COPD, indicating that in some instances, their presence in decompensated COPD represents an epiphenomenon. On the other hand, the acquisition of a new strain of a bacterial

TABLE 113.3 COPD Assessment Test (CAT)

	Likert scale	
I never cough	0 1 2 3 4 5	I cough all the time
I have no phlegm (mucus) in my chest at all	0 1 2 3 4 5	My chest is full of phlegm (mucus)
My chest does not feel tight at all	0 1 2 3 4 5	My chest feels very tight
When I walk up a hill or one flight of stairs I am not breathless	0 1 2 3 4 5	When I walk up a hill or one flight of stairs I am very breathless
I am not limited doing any activities at home	0 1 2 3 4 5	I am very limited doing activities at home
I am confident leaving my home despite my lung condition	0 1 2 3 4 5	I am not at all confident leaving my home because of my lung condition
I sleep soundly	0 1 2 3 4 5	I do not sleep soundly because of my lung condition
I have lots of energy	0 1 2 3 4 5	I have no energy at all

For each question, the patients have to choose one score (from 0 to 5) that best describes their condition. The total score thus ranges from 0 to 40. Available from: http://www.catestonline.org/english/indexEN.htm

TABLE 113.5 Combined Assessment Using Symptoms, Breathlessness, Spirometric Classification, and Risk of Exacerbations According to GOLD

Airflow limitation	4	**C**	**D**	≥2	or	**Exacerbation history**
(see Table 113.4)	3			≥1	with hospitalization	
	2	**A**	**B**	1		
	1			0		
		CAT <10	CAT ≥10			
		Symptoms (see Table 113.3)				
		OR				
		mMRC 0–1	mMRC ≥2			
		Breathlessness (see Table 113.2)				

species colonized with a pathogenic bacteria might lead to an exacerbation in stable COPD patients (14). All things considered, the best predictor of future exacerbations is having treated an exacerbation in the past, suggesting the existence of a frequent exacerbation phenotype (15). Other predictors of exacerbation include decreasing lung function, worsening quality of life, a history of gastroesophageal reflux, and an increased white-cell count (14). All exacerbations should be evaluated carefully for their potential to require hospitalization as a result of respiratory failure, which is associated with poor prognosis and increased risk of death. In the following section, we discuss the hospital treatment of COPD exacerbations.

Assessment and Treatment of Exacerbations

The goals of the treatment of COPD exacerbations are to eliminate or control the cause of the exacerbation, provide optimum bronchodilator therapy, assure adequate oxygenation, and correct respiratory acidemia, all the while avoiding tracheal intubation when possible. Most patients with mild exacerbations can be treated at home, but those with a more severe presentation require hospitalization. Signs of severity include use of accessory muscles, paradoxical breathing pattern, hemodynamic instability, and decreased level of consciousness (1). In-hospital mortality in those with severe exacerbations is approximately 10% to 24% and can reach 59% at 1 year (16,17).

Admission criteria according to the American Thoracic Society/European Respiratory Society guidelines (18) include:

- High-risk comorbidities including pneumonia, cardiac arrhythmia, congestive heart failure, diabetes mellitus, renal failure, or liver failure
- Inadequate response of symptoms to outpatient management
- Marked increase in dyspnea
- Inability to eat or sleep because of symptoms
- Worsening hypoxemia
- Worsening hypercapnia
- Changes in mental status
- Inability to care for oneself (i.e., lack of home support)
- Uncertain diagnosis

Pharmacologic Treatment

The mainstay of pharmacologic treatment is the use of bronchodilators, corticosteroids, and antibiotics, all of which are discussed below.

Bronchodilators

1. β_2-Agonists: The bronchodilators most commonly used are the inhaled short-acting β_2-agonists because of their rapid onset of action. They can be administered via a nebulizer or through metered dose inhalers (MDIs). Typically, two puffs of albuterol or salbutamol are given every 4 hours, or an equivalent dose via nebulizer. During mechanical ventilation, the use of a spacer interposed in the circuit between the tube and the Y-piece is recommended. An unresolved issue relates to dosage when MDIs are used with intubated patients. Fernandez et al. (19) used two puffs, Gay et al. (20) used three puffs, and Fuller et al. (21) used four puffs in their studies. Because the MDI dose deposited in the lungs of intubated patients is, at best, half of the dose deposited in the lungs of ambulatory patients, it seems reasonable to at least double the number of MDI puffs in intubated patients (i.e., at least four puffs). In some patients, this dose will be inadequate, and a greater number of puffs (e.g., 10–20) can be safe and effectively used. In such circumstances, tachycardia—a common and dose-dependent side effect of bronchodilators—should be monitored to avoid β_2-agonists overdose. Other potential side effects should be closely followed, such as agitation, tremulousness, hyperlactatemia, hypokalemia, and hyperglycemia.

   Long-acting β_2-agonists can also be considered. Subcutaneous or intravenous administration should not be used unless there is contraindication for the inhaled route because of their increased systemic effects.
2. Anticholinergics: Ipratropium bromide can be used in association with the β_2-agonists as needed. It is available both via nebulization (500 μg) or MDI (two puffs every 2–4 hours). There are no clinical studies that have evaluated the use of the long-acting anticholinergic tiotropium bromide during COPD exacerbations.
3. Methylxanthines: Methylxanthines are currently not indicated in the treatment of exacerbations of COPD.

Corticosteroids. Steroids are usually recommended for exacerbations of COPD. If feasible, prednisone can be given orally at a dose of 30 to 40 mg/day for 5 days (22). If the oral route is not an option, hydrocortisone or methylprednisolone can be substituted in equivalent doses. Some investigators advocate the use of much higher doses (methylprednisolone, 125 mg intravenously four times daily) (23), but as no studies have been designed to find the optimal dose, we favor the lower dose. The inhaled route can be an option (24,25). The combination of salmeterol, 50 μg, and fluticasone, 500 μg, given twice daily, has been compared with placebo and resulted in a reduction in mortality of 3 years ($p = 0.052$), fewer exacerbations, and improved health status and lung function. Nebulized budesonide, 1,500 μg four times daily, was compared with prednisolone 40 mg and demonstrated equal efficacy and potentially fewer side effects, especially less hyperglycemia.

Antibiotics. Antibiotics decrease mortality during exacerbations. These agents are indicated when there is increased production or change in the color of the sputum. For mild exacerbations, amoxicillin, sulfamethoxazole-trimethoprim, or doxycycline for 7 to 10 days is usually adequate. Patients requiring hospitalizations should receive penicillin/penicillinase (e.g., amoxicillin/clavulanate), a respiratory quinolone (levofloxacin, moxifloxacin), or a third-generation cephalosporin together with a macrolide (e.g., ceftriaxone plus clarithromycin). In addition to their antimicrobial activity, macrolides possess anti-inflammatory and mucoregulatory properties that may confer beneficial effects to patients with COPD (26).

Respiratory Support

The goal of respiratory support in patients with exacerbations of COPD is to correct hypoxemia/acidemia and reduce the respiratory work, thus avoiding respiratory muscle fatigue (27,28). In the acute setting, oxygen therapy alone is able to resolve hypoxemia, but not acidemia and respiratory distress. For this reason, invasive or noninvasive mechanical ventilation is frequently needed (2,28).

Oxygen Therapy. To improve the hypoxemia commonly present in exacerbations of COPD, controlled oxygen therapy is the cornerstone of hospital treatment (2). Long-term oxygen therapy is established as the standard of care for selected patients with advanced chronic stable hypoxemia due to COPD (29,30). However, in the acute setting, some patients have an impaired response to hypercapnia when treated with supplementary oxygen, leading to worsening of CO_2 retention (31,32). The precise mechanism of this impairment is not well understood, but ventilation/perfusion (33–37) and respiratory drive (34,38) disturbances have been implicated. Some evidence suggests that blunting of the hypoxic vasoconstriction response due to the higher oxygen content in poorly ventilated areas may be the culprit of the acute CO_2 retention. The increased perfusion of such poorly ventilated, previously hypoxic areas might suddenly increase the shunt effect, transferring a great part of the venous CO_2 content directly to the arterial compartment, causing some worsening of hypercapnia and sometimes deterioration of mental status.

There is no individual risk factor that identifies patients with COPD who will evolve to hypercapnia after oxygen exposure (2,31,32); therefore, the National Heart, Lung, Blood Institute/World Health Organization Global Initiative for Chronic Obstructive Lung Disease (GOLD) Workshop summary has recommended controlled oxygen therapy for the exacerbations, where adequate levels of oxygenation—PaO_2 of at least 60 mmHg or SaO_2 of at least 90%—are easy to achieve in uncomplicated exacerbations. Notwithstanding, CO_2 retention can occur insidiously with little change in symptoms; hence, measuring arterial blood gases 30 minutes after the start of oxygen therapy is recommended. Venturi masks are more accurate sources of oxygen than are nasal prongs, but are more likely to be removed by the patient (2). Controlled oxygen therapy must be started at a low inspiratory oxygen fraction—0.24 to 0.28—and titrated upward to reach a PaO_2 of at least 60 mmHg or SaO_2 of at least 90% without significant retention of CO_2. A clinically significant increase in $PaCO_2$ has been arbitrarily defined as a raise in CO_2 of 6.5 mmHg, especially if mental status deteriorates (32).

One must always remember that most of these patients have some degree of chronic vascular disease associated with their smoking history, and cardiovascular complications may be frequent during prolonged hypoxic episodes; for example, acute coronary syndromes, atrial fibrillation, cerebral ischemia, and pulmonary congestion. Therefore, the quick reversal of severe hypoxemia is frequently a priority.

Noninvasive Mechanical Ventilation. Patients with COPD are prone to acute hypercapnic respiratory failure, often resulting in emergency admission to the hospital. Between 20% and 30% of patients admitted with hypercapnic respiratory failure secondary to acute exacerbation of COPD will die in the hospital (39–42). Traditionally, patients who do not respond to conventional treatment are given invasive mechanical ventilation despite its well-known risks. Tracheal intubation and assisted ventilation have been associated with high morbidity and mortality rates, in addition to the difficulties during the weaning process from the ventilator (43,44). Many clinical complications seem to arise from the intubation procedure itself, or during the course of mechanical ventilation. The most common complications have been nosocomial infections, aspiration, pulmonary embolism, muscle atrophy, polyneuropathies, electrolyte imbalances, and gastrointestinal bleeding, as well as prolonging the stay in the intensive care unit (45,46).

In view of such difficulties, noninvasive positive pressure ventilation is an alternative treatment for patients admitted to the hospital with hypercapnic respiratory failure secondary to acute exacerbations of COPD. With this ventilatory modality, the patient receives air, or a mixture of air and oxygen, from a flow generator or a special ventilator through a facial/nasal mask, thus avoiding the need for tracheal intubation (40–42,47–49). Many studies have shown that noninvasive positive pressure ventilation increases pH, reduces $PaCO_2$, reduces the severity of breathlessness in the first 4 hours of treatment, and decreases the length of hospital stay (40–42). More importantly, mortality and the intubation rate are consistently reduced by this intervention (40–42). Some studies suggest that the use of proper noninvasive ventilation can reduce the chances of an eventual endotracheal intubation to less than half (0.42, 95% confidence interval [CI] of 0.31 to 0.59) when compared with the conventional treatment with oxygen mask. This alternative has been also associated to a reduced mortality rate (0.41, 95% CI 0.26 to 0.64). In clinical-physiological terms, the expected elevation of pH after 1 hour of treatment should be around 0.03 (95% CI 0.02 to 0.04) and the expected reduction in $PaCO_2$ in the same interval around –3.0 mmHg (95% CI –5.1 to –0.2) (50).

Unfortunately, noninvasive ventilation is not appropriate for all patients (2). Failure rates between 9% and 50% have been reported (51,52). One important signal that this procedure is not working for a patient is the progression—even if slight—of hypercapnia or acidosis 30 to 60 minutes after the procedure, and deterioration of the mental status.

The classic indications for noninvasive mechanical ventilation in exacerbated COPD patients are (1) respiratory distress with respiratory rate above 35 breaths/min; (2) respiratory acidosis with a pH below 7.35, and with normal or high standard base excess; and (3) a PaO_2 below 45 mmHg. These measurements are made after the patient has been breathing room air for at least 10 minutes (40,41,53). Noninvasive mechanical ventilation is contraindicated for patients with profound bradypnea, defined as a respiratory rate below 12 breaths/min, severe hypercapnic encephalopathy with Glasgow Coma Scale score below 10, cardiac and/or respiratory arrest, and hemodynamic instability (40,41,53). Some authors, however, have successfully applied noninvasive mechanical ventilation in comatose COPD patients with a Glasgow Coma Scale score below 8, with other causes of coma being ruled out (54). This latter use of noninvasive mechanical ventilation is not a consensus (53), but could be applied during a short-term trial (typically of 30–60 minutes) under continuous surveillance at the bedside. If the respiratory drive is blunted due to narcosis, the addition of mandatory breaths can be helpful.

Recommended settings of noninvasive ventilation vary among the studies. Few authors used an exclusive inspiratory pressure support (41) or inspiratory volume support (40). However, most physicians would recommend the use of positive end-expiratory pressure (PEEP) or continuous positive airway pressure (CPAP). This recommendations is based on the rationale that the use of PEEP/ CPAP further reduces the inspiratory work in patients with COPD exacerbation, especially the extra load generated by high levels of intrinsic PEEP (55–57).

There are many approaches to set the noninvasive ventilation. An easy way is to set the expiratory pressure at 5 cm H_2O, the inspiratory pressure at 10 cm H_2O—resulting in a "delta P" of 5 cm H_2O—and to increase the delta P in increments of 5 cm H_2O, up to 20 to 25 cm H_2O or the maximum tolerated, over 1 hour (49). An alternative approach is to adjust the inspiratory pressure in order to obtain a tidal volume of 6 to 8 mL/kg and a respiratory rate of 25 to 30 breaths/min, setting the end-expiratory pressure to 5 cm H_2O to offset the inspiratory threshold induced by intrinsic PEEP. Close observation of inspiratory time is very important for the success of this strategy, whatever the mode of ventilation. Too short, but especially too long inspiratory time causes great discomfort. Typically, inspiratory time should be set in the range of 0.7 to 1 second. In pressure support mode (PSV), inspiratory time can be optimized by adjusting the cycling-off criterion (automatically adjusted in some mechanical ventilators). Typical settings of this parameter lie within the range of 30% to 50% of peak inspiratory flow.

If inspiratory comfort is not achieved, asynchrony with the ventilator is often observed, with the patient often not able to trigger the assisted breath. Trials of 2 cm H_2O elevations in the PEEP/CPAP levels should be performed in order to further reduce the extra load imposed by the intrinsic PEEP. During these trials of augmentation of external PEEP, the minimum inspiratory pressure should be provided to maintain a stable tidal volume (58). Oxygen should be offered to keep oxygen saturation above 85% to 90% (2,49,58).

Theoretically, pure CPAP support in these patients might be of some help, offsetting part of the inspiratory threshold load imposed on COPD patients, caused by intrinsic PEEP. The appeal of such a strategy is the possibility of using low-cost CPAP systems. This approach, however, has not been tested systematically and should be reserved for very special conditions under close supervision. Whenever possible, some level of inspiratory support should always be added to a CPAP strategy, unloading also part of the resistive workload.

Success rates of noninvasive mechanical ventilation for COPD exacerbations can be in the order of 80% to 85% (53). Close monitoring after the start of noninvasive ventilation is very important to recognize early the minority of patients who will fail. Confalonieri et al. (59) evaluated the risk of failure of noninvasive ventilation in 1,033 consecutive patients with exacerbation of COPD admitted to experienced hospital units. In that study, some factors found on admission were associated with a failed attempt at noninvasive ventilation. These risk factors included a Glasgow Coma Scale score <11, an Acute Physiology and Chronic Health Evaluation (APACHE) II score >28, respiratory rate >30 breaths/min, and arterial pH <7.25. The presence of all these risk factors resulted in a predicted risk of failure greater than 70%. An arterial pH below 7.25 after 2 hours of ventilation greatly increased the risk of failure to over 90%. All these numbers and thresholds should be taken as relative reference points, because the success of noninvasive mechanical ventilation depends on a learning curve of the whole staff. The less experienced the staff, the more conservative they should be with these limits, not waiting for further deterioration of the patient before deciding to intubate.

After hospital admission, the correct timing for starting noninvasive ventilatory support is either immediately or at any time the patient shows worsening of the respiratory distress, a fall in PaO_2, or an increase in $PaCO_2$ (49,58). Noninvasive ventilatory support can be applied in any area of the hospital where close monitoring of the patient by trained personnel is available, such as intensive care units, emergency departments, high-dependency units, and respiratory wards. The duration of the noninvasive ventilation and the number of possible interruptions for oral and facial cleaning varies according to the patient need. Ventilatory periods lasting at least 40 minutes are warranted (41), and some patients will require uninterrupted use (49,58).

The choice for an appropriate mask is an important aspect of noninvasive mechanical ventilation. In general, patients benefit from a facial mask that covers the mouth and the nose; this is more efficient than the nasal type to deliver effective inspiratory pressures. Leaks directed at the eyes, sores in the nasal area, and dry mouth are frequent causes of extreme discomfort to patients. The total face mask may be better tolerated by some patients, but not all, and greatly reduces skin sores. However, one has to be aware that the anatomic dead space increases with this type of mask, which also imposes some challenges to the mechanical ventilator in terms of synchrony and PEEP maintenance.

High-Flow Oxygen Therapy. By delivering a high flow (typically 20 to 60 L/min) of heated and humidified air through a special nasal prong, at controlled inspiratory fractions (typically from 30% to 80% oxygen), recent studies in patients with acute lung injury (60) have shown benefits that may exceed the benefits of conventional oxygen therapy, or even the benefits of noninvasive ventilation. Studies are under way to prove the specific benefits of this strategy in patients with hypercapnic respiratory failure, and there is a good rationale to expect future benefits also extended to this population of patients with COPD exacerbation. Among the proven physiologic effects of this strategy, which forces some fresh air to flow from the nasal cavity toward the mouth, passing through the pharynx, studies demonstrated: (a) a decrease in the dead space, due to the washout of CO_2 accumulated in the nasal cavity, retropalatal cavity, pharynx, and mouth; (b) a CPAP effect that amounts to 3 to 7 cm H_2O depending on the flow settings, anatomy of airways, and the maintenance (or not) of a closed mouth; (c) a decrease in minute ventilation demands, which may be related to central effects or just to a decrease in dead space; and (d) an improvement in patient comfort (when compared to pure oxygen or to mask ventilation). Although promising, future trials will provide us with more information about safety and benefits of this new strategy, when compared to the traditional noninvasive ventilation, as described above.

Invasive Mechanical Ventilation. Invasive mechanical ventilation can be either the initial choice in patients with COPD exacerbation or the strategy to be applied after failure of a trial of noninvasive ventilation (2). Mechanical ventilation can reduce or eliminate the work of breathing and improve gas exchange, while allowing the respiratory function to return to baseline through the treatment of the precipitating causes of the acute decompensation (4).

Assuming that all appropriate measures to improve airflow obstruction have already been taken, minimization of dynamic hyperinflation is a key objective of the ventilatory support of these COPD patients. At the bedside, dynamic hyperinflation is typically detected by the presence of nonzero end-expiratory flow in the flow–time curve, or by effectively measuring the end-expiratory pressure (auto-PEEP) after an expiratory pause. Precise quantification of the auto-PEEP, however, is problematic in patients with spontaneous breathing efforts (61).

In some patients, especially in those with predominant emphysema, the airway obstruction in the expiratory phase is disproportionally higher than in the inspiration. In these patients, the measured auto-PEEP is higher than expected when considering the calculated inspiratory airway resistance. This situation can be anticipated by looking at the flow–volume curve available on most ventilators. During pressure-controlled ventilation, the slopes of the inspiratory and expiratory curves are proportional to the time constant of the respiratory system (a higher slope meaning lower resistance), and the differences between inspiratory and expiratory airway resistances can thus be determined (Fig. 113.1) (62).

To reduce the hyperinflation, several concepts should be employed alone or in combination (4,63). The most effective strategy is controlled hypoventilation (64), which decreases dynamic hyperinflation through the reduction of the minute volume. Hypoventilation, with a fixed inspiratory time, decreases the expiratory flow requirement and consequently reduces air trapping and plateau pressures (64–66). An appropriate clinical goal at present is to keep the plateau pressures no higher than 30 cm H_2O, a strategy associated with lower rates (4%) of barotrauma (67,68). Adequate sedation and analgesia help by lowering the production of CO_2 and allowing further reduction of the minute volume (4). At the bedside, the general rules to minimize hyperinflation are to keep the minute volume 8 L/min or less and to keep the expiratory time at at least 4 seconds; low respiratory rates should be used, for example, 8 to 10 breaths/min, with 5 to 8 mL/kg of tidal volume. Once these goals have been achieved, there is probably little gain from further adjusting the ventilator. For example, Leatherman et al. (69) showed that halving minute ventilation from 7.4 to 3.7 L/min, and

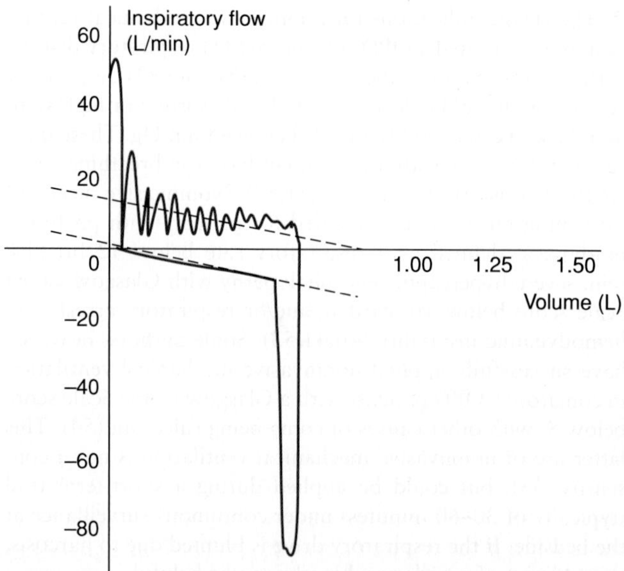

FIGURE 113.1 Example of a flow–volume curve of a patient mechanically ventilated with severe and equivalent inspiratory and expiratory flow limitation. The *dashed lines* represent the slope of the curves and are proportional to the inspiratory and expiratory time constants.

more than doubling expiratory time from 4.5 to 9.5 seconds had no significant effect on auto-PEEP and plateau pressure (63). Although controlled hypoventilation is the most effective measure to decrease hyperinflation, this ventilatory strategy frequently worsens CO_2 retention. The hypercapnia and acidosis are generally well tolerated and considered acceptable by most clinicians (4,63,64), provided that such levels of hypoventilation are essential to keep plateau pressures below 30 cm H_2O.

Metabolic acidosis may also accompany the respiratory acidosis seen in COPD exacerbations, resulting in amplification of the acidemia (70). The underlying mechanism of such acidosis is not clear (70), but its buffering may accentuate coexistent pulmonary injury in hypoxemic patients (71). The treatment of metabolic acidosis in these hypercapnic patients should be directed to the etiology of the process and not to the metabolic acidosis per se.

There is no optimal ventilation modality to support exacerbated COPD patients (63). The peak airway pressure may reach high values in the volume-controlled mode (69), but this is of limited clinical relevance because most of this pressure is dissipated in the orotracheal tube and large airways. Consequently, alveolar pressure is usually considerably lower than peak airway pressure (68). Caution is needed when monitoring the plateau pressure during this mode, as the use of an inspiratory pause every breath may worsen dynamic hyperinflation, by shortening expiratory time. On the other hand, in the pressure-controlled mode, conditions of fluctuating airway resistance and auto-PEEP entail the risk of variable tidal volumes, with sometimes unacceptably low alveolar ventilation. Furthermore, with this latter mode, severe respiratory alkalosis may develop if airway obstruction subsides rapidly (63).

Although there is no clear advantage of one over the other, volume-controlled ventilation is currently the preferred mode by most investigators (63,64,66,68,69). When using volume-controlled ventilation, the flow waveform should also be adjusted. The square waveform usually results in higher peak pressures, frequently triggering the high-pressure alarm, which should not be of much concern, as previously discussed (68,71). On the other hand, the decelerating flow waveform usually minimizes peak pressure, allowing full delivery of the tidal volume, with less interruption by opening of the pop-off safety valve (63). By forcing a slower flow at the end of inspiration, this flow waveform could result in two theoretical benefits: (1) less overdistension of alveoli distal to the least obstructed airways, and (2) slightly better CO_2 exchange. Whenever possible, and provided that peak pressures are effectively reduced (this must be tested), this flow pattern thus should be preferred. During controlled mechanical ventilation with volume-controlled ventilation, the inspiratory pause should be used with extreme caution. If applied continuously, a pause time between 0.25 and 0.5 second is advisable, not enough for full equilibration of pressures (due to marked pendelluft in those patients), but enough for monitoring purposes (to check whether hyperinflation is improving) and to enhance CO_2 removal. During the inspiratory pause, CO_2 diffuses into the larger airways thus lowering the anatomical dead space (72). It should be remembered that the efficacy of the inspiratory pause for CO_2 removal is mild, in the order of 10% at most, and the risks should always be balanced if used for this purpose: a quick test of its effects on hyperinflation should be performed.

When initiating mechanical ventilation in the pressure-controlled mode, one must keep in mind that the inspiratory time should be set in proportion to the inspiratory time constant in order to deliver the desired tidal volume with the lowest possible plateau pressure (73). Thus, patients with increased inspiratory resistance will need a longer inspiratory time. For a fixed respiratory rate, the increase in inspiratory time always occurs at the expense of a shortening of the expiratory time, which might aggravate pulmonary hyperinflation. Therefore, the ideal inspiratory time would optimize delivery of tidal volume without increasing air trapping. That will occur if, when looking at the flow–volume curve, both end-inspiratory and end-expiratory flows are equal or close to zero (4,63,68).

After choosing the best respiratory rate and inspiratory and expiratory times, the physician has to decide on how much PEEP to apply. During controlled mechanical ventilation, PEEP can be detrimental to paralyzed patients with severe airflow obstruction, raising the functional residual capacity (74). Based on this information, some authors have advocated the use of zero PEEP or no more than 5 cm H_2O (63,74). Another study showed that there are three typical responses to PEEP in those patients, suggesting that an individual approach is necessary. Some patients show a paradoxical response to an increase in PEEP, with relief of the air trapping (Fig. 113.2); in these patients, PEEP is generally advantageous. Some other patients may show no worsening of hyperinflation up to moderate PEEP levels (75), presenting the so-called water-fall response.

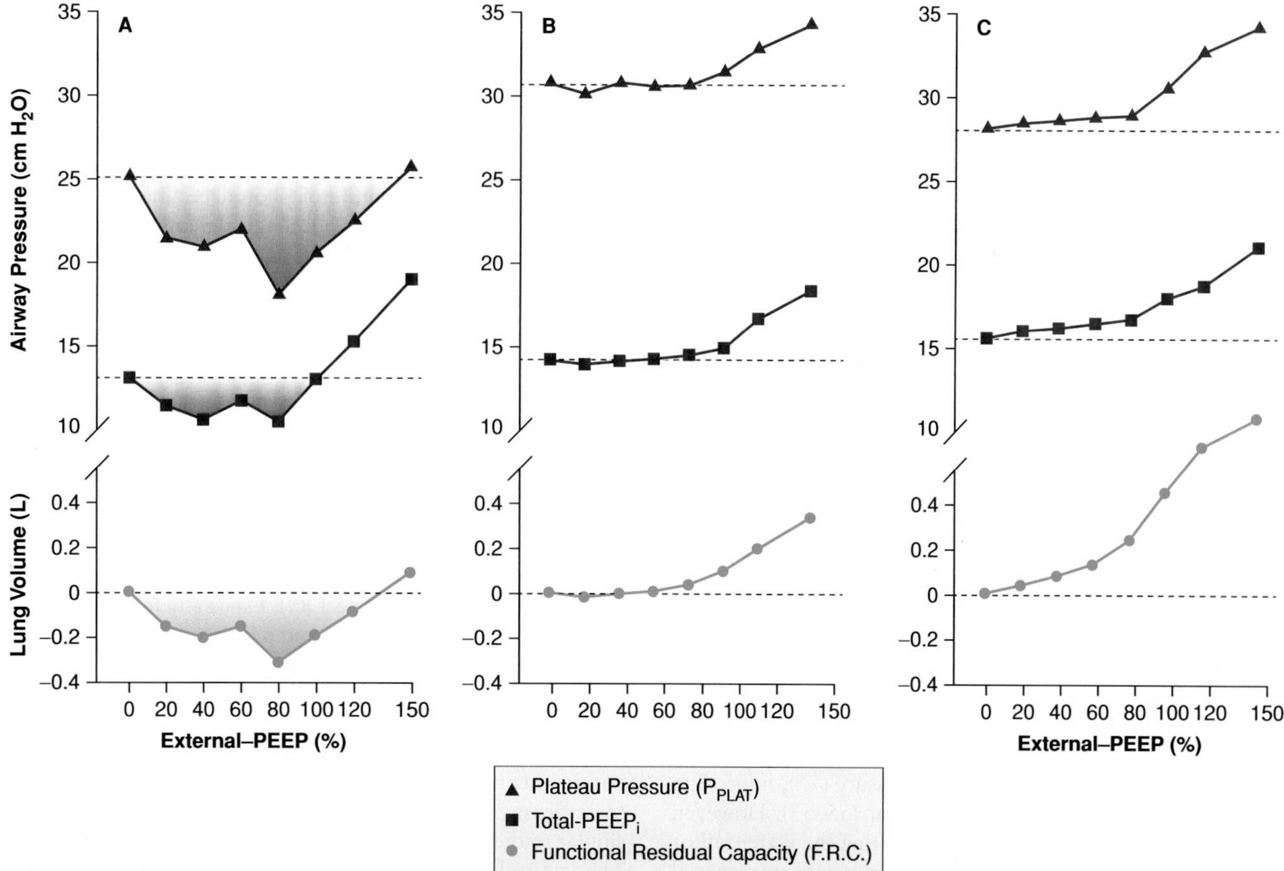

FIGURE 113.2 Three of the possible responses observed in plateau pressure (P_{PLAT}), total intrinsic positive end-expiratory pressure ($PEEP_i$), and functional residual capacity (FRC) with the application of external-PEEP (represented as percentage of $PEEP_i$ measured at zero external-PEEP). The FRC measured at zero external-PEEP was considered as the reference. **A**: Paradoxical response (patient 4), observed with a tidal volume (V_T) of 6 mL/kg and respiratory rate (RR) of 9 breaths/min. **B**: Biphasic response (patient 7), observed with V_T of 9 mL/kg and RR of 6 breaths/min. **C**: Classic overinflation response (patient 5), observed with a V_T of 9 mL/kg and RR of 9 breaths/min. (Adapted from Caramez MP, Borges JB, Tucci MR, et al. Paradoxical responses to positive end-expiratory pressure in patients with airway obstruction during controlled ventilation. *Crit Care Med.* 2005;33:1519–1528, with permission.)

This second group may still present some mild improvement in gas exchange or in hemodynamics after external PEEP application, but, in fact, they will actually benefit during the transitioning to assisted ventilation, improving their synchrony with the ventilator. And finally there is a third group, probably those with more fixed obstruction, in which every increment in external PEEP causes marked hyperinflation. For this third group, maybe ZEEP would be the best option, or some minimum PEEP just to maintain ventilator performance (2–4 cm H_2O).

We propose two alternative bedside procedures to characterize the typical patient response, according to the three possible types described above:

1. Using volume-control mode, with an inspiratory pause of 0.5 to 0.8 second, tidal volume of 5 to 8 mL/kg, and a respiratory rate of 10 breaths/min (with the lowest inspiratory:expiratory ratio possible, e.g., <1:4), increase the external PEEP in steps of 1–2 cm H_2O every 10 to 20 respiratory cycles, starting from ZEEP (baseline). In patients with paradoxical response, some PEEP level above ZEEP will cause plateau pressures to drop below baseline. The PEEP causing the lowest plateau should be used. In those with typical water-fall behavior, there will be a few PEEP levels above ZEEP in which plateau pressures will stay equal to baseline. In this latter case, we should choose the highest PEEP in which plateau is equal to baseline. And finally, the third group of patients will present marked elevation of plateau pressures (above baseline), right after the first increments in external PEEP. Probably ZEEP should be used for them.
2. If in pressure-control mode, start with ZEEP, driving pressure, and inspiratory time to achieve a tidal volume of 5 to 8 mL/g. Raise the external PEEP in steps of 1 to 2 cm H_2O every 10 to 20 respiratory cycles, keeping the plateau pressure constant (thus delta-P above PEEP will decrease). If there is an increase in tidal volume during the upward PEEP titration, it means there was recruitment of airways. PEEP should be kept at the level generating the highest tidal volume (in those with paradoxical response) or at the highest level before the tidal volume begins to fall (in those with typical water-fall behavior). Finally, if tidal volume drops markedly after each increment in external PEEP, this patient is not going to benefit from external PEEP.

There are no objective indicators of the best moment to start assisted ventilation; therefore, at least daily trials of assisted ventilation should be made, with close monitoring of patient comfort and plateau pressure (4,63). Adding external PEEP during assisted ventilation can reduce the inspiratory work by means of eliminating the offset of inspiratory pressure threshold induced by auto-PEEP (4). Appendini et al. (76) demonstrated that 41% of the inspiratory muscle effort was expended to overcome auto-PEEP in patients with COPD during spontaneous breathing. Adding external PEEP at an average of 80% of the measured auto-PEEP is well tolerated, with no increase of total PEEP or plateau pressure (77), improving synchrony between patient and ventilator (55–57). However, this is only true for those patients presenting the water-fall or the paradoxical response. Frequent reassessments are essential to ensure that the patient is not presenting a hyperinflation response, or that the level of external PEEP is still adequate to patient's mechanics and ventilatory requirements.

Many physicians prefer to change to PSV at this stage, trying to improve patient comfort and synchrony with the ventilator, assuming that the transition to weaning is going to be long. By increasing the patient's freedom to choose different ventilation patterns, the PSV typically provides an inspiratory flow and tidal volume better matching the patient's demands, providing also greater freedom for the patient to choose his inspiratory time. When pressure support is not properly adjusted it tend to overassist the patients, resulting in higher tidal volume than needed and increasing lung overinflation and intrinsic PEEP and asynchrony. General principles and targets when using this mode in COPD patients should be as follows: (a) inspiratory pressures just enough to achieve a tidal volume of 5.5 to 6.5 mL/kg (PBW) (78); (b) respiratory rates around 25 to 30 breaths/min (never below 20); and (c) inspiratory time between 0.6 and 1 second (thus changing cycling-off criteria from 25% of peak flow to around 30%–45%) (78). Alternative modes like proportional assisted ventilation (PAV) have been used with success in this population during this transition phase until weaning. In difficult cases, comfort and synchrony during mechanical ventilation can be improved by this mode, especially in weak and distressed patients, consumed by disease. Thus, a trial of PAV is advisable in cases in which the optimization of pressure support as described above did not work, particularly in those patients presenting clear signs of distress and discomfort during mechanical ventilation.

Humidification should be achieved with a heated humidifier, not with heat and moisture exchangers. The latter devices are undesirable for three reasons: (1) they increase expiratory airway resistance, which would hardly be of any help to reduce hyperinflation (79); (2) placed between the tracheal tube and the Y-piece of ventilator tubing, they increase dead space and therefore contribute unnecessarily to hypercapnia (80,81); and (3) the efficacy of any inhalational medication will be blunted by the heat and moisture exchanger (63).

Weaning from the ventilator should be initiated as soon as possible in order to avoid mechanical ventilator-associated complications (82). Roughly one-fifth of patients with COPD exacerbations remain partially dependent on the ventilator (83,84). In one study, the classic rapid shallow breathing criterion (<80 breaths/min/L) was met by 56% of COPD patients who failed the weaning trial (85). General patient condition and subjective dyspnea seemed to be more effective predictors of success of extubation than quantifiable indexes (86). Using spontaneous breathing trials or progressive reduction in pressure support is equally effective to wean the patient from the ventilator (87). Automatic algorithms for pressure support reduction are available today, which resulted in a faster, or at least equivalent, weaning process when compared with the physician-driven approach (88,89). Especially for centers with a low ratio between caregivers and patients, the automatic systems may present some advantage.

If the spontaneous breathing trial is chosen, it can be applied for at least 30 minutes, up to 2 hours, once a day (44). After tracheal decannulation, the use of intermittent or continuous support with noninvasive mechanical ventilation for at least 24 hours is strongly recommended, using settings similar to those used during conventional ventilation weaning. The last technique is associated with higher rates of extubation success, lower length of stay in the intensive care unit and/or hospital, and a lower mortality at 60 days (90,91). Nava et al. (92) have described a strategy in which patients are ventilated and sedated for 6 to 8 hours after intubation; an assisted mode is subsequently started using pressure support.

After 48 hours of conventional mechanical ventilation, in the absence of hypersecretion or hemodynamically instability, the patient is extubated and supported with noninvasive mechanical ventilation using the same ventilatory settings as before tracheal decannulation. This approach is associated with less ventilator-associated pneumonia, a shorter length of stay in the intensive care unit, and a lower mortality rate.

SEDATION AND NEUROMUSCULAR BLOCKADE

Benzodiazepines, often given with narcotics, are widely accepted (4,63,68). Benzodiazepines, especially when associated with opiates, are effective in facilitating the controlled hypoventilation in hypercapnic patients without the need of high doses (93). Propofol may also be used because of its bronchodilating action (63), but generally requires high infusion rates (93). Especially for patients presenting moderate airway resistance (≤25 cm H_2O/L/sec) during invasive mechanical ventilation, short-acting agents like propofol are preferable, since such numbers suggest that the cause of respiratory failure was acute and reversible, and that the weaning can be started soon. When patient–ventilator asynchrony cannot be suppressed by increasing the opioid dose, neuromuscular blocking agents should be given as intermittent intravenous boluses rather than as a continuous infusion in order to reduce the dose and duration of administration (4,63,68). Long muscle resting is not currently recommended (94); however, muscle unloading for a short time—about 12 hours—has been advocated for muscular recuperation after the fatigue of acute stress (63). Ideally, if the patient is going to stay for a long time during assisted mechanical ventilation, the level of muscle effort should be kept at low levels, typically with pressure swings in between 4 and 8 cm H_2O (driving muscle pressure), enough to prevent muscle atrophy, but providing adequate comfort for the patient.

SUMMARY

Respiratory failure in COPD is an exceptionally difficult disorder to manage. Better management during invasive mechanical ventilation and especially new possibilities to avoid invasive mechanical ventilation are already a reality and have contributed to a decreased mortality. Promising future developments include: new noninvasive ventilation techniques, high-flow oxygen systems, and new techniques for low-flow external removal of CO_2. All those techniques will make it possible to decrease the extra load to the respiratory muscles during the acute phase of the disease, without causing additional clinical problems as observed in the past.

Key Points

- COPD exacerbation is defined as acute worsening of dyspnea, cough, or sputum that requires therapy.
- Pharmacologic treatment is based on bronchodilators, corticosteroids, and antibiotics.
- Oxygen therapy should target low-normal levels (SpO_2 88%–92%) to avoid the risk of worsening hypercapnia.
- Noninvasive ventilation plays an important role and is associated with reduced endotracheal intubations and reduced mortality.
- Tidal volumes should be kept low (6–8 mL/kg) to avoid worsening of intrinsic PEEP and to minimize missed efforts.
- Close monitoring after the initiation of noninvasive ventilation is important to identify early those patients who will require endotracheal intubation.
- The goals of invasive ventilation are to reduce the work of breathing, restore pH levels to normal, and avoid intrinsic PEEP.
- As soon as possible, assisted modes should be employed to avoid ventilator-induced diaphragmatic dysfunction.
- When the patient condition is stable, spontaneous breathing trials should be applied daily to shorten the duration of invasive mechanical ventilation.
- After extubation, noninvasive ventilation should be used for at least 24 hours.

References

1. Rabe KF, Hurd S, Anzueto A, et al. Global strategy for the diagnosis, management, and prevention of chronic obstructive pulmonary disease: GOLD executive summary. *Am J Respir Crit Care Med.* 2007;176(6):532–555.
2. Pauwels RA, Buist AS, Calverley PM, et al. Global strategy for the diagnosis, management, and prevention of chronic obstructive pulmonary disease. NHLBI/WHO Global Initiative for Chronic Obstructive Lung Disease (GOLD) Workshop summary. *Am J Respir Crit Care Med.* 2001;163(5): 1256–1276.
3. Barnes PJ. Chronic obstructive pulmonary disease. *N Engl J Med.* 2000; 343(4):269–280.
4. Peigang Y, Marini JJ. Ventilation of patients with asthma and chronic obstructive pulmonary disease. *Curr Opin Crit Care.* 2002;8(1):70–76.
5. Rossi A, Ganassini A, Polese G, Grassi V. Pulmonary hyperinflation and ventilator-dependent patients. *Eur Respir J.* 1997;10(7):1663–1674.
6. Marchand E, Decramer M. Respiratory muscle function and drive in chronic obstructive pulmonary disease. *Clin Chest Med.* 2000;21(4):679–692.
7. Perez T, Becquart LA, Stach B, et al. Inspiratory muscle strength and endurance in steroid-dependent asthma. *Am J Respir Crit Care Med.* 1996;153(2): 610–615.
8. Lundback B, Lindberg A, Lindstrom M, et al. Not 15 but 50% of smokers develop COPD? Report from the Obstructive Lung Disease in Northern Sweden Studies. *Respir Med.* 2003;97(2):115–122.
9. Eriksson S. Pulmonary emphysema and alpha1-antitrypsin deficiency. *Acta Med Scand.* 1964;175:197–205.
10. Burchfiel CM, Marcus EB, Curb JD, et al. Effects of smoking and smoking cessation on longitudinal decline in pulmonary function. *Am J Respir Crit Care Med.* 1995;151(6):1778–1785.
11. Klooster K, ten Hacken NH, Hartman JE, et al. Endobronchial valves for emphysema without interlobar collateral ventilation. *N Engl J Med.* 2015;373(24):2325–2335.
12. Schuhmann M, Raffy P, Yin Y, et al. Computed tomography predictors of response to endobronchial valve lung reduction treatment: comparison with Chartis. *Am J Respir Crit Care Med.* 2015;191(7):767–774.
13. Rodriguez-Roisin R. Toward a consensus definition for COPD exacerbations. *Chest.* 2000;117(5 Suppl 2):398S–401S.
14. Sethi S, Evans N, Grant BJ, Murphy TF. New strains of bacteria and exacerbations of chronic obstructive pulmonary disease. *N Engl J Med.* 2002;347(7):465–471.
15. Hurst JR, Vestbo J, Anzueto A, et al. Susceptibility to exacerbation in chronic obstructive pulmonary disease. *N Engl J Med.* 2010;363(12):1128–1138.
16. Connors AF Jr., Dawson NV, Thomas C, et al. Outcomes following acute exacerbation of severe chronic obstructive lung disease. The SUPPORT investigators (Study to Understand Prognoses and Preferences for Outcomes and Risks of Treatments). *Am J Respir Crit Care Med.* 1996;154(4 Pt 1):959–967.
17. Seneff MG, Wagner DP, Wagner RP, et al. Hospital and 1-year survival of patients admitted to intensive care units with acute exacerbation of chronic obstructive pulmonary disease. *JAMA.* 1995;274(23):1852–1857.

18. Celli BR, MacNee W, Force AET. Standards for the diagnosis and treatment of patients with COPD: a summary of the ATS/ERS position paper. *Eur Respir J*. 2004;23(6):932–946.
19. Fernandez A, Lazaro A, Garcia A, et al. Bronchodilators in patients with chronic obstructive pulmonary disease on mechanical ventilation: utilization of metered-dose inhalers. *Am Rev Respir Dis*. 1990;141(1):164–168.
20. Gay PC, Patel HG, Nelson SB, et al. Metered dose inhalers for bronchodilator delivery in intubated, mechanically ventilated patients. *Chest*. 1991; 99(1):66–71.
21. Fuller HD, Dolovich MB, Turpie FH, Newhouse MT. Efficiency of bronchodilator aerosol delivery to the lungs from the metered dose inhaler in mechanically ventilated patients: a study comparing four different actuator devices. *Chest*. 1994;105(1):214–218.
22. Leuppi JD, Schuetz P, Bingisser R, et al. Short-term vs conventional glucocorticoid therapy in acute exacerbations of chronic obstructive pulmonary disease: the REDUCE randomized clinical trial. *JAMA*. 2013; 309(21):2223–2231.
23. Erbland ML, Deupree RH, Niewoehner DE. Systemic Corticosteroids in Chronic Obstructive Pulmonary Disease Exacerbations (SCCOPE): rationale and design of an equivalence trial. Veterans Administration Cooperative Trials SCCOPE Study Group. *Control Clin Trials*. 1998;19(4):404–417.
24. Calverley PM, Anderson JA, Celli B, et al. Salmeterol and fluticasone propionate and survival in chronic obstructive pulmonary disease. *N Engl J Med*. 2007;356(8):775–789.
25. Gunen H, Hacievliyagil SS, Yetkin O, et al. The role of nebulised budesonide in the treatment of exacerbations of COPD. *Eur Respir J*. 2007;29(4):660–667.
26. Gotfried MH. Macrolides for the treatment of chronic sinusitis, asthma, and COPD. *Chest*. 2004;125(2 Suppl):52S–60S.
27. Calverley PM, Walker P. Chronic obstructive pulmonary disease. *Lancet*. 2003;362(9389):1053–1061.
28. Wouters EF. Management of severe COPD. *Lancet*. 2004;364(9437):883–895.
29. Continuous or nocturnal oxygen therapy in hypoxemic chronic obstructive lung disease: a clinical trial. Nocturnal Oxygen Therapy Trial Group. *Ann Intern Med*. 1980;93(3):391–398.
30. Long term domiciliary oxygen therapy in chronic hypoxic cor pulmonale complicating chronic bronchitis and emphysema. Report of the Medical Research Council Working Party. *Lancet*. 1981;1(8222):681–686.
31. Calverley PM. Oxygen-induced hypercapnia revisited. *Lancet*. 2000; 356(9241):1538–1539.
32. Moloney ED, Kiely JL, McNicholas WT. Controlled oxygen therapy and carbon dioxide retention during exacerbations of chronic obstructive pulmonary disease. *Lancet*. 2001;357(9255):526–528.
33. Aubier M, Murciano D, Milic-Emili J, et al. Effects of the administration of O2 on ventilation and blood gases in patients with chronic obstructive pulmonary disease during acute respiratory failure. *Am Rev Respir Dis*. 1980; 122(5):747–754.
34. Dunn WF, Nelson SB, Hubmayr RD. Oxygen-induced hypercarbia in obstructive pulmonary disease. *Am Rev Respir Dis*. 1991;144(3 Pt 1):526–530.
35. Hanson CW III, Marshall BE, Frasch HF, Marshall C. Causes of hypercarbia with oxygen therapy in patients with chronic obstructive pulmonary disease. *Crit Care Med*. 1996;24(1):23–28.
36. Robinson TD, Freiberg DB, Regnis JA, Young IH. The role of hypoventilation and ventilation-perfusion redistribution in oxygen-induced hypercapnia during acute exacerbations of chronic obstructive pulmonary disease. *Am J Respir Crit Care Med*. 2000;161(5):1524–1529.
37. Sassoon CS, Hassell KT, Mahutte CK. Hyperoxic-induced hypercapnia in stable chronic obstructive pulmonary disease. *Am Rev Respir Dis*. 1987;135(4):907–911.
38. Dick CR, Liu Z, Sassoon CS, et al. O_2-induced change in ventilation and ventilatory drive in COPD. *Am J Respir Crit Care Med*. 1997;155(2):609–614.
39. Ambrosino N, Foglio K, Rubini F, et al. Non-invasive mechanical ventilation in acute respiratory failure due to chronic obstructive pulmonary disease: correlates for success. *Thorax*. 1995;50(7):755–757.
40. Bott J, Carroll MP, Conway JH, et al. Randomised controlled trial of nasal ventilation in acute ventilatory failure due to chronic obstructive airways disease. *Lancet*. 1993;341(8860):1555–1557.
41. Brochard L, Mancebo J, Wysocki M, et al. Noninvasive ventilation for acute exacerbations of chronic obstructive pulmonary disease. *N Engl J Med*. 1995;333(13):817–822.
42. Foglio C, Vitacca M, Quadri A, et al. Acute exacerbations in severe COLD patients: treatment using positive pressure ventilation by nasal mask. *Chest*. 1992;101(6):1533–1538.
43. Brochard L, Rauss A, Benito S, et al. Comparison of three methods of gradual withdrawal from ventilatory support during weaning from mechanical ventilation. *Am J Respir Crit Care Med*. 1994;150(4):896–903.
44. Esteban A, Frutos F, Tobin MJ, et al. A comparison of four methods of weaning patients from mechanical ventilation. Spanish Lung Failure Collaborative Group. *N Engl J Med*. 1995;332(6):345–350.
45. Guerin C, Girard R, Chemorin C, et al. Facial mask noninvasive mechanical ventilation reduces the incidence of nosocomial pneumonia: a prospective epidemiological survey from a single ICU. *Intensive Care Med*. 1997;23(10):1024–1032.
46. Nourdine K, Combes P, Carton MJ, et al. Does noninvasive ventilation reduce the ICU nosocomial infection risk? A prospective clinical survey. *Intensive Care Med*. 1999;25(6):567–573.
47. Celikel T, Sungur M, Ceyhan B, Karakurt S. Comparison of noninvasive positive pressure ventilation with standard medical therapy in hypercapnic acute respiratory failure. *Chest*. 1998;114(6):1636–1642.
48. Meduri GU, Abou-Shala N, Fox RC, et al. Noninvasive face mask mechanical ventilation in patients with acute hypercapnic respiratory failure. *Chest*. 1991;100(2):445–454.
49. Plant PK, Owen JL, Elliott MW. Early use of non-invasive ventilation for acute exacerbations of chronic obstructive pulmonary disease on general respiratory wards: a multicentre randomised controlled trial. *Lancet*. 2000;355(9219):1931–1935.
50. Lightowler JV, Wedzicha JA, Elliott MW, Ram FS. Non-invasive positive pressure ventilation to treat respiratory failure resulting from exacerbations of chronic obstructive pulmonary disease: Cochrane systematic review and meta-analysis. *BMJ*. 2003;326(7382):185.
51. Kramer N, Meyer TJ, Meharg J, et al. Randomized, prospective trial of noninvasive positive pressure ventilation in acute respiratory failure. *Am J Respir Crit Care Med*. 1995;151(6):1799–1806.
52. Soo Hoo GW, Santiago S, Williams AJ. Nasal mechanical ventilation for hypercapnic respiratory failure in chronic obstructive pulmonary disease: determinants of success and failure. *Crit Care Med*. 1994;22(8):1253–1261.
53. Evans TW. International Consensus Conferences in Intensive Care Medicine: non-invasive positive pressure ventilation in acute respiratory failure. Organised jointly by the American Thoracic Society, the European Respiratory Society, the European Society of Intensive Care Medicine, and the Societe de Reanimation de Langue Francaise, and approved by the ATS Board of Directors, December 2000. *Intensive Care Med*. 2001;27(1):166–178.
54. Diaz GG, Alcaraz AC, Talavera JC, et al. Noninvasive positive-pressure ventilation to treat hypercapnic coma secondary to respiratory failure. *Chest*. 2005;127(3):952–960.
55. Appendini L, Patessio A, Zanaboni S, et al. Physiologic effects of positive end-expiratory pressure and mask pressure support during exacerbations of chronic obstructive pulmonary disease. *Am J Respir Crit Care Med*. 1994;149(5):1069–1076.
56. Goldberg P, Reissmann H, Maltais F, et al. Efficacy of noninvasive CPAP in COPD with acute respiratory failure. *Eur Respir J*. 1995;8(11):1894–1900.
57. Smith TC, Marini JJ. Impact of PEEP on lung mechanics and work of breathing in severe airflow obstruction. *J Appl Physiol (1985)*. 1988;65(4):1488–1499.
58. Conti G, Antonelli M, Navalesi P, et al. Noninvasive vs. conventional mechanical ventilation in patients with chronic obstructive pulmonary disease after failure of medical treatment in the ward: a randomized trial. *Intensive Care Med*. 2002;28(12):1701–1707.
59. Confalonieri M, Garuti G, Cattaruzza MS, et al. A chart of failure risk for noninvasive ventilation in patients with COPD exacerbation. *Eur Respir J*. 2005;25(2):348–355.
60. Frat JP, Thille AW, Mercat A, et al. High-flow oxygen through nasal cannula in acute hypoxemic respiratory failure. *N Engl J Med*. 2015;372(23): 2185–2196.
61. Gladwin MT, Pierson DJ. Mechanical ventilation of the patient with severe chronic obstructive pulmonary disease. *Intensive Care Med*. 1998;24(9): 898–910.
62. Dhand R. Ventilator graphics and respiratory mechanics in the patient with obstructive lung disease. *Respir Care*. 2005;50(2):246–261.
63. Oddo M, Feihl F, Schaller MD, Perret C. Management of mechanical ventilation in acute severe asthma: practical aspects. *Intensive Care Med*. 2006;32(4):501–510.
64. Darioli R, Perret C. Mechanical controlled hypoventilation in status asthmaticus. *Am Rev Respir Dis*. 1984;129(3):385–387.
65. Darioli R, Domenighetti G, Perret C. [Mechanical ventilation in the treatment of acute respiratory insufficiency in asthma]. *Schweiz Med Wochenschr*. 1981;111(6):194–196.
66. Tuxen DV. Permissive hypercapnic ventilation. *Am J Respir Crit Care Med*. 1994;150(3):870–874.
67. Leatherman J. Life-threatening asthma. *Clin Chest Med*. 1994;15(3):453–479.
68. Leatherman JW. Mechanical ventilation in obstructive lung disease. *Clin Chest Med*. 1996;17(3):577–590.

69. Leatherman JW, McArthur C, Shapiro RS. Effect of prolongation of expiratory time on dynamic hyperinflation in mechanically ventilated patients with severe asthma. *Crit Care Med.* 2004;32(7):1542–1545.
70. Mountain RD, Heffner JE, Brackett NC Jr, Sahn SA. Acid-base disturbances in acute asthma. *Chest.* 1990;98(3):651–655.
71. Laffey JG, Engelberts D, Kavanagh BP. Buffering hypercapnic acidosis worsens acute lung injury. *Am J Respir Crit Care Med.* 2000;161(1):141–1416.
72. Astrom E, Uttman L, Niklason L, et al. Pattern of inspiratory gas delivery affects CO2 elimination in health and after acute lung injury. *Intensive Care Med.* 2008;34(2):377–384.
73. Marini JJ, Crooke PS III, Truwit JD. Determinants and limits of pressure-preset ventilation: a mathematical model of pressure control. *J Appl Physiol (1985).* 1989;67(3):1081–1092.
74. Tuxen DV. Detrimental effects of positive end-expiratory pressure during controlled mechanical ventilation of patients with severe airflow obstruction. *Am Rev Respir Dis.* 1989;140(1):5–9.
75. Caramez MP, Borges JB, Tucci MR, et al. Paradoxical responses to positive end-expiratory pressure in patients with airway obstruction during controlled ventilation. *Crit Care Med.* 2005;33(7):1519–1528.
76. Appendini L, Purro A, Patessio A, et al. Partitioning of inspiratory muscle workload and pressure assistance in ventilator-dependent COPD patients. *Am J Respir Crit Care Med.* 1996;154(5):1301–1309.
77. Guerin C, Milic-Emili J, Fournier G. Effect of PEEP on work of breathing in mechanically ventilated COPD patients. *Intensive Care Med.* 2000;26(9): 1207–1214.
78. Thille AW, Cabello B, Galia F, et al. Reduction of patient-ventilator asynchrony by reducing tidal volume during pressure-support ventilation. *Intensive Care Med.* 2008;34(8):1477–1486.
79. Verkerke GJ, Geertsema AA, Schutte HK. Airflow resistance of heat and moisture exchange filters with and without a tracheostoma valve. *Ann Otol Rhinol Laryngol.* 2002;111(4):333–337.
80. Hinkson CR, Benson MS, Stephens LM, Deem S. The effects of apparatus dead space on P(aCO2) in patients receiving lung-protective ventilation. *Respir Care.* 2006;51(10):1140–1144.
81. Moran I, Bellapart J, Vari A, Mancebo J. Heat and moisture exchangers and heated humidifiers in acute lung injury/acute respiratory distress syndrome patients. Effects on respiratory mechanics and gas exchange. *Intensive Care Med.* 2006;32(4):524–531.
82. Pingleton SK. Complications of acute respiratory failure. *Am Rev Respir Dis.* 1988;137(6):1463–1493.
83. Bagley PH, Cooney E. A community-based regional ventilator weaning unit: development and outcomes. *Chest.* 1997;111(4):1024–1029.
84. Dasgupta A, Rice R, Mascha E, et al. Four-year experience with a unit for long-term ventilation (respiratory special care unit) at the Cleveland Clinic Foundation. *Chest.* 1999;116(2):447–455.
85. Purro A, Appendini L, De Gaetano A, et al. Physiologic determinants of ventilator dependence in long-term mechanically ventilated patients. *Am J Respir Crit Care Med.* 2000;161(4 Pt 1):1115–1123.
86. Afessa B, Hogans L, Murphy R. Predicting 3-day and 7-day outcomes of weaning from mechanical ventilation. *Chest.* 1999;116(2):456–461.
87. Vitacca M, Vianello A, Colombo D, et al. Comparison of two methods for weaning patients with chronic obstructive pulmonary disease requiring mechanical ventilation for more than 15 days. *Am J Respir Crit Care Med.* 2001;164(2):225–230.
88. Bouadma L, Lellouche F, Cabello B, et al. Computer-driven management of prolonged mechanical ventilation and weaning: a pilot study. *Intensive Care Med.* 2005;31(10):1446–1450.
89. Lellouche F, Mancebo J, Jolliet P, et al. A multicenter randomized trial of computer-driven protocolized weaning from mechanical ventilation. *Am J Respir Crit Care Med.* 2006;174(8):894–900.
90. Ferrer M, Valencia M, Nicolas JM, et al. Early noninvasive ventilation averts extubation failure in patients at risk: a randomized trial. *Am J Respir Crit Care Med.* 2006;173(2):164–170.
91. Nava S, Gregoretti C, Fanfulla F, et al. Noninvasive ventilation to prevent respiratory failure after extubation in high-risk patients. *Crit Care Med.* 2005;33(11):2465–2470.
92. Nava S, Ambrosino N, Clini E, et al. Noninvasive mechanical ventilation in the weaning of patients with respiratory failure due to chronic obstructive pulmonary disease: a randomized, controlled trial. *Ann Intern Med.* 1998;128(9):721–728.
93. Vinayak AG, Gehlbach B, Pohlman AS, et al. The relationship between sedative infusion requirements and permissive hypercapnia in critically ill, mechanically ventilated patients. *Crit Care Med.* 2006;34(6):1668–1673.
94. Vassilakopoulos T, Zakynthinos S, Roussos C. Bench-to-bedside review: weaning failure—Should we rest the respiratory muscles with controlled mechanical ventilation? *Crit Care.* 2006;10(1):204.

CHAPTER

114

Pulmonary Embolism

KENNETH E. WOOD and AARON M. JOFFE

INTRODUCTION

Despite significant advances in prophylaxis, diagnostic approaches, and therapeutic modalities for pulmonary embolism (PE), this disease process still remains an under recognized and lethal entity. Contemporary estimates suggest that PE affects more than 600,000 patients per year in the United States and reportedly causes or contributes to 50,000 to 200,000 deaths. The incidence of PE causing, contributing to, or accompanying death in hospitalized patients has remained relatively constant at 15% for the past 40 years. Disconcertingly, the antemortem diagnosis of fatal PE has remained fixed at approximately 30% over the same time period. Large observational studies of PE have reported unexpectedly high mortality rates. In the Management Strategies and Determinants of Outcome in Acute Major PE (MAPPET) series, the overall 3-month mortality in patients with PE was 17% with an in-hospital mortality of 31% when PE was associated with hemodynamic instability; PE-attributable mortality was 45% and 91% in the respective groups (1). In the International Cooperative Pulmonary Embolism Registry (ICOPER), the 90-day mortality was 14.5% in hemodynamically stable PE patients and 51.9% in those with hemodynamic instability; PE-attributable mortality was 34% and 62.5% in the respective groups (2).

In fatal cases of PE, it has long been appreciated that two-thirds of PE deaths will occur within 1 hour of presentation and that anatomically massive PE will account for only one-half of the deaths, as the remainder can be attributed to smaller submassive or recurrent emboli. There are several important implications of these observations. First, an evidenced-based approach is nearly impossible to define for hemodynamically unstable PE. Second, it is reasonable to propose that outcome from PE is related to the size of the embolism and the underlying cardiopulmonary function. There is a dynamic interaction between the patient's underlying cardiopulmonary status and the embolism size; similar hemodynamic and clinical outcomes will manifest from an anatomically massive PE in a patient with normal cardiopulmonary function and an anatomically submassive embolism in a patient with impaired cardiopulmonary function. Third, an implicit understanding of the physiology of PE will allow for the application of physiologic risk stratification that can be used for diagnostic evaluation and therapeutics. Figure 114.1 represents a proposed risk stratification model defined by the relationship between mortality and severity characterized by the integration of cardiopulmonary status and embolism size. The combination of embolism size and underlying cardiopulmonary status that produces cardiac arrest is associated with a predicted mortality of 70%; this implies that 30% of arrested PE patients will survive and warrants continued use of chest compressions to mechanically fracture the embolism and consideration toward thrombolysis or embolectomy even without a definitive diagnosis when PE is highly suspected. At the opposite extreme, the combination of embolism size and cardiopulmonary status that fails to produce right ventricular (RV) dilatation is associated with 0% to 1% mortality provided therapeutic anticoagulation is achieved. The combination of embolism size and cardiopulmonary status that produces hemodynamic instability or shock is associated with a 30% mortality rate. Consequently, the presence of shock has traditionally defined the threshold for thrombolysis. As depicted in Figure 114.1, there is likely a broad spectrum of PE patients that are hemodynamically stable with RV dysfunction ranging from those with a minimal embolic burden and a low predicted mortality to patients with incipient shock and a predicted mortality just under 30%. The use of thrombolytics in this heterogeneous group is controversial as the constitutive characteristics of the mortality inflection point remain elusive. Syncope represents an intermediary position between shock and cardiac arrest as failure to recover consciousness results in cardiac arrest, and patients who regain consciousness have a high incidence of hemodynamic instability. The outcomes and mortality associated with emboli in transit and PE patients with a patent foramen ovale (PFO) have not been well reported and likely have severity as depicted in Figure 114.1.

The spectrum of PE most likely to confront the intensivist is predominantly confined to two situations; first, the patient presenting with undifferentiated shock or respiratory failure, and second, an established hospital patient or one in the intensive care unit (ICU) who develops PE after admission. In either situation, the diagnostics and therapeutics are challenging. Differentiating PE from other life-threatening cardiopulmonary disorders can be exceedingly difficult; logistic constraints can jeopardize definitive diagnostic testing, and hemorrhagic risks in the critically ill can significantly alter the therapeutic approach and compromise the ability to anticoagulate or institute thrombolytic therapy. This chapter will review a structured physiologic approach to diagnostic, resuscitative, and management strategies as well as discuss prophylaxis and ICU-specific PE issues.

PREVENTION OF VENOUS THROMBOEMBOLISM

Principles of Prophylaxis

Prophylaxis is defined as any measure "designed to preserve health and prevent the spread of disease." Insofar as venous thromboembolic disease (VTE) is prevalent among acutely ill hospitalized patients, and unprevented VTE may lead to adverse consequences, the use of pharmacologic, mechanical, or vena caval interruption as a means for reducing the occurrence of VTE certainly qualifies as a measure intended to preserve health. In fact, based on strength of evidence, the Agency for Healthcare Research and Quality (AHRQ) has identified

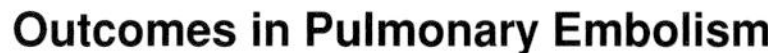

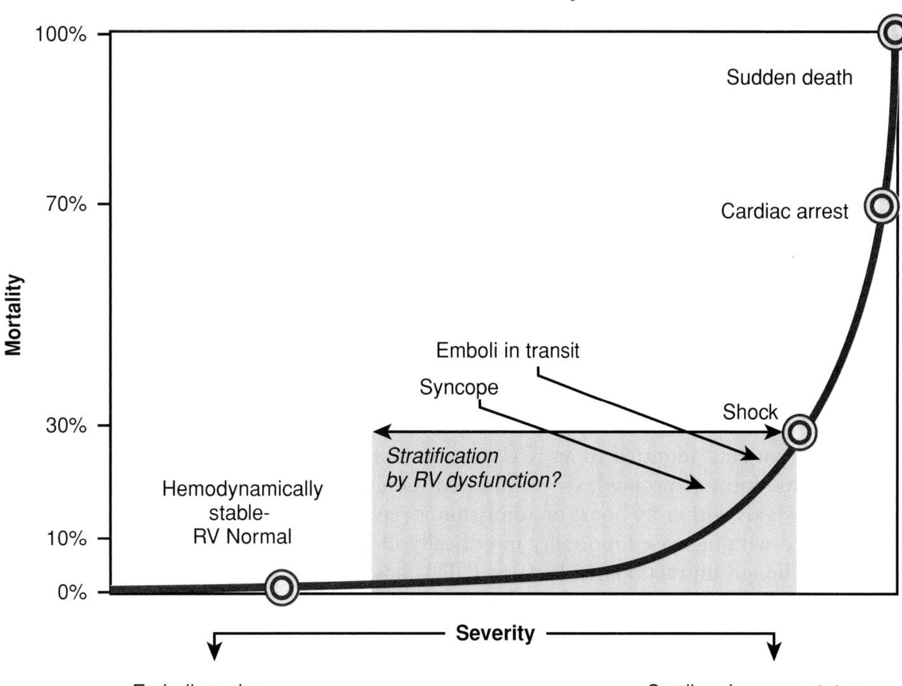

FIGURE 114.1 Outcomes in pulmonary embolism. RV, right ventricle.

"appropriate use of prophylaxis to prevent VTE in patients at risk" as the number one opportunity for improvement of patient safety, supporting more widespread implementation (3). The choice of primary prophylaxis is based on the patient's risk of bleeding and thrombosis and is presented in Table 114.1.

Risk Factors

The Virchow triad of stasis, vessel trauma, and hypercoagulability remain fundamental risk factors for VTE. Furthermore, risk factors can be considered clinical (i.e., multiple trauma or major abdominal surgery, acute myocardial infarction or stroke, need for mechanical ventilation) or patient-related (prior history of VTE, malignancy, inherited coagulopathy).

With respect to lower extremity deep venous thrombosis (DVT), observational studies of medical–surgical ICU patients have identified mechanical ventilation, treatment with neuromuscular blockers, and presence of a central venous catheter (CVC) as risk factors for DVT (4). Central venous catheterization, in particular, has been reported to confer an increased relative risk (RR) of 1.04 for each day the catheter was in place (5). Among 261 medical–surgical ICU patients, multivariate regression analysis defined exposure to platelet transfusions and the use of vasopressors to be independent risk factors for ICU-acquired DVT (6).

The two most powerful patient-related risk factors are a prior history of VTE and malignancy. Malignancy is perhaps the most common acquired hypercoagulable state encountered in the ICU and likely will become more prevalent as the general population continues to age. Additionally, end-stage renal disease has been identified as an independent risk factor for ICU-acquired DVT (6). Activated protein C resistance from factor V Leiden (FVL) is the most common hereditary defect predisposition for DVT. In order of descending prevalence among the general population, prothrombin gene mutation 20210A, antithrombin, protein C and S deficiency, elevations in homocysteine, and coagulation factors VIII, IX, and XI may predispose the patient to developing DVT (4). Although uncommon, heparin-induced thrombocytopenia (HIT), an acquired platelet disorder, results in increased risk of both venous and arterial thrombosis (7).

Cancer and the presence of a CVC are the two most powerful risk factors for upper extremity DVT (UEDVT). In the report of Mustafa et al., a CVC at the site of the UEDVT was present in 60% of patients and 46% were diagnosed with cancer. Underscoring the possible additive nature of these two risk factors, 76% of the patients with cancer also had an indwelling CVC (8). In a review of cancer patients who had an indwelling CVC, the reported prevalence of UEDVT, either symptomatic or asymptomatic, ranged from 6.7% to 48% (9). In a prospective registry of 592 patients with UEDVT, the presence of an indwelling CVC was the strongest independent predictor of occurrence (odds ratio [OR], 7.3) (10). It is important

TABLE 114.1 Venous Thromboembolism Prophylaxis of Critical Care Patient

Bleeding Risk	Thrombosis Risk	Prophylaxis Recommendation
Low	Moderate	LDH 5,000 units sq bid
Low	High	LMWH • Dalteparin • Enoxaparin
High	Moderate	GCS or IPC → LMWH when bleeding risk subsides
High	High	GCS or IPC → LMWH when bleeding risk subsides

LDH, low-dose unfractionated heparin; LMWH, low-molecular-weight heparin; GCS, graded compression stockings; IPC, intermittent pneumatic compression devices.

Adapted from Geerts W, Selby R. Prevention of venous thromboembolism in the ICU. *Chest.* 2003;124(6 Suppl):357S–363S.

to note that nearly 30% of patients will develop an UEDVT with no apparent cause. In these patients, inherited thrombophilia, particularly FVL, prothrombin G20210A mutation, and anticoagulant protein deficiencies may be causative. Evaluated prospectively for a median follow-up of 5.1 years, recurrence of primary UEDVT was reported to be 4.4% in those with inherited thrombophilia compared to 1.6% in those without (11).

Prevalence/Incidence

Critically ill patients are at substantial risk of developing DVT and accompanying PE as frequently all three components of Virchow triad of stasis, hypercoagulability, and intimal vessel damage are impacted by disease states and treatments. In the absence of prophylaxis, it is reported that the incidence of VTE ranges from 13% to 30% (12). As a consequence, virtually all patients admitted to an ICU are considered high risk and some form of prophylaxis is indicated. Omission of DVT prophylaxis within 24 hours of admission is reported to be associated with increased mortality in critically ill patients (13) and although unfractionated heparin (UFH) has proven to be effective in diminishing the rate of DVT, significant failure rates of up to 15% have been reported (6,14,15).

Patients undergoing major general surgery have an event rate of 25% without DVT prophylaxis; 9% of patients will have clinically detectable DVT, and 7% will have proximal DVT. In a study of trauma patients who did not receive prophylaxis, 58% of patients developed a DVT, one-third of which were proximal. Similarly, in patients undergoing elective hip surgery and not receiving prophylaxis, the incidence of DVT is 50%, with 23% being clinically detectable and 20% proximal (16). The pooled incidence of detectable DVT in neurosurgical patients is 22%, and the incidence in acute spinal cord injury patients is as high as 90% when prophylaxis is not used (4). The incidence of DVT in critically ill medical patients is reported to be 1% to 15% depending on which screening technique was used. No studies specific to the critically ill have been performed regarding UEDVT, and no prospective studies using systematic screening techniques are available to assess the prevalence or incidence. Nonetheless, there has been an increase over the last several decades attributed to the greater use of transvenous pacemakers and CVCs. Symptomatic PE is reported to occur in 7% to 9% of these patients (17,18), and studies using systematic ventilation/perfusion scanning in those previously diagnosed with UEDVT have reported high-probability scans in 13% (19).

Pharmacologic Prophylaxis

Four randomized controlled trials have evaluated the efficacy of UFH and/or low–molecular-weight heparin (LMWH) compared to placebo in critically ill patients (20–23). A systematic review that included these trials reported that UFH- or LMWH-prophylaxed patients had a significantly decreased relative risk for DVT (RR) 0.51 and PE (RR 0.52), with similar risk of bleeding compared to placebo (24). Three RCTs compared LMWH to UFH (25–27) and did not report significant differences in the incidence of DVT. Meta-analysis of similar data reported that LMWH decreased the incidence of PE compared to UFH (24).

Questions have been raised, whether subcutaneous (SQ) administration of LMWH has sufficient bioavailability to achieve therapeutic plasma levels (≥0.3 IU/mL) in the critically ill. A prospective, controlled, open-labeled study of enoxaparin, 40 mg once daily, in critically ill patients with normal renal function demonstrated significantly lower anti-Xa levels when compared with medical patients in the normal ward (28). This difference does not appear to be associated with vasopressor administration. These findings call into question whether once-daily dosing is appropriate for the critically ill.

Fondaparinux, a synthetic factor Xa inhibitor, in doses of 2.5 mg SQ daily has been reported to decrease VTE rates by half as compared to placebo in older, acutely ill medical patients (ARTEMIS) (29); to be more effective than enoxaparin, 30 mg twice daily, for VTE prophylaxis after elective major knee surgery (30); and equivalent to dalteparin, 5,000 IU daily, for the prevention of VTE in high-risk abdominal surgery (PEGASUS) (31). Of note, patients requiring mechanical ventilation and those with severe sepsis and septic shock were excluded from these trials, and most were not in the ICU. Nevertheless, the notion that these drugs are superior to placebo in the prevention of VTE is indeed supported. Although meta-analysis of DVT prophylaxis in critically ill patients did not report evidence of increased bleeding with pharmacologic prophylaxis compared to placebo, the risk benefit ratio should be reviewed for all patients; when bleeding risks are high, mechanical prophylaxis should be instituted.

Mechanical Prophylaxis

Graded compression stockings, intermittent pneumatic compression (IPC) devices, and venous foot pumps (VFPs) are attractive insofar as they are without bleeding risk. Compression stockings are reported to be less effective than pharmacoprophylaxis, and their utility as an independent prophylactic agent is uncertain (32). Two RCTs of mechanical prophylaxis reported IPCs combined with pharmacoprophylaxis; one reported a synergistic effect in decreasing DVT (33) and one reported no differences between IPC and Compression stockings (34).

In summary, all critically ill patients should receive DVT prophylaxis. Pharmacoprophylaxis is recommended in the absence of a bleeding contraindication and, when precluded, mechanical prophylaxis should be instituted (35). In an unblended study of 422 trauma patients, more DVT occurred in patients in whom IPC devices were used than with LMWH (2.7% vs. 0.5%) (36). Only a trend toward significance was found among 2,551 consecutive patients undergoing cardiac surgery treated with either UFH, 5,000 U SQ twice daily, or a combined prophylactic regimen of IPC and UFH; the incidence of objectively confirmed PE decreased from 4% to 1.5% (37). Use of IPC did not appear to have any additional benefit when used with either UFH or LMWH in a randomized pilot trial for VTE prophylaxis in patients undergoing craniotomy (38). IPC was less effective in preventing PE when used in addition to UFH versus LMWH alone in a prospective, randomized, multicenter trial involving acute spinal cord injury patients (39).

IVC Filters

The idea of interrupting the inferior vena cava (IVC) to prevent transit of lower extremity thromboses to the pulmonary circulation is attributed to Trousseau in 1868 (40). Today, IVC interruption is most often carried out by percutaneous insertion of a filter or "umbrella" via the femoral or jugular vein. As a result of technical refinements and ever-increasing expertise in performing the procedure, this one-time surgical technique is performed nearly 50,000 times a year (41). Categorical indications for IVC filter (IVCF) placement include contraindications to anticoagulation (absolute or relative), complications of previously instituted anticoagulation (failure, bleeding, thrombocytopenia, drug reactions), as a prophylactic adjunct to anticoagulation in patients thought to be unable to withstand another embolic event, failure of a previous IVCF, or in association with another procedure (thrombectomy, embolectomy, or thrombolysis). Unfortunately, methodologically sound literature in support of specific indications for filter placement is lacking.

Decousus et al. (42) reported one of the first RCTs of IVCFs for the prevention of PE in patients with documented proximal LEDVT. Patients were followed for 2 years in the initial report, and results of a longer-term follow-up in the same patients were reported after 8 years (43). In the initial report, 400 patients were randomized to receive a filter or no filter in addition to anticoagulation with UFH or LMWH. At 12 days, fewer patients suffered symptomatic or asymptomatic PE in the filter group while bleeding and mortality were unaffected. At 2 years, the number of patients suffering symptomatic PE was no longer significantly different (as a result of more symptomatic PE between years 1 and 2 in the filter group), and the recurrence of DVT was significantly higher in the filter group; placement of an IVCF had no effect on survival. At 8-year follow-up, patients with filters still had higher DVT rates, but symptomatic PE was lower than in patients without a filter; mortality was still unaffected. These reports suggest that DVT patients with or without PE may derive limited benefit from an IVCF in addition to anticoagulation alone. Placement of a filter in PE patients who have failed anticoagulation are at higher risk for a decrease in IVC patency or frank occlusion over time when compared to those with other indications for filter placement (44). However, no differences in edema formation, occurrence of varicose veins, trophic disorders, ulcer formation, or postthrombotic syndrome have been shown between those with and without a filter (43). Percutaneous filter placement in the superior vena cava may also be considered for prevention of symptomatic PE due to acute UEDVT in patients in whom therapeutic anticoagulation has failed or is contraindicated. Limited observational data support its safety and efficacy in this setting (45,46).

IVCF use has not been systematically studied in critical care outside the setting of major trauma, where the deployment of retrievable IVCFs (R-IVCF) has been favored. Allen et al. (47) reported that retrievable filters are safe and effective in the prevention of PE in high-risk trauma patients with contraindications to anticoagulation. Interpretation of their findings is hampered by several factors: lack of anticoagulated patients as a comparator, small numbers (53 devices placed in 2,426 patients), and a low overall incidence of thromboembolic events (2.1% with DVT, 0.2% with nonfatal PE, no fatal PE). Others have cautioned that liberal application of these filters in the trauma population does not alter rates of VTE and may lead to a greater incidence of filter and retrieval-related complications (48). Furthermore, two studies reported that only about one in five of these devices is, in fact, retrieved, suggesting that they have simply become permanent filters (48,49). Although there is limited data specifically referable to IVCs in critical care, a large retrospective analysis of IVC filters in patients showed that placement of IVCs in unstable PE patients decreased in-hospital all-cause mortality (24.5% vs. 42.0%). In unstable PE patients receiving thrombolytic therapy and an IVC, the mortality was 7.6% compared to 51.5% in those that received neither (50,51). The PREPIC 2 study evaluated the efficacy and safety of R-IVCFs versus anticoagulation in patients with the severity criterion (age >75 years, active cancer, chronic cardiac or respiratory disease, ischemic stroke with paralysis, DVT with iliocaval involvement) or evidence of right ventricular dysfunction and/or myocardial injury. At 3 and 6 months, there was no difference between the groups in recurrent PE, symptomatic DVT, major bleeding, or death (52). The preceding studies suggest that there is benefit in unstable PE patients but little support for filter placement in stable PE patients that can tolerate full anticoagulation.

DVT

Diagnosis

Validated prediction rules have been published and are useful in patients able to communicate their symptoms. However, many ICU patients will be incapable of effectively communicating any symptoms due to altered mental status, requirement for mechanical ventilation, and/or infusions of sedatives, analgesics, or neuromuscular blocking drugs; physical examination is equally unhelpful.

The gold standard for DVT is lower limb venography (53). When adequately performed, it is able to detect all clinically important forms of DVT, including calf thrombosis, thrombosis of the pelvis, and the IVC. Because of the technical nature of the test, risk of radiocontrast-induced nephrotoxicity, and need to transport the patient from the ICU, it is rarely performed outside research settings. Consequently, compression ultrasound (CUS) is the most commonly reported method of detecting DVT in the ICU setting (54). For symptomatic patients, the reported pooled sensitivity for CUS in excluding a proximal DVT is 97%, but only 62% in asymptomatic patients. Furthermore, CUS lacks sensitivity in the detection of distal DVT, yielding pooled sensitivities of 73% and 53% for symptomatic and asymptomatic patients, respectively (55). Negative serial CUS over a 7- to 10-day period may effectively rule out clinically important DVT, but thus far has only been validated in symptomatic outpatients (53). An alternative to both venography and CUS is computed tomography venography (CTV) of the lower extremities and the pelvic veins as a continuation of CT angiography of the pulmonary arteries. In the setting of diagnostic workup for PE, CTV has a reported sensitivity and specificity of 70% and 96%, respectively, for all DVT, comparable to CUS in one study (56) and was superior to CUS for detection of iliofemoral DVT in a second report, yielding 100% sensitivity and specificity (57). The PIOPED investigators reported that CTV and CUS are diagnostically equivalent, reporting a 95.5% concordance between CTV and CUS for diagnosis or exclusion of LEDVT (58). Thus the choice of imaging technique can be made on the basis of safety, expense, and time constraints. Limitations of the test are the same as for those previously mentioned for CT angiography of the pulmonary arteries.

In the case of UEDVT, the first-line diagnostic test is color duplex ultrasound with a three-step protocol involving compression, color, and color Doppler with reported sensitivity and specificity ranging from 78% to 100% and 82% to 100%, respectively (9). In the event of vessel incompressibility but in the presence of isolated flow abnormalities in combination with persistent clinical likelihood, contrast venography should be considered. Magnetic resonance venography (MRV) has been studied but with disappointing results. Reported sensitivities are 50% and 71% for MRV with and without gadolinium enhancement, respectively (57).

Treatment

The mainstay of therapy for all forms of VTE is anticoagulation. The reader is referred to the section for treatment of PE for further details. For larger clot burden involving the iliofemoral system, some suggest administration to thrombolytics. Indeed, a Cochrane review concluded that thrombolysis reduces postthrombotic syndrome and maintains venous patency after DVT when compared to traditional anticoagulation (59). However, the optimum drug, dose, and route of administration have yet to be determined. Endovascular catheter-directed thrombolysis is another promising treatment for acute iliofemoral thrombosis.

PULMONARY EMBOLISM

Contemporary risk stratification for the diagnosis, resuscitation, and treatment of PE is predicated on an implicit understanding of the pathophysiology of PE. The vicious pathophysiologic sequence of events related to the impaction of the embolic material on the pulmonary outflow is depicted in Figure 114.2. The combination of mechanical obstruction and neurohumoral factors, combined with the patients underlying cardiopulmonary status, results in an increase in pulmonary vascular impedance and the induction of pressure load on the right ventricle. Although the impact of the mechanical obstruction is well appreciated, the effect of neurohumoral influence is significantly underappreciated. The release of factors from platelets in the imbedded clot, which include serotonin, adenosine diphosphate (ADP), and thrombin, all precipitate vasoconstriction in the pulmonary artery system (60). The development of a pressure load will precipitate right ventricular decompensation, which decreases right ventricular output. Because the heart is two hydraulic pumps linked in series, diminished output of the right ventricle will result in diminished left ventricular preload. The consequence of diminished left ventricular preload is a decrease in cardiac output (CO) and a resultant loss of mean arterial pressure. The perfusion pressure gradient for the right ventricular subendocardium is the difference between the mean arterial pressure and the right ventricular end-diastolic pressure. PE precipitates an increase in right ventricular end-diastolic pressure through the induction of a right ventricular pressure load and the development of right ventricular decompensation. This increases right ventricular myocardial oxygen demands, which, because of the diminished gradient between the mean arterial pressure and the right ventricular subendocardium, induces further right ventricular decompensation and resultant right ventricular ischemia. The right ventricle compensates through the use of the Starling mechanism and increases right ventricular volume. This results in leftward shift of the intraventricular septum, further jeopardizing of left ventricular filling. Pericardial restraint further limits of left ventricular filling, and impairments of left ventricular distensibility additionally decreasing left ventricular preload. This pathophysiologic sequence results in a vicious cycle of ventricular decompensation that manifests as hemodynamic instability and shock.

Recent autopsy and laboratory investigations suggest that the pathophysiology of PE is strongly linked to an inflammatory

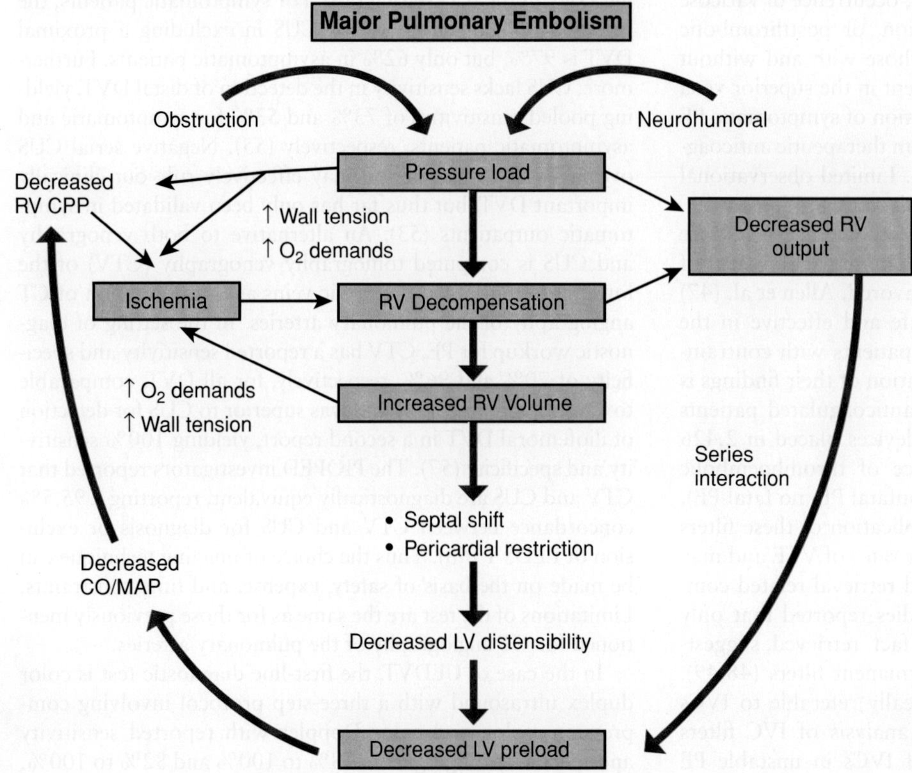

FIGURE 114.2 Pathophysiology of pulmonary embolism. CO/MAP, cardiac output/mean arterial pressure; CPP, cardiopulmonary pressure; LV, left ventricular; RV, right ventricular.

state induced by the preceding pressure-volume overload phenomena. An autopsy study of patients with fatal PE and no underlying cardiopulmonary disease reported inflammatory infiltrates composed of predominantly macrophages, T cells, and frequent neutrophilic inflammation with myocyte necrosis identified in association with the necrosis in 64% of cases; this was associated with a 6.1-fold increase in right ventricular fibrosis compared to controls (61). These inflammatory changes differed from the traditionally proposed ischemic mechanisms of RV dysfunction as they were multifocal rather than zonal, suggesting direct cellular injury resulting in fibrosis that may be a significant contributor to the persistent RV dysfunction observed in some patients. Animal laboratory investigations report that RV injury is related to both mechanical stress forces and RV ischemia that combine to promote a cytokine and chemokine-mediated inflammatory injury (62). Metalloproteinases (MMPs), important for remodeling of the cardiac extracellular matrix in both the developing and damaged heart, are reported to be activated by the pressure overload, and have been implicated as a cause of contractile dysfunction and troponin leaks (63). In animal models, inhibition of MMPs activity by doxycycline, tetracycline, and atorvastatin has been shown to attenuate MMP effects resulting in improvements in hemodynamics and CO, and decreases in pulmonary vascular resistance (PVR), RV dilatation troponin levels, and animal mortality (63,64). It is important to recognize that PE is a spectrum of presentations and that the most extreme form of PE will result in gross hemodynamic instability and cardiac arrest. Figure 114.3 illustrates a diagrammatic overview of the sequence of events that occur in PE.

The care of the critically ill patient often proceeds along two parallel pathways: physiologic resuscitation and generation of a differential diagnosis that eventually leads to a definitive diagnosis and treatment. Consequently, the use of a universally applicable model of the circulatory system is of substantial utility in characterizing the physiologic elements for resuscitation and assisting in the differential diagnosis generation. Figure 114.4 represents a three-compartmental model of the circulatory system that is characterized by two hydraulic pumps linked in series; each hydraulic pump has its own capacitance (volume reservoir) and impedance (resistive element) system. Insofar as the pumps are aligned in series, the output of one pump can never exceed the output of the other; consequently, hydraulic pumps may be conceptualized as a single hydraulic unit. Using this model, the circulatory system can be viewed as a venous capacitance reservoir that provides volume to a hydraulic pump that generates flow into an impedance bed. Any hemodynamic abnormality, such as hypovolemia, ventricular failure, sepsis, or major PE, may be characterized by defining one or more of the variables in this hydraulic pump. The surrogates for venous capacitance pressure, hydraulic pump function, and impedance are right atrial pressure (RAP), CO, and systemic venous resistance (SVR), respectively. Oftentimes invasive monitoring or echocardiographic assessment is not immediately available on patient presentation in the ICU. Consequently, it is frequently necessary to assess the model elements from physical examination; the venous capacitance reservoir may be estimated from examination the right internal jugular vein, and the pulse character and temperature of extremities maybe relied on

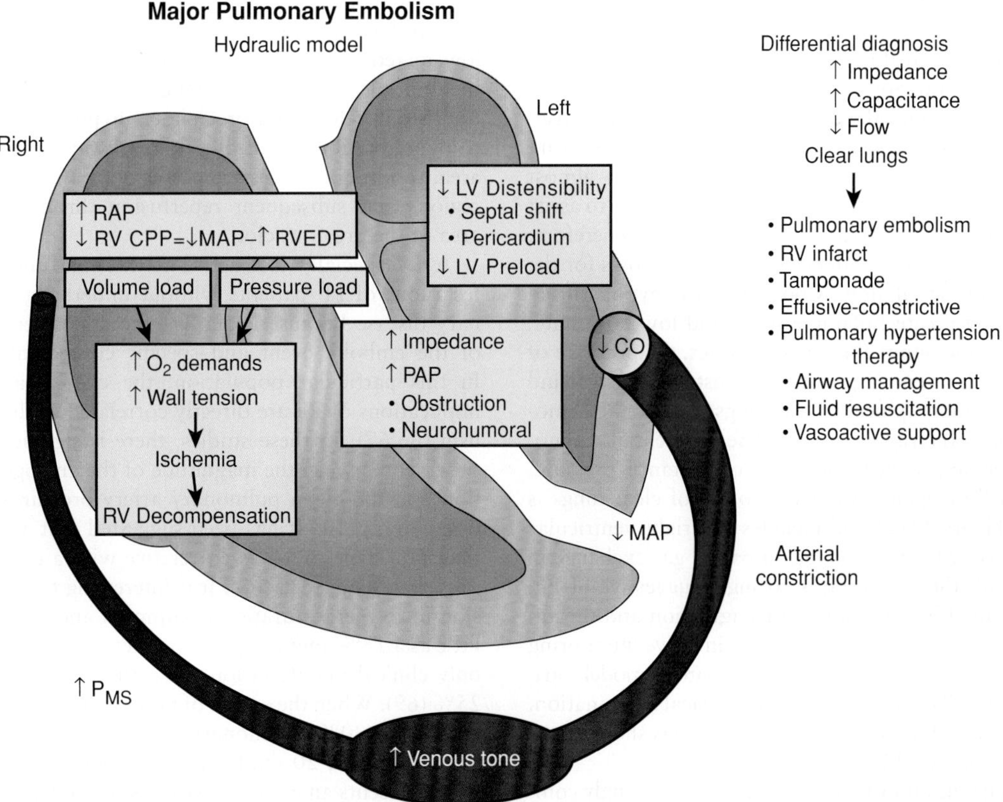

FIGURE 114.3 Pathophysiology and differential diagnosis of pulmonary embolism. CO, cardiac output; CPP, cardiopulmonary pressure; LV, left ventricular; MAP, mean arterial pressure; P_{MS}, PAP, pulmonary artery pressure; RAP, right atrial pressure; RV, right ventricular; RVEDP, RV end-diastolic pressure.

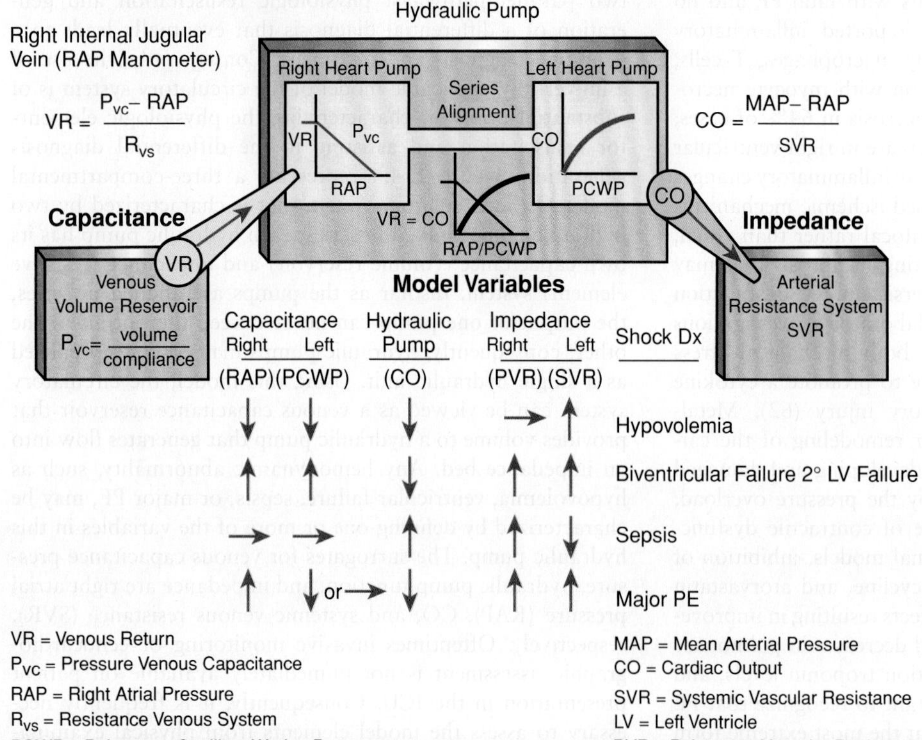

FIGURE 114.4 Three-compartment circulatory shock model.

to approximate the arterial impedance. Characteristically, a reciprocal relationship between flow and impedance is present in most disease states. Warm flushed extremities with a very wide pulse pressure indicate low vascular impedance and a correspondingly high flow state, whereas cool constricted extremities with a thready narrow pulse pressure suggest a state of high vascular impedance resulting from the compensatory increase in catecholamines to maintain perfusion pressure gradients. Recognizing that flow and impedance are almost uniformly reciprocal, one can exploit this relationship to assist with the differential diagnosis of shock patients. Therefore, the initial assessment of impedance (resistance) allows for the inferential derivation of flow. Cool, clamped hypoperfused extremities reflect a catecholamine surge and low flow state. Given the hydraulic pump alignment in series, the presence of an elevated jugular venous pressure against the background of clinical and radiographically clear lungs isolates the hemodynamic lesion to the right ventricle. The differential diagnosis of increased impedance, increased capacitance pressure, and decreased flow against the background of clear lungs is illustrated in Figure 114.3 and includes PE, right ventricular infarct, and pericardial tamponade. Impaired gas exchange in conjunction with the preceding is strongly suggestive of PE. Given the potential likelihood of anticoagulation and thrombolytic therapy in this patient population, invasive monitoring should be selectively used when the circulatory model variables cannot be well characterized from physical examination. A characterization of model variables for various shock states are depicted in Figure 114.4.

The gas exchange abnormalities in PE are exceedingly complex and a function of the size and character of the embolic material, the magnitude of the occlusion against the background of the patients underlying cardiopulmonary status, and the interval time since the embolic event (65). The multiple causes of hypoxia have been attributed to an increase in alveolar dead space, ventilation–perfusion (V/Q) abnormalities, right-to-left shunting and, in the case of cardiogenic shock, a low mixed venous O_2. Although seemingly counterintuitive, the multiple inert gas technique suggests that a low V/Q relationship develops and precipitates hypoxia in PE consequent to the redistribution of blood flow away from the embolized area, resulting in excessive perfusion in the unembolized lung regions and subsequent reperfusion through the atelectatic area of the previous clot.

It is especially instructive to examine the clinical manifestations of PE patients without underlying cardiac pulmonary disease because it permits the assessment of the effects of the embolic event and specific compensatory responses. In this particular population, the clinical and physiologic implications of PE are directly correlated to the size of embolism (66,67). In these studies, there is significant correlation observed between the magnitude of the angiographic obstruction and the mean pulmonary artery pressure (mPAP), RAP, PaO_2, and pulse. It has been suggested that a PVR of greater than 500 dyne-s-cm^{-5} is correlative with a degree of obstruction exceeding 50% (68). It is interesting to note that depression in oxygen saturation is common and may occur with as little as a 13% angiographic obstruction and, commonly, is the only clinical manifestation when the obstruction is less than 25% (69). When the extent of pulmonary vascular obstruction is 25% to 30%, pulmonary hypertension begins to develop (normal mPAP, 20 mmHg). It is important to recognize that this represents an increase in excess of similarly described nonembolic experimental obstruction, which further illustrates the relative contribution of the neurohumoral mechanism to pulmonary vascular impedance. Patients without underlying cardiopulmonary disease are unable to generate an mPAP in excess of 40 mmHg, which is reported to be the maximal pressure that a healthy ventricle can generate. In patients without underlying cardiopulmonary disease, either a large single embolus or the cumulative incremental effects of multiple recurrent emboli generating obstructions over 50% are needed to precipitate right ventricular failure. Consequently, mPAP in excess of 40 mmHg represents either significant underlying cardiopulmonary disease or the effects of multiple embolic events that have occurred over a prolonged time period, enabling the development of the right ventricular hypertrophy. It is important to recognize that the relationship between PVR and the extent of anatomic obstruction is hyperbolic and not linear. Direct increases in PVR occur when anatomic obstruction exceeds 60% (70). In the population with no underlying cardiopulmonary disease, an increase in RAP in the setting of PE is almost uniformly indicative of severe pulmonary vascular obstruction. The RAP is characteristically related to the mPAP, but is generally not elevated until the latter exceeds 30 mmHg and anatomic obstruction exceeds 35% to 40%. RAP can be elevated without a decrease in CO in patients with PE. However, a decrease in CO without an increase in RAP should suggest an alternative non–PE-related diagnosis.

In contrast to patients without an underlying cardiopulmonary disease, patients with previous cardiopulmonary disease characteristically will manifest a significantly greater degree of cardiovascular impairment with less anatomic vascular obstruction (71). This is perhaps best exemplified in the European Pulmonary Embolism Trial where 90% of the patients who presented in shock had prior cardiopulmonary disease and 56% of those with prior cardiopulmonary disease presented in shock compared to only 2% of patients without cardiopulmonary disease (72). In this population of patients with prior cardiac disease, the level of mPAP is disproportionately elevated compared to that of anatomic obstruction, which strongly suggests that underlying cardiopulmonary hemodynamics dominates the presentation process. With a mean angiographic obstruction of only 23%, significant elevations in mPAP were reported in a population with previous cardiopulmonary disease, and the increment in the mPAP was directly related to the pulmonary capillary wedge pressure (PCWP) (71). This level of anatomic obstruction would be below the threshold to elicit an increase in mPAP in patients without cardiopulmonary disease. In patients with prior cardiopulmonary disease, the RAP was reported to be an unreliable indicator of the magnitude of the embolic event and limited its usefulness in the assessment of extensive vascular obstruction and life-threatening disease. Therefore, it appears that there is no consistent relationship between the extent of embolic obstruction and right ventricular impairment in patients with previous cardiopulmonary disease. Hemodynamic and right ventricular function can be misleading as measurements of the effect of the embolic event, which clearly underscores that the assessment of the severity is predicated on the pre-embolic status of the patient as illustrated in Figure 114.1.

Readily Available Diagnostic Studies

The development of a differential diagnosis in the case of the undifferentiated shock patient or existing patients in the ICU is usually predicated on elements derived from the history, physical findings, and readily available diagnostic studies to include a chest x-ray (CXR) study, arterial blood gas (ABG) analysis, and electrocardiogram (ECG). It is important to recognize the physiologic footprint that PE makes on these readily available studies to ensure that PE is hierarchically incorporated into the differential diagnosis of the unstable patient. Generating this differential diagnosis is often difficult in the critical care environment, given the inability to obtain a current history from the patient, multiple comorbidities masking physical findings, and coexistent disease that already compromises existing laboratory variables. Although multiple risk factors are additive, admission to an ICU by itself denotes a significant risk factor for VTE. In patients presenting to the ICU with undifferentiated shock or respiratory failure, it is imperative to review each specific case for risk factors that may contribute to the development of PE. The previously defined hydraulic model of the circulation allows for a physiologic characterization of the differential diagnosis. The constellation of elevated RAP with cool clamped extremities, indicative of low flow, against the background of relatively clear lungs and CXR isolates the hydraulic lesion to the right ventricle with a very limited differential diagnosis as illustrated in Figure 114.3. Occasionally, invasive hemodynamic measurements will be available, which should reflect an increase in the RAP, a low CO state in the shock population, associated with a low PCWP, and a high SVR.

Electrocardiogram

Since the sentinel description in 1935 by McGinn and White (73) of the $S_1Q_3T_3$ pattern in a limited number of patients with PE-induced cor pulmonale, a plethora of ECG manifestation have been reported. However, several important points from large series regarding the ECG findings for PE may be helpful: First, a normal ECG is distinctly unusual, being reported in only a minority of patients in the UPET Trial without cardiopulmonary disease (14%) (74); a normal ECG was similarly appreciated in only 30% of patients in the PIOPED Trial (75). Rhythm disturbances are uncommon, and the incidence of atrial fibrillation and flutter as a presenting component of PE is exceedingly small as are first-, second-, or third-degree heart blocks. The most common ECG findings are related to abnormalities in the ST–T-wave segment. In UPET (74) and PIOPED (75), these changes occurred in 42% and 49% of patients, respectively. Recently, it has been shown that anterior T-wave inversion pattern is the most common abnormality in PE, occurring in 68% of patients. It was the ECG sign that was most correlative with the severity of the underlying embolic event, as 90% of the patients with anterior T-wave inversion had a Miller Score exceeding 50% (mean 60%), and 81% of those had an mPAP elevation exceeding 30 mmHg. The early appearance of the T-wave inversion was reported to be an even stronger marker of the severity of the event and similarly correlative with the efficacy of thrombolytic therapy given the T-wave normalization that occurred in patients who had successful thrombolytic therapy (76).

Chest Radiograph

Although the chest radiograph (CXR) cannot be effectively used to include and exclude PE, it is helpful in contributing to the diagnostic assessment by excluding other diseases that may mimic PE and defining abnormalities that necessitate further evaluation; further, it may provide a crude assessment of severity (77). Similar to the ECG, a normal CXR in patients with angiographic-proven PE is unusual, occurring in only 16% and 34% of patients in the PIOPED (75) and UPET (78), respectively, who did not have cardiopulmonary disease. In PIOPED, there appeared to be an association between severity of the thromboembolic event and the radiographic findings defined by the relationships between PAP, oxygen saturation, and CXR findings when normal CXR views were compared to those with parenchymal and vascular abnormalities (77). Vascular abnormalities, including relative oligemia in the area of embolic event, were correlative with the severity of PE. Other findings on CXR suggestive of PE include abrupt cutoff of the pulmonary artery, relative or focal oligemia, and distention of the proximal portion of the pulmonary artery.

Arterial Blood Gas

It is important to recognize that hypoxia in PE is not uniform, as PaO_2 readings greater than 80 mmHg were seen in approximately 12% of UPET patients and 19% of PIOPED patients (78,79). It is similarly important to recognize that a normal PaO_2 does not exclude PE, occurring in approximately 14% of patients in the PIOPED Trial (80). In patients without underlying cardiopulmonary disease, it is likely that these small changes in oxygen saturation reflect low levels of severity in PE. In contrast to the almost linear relationship between PE severity and arterial oxygen saturation levels in patients without cardiopulmonary disease, there appears to be no correlation between the arterial oxygen saturation or PaO_2 and magnitude of the embolic event in patients with cardiopulmonary disease. Given that many patients in ICUs have significant gas impairment and are maintained on mechanical ventilation, it is the change in the oxygen saturation or the requirement of escalating FiO_2 that should prompt the consideration toward evaluation for PE. In ICUs that are capable of measuring dead space (Vd/Vt) or end-tidal CO_2, these should similarly be used given the physiologic imprint of increased dead space with PE.

DIAGNOSTIC/THERAPEUTIC APPROACH

Risk Stratification

The contemporary approach to physiologic risk stratification is depicted in Figure 114.1. The combination of underlying cardiopulmonary status and embolic size that precipitates cardiac arrest is surprisingly associated with a mortality of only 70% in reported series. This underscores the necessity of aggressively pursuing patients with suspected underlying PE presenting with cardiac arrest, because approximately 30% of those patients with PE and cardiac arrest will survive. At the other extreme, it is equally underappreciated that the predicted mortality of patients with hemodynamically stable PE and normal right ventricle is very low when treated with appropriate anticoagulation. The combination of embolic size and cardiopulmonary status that precipitates decompensation resulting in shock is associated with 30% mortality. Although not well reported, syncope and emboli in transit have predicted mortalities just below that of a shock patient. Echocardiography is frequently used to risk-stratify patients with PE who are hemodynamically stable. However, it is important to recognize that the overwhelming majority of patients with right ventricular dysfunction and hemodynamic stability will do well with anticoagulation alone. As is evident in Figure 114.1, there is a spectrum of presentations related to hemodynamically stable patients with PE that may include patients with incipient shock and those with insignificant dilatation of the right heart. It is important to recognize that an anatomic obstruction of approximately 30% is necessary to provoke elevations in PAP. Similarly, literature related to echocardiography reveals that an obstruction of 30% is needed to precipitate right ventricular dilatation.

The presence of hemodynamic deterioration or shock in a patient with PE represents the failure of both compensatory mechanisms to maintain forward flow and is associated with significant increases in mortality. Consequently, the presence of shock has traditionally been used as a discriminator to define the likelihood of survivorship from PE. The presence of shock in patients with PE is associated with a threefold to sevenfold increase in mortality (81,82). It is underappreciated that the vast majority of patients with anatomically massive PE do not present in shock. Case series have reported a majority of patients without underlying cardiopulmonary disease and associated anatomically massive PE present with a normal CO (83). Similarly, it is important to recognize that hemodynamically stable patients who are not in shock, who have experienced submassive or massive PE, have similar mortality rates (81,82). An anatomically massive PE, unless accompanied by physiologic decompensation resulting in shock and hemodynamic instability, does not appear to be associated with increased mortality.

Figure 114.5 represents a diagnostic/therapeutic algorithm based on the presence or absent of shock. In all patients presenting with PE, therapeutic anticoagulation should be undertaken on presentation provided there are no contradictions to anticoagulation. The therapeutic effect of heparin is related to the ability to prevent further clot propagation and the prevention of recurrent of PE. Insofar as the risk of recurrent thromboembolic event is highest in the period immediately after PE, and because recurrent thromboembolic events are the most common cause of death in hemodynamic stable patients, it is pivotal to adequately and appropriately achieve a therapeutic level of anticoagulation as soon as feasible. Given the risks of bleeding associated with critical illness, unfractionated intravenous heparin is recommended because of the short half-life and the ability to reverse the therapeutic effect of heparin with protamine. ***Low-molecular-weight heparin, although appealing in the outpatient treatment of DVT and stable PE patients cannot be readily reversed.***

In patients without evidence of hemodynamic stability, spiral CT scanning has supplanted V/Q scanning as a diagnostic modality of choice in PE. In patients with elevated creatinine or inability to tolerate a CT scan, V/Q scanning represents a reasonable alternative given previous experience using this technique. Pretest probability characterizations are pivotal in the diagnosis of PE whether CT or V/Q scanning are used. Pretest probability can be characterized by the use of scoring systems or based on clinical judgment. The combination of a high pretest probability with a high-probability V/Q scan confirms the diagnosis of PE. Similarly, a low-probability V/Q scan in conjunction with a low clinical pretest probability effectively excludes PE. Any other combination of pretest probability and scan probability usually requires further testing to

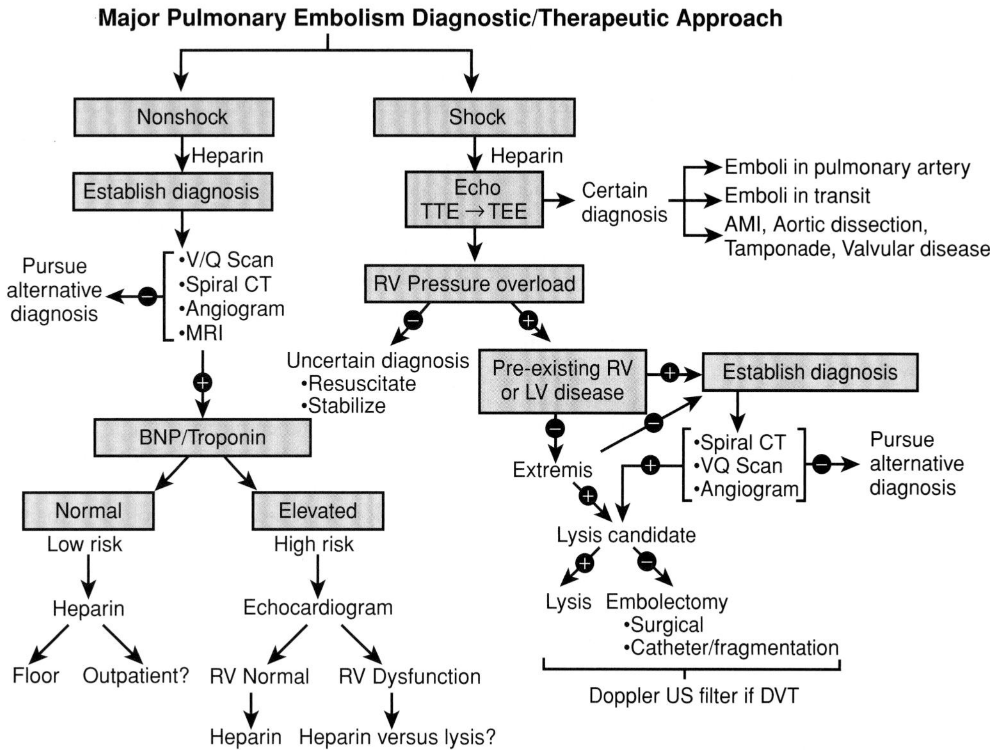

FIGURE 114.5 Diagnostic therapeutic approach to pulmonary embolism. AMI, acute mesenteric ischemia; CT, computed tomography; DVT, deep vein thrombus; LV, left ventricle; RV, right ventricle; TEE, transesophageal echocardiography; TTE, transthoracic echocardiography; US, ultrasound; V/Q, ventilation/perfusion.

include and exclude PE. Although spiral CT scanning has been used to either exclude or confirm PE, there is an evolving literature that suggests spiral CT scanning can be used to define the severity of PE. Recent reports have been able to characterize the extent of pulmonary artery obstruction (84,85). Similar to the Miller and Walsh scores, which defined the extent of anatomic obstruction, there has been variability in reports of outcome related to the extent of obstruction. Measurements that are available from the CT scan include the calculation of the RV/LV axis ratio, the diameter of the right ventricular chamber, assessment of pulmonary artery diameter, and reflux of contrast material into the IVC (86). The predictive value of CT for acute PE was recently evaluated in a systematic review and meta-analysis of 14 studies with 13,612 patients undergoing diagnostic CT imaging for PE. An abnormally increased RV/LV diameter ratio measured on the transverse section was associated with a 2.5 OR for increased all-cause mortality, 5.0 OR for PE-related mortality, and 2.3 OR for adverse outcome. Thrombus load (OR 1.6) and central location (OR 1.7) were not predictive of all-cause mortality, although associated with adverse clinical outcomes (87). Similar to RV dilatation on echocardiography, it would appear that RV dilatation on CT is very sensitive but not specific for mortality outcome, as the vast majority of patients with RV dilatation will survive with appropriate anticoagulation. With spiral CT scanning as the modality of choice for the diagnosis of PE, CT severity stratification will more frequently be used to define risk stratification.

Further risk stratification of hemodynamically stable patients with PE may be undertaken using brain natriuretic peptide (BNP) and troponin levels. In patients with hemodynamic stability and confirmed PE, presenting with a normal BNP and troponin levels, the predicted outcomes are excellent, and many of these patients may be treated as outpatient in the future. The presence of elevation in BNP and troponin define a high-risk population of patients with hemodynamic stability and warrant admission and close observation. The approach to this population will be discussed subsequently in this chapter.

In contrast to the patient presenting without hemodynamic instability, patients with suspected PE and hemodynamic instability are at high risk for rapid deterioration and sudden death. This demands an expeditious approach to the diagnosis, resuscitation, and therapy of this population. Echocardiography is an ideal first assessment of the hemodynamically unstable patient because it is readily available, an integral part of critical care medicine, repeatable, and useful in recognition and differentiation of PE along with assessing the severity of the embolic event and the patient's response to therapy (88–90). Characteristic findings suggestive of PE include right-sided thrombi, right ventricular dilatation, hypokinesis, tricuspid regurgitation, and paradoxical shifting of the ventricular septum. Similarly, the echocardiographic findings of acute myocardial infarction, tamponade, aortic dissection, or valvular disease may be equally useful in confirming the diagnosis and excluding PE. In patients without underlying cardiopulmonary disease, the magnitude of the abnormalities seen on echocardiogram correlate with the degree of pulmonary artery outflow obstruction (91). Consistent with the original data related to angiographic measurement of pressure generation with PE, it appears that an obstruction of 30% is necessary to produce right ventricular dilatation. Degrees of obstruction less than 30% will not characteristically present with right ventricular dilatation. Consequently, right ventricular dilatation has been used for severity stratification as the outcome of patients who do not have right ventricular dysfunction is excellent with therapeutic anticoagulation. It is crucial to recognize that the presence of right ventricular function is not specific for PE. Patients with previous cardiopulmonary disease may have evidence of right ventricular dysfunction at baseline. In this setting, right ventricular function might be a representative of a spectrum of diseases that range from RV infarct with cardiomyopathy to cor pulmonale and antecedent pulmonary hypertension. Several echocardiographic findings have been reported to be useful in differentiating PE from non-PE events: Patients with baseline cor pulmonale or recurrent PE characteristically have evidence of hypertrophy of the right ventricle with a thickness measuring greater than 5 mm (90,92) and minimal septal shift, whereas acute right ventricular failure secondary to PE should not be associated with right ventricular hypertrophy nor accompanied by a septal shift unless there is significant pulmonary hypertension (91,93). In patients with pre-existing cardiopulmonary disease, it is imperative to establish the diagnosis of PE, which may be undertaken with diagnostic studies previously discussed in a nonshock patient. Spiral CT scanning has supplanted V/Q scans in the critically ill population. In patients with evidence of PE that is confirmed on the diagnostic studies, candidacy for either medical thrombectomy with thrombolytic therapy or surgical embolectomy should be considered. It is crucial to recognize that the absence of right ventricular pressure overload on echocardiogram in the unstable patient when PE is being considered, effectively excludes PE as a culprit cause of the hemodynamic instability. Occasionally, and in the appropriate clinical context, patients without underlying cardiopulmonary disease in extremis and with anticipated arrest with evidence of right ventricular dilatation and high pretest probability for PE, may be considered as candidates for medical embolectomy with thrombolytic therapy or surgical embolectomy, as the time necessary to perform confirmatory studies may jeopardize effective treatment.

Resuscitation and Stabilization

Throughout the diagnostic evaluation, patients with suspected PE often require aggressive resuscitation and attempts at stabilization. In these patients, marginal hemodynamic stability is often maintained by an intense catecholamine surge. Frequently, escalating oxygen requirements necessitate intubation and mechanical ventilation. Intubation may precipitate cardiovascular collapse in patients with major PE for several reasons: sedative hypnotics that are used for intubation can mitigate the catecholamine surge upon which the patient is dependent and similarly produce vasodilatation, which impairs the perfusion pressure gradient to the right ventricular subendocardium, provoking further ischemia and cardiac decompensation. Excessive ventilation on initial intubation may create air trapping and diminish venous return. Initiation of mechanical ventilation can increase the PVR and further jeopardize right ventricular function. Consequently, intubation should be carefully undertaken, weighing the risk and benefits of a conscious awake technique with topical or local anesthesia in conjunction with a rapid-sequence approach using neuromuscular blockade and/or fiberoptic intubation. Etomidate is an ideal sedative hypnotic insofar as it preserves hemodynamic status.

Conventionally, volume expansion with 1 to 2 L of crystalloid solution is initial treatment for hypotension in patients with undifferentiated shock. However, in patients with PE-related shock, increases in right ventricular pressure and volume can generate significant increases in systolic wall stress, provoking further myocardial ischemia. Excessive fluid resuscitation further dilates the right ventricle and produces increased wall stress, resulting in further right ventricular decompensation. In patients with anatomically massive PE and low CO who were normotensive and required vasopressors on presentation, Mercat et al. (94) reported increases in CO with a 500-mL fluid challenge. The authors reported that the increase in CO was consistently proportional to the baseline right ventricular end-diastolic volume index. Therefore, fluid may be used judicially in normotensive patients without evidence of significant right ventricular dysfunction. In patients with echocardiographic evidence of severe right ventricular dysfunction, fluid resuscitation may provoke increased wall stress, ischemia, and right ventricular dysfunction. When measured right ventricular pressures are high or there is evidence of severe right ventricular dysfunction, early consideration should be given to vasopressor therapy.

Although there are no controlled human trials related to vasoactive support in PE, extrapolation from animal models suggests that norepinephrine improves right ventricular dysfunction through vasoconstriction that augments mean arterial pressure and enhances perfusion pressure gradients to the right ventricular subendocardium. In addition, norepinephrine possesses modest inotropic properties that have been shown to provide complementary enhancement of right ventricular function (95,96). Given the previously described vasoconstrictive effects of the neurohumoral response to PE, it may be reasonable to consider the use of inhaled nitric oxide to decrease pulmonary vascular afterload in patients with evidence of severe right ventricular dysfunction who are pressor dependent. Small reports have suggested that inhaled prostacyclin and nitric oxide will increase CO, decrease pulmonary artery pressures, and improve gas exchange in cases of shock-related PE (97,98).

The presence of shock or hemodynamic decompensation in patients with proven PE is an indication for either medical embolectomy with thrombolytic therapy or surgical embolectomy. Although the use of thrombolytic therapy is controversial in patients who are hemodynamically stable, it is acknowledged as the therapeutic choice in hemodynamically unstable patients in whom there is no contraindication to thrombolytic therapy. The PIOPED investigators considered thrombolytic therapy the standard of care for patients with "shock or major disability" and considered it unethical to treat patients with hemodynamic stability with heparin alone in the research trial (99). Several points regarding the use of thrombolytic therapy in PE patients should be emphasized. First, in virtually all studies, there is greater rapidity in the rate of resolution when comparing heparin to thrombolytic therapy in terms of the percent resolution detected by perfusion scanning and angiography. Second, no reported clinical trial has defined any difference in the degree of embolic resolution after day 7. This is perhaps best illustrated in the original UPET Trial conducted in 1970 (81). In this landmark publication related to the use of thrombolytic therapy and PE, the baseline angiographic defect in the heparin group was 25% and that in the urokinase group was 26%. Within the first 24 hours, the percent of angiographic resolution in the heparin group was 8.1%, with 22.1% in the urokinase-treated group. However, by day 5, the extent of angiographic resolution in the heparin and urokinase groups was equivalent at 36% and 40%, respectively. By 1 year, the extent of angiographic resolution was 77% in the heparin group and

TABLE 114.2 Rate and Extent of Perfusion Scan Resolution in Urokinase Pulmonary Embolism Trial (UPET)

	Heparin (81)		Urokinase (77)	
	25.4%		26.2%	
	Absolute Resolution	% Resolution	Absolute Resolution	% Resolution
24 hrs	2.7%	8.1%	6.2%	22.1%
Day 2	4.9%	17%	8.0%	25.8%
Day 5	9.3%	35.5%	11.3%	40.6%
Day 14	14.7%	58.2%	14.9%	52.0%
1 yr		77.2%		78.8%
No CPD 90% resolution		91% of patients		88% of patients
CPD 90% resolution		72% of patients		77% of patients

CPD, cardiopulmonary disease.
Data from Urokinase pulmonary embolism trial. Phase 1 results: a cooperative study. *JAMA*. 1970;214:2163–2172; and Urokinase pulmonary embolism trial. *Circulation*. 1973;47(Suppl):1–108.

78% in the urokinase group (Table 114.2). A comparison of clinical trials conducted comparing lytic therapy to heparin reveals similar findings as there is no reported difference in any physiologic or imaging modality after day 5 when comparing the two therapeutic options (Table 114.3). Third, there does not appear to be any difference related to the effectiveness of thrombolytic agents provided that they are given in equivalent doses over a similar time frame (83,100). This is best exemplified in trials that compared rT-PA given over 2 hours and urokinase given in the same time interval (83). Fourth, bleeding complications from thrombolytic therapy remain a substantial concern with major hemorrhage occurring in approximately 12%, and fatal hemorrhage occurring in 1% to 2%, of patients (101). Intracranial hemorrhage rates have been reported from 1.2% to 2.1% (102); these are fatal in at least half of the cases (103). Two recent meta-analyses of systemic thrombolytic therapy compared to heparin alone in PE evaluated the potential benefits and risks with similar findings and conclusions. Marti reported that thrombolytic therapy was associated with a significant reduction in the combined end point of death or treatment escalation (OR 0.34), PE mortality (OR 0.29) and PE recurrence (0.50), but with significant risks of major hemorrhage (OR 2.91) and fatal or intracranial bleeding (OR 3.18). No significant benefit was seen in hemodynamically stable patients with acute PE (104). Chatterjee reported similar outcomes except that major bleeding was not increased in patients less than 65 years of age and there was a mortality benefit in the intermediate risk group characterized by hemodynamically stable patients with RV dysfunction (105). These meta-analyses suggest the clinical benefits in patients without contraindications to thrombolytic therapy need to be balanced against the risks of bleeding.

Assessing the efficacy of thrombolytic therapy can be difficult in the first several hours. Echocardiographic studies undertaken prior to the use of thrombolytic therapy have suggested that there are two types of morphologic characteristics of PE that may assist in defining the efficacy of therapy. Thrombi that are long, mobile, and hypoechoic/heterogeneous seem to be more susceptible to thrombolytic therapy. In contrast, echocardiographically defined emboli that are immobile and hyperechoic/homogeneous seem less susceptible to thrombolytic therapy. In a small case report series of patients who received thrombolytic therapy and had the previous characterizations made by echocardiography, long mobile hypoechoic emboli had higher COs, lower central venous pressures, and diminished peripheral vascular resistance compared to the group with echocardiographically defined immobile embolism after the use of thrombolytic therapy. It is important to note that the mortality in the group that underwent successful embolectomy was 0% compared to 30% mortality in the group that failed to respond to thrombolytic therapy in this study (106). Monitoring the efficacy of thrombolytic therapy can similarly be challenging, as continuous echocardiography and imaging studies are not always available, nor feasible. Monitoring of end-tidal CO_2 has been proposed to monitor the efficacy of thrombolytic therapy. End-tidal CO_2 was found

TABLE 114.3 Randomized Trials: Lysis versus Heparin

	Early				
Study	Angio	Scan	Hemodyn	Echo	Late
UPET 1970	↑ 24 hrs	↑ 24 hrs	↑ 24 hrs	—	Scan, day 5; pulmonary HTN
Tibbutt 1974	↑ 72 hrs	—	↑ 72 hrs	—	Limited
Arnesen 1978	↑ 72 hrs	—	—	—	—
Ly 1978	↑ 72 hrs	—	—	—	—
Marini 1988	→ 7 days	→ 24 hrs	→ 7 days	—	No difference, 1 yr
PIOPED 1990	→ 2 hrs	→ 24, 48 hrs	↑ PVR 1.5 days	—	No difference
Giuntini 1984	—	↑ 24 hrs	—	—	Scan, day 3
Levine 1990	—	↑ 24 hrs	—	—	Scan, day 7
PAIMS 1992	↑ 2 hrs	→ 7 days	↑ 2 hrs PAP/CI	—	Scan/angio, day 7
Goldhaber 1993	—	↑ 24 hrs	—	↑ 3, 24 hrs	—

HTN, hypertension; PVR, pulmonary vascular resistance; PAP/CI, pulmonary artery pressure/cardiac index.

to be significantly increased in patients who survived with thrombolytic therapy compared nonsurvivors with no appreciable change in end-tidal CO_2 measurements. This would suggest that continuous monitoring of end-tidal CO_2 enables assessment of the efficacy of thrombolytic therapy and may be used as a barometer to define the need of subsequent thrombolytic or embolectomy in cases of failed thrombolytic therapy (107). Unsuccessful thrombolysis is reported to occur in approximately 8% of patients undergoing therapy; this may be defined as persistent clinical instability or significant residual echocardiographic dysfunction. In the limited literature that compares repeat thrombolysis to surgical thromboembolectomy, there appears to be significant survival benefit in undertaking surgical embolectomy. The mortality in patients undergoing surgical embolectomy after failed thrombolytic therapy was reported to be 7% compared to 38% of patients who underwent repeat thrombolysis. Recurrent PE was significantly higher in patients who underwent repeat thrombolysis and was the cause of death in a significant number of patients. It should be noted that patients who underwent surgical thromboembolectomy also had the placement of vena cava filters (108).

The long-term outcome of patients with thrombolytic therapy is not well described, but it appears that most patients undergo an uneventful course with mortality approximating 8%, major bleeding 9.6%, and recurrent PE in 7.6%. The mean vascular obstruction diminished from 64% to 29% within 48 hours, and right ventricular function was reversible within 48 hours in 80% of the patients, while lung scan improved by 45% within 6 to 8 days of therapy. This review of thrombolytic therapy similarly reported that predictive indicators of a poor hospital course in patients receiving thrombolytic therapy were an initial pulmonary vascular obstruction greater than 70% and hemodynamic instability at presentation associated with persistence of paradoxical septal motion on echocardiography. Long-term mortality was related to older age, persistence of vascular obstruction more than 30% after thrombolytic therapy, and cancer (109).

Attempts to reconcile the benefits of thrombolytic therapy with significant bleeding risks have led to the development of endovascular therapies that utilize a pharmacomechanical approach via percutaneous catheters. In a meta-analysis of 594 patients with hemodynamically unstable PE that defined clinical success by hemodynamic stabilization, resolution of hypoxia, and survival to discharge, success was achieved in 86%. A third of the cases were treated with mechanical disruption alone, with complications occurring in only 2.9% (110). Recent pharmacomechanical catheter-directed trials utilizing low-dose intrapulmonary thrombolytic therapy have reported significant clinical success evidenced by hemodynamic stabilization, improvement in RV strain and pulmonary hypertension, and survival with no major procedural complications, major hemorrhages, or hemorrhagic strokes (111,112). As this literature unfolds, catheter-directed therapy may evolve to the treatment of choice for hemodynamically unstable PE and potentially for stable patients with RV dysfunction if supported by longitudinal studies.

Surgical embolectomy is indicated for patients presenting in shock or cardiopulmonary instability and an inability to tolerate thrombolytic therapy. Ideally, these emboli are large and located centrally; consideration of embolectomy is undertaken prior to cardiac arrest. This requires preoperative localization via CT documentation and, ideally, echocardiographic of right heart function (113). In the era of modern surgical embolectomy, outstanding results have been reported by multiple investigators. In a study that undertook surgical embolectomy with most patients having a contraindication to thrombolytic therapy and significant right ventricular dysfunction, there was a 6% operative mortality and only 12% late deaths from disease other than PE (114). The overall improvement in operative mortality related to surgical thromboembolectomy most likely relates to preoperative selection of patients who had not experienced cardiac arrest, and the use of cardiopulmonary bypass (115). The precursor to extracorporeal membrane oxygenation (ECMO), the artificial heart and lung extracorporeal blood circuit, was developed by Gibbon over a 20-year period after watching a post-op gall bladder patient succumb to a massive PE in 1931 (116); the first successful use of cardiopulmonary bypass for embolectomy was reported by Cooley in 1961 (117). Although there are no randomized controlled trials utilizing ECMO, an extensive number of case reports suggest that there is potential benefit for select patients at centers familiar with utilizing VA ECMO and with embolectomy capabilities (118).

In summary, PE remains a common and lethal problem that usually confronts the intensivist in the form of undifferentiated respiratory failure and shock. Diagnosis is difficult and challenging in the ICU because of the patient complexity and coexistent illnesses. The use of spiral CT scans and echocardiography is evolving to define severity stratification in the ICU population and facilitate the timely diagnosis of PE. It is imperative to incorporate PE into the differential diagnosis of patients with undifferentiated shock, and the use of a structure model for shock diagnosis and therapy is helpful to ensure that PE is expeditiously diagnosed and optimal treatment is undertaken. Medical embolectomy with thrombolytic therapy or surgical embolectomy are recognized as the treatment of choice for hemodynamically unstable patients with an evolving use of catheter-directed pharmacomechanical techniques to be defined by further trials, and the optimal approach to the hemodynamically stable patient with right ventricular dysfunction remains to be defined.

Key Points

- All patients in a critical care unit are at high risk for VTE and should receive pharmacoprophylaxis or, if contraindicated, mechanical prophylaxis.
- PE should be incorporated in the differential diagnosis of patients with undifferentiated shock and/or respiratory failure.
- A normal RV on echocardiogram should effectively exclude PE as a cause of shock.
- IVC filters should be strongly considered in unstable patients receiving thrombolytic therapy or embolectomy.
- Aggressive fluid resuscitation in patients with echocardiographically documented RV dysfunction should be done with caution and strong consideration given to pulmonary afterload reduction with nitric oxide.
- Hemodynamically unstable PE patients should receive thrombolytic therapy with strong consideration to a catheter pharmacomechanical approach or, when contraindicated, traditional surgical embolectomy.
- Select cases in specialized centers should consider ECMO.

References

1. Kasper W, Konstantinides S, Geibel A, et al. Management strategies and determinants of outcome in acute major pulmonary embolism: results of a multicenter registry. *J Am Coll Cardiol.* 1997;30:1165–1171.
2. Goldhaber SZ, Visani L, De Rosa M. Acute pulmonary embolism: clinical outcomes in the International Cooperative Pulmonary Embolism Registry (ICOPER). *Lancet.* 1999;353:1386–1389.
3. Quality AfHRa. Agency for Healthcare Research and Quality (US). Making health care safer: a critical analysis of patient safety practices. April 28, 2008.
4. Cook DJ, Crowther MA, Meade MO, Douketis J; VTE in the ICU Workshop Participants. Prevalence, incidence, and risk factors for venous thromboembolism in medical-surgical intensive care unit patients. *J Crit Care.* 2005;20:309–313.
5. Ibrahim EH, Iregui M, Prentice D, et al. Deep vein thrombosis during prolonged mechanical ventilation despite prophylaxis. *Crit Care Med.* 2002;30:771–774.
6. Cook D, Crowther M, Meade M, et al. Deep venous thrombosis in medical-surgical critically ill patients: prevalence, incidence, and risk factors. *Crit Care Med.* 2005;33:1565–1571.
7. Warkentin TE, Greinacher A. Heparin-induced thrombocytopenia and cardiac surgery. *Ann Thorac Surg.* 2003;76:638–648.
8. Mustafa S, Stein PD, Patel KC, et al. Upper extremity deep venous thrombosis. *Chest.* 2003;123:1953–1956.
9. Gaitini D, Beck-Razi N, Haim N, Brenner B. Prevalence of upper extremity deep venous thrombosis diagnosed by color Doppler duplex sonography in cancer patients with central venous catheters. *J Ultrasound Med.* 2006;25:1297–1303.
10. Joffe HV, Kucher N, Tapson VF, Goldhaber SZ; Deep Vein Thrombosis (DVT) FREE Steering Committee. Upper-extremity deep vein thrombosis: a prospective registry of 592 patients. *Circulation.* 2004;110:1605–1611.
11. Martinelli I, Battaglioli T, Bucciarelli P, et al. Risk factors and recurrence rate of primary deep vein thrombosis of the upper extremities. *Circulation.* 2004;110:566–570.
12. Geerts W, Cook D, Selby R, Etchells E. Venous thromboembolism and its prevention in critical care. *J Crit Care.* 2002;17(2):95–104.
13. Ho KM, Chavan S, Pilcher D. Omission of early thromboprophylaxis and mortality in critically ill patients: a multicenter registry study. *Chest.* 2011;140(6):1436–1446.
14. Ribic C, Lim W, Cook D, Crowther M. Low-molecular weight heparin thromboprophylaxis in medical-surgical critically ill patients: a systematic review. *J Crit Care.* 2009;24(2):197–205.
15. Khouli H, Shapiro J, Pham VP, et al. Efficacy of deep venous thrombosis prophylaxis in medical intensive care unit. *J Intensive Care Med.* 2006;21(6):352–358.
16. Murray MT, Coursin DB, Pearl RG, et al., eds. *Critical Care Medicine: Perioperative Management.* 2nd ed. Philadelphia, PA: Lippincott Williams & Wilkins; 2002.
17. Becker DM, Philbrick JT, Walker FB 4th. Axillary and subclavian venous thrombosis: prognosis and treatment. *Arch Intern Med.* 1991;151:1934–1943.
18. Hingorani A, Ascher E, Lorenson E, et al. Upper extremity deep venous thrombosis and its impact on morbidity and mortality rates in a hospital-based population. *J Vasc Surg.* 1997;26:853–860.
19. Monreal M, Lafoz E, Ruiz J, et al. Upper-extremity deep venous thrombosis and pulmonary embolism: a prospective study. *Chest.* 1991;99:280–283.
20. Fraisse F, Holzapfel L, Couland JM, et al. Nadroparin in the prevention of deep vein thrombosis in acute decompensated COPD: the Association of Nonuniversity Affiliated Intensive Care Specialist Physicians of France. *Am J Resp Crit Care Med.* 2000;161:1109–1114.
21. Cade JF. High risk of critically ill for venous thrombo-embolism. *Crit Care Med.* 1982;10:448–450.
22. Kappor M, Kupfer YY, Tessler S. Subcutaneous heparin prophylaxis significantly reduces the incidence of venous thromboembolic events in the critically ill. *Crit Care Med.* 1999;27:A69.
23. Shorr AF, Williams MD. Venous thromboembolism in critically ill patients. Observations from a randomized trial in sepsis. *Thromb Haemost.* 2009;101(1):139–144.
24. Alhazzani W, Lim W, Jaeschke RZ, et al. Heparin thromboprophylaxis in medical–surgical critically ill patients: a systematic review and meta-analysis of randomized trails. *Crit Care Med.* 2013;41(9):2088–2098.
25. De A, Roy P, Garg VK, Pandey NK. Low-molecular weight heparin and unfractionated heparin in prophylaxis against deep vein thrombosis in critically ill patients undergoing major surgery. *Blood Coag Fibrin.* 2010; 21(1):57–61.
26. Cook D, Meade M, Guyatt G, et al. PROTECT Investigations for the Canadian Critical Care Trials Group and the Australian and New Zealand Intensive Care Society Clinical Trials Group. Dalteparin versus unfractionated heparin in critically ill patients. *N Engl J Med.* 2011;364(14): 1305–1314.
27. Goldhaber SZ, Kett DH, Cusumano CJ, et al. Low molecular weight heparin versus mini dose unfractionated heparin for prophylaxis against venous thromboembolism in medical intensive care unit patients: a randomized controlled trial. *J Am Call Cardiol.* 2000;35(Suppl):325A.
28. Priglinger U, Delle Karth G, Geppert A, et al. Prophylactic anticoagulation with enoxaparin: Is the subcutaneous route appropriate in the critically ill? *Crit Care Med.* 2003;31:1405–1409.
29. Cohen AT, Davidson BL, Gallus AS, et al.; ARTEMIS Investigators. Efficacy and safety of fondaparinux for the prevention of venous thromboembolism in older acute medical patients: randomised placebo controlled trial. *BMJ.* 2006;332:325–329.
30. Bauer KA, Eriksson BI, Lassen MR, Turpie AG; Steering Committee of the Pentasaccharide in Major Knee Surgery Study. Fondaparinux compared with enoxaparin for the prevention of venous thromboembolism after elective major knee surgery. *N Engl J Med.* 2001;345:1305–1310.
31. Agnelli G, Bergqvist D, Cohen AT, Gallus AS, Gent M; PEGASUS investigators. Randomized clinical trial of postoperative fondaparinux versus perioperative dalteparin for prevention of venous thromboembolism in high-risk abdominal surgery. *Br J Surg.* 2005;92:1212–1220.
32. Limpus A, Chaboyer W, McDonald E, Thalib L. Mechanical thromboprophylaxis in critically ill patients: a systematic review and meta-analysis. *Am J Crit Care.* 2006;15(4):402–410; quiz/discussion, 411–412.
33. Arabi YM, Khedr M, Dara SI, et al. Use of Intermittent pneumatic compression and not graduated compression stocking's is associated with lower incident VTE in critically ill patients: a multiple propensity scores adjusted analysis. *Chest.* 2013;144(1):152–159.
34. Vignon P, Deguin PF, Renault A, et al. Clinical Research in Intensive Care and Sepsis Group (CRIS Group). Intermittent pneumatic compression to prevent venous thromboembolism in patients with high risks of bleeding hospitalized in intensive care units: the CIREA randomized trial. *Intensive Care Med.* 2013;39(5):872–880.
35. Boonyowat K, Crowther MA. Venous thromboembolism prophylaxis in critically ill patients. *Semin Thromb Haemost.* 2015;41:68–74.
36. Ginzburg E, Cohn SM, Lopez J, et al.; Miami Deep Vein Thrombosis Study Group. Randomized clinical trial of intermittent pneumatic compression and low molecular weight heparin in trauma. *Br J Surg.* 2003;90: 1338–1344.
37. Ramos R, Salem BI, De Pawlikowski MP, et al. The efficacy of pneumatic compression stockings in the prevention of pulmonary embolism after cardiac surgery. *Chest.* 1996;109:82–85.
38. Macdonald RL, Amidei C, Baron J, et al. Randomized, pilot study of intermittent pneumatic compression devices plus dalteparin versus intermittent pneumatic compression devices plus heparin for prevention of venous thromboembolism in patients undergoing craniotomy. *Surg Neurol.* 2003;59:363–372; discussion 372–374.
39. Spinal Cord Injury Thromboprophylaxis Investigators. Prevention of venous thromboembolism in the acute treatment phase after spinal cord injury: a randomized, multicenter trial comparing low-dose heparin plus intermittent pneumatic compression with enoxaparin. *J Trauma.* 2003;54:1116–1124; discussion 1125–1126.
40. Trousseau A. Phlegmatia alba dolens: clinique medicale de l'hotel-dieu de paris. *JB Baillere Fils.* 1868:652–695.
41. Ansell J. Vena cava filters: Do we know all that we need to know? *Circulation.* 2005;112:298–299.
42. Decousus H, Leizorovicz A, Parent F, et al. A clinical trial of vena caval filters in the prevention of pulmonary embolism in patients with proximal deep-vein thrombosis. Prévention du Risque d'Embolie Pulmonaire par Interruption Cave Study Group. *N Engl J Med.* 1998;338:409–415.
43. PREPIC Study Group. Eight-year follow-up of patients with permanent vena cava filters in the prevention of pulmonary embolism: the PREPIC (Prévention du Risque d'Embolie Pulmonaire par Interruption Cave) randomized study. *Circulation.* 2005;112:416–422.
44. Crochet DP, Stora O, Ferry D, et al. Vena Tech-LGM filter: long-term results of a prospective study. *Radiology.* 1993;188:857–860.
45. Ascher E, Hingorani A, Tsemekhin B, et al. Lessons learned from a 6-year clinical experience with superior vena cava Greenfield filters. *J Vasc Surg.* 2000;32:881–887.
46. Spence LD, Gironta MG, Malde HM, et al. Acute upper extremity deep venous thrombosis: safety and effectiveness of superior vena caval filters. *Radiology.* 1999;210:53–58.

47. Allen TL, Carter JL, Morris BJ, et al. Retrievable vena cava filters in trauma patients for high-risk prophylaxis and prevention of pulmonary embolism. *Am J Surg.* 2005;189:656–661.
48. Antevil JL, Sise MJ, Sack DI, et al. Retrievable vena cava filters for preventing pulmonary embolism in trauma patients: a cautionary tale. *J Trauma.* 2006;60:35–40.
49. Karmy-Jones R, Jurkovich GJ, Velmahos GC, et al. Practice patterns and outcomes of retrievable vena cava filters in trauma patients: an AAST multicenter study. *J Trauma.* 2007;62:17–24; discussion 24–25.
50. Stein PD, Matta F, Keyes DC, Willyerd GL. Impact of vena cava filters on in-hospital case fatality rate from pulmonary embolism. *Am J Med.* 2012;125:478–484.
51. Dalen JE. Thrombolytics and vena cava filters decrease mortality in patients with unstable pulmonary embolism. *Am J Med.* 2012;25:429–430.
52. Mismetti P, Laporte S, Pellerin O; PREPIC2 Study Group. Effect of retrievable inferior vena cava filter plus anticoagulation vs. anticoagulation alone on risk of recurrent pulmonary embolism: a randomized clinical trial. *JAMA.* 2015;313(16):1627–1635.
53. Cook D, Douketis J, Crowther MA, et al. The diagnosis of deep venous thrombosis and pulmonary embolism in medical-surgical intensive care unit patients. *J Crit Care.* 2005;20:314–319.
54. Cook D, McMullin J, Hodder R, et al.; Canadian ICU Directors Group. Prevention and diagnosis of venous thromboembolism in critically ill patients: a Canadian survey. *Crit Care (Lond).* 2001;5:336–342.
55. Kearon C, Gent M, Hirsh J, et al. A comparison of three months of anticoagulation with extended anticoagulation for a first episode of idiopathic venous thromboembolism. *N Engl J Med.* 1999;340:901–907.
56. Taffoni MJ, Ravenel JG, Ackerman SJ. Prospective comparison of indirect CT venography versus venous sonography in ICU patients. *AJR Am J Roentgenol.* 2005;185:457–462.
57. Lim KE, Hsu WC, Hsu YY, et al. Deep venous thrombosis: comparison of indirect multidetector CT venography and sonography of lower extremities in 26 patients. *Clin Imaging.* 2004;28:439–444.
58. Goodman LR, Stein PD, Beemath A, et al. CT venography for deep venous thrombosis: continuous images versus reformatted discontinuous images using PIOPED II data. *AJR Am J Roentgenol.* 2007;189:409–412.
59. Watson LI, Armon MP. Thrombolysis for acute deep vein thrombosis. *Cochrane Database Syst Rev.* 2004(4):CD002783.
60. Stratmann G, Gregory GA. Neurogenic and humoral vasoconstriction in acute pulmonary thromboembolism. *Anesth Analg.* 2003;97:341–354.
61. Orde MM, Puranik R, Morrow PL, Duflon J. Myocardial pathology in pulmonary thromboembolism. *Heart.* 2011;97:1695–1699.
62. Watts JA, Marchick MR, Kline JA. Right ventricular heart failure from pulmonary embolism: key distinctions from chronic pulmonary hypertension. *J Card Fail.* 2010;16(3):250–259.
63. Neto-Neves EM, Kiss T, Muhl D, Tanus-Santos JE. Matrix metalloproteinases as drug targets in acute pulmonary embolism. *Curr Drug Targets.* 2013;14:344–352.
64. Cau SB, Barato RC, Celes MR, et al. Doxycycline prevents acute pulmonary embolism induced mortality and right ventricular deformation in rats. *Cardiovasc Drugs Ther.* 2013;27(4):259–267.
65. D'Alonzo GE, Dantzker DR. Gas exchange alterations following pulmonary thromboembolism. *Clin Chest Med.* 1984;5:411–419.
66. Dalen JE, Banas JS Jr, Brooks HL, et al. Resolution rate of acute pulmonary embolism in man. *N Engl J Med.* 1969;280:1194–1199.
67. McDonald IG, Hirsh J, Hale GS, O'Sullivan EF. Major pulmonary embolism, a correlation of clinical findings, haemodynamics, pulmonary angiography, and pathological physiology. *Br Heart J.* 1972;34:356–364.
68. Dalen JE, Grossman W. *Profiles in Pulmonary Embolism: Cardiac Catheterization and Angiography.* Philadelphia, PA: Lea & Febiger; 1980.
69. McIntyre KM, Sasahara AA. The hemodynamic response to pulmonary embolism in patients without prior cardiopulmonary disease. *Am J Cardiol.* 1971;28:288–294.
70. Petitpretz P, Simmoneau G, Cerrina J, et al. Effects of a single bolus of urokinase in patients with life-threatening pulmonary emboli: a descriptive trial. *Circulation.* 1984;70:861–866.
71. McIntyre KM, Sasahara AA. Determinants of right ventricular function and hemodynamics after pulmonary embolism. *Chest.* 1974;65:534–543.
72. The UKEP study: multicentre clinical trial on two local regimens of urokinase in massive pulmonary embolism. The UKEP Study Research Group. *Eur Heart J.* 1987;8:2–10.
73. McGinn S, White P. Acute cor pulmonale resulting from pulmonary embolism. *JAMA.* 1935;104:1473–1480.
74. Stein PD, Dalen JE, McIntyre KM, et al. The electrocardiogram in acute pulmonary embolism. *Prog Cardiovasc Dis.* 1975;17:247–257.
75. Stein PD, Terrin ML, Hales CA, et al. Clinical, laboratory, roentgenographic, and electrocardiographic findings in patients with acute pulmonary embolism and no pre-existing cardiac or pulmonary disease. *Chest.* 1991;100:598–603.
76. Ferrari E, Imbert A, Darcourt J. No scintigraphic evidence of myocardial abnormality in severe pulmonary embolism with electrocardiographic signs of anterior ischemia. *Eur Heart J.* 1995;16(Suppl):269 abstract.
77. Stein PD, Athanasoulis C, Greenspan RH, Henry JW. Relation of plain chest radiographic findings to pulmonary arterial pressure and arterial blood oxygen levels in patients with acute pulmonary embolism. *Am J Cardiol.* 1992;69:394–396.
78. Urokinase pulmonary embolism trial. *Circulation.* 1973;47(Suppl):1–108.
79. Stein PD, Goldhaber SZ, Henry JW, Miller AC. Arterial blood gas analysis in the assessment of suspected acute pulmonary embolism. *Chest.* 1996;109:78–81.
80. Stein PD, Goldhaber SZ, Henry JW. Alveolar-arterial oxygen gradient in the assessment of acute pulmonary embolism. *Chest.* 1995;107:139–143.
81. Urokinase pulmonary embolism trial. Phase 1 results: a cooperative study. *JAMA.* 1970;214:2163–2172.
82. Alpert JS, Smith R, Carlson J, et al. Mortality in patients treated for pulmonary embolism. *JAMA.* 1976;236:1477–1480.
83. Meneveau N, Schiele F, Metz D, et al. Comparative efficacy of a two-hour regimen of streptokinase versus alteplase in acute massive pulmonary embolism: immediate clinical and hemodynamic outcome and one-year follow-up. *J Am Coll Cardiol.* 1998;31:1057–1063.
84. Mastora I, Remy-Jardin M, Masson P, et al. Severity of acute pulmonary embolism: evaluation of a new spiral CT angiographic score in correlation with echocardiographic data. *Eur Radiol.* 2003;13:29–35.
85. Qanadli SD, El Hajjam M, Vieillard-Baron A, et al. New CT index to quantify arterial obstruction in pulmonary embolism: comparison with angiographic index and echocardiography. *AJR Am J Roentgenol.* 2001;176:1415–1420.
86. Ghaye B, Ghuysen A, Willems V, et al. Severe pulmonary embolism: pulmonary artery clot load scores and cardiovascular parameters as predictors of mortality. *Radiology.* 2006;239:884–891.
87. Meinel FG, Nance JW Jr, Schoepf UJ, et al. Predictive value of computed tomography in acute pulmonary embolism: systematic review and meta-analysis. *Am J Med.* 2015;128:747–759.e2.
88. Come PC. Echocardiographic evaluation of pulmonary embolism and its response to therapeutic interventions. *Chest.* 1992;101(Suppl 4):151S–162S.
89. Konstantinides S, Geibel A, Kasper W. Role of cardiac ultrasound in the detection of pulmonary embolism. *Semin Respir Crit Care Med.* 1996;17:39–49.
90. Torbicki A, Tramarin R, Morpurgo M. Role of echo/Doppler in the diagnosis of pulmonary embolism. *Clin Cardiol.* 1992;15:805–810.
91. Jardin F, Dubourg O, Bourdarias JP. Echocardiographic pattern of acute cor pulmonale. *Chest.* 1997;111:209–217.
92. Kasper W, Geibel A, Tiede N, et al. Distinguishing between acute and subacute massive pulmonary embolism by conventional and Doppler echocardiography. *Br Heart J.* 1993;70:352–356.
93. Kasper W, Geibel A, Tiede N, et al. Echocardiography in the diagnosis of lung embolism [in German]. *Herz.* 1989;14:82–101.
94. Mercat A, Diehl JL, Meyer G, et al. Hemodynamic effects of fluid loading in acute massive pulmonary embolism. *Crit Care Med.* 1999;27:540–544.
95. Angle MR, Molloy DW, Penner B, et al. The cardiopulmonary and renal hemodynamic effects of norepinephrine in canine pulmonary embolism. *Chest.* 1989;95:1333–1337.
96. Hirsch LJ, Rooney MW, Wat SS, et al. Norepinephrine and phenylephrine effects on right ventricular function in experimental canine pulmonary embolism. *Chest.* 1991;100:796–801.
97. Capellier G, Jacques T, Balvay P, et al. Inhaled nitric oxide in patients with pulmonary embolism. *Intensive Care Med.* 1997;23:1089–1092.
98. Webb SA, Stott S, van Heerden PV. The use of inhaled aerosolized prostacyclin (IAP) in the treatment of pulmonary hypertension secondary to pulmonary embolism. *Intensive Care Med.* 1996;22:353–355.
99. Tissue plasminogen activator for the treatment of acute pulmonary embolism: a collaborative study by the PIOPED investigators. *Chest.* 1990;97:528–533.
100. Goldhaber SZ, Kessler CM, Heit JA, et al. Recombinant tissue-type plasminogen activator versus a novel dosing regimen of urokinase in acute pulmonary embolism: a randomized controlled multicenter trial. *J Am Coll Cardiol.* 1992;20:24–30.
101. Levine MN. Thrombolytic therapy for venous thromboembolism: complications and contraindications. *Clin Chest Med.* 1995;16:321–328.
102. Dalen JE, Alpert JS, Hirsh J. Thrombolytic therapy for pulmonary embolism: Is it effective? Is it safe? When is it indicated? *Arch Intern Med.* 1997;157:2550–2556.

103. Arcasoy SM, Kreit JW. Thrombolytic therapy of pulmonary embolism: a comprehensive review of current evidence. *Chest.* 1999;115:1695–1707.
104. Marti C, John G, Konstantinides S, et al. Systemic thrombolytic therapy for acute pulmonary embolism: a systemic review and meta-analysis. *Eur Heart J.* 2015;36:605–614.
105. Chatterjee S, Chakraborty A, Weinberg I, et al. Thrombolysis for pulmonary embolism and risk of all-cause mortality, major bleeding and intracranial hemorrhage: a meta-analysis. *JAMA.* 2014;311(23):2414–2421.
106. Podbregar M, Krivec B, Voga G. Impact of morphologic characteristics of central pulmonary thromboemboli in massive pulmonary embolism. *Chest.* 2002;122(3):973–979.
107. Wiegand UK, Kurowski V, Giannitsis E, et al. Effectiveness of end-tidal carbon dioxide tension for monitoring thrombolytic therapy in acute pulmonary embolism. *Crit Care Med.* 2000;28:3588–3592.
108. Meneveau N, Seronde MF, Blonde MC, et al. Management of unsuccessful thrombolysis in acute massive pulmonary embolism. *Chest.* 2006;129:1043–1050.
109. Meneveau N, Ming LP, Seronde MF, et al. In-hospital and long-term outcome after sub-massive and massive pulmonary embolism submitted to thrombolytic therapy. *Eur Heart J.* 2003;24:1447–1454.
110. Kuo WT, Gould MK, Louie JD, et al. Catheter directed therapy for the treatment of massive pulmonary embolism: systematic review and meta-analysis of modern techniques. *J Vasc Interv Radiol.* 2009;20:1431–1440.
111. Kuo WT, Banerjee A, Kim PS, et al. Pulmonary embolism response to fragmentation, embolectomy and catheter thrombolysis (PERFECT): initial results from a prospective multicenter registry. *Chest.* 2015;148(3):667–673.
112. Piazza G, Hohlfelder B, Jaff MR, et al.; SEATTLE II Investigators. A prospective, single-arm, multi-center trial of ultrasound facilitated catheter directed, low dose fibrinolysis for acute massive and sub-massive pulmonary embolism: The SEATTLE II Study. *JACC.* 2015;8(10):1382–1392.
113. Aklog L. Emergency surgical pulmonary embolectomy. *Semin Vasc Med.* 2001;1:235–246.
114. Leacche M, Unic D, Goldhaber SZ, et al. Modern surgical treatment of massive pulmonary embolism: results in 47 consecutive patients after rapid diagnosis and aggressive surgical approach. *J Thor Cardiovasc Surg.* 2005;129:1018–1023.
115. He C, Von Seqessed LK, Kappetein PA, et al. Acute pulmonary embolectomy. *Eur J Cardiothorac Surg.* 2013;43:1087–1095.
116. Gibbon JM Jr. Development of the artificial heart and lung extracorporeal blood circuit. *JAMA.* 1968;206(9):1983–1986.
117. Cooley DA, Beall AC Jr, Alexander JK. Acute massive pulmonary embolism. *JAMA.* 1961;177(5):283–286.
118. Yusulf HO, Zochios V, Vuylsteke A. Extracorporeal membrane oxygenation in acute massive pulmonary embolism: a systematic review. *Perfusion.* 2015;30(8):611–615.

CHAPTER

115

Pleural Disease in the Intensive Care Unit

HIREN J. MEHTA and MICHAEL A. JANTZ

INTRODUCTION

Pleural disease in itself is an unusual cause for admission to the intensive care unit (ICU). Conditions potentially requiring ICU admission include a large pleural effusion causing acute respiratory failure, hemothorax producing respiratory or hemodynamic compromise, secondary spontaneous pneumothorax with respiratory failure, empyema with sepsis, and reexpansion pulmonary edema. Pleural complications of disease processes and procedures performed in the ICU are common, however, and the changes in respiratory physiology are additive to that of the underlying lung disease. The development of a pneumothorax in a critically ill patient, particularly in mechanically ventilated patients, may be a life-threatening event. Pleural effusions may be overshadowed by the illness requiring ICU admission in the critically ill patient. Pleural effusions and pneumothoraces may not be detected on chest radiographs because the radiologic appearance may differ in the supine patient.

PLEURAL EFFUSIONS IN THE INTENSIVE CARE UNIT

Radiologic Evaluation

In the normal pleural space, air and fluid tend to distribute following gravitational influences, with air initially accumulating between the superior portion of the lung and the apex of the thorax, while fluid accumulates between the inferior margin of the lung and the diaphragm. Pleural air and fluid collections shift location when radiographs are obtained in positions other than the erect position. Because radiographs in critically ill patients are taken in the supine or semierect position, the radiographic appearance of air and fluid in the pleural space may thus change.

In normal humans in the supine position, the radiolucency of the lung base is equal to or greater than that of the lung apex due to the anteroposterior diameter of the lung being greatest at the lung base. In addition, in the supine patient, breast and pectoral tissues will tend to move laterally away from the lung base. A pleural effusion should be suspected when increased homogeneous density is present over the lower lung fields as compared with the upper lung fields. Patient rotation, an off-center x-ray beam, prior lobectomy, or a pleural or chest wall mass may produce a unilateral homogeneous density that simulates the appearance of a pleural effusion (1). Cardiomegaly, a prominent epicardial fat pad, and lobar collapse or consolidation may obscure the detection of a pleural effusion on a supine radiograph.

Approximately 175 to 525 mL of pleural fluid will produce blunting of the costophrenic angle on an erect chest radiograph (2). This quantity of pleural fluid can usually be detected on a supine radiograph as an increased density over the lower lung zone. Blunting of the costophrenic angle (meniscus sign), silhouetting of the hemidiaphragm, and apical capping may be seen with larger effusions (3). An apparent elevation of the hemidiaphragm may be secondary to a subpulmonic collection of pleural fluid. A diffuse increase in the radiodensity of the hemithorax, or "veiling," may be seen with very large effusions in the supine radiograph. Thus, the major radiographic finding of a pleural effusion in the supine patient is an increased homogeneous density over the lower lung field that does not obliterate normal bronchovascular markings, does not demonstrate air bronchograms, and does not produce hilar or mediastinal displacement until the effusion is massive. If a pleural effusion is suspected in the supine patient, obtaining an erect or lateral decubitus radiograph may be helpful.

Because the critically ill patient often has underlying parenchymal lung disease, the diagnosis of pleural effusion can be problematic. Ultrasound (US) helps to diagnose, quantify, and guide drainage of pleural fluid and can be performed at bedside. Small-sized pleural effusions are common in the ICU; occasionally, they might be large enough to necessitate drainage (4). Pleural effusions appear on ultrasound as hypoechoic areas between the parietal and visceral pleura. If the fluid collection is sufficiently large, the lung may be seen floating on it like a "jelly fish" (5). Effusions may be echogenic and septate if exudative in nature; hemothorax and pyothorax are typically hyperechoic on ultrasound (6,7). The approximate volume of pleural effusion may be estimated by measuring the distance between the parietal and visceral pleura at the lung base with the breath held in midexpiration. In one study of 74 ICU patients evaluated by both chest radiograph and US, the latter detected a pleural effusion that was not appreciated on chest radiograph in 10 additional patients (29% of patients determined to have a pleural effusion) (4). In another study, US was helpful in making a diagnosis in 27 of 41 (66%) patients and influenced treatment planning in 17 of 41 critically ill patients (41%) (8). US-guided thoracentesis at the bedside was successful in 24 of 25 patients in that same study. Other studies have noted the usefulness of US to safely guide bedside thoracentesis in mechanically ventilated patients (9–11). The presence of complex septated, complex nonseptated, and homogeneously echogenic patterns within pleural fluid collections are typically indicative of an exudative pleural effusion (12). Homogeneously echogenic effusions suggest hemorrhagic effusions or empyemas, whereas US evidence of fibrin septae suggests a parapneumonic effusion, empyema, hemothorax, or malignant effusion (12). Disadvantages of US include impedance of the ultrasound wave by air in the lung or pleural space, a restricted field of view, inferior evaluation of the lung parenchyma compared to computed tomography (CT), and operator dependence (1).

CT may also be helpful in assessing pleural processes in the critically ill patient, and has the advantages of better lung parenchymal imaging, evaluation of the mediastinum, and ability to distinguish pleural from parenchymal abnormalities (1). On CT, free-flowing pleural fluid produces a sickle-shaped opacity in the most dependent part of the thorax (13). Loculated pleural fluid collections are seen as lenticular or rounded opacities in a fixed position with a relatively homogeneous water density (13). CT may be particularly helpful in the diagnosis and management of loculated pleural effusions (14). The most reliable sign of empyema, the split pleura sign, is usually identified during the organizing phase. Following administration of intravenous contrast, the parietal and visceral pleura will be thickened and enhanced and will be noted to be separated, and the extrapleural fat between the empyema and the chest wall may be increased in size (15,16). In one study, this sign was present in only 68% of patients, however (15). CT may be helpful in assessing inadequately drained fluid collections in patients with persistent fevers or sepsis due to malpositioned chest tubes (17). CT is much more sensitive at detecting pleural fluid, and in one study chest CT identified a pleural effusion in 13% of patients in the ICU which were missed by CXR (18).

Diagnostic Thoracentesis

Pleural effusions are common in the ICU. In one prospective study of 100 consecutive patients admitted to a medical ICU, pleural effusions were found on chest radiographs and/or by US in 62% of patients (4). Patients with a pleural effusion provide the opportunity to diagnose, at least presumptively, the underlying process responsible for the accumulation of pleural fluid. Although disease of any organ system can cause a pleural effusion in critically ill patients, the diagnoses listed in Table 115.1 represent the most common causes in the ICU.

When a pleural effusion is suspected on physical examination and confirmed radiologically, a diagnostic thoracentesis should be considered to establish the cause of the effusion. Observation alone may be reasonable in situations in which the clinical diagnosis is reasonably secure and a small amount of pleural fluid is present, such as in atelectasis or uncomplicated heart failure (19). Thoracentesis should be performed, however, if the patient's clinical condition changes. When the distance from the pleural fluid line to the inside of the chest wall is less than 1 cm on lateral decubitus radiograph, the risk of thoracentesis probably outweighs the value of pleural fluid analysis. If the underlying disease causing the pleural effusion becomes clinically problematic, the effusion will often increase in size and allow for safe thoracentesis. When sampling of a small-volume pleural effusion is indicated, thoracentesis should be performed with US guidance. Several studies (20,21) suggest that US-guided diagnostic thoracentesis can be successfully performed in up to 88% of patients after unsuccessful clinically guided thoracentesis.

TABLE 115.1 Causes of Pleural Effusions in ICU Patients

- Abdominal surgery
- Acute respiratory distress syndrome (ARDS)
- Atelectasis
- Chylothorax
- Congestive heart failure
- Coronary artery bypass surgery
- Empyema
- Esophageal rupture
- Esophageal sclerotherapy
- Hemothorax
- Hepatic hydrothorax
- Hypoalbuminemia
- Iatrogenic
  - Central venous catheter placement
  - Nasogastric tube placement
  - Vascular erosion by central venous catheter
- Intra-abdominal abscess
- Malignancy
- Pancreatitis/pancreatic pseudocyst
- Pneumonia
- Postcardiac injury syndrome
- Pulmonary embolism
- Uremia

The indications for diagnostic thoracentesis are not different in the ICU patient, and receiving mechanical ventilation is not a contraindication. Establishing the diagnosis quickly in critically ill patients may be more important than in the noncritically ill. The reported incidence of pneumothorax in nonventilated patients ranges from 4% to 30% (22–25). Various risk factors for developing a pneumothorax after thoracentesis have been reported, although operator inexperience, baseline lung disease, and use of positive pressure mechanical ventilation appear to be the most established risk factors. Several earlier studies have demonstrated that the incidence of pneumothorax after blind thoracentesis in mechanically ventilated patients, 5% to 10%, is similar to that of nonventilated patients, and it is thus safe to perform blind thoracentesis in mechanically ventilated patients (26,27). If the patient on mechanical ventilation does develop a pneumothorax, however, a significant risk of progression to a life-threatening tension pneumothorax exists. As such, some authors have advocated the routine use of ultrasound guidance for all thoracentesis procedures in mechanically ventilated patients, given the observed pneumothorax rates of 0% to 3% with ultrasound guidance in nonventilated patients (25,28), as well as in patients receiving mechanical ventilation (9–11). Strong consideration should be given to using US guidance in patients with small or moderate effusions. US or CT guidance should be used to sample loculated pleural fluid collections. There are no absolute contraindications to diagnostic thoracentesis; the major relative contraindications are a bleeding diathesis or anticoagulation. In one study of 207 patients requiring thoracentesis with mild to moderate coagulopathy, defined as a prothrombin time (PT) or partial thromboplastin time (PTT) up to twice normal, or a platelet count from 50,000 to 100,000 cells/μL, no increase in bleeding complications was noted (29). Thoracentesis should not be performed through an area of active skin infection. Analysis of pleural fluid in the ICU patient is similar to that in other settings and is beyond the scope of this chapter.

Therapeutic Thoracentesis and Physiologic Effects

The primary indication for therapeutic thoracentesis or chest tube drainage of a pleural effusion is relief of dyspnea, although pulmonary mechanics and oxygenation may be improved in some patients (30). Contraindications to and complications of therapeutic thoracentesis are similar to those of diagnostic thoracentesis, with the additional complications of hypoxemia, reexpansion pulmonary edema, and hypovolemia. An increased risk of pneumothorax has been noted with therapeutic thoracentesis in some studies (24,25,31) although not others (32,33). We would recommend the use of a catheter-over-needle system in performing therapeutic thoracentesis to reduce the risk of developing a pneumothorax. In patients with pleural effusion and ipsilateral shift suggesting endobronchial obstruction, chronic atelectasis, or a trapped lung, the risk of reexpansion pulmonary edema may be increased, and the patient may be less likely to experience a beneficial effect. In addition, patients with initial negative pleural pressures and those with more precipitous falls in pleural pressures with fluid removal also likely have trapped lung or endobronchial obstruction and are less likely to benefit from therapeutic thoracentesis (34).

Pleural effusions compress the lung, causing atelectasis, ventilation/perfusion mismatch, and shunt physiology with resultant hypoxemia (35). Pleural fluid tends to enlarge the volume of the hemithorax more than it compresses lung volume. Studies in humans have shown that total lung capacity following thoracentesis increases by only approximately one-third of the thoracentesis fluid volume, and forced vital capacity increases by approximately half of the increase in total lung capacity. Studies evaluating gas exchange in nonventilated patients have been mixed. One found a decrease in PaO_2 (36), while another found no change in PaO_2 (37), and a third showed a mild increase in PaO_2 (38). More recent studies have also shown variable results, with one study reporting a small increase in PaO_2 and decrease in alveolar-arterial O_2 gradient (39), although another noted no change in PaO_2, alveolar-arterial O_2 gradient or shunt, while the amount of blood flow to low ventilation/perfusion units increased slightly (35).

Despite these mixed results, some patients requiring mechanical ventilation may benefit from pleural fluid drainage. Talmor et al. (30) reported that 19 patients with acute respiratory failure and pleural effusions who had a poor response to positive end-expiratory pressure (PEEP), defined as the inability to wean FiO_2 to 0.5 with PEEP up to 20 cm H_2O, benefited from chest tube drainage of the pleural effusions. The PaO_2 increased from 125 to 199 mmHg, and the PaO_2/FiO_2 ratio increased from 151 to 254. Fourteen patients had a unilateral effusion, and five patients had bilateral effusions necessitating bilateral chest tube placement. More recently, Doelken et al. (40) studied the effects of thoracentesis on respiratory mechanics and gas exchange in eight mechanically ventilated patients. Following removal of 800 to 1,950 mL (mean 1,495 mL), no significant change in PaO_2 or dead space ventilation was observed. No significant changes were noted for peak and plateau pressures, dynamic and effective static compliance, respiratory system resistance, and intrinsic PEEP. Mean work performed by the ventilator did significantly decrease, however. A recent study of 20 patients showed that drainage of more than 500 mL of pleural fluid in mechanically ventilated patients improved respiratory mechanics with a decrease in plateau pressure and a large increase in end-expiratory transpulmonary pressure. Improvement in the PaO_2/FiO_2 ratio from baseline to 24 hours post drainage was positively correlated with the increase in end-expiratory lung volume but not with the amount of fluid drained. There was no significant effect of large volume thoracentesis on patient hemodynamics (41).

Further studies are required to confirm these results. In patients who are difficult to wean from mechanical ventilation, we would consider a trial of therapeutic thoracentesis.

COMMON CAUSES OF PLEURAL EFFUSIONS IN THE ICU

Abdominal Surgery

Approximately one-half of patients undergoing abdominal surgery will develop small unilateral or bilateral pleural effusions 24 to 48 hours following surgery (42,43). The incidence of pleural effusions is higher in procedures involving the upper abdomen, in patients having ascitic fluid at time of surgery, and in patients who have postoperative atelectasis (34). Larger left-sided effusions are common following splenectomy. The effusion after abdominal surgery is usually exudative* with a normal glucose level, pH more than 7.40, and less than 10,000 nucleated cells/μL (42). Small effusions generally do not require diagnostic thoracentesis and resolve spontaneously without becoming clinically significant. Thoracentesis is indicated to exclude empyema if the effusion is relatively large or loculated or if the possibility of a subdiaphragmatic abscess related to the surgery exists.

Acute Respiratory Distress Syndrome

The presence of pleural effusions in acute respiratory distress syndrome (ARDS) has not been well appreciated or studied. In a retrospective study of 25 patients with ARDS, 36% were found to have pleural effusions (44). All patients had extensive alveolar infiltrates in addition to pleural effusions. Pleural effusions have been observed in animal models of ARDS using α-naphthylthiourea, oleic acid, and ethchlorvynol (45,46). In the oleic acid model, 35% of the excess lung water collected in the pleural spaces (45). Effusions are likely underdiagnosed in ARDS because the patient has bilateral alveolar infiltrates and the radiograph is taken in the supine position. In experimental models of ARDS, the effusions are serous to serosanguineous with a predominance of polymorphonuclear leukocytes (PMNs) (46). In a post hoc analysis of a study looking at the effect of large volume thoracentesis in mechanically ventilated patients, no significant improvement in PaO_2/FiO_2 ratio was observed in patients with ARDS (41). These effusions resolve as the ARDS resolves and require no specific therapy.

Atelectasis

Atelectasis is a common cause of small pleural effusions in the ICU due to patients being immobile (4). Atelectasis and small effusions are commonly observed following cardiothoracic or abdominal surgery; other potential causes include endobronchial obstruction from tumor, foreign body, or mucus plugging as well as extrinsic airway compression from malignancy. With lung collapse, local areas of increased negative pressure are created by

*Effusions are termed exudative—or not—by lactate dehydrogenase (LDH) and protein criteria. Only LDH and protein values are used in the Light criteria although cholesterol level is used by some. pH, glucose, and cell counts are not part of the classification of transudate versus exudate.

the separation of the lung and chest wall. The decrease in pleural pressure favors the movement of fluid into the pleural space, presumably from the surface of the parietal pleura (19).

Pleural effusions from atelectasis are serous transudates with a few mononuclear cells, a glucose concentration equal to serum, and a pH of 7.45 to 7.55. The pleural effusions dissipate over several days when the atelectasis resolves.

Chylothorax

A chylothorax is defined as the accumulation of chyle in the pleural space. The predominant mechanisms of chylothorax formation include disruption of the thoracic duct, extravasation from pleural lymphatics, and transdiaphragmatic efflux from chylous ascites (47). The most common cause of chylothorax is lymphoma, accounting for 37% of chylothoraces in a series of 191 patients (48); the second most frequent cause is surgical trauma, which represented 25% of cases in the same series of 191 patients (48). The incidence of chylothorax following thoracic surgery has been reported to be 0.36% to 0.42% (49,50) and 1.9% following lower neck surgery (46). A higher proportion of chylothoraces are noted following esophagectomy. Virtually all intrathoracic surgical procedures, including lobectomy, pneumonectomy, and coronary artery bypass grafting, have been reported to cause chylothorax (48). Nonsurgical trauma, including blunt and penetrating injuries to the neck, thorax, and upper abdomen as well as obstruction of the superior vena cava or thrombosis of the left subclavian vein from indwelling central venous catheters (CVCs), may produce chylothoraces in ICU patients (51).

The patient may be asymptomatic if the effusion is small and unilateral, or may be dyspneic with a large unilateral effusion or bilateral effusions. The pleural fluid is usually milky but can be serous, serosanguineous, or bloody. The fluid may not have a milky appearance if the patient is malnourished or not eating (52). The pleural fluid typically has less than 7,000 nucleated cells/μL, which are over 80% lymphocytes. The pH is alkaline (7.40–7.80), and the triglyceride levels exceed plasma levels (19). A pleural fluid triglyceride concentration greater than 110 mg/dL makes the diagnosis of chylothorax highly likely, whereas a concentration below 50 mg/dL makes the diagnosis highly unlikely. With triglyceride concentrations of 50 to 110 mg/dL, lipoprotein electrophoresis is indicated to demonstrate the presence of chylomicrons, which confirms the diagnosis of chylothorax (52).

Up to 2 to 3 L of chyle may drain daily, causing loss of fluid, electrolytes, protein, fat, fat-soluble vitamins, and lymphocytes. Severe nutritional depletion and immunodeficiency may result if these losses are not addressed. In addition to chest tube drainage, initial conservative management consists of intravenous hydration and a nonfat, high-protein, high-calorie diet with medium-chain triglycerides, which are absorbed directly into the portal system, or discontinuing all oral feeding and initiating total parenteral nutrition. If the chylothorax fails to resolve with conservative measures after 7 to 14 days, then surgery with thoracic duct ligation may be considered (53), although pleuroperitoneal shunting has also been used.

Congestive Heart Failure

Congestive heart failure (CHF) is the most common cause of all transudative pleural effusions and in one study was the most common cause of pleural effusions in a medical ICU (4). Pleural effusions due to CHF are associated with increases in pulmonary venous pressure. In a study of 37 patients admitted for CHF, the mean pulmonary capillary wedge pressure (PCWP) was higher in patients with pleural effusions than in those without—24.1 versus 17.2 mmHg, respectively (54). Isolated increases in right heart pressures were not associated with pleural effusions. Patients with chronic obstructive pulmonary disease (COPD) and cor pulmonale, in the absence of left ventricular dysfunction, thus, rarely have pleural effusions, and other causes for pleural effusions should be sought in these patients.

Most patients with pleural effusion secondary to CHF have the usual signs and symptoms. The chest radiograph classically demonstrates cardiomegaly and bilateral small to moderate pleural effusions of similar size, with right-sided effusions often being slightly greater than the left. Radiographic evidence of pulmonary edema is usually present, with the severity of pulmonary edema correlating with the presence of effusions. In patients who have been hospitalized, records will usually show intake greater than output for several days, weight gain, an increasing alveolar-arterial O_2 gradient, and decreasing compliance in those patients requiring mechanical ventilation. Some patients without a history of CHF may not be suspected of having CHF until intravenous hydration produces pleural effusions and subsequent echocardiograms demonstrate left ventricular dysfunction (4).

Pleural effusions from CHF are transudates and have less than 1,000 nucleated cells/μL, which are mainly mesothelial cells and lymphocytes. Acute diuresis may increase the protein concentration of the pleural fluid and thus change the classification of the fluid from transudative to exudative in 8% to 38% of patients (55). In the afebrile patient with clinical CHF and cardiomegaly with bilateral effusions of relatively equal size on chest radiograph, the diagnosis is reasonably secure and observation is appropriate. Thoracentesis should be considered in patients who are febrile, have pleuritic chest pain, or are noted on chest radiograph to have effusions of disparate size, unilateral effusions, a larger effusion on the left than the right, or absence of cardiomegaly.

Treatment consists of decreasing preload and improving cardiac output with diuretics, inotropes, and afterload-reducing agents. With appropriate management, the pleural effusions will resolve over days to weeks.

Coronary Artery Bypass Surgery

A small left pleural effusion is virtually always present following coronary artery bypass surgery (CABG). The effusion is associated with left lower lobe atelectasis and elevation of the left hemidiaphragm on chest radiograph. Approximately 10% of patients will have a larger effusion occupying more than 25% of the hemithorax. These large effusions can be separated into *early effusions* occurring within the first 30 days of surgery that are bloody exudates with a high percentage of eosinophils, and *late effusions* occurring more than 30 days after surgery that are clear yellow lymphocytic exudates (56). Factors associated with higher incidence of *post*-CABG effusions and large effusions are internal mammary artery grafting, on pump surgery, and topical cardiac hypothermia with cold saline.

Rarely, a loculated hemothorax may develop with a trapped lung, resulting in clinically significant restriction (57). If a large effusion that qualifies as a hemothorax is present, the fluid should be drained by tube thoracostomy. It is unclear if a large hemorrhagic effusion with a pleural fluid/blood hematocrit less than 50% needs to be drained to avoid later necessity for decortication. If the effusion is small and the patient is asymptomatic, no treatment is necessary. Treatment with anti-inflammatory agents and possibly chemical pleurodesis may be required for patients with recurrent nonbloody effusions (56).

Esophageal Rupture

Spontaneous esophageal rupture—Boerhaave syndrome—is a potentially life-threatening event and requires immediate diagnosis and therapy. Esophageal rupture or perforation may rarely occur with blunt thoracic trauma or as a complication of endoscopy and nasogastric/orogastric tube placement. The history in spontaneous esophageal rupture is usually severe retching or vomiting; however, activities that generate a Valsalva maneuver can cause esophageal rupture, and in some patients the perforation may be silent (58). The findings on chest radiograph may vary depending on the time between perforation and obtaining of the chest radiograph, the site of perforation, and integrity of the mediastinal pleura. Mediastinal emphysema is present in less than half of patients, and may take 1 to 2 hours to be observed, whereas mediastinal widening may take several hours. Pneumothorax, indicating rupture of the mediastinal pleura, is present in 75% of patients; 70% of pneumothoraces are on the left, 20% are on the right, and 10% are bilateral (59). Pleural effusion, with or without associated pneumothorax, occurs in 75% of patients. A presumptive diagnosis should be confirmed radiographically with an esophagram as soon as possible. Because rapid passage of the contrast in the upright patient that may not demonstrate a small perforation, the study should be done with the patient in the appropriate lateral decubitus position.

Pleural fluid findings depend on the degree of perforation and the timing of thoracentesis. Early thoracentesis without mediastinal perforation shows a sterile serous exudate with a predominance of PMNs and a pH greater than 7.30. Amylase of salivary origin appears in the fluid in high concentration following disruption of the mediastinal pleura. With the seeding of the pleural space by anaerobic bacteria, the pH falls rapidly and progressively to approach 6.00. The presence of food particles and squamous epithelial cells in the pleural fluid also suggests esophageal rupture (60). Management is usually operative intervention in conjunction with pleural space drainage and antibiotics. Nonoperative therapy with antibiotics and chest tube drainage alone may be considered in a nontoxic patient with small perforations due to instrumentation.

Esophageal Sclerotherapy

Pleural effusions are found in approximately 50% of patients 48 to 72 hours following esophageal sclerotherapy (61). Effusions may be unilateral or bilateral, with no predilection for side. The effusions tend to be small serous exudates with variable nucleated (38,000–90,000 cells/μL) and red cell counts (126,000–160,000 cells/μL) and glucose concentrations similar to serum. The mechanism for development of these effusions is likely extravasation of the sclerosant beyond the esophageal mucosa, resulting in mediastinal and mediastinal pleural inflammation. An effusion that is not associated with fever, chest pain, or signs of perforation is not important clinically, and will usually resolve over several days to weeks without specific therapy. A diagnostic thoracentesis should be performed and an esophagram considered in patients with symptomatic effusions for 24 to 48 hours to exclude empyema and esophageal perforation.

Hemothorax

Hemothorax needs to be differentiated from a hemorrhagic pleural effusion, as the latter can be the result of only a few drops of blood in serous pleural fluid. The arbitrary definition of a hemothorax is a pleural fluid to blood hematocrit ratio greater than 50%. Hemothorax can be divided into three categories based on etiology: spontaneous, iatrogenic, and traumatic hemothorax; most hemothoraces result from blunt or penetrating thoracic trauma (62). Other etiologies include invasive procedures, pulmonary infarction, malignancy, and ruptured aortic aneurysms. Anticoagulation therapy or coagulopathy may rarely cause a spontaneous hemothorax. Hemothorax should be suspected in any patient with blunt or penetrating chest trauma with a pleural effusion on chest radiograph. Chest tube thoracostomy with a 28-Fr chest tube, or larger, should be performed in these patients and pleural fluid hematocrit measured. In patients with suspected iatrogenic or spontaneous hemothorax, thoracentesis should be performed first, and if positive, a chest tube should be inserted. Chest tube drainage allows the monitoring of the rate of bleeding, may potentially tamponade the bleeding, and will evacuate the pleural space, thus decreasing the risk of developing empyema or a subsequent fibrothorax (62,63). Prophylactic use of antibiotics (usually a first-generation cephalosporin) for at least 24 hours after the start of chest tube drainage for traumatic hemothorax, reduces the incidence of pneumonia and empyema (64). Whether antibiotic prophylaxis is useful for spontaneous hemothorax has not been investigated accurately.

Intrapleural fibrinolytic therapy can be applied in an attempt to evacuate residual blood clots and breakdown adhesions when initial chest tube drainage is inadequate. The dose, time to initiate, frequency, and duration of fibrinolytic use is unclear from existing literature. Generally, it is advised to evacuate the clotted hemothorax within 7 to 10 days. We recommend 5 to 10 mg of tissue plasminogen activator (tPA) in 50 mL of normal saline given intrapleurally once daily for 3 days starting on day 4 or later of the development of the hemothorax and evaluating the response at the end of 3 days with a chest CT. Indications for surgical exploration vary between clinicians, but general guidelines are hemodynamic instability despite adequate resuscitation, initial drainage greater than 1,500 mL, continued bleeding of more than 200 mL/hr for 3 consecutive hours, continued bleeding of more than 1,500 mL/day, and radiographic evidence of significant retained clot despite adequate noninvasive management as mentioned above (greater than one-third of the pleural space).

Hepatic Hydrothorax

Pleural effusions are present in approximately 6% of patients with cirrhosis and clinically apparent ascites (65,66). The effusions result from movement of ascitic fluid through congenital or acquired diaphragmatic defects. Rarely, a hepatic hydrothorax may be found in a patient without clinical ascites but with ascites demonstrated only by US, implying the presence of a large diaphragmatic defect. With a small pleural effusion, the patient may be asymptomatic, whereas with large to massive effusions, the patient may have varying degrees of dyspnea. The chest radiograph usually demonstrates a normal cardiac silhouette and a right-sided pleural effusion in 70% of patients, which can vary from small to massive. Effusions are less commonly isolated to the left pleural space (15%) or are bilateral (15%). The pleural fluid is a serous transudate with a low nucleated cell count and a predominance of mononuclear cells, pH greater than 7.40, a glucose level similar to serum, and an amylase less than serum amylase (19). The diagnosis is substantiated by demonstrating that the pleural fluid and ascitic fluid have similar chemistries. If the diagnosis is still in question, injection of a radionuclide into the ascitic fluid with subsequent detection on chest imaging supports the diagnosis (67).

Treatment of hepatic hydrothorax is directed at resolution of the ascites with sodium restriction, diuretics, and paracentesis. It is not uncommon for the effusion to persist until all of the ascitic fluid is mobilized. If the patient is acutely dyspneic or hypoxemic, therapeutic thoracentesis may be done as a temporizing measure. Chest tube drainage should be avoided, as it can cause infection of the fluid, and the prolonged drainage can lead to volume depletion, protein and lymphocyte depletion, and may precipitate renal failure. Chemical pleurodesis is usually unsuccessful due to rapid movement of ascitic fluid into the pleural space. Transjugular intrahepatic portal systemic shunt (TIPS) has been used to treat symptomatic hepatic hydrothorax refractory to medical management (65,66), as has video-assisted thoracoscopic surgery to patch the diaphragmatic defect followed by pleural abrasion or talc poudrage (68).

Hepatic hydrothorax may occasionally be complicated by spontaneous bacterial empyema (SBE), also known as spontaneous bacterial pleuritis, in 13% to 16% of the cases (69). The formation of SBE is a result of either bacterial translocation from infected ascitic fluid or bacteremia and seeding of a hepatic hydrothorax. However, in approximately 40% of cases, SBE can occur in the absence of spontaneous bacterial peritonitis (SBP) and even in the absence of ascites (70). The diagnostic criteria for SBE are similar to those for SBP, requiring a serum/pleural fluid albumin gradient greater than 1.1, a PMN count more than 250 cells/μL with a positive culture, or a PMN count greater than 500 cells/μL with negative cultures and exclusion of contiguous infections. The treatment for SBE is a third-generation cephalosporin given IV for 7 to 10 days. Given the significant mortality rate and its proven benefit in SBP, IV albumin 1.5 mg/kg on day 1 and 1 mg/kg on day 3 post diagnosis is recommended, although albumin use has not been specifically studied in SBE. Chest tube is generally not recommended in SBE unless frank pus is present, because it can lead to life-threatening fluid depletion, protein loss, and electrolyte imbalance (71).

Hypoalbuminemia

Many patients admitted to the medical ICU have chronic illnesses and associated hypoalbuminemia. Pleural effusions may be observed when the serum albumin is less than 1.8 g/dL. In one study evaluating the association of pleural effusions with hypoalbuminemia, 3 of 21 (14%) patients with serum albumin less than 2.0 g/dL had pleural effusions (72). Since the normal pleural space has an effective lymphatic drainage system, pleural fluid tends to be the last site of collection of extravascular fluid in patients with low oncotic pressure. It is, therefore, unusual to find a pleural effusion solely due to hypoalbuminemia in the absence of anasarca. The chest radiograph usually shows small to moderate bilateral effusions with a normal heart size. The pleural fluid is a serous transudate with pH ranging from 7.45 to 7.55, and the glucose level is similar to serum. Since hypoalbuminemia is an extremely rare cause of pleural effusion, recognition in these patients should prompt careful clinical evaluations to identify other potential causes for the effusion. The effusions resolve when the hypoalbuminemia is corrected.

Iatrogenic

Insertion of a CVC or extravascular migration of a CVC into the pleural space can cause a pneumothorax, hemothorax, chylothorax, or transudative pleural effusion (73,74). The incidence of this complication appears to be approximately 0.4% to 1.0% of catheter placements, but it may be higher considering that some cases remain unrecognized. It is more common with insertion into the left subclavian and internal jugular veins due to the horizontal orientation of the left brachiocephalic vein in relation to the superior vena cava (58). Catheterization via the internal jugular vein may result in fewer malpositions than catheterization via the subclavian vein (75). The postprocedure chest radiograph should always be assessed for proper catheter placement, with catheter positioning parallel to the long axis of the superior vena cava and tip positioning at the right tracheobronchial angle indicating proper placement (76).

Symptoms include chest pain and dyspnea in the conscious patient. Depending on the volume and rate of infusion of fluid into the mediastinum, tachypnea, respiratory distress, and cardiac tamponade may occur. The chest radiograph demonstrates the catheter tip in an abnormal position, a widened mediastinum, and unilateral or bilateral effusions. The effusion can have characteristics similar to the infusate (milky if lipid is being given), and may be hemorrhagic and neutrophil predominant due to trauma and inflammation. If a glucose-containing solution is being infused, the pleural fluid to serum glucose ratio is greater than 1.0 (74). The CVC should be removed immediately. Observation is sufficient if the effusion is small; if the effusion is large or causes respiratory distress, thoracentesis or tube thoracostomy should be performed. If a hemothorax is discovered, a chest tube should be placed.

Pancreatitis

Pleural effusions are commonly associated with pancreatitis due to the close proximity of the pancreas to the diaphragm. Pleural effusions have been noted in 3% to 20% of patients with pancreatitis (77). They are usually small to moderate left-sided effusions (60%), although effusions may be isolated to the right side (30%) or occur bilaterally (10%) (78). Pleural effusions related to acute pancreatitis have been shown to be an independent negative prognostic factor as well as a predictor of subsequent pseudocyst development (77–79). The diagnosis is confirmed by an elevated pleural fluid amylase concentration that is greater than serum, although a normal pleural fluid amylase may be found early in the course of acute pancreatitis. The pleural fluid is an exudate with 10,000 to 50,000 nucleated cells/μL, predominantly PMNs. The pleural fluid pH is usually 7.30 to 7.35, and the glucose level is similar to serum (19). No specific treatment is necessary for pleural effusions associated with acute pancreatitis. The effusion resolves as the pancreatic inflammation subsides; if the pleural effusion does not resolve in 2 to 3 weeks, pancreatic abscess or pseudocyst should be suspected.

As opposed to acute pancreatitis, pleural effusion due to a pancreaticopleural fistula is extremely unusual, with a frequency of 0.4% to 7% in chronic pancreatitis patients and 6% to 14% in patients with a pseudocyst. These effusions are large, recurrent, and often left sided (76%) (80). The underlying pancreatic disease is often asymptomatic, and therefore the diagnosis can be missed. Pleural fluid analysis reveals an extremely elevated pleural fluid amylase level (normal <150 IU/L), lipase, and high albumin content (>3 g/dL) (81). Serum amylase, is usually only mildly elevated. CT of the abdomen may demonstrate the fistulous tract and/or a pseudocyst. Magnetic resonance cholangiopancreaticography (MRCP) is reported to be particularly useful in demonstrating the presence of a pancreatic fistula. Endoscopic retrograde cholangiopancreaticography (ERCP) leads to diagnosis in 80% of cases and demonstrates the fistulous tract in 59% to 74% of the cases. Early endoscopic intervention with pancreatic duct stent placement is recommended given its high success rate in fistula closure. Medical therapies are useful adjuncts to endoscopic therapy but, alone, rarely result in pancreaticopleural fistula closure. Surgical interventions should only be considered after failure of endoscopic and medical therapies (82,83).

Parapneumonic Effusions and Empyema

Pleural effusions are a common finding in patients with pneumonia. More than 40% of patients with bacterial pneumonia, and 60% of patients with pneumococcal pneumonia, develop parapneumonic effusions. While treatment with antibiotics leads to resolution in most patients, some patients develop a more fibrinous reaction, with the presence of frank pus in the most severe cases. An *empyema* is defined as the presence of pus in the pleural space, although many clinicians extend the definition to include pleural fluid that has a positive Gram stain for bacteria or a positive bacterial culture. *Complicated parapneumonic effusions* are defined as pleural effusions in the setting of pneumonia that have either a pH below 7.2, glucose less than 60 mg/dL, lactate dehydrogenase (LDH) more than 1,000 IU/L, or septations or loculations, whereas *uncomplicated parapneumonic effusions* are the ones which do not meet the criteria for complicated parapneumonic effusion or empyema (84–87).

The usual presentation is similar to the non-ICU patient with fever, dyspnea, chest pain, purulent sputum, leukocytosis, and a new alveolar infiltrate on chest radiograph. In the elderly, debilitated, or immunosuppressed patient, however, many of these findings may be absent. Although pleural space infections most commonly occur in association with pneumonia, it should also be recognized that pleural space infections may result from thoracic surgery, chest tube placement, penetrating chest trauma, esophageal perforation, mediastinitis, subdiaphragmatic abscesses, SBP, and bacteremic seeding of a pre-existing effusion (84).

Once the diagnosis of parapneumonic effusion or empyema has been made, treatment options should be considered, which center around antibiotic therapy and pleural drainage. Pleural drainage can include therapeutic thoracentesis, image-guided catheter placement, tube thoracostomy, and surgical drainage procedures. There are multiple consensus guidelines to aid clinician with decisions regarding pleural drainage (88). In essence, free-flowing effusions less than 10 cm on lateral decubitus can be managed with antibiotics and close observation. For small to moderate effusions the fluid should be sampled, but further drainage procedures are not necessary in absence of empyema or evidence of complicated parapneumonic effusion, as diagnostic thoracentesis can completely drain the pleural space, and thus also serve a therapeutic role. In patients with complicated parapneumonic effusion or empyema, formal pleural drainage with a chest tube is indicated. Considerable controversy exists about what size chest tube is appropriate in which clinical settings. Typically, chest tubes are divided into small-bore (≤14 Fr) versus large-bore (≥14 Fr) tubes with smaller tubes generally placed by percutaneous Seldinger approaches and larger-bore tubes by open incision. Prospective evaluation of the outcomes relative to quartiles of chest tube size (<10 Fr, 10–14 Fr, 15–20 Fr, or >20 Fr) was performed in one study and demonstrated no difference in mortality or need for surgery based on chest tube size (89). In general, a larger-bore catheter has a theoretical advantage of facilitating effective drainage. However, this must be balanced against the increased pain associated with larger-bore tube insertion, which could compromise a patient with a tenuous respiratory status. When using smaller-bore tubes, the authors urge all practitioners to develop protocols to assure catheter patency. This approach would include routine checks to identify catheter kinking including careful anchoring at the entry site, routine catheter flushes, and connection to a closed pleural drainage system with continuous, regulated suction.

Evidence of pus, loculations, pleural thickening, and progressive organization in the chest would suggest that less invasive drainage procedures may be unsuccessful. These are the patients in whom intrapleural fibrinolytic therapy should be considered based on the results of the MIST2 trial, a four-arm double-blinded, double-dummy study of tPA plus placebo, deoxyribonuclease (DNase) plus placebo, combined tPA and DNase, or double placebo. Unlike the outcome in the MIST1 trial, the MIST2 study demonstrated improvement in pleural opacity in the tPA–DNase group compared with either agent alone or placebo. Combined therapy also demonstrated a reduction in surgical referral and length of hospital stay (90). Consequently, we recommend that, in a stable patient, chest tube drainage including fibrinolytic and DNase therapy (twice daily intrapleurally for 3 days) be considered first, reserving surgical intervention for clinical or radiographic fibrinolytic failure (72–75).

Postcardiac Injury Syndrome

Postcardiac injury syndrome (PCIS) is characterized by the onset of fever, pleuropericarditis, and parenchymal infiltrates typically 3 weeks (2–86 days) following injury to the myocardium or pericardium (91,92). PCIS includes different pleuropericardial syndromes that are elicited by an initial traumatic trigger affecting the pericardium/myocardium and/or pleura after cardiac surgery, an invasive percutaneous intervention, myocardial infarction, or chest trauma. The incidence following myocardial infarction has been estimated at up to 4%, and up to 30% following cardiac surgery. Based on available data, it appears that PCIS results from an autoimmune reaction following myocardial or pericardial injury (93).

Pleuritic chest pain is reported by virtually all patients, whereas one-half of patients are noted to have dyspnea, fever, pericardial rub, and rales. Half of the patients have a leukocytosis, and almost all have an elevated erythrocyte sedimentation rate. The chest radiograph is abnormal in most patients, with the most common abnormality being left-sided or bilateral pleural effusions (92). Pulmonary infiltrates are present in 75% of patients and are most commonly seen in the left lower lobe (91). The pleural fluid is a serosanguineous or bloody exudate with pH greater than 7.30 and glucose level greater than 60 mg/dL. Nucleated cells range from 500 to 39,000 cells/μL, with a predominance of PMNs early in the course (19). The finding of pericardial fluid on echocardiogram suggests PCIS. The diagnosis is made clinically after pulmonary embolism and parapneumonic effusion have been excluded. An antimyocardial antibody titer in pleural fluid greater than in serum further supports the diagnosis (94).

PCIS is usually self-limited and may not require treatment if symptoms are minor. Spontaneous recovery occurs in 66% of patients. Horneffer et al. conducted a trial for treatment of PCIS, comparing ibuprofen 600 mg orally four times per day, indomethacin 25 mg orally four times per day, or placebo for 10 days. The rate of resolution of the postpericardiotomy syndrome was 90% in the ibuprofen group, 89% in the indomethacin group, and 63% in the placebo group (p = 0.003), while recurrences at 30 days were 25% in the ibuprofen and indomethacin groups, and 50% in the placebo group (95). Corticosteroid therapy at low doses (i.e., prednisone 0.2–0.5 mg/kg/day) is useful when aspirin/NSAID are either contraindicated or not well tolerated, and to reduce the possible interference of aspirin/NSAID therapy with oral anticoagulant therapy (96); adjunctive colchicine is also advised in such cases. Following treatment, the pleural effusion resolves within 1 to 3 weeks. It is important to not misdiagnose PCIS as a pulmonary embolism, as anticoagulation therapy may lead to pericardial hemorrhage and tamponade.

Pulmonary Embolism

Pleural effusions occur in up to 50% of patients with pulmonary embolism (86). Pulmonary embolism has been established to be the fourth main cause of pleural effusion in the United States after congestive heart failure, parapneumonic effusion, and malignant effusion (97). The pathogenesis of pleural effusions in pulmonary embolism includes ischemia and inflammatory mediator-induced increased pleural capillary permeability, imbalance in microvascular and pleural space hydrostatic pressures, pleuropulmonary hemorrhage, and atelectasis. With pulmonary infarction, necrosis and hemorrhage into the lung and pleural space may result. More than 80% of patients with pulmonary infarction will have bloody pleural effusions, while up to 40% of patients without radiographic evidence of infarction will also have hemorrhagic fluid (98). Ipsilateral pleuritic chest pain occurs in most patients with pleural effusions complicating pulmonary embolism. A coexistent pulmonary infiltrate is noted on chest radiograph in approximately half of patients with pulmonary embolism and pleural effusion.

Pleural fluid analysis is variable and may demonstrate either an exudate or a transudate (19,99). A bloody pleural effusion in the absence of chest trauma, recent cardiac injury, asbestos exposure, or malignancy should increase the suspicion of pulmonary embolism. The pleural fluid is hemorrhagic in two-thirds of patients, although the number of red blood cells exceeds 100,000 cells/μL in less than 20% (19). The nucleated cell count ranges from less than 100 (presumably atelectatic transudates) to 50,000 cells/μL (pulmonary infarction). When thoracentesis is performed near the time of acute symptoms, PMNs are predominant; with later thoracentesis, lymphocytes represent the majority of cells, and eosinophils may be present as well. The effusion from pulmonary embolism is usually apparent (92%) on the initial chest radiograph and reaches a maximum volume during the first 72 hours. In patients who demonstrate progression of effusions after 72 hours of therapy, recurrent embolism, hemothorax secondary to anticoagulation, an infected infarction, or an alternative diagnosis should be considered. The effusions usually resolve in 1 week in the absence of an infiltrate on chest radiograph. When an infiltrate is present, presumably representing a pulmonary infarction, the resolution time is longer, typically 2 to 3 weeks (98).

The association of a pleural effusion with pulmonary embolism does not alter therapy. The presence of a bloody effusion is not a contraindication to full-dose anticoagulation, since hemothorax is a rare complication of heparin therapy for pulmonary embolism (100,101). An enlarging pleural effusion on therapy necessitates thoracentesis to exclude hemothorax, empyema, or another cause. The development of a hemothorax during therapy requires discontinuation of anticoagulation, chest tube thoracostomy, and placement of a vena cava filter.

Uremia

Uremic pleural effusions have been reported in 3% to 5% of patients undergoing chronic dialysis (102). In one study evaluating the cause of pleural effusions in 100 patients requiring long-term hemodialysis, uremic pleurisy accounted for 16% of cases (103). Patients may manifest fever, cough, chest pain, and pleural friction rubs. The chest radiograph usually shows a moderate unilateral effusion, although massive and bilateral pleural effusions have been reported (104–106). The pleural effusion is a serosanguineous or bloody exudate, with less than 1,500 nucleated cells/μL, predominantly lymphocytes. The creatinine concentration is high, although the pleural fluid to serum creatinine ratio is less than 1.0, unlike that seen in urinothorax (19). The effusions generally resolve with continued dialysis over several weeks but may recur. Uremic pleuritis may cause pleural fibrosis and restriction, requiring decortication in some patients (107,108).

PNEUMOTHORAX IN THE INTENSIVE CARE UNIT

Pneumothorax is defined as air identified within the pleural space and is a commonly encountered problem in the critical care setting. The prevalence of pneumothorax in ICU patients requiring mechanical ventilation ranges from 4% to 15%, (109,110) and it remains one of the most serious complications of positive pressure ventilation. Fortunately, if identified in a timely fashion, pneumothoraces in the ICU can be treated effectively with pleural drainage, minimizing both acute and long-term adverse sequelae. Three pathologic processes may give rise to extra-alveolar air: (a) generation by gas-forming microorganisms during an infectious process, (b) direct introduction following trauma to cutaneous or mucosal barriers, and (c) alveolar rupture due to pressure gradients between alveoli and the surrounding interstitial space (barotrauma) (111).

The mechanisms of spontaneous generation of extra-alveolar air were first delineated by Macklin and Macklin (112). In situations in which intra-alveolar pressure is increased, a gradient is produced between the alveolus and the adjacent vascular sheath, causing the alveoli to rupture at their bases. Following rupture, air is introduced in the perivascular adventitia, resulting in interstitial emphysema. The air then dissects proximally to the lung hilum and mediastinum due to a lower mean pressure in the mediastinum compared to that of the lung parenchyma. Once in the mediastinum, the accumulated air may decompress along paths of least resistance into the subcutaneous tissues or, less commonly, into the pericardium, peritoneum, and retroperitoneum. If mediastinal pressure increases abruptly or if decompression via these routes is not sufficient, the mediastinal parietal pleura may rupture, resulting in pneumothorax. Alternatively, air from ruptured alveoli may dissect to the periphery of the lung and rupture via subpleural blebs through the visceral pleura into the pleural space (113).

Pneumothoraces are classified as spontaneous, which occur without preceding trauma or other obvious causes, and traumatic, which occur as a result of direct or indirect trauma to the chest. Spontaneous pneumothoraces can be subdivided into primary spontaneous, which occur in otherwise healthy patients without clinical lung disease, and secondary spontaneous, which occur in patients with underlying lung disease. Traumatic pneumothoraces can be subdivided into the categories of iatrogenic and related to blunt or penetrating chest trauma. In addition, pneumothoraces can be classified as simple or complicated, with complicated pneumothoraces consisting of tension pneumothorax, hemopneumothorax, pyopneumothorax, and open pneumothorax in which the integrity of the chest wall is disrupted. The potential causes of pneumothoraces in critically ill patients are listed in Table 115.2. We will focus mainly on iatrogenic pneumothoraces and pneumothoraces resulting from barotrauma, as these are the most common causes of pneumothoraces in ICU patients.

TABLE 115.2 Causes of Pneumothoraces in ICU Patients

Secondary Spontaneous
- Airway diseases
  - Chronic obstructive pulmonary disease (COPD)
  - Status asthmaticus
  - Cystic fibrosis
- Parenchymal lung diseases
  - Idiopathic pulmonary fibrosis
  - Sarcoidosis (stage IV)
  - Langerhans cell histiocytosis (histiocytosis-X)
  - Malignancy
- Pulmonary infections
  - *Pneumocystis jirovecii*
  - Necrotizing bacterial pneumonia
  - Tuberculosis
  - Fungal pneumonia

Barotrauma/Volutrauma
- Mechanical ventilation
  - Acute respiratory disease syndrome (ARDS)
  - Status asthmaticus
  - COPD
- Inhalational drug usage
- Decompression injury

Trauma
- Blunt chest trauma
- Penetrating chest trauma
- Tracheobronchial injuries
- Rib fractures
- Esophageal rupture

Iatrogenic
- Endotracheal intubation
- Tracheostomy
- Central venous catheter placement
- Thoracentesis
- Nasogastric tube placement
- Bronchoscopy with bronchoalveolar lavage (BAL) or biopsies
- Postoperative
- Bag/valve/mask ventilation
- Cardiopulmonary resuscitation

Diagnostic Evaluation

The diagnosis of pneumothorax in the critically ill patient can sometimes be made with information from the history and physical examination, noting acute onset of dyspnea or chest pain, tachycardia, hypotension, decreased breath sounds, pulsus paradoxus, and contralateral tracheal deviation. Although clinical features can be used to diagnose the presence of a pneumothorax, it should be noted that many of these findings are nonspecific and have not been a reliable indicator of size. As a result, radiologic data remains the gold standard for the diagnosis of pneumothorax (114). Chest radiographs have traditionally been the first test ordered for suspected pneumothorax. In the critically ill, the traditional erect posterior–anterior expiratory film is not practical and thus, the supine or semirecumbent anterior–posterior film is frequently obtained. The radiographic signs of pneumothorax in the supine patient frequently differ from the classic visceral pleural line seen on erect views. In a review of 88 critically ill patients with 112 pneumothoraces, only 22% of pneumothoraces were in the classic apicolateral location (115). In this same study, 30% of pneumothoraces were not detected initially, and of these, half progressed to a tension pneumothorax. The anteromedial position is the most common location for pneumothoraces in the supine patient since this area is the least dependent pleural recess (116). With anteromedial collections of air above the level of the pulmonary hilum, the lucency sharply outlines adjacent vascular structures such as the ascending aorta, superior vena cava, and azygos vein. Below the hilum, the lateral cardiac borders are sharply outlined and paralleled by zones of radiolucency. Increased lucency in the region of the anterior cardiophrenic sulcus may also result from air below the hilar level. Alternatively, air may collect laterally in the costophrenic angle resulting in the classic deep sulcus sign (116).

An erect or decubitus radiograph should be obtained if possible to confirm or refute the presence of a pneumothorax; in problematic cases, CT or US can be diagnostic. CT scan is the gold standard test for both the diagnosis and sizing of a pneumothorax. Several studies have demonstrated the presence of pneumothoraces on CT that were not apparent or not appreciated on conventional radiographs (17,117). Occasionally, a pneumothorax may be confused with a large bulla in patients with COPD and other pulmonary diseases that generate cystic changes. In these instances, a CT may be helpful in making the correct diagnosis (113). Ultrasonographic assessment of pneumothorax has emerged recently as an alternative modality in facilities with physicians trained in bedside ultrasonography (US). US is the preferred first-line diagnostic test to exclude pneumothorax in the ICU. Because pleural air would block the visualization of the underlying lung, the presence of B lines and lung sliding rules out a pneumothorax with a negative predictive value of 100% in the location of the chest probe. The lung point (area where normal lung sliding meets an area where no lung sliding is seen) can be visualized with both B-mode and M-mode ultrasonography, and when seen, has 100% specificity for pneumothorax (118). A study comparing ultrasonography to CT scan and chest radiographs for the diagnosis of occult pneumothorax showed that the use of US detected 92% of occult pneumothoraces diagnosed with CT scan (119).

Primary and Secondary Spontaneous Pneumothorax

Patients with pneumothorax have a decrease in vital capacity and an increase in the alveolar-arterial O_2 gradient, with hypoxemia being present in some patients. The hypoxemia is thought to be secondary to development of both anatomic shunts and areas of low ventilation/perfusion in the atelectatic lung. Patients with primary spontaneous pneumothorax rarely require admission to the ICU, as the contralateral lung can maintain the necessary alveolar ventilation and hypoxemia can be managed with supplemental oxygen. Patients with secondary spontaneous pneumothoraces may need ICU admission because the gas exchange abnormality caused by the pneumothorax is superimposed on pre-existing gas exchange abnormalities and, thus, severe hypoxemia can occur. Patients with secondary spontaneous pneumothoraces are more likely to develop hypercapnic respiratory failure than are patients with primary spontaneous pneumothorax (120,121).

Iatrogenic Pneumothorax

As the number of operative procedures performed for diagnostic and therapeutic purposes increase in training and research hospitals, iatrogenic pneumothorax will become the most encountered type of pneumothorax after traumatic pneumothorax. This complication prolongs the hospitalization period, worsens the patients' physical condition and increases morbidity and mortality, especially in patients who develop barotrauma due to mechanical ventilation. Insertion of CVCs is the most common cause of iatrogenic pneumothoraces in the ICU. In two studies of mechanical complications of CVCs, 1.1% of 534 patients and 1.0% of 713 patients suffered a pneumothorax (122,123). Cannulation of the subclavian vein is associated with a higher risk of pneumothorax than cannulation of the internal jugular vein (124,125). Most pneumothoraces occur at the time of the procedure from direct lung puncture, but delayed pneumothoraces have been noted. Bilateral pneumothoraces have been reported to occur from unilateral cannulation attempts (126).

The second most frequent cause of iatrogenic pneumothorax is thoracentesis; the reported incidence is between 3% and 19% (32,22). Risk factors in thoracentesis are the experience of the personnel, coughing of the patient during the procedure, the underlying lung disease, and the number of passes performed. When the procedure is performed with the assistance of ultrasound, the rate of complications decreases to 2% to 3%. Ultrasound is especially beneficial when there is a very low amount of fluid present and for loculated fluids (22).

Cardiopulmonary resuscitation has been reported as a cause of iatrogenic pneumothorax. Pneumothorax in this setting may arise either from barotrauma as a consequence of bag-ventilation or from rib fractures sustained during the resuscitation. Hillman and Albin (127) described three patients who developed subcutaneous emphysema and pneumothoraces, one of whom had bilateral pneumothoraces following cardiopulmonary resuscitation with bag-ventilation. Shulman et al. (128) reported two patients in whom barotrauma was observed following resuscitation. One of the patients was ventilated with a self-inflating bag, whereas the other was ventilated with a positive pressure demand valve. Other cases of pneumothorax related to cardiopulmonary resuscitation or malfunctioning valves in self-inflating bags have been reported (129,130).

Pneumothoraces may rarely occur following endotracheal intubation, usually due to rupture of the posterior membranous portion of the trachea (131). In a prospective study of translaryngeal intubation in 297 critically ill patients in a teaching hospital, pneumothorax occurred in 1% of patients (132). Pneumothoraces may also result from tracheostomy, either from open procedures or bedside percutaneous dilatational tracheostomy (133). The incidence of pneumothorax after tracheostomy in adults has been reported to be between 0% and 4% (134).

Bronchoscopy in critically ill patients may also cause pneumothoraces. The risk is higher when transbronchial biopsies are obtained, although the degree of increased risk compared to nonventilated patients and the influence of high airway pressures and PEEP are unknown. It should be recognized that performing bronchoalveolar lavage (BAL) alone may produce a pneumothorax (135–137).

Pneumothorax is a frequent, potentially lethal complication of mechanical ventilation–induced barotrauma. The patient requiring mechanical ventilation usually becomes symptomatic after developing a pneumothorax because of the underlying lung parenchymal disease, and this complication should be suspected whenever a sudden clinical deterioration occurs. If conscious, the patient becomes dyspneic and tachypneic, and may become dyssynchronous with the ventilator; worsening oxygenation is often seen. Peak inspiratory pressures may increase with a coexisting decrease in lung compliance; a significant percentage of patients will develop a tension pneumothorax. There are multiple risk factors for acquiring a pneumothorax in mechanically ventilated patients in the ICU. Studies in mechanically ventilated patients with acute lung injury or ARDS have reported pneumothorax occurrence rates between 7% and 42% (128–133). A recent study by Papazian et al. (138) showed a significant reduction in pneumothoraces in patients with severe ARDS who were randomized to receive 48 hours of paralysis. An study in the pediatric population showed that the prevalence of pneumothorax in ventilated patients was significantly higher in the era before protective lung strategies with low tidal volumes were the standard of care (139). A higher prevalence of pneumothorax is seen in patients with ARDS, but not in those treated with prone positioning or different ventilatory strategies related to airway pressures alone. The patient requiring mechanical ventilation usually becomes symptomatic after developing a pneumothorax because of the underlying lung parenchymal disease, and this complication should be suspected whenever a sudden clinical deterioration occurs. A significant percentage of patients will develop a tension pneumothorax. A heightened suspicion for development of a pneumothorax should be maintained in patients who exhibit other forms of barotrauma, such as subcutaneous emphysema, pneumomediastinum, and subpleural air cysts.

Tension Pneumothorax

A tension pneumothorax occurs when intrapleural pressure exceeds atmospheric pressure throughout expiration, and often inspiration as well. This develops when a break in the visceral or parietal pleura produces a one-way valve that is open during inspiration, allowing air to enter the pleural space, but is closed during expiration, preventing the egress of air collecting in the pleural space (103). Tension pneumothoraces most commonly develop as a complication of mechanical ventilation—barotrauma or volutrauma—or as a result of blunt and penetrating thoracic trauma, although tension pneumothoraces can occur in 1% to 4% of patients with spontaneous pneumothoraces (140,141).

Tension pneumothorax usually presents as an acute cardiopulmonary emergency beginning with respiratory distress and, if unrecognized and untreated, progresses to cardiovascular collapse and death. Patients with tension pneumothorax often exhibit decreased ipsilateral breath sounds, hyperresonance to percussion, distended neck veins, tracheal deviation to the contralateral side, and hypotension. The absence of physical examination findings, however, does not completely exclude the diagnosis of a tension pneumothorax and when suspected should be treated as such without any confirmatory tests.

On the chest radiograph in a patient with tension pneumothorax, in addition to the pneumothorax, there is often shift of the trachea and mediastinum to the contralateral side, ipsilateral diaphragmatic depression, and increased distance between contiguous ribs compared to the unaffected side. It should be emphasized, however, that tension pneumothorax is a clinical diagnosis, and these radiographic findings may be observed in patients without physiologic evidence of a tension pneumothorax. It should also be noted that patients may have cardiopulmonary compromise due to a tension pneumothorax without observing tracheal or mediastinal shift on chest radiograph (142,143).

In one study of 16 ARDS patients with tension pneumothorax, only 5 patients had subtle mediastinal shift (142). Of these 16 patients, 11 had flattening of the diaphragm and 8 had depression of the diaphragm. Diaphragmatic abnormalities may therefore be a more sensitive indicator of tension pneumothorax in patients with ARDS. In 15 of the 16 patients, the location of a loculated tension pneumothorax was subpulmonic or paracardiac. Potential explanations for these observations include the presence of adhesions between the parietal and visceral pleura and the noncompliance of lungs in patients with ARDS which may prevent collapse of the ipsilateral lung and compression of the contralateral lung, allowing a small volume of air to significantly increase intrapleural pressure (142,143).

It is important to note that patients with ARDS can develop tension pneumothoraces despite the presence of a chest tube on the ipsilateral side having been placed for a previous pneumothorax (142–145). In the 16 patients reported by Gobien et al. (142) and the 3 patients reported by Ross et al. (143), all patients had a functional ipsilateral chest tube and had localized pneumothoraces. In a study by Heffner et al. (144), 14 patients had recurrent pneumothoraces despite ipsilateral chest tubes, with 9 of the 14 having tension pneumothoraces, and all nine of these chest tubes being horizontally placed. In the latter study, 12 of the 14 chest tubes had horizontal as opposed to vertical placement on chest radiograph. Seven of the 14 patients had subsequent CT scans, with the finding that all seven chest tubes were placed within interlobar fissures. Thus, chest tubes placed into interlobar or posterior locations may not drain anterior gas loculations, the most common location of pneumothoraces in ARDS patients (115,146), allowing for development of localized tension pneumothoraces. In the patient reported by McConaghy and Kennedy (145), the chest tube was intraparenchymal.

Management of Pneumothoraces and Tension Pneumothoraces

Most critically ill patients in the ICU will have poor cardiopulmonary reserve and may be unable to tolerate a pneumothorax, even in the absence of tension physiology. In nonventilated patients who are hemodynamically stable and have adequate oxygenation and ventilation, simple pneumothoraces that occur as a result of a procedure and are small may reasonably be managed with close observation and monitoring with serial radiographs. Patients with secondary pneumothoraces who require ICU care will usually require chest tube placement because of their poor pulmonary reserve. Patients who are not receiving positive pressure ventilation, but are hemodynamically unstable, should be treated with chest tube thoracostomy, since the additive effects of development of hypoxia or early tension physiology could quickly precipitate cardiopulmonary arrest. The role of manual aspiration in ventilated patients has not been studied, and there are currently no expert guidelines to suggest that manual aspiration has a role in the management of these patients.

In general, chest tube thoracostomy should be performed in mechanically ventilated patients with a pneumothorax of any size given the significant risk of progression to a tension pneumothorax. A wide variety of chest tube sizes exist, ranging from 6 Fr to 40 Fr. Traditionally, large-bore chest tubes were used for pneumothorax, but more recently, smaller-bore tubes inserted via a modified Seldinger technique have become widely available and have become commonly used in nonintubated patients. The risk of serious complications associated with small-bore catheters is minimal, with a frequency of injury of 0.2% and a malposition rate of 0.6%. The biggest risk is drain blockage, with a rate of 8.1%, and this is easily prevented with scheduled sterile flushing to maintain patency (147). A retrospective review by Lin et al. of 62 ventilated patients who underwent small-bore chest tube drainage as the primary management of pneumothorax found a 68.6% overall success rate, defined as no residual air seen in the follow-up chest radiograph, with no major complications (148). Based upon this study, some clinicians have suggested that small-bore catheters may be used as first-line therapy for pneumothorax in mechanically ventilated patients (149). In the study of Lin, however, the success rate for the subset of patients with iatrogenic pneumothorax was 87.5% versus 43.3% for patients with pneumothorax related to barotrauma (148). With this in mind, the authors as well as others would suggest that small tubes may be used for iatrogenic pneumothoraces while on mechanical ventilation, but large-bore chest tubes should be used when related to barotrauma (150).

Attempts to decrease plateau airway pressures, tidal volumes, and PEEP should be considered if possible after development of a pneumothorax in patients receiving mechanical ventilation. Controlled hypoventilation with the use of neuromuscular blockers or deep sedation may be required in some patients to achieve these goals. For patients with ARDS and recurrent pneumothoraces, the chest tube attempts should be made to place anteriorly where the loculation is most likely to occur. In those patients with recurrent loculated pneumothoraces who are stable for transport to the radiology department, we advocate the use of CT-guided percutaneous drainage, as blind placement of chest tubes into loculi may be difficult (151,152). When extra-alveolar gas is observed (subcutaneous emphysema, pneumopericardium, or mediastinal emphysema) in the absence of a pneumothorax, similar attempts to decrease plateau pressure, tidal volume, and PEEP should be considered. No evidence exists that placement of "prophylactic" chest tubes will prevent these patients from suffering a subsequent pneumothorax. These patients should be closely monitored for development of a tension pneumothorax, and equipment to perform an emergent bedside tube thoracostomy should be available.

The development of a tension pneumothorax represents a medical emergency, and the deteriorating patient should be treated based on clinical presentation without waiting for radiographic or US confirmation. In one series of 74 patients with tension pneumothorax, a diagnosis was made clinically in 45 patients (61%), and these patients had an attributable mortality of 7%. In the remaining 29 patients, diagnosis was delayed between 30 minutes and 8 hours; 31% of these patients died of pneumothorax (153). If a chest tube is not immediately available, a large-bore needle (14–16 gauge) or intravenous catheter should be inserted into the pleural space through the second intercostal space at the midclavicular line. Escape of air from the needle confirms the diagnosis. After decompression, the needle or catheter should be left in place and in communication with the atmosphere until definitive chest tube thoracostomy is performed. As previously mentioned, a high index of suspicion for tension pneumothorax should be maintained for patients who are in cardiac arrest and exhibit pulseless electrical activity.

BRONCHOPLEURAL FISTULA IN THE INTENSIVE CARE UNIT

A bronchopleural fistula (BPF) represents a communication between the bronchial tree and the pleural space. BPFs most commonly result from surgical procedures including pneumonectomy, segmentectomy, and wedge resections of the lung, with an incidence of 1.6% to 6.8% (154). The mortality in patients with BPFs following surgical resection is reported to be between 23% and 71%, usually due to infectious complications (154–156). BPFs may also result from blunt or penetrating chest trauma, pulmonary infarction, and as a complication of pulmonary and pleural infections such as tuberculosis, necrotizing pneumonia, lung abscess, or empyema (157,158). Last, BPFs may result as a complication of mechanical ventilation for acute respiratory failure, particularly in patients with ARDS, and, as such, represent a form of barotrauma/volutrauma (22,158,159). For this discussion, we will focus primarily on BPFs in the setting of patients requiring mechanical ventilation.

BPF in the ventilated patient is defined as an air leak that persists for more than 24 hours following placement of a chest tube. BPFs in patients receiving mechanical ventilation may present acutely with the development of a pneumothorax, with or without tension, or with sudden expectoration of potentially infected material from the pleural space, with flooding of the ipsilateral and contralateral airways leading to respiratory compromise.

Several potential adverse effects of a BPF in the mechanically ventilated patient have been noted. Depending on the size of the fistula, flow resistance through the fistula versus the airways and lung parenchyma, and pressure gradient between the airways and pleural space, air may be redirected from normal intrapulmonary routes to the BPF (160). This can cause loss of effective tidal volume, which may lead to difficulty in oxygenating and ventilating the patient and subsequent development of life-threatening hypoxemia and respiratory acidosis (159). If incomplete lung expansion due to the BPF is present, ventilation/perfusion mismatching and shunt may occur. There may be difficulty in maintaining PEEP with further decrements in oxygenation (161,162). If a high level of chest tube suction is used, the negative pressure may be transmitted to the proximal airways, causing inappropriate ventilator cycling (161–163). Finally, BPFs may cause pleural space infection or contamination of the airways.

The amount of air flow through a BPF is typically estimated by subtracting the expired tidal volume from the inspired tidal volume as measured by the ventilator. This method, however, becomes increasingly inaccurate as the size of the leak decreases, particularly when the size of the leak is less than 200 mL/breath. More accurate, albeit cumbersome, methods have been developed to quantify the amount of flow through a BPF (164–167). Air flows through BPFs have been reported up to 22 L/min (164). It has been recognized that the air escaping from a BPF does not flow passively from the airways into the pleural space, but instead participates to some degree in physiologic gas exchange. In two studies evaluating CO_2 excretion by BPF in 15 patients, the percentage of minute ventilation lost through the BPF ranged from 4% to 53%, with 3% to 44% of CO_2 excretion occurring via the BPF (168).

The development of a BPF has been regarded as a serious and life-threatening complication of mechanical ventilation. In one of the largest series reported—1,700 consecutive patients receiving mechanical ventilation—Pierson et al. (159) observed that 39 (2.3%) patients developed a BPF. In that study, overall mortality in patients with BPF was 67%; mortality was higher in patients who developed a BPF late in their illness (94%) than when it occurred within 24 hours of admission (45%). Patients with air leaks greater than 500 mL/breath had a mortality of 100% compared with a mortality of 57% in patients with air leaks less than 500 mL/breath. Mortality was also higher in patients with ARDS than in patients without—81% versus 50%—and in patients with pleural space infections compared to those without said infection—87% versus 54%. A study of patients with ARDS by Weg et al. (169), however, suggested that mortality was not different between patients with or without air leaks, 46% versus 39%, respectively. In that study, however, the duration of mechanical ventilation was 4.3 ± 1.3 days, which may not be typical for many patients with BPF, and the subset of patients with BPF was not analyzed separately. It may be that the presence of a BPF is a marker for severity of lung injury and by itself does not directly contribute to mortality.

Management of Bronchopleural Fistulae

Numerous interventions, listed in Table 115.3, have been proposed in the management of BPFs. Many of these are based on the concept of decreasing the pressure gradient between the airways and the pleural space, with decreased air flow through the fistula allowing for earlier closure. Although the various manipulations theoretically make sense, they have not been evaluated in controlled trials. The suggested changes in ventilator settings may actually worsen oxygenation and ventilation in some patients with ARDS. We will discuss those interventions for which some data are available in the following section. In the absence of difficulty oxygenating or ventilating the patient, it is unknown if active measures to close the BPF affect outcome. Definitive therapy for BPFs includes surgical procedures such as bronchial stump closure with thoracoplasty, myoplasty, or omentoplasty, or completion pneumonectomy (154,156). Unfortunately, most critically ill patients will not be sufficiently stable to undergo these procedures and must be managed medically. Adequate pleural space drainage, antibiotic therapy for pleural space infections, and support of nutritional status is vital in these patients.

TABLE 115.3 Potential Options for Management of Bronchopleural Fistula in Mechanically Ventilated Patients

Chest Tube Drainage
- Adequate size chest tube
- Drainage system with adequate ability to handle air leak
- Additional chest tube placement if lung not fully expanded

Reduce Airway Pressures
- Reduce delivered tidal volume
- Use synchronized intermittent mandatory ventilation (SIMV) instead of assist-control mode
- Decrease level of positive end-expiratory pressure (PEEP)
- Decrease inspiratory time (I:E ratio)
- Avoid inspiratory pause
- Minimize auto-PEEP

Alternative Modes of Mechanical Ventilation

High-frequency jet ventilation
High-frequency oscillatory ventilation
Independent lung ventilation

Chest Tube Manipulation

Decrease chest tube suction
Apply PEEP to chest tube
Inspiratory chest tube occlusion

Direct Closure/Occlusion of Bronchopleural Fistula (BPF)
- Surgical closure or resection
- Endobronchial occlusion of BPF
- Cyanoacrylate-based tissue adhesives
- Fibrin sealants
- Synthetic hydrogel
- One-way endobronchial valves
- Stent placement
- Pleurodesis
- Blood patch
- Talc
- Doxycycline

Adequate chest tube drainage and full expansion of the lung should be assessed in patients with BPF. An appropriately sized chest tube should be placed, recognizing that air flow through a chest tube is inversely proportional to the length and radius to the fourth power of the tube. It has been suggested that a tube with an internal diameter of 6 mm (18 Fr) is the smallest acceptable size because it will allow a maximum possible flow rate of 15 L/min at −10 cm H_2O (170). Our preference is to use at least a 28-Fr chest tube in these patients. Placement of additional chest tubes or CT-guided percutaneous catheters—if the pleural space is complicated—should be considered if the lung is not fully expanded. As with the chest tube, resistance to flow of air through a chest tube drainage system may need to be considered. In an animal model of BPF, when the size of air leak reached 4 to 5 L/min, the Thora-Klex and Sentinel Seal systems become clinically impractical. The Pleur-Evac system can handle flow rates up to 34 L/min, although its use with rates greater than 28 L/min is impractical due to intense bubbling in the control chamber. The Emerson pump, which can be set to deliver chest tube suction greater than −20 cm H_2O, is capable of handling air flows up to 35 L/min and is the system of choice for BPFs with extremely high flow rates (170).

Manipulation of the level of chest tube suction may affect BPF air flow, and some authors have suggested using the least amount of suction that maintains lung inflation (159,160). An animal model demonstrated that increasingly negative intrapleural pressures increased air flow in large BPFs but had no effect on small BPFs (171). Roth et al. (167) reported that increasing chest tube suction from 0 to 22.5 cm H_2O increased BPF flow in a patient from 24.6 to 26.7 L/min. In a study of six patients by Powner et al. (165), increasing chest tube suction from 0 to 25 cm H_2O increased BPF flow in two patients, had no effect in two patients, and decreased flow in two patients. To decrease air loss through the BPF when there is applied PEEP, some investigators have applied PEEP to the chest tube (162,172), while others have devised systems to synchronously occlude the chest tube during inspiration (173,174); a lack of success using these methods has been noted by other investigators, however (159). These techniques may pose a risk of increasing the size of the pneumothorax or causing a tension pneumothorax; thus, the patient should be closely monitored.

The goals of mechanical ventilation in patients with a BPF are to maintain adequate oxygenation and ventilation while reducing fistula flow. In general, strategies for conventional mechanical ventilation that limit airway pressure and tidal volumes may reduce the amount of air flow escaping through the BPF and allow the fistulous site to heal. As such, it has been recommended to use the lowest possible tidal volume, fewest mechanical breaths/min, lowest level of PEEP, and shortest inspiratory time.

Alternative methods of mechanical ventilation have been used in a few patients. High-frequency jet ventilation (HFJV) and high-frequency oscillatory ventilation (HFOV) have been used based on the principle that lower airway pressures may be generated in these modes of ventilation and should, therefore, decrease BPF air flow. In one animal model of BPF, an increase in fistula flow was seen with increasing mean airway pressures, and effects on flow were similar whether mean airway pressure was changed by manipulating peak inspiratory pressure, PEEP, or inspiratory:expiratory (I:E) ratios (171). In another animal model, a nonsignificant trend toward increasing BPF flow with increasing peak inspiratory pressures, and a significant increase in BPF flow with increasing PEEP was observed (175).

Several studies comparing HFJV and HFOV with conventional ventilation using animal models have shown less BPF air flow during HFJV and HFOV (176–179), although one study using HFJV demonstrated no difference (180). In studies reporting blood gases, improved oxygenation was seen during HFJV and HFOV compared with conventional ventilation (177–179). Increasing levels of PEEP were also noted to increase BPF flow in two studies (176,180). It is problematic to extrapolate these studies to patients in the ICU because the animal models were cannulated in more proximal bronchi and the lung parenchyma was relatively normal.

Other modes of mechanical ventilation have also been used in patients with BPF. Case reports have reported independent lung ventilation to be of benefit (181–183). Case reports of combining independent lung ventilation with high-frequency, low tidal volume ventilation of the affected lung (184) and HFJV of the affected lung have been published (185,186). Differential lung ventilation using a single ventilator and a variable resistance valve attached to one lumen of a bifurcated endotracheal tube has also been described (187,188). Discussion of the techniques of independent lung ventilation and its attendant difficulties is beyond the scope of this chapter, and the reader is referred to other reviews (189,190).

Because many critically ill patients are unable to tolerate a major thoracic procedure, bronchoscopic techniques may provide viable alternatives for closure of BPFs. Endobronchial occlusion of BPFs has been reported with cyanoacrylate-based tissue adhesives (Histoacryl, Bucrylate), fibrin sealants (Tisseal, Hemaseal), thrombin plus fibrinogen or cryoprecipitate, synthetic hydrogel (CoSeal), absorbable gelatin sponge (Gelfoam), vascular occlusion coils, doxycycline and blood, Nd:YAG laser, silver nitrate, and lead shot (191–193). The agent initially seals the leak by acting as a plug and subsequently induces an inflammatory process with fibrosis and mucosal proliferation, permanently sealing the area. Of these techniques, the uses of cyanoacrylate tissue adhesives and fibrin sealants have been most widely reported. Airway stents may be used to cover and seal the fistula in selected patients depending on the location of the fistula. BPFs due to breakdown of a stump after lobectomy or pneumonectomy, or bronchial dehiscence after lung transplantation or bronchoplastic procedures are the most amenable to successful closure with airway stenting. Successful closure of BPFs using bronchoscopic placement of endobronchial valves designed for emphysema has been described (194–196). More recently, synthetic hydrogel (CoSeal) was used to successfully seal the air leak in patients with BPF in a single center study (191).

Pleurodesis with various agents has also been tried to effect closure of BPFs. Autologous "blood patch" pleurodesis has been described to be effective in some patients (197–199). Pleurodesis with fibrin glue has also been reported (200,201). However, none of these patients was undergoing mechanical ventilation at the time of pleurodesis.

Key Points

- The major radiographic finding of a pleural effusion in the supine patient is an increased homogeneous density over the lower lung field that does not obliterate normal bronchovascular markings, does not demonstrate air bronchograms, and does not produce hilar or mediastinal displacement until the effusion is massive.
- The radiographic signs of pneumothorax in the supine patient frequently differ from the classic visceral pleural line seen on erect views. The anteromedial position is the most common location for pneumothoraces in the supine patient since this area is the least dependent pleural recess. The lucency sharply outlines adjacent vascular structures such as the ascending aorta, superior vena cava, and azygos vein.
- Ultrasonographic assessment of pneumothorax has emerged as a first-line diagnostic modality for physicians trained in bedside ultrasonography.
- Patients with ARDS can develop tension pneumothoraces despite the presence of a chest tube on the ipsilateral side being placed for a previous pneumothorax.
- In patients with complicated parapneumonic effusion or empyema, formal pleural drainage with a chest tube is indicated.
- Evidence of pus, loculations, pleural thickening, and progressive organization in the chest would suggest that patients would benefit from intrapleural fibrinolytic therapy.

References

1. Wiener MD, Garay SM, Leitman BS, et al. Imaging of the intensive care unit patient. *Clin Chest Med.* 1991;12:169–198.
2. Collins JD, Burwell D, Furmanksi S, et al. Minimal detectable pleural effusions: a roentgen pathology model. *Radiology.* 1972;105:51–53.
3. Woodring JH. Recognition of pleural effusion on supine radiographs: how much fluid is required? *AJR Am J Roentgenol.* 1984;142: 59–64.
4. Mattison LE, Coppage L, Alderman DF, et al. Pleural effusions in the medical ICU: prevalence, causes, and clinical implications. *Chest.* 1997;111: 1018–1023.
5. Joseph MX, Disney PJ, Da Costa R, Hutchison SJ. Transthoracic echocardiography to identify or exclude cardiac cause of shock. *Chest.* 2004;126: 1592–1597.
6. Koh DM, Burke S, Davies N, Padley SP. Transthoracic US of the chest: clinical uses and applications. *Radiographics.* 2002;22:e1.
7. Koegelenberg CF, Bolliger CT, Plekker D, et al. Diagnostic yield and safety of ultrasound-assisted biopsies in superior vena cava syndrome. *Eur Respir J.* 2009;33:1389–1395.
8. Yu CJ, Yang PC, Chang DB, Luh KT. Diagnostic and therapeutic use of chest sonography: value in critically ill patients. *AJR Am J Roentgenol.* 1992; 159:695–701.
9. Mayo PH, Goltz HR, Tafreshi M, Doelken P. Safety of ultrasound-guided thoracentesis in patients receiving mechanical ventilation. *Chest.* 2004; 125:1059–1062.
10. Lichtenstein D, Hulot JS, Rabiller A, et al. Feasibility and safety of ultrasound-aided thoracentesis in mechanically ventilated patients. *Intensive Care Med.* 1999;25:955–958.
11. Petersen S, Freitag M, Albert W, et al. Ultrasound-guided thoracentesis in surgical intensive care patients. *Intensive Care Med.* 1999;25:1029.
12. Yang PC, Luh KT, Chang DB, et al. Value of sonography in determining the nature of pleural effusion: analysis of 320 cases. *AJR Am J Roentgenol.* 1992;159:29–33.
13. McLoud TC, Flower CD. Imaging the pleura: sonography, CT, and MR imaging. *AJR Am J Roentgenol.* 1991;156:1145–1153.
14. McLoud TC. CT and MR in pleural disease. *Clin Chest Med.* 1998;19: 261–276.

15. Stark DD, Federle MP, Goodman PC, et al. Differentiating lung abscess and empyema: radiography and computed tomography. *AJR Am J Roentgenol.* 1983;141:163–7.
16. Waite RJ, Carbonneau RJ, Balikian JP, et al. Parietal pleural changes in empyema: appearances at CT. *Radiology.* 1990;175:145–150.
17. Mirvis SE, Tobin KD, Kostrubiak I, Belzberg H. Thoracic CT in detecting occult disease in critically ill patients. *AJR Am J Roentgenol.* 1987; 148:685–689.
18. Awerbuch E, Benavides M, Gershengorn HB. The impact of computed tomography of the chest on the management of patients in a medical intensive care unit. *J Intensive Care Med.* 2015;30:505–511.
19. Sahn SA. State of the art: the pleura. *Am Rev Respir Dis.* 1988;138:184–234.
20. Kohan JM, Poe RH, Israel RH, et al. Value of chest ultrasonography versus decubitus roentgenography for thoracentesis. *Am Rev Respir Dis.* 1986;133:1124–1126.
21. Weingardt JP, Guico RR, Nemcek AA Jr, et al. Ultrasound findings following failed, clinically directed thoracenteses. *J Clin Ultrasound.* 1994; 22:419–426.
22. Bartter T, Mayo PD, Pratter MR, et al. Lower risk and higher yield for thoracentesis when performed by experienced operators. *Chest.* 1993;103:1873–1876.
23. Seneff MG, Corwin RW, Gold LH, Irwin RS. Complications associated with thoracocentesis. *Chest.* 1986;90:97–100.
24. Collins TR, Sahn SA. Thoracocentesis. Clinical value, complications, technical problems, and patient experience. *Chest.* 1987;91:817–822.
25. Grogan DR, Irwin RS, Channick R, et al. Complications associated with thoracentesis. A prospective, randomized study comparing three different methods. *Arch Intern Med.* 1990;150:873–877.
26. Godwin JE, Sahn SA. Thoracentesis: a safe procedure in mechanically ventilated patients. *Ann Intern Med.* 1990;113:800–802.
27. McCartney JP, Adams JW 2nd, Hazard PB. Safety of thoracentesis in mechanically ventilated patients. *Chest.* 1993;103:1920–1921.
28. Jones PW, Moyers JP, Rogers JT, et al. Ultrasound-guided thoracentesis: Is it a safer method? *Chest.* 2003;123:418–423.
29. McVay PA, Toy PT. Lack of increased bleeding after paracentesis and thoracentesis in patients with mild coagulation abnormalities. *Transfusion.* 1991;31:164–171.
30. Talmor M, Hydo L, Gershenwald JG, Barie PS. Beneficial effects of chest tube drainage of pleural effusion in acute respiratory failure refractory to positive end-expiratory pressure ventilation. *Surgery.* 1998;123:137–143.
31. Raptopoulos V, Davis LM, Lee G, et al. Factors affecting the development of pneumothorax associated with thoracentesis. *AJR Am J Roentgenol.* 1991;156:917–920.
32. Colt HG, Brewer N, Barbur E. Evaluation of patient-related and procedure-related factors contributing to pneumothorax following thoracentesis. *Chest.* 1999;116:134–138.
33. Petersen WG, Zimmerman R. Limited utility of chest radiograph after thoracentesis. *Chest.* 2000;117:1038–1042.
34. Light RW, Jenkinson SG, Minh VD, George RB. Observations on pleural fluid pressures as fluid is withdrawn during thoracentesis. *Am Rev Respir Dis.* 1980;121:799–804.
35. Agusti AG, Cardús J, Roca J, et al. Ventilation-perfusion mismatch in patients with pleural effusion: effects of thoracentesis. *Am J Respir Crit Care Med.* 1997;156:1205–1209.
36. Brandstetter RD, Cohen RP. Hypoxemia after thoracentesis: a predictable and treatable condition. *JAMA.* 1979;242:1060–1061.
37. Karetzky MS, Kothari GA, Fourre JA, Khan AU. Effect of thoracentesis on arterial oxygen tension. *Respiration.* 1978;36:96–103.
38. Brown NE, Zamel N, Aberman A. Changes in pulmonary mechanics and gas exchange following thoracocentesis. *Chest.* 1978;74:540–542.
39. Wang JS, Tseng CH. Changes in pulmonary mechanics and gas exchange after thoracentesis on patients with inversion of a hemidiaphragm secondary to large pleural effusion. *Chest.* 1995;107:1610–1614.
40. Doelken P, Abreu R, Sahn SA, Mayo PH. Effect of thoracentesis on respiratory mechanics and gas exchange in the patient receiving mechanical ventilation. *Chest.* 2006;130:1354–1361.
41. Razazi K, Thille AW, Carteaux G, et al. Effects of pleural effusion drainage on oxygenation, respiratory mechanics, and hemodynamics in mechanically ventilated patients. *Ann Am Thorac Soc.* 2014;11:1018–24.
42. Light RW, George RB. Incidence and significance of pleural effusion after abdominal surgery. *Chest.* 1976;69:621–625.
43. Nielsen PH, Jepsen SB, Olsen AD. Postoperative pleural effusion following upper abdominal surgery. *Chest.* 1989;96:1133–1135.
44. Aberle DR, Wiener-Kronish JP, Webb WR, Matthay MA. Hydrostatic versus increased permeability pulmonary edema: diagnosis based on radiographic criteria in critically ill patients. *Radiology.* 1988;168:73–79.
45. Wiener-Kronish JP, Broaddus VC, Albertine KH, et al. Relationship of pleural effusions to increased permeability pulmonary edema in anesthetized sheep. *J Clin Invest.* 1988;82:1422–1429.
46. Miller KS, Harley RA, Sahn SA. Pleural effusions associated with ethchlorvynol lung injury result from visceral pleural leak. *Am Rev Respir Dis.* 1989;140:764–770.
47. Doerr CH, Miller DL, Ryu JH. Chylothorax. *Semin Respir Crit Care Med.* 2001;22:617–626.
48. Valentine VG, Raffin TA. The management of chylothorax. *Chest.* 1992; 102:586–591.
49. Ferguson MK, Little AG, Skinner DB. Current concepts in the management of postoperative chylothorax. *Ann Thorac Surg.* 1985;40:542–545.
50. Spiro JD, Spiro RH, Strong EW. The management of chyle fistula. *Laryngoscope.* 1990;100:771–774.
51. Teba L, Dedhia HV, Bowen R, Alexander JC. Chylothorax review. *Crit Care Med.* 1985; 13:49–52.
52. Staats BA, Ellefson RD, Budahn LL, et al. The lipoprotein profile of chylous and nonchylous pleural effusions. *Mayo Clin Proc.* 1980;55:700–704.
53. Cerfolio RJ, Allen MS, Deschamps C, et al. Postoperative chylothorax. *J Thorac Cardiovasc Surg.* 1996;112:1361–1365.
54. Wiener-Kronish JP, Matthay MA, Callen PW, et al. Relationship of pleural effusions to pulmonary hemodynamics in patients with congestive heart failure. *Am Rev Respir Dis.* 1985;132:1253–1256.
55. Shinto RA, Light RW. Effects of diuresis on the characteristics of pleural fluid in patients with congestive heart failure. *Am J Med.* 1990;88:230–234.
56. Light RW, Rogers JT, Cheng D, Rodriguez RM. Large pleural effusions occurring after coronary artery bypass grafting. Cardiovascular Surgery Associates, PC. *Ann Intern Med.* 1999;130:891–896.
57. Kollef MH. Trapped-lung syndrome after cardiac surgery: a potentially preventable complication of pleural injury. *Heart Lung.* 1990;19: 671–675.
58. Henderson JA, Peloquin AJ. Boerhaave revisited: spontaneous esophageal perforation as a diagnostic masquerader. *Am J Med.* 1989;86:559–567.
59. O'Connell ND. Spontaneous rupture of the esophagus. *Am J Roentgenol Radium Ther Nucl Med.* 1967;99:186–203.
60. Drury M, Anderson W, Heffner JE. Diagnostic value of pleural fluid cytology in occult Boerhaave's syndrome. *Chest.* 1992;102:976–978.
61. Bacon BR, Bailey-Newton RS, Connors AF Jr. Pleural effusions after endoscopic variceal sclerotherapy. *Gastroenterology.* 1985;88:1910–1914.
62. Symbas PN. Cardiothoracic trauma. *Curr Probl Surg.* 1991;28:741–797.
63. Feliciano DV. The diagnostic and therapeutic approach to chest trauma. *Semin Thorac Cardiovasc Surg.* 1992;4:156–162.
64. Wilson RF, Nichols RL. The EAST practice management guidelines for prophylactic antibiotic use in tube thoracostomy for traumatic hemopneumothorax: a commentary. Eastern Association for Trauma. *J Trauma.* 2000;48:758–759.
65. Gur C, Ilan Y, Shibolet O. Hepatic hydrothorax: pathophysiology, diagnosis and treatment—review of the literature. *Liver Int.* 2004;24:281–284.
66. Cardenas A, Arroyo V. Management of ascites and hepatic hydrothorax. *Best Pract Res Clin Gastroenterol.* 2007;21:55–75.
67. Verreault J, Lepage S, Bisson G, Plante A. Ascites and right pleural effusion: demonstration of a peritoneo-pleural communication. *J Nucl Med.* 1986;27:1706–1709.
68. Mouroux J, Perrin C, Venissac N, et al. Management of pleural effusion of cirrhotic origin. *Chest.* 1996;109:1093–1096.
69. Xiol X, Castellví JM, Guardiola J, et al. Spontaneous bacterial empyema in cirrhotic patients: a prospective study. *Hepatology.* 1996;23:719–723.
70. Allam NA. Spontaneous bacterial empyema in liver cirrhosis: an underdiagnosed pleural complication. *Saudi J Gastroenterol.* 2008;14:43–45.
71. Chen CH, Shih CM, Chou JW, et al. Outcome predictors of cirrhotic patients with spontaneous bacterial empyema. *Liver Int.* 2011;31:417–424.
72. Eid AA, Keddissi JI, Kinasewitz GT. Hypoalbuminemia as a cause of pleural effusions. *Chest.* 1999;115:1066–1069.
73. Scott WL. Complications associated with central venous catheters: a survey. *Chest.* 1988;94:1221–1224.
74. Duntley P, Siever J, Korwes ML, et al. Vascular erosion by central venous catheters. Clinical features and outcome. *Chest.* 1992;101:1633–1638.
75. Dunbar RD, Mitchell R, Lavine M. Aberrant locations of central venous catheters. *Lancet.* 1981;1:711–715.
76. Aslamy Z, Dewald CL, Heffner JE. MRI of central venous anatomy: implications for central venous catheter insertion. *Chest.* 1998;114:820–826.
77. Maringhini A, Ciambra M, Patti R, et al. Ascites, pleural, and pericardial effusions in acute pancreatitis: a prospective study of incidence, natural history, and prognostic role. *Dig Dis Sci.* 1996;41:848–852.
78. Kaye MD. Pleuropulmonary complications of pancreatitis. *Thorax.* 1968;23: 297–306.

79. Lankisch PG, Droge M, Becher R. Pleural effusions: a new negative prognostic parameter for acute pancreatitis. *Am J Gastroenterol.* 1994; 89:1849–1851.
80. Rockey DC, Cello JP. Pancreaticopleural fistula: report of 7 patients and review of the literature. *Medicine (Baltimore).* 1990;69:332–344.
81. Dhebri AR, Ferran N. Nonsurgical management of pancreaticopleural fistula. *JOP.* 2005;6:152–161.
82. Neher JR, Brady PG, Pinkas H, Ramos M. Pancreaticopleural fistula in chronic pancreatitis: resolution with endoscopic therapy. *Gastrointest Endosc.* 2000;52:416–418.
83. Pottmeyer EW 3rd, Frey CF, Matsuno S. Pancreaticopleural fistulas. *Arch Surg.* 1987;122:648–654.
84. Strange C, Sahn SA. The definitions and epidemiology of pleural space infection. *Semin Respir Infect.* 1999;14:3–8.
85. Rahman NM, Chapman SJ, Davies RJ. The approach to the patient with a parapneumonic effusion. *Clin Chest Med.* 2006;27:253–266.
86. Schiza S, Siafakas NM. Clinical presentation and management of empyema, lung abscess and pleural effusion. *Curr Opin Pulm Med.* 2006;12:205–211.
87. Light RW. Parapneumonic effusions and empyema. *Proc Am Thorac Soc.* 2006;3:5–80.
88. Colice GL, Curtis A, Deslauriers J, et al. Medical and surgical treatment of parapneumonic effusions : an evidence-based guideline. *Chest.* 2000;118: 1158–1171.
89. Rahman NM, Maskell NA, Davies CW, et al. The relationship between chest tube size and clinical outcome in pleural infection. *Chest.* 2010;137: 536–543.
90. Rahman NM, Maskell NA, West A, et al. Intrapleural use of tissue plasminogen activator and DNase in pleural infection. *N Engl J Med.* 2011;365:518–526.
91. Dressler W. The post-myocardial-infarction syndrome: a report on forty-four cases. *AMA Arch Intern Med.* 1959;103:28–42.
92. Stelzner TJ, King TE Jr, Antony VB, Sahn SA. The pleuropulmonary manifestations of the postcardiac injury syndrome. *Chest.* 1983;84:383–387.
93. Khan AH, The postcardiac injury syndromes. *Clin Cardiol.* 1992;15:67–72.
94. Kim S, Sahn SA. Postcardiac injury syndrome: an immunologic pleural fluid analysis. *Chest.* 1996;109:570–572.
95. Horneffer PJ, Miller RH, Pearson TA, et al. The effective treatment of postpericardiotomy syndrome after cardiac operations: a randomized placebo-controlled trial. *J Thorac Cardiovasc Surg.* 1990;100:292–296.
96. Imazio M, Brucato A, Cumetti D, et al. Corticosteroids for recurrent pericarditis: high versus low doses: a nonrandomized observation. *Circulation.* 2008;118:667–671.
97. Light RW. Clinical practice: pleural effusion. *N Engl J Med.* 2002;346: 1971–1977.
98. Bynum LJ, Wilson JE 3rd. Radiographic features of pleural effusions in pulmonary embolism. *Am Rev Respir Dis.* 1978;117:829–834.
99. Bynum LJ, Wilson JE 3rd. Characteristics of pleural effusions associated with pulmonary embolism. *Arch Intern Med.* 1976;136:159–162.
100. Simon HB, Daggett WM, DeSanctis RW. Hemothorax as a complication of anticoagulant therapy in the presence of pulmonary infarction. *JAMA.* 1969;208:1830–1834.
101. Brathwaite CE, Mure AJ, O'Malley KF, et al. Complications of anticoagulation for pulmonary embolism in low risk trauma patients. *Chest.* 1993;104:718–720.
102. Berger HW, Rammohan G, Neff MS, Buhain WJ. Uremic pleural effusion: a study in 14 patients on chronic dialysis. *Ann Intern Med.* 1975;82: 362–364.
103. Jarratt MJ, Sahn SA. Pleural effusions in hospitalized patients receiving long-term hemodialysis. *Chest.* 1995;108:470–474.
104. Galen MA, Steinberg SM, Lowrie EG, et al. Hemorrhagic pleural effusion in patients undergoing chronic hemodialysis. *Ann Intern Med.* 1975;82: 359–361.
105. Bakirci T, Sasak G, Ozturk S, et al. Pleural effusion in long-term hemodialysis patients. *Transplant Proc.* 2007;39:889–891.
106. Yoshii C, Morita S, Tokunaga M, et al. Bilateral massive pleural effusions caused by uremic pleuritis. *Intern Med.* 2001;40:646–649.
107. Rodelas R, Rakowski TA, Argy WP, Schreiner GE. Fibrosing uremic pleuritis during hemodialysis. *JAMA.* 1980;243:2424–2425.
108. Maher JF. Uremic pleuritis. *Am J Kidney Dis.* 1987;10:19–22.
109. Strange C. Pleural complications in the intensive care unit. *Clin Chest Med.* 1999;20:317–327.
110. de Latorre FJ, Tomasa A, Klamburg J, et al. Incidence of pneumothorax and pneumomediastinum in patients with aspiration pneumonia requiring ventilatory support. *Chest.* 1977;72:141–144.
111. Maunder RJ, Pierson DJ, Hudson LD. Subcutaneous and mediastinal emphysema: pathophysiology, diagnosis, and management. *Arch Intern Med.* 1984;144:1447–1453.
112. Macklin MT, Macklin CC. Malignant interstitial emphysema of the lungs and mediastinum as an important occult complication in respiratory diseases and other conditions: an interpretation of the clinical literature in the light of laboratory experiment. *Medicine.* 1944;23:281–358.
113. Jantz MA, Pierson DJ. Pneumothorax and barotrauma. *Clin Chest Med.* 1994;15:75–91.
114. Rankine JJ, Thomas AN, Fluechter D. Diagnosis of pneumothorax in critically ill adults. *Postgrad Med J.* 2000;76:399–404.
115. Tocino IM, Miller MH, Fairfax WR. Distribution of pneumothorax in the supine and semirecumbent critically ill adult. *AJR Am J Roentgenol.* 1985;144:901–905.
116. Buckner CB, Harmon BH, Pallin JS. The radiology of abnormal intrathoracic air. *Curr Probl Diagn Radiol.* 1988;17:37–71.
117. McGonigal MD, Schwab CW, Kauder DR, et al. Supplemental emergent chest computed tomography in the management of blunt torso trauma. *J Trauma.* 1990;30:1431–1434.
118. Maury E, Guglielminotti J, Alzieu M, et al. Ultrasonic examination: an alternative to chest radiography after central venous catheter insertion? *Am J Respir Crit Care Med.* 2001;164:403–405.
119. Soldati G, Testa A, Sher S, et al. Occult traumatic pneumothorax: diagnostic accuracy of lung ultrasonography in the emergency department. *Chest.* 2008;133:204–211.
120. Dines DE, Clagett OT, Payne WS. Spontaneous pneumothorax in emphysema. *Mayo Clin Proc.* 1970;45:481–487.
121. George RB. Herbert SJ, Shames JM, et al. Pneumothorax complicating pulmonary emphysema. *JAMA.* 1975;234:389–393.
122. Hagley MT, Martin B, Gast P, Traeger SM. Infectious and mechanical complications of central venous catheters placed by percutaneous venipuncture and over guidewires. *Crit Care Med.* 1992;20:1426–1430.
123. Giuffrida DJ, Bryan-Brown CW, Lumb PD, et al. Central vs peripheral venous catheters in critically ill patients. *Chest.* 1986;90:806–809.
124. Eerola R, Kaukinen L, Kaukinen S. Analysis of 13 800 subclavian vein catheterizations. *Acta Anaesthesiol Scand.* 1985;29:193–197.
125. Tyden H. Cannulation of the internal jugular vein—500 cases. *Acta Anaesthesiol Scand.* 1982;26:485–488.
126. Weiner P, Sznajder I, Plavnick L, et al. Unusual complications of subclavian vein catheterization. *Crit Care Med.* 1984;12:538–539.
127. Hillman K, Albin M. Pulmonary barotrauma during cardiopulmonary resuscitation. *Crit Care Med.* 1986;14:606–609.
128. Shulman D, Beilin B, Olshwang D. Pulmonary barotrauma during cardiopulmonary resuscitation. *Resuscitation.* 1987;15:201–207.
129. Myers DP, de Leon-Casasola OA, Bacon DR, et al. Bilateral pneumothoraces from a malfunctioning resuscitation valve. *J Clin Anesth.* 1993;5:433–435.
130. Silbergleit R, Lee DC, Blank-Reid C, McNamara RM. Sudden severe barotrauma from self-inflating bag-valve devices. *J Trauma.* 1996;40:320–322.
131. McCulloch TM, Bishop MJ. Complications of translaryngeal intubation. *Clin Chest Med.* 1991;12:507–521.
132. Schwartz DE, Matthay MA, Cohen NH. Death and other complications of emergency airway management in critically ill adults: a prospective investigation of 297 tracheal intubations. *Anesthesiology.* 1995;82:367–376.
133. Berrouschot J, Oeken J, Steiniger L, Schneider D. Perioperative complications of percutaneous dilational tracheostomy. *Laryngoscope.* 1997;107:1538–1544.
134. Myers EN, Carrau RL. Early complications of tracheotomy: incidence and management. *Clin Chest Med.* 1991;12:589–595.
135. Steinberg KP, Mitchell DR, Maunder RJ, et al. Safety of bronchoalveolar lavage in patients with adult respiratory distress syndrome. *Am Rev Respir Dis.* 1993;148:556–561.
136. Ruiz F, Casado T, Monso E. Pneumothorax during bronchoalveolar lavage. *Chest.* 1989;96:1441–1442.
137. Gammon RB, Shin MS, Buchalter SE. Pulmonary barotrauma in mechanical ventilation: patterns and risk factors. *Chest.* 1992;102:568–572.
138. Papazian L, Forel JM, Gacouin A, et al; ACURASYS Study Investigators. Neuromuscular blockers in early acute respiratory distress syndrome. *N Engl J Med.* 2010;363:1107–1116.
139. Miller MP, Sagy M. Pressure characteristics of mechanical ventilation and incidence of pneumothorax before and after the implementation of protective lung strategies in the management of pediatric patients with severe ARDS. *Chest.* 2008;134:969–973.
140. Moxon RK. Spontaneous pneumothorax; observations on 26 cases. *U S Armed Forces Med J.* 1950;1:1157–1161.
141. Myers JA. Simple spontaneous pneumothorax. *Dis Chest.* 1954;26:420–441.
142. Gobien RP, Reines HD, Schabel SI. Localized tension pneumothorax: unrecognized form of barotrauma in adult respiratory distress syndrome. *Radiology.* 1982;142:15–19.
143. Ross IB, Fleiszer DM, Brown RA. Localized tension pneumothorax in patients with adult respiratory distress syndrome. *Can J Surg.* 1994;37:415–419.

144. Heffner JE, McDonald J, Barbieri C. Recurrent pneumothoraces in ventilated patients despite ipsilateral chest tubes. *Chest.* 1995;108:1053–1058.
145. McConaghy PM, Kennedy N. Tension pneumothorax due to intrapulmonary placement of intercostal chest drain. *Anaesth Intensive Care.* 1995;23:496–498.
146. Tagliabue M, Casella TC, Zincone GE, et al. CT and chest radiography in the evaluation of adult respiratory distress syndrome. *Acta Radiol.* 1994;35:230–423.
147. Light RW. Tension pneumothorax. *Intensive Care Med.* 1994;20:468–469.
148. Lin YC, Tu CY, Liang SJ, et al. Pigtail catheter for the management of pneumothorax in mechanically ventilated patients. *Am J Emerg Med.* 2010;28:466–471.
149. Yarmus L, Feller-Kopman D. Pneumothorax in the critically ill patient. *Chest.* 2012;141:1098–1105.
150. Light RW. Pleural controversy: optimal chest tube size for drainage. *Respirology.* 2011;16:244–248.
151. Kaplan, LJ, Trooskin SZ, Santora TA, Weiss JP. Percutaneous drainage of recurrent pneumothoraces and pneumatoceles. *J Trauma.* 1996;41: 1069–1072.
152. Klein JS, Schultz S, Heffner JE. Interventional radiology of the chest: image-guided percutaneous drainage of pleural effusions, lung abscess, and pneumothorax. *AJR Am J Roentgenol.* 1995;164:581–588.
153. Steier M, Ching N, Roberts EB, Nealon TF Jr. Pneumothorax complicating continuous ventilatory support. *J Thorac Cardiovasc Surg.* 1974;67:17–23.
154. Gall SA Jr, Wolfe WG. Management of microfistula following pulmonary resection. *Chest Surg Clin North Am.* 1996;6:543–565.
155. Hollaus PH, Lax F, el-Nashef BB, et al. Natural history of bronchopleural fistula after pneumonectomy: a review of 96 cases. *Ann Thorac Surg.* 1997;63:1391–1396; discussion 1396–1397.
156. Puskas JD, Mathisen DJ, Grillo HC, et al. Treatment strategies for bronchopleural fistula. *J Thorac Cardiovasc Surg.* 1995;109:989–995; discussion 995–996.
157. Baumann MH, Sahn SA. Medical management and therapy of bronchopleural fistulas in the mechanically ventilated patient. *Chest.* 1990;97:721–728.
158. Calhoon JH, Grover FL, Trinkle JK. Chest trauma: approach and management. *Clin Chest Med.* 1992;13:55–67.
159. Pierson DJ, Horton CA, Bates PW. Persistent bronchopleural air leak during mechanical ventilation: a review of 39 cases. *Chest.* 1986;90:321–333.
160. Powner DJ, Grenvik A. Ventilatory management of life-threatening bronchopleural fistulae: a summary. *Crit Care Med.* 1981;9:54–58.
161. Zimmerman JE, Colgan DL, Mills M. Management of bronchopleural fistula complicating therapy with positive end expiratory pressure (PEEP). *Chest.* 1973;64:526–529.
162. Downs JB, Chapman RL Jr. Treatment of bronchopleural fistula during continuous positive pressure ventilation. *Chest.* 1976;69:363–366.
163. Tilles RB, Don HF. Complications of high pleural suction in bronchopleural fistulas. *Anesthesiology.* 1975;43:486–487.
164. Ritz R, Benson M, Bishop MJ. Measuring gas leakage from bronchopleural fistulas during high-frequency jet ventilation. *Crit Care Med.* 1984;12:836–837.
165. Powner DJ, Cline CD, Rodman GH Jr. Effect of chest-tube suction on gas flow through a bronchopleural fistula. *Crit Care Med.* 1985;13:99–101.
166. Albelda SM, Hansen-Flaschen JH, Taylor E, et al. Evaluation of high-frequency jet ventilation in patients with bronchopleural fistulas by quantitation of the airleak. *Anesthesiology.* 1985;63:551–554.
167. Roth MD, Wright JW, Bellamy PE. Gas flow through a bronchopleural fistula. Measuring the effects of high-frequency jet ventilation and chest-tube suction. *Chest.* 1988;93:210–213.
168. Bishop MJ, Benson MS, Pierson DJ. Carbon dioxide excretion via bronchopleural fistulas in adult respiratory distress syndrome. *Chest.* 1987;91:400–402.
169. Weg JG, Anzueto A, Balk RA, et al. The relation of pneumothorax and other air leaks to mortality in the acute respiratory distress syndrome. *N Engl J Med.* 1998;338:341–346.
170. Rusch VW, Capps JS, Tyler ML, Pierson DL. The performance of four pleural drainage systems in an animal model of bronchopleural fistula. *Chest.* 1988;93:859–863.
171. Walsh MC, Carlo WA. Determinants of gas flow through a bronchopleural fistula. *J Appl Physiol (1985).* 1989;67:1591–1596.
172. Phillips YY, Lonigan RM, Joyner LR. A simple technique for managing a bronchopleural fistula while maintaining positive pressure ventilation. *Crit Care Med.* 1979;7:351–353.
173. Blanch PB, Koens JC Jr, Layon AJ. A new device that allows synchronous intermittent inspiratory chest tube occlusion with any mechanical ventilator. *Chest.* 1990;97:1426–1430.
174. Gallagher TJ, Smith RA, Kirby RR, Civetta JM. Intermittent inspiratory chest tube occlusion to limit bronchopleural cutaneous airleaks. *Crit Care Med.* 1976;4:328–332.
175. Dennis JW, Eigen H, Ballantine TV, Grosfeld JL. The relationship between peak inspiratory pressure and positive end expiratory pressure on the volume of air lost through a bronchopleural fistula. *J Pediatr Surg.* 1980;15:971–976.
176. Barringer M, Meredith J, Prough D, et al. Effectiveness of high-frequency jet ventilation in management of an experimental bronchopleural fistula. *Am Surg.* 1982;48:610–613.
177. Sjostrand UH, Smith RB, Hoff BH, et al. Conventional and high-frequency ventilation in dogs with bronchopleural fistula. *Crit Care Med.* 1985;13:191–193.
178. Orlando R 3rd, Gluck EH, Cohen M, Mesologites CG. Ultra-high-frequency jet ventilation in a bronchopleural fistula model. *Arch Surg.* 1988;123:591–593.
179. Mayers I, Long R, Breen PH, Wood LD. Artificial ventilation of a canine model of bronchopleural fistula. *Anesthesiology.* 1986;64:739–746.
180. Spinale FG, Linker RW, Crawford FA, Reines HD. Conventional versus high frequency jet ventilation with a bronchopleural fistula. *J Surg Res.* 1989;46:147–151.
181. Dodds CP, Hillman KM. Management of massive air leak with asynchronous independent lung ventilation. *Intensive Care Med.* 1982;8:287–290.
182. Wendt M, Hachenberg T, Winde G, Lawin P. Differential ventilation with low-flow CPAP and CPPV in the treatment of unilateral chest trauma. *Intensive Care Med.* 1989;15:209–211.
183. Lohse AW, Klein O, Hermann E, et al. Pneumatoceles and pneumothoraces complicating staphylococcal pneumonia: treatment by synchronous independent lung ventilation. *Thorax.* 1993;48:578–580.
184. Feeley TW, Keating D, Nishimura T. Independent lung ventilation using high-frequency ventilation in the management of a bronchopleural fistula. *Anesthesiology.* 1988;69:420–422.
185. Crimi G, Candiani A, Conti G, et al. Clinical applications of independent lung ventilation with unilateral high-frequency jet ventilation (ILV-UHFJV). *Intensive Care Med.* 1986;12:90–94.
186. Mortimer AJ, Laurie PS, Garrett H, Kerr JH. Unilateral high frequency jet ventilation. Reduction of leak in bronchopleural fistula. *Intensive Care Med.* 1984;10:39–41.
187. Charan NB, Carvalho CG, Hawk P, et al. Independent lung ventilation with a single ventilator using a variable resistance valve. *Chest.* 1995;107:256–260.
188. Carvalho P, Thompson WH, Riggs R, et al. Management of bronchopleural fistula with a variable-resistance valve and a single ventilator. *Chest.* 1997;111:1452–1454.
189. Thomas AR, Bryce TL. Ventilation in the patient with unilateral lung disease. *Crit Care Clin.* 1998;14:743–773.
190. Ost D, Corbridge T. Independent lung ventilation. *Clin Chest Med.* 1996; 17:591–601.
191. Mehta HJ, Malhotra P, Begnaud A, et al. Treatment of alveolar-pleural fistula with endobronchial application of synthetic hydrogel. *Chest.* 2015;147: 695–699.
192. McManigle JE, Fletcher GL, Tenholder MF. Bronchoscopy in the management of bronchopleural fistula. *Chest.* 1990;97:1235–1238.
193. Lois M, Noppen M. Bronchopleural fistulas: an overview of the problem with special focus on endoscopic management. *Chest.* 2005;128:3955–3965.
194. Toma TP, Kon OM, Oldfield W, et al. Reduction of persistent air leak with endoscopic valve implants. *Thorax.* 2007;62:830–833.
195. Feller-Kopman D, Bechara R, Garland R, et al. Use of a removable endobronchial valve for the treatment of bronchopleural fistula. *Chest.* 2006;130:273–275.
196. Ferguson JS, Sprenger K, Van Natta T. Closure of a bronchopleural fistula using bronchoscopic placement of an endobronchial valve designed for the treatment of emphysema. *Chest.* 2006;129:479–481.
197. Andreetti C, Venuta F, Anile M, et al. Pleurodesis with an autologous blood patch to prevent persistent air leaks after lobectomy. *J Thorac Cardiovasc Surg.* 2007;133(3)759–762.
198. Droghetti A, Venuta F, Anile M, et al. Autologous blood patch in persistent air leaks after pulmonary resection. *J Thorac Cardiovasc Surg.* 2006;132:556–559.
199. Lang-Lazdunski L, Coonar AS. A prospective study of autologous 'blood patch' pleurodesis for persistent air leak after pulmonary resection. *Eur J Cardiothorac Surg.* 2004;26:897–900.
200. Matar AF, Hill JG, Duncan W, et al. Use of biological glue to control pulmonary air leaks. *Thorax.* 1990;45:670–674.
201. Nicholas JM, Dulchavsky SA. Successful use of autologous fibrin gel in traumatic bronchopleural fistula: case report. *J Trauma.* 1992;32:87–88.

CHAPTER

116

Interventional Bronchoscopy and Massive Hemoptysis

HIREN J. MEHTA and MICHAEL A. JANTZ

INTRODUCTION

Hemoptysis is defined as the expectoration of blood that originates from the lower respiratory tract. Pseudohemoptysis is the expectoration of blood from a source other than the lower respiratory tract such as the nares, oropharynx, larynx, or the gastrointestinal tract. Massive hemoptysis is defined as expectoration of blood exceeding 200 to 1,000 mL over a 24-hour period, with expectoration of more than 600 mL in 24 hours being the most commonly used definition (1).

In practice, the rapidity of bleeding and ability to maintain a patent airway are critical factors; life-threatening hemoptysis can alternatively be defined as the amount of bleeding that compromises ventilation (2). Only 3% to 5% of patients with hemoptysis have a massive bleed, with the mortality rate ranging from 20% to as high as 80% in some case series (3–5). Most patients who die from massive hemoptysis do so from asphyxiation secondary to airway occlusion by clot and blood—not from exsanguination. Prognostic factors associated with an increased risk of death from massive hemoptysis include bleeding in excess of 1,000 mL/24 hr, hemoptysis due to neoplasms, radiographic evidence of aspiration, and hemodynamic instability (3,6).

ETIOLOGY OF MASSIVE HEMOPTYSIS

Hemoptysis has multiple causes usually categorized under parenchymal diseases, airway diseases, and vascular diseases. Bleeding may originate from small or large lung vessels. The causes of massive hemoptysis are listed in Table 116.1. Virtually all causes of hemoptysis may result in massive hemoptysis. Infections associated with bronchiectasis, tuberculosis, lung abscess, and necrotizing pneumonia are commonly responsible for the massive bleeding. Other common causes include bronchogenic carcinoma, mycetoma, invasive fungal diseases, chest trauma, cystic fibrosis, pulmonary infarction, and coagulopathy. Although massive hemoptysis is usually due to bleeding from the bronchial circulation, alveolar hemorrhage due to conditions such as granulomatosis with polyangiitis (Wegener's) granulomatosis and Goodpasture syndrome may occasionally cause massive hemoptysis (Table 116.2).

ANATOMIC SOURCES OF HEMOPTYSIS

The sources of lower respiratory tract bleeding include the pulmonary and bronchial circulations. Two arterial vascular systems supply blood to the lungs: the pulmonary and the bronchial arteries. The pulmonary arteries provide 99% of the arterial blood to the lungs and are involved in gas exchange. The pulmonary circulation is a low pressure circuit under normal circumstances. The bronchial arteries serving the intrapulmonary airways and lung parenchyma arise from the thoracic aorta at the level of the third through the eighth thoracic vertebrae, originating most commonly at the level of the fifth and sixth vertebrae and drain through the bronchopulmonary anastomosis into the pulmonary veins, which empty into the left side of the heart. Bronchial circulation supplies nourishment to the extra- and intrapulmonary airways and to the pulmonary arteries (vasa vasorum), without being involved in the gas exchange (7). Complex capillary anastomoses exist between the pulmonary arteries and the systemic bronchial arteries. When the pulmonary circulation is compromised (e.g., in thromboembolic disease, vasculitic disorders, or in hypoxic vasoconstriction), the bronchial supply gradually increases, causing a hyperflow in the anastomotic vessels, which become hypertrophic with thin walls and tend to break into the alveoli and bronchi, giving rise to hemoptysis. Likewise, in chronic inflammatory disorders, such as bronchiectasis, chronic bronchitis, tuberculosis, mycotic lung diseases, and lung abscess, as well as in neoplastic diseases, the release of angiogenic growth factors promote neovascularization and pulmonary vessel remodeling, with engagement of collateral systemic vessels (8). These new and collateral vessels are fragile and prone to rupture into the airways.

Angiographic studies of patients with active hemoptysis have demonstrated that bleeding originates from bronchial and pulmonary arteries in 90% and 5% of cases, respectively (1,9). In the remaining 5% of cases, hemoptysis may derive from nonbronchial systemic arteries (9). Very rarely, hemoptysis has been reported originating from pulmonary and bronchial veins (10) and capillaries (11). A recent study by Noe et al. (12) shows that bleeding from bronchial arteries can coexist with bleeding from nonbronchial and pulmonary arteries in the same patient.

INITIAL EVALUATION

A detailed history and physical examination should be performed. Patients with a history of tuberculosis may have bleeding from rupture of a pulmonary artery aneurysm in the cavity lumen, known as a Rasmussen aneurysm, or by breakdown of bronchopulmonary anastomoses within the wall of old cavities. Bronchogenic carcinoma should be suspected in smokers older than 40 years of age. Repeated episodes of hemoptysis over months to years suggest bronchiectasis or a carcinoid tumor. Chronic sputum production predating the

TABLE 116.1 Potential Causes of Massive Hemoptysis

Neoplasm
Bronchogenic cancer
Metastasis (parenchymal or endobronchial)
Carcinoid
Leukemia
Infectious
Lung abscess
Bronchiectasis
Tuberculosis
Necrotizing pneumonia
Fungal pneumonia
Septic pulmonary emboli
Mycetoma (aspergilloma)
Pulmonary Parenchyma
Bronchiectasis
Cystic fibrosis
Sarcoidosis (fibrocavitary)
Diffuse alveolar hemorrhage
Airway foreign body
Cardiac/Vascular
Mitral stenosis
Pulmonary embolism/infarction
Arteriovenous malformation
Bronchoarterial fistula
Ruptured aortic aneurysm
Bronchial artery aneurysm
Congestive Heart Failure
Pulmonary arteriovenous fistula
Iatrogenic/Traumatic
Blunt or penetrating chest trauma
Tracheal/bronchial tear or rupture
Tracheoinnominate artery fistula
Bronchoscopy
Pulmonary artery rupture from pulmonary artery catheter
Endotracheal tube suctioning trauma
Hematologic
Coagulopathy
Disseminated intravascular coagulation
Thrombocytopenia
Drugs/Toxins
Anticoagulants
Antiplatelet agents
Thrombolytic agents
Crack cocaine

TABLE 116.2 Causes of Alveolar Hemorrhage

Goodpasture syndrome
Vasculitis/collagen vascular disease
Wegener granulomatosis
Microscopic polyangiitis
System lupus erythematosus
Mixed connective tissue disorder
Systemic sclerosis (scleroderma)
Rheumatoid arthritis
Henoch–Schonlein purpura
Mixed cryoglobulinemia
Behçet syndrome
Diffuse alveolar damage
Antiphospholipid syndrome
Idiopathic pulmonary hemosiderosis
Hematopoietic stem cell/bone marrow transplantation
Coagulopathy
Mitral stenosis
Lymphangioleiomyomatosis
Drugs/toxins
Isocyanates
Trimellitic anhydride
D penicillamine
Nitrofurantoin
All trans retinoic acid
Crack cocaine

hemoptysis implies a diagnosis of chronic bronchitis, bronchiectasis, or cystic fibrosis. Pulmonary embolism should be suspected in patients with a history of deep venous thrombosis or risk factors for pulmonary thromboembolism. A febrile illness with sputum production, night sweats, and weight loss suggests a lung abscess or tuberculosis. Excessive anticoagulation, thrombolytic therapy, and coagulopathy may also cause hemoptysis (13,14). In children with hemoptysis, the most likely diagnoses are carcinoid tumors, vascular anomalies, and aspiration of foreign bodies (15,16). Alveolar hemorrhage should be suspected in patients with dyspnea, hypoxemia, and diffuse pulmonary infiltrates. The triad of upper airway disease, lower airway disease, and renal disease suggests granulomatosis with polyangiitis (Wegener granulomatosis) (17). Goodpasture syndrome should be suspected in young men with alveolar hemorrhage and microscopic or macroscopic hematuria (18). Patients with a history of systemic lupus erythematosus (SLE) may develop alveolar hemorrhage at any time during the course of their disease, and alveolar hemorrhage may be the initial manifestation (19). Alveolar hemorrhage should be considered in patients with diffuse pulmonary infiltrates who have recently undergone hematopoietic stem cell or bone marrow transplantation (20). Although uncommon, tracheoinnominate artery fistula is an important consideration in patients with tracheostomy presenting with massive hemoptysis (21,22). The peak incidence is between the first and second week, although hemorrhage can occur as early as 48 hours and as late as 18 months after the procedure. A sentinel self-limited bleed is observed in 35% to 50% of patients. Trauma from suctioning, particularly in the setting of abnormal coagulation, may also cause hemoptysis in patients with a tracheostomy tube or in those who have an endotracheal tube (ET) in place. The possibility of traumatic rupture of a pulmonary artery should be considered in patients with a pulmonary artery catheter in place (23,24).

Physical Examination

The physical examination may provide clues to the diagnosis of massive hemoptysis. A saddle nose deformity and/or septal perforation suggest Wegener granulomatosis. Stridor or unilateral wheezing indicates a possible laryngeal tumor, tracheobronchial tumor, or airway foreign body. Pulmonary embolism should be considered in patients with tachypnea, a pleural friction rub, and lower extremity phlebitis. Diffuse rales on examination raises the possibility of diffuse alveolar hemorrhage, diffuse parenchymal lung disease, or cardiac disease as the cause of the hemoptysis. The presence of telangiectasias of the skin or mucous membranes suggests hereditary hemorrhagic telangiectasia or a connective tissue disease as the cause. Ecchymoses or petechiae suggest a hematologic abnormality or coagulopathy. Clubbing of the fingers may be a sign of a lung carcinoma, bronchiectasis, and cystic fibrosis. The finding of pulsation of the tracheostomy tube is of concern for the development of a tracheoinnominate fistula.

Laboratory Studies

Laboratory studies, including a complete blood count (CBC), coagulation studies, urinalysis, and chest radiograph, should be obtained in all patients. The CBC may suggest an infectious process or hematologic disorder as the cause of hemoptysis and indicate the need for blood transfusion. Coagulation studies may provide evidence for a hematologic disorder as the cause for the hemoptysis, or may identify a coagulopathy that is causing or contributing to the bleeding from another disease. Hematuria may be noted on urinalysis, which suggests the diagnosis of Goodpasture syndrome, Wegener granulomatosis, or another systemic vasculitis.

Chest Radiograph

The chest radiograph is an important study to identify the cause and side of bleeding. The chest radiograph may demonstrate abnormalities such as lung masses, cavitary lesions, atelectasis, focal infiltrates, and diffuse infiltrate. Single or multiple pulmonary cavities suggest neoplasm, tuberculosis, fungal disease, lung abscess, septic pulmonary emboli, parasitic infection, or Wegener granulomatosis as the cause for hemoptysis. The presence of a mass within a cavitary lesion indicates a possible mycetoma (aspergilloma). The appearance of a new air–fluid level in a cavity or infiltrate around a cavity is suggestive of the site of bleeding. A solitary pulmonary nodule that has vessels going toward the nodule may be an arteriovenous malformation. Diffuse pulmonary infiltrates suggest diffuse alveolar hemorrhage (Table 116.2), bleeding from coagulopathy, lung contusions from blunt chest trauma, hemorrhage with multiple areas of aspiration, or pulmonary edema with a cardiac cause for hemoptysis. Chest radiographs may be normal or nonlocalizing in 20% to 45% of patients (25,26). Therefore, in patients presenting with hemoptysis, a negative CXR warrants other diagnostic studies.

Computed Tomography

Computed tomography (CT) represents a noninvasive and highly useful imaging tool in the clinical context of hemoptysis, allowing a comprehensive evaluation of the lung parenchyma, airways, and thoracic vessels by using contrast material. Multidetector CT (MDCT) may identify the bleeding site in 63% to 100% of patients with hemoptysis (27); the role of CT in the management of massive hemoptysis is however somewhat controversial. CT may demonstrate abnormalities that are not visible on the chest radiograph. It is helpful in the diagnosis of bronchiectasis (28), although abnormalities from bronchiectasis can usually be appreciated on the chest radiograph. CT with contrast may detect pulmonary emboli, thoracic aneurysms, or arteriovenous malformations. CT scans may also demonstrate cavitation with a surrounding infiltrate, the halo sign, which suggests a necrotizing infection such as aspergillosis or mucormycosis (29,30). Some studies have noted that CT scanning before bronchoscopy may increase the yield of bronchoscopy (31). In one retrospective study of 80 patients with large or massive hemoptysis, chest CT was superior to chest radiograph or bronchoscopy in determining the cause of bleeding, and was similar to bronchoscopy in successfully localizing the site of bleeding (32). CT is useful to create a detailed and accurate map of the thoracic vasculature that may guide further treatment, depicting the number and origin of bronchial arteries and the coexistence of an additional nonbronchial arterial supply. CT can thus assist in choosing ectopic vessels amenable to embolization, preventing recurrence after initial successful embolization, reducing angiography procedure time, fluoroscopy radiation dose, contrast load, and decreasing iatrogenic complications (12). Some authors have argued that transport of the potentially unstable patient with massive hemoptysis may not be judicious, however; thus, the patient should be adequately stabilized prior to obtaining a chest CT.

Angiography

Angiography can determine the site of bleeding in 90% to 95% of cases. However, in one case series, routine use of diagnostic angiography provided a diagnosis not identified on bronchoscopy in only 4% of patients (33). Angiography can be helpful in detecting a pseudoaneurysm that has formed after healing of a pulmonary artery tear from pulmonary artery catheterization (34). As previously noted, the bronchial arteries and other collateral systemic arteries account for the source of bleeding in most cases with massive hemoptysis. Pulmonary angiography is usually performed only when there is suspicion for pulmonary aneurysms, arteriovenous malformations, and pulmonary embolism. Technetium labeled red blood cell or colloid studies rarely provided any information that is not obtained by bronchoscopy and chest CT. The use and timing of bronchoscopy will be discussed in a subsequent section.

Bronchoscopy

Bronchoscopy, performed with either a rigid or flexible endoscope, is helpful for identifying active bleeding and for checking the airways in patients with massive hemoptysis. The capability and success of bronchoscopy in localizing the bleeding site may vary according to the rate and severity of the hemorrhage. Hirshberg et al. (4) found that bronchoscopy was more effective in finding the bleeding site in patients with moderate to severe hemoptysis (64% and 67%) than in those with mild hemoptysis (49%). Bronchoscopy has an overall lower sensitivity than MDCT in detecting the underlying causes of bleeding (25,27,31). Nevertheless, bronchoscopy yields additional information on endobronchial lesions and allows samples for tissue diagnosis and microbial cultures.

Other Studies

Depending on the suspected causes of massive hemoptysis, additional studies may be indicated. Echocardiography may be performed if a cardiac cause is considered. If diffuse alveolar hemorrhage syndromes are suspected, laboratory testing, including antiglomerular basement membrane antibody, antineutrophilic cytoplasmic antibody, antinuclear antibody, rheumatoid factor, complement levels, cryoglobulins, and antiphospholipid antibodies, should be performed, depending on the causes that are being considered. Transbronchial lung biopsy, open lung biopsy, or kidney biopsy may be indicated in some cases of alveolar hemorrhage to establish a diagnosis.

MANAGEMENT OF MASSIVE HEMOPTYSIS

Airway Protection and Stabilization

Once the diagnosis of massive hemoptysis is established, the initial priorities are to protect the airway and stabilize the patient. In general, the patient with massive hemoptysis should be monitored in the ICU setting, even if intubation and mechanical ventilation are not required. Large bore IV access should be established and supplemental oxygen provided. Blood should be drawn for a CBC, arterial blood gas analysis, coagulation studies, electrolytes, renal function tests, and liver function tests. The patient should be type and cross-matched for blood, with 4 to 6 units of packed red blood cells always available. Correction of thrombocytopenia and coagulopathy, if present, with appropriate blood products should be considered. Attempts to lateralize the site of bleeding should be made in anticipation of steps to prevent aspiration into the nonbleeding lung; the patient may be positioned in a lateral decubitus position with the bleeding lung down.

Airway patency must be ensured in patients with massive hemoptysis, as deaths from this process are predominantly due to asphyxiation. Most patients with ongoing massive hemoptysis will require intubation and mechanical ventilation, although select patients who are not hypoxemic and are able to keep the airway clear on their own may not require intubation. Although intubation generally preserves oxygenation and facilitates blood removal from the lower respiratory tract, the ET can become obstructed by blood clots, leading to the inability to oxygenate and ventilate the patient. The largest possible ET should be inserted to allow the use of bronchoscopes with a 2.8- to 3.0-mm working channel for more effective suctioning and to allow for better ventilation with the bronchoscope in the airway for prolonged periods of time. In severe cases, the mainstem bronchus of the nonbleeding lung can be selectively intubated under bronchoscopic guidance to preserve oxygenation and ventilation from the normal lung.

Some authors have recommended the use of a double-lumen ET to isolate the normal lung and permit selective intubation. Although double-lumen ETs have been used successfully in the airway management of massive hemoptysis, there are several potential pitfalls. First, placement of a double-lumen ET is difficult for less experienced operators, particularly with a large amount of blood in the larynx and oropharynx. Second, the individual lumens of the ET are significantly smaller than a standard ET and are at significant risk of being occluded by blood and blood clots. Last, positioning of the double-lumen ET and subsequent bronchoscopic suctioning of the distal airways require a small pediatric bronchoscope with working channels of 1.2 to 1.4 mm. Adequate suctioning of large amounts of blood and blood clots through such bronchoscopes is extremely problematic. In one series of 62 patients with massive hemoptysis, death occurred in four of seven patients managed with a double-lumen ET due to loss of tube positioning and aspiration (35). In general, we do not recommend the use of double-lumen ETs for airway management in massive hemoptysis. As an alternative to selective mainstem bronchial intubation or intubation with a double-lumen ET, an ET that incorporates a bronchial blocker, such as the Univent tube, may be used.

Localization of Source and Cause of Hemoptysis

Once the patient is stabilized and airway patency is achieved, the source of bleeding should be localized as precisely as possible, and the cause of bleeding determined. Identification of the cause and location of the bleeding potentially allows for more specific therapy. Methods of localization include patient history, physical examination, chest radiograph, chest CT, bronchoscopy, and angiography. In one study of 105 patients with hemoptysis, patients themselves were able to localize the side of bleeding in 10% of cases, but with an accuracy of 70% when able to do so (36); localization by a physical examination performed by a physician was possible in 43% of patients. Chest radiographs were able to localize bleeding in 60% of cases. Bronchoscopy was accurate in localizing the source of bleeding in 86% of patients. In another study, 9 of 24 patients were able to accurately localize the side of their bleeding (37). Chest radiographs should be routinely obtained to help localize the source of bleeding and determine the cause. As discussed earlier, chest CT may provide additional information beyond the chest radiograph, and may be more accurate in localizing the bleeding and determining the cause, although concerns about transporting a potentially unstable patient out of the ICU exist (7,38). Bronchoscopy and angiography remain the modalities for localizing the source of hemoptysis and offer potential therapeutic intervention.

Early—rather than delayed—bronchoscopy should be performed to increase the likelihood of localizing the source of bleeding. Bronchoscopy performed within 48 hours of bleeding onset successfully localized bleeding in 34% to 91% of patients, depending on the case series, as compared to successful localization in 11% to 52% of patients if delayed bronchoscopy was performed (39). Bronchoscopy performed within 12 to 24 hours may provide an even higher yield. Bedside flexible bronchoscopy should not be performed to establish a diagnosis of a tracheoarterial fistula such as a tracheoinnominate fistula (21,40).

Bronchoscopic Therapies to Control Hemoptysis

Rigid bronchoscopy is the most efficient means of clearing the airways from blood clots and secretions, ensuring effective tamponade of the bleeding airway and safe isolation of the nonaffected lung, thereby preventing asphyxia and preserving ventilation. However, it requires a trained bronchoscopist, who is not always readily available. A variety of maneuvers can be performed with the flexible bronchoscope to control bleeding.

Balloon Tamponade

Endobronchial tamponade via flexible bronchoscopy can prevent aspiration of blood into the contralateral lung and preserve gas exchange in patients with massive hemoptysis. Endobronchial tamponade can be achieved with a 4-Fr Fogarty balloon-tipped catheter. The catheter may be passed directly through the working channel of the bronchoscope, or the catheter can be grasped with biopsy forceps placed though the working channel of the bronchoscope prior to introduction into the airway of the bronchoscope and catheter. The catheter is held in place adjacent to the bronchoscope by the biopsy forceps, and both are then inserted as a unit into the airway. The catheter tip is inserted into the bleeding segmental orifice, and the balloon is inflated. If passed through the suction channel, the proximal end of the catheter is clamped with a hemostat, the hub cut off, and a straight pin inserted into the catheter channel proximal to the hemostat to maintain inflation of the balloon catheter. The clamp is removed, and the bronchoscope is carefully withdrawn (41–43). The catheter can safely remain in position between 15 minutes and 1 week, until hemostasis is ensured by surgical resection of the bleeding segment or bronchial artery embolization. It should be deflated for a few minutes three times a day, in order to preserve mucosal viability and to check for bleeding recurrence. Right heart balloon catheters have been used in a similar fashion (44). A modified technique for placement of a balloon catheter has been described using a guidewire for insertion. A 0.035-in soft-tipped guidewire is inserted through the working channel of the bronchoscope into the bleeding segment. The bronchoscope is withdrawn, leaving the guidewire in place. A balloon catheter is then inserted over the guidewire and placed under direct visualization after reintroduction of the bronchoscope (45). The use of endobronchial blockers developed for unilateral lung ventilation during surgery may hold promise for management of massive hemoptysis in tamponading bleeding and preventing contralateral aspiration of blood (46). The Arndt endobronchial blocker is placed through a standard ET and directly positioned with a pediatric bronchoscope. Suctioning and injection of medications can be performed through the lumen of the catheter after placement. The Cohen tip deflecting endobronchial blocker is also placed through a standard ET and directed into place with a self-contained steering mechanism under bronchoscopic visualization. At this time, there is limited published experience with these blockers in the setting of massive hemoptysis, although the author has successfully used them for this application.

Other Bronchoscopic Techniques

Additional bronchoscopic techniques may be useful as temporizing measures in patients with massive hemoptysis. Bronchoscopically administered topical therapies, such as iced sterile saline lavage or topical 1:10,000 or 1:20,000 epinephrine solution, may be helpful (47). Direct application of a solution of thrombin or a fibrinogen–thrombin combination solution has been used (48). The use of bronchoscopy-guided topical hemostatic tamponade therapy using oxidized regenerated cellulose mesh has recently been described (49). Endobronchial placement of a silicone spigot can prove adequate for temporary control of bleeding, allowing patients to stabilize before endovascular embolization (50). Successful tamponade and isolation of the bleeding site in patients with massive hemoptysis can be achieved by the placement of covered self-expanding airway stents blocking the orifice of the bleeding airway (51). Although anecdotal, the author has had success with topical application of a sodium bicarbonate solution.

For patients who have hemoptysis due to endobronchial lesions, particularly endobronchial tumors, hemostasis may be achieved with the use of neodymium:yttrium aluminum garnet (Nd:YAG) laser phototherapy, electrocautery, argon plasma coagulation (APC), or cryotherapy via the bronchoscope.

Angiography and Embolization

Angiography can identify the bleeding site in more than 90% of cases. As noted, the bronchial arteries are the most frequent source of bleeding in massive hemoptysis. In some cases, systemic vessels other than the bronchial arteries can be the source of bleeding (52). The pulmonary arteries may be the source for massive hemoptysis in 8% to 10% of cases (53). Visualization of extravasated dye from a vessel is relatively uncommon. Signs suggesting a particular vessel is the source of bleeding include vessel tortuosity, increased vessel diameter, and aneurysmal dilatation.

Bronchial artery embolization has been widely used to control massive hemoptysis, as a temporary measure to stabilize patients before surgical resection or medical treatment (antibiotics/antituberculous drugs) or as a definitive therapeutic approach in patients who refuse surgery, who are not considered as candidates for surgery (poor lung function, bilateral pulmonary disease, comorbidities), or patients in whom surgery is contraindicated. Bronchial artery embolization is considered the most effective nonsurgical modality for treatment of massive hemoptysis. The immediate success rates from bronchial artery embolization range from 51% to 100% (3,9,37,54–66). This wide range of success rates across multiple studies can be partially attributed to heterogeneity with regard to analysis of results with some series, including patients in whom bronchial artery cannot be canalized or that spinal artery was seen coming off the bronchial vessel preventing embolization in the final analysis (61). Embolization has been performed with Gelfoam, polyurethane particles, polyvinyl alcohol particles, and vascular coils. Sclerosing agents may cause subsequent lung necrosis and should be avoided. Recurrence of bleeding, although usually nonmassive, has been noted in 16% to 46% of patients (9,54). Recurrence of hemoptysis may be due to incomplete embolization of the bronchial vessels, recanalization of the embolized arteries, presence of nonbronchial systemic arteries, or development of collateral circulation in response to continuing pulmonary inflammation (60,67). Repeat embolization may be required in some patients (37,59,63,68). Complications include chest pain, fever, vessel perforation and intimal tears, and embolization of material to mesenteric and extremity arteries. The most serious complication is embolization of the anterior spinal artery, which may arise from the bronchial artery, with subsequent spinal artery infarction and paraparesis; the risk of this occurrence is less than 1%.

Rupture of the Pulmonary Artery

The pulmonary artery may potentially be ruptured from right heart catheterization. This complication should be suspected in patients who develop hemoptysis with a pulmonary artery catheter in place. Balloon tamponade and contralateral selective intubation should be performed (69). The catheter should be withdrawn 5 cm with the balloon deflated, and the balloon then reinflated with 2 mL of air and allowed to float back into the ruptured vessel to occlude it. Patients who stop bleeding should undergo angiographic evaluation to localize the tear and identify the formation of a pseudoaneurysm (34,70). If a pseudoaneurysm is identified, embolization of the affected vessel should be considered to prevent subsequent hemorrhage.

Surgery

Emergency surgery for control of massive hemoptysis is performed less often due to the advent of bronchial artery embolization. Mortality rates for surgical management of massive hemoptysis range from 1% to 50% (3,71–76). Surgical resection of the source of bleeding offers definitive treatment as long as the lesion can be completely resected and the patient is able to tolerate resectional surgery. It is often difficult to accurately determine if these patients will be able to tolerate surgery, as they are often too ill to undergo pulmonary function tests, or are intubated and thus unable to perform pulmonary function tests. Surgical resection may be considered in patients when bronchial artery embolization is unavailable, if bleeding continues despite embolization, or if the cause of the hemoptysis is unlikely to be controlled with embolization.

Surgery also remains the strategy of choice for the management of massive hemoptysis caused by diffuse and complex arteriovenous malformations, iatrogenic PA rupture, chest trauma, and mycetoma not responding to other therapeutic strategies, or associated with recurrent life-threatening hemoptysis as outlined above. Bronchovascular fistulae—with ensuing massive bleeding, is most often encountered following surgery, local infection, associated with vascular aneurysms and, less frequently, following lung transplantation surgery—are also managed by surgical repair once the patient is stabilized (1).

Diffuse Alveolar Hemorrhage

Patients with diffuse alveolar hemorrhage syndromes are not candidates for bronchial artery embolization or surgery; treatment for these groups of patients is pharmacologic. Corticosteroids are typically used and are effective for a wide range of the alveolar hemorrhage syndromes (77). Doses of 1 to 2 mg/kg/day of methylprednisolone have been most commonly used. For life-threatening alveolar hemorrhage, initial doses of 500 to 1,000 mg/day of methylprednisolone have been recommended. For Goodpasture disease, granulomatosis polyangiitis, and other vasculitides, adjunctive cytotoxic therapy or plasmapheresis may be considered.

PROGNOSIS

Factors associated with high mortality in patients with massive hemoptysis include a bleeding rate of at least 1,000 mL within a 24-hour period, aspiration of blood in the contralateral lung, massive bleeding requiring single lung ventilation, and bronchogenic carcinoma as an underlying etiology (3,6). Patients seem to fare better when tuberculosis, bronchitis, or bronchiectasis are responsible for the massive hemoptysis. Patients who experience recurrent bleeding following embolization for massive hemoptysis have significantly higher mortality (78). Overall mortality rates for massive hemoptysis range from 9% to 38% (58,61,79), with significant reduction in mortality in recent years since bronchial artery embolization is considered as first-line therapy.

INTERVENTIONAL BRONCHOSCOPY

Interventional bronchoscopy is a field that utilizes minimally invasive techniques for the management of a variety of tracheobronchial disorders. There are a number of circumstances for which interventional bronchoscopy has application in the ICU. The most common need for such procedures arises from central airway obstruction (CAO), both malignant and benign in etiology. Other potential situations that interventional bronchoscopy may be of benefit include management of hemoptysis and management of persistent airleaks.

Malignant Airway Obstruction

CAO from malignancy may arise from endoluminal tumor, submucosal tumor infiltration, extrinsic compression by a tumor mass, extrinsic compression by malignant mediastinal adenopathy, or a combination of these pathologies. Bronchogenic carcinoma is the most common cause of malignant airway obstruction. The exact prevalence of airway obstruction in patients with lung cancer is not clear although it has been estimated that 20% to 30% of patients will develop large airway obstruction (80). Patients with other malignancies may also develop endobronchial metastases. Cancers of the thyroid, colon, breast, kidney, and esophagus as well as melanoma have been most commonly noted to cause endobronchial metastases. As a result of the airway obstruction, patients may experience respiratory distress, hypoxemia, or frank respiratory failure requiring mechanical ventilation. Postobstructive pneumonia may also occur.

Benign Airway Obstruction

Patients may develop tracheal stenosis or tracheal webs following endotracheal intubation. The reported incidence ranges from 10% to 22%, although only 1% to 2% of patients are symptomatic or have severe stenosis (81). Most stenoses occur at the site of the ET cuff, thought to be due to decreased regional blood flow as a result of pressure of the cuff on the tracheal wall. A similar incidence has been reported following tracheostomy tube placement (82). While patients may develop stenoses or webs at the site of the tracheostomy tube cuff, tracheal stenosis following tracheostomy tube placement typically occurs around the tracheal stomal site. This is thought secondary to abnormal wound healing with excess granulation tissue formation around the tracheal stoma (81). In addition, patients may develop focal tracheomalacia at the level of the stoma secondary to cartilaginous damage (dynamic A-shaped tracheal stenosis) (83). Patients may also develop airway obstruction secondary to granulation tissue above the tracheostomy tube and at the tip of the tracheostomy tube. Finally, patients may also develop tracheal or bronchial stenosis as a consequence of systemic disease, such as granulomatous polyangiitis (Wegener granulomatosis), relapsing polychondritis, sarcoidosis, and tracheobronchial amyloidosis. In about 3% to 5% of cases of tracheal stenosis, there is no known inciting process for the development of the stenosis and such cases are labeled idiopathic (84).

Expiratory central airway collapse—comprises two separate entities: tracheobronchomalacia (TBM), characterized by weakness of the airway cartilages, and excessive dynamic airway collapse (EDAC)—which is defined as excessive bulging of the posterior membrane into the airway lumen during expiration without cartilage collapse—may produce significant airway obstruction (85). Focal tracheomalacia may result from prolonged intubation, tracheostomy tube placement, vascular abnormalities such as vascular rings, and space occupying lesions of the mediastinum such as a large thyroid goiter. Focal tracheomalacia and bronchomalacia can occur following radiation therapy; diffuse TBM can result from relapsing polychondritis, and EDAC is associated with COPD, asthma, and obesity.

History and Evaluation

Symptoms depend on the location and degree of airway narrowing as well as concurrent thoracic pathology. Dyspnea is the most common symptom. Dyspnea on exertion typically occurs when the tracheal diameter is reduced to 8 mm; stridor may be noted when the tracheal diameter decreases to 5 mm (86). Airway narrowing of this degree increases susceptibility to acute obstruction from mucus plugs or blood clots. This is thought to be the reason why 50% of these patients present with acute respiratory distress. CT may be used as the initial evaluation modality for tracheobronchial obstruction. MDCT with thin collimation (0.6–1.5 mm) over the entire chest during a single breath hold at full inspiration allows acquisition of volumetric high resolution data sets. Reconstruction of axial overlapped thin slices permits multiplanar reformations of high quality. CT is useful for diagnosing the nature of the obstruction, identifying the precise anatomical location, the characteristics of the lesion, and the extent of disease, including distal airway patency and local vascular anatomy (87,88). Multiplanar reformations in sagittal, coronal, or oblique planes eliminate the known limitation of axial images including detection of subtle airway stenoses, underestimation of the longitudinal extent of narrowing, inadequate evaluation of the airways oriented obliquely to the axial plane, and the difficulty in displaying complex three-dimensional anatomy of the airways. In addition, virtual bronchoscopy imaging can be performed using CT images constructed during postprocessing. Flexible bronchoscopy can be used as a diagnostic modality although ideally bronchoscopy, either flexible or rigid, is performed in conjunction with a bronchoscopic therapeutic intervention. Caution should be taken in performing bronchoscopy in high-grade tracheal or bilateral mainstem obstruction if an interventional pulmonologist/thoracic surgeon is not available as a diagnostic bronchoscopy may precipitate acute, complete airway occlusion.

Interventional Bronchoscopy Techniques

Various interventional bronchoscopy modalities are available to manage malignant or benign CAO. Mechanical debulking and dilatation may be performed with a rigid bronchoscope to relieve obstruction from endoluminal tumor as well as benign stenoses. Rigid bronchoscopy may also be used in conjunction with other ablative modalities, and has some advantages over interventions performed via flexible bronchoscopy including the ability to ventilate the patient through the rigid bronchoscope, use of larger suction catheters to manage blood in the airway, and use of larger forceps to remove tumor and debris.

A variety of ablative techniques are available for relieving obstruction from endoluminal tumor (Table 116.3). Laser, electrocautery, and APC utilize heat thermal energy for tissue destruction. Microdebriders have been used in conjunction with rigid bronchoscopy for mechanical debulking; these

TABLE 116.3 Comparison of Ablative Modalities

Therapy	Mechanism of Action	Advantages	Disadvantages
Nd:YAG laser	Noncontact, thermal energy from laser light	Deep tissue penetration and hemostasis, good for major tissue debulking	Potential damage to adjacent tissue
Nd:YAP laser	Noncontact, thermal energy from laser light	Better hemostasis than that of Nd:YAG laser	Less tissue penetration than that of Nd:YAG laser
Carbon dioxide laser	Noncontact, thermal energy from laser light	More precise ablation than that of other lasers, shallow penetration	Minimal hemostasis, bulky equipment limits use in airways
Argon plasma coagulation	Noncontact, thermal energy from ionized argon gas	Good hemostasis, preferential flow to uncoagulated tissue, bends around corners	Shallow penetration, not ideal for major tissue debulking
Electrocautery	Contact, thermal electrical energy	Inexpensive, multiple accessory types for different situations, good hemostasis	Requires frequent cleaning of contact device, less precision than laser
Cryotherapy	Repeated cycles of freezing and thawing	Good for foreign body removal, no risk of airway fire	Not for acute airway use due to delayed tissue destruction, requires follow-up bronchoscopic tissue removal
Brachytherapy	Direct implantation of radiation source into/next to target lesion	Concentrated, long lasting, localized tissue effect	Not for acute airway use due to delayed tissue destruction, higher risk of hemorrhage and other complications
Photodynamic therapy	Preferential uptake of photosensitizer by malignant cells with nonthermal laser-activated phototoxic reaction	Potentially curative for early mucosal squamous cell cancers	Not for acute airway use due to delayed tissue destruction, requires follow-up bronchoscopic tissue removal, 4–6 wks of skin photosensitivity
Microdebrider	Mechanical removal of tissue by rotating blade and suction	No risk of airway fire	Device length limits to proximal airway use

Nd:YAG, neodymium:yttrium aluminum garnet; Nd:YAP, neodymium:yttrium aluminum perovskite. Adapted from Hsia D, Musani AI. Interventional pulmonology. *Med Clin North Am.* 2011;95(6):1095–1114.

TABLE 116.4 Results of Interventional Pulmonary Procedures in Patients Requiring Mechanical Ventilation

Author	Number of Patients on MV	Cause of CAO	Interventional Modality	Successfully Liberated from MV
Stanopoulos et al., 1993 (98)	17	Malignant	Laser	9/17
Saad et al., 2003 (99)	16	Malignant 8 Benign 8	Stent	14/16
Zannini et al., 1994 (100)	6	Malignant 1 Benign 5	Stent	6/6
Colt and Harrell, 1997 (101)	19	Malignant 11 Benign 8	Laser and/or dilatation and/or stent	10/19
Shaffer and Allen, 1998 (102)	8	Malignant 6 Benign 2	Stent	7/8
Chan et al., 2002 (103)	4	Malignant	Stent	4/4
Lippman et al., 2002 (104)	3	Malignant 2 Benign 1	Stent	3/3
Lin et al., 2008 (105)	26	Malignant 21 Benign 5	Stent	14/26
Razi et al., 2010 (106)	7	Malignant	Stent ± electrocautery	3/7
Murgu et al., 2012 (107)	12	Malignant	Laser and/or stent	9/12

CAO, central airway obstruction; MV, mechanical ventilation.

debriders are composed of a serrated blade rotating at 1,000 to 3,000 rpm attached to a hollow suction tube (89). These modalities, as well as mechanical debulking with the rigid bronchoscope, have the advantage of achieving immediate airway patency. Either silicone or self-expanding metal stents will often be placed to maintain airway patency once the airway is de-obstructed. Other techniques such as standard cryotherapy, brachytherapy, and photodynamic therapy have the disadvantages of not achieving immediate airway patency and thus would not be the procedures of choice for patients in the ICU with CAO. A modification of the method of cryotherapy, referred to as cryorecanalization, is able to achieve immediate airway patency, however (90).

For benign tracheal or bronchial stenosis, dilatation with the rigid bronchoscope or balloon bronchoplasty via rigid or flexible bronchoscopy may be performed (91). In some cases laser, electrocautery, or APC may be used as an adjunct to mechanical/balloon dilatation (92,93); some patients may require future repeat procedures. For patients who require repeated dilatation procedures, surgical intervention should be considered (94). If surgery is not feasible or contraindicated due to medical comorbidities, stent placement may be considered, although some clinicians prefer a trial of temporary stent placement before considering surgery. In general, silicone stents should be used for benign stenoses although the authors have had good success with the use of fully covered, self-expanding, metal stents that can be easily removed, similar to silicone stents.

For patients with TBM and EDAC causing respiratory failure, stent insertion can be considered to allow liberation from mechanical ventilation. Complications related to long-term stent placement in these patient populations are not insignificant however. Self-expanding metal stents can potentially fracture and cause granulation tissue. If uncovered metallic stents are used, removal at a later time if complications develop can be challenging. Silicone stents do not have issues with fracturing, but can cause granulation tissue and can migrate if a standard tracheal stent is used; a silicone Y stent is most commonly used in these patients. Consideration should be given for surgical management with tracheobronchoplasty once the patient is stabilized (85). Patients with focal tracheal cartilaginous malacia due to prolonged intubation or tracheostomy tube should typically not be managed with stent placement, as the need for the stent will be lifelong, and eventual complications are likely. Patients should be evaluated for resection of the pathologic segment and end-to-end anastomosis (95). If the patient is not a candidate for surgery, placement of a tracheostomy tube to bypass the segment may be required.

Outcomes for Airway Interventions in the ICU

Interventional bronchoscopy procedures can be successful in allowing patients to be liberated from mechanical ventilation (Table 116.4). Likewise, in a study by Noppen et al. 15 patients, who were ventilator/artificial airway dependent patients, were treated for airway obstruction after being referred for failed attempts at weaning from mechanical ventilation or from their tracheostomy cannula (96). All patients had benign disease, with most patients having postintubation tracheal stenosis or tracheomalacia. Median duration of mechanical ventilation prior to referral was 30 days (range, 7–105 days); 14 of the 15 patients were extubated/decannulated immediately following the intervention. Similarly, 36 patients with respiratory failure or impending respiratory failure due to malignant airway obstruction were treated emergently by Jeon et al. (97); of the 36 patients, 34 had a successful outcome. Overall survival ranged from 3 days to 69 months with a median of 23.6 months. Interventional bronchoscopy can have a significant impact on critically ill patients with CAO and may allow for successful withdrawal from mechanical ventilation, hospitalization in a lower level of care environment, relief of symptoms, and extended survival.

Key Points

- Massive hemoptysis is defined as expectoration of blood exceeding 200 to 1,000 mL in 24 hours.
- Bleeding in massive hemoptysis originates from bronchial and pulmonary arteries in 90% and 5% of cases respectively.

- CT scan with contrast helps localize bleeding in 63% to 100% of cases with massive hemoptysis and should be the investigation of choice if patients can tolerate the transport and are stable enough.
- The initial priority in management should be to protect the airway and stabilize the patient.
- Endobronchial balloon tamponade can be used to prevent aspiration of blood into the contralateral lung, preserve gas exchange, and can be used as a temporizing measure until more definitive management is instituted.
- Bronchial artery embolization is the most effective nonsurgical modality for treatment of massive hemoptysis, with success rates varying between 51% and 100%.
- Mortality rates for surgical management of massive hemoptysis range from 1% to 50% and should be considered only as a salvage therapy in the current era of minimally invasive approaches, that is, embolization and advanced bronchoscopic therapies.
- Caution should be taken in performing bronchoscopy in high-grade tracheal or bilateral mainstem obstruction if an interventional pulmonologist/thoracic surgeon is not available, as a diagnostic bronchoscopy may precipitate acute, complete airway occlusion.
- Interventional bronchoscopy can have a significant impact on critically ill patients with CAO and may allow for successful withdrawal from mechanical ventilation, hospitalization in a lower level of care environment, relief of symptoms, and extended survival.

References

1. Jean Baptiste E. Clinical assessment and management of massive hemoptysis. *Crit Care Med.* 2000;28(5):1642–1647.
2. Garzon AA, Cerruti MM, Golding ME. Exsanguinating hemoptysis. *J Thorac Cardiovasc Surg.* 1982;84(6):829–833.
3. Corey R, Hla KM. Major and massive hemoptysis: reassessment of conservative management. *Am J Med Sci.* 1987;294(5):301–309.
4. Hirshberg B, Biran I, Glazer M, Kramer MR. Hemoptysis: etiology, evaluation, and outcome in a tertiary referral hospital. *Chest.* 1997;112(2): 440–444.
5. Johnston H, Reisz G. Changing spectrum of hemoptysis: underlying causes in 148 patients undergoing diagnostic flexible fiberoptic bronchoscopy. *Arch Intern Med.* 1989;149(7):1666–1668.
6. Garzon AA, Gourin A. Surgical management of massive hemoptysis: a ten year experience. *Ann Surg.* 1978;187(3):267–271.
7. Bruzzi JF, Rémy-Jardin M, Delhaye D, et al. Multi detector row CT of hemoptysis. *Radiographics.* 2006;26(1):3–22.
8. McDonald DM. Angiogenesis and remodeling of airway vasculature in chronic inflammation. *Am J Respir Crit Care Med.* 2001;164(10 Pt 2): S39–S45.
9. Yoon W, Kim JK, Kim YH, et al. Bronchial and nonbronchial systemic artery embolization for life threatening hemoptysis: a comprehensive review. *Radiographics.* 2002;22(6):1395–1409.
10. Jaitovich A, Harmath C, Cuttica M. Pulmonary vein stenosis and hemoptysis. *Am J Respir Crit Care Med.* 2012;185(9):1023.
11. Park MS. Diffuse alveolar hemorrhage. *Tuberc Respir Dis (Seoul).* 2013; 74(4):151–162.
12. Noe GD, Jaffe SM, Molan MP. CT and CT angiography in massive haemoptysis with emphasis on pre embolization assessment. *Clin Radiol.* 2011;66(9):869–875.
13. Adelman M, Haponik EF, Bleecker ER, et al. Cryptogenic hemoptysis: clinical features, bronchoscopic findings, and natural history in 67 patients. *Ann Intern Med.* 1985;102(6):829–834.
14. Chang YC, Patz EF Jr, Goodman PC, Granger CB. Significance of hemoptysis following thrombolytic therapy for acute myocardial infarction. *Chest.* 1996;109(3):727–729.
15. al-Majed SA, Ashour M, al-Mobeireek AF, et al. Overlooked inhaled foreign bodies: late sequelae and the likelihood of recovery. *Respir Med.* 1997;91(5):293–296.
16. Thompson JW, Nguyen CD, Lazar RH, et al. Evaluation and management of hemoptysis in infants and children: a report of nine cases. *Ann Otol Rhinol Laryngol.* 1996;105(7):516–520.
17. Frankel SK, Cosgrove GP, Fischer A, et al. Update in the diagnosis and management of pulmonary vasculitis. *Chest.* 2006;129(2):452–465.
18. Ball JA, Young KR Jr. Pulmonary manifestations of Goodpasture's syndrome. Antiglomerular basement membrane disease and related disorders. *Clin Chest Med.* 1998;19(4):777–791, ix.
19. Zamora MR, Warner ML, Tuder R, Schwarz MI. Diffuse alveolar hemorrhage and systemic lupus erythematosus: clinical presentation, histology, survival, and outcome. *Medicine (Balt).* 1997;76(3):192–202.
20. Afessa, B, Tefferi A, Litzow MR, et al. Diffuse alveolar hemorrhage in hematopoietic stem cell transplant recipients. *Am J Respir Crit Care Med.* 2002;166(5):641–645.
21. Allan JS, Wright CD. Tracheoinnominate fistula: diagnosis and management. *Chest Surg Clin North Am.* 2003;13(2):331–341.
22. Epstein SK. Late complications of tracheostomy. *Respir Care.* 2005;50(4): 542–549.
23. Bussieres JS. Iatrogenic pulmonary artery rupture. *Curr Opin Anaesthesiol.* 2007;20(1):48–52.
24. Abreu AR, Campos MA, Krieger BP. Pulmonary artery rupture induced by a pulmonary artery catheter: a case report and review of the literature. *J Intensive Care Med.* 2004;19(5):291–296.
25. Naidich DP, Funt S, Ettenger NA, Arranda C. Hemoptysis: CT bronchoscopic correlations in 58 cases. *Radiology.* 1990;177(2):357–362.
26. Marshall TJ, Flower CD, Jackson JE. The role of radiology in the investigation and management of patients with haemoptysis. *Clin Radiol.* 1996; 51(6):391–400.
27. Hsiao EI, Kirsch CM, Kagawa FT, et al. Utility of fiberoptic bronchoscopy before bronchial artery embolization for massive hemoptysis. *AJR Am J Roentgenol.* 2001;177(4):861–867.
28. Stanford W, Galvin JR. The diagnosis of bronchiectasis. *Clin Chest Med.* 1988;9(4):691–699.
29. Lee YR, Choi YW, Lee KJ, et al. CT halo sign: the spectrum of pulmonary diseases. *Br J Radiol.* 2005;78(933):862–865.
30. Franquet T, Müller NL, Giménez A, et al. Spectrum of pulmonary aspergillosis: histologic, clinical, and radiologic findings. *Radiographics.* 2001; 21(4):825–837.
31. McGuinness G, Beacher JR, Harkin TJ, et al. Hemoptysis: prospective high resolution CT/bronchoscopic correlation. *Chest.* 1994;105(4):1155–1162.
32. Revel MP, Fournier LS, Hennebicque AS, et al. Can CT replace bronchoscopy in the detection of the site and cause of bleeding in patients with large or massive hemoptysis? *AJR Am J Roentgenol.* 2002;179(5):1217–1224.
33. Saumench J, Escarrabill J, Padró L, et al. Value of fiberoptic bronchoscopy and angiography for diagnosis of the bleeding site in hemoptysis. *Ann Thorac Surg.* 1989;48(2):272–274.
34. Bartter T, Irwin RS, Phillips DA, et al. Pulmonary artery pseudoaneurysm. A potential complication of pulmonary artery catheterization. *Arch Intern Med.* 1988;148(2):471–473.
35. Gourin A, Garzon AA. Operative treatment of massive hemoptysis. *Ann Thorac Surg.* 1974;18(1):52–60.
36. Pursel SE, Lindskog GE. Hemoptysis. A clinical evaluation of 105 patients examined consecutively on a thoracic surgical service. *Am Rev Respir Dis.* 1961;84:329–336.
37. Brinson GM, Noone PG, Mauro MA, et al. Bronchial artery embolization for the treatment of hemoptysis in patients with cystic fibrosis. *Am J Respir Crit Care Med.* 1998;157(6 Pt 1):1951–1958.
38. Khalil A, Fartoukh M, Tassart M, et al. Role of MDCT in identification of the bleeding site and the vessels causing hemoptysis. *AJR Am J Roentgenol.* 2007;188(2):W117–W125.
39. Dweik RA, Stoller JK. Role of bronchoscopy in massive hemoptysis. *Clin Chest Med.* 1999;20(1):89–105.
40. Ridley RW, Zwischenberger JB. Tracheoinnominate fistula: surgical management of an iatrogenic disaster. *J Laryngol Otol.* 2006;120(8):676–680.
41. Gottlieb LS, Hillberg R. Endobronchial tamponade therapy for intractable hemoptysis. *Chest.* 1975;67(4):482–483.
42. Saw EC, Gottlieb LS, Yokoyama T, Lee BC. Flexible fiberoptic bronchoscopy and endobronchial tamponade in the management of massive hemoptysis. *Chest.* 1976;70(5):589–591.
43. Lee SM., Kim HY, Ahn Y. Parallel technique of endobronchial balloon catheter tamponade for transient alleviation of massive hemoptysis. *J Korean Med Sci.* 2002;17(6):823–825.

44. Jolliet P, Soccal P, Chevrolet JC. Control of massive hemoptysis by endobronchial tamponade with a pulmonary artery balloon catheter. *Crit Care Med.* 1992;20(12):1730–1732.
45. Kato R, Sawafuji M, Kawamura M, et al. Massive hemoptysis successfully treated by modified bronchoscopic balloon tamponade technique. *Chest.* 1996;109(3):842–843.
46. Kabon B, Waltl B, Leitgeb J, et al. First experience with fiberoptically directed wire guided endobronchial blockade in severe pulmonary bleeding in an emergency setting. *Chest.* 2001;120(4):1399–1402.
47. Conlan AA, Hurwitz SS. Management of massive haemoptysis with the rigid bronchoscope and cold saline lavage. *Thorax.* 1980;35(12):901–904.
48. Tsukamoto T, Sasaki H, Nakamura H. Treatment of hemoptysis patients by thrombin and fibrinogen thrombin infusion therapy using a fiberoptic bronchoscope. *Chest.* 1989;96(3):473–476.
49. Valipour A, Kreuzer A, Koller H, et al. Bronchoscopy guided topical hemostatic tamponade therapy for the management of life threatening hemoptysis. *Chest.* 2005;127(6):2113–2118.
50. Dutau, H, Palot A, Haas A, et al. Endobronchial embolization with a silicone spigot as a temporary treatment for massive hemoptysis: a new bronchoscopic approach of the disease. *Respiration.* 2006;73(6):830–832.
51. Brandes JC, Schmidt E, Yung R. Occlusive endobronchial stent placement as a novel management approach to massive hemoptysis from lung cancer. *J Thorac Oncol.* 2008;3(9):1071–1072.
52. Keller FS, Rosch J, Loflin TG, et al. Nonbronchial systemic collateral arteries: significance in percutaneous embolotherapy for hemoptysis. *Radiology.* 1987;164(3):687–692.
53. Rabkin JE, Astafjev VI, Gothman LN, Grigorjev YG. Transcatheter embolization in the management of pulmonary hemorrhage. *Radiology.* 1987;163(2):361–365.
54. Hsu AA. Thoracic embolotherapy for life threatening haemoptysis: a pulmonologist's perspective. *Respirology.* 2005;10(2):138–143.
55. Park HS, Kim YI, Kim HY, et al. Bronchial artery and systemic artery embolization in the management of primary lung cancer patients with hemoptysis. *Cardiovasc Intervent Radiol.* 2007;30(4):638–643.
56. Poyanli A, Acunas B, Rozanes I, et al. Endovascular therapy in the management of moderate and massive haemoptysis. *Br J Radiol.* 2007; 80(953):331–336.
57. Vidal V, Therasse E, Berthiaume Y, et al. Bronchial artery embolization in adults with cystic fibrosis: impact on the clinical course and survival. *J Vasc Interv Radiol.* 2006;17(6):953–958.
58. Ong TH, Eng P. Massive hemoptysis requiring intensive care. *Intensive Care Med.* 2003;29(2):317–320.
59. Yu Tang Goh P, Lin M, Teo N, En Shen Wong D. Embolization for hemoptysis: a six year review. *Cardiovasc Intervent Radiol.* 2002;25(1):17–25.
60. Swanson KL, Johnson CM, Prakash UB, et al. Bronchial artery embolization: experience with 54 patients. *Chest.* 2002;121(3):789–795.
61. Mal H, Rullon I, Mellot F, et al. Immediate and long term results of bronchial artery embolization for life threatening hemoptysis. *Chest.* 1999;115(4):996–1001.
62. Tanaka N, Yamakado K, Murashima S, et al. Superselective bronchial artery embolization for hemoptysis with a coaxial microcatheter system. *J Vasc Interv Radiol.* 1997;8(1 Pt 1):65–70.
63. Ramakantan R, Bandekar VG, Gandhi MS, et al. Massive hemoptysis due to pulmonary tuberculosis: control with bronchial artery embolization. *Radiology.* 1996;200(3):691–694.
64. Zhang JS, Cui ZP, Wang MQ, Yang L. Bronchial arteriography and transcatheter embolization in the management of hemoptysis. *Cardiovasc Intervent Radiol.* 1994;17(5):276–279.
65. Hayakawa K, Cui ZP, Wang MQ, et al. Bronchial artery embolization for hemoptysis: immediate and long term results. *Cardiovasc Intervent Radiol.* 1992;15(3):154–158.
66. Uflacker R, Kaemmerer A, Picon PD, et al. Bronchial artery embolization in the management of hemoptysis: technical aspects and long term results. *Radiology.* 1985;157(3):637–644.
67. Cremaschi P, Nascimbene C, Vitulo P, et al. Therapeutic embolization of bronchial artery: a successful treatment in 209 cases of relapse hemoptysis. *Angiology.* 1993;44(4):295–299.
68. Katoh O, Kishikawa T, Yamada H, et al. Recurrent bleeding after arterial embolization in patients with hemoptysis. *Chest.* 1990;97(3):541–546.
69. Thomas R, Siproudhis L, Laurent JF, et al. Massive hemoptysis from iatrogenic balloon catheter rupture of pulmonary artery: successful early management by balloon tamponade. *Crit Care Med.* 1987;15(3):272–273.
70. Dieden JD, Friloux LA 3rd, Renner JW. Pulmonary artery false aneurysms secondary to Swan Ganz pulmonary artery catheters. *AJR Am J Roentgenol.* 1987;149(5):901–906.
71. Garzon AA, Cerruti M, Gourin A, Karlson KE. Pulmonary resection for massive hemoptysis. *Surgery.* 1970;67(4):633–638.
72. Gourin A, Garzon AA. Control of hemorrhage in emergency pulmonary resection for massive hemoptysis. *Chest.* 1975;68(1):120–121.
73. Sehhat, S, Oreizie M, Moinedine K. Massive pulmonary hemorrhage: surgical approach as choice of treatment. *Ann Thorac Surg.* 1978;25(1): 12–15.
74. Endo S, Otani S, Saito N, et al. Management of massive hemoptysis in a thoracic surgical unit. *Eur J Cardiothorac Surg.* 2003;23(4):467—472.
75. Jougon J, Ballester M, Delcambre F, et al. Massive hemoptysis: what place for medical and surgical treatment. *Eur J Cardiothorac Surg.* 2002;22(3): 345–351.
76. Lee TW, Wan S, Choy DK, et al. Management of massive hemoptysis: a single institution experience. *Ann Thorac Cardiovasc Surg.* 2000;6(4): 232–235.
77. Jantz MA, Sahn SA. Corticosteroids in acute respiratory failure. *Am J Respir Crit Care Med.* 1999;160(4):1079–1100.
78. van den Heuvel MM, Els Z, Koegelenberg CF, et al. Risk factors for recurrence of haemoptysis following bronchial artery embolisation for life threatening haemoptysis. *Int J Tuberc Lung Dis.* 2007;11(8): 909–914.
79. Knott Craig CJ, Oostuizen JG, Rossouw G, et al. Management and prognosis of massive hemoptysis: recent experience with 120 patients. *J Thorac Cardiovasc Surg.* 1993;105(3):394–397.
80. Ginsberg RJ, Ruben A. Non–small cell lung cancer. In: DeVita VT, Hellman S, Rosenberg SA, eds. *Cancer Principles and Practice of Oncology.* Philadelphia, PA: Lippincott Raven; 1997:858–911.
81. Zias N, Chroneou A, Tabba MK, et al. Post tracheostomy and post intubation tracheal stenosis: report of 31 cases and review of the literature. *BMC Pulm Med.* 2008;8:18.
82. Walz MK, Peitgen K, Thürauf N, et al. Percutaneous dilatational tracheostomy: early results and long term outcome of 326 critically ill patients. *Intensive Care Med.* 1998;24(7):685–690.
83. Plojoux J, Laroumagne S, Vandemoortele T, et al. Management of benign dynamic "A shape" tracheal stenosis: a retrospective study of 60 patients. *Ann Thorac Surg.* 2015;99(2):447–453.
84. Perotin JM, Jeanfaivre T, Thibout Y, et al. Endoscopic management of idiopathic tracheal stenosis. *Ann Thorac Surg.* 2011;92(1):297–301.
85. Murgu S, Colt H. Tracheobronchomalacia and excessive dynamic airway collapse. *Clin Chest Med.* 2013;34(3):527–555.
86. Hollingsworth HM. Wheezing and stridor. *Clin Chest Med.* 1987;8(2): 231–240.
87. Grenier PA, Beigelman-Aubry C, Brillet PY. Nonneoplastic tracheal and bronchial stenoses. *Radiol Clin North Am.* 2009;47(2):243–260.
88. Ferretti GR, Bithigoffer C, Righini CA, et al. Imaging of tumors of the trachea and central bronchi. *Radiol Clin North Am.* 2009;47(2): 227–241.
89. Lunn W, Garland R, Ashiku S, et al. Microdebrider bronchoscopy: a new tool for the interventional bronchoscopist. *Ann Thorac Surg.* 2005; 80(4):1485–1488.
90. Schumann C, Hetzel M, Babiak AJ, et al. Endobronchial tumor debulking with a flexible cryoprobe for immediate treatment of malignant stenosis. *J Thorac Cardiovasc Surg.* 2010;139(4):997–1000.
91. Shitrit D, Kuchuk M, Zismanov V, et al. Bronchoscopic balloon dilatation of tracheobronchial stenosis: long term follow up. *Eur J Cardiothorac Surg.* 2010;38(2):198–202.
92. Cavaliere S, Bezzi M, Toninelli C, et al. Management of post intubation tracheal stenoses using the endoscopic approach. *Monaldi Arch Chest Dis.* 2007;67(2):73–80.
93. Galluccio G, Lucantoni G, Battistoni P, et al. Interventional endoscopy in the management of benign tracheal stenoses: definitive treatment at long term follow up. *Eur J Cardiothorac Surg.* 2009;35(3):429–433.
94. Wain JC Jr. Postintubation tracheal stenosis. *Semin Thorac Cardiovasc Surg.* 2009. 21(3):284–289.
95. Stoelben E, Koryllos A, Beckers F, Ludwig C. Benign stenosis of the trachea. *Thorac Surg Clin.* 2014;24(1):59–65.
96. Noppen M, Stratakos G, Amjadi K, et al. Stenting allows weaning and extubation in ventilator or tracheostomy dependency secondary to benign airway disease. *Respir Med.* 2007;101(1):139–145.
97. Jeon K, Kim H, Yu CM, et al. Rigid bronchoscopic intervention in patients with respiratory failure caused by malignant central airway obstruction. *J Thorac Oncol.* 2006;1(4):319–23.
98. Stanopoulos IT, Beamis JF Jr, Martinez FJ, et al. Laser bronchoscopy in respiratory failure from malignant airway obstruction. *Crit Care Med.* 1993;21(3):386–391.

99. Saad CP, Murthy S, Krizmanich G, et al. Self expandable metallic airway stents and flexible bronchoscopy: long term outcomes analysis. *Chest.* 2003;124(5):1993–1999.
100. Zannini P, Melloni G, Chiesa G, Carretta A. Self expanding stents in the treatment of tracheobronchial obstruction. *Chest.* 1994;106(1):86–90.
101. Colt HG, JH Harrell. Therapeutic rigid bronchoscopy allows level of care changes in patients with acute respiratory failure from central airways obstruction. *Chest.* 1997;112(1):202–206.
102. Shaffer JP, Allen JN. The use of expandable metal stents to facilitate extubation in patients with large airway obstruction. *Chest.* 1998;114(5): 1378–1382.
103. Chan KP, Eng P, Hsu AA, et al. Rigid bronchoscopy and stenting for esophageal cancer causing airway obstruction. *Chest.* 2002;122(3):1069–1072.
104. Lippman M, Eiger G. Utility of tracheobronchial stents in mechanically ventilated patients with central airway obstruction. *J Bronchol Interv Pulmonol.* 2002;9:301–305.
105. Lin SM, Lin TY, Chou CL, et al. Metallic stent and flexible bronchoscopy without fluoroscopy for acute respiratory failure. *Eur Respir J.* 2008;31(5):1019–1023.
106. Razi SS, Lebovics RS, Schwartz G, et al. Timely airway stenting improves survival in patients with malignant central airway obstruction. *Ann Thorac Surg.* 2010;90(4):1088–1093.
107. Murgu S, Langer S, Colt H. Bronchoscopic intervention obviates the need for continued mechanical ventilation in patients with airway obstruction and respiratory failure from inoperable non small cell lung cancer. *Respiration.* 2012;84(1):55–61.

CHAPTER
117

Neurologic Injury: Prevention and Initial Care

CHERYLEE W. J. CHANG

INTRODUCTION

Traumatic Brain Injury

Traumatic brain injury (TBI) is defined as a disruption in the normal function of the brain or other evidence of brain pathology caused by an external force including a bump, blow, acceleration or deceleration forces, blast, or penetrating injury (1–3). Worldwide, TBI is the leading cause of death and disability in children and young adults and is involved in nearly half of all trauma-related deaths (1).

In the United States, unintentional injury is also the leading cause of death between age 1 and 44 years (4). In 2010, 2.5 million people sustained a TBI (2); of those, an estimated 280,000 were hospitalized, and over 50,000 died. Over the period of 2001 to 2010 in the United States, TBI-related emergency department (ED) visits increased by 70%, although the hospitalization rate only increased by 11%, and death rates decreased by 7% (5). Estimates of the global incidence of hospitalizations due to TBI is highest in Sweden with approximately 450, Brazil with 360, South Africa with 320, the United States with 92, and Pakistan with 50 cases/100,000 people/yr (6). A meta-analysis of reports from 23 European countries reported an incidence of 235 cases/100,000 people/yr (7).

The average TBI-associated mortality rate in Europe is estimated to be 15 deaths/100,000 population/yr (7) compared to 10 in Scandinavia, 20 in India, 30 in the United States, 38 in the Province of Taiwan in China, 81 in South Africa, and 120 in Columbia (8).

Globally, males have at least double the risk of TBI compared to females (1,9). In the United States in 2010, the rate of TBI-related death was more than two times higher in men than in women (25.4 in males vs. 9.0/100,000 in females). Death rates were highest in persons aged 65 years or older at 45.2/100,000 population (10).

Worldwide, the leading cause of head injury is road traffic accidents, which account for 40% to 50% of hospitalizations due to TBI (1). The World Health Organization (WHO) estimates that 3,000 people die daily and 30,000 people are seriously injured on the roads and nearly half suffer head injury; most are from low- or middle-income countries and are pedestrians, cyclists, motorcyclists, and bus passengers (11). In Australia, India, Northern Europe, and the United States, the leading causes of TBI are due to falls (7,12). In the United States, falls account for 40.5% of TBI; while 15.5% of TBI are due to "struck by/against" events, which include colliding with a moving or stationary object; 14.3% are from motor vehicle crashes (MVC) and 10.7% from assault; the remainder are not documented (13). The youngest (age 0–4 years) and oldest (age >65 years) are at highest risk for falls at 72.8% and 81.8% respectively (13).

The leading cause of TBI-related death also varies by age. In the United States, falls were the leading cause of death for persons over 65 years, assault for those under 4 years, and MVC for those between 5 and 24 years (13). For mechanism of injury, firearm-inflicted TBI has the highest mortality at 90.4% compared with 10.2% associated with falls (14,15).

In the military population, mild TBI or concussion is the most common traumatic injury with most occurring in the garrison or home station environment (16). However, during combat, TBI is often due to blast injuries with concussion, contusion, subdural hematoma (SDH), and axonal shear injury as a result (17). During the recent wars, 81% of injuries in Afghanistan and Iraq were explosion related compared to 65% in Vietnam, and 73% during World War II (18).

The economic impact includes the direct cost of hospitalization, outpatient and rehabilitation, and indirect costs for lost productivity both of the patient and caregiver. There are other less tangible social and psychological costs to the patient, family and friends related to death or the reduced quality of life. Over 5.3 million Americans require assistance with activities of daily living (ADL) as a consequence of the long-term effects on cognition and behavior with emotional and physical impairment following TBI (2,19,20). In the United States, lifetime costs of TBI, including medical costs and lost productivity, have been estimated at $60 billion annually (21).

Acute Spinal Cord Injury

Acute spinal cord injury (ASCI) represents another form of neurologic injury that can result in significant disability. The incidence of ASCI averages 54 cases/million population/yr, or about 17,000 new cases yearly in the United States (22). The highest incidence has been reported in Mississippi (93 cases/million/yr) (23) Alaska (83 cases/million/yr) (24), and lowest in Kentucky at 29.4 cases/million/yr (25). Approximately half of all injuries occur between the ages of 16 to 30. Previously, the average age was 28.7 years but, currently it is 42.6 years. Over 75% of injuries occur in males, involving alcohol in 38% to 50% of cases (24,26,27,28).

The WHO estimates that every year around the world, between 250,000 and 500,000 people suffer ASCI (27). The annual incidence has been reported to be lowest at 8.0 cases/million in Spain, 12.7 in France, 16.9 in Turkey, 19.5 in Sweden, and the highest in New Zealand at 49.1 (28).

In the United States, 38% of ACSI are related to motor vehicle collisions, followed by falls (30.5%), acts of violence such as gunshot wounds (13.5%), and sports injury (9%) (22). Of all patients with ASCI in the 2010 US database, 13.3% were discharged with complete tetraplegia, 45% with incomplete tetraplegia, 20% with complete paraplegia, and 21.3% with incomplete paraplegia; less than 1% had complete neurologic recovery (22). Globally, the most common cause of ASCI is also related to road traffic accidents followed by falls (29). In some countries, such as Malaysia and Bangladesh, 20% of SCIs result from falls while carrying heavy loads, particularly on the head (30).

The level and severity of injury impact mortality and cost. The mortality rate is highest in the first year. In the United States, for those who survive the first 24 hours, if the ASCI is incurred at age 20 years, lifespan is shortened from the normal life expectancy of 79 years by approximately 14 years for a paraplegic, by 19 to 23 years if tetraplegic, and by 33 years if ventilator-dependent at 1 year after injury (22).

The estimated economic burden is reflected in the cost of an estimated Canadian Dollar (CAD) $1.47 million/person with incomplete paraplegia and CAD $3.03 million/person for complete tetraplegia (31). In the United States in 2010, the estimated lifetime cost for a 25 year old at age of injury was $2.3 million with paraplegia and $4.7 million with complete tetraplegia (22).

Outcome following both TBI and ASCI is chiefly determined by the severity of the initial injury, age at time of injury, and comorbidities; however, careful attention to prevent complications and prevent secondary central nervous system injury from hypotension, hypoxia, hyperthermia, and hyperglycemia may help decrease morbidity and mortality.

Prevention

Given the lack of effective treatments able to reverse injury, primary prevention of TBI and ASCI is paramount. Prevention of neurologic injury includes strategies to increase public awareness to wear seat belts, use child safety seats, wear helmets, avoid driving while intoxicated or distracted such as using a phone with texting or talking, and install window guards and safety gates. To also prevent ASCI, it is recommended never to dive into water that is not clear and the depth is shallow or cannot be assessed.

The mechanism of injury may contain opportunities for prevention. From 2001 to 2009 in the United States, the rate of ED visits for sports or recreation-related brain injury rose 57% in children age 19 or younger (32). The US Centers for Disease Control and Prevention (CDC) has partnered with many national, state, and local organizations to launch a "HEADS UP" campaign to educate children, parents, school professionals, coaches, and sports officials as to the importance of concussion recognition and management (33).

For the elderly, the CDC has a Stopping Elderly Accidents, Deaths and Injuries (STEADI) program that provides tools and educational material based on the American and British Geriatric Societies clinical practice guidelines to screen for fall risk and provide interventions to reduce risk (34). Interventions include exercise programs, minimizing medications, particularly psychoactive medications, and modification of the home environment including appropriate lighting, and handrails (35,36).

Worldwide, road traffic crashes are the leading cause of all injury deaths and the tenth leading cause of all deaths (37); most are due to head injury. The WHO estimated the economic cost to developing countries alone is greater than $100 billion annually and $518 billion globally (38). It predicts that by 2015, the leading cause of premature death and disability for children age 5 and up will be due to road crashes, and that road traffic injuries will become the third largest contributor to the global burden of disease by 2020. In 2009, the United Nations General Assembly, with the sponsorship of more than 90 countries, launched a "Decade of Action for Road Safety 2011–2020" with the goal to decrease road deaths and injuries through road safety management, safer roads, safer vehicles, safer road users, and improved postcrash care (39).

PATHOPHYSIOLOGY

Primary Brain Injury

Primary focal neurologic injury following TBI includes hemorrhage into the subdural or epidural spaces, intraparenchymal hemorrhage (IPH), and cerebral contusions and lacerations. Primary diffuse injury includes subarachnoid (SAH) and intraventricular hemorrhage (IVH), diffuse axonal injury (DAI), and diffuse edema (40).

Subdural Hematoma

SDHs are more common than epidural hematomas (EDHs) and were seen in 25% of patients with severe head injury entered into the Traumatic Coma Data Bank (TCDB) supported by the National Institute of Neurological Disorders and Stroke (NINDS) between 1980 and 1988 (41,42). SDH typically results from tearing of the bridging veins between the brain and the draining venous sinuses. The mechanism usually involves high-velocity acceleration and deceleration forces.

Imaging shows a crescent-shaped hyperdensity that follows the contours of the brain. Hyperacute hemorrhages or SDH in anemic patients are isointense on initial CT and may be overlooked. Acute SDH carries a poor prognosis and is one of the most lethal of all head injuries. Fifty to 60% of patients with SDH die, and only 19% to 38% will achieve functional recovery despite surgical treatment (43,44). Early evacuation within the first 4 hours of injury decreased mortality from 90% to 30% in a single study of 82 consecutive comatose patients. This suggested that preventable secondary injury was the cause of the high mortality; however, multiple studies have not replicated these results. The high mortality following SDH is likely the result of the severity of initial forces from the primary mechanism of injury (45,46).

Epidural Hematomas

EDH was found in 9% of 1,030 patients in the TCDB (47). An EDH requires a great impact force and is often associated with a skull fracture that disrupts the middle meningeal artery in the supratentorial space or, if in the posterior fossa, is more likely due to injury of the venous sinuses (48). Classically, patients present awake and alert, a period known as the lucid interval, and quickly lapse into unconsciousness; imaging shows a lenticular-shaped hyperdensity. With rapid evacuation, EDH has a relatively good prognosis, with a mortality rate of 5% to 10% (49). Factors determining mortality and functional outcome include age, best motor response on the Glasgow Coma

Scale (GCS), hematoma volume, and degree of midline shift (49–51). In patients with EDH who are comatose, with either a very short or no period of wakefulness following injury, mortality can be as high as 40%. The motor score immediately before surgical evaluation is predictive; two-thirds of patients with scores of 3 or less become vegetative or die (52).

Cerebral Contusions

Cerebral contusions result from direct impact of the brain on the skull; these are known as *coup* injuries. Alternatively, acceleration/deceleration injury of the brain against the contralateral side of the direct impact causes *contrecoup* injuries. The most common areas of contusion are the frontal, temporal lobes and occipital regions. These lesions typically are hyperintense areas within the parenchyma on CT scan and are more diffuse than IPH. As discussed below, secondary injury can result when contusions enlarge, which causes cerebral edema and intracranial hypertension (53). Clinical deterioration or elevation in intracranial pressure (ICP) requires urgent repeat cerebral imaging.

Intraparenchymal Hemorrhage

Intraparenchymal hemorrhage (IPH), similar to a contusion, is hyperintense on CT scan. It is a focal process and less diffuse than a contusion as it is caused by direct vascular injury or by stretching of the vessels with brain shift and distortion. Hemorrhage in the upper brainstem (midbrain and pons), known as Duret hemorrhages, can also occur with rapidly evolving transtentorial herniation and may be due to stretching of the perforating arterioles or from venous thrombosis and infarction. Spontaneous causes of IPH are hypertensive hemorrhagic stroke, or hemorrhaging due to arteriovenous malformation, aneurysm, amyloid angiopathy, or tumor. In the setting of hemorrhage in the basal ganglia, cerebellum, or thalamus, the clinician should consider the differential of spontaneous IPH as a possible cause of the traumatic event, rather than the result.

Subarachnoid Hemorrhage

Trauma is the most common cause of subarachnoid hemorrhage, occurring in 21% to 53% of patients with severe TBI and causes worsened outcome (54,55). In contrast to aneurysmal SAH (aSAH), traumatic SAH (tSAH) is less likely concentrated in the basal cisterns and is usually found over the hemispheric convexities. The presence of tSAH in the basal cisterns carries a positive predictive value of unfavorable outcome of up to 70% (56).

Intraventricular Hemorrhage

IVH in isolation is not commonly seen in TBI. However, like tSAH, it has been associated with worsened outcome (55). Obstructive hydrocephalus may result and may require cerebrospinal fluid (CSF) diversion by external ventricular drainage (EVD).

Diffuse Axonal Injury

DAI occurs in approximately half of patients with severe TBI (57). Sudden acceleration–deceleration impact causes rotational forces and shear injury to axons; the axon may not be entirely transected, but axoplasmic transport is disrupted causing swelling and disconnection (58,59). The result is formation of a retraction ball with the axon undergoing Wallerian degeneration. Since axonal degeneration may be a secondary injury process, pharmacologic strategies to intervene may eventually be developed. Outcome is worsened with severe DAI (60–62). Although microscopic neuronal injury cannot be seen on imaging studies, the diagnosis is best made with MR imaging with gradient echo or susceptibility-weighted sequences that detect blood products from the capillary injury and leak that accompanies DAI (63).

PHYSIOLOGIC PRINCIPLES

The Monro–Kellie hypothesis describes the skull as a semiclosed compartment containing brain and interstitial fluid (80%), CSF (10%), and blood (10%). Compensatory mechanisms to decrease cerebral blood or CSF volume become active in pathologic conditions where intracranial volume and pressure increase. For example, with hemorrhage or edema after TBI, reductions in CSF production and cerebral blood flow (CBF) are seen. Once these compensatory mechanisms are overwhelmed, depending on the compliance (volume/pressure relationship) of the intracranial contents, pressure will increase. Patients with atrophy are able to tolerate larger volumes before the ICP increases. A young patient without much atrophy has low cerebral compliance, which increases the risk for early intracranial hypertension and potential cerebral herniation.

Cerebral perfusion pressure (CPP) is determined as the difference of the mean arterial pressure (MAP) and ICP. When ICP monitoring is used, the CPP supplants MAP goals in the intensive care unit (ICU). Normal ICP is less than 10 mmHg. In a study in which ICP and CPP were closely evaluated with respect to outcome, the most powerful predictor of neurologic worsening was the presence of intracranial hypertension, defined as an ICP of 20 mmHg or greater. As long as CPP was maintained greater than 60 mmHg, CPP did not correlate with neurologic worsening (64). Current Brain Trauma Foundation (BTF) guidelines recommend initiation of treatment of an ICP above 22 mmHg (65) and avoidance of aggressive therapy to maintain CPP above 70 mmHg with fluids and pressors because of an increased risk of acute respiratory distress syndrome (ARDS) (66); recommendations target a CPP between 60 and 70 mmHg and acknowledge that patients with intact pressure autoregulation tolerate higher CPP values. If cerebral autoregulation is not intact, increasing CPP may result in higher ICP and increased edema (67). Prior to placement of an intracranial monitor, recommendations are to maintain a systolic blood pressure (SBP) of 100 mm Hg or greater for patients 50-69 years of age or 110 mm Hg or above for patients 15 to 49 or over 70 years of age to decrease mortality and improve outcomes (68).

DIAGNOSIS

On arrival to the ICU, the initial focus is on respiratory and hemodynamic stability; this will be discussed below. In addition to the usual general examination, in the neurologically injured patient the evaluation includes an examination of the head for scalp lacerations, which can be a major source of bleeding and orbital, facial, and depressed skull fractures. Evidence for basilar skull fractures include periorbital ecchymoses (raccoon eyes) indicative of frontal skull base injury or

TABLE 117.1 Glasgow Coma Scale Scoring

Score	Eye Opening	Best Verbal	Best Motor
1	No response	No response	No response
2	To pain	Incomprehensible	Extensor
3	To speech	Inappropriate	Flexor
4	Spontaneous	Disoriented	Withdraws to pain
5	—	Oriented	Localizes pain
6	—	—	Obeys command

From Chesnut RM, Ghajar J, Maas AIR, et al. Early indicators of prognosis in severe traumatic brain injury: Glasgow Coma Scale Score. In: *Management and Prognosis of Severe Traumatic Brain Injury*. New York: Brain Trauma Foundation; 2000:163–173.

postauricular ecchymosis (the Battle sign) seen with middle fossa or temporal bone fractures. Cervical spine precautions are maintained in these patients and will be discussed later.

During the evaluation and observation of the TBI patient, repeated neurologic monitoring includes the vital signs with special attention to extremes in blood pressure. Hypotension may result in secondary injury, whereas hypertension, not always associated with bradycardia, can be a sign of impending cerebral herniation. If ICP rises, cerebral autoregulation elevates MAP to maintain an adequate CPP.

A rapid neurologic assessment includes level of consciousness and ability to speak or understand language by assessing the ability to follow simple commands or to at least mimic clear hand signals. The GCS score (Table 117.1), first developed and introduced in 1974 to help monitor the depth and duration of impaired consciousness, provides a standard, rapid, and reproducible score utilizing eye opening, verbal output, and motor movement (68). The severity of head injury based on the GCS has been divided into three categories: (i) Mild or minor: GCS 13 to 15; (ii) Moderate: GCS of 9 to 12, and (iii) Severe: GCS of 8 or less. Interrater variability is usually minimal, but can exist (69).

A patient's best GCS score following adequate fluid resuscitation and stabilization is predictive of outcome (70). A GCS of 3, reflecting no eye opening or motor movement to pain and no verbal output, has a 65% mortality compared to mortality of 10% to 15% in patients with a GCS of 7 to 13 (71). Additionally, when measured repetitively without effects of pharmacologic sedation or hemodynamic or pulmonary instability, a decreasing score can portend poor outcome (71,72).

Vision is assessed by asking the patient to count fingers placed in the right or left visual field with one eye covered, or to mimic finger movements. In patients with a lower level of consciousness, vision is assessed by blinking to a visual threat. Pupillary response to light (cranial nerves [CN] II, III), corneal reflex (CN V, VII), and gag and cough (CN IX, X) responses assess cranial nerve and brainstem function. Oculocephalic maneuvers (CN III, VI, VIII) should not be performed in patients who have a risk of cervical spine fracture. Ice water caloric response (CN III, VI, VIII) can be performed if the tympanic membranes are intact: the head of the bed (HOB) should be kept at 30 degrees, and 60 to 90 mL of ice water is instilled into the otic canal. A normal response is a slow lateral deviation to the side stimulated with ice water and nystagmus with the fast phase to the opposite side; absence of this response may be caused by medications or brainstem injury.

Motor response is assessed by verbal commands to move the limbs. In patients with lower levels of consciousness, motor responses are elicited by painful stimuli delivered to the sternum or fingernail bed. During painful stimulation, the examiner should also reassess facial movement for asymmetry. If flexion is noted, pain is applied to the supraorbital ridge or by trapezius squeeze to test for localization. In the lower extremities, it is important to recognize a triple flexion response, which is described by the flexion of the ankle, knee, and hip. The triple reflex is a spinal reflex to painful stimulation of the legs or feet. It is stereotyped in appearance, independent of the location of pain delivery on the lower extremity, and does not reflect brainstem or upper spinal cord function. Patients who are brain dead or who have higher complete spinal cord lesions can triple-flex lower extremities.

Laboratory evaluation of patients with head injury includes complete blood count with platelet counts, activated partial thromboplastin time (aPTT), prothrombin time (PT), electrolytes with blood urea nitrogen, creatinine, glucose, and liver function tests to assess for liver dysfunction which may impair clotting ability. Thrombin time or ecarin clotting time has recently been added by some to trauma-related admission panels due to new oral anticoagulants that are not reflected by the PT and aPTT (73). A toxicology screen including a blood alcohol level is essential to assist in evaluating for other causes of altered mental status and to determine whether delirium tremens may be a factor in the following days of ICU care. Arterial blood gas (ABG) and lactic acid levels help assess volume status and whether ventilation is adequate.

Imaging

The initial imaging, often coupled with the neurologic examination, determines the need for acute neurosurgical intervention. Neurosurgical guidelines have been established for focal intracranial lesions (74–76). Noncontrast head CT is the fastest, most widely available noninvasive imaging technique to determine this. All patients with altered mental status and/or focal neurologic findings should have an initial CT scan performed. In minor head injury, a CT scan may not be necessary if the examination is normal and the GCS is 15, unless the patient is older than 60 years, has a headache, emesis, drug or alcohol intoxication, deficits in short-term memory, physical evidence of trauma above the clavicles, coagulopathy, or seizures (77).

Evolving Injury and Repeat Head CT

Progressive intracranial hemorrhage consistent with an evolving contusion is seen in 14% to 38% of patients (57,78,79). Although worsening CT findings does not necessarily require treatment, up to 54% of patients may require neurosurgical intervention including ICP monitoring or craniotomy subsequent to the findings on a repeat scan (53,80–85). A significant risk factor is early initial imaging within 2 hours of injury (54,78,85,86). Often community standards are to repeat a CT scan within 12 to 24 hours of the initial imaging.

In stable patients without clinical neurologic deterioration, the utility of repeat imaging is debated and many believe it is unnecessary since it is unlikely that neurosurgical intervention will be required (54,82,85,86). Other independent risk factors for progression include associated tSAH, SDH, older age, and prolonged partial thromboplastin (53,57,78,85,86). A large initial contusional or IPH size and effacement of cisterns are strongly predictive of failure of nonoperative management (57).

TREATMENT

Following immediate impact and anatomic damage, secondary damage at the cellular level from inflammation, edema, free radicals, and excitatory neurotransmitters can worsen outcome. Contributing factors include hypoxemia, hypotension, seizures, fever, and intracranial hypertension. Immediate postinjury care focuses on the prevention of these problems.

Hypoxemia and Respiratory Management

Hypoxemia, defined as a PaO_2 less than 60 mmHg or O_2 saturation less than 90%, can independently increase mortality from 27% to 50% and increase poor outcome from 28% to 71% (87,88). Early intubation can prevent aspiration and minimize hypoxic and hypercapnic events (89), and is recommended by the Eastern Association for the Surgery of Trauma (EAST) (90), Advanced Trauma Life Support (ATLS) guidelines from the American College of Surgeons (91), and the Brain Trauma Foundation Traumatic Brain Injury prehospital guidelines (92). A GCS of 8 or less is the usual threshold for endotracheal intubation.

There are caveats to intubation of which the practitioner should be aware. In the prehospital setting, rapid sequence intubation has been associated with increased mortality (93–95). This may be a result of decreased cerebral perfusion due to hyperventilation-induced hypocapnia. Positive pressure ventilation may cause hypotension in a hypovolemic patient if central venous return is impeded by high intrathoracic pressures (96). Intubation is a high-risk procedure which may cause secondary neurologic injury. Sedative/hypnotic medications and bag/mask ventilation with positive pressure ventilation contribute to hypotension and hypercapnia and hypocapnia, respectively, during induction. In addition, direct laryngoscopy causes a marked, transient increase in ICP. Intravenous lidocaine may blunt this ICP response (97,98).

Hyperventilation with resultant hypocapnia causes cerebral vasoconstriction and a reduction in CBF (99–101). Prolonged hypocapnia appears to slow neurologic recovery (102). Prophylactic hyperventilation of $PaCO_2$ less than 35 mmHg should be avoided, although $PaCO_2$ as low as 30 mmHg may be necessary for brief periods for immediate treatment of intracranial hypertension. Options to identify cerebral ischemia in the setting of hyperventilation include the use of jugular venous oxygen saturation, arterial jugular venous oxygen content differences, brain tissue oxygen monitoring or CBF monitoring (103).

To achieve adequate ventilation, positive end-expiratory pressure (PEEP) may be necessary. PEEP affects CPP and ICP when the lung is compliant and the chest wall is not. The high lung compliance allows for an increased intrathoracic volume which, in the setting of a low compliant chest wall, increases intrathoracic pressures. The high intrathoracic pressure decreases cerebral venous outflow, which will increase ICP (104,105). Additionally, if intrathoracic pressure is elevated, cardiac venous return is diminished and results in lowered MAP and CPP.

Pulmonary infections were seen in 41% of patients registered in the TCDB and were an independent predictor of unfavorable outcome (106). Bedside management includes adequate pulmonary toilet and strategies such as elevation of the HOB to decrease the risk for ventilator-associated pneumonia (VAP). In patients with intracranial hypertension, during endotracheal suctioning, adequate sedation is necessary to prevent an increase in ICP (107).

Neurogenic Pulmonary Edema

In addition to hypoventilation and aspiration from poor airway protection, a less frequently recognized cause of hypoxemia following TBI is neurogenic pulmonary edema (NPE) (108), resulting from central sympathetic stimulation. Pretreatment with adrenergic-blocking agents prevents experimental NPE (109). Experimental lesions in the hypothalamus (110), bilateral nucleus tractus solitarius (111), and the ventrolateral medulla (112) can produce NPE. TBI causes a sympathetic discharge, which increases systemic and pulmonary vascular pressures; the resultant increase in pulmonary capillary pressure increases the hydrostatic pressure and causes pulmonary capillary injury. This, in turn, causes leakage of fluid and protein and pulmonary hemorrhages (113–115).

Clinical signs include dyspnea, tachypnea, tachycardia, and chest pain if the patient is awake; rales are present on chest auscultation. Laboratory results show hypoxemia and a mild leukocytosis, with chest radiograph showing a bilateral alveolar filling process (116). Pulmonary capillary wedge pressures and pulmonary artery pressures can be elevated or normal. There are two distinct forms of NPE: the classic form appears early, within minutes to a few hours after acute brain injury; a delayed form of NPE slowly progresses over 12 to 72 hours following injury. Treatment is supportive and often requires supplemental oxygen and positive pressure ventilation. Dobutamine may be effective by decreasing cardiac afterload and increasing cardiac contractility (117).

Hypotension

Hypotension, defined as SBP less than 90 mmHg, independently worsens mortality (118,119). The TCDB reports hypotension was present in 29% of patients and doubled mortality from 27% to 55% (106,118). In patients whose SBP were less than 90 mm Hg, mortality was 65% independent of age, admission GCS motor score, hypoxia, or associated severe extracranial trauma. Adequate fluid resuscitation with euvolemia is essential. Independent of ICP, MAP, or CPP, a negative fluid balance of approximately 600 mL was associated with poorer outcome (120). Guidelines recommend adequate fluid resuscitation and have been updated to recommend SBP 100 mm Hg or greater in patients 50 to 69 years old and 110 mm Hg or greater in patients 15 to 49 or greater than 70 years old. Blood pressure support to maintain SBP greater than 90 mmHg (67). Once an ICP monitor is placed, the optimal blood pressure is determined by that required to keep the CPP 60 to 70 mmHg (67).

Contraction Band Necrosis

Following head trauma, SAH, seizures, or stroke, patients may have cardiogenic shock with global hypokinesis associated with transient cardiac dysrhythmias and repolarization changes (121–124). Dysrhythmias may include supraventricular tachycardias, sinus bradycardia, atrioventricular (AV) block, AV dissociation, nodal rhythms, and paroxysmal ventricular tachycardia. These changes are cerebrally mediated and are recognized as myofibrillar degeneration (also known as contraction band necrosis [CBN] or coagulative myocytolysis). The histologic appearance of CBN contrasts to the coagulation necrosis seen with ischemic injury where there are cytoplasmic degenerative changes with cloudy swelling, hyaline droplets, and fatty change. With CBN, the myocardium instead shows loss of definition of the linear arrangement of myofibrils and the appearance of prominent dense eosinophilic transverse bands (contraction bands), and intervening granularity throughout the cytoplasm (125). This injury pattern was first described with pheochromocytoma and has been associated with the administration of catecholamines, including cocaine abuse (126,127). It is postulated that centrally mediated sympathetic or exogenous catecholamine stimulation of the myocardium results in cellular calcium overload and results in the formation of the contraction bands (128). CBN is predominantly located in the subendocardium with the cardiac conducting system, which results in the associated arrhythmias (129).

In CBN, cardiac enzymes are often elevated and may be difficult to differentiate from an acute coronary syndrome. However, the treatment for CBN is vastly different and typically includes observation for dysrhythmias and blood pressure support in contrast to reperfusion therapy with an acute ischemic myocardial infarction. Clinical differentiation typically relies on the recognition of patients with higher risk for coronary artery disease such as older age, hypertension, diabetes, and hyperlipidemia rather than a young patient with massive head injury.

Posttraumatic Vasospasm

Following TBI, posttraumatic vasospasm can occur in as many as 24% to 36% of adults and children (130–132) and causes focal ischemia with lateralizing neurologic deficits such as hemiparesis and aphasia between 2 to 37 days following injury (132–134). In patients with severe TBI, small studies have reported incidences as high as 82% (135). Explosive blast TBI is especially associated with early cerebral edema and cerebral vasospasm (136). Disruption of cerebrovascular tone may be a result of inflammatory and other vascular changes (137). Some mechanisms include an increased expression of an inducible isoform of nitric oxide synthase (138) and a hypercontraction-induced phenotypic switch that potentiates vascular remodeling (139). Transcranial Doppler, while reasonably specific, is not a sensitive test for vasospasm. If vasospasm is suspected, cerebral angiography can confirm the diagnosis. The effectiveness of treatment of posttraumatic vasospasm with modalities used following aSAH (e.g., hypervolemic, hypertensive therapy, or nimodipine) has not been assessed.

Hyperthermia

Hyperthermia accelerates neuronal injury by increasing basal energy requirements (neuronal discharges), excitatory neurotransmitters, free radial production, calcium-dependent protein phosphorylation, ICAM-1 and inflammatory responses, DNA fragmentation, and apoptosis, causing blood–brain barrier changes as seen by extravasation of protein tracers (140,141). Despite this, multiple TBI studies of prophylactic moderate hypothermia (32° to 33°C) and their meta-analyses have not shown improved outcome (142–144). This may be due to significant intercenter variability in the management of MAP, CPP, fluids, and vasopressors (145,146).

In the individual patient, therapeutic hypothermia lowers ICP by reducing the cerebral metabolic rate 7% for each degree Celsius decrease. This treatment can be lifesaving and result in reasonable neurologic recovery (144,147). Pentobarbital coma and/or neuromuscular blockade (NMB) may be necessary to achieve cooling without shivering. Various techniques for intravascular and topical cooling are available. Although complications of hypothermia can include increased risk of cardiac dysrhythmias, hypotension, bradycardia, thrombocytopenia, and pneumonia, in studies evaluating hypothermia in cardiac arrest patients, there was no statistical increase in these adverse events (148,149).

Hyperglycemia

Hyperglycemia can cause brain tissue acidosis (150), and early hyperglycemia has been associated with worsened neurologic outcome following TBI (151,152). Persistent hyperglycemia following severe TBI in one study was an independent risk factor of mortality with a 4.9 times increase in risk of death (153). It is not fully understood whether the hyperglycemia is causative or is a marker for severity of injury and subsequent poor outcome; however, control of hyperglycemia following TBI is theoretically reasonable.

In the ICU setting, where glycemic control often uses insulin infusion or injection, patients with acutely altered mental status should be urgently evaluated for hypoglycemia.

Coagulopathy

Brain is rich in tissue thromboplastin and following head injury, increased tissue thromboplastin activity in the frontal, parietal, and temporal lobes activates the coagulation cascade and causes a disseminated intravascular coagulopathy (DIC) (154). The TCDB reported that 19% of patients were coagulopathic (106). In children, the incidence of coagulopathy increased with worsening severity of head injury reflected by the head Abbreviated Injury Scale score and was as high as 40% (155). Although initial evaluation may show thrombocytopenia in 14% and coagulopathy in 21% of TBI patients, in ensuing days, DIC can be seen in 41% to 60% of patients with blunt brain injury (156,157). It is more common in patients with penetrating head trauma (158).

Abnormalities in PT, PTT, or platelet count have been associated with 55% of patients who have progressive intracranial hemorrhage after TBI (159,160). Associated coagulopathy and thrombocytopenia increases mortality in TBI (156,157,160,161). Some centers are using thromboelastometry and portable coagulometers to detect coagulopathy in the ED. Typically, fresh frozen plasma is transfused for an elevated aPTT or a PT international ratio (INR) of 1.5 or more. Current European guidelines for TBI patients recommend transfusion of platelets for values below 100,000 cells/μL or for patients receiving antiplatelet agents (162). Other alternatives such as activated factor VII or prothrombin complex concentrate (PCC) may be effective emergently (158); PCC is recommended in the European guidelines for emergency reversal of vitamin K-dependent and oral antifactor Xa agents such as rivaroxaban, apixaban, or edoxaban (162).

Intracranial Pressure Monitoring and Management

Normal ICP is less than 10 mmHg; the TCDB reports that 72% of patients with severe TBI had ICPs above 20 mmHg (163). Since multiple studies show worsened outcome with

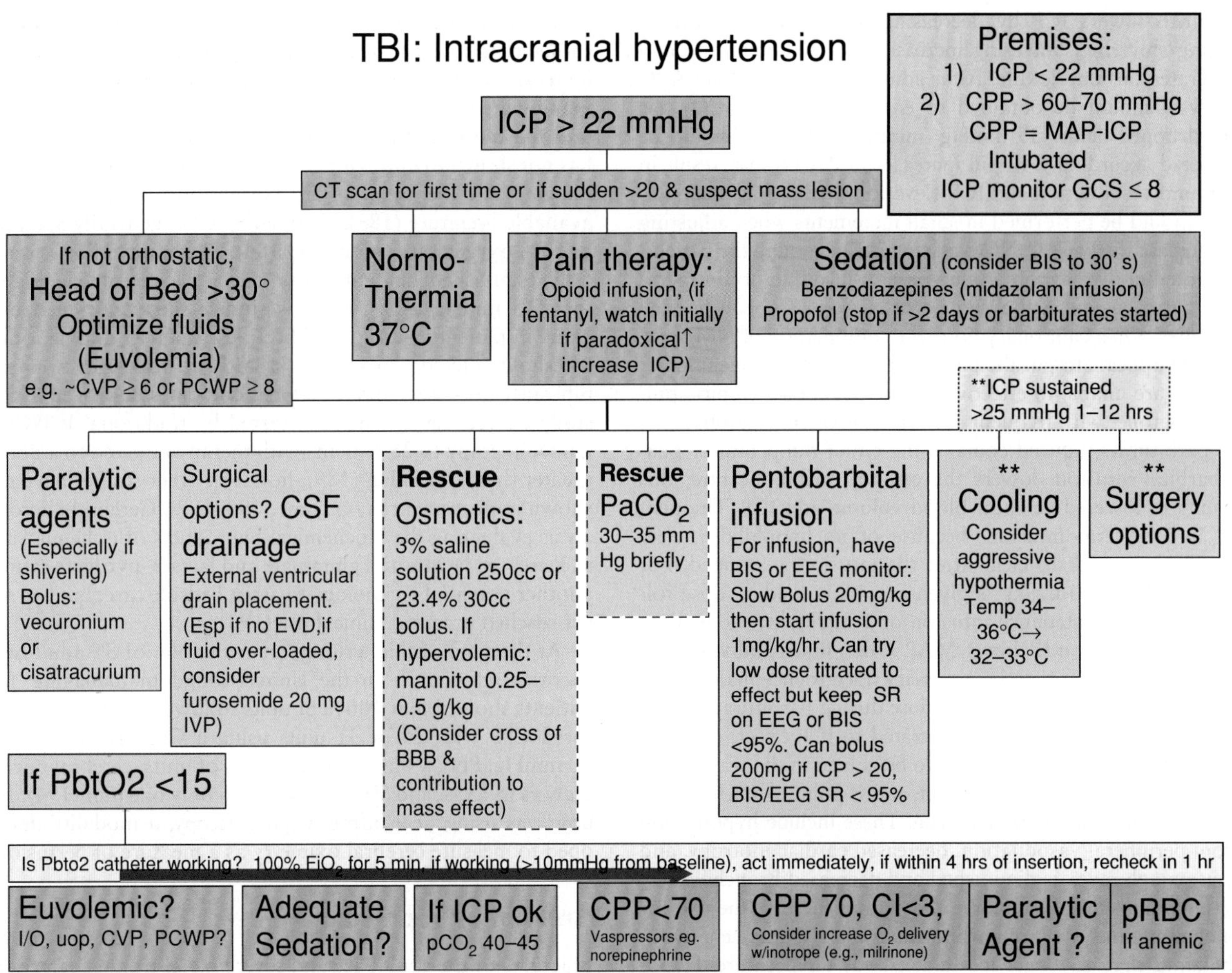

FIGURE 117.1 Algorithm for management of intracranial hypertension. CI, cardiac index L/min/m^2; pRBC, packed red blood cells; SR, suppression ratio.

ICP above 20 to 25 mmHg, published guidelines use this as the threshold to treat (65).

Maneuvers for management of ICP begin with those with fewer potential side effects and progress to more invasive treatments with higher complication risk (Fig. 117.1). Elevation of the head of bed to more than 30 to 45 degrees not only decreases the risk of VAP but can facilitate cerebral venous drainage and lower ICP. In orthostatic, hypovolemic patients, however, head of bed elevation can lower MAP; adequate fluid resuscitation is necessary. Adequate pain therapy with opioids and adequate sedation with sedative-hypnotics decrease ICP. Constant infusion may be hemodynamically better tolerated than bolus administration. Prophylactic or sustained hyperventilation of $PaCO_2$ less than 35 mmHg may be harmful and should be avoided (101–104). In the situation of impending herniation or refractory intracranial hypertension, decreasing $PaCO_2$ to 30 mmHg for transient "rescue" therapy will give the practitioner time to initiate other maneuvers to lower ICP.

Osmotic therapy is a mainstay in ICP management. Mannitol and hypertonic saline are both effective (164–166). However, repetitive dosing by the above agents may eventually shift fluid into the injured brain across the damaged blood–brain barrier and thereby increase the volume of injured brain and elevate ICP (167–169). To avoid this, osmotic therapy, similar to hyperventilation, might be best used as rescue therapy until more definitive therapy is implemented. Doses of 0.25 to 1 g/kg of mannitol are effective. The lower dose drops ICP and may decrease the risk of vasogenic edema seen with multiple dosing (167). High serum concentrations of mannitol may cause renal failure. Maximal mannitol dosing traditionally has been when serum osmolarity reaches 320 mOsm/kg, but with the increased use of hypertonic saline, an osmolar gap is now being used. The difference of measured to calculated serum osmolarity is a surrogate marker for mannitol concentration as an "unmeasured" osmole. A rising osmolar gap of greater than 10 from baseline may be a better indicator of maximized mannitol administration (170,171). Hypertonic saline may be more effective and have a longer duration of action on lowering ICP than mannitol (169,172,173). Usual doses include 250 mL of 3% or 30 mL of 23% saline which have equimolar amounts of sodium chloride (174). The concentration used usually depends on volume status, with the lower volume 23% saline used when the patient is hypervolemic. Osmotic therapy is best administered through a central venous access as it may sclerose veins. When deciding which osmotic agent to use, elevated ICP with low fluid status would be best treated with hypertonic saline. Studies evaluating the prophylactic use of hypertonic saline compared to conventional fluids for prehospital or ED resuscitation have not shown outcome improvement (175,176).

NMB lowers ICP by decreasing muscle tone, especially during shivering. Shivering increases the metabolic rate and generates carbon dioxide. After administering NMB, an ABG analysis should be obtained to ensure that the $PaCO_2$ has not dropped below 35 mmHg; minute ventilation should be adjusted accordingly. Rapid increases in $PaCO_2$ may result in rebound vasodilation and ICP elevation. Ventilator manipulation should be performed in small increments when adjusting to increase the $PaCO_2$. NMB also assists in cooling the patient. As noted above, hypothermia is useful in refractory intracranial hypertension. Temperatures of 32° to 33°C can be well tolerated. On a cautionary note, the combination of NMB and cooling appears to put the patient at high risk for pneumonia, as they are unable to effectively clear secretions; empiric pulmonary toilet with frequent suctioning is often necessary.

Barbiturate-induced coma, using either thiopental or pentobarbital infusion, lowers the cerebral metabolic rate; this results in lowered cerebral blood volume and ICP. Thiopental in long-term infusion, because of its lipophilicity, may take over a week to clear after the infusion is stopped. For pentobarbital, 20 mg/kg is given as a slow loading dose followed by a maintenance infusion of 1 mg/kg/hr; the loading dose may significantly lower MAP. Often fluids and vasopressor administration may be necessary. Electroencephalography (EEG) is critical to titrating the dose during barbiturate coma. Although the infusion can be titrated to ICP effect, once the EEG is isoelectric, there is little to be gained in the way of ICP control by increasing the infusion; at this point, worsening side effects result from increased drug. These include hypotension from peripheral vasodilation, decreased cardiac inotropy, and ileus; cough reflex is diminished and decreased bronchociliary activity and slowed leukocyte chemotaxis increase the risk for pneumonia. A benefit of barbiturate coma is a quiescent hypothalamus that no longer modulates body temperature. Hypothermia can often be achieved without the need for NMB since shivering is diminished.

Loop diuretics have been used to help manage ICP by decreasing CSF production in the choroids plexus (177). Loop diuretics will decrease volume status, thus unless the patient is hypervolemic, CSF diversion is a more effective method of lowering ICP.

Other therapy for refractory intracranial hypertension requires neurosurgical intervention. Placement of an EVD allows for CSF drainage. Hemicraniectomy may be life-saving and a viable option depending on the patient; case series of 19, 23, and 51 children at three different centers had mortalities of 30% to 31.4%. Favorable outcome with return to school and functional independence was reported in 68% to 81%; 18% to 21% were severely disabled and dependent on caregivers (178–180). In a randomized trial of adults with diffuse brain injury, early bilateral frontotemporoparietal decompressive craniectomy decreased ICP and the ICU length of stay, but was associated with worsened neurologic outcome (181).

Brain Tissue Oxygenation

To monitor and help prevent the secondary damage seen with hypoxic brain injury, new modalities to evaluate cerebral oxygenation have been developed. Jugular bulb oximetry ($SjvO_2$) is a global measure of the balance between oxygen delivery to the brain and oxygen consumption. Local brain tissue partial pressure oxygen ($PbtO_2$) can be measured either by a quenching process by fluorescence or by a polarographic Clark-type microcatheter. An increase in cerebral oxygen delivery is reflected by increases in $SjvO_2$ and $PbtO_2$. Oxygen delivery to the brain is manipulated by increases in blood pressure, cardiac output, and red blood cell transfusion (182). Normobaric hyperoxia has not shown to improve cerebral oxygen metabolism on PET imaging, and the use of 100% oxygen is not supported by the available literature (183). Optimal $SjvO_2$ is generally accepted as 50% oxygen saturation (103,184). The optimal $PbtO_2$ is not fully established but guidelines currently recommend higher than 15 mmHg (103). Various studies show worsened outcome in patients with mean $PbtO_2$ less than 15 mmHg; other thresholds include 25 mmHg (185–188). Mortality was significantly decreased and functional outcomes improved in one study comparing 25 patients treated by traditional ICP/CPP-guided therapy to 28 patients with therapy targeted to a $PbtO_2$ greater than 25 mmHg (189); however, other studies have not shown improvement in outcome (190–192). Cerebral microdialysis evaluating the biochemical byproducts of ischemia such as increased lactate and glutamate and lactate–pyruvate ratio is another potential technology to assist bedside care, but has not yet reached practical clinical use (193).

At the time of this writing, an evaluation of 31 adult neurocritical care units in the United Kingdom managing TBI patients showed that 100% of units followed ICP; 97% monitored CPP with 25 of 31 units using a CPP target of 60 to 70 mmHg; $PbtO_2$ was utilized in 26% of units, cerebral microdialysis in 13%, and $SjvO_2$ was used in only one unit (194). No unit was using near-infrared spectroscopy, a modality developed to measure cerebral oximetry as a measure of perfusion.

Antibiotic Prophylaxis

Fractures of the skull base and severe facial trauma can result in a CSF leak. Various studies report incidences of 2.6% to 4.6% of all patients with basilar or facial fractures (195,196). In one study, otorrhea was three times more common than rhinorrhea (195). Approximately 50% of CSF leaks stop within 5 days (197); the risk of bacterial meningitis is approximately 12% to 21%. Studies conflict as to whether prophylactic antibiotics decrease the risk of infection and meta-analyses suggest no benefit, hence, there are no guidelines or recommendations regarding antibiotics in this setting (197–199); constant surveillance for meningitis is essential.

In the setting of CSF leak, if the spine is stable and blood pressure is adequate, the HOB should be elevated to facilitate leak closure. Stool softeners help avoid vigorous Valsalva maneuvers that may worsen the leak. Neurosurgical intervention with CSF diversion (i.e., lumbar drain or EVD) or surgical closure may be necessary if the leak persists. Following penetrating head trauma, a CSF leak is the primary predictor of intracranial infection. Infection is seen in 38% to 63% of CSF leaks after military-related penetrating cerebral injury (200–202). Current recommendations advise treatment for 5 to 14 days with empiric broad-spectrum antibiotics immediately following penetrating brain injury (202–205).

For clean neurosurgical procedures, such as twist drill craniostomy for EVD or ICP monitor placement, burr holes, or craniotomy, guidelines have been established by the Surgical Infection Prevention and Surgical Care Improvement Projects that recommend an intravenous first-generation cephalosporin within 1 hour prior to surgical incision (206).

Posttraumatic Seizures

Early posttraumatic seizures occur within 7 days of injury; 3% to 6% of patients with closed head injury suffer early posttraumatic seizures, compared to 8% to 10% with penetrating brain injury (207–209). Late posttraumatic seizure by definition manifests at least 7 days postinjury and is seen in 30% of patients with penetrating brain injury; these late posttraumatic seizures may occur up to 5 years after injury. There is adequate evidence to recommend antiseizure medications, for example, phenytoin and carbamazepine, for the first week after closed and penetrating brain injury to prevent early posttraumatic seizures (210–213). Of note, valproate showed no benefit for seizures following brain injury and had a trend to higher mortality (214). Levetiracetam, compared to phenytoin, shows equal efficacy in post-TBI seizure prevention (215,216) and has fewer complications, such as hypotension, and does not require monitoring of therapeutic levels, although dosing should be adjusted in renal failure. There is no evidence that continuing prophylactic antiseizure medications beyond a week prevents late posttraumatic seizures, and it is not recommended for closed or penetrating head injury beyond 7 days of injury (210,213).

Thromboprophylaxis

In the general postoperative neurosurgical population, the risk for deep venous thrombosis (DVT) is 3% to 14% (217–220); following major head injury, the risk for DVT is as high as 54% (221). The BTF recommends the use of graduated compression stockings or intermittent pneumatic compression (IPC) stockings in combination with low–molecular-weight (LMWH) or low-dose unfractionated heparin (LDUH) with the warning that this may result in intracranial hemorrhage expansion; there were no specific recommendations for a preferred agent, dose, or timing of treatment (222). The American College of Chest Physicians (ACCP) 9th edition has similar recommendations for major trauma patients with TBI, ASCI, or spinal surgery for trauma (Grade 2C). The Neurocritical Care Society recommends initiating LMWH or UFH for VTE prophylaxis within 24-48 hours of presentation or 24 hours after craniotomy (223). If LMWH and LDUH are considered contraindicated, mechanical prophylaxis, preferably with IPC devices, should be utilized until the risk of bleeding diminishes and contraindication to chemoprophylaxis resolves (Grade 2C). Inferior vena cava (IVC) filters are not considered acceptable primary prophylaxis in trauma patients (Grade 2C) (220).

Nutrition

Following severe TBI, patients enter a hypermetabolic, catabolic state with rapid weight loss associated with a negative nitrogen balance and protein wasting. In experimental models of TBI, 3 hours after injury morphologic changes are seen in the gut mucosa that include shedding of epithelial cells, fracture of villi, focal ulcers, fusion of adjacent villi, mucosal atrophy, and edema in the villous interstitium and lamina propria. On electron microscopy, there is a loss of tight junctions between enterocytes, damage of mitochondria and endoplasm, and apoptosis of epithelial cells (224). These changes in gut permeability increase bacteria translocation and endotoxin, which increases the risk of the systemic inflammatory response; the amino acids arginine and glutamine modulate gut permeability.

Early parenteral or enteral nutrition within 24 to 72 hours can speed neurologic recovery and decrease disability and mortality (225–228). Early enteral feeding may have benefit over parenteral feeding by protecting against intestinal apoptosis and atrophy (229) and decreasing infection clinically (230). Early enteral nutrition with glutamine and probiotics may decrease the infection rate and length of ICU stay (231,232). There is some theoretical concern that glutamine should not be used in brain injury patients due to the potential increase in cerebral glutamate with neuroexcitatory properties and cell damage, although there are no data to date to support this concern.

Fasted TBI patients lose nitrogen at a rate that reduces weight by 15% per week. Replacement of resting energy expenditure (REE) by 100% to 140%, with 15% to 20% nitrogen calories may reduce nitrogen loss; therefore, BTF guidelines recommend that full (100% REE) nutritional replacement be achieved within 7 days after injury (233). An Institute of Medicine (IOM) report was more aggressive and recommended the provision of early (i.e., within 24 hours of injury) nutrition of more than 50% of total energy expenditure and 1 to 1.5 g/kg protein for the first 2 weeks after injury (232,234).

Stress Gastritis

Stress gastritis was seen in 91% of 44 comatose mechanically ventilated patients within 24 hours of head injury; lesions were most commonly seen in the fundus and body of the stomach (235). Mucosal ulceration is typically prevented by maintaining intraluminal pH above 5 or by H_2 receptor blockade (236). In TBI patients, stress ulcer bleeding prophylaxis with proton pump inhibitors or H_2 antagonists is recommended. Neither is recommended over the other, but the practitioner should be aware that one retrospective study in neurosurgery patients showed a statistically significant increased incidence of thrombocytopenia of 50 patients on famotidine compared to 98 of those not treated (34% vs. 11.2%) (237).

Prognosis

Survivors of TBI variably suffer from long-term cognitive, motor, sensory, and emotional deficits. These manifest as weakness, incoordination, emotional lability, impulsivity, and difficulty with vision, concentration, memory, judgment, and mood. Nearly 5.3 million in the United States live with disabilities as a result of TBI (14). When the postresuscitation GCS is not complicated by medications or intubation, approximately 20% of patients with GCS 3 will survive and 8% to 10% will have moderate to good recovery such that they are able to live independently (238). Despite this, 34% to 47% of "minor" head injury patients cannot return to work or their previous lifestyle (239,240). Independent predictors of outcome include older age at time of injury, the postresuscitation Glasgow coma score, injury severity score (ISS), pupillary response on admission, and CT scan findings of diffuse edema, tSAH, SDH, partial obliteration of the basal cisterns, or midline shift (241–246). The TCDB reports a postresuscitation mortality rate of severe TBI patients of 76% and 18%, for patients with postresuscitation GCS of 3 and 6 to 8, respectively. Overall mortality was 36% in 746 patients (42). In another study of 1,311 head-injured patients, the highest mortality was associated with spinal cord injury, obstructed airway, difficulty breathing, and shock, although none of these was independently predictive of survival when adjusted for GCS (247). There are on-going trials to find medications to improve outcome following TBI; studies to date, with agents such as free radical scavengers (248) and progesterone (249) have been unsuccessful.

ACUTE SPINAL CORD INJURY

Pathophysiology

Primary spinal cord injury results from cord compression from discs, bone, ligament, or hematoma, or from distractional forces such as flexion, extension, dislocation, or rotation, which cause shearing of the neuronal axons or vasculature with intramedullary hemorrhage. Similar to head injury, the spinal cord undergoes both primary and secondary injury. Secondary injury can result from additional mechanical injury if the spine is manipulated when it is unstable or as a result from systemic and local vascular insults, which may be a result of hypotension, electrolytes changes, edema, and excitotoxicity (250).

Diagnosis

Examination

The physical examination includes a general examination to survey for other injuries; the quality of the patient's breathing should be assessed to ensure adequate ventilatory effort. The neurologic examination should include a mental status evaluation as concomitant head injury may occur. A complete cranial nerve examination assesses for evidence of cranial neuropathies or nystagmus suggestive of brainstem or cerebellar ischemia that may result from vertebral artery injury. In 1982, the American Spinal Injury Association (ASIA) developed the International Standards for Neurological Classification of Spinal Cord Injury (ISNCSCI) (Fig. 117.2) (251) to improve precision in determining the level and extent of neurologic injury for the National SCI Statistical Center Database (252). These have been updated since that time, have good interrater reliability (253,254), and are recommended as the preferred neurologic examination tool (255). The ASIA Impairment Scale standardizes language used to describe severity SCI (Table 117.2) (251). The single neurologic level of injury is

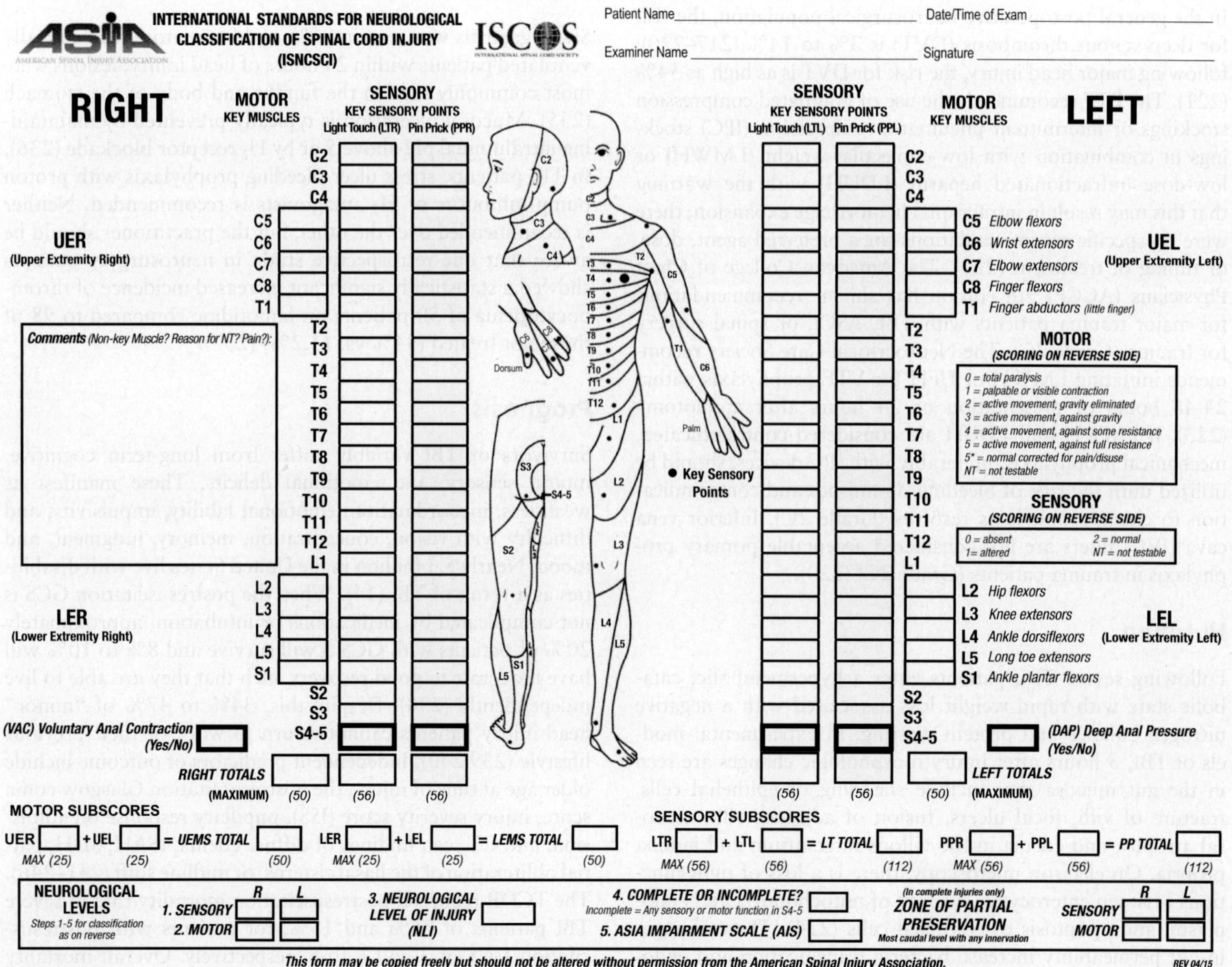

ASIA — AMERICAN SPINAL INJURY ASSOCIATION
INTERNATIONAL STANDARDS FOR NEUROLOGICAL CLASSIFICATION OF SPINAL CORD INJURY (ISNCSCI)
ISCOS — INTERNATIONAL SPINAL CORD SOCIETY

Patient Name ________ Date/Time of Exam ________
Examiner Name ________ Signature ________

RIGHT — MOTOR KEY MUSCLES; SENSORY KEY SENSORY POINTS: Light Touch (LTR), Pin Prick (PPR)

LEFT — SENSORY KEY SENSORY POINTS: Light Touch (LTL), Pin Prick (PPL); MOTOR KEY MUSCLES

C2, C3, C4

UER (Upper Extremity Right) / UEL (Upper Extremity Left):
C5 Elbow flexors
C6 Wrist extensors
C7 Elbow extensors
C8 Finger flexors
T1 Finger abductors (little finger)

T2, T3, T4, T5, T6, T7, T8, T9, T10, T11, T12, L1

LER (Lower Extremity Right) / LEL (Lower Extremity Left):
L2 Hip flexors
L3 Knee extensors
L4 Ankle dorsiflexors
L5 Long toe extensors
S1 Ankle plantar flexors

S2, S3, S4-5

Comments (Non-key Muscle? Reason for NT? Pain?):

● Key Sensory Points

MOTOR (SCORING ON REVERSE SIDE)
0 = total paralysis
1 = palpable or visible contraction
2 = active movement, gravity eliminated
3 = active movement, against gravity
4 = active movement, against some resistance
5 = active movement, against full resistance
5* = normal corrected for pain/disuse
NT = not testable

SENSORY (SCORING ON REVERSE SIDE)
0 = absent 2 = normal
1= altered NT = not testable

(VAC) Voluntary Anal Contraction (Yes/No)
(DAP) Deep Anal Pressure (Yes/No)

RIGHT TOTALS (MAXIMUM) (50) (56) (56)
LEFT TOTALS (56) (56) (50) (MAXIMUM)

MOTOR SUBSCORES
UER ☐ + UEL ☐ = UEMS TOTAL ☐ MAX (25) (25) (50)
LER ☐ + LEL ☐ = LEMS TOTAL ☐ MAX (25) (25) (50)

SENSORY SUBSCORES
LTR ☐ + LTL ☐ = LT TOTAL ☐ MAX (56) (56) (112)
PPR ☐ + PPL ☐ = PP TOTAL ☐ MAX (56) (56) (112)

NEUROLOGICAL LEVELS — Steps 1-5 for classification as on reverse
1. SENSORY R ☐ L ☐
2. MOTOR R ☐ L ☐
3. NEUROLOGICAL LEVEL OF INJURY (NLI) ☐
4. COMPLETE OR INCOMPLETE? ☐ Incomplete = Any sensory or motor function in S4-5
5. ASIA IMPAIRMENT SCALE (AIS) ☐
ZONE OF PARTIAL PRESERVATION (In complete injuries only) — Most caudal level with any innervation: SENSORY R ☐ L ☐; MOTOR R ☐ L ☐

This form may be copied freely but should not be altered without permission from the American Spinal Injury Association. REV 04/15

FIGURE 117.2 International Standards for Neurological Classification of Spinal Cord Injury (ISNCSCI). (From American Spinal Injury Association. *International Standards for Neurological Classification of Spinal Cord Injury, revised 2011*; Atlanta, GA. Updated 2015. Courtesy of the American Spinal Injury Association.)

Muscle Function Grading

0 = total paralysis
1 = palpable or visible contraction
2 = active movement, full range of motion (ROM) with gravity eliminated
3 = active movement, full ROM against gravity
4 = active movement, full ROM against gravity and moderate resistance in a muscle specific position
5 = (normal) active movement, full ROM against gravity and full resistance in a functional muscle position expected from an otherwise unimpaired person
5* = (normal) active movement, full ROM against gravity and sufficient resistance to be considered normal if identified inhibiting factors (i.e. pain, disuse) were not present
NT = not testable (i.e. due to immobilization, severe pain such that the patient cannot be graded, amputation of limb, or contracture of > 50% of the normal ROM)

Sensory Grading

0 = Absent
1 = Altered, either decreased/impaired sensation or hypersensitivity
2 = Normal
NT = Not testable

When to Test Non-Key Muscles:

In a patient with an apparent AIS B classification, non-key muscle functions more than 3 levels below the motor level on each side should be tested to most accurately classify the injury (differentiate between AIS B and C).

Movement	Root level
Shoulder: Flexion, extension, abduction, adduction, internal and external rotation **Elbow:** Supination	C5
Elbow: Pronation **Wrist:** Flexion	C6
Finger: Flexion at proximal joint, extension. **Thumb:** Flexion, extension and abduction in plane of thumb	C7
Finger: Flexion at MCP joint **Thumb:** Opposition, adduction and abduction perpendicular to palm	C8
Finger: Abduction of the index finger	T1
Hip: Adduction	L2
Hip: External rotation	L3
Hip: Extension, abduction, internal rotation **Knee:** Flexion **Ankle:** Inversion and eversion **Toe:** MP and IP extension	L4
Hallux and Toe: DIP and PIP flexion and abduction	L5
Hallux: Adduction	S1

ASIA Impairment Scale (AIS)

A = Complete. No sensory or motor function is preserved in the sacral segments S4-5.

B = Sensory Incomplete. Sensory but not motor function is preserved below the neurological level and includes the sacral segments S4-5 (light touch or pin prick at S4-5 or deep anal pressure) AND no motor function is preserved more than three levels below the motor level on either side of the body.

C = Motor Incomplete. Motor function is preserved at the most caudal sacral segments for voluntary anal contraction (VAC) OR the patient meets the criteria for sensory incomplete status (sensory function preserved at the most caudal sacral segments (S4-S5) by LT, PP or DAP), and has some sparing of motor function more than three levels below the ipsilateral motor level on either side of the body.
(This includes key or non-key muscle functions to determine motor incomplete status.) For AIS C – less than half of key muscle functions below the single NLI have a muscle grade ≥ 3.

D = Motor Incomplete. Motor incomplete status as defined above, with at least half (half or more) of key muscle functions below the single NLI having a muscle grade ≥ 3.

E = Normal. If sensation and motor function as tested with the ISNCSCI are graded as normal in all segments, and the patient had prior deficits, then the AIS grade is E. Someone without an initial SCI does not receive an AIS grade.

Using ND: To document the sensory, motor and NLI levels, the ASIA Impairment Scale grade, and/or the zone of partial preservation (ZPP) when they are unable to be determined based on the examination results.

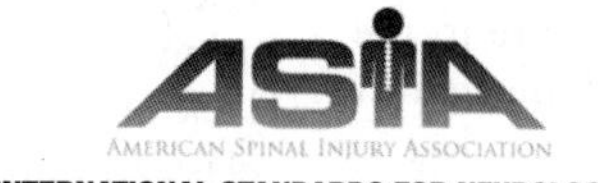

INTERNATIONAL STANDARDS FOR NEUROLOGICAL CLASSIFICATION OF SPINAL CORD INJURY

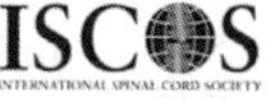

Steps in Classification

The following order is recommended for determining the classification of individuals with SCI.

1. Determine sensory levels for right and left sides.
The sensory level is the most caudal, intact dermatome for both pin prick and light touch sensation.

2. Determine motor levels for right and left sides.
Defined by the lowest key muscle function that has a grade of at least 3 (on supine testing), providing the key muscle functions represented by segments above that level are judged to be intact (graded as a 5).
Note: in regions where there is no myotome to test, the motor level is presumed to be the same as the sensory level, if testable motor function above that level is also normal.

3. Determine the neurological level of injury (NLI)
This refers to the most caudal segment of the cord with intact sensation and antigravity (3 or more) muscle function strength, provided that there is normal (intact) sensory and motor function rostrally respectively.
The NLI is the most cephalad of the sensory and motor levels determined in steps 1 and 2.

4. Determine whether the injury is Complete or Incomplete.
(i.e. absence or presence of sacral sparing)
If voluntary anal contraction = ***No*** *AND all S4-5 sensory scores =* ***0*** *AND deep anal pressure =* ***No,*** *then injury is* ***Complete.***
Otherwise, injury is ***Incomplete.***

5. Determine ASIA Impairment Scale (AIS) Grade:
Is injury Complete? **If YES, AIS=A** and can record ZPP (lowest dermatome or myotome on each side with some preservation)
NO ↓
Is injury Motor Complete? **If YES, AIS=B**
NO ↓ (No=voluntary anal contraction OR motor function more than three levels below the motor level on a given side, if the patient has sensory incomplete classification)

Are at least half (half or more) of the key muscles below the neurological level of injury graded 3 or better?

If sensation and motor function is normal in all segments, AIS=E
Note: AIS E is used in follow-up testing when an individual with a documented SCI has recovered normal function. If at initial testing no deficits are found, the individual is neurologically intact; the ASIA Impairment Scale does not apply.

FIGURE 117.2 *(Continued)*

defined as the most caudal segment of the cord with intact sensation and antigravity muscle function strength.

Radiologic Evaluation

No cervical radiologic evaluation is recommended in an awake, alert, nonintoxicated trauma patient who has no neck pain or tenderness and is neurologically normal unless there are significant associated injuries that would interfere with the history and physical examination. In this setting, cervical immobilization can be discontinued without imaging. However, in patients with neck pain or tenderness, a high-quality cervical spine CT should be performed. The CT scan is better than MRI for evaluating bones; however, for ligamentous injury, dynamic flexion/extension radiographs in an awake patient are preferred. Alternatively, an MRI within 48 hours of injury can also detect ligamentous injury (256). Newer-generation CT scanners are sensitive, and routine three-view (anteroposterior, lateral, and odontoid) cervical spine radiographs are not recommended unless high-quality CT imaging is not available. In obtunded patients, again, high-quality cervical CT is recommended to rule out clinically significant injury (257). However caution is taken before removing and immobilizing collar since an obtunded patient cannot report pain associated with ligamentous injury and instability. Options to remove the collar include: (1) waiting until the patient is awake and asymptomatic; (2) a normal MRI obtained within 48 hours of injury (although this is considered level III evidence with

TABLE 117.2 American Spinal Injury Association Impairment Scale

Grade	Classification	Description
A	Complete	No motor or sensory function preserved in S4-S5
B	Incomplete	Sensory but not motor function preserved below neurologic level, including S4-S5
C	Incomplete	Motor function preserved below neurologic level; ≥50% of key muscles below the neurologic level have muscle grade <3
D	Incomplete	Motor function preserved below neurologic level; ≥50% of key muscles below the neurologic level have muscle grade ≥3
E	Normal	Normal motor and sensory function

Data from *International Standards for Neurological Classification of Spinal Cord Injury*, revised 2011; Atlanta, GA: American Spinal Injury Association; 2015.

limited or conflicting data); (3) at the discretion of the treating physician (256) or 4) more recent guidelines recommend the removal of the collar following a normal high quality CT scan defined as 3 mm slices or less (258).

MRI is recommended for patients with cervical fracture-dislocation injuries if they cannot be examined during closed reduction. An MRI is performed to evaluate for disrupted or herniated intervertebral discs, which are found in up to 33% to 50% of patients with facet subluxation injuries (259). MRI is also recommended for patients with occipital condyle fractures to assess the integrity of the craniocervical ligaments (260).

Treatment

Immobilization

If the unstable spine is manipulated, 3% to 25% of spinal cord injuries may occur after the initial traumatic event. Additionally, nearly 20% of ASCIs include multiple noncontiguous vertebral levels (261,262). For this reason, early management of patients with SCI includes immediate prehospital immobilization of the entire spine with a rigid cervical collar with supportive blocks for head immobilization on a rigid backboard with straps (263). To prevent decubitus ulcers, it is recommended that the patient be transferred off the hard board as soon as possible; if the patient is awaiting transfer to another institution, they should be removed during the interim and replaced on the board for actual transport. Padded boards or bean bag boards are recommended to reduce pressure to the occiput and sacrum. Current recommendations advise against the use of sandbags and tape (264).

Hemodynamic Support

Systemic hypotension, which contributes to secondary spinal cord injury, can result from trauma-related hypovolemia and from neurogenic shock (265–267). Neurogenic shock is defined as the loss of sympathetic innervation that causes loss of peripheral vasoconstriction and cardiac compensatory mechanisms of tachycardia and increased stroke volume and cardiac output. In experimental models, microvascular spasm, thrombosis, and rupture will disrupt spinal cord vascular autoregulation and make the spinal cord more susceptible to systemic hypotension. This worsens spinal cord ischemia several hours after injury (267). MAP augmentation to 85 to 90 mmHg for 5 to 7 days after injury has been shown to reduce morbidity and mortality and shorten length of stay and are recommended by the recent 2013 guidelines (268–272).

Treatment typically includes volume resuscitation with crystalloid or red blood cell transfusion if the patient is anemic. Volume-resistant hypotension is fivefold more common among patients with complete spinal cord injury above the thoracic sympathetic innervation (269); vasoactive medications such as norepinephrine, dopamine, and phenylephrine may be required. In the subset of patients requiring vasopressors and inotropes, central venous catheters and invasive monitoring with arterial catheters should be used.

Surgical Intervention

The timing of surgical decompression, reduction of bony structures, and fusion in the treatment of ASCI have been debated. Earlier "practice options" included surgical intervention on patients with incomplete injury with persisting compression from dislocation with bilateral locked facets, burst fracture, or disc rupture, especially in patients with neurologic deterioration (273). Recent data suggest that early surgery, within 24 hours, has a beneficial effect on motor recovery (274) and current guidelines from 2013 are more definitive regarding recommendations with the goal of decompression of the spinal cord with restoration of the spinal canal (275). Recommendations include early (as rapidly as possible after injury) closed reduction of cervical spinal fracture/dislocation injury (259), and early reduction of fracture-dislocation injuries in the setting of acute traumatic central cord syndrome (CCS) with surgical decompression of the compressed spinal cord, particularly if the compression is focal and anterior (276). Overall, early surgery, possibly because of the ability to mobilize the patient earlier, appears to shorten hospital length of stay and reduce pulmonary complications (273,274,277–279).

Pharmacologic Intervention

Following ASCI, a cascade of biochemical processes is activated that produces excitatory amino acids, calcium fluxes, free radicals, acidosis, protein phosphorylation, phospholipases, and apoptosis, which can further injure surrounding tissue (267). Pharmacologic agents targeted to interrupt this cascade may provide neuroprotection by preventing secondary injury; however, similar to TBI, no agent has yet shown benefit (280).

Naloxone, GM-1 ganglioside, and methylprednisolone have undergone randomized clinical trials to examine their effects following spinal cord injury. After multiple trials evaluating the use of methylprednisolone (281–284), based on the lack of class I or class II evidence of benefit and inconsistent class III data, current neurosurgical and ATLS guidelines do not recommend the use of methylprednisolone after ASCI (91). Guidelines note that there are class I, II, and III evidence that high-dose steroids are associated with harmful side effects including pneumonia, gastrointestinal hemorrhage, sepsis and result in longer hospital stays, and death (281,285–287).

Pulmonary Support

The most common cause of death in patients with spinal cord injury is due to pneumonia, pulmonary emboli, and septicemia (22). In patients with tetraplegia, pneumonia and other respiratory complications occur in 40% to 70% of patients (288,289); aggressive pulmonary toilet is, therefore, essential.

Patients with high-level cervical injuries (C3–5) may fatigue over the first few hours to days. Pulmonary compromise can also be seen in patients with lower cervical cord injuries. Although diaphragmatic innervation arises from the cervical levels of three through five (C3–5), an effective cough and deep inspiration requires intercostal musculature and thoracic innervation to splint the chest wall while the diaphragm descends. Additionally, patients who are smokers with increased pulmonary secretions or those who have aspirated fluid such as blood, water, or stomach contents may have difficulty clearing their airway and should be monitored closely for failing pulmonary reserve.

Bedside evaluation with deep inspiration will frequently show a "functional flail chest," wherein, with deep inspiration, the diaphragm descends, the abdomen rises, but the chest wall does not rise, but collapses or is immobile. Of the pulmonary function tests, vital capacity (VC) appears to be the single global measure of ventilatory status that best correlates with other pulmonary function tests (290). Serial measurements of bedside VC can indicate the need for elective endotracheal intubation if the VC is less than 20 mL/kg or decreasing rapidly. Hypoxia and hypercapnia are late signs of respiratory failure, and intubation should not await these findings.

Associated Vascular Injury

Blunt cervical spinal trauma can result in vascular injury and cause cerebral ischemia (291). Incidence varies from 0.03% to 4.8% and likely depends on the screening method (292–294). Mortality ranges from 23% to 28%, while 48% to 58% of survivors have significant neurologic deficits (295). The most common mechanism of blunt cerebrovascular injury (BCVI) is MVC, followed by falls, and pedestrian and motorcycle crashes. Many institutions use modifications of the Denver Screening Criteria for BCVI based on risk factors to determine whom to screen (296). Risk factors include cervical fractures with subluxation or with a fracture through the transverse foramen, displaced or complex midface or mandibular fracture (LeForte II or III), a basilar skull fracture involving the carotid canal or sphenoid sinus, near-hanging resulting in cerebral hypoxia, and cervical vertebral body fraction or distraction injury, a seatbelt sign or tissue injury of the anterior neck, and massive epistaxis or a cervical hematoma (292). Suspicion should be high if the patient develops a lateralizing neurologic deficit with an initially normal CT scan, or evidence of a recent ischemic stroke on cerebral imaging. CT angiography (CTA) is sensitive for BCVI and has taken the place of conventional cerebral angiography as the recommended screening tool unless CTA is not available or endovascular treatment is anticipated (297–300). In a patient with a vertebral subluxation or complete spinal cord injury, MRI is the recommended diagnostic modality (300).

A grading system of injury has been described by Biffl (301) (Table 117.3). Fifty-seven percentage of grade I injuries heal spontaneously in 10 days independent of therapy (302); therefore, they can be treated with aspirin. Retrospective studies of grade II through IV injuries show no difference between antiplatelet agent or heparin therapy although heparinization increases hemorrhage risk (303,304). Current recommendations suggest individualized therapy dependent on the vascular injury, associated injuries, and the risk of hemorrhage. Options include no treatment, antiplatelet therapy, or anticoagulation. No recommendations regarding endovascular therapy can yet be made (300).

Thromboprophylaxis

DVT detection with ^{131}I-fibrinogen scans of patients with ASCI and paralysis ranges as high as 100% (305). Recommended diagnostic tests include: duplex Doppler ultrasound, impedance plethysmography, venous occlusion plethysmography, venography, and the clinical examination (306).

Prophylactic LMWH or LDUFH, in conjunction with mechanical prophylaxis such as pneumatic compression stockings or electrical stimulation, is recommended for patients with ASCI by both the American College of Chest Physicians, the Neurocritical Care Society, and Congress of Neurological Surgeons (221,224). Notably, neurosurgery Level II guidelines recommend that low-dose heparin therapy alone or oral anticoagulation alone is not recommended as a prophylactic treatment strategy. The period of highest risk for DVT is in the first few months following injury. Guidelines recommend early administration within 72 hours of injury and continued for 3 months (306).

By both guidelines, IVC filters are not recommended as primary prophylaxis against pulmonary embolus, but are recommended in patients who fail anticoagulation or who are not candidates for anticoagulation and/or mechanical devices. These may include those with concurrent severe head injury (307). "Quad" coughing is a Heimlich maneuver used for pulmonary toilet to clear secretions in SCI patients with a poor cough; IVC filters have been reported to embolize or perforate with quad coughing (308,309). In one series, the majority of patients with these complications received vigorous pulmonary toilet (46%) including quad coughing. Quad coughing probably should be avoided until the IVC filter is removed.

Following trauma, there may be patients who have undergone spinal surgery and require full anticoagulation due to an acute pulmonary embolism, or myocardial ischemia or infarction. There are no prospective randomized studies of the safety of anticoagulation following spinal surgery for ASCI (310). In this setting, an open discussion of the risks and benefits with the patient and his or her decision makers is necessary. If anticoagulation is used, close neurologic checks are essential as early evacuation of an acute EDH can impact neurologic outcome if the injury to the spinal cord is incomplete (311,312).

TABLE 117.3 Grading Scale for Blunt Cervical Vascular Injury

Grade	Description
I	Luminal irregularity or dissection <25% luminal narrowing
II	Dissection or intramural hematoma with ≥25% luminal narrowing, intraluminal thrombus, or raised intimal flap
III	Pseudoaneurysm
IV	Occlusion
V	Transection with free extravasation

Adapted from Biffl WL, Moore EE, Offner PJ, et al. Blunt carotid arterial injuries: implications of a new grading scale. *J Trauma.* 1999;47:845–853.

Nutritional Support

As described above, TBI is associated with a hypermetabolic, catabolic state with nitrogen loss. In spinal cord injury victims, indirect calorimetry will be more accurate than the Harris–Benedict equation to determine metabolic needs and is recommended (225,313). Although metabolic needs may be clevidipine, increased, the REE may be lower than expected.

Autonomic Dysreflexia

Autonomic dysreflexia is a life-threatening hypertensive emergency that typically occurs in patients with motor-complete SCI above the T6 neurologic level (314,315). Autonomic dysreflexia is typically seen in the rehabilitative phase of SCI; however, it has been recognized as early as 4 days after injury (316). Noxious stimuli including fecal impaction, bladder distention, or pain to the lower extremities increases sympathetic outflow below the injury level. Resultant vasoconstriction of the splanchnic bed forces blood into the system circulation and increases blood pressure. Reflex parasympathetic outflow rostral to the injury allows flushing of the skin above the level of the lesion and bradycardia. Recognition of this entity, and detection and removal of the inciting noxious stimulus is primary. Blood pressure treatment traditionally included ganglionic blockers, although intravenous antihypertensives such as clevidipine, nicardipine or nitroprusside can be effective.

Prognosis

Determinants of outcome following ASCI include the level and severity of injury, age, initial motor strength, and MRI findings. The ASIA Spinal Cord Injury Classification is useful for studies and comparison of outcome (317). Incomplete injury has a better prognosis than those that are complete. The ASIA Impairment Scale severity on presentation of injury is one of the strongest predictors for outcome (318,319). Those in group A are unlikely to have significant recovery (319) whereas those in groups C and D recover better than those in B. Most recovery occurs in the first 6 months after injury with the greatest rate of improvement in the first 3 months (22).

MRI shows that complete spinal cord injury is typically associated with more substantial maximum canal compromise, spinal cord compression, increased length of lesion, hemorrhage, and cord edema. Substantial canal compromise, intramedullary hemorrhage, and cord edema at time of presentation can be predictive of a poorer prognosis (320).

Two clinical entities described in ASCI are pertinent to prognosis. The first, spinal shock, is a transient loss of spinal cord sensorimotor function. Patients present with flaccid paralysis and loss of all spinal cord reflexes including the bulbocavernosus, cremasteric, and deep tendon reflexes. Priapism can be seen due to local unopposed parasympathetic outflow. If there is no anatomic injury, function returns within hours to days.

The second is the CCS in which the motor deficit in the upper extremities is disproportionately worse than that in the lower extremities, with bowel and bladder dysfunction and variable sensory loss below the level of injury (321,322). Most patients with CCS improve neurologically, although many have significant persistent neurologic deficits. Typically, CCS results from hyperextension injury without a fracture in older patients as a result of a stenotic spondylotic cervical canal (323). It is also seen in a younger population with acute cervical disc herniation or spinal instability which may require early surgical decompression and stabilization (276). Motor recovery is improved when there is a higher motor score at the time of injury (322).

CONTROVERSIES

- Current controversies with head injury typically involve imaging and monitoring. Since changes on repeat CT imaging that require clinical intervention are accompanied by changes in the neurologic examination, it would seem that close neurologic monitoring rather than routine repeat imaging should be adopted. It is a costly modality with some risk to the patient including radiation exposure and transport. Yet the possible consequence of a missed injury leads to the practice of unnecessary routine repeat imaging.
- While calculating CPP, there continues to be a lack of standardization of nursing practice of the measurement of MAP with regard to establishing the reference point for the transducer of the invasive arterial monitor. If the patient is being nursed in high Fowler position (HOB elevated) rather than supine, then the MAP relative to the brain will be lower than the MAP when the arterial transducer is zeroed to the heart (i.e., phlebostatic axis at the midaxillary line). When measuring MAP to calculate CPP, the reference point for the arterial transducer should be at the midbrain (i.e., level of the tragus); however, this is rarely the practice. A recent survey noted that of 34 neurocritical care centers, 74% reported used the heart and 16% used the midbrain (324). The same study reviewed 32 articles reporting CPP data. The reference point for MAP was reported in 16 of the studies with 10 using the heart, and 6 using the midbrain. To date, no standardized clinical practice has been achieved (324,325).
- Multimodality monitoring including cerebral blood oximetry, microdialysis, and near-infrared spectroscopy are available commercially. However, it is still unknown as to whether establishing target parameters with aggressive goal-directed therapy improves patient outcome.
- Screening for BCVI can be performed, but if injury is found the evidence base for the most effective and safe therapy especially after traumatic injury does not yet exist. Similarly, if there is an indication for full anticoagulation in a patient, the optimal timing in the setting of intracranial or spinal injury is not yet known.
- Following ASCI, controversies include the timing of surgery. There is no clear definition as to whether "early" surgery translates to 24, 48, or 72 hours or even earlier. The practicality of early surgery can be difficult in many settings and if outcome is poor after surgery, litigious individuals might consider the operative intervention to be causative. For this reason, despite the guidelines for early surgery, surgeons may be extremely conservative as to early operative approach.
- Also, despite guidelines evaluating the existing evidence that recommend that steroids may have more adverse effects than benefit following ASCI, some practitioners still choose to administer steroids in this setting.
- Although advances are being made in the area of the management of neurologically critically ill patients, much more work is needed to improve outcomes for these patients.

Key Points

- Primary prevention and avoidance of neurologic injury is essential to decrease neurologic injury. National and global efforts are underway, particularly to improve road traffic safety.
- Head injury: perform a rapid assessment of GCS score to determine severity of injury and need for endotracheal intubation or ICP monitoring.
- Spinal cord injury: early evaluation of the strength of pulmonary mechanics with visual examination of chest excursion with deep breathing and bedside VC measurement to determine need for intubation.
- Initial and serial neurologic bedside examination to assess alteration in mental status, cranial neuropathies, motor and sensory deficits in all patients.
- Emergent CT scan of the brain and spinal column following traumatic injury.
- CTA of the neck and brain to assess for BCVI following trauma in selected patients.
- Recognition of early signs of intracranial hypertension including systemic hypertension.

- To prevent secondary neurologic injury maintain:
  - Adequate oxygenation with PaO_2 above 60 mmHg and O_2 saturation above 90%.
  - Adequate perfusion following head injury with a SBP 100 mm Hg or greater in patients 50 to 69 years old and 110 mm Hg or greater in patients 15 to 49 or greater than 70 years old; or CPP 60 to 70 mmHg, and MAP equal or greater than 85 mm after ASCI.
- Euvolemia, euglycemia, and normothermia.
- ICP monitoring should be performed in patients with GCS of 8 or less.
- Steroids are not indicated for brain or spinal cord traumatic injury.
- Age and severity at time of brain or spinal cord injury and level of spinal cord injury are significant determinants of outcome.

References

1. Basso A, Previgliano I, Servadei F. Traumatic brain injuries. In: Aarli JA, Dua T, Janca A, Muscetta A, eds. *Neurological Disorders: Public Health Challenges*. Geneva, Switzerland: World Health Organization; 2006:164–175.
2. Bell JM, Jenkins EL, Brelding M, Haarbauer-Krupa J, Llonbarger MR, eds. *Report to Congress: Traumatic Brain Injury in the United States: Epidemiology and Rehabilitation.* Atlanta, GA: Centers for Disease Control and Prevention, National Center for Injury Prevention and Control, Division of Unintentional Injury Prevention; 2014.
3. Menon DK, Schwab K, Wright DW, Maas AI; Demographics and Clinical Assessment Working Group of the International and Interagency Initiative Toward Common Data Elements for Research on Traumatic Brain Injury and Psychological Health. Position statement: definition of traumatic brain injury. *Arch Phys Med Rehabil.* 2010;91:1637–1640.
4. Office of Statistics and Programming, National Center for Injury Prevention and Control, Centers for Disease Control. *Ten Leading Causes of Death by Age Group, United States—2010*. Atlanta, GA: National Vital Statistics System, National Center for Health Statistics; 2010.
5. Faul M, XU L, Wald MM, Coronado VG. *Traumatic Brain Injury in the United States: Emergency Department Visits, Hospitalizations, and Deaths*. Atlanta, GA: Center for Disease Control and Prevention, National Center for Injury Prevention and Control; 2010.
6. Roozenbeek B, Maas AI, Menon DK. Changing patterns in the epidemiology of traumatic brain injury. *Nat Rev Neurol.* 2013;9:231–236.
7. Tagliaferri F, Compagnone C, Korsic M, et al. A systematic review of brain injury epidemiology in Europe. *Acta Neurochir (Wien)*. 2006;148:255–268.
8. Berg J, Tagliaferri F, Servadei F. Cost of trauma in Europe. *Eur J Neurol.* 2005;12 (Suppl 1):85–90.
9. Langlois JA, Rutland-Brown W, Thomas KE. *Traumatic Brain Injury in the United States: Emergency Department Visits, Hospitalizations, and Deaths*. Atlanta, GA: Centers for Disease Control and Prevention, National Center for Injury Prevention and Control; 2004.
10. National Center for Injury Prevention and Control, Division of Unintentional Injury Prevention. *Rates of TBI-Related Deaths by Sex—United States, 2001–2010*. Centers for Disease Control and Prevention website. Available at: www.cdc.gov/traumaticbraininjury/data/rates_deaths_bysex.html. Accessed June 12, 2015.
11. Roberts I, Mohan D, Abassi K. War on the roads. *BMJ*. 2002;324(7346):1107–1109.
12. National Center for Injury Prevention and Control. *Traumatic Brain Injury in the United States: Fact Sheet*. Centers for Disease Control and Prevention website. Available at: www.cdc.gov/traumaticbraininjury/get_the_facts.htm. Accessed June 12, 2015.
13. National Center for Injury Prevention and Control, Division of Unintentional Injury Prevention. *Percent Distributions of TBI-related Emergency Department Visits by Age Group and Injury Mechanism—United States, 2006–2010*. Centers for Disease Control and Prevention website. Available at: www.cdc.gov/traumaticbraininjury/data//dist_ed.html. Accessed June 12, 2015.
14. Thurman D, Alverson C, Dunn K, et al. Traumatic brain injury in the United States: a public health perspective. *J Head Trauma Rehabil.* 1999;14:602–615.
15. National Center for Injury Prevention and Control. *Report to Congress: Traumatic Brain Injury in the United States*. Centers for Disease Control and Prevention website. Available at: http://www.cdc.gov/traumaticbrain injury/pubs/tbi_report_to_congress.html. Published 1999; Accessed June 12, 2015.
16. Helmick KM, Spells CA, Malik SZ, et al. Traumatic brain injury in the US military: epidemiology and key clinical and research programs. *Brain Imaging Behav.* 2015;9(3):358–366.
17. Warden D. Military TBI during the Iraq and Afghanistan wars. *J Head Trauma Rehabil.* 2006;21:398–402.
18. Owens BD, Kragh JF Jr, Wenke JC, et al. Combat wounds in operation Iraqi freedom and operation enduring freedom. *J Trauma*. 2008;65:295–299.
19. Zaloshnja E, Miller T, Langlois JA, Selassie AW. Prevalence of long-term disability from traumatic brain injury in the civilian population of the United States, 2005. *J Head Trauma Rehabil.* 2005;23:394–400.
20. Selassie AW, Zaloshnja E, Langolis JA, Miller T, et al. Incidence of long-term disability following traumatic brain injury hospitalization, United States, 2003. *J Head Trauma Rehabil.* 2008;23:123–131.
21. Finkelstein E, Corso P, Miller T. *The Incidence and Economic Burden of Injuries in the United States.* New York: Oxford University Press; 2006.
22. National Spinal Cord Injury Statistical Center. *Spinal Cord Injury (SCI) Facts and Figures at a Glance*. Birmingham, AL: University of Alabama at Birmingham; 2016.
23. Surkin J, Smith M, Penman A, et al. Spinal cord injury incidence in Mississippi: a capture–recapture approach. *J Trauma Injury Infection Crit Care.* 1998;5:502–504.
24. Warren S, Moore M, Johnson MS. Traumatic head and spinal cord injuries in Alaska (1991–1993). *Alaska Med.* 1995;37:11–19.
25. Burke DA, Linden RD, Zhang YP, et al. Incidence rates and populations at risk for spinal cord injury: a regional study. *Spinal cord.* 2001;39:274–278.
26. Garrison A, Clifford K, Gleason SF, et al. Alcohol use associated with cervical spinal cord injury. *J Spinal Cord Med.* 2004;27:111–115.
27. World Health Organization. *Spinal Cord Injury. Fact Sheet Number 384.* Available at: www.who.int/mediacentre/factsheets/fs384/en/. Published 2013, Accessed June 13, 2015.
28. Singh A, Tetreault L, Kalsi-Ryan S, et al. Global prevalence and incidence of traumatic spinal cord injury. *Clin Epidemiol.* 2014;6:309–331.
29. Cripps RA, Lee BB, Wing P, et al. A global map for traumatic spinal cord injury epidemiology: towards a living data repository for injury prevention. *Spinal Cord.* 2011;49:493–501.
30. Asia Spinal Cord Network. *Guidelines for Prevention of Spinal Cord Injuries.* Dhalko, Kathmandu: New Sandesh Printers; 2008
31. Lenehan B, Street J, Kwon BK, et al. The epidemiology of traumatic spinal cord injury in British Columbia, Canada. *Spine.* 2012;37:321–329.
32. Centers for Disease Control and Prevention. Nonfatal traumatic brain injuries related to sports and recreation activities among persons aged ≤19 years—United States, 2001–2009. *MMWR Morb Mortal Wkly Rep.* 2011;60:1337–1342.
33. Centers for Disease Control and Prevention. *Heads Up.* Available at: www.cdc.gov/HEADSUP/. Accessed June 13, 2015.
34. Stevens JA, Phelan EA. Development of STEADI: a fall prevention resource for health care providers. *Health Promot Pract.* 2013;14:706–714.
35. Gardner MM, Robertson MC, Campbell AJ. Exercise in preventing falls and fall related injuries in older people: a review of randomised controlled trials. *Br J Sports Med.* 2000;34:7–17.
36. Moyer VA. Prevention of falls in community-dwelling older adults: US Preventive Services Task Force Recommendation Statement. *Ann Int Med.* 2012;157:197–204.
37. World Health Organization. *Injury: A Leading Cause of the Global Burden of Disease.* Geneva, Switzerland: WHO; 2002.
38. Peden M, Scurfield R, Sleet D et al, eds. *World Report on Road Traffic Injury Prevention.* Geneva: World Health Organization; 2004.
39. Peden M. UN General Assembly calls for decade of action for road safety. *Inj Prev.* 2010;15:213.
40. Saatman KE, Duhaime AC, Bullock R, et al. Classification of traumatic brain injury for targeted therapies. *J Neurotrauma.* 2008;25:719–738.
41. Hlatky R, Valadka AB, Goodman JC, Robertson CS. Evolution of brain tissue injury after evacuation of acute traumatic subdural hematomas. *Neurosurgery.* 2004;55:1318–1324.
42. Marshall LF, Gautille T, Klauber MR, et al. The outcome of severe closed head injury. *J Neurosurg.* 1991;75:S28–S39.
43. Koc RK, Akdemir H, Oktem IS, et al. Acute subdural hematoma: outcome and outcome prediction. *Neurosurg Rev.* 1997;20:239–244.
44. Seelig JM, Becker DP, Miller JD, et al. Traumatic acute subdural hematoma: major mortality reduction in comatose patients treated within four hours. *N Engl J Med.* 1981;304:1511–1518.

45. Jamieson KG, Yelland JD. Surgically treated subdural hematomas. *J Neurosurg.* 1972;37:137–149.
46. Wilberger JE, Harris M, Diamond DL. Acute subdural hematoma: morbidity, mortality, and operative timing. *J Neurosurg.* 1991;74:212–218.
47. Foulkes MA, Eisenberg HM, Jane JA, et al. The Traumatic Coma Data Bank: design, methods and baseline characteristics. *J Neurosurg.* 1991;75:S8–S13.
48. Ford LE, McLaurin RL. Mechanisms of extradural hematomas. *J Neurosurg.* 1963;20:760–769.
49. Servadei F, Piazza G, Seracchioli A, et al. Extradural haematomas: an analysis of the changing characteristics of patients admitted from 1980 to 1986. Diagnostic and therapeutic implications in 158 cases. *Brain Inj.* 1988;2:87–100.
50. Servadei F. Prognostic factors in severely head injured adult patients with epidural haematomas. *Acta Neurochir (Wien).* 1997;139:273–278.
51. Lee EJ, Hung YC, Wang LC, et al. Factors influencing the functional outcome of patients with acute epidural hematomas: analysis of 200 patients undergoing surgery. *J Trauma.* 1998;45:946–952.
52. Seelig JM, Marshall LF, Toutant SM, et al. Traumatic acute epidural hematoma: unrecognized high lethality in comatose patients. *Neurosurgery.* 1984;15:617–620.
53. Oertel M, Kelly DF, McArthur D, et al. Progressive hemorrhage after head trauma: predictors and consequences of the evolving injury. *J Neurosurg.* 2002;96:109–116.
54. Kaups KL, Davis JW, Parks SN. Routinely repeated computed tomography after blunt head trauma: Does it benefit patients? *J Trauma.* 2004;56:475–481.
55. Maas A, Hukkelhoven C, Marshall LF, Steyerberg EW. Prediction of outcome in traumatic brain injury with computed tomographic characteristics: a comparison between the computed tomographic classification and combinations of computed tomographic predictors. *Neurosurgery.* 2005;57:1173–1182.
56. Chestnut R, Ghajar J, Maas A, et al. Early indicators of prognosis in severe traumatic brain injury. *J Neurotrauma.* 2000;17:535–627.
57. Chang EF, Meeker M, Holland MC, et al. Acute traumatic intraparenchymal hemorrhage: risk factors for progression in the early post-injury period. *Neurosurgery.* 2006;58:647–656.
58. Povlishock JT. Pathobiology of traumatically induced axonal injury in animals and man. *Ann Emerg Med.* 1993;22:980–986.
59. Davceva N, Basheska N, Balazic J. Diffuse axonal injury—A distinct clinicopathological entity in closed head injuries. *Am J Forensic Med Pathol.* 2015;36(3):127–133.
60. Jennett B, Adams JH, Murray LS, Graham DI. Neuropathology in vegetative and severely disabled patients after head injury. *Neurology.* 2001;56:486–490.
61. de la Plata CM, Ardelean A, Koovakkattu D, et al. Magnetic resonance imaging of diffuse axonal injury: quantitative assessment of white matter lesion volume. *J Neurotrauma.* 2007;24:591–598.
62. Yuan L, Wei X, Xu C, et al. Use of multisequence 3.0T MRI to detect severe traumatic brain injury and predict the outcome. *Br J Radiol.* 2015;88:20150129.
63. Ezaki Y, Tsutsumi K, Morikawa M, Nagata I. Role of diffusion-weighted magnetic resonance imaging in diffuse axonal injury. *Acta Radiol.* 2006;47:733–740.
64. Juul N, Morris GF, Marshall SB, Marshall LF. Intracranial hypertension and cerebral perfusion pressure: influence on neurological deterioration and outcome in severe head injury. The Executive Committee of the International Selfotel Trial. *J Neurosurg.* 2000;92:1–6.
65. Carney N, Totten AM, O'Reilly C, et al. Guidelines for the management of severe traumatic brain injury. Fourth Edition. *Neurosurg* 2017; 80:6–15.
66. Robertson CS, Valadka AB, Hannay HJ, et al. Prevention of secondary ischemic insults after severe head injury. *Crit Care Med.* 1999;27:2086–2095.
67. Guidelines for the management of severe traumatic brain injury. 4th Edition. https://www.braintrauma.org/coma/guidelines. Accessed May 26, 2017.
68. Teasdale G, Jennett B. Assessment of coma and impaired consciousness: a practical scale. *Lancet.* 1974;2:81–84.
69. Marion DM, Carlier PM. Problems with initial Glasgow Coma Scale assessment caused by prehospital treatment of patients with head injuries: results of a national survey. *J Trauma.* 1994;36:89–95.
70. Gennarelli TA, Champion HR, Copes WS, Sacco WJ. Comparison of mortality, morbidity, and severity of 59,713 head injured patients with 114,447 patients with extracranial injuries. *J Trauma.* 1994;37:962–968.
71. Chesnut RM, Ghajar J, Maas AI, et al. Early indicators of prognosis in severe traumatic brain injury: Glasgow Coma Scale Score. In: *Management and Prognosis of Severe Traumatic Brain Injury.* New York: Brain Trauma Foundation; 2000:163–173. https://www.braintrauma.org. Accessed May 26, 2017.
72. Jiang JY, Gao GY, Li WP, et al. Early indicators of prognosis in 846 cases of severe traumatic brain injury. *J Neurotrauma.* 2002;19:869–874.
73. Dager WE, Gosselin RC, Kitchen S, Dwyre D. Dabigatran effects on the international normalized ratio, activated partial thromboplastin time, thrombin time, and fibrinogen: a multicenter, in vitro study. *Ann Pharmacother.* 2012;46:1627–1636.
74. Bullock MR, Chestnut R, Ghajar J, et al; Surgical Management of Traumatic Brain Injury Author Group. Surgical management of acute epidural hematomas. *Neurosurgery.* 2006;58(3 Suppl):S7–S15.
75. Bullock MR, Chestnut R, Ghajar J, et al; Surgical Management of Traumatic Brain Injury Author Group. Surgical management of acute subdural hematomas. *Neurosurgery.* 2006;58(3 Suppl):S16–S24.
76. Bullock MR, Chestnut R, Ghajar J, et al; Surgical Management of Traumatic Brain Injury Author Group. Surgical management of traumatic parenchymal lesions. *Neurosurgery.* 2006;58(3 Suppl):S25–S46.
77. Haydel MJ, Preston CA, Mills TJ, et al. Indication for computed tomography in patients with minor head injury. *N Engl J Med.* 2000;343:100–105.
78. Servadei F, Murray GD, Penny K, et al. The value of the "worst" computed tomographic scan in clinical studies of moderate and severe head injury. *Neurosurgery.* 2000;46:70–77.
79. Lee TT, Aldana PR, Kirton OC, Green BA. Follow-up computerized tomography (CT) scans in moderate and severe head injuries: correlation with Glasgow Coma scores (GCS) and complication rate. *Acta Neurochir (Wien).* 1997;139:1042–1048.
80. Hurst JM, Davis K, Johnson DJ, et al. Cost and complications during in-hospital transport of critically ill patients: a prospective cohort study. *J Trauma.* 1992;33:582–585.
81. Givner A, Guerney J, O'Connor D, et al. Reimaging in pediatric neurotrauma: factors associated with progression of intracranial injury. *J Pediatr Surg.* 2002;37:381–385.
82. Sifri ZC, Homnick AT, Vaynman A, et al. A prospective evaluation of the value of repeat cranial computed tomography in patients with minimal head injury and an intracranial bleed. *J Trauma.* 2006;61:862–867.
83. Schuster R, Waxman K. Is repeated head computed tomography necessary for traumatic intracranial hemorrhage? *Am Surg.* 2005;71:701–704.
84. Wang MC, Linnau KF, Tirschwell DL, Hollingworth W. Utility of repeat head computed tomography after blunt head trauma: a systematic review. *J Trauma.* 2006;61:226–233.
85. Velmahos GC, Gervasini A, Petrovick L, et al. Routine repeat head CT for minimal head injury is unnecessary. *J Trauma.* 2006;60:494–501.
86. Almenawer SA, Bogza I, Yarascavitch B, et al. The value of scheduled repeat cranial computed tomography after mild head injury. *Neurosurg.* 2013;72:56–64.
87. Chestnut RM, Marshall LF, Klauber MR, et al. The role of secondary brain injury in determining outcome from severe head injury. *J Trauma.* 1993;34:216–222.
88. Chi JH, Knudson MM, Vassar MJ, et al. Prehospital hypoxia affects outcome in patients with traumatic brain injury: a prospective multicenter study. *J Trauma.* 2006;61:1134–1141.
89. Singbartl G. Significance of preclinical emergency treatment for the prognosis of patients with severe craniocerebral trauma [in German]. *Anasth Intensivther Notfallmed.* 1985;20:251–260.
90. Mayglothling J, Duane TM, Gibbs M, et al. Emergency tracheal intubation immediately following traumatic injury: An Eastern Association for the Surgery of Trauma practice management guideline. *J Trauma Acute Care Surg.* 2012;73:S333–S340.
91. Committee on Trauma of the American College of Surgeons. *Advanced Trauma Life Support.* 9th ed. Chicago, IL: American College of Surgeons; 2012.
92. Gabriel EJ, Ghajar J, Jacoda A, et al. *Guidelines for Prehospital Management of Traumatic Brain Injury.* New York: Brain Trauma Foundation, U. S. Department of Transportation National Highway Traffic Safety Administration; 2000.
93. Bernard SA. Paramedic intubation of patients with severe head injury: a review of current Australian practice and recommendations for change. *Emerg Med Australas.* 2006;18:221–228.
94. Davis DP, Fakhry SM, Wang HE, et al. Paramedic rapid sequence intubation for severe traumatic brain injury: perspectives from an expert panel. *Prehosp Emerg Care.* 2007;11:1–8.
95. Davis DP, Koprowicz KM, Newgard CD, et al. The relationship between out-of-hospital airway management and outcome among trauma patients with Glasgow coma scale scores of 8 or less. *Prehosp Emerg Care.* 2011;15:184–192.
96. Shafi S, Gentilello L. Pre-hospital endotracheal intubation and positive pressure ventilation is associated with hypotension and decreased survival

in hypovolemic trauma patients: an analysis of the National Trauma Data Bank. *J Trauma*. 2005;59:1140–1147.
97. Hamill JF, Bedford RF, Weaver DC, Colohan AR. Lidocaine before endotracheal intubation: intravenous or laryngotracheal? *Anesthesiology*. 1981; 55:578–581.
98. Yano M, Nishiyama H, Yokota H, et al. Effect of lidocaine on ICP response to endotracheal suctioning. *Anesthesiology*. 1986;64:651–653.
99. Coles JP, Minhas PS, Fryer TD, et al. Effect of hyperventilation on cerebral blood flow in traumatic head injury: clinical relevance and monitoring correlates. *Crit Care Med*. 2002;30:1950–1959.
100. Diringer MN, Videen TO, Yundt K, et al. Regional cerebrovascular and metabolic effects of hyperventilation after severe traumatic brain injury. *J Neurosurg*. 2002;96:103–108.
101. Imberti R, Bellinzona G, Langer M. Cerebral tissue PO2 and SjvO2 changes during moderate hyperventilation in patients with severe traumatic brain injury. *J Neurosurg*. 2002;96:97–102.
102. Muizelaar JP, Marmarou A, Ward JD, et al. Adverse effects of prolonged hyperventilation in patients with severe head injury: a randomized clinical trial. *J Neurosurg*. 1991;75:731–739.
103. Brain Trauma Foundation; American Association of Neurological Surgeons; Joint Section on Neurotrauma and Critical Care; Bratton SL, Chestnut RM, Ghajar J. Guidelines for the management of severe head injury: Brain oxygen monitoring and thresholds. *J Neurotrauma*. 2007;24(Suppl I):S65–S70.
104. Luce JM, Huseby JS, Kirk W, et al. Mechanism by which positive end-expiratory pressure increases cerebrospinal fluid pressure in dogs. *J Appl Physiol*. 1982;52:231–235.
105. Huseby JS, Pavlin EG, Butler J. Effect of positive end-expiratory pressure on intracranial pressure in dogs. *J Appl Physiol*. 1978;44:25–27.
106. Piek J, Chestnut RM, Marshall LF, et al. Extracranial complications of severe head injury. *J Neurosurg*. 1992;77:901–907.
107. Gemma M, Tommasino C, Cerri M, et al. Intracranial effects of endotracheal suctioning in the acute phase of head injury. *J Neurosurg Anesthesiol*. 2002;14:50–54.
108. Davison DL, Terek M, Chawla LS. Neurogenic pulmonary edema. *Crit Care*. 2012;16:212.
109. Bean JW, Beckman DL. Centrogenic pulmonary pathology in mechanical head injury. *J Appl Physiol*. 1969;27:807–812.
110. Marie FW, Patton HD. Neural structures involved in the genesis of preoptic pulmonary edema, gastric erosions, and behavior changes. *Am J Physiol*. 1956;184:345–350.
111. Talman WT, Perrone MH, Reis DJ. Acute hypertension after the local injection of kainic acid in to the nucleus tractus solitarii of rats. *Circulation Res*. 1981;48:292–298.
112. Blessing WW, West MJ, Chalmers J. Hypertension, bradycardia and pulmonary edema in the conscious rabbit after brainstem lesions coinciding with the A1 group of catecholamine neurons. *Circulation Res*. 1981;49: 949–958.
113. Schraufnagel DE, Patel KR. Sphincters in pulmonary veins. *Am Rev Respir Dis*. 1990;141:721–726.
114. Simon RP. Neurogenic pulmonary edema. *Neurol Clin*. 1993;11:309–323.
115. Theodore J, Robin ED. Speculation on neurogenic pulmonary edema (NPE). *Am Rev Resp Dis*. 1976;113:405–411.
116. Colice GL. Neurogenic pulmonary edema. *Clin Chest Med*. 1985;6: 473–489.
117. Knudsen F, Jensen HP, Petersen PL. Neurogenic pulmonary edema: treatment with dobutamine. *Neurosurgery*. 1991;29:269–270.
118. Chestnut RM, Marshall SB, Piek J, et al. Early and late systemic hypotension as a frequent and fundamental source of cerebral ischemia following severe brain injury in the Traumatic Coma Data Bank. *Acta Neurochir Suppl (Wien)*. 1993;59:121–125.
119. Manley G, Knudson MM, Morabito D, et al. Hypotension, hypoxia, and head injury. frequency, duration, and consequences. *Arch Surg*. 2001;136: 1118–1123.
120. Clifton GL, Miller ER, Choi SC, Levin HS. Fluid thresholds and outcome from severe brain injury. *Crit Care Med*. 2002;30:739–745.
121. Britton M, de Faire U, Helmers C, et al. Arrhythmias in patients with acute cerebrovascular disease. *Acta Med Scand*. 1979;205:425–428.
122. Andreoli A, di Pasquale G, Pinelli G, et al. Subarachnoid hemorrhage: frequency and severity of cardiac arrhythmia: a survey of 70 cases studied in the acute phase. *Stroke*. 1987;18:558–564.
123. Blumhardt LD, Smith PE, Owen L. Electrocardiographic accompaniments of temporal lobe epileptic seizures. *Lancet*. 1986;8489:1051–1056.
124. Jachuck SJ, Ramani PS, Clark F, Kalbag RM. Electrocardiographic abnormalities associated with raised intracranial pressure. *Br Med J*. 1975;1:242–244.
125. Reichenbach DD, Benditt EP. Catecholamines and cardiomyopathy: the pathogenesis and potential importance of myofibrillar degeneration. *Hum Pathol*. 1970;1:125–150.
126. Fineschi V, Wetli CV, Di Paolo M, Baroldi G. Myocardial necrosis and cocaine. A quantitative morphologic study in 26 cocaine-associated deaths. *Int J Legal Med*. 1997;110:193–198.
127. Kline IK. Myocardial alterations associated with pheochromocytomas. *Am J Pathol*. 1961;38:539–551.
128. Arnold G, Fischer R. Myocardial "contraction bands." *Hum Pathol*. 1987;18:99–101.
129. Samuels MA. Neurogenic heart disease: a unifying hypothesis. *Am J Cardiol*. 1987;60:15J–19J.
130. Taneda M, Kataoka K, Akai F, et al. Traumatic subarachnoid hemorrhage as a predictable indicator of delayed ischemic symptoms. *J Neurosurg*. 1996;84:762–768.
131. Zubkov AY, Pilkington AS, Parent AD, Zhang J. Morphological presentation of posttraumatic vasospasm. *Acta Neurochir Suppl*. 2000;76: 223–226.
132. O'Brien NF, Maa T, Yeates KO. The epidemiology of vasospasm in children with moderate-to-severe traumatic brain injury. *Crit Care Med*. 2015;43:674–685.
133. Martin NA, Doberstein C, Alexander M, et al. Posttraumatic cerebral arterial spasm. *J Neurotrauma*. 1995;12:897–901.
134. Kohta M, Minami H, Tanaka K, et al. Delayed onset massive oedema and deterioration in traumatic brain injury. *J Clin Neurosci*. 2007;14:167–170.
135. Gomez CR, Backer RJ, Bucholz RD. Transcranial Doppler ultrasound following closed head injury: vasospasm or vasoparalysis. *Surg Neurol*. 1991;35:30–35.
136. Magnuson J, Leonessa F, Ling GS. Neuropathology of explosive blast traumatic brain injury. *Curr Neurol Neurosci Rep*. 2012;12:570–579.
137. Elder GA, Gama Sosa MA, DeGasperi R, et al. Vascular and inflammatory factors in the pathophysiology of blast-induced brain injury. *Front Neurol*. 2015;6:1–22.
138. Villalba N, Sonkursare SK, Longden TA, et al. Traumatic brain injury disrupts cerebrovascular tone through endothelial inducible nitric oxide synthase expression and nitric oxide gain of function. *J Am Heart Assoc*. 2014;3:e001474.
139. Alford PW, Dabiri BE, Goss JA, et al. Blast-induced phenotypic switching in cerebral vasospasm. *Proc Natl Acad Sci USA*. 2011;108:12705–12710.
140. Noor R, Wang CX, Shuaib A. Effects of hyperthermia on infarct volume in focal embolic model of cerebral ischemia in rats. *Neurosci Lett*. 2003;349:130–132.
141. Olsen TS, Weber UJ, Kammersgaard LP. Therapeutic hypothermia for acute stroke. *Lancet Neurol*. 2003;2:410–416.
142. Clifton GL, Valadka A, Zygun D, et al. Very early hypothermia induction in patients with severe brain injury (the National Acute Brain Injury Study: Hypothermia II): a randomized trial. *Lancet Neurol*. 2011;10:131–139.
143. Adelson PD, Wisniewski SR, Beca J, et al. Paediatric Traumatic Brain Injury Consortium Comparison of hypothermia and normothermia after severe traumatic brain in children (Cool Kids): a phase 3 randomised controlled trial. *Lancet Neurol*. 2013;12:546–553.
144. Sandestig A, Romner B, Grände PO. Therapeutic hypothermia in children and adults with severe brain injury. *Ther Hypothermia Temp Manag*. 2014;4:10–20.
145. Clifton GL, Miller E, Choi SC, et al. Lack of effect of induction of hypothermia after acute brain injury. *N Engl J Med*. 2001;344:556–563.
146. Clifton GL, Choi SC, Miller ER, et al. Intercenter variance in clinical trials of head trauma—experience of the National Acute Brain Injury Study: Hypothermia. *J Neurosurg*. 2001;95:751–755.
147. Shiozaki T, Sugimoto H, Eaneda M, et al. Effect of mild hypothermia on uncontrollable intracranial hypertension after severe head injury. *J Neurosurg*. 1993;79:363–368.
148. Bernard SA, Gray TW, Buist MD, et al. Treatment of comatose survivors of out-of-hospital cardiac arrest with induced hypothermia. *N Engl J Med*. 2002;346:557–563.
149. The Hypothermia after Cardiac Arrest Study Group. Mild therapeutic hypothermia to improve the neurologic outcome after cardiac arrest. *N Engl J Med*. 2002;346:549–556.
150. Zygun DA, Steiner LA, Johnston AJ, et al. Hyperglycemia and brain tissue pH after traumatic brain injury. *Neurosurgery*. 2004;55:877–882.
151. Cochran A, Scaife ER, Hansen KW, Downey EC. Hyperglycemia and outcomes from pediatric traumatic brain injury. *J Trauma*. 2003;55: 1035–1038.
152. Jeremitsky E, Omert LA, Dunham CM, et al. The impact of hyperglycemia on patients with severe brain injury. *J Trauma*. 2005;58:47–50.

153. Salim A, Hadjizacharia P, Dubose J, et al. Persistent hyperglycemia in severe traumatic brain injury: an independent predictor of outcome. *Am Surg.* 2009;75:25–29.
154. Ashis P, Marwaha DS, Singh D, et al. Change in tissue thromboplastin content of brain following trauma. *Neurology India.* 2005;53:178–182.
155. Talving P, Lustenberger T, Lam L, et al. Coagulopathy after isolated severe traumatic brain injury in children. *J Trauma.* 2011;71:1205–1210.
156. Carrick MM, Tyrock AH, Youens CA, et al. Subsequent development of thrombocytopenia and coagulopathy in moderate and severe head injury: support for serial laboratory examination. *J Trauma.* 2005;58:725–730.
157. Hulka F, Mullins RJ, Frank EH. Blunt brain injury activates the coagulation process. *Arch Surg.* 1996;131:923–928.
158. Aiyagari V, Menendez JA, Diringer MN. Treatment of severe coagulopathy after gunshot injury to the head using recombinant activated factor VII. *J Crit Care.* 2005;20:176–180.
159. Stein S, Young G, Talucci R, et al. Delayed brain injury after head trauma: significance of coagulopathy. *Neurosurgery.* 1992;30:160–165.
160. Engstrom M, Romner B, Schalen W, Reinstrup P. Thrombocytopenia predicts progressive hemorrhage after head trauma. *J Neurotrauma.* 2005;22: 291–296.
161. Chabra G, Sharma S, Subramanian A, et al. Coagulopathy as prognostic marker in acute traumatic brain injury. *J Emerg Trauma Shock.* 2013;6: 180–185.
162. Spahn DR, Bouillon B, Cerny V, et al. Management of bleeding and coagulopathy following major trauma: an updated European guideline. *Crit Care.* 2013;17:R76.
163. Marmarou A, Anderson RL, Ward JD, et al. NINDS Traumatic Coma Data Bank: intracranial pressure monitoring methodology. *J Neurosurg.* 1991;75:S21–S27.
164. Wakai A, McCabe A, Roberts I, Schierhout G. Mannitol for acute traumatic brain injury. *Cochrane Database Syst Rev.* 2013;(8):CD001049.
165. Francony G, Fauvage B, Falcon D, et al. Equimolar doses of mannitol and hypertonic saline in the treatment of increased intracranial pressure. *Crit Care Med.* 2008;36:795–800.
166. Rickard AC, Smith JE, Newell P, et al. Salt or sugar for your injured brain? A meta-analysis of randomised controlled trials of mannitol versus hypertonic sodium solutions to manage raised intracranial pressure in traumatic brain injury. *Emerg Med J.* 2014;31:679–683.
167. Kaufmann AM, Cardoso ER. Aggravation of vasogenic cerebral edema by multiple-dose mannitol. *J Neurosurg.* 1992;77:584–589.
168. Bhardwaj A, Harukuni I, Murphy SJ, et al. Hypertonic saline worsens infarct volume after transient focal ischemia in rats. *Stroke.* 2000;31:1694–1701.
169. Wakai A, Roberts I, Schierhout G. Mannitol for acute traumatic brain injury. *Cochrane Database Syst Rev.* 2007;(1):CD001049.
170. Kruse JA, Cadnapaphornchai P. The serum osmole gap. *J Crit Care.* 1994; 9:185–197.
171. Garcia-Morales EJ, Cariappa R, Parvin CA, et al. Osmole gap in neurologic-neurosurgical intensive care unit: its normal value, calculation, and relationship with mannitol serum concentrations. *Crit Care Med.* 2004;32:986–991.
172. Mirski AM, Denchev ID, Schnitzer SM, et al. Comparison between hypertonic saline and mannitol in the reduction of elevated intracranial pressure in a rodent model of acute cerebral injury. *J Neurosurg Anesthesiol.* 2000;12:334–344.
173. Mortzavi MM, Romeo AK, Deep A, et al. Hypertonic saline for treating raised intracranial pressure: literature review with meta-analysis. *J Neurosurg.* 2012;116:210–221.
174. Harutjunyan L, Holz C, Rieger A, et al. Efficiency of 7.2% hypertonic saline hydroxyethyl starch 200/0.5 versus mannitol 15% in the treatment of increased intracranial pressure in neurosurgical patients—a randomized clinical trial. *Crit Care.* 2006;9:R530–R540.
175. Shackford SR, Bourguignon PR, Wald SL, et al. Hypertonic saline resuscitation of patients with head injury: a prospective, randomized clinical trial. *J Trauma.* 1998;44:50–58.
176. Cooper DJ, Myles PS, McDermott FT, et al. Prehospital hypertonic saline resuscitation of patients with hypotension and severe traumatic brain injury: a randomized controlled trial. *JAMA.* 2004;291:1350–1357.
177. Melby JM, Miner LC, Reed DJ. Effect of acetazolamide and furosemide on the production and composition of cerebrospinal fluid from the cat choroid plexus. *Can J Physiol Pharmacol.* 1982;60:405–409.
178. Kan P, Amini A, Hansen K, et al. Outcomes after decompressive craniectomy for severe traumatic brain injury in children. *J Neurosurg.* 2006; 105:337–342.
179. Jagannathan J, Okonkwo DO, Dumont AS, et al. Outcome following decompressive craniectomy in children with severe traumatic brain injury: a 10-year single-center experience with long-term follow up. *J Neurosurg.* 2007;106(Suppl 4):268–275.
180. Skoglund TS, Eriksson-Ritzen C, Jensen C, Rydenhag B. Aspects on decompressive craniectomy in patients with traumatic head injuries. *J Neurotrauma.* 2006;23:1502–1509.
181. Cooper DJ, Rosenfeld JV, Murray L, et al; DECRA Trial Investigators; Australian and New Zealand Intensive Care Society Clinical Trials Group. Decompressive craniectomy in diffuse traumatic brain injury. *N Engl J Med.* 2011;364:1493–1502.
182. Nortje J, Gupta AK. The role of tissue oxygen monitoring in patients with acute brain injury. *Br J Anaesth.* 2006;97:95–106.
183. Diringer MN, Aiyagari V, Zazulia AR, et al. Effect of hyperoxia on cerebral metabolic rate for oxygen measured using positron emission tomography in patients with acute severe head injury. *J Neurosurg.* 2007;106:526–529.
184. Kiening KL, Unterberg AW, Bardt TF, et al. Monitoring of cerebral oxygenation in patients with severe head injuries: brain tissue PO2 versus jugular vein oxygen saturation. *J Neurosurg.* 1996;85:751–757.
185. Doppenberg EM, Zauner A, Bullock PD, et al. Correlations between brain tissue oxygen tension, carbon dioxide tension, pH, and cerebral blood flow—a better way of monitoring the severely injured brain? *Surg Neurol.* 1998;49:650–654.
186. Zauner A, Doppenberg EM, Woodward JJ, et al. Continuous monitoring of cerebral substrate delivery and clearance: initial experience in 24 patients with severe acute brain injuries. *Neurosurgery.* 1997;41:1082–1091.
187. Vladka AB, Gopinath SP, Contant CF, et al. Relationship of brain tissue PO2 to outcome after severe head injury. *Crit Care Med.* 1998;26:1576–1581.
188. van den Brink WA, van Santbrink H, Steyerberg EW, et al. Brain oxygen tension in severe head injury. *Neurosurgery.* 2000;46:868–876.
189. Stiefel MF, Spiotta A, Gracias VH, et al. Reduced mortality rate in patients with severe traumatic brain injury treated with brain tissue oxygen monitoring. *J Neurosurg.* 2005;103:805–811.
190. Meixensberger J, Jaeger M, Väth A, et al. Brain tissue oxygen guided treatment supplementing ICP/CPP therapy after traumatic brain injury. *J Neurol Neurosurg Psychiatry.* 2003;74:760–764.
191. Martini RP, Deem S, Yanez ND, et al. Management guided by brain tissue oxygen monitoring and outcome following severe traumatic brain injury. *J Neurosurg.* 2009;111:644–649.
192. Green JA, Pellegrini DC, Vanderkolk WE, et al. Goal directed brain tissue oxygen monitoring versus conventional management in traumatic brain injury: an analysis of in hospital recovery. *Neurocrit Care.* 2013;18:20–25.
193. Sarrafzadeh AS, Sakowitz OW, Callsen TA, et al. Bedside microdialysis for early detection of cerebral hypoxia in traumatic brain injury. *Neurosurg Focus.* 2000;9:e2.
194. Wijayatilake DS, Talati C, Panchatsharam S. The monitoring and management of severe traumatic brain injury in the United Kingdom: Is there a consensus? A National Survey. *J Neurosurg Anesthesiol.* 2015;27:241–245.
195. Bell RB, Dierks EJ, Homer L, Potter BE. Management of cerebrospinal fluid leak associated with craniomaxillofacial trauma. *J Oral Maxillofac Surg.* 2004;62:676–684.
196. Bernal-Sprekelsen M, Bleda-Vazquez C, Carrau RL. Ascending meningitis secondary to traumatic cerebrospinal fluid leaks. *Am J Rhinol.* 2000;14: 257–259.
197. Friedman JA, Ebersold MJ, Quast LM. Post-traumatic cerebrospinal fluid leakage. *World J Surg.* 2001;25:1062–1068.
198. Choi D, Spann R. Traumatic cerebrospinal fluid leakage: risk factors and the use of prophylactic antibiotics. *Br J Neurosurg.* 1996;10:571–575.
199. Ratilal BO, Costa J, Pappamikail L, Sampaio C. Antibiotic prophylaxis for preventing meningitis in patients with basilar skull fractures. *Cochrane Database Syst Rev.* 2015;(4):CD004884.
200. Arendall RE, Meirowsky AM. Air sinus wounds: an analysis of 163 consecutive cases incurred in the Korean War: 1950–1952. *Neurosurgery.* 1983;13:377–380.
201. Gonul E, Baysefer A, Kahraman S, et al. Causes of infections and management results in penetrating craniocerebral injuries. *Neurosurg Rev.* 1997;20:177–181.
202. Meirowsky AM, Caveness WF, Dillon JD, et al. Cerebrospinal fluid fistulas complicating missile wounds of the brain. *J Neurosurg.* 1981;54:44–48.
203. Antibiotic prophylaxis for penetrating brain injury. *J Trauma.* 2001; 51(Suppl 2):S34–S40.
204. Bayston R, de Louvois J, Brown EM, et al. Use of antibiotics in penetrating craniocerebral injuries. "Infection in Neurosurgery" Working Party of British Society for Antimicrobial Chemotherapy. *Lancet.* 2000;355: 1813–1817.
205. Kazim SF, Sharmim MS, Tahir MZ, et al. Management of penetrating brain injury. *J Emerg Trauma Shock.* 2011;4:395–402.

206. Bratzler DW, Hunt DR. The Surgical Infection Prevention and Surgical Care Improvement Projects: national initiatives to improve outcomes for patients having surgery. *Clin Infect Dis.* 2006;43:322–330.
207. Lee S, Lui T. Early seizures after mild closed head injury. *J Neurosurg.* 1992;76:435–439.
208. Jennett B. Early traumatic epilepsy: incidence and significance after non-missile injuries. *Arch Neurol.* 1974;30:394–398.
209. Annegers JF, Hauser WA, Coan SP, Rocca WA. A population-based study of seizures after traumatic brain injuries. *N Engl J Med.* 1998;338:20–24.
210. Brain Trauma Foundation; American Association of Neurological Surgeons; Joint Section on Neurotrauma and Critical Care. Guidelines for the management of severe head injury. XIII. Antiseizure prophylaxis. *J Neurotrauma.* 2007;24(Suppl 1):S83–S86.
211. Temkin NR, Dikmen SS, Wilensky AJ, et al. A randomized, double-blind study of phenytoin for the prevention of post-traumatic seizures. *N Engl J Med.* 1990;323:497–502.
212. Temkin NR. Antiepileptogenesis and seizure prevention trials with anti-epileptic drugs: meta-analysis of controlled trials. *Epilepsia.* 2001;42: 515–524.
213. Antiseizure prophylaxis for penetrating brain injury. *J Trauma.* 2001;51: S41–S43.
214. Temkin NR, Dikmen SS, Anderson GD, et al. Valproate therapy for prevention of posttraumatic seizures: a randomized trial. *J Neurosurg.* 1999;91:593–600.
215. Zafar SN, Khan AA, Ghauri AA, Shamim MS. Phenytoin versus levetiracetam for seizure prophylaxis after brain injury- a meta-analysis. *BMC Neurol.* 2012;12:30.
216. Inaba K, Menaker J, Branco BC, et al. A prospective multicenter comparison of levetiracetam versus phenytoin for early posttraumatic seizure prophylaxis. *J Trauma Acute Care Surg.* 2013;74:766–771.
217. Dickinson LD, Miller LD, Patel CP, et al. Enoxaparin increases the incidence of postoperative intracranial hemorrhage when initiated preoperatively for deep venous thrombosis prophylaxis in patients with brain tumors. *Neurosurgery.* 1998;43:1074–1079.
218. Constantini S, Kornowski R Pomeranz S, Rappaport ZH. Thromboembolic phenomena in neurosurgical patients operated upon for primary and metastatic brain tumors. *Acta Neurochir (Wien).* 1991;109:93–97.
219. Auguste KI, Quinones-Hinojosa A, Gadkary C, et al. Incidence of venous thromboembolism in patients undergoing craniotomy and motor mapping for glioma without intraoperative mechanical prophylaxis to the contralateral leg. *J Neurosurg.* 2003;99:680–684.
220. Guyatt GH, Aki EA, Crowther M, et al. Executive summary: Antithrombotic Therapy and Prevention of Thrombosis, 9th ed: American College of Chest Physicians Evidence-Based Clinical Practice Guidelines. *Chest.* 2012;141(2 Suppl):7S–47S.
221. Geerts WH, Code KI, Jay RM, et al. A prospective study of venous thromboembolism after major trauma. *N Engl J Med.* 1994;331:1601–1606.
222. Brain Trauma Foundation; American Association of Neurological Surgeons; Joint Section on Neurotrauma and Critical Care. Guidelines for the management of severe head injury. Deep vein thrombosis prophylaxis. *J Neurotrauma.* 2007;24(Suppl 1):S32–S36.
223. Nyquist P, Bautista, Jichici D, et al. Prophylaxis of venous thrombosis in neurocritical care patients: an evidence-based guideline: A Statement for Healthcare Professionals from the Neurocritical Care Society. *Neurocrit Care* 2016;24:47–60.
224. Hang C, Shi J, Li J, et al. Alterations of intestinal mucosa structure and barrier function following traumatic brain injury in rats. *World J Gastroenterol.* 2003;9:2776–2781.
225. Young B, Ott L, Twyman D, et al. The effect of nutritional support on outcome from severe head injury. *J Neurosurg.* 1987;67:668–676.
226. Rapp RP, Young B, Twyman D, et al. The favorable effect of early parenteral feeding on survival in head-injured patients. *J Neurosurg.* 1983;58: 906–912.
227. Perel P, Yanagawa T, Bunn F, et al. Nutritional support for head-injured patients. *Cochrane Database Syst Rev.* 2006;(4):CD001530.
228. Grahm TW, Zadrozny DB, Harrington T. The benefits of early jejunal hyperalimentation in the head-injured patient. *Neurosurgery.* 1989;25: 729–735.
229. Aydin S, Ulusoy H, Usul H, et al. Effects of early versus delayed nutrition on intestinal mucosal apoptosis and atrophy after traumatic brain injury. *Surg Today.* 2005;35:751–759.
230. Taylor SJ, Fettes SB, Jewkes C, Nelson RJ. Prospective, randomized, controlled trial to determine the effect of early enhanced enteral nutrition on clinical outcome in mechanically ventilated patients suffering head injury. *Crit Care Med.* 1999;27:2525–2531.
231. Falcao de Arruda IS, de Aguilar-Nascimento JE. Benefits of early enteral nutrition with glutamine and probiotics in brain injury patients. *Clin Sci (Lond).* 2004;106:287–292.
232. Scrimgeour AG, Condlin ML. Nutritional treatment for traumatic brain injury. *J Neurotrauma.* 2014;31:989–999.
233. Brain Trauma Foundation; American Association of Neurological Surgeons; Joint Section on Neurotrauma and Critical Care. Guidelines for the management of severe head injury. XII. Nutrition. *J Neurotrauma.* 2007;24(Suppl 1):S77–S82.
234. Food and Nutrition Board. *Nutrition and Traumatic Brain Injury-Improving Acute and Subacute Health Outcomes in Military Personnel.* Washington, DC: National Academies Press; 2011.
235. Brown TH, Davidson PF, Larson GM. Acute gastritis occurring within 24 hours of severe head injury. *Gastrointest Endosc.* 1989;35:37–40.
236. Thompson JC, Walker JP. Indications for the use of parenteral H2-receptor antagonists. *Am J Med.* 1984;77:111–115.
237. Ecker RD, WIjdicks EF, Wix K, McClelland R. Does famotidine induce thrombocytopenia in neurosurgical patients? *J Neurosurg Anesthesiol.* 2004;16:291–293.
238. The Brain Trauma Foundation. The American Association of Neurological Surgeons. The Joint Section on Neurotrauma and Critical Care. Glasgow Coma scale score. *J Neurotrauma.* 2000;17:563–571.
239. Rimel RW, Giordani B, Barth JT, et al. Disability caused by minor head injury. *Neurosurgery.* 1981;9:221–228.
240. Thornhill S, Teasdale GM, Murray GD, et al. Disability in young people and adults one year after head injury: prospective cohort study. *BMJ.* 2000;320:1631–1635.
241. Marshall LF, Marshall SB, Kauber MR, et al. A new classification of head injury based on computerized tomography. *J Neurosurg.* 1991; 75(Suppl):S14–S20.
242. Mosenthal AC, Lavery RF, Addis M, et al. Isolated traumatic brain injury: age is an independent predictor of mortality and early outcome. *J Trauma.* 2002;52:907–911.
243. Livingston DH, Lavery RF, Mosenthal AC, et al. Recovery at one year following isolated traumatic brain injury: a Western Trauma Association prospective multicenter trial. *J Trauma.* 2005;59:1298–1304.
244. Fearnside MR, Cook RJ, McDougall P, McNeil RJ. The Westmead head injury project outcome in severe head injury: a comparative analysis of pre-hospital, clinical and CT variables. *Br J Neurosurg.* 1993;7:267–279.
245. Wardlaw JM, Easton VJ, Statham P. Which CT features help predict outcome after head injury? *J Neurol Neurosurg Psychiatry.* 2002;72:188–192.
246. Maas AI, Steyerberg EW, Butcher I, et al. Prognostic value of computerized tomography scan characteristics in traumatic brain injury: results from the IMPACT study. *J Neurotrauma.* 2007;24:303–314.
247. Klauber MR, Marshall LR, Barrett-Connor E, Bowers SA. Prospective study of patients hospitalized with head injury in San Diego County 1978. *Neurosurgery.* 1981;9:236–241.
248. Marshall LF, Maas AI, Marshall SB, et al. A multicenter trial on the efficacy of using tirilazad mesylate in cases of head injury. *J Neurosurg.* 1998;89:519–525.
249. Skolnick BE, Maas AI, Narayan RK, et al. A clinical trial of progesterone for severe traumatic brain injury. *N Engl J Med.* 2014;371:2467–2476.
250. AANS/CNS Joint Committee on Acute Spinal Cord Injury. Guidelines for management of acute spinal cord injuries. *Neurosurgery.* 2002;50:S1–S179.
251. *International Standards for Neurological Classification of Spinal Cord Injury, revised 2011.* Atlanta, GA: American Spinal Injury Association; 2015.
252. Waring WP 3rd, Biering-Sorensen F, Burns S, et al. 2009 review and revisions of the international standards for the neurological classification of spinal cord injury. *J Spinal Cord Med.* 2010;33:346–352.
253. Mulcahey MJ, Gaughan JP, Chafetz RS, et al. Interrater reliability of the international standards for neurological classification of spinal cord injury in youths with chronic spinal cord injury. *Arch Phys Med Rehabil.* 2011;92:1264–1269.
254. Marino RJ, Jones L, Kirshblum S, et al. Reliability and repeatability of the motor and sensory examination of the international standards for neurological classification of spinal cord injury. *J Spinal Cord Med.* 2008;31:166–170.
255. Hadley MN, Walters BC, Bizhan A, et al. Clinical assessment following acute cervical spinal cord injury. *Neurosurgery.* 2013;72:40–53.
256. Ryken TC, Hadley MN, Walters BC, et al. Radiographic Assessment. *Neurosurgery.* 2013:72:54–72.
257. Inaba K, Bush BS, Martin MJ, et al. Cervical spine clearance: A prospective Western Trauma Association multi-institutional trial. *J Trauma Acute Care Surg.* 2016;81:1122–1130.

258. Patel MB, Humble SS, Culliane DC, et al. Cervical spine collar clearance in the obtunded adult blunt trauma patient: a systematic review and practice management guideline from the Eastern Association for the Surgery of Trauma. *J Trauma Acute Care Surg.* 2015;78:430–441.
259. Gelb DE, Hadley MN, Aarabi B, et al. Initial closed reduction of cervical spinal fracture-dislocation injuries. *Neurosurgery.* 2013;72:73–83.
260. Theodore N, Aarabi B, Dhall SS, et al. Occipital condyle fractures. *Neurosurgery.* 2013;72:106–113.
261. Cervical spine immobilization before admission to the hospital. *Neurosurgery.* 2002;50:S7–S17.
262. Hachen HJ. Emergency transportation in the event of acute spinal cord lesion. *Paraplegia.*1974;12:33–37.
263. Ahn H, Singh J, Nathens A, et al. Pre-hospital care management of a potential spinal cord injured patient: A systematic review of the literature and evidence-based guidelines. *J Neurotrauma.* 2011;28:1341–1361.
264. Theodore N, Hadley MN, Aarabi B, et al. Prehospital cervical spinal immobilization after trauma.*Neurosurg.* 2013;72:22–34.
265. Tator CH. Experimental and clinical studies on the pathophysiology and management of acute spinal cord injury. *J Spinal Cord Med.* 1996; 19:206–214.
266. Tator CH, Fehlings, MG. Review of the secondary injury theory of acute spinal cord trauma with emphasis on vascular mechanisms. *J Neurosurg.* 1991;75:15–26.
267. Amar AP, Levy ML. Pathogenesis and pharmacological strategies for mitigating secondary damage in acute spinal cord injury. *Neurosurgery.* 1999;44:1027–1040.
268. Levi L, Wolf A, Rigamonti D, et al. Anterior decompression in cervical spine trauma: Does the timing of surgery affect the outcome? *Neurosurgery.* 1991;29:216–222.
269. Levi L, Wolf A, Belzberg H. Hemodynamic parameters in patients with acute cervical cord trauma: description, intervention and prediction of outcome. *Neurosurgery.* 1993;33:1007–1017.
270. Vale FL, Burns J, Jackson AB, et al. Combined medical and surgical treatment after acute spinal cord injury: results of a prospective pilot study to assess the merits of aggressive medical resuscitation and blood pressure management. *J Neurosurg.* 1997;87:239–246.
271. Wolf A, Levi L, Mirvis S, et al. Operative management of bilateral facet dislocation. *J Neurosurg.* 1991;75:883–890.
272. Ryken TC, Hurlbert RJ, Hadley MN, et al. The acute cardiopulmonary management of patients with cervical spinal cord injuries. *Neurosurgery.* 2013;72:84–92.
273. Tator CH. Review of treatment trials in human spinal cord injury: issues, difficulties, and recommendations. *Neurosurgery.* 2006;59:957–987.
274. Dvorak MF, Noonan VK, Fallah N, et al; RHSCIR Network. The influence of time from injury to surgery on motor recovery and length of hospital stay in acute traumatic spinal cord injury: an observational Canadian cohort study. *J Neurotrauma.* 2015;32:645–654.
275. Gelb DE, Aarabi B, Dhall SS, et al. Treatment of subaxial cervical spinal injuries. *Neurosurgery.* 2013;72:187–194.
276. Aarabi B, Hadley MN, Dhall SS, et al. Management of acute traumatic central cord syndrome (ATCCS). *Neurosurgery.* 2013;72:195–204.
277. Duh MS, Shepard MJ, Wilberger JE, et al. The effectiveness of surgery on the treatment of acute spinal cord injury and its relation to pharmacological treatment. *Neurosurgery.* 1994;35:240–248.
278. McKinley W, Meade MA, Kirshblum S, Barnard B. Outcomes of early surgical management versus late or no surgical intervention after acute spinal cord injury. *Arch Phys Med Rehabil.* 2004;85:1818–1825.
279. Kerwin AJ, Frykberg ER, Schinco MA, et al. The effect of early spine fixation on non-neurologic outcome. *J Trauma.* 2005;58:15–21.
280. Pointillart V, Petitjean ME, Wiart L, et al. Pharmacological therapy of spinal cord injury during the acute phase. *Spinal Cord.* 2000;38:71–76.
281. Short DJ, El Masry WS, Jones PW: High dose methylprednisolone in the management of acute spinal cord injury: a systematic review from a clinical perspective. *Spinal Cord.* 2000;38:273–286.
282. Bracken MB. Steroids for acute spinal cord injury. *Cochrane Database Syst Rev.* 2002;3:CD001046.
283. Bracken MB, Shepard MJ, Collin, et al. A randomized, controlled trial of methylprednisolone or naloxone in the treatment of acute spinal-cord injury. Results of the Second National Acute Spinal Cord Injury Study. *N Engl J Med.* 1990;322:1405–1411.
284. Bracken MB, Shepard MJ, Holford TR, et al. Administration of methylprednisolone for 24 or 48 hours or tirilazad mesylate for 48 hours in the treatment of acute spinal cord injury. Results of the Third National Acute Spinal Cord Injury Randomized Controlled Trial. National Acute Spinal Cord Injury Study. *JAMA.* 1997;277:1597–1604.
285. Galandiuk S, Raque G, Appel S, Polk HC Jr. The two-edged sword of large-dose steroids for spinal cord trauma. *Ann Surg.* 1993;218:419–427.
286. Gerndt SJ, Rodriguez JL, Pawlik JW, et al. Consequences of high-dose steroid therapy for acute spinal cord injury. *J Trauma.* 1997;42:279–284.
287. Hurlbert RJ, Hadley MN, Walters BC, et al. Pharmacological therapy for acute spinal cord injury. *Neurosurgery.* 2013;72:93–105.
288. Bellamy R, Pitt RW, Stauffer ES. Respiratory complications in traumatic quadriplegia. *J Neurosurg.* 1973;39:596–600.
289. Kiwerski J. Respiratory problems in patients with high lesion quadriplegia. *Int J Rehabil Res.* 1992;15:49–52.
290. Roth EJ, Nussbaum SB, Berkowitz M, et al. Pulmonary function testing in spinal cord injury: correlation with vital capacity. *Paraplegia.* 1995;33:454–457.
291. Management of vertebral artery injuries after nonpenetrating cervical trauma. *Neurosurgery.* 2002;50:S173–S178.
292. Biffl WL. Diagnosis of blunt cerebrovascular injuries. *Curr Opin Crit Care.* 2003;9:530–534.
293. Mayberry JC, Brown CV, Mullins RJ, et al. Blunt carotid artery injury: the futility of aggressive screening and diagnosis. *Arch Surg.* 2004;139: 609–613.
294. Harrigan MR, Falola MI, Shannon CN, et al. Incidence and trends in the diagnosis of traumatic extracranial cerebrovascular injury in the nationwide inpatient sample database, 2003–2010. *J Neurotrauma.* 2014;31: 1056–1062.
295. Biffl WL, Moore EE, Ryu RK, et al. The unrecognized epidemic of blunt carotid arterial injuries: early diagnosis improves neurologic outcome. *Ann Surg.* 1998;228:462–470.
296. Biffl WL, Moore EE, Offner PJ, et al. Optimizing screening for blunt cerebrovascular injuries. *Am J Surg.* 1999;178:517–522.
297. Schneidereit NP, Simons R, Nicolaou S, et al. Utility of screening for blunt vascular neck injuries with computed tomographic angiography. *J Trauma.* 2006;60:209–215.
298. Eastman A, Chason D, Perez CL, et al. Computed tomographic angiography for the diagnosis of blunt cervical vascular injury: Is it ready for prime time? *J Trauma.* 2006;60(5):925–929.
299. Biffl WL, Egglin T, Gibbs F. Sixteen-slice CT-angiography is a reliable noninvasive test that allows liberal screening for blunt cerebrovascular injuries. *J Trauma.* 2006;60(4):745–751.
300. Harrigan MR, Hadley MN, Dhall SS, et al. Management of vertebral artery injuries following non-penetrating cervical trauma. *Neurosurgery.* 2013;72:234–243.
301. Biffl WL, Moore EE, Offner PJ, et al. Blunt carotid arterial injuries: implications of a new grading scale. *J Trauma.* 1999;47:845–853.
302. Biffl WL, Ray CE, Moore EE, et al. Treatment-related outcomes from blunt cerebrovascular injuries: importance of routine follow-up arteriography. *Ann Surg.* 2002;235:699–707.
303. Wahl WL, Brandt MM, Thompson BG, et al. Antiplatelet therapy: an alternative to heparin for blunt carotid injury. *J Trauma.* 2002;52:896–901.
304. Eachempati SR, Vaslef SN, Sebastian MW, Reed RL 2nd. Blunt vascular injuries of the head and neck: Is heparinization necessary? *J Trauma.* 1998;45:997–1004.
305. Myllynen P, Kammonen M, Rokkanen P, et al. Deep venous thrombosis and pulmonary embolism in patients with acute spinal cord injury: a comparison with nonparalyzed patients immobilized due to spinal fractures. *J Trauma.* 1985;25:541–543.
306. Dhall SS, Hadley MN, Aarabi B, et al. Deep venous thrombosis and thromboembolism in patients with cervical spinal cord injuries. *Neurosurgery.* 2013;72:244–254.
307. Johns JS, Nguyen C, Sing RF. Vena cava filters in spinal cord injuries: evolving technology. *J Spinal Cord Med.* 2006;29:183–190.
308. Kinney TB, Rose SC, Valji K, et al. Does cervical spinal cord injury induce a higher incidence of complications after prophylactic Greenfield interior vena cava filter usage? *J Vasc Interv Radiol.* 1996;7:907–915.
309. Balshi JD, Cantelmo NL, Menzoian JO. Complications of caval interruption by Greenfield filter in quadriplegics. *J Vasc Surg.* 1989;9: 558–562.
310. Barnes B, Alexander JT, Branch CL Jr. Postoperative level I anticoagulation therapy and spinal surgery: practical guidelines for management. *Neurosurg Focus.* 2004;17:E5.
311. Lawton MT, Porter RW, Heiserman JE, et al. Surgical management of spinal epidural hematoma: relationship between surgical timing and neurological outcome. *J Neurosurg.* 1995;83:1–7.
312. Spanier DE, Stambough JL. Delayed postoperative epidural hematoma formation after heparinization in lumbar spinal surgery. *J Spinal Disord.* 2000;13:46–49.

313. Dhall SS, Hadley MN, Aarabi B, et al. Nutritional support after spinal cord injury. *Neurosurgery.* 2013;72:255–259.
314. Khastgir J, Drake MJ, Abrams P. Recognition and effective management of autonomic dysreflexia in spinal cord injuries. *Expert Opin Pharmacother.* 2007;8:945–956.
315. Helkowski WM, Ditunno JF Jr, Boninger M. Autonomic dysreflexia: incidence in persons with neurologically complete and incomplete tetraplegia. *J Spinal Cord Med.* 2003;26:244–247.
316. Krassioukov AV, Furlan JC, Fehlings MG. Autonomic dysreflexia in acute spinal cord injury: an under-recognized clinical entity. *J Neurotrauma.* 2003;20:707–716.
317. Savic G, Bergstrom EM, Frankel HL, et al. Inter-rater reliability of motor and sensory examinations performed according to American Spinal Injury Association standards. *Spinal Cord.* 2007;45(6):444–451.
318. Cifu DX, Huang ME, Kolakowsky-Hayner SA, Seel RT. Age, outcome, and rehabilitation costs after paraplegia caused by traumatic injury of the thoracic spinal cord, conus medullaris, and cauda equina. *J Neurotrauma.* 1999;16:805–815.
319. Coleman WP, Geisler FH. Injury severity as primary predictor of outcome in acute spinal cord injury: retrospective results from a large multicenter clinical trial. *Spine J.* 2004;4:373–378.
320. Miyanji F, Furlan JC, Aarabi B, et al. Acute cervical traumatic spinal cord injury: MR imaging findings correlated with neurologic outcome—prospective study with 100 consecutive patients. *Radiology.* 2007;243:820–827.
321. Schneider RC, Cherry G, Pantek H. The syndrome of acute central cervical spinal cord injury, with special reference to the mechanisms involved in hyperextension injuries of cervical spine. *J Neurosurg.* 1954;11:546–577.
322. Dvorak MF, Fisher CG, Hoekema J, et al. Factors predicting motor recovery and functional outcome after traumatic central cord syndrome: a long-term follow-up. *Spine.* 2005;30:2303–2311.
323. Harrop JS, Sharan A, Ratliff J. Central cord injury: pathophysiology, management and outcomes. *Spine J.* 2006;6:198S–206S.
324. Kosty JA, Leroux PD, Levine J, et al. Brief report: a comparison of clinical and research practices in measuring cerebral perfusion pressure: a literature review and practitioner survey. *Anesth Analg.* 2013;117:694–698.
325. Jones HA. Arterial transducer placement and cerebral perfusion pressure monitoring: a discussion. *Nurs Crit Care.* 2009;14:303–310.

CHAPTER 118

Elevated Intracranial Pressure

G. DUEMANI REDDY, SHANKAR GOPINATH, and CLAUDIA ROBERTSON

INTRODUCTION

Intracranial pressure (ICP), defined as the pressure of the cranial contents inside the skull, has been a closely monitored physiologic parameter in a variety of acute neurologic conditions since the pioneering work of Guillaume, Janny, and Lundberg first described methods for its measure (1,2). Elevations in this pressure can be caused by any number of mechanisms that result in the volume expansion of any space within the skull. For example, brain tumors are mass lesions that can directly occupy volume within either the intraparenchymal, intradural, or extradural space. Head trauma can result in a mass lesion such as an intraparenchymal, subdural, or epidural hemorrhage as well as diffuse cytotoxic brain edema. Ischemic or hemorrhagic strokes can also result in mass lesions and cellular edema. Even more systemic conditions, such as hepatic or renal failure can cause significant cerebral edema, thus elevating ICP. This increased pressure can in turn have dramatic consequences, including decreased blood flow, decreased oxygen delivery to the brain, global ischemia, and herniation of the brain with compression of vital structures, leading to death. A through understanding of the pathophysiology behind elevations in ICP as well as methods for diagnosing and treating it are crucial for effective neurologic critical care management. This chapter will discuss these issues, with a focus on elevated ICP secondary to traumatic brain injury (TBI).

PATHOPHYSIOLOGY

Physiology of the Intracranial Space

Monro–Kellie Doctrine

In the late 18th century Scottish physician Alexander Monro proposed that since the skull was a rigid container and the brain a nearly incompressible solid, any increase in volume of the skull's contents must be compensated by an equivalent volume loss in another intracranial compartment. His work was further confirmed by the experimental observations of his student, George Kellie approximately 40 years later and this principle has since become known as the Monro–Kellie doctrine. While more modern studies have shown that this principle does not fully account for the complex nature of ICP (3), it remains a highly useful conceptual tool.

The major components ("spaces") contained within the intracranial space are the brain, blood, and cerebrospinal fluid (CSF). However, a mass lesion such as a hematoma or a tumor can also contribute to the volume of the intracranial space. By the Monro–Kellie doctrine, as the volume of edema in the brain or an expanding mass lesion increases, the CSF and blood volume must decrease. Continued expansion of intracranial volume after these compensatory mechanisms are exhausted causes a rapid increase in ICP and herniation of the brain. To fully understand this process requires an understanding of both the CSF and cerebral vascular pathways, as well as how they interact to influence cerebral blood flow (CBF) and brain metabolism.

Circulation of Cerebrospinal Fluid

As mentioned above, CSF acts as a buffer against increased ICP. It is primarily secreted by the choroid plexus of the lateral and the tela choroidea of the third and fourth ventricles, with a smaller contribution from the extracellular fluid and cerebral capillaries across the blood–brain barrier (4). CSF drains from lateral ventricles through the two foramina of Monro into the third ventricle and from there it drains via the cerebral aqueduct into the fourth ventricle. From the fourth ventricle CSF drains via the two lateral foramina of Luschka and the median foramen of Magendie into the central canal of the spinal cord and subarachnoid space, where it is reabsorbed into the venous system via the arachnoid villi. Multiple studies have also shown absorption via extra-arachnoid pathways, including the extracranial lymphatic system and the meningeal sheaths surrounding cranial and spinal nerves, although these pathways are less understood (4–6). The normal total CSF volume in an adult is estimated to be approximately 150 mL, with 25 mL in the ventricles and 125 mL in the subarachnoid space. In a day, approximately 400 to 600 mL of CSF is secreted; thus in a young adult, the CSF volume is circulated about four times per day (4). Increased secretion or decreased absorption can cause communicating hydrocephalus and blockage of the circulation of CSF can cause obstructive hydrocephalus, both of which lead to direct elevations in ICP by increasing the intracranial volume occupied by the CSF space. Because compression of the CSF spaces is one compensatory mechanism for expanding volume within other spaces within the brain, hydrocephalus reduces the ability to compensate for an expanding mass lesion or worsening cerebral edema.

Circulation of Intracerebral Blood

In addition to the CSF, circulating intravascular blood volume is another space playing an important role in regulating ICP. While a complete description of the complex cerebrovasculature system is beyond the scope of this chapter, and not particularly relevant for posttraumatic ICP elevations, it is important to have a general concept of the intracerebral circulation. The blood supply to the anterior portion of the brain is primarily from branches of paired internal carotid arteries, which supply the frontal, parietal, and temporal lobes, as well as the thalamus and basal ganglia. Similarly the posterior portion of the brain is supplied by branches of the paired vertebral arteries, which merge to form the basilar artery. Together these vessels supply the brainstem, cerebellum, and occipital lobes. The anterior communicating artery connects the two internal carotid arteries, which are in turn connected to branches of the basilar artery through the posterior communicating arteries.

This anatomic connection between the anterior and posterior circulation is known as the Circle of Willis, and it provides for important collateral intracranial circulation if individual vessels are compromised. Venous drainage of blood is through cortical, as well as deep, veins to the sinuses, which then drain out of the intracranial vault through the internal jugular veins. Obstruction of the arterial circulation to the brain can lead to elevated ICP through ischemia and associated cytotoxic edema. Similarly, obstruction in the venous drainage results in elevations in ICP by increasing the intracerebral volume.

ICP Pressure–Volume Curve

The relationship between ICP and intracranial volume is a nonlinear one, typically characterized by three separate phases (7). An early increase in intracranial volume displaces CSF, which, as mentioned above, acts as a buffer and minimizes an associated increase in ICP. Once the maximal amount of CSF has been displaced from the intracranial compartment however, the ICP increases exponentially (Fig. 118.1). As ICP increases, cerebral perfusion pressure (CPP) decreases, as does blood flow to the brain, with the result that at high levels of ICP, there is terminal disruption of blood flow to the brain, compression of the vasculature, and a second plateau in the volume–pressure relationship (7,8). The overall shape of this relationship is thus sigmoidal.

Cerebral Perfusion Pressure

CPP is the driving force for blood flow to the brain and is defined as the mean arterial pressure (MAP) minus the ICP. Under normal physiologic conditions, the cerebral vasculature is able to maintain a relatively constant CBF by dynamically dilating or constricting its smooth muscle in response to transmural pressure changes. This process is known as cerebral pressure autoregulation and, under normal conditions, it maintains an adequate CBF at MAP values ranging from approximately 50 to 150 mmHg (9). However, autoregulation is commonly impaired, or even absent, in the injured brain (10–12). Such circumstances require a careful maintenance of a sufficient MAP and adequate control of ICP, as these patients have a higher risk of cerebral ischemia if hypoperfused. Additionally, sudden elevations in MAP should also be avoided as this may be directly transmitted into the microcirculation, leading to secondary hemorrhage and edema (12).

Brain Metabolism

The brain consumes a significant fraction of the body's blood, glucose, and oxygen. Normal CBF varies, but averages approximately 50 mL/100 g of brain tissue per minute with a minimum requirement of at least 20 mL/100 g/min for normal brain function (13,14). Studies have shown that between CBF values of 8 to 20 mL/min, the brain undergoes temporary neuronal dysfunction and below 8 mL/min, irreversible neuronal damage occurs (15).

These CBF thresholds were determined in normal brain, but seem to hold true for brain-injured patients, as well. As a result, a low CBF, particularly in the early postinjury period, is highly predictive of a poor outcome. Indeed, TBI patients with CBFs of less than 18 mL/100 g/min have a significantly worse outcome compared to patients with higher CBF (16) and within 12 hours of injury, every 10 mL/100 g/min increase in CBF was associated with a threefold increase in the probability of surviving the injury (17).

Brain oxygenation and cerebral perfusion can be monitored with both invasive and noninvasive techniques (7). For example, snapshots of oxygenation or perfusion can be acquired noninvasively using positron emission tomography (PET) or xenon computed tomography (CT) imaging, respectively. Similarly, qualitative assessments of CBF can be gathered from transcranial Doppler recordings, assuming that there is no appreciable change in the size of the measured vessel or the angle of measurement. On the other hand, invasive techniques can be used to continuously assess brain oxygenation and perfusion. For example, global assessment of both oxygenation and perfusion can be performed through combined monitoring of arterial oxygen saturation (SaO_2) and the oxygen saturation in the jugular bulb (SjO_2). This allows the calculation of the arteriojugular oxygen content difference ($AJDO_2$), which is dependent on the amount of oxygen consumed by the brain ($CMRO_2$) and on CBF by the formula $CMRO_2$/CBF. Thus, an increased $AJDO_2$ indicates a deficiency of flow relative to the metabolic needs of the brain. Brain oxygenation can also be monitored continuously in a local region of the brain by inserting an invasive probe to measure the brain tissue oxygen tension (PbO_2). While continuous global monitoring provides an overall assessment of brain oxygenation, it can miss local changes (18). On the other hand, continuous local monitoring with an invasive probe provides information on a specific portion of the brain but is dependent on probe location and may not reflect overall brain perfusion (19).

DIAGNOSIS

Identification of Patients with Increased ICP

Symptoms of elevated ICP are progressive. For example, a patient with mildly increased ICP can present with complaints

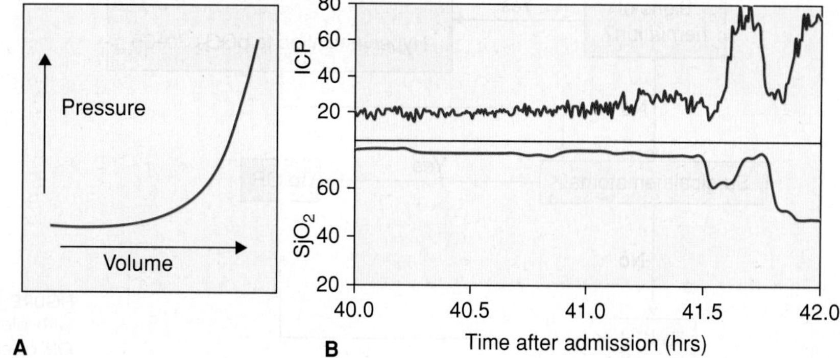

FIGURE 118.1 A: Nonlinear nature of the relationship between the volume of intracranial contents and intracranial pressure. B: Actual intracranial pressure (ICP) and jugular venous oxygen saturation (SjO_2) tracings in a patient who developed a delayed intracranial hematoma. Initially the rise in ICP was minimal as the brain was able to compensate for the increasing volume from the hematoma. Later when these compensatory mechanisms were exhausted, there was a very rapid increase in ICP associated with compromise of cerebral blood flow and a decrease in SjO_2.

of only headache and blurred vision; further increases in ICP are associated with decreased level of consciousness. If the ICP continues to climb, this may be associated with signs of brain herniation. Herniation of the temporal lobe over the edge of the tentorium can compress cranial nerve III and cause ipsilateral pupillary dilation. It can also directly compress the brainstem and cause contralateral posturing or hemiparesis. However, if the brainstem is displaced and compressed against the opposite side of the tentorium, there may be ipsilateral symptoms. This is known as *Kernohan notch phenomenon.* Further symptoms of herniation are hypertension, bradycardia, and widening pulse pressure, which are classically known as the *Cushing triad.* Respiratory abnormalities may be also present, including Cheyne–Stokes respiration, hypoventilation, or central neurogenic hyperventilation. Any patient in whom elevated ICP is suspected should undergo an emergent noncontrast CT scan of the brain to evaluate for mass lesions, hydrocephalus, subarachnoid hemorrhage, or other treatable causes.

For TBI patients, a degree of suspicion can be made based on the initial Glasgow coma score (GCS). A patient with a GCS of 13 to 15, defined as a mild head injury, has minimal risk of deteriorating or developing elevated ICP. Patients with GCSs that range from 9 to 12, defined as moderate head injury, have a higher chance of deteriorating and developing elevated ICP. Finally patients with a GCS of 8 or less, defined as severe head injury, have the highest risk of developing elevated ICP, and should undergo ICP monitoring, particularly if they have an abnormal head CT or if they meet two of the three criteria of age older than 40 years, unilateral or bilateral motor posturing, or SBP below 90 mmHg (20).

TREATMENT

Initial Stabilization and Management of Patients with Elevated ICP

The initial steps in managing any patient with elevated ICP (Fig. 118.2) follow the ABCs of trauma resuscitation. First and foremost, airway protection is crucial and current guidelines recommend that an appropriate airway should be established in any patient with a GCS less than 9, the inability to maintain an airway, or hypoxemia not corrected with supplemental oxygen. While some studies have shown that intubation in field to accomplish this goal leads to lower mortality rates (21), others have suggested that the rapid sequence intubation (RSI) techniques used by paramedics result in higher mortality rates and poorer outcomes (22). In general, the routine use of neuromuscular blocking agents (NMBAs) for RSI is not recommended in spontaneously breathing patient maintaining saturations above 90%. It is also recommended that if a patient is intubated in the field, it should be performed by a well trained paramedic, hyperventilation should be avoided unless signs of herniation are evident (23), and end tidal CO_2 monitors should be used to confirm placement of the tube in the airway when available (24,25).

Maintaining adequate blood oxygenation and pressure are also critical in patients with TBI. Episodes of hypoxemia (arterial PaO_2 <60 mmHg) or hypotension (systolic blood pressure <90 mmHg) have been associated in numerous studies with significantly worse outcome in these patients (26–30) and rapid correction is associated with increased survival (31). While hypotension can be secondary to brain injury, it should not be thus attributed unless all other possible causes have been excluded. Hemodynamic resuscitation should begin in the emergency department with the placement of two large-bore IVs or a femoral line. A radial arterial blood pressure catheter is also useful for continuous blood pressure recording and volume resuscitation with 0.9% normal saline or blood is the first step for managing hypotension. If a vasopressor is required, norepinephrine is preferred as it produces the most consistent improvement in blood pressure and cerebral profusion.

Once resuscitation has been initiated, management of ICP should be addressed as soon as possible. Multiple studies have shown improved survival if patients with suspected elevated ICP are taken to a center with immediately available CT scanning, neurosurgical care, and the ability to monitor ICP in an ICU setting (32–34). Initiation of osmotic therapy with

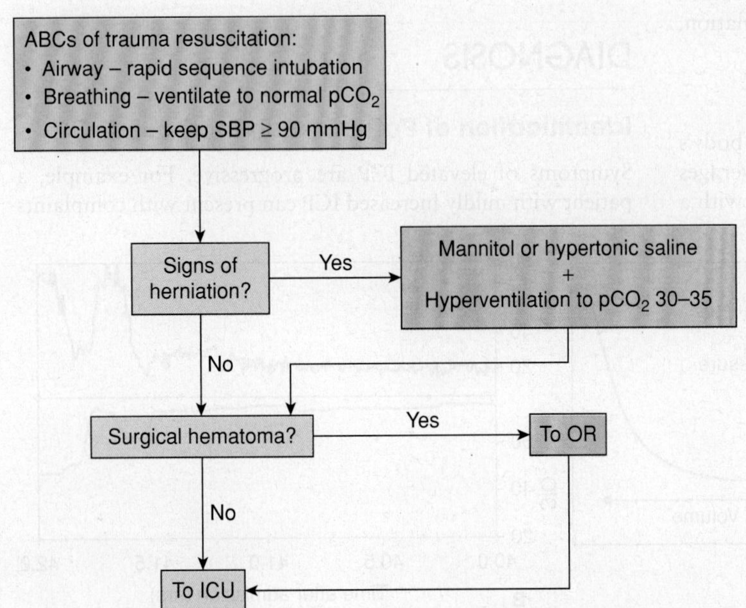

FIGURE 118.2 Algorithm for initial management of patient with elevated intracranial pressure. ICU, intensive care unit; OR, operating room; SBP, systolic blood pressure.

mannitol is effective at controlling raised ICP. However, ideally mannitol therapy is restricted to patients with ICP monitors or those who have signs of transtentorial herniation or progressive neurologic deterioration not attributable to other causes. Effective doses for mannitol range from 0.25 to 1 g/kg, with a 1 g/kg bolus being the standard dose. However, studies have shown improved outcome with preoperative doses as high as 1.4 g/kg in patients with signs of herniation secondary to subdural hematoma (35). Mannitol should only be given once fluid resuscitation has been completed as it does result in an osmotic diuresis and can cause hypotension in the incompletely resuscitated patient. Alternatively, hypertonic saline is another osmotic agent that can be used and has an advantage in a hypotensive patient since it does not cause diuresis.

Surgery

If a surgical lesion is identified, the patient should be taken immediately to the operating room for evacuation. Invasive monitoring devices can be inserted in the operating room if required; at a minimum, an ICP monitor should be inserted. Other monitoring devices that can be used if available include PbO_2 and SjO_2 catheters. An arterial line should also be placed and a central venous catheter may be needed, especially if hypotension is present or large doses of mannitol are required.

Commonly Monitored Parameters in Patients with Elevated ICP

Intracranial Pressure

Normal ICP in a healthy supine adult ranges between 7 and 15 mmHg (36). In a head-injured patient, several studies have demonstrated worse outcomes with ICP values greater than 20 mmHg (26,37–39) and values above 40 mmHg indicate severe life-threatening intracranial hypertension. Thus, the goal of treatment should be to maintain ICP values below 20 mmHg.

The gold standard for monitoring ICP is a ventriculostomy catheter inserted into one of the lateral ventricles and connected to an external strain gauge and drainage bag. This system provides the most accurate measurement of ICP and is stable over time (40). It can also be used to drain CSF and treat elevated ICP if needed. CSF should be intermittently drained to treat ICP except in cases that are associated with hydrocephalus, where continuous CSF drainage is optimal. In such cases, one of the secondary ICP monitors described below should be additionally used to continuously record ICP while the CSF is being drained. The main risk of ventriculostomy is infection, with rates ranging up to 20% (41). Antibiotic-impregnated ventriculostomy catheters, however, can reduce this risk significantly to around 1.5% (42) and thus should preferentially be used. Other problems often associated with ventriculostomy catheters, although to a much smaller degree, include obstruction, malposition, infection, and malfunction.

Other invasive monitors for measuring ICP include intraparenchymal, subarachnoid, and epidural monitors. The advantage of theses probes is they do not require insertion into the ventricle, which not only lowers the infection rate (41), but is also useful when the ventricle is collapsed or displaced by significant midline shift. However, these probes are less accurate and tend to drift over time (7). Of these monitors, intraparenchymal probes are arguably the most accurate with the least amount of drift, thus offering the best alternative to ventriculostomy (43).

Cerebral Perfusion Pressure

CPP is defined as the MAP minus the ICP and is a second major parameter that can be both monitored and treated in the patient with elevated ICP. CPPs below 50 mmHg should be avoided and can be supported by maintaining MAP and by lowering ICP, however, aggressive attempts to maintain CPPs above 70 mmHg using fluids and vasopressors should also be avoided secondary to the risk of acute respiratory distress syndrome (ARDS). Also, while patients with intact autoregulation can tolerate CPPs of 70 mmHg, patients with impaired autoregulation risk malignant hyperemia with CPPs above 60 mmHg (44). For most patients, a CPP of 60 mmHg is adequate (45) and guidelines recommend a range between 50 and 70 mmHg.

Brain Oxygenation

As describe above, brain tissue oxygenation can either be measured globally at a single time point using PET imaging techniques or continuously and locally by using probes to monitor PbO_2 and/or SjO_2. PET has provided important insights in TBI research, but is not widely available for ICU patients. In contrast, PbO_2 and SjO_2 monitoring can be used in any ICU setting.

Brain Tissue Oxygen Tension. PbO_2 monitoring is accomplished by inserting an oxygen-sensing probe into brain tissue. The location of the probe is critical and determines the nature of the PbO_2 information that will be obtained (Fig. 118.3). For example, if the probe is inserted near a focal lesion, oxygenation can be monitored in the tissue at greatest risk. In contrast, insertion of the probe in uninjured brain allows monitoring of a local area that should be representative of the overall less-injured oxygenation status of the brain (19). While normal values of brain PbO_2 are not well established, multiple studies have shown associated time-dependent worse outcomes with PbO_2 values lower than 10 to 15 mmHg (46–48) and values of less than 6 mmHg are also associated with poorer outcomes in a time-independent fashion (46). While some studies have shown reduced mortality when brain PbO_2 values are kept around 25 mmHg (49) or 20 mmHg (50), in general the recommended treatment threshold is less than 15 mmHg.

Jugular Venous Oxygen Saturation. SjO_2 is a measure of the oxygen saturation in the jugular bulb and can be monitored by inserting a catheter into the internal jugular vein and advancing toward the skull base. This allows measurement of the oxygen saturation of the blood exiting the brain, which provides information on the adequacy of CBF and oxygen delivery to the brain (18). Normal values for SjO_2 are better studied than PbO_2 values but are still not well established, with typical values from older series ranging from 55% to 71% (51). However, newer studies suggest that normal SjO_2 values may be as low as 45% (52). Despite this, episodes of SjO_2 desaturations to values less than 50% are associated with worse outcome (53) and should be treated. Increased SjO_2 of greater than 75% may indicate decreased oxygen uptake in the brain (54) and is also an indicator of poor outcome. While it is a useful tool for global cerebral oxygenation assessment, the major limitation to SjO_2 monitoring is that unlike brain PbO_2, it cannot detect local ischemia within the brain.

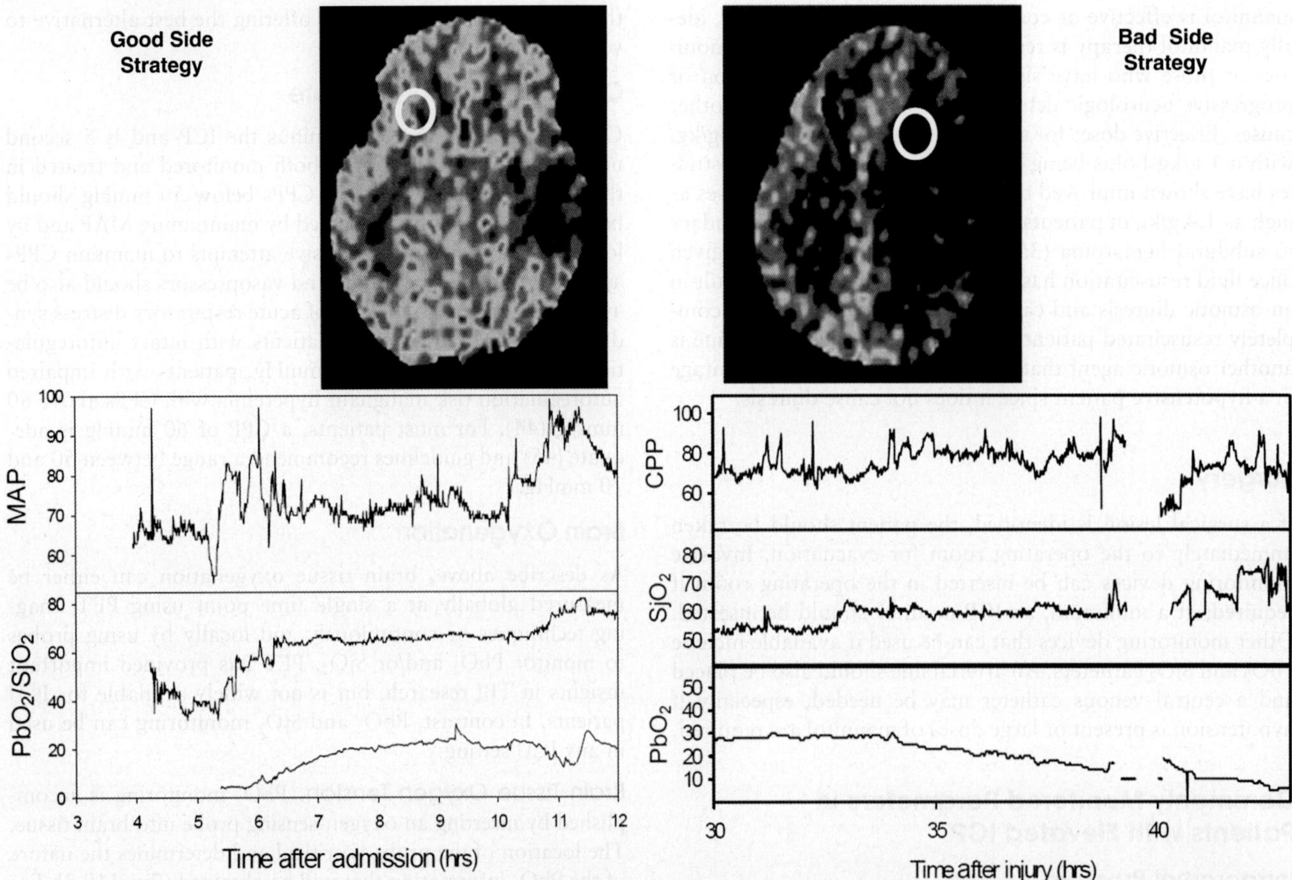

FIGURE 118.3 Location of the brain tissue oxygen tension (PbO_2) catheter relative to the injured brain determines the nature of the pO_2 information that will be obtained. On the left is a patient where the PbO_2 catheter was placed in relatively normal brain opposite a temporal contusion. The PbO_2 reflected the global oxygenation of the brain measured with jugular venous oxygen saturation (SjO_2). On the right is a patient where the PbO_2 catheter was placed near a contusion. As this contusion evolved, the PbO_2 decreased even though the global measures (SjO_2 and cerebral perfusion pressure (CPP)) remained unchanged. MAP, mean arterial pressure.

Treatment of Elevated ICP: Principles of CNS Resuscitation

Principles of management of intracranial hypertension (Fig. 118.4) include general measures that are used in all patients to minimize factors that exacerbate ICP rise, first-line therapies that are applied to patients who subsequently have elevated ICP, and additional treatments that can be used if elevated ICP is refractory to these first-line measures.

General Measures

Prevention or treatment of factors that may aggravate or precipitate intracranial hypertension is the cornerstone of central nervous system (CNS) resuscitation. Specific factors that may aggravate intracranial hypertension include the obstruction of venous return, hypoxia, hypercapnia, fever, severe hypertension, hyponatremia, anemia, and seizures. Routine critical care management of the patient at risk for intracranial hypertension should include measures to prevent these factors as much as possible. Also important are general strategies for maintaining normal brain oxygenation and CPP.

Minimize Obstruction to Venous Return

Head of the bed elevation to 30 degrees and neutral head positioning maximize venous return from the brain and has been standard neurosurgery practice for management of ICP. While some studies initially suggested that this resulted in a decrease in CPP (55), other studies designed to specifically address this question found no significant reduction in CPP, CBF, or regional microcirculation in most patients (56,57). If head elevation is used, it is important to remember that both the ICP and blood pressure transducers should be zeroed at the same level (i.e., at the level of the foramen of Monro) to get accurate measurements of CPP. It is also important to look for other potential causes of elevated ICP in patients refractory to standard therapies. For example, in patients with abdominal injury, an increased intra-abdominal pressure may also impede venous return from the brain and increase ICP. In such cases, abdominal decompression can improve an otherwise refractory ICP (58).

Prevent Fever

Fever is common during the recovery from a head injury. Fever is a potent cerebral vasodilator and has been associated with increased intracranial temperature, metabolic requirements, and ICP (59,60). As a result, it is also associated with longer hospital stays and worse outcomes (61). Efficient external cooling systems as well as intravascular cooling devices are available and can maintain normal body temperature when needed. However, more importantly, when fever occurs, infectious causes should be investigated with appropriate cultures and treated with antibiotics.

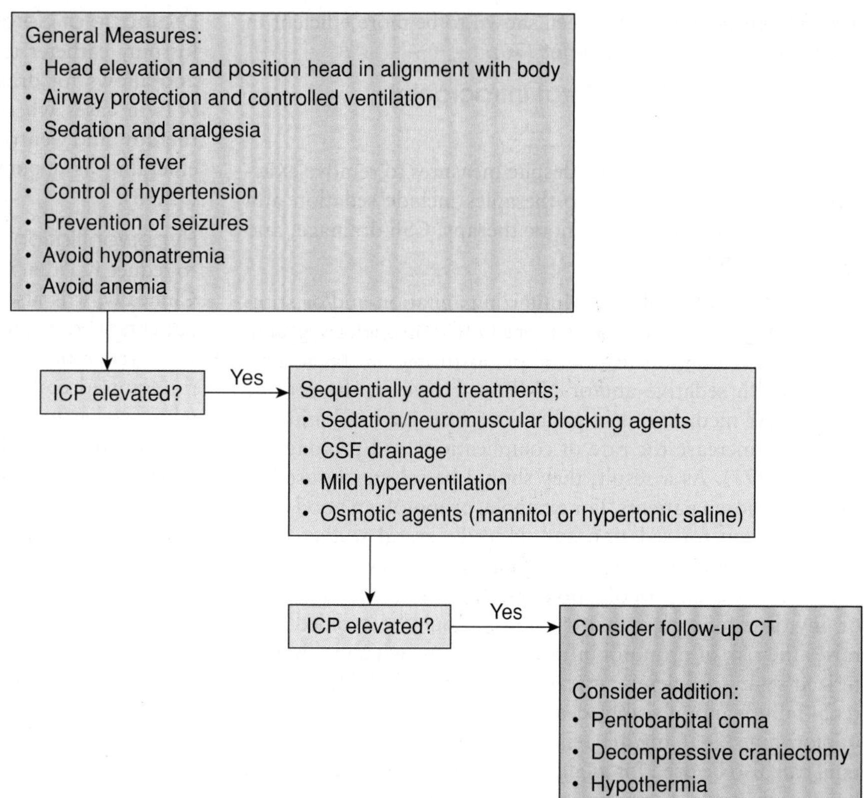

FIGURE 118.4 Algorithm for treatment of elevated intracranial pressure (ICP). CT, computed tomography; CSF, cerebrospinal fluid.

Prevent Seizures

Posttraumatic seizures (PTS) are not uncommon after TBI. While upward of 11% of civilian patients with TBI can have a seizure within 5 years (62), the number who will have early PTS, characterized as seizures within the first week of injury, is closer to 3% (63). This incidence is strongly dependent upon the severity of the injury (64). Unfortunately, severe TBI patients, who have the highest risk of seizure—which approximates 22%—are often pharmacologically sedated and paralyzed to treat intracranial hypertension, rendering clinical monitoring ineffective. For these high-risk patients, continuous electroencephalogram (EEG) monitoring may be particularly useful (65,66) and is recommended for 48 to 72 hours. Continuous monitoring of EEG should also be done in patients who clinically deteriorate or develop worsened ICP or brain oxygenation without an obvious explanation.

Based on large randomized control trials, prophylaxis with phenytoin has been shown to be effective in reducing early, but not late, PTS (67). Similar reductions in PTS have been found with both valproic acid (68) and levetiracetam (69), though mortality was higher in those treated with valproic acid. However, while these seizures can precipitate adverse effects in the acute phase by increasing cerebral metabolic rates, studies have shown that early PTS did not significantly influence neurologic recovery at 6 months (63). Thus, routine use of anti-seizure prophylax for PTS is controversial and is recommended only for one week to prevent early seizures. If it is used, it should be discontinued after 7 days if there is no evidence of a seizure.

Maintain Brain Oxygenation

Oxygen delivery to the brain is dependent on CBF as well as the oxygen content of the blood. Thus, while there has been no strong clinical evidence directly linking hypoxemia with increased morbidity or mortality, clinical intuition would suggest that TBI patients who also have episodes of hypoxemia should have poorer outcomes. While some studies have shown worse outcomes with early hypoxemia (70,71), at least one study has shown no relationship (72). In general, however, current guidelines recommend avoiding hypoxemia, which is typically defined as an oxygen saturation of less than 90% or a PaO_2 of less than 60 mmHg. As most oxygen content in the blood is bound to hemoglobin, avoiding anemia, common in TBI patients, should conceptually be beneficial in maintaining brain oxygenation. However, while there are data that transfusion improves brain oxygenation in some patients (73), a recent randomized control trial showed no significant benefit in outcome if hemoglobin values were kept greater than 10 g/dL versus 7 g/dL (74).

Maintain Cerebral Perfusion Pressure

Several studies have shown poorer outcomes in the TBI patient with episodes of early hypotension (26–28). As such, initial recommendations are to avoid hypotension, as characterized by systolic blood pressure of less than 90 mmHg. Once an ICP monitor is in place, further blood pressure management should be aimed at maintaining a CPP of at least 50 mmHg, and preferentially around 60 mmHg (45). Increasing CPP higher than 70 mmHg increases the risk of ARDS and does not improve outcome (45,75). Boluses of intravenous fluid can be used as initial treatment of low CPP. All intravenous fluids given should at least be isotonic to avoid worsening cerebral edema and there are data showing improved results with hypertonic solutions (31). If fluid resuscitation is not sufficient to maintain CPP, treatment with vasopressors should be initiated with norepinephrine, which has been shown to be more efficient in augmenting CPP than dopamine (76).

First-line Therapies to Treat Intracranial Hypertension

When ICP becomes elevated despite measures to remove exacerbating factors, the first-line therapies include sedation and neuromuscular blockade, osmotic therapy, CSF drainage, and hyperventilation.

Sedation and Paralysis. Minimizing agitation and/or stimuli that may contribute to elevations in ICP through coughing, controlled ventilation resistance, or posturing can be accomplished with sedative and/or NMBAs. However, the routine use of these medications in patients with severe head injury is known to increase the rate of complications and prolong the ICU stay (77). As a result, they should be selectively used in carefully chosen patients. For example, propofol is a good temporary option for sedation and, indeed, several studies have shown no significant changes in ICP with propofol infusion (78,79). However, propofol dosages of greater than 5 mg/kg/hr or any dose for longer than 48 hours should be avoided as it raises the risk of propofol infusion syndrome which is characterized by hyperkalemia, metabolic acidosis, rhabdomyolysis, renal failure and, possibly, death (80). Alternatively, infusions of morphine (2–10 mg/hr), fentanyl (100–200 μg/hr), or sufentanil can also be used for analgesia. A randomized control trial has shown similar outcome results to propofol with morphine infusion (81). While boluses of fentanyl or sufentanil have been shown to cause an elevation in ICP (82), (83), this can be avoided with slow titration (84). In patients in whom an NMBA is needed, cisatracurium has been shown to cause no significant changes in ICP when used in conjunction with sufentanil and midazolam, the latter agents for continuous sedation (85), and is the preferred neuromuscular blocker. Since the neurologic examination cannot be closely monitored while the patient is pharmacologically paralyzed, these medications should be withheld once a day, usually before morning rounds, to obtain a brief neurologic examination.

Osmotic Therapy to Reduce Intracranial Pressure. One of the mainstays of treatment of elevated ICP is osmotic therapy with either mannitol or hypertonic saline. Mannitol can be given in a single dose of 1 to 1.5 g/kg for short-term effect, particularly in patients without an ICP monitor who have clinical signs of active brain herniation (86). Once an ICP monitor has been inserted, it can also be used for prolonged therapy for patients with persistently elevated ICPs greater than 20 to 25 mmHg, either with intermittent boluses between 0.25 and 0.5 g/kg every 2 to 3 hours or with a continuous infusion, however there is little clinical evidence regarding this approach (87). The serum osmolality in either approach should be monitored and kept less than 320 mOsm/kg H_2O. Dosing to a serum osmolality of greater than 320 has not been demonstrated to improve outcome and increases the risk of acute renal failure (88).

Although mannitol has been more widely studied, some studies have suggested that boluses of 7.5% hypertonic saline are more effective at lowering ICP (89). Other variations of hypertonic saline that have shown improvements over mannitol include hypertonic saline/hetastarch (90) and hypertonic saline/dextran (91). However, further large randomized controlled studies are necessary to define the role of hypertonic saline in the treatment of increased ICP.

Drainage of Cerebrospinal Fluid. Placement of a ventriculostomy catheter is a mainstay of therapy for hydrocephalus and allows for drainage of CSF during episodes of increased ICP. In cases where ICP remains refractory to both medical therapy and ventriculostomy, additional lumbar drainage is emerging as a potential secondary source for CSF drainage (92,93).

Hyperventilation. Hyperventilation is a temporizing measure to reduce ICP that works by inducing cerebral vasoconstriction. Clinically, it is also known to reduce CBF (94). Thus, in TBI patients who already have lowered levels of CBF (95), aggressive hyperventilation risks precipitating ischemia and, indeed, randomized control trials show poorer outcomes in patients who receive *prophylactic* hyperventilation (96). As a result, current guidelines do not recommend prophylactic hyperventilation, as defined by $PaCO_2$ levels of 25 mmHg or less.

However, far less is known about the effects of moderate hyperventilation, as characterized by $PaCO_2$ values between 30 and 35 mmHg, and in general this is considered a possible treatment strategy for patients with refractory ICP. It is important to withdraw chronic hyperventilation over several days as abruptly returning the $PaCO_2$ to normal can result in a dramatic increase in ICP.

Additional Treatments for Refractory Intracranial Hypertension. All of the treatments outlined in this category have been shown in clinical studies to significantly reduce otherwise refractory ICP. However, none has demonstrated improved outcome. There are also no data to suggest which of these treatments is most effective or has the least morbidity. For these reasons, they are applied selectively to patients who are judged to have some potential for recovery if their ICP can be controlled. However, if ICP remains refractory, it is also important to consider whether a delayed intracranial hematoma may have developed. A follow-up CT scan may be indicated before advancing to these additional treatments and any surgical intracranial hematoma should be evacuated.

Pentobarbital Coma. The administration of pentobarbital coma has been shown in a randomized multicenter control trial to double the likelihood of ICP control in otherwise refractory patients (97). However, given its strong side effect profile, most notably for causing significant hypotension—which can significantly influence outcome (98)—its use should be restricted to those who are truly refractory to other methods. It has also been shown ineffective as a *prophylactic* treatment for all severe TBI patients with a poor examination (99), or as a first-line treatment for elevated ICP (100) and can be detrimental in these situations.

A simple paradigm for induction is a loading dose of 10 mg/kg intravenously (IV) over 30 minutes followed by 5 mg/kg/hr for three doses followed by a maintenance dose of 1 mg/kg/hr (97). The initial loading dose should be given by slow intravenous push with close monitoring of the blood pressure. While this dosing regimen is based upon titrating the maintenance dose to achieve a serum level of 3 to 4 mg/dL (30–40 μg/mL), there is poor correlation between serum levels of pentobarbital and benefit. Instead burst suppression on continuous electroencephalographic recording is a more accurate indicator of effect (101).

The goal of treatment is to reduce ICP to below 20 to 25 mmHg. After ICP has been controlled for 24 to 48 hours, pentobarbital can be weaned and stopped; if ICP increases during reduction of pentobarbital, stop the downtitration and increase the dose until ICP is controlled. It should be noted that in addition to risk of hypotension, which should be closely monitored and corrected with fluid boluses and vasopressors as needed, pentobarbital coma also increases the risk of hospital-acquired complications, including pneumonia, pressure ulcers, and paralytic ileus. Given this side effect profile, several studies have tried to identify the subgroup of TBI patients most likely to respond to pentobarbital coma. Some characteristics that have been identified include younger age, diffuse rather than focal brain injury, and a high pretreatment level of brain electrical activity (102). Other factors associated with a positive outcome include a lack of overwhelming injuries that would drastically reduce the cerebral metabolic rate and a lack of significant hypotension that would limit the amount of barbiturate that can be given (103). Preservation of the cerebrovascular reactivity to CO_2 has also predicted a good ICP response to barbiturates (104).

Decompressive Craniectomy. This therapeutic modality has a long and controversial history since its initial description by Kocher in the early 20th century. Indeed, its efficacy in trauma has been questioned for several issues, including early studies debating its usefulness in the evacuation of subdural hematomata (105,106) and more recent studies debating the effectiveness in managing refractory ICP (107,108). A recent multicenter randomized control trial has demonstrated that early decompressive craniectomy does decrease ICP, but is associated with more unfavorable outcomes (109). However, the patients in this trial only needed elevations in ICP of greater than 20 mmHg for 15 nonconsecutive minutes in a 1-hour period to be included. The results from patients with longer elevations in ICP is currently being evaluated in another multicenter randomized trial (110). In general, craniectomy for refractory ICP management in patients without an underlying surgically addressable lesion is only considered when CSF drainage, osmotic therapy, hyperventilation, and sedation have failed and ICP remains elevated for an extended period of time.

When performing a decompressive craniectomy, multiple technical considerations must be considered (111). Most notably in these considerations is the location. For example, if the injury primarily involves a single hemisphere of the brain, a hemicraniectomy in which a large bone flap over one hemisphere is removed with particular focus paid to visualization of the middle fossa floor and anterior temporal lobe can provide adequate decompression. Diffuse injury involving both hemispheres may necessitate bifrontal craniectomy, with decompression of both temporal and frontal lobes. Similarly, the size of the craniectomy has also been shown to significantly affect the degree of ICP reduction (111,112), with studies showing very poor outcomes with sizes less than 10 cm (112).

Hypothermia. This therapy has, conceptually, several potential neuroprotective effects, including reducing cerebral metabolism and decreasing ICP. However, the results from randomized control trials have been mixed, with some studies showing a positive benefit on outcome (113–116) and at least one large study showing no benefit (117) despite a reduction in ICP. Part of this difference in results might be secondary to differing levels of hypothermia and differing lengths of treatment in each trial. As a result, while avoiding hyperthermia (>38°C) is recommended, routine induction of hypothermia is not recommended, but it may be an effective adjunctive treatment for increased ICP refractory to other treatments.

Contraindicated Therapies (Therapies with No Beneficial Effect)

There is no demonstrated benefit in treating TBI patients with steroids. A multicenter randomized control trial was halted early after an observed increased risk of death in patients receiving methylprednisolone for 48 hours after injury (118). As a result, steroids are contraindicated for treatment of head injury. However, they can be given for other indications in TBI patients, including hypothalamic/pituitary dysfunction or a prior outpatient condition requiring steroid use, such as asthma.

Completion of Treatment

Treatment should be titrated off once ICP has been controlled below 20 mmHg for 24 to 48 hours. ICP monitors can be removed if ICP is stable below 20 mmHg for 24 to 48 hours after therapy has been stopped. It is important to remember that patients may develop delayed increase in ICP secondary to blossoming of contusions, evolution of a stroke, or development of new mass lesions.

CONTROVERSIES

Benefit of ICP Monitoring?

No study clearly demonstrates that monitoring and treating ICP improves neurologic outcome. On the one hand, there are strong associations between intracranial hypertension and a poor outcome, and the development of refractory intracranial hypertension has a very high mortality rate (26,37–39,97,100). Historically, institution of treatment protocols aimed at controlling elevated ICP has significantly improved outcome in TBI. For example, in 1977 Jennett et al. (119) reported a mortality rate of 50% in comatose patients (GCS <8) in a cohort treated without ICP monitoring. By way of contrast, Becker et al. (120) reported significantly lower mortality of 30% in a similar patient cohort in whom ICP monitoring was used. Additionally, mortality rates at 30 days for patients with severe brain injury have been slowly declining with an increase in treatment strategies designed to control ICP. The mortality of patients in the Traumatic Coma Data Bank decreased from 39% in 1984 to 27% in 1996 (121). On the other hand, the recent multicenter randomized control BEST-TRIP trial comparing ICP monitored care to care based on clinical and imaging without ICP monitoring found no difference in survival, functional status at 6 months, or neuropsychological outcome at 6 months (122).

The availability of multiple monitoring modalities has provided more information on the status of patients in whom poor outcomes develop, and has provided treatment goals. Treatment strategies are aimed at maintaining ICP less than 20 to 25 mmHg, maintaining CPP greater than 60 mmHg, and maintaining brain tissue oxygenation at greater than 10 mmHg. Even with these advances in treatment, TBI is still associated with significant morbidity and mortality in both the short and long term.

What Is the Most Important Physiologic End Point: ICP, CPP, or Brain Oxygenation?

As it has become possible to measure additional brain-specific physiologic parameters in the ICU, different management

TABLE 118.1 Normal Values and Treatment Thresholds for Physiologic Parameters

	Normal	Treatment Threshold
ICP	0–10 mmHg	20–25 mmHg
CPP	50 mmHg	60 mmHg
SjO_2	55–71%	50%
PbO_2	20–40 mmHg	15 mmHg

ICP, intracranial pressure; CPP, cerebral perfusion pressure; SjO_2, jugular venous oxygen saturation; PbO_2, brain tissue oxygen tension.

strategies have evolved that place special emphasis on parameters other than ICP. For example, some have advocated that ICP is not important as long as CPP is maintained. This philosophy led to the use of CPP-directed therapy where induced hypertension was used to drive CPP to high levels even though ICP was also increased by the therapy (55). However, all of these physiologic parameters are related to outcome, and there is no clear evidence that one parameter is more important than the others. Table 118.1 presents normal values and treatment thresholds for these parameters.

The best circumstance occurs when ICP, CPP, and brain oxygenation are all maintained in normal ranges, and this should probably be the goal of management. When this is not possible, it is important to understand the limitations of each of the monitors when making therapeutic decisions. Additionally, clinical studies are needed to demonstrate what management strategies may best improve neurologic outcome.

Key Points

- The volume of the intracranial space is fixed by the skull. An increase in volume of any component within the skull must be compensated, initially by displacement of CSF. Once this reserve is exhausted, ICP increases rapidly.
- CPP is defined as MAP minus ICP. CPP can be increased by lowering ICP or by raising MAP.
- Elevated ICP can be caused by multiple injuries, including stroke, subarachnoid hemorrhage, mass lesion, hydrocephalus, and TBI.
- Initial management of the patient with elevated ICP should focus on the ABCs of the Advanced Trauma Life Support (ATLS) system. When signs of herniation are present, mannitol or hypertonic saline should be given. Surgical mass lesions should be identified and promptly evacuated.
- CBF must be maintained at levels high enough to deliver sufficient oxygen, particularly in the injured brain.
- A ventriculostomy catheter placed into one of the lateral ventricles is the gold standard for ICP monitoring. ICP should be maintained at less than 20 mmHg in TBI patients.
- Brain oxygenation can be measured globally at a single time point using PET imaging or continuously using a catheter inserted into the internal jugular vein to measure the oxygen saturation of venous blood from the brain. Local brain oxygen tension can be measured continuously by inserting a PO_2 probe directly into the brain parenchyma.
- Surgical mass lesions should be identified and evacuated.
- Symptoms concerning for elevated ICP include decreased level of consciousness, a fixed and dilated pupil, decorticate or decerebrate posturing, and/or hemiparesis.
- Osmotic therapy is one of the mainstays of treatment for elevated ICP. Mannitol can be dosed with an initial bolus of 1 g/kg. Further bolus doses of 0.25 to 0.5 g/kg can be given as necessary. Hypertonic saline is another agent that can be used.
- Initial treatments of elevated ICP include sedation and paralysis, drainage of CSF, mild hyperventilation, and bolus administration of osmotic agents such as mannitol.
- If ICP is not controlled with these measures, additional treatments including pentobarbital coma, decompressive craniectomy, or hypothermia can be considered. Other parameters that can be monitored and treated include jugular venous oxygen saturation and brain tissue oxygenation.
- If CSF drainage and osmotic therapy are not sufficient to control elevated ICP, barbiturate coma has been shown to double the chances of controlling ICP. Hypotension is the most common complication of barbiturate coma and should be closely monitored and corrected with fluid boluses and vasopressors as needed.
- Therapy should be continued until ICP is controlled at less than 20 mmHg for 24 to 48 hours.
- Mortality rates for severe head injury have shown a steady decrease but are still greater than 20% (121,123).

References

1. Guillaume J, Janny P. Continuous intracranial manometry; importance of the method and first results. *Rev Neurol (Paris)*. 1951;84:131–142.
2. Lundberg N. Continuous recording and control of ventricular fluid pressure in neurosurgical practice. *Acta Psychiatr Scand Suppl*. 1960;36:1–193.
3. Schaller B, Graf R. Different compartments of intracranial pressure and its relationship to cerebral blood flow. *J Trauma*. 2005;59:1521–1531.
4. Sakka L, Coll G, Chazal J. Anatomy and physiology of cerebrospinal fluid. *Eur Ann Otorhinolaryngol Head Neck Dis*. 2011;128:309–316.
5. Kapoor KG, Katz SE, Grzybowski DM, Lubow M. Cerebrospinal fluid outflow: an evolving perspective. *Brain Res Bull*. 2008;77:327–334.
6. Pollay M. Overview of the CSF dual outflow system. *Acta Neurochir Suppl*. 2012;113:47–50.
7. Steiner LA, Andrews PJ. Monitoring the injured brain: ICP and CBF. *Br J Anaesth*. 2006;97:26–38.
8. Lofgren J, von Essen C, Zwetnow NN. The pressure-volume curve of the cerebrospinal fluid space in dogs. *Acta Neurol Scand*. 1973;49:557–574.
9. Lassen Na. Cerebral blood flow and oxygen consumption in man. *Physiol Rev*. 1959;39:183–238.
10. Hlatky R, Furuya Y, Valadka AB, et al. Dynamic autoregulatory response after severe head injury. *J Neurosurg*. 2002;97:1054–1061.
11. Bouma GJ, Muizelaar JP, Bandoh K, Marmarou A. Blood pressure and intracranial pressure-volume dynamics in severe head injury: relationship with cerebral blood flow. *J Neurosurg*. 1992;77:15–19.
12. Rangel-Castilla L, Gasco J, Nauta HJ, et al. Cerebral pressure autoregulation in traumatic brain injury. *Neurosurg Focus*. 2008;25:E7.
13. Melamed E, Lavy S, Bentin S, et al. Reduction in regional cerebral blood flow during normal aging in man. *Stroke*. 1980;11:31–35.
14. Astrup J, Siesjo BK, Symon L. Thresholds in cerebral ischemia: the ischemic penumbra. *Stroke*. 1981;12:723–725.
15. Furlan M, Marchal G, Viader F, et al. Spontaneous neurological recovery after stroke and the fate of the ischemic penumbra. *Ann Neurol*. 1996;40:216–226.

16. Bouma GJ, Muizelaar JP, Choi SC, et al. Cerebral circulation and metabolism after severe traumatic brain injury: the elusive role of ischemia. *J Neurosurg.* 1991;75:685–693.
17. Hlatky R, Contant CF, Diaz-Marchan P, et al. Significance of a reduced cerebral blood flow during the first 12 hours after traumatic brain injury. *Neurocrit Care.* 2004;1:69–83.
18. Robertson CS, Gopinath SP, Goodman JC, et al. SjvO2 monitoring in head-injured patients. *J Neurotrauma.* 1995;12:891–896.
19. Gopinath SP, Valadka AB, Uzura M, Robertson CS. Comparison of jugular venous oxygen saturation and brain tissue PO_2 as monitors of cerebral ischemia after head injury. *Crit Care Med.* 1999;27:2337–2345.
20. Narayan RK, Kishore PR, Becker DP, et al. Intracranial pressure: to monitor or not to monitor? A review of our experience with severe head injury. *J Neurosurg.* 1982;56:650–659.
21. Winchell RJ, Hoyt DB. Endotracheal intubation in the field improves survival in patients with severe head injury. Trauma Research and Education Foundation of San Diego. *Arch Surg.* 1997;132:592–597.
22. Davis DP, Hoyt DB, Ochs M, et al. The effect of paramedic rapid sequence intubation on outcome in patients with severe traumatic brain injury. *J Trauma.* 2003;54:444–453.
23. Davis DP, Fakhry SM, Wang HE, et al. Paramedic rapid sequence intubation for severe traumatic brain injury: perspectives from an expert panel. *Prehosp Emerg Care.* 2007;11:1–8.
24. Helm M, Schuster R, Hauke J, Lampl L. Tight control of prehospital ventilation by capnography in major trauma victims. *Br J Anaesth.* 2003;90:327–332.
25. Silvestri S, Ralls GA, Krauss B, et al. The effectiveness of out-of-hospital use of continuous end-tidal carbon dioxide monitoring on the rate of unrecognized misplaced intubation within a regional emergency medical services system. *Ann Emerg Med.* 2005;45:497–503.
26. Marmarou A, Anderson RL, Ward JD, et al. Impact of ICP instability and hypotension on outcome in patients with severe head trauma. *Special Suppl.* 1991;75:S59–S66.
27. Fearnside MR, Cook RJ, McDougall P, McNeil RJ. The Westmead Head Injury Project outcome in severe head injury. A comparative analysis of pre-hospital, clinical and CT variables. *Br J Neurosurg.* 1993;7:267–279.
28. Chesnut RM, Marshall LF, Klauber MR, et al. The role of secondary brain injury in determining outcome from severe head injury. *J Trauma.* 1993;34:216–222.
29. Miller JD. Head injury and brain ischaemia–implications for therapy. *Br J Anaesth.* 1985;57:120–130.
30. Pigula FA, Wald SL, Shackford SR, Vane DW. The effect of hypotension and hypoxia on children with severe head injuries. *J Pediatr Surg.* 1993;28:310–314.
31. Vassar MJ, Fischer RP, O'Brien PE, et al. A multicenter trial for resuscitation of injured patients with 7. 5% sodium chloride: the effect of added dextran 70. The Multicenter Group for the Study of Hypertonic Saline in Trauma Patients. *Arch Surg.* 1993;128:1003–1011.
32. Lee A, Garner A, Fearnside M, Harrison K. Level of prehospital care and risk of mortality in patients with and without severe blunt head injury. *Injury.* 2003;34:815–819.
33. Hannan EL, Farrell LS, Cooper A, et al. Physiologic trauma triage criteria in adult trauma patients: Are they effective in saving lives by transporting patients to trauma centers? *J Am Coll Surg.* 2005;200:584–592.
34. Hunt J, Hill D, Besser M, et al. Outcome of patients with neurotrauma: the effect of a regionalized trauma system. *Aust N Z J Surg.* 1995;65: 83–86.
35. Cruz J, Minoja G, Okuchi K. Improving clinical outcomes from acute subdural hematomas with the emergency preoperative administration of high doses of mannitol: a randomized trial. *Neurosurgery.* 2001;49:864–871.
36. Czosnyka M, Pickard JD. Monitoring and interpretation of intracranial pressure. *J Neurol Neurosurg Psychiatry.* 2004;75:813–821.
37. Marshall LF, Smith RW, Shapiro HM. The outcome with aggressive treatment in severe head injuries. Part I: the significance of intracranial pressure monitoring. *J Neurosurg.* 1979;50:20–25.
38. Miller JD, Butterworth JF, Gudeman SK, et al. Further experience in the management of severe head injury. *J Neurosurg.* 1981;54:289–299.
39. Saul TG, Ducker TB. Effect of intracranial pressure monitoring and aggressive treatment on mortality in severe head injury. *J Neurosurg.* 1982;56:498–503.
40. Bullock R, Chesnut RM, Clifton G, et al. Guidelines for the management of severe head injury. Brain Trauma Foundation. *Eur J Emerg Med.* 1996;3:109–127.
41. Aucoin PJ, Kotilainen HR, Gantz NM, et al. Intracranial pressure monitors. Epidemiologic study of risk factors and infections. *Am J Med.* 1986;80:369–376.
42. Zabramski JM, Whiting D, Darouiche RO, et al. Efficacy of antimicrobial-impregnated external ventricular drain catheters: a prospective, randomized, controlled trial. *J Neurosurg.* 2003;98:725–730.
43. Gopinath SP, Robertson CS, Contant CF, et al. Clinical evaluation of a miniature strain-gauge transducer for monitoring intracranial pressure. *Neurosurgery.* 1995;36:1137–1140.
44. Bratton SL, Chestnut RM, Ghajar J, et al. Guidelines for the management of severe traumatic brain injury. IX. Cerebral perfusion thresholds. *J Neurotrauma.* 2007;24(Suppl 1):S59–S64.
45. Robertson CS, Valadka AB, Hannay HJ, et al. Prevention of secondary ischemic insults after severe head injury. *Crit Care Med.* 1999;27:2086–2095.
46. Valadka AB, Gopinath SP, Contant CF, et al. Relationship of brain tissue PO2 to outcome after severe head injury. *Crit Care Med.* 1998;26:1576–1581.
47. Bardt TF, Unterberg AW, Hartl R, et al. Monitoring of brain tissue PO2 in traumatic brain injury: effect of cerebral hypoxia on outcome. *Acta Neurochir Suppl.* 1998;71:153–156.
48. van den Brink WA, van Santbrink H, Steyerberg EW, et al. Brain oxygen tension in severe head injury. *Neurosurgery.* 2000;46:868–876.
49. Stiefel MF, Spiotta A, Gracias VH, et al. Reduced mortality rate in patients with severe traumatic brain injury treated with brain tissue oxygen monitoring. *J Neurosurg.* 2005;103:805–811.
50. Narotam PK, Morrison JF, Nathoo N. Brain tissue oxygen monitoring in traumatic brain injury and major trauma: outcome analysis of a brain tissue oxygen-directed therapy. *J Neurosurg.* 2009;111:672–682.
51. Gibbs EL, Lennox WG, Nims LF, et al. Arterial and cerebral venous blood arterial-venous differences in man. *J Biol Chem.* 1942;144:325–332.
52. Chieregato A, Calzolari F, Trasforini G, et al. Normal jugular bulb oxygen saturation. *J Neurol Neurosurg Psychiatry.* 2003;74:784–786.
53. Gopinath SP, Robertson CS, Contant CF, et al. Jugular venous desaturation and outcome after head injury. *J Neurol Neurosurg Psychiatry.* 1994;57:717–723.
54. Cormio M, Valadka AB, Robertson CS. Elevated jugular venous oxygen saturation after severe head injury. *J Neurosurg.* 1999;90:9–15.
55. Rosner MJ, Coley IB. Cerebral perfusion pressure, intracranial pressure, and head elevation. *J Neurosurg.* 1986;65:636–641.
56. Feldman Z, Kanter MJ, Robertson CS, et al. Effect of head elevation on intracranial pressure, cerebral perfusion pressure, and cerebral blood flow in head-injured patients. *J Neurosurg.* 1992;76:207–211.
57. Meixensberger J, Baunach S, Amschler J, et al. Influence of body position on tissue-pO_2, cerebral perfusion pressure and intracranial pressure in patients with acute brain injury. *Neurol Res.* 1997;19:249–253.
58. Bloomfield GL, Dalton JM, Sugerman HJ, et al. Treatment of increasing intracranial pressure secondary to the acute abdominal compartment syndrome in a patient with combined abdominal and head trauma. *J Trauma.* 1995;39:1168–1170.
59. Rossi S, Zanier ER, Mauri I, et al. Brain temperature, body core temperature, and intracranial pressure in acute cerebral damage. *J Neurol Neurosurg Psychiatry.* 2001;71:448–454.
60. Soukup J, Zauner A, Doppenberg EM, et al. The importance of brain temperature in patients after severe head injury: relationship to intracranial pressure, cerebral perfusion pressure, cerebral blood flow, and outcome. *J Neurotrauma.* 2002;19:559–571.
61. Diringer MN, Reaven NL, Funk SE, Uman GC. Elevated body temperature independently contributes to increased length of stay in neurologic intensive care unit patients. *Crit Care Med.* 2004;32:1489–1495.
62. Annegers JF, Grabow JD, Groover RV, et al. Seizures after head trauma: a population study. *Neurology.* 1980;30:683–689.
63. Lee ST, Lui TN, Wong CW, et al. Early seizures after severe closed head injury. *Can J Neurol Sci.* 1997;24:40–43.
64. Annegers JF, Hauser WA, Coan SP, Rocca WA. A population-based study of seizures after traumatic brain injuries. *N Engl J Med.* 1998;338:20–24.
65. Vespa PM, Nenov V, Nuwer MR. Continuous EEG monitoring in the intensive care unit: early findings and clinical efficacy. *J Clin Neurophysiol.* 1999;16:1–13.
66. Vespa P. Continuous EEG monitoring for the detection of seizures in traumatic brain injury, infarction, and intracerebral hemorrhage: "to detect and protect". *J Clin Neurophysiol.* 2005;22:99–106.
67. Temkin NR, Dikmen SS, Wilensky AJ, et al. A randomized, double-blind study of phenytoin for the prevention of post-traumatic seizures. *N Engl J Med.* 1990;323:497–502.
68. Temkin NR, Dikmen SS, Anderson GD, et al. Valproate therapy for prevention of posttraumatic seizures: a randomized trial. *J Neurosurg.* 1999;91:593–600.
69. Caballero GC, Hughes DW, Maxwell PR, et al. Retrospective analysis of levetiracetam compared to phenytoin for seizure prophylaxis in adults with traumatic brain injury. *Hosp Pharm.* 2013;48:757–761.

70. Cooke RS, McNicholl BP, Byrnes DP. Early management of severe head injury in Northern Ireland. *Injury.* 1995;26:395–397.
71. Stocchetti N, Furlan A, Volta F. Hypoxemia and arterial hypotension at the accident scene in head injury. *J Trauma.* 1996;40:764–767.
72. Manley G, Knudson MM, Morabito D, et al. Hypotension, hypoxia, and head injury: frequency, duration, and consequences. *Arch Surg.* 2001;136: 1118–1123.
73. Zygun DA, Nortje J, Hutchinson PJ, et al. The effect of red blood cell transfusion on cerebral oxygenation and metabolism after severe traumatic brain injury. *Crit Care Med.* 2009;37:1074–1078.
74. Robertson CS, Hannay HJ, Yamal JM, et al. Effect of erythropoietin and transfusion threshold on neurological recovery after traumatic brain injury: a randomized clinical trial. *JAMA.* 2014;312:36–47.
75. Contant CF, Valadka AB, Gopinath SP, et al. Adult respiratory distress syndrome: a complication of induced hypertension after severe head injury. *J Neurosurg.* 2001;95:560–568.
76. Steiner LA, Johnston AJ, Czosnyka M, et al. Direct comparison of cerebrovascular effects of norepinephrine and dopamine in head-injured patients. *Crit Care Med.* 2004;32:1049–1054.
77. Hsiang JK, Chesnut RM, Crisp CB, et al. Early, routine paralysis for intracranial pressure control in severe head injury: Is it necessary? *Crit Care Med.* 1994;22:1471–1476.
78. Farling PA, Johnston JR, Coppel DL. Propofol infusion for sedation of patients with head injury in intensive care: a preliminary report. *Anaesthesia.* 1989;44:222–226.
79. Pinaud M, Lelausque JN, Chetanneau A, et al. Effects of propofol on cerebral hemodynamics and metabolism in patients with brain trauma. *Anesthesiology.* 1990;73:404–409.
80. Kang TM. Propofol infusion syndrome in critically ill patients. *Ann Pharmacother.* 2002;36:1453–1456.
81. Kelly DF, Goodale DB, Williams J, et al. Propofol in the treatment of moderate and severe head injury: a randomized, prospective double-blinded pilot trial. *J Neurosurg.* 1999;90:1042–1052.
82. Albanese J, Durbec O, Viviand X, et al. Sufentanil increases intracranial pressure in patients with head trauma. *Anesthesiology.* 1993;79:493–497.
83. Sperry RJ, Bailey PL, Reichman MV, et al. Fentanyl and sufentanil increase intracranial pressure in head trauma patients. *Anesthesiology.* 1992;77:416–420.
84. Lauer KK, Connolly LA, Schmeling WT. Opioid sedation does not alter intracranial pressure in head injured patients. *Can J Anaesth.* 1997;44:929–933.
85. Schramm WM, Jesenko R, Bartunek A, Gilly H. Effects of cisatracurium on cerebral and cardiovascular hemodynamics in patients with severe brain injury. *Acta Anaesthesiol Scand.* 1997;41:1319–1323.
86. Cruz J, Minoja G, Okuchi K, Facco E. Successful use of the new high-dose mannitol treatment in patients with Glasgow Coma Scale scores of 3 and bilateral abnormal pupillary widening: a randomized trial. *J Neurosurg.* 2004;100:376–383.
87. Roberts I, Schierhout G, Wakai A. Mannitol for acute traumatic brain injury. *Cochrane Database Syst Rev.* 2003;(2):CD001049
88. Becker DP, Vries JK. The alleviation of increased intracranial pressure by the chronic administration of osmotic agents. In: Brock M, Dietz H, eds. *Intracranial Pressure.* New York: Springer; 1972:309–315.
89. Vialet R, Albanese J, Thomachot L, et al. Isovolume hypertonic solutes (sodium chloride or mannitol) in the treatment of refractory posttraumatic intracranial hypertension: 2 mL/kg 7.5% saline is more effective than 2 mL/kg 20% mannitol. *Crit Care Med.* 2003;31:1683–1687.
90. Harutjunyan L, Holz C, Rieger A, et al. Efficiency of 7.2% hypertonic saline hydroxyethyl starch 200/0.5 versus mannitol 15% in the treatment of increased intracranial pressure in neurosurgical patients: a randomized clinical trial [ISRCTN62699180]. *Crit Care.* 2005;9:R530–R540.
91. Battison C, Andrews PJ, Graham C, Petty T. Randomized, controlled trial on the effect of a 20% mannitol solution and a 7.5% saline/6% dextran solution on increased intracranial pressure after brain injury. *Crit Care Med.* 2005;33:196–202.
92. Murad A, Ghostine S, Colohan AR. Controlled lumbar drainage in medically refractory increased intracranial pressure: a safe and effective treatment. *Acta Neurochir Suppl.* 2008;102:89–91.
93. Murad A, Ghostine S, Colohan AR. A case for further investigating the use of controlled lumbar cerebrospinal fluid drainage for the control of intracranial pressure. *World Neurosurg.* 2012;77:160–165.
94. Raichle ME, Plum F. Hyperventilation and cerebral blood flow. *Stroke.* 1972;3:566–575.
95. Bouma GJ, Muizelaar JP, Stringer WA, et al. Ultra-early evaluation of regional cerebral blood flow in severely head-injured patients using xenon-enhanced computerized tomography. *J Neurosurg.* 1992;77:360–368.
96. Muizelaar JP, Marmarou A, Ward JD, et al. Adverse effects of prolonged hyperventilation in patients with severe head injury: a randomized clinical trial. *J Neurosurg.* 1991;75:731–739.
97. Eisenberg HM, Frankowski RF, Contant CF, et al. High-dose barbiturate control of elevated intracranial pressure in patients with severe head injury. *J Neurosurg.* 1988;69:15–23.
98. Roberts I, Sydenham E. Barbiturates for acute traumatic brain injury. *Cochrane Database Syst Rev.* 2012;12:CD000033.
99. Ward JD, Becker DP, Miller JD, et al. Failure of prophylactic barbiturate coma in the treatment of severe head injury. *J Neurosurg.* 1985;62: 383–388.
100. Schwartz ML, Tator CH, Rowed DW, et al. The University of Toronto head injury treatment study: a prospective, randomized comparison of pentobarbital and mannitol. *Can J Neurol Sci.* 1984;11:434–440.
101. Kassell NF, Hitchon PW, Gerk MK, et al. Alterations in cerebral blood flow, oxygen metabolism, and electrical activity produced by high dose sodium thiopental. *Neurosurgery.* 1980;7:598–603.
102. Miller JD, Piper IR, Dearden NM. Management of intracranial hypertension in head injury: matching treatment with cause. *Acta Neurochir Suppl (Wien).* 1993;57:152–159.
103. Cormio M, Gopinath SP, Valadka A, et al. Cerebral hemodynamic effects of pentobarbital coma in head-injured patients. *J Neurotrauma.* 1999;16:927–936.
104. Messeter K, Nordstrom CH, Sundbarg G, et al. Cerebral hemodynamics in patients with acute severe head trauma. *J Neurosurg.* 1986;64: 231–237.
105. Ransohoff J, Benjamin V. Hemicraniectomy in the treatment of acute subdural haematoma. *J Neurol Neurosurg Psychiatry.* 1971;34:106.
106. Cooper PR, Rovit RL, Ransohoff J. Hemicraniectomy in the treatment of acute subdural hematoma: a re-appraisal. *Surg Neurol.* 1976;5:25–28.
107. Aarabi B, Hesdorffer DC, Ahn ES, et al. Outcome following decompressive craniectomy for malignant swelling due to severe head injury. *J Neurosurg.* 2006;104:469–479.
108. Sahuquillo J, Arikan F. Decompressive craniectomy for the treatment of refractory high intracranial pressure in traumatic brain injury. *Cochrane Database Syst Rev.* 2006;(1):CD003983.
109. Cooper DJ, Rosenfeld JV, Murray L, et al. Decompressive craniectomy in diffuse traumatic brain injury. *N Engl J Med.* 2011;364:1493–1502.
110. Hutchinson PJ, Corteen E, Czosnyka M, et al. Decompressive craniectomy in traumatic brain injury: the randomized multicenter RESCUEicp study (www.RESCUEicp.com). *Acta Neurochir Suppl.* 2006;96:17–20.
111. Skoglund TS, Eriksson-Ritzen C, Jensen C, Rydenhag B. Aspects on decompressive craniectomy in patients with traumatic head injuries. *J Neurotrauma.* 2006;23:1502–1509.
112. Sedney CL, Julien T, Manon J, Wilson A. The effect of craniectomy size on mortality, outcome, and complications after decompressive craniectomy at a rural trauma center. *J Neurosci Rural Pract.* 2014;5:212–217.
113. Qiu WS, Liu WG, Shen H, et al. Therapeutic effect of mild hypothermia on severe traumatic head injury. *Chin J Traumatol.* 2005;8:27–32.
114. Marion DW, Penrod LE, Kelsey SF, et al. Treatment of traumatic brain injury with moderate hypothermia. *N Engl J Med.* 1997;336:540–546.
115. Jiang J, Yu M, Zhu C. Effect of long-term mild hypothermia therapy in patients with severe traumatic brain injury: 1-year follow-up review of 87 cases. *J Neurosurg.* 2000;93:546–549.
116. Aibiki M, Maekawa S, Yokono S. Moderate hypothermia improves imbalances of thromboxane A2 and prostaglandin I2 production after traumatic brain injury in humans. *Crit Care Med.* 2000;28:3902–3906.
117. Clifton GL, Miller ER, Choi SC, et al. Lack of effect of induction of hypothermia after acute brain injury. *N Engl J Med.* 2001;344:556–563.
118. Edwards P, Arango M, Balica L, et al. Final results of MRC CRASH, a randomised placebo-controlled trial of intravenous corticosteroid in adults with head injury-outcomes at 6 months. *Lancet.* 2005;365:1957–1959.
119. Jennett B, Teasdale G, Galbraith S, et al. Severe head injuries in three countries. *J Neurol Neurosurg Psychiatry.* 1977;40:291–298.
120. Becker DP, Miller JD, Ward JD, et al. The outcome from severe head injury with early diagnosis and intensive management. *J Neurosurg.* 1977;47: 491–502.
121. Lu J, Marmarou A, Choi S, et al. Mortality from traumatic brain injury. *Acta Neurochir Suppl.* 2005;95:281–285.
122. Chesnut RM, Temkin N, Carney N, et al. A trial of intracranial-pressure monitoring in traumatic brain injury. *N Engl J Med.* 2012;367: 2471–2481.
123. Stein SC, Georgoff P, Meghan S, et al. 150 years of treating severe traumatic brain injury: a systematic review of progress in mortality. *J Neurotrauma.* 2010;27:1343–1353.

CHAPTER

119

Brain Death and Management of the Potential Organ Donor

DAVID S. GLOSS II, KENNETH E. WOOD, and A. JOSEPH LAYON

INTRODUCTION

Management of the potential organ donor in the intensive care unit (ICU) represents a significant part of the solution to the ongoing crisis in organ donation. Ensuring maximal utilization and optimal management of the existing donor pool significantly increases the number of donors available for procurement and enables transplantation to save the lives—and enhance quality of life—of those with end-stage disease. As in other areas in medicine, standardization and the elimination of inappropriate variation in the management of the potential organ donor leads to higher procurement rates, improved quality of organs procured, and improved recipient outcomes. The standardized approach to the management of the potential organ donor begins with surveillance to identify patients with severe neurologic injury that will likely progress to brain death, and identification of potential candidates for donation after cardiac death (DCD). The Organ Procurement Organization (OPO) notification process should, in addition, be standardized and utilize accepted clinical triggers such as the recognition of a nonsurvivable neurologic injury, initiation of end-of-life (EOL) discussions with a family, or the consideration of a formal brain death examination. The methodology to diagnose brain death should be standardized and followed by a uniform request for consent in all cases in which brain death occurs.

In the interval between the suspicion of brain death and its declaration, it is imperative that the patient be supported such that the brain death examination can be undertaken. Similarly, the brain-dead, potential organ donor should be fully supported in the interval between declaration and attempting to secure consent from the donor's family. The Centers for Medicare and Medicaid Services (CMS) Conditions of Participation requires that potential organ donors be supported during this interval and that formal request for donation be made in all cases of brain death. While the patient is fully supported during this interval, formal donor management commences only after consent is obtained. Donor management necessitates an intensity of care that is, actually, indistinguishable from the management of any other critically ill patient in our ICU. However, the focus shifts away from the previously undertaken cerebral protective strategies to those resulting in optimization of transplantable donor organs. This is a crucial management period: (a) it facilitates donor somatic survivorship such that procurement may be undertaken; (b) it maintains the donor organs in the best possible condition; and (c) it mitigates ongoing ischemia–reperfusion (IR) injury. The latter has been linked to an inflammatory response, creating an immunologic continuum between the donor and recipient, which may jeopardize organ function in the recipient. Management of the potential organ donor is effectively the simultaneous medical management of the seven potential recipients of the donor organs. The cornerstone of donor management is hemodynamic and cardiovascular maintenance, upon which we primarily focus.

BRAIN DEATH PHYSIOLOGY

Cushing's landmark manuscript, published in 1902, described the "Experimental and Clinical Observations Concerning States of Increased Intracranial Tension" (1). Utilizing an animal model and differentiating local compression from a general compression of the brain, Cushing examined the physiology of intracranial hypertension and its effect upon systemic hemodynamics, now known as Cushing triad—irregular respirations, decreased heart rate, and increased blood pressure. In contrast to Cushing model, where the experimentation is undertaken in a controlled setting, the physiology of human brain death remains challenging. For example, the time of actual brain death maybe significantly different from the certification time with significant physiologic changes occurring in the interval; treatment of the patient in the period antecedent to brain death and in the immediate postbrain death period may result in abnormalities independent of brain death; and lastly, there will never be a human model of brain death (2). Consequently, our understanding of brain death physiology is derived from animal models and inferential data from human case series.

Similarly, management of the potential organ donor requires an implicit understanding of the pathophysiology of brain death as well as an appreciation of the traumatic or physiologic events that contributed to, or precipitated, brain death, and which may act synergistically with brain death physiology to impair organ function during the management period. This is best exemplified in the cardiovascular system, in which hemodynamic instability in the potential organ donor is likely reflective of a series of events conspiring to produce coincident cardiac dysfunction and vasodilatation. It is recognized that brain injury may lead to cardiac dysfunction, reflected in ECG abnormalities and cardiac enzymatic elevations (3). However, recent studies of survivors of severe brain injury have revealed significant cardiovascular dysfunction consequent to that injury, best exemplified in the subarachnoid hemorrhage (SAH) patient population. Recognizing that the degree of injury in the brain-dead, potential organ donor is far greater than in survivors of severe neurologic injury, it is reasonable to assume that events predating brain death may precipitate cardiac dysfunction to which the brain death event is additive.

In patients with SAH, the initial event's severity has been shown to predict the magnitude of cardiac dysfunction (4–6). Eighty percent of Hunt Hess Grade 5 SAH patients will exhibit a troponin release compared to less than 10% of those with a

Hunt Hess Grade 1 SAH. Temporally, this release occurs in the early days after the bleed. In this population, left ventricular systolic dysfunction is reported to occur in 10% to 28%, and diastolic dysfunction in 70% of patients. Diastolic impairment and the associated distortion in the pressure volume relationship of the left ventricle will assume an important role in the volume resuscitation of organ donors and potentially contribute to increased extravascular lung water. The pattern of wall motion abnormalities reported differs appreciably from those related to coronary artery disease, with a pattern of unique apical sparing and frequent involvement of the basal and mid-ventricular portions of the anteroseptal and anterior walls and the mid-ventricular portions for the inferoseptal and anterolateral walls; this myocardial dysfunction is reversible over time which may have implications for the echocardiographic assessment of potential organ donors. In a study comparing sympathetic innervation evaluated with MIBG scanning (meta{123} iodobenzylguanidine) to myocardial vascular perfusion assessed with MIBI scanning (technetium sestamibi) in SAH patients with cardiac dysfunction, an association between regions of contractile dysfunction and abnormalities in sympathetic innervation with normal perfusion was noted. Patients with evidence of global cardiac denervation manifested the lowest cardiac ejection fraction (EF) and worst regional wall motion scores compared to patient's without evidence of cardiac denervation, whose EF and wall motion scores were preserved (7). The preceding is at least partially explained by a catecholamine release hypothesis related to severe brain injury with the resultant effect upon cardiac function. Although not well studied, it appears that similar neurocardiac associations occur in other forms of severe brain injury such as traumatic brain injury (TBI). Insofar as severely brain-injured patients that ultimately die undoubtedly have a more severe form of brain injury than those surviving, it would be reasonable to conclude that the antecedent brain injury, in conjunction with the brain death process described below, will significantly impact upon cardiac function.

Similar to the above recognition of a neurocardiac axis, there is evidence of endocrine dysfunction in patients with severe brain injury. Given the controversial use of hormone resuscitation therapy (HRT) in the management of potential organ donors, it is important to appreciate that antecedent endocrine dysfunction may be present in advance of brain death and contribute to the instability of potential organ donors. Prebrain death endocrine dysfunction may be precipitated by direct injury to the hypothalamic pituitary axis, neuroendocrine effects from catecholamines and cytokines, disruption of the vascular supply, or from systemic infection or inflammation. In a review of endocrine failure after TBI in adults, the estimated incidence of hormonal reduction was adrenal 15%, thyroid 5% to 15%, growth hormone 18%, vasopressin 3% to 37%, and gonadal 25% to 80%; hyperprolactinemia was present in more than 50% of patients. The authors concluded that severe TBI, when accompanied by basilar skull fracture, hypothalamic edema, prolonged unresponsiveness, hyponatremia, and/or hypotension, was associated with a high incidence of endocrinopathy (8,9). As with antecedent cardiac dysfunction, it would seem reasonable that prebrain death endocrine dysfunction, in conjunction with the brain death process, may contribute to instability during the donor management period.

In concert with the previously described prebrain death physiology associated with severe brain injury, the process of brain death results in significant pathophysiologic changes in all organ systems with the cardiovascular system being most impacted. The rostrocaudal progression of ischemia, contemporarily known as coning is illustrated in Figure 119.1.

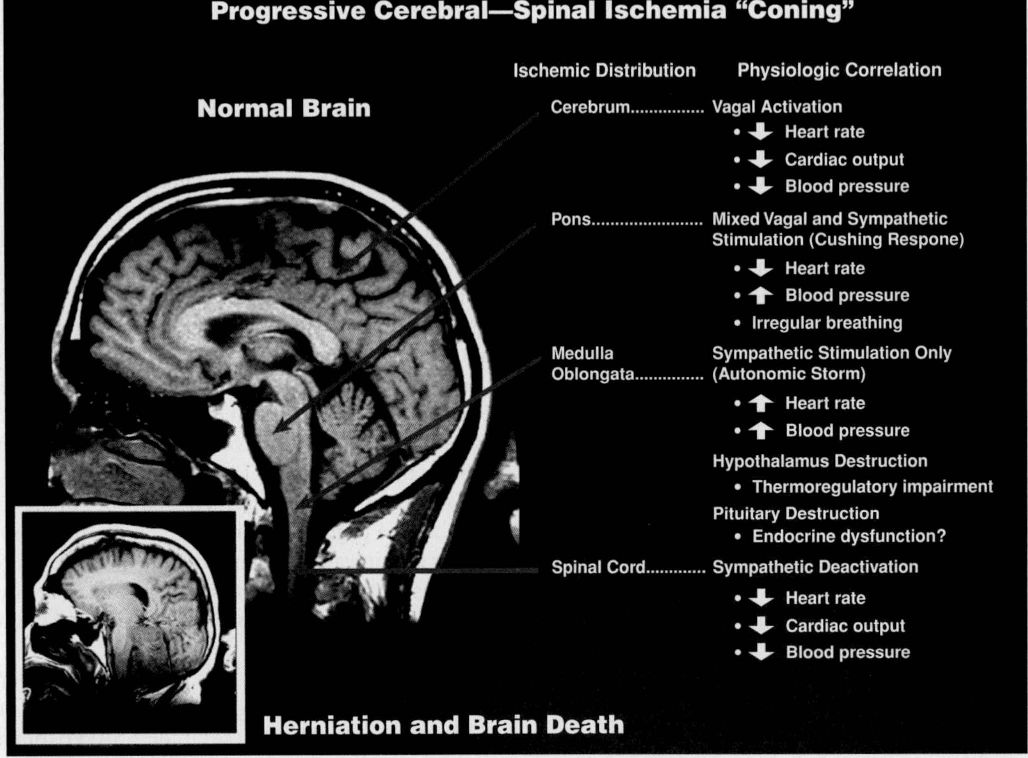

FIGURE 119.1 The rostrocaudal progression of ischemia contemporarily known as coning.

TABLE 119.1 Central Herniation

Stage of Herniation	Diencephalon	Midbrain to Upper Pons	Lower Pons	Medulla
Consciousness	Lethargy (early), agitation, progresses to coma (late)	Coma	Coma	Coma
Pupils	Small (1–3 mm), Sluggishly reactive	Mid-position (3–5 mm), Sluggish to not reactive	Mid-position, not reactive	Dilated, not reactive
Respirations	Pauses, sighs, Cheyne–Stokes	Central neurogenic hyperventilation, Cheyne–Stokes	Central neurogenic hyperventilation	Ataxic (i.e., irregular), apneas
Eyes	Doll's eyes and cold water calorics intact	Doll's eyes and cold water calorics impaired	Doll's eyes and cold water calorics impaired	Doll's eyes and cold water calorics impaired
Motor function	Gegenhalten ipsilaterally (early), decorticate (late)	Decorticate, decerebrate	No response except triple flexion	No response except triple flexion
Survivability	Often reversible	Rarely reversible, only 3% of trauma patents recover after having bilaterally fixed pupils (12)	Unlikely to survive	Terminal

Adapted from Plum F, Posner JB. *Diagnosis of Stupor and Coma*. Philadelphia, PA: FA Davis & Co; 1966.

Ischemia at the cerebral level produces vagal activation associated with a decreased heart rate, decreased cardiac output (CO), and decreased blood pressure. Although underappreciated, the first signs of incipient central herniation may simply be bradycardia in a severely brain-injured patient. Ischemia at the pons level produces the mixed vagal and sympathetic stimulation known as the Cushing response characterized by bradycardia and hypertension associated with irregular breathing. Further progression of the coning process to involve ischemia of the medulla oblongata is associated with a sympathetic stimulation termed the autonomic storm; Table 119.1 details the progression of central herniation. During this period, dramatic increases in catecholamines are reported with significant tachycardia and elevations in blood pressure. This represents the severely brain-injured patient's attempt to maintain cerebral perfusion pressure (CPP) gradients in the face of elevated increased intracranial pressure (ICP) and evolving herniation. During this period, there is ischemic destruction of the hypothalamic pituitary axis resulting in thermoregulatory impairment and purported endocrine dysfunction. Further progression of ischemia results in spinal cord destruction with herniation and sympathetic deactivation characterized by bradycardia, vasodilatation, and a low CO state. Somatic death after clinical brain death will inevitably occur in the absence of aggressive support. In an era when brain death was not accepted, prolonged survivorship, with a mean duration of 23 days, was noted in a study that aggressively maintained brain-dead patients (10). Autopsy studies of patients that were declared brain dead revealed histopathologic evidence of necrosis and liquefaction (11).

The catecholamine surge or autonomic storm produces multiple ECG and hemodynamic abnormalities along with biochemical and histologic changes in the cardiac system. In a series of sentinel observations and experiments, Novitzky (13–18) initially defined the cardiovascular pathophysiology associated with brain death. Catecholamines induce a sudden increase in cytosolic calcium, which jeopardizes ATP production and activates lipases, proteases, and endonucleases. Xanthine oxidase activation reportedly produces free radicals, further impairing organ function. Histopathologic changes reported in experimental animals reveal various degrees of focal myocyte necrosis located predominantly in the subendocardial area consisting of contraction bands and myocytolysis with mononuclear cell infiltrates precipitating edema proximate to the necrotic areas. Contraction bands were observed in the smooth muscle of coronary arteries, and electron microscopy revealed a hypercontractile state of the sarcomere visualizing mitochondrial deposition of electron-dense material and secondary lysosome containing injured mitochondrial. The loss of ATP production jeopardizes myocardial energy stores and mediates the transition from the aerobic to anaerobic metabolism compromising myocardial function.

Animal data and observations from human series have defined multiple abnormalities related to the catecholamine surge and brain death including impaired coronary endothelial dysfunction (19), selective expression of inflammatory molecules (20), downregulation of myocardial contractility (21), abnormalities in loading conditions and impaired coronary perfusion (22), abnormalities of left ventricular myocardial gene expression (23), and changes in myocardial beta-adrenergic receptor function and high-energy phosphates along with beta-adrenergic receptor deregulation (24,25). From animal models, it appears that a sudden rise in ICP is more provocative of the hyperdynamic–hemodynamic response, with significantly higher catecholamine levels, and is associated with greater histopathologic damage. A more gradual increase in ICP resulting in brain death is associated with a milder hyperdynamic response, less catecholamine release, and milder ischemic changes in the myocardium (26). Clinically, this has been correlated with the development of cardiac allograft vasculopathy in the recipient. The coronary artery vasoconstriction, subendocardial ischemia, and focal myocardial necrosis associated with the autonomic storm have been reported to be associated with a high incidence of intimal thickening of the transplanted heart coronary arteries, myocardial infarction, and the need for subsequent revascularization surgery (27).

The hemodynamic abnormalities and their impact are illustrated in a study comparing postbrain death cardiac function in a group of potential organ donors whose autonomic storm was attenuated with donors whose autonomic system storm was untreated. Using a definition of autonomic storm characterized by a systolic blood pressure ≥200 mmHg and tachycardia with heart rates >140 beats per minute, the authors treated this hemodynamic response in the study group, which was observed in 63% of donors for a mean duration of 1.2 hours, with beta-blockers. Treatment resulted in a significantly higher postbrain death left ventricular ejection fraction (LVEF) (63.9% vs. 49.0%), a higher rate of cardiac transplantation (91.7% vs. 41.2%), and better heart recipient survival at 2 months (100% vs. 43%). The investigators concluded that treatment of the autonomic storm enabled better cardiac function postbrain death, higher rates of cardiac transplantation, and better recipient outcomes (28). Recommendations regarding the treatment of the autonomic surge should be viewed with caution, as this physiologic compensatory mechanism represents the patient's attempt to maintain cerebral perfusion in the face of herniation. Abolition of this response constitutes active intervention and donor management in patients who have not been declared brain dead which raises significant ethical concerns.

Globally, the intense systemic vasoconstriction of the autonomic storm compromises blood flow to various organs. Subsequently, with herniation/brain death and associated denervation with vasodilatation, there is reperfusion which forms the basis of the global IR injury, thought to contribute significantly to organ dysfunction in the donor, and facilitate the development of an immunologic continuum between the donor and recipient. In addition to the IR injury that occurs with the brain death process, IR may occur antecedent to the brain death event during resuscitation from the initial trauma, or may follow brain death during the periods of cold storage and transplantation. Ischemia precipitates the loss of aerobic oxidative metabolism, associated cellular energy loss along with changed ion gradients which promote calcium influx. With reperfusion of oxygen-rich blood, there is generation of oxygen radicals, lipid peroxidation, and further membrane permeability to calcium. IR activates the vascular endothelium and donor leukocytes with resultant cytokine expression. This precipitates local inflammation, which is thought to contribute to graft immunogenicity by producing major histocompatibility antigens and adhesion molecules.

In concert with the above, there is substantial animal and some human data to support that hypothalamic pituitary destruction produces an endocrinopathy of brain death which is additive to the above. Dominated by the thyroid and adrenal deficiencies, it is proposed that the absence of these key hormones contributes to cellular dysfunction, metabolic abnormalities, and hemodynamic deterioration. Deficiency of thyroid hormone is proposed to impair mitochondrial function and consequently diminishes energy substrate with the resultant transition from aerobic to anaerobic metabolism. Proponents of HRT propose that diminished cardiac contractility consequent to low thyroid hormone levels can be reversed with exogenous hormone supplementation. However, significant disparities exist related to hypothalamic–pituitary axis dysfunction when comparing animal and human studies. An abundance of animal data suggests that low-circulating thyroid hormone levels are responsible for abnormal energy sources, impaired cardiac function, and hemodynamic instability (15,16,29). Animal studies and some human reports suggest that there is a dramatic reversal of the anaerobic metabolism, improvement in cardiovascular stability, and normalization of laboratory parameters and EKG changes, as well as improved organ suitability for transplantation when the exogenous hormonal therapy is employed (15,16).

Nonetheless, several studies have failed to define the presence of endocrine dysfunction (30–32), show improvement with the addition of exogenous hormones (33,34), or correlate hemodynamic instability with hormone levels (31,32). Consequently, the use of HRT remains controversial; this is further discussed under cardiovascular management.

The impact of brain death upon graft function and transplanted organs was first recognized in the early 1980s. Cooper et al. (29) observed that hearts procured from healthy anesthetized baboons and stored for 48 hours, when subsequently transplanted functioned immediately with no evidence of cardiac dysfunction. However, hearts procured from brain-dead donors and stored in a similar fashion required several hours to achieve adequate function. These investigators recognized that the only difference between the two groups was brain death, and determined that the brain death process was a risk factor for poor outcomes after transplantation. These observations began to establish that the brain death process was not static, and that the graft not biologically inert. Tilney et al. (35,36) proposed the existence of an immunologic continuum between donors and recipients as a mechanism to understand the influence of brain death on recipient organ function. Utilizing this model, they hypothesize that IR events associated with brain death and pre/postbrain death events precipitate immunologic and nonimmunologic injuries that impact upon short- and long-term graft function. A major component of the immunologic continuum is the IR injury, proposed to initiate a significant inflammatory response, which triggers and amplifies the acute postimmunologic activity, impacting multiple organs and contributing to their dysfunction in the short and long terms.

It has been noted that increased plasma IL-6 levels in donors is associated with lower recipient hospital-free survival after cadaveric organ transplantation (37). Similarly, elevated plasma IL-6 levels in donors were associated with greater degrees of preload responsiveness that correlated with fewer organs transplanted (38). In cardiac donors, serum and myocardial levels of tumor necrosis factor-alpha (TNF-α) and IL-6 were elevated in all, but were more markedly elevated in the dysfunctional unused donor hearts (39). An intense inflammatory environment defined by elevated levels of IL-1, IL-6, TNF-α, C-reactive protein (CRP), and procalcitonin (PCT) has been reported in potential heart and lung donors. In this series, elevated PCT levels were correlated with worse cardiac function and, potentially, thought to attenuate any improvement in cardiac function gained by donor management (40). Similar elevations of inflammatory markers have been reported in liver transplantation. In a comparison study of hepatic tissue from brain-dead and living donors, investigators reported significant elevations in inflammatory cytokines in brain-dead, as compared to living, donors. Cellular infiltrates were appreciably increased in parallel to the cytokine levels; this correlated with elevated liver enzymes, bilirubin levels, and increased rates of rejection and primary graft nonfunction (41). Attenuation of the increased inflammatory response with methylprednisolone was shown to significantly decrease soluble interleukins and the inflammatory response, which significantly ameliorated IR injury in the posttransplant course, and was accompanied by a decreased incidence of acute rejection (42). In summary, there is appreciable evidence that brain death and the associated inflammatory response have a substantial impact upon the transplanted organs. Future strategies will likely seek to preserve not simply organs, but to attenuate the donor inflammatory response.

BRAIN DEATH DECLARATION

After the 1959 description of "Le coma depasse" by Mollarat and Goulon, the description and understanding of coma and death were forever changed (43). These authors presented 23 cases from their Paris hospital in which they described irreversible or "irretrievable coma." This coma was associated with a lack of cognitive and vegetative functions, going beyond any coma previously described. This case series formed the basis of what is contemporarily recognized as brain death. The investigators noted the necessity of considering the circumstances of the injury, the role of the neurologic examination, the results of electroencephalography (EEG), and the consequence of brain death on other organs. They found that the majority of injuries to the brain were confined to trauma, SAH, meningitis, cerebral venous thrombosis, massive stroke, and brain death after craniotomy for posterior fossa tumor. The investigators detailed problems including deterioration of pulmonary function, polyuria, hyperglycemia, and tachycardia. It is intriguing that this paper, even though published in a relatively well-known European journal, took more than 15 years before it became known in the United States and Great Britain.

Interestingly, Mollart and Goulan's paper was not the first description of brain death (43). Lofstedt and von Reis (44) described six mechanically ventilated patients with absent reflexes, apnea, hypotension, hypothermia, and polyuria associated with absent angiographic cerebral blood flow; death was declared when cardiac arrest occurred, between 2 and 26 days after the clinical examination. In 1963, Schwab and associates (45) reported EEG as an adjunct for determining death when cardiac activity was present. These authors proposed the following criteria to determine death: (1) absence of spontaneous respiration for 30 minutes; (2) no tendon reflexes of any type; (3) no pupillary reflexes; (4) absence of the occulocardiac reflex; and (5) 30 minutes of an isoelectric EEG.

This corpus of research, and the recommendations contained therein, generated substantial controversy in the organ transplant community, as some were uncomfortable procuring organs for transplantation from donors that were pronounced dead using brain death criteria. Nonetheless, in 1968, Harvard Anesthesiologist Henry Beecher chaired a committee at Harvard Medical School which attempted to define irreversible coma as new criteria for death. The committee defined death as the irreversible loss of all brain functions and proposed the criteria necessary to make that determination (46). The Harvard criteria included nonreceptivity and unresponsiveness, no movements or breathing, no reflexes, and a flat EEG. The committee suggested that the tests be repeated at 24 hours and, in the absence of hypothermia and central nervous system depressants and with no change in examination, the patient would fulfill criteria for the diagnosis of brain death.

Subsequently, concern regarding the relevance of EEG unfolded and, the Conference of the Royal Colleges and Faculties of the United Kingdom published the *Diagnosis of Brain Death* first in 1976 and again in 1995, altering the definition from brain death to brain stem death (47). They determined that if the brain stem was dead, the brain was dead, and if the brain was dead, the patient was dead. The conference required that the etiology of the condition that led to coma be established, and a search for reversible factors be undertaken. Examples of "reversible factors" included central nervous system depressant drugs, neuromuscular blocking agents, respiratory depressants, and metabolic or endocrine disturbances. A period of observation was recommended and the technique for apnea testing was described (47,48).

The Quality Standards Subcommittee of the American Academy of Neurology formally redefined brain death in 1993, utilizing an evidence-based approach. They defined criteria for evaluating brain death as the presence of coma and evidence for the cause of the coma, with the absence of the following confounding factors: hypothermia, intoxication, sedative drugs, neuromuscular blocking agents, severe electrolyte disturbances, severe acid–base abnormalities, endocrine crises. Fulfilling the preceding criteria, brainstem reflexes and motor responses needed to be absent, and a positive apnea test established the clinical diagnosis of brain death. An apnea test was finally established as a criterion and part of the examination to define brain death. The subcommittee recommended a repeat evaluation 6 hours after the initial evaluation, but recognized that the time was arbitrary and suggested that confirmatory studies should only be required when specific components of clinical testing could not be reliably evaluated (49). With the 2010 update, the subcommittee recognizes there is insufficient evidence for determination of the minimally acceptable time for an observation period (50).

The 1977 NIH-sponsored study (51) is the only prospective attempt to develop comprehensive guidelines for determination of brain death based on neurologic criteria. Enrollment required demonstration of cerebral unresponsiveness and apnea, and at least one isoelectric EEG. This group recommended examinations at least 6 hours after the onset of coma and apnea. The examination required demonstration of cerebral unresponsiveness, dilated pupils, absent brain stem reflexes, apnea, and an isoelectric EEG. The apnea examination, as defined in this study, only required that the patient not make any effort to breath over the ventilator. In the United States today, most institutional policies are modeled after the Quality Standards Subcommittee of the American Academy of Neurology (50).

Examination to Determine Brain Death

When the diagnosis of brain death is considered in the appropriate clinical context, a very careful physical examination must be performed. Brain death testing requires first, definitive evidence of an acute catastrophic event that involves both cerebral hemispheres or the brain stem in the appropriate clinical context so that irreversibility is assured; second, complicating medical conditions that could potentially compromise the clinical assessment must be ruled out. These include electrolyte, acid–base, and endocrine disturbances. There should be no evidence of drug intoxication, neuromuscular blocking agent use, poisoning, or any other agent that might compromise the clinical examination. Additionally, hypothermia needs to be corrected; ideally, the patient should have a core temperature between 35° and 38°C. Frequently, the computerized tomographic (CT) scan of the head will provide evidence for the magnitude of the brain injury. These injuries may include massive intraparenchymal hemorrhage or SAH, and/or epidural or subdural hemorrhage with mass effect. The CT scan may also appear slightly less dramatic after a cardiac arrest. Findings may be limited to the loss of sulci and the gray matter–white mater differentiation, effacement of the basilar cisterns, all of which reflect cerebral edema.

The patient must exhibit lack of consciousness. Determining unresponsiveness usually implies the administration of some painful stimuli. While there are multiple approaches—sternal rubbing, rubbing knuckles on ribs, twisting nipples, and pin prick—we consider these to be somewhat abusive. Perhaps more appropriate, although not accepted as the standard, is to utilize an instrument such as a pen, pencil, or the tip of a Kelly clamp to apply pressure at the lunula (junction of the cuticle and skin of the digit). This pressure will consistently elicit a response in patients with an intact nervous system and it is not construed as potentially "violent" as pin prick or nipple twisting. Furthermore, it does not leave bruising that nipple twisting does and will not cause skin abrasions in the fragile skin of the elderly.

When painful stimulation is applied, there should be no responses such as eye opening or withdrawal and grimacing, although there may be an occasional "spinal" reflex with this stimulus; this spinal reflex is neither reproducible nor purposeful. Spinal movements have been described by Wijdicks (52) as brief, slow movements in upper limbs, flexion of the finger, and arm lifting that is not a decerebrate or decorticate response; these movements are not persistent and usually not reproducible. The precise reflex pathway(s) is not understood; however, these are recognized as spinal reflexes. Moreover, triple flexion (flexion of foot, knee, and hip) should be carefully considered whether it is withdrawal, or just represents a spinal reflex. In the examination for brain death, there should be no uncertainty, so triple flexion can lead to diagnostic uncertainty.

Each patient needs to be examined as prescribed by institutional and state standards which vary. Please be aware of your local standards. We give an accurate general description, but make no attempt to include local standards.

Brain Stem Reflexes

Pupillary Response

The pupillary response to light should be absent in both eyes. The pupils in brain-dead patients are most often dilated, midposition, usually 4 to 6 mm. It is important to ensure that there is no pre-existing ocular abnormalities and that topical ocular agents have not been instilled. Wijdicks (52) suggests that neuromuscular blocking agents may cause a nonreactive light reflex, although in our experience this is quite rare. The cranial nerves (CrNs) evaluated in the pupil light response are CrN II and III.

Ocular Testing

In the presence of brain death, there should be no ocular movements either to brisk movement of the head from side to side (absence of dolls' eyes) nor to instillation of cold water into the auditory canals. The nerves stimulated by these maneuvers include CrN VIII (efferent) with CrN III and VI (afferents). Prior to stimulating the oculocephalic reflex, one must ensure that the cervical spine is intact and the test should not be performed when there is known or suspected cervical spine injury. With the head in neutral position, the head is briskly moved, first to the left and held there for approximately 30 seconds; if the CrNs are intact, the eyes will move from the direct frontal gaze, to the left and then back toward the previous midline focus. The same is true when head is moved to the right, if the nerves are intact, the eyes will move from the direct frontal gaze to the right, and then back to the previous midline frontal gaze. In the presence of brain death, the eyes will remain in the direction the head is moved.

Even though cold water calorics test the same nerves, they also need to be tested on both sides. Prior to the instillation of iced saline into the auditory canal, one must ensure that the tympanic membranes are intact and that there is no occlusion of the auditory canal. Approximately 50 mL of iced saline is instilled into the auditory cannel. The cold stimulus results in sedimentation of the endolymph and stimulation of hair cells in the vestibular apparatus; the response in a comatose patient with an intact neurologic system is a slow deviation of the eyes toward the cold stimulus. In the presence of brain death, the eyes stay fixed in midline position. Drugs such as aminoglycosides, tricyclic antidepressants, anticholinergic agents, any antiepileptic drug, and some chemotherapeutic agents may ablate or abolish this caloric response in the presence of an intact brain stem (52). Basilar fracture may abrogate the response unilaterally on the side of the fracture. Nurses appreciate placement of towels to capture the water which spills out. Cold water caloric testing is often performed immediately prior to apnea testing.

Corneal Reflexes

Corneal reflexes should be evaluated by carefully using a sterile cotton-tipped swab. Blinking requires an intact brain stem, but care must be taken so that the eyelashes are not stimulated. The CrNs involved are V (afferent) and VII (efferent). Blinking that occurs with stimulation of the cornea is not compatible with brain death. Severe facial and ocular trauma can compromise the interpretation of these findings.

Pharyngeal and Tracheal Reflexes

In the intact brainstem, pharyngeal and tracheal reflexes—cough, gag—may be stimulated by passing a catheter through the endotracheal tube into the trachea and suctioning for several seconds. The CrNs involved are IX and X; CrN IX is the afferent to the trachea and CrN X is the efferent from the brain stem back to the trachea. The presence of a cough reflex is not compatible with brain death; the gag response may be difficult to interpret and is unreliable in an intubated patient (52).

Apnea Study

The apnea study is usually the final portion of the clinical examination to determine brain death. In principle, the arterial partial pressure of CO_2 ($PaCO_2$) must rise to at least 60 or 20 mmHg greater than the patient's baseline. This relatively rapid rise in $PaCO_2$ results in a decrease in the cerebral spinal fluid pH, which is sensed by the medullary respiratory center. When the respiratory center is functional, respiratory efforts will result; in the presence of brain death, there will be no respiratory effort.

Initially, one ensures that the patient's core temperature is between 35° and 38°C, preferably normothermic. The patient is denitrogenated ("pre-oxygenated") and stabilized, ensuring correction of any hemodynamic or electrolyte abnormalities.

This is especially true when the technique used for the apnea study is the removal of the patient from the ventilator with no continuous positive airway pressure (CPAP). Denitrogenation usually requires 10 minutes of breathing an FiO_2 of 1.0. Prior to initiation of the procedure, an arterial blood gas (ABG) analysis must be obtained both to ensure adequate oxygenation and to define a baseline arterial CO_2 value. With the baseline arterial CO_2 value, one can calculate the apnea time required for the $PaCO_2$ to rise to 60 mmHg.

The technique is as follows: The measured $PaCO_2$ value from the ABG is subtracted from 60 mmHg (delta-CO_2). It is recognized that $PaCO_2$ will climb approximately 3 mmHg, in the first minute of apnea and thereafter, it will climb by approximately 2 mmHg/min. Therefore, dividing the delta-CO_2 by the lower value of 2 mmHg increase per minute will ensure an adequate apnea time, allowing the $PaCO_2$ to achieve the minimal value of 60 mmHg in the presence of brain death–associated apnea, or a 20 mmHg rise from baseline.

Once the time required to achieve the delta value is determined, there are three techniques that may be used for the apnea study. These include (1) simply removing the patient from mechanical ventilation, and placing a catheter through the ETT while insufflating O_2 at approximate 6 L/min. This will most often ensure adequate apneic oxygenation. (2) Set the mechanical ventilator to spontaneous mode with no backup apneic mode. With this approach, the patient can be maintained on a low level of CPAP to preserve oxygenation. The monitoring modalities of the mechanical ventilator can be used to visualize respiratory efforts if these were to occur. (3) The patient may be taken off mechanical ventilation, and connected to a Mapleson D circuit with a Wright spirometer placed in line. With fresh O_2 flow of 6 to 10 L/min, one can partially close the Mapleson D circuit pop-off valve, ensure that there is some CPAP, and then watch both the bag of the circuit and the Wright spirometer for respiratory efforts.

Whichever technique is used, the patient is kept off mechanical ventilation for the calculated time to achieve the delta CO_2 value; pulse oximetric saturation is followed to ensure that desaturation does not occur. Desaturations, hemodynamic instability, or significant rhythm disturbances necessitate immediate replacement of full mechanical ventilation. Ideally, an ABG should be drawn at the onset of instability and used for assessment. A $PaCO_2$ >60 mmHg is consistent with a failed apnea test. Failure to achieve a PCO_2 ≥60 mmHg, in the absence of any respiratory efforts, suggests inadequate time for CO_2 production to achieve threshold. In this case, the test may be reperformed after correcting metabolic/physiologic abnormalities or moving directly to a confirmatory study. At the end of the newly calculated time period, an ABG is obtained. If the $PaCO_2$ value is ≥60 mmHg, or has increased >20 mmHg above the patients known baseline value, and there have been no respiratory efforts, the result is compatible with brain death.

After the second ABG is drawn, the patient is reconnected to the mechanical ventilator and, if the $PaCO_2$ from the previous sample is ≥60 mmHg, the family is notified that the examination is consistent with brain death. With a "failed" apnea study, the patient is pronounced clinically brain dead.

Common complications of the apnea study are hypotension and cardiac dysrhythmias. If one is unable to adequately perform the apnea study because of these complications or because of hypoxia, confirmatory tests, such as a radionuclear cerebral blood flow study or a four-vessel angiogram, will be required. Taylor et al. (53), in a meta-analysis of CT angiography as a confirmatory study in the setting of clinical brain death, found that based upon the extant data, CTA had a sensitivity, after the clinical determination of brain death, of only 85%. They suggest that this study not be used as a confirmatory study as approximately 15% of patients clinically dead will not have this diagnosis confirmed; other studies—as above—are more appropriate. Finally, a single apnea examination will suffice (43) for the declaration of brain death; when a repeat clinical examination is performed, a repeat apnea study is not an absolute requirement, although it is imperative to ensure that institution and state regulations are followed.

EXCLUSIONS AND CONTRAINDICATIONS

Given the shortage of organs available for donation, exclusions and contraindications should be viewed as absolutely relative or relatively absolute (54). Consequently, all cases should be reviewed in conjunction with the OPO coordinator to determine suitability. Successful procurement has been undertaken in a broad array of cases that were previously deemed unsuitable including patients with sepsis and bacterial meningitis, provided appropriate anti-infective treatment is undertaken. However, organs should not be procured from potential donors when the etiology of the purported infection has not been determined. An evolving literature suggests that organ procurement from patients with known meningitis that has been appropriately treated has not resulted in significant transmission of the infectious agent nor organ compromise in the recipient (55). In a retrospective study performed over 10 years in 39 patients undergoing heart and lung transplantation, undertaken with organs from cadaveric donors with bacterial meningitis defined by either positive blood or cerebral spinal fluid cultures and associated clinical signs and symptoms, no contraindications could be defined because none of the recipients died of infection-related causes. Common organisms in the donor were reported to be *Neisseria meningitides,* 53.8%; *Streptococcus pneumonia,* 41%; and *Haemophilus influenza,* 5.2%. Importantly, adequate antibiotic therapy was initiated before organ retrieval and continued after transplantation (56). Similarly, Satoi (57) reported that liver transplantation from donors with bacterial meningitis was safe, provided the donor and recipient received adequate antimicrobial therapy. In this study of 34 recipients, there were no infectious complications caused by the meningeal pathogens. Although recommendations are difficult to establish, treatment of the donor for 24 to 48 hours and a minimum 7 to 10 days for the recipient appears to be adequate.

Frequently, potential organ donors in the ICU are bacteremic; similar to the above literature for donors with meningitis, procurement of organs from bacteremic patients has been successfully undertaken and the presence of bacteremia should not preclude donor evaluation. In a study that reviewed heart transplantation from donors that expired from community-acquired infections with severe septic shock, meningitis, and/or pneumonia, no evidence of donor-associated infection and sepsis or rejection was observed in the recipient (58). In a report of transplantation from bacteremic donors with gram-negative septic shock, all recipients were alive with good graft function 60 days following transplantation with no infectious complications. It is recommended that appropriate antibiotics be given for at least 48 hours prior to organ retrieval and that recipients receive 7 days of culture specific antibiotics posttransplantation (59).

Patients with human immunodeficiency virus (HIV) represent an absolute contraindication to donation. However, the occasional patient engaging in high-risk social behavior, but remaining HIV seronegative, may be considered for possible organ donation. In this circumstance, there should be an extensive review of the medical record, interviews with the family, and active communication with OPO. It is recommended, however, that information about the donor's high-risk behavior be conveyed to the transplant center, which ought to inform the potential recipient of the risks and benefits of donation from this individual.

Donor malignancy represents another area of concern that warrants careful evaluation when a donor is considered for procurement. Any active noncentral nervous system malignancy is viewed as an absolute contraindication to donation. A previous history of choriocarcinoma, lung cancer, melanoma, and patients with previous colon, breast, or kidney cancer are, similarly, precluded. Donors with a previous history of nonmelanoma skin cancers and a select group of patients with cancer defined *in situ* or with very low-grade levels of malignancy may be considered as can be patients with a history of previous curative therapy; these cases should be discussed on an individual basis with the OPO and the transplant center. Central nervous system malignancies are not uncommon in the potential organ donor population. Given their rare metastasis and low incidence of development in the recipient, procurement is frequently undertaken. Potential donors with a low-grade tumor, absent craniotomy, and no ventricular shunts are better candidates than those donors with previously defined high-grade malignancy, craniotomy, and shunt placement.

CONSENT

Approaching and obtaining consent from the potential donor's family is an absolute requirement for organ donation. In the case of previously defined, first-person consent, in which an individual firmly establishes their desire to donate *via* a driver's license or donor card, it is imperative that the first-person consent be honored and recognized as the basis for consent. In 1998, the CMS established several parameters governing the organ donation process through the Federal Conditions of Participation. A change in the Conditions of Participation required timely notification of the OPO when death is imminent to ensure that families were provided the opportunity to discuss the option of organ and tissue donation. Similarly, the Conditions of Participation mandated that individuals specially trained in requesting, termed "designated requestors" be responsible for making the request, and required that all individuals discussing organ donation with families receive the appropriate training.* The intent of this mandate was to ensure that individuals approaching families and discussing organ donation were trained and sensitive to the family situation. Initially, this was interpreted by some to imply that physicians would be excluded from the request process and only OPO-designated requestors could approach the family. Subsequent discussion and policy recommendations adopted by the American Medical Association suggested that the designated requestor contacts the attending physician before organ donation requests and includes the attending physician in the discussion with the family. It is important to appreciate that OPO coordinators, physicians, and nurses may be defined as designated requestors, provided they undertake the appropriate training (60).

Family characteristics and the approach to the consent process have been shown to significantly impact upon the decision to donate. Nondonor families tend to be less satisfied with the quality of care, have a lesser degree of understanding of brain death, and remain under the impression that brain-dead patients could survive. These families felt that there was insufficient time and privacy during the request process and that the requestor was not sensitive to their needs. Alternatively, consenting families had a much clearer understanding of brain death and were more satisfied with the overall consent process and their decision-making (61). Siminoff (62) evaluated the roles of prerequest factors and decision process variables in the consent process in a large study of 11,555 deaths; of 741 potential donors and a family request rate of 80%, the final consent rate was 48%. Decisions were made early, with 55% of families making their decision during the initial request. Of those families with an initial favorable view of consent (58%), 81% went on to complete the consent with consent not obtained in 19%. In families who initially had an unfavorable view of the donation process (25%), consent was eventually obtained in 9% and no consent was sustained in the remaining 91%. In the 17% of families that were undecided during the initial donation request, 47% went on to consent and consent was not obtained in 53%. The initial response predicted a final donation decision in 70% of families. Prerequest factors that were associated with successful consent included patient characteristics of young, white males dying from trauma and family beliefs in donation, prior knowledge of organ donation, the presence of a donor card, explicit discussions, and a belief that the patient would have wished to donate and that the information provided was adequate and the health care provider was comfortable with questions. There was no association noted between family education and income levels, hospital environmental factors, health care practitioner–associated demographics or the health care practitioner's attitude toward donation. Decision process variables that correlated with donation were the correct initial assessment by the health care provider, instances when the family raised the donation issue, conversations and time spent with the OPO coordinator, and clear, unambiguous discussions related to cost, funeral homes, and choices. Decision process variables that had a negative correlation with donation included perceptions that the health care provider was not caring, surprise by the family when the request was made, or feeling harassed and pressured to make a decision. No correlation was found with the overall satisfaction of care, the timing of the request, or the belief that the patient was alive after the declaration of brain death. Hazard ratios for factors that directly related to donation included prerequest characteristics (7.68), optimal request pattern with the health care provider being a nonphysician and the OPO coordinator (2.96), OPO-related factors (3.08), and the topics discussed (5.22).

The request for organ donation has undergone an evolutionary process from random or inconsistent requesting to the

*(COP) (42CFR Part 482 {HCFA-3005-F} RIN:0938-A195).

use of designated requestors to the use of an effective requestor to the currently recommended process of effective requesting. Key elements of the requesting process recommended by the Institute of Medicine (IOM) include a focus on the family and the continuation of compassionate care with an acknowledgement of the uniqueness of each family and avoiding scripted statements. A determination of the most appropriate requestor and the timing of the request should be individualized and done on a case-by-case basis. Families of patients with protracted ICU stays frequently develop close associations with specific physicians or nurses, and may be willing to accept discussions related to impending death and donation at times earlier in the course than families with an acute crisis. The IOM panel recommended that donation be discussed as an opportunity, utilizing language that emphasizes the benefit to the transplant recipient and the potential of healing for the donor family. Importantly, the panel recommended that excellent EOL care be continued for the family, independent of the donation decision (63).

Although there is some variability, it has generally been accepted that decoupling or separating the request for donation from the declaration of brain death notification be used as the model for requests (64,65). In this model, the notification of brain death is both temporally and geographically segregated from the organ donation request. This provides the opportunity for the family to process the notification of brain death before the request is made for consent, although it has been suggested that consent may occur after the family has accepted that further care is futile (66). In conjunction with the decoupling process, factors that have been associated with a successful consent rate include making the request in a private setting, and ensuring the engagement of the OPO Transplant Coordinator. When all three elements are present, the consent rate was reported to be 2.5 times greater than when none of the elements were present (64). The Council on Scientific Affairs for the American Medical Association recommended that the process focuses upon supporting the family of all potential donors, be consistent with quality EOL principles, decouple discussions of brain death from the organ donation requests, ensure that the opportunity to donate is presented to all families, and do so in a private setting. Ensuring that thc OPO Transplant Coordinator is involved and assists with coordinating the efforts in the ICU was strongly recommended; for those wishing to participate in the request process, special training should be undertaken, and certification as a designated requestor obtained.

MEDICAL MANAGEMENT

Hemodynamic and cardiovascular management form the cornerstone of potential organ donor management (ODM). A standardized and structured approach to hemodynamic management ensures that the donor somatically survives for procurement and maintains the remainder of potential organs in the best possible condition. Similar to the care of any critical patient, a collaborative approach utilizing the skills of physicians, nursing, respiratory therapists, and the OPO coordinator is pivotal for optimum management. Standardization of donor management from the referral process through consent, followed by management and recovery has been shown to significantly increase the number of organs recovered and organs transplanted. A 10.3% increase in organs recovered per 100 donors and a 3.3% increase in total organs transplanted per 100 donors was reported by Rosendale in a study that emphasized standardization of general medical management, eliminating variability in laboratory and diagnostic studies, along with standardization of respiratory therapy, and IV fluids and medications (67). The Surgical Trauma Group at the University of Southern California has been instrumental in pioneering the standardized approach to ODM. The development of an aggressive ODM program was reported to significantly increase the number or organs available for transplantation. Employing a critical care team that accepted potential organ donors for management utilizing pulmonary artery catheters (PAC), fluid resuscitation and use of vasopressors, prevention and treatment of complications associated with brain death, and liberal use of thyroid hormone in unstable donors, resulted in a 57% increase in total referrals, a 19% increase in potential donors, an 82% increase in the number of actual donors and an 87% decrease in the number of donors lost to hemodynamic instability. Overall, the implementation of this aggressive donor management team resulted in a 71% increase in the number of organs recovered (68). In a follow-up study by the same group utilizing an aggressive approach to ODM, the authors evaluated the impact of the complications of brain death upon organ retrieval. They hypothesized that brain death–related complications would have no significant impact on the number of organs donated, provided there was an aggressive ODM protocol in place. With complications defined as the requirement for vasoactive support which occurred in 97.1%, coagulopathy in 55.1%, thrombocytopenia in 53.6%, diabetes insipidus in 46.4%, cardiac ischemia in 30.4%, lactic acidosis in 24%, renal failure in 20.3%, and adult respiratory distress syndrome noted in 13%, there was no appreciable impact of the complications on the average number of organs procured. Additional benefits included a dramatic diminution in the number of donors lost to cardiovascular collapse, and improvement in conversion rates (69). In a comparison with other Level I trauma centers that did not utilize an aggressive donor management protocol, dramatic benefits were similarly reported which included a significant decrease in the incidence of cardiovascular collapse, and the number of organs procured per potential donor (69).

Although the traditional management of the potential organ donor has been taken by the OPO transplant coordinator, there has been an evolution toward a collaborative approach between the Intensivist/critical care community and the OPO, as reflected in the above-mentioned studies. Intensivist-led management of potential organ donors has been reported to increase the organs recovered for transplantation. In a study that evaluated the implementation of an Intensivist-led donor management program, the overall number of organs recovered for transplantation increased significantly (44% vs. 31%), which was largely reflective of an increase in the number of lungs procured and transplanted (24% vs. 11%). No appreciable change occurred in the number of hearts and livers recovered for transplantation. This study is reflective of the enormous impact that a collaborative and partnered approach between Intensivists and OPO coordinators can have upon donor management (70).

Although no clear current consensus exists, the traditional approach to ODM was to minimize the time between brain death and procurement because of the perception that prolonged management was detrimental to the donor organs and bed utilization in busy ICUs necessitated admission for salvageable patients. However, this concept has recently been challenged as evolving literature reports that a longer period of donor management may be beneficial (71). In a retrospective study with a mean time from brain death to procurement of 35 hours, it was reported that there was no decrease in the procurement to consented ratio with increasing time after brain death. When individual organs were analyzed separately, heart and pancreas procurement improved with an increased management period after brain death and some organs were successfully procured greater than 60 hours after brain death (72). Similarly, in a study of 100 consecutive organ donors whose mean donor management time was 23 hours, it was reported that donors managed in excess of 20 hours resulted in significantly more heart and lung procurements, more organs procured per donor (4.2 vs. 3.2) and more organs transplanted per donor (3.7 vs. 2.6). Interestingly, there was no significant difference noted in the obtainment of donor management goals (73).

Specific donor management goals during the donor management period have evolved as a standard. Attainment of these management goals has resulted in a significant increase in the number of organs procured and transplanted per donor. In an initial report by Hagan, consensus was developed for six specific donor management goals among six OPO organizations. The following management goals were derived: mean arterial pressure greater than 60 mmHg, CVP less than 10 mmHg (or serum osmolarity 285 to 295 mOsm/kg), sodium less than 155 mMol/L, pH 7.25 to 7.5, pressors (1 or none—1 pressor plus vasopressin for diabetes insipidus was deemed appropriate), and PaO_2 greater than 300 mmHg while on 100% oxygen. These donor management goals were considered a bundle with compliance defined as achieving a minimum of five goals. The number of organs transplanted per donor was 4.87 in those meeting goals and 3.19 in those donors failing to meet the bundle goals for standard criteria donors. No significant change was noted for extended criteria donors (74). In a similar consensus-driven study, eight common goals were defined: mean airway pressure, CVP, pH, PaO_2, sodium, glucose, vasopressor use, and urine output. Throughout the study period, there was a dramatic increase in the compliance with donor management goals, which was associated with a significant improvement in organs transplanted per donor. The authors reported that the success of transplantation was predominantly associated with limitations in vasopressor use and achieving adequate PaO_2. Thoracic organs were most sensitive to the donor management goals as there was a dramatic increase in lung transplantation with higher levels of PaO_2. Interestingly, mean arterial pressure, CVP, pH, sodium, and urine output had little effect on the transplantation rate. The authors concluded that goals and standardization of endpoints of donor management are associated with increased rates of transplantation. However, it was evident that not all standard goals are necessary with the most significant parameters being the low use of vasopressors and ensuring adequate oxygenation, which should form the focus of donor management (75). Similarly, in a study that evaluated 10 donor management goals and defined success as the achievement of eight goals, the authors used binary logistic regression to determine the independent predictors of more than four organs transplanted per donor. The authors reported that donors meeting donor management goals had more organs transplanted per donor (4.4 vs. 3.3). Independent predictors of transplanting more than four organs were age, serum creatinine, thyroid hormone, and meeting donor management goals. Among the individual donor management goals, odds ratios (ORs) were higher for CVP 4 to 10 mmHg (OR = 1.9), EF greater than 50% (OR = 4.0), PaO_2/FiO_2 greater than 300 (OR = 4.6), and a serum sodium 135 to 168 mEq/L (OR = 3.4) (75,76). The impact of a structured and standardized approach to ODM has similarly been reported to dramatically increase the retrieval rate of lungs and hearts for transplantation. In a study where potential lung donors were aggressively managed through protocol-guided optimization of ventilatory and hemodynamic strategies that consisted of measurements of extravascular lung water, bronchoscopy, and invasive monitoring, a dramatic increase in the rate of lung procurement was reported (40% vs. 27%) (77). Similarly, an aggressive and structured approach to the management of potential heart donors reported a significant increase in the numbers of hearts procured with a standardized approach using invasive monitoring and critical care management techniques (78). It appears that over the past decade, there has been an overall increase in available donors and organs, as well as a moderate increase in the mean number of organs per TBI donor. Additionally, the increased use of hormone replacement therapy (HRT) appears to be key to the successful conversion of marginal donors and enhanced recovery from certain subsets leading to decreased transplant wait times (79). For example, in the decade studied by Callahan and colleagues (79) using the Organ Procurement and Transplant Network's (OPTN) organ donor and thoracic recipient dataset (from July 1, 2001 to June 30, 2012), the most common causes of donor death were cerebrovascular disease (31,804 cases, 42.9%) and TBI (28,142 cases, 37.9%). A slow but significant increase in the raw number of donors per year, from 5,857 in 2002 to 6,945 in 2012 ($p < 0.001$) was noted, as was an increase in the raw number of total organs procured, from 20,558 to 24,308 ($p < 0.001$). These increases coincide with the increased use of HRT in donor management, from 25.1% to 72.3% ($p < 0.001$); high-yield donors showed a similar increase in the use of HRT, from 33% in 2002 to 76.6% in 2012 ($p < 0.001$) (79).

Finally, recent data (80) suggest that elevated glucose is common in patients who donate after determination of neurologic death. Glucose levels above 180 mg/dL are associated with lower organ transplantation rates and worse graft outcomes. It is recommended that serum glucose levels be targeted to a glucose of 180 mg/dL or less; in our practice, we aim for 150 to 180 mg/dL.

Cardiovascular and Fluid Goals

An algorithmic approach to the cardiovascular and hemodynamic management of the potential organ donor is suggested (Fig. 119.2). As depicted in the figure, age plays a major role in the initial cardiac evaluation. Traditionally, cardiac catheterization has been required for potential organ donors over 40 years of age. Given the significant myocardial stress associated with brain death, echocardiography should not be performed immediately after brain death declaration as this may provide misleading information related to cardiac function. Initial attempts at stabilization should include normalizing blood pressure, metabolic abnormalities, and electrolyte disturbances. Transthoracic echocardiography (TTE) should be

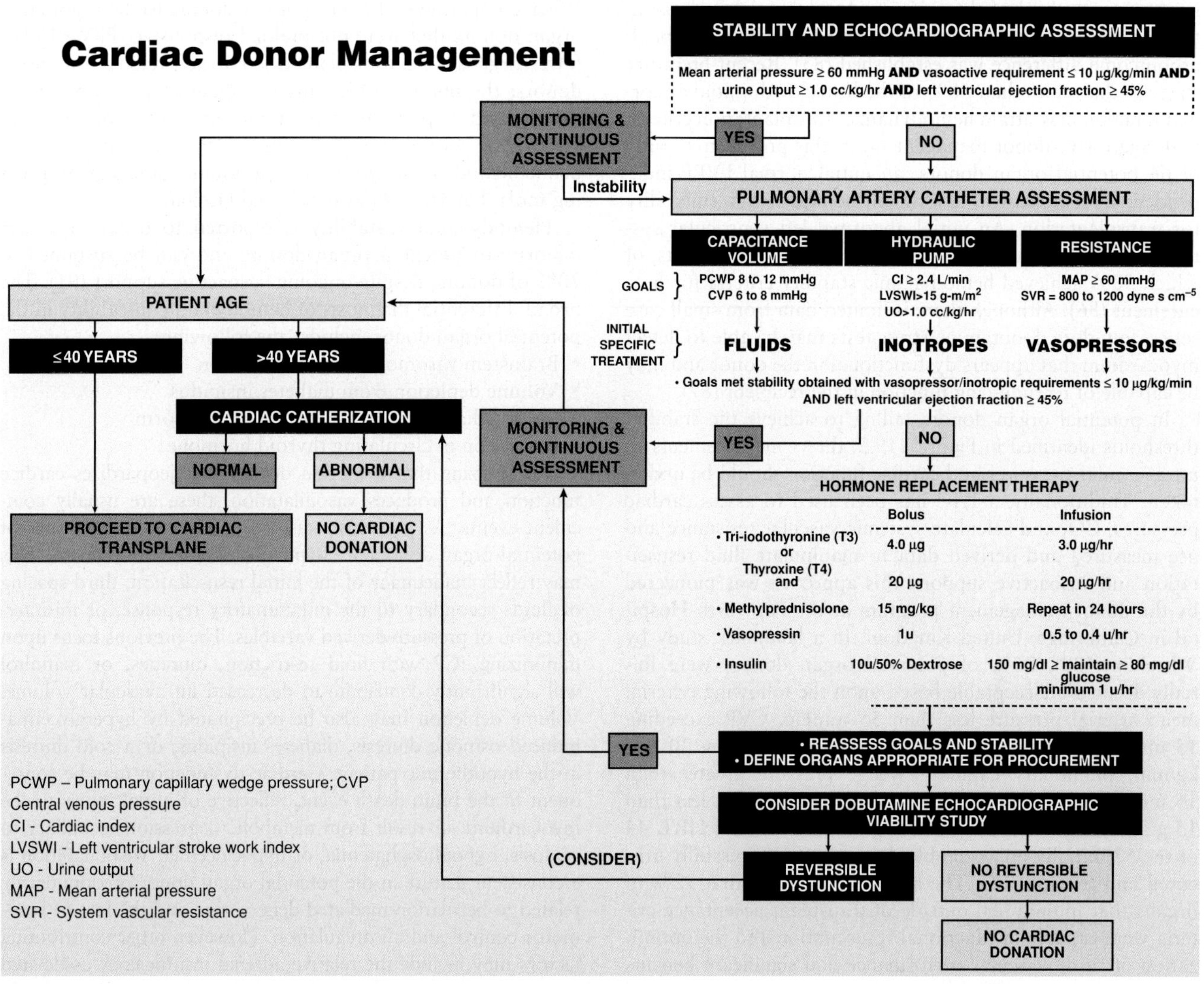

FIGURE 119.2 Algorithmic approach to the cardiovascular and hemodynamic management of the potential organ donor.

performed in all patients to evaluate structural abnormalities that may preclude cardiac donation and evaluate the LVEF. Since first reported in the evaluation of potential organ donors in 1988, TTE has proven invaluable for evaluation of cardiac function, particularly in circumstances where clinical events might have precluded cardiac utilization. In the original study, 29% of donor hearts that would have been previously excluded on clinical criteria were procured and successfully transplanted (81). Echocardiographic abnormalities are reported to be responsible for 26% of nonused hearts with an OR of 1.48 per 5% decrease in EF (82). Although instrumental in the evaluation of cardiac function in the potential organ donor, several issues warrant consideration regarding echocardiographic evaluation. These include the difficulty in securing the test, technical challenges with imaging in critically ill patients, and the accuracy and impact of the echocardiographic interpretation. Similarly, it is important to appreciate that LVEF is a load-dependent measure of contractility with variance noted when there are changes in preload and afterload (83). It is also important to recognize that temporal changes occur in left ventricular systolic function. In a study that evaluated sequential echocardiograms in potential organ donors, with EFs less than 50% or regional wall motion abnormalities on the initial cardiogram, 12 of 13 patients improved after donor management. Utilizing a strategy that employed high-dose corticosteroids and dopamine without the use of thyroid hormone, these 12 donor hearts were transplanted with a survival rate of 92% with an average follow-up of 16 months (84). In a series that evaluated clinical characteristics, echocardiographic and pathologic findings of myocardial dysfunction in potential donors, echocardiographic evidence of systolic dysfunction was appreciated in 42% of potential organ donors; this was not predicted by clinical findings, the EKG findings, or the type of neurologic injury. Histopathologically, there was a very limited correlation to the area of echocardiographic dysfunction in the histopathology of hearts that were not procured, suggesting, again, that brain death is associated with significant myocardial dysfunction and the potential for reversibility needs to be appreciated. Consequently, no heart should be rejected on the basis of a first initial abnormal echocardiogram. In instances where TTE evaluation is difficult, consideration should be given to the use of transesophageal echocardiography (TEE); limited literature comparing TTE with TEE suggests that the TTE assessment may be inadequate in almost one-third of the patients. A substantial increase in the number of abnormalities was detected with TEE, although no outcome difference was established (85). Recent literature suggests that more than 50% of the hearts with initial abnormal function may attain hemodynamic transplantation criteria with aggressive donor management. In this prospective study of 66 potential organ donors, an initial normal LVEF independently predicted end assessment hemodynamic suitability for transplantation. An initial abnormal left ventricular systolic function was identified in almost half of donor hearts, of which 58% achieved hemodynamic stability criteria for procurement (86). Although there is limited data from small case series, low-dose dobutamine stress tests may be able to detect myocardium that appears dysfunctional in the donor and may be capable of recrudescing function in the recipient (87).

In potential organ donors failing to achieve the stability thresholds identified in Figure 119.2, direct measurements of intravascular pressures and cardiac function should be undertaken. Traditionally, a PAC has been used to assess cardiac pressures, CO, and calculate systemic vascular resistance and use measured and derived data to manipulate fluid resuscitation and vasoactive support; this approach was pioneered by the donor management program at the Papworth Hospital in Cambridge, United Kingdom. In a landmark study by Wheeldon (88), 35% of potential organ donors were initially deemed unacceptable based upon the following criteria: mean arterial pressure less than 55 mmHg, CVP exceeding 15 mmHg, inotropic support requirement exceeding 20 mg/kg/min, pulmonary capillary wedge pressure greater than 15 mmHg and a left ventricular stroke work index less than 15 g. Utilizing invasive monitoring with a PAC and HRT, 44 of the 52 initially unacceptable donors were successfully procured and transplanted. The authors concluded that 92% of organs that initially fell outside of transplant acceptance criteria were capable of functional resuscitation and the optimization of cardiovascular performance had significant benefits for the viability of all organs. Given the current speculation regarding the use of PACs, it may be that the dramatic success seen in this and other studies reflect the time, effort, and vigilant commitment to the donor management process as much as the placement of a PAC. Recently, the commonly accepted practice of inferring volume status from pressure measurements has been questioned. In a systematic review of the literature assessing the accuracy of CVP to predict fluid responsiveness found an exceedingly poor correlation between CVP and blood volume. The inability of the CVP/change in CVP with fluid challenge to predict a hemodynamic response led to the conclusion that CVP should not be used to make decisions regarding fluid management (89). Consequently, other measurements have been proposed to evaluate intravascular volume and fluid responsiveness in critically ill patients, which are equally applicable to the management of the potential organ donor. Dynamic changes in the arterial waveform–derived variables have been shown to be an accurate predictor of fluid responsiveness in mechanically ventilated patients (90) and has been applied to the management of potential organ donors (38). In a study that utilized a pulse pressure variation (PPV) greater than 13% to define preload responsiveness, 48% of potential organ donors were characterized as preload responsive. IL-6 and TNF concentrations were greater in preload responsive donors, suggesting that there was inadequate volume resuscitation in the early phase donor management. When comparing preload responsive donors to those potential organ donors that were not preload responsive (PPV <13%), fewer organs were transplanted from the preload responsive donors; the number of organs transplanted per donor from the preload responsive versus unresponsive donors was 1.8 versus 3.7. As illustrated in Figure 119.2, it is important to define hemodynamic profiles for optimum management utilizing tools that are both available and familiar.

Hemodynamic instability is reported to occur in a vast majority of potential organ donors and can be sustained in 20% of donors, despite ongoing vasoactive support (91). The broad differential diagnosis of hemodynamic instability in the potential organ donor includes the following:

- Brainstem vasomotor center infarction
- Volume depletion from diabetes insipidus
- Myocardial injury from catecholamine storm
- Reduction in circulating thyroid hormone

Recognizing that the brain death event jeopardizes cardiac function and produces vasodilatation, these are usually coincident events. As previously discussed, a significant number of potential organ donors are hypovolemic after brain death. This may reflect inadequacy of the initial resuscitation, third spacing of fluids secondary to the inflammatory response, or misinterpretation of pressure-derived variables. The previous focus upon minimizing ICP with fluid restriction, diuretics, or mannitol will significantly contribute to decreased intravascular volume. Volume depletion may also be precipitated by hyperglycemia-induced osmotic diuresis, diabetes insipidus, or a cold diuresis in the hypothermic patient. Cardiac dysfunction may be consequent to the brain death event, reflective of initial injury to the myocardium, or result from metabolic depression secondary to acidosis, hypophosphatemia, or hypocalcemia. Vasodilatation is a consistent feature in the potential organ donor predominantly related to herniation-mediated denervation and the loss of vasomotor control and autoregulation. However, other contributing factors may include the relative adrenal insufficiency associated with trauma/critical illness, the endocrinopathy of brain death, or a superimposed/acquired sepsis. Ongoing hypotension further compounds the initial IR injury, which may result in cardiac arrest and loss of the potential organ donor. Consequently, an aggressive approach to defining the adequacy of intravascular volume, cardiac function, and the degree of vasodilatation is of paramount importance in managing the potential organ donor. Whenever possible, fluid resuscitation in the potential organ donor should be guided by objective measurements and defined endpoints. Traditionally, normal saline has been used as the initial fluid for volume resuscitation to achieve either the previously described central venous pressure endpoints or abolition of preload responsiveness determined by PPV. Inadequacy of initial volume resuscitation has been shown to precipitate a significant increase in inflammatory mediators with fewer organs procured and transplanted (38). Diabetes insipidus is common in potential organ donors and predisposes toward hypernatremia. After achieving intravascular volume repletion, a transition to more hypotonic solutions such as dextrose and water may be undertaken to ensure correction of the serum sodium. Serum sodium levels greater than 155 mMol/L have been shown to adversely affect liver transplantation with a higher incidence of graft loss and metabolic abnormalities. Totsuka (92) reported that a serum sodium above 155 was associated with a higher incidence of graft loss, compared to donors whose serum sodium was below 155 mMol/L. In patients who initially had a serum sodium exceeding

155 mMol/L and were effectively treated to achieve a preprocurement sodium less than 155 mMol/L, graft dysfunction was minimized. Therefore, cautious attention to correcting the serum sodium and appropriately transitioning from normal saline to a hypotonic solution is appropriate once intravascular volume has been replete and there is evidence of adequate perfusion. Similarly, it is important to recognize that the infusion of significant amounts of hypotonic solutions containing dextrose, which are frequently used to treat diabetes insipidus, may precipitate hyperglycemia, osmotic diuresis, and hyperglycemia-mediated immune dysfunction. Similar to other critical care scenarios, the use of colloid for resuscitation remains controversial. Initial reports suggested that the use of colloid may facilitate minimizing extravascular lung water, and result in an increased rate of lung procurement (93). In the context of marginal donors and potential hepatic dysfunction, Oliver et al. (94) conducted a case-control study of brain-dead donors (BDDs) at a single OPO to evaluate the clinical characteristics of BDDs undergoing percutaneous prerecovery liver biopsy (PLB), whether PLB delays organ recovery, the safety of PLB, the concordance between donor hospital and transplant center pathologists in the interpretation of PLB, and whether PLB decreases futile liver recovery and increases the utilization of livers. With each case (n = 23) matched to sequential (n = 48) and clinical (n = 69) controls, the investigators found that PLB cases had no difference in primary or secondary complications as compared to the two control groups; the interval from commencement of donor management to organ recovery was significantly longer in the cases (22.4 ± 8.5 hours) as compared to the controls (sequential 16.5 + 8.8, clinical 15.9 ± 7 hours) (p = 0.01 for both comparisons). While the proportions of livers transplanted in the study and clinical control groups were similar (60.9% vs. 59.4%), the proportion of livers for which recovery was ruled out was higher for cases as compared to the clinical controls (30.4% vs. 8.7%) and, as expected, the proportion of liver recoveries without transplantation was lower for the cases versus the controls (8.7% vs. 31.9%) (p = 0.009). The implication of this work is that PLB patients at risk for liver pathology is safe, and that its use minimizes futile recovery (94). The duration of "brain death time" before procurement and transplant does not seem to impact outcome in a major way (94,95).

Frequently, there are antagonistic and competing strategies related to fluid resuscitation in the potential organ donor. Excessive fluid resuscitation with the resultant increase in extravascular lung water has been reported to be the single largest reason for lung procurement failure. In a study of potential organ donors with a lung procurement rate of 17.1%, progressive pulmonary dysfunction occurred in 31% of donors who had a significant positive fluid balance of approximately 7,000 mL (96). Traditionally, there has been an emphasis upon overhydration to maximize renal function; this stems from a large body of literature originating during the renal transplantation surgery in the recipient, which has emphasized significant positive fluid balance, as evidenced in the following study that evaluated the impact of the timing of maximal crystalloid hydration on early graft function during renal transplantation. Early graft dysfunction was minimized when intraoperative CVP was maintained at 15 mmHg and 3 L of fluid was given with an average infusion rate of 48.3 mL/min during the 48 minutes of renal ischemia. Older donor management literature suggested that urine output greater than 100 mL/hr during the hour prior to explanation and a decrease in the creatinine, reflective of increased hydration, were associated with improved renal function in the recipient (97). Consequent to these and multiple other studies, there has been an emphasis upon maximal hydration for below-the-diaphragm organs, which contrasts with the more minimalist volume resuscitation approach believed to enhance lung procurement. Recently, several studies have sought to clarify the approach to an appropriate fluid balance that will ensure the optimum procurement of both lungs and kidneys. In a study that compared the relationship between HRT and CVP on increasing organs for transplantation, the authors reported that when HRT was infused for greater than 15 hours and a CVP was maintained at less than 10 mmHg, there was a dramatic increase in the number of hearts and lungs procured. When a final CVP was less than 10 mmHg, 44% more hearts, 95% more lungs, and 13% more kidneys were transplanted (98). A similar retrospective study sought to evaluate the impact of a restrictive fluid balance that focused upon increasing lung procurement and evaluating renal function after kidney transplantation. The authors reported that a negative or equal fluid balance with a CVP less than or equal to 6 mmHg had no effect on kidney recipient graft function or the development of delayed graft function. A positive fluid balance between the brain death event and organ procurement did not reduce the risk of graft survivorship of delayed graft function. The authors concluded that a restrictive fluid management approach, focused upon enhancing lung procurement with a CVP less than 6 mmHg avoided volume overload, minimized the effects of neurogenic pulmonary edema, and increased the rate of lung procurement without an adverse effect on either kidney graft survivorship or delayed graft function (99). In summary, fluid resuscitation should be guided by objective measurements and defined endpoints similar to that used in the management of other critically ill patients. Previous strategies that focused upon aggressive overhydration to enhance renal perfusion have been shown to jeopardize pulmonary function and preclude procurement. A moderate or restrictive fluid resuscitative strategy is appropriate for both lung procurement and maintenance of renal function similar to the management approach for other critically ill patients.

In patients failing to achieve stability and defined endpoints in Figure 119.2, vasopressors are frequently necessary to maintain perfusion pressures and are used in a majority of potential organ donors. Clear recommendations regarding the choice of vasopressors remain handicapped by an absence of controlled trials and perceived negative effects of catecholamines from studies that did not reliably measure the adequacy of intravascular volume. When employed, vasopressor and the endpoints of therapy should be clearly defined and vasopressor use titrated to specific physiologic abnormalities. Once intravascular volume resuscitation has been adequately undertaken, the choice of vasoactive support depends upon the predominant physiologic abnormalities in organ donors. In those with predominant myocardial dysfunction and inadequate flow, despite adequate volume resuscitation, dobutamine should be used for inotropic support. In potential organ donors whose hemodynamic instability is dominated by vasodilatation, vasopressors should be used to maintain mean arterial pressure and ensure adequacy of perfusion pressure gradients. Traditionally, alpha agents such as phenylephrine or norepinephrine were used to maintain vascular tone in the face of brain death–induced vasodilatation. However, recent recommendations have supported the use of vasopressin as a first-line agent to maintain vascular tone (100). In one of the few large randomized prospective controlled trials of HRT in potential organ donors, the transition from norepinephrine to vasopressin was associated with a significant increase in CO (3.18 to 3.72 L/min/m^2) and a fall in systemic vascular resistance (1,190 to 964 Dyne cm sec). Consequently, vasopressin has begun to supplant the use of phenylephrine and norepinephrine for patients whose hemodynamic profile is dominated by vasodilatation.

Although not well appreciated, catecholamines have immunomodulatory properties. A large retrospective study conducted by Schnuelle (101,102), reported that the donor use of dopamine and/or norepinephrine was associated with beneficial results related to acute rejection that were attributed to the immunomodulatory ability of catecholamines. This benefit was dominantly confined to renal graft survivorship, although a potential negative impact of norepinephrine was noted on heart transplantation. Recent literature suggests that the use of low-dose dopamine (4 µg/kg/min), independent of hemodynamic instability, was associated with a decrease in the need for dialysis after kidney transplantation (103). Similarly, a recent review of donor pretreatment with dopamine on survivorship after heart transplant was reported. In this study, donor dopamine was associated with an improved survival after 3 years (87% vs. 67.8%). The authors concluded that fewer recipients of a pretreated graft required hemofiltration after transplantation (21.7% vs. 40.4%), and that treatment of potential brain-dead donors with dopamine of 4 µg/kg/min did not harm cardiac allographs and improved the clinical course of the recipient (104).

The use of HRT is predicated upon the assumption that the ischemic damage to the hypothalamic pituitary axis occurring with brain death creates an endocrinopathy dominated by the absence of thyroid and adrenal hormones that contribute to donor instability. Although beyond the scope of the textbook chapter to review in great detail, it is important to recognize that the anterior pituitary and posterior pituitary have distinct differences in blood supply, innervation, and hormonal production. There is no specific direct arterial blood supply to the anterior pituitary, which receives its blood supply via drainage from the hypothalamus. Blood emerging from the hypothalamus empties into a portal system that bathes the anterior pituitary. Blood supply for the posterior pituitary is via the inferior hypophyseal artery and the connection to the hypothalamus is predominantly neuronal. HRT proposes that there is significant damage to the blood supply to the hypothalamic and pituitary areas that precipitate an endocrinopathy with the attendant physiologic sequelae of a low thyroid hormone state and adrenal insufficiency. As previously discussed, there is substantial animal data and some human data to support a state of profound thyroid/adrenal depletion with exogenous supplementation reported to dramatically improve hemodynamic instability and suitability for transplantation (15). In the original work utilizing HRT, which consisted of thyroid hormone, corticosteroids, and insulin, dramatic improvements in organ donor stability was achieved resulting in significant improvements in transplant suitability, diminutions in the requirements for vasoactive support and dramatic improvements in cardiac function (16). Large retrospective reviews of brain-dead donors reported significant benefit through the use of steroids, vasopressin, and utilization of either triiodothyronine or thyroxine. In the group of potential organ donors that received HRT, the number of organs procured was significantly higher than the donors that did not receive HRT. This resulted in a 23% increase in the number of organs procured with dramatic improvements in the likelihood of an organ being transplanted (105). However, a review of thyroid hormone administration during adult donor care concluded that no publications support the routine administration of thyroid hormone for all donors. Rescue replacement for cardiac inotropic support was supported by some studies, although the methodologic designs were not detailed enough to support a recommendation for routine use (106). In one of the few prospective randomized double-blind trials, 80 potential cardiac donors were allocated to receive triiodothyronine (0.8 mg/kg/ bolus followed by a 0.113 mg/kg/hr infusion), methylprednisolone 1,000 mg bolus, both drugs, or placebo following an initial hemodynamic assessment. Independent of the use of HRT, an explicit donor management algorithm with optimization variables was initiated that used vasopressin as the primary vasoactive agent. During the 6-hour management period, cardiac index was noted to significantly increase in virtually all donors. However, the administration of thyroid hormone and methylprednisolone, either alone or in combination, did not affect the hemodynamics nor have any impact upon heart retrieval. Importantly, 35% of the hearts initially deemed marginal or dysfunctional were suitable for transplantation at the end of the assessment. The authors concluded that donor circulatory status can be improved by active management with the potential to increase transplantable hearts when organ acceptance is deferred until a period of resuscitation and assessment is completed. Hemodynamic management utilizing a PAC was felt to be the cornerstone of donor management and the introduction of hormonal therapy was not a substitute for a detailed hemodynamic assessment and management optimization approaches (78). Consequently, the use of HRT in potential ODM remains controversial and of uncertain benefit. Pragmatically, it would appear that this therapy should be utilized in hemodynamically unstable donors with ongoing instability, despite aggressive optimization management.

Pulmonary Status

Management of the potential organ donor with a focus upon optimizing the respiratory status has assumed a greater degree of importance as the overall lung procurement ratings are usually below 20%. The overall poor procurement rate may be explained by many factors such as an unknown past history, multiple associations with the causative brain death event, including aspiration, pulmonary contusion, shock, and resuscitation, or the complications of mechanical ventilation to include atelectasis, barotrauma, and oxygen toxicity. However, it is important to recognize that several recent studies have shown dramatic increases in the rate of lung procurement when an aggressive strategy focused upon ventilator management and respiratory care was employed.

Pathophysiologically, multiple factors conspire to jeopardize pulmonary function. These include the aforementioned events that transpire before brain death, and similar to the cardiovascular consequences of brain death, pulmonary consequences have been increasingly recognized. Traditionally, this has been dominated by neurogenic pulmonary edema consisting of the initial blast injury associated with brain death. Consequent to the catecholamine surge, there are significant elevations in systemic vascular resistance that result in elevations in left arterial pressure. This represents a transient massive hydrostatic pressure gradient generating fluid flux into the lung that is coupled with structural damage to the capillary endothelium. Against this background of capillary permeability, ongoing fluid resuscitation is purported to increase extravascular lung water, which is associated with changes in the chest x-ray appearance and diminution in lung function which have precluded procurement. Initial work in animal models revealed a dramatic distribution of blood to the right atrium and right ventricle consequent to venoconstriction and augmentation of venous return. Increases in pulmonary artery pressure were reported that resulted in 72% of the effective circulating volume contained in the lungs for several minutes during the brain death event (17). Subsequent to this hydrostatic and capillary burst injury pattern associated with brain death, Fisher (107) recognized the presence of an inflammatory response associated with brain death. In a study that compared inflammatory signals in brain-dead patients to controls, dramatic increases in neutrophil concentration and lavage concentrations of IL-8 were reported. In a subsequent study by Fisher et al. (108), the magnitude of the inflammatory response in the donor was evaluated in the recipient. The IL-8 signal in the donor was found to be correlative with the degree of impairment in graft oxygenation, the development of severe early graft dysfunction, and early recipient mortality. Avlonitis (109,110) has proposed that a combination of hydrostatic forces and inflammatory responses conspire to jeopardize pulmonary function during the donor management period. The inflammatory response is derived from events that are antecedent to brain death in conjunction with IR injury of brain death. Allowing time for the lung to recover in the immediate brain death period could potentially mitigate the reperfusion injury, hemodynamic mechanisms of lung injury, and systemic response following brain death to the transplant donor.

The criteria for ideal lungs suitable for procurement were defined during the early phase of transplantation and included a PaO_2/FiO_2 ratio greater than 300 mmHg, a clear chest x-ray, positive end-expiratory pressure (PEEP) requirements of no more than 5 cm of H_2O, age less than 55 years, minimal tobacco abuse, and the absence of significant chest trauma, pulmonary secretions, or aspiration. However, there has been a liberalization of these criteria, which were thought to be excessively stringent and capricious. In a large autopsy series of potential donors, 47% of those potential donors deemed suitable for lung procurement but not procured, had significant pulmonary disease, and 25% had bronchopneumonia. In those potential donors that were deemed not suitable, only 15% had minor pulmonary abnormalities (111). Similarly, autopsy assessment of lungs rejected for transplantation reveals that 41% of rejected lungs were potentially suitable for transplantation. In this case-matched study of lungs rejected for donation, 83% were found to have absent or mild pulmonary edema, 74% had an intact alveolar fluid clearance, and 62% had normal or only mildly abnormal cystopathology (112). Additionally, Fisher (113) reported the traditional criteria were poor discriminators of pulmonary injury and infection, which led to the exclusion of potentially usable lungs. Utilizing bronchial alveolar lavage samplings of inflammatory mediators, there was no difference between those lungs that were accepted and those excluded by clinical criteria. Finally, Shafaghi and colleagues (105a) found that 27/30 (90%) brain-dead patients, on whom bronchoalveolar lavage (BALs) were performed, had positive bacterial and fungal cultures. They suggest that such patients—donors and recipients—must be more aggressively managed if the lungs are to be used; for example, combined intravenous and aerosolized antibiotics in donors and recipients can reduce the incidence of recipient pneumonia. Nonetheless, recipients would be expected to have longer ICU length of stay and ventilator days, as well as decreased survival.

Traditionally, donor lung ventilator management was not aggressively pursued and frequently suboptimal for preservation of lung function. This is illustrated in a study of 34 brain-dead patients, of whom 11 were considered eligible lung donors, yet only two donated lungs. In this potential lung donor population, no ventilator changes were made after confirmation of brain death, no recruitment maneuvers were undertaken to preserve gas exchange, saline infusion was increased from 187 to 275 mL/hr, and CVP was permitted to increase; 45% of the potential lung donors experienced decrements in the PaO_2/FiO_2 ratio, making them ineligible for donation.

In contrast, several studies that focused upon optimization of donor lungs have reported dramatic improvement in the rate of lung procurement. In one of the original studies of lung donor management that included antibiotic therapy, strict fluid management, physiotherapy, bronchoscopy, and pulmonary toilet, along with alterations in ventilator status including the initiation of pressure ventilation, dramatic improvements in lung procurement were reported. In a study population with an initial PaO_2/FiO_2 ratio less than 300 mmHg, 31% of lungs were clearly unsuitable and were not subjected to aggressive donor management. However, the remaining 69% were aggressively managed to include manipulations in mechanical ventilation, adjustments in PEEP, and bronchoscopy; 49% of those subjected to aggressive donor management were able to achieve a PaO_2/FiO_2 ratio higher than 300 mmHg and were successfully transplanted with outcomes indistinguishable from those with an initially acceptable ratios. Similar outcomes between the ideal and donor management lungs were achieved related to postoperative gas exchange, ICU length of stay, and short- or medium-term mortality (114). A subsequent study similarly reported the results of an aggressive donor management program to improve the rate of lung procurement. The San Antonio Lung Transplant (SALT) Donor Management Protocol hypothesized that the implementation of a donor lung management program would increase the rate of lung procurement without adversely impacting the overall survival rate of lung transplant recipients. Elements of the protocol included educational activity to enhance the interaction between transplant pulmonologists and OPO staff related to donor selection and management, emphasis upon every donor as a lung donor, ensuring requests for donation for donation, and educating organ procurement coordinators about donor management strategies. These included the use of recruitment maneuvers which were defined as maintenance of a pressure-controlled ventilation of 25 cm of H_2O and a PEEP of 15 cm of H_2O for 2 hours with subsequent transition to conventional volume control ventilation with a tidal volume of 10 mL/kg and a PEEP of 5 cm of H_2O. Fluid balance focused upon minimizing the use of crystalloid solutions, and diuretics to maintain a neutral or negative fluid balance. Aspiration risk was minimized by elevating the head of the bed to 30 degrees and inflating the endotracheal balloon to

25 cm of H_2O. Additionally, bronchoscopy with bronchial alveolar lavage was performed on all patients to evaluate the chest x-ray area of infiltrate. Despite poor donors accounting for 76% of the total donors during the trial period, a dramatic increase in actual lung donors (98 vs. 38) and a significant increase in lung transplantations (121 vs. 53) resulted. The authors concluded that an aggressive protocol focused on lung donor management significantly increased the number of lung donors and transplant procedures without compromising lung function, length of stay, or survival of the recipients (115).

In a recent comparison trial of lung donor management, a significant increase in the rate of lung procurement was reported—40% versus 27%—with an aggressive lung donor management strategy. In the control group, donor management commenced within 2 hours of consent for donation and continued for approximately 7 hours. Management strategies included early bronchoscopy, tidal volumes of 10 mL/kg with a PEEP of 5 cm of H_2O, frequent suctioning and volume recruitment enabled by turning the potential donor every 2 hours. A specific hemodynamic algorithm titrating vasoactive support and fluid resuscitation to a cardiac index of greater than 2.5 L/min/m^2, focusing on a low CVP and pulmonary capillary wedge pressures was employed. Fluid resuscitation was minimized and colloid solution was preferentially utilized. Donor lungs subjected to this aggressive management approach resulted in a procurement rate of 40% (77).

Miñambres and colleagues (116) showed in a before–after series that use of an aggressive lung management protocol led to a quadrupling of lung donors (transplanted lungs) with no change in postgraft dysfunction. These investigators followed a seven-step protocol:

1. Apnea test performed with ventilator in the continuous positive-pressure mode
2. Mechanical ventilation with PEEP of 8 to 10 cm H_2O and tidal volume of 6 to 8 mL/kg
3. Recruitment maneuvers once per hour and after any disconnection from the ventilator
4. Bronchoscopy with bilateral bronchoalveolar lavage
5. Hemodynamics closely monitored with the PICCO system, with a goal of extravascular lung water of 10 mL/kg or less, administering diuretics if needed, and a CVP of 6 to 8 mmHg
6. Methylprednisolone, 15 mg/kg after brain death declaration
7. Alveolar recruitment with controlled ventilation—peak pressure limit of 35 mmHg with PEEP of 18 to 20 cm H_2O for 1 minute and decreased 2 cm H_2O each minute—after that tidal volumes were increased by 50% for 10 breaths

They attributed their success at increasing lung donors to this protocol, as other issues remained unchanged.

Although a lung protective strategy has been adopted by the intensive care community for patients with acute lung injury (ALI), traditional donor management has utilized relatively high tidal volumes in an effort to minimize de-recruitment and improve gas exchange. In all likelihood, hyperinflation has cosmetically improved the chest x-ray, which is one of the traditional criteria for procurement. However, these traditional concepts were recently challenged in a randomized controlled trial comparing the outcomes of conventional ventilator strategies with tidal volumes of 10 to 12 mL/kg, PEEP maintenance with 3 to 5 cm of H_2O and the performance of apnea tests by disconnecting the ventilator with an open suction to a protective ventilator strategy with tidal volumes of 6 to 8 mL/kg, PEEP of 8 to 10 cm of H_2O with apnea tests performed by using CPAP and closed circuit for suction. In the conventional strategy group, only 54% of potential donors met lung donor eligibility after a 6-hour observation period compared to 95% in the protective strategy group. Only 27% of lungs were procured from donors in the conventional strategy group compared to a procurement rate of 54% in the protective strategy group. Six-month survivorship did not differ between those recipients receiving lungs from either category. Similar to data from patients with ALI, a significantly higher level of inflammatory mediators was reported in the conventional ventilator strategy compared to the protective ventilator strategy. This study strongly suggests that hyperinflation has an adverse effect on lung function, compromises eligibility of lung donors, and should be replaced by a protective ventilator strategy similar to patients with acute lung injury. Similar to the evidence supporting aggressive donor cardiac management, an aggressive approach to lung donor management will result in a higher level of lung donor procurement, and no donor lung should be rejected upon the initial evaluation. Ongoing assessments for suitability are required in conjunction with aggressive donor management (117). Recent evidence suggests that the use of airway pressure release ventilation (APRV), as compared to assist control ventilation (ACV), results in a higher PaO_2/FiO_2 ratio (mean [SD], 498 [43] vs. 334 [104] mmHg, respectively; $p < 0.001$) after 100% O_2 challenge. The ACV group ultimately donated 7 of 40 potential lungs (18%) compared with 42 of 50 potential lungs (84%) in the APRV group ($p < 0.001$) (118).

Supportive Care

Hemodynamic management forms the cornerstone of potential ODM. Ensuring adequate perfusion to all organs is the best approach to support liver, kidney, pancreas, and small bowel function, anticipating possible procurement. This requires ongoing hemodynamic measurements using the previously described donor management endpoints. A recent paper by Smith and colleagues (119) reported—in a prospective but nonrandomized study—that direct peritoneal resuscitation (DPR), using of 2.5% glucose-based clinical peritoneal dialysis solution, reduced IV fluid requirement and pressor use, increased hepatic blood flow, and organs transplanted per donor. The mechanism of action is thought to be its action as a nonpharmacologic vasodilator, increasing microcirculatory flow, as well as creating an osmotic gradient with the extracellular space that reduces cellular edema. The anti-inflammatory cytokine, IL-10, was significantly upregulated compared to controls. While DPR appears to be a safe, effective method to augment organ donor resuscitation, its use needs to be further studied.

Although there are extremely limited data, there is speculation that hepatic glycogen stores may be depleted in the brain death period and that support with enteral nutrition may play an important role in modulating organ function after transplantation (120). In the absence of contraindications, it is appropriate to continue enteral nutrition carefully following for any evidence of hyperglycemia. As previously mentioned, the liver is explicitly sensitive to hypernatremia, so serum sodium level should be corrected to less than 155 mEq/L. Diabetes insipidus is a frequent complication of brain death secondary to a deficiency of vasopressin after pituitary destruction. Vasopressin absence can contribute to multiple donor management issues, including hyperosmolarity, electrolyte disturbances, and intravascular volume depletion. It is important to differentiate diabetes insipidus from mannitol-induced osmotic diuresis. Diabetes insipidus is generally associated with serum sodium greater than 150 mEq/L, an elevated serum osmolarity, a urine output exceeding 300 mL/hr, and a urine osmolarity usually less than 200 mOsm/L with an associated normal serum osmolar gap. The preceding serves to differentiate diabetes insipidus from mannitol-induced polyuria. Diabetes insipidus should be treated with hypotonic solutions and, frequently, 5% dextrose in water is used to match urine output mL for mL. In instances of urine output greater than 200 to 300 mL/hr, desmopressin acetate (DVAVP) or arginine vasopressin may be utilized. Vasopressin exerts its effect on three receptors: V1 receptors on the smooth muscle and is responsible for vasopressor effects, V2 receptors located in the kidney which promote the antidiuretic effect, and V3 receptors in the pituitary which regulate corticotropin-releasing hormone. Arginine vasopressin has antidiuretic and vasopressor effects, whereas DVAVP has greater affinity for the V2 receptor and consequently a predominant antidiuretic affect. Clinically, 1 to 4 μg of DDAVP is given intravenously, following urine osmolarity, urine output, and serum sodium closely. Subsequent dosing is dependent upon the response. In the setting of hypotension, arginine vasopressin is preferred at a dose between 0.01 and 0.04 IU/min. Hyperglycemia is frequent in potential organ donors and often necessitates the use of insulin for control. Although the effects of hyperglycemia are not well established, hyperglycemia is believed to impair organ function. Consequently, hyperglycemia should be treated similarly to critically ill patients using an empiric level of 150 mg/dL to initiate therapy. Coagulation abnormalities are common in potential organ donors and ongoing assessment of coagulopathy and hemoglobin are necessary during the course of donor management. Although there is no outcome data for potential organ donors, the approach advocated is similar to that of other critically ill patients utilizing a transfusion threshold for hemoglobin of 8 mg/dL and normalization of coagulation parameters. Pituitary injury predisposes to thermoregulatory impairment and it is imperative that the donor receives warmed fluids and body temperature be monitored routinely, as hypothermia can further impair coagulation and predispose to cardiac rhythm disturbances. Nonetheless, there is at least speculation that when ODM is properly applied, additional benefit of previously recommended drugs and hormones may be marginal (121).

DONATION AFTER CARDIAC DEATH

DCD refers to the recovery of organs from patients that are not brain dead, but die secondary to cardiopulmonary causes. This was previously known as a nonheart-beating donor. Donation may occur in several circumstances that are either controlled or uncontrolled. The vast majority of DCD occurs during controlled situations when care is withdrawn and the patient is pronounced dead from cardiopulmonary arrest. Uncontrolled DCD is far less common and occurs in emergent circumstances such as death from an acute trauma. Prior to 1968, there was no legal definition for brain death and DCD was the primary method for obtaining organs for transplantation. After the acceptance of brain death, donation from brain-dead donors has significantly exceeded those from DCD. The IOM formally evaluated the DCD practice into separate reports (122,123). Specifically, the IOM stipulated that the decision to withdraw or withhold care be undertaken based upon the patient's wishes and not influenced by any potential for organ donation. It was further recommended that a separate team provides EOL care that was distinct from the transplant team. DCD must adhere to the dead donor rule, which stipulates that donor organs may only be procured from dead patients. When undertaking DCD, the withdrawal of care should be indistinguishable from the withdrawal of care in any other critically ill patient. Death is declared when there is cessation of cardiopulmonary function and after a period of time to ensure that there is no spontaneous recrudescence of respiratory function. Although the initial 1997 recommendation from the IOM was a 5-minute period between the diagnosis of death and the initiation of organ recovery, it is currently recommended that this period be at least 2 minutes and no more than 5 minutes (124).

Key Points

- Care must be taken in the ICU so that early identification of potential donors is made, the OPO is informed, and donor loss prevented.
- Patients who have become potential organ donors demand the same high-quality critical care as was given while they were alive.
- Intensivist involvement and protocolized/standardized care are the most important components of ODM.
- When ODM is properly applied, the additional benefit of previously recommended drugs and hormones may be limited.

References

1. Cushing H. Some experimental and clinical observations concerning states of increased intracranial tension. *Am J Med Sci.* 1901;124:375–400.
2. Power BM, van Heerden PV. The physiological changes associated with brain death—current concepts and implications for treatment of the brain dead organ donor. *Anaesth Intensive Care.* 1995;23:26–36.
3. Kopelnik A, Zaroff JG. Neurocardiogenic injury in neurovascular disorders. *Crit Care Clin.* 2006;22:733–752.
4. Banki NM, Zaroff JG. Neurogenic cardiac injury. *Curr Treat Options Cardiovasc Med.* 2003;5:451–458.
5. Banki NM, Kopelnik A, Dae MW, et al. Acute neurocardiogenic injury after subarachnoid hemorrhage. *Circulation.* 2005;112:3314–3319.
6. Tung P, Kopelnik A, Banki N, et al. Predictors of neurocardiogenic injury after subarachnoid hemorrhage. *Stroke.* 2004;35:548–551.
7. Banki NM, Parmley WW, Foster E, et al. Reversibility of left ventricular systolic dysfunction in humans with subarachnoid hemorrhage (abstracted). *Circulation.* 2001;104:11.
8. Powner DJ, Boccalandro C, Alp MS, Vollmer DG. Endocrine failure after traumatic brain injury in adults. *Neurocrit Care.* 2006;5:61–70.
9. Schneider HJ, Kreitschmann-Andermahr I, Ghigo E, et al. Hypothalamopituitary dysfunction following traumatic brain injury and aneurysmal subarachnoid hemorrhage: a systematic review. *JAMA.* 2007;298:1429–1438.
10. Yoshioka T, Sugimoto H, Uenishi M, et al. Prolonged hemodynamic maintenance by the combined administration of vasopressin and epinephrine in brain death: a clinical study. *Neurosurgery.* 1986;18:565–567.
11. Black PM. Brain death (first of two parts). *N Engl J Med.* 1978;299:338–344.
12. Andrews BT, Pitts LH. Functional recovery after traumatic transtentorial herniation. *Neurosurgery.* 1991;29:227–231.
13. Novitzky D. Donor management: state of the art. *Transplant Proc.* 1997; 29:3773–3775.

14. Novitzky D, Cooper DK, Chaffin JS, et al. Improved cardiac allograft function following triiodothyronine therapy to both donor and recipient. *Transplantation.* 1990;49:311–316.
15. Novitzky D, Cooper DK, Morrell D, Isaacs S. Change from aerobic to anaerobic metabolism after brain death, and reversal following triiodothyronine therapy. *Transplantation.* 1988;45:32–36.
16. Novitzky D, Cooper DK, Reichart B. Hemodynamic and metabolic responses to hormonal therapy in brain-dead potential organ donors. *Transplantation.* 1987;43:852–854.
17. Novitzky D, Wicomb WN, Rose AG, et al. Pathophysiology of pulmonary edema following experimental brain death in the chacma baboon. *Ann Thorac Surg.* 1987;43:288–294.
18. Novitzky D, Wicomb W, Cooper AG, Rose. Electrocardiographic, hemodynamic & endocrine changes occurring during experimental brain death in the chacma baboon. *Heart Transplant.* 1984;IV:63–69.
19. Szabo G, Buhmann V, Bahrle S, et al. Brain death impairs coronary endothelial function. *Transplantation.* 2002;73:1846–1848.
20. Segel LD, vonHaag DW, Zhang J, Follette DM. Selective overexpression of inflammatory molecules in hearts from brain-dead rats. *J Heart Lung Transplant.* 2002;21:804–811.
21. Szabo G, Hackert T, Buhmann V, et al. Downregulation of myocardial contractility via intact ventriculo–arterial coupling in the brain dead organ donor. *Eur J Cardiothorac Surg.* 2001;20:170–176.
22. Szabo G, Hackert T, Buhmann V, et al. Myocardial performance after brain death: studies in isolated hearts. *Ann Transplant.* 2000;5:45–50.
23. Yeh T Jr, Wechsler AS, Graham LJ, et al. Acute brain death alters left ventricular myocardial gene expression. *J Thorac Cardiovasc Surg.* 1999;117:365–374.
24. Bittner HB, Chen EP, Milano CA, et al. Myocardial beta-adrenergic receptor function and high-energy phosphates in brain death–related cardiac dysfunction. *Circulation.* 1995;92:472–478.
25. D'Amico TA, Meyers CH, Koutlas TC, et al. Desensitization of myocardial beta-adrenergic receptors and deterioration of left ventricular function after brain death. *J Thorac Cardiovasc Surg.* 1995;110:746–751.
26. Shivalkar B, Van Loon J, Wieland W, et al. Variable effects of explosive or gradual increase of intracranial pressure on myocardial structure and function. *Circulation.* 1993;87:230–239.
27. Mehra MR, Uber PA, Ventura HO, et al. The impact of mode of donor brain death on cardiac allograft vasculopathy: an intravascular ultrasound study. *J Am Coll Cardiol.* 2004;43:806–810.
28. Audibert G, Charpentier C, Seguin-Devaux C, et al. Improvement of donor myocardial function after treatment of autonomic storm during brain death. *Transplantation.* 2006;82:1031–1036.
29. Cooper DK, Novitzky D, Wicomb WN. The pathophysiological effects of brain death on potential donor organs, with particular reference to the heart. *Ann R Coll Surg Engl.* 1989;71:261–266.
30. Gramm HJ, Meinhold H, Bickel U, et al. Acute endocrine failure after brain death? *Transplantation.* 1992;54:851–857.
31. Howlett TA, Keogh AM, Perry L, et al. Anterior and posterior pituitary function in brain-stem-dead donors. A possible role for hormonal replacement therapy. *Transplantation.* 1989;47:828–834.
32. Powner DJ, Hendrich A, Lagler RG, et al. Hormonal changes in brain dead patients. *Crit Care Med.* 1990;18:702–708.
33. Goarin JP, Cohen S, Riou B, et al. The effects of triiodothyronine on hemodynamic status and cardiac function in potential heart donors. *Anesth Analg.* 1996;83:41–47.
34. Randell TT, Hockerstedt KA. Triiodothyronine treatment in brain-dead multiorgan donors—a controlled study. *Transplantation.* 1992;54:736–738.
35. Gasser M. Organ transplantation from brain dead donors: its impact on short and long term outcome revisited. *Transplant Rev.* 2001;15:1–10.
36. Pratschke J, Wilhelm MJ, Kusaka M, et al. Brain death and its influence on donor organ quality and outcome after transplantation. *Transplantation.* 1999;67:343–348.
37. Murugan R, Venkataraman R, Wahed AS, et al. Increased plasma interleukin-6 in donors is associated with lower recipient hospital-free survival after cadaveric organ transplantation. *Crit Care Med.* 2008;36:1810–1816.
38. Murugan R, Venkataraman R, Wahed AS, et al. Preload responsiveness is associated with increased interleukin-6 and lower organ yield from brain-dead donors. *Crit Care Med.* 2009;37:2387–2393.
39. Birks EJ, Burton PB, Owen V, et al. Elevated tumor necrosis factor-alpha and interleukin-6 in myocardium and serum of malfunctioning donor hearts. *Circulation.* 2000;102:352–358.
40. Venkateswaran RV, Dronavalli V, Lambert PA, et al. The proinflammatory environment in potential heart and lung donors: prevalence and impact of donor management and hormonal therapy. *Transplantation.* 2009;88:582–588.
41. Weiss S, Kotsch K, Francuski M, et al. Brain death activates donor organs and is associated with a worse I/R injury after liver transplantation. *Am J Transplant.* 2007;7:1584–1593.
42. Kotsch K, Ulrich F, Reutzel-Selke A, et al. Methylprednisolone therapy in deceased donors reduces inflammation in the donor liver and improves outcome after liver transplantation: a prospective randomized controlled trial. *Ann Surg.* 2008;248:1042–1050.
43. Mollaret P, Goulon M. [The depassed coma (preliminary memoir)]. *Rev Neurol (Paris).* 1959;101:3–15.
44. Lofstedt S. Intracranial lesions with abolished passage of x-ray contrast throughout the internal carotid arteries. *Pacing Clin Electrophysiol.* 1956;8:199–202.
45. Schwab R. EEG as an aid in determining death in the presence of cardiac acuity. *Electroencephalogr Clin Neurophys.* 1963;15:147.
46. A definition of irreversible coma. Report of the Ad Hoc Committee of the Harvard Medical School to Examine the Definition of Brain Death. *JAMA.* 1968;205:337–340.
47. Diagnosis of brain death. Statement issued by the honorary secretary of the Conference of Medical Royal Colleges and their Faculties in the United Kingdom on 11 October 1976. *Br Med J.* 1976;2:1187–1188.
48. Criteria for the diagnosis of brain stem death. Review by a working group convened by the Royal College of Physicians and endorsed by the Conference of Medical Royal Colleges and their Faculties in the United Kingdom. *J R Coll Phys Lond.* 1995;29:381–382.
49. Practice parameters for determining brain death in adults (summary statement). The Quality Standards Subcommittee of the American Academy of Neurology. *Neurology.* 1995;45:1012–1014.
50. Wijdicks EF, Varelas PN, Gronseth GS, Greer DM; American Academy of Neurology. Evidence-based guideline update: determining brain death in adults: report of the Quality Standards Subcommittee of the American Academy of Neurology. *Neurology.* 2010;74:1911–1918.
51. An appraisal of the criteria of cerebral death. A summary statement. A collaborative study. *JAMA.* 1977;237:982–986.
52. Wijdicks EF. Clinical diagnosis and confirmatory testing of brain death in adults. In: *Brain Death*. Philadelphia, PA: Lippincott Williams & Wilkins; 2001:61–90.
53. Taylor T, Dineen RA, Gardiner DC, et al. Computed tomography (CT) angiography for confirmation of the clinical diagnosis of brain death. *Cochrane Database Syst Rev* 2014;(3):CD009694. doi: 10.1002/14651858.CD009694.pub2.
54. Lutz-Dettinger N, de Jaeger A, Kerremans I. Care of the potential pediatric organ donor. *Pediatr Clin North Am.* 2001;48:715–749.
55. Lopez-Navidad A, Domingo P, Caballero F, et al. Successful transplantation of organs retrieved from donors with bacterial meningitis. *Transplantation.* 1997;64:365–368.
56. Bahrami T, Vohra HA, Shaikhrezai K, et al. Intrathoracic organ transplantation from donors with meningitis: a single-center 20-year experience. *Ann Thorac Surg.* 2008;86:1554–1556.
57. Satoi S, Bramhall SR, Solomon M, et al. The use of liver grafts from donors with bacterial meningitis. *Transplantation.* 2001;72:1108–1113.
58. Kubak BM, Gregson AL, Pegues DA, et al. Use of hearts transplanted from donors with severe sepsis and infectious deaths. *J Heart Lung Transplant.* 2009;28:260–265.
59. Cohen J, Michowiz R, Ashkenazi T, et al. Successful organ transplantation from donors with Acinetobacter baumannii septic shock. *Transplantation.* 2006;81:853–855.
60. Williams MA. Lipsett PA, Rushton CH, et al. The physician's role in discussing organ donation with families. *Crit Care Med.* 2003;31:1568–1573.
61. DeJong W, Franz HG, Wolfe SM, et al. Requesting organ donation: an interview study of donor and nondonor families. *Am J Crit Care.* 1998;7:13–23.
62. Siminoff LA, Gordon N, Hewlett J, Arnold RM. Factors influencing families' consent for donation of solid organs for transplantation. *JAMA.* 2001;286:71–77.
63. James FC, Catharyn TL. *Organ Donation.* Washington, DC: The National Academies Press; 2006.
64. Gortmaker SL, Beasley CL, Sheehy E, et al. Improving the request process to increase family consent for organ donation. *J Transpl Coord.* 1998;8:210–217.
65. Garrison RN, Bentley FR, Raque GH, et al. There is an answer to the shortage of organ donors. *Surg Gynecol Obstet.* 1991;173:391–396.
66. Siminoff LA, Lawrence RH, Zhang A. Decoupling: what is it and does it really help increase consent to organ donation? *Prog Transplant.* 2002;12:52–60.
67. Rosendale JD, Chabalewski FL, McBride MA, et al. Increased transplanted organs from the use of a standardized donor management protocol. *Am J Transplant.* 2002;2:761–768.

68. Salim A, Velmahos GC, Brown C, et al. Aggressive organ donor management significantly increases the number of organs available for transplantation. *J Trauma.* 2005;58:991–994.
69. Salim A, Martin M, Brown C, et al. The effect of a protocol of aggressive donor management: Implications for the national organ donor shortage. *J Trauma.* 2006;61:429–433.
70. Singbartl K, Murugana R, Kaynara AM, et al. Intensivist-led management of brain-dead donors is associated with an increase in organ recovery for transplantation. *Am J Transplant.* 2011;11:1517–1521.
71. Wauters S, Verleden GM, Belmans A, et al. Donor cause of brain death and related time intervals: does it affect outcome after lung transplantation? *Eur J Cardio-Thoracic Surg.* 2011;39:e68–e76.
72. Inaba K, Branco BC, Lam L, et al. Organ donation and time to procurement: late is not too late. *J Trauma.* 2010;68:1362–1366.
73. Christmas AB, Bogart TA, Etson KE, et al. The reward is worth the wait: a prospective analysis of 100 consecutive organ donors. *Am Surg.* 2012;78:296–299.
74. Hagan ME, McClean D, Falcone CA, et al. Attaining specific donor management goals increases number of organs transplanted per donor: a quality improvement project. *Prog Transplant.* 2009;19:227–231.
75. Franklin GA, Santos AP, Smith JW, et al. Optimization of donor management goals yields increased organ use. *Am Surg.* 2010;76:587–594.
76. Malinoski DJ, Daly MC, Patel MS, et al. Achieving donor management goals before deceased donor procurement is associated with more organs transplanted per donor. *J Trauma.* 2011;71:990–995.
77. Venkateswaran RV, Patchell VB, Wilson IC, et al. Early donor management increases the retrieval rate of lungs for transplantation. *Ann Thorac Surg.* 2008;85:278–286.
78. Venkateswaran RV, Steeds RP, Quinn DW, et al. The haemodynamic effects of adjunctive hormone therapy in potential heart donors: a prospective randomized double-blind factorially designed controlled trial. *Eur Heart J.* 2009;30:1771–1780.
79. Callahan DS, Kim D, Bricker S, et al. Trends in organ donor management: 2002 to 2012. *J Am Coll Surg.* 2014;219:752–756.
80. Sally MB, Ewing T, Crutchfield M, et al. Determining optimal threshold for glucose control in organ donors after neurologic determination of death: A United Network for Organ Sharing Region 5 Donor Management Goals Workgroup prospective analysis. *J Trauma Acute Care Surg.* 2014;76:62–69.
81. Gilbert EM, Krueger SK, Murray JL, et al. Echocardiographic evaluation of potential cardiac transplant donors. *J Thorac Cardiovasc Surg.* 1988;95:1003–1007.
82. Zaroff JG, Babcock WD, Shiboski SC. The impact of left ventricular dysfunction on cardiac donor transplant rates. *J Heart Lung Transplant.* 2003;22:334–337.
83. Zaroff J. Echocardiographic evaluation of the potential cardiac donor. *J Heart Lung Transplant.* 2004;23:S250–2.
84. Zaroff JG, Babcock WD, Shiboski SC, et al. Temporal changes in left ventricular systolic function in heart donors: results of serial echocardiography. *J Heart Lung Transplant.* 2003;22:383–388.
85. Stoddard MF, Longaker RA. The role of transesophageal echocardiography in cardiac donor screening. *Am Heart J.* 1993;125:1676–1681.
86. Venkateswaran RV, Townend JN, Wilson IC, et al. Echocardiography in the potential heart donor. *Transplantation.* 2010;89:894–901.
87. Kouo T, Nishina T, Morita H, et al. Usefulness of low dose dobutamine stress echocardiography for evaluating reversibility of brain death-induced myocardial dysfunction. *Am J Cardiol.* 1999;84:558–582.
88. Wheeldon DR, Potter CD, Oduro A, et al. Transforming the "unacceptable" donor: outcomes from the adoption of a standardized donor management technique. *J Heart Lung Transplant.* 1995;14:734–742.
89. Marik PE, Baram M, Vahid B. Does central venous pressure predict fluid responsiveness? A systematic review of the literature and the tale of seven mares. *Chest.* 2008;134:172–178.
90. Marik PE, Cavallazzi R, Vasu T, Hirani A. Dynamic changes in arterial waveform derived variables and fluid responsiveness in mechanically ventilated patients: a systematic review of the literature. *Crit Care Med.* 2009;37:2642–2647.
91. Whelchel J, Diethelm A, Phillips M. The effect of high dose dopamine in cadaveric donor management in delayed graft function and graft survival following renal transplant. *J Transplant Proc.* 1986;18:523–527.
92. Totsuka E, Dodson F, Urakami A, et al. Influence of high donor serum sodium levels on early postoperative graft function in human liver transplantation: effect of correction of donor hypernatremia. *Liver Transplant Surg.* 1999;5:421–428.
93. Follette D, Rudich S, Bonacci C, et al. Importance of an aggressive multidisciplinary management approach to optimize lung donor procurement. *Transplant Proc.* 1999;31:169–170.
94. Oliver JB, Peters S, Bongu A, et al. Prerecovery liver biopsy in the brain-dead donor: a case-control study of logistics, safety, precision, and utility. *Liver Transpl.* 2014;20:237–244.
95. Nijboer WN, Moers C, Leuvenink HG, Ploeg RJ. How important is the duration of the brain death period for the outcome in kidney transplantation? *Transplant Int.* 2011;24:14–20.
96. Reilly P, Morgan L, Grossman MD, et al. Lung procurement from solid organ donors – role of fluid resuscitation in procurement failures. *Internet J Emerg Intensive Care Med.* 1999;3(2). [serial online]. Available at: http://www.ispub.com/journals/IJEICM/VOl3N2/organ.htm.
97. Lucas BA, Vaughn WK, Spees EK, Sanfilippo F. Identification of donor factors predisposing to high discard rates of cadaver kidneys and increased graft loss within one year posttransplantation–SEOPF 1977–1982. South-Eastern Organ Procurement Foundation. *Transplantation.* 1987;43:253–258.
98. Abdelnour T, Rieke S. Relationship of hormonal resuscitation therapy and central venous pressure on increasing organs for transplant. *J Heart Lung Transplant.* 2009;28:480–485.
99. Minambres E, Rodrigo E, Ballesteros MA, et al. Impact of restrictive fluid balance focused to increase lung procurement on renal function after kidney transplantation. *Nephrol Dial Transplant.* 2010;25:2352–2356.
100. Shemie SD, Ross H, Pagliarello J, et al. Organ donor management in Canada: recommendations of the forum on Medical Management to Optimize Donor Organ Potential. *CMAJ.* 2006;174:S13–32.
101. Schnuelle P, Lorenz D, Mueller A, et al. Donor catecholamine use reduces acute allograft rejection and improves graft survival after cadaveric renal transplantation. *Kidney Int.* 1999;56:738–746.
102. Schnuelle P, Berger S, de Boer J, et al. Effects of catecholamine application to brain-dead donors on graft survival in solid organ transplantation. *Transplantation.* 2001;72:455–463.
103. Schnuelle P, Gottmann U, Hoeger S, et al. Effects of donor pretreatment with dopamine on graft function after kidney transplantation: a randomized controlled trial. *JAMA.* 2009;302:1067–1075.
104. Benck U, Hoeger S, Brinkkoetter PT, et al. Effects of donor pre-treatment with dopamine on survival after heart transplantation: a cohort study of heart transplant recipients nested in a randomized controlled multicenter trial. *J Am Coll Cardiol.* 2011;58:1768–1777.
105. Rosendale JD, Kauffman HM, McBride MA, et al. Aggressive pharmacologic donor management results in more transplanted organs. *Transplantation.* 2003;75:482–487.
105a. Shafaghi S, Dezfuli AA, Makki SS, et al. Microbial pattern of bronchoalveolar lavage in brain dead donors. *Transplant Proc.* 2011;43(2):422–423.
106. Powner DJ, Hernandez M. A review of thyroid hormone administration during adult donor care. *Progr Transplant.* 2005;15:2002–2007.
107. Fisher AJ, Donnelly SC, Hirani N, et al. Enhanced pulmonary inflammation in organ donors following fatal non-traumatic brain injury. *Lancet.* 1999;353:1412–1413.
108. Fisher A, Donnelly SC, Mirani N, et al. Elevated levels of interleukin-8 in donor lungs is associated with early graft failure after lung transplantation. *Am J Resp Crit Care Med.* 2001;163:259–265.
109. Avlonitis VS, Wigfield CH, Golledge HD, et al. Early hemodynamic injury during donor brain death determines the severity of primary graft dysfunction after lung transplantation. *Am J Transplant.* 2007;7:83–90.
110. Avlonitis VS, Wigfield CH, Kirby JA, Dark JH. The hemodynamic mechanisms of lung injury and systemic inflammatory response following brain death in the transplant donor. *Am J Transplant.* 2005;5:684–693.
111. Finfer S, Bohn D, Colpitts D, et al. Intensive care management of paediatric organ donors and its effect on post-transplant organ function. *Intensive Care Med.* 1996;22:1424–1432.
112. Ware LB, Wang Y, Fang X, et al. Assessment of lungs rejected for transplantation and implications for donor selection. *Lancet.* 2002;360:619–620.
113. Fisher AJ, Donnelly SC, Pritchard G, et al. Objective assessment of criteria for selection of donor lungs suitable for transplantation. *Thorax.* 2004;59:434–437.
114. Gabbay E, Williams TJ, Griffiths AP, et al. Maximizing the utilization of donor organs offered for lung transplantation. *Am J Respir Crit Care Med.* 1999;160:265–271.
115. Angel LF, Levine DJ, Restrepo MI, et al. Impact of a lung transplantation donor-management protocol on lung donation and recipient outcomes. *Am J Respir Crit Care Med.* 2006;174:710–716.
116. Miñambres E, Coll E, Duerto J, et al. Effect of an intensive lung donor-management protocol on lung transplantation outcomes. *J Heart Lung Transplant.* 2014;33:178–184.
117. Mascia L, Pasero D, Slutsky AS, et al. Effect of a lung protective strategy for organ donors on eligibility and availability of lungs for transplantation: a randomized controlled trial. *JAMA.* 2010;304:2620–2627.

118. Hanna K, Seder CW, Weinberger JB, et al. Airway pressure release ventilation and successful lung donation. *Arch Surg.* 2011;146(3):325–328.

119. Smith JW, Matheson PJ, Morgan G, et al. Addition of direct peritoneal lavage to human cadaver organ donor resuscitation improves organ procurement. *J Am Coll Surg.* 2015;220:539–547.

120. Singer P, Cohen J, Cynober L. Effect of nutritional state of brain-dead organ donor on transplantation. *Nutrition.* 2001;17:948–952.

121. McKeown DW, Ball J. Treating the Donor. *Curr Opin Organ Transplant.* 2014;19:85–91.

122. *Institute of Medicine, National Academy of Sciences.* Washington, DC: National Academy Press; 1997.

123. *Institute of Medicine, National Academy of Sciences.* Washington, DC: National Academy Press; 2000.

124. Ethics Committee, American College of Critical Care Medicine; Society of Critical Care Medicine. Recommendations for non-heartbeating organ donation: a position paper by the Ethics Committee, American College of Critical Care Medicine, Society of Critical Care Medicine. *Crit Care Med.* 2001;29:1826–1831.

CHAPTER
120
Altered Consciousness and Coma in the Intensive Care Unit

JOSEPH ZACHARIAH and EELCO F. M. WIJDICKS

INTRODUCTION

Impaired consciousness is a common neurologic problem in the intensive care unit (ICU). Neurologists are commonly consulted for "altered mental status," often after sedation has been discontinued, after cardiopulmonary resuscitation and failure to awaken, and in patients with multisystem trauma to address the extent of traumatic brain injury and assist in management. With the emergence of transplantation ICUs, neurologic complications have surfaced with many involving altered awareness.

The assessment of impaired consciousness or coma is a complex undertaking. Obviously, there are multiple factors in play, but simply denoting the cause of impaired consciousness as multifactorial would be counterproductive and, most likely, inaccurate. Some patterns, however, are apparent. First, prolonged accumulation of sedative agents in patients with impaired renal or hepatic function is common, and allowance of time for these agents to metabolize would lead to improvement. Second, hypoxic/ischemic injury to the brain is probably more likely than commonly appreciated. In the ICU, the circumstances for episodic hypoxemia and shock are commonly present, and therefore, the brain is at risk. Third, the clinical spectrum of the neurologic aspect of critical illness has become better defined. In many circumstances, with a plethora of potential causes of coma, it is possible to localize the lesion and diagnose the cause of coma. The more frequent use of magnetic resonance imaging (MRI) technology has increased, providing not only important diagnostic findings, but also prognostic pointers. This chapter provides the essentials of neurologic examination and places it into the context of the different ICUs.

ANATOMY

Consciousness is thought to arise from a network of neurons known as the reticular activating system (RAS) fibers connecting the thalamus with the cortex and dorsal forebrain. The RAS originates from various nuclei in the brainstem and receives input of several sensory pathways. In order to disturb consciousness, it is well known that the insult will either need to occur in the brainstem affecting the RAS pathway or result from a bihemispheric etiology. A patient with a chronic left-sided lesion can become transiently comatose with an acute right-sided insult. A unilateral lesion if large enough to cause either midline shift or affect the RAS pathway can also lead to altered consciousness. The RAS can also be affected by acute obstructive hydrocephalus typically noted in subarachnoid hemorrhage (SAH). Alternatively, electrolyte derangements or toxometabolic factors such as hyperammonemia from liver failure are also thought to contribute to a structural etiology by means of cerebral edema (1).

DEFINITIONS

There are various terms used to describe altered mental status. The term *unresponsive* has become a tired label which is disliked by many neurologists mostly because it can describe a variety of conditions ranging from awake and not responding to comatose or brain dead. Level of alertness is generally categorized into *alert, drowsy, somnolent,* and *comatose*. An *alert* patient is one who is awake and needs no further definition. *Drowsiness* is described as a patient who fluctuates in and out of alertness requiring mild to moderate amount of stimuli to awaken. A *stuporous* patient requires considerable stimuli, frequently painful stimuli, to transiently arouse and a *comatose* patient will not awake to any stimuli.

In addition to the level of alertness, consciousness can also be described with the content of awareness. A patient in an *acute confusional state*, frequently seen in drug intoxications, is one with profound impairments of memory, orientation, attention span, and difficulty following commands. Patients are described as *delirious* when they suffer hallucinations and autonomic hyperactivity such as tachycardia, hypertension, and hyperhidrosis in addition to their acute confusional state. *Delirium tremens* which occurs in the setting of alcohol or benzodiazepine withdrawal will present with hypertension, tachypnea, tachycardia, fever, and seizures. The seizure in the setting of delirium tremens is frequently generalized, but can frequently be focal in the presence of a pre-existing unilateral lesion. Coma and delirium in itself is an independent predictor of poor outcome.

Patients in a coma for a prolonged period of time start to develop sleep–wake cycles. Some eventually open their eyes and even follow minimal commands described as *minimally conscious*. On the other hand, those patients who remain comatose with the caveat of intact brainstem reflexes are described to be in a *persistent vegetative state*. Once these patients continue unchanged past 3 months for anoxic injury or 12 months for traumatic injury, chances of further recovery becomes bleak and the term *permanent vegetative state* should be used. Once all brain function ceases, *brain death* criteria should be considered and addressed. Further explanation of the *brain death* criteria is discussed toward the end of this chapter.

SCORING SYSTEMS

The two main standardized scales that are commonly used for patients in coma are the Glasgow Coma Scale (GCS) and the FOUR (Full Outline of UnResponsiveness) score (Table 120.1). These scoring systems have been validated across several different ICU and emergency departments. Scoring systems are invaluable in interphysician communication, and offer rough estimations of prognostication as well as therapeutic decision

TABLE 120.1 Comparison of the FOUR Score and the Glasgow Coma Scale

FOUR Score	Glasgow Coma Scale
Eye response	Eye response
4 = eyelids open or opened, tracking, or blinking to command	4 = eyes open spontaneously
3 = eyelids open but not tracking	3 = eye opening to verbal command
2 = eyelids closed but open to loud voice	2 = eye opening to pain
1 = eyelids closed but open to pain	1 = no eye opening
0 = eyelids remain closed with pain	Motor response
Motor response	6 = obeys commands
4 = thumbs up, fist, or peace sign	5 = localizing pain
3 = localizing to pain	4 = withdrawal from pain
2 = flexion response to pain	3 = flexion response to pain
1 = extension response to pain	2 = extension response to pain
0 = no response to pain or generalized myoclonus status	1 = no motor response
Brainstem reflexes	Verbal response
4 = pupil and corneal reflexes present	5 = oriented
3 = one pupil wide and fixed	4 = confused
2 = pupil or corneal reflexes absent	3 = inappropriate words
1 = pupil and corneal reflexes absent	2 = incomprehensible sounds
0 = absent pupil, corneal, and cough reflex	1 = no verbal response
Respiration	
4 = not intubated, regular breathing pattern	
3 = not intubated, Cheyne–Stokes breathing pattern	
2 = not intubated, irregular breathing	
1 = breathes above ventilator rate	
0 = breathes at ventilator rate or apnea	

FOUR, Full Outline of UnResponsiveness.
From Fischer M, Rüegg S, Czaplinski A, et al. Inter-rater reliability of the Full Outline of UnResponsiveness score and the Glasgow Coma Scale in critically ill patients: a prospective observational study. *Crit Care.* 2010;14(2):R64. Copyright © 2010 Fischer et al.

making; GCS under 8, intubate. The downside with GCS lies in intubated patients where the verbal component which makes up a third of the score cannot be reliably assessed. The advantage in the FOUR score system is that it can also point toward locked in syndrome, brainstem dysfunction, breathing patterns, increased intracranial pressure (ICP), or uncal herniation (2). See Chapters 118 and 119 for further information on these scoring systems.

CLINICAL EXAMINATION

The neurologic coma examination, admittedly limited, is still able to offer several localizing clues. The examination includes an assessment of mental status as described earlier, brainstem reflex testing, motor responses, tone, reflexes, and documentation of adventitious movements.

Brainstem Testing

Pupillary reflexes in themselves can point to the etiology of coma. Bilateral miotic pupils are most commonly the result of a pontine lesion or intoxication with drugs of abuse such as opiates or cocaine. On the other hand, bilateral mydriasis can be due to opiate withdrawal or intoxication with anticholinergics or drugs of sedating properties. Pupillary asymmetry can be the result of pathology to either the larger pupil in the setting of herniation causing blown pupil, or pathology to the smaller pupil in Horner syndrome. An acute Horner syndrome in the ICU is typically the result of damage to the third-order sympathetic chain fibers from internal jugular vein central line placement or to the second-order sympathetic fibers during thoracic surgery. Unilateral pupillary dilation in the setting of aerosolized anticholinergics for respiratory conditions or a scopolamine patch for nausea can commonly raise alarms and lead to unnecessary brain imaging. A unilateral blown pupil in an individual who is neurologically otherwise intact and able to converse normally should raise suspicion for topical drug-related mydriasis.

An acute oval pupil implies either midbrain disease or increased ICP with impending herniation. Chronic oval or irregular pupils reflect intrinsic eye disease or previous ocular surgery (2). Hippus is an intriguing, but normal, cyclic pupillary constriction and dilation to ongoing illumination which can catch the eye of the astute observer.

Forced gaze deviation can be seen in a multitude of etiologies and do not necessarily point toward a structural focus. Gaze preference on the other hand implies injury to the ipsilateral hemisphere in either frontal, parietal, or occipital gaze centers. Intermittent gaze preference would point toward an epileptic etiology. Downward gaze can occur in a lesion to the thalamus or dorsal midbrain as a result of either hypoxic/ischemic injury, increased ICP, or acute hydrocephalus. Upward gaze on the other hand is poorly localized, indicative of bihemispheric damage and seen especially in the setting of considerable anoxic injury. Skew deviation is the vertical malalignment of the eyes and indicates damage to either the brainstem or the cerebellum. Roving eye movements are constant spontaneous horizontal back and forth eye movements which are frequently seen in severe encephalopathy of any cause. Ping pong gaze is also spontaneous horizontal gaze that alternates every few seconds and has been seen in toxometabolic encephalopathy, strokes, and hemorrhages (3). Ocular bobbing is spontaneous rapid downward nystagmus with slow upward correction whereas ocular dipping is rapid upward nystagmus with slow downward correction, both indicating pontine damage. Finally, convergence nystagmus occurs with ocular divergence followed by rapid convergence. Most of the gaze findings with the exception of roving eye movements and forced gaze deviation are indicative of structural brain lesions.

Corneal reflexes test the integrity of ipsilateral cranial nerve (CN) V to bilateral CN VII. The examiner can squirt a small amount (about 2–3 mL) of normal saline into the eye and test for a blink response. This is advised in order to avoid corneal trauma via repeated scratch testing. Please take care in wiping tears of patients with infections transmissible via mucous membranes such as hepatitis C. If saline does not trigger a blink, one should proceed with a cotton wisp or the edge of a tissue and slightly touch the side of the cornea. Please keep in mind that corneal reflexes might not be consistent when patients develop corneal edema frequently seen in prolonged ICU admissions.

The facial nerve can be assessed grossly in the intubated patient by examining the symmetry of grimacing to painful stimuli. Vestibuloocular or oculocephalic reflexes test the reflex arc between CN VIII and CN III and VI. This test should be substituted with cold calorics if the patient is in a neck collar. Frequent missteps while performing the cold calorics testing include neglecting to examine the tympanic membrane for perforation and insufficient coldness to the water used.

Gag testing should be completed with a gloved hand physically gagging the comatose patient with the other hand over the diaphragm to assess for minimal responses. Reflex arcs for gag include CN V to CN X when stimulated on the soft palate and CN IX to CN X when assessed posteriorly by the pharynx. Cough reflex is stimulated by introducing a suction catheter into the endotracheal tube. One should note the depth of catheter advancement required to stimulate a cough reflex. The examiner should also note the ability of the patient to take independent breaths above the ventilator setting, so-called "breathing over the vent." This assessment can be tricky for several reasons. When patients are hyperventilated with a ventilator rate set at or above 18 breaths/min, there is usually no physiologic drive to breathe over the set rate. These patients would commonly be labeled as not breathing over the vent. On the other hand, the sensitivity of the ventilator in picking up an initial breath might be set so low that random movements can be misconstrued by the machine as an attempt to breath. These patients will falsely be labeled as breathing over the ventilator. There are several ways to assess for independent breathing including switching ventilation to spontaneous mode, disconnecting the ventilator transiently, or setting the respiratory rate low and the sensitivity high. In conclusion, a good coma brainstem examination can assess for CN II, III, V, VI, VII, VIII, IX, and X.

Motor Testing

Motor testing in an uncooperative patient can be difficult. Much of the testing is done by observation of spontaneous movements. Restraints on a patient can offer a good starting point of motor assessment. If a patient does not require restraints on his right arm, one would suspect paresis. Tone is a valuable component of the coma examination which is unfortunately frequently overlooked. Asymmetric tone is suspicious for hemiparesis whereas diffuse hypertonia raises suspicion for tetany or neuroleptic malignant syndrome (NMS). Tone predominantly increased in the lower extremities is a common presentation of serotonin syndrome (SS). Meningeal signs should also be tested with nuchal rigidity and Kernig and Brudzinski signs. Marked acute flaccidity might point to poisoning or drug intoxication whereas flaccidity in the setting of a prolonged ICU admission implies critical illness myopathy.

Miscellaneous Testing

Adventitious movements should be noted, especially fine rhythmic movements such as flickering of eyelids, continuous low amplitude jerking of any limb, or continued nystagmus which should raise alarm for nonconvulsive status epilepticus (NCSE). Asterixis or negative myoclonus, if noted, can point toward a hepatic or renal encephalopathy. Asterixis is seen not only in the failure to maintain extension of the hand at the wrist but also with the inability to sustain lip puckering or a flexion–abduction position at the hip.

LOCALIZATION

General Care Principles

The following subsections discuss the most common causes of altered awareness within each subset of patients. There is a plethora of causes for mental status changes and any of these etiologies can be found in any patient. Tables 120.2 and 120.3 review common items in a differential diagnosis of encephalopathy, separated by history, location, general examination findings, neurologic examination findings, laboratory results, and electrophysiologic testing and imaging.

Coma in the Infected Patient

Meningoencephalitis can undoubtedly result in mental status changes. With any suspicion for a meningeal infection, blood cultures should be drawn before antibiotics are administered, as long as doing so does not delay the dosing. Acyclovir should be added to the meningeal antimicrobial regimen until herpes simplex virus has been ruled out by cerebrospinal fluid (CSF) analysis.

Systemic infections resulting sepsis or septic shock commonly give rise to mental status changes largely as a result of hypoxic–ischemic conditions (4). One should be cautious in attributing altered mental status to a urinary tract infection unless in the setting of overt pyuria or urosepsis.

Altered consciousness can be triggered by not only systemic infections, but also by antibiotics or other drugs prescribed by medical practitioners (Table 120.4). The main culprits for antibiotic-induced encephalopathy are cefepime and metronidazole. Cefepime-related encephalopathy can be quite severe and has even been noted to present almost like brain death (5). Withdrawal of these antimicrobials should result in gradual mental status improvement.

Coma in the Risk-Taking Patient

Patients in this cohort are those who partake in substance abuse, either alcohol, illicit medications, or prescription medication. Performing toxicology screens are absolutely essential in the workup of patient with altered mental status; one needs be familiar with the various toxicology screens available in their institution between urine and serum analysis. Alcohol intoxication and withdrawal are obvious causes of mental status changes and will

TABLE 120.2 Common Considerations in a Differential Diagnosis of Encephalopathy

History

- Trauma
  - Concussion
  - Contusion
  - Intraparenchymal hemorrhage
  - SAH/SDH/epidural hemorrhage
  - Diffuse axonal injury
  - Herniation
  - Fat emboli
- Infected
  - Meningitis
  - Encephalitis
  - Sepsis
  - Antibiotics related
- Transplant
  - Hyperammonemia
  - Immunosuppressant toxicity
  - Opportunistic infections
- Cancer
  - Chemo neurotoxicity
  - Brain metastasis–induced seizure
  - Hemorrhagic brain metastasis
  - Carcinomatous meningitis
- Psychiatric/abuse
  - NMS/SS
  - Akinetic mutism
  - Benzodiazepine withdrawal
  - Psychogenic coma
  - Substance abuse
  - Delirium tremens
  - Wernicke encephalopathy

Location

- Medical ICU
  - Electrolyte imbalance
  - Acid–base disorder
  - Hypoglycemia
  - Hypoxia
  - PRES
  - Seizure
  - Adrenal insufficiency
- Cardiac ICU
  - Cardioembolic stroke
  - Hypoxic–ischemic injury
- Surgical ICU
  - Anesthesia clearance
  - Hypoxic–ischemic injury
  - Stroke
  - Serotonin syndrome
- Transplant ICU
  - Similar to surgical ICU
  - Electrolyte imbalance
  - Hyperammonemia
  - Immunosuppressant toxicity
  - Opportunistic infections

General Examination

- Fever
  - Meningitis
  - Sepsis
  - NMS/SS
  - SAH
  - PCP/ketamine
- Hypothermia
  - Environmental
  - Alcohol/opiates
  - Sedatives
  - Sepsis
  - Adrenal crisis
- Hypertension
  - Hypertensive encephalopathy
  - PRES
  - Stimulant intoxication
  - SAH
  - Eclampsia
- Hypotension
  - Sepsis
  - Sedative intoxication
- Tachycardia
  - Sepsis
  - Stimulant intoxication
  - Afib RVR
- Bradycardia
  - Sedative intoxication
  - Increased intracranial pressure
  - Organophosphates
- Breath
  - Fruity: ketoacidosis
  - Garlic: organophosphates
- Tachypnea
  - Sepsis
  - Metabolic acidosis
  - Brainstem damage
- Slow respirations
  - Sedatives
  - Brainstem damage
  - Organophosphates
- Ataxic breathing
  - Brainstem damage
- Skin
  - Jaundice + hepatomegaly, ascites, caput medusa
    - Hepatic encephalopathy
- Hyperhidrosis
  - NMS/SS
  - Organophosphates
  - Sympathetic storm
  - Hypoglycemia

Neurologic Examination

- Pupils
  - Miosis
    - Narcotics
    - Pontine lesion
  - Mydriasis
    - Stimulant overdose
    - Delirium or pain in neuromuscular blockade
  - Oval
    - Increased intracranial pressure
    - Eye surgery history
    - Midbrain injury
    - Intrinsic eye disease
  - Asymmetric
    - Herniation
    - Horner's
    - Topical drug-related mydriasis
- Gaze
  - Gaze preference
    - Persistent: contralateral gaze center lesion
    - Intermittent: seizure
  - Downgaze
    - Thalamus
    - Midbrain
    - Acute hydrocephalus
    - Increased intracranial pressure
  - Upgaze
    - Bihemispheric damage
  - Skew
    - Brainstem
    - Cerebellum
  - Bobbing
  - Dipping
    - Pontine
  - Forced deviation or roving
    - Nonlocalizing
- Strength
  - Asymmetric
    - Contralateral lesion
    - Ipsilateral false localizing sign
- Tone
  - Increased
    - Tetanus
    - NMS
    - Intoxication
    - Increased
    - Legs > arms: SS
  - Decreased
    - Intoxication
    - Critical illness myopathy
  - Asymmetric
    - Stroke
  - Meningismus
    - Meningitis
- Miscellaneous
  - Fine movements
    - Seizure
    - Tremor
  - Asterixis
    - Renal disease
    - Hepatic disease

Laboratory Studies

- Hypoglycemia
  - Excessive insulin
  - Cortisol deficiency
  - Sepsis
  - Alcohol
  - Insulinoma
- Hyperglycemia
  - Diabetic ketoacidosis
  - HONK

TABLE 120.2 Common Considerations in a Differential Diagnosis of Encephalopathy (*Continued*)

- Hyponatremia
  - Carbamazepine
  - Oxcarbazepine
  - Beer potomania
  - Thiazides
  - SIADH/CSW
- Hypernatremia
  - Hypovolemia
  - Insensible losses
  - Diabetes insipidus
- Hypomagnesemia
  - GI losses
  - Diuretics
  - Primary hyperparathyroidism
  - Uncontrolled diabetes
- Hypocalcemia
  - CKD
  - Sepsis
  - Drug induced
  - PTH abnormalities
  - Acid–base derangement
  - Pancreatitis
- Hypercalcemia
  - CKD
  - Malignancy
  - Adrenal insufficiency
  - Thiazides
  - Lithium
- Hyperammonemia
  - Liver disease
  - Urea cycle d/o
  - Valproic acid
  - Lung transplant
- Metabolic acidosis
  - MUDPILES
- Metabolic alkalosis
  - Vomiting
  - Diuretics
  - Contraction alkalosis
- Respiratory acidosis
  - Sedatives
  - Hypercarbic respiratory failure
- Respiratory alkalosis
  - Salicylate
  - Central hyperventilation
  - Pneumonia

Electrocardiography

- Prolonged QTc interval
  - Psychiatric medications
  - Electrolyte imbalance
  - Hypothermia
  - Structural brain damage
- Inverted T waves
  - SAH
  - Intraparenchymal hemorrhage
  - Increased ICP

Electroencephalography

- Triphasic waves
  - Hepatic disease
  - Renal disease
  - Metabolic causes
  - Hypoxia
- Diffuse slowing
  - Nonlocalizing
- Focal slowing or PLEDs
  - Focal lesion
  - HSV
- GPEDs
  - Anoxic injury
  - Metabolic causes
  - Infections
- Burst suppression
  - Anesthetics
  - Anoxia
- Seizures
  - Convulsive seizures
  - Nonconvulsive status epilepticus
- Alpha coma
  - Hypoxia
  - Drug overdose
- Excessive beta
  - Benzodiazepine
  - Barbiturates
- Inactive
  - Hypothermia
  - Sedatives
  - Brain death
- Normal
  - Infratentorial lesion
  - Brainstem lesion
  - Alcohol withdrawal
  - Locked in syndrome
  - Psychogenic

Neuroimaging

- Cortical lesions
  - Neoplasm
  - Stroke
  - Infectious
  - Prolonged seizure
- White matter lesions
  - Stroke
  - Toxin/drug induced
  - Infectious
  - Fat emboli
  - Neoplasm
  - Prolonged seizure
- Hydrocephalus
  - Intraventricular hemorrhage
  - Meningitis
  - Carcinomatous meningitis
- PRES
  - Hypertension
  - Toxin/drug induced
- Hemorrhage
  - SAH
  - Intraparenchymal
  - SDH
  - Epidural hemorrhage
  - Contusion
- Extra-axial
  - Tumor
  - SDH
  - Epidural hemorrhage
- Herniation
  - Tumor
  - Large infarct
  - Large hemorrhage
  - Large abscess
- Normal
  - See Table 120.3

not be discussed further. Please see *Definitions* section on *delirium tremens*. With any suspicion for alcohol history, administer thiamine prior to glucose in order to avoid depletion of thiamine stores and precipitation of Wernicke encephalopathy.

Drug intoxication, be it illicit or prescription overdose, can be difficult to confirm at times. The metabolic rate to clear massive overdoses might be unpredictable and daily toxicology screens might be required to assure clearance of the offending agent. Of note, several of the newer synthetic illicit substances do not surface in conventional drug screens.

Coma in the Neurologic Patient

In addition to the etiologies listed in these subcategories, neurologic patients can present with abrupt mental status changes in the setting of certain infarcts, acute hydrocephalus, postictal periods, and herniation syndromes. Strokes causing altered awareness without focal findings include diffuse embolic shower commonly seen in patients with atrial fibrillation, a temporal lobe infarct, or a thalamic infarct. Keep in mind that not all strokes result in a focal finding; among infarcts, a strategic infarct of the pons can result in a locked in state in which patients have movement limited only to eyes. These patients appear to be comatose but are locked in with intact awareness as the RAS arc is spared. They have an intact ability to communicate via eye blinking and should not be classified as comatose.

Acute hydrocephalus in the setting of SAH can present as a brain dead patient. With confirmation via computerized tomography (CT) of the head, prompt CSF drainage can result in rapid improvement of mental status.

TABLE 120.3 Altered Mental Status with Normal CT/MRI of the Head

CT Scan
General
Electrolyte imbalance
Hepatic or uremic encephalopathy
Hypoglycemia
Meningitis
Carcinomatous meningitis
Most drug-induced encephalopathy
Intoxication or withdrawal syndromes
SAH
Wernicke encephalopathy
Early encephalitis
Early PRES
Amniotic fluid embolus
Psychiatric
NMS/SS
Psychogenic coma
Trauma
Concussion
Early diffuse axonal injury
Neurologic
Seizure or nonconvulsive status epilepticus
Early hypoxic–ischemic injury
Diffuse small embolic shower
Fat emboli
Early ischemic infarct
MRI
General
Electrolyte imbalance
Hepatic or uremic encephalopathy
Hypoglycemia (unless severe)
Meningitis (requires contrast)
Carcinomatous meningitis (requires contrast)
Most drug-induced encephalopathy
Intoxication or withdrawal syndromes
Psychiatric
NMS/SS
Psychogenic coma
Trauma
Concussion
Neurologic
Seizure or nonconvulsive status epilepticus (unless prolonged)
Early hypoxic–ischemic injury

Patients with a history of seizures presenting with altered awareness should point to a postictal state. Look for clues of seizure such as Todd paresis or tongue trauma. Prolactin is released when a seizure focus runs through the thalamus. Levels are elevated only in cases of status epilepticus, generalized and complex partial seizures, not in focal or non convulsive seizures. Utility of prolactin levels is limited to distinguishing an epileptic convulsion from a pseudoseizure. An electroencephalogram (EEG) can be useful to rule out NCSE in patients with a prolonged postictal state with occasional adventitious movements described above.

TABLE 120.4 Causes of Drug-Induced Encephalopathy

Antibiotics
Cefepime
Metronidazole
Linezolid (rare)
Clarithromycin (rare)
Anesthetics
Bupivacaine
Morphine
Neuroleptics
Haldol
Lithium
Clozapine
Amitriptyline
Most antiepileptic medications
Immunosuppressants
IVIg
Antineoplastic
Tacrolimus
Capecitabine
Cisplatin (rare)
Ifosfamide
Vincristine
Cyclosporine
Methotrexate

From Hansen N. Drug-induced encephalopathy. In: Tanasescu R, ed. *Miscellanea on Encephalopathies: A Second Look.* Intech Open Access website. http://www.intechopen.com/books/miscellanea-on-encephalopathies-a-second-look/drug-induced-encephalopathy. Published April 25, 2012; accessed March 15, 2015.

Any of the herniation syndromes can result in altered awareness, if not coma. These patients exhibit Cushing reflex—bradycardia and hypertension—prior to having respiratory compromise, which completes the triad of Cushing. Interventions to lower intracerebral pressure such as hyperosmolar or hypertonic therapy, transient hyperventilation, and head of bed elevation to 30 degrees should be rapidly instituted. Treatment specifics for increased ICP are discussed in Chapter 118.

Coma in the Psychiatric Patient

Altered awareness in the psychiatric patient can result from NMS, SS, akinetic mutism, or benzodiazepine withdrawal, to name but a few of the causes.

NMS and SS should be at the top of the physician's differential diagnostic list for psychiatric patients. There are numerous medications that can precipitate either of the syndromes and it is imperative to abort the offending agent as soon as it is discovered. NMS can present with many of the same signs and symptoms as SS. Both syndromes can cause altered awareness to varying degrees, fever, hypertonicity, and autonomic dysfunction. The onset of NMS is generally slower taking days to weeks whereas SS can occur abruptly. SS can also be differentiated by the presence of shivering and marked hypertonicity of the lower extremities compared to NMS which presents with symmetric hypertonicity. Hyporeflexia can be seen with NMS as opposed to hyperreflexia with SS. In either syndrome, the offending agent should be discontinued and benzodiazepine started, making the point that differentiating between the two syndromes is nowhere as important as implementing medication changes.

Patients with advanced psychiatric conditions can also present with akinetic mutism when falling ill with another medical condition. In this syndrome, patients appear locked in, only capable of moving their eyes, but have an unremarkable neurologic examination. Yet another issue is that scheduled benzodiazepines are frequently in a psychiatric patient's outpatient medication regimen. Many of these medications are not continued for various reasons during an admission, which may result in benzodiazepine withdrawal gradually occurring.

Malingering patients can present with psychogenic coma, a diagnosis of exclusion. In addition to appearing to be in a coma, these patients resist and avoid various stimuli ranging from mildly irritating to noxious. The classic test of dropping the arm over the face will result in the patient swinging it down to avoid the face. Performing a cold caloric vestibuloocular test in a nonorganic coma patient might be the ultimate noxious stimuli resulting in emesis and rapid reversal of coma.

Coma in the Medical Care Unit

The medical intensive care unit (MICU) encounters its fair share of patients with altered mental status. In addition to the several etiologies discussed earlier in this chapter, the most common causes of encephalopathy in the MICU includes metabolic causes such as electrolyte imbalances, acid–base disturbances, blood sugar derangements, hypoxia, and drug-induced encephalopathy; Table 120.4 lists medications frequently resulting in encephalopathy.

Patients with renal, hepatic, or gastrointestinal comorbidities affecting absorption frequently have electrolyte imbalances. The main electrolytes at play for encephalopathy include sodium, magnesium, and calcium. Hepatic failure can result in hyperammonemia, which improves with lactulose. Renal failure, when severe, can cause mental status changes due to acidemia, further electrolyte changes, or uremic encephalopathy; the initial dialysis session can also trigger encephalopathy due to osmotic shifts with the initial dialysis, a condition known as dialysis disequilibrium syndrome.

Endocrine-related etiologies of mental status changes include severe hypothyroidism known as Hashimoto encephalopathy, as well as severe hypo- or hyperglycemia from poor insulin management. Acute adrenal insufficiency, Addison disease, can present due to either insufficient steroid supplementation at times of physical stress—such as surgery—or sepsis. As the adrenal crisis progress, patients can become profoundly encephalopathic, although, if treated appropriately, prognosis is good. Acidosis and hypoxia are very common in the MICU from various respiratory causes. Mental status changes resulting from severe hypoxia have a grim prognosis with respect to recovery; further details are discussed in the cardiac patient subcategory. The clinical spectrum of acidosis can range from neurologically intact to seizures and coma.

Patients with uncontrolled hypertension can develop posterior reversible encephalopathy syndrome (PRES). MRI of the brain shows white matter changes in posterior lobes, but these changes can also be found in the rest of the brain. When the high blood pressure is addressed, patients generally return to their baseline unless the PRES lesions resulted in ischemic or hemorrhagic complications.

Coma in the Pregnant Patient

Pregnant patients with preeclampsia are routinely subject to PRES, described above. One frequently overlooked detail is the patient's baseline blood pressure. Pregnant women usually have low blood pressures and a sudden rise of systolic pressures to 160 or 170 might be high enough to trigger PRES. Seizures can result with eclampsia and should be treated immediately with magnesium. Seizures and altered mental status may also be the result of HELLP syndrome which is composed of hemolysis, elevated liver enzymes, and low platelets. With thrombocytopenia, widespread bleeding can occur including SAH. Treatment includes antihypertensives, platelet transfusions, and prompt delivery of the baby. Peripartum abrupt mental status changes are alarming, and usually due to either pituitary apoplexy or amniotic fluid embolism, both of which can have grim prognoses.

Coma in the Cardiac Care Unit

Consultations from the cardiac ICU for encephalopathy are mostly resultant to either cardioembolic infarcts or postresuscitative mental status changes; see the subsection on coma in neurologic patients for details on stroke-related encephalopathy.

With layperson CPR becoming commonplace, the survival of patients who suffer cardiac arrest has increased. Prognosis after cardiac arrest has become increasingly difficult in the era of hypothermia. Several of the previously known factors pointing toward poor prognosis are now noted to have higher false-positive rates (FPRs). Absence of pupillary reactivity, myoclonic jerks on the first day of arrest, absent somatosensory responses, and serum neuron–specific enolase (NSE) value more than 33 ng/mL previously had very low individual FPRs. Several case series have been published in regard to each of these prognostication markers with higher FPRs (6–9). It is important to consider these factors together for accurate prognostication after cardiac arrest in order to avoid the self-fulfilling prophecy that results from withdrawal of care.

Coma in the Postoperative Patient

The most common reasons for coma or altered awareness in a postoperative patient include delayed anesthesia clearance, hypoxic or ischemic injury suffered during surgery, or fentanyl-related SS. A patient's baseline cognitive status can help predict the rate of recovery from anesthesia. A patient that is demented will take longer to recover than a cognitively healthy individual. If a cognitive baseline is not available, a CT of the head showing considerable atrophy can be of help in determining the cause for slow emergence. Delayed clearance of anesthetics can also occur in patients with pre-existing hepatic or renal failure. To add to this, complicated surgeries can require patients to be placed under sedation for days to recover purely from a surgical standpoint. It is near impossible to predict when prolonged and continuous sedation will be completely metabolized. Finally, as surgical procedures are being performed in an increasingly aging population, it is not uncommon for patients to emerge from anesthesia after surgery with a stroke. Hypoxic/anoxic injury after surgery, resultant from prolonged esophageal intubation, is thankfully rare given the monitoring changes implemented in modern operating suites and driven by anesthesiology, such as pulse oximetry and capnography, among others.

Fentanyl is commonly used in the operating room, and patients on concomitant psychotropic medications with renal failure can be prone to SS. When patients are in the recovery room, altered mental status may not be recognized, and shivering from SS sets in; meperidine is frequently given for postoperative shivering which turns out to be another precipitant of SS. Unfortunately, SS is often not recognized, and patients can decline secondary to this failure to recognize. It requires an astute observer to note hypertonicity in the legs greater than arms to introduce SS into the differential diagnosis.

Coma in the Posttransplant Patient

Much related to coma in the posttransplant patients is shared with postoperative patients. However, in addition to the previously mentioned causes, the posttransplant patients also suffer from electrolyte derangements, hyperammonemia, neurotoxicity from potent immunosuppressive agents, and opportunistic infections.

Among opportunistic agents, cytomegalovirus, *Cryptococcus neoformans,* or *Aspergillus fumigatus* are common players. Cytomegalovirus, although the most common systemic posttransplant opportunistic infection, rarely triggers encephalitis. Fungi, on the other hand, can result in numerous brain abscesses which are both generators of seizures and may also result in intracranial hemorrhage. Aspergillosis should be considered in a posttransplant patient with multiple simultaneous intracranial hemorrhages.

Toxicity from either chemotherapeutic or immunosuppressant agents usually results in a gradual alteration of consciousness. MRI generally reveals diffuse white matter lesions, which are fully reversible with discontinuation of the medication. Tacrolimus and cyclosporine commonly cause neurotoxicity, whereas sirolimus is generally well tolerated from a neurologic standpoint (9). Seizures occur in up to 39% of cardiac transplant patients, most frequently due to immunosuppressive medications.

Coma in the Cancer Patient

Cancer patients are unfortunately subject to neurotoxicity from chemotherapeutics, seizures from cerebral metastasis, and intracerebral hemorrhage of metastases or carcinomatous meningitis.

Methotrexate is an agent notorious for causing encephalopathy. MRI usually demonstrates widespread white matter changes, not necessarily reversible if the agent is not discontinued promptly. Cerebral metastasis or primary neoplasms frequently bleeding include glioblastoma multiforme, renal cell carcinoma, small cell cancer of the lung, melanoma, and choriocarcinoma. These tumors have a higher incidence of bleeding as they are highly vascular or tend to erode into vasculature, as in the case of choriocarcinoma (10). Tumors that trigger seizures are usually slow growing primary brain tumors such as gliomas or a metastasis to the cortical surface. Typical cerebral metastasis that induce seizures include melanoma and lung and breast cancers (11). Lamotrigine, valproic acid, and topiramate are first-line antiepileptic treatments of choice (12).

Carcinomatous meningitis can be a difficult entity to diagnose, often requiring a high-quality MRI and several spinal fluid samples. The sensitivity for CSF cytology can be as low as 50% (13), with modest gains on repeat taps. Patients usually present with subacute signs very similar to meningoencephalitis, but may also acutely decompensate if hydrocephalus develops.

Coma in the Trauma Patient

Altered consciousness in the trauma patient is self-evidently due to damage to the structural integrity of the brain. The etiologies are most commonly contusion, concussion, and/or hemorrhage, be it subarachnoid, epidural, subdural, or intraparenchymal and, in severe cases, diffuse axonal injury (DAI) or herniation. If the patient has a poor coma scale score, demonstrated by either GCS or FOUR systems, an ICP monitor should be placed. Patients should be examined for periorbital or mastoid ecchymosis known as raccoon and Battle signs, respectively, both indicating skull fractures; CSF otorrhea and rhinorrhea can be noted in these cases.

Depending on the severity of injury, patients can have either concussions or contusions. Any of the different types of hemorrhage can present with coma depending on the degree of mass effect, brain shift, and subsequent swelling. Neurosurgery's timely drainage or decompression of the lesion determines the best outcome. If this drainage does not occur, and if patients undergo uncal herniation, the mesial temporal lobe can cause mass effect and push the brainstem over to the contralateral side. As the contralateral cerebral peduncle is pushed against the tentorium, the patient develops paresis of the ipsilateral side to the primary brain injury. Hence, a patient with injury to the left temple can have left hemiparesis. This is known as the Kernohan notch phenomenon or the "uncal herniation false localizing sign" and is a frequent cause of misdiagnosis.

Fat embolus is a rare etiology for altered awareness in the setting of long bone injury after trauma. The fat emboli can cause pulmonary edema, marked hypoxia, and subconjunctival or axillary petechiae. These patients have a star-speckled pattern of diffusion changes on MRI of the brain, which slowly resolves over 3 to 4 weeks; these patients generally have an excellent recovery. Unfortunately, after the trauma patient is stabilized, some do not awaken. These patients should be considered to have, and worked up for severe DAI. DAI is known to occur mostly in younger patients, in whom trauma may disrupt nerve fiber integrity in a global fashion. Recovery from DAI is grim; follow-up scans will demonstrate widespread atrophy of injured regions.

EXAMPLE CASES

Case 1

A middle-aged patient with a history of seizures and hypertension presents in a comatose state. There is no additional history or witnesses available. Vital signs demonstrate a normotensive and afebrile individual with slow breaths, bradycardia, and desaturations while on supplemental oxygen, which leads to endotracheal intubation (ETI). The differential diagnosis is broad at this point with a high suspicion for seizures. General and neurologic examinations are unrevealing apart from roving eye movements, which are nonlocalizing. Laboratory studies, including toxicology screen, are unremarkable except for an arterial blood gas analysis, performed prior to ETI, consistent with respiratory acidosis. An EEG is obtained and the report states "excessive beta activity without seizures"; a CT of the head is unremarkable. In keeping with Table 120.2, the differential diagnosis in this case leads to either benzodiazepine or barbiturate overdose; diligent review of the patient's medication regimen reveals phenobarbital and a laboratory study confirms overdose.

Case 2

An elderly, anxious, individual is evaluated for, cleared for, and undergoes a liver transplant. The surgery is a success and the patient does well, about to be discharged on postoperative day 4. On the morning of discharge, the nurse pulls you aside to state that the patient has become quite agitated. Examination reveals a restless and tremulous individual with tachycardia, tachypnea, elevated blood pressure, and diaphoresis. Halfway through the examination, the patient suffers a generalized tonic–clonic seizure, without localizing signs. Laboratory studies and CT imaging of the head are unrevealing, and EEG demonstrates mild diffuse slowing, commonly seen after seizure. Careful review of the patient's medications reveal that he takes 2 mg of lorazepam orally three times daily for anxiety, which had not been continued during his admission. This presentation is of benzodiazepine withdrawal, unfortunately a common scenario. The importance of scrutinizing medications cannot be overstated.

Case 3

A middle aged patient with no known medical history presents in a confused state with bloody emesis. Examination reveals tachycardia, the odor of alcohol on patient's breath, ascites, and *caput medusa*. Neurologic examination shows roving eye movements, decreased muscle tone, and asterixis. Laboratory studies of hepatic function and ammonia confirm a suspicion for hepatic encephalopathy and the patient was treated with lactulose.

MANAGEMENT

The initial evaluation of the patient with altered mental status should include a brief history, assessing airway, breathing, vital signs, obtaining a coma scale score, and general and neurologic examination, basic laboratory studies including electrolyte panel, magnesium, ammonia, liver function studies, blood glucose, blood and urine toxicology screens including alcohol level. A list of the basic steps for initial management is listed in Table 120.5. The most important step is the diligent screening of both outpatient and inpatient medication regimens. Needless to say, the etiologies for encephalopathy are so diverse such that treatment regimen relies heavily on accurate diagnosis.

TABLE 120.5 Workup of Altered Mental Status

- *Accurate* medication list—both inpatient and outpatient regimens
- Assess for drug interactions
- Laboratory studies
  - Electrolyte panel including calcium, magnesium, creatinine
  - Complete blood count
  - Liver function panel
  - Ammonia
  - Urine and blood toxicology screen
  - Blood alcohol level
  - Blood sugar
  - Drug levels where appropriate
  - Blood and urine cultures
  - Thyroid function tests
  - Arterial blood gas analysis
- Other studies
  - CT head
  - MRI head
  - Lumbar puncture
  - EEG

TABLE 120.6 Head Imaging Not Required

- Hypoglycemia
- Hyperammonemia
- Drug or alcohol intoxication (unless cocaine)
- Electrolyte derangements

If appropriate, CT or MRI of the brain should be obtained. Not all conditions, however, necessitate neuroimaging (Table 120.6), and there are numerous etiologies of altered consciousness where neuroimaging will not reveal a diagnosis (Table 120.3); nonetheless, despite obvious laboratory findings, certain situations warrant further imaging (Table 120.7).

Lumbar puncture and EEG can be considered in the situations outlined in Table 120.8 has become available, the use of EEG has been limited to ruling out NCSE. A certain degree of slowing is an expected EEG finding in the setting of encephalopathy of any cause; triphasic waves, on the other hand, indicate encephalopathy related to either hepatic or renal failure. Burst suppression and a lack of reactivity can be associated with poor outcome unless in the setting of sedation, hypothermia, or drug intoxication. Further details of EEG results are outlined late in Table 120.2.

With increased ICP, neurosurgery can assist with either placement of a ventriculostomy drain, removal of the mass lesion, or performing a craniotomy. Medical management of increased ICP will be discussed in Chapter 118.

Delirium

Typical antipsychotics, such as haloperidol and chlorpromazine, have been traditionally used due to their more desirable adverse effect profile. In recent years, atypical antipsychotics such as quetiapine or olanzapine have gained traction as first-line medication with less extrapyramidal effects; with pre-existing prolonged QTc, aripiprazole should be used instead. Benzodiazepines should only be used for benzodiazepine withdrawal, NMS, or SS and signs of respiratory depression should be monitored.

Nonpharmacologic interventions can also significantly assist in abating delirium. These techniques include frequent reorientation, offering visual or auditory assist devices to prevent sensory deprivation, sleep enhancement, ensuring optimal sleep–wake cycle, and using the presence of family members or placement of familiar photographs in the room. Bodily restraints should be kept to a minimum. See Chapter 123 for further information.

Prognosis

Prognosis of alterations of mental status is understandably related to the etiology. A judgment of prognosis cannot be

TABLE 120.7 Head Imaging Recommended Despite Obvious Laboratory Abnormality

- Cocaine intoxication—not uncommonly cause hemorrhage or infarcts
- Any laboratory finding with focality in examination or focality in seizure
- Mental status not improving despite corrected abnormality.

TABLE 120.8 Instrumentation versus EEG

Consider lumbar puncture
With fever, new or severe headache, meningismus, or unclear etiology
Without focal mass lesion on imaging
Send the following studies: Gram stain, cell count with differential, culture, cytology, flow cytometry
Consider EEG
Fluctuations in consciousness or fine motor movements noted

made if a patient's encephalopathy is stated as multifactorial. Most etiologies of mental status changes have very good potential if discovered early. The longer the patient goes undiagnosed, the bleaker the recovery. The causes of encephalopathy with poor prognosis include TBI, cardiac arrest, and severe cerebral structural damage such as large hemorrhages, multifocal hemorrhages, or infarcts or basilar thrombosis.

Important prognostic factors in cardiac arrest include time without circulation and the presence of poor prognostication signs such as early myoclonus, absent pupillary and corneal reflexes, absent somatosensory evoked potentials, and elevated NSE values. Prognosis for TBI patients is determined by prehospital hypoxemia and the extent of injury. Improvements in TBI patients can commence up to 12 months from initial injury and so medical providers should be wary of offering an early prognosis.

Brain Death

The topic of brain death commonly provokes a certain degree of unrest in those inexperienced in the subject, especially in light of recent public misconceptions of brain dead individuals. Once a patient suffers a catastrophic brain injury and brain death criteria are fulfilled, the patient should be declared dead. Although brain dead, some patients continue to demonstrate movements either spontaneously or with stimuli. This is known as the Lazarus sign and can cause great uncertainty in the family and uneasiness in the medical staff. Family should be warned of possible spinal reflexes that might continue to occur for a short period of time after brain death (see Chapter 119).

Withdrawal of Care

Once a poor prognosis is recognized, many families opt to withdraw care, rightfully so based on the patient's preferences or established directives of care. The presence of the neurointensivist at family discussions is often useful, especially in discussions of withdrawal of care. Family members should be comforted in that patients will pass without pain or suffering under the guidance of the ICU and palliative care teams. Seizure medications should not be withdrawn with the rest of the patient's medications as a seizure during active withdrawal of care would be haunting in the eyes of mourning family at bedside. The deciding family member delivering the final withdrawal of care decision should be repeatedly consoled as they can become overconsumed by guilt in the coming months.

Key Points

- Precise diagnosis of the cause of altered mental status should be found.
- Avoid the label of multifactorial mental status changes.
- *Scrutinize* the patients drug regimen, both outpatient and inpatient.
- The general examination and neurologic examination can be invaluable even in a comatose patient.
- Be aware of situations where neuroimaging is recommended despite discovery of seemingly obvious etiology.
- Be knowledgeable in etiologies that result in unrevealing CT or MRI.
- Be diligent in obtaining further studies such as EEG and LP.
- A favorable prognosis frequently depends on early and accurate diagnosis.

References

1. Wijdicks EF. Clinical scales for comatose patients: the Glasgow Coma Scale in historical context and the new FOUR Score. *Rev Neurol Dis.* 2006;3(3):109–117.
2. Mittal MK, Rabinstein AA, Wijdicks EF. Pearls & oy-sters: oval pupil: two observations. *Neurology.* 2013;81(17):e124–e125.
3. Kuroiwa Y, Toda H. [Clinical aspects of abnormal eye movements]. *Rinsho Shinkeigaku.* 2003;43(11):765–768.
4. Wijdicks EF, Stevens M. The role of hypotension in septic encephalopathy following surgical procedures. *Arch Neurol.* 1992;49(6):653–656.
5. Fugate JE, Kalimullah EA, Hocker SE, et al. Cefepime neurotoxicity in the intensive care unit: a cause of severe, underappreciated encephalopathy. *Crit Care.* 2013;17(6):R264.
6. Daubin C, Quentin C, Allouche S, et al. Serum neuron-specific enolase as predictor of outcome in comatose cardiac-arrest survivors: a prospective cohort study. *BMC Cardiovasc Disord.* 2011;11:48.
7. Fugate JE, Wijdicks EF, Mandrekar J, et al. Predictors of neurologic outcome in hypothermia after cardiac arrest. *Ann Neurol.* 2010;68(6):907–914.
8. Rossetti AO, Oddo M, Logroscino G, Kaplan PW. Prognostication after cardiac arrest and hypothermia: a prospective study. *Ann Neurol.* 2010; 67(3):301–307.
9. Wijdicks EF. Neurotoxicity of immunosuppressive drugs. *Liver Transpl.* 2001;7(11):937–942.
10. van den Doel EM, van Merrienboer FJ, Tulleken CA. Cerebral hemorrhage from unsuspected choriocarcinoma. *Clin Neurol Neurosurg.* 1985; 87(4):287–290.
11. Gavrilovic IT, Posner JB. Brain metastases: epidemiology and pathophysiology. *J Neurooncol.* 2005;75(1):5–14.
12. van Breemen MS, Wilms EB, Vecht CJ. Epilepsy in patients with brain tumours: epidemiology, mechanisms, and management. *Lancet Neurol.* 2007;6(5):421–430.
13. Gomes HR. Cerebrospinal fluid approach on neuro-oncology. *Arq Neuropsiquiatr.* 2013;71(9B):677–680.

CHAPTER
121
Status Epilepticus

DAVID S. GLOSS II

INTRODUCTION

Definitions and Classifications

The classification system used by the International League Against Epilepsy (ILAE) is probably the most commonly used system for epilepsy. Herein, I talk about status epilepticus (SE) using parts of their more recent classification documents (1,2), except for that which does not address SE (3).

The definition of SE is, itself, embroiled in controversy. The 1993 ILAE guidelines for epidemiologic studies give a definition of SE as a seizure lasting more than 30 minutes, or more than one epileptic seizures where function has not been regained for more than 30 minutes (4). In certain animal models, 30 minutes is the time in which neuronal injury occurs, so there is logic to the 30-minute window; unfortunately, none of the American Academy of Neurology (AAN) class I trials on SE use the 30-minute definition. The Veterans Administration SE cooperative trial, for example, used 10 minutes as its inclusion criteria; others have suggested time periods ranging from 5 to 15 minutes (5). In keeping with this definitional controversy, a Yale University study of patients with complex partial status epilepticus found no significant difference between episodes of SE lasting more or less than 30 minutes (6). This has led some to create an operational, or impending, definition of SE, in which a seizure is treated as if it were SE after 5 minutes, even if it cannot be formally diagnosed until 30 minutes.

The classification of SE contains 11 different types and subtypes:

1. Epilepsia partialis continua (EPC) of Jevnikov: This is a combination of focal seizures with ongoing twitching of the same area. There are three subtypes of EPC.
   a. Rasmussen syndrome—EPC with Rasmussen syndrome has focal myoclonus and focal seizures emanating from the same hemisphere. There is variability to the EEG correlate of the myoclonic jerks, and there is persistence of the jerks in sleep. The EEG shows progressive background slowing in the affected hemisphere. Antiepileptic drugs (AEDs) are largely ineffective for the treatment of Rasmussen-related EPC (7). The definitive treatment for Rasmussen syndrome, in general, is surgical.
   b. Focal lesions—EPC with focal lesions have jerks affecting the same area as the focal seizures, but do not persist in sleep. These can persist for days to months and may also be seen with nonketotic hyperglycemia. Treatment is generally with AEDs and discovering the underlying cause. Focal lesions do not represent the same kind of emergency as generalized convulsive SE. One group noted that the range of EPC lasted from 1 hour to 48 months (8). In their series, there were 26 patients in whom seizures remained uncontrolled; only three died. In another series of 46 patients with EPC, four died due to underlying infarction, nine had morbidity: six due to underlying cause, one due to the status, and two of unclear etiology (9).
   c. Inborn errors of energy metabolism—EPC with inborn errors of metabolism have unilateral then bilateral rhythmic jerks, which persist in sleep, with an EEG correlate. These inborn errors of metabolism for which EPC occurs are the ones affecting energy metabolism, like MERRF (myoclonic epilepsy with ragged red fibers) or Alpers syndrome. These cases are quite rare, and there are only case reports and small case series of published experience. In general, expert consultation is advised, and treatment is not particularly likely to be successful. It is probably best to avoid the use of valproic acid in these patients (10).
2. Supplementary motor area (SMA): There are two subtypes of SMA.
   a. Subgroup 1 is composed of individual tonic motor seizures that occur every few minutes through the night.
   b. Subgroup B is composed of repetitive seizures, which evolve to a bilateral, convulsive seizure, which then become repetitive asymmetrical tonic motor seizures with impairment of consciousness.
3. Aura continua: These involve seizure episodes without impairment of consciousness, with symptoms—depending upon localization—which wax and wane, often for hours. Symptoms may include a motor component, dysesthesia, painful sensations, or visual changes. Perhaps the most common form is limbic aura continua, which may include fear, epigastric rising, or other limbic features, which recur every few minutes for hours or longer; EEG correlation is variable and these can evolve into, or alternate with, dyscognitive focal status (see below section 4). In such cases, the seizures are categorized as dyscognitive focal seizures. Treatment depends upon etiology; if the seizure develops after a neurosurgical procedure, it may explain hemiparesis or aphasia of unknown etiology, even days after surgery, and can be treated with an AED (11). If the etiology is related to a nonsurgical cause of epilepsy, the condition is typically chronic, and treatment is meant to provide symptomatic relief (12); in these cases, there is no emergency.
4. Dyscognitive focal (focal seizures with impairment of consciousness or awareness leading to status epilepticus). These are most commonly called complex partial seizures and are divided into two types.
   a. Mesial temporal dyscognitive focal SE are a series of dyscognitive focal seizures without clear return of consciousness between events. Electrographic onset can be unilateral, or can alternate sides.
   b. Neocortical dyscognitive focal status epilepticus is unpredictable. It may mimic absence status, generalized tonic–clonic status, or repetitive discrete seizures; the

symptoms may reflect the localization. Complex partial status epilepticus represents about 20% of all cases of SE (13). It is generally thought to be a relatively benign condition, although in cases where it persists for 36 hours or longer, it can cause significant neurologic deficits or death (14). In general, complex partial SE is treated initially as is generalized convulsive status epilepticus (GCSE) with some variation (15).

5. Tonic–clonic seizures are what people generally think about when they consider status epilepticus, but the more proper term is generalized convulsive status epilepticus (GCSE); some use the term status epilepticus to mean GCSE, but this is confusing, and should be avoided. GCSE may appear as a primary generalized event from genetic and structural/metabolic causes, commonly (but not always) evolving into bilateral, convulsive seizures from a focal start; sometimes the process is unilateral. There are several important features that are not mentioned in the ILAE classification. For example, with GCSE there is always profound impairment of consciousness. There can be variable combinations of tonic, clonic, or tonic–clonic seizures in an episode of SE. It is important to note that, at least for focal-onset tonic–clonic seizures, they are in a dynamic state. If SE continues, the motor manifestations may wane, until there are only subtle movements, often termed subtle status (see below section 9) Before the motor manifestations wane, there will be a clear ictal EEG component which ends abruptly when the seizure ends. If the patient does not fully return to baseline before the next tonic–clonic seizure starts, it is termed tonic–clonic SE. Treatment of GCSE will be dealt with in a later section.

   Genetic epilepsy is one in which a known or presumed genetic defect(s) results in seizures which are the core symptom of the disorder. A structural/metabolic epilepsy is one in which there is a demonstrated increased risk of epilepsy with the structural or metabolic condition.

6. Typical and atypical absence seizures: Absence and atypical absence may actually be several different types of SE, which have a similar presentation. Both absence and atypical absence may be seen in genetic epilepsies, and are terminated by AEDs. In generalized structural/metabolic epilepsies, there may be overlap with focal SE, due to frontal focal lesions. In the elderly, new-onset absence SE may be seen; there are also drug-induced, and drug-withdrawal versions of absence SE. The ILAE terminology does not capture some significant details of these events, which make them appear to be different phenomena. However, there are five well-described versions of absence seizures, given below.
   a. Absence status epilepticus is typically considered to be a component of genetic epilepsy, with impairment of consciousness. The level of impairment is often "individual-variable," with about 20% having slight clouding of consciousness, about 60% a confusional state in which the patient is typically calm but does not interact with the environment, and about 20% with more severe impairment; there are sometimes accompanying subtle jerks of the eyelids during the event. The EEG correlate is bilateral and symmetric, typically bifrontally predominant, spike or polyspike and wave complexes at least 2.5 Hz, at least initially during the event; other patterns are also possible. This type of status recurs in most patients, and rarely can occur frequently (16). Neuronal damage is unlikely to occur with this type of status, and as such, aggressive treatment is not recommended (17). Most commonly, intravenous benzodiazepines will terminate the event. If ineffective, one may consider using intravenous valproic acid (18). Additionally, valproic acid may be effective in reducing recurrent events in patients with multiple episodes of absence status.
   b. Atypical absence status is more commonly encountered in patients with structural/metabolic epilepsy, presenting with a fluctuating level of consciousness; it is also seen in patients with genetic epilepsy. This fluctuating confusional state is different than absence SE, which usually has a certain level of impairment. The ictal semiology is quite different than absence status, because it can include tonic, atonic, myoclonic, or otherwise lateralized phenomena. The EEG is spike, and polyspike and wave complexes, which are irregular, but even when quasirhythmic, occur at less than 2.5 Hz; these episodes may recur. The atypical episodes are generally not amenable to benzodiazepine treatment. In patients with recurrent atypical absence SE with an underlying genetic epilepsy, valproic acid may be particularly helpful in reducing recurrences. Atypical absence SE is likely a form of status not causing neuronal damage (19).
   c. Absence SE with focal features is most typically encountered in frontal lobe localization-related epilepsy. There is impairment of consciousness, but the level of impairment may be individual dependent. The EEG is typically bilateral, but asymmetric and may develop into one looking like absence SE later in the episode. Treatment response varies with individual.
   d. Late-onset, de novo absence SE occurs in older adults, with an underlying toxic or metabolic issue leading to seizures. Such patients can have repeated episodes with recurrent toxic/metabolic issues causing further episodes of SE. The preferred treatment is to deal with—including prevention—the underlying toxic/metabolic cause, but the individual episode can be typically easily terminated with benzodiazepines (18). Of note, there may not be a need to treat these patients with long-term AED therapy (20).
   e. Myoclonic absence seizures are proximal, predominantly upper extremity myoclonic jerks synchronized to the 3 Hz spike and wave seen on the EEG during the SE. These can last for hours or days, and are most commonly refractory to therapy. Treatment is possible for some patients, and, in particular, withdrawal of agents known to aggravate idiopathic generalized epilepsies (like carbamazepine) may be beneficial (21).

7. Myoclonic seizures do not cause a change in consciousness. There is irregular, typically bilateral, myoclonic jerking which may persist for hours. Seen in conjunction with Dravet syndrome, myoclonic astatic epilepsy, nonprogressive myoclonic epilepsy in infancy (especially Angelman syndrome), and incompletely controlled juvenile myoclonic epilepsy. It can be benign, without untoward sequelae (22).

   The ILAE report makes no mention as to whether negative myoclonic status, like that which may be seen in continuous spike-wave in slow wave sleep qualifies as myoclonic seizures; there is a logic to including it in this part of the classification schema. In myoclonic SE, there is a limb, often in the upper extremity, which becomes paralyzed, but has continued, brief atonic episodes. There can be alteration of consciousness with these events, which can appear during the episode, with risk that the abnormalities may persist after the episode ends. Myoclonic seizures are associated with anoxic encephalopathy. In the era before induced hypothermia was used, the appearance of these seizures heralded a dire prognosis; this may no longer be the case.

8. In tonic SE, the patient will have brief tonic spasms, which can continue for hours, interspersed with periods of apparent calm. Most typically, if the patient is lying down, the neck and arms are flexed. Tonic SE may occur with both structural/metabolic and genetic epilepsies; with structural/metabolic seizures, the duration can be longer than hours.
9. Subtle SE is the end result of uncontrolled tonic–clonic SE, with focal or multifocal myoclonias, coma, periodic lateralized epileptiform discharges (PLEDs), and a slow suppressed background EEG (23,24); the myoclonias may not be epileptic in nature. The ILAE guidelines do not provide details of the myoclonias, but they are typically in the form of subtle twitches of the trunk or extremities, and can also present as nystagmus. The EEG typically is composed of ictal, but asymmetrically bilateral, rhythmic discharges. While the ILAE guidelines are silent about progression, eventually, there is complete loss of motor component, with only ongoing ictal EEG activity; electrocerebral silence ensues if the seizure is not controlled.
10. Nonconvulsive status epilepticus (NCSE) is not part of the ILAE definition, yet is likely more frequently encountered in properly monitored ICU patients than all other forms of SE. While NCSE rarely appears as the end stage of tonic–clonic SE, it is far more frequently found in ICU patients with unexplained mental status. While NCSE is an area of ongoing investigation, a frequently quoted definition is given as follows (25).
    a. In patients without a known epileptic encephalopathy:
        i. Rhythmic spikes, polyspikes, sharp waves, sharp and slow wave complexes of greater than 2.5 Hz
        ii. Rhythmic spikes, polyspikes, sharp waves, sharp and slow wave complexes of less than 2.5 Hz, or rhythmic delta/theta activity of greater than 0.5 Hz with one or more of the following.
            1. Intravenous AEDs result in improvement of both clinical status and EEG.
            2. During the EEG pattern above, there are subtle clinical ictal phenomena.
            3. There is an increase in voltage and change in frequency at onset, with a change in frequency by more than 1 Hz and/or change in location/spread during event, or a change in voltage or frequency on termination of the event.
    b. In patients with known epileptic encephalopathy:
        i. There is an increase in prominence or frequency in the features mentioned in 10A (above), with both an observable change in clinical status and a change from baseline at the same time.
        ii. Intravenous AEDs cause improvement of both clinical status and EEG status. It is an open question as to how aggressively NCSE should be treated.
11. Febrile SE was included in the 1993 ILAE report, but is not mentioned in the 2006 report, in which the ILAE explicitly classifies SE. We include it herein for purposes of completeness. Febrile SE is defined as seizure during a febrile illness without a central nervous system (CNS) infection or acute electrolyte imbalance in a child older than 1 month of age, without previous febrile seizures, in which there are 30 minutes of continuous seizure activity, or intermittent activity lasting at least 30 minutes without return to baseline consciousness. There is evidence that outcome is related to the duration of the seizure; in particular, seizure duration longer than 120 minutes is associated with poor outcome (26).

EPIDEMIOLOGY

The incidence of SE ranges from 10 to 41 per 100,000 individuals per year (27–30). All studies showed a significantly higher incidence in the elderly, especially after 60 years of age, raising a concern that the overall incidence may rise as the population ages. In addition, only 40% to 50% of patients presenting with first-time SE have a previous diagnosis of epilepsy (28,29). NCSE represents about 30% to 40% of all cases of SE, with an estimated incidence of 5 to 9 per 100,000 individuals per year. However, the true incidence of NCSE may be underestimated. In fact, in various studies the reported incidence of NCSE in ICU patients with altered mental status ranged from 8% to 37% (31–35). Diagnosis requires clinical suspicion and long-term EEG monitoring, which is not routinely performed on critically ill patients in many institutions.

Mortality from SE, estimated in most studies at 10% to 20%, rises significantly with age (36), reaching 38% in the elderly (60 years of age or greater) (27). One of the primary predictors of poor outcome is prolonged seizure; a seizure lasting more than 1 hour has mortality reaching 32%, compared to 2.7% with shorter seizures (36,37). Mortality from NCSE seems to be higher, averaging 50% (38).

ETIOLOGY

In about 30% of cases, SE occurs in patients with chronic epilepsy and is due to withdrawal, or low blood concentrations, of AEDs (37,39,40). In the majority of cases, SE occurs in patients with no history of epilepsy and may be due to a variety of causes, most commonly intracranial pathology, such as ischemic stroke, intracerebral (ICH) and subarachnoid hemorrhage (SAH), CNS infections, head trauma, and brain tumors. Other etiologies include cardiac arrest and hypoxic/anoxic brain injury, alcohol-withdrawal, metabolic disturbances, and toxic causes. In some patients, no cause is identified (39,40).

Both acute and chronic intracranial pathology can cause seizures. Seizures and SE may actually be the presenting signs of several neurologic conditions. This is true for intracranial hemorrhage, including SAH and ICH, acute embolic stroke, and brain tumors. Approximately 50% of patients with brain tumors experience seizures (41,42), and a seizure is the presenting sign of a tumor in 23% of cases (43). Seizures can also be the presenting sign of an acute stroke (44) and frequently occur in the first 2 weeks after a stroke. It is estimated that seizures occur in up to 6% of patients with ischemic stroke, up to 18% of patients with ICH, and up to 26% of patients with SAH (44,45). Up to 2.8% of patients with stroke go into SE either at presentation, or within 2 weeks, of their stroke (46). The risk of chronic epilepsy is 17 times higher after an ischemic stroke than the general population (47), and the risk of having a seizure or developing chronic epilepsy after any type of stroke is 11.5% (48). In SAH, generalized tonic–clonic seizures have been reported in up to 26% of patients at the time of onset or shortly after onset (45,49), and NCSE occurred in 8% of patients who survived the first 48 hours and had an unexplained decline in their level of consciousness (50).

Metabolic disturbances that may cause seizures include hyponatremia, hypoglycemia, hypocalcemia, hypomagnesemia, uremia, hepatic encephalopathy, and hyperosmolar states (50). However, it is important to note that metabolic encephalopathies can frequently cause EEG abnormalities that can be difficult to distinguish from subtle seizure activity, such as high-amplitude slowing and triphasic waves. Therefore, extra care should be taken to avoid both over- and underdiagnosing patients as having SE when they have a clear metabolic dysfunction; response to treatment may be critical in these situations.

Several drugs can cause seizures at toxic levels, including some analgesics such as meperidine, propoxyphene, and tramadol; some psychiatric medications such as bupropion, tricyclic antidepressants, lithium, olanzapine, selective serotonin reuptake inhibitors (SSRIs), venlafaxine, and clozapine. Theophylline, isoniazid, lidocaine, phenothiazines, and some antibiotics such as imipenem/cilastatin, penicillins, and ciprofloxacin may also induce seizures. Furthermore, several commonly abused drugs can cause seizures, most notably cocaine, amphetamines, phencyclidine, and γ-hydroxybutyric acid (51,52).

PATHOPHYSIOLOGY AND MECHANISMS

The great majority of seizures stop spontaneously in less than 2 minutes (53). This is most likely due to inhibitory mechanisms that attempt to deter any excessive, abnormal neuronal activity. This inhibition is evident on the EEG as postictal slowing and attenuation. It is believed that SE occurs when inhibitory mechanisms fail, resulting in a self-sustaining and prolonged seizure activity; the exact cause of this failure is not well understood. A large number of elegant experiments done on animal models of SE have attempted to shed light on the underlying mechanisms causing SE. Review of these studies is beyond the scope of this chapter; however, two points are worth discussing, since they have important implications on treatment strategy.

Self-sustaining SE can be easily triggered in animal models using electrical stimulation (54). However, this can be blocked by many drugs that increase inhibition or reduce excitation only if administered early, prior to the development of a self-sustained seizure (55). In contrast, once a self-sustaining state is established, it becomes more difficult to stop the seizure (56), and much higher dosages of inhibitory drugs are required, leading to significant toxicity, including cardiovascular depression (57). Another important feature of self-sustaining SE is the progressive development of resistance to AEDs. The anticonvulsant potency of benzodiazepines can decrease by 20 times within 30 minutes of self-sustaining SE (58). The same phenomenon was observed with other anticonvulsants, such as phenytoin; however, the decline in potency was slower (59).

Pathophysiologically, SE produces a number of neurologic and systemic changes. Primary neurologic complications occur in both convulsive and some forms of nonconvulsive SE, and are time dependent and probably preventable with early termination of the seizure. In animal models of SE, neuronal injury occurs even in the absence of convulsive activity (60,61), and cell death is thought to result from excessive neuronal firing through excitotoxic mechanisms (62). It is impossible to replicate these experiments in human beings; however, there is widespread belief—supported by some anecdotal evidence—that neuronal injury and death occur after prolonged seizures. For example, brain damage and decreased hippocampal neuronal density are often seen in patients who die from SE (63,64). Furthermore, cerebral edema and chronic brain atrophy seen on neuroimaging studies have been reported after SE (65–68).

Systemic complications of prolonged seizures are seen primarily in GCSE, and are due to autonomic hyperactivity and excessive muscle activity. Therefore, systemic complications can potentially be prevented, or minimized, with early termination of seizure activity or induction of muscle paralysis and artificial ventilation (61). Pathophysiologic manifestations include increased systemic blood pressure, tachycardia, and cardiac arrhythmias; increased pulmonary blood pressure; increase in cerebral blood flow; elevation of body temperature; increased peripheral white cell count; transient pleocytosis in the spinal fluid; and a marked metabolic acidosis (60,69,70). Epinephrine levels are elevated and reach the dysrhythmogenic range; these may play a role in sudden death (70). With prolonged convulsive SE—defined as lasting 30 minutes or more–systemic blood pressure and cerebral blood flow can drop significantly (60). Additionally, blood glucose is initially elevated in response to excessive adrenergic stimulation; however, after 30 minutes of GCSE, hypoglycemia may occur (60). Both hypoglycemia and decreased cerebral blood flow contribute to further neuronal injury (71). Excessive muscle contraction often causes severe metabolic acidosis, breakdown of muscle tissue, and hyperkalemia (60,61,69). Arterial pH has been reported to fall below 7.0 (72) and contribute, along with hyperkalemia, to cardiac dysrhythmias. Rhabdomyolysis and myoglobinuria can also occur and may lead to acute renal failure (73).

EVALUATION

Clinical Presentation

Obtaining a focused history and examination may be very helpful for diagnosis and management (Table 121.1). Convulsive and nonconvulsive SE have very different clinical presentations, and their treatment is quite different. Convulsive SE frequently occurs outside the hospital, and management may start in the ambulance before patients arrive to the emergency room. The diagnosis is usually evident, unless there is a strong clinical suspicion of psychogenic nonepileptic seizure (PNES). Convulsive SE often starts as a focal seizure with secondary generalization. Rarely, primary generalized seizures evolve

TABLE 121.1 History and Physical Examination

Parameter	Comment
History of epilepsy	Current antiepileptic drugs, missed doses, compliance, recent gastrointestinal illness
List of current medications	Toxic ingestion of medications or other agents
History of psychiatric illness	Suicidal ideations or attempts
Trauma	Evidence of scalp laceration and bruises
Medical history	Previous stroke, traumatic brain injury, abscess
Focal neurologic signs	May be difficult to assess: look for obvious signs
Signs of medical illness	Hepatic or renal disease, infection, hypoxia, hypertensive emergency, meningitis
Signs of substance abuse	Alcohol withdrawal or intoxication, cocaine intoxication
	Opioid, benzodiazepine, or barbiturate withdrawal

Adapted from Brophy GM, Bell R, Claasen J, et al. Guidelines for the evaluation and management of status epilepticus. *Neurocrit Care.* 2012;17:3–23.

into SE. The generalized convulsion either becomes continuous, or stops and recurs before the patient regains full consciousness. In either case, the tonic–clonic activity changes in character with time and often patients go into a continuous clonic phase where clonic activity persists and gradually slows down and becomes more subtle. With time, the only persistent motor activity may consist of small-amplitude twitching of the face, hands, or feet or nystagmoid jerking of the eyes (74,75). Sometimes the motor activity subsides completely, and patients remain stuporous or comatose; in this case, patients evolve from convulsive to NCSE (33).

By the time patients arrive to the emergency department (ED), they may already be in established SE. If there is strong clinical suspicion of PNES, an EEG is essential to confirm the diagnosis. The average duration of a PNES in one study was 5 minutes (76); however, they can be protracted and may mimic convulsive SE. Another study of patients in an epilepsy monitoring unit had nearly 20% of PNES patients, with PNES mimicking SE (77). Additionally, patients with PNES may also have epilepsy, making it all the more difficult to know how to treat.

NCSE has a different clinical presentation, with unexplained decline in mental status that cannot be completely explained by other causes. It may occur either outside the hospital or, frequently, in the hospital, in patients already admitted for other reasons such as stroke, intracranial hemorrhage, brain tumors, or metabolic disturbances. Frequently, the underlying etiology may account in part for the impairment in consciousness; however, patients frequently have an unexplained decline of mental status after a period of clinical improvement. Therefore, clinical suspicion should be strong, and evaluation for NCSE should be undertaken in any patient with unexplained impairment in mental status.

Electroencephalogram

The EEG is the only diagnostic tool that can confirm or refute the diagnosis of SE. In GCSE, an EEG may not be necessary initially, unless PNES must be excluded. However, if convulsive activity stops and patients do not recover their baseline level of consciousness, evaluation with an EEG is important to exclude the continuous presence of seizure activity. In NCSE, the EEG is essential. However, a single routine EEG of 20 minutes' duration may not be adequate and may only capture seizure activity in 20% of cases. A longer EEG recording of at least 1 hour increases the sensitivity to 50%. More prolonged EEG monitoring is recommended if shorter-duration EEGs are nondiagnostic. Long-term EEG monitoring of 24 to 48 hours can increase the diagnostic accuracy to over 90% (35). Several EEG patterns have been described during SE, probably reflecting different stages of brain activity (75). In addition, several patterns have been described in NCSE. Discussion of these different EEG patterns is beyond the scope of this chapter; however, an important issue needs to be emphasized. Some EEG patterns can be difficult to distinguish from epileptiform activity, such as diffuse triphasic waves in metabolic encephalopathies (Fig. 121.1) and breach rhythms after a craniotomy (Fig. 121.2). These patterns can be very deceiving and can often be misinterpreted as epileptiform. Therefore, it is very important for the EEG to be interpreted by an experienced electroencephalographer.

Neuroimaging

Neuroimaging studies are always recommended to assess for the presence of intracranial pathology. Even in patients with known pathologies, such as tumors or stroke, repeat imaging is recommended to exclude progression or complications of the underlying disease. For example, a stable tumor can become necrotic or hemorrhagic, or a stable acute or subacute infarct can turn hemorrhagic. Unenhanced computed tomography (CT) of the brain is adequate in the acute setting; however, magnetic resonance imaging (MRI) is much more sensitive and may detect lesions not seen on CT.

Laboratory Evaluation

Full laboratory evaluation is always recommended (Table 121.2), including blood cell count, renal function, liver function, electrolytes, calcium, magnesium, and AED levels. Toxicology should be performed when there is a clinical suspicion of intoxication or substance abuse. This is especially important in patients with a psychiatric illness at risk of suicide and in children who may have access to adult medications. Lumbar puncture is indicated if there is ***any*** consideration of an infectious etiology. Also, a lumbar puncture should be considered when SAH, not seen on CT scan, is suspected. However, in the presence of any sign of intracranial hypertension, lumbar puncture should be avoided, since it may increase the risk of transtentorial herniation. It is important to note that patients with convulsive SE often exhibit clinical features suggestive of meningitis, such as elevated temperatures, increased peripheral white blood cell counts, and pleocytosis in the cerebrospinal fluid (CSF) (70). These abnormalities have been reported in up to 18% of patients with convulsive SE, without any evidence of infection (70), and are thought to result from breakdown of the blood–brain barrier. Usually, the total white blood cell count in the CSF remains under 100 and glucose level remains normal. Treatment with antimicrobials should be initiated if there is clinical suspicion for a CNS infection.

TREATMENT

General Rubric

The most important thing to know is that this is a very complicated subject. Each of the 11 different kinds of status is considered differently. It can be confusing, when looking at papers on this subject, because there is often the assumption that when an author talks about SE, he or she means generalized convulsive SE.

Generalized Convulsive Status Epilepticus

Treatment Principles

GCSE is a medical emergency and should be dealt with as such. Therapies are aimed at early termination of seizure activity, identification and correction of the cause, prevention of seizure recurrence, and treatment of pathophysiologic complications. There is ample evidence that delayed treatment leads to poor outcome (36,78). In addition, there is a time-dependent loss of efficacy of anticonvulsant medications (58,59). Therefore, early initiation of aggressive treatment is essential in the management of GCSE. It is highly recommended that every ED and ICU have a well-defined and clear treatment protocol. This helps avoid many of the pitfalls leading to delayed and insufficient treatment of SE (79).

Prehospital Management

In many cases, patients with convulsive SE are brought into the ED by ambulance, making prehospital treatment possible. Initiation of treatment in the ambulance is highly recommended, when possible, given the importance of early intervention. Both rectal diazepam (80,81) and intravenous diazepam and lorazepam (82) can be safely and effectively used. In one randomized, double-blind, prospective study (82), seizures terminated before arrival to the ED in 59% of patients who received intravenous lorazepam, 43% of those who received intravenous diazepam, and 21% of those who received placebo. The safety profile was also good, with more patients having respiratory or circulatory complications in the placebo group than the treatment groups. Treatment in the ambulance with intravenous benzodiazepines should only be initiated if the paramedical team transporting the patient has the training and equipment to perform endotracheal intubation and artificial ventilation, in case of respiratory depression.

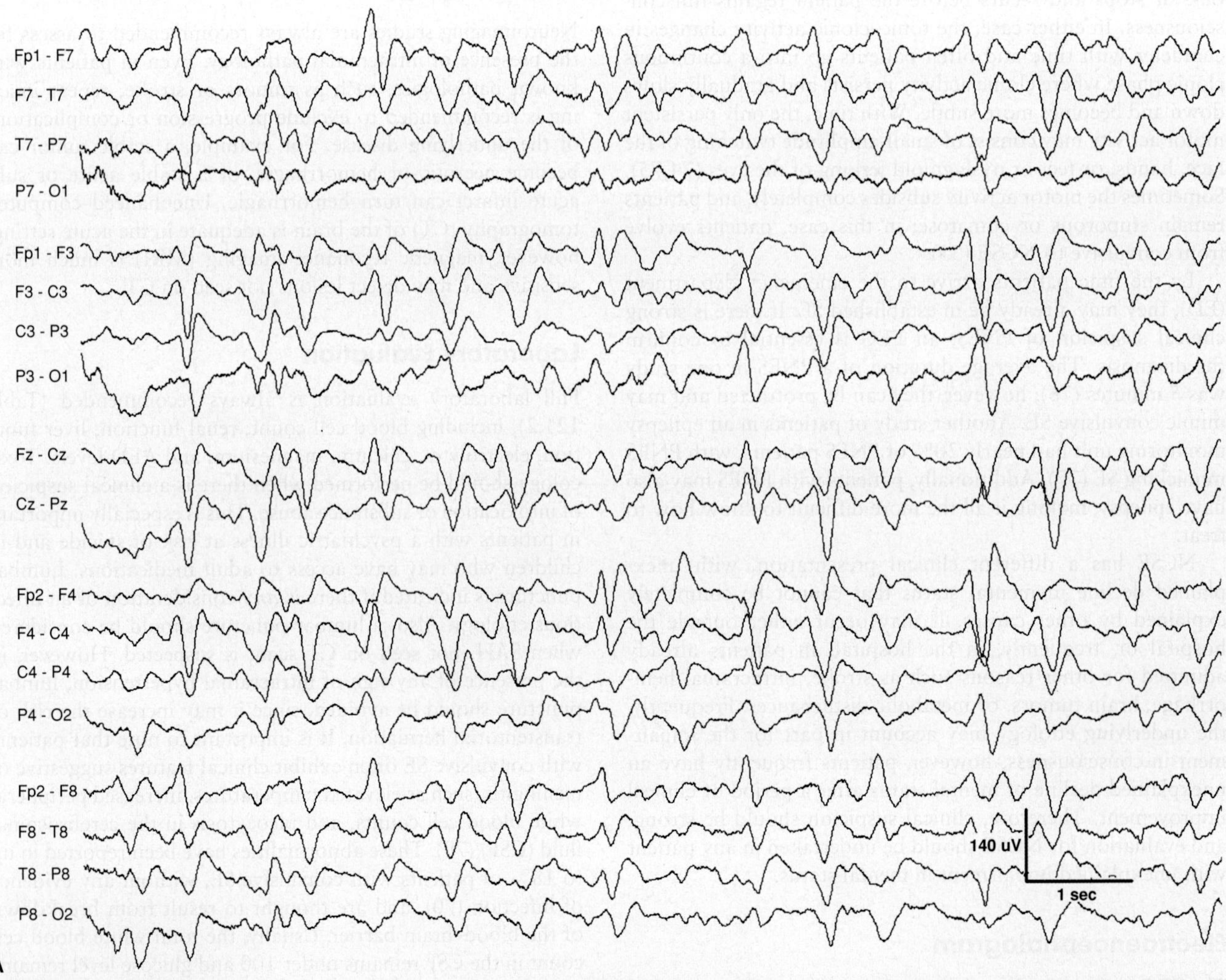

FIGURE 121.1 Generalized status versus generalized slowing with triphasic waves. A: Electroencephalogram (EEG) of a patient in hepatic encephalopathy showing diffuse background slowing and prominent triphasic waves.

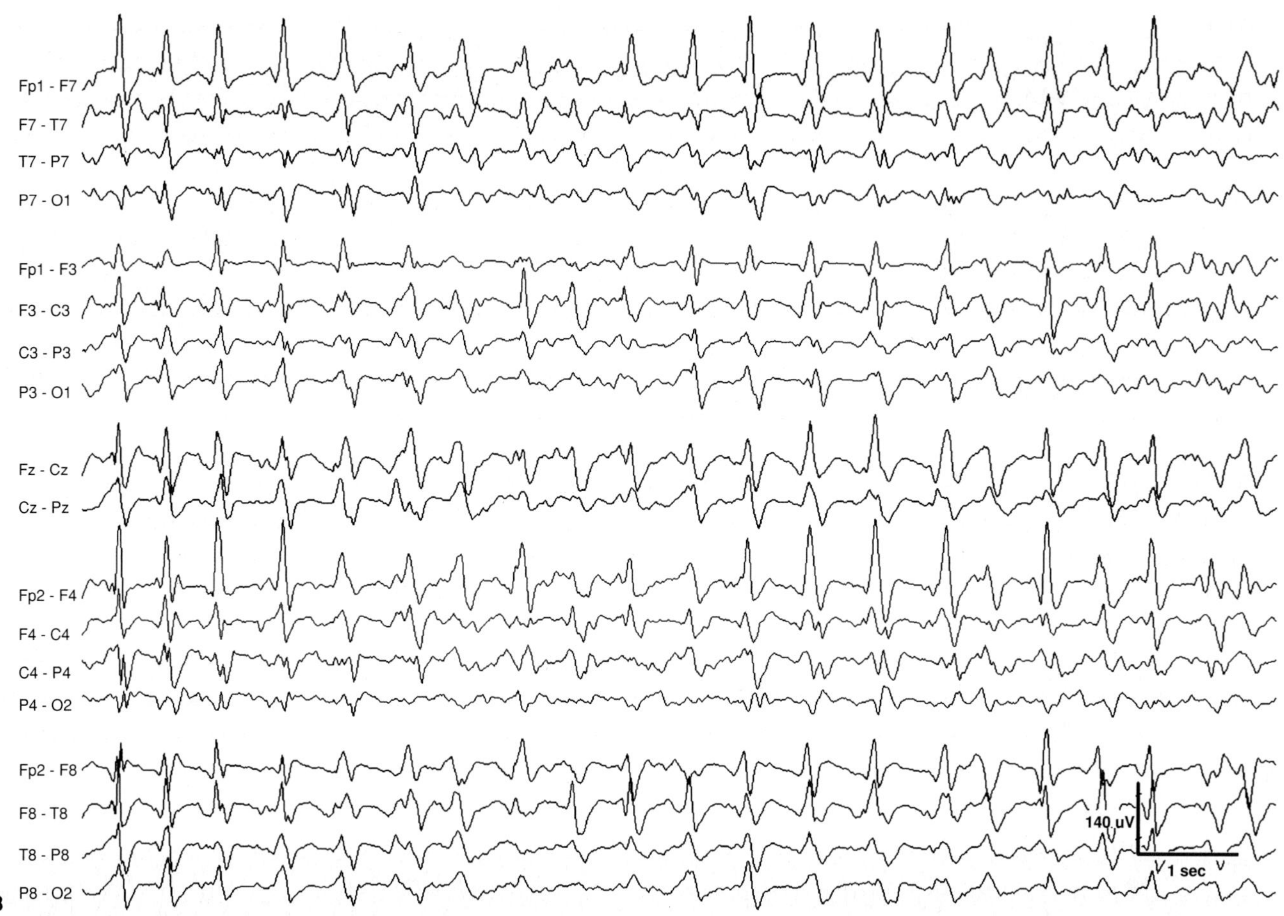

FIGURE 121.1 (*Continued*) **B**: EEG of a patient in generalized nonconvulsive status epilepticus. The two patterns can be difficult to distinguish and occasionally the pattern shown in (A) may be seen in long-standing status. The history and laboratory evaluation are sometimes helpful in distinguishing between the two patterns.

Medical Management

Medical management should focus on the prevention and reversal of medical complications (Table 121.3) (83). As in any other medical emergency, basic life support should always be the initial step in management, including maintenance of airways and blood pressure. Vital signs should be continuously monitored, including pulse oximetry. Oxygen at an FiO_2 of 1.0 should be given by nonrebreather mask. Endotracheal intubation should be considered if there is evidence of respiratory failure, including hypoxemia and/or respiratory acidosis. Pharmacologic paralysis for intubation should be avoided if possible, since it can result in the false impression that the seizure has stopped. If the use of a paralytic agent is necessary, continuous EEG monitoring should be performed. Large-bore intravenous access should be established for the administration of intravenous medications. Hyperthermia is believed to contribute to neuronal damage and should be corrected (84,85). Systolic blood pressure should be maintained above 120 mmHg if possible, but definitely not lower than 90 mmHg, to ensure adequate cerebral blood flow (39). Correction of acidosis with intravenous bicarbonate remains controversial. Many experts recommend treatment if the patient becomes hypotensive and arterial pH falls below 7 (39). Results of laboratory abnormalities should guide further medical treatment, including electrolyte abnormalities, blood sugar levels, and AED levels. Mild hyperglycemia is frequently seen and usually does not require intervention (86). If hypoglycemia is present, or if the blood sugar level is not available, patients should receive 100 mg thiamine followed by 50 mL 50% glucose solution intravenously (87). If a metabolic abnormality is present, such as hyponatremia or hypoglycemia, the most effective treatment of status is correction of the underlying problem.

Pharmacologic Treatment

Treatment with AEDs should be started after 5 minutes of continuous generalized, convulsive seizure activity. Early initiation of treatment can potentially lead to a better response and prevent GCSE from becoming refractory. In fact, when treatment is started within 30 minutes of onset, up to 80% of patients achieve control, compared to only 40% achieving control when treatment is started after 2 hours of onset (40,88). The choice of initial treatment largely depends on the institution, with different protocols being used by various institutions and specialists (80,89). This is due primarily to the lack of sufficient class I evidence. Three controlled clinical trials on the treatment of SE have been published. One study compared diazepam to lorazepam and found no significant difference (90). The second compared four treatment protocols: phenytoin alone, phenytoin with diazepam, lorazepam alone, and phenobarbital alone. The highest percentage of responders was in the lorazepam arm; however, the only significant difference was between lorazepam alone and phenytoin

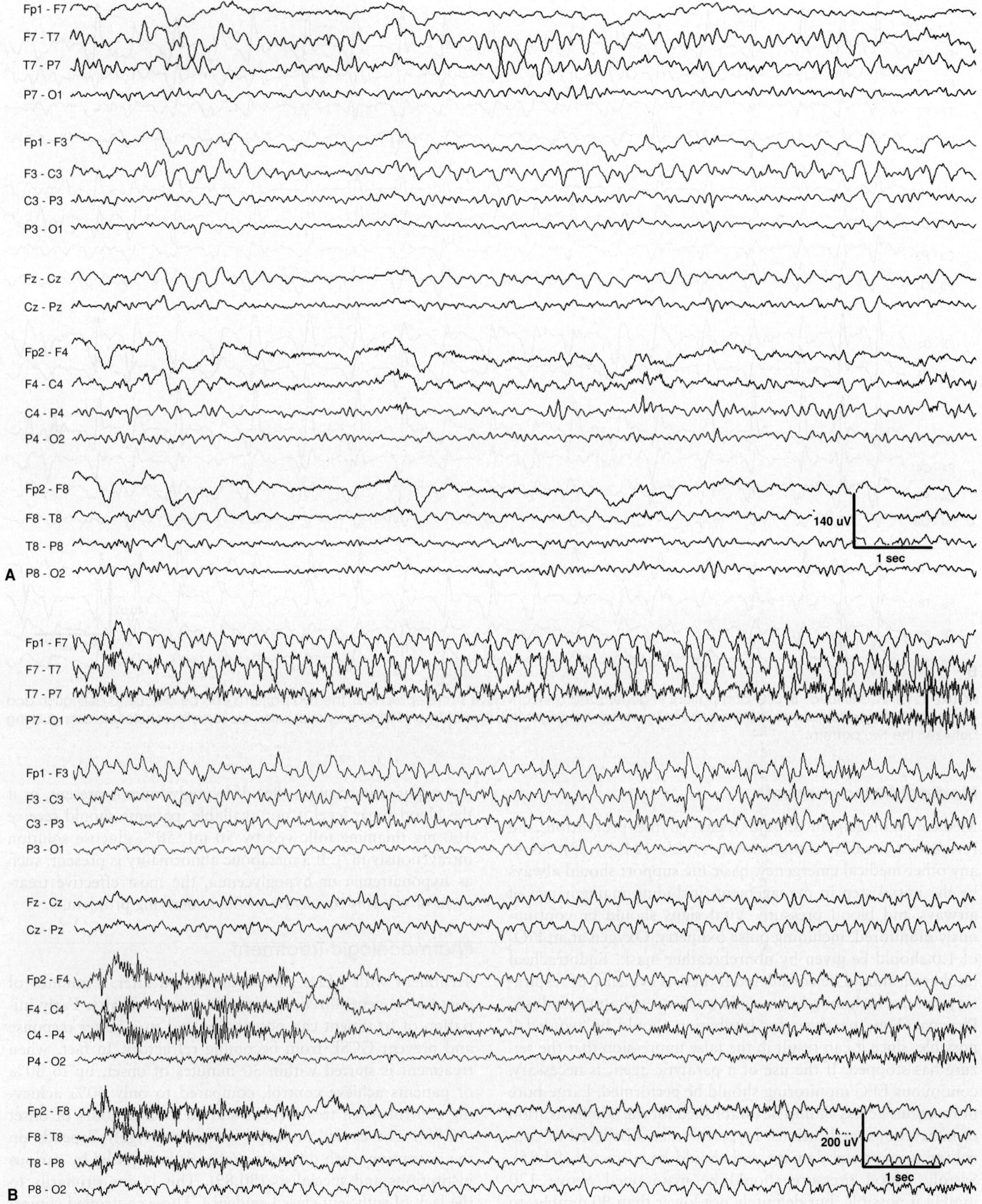

FIGURE 121.2 Focal status versus focal slowing and breach rhythm. A: Electroencephalogram (EEG) of a patient with a history of left temporal benign tumor, surgically resected several years ago. The high-amplitude slowing seen focally from the left temporal and frontal regions represents a breach rhythm, believed to result from the loss of resistance to electrical flow after a craniotomy. B: EEG of a patient having a left temporal lobe seizure. Note the presence of well-organized rhythmic activity compared to A, where the rhythmic slowing is more random and intermittent.

TABLE 121.2 Laboratory Evaluation

- Fingerstick glucose
- Complete blood count
- Electrolytes, calcium, and magnesium
- Liver function studies
- Renal function studies
- Toxicology for drugs of abuse and alcohol
- Serum antiepileptic drug levels
- Continuous video-EEG monitoring
- CT brain imaging as soon as possible
- More comprehensive imaging by MRI including MRA or MRV, if there remains clinical concern
- Lumbar puncture if strong suspicion of meningitis/encephalitis
- If worrisome for toxidrome, consider testing for toxins that are associated with seizures: isoniazid, tricyclic antidepressants, organophosphates, and cyclosporine

Adapted from Brophy GM, Bell R, Claasen J, et al. Guidelines for the evaluation and management of status epilepticus. *Neurocrit Care.* 2012;17:3–23.

alone (91). The third study compared prehospital treatment with diazepam, lorazepam, and placebo, and found that both lorazepam and diazepam were efficacious (83).

Regardless of the choice of initial therapy, the rapid sequential use of several agents is strongly recommended until seizure activity is terminated (Table 121.4). The caveat of this approach is that the use of agents with long elimination half-life may lead to cumulative adverse effects, with high risk of inducing respiratory and cardiovascular depression. However, it is important to keep in mind that both respiratory and cardiovascular depression are usually easily treatable in the ED or ICU settings, while prolonged SE may lead to irreversible neuronal injury. This formula should be kept in mind when making important therapeutic decisions. In the Veterans Affairs Cooperative Study (91), 60% of patients, on average, responded to the first drug; an additional 7.3% responded to the second drug; and only 2% responded to the third drug. Although these numbers seem discouraging, the number of drugs currently available has significantly increased, providing more options for treatment and potentially a better response rate. However, more clinical trials are needed to study the efficacy of newer agents.

TABLE 121.3 Initial Management of Status Epilepticus

ABC	Airways, vital signs, pulse oximetry, and cardiac rhythm. Establish peripheral IV access (preferably at least 2—at least one should be large bore so that fluid resuscitation can be performed)
Blood glucose	Intravenous infusion of thiamine 100 mg followed by 50 mL of glucose 50%
Antiepileptic drugs	See Table 121.4
Evaluation	History and examination (see Table 121.1) and laboratory tests (see Table 121.2)

Adapted from Brophy GM, Bell R, Claasen J, et al. Guidelines for the evaluation and management of status epilepticus. *Neurocrit Care.* 2012;17:3–23.

The ideal initial drug would be easy to administer, have an immediate and long-lasting seizure-suppressing action, and be free of serious adverse effects on cardiorespiratory function and level of consciousness. Unfortunately, the ideal drug does not exist. Benzodiazepines and barbiturates depress consciousness and respiratory drive and may lower blood pressure; phenytoin can cause hypotension and cardiac arrhythmias, which limits the rate of intravenous infusion.

TABLE 121.4 Suggested Protocol for Antiepileptic Drug Treatment

Step	Medication	Dosage	Route	Maximum Rate	Comment
1	Lorazepam	0.1 mg/kg	IV bolus	2 mg/min	May repeat once if seizure activity continues after 5 min If seizure activity stops, additional medications may not be required
2	Phenytoin	20 mg/kg	IV bolus	50 mg/min	May give additional 5–10 mg/kg if seizure continues
	Fosphenytoin	20 mg/kg PE	IV bolus	150 mg/min	Consider valproate in patients with epilepsy on valproate, especially with subtherapeutic level
3	Phenobarbital	20 mg/kg	IV bolus	50 mg/min	Skip this stage and go straight to general anesthesia if status started more than 60 min ago
	Valproate	25 mg/kg	IV bolus	200 mg/min	May give additional 5–10 mg/kg if seizure continues
4	Pentobarbital				
	Initial bolus	5–10 mg/kg	IV bolus	50 mg/min	Repeat 5 mg/kg every 5–10 min until seizures stop
	Maintenance	1 mg/kg/hr	IV infusion		Titrate up to 10 mg/kg/hr, until desired EEG pattern attained[a]
	Midazolam				
	Initial bolus	0.2 mg/kg	IV bolus	—	Repeat 0.2–0.4 mg/kg every 5 min until seizures stop, maximum 2 mg/kg
	Maintenance	0.1 mg/kg/hr	IV infusion		Titrate up to 2 mg/kg/hr until desired EEG pattern attained[a]
	Propofol				
	Initial bolus	1 mg/kg	IV bolus	—	Repeat 1–2 mg/kg every 5 min until seizures stop, maximum 10 mg/kg
	Maintenance	1 mg/kg/hr	IV infusion		Titrate up to 1 mg/kg/hr = 16 µg/kg/min, until desired EEG pattern attained[a]
5	Ketamine	0.5mg/kg/hr	IV infusion	2 mg/kg/hr	Titrate to burst suppression on continuous EEG. Maximum daily dose, 4,000 mg
	Inhalation anesthetic	Up to 1.0 MAC	Inhalational anesthetic		Consider titration to burst suppression on continuous EEG

[a]Usually burst-suppression pattern.

PE, phenytoin equivalent; EEG, electroencephalogram; MAC, minimal alveolar concentration.

Benzodiazepines are the most commonly used first-line agents due to their potency and fast-acting effect. Pharmacologically, they enhance inhibitory γ-aminobutyric acid (GABA) transmission. The three most commonly used agents are lorazepam, diazepam, and midazolam. Direct comparison between lorazepam and diazepam revealed no significant difference (78). Diazepam is more lipid soluble, and may cross the blood–brain barrier and reach higher concentrations in the CSF more rapidly than lorazepam. However, this increased lipid solubility may be disadvantageous, and leads to a higher rate of redistribution in peripheral adipose tissue. Therefore, despite having a longer elimination half-life of 48 hours, the effective duration of action of diazepam is actually shorter—15 to 30 minutes—than that of lorazepam, which has a duration of action of 12 to 24 hours. This may lead to increased incidence of seizure recurrence after initial termination of SE when diazepam is used alone. The rapid onset of action and prolonged duration of seizure-suppressing effect has made lorazepam the preferred first-line agent by many neurologists. Midazolam has never been used in a double-blind study. Like diazepam and lorazepam, midazolam has a rapid onset of action, but its extremely short elimination half-life makes it more appropriately used as a continuous intravenous infusion in refractory SE.

The routine concomitant or sequential use of a second agent is advocated by many experts. It is recommended to use an agent with a different mechanism of action, such as phenytoin or fosphenytoin. However, as shown by the Veterans Affairs Cooperative Study (91), lorazepam alone may be sufficient in many cases, especially when SE is caused by a known and reversible process, such as low serum concentration of AEDs or acute metabolic disturbances. Some experts argue that the early use of phenytoin or fosphenytoin is important to prevent seizure recurrence. This is based on the experimental evidence that benzodiazepines are subject to rapid time-dependent loss of potency as opposed to phenytoin, which loses its potency at a much slower rate (58,59); this claim, however, remains to be proven in controlled clinical trials.

The recommended dose of intravenous phenytoin is 20 mg/kg total body weight. The common practice of administering a standard loading dose of 1,000 mg of phenytoin is inadequate for most patients, and some patients require as much as 30 mg/kg to stop seizure activity (92). Phenytoin should be administered at a maximum infusion rate of 50 mg/min. A faster administration rate may result in cardiovascular complications, including hypotension, bradycardia, and ectopic beats. These effects are more common in elderly patients and patients with pre-existing cardiac disease. Cardiovascular complications are not due to phenytoin itself, but to the propylene glycol diluent (93). For this reason, fosphenytoin, a water-soluble prodrug of phenytoin, was introduced and has gained broad popularity. Fosphenytoin is rapidly converted to phenytoin, and is dosed in phenytoin equivalents. Because of its water solubility, fosphenytoin can be administered at a much faster infusion rate than phenytoin—up to 150 mg/min. Theoretically, the risk of cardiovascular adverse effects should be lower with fosphenytoin; however, this was never proven in clinical trials. In fact, in one study, the rate of complications was similar for intravenous phenytoin and fosphenytoin (94) as long as the recommended maximum rate of administration is followed, although infusion site reactions (phlebitis and soft tissue damage) were less common with fosphenytoin. The main advantage of fosphenytoin in the treatment of SE seems to be related to the rapidity of infusion. The question of whether fosphenytoin reaches its peak concentration in the brain faster than phenytoin is not known. Fosphenytoin has to be hepatically converted to phenytoin, a process that may delay its true bioavailability. One study found that when phenytoin or fosphenytoin are administered at the maximum recommended infusion rate, the therapeutic serum concentration of phenytoin for either drug is attained within 10 minutes (95). Thus, fosphenytoin and phenytoin may very well have an equivalent onset of action; however, this will need to be studied in controlled clinical trials.

Phenobarbital is another effective treatment for SE; however, because of its powerful depressant effect on respiratory drive, level of consciousness, and blood pressure, it should be used only after benzodiazepines and phenytoin fail. The usual recommended loading dose is 20 mg/kg at an infusion rate of 50 mg/minute.

Intravenous valproic acid is another viable option for the acute treatment of SE, and may offer a significant advantage over phenobarbital, with a much safer side effect profile (96). Although the recommended infusion rate is 20 mg/minute, much faster infusion rates up to 555 mg/min have been safely used (97). Several anecdotal reports and uncontrolled trials were initially published, suggesting a potential usefulness for valproate in the treatment of SE (98–100). A single, double-blind controlled trial was published comparing phenytoin to valproic acid in acute convulsive SE (101), and found a higher rate of seizure termination with valproic acid as a first-line agent (66% vs. 43% for phenytoin). After failure of the first agent, valproic acid was also superior to phenytoin when used as a second agent. The current evidence and clinical experience are insufficient to recommend valproate as first-line treatment for SE; however, it may be safely and effectively used as a third- or fourth-line treatment when other agents are unsuccessful and before resorting to general anesthesia (102). The question of whether intravenous valproic acid should replace phenytoin as a second-line agent remains unanswered.

Topiramate has been reported to be useful in some patients with refractory SE (103,104), including children (105). It is administered as suspension via a nasogastric tube, with a good rate of seizure termination and an excellent safety profile. Although intravenous formulations are most likely more effective, topiramate may be a safe alternative to more aggressive treatments. Controlled clinical trials are needed to establish its efficacy and safety in this setting.

Intravenous levetiracetam was recently introduced and seems to have a good safety profile (106). There are no published studies about its use in SE, and therefore, no recommendations can be made. Levetiracetam has, overall, very good pharmacokinetic properties and a good safety profile, and may offer another option for the treatment of SE in the future.

Refractory Generalized Convulsive Status Epilepticus

GCSE is considered refractory if it does not respond to two or three first-line treatments (107). In practice, if seizure activity continues after the administration of a benzodiazepine, phenytoin, or phenobarbital, status is considered refractory and more aggressive treatment should be pursued. In the Veterans

Affairs Cooperative Study (91), failure of the first two agents was seen in 38% of patients presenting with convulsive SE and 82% of patients presenting with subtle SE. Patients with refractory SE are at higher risk of developing complications (108), including respiratory failure, fever, pneumonia, hypotension, sepsis, and requiring blood transfusion. In addition, the clinical outcome is worse than nonrefractory SE, with a mortality of 23% compared with 14% in nonrefractory cases (108).

In a survey conducted among neurologists (89), there was strong agreement for the use of benzodiazepines and phenytoin or fosphenytoin as first- and second-line therapies for SE. However, there was less consistency for the choice of third- and fourth-line therapy. Treatment options include intravenous phenobarbital or valproate, or continuous infusion of pentobarbital, propofol, or midazolam. It is important to note that once the choice of continuous infusion of antiseizure medication—often termed "general anesthesia," although this is a serious misnomer—is made, patients are committed to undergo endotracheal intubation and artificial ventilation for a period of time. While it is extremely important to terminate seizure activity as rapidly as possible, intubation and ventilation are not, of course, complication free, which should be kept in mind when making such a decision. Although there is no consensus agreement on the treatment approach, one approach is to attempt a third-line agent before resorting to general anesthesia, especially given the safety profiles of intravenous valproate and levetiracetam.

Continuous intravenous infusion of pentobarbital, propofol, and midazolam at anesthetic doses is the treatment of choice for refractory SE. A published meta-analysis provides useful information on the relative advantages and disadvantages of each drug (107). Overall, pentobarbital appears to be more effective in stopping seizures and preventing seizure recurrence. However, pentobarbital is associated with more severe hemodynamic instability and hypotension, often requiring the use of vasopressors and, even in young individuals, mandating the placement of invasive monitoring devices to manage the significant negative inotropic state-induced inadequate oxygen delivery. Of importance, there is no difference in mortality among the three treatments. Propofol and midazolam have become the preferred agents for refractory SE mainly because of their rapid onset of action and short half-life, with rapid clearance. However, a number of articles reporting data about the use of propofol in refractory SE raised several concerns about the safety of propofol in this setting (109). In contrast, more recent emerging evidence suggests propofol to be superior and safer than pentobarbital (110), even in children (111).

Once continuous infusion of an anesthetic agent is initiated, a multidisciplinary approach, including an experienced neurologist and a critical care team, is crucial to ensure adequate treatment. Continuous EEG monitoring is strongly recommended, and can provide online information about the presence of seizure activity and the success of treatment. This is especially true if convulsive activity stops, since often patients continue to have NCSE after the cessation of motor activity. Once seizure activity is completely suppressed and the desired level of anesthesia is attained—most often a 90% burst-suppression pattern on EEG—the infusion is maintained for 12 to 24 hours and is then gradually withdrawn. It is extremely important to make sure that patients are on adequate standing dosages and have adequate serum levels of other AEDs prior to withdrawal of the coma-inducing agent(s). If seizure activity recurs, therapy should be resumed for progressively longer periods, and the depth of anesthesia may be increased. In this situation, some experts advocate, but this is controversial, that attaining electrocerebral silence in severely refractory cases is helpful. If infusion of one agent is not successful in stopping seizure activity despite high dosages, and significant side effects, then a second agent should be tried, either alone or in combination. Prolonged treatment with midazolam may lead to tachyphylaxis, leading to the need of very high dosages.

Other treatment options for refractory status epilepticus include inhalation anesthetic agents and ketamine. Both isoflurane and desflurane have been reported to rapidly suppress all electrographic seizure activity in patients who failed treatment with propofol, midazolam, and pentobarbital (112). However, the risk of complications is high and these agents should only be used as a last resort. Ketamine is another agent that has been advocated as a potential treatment option for patients with refractory SE (113). While ketamine can lower the seizure threshold, it has a novel mechanism of action: a noncompetitive glutamate antagonist acting at the NMDA receptor, which may be helpful in refractory status. Ketamine offers the advantage of being neuroprotective and can increase blood pressure due to its sympathomimetic properties (79). The clinical experience with ketamine is very limited, and the potential for serious complications is unknown (114).

PROGNOSIS

Status epilepticus is associated with significant morbidity and mortality. Several factors influence outcome, including etiology, age, and the duration of seizure activity (36,72). The overall mortality rate among adults is approximately 20% but rises significantly with age (36), reaching 38% in those older than 60 (27). Longer duration of SE usually leads to worse outcome, especially in the presence of severe physiologic disturbances. Mortality for seizures lasting more than 1 hour is 32%, compared to 2.7% when seizures are less than 1 hour long (36,37). Among survivors, the risk of developing chronic epilepsy and subsequent episodes of status is very high (88).

Patients with refractory GCSE tend to have a worse outcome (79). This is likely due to a combination of factors, including a more serious etiology and longer duration of seizure activity, which usually leads to increased duration of stay in the ICU, and subsequently, an increased rate of complications (95,115). Furthermore, patients with refractory GCSE are at significantly higher risk of developing chronic epilepsy than those with nonrefractory GCSE (115).

Patients with acute neurologic disease, such as infection, stroke, intracranial hemorrhage, or trauma, and patients with concomitant systemic illnesses tend to have worse outcomes (116); patients with anoxic brain injury have a very poor outcome (117). However, in these patients, the etiology and comorbid conditions are most likely the major determinants of outcome, with SE playing an additional complicating role. There is a scoring system that can be considered for help in determining likelihood of prognosis (118).

Key Points

- Status epilepticus is defined as continuous or rapidly repeating seizures.
- Any seizure type can turn into status epilepticus.
- Every institution should have a well-defined treatment protocol to avoid delays and inadequate treatment.
- In the majority of cases, status epilepticus develops in patients without any history of seizures or epilepsy.
- In patients with a history of epilepsy, the most common cause is low serum concentration of AEDs.
- Intracranial pathology and metabolic disturbances can cause status epilepticus.
- When possible, correction of the underlying etiology is the most effective treatment.
- GCSE is a medical emergency requiring aggressive and immediate therapeutic intervention; other kinds of status are not necessarily an emergency.
- Mortality and morbidity increase significantly if generalized convulsive seizure activity persists longer than 60 minutes.
- Delayed treatment may cause the generalized convulsive status to become refractory to therapy.
- Rapid sequential use of several anticonvulsive medications is strongly recommended.
- In refractory cases, general anesthesia is the recommended therapy.
- NCSE is frequently underdiagnosed in comatose patients, especially those with acute neurologic injury.
- Continuous EEG monitoring is strongly recommended in most cases.

ACKNOWLEDGMENT

I would like to thank G.A. Ghacibeh for doing the chapter for the 4th edition. While some of the chapter was updated, much remains his work.

References

1. Berg AT, Berkovic SF, Brodie MJ, et al. Revised terminology and concepts for organization of seizures and epilepsies: report of the ILAE Commission and Terminology, 2005–2009. *Epilepsia*. 2010;51(4):676.
2. Engel JE. Report of the ILAE Classification Core Group. *Epilepsia*. 2006;47(9):1558.
3. Panayiotopoulos CP. The new ILAE report on terminology and concepts for organization of epileptic seizures: a clinician's critical view and contribution. *Epilepsia*. 2011;52(12):2155.
4. Commission on Epidemiology and Prognosis, International League Against Epilepsy. Guidelines for epidemiologic studies on epilepsy. *Epilepsia*. 1993;34(4):592.
5. Lowenstein DH, Bleck T, Macdonald RM. It's time to revise the definition of status epilepticus. *Epilepsia*. 1999;40(1):120.
6. Williamson PD, Spencer DD, Spencer SS, et al. Complex partial status epilepticus: a depth-electrode study. *Ann Neurol*. 1985;8:647.
7. Bien CG, Granata T, Antozzi C, et al. Pathogenesis, diagnosis and treatment of Rasmussen encephalitis: a European consensus statement. *Brain*. 2005;128:454.
8. Sinha S, Satishchandra P. Epilepsia Partialis Continua over the last 14 years: Experience from a tertiary care center from south India. *Epilep Res*. 2007;74(1):55.
9. Scholtes FB, Reier WO, Meinardi H. Simple partial status epilepticus: causes, treatment, and outcome in 47 patients. *J Neurol Neurosurg Psychiatr*. 1996;61:90.
10. Silva MFB, Aires CCP, Luis PBM. Valproic acid metabolism and its effects on mitochondrial fatty acid oxidation: a review. *J Inherit Metab Dis*. 2008;31:205.
11. Armon C, Radtke RA, Friedman AH. Inhibitory simple partial (non-convulsive) status epilepticus after intracranial surgery. *J Neurol Neurosurg Psychiatr*. 2000;69:18.
12. Sessia SS and McLachlan RS. Aura continua. *Epilepsia*. 2005;46(3):454.
13. Celesia GG. Modern concepts of status epilepticus. *JAMA*. 1976;235:1571.
14. Krumholz A, Sung GY, Fisher RS, et al. Complex partial status epilepticus accompanied by serious morbidity and mortality. *Neurology*. 1996;45:1499.
15. Meierkord H, Boon P, Engelsen B, et al. EFNS guideline on the management of status epilepticus in adults. *Eur J Neurol*. 2010;17:348.
16. Baykan B, Gokyigit A, Gurses C, et al. Recurrent absence status epilepticus: clinical and EEG characteristics. *Seizure*. 2002;11:310.
17. Korff CM, Nordlii DR Jr. Diagnosis and management of nonconvulsive epilepticus in children. *Nat Clin Pract Neurol*. 2007;3:505.
18. Shorvon S, Walker M. Status epilepticus in idiopathic generalized epilepsies. *Epilepsia*. 2005;46(S9):73.
19. Shirasaka Y. Lack of neuronal damage in atypical absence status epilepticus. *Epilepsia*. 2002;43:1498–1501.
20. Thomas P, Beaumanoir A, Genton P, Chatel M. "De novo" absence status of late onset: report of 11 cases. *Neurology*. 1992;42:104.
21. Thomas P, Valton L, Genton P. Absence and myoclonic status epilepticus precipitated by antiepileptic drugs in idiopathic generalized epilepsy. *Brain*. 2006;129:1281.
22. Jumao-as A, Brenner RP. Myoclonic status epilepticus: a clinical and electroencephalographic study. *Neurology*. 1990;40:1199.
23. Treiman DM, Walton NY, Kendrick C. A progressive sequence of electroencephalographic changes during generalized convulsive status epilepticus. *Epilepsy Res*. 1990;5:49.
24. Pender RA, Losey TE. A rapid course through the five electrographic stages of status epilepticus. *Epilepsia*. 2012;53(11):e193.
25. Beniczky S, et al. Unified EEG terminology and criteria for nonconvulsive status epilepticus. *Epilepsia*. 2013;54(S6):28.
26. Nishiyama M, Nagase H, Trinka T, et al. Demographics and outcomes of patients with pediatric febrile convulsive status epilepticus. *Pediatr Neurol*. 2015;52(5):499.
27. DeLorenzo RJ, Hauser WA, Towne AR, et al. A prospective, population-based epidemiologic study of status epilepticus in Richmond, Virginia. *Neurology*. 1996;46:1029.
28. Knake S, Rosenow F, Vescovi M, et al. Incidence of status epilepticus in adults in Germany: a prospective, population-based study. *Epilepsia*. 2001;42:714.
29. Coeytaux A, Jallon P, Galobardes B, et al. Incidence of status epilepticus in French-speaking Switzerland: (EPISTAR). *Neurology*. 2000;55:693.
30. Hesdorffer DC, Logroscino G, Cascino G, et al. Incidence of status epilepticus in Rochester, Minnesota, 1965–1984. *Neurology*. 1998;50:735.
31. Towne AR, Waterhouse EJ, Boggs JG, et al. Prevalence of nonconvulsive status epilepticus in comatose patients. *Neurology*. 2000;54:340.
32. Privitera M, Hoffman M, Moore JL, et al. EEG detection of nontonic-clonic status epilepticus in patients with altered consciousness. *Epilepsy Res*. 1994;18:155.
33. DeLorenzo RJ, Waterhouse EJ, Towne AR, et al. Persistent nonconvulsive status epilepticus after the control of convulsive status epilepticus. *Epilepsia*. 1998;39:833.
34. Vespa PM, O'Phelan K, Shah M, et al. Acute seizures after intracerebral hemorrhage: a factor in progressive midline shift and outcome. *Neurology*. 2003;60:1441.
35. Claassen J, Mayer SA, Kowalski RG, et al. Detection of electrographic seizures with continuous EEG monitoring in critically ill patients. *Neurology*. 2004;62:1743.
36. Towne AR, Pellock JM, Ko D, et al. Determinants of mortality in status epilepticus. *Epilepsia*. 1994;35:27.
37. Lawn ND, Wijdicks EF. Progress in clinical neurosciences: status epilepticus: a critical review of management options. *Can J Neurol Sci*. 2002;29:206.
38. Ruegg SJ, Dichter MA. Diagnosis and treatment of nonconvulsive status epilepticus in an intensive care unit setting. *Curr Treat Options Neurol*. 2003;5:93.
39. Chen JW, Wasterlain CG. Status epilepticus: pathophysiology and management in adults. *Lancet Neurol*. 2006;5:246.
40. Lowenstein DH, Alldredge BK. Status epilepticus at an urban public hospital in the 1980s. *Neurology*. 1993;43:483.
41. Schaller B, Ruegg SJ. Brain tumor and seizures: pathophysiology and its implications for treatment revisited. *Epilepsia*. 2003;44:1223.
42. Sperling MR, Ko J. Seizures and brain tumors. *Semin Oncol*. 2006;33:333.
43. Liigant A, Haldre S, Oun A, et al. Seizure disorders in patients with brain tumors. *Eur Neurol*. 2001;45:46.

44. Labovitz DL, Hauser WA, Sacco RL. Prevalence and predictors of early seizure and status epilepticus after first stroke. *Neurology*. 2001;57:200.
45. Hart RG, Byer JA, Slaughter JR, et al. Occurrence and implications of seizures in subarachnoid hemorrhage due to ruptured intracranial aneurysms. *Neurosurgery*. 1981;8:417.
46. Afsar N, Kaya D, Aktan S, et al. Stroke and status epilepticus: stroke type, type of status epilepticus, and prognosis. *Seizure*. 2003;12:23.
47. So EL, Annegers JF, Hauser WA, et al. Population-based study of seizure disorders after cerebral infarction. *Neurology*. 1996;46:350.
48. Burn J, Dennis M, Bamford J, et al. Epileptic seizures after a first stroke: the Oxfordshire Community Stroke Project. *BMJ*. 1997;315:1582.
49. Hasan D, Schonck RS, Avezaat CJ, et al. Epileptic seizures after subarachnoid hemorrhage. *Ann Neurol*. 1993;33:286.
50. Dennis LJ, Claassen J, Hirsch LJ, et al. Nonconvulsive status epilepticus after subarachnoid hemorrhage. *Neurosurgery*. 2002;51:1136.
51. Kunisaki TA, Augenstein WL. Drug- and toxin-induced seizures. *Emerg Med Clin North Am*. 1994;12:1027.
52. Wills B, Erickson T. Drug- and toxin-associated seizures. *Med Clin North Am*. 2005;89:1297.
53. Jenssen S, Gracely EJ, Sperling MR. How long do most seizures last? A systematic comparison of seizures recorded in the epilepsy-monitoring unit. *Epilepsia*. 2006;47:1499.
54. Vicedomini JP, Nadler JV. A model of status epilepticus based on electrical stimulation of hippocampal afferent pathways. *Exp Neurol*. 1987;96:681.
55. Wasterlain CG, Mazarati AM, Naylor D, et al. Short-term plasticity of hippocampal neuropeptides and neuronal circuitry in experimental status epilepticus. *Epilepsia*. 2002;43(Suppl 5):20.
56. Mazarati AM, Wasterlain CG. N-methyl-D-aspartate receptor antagonists abolish the maintenance phase of self-sustaining status epilepticus in rat. *Neurosci Lett*. 1999;265:187.
57. Krishnamurthy KB, Drislane FW. Relapse and survival after barbiturate anesthetic treatment of refractory status epilepticus. *Epilepsia*. 1996;37:863.
58. Kapur J, Macdonald RL. Rapid seizure-induced reduction of benzodiazepine and Zn^{2+} sensitivity of hippocampal dentate granule cell $GABA_A$ receptors. *J Neurosci*. 1997;17:7532.
59. Mazarati AM, Baldwin RA, Sankar R, et al. Time-dependent decrease in the effectiveness of antiepileptic drugs during the course of self-sustaining status epilepticus. *Brain Res*. 1998;814:179.
60. Meldrum BS, Horton RW. Physiology of status epilepticus in primates. *Arch Neurol*. 1973;28:1.
61. Meldrum BS, Vigouroux RA, Brierley JB. Systemic factors and epileptic brain damage. Prolonged seizures in paralyzed, artificially ventilated baboons. *Arch Neurol*. 1973;29:82.
62. Sloviter RS. Decreased hippocampal inhibition and a selective loss of interneurons in experimental epilepsy. *Science*. 1987;235:73.
63. Corsellis JA, Bruton CJ. Neuropathology of status epilepticus in humans. *Adv Neurol*. 1983;34:129.
64. DeGiorgio CM, Correale JD, Gott PS, et al. Serum neuron-specific enolase in human status epilepticus. *Neurology*. 1995;45:1134.
65. Chu K, Kang DW, Kim JY, et al. Diffusion-weighted magnetic resonance imaging in nonconvulsive status epilepticus. *Arch Neurol*. 2001;58:993.
66. Walker MT, Lee SY. Profound neocortical atrophy after prolonged, continuous status epilepticus. *AJR Am J Roentgenol*. 1999;173:1712.
67. Lansberg MG, O'Brien MW, Norbash AM, et al. MRI abnormalities associated with partial status epilepticus. *Neurology*. 1999;52:1021.
68. Lazeyras F, Blanke O, Zimine I, et al. MRI, (1)H-MRS, and functional MRI during and after prolonged nonconvulsive seizure activity. *Neurology*. 2000;55:1677.
69. Wasterlain CG. Mortality and morbidity from serial seizures: an experimental study. *Epilepsia*. 1974;15:155.
70. Simon RP. Physiologic consequences of status epilepticus. *Epilepsia*. 1985;26(Suppl 1):S58.
71. Meldrum BS, Brierley JB. Prolonged epileptic seizures in primates: ischemic cell change and its relation to ictal physiological events. *Arch Neurol*. 1973;28:10.
72. Aminoff MJ, Simon RP. Status epilepticus. Causes, clinical features and consequences in 98 patients. *Am J Med*. 1980;69:657.
73. Winocour PH, Waise A, Young G, et al. Severe, self-limiting lactic acidosis and rhabdomyolysis accompanying convulsions. *Postgrad Med J*. 1989;65:321.
74. Treiman DM, Walton NY, Kendrick C. A progressive sequence of electroencephalographic changes during generalized convulsive status epilepticus. *Epilepsy Res*. 1990;5:49.
75. Lowenstein DH, Aminoff MJ. Clinical and EEG features of status epilepticus in comatose patients. *Neurology*. 1992;42:100.
76. Jedrzejczak J, Owczarek K, Majkowski J. Psychogenic pseudoepileptic seizures: clinical and electroencephalogram (EEG) video-tape recordings. *Eur J Neurol*. 1999;6:473.
77. Dworetzky BA, Mortati KA, Rossetti AO, et al. Clinical characteristics of psychogenic nonepileptic seizures. *Epilepsy Behav*. 2006;9(2):35–38.
78. Lowenstein DH. The management of refractory status epilepticus: an update. *Epilepsia*. 2006;47(Suppl 1):35.
79. Walker MC, Smith SJ, Shorvon SD. The intensive care treatment of convulsive status epilepticus in the UK. Results of a national survey and recommendations. *Anaesthesia*. 1995;50:130.
80. Cloyd JC, Lalonde RL, Beniak TE, et al. A single-blind, crossover comparison of the pharmacokinetics and cognitive effects of a new diazepam rectal gel with intravenous diazepam. *Epilepsia*. 1998;39:520.
81. Collins M, Marin H, Rutecki P, et al. A protocol for status epilepticus in a long-term care facility using rectal diazepam (Diastat). *J Am Med Dir Assoc*. 2001;2:66.
82. Alldredge BK, Gelb AM, Isaacs SM, et al. A comparison of lorazepam, diazepam, and placebo for the treatment of out-of-hospital status epilepticus. *N Engl J Med*. 2001;345:631.
83. Brophy GM, Bell R, Claasen J, et al. Guidelines for the evaluation and management of status epilepticus. *Neurocrit Care*. 2012;17:3.
84. Lundgren J, Smith ML, Blennow G, et al. Hyperthermia aggravates and hypothermia ameliorates epileptic brain damage. *Exp Brain Res*. 1994; 99:43.
85. Liu Z, Gatt A, Mikati M, et al. Effect of temperature on kainic acid-induced seizures. *Brain Res*. 1993;631:51.
86. Swan JH, Meldrum BS, Simon RP. Hyperglycemia does not augment neuronal damage in experimental status epilepticus. *Neurology*. 1986;36: 1351.
87. Pang T, Hirsch LJ. Treatment of convulsive and nonconvulsive status epilepticus. *Curr Treat Options Neurol*. 2005;7:247.
88. Lowenstein DH, Alldredge BK. Status epilepticus. *N Engl J Med*. 1998;338: 970.
89. Claassen J, Hirsch LJ, Mayer SA. Treatment of status epilepticus: a survey of neurologists. *J Neurol Sci*. 2003;211:37.
90. Leppik IE, Derivan AT, Homan RW, et al. Double-blind study of lorazepam and diazepam in status epilepticus. *JAMA*. 1983;249:1452.
91. Treiman DM, Meyers PD, Walton NY, et al. A comparison of four treatments for generalized convulsive status epilepticus. Veterans Affairs Status Epilepticus Cooperative Study Group. *N Engl J Med*. 1998;339:792.
92. Osorio I, Reed RC. Treatment of refractory generalized tonic–clonic status epilepticus with pentobarbital anesthesia after high-dose phenytoin. *Epilepsia*. 1989;30:464.
93. Cranford RE, Leppik IE, Patrick B, et al. Intravenous phenytoin: clinical and pharmacokinetic aspects. *Neurology*. 1978;28:874.
94. Coplin WM, Rhoney DH, Rebuck JA, et al. Randomized evaluation of adverse events and length-of-stay with routine emergency department use of phenytoin or fosphenytoin. *Neurol Res*. 2002;24:842.
95. Kugler A, Knapp L, Eldon M. Attainment of therapeutic phenytoin concentration following administration of loading doses of fosphenytoin: a meta-analysis [abstract]. *Neurology*. 1996;46(Suppl):A176.
96. Ramsay RE, Cantrell D, Collins SD, et al. Safety and tolerance of rapidly infused Depacon: a randomized trial in subjects with epilepsy. *Epilepsy Res*. 2003;52:189.
97. Limdi NA, Faught E. The safety of rapid valproic acid infusion. *Epilepsia*. 2000;41:1342.
98. Limdi NA, Shimpi AV, Faught E, et al. Efficacy of rapid IV administration of valproic acid for status epilepticus. *Neurology*. 2005;64:353.
99. Sinha S, Naritoku DK. Intravenous valproate is well tolerated in unstable patients with status epilepticus. *Neurology*. 2000;55:722.
100. Yu KT, Mills S, Thompson N, et al. Safety and efficacy of intravenous valproate in pediatric status epilepticus and acute repetitive seizures. *Epilepsia*. 2003;44:724.
101. Misra UK, Kalita J, Patel R. Sodium valproate vs. phenytoin in status epilepticus: a pilot study. *Neurology*. 2006;67:340.
102. Hodges BM, Mazur JE. Intravenous valproate in status epilepticus. *Ann Pharmacother*. 2001;35:1465.
103. Towne AR, Garnett LK, Waterhouse EJ, et al. The use of topiramate in refractory status epilepticus. *Neurology*. 2003;60:332.
104. Bensalem MK, Fakhoury TA. Topiramate and status epilepticus: report of three cases. *Epilepsy Behav*. 2003;4:757.
105. Perry MS, Holt PJ, Sladky JT. Topiramate loading for refractory status epilepticus in children. *Epilepsia*. 2006;47:1070.
106. Ramael S, Daoust A, Otoul C, et al. Levetiracetam intravenous infusion: a randomized, placebo-controlled safety and pharmacokinetic study. *Epilepsia*. 2006;47:1128.

107. Claassen J, Hirsch LJ, Emerson RG, et al. Treatment of refractory status epilepticus with pentobarbital, propofol, or midazolam: a systematic review. *Epilepsia.* 2002;43:146.
108. Mayer SA, Claassen J, Lokin J, et al. Refractory status epilepticus: frequency, risk factors, and impact on outcome. *Arch Neurol.* 2002;59:205.
109. Niermeijer JM, Uiterwaal CS, Van Donselaar CA. Propofol in status epilepticus: little evidence, many dangers? *J Neurol.* 2003;250:1237.
110. Rossetti AO, Reichhart MD, Schaller MD, et al. Propofol treatment of refractory status epilepticus: a study of 31 episodes. *Epilepsia.* 2004;45:757.
111. van Gestel JP, Blusse van Oud-Alblas HJ, Malingre M, et al. Propofol and thiopental for refractory status epilepticus in children. *Neurology.* 2005;65:591.
112. Mirsattari SM, Sharpe MD, Young GB. Treatment of refractory status epilepticus with inhalational anesthetic agents isoflurane and desflurane. *Arch Neurol.* 2004;61:1254.
113. Sheth RD, Gidal BE. Refractory status epilepticus: response to ketamine. *Neurology.* 1998;51:1765.
114. Ubogu EE, Sagar SM, Lerner AJ, et al. Ketamine for refractory status epilepticus: a case of possible ketamine-induced neurotoxicity. *Epilepsy Behav.* 2003;4:70.
115. Holtkamp M, Othman J, Buchheim K, et al. Predictors and prognosis of refractory status epilepticus treated in a neurological intensive care unit. *J Neurol Neurosurg Psychiatry.* 2005;76:534.
116. Shneker BF, Fountain NB. Assessment of acute morbidity and mortality in nonconvulsive status epilepticus. *Neurology.* 2003;61:1066.
117. Drislane FW, Schomer DL. Clinical implications of generalized electrographic status epilepticus. *Epilepsy Res.* 1994;19:111.
118. Rossetti A, Logroscino G, Bromfield EB. A clinical score for prognosis of status epilepticus in adults. *Neurology.* 2006;66:1736–1738.

CHAPTER

122

Neuromuscular Disorders

SANAM BAGHSHOMALI, SWARNA RAJAGOPALAN, and ATUL KALANURIA

INTRODUCTION

Neuromuscular disorders are commonly encountered in the critical care setting. Patients with known neuromuscular disorders, such as Guillain–Barré syndrome (GBS) or myasthenia gravis (MG), are admitted when muscle weakness compromises the patient's ability to protect his or her airway or threatens respiratory failure. Patients admitted with respiratory failure of unknown cause may be diagnosed with a neuromuscular disorder such as amyotrophic lateral sclerosis (ALS) or myasthenia gravis. Rarely, treatment may unmask a pre-existing neuromuscular disorder, as when drugs with neuromuscular blocking properties are given to patients with myasthenia gravis. Finally, patients with nonneuromuscular critical illnesses frequently develop neuromuscular weakness as a result of their illness or its treatment (1).

Intensive care physicians need to be familiar with the underlying diagnosis and management of patients with neuromuscular disease. Because electrophysiologic testing is often necessary to diagnose neuromuscular disorders in the intensive care setting, they should also have a basic appreciation of the techniques and indications for these studies. GBS and myasthenia gravis are considered in some detail because they are prevalent and treatable, and because, with proper treatment, they often carry a favorable prognosis. Finally, the intensive care physician will be responsible for recognizing and managing neuromuscular disorders that result from critical illness, which are now the neuromuscular disorders most commonly encountered in the intensive care setting (2).

CLINICAL PRESENTATION AND LOCALIZATION

As with central nervous system (CNS) disorders, the first step in the diagnosis of neuromuscular disorders is localization. Neuromuscular disorders comprise disorders of the anterior horn cell, the peripheral nervous system (PNS), the neuromuscular junction, and muscle (Fig. 122.1). Localization of the PNS is further subdivided into roots, plexus, and peripheral nerve; and disorders of peripheral nerve are further subdivided into focal neuropathies, multifocal neuropathies, and polyneuropathies which can be either length dependent or non–length dependent. Each of these nine major localizations has a characteristic pattern of symptoms and physical findings (Table 122.1) and allows the physician to narrow the range considerably of likely diagnoses (see Fig. 122.1). For example, if deficits are restricted to the distribution of a single nerve, the diagnosis is probably nerve entrapment, compression, or trauma. Multiple individual peripheral nerve involvement, in the absence of multiple trauma, should suggest an autoimmune neuropathy, often a vasculitis. Length-dependent polyneuropathy affects the longest nerves first, and consequently presents with deficits in the feet and legs before affecting the hands. Proximal strength is preserved until late. The differential diagnosis is wide, but comprises principally metabolic, toxic, or inherited neuropathies. Non–length-dependent localization is suggested when proximal weakness is greater than would be expected with a length-dependent polyneuropathy. Non–length-dependent polyneuropathies are overwhelmingly caused by autoimmune processes, including GBS. Critical illness polyneuropathy (CIP) may also be considered non–length dependent.

Neuromuscular problems are first suspected when patients recovering from critical illness cannot be weaned from the ventilator or appear extremely weak; both central and neuromuscular causes of weakness need to be considered. This can be straightforward in patients who can give a history of their illness, and who can be adequately examined, however it can be quite challenging in critically ill patients, since these patients are often unable to provide a history or to cooperate with the examination. Central causes of weakness may be suggested by the history and physical examination. Hemiparesis should always suggest a central localization; however, bilateral weakness can also result from central causes. A history of severe hypotension suggests the possibility of bilateral watershed infarction (3); rapid correction of hyponatremia predisposes to central pontine myelinolysis (CPM), an osmotic demyelination syndrome that presents with bulbar weakness and quadriparesis (4); patients after cardiac surgery may have multiple cerebral emboli; patients with aortic dissection may suffer spinal cord infarction.

If the problem is exclusively neuromuscular, features suggestive of CNS localization should be absent. These include mental status changes, hemibody weakness, or numbness suggestive of hemispheric or lateralized brainstem lesions; truncal motor or sensory level suggestive of spinal cord localization; increased muscle tone; hyperactive tendon reflexes; and pathologic reflexes such as the Babinski response. Features consistent with localization to the PNS include weakness, atrophy, decreased or absent tendon reflexes, and sensory loss. Most acquired myopathies present with symmetric proximal weakness, and sensory loss is not a feature of either myopathy or disorders of neuromuscular transmission. Fatigable ptosis, weakness of extraocular movement, dysphagia, dysarthria, and neck, respiratory, and proximal limb weakness should suggest myasthenia gravis, the most common nonpharmacologic disorder of neuromuscular transmission.

Rarely, the presentation of a neuromuscular disorder may be so restricted as to first suggest a nonneurologic problem. Acute pan dysautonomia presents with autonomic failure that can mimic cardiovascular, gastrointestinal, or urinary disorders (5). Diabetic truncal neuropathy can present with abdominal pain that often leads to extensive evaluation for nonneurologic abdominal disorders, including exploratory

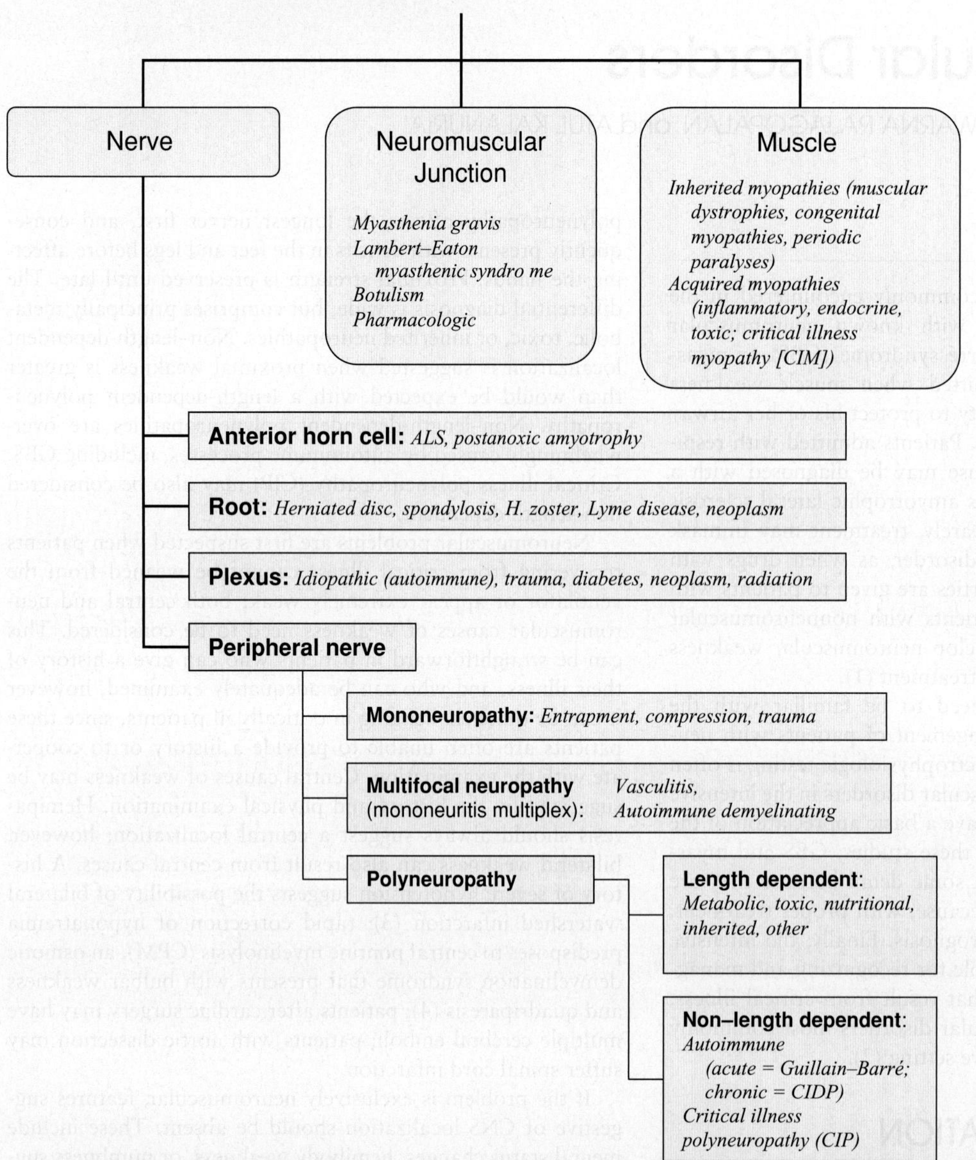

FIGURE 122.1 Localization of neuromuscular disorders, with the most important exemplars for each of the nine localizations. ALS, amyotrophic lateral sclerosis; CIDP, chronic inflammatory demyelinating polyneuropathy.

TABLE 122.1 Salient Features of Neuromuscular Disorders

Localization	Pain	Sensory Loss	Tendon Reflexes	Distribution of Weakness
Muscle	Variable (myalgia)	*No*	Normal or ↓	Symmetric, proximal
Neuromuscular junction				
Myasthenia gravis	*No*	*No*	Normal	EOM, bulbar, respiratory, proximal
Lambert–Eaton	*No*	*No*	↓	Bulbar, proximal
Nerve				
Anterior horn cell	*No*	*No*	↓, (↑ *in ALS*)	*Diffuse (begins focally); spares EOMs, bladder*
Root	Yes	Variable	Focally ↓	*Root*
Plexus	Yes	Variable	Focally ↓	*Plexus*
Mononeuropathy	Variable	Usual	Often normal	*Single nerve*
Multiple mononeuropathy	Variable	Usual	Often normal	*Two or more single nerves*
Length-dependent polyneuropathy	Variable	Usual	Ankle jerks ↓	*Distal (feet → legs → hands)*
Non–length-dependent polyneuropathy	Variable	Variable	Often areflexic	*Proximal as well as distal*

ALS, amyotrophic lateral sclerosis; EOM, extraocular muscle.
The most important features are indicated in italics.

TABLE 122.2 Electrodiagnostic Features in Nonfocal Neuromuscular Disorders

	Anterior Horn Cell	Axonal Neuropathy	Demyelinating Neuropathy	Neuromuscular Junction Disorder	Myopathy
Motor nerve conduction studies					
CMAP amplitude to distal stimulation	Small	*Small*	*Larger than to proximal stimulation*	Normal (MG) or small (MG, LEMS)	Normal or small
CMAP amplitude to proximal stimulation	Same as to distal stimulation	Same as to distal stimulation	*Smaller than to distal stimulation*	Same as to distal stimulation	Same as to distal stimulation
Conduction velocity	Over 70% LLN	*Over 70% LLN*	*Can be <70% LLN*	Normal	Normal
F-wave studies					
F-wave latency	Normal or increased latency	Normal or increased latency	Absent or increased latency	Normal	Normal
Sensory nerve conduction studies					
Sensory nerve action potentials	*Normal*	*Can be reduced or absent (normal in pure motor forms)*	Often reduced or absent (normal in pure motor forms)	*Normal*	*Normal*
Needle EMG					
Spontaneous activity	*Increased*	Increased	Normal	Normal	Normal or increased
MUP morphology	*Normal or large*	Normal or large	Normal or large	Variable MUP morphology	*Small amplitude, polyphasic*
Recruitment	*Decreased*	Decreased	Decreased	Normal or "increased"	*Full recruitment produces little force*
Repetitive stimulation					
2–3 Hz stimulation	Usually normal	Usually normal	Usually normal	*>10% decrement in MG, LEMS*	Usually normal
20–50 Hz stimulation	Normal	Normal	Normal	*>50% increment in LEMS*	Normal

CMAP, compound muscle action potential (the potential recorded in motor nerve conduction studies); EMG, electromyography; MG, myasthenia gravis; LLN, lower limits of normal; LEMS, Lambert–Eaton myasthenic syndrome; MUP, motor unit potential.
The most important features for each localization are indicated in italics.

surgery (6). Respiratory failure can be the presenting feature of a number of neuromuscular diseases, including ALS (7,8), myasthenia gravis (9), and myopathies such as adult-onset acid maltase deficiency (10). These patients may be admitted for respiratory support before the cause is understood; it is left to the intensive care physician to suspect the correct diagnosis.

Brain imaging may help establish a diagnosis in stroke or CPM; in other conditions, such as hypoxia or even acute spinal cord ischemia, imaging may be normal or nondiagnostic. If the cause of apparent weakness remains in question, electrodiagnostic testing is of value in suggesting or helping to exclude a neuromuscular localization.

ELECTRODIAGNOSTIC STUDIES

Nerve conduction studies (NCSs), late wave analysis, needle electromyography (EMG), and repetitive stimulation are the standard procedures available to assist in the diagnosis of neuromuscular disorders, and can be performed using portable equipment in the intensive care setting. Table 122.2 summarizes the typical electrodiagnostic findings in disorders of nerve, neuromuscular junction, and muscle.

Nerve Conduction Studies

Motor nerves that are usually tested by NCSs include the tibial, peroneal, and ulnar nerves (11). Figure 2A illustrates the typical motor nerve conduction procedure and normal response from stimulation of the tibial nerve. The nerve is stimulated at two or more sites, and the response is recorded with surface electrodes over a muscle innervated by that nerve. The muscle response is called a *compound muscle action potential* (CMAP), because it is the sum of all muscle fiber action potentials activated by nerve stimulation. The stimulus at each site is gradually increased until no further increase in CMAP amplitude is seen. This indicates that all of the motor neurons capable of generating an action potential have been activated. The latency to the onset of the CMAP reflects the speed of conduction in the fastest nerve fibers. Motor nerve conduction velocity is calculated by measuring the distance between the sites of stimulation, and dividing that distance by the proximal minus the distal latency, which is the time it takes for the stimulus to traverse that nerve segment. By itself, motor nerve conduction can be diagnostic of focal or generalized demyelinating neuropathy (see Fig. 2C,D). Interpreting a low-amplitude response (see Fig. 2B) requires additional studies, since low CMAP amplitude can reflect not only loss of nerve axons or conduction block, but also defective neuromuscular transmission or loss of muscle fibers.

Sensory nerves are mostly evaluated on electrodiagnostic studies are radial, ulnar and sural nerves (11). In orthodromic sensory NCSs, the skin is stimulated and a response is recorded over the nerve. Antidromic studies are more commonly performed by stimulating the nerve and recording over the skin. The result in either case is a sensory nerve action potential

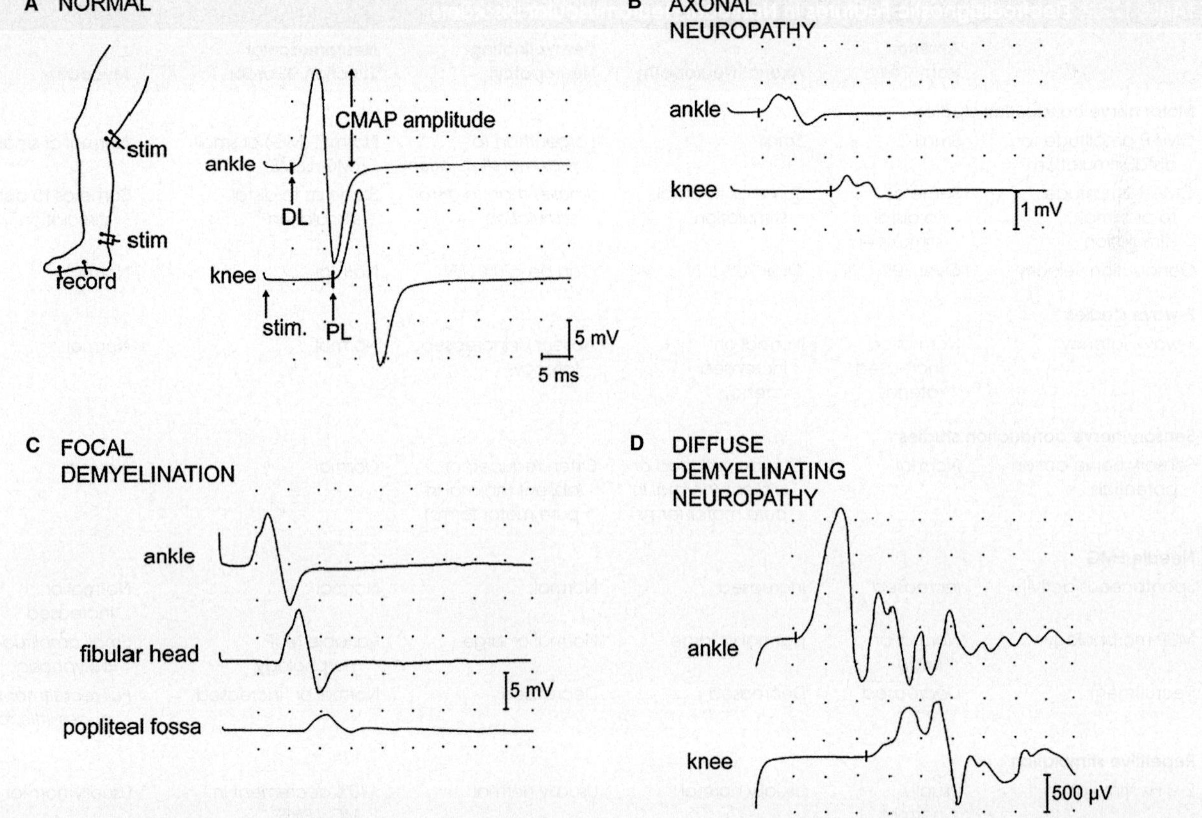

FIGURE 122.2 Typical motor nerve conduction findings. The sweep speed is 5 ms/div in all traces, but the gain is 5 mV/div in (A) and (C), 1 mV/div in (B), and 500 μV/div in (D). **A:** Tibial motor nerve conduction in a normal subject. The drawing shows the two sites of stimulation over the posterior tibial nerve at the ankle and knee, and the sites of surface electrodes recording the response of the medial plantar muscle group. The two waveforms are the responses to stimulation at the ankle and knee. Conduction velocity is calculated as the distance between proximal and distal sites of stimulation divided by the time it takes for the stimulus to travel between the sites of stimulation (PL minus DL). **B:** Tibial motor nerve conduction in a patient with axonal sensorimotor neuropathy. CMAP amplitudes are less than 2 mV, with normal being greater than 4 mV. The amplitudes are similar with proximal (knee) and distal (ankle) stimulation. The conduction velocity is slightly slow, but is greater than 80% of the lower limits of normal. **C:** Peroneal motor nerve conduction study in focal nerve compression. CMAP amplitude drops sharply with nerve stimulation above the site of compression, at the fibular head. This conduction block is caused by focal nerve demyelination. Because there is no damage to axons, the nerve responds normally to stimulation distal to the area of demyelination. Conduction velocity is slow across the fibular head. **D:** Acquired diffuse demyelinating polyradiculoneuropathy. Multifocal demyelination affects some neurons more than others, resulting in prolonged and irregular CMAPs. Conduction velocities less than 70% of the lower limits of normal are also diagnostic of demyelination. DL, distal latency; PL, proximal latency; CMAP, compound muscle action potential.

(SNAP), with a latency that reflects conduction in the fastest nerve fibers, and an amplitude that is proportional to the number of functioning nerve fibers. The normal SNAP amplitude is small and measured in microvolts. Abnormal SNAPs are indicative of pathology distal to dorsal root ganglion—either plexopathy or neuropathy. SNAPs are normal in radiculopathy if the pathology spares the dorsal root ganglia in CNS disorders as well as in disorders of neuromuscular transmission and muscle. In a patient with weakness and abnormal motor NCSs, small or absent SNAPs suggest sensorimotor neuropathy or plexopathy.

Action potentials in motor neurons, called F waves, are normally generated at the axon hillock and travel distally to nerve terminals in muscle; when the nerve is stimulated in the course of NCSs, action potentials travel both orthodromically (distally) and antidromically (proximally) from the point of stimulation. The antidromic action potential depolarizes the axon hillock and, in a minority of neurons, this depolarization generates another action potential that travels orthodromically down the nerve. F wave are small and late muscle action potential can be recorded from most muscles. Increased F-wave latency, when combined with normal distal motor nerve conduction, indicates disease in the proximal portions of the nerve. Abnormal or absent F waves are the earliest electrophysiologic manifestation of GBS (12,13).

In patients whom a neuropathic process is suspected, electrodiagnostic studies begin with NCSs in bilateral lower extremities and one upper extremity preferably on the side that is more symptomatic if the symptoms are asymmetric. In myopathies, NCSs are not necessary and are only required when there is severe atrophy of distal muscles of the affected limb. In disease processes where there is damage to myelin sheath (demyelination), general findings on NCSs include decrease conduction velocity, prolonged F wave, prolonged distal latency, reduced SNAP, and reduce/absence of CMAP. There are two other measures; temporal dispersion and conduction block that help differentiate between a uniform and a segmental process. In uniform demyelinating processes (Hereditary Neuropathies) conduction block and temporal dispersion are not seen.

EMG entails inserting a recording needle electrode into a muscle and observing (a) insertional activity consisting of action potentials generated by mechanical deformation of muscle fibers; (b) resting activity, which in normal muscles is only seen when the needle is near an end plate; and (c) voluntary activity, which consists of motor unit action potentials (MUAPs). The motor unit consists of a motor neuron and all the muscle fibers innervated by it. The MUP is the sum of action potentials of all the muscle fibers in the vicinity of the recording needle electrode that are activated by a single motor neuron. Insertional and resting activity does not require patient cooperation, and can be observed in comatose or uncooperative patients. One to 3 weeks after denervation associated with axon damage, denervated muscle membranes become hypersensitive and discharge both spontaneously and in response to needle insertion, causing increased insertional activity and the of positive sharp waves and fibrillations, which are spontaneous or needle movement–induced discharges of single muscle fibers. Similar abnormal spontaneous activity can be seen in disorders of muscle, particularly in the inflammatory myopathies, perhaps as a result of functional denervation caused by muscle fiber damage. If the patient is cooperative or happens to activate the muscle during the needle EMG study, additional information can be obtained by observing MUP activity. MUP morphology is of diagnostic value: high-amplitude, long-duration motor unit potentials indicate denervation with reinnervation, and low-amplitude, polyphasic motor unit potentials suggest primary disease of muscle or neuromuscular junction. Observation of motor unit recruitment with increasing effort can be diagnostic of denervation in the absence of any other abnormality. With denervation, MUP firing frequency increases with increasing effort, but insufficient numbers of different MUPs are recruited. Conversely, rapid recruitment of small polyphasic MUPs suggests myopathy or a disorder of neuromuscular transmission. Increased variability of the shape of a single MUP suggests a disorder of neuromuscular transmission.

EMG in neuropathic processes should begin with distal muscles since those muscles are affected earlier in the course of the disease. If a motor neuron disease is of concern, both distal and proximal muscles of upper and lower extremities should be evaluated (11). Electrodiagnostic findings in motor neuron disease include low motor amplitude, normal distal motor latencies, normal conduction velocities, and normal sensory NCS. On EMG, patients have spontaneous muscle activity, for example, fibrillation, fasciculation, or positive sharp waves with small or large MUAPs (EMG-NCV). In neuromuscular junction disorders MUAPs can be normal or polyphasic with small duration and low amplitude which is secondary to decrease in neuromuscular transmission (11).

Disorders of neuromuscular transmission may be postsynaptic, as is the case in myasthenia gravis or most pharmacologic neuromuscular blocking agents, or presynaptic, as in Lambert–Eaton myasthenic syndrome (LEMS) and with exposure to botulinum toxin. Repetitive nerve stimulation (RNS) results are dependent on safety factor of the neuromuscular junction. Safety factor is the number of activated acetylcholine receptors required to produce an action potential, large enough to depolarize the membrane and subsequently muscle contraction (14). In presynaptic disorders, acetylcholine release from the presynaptic membrane is not enough to activate the postsynaptic receptors available. On the opposite side, in postsynaptic disorders, there is enough acetylcholine released from presynaptic membrane but not enough receptors available in postsynaptic membrane to be activated and generate the action potential required for muscle contraction. RNS studies are helpful in distinguishing these two categories. RNS is performed at a slow rate (2–3 Hz) and a fast rate (20–30 Hz) (11). Repetitive supramaximal stimulation of a motor nerve at a constant rate for five to ten stimuli is a simple way to assess for deficits of neuromuscular transmission. The resultant CMAP amplitudes should be constant. In patients with neuromuscular disorders, given multiple slow stimulations repetitively, the amount of acetylcholine released from presynaptic membrane decreases with each stimulation, with subsequent lower CMAPs and NMJ block (11).

Progressive decrements in amplitude across the first four to five responses with 3-Hz stimulation are seen in both postsynaptic and presynaptic disorders of neuromuscular transmission. Progressive increments in response at rates of stimulation above 20 Hz suggest a presynaptic neuromuscular block, as in LEMS, or botulism. An alternative—and more tolerable—means to look for this incremental response is to stimulate the nerve supramaximally just before and just after 10 to 60 seconds of sustained voluntary contraction of the muscle being tested. An increase in amplitude after exercise—postexercise facilitation—is seen in pre- and postsynaptic disorders; however, increases greater than 100% are seen only in presynaptic disorders (15). Repetitive stimulation is important in documenting residual neuromuscular blockade as a cause of weakness in ICU patients. RNS should not be performed close to central venous catheters or pacemakers.

CLINICAL MANAGEMENT

Prehospital Management

Neuromuscular disorders can present acutely as a neurologic emergency. The first responder priority is to assess the patency and stability of the patient's airway, breathing, and circulation (ABC's). A brief neurologic assessment must be made in order to rule out major neurologic disorders such as acute strokes, subarachnoid hemorrhage, seizures, toxin exposures, etc.

A detailed history helps formulating a diagnosis by localizing the disorder and understanding the underlying pathophysiology. Patient should be interviewed regarding presenting symptoms, the pace of progression, the pattern of weakness (ascending vs. descending), and diurnal variation and fatigability (steady progression vs. fluctuating pattern). The emergency neurological life support (ENLS) algorithm is a useful guide to assist the physician with deducing the level of the lesion (16).

Evaluation for Intensive Care Unit Admission

Indications for intensive care of patients with neuromuscular disorders include airway protection, respiratory failure, and autonomic instability. It is worth pointing out that many of the signs typically associated with respiratory failure in patients with obstructive pulmonary disorders, such as increased respiratory excursion, may not be seen in patients with neuromuscular causes of respiratory failure. Instead, difficulty clearing secretions, staccato speech and repiratory symptoms such as air hunger, tachypnea and shallow breathing are characteristic. An inability to lay supine and paradoxical respirations are manifestations of severe diaphragmatic weakness. Confusion and somnolence with rising partial pressure of carbon dioxide

($PaCO_2$) may lessen respiratory distress and make recognition of respiratory insufficiency more difficult. Bedside tests of respiratory function that indicate a need for respiratory support include the inability to count to 20 on one breath, a forced vital capacity of less than 15 mL/kg, a negative inspiratory force of less than 25 cm H_2O, and a positive expiratory force of less than 40 cm H_2O (17–20). Patients with facial weakness may have difficulty performing bedside tests, necessitating greater reliance on blood gas monitoring. Intubation may be required earlier in patients with dysphagia in order to protect the airway.

Autonomic dysfunction and pain can be features of the GBS and are discussed under that topic below. Patients who are immobile from weakness or other causes may suffer compressive neuropathies. The peroneal nerve at the head of the fibula and the ulnar nerve at the elbow are especially vulnerable. Constant attention to positioning is required to prevent pressure palsies. Pneumatic compression devices should not cover the proximal fibula.

Neuromuscular disorders do not affect mentation, and it is important to maintain communication to inquire about discomfort and pain, involve patients in care and decision making, and support them through what can be a terrifying experience. Bowes, a physician who recovered from ventilator-dependent GBS, gives a personal account of her experience that is instructive for caregivers (21). Additional aspects of the intensive care of neuromuscular disorders are discussed below with reference to specific disorders.

Table 122.3 lists some of the neuromuscular conditions that can cause respiratory failure. Weakness can develop gradually, and initial management might not require immediate need for intensive care, except when intercurrent illness, such as aspiration pneumonia, complicates the hospital course. ALS inevitably leads to respiratory failure. In a minority of patients with ALS respiratory insufficiency is the presenting symptom, and leads to intensive care admission before the diagnosis is made. The diagnosis is suggested by finding fasciculations, atrophy, weakness, and hyperactive reflexes in the absence of sensory loss, extraocular muscle weakness, or autonomic dysfunction, and by excluding alternative causes, such as spinal cord compression or neuropathy. Electrophysiologic studies can be helpful. NCSs document normal SNAPs, and needle EMG reveals denervation in muscle of three or more extremities or two extremities and bulbar muscles. Needle EMG can also document diaphragm denervation. Early in the course, clinical and electrophysiologic findings may not suffice for definitive diagnosis.

Respiratory weakness is seen in some muscle disorders, and is a terminal event in Duchenne muscular dystrophy. Respiratory weakness can be the presenting feature of adult-onset acid maltase deficiency, a glycogen storage disease (22), and it is a feature of some of the congenital myopathies and muscular dystrophies. Respiratory weakness can occur in inflammatory myopathies in the context of severe proximal limb weakness, and polymyositis associated with Jo-1 antibodies can be associated with interstitial pulmonary disease (23).

TABLE 122.3 Neuromuscular Causes of Respiratory Failure

Disorders of Nerve

- Amyotrophic lateral sclerosis (ALS)
- Guillain–Barré syndrome
- Toxic neuropathies
- Critical illness polyneuropathy
- Phrenic neuropathy (brachial plexus neuropathy, radiation trauma, postthoracotomy)
- Vasculitic neuropathy and collagen vascular diseases (e.g., in SLE, systemic vasculitis)
- Acute intermittent porphyria
- Transverse myelitis
- Spinal cord infarction, Brown-Séquard syndrome
- Acute diabetic neuropathy
- Viral illness mediated (e.g., West Nile virus infection, polio)
- Nerve compression
- Polyneuropathy, organomegaly, endocrinopathy, monoclonal gammopathy, skin changes (POEMS) syndrome

Disorders of Neuromuscular Junction

- Myasthenia gravis
- Acetylcholine receptor antibody associated
- Muscle-specific kinase (MuSK) antibody associated
- Lambert–Eaton myasthenic syndrome (LEMS)
- Tetanus and botulism
- Pharmacologic neuromuscular blockade
- Animal/insect bite with envenomation (snake bite, tick paralysis)
- Toxin mediated, poisoning (e.g., organophosphate poisoning, heavy metal toxicity, nerve gas exposure)
- Hypermagnesemia

Disorders of Muscle

- Polymyositis/dermatomyositis
- Muscular dystrophies (dystrophinopathies, limb girdle types 2A and 2I, myotonic muscular dystrophy, myofibrillar myopathies)
- Congenital myopathies (nemaline rod, centronuclear)
- Glycogen storage disorders (acid maltase deficiency, debrancher enzyme deficiency)
- Other inherited myopathies (mitochondrial myopathies, distal muscular dystrophy with respiratory weakness)
- Metabolic myopathies (e.g., acid maltase deficiency, mitochondrial myopathy, deficiency of β-oxidation or fatty acid transport enzymes)
- Endocrine disorders (hyperthyroidism/hypothyroidism, hypoadrenalism/hyperadrenalism, hyperparathyroidism)
- Periodic paralysis
- Medication induced (e.g., antiretroviral drugs, corticosteroids, HMG-CoA reductase inhibitors, colchicine)
- Toxic myopathies (alcohol, cocaine, heroin)
- Hypophosphatemia

RESPIRATORY FAILURE

The main cause of respiratory failure in patients with neuromuscular disorders is muscle weakness, which can be significant in respiratory muscles, or causes inability to protect ones airway. In most causes this leads to intrathoracic infections, notably pneumonia. Although uncommon, respiratory failure can be the only presenting symptom in some of the neuromuscular disorders, however in most causes, it develops during the course of the disease (24–26).

Three groups of muscles aid with inspiration; the diaphragm, which is responsible for 70% of inspiratory tidal volume and is innervated by phrenic nerve (C3–5): external intercostal muscles: accessory muscles.

Exhalation is assisted through two groups of muscles; internal intercostal muscles and abdominal muscles. Bulbar muscles are responsible for speech and swallowing (24).

Weakness of respiratory muscles prevents patients from taking deep breaths causing a decline in tidal volume and subsequently CO_2 retention and hypercapnic/hypoxic respiratory failure.

Patients with neuromuscular disorders have reduced respiratory reserve and can decompensate quickly with any additional respiratory load.

In patients with skeletal abnormalities related to the underlying disease (kyphoscoliosis in some of muscular dystrophies) respiratory failure can appear early (24).

Upon assessing patients for respiratory status, it is important to identify which muscles are weak and the degree of weakness. Bulbar muscles weakness causes difficulty in mastication, swallowing, and maintaining airway, which increases the risk of aspiration pneumonia. Weakness of respiratory muscles, in particular the diaphragm, causes a decrease in inspiratory tidal volume causing atelectasis and eventually pneumonia.

Accurate diagnostic evaluation includes the following evaluation.

- Detailed history regarding similar symptoms in the past, prior intubation for respiratory failure secondary to muscle weakness, diplopia, swallowing difficulties, recent changes in voice.
- Detailed cranial nerve examination for evaluation gag reflex, cough, and tongue movements/strength as well as signs of swallowing difficulty like dystonia and drooling.
- Abdominal examination to evaluate paradoxical abdominal movements as a sign of diaphragm weakness and pending respiratory failure.
- Continuous pulse oximetry evaluation.
- Chest x-ray for evaluation of underlying pulmonary diseases.
- ABG: provides PO_2 and PCO_2 measures that help in assessing oxygenation and ventilation.
- Serial bedside spirometry to assess the progression of muscle weakness. Forced vital capacity, Maximum inspiratory pressure (also know as negative inspiratory pressure) and maximum expiratory pressure assess diaphragmatic strength, with a vital capacity of less than 15 mL/kg indicating an immediate risk of respiratory failure. Patient's lack of cooperation for an accurate measurement can cause variable values reduced accuracy of measurement.

Noninvasive positive pressure ventilation (NIPPV) can be attempted in cases of mild respiratory dysfunction but only if rapid improvement in respiratory symptoms is expected with therapy (e.g., myasthenia gravis). Rapid sequence intubation is preferred for patients requiring an advanced airway. Succinylcholine may be ineffective at standard doses and no agents or short acting nondepolarizing agents are usually used (e.g., progressive muscular weakness). Autonomic instability might follow intubation and should be promptly treated (e.g., in GBS). Glycopyrrolate and atropine in sequence should be available to treat severe bradyarrhythmias (16,27).

The two neuromuscular disorders that most commonly lead to admission for intensive care are Guillain–Barré and myasthenia gravis. They are both autoimmune disorders and can cause rapidly progressive weakness and treatable. They will be examined in detail in this chapter.

GUILLAIN–BARRÉ SYNDROME

In 1859, Landry (28) described a syndrome of ascending paralysis progressing to respiratory paralysis and death. Guillain, Barré, and Strohl described the classic features of progressive weakness, sensory symptoms, and loss of tendon reflexes. They also described increased cerebrospinal fluid (CSF) protein without cells (albuminocytologic dissociation), a finding that distinguishes this disorder from poliomyelitis (29). An association with prior infection was established (30,31), and the concept that the disease was of autoimmune pathogenesis was supported by the development of an animal model—experimental allergic neuritis (EAN), in which inflammation and demyelination of peripheral nerves followed exposure to components of peripheral nerves (32).

Definition and Subtypes

GBS is an autoimmune disorder of peripheral nerves with progression over less than 4 weeks, which is manifested by weakness, reduced or absent tendon reflexes, and variable sensory and autonomic dysfunction (33). Subtypes have been distinguished based on the presence or absence of motor, sensory, and/or autonomic involvement, and on whether the predominant damage is to myelin sheaths or axons. Acute inflammatory demyelinating polyradiculoneuropathy (AIDP) is by far the most common subtype, accounting for more than 85% of cases in the United States (34). Patients have weakness and reflex loss, with varying degrees of sensory and autonomic involvement, and there is electrophysiologic and pathologic evidence of peripheral nerve demyelination. Patients who have no sensory loss and electrodiagnostic studies suggesting axonal rather than demyelinating pathology have acute motor axonal neuropathy (AMAN). This variety of GBS was first described in Asia, where it occurs epidemically following gastroenteritis caused by *Campylobacter jejuni* (35). Acute motor sensory axonal neuropathy (AMSAN) is diagnosed when there is both motor and sensory involvement and NCSs are consistent with early axonal dysfunction (36). The axonal forms of Guillain–Barré comprise less than 5% of cases in Europe and North America, but up to 47% of cases in China, Japan, and Central and South America (37). Acute dysautonomic dysfunction (5,38) and some forms of acute sensory neuropathy (39) are sometimes considered to be subtypes of GBS even though weakness is not a feature, since they run a similar time course, and are presumed to be autoimmune. The Miller–Fisher variant of GBS features ophthalmoplegia, ataxia, and areflexia (40). The Miller–Fisher variant may overlap with other forms of GBS (37,41).

Epidemiology and Pathogenesis

The incidence of Guillain–Barré is less than 1 in 100,000 in children, averages 1 to 2 per 100,000 in adults, and increases to 4 in 100,000 in adults over 75 years of age (42,43). In about two-thirds of patients, the disease follows an infection, most often a flu-like syndrome or gastroenteritis, by 1 to 8 weeks (44). When serologic studies are performed, evidence of infection with *C. jejuni,* cytomegalovirus, Epstein–Barr virus, *Haemophilus influenzae,* and *Mycoplasma pneumoniae* are found to account for the majority of cases (45,46); 5% follow surgery (31). Although 3% of cases are attributed to vaccination (44), only rabies vaccine is associated with a definite increase in the incidence of Guillain–Barré (47); influenza vaccination increase is minimal (47,48).

The pathology of AIDP consists of a multifocal inflammation of peripheral nerves, in which macrophages destroy the myelin sheath (49–52). This response is mediated by activated T cells (53). Direct binding of antibodies to Schwann cell membranes with subsequent complement-mediated destruction and secondary macrophage invasion may also play a role (54). Similar pathologic findings characterize EAN, which is considered to be a good experimental model for GBS (55). EAN can be initiated by injections of several myelin components, including myelin proteins P0 and P2, myelin basic protein, peripheral myelin protein-22 (PMP-22), and myelin-associated glycoprotein (MAG) (53). No specific myelin antibodies have been identified in the pathogenesis of AIDP.

The pathology of AMAN differs from that of AIDP in that macrophages target the axonal membrane in ventral (motor) roots and nerves at nodes of Ranvier, resulting in axonal rather than myelin damage (56,57). The pathology in AMSAN is similar to that of AMAN, except that the disorder affects both motor and sensory roots and nerves (36). Recent evidence suggests that AMAN may result from molecular mimicry. The capsule of the strains of *C. jejuni* implicated in patients with GBS contains a lipopolysaccharide with a structure similar to the GM_1 ganglioside present in peripheral nerves. Antibodies to these strains of *C. jejuni* cross-react with peripheral nerve GM_1 ganglioside, resulting in axonal dysfunction in experimental animals (58). Similarly, many patients with the Miller–Fisher variant have GQ1b and GT1a antibodies (59) that cross-react with *Campylobacter* lipopolysaccharides (60,61). Anti-GD1b antibodies have been associated with acute and chronic sensory neuropathies (37). Although there is evidence that molecular mimicry is a plausible explanation for some patients with Guillain–Barré polyneuropathy, the relationships are complex. Patients may have antibodies to several gangliosides, antibodies to a particular ganglioside can be associated with several different types of neuropathy, and infections with a specific organism may be followed by more than one kind of neuropathy (37).

Clinical Presentation and Differential Diagnosis

GBS is a subacute process. AIDP, the most common form of Guillain–Barré, presents with weakness and decreased or absent tendon reflexes. It is a non–length-dependent polyneuropathy, with proximal as well as distal weakness that usually begins in the legs and ascends, but can affect other regions first. Bilateral facial weakness occurs in half of the patients. Since symptoms can progress to oropharyngeal and respiratory weakness in 33% of patients, all patients require careful monitoring, as discussed below. Eye movements are usually spared, the exception being the Miller–Fisher variant. Sensory symptoms occur in 80% of patients. Sensory signs are less frequent and often mild, but, when prominent, can contribute significantly to disability (62). Pain and temperature sensation mediated by small unmyelinated neurons may be affected less than position and vibratory sensation, mediated by large myelinated fibers. Fifty percent have pain, either back and muscle pain that can be aggravated by movement, or neuropathic pain, such as burning paresthesias, sometimes with allodynia (pathologic sensitivity to touch). Tendon reflexes are lost early in the course of the disease; indeed, the diagnosis should be questioned if reflexes are retained. Autonomic dysfunction is present in 66% of patients, and can manifest with tachyarrhythmias or bradyarrhythmias, spontaneous or orthostatic hypotension, paroxysmal hypertension, abnormalities of sweating, urinary retention, or ileus (63). Fifty percent of patients stop progressing in less than 2 weeks, 80% by 3 weeks, and more than 90% by 4 weeks (64).

The differential diagnosis of patients presenting with subacute weakness includes disorders of the CNS, PNS, neuromuscular junction, and muscle. Although Babinski responses, brisk reflexes, and sensory level will usually distinguish spinal cord from peripheral nerve diseases, there is overlap because reflexes may be depressed acutely in CNS disorders; bladder dysfunction, while suggestive of CNS lesions, can be seen in Guillain–Barré; and CNS demyelination may occasionally accompany GBS (65). Conversely, GBS should be in the differential of patients with the locked-in syndrome when tendon reflexes are depressed. Toxic, drug-induced, and metabolic neuropathies may occasionally present over a similar time course as GBS. In patients without sensory disturbances, disorders of neuromuscular junction and muscle should be considered. Muscle disorders that can present with severe subacute or acute weakness include the periodic paralyses, hypokalemic myopathy, drug-induced myopathies, and inflammatory myopathies.

Diagnostic Workup

Evaluation should include appropriate imaging to exclude CNS disorders, routine laboratory studies, and lumbar puncture. Upper motor neuron signs should prompt an magnetic resonance imaging (MRI) study of the spine to rule out structural lesions (66). The CSF is normal during the first days of illness, after which there is a transient elevation of protein with minimal or no pleocytosis. Although this diagnostic finding can be very helpful, the increases in CSF protein levels can be delayed until the second week of the illness, allowing for a normal LP. A repeat LP should be considered if there are high suspicions regarding the diagnosis (67). A significant pleocytosis should raise the question of infection such as Lyme disease or West Nile virus (68); when the clinical picture is otherwise classic for Guillain–Barré, CSF pleocytosis should suggest human immunodeficiency virus (HIV) infection in which immune dysregulation increases the incidence of autoimmune disorders (69). Blood tests are mainly done to rule out other underlying causes of weakness that can mimic GBS (67). Blood should be sent for basic metabolic profile, B_{12}, porphyrins, tests for Lyme disease and HIV, and heavy metal levels. Recently, the association between antiganglioside antibodies and GBS (acute motor axonal variant), mainly GM1a, GM1b, GD1a, GalNac-GD1a, and GQ1b has been used to increase diagnostic accuracy (67). This is especially true for GQ1b and the Miller–Fisher variant of GBS.

Electrodiagnostic studies must be interpreted in the context of the clinical findings. Early in Guillain–Barré, nerve conduction and F-wave studies may be normal if recorded from a limb without severe weakness. Delayed or absent F waves, sometimes replaced by axon reflex waves, are the earliest abnormalities (70). Conduction blocks are seen in the later stages of the disease (67). The much less common axonal variants of Guillain–Barré are distinguished from AIDP by electrophysiologic studies. NCSs should show low-amplitude motor CMAPs without marked conduction slowing, conduction block, or dispersion in both AMAN and AMSAN. AMAN is distinguished from AMSAN by preservation of SNAP amplitudes (71). If axons of the motor neurons are involved (AMAN) then motor nerve action potential amplitudes are reduced. If sensory axons are affected as well (AMSAN) a decrease in sensory amplitudes is also noted (67). When recorded from a paralyzed muscle, normal motor NCSs with normal F waves indicate that the weakness does not result from a peripheral cause, and should direct attention toward an alternative diagnosis with localization to the CNS.

Management

Patients with GBS should be admitted and carefully monitored for respiratory failure, swallowing ability, and autonomic function. Specific treatment can hasten recovery and reduce hospital costs, and is recommended for all patients whose weakness threatens loss of ambulation (72). Plasma exchange was the first treatment demonstrated to be effective in GBS. Treated patients demonstrated greater improvement at 4 weeks than untreated controls, and treatment reduced the proportion of patients requiring mechanical ventilation at 4 weeks from 27% to 14% (35,73–75). Every-other-day treatment to a total of five plasma volumes is usually employed. Complications include pneumothorax and sepsis related to central venous access, hypocalcemia, coagulopathy, and hypotension. Intravenous immunoglobulin (IVIG) treatment was shown to be equally effective as plasma exchange in controlled trials (76), and has become the preferred treatment because of greater ease of administration and lesser risk of serious complications. The usual dose is 0.4 g/kg/day infused slowly for 5 days to a total dose of 2 g/kg. Complications include hypersensitivity in patients with immunoglobulin A (IgA) deficiency, acute renal failure, congestive failure, hypercoagulable state, and aseptic meningitis. Treatment is indicated in all but the mildest cases, and is best instituted early in the course of the disease. Treatment after 4 weeks is unlikely to be of benefit. High-dose corticosteroids are of no proven benefit, and in several trials treated patients had more disability than controls (77).

Autonomic instability is common and usually not life threatening, unless it is manifested by asystole or ventricular fibrillation. Hypertension should be treated cautiously, as patients may be unusually sensitive to antihypertensive medications. Paroxysmal hypertension may sometimes be a manifestation of pain, in which case adequately treating the pain can be curative. Neuropathic pain can be treated with antiepileptic medications such as gabapentin (78), antidepressants such as amitriptyline, or analgesics.

The prognosis for recovery is good in all types of GBS, but is poorest for patients with severe AMSAN. Poor recovery is correlated with age, severity of deficits at the nadir of the disease, more rapid progression of deficits (37), and, in some studies, evidence of axonal damage on electrophysiologic studies (79); however, even the most severely afflicted patients may recover fully. About half of patients with otherwise good recovery are left with mild sensory disturbances (62,80,81).

Patients with rapidly progressive weakness should be transferred to the ICU. Respiratory failure is often preceded by progression of weakness to involve the upper extremities, shoulders, neck, and face, but may occur before this weakness is evident. Tachypnea, paradoxical respirations, hypophonia, staccato speech, and a marked decrease in minute ventilation when supine are clinical indications of respiratory failure (17).

MYASTHENIA GRAVIS

The first description of myasthenia gravis is credited to Wilks in 1867 or to Erb in 1879, although Sir Thomas Willis provided a description of the symptoms more than 200 years earlier (82). Freidreich Jolly, who first described the decremental response to repetitive stimulation, called this disorder myasthenia gravis pseudoparalytica (83). Mary Walker, a physician working at St. Alfege's Hospital in Greenwich, was the first to use acetylcholinesterase inhibitors to treat myasthenic patients (84). The dramatic, albeit temporary, reversal of weakness by physostigmine was called the "Miracle of St. Alfege's Hospital." The transient weakness manifested by infants born to myasthenic mothers, and the association of myasthenia with thymic tumors and with thyroiditis, led to the theory that myasthenia was an autoimmune disease (85). This was confirmed in the early 1970s with the demonstration that animals injected with concentrated acetylcholine receptor produced antibodies that caused weakness (86), as well as with the discovery of antibodies to acetylcholine receptors in the sera of myasthenic patients (87). Immunotherapy and improved critical care have lessened overall mortality from 20% to 30% in the 1950s (88) to nearly zero (89).

Myasthenia gravis has a current prevalence of about 20 per 100,000 population. There are about 60,000 patients with myasthenia in the United States (90). Myasthenia gravis occurs throughout life with bimodal peaks in the second and third decade in women and in the fifth and six decades in men (91). As the population ages, the average age of onset has increased and men are now more often affected than women (90). Myasthenic crisis occurs in about 20% of patients with myasthenia; almost 33% of these patients can experience a second crisis (92,93).

Pathophysiology

The neuromuscular junction is composed of a presynaptic motor neuron membrane, the synaptic cleft, and the postsynaptic muscle membrane. In the normal neuromuscular junction, the arrival of an action potential at the nerve terminal leads to the influx of calcium through voltage-gated calcium channels, which triggers release of acetylcholine into the synaptic cleft (94). Acetylcholine diffuses across the synaptic cleft to bind with acetylcholine receptors on the postsynaptic muscle membrane. This binding generates end-plate potentials that depolarize the muscle membrane. When the depolarization exceeds threshold, a muscle action potential is generated, which leads to a cascade of events that results in muscle contraction (95). Neuromuscular transmission fails if the end-plate potential fails to reach the threshold for muscle action potential generation. In LEMS, the end-plate potential is small because antibodies to voltage-gated calcium channels on the presynaptic membrane interfere with acetylcholine release. In myasthenia gravis, the end-plate potential is small because antibodies to the acetylcholine receptor or related sites on the postsynaptic membrane decrease the depolarization caused by normal amounts of acetylcholine.

The acetylcholine receptor is composed of four subunits (96). Antibodies to the acetylcholine receptor can be found in 80% to 90% of patients with generalized myasthenia (97). These antibodies can cause neuromuscular transmission failure by binding to the acetylcholine receptor and altering function, by increasing the rate of degradation of the receptors, and by complement-mediated destruction of the postsynaptic membrane (98). About 30% of patients with generalized myasthenia who are seronegative for acetylcholine receptor antibodies have antibodies to muscle-specific kinase (MuSK) (99). Patients with MuSK antibodies demonstrate more severe disease than patients with antibodies against the acetylcholine receptor (100). MuSK-positive patients have a higher female predominance and higher rates of facial and bulbar weakness with shoulder and neck involvement (101,102,103).

Recent studies have shown that 3% to 50% of patients who are seronegative for AChl receptor and MuSk antibody are positive for a newly found protein called low-density lipoprotein receptor–related protein 4 (Lrp4) which is responsive for retrograde signaling from muscle to presynaptic nerve terminals (101,104,105).

The thymus gland has been implicated in the pathogenesis of myasthenia gravis. Thymic abnormalities are seen in 75% of patients with myasthenia gravis. Of these, 75% have lymphoid follicular hyperplasia and 15% have thymomas (106). Acetylcholine receptors are found on myoid cells of the thymus (107). The majority of myasthenic thymuses contain B cells that can produce antibodies to the acetylcholine receptor (108). Antistriated muscle antibodies in patients with myasthenia gravis correlate highly with thymoma (109).

Patients with myasthenia gravis often have other autoimmune disorders, including thyroiditis, scleroderma, Sjögren syndrome, rheumatoid arthritis, pernicious anemia, polymyositis, and lupus erythematosus (110).

Clinical Presentation

Patients with myasthenia gravis present with fluctuating weakness that improves with rest. The most common complaints are ocular—namely, ptosis and diplopia related to weakness of the levator palpebrae and the extraocular muscles, respectively. Ptosis is the presenting symptom in 50% to 90% of patients, and 90% to 95% of patients complain of diplopia during the disease. Weakness can remain purely ocular in up to 15% of cases, but the majority of patients with myasthenia gravis develop generalized symptoms (83). Dysarthria and dysphagia are common complaints. Neck extensors and flexors are often more involved than other muscles in generalized disease (83). Patients may have to support their chin with their hand to prevent head drop because of neck extensor weakness or to keep their jaw shut because of weakness of the temporalis and masseter muscles. Proximal limb weakness is usually present when the disease is not purely ocular. It is sometimes asymmetric, is occasionally very focal, and can affect distal muscles. In less than 10% of cases, myasthenia presents with proximal weakness without bulbar or ocular weakness.

Myasthenic crisis is diagnosed when weakness progresses to cause dysphagia with loss of airway protection or hypoventilation. Myasthenic crisis can be precipitated by infection, surgical procedures, pregnancy, treatment with corticosteroids, sepsis, cholinergic crisis, and the rapid withdrawal of immune-suppressing medications (93). Pulmonary system infection, including aspiration pneumonia, is the most common identifiable precipitating factor (93). Many medications can also worsen myasthenic symptoms (111), often because they impair neuromuscular transmission. Aminoglycoside antibiotics, quinidine, and procainamide are particularly likely to cause weakness, and should be avoided in patients with myasthenia. Limited experience with telithromycin suggests that it should also be avoided (112). Penicillamine and α-interferon may cause autoimmune myasthenia. Evidence that other medications exacerbate myasthenia gravis is less convincing, but in patients with increasing weakness, all medications must be scrutinized against the long list of potentially offending agents (111).

Myasthenic crisis can involve muscles of inspiration, including the diaphragm and the external intercostals, along with accessory muscles of inspiration, including the scalene and sternocleidomastoid muscles. Respiratory strength can be measured by vital capacity and negative inspiratory force (113). As respiratory weakness leads to ventilatory failure, tidal volumes decline. Patients in myasthenic crisis have an intact respiratory drive, and therefore respond to the decrease in tidal volume with an increase in respiratory rate (114). Oropharyngeal muscle weakness may result in obstruction with upper airway collapse. Secretions can be difficult to control and can also obstruct the airway and lead to aspiration. In the 1950s and 1960s, mortality from myasthenic crisis was as high as 70% to 80% (115,116). In more recent reports, mortality is closer to 4% (85,86), related to improvements in intensive care as well as effective immunomodulatory treatment.

Diagnosis

The history and examination often strongly suggest the diagnosis. A history of fluctuating ptosis, diplopia, fatigable dysarthria, dysphagia, and neck weakness are highly suggestive. Sometimes the presentation may be misleading, as when ocular myasthenia presents with isolated eye muscle weakness or with a pattern of eye movements that mimics internuclear ophthalmoplegia from brainstem lesions, or when patients have proximal limb weakness without eye or bulbar weakness, suggesting a primary disorder of muscle. Conversely, patients with purely ocular findings should be worked up for other causes of ophthalmoplegia, including thyroid eye disease and retrobulbar or cavernous sinus lesions. ALS may present with bulbar symptoms, but patients with ALS do not have ptosis or eye movement weakness, and often have pseudobulbar dysarthria, characterized by slow labored speech and poorly modulated emotional expression, with laughing or crying that is disproportionate to the situation.

Many tests are available to confirm the diagnosis of myasthenia. Definitive diagnosis is important, as most patients will require years of immunomodulatory therapy. The "ice pack test" can be done at bedside to help with diagnosis of MG when improvement in ptosis is seen after applying ice pack to the eyelids (16). Pharmacologic testing with edrophonium (Tensilon), a rapid-acting, short-duration acetylcholinesterase, can result in transient increase in strength. Caution should be used in using edrophonium because anticholinergic side effects, such as bradycardia and bronchospasm, can develop. A test dose of 2 mg of edrophonium, given intravenously, should be administered, followed by increments of 2 mg, for a total dose of 10 mg. Atropine should be available to counteract muscarinic side effects (117). Definite improvement in strength, as demonstrated by improvement in ptosis, dysarthria, or resistance against the examiner's testing, is supportive of the diagnosis. The test is, therefore, most helpful in patients with clear weakness that can be evaluated in an objective manner (117). In patients with cardiac disease, especially those on β-blockers or drugs that cause atrioventricular block, edrophonium should be avoided, as it can cause asystole (118). Fortunately, there are many alternative tests to confirm the diagnosis of myasthenia.

Serum acetylcholine receptor antibodies are found in 80% to 90% of patients with generalized myasthenia gravis, and have very high diagnostic specificity. Increased titers are also found in patients with thymoma without myasthenia, and rarely in other diseases, including systemic lupus, ALS, liver disease, and inflammatory neuropathies, and in patients with LEMS (119). Antibodies to striated muscle are present in about 30% of patients with myasthenic gravis, and are highly associated with thymoma (120). About 30% of patients with myasthenia gravis who lack antibodies to acetylcholine receptor have antibodies to MuSK. Other antibodies directed against muscle antigens can be found in patients with myasthenia gravis (121).

Patients diagnosed with myasthenia should have additional testing for associated conditions. Computed tomography (CT) or MRI of the chest is required to evaluate for thymoma (89). Tests of thyroid function are important, because about 10% of myasthenics have associated autoimmune thyroid disease, and because proximal weakness and restriction of extraocular movements can be caused by thyroid disease. Antinuclear antibody (ANA) and rheumatoid factor may detect much less commonly associated autoimmune disorders. Tuberculin test and fasting glucose should be obtained prior to treatment with steroids.

Electrodiagnostic Studies

Sensory and motor NCSs are normal except decreased CMAP amplitudes in severely weak muscles (11). The pattern seen in MG with EMG is a decrement in CMAP amplitude with slow repetitive stimulation that improves immediately after exercise and worsens again 2 to 4 minutes after exercise (11).

RNS can be performed to rule out a decrement in the amplitude or area of the fourth or fifth potential compared to the first potential. A train of 5 to 10 stimuli is delivered at a rate of 2 to 3 Hz. If the decrement is more than 10%, it is considered abnormal. The yield can be increased by testing clinically weak muscles and with repeat testing after exercise of the specific muscle. Because typically myasthenia affects proximal more than distal muscles, the test is more likely to be abnormal when testing proximal or facial muscles than when testing hand muscles (122).

The most significant finding on EMG is moment to moment variation in MUAPs amplitude (11).

Single-fiber EMG is abnormal in nearly all patients with generalized myasthenia (123), but it is not widely available because it is time consuming, is technically demanding, and requires expensive needle electrodes.

Anticholinesterase antibodies have to be discontinued 12 hours prior to RNS studies for an accurate result (11).

LEMS is an example of a presynaptic neuromuscular disorder. NCSS can be normal but frequently LEMS is caused by a malignancy and there is an associated paraneoplastic sensory or sensorimotor neuropathy, which results in abnormal values in NCS. Motor NCSS show primarily a low CMAP amplitude increasing by over 100% after 10 to 20 seconds of exercise secondary to increased accumulation of calcium and release of acetylcholine (11).

Clinical Management

The majority of myasthenic patients respond well to anticholinesterase and immunomodulatory treatment and rarely require intensive care. While these treatments can produce dramatic improvement in strength, they do not address the underlying autoimmune pathogenesis of the disease, and tend to become ineffective as the disease progresses.

Treatment

Symptomatic

Pyridostigmine, an anticholinesterase, is used for symptomatic treatment. The dose and frequency of this drug is greatly dependent on the patient's level of weakness and the potential for side effects. Pyridostigmine does not cross the blood–brain barrier and is the most commonly used oral agent. Sustained-release pyridostigmine is appropriate for use at bedtime to mitigate weakness during the night and in the morning. Multiple daytime doses of sustained-release preparations should be avoided, as accumulation may lead to cholinergic weakness.

Immunosuppressive

Oral prednisone is the most commonly used agent to induce remission in myasthenic patients, and is effective in 80% to 90% of patients. High-dose prednisone—60 to 100 mg/day—may cause transient worsening of myasthenia, and should not be initiated unless patients can be closely observed. Lower doses appear safer, but are not entirely free from this complication. Most patients experience gradual improvement in strength beginning 2 or 3 weeks after initiation of therapy. Once a good response has been achieved, the dose can be tapered over several months to low-dose alternate-day treatment. Doses less than 40 mg every other day are generally well tolerated. Doses of 40 mg or above every other day are associated with many long-term side effects, including diabetes, hypertension, cataracts, avascular necrosis, and increased susceptibility to infection. Azathioprine may reduce steroid dependence. Physicians should consider initiation of non-steroidal immunosuppressants such as azathioprine during the acute phase, to help with tapering steroids.

Rituximab, a monoclonal CD20 antibody (causing depletion of B lymphocytes), used in some retrospective case series for treatment of refractory MG has shown 78% to 100% improvement in clinical symptoms and a reduction in steroids or other immunosuppressant dosage when repeated in cycles over a 6 months period or more (124–126).

Treatment with IVIG can produce rapid improvement in strength, and may be useful to provide short-term improvement while waiting for steroids to become effective.

Plasma exchange has been shown to be effective for the treatment of myasthenic crisis and to prepare patients for surgery (127). Many different protocols are used, but a series of five to six exchanges of 2 to 4 L every other day is most commonly employed. Improvement can usually be seen in 3 to 4 days and can last for several weeks, but is not sustained without the addition of an immunosuppressant agent. Side effects of plasma exchange, which can be life threatening, include hypotension, bradycardia, congestive heart failure, venous thrombosis, infection, and dramatic shifts in electrolytes, including calcium. Controlled randomized trials have demonstrated that IVIG is as effective as plasma exchange in patients with myasthenic crises (128). This trial used 1.2 and 2.0 g/kg of IVIG over 2 to 5 days. Patients who fail to respond to IVIG may subsequently respond to plasma exchange (PLEX) (129). Although patients treated with PLEX may have rapid improvement in their symptoms compared to IVIG, patients receiving IVIG have fewer adverse events. This cannot be extrapolated to all patient groups though. Clinical response rates for IVIG and PLEX are usually similar and range between 55% and 65% (128) (130).

Based on current data, IVIG and PLEX can both be used in treatment of severe MG and MG exacerbation with similar efficacy but it is believed that in patients with MG crisis with respiratory failure requiring ventilator support, PLEX may be superior to IVIG. However IVIG is easier to administer, may have less complications, is readily available and may lower health care costs. Hence, decision on treatment is based on the individual patient, drug availability, and patient's comorbidities (101).

Intravenous steroids have been used in high doses in myasthenic crisis in patients who do not respond to IVIG or plasma exchange (131), but this may be complicated by transient worsening of myasthenic weakness that may precipitate the need for, or prolong, mechanical ventilation. Other immunosuppressant medications can be useful as steroid-sparing drugs and as sole therapy for myasthenia, but they take weeks or months to produce improvement, and therefore are not appropriate choices to treat myasthenic crisis.

AAN guidelines published in 2000 considers thymectomy as an option for treatment of MG based on a 28 case series showing higher rates of medication-free remission and improvement in patients who underwent thymectomy (132).

Thymectomy is indicated in patients with thymoma, and is also accepted therapy for myasthenia gravis without thymoma, particularly in younger patients without thymic involution. However, the absence of class I evidence and the shortcomings of existing case-control or cohort trials have led to a call for prospective randomized controlled clinical trials (132).

Airway Management

Myasthenia crisis is defined by development of respiratory failure and a need for ventilator support by noninvasive or invasive mechanical ventilation. It is usually seen in 15% to 25% of patients with MG and is mostly seen in patients with known diagnosis of the disease. It can be triggered by a variety of stressors, including surgery, infections, changes in medication, etc. (66,101).

Myasthenic weakness can progress very rapidly; therefore, patients with worsening myasthenic symptoms should be hospitalized for definitive management. Patients with progressive bulbar weakness who have difficulty controlling secretions, an ineffective cough, or vital capacities less than 20 to 25 mL/kg should be admitted to the ICU (133,134). Unlike patients with GBS who would not benefit from noninvasive ventilation, patients with MG benefit greatly from noninvasive modes of ventilation in particular BiPAP which can prevent patients from reaching the point of intubation and mechanical ventilation. It is imperative to initiate supportive care with BiPAP as soon as the patient is admitted to ICU since respiratory failure rates, pulmonary complications, and pneumonia rates may increase if there is delay in treatment (67). When the vital capacity reaches 15 mL/kg, endotracheal intubation should be strongly considered. Elective intubation can help patients avoid abrupt respiratory failure and mucous plugging (135). Intermittent mandatory ventilation with pressure support is used to reduce alveolar collapse or atelectasis. Positive end-expiratory pressure can reduce complications related to atelectasis (136). If mechanical ventilation is required for more than 2 weeks, tracheostomy should be considered. The most common complications of myasthenic crisis are fever, pneumonia, and atelectasis (93). Aggressive respiratory treatment with suctioning, bronchodilator treatments, sighs, chest physiotherapy, and intermittent positive pressure can reduce the complications of mechanical ventilation and shorten the period that patients are in the intensive care unit (137). Weaning trials should be attempted with patients who show clear improvement of respiratory muscle strength, with the goal to eliminate mandatory ventilation and then reduce the amount of pressure support. If oral and respiratory secretions are concerning, the dose of pyridostigmine can be either decreased or the medication is completely stopped after intubation, and should be reintroduced prior to weaning trials. In patients on noninvasive ventilation, pyridostigmine should not be discontinued if possible.

Perioperative Care

Myasthenic crisis is common in patients undergoing surgical procedures. The main risk factors for postoperative complications include severe bulbar weakness, chronic myasthenia, respiratory illness, and decreased vital capacity preoperatively (138). Whenever possible, preoperative treatment to improve strength should be undertaken. Plasma exchange or IVIG can be performed preoperatively in patients with bulbar weakness or generalized myasthenia. A response is often seen within 3 to 6 days, although preoperative IVIG has shown a variable time to maximal response (1,139). Preoperative pulmonary function testing can be performed to assess respiratory function.

CRITICAL ILLNESS POLYNEUROPATHY AND MYOPATHY

Although limb and respiratory muscle weakness in critically ill patients was noted in 1892 by Osler (140), it was initially attributed to catabolic myopathy and diaphragmatic fatigue. Recognition that critically ill patients frequently develop new neuromuscular dysfunction was not widespread until the final decades of the 20th century. In 1984, Bolton et al. (1) described five patients who failed to wean from the ventilator after treatment of sepsis, and were found to have neuromuscular weakness related to an axonal sensorimotor polyneuropathy. They called this *critical illness polyneuropathy* (CIP). In 1992, Sagredo et al. (141) attributed prolonged paralysis, seen in patients in whom vecuronium had been weaned, to persistent plasma levels of vecuronium metabolites in those patients with impaired renal function. Hirano et al. (142) described severe weakness in two critically ill asthmatic patients treated with steroids and nondepolarizing blocking agents. Muscle biopsy demonstrated depletion of thick myosin filaments. They called this *acute quadriplegic myopathy.* Other terms for the same or similar illness have included hydrocortisone myopathy, necrotizing myopathy, thick filament myopathy, postparalysis syndrome, and acute myopathy of intensive care; we will refer to it by the most common designation: critical illness myopathy (CIM). The term *critical illness neuromyopathy* (CINM) is used to refer to patients in whom both neuropathy and myopathy coexist, or when it is uncertain which condition is causing the patient's weakness. The term CINM could also be applied to patients with persistent neuromuscular blockade; however, electrophysiologic studies should exclude this as a contributing factor in most patients.

Epidemiology

The incidence of CINM is estimated to be as high as 70% of mechanically ventilated ICU patients with sepsis and multiorgan failure. Witt et al. (143) found, in a prospective study, that 70% of 43 ICU patients with sepsis and failure of more than two organs developed electrophysiologic evidence of peripheral neuropathy, and half of these patients had clinically evident neuropathy with difficulty being weaned from the ventilator. De Jonghe et al. (144) found that 25.3% of ICU patients intubated for 7 or more days developed neuromuscular weakness. All had sensorimotor axonopathy, and all who were biopsied also had myopathy. Bednarik et al. (145) prospectively studied 61 ICU patients with evidence of multiorgan failure; 27% had clinical and 54% electrophysiologic evidence for CINM. Bercker et al. (146) found that 60% of 50 consecutive patients with acute respiratory distress syndrome (ARDS) studied retrospectively developed CINM.

Pathophysiology

Critically ill ICU patients can develop severe weakness of limb and respiratory muscles from an axonal polyneuropathy (CIP) or a myopathy (CIM). They often coexist, thus the term critical illness neuromyopathy or a more recently coined term, ICU-acquired weakness is used to describe the entity of clinically detected weakness with no plausible cause other than critical illness (147). They may occur in approximately 50% of patients that have severe sepsis, multiorgan failure, or are mechanically ventilated for 3 or more days and can be a common cause of failure to wean from mechanical ventilation in these patients (148).

Critical Illness Polyneuropathy

Sepsis and multiorgan failure are the major risk factors for CIP (145,149,150,151); other risk factors include duration of mechanical ventilation, hyperglycemia, hyperosmolality, and hypoalbuminemia (143). The PNS is one of the organ systems damaged in systemic inflammatory response syndrome (SIRS) which can cause cytokine release. There is speculation that endothelial cell activation, increased permeability of the microcirculation, nerve ischemia and mitochondrial injury play a role in pathogenesis. A high catabolic state due to systemic inflammation and oxidative stress is also associated with skeletal muscle wasting, and diaphragmatic weakness was seen as early as 6 days in mechanically ventilated patients (152). Decreased nutrient supply, increased demand, decreased clearance of toxic substances, and tissue edema can ultimately terminate in neuronal injury and axonal degeneration. Pathologically, there is axonal degeneration without inflammation, and there is an increase in adhesion molecule expression in nerve (149).

Critical Illness Myopathy

Risk factors for CIM overlap with those for CIP; however, there is more emphasis on primary pulmonary disease (asthma and ARDS) and on the use of neuromuscular blocking agents and corticosteroids (144,153). High corticosteroid levels may increase expression of ubiquitin, leading to increased proteolytic activity (154). Muscle inactivity in itself can act as a potent stimulus of the ubiquitin-proteasome pathway of proteolysis and can cause muscle wasting. Denervation from coexisting CIP may make the muscle more susceptible. Muscle biopsy shows loss of thick (myosin) filaments; there may also be fiber-type atrophy and/or necrosis (142,155). Whether the different pathologies represent a spectrum of severity or different entities remain unsettled.

Most patients on ventilators are given neuromuscular blocking agents. Normally, the effects of these agents wear off within hours of discontinuation; however, it is not unusual for residual blockade to last 1 to 2 days (141). Early reports of more prolonged weakness after neuromuscular blockade did not consider the effects of CIP and CIM. In a recent review, Murray et al. (153) concluded that nondepolarizing neuromuscular blocking agents may potentiate muscle weakness by a number of mechanisms, including upregulation of acetylcholine receptors with fetal-type receptors that are less responsive to acetylcholine, presynaptic inhibition of exocytosis of acetylcholine, and potentiation of muscle damage by corticosteroids and by sepsis-induced ischemia.

Clinical Presentation

CIP is often preceded by SIRS, severe sepsis, or multiorgan failure. CIM may have similar antecedents, but is more likely in the setting of ventilatory failure from asthma (142,155) or ARDS (146). The use of neuromuscular blocking agents (156) and corticosteroids (144 appears to predispose to CIM, although CIM has been reported without either one (157).

CIP or CIM are most often diagnosed when sedation is weaned or sepsis and encephalopathy improve in a mechanically ventilated patient, revealing a profound generalized weakness. Neurologic examination can reveal a normal mental status and cranial nerves with generalized flaccid weakness which is sometimes worse distally and failure to wean from the ventilator. Hyporeflexia, areflexia, and muscle atrophy can be seen in CIP where reflexes are usually preserved or hypoactive in CIM. Distal sensory loss may be present in majority of patients with CIP, but is not always reported or amenable to testing (158). Sensation is normal in CIM if neuropathy does not coexist, but often encephalopathy and poor communication make this difficult to assess. Electrodiagnostic studies can therefore be key to diagnosis.

Diagnosis

The diagnosis is likely in patients with risk factors, particularly sepsis, SIRS, multiorgan failure, prolonged artificial ventilation, hyperglycemia, and exposure to neuromuscular blocking agents or corticosteroids (159). Alternative causes for weakness in the ICU must be considered and, if possible, excluded. These include medications that cause myopathy, neuromuscular blockade, or neuropathy; electrolyte disorders such as hypokalemia or hypophosphatemia; undiagnosed neuromuscular disorders such as myasthenia gravis, GBS, or ALS; and a variety of CNS disorders, including ischemic myelopathy, anterior horn cell loss from hypoxia (160), CPM that most often follows rapid correction of hyponatremia, and hemispheric stroke from hypotension, emboli, or hemorrhage (161). West Nile encephalitis (WNE) should be considered in patients who present with fever and encephalopathy, and in those who develop neuromuscular weakness, since WNE can affect anterior horn cells and, less often, peripheral nerves (162). Depending on clinical suspicions, imaging of the brain and spinal cord may be appropriate. If clinical findings suggest neuromuscular weakness rather than a CNS disorder, it may be more efficient to confirm with electrodiagnostic studies than to pursue studies for CNS disorders.

Laboratory studies can help to exclude mimicking disorders. They should include a basic metabolic profile to assess blood sugar and electrolytes. Elevation of creatine kinase (CK) may suggest myopathy, and very high CK could suggest rhabdomyolysis. Normal CK does not exclude CIM, and mild elevations in CK can be seen with acute denervation. Tests for myasthenia (see Myasthenia Gravis, above) are indicated when there is a clinical suspicion. Spinal fluid findings are not often reported in CIP. Lumbar puncture is indicated principally if there is clinical suspicion of infection.

Electrophysiologic testing and muscle biopsy can help confirm the clinical suspicion of CIM or CIP and help to distinguish them from each other as well as other disorders of nerve, neuromuscular junction, and muscle (for a more detailed synopsis, see Dhand (163)). NCSs may be difficult to perform and interpret due to multiple artifacts, extremities may be cool and difficult to warm and they may be confounded by tissue edema. EMG may not be useful when patients are not awake or unable to contract muscles to command. Nonetheless, they are usually diagnostic (159).

NCSs in CIP show a very decreased amplitude of CMAP and SNAPs without significant slowing of conduction velocities or increased CMAP durations. The abnormalities are usually length dependent. NCS findings are generally present by day 14 of critical illness, but low amplitudes may be noted within a week and as early as 72 hours after onset of sepsis (159). In patients with CIM, the CMAP is also of low amplitude, but unlike CIP, CMAP duration may be prolonged due to slowing of muscle fiber conduction velocity and reduced excitability of the sarcolemmal membrane (164,165). These changes occur within 2 weeks of critical illness (165). SNAPs should be normal in CIM, unless there is coexistent CIP. It should be kept in mind that pre-existing neuropathy may account for some of the deficits found on electrophysiologic testing, as, for example, in patients with diabetic neuropathy. Needle EMG studies may show fibrillation potentials and positive sharp waves in a multifocal pattern generally after 2 weeks but have been reported as early as 7 days after initiation of mechanical ventilation (150). Voluntary activity may be difficult to study in poorly cooperative patients and reduced response on direct muscle stimulation can be suggestive of CIM. When the patient can provide good effort, there is reduced recruitment in CIP and small polyphasic motor unit potentials in myopathy, helping to differentiate CIP from CIM.

Guillain–Barré polyneuropathy can follow surgery or trauma, and could therefore occur in settings similar to the critical illness neuromyopathies. Electrophysiologic findings diagnostic of demyelinating neuropathy—not found in CIP or CIM—would suggest this possibility. In theory, an axonal form of Guillain–Barré would be electrophysiologically indistinguishable from CIP. This highly unlikely occurrence should be considered in patients who lack the usual risk factors for CIP.

Additional electrodiagnostic studies that may be useful in diagnosis include phrenic nerve stimulation, diaphragmatic EMG, and direct muscle stimulation. While these studies do not require specialized equipment, many electromyographers do not have sufficient experience with them to be confident in their performance or interpretation. Phrenic nerve stimulation in the neck with surface recording over the diaphragm shows a normal response in patients with pulmonary causes of respiratory failure, but a low amplitude or absent response in patients with neuromuscular respiratory weakness. Needle EMG of the diaphragm can be done in patients without severe chronic obstructive pulmonary disease (COPD), ileus, or coagulopathy, and may diagnose denervation or myopathy affecting the diaphragm (166). CIP and CIM may be distinguished by comparing the muscle response to direct muscle stimulation with the response to nerve stimulation. If the response to muscle stimulation is larger than to nerve stimulation, CIP is likely; when both are small, CIM is likely (167,168).

Muscle biopsy in CIP may show signs of acute denervation with atrophy of types 1 and 2 fibers and grouped atrophy may be seen in severe cases. Nerve biopsy in CIP shows signs of axonal neuropathy. Muscle biopsy in CIM shows a selective loss of thick (myosin) filaments with degree of muscle necrosis directly proportional to disease severity. Although muscle and nerve biopsies may be diagnostic, they often only change management if they demonstrate an alternative diagnosis that may be amenable to treatment, such as a demyelinating or vasculitic neuropathy, or an inflammatory myopathy. In patients whose neuromuscular deficits are clearly related to the usual risk factors for CINM, treatable conditions are not sufficiently likely to warrant biopsy (169).

Management

Treatment of hyperglycemia, early physical rehabilitation and minimization of sedation have been demonstrated to improve functional outcomes, reduce delirium and increase ventilator-free days in critically ill patients. These interventions are likely beneficial but no specific therapy for CINM exists (170). Of the factors that may contribute to the development of CINM, many—like the response to sepsis and the incidence of multiorgan failure—are related to the severity of the presenting critical illness, and are not easily modifiable. It remains to be demonstrated whether the reduced use of corticosteroids or neuromuscular blocking agents will result in a decreased incidence of CIM. Intensive insulin therapy to maintain strict normoglycemia was shown to reduce the incidence of CIP by 49% in a single-center study (171), but this practice has been shown to increase mortality in patients who are critically ill (172). Therefore, control of sustained hyperglycemia is reasonable, but aggressive insulin protocols and any hypoglycemic episodes should be avoided (172–174). Neurotoxic medications should also be avoided. Patients with neuropathy are more prone to pressure palsies, and thus, great care must be taken in positioning and support to avoid this complication. In patients that are unable to participate in strengthening exercises, early physical therapy should be directed toward prevention of contractures and improvement of functional outcome (170).

Prognosis

Long-term prognosis in CINM is still not fully studied but the initial mortality is high (152). Patients with CINM who survive the acute illness will slowly recover over weeks to months. A subset of patient with prolonged severe illness and CINM will never fully recover. Patients with CINM who fail to show clinical improvement in strength should be evaluated with periodical electrophysiologic testing. Patients with evidence of severe axonal loss, small or absent responses to nerve stimulation, and abundant positive waves and fibrillations on needle EMG are likely to have residual deficits (2,143,151,165,175–177). CIM seems to have a better functional recovery than CINM at 1-year follow-up (178).

SUMMARY

Neuromuscular diseases may necessitate admission for intensive care to provide airway protection and respiratory support. Disorders such as GBS and myasthenia gravis can lead to life-threatening precipitous weakness. Management must also address autonomic dysfunction, sensory loss, pain, and psychological distress. Neuromuscular disorders of autoimmune pathogenesis often respond to specific treatments, and a favorable outcome can be expected for the majority of such patients. Critical illness neuromyopathies have become the most common cause of weakness that develop in the intensive care setting, requiring critical care physicians to be familiar with their presentation, diagnosis, and management. Although no specific treatment is currently available for CINM, most patients improve with supportive care and intensive physiotherapy. A minority, however, are left with irreversible weakness.

Key Points

- The pattern of neuromuscular disorders differs between individuals and carries importance in differentiating one disease process from another.
- Care of the patient suffering from acute neuromuscular disease often begins in the prehospital setting.
- Neuromuscular emergencies can follow an acute condition or the worsening of a chronic neuromuscular illness.
- Respiratory failure is the most important complication observed in patients suffering from an acute neuromuscular disorder.
- NIPPV is gaining importance in the management of respiratory symptoms in myasthenia gravis, particularly in the initial stage of symptoms.
- Early diagnosis can be achieved with an accurate clinical history, physical examination, laboratory and radiologic testing.
- IVIG and plasma exchange are the cornerstones of treating GBS.
- Critical illness neuropathy and myopathy are increasingly being diagnosed as a sequela of prolonged hospitalization in critically ill patients.
- Electrophysiologic studies can provide valuable information for diagnosing the underlying disorder.

References

1. Bolton CF, Gilbert JJ, Hahn AF, Sibbald WJ. Polyneuropathy in critically ill patients. *J Neurol Neurosurg Psychiatry.* 1984;47:1223–1231.
2. Lacomis D, Petrella JT, Giuliani MJ. Causes of neuromuscular weakness in the intensive care unit: a study of ninety-two patients. *Muscle Nerve.* 1998;21:610–617.
3. Mohr JP. Distal field infarction. *Neurology.* 1969;12:279.
4. Riggs JE. Neurologic manifestations of electrolyte disturbances. *Neurol Clin.* 2002;20:227–239, vii.
5. Young RR, Asbury AK, Corbett JF, Adams RD. Pure pandysautonomia with recovery: description and discussion of diagnostic criteria. *Brain.* 1975; 98:613–636.
6. Waxman SG, Sabin TD. Diabetic truncal polyneuropathy. *Arch Neurol.* 1981;38:46–47.
7. Fromm GB, Wisdom PJ, Block AJ. Amyotrophic lateral sclerosis presenting with respiratory failure: diaphragmatic paralysis and dependence on mechanical ventilation in two patients. *Chest.* 1977;71:612–614.
8. Chen R, Grand'Maison F, Strong MJ, et al. Motor neuron disease presenting as acute respiratory failure. A clinical and pathological study. *J Neurol Neurosurg Psychiatry.* 1996;60:455–458.
9. Dushay KM, Zibrak JD, Jensen WA. Myasthenia gravis presenting as isolated respiratory failure. *Chest.* 1990;97:232–234.
10. Rosenow EC 3rd, Engel AG. Acid maltase deficiency in adults presenting as respiratory failure. *Am J Med.* 1978;64:485–491.
11. Lipa BM, Han JJ. Electrodiagnosis in neuromuscular disease. *Phys Med Rehabil Clin N Am.* 201223:565–587.
12. Kimura J, Butzer JF. F-wave conduction velocity in Guillain-Barré syndrome. Assessment of nerve segment between axilla and spinal cord. *Arch Neurol.* 1975;32:524–529.
13. Kuwabara S, Ogawara K, Mizobuchi K, et al. Isolated absence of F waves and proximal axonal dysfunction in Guillain-Barré syndrome with antiganglioside antibodies. *J Neurol Neurosurg Psychiatry.* 2000;68:191–195.
14. Dumitru D. Neuromuscular junction disorders. In: Dumitru D, ed. *Electrodiagnostic Medicine.* Philadelphia, PA: Hanley & Belfus; 2002:1127–1228.
15. Maddison P, Newsom-Davis J, Mills KR. Distribution of electrophysiological abnormality in Lambert-Eaton myasthenic syndrome. *J Neurol Neurosurg Psychiatry.* 1998;65:213–217.
16. Flower O, Wainwright MS, Caulfield AF. Emergency neurological life support: acute non-traumatic weakness. *Neurocrit Care.* 2015;23:S23–S47.
17. Chalela JA. Pearls and pitfalls in the intensive care management of Guillain-Barré syndrome. *Semin Neurol.* 2004;21:399–405.
18. Borel CO, Guy J. Ventilatory management in critical neurologic illness. In: Jordan KG, ed. *Neurologic Clinics.* Philadelphia, PA: WB Saunders; 1995:627.
19. Ropper AJ, Wijdicks EFM, Truax BT. General care. In: Ropper AH, Wijdicks EFM, Truax BT, eds. *Guillain-Barré Syndrome.* Philadelphia, PA: FA Davis; 1991:237.
20. Fulgham JR, Wijdicks EFM. Guillain-Barré syndrome. In: Diringer M, ed. *Critical Care Clinics: Update on Neurologic Critical Care.* Philadelphia, PA: WB Saunders; 1997:1.
21. Bowes D. The doctor as a patient: an encounter with Guillain-Barré syndrome. *Can Med Assoc J.* 1984;131:1343–1348.
22. Winkel LP, Hagemans ML, van Doom PA, et al. The natural course of non-classic Pompe's disease; a review of 225 published cases. *J Neurol.* 2005;252:875–884.
23. Dalakas MC, Hohlfeld R. Polymyositis and dermatomyositis. *Lancet.* 2003;362:1762.
24. Mangera Z, Panesar G, Makker H. Practical approach to management of respiratory complications in neurological disorders. *Int J Gen Med.* 2012:5:255–263.
25. Kim WH, Kim JH, Kim EK, et al. Myasthenia gravis presenting as isolated respiratory failure: A case report. *Korean J Intern Med.* 2010;25:101–104.
26. Qureishi AI, Choundry MA, Mohammad Y, et al. Respiratory failure as a first presentation of myasthenia gravis. *Med Sci Monit.* 2005;10: CR684–689.
27. Abel M, Eisenkraft JB. Anesthetic implications of myasthenia gravis. *Mt Sinai J Med.* 2002;69:31–37.
28. Landry O. Note sur la paralysie ascendante aiguë. *Gaz Hebd Med Paris.* 1859;6:472.
29. Guillain G, Barré JA, Strohl A. Sur un syndrome de radiculonévrite avec hyperalbuminose du liquide céphalo-rachidien sans réaction cellulaire. Remarques sur les caractéres cliniques et graphiques des réflexes tendineux. *Bull Mem Soc Med Hop Paris.* 1916;40:1462–1470.
30. Melnick SC, Flewett TH. Role of infection in the Guillain-Barre syndrome. *J Neurol Neurosurg Psychiatry.* 1964;27:395–407.

31. Hurwitz ES, Holman RC, Nelson DB, Schonberger LB. National surveillance for Guillain-Barre syndrome: January 1978–March 1979. *Neurology.* 1983;33:150–157.
32. Waksman BH, Adams RD. A comparative study of experimental allergic neuritis in the rabbit, guinea pig, and mouse. *J Neuropathol Exp Neurol.* 1956;15:293–334.
33. National Institute of Neurological and Communicative Disorders and Stroke ad hoc Committee (NINCDS). Criteria for diagnosis of Guillain-Barré syndrome. *Ann Neurol.* 1978;3:565–566.
34. Griffin JW, Sheikh K. The Guillain-Barré syndromes. In: Dyck PJ, Thomas PK, eds. *Peripheral Neuropathy.* 4th ed. Philadelphia, PA: Elsevier Saunders; 2005:2197.
35. McKhann GM, Cornblath DR, Griffin JW, et al. Acute motor axonal neuropathy: a frequent cause of acute flaccid paralysis in China. *Ann Neurol.* 1993;33:333–342.
36. Griffin JW, Li CY, Ho TW, et al. Pathology of the motor-sensory axonal Guillain-Barré syndrome. *Ann Neurol.* 1996;39:17–28.
37. Hughes RA, Cornblath DR. Guillain-Barré syndrome. *Lancet.* 2005; 366:1653–1666.
38. Young RR, Asbury AK, Adams RD, Corbett JL. Pure pandysautonomia with recovery. *Trans Am Neurol Assoc.* 1969;94:355–357.
39. Pan CL, Yuki N, Koga M, et al. Acute sensory ataxic neuropathy associated with monospecific anti-GD1b IgG antibody. *Neurology.* 2001;57: 1316–1318.
40. Fisher CM. An unusual variant of acute idiopathic polyneuritis: (syndrome of ophthalmoplegia, ataxia and areflexia). *N Engl J Med.* 1956;255:57–65.
41. Shimamura H, Miura H, Iwaki Y, et al. Clinical, electrophysiological, and serological overlap between Miller Fisher syndrome and acute sensory ataxic neuropathy. *Acta Neurol Scand.* 2002;105:411–413.
42. Chio A, Cocito D, Leone M, et al. Guillain-Barré syndrome: a prospective, population-based incidence and outcome survey. *Neurology.* 2003;60:1146–1150.
43. Alter M. The epidemiology of Guillain-Barré syndrome. *Ann Neurol.* 1990;27(Suppl):S7–S12.
44. Hadden RD, Karch H, Hartung HP, et al. Preceding infections, immune factors, and outcome in Guillain-Barre syndrome. *Neurology.* 2001;56: 758–765.
45. Van Koningsveld R, Schmitz PI, Ang CW, et al. Infections and course of disease in mild forms of Guillain-Barre syndrome. *Neurology.* 2002;58: 610–614.
46. Hemachudha T, Griffin DE, Chen WW, Johnson RT. Immunologic studies of rabies vaccination-induced Guillain-Barré syndrome. *Neurology.* 1988;38:375–378.
47. Kaplan JE, Katona P, Hurwitz ES, Schonberger LB. Guillain-Barré syndrome in the United States, 1989–1980 and 1980–1981. Lack of an association with influenza vaccination. *JAMA.* 1982;248:698–700.
48. Lasky T, Terracciano GJ, Magder L, et al. The Guillain-Barré syndrome and the 1992–1993 and 1993–1994 influenza vaccines. *N Engl J Med.* 1998;339:1797–1802.
49. Asbury AK, Arnason BG, Adams RD. The inflammatory lesion in idiopathic polyneuritis. Its role in pathogenesis. *Medicine (Baltimore).* 1969;48: 173–215.
50. Prineas JW. Acute idiopathic polyneuritis. An electronmicroscope study. *Lab Invest.* 1972;26:133–147.
51. Prineas JW. Pathology of the Guillain-Barré syndrome. *Ann Neurol.* 1981;9(suppl):6.
52. Lampert PW. Electron microscopic studies on ordinary and hyperacute experimental allergic encephalomyelitis. *Acta Neuropathol.* 1967;9:99–126.
53. Kieseier BC, Kiefer R, Gold R, et al. Advances in understanding and treatment of immune-mediated disorders of the peripheral nervous system. *Muscle Nerve.* 2004;30:131–156.
54. Waksman NH, Adams RD. Allergic neuritis: an experimental disease in rabbits induced by the injection of peripheral nervous tissue and adjuvant. *J Exp Med.* 1955;102:213–236.
55. Hafer-Macko CE, Sheikh KA, Li CY, et al. Immune attack on the Schwann cell surface in acute inflammatory demyelinating polyneuropathy. *Ann Neurol.* 1996;39:625–635.
56. Griffin JW, Li CY, Macko C, et al. Early nodal changes in the acute motor axonal neuropathy pattern of the Guillain-Barré syndrome. *J Neurocytol.* 1996;25:33–51.
57. Hafer-Macko C, Hsieh ST, Li CY, et al. Acute motor axonal neuropathy: an antibody-mediated attack on axolemma. *Ann Neurol.* 1996;40:635–644.
58. Yuki N, Susuki K, Koga M, et al. Carbohydrate mimicry between human ganglioside GM1 and Campylobacter jejuni lipooligosaccharide causes Guillain-Barré syndrome. *Proc Natl Acad Sci U S A.* 2004;101:11404–11409.
59. Chiba A, Kusunoki S, Shimizu T, Kanazawa I. *Ann Neurol.* 1992;31: 677–679.
60. Willison HJ. The immunobiology of Guillain-Barre syndromes. *J Peripher Nerv Syst.* 2005;10:94–112.
61. Koga M, Gilbert M, Li J, et al. Antecedent infections in Fisher syndrome: a common pathogenesis of molecular mimicry. *Neurology.* 2005;64: 1605–1611.
62. Bernsen RA, Jager AE, Schmitz PI, van der Meché FG. Long-term sensory deficit after Guillain-Barré syndrome. *J Neurol.* 2001;248:483–486.
63. Ropper AH, Wijdicks EFM, Truax BT. *Guillain-Barré Syndrome.* Philadelphia, PA: FA Davis; 1991.
64. Masucci EF, Kurtzke JG. Diagnostic criteria for the Guillain-Barré syndrome. An analysis of 50 cases. *J Neurol Sci.* 1971;13:483–501.
65. Maier H, Schmidbauer M, Pfausler B, et al. Central nervous system pathology in patients with the Guillain-Barré syndrome. *Brain.* 1997;120: 451–464.
66. Bucelli R, Harms MB. Neuromuscular emergencies. *Semin Neurol.* 2015; 35(6):683–689.
67. Rabinstein AA. Acute neuromuscular respiratory failure. *Continuum (Minneap Minn).* 2015;21(5):1324–1345.
68. Jeha LE, Sila CA, Lederman RJ, et al. West Nile virus infection: a new acute paralytic illness. *Neurology.* 2003;61:55–59.
69. Brannagan TH 3rd, Zhou Y. HIV-associated Guillain-Barré syndrome. *J Neurol Sci.* 2003;208:39–42.
70. Olney RK, Aminof MJ. Electrodiagnostic features of the Guillain-Barré syndrome: the relative sensitivity of different techniques. *Neurology.* 1990;40: 471–475.
71. Kuwabara S, Ogawara K, Misawa S, et al. Sensory nerve conduction in demyelinating and axonal Guillain-Barre syndromes. *Eur Neurol.* 2004;51: 196–198.
72. Hughes RA, Wijdicks EF, Barohn RJ, et al. Practice parameter: immunotherapy for Guillain-Barré syndrome: report of the Quality Standards Subcommittee of the American Academy of Neurology. *Neurology.* 2003;61:736–740.
73. Osterman PO, Fagius J, Lundemo G, et al. Beneficial effects of plasma exchange in acute inflammatory polyradiculoneuropathy. *Lancet.* 1984;2: 1296–1299.
74. Humphrey JG, Ropper AH, Feasby TE, et al. Plasmapheresis and acute Guillain-Barré syndrome. The Guillain-Barré Syndrome Study Group. *Neurology.* 1985;35:1096–1104.
75. Raphaël JC, Chevret S, Hughes RA, Annane D. Plasma exchange for Guillain-Barré syndrome. *Cochrane Database Syst Rev.* 2002;2:CD001798.
76. van der Meché FG, Schmitz PI. A randomized trial comparing intravenous immune globulin and plasma exchange in Guillain-Barré syndrome. Dutch Guillain-Barré Study Group. *N Engl J Med.* 1992;326:1123–1129.
77. Hughes RA, van der Meché FG. Corticosteroids for treating Guillain-Barré syndrome. *Cochrane Database Syst Rev.* 2000;(2):CD001446.
78. Pandey CK, Bose N, Garg G, et al. Gabapentin for the treatment of pain in Guillain-Barré syndrome: a double-blinded, placebo-controlled, crossover study. *Anesth Analg.* 2002;95:1719–1723.
79. Cornblath DR, Mellits ED, Griffin JW, et al. Motor conduction studies in Guillain-Barré syndrome: description and prognostic value. *Ann Neurol.* 1988;23:354–359.
80. Dornonville De la Cour C, Jakobsen J. Residual neuropathy in long-term population-based follow-up of Guillain-Barré syndrome. *Neurology.* 2005;64:246–253.
81. Forsberg A, Pressc R, Einarssonb U, et al. Impairment in Guillain-Barré syndrome during the first 2 years after onset: a prospective study. *J Neurol Sci.* 2004;227:131–138.
82. Pearce JM. Mary Broadfoot Walker (1888–1974): a historic discovery in myasthenia gravis. *Eur Neurol.* 2005;53:51–53.
83. Drachman DB. Myasthenia gravis: an illustrated history (book review). *N Engl J Med.* 2003;348:181–182.
84. Walker MB. Treatment of myasthenia gravis with physostigmine. *Lancet.* 1934;223:1200–1201.
85. Simpson JA. Immunological disturbances in myasthenia gravis with a report of Hashimoto's disease developing after thymectomy. *J Neurol Neurosurg Psychiatry.* 1964;27:485–492.
86. Patrick J, Lindstrom J. Autoimmune response to acetylcholine receptor. *Science.* 1973;180:871–872.
87. Almon RR, Andrew CG, Appel SH. Serum globulin in myasthenia gravis: inhibition of a-bungarotoxin binding to acetylcholine receptors. *Science.* 1974;186:55–57.
88. Oosterhuis HJ. The natural course of myasthenia gravis: a long-term follow-up study. *J Neurol Neurosurg Psychiatry.* 1989;52:1121–1127.
89. Drachman DB. Myasthenia gravis. *N Engl J Med.* 1994;330:1797–1810.

90. Phillips LH 2nd. The epidemiology of myasthenia gravis. *Ann N Y Acad Sci.* 2003;998:407–412.
91. Richman DP, Agius MA. Myasthenia gravis: pathogenesis and treatment. *Semin Neurol.* 1994;14:106–110.
92. Gracy DR, Divertie MB, Howard FM Jr. Mechanical ventilation for respiratory failure in myasthenia gravis: two-year experience with 22 patients. *Mayo Clin Proc.* 1983;58:597–602.
93. Thomas CE, Mayer SA, Gungor Y, et al. Myasthenic crisis: clinical features, mortality, complications, and risk factors for prolonged intubation. *Neurology.* 1997;48:1253–1260.
94. Engel AG. Anatomy and molecular architecture of the neuromuscular junction. In: Engel AG, ed. *Myasthenia Gravis and Myasthenic Disorders.* Oxford: Oxford University Press; 1999:2.
95. Ruff RL. Neurophysiology of the neuromuscular junction: overview. *Ann N Y Acad Sci.* 2003;998:1–10.
96. Lindrstrom J. Acetylcholine receptor structure. In: Kaminiski HL, ed. *Myasthenia Gravis and Related Disorders.* Totowa, NJ: Humana Press; 2003:15.
97. Lindstrom JM, Seybold MD, Lennon VA, et al. Antibody to acetylcholine receptor in myasthenia gravis: prevalence, clinical correlates, and diagnostic value. *Neurology.* 1976;26:1054–1059.
98. Drachman D, Angus CW, Adams RN, Kao I, et al. Effect of myasthenic patients' immunoglobulin on acetylcholine receptor turnover: selectivity of degradation process. *Proc Natl Acad Sci USA.* 1978;75:3422–3426.
99. Hoch W, McConville J, Helms S, et al. Auto-antibodies to the receptor tyrosine kinase MuSK in patients with myasthenia gravis without acetylcholine receptor antibodies. *Nat Med.* 2001;7:365–368.
100. Evoli A, Tonali PA, Padua L, et al. Clinical correlates with anti-MuSk antibodies in generalized myasthenia gravis. *Brain.* 2003;126:2304–2311.
101. Statland JM, Ciafaloni E. Myasthenia gravis: five new things. *Neurol Clin Pract.* 2013;3(2):126–133.
102. Pasnoor M, Wolfe GI, Nations S, et al. Clinical findings in MuSK-antibody positive myasthenia gravis: a U.S. experience. *Muscle Nerve.* 2010;41:370–374.
103. Guptill JT, Sanders DB, Evoli A. Anti-MuSK antibody myasthenia gravis: clinical findings and response to treatment in two large cohorts. *Muscle Nerve.* 2011;44:36–40.
104. Pevzner A, Schoser B, Peters K, et al. Anti-LRP4 autoantibodies in AChR- and MuSK-antibody-negative myasthenia gravis. *J Neurol.* 2012;259: 427–435.
105. Jacob S, Viegas S, Leite MI, et al. Presence and pathogenic relevance of antibodies to clustered acetylcholine receptor in ocular and generalized myasthenia gravis. *Arch Neurol.* 2012;69:994–1001.
106. Hohlfeld R, Wekerle H. The thymus in myasthenia gravis. *Neurol Clin.* 1994;12:331–342.
107. Kao I, Drachman DB. Thymic muscle cells bear acetylcholine receptors: possible relation to myasthenia gravis. *Science.* 1977;195:74–75.
108. Kaminski HJ, Fenstermaker RA, Abdul-Karim FW, et al. Acetylcholine receptor subunit gene expression in thymic tissue. *Muscle Nerve.* 1993;16:1332–1337.
109. Iwasa K. Striational autoantibodies in myasthenia gravis mainly react with ryanodine receptor. *Muscle Nerve.* 1997;20:753–756.
110. Behan PO. Immune disease and HLA associations with myasthenia gravis. *J Neurol Neurosurg Psychiatry.* 1980;43:611–621.
111. Pascuzzi RM. *Medications and Myasthenia Gravis: A Reference for Health Care Professionals. Myasthenia Gravis Foundation of America website.* Available at: http://www.myasthenia.org/portals/0/draft_medications_and_myasthenia_gravis_for_MGFA_website_8%2010%2012.pdf. Dated August 2012; accessed August 2, 2016.
112. Perrot X, Bernard N, Vial C, et al. Myasthenia gravis exacerbation or unmasking associated with telithromycin treatment. *Neurology.* 2006;67: 2256–2258.
113. Garrity ER. Respiratory failure due to disorders of the chest wall and respiratory muscles. In: MacDonnell KF, Fahey PJ, Segal MS, eds. *Respiratory Intensive Care.* Boston, MA: Little Brown; 1987:312.
114. Borel CO, Teitelbaum JS, Hanley DF. Ventilatory failure and carbon monoxide response in ventilatory failure due to myasthenia gravis and Guillain-Barre syndrome. *Crit Care Med.* 1993;21:1717–1726.
115. Tether JE. Management of myasthenic and cholinergic crisis. *Am J Med.* 1955;19:740–742.
116. Ashworth B, Hunter AR. Respiratory failure in myasthenia gravis. *Proc R Soc Med.* 1971;64:489–490.
117. Daroff RB. The office Tensilon test for ocular myasthenia gravis. *Arch Neurol.* 1986;43:843–844.
118. Okun MS, Charriez CM, Bhatti MT, et al. Asystole induced by edrophonium following beta blockade. *Neurology.* 2001;57:739.
119. Lennon VA. Serological diagnosis of myasthenic gravis and Lambert-Eaton myasthenic syndrome. In: Lisak RP, ed. *Handbook of Myasthenic Gravis and Myasthenic Syndromes.* New York: Marcel Dekker; 1994:149.
120. Cikes N, Momi MY, Williams CL, et al. Striational autoantibodies: quantitative detection by enzyme immunoassay in myasthenia gravis, thymoma, and recipients of D-penicillamine or allogenic bone marrow. *Mayo Clin Proc.* 1998;63:474–481.
121. Skeie Go, Romi F, Aarli JA, et al. Pathogenesis of myositis and myasthenia associated with titin ryanodine receptor antibodies. *Ann N Y Acad Sci.* 2003;998:343–350.
122. Howard JF Jr, Sanders DB, Massey JM. The electrodiagnosis of myasthenia gravis and the Lambert-Eaton myasthenic syndrome. *Neurol Clin.* 1994;12:305–330.
123. Oh SJ, Kim DE, Kuruoglu R, et al. Diagnostic sensitivity of the laboratory tests in myasthenia gravis. *Muscle Nerve.* 1992;15:720–724.
124. Blum S, Gillis D, Brown H, et al. Use and monitoring of low dose rituximab in myasthenia gravis. *J Neurol Neurosurg Psychiatry.* 2011;82:659–663.
125. Diaz-Manera J, Martinez-Hernandez E, Querol L, et al. Long-lasting treatment effect of rituximab in MuSK myasthenia. *Neurology.* 2012;78: 189–193.
126. Nowak RJ, Dicapua DB, Zebardast N, Goldstein JM. Response of patients with refractory myasthenia gravis to rituximab: a retrospective study. *Ther Adv Neurol Disord.* 2011;4:259–266.
127. Antozzi C, Gemma M, Regi B, et al. A short plasma exchange protocol is effective in severe myasthenia gravis. *J Neurol.* 1991;238:103–107.
128. Gajdos P, Chevert S, Clair B, et al. Clinical trial of plasma exchange and high-dose intravenous immunoglobulin in myasthenia gravis. Myasthenia Gravis Clinical Study Group. *Ann Neurol.* 1997;41:789–796.
129. Stricker RB, Kwiatkowska BJ, Habis JA, Kiprov DD. Myasthenic crisis: response to plasmapheresis following failure of intravenous gamma-globulin. *Arch Neurol.* 1993;50:837–840.
130. Barth D, Nabavi Nouri M, Ng E, et al. Comparison of IVIg and PLEX in patients with myasthenia gravis. *Neurology.* 2011;76:2017–2023.
131. Arsura E, Brunner NG, Namba T, Grob D. High-dose intravenous methylprednisolone in myasthenia gravis. *Arch Neurol.* 1985;42:1149–1153.
132. Gronseth GS, Barohn RJ. Practice parameter: thymectomy for autoimmune myasthenia gravis (an evidence-based review): report of the Quality Standards Subcommittee of the American Academy of Neurology. *Neurology.* 2000;55:7–15.
133. Bedlack RS, Sanders DB. On the concept of myasthenic crisis. *J Clin Neuromusc Dis.* 2002;4:40–42.
134. Rabinstein AA, Wijdicks EF. Warning signs of imminent respiratory failure in neurological patients. *Semin Neurol.* 2003;23:97–104.
135. Bennet DA, Bleck TP. Recognizing impending respiratory failure from neuromuscular causes. *J Crit Illness.* 1998;3:46.
136. Juel VC. Myasthenia gravis: management of myasthenic crisis and perioperative care. *Semin Neurol.* 2004;24:75–81.
137. Varelas PN, Chua HC, Natterman J, et al. Ventilatory care in myasthenia gravis crisis: assessing the baseline adverse event rate. *Crit Care Med.* 2002;30:2663–2668.
138. Leventhal SR, Orkin FK, Hirsh RA. Prediction for postoperative mechanical ventilation in myasthenia gravis. *Anesthesiology.* 1980;53:26–30.
139. Huang CS, Hsu HS, Kao KP, et al. Intravenous immunoglobulin in the preparation of thymectomy for myasthenia gravis. *Acta Neurol Scand.* 2003;108:136–138.
140. Osler W. New York: D. Appleton & Co; 1892. The Principles and Practice of Medicine.
141. Sagredo V, Caldwell JE, Matthay MA, et al. Persistent paralysis in critically ill patients after long-term administration of vecuronium. *N Engl J Med.* 1992;327:524–528.
142. Hirano M, Ott BR, Raps EC. Acute quadriplegic myopathy: complication of treatment with steroids, nondepolarizing blocking agents, or both. *Neurology.* 1992;42:2082–2087.
143. Witt NJ, Zochodne DW, Bolton CF, et al. Peripheral nerve function in sepsis and multiple organ failure. *Chest.* 1991;99:176–184.
144. De Jonghe B, Sharshar T, Lefaucheur J-P, et al. Paresis acquired in the intensive care unit: a prospective multicenter study. *JAMA.* 2002;288: 2859–2867.
145. Bednarik J, Vondracek P, Dusek L, et al. Risk factors for critical illness polyneuromyopathy. *J Neurol.* 2005;252:343–351.
146. Bercker S, Weber-Carstens S, Deja M, et al. Critical illness polyneuropathy and myopathy in patients with acute respiratory distress syndrome. *Crit Care Med.* 2005;33:711–715.
147. Kress JP, Hall JB. ICU-acquired weakness and recovery from critical illness. *N Engl J Med.* 2014;370:1626–1635.

148. Stevens RD, Dowdy DW, Michaels RK, et al. Neuromuscular dysfunction acquired in critical illness: a systematic review. *Intensive Care Med.* 2007;33(11):1876–1891.
149. Zochodne DW, Bolton CF, Wells GA, et al. Critical illness polyneuropathy: a complication of sepsis and multiple organ failure. *Brain.* 1987;110: 819–841.
150. de Letter MA, Schmitz PI, Visser LH, et al. Risk factors for the development of polyneuropathy and myopathy in critically ill patients. *Crit Care Med.* 2001;29:2281–2286.
151. Leijten FS, De Weerd AW, Poortvliet DC. Critical illness polyneuropathy in multiple organ dysfunction syndrome and weaning from the ventilator. *Intensive Care Med.* 1996;22:856–861.
152. Jaber S, Petrof BJ, Jung B, et al. Rapidly progressive diaphragmatic weakness and injury during mechanical ventilation in humans. *Am J Respir Crit Care Med.* 2011;183:364–371.
153. Murray MJ, Brull SJ, Bolton CF. Brief review: nondepolarizing neuromuscular blocking drugs and critical illness myopathy. *Can J Anesth.* 2006;53:1148–1156.
154. Minetti C, Hirano M, Morreale G, et al. Ubiquitin expression in acute steroid myopathy with loss of thick myosin filaments. *Muscle Nerve.* 1996;19:94–96.
155. Danon MJ, Carpenter S. Myopathy and thick filament (myosin) loss following prolonged paralysis with vecuronium during steroid treatment. *Muscle Nerve.* 1991;14:1131–1139.
156. Adnet F, Dhissi G, Borron SW, et al. Complication profiles of adult asthmatics requiring paralysis during mechanical ventilation. *Intensive Care Med.* 2001;27(11):1729–1736.
157. Hoke A, Rewcastle NB, Zochodne DW. Acute quadriplegic myopathy unrelated to steroids or paralyzing agents: quantitative EMG studies. *Can J Neurol Sci.* 1999;26:325–329.
158. Lacomis D. Electrophysiology of neuromuscular disorders in critical illness. *Muscle Nerve.* 2013;47(3):452–463.
159. Deem S. Intensive-care-unit-acquired muscle weakness. *Respir Care.* 2006;51:1042–1052; discussion 1052–1053.
160. Azzarelli B, Roessmann U. Diffuse "anoxic" myelopathy. *Neurology.* 1977;27:1049–1052.
161. Maramattom BV, Wijdicks EF. Acute neuromuscular weakness in the intensive care unit. *Crit Care Med.* 2006;34:2835–2841.
162. Glass JD, Samuels O, Rich MM. Poliomyelitis due to West Nile virus. *N Engl J Med.* 2002;347:1280–1281.
163. Dhand UK. Clinical approach to the weak patient in the intensive care unit. *Respir Care.* 2006;51:1024–1040; discussion 1040–1041.
164. Parak EJ, Nishida T, Sufit RL, Minieka MM. Prolonged compound muscle action potential duration in critical illness myopathy: report of nine cases. *J Clin Neuromusc Dis.* 2004;5:176–183.
165. Latronico N, Fenzi F, Boniotti C,Guarneri B. Acute reversible paralysis in critically ill patients. *Acta Anaesthesiol Ital.* 1993;44:157.
166. Bolton CF. AAEM minimonograph #40: clinical neurophysiology of the respiratory system. *Muscle Nerve.* 1993;16:809–818.
167. Rich MM, Teener JW, Raps EC, et al. Muscle is electrically inexcitable in acute quadriplegic myopathy. *Neurology.* 1996;46:731–736.
168. Lefaucheur JP, Nordine T, Rodriguez P, Brochard L. Origin of ICU acquired paresis determined by direct muscle stimulation. *J Neurol Neurosurg Psychiatry.* 2006;77:500–506.
169. Lacomis D, Zochodne DW, Bird SJ. Critical illness myopathy. *Muscle Nerve.* 2000;23:1785–1788.
170. Schweickert WD, Pohlman MC, Pohlman AS, et al. Early physical and occupational therapy in mechanically ventilated, critically ill patients: a randomised controlled trial. *Lancet.* 2009;373(9678):1874–1882.
171. Van den Berghe G, Schoonheydt K, Becx P, et al. Insulin therapy protects the central and peripheral nervous system of intensive care patients. *Neurology.* 2005;64:1348–1353.
172. NICE-SUGAR Study Investigators, Finfer S, Chittock DR, et al. Intensive versus conventional glucose control in critically ill patients. *N Engl J Med.* 2009;360(13):1283–1297.
173. Malhotra A. Intensive insulin in intensive care. *N Engl J Med.* 2006; 354:516–518.
174. Brunkhorst FM, Kuhnt E, Engel C, et al. Intensive insulin therapy in patient with severe sepsis and septic shock is associated with an increased rate of hypoglycemia: results from a randomized multicenter study (VISEP). *Infection.* 2005;33(Suppl):19.
175. Zifko UA. Long-term outcome of critical illness polyneuropathy. *Muscle Nerve Suppl.* 2000;9:S49–S52.
176. Latronico N, Shehu I, Seghelini E. Neuromuscular sequelae of critical illness. *Curr Opin Crit Care.* 2005;11:381–390.
177. Latronico N, Fenzi F, Recupero D, et al. Critical illness myopathy and neuropathy. *Lancet.* 1996;347:1579–1582.
178. Guarneri B, Bertolini G, Latronico N. Long-term outcome in patients with critical illness myopathy or neuropathy: the Italian multicentre CRIMYNE study. *J Neurol Neurosurg Psychiatry.* 2008;79(7):838–841.

CHAPTER
123

Delirium and Behavioral Disturbances

KAREN A. KORZICK and E. WESLEY ELY

INTRODUCTION

There are a wide variety of central nervous system (CNS)-mediated neuropsychological responses to severe, acute illness: delirium, pain, fever, anxiety, depression, anhedonia, fatigue, sleepiness, cognitive slowing, memory changes, and social withdrawal (1,2); delirium is the most problematic and life-threatening neuropsychological complication of intensive care unit (ICU) patients. Delirium is present when all of the following diagnostic criteria have been met:

- Inattention
- Acute change in baseline cognitive function due to acute dysfunction in one or more cognitive domains such as orientation, memory, perception (visual, auditory, tactile hallucinations), language, cognitive processing speed, judgment
- Acute onset with a fluctuating time course over hours or days
- Concurrent systemic illness (3,4)

Subsyndromal delirium exists when a patient has one or more components of delirium but never develops all four components (3,5).

Delirium rates in the ICU vary depending on the population studied, ranging from 16% to over 80% (6–21). Regardless of age, about 30% to 40% of adults may be delirious during their ICU stay (6,22). Delirium in the ICU is associated with statistically significant increases in ICU and hospital lengths of stay (LOS), days on mechanical ventilation (5,7,13,15,17–24), as well as unintended removal of medical devices and failed extubation (25). In the elderly, delirium is associated with a two to three times increased risk of institutionalization, higher rates of readmissions, falls, deep tissue injuries, and unintended removal of medical devices (6,26).

Delirium is a significant risk factor for death while in the ICU, after discharge from the ICU while still hospitalized, and after discharge from the hospital, with reported mortality hazard ratios ranging from 1.67 to 3.2. (5,11,13,17–19,23,27,28). In a patient cohort with 3 delirious days (median), the hazard ratio for death associated with delirium was 1.10 (95% CI 1.02 to 1.18); for each additional ICU day spent in delirium, the mortality hazard risk increased by 10% (28). Delay in treating ICU delirium may increase mortality (29), while a recent meta-analysis of 17 studies evaluating 2,849 delirious patients found no short-term mortality reduction associated with treating delirium once it has occurred (30). More data are needed from large, robustly designed studies.

Delirium imposes significant economic burdens on patients, families, and health care delivery systems. Delirium increases the costs of medical care due to prolonged ICU and hospital LOS, increased time on mechanical ventilation, and increased need for prolonged care after hospital discharge (4,26,31–33). The cost of ICU care for a delirious mechanically ventilated patient is 39% more than a nondelirious, mechanically ventilated ICU patient; total hospital cost of care for the former group of patients is 31% higher than the latter (31). Conservative methodology suggests that ICU delirium consumes $300 million to $4 billion of health care expenditure yearly in the USA; using less restrictive assumptions, the cost of delirium may range from $6.5 to $20.4 billion yearly (4).

Patients employed prior to an admission complicated by delirium may be delayed in return to work due to persistent cognitive difficulties, causing significant negative financial impact on their families. Care providers report decreased income, and in some cases, loss of employment, in order to stay home to care for a survivor of delirium (1).

Delirium that begins in the ICU can persist through the hospital discharge and may be a predictor of long-term cognitive and psychiatric impairment in survivors of critical illness. Cognitive deficits may include impairment in memory, attention, and executive function, and may last for weeks, months, years, or may even be permanent (3,15,19,26,33–45). Psychiatric impairments include increased risk for depression and posttraumatic stress disorder (PTSD) (40,44). The relationship between delirium and dementia is recognized, but poorly understood; the two diseases may represent stages on a continuum of neurologic injury (33,34). Pre-existing dementia is a risk factor for developing delirium, and delirium has been associated with a two- to threefold increase in the risk of being diagnosed with dementia up to 2 years after discharge from an inpatient admission with incident delirium and no pre-existing diagnosis of dementia (6,26,33,34). Increased duration of ICU delirium is an independent risk factor for long-term cognitive impairment after critical illness (35–37). (See Chapter 12 for a discussion of the long-term neurocognitive and functional consequences of ICU delirium.)

PATHOPHYSIOLOGY

The pathophysiology of delirium has been studied in experimental animal models and clinically in humans for more than five decades, but remains poorly understood (1,2,46–50). Contemporary thought is that delirium is a complex process triggered by a wide variety of stimuli which result in the activation of one or more pathophysiologic mechanisms, resulting in acute brain dysfunction that presents clinically as delirium. There are seven prominent pathophysiologic theories for the etiology of delirium (46). It is generally agreed upon that a single theory cannot adequately explain the etiology of delirium; rather, the numerous etiologies of delirium are interrelated, can occur in various combinations from patient to patient, and may vary over time during the clinical course of delirium in any one patient (Fig. 123.1) (46).

Neuroinflammatory Hypothesis

Activation of acute peripheral inflammation induced by a variety of systemic events results in activation of brain parenchymal

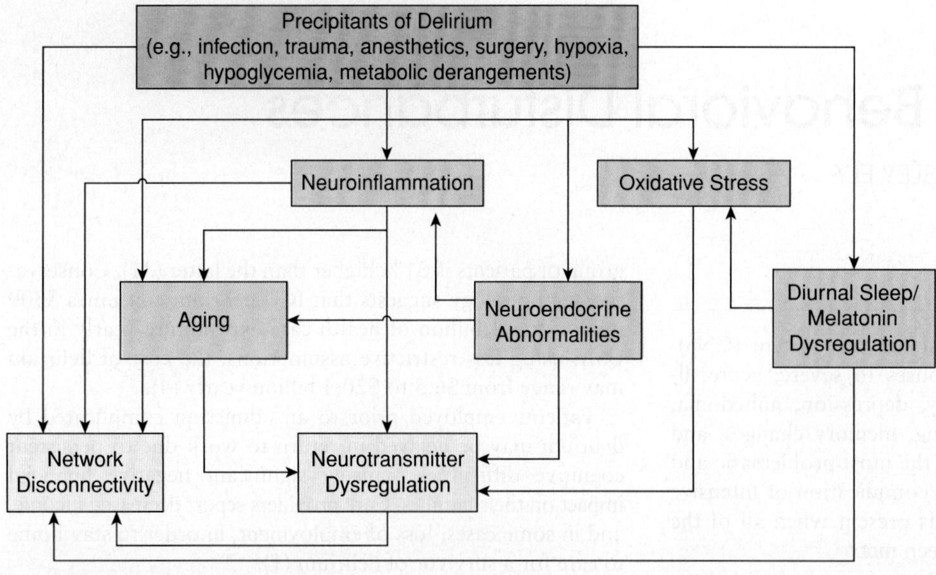

FIGURE 123.1 Etiologic theories of delirium and their relationship to each other. (Adapted from Maldonado JR. Neuropathogenesis of delirium: review of current etiologic theories and common pathways. *Am J Geriatr Psychiatry*. 2013;21:1190–1222; with permission.)

cells, which produce pro-inflammatory cytokines and inflammatory mediators within the CNS, causing neuronal and synaptic dysfunction, ischemia, and neuronal apoptosis resulting in acute brain dysfunction presenting clinically as delirium (46–48,51–53). Systemic inflammatory mediators can reach the brain by one of two routes, the slower humoral route and/or the faster neural route (1,46). The humoral route has three possible mechanisms by which these mediators can affect brain function (1):

- Circulating cytokines activate macrophage-like cells in the circumventricular organs of the CNS, where a functional blood–brain barrier is absent, to secrete high levels of cytokines which then enter the brain by volume diffusion.
- Some cytokines may be able to cross the blood–brain barrier by saturable transport mechanisms.
- By a direct effect of humoral cytokines on brain vascular endothelium, with subsequent alterations in the blood–brain barrier.

The neural route is suggested by animal studies of abdominal sepsis showing that vagal nerve activation by peripheral inflammatory mediators in the abdominal cavity provide afferent input into the brain, with subsequent activation of inflammatory mediators within the brain; the CNS inflammatory response to intra-abdominal inflammatory mediators can be ablated by transecting the vagal nerve (1). The brain may be primed by inflammatory signals that first reach it via the neural route; this then sensitizes the brain to subsequent input from the slower humoral routes (1).

Neuronal Aging Hypothesis

Numerous studies in ICU and non-ICU patient populations have identified age as an independent risk factor for delirium (4,13,15,25,26,38,46,50). The physiologic and anatomic changes associated with aging in the brain may render it more susceptible to exogenous insults known to trigger delirium, such as acute inflammatory states in the body (neuroinflammatory hypothesis [NIH]). Additionally, the aging brain may mount a more exuberant CNS inflammatory response, as compared to a younger brain, when stimulated by peripheral inflammatory states. The presence of the apolipoprotein E (APOE) A4 allele has been associated with an increased risk of postoperative cognitive dysfunction and delirium in the elderly, possibly through increased inflammation and/or decreased cholinergic activity in the brain (54,55).

Neurotransmitter Hypothesis

Abnormal levels and/or relative imbalances of systems of neurotransmitters—including acetylcholine, dopamine, tryptophan, serotonin, noradrenaline, gamma-butyric acid (GABA), glutamate, and histamine—have all been implicated in the etiology of delirium (46,47,56–60). Debate continues on whether there is a common final pathway for any etiology of delirium, mediated by any of a variety of the neurotransmitters noted above (46–49,55,56). Acetylcholine deficiency is the most often cited candidate neurotransmitter for a common final pathway (49,55,56). Genetics may also play a role in neurotransmitter function in the CNS, via control of the types and expression of neurotransmitter receptors (55).

Oxidative Stress Hypothesis

Many stimuli can increase oxygen consumption in and/or decrease oxygen delivery to the CNS, causing increased CNS energy expenditure and reduced cerebral oxidative metabolism resulting in CNS dysfunction (46). Metabolic derangements induced by oxidative stress are one mechanism by which neurotransmitter imbalances can occur (neurotransmitter hypothesis [NTH]) (46,56). Nutritional deficiencies leading to further derangements of CNS tissue metabolism may play a role in the pathogenesis of delirium (61).

Neuroendocrine Hypothesis

Delirium may be caused by neuronal damage mediated by high levels of glucocorticoids in the CNS, due either to activation of the hypothalamic–pituitary–adrenal axis in response to physiologic stressors such as infection, surgery, or trauma (2,46,47,50,62), or by the administration of exogenous glucocorticoids (63). Chronically high levels of physiologic stress are also associated with increased levels of inflammation in the body, connecting the NIH and neuroendocrine hypothesis (NEH) theories of delirium (2,46,50,52).

Diurnal Dysregulation or Melatonin Dysregulation Hypothesis

Delirium may be caused by disruptions in circadian cycles, most notably induced by sleep deprivation; obstructive sleep apnea is also associated with delirium (46,64–70). Derangements in melatonin levels may cause delirium, due to its central role in the regulation of circadian rhythm and sleep–wake cycles (46,64–67). Other CNS neurotransmitters implicated in diurnal dysregulation include acetylcholine, dopamine, GABA, tryptophan, serotonin, and cortisol (64–66). Sleep deprivation has been associated with increased levels of inflammatory substances, connecting the diurnal dysregulation or melatonin dysregulation hypothesis (DDH) and NIH theories of delirium (64).

Network Disconnectivity Hypothesis

The proper function of the brain depends on the rich connection between different regions of the brain in neural networks, mediated by specific neurotransmitter activity (NTH) across that particular neural network. A variety of insults to the brain may result in the loss of the proper function of any of these neural networks, disconnecting the component parts of the network from each other, altering normal brain function and resulting in delirium (46). The network disconnectivity hypothesis (NDH) postulates that the clinical forms of delirium, hypoactive versus hyperactive, may be determined by which neural networks break down in response to stressors such as aging (NAH), sleep deprivation (DDH), infection/inflammation (NTH), or medication exposure (NTH). How they will break down in the face of a particular stressor is thought to be related to the degree of baseline network connectivity and the level of inhibitory tone, mediated by GABA levels (NTH), in that particular neural network (46).

DIAGNOSIS

Delirium is a clinically established diagnosis requiring a thorough history and physical exam to identify risk factors, including a detailed review of outpatient and inpatient medication records with attention to those drugs whose administration or abrupt withdrawal are associated with delirium (47) (Table 123.1). The impression of the ICU physician as to whether or not their patient has delirium is very inaccurate, with a sensitivity of only 29% (71), and subjective assessment for delirium by ICU nurses missed 6.4% of patients found to have delirium using objective assessment methods (72). Hypoactive and mixed delirium, the most common forms of delirium in the ICU, may be missed without the use of delirium detection tools (22,71,73). Therefore, a cognitive function assessment using a delirium detection tool validated for use in ICU populations is a critical component of the examination of the delirious patient.

Six tools have been developed and validated for use in ICU populations: the Confusion Assessment Method ICU (CAM-ICU), the Delirium Detection Score (DDS), the Intensive Care Delirium Screening Checklist (ICDSC), the Cognitive Test for Delirium (CTD), the Abbreviated Cognitive Test for Delirium, the Neelson and Champagne Confusion Scale (NEECHAM), and the Nursing Delirium Screening Scale (NuDESC) (9,10,12,74–79). The Society of Critical Care Medicine Task Force on pain, agitation, and delirium recommends the use of either the CAM-ICU or the ICDSC for daily ICU delirium detection and monitoring (73). Of these, the CAM-ICU has been shown to have superior pooled sensitivity (80.0%, 95% CI 77.1% to 82.6%) and pooled specificity (95.9%, 95% CI 94.8% to 96.8%), while the ICDSC has moderate pooled sensitivity (74%, 95% CI 65.3% to 81.5%) and good pooled specificity (81.9%, 95% CI 8.51% to 54.4%) (79). The

TABLE 123.1 Pharmacologic Agents Associated with Delirium

Medications that, when administered, may cause delirium, either by direct effect or drug–drug interaction
ACE inhibitors
Alpha-blockers
Amantadine
Aminophylline
Amiodarone
Anticholinergics
Antiemetics (anticholinergic effects)
Antiepileptics
Antihistamines (anticholinergic effects)
Antineoplastics
Antipsychotics with anticholinergic properties: chlorpromazine, clozapine, mesoridazine, olanzapine, quetiapine, thioridazine
Antispasmodics (anticholinergic effects)
Barbiturates
Benzodiazepines
Beta-blockers
Calcium channel blockers
Carbidopa/levodopa, dopaminergic drugs
Carisoprodol
Cefepime
Corticosteroids
Digoxin
Diuretics
Fluoroquinolones
Immunosuppressants
Lidocaine
Lithium
Monoamine oxidase inhibitors
Nonsteroidal anti-inflammatory drugs
Opioids
Pregabalin
Quinidine
Tricyclic antidepressants (anticholinergic effects)
Zolpidem and related hypnotics
Medications that, when abruptly withdrawn in chronic users, may cause delirium
Antiepileptics
Antipsychotics/neuroleptics
Barbiturates
Benzodiazepines
Carisoprodol
Opioids
Selective serotonin reuptake inhibitors
Tricyclic antidepressants
Zolpidem and related hypnotics
Substances of abuse that, when abruptly withdrawn in chronic users, may cause delirium
Alcohol
Benzodiazepines
Cocaine
Methamphetamines
Nicotine
Opioids

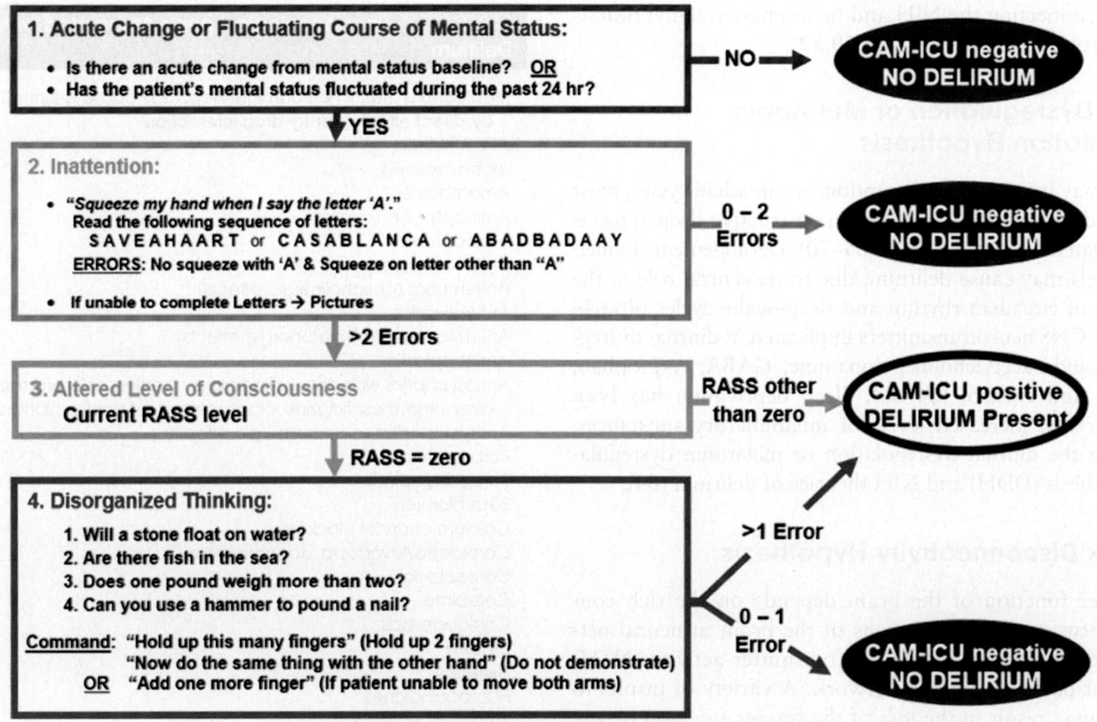

FIGURE 123.2 CAM-ICU algorithm. (Copyright © 2002, E. Wesley Ely, MD, www.icudelirium.org.)

CAM-ICU also has superior interrater reliability ($k = 0.91$) (Fig. 123.2, Table 123.2) (76).

The ICDSC and CAM-ICU have their differences and their limitations, and a more detailed cognitive evaluation may be required to detect subsyndromal delirium or hypoactive delirium in some ICU patients (80). Sensitivity of the CAM-ICU has been shown to be lower in nonresearch clinical practice settings as compared to clinical research settings (76,81–85). CAM-ICU and ICDSC sensitivity is decreased when used in nonintubated postoperative geriatric patients and noncritically ill oncology patients, suggesting that their use in detecting delirium in patients who are admitted to the ICU, but not intubated or with lower severity of illness scores as their illnesses improve, may be limited (86,87). There are limited data on the diagnostic accuracy of the ICU delirium detection tools when applied to patients with pre-existing dementia (9,10,88). The

TABLE 123.2 Intensive Delirium Screening Checklist

The scale is completed based on information collected from each entire 8-hr shift or from the previous 24 hr. Obvious manifestation of an item = 1 point; no manifestation of an item or no assessment possible = 0 point. The score of each item is entered in the corresponding empty box and is 0 or 1.

1. Altered level of consciousness

   A/B: No response (A) or the need for vigorous stimulation (B) in order to obtain any response signified a severe alteration in the level of consciousness precluding evaluation. If there is coma (A) or stupor.

   (B) most of the time period then a dash (–) is entered, and there is no further evaluation during that period.

   C: Drowsiness or requirement of a mild-to-moderate stimulation for a response implies an altered level of consciousness and scores 1 point.

   D: Wakefulness or sleeping state that could easily he aroused is considered normal and scores no point.

   E: Hypervigilance is rated as an abnormal level of consciousness and scores 1 point.
2. Inattention: Difficulty in following a conversation or instructions. Easily distracted by external stimuli. Difficulty in shifting focuses. Any of these scores 1 point.
3. Disorientation: Any obvious mistake in time, place, or person scores 1 point.
4. Hallucination, delusion or psychosis: The unequivocal clinical manifestation of hallucination or of behavior probably due to hallucination (e.g., trying to catch a nonexistent object) or delusion; gross impairment in reality testing. Any of these scores 1 point.
5. Psychomotor agitation or retardation: Hyperactivity requiring the use of additional sedative drugs or restraints in order to control potential danger to oneself or others (e.g., pulling out intravenous lines, hitting staff); hypoactivity or clinically noticeable psychomotor slowing. Any of these scores 1 point.
6. Inappropriate speech or mood: Inappropriate, disorganized, or incoherent speech; inappropriate display of emotion related to events or situation. Any of these scores 1 point.
7. Sleep/wake cycle disturbance: Sleeping less than 4 hr or waking frequently at night (do not consider wakefulness initiated by medical staff or loud environment); sleeping during most of the day. Any of these scores 1 point.
8. Symptom fluctuation: Fluctuation in the manifestation of any item or symptom over 24 hr (e.g., from one shift to another) scores 1 point.

From Devlin JW, Fong JJ, Fraser GL, Riker RR. Delirium assessment in the critically ill. *Intensive Care Med.* 2007;33:929–940, with permission.

TABLE 123.3 Biomarkers Associated with Delirium (1,47,54,95,96,98,99)

Serum/Plasma Biomarkers of Delirium Risk			
Apolipoprotein A4 allele		A9 allele of the dopamine transporter	
Serum/plasma Biomarkers of Delirium Disease Activity			
Cytokines	**Inflammatory mediators**	**Markers of brain injury**	**Other**
IL-1 beta	Matrix metalloproteinase 9	Neuron-specific enolase	Phenylalanine
IL-6	C reactive protein	S-100 beta	Trypytophan
IL-8	Protein C	Neuronal tau protein	Melatonin
IL-RA	Procalcitonin		Cortisol
TNF-alpha			Serum anticholinergic activity (SSA)
sTNFR1			
IFN-alpha			
IFN-gamma			
IGF-1			
CSF Biomarkers			
Elevated levels associated with delirium		**Reduced levels associated with delirium**	
Serotonin metabolites		Acetylcholine	
IL-8		Somatostatin	
Cortisol		Beta endorphin	
Lactate		Neuron-specific enolase	
Protein			
Acetylcholinesterase—associated with poor long-term outcome			
Dopamine metabolites—associated with psychotic features			

CAM-ICU identifies if delirium is present, but does not allow for an assessment of the severity of delirium (89). The ICDSC evaluates more symptoms of delirium than the CAM-ICU and it can detect patients with subsyndromal delirium (90). The ability of these tools to detect ICU delirium accurately could be decreased by the effects of sedation and by the time interval between interruption of sedation and delirium assessment (91–94). Delirium assessment should occur after sedation interruption with enough time allowed for sedation effects to clear; but how long that time should be is unclear (94,95).

In addition to cognitive assessment, the delirium-oriented physical examination should include a bedside visual acuity examination to exclude new visual deficits and an examination of the external auditory canals to exclude cerumen impaction resulting in decreased hearing acuity. The neck should be examined for evidence of unrecognized thyroid disease, and the abdominal examination should assess for evidence of bladder retention/distension and bowel dysfunction from ileus or obstipation, as these can be factors causing delirium, particularly in patients with spinal cord injuries and the elderly. A thorough search for sources of infection, including the inspection of all insertion sites of catheters, drains, and the removal of surgical dressings for direct inspection of all surgical sites for evidence of infection, is required in the evaluation of a newly delirious ICU patient.

Serum chemistry, complete blood count (CBC), and lactate should be evaluated for electrolyte, metabolic, and glucose abnormalities, as well as infection and acute, severe anemia. Liver function tests should be evaluated for evidence of developing liver failure. Assessment of arterial blood gas for evidence of respiratory failure as well as thyroid and hypothalamic–pituitary–adrenal axis function screening may be appropriate in selected patients. If the history, the examination, and/or the lab findings are suggestive of infection, additional studies including chest x-ray, urinalysis, blood cultures, and advanced imaging may be required. In some patients, it may be appropriate to order organ-specific testing if there is clinical evidence of new organ dysfunction, such as an echocardiogram for suspected heart failure. A limited number of ICU patients may require CNS imaging or electroencephalography (EEG) as part of their assessment for delirium.

Due to the limitations of the validated clinical tools used to assess for ICU delirium, interest exists in identifying adjunctive tools to increase the accuracy of diagnosing ICU delirium. Serum biomarkers associated with delirium, including a variety of cytokines, inflammatory markers, and genes, may play a role in the pathogenesis of delirium or may be useful in clinical research studies to identify those at risk for delirium or prolonged neurocognitive injury after an episode of delirium. However, at present, none are ready for routine use in daily clinical practice (Table 123.3) (1,2,46–48,50–55,96–101).

There is no neuroimaging modality that can, as a standalone study, confirm or exclude the diagnosis of delirium. Imaging modalities such as CT or MRI of the brain may be useful in select patients who present with fever, stiff neck, focal motor deficits, history of trauma, acute onset of severe headache, or no other identifiable cause or risk factor for delirium (26,33,102). MRI in survivors of ICU delirium demonstrates a correlation between duration of ICU delirium, the degree of white matter disruption, smaller brain volumes seen on MRI, and the degree of cognitive dysfunction up to 12 months post-ICU discharge (103,104), but no difference in brain region activity during cognitive tasks (105). Specialized neurophysiologic studies such as cerebral blood flow (CBF), single-photon emission computed tomography (SPECT), positron emission tomography (PET), amyloid PET imaging, and specialized MRI techniques have been reported or suggested as possible tools to study the brain in the setting of delirium research (102). EEG to exclude subclinical seizures may be appropriate in selected delirious ICU patients for whom no other explanation for their delirium exists, or in patients who fail to respond to therapy for treatable causes of delirium. Several research groups have used EEG in the detection and monitoring of delirious ICU patients; however, routine use of EEG monitoring of delirious ICU patients has no role, currently, in routine clinical practice (106–111).

TREATMENT

The optimal pharmacologic treatment for delirium is currently unknown. This reality should prompt caregivers to remember that the treatment of underlying medical conditions and attention to nonpharmacologic issues like noise, light, sleep, and mobility are critical aspects of delirium management. Given the complex interplay of multiple risk factors, CNS anatomy and physiology, and the diversity of potential pathophysiologic mechanisms leading to the development of delirium in any individual patient, the optimal treatment for delirium will require customization to each individual patient and will involve multiple therapeutic modalities, both nonpharmacologic and pharmacologic.

When an ICU patient is diagnosed with delirium, a comprehensive clinical assessment to identify the contributing delirium risk factors and to exclude other diagnoses in the differential diagnosis of ICU delirium must be undertaken (80). In patients with few risk factors for delirium, a greater insult is likely needed to trigger delirium, while for patients with a large number of risk factors, it may take a trivial insult to precipitate delirium (4,49). Three or more risk factors for the development of delirium raises the likelihood of developing delirium to 60% or more (4). Delirious ICU patients have been shown to have in excess of 10 identified risk factors for the development of this disorder (4,24); multiple classification systems for delirium risk factors exist (16,25,112–115). Regardless of the risk factor classification scheme used, the most important issue is to identify those risk factors that are modifiable, as these represent targets for intervention. There is a wide heterogeneity of ICU and non-ICU populations which have been studied to identify risk factors for delirium, resulting in a large number of reported risk factors (Table 123.4). The pre-existing risk factors at the time of ICU admission that are highly associated with developing ICU delirium include pre-existing history of dementia, hypertension, alcoholism, and high severity of illness at ICU admission (73). Any identified modifiable risk factor for delirium requires intervention to neutralize that factor and remove it as a cause of delirium.

Once a diagnosis of delirium is established, it may be useful to consider ICU delirium by motorific subtype: hyperactive, hypoactive, and mixed (22,117,118). Motor subtype of delirium may be predictive of the cause of the delirium. Hyperactive delirium is associated with substance withdrawal (alcohol,

TABLE 123.4 Delirium Risk Factors in ICU Studies[a]

ICU Type	Nonmodifiable	Modifiable/Potentially Modifiable
SICU/trauma (8)		Pain Benzodiazepines Fentanyl
Cardiovascular surgery ICU (14–16,18)	Age Preoperative cognitive impairment Ongoing major depression Cerebrovascular disease Peripheral vascular disease Euroscore ≥ 5 Diabetes NYHA CHF Class Canadian Cardiovascular Society degree Type of CV surgery Intraoperative hemofiltration Reoperation Educational background Marital status Chronic renal disease Emergency cardiac surgery MI within past 90 d	Benzodiazepines Physical restraints Anemia Atrial fibrillation Prolonged intubation Postoperative hypoxia Cardiogenic shock Hypoalbuminemia Acute infection Acute Renal failure Duration of surgery Duration of perfusion Duration of reperfusion Duration of aortic cross clamp time $PaCO_2$ > 45 mmHg PaO_2 4 units (1 L) Plasma transfusion > 1 unit Body temperature 12 hr Duration of mechanical ventilation Myocardial infarction
Med-surg ICUs (17,18,20,21,116[b])	Age Hypertension APACHE II score on ICU admission APACHE IV score Male Type of admission: medical, surgical, trauma Type of ICU Preferred language non-English Charlson comorbidity Index score Dementia Primary admitting diagnosis to ICU Severe sepsis Respiratory failure	Active tobacco use Active alcohol use Active drug abuse Epidural catheter use Opioids Benzodiazepines Propofol Indomethacin Steroids Coma Pain Physical restraint Central venous or arterial catheter ARDS

[a]Including univariate and multivariate analysis results with $p \le 0.05$.
[b]Meta-analysis of cigarette smoking in hospitalized and ICU patients was inconclusive.

nicotine, illicit substances, and prescribed medications with CNS activity such as benzodiazepines, narcotics, neuroleptics), while hypoactive delirium is associated with organ system dysfunction (respiratory failure, renal failure, liver failure) or metabolic abnormalities (22,118).

Evaluation of the literature on pharmacologic treatment of ICU delirium is complicated because of the small number of ICU specific studies, the clinical diversity of ICU patient populations studied, the diversity of the pharmacologic agents used, heterogeneity in how delirium was measured, small sample sizes, and study design variations (119). Multiple classes of pharmacologic agents including benzodiazepines, antipsychotics, central alpha-2 agonists (dexmedetomidine), and cholinesterase inhibitors have been studied in the treatment of ICU delirium. Of these, antipsychotics and dexmedetomidine are frequently used to control the symptoms of ICU delirium. However, to date, no pharmacologic agent has been definitively proven to be effective in treating ICU delirium (73,119). When needed, the selection of pharmacologic agent(s) to treat ICU delirium must be individualized to each patient and their clinical circumstances (73,119–124). It is extremely important for clinicians to understand that, by administering a medication, they may not be treating delirium, but instead may only be controlling the undesired effects of delirium, particularly agitated delirium. It is also important to recognize that many of the drugs commonly used to control agitation not responsive to adequate analgesia have been implicated as causes of delirium (8,14,20,73,125–131).

Discussion continues as to whether the benzodiazepine class of medications are an independent risk factor for delirium, with most studies suggesting they are (8,14,20,125–128), while a smaller number of studies found no association between the administration of benzodiazepines and the development of delirium in various ICU populations (15,16,36,101). Current guidelines for delirium management recommended the avoidance of benzodiazepines to treat ICU delirium except in those patients whose delirium is caused by acute ETOH or benzodiazepine withdrawal (73,132).

Antipsychotic agents, including haloperidol, risperidone, quetiapine, and olanzapine, have been studied with varying results in terms of their effect on ICU delirium (119,124,133–139). Haloperidol use in the ICU is safe with QTc monitoring, but has not been shown to be effective in treating delirium (137,138). Two small studies using quetiapine have shown efficacy in treating ICU delirium, but further study is needed before the routine use of quetiapine in the ICU can be recommended (136,139). Antipsychotic agents should be used with caution in patients with Parkinson's disease or Lewy Body disease, as the use of these agents in these patient subgroups can precipitate life-threatening parkinsonian crisis. There has been no reported increased ICU mortality associated with the short-term use of antipsychotics in the ICU (137,138), although there is evidence of increased mortality risk and other adverse outcomes with the prolonged use of antipsychotics in the elderly, particularly those with dementia (135,140–142). If prescribed for ICU delirium, the optimum treatment duration with antipsychotics is unknown (131,143). In the study by Devlin et al. (136), quetiapine was stopped either at physician discretion or upon ICU discharge. In 14 days of follow-up post-ICU discharge, 20% of the quetiapine group and 56% of the placebo group had one or more days of delirium. The MIND trial investigators tapered antipsychotics to off over 48 hours after delirium cleared (137). Further study is required to determine an optimal length of therapy, but due to safety concerns for long-term use of antipsychotics, particularly in the elderly, it is suggested that antipsychotics started in the hospital should not be continued after discharge. If they are continued after discharge, the patient should be closely monitored with strong consideration of referral to qualified psychiatric or geriatric health care experts.

Multiple studies have suggested that dexmedetomidine is a promising agent to treat ICU delirium, either by decreasing incidence rates of the disorder or reducing delirious days (126,127,144–152). Dexmedetomidine use may be limited by the presence of hypotension or cardiac conduction abnormalities, both of which are frequently encountered in ICU patient populations. As with the antipsychotics, further research on dexmedetomidine and its role in the treatment of ICU delirium is required (153).

Rivastigmine was studied for the treatment of ICU delirium, but due to increased mortality in the first interval data analysis, the study was stopped (154). Rivastigmine and other cholinesterase inhibitors are not recommended in the treatment of ICU delirium (73,154).

There is an important connection between pain, analgesia, sedation, short- and long-term cognitive functions, mobility, and delirium in the ICU (73,112,119,123,155). Poorly controlled pain is a frequent cause of agitation in ICU patients (49,75) and prolonged pain is a risk factor for delirium (7,8,73). The use of opioids to control pain and their relationship to delirium is complex. Continuous infusion fentanyl was shown to be associated with increased delirium, while bolus dosing of morphine was shown to be protective for delirium in surgical/trauma ICU patients (7,8). Opioid use is frequently implicated as a cause of delirium in the elderly (26,33); sedatives, including benzodiazepines (8,14,123,125–128), propofol (129), and dexmedetomidine (130,131) have also been implicated as causal of delirium. Prolonged deep sedation interferes with the ability to accurately assess the patient for delirium and is associated with increased levels of cognitive dysfunction both in the ICU and postdischarge (91,93,94,119,120,123). In addition, prolonged, deep sedation interferes with the ability to extubate and to mobilize the patient as early as possible during their ICU stay (156). While implementation of ICU sedation strategies including daily awakening trials or targeted sedation goals have many important benefits to ICU patients, such as reduced mortality and shorter ICU stays, these strategies have not been shown to consistently reduce ICU delirium (119,128,150,155,157–168); however, they may decrease subsyndromal delirium (169).

One ICU care modality that has been consistently shown to decrease ICU delirium rates is early exercise and mobility in the ICU, including the ambulation of appropriately selected intubated ICU patients (119,170–172). To optimize overall ICU patient outcomes and to allow for early mobility, current pain and sedation guidelines recommend a multimodality, stepped approach (73,119). The first level uses nonpharmacologic and nonopioid pharmacologic modalities. If the first level provides inadequate analgosedation, the second level adds opioids, with bolus dosing preferred over continuous infusion, whenever possible. If inadequate analgosedation remains, the third level adds sedatives with bolus dosing preferred over continuous infusion whenever possible.

In addition to early mobility, sleep hygiene has received increased attention in the treatment and prevention of ICU delirium. Two studies have now been published showing statistically significant reductions in ICU delirium incidence rates and decreased delirious ICU days when ICU care bundles to improve sleep hygiene were implemented in medical and medical/surgical ICU populations (173,174).

PREVENTION

Due to the difficulty in treating ICU delirium once it occurs, as well as the long-term cognitive and psychiatric deficits, and increased mortality, associated with ICU delirium, the prevention of this disorder is important. Prevention is achievable through both nonpharmacologic and pharmacologic prevention protocols (115,175,176).

Nonpharmacologic prevention begins with screening patients at ICU admission for their risk of developing delirium. A prediction model for the risk of developing ICU delirium has been published, identifying 10 risk factors that can be identified within the first 24 hours of ICU admission, allowing for targeted delirium prevention strategies for those patients at high risk of developing ICU delirium (115,177). There is increasing awareness of how ICU culture and patterns of care delivered to ICU patients can increase or decrease the risk of ICU delirium (156,167,168,178,179). ICU cultures that tolerate the use of continuous deep sedation, prolonged bed rest, and poor nocturnal sleep hygiene are increasingly recognized as harmful to ICU patients. Provision of adequate analgesia for pain control, targeted sedation strategies, daily spontaneous breathing trials for intubated patients, routine screening for ICU delirium, and early mobilization of ICU patients are the hallmarks of high-quality, safe ICU patient care and ICU culture (115,120,156). Avoidance of sensory deprivation by the provision of glasses and hearing aids if used at home; cognitive stimulation by frequent reorientation and the provision of music during daytime; circadian cycle promotion by control of window blinds, nocturnal ICU noise and light reduction strategies and the bundling of nocturnal ICU nursing care to avoid frequent nocturnal stimulation of patients; family involvement in patient care; and, family/nursing staff education on the importance of ICU culture are the components of multi-intervention ICU nursing care bundles that, when implemented in various combinations by ICU care teams, have prevented ICU delirium (173,174,176,180,181).

Interpretation of the literature on pharmacologic prevention of ICU delirium is complicated by many of the same issues complicating the literature on pharmacologic treatment of ICU delirium: diverse patient populations studied, diversity of pharmacologic agents used, variations in severity of illness scores, small sample sizes, methods of delirium assessment, and study design (119,121,122). Antipsychotics for delirium prophylaxis, including haloperidol and risperidone, have been studied in cardiac surgery patients, with some evidence of effectiveness in preventing delirium in the postsurgery period (182,183). The MIND study showed no difference in delirium incidence or severity measures among ICU patients treated with haloperidol, ziprasidone, or placebo (137), though it was only designed as a pilot feasibility study. A study using haloperidol prophylaxis in ICU patients at high risk to develop delirium decreased delirium incidence in the prophylaxis group (184). Dexmedetomidine has conflicting results in delirium prevention in various ICU populations, with one study showing increased delirium (129), four studies showing reduced delirium (126,127,146,152), and three studies showing no effect (145,147,150), though these later studies did not study the outcome in a granular fashion. Prophylaxis with ramelteon, a melatonin agonist, resulted in reduced delirium in an elderly patient population admitted to ICUs in Japan (185,186). Of note, the majority of patients in this study were not intubated and the APACHE II mean score was 14 to 15. Statin use has been associated with decreased rates of postoperative delirium in cardiac surgery patients and mixed medical/surgical ICU patients (187,188).

Similar to the use of rivastigmine to treat ICU delirium, there is no role for rivastigmine as a prophylactic agent to prevent ICU delirium (189). Cardiac surgery patients who received a single dose of ketamine as part of their induction anesthesia had a statistically significant reduction in postoperative delirium, 3% versus 31%, $p = 0.01$ (190). At the present time, there is no recommendation for the routine use of pharmacologic ICU delirium prophylaxis (73,119). Further research is required to study pharmacologic ICU delirium prophylaxis before it can be recommended for routine use.

Early mobilization and ICU sleep hygiene protocols have both been shown to prevent ICU delirium (119,170–174). Both approaches have been shown to be safe when used in properly selected patients, can be easily and safely implemented, and should be a routine part of daily ICU care (180).

CONTROVERSIES

One controversy in ICU delirium is whether it is the choice of pharmacologic agent used for ICU sedation, when sedation is needed, versus the manner in which the drug is administered and titrated, which places a patient at risk for delirium (8,14–17,20,36,101,125–128,191–195). There is a body of literature that suggests delirium may be related mostly to the depth and duration of sedation, and not necessarily the agent(s) used (17,112,119,157,160,192,195). Research continues on the relationship between sedation depth, drugs used, and both short- and long-term neurocognitive deficits including delirium.

A second controversy is whether there are different subtypes of delirium along a delirium spectrum, and whether these subtypes portend different outcomes or may warrant different approaches to the detection of delirium, prevention, and treatment (5,93,94,169,196–204). The ICDSC can detect patients with subsyndromal delirium by using a score range of 1 to 3. Using this score range, Ouimet (5) demonstrated worse outcomes in mortality and ICU LOS for patients with subsyndromal delirium. Skrobik et al. (169) demonstrated reduced subsyndromal delirium, but no reduction in full-syndrome delirium, when protocolized management of analgesia, sedation, and delirium management was implemented. Patel et al. (93) demonstrated clinically relevant differences in mortality, ventilator-free days, hospital LOS, and discharge home rates in patients with rapidly reversible sedation-related delirium as compared to patients with persistent ICU delirium. To date, few studies of postanesthesia emergence delirium have been conducted in adults (200–204). Additional research on the significance of postanesthesia emergence delirium, rapidly reversible sedation-related delirium, subsyndromal delirium, and persistent ICU delirium will be required to further understand these subtypes of delirium and their implications for detection, prevention, treatment, and outcomes.

Key Points

- ICU delirium is an acute CNS disease that represents acute brain dysfunction and should be treated with the same sense of urgency as we do any other acute, life-threatening organ system dysfunctions. For example, delirium may be due to under-resuscitation and brain perfusion issues, or due to undiagnosed sepsis and its attendant systemic inflammatory and thrombophilic abnormalities, or to errant receipt of psychoactive medications, all of which should prompt acute response by clinicians to diagnose and intervene.
- Patients should be assessed for ICU delirium risk at the time of ICU admission and an appropriate care plan for risk reduction, most of which is covered within the concepts of the ABCDEF bundle, derived from over 150 references and now being used to implement the SCCM's PAD guidelines, should be implemented. For further details, see the ICU Liberation Collaborative, www.iculiberation.org.
- Daily screening of all ICU patients for the presence of delirium using a valid and reliable delirium assessment tool should be performed.
- The treatment of ICU delirium requires a diligent, methodical clinical assessment for the treatable/reversible causes of delirium with the expectation that multiple factors contributing to delirium will be present in any single delirious patient.
- Given the multiple risk factors present in any patient, and the diversity of risk factor variation from patient to patient, the treatment plan for ICU delirium must be individualized for each patient and will vary over the clinical course and evolution of delirium for each patient.
- Nonpharmacologic approaches should be the mainstay and first-line management for delirium in the critically ill, including early mobility and sleep hygiene bundles which have been proven safe and effective in preventing ICU delirium, and should be part of the standard care of ICU patients.
- There is currently no consensus as to the best pharmacologic agent to prevent or treat the symptoms of acute ICU delirium, but the SCCM's PAD guidelines found that quetiapine and dexmedetomidine appear to be safe and may be effective when used to treat ICU delirium. More data on both these drugs are on the horizon.

ACKNOWLEDGMENTS

Dr. Ely has received honoraria for CME activity sponsored by Abbott, Hospira, Orion, and Pfizer. He has NIH and VA funding for ongoing research studies. The authors would like to thank Margaret Pan, Annachiara Marra, MD, and Kwame Frimpong, MD, for their review of, and editorial assistance with, the manuscript. In addition, we would like to thank the staff at the Geisinger Health Sciences Library for their assistance in the literature search for this chapter.

References

1. Poon DC, Ho YS, Chiu K, Chang RC. Cytokines: how important are they in mediating sickness? *Neurosci Biobehav Rev.* 2013;37:1–10.
2. Cunningham C, Maclullich AM. At the extreme end of the psychoneuorimmmunological spectrum: delirium as a maladaptive sickness behavior response. *Brain Behav Immun.* 2013;28:1–13.
3. Morandi A, Pandharipande PP, Jackson JC, et al. Understanding terminology of delirium and long-term cognitive impairment in critically ill patients. *Best Prac Res Clin Anaesthesiol.* 2012;26:267–276.
4. Pandharipande P, Jackson J, Ely EW. Delirium: acute cognitive dysfunction in the critically ill. *Curr Opin Crit Care.* 2005;11:360–368.
5. Ouimet S, Riker R, Bergeon N, et al. Subsyndromal delirium in the ICU: evidence for a disease spectrum. *Intensive Care Med.* 2007;33:1007–1013.
6. McNicoll L, Pisani MA, Zhang Y, et al. Delirium in the intensive care unit: occurrence and clinical course in older patients. *J Am Geriatr Soc.* 2003;51:591–598.
7. Lat I, McMillian W, Taylor S, et al. The impact of delirium on clinical outcomes in mechanically ventilated surgical and trauma patients. *Crit Care Med.* 2009;37(6):1898–1905.
8. Pandharipande P, Cotton BA, Shintani A, et al. Prevalence and risk factors for development of delirium in surgical and trauma intensive care unit patients. *J Trauma.* 2008;65:34–41.
9. Ely EW, Inouye SK, Bernard GR, et al. Delirium in mechanically ventilated patients: validity and reliability of the confusion assessment method for the intensive care unit (CAM-ICU). *JAMA.* 2001;286(21):2703–2710.
10. Ely EW, Margolin R, Francis J, et al. Evaluation of delirium in critically ill patients: validation of the confusion assessment method for the intensive care unit (CAM-ICU). *Crit Care Med.* 2001;29(7):1370–1379.
11. Lin SM, Liu CY, Wang CH, et al. The impact of delirium on the survival of mechanically ventilated patients. *Crit Care Med.* 2004;32(11):2254–2259.
12. Mitasova A, Kostalova M, Bednarik J, et al. Poststroke delirium incidence and outcomes: validation of the confusion assessment method for the intensive care unit (CAM-ICU). *Crit Care Med.* 2012;40(2):484–490.
13. Pauley E, Lishmanov A, Schumann S, et al. Delirium is a robust predictor of morbidity and mortality among critically ill patients treated in the cardiac intensive care unit. *Am Heart J.* 2015;170(1):79–86.
14. McPherson JA, Wagner CE, Boehm LM, et al. Delirium in the cardiovascular ICU: exploring modifiable risk factors. *Crit Care Med.* 2013; 41(2):405–413.
15. Kazmierski J, Kowman M, Banach M, et al.; IPDACS Study. Incidence and predictors of delirium after cardiac surgery: results from the IPDACS study. *J Psychosom Res.* 2010;69:179–185.
16. Chang YL, Tsai YF, Lin PJ, et al. Prevalence and risk factors for postoperative delirium in a cardiovascular intensive care unit. *Am J Crit Care.* 2008;17(6):567–575.
17. Ouimet S, Kavanagh BP, Gottfried SB, Skrobik J. Incidence, risk factors and consequences of ICU delirium. *Intensive Care Med.* 2007;33:66–73.
18. Norkiene I, Ringaitiene D, Misiuriene I, et al. Incidence and precipitating factors of delirium after coronary artery bypass grafting. *Scand Cardiovasc J.* 2007;41:180–185.
19. Salluh JI, Wang H, Schneider EB, et al. Outcome of delirium in critically ill patients: systematic review and meta-analysis. *BMJ.* 2015;350:h2538.
20. Mehta S, Cook D, Devlin JW, et al.; SLEAP Investigators; Canadian Critical Care Trials Group. Prevalence, risk factors, and outcomes of delirium in mechanically ventilated adults. *Crit Care Med.* 2015;43(3):557–566.
21. Hsieh SJ, Soto GJ, Hope AA, et al. The association between acute respiratory distress syndrome, delirium, and in-hospital mortality in intensive care unit patients. *Am J Resp Crit Care Med.* 2015;191(1):71–78.
22. Peterson JF, Pun BT, Dittus RS, et al. Delirium and its motoric subtypes: a study of 614 critically ill patients. *J Am Geriatr Soc.* 2006;54:479–484.
23. Ely EW, Shintani A, Truman B, et al. Delirium as a predictor of mortality in mechanically ventilated patients in the intensive care unit. *JAMA.* 2004;291(14):1753–1762.
24. Ely EW, Gautam S, Margolin R, et al. The impact of delirium in the intensive care unit on hospital length of stay. *Intensive Care Med.* 2001;27: 1892–1900.
25. Girard TD, Pandharipande PP, Ely EW. Delirium in the intensive care unit. *Crit Care.* 2008;12(Suppl 3):S3.
26. Saxena S, Lawley D. Delirium in the elderly: a clinical review. *Postgrad Med J.* 2009;85:405–413.
27. Gottesman RF, Grega MA, Bailey MM, et al. Delirium after coronary artery bypass graft surgery and late mortality. *Ann Neurol.* 2010;67:338–344.
28. Pisani MA, Kong SY, Kasl SV, et al. Days of delirium are associated with 1-year mortality in an older intensive care unit population. *Am J Respir Crit Care Med.* 2009;180:1092–1097.
29. Heyman A, Radtke F, Schiemann A, et al. Delayed treatment of delirium increases mortality rate in intensive care unit patients. *J Int Med Res.* 2010; 38:1584–1595.
30. Al-Qadheeb, NS, Balk EM, Fraser GL, et al. Randomized ICU trials do not demonstrate an association between interventions that reduce delirium duration and short-term mortality: a systematic review and meta-analysis. *Crit Care Med.* 2014;42(6):1442–1454.

31. Milbrandt EB, Deppen S, Harrison PL, et al. Costs associated with delirium in mechanically ventilated patients. *Crit Care Med.* 2004;32(4):955–962.
32. Leslie DL, Marcantonio ER, Zhang Y, et al. One-year health care costs associated with delirium in the elderly population. *Arch Intern Med.* 2008;168(1):27–32.
33. Inouye SK. Delirium in older persons. *N Engl J Med.* 2006;354(11): 1157–1165.
34. Jackson JC, Gordon SM, Hart RP, et al. The association between delirium and cognitive decline: a review of the empirical literature. *Neuropsych Rev.* 2004;14(2):87–98.
35. Girard TD, Jackson JC, Pandharipande PP, et al. Delirium as a predictor of long-term cognitive impairment in survivors of critical illness. *Crit Care Med.* 2010;38(7):1513–1520.
36. Pandharipande PP, Girard TD, Jackson JC, et al.; BRAIN-ICU Study Investigators. Long-term cognitive impairment after critical illness. *N Engl J Med.* 2013;369(14):1306–1316.
37. Brummel NE, Jackson JC, Pandharipande PP, et al. Delirium in the ICU and subsequent long-term disability among survivors of mechanical ventilation. *Crit Care Med.* 2013;42(2):369–377.
38. Pisani MA, Murphy TE, Araujo KL, Van Ness PH. Factors associated with persistent delirium after intensive care unit admission in an older medical patient population. *J Crit Care.* 2010;25:540e1–540e7.
39. Dasgupta M, Hillier LM. Factors associated with prolonged delirium: a systematic review. *Int Psychogeriatr.* 2010;22(3):373–394.
40. Jones C, Backman C, Capuzzo M, et al. Precipitants of post-traumatic stress disorder following intensive care: a hypothesis generating study of diversity of care. *Intensive Care Med.* 2007;33:978–985.
41. van den Boogaard M, Schoonhoven L, Evers AW, et al. Delirium in critically ill patients: impact on long-term health-related quality of life and cognitive functioning. *Crit Care Med.* 2012;40(1): 112–118.
42. Brummel NE, Jackson JC, Girard TD, et al. A combined early cognitive and physical rehabilitation program for people who are critically ill: the activity and cognitive therapy in the intensive care unit (ACT-ICU) trial. *Phys Ther.* 2012;92(12):1580–1592.
43. Jackson JC, Ely EW, Morey MC, et al. Cognitive and physical rehabilitation of intensive care unit survivors: results of the RETURN randomized controlled pilot investigation. *Crit Care Med.* 2012;40(4):1088–1097.
44. Jackson JC, Pandharipande PP, Girard TD, et al.; Bringing to light the Risk Factors And Incidence of Neuropsychological dysfunction in ICU survivors (BRAIN-ICU) study investigators. Depression, post-traumatic stress disorder, and functional disability in survivors of critical illness in the BRAIN-ICU study: a longitudinal cohort study. *Lancet Respir Med.* 2014;2;369–379.
45. Brummel NE, Balas MC, Morandi A, et al. Understanding and reducing disability in older adults following critical illness. *Crit Care Med.* 2015;43: 1265–1275.
46. Maldonado JR. Neuropathogenesis of delirium: review of current etiological theories and common pathways. *Am J Geriatr Psychiatry.* 2013;2(12): 1190–1222.
47. Maldonado JR. Pathoetiological model of delirium: a comprehensive understanding of the neurobiology of delirium and an evidence-based approach to prevention and treatment. *Crit Care Clin.* 2008;24: 789–856.
48. Gunther ML, Morandi A, Ely EW. Pathophysiology of delirium in the intensive care unit. *Crit Care Clin.* 2008;24:45–65.
49. Steiner LA. Postoperative delirium. Part 1: pathophysiology and risk factors. Eur J Anaesthesiol. 2011;28:628–636.
50. MacLullich AM, Ferguson KJ, Miller T, et al. Unravelling the pathophysiology of delirium: a focus o the role of aberrant stress responses. *J Psychosoma Res.* 2008;65(3):229–238.
51. Cerejeira J, Firmino H, Vaz-Serra A, Mukaetova-Ladinska EB. The neuroinflammatory hypothesis of delirium. *Acta Neuropathol.* 2010;119:737–754.
52. Simone MJ, Tan ZS. The role of inflammation in the pathogenesis of delirium and dementia in older adults: a review. *CNS Neurosci Ther.* 2011:17:506–513.
53. Zampieri FG, Park M, Machado FS, Azevedo LC. Sepsis-associated encephalopathy: not just delirium. *Clinics (Sao Paulo).* 2011;66(10):1825–1831.
54. Ely EW, Girard TD, Shintani AK, et al. Apolipoprotein E4 polymorphism as a genetic predisposition to delirium in critically ill patients. *Crit Care Med.* 2007;35(1):112–117.
55. van Munster BC, de Rooij SE, Korevaar JC. The role of genetics in delirium in the elderly patient. *Dement Geriatr Cogn Disord.* 2009;28:187–195.
56. Hshieh TT, Fong TG, Marcatonio ER, Inouye SK. Cholinergic deficiency hypothesis in delirium: a synthesis of current evidence. *J GerontolA Biol Sci Med Sci.* 2008;63(7):764–772.
57. Gaudreau JD, Gagnon P. Psychotropic drugs and delirium pathogenesis: the central role of the thalamus. *Med Hypotheses.* 2005;64:471–475.
58. Gonzalez-Lopez A, Lopez-Alonso I, Aguirre A, et al. Mechanical ventilation triggers hippocampal apoptosis by vagal and dopaminergic pathways. *Am J Respir Crit are Med.* 2013;188(6):693–702.
59. Adams Wilson JR, Morandi A, Girard TD, et al. The association of the kynurenine pathway of tryptophan metabolism with acute brain dysfunction during critical illness. *Crit Care Med.* 2012;40(3):835–841.
60. Devlin JW, Skrobik Y. The kynurenine pathway: a metabolinomic pathway for intensive care unit delirium? *Crit Care Med.* 2012;40(3):1001–1002.
61. Sanford AM, Flaherty JH. Do nutrients play a role in delirium? *Curr Opin Clin Nutr Metab Care.* 2014;17:45–50.
62. Mu D, Wang DX, Li LH, et al. High serum cortisol level is associated with increased risk of delirium after coronary artery bypass graft surgery: a prospective cohort study. *Crit Care.* 2010;14:R238.
63. Schreiber MP, Colantuoni E, Bienvenu OJ, et al. Corticosteroids and transition to delirium in patients with acute lung injury. *Crit Care Med.* 2014;42(6):1480–1486.
64. Fitzgerald JM, Adamis D, Trzepacz PT, et al. Delirium: a disturbance of circadian integrity? *Med Hypotheses.* 2013;81:568–576.
65. Weinhouse GL, Schwab RJ, Watson PL, et al. Bench-to-bedside review: delirium in ICU patients–importance of sleep deprivation. *Crit Care.* 2009;13:234.
66. Figueroa-Ramos MI, Arroyo-Novoa CM, Lee KA, et al. Sleep and delirium in ICU patients: a review of mechanisms and manifestations. *Intensive Care Med.* 2009;35:781–795.
67. Drouot X, Cabello B, d'Ortho MP, Brochard L. Sleep in the intensive care unit. *Sleep Med Rev.* 2008;12:391–403.
68. Kamdar BB, Needham DM, Collop NA. Sleep deprivation in critical illness: its role in physical and psychological recovery. *J Intensive Care Med.* 2012; 27(2):97–111.
69. Mirrakhimov AE, Brewbaker CL, Krystal AD, Kwatra MM. Obstructive sleep apnea and delirium: exploring possible mechanisms. *Sleep Breath.* 2014;18:19–29.
70. de Rooij SE, van Munster BC. Melatonin deficiency hypotheses in delirium: a synthesis of current evidence. *Rejuv Res.* 2013;16(4):273–278.
71. van Eijk MM, van Marum RJ, Klijn IA, et al. Comparison of delirium assessment tools in a mixed intensive care unit. *Crit Care Med.* 2009;37(6): 1881–1885.
72. Guenther U, Weykam J, Andorfer U, et al. Implications of objective vs subjective delirium assessment in surgical intensive care patients. *Am J Crit Care.* 2012;21(1):e12–e20.
73. Barr J, Graser GL, Puntillo K, et al.; American College of Critical Care Medicine. Clinical practice guidelines for the management of pain, agitation, and delirium in adult patients in the intensive care unit. *Crit Care Med.* 2013;41(1):263–306.
74. Bergeron N, Dubois MJ, Dumont M, et al. Intensive care delirium screening checklist: evaluation of a new screening tool. *Intensive Care Med.* 2001;27:859–864.
75. Devlin JW, Fong JJ, Fraser GL, Riker RR. Delirium assessment in the critically ill. *Intensive Care Med.* 2007;33:929–940.
76. Luetz A, Heymnn A, Radtke FM, et al. Different assessment tools for intensive care unit delirium: which score to use? *Crit Care Med.* 2010;38(2):409–418.
77. Matarese M, Generoso S, Ivziku D, et al. Delirium in older patients: a diagnostic study of NEECHAM Confusion Scale in surgical intensive care unit. *J Clin Nurs.* 2012;22:2849–2857.
78. Yu A, Teitelbaum J, Scott J, et al. Evaluating pain, sedation, and delirium in the neurologically critically ill–feasibility and reliability of standardized tools: a multi-institutional study. *Crit Care Med.* 2013;41(8):2002–2007.
79. Gusmao-Flores D, Salluh JI, Chalhub RA, Quarantini LC. The confusion assessment method for the intensive care unit (CAM-ICU) and intensive care delirium screening checklist (ICDSC) for the diagnosis of delirium: a systematic review and meta-analysis of the literature. *Crit Care.* 2012;16:R115.
80. Hipp D, Ely EW. Pharmacological and nonpharmacological management of delirium in critically ill patients. *Neurotherapeutics.* 2012;9:158–175.
81. van Eijk MM, van der Boogarrd M, van Marum RJ, et al. Routine use of the Confusion Assessment Method for the intensive care unit: a multicenter study. *Am J Respir Crit Care Med.* 2011;184:340–344.
82. Reade MC, Eastwood GM, Peck L, et al. Routine use of the confusion assessment method for the intensive care unit (CAM-ICU) by bedside nurses may underdiagnose delirium. *Crit Care Resusc.* 2011;13:217–224.
83. Patel SB, Kress JP. Accurate identification of delirium in the ICU. *Am J Respir Crit Care Med.* 2011;184:287–288.
84. Vasilevskis EE, Girard TD, Ely EW. The bedside diagnosis of ICU delirium: specificity is high, let's optimize sensitivity. *Am J Respir Crit Care Med.* 2012;185:107–108.

85. van Eijk MM, Slooter AJ. From the authors. *Am J Respir Crit Care Med.* 2012;185:108.
86. Neufeld KJ, Hayat MJ, Coughlin JM, et al. Evaluation of two intensive care delirium screening tools for non-critically ill hospitalized patients. *Psychosomatics.* 2011;52(2):133–140.
87. Neufeld KJ, Leoutsakos JS, Sieber FE, et al. Evaluation of two delirium screening tools for detecting post-operative delirium in the elderly. *Br J Anesth.* 2013;111(4):612–618.
88. Morandi A, McCurley J, Vasilevskis EE, et al. Tools to detect delirium superimposed on dementia: a systematic review. *J Am Geriatr Soc.* 2012; 60:2005–2013.
89. Pisani MA. Delirium assessment in the intensive care unit: patient population matters. *Crit Care.* 2008;12:131.
90. Pun BT, Devlin JW. Delirium monitoring in the ICU: Strategies for initiating and sustaining screening efforts. *Semin Respir Crit Care Med.* 2013;34: 179–188.
91. Can delirium Assessments Be Accurately Labelled (CABAL) Investigators group, Devlin JW, Fraser GL, et al. The accurate recognition of delirium in the ICU: the emperor's new clothes? *Intensive Care Med.* 2013;39:2196–2199.
92. Haenggi M, Blum S, Brechbuehl R, et al. Effect of sedation level on the prevalence of delirium when assessed with the CAM-ICU and ICDSC. *Intensive Care Med.* 2013;39:2171–2179.
93. Brummel NE, Ely EW. Sedation level and the prevalence of delirium. *Intensive Care Med.* 2014;40:135.
94. Patel SB, Poston JT, Pohlman A, et al. Rapidly reversible, sedation-related delirium versus persistent delirium in the intensive care unit. *Am J Respir Crit Care Med.* 189(6):658–665.
95. Takala J. Of delirium and sedation. *Am J Respir Crit Care Med.* 2014;189(6): 622–624.
96. Marcantonio ER, Rudolph JL, Culley D, et al. Serum Biomarkers for Delirium. *J Gerontol A Biol Sci Med Sci.* 2006;61(12):1281–1286.
97. van Munster BC, Korevaar JC, Zwinderman AH, et al. Time-course of cytokines during delirium in elderly patients with hip fractures. *J Am Geriatr Soc.* 2008;56:1704–1709.
98. Hall RJ, Shenkin SD, MacLullich AM. A systematic literature review of cerebrospinal fluid biomarkers in delirium. *Dement Geriatr Cogn Disord.* 2011;32:79–93.
99. McGrane S, Girard TD, Thompson JL, et al. Procalcitonin and C-reactive protein levels at admission as predictors of duration of acute brain dysfunction in critically ill patients. *Crit Care.* 2011;15:R78.
100. Girard TD, Ware LB, Bernard GR, et al. Associations of markers of inflammation and coagulation with delirium during critical illness. *Intensive Care Med.* 2012;38:1965–1973.
101. Skrobik Y, Leger C, Cossette M, et al. Factors predisposing to coma and delirium: fentanyl and midazolam exposure; CYP3A5, ABCB1, and ABCG2 genetic polymorphisms; and inflammatory factors. *Crit Care Med.* 2013;41:999–1008.
102. Alsop DC, Fearing MA, Johnson K, et al. The role of neuroimaging in elucidating delirium pathophysiology. *J GerontolA Biol Sci Med Sci.* 2006;61(12):1287–1293.
103. Morandi A, Rogers BP, Gunther ML, et al. The relationship between delirium duration, white matter integrity, and cognitive impairment in intensive care unit survivors as determined by diffusion tensor imaging: the VISIONS prospective cohort magnetic imaging study. *Crit Care Med.* 2012;40(7):2182–2189.
104. Gunther ML, Morandi A, Krauskopf E, et al. The association between brain volumes, delirium duration, and cognitive outcomes in intensive care unit survivors: the VISIONS cohort magnetic resonance imaging study. *Crit Care Med.* 2012;40(7):2022–2032.
105. Jackson JC, Morandi A, Girard TD, et al. Functional brain imaging in survivors of critical illness: a prospective feasibility study and exploration of the association between delirium and brain activation patterns. *J Crit Care.* 2015;30:653e1–653e7.
106. Plaschke K, Hill H, Engelhardt R, et al. EEG changes and serum anticholinergic activity measured in patients with delirium in the intensive care unit. *Anesthesia.* 2007;62:1217–1223.
107. Thomas C, Hestermann U, Walther S, et al. Prolonged activation EEG differentiates dementia with and without delirium in frail elderly patients. *J Neurol Neurosurg Psychiatry.* 2008;79:119–125.
108. Plaschke K, Fichtenkamm P, Shcramm C, et al. Early postoperative delirium after open-heart cardiac surgery is associated with decreased bispectral EEG and increased cortisol and interleukin-6. *Intensive Care Med.* 2010;36:2081–2089.
109. van der Kooi AW, Leijten FS, van der Wekken RJ, Slooter AJ. What are the opportunities for EEG-based monitoring of delirium in the ICU? *J Neuropsychiatry Clin Neurosci.* 2012;24(4):472–477.
110. Semmler A, Widmann CN, Okulla T, et al. Persistent cognitive impairment, hippocampal atrophy and EEG changes in sepsis survivors. *J Neurol Neurosurg Psychiatry.* 2013;84:62–70.
111. Andresen JM, Girard TD, Pandharipande PP, et al. Burst suppression on processed electroencephalography as a predictor of postcoma delirium in mechanically ventilated ICU patients. *Crit Care Med.* 2014;42(10): 2244–2251.
112. Hughes CG, Pandharipande PP. Review articles: the effects of perioperative and intensive care unit sedation on brain organ dysfunction. *Anesth Analg.* 2011;112:1212–1217.
113. Allen J, Alexander E. Prevention, recognition, and management of delirium in the intensive care unit. *AACN Advanced Critical Care.* 2012;23(1):5–11.
114. Maclullich AM, Anand A, Davis DH, et al. New horizons in the pathogenesis, assessment and management of delirium. *Age Ageing.* 2013;42:667–674.
115. Hsieh SJ, Ely EW, Gong MN. Can intensive care unit delirium be prevented and reduced? *Ann Am Thorac Soc.* 2013;10(6):648–656.
116. Hsieh SJ, Shum M, Lee AN, et al. Cigarette smoking as a risk factor for delirium in hospitalized and intensive care unit patients. A systematic review. *Ann Am Thorac Soc.* 2013;10(5):496–503.
117. Meagher D, Moran M, Raju B, et al. A new data-based motor subtype schema for delirium. *J Neuropsychiatry Clin Neurosci.* 2008 Spring;20(2): 185–193.
118. Meagher D. Motor subtypes of delirium: past, present and future. *Intensive Rev Psych.* 2009;21(1):59–73.
119. Devlin JW, Fraser GL, Ely EW, et al. Pharmacologic management of sedation and delirium in mechanically ventilated ICU patients: remaining evidence gaps and controversies. *Semin Respir Crit Care Med.* 2013;34: 201–215.
120. King MS, Render ML, Ely EW, Watson PL. Liberation and animation: strategies to minimize brain dysfunction in critically ill patients. *Semin Respir Crit Care Med.* 2010;31:87–96.
121. Devlin JW, Al-Qadhee NS, Skrobik Y. Pharmacologic prevention and treatment of delirium in critically ill and non-critically ill hospitalized patients: a review of data from prospective, randomized studies. *Best Prac & Res Clin Anaesth.* 2012;26:289–309.
122. Bledowski J, Trutia A. A review of pharmacologic management and prevention strategies for delirium in the intensive care unit. *Psychosomatics.* 2012;53:203–211.
123. Reade MC, Finfer S. Sedation and delirium in the intensive care unit. *NEJM.* 2014;370(5):444–454.
124. Mu JL, Lee A, Joynt GM. Pharmacologic agents for the prevention and treatment of delirium in patients undergoing cardiac surgery: systematic review and meta-analysis. *Crit Care Med.* 2015;43(1):194–204.
125. Pandharipande P, Shintani A, Peterson J, et al. Lorazepam is an independent risk factor for transitioning to delirium in intensive care unit patients. *Anesthesiology.* 2006;104:21–26.
126. Pandharipande PP, Pun BT, Herr DL, et al. Effect of sedation with dexmedetomidine v lorazepam on acute brain dysfunction in mechanically ventilated patients. *JAMA.* 2007;298(22):2644–2653.
127. Riker RR, Shehabi Y, Boikesch PM, et al.; SEDCOM (Safety and Efficacy of Dexmedetomidine Compared With Midazolam) Study Group. Dexmedetomidine vs midazolam for sedation of critically ill patients. *JAMA.* 2009;301(5):489–499.
128. Seymour CW, Pandharipande PP, Koestner T, et al. Diurnal sedative changes during intensive care: impact on liberation from mechanical ventilation and delirium. *Crit Care Med.* 2012;40(10):2788–2796.
129. Brown KE, Mirrakhimov, AE, Yeddula K, Kwatra MM. Propofol and the risk of delirium: exploring the anticholinergic properties of propofol. *Med Hypotheses.* 2013; 81:536–539.
130. Ruokonen E, Parviainen I, Jakob SM, et al.; "Dexmedetomidine for Continuous Sedation" Investigators. Dexmedetomidine versus propofol/midazolam for long-term sedation during mechanical ventilation. *Intensive Care Med.* 2009;35:282–290.
131. Flannery AH, Flynn JD. More questions than answers in ICU delirium: pressing issues for future research. *Ann Pharmacother.* 2013;47(11): 1558–1561.
132. Awissi D, Lebrun G, Fagnan M, et al. Alcohol, nicotine, and iatrogenic withdrawals in the ICU. *Crit Care Med.* 2013;41(9 Suppl 1):S57–S68.
133. Skrobik YK, Bergeron M, Dumont M, Gottfried SB. Olanzapine vs haloperidol: treating delirium in a critical care setting. *Intensive Care Med.* 2004;30:444–449.
134. Sockalingam S, Parekh N, Bogoch II, et al. Delirium in the postoperative cardiac patient: a review. *J Card Surg.* 2005;20:560–567.
135. Alici-Evcimen Y, Breitbart W. An update on the use of antipsychotics in the treatment of delirium. *Palliat Support Care.* 2008;6:177–182.

136. Devlin JW, Roberts RJ, Fong JJ, et al. Efficacy and safety of quetiapine in critically ill patients with delirum: a prospective, multicenter, randomized, double-blind, placebo-controlled pilot study. *Crit Care Med.* 2010;38(2):419–427.
137. Girard TD, Pandharipande PP, Carson SS, et al.; MIND Trial Investigators. Feasibility, efficacy, and safety of antipsychotics for intensive care unit delirium: the MIND randomized, placebo-controlled trial. *Crit Care Med.* 2010;38(2):428–437.
138. Page VJ, Ely EW, Gates S, et al. Effect of intravenous haloperidol on the duration of delirium and coma in critically ill patients (Hope-ICU): a randomized, double-blind, placebo-controlled trial. *Lancet Respir Med.* 2013;1:515–523.
139. Michaud CJ, Bullard HM, Harris SA, Thomas WL. Impact of quetiapine treatment on duration of hypoactive delirium in critically ill adults: a retrospective analysis. *Pharmacotherapy.* 2015;35(8):731–739.
140. Wang PS, Schneeweiss S, Avorn J, et al. Risk of death in elderly users of conventional vs. atypical antipsychotic medications. *N Engl J Med.* 2005;353(22):2335–2341.
141. Schneider L, Dagerman KS, Insel P. Risk of death with atypical antipsychotic drug treatment for dementia. *JAMA.* 2005;294(15):1934–1943.
142. Hwang YJ, Dixon SN, Reiss JP, et al. Atypical antipsychotic drugs and the risk for acute kidney injury and other adverse outcomes in older adults. *Ann Intern Med.* 2014;161:242–248.
143. Jasiak KD, Middleton EA, Camamo JM, et al. Evaluation of discontinuation of atypical antipsychotics prescribed for ICU delirium. *J Pharm Pract.* 2012;26(3):253–256.
144. Siobal MS Kallet RH, Kivett VA, Tang JF. Use of dexmedetomidine to facilitate extubation in surgical intensive-care-unit patients who failed previous weaning attempts following prolonged mechanical ventilation: a pilot study. *Resp Care.* 2006;51(5);492–496.
145. Shehabi Y, Grant P, Wolfende H, et al. Prevalence of delirium with dexmedetomidine compared with morphine based therapy after cardiac surgery. *Anesthesiology.* 2009;111(5):1075–1084.
146. Maldonado JR, Wysong A, van der Starre PJ, et al. Dexmedetomidine and the reduction of postoperative delirium after cardiac surgery. *Psychosomatics.* 2009;50(3):206–217.
147. Reade MC, O'Sullivan K, Bates S, et al. Dexmedetomidine vs. haloperidol in delirious, agitated, intubated patients: a randomized open-label trial. *Crit Care.* 2009;13:R75.
148. Tan JA, Ho KM. Use of dexmedetomidine as a sedative and analgesic agent in critically ill adult patients: a meta-analysis. *Intensive Care Med.* 2010;36:926–939.
149. Yapici N, Coruh T, Kahlibar T, et al. Dexmedetomidine in cardiac surgery patients who fail extubation and present with a delirium state. *Heart Surg Forum.* 2011;E93–E98.
150. Jakob SM, Ruokonen E, Grouns RM, et al.; Dexmedetomidine for Long-Term Sedation Investigators. Dexmedetomidine vs midazolam or propofol for sedation during prolonged mechanical ventilation. *JAMA.* 2012;307(11): 1151–1160.
151. Mo Y, Zimmerman AE. Role of dexmedetomidine for the prevention and treatment of delirium in intensive care unit patients. *Ann Pharm.* 2013 47:869–876.
152. Ji F, Li Z, Nguyen H, et al. Perioperative dexmedetomidine improves outcomes of cardiac surgery. *Circulation.* 2013;127:1576–1584.
153. Pandharipande P. The MENDS II study, maximizing the efficacy of sedation and reducing neurological dysfunction and mortality in septic patients with respiratory failure. Available: https://www.clinicaltrials.gov/ct2/show/NCT01739933.
154. van Eijk MM, Roes KC, Honing ML, et al. Effect of rivastigimine as an adjunct to usual care with haloperidol on duration of delirium and mortality in critically ill patients: a multicenter, double-blind, placebo-controlled randomized trial. *Lancet.* 2010;376:1829–1837.
155. Hager DN, Dinglas VD, Subhas S, et al. Reducing deep sedation and delirium in acute lung injury patients: a quality improvement project. *Crit Care Med.* 2013;41:1435–1442.
156. Pandharipande P, Banerjee A, McGrane S, Ely EW. Liberation and animation for ventilated ICU patients: the ABCDE bundle for the back-end of critical care. *Crit Care.* 2010;14:157. Available: http://ccforum.com/content/14/3/157.
157. Samuelson KA, Lundberg D, Fridlund B. Light vs. heavy sedation during mechanical ventilation after oesophagectomy—a pilot experimental study focusing on memory. *Acta Anaesthesiol Scand.* 2008;52:1116–1123.
158. Girard TD, Kress JP, Fuchs BD, et al. Efficacy and safety of a paired sedation and ventilator weaning protocol for mechanically ventilated patients in intensive care (awakening and breathing controlled trial): a randomized controlled trial. *Lancet.* 2008;371:126–134.
159. de Wit M, Gennings C, Jenvey WI, Epstein SK. Randomized trial comparing daily interruption of sedation and nursing-implemented sedation algorithm in medical intensive care unit patients. *Crit Care.* 2008; 12:R70.
160. Treggiari MM, Romand J, Yanez ND, et al. Randomized trial of light versus deep sedation on mental health after critical illness. *Crit Care Med.* 2009;37(9):2527–2534.
161. Strom T, Martinussen T, Toft P. A protocol of no sedation for critically ill patients receiving mechanical ventilation: a randomised trial. *Lancet.* 2010;375:475–480.
162. Mirski MA, Lewin JJ, LeDroux S, et al. Cognitive improvement during continuous sedation in critically ill, awake and responsive patients: the Acute Neurological ICU Sedation Trial (ANIST). *Intensive Care Med.* 2010;36:1505–1513.
163. Awissi DK, Begin C, Moisan J, et al. I-SAVE Study: impact of sedation, analgesia, and delirium protocols evaluated in the intensive care unit: an economic evaluation. *Ann Pharmacother.* 2012;46:21–28.
164. Shehabi Y, Bellomo R, Reade MC, et al.; Sedation Practice in Intensive Care Evaluation (SPICE) Study Investigators; ANZICS Clinical Trials Group. Early intensive care sedation predicts long-term mortality in ventilated critically ill patients. *Am J Respir Crit Care Med.* 2012;186(8): 724–731.
165. Mehta S, Burry L, Cook D, et al.; Canadian Critical Care Trials Group. Daily sedation interruption in mechanically ventilated critically ill patients cared for with a sedation protocol: a randomized controlled trial. *JAMA.* 2012;308(19):1985–1992.
166. Shehabi Y, Bellomo R, Reade MC, et al.; Sedation Practice in Intensive Care Evaluation Study Investigators; Australian and New Zealand Intensive Care Society Clinical Trials Group. Early goal-directed sedation versus standard sedation in mechanically ventilated critically ill patients: a pilot study. *Crit Care Med.* 2013;41:1983–1991.
167. Balas MC, Vasilevskis EE, Olsen KM, et al. Effectiveness and safety of the awakening and breathing coordination, delirium monitoring/management, and early exercise/mobility bundle. *Crit Care Med.* 2014;42:1024–1036.
168. Khan BA, Fadel WF, Tricker JL, et al. Effectiveness of implementing a wake up and breathe program on sedation and delirium in the ICU. *Crit Care Med.* 2014;42:e791–e795.
169. Skrobik Y, Ahern S, Leblanc M, et al. Protocolized intensive care unit management of analgesia, sedation, and delirium improves analgesia and subsyndromal delirium rates. *Anesth Analg.* 2010;111:451–463.
170. Schweickert WD, Pohlman MC, Pohlman AS, et al. Early physical and occupational therapy in mechanically ventilated, critically ill patients: a randomized controlled trial. *Lancet.* 2009;373:1874–1882.
171. Needham DM, Korupolu R, Zanni JM, et al. Early physical medicine and rehabilitation for patients with acute respiratory failure: a quality improvement project. *Arch Phys Med Rehabil.* 2010;91:536–542.
172. Banerjee A, Girard TD, Pandharipande P. The complex interplay between delirium, sedation, and early mobility during critical illness: applications in the trauma unit. *Curr Opin Anesthesiol.* 2011;24: 195–201.
173. Kamdar BB, King LM, Collop NA, et al. The effect of a quality improvement intervention on perceived sleep quality and cognition in a medical ICU. *Crit Care Med.* 2013;41(3):800–809.
174. Patel J, Baldwin J, Bunting P, Laha S. The effect of a multicomponent multidisciplinary bundle of interventions on slep and delirium in medical and surgical intensive care patients. *Anaesthesia.* 2014;69:540–549.
175. Vasilevskis EE, Pandharipande PP, Girard TD, Ely EW. A screening, prevention, and restoration model for saving the injured brain in intensive care unit survivors. *Crit Care Med.* 2010;38(Suppl):S683–S691.
176. Martinez F, Tobar C, Hill N. Preventing delirium: should non-pharmacologcal, multicomponent interventions be used? A systematic review and meta-analysis of the literature. *Age and Ageing.* 2015;44:196–204.
177. van den Boogaard M, Pickkers P, Slooter AJ, et al. Development and validation of PRE-DELIRIC (PREdiction of DELIRium in ICu patients) delirium prediction model for intensive care patients: observational multicentre study. *BMJ.* 2012;344:e420.
178. Jackson JC, Santoro MJ, Ely TM, et al. Improving patient care through the prism of psychology: application of Maslow's hierarchy to sedation, delirium, and early mobility in the intensive care unit. *J Crit Care.* 2014;29:438–444.
179. Bassett R, Adams KM, Danesh V, et al. Rethinking critical care: decreasing sedation, increasing delirium monitoring, and increasing patient mobility. *Jt Comm J Qual Patient Saf.* 2015;41(2):62–74.
180. Riovsecchi RM, Smithburger PL, Svec S, et al. Nonpharmacological interventions to prevent delirium: an evidence-based systematic review. *Crit Care Nurse.* 2015;35(1):39–49.
181. Melville NA. Establishing familiar routines in ICU reduces delirium. *Medscape.* 2015.

182. Prakanrattana U, Prapaitrakool S. Efficacy of risperidone for prevention of postoperative delirium in cardiac surgery. *Anaesth Intensive Care.* 2007; 35:714–719.
183. Wang W, Li HL, Wang DX, et al. Haloperidol prophylaxis decreases delirium incidence in elderly patients after noncardiac surgery: a randomized controlled trial. *Crit Care Med.* 2012;40(3):731–739.
184. van den Boogaard M, Schoonhoven L, van Achterberg T, et al. Haloperidol prophylaxis in critically ill patients with a high risk for delirium. *Crit Care.* 2013;17:R9. Available: http://ccforum.com/content/17/1/R9.
185. Hatta K, Kishi Y, Wada K, et al. Preventive effects of ramelteon on delirium a randomized placebo-controlled trial. *JAMA Psychiatry.* 2014;71(4):397–403.
186. de Rooij SE, van Munster BC, de Jonghe A. Melatonin prophylaxis in delirium panacea or paradigm shift? *JAMA Psychiatry.* 2014;71(4):364–365.
187. Katznelson R, Djaiani GN, Borger MA, et al. Preoperative use of statins is associated with reduced early delirium rates after cardiac surgery. *Anesthesiology.* 2009;110(1):67–73.
188. Page VJ, Davis D, Zhao XB, et al. Statin use and risk of delirium in the critically ill. *Am J Respir Crit Care Med.* 2014;189(6):666–673.
189. Gamberini M, Bolliger D, Lurati Buse GA, et al. Rivastigmine for the prevention of postoperative delirium in elderly patients undergoing elective cardiac surgery—a randomized controlled trial. *Crit Care Med.* 2009;37(5):1762–1768.
190. Hudetz JA, Patterson KM, Iqbal Z, et al. Ketamine attenuates delirium after cardiac surgery with cardiopulmonary bypass. *J Cardiothor Vasc Anesth.* 2009;23(5):651–657.
191. Ely EW, Dittus RS, Girard TD. Point: should benzodiazepines be avoided in mechanically ventilated patients? Yes. *Chest.* 2012;142(2):281–284; discussion 289–290.
192. Skrobik Y. Counterpoint: should benzodiazepines be avoided in mechanically ventilated patients? No. *Chest.* 2012;142(2):284–287; discussion 287–289.
193. Ely WE, Dittus RS, Girard TD. Rebuttal from Dr. Ely et al. *Chest.* 2012; 142(2):287–289.
194. Skrobik Y. Rebuttal from Dr. Skrobik. *Chest.* 2012;142(2):289–290.
195. Fraser GL, Riker RR. Comfort without coma: changing sedation practices. *Crit Care Med.* 2007;35(2):635–637.
196. Ely EW. Our enlightened understanding of the risks of persistent delirium. *Am J Respir Crit Care Med.* 2014;189(11):1442–1443.
197. Pandharipande PP, Girard TD. Only a small subset of sedation-related delirium is innocuous: we cannot let our guard down. *Am J Respir Crit Care Med.* 2014;189(11):1443–1444.
198. Takala J. Reply: is the glass of delirium half full or half empty? *Am J Respir Crit Care Med.* 2014;189(11):1444.
199. Kress JP. Patel SB, Hall JB. Reply: the importance of determining the reason for intensive care unit delirium. *Am J Respir Crit Care Med.* 2014;189(11):1444–1445.
200. Lepousse C, Lautner CA, Liu L, et al. Emergence delirium in adults in the post-anaesthesia care unit. *Br J Anaesth.* 2006;96(6):747–753.
201. Radtk FM, Franck M, Hagemann L, et al. Risk factors for inadequate emergence after anesthesia: emergence delirium and hypoactive emergence. *Minerva Anestesiol.* 2010;76(6):394–404.
202. Bilotta F, Doronzio A, Stazi E, et al. Postoperative cognitive dysfunction: toward the Alzheimer's disease pathomechanism hypothesis. *J Alzheimers Dis.* 2010;22:S81–S89.
203. Bilotta F, Doronzio A, Stazi E, et al. Early postoperative cognitive dysfunction and postoperative delirium after anaesthesia with various hypnotics: study protocol for a randomized controlled trial–the PINOCCHIO trial. *Trials.* 2011;12:170.
204. Card E, Pandharipande P, Tomes C, et al. Emergence from general anaesthesia and evolution of delirium signs in the post-anaesthesia care unit. *Br J Anaesth.* 2015;411–417.

CHAPTER

124

Central Nervous System Vascular Disease

GANESH ASAITHAMBI, BRIAN L. HOH, and MICHAEL F. WATERS

INTRODUCTION

Strokes may be ischemic, resulting from the occlusion of small or large arteries, or hemorrhagic, resulting from the rupture of a conducting artery or an intraparenchymal arteriole. An abrupt focal lateralizing neurologic deficit attributable to a cerebrovascular distribution is the hallmark of ischemic stroke. A depressed level of consciousness is rarely the presenting symptom of ischemic stroke and much more commonly occurs in the setting of a hemorrhagic event. Patients with acute ischemic stroke may be candidates for thrombolytic therapy, but the therapeutic window is extremely narrow, so timely diagnosis and evaluation is of the utmost importance.

DIFFERENTIAL DIAGNOSIS

Most patients who suddenly develop a lateralized focal neurologic problem have, in fact, had a stroke. It is by far the most common acute, focal, nontraumatic brain disease. When the presentation differs from this definition, further investigation and supportive evidence should be sought before establishing the diagnosis. As shown in Table 124.1, there are many stroke symptoms that may occur alone, unaccompanied by other evidence of neurologic damage, that are not an expression of vascular disease. Most of the errors in the diagnosis of stroke occur in patients with altered mental status. Beware of attributing such nonfocal symptoms to strokes without corroborating historic or diagnostic evidence.

Table 124.2 lists the diseases most commonly mistaken for stroke. Epilepsy mimics stroke more often than any other condition. In one study of 821 consecutive patients admitted to a stroke unit, only 13% had a disease other than stroke, but almost 40% of these misdiagnosed patients had seizures (1). Focal onset seizures may leave a portion of the ictal brain dysfunctional for a prolonged period (hours or more), and the deficits may be indistinguishable from those of ischemic stroke. Often, the only clues will be a history of seizures or absence of diagnostic evidence of ischemia.

Intracranial hemorrhage, encephalitis, or other structural brain lesions, such as tumors, may produce focal deficits identical to ischemic stroke. However, headache and altered or depressed level of consciousness are more likely to be the primary complaint in these cases. Findings consistent with infection or demonstration of a hemorrhage on computed tomography (CT) are usually all that is required to differentiate these disorders from ischemic stroke. The next largest group of mistaken diagnoses occurs in patients suffering confusion and neurologic deficits from drug intoxication, alcohol, or metabolic abnormalities. Extreme electrolyte or serum glucose derangements can produce temporary focal deficits.

Migraine may produce several transient neurologic symptoms that may be misinterpreted as stroke. Visual phenomena, such as bright lines, and blurriness or loss of vision are commonly described. Sensory disturbances, and particularly well-demarcated regions on the upper extremity and periorally, often occur. These symptoms may occur with or without the associated head pain but do not respect laterality or vascular territories as ischemic strokes do. People who suffer migraines, however, are at increased risk for ischemic stroke, so a thorough evaluation is warranted before dismissing the symptoms, particularly if it is the first occurrence. Motor deficits only very rarely result from migraine, so they should be attributed to stroke until proven otherwise.

Occasionally, peripheral nerve lesions, such as Bell palsy, may appear suddenly and mimic an ischemic stroke. Careful differentiation between upper and lower motor signs will most often clarify the diagnosis, but incomplete presentations can be confusing. In general, dense paralysis in the absence of other neurologic signs or complaints is more likely the result of a peripheral lesion. Although uncommon, stroke may present with bizarre or otherwise unbelievable symptoms, so the diagnosis of a psychogenic disorder should remain one of exclusion.

Establishing a correct diagnosis of these stroke mimics usually depends heavily on the patient's history, and the physician must specifically probe for characteristics of these diseases. A thorough history and physical examination, combined with appropriate laboratory testing and brain imaging such as magnetic resonance imaging (MRI) or CT scan, can usually exclude most conditions that mimic a stroke.

ISCHEMIC STROKE

Pathogenesis

Ischemic stroke occurs when the supply of blood to brain tissue is acutely interrupted. Normal cerebral blood flow in gray matter is about 80 mL/100 g tissue/min, whereas white matter is about 20 mL/100 g tissue/min. A global average in cortical mantle (assuming a 50:50 mix of gray and white matter) is about 50 mL/100 g tissue/min. Modest perturbations of the amount of cerebral blood flow can be accommodated by the autoregulatory capacity of the cerebral vasculature. When systemic blood pressure drops, resistance vessels in the brain dilate to increase flow. Once these vessels are maximally dilated, further drops in systemic pressure will reduce cerebral blood flow. If the average cerebral blood flow drops below 35 mL/100 g tissue/min, protein synthesis stops; below 20 mL/100 g tissue/min, synaptic failure occurs and neurons cease to function. As this threshold is crossed, patients become suddenly symptomatic. When cerebral blood flow drops below 10 mL/100 g tissue/min, metabolic failure and irreversible cell death occur.

Disruption of blood flow to the brain does not affect all tissues within the vascular distribution equally. Most often, there is a region with markedly reduced flow that quickly undergoes

TABLE 124.1 Symptoms Seldom Resulting from Cerebrovascular Disease

- Vertigo alone
- Dysarthria alone
- Dysphagia alone
- Diplopia alone
- Headache
- Tremor
- Tonic–clonic motor activity
- Confusion
- Memory loss
- Delirium
- Coma
- Syncope
- Incontinence
- Tinnitus

infarction; surrounding that area are regions with diminished flow that will survive longer, but not indefinitely. This potentially salvageable area is referred to as the *penumbra*. The purpose of acute stroke therapies is to salvage the penumbra.

In the general adult population, the causes of disruptions of arterial flow can be separated into three major categories based on cause: large vessel atherothrombotic disease (small vessel (lacunar) infarction, and cardiogenic embolism. This categorization will focus the diagnostic evaluation and therapy and has prognostic implications. Determining the cause will also guide the clinician in administering the appropriate level of care based on the possibility of progression and anticipated complications. For example, subtle speech changes and right-hand weakness could be the presenting symptoms of any of the three stroke subtypes outlined above. If a lacunar infarction is the cause, symptoms will most likely be maximal at onset and rarely will the patient experience complications compromising respiration or circulation. The volume of brain tissue involved is by definition small, and the risk for progression or recurrence in the acute period is quite small. A cardiogenic embolus would also be expected to cause symptoms maximal at onset, but the infarct volume could be large enough to cause mass effect and, depending on the underlying cardiac pathology, the risk for complications could be substantial.

Large Vessel Atherothrombosis

Large vessel atherothrombosis encompasses approximately 15% of all strokes; of these, two-thirds are of extracranial internal carotid artery (ICA) origin, and one-third are due to intracranial atheromatous disease (2). Atheromatous disease of large vessels is a slowly degenerative process, but as the disease progresses, the chance for lesion instability increases. Vascular plaques may fragment, exposing an ulcerated surface that is highly thrombogenic and leading to local occlusion or creation of emboli material. Thus, in large vessel disease, thrombosis or artery-to-artery embolism are often parts of the same underlying pathologic process. Atherosclerotic lesions tend to occur at bifurcations or sharp turns in the vessel, both of which are associated with increased blood flow turbulence. The prototypic example of this is carotid stenosis at the origin of the ICA. Other common extracranial sites include the origin of the vertebral artery and the other great vessels. Intracranially, common sites include the distal vertebral artery, the mid-basilar artery, the siphon of the ICA, and the proximal middle cerebral artery (MCA).

TABLE 124.2 Conditions Most Frequently Mistaken for Stroke

- Seizures
- Metabolic encephalopathy
- Cerebral tumor
- Subdural hematoma
- Cerebral abscess
- Vertigo, Meniere disease
- Peripheral neuropathy and Bell palsy
- Multiple sclerosis
- Hypoglycemia
- Encephalitis
- Migraine
- Psychogenic illness

Lacunar Strokes

Lacunar strokes represent approximately one-quarter of all such events. They are caused by occlusion of a single perforating arteriole, such as those that supply deep brain structures like the thalamus, pons, or basal ganglia (Fig. 124.1). The result is a small infarction—by most definitions, less than 1 cm^3—that undergoes liquefaction necrosis with time, leaving a tiny fluid-filled space for which they are named. The primary risk factor for lacunar infarction is hypertension, which results in lipohyalinosis of the vessel wall with progressive concentric stenosis and eventual thrombosis (3).

Cardiogenic Embolism

Approximately 60% of all ischemic strokes are caused by cerebral embolism, of which only one-third have a definitively known clinical source (4). Cerebral emboli may be composed of atherosclerotic plaque material, clotted blood, or, in rare cases, air or fat. Once free in the arterial circulation, the emboli will tend to follow the straightest path formed by the most blood. Therefore, most emboli will affect distal branches of the MCA, although other locations are possible; the larger the embolus, the more proximal it will lodge.

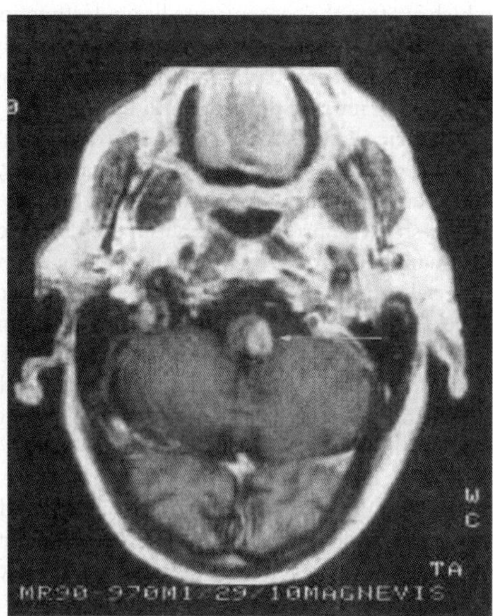

FIGURE 124.1 Intracerebral hemorrhage of the left basal ganglia. Hyperdense appearance of blood on the CT scan easily defines the extent of hemorrhage.

Cerebral emboli may originate from atheromatous disease of more proximal large vessels, such as the aortic arch, as outlined above, or the heart (5). Atrial fibrillation is the most common cardiac cause, but others include valvular heart disease, intracardiac thrombus, atrial myxoma, dilated cardiomyopathy, patent foramen ovale (PFO), especially when accompanied by an atrial septal defect, and endocarditis. Air emboli are usually iatrogenic and result when a large amount of air enters the venous circulation (e.g., through a central venous catheter) and bypasses the lungs through a PFO, thereby entering the arterial circulation. Fat emboli are generally the result of long-bone fractures in severe trauma. It is important to seek out the definitive source whenever possible, as it may have a profound impact on the management of secondary stroke prevention. For example, although most sources of cardiogenic emboli are treated with oral anticoagulation, several conditions may contraindicate it, such as bacterial endocarditis (6) or atrial myxoma (7).

Arterial Dissections

Although arterial dissections may occur at any age, they are probably the most common cause of stroke in young patients (<50 years old) who are unlikely to have typical risk factors. Arterial dissections may arise spontaneously or following a traumatic head or neck injury (8). These lesions typically arise at the petrous portion of the ICA or at the C1–2 level in the vertebral artery. Thrombus may form at the site of intimal tear, extending into the media, with subsequent artery-to-artery embolism. If a large intimal flap or intramural hematoma forms, occlusion of the affected vessel may occur. Dissection may also lead to subarachnoid hemorrhage (SAH) when a pseudoaneurysm forms after the artery passes intradurally (9).

Clinical Evaluation

History

The history, when available, is the key instrument in diagnosing neurologic disease. If the patient is unable to provide a reliable history, which is often the case in acute brain dysfunction, then historic details should be sought from witnesses, family, EMS records, or whatever sources are available; no other diagnostic tool will so quickly narrow the differential diagnosis.

The key historic element in ischemic cerebrovascular disease is *sudden* onset of symptoms, which are typically maximal at onset. Under certain circumstances, the symptoms may follow a stuttering or stepwise progression, but in each instance there is a sudden change. Contrast this with the waxing and waning character of delirium or the symptoms that may develop over days to weeks from a brain tumor. There is an unfortunate tendency to dismiss symptoms of short duration, but this is a serious mistake, as the duration of the symptoms speaks little to the underlying pathogenesis. For example, a patient with occult atrial fibrillation may suffer transient neurologic deficits from an embolus that happens to spontaneously lyse before infarction has completed. Without addressing the underlying cause, the patient is unlikely to continue to be so fortunate, and an opportunity to prevent a devastating neurologic injury will have been lost.

If the ictal event is consistent with a stroke, the remainder of the initial history should be focused on determining if the patient is a candidate for thrombolytic therapy and identifying possible risk factors. Whereas other details not elucidated in the initial history can be revisited at a later time, it is of the utmost importance to obtain the exact time of symptom onset, as current acute stroke treatment protocols depend on this for inclusion. If the onset was not witnessed, then the time when last known to be normal is used. For example, if the patient awakens with symptoms, then the time when the patient retired is used (assuming he or she was asymptomatic then). The reason time of onset is so important is that it is used as a surrogate marker for the likelihood that salvageable tissue remains. Additionally, the risk of intracerebral hemorrhage (ICH) associated with thrombolytics increases with time after onset of symptoms. Current research is focused on using multimodal imaging to generate physiologic data that may be used *in lieu* of time to identify patients with a salvageable penumbra, but these techniques have yet to mature.

Aside from time of onset, factors that may place the patient at increased risk for bleeding must be sought. Tables 124.3 to 124.6 list common inclusion and exclusion criteria for intravenous (IV) tissue plasminogen activator (tPA), which are based on those used in the pivotal trials. Most institutions have their own protocols, which may vary somewhat from those used in the trials.

TABLE 124.3 Inclusion Criteria for Tissue Plasminogen Activator Use within 3 Hours from Symptom Onset

- Symptoms consistent with acute ischemic stroke, with a clearly defined onset of less than 3 hr before rtPA will be given (if the onset was not witnessed, the ictus is measured from the time the patient was last seen to be at baseline)
- A significant neurologic deficit is expected to result in long-term disability
- Noncontrast computed tomography with no evidence of hemorrhage or well-established infarction
- Age ≥ 18 yr

Data from Jauch EC, Saver JL, Adams HP Jr, et al. Guidelines for the early management of adults with ischemic stroke: a guideline from the American Heart Association/American Stroke Association. *Stroke.* 2013;44(3):870–947.

TABLE 124.4 Absolute Contraindications to Tissue Plasminogen Activator Use

- Significant head trauma or prior stroke in previous 3 mo
- Hemorrhage on CT, well-established acute infarct on CT, or any other CT diagnosis that contraindicates treatment, including abscess or tumor (excluding small meningiomas)
- Symptoms suggest subarachnoid hemorrhage
- Arterial puncture at noncompressible site within 7 d
- History of previous intracranial hemorrhage
- Intracranial neoplasm, aneurysm, or arteriovenous malformation
- Recent intracranial or spinal surgery
- Elevated blood pressure (systolic >185 mmHg or diastolic >110 mmHg) despite use of antihypertensive agents
- Active internal bleeding
- Acute bleeding diathesis
- Platelet count <100,000/mm^3
- Heparin received within 48 hr, resulting in abnormally elevated aPTT greater than the upper limit of normal
- Current use of anticoagulant with INR >1.7 or PT >15 s
- Current use of direct thrombin inhibitors or direct factor Xa inhibitors with elevated sensitive laboratory tests (such as aPTT, INR, platelet count, and ECT; TT; or appropriate factor Xa activity assays)
- Blood glucose concentration <50 mg/dL

CT, computed tomography; CNS, central nervous system.
Data from Jauch EC, Saver JL, Adams HP Jr, et al. Guidelines for the early management of adults with ischemic stroke: a guideline from the American Heart Association/American Stroke Association. *Stroke* 2013;44(3):870–947.

TABLE 124.5 Relative Contraindications to Tissue Plasminogen Activator Use

- Minor or rapidly improving stroke symptoms
- Seizure at onset with postictal residual neurologic impairments
- Major surgery within the past 14 d
- Pregnancy (and ≤10 d postpartum)
- Gastrointestinal, urologic, or respiratory hemorrhage within past 21 d
- Major surgery or trauma within past 14 d
- Recent acute myocardial infarction within past 3 mo

Data from Jauch EC, Saver JL, Adams HP Jr, et al. Guidelines for the early management of adults with ischemic stroke: a guideline from the American Heart Association/American Stroke Association. *Stroke.* 2013;44(3):870–947.

Once a decision regarding acute treatment has been made, attention can be directed to identifying conditions that may have caused the patient's stroke. Cerebrovascular and cardiovascular diseases share many of the same risk factors, including hypertension, hyperlipidemia, diabetes mellitus, cigarette smoking, and obesity. Other risk factors that may be important include obstructive sleep apnea, migraine headaches with an aura, and drug abuse. Family history may provide insight into heritable causes of stroke such as cerebral autosomal dominant arteriopathy with subcortical infarcts and leukoencephalopathy (CADASIL) or Fabry disease.

Neurologic Examination

The neurologic examination will allow the clinician to quickly determine which brain areas are dysfunctional and further narrow the differential diagnosis. The neurologic deficits caused by ischemic cerebrovascular disease are expected to be lateralizing and confined to a vascular distribution. For example, the triad of language disturbance and right face and arm motor deficits is typical for occlusion of the left MCA. However, sudden-onset motor and sensory deficit of both arms is not lateralizing, nor readily explained by a cerebrovascular occlusion, and thus is more likely due to spinal cord pathology.

The first step in localization of vascular lesions is determining, based on the signs and symptoms, whether they arise from the anterior circulation (carotid artery and its main branches, the anterior and middle cerebral arteries) or the posterior circulation (vertebral, basilar, and posterior cerebral arteries). This finding will guide the remainder of the diagnostic evaluation, therapy, and prognosis. Ideally, these two separate circulations would be robustly connected such that a failure in one could be compensated by the other, but this is rarely the case.

TABLE 124.6 Additional Inclusion and Exclusion Criteria for the Use of IV tPA within 3 and 4.5 Hours from Symptom Onset

Inclusion

1. Diagnosis of ischemic stroke causing neurologic deficit
2. Onset of symptoms within 3 and 4.5 hr from onset

Relative Exclusion Criteria

1. Age > 80 yr
2. Severe stroke (NIHSS >25)
3. Use of oral anticoagulation regardless of INR value
4. History of both diabetes and prior ischemic stroke

Data from Jauch EC, Saver JL, Adams HP Jr, et al. Guidelines for the early management of adults with ischemic stroke: a guideline from the American Heart Association/American Stroke Association. *Stroke.* 2013;44(3):870–947.

The two symptoms that most accurately reflect carotid circulation disease are aphasia and monocular blindness. Aphasia is a deficit in either the expression or comprehension of language and may involve both in the acute period. Aphasia must be distinguished from dysarthria, which is the inability to correctly produce words due to motor impairment of facial, lingual, or pharyngeal muscles; dysarthria may result from either anterior or posterior circulation infarcts. The areas responsible for language reside in the dominant (nearly always left) hemispheric cortex, within the territory of the MCA; a stroke causing aphasia must, therefore, involve this circulation. Similarly, the blood supply of the eye arises largely from the ophthalmic artery, a direct branch from the carotid artery, and monocular ischemia, therefore, implicates the carotid circulation. The prototypic example of this process is amaurosis fugax, or transient monocular blindness, in which vision is lost in *one eye* for minutes. This must be contrasted with a visual field deficit, which affects one field of *both eyes,* as this is more likely the result of posterior circulation ischemia. Pain is rarely a significant complaint, but when present, especially if following the course of a major blood vessel, arterial dissection should be considered. Involvement of the carotid artery may cause Horner syndrome.

Because of the density of discrete populations of neurons supplied by the posterior circulation, the clinical syndromes that result from strokes in this area are usually more complex than those in the cerebral hemispheres. The medulla, pons, midbrain, cerebellum, parts of the thalami, and the visual cortices are the major structures involved. Strokes involving the brainstem often manifest with cranial nerve dysfunction (dysarthria, dysphagia, diplopia). Crossed signs, with motor or sensory deficits affecting one side of the face and the opposite side of the body, may occur as major decussations in these pathways and occur in the pons and medulla. The unique vascular anatomy of the basilar artery, with a single midline vessel supplying both sides of the pons and the posterior cerebral arteries, may lead to bilateral neurologic deficits.

Lacunar infarctions also have a set of clinical features that may be used to differentiate them from other stroke subtypes. Classic lacunar syndromes include pure motor hemiparesis (caused by infarction in the internal capsule or *basis pontis*), pure hemisensory symptoms (caused by infarction in the ventral posterolateral [VPL] thalamic nucleus), dysarthria–clumsy hand syndrome (with pontine or internal capsule infarcts), and ataxia–hemiparesis (pontine infarct).

Vascular System Examination

Physical examination of the vascular system itself is usually surprisingly unrewarding. Atherosclerosis may present few outward signs. Although carotid bruits were classically emphasized, modern ultrasound techniques have proven them to be of low sensitivity and specificity for predicting vascular disease. No characteristic feature, including the volume, pitch, or duration of the bruit, reliably indicates the degree or the nature of constriction of the vascular lumen. Many bruits reflect benign conditions. The clinical significance of carotid bruits is minimized because they are audible in many asymptomatic persons without atherosclerosis who never suffer from cerebrovascular disease, but may be absent in severely diseased vessels. Therefore, even if a carotid bruit is detected, it may be difficult to decide whether it is relevant to the patient's symptoms, and it should not be given undue emphasis in the overall evaluation. Clinical decisions should be based on definitive assessment of blood vessels using ultrasound or angiography.

Examination of the heart should focus on detecting thrombogenic diseases, including myocardial infarction (MI), congestive heart failure, arrhythmias, prosthetic valves, and bacterial endocarditis. Heart disease is a key risk factor for stroke and may complicate the acute period. Patients with stroke may also present concurrently with a MI and, without careful examination, the less dramatic of the two may go undetected. Elevation of serum troponin levels is a very sensitive and specific indicator of an MI. Isolated creatine kinase (CK)-MB elevations should be interpreted with caution, however, as the MB fraction is expressed in brain tissue, and small elevations are not uncommon in stroke (10).

Laboratory Studies

Laboratory studies will also help narrow the differential diagnosis and may reveal relevant comorbid conditions. Some studies need to be obtained immediately to determine a patient's candidacy for thrombolytic therapy, including an electrolyte battery, glucose, platelet count, cardiac enzymes, beta-human chorionic gonadotropin (β-HCG), and coagulation parameters. Severe electrolyte (specifically hyponatremia or hypernatremia) or glucose disturbances can cause neurologic dysfunction that may mimic stroke. Cardiac enzymes will determine if cardiac ischemia is part of the current presentation, and a β-HCG will reveal occult pregnancy, both of which may be contraindications to systemic thrombolytics. Coagulation parameters and a platelet count will identify patients who may be at greater risk for bleeding.

Other laboratory studies will help determine the cause and identify risk factors but do not need to be obtained immediately. A fasting lipid profile should be obtained for potential vascular risk factor modification. In patients more than 50 years of age, an erythrocyte sedimentation rate and C-reactive protein are essential if giant cell arteritis is suspected. In patients for whom an unusual cause of stroke is suspected (young patients or minimal vascular risk factors), laboratory investigation of prothrombotic states could be considered. The interpretation of these tests is very complex and should be performed in consultation with a hematologist (11). Toxicology screening should be performed on hospital admission, with attention directed to amphetamines, phencyclidine, ephedrine, and cocaine.

Imaging Studies

CT Scan

Several imaging studies are used in the evaluation of acute stroke. A noncontrasted CT scan of the brain is the standard initial evaluation for stroke. CT is very sensitive to the presence of hemorrhage, which is the primary reason for its use in the acute setting, and is the only radiologic test necessary to determine eligibility for IV-tPA. CT is not sensitive for the detection of an acute cerebral infarction (Fig. 124.2), and the lack of abnormality within the first 24 hours should be expected. The view of the posterior fossa is also quite limited, and any changes (with the exception of hemorrhage) seen within the brainstem or cerebellum should be confirmed with MRI. When available, CT angiography (CTA) and perfusion (CTP) studies can be obtained with very little additional time and provide valuable additional information regarding the patency of blood vessels and blood flow to individual large vessel territories. Pathologic changes on these studies are visible immediately, but they require iodinated contrast, which may be a limiting factor for some patients. The angiographic results from CTA are closest to the traditional gold standard examination: digital subtraction catheter angiography (DSA). When examining the carotid arteries, the results from CTA are often sufficient to differentiate a high-grade stenosis (60% to 99%) that is treatable from complete occlusion that is not. Use of CTP in conjunction with noncontrasted CT brain and CTA can help determine tissue that is potentially salvageable with reperfusion strategies.

MRI

MRI is far more sensitive for acute infarction than CT. Diffusion MR sequences can detect ischemia within, perhaps,

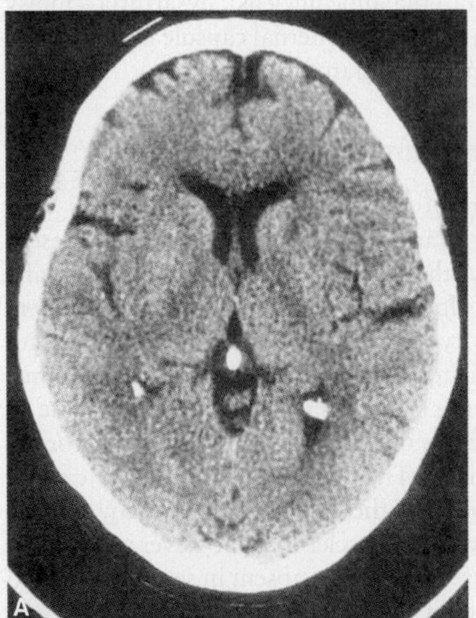

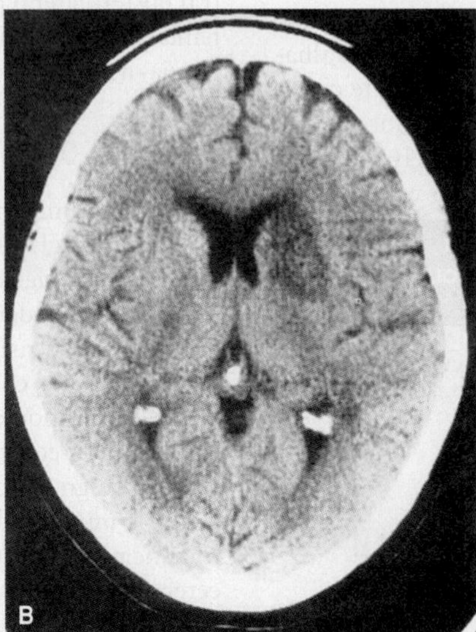

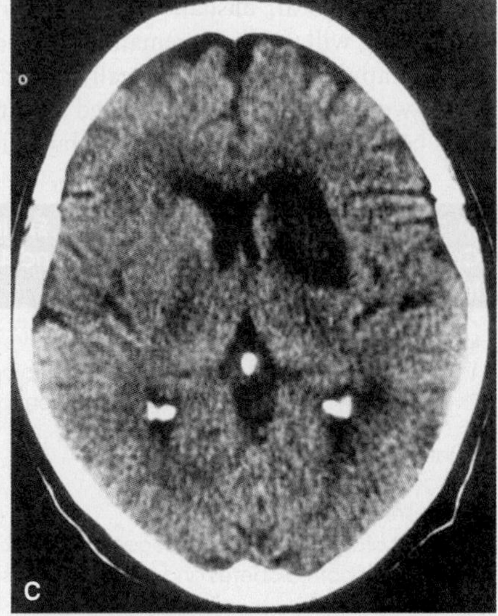

FIGURE 124.2 Evolving radiographic evidence of cerebral infarction. A: CT scan at 3 hours shows little evidence of acute ischemia. B: At 3 days, damaged brain is indicated by hypodensity in the left subcortical region. C: At 8 days, frank infarction is now clearly demonstrated by CT.

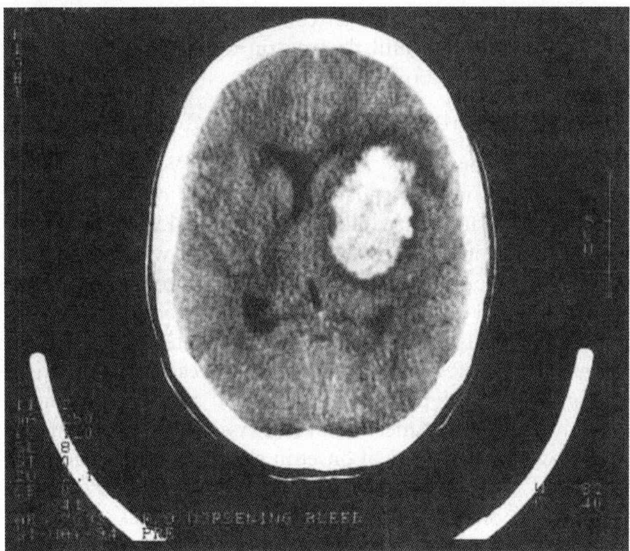

FIGURE 124.3 MRI demonstrates enhancing left lateral medullary infarction in a patient with Wallenberg syndrome.

minutes of onset. MRI is of special value in brainstem and posterior circulation strokes, since the images it produces are not obscured by bony artifacts as with CT (Fig. 124.3). The combination of multiple MRI sequences allows for much more specific differentiation between ischemic brain and other structural abnormalities. In addition, MRI can display flow-related enhancement of the vasculature, resulting in a magnetic resonance angiogram (MRA). The resulting image can be manipulated in three dimensions, allowing for more accurate interpretation of small abnormalities. MRA uses gadolinium as a contrast agent instead of an iodinated material, making the study available to more patients. Perfusion studies, very similar to those performed with CT, may also be obtained if the right equipment is available. Disadvantages of MRI and MRA include reduced availability and substantially longer scanning times, which place some limitations on their use.

DSA

DSA is an invasive imaging technique in which the artery of interest is selectively catheterized under fluoroscopy and dye injection enables a high-resolution view of the vessel that can be obtained in multiple planes. As the quality of noninvasive imaging techniques has improved and the associated morbidity is approximately 1% (12), DSA is no longer used as a routine screening test. Indications now include precisely delimiting critical vascular stenoses and examination of arterial dissections, arteriovenous malformations (AVMs), and aneurysms.

Carotid Ultrasound

Carotid ultrasound provides a rapid noninvasive assessment of carotid artery disease, based on abnormalities of either flow (Doppler) or morphology (B-mode). As with any ultrasound technique, sensitivity is to some degree operator-dependent, but with experienced technicians and interpreters, duplex scanning provides a reproducible, accurate screening examination for carotid disease. However, this technique suffers from the same limitation as MRA in differentiating high-grade stenosis and occlusion. Lesions of the more distal ICA may also be difficult to visualize in some patients.

Transcranial Doppler

Transcranial Doppler (TCD) allows rapid bedside assessment of abnormal flow within the distal ICA and major intracranial arteries. It is primarily a functional study that provides information about blood flow velocity and vascular resistance rather than structural features. The 2-MHz ultrasonic signal can penetrate various bony "windows" in most patients, and its gated character allows identification of arteries by "depth" of the reflected signal. TCD can examine proximal portions of all major branches of the circle of Willis, but is insensitive for pathology beyond the A1, M1, or P1 segments. Newer applications include detection of microemboli and online monitoring of arterial flow during invasive procedures, such as carotid endarterectomy (Fig. 124.4). TCD may also be useful as an adjunctive therapy to tPA, as continuous insonation may enhance thrombolysis (13). Disadvantages include major dependency on operator skill and the prevalence of acoustically inadequate bony windows.

Transthoracic Echocardiography

Transthoracic echocardiography (TTE) is essential to evaluate cardiac function. Physicians must attend not only to a visualized thrombus, but also to other pathologic states associated with systemic embolization, including left ventricular wall motion abnormalities, chamber dilatation, valvular disease, ejection fraction, and septal defects. TTE can be routinely performed and is a superior study for the detection of ventricular apex pathology, left ventricle thrombus, and views of prosthetic valves. Transesophageal echocardiography (TEE) provides much greater resolution and is more sensitive for pathology of the left atrial appendage, interatrial septum, atrial aspect of mitral–tricuspid valves, and the ascending aorta. TEE is an invasive procedure that requires sedation but can be performed safely on most patients (14).

MANAGEMENT

Acute Therapy

As with any acutely ill patient, attention should initially be focused on the evaluation of airway, breathing, and circulation. A secure airway should be established for patients with depressed levels of consciousness. Supplemental oxygen or mechanical ventilation should be used as needed to treat any degree of hypoxia. Circulation assessment includes evaluation of blood pressure and cardiac electrical activity with an ECG, as coexistent MI is not uncommon. Patients with acute stroke are often markedly hypertensive, and one should be cautious in aggressively treating elevated blood pressure before a more complete assessment of the patient has been completed. Blood pressure goals are determined by type of stroke, cause, and the presence of comorbid conditions, such as coronary artery disease; this will be discussed in the following sections.

The immediate goal will be to determine if the patient is a candidate for thrombolytic therapy; thus attention should be focused on obtaining the relevant history and performing a neurologic examination. The care of patients who will ultimately not receive thrombolytic therapy will be discussed below (see Supportive Care). Crucial for therapy is the proper determination of the exact time of onset of the stroke. The patient must be witnessed to have had an abrupt change in

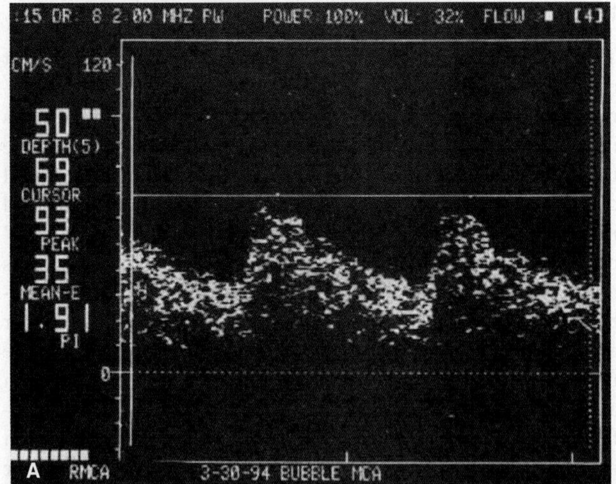

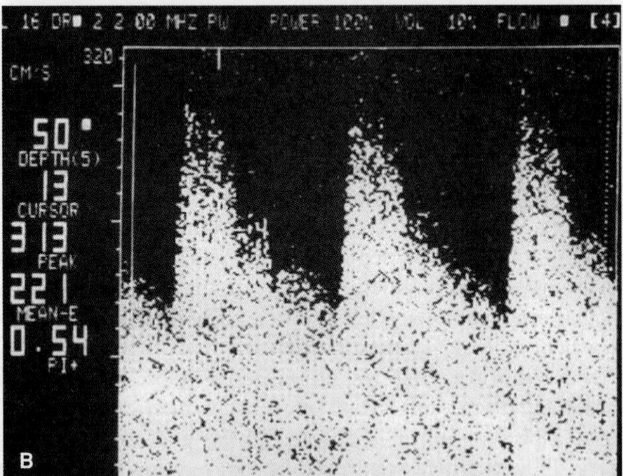

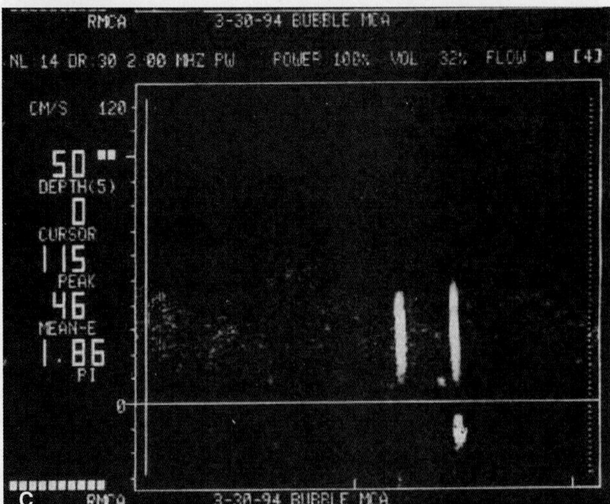

FIGURE 124.4 Transcranial Doppler. **A**: The normal flow-velocity profile through the middle cerebral artery (velocity plotted over time during three cardiac cycles) is demonstrated. **B**: Elevated flow velocities as a result of the arterial spasm associated with subarachnoid hemorrhage is demonstrated. **C**: Two microemboli are detected through the middle cerebral artery as transient high-intensity signals.

neurologic status by a reliable observer; otherwise the time of onset, by default, must be the last time the patient was seen at his or her baseline level of neurologic function. All patients should be evaluated with the National Institutes of Health Stroke Scale (NIHSS), which can help to exclude a patient from potentially harmful therapy on the basis of the stroke being too small or too severe.

Thrombolytic Therapy

Currently, thrombolytic treatment with IV-tPA in eligible stroke patients is the standard of care based on the results of several large randomized controlled trials (15–22). The collective results indicate that patients treated with tPA within 4.5 hours of onset had significantly higher odds of a good stroke outcome (23). The average disability across all groups was, additionally, decreased in the treatment group. The benefit seen by the tPA-treated group existed regardless of patient age or stroke subtype. It is important to acknowledge, however, that while the American Stroke Association recommends IV-tPA within 4.5 hours of onset in eligible patients, the Food and Drug Association has only approved the use of tPA within 3 hours of onset (24,25). Table 124.6 provides additional inclusion and relative exclusion criteria for use of tPA in the 3- to 4.5-hour window.

To maximize the possible benefit and minimize the risk for hemorrhage, the National Institute of Neurological Disorders and Stroke (NINDS) study helped to establish strict inclusion criteria for the administration of thrombolytic therapy in acute stroke patients, which are outlined in Table 124.3 (15). Absolute exclusion criteria have been established as well (see Table 124.4). In addition, there is a list of *relative* contraindications to thrombolytic therapy (see Table 124.5), which often vary slightly in institutional protocols. These can be summarized as risks for bleeding from a noncompressible site, the presence of potential stroke mimics, or uncontrollable hypertension. The rationale for excluding patients with improving symptoms is to avoid giving a potentially harmful treatment to patients with epileptic postictal presentations or spontaneous recovery.

When the protocol is followed, the administration of tPA is safe relative to other commonly accepted treatments. Several studies have attempted to examine the risk, but perhaps the most clinically relevant is the number needed to harm. For every 100 patients treated with tPA who match the NINDS trials populations across all levels of final global disability, approximately 32 will receive benefit and 3 will be harmed (26). The risk–benefit ratio, thus, strongly favors treatment. Many of the hemorrhages that occur are asymptomatic, and of those that are symptomatic, not all symptoms persist to discharge. Most patients who experience ICH after tPA therapy have severe baseline insults and were already destined for a poor outcome; thus the hemorrhage does little to alter the final outcome (27). One should keep in mind that, although excluding a patient from treatment will mitigate the risk for hemorrhage, it also denies the patient a significantly better chance of recovery.

The dose of tPA is 0.9 mg/kg, with a maximum dose of 90 mg; 10% is given as a bolus over 1 minute, and the remaining 90% is infused over 60 minutes. Following treatment, patients should be monitored in an intensive care unit (ICU) for at least 24 hours. While many post-tPA patients will not need ventilatory or vasopressor support, as do many other patients in the ICU, blood pressure monitoring and frequent neurologic examinations are critical for a favorable outcome, as hypertension dramatically increases the risk for hemorrhage. Blood pressure must initially be monitored noninvasively as arterial puncture is contraindicated for 24 hours after the administration of tPA. All other invasive procedures, such

TABLE 124.7 Management of Blood Pressure During and After Treatment with Tissue Plasminogen Activator or Other Acute Reperfusion Intervention

- Monitor blood pressure (BP must be <180/105) every 15 min during treatment and then for another 2 hr, then every 30 min for 6 hr, and then every hour for 16 hr.
- For systolic 180–230 mmHg or diastolic 105–120 mmHg:
- Labetalol 10 mg IV followed by continuous IV infusion 2–8 mg/min; or
- Nicardipine 5 mg/hr IV, titrate up to desired effect by 2.5 mg/hr every 5–15 min, maximum 15 mg/hr
- For BP not controlled or diastolic >140 mmHg, consider IV sodium nitroprusside.

Data from Jauch EC, Saver JL, Adams HP Jr, et al. Guidelines for the early management of adults with ischemic stroke: a guideline from the American Heart Association/American Stroke Association. *Stroke.* 2013;44(3):870–947.

as placement of nasogastric tubes, urinary bladder catheters, central venous lines, intramuscular injections, and rectal temperature, should be avoided for 24 hours as well. Also, any drug that impairs hemostasis such as heparin, or antiplatelet or nonsteroidal anti-inflammatory agents is contraindicated during this 24-hour period.

Vital Signs

Vital signs should be checked every 15 minutes for the first 2 hours, then every 30 minutes for 6 hours, and then every hour for 16 hours. Blood pressure should be strictly controlled for 24 hours, keeping the systolic blood pressure less than 180 mmHg and the diastolic blood pressure less than 105 mmHg (Table 124.7). Labetalol is recommended for control of hypertension; 10 mg should be given intravenously over 1 to 2 minutes, and the dose repeated or doubled every 10 to 20 minutes, up to a total of 150 mg. If the blood pressure remains refractory despite these measures, consideration can be given to a continuous infusion of nicardipine or sodium nitroprusside. Neurologic evaluation should be performed every hour. Oxygenation should be checked by continuous pulse oximetry and oxygen provided to keep saturation >95%. The benefit of therapeutic hypothermia is yet to be confirmed, but euthermia is clearly associated with better outcome (28). Acetaminophen, 650 mg every 4 hours orally or rectally, should be given for any temperature higher than 37.4°C, and a cooling blanket used for temperatures over 38.9°C.

STAT Head CT

A STAT head CT should be performed for any worsening neurologic status. Should an ICH develop following thrombolysis, several steps must be taken emergently. Neurosurgery should be contacted for possible hematoma evacuation, and thrombolytics should be reversed based on local hospital protocols.

Intra-arterial Approach for Thrombolytic Therapy

The use of thrombolytic interventions outside of the 4.5-hour time window is controversial. However, there have been several attempts to prove the benefit of catheter-directed therapy via an intra-arterial approach for focal clot lysis. The most studied agent was prourokinase (29), but it was removed from the market in 1999 due to concerns with its preparation. The agent most commonly used today is tPA.

Theoretically, there are several potential benefits to treatment of stroke via an intra-arterial approach. First, angiographic confirmation of vessel occlusion can be obtained at the time of treatment. Second, high concentrations of thrombolytic agents can be given directly at the site of thrombosis, thereby minimizing systemic exposure. Third, the response to lysis can be monitored by direct visualization. Fourth, mechanical disruption of the clot (e.g., via balloon angioplasty, thrombectomy device) may accelerate thrombolysis (30).

While some studies have shown overall ineffectiveness (31–33), more recently, there has been promise especially when intra-arterial methods (particularly with thrombectomy devices) are combined with IV-tPA. Patients who undergo intra-arterial thrombectomy within 6 hours of symptom onset and with proof of distal ICA or proximal MCA occlusion by CTA have significantly higher changes of favorable outcomes. In almost all patients studied, intra-arterial thrombectomy was preceded by IV-tPA; therefore, IV-tPA should never be withheld from eligible patients (34–38). While CTP was not used in these recent trials, data has shown support for its utilization in patients who may not otherwise be eligible for intra-arterial therapy based on time of onset. By measuring volume of infarct in comparison to volume of salvageable tissue, patients who wake up with stroke symptoms or present past 6 hours of symptom onset may be eligible for intra-arterial therapies if determined to be safe (39).

Based on the most recent intra-arterial stroke trials, the American Stroke Association has strongly recommended the use of intra-arterial thrombectomy devices among eligible patients with proximal large vessel occlusions. The availability of intra-arterial treatment should not preclude the administration of IV-tPA in otherwise eligible patients. Treatment requires immediate access to cerebral angiography and qualified interventionists (40).

Supportive Care

Supportive care lacks the excitement and drama of acute therapy, but nonetheless is critical to patient outcomes. Since the 1970s, mortality from stroke has markedly diminished from a rate of 156 to 56/100,000 cases (41), with only 3% to 10% of stroke patients receiving thrombolytic therapy; this trend cannot be explained by tPA (42,43). Rather, it is the advancements made in the prevention of medical complications that has reduced mortality.

Motor Deficits

Dysphagia is common after stroke, whether it be from upper or lower motor neuron deficits. All patients with stroke should be screened for dysphagia before being allowed to take anything by mouth, as aspiration pneumonia is a substantial contributor to mortality after stroke (44). Any impairment in level of consciousness or motor function of mouth, tongue, palate, or muscles of facial expression should alert the physician to a high risk for dysphagia. Coarse breath sounds may indicate that aspiration has already occurred. A preserved gag reflex may not indicate safety with swallowing (45). If any of these signs are present, a formal swallowing evaluation is indicated. Enteral access can be achieved by placement of a nasogastric or Dobhoff tube. Feeding and hydration should be initiated immediately (46). Dysphagia often improves rapidly, but placement of a percutaneous endoscopic gastrostomy (PEG) tube may be necessary for prolonged feeding.

Before the advent of routine prophylaxis, deep vein thromboses (DVTs) and resulting pulmonary emboli were common in stroke patients who frequently have profound lower extremity immobility; pulmonary embolism presently accounts for approximately 10% of deaths in stroke patients (47). Recent trials, including PREVAIL (48), have shown low–molecular-weight heparin to be safe and more effective than unfractionated heparin. Early mobilization not only prevents DVTs, but also speeds rehabilitation.

Early initiation of physical, occupational, and speech therapy services hastens functional recovery from stroke. Each patient requires individualized assessment for potential benefit from these services. Speech therapists are also commonly involved in formal assessment of aspiration risk. A video fluoroscopy swallowing study is the most sensitive measure and should be a consideration for most patients with a stroke. At the least, bedside swallowing function should be observed by a trained technician, nurse, or physician before oral intake is resumed.

Blood Pressure Maintenance

Blood pressure goals in the acute period after ischemic stroke are often a source of confusion for many practitioners. Ischemic stroke patients are often quite hypertensive, and, while the reflex may be to aggressively lower the blood pressure, this may cause more harm than benefit. When blood flow is impaired, the resulting change in pressure gradients will allow circulation through alternative or collateral paths. Through autoregulation, these collateral vessels maximally dilate, and thus flow becomes entirely dependent on cerebral perfusion pressure. Some even advocate the induction of therapeutic hypertension with vasopressors, but insufficient evidence exists to recommend this practice. Therefore, lowering blood pressure potentially reduces blood flow to the potentially salvageable penumbra. Determining the exact pressure required for adequate blood flow is not readily accomplished, so one must err on the side of hypertension. For most stroke patients with acute hypertension, the general practice is to refrain from intervening until the pressure exceeds an arbitrary limit of 220 mmHg systolic or 120 mmHg diastolic (49). Patients with coronary artery disease or those with another comorbidity that may preclude tolerance of such pressures may require a careful decrement in blood pressure. In these cases, it is recommended that blood pressure be lowered slowly, using frequent smaller doses of drug rather than larger ones that may cause rapid changes; patients should be carefully observed for acute worsening as pressure is lowered. In patients having received thrombolytics, the tolerable limit is lower, as the risk for ICH increases with increasing blood pressure. In this case, pressures greater than 180 mmHg systolic or greater than 105 mmHg diastolic require treatment according to the protocol (see Table 124.7).

Hyperglycemia

Hyperglycemia will be detected on admission in approximately one-third of patients with stroke (50). Predictions for patients with persistent hyperglycemia (blood glucose level >200 mg/dL) during the first 24 hours after stroke are expansion of the volume of ischemic stroke and poor neurologic outcomes (51). Our practice is to aggressively control glucose—keeping it between 80 and 140 mg/dL—but care must be taken to avoid hypoglycemia, as the morbidity from that may abolish the benefit obtained from treating hyperglycemia.

Although most patients eventually improve substantially after a stroke, early clinical deterioration is not uncommon. Neurologic causes of clinical deterioration include progressive or recurrent stroke, hemorrhagic transformation of the infarct, and local cerebral edema. The latter is the most common cause of deterioration, and may well cause fatal herniation in large MCA infarctions, especially in the young, women, and in patients with involvement of additional vascular territories (52). Brain swelling typically appears about 4 days after the stroke onset (53). Dramatic early swelling has been described; the term *malignant MCA infarction* is used to delineate a group of patients with large territorial infarcts that swell within 24 hours (54).

Ischemia-related edema is cytotoxic and unresponsive to treatments useful for vasogenic edema. Corticosteroids, in particular, do not appear helpful, and hyperglycemia associated with their use may worsen clinical outcome (49,55,56). Although no evidence exists that ultimate outcome is improved, certain treatments are often used to reduce intracranial pressure (ICP): mannitol (1 g/kg bolus, then 0.3 g/kg every 6 hours) dehydrates viable brain tissue (57) to create more space for swelling tissue, and is primarily useful as a temporizing measure for patients destined for decompressive surgery, as the effects of this medication are transient and associated with eventual rebound. Other measures such as mechanical hyperventilation (to a $PaCO_2$ of 25 to 30 mmHg), or use of albumin and furosemide to raise colloid oncotic pressure (to 25 to 30 mmHg) are used, but, again, their efficacy in improving outcome remains to be demonstrated.

Decompressive Surgery

Decompressive surgery, including hemicraniectomy and durotomy with temporal lobe resection, for treatment of brain edema after stroke has been a controversial topic. Many studies in the past have shown conflicting results, but these trials enrolled mixed age groups and surgery was often not performed until symptomatic herniation occurred (58). Three large European trials (HAMLET, DESTINY, and DECIMAL) (59–61) enrolled patients younger than 60 years of age and were prematurely terminated after it became clear that decompressive craniotomy was associated with a dramatic outcome benefit. Upon pooled analysis of these studies, young patients with malignant MCA syndromes who underwent decompressive surgery within 48 hours had reduced rates of mortality and higher rates of favorable functional outcomes (62). In elderly patients, the results have generally shown that, while mortality may be decreased, outcomes remained poor (63).

Hemorrhagic Transformation

The likelihood of hemorrhagic transformation of a stroke increases as stroke volume increases. Often, this transformation may be limited to petechial transudation of blood products into the ischemic tissue bed. Generally, this phenomenon occurs in a delayed fashion with no associated clinical deterioration. Specific therapy is not usually required, although any ongoing anticoagulation is generally held for 1 to 2 weeks. If the hemorrhage is associated with clinical deterioration, management should follow those principles outlined in the Intracerebral Hemorrhage section.

INTRACEREBRAL HEMORRHAGE

Pathogenesis

In contrast to ischemic stroke, primary ICH involves bleeding, usually of arterial origin, into normally perfused brain, and thus must be distinguished from hemorrhagic transformation of an initially ischemic stroke. The expanding hematoma causes direct injury to local brain tissue and dysfunction in surrounding regions. The onset is typically very sudden, although continued bleeding often progresses over minutes or hours. Very often, there is either depression or loss of consciousness due to an abrupt increase in ICP from the sudden outpouring of blood into the brain. In addition to the initial cerebral insult caused by the hemorrhage, secondary injury can occur by various means, including seizures, hydrocephalus, and edema, all of which can lead to a further increase in ICP.

In younger patients, hypertension is by far the more common cause, and, as such, ICH tends to occur in the same brain areas where other hypertensive pathologies occur, specifically brainstem, cerebellum, and deep supratentorial structures (64). In contrast, lobar ICHs occur more commonly in the elderly population and are often associated with cerebral amyloid angiopathy in the absence of hypertension (65). ICH may also occur in the setting of trauma, use of illicit drugs (e.g., cocaine) or over-the-counter medications (e.g., phenylpropanolamine) (66), excessive alcohol consumption (67), an underlying vascular abnormality (e.g., AVM, cerebral aneurysm), brain tumor (primary or secondary), or a bleeding diathesis.

ICH causes approximately 10% of first-time strokes. The 30-day mortality rate is high at 35% to 50%, with half of the deaths occurring within the first 2 days (68). Outcome in ICH is dependent on several factors, including the location and size of the hemorrhage (69), the age of the patient, the Glasgow Coma Scale (GCS) on presentation (70), and the cause of the hemorrhage. When intraventricular blood is present, the mortality substantially increases (71) and worsens further with increasing volume (72). The presence of hydrocephalus also confers a poor prognosis (73).

Clinical Evaluation

Rapid diagnosis of ICH is essential, as progression during the first several hours is the norm. The hallmark is sudden-onset focal neurologic deficit, which progresses over minutes to hours. Steady symptomatic progression of a focal deficit is rare in either ischemic stroke or SAH. Headache, increased blood pressure, and impaired level of consciousness are common features that complete the presentation. History gathering should be directed at elucidating the presence of risk factors as outlined above. Other considerations include the use of antithrombotic medications (e.g., aspirin or warfarin) or hematologic disorders that predispose to bleeding, such as severe liver disease. The initial physical examination is similar to that of patients with ischemic stroke, focusing on airway, breathing, and circulation before assessing the level of consciousness and neurologic deficits. The patient's coagulation parameters should be checked immediately and corrected if abnormal.

Once stabilized, the patient should undergo a noncontrast head CT immediately to verify brain hemorrhage. CTA may also be helpful in detecting aneurysms, AVMs, underlying tumors, or abscesses. Contrast extravasation into the hematoma is thought to represent ongoing bleeding (74). MRI will also provide information about the hemorrhage but is time consuming and potentially dangerous for an unstable patient. When it can be obtained safely, MRI is most useful for dating the time course of the hemorrhage if the history is in doubt, detecting areas of prior hemorrhage (with the use of gradient-echo imaging) (75), and diagnosing cavernous malformations. DSA should be considered in a young patient with an ICH and no history of hypertension, as an occult AVM or aneurysm may be responsible.

Cardiac arrhythmias represent another potentially catastrophic secondary complication of ICH, especially those that occur in the right hemisphere insular region. Dysfunction of this area has a propensity for causing abnormal cardiac electrical activity and "cerebrogenic sudden death" (76). Patients with such lesions must have close cardiac monitoring in the ICU during their first several days after hemorrhage.

Management

The mainstays of medical treatment of acute ICH are correction of any coagulopathy and avoidance of hypertension. Most studies suggest that hematoma expansion occurs within the first several hours of onset, and therefore, treatment must begin as soon as possible (77). If the patient recently received heparin, protamine sulfate (1 mg/100 units of heparin) should be administered; this drug is given carefully to avoid hypotension. Patients anticoagulated with warfarin with an elevated international normalized ratio (INR) should be reversed with vitamin K (10 mg intravenously administered over 15 to 20 minutes to prevent anaphylactoid reaction); prothrombin complex concentrates (PCCs) are being favored over fresh frozen plasma due to quicker reversal of anticoagulation and fewer adverse effects, but it remains unclear if outcomes differ (78). Now there is increasing use of novel oral anticoagulants, including dabigatran (a direct thrombin inhibitor) and apixaban and rivaroxaban (both factor Xa inhibitors), for nonvalvular atrial fibrillation; however, there are no clear antidotes should hemorrhagic complications arise, but PCCs are being used controversially (79).

Beyond the first few hours after onset, aggressive lowering of blood pressure may be potentially harmful. Large hemorrhages will lead to increased ICP, and attention must be focused on maintaining the cerebral perfusion pressure (subtracting the ICP from the mean arterial pressure [MAP – ICP]) >70 mmHg to avoid secondary ischemia. Based on available evidence, the American Stroke Association recommends for ICH patients presenting with elevated systolic blood pressures between 150 and 220 mmHg, lowering blood pressures to 140 mmHg is safe (78); commonly used anti-hypertensives include labetalol and nicardipine.

Seizures—occasionally nonconvulsive—occur commonly after ICH. The published incidence rates vary from 4% in unmonitored populations (80) to 28% in patients with continuous electrophysiologic monitoring in a neurocritical care unit (81). Prophylactic anticonvulsant medications, though not routinely recommended, may be considered for patients with cortical involvement. If seizures are confirmed, they should be treated aggressively. Phenytoin remains the preferred first-line agent, as it is nonsedating, and loading doses can be given intravenously. Loading doses are 15 to 20 mg/kg and should be given as fosphenytoin if needed quickly to avoid hypotension and potential toxic infusion reactions. Maintenance doses are often 4 to 5 mg/kg/d and may be given slowly. Total serum levels of phenytoin should be followed daily, at least initially. Free levels may be necessary, as phenytoin is protein bound, and critically ill patients are very frequently protein depleted. Additional anticonvulsants should be added as necessary. The duration of therapy with anticonvulsants is unclear, but in seizure-free nonepileptic patients, anticonvulsant medications are often arbitrarily withdrawn after 4 to 6 weeks of therapy.

Other general supportive care measures are similar to those described above for ischemic stroke, including attention to DVT prophylaxis, and treatment of hyperthermia and hyperglycemia. Patients with increased ICP often develop disturbances of free-water homeostasis in the form of either hyponatremia or hypernatremia. As with ischemic stroke, corticosteroids for treatment of edema are of no benefit and actually increase morbidity (82).

Treatment of increased ICP should initially focus on more conservative noninvasive measures, such as keeping the head of the bed at 30 degrees, hyperventilation if intubated, and osmolar therapy with hypertonic saline or mannitol. An implanted ICP monitor should be considered for those patients with large hematomas. This will inform the decision to place an intraventricular drain or perform a surgical evacuation.

In general, patients with a GCS of 4 or more have a uniformly poor outcome, whether or not surgery is performed, and thus these patients should be treated medically. Patients with cerebellar hemorrhages >3 cm in diameter should be considered for emergency decompression, especially if there are signs of brainstem compression, hydrocephalus, or neurologic deterioration (78); whether surgery is indicated in most other patients is not clear. Clinicians treating patients who deteriorate despite maximal medical therapy may turn to hematoma evacuation via surgical decompression or minimally invasive means, but results from clinical trials have been mixed (83–86). Patients with lobar hemorrhages secondary to amyloid angiopathy have exceptionally friable cortical blood vessels and are poor surgical candidates.

ANEURYSMAL SUBARACHNOID HEMORRHAGE

SAH is a relatively uncommon but often devastating type of stroke. Incidence is estimated at 30,000 patients per year in the United States, with a mortality that exceeds 50%. Whereas head trauma is the most frequent cause of SAH, aneurysmal rupture results in the greatest morbidity and mortality. Clinically, this is an apoplectic disorder. Most commonly, patients perceive a sudden severe headache with rapid impairment of consciousness, both symptoms related to the sudden release of irritating blood products into the meningeal spaces surrounding the brain. Focal neurologic symptoms such as hemiparesis, sensory loss, or diplopia may occur if loculation of subarachnoid blood or intraparenchymal extension of the hemorrhage develops. The most important features of the neurologic examination are the assessment of level of consciousness, cranial nerve function, and motor function. Clinical severity of SAH is graded on these findings (87) (grades I to V) and can be a rough prognostic indicator.

Diagnosis

Diagnosis of SAH is based on neuroimaging or cerebrospinal fluid (CSF) analysis. Brain CT scan is a very sensitive indicator of the presence of subarachnoid blood, although close examination must be paid to the subarachnoid spaces surrounding the brainstem and over the cerebral convexities (Fig. 124.5). Brain parenchyma itself most commonly displays no acute

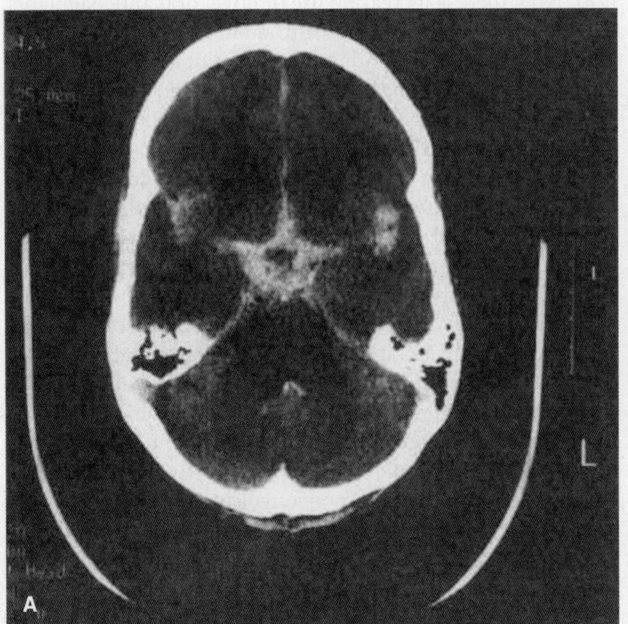

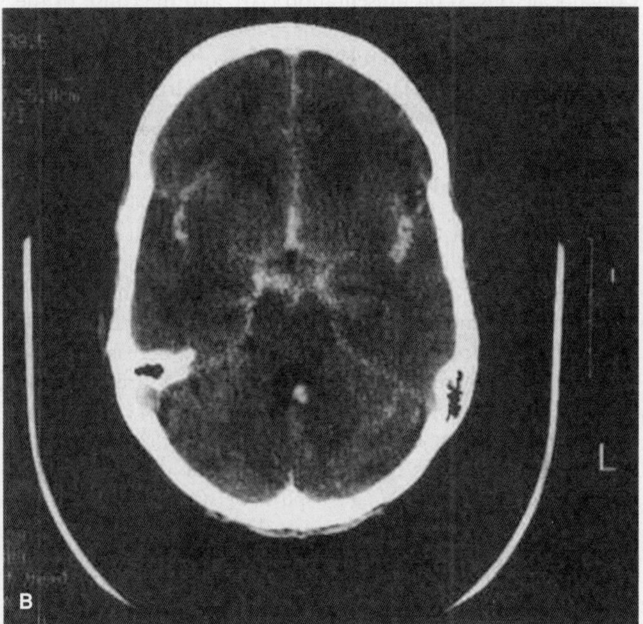

FIGURE 124.5 Subarachnoid hemorrhage. Blood is imaged as hyperdense fluid within the cisterns surrounding the brainstem and within bilateral Sylvian fissures.

abnormalities. Erythrocyte concentration in CSF below approximately 30,000 cells/µL may not result in the diagnostic increased density within CSF on CT scans. In approximately 10% of patients, diagnosis therefore requires CSF analysis through lumbar puncture. In addition to elevated erythrocyte count, CSF xanthochromia and elevation of CSF D-dimer can often be detected in true SAH. The latter two findings may help distinguish bloody CSF from a "traumatic tap," as these serve as markers of the breakdown of thrombosis or blood products. Serial cell counts should always be obtained, however, whenever SAH is suspected. Cell counts in SAH should be roughly equivalent in all tubes, whereas a declining count is usual in traumatic punctures. It should be stressed that lumbar puncture should be avoided in any patient with a depressed level of consciousness until CT scan excludes a focal mass (such as intraparenchymal or subdural hemorrhage). If bacterial meningitis is a concern, blood cultures should be obtained and antibiotics started while awaiting results of the CT scan.

Management

Patients with acute SAH are at high risk for a multitude of complications (Table 124.8) (88) that usually mandate admission to an intensive care facility. All patients should be placed on strict bed rest, with appropriate precautions for DVT and aspiration. Patients with progressive lethargy may require intubation for airway protection and mechanical ventilation. Until the aneurysm has been ablated, blood pressure should be kept in the normotensive range, and isotonic IV fluids should be used to maintain normovolemia. All patients should be started on nimodipine at 60 mg every 4 hours (duration 21 days), either orally or through a nasogastric tube, for prevention of vasospasm (see below).

Clinical seizures occur in less than 7% of patients with SAH and are often the result of re-rupture from an unsecured aneurysm (89). Historically, patients were placed on prophylactic anticonvulsants, but this practice has recently come into question, as patients who were on prophylactic anticonvulsants had significantly more in-hospital complications and worse clinical outcomes (90). If prophylactic anticonvulsant therapy is ultimately used, it has been recommended that it be discontinued after 7 days. Continuous electroencephalography should be utilized to detect sublinical seizures, especially among those with poor-grade SAH and those with an undetermined cause for neurologic decline (89).

ECG changes and elevations in cardiac enzymes, troponin, and CK-MB are commonly seen in SAH patients and may represent the phenomenon of stunned myocardium, in which case management should be aimed at optimizing left ventricular function to support cardiovascular and cerebrovascular perfusion (91–94). Serum electrolytes are closely monitored, as hyponatremia may be seen in more than 30% of patients after SAH; however, hypernatremia can occur as well and is significantly associated with clinical outcome (95). The cause of hyponatremia after SAH is most commonly reported to be due to syndrome of inappropriate antidiuretic hormone (SIADH) but can also be due to cerebral salt-wasting (CSW) syndrome and other causes (96). It is intuitive that SIADH and CSW are *not* treated in the same manner.

Serum glucose levels should also be closely monitored, as hyperglycemia has been significantly associated with mortality and poor functional outcome in SAH patients (97). Because fever in SAH patients has been associated with mortality and poor clinical outcome (96), and has even been linked to vasospasm (98), patients should be kept normothermic. Platelet levels should be monitored, as a relatively significant incidence of heparin-induced thrombocytopenia has been reported in SAH patients (99).

Rebleeding

In those patients surviving the initial hemorrhage, *the leading factor associated with mortality is rebleeding from the aneurysm.* A second bleed from an aneurysm is associated with a 74% mortality rate (100). Untreated aneurysms rebleed at a rate of 5% to 10% over the first 72 hours after initial hemorrhage (89). Thus, early treatment to secure a ruptured aneurysm is critical (101). We have adopted a protocol of treating aneurysms in the ultra-early period (less than 24 hours after presentation). Early treatment of the ruptured aneurysm also allows aggressive management of vasospasm, which requires manipulations that would increase the risk of rebleeding from an unsecured aneurysm.

Vasospasm

After rebleeding, vasospasm is the next leading cause of mortality and morbidity from an SAH (102). The exact cause of arterial vasospasm following SAH is unknown, but its incidence does appear to be correlated with the density of blood products seen

TABLE 124.8 Complications of Subarachnoid Hemorrhage

Complication	Clinical Features	Diagnostic Tests	Therapy
Increased ICP	Decreased alertness, worsened headache, herniation syndrome	ICP monitor	Mannitol, steroids, hyperventilation
Hydrocephalus	Decreased alertness, worsened headache, herniation syndrome	CT scan	Ventriculostomy drainage or shunt
Vasospasm	Delayed focal neurologic deficit	TCD, angiography	Nimodipine, hypervolemia, hypertension, angioplasty
Rebleed	Worsened neurologic condition, especially level of consciousness	CT scan, lumbar puncture	Ablation of aneurysm
Seizure	Sudden behavioral change or uncontrolled motor activity	EEG	Anticonvulsants
Hyponatremia	Confusion, seizure	Serum electrolytes	Isotonic fluids to achieve euvolemia or hypervolemia
Infection	Confusion, lethargy	Panculture, chest radiograph, urinalysis	Appropriate antibiotic

ICP, intracranial pressure; CT, computed tomography; TCD, transcranial Doppler; EEG, electroencephalogram.

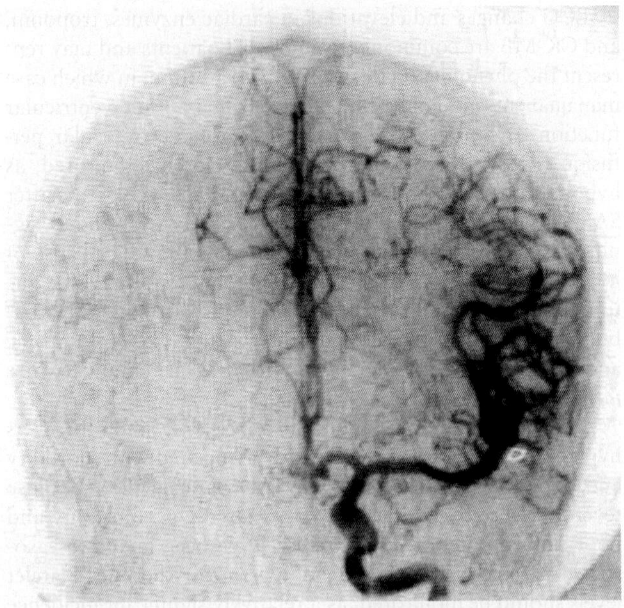

FIGURE 124.6 Aneurysm at the bifurcation of the left middle cerebral artery demonstrated by angiography. (Courtesy of R. Nick Bryan, MD, Baylor College of Medicine, Houston, TX.)

on CT scan, the basis for the Fisher score to predict vasospasm (103,104). Severe vasospasm may result in cerebral infarction within the vascular distribution of the involved artery. The risk for vasospasm begins about 3 days after the bleed and may persist for 3 weeks. TCD is a sensitive, noninvasive indicator of the presence and degree of vasospasm within proximal arteries, although it may not detect vasospasm restricted to smaller peripheral vessels. This technique may be used daily to guide and monitor management strategies. Modern techniques, such as CTA and CTP studies, have been reported to be successful in diagnosing vasospasm (Fig. 124.6) (105).

Nimodipine, a calcium channel blocker, has been shown to improve outcomes after aneurysmal SAH by limiting delayed cerebral ischemia from vasospasm (106). Trials with magnesium sulfate have yielded promising results in reducing vasospasm (107–109) or achieving better clinical outcomes in patients (110) but its use still remains investigational. Studies with statin therapy (HMG Co-A inhibitors), such as pravastatin and simvastatin, have demonstrated promising results with reduced rates of vasospasm and better clinical outcomes (111–114).

Once the aneurysm is secured, vasospasm can be managed aggressively. Previously, triple-H therapy—hypertension, hypervolemia, hemodilution—was the first-line therapy against vasospasm but has fallen out of favor. The maintenance of euvolemia has been practiced in order to prevent cardiac and pulmonary complications from hypervolemic treatment. Blood pressure can be augmented if symptomatic vasospasm occurs with the assistance of vasopressors (e.g., phenylephrine, 0.1 to 5 μg/kg/min or vasopressin, 0.01 to 0.04 units/min), targeting MAPs of 120 to 140 mmHg (or systolic blood pressures 180 to 200 mmHg). Close cardiac monitoring should be undertaken including that of cardiac output and risk of ischemia. The use of hemodilution is only supported in the presence of erythrocythemia (93).

For symptomatic vasospasm refractory to these therapies, endovascular interventions can be performed, such as percutaneous transluminal balloon angioplasty and/or intra-arterial administration of calcium channel blockers or other vasodilating agents (115,116) may be considered in experienced hands. Even using the most aggressive management strategies, vasospasm remains a leading cause of morbidity and mortality after SAH.

Acute Hydrocephalus

Acute hydrocephalus occurs in approximately 20% of survivors of SAH, either as a result of direct obstruction of CSF channels or by impeding CSF absorption at arachnoid granulations. The likelihood of hydrocephalus increases with worsening grade of hemorrhage. Ventriculostomy drainage is recommended for patients with acute hydrocephalus and decreased level of consciousness; improvement can be expected in over 50% of patients.

Key Points

- The first concern is to establish the diagnosis of stroke and determine if the patient is a candidate for thrombolytic therapy.
- Strokes may be ischemic, resulting from the occlusion of small or large arteries, or hemorrhagic, resulting from the rupture of a conducting artery or an intraparenchymal arteriole.
- An abrupt focal lateralizing neurologic deficit attributable to a cerebrovascular distribution is the hallmark of ischemic stroke.
- A depressed level of consciousness is rarely the presenting symptom of ischemic stroke and much more commonly occurs in the setting of a hemorrhagic event.
- Patients with acute ischemic stroke may be candidates for thrombolytic therapy, but the therapeutic window is extremely narrow, so timely diagnosis and evaluation is of the utmost importance.
- A CT scan of the brain is critical for the initial evaluation and management of the stroke patient. Additionally, when available, CTA and CTP studies may aid in diagnosis and management.
- MRI is more sensitive than CT, but it is usually less available urgently, and patients must remain still for a much longer period of time.
- Vascular ultrasound allows rapid bedside assessment of abnormal flow within the major intracranial and extracranial arteries and can provide valuable immediate information about the vascular physiology to supplement the anatomic information provided by the CT scan.
- A transthoracic or transesophageal echocardiogram may identify potential cardiac sources of cerebral emboli.
- An electrocardiogram (ECG) followed by continuous cardiac telemetry monitoring is often necessary to identify arrhythmias associated with stroke.
- A lumbar puncture may be necessary to rule out SAH in patients in whom the diagnosis is strongly suspected but CT is unrevealing.
- Thrombolytics are the mainstay of treatment of acute ischemic stroke in eligible patients.
- Careful attention to blood pressure may reduce complications such as hemorrhage.

- Supportive care, with special attention paid to prevention of aspiration pneumonia and DVT, is essential to reduce mortality associated with stroke.
- Rapid initiations of secondary preventive therapies are effective in reducing risk for recurrent stroke.
- Certain patients, such as those with large ischemic or hemorrhagic strokes, will require monitoring of ICP and, potentially, decompressive surgery.

References

1. Norris JW, Hachinski VC. Misdiagnosis of stroke. *Lancet.* 1982;1(8267):328–331.
2. Inzitari D, Eliasziw M, Gates P, et al. The causes and risk of stroke in patients with asymptomatic internal-carotid-artery stenosis. North American Symptomatic Carotid Endarterectomy Trial Collaborators. *N Engl J Med.* 2000;342(23):1693–1700.
3. Fisher CM. The arterial lesions underlying lacunes. *Acta Neuropathol.* 1968;12(1):1–15.
4. Bogousslavsky J, Van Melle G, Regli F. The Lausanne Stroke Registry: analysis of 1,000 consecutive patients with first stroke. *Stroke.* 1988;19(9):1083–1092.
5. Mohr JP, Caplan LR, Melski JW, et al. The Harvard Cooperative Stroke Registry: a prospective registry. *Neurology.* 1978;28(8):754–762.
6. Pruitt AA, Rubin RH, Karchmer AW, Duncan GW. Neurologic complications of bacterial endocarditis. *Medicine (Baltimore).* 1978;57(4):329–343.
7. Roeltgen DP, Weimer GR, Patterson LF. Delayed neurologic complications of left atrial myxoma. *Neurology.* 1981;31(1):8–13.
8. Bogousslavsky J, Pierre P. Ischemic stroke in patients under age 45. *Neurol Clin.* 1992;10(1):113–124.
9. Kalb R. Spontaneous dissection of the carotid and vertebral arteries. *N Engl J Med.* 2001;345(6):467.
10. Ay H, Arsava EM, Saribas O. Creatine kinase-MB elevation after stroke is not cardiac in origin: comparison with troponin T levels. *Stroke.* 2002;33(1):286–289.
11. Hankey GJ, Eikelboom JW, van Bockxmeer FM, et al. Inherited thrombophilia in ischemic stroke and its pathogenic subtypes. *Stroke.* 2001;32(8):1793–1799.
12. Hankey GJ, Warlow CP, Sellar RJ. Cerebral angiographic risk in mild cerebrovascular disease. *Stroke.* 1990;21(2):209–222.
13. Alexandrov AV, Molina CA, Grotta JC, et al.; CLOTBUST Investigators. Ultrasound-enhanced systemic thrombolysis for acute ischemic stroke. *N Engl J Med.* 2004;351(21):2170–2178.
14. DeRook FA, Comess KA, Albers GA, Popp RL. Transesophageal echocardiography in the evaluation of stroke. *Ann Intern Med.* 1992;117(11):922–932.
15. Tissue plasminogen activator for acute ischemic stroke. The National Institute of Neurological Disorders and Stroke rt-PA Stroke Study Group. *N Engl J Med.* 1995;333(24):1581–1587.
16. Hacke W, Kaste M, Fieschi C, et al. Intravenous thrombolysis with recombinant tissue plasminogen activator for acute hemispheric stroke. The European Cooperative Acute Stroke Study (ECASS). *JAMA.* 1995;274(13):1017–1025.
17. Hacke W, Kaste M, Fieschi C, et al. Randomised double-blind placebo-controlled trial of thrombolytic therapy with intravenous alteplase in acute ischaemic stroke (ECASS II). Second European-Australasian Acute Stroke Study Investigators. *Lancet.* 1998;352(9136):1245–1251.
18. Clark WM, Albers GW, Madden KP, Hamilton S. The rtPA (alteplase) 0- to 6-hour acute stroke trial, part A (A0276g): results of a double-blind, placebo-controlled, multicenter study. Thrombolytic therapy in acute ischemic stroke study investigators. *Stroke.* 2000;31(4):811–816.
19. Clark WM, Wissman S, Albers GW, et al. Recombinant tissue-type plasminogen activator (Alteplase) for ischemic stroke 3 to 5 hours after symptom onset. The ATLANTIS Study: a randomized controlled trial. Alteplase Thrombolysis for Acute Noninterventional Therapy in Ischemic Stroke. *JAMA.* 1999;282(21):2019–2026.
20. Hacke W, Kaste M, Bluhmki E, et al.; ECASS Investigators. Thrombolysis with alteplase 3 to 4.5 hours after acute ischemic stroke. *N Engl J Med.* 2008;359:1317–1329.
21. Davis SM, Donnan GA, Parsons MW, et al.; EPITHET investigators. Effects of alteplase beyond 3 h after stroke in the Echoplanar Imaging Thrombolytic Evaluation Trial (EPITHET): a placebo-controlled randomised trial. *Lancet Neurol.* 2008;7:299–309.
22. IST-3 Collaborative Group, Sandercock P, Wardlaw JM, et al. The benefits and harms of intravenous thrombolysis with recombinant tissue plasminogen activator within 6 h of acute ischemic stroke (the third international stroke trial [IST-3]): a randomised controlled trial. *Lancet.* 2012;379:2352–2363.
23. Emberson J, Lees KR, Lyden P, et al.; Stroke Thrombolysis Trialists' Collaborative Group. Effect of treatment delay, age, and stroke severity on the effects of intravenous thrombolysis with alteplase for acute ischemic stroke: a meta-analysis of individual patient data from randomised trials. *Lancet.* 2014;384(9958):1929–1935.
24. del Zoppo GJ, Saver JL, Jauch EC, Adams HP Jr; American Heart Association Stroke Council. Expansion of the time window for treatment of acute ischemic stroke with intravenous tissue plasminogen activator. A Science Advisory from the American Heart Association/American Stroke Association. *Stroke.* 2009;40:2945–2948.
25. Wechsler LR, Jovin TG. Intravenous recombinant tissue-type plasminogen activator in the extended time window and the US Food and Drug Administration: confused about the time. *Stroke.* 2012;43(9):2517–2519.
26. Saver JL. Number needed to treat estimates incorporating effects over the entire range of clinical outcomes: novel derivation method and application to thrombolytic therapy for acute stroke. *Arch Neurol.* 2004;61(7):1066–1070.
27. Saver JL. Hemorrhage after thrombolytic therapy for stroke: the clinically relevant number needed to harm. *Stroke.* 2007;38(8):2279–2283.
28. Olsen TS, Weber UJ, Kammersgaard LP. Therapeutic hypothermia for acute stroke. *Lancet Neurol.* 2003;2(7):410–416.
29. del Zoppo GJ, Higashida RT, Furlan AJ, et al. PROACT: a phase II randomized trial of recombinant pro-urokinase by direct arterial delivery in acute middle cerebral artery stroke. PROACT Investigators. Prolyse in acute cerebral thromboembolism. *Stroke.* 1998;29(1):4–11.
30. Smith WS, Sung G, Starkman S, et al.; MERCI Trial Investigators. Safety and efficacy of mechanical embolectomy in acute ischemic stroke: results of the MERCI trial. *Stroke.* 2005;36(7):1432–1438.
31. Broderick JP, Palesch YY, Demchuk AM, et al.; Interventional Management of Stroke (IMS) III Investigators. Endovascular therapy after intravenous t-PA versus t-PA alone for stroke. *N Engl J Med.* 2013;368(10):893–903.
32. Ciccone A, Valvassori L, Nichelatti M, et al.; SYNTHESIS Expansion Investigators. Endovascular treatment for acute ischemic stroke. *N Engl J Med.* 2013;368(10):904–913.
33. Kidwell CS, Jahan R, Gornbein J et al.; MR RESCUE Investigators. A trial of imaging selection and endovascular treatment for ischemic stroke. *N Engl J Med.* 2013;368(10):914–923.
34. Berkhemer OA, Fransen PS, Beumer D et al.; MR CLEAN Investigators. A randomized trial of intraarterial treatment for acute ischemic stroke. *N Engl J Med.* 2015;372(1):11–20.
35. Goyal M, Demchuk AM, Menon BK, et al.; ESCAPE Trial Investigators. Randomized assessment of rapid endovascular treatment of ischemic stroke. *N Engl J Med.* 2015;372(11):1019–1030.
36. Campbell BC, Mitchell PJ, Kleinig TJ et al.; EXTEND-IA Investigators. Endovascular therapy for ischemic stroke with perfusion-imaging selection. *N Engl J Med.* 2015;372(11):1009–1018.
37. Saver JL, Goyal M, Bonafe A et al.; SWIFT PRIME Investigators. Stent-retriever thrombectomy after intravenous t-PA vs. t-PA alone in stroke. *N Engl J Med.* 2015;372:2285–2295.
38. Jovin TG, Chamarro A, Cobo E et al.; REVASCAT Trial Investigators. Thrombectomy within 8 Hours after Symptom Onset in Ischemic Stroke. *N Engl J Med.* 2015;372:2296–2306.
39. Amenta PS, Ali MS, Dumont AS, et al. Computed tomography perfusion-based selection of patients for endovascular recanalization. *Neurosurg Focus.* 2011;30(6):E6.
40. Powers WJ, Derdeyn CP, Biller J, et al.; American Heart Association Stroke Council. 2015 American Heart Association/American Stroke Association Focused Update of the 2013 Guidelines for the early management of patients with acute ischemic stroke regarding endovascular treatment. *Stroke.* 2015;46:3020–3035.
41. Jemal A, Ward E, Hao Y, Thun M. Trends in the leading causes of death in the United States, 1970–2002. *JAMA.* 2005;294(10):1255–1259.
42. Heuschmann PU, Berger K, Misselwitz B, et al. Frequency of thrombolytic therapy in patients with acute ischemic stroke and the risk of in-hospital mortality: The German Stroke Registers Study Group. *Stroke.* 2003;34(5):1106–1112.
43. Koennecke HC, Nohr R, Leistner S, Marx P. Intravenous tPA for ischemic stroke team performance over time, safety, and efficacy in a single-center, 2-year experience. *Stroke.* 2001;32(5):1074–1078.
44. Aslanyan S, Weir CJ, Diener HC, et al.; GAIN International Steering Committee and Investigators. Pneumonia and urinary tract infection after acute

ischaemic stroke: a tertiary analysis of the GAIN International trial. *Eur J Neurol.* 2004;11(1):49–53.
45. Addington WR, Stephens RE, Gilliland KA. Assessing the laryngeal cough reflex and the risk of developing pneumonia after stroke: an interhospital comparison. *Stroke.* 1999;30(6):1203–1207.
46. Choi-Kwon S, Yang YH, Kim EK, et al. Nutritional status in acute stroke: undernutrition versus overnutrition in different stroke subtypes. *Acta Neurol Scand.* 1998;98(3):187–192.
47. Wijdicks EF, Scott JP. Pulmonary embolism associated with acute stroke. *Mayo Clin Proc.* 1997;72(4):297–300.
48. Sherman DG, Albers GW, Bladin C, et al.; PREVAIL Investigators. The efficacy and safety of enoxaparin versus unfractionated heparin for the prevention of venous thromboembolism after acute ischaemic stroke (PREVAIL Study): an open-label randomised comparison. *Lancet.* 2007;369(9570):1347–1355.
49. Jauch EC, Saver JL, Adams HP Jr, et al. Guidelines for the early management of adults with ischemic stroke: a guideline from the American Heart Association/American Stroke Association. *Stroke.* 2013;44(3):870–947.
50. Williams LS, Rotich J, Qi R, et al. Effects of admission hyperglycemia on mortality and costs in acute ischemic stroke. *Neurology.* 2002;59(1):67–71.
51. Baird TA, Parsons MW, Phan T, et al. Persistent poststroke hyperglycemia is independently associated with infarct expansion and worse clinical outcome. *Stroke.* 2003;34(9):2208–2214.
52. Maramattom BV, Bahn MM, Wijdicks EF. Which patient fares worse after early deterioration due to swelling from hemispheric stroke? *Neurology.* 2004;63(11):2142–2145.
53. Ropper AH, Shafran B. Brain edema after stroke. Clinical syndrome and intracranial pressure. *Arch Neurol.* 1984;41(1):26–29.
54. Qureshi AI, Suarez JI, Yahia AM, et al. Timing of neurologic deterioration in massive middle cerebral artery infarction: a multicenter review. *Crit Care Med.* 2003;31(1):272–277.
55. Tellez H, Bauer RB. Dexamethasone as treatment in cerebrovascular disease. 1. A controlled study in intracerebral hemorrhage. *Stroke.* 1973;4(4):541–546.
56. Bauer RB, Tellez H. Dexamethasone as treatment in cerebrovascular disease. 2. A controlled study in acute cerebral infarction. *Stroke.* 1973;4(4):547–555.
57. Videen TO, Zazulia AR, Manno EM, et al. Mannitol bolus preferentially shrinks non-infarcted brain in patients with ischemic stroke. *Neurology.* 2001;57(11):2120–2122.
58. Gupta R, Connolly ES, Mayer S, Elkind MS. Hemicraniectomy for massive middle cerebral artery territory infarction: a systematic review. *Stroke.* 2004;35(2):539–543.
59. Hofmeijer J, Kappelle LJ, Algra A, et al. Surgical decompression for space-occupying cerebral infarction (the Hemicraniectomy After Middle Cerebral Artery infarction with Life-threatening Edema Trial [HAMLET]): a multicentre, open, randomised trial. *Lancet Neurol.* 2009;8(4):326–333.
60. Vahedi K, Vicaut E, Mateo J, et al.; DECIMAL Investigators. Sequential-design, multicenter, randomized, controlled trial of early decompressive craniectomy in malignant middle cerebral artery infarction (DECIMAL Trial). *Stroke.* 2007;38(9):2506–2517.
61. Juttler E, Schwab S, Schmiedek P, et al.; DESTINY Study Group. Decompressive surgery for the treatment of malignant infarction of the middle cerebral artery (DESTINY): a randomized, controlled trial. *Stroke.* 2007;38(9):2518–2525.
62. Vahedi K, Hofmeijer J, Juettler E, et al.; DECIMAL, DESTINY, and HAMLET investigators. Early decompressive surgery in malignant infarction of the middle cerebral artery: a pooled analysis of three randomised controlled trials. *Lancet Neurol.* 2007;6:215–222.
63. Holtkamp M, Buchheim K, Unterberg A, et al. Hemicraniectomy in elderly patients with space occupying media infarction: improved survival but poor functional outcome. *J Neurol Neurosurg Psychiatry.* 2001;70(2):226–228.
64. Flaherty ML, Woo D, Haverbusch M, et al. Racial variations in location and risk of intracerebral hemorrhage. *Stroke.* 2005;36(5):934–937.
65. Tonk M, Haan J. A review of genetic causes of ischemic and hemorrhagic stroke. *J Neurol Sci.* 2007;257(1–2):273–279.
66. Yoon BW, Bae HJ, Hong KS, et al.; Acute Brain Bleeding Analysis (ABBA) Study Investigators. Phenylpropanolamine contained in cold remedies and risk of hemorrhagic stroke. *Neurology.* 2007;68(2):146–149.
67. Monforte R, Estruch R, Graus F, et al. High ethanol consumption as risk factor for intracerebral hemorrhage in young and middle-aged people. *Stroke.* 1990;21(11):1529–1532.
68. Anderson CS, Chakera TM, Stewart-Wynne EG, Jamrozik KD. Spectrum of primary intracerebral haemorrhage in Perth, Western Australia, 1989–90: incidence and outcome. *J Neurol Neurosurg Psychiatry.* 1994;57(8):936–940.
69. Broderick JP, Brott TG, Duldner JE, et al. Volume of intracerebral hemorrhage. A powerful and easy-to-use predictor of 30-day mortality. *Stroke.* 1993;24(7):987–993.
70. Tuhrim S, Dambrosia JM, Price TR, et al. Prediction of intracerebral hemorrhage survival. *Ann Neurol.* 1988;24(2):258–263.
71. Tuhrim S, Horowitz DR, Sacher M, Godbold JH. Validation and comparison of models predicting survival following intracerebral hemorrhage. *Crit Care Med.* 1995;23(5):950–954.
72. Tuhrim S, Horowitz DR, Sacher M, Godbold JH. Volume of ventricular blood is an important determinant of outcome in supratentorial intracerebral hemorrhage. *Crit Care Med.* 1999;27(3):617–621.
73. Diringer MN, Edwards DF, Zazulia AR. Hydrocephalus: a previously unrecognized predictor of poor outcome from supratentorial intracerebral hemorrhage. *Stroke.* 1998;29(7):1352–1357.
74. Becker KJ, Baxter AB, Bybee HM, et al. Extravasation of Radiographic Contrast Is an Independent Predictor of Death in Primary Intracerebral Hemorrhage. *Stroke.* 1999;30(10):2025–2032.
75. Greenberg SM, Finklestein SP, Schaefer PW. Petechial hemorrhages accompanying lobar hemorrhage: detection by gradient-echo MRI. *Neurology.* 1996;46(6):1751–1754.
76. Cheung RT, Hachinski V. The insula and cerebrogenic sudden death. *Arch Neurol.* 2000;57(12):1685–1688.
77. Kazui S, Naritomi H, Yamamoto H, et al. Enlargement of spontaneous intracerebral hemorrhage. Incidence and time course. *Stroke.* 1996;27(10):1783–1787.
78. Hemphill JC 3rd, Greenberg SM, Anderson CS, et al. Guidelines for the management of spontaneous intracerebral hemorrhage: a guideline for professionals from the American Heart Association/American Stroke Association. *Stroke.* 2015;46:2032–2060.
79. Aguilar MI, Kuo RS, Freeman WD. New anticoagulants (dabigatran, apixaban, rivaroxaban) for stroke prevention in atrial fibrillation. *Neurol Clin.* 2013;31(3):659–675.
80. Passero S, Rocchi R, Rossi S, et al. Seizures after spontaneous supratentorial intracerebral hemorrhage. *Epilepsia.* 2002;43(10):1175–1180.
81. Vespa PM, O'Phelan K, Shah M, et al. Acute seizures after intracerebral hemorrhage: a factor in progressive midline shift and outcome. *Neurology.* 2003;60(9):1441–1446.
82. Poungvarin N, Bhoopat W, Viriyavejakul A, et al. Effects of dexamethasone in primary supratentorial intracerebral hemorrhage. *N Engl J Med.* 1987;316(20):1229–1233.
83. Morgenstern LB, Frankowski RF, Shedden P, et al. Surgical treatment for intracerebral hemorrhage (STICH): a single-center, randomized clinical trial. *Neurology.* 1998;51(5):1359–1363.
84. Auer LM, Deinsberger W, Niederkorn K, et al. Endoscopic surgery versus medical treatment for spontaneous intracerebral hematoma: a randomized study. *J Neurosurg.* 1989;70(4):530–535.
85. Mould WA, Carhuapoma JR, Muschelli J et al.; MISTIE Investigators. Minimally invasiave surgery plus recombinant tissue-type plasminogen activator for intracerebral hemorrhage evacuation decreases perihematomal edema. *Stroke.* 2013;44(3):627–634.
86. Mendelow AD, Gregson BA, Rowan EN et al.; STICH II Investigators. Early surgery versus initial conservative treatment in patients with spontaneous supratentorial lobar intracerebral haematomas (STICH II): a randomised trial. *Lancet.* 2013;382(9890):397–408.
87. Hunt WE, Hess RM. Surgical risk as related to the time of intervention in the repair of intracranial aneurysms. *J Neurosurg.* 1968;28:14–20.
88. Connolly ES Jr, Rabinstein AA, Carhuapoma JR, et al. Guidelines for the management of aneurysmal subarachnoid hemorrhage: a guideline for healthcare professionals from the American Heart Association/American Stroke Association. *Stroke.* 2012;43(6):1711–1737.
89. Diringer MN, Bleck TP, Claude Hemphill J 3rd, et al.; Neurocritical Care Society. Critical care management of patients following aneurysmal subarachnoid hemorrhage: recommendations from the Neurocritical Care Society's Multidisciplinary Consensus Conference. *Neurocrit Care.* 2011;15(2):211–240.
90. Rosengart AJ, Huo JD, Tolentino J, et al. Outcome in patients with subarachnoid hemorrhage treated with antiepileptic drugs. *J Neurosurg.* 2007;107:253–260.
91. Urbaniak K, Merchant AI, Amin-Hanjani S, Roitberg B. Cardiac complications after aneurysmal subarachnoid hemorrhage. *Surg Neurology.* 2007;67:21–28.
92. Banki NM, Kopelnik A, Dae MW, et al. Acute neurocardiogenic injury after subarachnoid hemorrhage. *Circulation.* 2005;112:3314–3319.
93. Naidech AM, Kreiter KT, Janjua N, et al. Cardiac troponin elevation, cardiovascular morbidity, and outcome after subarachnoid hemorrhage. *Circulation.* 2005;112:2851–2856.

94. Deibert E, Barzilai B, Braverman AC, et al. Clinical significance of elevated troponin I levels in patients with nontraumatic subarachnoid hemorrhage. *J Neurosurg.* 2003;98:741–746.
95. Qureshi AI, Suri MF, Sung GY, et al. Prognostic significance of hypernatremia and hyponatremia among patients with aneurysmal subarachnoid hemorrhage. *Neurosurgery.* 2002;50:749–755.
96. Sherlock M, O'Sullivan E, Agha A, et al. The incidence and pathophysiology of hyponatremia after subarachnoid haemorrhage. *Clin Endocrinol (Oxf).* 2006;64:250–254.
97. Wartenberg KE, Schmidt JM, Claassen J, et al. Impact of medical complication on outcome after subarachnoid hemorrhage. *Crit Care Med.* 2006;34:617–623.
98. Oliveira-Filho J, Ezzeddine MA, Segal AZ, et al. Fever in subarachnoid hemorrhage—relationship to vasospasm and outcome. *Neurology.* 2001; 56:1299–1304.
99. Hoh BL, Aghi M, Pryor JC, Ogilvy CS. Heparin-induced thrombocytopenia Type II in subarachnoid hemorrhage patients—incidence and complications. *Neurosurgery.* 2005;57:243–248; discussion 243–248.
100. Juvela S. Rebleeding from ruptured intracranial aneurysms. *Surgical Neurol.* 1989;32:323–326.
101. Lawson MF, Chi YY, Velat GJ, et al. Timing of aneurysm surgery: the International Cooperative Study revisited in the era of endovascular coiling. *J Neurointerv Surg.* 2010;2(2):131–134.
102. Hoh BL, Topcuoglu MA, Singhal AB, et al. Effect of clipping, craniotomy, or intravascular coiling on cerebral vasospasm and patient outcome after aneurysmal subarachnoid hemorrhage. *Neurosurgery.* 2004;55:779–786; discussion 786–789.
103. Fisher CM, Kistler JP, Davis JM. Relation of cerebral vasospasm to subarachnoid hemorrhage visualized by computer tomographic scanning. *Neurosurgery.* 1980;6:1–9.
104. Kistler JP, Crowell RM, Davis KR, et al. The relation of cerebral vasospasm to the extent and location of subarachnoid blood visualized by CT scan—a prospective study. *Neurology.* 1983;33:424–436.
105. Binaghi S, Colleoni ML, Maeder P, et al. CT angiography and perfusion CT in cerebral vasospasm after subarachnoid hemorrhage. *AJNR Am J Neuroradiol.* 2007;28:750–758.
106. Velat GJ, Kimball MM, Mocco JD, Hoh BL. Vasospasm after aneurysmal subarachnoid hemorrhage: review of randomized controlled trials and meta-analysis in the literature. *World Neurosurg.* 2011;76(5):446–454.
107. van den Bergh WM, Algra A, van Kooten F, et al.; MASH Study Group. Magnesium sulfate in aneurysmal subarachnoid hemorrhage—a randomized controlled trial. *Stroke.* 2005;36:1011–1015.
108. Stippler M, Crago E, Levi EI, et al. Magnesium infusion for vasospasm prophylaxis after subarachnoid hemorrhage. *J Neurosurg.* 2006;105: 723–729.
109. Schmid-Elsaesser R, Kunz M, Zausinger S, et al. Intravenous magnesium versus nimodipine in the treatment of patients with aneurysmal subarachnoid hemorrhage—a randomized study. *Neurosurgery.* 2006;58:1054–1065.
110. Muroi C, Terzic A, Fortunati M, et al. Magnesium sulfate in the management of patients with aneurysmal subarachnoid hemorrhage—a randomized, placebo-controlled, dose-adapted trial. *Surg Neurol.* 2008;69:33–39; discussion 39.
111. McGirt MJ, Blessing R, Alexander MJ, et al. Risk of cerebral vasospasm after subarachnoid hemorrhage reduced by statin therapy. A multivariate analysis of an institutional experience. *J Neurosurg.* 2006;105:671–674.
112. Lynch JR, Wang H, McGirt MJ, et al. Simvastatin reduces vasospasm after aneurysmal subarachnoid hemorrhage—results of a pilot randomized clinical trial. *Stroke.* 2005;36:2024–2026.
113. Tseng MY, Czosnyka M, Richards H, et al. Effects of acute treatment with pravastatin on cerebral vasospasm, autoregulation and delayed ischemic deficits after aneurysmal subarachnoid hemorrhage: a phase II randomized, placebo controlled trial. *Stroke.* 2005;36:1627–1632.
114. Tseng MY, Hutchinson PJ, Czosnyka M, et al. Effects of acute pravastatin treatment on intensity of rescue therapy, length of inpatient stay, and 6 month outcome in patients after aneurysmal subarachnoid hemorrhage. *Stroke.* 2007;38:1545–1550.
115. Hoh BL, Ogilvy CS. Endovascular treatment of cerebral vasospasm—transluminal balloon angioplasty, intra-arterial papaverine, and intra-arterial nicardipine. *Neurosurg Clin North Am.* 2005;16:501–516.
116. Kimball MM, Velat GJ, Hoh BL. Critical care guidelines on the endovascular management of cerebral vasospasm. *Neurocrit Care.* 2011;15(2): 336–341.

SECTION 13 GASTROINTESTINAL DISEASE AND DYSFUNCTION

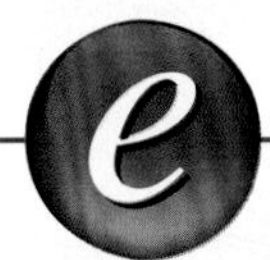

This chapter can be accessed in the accompanying eBook (see inside front cover for access instructions).

CHAPTER
125

Upper Gastrointestinal Bleeding

GÖKHAN M. MUTLU and ECE A. MUTLU

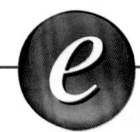

This chapter can be accessed in the accompanying eBook (see inside front cover for access instructions).

CHAPTER
126

Approach to Lower Gastrointestinal Bleeding

HSIU-PO WANG

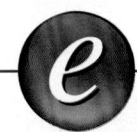

This chapter can be accessed in the accompanying eBook (see inside front cover for access instructions).

CHAPTER
127

Liver Failure: Acute and Acute-on-Chronic

CONSTANTINE KARVELLAS and R. TODD STRAVITZ

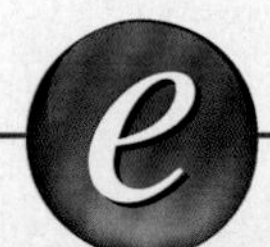

This chapter can be accessed in the accompanying eBook (see inside front cover for access instructions).

CHAPTER 128

Pancreatic Disease

FRANCISCO IGOR MACEDO and DANNY SLEEMAN

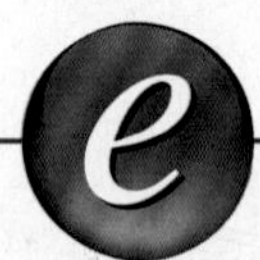

This chapter can be accessed in the accompanying eBook (see inside front cover for access instructions).

CHAPTER 129

Inflammatory Bowel Disease and Toxic Megacolon

SARAH FLORES and NIMISHA K. PAREKH

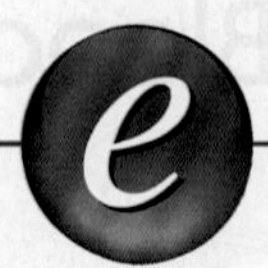

This chapter can be accessed in the accompanying eBook (see inside front cover for access instructions).

CHAPTER 130

Esophageal Disorders

PHILLIP K. HENDERSON and JACK A. DIPALMA

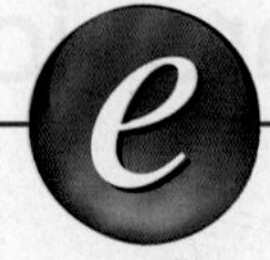

This chapter can be accessed in the accompanying eBook (see inside front cover for access instructions).

CHAPTER 131

Mesenteric Ischemia

THOMAS S. HUBER and JAVAIRIAH FATIMA

CHAPTER 132

Acute Renal Injury

RASHID ALOBAIDI, RINALDO BELLOMO, and SEAN M. BAGSHAW

INTRODUCTION

Acute kidney injury (AKI) remains a major diagnostic and therapeutic challenge for the critical care physician. The term, *AKI*, describes a syndrome characterized by a rapid decrease—that is, hours to days—in the kidney's ability to eliminate metabolic waste and maintain volume homeostasis. Such loss of function is clinically manifested by the accumulation of end products of nitrogen metabolism such as urea and creatinine. Other typical clinical manifestations include decreased urine output (although this is not always present), accumulation of nonvolatile acids, an increased concentration of potassium and phosphate, and extravascular fluid accumulation.

CONSENSUS DEFINITIONS OF AKI

There have been longstanding challenges for arriving at a unified definition of AKI. In response, a consensus definition and classification for AKI has been developed and validated in hospitalized and critically ill patients. The RIFLE classification scheme provides an operational definition for AKI and stratifies it into categories of severity (risk, injury, failure, and end-stage kidney disease) (1–3). Recently, the Kidney Disease: Improving Global Outcomes (KDIGO) AKI group proposed further refinement to this classification scheme. The KDIGO classification defines AKI as the rapid deterioration of kidney function that is associated with (a) an increase in serum creatinine by at least 0.3 mg/dL (26.5 µmol/L) within 48 hours; (b) an increase in serum creatinine at least 1.5 times above baseline over 7 days; and/or (c) oliguria with urine output below 0.5 mL/kg/hr over 6 hours (Table 132.1) (4). The KDIGO classification utilizes absolute and relative changes in serum creatinine level and urine output to define and assess the severity of kidney injury. While the KDIGO classification is an important advance in the field of AKI, the use of creatinine and urine output have limitations that will be discussed in the next section.

ASSESSMENT OF RENAL FUNCTION

Renal function is complex, involving acid–base balance, water balance, tonicity control, regulation of calcium and phosphate, erythropoiesis, disposal of selected cytokines, lactate removal, and so forth. In the clinical context, however, monitoring of renal function is reduced to the indirect assessment of glomerular filtration rate (GFR) by the measurement of serum creatinine and urea. These waste products are insensitive markers of GFR and are heavily modified by numerous factors such as age, sex, muscle mass, nutritional status, the use of steroids, the presence of gastrointestinal blood, or muscle injury. They start becoming abnormal only when GFR is reduced by over 50%, and they fail to reflect dynamic changes in GFR and can be grossly modified by aggressive fluid resuscitation. Moreover, changes to serum creatinine are often delayed, requiring more than 24 hours to reach a new steady state after acute changes to GFR (5,6). The use of creatinine clearance via a 2- or 4-hour urine collection or of calculated clearance by means of formulae might increase the accuracy of GFR estimation but rarely changes clinical management. The use of more sophisticated radionuclide-based tests is cumbersome in the ICU and useful only for research purposes.

Urine output is another commonly measured parameter of renal function and is often more sensitive to changes in renal hemodynamics than biochemical markers of solute clearance. However, urine output alone is also of limited value, with patients capable of developing severe AKI, as detected by a markedly elevated serum creatinine, while maintaining normal urine output (so-called nonoliguric AKI). Some data suggest that the use of urine output of 0.5 mL/kg/hr might be too sensitive in detecting AKI, and that lower threshold of 0.3 mL/kg/hr may better correlate with outcome (7). While an episode of oliguria may not always be followed by increments in serum creatinine consistent with AKI, oliguria still remains a valuable bedside predictor of early changes on kidney function (8,9). Recent evidence has shown a strong association between the duration and frequency of episodes of oliguria and increased risk for mortality (10,11).

Classic urine biochemistry and derived indices such as measurement of urinary sodium, fractional excretion of sodium and urea, have been promoted to help clinicians identify and classify AKI (Table 132.2). Unfortunately, their accuracy and significance are questionable (Fig. 132.1) (12–15). The clinical value of these tests in ICU patients who receive vasopressors, massive fluid resuscitation, and loop diuretics is low. Instead, recent evidence suggests urinary sediment for renal epithelial cells and casts can provide prognostic information about the risk for worsening AKI (Table 132.3). A higher urinary sediment score, defined by a greater quantity of measured cells and casts in the urine, can help discriminate AKI severity and better inform a patients' risk for worsening AKI (16).

The precise role of novel kidney damage biomarkers (e.g., cystatin C; neutrophil gelatinase-associated lipocalin [NGAL]; insulin-like growth factor-binding protein 7 [IGFBP7] and tissue inhibitor of metalloproteinases-2 [TIMP-2]; kidney injury

TABLE 132.1 KDIGO AKI Staging

Stage	Serum Creatinine	Urine Output
1	1.5–1.9 times baseline *or* Increase of ≥0.3 mg/dL (≥26.5 mmol/L)	<0.5 mL/kg/hr for 6–12 hr
2	2.0–2.9 times baseline	<0.5 mL/kg/hr for ≥12 hr
3	3.0 times baseline *or* Increase of ≥4.0 mg/dL (≥353.6 mmol/L) *or* Initiation of renal replacement therapy *or* In patients <18 yr, decrease in eGFR to <35 mL/min per 1.73 m²	<0.3 mL/kg/hr for ≥24 hr *or* Anuria for ≥12 hr

molecule-1 [KIM-1]; interleukin-18 [IL-18]; L-type fatty acid binding protein (L-FABP]) detectable in the blood and urine, while very promising for the earlier detection of patients at risk for developing AKI and for the earlier diagnosis of kidney damage, are still undergoing investigation to optimally understand their use to inform bedside clinical decision support (i.e., when to start renal replacement therapy [RRT]).

EPIDEMIOLOGY

In a recent systematic review of 312 studies including 49 million patients, the syndrome of AKI (according to KDIGO definition) was found to affect 1 in 5 adults and 1 in 3 children during hospital admission (17). A degree of acute renal injury (manifested by release of NGAL, albuminuria, loss of small tubular proteins, or inability to excrete a water load, sodium load or an amino acid load, or any combination of the above) can be demonstrated in most ICU patients. Using the RIFLE classification, the incidence of at least some degree of AKI has been reported as high as 67% in a study of more than 5,000 critically ill patients (3). The development of AKI with a maximum RIFLE category Failure has been reported in up to 28% of critically ill patients and is associated with a several fold increased risk of in-hospital death (2,3). Recent trends have suggested that the incidence of AKI may be increasing, in particular in critically ill patients. This may be attributable to improved recognition and reporting with the introduction of consensus definitions; however, this is also likely attributable

TABLE 132.2 Laboratory Tests to Differentiate Prerenal AKI from Established AKI

Test	Prerenal AKI	Established AKI
Urine sediment	Normal	Epithelial casts
Specific gravity	High: >1.020	Low: <1.020
Urine sodium (mmol/L)	Low: <10	High: >20
Fractional excretion of sodium	<1%	>1%
Fractional excretion of urea	<35%	>35%
Urine osmolality (mOsm/kg H_2O)	High: >500	Near serum: <300
Urine/Plasma creatinine ratio	High: >40	Low: <10
Plasma urea:creatinine ratio	High	Normal

to changes in population demographics, baseline susceptibilities, and comorbid diseases, and greater exposure to more complex and technologically advanced procedures and treatments (i.e., immune suppression; chemotherapy; organ transplantation; cardiac surgery).

Several risk factors for AKI in ICU patients have been identified including baseline (nonmodifiable) susceptibilities and potentially modifiable events or factors. These risk factors include older age, male sex, preexisting comorbid illness, a diagnosis of sepsis, cardiogenic shock, major surgery (specifically cardiac surgery), hypovolemia, and exposure to nephrotoxic drugs (18,19). In addition, multiorgan dysfunction, specifically concomitant acute circulatory, pulmonary, and hepatic organ dysfunction, is commonly associated with AKI (Table 132.4) (20–22).

PRESENTATION AND CLINICAL CLASSIFICATION

The clinical presentation of AKI may vary according to the etiology and the severity. AKI may be clinically silent until there are overt changes to serum creatinine (which is dependent on serum creatinine being routinely monitored in "at-risk" patients) and/or urine output. Urine output is often, but not always, decreased. As kidney function worsens, electrolyte disturbances such as hyperkalemia, hyperphosphatemia, metabolic acidosis due to diminished clearance of acid, and fluid accumulation occur. In those patients not carefully monitored or untreated, disruption of metabolic and fluid balance homeostasis can lead to life-threatening complications such as ventricular dysrhythmias and pulmonary edema.

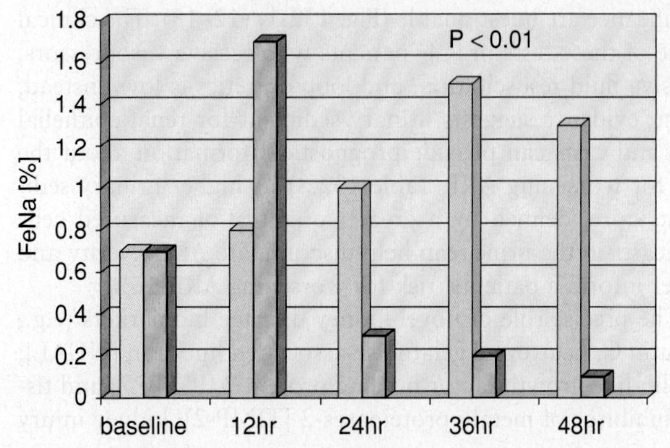

FIGURE 132.1 Histogram showing the effect of experimental sepsis in sheep on the fractional excretion of sodium (FeNa). FeNa decreased in sepsis as would be expected during decreased perfusion. In fact, all experimental animals had a twofold to threefold increase in renal blood flow, providing proof of the concept that FeNa cannot be used to infer renal hypoperfusion.

TABLE 132.3 Urinary Sediment Scoring System (16)

Score	Description
1	RTE cells 0 and granular casts 0
2	RTE cells 0 and granular casts 1–5, *or* RTE cells 1–5 and granular casts 0
3	RTE cells 1–5 and granular casts 1–5 or RTE cells 0 and granular casts 6–10, *or* RTE cells 6–20 and granular casts 0

RTE, renal tubular epithelial.

The contributing factors for AKI can largely be categorized into conditions that alter renal hemodynamics, conditions that cause direct kidney injury, or conditions that contribute to the obstruction of urine flow. Often patients will present with multiple concurrent and temporally associated contributing factors for AKI. The early identification of precipitating causes is essential for limiting the extent of ongoing injury and promoting repair and recovery.

Alternation to kidney hemodynamics, due to either or both systemic and regional factors, is likely the most common etiology for AKI in the ICU. These include events that affect systemic hemodynamics by causing decrease of extracellular volume (i.e., hypovolemia, dehydration, hemorrhage, burns), redistribution of that volume (i.e., capillary leak in sepsis, pancreatitis, or hepatic failure), events associated with decreased cardiac output (i.e., myocardial infarction, heart failure, septic cardiomyopathy), or those associated with low perfusion pressure (i.e., anaphylaxis). Kidney function can also be impacted by alterations to regional kidney hemodynamics. Processes that alter afferent (i.e., nonsteroidal anti-inflammatory drugs) and/or efferent arteriolar tone (i.e., ACE inhibitors/ARB) can adversely impact glomerular filtration.

Less commonly, AKI can present where the principal source of damage is within the kidney and where typical structural changes can be seen on microscopy. Numerous disorders, which affect the glomerulus or the tubule, may be responsible. Among these, nephrotoxins are particularly important, especially in hospitalized patients (23). The most common nephrotoxic drugs affecting ICU patients are listed in Table 132.5. Many cases of drug-induced AKI rapidly improve upon removal of the offending agent. Accordingly, a careful history of drug administration is essential in all patients with AKI.

TABLE 132.4 AKI Risk Factors

Baseline Susceptibilities

- Older age
- Male sex
- Black race
- Pre-existing chronic kidney disease
- Proteinuria
- Hypertension
- Diabetes mellitus
- Heart failure
- Chronic liver disease
- Peripheral vascular disease
- Malignancy
- Obesity

Modifiable Risk Factors

- Anemia
- Critical illness
- Sepsis
- Trauma
- Cardiopulmonary bypass
- Major noncardiac surgery
- Rhabdomyolysis
- Exposure to radiocontrast agents
- Nephrotoxic drugs
- Fluid accumulation/overload
- High-risk emergency procedures
- Intra-abdominal hypertension

TABLE 132.5 List of Medications Known to Be Associated with Nephrotoxicity (26)

Acyclovir	Enalaprilat	Mesalamine
Ambisome	Foscarnet	Methotrexate
Amikacin	Gadopentetate	Nafcillin
Amphotericin B	Gadoxetate	Piperacillin/tazobactam
Captopril	Ganciclovir	Piperacillin
Carboplatin	Gentamicin	Sirolimus
Cefotaxime	Ibuprofen	Sulfasalazine
Ceftazidime	Ifosfamide	Tacrolimus
Cefuroxime	Iodixano	Ticarcillin/clavulanic acid
Cidofovir	Iohexo	Tobramycin
Cisplatin	Iopamido	Topiramate
Colistimethate	Ioversol	Valacyclovir
Cyclosporine	Ketorolac	Valganciclovir
Dapsone	Lisinopril	Vancomycin
Enalapril	Lithium	Zonisamide

More than a third of patients who develop AKI in ICU have chronic kidney disease (CKD) due to factors such as age-related changes in nephron mass, longstanding hypertension, diabetes mellitus, or atheromatous disease of the renal vessels. Such CKD may be manifest by a prehospital elevation in serum creatinine or evidence of proteinuria; however, this may not be universally evident or known. Often, what may seem to the clinician as a relatively trivial kidney insult may unmask more significant AKI due to a lack of renal functional reserve related to subclinical pre-existing CKD.

Obstruction to urine outflow is a common cause of functional AKI in the community (24), but is uncommon in the ICU. The pathogenesis of obstructive AKI involves several humoral responses as well as mechanical factors. Typical causes of obstructive AKI include bladder neck obstruction from an enlarged prostate, ureteric obstruction from pelvic tumors or retroperitoneal fibrosis, papillary necrosis, or large calculi. The clinical presentation of obstruction may be acute or acute-on-chronic in patients with longstanding renal calculi. It may not always be associated with oliguria. If obstruction is suspected, ultrasonography can be easily performed at the bedside. However, not all cases of acute obstruction have an abnormal ultrasound and, in many cases, obstruction occurs in conjunction with other renal insults (e.g., staghorn calculi and severe sepsis of renal origin). The use of medications that lead to urinary retention in those without an indwelling urinary catheter may exacerbate the presentation. Assessment of the role of each factor and overall management should be conducted in conjunction with an urologist. Finally, the sudden and unexpected development of anuria in an ICU patient should always suggest obstruction of the urinary catheter as the cause. Appropriate flushing or changing of the catheter should be implemented in this setting.

Clinical risk prediction tools can be utilized to identify patients at greater risk of AKI. Those at high-risk patients can be monitored closely for development of AKI including frequent assessments of serum creatinine, continuous urine

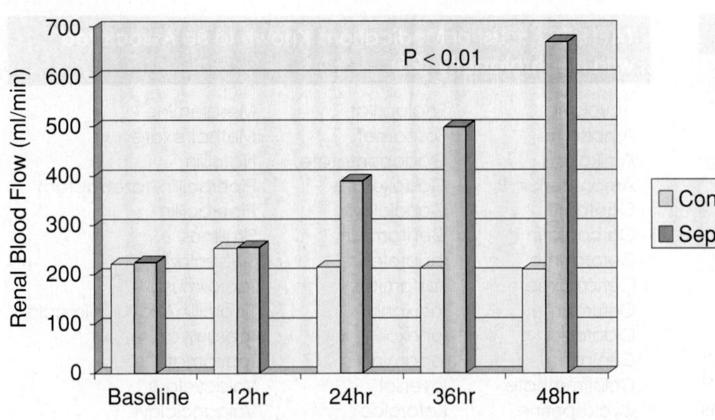

FIGURE 132.2 Histogram showing the effect on renal blood flow of experimental sepsis in sheep. Renal blood flow increased threefold while creatinine increased from 80 to 400 μmol/L, providing evidence that acute renal failure in sepsis can occur during renal hyperemia.

output monitoring, and strict avoidance of nephrotoxins. For example, Kheterpal et al. (25) developed and validated a clinical risk score for AKI for patients undergoing general surgery. Five classes of risk were created based on the presence of 11 preoperative risk factors. The risk index showed progressively greater AKI risk with higher class, with a 9% risk in those in Class V (at least six risk factors) compared to a 0.2% risk in those with Class I (up to two risk factors).

Modern clinical information systems can be designed to trigger alerts to clinicians for "at-risk" patients who are developing early AKI or who are exposed to unnecessary nephrotoxins. Recently, the use of automated alerting from clinical information systems that can integrate bedside information such as urine output, laboratory information such as absolute and relative changes in serum creatinine, and pharmacy information, such as potential nephrotoxin exposure have been shown to improve the recognition of AKI in hospitalized patients. Electronic alerting has been shown to translate into earlier interventions, reduce severity among those developing AKI, and improve outcomes (26,27).

PATHOGENESIS OF SPECIFIC SYNDROMES

Septic AKI

Sepsis is a leading predisposing factor to AKI in critically ill patients (19). Epidemiologic studies estimate between 45% and 70% of all AKI encountered in the ICU is associated with sepsis (18,19,28). The distinction between septic and nonseptic AKI may have particular clinical relevance considering recent evidence to suggest that septic AKI may be characterized by a unique pathophysiology (29–32).

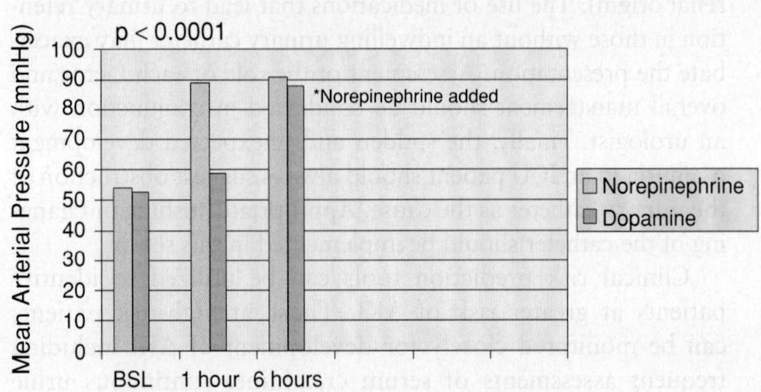

The classic teaching is that sepsis brings about hypotension, leading to a reduction in critical organ blood flow including in the kidney, causing ischemic injury and AKI. Furthermore, sepsis would lead to activation of the sympathetic nervous system, stimulating the release of potent vasoconstrictors that induce renal vasoconstriction and aggravate kidney ischemia, thus worsening AKI. However, growing evidence questions this ischemic-induced paradigm of septic AKI (29,30,32). An experimental study in a large mammalian model of hyperdynamic sepsis found that RBF was marked increased above baseline despite significant reductions in kidney excretory function (Fig. 132.2) (31). These findings are supported by small clinical studies of resuscitated patients with septic AKI that also show increases in RBF (33–35). The implications are that in hyperdynamic sepsis, AKI is hyperemic, rather than ischemic, with global RBF considerably increased. Moreover, experimental studies have shown that regional cortical and medullary RBF are preserved in sepsis and can be further augmented by infusion of norepinephrine (Fig. 132.3) (36). This concept of hyperemic AKI in sepsis is consistent with the relative paucity of renal histopathologic evidence of tubular necrosis in patients with septic AKI (37).

Thus, evolving evidence suggests that the pathogenesis of septic AKI predominantly involves toxic and immune-mediated mechanisms. Sepsis is known to release a vast array of pro- and anti-inflammatory mediators such as cytokines (damage-associated molecular proteins [DAMPs] and pathogen-associated molecular proteins [PAMPs], arachidonic acid metabolites, and thrombogenic agents that all may participate in the development of AKI (38). Similarly, experimental studies have found evidence of renal tubular cell apoptosis in response to inflammatory mediators in endotoxemia (39,40). Renal tubular apoptosis may prove an important mechanism of septic AKI in critically ill patients (37,41,42). No studies exist to

FIGURE 132.3 Histogram showing the effect of norepinephrine on mean arterial blood pressure (MAP) compared to high-dose dopamine in a randomized controlled trial in humans. MAP is more reliably restored using norepinephrine when given alone as an alternative to high-dose dopamine or after high-dose dopamine has failed. BSL, baseline.

tell us which of the above mechanisms are most important and when they might be active in the course of an episode of septic AKI. However, interventions with antiapoptotic properties, such as with selective caspase inhibitors, may theoretically aid in attenuating kidney injury and promote recovery of function (38). To date, however, no human randomized controlled trials have assessed the impact of these interventions on kidney function and their value is unknown.

AKI in Association with Major Surgery

AKI is a common complication following major surgery (19, 43). The incidence is variable and dependent on the prevalence of pre-existing comorbid illnesses, preoperative kidney function, and the type and urgency of surgery being performed. Numerous intraoperative events can act to negatively affect kidney function, including the following:

- Hemodynamic instability (e.g., intravenous or inhaled anesthetic agents)
- Hypovolemia due to blood loss or third spacing
- Details of the operative field (e.g., aortic cross-clamping in major vascular surgery)
- Increases in intra-abdominal pressure (e.g., laparoscopic insufflation of CO_2)
- Concomitant sepsis
- Use of nephrotoxin drugs

Any of these factors, alone or in combination, may contribute to a critical reduction in RBF and ischemia, impaired oxygen delivery, and toxin- or inflammatory-mediated injury. Postoperative AKI is believed to be, in part, mediated by proinflammatory mechanisms such as increased endothelial cell adhesion, tubular cell infiltration, generation of reactive oxygen species, proinflammatory cytokines, and reperfusion injury (44,45). Cardiac surgery with cardiopulmonary bypass (CPB) commonly induces early postoperative AKI. The mechanisms whereby CPB causes injury are incompletely understood, although there is a suggestion that CPB is proinflammatory, activating components of the nonspecific immune system. In turn, this leads to oxidative stress with the generation of oxygen-free radical species and serum lipid peroxidation products (46). In addition, CPB has been shown to deplete serum antioxidative capacity for a prolonged duration after surgery. Such oxidant stress has been shown to directly induce kidney injury in experimental studies (47).

Surgery-specific clinical prediction tools have been developed and validated to assess risk and predict AKI after surgery. Such tools can be utilized to identify patients at greater risk of perioperative AKI prior to planned procedures or among those requiring urgent or emergent procedures. These patients can be triaged to higher levels of perioperative monitoring if indicated (i.e., high-dependency units or intensive care; frequent assessments of serum creatinine; continuous urine output monitoring; strict avoidance of nephrotoxins).

Hepatorenal Syndrome

This condition is a form of AKI, which typically occurs in the setting of advanced cirrhosis; however, it can occur with severe liver dysfunction due to alcoholic hepatitis or other forms of acute hepatic failure (48). The recent consensus definition of HRS includes any form of kidney disease occurring in patients with cirrhosis regardless of etiology (Table 132.6) (49). The pathogenesis of hepatorenal syndrome (HRS) is incompletely understood; however, there are several potential mechanisms that may contribute to HRS, including activation of the renin–angiotensin system in response to systemic hypotension, activation of the sympathetic nervous system in response to systemic hypotension and increased intrahepatic sinusoidal pressure, increased release of arginine vasopressin due to systemic hypotension, and reduced hepatic clearance of various vascular mediators such as endothelin, prostaglandins, and endotoxin (48,50).

TABLE 132.6 Summary of the Diagnostic Criteria for Kidney Dysfunction in Chronic Liver Disease and Hepatorenal Syndrome (49)

Diagnosis	Definition
AKI	• ↑ in SCr ≥50% from baseline or ↑ SCr >0.3 mg/dL (26.5 μmol/L) • Type-1 HRS is a specific form of AKI
CKD	• GFR <60 mL/min for >3 mo calculated using MDRD-6 formula
Acute on CKD	• ↑ in SCr ≥50% from baseline or ↑ SCr >0.3 mg/dL (26.5 μmol/L) in a patient with cirrhosis whose GFR is <60 mL/min for >3 mo calculated using MDRD-6 formula
Hepatorenal syndrome	• Confirmed diagnosis of cirrhosis with ascites • SCr >1.5 mg/dL (132.6 μmol/L) • No improvement in SCr (<1.5 mg/dL (132.6 μmol/L)) after 2 d of diuretic withdrawal and volume expansion • Absence of shock • No current or recent exposure with nephrotoxin medications • Absence of parenchymal kidney disease as indicated by proteinuria > 0.5 g/d, microhematuria (>50 cells/hpf) and/or abnormal ultrasonography

AKI, acute kidney injury; CKD, chronic kidney disease; SCr, serum creatinine.
MDRD-6: GFR = 170 × Scr (mg/dL) − 0.999 × age − 0.176 × 1.180 (if black) × 0.762 (if female) × serum urea nitrogen − 0.170 × albumin 0.138.

Although HRS can occur spontaneously in patients with advanced cirrhosis, it is important to recognize that other precipitants are much more common. These include sepsis, specifically spontaneous bacterial peritonitis (SBP), raised intra-abdominal pressure due to tense ascites, bile acid nephropathy in those with severe hyperbilirubinemia, gastrointestinal bleeding, and hypovolemia due to paracentesis, diuretics and/or lactulose, or any combination of these factors. Likewise, other contributing factors to AKI should be routinely assessed for including cardiomyopathy due to alcoholism, nutritional deficiencies or viral infection, and exposure to nephrotoxins.

Typically, HRS develops in patients with advanced cirrhosis and evidence of portal hypertension with ascites in the absence of other apparent causes of AKI. It generally presents as oligo-anuria with progressive increases in serum creatinine and/or urea and bland urinary sediment. These patients develop profound sodium and water retention with evidence of hyponatremia, a urine osmolality higher than that of plasma, and a very low urinary sodium concentration (<10 mmol/L).

Management of the patient with HRS can be challenging. However, it should include the systematic identification and prompt treatment of potential reversible precipitants (i.e., sepsis). The avoidance of hypovolemia by albumin administration in patients with SBP has been shown to decrease the incidence of AKI in a randomized controlled trial (51). These causes must be looked for and promptly treated. Some studies suggest that vasopressin derivatives (i.e., terlipressin) may improve GFR in this condition (52,53). Other treatment options include oral α-adrenergic agonist midodrine with subcutaneous octreotide or referral for albumin-based extracorporeal therapies. Placement of a transjugular intrahepatic portosystemic stent-shunt (TIPS) has been associated with modest improvements in kidney function in those with HRS, may improve outcome and represent a measure for those who are not a candidate for or awaiting transplant (54,55). In general, the ideal solution for reversal of AKI in these patients is either improvement in hepatic function by therapy for the underlying primary liver disease and/or referral for and successful liver transplantation.

AKI with Rhabdomyolysis

The incidence of rhabdomyolysis-induced AKI is estimated at 1% in hospitalized patients but it may account for close to 5% to 7% of cases of AKI in critically ill patients depending on the setting (23,28). Its pathogenesis involves the interplay of prerenal, intrarenal, and postrenal factors including concurrent hypovolemia, ischemia, direct tubular toxicity mediated by the heme pigment in myoglobin, and intratubular obstruction (56). The causes of muscle injury that can result in rhabdomyolysis include major trauma, burns, drug overdose (i.e., narcotics, cocaine, or other stimulants), vascular embolism, prolonged seizures, neuroleptic malignant syndrome, various infections (i.e., pyomyositis, necrotizing fasciitis, influenza, HIV), severe exertion, impaired cellular energy production (i.e., hereditary enzyme disorders, toxins), increased calcium influx (i.e., malignant hyperthermia), alcoholism, and in response to a variety of agents which can interact to induce major muscle injury (i.e., combination of macrolide antibiotics or cyclosporin and statins). The clinical manifestations of rhabdomyolysis include an elevated serum creatine kinase and evidence of pigmented granular casts and red to brown coloring of the urine. Patients can also have various electrolyte disorders as a result of muscle breakdown including hyperphosphatemia, hyperkalemia, hypocalcemia, and hyperuricemia.

The principles of prevention of AKI include identification and elimination of potential causative agents and/or correction of underlying compartment syndromes; prompt and aggressive fluid resuscitation and maintenance of polyuria (i.e., ≥1.5 to 2 mL/kg ideal or adjusted body weight per hour, usually more than about 300 mL/hr to restore vascular volume and potentially flush obstructing cellular casts); and urine alkalinization to a goal pH above 6.5 in order to reduce renal toxicity by myoglobin-induced lipid peroxidation and improve the solubility of myoglobin (56). Experimental studies have suggested mannitol may act as a scavenger of free radicals and reduce cellular toxicity; however, the role of forced diuresis with mannitol remains controversial. Other controversial therapies include allopurinol; deferoxamine; dantrolene, and glutathione, and high volume and/or high cut-off membrane hemofiltration.

AKI due to Nephrotoxins

Several mechanisms have been reported to play a role in the development of kidney injury after exposure to nephrotoxins. Particular drugs can often invoke a variety of pathophysiologic effects on the kidney that collectively contribute to AKI. Alterations in intra-renal hemodynamics are an important initial consequence of many nephrotoxins. These changes to regional renal blood flow may occur through increased activity of local vasoconstrictors such as angiotensin II, endothelin, adenosine; at the same time, there is diminished activity of important vasodilators (i.e., nitric oxide and prostaglandins). This imbalance can lead to renal vasoconstriction and ischemia, particularly to susceptible regions such as the outer medulla, for example, in response to radiocontrast media, or can induce humorally mediated vasoconstriction of afferent arterioles as a result of exposure to NSAIDs and cyclosporine. The end result of a reduction in regional blood flow is a critical reduction in oxygen delivery, thus predisposing to tubular hypoxia (57). In addition, nephrotoxins can directly contribute to impaired tubular metabolism and oxygen utilization. They lead to generation of radical oxygen species including superoxide anions, hydrogen peroxide, hydroxyl radicals, reduction in intrinsic antioxidant enzyme activity, accumulation of intracellular calcium, mitogen-activated protein kinases, and phospholipase A2, for example, after exposure to aminoglycosides (58–60).

These responses to nephrotoxins can induce tubular cell vacuolization, interstitial inflammation, altered cell membrane properties, and disruption of normal tubular adhesion to basement membranes. Failure of these mechanisms contributes to tubular cell apoptosis, necrosis and tubular sloughing into the luminal space, cast formation, and obstruction (58). Raised intraluminal pressures due to obstruction, altered cellular permeability, and interstitial inflammation can contribute back diffusion of fluid and secondary edema formation.

Radiocontrast media and aminoglycosides are leading agents contributing to nephrotoxin-induced AKI (61,62). Radiocontrast media–induced toxicity is believed to occur from the interplay of alterations in renal hemodynamics due to vasoconstriction, increased intravascular viscosity and erythrocyte aggregation, direct tubular epithelial cell toxicity, and concomitant atheroembolic microshowers in the renovasculature. Aminoglycosides are taken up via organic anion transport systems in the proximal tubules where they accumulate and generate radical oxygen species, increased intracellular calcium, which lead to tubular apoptosis, necrosis, and nonoliguric AKI.

Radiocontrast-Induced Nephropathy

Radiocontrast-induced nephropathy (RCIN) is the leading cause of iatrogenic AKI in hospitalized patients and results in prolonged hospitalization, higher mortality rates, excessive health care costs, and potentially long-term kidney impairment (23). RCIN presents with an acute rise in serum creatinine within 24 to 48 hours following injection of radiocontrast media. The serum creatinine level generally peaks within 3 to 5 days and returns toward baseline within 7 to 10 days; however, in some patients kidney function may not return to baseline and a persistent reduction in function may occur. RCIN is often associated with pre-existing risk factors, in particular pre-existing CKD (GFR <60 mL/min/1.73 m^2), a diagnosis of diabetes mellitus, and use of large quantities of radiocontrast media.

There are few effective prophylactic or therapeutic interventions with evidence for reducing the occurrence of radiocontrast nephropathy and no therapy has proven effective once it is established (63). Strategies for prevention include early identification of patients at risk, consideration to either delay of the investigation, or using alternative modality until kidney function can be optimized. Likewise, every effort should be made correct volume depletion and discontinue potential nephrotoxins. There is no evidence to support the routine use of diuretics, mannitol or dopamine. Studies have shown that periprocedure hydration and use of nonionic iso-osmolar (e.g., iodixanol) radiocontrast media can reduce the risk (64–67). Several randomized trials and meta-analyses have suggested potential benefit with the use of *N*-acetylcysteine or sodium bicarbonate; however, further definitive evidence is pending (68,69). Their effectiveness in already fluid-resuscitated ICU patients, however, remains unknown.

AKI in Association with Mechanical Ventilation

Most critically ill patients require mechanical ventilation (MV), either for disease-specific indications such as acute respiratory distress syndrome (ARDS) or simply for routine postoperative care. The application of positive pressure MV, particularly with positive end-expiratory pressure (PEEP), can have important physiologic effects on kidney function. Experimental and clinical studies have clearly established an association between MV and PEEP and alterations in kidney function. This can occur through several mechanisms, including alterations in cardiovascular function, alterations in neurohormonal activation, abnormalities in gas exchange, and alterations in systemic inflammatory mediators (70,71).

The positive pressure applied during MV acts to increase intrathoracic, intrapleural, and intra-abdominal pressures, both during inspiration and for the duration of the respiratory cycle. This increase in intrathoracic pressure, monitored clinically by changes in mean airway pressure, can act to reduce intrathoracic blood volume, decrease transmural pressure, reduce right ventricular preload, increase right ventricular afterload, exert alterations to pulmonary vascular resistance and volume, and contribute to changes in left ventricular filling and geometry. The result of these effects may be a decrease in cardiac output and renal perfusion. Similarly, raised intrathoracic pressure, by altering transmural pressures and reducing cardiac output, can act to unload intrathoracic baroreceptors. This initiates a cascade of compensatory neurohormonal events characterized by increased systemic and renal sympathetic nervous activity, increased activation of the renin–angiotensin–aldosterone system, increased secretion of vasopressin, and a reduction in release of atrial natriuretic peptide. These culminate in altered renal perfusion and kidney excretory function. Renal function may not be impaired *per se* with MV, but rather, may appropriately respond to stimuli by reducing osmolar, sodium, and water clearance. In addition, acute hypoxemia and/or hypercapnia, both commonly encountered in patients with ARDS, can act to alter systemic hemodynamics and increase systemic inflammation, both of which may exert negative effects on renal perfusion and function. Particular strategies of MV, specifically in ARDS, are now recognized to contribute to or provoke ventilator-induced lung injury (VILI). Evidence now suggests that the pathophysiology of VILI is multifactorial and results from the combined effects of volutrauma (excessive tidal or end-expiratory volumes), barotrauma (excessive end-inspiratory peak and plateau pressures), atelectatic trauma (cyclical opening and closing of alveolar units), and biotrauma (local release of inflammatory mediators from injured lung) (72). Such injurious MV can initiate a cascade of events that increases systemic inflammation and adversely impact kidney function (73).

AKI in Association with Intra-Abdominal Hypertension/Abdominal Compartment Syndrome

Intra-abdominal hypertension (IAH) and abdominal compartment syndrome (ACS) can worsen kidney function and precipitate AKI. Mechanical compression on abdominal and thoracic vessels results in diminished venous return, congestion, increased renal venous pressure, which leads to renal interstitial edema. This coupled with renal arterial vasoconstriction due to compensatory renin–angiotensin–aldosterone system activation contributes to impaired perfusion pressure across the renal circulation. Patients with IAH progressing to ACS commonly present with marked abdominal distension, measured IAP above 15 mmHg, and increasing serum creatinine and oliguria. ACS is commonly associated with major trauma or large burn injuries, complex intra-abdominal surgeries, pancreatitis or ruptured aneurysms, and in patients receiving large volume resuscitation.

Identification of IAH/ACS requires a high index of suspicion among susceptible patients, and should include the routine measurement of bladder pressures. Management is generally supportive and includes optimization of sedation, neuromuscular blockade, patient repositioning, nasogastric and rectal decompression, draining fluid collections and optimizing fluid balance through minimizing nonessential fluid, administration of diuretics or if necessary, initiation of RRT. In those with refractory ACS and sustained IAH above 20 mmHg, surgical decompression should be considered (74).

GENERAL MANAGEMENT

The most common clinical picture seen in the ICU is that of a patient who has sustained or is experiencing a major systemic insult such as trauma, sepsis, myocardial infarction, severe hemorrhage, cardiogenic shock, or major surgery. When the patient arrives in the ICU, resuscitation is typically well underway, or surgery may have just been completed. Despite such efforts, the patient is already anuric or profoundly oliguric, and the serum creatinine is rising, and a metabolic acidosis is developing; serum potassium and phosphate levels may be rapidly rising as well. In these critically ill patients with AKI, multiple organ dysfunction—with the need for MV and vasoactive drugs—is common. Fluid resuscitation is typically undertaken in the ICU with the guidance of invasive hemodynamic monitoring. Vasoactive drugs are often used to restore mean arterial pressure (MAP) to acceptable levels, typically greater than 65 to 70 mmHg (see Figure 132.3). The patient may improve over time, and urine output may return with or without the assistance of diuretic agents (Fig. 132.4). If urine output does not return, however, RRT needs to be considered. If the cause of AKI has been removed, and the patient has become physiologically stable, slow recovery occurs within 4 to 5 days to as long as 3 or 4 weeks. In some cases, urine output can be above normal for several days. If the cause of AKI has not been adequately remedied, the patient remains gravely ill, the kidneys do not recover, and death from multiorgan failure may occur.

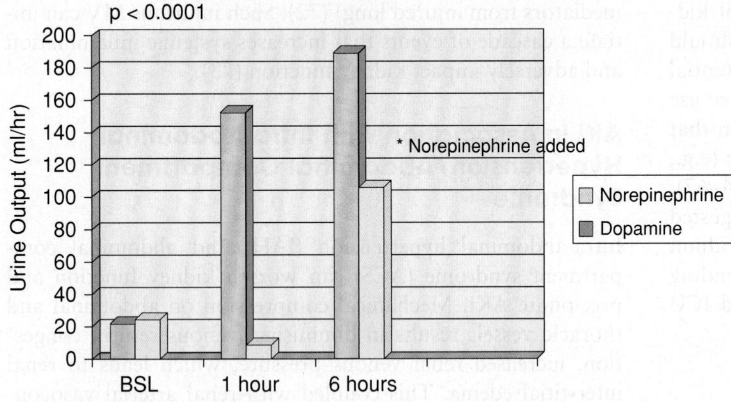

FIGURE 132.4 Diagram showing the effect of norepinephrine on urine output compared to high-dose dopamine in patients in septic shock. Urine output is more effectively restored with norepinephrine infusion when given alone as an alternative to high-dose dopamine or after high-dose dopamine has failed. BSL, baseline.

Fluid Resuscitation

Intravascular volume must be maintained or rapidly restored, and this is often best done using invasive hemodynamic monitoring such as with central venous catheter, arterial cannula, and pulmonary artery catheter or pulse contour cardiac output catheters. Oxygenation must be maintained. An adequate hemoglobin concentration, usually at least more than 7.0 g/dL must be maintained or immediately restored. Once intravascular volume has been restored, some patients remain hypotensive with MAP less than 70 mmHg. In these patients, autoregulation of RBF may be lost. Restoration of MAP to near-normal levels may increase GFR (75–77). Such elevations in MAP, however, require the addition of vasopressor drugs (75–77). In patients with pre-existing hypertension or renovascular disease, a MAP of 75 to 80 may still be inadequate. Experimental evidence suggests that vasopressor support in hypotensive sepsis increases renal blood flow (Fig. 132.5) and renal medullary blood flow (Fig. 132.6). The renal protective role of additional fluid therapy in a patient with a normal or increased cardiac output and blood pressure is questionable. Despite these resuscitation measures, renal failure may still develop if cardiac output is inadequate. This may require a variety of interventions from the use of inotropic drugs to the application of ventricular assist devices.

Fluid Therapy

Fluid therapy is the cornerstone of resuscitation of the critically ill patient, and is the primary strategy for preservation of kidney function in the setting of increases in serum creatinine and/or urea, and oliguria. However, evolving evidence has suggested there may be negative consequences to overly aggressive fluid therapy for both renal and nonrenal organ function. A large multicentre study found no significant difference in the incidence of AKI when comparing fluid resuscitation with crystalloid to albumin in critically ill patients (78). However, some synthetic colloid therapies, such as hydroxyethyl starches (HES), are associated with higher risk of AKI and need for RRT in critically ill patients (79,80). Although the exact mechanism(s) remain uncertain, HES solutions may influence intrarenal hemodynamics or glomerular filtration through alterations in vascular oncotic pressure. Recent data have also focused on the composition of crystalloid solutions and the risk of adverse events. The preferential use of balanced crystalloid solutions such as Ringer's lactate and plasmalyte have been shown to reduce the risk of iatrogenic metabolic acidosis, and AKI, including severe AKI requiring RRT (81).

In critically ill patients, once apparent optimization of hemodynamics and intravascular volume status has been achieved, there is little evidence to support continued aggressive fluid resuscitation to improve kidney function. Rather, fluid overload in AKI is associated with less favorable outcomes, including higher utilization of RRT, higher mortality, and reduced likelihood of renal recovery (82,83). Additionally, there is evidence to suggest that such continued fluid administration and a positive cumulative balance can contribute to notable deteriorations in nonrenal organ function, in particular, lung function (84,85). The ARDS Clinical Trials Network completed the largest randomized trial assessing fluid therapy in patients with acute lung injury (ALI) (86). This trial compared restrictive and liberal strategies for fluid management in 1,000 critically ill patients, mostly with pneumonia or sepsis, and evidence of with ALI. At 72 hours, those receiving a restrictive

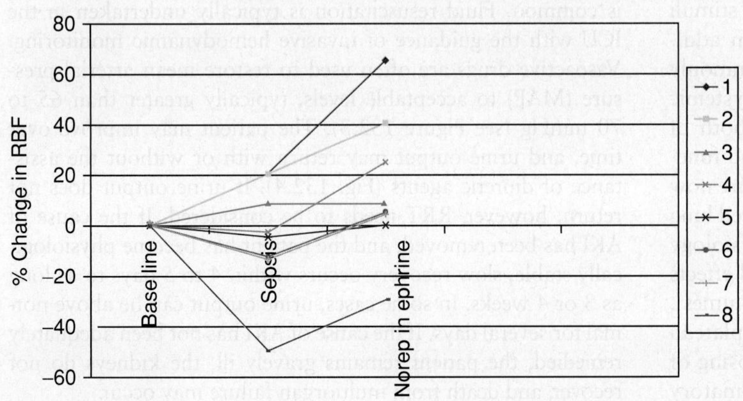

FIGURE 132.5 Diagram showing the changes in renal blood flow (RBF) during experimental *E. coli*–induced septic shock in sheep. The addition of norepinephrine increased renal blood flow.

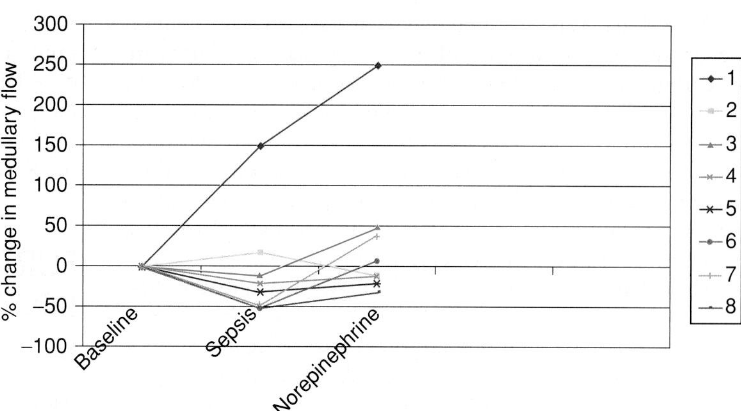

FIGURE 132.6 Diagram showing the changes in medullary renal blood flow during experimental septic shock in sheep induced by *E. coli* administration. The addition of norepinephrine increased medullary blood flow.

fluid strategy had a near neutral fluid balance, whereas those in the liberal strategy were positive above 5 L. While the study failed to show a difference in mortality between the strategies, a restrictive strategy improved lung function, increased in ventilator-free days, and reduced ICU length of stay. Moreover, those in the restrictive group had a trend toward a reduced utilization of RRT.

Avoidance of Nephrotoxins

In patients with established AKI, as well in those at increased risk, avoidance of nephrotoxins is a priority to prevent iatrogenic overt or worsening AKI and delay of renal recovery. In circumstances where there are no options other than to use a nephrotoxin, for example, with certain antimicrobials or calcineuron inhibitors, therapeutic drug monitoring and careful dose adjustment, in multidisciplinary consultation with pharmacy, should be undertaken. The perceived benefits and risks of receiving contrast media for diagnostic imaging should be carefully evaluated; and where applicable, delay or choosing alternative imaging modalities should be undertaking in those at high risk where possible.

Renal Protective Drugs

Following acute resuscitation, hemodynamic optimization, and attention to nephrotoxin use, it is unclear whether the use of additional pharmacologic measures is of further benefit to the kidneys.

Renal Dose or Low-Dose Dopamine

Evidence of the efficacy or safety of its administration in critically ill patients is lacking. However, this agent is a tubular diuretic and occasionally increases urine output. This may be incorrectly interpreted as an increase in GFR. Furthermore, a large phase III trial in critically ill patients showed low-dose dopamine to be as effective as placebo in the prevention of AKI (87).

Mannitol

A biologic rationale exists for its use, as is the case for dopamine. However, no controlled human data exist to support its clinical use. The effect of mannitol as a renal protective agent remains questionable.

Loop Diuretics

These agents may protect the loop of Henle from ischemia by decreasing its transport-related workload. Animal data are encouraging, as are *ex vivo* experiments. There are no double-blind randomized controlled studies of suitable size to prove that these agents reduce the incidence of AKI. However, there are some studies, which support the view that loop diuretics may decrease the need for RRT in patients developing AKI (88). They appear to achieve this by inducing polyuria, which allows for easier control of volume overload, acidosis, and hyperkalemia, three major triggers for RRT in the ICU. Because avoiding RRT simplifies treatment and reduces cost of care, loop diuretics are commonly used in patients with AKI, especially in the form of continuous infusion.

Other Agents

Other agents such as theophylline, urodilatin, and anaritide (a synthetic atrial natriuretic factor) have also been proposed. Studies so far, however, have been either been experimental, too small, or have shown no beneficial effect. In a randomized double-blind, placebo-controlled trial, fenoldopam has been shown to attenuate the deterioration in serum creatinine typically seen in septic patients (89). Studies of fenoldopam in other situations, however, have failed to show a benefit (90). Thus, its role in AKI remains uncertain. Similarly, in a single-center study, rhANF has been shown to attenuate renal injury in higher-risk patients having cardiac surgery (91), but a large multicenter study of AKI failed to show a benefit (92). Many more investigations are urgently needed in this field.

MANAGEMENT OF ESTABLISHED AKI

The principles of management of established AKI should always include the following:

- Confirmation of probable cause
- Elimination of potential contributors
- Institution of disease-specific therapy if applicable
- Prevention and management of AKI-related complications with maintenance of physiologic homeostasis while allowing recovery to occur

Complications such as encephalopathy, pericarditis, myopathy, neuropathy, electrolyte disturbances, or other major electrolyte, fluid, or metabolic derangements should never occur in a modern ICU. They can be prevented by several measures, which vary in complexity from fluid restriction to the initiation of RRT.

Nutritional support should be started early and contain adequate calories, around 30 to 35 kcal/kg/d, as a mixture of carbohydrates and lipids. Sufficient protein of at least 1 to 2 g/kg/d must be administered. There is no evidence that specific renal nutritional solutions are useful. Vitamins and trace elements should be administered at least according to their recommended daily allowance. The role of newer immunonutritional solution remains controversial. The enteral route is preferred to the use of parenteral nutrition.

Hyperkalemia—a serum potassium level of greater than 6 mmol/L—must be promptly treated either with insulin and dextrose administration, the infusion of bicarbonate if acidosis is present, the administration of nebulized salbutamol, or all of the above combined. If the "true" serum potassium is more than 7 mmol/L, or if electrocardiographic signs of hyperkalemia appear, calcium gluconate—10 mL of 10% solution administered IV—should also be used. The above measures are temporizing actions while RRT is being arranged. The presence of hyperkalemia is a major life-threatening indication for the immediate institution of RRT.

Metabolic acidosis is almost always present but rarely requires treatment per se. Anemia requires correction to maintain a hemoglobin of at least 70 g/L. More aggressive transfusion needs individual patient assessment (93). Drug therapy must be adjusted to take into account the effect of the decreased clearances associated with loss of kidney function. Stress ulcer prophylaxis is advisable and should be based on H2-receptor antagonists or proton pump inhibitors in selected cases. Assiduous attention should be paid to the prevention of infection.

Fluid overload can be prevented by the avoidance of administration of nonessential fluids and the judicious use of loop diuretics. However, if the patient is oliguric, the only way to avoid fluid overload is to institute RRT at an earlier stage. Marked azotemia, defined as a urea more than 40 mmol/L (BUN [blood urea nitrogen] of 112 mg/dL) or a creatinine level more than 400 μmol/L (4.5 mg/dL) is undesirable and should probably be treated with RRT unless recovery is imminent or already under way and a return toward normal values is expected within 24 to 48 hours.

In critically ill patients with life-threatening complications from AKI, referral for RRT should occur without delay. In general, relative few patients develop these severe complications. Accordingly, the decision to start RRT is often more complex and occurs amid a number of factors such as conservative therapy to manage fluid accumulation is failing coupled with evidence of worsening electrolyte disorders, acidosis or azotemia. Whether the early initiation of RRT in the absence of these indications improves survival remains unproven (94); however, it is advisable to start RRT in anticipation of complications rather need to urgently rescue patients. Indeed, recent data have shown these complications have an independent and attributable contribution to mortality to critically ill patients with AKI. The ideal modality to support critically ill patients with AKI remains unresolved. In general, in hemodynamically or physiologically unstable patients, patients should be preferentially treated initially with continuous renal replacement therapy (CRRT) rather than intermitted forms of hemodialysis (IHD) in an ICU setting. While no definitive evidence has shown a survival advantage with one particular modality, recent data support the greater likelihood of recovery of kidney function and dialysis independence among those initially treated with CRRT (95). Evidence from two large multicenter randomized trials showed no added benefit higher intensity-dose RRT compared to lower intensity-dose RRT with fewer metabolic complications (96,97). For a more comprehensive evidence-based review of the principles of RRT in AKI, review the KDIGO Clinical Practice Guidelines for AKI (4).

FURTHER DIAGNOSTIC INVESTIGATIONS

An etiologic diagnosis of AKI must always be established. Although such diagnosis may be obvious on clinical grounds, in many patients it is best to consider all possibilities and exclude common treatable causes by simple investigations. One such investigation includes microscopic examination of the urinary sediment. Urinalysis is a simple and noninvasive test that yields important diagnostic information and patterns suggestive of specific syndromes. The finding of dysmorphic red blood cells (RBC) or RBC casts is virtually diagnostic of active glomerulonephritis or vasculitis. Heavy proteinuria suggests some form of glomerular disease. White blood cell casts can suggest either interstitial nephropathy or infection. Similarly, a normal urinalysis can provide important information and can suggest that AKI is more likely to be transient or due to an obstructive cause. Finally, examination of urine will provide evidence of whether a urinary tract infection is present.

Several additional investigations may be necessary to establish the diagnosis. Evidence of marked anemia in the absence of blood loss may suggest acute hemolysis, thrombotic microangiopathy, or paraproteinemia related to malignancy. In microangiopathic hemolytic anemia, a peripheral blood smear will typically show evidence of hemolysis with the presence of schistocytes; the additional measurement of lactic dehydrogenase, haptoglobin, unconjugated bilirubin, and free hemoglobin are needed. If paraproteinemia due to multiple myeloma or lymphoma is suspected, serum and urine protein electrophoresis and serum calcium should be measured. A history of recent cancer diagnosis or chemotherapy should prompt the measurement of uric acid for tumor lysis syndrome.

In patients with a possible mechanism for muscle injury, creatinine kinase and free myoglobin for possible rhabdomyolysis should be determined. If an elevated anion gap metabolic acidosis is present with suggestion of a toxic ingestion, ethylene glycol, methanol, and salicylates should be measured.

Systemic eosinophilia may be a clue suggesting systemic vasculitis, allergic interstitial nephritis, or atheroembolic disease. The measurement of specific antibodies—antiglomerular basement membrane (GBM), antineutrophil cytoplasmic antibodies (ANCA), antinuclear antibodies (ANA), anti-DNA, antismooth muscle, and so forth—or cryoglobulins are extremely useful screening tests to support the diagnosis of vasculitis or certain types of collagen vascular diseases or glomerulonephritis.

Imaging by renal ultrasonography is a rapid noninvasive investigation principally designed to rule out evidence of obstruction, stones, cysts, masses, or overt renovascular disease. A chest radiograph may be important both to assess for pulmonary complications of AKI and if a diagnosis of systemic vasculitis is considered. In the occasional patient, a percutaneous renal biopsy becomes necessary to confirm the diagnosis, determine the severity of renal injury, guide therapy, and evaluate prognosis and potential for recovery (98). A renal biopsy is indicated when a thorough noninvasive investigation has failed to yield the diagnosis, when transient and postrenal causes have been excluded, and prior to the administration of potentially toxic immunosuppressive therapy. A renal biopsy can be performed under ultrasound guidance with local anesthetic in critically ill patients undergoing MV without additional risks when compared to standard conditions.

PROGNOSIS

AKI can independently influence both short- and long-term prognosis. In hospitalized patients, mortality is estimated at 20% among all those developing AKI; however, this rate is greatly influenced by the severity of renal injury. The prognosis is worse for critically ill patients and those where RRT becomes necessary. The in-hospital mortality for critically ill patients with AKI is estimated at 50% to 60% (yet can range between 30% and 80% depending on the case-mix) (18,19,99–102). It is frequently stated that patients die *with* AKI rather than *of* AKI. However, growing evidence suggests that better uremic control and more intensive artificial kidney support may improve survival by perhaps 30% (103–105). Such evidence supports a careful and proactive approach to the treatment of critically ill patients with AKI, which is based on the prevention of uncontrolled uremia, and fluid overload.

AKI is also associated with significant morbidity. AKI is associated with greater susceptibility to infection/sepsis, prolonged duration and delayed weaning from MV, and longer or unanticipated stays in ICU and hospital. Perhaps more importantly, AKI is a clear risk factor for development of CKD. In addition to CKD, recent data have also suggested survivors of AKI remain at increased long-term risk infection, major cardiovascular events, malignancy, and higher health services use (18,19,106).

Failure to recover function can have both individual patient and broader health care implications. Persistent CKD or need for long-term RRT can negatively influence the health status and quality of life of patients, and contribute to considerable annual health care expenditures. Recovery to independence from RRT occurs in an estimated 68% to 85% of critically ill patients by hospital discharge and generally peaks by 90 days (18,19). Studies have shown that older patients and those with pre-existing comorbid illnesses such as CKD or advanced cardiovascular disease are less likely to recover function whereas those with septic AKI may be more likely to recover function. Several other potentially modifiable factors have been linked with improved rates of recovery including timely initiation of RRT when indicated, initial use of continuous rather than intermittent RRT, early and adequate nutritional support. Whether adjuvant erythropoietin and routine use of loop diuretics can influence kidney prognosis and promote early recovery remain controversial.

In those who survive an episode of AKI, the long-term health status, including quality of life, functional status, and hospital discharge location, are also now considered important indicators of morbidity. These patients frequently describe limitations in daily activities, difficulties with mobility, and high levels of sleep disturbance, fatigue, anxiety, and depression. However, quality of life is often described as being generally good and perceived as acceptable, despite evidence of being considerably lower than that of the general population (107–110).

Key Points

- Restoring MAP within the autoregulatory range for blood flow to the kidney—65 to 110 mmHg—is important in maintaining the GFR. Once the patient has been adequately fluid resuscitated, and the cardiac output is known to be adequate, MAP should be corrected within autoregulation with the use of norepinephrine.
- Low-dose dopamine has been extensively studied, meta-analyzed, and assessed for the prevention and treatment of AKI. Although it probably increases urine output through its tubular diuretic effect, it does not maintain or improve the GFR or improve outcome.
- In an adequately fluid-resuscitated patient as described above, if the cardiac output is adequate or high, and the MAP is adequate or normal, there is no "renal" benefit to be gained by giving additional intravenous fluids. Such fluids often precipitate extravascular complications and have no appreciably beneficial effect on GFR. In these circumstances, support with RRT should be considered.

ACKNOWLEDGMENTS

Dr. Bagshaw is supported by a Canada Research Chair in Critical Care Nephrology.

References

1. Bellomo R, Ronco C, Kellum JA, et al. Acute Dialysis Quality Initiative with acute renal failure: definition, outcome measures, animal models, fluid therapy and information technology needs. The Second International Consensus Conference of the Acute Dialysis Quality Initiative (ADQI) Group. *Crit Care.* 2004;8(4):R204–R212.
2. Uchino S, Bellomo R, Goldsmith D, et al. An assessment of the RIFLE criteria for acute renal failure in hospitalized patients. *Crit Care Med.* 2006;34:1913–7.
3. Hoste EA, Clermont G, Kersten A, et al. RIFLE criteria for acute kidney injury are associated with hospital mortality in critically ill patients: a cohort analysis. *Crit Care.* 2006;10(3):R73.
4. KDIGO. KDIGO clinical practice guidelines on acute kidney injury. *Kidney Int.* 2012;2(1):8–12.
5. Pickering JW, Endre ZH. GFR shot by RIFLE: errors in staging acute kidney injury. *Lancet.* 2009;373(9672):1318–1319.
6. Doi K, Yuen PS, Eisner C, et al. Reduced production of creatinine limits its use as marker of kidney injury in sepsis. *J Am Soc Nephrol.* 2009;20(6):1217–1221.
7. Ralib A, Pickering JW, Shaw GM, Endre ZH. The urine output definition of acute kidney injury is too liberal. *Crit Care.* 2013;17(3):R112.
8. Prowle JR, Liu YL, Licari E, et al. Oliguria as predictive biomarker of acute kidney injury in critically ill patients. *Crit Care.* 2011;15(4):R172.
9. Macedo E, Malhotra R, Claure-Del Granado R, et al. Defining urine output criterion for acute kidney injury in critically ill patients. *Nephrol Dial Transpl.* 2011;26(2):509–515.
10. Mandelbaum T, Lee J, Scott DJ, et al. Empirical relationships among oliguria, creatinine, mortality, and renal replacement therapy in the critically ill. *Intensive Care Med.* 2013;39(3):414–419.
11. Macedo E, Malhotra R, Bouchard J, et al. Oliguria is an early predictor of higher mortality in critically ill patients. *Kidney Int.* 2011;80(7):760–767.
12. Bagshaw SM, Langenberg C, Bellomo R. Urinary biochemistry and microscopy in septic acute renal failure: a systematic review. *Am J Kidney Dis.* 2006;48(5):695–705.

13. Langenberg C, Wan L, Bagshaw SM, et al. Urinary biochemistry in experimental septic acute renal failure. *Nephrol Dial Transplant.* 2006;21(12):3389–3397.
14. Kanbay M, Kasapoglu B, Perazella MA. Acute tubular necrosis and pre-renal acute kidney injury: utility of urine microscopy in their evaluation: a systematic review. *Int Urol Nephrol.* 2010;42(2):425–433.
15. Carvounis CP, Nisar S, Guro-Razuman S. Significance of the fractional excretion of urea in the differential diagnosis of acute renal failure. *Kidney Int.* 2002;62(6):2223–2229.
16. Perazella MA, Coca SG, Hall IE, et al. Urine microscopy is associated with severity and worsening of acute kidney injury in hospitalized patients. *Clin J Am Soc Nephrol.* 2010;5(3):402–408.
17. Susantitaphong P, Cruz DN, Cerda J, et al. World incidence of AKI: a meta-analysis. *Clin J Am Soc Nephrol.* 2013;8(9):1482–1493.
18. Bagshaw SM, Laupland KB, Doig CJ, et al. Prognosis for long-term survival and renal recovery in critically ill patients with severe acute renal failure: a population-based study. *Crit Care.* 2005;9(6):R700–R709.
19. Uchino S, Kellum JA, Bellomo R, et al. Acute renal failure in critically ill patients: a multinational, multicenter study. *JAMA.* 2005;294(7):813–818.
20. de Mendonca A, Vincent JL, Suter PM, et al. Acute renal failure in the ICU: risk factors and outcome evaluated by the SOFA score. *Intensive Care Med.* 2000;26(7):915–921.
21. McCarthy JT. Prognosis of patients with acute renal failure in the intensive-care unit: a tale of two eras. *Mayo Clin Proc.* 1996;71(2):117–126.
22. Tran DD, Cuesta MA, Oe PL. Acute renal failure in patients with severe civilian trauma. *Nephrol Dial Transpl.* 1994;9(Suppl 4):121–125.
23. Nash K, Hafeez A, Hou S. Hospital-acquired renal insufficiency. *Am J Kidney Dis.* 2002;39(5):930–936.
24. Feest T, Round A, Hamad S. Incidence of severe acute renal failure in adults: results of a community based study. *BMJ.* 1993;306:481–483.
25. Kheterpal S, Tremper KK, Heung M, et al. Development and validation of an acute kidney injury risk index for patients undergoing general surgery: results from a national data set. *Anesthesiology.* 2009;110(3):505–515.
26. Goldstein SL, Kirkendall E, Nguyen H, et al. Electronic health record identification of nephrotoxin exposure and associated acute kidney injury. *Pediatrics.* 2013;132(3):e756–e767.
27. Selby NM, Crowley L, Fluck RJ, et al. Use of electronic results reporting to diagnose and monitor AKI in hospitalized patients. *Clin J Am Soc Nephrol.* 2012;7(4):533–540.
28. Silvester W, Bellomo R, Cole L. Epidemiology, management, and outcome of severe acute renal failure of critical illness in Australia. *Critical Care Med.* 2001;29(10):1910–1915.
29. Langenberg C, Bellomo R, May C, et al. Renal blood flow in sepsis. *Crit Care.* 2005;9(4):R363–R374.
30. Langenberg C, Bellomo R, May CN, et al. Renal vascular resistance in sepsis. *Nephron Physiol.* 2006;104(1):p1–p11.
31. Langenberg C, Wan L, Egi M, et al. Renal blood flow in experimental septic acute renal failure. *Kidney Int.* 2006;69(11):1996–2002.
32. Gomez H, Ince C, De Backer D, et al. A unified theory of sepsis-induced acute kidney injury: inflammation, microcirculatory dysfunction, bioenergetics, and the tubular cell adaptation to injury. *Shock.* 2014;41(1):3–11.
33. Lucas CE, Rector FE, Werner M, Rosenberg IK. Altered renal homeostasis with acute sepsis: clinical significance. *Arch Surg.* 1973;106(4):444–449.
34. Rector F, Goyal S, Rosenberg IK, Lucas CE. Renal hyperemia in associated with clinical sepsis. *Surg Forum.* 1972;23(0):51–53.
35. Brenner M, Schaer GL, Mallory DL, et al. Detection of renal blood flow abnormalities in septic and critically ill patients using a newly designed indwelling thermodilution renal vein catheter. *Chest.* 1990;98(1):170–179.
36. Di Giantomasso D, Morimatsu H, May CN, Bellomo R. Intrarenal blood flow distribution in hyperdynamic septic shock: effect of norepinephrine. *Crit Care Med.* 2003;31(10):2509–2513.
37. Hotchkiss RS, Swanson PE, Freeman BD, et al. Apoptotic cell death in patients with sepsis, shock, and multiple organ dysfunction. *Crit Care Med.* 1999;27(7):1230–1251.
38. Wan L, Bellomo R, Di Giantomasso D, Ronco C. The pathogenesis of septic acute renal failure. *Curr Opin Crit Care.* 2003;9(6):496–502.
39. Jo SK, Cha DR, Cho WY, et al. Inflammatory cytokines and lipopolysaccharide induce Fas-mediated apoptosis in renal tubular cells. *Nephron.* 2002;91(3):406–415.
40. Messmer UK, Briner VA, Pfeilschifter J. Tumor necrosis factor-alpha and lipopolysaccharide induce apoptotic cell death in bovine glomerular endothelial cells. *Kidney Int.* 1999;55(6):2322–2337.
41. Bonegio R, Lieberthal W. Role of apoptosis in the pathogenesis of acute renal failure. *Curr Opin Nephrol Hypertens.* 2002;11(3):301–308.
42. Imai Y, Parodo J, Kajikawa O, et al. Injurious mechanical ventilation and end-organ epithelial cell apoptosis and organ dysfunction in an experimental model of acute respiratory distress syndrome. *JAMA.* 2003;289(16):2104–2112.
43. Bastin AJ, Ostermann M, Slack AJ, et al. Acute kidney injury after cardiac surgery according to Risk/Injury/Failure/Loss/End-stage, Acute Kidney Injury Network, and Kidney Disease: Improving Global Outcomes classifications. *J Crit Care.* 2013;28(4):389–396.
44. Gueler F, Rong S, Park JK, et al. Postischemic acute renal failure is reduced by short-term statin treatment in a rat model. *J Am Soc Nephrol.* 2002;13(9):2288–2298.
45. Noiri E, Nakao A, Uchida K, et al. Oxidative and nitrosative stress in acute renal ischemia. *Am J Physiol Renal Physiol.* 2001;281(5):F948–F957.
46. Starkopf J, Zilmer K, Vihalemm T, et al. Time course of oxidative stress during open-heart surgery. *Scand J Thorac Cardiovasc Surg.* 1995;29(4):181–186.
47. Ishizuka S, Nagashima Y, Numata M, et al. Regulation and immunohistochemical analysis of stress protein heme oxygenase-1 in rat kidney with myoglobinuric acute renal failure. *Biochem Biophys Res Commun.* 1997;240(1):93–98.
48. Gines P, Guevara M, Arroyo V, Rodes J. Hepatorenal syndrome. *Lancet.* 2003;362(9398):1819–1827.
49. Nadim MK, Kellum JA, Davenport A, et al. Hepatorenal syndrome: the 8th International Consensus Conference of the Acute Dialysis Quality Initiative (ADQI) Group. *Crit Care.* 2012;16(1):R23.
50. Arroyo V, Guevara M, Gines P. Hepatorenal syndrome in cirrhosis: pathogenesis and treatment. *Gastroenterology.* 2002;122(6):1658–1676.
51. Sort P, Navasa M, Arroyo V, et al. Effect of intravenous albumin on renal impairment and mortality in patients with cirrhosis and spontaneous bacterial peritonitis. *N Engl J Med.* 1999;341(6):403–409.
52. Guevara M, Gines P, Fernandez-Esparrach G, et al. Reversibility of hepatorenal syndrome by prolonged administration of ornipressin and plasma volume expansion. *Hepatology.* 1998;27(1):35–41.
53. Fabrizi F, Dixit V, Martin P. Meta-analysis: terlipressin therapy for the hepatorenal syndrome. *Aliment Pharmacol Ther.* 2006;24(6):935–944.
54. Guevara M, Gines P, Bandi JC, et al. Transjugular intrahepatic portosystemic shunt in hepatorenal syndrome: effects on renal function and vasoactive systems. *Hepatology.* 1998;28(2):416–422.
55. Brensing KA, Textor J, Perz J, et al. Long term outcome after transjugular intrahepatic portosystemic stent-shunt in non-transplant cirrhotics with hepatorenal syndrome: a phase II study. *Gut.* 2000;47(2):288–295.
56. Holt SG, Moore KP. Pathogenesis and treatment of renal dysfunction in rhabdomyolysis. *Intensive Care Med.* 2001;27(5):803–811.
57. Heyman SN, Brezis M, Reubinoff CA, et al. Acute renal failure with selective medullary injury in the rat. *J Clin Invest.* 1988;82(2):401–412.
58. Bonventre JV. Mechanisms of ischemic acute renal failure. *Kidney Int.* 1993;43(5):1160–1178.
59. di Mari JF, Davis R, Safirstein RL. MAPK activation determines renal epithelial cell survival during oxidative injury. *Am J Physiol.* 1999;277(2 Pt 2):F195–F203.
60. Portilla D, Mandel LJ, Bar-Sagi D, Millington DS. Anoxia induces phospholipase A2 activation in rabbit renal proximal tubules. *Am J Physiol.* 1992;262(3 Pt 2):F354–F360.
61. Bennett WM, Luft F, Porter GA. Pathogenesis of renal failure due to aminoglycosides and contrast media used in roentgenography. *Am J Med.* 1980;69(5):767–774.
62. Cunha MA, Schor N. Effects of gentamicin, lipopolysaccharide, and contrast media on immortalized proximal tubular cells. *Renal Failure.* 2002;24(6):687–690.
63. Bagshaw SM, Culleton BF. Contrast-induced nephropathy: epidemiology and prevention. *Minerva Cardioangiol.* 2006;54(1):109–129.
64. Aspelin P, Aubry P, Fransson SG, et al. Nephrotoxic effects in high-risk patients undergoing angiography. *N Engl J Med.* 2003;348(6):491–499.
65. Merten GJ, Burgess WP, Gray LV, et al. Prevention of contrast-induced nephropathy with sodium bicarbonate: a randomized controlled trial. *JAMA.* 2004;291(19):2328–2334.
66. Mueller C, Seidensticker P, Buettner HJ, et al. Incidence of contrast nephropathy in patients receiving comprehensive intravenous and oral hydration. *Swiss Med Wkly.* 2005;135(19–20):286–290.
67. Stevens MA, McCullough PA, Tobin KJ, et al. A prospective randomized trial of prevention measures in patients at high risk for contrast nephropathy: results of the P.R.I.N.C.E. Study. Prevention of Radiocontrast Induced Nephropathy Clinical Evaluation. *J Am Coll Cardiol.* 1999;33(2):403–411.
68. Bagshaw SM, Ghali WA. Acetylcysteine for prevention of contrast-induced nephropathy after intravascular angiography: a systematic review and meta-analysis. *BMC Med.* 2004;2:38.

69. Tepel M, van der Giet M, Schwarzfeld C, et al. Prevention of radiographic-contrast-agent-induced reductions in renal function by acetylcysteine. *N Engl J Med*. 2000;343(3):180–184.
70. Kuiper JW, Groeneveld AB, Slutsky AS, Plotz FB. Mechanical ventilation and acute renal failure. *Crit Care Med*. 2005;33(6):1408–1415.
71. Pannu N, Mehta RL. Mechanical ventilation and renal function: an area for concern? *Am J Kidney Dis*. 2002;39(3):616–624.
72. Ricard JD, Dreyfuss D, Saumon G. Ventilator-induced lung injury. *Curr Opin Crit Care*. 2002;8(1):12–20.
73. Ranieri VM, Suter PM, Tortorella C, et al. Effect of mechanical ventilation on inflammatory mediators in patients with acute respiratory distress syndrome: a randomized controlled trial. *JAMA*. 1999;282(1):54–61.
74. Mohmand H, Goldfarb S. Renal dysfunction associated with intra-abdominal hypertension and the abdominal compartment syndrome. *J Am Soc Nephrol*. 2011;22(4):615–621.
75. Albanese J, Leone M, Garnier F, et al. Renal effects of norepinephrine in septic and nonseptic patients. *Chest*. 2004;126(2):534–539.
76. Bellomo R, Kellum JA, Wisniewski SR, Pinsky MR. Effects of norepinephrine on the renal vasculature in normal and endotoxemic dogs. *Am J Resp Crit Care Med*. 1999;159(4 Pt 1):1186–1192.
77. Bourgoin A, Leone M, Delmas A, et al. Increasing mean arterial pressure in patients with septic shock: effects on oxygen variables and renal function. *Crit Care Med*. 2005;33(4):780–786.
78. Finfer S, Bellomo R, Boyce N, et al. A comparison of albumin and saline for fluid resuscitation in the intensive care unit. *N Engl J Med*. 2004;350(22):2247–2256.
79. Myburgh JA, Finfer S, Bellomo R, et al. Hydroxyethyl starch or saline for fluid resuscitation in intensive care. *N Engl J Med*. 2012;367(20):1901–1911.
80. Perner A, Haase N, Guttormsen AB, et al. Hydroxyethyl starch 130/0.42 versus Ringer's acetate in severe sepsis. *N Engl J Med*. 2012;367(2):124–134.
81. Chowdhury AH, Cox EF, Francis ST, Lobo DN. A randomized, controlled, double-blind crossover study on the effects of 2-L infusions of 0.9% saline and plasma-lyte(R) 148 on renal blood flow velocity and renal cortical tissue perfusion in healthy volunteers. *Ann Surg*. 2012;256(1):18–24.
82. Payen D, de Pont AC, Sakr Y, et al. A positive fluid balance is associated with a worse outcome in patients with acute renal failure. *Crit Care*. 2008;12(3):R74.
83. Grams ME, Estrella MM, Coresh J, et al. Fluid balance, diuretic use, and mortality in acute kidney injury. *Clin J Am Soc Nephrol*. 2011;6(5):966–973.
84. Sakr Y, Vincent JL, Reinhart K, et al. High tidal volume and positive fluid balance are associated with worse outcome in acute lung injury. *Chest*. 2005;128(5):3098–3108.
85. Simmons RS, Berdine GG, Seidenfeld JJ, et al. Fluid balance and the adult respiratory distress syndrome. *Am Rev Resp Dis*. 1987;135(4):924–929.
86. Wiedemann HP, Wheeler AP, Bernard GR, et al. Comparison of two fluid-management strategies in acute lung injury. *N Engl J Med*. 2006;354(24):2564–2575.
87. Bellomo R, Chapman M, Finfer S, et al. Low-dose dopamine in patients with early renal dysfunction: a placebo-controlled randomised trial. Australian and New Zealand Intensive Care Society (ANZICS) Clinical Trials Group. *Lancet*. 2000;356(9248):2139–2143.
88. Shilliday IR, Quinn KJ, Allison ME. Loop diuretics in the management of acute renal failure: a prospective, double-blind, placebo-controlled, randomized study. *Nephrol Dial Transpl*. 1997;12(12):2592–2596.
89. Morelli A, Ricci Z, Bellomo R, et al. Prophylactic fenoldopam for renal protection in sepsis: a randomized, double-blind, placebo-controlled pilot trial. *Crit Care Med*. 2005;33(11):2451–2456.
90. Bove T, Landoni G, Calabro MG, et al. Renoprotective action of fenoldopam in high-risk patients undergoing cardiac surgery: a prospective, double-blind, randomized clinical trial. *Circulation*. 2005;111(24):3230–3235.
91. Sward K, Valsson F, Odencrants P, et al. Recombinant human atrial natriuretic peptide in ischemic acute renal failure: a randomized placebo-controlled trial. *Crit Care Med*. 2004;32(6):1310–1315.
92. Chertow GM, Lazarus JM, Paganini EP, et al. Predictors of mortality and the provision of dialysis in patients with acute tubular necrosis. The Auriculin Anaritide Acute Renal Failure Study Group. *J Am Soc Nephrol*. 1998;9(4):692–698.
93. Hebert PC, Wells G, Blajchman MA, et al. A multicenter, randomized, controlled clinical trial of transfusion requirements in critical care. Transfusion Requirements in Critical Care Investigators, Canadian Critical Care Trials Group. *N Engl J Med*. 1999;340(6):409–417.
94. Karvellas CJ, Farhat MR, Sajjad I, et al. A comparison of early versus late initiation of renal replacement therapy in critically ill patients with acute kidney injury: a systematic review and meta-analysis. *Crit Care*. 2011;15(1):R72.
95. Schneider AG, Bellomo R, Bagshaw SM, et al. Choice of renal replacement therapy modality and dialysis dependence after acute kidney injury: a systematic review and meta-analysis. *Intensive Care Med*. 2013;39(6):987–997.
96. VA/NIH ATN Trial Investigators, Palevsky PM, Zhang JH, et al. Intensity of renal support in critically ill patients with acute kidney injury. *N Engl J Med*. 2008;359(1):7–20.
97. RENAL Trial Investigators, Bellomo R, Cass A, et al. Intensity of continuous renal-replacement therapy in critically ill patients. *N Engl J Med*. 2009;361(17):1627–1638.
98. Korbet SM. Percutaneous renal biopsy. *Semin Nephrol*. 2002;22(3):254–267.
99. Liano F, Junco E, Pascual J, et al. The spectrum of acute renal failure in the intensive care unit compared with that seen in other settings. The Madrid Acute Renal Failure Study Group. *Kidney Int Suppl*. 1998;66:S16–S24.
100. Mehta RL, Pascual MT, Soroko S, et al. Spectrum of acute renal failure in the intensive care unit: the PICARD experience. *Kidney Int*. 2004;66(4):1613–1621.
101. Ympa YP, Sakr Y, Reinhart K, Vincent JL. Has mortality from acute renal failure decreased? A systematic review of the literature. *Am J Med*. 2005;118(8):827–832.
102. Nisula S, Kaukonen KM, Vaara ST, et al. Incidence, risk factors and 90-day mortality of patients with acute kidney injury in Finnish intensive care units: the FINNAKI study. *Intensive Care Med*. 2013;39(3):420–428.
103. Ronco C, Bellomo R, Homel P, et al. Effects of different doses in continuous veno-venous haemofiltration on outcomes of acute renal failure: a prospective randomised trial. *Lancet*. 2000;356(9223):26–30.
104. Schiffl H, Lang SM, Fischer R. Daily hemodialysis and the outcome of acute renal failure. *N Engl J Med*. 2002;346(5):305–310.
105. Saudan P, Niederberger M, De Seigneux S, et al. Adding a dialysis dose to continuous hemofiltration increases survival in patients with acute renal failure. *Kidney Int*. 2006;70(7):1312–1317.
106. Coca SG, Singanamala S, Parikh CR. Chronic kidney disease after acute kidney injury: a systematic review and meta-analysis. *Kidney Int*. 2012;81(5):442–448.
107. Ahlstrom A, Tallgren M, Peltonen S, et al. Survival and quality of life of patients requiring acute renal replacement therapy. *Intensive Care Med*. 2005;31(9):1222–1228.
108. Korkeila M, Ruokonen E, Takala J. Costs of care, long-term prognosis and quality of life in patients requiring renal replacement therapy during intensive care. *Intensive Care Med*. 2000;26(12):1824–1831.
109. Maynard SE, Whittle J, Chelluri L, Arnold R. Quality of life and dialysis decisions in critically ill patients with acute renal failure. *Intensive Care Med*. 2003;29(9):1589–1593.
110. Morgera S, Kraft AK, Siebert G, et al. Long-term outcomes in acute renal failure patients treated with continuous renal replacement therapies. *Am J Kidney Dis*. 2002;40(2):275–279.

CHAPTER

133

Renal Replacement Therapy

CLAUDIO RONCO, ZACCARIA RICCI, and STEFANO ROMAGNOLI

INTRODUCTION

Despite recent advances in acute kidney injury (AKI) definition, diagnosis, and treatment, many aspects remain subject to controversy. Renal replacement therapies (RRTs) currently remain the most important part of AKI treatment and, although modern technology has made a vast pool of different strategies of extracorporeal renal support easily available, it is still not clear which one is superior to the others in terms of efficacy and outcome. Moreover, evidence-based medicine has not yet defined the best time to prescribe RRT and when and how patients should be weaned from this therapy. This chapter will review most of these aspects, and will provide some theoretical and practical bases for RRT prescription with the goal of helping intensive care unit (ICU) clinicians to understand critical care nephrology.

Acute Kidney Injury and the Critically Ill Patient

A consensus document from the Kidney Disease Improving Global Outcome (KDIGO) Workgroup (1) pointed out all aspects related to AKI definition, diagnosis, and treatment. AKI is now defined and classified according to KDIGO classification: it identifies three different AKI severity levels that should allow the clinicians to uniformly identify and eventually treat this deadly syndrome (Table 133.1). This document also clearly specifies all the supportive measures that can be adopted in case of AKI but also, for the first time, tries to associate AKI staging with a progressively increasing treatment effort: according to these authors, RRT should be at least considered when AKI severity reaches the KDIGO stage II. Before this classification was available, a milestone multinational observational study on about 30,000 critically ill patients found that, worldwide, AKI incidence is around 6% and that 75% of these underwent a dialytic treatment (2) with an overall hospital mortality of 60.3%. What significantly changed since the publication of that paper is the clinician's capacity to identify AKI according to the new standard approach that probably increased awareness of AKI incidence, today reaching 25% of critically ill patients in the ICU (3). Unfortunately crude mortality has remained high and it has not significantly changed in the last 30 years. Nevertheless, a much greater illness severity and multiorgan failure (much different from isolated acute kidney failure) is currently the main characteristic of RRT patients. The techniques of artificial renal support have evolved markedly (4). It is likely, however, that the 50% to 60% crude mortality associated with AKI will remain unchanged into the next decade. In fact, as therapeutic capability improves and the system continues to accept a mortality of 50% as reasonable for these very sick patients, the health care system will progressively admit and treat sicker and sicker patients with AKI.

From Kramer's initial description of continuous arteriovenous hemofiltration (CAVH) in 1977 (5), RRT has progressively evolved in the ICU from a last-chance therapy for AKI to a standardized, widely used, fully independent form of artificial kidney support. Hardware and software technology supporting the application of RRT has greatly improved. The trend of this evolution and the potential of RRT have grown to a point in which multiple organ support therapy (MOST) is envisaged as a possible therapeutic approach in the critical care setting.

Thus, AKI and the requirement for acute RRT have become established realities. It is estimated that the incidence of AKI requiring extracorporeal support is 11 per 100,000 population per year; mortality is 7.3 per 100,000 residents per year, with the highest rates in males over 65 years. Renal recovery occurs in 78% (68/87) of survivors at 1 year, meaning that, although a great number of patients with severe AKI die, most survivors will become independent from RRT within a year (6).

The number of acute dialytic treatments has grown with the development of a new specialized branch of nephrology—critical care nephrology—in the last 10 years. However, a critically ill patient with AKI is not a patient with isolated renal dysfunction. AKI requires a multidisciplinary approach with intensivists and nephrologists sharing their respective knowledge. Fluid balance, vasopressors dosage, mechanical ventilation support, and arterial blood gas exchange—including PaO_2/FiO_2 ratio—need to be correlated with the RRT prescription, dialysis dose, ultrafiltration requirement, and anticoagulation strategy; younger ICU clinicians need to understand in depth in their routine practice all theoretical and technical aspects of critical care nephrology.

Indications for Initiation and Cessation

When to Start

Whether and when to start RRT are among the top priorities and most debated issues in the field of severe AKI, and there is no consensus between nephrologists and intensivists. RRT has the following targets when applied in patients with AKI: (1) to optimize fluid balance; (2) to guarantee electrolyte, acid–base, and solute homeostasis; (3) to prevent further injuries to the kidney; (4) to potentially "unload" the injured kidney thus facilitating renal recovery. Current indications for urgent/emergency RRT in clinical practice are well defined: fluid overload, hyperazotemia, hyperkalemia, severe acidosis, and intoxication (Table 133.2) (1). On the other hand, in the absence of these unquestioned indications, there is a global tendency to delay RRT in order to limit potential complications related to the extracorporeal application: biocompatibility, anticoagulation, vascular access, loss of beneficial molecules. Outside the urgent/emergency conditions listed above, a decision for RRT initiation cannot be based solely on azotemia (serum creatinine and/or urea) and a global evaluation including the clinical

TABLE 133.1 KDIGO Classification of Acute Kidney Inury

	Stage 1	Stage 2	Stage 3
Serum creatinine*	≥0.3 mg/dL (≥26.5 μmol/L) increase *or* 1.5–1.9× baseline	2.0–2.9 × baseline	Increase to ≥4.0 mg/dL (≥353.6 μmol/L) *or* ≥3.0× baseline or more *or* Initiation of RRT *or* In pediatric patients, decrease in eGFR to <35 mL/min/1.73 m^2
Urine output	<0.5 mL/kg/hr for 6–12 h	<0.5 mL/kg/hr for ≥12 hr	<0.3 mL/kg/hr for ≥24 hr *or* Anuria for ≥12 hr

*Timeframe for serum creatinine increase: either 0.3 mg/dL within 48 hr or 1.5 × increase within a wk.
eGFR, estimated glomerular filtration rate; eGFR, estimated GFR; RRT, renal replacement therapy.
Adapted from Kidney Disease: Improving Global Outcomes (KDIGO) Acute Kidney Injury Work Group. KDIGO clinical practice guideline for acute kidney injury. *Kidney Int Suppl.* 2012;2:8.

context and the trend of laboratory tests, rather than single values, are recommended when deciding whether to start RRT (1). In light of this, the severity of the underlying disease and organ dysfunction—that may affect the recovery of kidney function and tolerance of fluid accumulation—the occurrence of solute burden such as rhabdomyolysis, and the need for nutrition or drug therapies, should be considered. In addition, when medical management—diuretics, bicarbonate, glucose–insulin solutions, beta$_2$-agonists, fluid and nutritional restriction—fails to prevent or treat renal dysfunction, treatment is usually escalated to RRT. Further, there is some interest in the role of biomarkers—neutrophil gelatinase–associated lipocalin, NGAL—as potential predictors of RRT requirement (7).

The timing between initiation of extracorporeal therapy and ICU admission is another issue that should be taken into account for classification purposes of early and late RRTs. Data available from the BEST kidney registry (8) reveal that, when timing was analyzed in relation to ICU admission, "late" RRT was associated with greater crude mortality, covariate-adjusted mortality, RRT requirement, and hospital length of stay (8). Although several studies have suggested a possible positive role of early RRT among AKI patients, contrasting results are available in literature. In 2002, Bouman et al. (9) showed no differences for ICU or hospital mortalities and for renal recovery among patients treated with an early or late RRT. However, if cumulatively considered in systematic review or meta-analysis, by parameters utilized to define the onset, an early initiation of RRT seems to be associated to an improved outcome (10). In a recent meta-analysis, including 15 unique studies published through 2010, comparing early and late initiation of renal support, Karvellas et al. have calculated an odds ratio for 28-day mortality of 0.45 associated with an early RRT (10). Similar results were obtained by Wang and colleagues (11) in a 2012 meta-analysis encompassing data from 2,955 patients; the results of this study have clearly demonstrated that an early initiation of both continuous and intermittent RRT may reduce the mortality of patients with AKI compared with late treatments.

TABLE 133.2 Indications for Renal Replacement Therapy[a]

General
Renal replacement
Life-threatening indications
Nonemergent indications
Renal support[b]
Specific pediatric indications
Specific
Little or no residual kidney function
Hyperkalemia/severe acidemia
Pulmonary edema, uremic complications
Solute control (hyperazotemia, hypercreatininemia), fluid removal, correction of acid-base abnormalities
Volume control, nutrition, drug delivery
Regulation of acid–base and electrolyte status
Solute modulation, sepsis syndrome
Inborn error of metabolism

[a]According to the KDIGO Workgroup, no standard evidence-based criteria for initiating dialysis currently exist in either pediatric or adult patients.
[b]Renal support implies a proactive utilization of RRT techniques as an adjunct to enhance kidney function, modify fluid balance, and control solute levels before they have reached "severity" criteria.
Data from Cruz DN, de Cal M, Garzotto F, et al. Plasma neutrophil gelatinase-associated lipocalin is an early biomarker for acute kidney injury in an adult ICU population. *Intensive Care Med.* 2010;36:444–451.

When to Stop

Once RRT has been started, timing for stopping is another field of uncertainty as the literature is scarce. Bedside evaluation of weaning RRT implies two fundamental clinical data elements: the state of renal function, and recovery from the morbidity that initially led to RRT. Current guidelines suggest discontinuing RRT when kidney function has recovered and is able to meets patient needs or, globally "is no longer consistent with the goals of care" (1). Many, but not all, patients receiving RRT will recover renal function, so daily evaluation of the appropriateness of treatment is necessary to identify weaning opportunities, including a modality transitions—e.g., from continuous to intermittent—or to decide to withdraw treatment for futility (12–13). The assessment of kidney function during RRT is a complex issue and clear recommendations are not available. From a practical clinical point of view, diuresis seems to be the most efficient predictor of RRT weaning success. A large prospective observational study, encompassing 529 patients, showed that urine output was the most significant predictor of successful termination of RRT (14). It is important to underline that, while diuretics increase urine output even in AKI patients, current guidelines suggest "not using diuretics to enhance kidney function recovery, or to reduce the duration or frequency of RRT" (1). In fact, diuretics increase urine output but do not seem to positively influence renal function.

Unanswered Research Topics

A number of issues remain unaddressed, warranting future research. The KDIGO guidelines recommend studies to establish reproducible criteria capable of suggesting optimal timing for initiation of RRT in AKI patients (1). Timing—early versus late initiation and criteria for weaning—should be correlated with outcome measures, taking into consideration all the variables: dose, modality, materials, and anticoagulation.

CONTINUOUS, INTERMITTENT, DIFFUSIVE, CONVECTIVE: AN ONGOING MATTER

Definitions

Renal replacement consists of the purification of blood by semipermeable membranes; a wide range of molecules—from water to urea to low–, middle–, and high–molecular-weight solutes—are transported across such membranes by the mechanism of ultrafiltration (water), convection, and diffusion (solutes) (Fig. 133.1).

During *diffusion*, movement of solute depends upon their tendency to reach the same concentration on each side of the membrane; the practical result is the passage of solutes from the compartment with the highest concentration to the compartment with the lowest. Other components of the semipermeable membrane deeply affect diffusion: thickness and surface, temperature, and diffusion coefficient. *Dialysis* is a modality of RRT and is predominantly based on the principle of diffusion: a dialytic solution flows through the filter in a manner counter (countercurrent) to blood flow in order to maintain the highest solute gradient from inlet to outlet port.

During *convection*, the movement of solute across a semipermeable membrane takes place in conjunction with significant amounts of *ultrafiltration* (water transfer across the membrane). In other words, as the solvent (plasma water) is pushed across the membrane in response to the transmembrane pressure (TMP) by ultrafiltration (UF), solutes are carried with it, as long as the porosity of the membrane allows the molecules to be sieved from blood. The process of UF is governed by the UF rate (Q_f), the membrane UF coefficient (Km), and the TMP gradient generated by the pressures on both sides of the membrane (see the legend of Fig. 133.1).

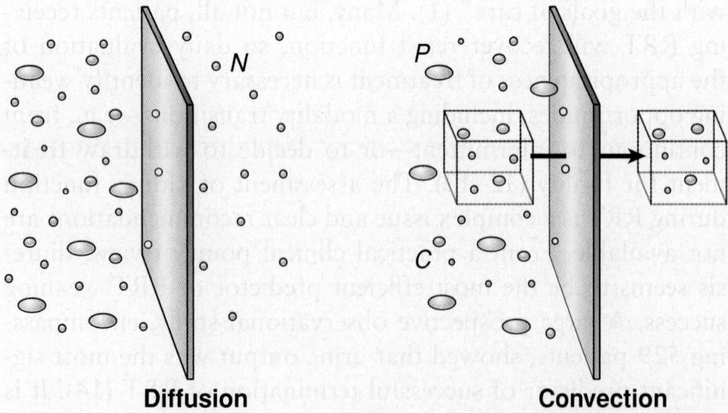

FIGURE 133.1 Diffusion and convection are schematically represented. During diffusion, solute flux (J_x) is a function of solute concentration gradient (dc) between the two sides of the semipermeable membrane, temperature (T), diffusivity coefficient (D), membrane thickness (dx) and surface area (A) according to the equation $J_x = D \times T \times A$ (dc/dx). Convective flux of solutes (J_f), however, requires a pressure gradient between the two sides of the membrane (transmembrane pressure; TMP): TMP = $(P_b - P_d) - \pi$, where P_b is blood hydrostatic pressure, P_d is hydrostatic pressure on ultrafiltrate side of the membrane, and π is blood oncotic pressure. This pressure gradient moves a fluid (plasma, water) with its crystalloid content, a process called ultrafiltration. The functionality of ultrafiltration is also dependent on the membrane permeability coefficient K_f, in that $J_f = K_f \times$ TMP. Colloids and cells will cross or not cross the semipermeable membrane, depending on the membrane's pore sizes.

The hydrostatic pressure in the blood compartment is dependent on blood flow (Q_b). The greater the Q_b, the greater the TMP. In modern RRT machines, UF control throughout the filter is obtained by the use of a pump, which generates suction to the UF side of the membrane. Modern systems are optimally designed in order to maintain a constant Q_f; it is worth noting that, when the filter is "fresh," the initial effect of the UF pump is to retard UF production, generating a positive pressure on the UF side. Thus, TMP is initially dependent only on Q_b. As the membrane fibers foul, a negative pressure is necessary to achieve a constant Q_f. In this case, a progressive increase of TMP can be observed up to a maximal level in which clotting is likely, membrane rupture may occur and, above all, solute clearance may be significantly compromised. In fact, if it is true that the size of molecules cleared during convection exceeds that during diffusion, because they are physically dragged to the UF side, it is also true that this feature is seriously limited by the protein layer that progressively closes filter pores during convective treatments (15). A peculiar membrane capacity, termed adsorption, has been shown to have a major role in higher–molecular-weight toxins (16); however, membrane adsorptive capacity is generally saturated in the first hours from the beginning of the treatment. This observation notes the scarce impact of the adsorption component on solute clearance and suggests relying only on the effects of mass separation processes such as diffusion and convection (17). As UF proceeds, and plasma water and solutes are filtered from blood, hydrostatic pressure within the filter is lost, and oncotic pressure is gained because blood concentrates and hematocrit increase. The fraction of plasma water that is removed from blood during UF is called filtration fraction; it should be kept in the range of 20% to 25% to prevent excessive hemoconcentration within the filtering membrane and to avoid the critical point where oncotic pressure is equal to TMP and a condition of filtration/pressure equilibrium is reached. Finally, replacing plasma water with a substitute solution completes the *hemofiltration* (HF) process and returns purified blood to the patient. The replacement fluid can be administered after the filter, a process called postdilution HF. Otherwise, the solution can be infused before the filter in order to obtain predilution HF, whereas predilution plus postdilution replacement is obtained on mixed infusion of substitution fluids both before and after filtering the membrane. While postdilution allows a urea clearance equivalent to therapy delivery (i.e., 2,000 mL/hr; see below) predilution, despite a theoretical reduced solute clearances, prolongs the circuit lifespan, and reduces hemoconcentration and protein-caking effects occurring within filter fibers. Conventional HF is performed with a highly permeable, steam-sterilized membrane with a surface area of about 1 m^2, and with a cutoff point of 30 kd (Fig. 133.2).

Concept of RRT Dose

The conventional view of RRT dose is that it is a measure of the quantity of blood purification achieved by means of extracorporeal techniques. As this broad concept is too difficult to measure and quantify, the *operative* view of RRT dose is that it is a measure of the quantity of a representative marker solute that is removed from a patient. This marker solute is considered to

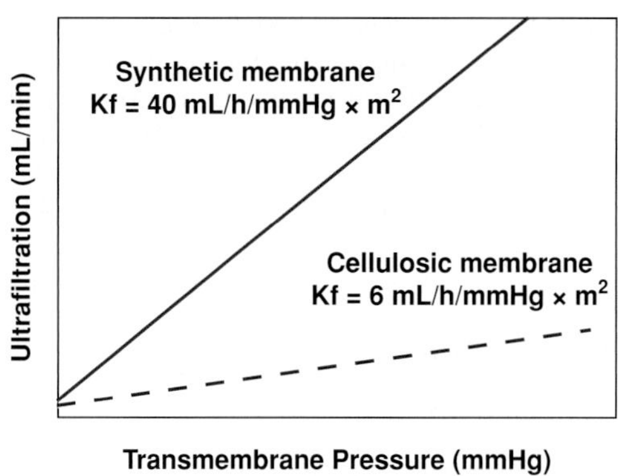

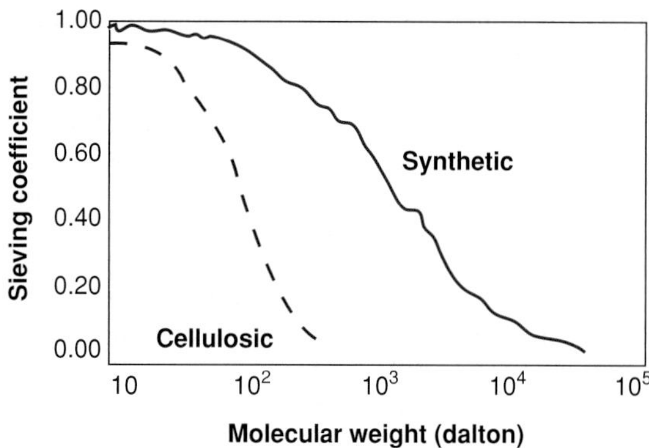

FIGURE 133.2 Membranes are classified based on their permeability or filtration coefficient (K_f; in mL/hr/mmHg) and their sieving coefficient. A high flux (synthetic membrane) will have higher permeability to water with optimal use during hemofiltration or hemodiafiltration (prevalently convective treatments) and bigger pore sizes in order to let higher molecular weight molecules cross the membrane.

be reasonably representative of similar solutes, which require removal for blood purification to be considered adequate. This premise has several major flaws: the marker solute cannot and does not represent all the solutes that accumulate in renal failure; its kinetics and volume of distribution are also different from such solutes; finally, its removal during RRT is not representative of the removal of other solutes. This is true both for end-stage renal failure and acute renal failure. However, a significant body of data in the end-stage renal failure literature (18–23) suggests that, despite all of the above major limitations, a single-solute marker assessment of dialysis dose appears to have a clinically meaningful relationship with patient outcome and, therefore, clinical utility. Nevertheless, the HEMO study, examining the effect of intermittent hemodialysis (IHD) doses, enforced the concept that "less dialysis is worse," but failed to confirm the intuition that "more dialysis is better" (23). Thus, if this premise seems useful in end-stage renal failure, it is accepted to be potentially useful in AKI for operative purposes. Hence, the amount (measure) of delivered dose of RRT can be described by various terms: efficiency, intensity, frequency, and clinical efficacy; each will be discussed below.

The *efficiency* of RRT is represented by the concept of clearance (K), i.e., the volume of blood cleared of a given solute over a given time. K does not reflect the overall solute removal rate (mass transfer) but, rather, its value normalized by the serum concentration. Even when K remains stable over time, the removal rate will vary if the blood levels of the reference molecule change. K depends on solute molecular size and transport modality—diffusion or convection—as well as circuit operational characteristics—blood flow rate (Q_b), dialysate flow rate (Q_d), ultrafiltration rate (Q_f), hemodialyzer type, and size. K can normally be used to compare the treatment dose during each dialysis session, but it cannot be employed as an absolute dose measure to compare treatments with different time schedules. For example, K is typically higher in IHD than in continuous renal replacement therapy (CRRT) and sustained low-efficiency daily dialysis (SLEDD). This is not surprising, since K represents only the instantaneous efficiency of the system. However, mass removal may be greater during SLEDD or CRRT. For this reason, the information about the time span during which K is delivered is fundamental to describe the effective dose of dialysis.

The *intensity* of RRT can be defined by the product "clearance × time" (K_t). K_t is more useful than K in comparing various RRTs. A further step in assessing dose must include frequency of the K_t application over a particular period (e.g., a week). This additional dimension is given by the product of intensity × frequency (K_t × treatment days/week = K_t d/w). K_t d/w is superior to K_t since it offers information beyond a single treatment—patients with AKI typically require more than one treatment. This concept of K_t d/w offers the possibility to compare disparate treatment schedules—intermittent, alternate-day, daily, continuous. However, it does not take into account the size of the pool of solute that needs to be cleared; this requires the dimension of efficacy.

The *efficacy* of RRT represents the effective solute removal outcome resulting from the administration of a given treatment to a given patient. It can be described by a fractional clearance of a given solute (K_t/V), where V is the volume of distribution of the marker molecule in the body. K_t/V is an established marker of adequacy of dialysis for small solutes correlating with medium-term (several years) survival in chronic hemodialysis patients (23). Urea is typically used as a marker molecule in end-stage kidney disease to guide treatment dose, and a K_t/V_{UREA} of at least 1.2 is currently recommended. As an example, we can consider the case of a 70-patient who is treated 20 hr/d with a postfilter HF of 2.8 L/hr at a zero balance. The patient's K_{UREA} will be 47 mL/min (2.8 L/hr = 2,800 mL/60 min) because we know that during postfilter HF, ultrafiltered plasmatic water will drag all urea across the membrane, making its clearance identical to UF flow. The treatment time (t) will be 1,200 minutes (60 minutes for 20 hours). The urea volume of distribution will be approximately 42,000 mL (60% of 70 kg, 42 L = 42,000 mL)—that is, roughly equal to total body water. Simplifying our patient's K_t/V_{UREA}, we will have 47 × 1,200/42,000 = 1.34.

However, K_t/V_{UREA} application to patients with AKI has not been rigorously validated. In fact, although the application of K_t/V to the assessment of dose in AKI is theoretically intriguing, many concerns have been raised because problems intrinsic to AKI can hinder the accuracy and meaning of such dose measurement. These include the lack of a metabolic steady state, uncertainty about the volume of distribution of urea (V_{UREA}), a high-protein catabolic rate, labile fluid volumes, and possible residual renal function, which changes dynamically during the course of treatment. Furthermore, delivery of prescribed dose in AKI can be limited by technical problems such as access recirculation, poor blood flows with temporary venous catheters, membrane clotting, and machine malfunction. Furthermore, clinical issues such as hypotension and vasopressor requirements can be responsible for solute disequilibrium within tissues and organs.

These aspects are particularly evident during IHD, less so during SLEDD, and even less so during CRRT. This difference is due to the fact that, after some days of CRRT, the patients' urea levels approach a real steady state. Access recirculation is also an issue of lesser impact during low-efficiency continuous techniques. Finally, because the therapy is applied continuously, the effect of compartmentalization of solutes is minimized and, from a theoretical point of view, single-pool kinetics can be applied (spK_t/V) with a reasonable chance of approximating true solute behavior. In a prospective study on continuous therapies, the value of clearance predicted by a simple excel software applying formulas for K calculation showed a significant correlation between estimated K and that obtained from direct blood and dialysate determinations during the first 24 treatment hours, irrespective of the continuous renal replacement modality used (24,25).

The major shortcoming of the traditional solute marker–based approach on dialysis dose lies beyond any methodologic critique of single-solute kinetics-based prescriptions: in patients with AKI, the majority of whom are in intensive care, a restrictive (solute-based only) concept of dialysis dose seems grossly inappropriate. In these patients, the therapeutic needs that can be or need to be affected by the "dose" of RRT are more than the simple control of small solutes as represented by urea. They include control of acid–base, tonicity, potassium, magnesium, calcium, phosphate, intravascular volume, extravascular volume, temperature, and the avoidance of unwanted side effects associated with the delivery of solute control. In the critically ill patient, it is much more important (e.g., in the setting of coagulopathic bleeding after cardiac surgery) for 10 units of fresh frozen plasma, 10 units of cyroprecipitate, and 10 units of platelets to be administered rapidly without inducing fluid overload (because 1 to 1.5 L of ultrafiltrate is removed in 1 hour) than for K_t/V to be of any particular value at all. A dose of RRT is about prophylactic volume control. In a patient with right ventricular failure, AKI, ARDS, who is receiving lung-protective ventilation with permissive hypercapnia and with acidemia, inducing a further life-threatening deterioration in pulmonary vascular resistance, the "dose" component of RRT that matters immediately is acid–base control and normalization of pH 24 hours a day. The K_t/V (or any other solute-centric concept of dose) is essentially a byproduct of such dose delivery. In a young man with trauma, rhabdomyolysis, and a rapidly rising serum potassium already at 7 mMol/L, the beginning dialysis dose is all about controlling hyperkalemia. In a patient with fulminant liver failure, AKI, sepsis, and cerebral edema awaiting urgent liver transplantation, and whose cerebral edema is worsening because of fever, RRT dose is centered on lowering the temperature without any tonicity shifts that might increase intracranial pressure. Finally, in a patient with pulmonary edema after an ischemic ventricular septal defect requiring emergency surgery, along with AKI, ischemic hepatitis, and the need for inotropic and intra-aortic balloon counterpulsation support, RRT dose mostly concerns removing fluid gently and safely so that the extravascular volume falls while the intravascular volume remains optimal. Solute removal is just a byproduct of fluid control. These aspects of dose must explicitly be considered when discussing the dose of RRT in AKI, for it is likely that patients die more often from incorrect "dose" delivery of this type than incorrect dose delivery of the K_t/V type. Although each and every aspect of this broader understanding of dose is difficult to measure, clinically relevant assessment of dose in critically ill patients with AKI should include all dimensions of such a dose, and not one dimension picked because of a similarity with end-stage renal failure. There is no evidence in the acute field that such solute control data are more relevant to clinical outcomes than volume control, acid–base control, or tonicity control.

RRT Prescription

Theoretical Aspects

Despite all the uncertainty surrounding its meaning and the gross shortcomings related to its accuracy in patients with AKI, the idea that there might be an optimal dose of solute removal continues to have a powerful hold in the literature. This is likely due to evidence from ESRD, where a minimum K_t/V of 1.2 thrice weekly is indicated as standard (23). However, the benefits of greater K_t/V accrue over years of therapy. In AKI, any difference in dose would apply for days to weeks. The view that it would still be sufficient to alter clinical outcomes remains somewhat optimistic. Nonetheless, the hypothesis that higher doses of dialysis may be beneficial in critically ill patients with AKI must be considered by analogy and investigated. Several reports exist in the literature dealing with this issue. Furthermore, the concept of predefined dose is a powerful tool to guide clinicians to a correct prescription and to, at least, avoid under treatment.

Brause et al. (26), using continuous venovenous hemofiltration (CVVH), found that higher K_t/V values (0.8 vs. 0.53) correlated with improved uremic control and acid–base balance; no clinically important outcome metric was affected. Investigators from the Cleveland clinic (27) retrospectively evaluated 844 patients with AKI requiring CRRT or IHD over a 7-year period. They found that, when patients were stratified for disease severity, dialysis dose did not affect outcome in patients with very high or very low scores, but did correlate with survival in patients with intermediate degrees of illness. A mean K_t/V greater than 1.0 or TAC_{UREA} below 45 mg/dL was associated with increased survival. This study was retrospective with a clear *post hoc* selection bias. Therefore, the validity of these observations remains highly questionable.

Daily IHD, compared to alternate-day dialysis, also seemed to be associated with improved outcome in a randomized trial (28). Daily hemodialysis resulted in significantly improved survival (72% vs. 54%, $p = 0.01$), better control of uremia, fewer hypotensive episodes, and more rapid resolution of AKI. However, several limitations limited this study: sicker, hemodynamically unstable patients were excluded, undergoing CRRT instead. Furthermore, according to the mean TAC_{UREA} reported, it appears that patients receiving conventional IHD were under-dialyzed. In addition, this was a single-center study with all the inherent limitations in regard to external validity. Finally, the second daily dialysis was associated with significant differences in fluid removal and dialysis-associated hypotension, suggesting that other aspects related to "dose," beyond solute control—such as inadequate and episodic volume control—may explain the findings. Clearly, further studies need be undertaken to assess the effect of dose of IHD on outcome.

In a randomized controlled trial of CRRT dose, continuous venovenous postdilution hemofiltration (CVVH) at 35 or 45 mL/kg/hr was associated with improved survival when compared to 20 mL/kg/hr in 425 critically ill patients with AKI (29). Applying K_t/V dose assessment methodology to CVVH, at a dose of 35 mL/kg/hr in a 70-kg patient treated for 24 hours, a treatment day would be equivalent to a K_t/V of 1.4 daily. Despite the uncertainty regarding the calculation of V urea, CVVH at 35 mL/kg/hr would still provide an effective *daily* delivery of 1.2, even in the presence of an underestimation of V_{UREA} by 20%. Many technical and/or clinical problems—including filter clotting, high filtration fraction in the presence of vascular access dysfunction with fluctuations in blood flow, circuit down-time during surgery or radiological procedures, and filter changes—can make it difficult, in routine practice, to apply such a strict protocol by pure postdilution HF. Equally important is the observation that this study was conducted over 6 years in a single center, uremic control was not reported, the incidence of sepsis was low compared to the typical populations reported to develop AKI in the world, and the final outcome was not the accepted 28- or 90-day mortality typically used in ICU trials. Thus, despite the interesting findings, the external validity of this study remains untested.

Another prospective randomized trial conducted by Bouman et al. (9) assigned patients to three intensity groups: early high-volume HF (72–96 L/24 hr); early low-volume HF (24–36 L/24 hr); and late low-volume HF (24–36 L/24 hr). These investigators found no difference in terms of renal recovery or 28-day mortality. Unfortunately, prescribed doses were not standardized by weight, causing a wide variability in RRT dose ultimately delivered to patients. Furthermore, the number of patients was small, making the study insufficiently powered and, again, the incidence of sepsis was low compared to the typical populations reported to develop AKI in the world.

Notwithstanding the problems we raise with these studies, they must be seen in light of an absolute lack of any previous attempt to adjust AKI treatment dose to specific target levels. The differences between delivered and prescribed dose in patients with AKI undergoing IHD were analyzed by Evanson and coworkers (30). The authors found that a high patient weight, male gender, and low blood flow were limiting factors affecting RRT administration, and that about 70% of dialysis delivered a K_t/V of less than 1.2. A retrospective study by Venkatarman et al. (31) also showed, similarly, that patients receive only 67% of prescribed CRRT therapy. These observations underline that RRT prescriptions for AKI patients in the ICU should be monitored closely if one wishes to ensure adequate delivery of prescribed dose.

Two recent large randomized trials, the Randomised Evaluation of Normal versus Augmented Level of Replacement Therapy (RENAL) (32) and the Acute Renal Failure Trial Network (ATN) (33) studies, seemed to definitely refute the concept that a "higher" dose is better. These two large multicenter, randomized controlled trials did not show improved outcome with a "more intensive dose" (40 and 35 mL/kg/hr, respectively) compared to a "less intensive dose" (25 and 20 mL/kg/hr, respectively). Based upon these findings, the current KDIGO guidelines recommend delivering an effluent volume of 20 to 25 mL/kg/hr for CRRT in patients with AKI (1). In addition, by comparing two multicenter CRRT databases, Uchino et al. (34) found that patients with AKI treated with low-dose CRRT did not have worse short-term outcome compared to patients treated with what is currently considered the standard (higher) dose. In particular, comparing patients from The Beginning and Ending Supportive Therapy (BEST) study (2) and from The Japanese Society for Physician and Trainees Intensive Care (JSEPTIC) Clinical Trial Group, the authors observed no differences between groups of patient treated with a doses of 14.3 and 20.4 mL/kg/hr (34). Finally, considering that high-dose CRRT could lead to electrolyte disorders, removal of nutrients and drugs (e.g., antibiotics) and high costs (35), but at the same time low dose may expose patients to undertreatment, potentially worsening outcome, seeking the range of adequate treatment dose is a crucial issue. At this time, a delivered dose (without downtime) between 20 and 35 mL/kg/hr may be considered clinically acceptable (36). A CRRT dose prescription below 20 mL/kg/hr and over 35 mL/kg/hr may be definitely identified as the dose-dependent range, where the dialytic intensity is likely to negatively affect outcomes, due to both under- and overdialysis. On the other hand, the prescriptions lying between these two limits can be considered as practice-dependent and variables such as timing, patients characteristics, comorbidities, or concomitant supportive pharmacologic therapies may have a significant role for patients' outcome and should trigger a careful prescription and a closest monitoring of dose delivery.

Practical Aspects

During RRT, clearance depends on circuit blood flow (Q_b), hemofiltration (Q_f), or dialysis (Q_d) flow, solute molecular weights, and hemodialyzer type and size. Q_b, as a variable in delivering RRT dose, is mainly dependent on vascular access and the operational characteristics of machines utilized in the clinical setting. Qf is strictly linked to Qb, during convective techniques, by filtration fraction. Filtration fraction does not limit Q_d, but when Q_d/Q_b ratio exceeds 0.3, it can be estimated that dialysate will not be completely saturated by blood-diffusing solutes. The search for specific toxins to be cleared, furthermore, has not been successful despite years of research, and urea and creatinine are generally used as reference solutes to measure renal replacement clearance for renal failure. While available evidence does not allow the direct correlation of the degree of uremia with outcome in chronic renal disease, in the absence of a specific solute, clearances of urea and creatinine blood levels are used to guide treatment dose. During UF, the driving pressure forces solutes, such as urea and creatinine, against the membrane and into the pores, depending on membrane sieving coefficient (SC) for that molecule. SC expresses a dimensionless value and is estimated by the ratio of the concentration of the solutes in the filtrate divided by that in the plasma water, or blood. An SC of 1.0, as is the case for urea and creatinine, demonstrates complete permeability, and a value of 0 reflects complete impermeability. Molecular size over approximately 12 kDa and filter porosity are the major determinants of SC. The K during convection is measured by the product of Q_f and SC. Thus, different from diffusion, there is a linear relationship between K and Q_f, the SC being the changing variable for different solutes. During diffusion, the linear relationship is lost when Q_d exceeds about one-third of Q_b. As a rough estimate, we can consider that during continuous slow-efficiency treatments, RRT dose is a direct expression of Q_f–Q_d, independent of which solute must be removed from blood. During continuous treatment, it has now been suggested to deliver at least a urea clearance of 2 L/hr, with the clinical evidence that 35 mL/kg/hr may be the best prescription (i.e., about 2.8 L/hr in a 70-kg patient). Other

TABLE 133.3 Algorithm for RRT Prescription

Clinical Variables	Operational Variables	Setting
Fluid balance	Net ultrafiltration	Continuous management of negative balance (100–300 mL/hr) is preferred in hemodynamically unstable patients. Complete monitoring (CVC, SG, arterial line, ECG, pulse oximeter) is recommended.
Adequacy and dose	Clearance/modality	2000–3000 mL/hr K (or 35 mL/kg/hr) for CRRT, consider first CVVHDF. If IHD is selected, a daily/ every 4-hr prescription is recommended. Prescribe a K_t/V >1.2.
Acid–base	Solution buffer	Bicarbonate buffered solutions are preferable to lactate buffered solutions in case of lactic acidosis and/or hepatic failure.
Electrolyte	Dialysate/replacement	Consider solutions without K^+ in case of severe hyperkalemia. Manage accurately Mg, PO_4.
Timing	Schedule	Early and intense RRT is suggested.
Protocol	Staff/machine	Well-trained staff should routinely utilize RRT monitors according to predefined institutional protocols.

CVC, central venous catheter; SG, Swan-Ganz catheter; ECG, electrocardiogram; CRRT, continuous renal replacement therapy; CVVHDF, continuous venovenous hemodiafiltration; IHD, intermittent hemodialysis.

authors suggest a prescription based on patient requirements, i.e., as a function of the urea generation rate and catabolic state of the single patient. It has been shown, however, that during continuous therapy, a clearance less than 2 L/hr will almost definitely be insufficient in an adult critically ill patient. For more exact estimations, simple computations have been shown to adequately estimate clearance (23,37). Tables 133.3 and 133.4 show a potential flow chart that could be followed each time an RRT prescription is indicated.

From Continuous to Intermittent: One Treatment Fits All?

Clearance-based dose quantification methods may not be adequate to compare effectiveness. For example, peritoneal dialysis (PD), traditionally providing less urea clearance per week than IHD, has comparable patient outcomes. Furthermore, when EKR_c (equivalent renal urea clearance corrected for urea volume) is used to compare intermittent and continuous therapies, it does not appear to be equivalent in terms of outcome; typically, PD patients have better comparable outcomes with less EKR_c than IHD patients (38). When the critical parameter is metabolic control, an acceptable mean blood urea nitrogen level of 60 mg/dL—easily obtainable in a 100-kg patient with a 2 L/hr CVVH in a computer-based simulation—has been shown to be very difficult to reach, even by intensive IHD regimens (37). In addition to the benefits specifically pertaining to the kinetics of solute removal, increased RRT frequency results in decreased ultrafiltration requirements per treatment. The avoidance of volume swings related to rapid ultrafiltration rates may also represent another dimension of dose where comparability is difficult.

Despite the development of new membranes, sophisticated dialysis machinery, tailored dialysate composition, and continuous dialysis therapies, a relationship between the frequency of RRT (continuous vs. intermittent) delivery has not been fully established. Most recently, the Surviving Sepsis Campaign guidelines for management of severe sepsis and septic shock (39) concluded that, based on the present scientific evidence, continuous RRT should be considered equivalent to IHD for the treatment of AKI. However, the use of continuous therapies to facilitate management of fluid balance in hemodynamically unstable septic patients was suggested (39). In a large comparative trial randomizing 166 critically ill patients with AKI to either CRRT or IHD (40), the authors found that the CRRT population, despite randomization, had significantly greater severity of illness scores. This could, in part, explain why, despite better control of azotemia and a greater likelihood of achieving the desired fluid balance, CRRT had increased mortality. Another more recent smaller trial at the Cleveland Clinic (41) failed to find a difference in outcome between one therapy and another. In recent years, a meta-analysis on this issue has been unable to solve the debate of continuous versus intermittent treatment. A meta-analysis of

TABLE 133.4 Schematic Example of a Possible Prescription for a Continuous Treatment in a 70-kg Patient

	Estimated Urea Clearance (K_{CALC})	Notes	Value of Q to Obtain 35 mL/kg/hr	Value of Q to Obtain a K_t/V of 1
CVVH postdilution	$K_{CALC} = Q_{rep}$	Always keep filtration fraction <20% (Q_b must be 5× Q_{rep})	Q_{rep}: 41 mL/min or 2,450 mL/hr	Q_{rep}: 29 mL/min or 1,750 mL/hr
CVVH predilution	$K_{CALC} = Q_{uf}/(1 + (Q_{rep}/Q_b))$	Filtration fraction computation changes (keep <20%)	For a Q_b of 200 mL/min: Q_{rep}: 53 mL/min or 3,200 mL/hr	For a Q_b of 200 mL/min: Q_{rep}: 35 mL/min or 2,100 mL/hr
i. CVVHD	$K_{CALC} = Q_{do}$	Keep Q_b ≥3× Q_d	Q_{do}: 41 mL/min or 2,450 mL/hr	Q_{do}: 29 mL/min or 1,750 mL/hr
ii. CVVHDF postdilution (50% convective and diffusive K)	$K_{CALC} = Q_{rep} + Q_{do}$	Consider both notes of CVVH and CVVHD	Q_{rep}: 20 mL/min + Q_{do}: 21 mL/min	Q_{rep}: 14 mL/min replacement solution + Q_{do}: 15 mL/min

Qb, blood flow rate; Qrep, replacement solution flow rate; Q_{uf}, ultrafiltration flow rate (Q_{uf}: $Q_{rep} + Q_{ne}$t); Qnet, patient's net fluid loss; Q_{do}, dialysate solution flow rate.
b) V_{UREA}: 42 L during an ideal session of 24 hr (1,440 min). Net ultrafiltration (patient fluid loss) is considered zero in K_{CALC} for simplicity.
- Urea volume of distribution, V (L): patient's body weight (kg) × 0.6.
- Estimated fractional clearance (K_t/V_{CALC}): K_{CALC} (mL/min) × prescribed treatment time (min)/V (mL).
- 35 mL/kg/hr roughly corresponds to a K_t/V of 1.4. A K_t/V of 1 approximately corresponds to 25 mL/kg/hr.
- Filtration fraction calculation (postdilution): $Q_{rep}/Q_b \times 100$; filtration fraction calculation (predilution): $Q_{rep}/Q_b + Q_{rep} \times 100$.

13 studies conducted by Kellum and coauthors, concluded that, after the stratification of 1,400 patients according to disease severity, when similar patients were compared, CRRT was associated with a significant decrease in the risk of death (42). However, when the same data were analyzed the same year by another group (43), no difference in outcome could be detected. Thus, it remains uncertain whether the choice of RRT modality (intermittent or continuous) actually matters to patient outcome. A recent randomized controlled trial comparing IHD and continuous venovenous hemodiafiltration (CVVHDF) concluded that, provided strict guidelines to improve tolerance and metabolic control are used, almost all patients who have AKI as part of their multiorgan dysfunction syndrome can be treated with IHD (44).

Given the lack of clear outcome data, the community of critical care nephrologists might then consider compromise solutions. One such solution could be represented by hybrid techniques such as SLEDD. Hybrid techniques have been given a variety of names such as slow, low-efficiency extended daily dialysis (SLEEDD), prolonged intermittent daily RRT (PDIRRT), extended daily dialysis (EDD), or simply extended dialysis (45–48), depending on variations in schedule and type of solute removal (convective or diffusive). Theoretically speaking, the purpose of such therapy would be the optimization of the advantages offered by either CRRT or IHD, including efficient solute removal with minimum solute disequilibrium, reduced ultrafiltration rate with hemodynamic stability, optimized delivery to prescribed ratio, low anticoagulant need, diminished cost of therapy delivery, efficiency of resource use, and improved patient mobility. Initial case series have shown the feasibility and high clearances potentially associated with such approaches. A single, short-term, single-center trial comparing hybrid therapies to CRRT has shown satisfying results in terms of dose delivery and hemodynamic stability. New technology which can be used in the ICU by nurses to deliver SLEDD with convective components offers further options from a therapeutic, logistic, and cost-effectiveness point of view.

One last aspect may be relevant: if short-term hard outcomes are not impacted by RRT modality, it may not be the case for long-term ones. In fact, IHD has been suspected to cause long-term chronic kidney disease in AKI patients. Two recent studies (49,50)—a meta-analysis and a retrospective analysis—noted that, compared with CRRT, IHD prescription for AKI treatment is significantly and strongly associated with a lower possibility of recovery of renal function. If these data are further confirmed, IHD should be abandoned for the treatment of AKI.

TECHNICAL NOTES

RRT Modalities: Description and Nomenclature

Apart from what evidence-based medicine dictates, continuous therapies are utilized in 80% of ICUs worldwide, while IHD (17%) and PD (3%) have less common utilization (2). In the 1980s, a passionate debate between simple CAVH and complex early CVVH lasted for the decade, stimulating the industries to produce increasingly effective equipment and monitoring systems. Accurate ultrafiltration control is now obtained by integrated roller volumetric pumps—for blood, replacement fluid, dialysate, and effluent—and scales. These monitors display pressure measurements of all crucial segments of the circuit: catheter inlet and outlet, filter inlet and outlet, UF, and dialysate ports. This information, integrated with adequate alarm systems, has allowed the ICU staff to increase filter efficiency and lengthen circuit patency, with the ability to detect potential sources of clotting, thereby improving patient safety. Complete monitoring of fluid balance is also provided by continuous recording of the history of the last 24 hours of treatment. When an alarm occurs, a "smart" message on the screen suggests the most appropriate intervention required. A complete range of ICU RRT therapeutic modalities includes IHD, slow continuous ultrafiltration (SCUF), CVVH, continuous venovenous hemodialysis (CVVHD), CVVHDF, and therapeutic plasma exchange (TPE) described in more detail in Table 133.5 and Figure 133.3.

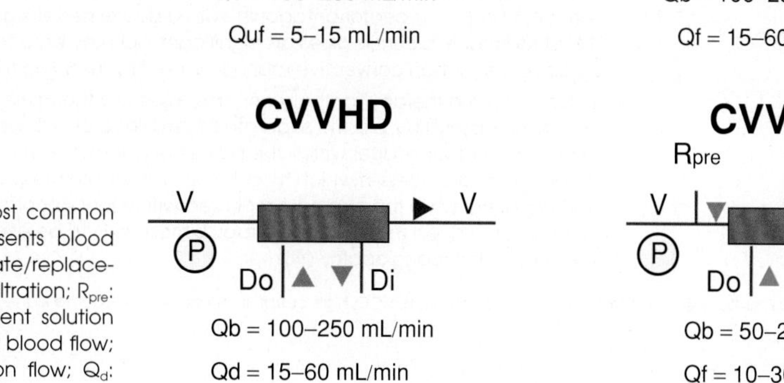

FIGURE 133.3 Schematic representation of most common continuous RRT set-ups. Black triangle represents blood flow direction; gray triangle indicates dialysate/replacement solutions flows. V-V: venovenous; Uf: ultrafiltration; R_{pre}: replacement solution prefilter; R_{post}: replacement solution post-filter; D_o: dialysate out; D_i: dialysate in; Q_b: blood flow; Q_{uf}: ultrafiltration flow; Q_f replacement solution flow; Q_d: dialysate solution flow.

TABLE 133.5 Extracorporeal Blood Purification Techniques

Nomenclature	Description
Intermittent hemodialysis (IHD)	A prevalently diffusive treatment in which blood and dialysate are circulated in counter current mode and, generally, a low permeability, cellulose-based membrane is employed. Dialysate must be pyrogen free but not necessarily sterile, since dialysate–blood contact does not occur. The UF rate is equal to the scheduled weight loss. This treatment can be typically performed 4 hr thrice weekly or daily. Q_b, 150–300 mL/min; Q_d, 300–500 mL/min.
Peritoneal dialysis (PD)	A predominantly diffusive treatment where blood, circulating along the capillaries of the peritoneal membrane, is exposed to dialysate. Access is obtained by the insertion of a peritoneal catheter, which allows the abdominal instillation of dialysate. Solute and water movement is achieved by the means of variable concentration and tonicity gradients generated by the dialysate. This treatment can be performed continuously or intermittently.
Slow continuous ultrafiltration (SCUF)	Technique where blood is driven through a highly permeable filter via an extracorporeal circuit in venovenous mode. The ultrafiltrate produced during membrane transit is not replaced and it corresponds to weight loss. It is used only for fluid control in overloaded patients (i.e., congestive heart failure resistant to diuretic therapy). Q_b, 100–250 mL/min; Q_{uf}, 5–15 mL/min (Fig. 133.2).
Continuous venovenous hemofiltration (CVVH)	Technique where blood is driven through a highly permeable filter via an extracorporeal circuit in venovenous mode. The ultrafiltrate produced during membrane transit is replaced in part or completely to achieve blood purification and volume control. If replacement fluid is delivered after the filter, the technique is defined postdilution hemofiltration. If it is delivered before the filter, the technique is defined predilution hemofiltration. The replacement fluid can also be delivered both pre and post filter. Clearance for all solutes is convective and equals UF rate. Q_b, 100–250 mL/min; Q_{uf}, 15–60 mL/min.
Continuous venovenous hemodialysis (CVVHD)	Technique where blood is driven through a low permeability dialyzer via an extracorporeal circuit in venovenous mode and a counter current flow of dialysate is delivered on the dialysate compartment. The ultrafiltrate produced during membrane transit corresponds to patient's weight loss. Solute clearance is mainly diffusive and efficiency is limited to small solutes only. Q_b: 100–250 mL/min; Q_d: 15–60 mL/min (Fig. 133.2).
Continuous venovenous hemodiafiltration (CVVHDF)	Technique where blood is driven through a highly permeable dialyzer via an extracorporeal circuit in venovenous mode and a countercurrent flow of dialysate is delivered on the dialysate compartment. The ultrafiltrate produced during membrane transit is in excess of the patient's desired weight loss. A replacement solution is needed to maintain fluid balance. Solute clearance is both convective and diffusive. Q_b, 100–250 mL/min; Q_d, 15–60 mL/min; Q_r, 15–60 mL/min (Fig. 133.2).
Hybrid techniques	Slow low efficiency daily dialysis (SLEDD), prolonged daily intermittent RRT (PDIRRT), extended daily dialysis (EDD), extended daily dialysis with filtration (EDDf), extended IHD.
Hemoperfusion (HP)	Blood is circulated on a bed of coated charcoal powder to remove solutes by adsorption. The technique is specifically indicated in cases of poisoning or intoxication with agents that can be effectively removed by charcoal. Polymixin hemoperfusion has been attempted for endotoxin removal in gram-negative septic AKI patients (44). This treatment may cause platelet and protein depletion.
Plasmapheresis (PP)	A treatment that uses specific plasma filters. Molecular weight cutoff of the membrane is much higher than that of hemofilters (100,000–1,000,000 kDa): plasma as a whole is filtered and blood is reconstituted by the infusion of plasma products such as frozen plasma or albumin. This technique is performed to remove proteins or protein bound solutes.
High-flux dialysis (HFD)	A treatment that uses highly permeable membranes in conjunction with an UF control system. Because of the characteristics of the membrane, UF occurs in the proximal part of the filter, that is counterbalanced by a positive pressure applied to the dialysate compartment: this causes in the distal part of the filter a phenomenon called back filtration, that consist in convective passage of the dialysate into the blood. Diffusion and convection are combined, but thanks to the use of a pyrogen-free dialysate replacement is avoided.
High-volume hemofiltration (HVHF)	A treatment that utilizes highly permeable membranes and hemofiltration with a high volume setting. Q_b, >200 mL/min; Q_r, >35 mL/kg/hr.
High-cutoff hemofiltration or hemodialysis	A technique aimed at removing inflammatory mediators (e.g., cytokines) in septic patients. HCO membranes are porous enough to achieve the removal of larger molecules (approximately 15–60 kD) by diffusion. Its ability to remove cytokines in ex vivo and in vivo studies has now been shown to be greater than that of any other technology so far (45) and has increased survival in experimental models of sepsis (46). HCO therapy seems to have beneficial effects on immune cell function and preliminary human studies using intermittent hemodialysis with HCO membranes have confirmed its ability to remove marker cytokines IL-6 and IL-1 receptor antagonist, with a decreased dosage of norepinephrine in patients with sepsis (47). Predictably, albumin losses are significant, but may be attenuated by using HCO membranes in a diffusive rather than convective manner while still preserving the effect on cytokine clearance.
Plasma Therapy	The term "plasma therapy" actually encompasses two therapies: plasma adsorption and plasma exchange. In plasma adsorption, plasma separated from blood cells flows along one or more columns that contain different adsorbents, after which the processed plasma is reinfused back to the patient. Plasma exchange is a single-step process in which blood is separated into plasma and cells and the cells are returned back to the patient while the plasma is replaced with either donor plasma or albumin. With respect to sepsis, it has been argued that plasma therapy is most likely to be effective in patients with sepsis-associated thrombotic microangiopathy (48).

Q_b, blood flow; Q_d, dialysis flow; Q_r, ultrafiltration rate; UF, ultrafiltration; HCO, high cutoff; IL, interleukin; AKI, acute kidney injury; ICU, intensive care unit.

Anticoagulation

The need for anticoagulation of the CRRT circuit arises from the fact that the contact between blood and the tubing of the circuit and the membrane of the filter induces activation of the coagulation cascade and platelets activation; this extracorporeal activation inevitably results in filter or circuit clotting. It is evident that the anticoagulation strategy will change depending on the prescribed RRT schedule, being a priority feature of continuous treatments where blood–artificial surface interaction is maximized. The aims of anticoagulation are maintenance of extracorporeal circuit and dialyzer patency; reduction of off-treatment time (down time) that could have a clinical impact in the overall RRT clearance; reduction of treatment cost by, as possible, the utilization of less material; and achievement of the above aims with minimal risk for the patient. In fact, continuous anticoagulation may represent an important drawback of RRT in some categories of patients. This last concept should perhaps be the first rule of anticoagulation management: under no circumstances should the patient be put at risk of bleeding in order to prolong circuit life. The general principle from KDIGO guidelines suggest that anticoagulation for RRT be weighted on assessment of the potential risks and benefits to the patient (1).

Circuit Setup Optimization and No Anticoagulation

Several technical features of RRT circuit are likely to affect the success of any anticoagulant approach. Vascular access has to be of adequate size; tubing kinking should be avoided; blood flow rate should exceed 100 mL/min; pump flow fluctuations must be prevented (in modern machines this event is mainly due to circuit increased resistances rather than flow rate inaccuracies); and a venous bubble trap—where air/blood contact occurs—must be accurately monitored. In this light, another component of circuit setup has to be addressed: plasma filtration fraction should be kept has far as possible below 20% and, when possible or considered correct, predilutional HF should be selected. There is evidence that, when the setup is perfectly optimized, anticoagulants are only a relatively minor component of circuit patency; in fact, whenever the patient's clinical has risk factors for bleeding—prolonged clotting times, thrombocytopenia—RRT can be safely performed without the utilization of any anticoagulant (51). In these cases, special attention is required to prolong filter survival: optimal vascular access (i.e., high blood flow), reduction of blood viscosity by saline boluses, predilution, and diffusive treatment. Alarm setting is clearly important to identify circuit problems, especially in these cases. Although potentially avoidable, the general indication is for the use of anticoagulation for patients without an increased bleeding risk and not already receiving systemic anticoagulation for his/her disease. In case of intermittent RRT, either low–molecular-weight heparin (LMWH) or unfractioned heparin (UFH) are recommended. LMWH, in patients with chronic IHD, is recommended in order to reduce the risk of heparin-induced thrombocytopenia (HIT), and of long-term side effects (abnormal serum lipids, osteoporosis, hypoaldosteronism) (1). For continuous treatments, regional citrate anticoagulation (in the absence of contraindications) is suggested; when citrate is contraindicated (see below), either UFH or LMWH should be administered (1).

Unfractioned Heparin

This agent is the most widely used anticoagulant during continuous RRT, although guidelines suggest citrate anticoagulation as a general rule. UFH is mostly administered as a prefilter infusion or as systemic infusion in specific cases. It is easy to use as there is a large experience in most centers, is not expensive, quick monitoring—aPTT or activated clotting time (ACT)—is readily available, has a short half-life, and an antagonist—protamine—exists. Heparin doses might range from 5 to 10 IU/kg/hr. In patients with very limited circuit duration, it can also be used in combination with protamine (regional heparinization), with a 1: 1 ratio (150 IU of UFH per mg of protamine) and strict aPTT monitoring. The problem with UFH is its relative unpredictable bioavailability (monitoring required), the narrow therapeutic index (risk of bleeding), the necessity for antithrombin (AT) level optimization, heparin resistance, and the occurrence of HIT. The balance between heparin dose, aPTT/ACT, filter survival, and potential/actual complications have to be considered during RRT.

Low–Molecular-Weight Heparins

Some centers have gained experience with LMWHs. These have some advantages—predictable kinetics, no monitoring required, reduced risk of HIT—that make this drug particularly efficient for intermittent RRT; a single predialysis dose may be sufficient. The main disadvantages are risk of accumulation in case of kidney failure, requiring dose adaptation or administration interruption; incomplete reversal by protamine; monitoring requires a laboratory test (anti-factor Xa) that might not be easily available, and the drug is certainly more expensive than UFH.

Prostacyclin

This agent is a potentially useful drug for RRT anticoagulation, being the most potent inhibitor of platelet aggregation with the shortest half-life. PGI_2 is infused at a dose of 4 to 8 ng/kg/hr, with or without the adjunct of low dose of UFH. PGI_2 appears to have a limited efficacy when used alone and hypotension may occur. Because of these drawbacks as well as its high cost, PGI_2 use during CRRT is not recommended (52).

Citrate

This form of regional anticoagulation depends on the ability of citrate to chelate calcium, thus stopping the coagulation cascade. Briefly, a calcium-free sodium citrate–containing replacement solution and/or dialysate solution is prepared and administered at the appropriate rate to achieve the desired aPTT (60 to 90 seconds). Citrate is rapidly metabolized in the liver, muscle, and kidney, liberating the calcium and producing bicarbonate (1 to 3 moles ratio). Calcium chloride is administered to replace chelated/dialyzed calcium and maintain normocalcemia. Regional citrate anticoagulation requires a strict protocol, adapted to the treatment modality. This approach is effective in maintaining excellent filter patency and compares favorably with heparin. It also avoids the risk for HIT and does not lead to systemic anticoagulation. The relative drawbacks of this anticoagulation management include the risk for hypocalcemia, hypercalcemia, hypernatremia, metabolic alkalosis—or metabolic acidosis for impaired capacity to metabolize citrate in shock states or liver failure, considered contraindications for citrate anticoagulation—and the cumbersome

TABLE 133.6 Anticoagulation Strategies

Drug	Pro	Con
No anticoagulation	Use in patients at high risk of bleeding	Relative shorter circuit lifespan
Unfractionated heparin	Routine	HIT
Low-molecular-weight heparin	Routine (alternative to UH)	HIT
Prostacycline	Improves circuit lifespan	Hypotension
Citrate	Routine/improves circuit lifespan	Hypocalcemia
Danaparoid	HIT	Insufficient data available
Argatroban	HIT	Insufficient data available
Irudine	HIT	Insufficient data available
Nafamostatmesilate	HIT	Insufficient data available
Heparin-coated circuits	Routine	Insufficient data available

HIT, heparin-induced thrombocytopenia.

replacement/dialysate fluid preparation (53). Guidelines suggest using regional citrate anticoagulation for patients with an increased bleeding risk, who are not receiving anticoagulation, and are without contraindications to the agent (1).

Other Strategies

Alternatives to the techniques presented above are here listed in Table 133.6 for completeness.

Unanswered Research Topics

Outcome variables including bleeding, renal recovery, mortality, incidence of HIT, circuit survival, efficiency of treatment, and metabolic complications, should be tested with RCTs designed to compare UFH to LMWH during IHD and CRRT. In addition, citrate should be compared with UFH and LMWH during CRRT. Finally, trials comparing strategies without anticoagulation versus different modalities of anticoagulation are lacking and should be considered in the future.

VASCULAR ACCESS

The fundamental role played by vascular access must be emphasized. In fact, circuit failure is more often due to vascular access inadequacy than insufficient anticoagulation; the optimal dialysis catheter can save the patient from inappropriate increases of the anticoagulation dose. Venovenous RRT relies on the use of a temporary double-lumen catheter. Such catheters are inserted in a central vein and available in different brands, shapes, and sizes. The site of insertion of double-lumen catheters implies a number of considerations (clinician expertise, body habitus of the patient, the presence of other intravenous catheters). The femoral vein is generally the first choice of vascular access; internal jugular or subclavian accesses are often associated with inadequate performance, and the inguinal puncture is safer and easier to perform in coagulopathic critically ill patients. A valid alternative may be achieved by cannulation of the right jugular internal vein with the tip of the catheter reaching the right atrium; circuit blood flow rates with this approach can reach 300 mL/min. Catheter size for adult patients range from 12 to 14 French and length from 16 to 25 cm; the larger and shorter the catheter, the higher the performance. Nonetheless, when the femoral vein is selected, a 20-cm-long catheter with its tip positioned close to the inferior vena cava allows optimal circuit flows. When inadequate blood flow or a catheter malfunction is suspected, venous and arterial lumens should be flushed with saline, with the goal of testing resistance to injection and aspiration. Clotting of a limb of the line versus kinking due to patient's position must be distinguished. In the first case, a heparin or urokinase lock can be tried for few hours; in the second case, switching of arterial and venous limbs can be attempted. This maneuver increases circuit recirculation, but clinical consequences are negligible. Another approach is a catheter exchange over a guide wire; this is generally not recommended unless vascular access is extremely difficult, as the risk of line infection is significant.

RRT FOR CHILDREN

There are some important differences in the RRT indications, methods, and prescription between children and adult patients; nevertheless, the technique is essentially the same. A priority indication includes the correction of water overload. Different from the adult setting, where solute control may play an key role, it has been shown that restoring an adequate water content in small children is the main independent variable for outcome prediction (54–55). This concept is much more important in critically ill, smaller children, where a relatively larger amount of fluid must be administered in order to deliver an adequate amount of drug infusion, parenteral/enteral nutrition, blood derivatives, and so forth. Corrections of acid–base imbalances and electrolyte disorders is also a strong indication for RRT prescription in children.

Catheter size ranges from 6.5 French (10 cm long) for less than 10-kg patients to 8 French (15 cm long) for 11- to 15-kg patients. Blood priming may be indicated if more than 8 mL/kg of patient's blood is necessary to fill an RRT circuit. Full anticoagulation must be always maintained in order to avoid excessive blood loss in case of circuit clotting. Predilution HF is generally the preferred modality and is delivered in a continuous fashion. Fluid balance requires strict monitoring and highest accuracy due to the risk of excessive patient dehydration. Prescription of RRT clearance should be titrated on the patient body surface area, an approach that will usually lead to relatively higher doses for small children with respect to adult patients when considered per kilogram (56). Critically ill children below 10 kg body weight and neonates with AKI are often treated with PD; discussion of this topic goes beyond the scope of this chapter. An important exception to this general approach is the case of children with AKI during an extracorporeal membrane oxygenation treatment (ECMO). In this case, the RRT circuit is placed in parallel to the ECMO circuit, and it is possible to let a significant blood flow run into the filter even in the smallest patients.

Recently, two dialysis monitors specifically dedicated to neonates and infants have been developed and clinically applied: the CARPEDIEM (CArdio Renal PEDIatric Emergency Machine) and the Nidus (Newcastle infant dialysis and ultrafiltration system). The first of these (57–59) is a miniaturized (13 kg) device featuring four mini-roller pumps, as well as all the other technical requirements of a third-generation machine. The monitor is equipped with three circuits with different priming volumes—27.2, 33.5, and 41.5 mL—and filter sizes—0.075, 0.147, and 0.245 m^2—to allow optimal adaptability for patients weighting less than 3 kg, from 3 to 6 kg, and from 6 to 10 kg, respectively. One of the most interesting aspects of CARPEDIEM monitor is its accurate management of fluid balance. The machine is equipped with a gravimetric control with a scale sensitivity of 1 g for both infusion and effluent bags. An automatic feedback system adjusts pump speed according to the prescribed and actual delivery of fluid, and the difference between prescribed and achieved fluid balance is always kept at less than 20 g/24 hr. The treatment is terminated if a fluid balance error of 50 g is reached within a single session. The NIDUS (59) is an original machine driven by syringes instead of roller pumps, providing single-needle vascular access. The circuit volume is only 13 mL, and its designers claim that there is no need for circuit blood-priming. Recently, Coulthard and co-workers successfully treated 10 babies weighing between 1.8 and 5.9 kg, with satisfactory results in terms of adequacy of clearance and machine accuracy (59). Further studies into these two interesting devices are anticipated, and there promises to be a significant outcome improvement for neonates with severe AKI requiring RRT.

PERSPECTIVE FOR THE FUTURE

The ideal RRT machine for the future should self-set the right RRT technique, modality, and prescription after the clinician has provided all the information for the specific patient. Monitors and material of the future will further increase ease of use, safety measures, and the accuracy of each component of the integrated system, reducing the labor involved. Unfortunately, there is no solution to the ill-conceived use of a perfect system. Furthermore, in the light of progressively increasing severity of critical illness, a monitor able to provide supportive treatment beyond the classic renal indications is currently awaited. In the near future, technical developments in extracorporeal devices will lead to the creation of MOSTs, so that comprehensive replacement or at least support can be provided to multiple organs simultaneously. New machines already include multiple platforms in which different circuits and filters can be used in combination to support renal, heart, liver and lung function. Such machines will ideally be able to automatically detect both "traditional" (urea) and "inflammatory" (cytokines) solutes in critically ill patients' plasma in order to automatically (or semiautomatically) tailor the therapy towards the "perfect blood purification" system (53).

CONCLUSIONS

The mechanisms involved in RRT are founded upon the principle of water and solute transport according to two fundamental mechanisms: diffusion and convection. These mechanisms can be applied into clinical practice as different techniques (intermittent, extended, or continuous RRT) and modalities (HF, hemodialysis, hemodiafiltration, plasmafiltration, hemoperfusion, coupled plasmafiltration, and adsorption). A precise understanding of technical and clinical implications of such therapies seems important to create a correct RRT prescription since, so far, no consensus exists about which modality should be administered to critically ill patients with AKI. Different RRT prescriptions, modalities, and schedules can be administered to critically ill patients with AKI. Clinical effects on critically ill patients depend on the selected RRT strategy and on the severity and complexity of the patient's clinical picture. Modern versatile machines and flexible operative prescriptions allow the operators to range from highly intermittent high-efficiency therapies to slow continuous HF, depending on the patient's hemodynamic stability, fluid balance needs, acid–base, and electrolyte derangements. A specific dose of RRT has not been adopted in clinical practice; a standard dose prescription and a strict control of delivered dose should be monitored if one wishes to ensure the adequate delivery of a prescribed dose. The best evidence to date supports an RRT dose in the range of 25 to 35 mL/kg/hr.

Key Points

- RRTs currently remain the most important part of AKI treatment. AKI is defined and classified according to KDIGO classification.
- Current indications for urgent/emergent RRT in clinical practice are well defined: fluid overload, hyperazotemia, hyperkalemia, severe acidosis, and intoxication; each of these parameters can be present at different levels of severity and can be differently evaluated by different clinicians at different centers. Outside these conditions (e.g., in case of sepsis), timing for the start of RRT is currently being debated.
- Once RRT has started, timing for cessation is another field of uncertainty as the literature is scarce.
- During *diffusion*, movement of solute depends upon their tendency to reach the same concentration on each side of the membrane; dialysis is a modality of RRT and is predominantly based on the principle of diffusion. During *convection*, the movement of solute across a semipermeable membrane takes place in conjunction with significant amounts of ultrafiltration (water transfer across the membrane).
- The current KDIGO guidelines recommend delivering an effluent volume of 20 to 25 mL/kg/hr for continuous RRT (CRRT) in patients with AKI (without downtime).
- The Surviving Sepsis Campaign guidelines for management of severe sepsis and septic shock suggest that CRRT should be considered equivalent to IHD for the treatment of AKI. However, the use of continuous therapies facilitates the management of fluid balance in hemodynamically unstable septic patients.
- The general principle from the KDIGO guidelines suggest that anticoagulation for RRT be weighted on assessment of the potential risks and benefits to the patient but, for continuous treatments, regional

citrate anticoagulation (in the absence of contraindications) is suggested; when citrate is contraindicated, either unfractioned heparin or LMWH should be administered.

- Different from the adult setting, where solute control may play a key role, it has been shown that restoring an adequate water content in small children is the main independent variable for outcome prediction.
- In the near future, technical developments in extracorporeal devices will lead to the creation of MOSTs, so that comprehensive replacement or at least support can be provided to multiple organs simultaneously.

References

1. Kidney disease: Improving global outcomes (KDIGO). Acute Kidney Injury Work Group. KDIGO clinical practice guideline for acute kidney injury. *Kidney Int Suppl.* 2012;2:1–138.
2. Uchino S, Kellum JA, Bellomo R, et al.; for the Beginning and Ending Supportive Therapy for the Kidney (BEST Kidney) Investigators. Acute renal failure in critically ill patients :a multinational, multicenter study. *JAMA.* 2005;294:813–818.
3. Tolwani A. Continuous renal-replacement therapy for acute kidney injury. *N Engl J Med.* 2012;367:2505–2514.
4. Bellomo R. The epidemiology of acute renal failure: 1975 versus 2005. *Curr Opin Crit Care.* 2006;12:557–560.
5. Kramer P, Wigger W, Rieger J, et al. Arterio-venous hemofiltration: a new simple method for treatment of overhydrated patients resistant to diuretics. *Klein Wschr.* 1977;55:1121.
6. Bagshaw SM, Laupland KB, Doig CJ, et al. Prognosis for long-term survival and renal recovery in critically ill patients with severe acute renal failure: a population-based study. *Crit Care.* 2005;9:R700–R709.
7. Cruz DN, de Cal M, Garzotto F, et al. Plasma neutrophil gelatinase-associated lipocalin is an early biomarker for acute kidney injury in an adult ICU population. *Intensive Care Med.* 2010;36:444–451.
8. Bagshaw SM, Uchino S, Bellomo R, et al. Timing of renal replacement therapy and clinical outcomes in critically ill patients with severe acute kidney injury. *J Crit Care.* 2009;24:129–140.
9. Bouman C, Oudemans-van Straaten H, Tijssen J, et al. Effects of early high-volume continuous venovenous hemofiltration on survival and recovery of renal function in intensive care patients with acute renal failure: a prospective randomized trial. *Crit Care Med.* 2002;30:2205–2211.
10. Karvellas CJ, Farhat MR, Sajjad I, et al. A comparison of early versus late initiation of renal replacement therapy in critically ill patients with acute kidney injury: a systematic review and meta-analysis. *Crit Care.* 2011;15:R72.
11. Wang X, Yuan WJ. Timing of initiation of renal replacement therapy in acute kidney injury: a systematic review and meta-analysis. *Renal Fail.* 2012;34:396–402.
12. Bagshaw SM, Mortis G, Godinez-Luna T, et al. Renal recovery after severe acute renal failure. *Int J Artif Org.* 2006;29:1023–1030.
13. Swartz R, Perry E, Daley J. The frequency of withdrawal from acute care is impacted by severe acute renal failure. *J Palliat Med.* 2004;7:676–682.
14. Uchino S, Bellomo R, Morimatsu H, et al. Discontinuation of continuous renal replacement therapy: a post hoc analysis of a prospective multicenter observational study. *Crit Care Med.* 2009;37:2576–2582.
15. Ronco C, Bellomo R. Principles of solute clearance during continuous renal replacement therapy. In: *Critical Care Nephrology.* 2nd ed. New York, NY: Kluwer Academic Publishers; 2008;1213–1223.
16. Cole L, Bellomo R, Davenport P, et al. Cytokine removal during continuous renal replacement therapy: an ex vivo comparison of convection and diffusion. *Int J Artif Organs.* 2004;27:388–397.
17. Ricci Z, Ronco C, Bachetoni A, et al. Solute removal during continuous renal replacement therapy in critically ill patients: convection versus diffusion. *Critical Care.* 2006;10:R67.
18. Owen W, Lew N, Liu Y, et al. The urea reduction ratio and serum albumin concentrations as predictors of mortality in patients undergoing hemodialysis. *N Engl J Med.* 1993;329:1001–1006.
19. Collins AJ, Ma JZ, Umen A, et al. Urea index and other predictors of long term outcome in hemodialysis patient survival. *Am J Kidney Dis.* 1994;23:272–282.
20. Hakim R, Breyer J, Ismail N, et al. Effects of dose of dialysis on morbidity and mortality. *Am J Kidney Dis.* 1994;23:661–669.
21. Parker T, Hushni L, Huang W, et al. Survival of hemodialysis patients in the United States is improved with a greater quantity of dialysis. *Am J Kidney Dis.* 1994;23:670–680.
22. Eknoyan G, Levin N. NKF-K/DOQI clinical practice guidelines: update 2000. *Am J Kidney Dis.* 2001;38:917.
23. Arabed G, Knoyan E, Erald G, et al. Effect of dialysis dose and membrane flux in maintenance hemodialysis. *N Engl J Med.* 2002;347:2010–2109.
24. Ricci Z, Salvatori G, Bonello M, et al. In vivo validation of the adequacy calculator for continuous renal replacement therapies. *Crit Care.* 2005;9:R266–R273.
25. Pisitkun T, Tiranathanagul K, Poulin S, et al. A practical tool for determining the adequacy of renal replacement therapy in acute renal failure patients. *Contrib Nephrol.* 2004;144:329–349.
26. Brause M, Nuemann A, Schumacher T, et al. Effect of filtration volume of continuous venovenous hemofiltration in the treatment of patients with acute renal failure in intensive care units. *Crit Care Med.* 2003;31:841–846.
27. Paganini EP, Tapolyai M, Goormastic M, et al. Establishing a dialysis therapy/patient outcome link in intensive care unit acute dialysis for patients with acute renal failure. *Am J Kidney Dis.* 1996;28(Suppl 3):S81–S89.
28. Schiffl H, Lang SM, Fischer R. Daily hemodialysis and the outcome of acute renal failure. *N Engl J Med.* 2002;346:305–310.
29. Ronco C, Bellomo R, Homel P, et al. Effects of different doses in continuous venovenous haemofiltration on outcomes of acute renal failure: a prospective randomised trial. *Lancet.* 2000;356:26–30.
30. Evanson JA, Himmelfarb J, Wingard R, et al. Prescribed versus delivered dialysis in acute renal failure patients. *Am J Kidney Dis.* 1998;32:731–738.
31. Venkataraman R, Kellum JA, Palevsky P. Dosing patterns for CRRT at a large academic medical center in the United States. *J Crit Care.* 2002;17:246–250.
32. RENAL Replacement Therapy Study Investigators, Bellomo R, Cass A, Cole L, et al. Intensity of continuous renal-replacement therapy in critically ill patients. *N Engl J Med.* 2009;361:1627–1638.
33. VA/NIH Acute Renal Failure Trial Network, Palevsky P, Zhang J, et al. Intensity of renal support in critically ill patients with acute kidney injury. *N Engl J Med.* 2008;359:7–20.
34. Uchino S, Toki N, Takeda K, et al. Validity of low-intensity continuous renal replacement therapy. *Crit Care Med.* 2013;41:2584–2591.
35. Rimmelé T, Kellum JA. Clinical review: blood purification for sepsis. *Crit Care.* 2011;15:205.
36. Ricci Z, Ronco C. Timing, dose and mode of dialysis in acute kidney injury. *Curr Opin Crit Care.* 2011;17:556–561.
37. Clark WR, Mueller BA, Kraus MA, et al. Renal replacement quantification in acute renal failure. *Nephrol Dial Transplant.* 1998;13(Suppl 6):86–90.
38. Depner TA. Benefits of more frequent dialysis: lower TAC at the same Kt/V. *Nephrol Dial Transplant.* 1998;13(Suppl 6):20–24.
39. Dellinger RP, Levy MM, Rhodes A, et al.; Surviving Sepsis Campaign Guidelines Committee including the Pediatric Subgroup. Surviving sepsis campaign: international guidelines for management of severe sepsis and septic shock. *Crit Care Med.* 2013;41:580–637.
40. Mehta RL, McDonald B, Gabbai FB, et al. A randomized clinical trial of continuous versus intermittent dialysis for acute renal failure. *Kidney Int.* 2001;60:1154–1163.
41. Augustine JJ, Sandy D, Seifert TH, Paganini EP. A randomized controlled trial comparing intermittent with continuous dialysis in patients with AKI. *Am J Kidney Dis.* 2004;44:1000–1007.
42. Kellum J, Angus DC, Johnson JP, et al. Continuous versus intermittent renal replacement therapy: a meta-analysis. *Intensive Care Med.* 2002;28:29–37.
43. Tonelli M, Manns B, Feller-Kopman D. Acute renal failure in the intensive care unit: a systematic review of the impact of dialytic modality on mortality and renal recovery. *Am J Kidney Dis.* 2002;40:875–885.
44. Vinsonneau C, Camus C, Combes A, et al. Hemodiafe Study Group. Continuous venovenous haemodiafiltration versus intermittent haemodialysis for acute renal failure in patients with multiple-organ dysfunction syndrome: a multicenter randomised trial. *Lancet.* 2006;368:379–385.
45. Marshall MR, Golper TA, Shaver MJ, et al. Urea kinetics during sustained low efficiency dialysis in critically ill patients requiring renal replacement therapy. *Am J Kidney Dis.* 2002;39:556–570.
46. Naka T, Baldwin I, Bellomo R, et al. Prolonged daily intermittent renal replacement therapy in ICU patients by ICU nurses and ICU physicians. *Int J Artif Organs.* 2004;27:380–387.
47. Kumar VA, Craig M, Depner T, et al. Extended daily dialysis: a new approach to renal replacement for acute renal failure in the intensive care unit. *Am J Kidney Dis.* 2000;36:294–300.
48. Kielstein JT, Kretschmer U, Ernst T, et al. Efficacy and cardiovascular tolerability of extended dialysis in critically ill patients: a randomized controlled study. *Am J Kidney Dis.* 2004;43:342–349.

49. Schneider AG, Bellomo R, Bagshaw SM, et al. Choice of renal replacement therapy modality and dialysis dependence after acute kidney injury: a systematic review and meta-analysis. *Intensive Care Med.* 2013;39:987–997.
50. Wald R, Shariff SZ, Adhikari NK, et al. The association between renal replacement therapy modality and long-term outcomes among critically ill adults with acute kidney injury: a retrospective cohort study. *Crit Care Med.* 2014;42:868–877.
51. Tan HK, Baldwin I, Bellomo R. continuous venovenous hemofiltration without anticoagulation in high-risk patients. *Intensive Care Med.* 2000;26: 1652–1657.
52. Fiaccadori E, Maggiore U, Rotelli C, et al. Continuous haemofiltration in acute renal failure with prostacyclin as the sole anti-haemostatic agent. *Intensive Care Med.* 2002;28:586–593.
53. Ronco C, Ricci Z, De Backer D, et al. Renal replacement therapy in acute kidney injury: controversy and consensus. *Crit Care.* 2015;19:146.
54. Goldstein SL, Currier H, Graf C, et al. Outcome in children receiving continuous venovenous hemofiltration. *Pediatrics.* 2001;107:1309–1312.
55. Foland JA, Fortenberry JD, Warshaw BL, et al. Fluid overload before continuous hemofiltration and survival in critically ill children: a retrospective analysis. *Crit Care Med.* 2004;32:1771–1776.
56. Brophy PD, Bunchman TE. References and overview for hemofiltration in pediatrics and adolescents. Available: www.pcrrt.com. Accessed June 25, 2006.
57. Ronco C, Garzotto F, Ricci Z. CA.R.PE.DI.E.M. (Cardio-Renal Pediatric Dialysis Emergency Machine): evolution of continuous renal replacement therapies in infants. A personal journey. *Pediatr Nephrol.* 2012;27: 1203–1211.
58. Ronco C, Garzotto F, Brendolan A, et al. Continuous renal replacement therapy in neonates and small infants: development and first-in-human use of a miniaturised machine (CARPEDIEM). *Lancet.* 2014;383:1807–1813.
59. Coulthard MG, Crosier J, Griffiths C, et al. Haemodialysing babies weighing <8 kg with the Newcastle infant dialysis and ultrafiltration system (Nidus): comparison with peritoneal and conventional haemodialysis. *Pediatr Nephrol.* 2014;29:1873–1881.

CHAPTER

134

Fluid and Electrolytes

STEVEN G. ACHINGER and JUAN CARLOS AYUS

INTRODUCTION

Fluid and electrolyte disorders are very common in critically ill patients. There are some circumstances in which a patient is placed in intensive care for the management of a specific electrolyte disturbance such as hyponatremia or hyperkalemia. The development of electrolyte disturbances among critically ill patients is also common due to breakdown of homeostatic mechanisms that prevent the development of electrolyte disturbances. These impairments in homeostatic function are numerous such as renal failure, use of diuretics, and nonosmotic release of antidiuretic hormone (ADH) due to nausea, pain, or other stimuli. In this chapter, the pathophysiology of electrolyte disturbances will be addressed with a focus on presentations common among intensive care unit (ICU) patients. Disorders of water balance (hyponatremia and hypernatremia) will be addressed in more detail due to the importance of these disorders as a cause of morbidity and mortality and the prevalence of impaired water balance in ICU patients.

In an average person without extremes of weight, approximately 60% of total body weight is water. Of this total body water, two-thirds (40% of total body weight) is in the intracellular (intracellular fluid [ICF]) space, and one-third (20% of total body weight) is outside the cells, i.e., extracellular (extracellular fluid [ECF]) space. Extracellular volume is divided into intravascular space and interstitial fluid (5% and 15% of total body weight, respectively). The intravascular space containing plasma is the most mobile fluid compartment and the first to be released to areas of injury and the first to be repleted through intravenous (IV) infusion. In the intravascular space are red cells in addition to plasma. Red cell volume plus plasma volume compose the blood volume (BV), which is estimated to be 7% of the total body weight. In a 70-kg person, total body water is 42 L (60% × 70 kg), circulating BV is 4.9 L (7% × 70 kg), ICF is 28 L (40% × 70 kg), and ECF is 14 L (20% × 70 kg). The percentage of weight used will vary depending on deviation from ideal body weight and sex (see Blood Volume chapter).

Water is freely permeable between body compartments and migrates to areas of higher solutes, but this takes time. Therefore, chronic hypotonic losses with ability to "borrow" from ICF (28 L) is better tolerated than acute isotonic losses, which has only the ECF (14 L) to borrow from. Osmolality (tonicity) defined as number of particles in solution is normally 280 to 300 mOsm/L in the serum.

The ICF concentration of solutes is vastly different from that of the ECF, and approximately 80% of adenosine triphosphate (ATP) generated is used to maintain this gradient. Some of the ECF cations are as follows: sodium (Na^+), 142 mEq/L; potassium (K^+), 4 mEq/L; calcium (Ca), 5 mEq/L; and magnesium (Mg), 3 mEq/L. The ICF cations are K^+, 150 mEq/L; Mg, 40 mEq/L; and Na^+, 10 mEq/L. Some of the ECF anions (in mEq/L) are chloride (Cl^-), 103; and bicarbonate, 27. The major ICF anions (in mEq/L) are phosphates, 107; proteins, 40; and sulfates, 43. This difference in ICF and ECF electrolyte composition explains the clinical observations that large amounts of certain electrolytes are needed to replete small deficiencies in the serum (ECF) if the ICF stores are depleted. One of our limitations is the inability to assess ICF electrolyte composition easily at the bedside.

Because water is freely permeable, the osmolality of all body compartments should be the same, but in reality, the protein concentration in the plasma to interstitial fluid is 16:1, generating an oncotic pressure difference between the two compartments. Starling forces describe net fluid flux between intravascular space and the interstitium:

$$Q = K_f \{(P_c - P_i) - \sigma (\pi_c - \pi_i)\}$$

where Q is the net fluid flux (mL/min), ($P_c - P_t$) is hydrostatic pressure difference between capillary (c) and interstitium (i), and ($\pi_c - \pi_i$) is the oncotic pressure difference between the capillary and interstitium. K_f is the filtration coefficient for that membrane (mL/min/mmHg), and is the product of capillary surface area and capillary hydraulic conductance, and σ is the permeability factor (i.e., reflection coefficient) with one being impermeable, and zero being completely permeable.

The permeability factor explains why, in times of capillary leak as in shock states, colloids cannot maintain an oncotic pressure difference and tend to leak out into the interstitium. The general principle of fluid resuscitation is that intravascular hypovolemia should be replaced with isotonic fluid, which tends to distribute in the ECF (3:1) intravascular:interstitium. Hypotonic fluid will distribute between all body compartments with only a small amount remaining in the intravascular space (since water is freely permeable). Maintaining intravascular blood volume is of primary importance to deliver nutrition (via plasma) and oxygen (via red cells) to the tissues. Frequently used isotonic solutions are 0.9% normal saline (154 mEq/L of Na^+ and Cl each) and lactated Ringer solution (130 mEq/L Na^+, 109 mEq/L Cl^-, 4 mEq/L K^+, 3 mEq/L Ca^{2+}, 28 mEq/L lactate).

The endpoint of fluid resuscitation continues to be an area of great debate since routine measurement of intravascular (plasma) volume is not the norm. Surrogate markers are used to assess adequate fluid resuscitation: blood pressure, heart rate, urine output, and parameters of perfusion and cardiac function. Although every clinician wants to treat patients to "euvolemia," there are only a few centers measuring intravascular volume using radioisotope studies (see Blood Volume chapter). Debate will continue on how much fluid to give until an easy method of measuring intravascular volume is available.

DISORDERS OF WATER METABOLISM

Dysnatremias (hyponatremia or hypernatremia) are among the most common electrolyte disturbances and usually are associated with poor outcomes. This problem persists due to failure to promptly recognize a life-threatening condition and initiate appropriate treatment. This chapter will focus on the pathogenesis, diagnosis, treatment, and prevention of dysnatremias.

Regulation of Water Balance

ECF tonicity is generally reflected in the concentration of sodium in the serum. The serum sodium is proportional to the total body exchangeable sodium (Na_e) plus the total body exchangeable potassium (K_e). This critical relationship is shown mathematically in Equation (1). Equation (1) is not used clinically; rather, it illustrates the relationship between total body solutes and total body water. Decreases in potassium often accompany hyponatremia, and replacement of intracellular solute losses can also be an important part of treating hyponatremia. As water intake and excretion are tightly regulated to maintain near-constant plasma osmolality (Fig. 134.1), disturbances in serum sodium indicate disorders in water balance, not gains or loss of sodium. This is a crucial point in understanding dysnatremias. The actions of ADH, also called arginine vasopressin (AVP) (1), on the kidney tightly regulates water excretion. To maintain water balance, an intact thirst mechanism and the ability of the kidneys to vary urinary concentration are required:

$$\frac{Na_e + K_e}{\text{Total body water}} \alpha \ Na_{pl} \qquad (1)$$

Renal Water Handling

The kidney can vary urinary concentration significantly and either excrete a large water load in very dilute urine or conserve water significantly such that the daily solute load is excreted in a small volume of urine. When the urinary filtrate passes into the cortical collecting duct, it is very dilute (as low as 50 mOsm/kg). As the urine moves through the cortical collecting duct into the collecting tubule, water reabsorption occurs in the presence of ADH. In the absence of ADH activity (as in diabetes insipidus), urine concentration will remain very low (50 to 80 mOsm/kg). When ADH activity is maximal, urinary concentration can be as high as 1,200 mOsm/kg. This ability to excrete very dilute or a very concentrated urine allows the body to achieve water balance across a very wide range of water intake (between approximately 0.8 and 15 L/d). Impairments of this hormonal system that links perturbations in serum osmolality as detected by osmoreceptors in the hypothalamus to variations in urinary concentration can lead to impairments in water balance. Administration of water to a patient with impaired water excretion (Table 134.1) can lead to hyponatremia.

TABLE 134.1 States of Impaired Water Excretion in the ICU Resulting in Hyponatremia

Volume-depleted states
- Volume depletion
- Diuretics

Normal-volume states
- Syndrome of inappropriate antidiuretic hormone
- Pain
- Postoperative state
- Nausea
- Hypothyroidism

Volume-expanded states
- Congestive heart failure
- Renal failure
- Cirrhosis

Electrolyte Free Water

Electrolyte free water is a useful concept in the approach to the patient with a disturbance in water balance. Electrolyte free water is a conceptual volume of a body fluid (usually urine) that represents the volume of that fluid that would be required to dilute the electrolytes contained within total volume of the

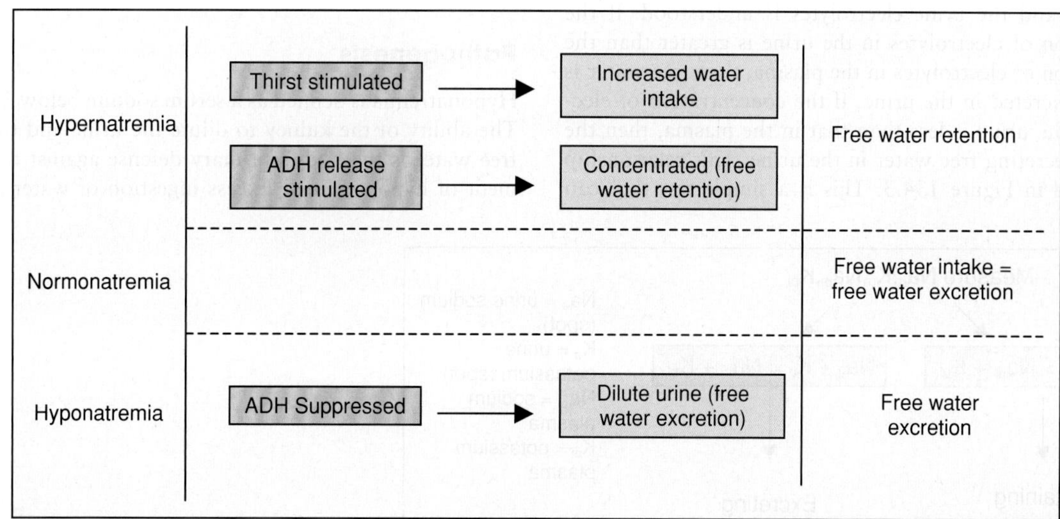

FIGURE 134.1 Water intake and excretion regulation. ADH, antidiuretic hormone.

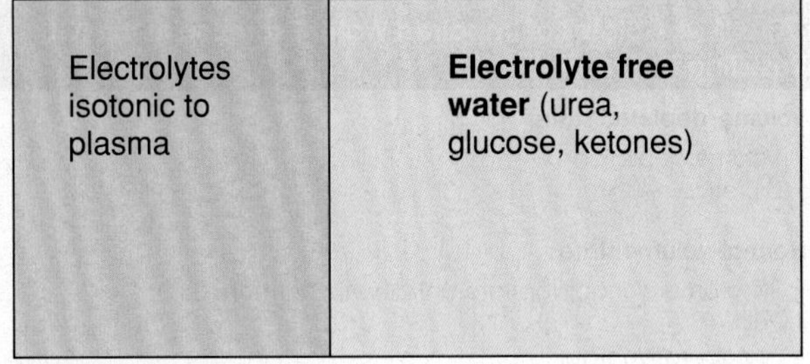

FIGURE 134.2 Electrolyte free water.

fluid to the same tonicity as plasma electrolytes (Fig. 134.2). The remainder of the volume (total volume minus electrolyte free water) can be thought of as containing the nonelectrolyte osmoles. This nonelectrolyte water excretion is the amount of water excreted above the excretion of electrolyte solutes, and thus if it is not replaced, will have an effect on the plasma sodium concentration. In other words, the osmolality of a solution is not important in determining if it contains "free water"; rather, it is the concentration of electrolytes that is important. An example of this is that the administration of dextrose solutions provides the same amount of free water as an equal volume of deionized water, whereas 0.45% normal saline contains approximately 50% less. Electrolyte free water clearance can be calculated as a convenient clinical tool in assessing water need in a patient. The amount of electrolyte free water in a body fluid (e.g., urine, sweat, nasogastric [NG] aspirate) is calculated by the following formula:

$$[1 - ([Na^+]_{fl} + [K^+]_{fl})/([Na^+]_{pl} + [K^+]_{pl}) \times \text{volume of fluid (mL)} = \text{electrolyte free water clearance} \quad (2)$$

where fl is the body fluid and pl is plasma.

Clinical Application of Electrolyte Free Water Clearance

The most important conceptual point to understand is that the urine electrolytes and *not* the urine osmolality determine the degree of free water excretion in the urine. It is not always necessary to calculate an exact value for the electrolyte free water clearance if the relationship between the plasma electrolytes and the urine electrolytes is understood. If the concentration of electrolytes in the urine is greater than the concentration of electrolytes in the plasma, then free water is not being excreted in the urine. If the concentration of electrolytes in the urine is less than that in the plasma, then the patient is excreting free water in the urine. This relationship is illustrated in Figure 134.3. This is a simple test that can allow for a quick assessment of the ongoing losses of water in the urine.

TABLE 134.2 Nonosmotic Causes of Arginine Vasopressin Excess (81)

Hemodynamic stimuli
Volume depletion
Hypotension
Congestive heart failure
Cirrhosis
Nephrotic syndrome
Adrenal insufficiency
Nonhemodynamic stimuli
Pain and stress
Nausea and voliting
Hypoxemia and hyercapnia
Hypoglycemia
Medications
Perioperative status
Inflammation
Cancer
Pulmonary disease
CNS disease

HYPONATREMIA

Hyponatremia commonly occurs in hospital settings and especially in the ICU setting (Table 134.2). Often the condition is minimally symptomatic, but hyponatremic encephalopathy (brain dysfunction due to cerebral edema in turn due to hyponatremia) can result (2–4). Hyponatremic encephalopathy is a life-threatening medical emergency, and it must be recognized and promptly treated as it can often lead to death or devastating neurologic complications (5,6). Differentiating between these two spectrums of the disease presentation is critical. Among risk factors for life-threatening hyponatremia are female gender of premenopausal age (7), children (5), and hypoxia (7). Research over the last two decades has elucidated the pathogenetic mechanisms that underlie these risk factors, and this has prompted new thinking and mandated shifts in the clinical approach to hyponatremia.

Pathogenesis

Hyponatremia is defined as a serum sodium below 135 mEq/L. The ability of the kidney to dilute the urine and thus excrete free water is the body's primary defense against the development of hyponatremia. Excess ingestion of water as the sole

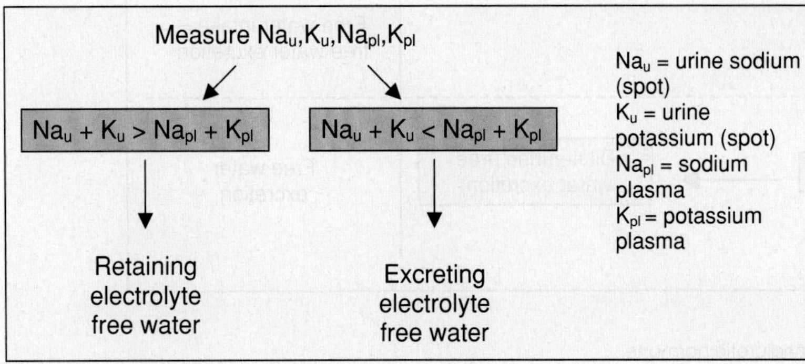

FIGURE 134.3 Relationship of electrolyte concentration in urine and plasma to the amount of free water excreted.

cause of hyponatremia is rare since the typical adult with normal renal function can excrete a massive free water load (15 L of free water per day). The combination of factors necessary for the development of hyponatremia are free water intake in the setting of an underlying condition that impairs free water excretion (see Table 134.1). The states that impair water excretion are usually states where ADH release is a physiologic response to a stimulus such as volume depletion, pain, nausea, postoperative state, or congestive heart failure (due to decreased circulating blood volume). In other instances, pathologic release of ADH occurs in syndrome of inappropriate ADH release (SIADH) and with certain medications such as thiazide diuretics and anticonvulsants.

Brain Defenses against Cerebral Edema

Hyponatremia induces an osmotic gradient that favors water movement into the brain leading to cerebral edema and neurologic injury. However, the brain is contained within a specialized compartment separated from the systemic circulation by the blood–brain barrier that impedes entry of water and has specialized mechanisms for handling water fluxes (8–10). The blood–brain barrier is a specialized structure with tight junctions between vascular endothelial cells (11–13) that interface with glial cells (astrocytes) on the brain side of the blood–brain barrier. Astrocytes form an important part of the microvascular compartment in the brain and project foot processes that abut the endothelial cells of the brain capillaries (14). This highly specialized cell performs many supporting functions in maintaining the fluid environment and the electrolyte milieu of the extracellular space of the brain (15,16). Among these functions is shunting of potassium from the microenvironment by uptake and release of potassium with water accompanying, in the perivascular space away from neurons. This function is accomplished through a concentration of aquaporin-4 water channels and Kir4.1 potassium channel located at the end-feet around the perivascular space (8). There is increasing evidence that glial cells also have an important role in brain water handling. The observation that glial cells (but not neurons) selectively swell following hypotonic stress presaged the existence of a glial-specific water pore, which has now been shown to be aquaporin 4. Mice lacking aquaporin 4 do not develop cerebral edema in response to hyponatremia, suggesting that these channels may have an important role not only in normal water regulation in the brain, but also in the pathogenesis of hyponatremia-induced cerebral edema (17). During states of cytotoxic brain edema, water is shunted through the astrocyte, which swells, and the neuron is protected from this influx of water. Therefore, astrocytes are the principal regulator of the brain water content as they comprise the bulk of the intracellular space, and the response of these cells following osmolar stress is an important determinant of the changes in brain volume during hyponatremia. This swelling of astrocytes is a principal factor in the development of cerebral edema during hyponatremic stress (Fig. 134.4).

The brain has several defenses against the development of cerebral edema. The first response is the shunting of cerebrospinal fluid (CSF) from within the brain, but this mechanism has a limited capacity to buffer volume changes (18). Immediately after a volume stress, cell volume regulatory mechanisms in the cerebral astrocytes play an important role in reducing brain volume through reduction in cellular osmolyte (mainly electrolyte) content. These are adaptive mechanisms that are used by multiple cell types to counteract an increase in cell volume; however, the astrocyte responds to cellular swelling differently than many other cells (18). In erythrocytes, white blood cells, and epithelial cells, swelling occurs due to a hypotonic environment and calcium influx that begins a series of events termed the *regulatory volume decrease* (RVD) mediated by activation of K^+ and Cl^- channels that allow these ions to be released into the extracellular environment. In glial cells this is not the predominant response. The glial cell uses ATP-dependent mechanisms (18) that require the Na^+/K^+ ATPase during which ions are extruded from the glial cell and water obligatorily follows the extruded ions, reducing brain volume and protecting from the development of cerebral edema. This response is ongoing, and in animal models of acute hyponatremia, brain water content is close to the baseline value 6 hours after induction of acute hyponatremia (19). The Na^+/K^+ ATPase is ubiquitous and plays an essential role in cellular ion homeostasis. In the brain, this enzyme is very important in the response of the cell to volume stress and hypotonic insult (20). The enzyme has binding domains for sodium, potassium, and cardiac glycosides and requires the hydrolysis of ATP to ADP to provide energy for moving these ions against concentration gradients (21). Therefore, *in vitro* evidence suggests that the actions of the sodium

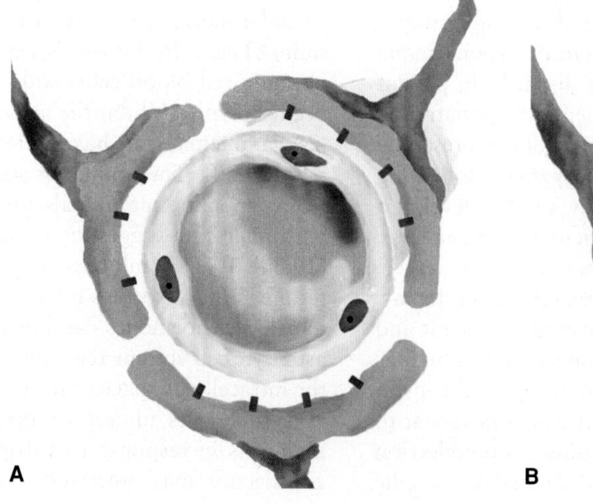

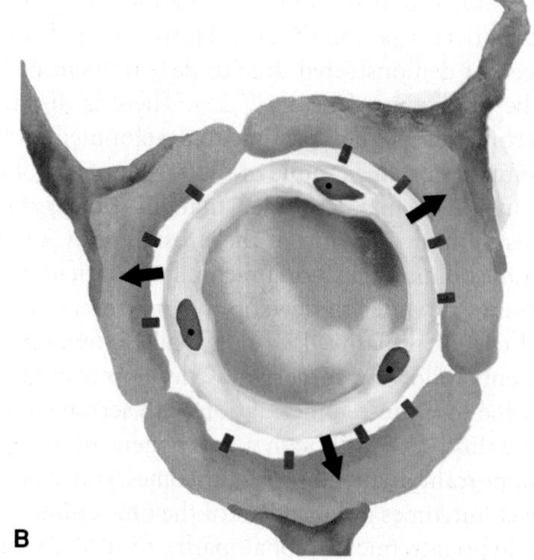

FIGURE 134.4 The pathogenesis of cerebral edema following hyponatremic stress. **A**: Aquaporin-4 (depicted in blue) expressed on the astrocyte foot process form an important component of the blood–brain barrier. **B**: During hyponatremic states, intracellular osmolality of the astrocytes exceeds that of the plasma and water follows it concentration gradient, through aquaporin-4 channels into the astrocytes leading to cerebral edema. (Courtesy of Sydney Achinger.)

potassium ATPase are the important immediate responses in determining the brain's response to hypo-osmolar stress.

In summary, during times of systemic hypo-osmolality, water enters the brain through aquaporin-4 channels located in the glial cell end-feet surrounding brain capillaries. This osmotic swelling may also allow sodium into the glial cell, and expansion of the glial cell quickly ensues. Immediate shunting of CSF accommodates some of this expansion, but this is a limited mechanism. The glial cell reduces the intracellular volume by energy-dependent extrusion of solutes via the Na^+/K^+ ATPase pump. Several clinical factors have been shown to impair these glial cell adaptive responses, resulting in poor patient outcomes.

Clinical Manifestations

Symptoms of hyponatremia are due to osmotic swelling of the brain that accompanies the decrease in plasma osmolality. Manifestations are varied, and they depend on the degree of central nervous system (CNS) adaptation to hypo-osmolality. Significant degrees of hyponatremia can be asymptomatic, such as chronic hyponatremia secondary to cirrhosis or heart failure. Conversely, hyponatremic encephalopathy is the clinical term for symptomatic cerebral edema secondary to hyponatremia, and this condition can have a fulminant presentation. Early signs are usually nonspecific—nausea, vomiting, headaches (22)—and often go unrecognized and are thought to be due to cerebral edema. When pressure is exerted on the skull by the brain, seizures may occur and if uncorrected, brainstem herniation with respiratory failure and death will follow (23). The triad of hypoxia, cerebral edema, and neurogenic pulmonary edema—which can be presenting signs of hyponatremia—can lead to the Ayus–Arieff syndrome in which hyponatremia produces cytotoxic cerebral edema, which in turn leads to a neurogenic pulmonary edema (24). Pulmonary edema leads to hypoxia, which impairs brain cell volume regulation resulting in a vicious cycle of worsening cerebral edema and pulmonary edema. This syndrome can be reversed by the prompt administration of 3% NaCl.

Risk Factors for Hyponatremic Encephalopathy

The time to development of hyponatremia (i.e., acute versus chronic) has previously been presumed to be an important risk factor in determining severity of symptoms. *In vitro* studies have shown that full brain adaptation to hypo-osmolar stress occurs over a period of days. However, epidemiologic studies have not demonstrated time to development of hyponatremia to be predictive of death (7,25). There is disparity in patient outcomes even when the time to development of hyponatremia is similar. For an example of the perplexing problem presented by hyponatremia, consider that an elderly male following transurethral resection of the prostate may acutely develop a serum sodium of 110 or a mentally ill patient may ingest large volumes of water to develop hyponatremia of similar degree, and encephalopathy does not result. However, young female patients following surgery may develop respiratory arrest and die due to brainstem herniation with serum sodium as high as 128 mEq/L (7). Although a component of acuity of the insult is important in affecting the outcomes, other factors appear to affect outcomes independent of the time course. A predilection for hyponatremic encephalopathy to affect females is a clue that patient-specific factors may be important in determining patient outcomes (7,26).

Neurologic symptoms of hyponatremic encephalopathy are due to pressure of the brain on the rigid skill. Brain size is determined by the incremental change in cell size due to osmotic influx of water, minus the RVD in response to hypo-osmolality. There are three major risk factors for poor outcomes following hyponatremic encephalopathy, which are discussed below. Patient factors play an important role in outcome.

In an epidemiologic study, being female of premenopausal age was shown to be the most important factor in predicting poor outcomes among post-surgical patients developing hyponatremia (7). Although male and female patients were equally likely to develop hyponatremia and hyponatremic encephalopathy postoperatively, permanent brain damage or death was 25 times more likely to occur in female patients (7). The degree of reduction in serum sodium and time to development of hyponatremia did not influence outcome. Comorbid conditions (coronary artery disease, chronic obstructive pulmonary disease, and peripheral vascular disease) were all more prevalent in male survivors than in female nonsurvivors with hyponatremic encephalopathy. Hypoxia at disease presentation was also identified as an important risk factor for hyponatremic encephalopathy. These findings have subsequently been verified in a general inpatient population (25). Therefore, three patient-related clinical factors—gender, age, and the presence of hypoxia—are more important in determining outcomes than the rate of development or the severity of hyponatremia. Children are another risk group for poor outcomes due to a high brain-to-cranial vault ratio as brain development is complete around age 6 years, but the skull is not fully grown until adulthood. The identification of risk factors for poor outcomes has been an important step leading to aggressive therapy and a high degree of vigilance.

Gender in Hyponatremic Encephalopathy

There are no significant anatomic differences that are known to exist between males and females that could explain this disparity in outcomes, and therefore, it was hypothesized that differences in brain adaptation to hypo-osmolar stress may exist. Estrogens have a similar core steroidal structure to ouabain and cardiac glycosides (such as digoxin), which are among the best known inhibitors of the sodium potassium ATPase (27). Ouabains bind to the α subunit of the Na^+/K^+ ATPase and inhibit the catalytic activity of the enzyme, and estrogen likely acts in a similar mechanism to reduce the activity of the sodium potassium ATPase. In diverse tissues such as mammalian heart, diaphragm, red blood cells, and liver, female sex hormones have been shown to inhibit the activity of the Na^+/K^+ ATPase pump (28), and female rats have increased morbidity from hyponatremia (29,30). The uptake of sodium by isolated synaptosomes from hyponatremic animals is increased in female rats compared with male rats suggesting an impairment in sodium extrusion (29,31). RVD is inhibited by the presence of estrogen/progesterone in rat astrocytes treated *in vitro* (32), demonstrating that female sex hormones can impair the critical energy-dependent astrocyte cell volume regulation that actively extrudes ions from the intracellular space of the edematous astrocytes.

Female rats undergo more intense vasoconstriction than male rats in response to vasopressin (30). This intense vasoconstriction may precipitate tissue hypoxia in the brain.

Role of Hypoxia in Hyponatremic Encephalopathy

Epidemiologic studies have shown that hypoxic patients fare much worse than patients without hypoxia, after adjustment for comorbid conditions in patients with hyponatremic encephalopathy (7,25). Recall that the glial cell is the primary cell involved in volume regulation in the brain. As estrogens had been shown to impair brain adaptive mechanisms through inhibition of the Na^+/K^+ ATPase, hypoxia may also impair brain adaptation as tissue hypoxia will impair energy-dependent mechanisms such as astrocyte cell volume regulation. In fact, impairment of energy use in the brain alone can lead to diffuse cerebral edema termed *cytotoxic cerebral edema* seen after asphyxiation or cardiac arrest. This impairment in volume regulatory mechanisms through hypoxia can lead to more severe cerebral edema and lead to worse patient outcomes.

The proposed mechanism for the association of hypoxia and poor outcomes is an impairment in brain adaptation due to insufficient RVD (33). Brain hypoxia can occur in two major settings: ischemia or systemic hypoxemia. Although the effect on tissue oxygenation is the same in these settings, cerebral blood flow is significantly different because brain blood flow increases in response to hypoxia. In response to hypoxia, there are many cellular adaptations that are aimed at preserving the levels of ATP (34). Cells activate pathways such as glycolysis that can produce ATP independent of cellular respiration, and there is downregulation of ATP-consuming processes. Activity of the Na^+/K^+ ATPase is downregulated through increased targeting of the enzyme for endocytosis; thus the cell favors maintenance of intracellular ATP levels over cell volume regulatory mechanisms. This may contribute to the glial cell impairment in volume regulation. Subsequent animal studies have shown that in brain hypoxia induced by either tissue ischemia or by systemic hypoxia, brain adaptation and survival are significantly impaired (33,35).

Hypoxia has been shown to develop in patients with hyponatremic encephalopathy through two mechanisms: hypercapneic respiratory failure and neurogenic pulmonary edema (36,37). Hypercapneic respiratory failure usually develops as a consequence of central respiratory depression and is the first sign of impending brain herniation. Neurogenic pulmonary edema is a well-described complication of cerebral edema from other causes as well as in hyponatremic encephalopathy (36,37). Neurogenic pulmonary edema is a complex disorder characterized by increased vascular permeability and increased catecholamine release (38) that occurs secondary to elevated intracranial pressure. Hypoxemia plays the role of both a risk factor and pathogenetic mechanism in severe cerebral edema. Whether hypoxia is present initially or develops as a consequence of hyponatremia through hypercapneic respiratory failure and/or neurogenic pulmonary edema (36,37), poor outcomes ensue (Fig. 134.5).

Approach to Hyponatremic Patient

The first step in working up the hyponatremic patient is to exclude hyperosmolar hyponatremia (Fig. 134.6). An osmotically active substance that is confined to the ECF (usually glucose or mannitol) will remove water from the intracellular space and will dilute the serum sodium concentration (translocational hyponatremia). To assess for a sodium disturbance in the setting of hyperglycemia, one must correct the serum sodium by adding 1.6 mEq/L for every 100 mg/dL increase of the serum glucose above 100 mg/dL. Significant hyperosmolality can exist in the setting of a normal or low serum sodium in cases of hyperglycemia. For example, a patient has a serum glucose of 650 mg/dL and a serum sodium of 130 mEq/L. Correct the serum sodium as follows:

$$\frac{650 \text{ mg/dL} - 100 \text{ mg/dL}}{100 \text{ mg/dL}} \times 1.6 \text{ mEq/L}$$
$$= 5.5 \times 1.6 \text{ mEq/L} = 8.8 \text{ mEq/L}$$

Thus the corrected serum sodium in this patient is 139 mEq/L.

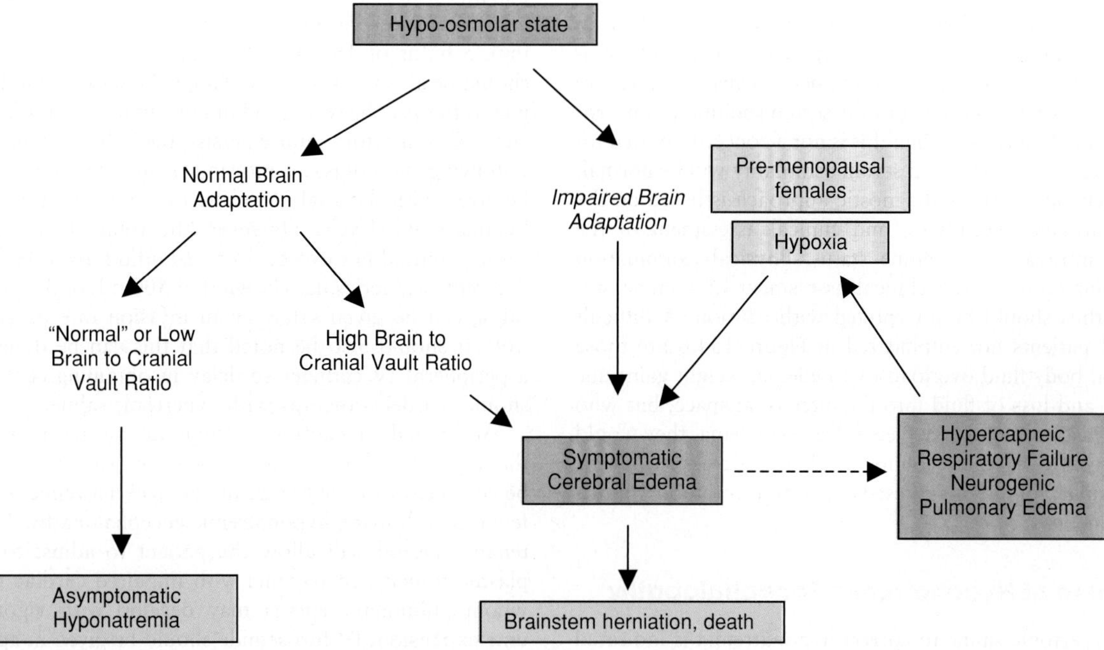

FIGURE 134.5 The role of hypoxia.

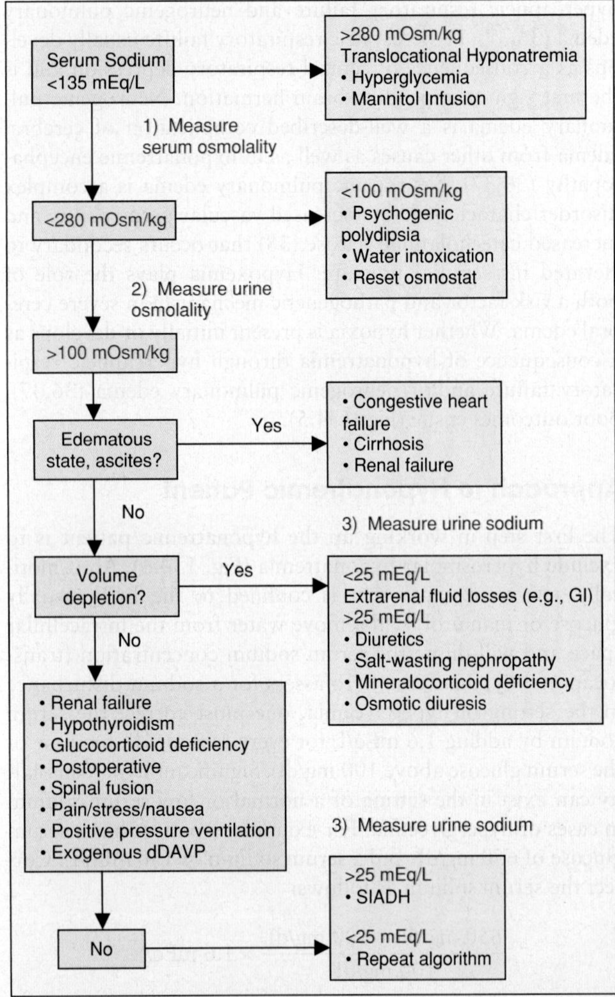

FIGURE 134.6 Diagnostic approach to hyponatremia. DDAVP, desmopressin; GI, gastrointestinal; SIADH, syndrome of inappropriate antidiuretic hormone.

The entity of pseudohyponatremia should also be kept in mind. Hyperproteinemia and hyperlipidemia can lead to spuriously low serum sodium measurements when *samples are diluted* prior to measurement of the serum sodium. If a potentiometric method is used, then this is not a concern. In pseudohyponatremia, the measured serum osmolality will be normal.

The remainder of the diagnostic approach is based on the history, urinary electrolytes, and clinical assessment of the patient's intravascular volume status. Physical examination can be unreliable in the clinical assessment of volume status and thus should be interpreted with caution. A difficult group of patients not emphasized in Figure 134.6 are those with total body fluid overload (with edema, weight gain) due to shock and loss of fluid into the interstitial space, but who are intravascular volume depleted. Despite edema, they would be categorized as the "volume depletion" group, and the intravascular volume may best be assessed by blood volume measurements.

Treatment of Hyponatremic Encephalopathy

Use of hypertonic saline to correct hyponatremia is indicated for patients with signs of hyponatremic encephalopathy. Also,

TABLE 134.3 Treatment of Hyponatremia (6)

High-risk groups for poor outcomes
- Menstruant females
- Children
- Hypoxic patients

Hyponatremic encephalopathy with evidence of cerebral edema (seizures, respiratory arrest, decreased mental status, headache, nausea, vomiting)
- Bolus, 100 mL of 3% NaCl over 10 min
- Can repeat bolus 1–2 times with the goal of increasing serum sodium 2–4 mEq/L or until clinical improvement
- A total of 500 mL of intravenous 3% sodium chloride can be given safely in the first 5 hr or therapy. This amount is likely to be sufficient for treatment of cerebral edema in the majority of cases. A lesser amount may also be sufficient.
- The goal should be to not correct the serum sodium more than 15–20 mEq/L *in the initial 48 hr of therapy*

Hyponatremia without clinical signs of cerebral edema
- Fluid restriction unless hypovolemia is suspected
- Demeclocycline
- Vasopressin V2 receptor antagonists

the serum osmolality should be measured prior to beginning therapy with hypertonic saline to verify that a hypotonic state exists (23). Fluid restriction alone is never appropriate to manage a patient with hyponatremic encephalopathy, especially in intravascular hypovolemic states. Early recognition of the problem and prompt therapy are the most important factors associated with successful intervention and good neurologic outcomes (22).

The rationale for treatment with hypertonic saline can be summarized as follows: Remove patients with severe manifestations of cerebral edema from immediate danger, correct serum sodium to a mildly hyponatremic level, and maintain this level of serum sodium to allow for the brain to adapt to the change in serum osmolality. Table 134.3 gives an overview of the approach to therapy. Prompt therapy should be instituted in all patients with hyponatremic encephalopathy. In patients with neurologic manifestations suggestive of cerebral edema (seizures, respiratory failure, headache, nausea, vomiting), a bolus of 100 mL 3% saline (given over 10 minutes) should be given to promptly change the serum osmolality. The goal is to raise the serum sodium by about 2 to 4 mEq/L. If seizures or respiratory failure persist, the bolus may be repeated. Following the bolus, an infusion of hypertonic saline should be given with the goal of raising the serum sodium to mildly hyponatremic levels. However, the total change in serum sodium should not exceed 15 to 20 mEq/L over 48 hours (6). A recent case series has shown that 500 mL of 3% hypertonic saline can be given safely at an infusion rate of 100 mL/hr (39). It should also be noted that this can be done through a peripheral IV catheter so delay in obtaining central access should not delay therapy with hypertonic saline.

Additional precautionary steps are necessary to prevent therapy-induced brain injury. The serum sodium should never be corrected to normonatremic or hypernatremic levels for a few days following hyponatremic encephalopathy. This maintenance period will allow the patient to adjust to the new plasma tonicity. In patients with impaired cardiac output in whom pulmonary edema may develop with vigorous volume expansion, IV furosemide should be given in addition to hypertonic saline to prevent volume overload.

There are formulas that have been advocated to calculate the infusion rate when giving hypertonic saline; however, we do not endorse their use. This practice can lead to patient injury when a calculated rate is used as a substitute for proper patient monitoring. Any patient receiving 3% saline should have the serum sodium checked at least every 2 hours until the patient and the serum sodium values are stable. All patients with severe manifestations must be placed in an intensive care setting. The rationale for close monitoring is that ongoing water losses cannot be predicted, and equations that calculate infusion rates assume a closed system (i.e., no ongoing water losses) and significant overcorrection can occur. To guide initial therapy, an infusion of 3% saline of 1 mL/kg will estimate an increase in serum sodium by approximately 1 mEq/L. Initial infusion rates should be adjusted based on repeated serum sodium values and the patient's clinical response.

Use of Desmopressin

Desmopressin (1-deamino-8-D-arginine vasopressin; DDAVP)-associated hyponatremia is a special case of drug-induced hyponatremia that warrants special mention. DDAVP is a synthetic vasopressin receptor agonist, is typically prescribed for central diabetes insipidus (CDI, von Willebrand's disease, and for enuresis in children and the elderly. This medication causes renal water retention via stimulation of the vasopressin-2 (V2) receptor in the collecting duct and through increased expression of aquaporins in the luminal membrane of the collecting duct, thereby increasing water reabsorption along the medullary interstitial concentration gradient. DDAVP-associated hyponatremia is a known complication of DDAVP therapy and is not an uncommon clinical encounter. This occurs when DDAVP is used and free water intake (either enteral or parenteral) is not appropriately restricted. When the use of DDAVP leads to severe, symptomatic hyponatremia with neurologic symptoms, the clinician faces a challenging clinical dilemma. The management of a patient with DDAVP-associated hyponatremia poses particular difficulties. This is because a patient with DDAVP-associated hyponatremia is initially in an antidiuretic state and the acutely symptomatic patient will need early treatment to bring up the serum sodium with hypertonic saline to prevent the complications of cerebral edema. However, if the DDAVP is discontinued, a state of water diuresis may occur where urinary dilution is now maximal and the patient will excrete copious amounts of free water. This can lead to put the patient at risk of autocorrection of the serum will ensue and significant overcorrection can occur, especially if IV saline is given at the time. Therefore, in the management of DDAVP-associated hyponatremia with neurologic symptoms, the drug should not be withheld and the medication should be continued, despite the presence of hyponatremia. Symptomatic individuals should be treated with hypertonic saline while continuing DDAVP, a 100-mL bolus of 3% saline can be used as initial therapy (Fig. 134.7). We feel that DDAVP should not be stopped as part of the initial management of this disorder to prevent overcorrection of the serum sodium and possible neurologic injury (40).

During the treatment of hyponatremia, the clinician needs to be vigilant to be sure that a free water diuresis does not occur. Clinical scenarios where this is more of concern are interruption of DDAVP therapy (as noted above), psychogenic polydipsia, and drug-induced hyponatremia when the offending agent is stopped. To prevent ongoing water losses in the urine and "autocorrection" of the serum sodium, DDAVP can be given to increase urinary concentration and reduce free water losses. This must be done carefully with the patient strictly fluid restricted or kept with no enteral intake in an ICU setting. If unrestricted fluid intake occurs during DDAVP administration, significant hyponatremia can develop. Consultation with an expert experienced in treating sodium disorders is mandatory in such cases. An increase in urine output is the first sign that a water diuresis is ensuing, and therefore, hourly urine output needs to be followed in all patients with hyponatremic encephalopathy. The difficulty in treating cases where autocorrection can occur is illustrated in the special case studies below.

Risk Factors for the Development of Cerebral Demyelination

Cerebral demyelination is a rare, serious complication associated with the correction of severe hyponatremia. When symptoms manifest, it is usually a delayed phenomenon occurring days to weeks following correction of hyponatremia and can

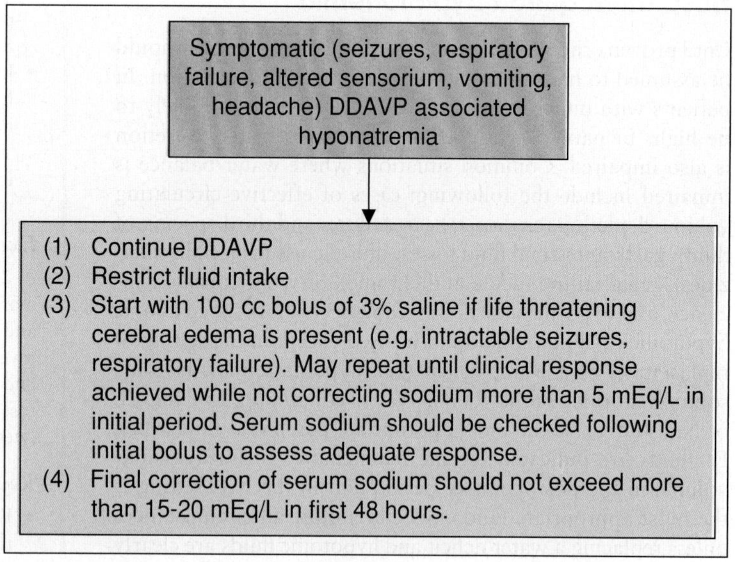

Symptomatic (seizures, respiratory failure, altered sensorium, vomiting, headache) DDAVP associated hyponatremia

↓

(1) Continue DDAVP
(2) Restrict fluid intake
(3) Start with 100 cc bolus of 3% saline if life threatening cerebral edema is present (e.g. intractable seizures, respiratory failure). May repeat until clinical response achieved while not correcting sodium more than 5 mEq/L in initial period. Serum sodium should be checked following initial bolus to assess adequate response.
(4) Final correction of serum sodium should not exceed more than 15-20 mEq/L in first 48 hours.

FIGURE 134.7 Treatment approach to DDAVP-associated hyponatremia. (Adapted from Achinger SG, Arieff AI, Kalantar-Zadeh K, Ayus JC. Desmopressin acetate (DDAVP)-associated hyponatremia and brain damage: a case series. *Nephrol Dial Transpl.* 2014;29(12):2310–2315.)

manifest as a pseudocoma with a locked-in stare. This condition can also be asymptomatic and, therefore, magnetic resonance imaging (MRI) (which is sensitive for the detection of demyelinating lesions) is necessary for the diagnosis. It is important to understand that the rate of correction of serum sodium alone does not predict the development of cerebral demyelination; rather, the absolute change in serum sodium over 48 hours is predictive (6). Other clinical factors such as liver disease and hypoxia increase the risk of demyelination, and care must be exercised in these groups. As noted above, the serum sodium can be quickly be corrected in an acutely symptomatic patient without increasing the risk of demyelination as long as the absolute change over 48 hours does not exceed 15 to 20 mEq/L and the patient is not corrected to normonatremic levels. *Patients with liver disease are particularly susceptible to cerebral demyelination, and caution should be exercised in this setting; the safe degree of correction over 48 hours in this group is not known.*

Management of Hyponatremia without Signs of Encephalopathy

Regardless of the cause and regardless of the absolute level of the serum sodium, hyponatremia without signs of encephalopathy does not require aggressive therapy, but the diagnostic approach to hyponatremia is similar (see Fig. 134.6), and treatment should be based on the cause. Fluid restriction can be used alone if hypovolemia is not suspected, but this will typically not result in resolution of the hyponatremia, especially in cases of SIADH where electrolyte free water excretion is negative. Precipitating medications such as thiazide diuretics and anticonvulsants should be stopped. If hyponatremia persists despite fluid restriction, demeclocycline can be used to lower osmolality and increase free water excretion. Vasopressin receptor (V2) blockers are new agents that show promise for the treatment of hyponatremia (41). There is currently limited experience with these medications. However, they may become the mainstay of therapy for hyponatremia without signs of encephalopathy in the future as demeclocycline has potential side effects.

Fluid Therapy and Prevention of Hospital-Acquired Hyponatremia

Until proven otherwise, a patient in a critical care setting should be assumed to have an impairment in free water excretion. In patients with intact kidney function, ADH levels are likely to be high. In patients with renal failure, free water excretion is also impaired. Common situations where water balance is impaired include the following: cases of effective circulating volume depletion (cirrhosis, heart failure, and third spacing of fluid), gastrointestinal fluid losses, diuretic use (especially thiazides), renal failure (acute and chronic), SIADH, cortisol deficiency, and hypothyroidism (see Table 134.1). As noted above, hypotonic IV fluids should not be used except in the setting of replacement of a water deficit (i.e., hypernatremia). Isotonic solution normal saline (0.9% NaCl) containing 154 mEq/L of Na^+ and Cl^- is the most appropriate parenteral fluid when IV fluids are indicated for the maintenance of intravascular volume in the postoperative period and in the ICU setting is the most appropriate fluid choice in almost all circumstances unless replacing a water deficit and hypotonic fluids are clearly needed (42). Also, any patient receiving fluid therapy should have the serum sodium measured at least daily.

Hospital-acquired hyponatremic encephalopathy occurs most commonly when hypotonic fluids are administered to a patient with an impairment of free water excretion. A clinical setting that merits specific discussion is the postoperative state. Approximately 1% of patients develop a serum sodium below 130 mEq/L following surgery, and clinically important hyponatremia complicates 20% of these cases. The postoperative state commonly includes multiple stimuli for ADH release including pain, stress, nausea, vomiting, narcotic medications, and volume depletion. Administration of a hypotonic IV fluid in the postoperative state or in other clinical settings characterized by impaired free water excretion can have disastrous consequences. The use of hypotonic fluids is reserved for treatment of a free water deficit, such as exists in the setting of hypernatremia.

Special Case Studies

Postoperative Hyponatremia

A 32-year-old female with no significant past medical history undergoes elective laparoscopic bilateral tubal ligation at 8:00 am; 5% dextrose, 1/4 normal saline is started by the anesthesiologist and maintained at 125 mL/hr. The patient remains in recovery until late in the afternoon and is kept because she is too sedated to leave. IV meperidine is given, with adequate pain relief. She does not tolerate oral intake, and the IV fluids are continued at the current rate. At 2:45 am the following day, the patient complains of headache and she is given Vicodin by the on-call physician. At 9:00 am, a nurse notifies the surgeon of a sodium of 129 mEq/L; no new orders are received, and IV fluids are continued. Later that morning the patient is noted to be lethargic, and the surgeon is notified by the nursing staff; an order is received to hold pain medications. At 3:30 pm, the patient has a generalized seizure and goes into respiratory failure. She is intubated and mechanical ventilation is initiated. Serum sodium at this time is 124 mEq/L.

Key Points

- This patient has multiple stimuli for ADH release and thus impaired free water excretion. Administration of a hypotonic fluid was not appropriate and placed the patient at risk for hyponatremia.
- The most important measure to prevent postoperative hyponatremia is to avoid the use of a hypotonic fluid in a postsurgical patient and administer 0.9% sodium chloride when parenteral fluids are indicated.
- In this case the clinicians failed to recognize the early signs of hyponatremic encephalopathy (headache, nausea, and vomiting), which occurred when the patient's sodium was 129 mEq/L. The presence or absence of symptoms of hyponatremic encephalopathy and not the absolute level of the serum sodium determines whether or not a life-threatening condition exists.

Exercise-Induced Hyponatremia

A 21-year-old woman collapses 30 minutes after completing a marathon and is brought to the emergency room. She is disoriented and significantly short of breath on arrival. Physical examination reveals a normal cardiac examination, crackles in all lung fields, and a nonfocal neurologic examination with depressed mental status. Chest radiograph reveals pulmonary edema. Serum electrolytes include sodium of 126 mEq/L and potassium of 3.1 mEq/L.

Key Points

- Exercise-associated hyponatremia has been described in marathon runners. Those who develop this problem consume large

amounts of water throughout the race, in excess of the water lost through sweating (36,40). The proposed mechanism is that significant portions of consumed water remains sequestered in the gut as there is divergence of blood flow from the splanchnic circulation during the race. Additionally, ADH is released secondary to the extreme physical exertion of the race. Following completion of the marathon, the ingested water is absorbed and acute hyponatremia ensues, which can be fatal.
- Noncardiogenic pulmonary edema induced by cerebral edema has been described in association with exercise-induced hyponatremia. Paradoxically, treatment with 3% saline leads to resolution of the pulmonary edema by treating the underlying cerebral edema (43).
- Limiting fluid intake is necessary as hypotonic electrolyte sports drinks or salt consumption during the race do not appear to be effective in prevention of this condition (44).

DDAVP Withdrawal

A 76-year-old nursing home patient with a history of urinary incontinence, following transurethral resection of the prostate, is treated with intranasal DDAVP, 10 μg each night. On a routine chemistry panel 1 week prior to admission, his sodium was 138 mEq/L and the patient was doing quite well. Two days prior to presentation he was started on DDAVP, 10 μg in the late morning. On the day of admission, the patient is found to be lethargic and unresponsive and is transported to an emergency room. His serum sodium is 104 mEq/L and serum potassium is 4.0 mEq/L. Urine sodium is 95 mEq/L and urine potassium is 45 mEq/L. He is treated with a 75-mL bolus, then infusion of 3% saline, and his neurologic status improves. Infusion of 3% saline is held when the serum sodium is 120 mEq/L. DDAVP has also been withheld because it is noted to have caused the hyponatremia. Urine output increases significantly over the ensuing night and on the following morning his serum sodium is 139 mEq/L, urine sodium is 17 mEq/L, and urine potassium is 11 mEq/L.

Key Points

- DDAVP alone will not induce hyponatremia. DDAVP will cause retention of free water, and thus the dosing needs to be titrated in conjunction with the patient's fluid intake. Proper patient instruction and close monitoring are essential during dose changes.
- If DDAVP is withheld, which is commonly done in cases of DDAVP-associated hyponatremia, a free water diuresis will ensue and dangerous overcorrection of the serum sodium hypernatremia may occur.
- The best approach to a patient with hyponatremic encephalopathy due to DDAVP-associated hyponatremia is to continue DDAVP and restrict all enteral fluid intake (40). Three percent NaCl should be used to correct the patient to the desired serum sodium level, then should be discontinued. A slow infusion of 0.9% can be continued if necessary to support volume status, and absolutely no hypotonic fluids should be administered (see Fig. 134.7). This will prevent overcorrection of the serum sodium secondary to a water diuresis. Consultation with a specialist is recommended in these complex cases.

NMDA-Associated Hyponatremia

A 19-year-old female college student with no past medical history presents early in the morning following an evening of NMDA (ecstasy) use and copious water drinking at a late night dance party. She did not have any particular symptoms prior to going to sleep at 4:00 am, though she was found unresponsive in her bed the following morning around 10:00 am by her dormitory roommate. On arrival in the emergency room she was to be poorly responsive with dilated, minimally responsive pupils, hypoxemic, and in respiratory distress and with evidence of pulmonary edema. Serum sodium was 117 mEq/L.

Key Points

- NMDA use has been associated with severe, symptomatic hyponatremia associated with noncardiogenic pulmonary edema.
- Optimal treatment of this condition involves prompt recognition of the role of hyponatremia in the pathogenesis of pulmonary edema. Administration of hypertonic saline and optimization of respiratory status. In patient's presenting with life-threatening symptoms (seizures, pulmonary edema, etc.), a bolus of 100 mL of 3% hypertonic saline should be administered.

HYPERNATREMIA

Hypernatremia, a serum sodium above 145 mEq/L, is commonly encountered in the ICU. Thirst is a powerful protective mechanism, and therefore, restricted access to water is nearly always necessary for the development of hypernatremia. Restricted access to water occurs in various settings, often at the extremes of age: patients who are debilitated by an acute or chronic illness, in neurologic impairment such as dementia, in infants, in moribund patients, or in those on mechanical ventilation with inability to drink water, or in any situation without free access to water. Hypernatremia can develop in essentially any critically ill patient with altered mental status or intubated for mechanical ventilation, because these patients have restricted access to fluids. In most patients in the ICU with hypernatremia, there is a combination of impaired access to water and ongoing free water losses. Renal water losses may occur secondary to solute diuresis (typically urea or glucose), renal concentrating defects (such as loop diuretics), excess hypertonic sodium bicarbonate administration, and gastrointestinal fluid losses (especially nasogastric suction and lactulose administration).

Pathogenesis

The thirst mechanism and the kidney's urinary concentrating ability that minimize water losses in the urine are the body's defenses against the development of hypernatremia. The common causes of hypernatremia in the ICU usually involve states of impaired water access in conjunction with excessive free water losses (Table. 134.4). Hypernatremia is a relatively uncommon diagnosis on admission to the ICU but frequently develops during critical illness, and the cause is nearly always iatrogenic. Failure to recognize significant electrolyte free water losses in the urine and to provide adequate replacement in either parenteral or enteral solutions

TABLE 134.4 Common Causes of Hypernatremia in the ICU

Common Causes of Hypernatremia in the ICU
Lack of water intake
• Decreased thirst (dementia, neurologic impairment)
• Mechanical ventilation
• Bowel rest, nasogastric suction
Increased water loss
• Solute diuresis (hyperglycemia, urea loading from tube feeds or hyperalimentation)
• Loop diuretics
• Gastrointestinal water losses
• Diabetes insipidus

is a common cause of hypernatremia in the intensive care setting.

During hypernatremic states, the brain is subject to osmolar stress that favors the movement of water out of the brain and can lead to significant brain damage. *In vivo* studies have shown that the brain adapts to hypernatremia through increases in osmotically active ions and *de novo* generation of osmotically active idiogenic osmoles. The osmotically active cations that are increased in the brain during hypernatremia are sodium and potassium. Idiogenic osmoles refer to a heterogeneous group of osmotically active substances such as myoinositol, glycerophosphocholine, choline, and sorbitol (45,46). This response is seen in the acute setting, and no further changes in brain osmolality are observed after 1 week of hypernatremia (47). These defenses preserve brain volume during elevations in the plasma osmolality and prevent significant decrease in brain size due to osmotic water losses in the brain. In correction of chronic hypernatremia, idiogenic osmoles do not dissipate quickly, and rapid correction of chronic hypernatremia over 24 hours can lead to cerebral edema (47).

Approach to the Hypernatremic Patient

A detailed history focusing on fluid intake and losses is the first step in the evaluation of the hypernatremic patient. Various sources of water losses in the critically ill patient are (Fig. 134.8) water losses in the urine, from the gastrointestinal tract (diarrhea and nasogastric suction), and insensible losses (fever, sepsis, massive diaphoresis, burns). These amounts should be calculated (when accurate counts are available) or estimated. In assessing urinary water losses, both the urine osmolality and electrolytes should be measured in evaluation of urinary concentrating ability and to assess urinary water losses. Caution should be exercised in the interpretation of the urine osmolality as this is an area where error is frequently made. The urine osmolality alone cannot be used to determine whether or not there is free water loss in the urine. This is because water is excreted with nonelectrolyte osmoles (which under physiologic conditions is typically urea) and with electrolyte osmoles. Both contribute to the osmolality of the urine but have differential effects on water balance. Water that is excreted with nonelectrolyte osmoles is water that is lost in excess of electrolyte loss. Recall that the serum sodium is proportional to total body electrolytes relative to total body water (Equation (1)). Therefore, loss of water with the nonelectrolyte osmoles will raise the serum sodium. By contrast, water that is excreted with electrolyte osmoles will not affect the serum sodium (as long as the concentration of electrolytes in the urine and serum are similar). This is because both the numerator and denominator of Equation (1) are decreasing, so the proportion is unchanged. In cases where there is a high urea or glucose load, significant amounts of water can be lost in the urine despite maximal urinary concentration. Failure to concentrate the urine in the face of hypernatremia should raise suspicion of a urinary concentrating defect. Renal failure, loop diuretics, tubulointerstitial renal disease, and diabetes insipidus are the main causes of urinary concentrating defects. In summary, all sources of water intake and water loss should be considered in assessing the water needs of a critically ill patient (see Fig. 134.8) as an imbalance favoring water loss over water intake will lead to hypernatremia.

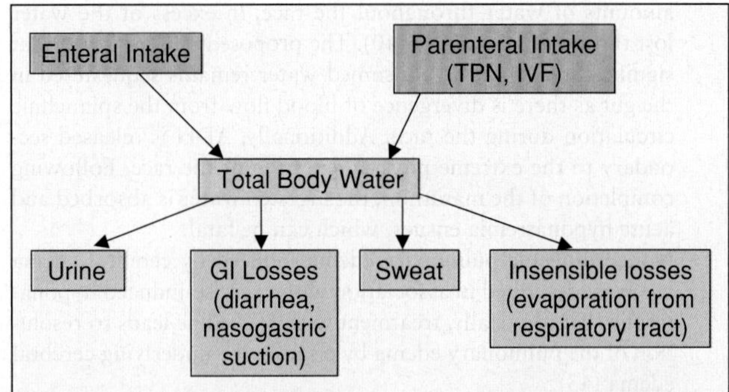

FIGURE 134.8 Sources of water intake and loss in the ICU. GI, gastrointestinal; IVF, intravenous fluid; TPN, total parenteral nutrition.

Clinical Manifestations

Hypernatremia leads to an efflux of fluid from the intracellular space to the extracellular space to maintain osmotic equilibrium across the cell membranes. The primary clinical manifestations are due to CNS depression as cerebral dehydration and cell shrinkage occurs. Hypernatremia carries an overall mortality between 40% and 70% in children (48). The elderly and patients with end-stage liver disease are at particular risk for complications from hypernatremia. Treatment of hepatic encephalopathy with lactulose frequently causes an osmotic diarrhea that leads to water losses in the stool. As a result, hypernatremia can quickly develop and lead to severe morbidity. Patients with liver disease are at high risk for cerebral demyelination in the setting of changes in serum sodium (6).

Central Diabetes Insipidus

CDI is a unique cause of hypernatremia that can be seen in the ICU and is most commonly in the setting of head injury, pituitary surgery, and cerebral hemorrhages. Specific therapy is indicated for this condition and therefore it needs to be recognized early. With polyuria secondary to water diuresis, severe hypernatremia can rapidly develop in an individual who has restricted access to fluids such as an ICU patient. Sodium-retentive mechanisms are intact in patients with CDI, and therefore, clinical volume depletion is not a characteristic feature. The diagnosis of CDI should be suspected if the urine is not concentrated in the setting of hypernatremia (49). In general, the plasma osmolality typically exceeds the urine osmolality in CDI. Formal diagnostic testing for diabetes insipidus is beyond the scope of this text and is usually undertaken in consultation with a nephrologist. A simple and reliable clinical test that can be used to distinguish CDI from nephrogenic diabetes insipidus is to administer a V2 receptor agonist, such as DDAVP. A 50% increase in urine osmolality following DDAVP administration strongly suggests CDI. Once the diagnosis is established, DDAVP can be given either subcutaneously or intranasally. When DDAVP is administered, water intake should be adjusted appropriately to avoid precipitation of significant hyponatremia, and serial serum electrolytes should be monitored during dose titration (23).

Treatment

The goal of treatment of hypernatremia is to achieve normal circulatory volume as patients typically have circulatory

TABLE 134.5 Treatment of Hypernatremia (82)

1. Replete intravascular volume with colloid solution, isotonic saline, or plasma.
2. Estimate water deficit. Deficit should be replaced over 48–72 hr, aiming for a correction of 1 mOsm/L/hr. In severe hypernatremia (>170 mEq/L), serum sodium should not be corrected to below 150 mEq/L in the first 48–72 hr. Replacement of ongoing water losses are given in addition to the deficit.
3. Hypotonic fluid should be used. Usual replacement fluid is 77 mEq/L (0.45 N saline). A lower sodium concentration may be needed if there is a renal concentrating defect or sodium overload. Glucose-containing solutions should be avoided, and an oral route of administration should be used.
4. Monitor plasma; electrolytes should be monitored every 2 hr until patient is neurologically stable.

volume depletion and then to correct the serum sodium with free water replacement (Table 134.5). The first step is to assess the ongoing water losses in the urine to determine if the water losses are renal in origin, or if the kidneys are appropriately conserving water. A simple method for assessing free water loss in the urine is displayed in Equation (3), which is Equation (2) but looking specifically at the urine:

$$\left(1-\frac{[\mathrm{Na}^+]_U+[\mathrm{K}^+]_U}{[\mathrm{Na}^+]_p+[\mathrm{K}^+]_p}\right)\times \text{urine output rate}$$
$$= \text{rate of urinary water loss} \qquad (3)$$

The degree of ongoing water losses in the urine will assist in determining the rate of fluid administration. In cases of extrarenal fluid losses, the fluid loss will need to be estimated. Fluid resuscitation with normal saline or colloid to replenish the circulating volume should precede correction of the water deficit (see Table 134.5). In hypernatremic states, insulin resistance has also been observed (50). This can lead to severe hyperglycemia and potential worsening of hyperosmolality during therapy with glucose-containing solutions. For this reason, glucose-containing solutions are potentially harmful and should be avoided if possible. If IV glucose solutions must be used (e.g., 5% dextrose in water), hourly measurement of the plasma glucose should be made and an insulin drip considered if plasma glucose becomes elevated. Oral hydration is preferable to parenteral and should be used when possible. Serial measurement of electrolytes every 2 hours is necessary until the patient is neurologically stable. In patients without evidence of hypernatremic encephalopathy, the serum sodium should not be corrected more quickly than 1 mEq/hr or 15 mEq/24 hr. In severe cases (>170 mEq/L), sodium should not be corrected to below 150 mEq/L in the first 48 to 72 hours (36).

Case Scenario: SOLUTE DIURESIS FROM EXCESS UREA LOAD

A 46-year-old man is admitted with severe necrotizing pancreatitis. He has a history of alcohol abuse, hepatitis C, and chronic liver disease. The patient weighs 76 kg. Admission labs are listed below. The patient is kept without enteral intake overnight and volume expanded with 6 L of normal saline. Twenty-four hours after admission, abdominal pain worsens and he is continued without enteral intake. Serum sodium is 145. Over the next 24 hours, urine output increases and isotonic saline is continued at 100 mL/hr. Total parenteral nutrition is initiated with a total volume of 2 L, 120 mEq of sodium, and high amino acid content. The chemistry and urine studies 48 hours after admission are listed.

	Admission	48 hr after admission
Sodium (mEq/L)	137	155
Potassium (mEq/L)	3.5	3.1
Chloride (mEq/L)	103	112
Bicarbonate (mmol/L)	21	24
Blood urea nitrogen (mg/dL)	23	53
Creatinine (mg/dL)	1.3	1.1
Urine output (mL/hr)	40	200
Urine sodium (mEq/L)	—	45
Urine potassium (mEq/L)	—	22
Urine osmolality (mOsm/kg)	—	610

What is the cause of the polyuria in this patient? Answer: Solute diuresis.

Key Point

- Solute diuresis secondary to a high urea load is a common cause of hypernatremia in the critical care setting.

This patient presents a typical example of a solute diuresis leading to hypernatremia in the critical care setting. By taking the ratio of the sodium plus potassium in the urine over the sodium plus potassium in the serum, urinary water losses can be assessed. The sodium plus potassium in the urine is lower than that in the blood. In this case, the ratio is 70/156 = 0.45. This means that 45% of his urine is electrolyte containing and conversely that 55% of the urine is electrolyte free water. At his current urine output, he is losing (0.55 × 200 mL/hr) = 110 mL of water per hour in the urine. Water replacement must be at least equal to this to replace his ongoing water losses in the urine. The urine osmolality is high due to ADH secretion, and this is increasing the urine concentration. The low urine sodium and potassium, at a time when the urine osmolality is high, signifies that there is a nonelectrolyte osmole in the urine that is obligating water loss. This is a classic presentation of an osmotic diuresis secondary to urea. The high urea load in this case is probably multifactorial, being secondary to the hypercatabolic state with muscle breakdown in addition to the necessarily high protein in the total parenteral nutrition.

Prevention

The prevention of hypernatremia is best accomplished by recognition of patients at risk for this disorder and at risk of a poor outcome. It is not necessary to memorize a list of conditions but to understand that hypernatremia requires at least one of the following to occur: impaired access to water (dementia, mental illness, encephalopathy, child/infant, critically ill patient, patient who is restricted in enteral intake or using a feeding tube) or a massive sodium load (improper infant formula mixture, administration of large amounts of hypertonic sodium solutions such as sodium bicarbonate or sodium phosphate) (23).

DISORDERS OF POTASSIUM BALANCE

Physiology of Potassium Homeostasis

Potassium is present mainly in the intracellular space (approximately 4,000 mEq of total body stores) and is sequestered in the intracellular space through the action of the Na^+/K^+ ATPase pump. The serum potassium level is tightly regulated so that the potential differences across membranes, especially cardiac, are not affected by alterations in potassium level. As the extracellular space contains very little of the total body potassium, shifting of potassium from one space to another is a major cause of both hyperkalemia and hypokalemia. The major influences that favor potassium movement into cells are insulin and β_2-adrenergic stimulation. Metabolic acidosis favors potassium movement out of cells as H^+ is exchanged for K^+ when H^+ moves intracellularly. However, this may have less importance in settings where an organic anion is generated as a result of the acidosis (such as lactic acidosis) as the organic ions may also move intracellularly and thus negate the electrogenic stimulus for potassium to move out of the cell.

Potassium excretion is tightly regulated, and the excretion of potassium can be varied such that potassium balance is maintained across a wide range of potassium intake. There are two main determinants of potassium excretion of clinical significance: flow of tubular filtrate into the distal nephron and secretion of potassium into the electronegative filtrate through epithelial potassium channels. The electronegativity of the tubular filtrate is determined by reabsorption of sodium from the filtrate at a faster rate than reabsorption of Cl^-. This reabsorption occurs through the epithelial sodium channel ENaC (51,52). The effect of aldosterone with sodium retention is the most important influence increasing the action of ENaC and therefore stimulates potassium excretion. Medications such as amiloride, triamterene, and trimethoprim (52) block ENaC and lead to decreased K^+ secretion and can lead to clinically important hyperkalemia. Decrease in the rate of tubular flow into the distal nephron stimulates the renin angiotensin system, which in turn stimulates release of aldosterone. The renin angiotensin axis, in addition to stimulating the release of aldosterone, also affects hemodynamic changes at the glomerular level, which act to maintain glomerular filtration rate (GFR) and therefore maintain distal flow into the nephron with the ability to excrete potassium. In summary, the renal excretion of potassium is enhanced during states of high tubular flow and also under the actions of aldosterone. Therefore, inhibition of either of these through a decrease in GFR (of any cause) or inhibition of the action of aldosterone (e.g., adrenal insufficiency or pharmacologic blockade) can lead to potassium retention.

Hyperkalemia

Pathophysiology

Hyperkalemia occurs through two major mechanisms: shifting of potassium from intracellular compartment to the ECF compartment or through total body excess (Table 134.6). Total body potassium excess nearly always implies a deficiency in renal potassium excretion as the kidney. It is difficult to overcome a normal kidney's ability to increase potassium

TABLE 134.6 Causes of Hyperkalemia (82)

Assess for increased potassium intake
- Low-sodium salt substitutes and potassium supplements

Assess for shift of potassium intracellular fluid to extracellular fluid
- Metabolic acidosis
- Tissue necrosis (rhabdomyolysis, bowel infarction, tumor lysis) or depolarization
- Insulin deficiency
- β_2-Blockade

Assess for reduced potassium excretion in urine
- Renal failure
- Low aldosterone action (typically drug-related, especially heparin, cyclosporine, tacrolimus, angiotensin-converting enzyme inhibitors, angiotensin receptor blockers)
- Decreased distal nephron flow rate

excretion by increasing potassium intake except in cases of a massive potassium load (rhabdomyolysis, tumor lysis syndrome). Chronic renal failure alone typically does not lead to hyperkalemia until the GFR falls below approximately 15 mL/min. Other mitigating factors will exacerbate hyperkalemia in the setting of chronic renal failure such as medications (Table 134.7). Hyperkalemia commonly complicates acute renal failure and is less tolerated in the acute setting. Hyperkalemia is most often encountered in unexpected development of acute renal failure such as in postsurgery (especially after cardiac or vascular surgery), post-IV contrast study, administration of nephrotoxic antibiotics (especially aminoglycosides), postcardiac catheterization. Other settings include end-stage renal disease, adrenal insufficiency, type IV renal tubular acidosis (RTA) (usually seen in diabetics), crush injury, diabetes, and massive blood transfusion. Medications are a very important risk factor for the development of hyperkalemia (see Table 134.7).

Management

The first step in the management of hyperkalemia is to differentiate life-threatening hyperkalemia from less urgent cases and then to identify the diagnosis. The absolute levels of the potassium cannot be reliably used to determine if a life-threatening condition exists, and the effect of elevated potassium on the cardiac membrane must be determined through an electrocardiogram. The management of emergent hyperkalemia is detailed in Table 134.8. As a temporizing measure, shifting of potassium intracellularly with insulin or β-agonists can be used until definitive removal therapy is instituted. If normal renal function is present, diuretics and IV saline can

TABLE 134.7 Medications That Cause Hyperkalemia (82)

Drugs that interfere with potassium excretion
- Interfere with renin–angiotensin–aldosterone axis
  - Angiotensin-converting enzyme inhibitors, angiotensin receptor blockers, aldosterone blockers, heparin (decrease aldosterone synthesis), β-blockers (decrease renin release)
- Interfere with tubular potassium handling
  - Potassium-sparing diuretics (amiloride, triamterene), trimethoprim, calcineurin inhibitors (cyclosporine, tacrolimus)

Drugs that shift potassium from intracellular fluid to extracellular
- β_2-Blockers, depolarizing paralytics (e.g., succinylcholine), digitalis

TABLE 134.8 Treatment of Hyperkalemia

Immediate actions

- Electrocardiogram. Look for peaked T waves, loss of p waves, widened QRS. Loss of p-wave and widened QRS suggest impending ventricular fibrillation.
- Send repeat serum potassium to confirm diagnosis (do not wait for confirmatory test to initiate emergency therapy).

Hyperkalemia with electrocardiographic (ECG) changes

- Stabilize cardiac membrane
  - IV calcium gluconate or chloride to stabilize cardiac membrane, may repeat in 5 min if ECG changes persist
  - Place patient on cardiac monitoring
- Shift potassium into cells
  - IV insulin (with IV dextrose if necessary to prevent hypoglycemia)
  - Albuterol, 10–20 mg by nebulization (caution in heart disease)
  - IV $NaHCO_3$ may be of benefit

Potassium removal

- Dialysis
- Diuretics (with IV saline if patient is not volume overloaded) if renal function is normal
- Cation exchange resins (caution with decreased gastrointestinal motility as bowel necrosis can occur)

Hyperkalemia without electrocardiographic changes

- Remove offending agents
- Otherwise follow same therapy as above with dialysis, diuretics, and/or cation exchange resins.

be used to remove potassium. Cation exchange resins can be used as an adjunctive therapy. In patients with renal failure, especially with oliguria, emergency dialysis is often necessary. Hyperkalemia not associated with electrocardiographic changes can sometimes be managed with discontinuation of the offending agent. Some medications causing hyperkalemia such as spironolactone can have a long half-life, and the effect can last for up to 1 to 2 weeks. Close follow-up is mandatory with serial measurements of serum potassium and renal function (53). If managed properly, hyperkalemia is usually associated with good long-term prognosis.

Case Scenario: HEPARIN-INDUCED HYPERKALEMIA

A 60-year-old female patient is 5-day post–total hip replacement for osteoarthritis. She has a history of diabetes, hypertension, and a seizure disorder and no known kidney disease. Her outpatient medications include insulin, metformin, atenolol, hydrochlorothiazide, and Dilantin. The surgery was uneventful, but on postsurgical day 2, she develops severe shortness of breath and chest pain. A pulmonary embolism is diagnosed, and she is placed on unfractionated heparin and transferred to the ICU. Following the surgery, she has additionally been receiving promethazine, 12.5 mg, as needed (prn) for nausea and vomiting, and meperidine, 25 mg prn, for pain. Her preoperative labs were all normal; today's chemistry panel (on postoperative day 4) is listed below:

Sodium (mEq/L)	138
Potassium (mEq/L)	5.9
Chloride (mEq/L)	102
Bicarbonate (mEq/L)	27
Blood urea nitrogen (BUN) (mg/dL)	18
Creatinine (mg/dL)	1.1
Glucose (mg/dL)	153

Which of the following best explains the development of hyperkalemia? Answer: Use of heparin.

Key Point

- Heparin can lead to hyperkalemia by decreasing aldosterone levels (54).

Heparin is a frequent cause of hyperkalemia in the hospital setting in both patients with normal renal function and in those with renal insufficiency. In this case, renal function appears to be normal. Heparin inhibits the synthesis of aldosterone and leads to impairment of renal potassium secretion in the distal tubule. Two major factors are necessary for potassium excretion to occur: distal flow of urine to the distal nephron (this is impaired in acute renal failure) and aldosterone action. The necessity for distal secretion of potassium to maintain potassium balance is because of the very low filtered load of potassium due to the low concentration of potassium in the blood. Aldosterone acts by promoting the exchange of potassium for sodium in the distal tubule. The GFR is normal in this case, but due to decreased distal secretion of potassium, potassium excretion is impaired.

HYPOKALEMIA

Pathophysiology

Hypokalemia can occur either through shifting from ECF to ICF or through total body potassium depletion via gastrointestinal losses (distal to the stomach) or urinary losses (Table 134.9). Gastric secretion contains only 10 mEq/L of K^+, but hypovolemia associated with vomiting/NG suction stimulates aldosterone with sodium retention and potassium excretion. Shifting of potassium into the intracellular compartment is a physiologic process that normally occurs in response to insulin secretion. Without this process, a meal could lead to a dangerously high potassium level since the total amount of potassium contained within the extracellular space is quite low. β_2-Adrenergic stimulation is another avenue for cellular uptake of potassium. This is clinically significant as β_2-agonists can be used to transiently treat hyperkalemia and possibly lead to hypokalemia in certain clinical settings.

Clinical Manifestations

The effects of hypokalemia are related to the effect of low potassium on neuromuscular transmission and conduction

TABLE 134.9 Common Causes of Hypokalemia (2)

Potassium shift into cells
  Alkalosis, recovery from diabetic ketoacidosis, β_2-agonists, insulin
Gastrointestinal potassium losses[a]
  Vomiting, nasogastric suction, diarrhea
Renal potassium losses
  Diuretics, hypomagnesemia, hyperaldosteronism, drugs (amphotericin B, cisplatin), proximal (type II) and distal (type I) renal tubular acidosis (RTA), Bartter and Gitelman syndromes.
Decreased potassium intake

[a]Intestinal secretion contains 30–60 mEq/L of potassium. Gastric secretion contains only 10 mEq/L of potassium, and hypokalemia may be a result of hypovolemia with stimulation of aldosterone. Aldosterone will lead to sodium retention and potassium excretion in the kidneys.

in the heart. A decrease in extracellular potassium makes the membrane less excitable and muscle weakness results. Hypokalemia can lead to arrhythmias (especially in patients on digitalis or with heart disease). Other effects include ileus, muscular cramps, augmented ammonia production in the kidney (which can potentiate hepatic encephalopathy), and rhabdomyolysis. Hypokalemia is often associated with hypomagnesemia, and serum magnesium status should be assessed in all patients with hypokalemia.

Management

Potassium can be replaced with potassium chloride (KCl). For severe hypokalemia, potassium chloride should be given intravenously (IV) at a rate of 10 to 20 mEq/hr. Hypomagnesemia should also be corrected if present. Total body potassium deficits are typically large (200 to 300 mmol for serum potassium of 3.0 mEq/L, i.e., for each 1 mEq below normal), and repeated replacements may be needed with serial measurements (53). Since K^+ is a major intracellular cation, serum levels may not reflect the severity of deficiency.

Case Scenario: HYPOKALEMIA ASSOCIATED WITH METABOLIC ACIDOSIS

A 21-year-old woman is admitted for a 1-week history of muscular weakness and shortness of breath. Her past medical history is insignificant except for a history of dental caries and dry eyes. Her admission laboratories are listed below:

Sodium (mEq/L)	137
Potassium (mEq/L)	1.8
Chloride (mEq/L)	115
Bicarbonate (mEq/L)	9
BUN (mg/dL)	16
Creatinine (mg/dL)	0.9
Glucose (mg/dL)	110
Arterial pH	7.09
PCO_2	14
PO_2	115

The patient is placed in the ICU on a cardiac monitor.

What is the most likely diagnosis? This is a dramatic presentation of distal RTA with profound hypokalemia. Her history is suggestive of Sjögren syndrome, which can be complicated by distal RTA (55).

What is the next appropriate step in electrolyte and acid-base management? Replete potassium with IV potassium chloride. It is important not to treat this patient initially with alkali therapy; this can lead to shifting of potassium intracellularly and fatal hypokalemia. Once her potassium has been corrected, she can be treated with IV sodium bicarbonate.

DISORDERS OF DIVALENT IONS

The divalent ions, phosphorus, calcium, and magnesium, play important roles in cellular function such as regulation of enzymes and energy metabolism. In critical illness, the homeostasis of these ions is often altered, and abnormal levels are commonly encountered. The best treatment of these conditions requires knowledge of the pathophysiology of the alterations in the levels in these ions.

Phosphate Homeostasis

Phosphate is important for many basic processes of cellular metabolism and bone metabolism. Clinically in the intensive care setting, the need for phosphate for proper cellular energy metabolism through high-energy phosphate compounds (e.g., ATP) is among the most important. Phosphate is obtained in the diet primarily through protein intake. The typical Western diet contains sufficient phosphate to meet metabolic demands; however, in patients with poor nutritional status, often seen in alcoholics, hypophosphatemia may develop. The phosphate excretion in the kidney is regulated by several factors that favor tubular phosphate reabsorption (such as insulin, prostaglandin E_2, and thyroid hormone) and factors that inhibit phosphate reabsorption (such as parathyroid hormone (PTH) and the newly characterized phosphaturic hormone FGF-23 that plays a role in hereditary and acquired phosphate-wasting disorders). Phosphate reabsorption is handled principally in the proximal tubule through the NPT2 sodium phosphate cotransporter. Therefore, disorders of the proximal tubule, such as Fanconi syndrome, may lead to renal phosphate wasting.

Hypophosphatemia

Pathophysiology

There are three major mechanisms of hypophosphatemia (Table 134.10): shifting of phosphate from the extracellular to the intracellular space, renal phosphate losses, and gastrointestinal losses. Very often the disorder occurs as a multifactorial disease with acid–base disturbances, decreased intake, and renal losses all contributing. Phosphate, like potassium and magnesium, is mainly an intracellular ion. Therefore, low serum phosphate usually represents significant total body phosphate

TABLE 134.10 Causes of Hypophosphatemia (82)

Decreased phosphate absorption, GI phosphate losses
- Alcoholism/poor nutrition
- Diarrhea
- GI tract surgery
- Ingestion of phosphate-binding medications or antacids
- TPN preparations with inadequate phosphorus
- Vitamin D deficiency
- Use of corticosteroids

Shifting of phosphate from extracellular space
- Refeeding syndrome
- Respiratory alkalosis
- Hungry bone syndrome
- High-grade lymphoma, acute leukemia
- Administration of glucagon, epinephrine

Increased renal losses of phosphate
- Hyperparathyroidism
- Fanconi syndrome (proximal tubular dysfunction seen in several diseases especially multiple myeloma)
- Diuretics, especially carbonic anhydrase inhibitors
- Acute volume expansion
- Amphotericin B
- Oncogenic osteomalacia
- Hypophosphatemic rickets (X-linked and AD)

AD, autosomal dominant; GI, gastrointestinal; TPN, total parenteral nutrition.

depletion. Hypophosphatemia commonly occurs in alcoholics and in hospitalized patients. The diagnosis is usually evident from the history; however, if the cause is in doubt, renal phosphate losses can be assessed by calculating the fractional excretion of phosphorus:

$$\left(\frac{[P]_u \times [Cr]_{pl}}{[P]_{pl} \times [Cr]_u}\right) \times \text{fractional excretion of phosphorus}$$

where P is phosphorus level, u is urine, pl is plasma, and Cr is creatinine level.

This will help discern if the phosphate losses are gastrointestinal (GI) in origin or if the losses are in the urine. The fractional excretion of phosphorus should be measured at a time when serum phosphorus is low, and if the fractional excretion of phosphorus is below 5%, the kidney is appropriately conserving phosphate and therefore the losses are extrarenal. In critically ill patients, there are many common conditions and circumstances that set the patient up to be at risk for hypophosphatemia. Alcoholism, nasogastric suction, malnutrition, extensive bowel resection, malignancy, low sun exposure, and diuretic use are among the conditions seen in ICU patients that are associated with hypophosphatemia.

Clinical Manifestations

Symptoms are often absent in mild cases. In severe depletion, muscular weakness (especially large muscle groups, proximal extremity weakness), arrhythmias, rhabdomyolysis, hypotension, hypoventilation, seizures, coma, and hemolytic anemia may occur. The most life threatening is cardiac and ventilatory failure. Other undesirable effects of hypophosphatemia are the following: shift of oxygen dissociation curve to the left from deficiency of 2,3,DPG; depressed immune function (chemotaxis, phagocytosis, bacteriocidal activity); platelet dysfunction (adhesion and aggregation); metabolic acidosis (impaired bicarbonate resorption and ammonia production); and abnormal glucose metabolism from decreased entry into the cell to make high-energy phosphates.

Treatment

Phosphorus replacement in asymptomatic patients should be oral and can be given as a potassium or sodium salt. Parenteral phosphorus administration should be undertaken in symptomatic patients or in patients with severe depletion (<1.0 mg/dL) or when the oral route is not appropriate. Parenteral phosphate preparations are generally ordered in millimoles. One millimole (mmol) of phosphate equals 31 mg of phosphorus. Since phosphate is administered as either a sodium salt or a potassium salt, intolerance to either of these should be considered in settings such as renal failure or congestive heart failure. Phosphate replacement should be judicious in patients with renal failure as significant hyperphosphatemia can occur.

Case Scenario: REFEEDING SYNDROME

A 37-year-old man with a long history of alcoholism is admitted to the ICU with severe pancreatitis. His friends state that for the last several weeks he has been drinking beer all day and has been eating very little except for salty snacks. Over the course of the next 3 days, his ICU course is complicated by development of sepsis and a pancreatic abscess that has required drainage. Five days into his hospital course he remains on mechanical ventilation and vasopressor support. On this day, his chemistry panel is given below:

Serum	
Sodium (mEq/L)	136
Potassium (mEq/L)	4.3
Chloride (mEq/L)	105
Bicarbonate (mEq/L)	22
BUN (mg/dL)	6
Creatinine (mg/dL)	0.6
Calcium (mg/dL)	7.0
Albumin (g/dL)	2.7
Phosphorus (mg/dL)	2.1
Magnesium (mg/dL)	2.0
Glucose (mg/dL)	98

He is started on total parenteral nutrition with 2,000 total calories, 20% from fat. There is 120 mEq of sodium and 80 mEq of potassium, and the total volume is 2 L a day.

This patient is at high risk for which complications following the institution of total parenteral nutrition? Answer: Refeeding syndrome and rhabdomyolysis.

Key Points

- Refeeding syndrome is a potential complication in patients who are malnourished and suddenly given a large calorie load.
- Rhabdomyolysis is a potentially severe complication of the refeeding syndrome.

This patient is at high risk for the refeeding syndrome, and therefore, the potential for rhabdomyolysis is a concern (56). His history and laboratory values (low BUN and albumin) suggest malnutrition, and thus phosphate depletion is likely present despite the close-to-normal value for serum phosphate. The phosphate is sequestered in the intracellular compartment, and it is the intracellular depletion of phosphate that is critical. Once this patient is supplied with calories, especially carbohydrates, oxidative phosphorylation, and generation of ATP will quickly deplete the intracellular phosphate and lead to rhabdomyolysis. The best means of preventing this complication from occurring is recognizing patients who are at high risk and monitoring serum phosphate closely.

Hyperphosphatemia

Pathophysiology

Hyperphosphatemia occurs primarily in the setting of impaired renal function and is not typically seen outside of iatrogenic causes in patients with normal kidney function. Significant phosphate loading can occur due to exogenous phosphate administration or as part of the tumor lysis syndrome (however, renal insufficiency also commonly complicates this condition). Occult sources of phosphate loading include sodium phosphate solutions (either orally or as an enema), which can produce significant and, in some rare cases, fatal outcomes. In renal failure, elevated serum phosphorus is associated with cardiovascular disease and cardiovascular mortality and should be avoided.

Clinical Manifestations

There are few overt symptoms of hyperphosphatemia, and the syndrome may be insidious. Nephrocalcinosis can complicate hyperphosphatemia and manifest as renal insufficiency. On rare occasions, acute dialysis may be indicated to treat hyperphosphatemia. Extended dialysis session (>4 hours) may be necessary as phosphorus mobilization is time dependent and phosphorus removal in short dialysis sessions is limited (57).

Case Scenario: HYPERPHOSPHATEMIA AS A COMPLICATION OF SODIUM PHOSPHATE ADMINISTRATION

An 85-year-old man with a history of hypertension is admitted to the ICU with refractory hypotension. His wife states that he had been complaining of constipation and had used several enemas at home over the past 48 hours. His wife then stated that he has become progressively lethargic throughout the day, and she called an ambulance because he fell after trying to get up from a chair and was severely confused. He takes only hydrochlorothiazide for hypertension and is otherwise without significant medical history. The physical examination is significant for blood pressure of 85/45 and pulse of 58; respirations are 8 breaths/min, and he is afebrile. The physical examination is otherwise significant only for Chvostek sign.

The chemistry panel on admission is given below:

Serum	
Sodium (mEq/L)	149
Potassium (mEq/L)	4.5
Chloride (mEq/L)	109
Bicarbonate (mEq/L)	20
BUN (mg/dL)	23
Creatinine (mg/dL)	1.7
Calcium (mg/dL)	4.8
Albumin (g/dL)	3.8
Phosphorus (mg/dL)	8.2
Magnesium (mg/dL)	2.0
Glucose (mg/dL)	98

What risk factor for hyperphosphatemia did this patient have? Answer: Renal insufficiency put this patient at risk. The creatinine level of 1.7 in a patient of his age is indicative of significant decrease in GFR (estimated at 41 mL/min). The use of hyperosmolar phosphate enemas is a risk in this population. The time that the solution is allowed to dwell determines the amount of phosphate absorbed. Fatal cases have been reported even in patients without renal failure (58). This patient is exhibiting signs of hypocalcemia, hypotension, and impending cardiovascular collapse that can occur with acute hyperphosphatemia.

Overview of Calcium Balance

Calcium concentration in plasma is tightly regulated. Intracellular calcium levels are very low whereas the total body calcium stores in the bone are plentiful. Calcium balance and the calcium concentration in the blood are maintained by regulatory processes that promote calcium influx into the ECF (mainly intestinal calcium absorption and release of calcium from bone demineralization) and remove calcium from the ECF (urinary calcium excretion and bone formation). Disturbances in serum calcium occur when there is an imbalance between these processes regulating calcium movement. The hormonal influences that regulate these processes are complex but involve the actions of two principal hormones: PTH and calcitriol. Calcium exists in the plasma as protein-bound calcium and ionized calcium, usually measured in mmol/L. Measurement of the total serum calcium reflects the aggregate amount of these two pools of plasma calcium. Ionized calcium is the active component and the more important physiologically.

The total measured serum calcium needs to take into account changes in the amount of albumin, which is the predominant calcium-binding protein in the circulation. A simple correction for the total calcium based on perturbations of the serum albumin is the following: a reduction in plasma albumin of a 1 g/L will decrease the serum total calcium by 0.8 mg/dL (59). If the decrease in total serum calcium is within the range as would be expected based on the decrease in albumin, then it can be surmised that the ionized serum calcium is probably normal. The validity of this correction in critical illness has been questioned, possibly due to factors that affect binding of calcium to albumin. Measurement of ionized calcium levels in critically ill patients is a good practice, and results may be available within minutes of using point-of-care testing.

Hypocalcemia

Pathophysiology

The causes of hypocalcemia can be divided into either efflux of calcium out of the extracellular space or by decreased entry of calcium into the extracellular space (Table 134.11) (60). Under normal circumstances, homeostatic mechanisms can maintain serum calcium levels despite low intake by increasing mobilization from the bone. Hypocalcemia can result from decreased calcium absorption and decreased calcium mobilization from bone stores in hypoparathyroidism and vitamin D deficiency. Increased calcium removal from the serum occurs in severe pancreatitis through saponification of fats and in osteoblastic metastatic disease. The ionized calcium is the important factor for determining severity, and conditions that alter protein binding of calcium in the blood may precipitate symptomatic hypocalcemia. Alkalemia will increase the affinity of albumin for calcium (through altering the net charge of the protein) and will lower the ionized calcium. Acute increases in total albumin may lower ionized calcium. Risk factors for hypocalcemia include the following: neck irradiation, parathyroid surgery, renal transplantation in patients with tertiary hyperparathyroidism, malignancy, alcoholism, low sun exposure, and malnutrition.

TABLE 134.11 Causes of Hypocalcemia (82)

- Hypoparathyroidism/pseudohypoparathyroidism
- Hyperphosphatemia
- Hypomagnesemia
- Vitamin D deficiency
  - Dietary deficit
  - Reduced sun exposure
  - Decreased 25-hydroxylation of vitamin D (liver disease, alcoholism)
  - Decreased vitamin D–sensitive rickets type 1 (1-α hydroxylase deficiency) and type 2 (receptor deficiency)
- Renal failure (reduced 1-hydroxylation of vitamin D)
- Osteoblastic metastases (prostate, breast)
- Saponification in severe pancreatitis
- Citrate load (blood transfusion)

Clinical Manifestations

The clinical manifestations include altered mental status and tetany (Chvostek and Trousseau signs). The association between hypocalcemia and sepsis is not well understood although it is now recognized that elevated intracellular calcium levels are a common mechanism for cell death. Possible mechanisms for the association of sepsis and hypocalcemia are PTH insufficiency, altered vitamin D metabolism, hypomagnesemia, chelation of calcium by lactate, and also calcitonin precursors (61–65). Hypocalcemia in critical illness is a common finding and is often asymptomatic.

Management

One of the first questions to be addressed in approaching a patient with altered levels of serum calcium is to what degree is the ionized calcium altered and why? If the ionized calcium is decreased due to chelation from hyperphosphatemia, treatment of the hypocalcemia can be dangerous as it can precipitate vascular calcification. In sepsis, hypocalcemia is common and treatment is not usually necessary unless cardiovascular collapse with ionized calcium levels of less than 0.8 mmol/L is present. Data from animal models suggest that it may be harmful to treat hypocalcemia in the setting of sepsis (66,67). There are no randomized clinical studies to guide treatment of hypocalcemia in sepsis, and treatment should be reserved for those with symptomatic hypocalcemia and/or severe hypocalcemia. Reflex treatment of hypocalcemia without consideration of the underlying cause (especially in the setting of hyperphosphatemia) can be detrimental: therefore, it is important to determine the cause and degree of symptoms before deciding to initiate therapy.

For acute symptomatic hypocalcemia, administer IV calcium chloride or calcium gluconate (59). Calcium gluconate is advantageous because it is less caustic to veins. Calcium should not be infused more rapidly than 2.5 to 5 mmol in 20 minutes because of the risk of cardiac abnormalities and asystole. IV calcium will transiently normalize the calcium level, and an infusion should be started following the bolus, especially in settings where there is an ongoing process such as the hungry bone syndrome following parathyroidectomy. Magnesium deficiency, by inducing resistance to the actions of PTH, can be an important cause of hypocalcemia in the critical care setting. If magnesium deficiency is the cause, calcium levels should return to normal once magnesium is replaced.

Case Scenario: HYPOCALCEMIA ASSOCIATED WITH SEPSIS

A 43-year-old man with end-stage liver disease secondary to chronic hepatitis C infection presents with shortness of breath and abdominal pain. He has significant ascites and has decreased urine output for the last week. His appetite has been very poor over the last week although he has no other complaints. His blood pressure is 71/50, pulse is 86, and temperature 98.4°F. Admission labs are given below:

Sodium (mEq/L)	131
Potassium (mEq/L)	4.9
Chloride (mEq/L)	108
Bicarbonate (mEq/L)	20
BUN (mg/dL)	24
Creatinine (mg/dL)	1.6
Albumin (mg/dL)	2.4
Calcium (mg/dL)	6.8
Phosphorus (mg/dL)	2.8
Glucose (mg/dL)	78

He is admitted to the ICU and treated with broad-spectrum antibiotics and vasopressor for presumed septic shock.

What considerations should be taken in determining if this hypocalcemia should be treated? Answer: The cause is an important factor. This is likely a case of mild hypocalcemia due to sepsis. Check the ionized calcium level, serum magnesium level, and assess the degree of symptoms including electrocardiogram. If the serum magnesium level is decreased, this should be treated. If the ionized calcium is <0.8 mmol/L or if the patient appears to be symptomatic, the patient may benefit from treatment with IV calcium.

Key Point

- Sepsis is a common cause of hypocalcemia. Check the level of ionized calcium and magnesium in critically ill patients with hypocalcemia.

Hypercalcemia

Pathophysiology

Hypercalcemia is caused by entrance of calcium into the intravascular space in excess of renal excretion and calcium incorporation into bone. Two sources of calcium influx into the intravascular space are intestinal absorption and bone reabsorption. The most common causes are primary hyperparathyroidism, malignancy, and granulomatous diseases. Other causes are listed in Table 134.12. Additionally, hypercalcemia can be caused by decreased renal excretion as occurs in primary hyperparathyroidism and thiazide diuretics. Total calcium must be corrected for serum albumin because of protein binding, and ionized calcium should be measured in hypercalcemic patients.

Clinical Manifestations

Hypercalcemia produces a decrease in neuromuscular excitability and decreased muscular tone. Clinical manifestations

TABLE 134.12 Causes of Hypercalcemia (82)

Excess calcium influx into vascular space
- Primary hyperparathyroidism (usually adenoma, gland hyperplasia; parathyroid malignancy is rare)
- Malignancy (multiple myeloma, carcinomas through production of PTH-related peptide, osteosarcomas)
- Immobilization
- Granulomatous disease (increased vitamin D production?)
  - Sarcoidosis
  - Tuberculosis
- Paget disease
- Milk-alkali syndrome
- Vitamin D intoxication
- Hyperparathyroidism (stimulation of osteoclasts)

Decreased calcium excretion
- Primary hyperparathyroidism
- Thiazide diuretics
- Familial hypocalciuric hypercalcemia

PTH, parathyroid hormone.

of hypercalcemia include lethargy, confusion, coma, nausea, constipation, polyuria, and hypertension. Hypercalcemia can lead to volume depletion, nephrolithiasis, and nephrogenic diabetes insipidus.

Approach to Diagnosis

The causes of hypercalcemia are listed in Table 134.12. The first step is to measure the PTH level. The normal response of the parathyroid gland in the presence of elevated ionized calcium levels is to decrease secretion of PTH. Failure to suppress PTH secretion in the face of hypercalcemia denotes hyperparathyroidism. Primary hyperparathyroidism is among the most common causes of hypercalcemia in the general population but typically does not result in severe, symptomatic hypercalcemia. In hypercalcemia of malignancy, PTH is usually suppressed (this is the normal response of the parathyroid gland). PTH-related peptide (PTHrp) should also be ordered if malignancy is suspected as many cancers express this protein product that stimulates PTH receptors (68). Additionally, 1,25-hydroxyvitamin D and 25-hydroxyvitamin D levels can be helpful if abnormal vitamin D metabolism is suspected. Certain granulomatous conditions lead to increased 1,25-vitamin D (69), and in cases of vitamin D intoxication, high levels of 25-OH vitamin D reflective of total body vitamin D stores may be seen (70).

Management

In most patients with symptomatic hypercalcemia, volume depletion occurs and one of the first steps is volume repletion with IV saline (0.9% saline is the treatment of choice). This replacement of the extracellular volume will increase calcium excretion in the urine. Caution is advised in infusing large amounts of saline to an oliguric patient. After fluid resuscitation, normal saline should be continued and furosemide can also be given to increase urinary calcium excretion. A common mistake is to administer furosemide at the same time as starting fluid resuscitation. Diuretics should not be given until the patient is completely volume resuscitated. The action of loop diuretics is distinct from that of thiazide diuretics. Loop diuretics act in the ascending limb of Henle and will promote calcium excretion in the urine. Thiazide diuretics act more distally in the nephron and will decrease calcium excretion. Bisphosphonates are good long-term treatment for hypercalcemia of malignancy by impairing bone reabsorption, but these agents must be used with caution in patients with renal insufficiency (Table 134.13). Calcitonin is usually effective in the short term, but tachyphylaxis develops. It is best used early in the management while waiting for diuresis to remove calcium from the body. In patients with renal failure, dialysis is usually necessary to treat symptomatic hypercalcemia.

TABLE 134.13 Treatment of Severe Hypercalcemia

- Replete intravascular volume with normal saline.
- Use intravenous furosemide to increase calcium excretion (after volume repletion).
- In hypercalcemia of malignancy, use bisphosphonates to decrease calcium reabsorption from the bone.
- Adjunctive therapy includes calcitonin (effect is usually short term; tachyphylaxis develops).
- Start hemodialysis.

Case Scenario: HYPERCALCEMIA OF MALIGNANCY

A 46-year-old man with a 1-year history of pain in his legs and back is brought to the emergency room for decreased mental status. His wife states that he is very active and works as an attorney, but he has been easily fatigable over the last several months. Over the last 12 hours, he has gotten progressively more lethargic and is difficult to arouse.

Sodium (mEq/L)	136
Potassium (mEq/L)	4.8
Chloride (mEq/L)	108
Bicarbonate (mEq/L)	16
BUN (mg/dL)	51
Creatinine (mg/dL)	5.8
Albumin (mg/dL)	3.8
Calcium (mg/dL)	16.8
Magnesium (mg/dl)	2.8
Phosphorus (mg/dL)	4.6
Glucose (mg/dL)	98

A Foley catheter is inserted, and the urine output is 50 mL. In the emergency room, he is administered 2 L of 0.9% NaCl IV, and over the next 2 hours there is no urine output.

What is the next appropriate step in management of hypercalcemia in this patient? Answer: This patient should undergo emergency hemodialysis, which can be used in cases of renal failure and severe hypercalcemia (71). From history, this patient likely has multiple myeloma with complications of this disorder: hypercalcemia and renal failure. It is appropriate to give a volume challenge with normal saline to treat prerenal azotemia. However, with no urine output after 2 L of saline, acute renal failure is likely, and hemodialysis offers the best treatment for severe hypercalcemia. The patient should be dialyzed on a hypocalcemic bath in an intensive care setting, with cardiac monitoring and very close monitoring of the ionized calcium.

Hypomagnesemia

Pathophysiology

Magnesium depletion occurs in many conditions (Table 134.14) and is common in critical illness (72). Hypomagnesemia, because of its effect on the myocardial membrane, is important to identify, especially in those with known (or at risk for) cardiac arrhythmias. Sources of magnesium loss can be through urinary losses or also in the GI tract. Often, inadequate intake in malnourished patients is the principal cause

TABLE 134.14 Causes of Hypomagnesemia (82)

Gastrointestinal losses

- Diarrhea
- Nasogastric suction
- Malabsorption
- Steatorrhea
- Extensive bowel resection
- Acute pancreatitis
- Intestinal fistula

Urinary losses

- Diuretics, aminoglycosides, cisplatin, alcohol
- Pentamidine, foscarnet, cyclosporine, amphotericin B
- Phosphorus depletion
- Metabolic acidosis

of the magnesium deficiency. High-risk patients at particular risk for hypomagnesemia include hospitalized patients, alcoholics, and ICU patients. Magnesium depletion has effects on the homeostasis of other ions, and therefore, magnesium depletion often occurs in the presence of hypokalemia and hypocalcemia. Magnesium depletion causes a potassium-wasting state, and patients with hypokalemia should be assessed for magnesium depletion. Hypomagnesemia induces a state of reduced PTH secretion and PTH resistance. Tissue magnesium depletion can be present in the absence of decreased serum magnesium levels (since most magnesium is in the intracellular space), and that tissue depletion can lead to adverse outcomes (73).

Decreased total serum magnesium levels are common in critically ill patients. This is often due to a decrease in serum albumin, which is the principal binding protein of magnesium, and many of these patients do not have decreased ionized magnesium levels (72). The correlation of ionized hypomagnesemia and mortality in ICU patients is controversial. Magnesium is not actively mobilized from a body pool (unlike calcium), and therefore, serum levels are very dependent on intake. If magnesium intake is exceeded by magnesium loss (e.g., urinary losses), then the serum magnesium levels will be decreased.

Clinical Manifestations

The most serious consequences of hypomagnesemia are its cardiovascular effects. Hypomagnesemia is associated with poor outcomes in acute myocardial infarction and may predispose to arrhythmias (74). Magnesium treatment may decrease arrhythmias after myocardial infarction, but studies conflict on whether outcomes are improved with magnesium treatment (75–77). Magnesium depletion increases the risk of torsades des pointes, a form of polymorphic ventricular tachycardia. IV magnesium is regarded as treatment for *torsades des pointes* and refractory ventricular tachycardia even in the absence of documented hypomagnesemia. Additionally, hypomagnesemia may contribute to atrial arrhythmias following cardiopulmonary bypass (78). Other manifestations include altered mental status, seizures, and muscular weakness. Magnesium is an important cofactor for multiple enzyme function (including ATPase) and an essential electrolyte.

Treatment

For acutely symptomatic patients, parenteral administration should be undertaken. In asymptomatic patients, the oral route should be used although absorption is variable. Parenterally administered magnesium inhibits magnesium reabsorption in the ascending limb of Henle, and much of a parenterally administered dose may be wasted in the urine. For patients with severe manifestations, 8 to 16 mEq should be administered IV in 5 to 10 minutes followed by 48 mEq over the next 24 hours.

Case Scenario: HYPOMAGNESEMIA AND ASSOCIATED ELECTROLYTE DISTURBANCES

A 56-year-old man is admitted to the surgical ICU after an emergency coronary artery bypass performed following the dissection of his left anterior descending artery during an attempted percutaneous coronary intervention. He has a history of hypertension, smoking, and alcohol abuse. His medications are atenolol and aspirin. His surgery was uncomplicated, and his urine output was 70 mL/hr. His chemistry panel on admission to the ICU is given:

Sodium (mEq/L)	138
Potassium (mEq/L)	3.1
Chloride (mEq/L)	106
Bicarbonate (mEq/L)	24
BUN (mg/dL)	22
Creatinine (mg/dL)	1.4
Albumin (mg/dL)	3.7
Calcium (mg/dL)	7.3
Magnesium (mg/dL)	1.3
Phosphorus (mg/dL)	2.4
Ionized calcium (mmol/L)	0.8
Glucose (mg/dL)	98

Treatment of hypomagnesemia in this patient is likely to improve which other electrolyte disorders in this patient? Answer: magnesium deficiency due to poor dietary intake is the most likely cause of both the hypokalemia and hypocalcemia. Treatment of the hypomagnesemia will likely lead to resolution of the hypocalcemia. Potassium replacement should be given as well, as hypomagnesemia has lead to renal potassium wasting.

Hypermagnesemia

Pathophysiology

Hypermagnesemia is not a common condition, and it is often iatrogenic. Magnesium is readily excreted by the kidney in patients with normal renal function, and this disorder is uncommon except in cases of large ingestions (Epsom salt and magnesium-containing cathartics). In the presence of gastrointestinal disease such as peptic ulcer disease, magnesium absorption can be enhanced, and magnesium-containing antacids in this setting can lead to toxic hypermagnesemia (79). Patients with renal failure are at highest risk for developing hypermagnesemia, and the administration of magnesium-containing cathartics to these patients can be fatal (80). Clinical manifestations of hypermagnesemia include hypotension, bradycardia, respiratory depression, decreased mental status, and ECG abnormalities.

Management

Removal of the offending agent may be sufficient in mild cases with normal renal function. In symptomatic hypermagnesemia, the neuromuscular membrane can be stabilized by administration of 1 g of calcium chloride IV over 5 to 10 minutes. Dialysis is usually necessary in the setting of renal insufficiency or severe toxicity.

Case Scenario: HYPERMAGNESEMIA AND RISK FACTORS FOR DEVELOPMENT

An 84-year-old man is brought in from a nursing home with decreased level of consciousness. He has a past medical history significant for hypertension and peptic ulcer disease. He was recently diagnosed with a gastric ulcer and erosive esophagitis by esophagogastroduodenoscopy, and he has been taking lansoprazole. He has had continuous heartburn and symptoms, and he has been taking antacids frequently according to his wife. His physical examination is significant for blood pressure of 85/40 and pulse of 72. Respiratory rate is 8 breaths/min.

Sodium (mEq/L)	138
Potassium (mEq/L)	4.0
Chloride (mEq/L)	106
Bicarbonate (mEq/L)	22
BUN (mg/dL)	23
Creatinine (mg/dL)	1.5
Albumin (mg/dL)	3.9
Calcium (mg/dL)	7.3
Magnesium (mg/dL)	6.8
Phosphorus (mg/dL)	2.2
Glucose (mg/dL)	91

Why did this patient develop severe hypermagnesemia? Answer: This patient has two risk factors that predisposed to the development of hypermagnesemia. He has chronic renal dysfunction, which was not appreciated by the treating physicians. He also has gastrointestinal disease, which can increase the absorption of magnesium from the gut, especially in magnesium-containing antacids.

References

1. Dunn FL, Brennan TJ, Nelson AE, Robertson GL. The role of blood osmolality and volume in regulating vasopressin secretion in the rat. *J Clin Invest.* 1973;52(12):3212–3219.
2. Arieff AI, Ayus JC. Endometrial ablation complicated by fatal hyponatremic encephalopathy. *JAMA.* 1993;270(10):1230–1232.
3. Arieff AI, Ayus JC. Pathogenesis of hyponatremic encephalopathy: current concepts. *Chest.* 1993;103(2):607–610.
4. Ayus JC, Levine R, Arieff AI. Fatal dysnatraemia caused by elective colonoscopy. *BMJ.* 2003;326(7385):382–384.
5. Arieff AI, Ayus JC, Fraser CL. Hyponatraemia and death or permanent brain damage in healthy children. *BMJ.* 1992;304(6836):1218–1222.
6. Ayus JC, Krothapalli RK, Arieff AI. Treatment of symptomatic hyponatremia and its relation to brain damage: a prospective study. *N Engl J Med.* 1987;317(19):1190–1195.
7. Ayus JC, Wheeler JM, Arieff AI. Postoperative hyponatremic encephalopathy in menstruant women. *Ann Intern Med.* 1992;117(11):891–897.
8. Nielsen S, Nagelhus EA, Amiry-Moghaddam M, et al. Specialized membrane domains for water transport in glial cells: high-resolution immunogold cytochemistry of aquaporin-4 in rat brain. *J Neurosci.* 1997;17(1):171–180.
9. Agre P, Preston GM, Smith BL, et al. Aquaporin CHIP: the archetypal molecular water channel. *Am J Physiol.* 1993;265(4 Pt 2):F463–F476.
10. Nielsen S, Smith BL, Christensen EI, Agre P. Distribution of the aquaporin CHIP in secretory and resorptive epithelia and capillary endothelia. *Proc Natl Acad Sci USA.* 1993;90(15):7275–7279.
11. Simard M, Arcuino G, Takano T, Liu QS, et al. Signaling at the gliovascular interface. *J Neurosci.* 2003;23(27):9254–9262.
12. Amiry-Moghaddam M, Ottersen OP. The molecular basis of water transport in the brain. *Nat Rev Neurosci.* 2003;4(12):991–1001.
13. Dolman D, Drndarski S, Abbott NJ, Rattray M. Induction of aquaporin 1 but not aquaporin 4 messenger RNA in rat primary brain microvessel endothelial cells in culture. *J Neurochem.* 2005;93(4):825–833.
14. Abbott NJ, Ronnback L, Hansson E. Astrocyte-endothelial interactions at the blood-brain barrier. *Nat Rev Neurosci.* 2006;7(1):41–53.
15. Simard M, Nedergaard M. The neurobiology of glia in the context of water and ion homeostasis. *Neuroscience.* 2004;129(4):877–896.
16. Paulson OB, Newman EA. Does the release of potassium from astrocyte endfeet regulate cerebral blood flow? *Science.* 1987;237(4817):896–898.
17. Manley GT, Fujimura M, Ma T, et al. Aquaporin-4 deletion in mice reduces brain edema after acute water intoxication and ischemic stroke. *Nat Med.* 2000;6(2):159–163.
18. Reulen HJ, Tsuyumu M, Tack A, et al. Clearance of edema fluid into cerebrospinal fluid: a mechanism for resolution of vasogenic brain edema. *J Neurosurg.* 1978;48(5):754–764.
19. Melton JE, Patlak CS, Pettigrew KD, Cserr HF. Volume regulatory loss of Na, Cl, and K from rat brain during acute hyponatremia. *Am J Physiol.* 1987;252(4 Pt 2):F661–F669.
20. Olson JE, Sankar R, Holtzman D, et al. Energy-dependent volume regulation in primary cultured cerebral astrocytes. *J Cell Physiol.* 1986;128(2):209–215.
21. Blanco G, Mercer RW. Isozymes of the Na-K-ATPase: heterogeneity in structure, diversity in function. *Am J Physiol.* 1998;275(5 Pt 2):F633–F650.
22. Moritz ML, Ayus JC. The pathophysiology and treatment of hyponatraemic encephalopathy: an update. *Nephrol Dial Transplant.* 2003;18(12):2486–2491.
23. Achinger SG, Moritz ML, Ayus JC. Dysnatremias: why are patients still dying? *South Med J.* 2006;99(4):353–362; quiz 363–354.
24. Moritz ML, Kalantar-Zadeh K, Ayus JC. Ecstacy-associated hyponatremia: why are women at risk? *Nephrol Dial Transplant.* 2013;28(9):2206–2209.
25. Nzerue CM, Baffoe-Bonnie H, You W, et al. Predictors of outcome in hospitalized patients with severe hyponatremia. *J Natl Med Assoc.* 2003; 95(5):335–343.
26. Arieff AI. Hyponatremia, convulsions, respiratory arrest, and permanent brain damage after elective surgery in healthy women. *N Engl J Med.* 1986;314(24):1529–1535.
27. Chen JQ, Contreras RG, Wang R, et al. Sodium/potassium ATPase (Na+, K+-ATPase) and ouabain/related cardiac glycosides: a new paradigm for development of anti- breast cancer drugs? *Breast Cancer Res Treat.* 2006;96(1):1–15.
28. Davis RA, Kern F Jr, Showalter R, et al. Alterations of hepatic Na^+,K^+-ATPase and bile flow by estrogen: effects on liver surface membrane lipid structure and function. *Proc Natl Acad Sci USA.* 1978;75(9):4130–4134.
29. Fraser CL, Kucharczyk J, Arieff AI, et al. Sex differences result in increased morbidity from hyponatremia in female rats. *Am J Physiol.* 1989;256(4 Pt 2):R880–R885.
30. Arieff AI, Kozniewska E, Roberts TP, et al. Age, gender, and vasopressin affect survival and brain adaptation in rats with metabolic encephalopathy. *Am J Physiol.* 1995;268(5 Pt 2):R1143–R1152.
31. Fraser CL, Sarnacki P. Na^+-K^+-ATPase pump function in rat brain synaptosomes is different in males and females. *Am J Physiol.* 1989;257(2 Pt 1):E284–E289.
32. Fraser CL, Swanson RA. Female sex hormones inhibit volume regulation in rat brain astrocyte culture. *Am J Physiol.* 1994;267(4 Pt 1):C909–C914.
33. Vexler ZS, Ayus JC, Roberts TP, et al. Hypoxic and ischemic hypoxia exacerbate brain injury associated with metabolic encephalopathy in laboratory animals. *J Clin Invest.* 1994;93(1):256–264.
34. Hochachka PW, Buck LT, Doll CJ, Land SC. Unifying theory of hypoxia tolerance: molecular/metabolic defense and rescue mechanisms for surviving oxygen lack. *Proc natl Acad Sci USA.* 1996;93(18):9493–9498.
35. Ayus JC, Armstrong D, Arieff AI. Hyponatremia with hypoxia: effects on brain adaptation, perfusion, and histology in rodents. *Kidney Int.* 2006; 69(8):1319–1325.
36. Ayus JC, Arieff AI. Pulmonary complications of hyponatremic encephalopathy. Noncardiogenic pulmonary edema and hypercapnic respiratory failure. *Chest.* 1995;107(2):517–521.
37. Ayus JC, Varon J, Arieff AI. Hyponatremia, cerebral edema, and noncardiogenic pulmonary edema in marathon runners. *Ann Intern Med.* 2000; 132(9):711–714.
38. McClellan MD, Dauber IM, Weil JV. Elevated intracranial pressure increases pulmonary vascular permeability to protein. *J Appl Physiol.* 1989;67(3):1185–1191.
39. Ayus JC, Caputo D, Bazerque F, et al. Treatment of hyponatremic encephalopathy with a 3% sodium chloride protocol: a case series. *Am J Kidney Dis.* 2015;65(3):435–442.
40. Achinger SG, Arieff AI, Kalantar-Zadeh K, Ayus JC. Desmopressin acetate (DDAVP)-associated hyponatremia and brain damage: a case series. *Nephrol Dial Transpl.* 2014;29(12):2310–2315.
41. Schrier RW, Gross P, Gheorghiade M, et al. Tolvaptan, a selective oral vasopressin V2-receptor antagonist, for hyponatremia. *N Engl J Med.* 2006; 355(20):2099–2112.
42. Moritz ML, Ayus JC. Prevention of hospital-acquired hyponatremia: a case for using isotonic saline. *Pediatrics.* 2003;111(2):227–230.
43. Ayus JC, Arieff AI. Noncardiogenic pulmonary edema in marathon runners. *Ann Intern Med.* 2000;133(12):1011.
44. Hew-Butler T, Almond C, Ayus JC, et al. Consensus statement of the 1st International Exercise-Associated Hyponatremia Consensus Development Conference, Cape Town, South Africa 2005. *Clin J Sport Med.* 2005; 15(4):208–213.
45. Heilig CW, Stromski ME, Blumenfeld JD, et al. Characterization of the major brain osmolytes that accumulate in salt-loaded rats. *Am J Physiol.* 1989;257(6 Pt 2):F1108–F1116.
46. Lien YH, Shapiro JI, Chan L. Effects of hypernatremia on organic brain osmoles. *J Clin Invest.* 1990;85(5):1427–1435.

47. Ayus JC, Armstrong DL, Arieff AI. Effects of hypernatraemia in the central nervous system and its therapy in rats and rabbits. *J Physiol.* 1996;492 (Pt 1):243–255.
48. Moritz ML, Ayus JC. The changing pattern of hypernatremia in hospitalized children. *Pediatrics.* 1999;104(3 Pt 1):435–439.
49. Moritz ML, Ayus JC. Dysnatremias in the critical care setting. *Contrib Nephrol.* 2004;144:132–157.
50. Ayus JC, Krothapalli R. Hyperglycemia assoicated with non-diabetic hypernatremia (NDH) patients. *J Am Soc Nephrol.* 1990;1:317A.
51. Halperin ML, Kamel KS. Potassium. *Lancet.* 1998;352(9122):135–140.
52. Schlanger LE, Kleyman TR, Ling BN. K(+)-sparing diuretic actions of trimethoprim: inhibition of Na+ channels in A6 distal nephron cells. *Kidney Int.* 1994;45(4):1070–1076.
53. Gennari FJ. Disorders of potassium homeostasis: hypokalemia and hyperkalemia. *Crit Care Clin.* 2002;18(2):273–288.
54. Leehey D, Gantt C, Lim V. Heparin-induced hypoaldosteronism: report of a case. *JAMA.* 1981;246(19):2189–2190.
55. al-Jubouri MA, Jones S, Macmillan R, et al. Hypokalaemic paralysis revealing Sjogren syndrome in an elderly man. *J Clin Pathol.* 1999;52(2):157–158.
56. Marinella MA. Refeeding syndrome and hypophosphatemia. *J Intensive Care Med.* 2005;20(3):155–159.
57. Achinger SG, Ayus JC. The role of daily dialysis in the control of hyperphosphatemia. *Kidney Int Suppl.* 2005;(95):S28–S32.
58. Pitcher DE, Ford RS, Nelson MT, Dickinson WE. Fatal hypocalcemic, hyperphosphatemic, metabolic acidosis following sequential sodium phosphate-based enema administration. *Gastrointest Endosc.* 1997;46(3):266–268.
59. Body JJ, Bouillon R. Emergencies of calcium homeostasis. *Rev Endocrine Metab Disord.* 2003;4(2):167–175.
60. Tohme JF, Bilezikian JP. Hypocalcemic emergencies. *Endocrinol Metab Clin North Am.* 1993;22(2):363–375.
61. Zaloga GP, Chernow B. The multifactorial basis for hypocalcemia during sepsis. Studies of the parathyroid hormone-vitamin D axis. *Ann Intern Med.* 1987;107(1):36–41.
62. Robertson GM Jr, Moore EW, Switz DM, et al. Inadequate parathyroid response in acute pancreatitis. *N Engl J Med.* 1976;294(10):512–516.
63. Weir GC, Lesser PB, Drop LJ, et al. The hypocalcemia of acute pancreatitis. *Ann Intern Med.* 1975;83(2):185–189.
64. Hersh T, Siddiqui DA. Magnesium and the pancreas. *Am J Clin Nutr.* 1973;26(3):362–366.
65. Cooper DJ, Walley KR, Dodek PM, et al. Plasma ionized calcium and blood lactate concentrations are inversely associated in human lactic acidosis. *Intensive Care Med.* 1992;18(5):286–289.
66. Zaloga GP, Sager A, Black KW, Prielipp R. Low dose calcium administration increases mortality during septic peritonitis in rats. *Circ Shock.* 1992;37(3):226–229.
67. Malcolm DS, Zaloga GP, Holaday JW. Calcium administration increases the mortality of endotoxic shock in rats. *Crit Care Med.* 1989;17(9):900–903.
68. Moseley JM, Kubota M, Diefenbach-Jagger H, et al. Parathyroid hormone-related protein purified from a human lung cancer cell line. *Proc Natl Acad Sci USA.* 1987;84(14):5048–5052.
69. Adams JS, Singer FR, Gacad MA, et al. Isolation and structural identification of 1,25-dihydroxyvitamin D3 produced by cultured alveolar macrophages in sarcoidosis. *J Clin Endocrinol Metab.* 1985;60(5):960–966.
70. Dusso AS, Brown AJ, Slatopolsky E. Vitamin D. *Am J Physiol Renal Physiol.* 2005;289(1):F8–F28.
71. Camus C, Charasse C, Jouannic-Montier I, et al. Calcium free hemodialysis: experience in the treatment of 33 patients with severe hypercalcemia. *Intensive Care Med.* 1996;22(2):116–121.
72. Soliman HM, Mercan D, Lobo SS, et al. Development of ionized hypomagnesemia is associated with higher mortality rates. *Crit Care Med.* 2003;31(4):1082–1087.
73. Ryzen E, Elkayam U, Rude RK. Low blood mononuclear cell magnesium in intensive cardiac care unit patients. *Am Heart J.* 1986;111(3):475–480.
74. Dyckner T. Serum magnesium in acute myocardial infarction: relation to arrhythmias. *Acta Med Scand.* 1980;207(1–2):59–66.
75. Woods KL, Fletcher S, Roffe C, Haider Y. Intravenous magnesium sulphate in suspected acute myocardial infarction: results of the second Leicester Intravenous Magnesium Intervention Trial (LIMIT-2). *Lancet.* 1992;339(8809):1553–1558.
76. ISIS-4: a randomised factorial trial assessing early oral captopril, oral mononitrate, and intravenous magnesium sulphate in 58,050 patients with suspected acute myocardial infarction. ISIS-4 (Fourth International Study of Infarct Survival) Collaborative Group. *Lancet.* 1995;345(8951):669–685.
77. Magnesium in Coronaries Trial I. Early administration of intravenous magnesium to high-risk patients with acute myocardial infarction in the Magnesium in Coronaries (MAGIC) Trial: a randomised controlled trial. *Lancet.* 2002;360(9341):1189–1196.
78. Maslow AD, Regan MM, Heindle S, et al. Postoperative atrial tachyarrhythmias in patients undergoing coronary artery bypass graft surgery without cardiopulmonary bypass: a role for intraoperative magnesium supplementation. *J Cardiothorac Vasc Anesth.* 2000;14(5):524–530.
79. Clark BA, Brown RS. Unsuspected morbid hypermagnesemia in elderly patients. *Am J Nephrol.* 1992;12(5):336–343.
80. Onishi S, Yoshino S. Cathartic-induced fatal hypermagnesemia in the elderly. *Intern Med.* 2006;45(4):207–210.
81. Moritz ML, Ayus JC. Maintenance intravenous fluids in acutely ill patients. *N Engl J Med.* 2015;373(14):1350–1360.
82. Epstein PE, Alguire PC, eds. *MKSAP 14—Medical Knowledge Self-Assessment Program.* Philadelphia, PA: American College of Physicians; 2006.

CHAPTER

135

Blood Gas Analysis and Acid–Base Disorders

STEVEN G. ACHINGER and JUAN CARLOS AYUS

INTRODUCTION

Acid–base physiology is among the most complex topics in clinical medicine. Disturbances of this system are common in the critically ill, and important clinical decisions based on measured acid–base parameters occur on a daily, even hourly basis. Therefore, a sound understanding of acid–base physiology is mandatory for the intensivist.

The field is full of complicated concepts and equations that, at times, have only limited applicability to the practicing clinician due to the failure of any current model to faithfully and completely recapitulate the complex buffering process *in vivo*. The purpose of this chapter is to provide a conceptual introduction to the current approach to acid–base physiology, while de-emphasizing calculations and formulas. We will review the body's clinically significant buffering systems and discuss acid–base disorders in the context of the "traditional model" that utilizes the familiar concepts of the anion gap and the Hendersen–Hasselbach relationship. We will also introduce the physiochemical model (Stewart model), which takes a broader, more quantitative definition of the body's buffering systems. The goal is not to know how to derive the commonly used formulas, but rather to understand the meaning of measured and derived acid–base parameters that are used clinically, and how they may—or may not—help in answering three essential questions in the critically ill patient with an acid–base disturbance:

- What acid–base disorder(s) is (are) present?
- How severe is the disturbance?
- What is the underlying cause of the derangements?

MAINTENANCE OF THE ARTERIAL pH AND ACID–BASE BALANCE: BUFFERING AND ACID EXCRETION

Buffering of acids is the first line of defense against perturbations in systemic pH. Recall that the pH is a logarithmic scale that is a function of the concentration of H_3O^+ species in solution (H^+ will be used interchangeably with H_3O^+ in this chapter). In neutral solution, $[H^+]$ is $\times\ 10^{-7}$ M and $[OH^-]$ is 10^{-7} M; this satisfies the dissociation constant for water:

$$[H_2O] \leftrightarrow [H^+] + [OH^-]\ Ksp = 10^{-14}$$

The pH, defined by Sorenson, is the negative log of the concentration of H^+. Therefore, in neutral solution, the pH is 7. This is a very small concentration of $[H^+]$, and therefore, addition of small amounts of $[H^+]$ to water will lead to significant fluctuations in pH. For example, we will consider an experiment performed by Jorgensen and Astrup (1) in which 1.25 mEq/L of HCl is added to hemolyzed human blood. Assuming that the blood contained no buffers (i.e., if the blood was imagined to be a container of water that starts at a neutral pH), the expected pH following such an infusion would be calculated by the following:

$$\begin{aligned} &1.25 \times 10^{-2} \text{ moles (number of moles of } H^+ \text{ added)} \\ &+ 1 \times 10^{-7} \text{ moles (number of moles of } H^+ \text{ in neutral water)} \\ &= 1.25 \times 10^{-2} \text{ moles/L} \end{aligned} \quad (1)$$

Taking the negative log yields a pH of 1.9; this would be the expected pH if there were not buffers available. However, following the infusion, the pH of the blood changed approximately 0.2 pH points. This means that less than 1/10,000th of the H^+ added remains unbound in the blood. This illustrates the tremendous buffering capacity of the blood. A buffer can be thought of as a substance that, when present in solution, takes up $[H^+]$ and therefore resists change in pH when $[H^+]$ is added. The overall buffering system of the body is complex and includes several components (Table 135.1). The most important system is the carbon dioxide–bicarbonate system, which is the principal buffer in the extracellular fluid (ECF). This buffering system is also very important clinically since it is the only buffering system where the two components (acid and conjugate base) are readily measurable in the ECF. Buffers work by binding the free H^+ as the conjugate base, which is a weak acid.

Buffers allow the body to resist acute changes in pH; however, buffering capacity will eventually be depleted if acid is continually added. For example, in humans, the fixed acid production is approximately 70 to 100 mmol/d. It is through the excretion of the daily acid load that ultimately allows the body to maintain acid–base balance. The excretion of the daily acid load occurs through two distinct mechanisms: the renal excretion of fixed acid, and the respiratory excretion of volatile acid (i.e., carbon dioxide). Through the interconversion of bicarbonate, carbonic acid, and carbon dioxide, fixed and volatile acids can be buffered until they can be excreted through the urine or respiration (Fig. 135.1). In the lung, CO_2 is released, which ultimately leads to more H^+ reacting with HCO_3^- to generate water and more CO_2. In the kidneys, the entire filtered load of bicarbonate is—in order to avoid losing base—reabsorbed. When the kidney excretes one H^+ in the urine, one "new" HCO_3^- is generated. These two processes are both important in the excretion of the acid load, and modulation of these processes is also important in compensating for acid–base disturbances.

Urinary Excretion of Fixed Acids

In the reabsorption of bicarbonate, the corresponding H^+ produced in the process must be excreted in the urine. As most bicarbonate reabsorption occurs in the proximal tubule, the renal secretion of H^+ is ten times greater in the proximal tubule—approximately 4,000 mmol/d—as compared

TABLE 135.1 Blood and Extracellular Fluid Buffers

Acid	Conjugate Base
H_2CO_3	HCO_3^-
Albumin-H	Albumin⁻
H_2PO_4	HPO_4^-
Hgb-H	Hgb⁻

with the distal tubule—approximately 400 mmol/d. However, in the distal tubule, there is a much higher luminal–intracellular H^+ gradient than that seen in the proximal tubule—a ratio of approximately 500:1. This high gradient is due to active secretion of H^+ into the tubule. If the excretion of acid occurred in the absence of buffers, the ability to excrete acid in the urine would be limited. In much the same way that the body can absorb large amounts of acid without much change in pH, the kidney accomplishes a similar task in the excretion of large amounts of fixed acid through the use of buffers in the urine with modestly acidic pH (approximately 5.5 under maximal conditions). The excretion of H^+ in the urine occurs with different conjugate bases, which are grouped as titratable acids—mostly phosphates—and nontitratable acids—ammonium. The excretion of titratable acid has a limit that is, for the most part, dependent on the filtered load of phosphate, as this is the main buffer for nontitratable acids. However, the kidney can generate its own buffer—ammonia; moreover, the renal capacity to generate ammonia and to excrete acid as ammonium under normal conditions is substantial. This capacity may be significantly upregulated in the face of systemic acidosis. Ammonia is produced in the kidney, traverses the plasma membrane, and is "trapped" in the tubular lumen because the low pH drives the following reaction to the right, as the plasma membrane is much less permeable to the charged species ammonium:

$$NH_3 + H^+ \leftrightarrow NH_4^+ \quad (2)$$

Therefore, ammonia–ammonium acts as a urinary buffer system, allowing the elimination of one H^+ for nearly every ammonia produced. The buffering of acid in the urine, especially via ammonium, allows for substantial amounts of acid to be excreted without generating excessively acidic urine.

Titratable acids make up a relatively small proportion of the acid excreted and do not increase to near the degree that

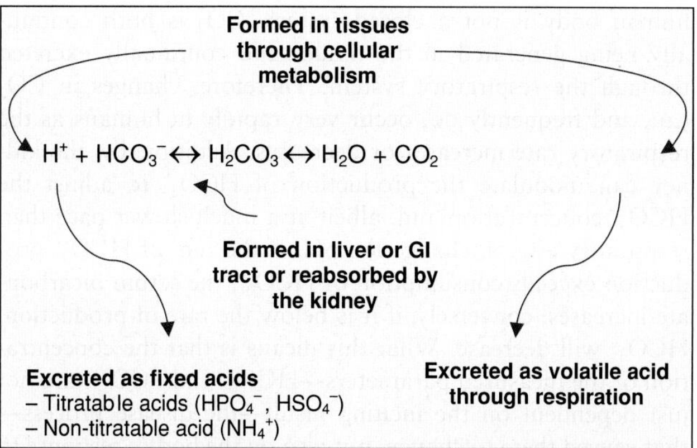

FIGURE 135.1 Normal acid–base homeostasis.

nontitratable acidity (ammonium) increases in the face of systemic acidosis.

The kidney, through active secretion of H^+ in the distal tubule, is able to achieve an H^+ concentration gradient of approximately 100:1 between the urine and the intracellular space of the tubular epithelial cells. This corresponds to the maximally acidic urine of approximately pH 5. Without any buffers, it would require 7,000 L of urine to excrete a daily load of 70 mEq of acid in buffer-free urine of pH 5.0! Therefore, urinary buffers are very important in allowing the body to excrete the daily fixed acid load. Chronic metabolic acidosis stimulates the renal production of ammonia as a physiologic response; this response reaches its maximum production after several days.

Assessing Urinary Acid Excretion

In the presence of systemic acidosis, the kidney will compensate by increasing the excretion of fixed acids, mainly in the nontitratable form (i.e., ammonium). The increase in ammonium—which is a cation; recall that ammonia is predominantly in the form of NH_4^+ at a pH of 7 or below—excretion results in a perturbation in the electrolytes present in the urine. This manifests as a change in the urine anion gap where ammonium is the unmeasured anion. The urinary anion gap is a useful clinical test that can be used to gauge the amount of ammonium excreted in the urine without directly measuring it (2). It may be used to indirectly estimate the amount of ammonium in the urine and is calculated using the following formula:

$$[Na^+] + [K^+] - [Cl^+] = \text{urinary anion gap} \quad (3)$$

The urine anion gap is assessed in patients with metabolic acidosis and is used to determine if the renal response to the systemic acidosis is appropriate. In other words, the urine anion gap answers the question: Are the kidneys excreting the acid load appropriately or are the kidneys part of the acid–base problem? If the kidneys are excreting the acid load appropriately, there must be a nonrenal source of the acidosis—for example, diarrhea. Because ammonium is not a measured cation in this equation, the presence of significant amounts of ammonium causes an abundance of chloride relative to the measured cationic constituents of the urine (sodium and potassium). Therefore, if there is a high level of ammonium in the urine, the urine anion gap will be negative. The relationship between the amount of ammonium in the urine and the urine anion gap is illustrated in Figure 135.2. As a general rule, a negative urinary anion gap suggests that the kidney is excreting ammonium in the urine. This is a continuous variable, and the more negative the value, the greater the renal response. In the face of systemic acidosis, if the renal response is appropriate, there will be a high amount of ammonium in the urine, and the urine anion gap will be highly negative. This is sometimes referred to as a *negative net urinary charge*; however, this is a bit misleading because the urine is, of course, electroneutral; it is simply because we are not considering the contribution of ammonium that the net urinary charge seems negative. A highly negative urine anion gap is strong evidence that the renal response to metabolic acidosis is normal. Conversely, an anion gap that is near zero or positive suggests that there is little or no ammonium in the urine, which is reflected by a paucity of

***Scenario 1**. Small amount of NH_4+ in the urine.*
<u>Urine anion gap</u> close to zero or positive

$$[Na^+] + [K^+] + [NH_4^+] \sim [Cl^-] \longrightarrow [Na^+] + [K^+] \sim [Cl^-]$$

***Scenario 2**. Large amount of NH_4+ in the urine.*
<u>Urine anion gap</u> very negative

$$[Na^+] + [K^+] + [NH_4^+] \sim [Cl^-] \longrightarrow [Na^+] + [K^+] < [Cl^-]$$

FIGURE 135.2 Effect of urine ammonium concentration on the urine anion gap.

chloride in the urine relative to the concentration of measured cations. This is evident that the kidney is not appropriately excreting ammonium in the urine and suggests a renal contribution to the acidosis. A caveat that is often clinically important is that the presence of unmeasured anions in the urine (such as β-hydroxybutyrate) may falsely depress the urinary anion gap, and therefore this test does have some limitations, such as during ketonuria.

RELATIONSHIP BETWEEN SYSTEMIC pH AND BUFFER CONCENTRATIONS: AN EVOLVING CONCEPT

We have previously noted that, because of the presence of buffers, addition of—or conversely, removal of—$[H^+]$ to the body does not produce the expected change in pH that would occur in unbuffered solutions. In this section, we will address the question of the relationship between pH and the concentrations of buffers.

Traditional Paradigm

One of the earliest observations in this field, and still very important clinically today, was the observation by Hendersen that the concentration of H^+ in the blood was dependent upon the concentration of CO_2, H_2CO_3, and HCO_3^-. The Henderson–Hasselbalch equation was later derived by using the Sorenson convention of expressing $[H^+]$ as pH. This relationship is usually expressed as:

$$pH = 6.1 + \log [HCO_3^-]/[H_2CO_3]$$

As the $[H_2CO_3]$ in plasma is related to the partial pressure of CO_2, this relationship can be rewritten as:

$$pH = 6.1 + \log ([HCO_3^-]/0.03 \times PCO_2) \quad (4)$$

This relationship became very meaningful clinically as the methodologies to measure the key variables pH, HCO_3^-, and PCO_2 were developed. Now the concentration of the constituents of the principal buffering system could be related to the systemic pH. This allowed, among other things, a framework around which to understand how much alkali must be added in order to affect systemic pH in an acidemic patient. However, it became apparent that the relationship between pH, HCO_3^-, and PCO_2 failed to completely describe the relative contributions of fixed acids and volatile acids (the respiratory component) to acidosis. This is because PCO_2 and HCO_3^- are not truly independent of each other, as changes in one will lead to changes in the other, as will be seen later, according to the relationship given in Equation (11). Additionally, it was noted that no single value accurately quantifies the degree of fixed acids present during metabolic acidosis or alkalosis. The degree of acidemia could be considered as simply the pH, as the pH is ultimately a composite of the net respiratory and metabolic components of the acid–base disturbance. However, because of the buffering capacity of the body, a quantification of the fixed acid derangement is not explained by this relationship alone.

Historically, several theoretical frameworks have been developed in an attempt to overcome this lack of exactitude in the concepts of quantification and etiology. The first obstacle to accurate quantification is the reality that the HCO_3^- system was not the only quantitatively important buffering system to be considered. The erythrocyte membrane is permeable to H^+, and therefore, H^+ can diffuse inside the cell and hemoglobin can act as an intracellular buffer. Other buffering systems, such as phosphate and circulating proteins, can act as clinically relevant buffers as well (see Table 135.1). By quantitative chemistry, the pH of a system is dependent on the relative concentrations of the acids and conjugate bases of all of the buffering systems present. Clinically, we measure accurately the concentration of the acid (CO_2) and conjugate base (HCO_3^-) of only one buffering system. Therefore, perturbations in the other buffering systems are not accounted for in the framework that only considers carbonate species.

Another major complicating factor is the fact that the human body is not a closed system. CO_2 is both continually being generated in the tissues and continually excreted through the respiratory system. Therefore, changes in CO_2 can, and frequently do, occur very rapidly in humans as the respiratory rate increases or decreases. Additionally, the kidney can modulate the production of HCO_3^- to adjust the HCO_3^- concentration and, albeit at a much slower pace than respiratory effects, change the pH. If the rate of HCO_3^- production exceeds consumption of HCO_3^-, the serum bicarbonate increases; conversely, if it is below the rate of production, HCO_3^- will decrease. What this means is that the concentration of the measured parameters—HCO_3^- and PCO_2—are not just dependent on the inciting insult—the disease process—that caused them to change, but also on the body's response to that change (i.e., compensation).

Base Excess and Standard Base Excess

The change in pH of a system is dependent on both the amount of acid (or base) added and that present on the buffering capacity. As acid is added to a buffered solution, for every H^+ that is buffered, one molecule of conjugate base of the buffer is consumed. Therefore, assessing changes in concentrations of the conjugate base is more helpful than the degree of change in the pH in quantifying the degree of fixed acids present. The difficulty in describing the buffering system of a patient is the inaccessibility for measurement of a fair proportion of the buffers (see Table 135.1), especially intracellular buffers. Several expressions have been proposed to quantify the degree of acid loading based on the change in body buffers. The most commonly used concept in this regard is the *base excess*. Siggaard-Andersen defined the base excess of blood as the number of mEq of acid (or base) needed to titrate 1 L of blood to a pH of 7.4 at 37°C with a PCO_2 of 40 mmHg; note that this is an experimentally arrived upon value. The standard base excess is the base excess corrected for changes in hemoglobin, recalling that hemoglobin is an important intracellular buffer. The base excess can be considered as a measurement of the "metabolic" portion of an acid–base disturbance since the concentration of CO_2 is being held constant at a normal level. The base excess has become a widely used parameter to characterize acid–base disturbances. One major drawback of the base excess is that it is a measured parameter of whole blood. However, *in vivo*, the blood is circulating and comes into contact with other tissues that can serve to provide buffering capacity. In clinical practice, however, the base excess is not measured by titration; rather, it is calculated from a nomogram that assumes normal nonbicarbonate buffers. This simplification, while allowing the widespread application of the base excess, has, in one sense, the drawback of losing the actual measurement of nonbicarbonate buffers that occurs when blood is directly titrated. Despite potential drawbacks, the base excess is very useful in describing the magnitude of a metabolic disturbance on the concentration of buffers and has become a widely used parameter to assess the degree of a metabolic disturbance.

The Anion Gap

The anion gap is calculated by taking the difference between the concentrations of the measured cations and the measured anion; it takes on a value of approximately 8 to 12 mEq/L in healthy individuals (3–5). The anion gap is an indirect estimation of the amount of "extra anions" in the circulation. The anion gap normally reflects the serum albumin (negatively charged at physiologic pH) (6), phosphate, and other minor anions (7). The unmeasured anions that may, under pathologic situations, lead to an increased anion gap can be either endogenous substances normally found in lower levels such as lactate or β-hydroxybutyrate or exogenous substances such as salicylates. The anion gap is calculated using the following formula:

$$[Na^+] - ([Cl^-] + [HCO_3^-]) \quad (5)$$

Metabolic acidosis is subdivided into anion gap and non-anion gap metabolic acidosis based on the value of the anion gap. In general, metabolic acidosis is caused either by the loss of bicarbonate—as in gastrointestinal (GI) losses or impaired renal acid excretion—or by a gain of acid associated with an unmeasured anion. The gain of acid is usually associated with the presence of an unmeasured anion (e.g., lactic acid); an exception might be intake of HCl. The extra base present—again, using the example of lactate—leads to a greater difference between the measured anions and cations, and therefore a greater anion gap. There is a wide range for the normal anion gap (4) and, in our experience, a normal anion gap is approximately 8 to 10 mEq/L—slightly lower than the value referenced above—but this may vary with methodologies in various labs; thus, checking with the local laboratory is imperative (4,8). When interpreting the anion gap, caution must be exercised, as there is significant variation in the anion gap and it can be influenced by many conditions other than metabolic acidosis.

Hypoalbuminemia is the most common condition that affects the normal anion gap since albumin normally contributes to the net negative charge of the blood (9). For every 1 mg/dL fall in the plasma albumin concentration, the anion gap should decrease by approximately 3 mEq/L (3). In plasma cell dyscrasias, such as multiple myeloma, the presence of cationic proteins in the serum is a cause for falsely depressing the anion gap (10), which has been attributed to an increased net positive charge due to the presence of net cationic immunoglobulins (11). Conditions that have been noted to increase the anion gap in the absence of metabolic acidosis are renal failure, volume depletion, metabolic alkalosis (12), and some penicillins. The anion gap can be lowered by hypoalbuminemia, hypercalcemia, and hyponatremia (13). Because of the wide variation in the anion gap and the variety of conditions that can affect it, it is best to directly measure "unmeasured anions" such as lactate whenever feasible.

Case #1: USE OF HENDERSON–HASSELBALCH EQUATION TO GUIDE VENTILATION

A 48-year-old morbidly obese patient is admitted to the hospital with shortness of breath and fever. In the emergency room, he is started on intravenous antibiotics. Over the next 3 hours, he becomes severely short of breath and develops a diminished level of consciousness. He is intubated and placed on mechanical ventilation. His past medical history is significant for diabetes mellitus and hypertension. Social history is significant for one pack per day tobacco abuse for 20 years. Current medications include amlodipine 5 mg PO daily, enalapril 5 mg PO bid, and hydrochlorothiazide 12.5 mg PO bid. Physical examination shows blood pressure of 156/88 mmHg, pulse 76 beats/min, and temperature 96°F. The patient is morbidly obese. Cardiovascular examination is normal. Lung examination reveals bilateral breath sounds with diffuse crackles on the right and egophony. The initial ventilator settings are synchronous intermittent mandatory ventilation (SIMV) with a rate of 20, tidal volume of 800 mL, and positive end-expiratory pressure (PEEP) of 5 cm H_2O, with an FiO_2 of 1.0. Thirty minutes after mechanical ventilation is initiated, the following labs are drawn:

Serum	
Sodium	141 mEq/L
Potassium	4.2 mEq/L
Chloride	100 mEq/L
Bicarbonate	34 mEq/L
BUN	13 mg/dL
Phosphorus	3.8 mg/dL
Creatinine	0.8 mg/dL
Albumin	3.8 g/dL
Glucose	152 mg/dL
Arterial blood gas	
pH	7.65
PO_2	340 mmHg
PCO_2	32 mmHg

- **What acid–base disorder is present in this patient?** This patient has an underlying respiratory acidosis with compensation (note elevated HCO_3^-). When a patient with chronic respiratory acidosis and appropriate renal compensation is placed on mechanical ventilation, he or she is at risk of developing severe alkalemia. This occurs because mechanical ventilation can remove PCO_2 from the blood quickly, hence increasing the pH precipitously. However, it takes time for the kidney to adapt to the change in blood pH. In time, the kidney can adapt by decreasing bicarbonate reabsorption, leading to loss of bicarbonate in the urine if the patient is not chloride depleted, but this does not happen in the acute setting. Following the start of mechanical ventilation in this patient, he has developed an iatrogenic respiratory alkalosis and a dangerously high arterial pH.
- **To correct the pH to 7.35, what goal CO_2 should be maintained?** The appropriate measure is to decrease the minute ventilation to allow the PCO_2 to rise to a level that would lead to a normal or slightly acidic pH. To determine the PCO_2 that corresponds to a pH of 7.35, use the Henderson–Hasselbalch relationship. In the acute setting, the HCO_3^- will not change since renal adjustments take several days to have full effect, and therefore the best way to change the pH is to adjust PCO_2.

$$7.35 = 6.1 + \log(34/0.03 * PCO_2)$$
$$PCO_2 = 64 \text{ mmHg}$$

Therefore, the ventilation rate should be decreased to maintain a PCO_2 of approximately 64 to achieve a pH of 7.35.

Newer Models of Acid-Base Quantification: Stewart Approach

The assumptions made in the traditional model are that acids behave as Brønsted/Lowry acids—that is, proton donors—and that the degree of a metabolic disturbance causes a decrease in buffers, which is best approximated by the decrease in serum bicarbonate. Therefore, every mole of H^+ added results in a reciprocal decrease in the concentration of buffers. This decrease in buffers occurs principally as a decrease in serum bicarbonate, but other unmeasured buffers, such as Hgb–H, are also decreased during acidosis. An approach that is gaining popularity, especially among critical care physicians, is the Stewart model, a deviation from the traditional approach to acid–base quantification, which makes different assumptions about the definition of acids and bases. In essence, in the Stewart model, an acid is defined as any substance that raises the $[H^+]$ of a solution, not necessarily limited to an H^+-donating species. Many excellent reviews have been written on this topic (14–17); discussion in this chapter will be limited to an introduction to the key-derived parameters of the Stewart model so that they can be contrasted with the standard approach. The most strikingly different concept of the Stewart model is that the serum bicarbonate is not used as the sole measure of buffering capacity present. This model uses the strong ion difference as a fundamental measure of the presence of buffers.

The Strong Ion Difference

Strong ions are the ions in the blood that can be considered as completely dissociated in solution (18). *The strong ion difference (SID) is analogous to the buffer base of a solution.* The SID is calculated as:

$$[SID] = \{[Na^+] + [K^+]\} - \{[Cl^-] - [lactate]\} \quad (6)$$

The remaining anions in solution are the buffers, which can be thought of as the bicarbonate plus the nonbicarbonate buffers, denoted $[A^-]$. $[A^-]$ is the sum of negative charge (buffering capacity) of albumin and phosphate:

$$[SID] = [HCO_3^-] + [A^-] \quad (7)$$

SID in the Stewart model is considered more reflective of the concentrations of buffers and not the serum bicarbonate. In fact, the Stewart equation describes the pH in terms of three independent variables: The strong ion difference [SID], $[A_{tot}]$, and PCO_2, where A_{tot} is the concentration of weak acids. This is in contrast to the Henderson–Hasselbalch equation, which relates pH to $[HCO_3^-]$ and PCO_2 (Equation (4)). In the Stewart model, bicarbonate concentration varies dependently on these other more fundamental parameters. The arguments for and against this claim are many, and are beyond the scope of this text. It can be stated, however, that the traditional approach to acid–base disturbances is still practiced most frequently, and the Stewart model has gained widest acceptance in the critical care field. This makes sense in that the Stewart model may have advantages in description of extreme acid–base conditions, especially when the assumption that noncarbonate buffers are constant may not be true, such as in critical illness. A high SID denotes metabolic alkalosis, and a low SID denotes metabolic acidosis. There are modifications of the standard model that attempt to take into account perturbations in noncarbonate species such as the correction of the anion gap for disturbances in serum albumin; this will be illustrated later in examples.

Expected and Apparent Strong Ion Difference. The SID under normal conditions can be thought as the sum of the buffer anions (bicarbonate and nonbicarbonate buffer anions) and should be about 40 mEq/L. As noted above, when the SID deviates from this value, a metabolic acid–base disturbance should be suspected. As noted above, the SID is one of three independent variables that determines $[H^+]$, and therefore, conversely, the SID can be related to the three fundamental values: pH, PCO_2, and $[A_{tot}]$. The expected SID (SID_e) is the SID that would be predicted based on the pH, PCO_2, and A_{tot} (in this case A_{tot} is approximated based on the albumin and phosphate). This relationship is given as follows:

$$[SID_e] = (1{,}000 \times 2.46 \times 10^{-11} \times PCO_2/10^{-pH}) + [albumin] \times (0.123 \times pH - 0.631) + [phosphate] \times (0.309 \times pH - 0.469) \quad (8)$$

The apparent SID (SID_a) is the strong ion difference considering the concentrations of the strong ions that are normally present in the serum: Na^+, K^+, and Cl^-. This definition is given as follows:

$$[SID_a] = \{[Na^+] + [K^+]\} - [Cl^-] \quad (9)$$

When the SID_a and SID differ, there is a strong anion gap, which is described below.

Strong Ion Gap

The strong ion gap (SIG) should be considered as an evaluation of unmeasured anions, analogous to the traditional anion gap. The strong anion gap is normally zero and is defined as:

$$SIG = \text{anion gap} - [A^-]$$

where A^- is the composite of nonbicarbonate buffers in the blood. $[A^-] = 2.8$ (albumin in g/dL) + 0.6 (phosphate in mg/dL) at a pH of 7.4.

$$SIG = [SID_e] - [SID_a] \quad (10)$$

When the SIG exceeds zero, there is an unmeasured anion present. This is analogous to the traditional anion gap, with a correction factor for the presence of hypoalbuminemia (19). The traditional anion gap is rarely corrected for disturbances in phosphate, although, as can be seen in the above formula for A^-, the contribution of deviations in phosphate is much smaller than that of albumin, reflecting that, quantitatively, albumin has much greater buffering capacity than phosphate.

The Stewart model has also been used to classify metabolic acid–base disorders based on the SID. An elevated SID is consistent with metabolic alkalosis, and a low SID is consistent with metabolic acidosis. The metabolic acidoses are further subdivided based on a high SIG (analogous in many ways to a high anion gap) and a low SIG (analogous to a low or normal anion gap). In this regard, the two approaches approximate each other. The use of the SIG may be advantageous over the use of the standard anion gap, given that the anion gap can have a wide range of values and is thus somewhat imprecise. This is especially true in settings where nonbicarbonate buffers deviate from normal—for example, the patient with acidosis, sepsis, and acute renal failure with serum albumin of 1.9, phosphorus of 7.0, and hemoglobin of 7.2 mg/dL. Clearly in this extreme, the assumption that only changes in serum bicarbonate species reflect the metabolic component of the acidosis may not hold true.

Stewart versus Traditional Approach

Despite the differences in these two approaches to acid–base quantification presented, it should be noted that they are quite similar. The advantage of the Stewart approach is that nonbicarbonate buffers are considered in quantifying acid–base disturbances and, as noted before, this is most likely to be pivotal in critical illness. However, accurate quantification of acid–base status is only part of managing acid–base disturbances. The traditional model focuses on the CO_2–bicarbonate buffering system and for the most part ignores the contribution of nonbicarbonate buffers. This assumption is valid enough in almost all clinical situations that the ultimate acid–base diagnosis is not affected. Correctly diagnosing acid–base disorders and treating them appropriately is the ultimate goal; in this regard, we do not find considerable advantage of the Stewart approach over more traditional methodologies, given the much more cumbersome calculations involved with the Stewart approach. It is important that the clinician understand the limitation of any of the acid–base models, such as understanding when perturbations in the anion gap are significant and when they are not. In the cases presented in this chapter, we have used a traditional approach to acid–base analysis, and we continue use this approach in our own practice.

Case #2: STRONG IONS AND INTERRELATIONSHIP OF ELECTROLYTES AND ACID–BASE STATUS [19]

A 31-year-old woman has gastroenteritis with vomiting. She is hypotensive and weak and admitted to the intensive care unit. Serum electrolytes show a sodium concentration of 125 mmol/L, potassium of 2.6 mmol/L, chloride of 72 mmol/L, and bicarbonate of 40 mmol/L. Arterial pH was 7.54, PCO_2 is 48 mmHg and urinary pH is 5.0.

The ECF volume, sodium, chloride, and potassium depletion in this patient activate mechanisms that work to maintain volume status and electrolyte balance. Angiotensin and aldosterone levels are increased. Mechanisms aimed at minimizing sodium and potassium losses also increase bicarbonate reabsorption.

- **What does this case illustrate?**
  Once bicarbonate reabsorption is nearly total, urinary pH drops, giving the paradoxical aciduria in the face of systemic alkalosis. Treatment of the alkalemia in this situation is through restoring the strong ion deficits. Once volume resuscitation and potassium repletion are complete, bicarbonate excretion through the kidney can ensue. The acid–base status is restored through the actions of the kidney. This case illustrates the principle that acid–base status can be dependent on the concentration of the strong ions.

Volatile Acidity

Up until now, we have dealt exclusively with fixed acids. Disturbances in fixed acids cause a change in available buffers and change in systemic pH. It is critical to note that volatile acidity plays a very important role in determining the systemic pH both in primary respiratory disturbances and in compensation to metabolic disturbances as will be discussed.

Carbon dioxide is soluble in water, and in solution, reacts with water molecules to form carbonic acid, which can then further react as the following:

$$CO_2 + H_2O \leftrightarrow H_2CO_3 \leftrightarrow H^+ + HCO_3^- \qquad (11)$$

H_2CO_3 is the acid portion of the bicarbonate buffer; however, its concentration is proportional to the partial pressure of CO_2, and therefore, its direct measurement is not necessary. By the equilibrium expressions above, it can be seen that primary changes in PCO_2 will alter the amount of H_2CO_3. A high PCO_2 will increase the concentration of H_2CO_3, and a low PCO_2 will decrease the concentration of H_2CO_3. By quantitative chemistry, as you increase the concentration of the conjugate acid, the pH of a buffered solution will increase, and as you decrease concentration of conjugate acid, the opposite occurs. The PCO_2 in the circulation is the sum of its production and excretion. The production of CO_2 is not frequently altered; however, the excretion of CO_2—occurring only through respiration—is variable based upon the minute ventilation.

Mechanisms of Compensation

The previous sections have detailed how buffering allows the body to absorb significant amounts of H^+ without large fluctuations in pH. These buffering systems allow pH to remain constant during physiologic changes in endogenous acid production, and they also form the first defense against an acid–base insult (see Table 135.1). The buffering systems and respiratory compensation are very rapid, whereas renal compensation may take days to become fully effective (20). The capacity of the body's buffering system is substantial, and therefore significant amounts of acid can be absorbed before a relatively small change in systemic pH occurs. Buffers act immediately and are thus the first line of defense.

In response to systemic changes in pH, compensatory mechanisms act to counteract the primary disturbance. Figure 135.3 gives an overview of the compensatory responses to the primary acid–base disturbances. In response to metabolic acidosis, there is increased ventilation to decrease PCO_2; the kidney responds by increasing the excretion of H^+, thereby generating more HCO_3^- (see Fig. 135.3A). The opposite response occurs during metabolic alkalosis, except that the kidneys are usually

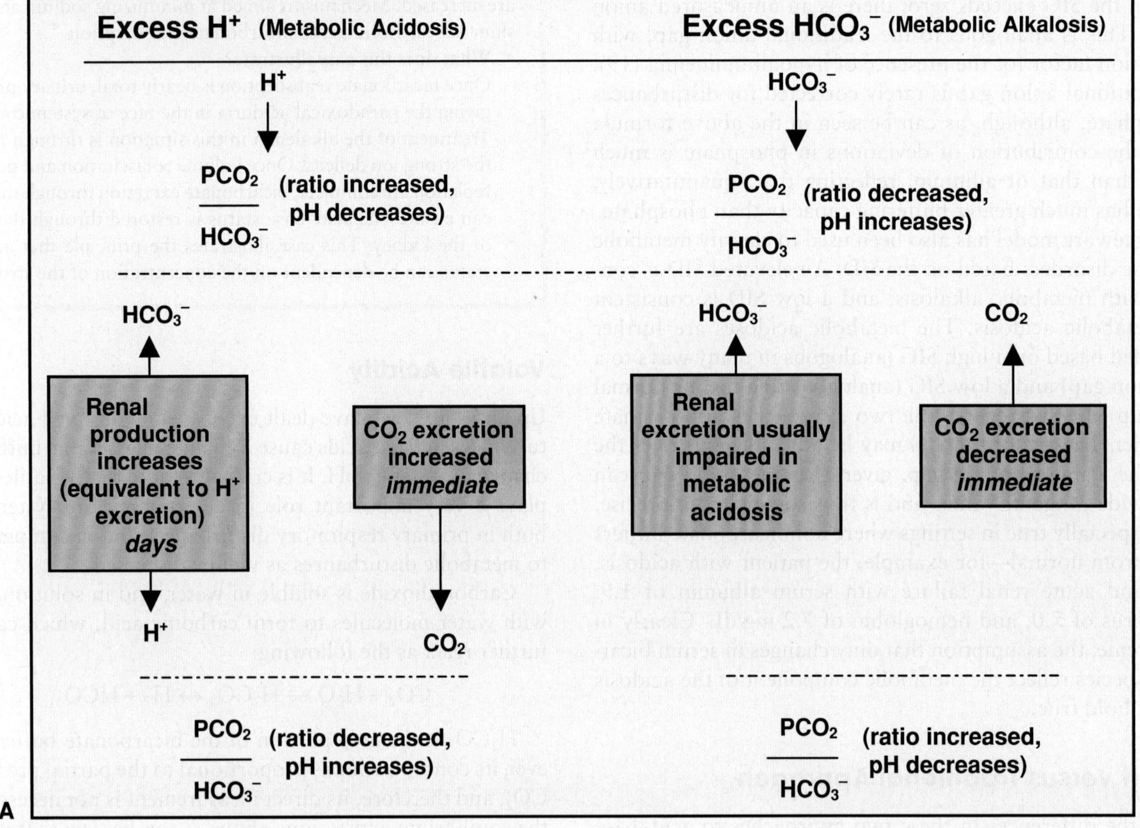

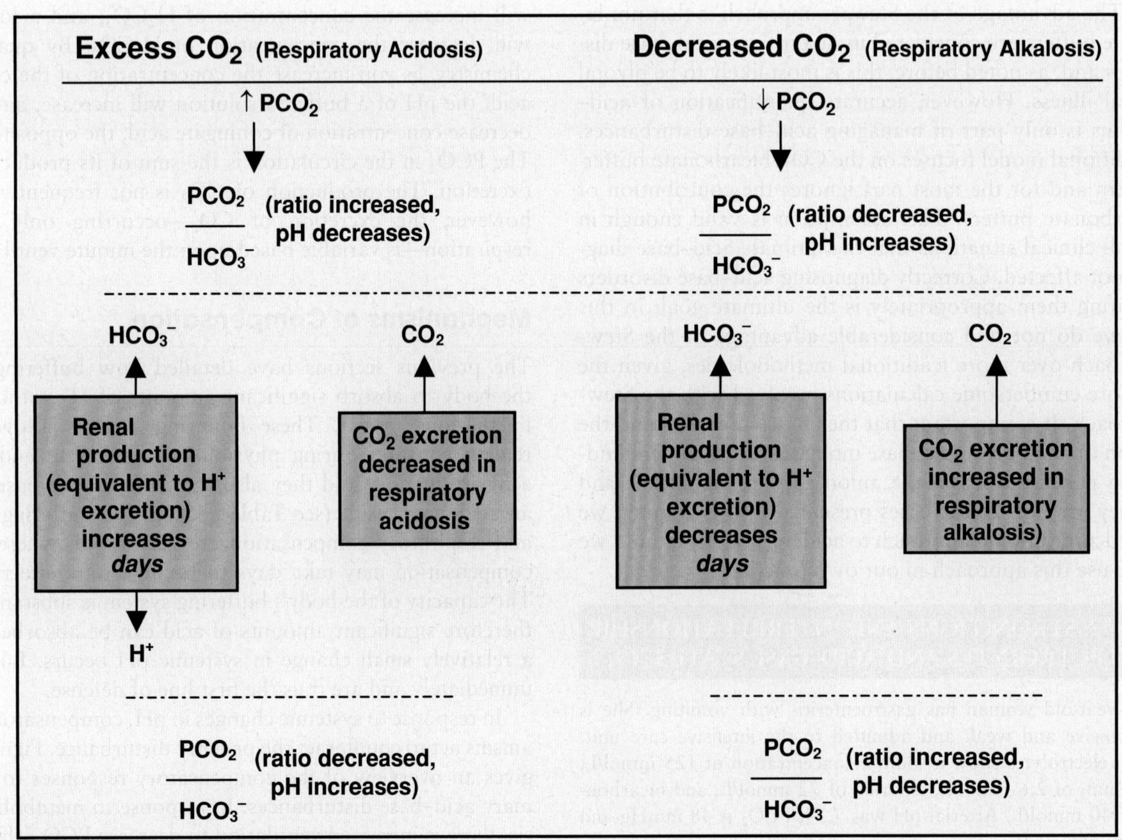

FIGURE 135.3 A: Primary metabolic acid–base disturbances and compensatory mechanisms. B: Primary respiratory acid–base disturbances and compensatory mechanisms.

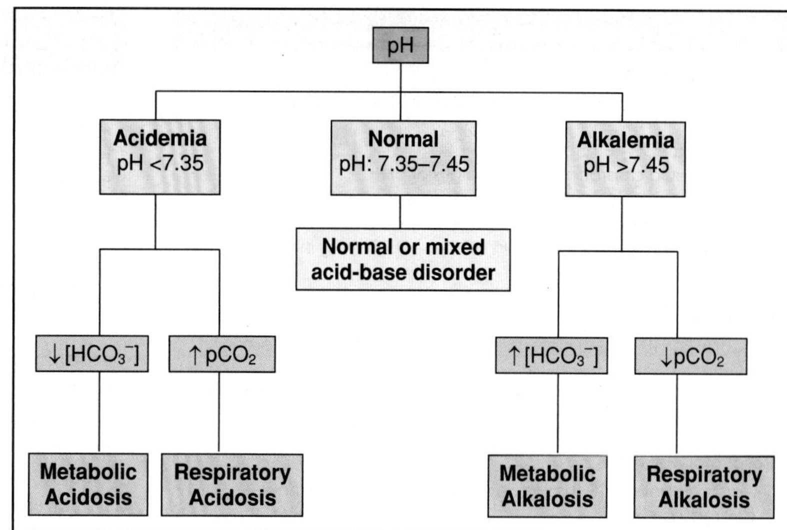

FIGURE 135.4 General approach to acid–base disorders. (From Ayus JC. Nephrology section. *Medical Knowledge Self-assessment Program—14.* Philadelphia, PA: American College of Physicians; 2006. Copyright by the American College of Physicians.)

not able to respond to the increase in HCO_3^- appropriately, as failure of the kidney to respond to elevated HCO_3^- is necessary for the development of metabolic alkalosis (this is described later). The response to elevated PCO_2 is to increase the renal excretion of H^+, which leads to increased HCO_3^- production (see Fig. 135.3B). In response to metabolic alkalosis, the excretion of H^+ decreases and less bicarbonate is produced, thereby decreasing serum bicarbonate. Each of the four primary disturbances leads to a perturbation of one of the carbonate species. Consequently, the main compensatory response is to alter the concentration of the conjugate species so that the ratio between the two can be maintained. The response to respiratory disorders has acute and chronic components. The acute response is related to immediate buffering, and the chronic phase of the response occurs as renal compensation takes place; only the chronic phase is depicted in Figure 135.3B. An important point to remember in determining the acid–base disturbances present in a patient is that a compensatory response will never normalize the serum pH or lead to a recovery of the pH past neutrality. If this has occurred, there must be another acid–base disturbance present.

Determining Which Acid-Base Disturbances Are Present

A systematic approach is important in correctly diagnosing acid–base disorders in critically ill patients. Because it is common to have mixed acid–base disorders with two or even three disorders present, it is important to evaluate the available information thoroughly and avoid quick judgments based on an incomplete picture.

The approach to acid–base disorders is summarized in Table 135.2 and Figure 135.4. A key is to identify the primary disturbance. This is best accomplished by analyzing acid–base data in conjunction with a good history. The physical examination is rarely helpful in determining the etiology of an acid–base disorder. It is also important to note that the algorithm in Figure 135.4 is useful in the case of single acid–base disorders. Mixed disturbances are discussed later. Once the primary disturbance is identified, the next step is to assess the adequacy of compensation. Table 135.3 gives the expected values of PCO_2 and HCO_3^- following compensations for primary disturbances. In the setting of respiratory disorders, acute compensation occurs over minutes, while the chronic compensation occurs over days. If there is only one disturbance, and the compensation is adequate, there is nothing more to do. On the other hand, if the compensation is inappropriate, then a second disorder is present. Recall that compensation will never normalize the pH or "compensate" past the point of neutrality (e.g., a primary metabolic acidosis as a single disorder cannot lead to a neutral or alkaline pH). In these cases, a mixed acid–base disorder is present. An additional clue that a mixed acid–base disorder is present is an elevated anion gap when a metabolic acidosis is not suspected. For this reason, it is good practice to calculate the anion gap in all critically ill patients.

CAUSES OF ACID–BASE DISORDERS

In determining the etiology, the clinician usually must rely on the history, clinical presentation, and, most importantly,

TABLE 135.2 Approach to the Critically Ill Patient with an Acid–Base Disorder

The first step is to determine which acid–base disorders are present, the cause of each disorder, and the degree of compensation, There are four important variables to look at when determining the acid–base status of a patient, and these should be evaluated in all critically ill patients.

- **Arterial pH:** Always the starting point. Avoid making judgments in the absence of a measured arterial pH. The pH is the negative logarithm of the concentration of H^+, with a physiologic of 7.38–7.44.
- **Arterial PCO_2:** Indicator of the amount of volatile acidity. The PCO_2 generally reflects the respiratory response or contribution to the acid–base disorder.
- **Serum bicarbonate:** Indicative of the degree of fixed acids present (lower means more fixed acids present). Normal is 34 mEq/L.
- **Serum anion gap** ($(Na^+) - \{(Cl^-) + (HCO_3^-)\}$): Measure of conjugate bases (anions) present above what is expected under normal" conditions. Has a wide variability; normal is usually 8–12 mEq/L.

TABLE 135.3 Compensations for Acid–Base Disorders

Metabolic acidosis
• For every 1 mmol/L decrease in HCO_3^- → 1 mmHg decrease in PCO_2
• Expected PCO_2 = 1.5 (HCO_3^-) + 8 ± 2
• PCO_2 should approach last two digits of pH
Metabolic alkalosis
• For every 1 mmol/L increase in HCO_3^- → 0.7 mmHg increase in PCO_2
Respiratory acidosis
• Acute: For 10 mmHg increase in PCO_2 → 1 mmol/L increase in HCO_3^-
• Chronic: For 10 mmHg increase in PCO_2 → 4 mmol/L increase in HCO_3^-
Respiratory alkalosis
• Acute: For every 10 mmHg decrease in PCO_2 → 2 mmol/L decrease in HCO_3^-
• Chronic: For every 10 mmHg decrease in PCO_2 → 4 mmol/L decrease in HCO_3^-

laboratory data in order to determine the inciting disease state (Fig. 135.5).

Metabolic Acidosis

Causes of Anion Gap Acidosis

The common etiologies of elevated anion gap metabolic acidosis are listed in Table 135.4.

Diabetic Ketoacidosis. Insulin is secreted and mediates the metabolism of carbohydrates and the storage of fat during times of normal enteral intake. Under fasting conditions, insulin secretion decreases. Diabetic ketoacidosis occurs when a deficit of insulin activity leads to altered cellular metabolism and glucose utilization is impaired. The deficiency of insulin causes the liberation of fatty acids and

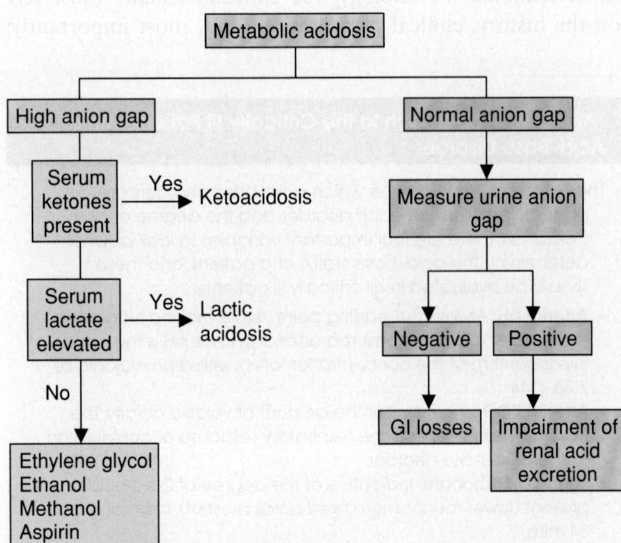

FIGURE 135.5 Diagnostic approach to metabolic acidosis. (From Ayus JC. Nephrology section. *Medical Knowledge Self-assessment Program—14.* Philadelphia, PA: American College of Physicians; 2006. Copyright by the American College of Physicians.)

TABLE 135.4 Common Causes of Elevated Anion Gap Metabolic Acidosis

Lactic acidosis
Diabetic ketoacidosis
Renal failure
Ingestions
• Methanol
• Ethylene glycol
• Paraldehydes
• Salicylates

pathophysiologic ketoacid production. The degree of increase in the anion gap is related to the amount of retained ketones, and therefore, diabetic ketoacidosis can be present with varying degrees of hyperchloremia (21). In addition to abnormal ketoacid production, diabetic ketoacidosis is typically also associated with hyperglycemia, a decrease in circulatory volume, and, oftentimes, free water deficits as well, in addition to hypokalemia and hypophosphatemia. Even though total body potassium stores are decreased, the serum potassium concentration is frequently elevated on presentation due to the effects of insulin deficiency, hyperglycemia, and acidosis on potassium distribution. The treatment of diabetic ketoacidosis includes re-expansion of the ECF volume, administration of insulin to halt acid production, and correction of potassium and phosphorus deficits, with close monitoring of plasma electrolytes.

Cerebral Edema Complicating Therapy of Diabetic Ketoacidosis. An emerging concept in the treatment of diabetic ketoacidosis warrants special attention. The developed of cerebral edema during DKA therapy is a severe, sometimes fatal complication. The proposed mechanism for the development of this form of cerebral edema is a relative imbalance between the intracellular effective osmolality and the effective osmolality of the ECF. Recall that the effective osmolality of plasma can be can be estimated by the following:

$$2 \times [\text{plasma sodium (mEq/L)}] + [\text{plasma glucose (mg/dL)}]/18 \quad (12)$$

Urea does not show up in the calculation of effective osmolality (compare to total osmolality, Equation (13)) since urea is rapidly transported across most cell membranes and maintains equal concentrations in both compartments (thus urea will contribute to *total* osmolality of the compartment, but does not contribute to *effective* osmolality). The rapid administration of large amounts of intravenous fluids, especially hypotonic fluids and possibly the administration if intravenous boluses of insulin are two purported iatrogenic factors that have been implicated in the development of this syndrome. The imbalance between effective osmoles in the intracellular compartment of the brain and the plasma is believed to develop as fluid therapy lower plasma osmolality rapidly and bolus insulin may increase intracellular sodium by stimulating cation exchangers in the brain (22). Current guidelines do not advise initial intravenous boluses of insulin in all children and the judicious use of fluids as well as a way of preventing this complication. Also, the use of hypotonic fluids should be avoided. The treatment of cerebral edema associated with diabetic ketoacidosis consists of hypertonic saline to raise the plasma osmolality and correct the imbalance between the effective osmolality in the intracellular compartment of the brain and plasma.

Lactic Acidosis. There are two types of lactic acidosis: Type A lactic acidosis is due to tissue hypoxia and the formation of excess lactic acid, and constitutes the majority of cases of lactic acidosis. This is frequently seen in sepsis, profound anemia, shock, hypotension, and bowel and limb ischemia. Lactate is formed in tissues under hypoxic conditions as it is a by-product of anaerobic cellular metabolism. Type A lactic acidosis is often associated with poor outcomes if the cause is not quickly reversed, usually due to the severity of the underlying condition, such as septic shock or bowel infarction.

Type B lactic acidosis occurs when there is insufficient liver metabolism of lactate. The normal metabolism of lactate leads to the generation of bicarbonate, and therefore, when this pathway is less operative, there is decreased bicarbonate and systemic acidosis. This condition can be seen in severe liver disease and/or other conditions that interfere with liver metabolism. Several commonly used medications have been associated with lactic acidosis including propofol, metformin, the nonnucleotide reverse transcriptase inhibitors, stavudine, didanosine, and zidovudine. Carbon monoxide poisoning can present with nonspecific symptoms and lead to lactic acidosis by inhibiting oxygen utilization in the tissues.

Toxic Ingestions Associated with Elevated Anion Gap Acidosis. Ingestions are important causes of acidosis in the critical care setting (23). Common ingestions that often lead to elevated anion gap metabolic acidosis are listed in Table 135.4. The presence of ingested alcohols or other solvents can be inferred by measurement of the osmolal gap when an ingestion is suspected.

The osmolal gap can be calculated using the following formula:

$$\text{(Measured serum osmolality)} - \text{(calculated serum osmolality)}$$

where the calculated serum osmolality is obtained as follows:

$$2 \times [\mathrm{Na}^+]\ (\mathrm{mEq/L}) \times \text{urea nitrogen (mg/dL)}/2.8 + \text{glucose (mg/dL)}/18 \quad (13)$$

The osmolal gap is normally approximately 10 mOsm/kg H_2O. The normal osmolal gap is a reflection of substances normally present in the serum that exert oncotic forces. These are plasma proteins and ions found in smaller quantities, such as calcium and magnesium. An elevated osmolal gap is an indication that an unmeasured osmole is present in the serum; in the intensive care setting, this is commonly due to ethanol. The osmolal gap can also be used to quantify the level of ethylene glycol or methanol, although direct measurement of these toxins is indicated if their presence is suspected; however, therapy should not be delayed while waiting for confirmation.

Case #3: SALICYLATE TOXICITY

A 68-year-old man presents to the emergency room following an intentional toxic ingestion. He was brought in by his son, who found him confused when he stopped by his (the patient's) house. One month prior to admission, he suffered the loss of his wife and has felt hopeless since that time. Upon presentation, he is lethargic and weak. His past medical history is significant for hypertension and gout. Past surgical history is significant for an appendectomy 20 years ago and coronary artery bypass graft (CABG) 2 years ago. He smokes one and a half packs of cigarettes a day and he denies the use of alcohol or illicit drugs. Physical examination is significant for blood pressure of 156/80 mmHg, pulse of 79 beats/min, respirations of 32 breaths/min, and temperature of 98°F. He is lethargic, in moderate respiratory distress, and oriented only to place and person. Cardiovascular examination is normal, and there is no wheezing on chest examination. Laboratory data are given below:

Serum	
Sodium	141 mEq/L
Potassium	3.9 mEq/L
Chloride	105 mEq/L
Bicarbonate	9 mEq/L
BUN	21 mg/dL
Creatinine	1.2 md/dL
Glucose	128 mg/dL
Arterial blood gas	
pH	7.40
PO_2	67 mmHg
PCO_2	15 mmHg

Salicylate toxicity is typically associated with an anion gap metabolic acidosis and respiratory alkalosis; this is the acid–base disorder present in this patient. In diagnosing the acid–base disturbance in this patient, the first step is to look at the serum pH. The pH is normal with low serum bicarbonate. This is the first clue that a complex disorder is present since a compensatory response to metabolic acidosis would not normalize the serum pH. We can determine that there is a metabolic acidosis present because of the elevated anion gap (anion gap = 27). Given the presence of a metabolic acidosis, we can then predict what the PCO_2 should be. Using the Winter formula, the expected PCO_2 is approximately 21 mmHg (see Table 135.3), and thus a respiratory alkalosis is present. This pattern is strongly suggestive of salicylate toxicity (24).

Case #4: LACTIC ACIDOSIS IN THE SETTING OF ABNORMAL LEVELS OF NONBICARBONATE BUFFERS

A 44-year-old woman with cirrhosis secondary to autoimmune hepatitis is admitted to the hospital for fever and abdominal pain. The patient is listed for an orthotopic liver transplantation and has been clinically stable for the past month. She noted abdominal pain and fever that have gotten progressively worse over the last 2 days. Her past medical history is otherwise nonsignificant. Current medications include spironolactone 100 mg PO bid, furosemide 80 mg PO bid, and lactulose 30 mL PO bid. Previous surgeries include the placement of a transjugular intrahepatic portosystemic shunt (TIPS) and a cholecystectomy. Physical examination is significant for blood pressure of 74/55 mmHg, pulse of 72 beats/min, temperature 100.8°F, and respiratory rate of 24 breaths/min. She appears cachectic. Cardiovascular and chest exams are normal. Her abdomen is distended and there is diffuse tenderness. She has 1+ pitting edema in the lower extremities. Spontaneous bacterial peritonitis is suspected, and the patient is admitted to the hospital. Admission labs are given below:

Serum	
Sodium	128 mEq/L
Potassium	5.1 mEq/L
Chloride	106 mEq/L
Bicarbonate	11 mEq/L
BUN	20 mg/dL
Creatinine	1.3 mg/dL
Phosphorus	2.1 mg/dL
Albumin	1.4 g/dL
Glucose	84 mg/dL

Arterial blood gas

pH	7.23
PO_2	78 mmHg
PCO_2	28 mmHg

- **What is the best characterization of the acid–base disturbance in this patient?**

The acid–base disorder is an anion gap metabolic acidosis, likely lactic acidosis. While the anion gap appears normal, the degree of hypoalbuminemia needs to be considered because the negative charge on albumin is a significant component of the "normal" unmeasured anions. For every 1 g/dL decrease in the serum albumin, the expected anion gap decreases by 2.5 mEq/L. Thus, in this patient, to consider her anion gap at a normal level, it should not exceed approximately 5 to 6 mEq/L. Again, caution should be used in interpreting the anion gap in these settings; if any suspicion exists for lactic acidosis, the serum lactate should be measured directly.

Nonanion Gap Acidosis

In a nonanion gap (hyperchloremic) acidosis, there is a primary decrease in the serum bicarbonate and an associated increase in the serum chloride. The serum bicarbonate decreases because of renal or extrarenal, GI losses (Table 135.5). One of the key etiologic questions to be answered in the approach to a patient with a nonanion gap acidosis is whether or not the kidney is appropriately responding to the acidosis by excreting the acid load or if the cause of the acidosis is improper acid excretion by the kidney. This allows one to differentiate renal from nonrenal causes of the acidosis. The urine anion gap, which is calculated using Eq. 3, is a convenient methodology to assess urinary acid excretion. If the urine anion gap is positive or close to zero, this suggests that there is very little ammonium in the urine (see Fig. 42.2) and that the kidney is not appropriately excreting acids. If the urine anion gap is highly negative, this suggests that there is a large amount of ammonium in the urine and that the kidney is excreting acids appropriately.

Causes of Nonanion Gap Metabolic Acidosis

Diarrhea. Severe diarrhea leads to nonanion gap metabolic acidosis through loss of bicarbonate, and is typically associated with volume depletion and hypokalemia. In very severe cases, circulatory collapse can occur, and an anion gap (lactic) acidosis may supervene upon the nonanion gap acidosis. Patients who chronically abuse laxatives may develop metabolic acidosis and hypokalemia. However, frequently, these patients also abuse diuretics and therefore can have an associated metabolic alkalosis. In order to determine if the renal response to the acidosis is normal, the urine anion gap should be measured.

TABLE 135.5 Causes of Nonanion Gap Metabolic Acidosis

Extrarenal source
- Gastrointestinal disorders
- Diarrhea
- Pancreatic and biliary fistulas
- Laxatives, cholestyramine
- Ureterointestinal diversions (ileal conduit)

Renal source
- Renal tubular acidosis
- Renal failure
- Hypoaldosteronism

Ureterointestinal Diversions. In a ureterointestinal diversion, urine in the intestine leads to reabsorption of chloride and water. Consequently, the absorption of chloride can induce secretion of bicarbonate into the intestine. Additionally, urease-positive bacteria in the intestine metabolizes the urea in the urine to form ammonium, which, when absorbed, liberates excess acid after it is metabolized in the liver. Also, chronic pyelonephritis is common in the diverted kidney, and a superimposed distal renal tubular acidosis (RTA) may occur.

Renal Tubular Acidosis. RTA is a heterogeneous mix of disorders that is characterized by defects in urinary acid excretion in the setting of intact renal function. Proximal (type 2) RTA is caused by a decrease in proximal bicarbonate reabsorption, whereas in distal (type 1) RTA, the primary defect is impairment of distal acidification (25,26). The net result is that the urine pH is not maximally acidified. The lack of acidification—in other words, secretion of H^+—leads to less ammonium trapping in the urine and therefore to an anion gap that is either positive or near zero. In the intensive care unit, RTA often presents with profound acidosis and hypokalemia. It is important to treat the hypokalemia first with potassium chloride before correcting the acidosis, as administration of bicarbonate in the setting of severe potassium depletion can lead to fatal hypokalemia as potassium is taken up by cells when H^+ exits the cells. Type 4 RTA is a clinical syndrome of hyperkalemia and hyperchloremic metabolic acidosis (27) caused by a lack of aldosterone effect on the kidney and is seen most commonly in the following settings: diabetes, advanced age, acquired immunodeficiency syndrome (AIDS), interstitial nephritis, obstructive uropathy, postrenal transplant status, use of angiotensin-converting enzyme inhibitors and heparin (both of which impair aldosterone production), and use of cyclosporine.

RTA should be suspected if the renal response to systemic acidemia is impaired as evidenced by a positive urine anion gap. The next step is to determine the type. The most practical starting point is to differentiate a proximal from a distal RTA. To understand this, some physiology must be discussed. Recall that bicarbonate is reabsorbed predominantly in the proximal tubule. Proximal RTA develops because of impaired reabsorption of bicarbonate. The lack of bicarbonate reabsorption in patients with normal serum bicarbonate leads to wasting of bicarbonate in the urine until a steady state is reached in which the serum bicarbonate drops to a level at which the reabsorptive capacity of the proximal tubule is no longer overwhelmed. At this point, there is no longer any bicarbonate in the urine. For this reason, in a patient with proximal RTA, the serum bicarbonate will be low; however, the urine pH will be low—this is because the distal acidification mechanisms are functional. If such a patient is given an alkali load, serum bicarbonate is temporarily increased, and bicarbonate "spills" into the urine because the filtered load of bicarbonate exceeds the reabsorptive threshold, which leads to an increase in the urine pH. Once the alkali load is stopped, serum bicarbonate drops, bicarbonate no longer appears in the urine, and the urine pH can now drop to its maximally acidic level of approximately 5.5. This is the basis for the provocative testing to demonstrate a proximal RTA, and also explains why these patients often have to take a tremendous amount of alkali in order to achieve normal serum pH.

Renal Failure. The kidneys have the capacity to excrete acids to such a degree that acid–base balance is maintained until kidney function deteriorates to below a glomerular filtration rate of approximately 20 mL/min. The resulting acidosis is of a mixed type and it is generally, but not universally, associated with an elevated anion gap. Chronic metabolic acidosis should be treated to prevent bone demineralization, which may occur with time. The goal of treatment is to maintain normal acid–base status.

Pancreatic or Biliary Fistula. These disorders can lead to the loss of bicarbonate-rich solutions through the GI tract and result in systemic acidosis. If correction of the underlying fistula is not possible, treatment with alkali salts can be helpful.

Hypoaldosteronism. Similar to type 4 RTA acidosis, hypoaldosteronism can lead to an impairment in renal acid excretion. Aldosterone activity in the kidney leads to hypokalemia and metabolic alkalosis; conversely, lack of this activity decreases aldosterone secretion and leads to hyperkalemia and metabolic acidosis.

Case #5: NONANION GAP METABOLIC ACIDOSIS: ASSESSING URINARY ACID EXCRETION

A 66-year-old man is seen in the emergency room. He has had 8 days of severe diarrhea, abdominal pain, and decreased food intake, but adequate intake of liquids. He believes that he became sick after babysitting his grandson who had similar symptoms. His medical history is significant for diabetes and hypertension. Surgical history only consists of coronary artery bypass grafting 3 years ago. His medications include enalapril 20 mg PO bid, aspirin 81 mg PO daily, atenolol 50 mg PO daily, hydrochlorothiazide 25 mg PO daily, and metformin 1 g PO bid. He has a family history of diabetes and premature coronary artery disease. He does not smoke or use drugs, and drinks alcohol occasionally. Physical examination is significant for blood pressure of 105/70 mmHg and a pulse of 72 beats/min; blood pressure drops to 90/50 mmHg when the patient stands. Temperature is 98.8°F, and respiratory rate is 32 breaths/min. There is a small amount of occult blood in the stool. Laboratory results are given below:

Serum	
Sodium	136 mEq/L
Potassium	3.9 mEq/L
Chloride	114 mEq/L
Bicarbonate	13 mEq/L
BUN	21 mg/dL
Creatinine	1.2 mg/dL
Albumin	4.0 g/dL
Glucose	128 mg/dL
Urine	
pH	6
Sodium	32 mEq/L
Potassium	21 mEq/L
Chloride	80 mEq/L
Arterial blood gas	
pH	7.27
PO_2	90 mmHg
PCO_2	30 mmHg

- **Which acid–base disorder is present and what is the likely etiology?**

  This patient has a nonanion gap metabolic acidosis from a nonrenal origin. The low pH and decreased serum bicarbonate indicate the presence of metabolic acidosis. Respiratory compensation is adequate, and therefore, there is no complex acid–base disorder present. The serum anion gap is not elevated. The urine electrolytes and the calculation of the urine anion gap are useful to distinguish between a renal source and a GI source of the acidosis. If GI losses are the cause of the acidosis and the renal response to the acidosis is normal, a significant amount of ammonium will be present in the urine. The presence (or absence) of ammonium can be inferred by calculating the urine anion gap. The formula for the urine anion gap is as follows: $[K^+] + [Na^+] - [Cl^-]$. If there is an unmeasured anion present, then $[Cl^-]$ exceeds $[K^+] + [Na^+]$ and the urine anion gap is significantly negative. When there is little or no unmeasured anion present, the urine anion gap will take on a positive value. In this case, the urine anion gap = 32 mEq/L + 21 mEq/L − 80 mEq/L = −27 mEq/L, and therefore, there is a significant amount of ammonium (NH_4^+) in the urine, which implies a normal renal response to the systemic acidosis—thereby designating an extrarenal cause of the acidosis.

Treatment of Metabolic Acidosis

Treatment of Anion Gap Metabolic Acidosis. The treatment of an anion gap metabolic acidosis is focused on reversing the pathogenesis of the endogenous acid production and eliminating excess acid. By far the most important aspect of treatment is to identify the source of the acidosis if it is not already apparent, such as in diabetic ketoacidosis or septic shock. Treatment of an anion gap acidosis with bicarbonate replacement therapy remains controversial, especially in lactic acidosis. It has been argued that bicarbonate may be used as a bridge until homeostatic mechanisms reverse the condition through the metabolism of endogenous bases, such as lactate and ketone bodies, and therefore bicarbonate regeneration. This approach of using alkali therapy assumes that there is a detriment to a low pH (or serum bicarbonate) above and beyond the harm caused by the underlying condition. However, evidence from animal models argues that bicarbonate therapy may have deleterious effects on pH, serum lactate levels, and cardiac function (28–30). Bicarbonate leads to the generation of CO_2 during buffering and, as CO_2 readily diffuses across cell membranes, intracellular acidosis has been shown to worsen during bicarbonate therapy. Worsening of cardiac function, which has been associated with intracellular acidosis, is the proposed mechanism for worsening of lactic acidosis following the administration of bicarbonate during lactic acidosis (31). Hemodialysis rapidly corrects acidosis and is typically necessary to treat acidosis in the setting of renal failure.

Treatment of Nonanion Gap Metabolic Acidosis. Bicarbonate therapy is generally indicated in nonanion gap acidosis since the primary disturbance is a decrease in bicarbonate. This is contrasted to anion gap acidosis where correction of the underlying cause is the primary concern. Oral bicarbonate or oral citrate solutions are agents for chronic therapy for nonanion gap acidosis. For acute presentations, especially in patients who may not be able to tolerate prolonged hyperventilation, intravenous bicarbonate therapy may be used.

Medications and Metabolic Acidosis

Medications are an increasingly important cause of severe acidosis and can be life threatening in many cases. Lactic acidosis has been reported with all nonnucleoside reverse transcriptase inhibitors used to treat human immunodeficiency virus (HIV); this effect is related to the drug's inhibition of mitochondrial function, with resultant anaerobic metabolism (32–35). The newer-generation anticonvulsant topiramate has also been associated with lactic acidosis (35). Metformin is also well known to lead to lactic acidosis, which can be treated with hemodialysis (36). The propofol infusion syndrome is a dangerous complication sometimes seen with the use of this drug; it is associated with head injury, use of propofol for more than 48 hours, use in children, and concomitant use of catecholamines and steroids (37–39).

Case #6: PROPOFOL INFUSION SYNDROME

A 25-year-old male is in the intensive care unit following a craniotomy for a traumatic head injury. He had suffered a depressed skull fracture to the left frontal bone from blunt trauma during an altercation. He has no known medical problems and takes no medications. Family members state that he occasionally uses intravenous cocaine and smokes cigarettes. Intraoperatively, he is given intravenous cefazolin and phenytoin. It is now postoperative day 2, and he is currently receiving propofol infusion at 8 μg/kg/min. Blood pressure is 155/90 mmHg, pulse 80 beats/min, temperature 97.4°F, and respiratory rate 12 breaths/min. He is currently mechanically ventilated on SIMV mode with bilateral breath sounds. He has a normal cardiac examination, and there is no peripheral edema. Laboratory data are as follows:

	Day 3	Day 6
Sodium (mEq/L)	136	137
Potassium (mEq/L)	3.9	4
Chloride (mEq/L)	104	103
Bicarbonate (mEq/L)	20	12
BUN (mg/dL)	18	19
Creatinine (mg/dL)	1.1	1.0
Albumin (g/dL)	4.0	4.0
Glucose (mg/dL)	128	112
Lactate (mMol/L)		7
pH	7.37	7.21
PCO_2 (mmHg)	38	32

- **What is the likely cause of the acidosis in this patient?**
  Propofol infusion syndrome is an important entity in the intensive care unit (38–41). The cause is thought to be related to mitochondrial respiratory chain inhibition or impaired mitochondrial fatty acid metabolism; it is associated with refractory bradycardia in the presence of lactic acidosis, rhabdomyolysis, hyperlipidemia, and fatty liver. The patients who appear to be at the greatest risk for the condition are those receiving prolonged infusions after suffering brain injury. Treatment for the condition appears to be discontinuation of propofol; hemofiltration has been used successfully (41,42). It is important to note that many fatalities have occurred when the condition is not recognized promptly, and thus early recognition is critical.

Metabolic Alkalosis

Metabolic alkalosis occurs when there is an excess of buffers present, raising the systemic pH. In metabolic alkalosis, there is a primary elevation in the serum bicarbonate. This condition is common in the intensive care setting and can have severe complications. As the primary problem is an increase in bicarbonate, metabolic alkalosis can be readily corrected by renal bicarbonate excretion. Under normal circumstances the potential for bicarbonate excretion is tremendous, and thus, alterations in the renal handling of bicarbonate must occur to maintain the alkalosis. Without an impairment of the renal capacity to excrete bicarbonate, the kidneys would simply excrete the bicarbonate load. The most common reason for impairment of renal excretion of bicarbonate is chloride deficiency and renal failure. In general, metabolic alkaloses are generated by either bicarbonate intake in excess of loss or by the primary loss of H^+ (Table 135.6).

TABLE 135.6 Causes of Alkalosis Generation

Excessive alkaline load
Bicarbonate infusion, hemodialysis
$CaCO_3$ supplements
Oral citrate solutions
Parenteral nutrition (acetate, glutamate)
Loss of hydrogen ions
Gastrointestinal losses: vomiting, nasogastric suction
Renal losses: diuretics, excessive mineralocorticoid

Chloride-Sensitive Metabolic Alkalosis

Nasogastric suction, vomiting, and diuretics are very frequent causes of metabolic alkalosis. Hypokalemia develops in the setting of vomiting or nasogastric suction not due to GI losses, as the stomach contents are not rich in potassium; rather, the losses of potassium are renal losses due to potassium bicarbonate excretion and secondary hyperaldosteronism. In these settings, renal losses of sodium and potassium are obligatory in order to excrete bicarbonate. As the disturbance progresses, increased sodium and potassium reabsorption in both the proximal tubule and the collecting duct leads to increased bicarbonate reabsorption until urinary bicarbonate becomes low and urinary pH decreases, thus leading to a paradoxically acidic urine in the face of a systemic alkalemia (19). In this situation, the urinary chloride (not the urinary sodium) better reflects the effective blood volume of the patient. Similar to the loss of gastric secretions, diuretic-induced ECF volume depletion stimulates aldosterone secretion. The action of aldosterone stimulates sodium reabsorption in the distal tubule, which is coupled with secretion of potassium and H^+. Therefore, urine that is paradoxically acidic is generated. Other causes of metabolic alkalosis that are sensitive to the administration of chloride include those occurring after hypercapnic and after diuretic use.

As noted above, in order to maintain the alkalosis, renal bicarbonate excretion must be impaired in some way. In the setting of chloride depletion, the kidney is unable to excrete the excess bicarbonate, and therefore, the alkalosis is maintained (Table 135.7) (43,44). Among patients with normal renal function and normal chloride status, attempting to raise the serum bicarbonate concentration 2 to 3 mEq/L above the normal value is virtually impossible because the kidneys can easily excrete the excess bicarbonate.

Chloride-Insensitive Metabolic Alkalosis

The chloride-insensitive metabolic alkalosis commonly encountered in the critical care setting is that occurring after the use of loop diuretics. The loss of large amounts of bicarbonate-free fluid in a patient with expanded ECF space—such as during therapy with a loop diuretic—is thought to lead to a reduction in the ECF space, with relative conservation of

TABLE 135.7 Classification of Metabolic Alkalosis by Chloride Handling

Chloride Sensitive (Urine Cl^-<20 mEq/L)	Chloride Resistant (Urine Cl^->40 mEq/L)
Gastrointestinal acid losses	**Hypertensive**
• Nasogastric suction, vomiting	• Renovascular hypertension
• Congenital Cl^- losses in stool?	• Hyperaldosteronism
• Rectal adenoma	• Liddle syndrome
	• Glycyrrhizic acid
Renal acid losses	**Normotensive**
• Penicillins, citrate	• Diuretics
• Postdiuretic	• Bartter and Gitelman syndromes
• Posthypercapnic	• Administration of alkali

bicarbonate concentration. This has been termed *contraction alkalosis*. In the physiochemical model, the explanation for the acid base disturbance that develops in this situation is that the change in relative content of the strong ions in the ECF compartment leads secondarily to changes in plasma bicarbonate. Recall that the ratio of sodium to chloride in the ECF compartment is typically 1.4:1 and the when the sodium, potassium chloride co-transporter is inhibited, the loss of sodium + potassium in the urine is in a stoichiometric ratio of 1:1. Other causes of chloride-insensitive metabolic alkalosis are hyperaldosteronism—both primary and secondary—such as might be seen with renovascular disease (see Table 135.7). Rare causes of chloride-insensitive metabolic alkalosis are Bartter and Gitelman syndromes.

Renal and Extrarenal Compensation

Immediately following the generation of metabolic alkalosis, buffering systems begin to decrease the effects of the alkaline load. Respiratory compensation for a metabolic alkalosis involves respiratory suppression and an increase in the PCO_2 (see Fig. 42.3A and Table 135.3). Respiratory compensation for severe metabolic alkalosis has practical limits, as respirations can be suppressed only to a certain degree. Without the effect of mitigating factors such as volume depletion, the kidney will respond to metabolic alkalosis through increasing the renal excretion of bicarbonate. Severe chloride depletion can theoretically inhibit this exchange and therefore inhibit bicarbonate secretion. Finally, hyperaldosteronism secondary to diuretic use stimulates the tubular secretion of potassium and H^+. The net effect is acidic urine that also helps to maintain the alkalosis. In patients with low urinary chloride, chloride replacement is indicated to allow bicarbonate excretion.

Treatment of Metabolic Alkalosis

The metabolic alkalosis seen in the intensive care unit often develops as a complication rather than a presenting disorder. The use of diuretics and nasogastric suctioning is commonplace in the intensive care unit and often leads to metabolic alkalosis. In patients with chloride-sensitive metabolic alkalosis, treatment usually consists of replacement of the chloride deficit—usually with normal saline since volume depletion is also often present. Potassium chloride is almost always indicated when hypokalemia is also present, although potassium concentrations may increase as the alkalosis is corrected. In severe, symptomatic metabolic alkalosis—a pH greater than 7.6—hemodialysis may be indicated and can be used to correct

TABLE 135.8 Treatment of Metabolic Alkalosis

Chloride sensitive
- IV normal saline volume expansion
- Discontinue diuretics if possible
- H_2 blockers or proton pump inhibitors in cases of nasogastric suction and vomiting

Chloride resistant
- Remove offending agent
- Replace potassium if deficient

Extreme alkalosis
- Hemodialysis
- NH_4Cl or HCl can also be used

alkalemia, especially when associated with renal failure (45). The use of acidic solutions is rarely indicated (Table 135.8).

Case #7: MIXED ACID–BASE DISTURBANCE: DIABETIC KETOACIDOSIS WITH CONCOMITANT METABOLIC ALKALOSIS—CLINICAL USE OF THE DELTA–DELTA GAP

A 21-year-old man presents to the emergency room with severely diminished mental status. He states that he has felt nauseated for the last few days and has been unable to eat well. This morning, he vomited several times and was brought to the emergency room by his girlfriend. His past medical history is negative for any chronic medical problems. He had a tonsillectomy as a child but no other surgeries. Physical examination is significant for blood pressure of 122/57 mmHg, pulse of 105 beats/min, respiratory rate of 28 breaths/min, and temperature of 99.3°F. He is thin and in moderate distress. Chest examination is normal. His abdomen is soft and nontender. Stool is negative for occult blood. In the emergency room, the patient begins to vomit large amounts, and he aspirates a significant amount of stomach contents and develops respiratory failure. He is intubated and started on mechanical ventilation. After 1 hour of mechanical ventilation, the following laboratory values are received:

Serum	
Sodium (mEq/L)	138 mEq/L
Potassium (mEq/L)	3.7 mEq/L
Chloride (mEq/L)	91 mEq/L
Bicarbonate (mEq/L)	16 mEq/L
BUN (mg/dL)	11 mg/dL
Creatinine (mg/dL)	1.7 mg/dL
Phosphorus (mg/dL)	2.2 mg/dL
Albumin (g/dL)	3.6 g/dL
Glucose (mg/dL)	980 mg/dL
Arterial blood gas	
pH	7.41
pO_2	67 mmHg
PCO_2	27 mmHg

- **What is the acid–base disturbance present in this patient?**
This patient has a mixed acid–base disorder, metabolic acidosis/metabolic alkalosis. The patient presents with diabetic ketoacidosis. The anion gap is 31, which signifies a large degree of ketoacid production. Because of the nausea and vomiting, he also has developed a metabolic alkalosis, and thus the bicarbonate level is higher than one would expect with this degree of acid production. This can be formalized by calculating the delta–delta anion gap. Another method of conceptualizing what is occurring is to take the difference of the anion gap and a normal anion gap. To illustrate how this works, we define the normal anion gap as 12 mEq/L. In this case, the difference between

the patient's anion gap and the normal anion gap is 31 − 12 = 19 mEq/L. This difference is often referred to as the delta–delta anion gap. If this number is added to the patient's bicarbonate, the result is 35. This significantly exceeds the normal bicarbonate of 24, which indicates that a metabolic alkalosis is present. What this tells us is that if all of the unmeasured anions—which are potentially bicarbonate—are converted back to bicarbonate, the patient would be considered to have a metabolic alkalosis.

Respiratory Acid-Base Disorders

Under normal conditions, through endogenous metabolism, approximately 15,000 mmol/d of CO_2 is produced. Carbon dioxide enters the plasma and forms carbonic acid, which subsequently dissociates to bicarbonate and H^+. The majority of this CO_2 generated is transported to the lungs in the form of bicarbonate. The H^+ produced in the process is exchanged across the erythrocyte cell membrane and is buffered intracellularly. In the alveoli, this process is reversed and the bicarbonate combines with H^+, liberating CO_2, which is then excreted through respiration. Carbon dioxide is the main stimulus for respiration, which is activated by small elevations in the PCO_2. Hypoxia is a minor stimulus for respiration and is typically effective when the PO_2 is in the range of 50 to 55 mmHg. Derangements in respiratory CO_2 excretion lead to alterations in the ratio of PCO_2 to bicarbonate in the serum and, therefore, alter systemic pH (recall the Henderson–Hasselbalch relationship, Equation 4).

Respiratory Acidosis

Respiratory acidosis results from the primary retention of carbon dioxide; a variety of disorders that reduce ventilation can lead to respiratory acidosis. The common etiologies of respiratory acidosis seen in intensive care unit patients are listed in Table 135.9.

The increase in the plasma PCO_2 decreases the pH by formation of carbonic acid (Equation 11). The principal compensatory defense mechanisms against respiratory acidosis are buffering and renal compensation. Recalling the Henderson–Hasselbalch relationship (Equation 4), the pH of the blood is dependent on the relative concentrations of CO_2 and bicarbonate. Therefore, when there is an increase in PCO_2, the renal response to increase HCO_3^- is an action to normalize this relationship (see Fig. 42.3B). In respiratory acidosis, the extracellular buffering capacity is severely limited because bicarbonate cannot buffer carbonic acid. Intracellular buffers—hemoglobin and other intracellular proteins—serve as the protection against acute rises in PCO_2. In circulating erythrocytes, the H^+ that is produced as carbonic acid is formed from CO_2 that is buffered by hemoglobin; bicarbonate then leaves the cell in exchange for chloride. The buffering response to an elevation of CO_2 occurs within 10 to 15 minutes.

Renal compensation occurs in response to chronic respiratory acidosis. Hypercapnia stimulates secretion of protons in the distal nephron. Additionally, the urinary pH decreases and urinary ammonium excretion is increased, as is titratable acid excretion and excretion of chloride. The net effect is enhanced reabsorption of bicarbonate. The kidney's response to an acute increase in PCO_2 through compensation takes 3 to 4 days to reach completion (see Table 135.3).

Aside from the compensatory mechanisms mentioned above, an increase in alveolar ventilation is ultimately required in order to eliminate excess CO_2 and therefore to re-establish equilibrium. If ventilation increases quickly during the acute period, the decrease in PCO_2 re-establishes equilibrium. However, following sustained hypercapnia that has elicited an appropriate renal response (i.e., a compensatory increase in serum bicarbonate), bicarbonaturia accompanies the return of the PCO_2 to normal. However, in order for this to occur, the chloride intake must be sufficient to replenish the deficit that developed during the renal compensation to the chronic respiratory acidosis, which induces a negative chloride balance. If chloride is deficient, the serum bicarbonate will remain persistently elevated, a phenomenon termed posthypercapnic metabolic alkalosis.

TABLE 135.9 Causes of Respiratory Acidosis

Airway obstruction
- Foreign body, aspiration
- Obstructive sleep apnea
- Laryngospasm or bronchospasm

Neuromuscular disorders of respiration

Acute
- Myasthenia gravis
- Guillain-Barré syndrome
- Botulism, tetanus, drugs
- Hypokalemia, hypophosphatemia (respiratory muscle impairment)
- Cervical spinal injury

Chronic
- Morbid obesity (aka Pickwickian syndrome)
- Central sleep apnea

Central respiratory depression
- Drugs (opiates, sedatives), anesthetics
- Oxygen administration in acute hypercapnia
- Brain trauma or stroke

Respiratory disorders

Acute
- Severe pulmonary edema
- Asthma or pneumonia
- Acute respiratory distress syndrome
- Chronic obstructive pulmonary disorder
- Pulmonary fibrosis

Chronic
- Chronic pneumonitis

Clinical Presentation. Acute respiratory acidosis can produce headaches, confusion, irritability, anxiety, and insomnia, although the symptoms are difficult to separate from concomitant hypoxemia. Symptoms may progress to asterixis, delirium, and somnolence. The severity of the clinical presentation correlates more closely with the rapidity of the development of the disturbance rather than the absolute PCO_2 level.

Treatment. The treatment of respiratory acidosis is focused on alleviating the underlying disorder. In patients with acute respiratory acidosis and hypoxemia, supplemental oxygen is appropriate. However, to treat the hypercapnia, an increase in effective alveolar ventilation is necessary through either reversal of the underlying cause or, if necessary, mechanical ventilation. The administration of bicarbonate in respiratory acidosis when a coexisting metabolic acidosis is not present is potentially harmful. Bicarbonate in the setting of acute respiratory acidosis may precipitate acute pulmonary edema, metabolic alkalosis, and augmented carbon dioxide production, leading to increased PCO_2 in patients with inadequate respiratory reserve (45).

During chronic respiratory acidosis, renal compensation leads to a near-normalization of the arterial pH. In treating chronic respiratory acidosis, the objective is to ensure adequate oxygenation and, if possible, to increase alveolar ventilation. The administration of excessive oxygen and use of sedatives should be avoided because these treatments can depress the respiratory drive. Mechanical ventilation may be indicated when there is an acute exacerbation of chronic hypercapnia. If mechanical ventilation is used, the PCO_2 should be decreased gradually, avoiding precipitous drops, as rapid correction may cause severe alkalemia. Also, this may increase the cerebrospinal fluid pH, because carbon dioxide rapidly equilibrates across the blood–cerebrospinal fluid barrier. This complication can lead to serious neurologic problems, including seizures and death.

Special Scenario: Permissive Hypercapnia. It has been shown that ventilator strategies to reduce ventilator-associated lung injury (VALI) improve intensive care unit outcomes (46–49). This strategy is referred to as permissive hypercapnia and may reduce VALI through several mechanisms: by reducing stretch trauma and associated release of cytokines, and by preventing translocation of endotoxin and bacteria across the alveolar capillary barrier (50–54). It is not known for certain if respiratory acidosis per se has a beneficial effect, though there are recent data to suggest such an effect (55). Primary elevation of PCO_2 is also suggested to be deleterious on cardiac function (27,28), though this may be outweighed by protective effects of hypercapnia on lung injury (56). Further studies will be needed to delineate the specific roles of low tidal volume and respiratory acidosis with or without buffering in the management of acute lung injury.

Case #8: RESPIRATORY ACIDOSIS

A 56-year-old morbidly obese patient is admitted to the hospital with severe cellulitis of the right lower extremity that fails to respond to intravenous antibiotics. On hospital day 3, he undergoes a right below-knee amputation and, although recovering well, complains of severe pain postoperatively. His blood cultures drawn at admission are negative. His past medical history is significant for diabetes mellitus and chronic lower extremity ulceration that is felt to be secondary to venous stasis. Current medications include hydrochlorothiazide 25 mg PO daily, amlodipine 10 mg PO daily, enalapril 10 mg PO bid, metformin 1,000 mg PO bid, and a fentanyl patch 25 μg/hr. Two days following the operation he is found to have diminished mental status and the following laboratory data are obtained:

Serum	
Sodium	140 mEq/L
Potassium	4.4 mEq/L
Chloride	98 mEq/L
Bicarbonate	34 mEq/L
BUN	19 mg/dL
Creatinine	1.2 mg/dL
Phosphorus	4.3 mg/dL
Albumin	3.7 g/dL
Glucose	180 mg/dL
Arterial blood gas	
pH	7.09
PO_2	55 mmHg
PCO_2	110 mmHg

- **Which medication contributed most to the acid–base disorder prior to initiation of mechanical ventilation?**

The laboratory values are consistent with acute respiratory acidosis, secondary to fentanyl, likely in the setting of a chronic respiratory acidosis, itself probably secondary to restrictive lung disease from obesity. The chronic respiratory acidosis is evidenced by the increased serum bicarbonate with a decreased pH. This is consistent with a history of obesity, which can lead to a restrictive pattern of lung disease characterized by chronic respiratory insufficiency. An acute respiratory acidosis is present because the expected degree of renal compensation is not present as it would be if the patient had a chronic elevation of the PCO_2 to levels of 110 mmHg. The acute respiratory failure is most likely secondary to narcotic overdose, and thus fentanyl is the most likely causative agent.

Respiratory Alkalosis

Pathophysiology. Respiratory alkalosis is due to a primary increase in ventilation, which leads to a decrease in the PCO_2 and occurs commonly in the intensive care unit either as a treatment (e.g., for elevated intracranial pressure), as an iatrogenic complication of mechanical ventilation, or as part of a disease presentation (Table 135.10) (57). The lowered PCO_2 in turn reduces carbonic acid levels, which decreases systemic pH. The buffering system and, ultimately, renal compensation are the counterregulatory measures that are directed at maintaining plasma pH in this setting. In the setting of acute respiratory alkalosis, proteins, phosphates, and hemoglobin liberate H^+. These liberated protons subsequently react with bicarbonate to form carbonic acid. At the level of the erythrocyte, a shift of chloride to the extracellular compartment ensues, as bicarbonate and cations enter in exchange for protons. The net effect of this buffering system reduces plasma pH and accounts for a 2 mEq/L decrease in the serum bicarbonate for every 10 mmHg decrease in the PCO_2 that occurs in the acute setting (see Table 135.3). Persistent respiratory alkalemia elicits the renal response, which leads to a net decrease in the secretion of H^+. This renal compensation causes a decrease in the proximal reabsorption of bicarbonate and a decrease in

TABLE 135.10 Causes of Respiratory Alkalosis

Hypoxia
- High altitude
- Congestive heart failure
- Severe V/Q mismatch

Lung diseases
- Pulmonary fibrosis
- Pulmonary edema
- Pneumonia
- Pulmonary embolism

Drugs
- Salicylates
- Progesterone
- Nicotine

Direct stimulation of respiratory drive
- Psychogenic hyperventilation
- Cirrhosis
- Gram-negative sepsis
- Pregnancy (progesterone)
- Excessive mechanical ventilation
- Neurologic disorders (e.g., pontine tumors)

the excretion of titratable acids and of ammonium. Recall that the excretion of one H^+ in the kidney leads to the regeneration of a HCO_3^- molecule; therefore, these renal changes decrease renal production of HCO_3^-. This compensatory response is maximal 3 to 4 days following the onset of alkalemia and leads to further decrease in serum HCO_3^-.

Clinical Presentation. Respiratory alkalosis may lead to a wide range of clinical manifestations ranging from alteration in consciousness, perioral paresthesias, and muscle spasms to cardiac arrhythmias. In addition, alkalemia also can affect metabolism of divalent ions. By stimulating glycolysis, alkalemia causes phosphate to shift from the extracellular space into the intracellular compartment as glucose-6-phosphate is formed. Additionally, the level of ionized calcium in the blood may also decrease due to increased binding of calcium to albumin.

Treatment. The underlying cause for respiratory alkalosis should be sought (see Table 135.10). Cirrhosis can lead to respiratory alkalosis through impaired clearance from the circulation of progesterones and estrogens, similar to pregnancy (58). This is a commonly seen acid–base disorder in the intensive care unit. In psychogenic hyperventilation, rebreathing air using a bag increases the systemic PCO_2 and can treat alkalemia. Specific therapy, other than treatment of the underlying cause, is typically not necessary.

Case #9: SEVERE ACUTE RESPIRATORY ALKALOSIS: A POTENTIAL COMPLICATION OF MECHANICAL VENTILATION

A 42-year-old patient with morbid obesity is admitted to the hospital with shortness of breath and fever. In the emergency room, he is started on intravenous antibiotics. Over the next 3 hours, he becomes severely short of breath and develops a diminished level of consciousness. He is intubated and placed on mechanical ventilation. His past medical history is significant for diabetes mellitus and hypertension. The social history is significant for one pack per day of smoking for 20 years. Current medications include amlodipine 5 mg PO daily, enalapril 5 mg PO bid, and hydrochlorothiazide 12.5 mg PO bid. Physical examination shows blood pressure of 156/80 mmHg, pulse of 70 beats/min, and temperature of 100.8°F. The patient is morbidly obese. The cardiovascular examination is normal. Lung examination reveals bilateral breath sounds with diffuse crackles on the right and egophony. Thirty minutes after mechanical ventilation laboratory studies are sent, with the following results:

Serum	
Sodium	140 mEq/L
Potassium	4.4 mEq/L
Chloride	97 mEq/L
Bicarbonate	35 mEq/L
BUN	15 mg/dL
Creatinine	0.9 mg/dL
Phosphorus	4.0 mg/dL
Albumin	3.9 g/dL
Glucose	146 mg/dL
Arterial blood gas	
pH	7.66
PO_2	340 mmHg
PCO^2	31 mmHg

- **What PCO_2 goal should be targeted in order to correct the acid–base disorder and attain a normal pH?**

The respiratory rate should be decreased to maintain the pH at a level of about 55 mmHg, as this will lead to a pH of approximately 7.4. When a patient with chronic respiratory acidosis and appropriate renal compensation is placed on mechanical ventilation, he or she is at risk of developing a posthypercapnic metabolic alkalosis, as occurred in this case. Quickly lowering the PCO_2 in a patient with an elevated bicarbonate can lead to a dangerous degree of alkalemia. This occurs because mechanical ventilation can remove PCO_2 from the blood quickly, thus increasing the pH precipitously. However, it takes time for the kidney to adapt to the change in blood pH. In time, the kidney can adapt by decreasing bicarbonate reabsorption, leading to loss of bicarbonate in the urine; but this does not happen quickly, usually requiring a minimum of 24 to 36 hours. The appropriate measure is to decrease the minute ventilation to allow the PCO_2 to rise to a level that would lead to a normal or slightly acidic pH. The target PCO_2 can be calculated by using the Henderson-Hasselbalch equation; however, this degree of precision is not always necessary. The minute ventilation can simply be decreased and titrated to achieve the desired pH.

MIXED ACID–BASE DISORDERS

Mixed acid–base disorders are more difficult to diagnose than simple acid–base disorders. A good general rule is to keep in mind that in patients with a known primary acid–base disorder, a mixed disorder needs to be suspected if the pH is normal or if the apparent "compensation" has led to a pH that is beyond the normal. For example, if a patient with metabolic acidosis has a pH of 7.47, this indicates an accompanying respiratory alkalosis since a compensation would not lead to an alkaline pH if the primary disorder is an acidosis.

Metabolic and Respiratory Acidosis

In this mixed disorder, respiratory compensation is insufficient for the degree of decrease in bicarbonate. The most extreme example of this mixed-condition disorder occurs following cardiopulmonary arrest. In this setting, there is a decrease in bicarbonate levels—a metabolic acidosis secondary to lactic acidosis—and retention of carbon dioxide secondary to respiratory arrest. The pH in this setting is very low. Mixed metabolic and respiratory acidosis is also commonly seen in patients with a primary metabolic acidosis and concomitant lung disease. The lung disease impairs the ability of the patient to increase the ventilatory rate to appropriately decrease the PCO_2. Furthermore, this combination of disorders can manifest as a patient with a chronically elevated PCO_2 and an inability to increase the serum bicarbonate. This would indicate a chronic respiratory acidosis and possibly a metabolic acidosis due to a "normalized" serum bicarbonate in a setting in which the bicarbonate would be expected to be elevated. Finally, the presence of an anion gap, despite a normal serum bicarbonate level, should raise the index of suspicion for this combination of conditions.

Metabolic and Respiratory Alkalosis

Acidemia is better tolerated than is alkalemia. For example, a pH of 7.2 is well tolerated, whereas a pH of greater than 7.6 is associated with significant mortality. Mixed metabolic and respiratory alkalosis can lead to a significant elevation in the pH and is therefore very serious. This condition typically occurs in patients on mechanical ventilation. Often, mechanical ventilation, by mandating a minimum minute ventilation, will not allow the patient to elevate the PCO_2 significantly in response to alkalemia. Frequently, the metabolic alkalosis in this setting is due to diuretic use, administration of bicarbonate solutions, or massive transfusions with a citrate load.

Respiratory Alkalosis and Metabolic Acidosis

Most commonly, this combination is seen in gram-negative sepsis, which can stimulate the respiratory drive—resulting in respiratory alkalosis—and also cause circulatory collapse with subsequent lactic acidosis. In the medical intensive care unit, salicylate intoxication classically leads to a mixed metabolic acidosis and respiratory alkalosis (23). Salicylates directly lead to an anion gap metabolic acidosis, and they also directly stimulate respiration.

Approach to Mixed Acid–Base Disorders

There is no simple algorithm to use in the approach to a mixed acid–base disorder. The approach outlined in Figure 135.4 assumes that only a single disorder is present. Complex acid–base problems should be suspected when the values cannot be explained by a single disorder and its compensation. An example of this might be a patient with lactic acidosis and an alkaline pH.

Case #10: MIXED ACID–BASE DISORDER: METABOLIC ACIDOSIS AND RESPIRATORY ACIDOSIS

A 64-year-old is admitted to the intensive care unit with pneumonia and septic shock. The patient states that he has had increasing shortness of breath and fever over the past 4 days. His past medical history is significant for hypertension. Surgical history is significant for a previous cholecystectomy. Medications include amlodipine and hydrochlorothiazide. Physical examination shows a blood pressure of 85/50 mmHg, pulse of 110 beats/min, respiratory rate of 22 breaths/min, and temperature of 101.8°F. The cardiovascular examination is significant for a 2/6 systolic murmur and there are crackles over his entire right lung field. There is trace pedal edema. Chemistry values on admission are given below:

Serum	
Sodium	135 mEq/L
Potassium	4.8 mEq/L
Chloride	103 mEq/L
Bicarbonate	10 mEq/L
BUN	22 mg/dL
Creatinine	1.4 mg/dL
Phosphorus	2.8 mg/dL
Albumin	3.8 g/dL
Glucose	115 mg/dL
Arterial blood gas	
pH	6.95
PO_2	51 mmHg
PCO_2	48 mmHg

- **What acid–base disorder(s) is (are) present in this patient?**
  The acid–base disorder is a mixed anion gap metabolic acidosis with a respiratory acidosis. The decrease in bicarbonate accompanied by an elevated anion gap is consistent with a primary metabolic acidosis. The expected PCO_2 using the Winter formula = 10(1.5) + 4 = 19. The PCO_2 is significantly elevated above this level, and thus a respiratory acidosis is present. The PCO_2 is much higher than would be expected based on the degree of acidemia, and thus a respiratory acidosis, secondary to inadequate ventilation from pneumonia, is present.

Key Points

- The buffering of acids allows the body to "absorb" large amounts of acid without significant disturbance in pH. It is through the excretion of the daily acid load, however, that the body is allowed to maintain acid–base balance. A highly negative urinary anion gap suggests that there is significant ammonium in the urine; in response to metabolic acidosis, this would indicate that the renal compensation is intact. A urinary anion gap that is near zero or positive suggests that there is little or no ammonium in the urine and, in the face of systemic acidosis, would indicate renal acid wasting.
- Bicarbonate is the principal buffer in the body; however, other buffers play an important role in maintaining systemic pH, and disturbances in nonbicarbonate buffers may be more important in critical illness than in other settings.
- Bicarbonate therapy is indicated for nonanion gap acidosis.
- The primary concern in anion gap acidosis is correction of the underlying cause.
- Metabolic alkalosis is often accompanied by a decrease in chloride such that the decrease offsets the incremental increase in bicarbonate.
- Metabolic alkalosis is caused by excessive bicarbonate intake or loss of H^+.
- Vomiting, nasogastric suction, and diuretics are the most frequent causes of metabolic alkalosis in the intensive care unit setting.
- In patients with metabolic alkalosis and low urinary chloride, normal saline is indicated to expand the extracellular space.
- In patients with a known primary acid–base disturbance, a mixed acid–base disorder should always be suspected if the pH is normal or the "compensation" has surpassed the normal pH.
- Mixed metabolic and respiratory acidosis occurs when the respiratory compensation is insufficient for the degree of decrease in bicarbonate.
- The presence of an increased anion gap despite normal serum bicarbonate levels should raise suspicion for mixed metabolic acidosis and metabolic alkalosis.
- Nonanion gap metabolic acidosis and anion gap metabolic acidosis can coexist.
- Gram-negative sepsis is a common cause of respiratory alkalosis and metabolic acidosis.
- Mixed metabolic acidosis and metabolic alkalosis occurs commonly in diabetic ketoacidosis.

References

1. Jorgensen K, Astrup P. Standard bicarbonate, its clinical significance, and a new method for its determination. *Scand J Clin Lab Invest.* 1957; 9(2):122–132.
2. Batlle DC, Hizon M, Cohen E, et al. The use of the urinary anion gap in the diagnosis of hyperchloremic metabolic acidosis. *N Engl J Med.* 1988;318(10):594–599.
3. Gabow PA. Disorders associated with an altered anion gap. *Kidney Int.* 1985;27(2):472–483.
4. Winter SD, Pearson JR, Gabow PA, et al. The fall of the serum anion gap. *Arch Intern Med.* 1990;150(2):311–313.
5. Sadjadi SA. A new range for the anion gap. *Ann Intern Med.* 1995; 123(10):807.
6. Figge J, Rossing TH, Fencl V. The role of serum proteins in acid–base equilibria. *J Lab Clin Med.* 1991;117(6):453–467.
7. Fencl V, Jabor A, Kazda A, et al. Diagnosis of metabolic acid–base disturbances in critically ill patients. *Am J Respir Crit Care Med.* 2000;162(6): 2246–2251.
8. Moe OW, Fuster D. Clinical acid–base pathophysiology: disorders of plasma anion gap. *Best Pract Res Clin Endocrinol Metab.* 2003;17(4):559–574.
9. Hassan H, Joh JH, Bacon BR, et al. Evaluation of serum anion gap in patients with liver cirrhosis of diverse etiologies. *Mt Sinai J Med.* 2004;71(4):281–284.
10. Schnur MJ, Appel GB, Karp G, et al. The anion gap in asymptomatic plasma cell dyscrasias. *Ann Intern Med.* 1977;86(3):304–305.
11. Murray T, Long W, Narins RG. Multiple myeloma and the anion gap. *N Engl J Med.* 1975;292(11):574–575.
12. Madias NE, Ayus JC, Adrogue HJ. Increased anion gap in metabolic alkalosis: the role of plasma-protein equivalency. *N Engl J Med.* 1979; 300(25):1421–1423.
13. Salem MM, Mujais SK. Gaps in the anion gap. *Arch Intern Med.* 1992;152(8):1625–1629.
14. Story DA, Kellum JA. New aspects of acid–base balance in intensive care. *Curr Opin Anaesthesiol.* 2004;17(2):119–123.
15. Corey HE. Stewart and beyond: new models of acid–base balance. *Kidney Int.* 2003;64(3):777–787.
16. Wooten EW. Science review: quantitative acid–base physiology using the Stewart model. *Crit Care.* 2004;8(6):448–452.
17. Story DA. Bench-to-bedside review: a brief history of clinical acid–base. *Crit Care.* 2004;8(4):253–258.
18. Kellum JA, Kramer DJ, Pinsky MR. Strong ion gap: a methodology for exploring unexplained anions. *J Crit Care.* 1995;10(2):51–55.
19. Feldman M, Soni N, Dickson B. Influence of hypoalbuminemia or hyperalbuminemia on the serum anion gap. *J Lab Clin Med.* 2005;146(6): 317–320.
20. Pierce NF, Fedson DS, Brigham KL, et al. The ventilatory response to acute base deficit in humans: time course during development and correction of metabolic acidosis. *Ann Intern Med.* 1970;72(5):633–640.
21. Adrogue HJ, Wilson H, Boyd AE III, et al. Plasma acid–base patterns in diabetic ketoacidosis. *N Engl J Med.* 1982;307(26):1603–1610.
22. Judge BS. Differentiating the causes of metabolic acidosis in the poisoned patient. *Clin Lab Med.* 2006;26(1):31–48, vii.
23. Krause DS, Wolf BA, Shaw LM. Acute aspirin overdose: mechanisms of toxicity. *Ther Drug Monit.* 1992;14(6):441–451.
24. Kurtzman NA. Disorders of distal acidification. *Kidney Int.* 1990; 38(4):720–727.
25. Narins RG, Goldberg M. Renal tubular acidosis: pathophysiology, diagnosis and treatment. *Dis Mon.* 1977;23(6):1–66.
26. DeFronzo RA. Hyperkalemia and hyporeninemic hypoaldosteronism. *Kidney Int.* 1980;17(1):118–134.
27. Arieff AI, Leach W, Park R, et al. Systemic effects of $NaHCO_3$ in experimental lactic acidosis in dogs. *Am J Physiol.* 1982;242(6):F586–F591.
28. Graf H, Leach W, Arieff AI. Evidence for a detrimental effect of bicarbonate therapy in hypoxic lactic acidosis. *Science.* 1985;227(4688):754–756.
29. Jeffrey FM, Malloy CR, Radda GK. Influence of intracellular acidosis on contractile function in the working rat heart. *Am J Physiol.* 1987;253(6 Pt 2): H1499–H1505.
30. Ayus JC, Krothapalli RK. Effect of bicarbonate administration on cardiac function. *Am J Med.* 1989;87(1):5–6.
31. Kalkut G. Antiretroviral therapy: an update for the non-AIDS specialist. *Curr Opin Oncol.* 2005;17(5):479–484.
32. Wohl DA, McComsey G, Tebas P, et al. Current concepts in the diagnosis and management of metabolic complications of HIV infection and its therapy. *Clin Infect Dis.* 2006;43(5):645–653.
33. Moyle GJ, Datta D, Mandalia S, et al. Hyperlactataemia and lactic acidosis during antiretroviral therapy: relevance, reproducibility and possible risk factors. *AIDS.* 2002;16(10):1341–1349.
34. Tebb Z, Tobias JD. New anticonvulsants–new adverse effects. *South Med J.* 2006;99(4):375–379.
35. Guo PY, Storsley LJ, Finkle SN. Severe lactic acidosis treated with prolonged hemodialysis: recovery after massive overdoses of metformin. *Semin Dial.* 2006;19(1):80–83.
36. Parke TJ, Stevens JE, Rice AS, et al. Metabolic acidosis and fatal myocardial failure after propofol infusion in children: five case reports. *BMJ.* 1992;305(6854):613–616.
37. Cremer OL, Moons KG, Bouman EA, et al. Long-term propofol infusion and cardiac failure in adult head-injured patients. *Lancet.* 2001;357(9250):117–118.
38. Perrier ND, Baerga-Varela Y, Murray MJ. Death related to propofol use in an adult patient. *Crit Care Med.* 2000;28(8):3071–3074.
39. Vasile B, Rasulo F, Candiani A, et al. The pathophysiology of propofol infusion syndrome: a simple name for a complex syndrome. *Intensive Care Med.* 2003;29(9):1417–1425.
40. Corbett SM, Moore J, Rebuck JA, et al. Survival of propofol infusion syndrome in a head-injured patient. *Crit Care Med.* 2006;34(9):2479–2483.
41. Wolf A, Weir P, Segar P, et al. Impaired fatty acid oxidation in propofol infusion syndrome. *Lancet.* 2001;357(9256):606–607.
42. Cray SH, Robinson BH, Cox PN. Lactic acidemia and bradyarrhythmia in a child sedated with propofol. *Crit Care Med.* 1998;26(12):2087–2092.
43. Luke RG, Galla JH. Chloride-depletion alkalosis with a normal extracellular fluid volume. *Am J Physiol.* 1983;245(4):F419–F424.
44. Galla JH, Bonduris DN, Luke RG. Effects of chloride and extracellular fluid volume on bicarbonate reabsorption along the nephron in metabolic alkalosis in the rat: reassessment of the classical hypothesis of the pathogenesis of metabolic alkalosis. *J Clin Invest.* 1987;80(1):41–50.
45. Ayus JC, Olivero JJ, Adrogue HJ. Alkalemia associated with renal failure: correction by hemodialysis with low-bicarbonate dialysate. *Arch Intern Med.* 1980;140(4):513–515.
46. Amato MB, Barbas CS, Medeiros DM, et al. Effect of a protective-ventilation strategy on mortality in the acute respiratory distress syndrome. *N Engl J Med.* 1998;338(6):347–354.
47. Hickling KG, Walsh J, Henderson S, et al. Low mortality rate in adult respiratory distress syndrome using low-volume, pressure-limited ventilation with permissive hypercapnia: a prospective study. *Crit Care Med.* 1994;22(10):1568–1578.
48. Brower RG, Rubenfeld GD. Lung-protective ventilation strategies in acute lung injury. *Crit Care Med.* 2003;31(4 Suppl):S312–S316.
49. Laffey JG, O'Croinin D, McLoughlin P, et al. Permissive hypercapnia–role in protective lung ventilatory strategies. *Intensive Care Med.* 2004; 30(3):347–356.
50. Maggiore SM, Jonson B, Richard JC, et al. Alveolar derecruitment at decremental positive end-expiratory pressure levels in acute lung injury: comparison with the lower inflection point, oxygenation, and compliance. *Am J Respir Crit Care Med.* 2001;164(5):795–801.
51. Boussarsar M, Thierry G, Jaber S, et al. Relationship between ventilatory settings and barotrauma in the acute respiratory distress syndrome. *Intensive Care Med.* 2002;28(4):406–413.
52. Slutsky AS, Tremblay LN. Multiple system organ failure. Is mechanical ventilation a contributing factor? *Am J Respir Crit Care Med.* 1998;157(6 Pt 1): 1721–1725.
53. Tremblay L, Valenza F, Ribeiro SP, et al. Injurious ventilatory strategies increase cytokines and c-fos m-RNA expression in an isolated rat lung model. *J Clin Invest.* 1997;99(5):944–952.
54. Murphy DB, Cregg N, Tremblay L, et al. Adverse ventilatory strategy causes pulmonary-to-systemic translocation of endotoxin. *Am J Respir Crit Care Med.* 2000;162(1):27–33.
55. Kregenow DA, Rubenfeld GD, Hudson LD, et al. Hypercapnic acidosis and mortality in acute lung injury. *Crit Care Med.* 2006;34(1):1–7.
56. Sinclair SE, Kregenow DA, Lamm WJ, et al. Hypercapnic acidosis is protective in an in vivo model of ventilator-induced lung injury. *Am J Respir Crit Care Med.* 2002;166(3):403–408.
57. Laffey JG, Kavanagh BP. Hypocapnia. *N Engl J Med.* 2002;347(1):43–53.
58. Lustik SJ, Chhibber AK, Kolano JW, et al. The hyperventilation of cirrhosis: progesterone and estradiol effects. *Hepatology.* 1997;25(1):55–58.

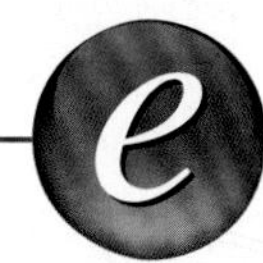

This chapter can be accessed in the accompanying eBook (see inside front cover for access instructions).

CHAPTER
136

Endocrinopathy in the ICU

ADRIEN BOUGLE and DJILLALI ANNANE

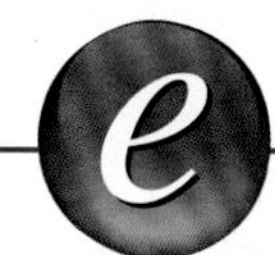

This chapter can be accessed in the accompanying eBook (see inside front cover for access instructions).

CHAPTER
137

Disordered Glucose Metabolism

ELAMIN M. ELAMIN and CHAKRAPOL SRIAROON

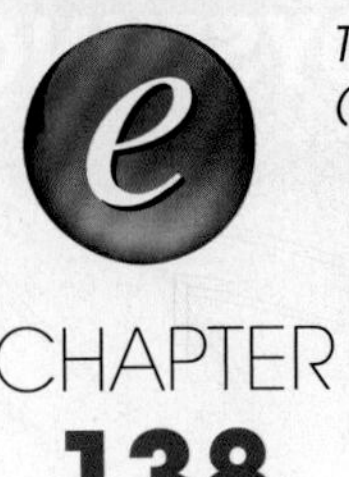

This chapter can be accessed in the accompanying eBook (see inside front cover for access instructions).

CHAPTER
138

The Adrenal Gland in Critical Illness

MARK COOPER

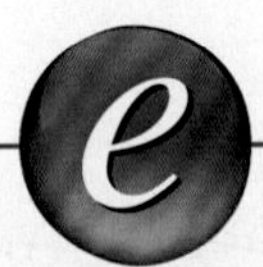

This chapter can be accessed in the accompanying eBook (see inside front cover for access instructions).

CHAPTER
139

Pheochromocytoma

DANIEL T. RUAN and QUAN-YANG DUH

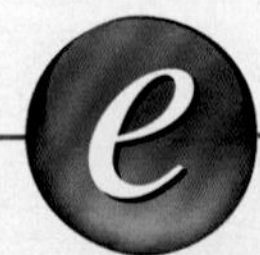

This chapter can be accessed in the accompanying eBook (see inside front cover for access instructions).

CHAPTER
140

Thyroid Disease in the Intensive Care Unit

WILLIAM CANCE

SECTION 16 SKIN, MUSCLE, AND BONE DISEASE AND DYSFUNCTION

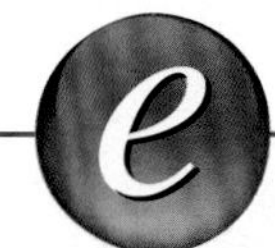

This chapter can be accessed in the accompanying eBook (see inside front cover for access instructions).

CHAPTER 141

Critical Care of Autoimmune and Connective Tissue Disorders: Rheumatologic Diseases in the Intensive Care Unit

YEHUDA

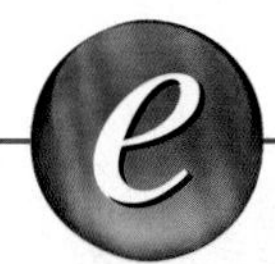

This chapter can be accessed in the accompanying eBook (see inside front cover for access instructions).

CHAPTER 142

Dermatologic Conditions/Prevention of Pressure Injuries in the Intensive Care Unit

LARRY CARUSO and JOSE JAVIER TRUJILLANO CABELLO

CHAPTER
143

Coagulation Issues

ROBERT I. PARKER

INTRODUCTION

This chapter focuses on a variety of pathophysiologic conditions associated with abnormal hemostasis or abnormal laboratory measurements of hemostasis. In order to understand how to approach a patient with a bleeding problem, this chapter will start with a brief overview of our current understanding of coagulation including an overview of the processes involved in the regulation of hemostasis and a brief discussion of the interactions of coagulation and inflammation. The coagulopathic conditions frequently encountered in the intensive care unit (ICU) can be arbitrarily divided into three categories: conditions associated with serious bleeding or a high probability of bleeding; thrombotic syndromes or conditions associated with a higher probability of thrombosis; and systemic diseases associated with acquired selective coagulation factor deficiencies. In addition, there are a few conditions associated with abnormal coagulation screening tests that represent laboratory phenomena that are not associated with an increased risk of bleeding. A topical listing of these conditions is included for review in Table 143.1. The order in which these categories are listed suggests their relative importance to the critical care practitioner. This chapter will then end by noting future directions in research and care of the critically ill patient with a hemostatic abnormality. While space limitation will not allow for a comprehensive discussion of all aspects of pathophysiology, clinical presentation, and management of hemorrhagic and thrombotic disorders encountered in the ICU, the goal is to provide a framework that will allow the reader to garner a basic understanding of the issues and direct him/her toward additional sources of information.

OVERVIEW OF COAGULATION

Traditionally, medical students have been taught that the process of blood clotting is divided into the "intrinsic," "extrinsic," and "common" pathways (Fig. 143.1), and students often come away with the thought that clotting occurs as the result of an orderly, sequential process. While this arbitrary segmentation of the clotting process may allow for a basic level of understanding, it obscures the fact that once initiated, clot production and clot destruction (fibrinolysis) occur simultaneously, and also minimizes the role platelets and the endothelium play in the overall process. This section of the chapter will try to clarify some of the newer thoughts on coagulation and the overall process of hemostasis.

While previously it was thought that the "intrinsic" pathway beginning with the activation of factor XII (F.XII) to activated factor XII (F.XIIa) in contact with some biologic or foreign surface was physiologically most important in the initiation of clot formation, we now know that the activation of F.X to F.Xa through the action of the F.VIIa/tissue factor (TF) complex is paramount in this regard (1,2). It is also evident that the various elements of the clotting cascade frequently act in concert; hence the use of the term "tenase" to describe the action of F.VIIa /TF complex along with the F.IXa/F.VIIIa complex on the activation of factor X to Xa, and the use of the term "prothrombinase" to describe the factor Xa/Va complex which cleaves prothrombin (factor II) to form thrombin (factor IIa). In addition, we now know that there is both "cross-talk" between the two arms of the clotting cascade and downstream effects of several clotting factors. Chief among these is the ability of F.VIIa to enhance the activation of F.IX (to F.IXa) and F.XI (to F.XIa) (further pointing out the central role F.VIIa and TF play *in vivo*) and the procoagulant effect of F.XI in activating F.V and F.VIII to their active forms (F.Va and factor VIIa) (3) (Fig. 143.2). Furthermore, there are various "feedback" loops, principally involving thrombin, that enhance the "upstream" activation and inhibition of the clotting process.

Tissue factor is present not only in the subendothelial matrix, but is also present circulating freely in plasma as soluble tissue factor and can be identified on cellular elements such as monocytes. However, clotting does not occur in free-flowing blood but rather on surfaces. Platelets, endothelial cells, the subendothelial matrix, and biologic polymers (e.g., catheters, grafts, stents, etc.) can provide these surfaces for clot formation and all play a critical role in clot formation.

Platelets not only initiate the clot formation through the formation of a platelet plug, but, more importantly, they bring specialized proteins that regulate the clotting response (e.g., F.VIII, inhibitors of fibrinolysis, etc.) to the area of bleeding, and provide a surface for the colocalization of clotting factors for efficient clot formation (Fig. 143.3). Platelets do not ordinarily adhere to the vascular endothelium, but when the endothelium is mechanically disrupted (e.g., cut) or activated by inflammation, platelets will then bind to the endothelial cell or subendothelial matrix via a von Willebrand factor (vWf)-dependent mechanism. Once adherent, the platelets become activated and secrete various molecules that further enhance

TABLE 143.1 Overview of Coagulation Disorders Seen in the ICU

Conditions associated with serious bleeding or a high probability of bleeding
Disseminated intravascular coagulation (DIC)
Liver disease/hepatic insufficiency
Vitamin K deficiency/depletion
Massive transfusion syndrome
Anticoagulant overdose (heparin, warfarin)
Thrombocytopenia (drug-induced, immunologic)
Acquired platelet defects (drug-induced, uremia)
Thrombotic clinical syndromes
Thombotic thrombocytopenia purpura/hemolytic uremic syndrome
Deep venous thrombosis
Pulmonary embolism
Coronary thrombosis/acute myocardial infarction
Laboratory abnormalities not associated with clinical bleeding
Lupus anticoagulant
Reactive hyperfibrinogenemia
Other selected clinical syndromes
Hemophilia (A and B)
Specific factor deficiencies associated with specific diseases
Amyloidosis–factor X, Gaucher's–factor IX, nephrotic syndrome–factor IX, antithrombin III
Cyanotic congenital heart disease (polycythemia, qualitative platelet defect)
Depressed clotting factor levels (newborns)

platelet adherence and aggregation, vascular contraction, clot formation, and wound healing (4).

The endothelium is a specialized organ that plays a central role in the regulation of clot formation (i.e., hemostasis) by presenting a nonthrombogenic surface to flowing blood and by enhancing clot formation when the endothelium is disrupted by trauma or injured by infection or inflammation (Fig. 143.4) (5,6). The normal endothelium produces inhibitors of blood coagulation and platelet activation and modulates vascular tone and permeability. Endothelial cells also synthesize and secrete the components of the subendothelial extracellular matrix including adhesive glycoproteins, collagen, fibronectin, and vWf. When disrupted, bleeding occurs. However, when injured, the endothelium often becomes a prothrombotic rather than an antithrombotic organ and unwanted clot formation may occur. The final phase in hemostasis, fibrinolysis, is also dependent on both plasma and endothelial cell factors (Fig. 143.5). None of these are measured in the traditional tests of coagulation (i.e., PT, aPTT) and, consequently, these tests will be normal unless the pace of fibrinolysis is such that clotting factor consumption is greater that replacement (i.e., a consumptive coagulopathy, DIC) (7). Fibrinolysis is initiated once thrombin is generated and will result in an increase in fibrin and fibrinogen fragments (D-dimer or FSPs/FDPs, respectively). Thrombin binding to thrombomodulin on the endothelial surface is a critical step in the thrombin-mediated activation of protein C (to produce activated protein C; aPC) and for the activation of thrombin-activatable fibrinolysis inhibitor (TAFI). However, activation or injury to endothelial cells frequently results in a shedding of surface expressed thrombomodulin (and an increase in plasma soluble thrombomodulin) and, therefore, a downregulation in intrinsic anticoagulation (i.e., decrease in aPC) and fibrinolysis inhibition (i.e., decreased TAFI), both of which will increase the risk of microvascular thrombosis and development of multiorgan dysfunction (8,9).

INTERACTION OF COAGULATION AND INFLAMMATION

There are multiple points of intersection between the biochemical events of inflammation and those of coagulation and fibrinolysis (10–12). While a full discussion of these points is beyond the scope of this chapter, the "cross-talk" between inflammation and coagulation likely takes place at the level of the endothelium, and is bidirectional wherein activation

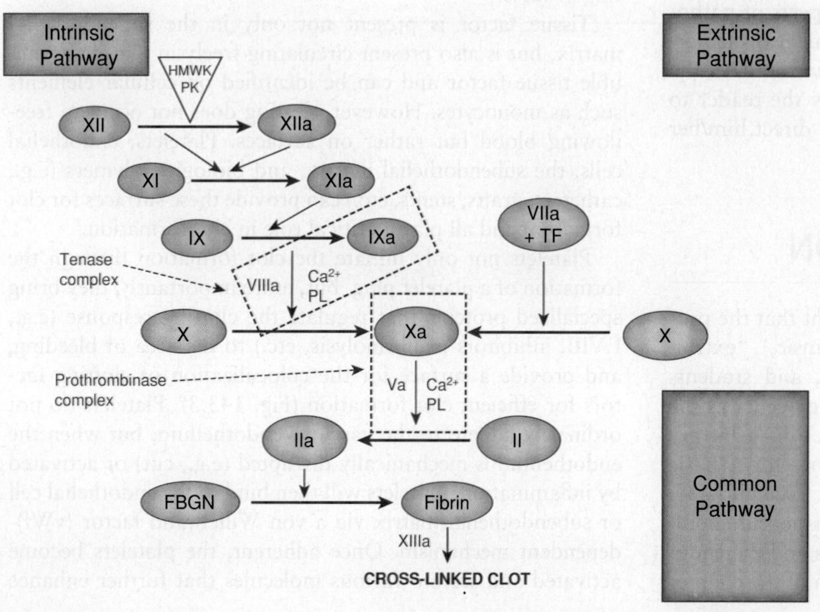

FIGURE 143.1 Classical coagulation pathway. Coagulation is initiated either through the intrinsic pathway by activation of factor XII by the generation of high-molecular-weight kininogen and kallekrein, or through activation of the extrinsic pathway by tissue factor. Roman numerals indicate zymogen clotting factors; "a" indicates activated forms of the clotting factors.

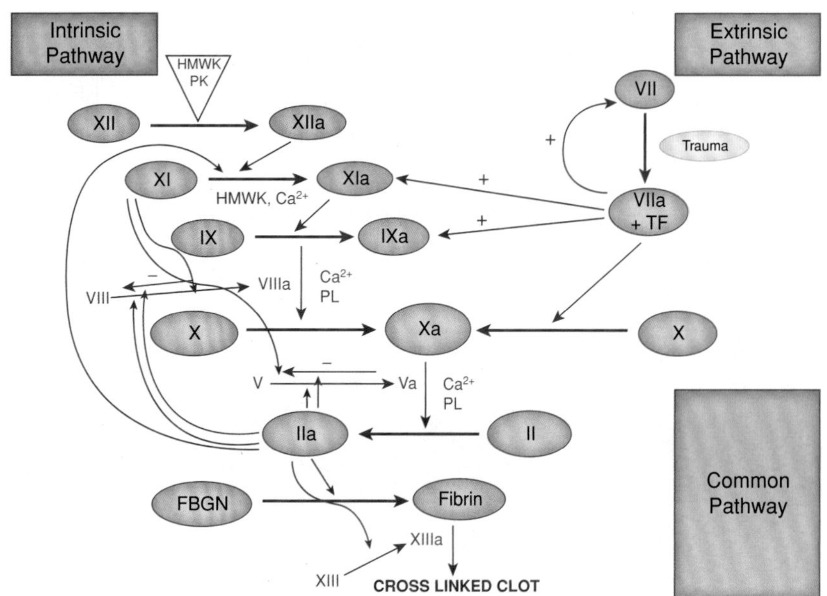

FIGURE 143.2 Modified clotting cascade indicating cross-talk between the intrinsic and extrinsic pathways by the action of VIIa/tissue factor (TF) enhancing the conversion of factor XI to activated factor XI (XIa) (*dotted lines*).

of either pathway affects the functioning of the other (10). While many different inflammatory cytokines have been identified as promoters of a procoagulant milieu, the interconnection of TF and tissue necrosis factor-α (TNF-α) may potentially be the most important of these (13). During sepsis, tissue factor expression is upregulated in activated monocytes and endothelial cells as a response to endotoxin, with the consequence being both the secretion of pro-inflammatory cytokines (e.g., IL-6, TNF) from activated mononuclear cells, and the activation of coagulation. This results in increased thrombin production which plays a central role in coagulation and inflammation through the induction of procoagulant, anticoagulant, inflammatory, and mitogenic responses (12). Thrombin results in the activation, aggregation and lysis of leukocytes and platelets, activation of endothelial cells with resultant increase in pro-inflammatory cytokines IL-6 and TNF expression. The net result of thrombin generation is to produce a pro-inflammatory and procoagulant state leading to the formation of fibrin and microvascular thrombosis. However, these pro-inflammatory effects of thrombin are counterbalanced by the anti-inflammatory effects of activated protein C (aPC) (see Fig. 143.4) (12).

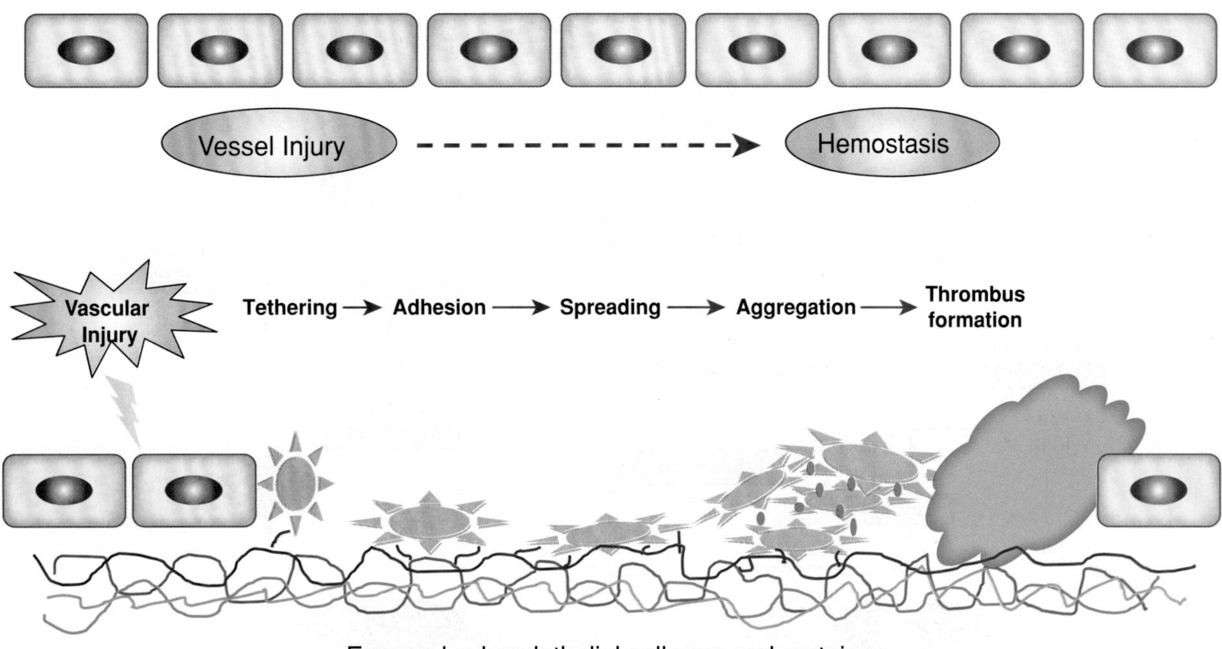

FIGURE 143.3 The role of platelets in mediating primary hemostasis at sites of vascular injury. Platelets are initially activated and express specific adhesion receptors on their surface followed by adhesion to activated endothelial cells and exposed subendothelial components (e.g., collagen, von Willebrand factor). Subsequent platelet aggregation occurs with the development of a primary platelet plug. Coagulation occurs on the developing platelet plug with the creation of a fibrin clot.

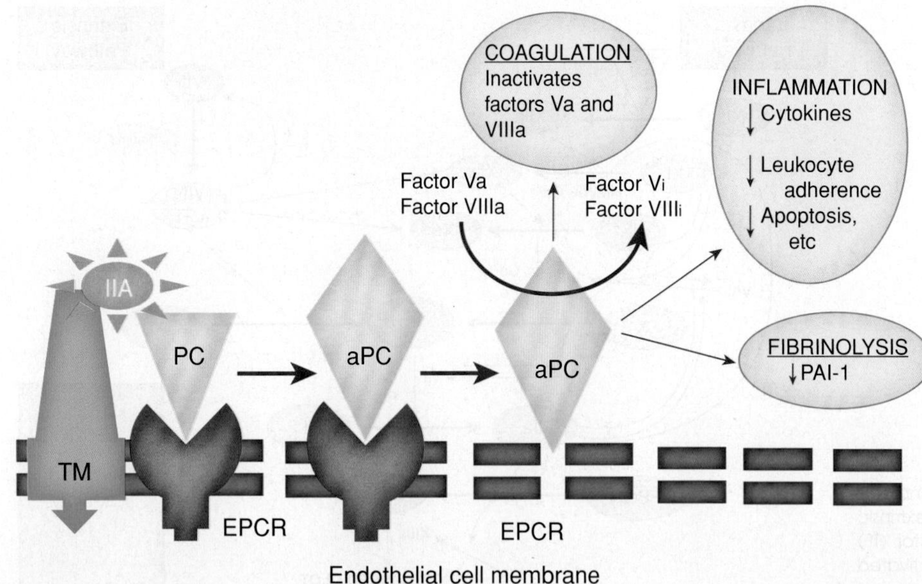

FIGURE 143.4 The interaction of the protein C system with the endothelium. Thrombin bound to thrombomodulin (TM) modifies protein C bound to the endothelial protein C receptor (EPCR) on the cell surface to generate activated protein C (aPC). aPC acts as a natural anticoagulant by inactivating activated factors V (fVa) and VIII (fVIIIa), modulates inflammation by down regulating the synthesis of pro-inflammatory cytokines, leukocyte adherence and apoptosis, and enhances fibrinolysis by inhibiting thrombin activatable fibrinolysis inhibitor (TAFI) and plasminogen activator inhibitor type-1 (PAI-1).

The second important point of connection of coagulation and inflammation is through the protein C system (14–16). While the anticoagulant effects of aPC and its cofactor protein S are well known, only recently have the anti-inflammatory roles of these proteins been appreciated. In experimental models, aPC has been shown to increase the secretion of anti-inflammatory cytokines, reduce leukocyte migration and adhesion, and protect endothelial cells from injury. Additionally, the balance between the anticoagulant and anti-inflammatory roles of aPC may be mediated by the relative distribution of free and C_4BP bound protein S (15,16). *In vitro*, aPC inhibits TNF-α elaboration from monocytes and blocks leukocyte adhesion to selectins, as well as influences apoptosis (12). The protein C pathway is engaged when thrombin binds to thrombomodulin on the surface of the endothelium. Binding of PC to the endothelial cell protein C receptor (EPCR) augments protein C activation by the thrombin–TM complex more than 10-fold *in vivo*. EPCR is shed from the endothelium through the action of inflammatory mediators and thrombin thereby down regulating aPC generation in sepsis and inflammation.

The third important link between inflammation and coagulation occurs at the level of fibrinolysis and also involves the protein C system. aPC is capable of neutralizing the fibrinolysis inhibitors plasminogen activator inhibitor type-1 (PAI-1) and thrombin activatable fibrinolysis inhibitor (TAFI). Consequently, depressed levels of aPC not only promote clot for-

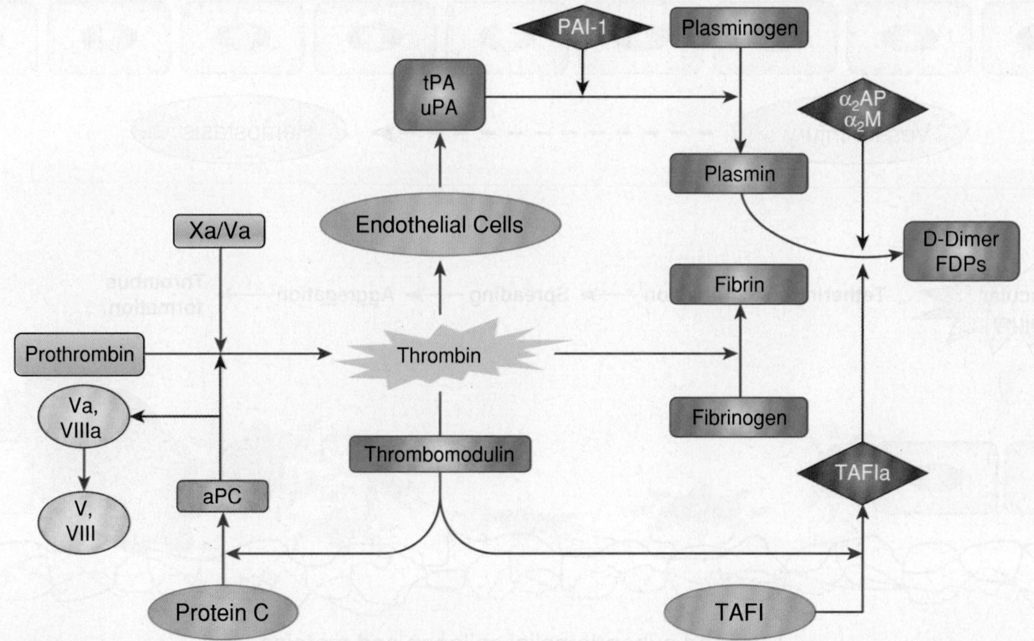

FIGURE 143.5 The generation of thrombin results in activation of endothelial cells with production of tissue-type plasminogen activator (tPA) and urothelial-type plasminogen activator (uPA). Plasminogen is converted to plasmin by tPA or uPA with resultant degradation of fibrin producing D-dimer fragments. Thrombin bound to thrombomodulin on the surface of endothelial cells activates protein C to activated protein C (aPC) and thrombin activatable fibrinolysis inhibitor (TAFI) to activated TAFI. TAFIa inhibits the action ofplasmin; additional inhibitors of plasmin are α_2-antiplasmin (α_2-AP) and α_2-macroglobulin (α_2M). Activated PC acts as an anticoagulant by degrading F.Va and F.VIIIa, and inhibiting the conversion of prothrombin to thrombin by the prothrombinase complex. Both tPA and uPA are inhibited by plasminogen activator inhibitor-type 1 (PAI-1).

mation by reducing the inactivation of the procoagulant molecule–activated factors V and VIII (F.Va, F.VIIIa) leading to increased generation of thrombin and fibrin clots, but also by limiting the fibrinolytic response needed to degrade clots. TAFI (also known as carboxypeptidase R) has also been shown to inactivate inflammatory peptides such as complement factors C3a and C5a which can play a role in the contact activation of coagulation. In addition, polymorphisms of the promoter region of the PAI-1 gene which lead to differences in PAI-1 production have been demonstrated to affect the prognosis in meningococcal sepsis in and multiple trauma pointing out the important role of this regulatory system (17). This finding points out the importance of our developing knowledge of how common polymorphisms of genes encoding important molecules affect our response to infection and injury. The importance of these interactions between coagulation and inflammation, the central role of protein C, and the importance gene polymorphisms play in host responses and clinical outcomes is further reinforced by a recent report demonstrating increased mortality and organ dysfunction and increased inflammation in patients who exhibited a specific polymorphism (1641AA) of the protein C gene (18).

AN APPROACH TO THE PATIENT WITH AN ACTUAL OR SUSPECTED COAGULATION DISORDER

Clinical History

Diagnostic assessment begins at the bedside. The medical history, both past and present, may lend some insight into the risk for significant bleeding (19,20). A prior history of prolonged or excessive bleeding or of recurrent thrombosis is important to elicit. Specific questions regarding bleeding should investigate the occurrence of any of the following: spontaneous, easy, or disproportionately severe bruising; intramuscular hematoma formation (either spontaneous or related to trauma); spontaneous or trauma-induced hemarthrosis; spontaneous mucous membrane bleeding; prior problems with bleeding related to surgery (including dental extractions, tonsillectomy, and circumcision); the need for transfusions in the past; menstrual history; and, finally, current medications. There are innumerable aspirin-containing medications available to the consumer, all of which can potentially interfere with platelet-mediated primary hemostasis. Many other drugs used in the ICU also are associated with bleeding abnormalities and are discussed later in this chapter. In situations involving trauma (either surgical or accidental), it is important to determine the severity of injury relative to the magnitude of bleeding that followed. A prior history of significant thrombosis (e.g., deep venous thrombosis, pulmonary embolus, stroke) also suggests the possibility that a hypercoagulable condition may be present. As thrombotic events are generally uncommon in younger adults, the occurrence of thrombotic events, particularly early cardiovascular events such as myocardial infarction, in young adult relatives should cause the clinician to consider the presence of a congenital thrombophilic abnormality in his patient. These include deficiencies of antithrombin III, protein C or protein S, the presence of the factor V Leiden R506Q mutation, and the prothrombin G20210A polymorphism/mutation. While the C677T mutation/polymorphism of the MTHFR (methylenetetrahydrofolate reductase) gene has previously been identified as a thrombotic risk factor, more recent evaluation of the available data suggests that the thrombophilic risk of this genetic may principally derive from the increase in serum homocysteine that can result from this mutation. Consequently, it may be that only in the presence of an elevated serum homocysteine is the C677T mutation of the MTHFR gene clinically relevant (21–23). In addition, vasculitis associated with an "autoimmune" disorder such as systemic lupus erythematosus (SLE) must always be considered in the evaluation of an individual with an unexplained pathologic clot. In all cases, the family history is important in trying to separate congenital from acquired disorders.

In a general sense, one can segregate defects into those involving primary or secondary hemostasis according to the nature of the bleeding. Patients with primary hemostatic defects tend to manifest "platelet- or capillary-type bleeding"—oozing from cuts or incisions, mucous membrane bleeding, or excessive bruising. This type of bleeding is seen in patients with quantitative or qualitative platelet defects or von Willebrand disease. In contrast, patients with deficits in secondary hemostasis tend to display "large-vessel bleeding" characterized by hemarthroses, intramuscular hematomas, and the like. This type of bleeding is most often associated with specific coagulation factor deficiencies or inhibitors.

Physical Examination

Development of generalized bleeding in critically ill ICU patients presents a special problem. Such bleeding is often associated with severe underlying multiple organ system dysfunction. Thus, correction of the coagulopathy usually requires improvement in the patient's overall clinical status. Supportive evidence or physical findings of other concurrent organ system dysfunction (e.g., oliguria or anuria, respiratory failure, hypotension) often are readily apparent. With the exception of massive transfusion syndrome (discussed later), generalized bleeding in critically ill patients is often caused by sepsis-related DIC (24,25). However, the clinician must also consider the coagulopathy of severe liver dysfunction, undiagnosed hemophilia, or, in the elderly or debilitated, vitamin K deficiency in the differential diagnosis (24–26).

The physical examination of the patient with a bleeding disorder should answer several basic questions. Is the process localized or diffuse? Is it related to an anatomic or surgical lesion? Is there mucosal bleeding? And finally, when appropriate, are there signs of thrombosis (either arterial or venous)? These answers may give clues to the cause of the problem (primary vs. secondary hemostatic dysfunction; anatomic bleeding vs. generalized coagulopathy).

During the course of the examination, particular attention should be paid to the presence of several specific physical findings that may be helpful in determining the etiology of a suspected hemostatic abnormality. For example, the presence of an enlarged spleen coupled with thrombocytopenia suggests that splenic sequestration may be a contributor to the observed thrombocytopenia. Further, evidence of liver disease (e.g., portal hypertension, ascites) points to decreased factor synthesis as a possible etiology of a prolonged PT or aPTT. When lymphadenopathy, splenomegaly, or other findings suggestive of disseminated malignancy are detected, acute or chronic DIC should be suspected as the cause of prolonged coagulation times, hypofibrinogenemia, and/or thrombocytopenia. Purpura that are palpable suggest capillary leak from vasculitis, whereas purpura associated with thrombocytopenia or qualitative platelet defects are generally not elevated and cannot be distinguished by touch. Finally, venous and arterial telangiectasia may be seen in von Willebrand disease and liver disease, respectively. When selective pressure is centrally applied to an arterial telangiectasia, the whole lesion fades, whereas a venous telangiectasia requires confluent pressure across the entire lesion (as with a glass slide) for blanching to occur.

Diagnostic Laboratory Evaluation

This section focuses on selecting appropriate tests to enable the clinician to sort out information from the history, physical examination, or previously obtained (and often confusing) laboratory data. Before we proceed, however, the importance of correct specimen collection for hemostatic evaluation must be emphasized. In the ICU, it is common for laboratory samples to be drawn through an indwelling arterial or central venous cannula, often because other access is no longer available. Heparin is, therefore, commonly present, either in solutions used to flush the cannula, to transduce a waveform, or as a component of the intravenous infusion. Depending on the concentration of heparin in the infusing fluid and the volume of blood withdrawn, several tests can be influenced. Fibrin degradation products (FDPs) can be falsely elevated and fibrinogen can be falsely low. Likewise, the PT, aPTT, and thrombin time (TT) can be spuriously prolonged. A minimum of 20 mL of blood in adolescents and adults (10 mL of blood in younger children) should therefore be withdrawn through the cannula and either discarded or used for other purposes before obtaining a specimen for laboratory hemostasis analysis (27). This practice should minimize any influence of heparin on the results. In some clinical situations, it may not be reasonable to withdraw this volume of blood and a peripheral venipuncture may be necessary. Because the aPTT is sensitive to the presence of small amounts of heparin, the presence of an unexpected prolonged aPTT obtained through a heparinized catheter should raise the suspicion of sample contamination. In this setting, the TT also will be prolonged but will normalize if the contaminating heparin is neutralized (e.g., with toluidine blue or protamine sulfate).

The presence of most suspected bleeding disorders can be confirmed using routinely available tests. These include evaluation of the peripheral blood smear (including an estimate of the platelet count and platelet and red blood cell morphologic features); measurement of the PT, aPTT, and the TT; and, finally, assays for fibrinogen or the presence of FDPs or the D-dimer fragment of polymerized fibrin. This latter test is more specific for the fibrinolytic fragment produced when polymerized fibrin monomer, produced through the action of thrombin on fibrinogen, is cleaved by the proteolytic enzyme plasmin (8). In contrast to the older assays for fibrin degradation or fibrin-split products (FDPs and FSPs) which will be positive even if fibrin is not produced and the fragments are the result of proteolytic degradation of native fibrinogen, the D-dimer assay is positive only if fibrinogen has been cleaved to fibrin by the action of thrombin. Discretion should be used in determining which of these tests are most appropriate for assessment; they need not be ordered as a blanket panel on all patients with known or suspected bleeding disorders. Table 143.2 summarizes several major categories of hemorrhagic disorders and the tests that are characteristically abnormal in each. In most instances, measurement of the platelet count, fibrinogen level, PT, aPTT, and TT should provide sufficient information for determining the correct diagnosis—or at least making an educated guess. By using these five screening tests and assessing other more specific tests only when an absolute diagnosis is necessary, inappropriate use of laboratory resources may be avoided. The use of thromboelastography as tool to both assess hemostasis and guide transfusion of blood products in patients is frequently employed in Europe but less often in North America. While this methodology (thromboelastography [TEG] or rotational thromboelastometry [ROTEM]) offers potential benefits over

TABLE 143.2 Hemorrhagic Syndromes and Associated Laboratory Findings

Clinical Syndrome	Screening Tests	Supportive Tests
DIC	Prolonged PT, aPTT, TT; decreased fibrinogen, platelets; microangiopathy	(+) FDPs, D-dimer; decreased factors V, VIII, and II (late)
Massive transfusion	Prolonged PT, aPTT; decreased fibrinogen, platelets ± prolonged TT	All factors decreased; (–) FDPs, D-dimer (unless DIC develops); (+) transfusion history
Anticoagulant overdose		
Heparin	Prolonged aPTT, TT; ± prolonged PT	Toluidine blue/protamine corrects TT; reptilase time normal
Warfarin (same as vitamin K deficiency)	Prolonged PT; ± prolonged aPTT (severe); normal TT, fibrinogen, platelets	Vitamin K–dependent factors decreased; factors V, VIII normal
Liver disease		
Early	Prolonged PT	Decreased factor VII
Late	Prolonged PT, aPTT; decreased fibrinogen (terminal liver failure); normal platelet count (if splenomegaly absent)	Decreased factors II, V, VII, IX, and X; decreased plasminogen; ± FDPs unless DIC develops
Primary fibrinolysis	Prolonged PT, aPTT, TT; decreased fibrinogen ± platelets decreased	(+) FDPs, (–) D-dimer; short euglobulin clot lysis time
TTP	Thrombocytopenia, microangiopathy with mild anemia; PT, aPTT, fibrinogen generally WNL/mildly abnormal	ADAMTS13 deficiency/inhibitor, unusually large vWf multimers between episodes; mild increase in FDPs or D-dimer
HUS	Microagniopathic hemolytic anemia, ± thrombocytopenia; PT, aPTT generally WNL	Renal insufficiency; FDPs and D-dimer generally (-)

PT, prothrombin time; aPTT, activated partial thromboplastin time; TT, thrombin time; DIC, disseminated intravascular coagulation; FDPs, fibrin degradation products; WNL, within normal limits.

plasma-based tests (e.g., aPTT, PT, TT), by simultaneously assessing the multiple elements of hemostasis in whole blood, adoption of this testing methodology has been sporadic as it has not yet been shown to be superior to the more traditional plasma-based tests of coagulation (28–30).

Evaluation of Thrombosis

Patients who present with a thrombotic event will generally not display abnormalities of usual "clotting" studies, that is, their PT, aPTT, TT, and fibrinogen will usually be within normal ranges. While hyperfibrinogenemia and persistent elevations of F.VIII have been associated with an increased risk of thrombosis, both may be elevated by acute inflammation and consequently the finding of elevations of these clotting factors is of limited usefulness in the evaluation of a thrombotic event in an acutely ill individual. Other studies such as TEG, ROTEM, measurement of endogenous thrombin potential (ETP), indirect markers of thrombin generation (e.g., prothrombin fragment F1+2, thrombin–antithrombin complexes [TAT], and markers of fibrinolysis activation and inhibition (e.g., plasmin–antiplasmin complexes [PAP], PAI-1 activity) may be more useful in identifying those patients most at risk for thrombotic events (31). However, most of these studies do not fall into the category of "routine" tests readily available with a rapid turnaround time that would facilitate acute care decision-making. Several inherited or acquired abnormalities that place an individual at increased risk for thrombosis have been identified and determination of these factors should be undertaken when a thrombotic event is suspected or documented. Prior to initiation of anticoagulation, plasma levels of protein C (antigen and activity), protein S (antigen and activity; total and free), and antithrombin III (antigen and activity) should be obtained. In addition, PCR analysis for mutations in the factor V (factor V Leiden; [Arg]R506Q[Gln]), and prothrombin ([Gly]G20210A[Ala]) genes should be performed; determination of the methylenetetrahydrofolate reductase (MTHFR; [Cys]C677T[Thr]) mutation can be deferred unless serum homocysteine is found to be elevated. Acquired thrombotic risk factors include the presence of "Lupus" anticoagulants, antiphospholipid and anticardiolipin antibodies which may be associated with underlying autoimmune disorders or with acute inflammation. In adult populations, approximately 40% of patients with thrombosis will not display one of the known thrombophilic risk factors. The intensivist must look for confounding clinical conditions such as severe dehydration with marked hemoconcentration (in the case of central venous sinus thrombosis), indwelling catheters, vascular compression (e.g., cervical ribs), type-II heparin-induced thrombocytopenia (see below), etc. in their evaluation of a patient with thrombosis.

CONDITIONS ASSOCIATED WITH SERIOUS BLEEDING OR A HIGH PROBABILITY OF BLEEDING

Disseminated Intravascular Coagulation

Pathogenesis

Because it often occurs in conjunction with more serious, life-threatening disorders, DIC is one of the most serious hemostatic abnormalities seen in the ICU. The clinical syndrome itself results from the activation of blood coagulation, which then leads to excessive thrombin generation. The final result of this process is the widespread formation of fibrin thrombi in the microcirculation, with resultant consumption of certain clotting factors and platelets. Ultimately, this consumption generally results in the development of significant bleeding as the rate of consumption outpaces the rate at which the clotting factors and platelets are produced (32). Table 143.3 reviews several specific conditions associated with the development of DIC. In general, the conditions associated with DIC are the same for either adult or pediatric populations. These include a wide variety of disorders that share as their common feature the ability to initiate coagulation to varying degrees. The mechanisms involved generally can be considered in two categories: (1) those intrinsic processes that enzymatically activate procoagulant proteins; and (2) those that cause the release of tissue factor, which then triggers coagulation. These are complex events that can lead to significant bleeding and often complicate the management of an already critically ill patient.

TABLE 143.3 Underlying Diseases Associated With Disseminated Intravascular Coagulation

Sepsis
Liver disease
Shock
Penetrating brain injury
Necrotizing pneumonitis
Tissue necrosis/crush injury
Intravascular hemolysis
Acute promyelocytic leukemia
Thermal injury
Freshwater drowning
Fat embolism syndrome
Retained placenta
Hypertonic saline abortion
Amniotic fluid embolus
Retention of a dead fetus
Eclampsia
Localized endothelial injury (aortic aneurysm, giant hemangiomata, angiography)
Disseminated malignancy (prostate, pancreatic)

Fibrinolysis invariably accompanies thrombin formation in DIC (32). Thrombin generation or release of tissue plasminogen activator usually initiates this process. Plasmin is generated which then digests fibrinogen and fibrin clots as they form. Plasmin also inactivates several activated coagulation factors and also impairs platelet aggregation. DIC represents an imbalance between the activity of thrombin, which leads to microvascular thrombi with coagulation factor and platelet consumption, and plasmin, which degrades these fibrin-based clots as they form. Therefore, thrombin-induced coagulation factor consumption, thrombocytopenia, and plasmin generation all contribute to the presence of bleeding.

In addition to bleeding complications, the presence of fibrin thrombi in the microcirculation also can lead to ischemic tissue injury. Pathologic data indicate that renal failure, acrocyanosis, multifocal pulmonary emboli, and transient cerebral ischemia may be related clinically to the presence of such thrombi. The fibrinopeptides A and B (resulting from enzymatic cleavage of fibrinogen) lead to pulmonary and systemic vasoconstriction, which can potentiate an existing ischemic injury. In a given patient with DIC, either bleeding or thrombotic tendencies may predominate; in most patients, bleeding is usually the predominant problem. In up to 10% of patients with DIC, however, the presentation is exclusively thrombotic (e.g., pulmonary emboli with pulmonary hypertension, renal insufficiency, altered mental status, acrocyanosis) without hemorrhage. Whether the presentation of DIC is thrombotic, hemorrhagic or "compensated" (i.e., laboratory results consistent with DIC without overt bleeding), microthrombosis probably contributes to the development and progression of multiorgan failure.

Clinical Presentation and Diagnosis

The suspicion that DIC is present usually stems from one of two situations: (1) unexplained, generalized oozing or bleeding; or (2) unexplained abnormal laboratory parameters of hemostasis. This usually occurs in the context of a suggestive clinical scenario or associated disease (see Table 143.3). While infection and multiple trauma are the most common underlying conditions associated with the development of DIC, certain other organ system dysfunctions predispose to DIC, including hepatic insufficiency and splenectomy (24,25). Both of these conditions are associated with impaired reticuloendothelial system function and consequent impaired clearance of activated coagulation proteins and fibrin/fibrinogen degradation fragments which may inhibit fibrin polymerization and clot formation.

The clinical severity of DIC frequently has been assessed by the severity of bleeding and coagulation abnormalities. Recently, scoring tools employing a panel of laboratory tests along with severity of illness scores to assess the likelihood and severity of DIC have been proposed in an attempt to determine prognosis and direct initial therapy at the time of diagnosis. A listing of the tests most commonly employed in many of these scoring systems for the diagnosis of DIC are found in Table 143.4. The use of these scoring systems for the early diagnosis and treatment of DIC does appear to have prognostic value, particularly in patients with sepsis (33–35). The systems suggested by Leclerc (36) (for children) and those developed by the International Society on Thrombosis and Hemostasis (ISTH) (37) and Japanese Association for Acute Medicine (JAAM) (38) are three of the more commonly employed scoring systems and may serve as a template for the diagnosis of DIC: a qualitative score (three out of tests positive; Leclerc) or a quantitative score (five points ISTH, four points JAAM) are strongly suggestive of a diagnosis of DIC. The combination of a prolonged PT, hypofibrinogenemia, and thrombocytopenia in the appropriate clinical setting is sufficient to suspect the diagnosis of DIC in most instances. Severe hepatic insufficiency (with splenomegaly and splenic sequestration of platelets) also can yield a similar laboratory profile and must be ruled out.

TABLE 143.4 Laboratory Tests for the Diagnosis of DIC

Test	Discriminator Value
Platelet count	<80,000–100,000 or a decrease of >50% from baseline
Fibrinogen	<100 mg/dL or a decrease of >50% from baseline
PT	>3 s prolongation above ULN
FDPs	>80 mg/dL
D-dimer	"Moderate" increase

In addition to liver disease, several other conditions have presentations similar to DIC and must be considered in the differential diagnosis:

Liver disease
Massive transfusion
Primary fibrinolysis
Thrombotic thrombocytopenic purpura (TTP)/hemolytic uremic syndrome (HUS)
Heparin therapy
Dysfibrinogenemia

With the exception of massive transfusion syndrome, these disorders generally have only two of the three characteristic laboratory findings of DIC; a comparison of the laboratory findings in these disorders is noted in Table 143.2. In order to confirm a diagnosis of suspected DIC, confirmatory tests indicating increased fibrinogen turnover (i.e., elevated FDPs or D-dimer assay) may be necessary. The D-dimer assay for the D–D fragment of polymerized fibrin has been shown to be both highly sensitive and specific for proteolytic degradation of polymerized fibrin (fibrin clot that has been produced in the presence of thrombin). Consequently, this test is being employed with increasing frequency in patients with suspected DIC. However, remembering that thrombin is produced whenever coagulation is activated in the presence of bleeding, the clinician must interpret a modest elevation of D-dimer in a postoperative or trauma patient with some degree of caution. The presence of a marked elevation of D-dimer in a nonbleeding patient essentially excludes primary fibrinogenolysis as the sole cause of measurable FDPs in the serum. The TT is a less sensitive test for DIC, but may be useful in cases of suspected heparin overdose because it corrects in the test tube with the addition of protamine sulfate or toluidine blue. Similarly, the euglobulin clot lysis time may not be sensitive to fibrinolysis associated with DIC but is significantly shortened in most cases of primary fibrinolysis. Other tests of purported value, such as soluble fibrin monomer or thrombin–antithrombin complex formation, either have problems with sensitivity or are impractical for widespread use outside of research settings.

TTP and HUS

Specific mention of TTP and HUS should be made. While neither generally produces a coagulopathic state, both are characterized by marked microangiopathy and microvascular thrombosis. While their similar clinical presentation suggests that these two diseases may represent different ends of the spectrum of end-organ dysfunction possible in microangiopathic states, our improved understanding of the pathophysiology in these two entities confirms that they are not merely differing clinical manifestations of a single-disease entity (39). TTP is characterized by the pentad of microangiopathic hemolytic anemia (MAHA), thrombocytopenia, neurologic symptoms, fever, and renal dysfunction. While only 40% of patients will display the full pentad, up to 75% will manifest a triad of MAHA, neurologic symptoms, and thrombocytopenia. This disorder is felt to be due to the congenital or acquired (often antibody-mediated) absence of a vWf cleaving protease (ADAMTS13) resulting in the circulation of unusually large vWf multimers which can induce or enhance the pathologic adhesion of platelets to the endothelium. The therapy of choice for TTP is plasma exchange by apheresis. While the literature is not consistent regarding routine (prophylactic) platelet transfusions in TTP or HUS, except in the case of major bleeding they are considered contraindicated by many as platelet transfusions have been associated with an increased risk of arterial occlusion including stroke (40–43).

HUS is more commonly seen in children and is characterized by a prodrome of fever and diffuse diarrhea (often bloody). Endemic cases of HUS are generally caused by verotoxin expressing enteropathic strains of *Escherichia coli* (O157:H7) or shigatoxin expressing strains of *Shigella*. Sporadic cases are generally not associated with diarrhea and have been associated with congenital or acquired defects in complement factor H (39). Therapy is supportive including renal replacement measures. In contrast to the experience with TTP, plasma infusion and plasma exchange do not generally produce a dramatic improvement in clinical manifestations in typical endemic HUS. While limited data suggests that plasmapheresis/plasma exchange may play a role in the treatment of aHUS, there is no clear consensus regarding how it should be employed (44). Additionally, in limited use, the anticomplement monoclonal antibody eculizumab has also been shown to be beneficial in atypical HUS (39,44).

Management of DIC

The primary treatment for DIC is correction of the underlying problem that led to its development. Specific therapy for DIC should not be undertaken unless the patient has significant bleeding or organ dysfunction secondary to DIC, significant thrombosis has occurred, or treatment of the underlying disorder (i.e., acute promyelocytic leukemia) is likely to increase the severity of DIC.

Supportive therapy for DIC includes the use of several component blood products (45). Packed red blood cells are given according to accepted guidelines in the face of active bleeding. Fresh whole blood (i.e., less than 24 to 48 hours old) also may be given to replete both volume and oxygen-carrying capacity, with the additional potential benefit of providing coagulation proteins, including fibrinogen, and platelets. Fresh frozen plasma (FFP) is of limited value for the treatment of significant hypofibrinogenemia because of the inordinate volumes required to produce any meaningful increase in plasma fibrinogen concentration. Infusion of fibrinogen concentrate, or if concentrate is not available, cryoprecipitate is the preferred product for the correction of significant hypofibrinogenemia (46). FFP infusions, however, may effectively replete other coagulation factors consumed with DIC such as protein C although the increase in these proteins may be quite small unless large volumes of FFP are infused. The use of cryoprecipitate, FFP, or other blood products in the treatment of DIC has, in the past, been open to debate because of concern that these products merely provide further substrate for ongoing DIC and thus increase the amount of fibrin thrombi formed. However, clinical (autopsy) studies have failed to confirm this concern.

The goal of blood component therapy is not to produce normal "numbers" but rather to produce clinical stability. If the serum fibrinogen level is less than 75 to 50 mg/dL, repletion with fibrinogen concentrate or cryoprecipitate to raise plasma levels to 100 mg/dL or higher is the goal. Fibrinogen concentrate dose is calculated based on a formula provided by the manufacturer in the package insert. For cryoprecipitate, a reasonable starting dose is one bag of cryoprecipitate for every 10 kg body weight every 8 to 12 hours. As cryoprecipitate is not a standardized component (i.e., its content varies from bag to bag), one should recheck the fibrinogen level after an infusion to document the increase in fibrinogen level. The amount and timing of the next infusion is then adjusted according to the results. Platelet transfusions also may be used when thrombocytopenia is thought to contribute to ongoing bleeding. Many of the fibrin/fibrinogen fragments produced in DIC have the potential to impair platelet function by inhibiting fibrinogen binding to platelets. This may be clinically significant at the concentration of FDPs achieved with DIC. Platelet transfusions in patients with DIC should be considered to maintain platelet counts up to 40,000 to 80,000/μL depending on the clinical specifics of the patient.

Pharmacologic therapy for DIC has two primary aims: to "turn off" ongoing coagulation so that repletion of coagulation factors may begin, and to impede thrombus formation and ensuing ischemic injury. Several recombinant blood products have been developed which have some potential usefulness in the treatment of DIC. The first of these was recombinant aPC, which was ultimately removed from the market due to lack of significant efficacy. The second new agent for the treatment of severe bleeding, including DIC, is recombinant activated factor VII (rhF.VIIa). While there are limited controlled trials of its use, and none in the pediatric age range with the exception of those patients with acquired inhibitors to F.VIII, it has been shown to be a potent agent for the control of bleeding in a number of medical and surgical settings, including DIC and other consumptive coagulopathies (47–49). This agent has also been shown to correct the hemostatic defect caused by the antiplatelet agents aspirin and clopidogrel (50). However, while control of bleeding can be effected with this agent, no studies have demonstrated a benefit in mortality (51). There have been reports that the use of rhF.VIIa may result in an increase in thrombosis and thromboembolic events, although the incidence appears to be small and the severity of most events mild (52). An additional recombinant agent under investigation is recombinant thrombomodulin. In limited use, it has been shown to decrease the severity of DIC and development of multiorgan failure (53). In addition to aPC, other anticoagulant molecules such as heparin and antithrombin III, and thrombolytic agents continue to be studied as therapy for DIC and sepsis (54,55).

Liver Disease and Hepatic Insufficiency

Abnormal Hemostasis in Liver Disease

Liver disease is a common cause of abnormal hemostasis in ICU patients, with abnormal coagulation studies or overt bleeding occurring in approximately 15% of patients with either clinical or laboratory evidence of hepatic dysfunction. It is a common cause of a prolonged PT or aPTT, often without any clinical sequelae. The hemostatic defect associated with liver disease is multifactorial with multiple aspects of hemostasis affected (56,57).

In liver disease, synthesis of several plasma coagulation proteins is impaired. These include factors II, V, VII, IX, and X. Fibrinogen synthesis by the liver usually can be maintained at levels that prevent bleeding until terminal liver failure supervenes. The physiologic action of fibrinogen synthesized by a diseased liver may not be normal owing to an increased carbohydrate content in its structure (sialic acid) which may result in a diminished hemostatic activity (i.e., a dysfibrinogen). Factor

XIII activity also is often decreased in the setting of hepatocellular disease. However, the clinical significance of this decrease in factor XIII is uncertain because levels as low as 3% provide for normal fibrin clot stabilization. Although factor VIII (i.e., factor VIII:C, AHF) is synthesized in the liver, recent data shows it to be in hepatic sinusoidal cells rather than hepatocytes (58). Consequently, synthesis seems to be independent of the state of hepatic function. Indeed, factor VIII levels may be increased in some types of liver disease. Plasma protein C and antithrombin III levels are low in many conditions of hepatic insufficiency, with variable effects.

In addition to these deficiencies in plasma coagulation protein synthesis, many patients with liver disease, particularly cirrhosis, have increased fibrinolytic activity. The mechanism for this heightened fibrinolytic state is not clear but may be related to the increased amounts of plasminogen activator often noted in these patients. It may be difficult to discern whether fibrinolysis occurs solely because of underlying severe liver disease or as a result of concurrent DIC as patients with cirrhosis are at increased risk for the development of DIC. The clinical distinction between primary DIC and a secondary hemostatic defect resulting from liver disease can be virtually impossible to make if active bleeding is present. In liver disease, levels of FDPs can be increased by both increased fibrinolysis and by decreased hepatic clearance. Finally, clinically significant fibrinolysis is a frequent occurrence in patients who undergo portacaval shunt procedures.

Thrombocytopenia may be present to a variable degree in patients with hepatic dysfunction. This is usually ascribed to splenic sequestration. It is rarely profound and generally does not produce clinically significant bleeding as a solitary defect. *In vitro* platelet aggregation may also be affected, however. Increased plasma concentrations of FDPs are a possible cause of these qualitative platelet abnormalities. The thrombocytopenia of liver disease in conjunction with other coagulation or hemostatic defects secondary to liver disease may result in bleeding that is difficult to manage clinically, particularly if all aspects of the problem are not addressed.

Patients with hepatocellular liver disease may also exhibit decreased synthesis of the vitamin K–dependent anticoagulant proteins, protein C and protein S, as well as antithrombin III (56). Decreased levels of these natural anticoagulants may increase the risk of thrombosis. Neither the PT, aPTT, nor TT will be affected by the levels of any of these naturally occurring anticoagulants.

Presentation

The hemostatic defect in liver disease is multifactorial, and each patient should be approached accordingly. The most common scenario is a patient with liver disease and a prolonged PT without overt bleeding in whom the potential for bleeding is a concern. In patients with liver disease and impaired synthetic capabilities, particularly those who are critically ill, factor VII activity levels are usually the first to decrease due to its short half-life of 4 to 6 hours and increased turnover. This results in a prolonged PT, and can be noted even when usual markers of hepatocellular injury or hepatic insufficiency remain relatively normal (56,57). A prolonged TT in the setting of liver disease may indicate the presence of dysfibrinogenemia as a result of altered hepatic fibrinogen synthesis, or may indicate an acquired defect in fibrin polymerization (e.g., increased FDPs). As the severity of liver disease increases, the aPTT also may be affected, reflecting more severely impaired synthetic function. In this setting, plasma concentrations of the vitamin K–dependent coagulation proteins decrease, as do those of factor V (which is not vitamin K–dependent). Although fibrinogen synthesis occurs in the liver, plasma levels of fibrinogen are generally maintained until the disease approaches end-stage. When fibrinogen levels are severely depressed, liver failure has typically reached the terminal phase. In contrast to the hypofibrinogenemia noted with consumptive coagulopathies, hypofibrinogenemia noted in liver disease is the result of decreased synthesis and is not accompanied by a marked increase in either FDPs or D-dimers.

In more severe forms of liver disease, fibrinolysis may complicate clinical management. The differentiation between concomitant DIC and fibrinolysis attributable to liver disease alone may be difficult (57). The D-dimer assay result should be negative in the patient who has liver disease and elevated FDPs but no active bleeding. Further clinical distinction usually is not possible.

Management

If the patient is not actively bleeding, no specific therapy is required, with certain provisos. In patients with a markedly prolonged PT who are in a postoperative state or are scheduled for an invasive procedure, correction of the PT should be attempted. FFP or a prothrombin complex concentrate (PCC) provides the most immediate source of specific coagulation factors (i.e., factors II, VII, IX, and X). While FFP usually corrects an isolated mild PT prolongation, it is less effective in correcting a more profound prolongation of the PT. Consequently, consensus is moving toward the use of a PCC, preferably a 4-factor PCC (4PCC) as the initial choice to correct a markedly prolonged PT due to the greater amount of F.VII contained in 4PCCs. For this reason, 4PCCs are also preferred over the use of rhFVIIa to correct a prolonged PT (59). Fibrinogen support in the form of fibrinogen concentrate or cryoprecipitate is required if fibrinogen levels are <50 to 100 mg/dL, or if there is documentation of a significant dysfibrinogenemia.. The routine correction of prolonged PT/INR in patients who are to undergo minor invasive procedures has not been shown to affect procedural blood loss (60).

Vitamin K deficiency also is relatively common in this patient population, and replacement may be needed. In contrast to patients with dietary vitamin K deficiency and normal liver function, correction of the PT in vitamin K–responsive critically ill patients typically requires longer than 12 to 24 hours. Patients with significant hepatic impairment may manifest a partial response or may not respond at all. Individuals with severe liver disease, or marked prolonged vitamin K deficiency, will demonstrate a prolongation of the aPTT in addition to a prolonged PT. This prolongation of the aPTT is the result of other clotting factors besides F.VII being low. In this setting, the use of rhFVII a will not provide adequate hemostatic support. If the prolongation of the aPTT is due solely to decreases in the vitamin K–dependent factors (II, VII, IX, X), infusion of a 4PCC is the treatment of choice. However, if other clotting factor deficiency is suspected, plasma (either FFP or commercial solvent/detergent-purified commercial product) is preferred. While recombinant human activated factor VII (rhF.VIIa) infusions have been shown to control the bleeding in severe liver disease, reduced reduction in mortality has not been demonstrated (51,59). The use of rhF.VIIa should be reserved for patients with poorly controlled bleeding that is unresponsive to other more established therapeutic modalities such as infusion of plasma or 4PCCs.

A comprehensive therapeutic approach is needed in the patient with active bleeding as a result of liver disease. Initially, a 4PCC at a dose calculated to increase F.VII to ≥50% of normal (i.e., 0.5 units/mL) should be administered. If a 4PCC is not available, plasma, 10 to 15 cc/kg body weight, may be given. Doses of 4PCC or plasma should be repeated every 6 to 8 hours until bleeding slows significantly, and should then be continued at maintenance levels as dictated by clinical status and coagulation studies. Recombinant human activated factor VII may be used in those patients unresponsive to FFP infusions (60). Cryoprecipitate should be infused for fibrinogen levels <50 to 100 mg/dL. Platelet transfusions also may be required if the platelet count is <40 to 80,000/μL, depending on the clinical situation. Vitamin K should be empirically administered on the presumption that part of the synthetic defect may result from a lack of this cofactor. However, one must anticipate a poor response to vitamin K in the presence of severe liver disease. Transfusions of packed cells are given as deemed appropriate by the clinician.

Vitamin K Deficiency

The most common cause of a prolonged PT in the ICU is vitamin K deficiency. Vitamin K is necessary for the gamma-carboxylation of factors II, VII, IX, and X, without which these factors cannot bind calcium and are not efficiently converted into their activated forms. Factor VII has the shortest half-life of these coagulation proteins; accordingly, the PT is the most sensitive early indicator of vitamin K deficiency.

Vitamin K deficiency is relatively common in critically ill patients for several reasons including the use of broad-spectrum antibiotics, poor nutrition preceding or subsequent to ICU admission, and the use of parenteral nutrition without vitamin K supplementation. Many of the second- and third-generation cephalosporins directly interfere with vitamin K absorption from the gut lumen. The metabolites of some of these antibiotics may even act as competitive inhibitors of vitamin K. In addition, these and other antibiotics may kill or inhibit the growth of gut bacteria and thus limit the amounts of vitamin K they normally produce and excrete into the gut lumen. While malnutrition also may contribute to the development of vitamin K deficiency, this usually requires 1 to 2 weeks to develop in the complete absence of vitamin K intake. However, the use of parenteral alimentation without vitamin K supplementation coupled with antibiotic use may result in rapid vitamin K depletion and prolongation of the PT can occur within only 2 to 3 days. Finally, fat malabsorption states, including cystic fibrosis, may be associated with vitamin K deficiency. Vitamin K is fat soluble and is not absorbed well in some conditions of biliary tract and intrinsic small bowel disease. In the ICU, vitamin K deficiency usually results from the interaction of several of these factors and is rarely limited to one of the conditions mentioned. It is the responsibility of the clinician to maintain an awareness of the potential for vitamin K deficiency and to treat accordingly.

The differential diagnosis of an isolated prolongation of the PT, with or without bleeding, includes both vitamin K deficiency and liver disease. The clinical presentation of these patients is often quite similar. In fact, the distinction sometimes can be made only on the basis of the response (or lack thereof) to empirical vitamin K therapy. Warfarin administration (either overt or covert) also should be excluded as a cause of a prolonged PT. Newer, long-acting vitamin K antagonist (VKA) rodenticides (so-called "super-warfarin"), which, when ingested, produce a profound, prolonged, vitamin K–resistant reduction in vitamin K–dependent clotting factors may produce an isolated prolongation of the PT initially. Treatment of poisoning with these agents requires aggressive prolonged use of vitamin K, and, in the bleeding patient, infusions of FFP or rhF.VIIa. Confirmation of warfarin exposure as the cause of a prolonged PT is possible by toxicologic methods to detect the drug and/or its metabolites, or one can identify the presence of noncarboxylated forms of vitamin K–dependent clotting factors in plasma (proteins induced by vitamin K antagonist; PIVKAs). In addition, the presence of a specific inhibitor or congenital deficiency of factor VII will also result in an isolated prolongation of the PT. Acquired inhibitors of factor VII are rare, and homozygous deficiency of factor VII has not been described. Individuals heterozygous for factor VII deficiency and those with certain polymorphisms of the promoter region of the factor VII gene tend to have factor VII levels in the 25% to 35% range and do not appear to be at significant increased risk for bleeding. Lupus-like anticoagulants resulting from inflammation may also result in an isolated prolongation of the PT; these are generally of no clinical significance and are not associated with an increased risk of bleeding. These patients are not at increased risk for bleeding.

The laboratory findings of an isolated vitamin K deficiency, in addition to a prolonged PT, include a normal fibrinogen level, platelet count, and factor V level. Factor V is not a vitamin K–dependent protein and should therefore be normal except in cases of DIC (consumption) or severe liver disease (decreased production). Prolongation of the aPTT from vitamin K deficiency, warfarin therapy, or from liver disease is a relatively late event and occurs initially as a result of factor IX depletion.

Management

The management of vitamin K deficiency consists primarily of its repletion, usually by intravenous or subcutaneous routes in critically ill patients. Therapy should not await the development of bleeding or oozing but should be administered when the PT abnormality is detected and vitamin K deficiency is thought to be responsible. As with other drugs administered subcutaneously (e.g., insulin), adequate blood pressure and subcutaneous perfusion are needed to ensure reliable absorption from the soft tissues. Concern about the possibility of anaphylactoid reactions with the intravenous use of vitamin K exists. This risk is almost completely negated when the drug is given as a piggyback infusion over 30 to 45 minutes in a small volume of fluid rather than as a bolus or "slow-push" dose. This is the preferred method of drug administration in hemodynamically unstable patients. The usual dose of vitamin K in adults is 10 to 15 mg intravenously or subcutaneously (1 to 5 mg in young children, up to 10 mg in larger children). In an otherwise healthy person, the PT should correct within 12 to 24 hours after this dose. Serial dosing of critically ill patients is often utilized, however, and the PT may require up to 72 hours to normalize. If the PT does not correct within 72 hours after three daily doses of vitamin K, intrinsic liver disease should be suspected. Further administration of vitamin K is of no additional benefit in this setting.

When the patient is actively bleeding, it is not sufficient to give vitamin K alone. A more immediate restoration of coagulation is required. FFP has traditionally been employed in this setting. To restore hemostasis to an acceptable level (30% to 50%) of normal enzyme activity, 10 to 15 cc/kg body weight of FFP is typically required. A similar approach is used in patients previously given warfarin. Recombinant human activated factor VII (rhF.VIIa) has been used with success to reverse the bleeding noted in vitamin K deficiency and in warfarin overdose (60,61).

Massive Transfusion Syndrome

Transfusion of large quantities of blood can result in a multifactorial hemostatic defect. The genesis of this problem is related to the "washout" of plasma coagulation proteins and platelets, and it may be exacerbated by the development of DIC with consequent factor consumption, hypothermia, acidosis or, rarely, by citrate toxicity or hypocalcemia. These variables often act in combination to cause a coagulopathic state (62).

A washout syndrome can result from the transfusion of large amounts of stored blood products devoid of clotting factors and platelets. This develops exclusively in patients who receive large volumes of packed RBCs (e.g., trauma victims, patients with massive gastrointestinal hemorrhage or hepatectomy, or those undergoing cardiopulmonary bypass) without also receiving FFP and platelets. Factors V and VII have short shelf half-lives and are often deficient in blood that has been banked longer than 48 hours. In addition, a qualitative platelet defect can be demonstrated in whole blood within hours of its storage, especially if an acid–citrate–dextrose solution is used. Consequently, transfusion of large quantities of stored whole blood may produce limited benefit in controlling the bleeding resulting from decreased clotting factors and platelets.

Massive transfusion had generally been defined, in adults, as the transfusion of >10 units of RBCs within 24 hours, >4 units of RBs in 1 hour, or >50% blood volume replacement within 3 hours. The development of a washout coagulopathy is directly dependent on the volume of blood transfused relative to the blood volume of the patient. As a general rule, residual plasma clotting activity after one-blood volume exchange falls to 18% to 37% of normal; whereas after a two-blood volume exchange, residual activity is only 3% to 14%; and after a three-blood volume exchange, less than 5% of normal clotting function remains.

As previously discussed, DIC may develop in many clinical settings, including some associated with major hemorrhage or massive transfusion. In the presence of hypotension associated with hypovolemia or hemorrhagic shock, DIC is a common sequela. Major trauma itself, especially with the release of tissue factors into the plasma, also can result in the development of DIC. Exsanguinating hemorrhage sometimes requires blood replacement faster than a type and crossmatch of each unit can be performed, and unmatched blood is given as a lifesaving measure. Donor–recipient incompatibility—even when the mismatch is only of the minor blood group systems—can lead to DIC. Human error resulting in major incompatibility can produce severe hemolysis and be lethal. Finally, microaggregates of blood cells that form within stored blood products also can cause DIC. The advent of smaller pore, more effective filtering systems for blood product administration, however, has essentially eliminated this as a source of problems.

The patient who is bleeding as a consequence of massive transfusion or washout presents with diffuse oozing and bleeding from all surgical wounds and puncture sites. Laboratory abnormalities include prolonged PT, aPTT, and TT. Fibrinogen levels and platelet counts are typically decreased; FDPs are not usually increased unless concurrent DIC is present (see Table 143.2). The likelihood that the clinicolaboratory picture is a direct result of the massive transfusion can be estimated from the amount of bleeding that has occurred and the blood volume administered relative to the patient's blood volume (i.e., the number of blood volume exchanges that have been given). The more stored blood (e.g., packed RBCs) transfused relative to the patient's blood volume, the greater the chance of the development of coagulopathy due to massive transfusion.

Management

The therapeutic approach to patients who develop a coagulopathy from massive transfusion is supportive. Platelets and FFP are given to replete the components of coagulation that are typically lacking (40). Platelet administration may help stem bleeding from anatomic wounds. Severe bleeding associated with thrombocytopenia alone is uncommon unless counts fall below 20,000 to 30,000/μL of blood. Because of the complex nature of bleeding seen with massive transfusion, patients may benefit from platelet transfusion at counts even as high as 80,000 to 100,000/μL. FFP is preferred over cryoprecipitate because it has a more complete coagulation protein composition. However, cryoprecipitate may be specifically given when fibrinogen depletion is thought to be a major contributor to the observed bleeding. Over the past 2 to 3 decades, the approach to transfusion support to individuals who require multiple blood transfusions acutely for the treatment of trauma or massive surgical hemorrhage has evolved from a policy of 1 unit of FFP and 1 unit of platelets for every 4 to 5 units of pRBCs transfused to a current 1:1:1 ratio of pRBC:FFP:platelets (63,64). However, the increased patient exposure to plasma with these new transfusion algorithms has also increased the risk for transfusion-related acute lung injury (TRALI) (65). Use of a commercially prepared solvent/detergent virally purified plasma produced form pooled fresh plasma has been shown to result in a decreased risk of TRALI in comparison to that with traditional single-donor plasma, and has also been shown to have a more consistent clotting factor profile than does the various forms of "fresh frozen" plasma available at hospitals (66,67).

Prospective identification of those at risk to develop a coagulopathy from massive transfusion is important. When the magnitude of the insult and the anticipated need for blood are large, both platelets and FFP should be given before a coagulopathy develops. Many institutions have developed infusion algorithms that include activating a "massive transfusion" protocol with their Transfusion Medicine service. These programs have generally resulted in more efficient utilization of blood products in the setting of trauma care (68,69). Use of a higher pRBC:plasma:platelet ratio transfusion regimen should prevent washout and its attendant bleeding. If the patient continues to bleed despite what should be adequate therapy for massive transfusion syndrome, other causes should be considered. Specifically, anatomic bleeding and the possibility of DIC should be investigated. Therapy in this setting may include rhF.VIIa infusion (49).

Anticoagulant Overdose

Anticoagulant therapy is not unusual in the ICU, and the possibility of errors in administration exists. Methods of prophylactic anticoagulant use, systemic anticoagulation, and thrombolytic therapy are sometimes poorly standardized and can lead to overdose.

Heparin

Heparin is a repeating polymer of two disaccharide glycosaminoglycans and is commercially prepared from either porcine intestinal mucosa or bovine lung. Heparin is currently found in two forms, unfractionated heparin (UH) and low–molecular-weight heparin (LMWH). It is important to understand the differences between these two forms of the drug as they have different mechanisms of action and associated precautions. Unfractionated heparin has an immediate effect on coagulation that is mediated primarily through its interaction with antithrombin III. The resulting heparin–antithrombin III complex possesses a much greater affinity for thrombin than does AT III alone and inactivates thrombin, thereby damping-down clot formation. In addition, heparin also has a direct effect inhibiting activated factor X (F.Xa). This anticoagulant effect of UH is relatively minor. Consequently, achieving a therapeutic aPTT with UH is very difficult in the face of low levels of AT III. The degree of anticoagulation produced by heparin has traditionally been monitored by the prolongation of the aPTT. In contrast, LMWH, produced by controlled enzymatic cleavage of heparin polymers, produces anticoagulation almost exclusively through inhibition of F.Xa. This produces a more stable degree of anticoagulation, and due to its longer half-life (approximately 3 to 5 hours) and biologic activity (approximately 24 hours), allows for intermittent bolus therapy (i.e., every 12 or 24 hours) while still maintaining steady-state effect. However, LMWH does not produce consistent prolongation of the aPTT and requires assay of anti-Xa activity for monitoring (if desired). Recently, a therapeutic range for the anti-Xa level achieved with UH infusions has been developed. As most hospital labs now routinely measure anti-Xa levels, some institutions/clinicians monitor UH therapy and adjust doses accordingly.

Heparin is metabolized in the liver by the "heparinase" enzyme in a dose-dependent fashion with excess heparin then being excreted through the kidneys. As the rate of heparin administration is increased, the half-life of the drug is prolonged due the increase in the percentage of the drug being excreted by the kidney. For example, when a 100 U/kg bolus of heparin is infused intravenously, the average half-life of the drug is 1 hour. If the bolus is increased to 400 or 800 U/kg, however, the half-life is prolonged to 2.5 and 5 hours, respectively. The nonlinear response results in greater drug effects on coagulation with smaller dosage increments. When one "reboluses" or increases a heparin infusion rate in response to insufficient anticoagulation (i.e., inadequate prolongation of the aPTT or anti-Xa level), a point will be reached when further small increments in the heparin infusion rate may result in a substantially greater prolongation of the aPTT. The risk of pathologic bleeding associated with heparin increases when the prolongation of the aPTT is beyond the therapeutic window (generally considered to be 1.5 to 2.5 times the patient's baseline aPTT, corresponding to a plasma heparin concentration of 0.2 to 0.4 units/mL, or 0.3 to 0.7 anti-Xa units/mL). As a corollary, administration of heparin as a continuous infusion rather than in an intermittent bolus dose regimen is less likely to be associated with pathologic bleeding.

Management

Serious bleeding associated with heparin overdose can be rapidly reversed by protamine sulfate. Protamine binds ionically with heparin to form a complex that lacks any anticoagulant activity. As a general rule, 1 mg of protamine neutralizes approximately 100 U of heparin (specifically, 90 USP units of bovine heparin or 115 USP units of porcine heparin). The dose of protamine needed is calculated from the number of units of active heparin remaining in the patient's system. This, in turn, is estimated from the original heparin dose and the typical half-life for that infusion rate. The aPTT is used to gauge the residual effects of heparin. Protamine itself potentially has anticoagulant effects, and precautions are necessary during its administration. The drug should be given by slow intravenous push over 8 to 10 minutes. A single dose should not exceed 1 mg/kg (50 mg maximum dose). This dose may be repeated, but no more than 2 mg/kg (100 mg maximum dose) should be given as a cumulative dose without rechecking coagulation parameters. The dose of protamine should always be monitored by coagulation studies. Significant side effects are most commonly seen in situations of overly rapid drug administration and include hypotension and anaphylactoid-like reactions. LMWH is not consistently neutralized by protamine, so invasive procedures should not be performed within 24 hours of administration. Bleeding following LMWH therapy has been treated effectively with rhF.VIIa.

Warfarin

Warfarin and vitamin K are structurally similar in their respective 4-hydroxycoumarin nucleus and naphthoquinone ring. The mechanism of action of warfarin is through inhibition of vitamin K epoxide reductase (VKOR; specifically the C1 subunit VKORC1) which is necessary to maintain a reduced form of vitamin K (vitamin K hydroquinone). Vitamin K hydroquinone is a necessary substrate of the γ-carboxylase which creates the calcium-binding site on the vitamin K–dependent clotting factors (factors II, VII, IX, X). This postsynthetic modification is necessary to produce a calcium-binding site on the molecule which, when occupied, allows for the efficient activation of the zymogen clotting factor into its enzymatically active form. When warfarin is present in sufficient plasma concentrations, there is depletion of reduced vitamin K (vitamin K hydroquinone) and consequent depletion of the active forms of vitamin K–dependent factors.

The PT, or more precisely the international normalized ratio (INR) calculated from the PT, is an accurate indicator of the intensity of anticoagulation with warfarin when its use has continued beyond 2 or 3 days. Factor VII has a half-life of only 4 to 6 hours and (the active form) is rapidly depleted after one or two doses of warfarin. The remainder of the vitamin K–dependent factors may take up to a week to become depleted. The PT becomes prolonged, and INR elevated, with factor VII depletion alone but does not reflect an overall state of anticoagulation until an equilibrium period of several days has passed. Over this time, the other vitamin K–dependent factors are depleted and PT prolongation (INR elevation) can then be used to assess the anticoagulant effects of warfarin. In severe cases of warfarin overdose, the aPTT also becomes prolonged as a result of depletion of the active forms of factors II, IX, and X. While the INR is calculated from the PT and is frequently used as a surrogate for the PT and in this manner used to assess bleeding risks, the INR has only been validated as an indicator of anticoagulant intensity with VKA therapy. While some retrospective studies have identified an INR 1.5 as being associated with an increased risk of bleeding, INR alone has not been shown to be a consistent indicator of bleeding risk with invasive procedures, in liver disease or other medical conditions (70–72).

Several drugs and pathophysiologic conditions are associated with potentiation of warfarin's effects on coagulation. Table 143.5 lists many of the drugs known to prolong the effects of warfarin. These drugs have a variety of mechanisms, which generally include either inhibition of function or competitive binding of the enzymes responsible for active warfarin metabolism. Aspirin does not seem to have any direct influence on warfarin metabolism but can so profoundly influence qualitative platelet function that it must be considered as a potentiator of warfarin's anticoagulant effects. The same is true for clofibrate. Ingestion of large quantities of aspirin may also impair prothrombin (factor II) synthesis, further increasing the effects of warfarin administration. Warfarin is metabolized by the liver. Conditions of acute and chronic hepatic dysfunction can alter warfarin metabolism and vitamin K–mediated γ-carboxylation of the vitamin K–dependent coagulation proteins. Broad-spectrum antibiotics also may limit vitamin K availability through their alteration of the gut flora (in addition to any direct effect on vitamin K metabolism). All of these factors may ultimately influence a patient's response to warfarin.

A clinical syndrome referred to as "warfarin (coumadin) necrosis" has been noted during the initial stages of anticoagulation with a VKA. It is characterized clinically by the development of skin and subcutaneous necrosis, particularly in areas of subcutaneous fat, and pathologically by the thrombosis of small blood vessels in the fat and subcutaneous tissues. This syndrome is caused by the rapid depletion of the vitamin K–dependent anticoagulant protein C prior to achieving depletion of procoagulant proteins and occurs predominantly in individuals heterozygous for protein C deficiency. While anticoagulation generally requires a decrease in procoagulant protein levels to approximately 20% to 25%, a prothrombotic milieu is created with protein C levels of 40% or less. Consequently, individuals who are heterozygous for protein C deficiency and have baseline protein C levels of 50% to 60% may develop a prothrombotic environment during the first few days of warfarin therapy. The risk of developing warfarin necrosis appears to be greater when an initial dose of warfarin greater than 10 to 15 mg is administered. The development of this syndrome generally can be avoided if heparin and warfarin therapy are overlapped until "coumadinization" is complete, and if large loading doses of warfarin are avoided.

TABLE 143.5 Drugs That Potentiate the Anticoagulant Effects of Warfarin

Antibiotics
Broad-spectrum antibiotics (especially cephalosporins)
Griseofulvin (oral)
Metronidazole
Sulfonamides
Trimethoprim–sulfamethoxazole
Anti-inflammatory drugs
Steroids (anabolic, in particular)
Acetylated salicylates
Phenylbutazone (oxyphenbutazone)
Sulfinpyrazone
Other drugs
Cimetidine
Clofibrate
Disulfiram
Phenytoin
Thyroxine (both D- and L-isomers)
Tolbutamide

Management

When over-anticoagulation with warfarin presents with bleeding, immediate reversal is usually mandated (38). Infusion of FFP or 4PCCs, which provide prompt restoration of the deficient vitamin K–dependent coagulation proteins, is preferred over rhF.VIIa infusions for the restoration of hemostatic function in patients on VKA therapy. The routine correction of prolonged PT/INR in patients who are to undergo minor invasive procedures has not been shown to affect procedural blood loss (59,73,74). A typical dose of 4PCC for correction of a prolonged INR secondary to VKA therapy in 15 IU F.VII/kg body weight; for correction with FFP, 10 to 15 cc/kg is usually sufficient to produce significant correction of the PT although repeat infusions of FFP may be needed to effect continued correction of the PT due to the short half-life of factor VII (40). Vitamin K also may be administered, particularly in situations that are less acute (see section "Vitamin K Deficiency") although this will make it more difficult to "re-coumadinize" the patient afterwards. For severe bleeding or bleeding not controlled by 4PCC or FFP infusions, an activated PCC or rhF.VIIa may be given.

Platelet Disorders

Platelets are necessary for efficient clot formation. They not only produce a physical barrier at the site of vascular injury (the so-called "platelet plug"), they also serve to focus the clotting process at the point of bleeding by delivering vasoconstrictors, clotting factors, and a surface on which clot development occurs to the bleeding site (see Fig. 143.3). Quantitative and qualitative platelet disorders are a common cause of clinical bleeding in the ICU. Table 143.6 presents an overview of platelet disorders based on this classification scheme.

Quantitative Platelet Disorders

A decrease in the number of circulating platelets reflects the presence of increased peripheral destruction/sequestration, decreased marrow production, or a combination of these factors. Examples of increased peripheral destruction include immune-mediated processes (both autoimmune and drug-induced), abnormal consumption (as in DIC), and mechanical destruction (e.g., cardiopulmonary bypass, hyperthermia). Autoimmune processes such as idiopathic thrombocytopenic purpura (ITP), SLE, or acquired immunodeficiency syndrome (AIDS) can result in increased peripheral destruction and increased splenic sequestration of platelets. Autoimmune destruction also may occur in conjunction with lymphocytic leukemia or lymphoma. The prototypic example of immune thrombocytopenia is ITP, in which immunoglobulin (generally

TABLE 143.6 Platelet Disorders Seen in the ICU

Quantitative	Qualitative
Increased destruction	**Drugs**
Immune	Anti-inflammatory agents
Idiopathic thrombocytopenic purpura	Aspirin (irreversible)
Systemic lupus erythematosus	Nonsteroidal anti-inflammatory agents
Acquired immunodeficiency syndrome	Corticosteroids
Drugs (gold salts, heparin, sulfonamides, quinidine, quinine)	Antibiotics
Sepsis	Penicillins (e.g., ampicillin, carbenicillin, ticarcillin, penicillin-G)
Nonimmune	Cephalosporins (e.g., cephalothin)
Thrombotic thrombocytopenic purpura/hemolytic uremic syndrome	Nitrofurantoin
Mechanical destruction (e.g., cardiopulmonary bypass, hyperthermia)	Chloroquine, hydroxychloroquine
Consumption (i.e., DIC)	Phosphodiesterase inhibitors
Decreased production	Dipyridamole
Marrow suppression	Methylxanthines (e.g., theophylline)
Chemotherapy	Other drugs
Viral illness (e.g., cytomegalovirus, Epstein–Barr virus, herpes simplex, parvovirus)	Antihistamines
Drugs (thiazides, ethanol, cimetidine)	α-blockers (e.g., phentolamine)
Marrow replacement	β-blockers (e.g., propranolol)
Tumor	Dextran
Myelofibrosis	Ethanol
Other conditions	Furosemide
Splenic sequestration	Heparin
Dilution (see massive transfusion syndrome)	Local anesthetics (e.g., lidocaine)
	Phenothiazines
	Tricyclic antidepressants
	Nitrates (e.g., sodium nitroprusside, nitroglycerin)
	Metabolic causes
	Uremia
	Stored whole blood
	Disseminated intravascular coagulation (i.e., FDP-mediated inhibition)
	hypothyroidism

IgG) directed against specific platelet antigens is thought to be responsible for platelet destruction. Acute ITP is usually self-limited, with life-threatening bleeding occurring only rarely. In contrast, chronic ITP generally requires some sort of immunosuppressive therapy. Steroids may be given (2 to 4 mg/kg day of prednisone or its equivalent). High doses of intravenous gamma globulin (1 to 2 g/kg given over 2 to 5 days), infusions of anti-RhD antigen antibody (WinRho; 25 to 60 μg/kg) are equally efficacious in producing at least transient elevations in platelet counts. Agents such as vincristine/vinblastine, cyclophosphamide, and most recently rituximab (Rituxin; anti-CD20 monoclonal antibody) also have been used as immunosuppressants, with variable success, although responses are generally not immediate. Splenectomy also may be required to avert serious bleeding complications in patients who do not respond to medical management, although this approach is chosen much less often in children than in adults. In ITP, the degree of bleeding attributed to the thrombocytopenia is generally less than that which is noted when thrombocytopenia results from decreased production. In general, severe bleeding is not noted until the platelet count is <10,000/μL, although levels below 40,000 to 50,000/μL may increase the risk of bleeding with invasive procedure.

Drug-induced immune-mediated platelet destruction is a cause of thrombocytopenia frequently considered in the thrombocytopenic ICU patient. Fortunately, when present it is usually reversible; withdrawal of the offending drug prevents further immune-mediated platelet destruction. The exact mechanism of platelet destruction seems to be related to the binding of a drug to the platelet membrane, with subsequent binding to the platelet, platelet–drug complex, or both, of a specific antibody. The resulting platelet–drug–antibody complexes then are cleared by the reticuloendothelial system (e.g., the spleen) and thrombocytopenia develops. Drugs used in the ICU that are most commonly associated with this clinical picture include quinidine, quinine, heparin, gold salts, various penicillin and cephalosporin antibiotics, and the sulfonamides. The anticonvulsant valproic acid (Depakote, Depakane) frequently produces a dose-dependent thrombocytopenia which, at least in part, is immunologic in nature.

A variety of drugs are associated with a nonimmune mechanism of thrombocytopenia by bone marrow suppression. Most cancer chemotherapeutic agents produce thrombocytopenia as a consequence of marrow suppression. The thiazide diuretics, cimetidine, ethanol, and several of the cephalosporin and penicillin antibiotics may suppress platelet production. Generalized infection, such as bacterial sepsis, and many viral illnesses also are associated with bone marrow suppression and thrombocytopenia, even if there is an element of immune platelet destruction. Disorders such as Gaucher disease may produce a mild-to-moderate thrombocytopenia as a result of marrow replacement by nonhematopoietic cells.

Consumption of platelets also can cause thrombocytopenia. Mechanical destruction invariably occurs during the use of cardiopulmonary bypass machines and it is not uncommon to note a 50% drop in platelet count postbypass when compared to preoperative platelet levels. Platelet counts may continue to decrease for 48 to 72 hours after bypass before recovering toward preoperative levels. Platelets may also be destroyed by the high body temperatures seen in severe hyperthermic syndromes, and are consumed during microvascular coagulation in DIC. In many of these circumstances, the thrombocytopenia may be the sole or a contributing cause of significant bleeding.

Heparin-Induced Thrombocytopenia

The special problems associated with heparin merit emphasis. Heparin use is ubiquitous in the ICU. Heparin-induced thrombocytopenia may develop in one of two ways. Acute nonidiosyncratic heparin-induced thrombocytopenia is seen in approximately 10% to 15% of patients receiving heparin. The degree of thrombocytopenia is usually mild and usually remits despite the continued use of the drug (type I HIT). The thrombocytopenia that develops has no clinical significance. Heparin need not be stopped in these patients. Idiosyncratic heparin-induced thrombocytopenia is of much greater clinical consequence. Although it is a less frequent occurrence (typically seen in fewer than 5% of patients receiving heparin), it has a much greater potential for clinical morbidity. Arterial thrombosis is the most significant risk of this form of heparin-induced thrombocytopenia (type II HIT) and may be life-threatening causing myocardial infarction, cerebrovascular accident, pulmonary embolism, or renal infarction. The mechanism of thrombosis is thought to be a consequence of the deposition of platelet aggregates in the microcirculation (75). Thrombocytopenia, like other immune-mediated drug reactions, seems to involve the formation of heparin-dependent IgG antibodies directed against a heparin–platelet factor-4 complex expressed on the platelet membrane. Binding of this antibody–heparin complex results in platelet activation with aggregation leading to microvascular thrombus. This process requires minuscule amounts of heparin. Clinical bleeding is an infrequent problem in these patients in spite of the often marked thrombocytopenia observed.

From a practical perspective, the diagnosis of heparin-induced thrombocytopenia is usually one of exclusion. Diagnostic markers do exist (e.g., heparin-dependent platelet antibodies, aggregation, or serotonin release), but these tests are best considered confirmatory and not exclusionary. An ELISA assay for heparin-dependent platelet antibodies is the most common test obtained to investigate a possible diagnosis of HIT, but because of a relatively high "false-positive" rate, it is generally recommended that a more specific heparin-induced platelet injury assay, such as a serotonin release assay, be performed for confirmation. The diagnosis may be difficult to confirm because coexisting clinical illnesses with the potential to cause thrombocytopenia also may be present. While heparin-induced thrombocytopenia may be more likely to be associated with the use of bovine lung heparin, it can occur after exposure to porcine heparin or, much less commonly, to LMWH. When type II HIT is suspected or confirmed, all exposure to heparin, including heparin flushes, heparin in TPN, and heparin-coated catheters, must be removed and anticoagulation with an alternate agent must be initiated because of the risk of delayed thrombosis which can occur up to 30 days after the removal of heparin exposure (75). Patients with type II HIT should receive continued anticoagulation with direct thrombin inhibitors (argatroban, bivalirudin) (76, 77). While other agents have been employed to provide anticoagulation in the past, production of the direct thrombin inhibitor lepirudin was discontinued in 2012 and the heparinoid. Danaparoid is not available in the United States. The direct thrombin inhibitors are preferred as they carry no risk of cross-reacting with the heparin-dependent antibodies already present (78). Argatroban is cleared by the liver and lepirudin by the kidney. Consequently, the choice and dose of drug may be affected by the presence of hepatic or renal insufficiency. Warfarin alone is not an adequate therapy for suspected type II HIT because of the risk of thrombosis from depression of protein C levels. However, warfarin can be utilized in conjunction with a direct thrombin inhibitor and subsequently continued as a single agent once therapeutic suppression of vitamin K–dependent clotting factors has been achieved. Platelet transfusions are contraindicated in type II HIT due to the risk of inducing vascular thrombosis (75).

Qualitative Platelet Disorders

Many of the drugs frequently used in the ICU have the potential to impair platelet function. Frequently, the sicker the patient, the greater the likelihood that he/she will be exposed to one of these drugs. These patients often have other underlying pathophysiologic conditions that in and of themselves can predispose to bleeding. Table 143.6 provides an abbreviated list of the drugs that can affect at least *in vitro* platelet function.

All unnecessary drugs should be viewed as suspect and discontinued in patients with evidence or a strong suspicion of qualitative platelet dysfunction. In most cases, terminating the offending drugs usually results in a restoration of normal platelet functional activity. Aspirin is the notable exception as it irreversibly inhibits platelet cyclo-oxygenase, resulting in a defect that lasts for the duration of the platelet life span (8 to 9 days). The effect is profound: a single 325 mg aspirin tablet results in a qualitative platelet defect that remains in 50% of the circulating platelets 5 days after its ingestion. Ideally, one would like to avoid all aspirin ingestion for at least 7 days prior to an elective invasive procedure.

Nonsteroidal anti-inflammatory agents (NSAIDs) such as ibuprofen or naproxen sodium similarly inhibit platelet cyclo-oxygenase. However, their effects are reversible, and normal platelet function is usually restored within 24 hours of the last dose. Under most circumstances, the degree of platelet inhibition produced by NSAIDs is not clinically significant and patients can receive these drugs for analgesia and fever control. It is reasonable, however, to minimize the use of NSAIDs in the bleeding severely thrombocytopenic patient. Other antiplatelet agents such as the thienopyridines clopidogrel and prasugrel, ticlopidine and dipyridamole can produce platelet inhibition that remains evident for several days after discontinuing the drug. The β-lactam antibiotics can sterically hinder the binding of a platelet aggregation agonist (e.g., ADP) to its specific platelet receptor, thus resulting in impaired platelet aggregation under circumstances of normal physiologic stimulation. This, too, is reversed on removal of the drug. Fortunately, only a minority of patients exposed to these antibiotics will exhibit clinically significant platelet inhibition.

In the ICU, one must also always consider the possibility that a patient with bleeding suggestive of a platelet defect might have an inherited disorder of platelet function. While rare, these disorders are encountered from time to time and include Glanzmann's thrombasthenia (abnormal platelet GPIIb/IIIa), Bernard–Soulier syndrome (abnormal GP Ib/IX), Wiskott–Aldrich syndrome, platelet storage pool deficiency (abnormal platelet dense bodies), and the Gray platelet disorder (abnormal platelet α-granules).

Management

Because many of the adverse drug-related platelet effects are reversible, all unnecessary medications should be discontinued promptly when platelet function seems impaired. The more controversial issue is deciding whether platelet transfusions are warranted in a particular patient. The relationship of thrombocytopenia to clinical bleeding is relative, that is, it is difficult to identify a specific, arbitrary platelet count (threshold) below which bleeding is likely to occur. Several conditions, such as massive transfusion syndrome and DIC, may respond to empirical platelet transfusion at counts as high as 80,000 or even 100,000 platelets/μL, although bleeding in the presence of a platelet count of 80,000/μL (or greater) is unlikely to be a result of the thrombocytopenia. With other causes, such as thrombocytopenia seen with cancer chemotherapy and bone marrow aplasia, therapy may not be required until counts fall below 10 to 20,000/μL. As previously stated, rhFVIIa has also been used to counteract the hemostatic defect caused by aspirin or clopidogrel (50).

The morbidity and mortality related to bleeding increase measurably in patients undergoing induction chemotherapy for acute leukemia when the platelet count falls below 10,000 to 20,000/μL. Empirical administration of platelets to these patients significantly limits both morbidity and mortality. This finding, however, has been generalized to virtually all patients with platelet counts in this range. The appropriateness of this approach is unclear. A major concern that should temper the empirical use of platelet transfusion is the development of alloimmunization to transfused platelets, potentially negating any future benefit from platelet transfusion in a time of need. Patients with acute leukemia typically have self-limited marrow aplasia resulting from chemotherapy. Therefore, the need for platelet transfusion is also limited and the chances for development of antiplatelet antibodies are greatly decreased. Patients with aplastic anemia, however, have an ongoing need for platelet transfusion, so their risk of alloimmunization is high. Autoimmune disorders associated with increased peripheral platelet destruction, disorders of splenic sequestration, and drug-related thrombocytopenia are unlikely to benefit from platelet transfusion. An exception is related to a planned invasive procedure associated with an increased risk of bleeding. In this situation, empirical platelet transfusion immediately before the procedure may be reasonable. As previously noted, platelet transfusions in the presence of type II HIT are contraindicated.

Uremia

Uremia is commonly seen in the ICU and is associated with an increased risk of bleeding (79,80). Uremia has been shown to cause a reversible impairment of platelet function, although the "toxin" responsible for this defect is not well defined. Some studies have demonstrated an impairment of platelet–vessel wall interactions and suggest defects in vWf. The degree of platelet impairment appears to be related to the severity of uremia for a given patient. In addition, thrombotic events are also increased in patients with uremia. These, too, appear to be multifactorial in etiology but in part reflect the increase in renal loss of antithrombin III and protein S in nephrotic range proteinuria (81).

Several therapeutic approaches may modulate the qualitative platelet defect associated with uremia. The primary therapy in this setting is dialysis. Cryoprecipitate, 1-deamino-8-D-arginine vasopressin (DDAVP; 0.3 μg/kg maximum dose 21 μg), and conjugated estrogens (10 mg/d in adults) have been given to patients with severe uremia and an acquired defect in primary hemostasis with good results. The benefit derived by treatment with cryoprecipitate or DDAVP appears to be related to the consequent increase in the plasma concentration of the large multimeric forms of vWF, thus greatly improving platelet adhesion. The durations of action of these agents, however, are limited, reaching their zenith between 2 and 6 hours. Additional doses of DDAVP during the same 24-hour period may result in a diminished response to the drug (tachyphylaxis) with little or no further benefit. Patients who exhibit tachyphylaxis to DDAVP may require 48 to 72 hours before again responding to this agent. The mechanism of action of the conjugated estrogens is not known. In contrast to the first two therapies described, the effect of estrogen is more protracted and does not diminish with repeat dosing although a benefit is not noted for 3 to 5 days after starting therapy.

THROMBOTIC SYNDROMES

Thrombotic events may often be the cause of admission to an ICU, particularly if one includes acute coronary syndromes in this category. The noncardiac thrombotic syndromes frequently encountered in the ICU include:

- Deep venous thrombosis (specifically in association with a central venous catheter)
- Heparin-induced thrombocytopenia
- Pulmonary embolism syndrome
- TTP/hemolytic-uremic syndrome
- Thrombotic DIC
- Stroke and central nervous system (CNS) venous sinus thrombosis (most commonly seen in infants and the elderly in association with marked dehydration)

Many of these conditions, particularly venous thromboembolic events, often develop while the patient is in the ICU and may be preventable. The intensivist should assess risk of DVT and risks of thromboprophylaxis in all patients and institute appropriate therapy on a case-by-case basis based on the assessed risk of thrombosis. In general, postoperative patients and those who will be immobilized for long periods of time are considered at risk and should be considered candidates for some sort of thromboprophylaxis (82). Approximately 10% of ICU patients will develop DVT while in the ICU in spite of receiving some sort of thromboprophylaxis, and up to 15% of these patients will experience a symptomatic pulmonary embolus (83,84). However, not all patients are at the same risk and not all respond to prophylactic measures equally. Consequently, recognition of patient risk factors and initiation of effective prophylaxis measures are critical for the care of these patients. Patients with multiple genetic thrombosis risk factors have been shown to have a greater risk for DVT or pulmonary emboli than do patients without any or only one identified risk factor (85).

Management

The initial management approach for a patient with a documented (or highly suspected) thrombotic event is generally anticoagulation with either UH or LMWH. The efficacy of either appears to be equivalent although some studies suggest that the incidence of severe bleeding is less with LMWH (86). The use of LMWH may produce a more stable level of anticoagulation which may result in fewer laboratory tests and dose adjustments. The choice of which agent to use is at the discretion of the intensivist. However, if repeated invasive procedures are anticipated, UH may be the preferred agent owing to its shorter half-life. Most patients may be started on UH with a bolus dose of 50 unit/kg followed by a continuous infusion of 10 units/kg/hr, these doses may be reduced for the elderly or frail patient. Once initiated, anticoagulation is adjusted to keep the aPTT roughly 1.5 to 2.5 times baseline values (corresponding to a plasma heparin concentration of 0.2 to 0.4 units/ml or anti-Xa level of 0.4 to 0.7 units/mL). Dosing of LMWH is weight based generally starting at 1 mg/kg every 12 or 24 hours depending on the clinical presentation. Doses are titrated to achieve an anti-Xa activity level of between 0.4 and 1.0 units/mL (determined 3 to 4 hours after a dose) depending on the intensity of anticoagulation desired. The dose of warfarin is titrated to maintain an INR of the PT between 1.5 and 4.0 depending on the intensity of anticoagulation desired.

SELECTED DISORDERS

Systemic Diseases Associated with Factor Deficiencies

Amyloidosis, Gaucher's disease, and the nephrotic syndrome are occasionally seen in the ICU. Each may have one or more associated factor deficiencies that may complicate patient management and result in bleeding. Patients with either amyloidosis or Gaucher's disease may develop factor IX deficiency. Factor X deficiency also has been associated with amyloidosis. These deficiencies generally result from the absorption of the specific clotting factor onto the abnormal proteins present with each disorder. In the nephrotic syndrome, factor IX deficiency also may develop. Although it was originally thought that proteinuria was responsible for the development of factor IX deficiency, this may not be the case. The deficiency typically remits with corticosteroid therapy. Finally, antithrombin III deficiency can be seen along with the nephrotic syndrome and may lead to thrombosis. The loss of antithrombin III does appear to be related to proteinuria.

Laboratory Disorders not Associated with Bleeding

Lupus Anticoagulants

The lupus anticoagulant has received much attention as a potential cause of bleeding by virtue of its name and its associated laboratory abnormalities. As an isolated hemostatic defect, thrombosis is the most likely problem (25% incidence rate), with bleeding in one series occurring in only 1 of 219 patients with the lupus anticoagulant (87–89).

The PT and aPTT assays depend on the interaction of various coagulation factors with either a lipoprotein or phospholipid to activate coagulation efficiently. The lupus anticoagulant is an antiphospholipid antibody directed against these phospholipids or lipoproteins and produces prolongation of the PT, aPTT, or the measured recalcification time of platelet-rich plasma. Prolongation of the aPTT occurs more commonly than prolongation of the PT, although an isolated prolongation of the PT can be seen. Twenty-five percent of patients with active SLE and the lupus anticoagulant also have associated thrombocytopenia or hypoprothrombinemia and are therefore at risk for bleeding in contrast to those patients with the lupus anticoagulant alone who are not at increased risk for bleeding. Although the lupus anticoagulant was originally described in patients with SLE, it is not limited to this class of diseases. Indeed, lupus anticoagulants or anticardiolipin antibodies, or both, have been demonstrated in large percentages of patients with human immunodeficiency virus infection, hemophilia A, or both. Lupus anticoagulants also are observed in disorders accompanied by chronic and acute inflammation.

Thrombotic events in patients who exhibit a lupus anticoagulant may occur independent of the underlying disorder and can be directly related to the lupus anticoagulant itself. The likelihood of thrombosis associated with a lupus anticoagulant appears to be the greatest when the lupus anticoagulant has specificity for β_2-glycoprotein I or for phosphatidylserine. Some forms of the disorder, such as that associated with pregnancy, do respond to anti-inflammatory drugs such as aspirin or prednisone. Thrombosis, when it occurs, is equally likely to be venous or arterial. Venous thrombosis is more common in the extremities while arterial thrombosis is more common in the CNS. Placental infarcts are frequently seen in placental specimens in those patients with repeated fetal wastage. Stroke, myocardial infarction, and pulmonary embolization are also well described in patients with the lupus anticoagulant.

Reactive Hyperfibrinogenemia

Hyperfibrinogenemia is defined as a plasma fibrinogen concentration greater than 800 mg/dL. In the clinical lab, fibrinogen is measured using a functional assay in which time to fibrin clot formation is the endpoint. Plasma from the patient is allowed to clot in the presence of excess thrombin. The time to clotting in this setting is proportional to the amount of fibrinogen present in the sample. When excessive amounts of fibrinogen are present, clotting is incomplete and fibrin fragments that inhibit further fibrin clot formation are formed. Other hematologic parameters, such as the aPTT, PT, and the TT, are consequently prolonged, suggesting a potential (artifactual) for bleeding despite a high fibrinogen level. This can be evaluated by diluting the plasma to a normal fibrinogen concentration using saline or defibrinated plasma. These same clotting studies will now be normal. Bleeding is not seen unless the fibrinogen also is a dysfibrinogen, although even in these patients, bleeding remains an uncommon problem. In patients with dysfibrinogenemia, clotting studies fail to correct when either saline or defibrinated plasma dilutions are undertaken, thus distinguishing them from patients with reactive hyperfibrinogenemia.

Future Directions

Current areas of active investigation include defining subsets of patients with acute illness-related coagulopathies to better identify appropriate therapeutic interventions that address specific pathophysiologic aberrations causing the coagulopathic state (e.g., complement activation, metabolic abnormalities, endothelial injury, etc.). Progress in this area will require continued investigation into endothelial function, the links between hemostasis (coagulation) and inflammation, and the various regulatory pathways involved in both hemostasis and inflammation. While we look for new drugs that address these issues, we must take care to not discard older drugs that may represent important therapies for some of these patient groups. While single-institution case series comparing new treatment strategies to historic outcomes may help identify potential treatments, large multi-institutional studies will be required to answer the questions. In a similar fashion, work to better define those patients most at risk for thrombosis in the ICU and prophylactic therapies to be employed continues. Thirdly, investigation into transfusion practices to maximize benefit and minimize risks and unnecessary transfusions need to continue. This, too, will require large, multi-institutional randomized studies.

Key Points

- Hemostasis is a dynamic process in which clot formation (coagulation) and clot lysis (thrombolysis) are active and balanced according to the needs of the patient.
- Bleeding may result from too little coagulation, too much fibrinolysis, or both.
- Localized bleeding generally indicates a local (anatomic) problem while a generalized hemostatic abnormality generally results in generalized bleeding.

- The routine tests of coagulation (aPTT, PT/INR) only provide a measure of *in vitro* clot formation and do not provide information on platelet function or fibrinolysis. Consequently, they are of limited value in determining bleeding risk.
- If HIT is suspected, all heparin exposure must be eliminated and alternate anticoagulation provided until the diagnosis is confirmed (or excluded).
- Use of blood product support (e.g., FFP, platelet concentrates, factor concentrates) should be directed to correct a known hemostatic deficit. FFP should not be utilized to provide intravascular volume in the absence of a plasmatic hemostatic abnormality.
- While DIC is the 800-lb gorilla of bleeding, it is frequently *not* in the room.

References

1. Palta S, Saroa R, Palta A. Overview of the coagulation system. *Indian J Anaesth*. 2014;58:515.
2. Eilertsen KE, Osterud B. Tissue factor: (patho)physiology and cellular biology. *Blood Coagul Fibrinolysis*. 2004;15:521.
3. Matafonov A, Cheng Q, Geng Y, et al. Evidence for factor IX-independent roles for factor XIa in blood coagulation. *J Thromb Haemost*. 2013;11:21187.
4. Hayward CP, Rao AK, Cattaneo M. Congenital platelet disorders: overview of their mechanisms, diagnostic evaluation and treatment. *Haemophilia*. 2006;12(Suppl 3):128.
5. Aird WC. The role of the endothelium in severe sepsis and the multiple organ dysfunction syndrome. *Blood*. 2003;23:23.
6. Levi M, ten Cate H, van der Poll T. Endothelium: Interface between coagulation and inflammation. *Crit Care Med*. 2002;30(Suppl):S220.
7. Chee YL. Coagulation. *J R Coll Physicians Edinb*. 2014;44:42.
8. Olson JD. D-dimer: an overview of hemostasis and fibrinolysis, assays, and clinical applications. *Adv Clin Chem*. 2015;69:1.
9. Draxler DF, Medcalf RL. The fibrinolytic system-more than fibrinolysis? *Transfus Med Rev*. 2015;29:102.
10. Lupu F, Keshari RS, Lambris JD, Coggeshall KM. Crosstalk between the coagulation and complement systems in sepsis. *Thromb Res*. 2014;133:S28.
11. Bergmann S, Hammerschmidt S. Fibrinolysis and host response in bacterial infections. *Thromb Haemost*. 2007;98:512.
12. Weiler H. Inflammation-associated activation of coagulation and immune regulation by protein C pathway. *Thromb Res*. 2014;133:S32.
13. Eilertsen KE, Osterud B. Tissue factor: (patho)physiology and cellular biology. *Blood Coagul Fibrinolysis*. 2004;15:521.
14. Liaw PCY. Endogenous protein C activation in patients with severe sepsis. *Crit Care Med*. 2004;32(Suppl):S214.
15. Joyce DE, Nelson DR, Grinnell BW. Leukocyte and endothelial cell interactions in sepsis: relevance of the protein C pathway. *Crit Care Med*. 2004; 32(Suppl):S280.
16. Rigby AC, Grant MA. Protein S: A conduit between anticoagulation and inflammation. *Crit Care Med*. 2004;32(Suppl):S336.
17. Hermans PW, Hazelzet JA. Plasminogen activator inhibitor type 1 gene polymorphism and sepsis. *Clin Infect Dis*. 2005;41(Suppl 7):S453.
18. Walley KR, Russell JA. Pretein C-1641 AA is associated with decreased survival and more organ dysfunction in severe sepsis. *Crit Care Med*. 2007; 35:12.
19. Lillicrap D, Nair SC, Srivastava A, et al. Laboratory issues in bleeding disorders. *Hemophilia*. 2006;12(Suppl 3):68.
20. Khair K, Liesner R. Bruising and bleeding in infants and children: a practical approach. *Br J Haematol*. 2006;133:221.
21. Brezovska-Kavrakova J, Krstevska M, Bosilkova G, et al. Hyperhomocysteinemia and of methylenetetrahydrofolate reductase (C677T) genetic polymorphism in patients with deep vein thrombosis. *Mater Sociomed*. 2013;25:170.
22. Li D, Zhou M, Peng X, Sun H. Homocysteine, methylenetetrahydrofolate reductase C677T polymorphism, and risk of retinal vein occlusion: an updated meta-analysis. *BMC Ophthalmol*. 2014;14:147.
23. Qi X, Yang Z, De Stefano V, Fan D. Methylenetetrahydrofolate reductase C677T gene mutation and hyperhomocysteinemia in Budd-Chiari syndrome and portal vein thrombosis: a systematic review and meta-analysis of observational studies. *Hepatol Res*. 2014;44:E480.
24. Oren H, Cingoz I, Duman M, et al. Disseminated intravascular coagulation in pediatric patients: clinical and laboratory features and prognostic factors influencing survival. *Pediatr Hematol Oncol*. 2005;22:679.
25. Chuansumrit A, Hotrakitya S, Sirinavin S, et al. Disseminated intravascular coagulation findings in 100 patients. *J Med Assoc Thai*. 1999;82(Suppl 1): S63.
26. Girolami A, Luzzatto G, Varvarikis C, et al. Main clinical manifestations of a bleeding diathesis: an often disregarded aspect of medical and surgical history taking. *Hemophilia*. 2005;11:193.
27. Barton JC, Poon MC. Coagulation testing of the Hickmann catheter blood in patients with acute leukemia. *Arch Intern Med*. 1986;146:2165.
28. Franz RC. ROTEM analysis: a significant advance in the field of rotational thromboelastometry. *S Afr J Surg*. 2006;47:2.
29. Hunt H, Stanworth S, Curry N, et al. Thromboelastography (TEG) and rotational thromboelastometry (ROTEM) for trauma induced coagulopathy in adult trauma patients with bleeding. *Cochrane Database Syst Rev*. 2015;2:CDC010438.
30. Haas T, Gorlinger K, Grassetto A, et al. Thromboelastometry for guiding bleeding management of the critically ill patient: a systematic review of the literature. *Minerva Anestesiol*. 2014;80:1320.
31. Lipets EN, Ataullakhanov FI. Global assays of hemostasis in the diagnosis of hypercoagulation and evaluation of thrombosis risk. *Thromb J*. 2015;13:4.
32. Bick RL, Arun B, Frenkel EP. Disseminated intravascular coagulation: clinical and pathophysiological mechanisms and manifestations. *Haemostasis*. 1999;29:111.
33. Voves C, Wuillemin WA, Zeerleder S. International Society on Thrombosis and Haemostasis score for overt disseminated intravascular coagulation predicts organ dysfunction and fatality in sepsis patients. *Blood Coagul Fibrinolysis*. 2006;17:445.
34. Cauchie P, Cauchie Ch, Boudjeltia KZ, et al. Diagnosis and prognosis of overt disseminated intravascular coagulation in a general hospital: meaning of the ISTH score system, fibrin monomers, and lipoprotein-C-reactive protein complex formation. *Am J Hematol*. 2006;81:414.
35. Gando S, Iba T, Eguchi Y, et al. A multicenter, prospective validation of disseminated intravascular coagulation diagnostic criteria for critically ill patients: comparing current criteria. *Crit Care Med*. 2006;34:625.
36. Leclerc F, Hazelzet J, Jude B, et al. Protein C and S deficiency in severe infectious purpura of children: a collaborative study of 40 cases. *Intensive Care Med*. 1992;18:202.
37. Taylor FB Jr, Toh CH, Hoots WK, et al. Scientific Subcommittee on Disseminated Intravascular Coagulation (DIC) of the International Society on Thrombosis and Haemostasis (ISTH): towards definition, clinical and laboratory criteria, and a scoring system for disseminated intravascular coagulation. *Thromb Haemost*. 2001;86:1327.
38. Gando S. The utility of a diagnostic scoring system for disseminated intravascular coagulation *Crit Care Clin*. 2012;28:373.
39. Verhave JC, Wetzels JF, van der Kar NC. Novel aspects of atypical haemolytic uremic syndrome and the role of eculizumab. *Nephrol Dial Transplant*. 2014;29:iv131.
40. Sarode R, Bandarenko N, Brecher ME, et al. Thrombotic thrombocytopenic purpura: 2012 American Society for Apheresis (AFSA) consensus conference on classification, diagnosis, management, and future research. *J Clin Apher*. 2014;29:148.
41. Goel R, Ness PM, Takemoto CM, et al. Platelet transfusions in platelet consumptive disorders are associated with arterial thrombosis and in-hospital mortality. *Blood*. 2015;26:1470.
42. Zhou A, Mehta RS, Smith RE. Outcomes of platelet transfusion in patients with thrombotic thrombocytopenic purpura: a retrospective case series study. *Ann Hematol*. 2015;94:467.
43. Otrock ZK, Liu C, Grossman BJ. Platelet transfusion in thrombotic thrombocytopenic purpura. *Vox Sang*. 2015;109(2):168.
44. Loriat C, Fakhouri F, Ariceta G, et al. An international consensus approach to the management of atypical hemolytic uremic syndrome in children. *Pediatr Nephrol*. 2016;31(1):15.
45. Kaplan BS, Ruebner RL, Spinnale JM, Copelovitch L. Current treatment of atypical hemolytic uremic syndrome. *Intract Rare Dis Res*. 2014;3:34.
46. Elliott BM, Aledort LM. Restoring hemostasis: fibrinogen concentrate versus cryoprecipitate. *Expert Rev Hematol*. 2013;6:277.
47. Sallah S, Husain A, Nguyen NP. Recombinant activated factor VII in patients with cancer and hemorrhagic disseminated intravascular coagulation. *Blood Coagul Fibrinolysis*. 2004;15:577.
48. Scarpelini S, Rizoli S. Recombinant factor VIIa and the surgical patient. *Curr Opin Crit Care*. 2006;12:351.

49. Boffard KD, Riou B, Warren B, et al. Recombinant factor VIIa as adjunctive therapy for bleeding control in severely injured trauma patients: two parallel randomized, placebo-controlled, double blind clinical trials. *J Trauma.* 2005;59:8.
50. Altman R, Scazziota A, De Lourdes Herrera M, Gonzalez C. Recombinant factor VIIa reverses the inhibitory effect of aspirin or aspirin plus clopidogrel on *in vivo* thrombin generation. *J Thromb Haemost.* 2006;4:2022.
51. Ganguly S, Spengel K, Tilzer LL, et al. Recombinant factor VIIa: unregulated continuous use in patients with bleeding and coagulopathy does not alter mortality and outcome. *Clin Lab Haematol.* 2006;28:309.
52. O'Connell KA, Ward JJ, Wise RP, et al. Thromboembolic adverse events after use of recombinant human coagulation factor VIIa. *JAMA.* 2006;295:293.
53. Yoshimura J, Yamakawa K, Ogura H, et al. Benefit profile of recombinant human soluble thrombomodulin in sepsis-induced disseminated intravascular coagulation: a multicenter propensity score analysis. *Crit Care.* 2015;19:78.
54. Gando S, Saitoh D, Ishikura M, et al. A randomized, controlled, multicenter trial of the effects of antithrombin on disseminated intravascular coagulation in patients with sepsis. *Crit Care.* 2013;17:R297.
55. Jaimes F, de la Rosa G, Arango C, et al. A randomized clinical trial of unfractionated heparin for treatment of sepsis (the HETRASE study): design and rationale. *Trials.* 2006;7:19.
56. Lisman T, Caldwell SH, Leebeck FW, Portes RJ. Hemostasis in chronic liver disease. *J Thromb Haemost.* 2006;4:2059.
57. Dasher K, Trotter JF. Intensive care unit management of liver-related coagulation disorders. *Crit Care Clin.* 2012;28:389.
58. Shahani T, Covens RK, Lavend'Homme N, et al. Human liver sinusoidal endothelial cells but not hepatocytes contain factor VIII. *J Thromb Haemost.* 2013;12:36.
59. Goodnough LT. A reappraisal of plasma, prothrombin complex concentrates, and recombinant factor VIIa in patient blood management. *Crit Care Clin.* 2012;28:413.
60. Muller MC, Arbous MS, Spoelstra-de Man AM, et al. Transfusion of fresh-frozen plasma in critically ill patients with a coagulopathy before invasive procedures: a randomized clinical trial (CME). *Transfusion.* 2015;55:26.
61. Dentali F, Ageno W, Crowther M. Treatment of coumarin-associated coagulopathy: a systemic review and proposed treatment algorithms. *J Thromb Haemost.* 2006;4:1853.
62. Hardy JF, de Moerloose P, Samama CM; members of the Groupe d'Interet en Hemostase Perioperatoire. Massive transfusion and coagulopathy: pathophysiology and implications for clinical management. *Can J Anaesth.* 2006;53(6 Suppl):S40.
63. Spinella PC, Holcomb JB. Resuscitation and transfusion principles for traumatic hemorrhagic shock. *Blood Rev.* 2009;23:231.
64. Ledgerwood AM, Blaisdell W. Coagulation challenges after severe injury with hemorrhagic shock. *J Trauma Acute Care Surg.* 2012;72:1714.
65. Hallet J, Lauzier F, Mailloux O, et al. The use of higher platelet:RBC transfusion ratio in the acute phase of trauma resuscitation: a systematic review. *Crit Care Med.* 2013;41:2800.
66. Hellstern P. Fresh-frozen plasma, pathogen-reduced single-donor plasma or biopharmaceutical plasma? *Transfus Apher Sci.* 2008;39:69.
67. Liumbruno GM, Marano G, Grazzini G, et al. Solvent/detergent-treated plasma: a tale of 30 years of experience. *Exp Rev Hematol.* 2015;8:3674.
68. Brown RE, Dorion RP, Trowbridge C, et al. Algorithmic and consultative integration of transfusion medicine and coagulation: a personalized medicine approach with reduced blood component utilization. *Ann Clin Lab Sci.* 2011;41:211.
69. Khan S, Allard S, Weaver A, et al. A major haemorrhagic protocol improves the delivery of blood component therapy and reduces waste in trauma massive transfusion. *Injury.* 2012;44:587.
70. Hsu JM, Hitos K, Fletcher JP. Identifying the bleeding trauma patient: predictive factors for massive transfusion in an Australasian trauma population. *J Trauma Acute Care Surg.* 2013;75:359.
71. Segal JB, Dzik WH. Paucity of studies to support that abnormal coagulation test results predict bleeding in the setting of invasive procedures: an evidence-based review. *Transfusion.* 2005;45:14
72. Keeling D. International normalized ratio in patients not on vitamin K antagonists. *J Thromb Haemost.* 2007;5:188.
73. Goldstein JN, Refaai MA, Milling TJ Jr, et al. Four-factor prothrombin complex concentrate versus plasma for rapid vitamin K antagonist reversal in patients needing urgent surgical or invasive interventions: a phase 3b, open-label, non-inferiority, randomized trial. *Lancet.* 2015;385(9982):2077.
74. Muller MC, Arbous MS, Spoelstra-de Man AM, et al. Transfusion of fresh-frozen plasma in critically ill patients with a coagulopathy before invasive procedures: a randomized clinical trial. *Transfusion.* 2015;55:26.
75. Warkentin TE, Kelton JG. A 14-year study of heparin-induced thrombocytopenia. *Am J Med.* 1996;101:502.
76. Bartholomew JR, Pratts J. Bivalirudin for the treatment of heparin-induced thrombocytopenia. In: Warkentin TE, Greinacher A, eds. *Heparin-Induced Thrombocytopenia.* Boca Raton, FL: CRC Press–Taylor and Francis Group; 2012:429.
77. Joseph L, Casanegra AI, Dhariwal M, et al. Bivalirudin for the treatment of patients with confirmed or suspected heparin-induced thrombocytopenia. *J Thromb Haemost.* 2014;12:1044.
78. Dager WE, White RH. Pharmacotherapy of heparin-induced thrombocytopenia. *Exp Opin Pharmacother.* 2003;4:919.
79. Sohal AS, Ganji AS, Crowther MA, Treleavan D. Uremic bleeding: pathophysiology and clinical risk factors. *Thromb Res.* 2006;118:417.
80. Boccardo P, Remuzzi G, Galbusera M. Platelet dysfunction in renal failure. *Semin Thromb Hemost.* 2004;30:579.
81. Molino D, DeLucia D, Gaspare de Santo N. Coagulation disorders in uremia. *Semin Nephrol.* 2006;26:46.
82. Geerts WH, Pineo GF, Heit JA, et al. Prevention of venous thromboembolism: the Seventh ACCP Conference on Antithrombotic and Thrombolytic Therapy. *Chest.* 2004;126(3 Suppl):338S.
83. Cook D, Crowther M, Meade M, et al. Deep venous thrombosis in medical-surgical critically ill patients: prevalence, incidence, and risk factors. *Crit Care Med.* 2005;33:1565.
84. Khouli H, Shapiro J, Pham VP, et al. Efficacy of deep venous thrombosis prophylaxis in the medical intensive care unit. *J Intensive Care Med.* 2006;21:352.
85. Simsek E, Yesilyurt A, Pinarli F, et al. Combined genetic mutations have remarkable effect on deep venous thrombosis and/or pulmonary embolism occurrence. *Gene.* 2014;536:171.
86. Kearon C, Ginsberg JS, Julian JA, et al. Comparison of fixed-dose weight-adjusted unfractionated heparin and low-molecular-weight heparin for acute treatment of venous thromboembolism. *JAMA.* 2006;296:935.
87. Giannakopoulos B, Krilis SA. The pathogenesis of the antiphospholipid syndrome. *N Engl J Med.* 2013;368:1033.
88. Galli M, Norbis F, Ruggeri L, et al. Lupus anticoagulants and thrombosis: clinical association of different coagulation and immunologic tests. *Thromb Haemost.* 2000;84:1012.
89. Willis R, Gonzalez EB, Brasier AR. The journey of antiphospholipid antibodies from cellular activation to antiphospholipid syndrome. *Curr Rheumatol Rep.* 2015;17:16.

CHAPTER

144

Transfusion Therapy: When to Use It and How to Minimize It

AMANDA WEHLER and SAMIR M. FAKHRY

INTRODUCTION

Physicians encounter a large spectrum of medical and surgical conditions that may require transfusion therapy, including acute blood loss, catastrophic illness in the critical care setting, diseases associated with chronic anemia, and a variety of congenital and acquired bleeding disorders. The modern-day care of the critically ill requires a thorough knowledge of the pathophysiology of blood loss and anemia, as well as an understanding of normal hemostatic mechanisms and the sometimes-complex disorders of coagulation encountered in these populations. The ability to administer blood products is a very important therapeutic modality in the care of the critically ill patients. When carried out with a thorough, up-to-date understanding of indications, risks, and benefits, blood transfusion can be reasonably safe and effective.

In this chapter, the basic concepts of anemia are discussed, and the indications for and use of blood components, potential risks of blood products, and alternatives to blood transfusion are reviewed. Because blood products are a limited resource with potential serious adverse side effects, knowledge of appropriate indications, potential risks, and available alternatives will allow clinicians to exercise judgment in using this treatment modality. Based on the accumulating evidence, special emphasis will be placed on minimizing transfusion in the critical care setting.

BLOOD AND BLOOD PRODUCT USE

Although blood product collection and transfusion has been decreasing since 2008, approximately 13.8 million units of whole blood/red blood cells (WB/RBC), 2.2 million apheresis-equivalent units of platelets, and 3.8 million units of plasma are transfused annually in the United States. The most recent National Blood Collection and Utilization Survey Report, published by the Department of Health and Human Services in 2011, showed that, compared to 2008, WB/RBC transfusions had decreased 8.2%, plasma transfusions decreased 13.4%, and total collections of blood products decreased 9.1%; the use of platelets was unchanged. Only 4.5% of the US population donated blood in 2011, a decrease from 5.4% in 2008. Transfusion rates in the United States for 2011 were estimated at 44.0 units of WB/RBC transfusion per 1,000 overall population. This fell from 48.8 per 1,000 population in 2008 and approaches rates reported in the 1990s (1). Efforts at blood management have targeted transfusion utilization in recent years and have changed projections in the available blood supply from one of shortage to one of surplus.

Despite trending decreases in blood collection and transfusion, the most common procedure performed during hospitalization in 2010 among all age groups, except infants, was blood transfusion; 11% of hospital stays that included a procedure—ranging from vaccination to parenteral nutrition to surgery—were transfused (2). Anemia is common in critically ill patients due to cumulative blood loss, diminished erythropoiesis, deficient erythropoietin, and hemolysis. Some estimates for the incidence of anemia in the intensive care unit (ICU) range as high as 95% (3). Not surprisingly, the transfusion rate is even higher in the critically ill, where various studies show 14.7% to 53.0% of ICU patients are transfused (4).

PATHOPHYSIOLOGY

Understanding Blood Product Collection, Preparation, and Storage

The historic origin of transfusion centered on whole blood transfusion. Modern-day blood banks have adopted component therapy both to optimize management of the blood supply and because the majority of patients do not require therapeutic red blood cells, platelets, and plasma all at once. There are two methods for blood collection: whole blood donation and apheresis collection. In whole blood donation, a unit of whole blood is collected from the donor and is then separated into its individual components—packed red blood cells (PRBCs), plasma, and platelets—to maximize the benefits of each donated unit. After collection, each whole blood unit is gently centrifuged to sediment or "pack" the red blood cells away from the platelet-rich plasma, which is then extracted off the red blood cells, yielding a unit of PRBCs and a platelet-rich plasma unit; the latter is centrifuged again to sediment the platelets. The platelet-poor plasma is extracted off the platelets and rapidly frozen to yield a unit of plasma. Finally, the platelets are then resuspended in the residual plasma, yielding a platelet concentrate. If cryoprecipitate is desired, the frozen plasma is allowed to thaw at 4°C and the precipitate that forms is collected to yield cryoprecipitate. Albumin and other proteins can then be extracted from the remaining cryoprecipitate-poor plasma.

Another option for the collection of blood erythrocytes, leukocytes, platelets, or plasma is through automated cell separators (apheresis). Whole blood is withdrawn from a donor and enters the apheresis instrument, which contains a centrifuge that separates whole blood into various components based on the specific gravity of the different cells. Erythrocytes, leukocytes, platelets, or plasma can selectively be removed, and the remaining blood is returned to the donor. Using this technique, multiple units of erythrocytes or platelets can be removed at a time.

In both whole blood collection and apheresis collection, blood is collected from donors into plastic bags containing a citrate anticoagulant solution that binds calcium, thus preventing coagulation. These anticoagulant solutions include citrate phosphate dextrose (CPD), citrate phosphate double dextrose (CP2D), and citrate phosphate dextrose adenine (CPDA-1). Additional solutions, called additive solutions (AS), are often added that extend the shelf-life of PRBC, and contain dextrose, adenine, sodium chloride, and either phosphate (AS-3) or mannitol (AS-1 and AS-5). In adults, the various types of anticoagulants and AS are not of clinical concern; however, in children, AS units should be used with caution in massive transfusion, cardiac surgery, exchange transfusion, and renal or hepatic insufficiency since the safety of large-volume transfusion of AS in children is unknown.

Storage and refrigeration create progressive changes in PRBCs, known as the *storage lesion.* During storage, glucose is consumed, 2,3-diphosphoglycerate (2,3-DPG) and adenosine triphosphate (ATP) decrease, and potassium increases. The decrease in 2,3-DPG causes a high-oxygen affinity state for hemoglobin, which decreases oxygen delivery to tissue until 2,3-DPG normalizes in the red cells after transfusion. Red blood cell morphology changes from biconcave disk to echinocyte to spherocyte, all of which reduce red blood cell flexibility and increase fragility, which can lead to hemolysis. Hemolysis can increase nitric acid consumption and induce inflammation. It is important to realize, however, that many of these changes are reversed shortly after transfusion.

Two recent randomized controlled trials (RCTs) have evaluated the effects of PRBC storage duration on ICU and cardiac surgery patient outcomes by randomizing patients to receive fresher or older PRBC units. Neither of these studies found any differences related to storage duration in primary or secondary outcomes to include mortality, organ function, infection, ischemic events, thrombosis, ventilator time, or length of stay (5,6). At least 16 additional studies have been completed in over 9,300 critically ill patients, ranging in type from retrospective to prospective, with and without randomization. The majority of these studies did not find adverse patient outcomes associated with longer blood storage, although few were conflicting on whether there is higher mortality and/or higher gastric mucosal pH in patients receiving older blood (7). Overall, there is a growing body of evidence that points toward no measurable adverse clinical effects related to red blood cell storage duration, including one RCT on pediatric patients (8).

Anemia Pathophysiology

The strictest definition of anemia is that of a decrease in red blood cell mass. The World Health Organization further specifies that anemia in males is a hemoglobin less than 13 g/dL and in females it is defined as a hemoglobin less than 12 g/dL. Anemia can be classified as absolute, related either to impaired red blood cell production or red blood cell loss, or it can be relative, such as in pregnancy or other fluid overload. Since red blood cell function centers on oxygen delivery from lung to tissue and carbon dioxide delivery from tissue to lung, a decrease in red blood cell mass theoretically impairs normal oxygen and carbon dioxide gas exchange and delivery.

Oxygen supply to tissue depends not only on hemoglobin concentration, but also on oxygen saturation and affinity. If there is blood loss, the degree and rate of change in blood volume also affect the oxygen supply. The physiologic response to anemia varies according to acuity and etiology. Gradual onset of anemia allows for compensatory mechanisms in patients without marked compromise in cardiovascular or pulmonary systems. The clinical manifestations of anemia include easy fatigability, dyspnea on exertion, feeling faint or weak, palpitation, or headache; patients may appear pale, tachycardic, and hypotensive. These changes occur due to an increase in cardiac output as compensation for the anemia. In severest cases, tissue hypoxia can result in shock, hypotension, coronary, or pulmonary insufficiency.

In the critically ill patient, tolerance to anemia is affected by volume status, physiologic reserve, and the etiology and rate of onset of the anemia. Anemia inherently causes a decrease in blood viscosity. Normovolemic patients, whose cardiac output is not compromised as it would be in hypovolemia, are often more capable of mounting tachycardia and increased myocardium contractility via the adrenergic response. Additional compensatory response includes preferential distribution of blood to vital organs primarily over the periphery and an increase in the oxygen extraction ratio, reflected as a decrease in mixed venous saturation. Acute anemia places the myocardium at special risk, as oxygen demand is increased with the increased myocardial work of tachycardia and increased contractility, yet oxygen extraction in the myocardium is already near maximal at rest. Patients with coronary artery disease, heart failure, or acute coronary syndrome may be unable to mount a physiologic response to anemia and, thus, experience myocardial ischemia, infarction, or dysrhythmia (4).

Iron deficiency is most common in gastrointestinal and cancer patients, but also affects patients with obstetric, renal, and immune disorders. Nearly all body systems are affected by iron deficiency: fatigue, depression, and impaired cognitive function in the central nervous system; anorexia and nausea in the gastrointestinal system; low skin temperature and pallor of skin, mucous membranes, and conjunctiva in the vascular system; impaired T-cell and macrophage function in the immune system; exertional dyspnea, tachycardia, palpitations, cardiac hypertrophy, and increased pulse pressure in the cardiorespiratory system; and menstrual problems and loss of libido in the genitourinary system.

DIAGNOSIS

Diagnosis of Anemia

Once a decreased hemoglobin level (anemia) is discovered, attention must be turned to the discovery of the etiology. As mentioned previously, absolute anemia is often broken into broad categories of impaired production of red blood cells or red blood cell loss. Relative anemia should first be excluded as a potential cause of the decreased hemoglobin, through an examination of clinical history for pregnancy or macroglobulinemia and review of fluid balance. If these are excluded, consider red blood cell loss and evaluate the patient for sources of obvious or occult bleeding. Hemolysis is another source of blood loss and can be evaluated with lactate dehydrogenase, haptoglobin, direct Coombs (or direct antiglobulin test), bilirubin (direct and indirect), urinalysis, and a peripheral blood smear. If the anemia is related to impaired production of red blood cells, diagnosis is often guided by the classic red

TABLE 144.1 Guidelines for Diagnosis of Anemia

Anemia	Cause	Common Laboratory Abnormality
Hypoproliferative, microcytic	Iron deficiency	Low ferritin, increased IBC, decreased serum iron, reduced Fe/TIBC ratio, generally increased RDW
Hypoproliferative, microcytic	Anemia of chronic disease	Generally high ferritin, normal IBC, decreased serum iron, normal Fe/TIBC ratio, generally normal RDW
Hyperproliferative, normocytic	Hemolytic anemia	Schistocytosis, increased reticulocytes, low haptoglobin, elevated carboxyhemoglobin, elevated LD, elevated indirect bilirubin, generally increased RDW
Hypoproliferative, normocytic	Aplastic anemia	Leukopenia, thrombocytopenia, hypocellular bone marrow, generally normal RDW
Hypoproliferative, normocytic	Renal failure	Elevated BUN and creatinine, low erythropoietin, burr cells, generally normal RDW
Hypoproliferative, macrocytic (megaloblastic)	B_{12} and/or folate deficiency	Low B_{12} and/or folate, hyperlobulated polymorphonuclear leukocytes, macro-ovalocytes, increased RDW
Hypoproliferative, macrocytic (non-megaloblastic)	Hypothyroidism	Elevated TSH, normal RDW

IBC, iron binding capacity; Fe, iron; TIBC, total IBC; RDW, red cell distribution width; LD, lactate dehydrogenase; BUN, blood urea nitrogen; TSH, thyroid stimulating hormone.
From Pincus MA, Abraham NZ. Interpreting laboratory results. In: McPherson RA, Pincus MR, eds. *Henry's Clinical Diagnosis and Management by Laboratory Methods.* 21st ed. Philadelphia, PA: WB Saunders; 2007:76–90.

blood cell morphology descriptions of normocytic, microcytic, or macrocytic. In a complete blood count (CBC) profile, the mean corpuscular volume (MCV) correlates to red blood cell size. When MCV is normal, decreased, or increased, red blood cells are considered normocytic, microcytic, or macrocytic, respectively. Generally microcytic anemia is often related to iron deficiency and thalassemia; normocytic anemia is often related to early blood loss or anemia of chronic disease; and macrocytic anemia is often related to vitamin B_{12} or folate deficiency or hematologic malignancy. The MCV can thus suggest additional laboratory tests or clinical assessment to further elucidate the cause of the anemia. Table 144.1 suggests diagnostic pathways for the diagnosis of anemia. Complete understanding of the cause of the anemia is required in order to determine treatment.

TREATMENT

Transfusion Decision-Making

Transfusion based on sound physiologic principles and an understanding of relative risks and benefits should give maximal benefit to the patient, with efficient use of a valuable and finite resource. Utilizing data from recent studies, it is increasingly possible to base transfusion practice on scientific grounds. The following transfusion guidelines are presented based on the best evidence currently available. Given the active ongoing investigations in this area, it is likely that frequent updates will be forthcoming.

Whole Blood

There have been few widely accepted indications for whole blood in modern transfusion practice. Storage of whole blood precludes the extraction of components and, from a systems perspective, is highly inefficient. As such, whole blood is not available from most blood banks in the United States. In theory, the goals of oxygen delivery and volume expansion can be achieved with PRBC and crystalloid solutions. Experience with the use of whole blood by the US military (9) has suggested that transfusion of warm fresh whole blood to combat-related trauma patients may have survival benefits versus similar patients receiving component therapy (10). The military experience with whole blood has not crossed into civilian medicine at this time (11), though it has launched discussion in related topics, such as appropriate PRBC/plasma/platelet ratio in massive hemorrhage resuscitation, limiting crystalloid infusion during hemorrhage resuscitation, and whether early plasma and platelet transfusion in hemorrhage conveys survival benefit.

Some pediatric cardiovascular surgeons use fresh whole blood for pediatric cardiovascular surgical patients. Cardiovascular surgery, especially cases involving cardiopulmonary bypass, instigates hemodilution and platelet dysfunction, which results in coagulopathy, as well as cytokine release and complement activation, which results in inflammation. Proponents of whole blood for pediatric cardiovascular surgery claim whole blood has improved hemostatic properties and induces less inflammation (12,13); however, this has been refuted by an RCT finding no clinical or biochemical advantage in fresh whole blood over component therapy in pediatrics undergoing cardiopulmonary bypass. In this study, fresh whole blood was actually associated with longer length of stay in ICU, fluid overload, and longer ventilator time (14).

Red Blood Cells

Packed red blood cells are the most commonly transfused blood product. The indications for transfusing PRBC are generally divided between two main categories of patients: those with and without acute hemorrhage. In both cases, PRBCs are transfused with the purported effects of increasing circulatory volume, transporting oxygen, and the rheologic effect of increasing blood flow/viscosity; in reality, these effects may not be demonstrated. Today, transfusions are not recommended for volume expansion, perhaps with the exception of massive hemorrhage, and may lead to transfusion-associated circulatory overload. Blood viscosity, while necessary to maintain microvascular circulation, may only benefit from rheologic support of transfusion in severe hemodilution, and a significant increase in blood viscosity may actually hinder perfusion

(15). Despite this, anemia is a more common indication for PRBC transfusion than active hemorrhage (4,16–22). Practitioners commonly assume that anemia confers a risk for ischemia due to decreased oxygen delivery and, similarly, assume that PRBC transfusion can improve oxygen delivery and mitigate the risk of ischemia. In actuality, anemia *may* increase the risk of ischemia, and a PRBC transfusion *may* improve tissue oxygenation in some cases of severe anemia but, in many situations, the risk of transfusing PRBC appears to be greater than the probability of benefit.

The decision to transfuse a nonhemorrhaging patient can generally be made according to substantial evidence in the literature. As of this writing, approximately 9,000 patients have been enrolled in multiple RCTs comparing practices of giving PRBC transfusions at restrictive hemoglobin thresholds (i.e., 7 to 8 g/dL) versus liberal hemoglobin thresholds (i.e., 9 to 10 g/dL). Four RCTs evaluating the patient outcomes of 30- or 60-day mortality, organ failure, ability to walk 10 feet, myocardial infarction, and revascularization events in various patient groups (ICU, coronary artery bypass graft or cardiac valve surgery, hip fracture with cardiovascular disease, acute coronary syndrome) found no significant difference in outcomes in patients transfused restrictively or liberally (23–26). Two RCTs evaluating patient outcomes of 30- or 45-day mortality, myocardial infarction, and revascularization events in various patient groups (acute coronary syndrome, upper gastrointestinal bleed) favored restrictive transfusion practice over liberal (27,28); one of these studies associated increased mortality with liberal transfusion. Conversely, one RCT in cardiac surgical patients associated slightly higher mortality with restrictive transfusion practice at hemoglobin threshold of 7.5 g/dL (29). The summation of this high-quality evidence supports the use of a restrictive transfusion threshold, such as hemoglobin of 7 g/dL in ICU patients and gastrointestinal bleeds and hemoglobin of 8 g/dL in cardiac surgery or acute coronary syndrome patients.

It is important to understand that, despite intention of giving PRBC transfusion to anemic patients to enhance oxygen utilization by tissue, this does not always occur (15,30–33). Global oxygen delivery (DO_2) is determined by the arterial content of oxygen as well as cardiac output ($DO_2 = CO \times CaO_2$; where CO is the cardiac output and CaO_2 is the arterial oxygen content). Arterial oxygen content is dependent on hemoglobin level and hemoglobin saturation. The ratio of oxygen delivery to global oxygen consumption (VO_2), or DO_2/VO_2, is known as the oxygen extraction ratio and can be measured by mixed venous saturation (SvO_2). The oxygen extraction ratio in a homeostatic patient is generally wide, around 20% to 30%, which allows for a broad margin of safety. With anemia or blood loss, as DO_2 decreases and the oxygen extraction ratio narrows, a critical DO_2 level is reached when DO_2 can no longer keep up with VO_2. A simple hypothesis postulates that a PRBC transfusion, by increasing both cardiac output and arterial oxygen content, would increase DO_2 and therefore VO_2. However, in actuality, VO_2 seems to demonstrate independence of DO_2 in circumstances where hypoxia is not severe. Studies show conflicting results on whether DO_2 is actually increased after PRBC transfusion (4,34,35). While a PRBC transfusion almost always causes a posttransfusion rise in hemoglobin, which in itself is often associated with increased DO_2, the VO_2 is not always increased and ischemia (measured in terms of blood lactate level) is rarely improved (15,32,34,36,37); the reasons for this are not entirely understood. One reason may be that the increase in hemoglobin after a PRBC transfusion, by increasing blood viscosity, dampens the sympathetic response to anemia, decreasing cardiac output (4,38,39). Other reasons may include inability of oxygen to dissociate from hemoglobin based on depleted 2,3-diphosphoglycerate in transfused red blood cells, decreased functional density of the microcirculation, or the belief that many patients whom receive PRBC transfusions do not have severe enough ischemia whereby their VO_2 is in the dependent phase with DO_2 (4,15,40–42).

The decision to transfuse PRBC in nonhemorrhaging patients should be based on clinical assessment and not solely on hemoglobin levels. Common symptoms of anemia may include shortness of breath, fatigue, and tachycardia, but hypovolemia can also cause these symptoms, and the latter can be easily treated with crystalloids. Additional consideration should be given to factors such as patient age, comorbidity, and evidence or risk of ischemia. Consider the possibility of systemic hypoperfusion when there is persistently high lactate or central or mixed venous saturation below 60%. If the combined laboratory and clinical assessment of the nonhemorrhaging patient meet evidence-based guidelines for transfusion, one unit of PRBC at a time should be transfused. Hemoglobin equilibrates 15 minutes after transfusion is completed, and one PRBC unit can be expected to increase hemoglobin by 1 g/dL and hematocrit by 3%. After one unit, hemoglobin and clinical reassessment should be repeated to determine if further PRBC transfusion is necessary. The ultimate goal of the PRBC transfusion should not be to maintain a hemoglobin number, but to improve patient outcome. Guidelines for PRBC transfusion can be found in Table 144.2.

Platelets

Most platelet transfusions are given prophylactically to reduce the risk for spontaneous bleeding in thrombocytopenic patients. As described earlier, platelets can be prepared from whole blood, where one single platelet concentrate comes from one whole blood donation, or from apheresis, where up to three units can be collected at a time from a single donor. Platelet concentrates from whole blood can be transfused singly, often to pediatric patients, but are more commonly pooled together in pools of four or six concentrates, commonly referred to as a "six-pack." Platelet units from apheresis donors are also known as "single-donor platelets." One apheresis unit is considered equivalent to one pooled platelet containing four to six concentrates from multiple donors; the transfusion of the apheresis type of platelets is on the rise (1). The administration of an apheresis unit of platelets is advantageous since it exposes the recipient to a set of foreign antigens from a single donor, whereas an equivalent dose of pooled platelet transfusion exposes the patient to four to six sets of foreign antigens, increasing the risk of alloimmunization, or

TABLE 144.2 Guidelines for Transfusion of Packed Red Blood Cells

- Active hemorrhage
- Hgb <7 g/dL
- Hgb <8 g/dL for cardiac surgery or acute coronary syndrome
- Systemic hypoperfusion (persistently high lactate or central or mixed venous saturation <60%)

antibody-formation, to foreign antigens such as human platelet antigens (HPA) or human leukocyte antigens (HLA). In addition, bacterial contamination is less likely with single-donor apheresis platelets. In cases of alloimmunization to HPA or HLA, platelet refractoriness can occur, potentially necessitating special laboratory evaluation and procurement of products such as crossmatched platelets or HLA-selected platelets. These are costly and time consuming and may cause delay in transfusion.

The efficacy of platelet transfusion may be assessed both by clinical parameters (improved hemostasis) and by following the platelet counts at 1 hour and 24 hours as an estimate of platelet survival. The platelet count at 1-hour posttransfusion of a unit of apheresis platelets (or apheresis-equivalent pooled platelets) should increase by 30,000 to 60,000 platelets/μL. Less pronounced responses should be expected with repeated transfusion and the development of alloimmunization, or in the presence of fever, sepsis, consumption, or splenomegaly. Failure of an appropriate rise in platelet count at 1-hour posttransfusion is suggestive of immune platelet refractoriness (i.e., alloimmunization), and failure to sustain increased platelet counts in 24-hour posttransfusion is suggestive of nonimmune platelet refractoriness (i.e., fever, sepsis, consumption, or splenomegaly) (43).

The evidence to support platelet transfusion decision-making ranges from low to moderate quality, as there are both observational studies and RCTs evaluating this concept (44). Three RCTs determined that prophylactic transfusions significantly reduced risk for spontaneous grade two or greater bleeding in inpatients with radiation and/or chemotherapy-associated hypoproliferative thrombocytopenia (45–48). Four RCTs determined the most appropriate platelet count threshold for prophylactic platelet transfusion to effectively reduce bleeding in therapy-associated hypoproliferative thrombocytopenia is 10,000 cells/μL (49–52). Transfusion of platelets at a 10,000 cells/μL threshold was associated with less platelet usage and fewer transfusion reactions, while transfusion at a 20,000 to 30,000 cells/μL threshold did not further decrease incidence of bleeding or bleeding-related mortality.

When the decision to transfuse platelets is made, dosing should commence with a single apheresis platelet or apheresis-equivalent single pool of platelets. Six RCTs have evaluated platelet dosing and determined that two apheresis platelet units does not decrease bleeding risk compared to one apheresis platelet unit (53,54), and that half of an apheresis platelet unit actually conveys the same prophylactic bleeding protection as one whole apheresis platelet unit (54–58).

Evidence supporting prophylactic platelet transfusion for invasive procedures is largely based on observational studies. A set of clinical practice guidelines on platelet transfusion from the AABB (formerly American Association of Blood Banks) suggests an appropriate platelet count for placement of central venous catheter is 20,000 cells/μL and for lumbar puncture or for major elective nonneuraxial surgery is 50,000 cells/μL (44). Guidelines for platelet transfusion can be found in Table 144.3.

TABLE 144.3 Guidelines for Transfusion of Platelets

Platelet Count	Plus
<10,000 cells/μL	Bone marrow failure
<50,000 cells/μL	Impending surgery or invasive procedure *or* Active bleeding
<100,000 cells/μL	Neurosurgical or ophthalmic procedure *or* Multiple trauma or cardiopulmonary bypass patient with intra-aortic balloon pump

Plasma

Plasma is used as a source of clotting factors in bleeding patients or patients requiring an invasive procedure with multiple coagulation factor deficiencies, such as those in liver dysfunction or consumptive or dilutional coagulopathy. An understanding of the half-life of clotting factors is necessary to help understand the appropriate use of plasma. Factor VII, the main clotting factor of the extrinsic pathway of the coagulation cascade, has the shortest half-life, in the range of 2 to 7 hours. Most factor VII is, therefore, depleted from plasma products before their manufacturing is complete, and thus plasma cannot correct a deficiency in factor VII, diagnosed by a prolonged prothrombin time (PT) and normal activated partial thromboplastin time (aPTT). The next factors with the shortest half-lives are factors V and VIII, with 15 to 36 and 8 to 12 hours, respectively. These factors also decline during plasma processing and storage, but not below the levels required for hemostasis. It is important to understand that normal hemostasis can be achieved with only 5% to 30% of normal clotting factor activity (59). The PT and the aPTT can be used to assess patients for need for plasma transfusion and to follow the efficacy of administered plasma. If both PT and aPTT are prolonged, consider a decrease in final common pathway clotting factors (prothrombin, fibrinogen, factor V, factor X) or a combined decrease in extrinsic and intrinsic factors, such as in vitamin K antagonists or liver disease. If aPTT alone is prolonged, consider a decrease in extrinsic clotting factors (factors VIII, IX, XI, and XII), such as with lupus anticoagulant.

Clinical practice for the evaluation of bleeding or bleeding risk often deviates from the assessment of PT and aPTT as described above, focusing rather on the international normalized ratio (INR). The INR is a calculated value meant to standardize commercial reagents against international standards, in order for patients on vitamin K antagonists to achieve accurate and standardized results assessing their therapeutic range of treatment regardless of which laboratory performs the test. Some argue that the INR should only be used for this purpose but many in clinical practice use the INR to evaluate bleeding risk or target the INR for "correction" with therapeutic intervention in bleeding patients.

Two main points must be emphasized: firstly, that an INR prolonged in the mild to moderate range (<2) is not predictive of bleeding, and, secondly, plasma does not "correct" a mild to moderate elevation in INR. Twenty-five published studies between 1966 and 1996 have addressed these points, with the preponderance of data showing that the PT/INR does not show any correlation with clinical bleeding in association with invasive procedures unless they are very abnormal and that prophylactic plasma does not attenuate bleeding risk (59–73). The actual INR measured on plasma products varies between 1.14 and 1.4. Appropriate prophylactic utilization of plasma can thus be considered for patients requiring an invasive procedure with an INR in the moderately prolonged range, conservatively between 1.7 and 2.0.

Additional indications for plasma include dilutional coagulopathy related to massive hemorrhage, factor deficiencies

TABLE 144.4 Guidelines for Transfusion of Plasma

- International normalized ratio >1.7 with an anticipated invasive procedure
- Postmassive transfusion to prevent development of coagulopathy
- Treatment of thrombotic thrombocytopenia purpura if plasmapheresis not available
- Single-factor deficiency where commercial concentrate is not available
- Warfarin reversal *only if* vitamin K and/or 4-factor prothrombinase complex concentrate are not available
- Treatment or prophylaxis of thromboembolism in antithrombin, protein C, or protein S deficiency

where commercial factor concentrates are unavailable (factor V, factor XI), vitamin K antagonist reversal if vitamin K and/or four-factor prothrombinase complex concentrate are not available, thrombotic thrombocytopenic purpura if plasmapheresis is not available, and treatment or prophylaxis of thromboembolism in deficiency of antithrombin, protein C, or protein S.

Plasma should be avoided for normalizing an INR below 1.7 in the absence of bleeding, blood volume expansion or nutrition support, coagulopathy that can be corrected with vitamin K administration, and single-factor deficiency where commercial factor concentrates are available.

The dosing of plasma varies according to the underlying disease process necessitating the transfusion. When plasma is given for clotting factor replacement, a dose of 10 to 20 mL/kg total body weight is often used, which would increase clotting factors approximately 20% immediately posttransfusion. Guidelines for plasma transfusion can be found in Table 144.4.

Cryoprecipitate

Cryoprecipitate was originally developed as treatment for hemophilia A, due to the factor VII content. Each unit of cryoprecipitate contains a minimum of 80 IU of factor VIIIC and 150 mg fibrinogen in 5 to 20 mL plasma; it also contains von Willebrand factor and factor XII. With technologic advances in recombinant factor development, cryoprecipitate is no longer used for its original purpose, but is instead used for acquired coagulopathy, such as in clinical settings associated with hemorrhage, or in consumptive disorders of fibrinogen. Solid clinical evidence for appropriate utilization and fibrinogen threshold for cryoprecipitate transfusion is lacking. Empirically, general guidelines for the transfusion of cryoprecipitate include bleeding patients with fibrinogen below 100 mg/dL or von Willebrand disease unresponsive to desmopressin when factor concentrates are unavailable. Cryoprecipitate has fallen out of favor, particularly in some European countries where it has been removed from the market, in lieu of fibrinogen concentrate, which delivers fibrinogen in a smaller volume and with a safer profile than a human donor blood product (74).

In adults, cryoprecipitate is often given in a pool of 5 to 10 individual units, resulting in a volume between 50 and 200 mL, dependent on individual blood banks; each unit in the pool will increase the fibrinogen by 5 to 10 mg/dL in an average-sized adult. In children, cryoprecipitate can be given in individual units at a dose of 1 to 2 units/10 kg, which can increase fibrinogen by up to 100 mg/dL. Guidelines for cryoprecipitate transfusion can be found in Table 144.5.

TABLE 144.5 Guidelines for Transfusion of Cryoprecipitate

- Diffuse active bleeding with fibrinogen <100 mg/dL
- Von Willebrand's disease unresponsive to desmopressin when factor concentrates are unavailable

Blood Component Modification

Once the decision to transfuse a patient with a blood product is made, attention must be turned to whether the patient requires modification to the blood product, such as leukoreduction, irradiation, or washing. Leukoreduction is a process that depletes the white blood cells in either a PRBC or platelet blood product, and this process can be completed prestorage or poststorage (i.e., pretransfusion). Prestorage leukoreduction is often preferred because earlier removal of white blood cells from the product decreases the possibility of cytokine leak from white blood cells into the product. In blood products collected by apheresis, leukoreduction is inherently performed by the mechanics of apheresis collection. Leukoreduced blood products are considered cytomegalovirus-safe ("CMV-safe"); the sites of CMV latency are thought to include progenitor cells that express CD34 and monocytes that express CD13 and CD14 antigens, thus leukoreduction of blood products decrease the transmission of CMV. One school of thought reasons that leukoreduced products are superior to CMV-seronegative products because, in early CMV infection, when the virus is solely intracellular, antibody tests used to connote a donor as seronegative would result as negative despite viral infection. In actuality, neither CMV-seronegative nor CMV-safe products equal "zero risk" to patients, as CMV transmission can occur at extremely low rates from both types of products (75). To combat acquisition of CMV from transfusion, patients in at-risk disease states should be transfused with leukoreduced blood products and then be monitored for CMV infection and/or treated with CMV prophylactic medication. CMV-seronegative blood products, while also effective at decreasing CMV transmission, are more difficult to acquire and cause delays in transfusion and potential costs to the health system. Overall, leukoreduction is indicated for decreased transmission of CMV, decreased incidence of febrile non-hemolytic transfusion reaction (HTR), and decreased likelihood of developing HLA alloimmunization in transplant patients or patients that are transfusion-dependent.

Irradiation is a process whereby gamma or x-ray irradiation causes DNA cross-linking in T-lymphocytes, rendering them inactive and unable to mount an immune response against the recipient. When T-lymphocytes do mount immune responses against immunocompromised transfusion recipients, the result is transfusion-associated graft versus host disease (TA-GVHD), which is nearly uniformly fatal. Indications for irradiated blood products include bone marrow or hematopoietic stem cell transplant candidate/recipient, congenital cellular immune deficiency, pediatric oncology on active chemotherapy, intrauterine transfusion, transfusion from blood relative, neonates less than 4 months of age, or patients receiving fludarabine, other purine analogues, or alemtuzumab chemotherapy. Caution should be exercised in pediatric patients receiving large-volume or rapid infusion of irradiated PRBC if the irradiation was performed more than 24 hours before the transfusion, as irradiation can damage red blood cells, leading to potassium leak into product supernatant and placing the patient at risk for hyperkalemia.

Washing is a process that removes most plasma/supernatant from PRBC or platelet products. The process of washing can remove up to 99% of the plasma/supernatant but also results in cellular loss of up to 33% of the red blood cells or platelets; it also causes increased red blood cell fragility, making them more susceptible to hemolysis, and can adversely affect platelet function. Washing decreases the shelf-life of the product, and, if performed in an open system, can increase the chance of bacterial contamination. The process is labor-intensive and can create over a 1-hour delay for transfusion. The indications for washed PRBC and platelets are in patients with IgA deficiency and anti-IgA antibody if no IgA-deficient products are available or in patients with history of severe anaphylactoid reactions to blood products.

Risks of Blood Transfusion

Even though a blood transfusion is a potentially life-saving intervention, significant risks are still involved in the administration of these products. Direct risks causally related to the transfusion range from mild, in the case of urticaria, to fatal and include transfusion-transmitted infection, transfusion reactions, volume overload, and potential for alloimmunization and mistransfusion. There are also plausible risks for increased morbidities such as increased infection, prolonged ventilator use, increased length of stay, and organ dysfunction, as well as increased mortality. A summary of blood transfusion risks can be found in Table 144.6.

The U.S. Food and Drug Administration (FDA) produces an annual report on fatalities related to blood transfusion.

TABLE 144.6 Risks of Blood Transfusion

Transfusion-Transmitted Infection
- Viral infection transmission
  - Hepatitis A
  - Hepatitis B
  - Hepatitis C
  - Human immunodeficiency virus 1 and 2
  - Human T-cell leukemia virus 1 and 2
  - Cytomegalovirus
  - West Nile virus
  - *Enterovirus* spp.
  - Human parvovirus B-19
  - Epstein–Barr virus
- Bacterial/protozoal/prion contamination of blood products
  - *Yersinia enterocolitica*
  - *Serratia marcescens*
  - *Staphylococcus* spp.
  - *Enterobacter cloacae*
  - *Escherichia coli*
  - Syphilis (*Treponema pallidum*)
  - Malaria (*Plasmodium* spp.)
  - Babesiosis (*Babesia* spp.)
  - Chagas disease (*Trypanosoma cruzi*)
  - Variant Creutzfeldt-Jakob disease

Transfusion reactions
Alloimmunization
Mistransfusion
Plausible risks
- Increased mortality
- Increased hospital and/or ICU length of stay
- Increased infection
- Prolonged ventilator time and/or systemic inflammatory response syndrome
- Renal failure
- Cardiac ischemia and/or atrial fibrillation

During the FDA fiscal year 2013 (October 1, 2012, to September 30, 2014), 65 transfusion recipient fatalities were reported to the FDA (76). Of the 65 deaths, 38 were directly related to the transfusion, and, in 21 deaths, the transfusion could not be ruled out as the cause of death. The majority of deaths were due to transfusion-related acute lung injury (TRALI) (14 deaths), followed by transfusion-associated circulatory overload (TACO) (13 deaths), non-ABO HTR (5 deaths), microbial infection (5 deaths), and ABO hemolytic-transfusion reaction (1 death). The leading causes of transfusion-related death over the past 5 years have remained primarily TRALI, followed by TACO. Physicians are bound by oath and duty to fully understand the risks of transfusion, along with the benefits, alternatives, and consequences of not transfusing, in order to engage patients in discussions regarding transfusion decision-making and to obtain informed consent.

Transfusion-Transmitted Infection

Infectious pathogens within blood products have been well-documented as posing a threat to public safety. Nearly all blood products are administered to recipients without sterilization or pathogen inactivation, and thus infectious pathogens that are not detected in the donor at the time of donation can be passed to the recipient. Pathogens range from bacterial to viral to parasitic to prion, some of which are highly tested for in donors but others of which rely on accurate answers and comprehension of donor screening questions in order to defer donors from donating potentially infectious blood.

Currently, tests are required on all blood donations for the detection of hepatitis B virus (HBV), hepatitis C virus (HCV), human immunodeficiency virus, types 1 and 2 (HIV-1/2), human T-cell lymphotropic virus, types I and II (HTLV-I/II), syphilis, west nile virus (WNV), and *Trypanosoma cruzi*. All of these pathogens have been documented to cause transfusion-transmitted infection. Technologic advances in many of the viral tests have become so advanced that, via detection of viral nucleic acid, transmission of HBV, HCV, and HIV through transfusion is nearly nonexistent. The rate of transmission of these is so low that risk is calculated only by theoretical modeling. There are still windows of time, however, immediately after infection occurs when even the highest quality tests cannot detect the virus. These periods of time, known as the "infectious window period," is 7.4 days for HCV, 9.1 days for HIV, and 26.5 to 18.5 days for HBV (77). Extensive questioning of donors on risk-associated behavior is also used to defer donors who have engaged in activities that may confer infection from these viruses.

Other than syphilis, there are no specific tests on donors for bacteria. Bacterial contamination occurs in approximately 1 in 3,000 blood products, and can cause anything from asymptomatic bacteremia in recipients to death. *Babesia microti* and *Staphylococcus aureus* have caused the most transfusion-transmitted infection fatalities over the past 5 years (76). Platelets do undergo blood culture prior to transfusion, although occasional culture-negative platelets have still caused transfusion–transmitted infection. The requirement for a secondary test for bacterial detection in platelet products is under current consideration by the FDA.

Transfusion–transmission of malarial protozoa and the prion responsible for variant-Creutzfeldt–Jakob disease have been documented. There are no FDA-approved tests for these pathogens and therefore donor screening questions help protect recipients from being at risk for these infections.

Transfusion Reactions

As discussed earlier, the noninfectious complications of transfusion are more likely to cause fatality than infectious ones, and the three leading causes of transfusion-associated mortality are TRALI, TACO, and HTR. Categories of adverse transfusion reactions and their management according to AABB are shown in Table 144.7. Transfusion reactions can be categorized broadly by timing and etiology into acute (<24 hours) or delayed (>24 hours) and immunologic or nonimmunologic. The responsibility for understanding transfusion reactions lies both with the physician ordering the transfusion, as he or she must discuss the risks with the patient, and with the transfusionist administering the blood product, as he or she must be vigilant for signs and symptoms of a reaction. Many common signs and symptoms of transfusion reactions are shared among the various types of reactions and generally include:

- Fever (defined as temperature ≥38°C and an increase of at least 1°C from pretransfusion value)
- Chills and/or rigor
- Skin manifestations such as urticaria, rash, flushing
- Hypo- or hypertension
- Respiratory distress such as tachypnea, dyspnea, wheezing, or coughing
- Pain at site of infusion or in abdomen, back, chest, or flank
- Jaundice (hyperbilirubinemia)
- Nausea/vomiting

TABLE 144.7 Transfusion Reactions: AABB Classification

Type and Incidence	Presentation	Treatment
Acute (<24 hr)—Immunologic		
Hemolytic ABO RH mismatch: 1 in 40,000 AHTR: 1 in 76,000 Fatal HTR: 1 in 1.8 million	Chills, fever, hypotension, renal failure, back pain, hemoglobinuria, pain along infusion vein, anxiety, DIC (oozing from IV sites)	Keep urine output >1 mL/kg/hr with fluids and IV diuretic (furosemide); analgesics; pressors (low-dose dopamine)
Febrile, nonhemolytic: 0.1–1% with universal leukoreduction products	Temperature elevation >1°C from baseline, chills and/or rigors, headache, vomiting	Antipyretics (acetaminophen)
Urticarial: 1:100–1:33 (1–3%)	Pruritus, urticaria, flushing	Antihistamine
Anaphylactic: 1:20,000–1:50,000	Hypotension, urticaria, bronchospasm, respiratory distress, wheezing, local edema, anxiety	Trendelenburg position; fluids; epinephrine; antihistamines; corticosteroids, beta-2 agonists
Transfusion-associated acute lung injury: 1:1,200–1,190,000	Hypoxemia, respiratory failure, hypotension, fever, bilateral pulmonary edema	Supportive care
Acute (<24 hr)—Nonimmunologic		
Transfusion-associated sepsis: incidence varies by component	Fever, chills, hypotension	Broad spectrum antibiotics; treat complications (e.g., shock)
Hypotension (associated with ACE inhibition): incidence dependent on clinical setting	Flushing, hypotension	Discontinue ACE inhibition; avoid albumin volume replacement for plasmapheresis; avoid bedside leukocyte filtration
Circulatory overload: <1%	Dyspnea, orthopnea, cough, tachycardia, hypertension, headache	Upright posture; oxygen; IV diuretic (furosemide); phlebotomy (250-mL increments)
Nonimmune hemolysis: rare	Hemoglobinuria. hemoglobinemia	Identify and eliminate cause
Air embolus : rare	Sudden dyspnea, acute cyanosis, pain, cough, hypotension, cardiac arrhythmia	Place patient on left side with legs elevated above chest and head
Hypocalcemia (i.e., ionized calcium) AKA citrate toxicity: incidence dependent on clinical setting	Paresthesia, tetany, arrhythmia	PO calcium supplement for mild symptoms during therapeutic apheresis procedures; slow calcium infusion in severe cases
Hypothermia: incidence dependent on clinical setting	Cardiac arrhythmia	Employ blood warmer
Delayed (>24 hr)—Immunologic		
Hemolytic: 1:2,500–1:11,000	Fever, decreasing hemoglobin, new positive antibody screening test, mild jaundice	Transfuse compatible PRBC as needed
Graft versus host disease: rare	Erythroderma, maculopapular rash, anorexia, nausea, vomiting, diarrhea, hepatitis, pancytopenia, fever	Corticosteroids, cytotoxic agents
Posttransfusion purpura: rare	Thrombocytopenic purpura, bleeding 8–10 days after transfusion	IVIG, plasmapheresis
Alloimmunization, human leukocyte antigens: 1:10 (10%)	Platelet refractoriness	Avoid unnecessary transfusions
Alloimmunization, red cell antigens: 1:100 (1%)	Positive blood group antibody screening test, delayed hemolytic reaction, hemolytic disease of the fetus/newborn	Avoid unnecessary transfusions
Delayed (>24 hr)—Nonimmunologic		
Iron overload Typically after 100 transfusions	Diabetes, cirrhosis, cardiomyopathy	Iron chelators

Adapted from Mazzei CA, Popovsky MA, Kopko PM. Noninfectious complications of blood transfusion. In: Fung MK, Grossman BJ, Hillyer CD, Westhoff CM, eds. *Technical Manual.* 18th edition. Bethesda, MD: AABB; 2014:665–696.

- Edema or erythema of mouth or periorbital area
- Urinary changes such as oliguria, anuria, hemoglobinuria

The diagnosis may be especially difficult in the patient under general anesthesia, and a high index of suspicion is needed in order to make a prompt diagnosis in such patients.

When a transfusion reaction is suspected, the infusion should be stopped immediately and the intravenous access line should be kept open with saline. A clerical recheck between the patient and the component must occur, to include review of all labels on the component and the patient's identification band. The only time a transfusion can be restarted is for a mild allergic transfusion reaction consistent of urticaria without respiratory involvement. Otherwise, the unit, including all intravenous solutions and tubing, should be sent promptly to the blood bank for examination, along with a patient blood sample drawn from a remote site.

Blood banks will vary in protocol and procedure for the workup of a transfusion reaction. Contacting your transfusion service for directions on investigating the cause of the reaction may be warranted. If an acute hemolytic transfusion reaction is suspected, a urinalysis should be completed along with tests for hemolysis (such as LD, haptoglobin, bilirubin). The blood bank testing will include a clerical recheck, repeat ABO testing on the patient and on the product, visual check for hemolysis, and direct Coombs (or direct antiglobulin test). Additional blood products, if required, can be given after acute hemolytic transfusion reaction is excluded. Recall that the signs and symptoms of a febrile, nonhemolytic transfusion reaction may mimic those of an HTR, so an increase in temperature must always be worked up as a transfusion reaction by the blood bank.

An *acute hemolytic transfusion reaction* is defined as acute lysis of red blood cells due to preformed antibodies against red cell antigens. This reaction can occur from as little as 10 mL of transfused incompatible blood product. The antibodies can be ABO or non-ABO, such as in cases of Rh antibodies (commonly anti-D, anti-c) or other blood groups (commonly anti-K). The preformed immunoglobulin attaches to red cell antigens and may also fix complement in order to destroy the red blood cell, either by intravascular hemolysis or extravascular hemolysis. The reaction varies from mild to severe, depending on the degree of complement activation and cytokine release and the total volume of incompatible blood transfused. Red cell destruction results in the release of vasoactive amines, kinins, and other mediators, which leads to hypotension, impaired renal function, activation of coagulation cascade, and, in more severe cases, disseminated intravascular coagulation (DIC) and shock. Aggressive fluid resuscitation should be initiated to maintain blood pressure, and urine output should also be maintained at high levels, which may require furosemide. The early development of hypotension and DIC is associated with increased mortality. The frequency of acute HTR due to ABO incompatibility is approximately 1:80,000 and results in fatality in approximately 1 in 1.8 million (78,79).

A *delayed hemolytic transfusion reaction* may occur days to months after transfusion of incompatible blood product. A transfused patient who develops an unexplained fall in hemoglobin or hematocrit, fever, or jaundice should be evaluated for the possibility of an HTR. Because the hemolysis is often extravascular, there is less risk for acute renal failure and DIC. The workup is similar to that for acute hemolytic reactions, and the need for clinical intervention is less likely.

Allergic transfusion reactions occur on a spectrum from mild, such as in urticaria, to fatal, such as in anaphylaxis. Symptoms can develop within minutes of the start of the transfusion and range up to 4-hour posttransfusion. Mechanisms behind allergic transfusion reactions are not fully understood. Some are hypersensitivity reactions to allergens in the product caused by preformed IgE in the recipient. Mast cell activation and degranulation causes release of secondary mediators, such as cytokines and lipids. The manifestations vary from a slight rash or urticaria to hemodynamic instability, with bronchospasm and anaphylaxis. Mild allergic reactions may be treated with antihistamines (e.g., diphenhydramine); more severe urticarial reactions may require methylprednisolone or prednisone. If anaphylactoid response occurs, epinephrine, oxygen, beta-2 agonists, and intubation may be required.

Febrile nonhemolytic transfusion reactions are defined according to temperature 38°C or higher and an increase of at least 1°C from pretransfusion value; other causes of fever should not be identifiable. This temperature change can occur during the transfusion up to 4 hours after the transfusion is complete. The etiology is thought to result from recipient antibodies against antigens on donor leukocytes or platelets or from accumulated cytokines in cellular blood components. Treatment consists of antipyretics and/or meperidine if rigors are present. These reactions can be prevented with transfusion of leukocyte-reduced blood components when pharmacotherapy fails.

TRALI is, by definition, a form of acute lung injury (ALI). ALI, as defined by the American–European Consensus Conference, includes acute hypoxemia with PaO_2/FiO_2 ratio up to 300 mmHg and bilateral pulmonary edema on frontal chest radiograph (80). Specific criteria for the diagnosis of TRALI were established by the Canadian Consensus conference (81):

- ALI with hypoxemia and PaO_2/FiO_2 up to 300 or SpO_2 below 90% on room air
- No pre-existing ALI before transfusion
- Onset of symptoms within 6 hours of transfusion
- No temporal relationship with an alternative risk factor for ALI

As such, signs and symptoms of TRALI typically are those of new-onset pulmonary edema (dyspnea, cyanosis, hypotension) and may include fever and chills. In one large study of TRALI patients, 100% required oxygen support and 72% required mechanical ventilation (82). The ALI in TRALI is often transient, and approximately 80% of patients improve within 48 to 96 hours; the remaining 20% may have a prolonged clinical course or fatality (78). Since the clinical syndrome is similar to many other conditions encountered in the critical care setting, the diagnosis of TRALI is made by exclusion and is likely underreported.

Transfusion-related ALI can occur secondary to the transfusion of all different kinds of blood components, but most commonly results from platelets and plasma. Like other etiologies of ALI, TRALI causes an increase in pulmonary microvascular permeability with increased protein levels in the edema fluid. The precise mechanism of TRALI is not fully elucidated. Two theories of the increased pulmonary microvascular permeability have been proposed in patients who develop TRALI. The first hypothesis suggests that leukocyte antibodies from the donor unit activate recipient leukocytes in the pulmonary circulation, leading to increased microvascular permeability and noncardiogenic pulmonary edema. Blood donations from multiparous women have been implicated as a contributing factor for TRALI, possibly because of increased leukocyte antibody levels. The second hypothesis assumes an initial predisposing event that primes the patient's neutrophils and sequesters them in the lung. Biologically active lipids and cytokines in the donor unit then further prime and activate the recipient's neutrophils, with resultant microvascular permeability and noncardiogenic pulmonary edema.

The treatment of TRALI is supportive and consists of appropriate hemodynamic and ventilatory support. Once TRALI is suspected, the transfusion should be terminated immediately and the blood bank notified. The donor unit can be tested for anti-HLA and/or antigranulocyte antibodies. Recently, regulatory bodies have required implementation of TRALI-reduction strategies by the blood donor industry, reducing the likelihood of presence of HLA antibodies in donor plasma.

TACO has a clinical presentation very similar to TRALI. The key distinction between TACO and TRALI relies in the etiology of the pulmonary edema. TACO results from cardiogenic pulmonary edema, while TRALI results from noncardiogenic pulmonary edema. The diagnosis of TACO, according to the Centers for Disease Control, requires new onset or exacerbation of three or more of the following within 6 hours after transfusion is completed (83):

- Acute respiratory distress (dyspnea, orthopnea, cough)
- Evidence of positive fluid balance
- Radiographic evidence of pulmonary edema
- Evidence of left heart failure
- Elevated central venous pressure (CVP)
- Elevated brain natriuretic peptide (BNP)

Patients at highest risk for TACO are very old and very young and those with congestive heart failure. The infusion of large volumes of blood products and other fluids most often precipitate TACO; however, it has also occurred secondary to modest volumes. Frequently a high flow rate is involved. As with all transfusion reactions, transfusion should be stopped as soon as symptoms develop. Several groups studying the pathophysiology of TACO suggest that it has a multiphasic spectrum, whereby pulmonary manifestations are later stage and earlier recognition can be made with trend monitoring of blood pressure and temperature, both of which have been shown to gradually increase in earlier stages of TACO (84,85). Treatment includes placing the patient in a seated position, providing oxygen, and reducing intravascular volume with diuretics. In severe cases, therapeutic phlebotomy may be indicated.

Alloimmunization and Compatibility

The blood bank plays a vital role in patient safety related to blood transfusion. This area of the laboratory performs under intense regulation for safe and quality practices and undergoes many inspections by regulatory personnel to ensure compliance. The process from the time a type and screen is drawn from a patient, through the testing that is performed in the blood bank and the assignment of blood products to the patient, to the bedside administration of the blood product is intensely scrutinized for appropriate patient identification and safety checks to ensure the right blood is transfused to the right patient. All of this is necessary because the risks of mistransfusion include fatality. Despite the highest level of safety and quality, patients may still have hemolytic transfusion reactions, both acute and delayed, if an antibody is not detected in the antibody screen, and every exposure to donor red blood cells poses a risk of alloimmunization, meaning antibody formation to a foreign red blood cell antigen.

While much of the process of an actual transfusion falls outside of the physician role (phlebotomist draws type and screen; laboratorian performs testing; tranfusionist administers product), occasionally the physician will be asked to make decisions on appropriate products for transfusion. A basic understanding of ABO and Rh blood groups and blood bank testing may help the physician make these decisions. Patients can safely receive ABO-compatible PRBC and plasma products without requiring ABO-identical products according to the physiologic nature of antigen expression and naturally occurring isoagglutinins or antibodies. For example, group O patients are the universal acceptor for all ABO groups of plasma products because there are no antigens expressed on group O red blood cells, and therefore, no donor antibody in plasma products will be able to recognize their target epitope in the recipient. However, group O patients can only receive type O PRBC because group O patients naturally have anti-A and anti-B isoagglutinins and will therefore destroy any non-group O PRBC transfused to them. ABO-incompatible plasma product transfusions are occasionally acceptable, however. Adults can safely receive up to two out-of-group platelets in a 24-hour period if the platelets are demonstrated to contain low-titer antibodies. Cryoprecipitate can be transfused without regard to ABO type because of the inherently low concentration of antibodies in the plasma. Trauma and other patients can receive ABO-incompatible plasma, although a limitation on the number of incompatible products, such as two to four units, is reasonable.

Part of the patient blood type reported by the blood bank includes the expression or absence of the D antigen. For example, a patient designated as O-positive expresses D antigen, and a patient designated as O-negative lacks the D antigen. The D antigen is one of the proteins categorized in the Rh group, along with C/c and E/e. Patients do not have natural converse immunity to Rh proteins as they do for ABO proteins. Therefore, a patient must be exposed to the D antigen in order to form anti-D. In general, the blood bank will strive to transfuse D antigen-negative PRBC to patients who do not express the D antigen in order to prevent alloimmunization and formation of anti-D. However, when it comes to blood products, D-negative PRBCs are a limited resource, and there are not enough of them to meet the transfusion needs of all D antigen–negative patients. Females of childbearing age are at the highest risk of consequence to carry an anti-D, due to anti-D's association with hemolytic disease of the fetus/newborn (HDFN). Therefore, in many large health systems, D-negative PRBCs are conserved for females of childbearing age and individuals who have anti-D. Older studies suggest that 80% of D antigen–negative individuals will form anti-D when exposed to D antigen–positive red blood cells (86), but newer studies suggest the rate is much lower, at about 22% particularly in cancer patients (87). The volume of red blood cells required for sensitization is extremely low, less than 0.1 mL, and therefore, platelet products (especially platelets manufactured from whole blood donations) can also cause anti-D alloimmunization due to slight red blood cell contamination. There are no Rh proteins on the platelets themselves. Again, the blood bank will often conserve platelet products from D-negative donors for females of childbearing age and for children. If a D-positive platelet is all that is available for transfusion to one of these patients, Rh-immune globulin can be given to prevent alloimmunization to D antigen.

When the blood bank performs a type and screen test on a patient in order to select a safe blood product, the screen portion of this test is only testing for antibodies against approximately 20 common red blood cell antigens. There are over 500 known red blood cell antigens, so many of these are not tested. The blood bank will also perform a crossmatch to evaluate for compatibility between the donor blood product and the recipient. If an antibody screen is positive, depending on the nature of the antibody, the blood bank may need to arrange for antigen-negative blood products. If the antigen is common in the donor population, the blood may be available immediately. If the antigen is not common or if the hospital is small, there may be several hours or days of delay locating the antigen-negative units. On rare occasions, crossmatch-incompatible PRBC can be transfused, such as in patients with warm or cold autoantibodies, where crossmatch compatibility is not achievable. In these cases, the transfused donor cells are likely to survive as long as the recipient's own red blood cells, e.g., if the warm autoantibody is causing brisk warm autoimmune hemolytic anemia in the patient, then the donor PRBC will also be briskly hemolyzed, but if the autoantibody lacks clinical significance, then transfused donor PRBC will not likely be affected.

Plausible Risks

Various adverse effects have been linked to blood transfusion beyond those direct risks of transfusion-transmitted infection and transfusion reaction. Several cohort studies have been published suggesting a link between transfusion and increased mortality (both short- and long-term), increased hospital and/or ICU length of stay, and higher incidence of various morbidities, including serious infections, prolonged ventilator time, renal failure, cardiac ischemia, atrial fibrillation, and/or systemic inflammatory response syndrome (15–17,88–105). The strength of evidence is low for these plausible links, however, with many of these studies being retrospective or observational. Of great interest is the fact that the majority of RCTs evaluating restrictive versus liberal transfusion practices show no difference in these types of outcomes (23–26,106), rather than an increased incidence of mortality or complications in patients receiving more PRBC. There are, of course, two notable exceptions where one RCT established increased mortality in gastrointestinal hemorrhage patients liberally transfused to maintain hemoglobin of 9 g/dL (27), and, conversely, where one RCT established increased mortality in cardiac surgical patients that were not transfused until a restrictive hemoglobin threshold of 7.5 g/dL (29).

Minimizing Transfusion

Given the known risks and the costs associated with blood transfusions, efforts should be made to minimize the use of transfusion whenever possible, and a comprehensive strategy of Patient Blood Management should be followed. Patient Blood Management is a multidisciplinary, patient-focused effort defined as "the timely application of evidence-based medical and surgical concepts designed to maintain hemoglobin concentration, optimize hemostasis and minimize blood loss in an effort to improve patient outcomes" (107). In patients with anemia, the need to correct anemia should be assessed (with emphasis on type and etiology of anemia), sources of ongoing blood loss should be controlled, and measures to enhance erythropoiesis should be entertained.

Minimizing Blood Loss

A significant amount of blood can be lost with repeated phlebotomy in the ICU, with some studies suggesting that up to 40 mL blood are being phlebotomized daily from a single patient (4,16); this is particularly significant in children with smaller blood volumes. Critical care practitioners should carefully consider the need for frequent phlebotomy in the ICU. A policy of obtaining laboratory results only when clinically indicated should be followed to avoid iatrogenic anemia. Consider eliminating standing laboratory orders, using microsampling techniques including bedside point-of-care testing, and limiting the practice of drawing the "rainbow" collection of specimen tubes without purposeful ordering.

Intraoperatively, there are multiple techniques that can be used to minimize blood loss. *Acute normovolemic hemodilution* is a technique whereby whole blood is removed from a patient at the beginning of a surgical procedure and crystalloid or colloid fluid is used to replace the blood volume removed, creating a relative anemia. Thus, when the patient undergoes operative bloodshed, the blood lost will contain fewer red blood cells. At the end of the procedure, the whole blood is returned to the patient. *Intraoperative blood recovery* (also known as cell salvage) is the process of collecting shed blood during surgery, anticoagulating it, and then washing and returning the erythrocytes to the patient. *Antifibrinolytic agents* (such as tranexamic acid or epsilon-aminocaproic acid) are utilized intravenously or topically at surgical sites such as the intrapericardial space or in a joint space to decrease the breakdown of fibrin and thus decrease bleeding. *Topical hemostatics and fibrin sealants* exist as various different commercial products or can be manufactured bedside, such as autologous platelet gel, and are used to close tissue defects and prevent excess blood loss via augmentation or stimulation of the coagulation cascade. Additional ancillary techniques to control intraoperative bleeding include bipolar cautery, deliberate hypotension, maintenance of normothermia, positioning, use of volume expanders, and selection of spinal or epidural anesthesia over general anesthesia when possible. It should be noted that preoperative autologous blood donation is no longer recommended due its provocation of iatrogenic anemia, creating a paradoxical increase in need for allogeneic transfusion. Also, a large number of preoperative autologous donated units were never transfused back to the patients who donated them.

Optimization of Red Cell Production

Erythropoiesis, the generation of red blood cells, is a process dependent on both iron and erythropoietin. Erythropoietin is essential early in the developmental progression from pluripotent stem cell to proerythroblast, while iron is essential in the developmental progression through the stages of erythroblast maturation. Iron is incorporated into the heme group, which serves as the site of attachment for oxygen.

If iron-deficiency anemia is confirmed, treatment must consist of addressing chronic or acute bleeding and may also consist of iron replacement. Oral iron therapy can take weeks to months to replete iron, has a number of adverse side effects, and is therefore not appropriate in the acute care setting. Also, hospitalized patients commonly demonstrate chronic inflammatory states, which may impede iron absorption that is inherently already low, and persistent blood loss can exceed the dosing of oral iron or gastrointestinal absorption rates. Intravenous iron therapy is faster, taking days to weeks to replete iron. However, there have been some associations of intravenous iron with hypersensitivity reactions, particularly in the high–molecular-weight formulations that have fallen out of common use, and also with increased infections, which has not been confirmed in clinical trials (108). Intravenous iron has demonstrated efficacy in anemia treatment, with multiple studies showing statistically significant increases in hemoglobin in diverse patient groups (109–123).

Erythropoiesis-stimulating agents (ESAs) are synthetic versions of the human hormone erythropoietin. ESAs are approved for the treatment of anemia secondary to chronic kidney disease, chemotherapy, and certain human immunodeficiency virus therapies, as well as to reduce the number of blood transfusions pre- and postsurgery. Studies and clinical trials have shown that the administration of ESAs can reduce need for blood transfusion and increase hemoglobin (124–130). Conversely, a number of other trials have shown adverse outcomes including thromboembolic events and decreased overall survival (131–143), which has resulted in an FDA black-box label for ESAs. Nonetheless, ESAs can be used safely in appropriate patient populations with appropriate dosing and as part of an overall treatment strategy, often incorporating intravenous iron (144,145).

Transfusion Alternatives

Broad concerns regarding the risks of blood transfusion, combined with the concern for a sufficient blood donor supply, have created a quest for an alternative solution to transfusion. Research and developmental investigations for a substance mimicking red blood cells that can transport oxygen from the lungs to the tissues have spanned seven decades (146–148). A variety of substances have been studied over the years, but, to date, no substance has been approved by the FDA for patient use. The first-generation substances were perfluorocarbons and stroma-free hemoglobin, but research on these has largely been abandoned due to problems with manufacturing, ease of use, and adverse effects (149–151). Current investigation is now focused on the hemoglobin-based oxygen carriers (HBOCs). The hemoglobin molecules in these products come from outdated human blood, animal blood, or recombinant DNA technology. Conceptually, HBOCs offer benefits that are superior to donor blood products, such as the fact that they are pathogen-free, have extended storage stability at room temperature, and lack antigenicity, therefore not requiring blood type or antibody screen prior to infusion. However, persistent safety concerns have stalled the development of HBOCs, which in clinical trials are causing vasoconstriction and hypertension in patients (152–155).

Refusal of Blood Transfusion

Critically ill patients who refuse transfusions for religious or personal reasons can present a challenging management problem. Honoring these beliefs requires modification of medical management strategies and presents a unique opportunity to question transfusion guidelines. The care of these patients requires early identification of transfusion preferences. All patients admitted to the critical care setting should have treatment preferences (including blood transfusion) discussed with them or their legal representative as soon as possible. Although transfusion may need to be administered in some emergent situations without the opportunity to obtain informed consent, in most circumstances the critical care practitioner should be able to discuss the risks, benefits, and potential complications of transfusion of various blood products with the patient or representative. Moreover, individual patients may have preferences—religious or otherwise—regarding some blood products but not others, so it is important to establish these preferences for each blood product available. Discussion with patients and family members should include a detailed explanation of each blood product, as the origin and technical aspects of these products may affect their acceptance. In the case of the Jehovah's Witness or other group with religious preferences, assistance from a church representative, or other religious leaders, may be extremely helpful to the family and the physician.

TABLE 144.8 Patient Blood Management Strategies

Tolerate low hemoglobin
- Restrictive transfusion strategy
- Transfuse of one unit at a time in nonhemorrhaging patients

Minimize blood loss
- Eliminate standing laboratory orders
- Consequential blood tests only
- Use microsampling techniques including bedside point-of-care testing
- Discontinue anticoagulants, antiplatelet drugs, herbal supplements
- Intraoperative
  - Acute normovolemic hemodilution
  - Antifibrinolytic agents (epsilon-aminocaproic acid, tranexamic acid)
  - Intraoperative blood recovery
  - Topical hemostatics and fibrin sealants
  - Bipolar cautery
  - Deliberate hypotension
  - Maintenance of normothermia
  - Positioning
  - Use of volume expanders
  - Selection of spinal or epidural anesthesia over general anesthesia when possible
- Other pharmaceuticals
  - Reversal agents (protamine, vitamin K)
  - Coagulation factor concentrates (prothrombin complex concentrates, recombinant factor VIIa)
  - Fibrinogen concentrate
  - Desmopressin
  - Proton pump inhibitors
  - Octrotide

Maximize oxygen delivery
- Maintain high oxygen saturation
- Minimize oxygen demand
  - Sedation
  - Mechanical ventilation
  - Neuromuscular blockade
  - Allow permissive hypercapnia/metabolic acidosis
- Hyperbaric oxygen

Optimization of red blood cell production
- Anemia screening and management
- Erythropoiesis-stimulating agents
- Intravenous iron therapy

One retrospective cohort study evaluated morbidity and mortality in 300 patients who declined transfusion despite postoperative hemoglobin levels up to 8 g/dL and found that the odds of death increased 2.5 times for each gram decrease in hemoglobin below 8 g/dL, with sharper rise in morbidity and mortality with hemoglobin level 5 to 6 g/dL (155). Nonetheless, exceedingly low hemoglobin levels have been associated with survival, as in the case of an injured patient who was a Jehovah's Witness and who survived without neurologic impairment despite extremely low hemoglobin and hematocrit levels (2.7 g/dL and 7.8%, respectively) (156). The implementation of Patient Blood Management strategies, as well as iron and erythropoietin, is an option in the management of these patients. Table 144.8 lists Patient Blood Management strategies that should be considered for all patients in the critical care setting to minimize the need for transfusion.

Key Points

- Anemia is common in hospitalized patients and is associated with morbidity and mortality. The most common etiology is iron deficiency, which is highly treatable.
- Transfusions pose extensive risks to patients with questionable benefit outside of patients with active hemorrhage. Direct risks include transfusion-transmitted infection, transfusion reactions, and alloimmunization. Indirect plausible risks include mortality, increased length of stay, infection, and organ dysfunction.
- Practice tolerance of low hemoglobin, using a restrictive transfusion strategy and transfusing one unit at a time in nonhemorrhaging patients when transfusion is necessary.
- A mild–moderate prolongation of the INR does not correlate to risk for hemorrhage, and plasma transfusion cannot reverse a mildly to moderately prolonged INR.
- Patient Blood Management strategies aimed at minimizing blood loss, maximizing oxygen delivery, and optimizing red blood cell production are an essential component of caring for all patients.

References

1. *The 2011 national blood collection and utilization survey report.* US Department of Health and Human Services website. Available: http://www.hhs.gov/ash/bloodsafety/nbcus/. Accessed March 31, 2015.
2. Pfuntner A, Wier L, Stocks C. *Most frequent procedures performed in U.S. Hospitals, 2010. Healthcare cost and utilization project statistical brief #149.* Agency for Healthcare Research and Quality website. Available: http://hcup-us.ahrq.gov/reports/statbriefs/sb149.jsp/ Published February 2013; accessed March 31, 2015.
3. DeBellis RJ. Anemia in critical care patients: Incidence, etiology, impact, management, and use of treatment guidelines and protocols. *Am J Health Syst Pharm.* 2007;64(3 Suppl 2):S14–21.
4. Lelubre C, Vincent JL. Red blood cell transfusion in the critically ill patient. *Ann Intensive Care.* 2011;1:43.
5. Lacroix J, Hébert PC, Fergusson DA, et al. Age of transfused blood in critically ill adults. *N Engl J Med.* 2015;372(15):1410–1418.
6. Steiner ME, Ness PM, Assmann SF, et al. Effects of red-cell storage duration on patients undergoing cardiac surgery. *N Engl J Med.* 2015;372:1419–1429.
7. Qu L, Triulzi DJ. Clinical effects of red blood cell storage. *Cancer Contr.* 2015;22(1):26–37.
8. Fergusson DA, Hébert P, Hogan DL, et al. Effect of fresh red blood cell transfusions on clinical outcomes in premature, very low-birth-weight infants: the ARIPI randomized trial. *JAMA.* 2012;308(14):1443–1451.
9. Kauvar DS, Holcomb JB, Norris GC, et al. Fresh whole blood transfusion: a controversial military practice. *J Trauma.* 2006;61(1):181–184.
10. Spinella PC, Perkins JG, Grathwohl KW, et al. Warm fresh whole blood is independently associated with improved survival for patients with combat-related traumatic injuries. *J Trauma.* 2009;66(4 Suppl):S69–S76.
11. Repine TB, Perkins JG, Kauvar DS, et al. The use of fresh whole blood in massive transfusion. *J Trauma.* 2006;60(Suppl 6):S59–S69.
12. Petäjä J, Lundström U, Leijala M, et al. Bleeding and use of blood products after heart operations in infants. *J Thorac Cardiovasc Surg.* 1995;109:524–529.
13. Pizarro C, Davis DA, Healy RM, et al. Is there a role for extracorporeal life support after stage I Norwood? *Eur J Cardiothorac Surg.* 2001;19:294–301.
14. Mou SS, Giroir BP, Molitor-Kirsch EA, et al. Fresh whole blood versus reconstituted blood for pump priming in heart surgery in infants. *N Engl J Med.* 2004;351:1635–1644.
15. Shander A, Gross I, Hill S, et al. A new perspective on best transfusion practices. *Blood Transfus.* 2013;11:193–202.
16. Vincent JL, Baron JF, Reinhart K, et al. Anemia and blood transfusion in critically ill patients. *JAMA.* 2002;288:1499–1507.
17. Corwin HL, Gettinger A, Pearl RG, et al. The CRIT study: anemia and blood transfusion in the critically ill: current clinical practice in the United States. *Crit Care Med.* 2004;32:39–52.
18. Rao MP, Boralessa H, Morgan C, et al. Blood component use in critically ill patients. *Anaesthesia.* 2002;57:530–534.
19. Walsh TS, Garrioch M, Maciver C, et al. Red cell requirements for intensive care units adhering to evidence-based transfusion guidelines. *Transfusion.* 2004;44:1405–1411.
20. Westbrook A, Pettila V, Nichol A, et al. Transfusion practice and guidelines in Australian and New Zealand intensive care units. *Intensive Care Med.* 2010;36:1138–1146.
21. Hebert PC, Wells G, Martin C, et al. Variation in red cell transfusion practice in the intensive care unit: a multicentre cohort study. *Crit Care.* 1999;3:57–63.
22. French CJ, Bellomo R, Finfer SR, et al. Appropriateness of red blood cell transfusion in Australasian intensive care practice. *Med J Aust.* 2002;177:548–551.
23. Hebert PC, Wells G, Blajchman M, et al. A multicenter, randomized, controlled clinical trial of transfusion requirement in critical care. *N Engl J Med.* 1999;340:409–417.
24. Hajjar LA, Vincent JL, Galas F, et al. Transfusion requirements after cardiac surgery, the TRACS randomized controlled trial. *JAMA.* 2010;304(14):1559–1567.
25. Carson JL, Terrin ML, Noveck H, et al. Liberal or restrictive transfusion in high-risk patients after hip surgery. *N Engl J Med.* 2011;365:2453–2462.
26. Carson JL, Brooks MM, Abbott JD, et al. Liberal versus restrictive transfusion thresholds for patients with symptomatic coronary artery disease. *Am Heart J.* 2013;165(6):964–971.
27. Villaneuva C, Colomo A, Bosch A, et al. Transfusion strategies for acute upper gastrointestinal bleeding. *N Engl J Med.* 2013;368:11–21.
28. Cooper HA, Rao SV, Greenberg MD, et al. Conservative versus liberal red cell transfusion in acute myocardial infarction (the CRIT Randomized Pilot Study). *Am J Cardiol.* 2011;108(8):1108–1111.
29. Murphy GJ, Pike K, Rogers CA, et al. Liberal or restrictive transfusion after cardiac surgery. *N Engl J Med.* 2015;372:997–1008.
30. Napolitano LM, Corwin HL. Efficacy of red blood cell transfusion in the critically ill. *Crit Care Clin.* 2004;20:255–268.
31. Madjdpour C, Spahn DR. Allogeneic red blood cell transfusion: physiology of oxygen transport. *Best Pract Res Clin Anaesthesiol.* 2007;21:163–171.
32. Vincent JL, Sakr Y, De Backer D, Van der Linden P. Efficacy of allogeneic red blood cell transfusions. *Best Pract Res Clin Anaesthesiol.* 2007;21:209–219.
33. Fernandes CJ Jr, Akamine N, De Marco FV, et al. Red blood cell transfusion does not increase oxygen consumption in critically ill septic patients. *Crit Care.* 2001;5:362–367.
34. Tinmouth A, Fergusson D, Yee IC, Hebert PC. Clinical consequences of red cell storage in the critically ill. *Transfusion.* 2006;46:2014–2027.
35. Shah DM, Gottlieb ME, Rahm RL, et al. Failure of red blood cell transfusion to increase oxygen transport or mixed venous PO2 in injured patients. *J Trauma.* 1982;22:741–746.
36. Hebert PC, Van der Linden P, Biro G, Hu LQ. Physiologic aspects of anemia. *Crit Care Clin.* 2004;20:187–212.
37. Napolitano LM, Kurek S, Luchette FA, et al. Clinical practice guideline: red blood cell transfusion in adult trauma and critical care. *Crit Care Med.* 2009;37:3124–3157.
38. English M, Ahmed M, Ngando C, et al. Blood transfusion for severe anaemia in children in a Kenyan hospital. *Lancet.* 2002;359:494–495.

39. Martini J, Carpentier B, Negrete AC, et al. Paradoxical hypotension following increased hematocrit and blood viscosity. *Am J Physiol Heart Circ Physiol.* 2005;289:H2136–2143.
40. Pape A, Stein P, Horn O, Habler O. Clinical evidence of blood transfusion effectiveness. *Blood Transfus.* 2009;7:250–258.
41. Tsai AG, Cabrales P, Intaglietta M. Microvascular perfusion upon exchange transfusion with stored red blood cells in normovolemic anemic conditions. *Transfusion.* 2004;44:1626–1634.
42. Zimrin AB, Hess JR. Current issues relating to the transfusion of stored red blood cells. *Vox Sang.* 2009;96:93–103.
43. Vassallo R. New paradigms in the management of alloimmune refractoriness to platelet transfusions. *Curr Opin Hematol.* 2007;14:655–663.
44. Kaufman RM, Djulbegovic B, Gernsheimer T, et al. Platelet transfusion: a clinical practice guideline from the AABB. *Ann Intern Med.* 2015;162(3): 205–213.
45. Stanworth SJ, Estcourt LJ, Powter G, et al. A no-prophylaxis platelet-transfusion strategy for hematologic cancers. *N Engl J Med.* 2013;368: 1771–1780.
46. Wandt H, Schaefer-Eckart K, Wendelin K, et al. Therapeutic platelet transfusion versus routine prophylactic transfusion in patients with haematological malignancies: an open-label, multicentre, randomised study. *Lancet.* 2012;380:1309–1316.
47. Murphy S, Litwin S, Herring LM, et al. Indications for platelet transfusion in children with acute leukemia. *Am J Hematol.* 1982;12:347–356.
48. Stanworth SJ, Estcourt LJ, Llewelyn CA, et al. Impact of prophylactic platelet transfusions on bleeding events in patients with hematologic malignancies: a subgroup analysis of a randomized trial (CME). *Transfusion.* 2014;54:2385–2393.
49. Diedrich B, Remberger M, Shanwell A, et al. A prospective randomized trial of a prophylactic platelet transfusion trigger of 10 × 10(9) per L versus 30 × 10(9) per L in allogeneic hematopoietic progenitor cell transplant recipients. *Transfusion.* 2005;45:1064–1072.
50. Heckman KD, Weiner GJ, Davis CS, et al. Randomized study of prophylactic platelet transfusion threshold during induction therapy for adult acute leukemia: 10,000/microL versus 20,000/microL. *J Clin Oncol.* 1997; 15:1143–1149.
51. Zumberg MS, del Rosario ML, Nejame CF, et al. A prospective randomized trial of prophylactic platelet transfusion and bleeding incidence in hematopoietic stem cell transplant recipients: 10,000/L versus 20,000/ microL trigger. *Biol Blood Marrow Transplant.* 2002;8:569–576.
52. Rebulla P, Finazzi G, Marangoni F, et al. The threshold for prophylactic platelet transfusions in adults with acute myeloid leukemia. Gruppo Italiano Malattie Ematologiche Maligne dell'Adulto. *N Engl J Med.* 1997;337:1870–1875.
53. Sensebe´ L, Giraudeau B, Bardiaux L, et al. The efficiency of transfusing high doses of platelets in hematologic patients with thrombocytopenia: results of a prospective, randomized, open, blinded end point (PROBE) study. *Blood.* 2005;105:862–864.
54. Slichter SJ, Kaufman RM, Assmann SF, et al. Dose of prophylactic platelet transfusions and prevention of hemorrhage. *N Engl J Med.* 2010; 362:600–613.
55. Guyatt GH, Oxman AD, Kunz R, et al. Going from evidence to recommendations. *BMJ.* 2008;336:1049–1051.
56. Heddle NM, Cook RJ, Tinmouth A, et al. A randomized controlled trial comparing standard- and low-dose strategies for transfusion of platelets (SToP) to patients with thrombocytopenia. *Blood.* 2009;113:1564–1573.
57. Tinmouth A, Tannock IF, Crump M, et al. Low-dose prophylactic platelet transfusions in recipients of an autologous peripheral blood progenitor cell transplant and patients with acute leukemia: a randomized controlled trial with a sequential Bayesian design. *Transfusion.* 2004;44:1711–1719.
58. Roy AJ, Jaffe N, Djerassi I. Prophylactic platelet transfusions in children with acute leukemia: a dose response study. *Transfusion.* 1973;13:283–290.
59. West KL, Adamson C, Hoffman M. Prophylactic correction of the international normalized ratio in neurosurgery: a brief review of a brief literature. *J Neurosurg.* 2011;114;9–18.
60. Tavares M, DiQuattro P, Nolette N, et al. Reduction in plasma transfusion after enforcement of transfusion guidelines (CME). *Transfusion.* 2011;51(4):754–761.
61. Spector I, Corn M, Ticktin H. Effect of plasma transfusions on the prothrombin time and clotting factors in liver disease. *N Engl J Med.* 1966;275:1032–1037.
62. Ewe K. Bleeding after liver biopsy does not correlate with indices of peripheral coagulation. *Dig Dis Sci.* 1981;26(5):388–393.
63. Ragni MV, Lewis JL, Spero JA, Hasiba U. Bleeding and coagulation abnormalities in alcoholic cirrhotic liver disease. *Alcohol Clin Exp Res.* 1982;6(2):267–274.
64. Friedman EW, Sussman II. Safety of invasive procedures in patients with the coagulopathy of liver disease. *Clin Lab Haemat.* 1989;11(3):199–204.
65. McVay PA, Toy P. Lack of increased bleeding after paracentesis and thoracentesis in patients with mild coagulation abnormalities. *Transfusion.* 1991;31(2):164–171.
66. Zins M, Vilgrain V, Gayno S, et al. US-guided percutaneous liver biopsy with plugging of the needle track: a prospective study in 72 high-risk patients. *Radiology.* 1992;184(3):841–843.
67. Foster PF, Moore LR, Sankary HN, et al. Central venous catheterization in patients with coagulopathy. *Arch Surg.* 1992;127:273–275.
68. Caturelli E, Squillante MM, Andriulli A, et al. Fine-needle liver biopsy in patients with severely impaired coagulation. *Liver.* 1993;13(5):270–273.
69. Kozak EA, Brath LK. Do "screening" coagulation tests predict bleeding in patients undergoing fiber optic bronchoscopy with biopsy? *Chest.* 1994; 106:703–705.
70. Inabnet WB, Deziel DJ. Laparoscopic liver biopsy in patients with coagulopathy, portal hypertension and ascites. *Am Surg.* 1995;61:603–606.
71. DeLoughery TG, Liebeer JM, Simonds V, Goodnight SH. Invasive line placement in critically ill patients: do hemostatic defects matter? *Transfusion.* 1996;36:827–831.
72. Gilmore IT, Burroughs A, Murray-Lyon IM, et al. Indications, methods, and outcomes of percutaneous liver biopsy in England and Wales: an audit by the British Society of Gastroenterology and the Royal College of Physicians of London. *Gut.* 1995;36:437–441.
73. Seeff LB, Everson GT, Morgan TR, et al. Complication rate of percutaneous liver biopsies among persons with advanced chronic liver disease in the HALT-C trial. *Clin Gastro Hepatol.* 2010;8(10):877–883.
74. Nascimento B, Goodnough LT, Levy JH. Cryoprecipitate therapy. *Br J Anaesth.* 2014;113(6):922–934.
75. Ziemann M, Juhl D, Görg S, Hennig H. The impact of donor cytomegalovirus DNA on transfusion strategies for at-risk patients. *Transfusion.* 2013;53(10):2183–2189.
76. *Fatalities reported to FDA following blood collection and transfusion: annual summary for fiscal year 2013.* FDA website. Available: http://www.fda.gov/BiologicsBloodVaccines/SafetyAvailability/ReportaProblem/TransfusionDonationFatalities/ucm391574.htm. Accessed April 2, 2015.
77. Galel S. Infectious disease screening. In: Fung MK, Grossman BJ, Hillyer CD, Westhoff CM, eds. *Technical Manual.* 18th ed. Bethesda, MD: AABB; 2014:179–212.
78. Mazzei CA, Popovsky MA, Kopko PM. Noninfectious complications of blood transfusion. In: Fung MK, Grossman BJ, Hillyer CD, Westhoff CM, eds. *Technical Manual.* 18th ed. Bethesda, MD: AABB; 2014:665–696.
79. Vamvakas EC, Blajchman MA. Transfusion-related mortality: the ongoing risks of allogeneic blood transfusion and the available strategies for their prevention. *Blood.* 2009;113:3406–3417.
80. Bernard GR, Artigas A, Brigham KL et al. The American-European consensus conference on ARDS. Definitions, mechanisms, relevant outcomes, and clinical trial coordination. *Am J Respir Crit Care Med.* 1994;149:818–824.
81. Kleinman S, Caulfield T, Chan P, et al. Toward an understanding of transfusion-related acute lung injury: Statement of a consensus panel. *Transfusion.* 2004;44:1774–1789.
82. Popovsky MA, Moore SB. Diagnostic and pathogenetic considerations in transfusion-related acute lung injury. *Transfusion.* 1985;25:573–577.
83. *National Healthcare Safety Network Biovigilance Component, Hemovigilance Module Surveillance Protocol v2.1.2.* Atlanta: Division of Healthcare Quality Promotion, National Center for Emerging and Zoonotic Infectious Diseases, Centers for Disease Control and Prevention; 2014.
84. Andrzejewski C Jr, Popovsky MA, Stec TC, et al. Hemotherapy bedside biovigilance involving vital sign values and characteristics of patients with suspected transfusion reactions assocuated with fluid challenges: can some cases of transfusion-associated circulatory overload have proinflammatory aspects? *Transfusion.* 2012;52(11):2310–2320.
85. Khawaja F, Wagholikor P, Clifford L, et al. Transfusion-associated circulatory overload: hints from the hemodynamics? [Abstract]. *Transfusion.* 2014;54(Suppl):51A.
86. Gunson HH, Stratton F, Cooper DG, Rawlinson VI. Primary immunization of Rh-negative volunteers. *Br Med J.* 1970;1:593–595.
87. Yazer M, Triulzi D. Detection of anti-D in D– recipients transfused with D+ red blood cells. *Transfusion.* 2007;47(12):2197–2201.
88. Leal-Noval SR, Rincon-Ferrari MD, Garcia-Curiel A, et al. Transfusion of blood components and postoperative infection in patients undergoing cardiac surgery. *Chest.* 2001; 119:1461–1468.
89. Wu WC, Rathore SS, Wang Y, et al. Blood transfusion in elderly patients with acute myocardial infarction. *N Engl J Med.* 2001;345:1230–1236.

90. Engoren MC, Habib RH, Zacharias A, et al. Effect of blood transfusion on long-term survival after cardiac operation. *Ann Thorac Surg.* 2002;74:1180–1186.
91. Malone DL, Dunne J, Tracy JK, et al. Blood transfusion, independent of shock severity, is associated with worse outcome in trauma. *J Trauma.* 2003;54:898–905; discussion 905–907.
92. Dunne JR, Malone DL, Tracy JK, Napolitano LM. Allogenic blood transfusion in the first 24 hours after trauma is associated with increased systemic inflammatory response syndrome (SIRS) and death. *Surg Infect (Larchmt).* 2004;5:395–404.
93. Innerhofer P, Klingler A, Klimmer C, et al. Risk for postoperative infection after transfusion of white blood cell-filtered allogeneic or autologous blood components in orthopedic patients undergoing primary arthroplasty. *Transfusion.* 2005;45:103–110.
94. Weber EW, Slappendel R, Hemon Y, et al. Effects of epoetin alfa on blood transfusions and postoperative recovery in orthopaedic surgery: the European Epoetin Alfa Surgery Trial (EEST). *Eur J Anaesthesiol.* 2005;22:249–257.
95. Koch CG, Li L, Van Wagoner DR, et al. Red cell transfusion is associated with an increased risk for postoperative atrial fibrillation. *Ann Thorac Surg.* 2006;82:1747–1756.
96. Koch CG, Li L, Duncan AI, et al. Morbidity and mortality risk associated with red blood cell and blood-component transfusion in isolated coronary artery bypass grafting. *Crit Care Med.* 2006;34:1608–1616.
97. Murphy GJ, Reeves BC, Rogers CA, et al. Increased mortality, postoperative morbidity, and cost after red blood cell transfusion in patients having cardiac surgery. *Circulation.* 2007;116:2544–2552.
98. Koch C, Li L, Figueroa P, et al. Transfusion and pulmonary morbidity after cardiac surgery. *Ann Thorac Surg.* 2009;88:1410–1418.
99. Pedersen AB, Mehnert F, Overgaard S, Johnsen SP. Allogeneic blood transfusion and prognosis following total hip replacement: a population-based follow up study. *BMC Musculoskelet Disord.* 2009;10:167.
100. Nikolsky E, Mehran R, Sadeghi HM, et al. Prognostic impact of blood transfusion after primary angioplasty for acute myocardial infarction: analysis from the CADILLAC (Controlled Abciximab and Device Investigation to Lower Late Angioplasty Complications) Trial. *JACC Cardiovasc Interv.* 2009;2:624–632.
101. Surgenor SD, Kramer RS, Olmstead EM, et al. The association of perioperative red blood cell transfusions and decreased long-term survival after cardiac surgery. *Anesth Analg.* 2009;108:1741–1746.
102. D'Ayala M, Huzar T, Briggs W, et al. Blood transfusion and its effect on the clinical outcomes of patients undergoing major lower extremity amputation. *Ann Vasc Surg.* 2010;24:468–473.
103. O'Keeffe SD, Davenport DL, Minion DJ, et al. Blood transfusion is associated with increased morbidity and mortality after lower extremity revascularization. *J Vasc Surg.* 2010;51:616–621.
104. van Straten AH, Kats S, Bekker MW, et al. Risk factors for red blood cell transfusion after coronary artery bypass graft surgery. *J Cardiothorac Vasc Anesth.* 2010;24:413–417.
105. Veenith T, Sharples L, Gerrard C, et al. Survival and length of stay following blood transfusion in octogenarians following cardiac surgery. *Anaesthesia.* 2010;65:331–336.
106. Carson JL, Carless PA, Hebert PC. Transfusion thresholds and other strategies for guiding allogeneic red blood cell transfusion. *Cochrane Database System Rev.* 2012;(4):CD002042.
107. *Society for the Advancement of Blood Management (SABM).* Available: www.sabm.org. Accessed April 13, 2015.
108. Auerbach M, Ballard H. Clinical use of intravenous iron: administration, efficacy, and safety. *Hematol Am Soc Hematol Educ Program.* 2010;2010: 338–347.
109. Shander A, Spence RK, Auerbach M. Can intravenous iron therapy meet the unmet needs created by the new restrictions on erythropoietic stimulating agents? *Transfusion.* 2010;50:719–732.
110. Bolger AP, Bartlett FR, Penston HS, et al. Intravenous iron alone for the treatment of anemia in patients with chronic heart failure. *J Am Coll Cardiol.* 2006;48:1225–1227.
111. Usmanov RI, Zueva EB, Silverberg DS, Shaked M. Intravenous iron without erythropoietin for the treatment of iron deficiency anemia in patients with moderate to severe congestive heart failure and chronic kidney insufficiency. *J Nephrol.* 2008;21:236–242.
112. Karkouti K, McCluskey SA, Ghannam M, et al. Intravenous iron and recombinant erythropoietin for the treatment of postoperative anemia. *Can J Anaesth.* 2006;53:11–9.
113. Theusinger OM, Leyvraz PF, Schanz U, et al. Treatment of iron deficiency anemia in orthopedic surgery with intravenous iron: efficacy and limits: a prospective study. *Anesthesiology.* 2007;107:923–927.
114. Breymann C, Richter C, Huttner C, et al. Effectiveness of recombinant erythropoietin and iron sucrose vs. iron therapy only, in patients with postpartum anaemia and blunted erythropoiesis. *Eur J Clin Invest.* 2000;30:154–161.
115. VanWyck DB, Martens MG, Seid MH, et al. Intravenous ferric carboxymaltose compared with oral iron in the treatment of postpartum anemia: a randomized controlled trial. *Obstet Gynecol.* 2007;110(2 Pt 1):267–278.
116. Wagstrom E, Akesson A, Van Rooijen M, et al. Erythropoietin and intravenous iron therapy in postpartum anaemia. *Acta Obstet Gynecol Scand.* 2007; 86:957–962.
117. Agarwal R, Rizkala A, Bastani B, et al. A randomized controlled trial of oral versus intravenous iron in chronic kidney disease. *Am J Nephrol.* 2006;26:445–454.
118. Gotloib L, Silverberg D, Fudin R, Shostak A. Iron deficiency is a common cause of anemia in chronic kidney disease and can often be corrected with intravenous iron. *J Neprol.* 2006;19:161–167.
119. Mircescu G, Gârneata L, Capusa C, Ursea N. Intravenous iron supplementation for the treatment of anaemia in pre-dialyzed chronic renal failure patients. *Nephrol Dial Transplant.* 2006;21;120–124.
120. Silverberg DS, Blum M, Agbaria Z, et al. The effect of IV iron alone or in combination with low dose erythropoietin in the rapid correction of anemia of chronic renal failure in the predialysis period. *Clin Nephrol.* 2001;55:212–219.
121. Silverberg D, Iaina A, Peer G, et al. Intravenous iron supplementation for the treatment of anemia of moderate to severe chronic renal failure patients not receiving dialysis. *Am J Kidney Dis.* 1996;27:234–238.
122. Auerbach M, Witt D, Toller W, et al. Clinical use of the total dose intravenous infusion of iron dextran. *J Lab Clin Med.* 1988;111:566–570.
123. Kim YT, Kim SW, Yoon BS, et al. Effect of intravenously administered iron sucrose on the prevention of anemia in the cervical cancer patients treated with concurrent chemoradiotherapy. *Gynecol Oncol.* 2007;105: 199–204.
124. Corwin HL, Gettinger A, Pearl R, et al. Efficacy of recombinant human erythropoietin in critically ill patients: a randomized controlled trial. *JAMA.* 2002;288(22):2827–2835.
125. Tonia T, Mettler A, Robert N, et al. Erythropoietin or darbepoetin for patients with cancer. *Cochrane Database Syst Rev.* 2012;12:CD003407.
126. Kotecha D, Ngo K, Walters JA, et al. Erythropoietin as a treatment of anemia in heart failure: systematic review of randomized trials. *Am Heart J.* 2011;161:822–831.
127. Palmer SC, Navaneethan SD, Craig JC, et al. Meta-analysis: erythropoiesis-stimulating agents in patients with chronic kidney disease. *Ann Intern Med.* 2010;153:23–33.
128. Glaspy J, Bukowski R, Steinberg D, et al. Impact of therapy with epoetin alfa on clinical outcomes in patients with nonmyeloid malignancies during cancer chemotherapy in community oncology practice. Procrit Study Group. *J Clin Oncol.* 1997;15:1218–1234.
129. Vansteenkiste J, Pirker R, Massuti B, et al. Double-blind, placebo-controlled, randomized phase III trial of darbepoetin alfa in lung cancer patients receiving chemotherapy. *J Natl Cancer Inst.* 2002;94:1211–1220.
130. Seidenfeld J, Piper M, Flamm C, et al. Epoetin treatment of anemia associated with cancer therapy: a systematic review and meta-analysis of controlled clinical trials. *J Natl Cancer Inst.* 2001;93:1204–1214.
131. Stowell CP, Jones SC, Enny C, et al. An open-label, randomized, parallel-group study of perioperative epoetin alfa versus standard of care for blood conservation in major elective spinal surgery: safety analysis. *Spine.* 2009;34:2479–2485.
132. Besarab A, Bolton WK, Browne JK, et al. The effects of normal as compared with low hematocrit values in patients with cardiac disease who are receiving hemodialysis and epoetin. *N Engl J Med.* 1998;339:584–590.
133. Singh AK, Szczech L, Tang KL, et al. Correction of anemia with epoetin alfa in chronic kidney disease. *N Engl J Med.* 2006;355:2085–2098.
134. Drueke TB, Locatelli F, Clyne N, et al. Normalization of hemoglobin level in patients with chronic kidney disease and anemia. *N Engl J Med.* 2006;355:2071–2084.
135. Pfeffer MA, Burdmann EA, Chen CY, et al. A trial of darbepoetin alfa in type 2 diabetes and chronic kidney disease. *N Engl J Med.* 2009;361: 2019–2032.
136. Hedenus M, Adriansson M, San Miguel J, et al. Efficacy and safety of darbepoetin alfa in anaemic patients with lymphoproliferative malignancies: a randomized, double-blind, placebo-controlled study. *Br J Haematol.* 2003;122:394–403.
137. Leyland-Jones B, Semiglazov V, Pawlicki M, et al. Maintaining normal hemoglobin levels with epoetin alfa in mainly nonanemic patients with metastatic breast cancer receiving first-line chemotherapy: a survival study. *J Clin Oncol.* 2005;23:5960–5972.

138. Untch M, Fasching PA, Konecny GE, et al. PREPARE trial: a randomized phase III trial comparing preoperative, dose-dense, dose-intensified chemotherapy with epirubicin, paclitaxel and CMF versus a standard-dosed epirubicin/cyclophosphamide followed by paclitaxel ± darbepoetin alfa in primary breast cancer—results at the time of surgery. *Ann Oncol.* 2011;22:1988–1998.
139. Overgaard J, Hoff C, Sand Hansen H, et al. Randomized study of the importance of novel erythropoiesis stimulating protein (Aranesp) for the effect of radiotherapy in patients with primary squamous cell carcinoma of the head and neck (HNSCC): the Danish Head and Neck Cancer Group DAHANCA 10 randomized trial. *Eur J Cancer.* 2007;5(6):7.
140. Thomas G, Ali S, Hoebers FJ, et al. Phase III trial to evaluate the efficacy of maintaining hemoglobin levels above 12.0 g/dL with erythropoietin vs above 10.0 g/dL without erythropoietin in anemic patients receiving concurrent radiation and cisplatin for cervical cancer. *Gynecol Oncol.* 2008;108:317–325.
141. Wright JR, Ung YC, Julian JA, et al. Randomized, double-blind, placebo-controlled trial of erythropoietin in non-small-cell lung cancer with disease-related anemia. *J Clin Oncol.* 2007;25:1027–1032.
142. Smith RE, Aapro MS, Ludwig H, et al. Darbepoetin alpha for the treatment of anemia in patients with active cancer not receiving chemotherapy or radiotherapy: results of a phase III, multicenter, randomized, double-blind, placebo-controlled study. *J Clin Oncol.* 2008;26:1040–1050.
143. Henke M, Laszig R, Rube C, et al. Erythropoietin to treat head and neck cancer patients with anaemia undergoing radiotherapy: randomised, double-blind, placebo-controlled trial. *Lancet.* 2003;362:1255–1260.
144. Goodnough LT, Shander A. Update on erythropoiesis-stimulating agents. *Best Pract Res Clin Anaesthesiol.* 2013;27:121–129.
145. Shander A, Ozawa S, Gross I, Henry D. Erythropoiesis-stimulating agents: friends or foes? *Transfusion.* 2013;53(9):1867–1872.
146. Sellards AW, Minot GR. Injection of hemoglobin in man and its relation to blood destruction, with special reference to the anemias. *J Med Res.* 1916;34:469–494.
147. Winslow RM. Current status of oxygen carriers (blood substitutes): 2006. *Vox Sang.* 2006;91(2):102–110.
148. Stowell CP. Hemoglobin-based oxygen carriers. *Curr Opin Hematol.* 2002;9:537–543.
149. Stowell CP, Levin J, Speiss BD, et al. Progress in the development of RBC substitutes. *Transfusion.* 2001;41:287–299.
150. Moore E. Blood substitutes: the future is now. *J Am Coll Surg.* 2003;196(1):1–17.
151. Scott MG, Kucik DF, Goodnough LT, et al. Blood substitutes: evolution and future applications. *Clin Chem.* 1997;43:1724–1731.
152. Alayash A. Blood substitutes: why haven't we been more successful? *Trends Biotechnol.* 2014;32(4):177–185.
153. Kim HW, Hai CM, Greenburg AG. Acellular hemoglobin-based oxygen carrier induced vasoactivity: a brief review of potential pharmacologic remedies. In: Kim HW, Greenburg AG, eds. *Hemoglobin-Based Oxygen Carriers as Red Cell Substitutes and Oxygen Therapeutics*. Berlin, Germany: Springer; 2013:713–733.
154. Varnado CL, Mollan TL, Birukou I, et al. Development of recombinant hemoglobin-based oxygen carriers. *Antioxid Redox Signal.* 2013;18(17), 2314–2328.
155. Carson JL, Noveck H, Berlin JA, Gould SA. Mortality and morbidity in patients with very low postoperative Hb levels who decline blood transfusion. *Transfusion.* 2002;42(7):812–818.
156. Vaziri K, Roland J, Robinson L, et al. Extreme anemia in an injured Jehovah's Witness: a test of our understanding of the physiology of severe anemia and the threshold for blood transfusion. *J Trauma Inj Infect Crit Care.* 2009;67:E11–13.

CHAPTER
145

Antithrombotic and Thrombolytic Therapy

GOHAR H. DAR and STEVEN R. INSLER

INTRODUCTION

The occurrence of venous and arterial thromboembolism has had a large impact on medical care and is a major cause of both morbidity and mortality. Arterial thromboembolism, commonly implicated in myocardial infarctions (MIs), stroke, and limb ischemia, is responsible for more deaths each year than the next seven leading causes of death combined (1,2). Venous thrombosis may lead to pulmonary embolism, right heart dysfunction, venous insufficiency, and postthrombotic syndrome (3). The incidence of patients in the intensive care unit developing venous thromboembolism ranges from 5% to 33% (4–6). There are an estimated 2 million cases of venous thromboembolism each year in the United States alone, with an annual estimated mortality of about 60,000 from pulmonary embolism (7–9). The ability to rapidly diagnose and initiate effective therapy is paramount. This chapter will briefly review the formation of arterial and venous thrombi, regulation of the coagulation cascade, and current antithrombotic and thrombolytic therapies.

THROMBOGENESIS AND COAGULATION

Deep venous thromboemboli are associated with many different clinical situations, and the stimulus for developing thrombi depends on the underlying clinical condition. A patient may have an underlying primary hypercoagulable predisposition to developing venous thrombosis secondary to decreased antithrombotic or increased prothrombotic proteins (thrombophilias) (10), increasing the relative risk of thrombosis up to 10-fold. Deep venous thrombosis (DVT) will form under conditions of low flow and are predominantly composed of fibrin and red blood cells. They usually originate in the muscular calf veins or in the valve cusps of the deep calf veins (1). The risk factors for DVT are listed in Table 145.1.

In vivo, coagulation in the veins is initiated by a complex of tissue factor (TF), a type I transmembrane protein—and the serine protease factor VIIa. Low levels of factor VIIa circulate in plasma so that the system will respond efficiently if vessel injury occurs and TF is exposed; the factor VIIa/TF complex activates factors IX and X. Activated factor X cleaves small amounts of prothrombin to generate thrombin. The low concentrations of thrombin generated are sufficient to activate factors V and VIII, essential steps for the propagation of the coagulation cascade (Fig. 145.1) (11–13).

Arterial thrombi typically form under high flow (shear) conditions, and are made up primarily of platelet aggregates held together by fibrin strands. Most arterial thrombi are superimposed on ruptured atherosclerotic plaques. Arterial plaque rupture exposes thrombogenic material in the lipid-rich core of the blood (14). When plaques rupture, subendothelial collagen and von Willebrand factor is exposed; collagen and von Willebrand factor provide a substrate for platelet adhesion (15,16). Collagen binds to platelets' glycoprotein Ia/IIa receptor complex; von Willebrand factor binds to glycoprotein Ib/IX/V receptor complex; and other exposed extracellular matrix, such as fibronectin and laminin bind to glycoprotein VI. These actions cause the up-regulation of platelet glycoprotein IIb/IIIa receptor complex, which in turn results in platelet aggregation. Glycoprotein IIb/IIIa accelerates platelet adhesion to the subendothelium by binding to fibrinogen and von Willebrand factor (17,18). Additionally, plaque rupture causes TF release, which accelerates the extrinsic coagulation cascade (Fig. 145.2).

Once coagulation is initiated in either veins or arteries, and TF has activated factor VII, converting it to factor VIIa, the factor VIIa/TF complex activates factors IXa and Xa, respectively. Factor IXa binds to factor VIIIa on the membrane surfaces to form intrinsic tenase, which activates factor X; by feedback activation of factor VII, factor Xa initiates and amplifies coagulation (19,20).

Factor Xa propagates coagulation by binding with factor Va, and in turn activates prothrombin to thrombin and, ultimately, to fibrin clot formation. If the thrombus is of sufficient size to disrupt blood flow, shear increases and promotes additional platelet and fibrin deposition.

Regulation of the Coagulation Cascade

Three inhibitory systems are involved in the regulation of the coagulation cascade. The pathway of TF inhibition interferes with the initiation of coagulation. The protein C pathway regulates thrombin generation and inhibits the propagation of coagulation. Antithrombin blocks the generation of thrombin and, subsequently, thrombin activity. Additionally, the fibrinolytic system promotes fibrin degradation.

Tissue Factor Pathway Inhibitor

The factor VIIa/TF complex is inhibited by the TF pathway inhibitor, most of which is bound to endothelium, in two steps. First, the TF pathway inhibitor binds and then inactivates factor Xa. This complex in turn inactivates factor VIIa, which is bound to TF (12).

Protein C Pathway

The protein C pathway is initiated when thrombin binds to thrombomodulin, which is found on endothelium. Once bound to thrombomodulin, thrombin undergoes a conformational change at its active site, which converts it from a procoagulant enzyme to a potent activator of protein C. Activated protein C, a vitamin K–dependent protein, acts as an anticoagulant by proteolytically degrading and inactivating factors Va and VIIIa, thus blocking thrombin generation (21).

TABLE 145.1 Potential Mechanisms by which Various Clinical Conditions May Facilitate Deep Venous Thrombosis (DVT)

	Increased Baseline Propensity for Thrombosis	Acute Insult
Hypercoagulability	*Genetic* Increased coagulants Prothrombin mutation G20210A Decreased anticoagulants AT deficiency Protein C deficiency Protein S deficiency Factor V Leiden *Acquired* Malignancy Hyperhomocysteinemia HRT/OCT (?) Pregnancy (hormone-related) Nephrotic syndrome (loss of AT) Antiphospholipid syndrome Increased levels of clotting factors	*Increased coagulants* Blood-borne tissue factor Malignancy (Trousseau syndrome) Congestive heart failure (?) Systemic infection (?) Exogenous administration of clotting factors rVIIa rVIII *Acute loss of anticoagulants* Nephrotic syndrome (loss of AT) Initial warfarin therapy without heparin
Direct vessel injury	Direct vessel injury most often represents an acute insult Examples of low-grade, chronic vessel injury that increase the baseline propensity for thrombosis may include: Endothelial injury secondary to chemotherapy Hyperhomocysteinemia Vasculitis Antiphospholipid syndrome	Intravascular catheters Trauma Surgery
Blood stasis	More commonly functioning as an acute insult Precipitating thrombosis, rather than increasing the baseline propensity for thrombosis: Age Obesity Pregnancy (gradual immobility/stasis) Sedentarism	Hospitalization/bedridden Pregnancy (stasis) Limb paralysis (e.g., stroke, plaster casts) Right heart failure Long-haul flights Vein compression (e.g., enlarged lymph node)

AT, antithrombin; HRT, hormone replacement therapy; OCT, oral contraceptives; ?, may or may not be effective.
Risk factors or clinical conditions that increase the risk of DVT can be classified as either increasing the baseline propensity for thrombosis or precipitating the thrombotic event acutely. Thrombosis may occur by one of three major mechanisms: inducing hypercoagulability, directly injuring the vessel wall, or causing blood stasis (low flow).
From Lopez JA, Kearon, Lee AY. Deep venous thrombosis. *Hematology*. 2004;1:442.

Antithrombin

Antithrombin inhibits thrombin, factor Xa, and other activated clotting factors, but in the absence of heparin, these reactions occur slowly. Heparin addition will increase the rate of inhibition of these reactions by 1,000-fold (22). Small amounts of the proteoglycan heparan sulfate located on the luminal surface may maintain intact endothelium in a nonthrombogenic state (23).

Fibrinolytic Degradation of Fibrin

This system is designed to remove intravascular fibrin and restore normal blood circulation. Fibrinolysis is initiated by plasminogen activators that convert plasminogen to plasmin, a trypsinlike protease. Plasmin degrades fibrin into soluble fibrin degradation products (24).

D-Dimers. D-Dimers are a specific fibrin degradation product formed only by plasmin degradation of fibrin and not by plasmin degradation of intact fibrinogen (Fig. 145.3). Thus, its presence indicates that fibrin has been formed. d-Dimer has been validated as a diagnostic tool to help in the exclusion of venous thrombosis and pulmonary embolism and is widely used in the emergency room setting for this purpose (25–27). Elevated d-dimer levels have been reported as a marker of risk for both multiple organ failure and death in critically ill patients (28).

ANTIPLATELET AGENTS

Platelet aggregation leading to a disruption of blood flow can have devastating outcomes, often causing permanent disability or death. The understanding of normal platelet function has led to the rational basis for the development of antiplatelet agents.

Aspirin

The efficacy of aspirin in acute coronary syndrome (ACS) has been established in numerous clinical trials. For example, the International Study of Infarct Survival (ISIS)-2 demonstrated that for acute MI, aspirin alone reduced mortality to a similar extent as did streptokinase alone, with an additive benefit when both agents were used (29). A recent meta-analysis by the Antiplatelet Trialists' Collaboration found that aspirin reduced the risk of MI, stroke, or death from 13.3% to 8.0% in patients with unstable angina (30). The meta-analysis also found that the greatest risk reduction occurred with a dose of 75 to 150 mg per day; higher doses such as 325 mg per day did not appear to confer any added benefit. In a subsequent investigation, the CURRENT/OASIS-7 (Clopidogrel optimal loading dose Usage to Reduce Recurrent EveNTs—Organization to Assess Strategies in Ischemic Syndromes) trial compared the effectiveness of double-dose clopidogrel versus a standard dose for 30 days

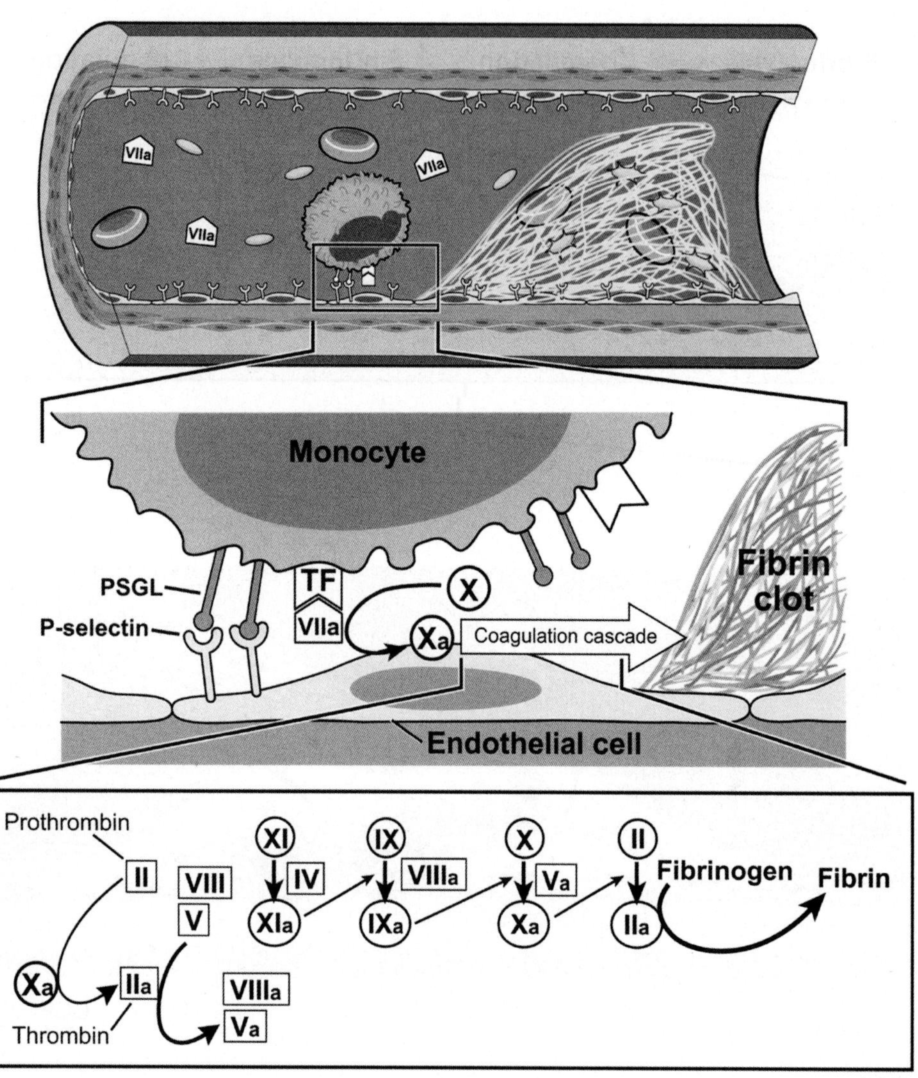

FIGURE 145.1 Model for venous thrombosis. Coagulation in veins is initiated by the tissue factor-VIIa complex which then activates factors IX and X. Factor II, prothrombin; factor IIa, thrombin; PSGL-1, p-selectin glycoprotein ligand-1.

coupled to an open label randomization to high (300 to 325 mg/day) versus a low dose (75 to 100 mg/day) of aspirin in 25,086 patients with ACSs undergoing invasive therapy. This study found no significant difference between either regimen with respect to the primary outcome of cardiovascular death, infarction, or stroke. It did however note a small increase in the incidence of major gastrointestinal bleeding among patients receiving the higher-dose aspirin regimen as compared to the lower dosage (47 patients [0.4%] vs. 29 patients [0.2%]; p = 0.04) (31). Aspirin therapy has, thus, become the standard for the secondary prevention of cardiovascular events in high-risk patients. The role of aspirin alone, versus other antithrombotic agents, in atrial fibrillation has been addressed in many studies, the results suggesting that the risk reduction of ischemic strokes associated with oral vitamin K–inhibiting anticoagulant therapy is greater than that provided by aspirin (32,33).

Aspirin Resistance

The efficacy of aspirin in the inhibition of platelet function differs between patients. Cardiovascular events occur preferentially in patients with low responses to aspirin therapy (34), referred to as *aspirin resistance.* The prevalence is reported to vary between 5% and 60%, depending on the laboratory studies used (35). Gum et al. (36), in a prospective study, followed 325 patients with stable coronary artery disease for 2 years, finding aspirin resistance in 5.5% of patients using optical platelet aggregability, and in 9.5% by using the Platelet Function Analyzer 100 (PFA-100). Aspirin-resistant patients were noted to have a 24% risk of death, MI, or stroke, as compared with a 10% risk for patients who were aspirin sensitive.

There are two aspects of resistance: biochemical and clinical. Biochemical resistance refers to the inability of aspirin to initiate platelet inhibition, whereas clinical resistance indicates an increased risk of cardiovascular events in patients receiving treatment with aspirin (37). Platelet receptor polymorphism is thought to be responsible for aspirin resistance (38).

The risk of hemorrhage, especially from the gastrointestinal tract, is a major concern when doses higher than 325 mg per day are used. The local effect of aspirin on the gastric mucosa is more prevalent with the higher doses, but patients with vascular malformations or mucosal lesions may bleed at lower doses. There is also a risk of cerebral hemorrhage in patients with prior stroke or with uncontrolled hypertension. In the event of hemorrhage, aspirin should be discontinued and the patient observed but, if needed, the patient may be

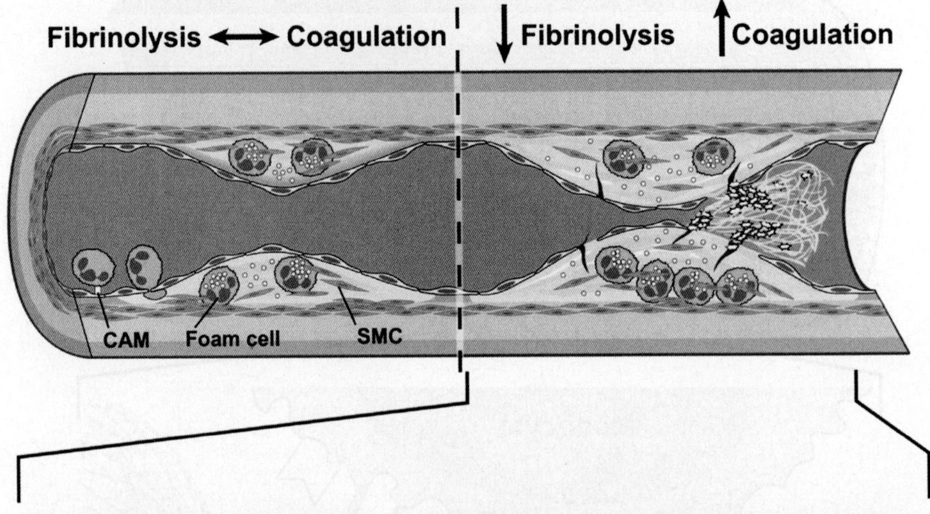

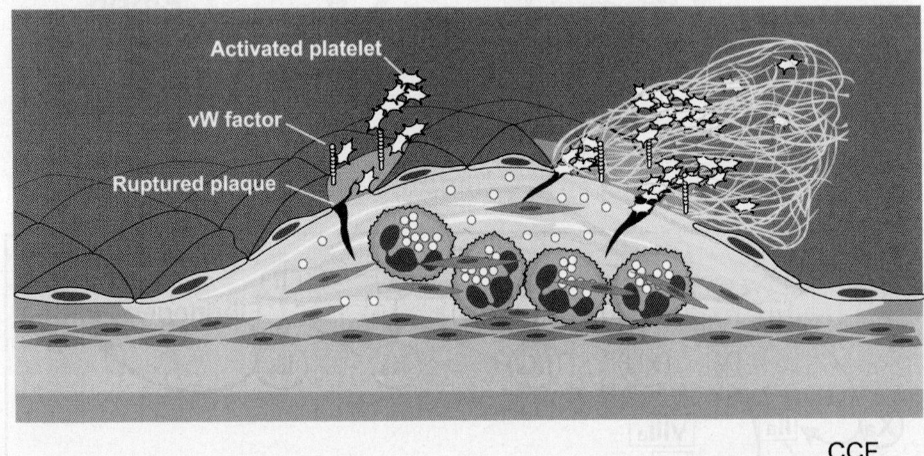

FIGURE 145.2 Arterial thrombi begin with a dysfunctional endothelium, resulting in monocyte infiltration and subsequent macrophage differentiation, foam cell lipid accumulation, and smooth muscle cell proliferation. Normally, there is a balance between blood fibrinolysis and coagulation. When plaques rupture, the balance between fibrinolysis and coagulation is shifted (greater thrombosis), and an occlusive thrombus may form. CAM, cellular adhesion molecule; SMC, smooth muscle cell; vW factor, von Willebrand factor.

treated with fresh platelet transfusion. For elective surgical procedures, aspirin should be stopped 5 days before the intervention (39). Aspirin is not recommended for venous thromboembolic prophylaxis (40); other forms of standard venous thromboembolism prophylaxis—for example, subcutaneous heparin and pneumatic compression devices—are preferred.

P2Y12 Receptor Antagonists

Adenosine diphosphate (ADP) interacts with two different receptors on platelets, known as P2Y1 and P2Y12. Interaction with P2Y1 receptors initiates the platelet response while interaction with P2Y12 receptors promotes the response. Blockade of the effects of ADP at either of these receptors results in a marked reduction in the overall effect of ADP on platelet function. The initial response to ADP is a change in the shape of the platelet; the disc-shaped cells will convert into a spherical form from which pseudopodia emerge. This change, mediated by the P2Y1 receptor, involves Ca^{2+} influx, intracellular Ca^{2+} mobilization, and actin polymerization. Interaction of ADP with the P2Y12 receptor results in inhibition of adenylate cyclase, which is accompanied by platelet aggregation (41,42). P2Y12 inhibition is recommended for patients undergoing antiplatelet therapy for the prevention of ischemic events.

The thienopyridine (ticlopidine, clopidogrel, and prasugrel) and nonthienopyridine (cangrelor and ticagrelor) class of antiplatelet agents have been approved for clinical use. These medications achieve their antiplatelet effect by irreversibly blocking the binding of ADP to the specific platelet receptor P2Y12, thus inhibiting adenyl cyclase and platelet aggregation (Fig. 145.4).

Clopidogrel

Clopidogrel, a member of the thienopyridine family, is a potent platelet inhibitor, working by irreversibly binding to low-affinity ADP receptors. It is rapidly absorbed and metabolized by the hepatic cytochrome P450 enzyme system to an active metabolite that selectively and irreversibly inhibits ADP-induced platelet aggregation. This metabolite also impairs the activation of glycoprotein (GP) IIb/IIIa complex and prevents fibrinogen binding to the platelets. Platelets exposed to this drug are affected for the remainder of their life span. Dose-dependent platelet inhibition can be seen within 2 hours after a single oral dose. For maximum effect, patients may be given a loading dose of 300 to 600 mg, followed by 75 mg per day. With repeated doses of 75 mg per day, maximum platelet inhibition can be achieved within 3 to 7 days (43).

When steady state is achieved, platelet aggregation is inhibited by 40% to 60% (44). Prolongation of bleeding time

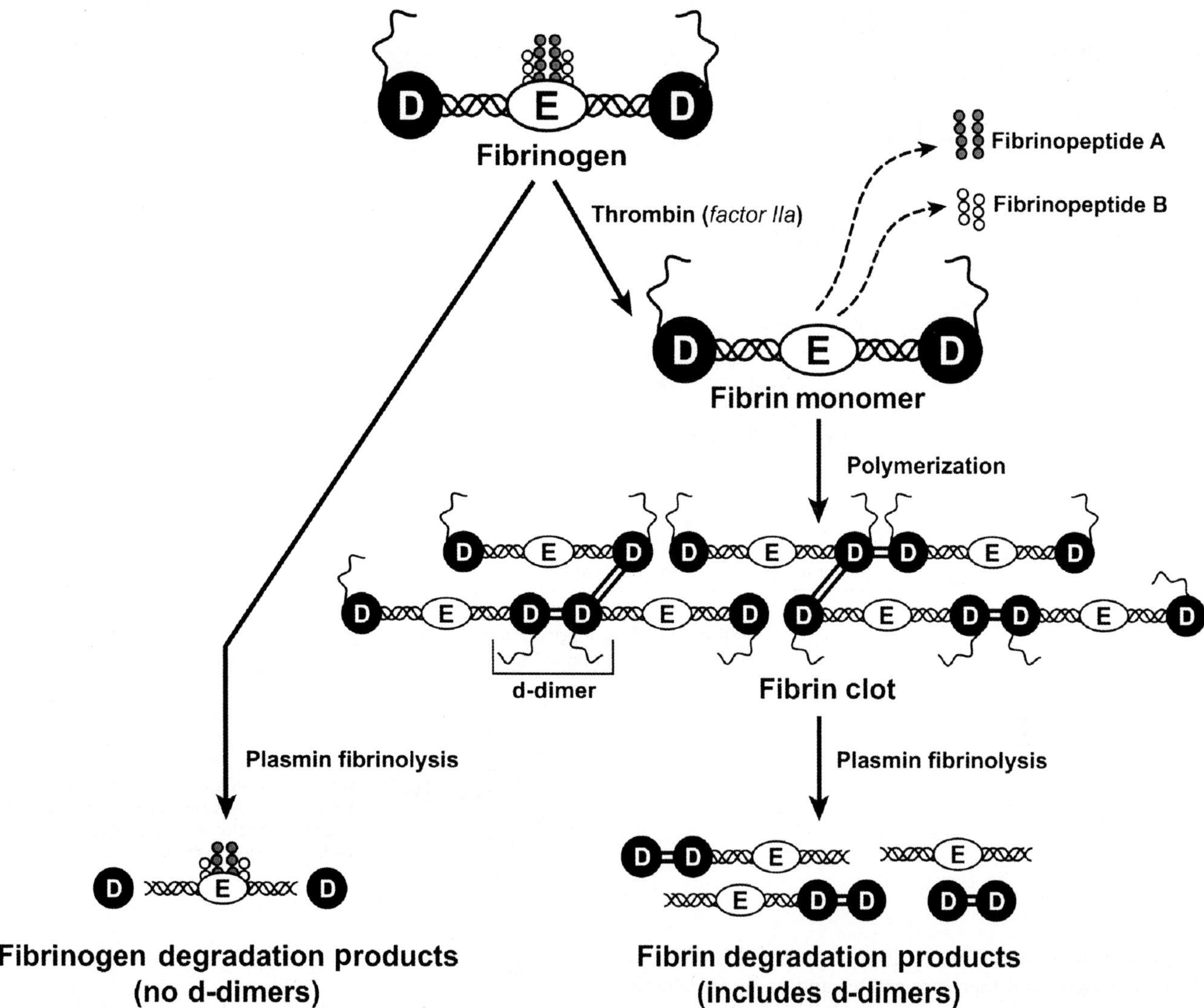

FIGURE 145.3 Fibrin clot formation and degradation. This figure shows the simplified conversion of fibrinogen into fibrin monomers called fibrinopeptides A and B. These monomers either polymerize to form fibrin clot or degrade into fibrinogen degradation products (without d-dimer formation). Fibrinolysis of a fibrin clot leads to formation of fibrin degradation products and d-dimers. Positive d-dimer assays are indicative of fibrin clot formation, followed by degradation by plasmin.

is independent of age, renal impairment, or gender. Platelet aggregation and bleeding time generally return to baseline about 5 days after discontinuation of clopidogrel. The CAPRIE trial was among the first to establish that clopidogrel is more effective than aspirin in reducing atherosclerotic events—including peripheral vascular disease, MI, and stroke—by 8.7% (45). The efficacy and safety of clopidogrel have been evaluated in ACS patients in the CURE trial, showing a 20% relative risk reduction in composite triple end points: nonfatal MI, death, or stroke (46). Clopidogrel, like ticlopidine, prolongs the bleeding time. While there was an incidence of neutropenia reported at 0.1% in the CAPRIE trial, there have been rare case reports of clopidogrel-associated thrombotic thrombocytopenic purpura. The incidence of gastrointestinal bleeding is less when compared to aspirin, but the incidence of bleeding is higher among patients requiring urgent surgical procedures who take clopidogrel (47). However, the clopidogrel effect can be reversed by transfusion of fresh platelets.

Ticlopidine

Ticlopidine, an older thienopyridine compound, inhibits platelet aggregation irreversibly and interferes with ADP-induced binding of fibrinogen to platelet receptors. It has fallen out of favor because of two major side effects: neutropenia and thrombotic thrombocytopenic purpura. Rare case reports of severe bone marrow toxicity limit ticlopidine use to patients who are intolerant or unresponsive to aspirin.

Prasugrel

Prasugrel, a third-generation thienopyridine, is an orally administered irreversible platelet P2Y12 receptor antagonist. It is a prodrug and requires metabolism via a cytochrome P450–dependent pathway into its active metabolite. Compared to clopidogrel, it has a more rapid onset of action after oral administration, it achieves and renders a more consistent and predictable platelet inhibition in individual patients (48).

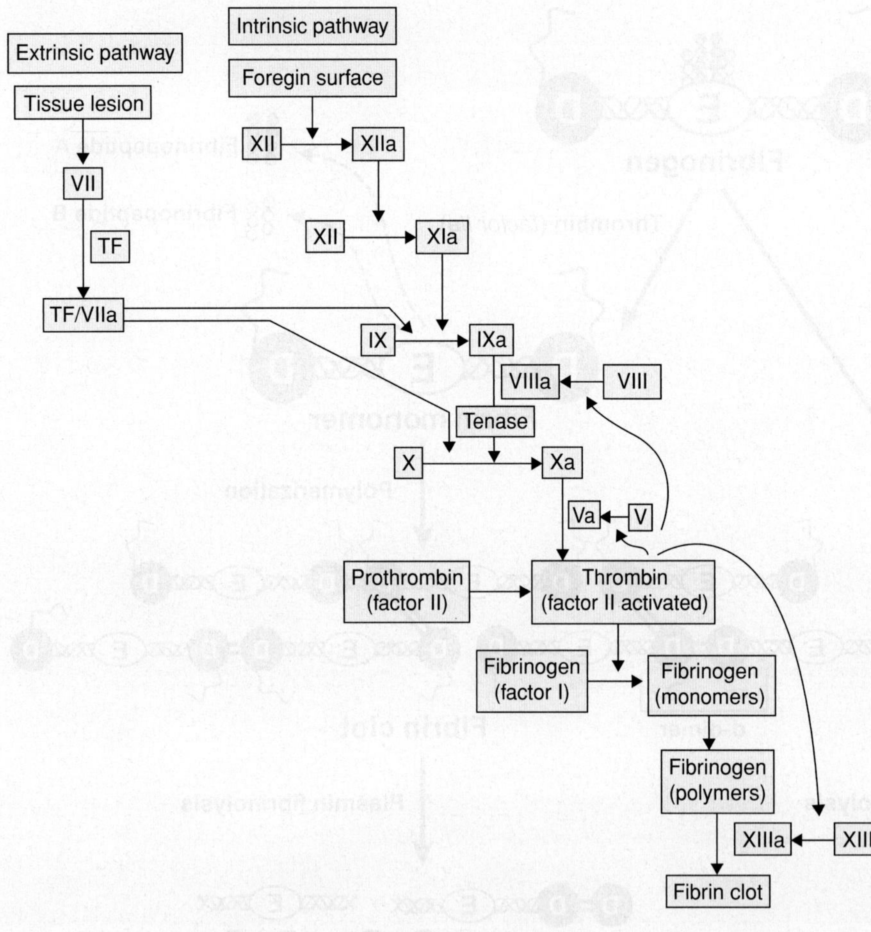

FIGURE 145.4 The coagulation cascade. The extrinsic pathway of coagulation is initiated by the factor VIIa/tissue factor complex, whereas the intrinsic pathway is initiated when factor XII contacts a foreign surface. Both pathways lead to factor IX and X activation. Activated factor IXa propagates coagulation by activating factor X in a reaction using activated factor VIIIa as a cofactor. Activated factor Xa combining with activated factor Va acts as a cofactor and converts prothrombin (factor II) to thrombin (factor IIa). Thrombin then converts fibrinogen to fibrin.

This occurs because the metabolism of prasugrel is different than clopidogrel and there are greater and more predictable amounts of active metabolite produced. This leads to longer recovery of platelet function (7 days for a 75% return to baseline platelet function as opposed to 5 days for clopidogrel). Surgical bleeding may be more problematic as a result (49).

In patients with ACSs undergoing percutaneous coronary intervention (PCI), prasugrel offers more effective antithrombotic therapy when compared to clopidogrel as shown in the TRITON-TIMI 38 study (trial to assess improvement in therapeutic outcomes by optimizing platelet inhibition with prasugrel-thrombolysis in MI 38) (48). This was a double-blinded, randomized controlled trial directly comparing prasugrel (60-mg loading dose followed by a 10-mg maintenance dose) and standard clopidogrel (300-mg loading dose followed by a 75-mg maintenance dose). The primary efficacy end point (cardiovascular death, nonfatal MI, or nonfatal stroke) occurred significantly less often in patients treated with prasugrel (9.9 vs. 12.1%; $p < 0.001$). The rate of probable stent thrombosis was significantly decreased in the prasugrel group (1.1 vs. 2.4%; $p < 0.001$). There was, however, a significant increased risk of bleeding associated with prasugrel in comparison to clopidogrel (2.4 vs. 1.8%; $p = 0.03$), most notable in patients with a prior history of stroke, age >75 years, and those with a body weight of <60 kg. Prasugrel effects are not modulated by aspirin dose or cytochrome interfering drugs including proton pump inhibitors. A washout period of 7 days is indicated for prasugrel-treated patients requiring surgery.

Ticagrelor

Ticagrelor is an orally administered cyclopentyltriazolopyrimidine, a new compound class very different from both clopidogrel and prasugrel, ticagrelor interacts with P2Y12 receptors on platelets, disabling their ability to interact with ADP. Although this compound is metabolized to an active agent, it is chemically very similar to the parent compound and metabolic conversion is not required for receptor interaction. It directly binds to the platelet receptor and allows for a faster onset of action, more intense, and consistent platelet inhibition than does clopidogrel (50). The reversible binding effects and the plasma half-life of 8 to 12 hours necessitate twice daily dosing (51). The ONSET/OFFSET study demonstrated ticagrelor exhibited greater platelet inhibition than clopidogrel. It looked at 123 patients with stable coronary artery disease on aspirin therapy and compared the addition of clopidogrel (600 mg load followed by 75 mg/day maintenance) or ticagrelor (180 mg load followed by 90 mg twice daily) or placebo. Analysis performed 2 hours after the loading doses demonstrated 90% of patients receiving ticagrelor achieved greater than 70% platelet inhibition as compared to 16% in the clopidogrel group. This effect was sustained at 6 weeks with patients taking ticagrelor (51).

Additionally, the PLATO trial (Platelet Inhibition and Patient Outcomes) examined the clinical benefit of ticagrelor (180-mg loading dose followed by 90 mg twice daily) compared to clopidogrel (300- to 600-mg loading dose followed by 75 mg daily) in 18,624 patients with ACSs randomized to receive either medication as soon as possible after hospital admission. The PLATO trial demonstrated that ticagrelor significantly reduced the rate of the primary end point (death from vascular causes, nonfatal myocardial infarct, or nonfatal stroke) at 12 months (9.8% vs. 11.7%; Hazard Ratio 0.84, $p = 0.0001$). There were no significant differences in the rate of major bleeding between either medication (11.6% vs. 11.2%, respectively), but ticagrelor was associated with a significantly higher rate of major bleeding not related to coronary artery bypass grafting (4.5% vs. 3.8%) (52).

Ticagrelor has been approved for clinical use and is indicated for the prevention of atherothrombotic events in patients with ACSs, including patients managed medically and invasively. In addition to being contraindicated in patients at high risk for bleeding, ticagrelor is contraindicated in patients with prior hemorrhagic stroke and severe hepatic dysfunction (50).

Cangrelor

Cangrelor is an intravenous, rapid onset, potent, and direct-acting platelet ADP P2Y12 inhibitor that has rapidly reversible effects. When a bolus of cangrelor is administered, the antiplatelet effect is immediate, and the effect can be maintained with a continuous infusion. The plasma half-life of cangrelor is approximately 3 to 5 minutes, and platelet function is restored within 1 hour after cessation of the infusion (53).

In the CHAMPION PHOENIX trial, 11,145 patients undergoing either urgent or elective percutaneous coronary intervention (PCI) were enrolled in a double-blind, placebo controlled manner to evaluate the impact of clopidogrel and cangrelor on outcome; patients received guideline-recommended therapy of a bolus and infusion of cangrelor or a loading dose of 600 mg or 300 mg of clopidogrel. The primary efficacy end point was a composite of death, MI, ischemia-driven revascularization, or stent thrombosis at 48 hours after randomization; the key secondary end point was stent thrombosis at 48 hours. The rate of the primary efficacy end point was 4.7% in the cangrelor group and 5.9% in the clopidogrel group (adjusted odds ratio with cangrelor, 0.78; 95% confidence interval [CI], 0.66 to 0.93; $p = 0.005$). The rate of the primary safety end point was 0.16% in the cangrelor group and 0.11% in the clopidogrel group (odds ratio, 1.50; 95% CI, 0.53 to 4.22; $p = 0.44$). Stent thrombosis developed in 0.8% of the patients in the cangrelor group and in 1.4% in the clopidogrel group (odds ratio, 0.62; 95% CI, 0.43 to 0.90; $p = 0.01$). The rates of adverse events related to the study treatment were low in both groups; the primary safety end point was severe bleeding at 48 hours (54). At the time of this writing the U.S. Food and Drug Administration (FDA) is continuing to evaluate cangrelor for approval.

Vorapaxar

In 2014, the FDA approved a new class of antiplatelet medication, to reduce the risk of MI or peripheral artery disease (PAD). This class of medication, considered a protease–activated-receptor 1 antagonist (PAR-1), is intended as part of a therapeutic regimen inclusive of aspirin and clopidogrel.

Approval of this medication was based on the Thrombin-Receptor Antagonist in Secondary Prevention of Atherothrombotic Ischemic Events (TRA 2 P TIMI-50) trial. Results of the trial ($n = 26{,}499$ patients) demonstrated cardiovascular death, MI, stroke, or urgent coronary revascularization was decreased by 13% in patients taking vorapaxar. When coronary revascularization was excluded, the secondary endpoint of cardiovascular death, MI, or stroke was also significantly reduced (55). Because of vorapaxar's antiplatelet effects, moderate or severe bleeding occurred in 3.4% of patients compared with 2.1% in the placebo-treated patients. Intracranial hemorrhage occurred in 0.6% of those taking vorapaxar compared with 0.4% taking placebo (55).

Glycoprotein IIb/IIIa Antagonists

Abciximab

This, the most successful GPIIb/IIIa antagonist, is a human-murine Fab chimeric monoclonal antibody fragment to the GPIIb/IIIa binding site; it is a large protein with a rapid and prolonged response, causing the bleeding time to remain elevated for 12 hours after injection. Abciximab is used in combination with aspirin and heparin in patients with unresponsive unstable angina or undergoing PCI. It has been demonstrated to deliver a 60% relative risk reduction in triple end points: MI, emergent revascularization, or cardiovascular deaths (56,57). The major complications of this agent include intracranial bleeding or a decrease in hemoglobin of more than 15%, reported as frequently as 10.5% (58). There is a high incidence of thrombocytopenia, which can be spurious (4%) due to platelet clumping, but true and severe thrombocytopenia may also develop, resulting in profound bleeding (59). In the event of profuse bleeding, platelet transfusions are required to normalize the platelet count. Desmopressin has been shown to normalize the bleeding time (60).

Eptifibatide

This disintegrin, derived from the southeastern pygmy rattlesnake, is rapidly bound and rapidly reversed, with a normalization of the bleeding time within 1 to 4 hours. This drug has been shown to be more effective in milder forms of ACSs (61).

Tirofiban

This is a small nonpeptide compound derived from tyrosine, which interacts with the arginine-glycine-aspartic acid fibrinogen receptor. Tirofiban has been used in unstable angina with mixed results (62).

Dipyridamole

Dipyridamole is a phosphodiesterase inhibitor, reversibly inhibiting platelet aggregation. As it increases c-AMP and c-GMP levels, through its inhibition of phosphodiesterases, it potentiates the effect of nitric oxide. It has been used adjunctively with aspirin to reduce stroke events in patients younger than 70 years (63).

ANTITHROMBOTIC THERAPY

Unfractionated Heparin

Unfractionated heparin (UH) is a naturally occurring acidic glycosaminoglycan. Its pentasaccharide sequence binds to antithrombin, causing a conformational change at the arginine reactive site that potentiates the effect of antithrombin,

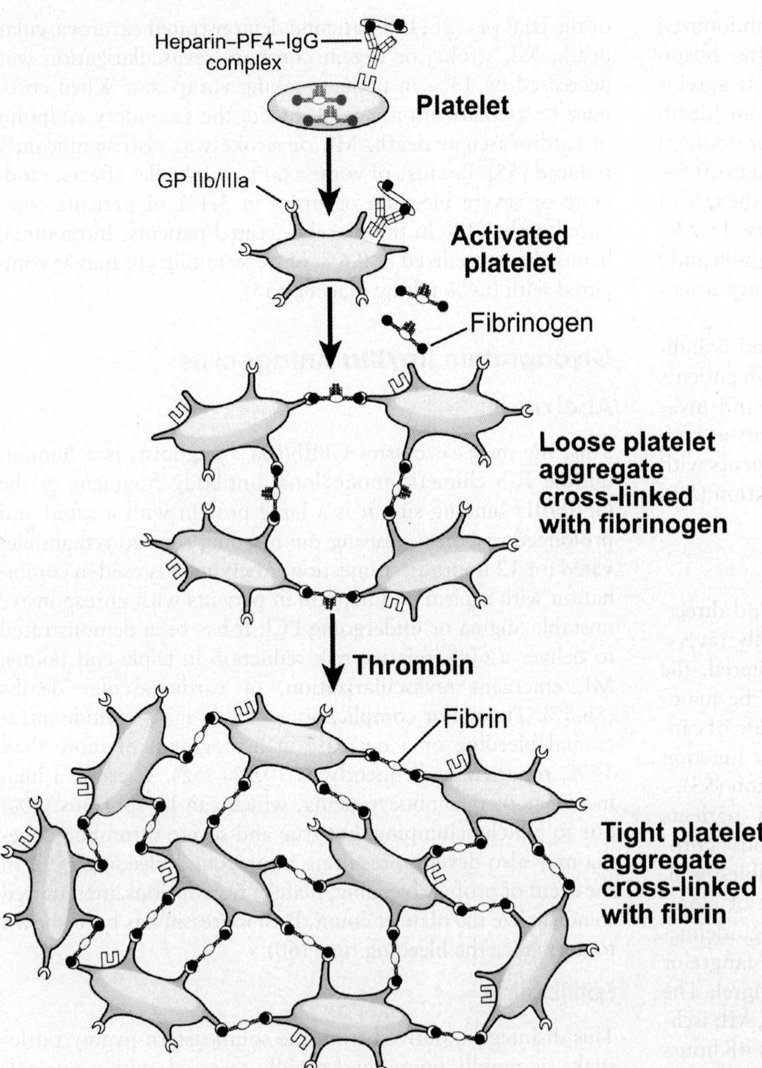

FIGURE 145.5 The immune-mediated platelet activation involves the binding of heparin–platelet factor 4–IgG complex to the platelets and brings about conformational changes, exposing GPIIb/IIIa to fibrinogen. This complex leads to further platelet activation, cross-linking them into platelet aggregates. Thrombin plays a major role in the conversion of fibrinogen to fibrin, forming tight platelet aggregates. PF 4, platelet factor 4; IgG, immunoglobulin G; GPIIb/IIIa, glycoprotein IIb/IIIa.

causing it to have an enhanced effect on inhibition of the coagulation enzymes, in particular thrombin (factor IIa) and factor Xa. Heparin also acts to inhibit activation of factors V and VIII by thrombin (Fig. 145.5) (64,65). The increase in inhibition of these enzymes in the presence of UH may be up to 2,000 times faster than in its absence. The molecular weight of UH is 3,000 to 35,000 daltons (d) on average, with a mean molecular weight of 15,000 d, composed of approximately 45 monosaccharide chains. Due to the variable size and structure of heparin, only about one-third of any given dose of heparin will demonstrate therapeutic anticoagulant activity. The different-sized molecules are cleared at different rates by the kidney, with the larger ones being cleared more rapidly. Thus, the combination of these factors leads to great variability in the anticoagulant effects on individuals, necessitating the need for monitoring with activated partial thromboplastin time (aPTT). Heparin is obtained from either bovine lung or porcine intestine and is available as a sodium or calcium salt.

The unit of heparin is measured in animals in a biologic assay, with the unit measurement being variable by as much as 50% on a weight basis. Therefore, UH is prescribed for patients on a unit basis/kg, not the weight of medication (66).

Uses of Unfractionated Heparin

Heparin is indicated for prophylaxis of venous thromboembolism. It is used in the treatment of DVT and pulmonary embolus, as well as for early treatment of patients suffering from ACSs.

Prevention of Thromboembolism. To prevent thromboembolism, UH at a fixed low dose of 5,000 units, subcutaneously every 8 to 12 hours, results in a 60% to 70% relative risk reduction for DVT and fatal pulmonary embolus (PE) (40,67). In high-risk surgical and acutely ill medical patients, the use of low–molecular-weight heparin (LMWH) is becoming the standard for prevention of thrombosis (68,69).

In the patient who is unable to tolerate any type of anticoagulation, the use of intermittent pneumatic compression is useful as a mechanical means for preventing DVT by intermittently squeezing the patient's calves, leading to increased blood flow through the venous system. Intermittent pneumatic compression may also stimulate fibrinolysis by stimulating the vascular endothelium (70).

Venous Thromboembolism and Pulmonary Embolus. Therapy for treating proximal or symptomatic distal venous thromboembolism and PE is aimed at preventing extension of the clot with further embolization and recurrence; anticoagulation has long been an effective strategy for the treatment of both conditions (71). Multiple studies have demonstrated the efficacy of heparin in reducing mortality in patients with venous thromboembolism (72,73), as well as the high mortality in patients with PE who are not anticoagulated (74). More recent clinical studies further demonstrated the benefit of treating DVT with continuous intravenous heparin and, in some cases, LMWH (75–77). Additionally, data show the effectiveness of using subcutaneous heparin as the initial treatment for DVT, as long as adequate doses are used and the aPTT is prolonged into the therapeutic range (78–80). Recently, Kearon et al. (81) demonstrated that administration of a fixed dose, weight-adjusted, UH was as effective and safe as the administration of LMWH in patients with acute DVT and may also be suitable for treatment in the outpatient setting.

Perhaps the most efficient method for initiating intravenous heparin therapy is using weight-adjusted nomograms. The important consideration is to maintain a therapeutic range when heparin anticoagulation therapy is initiated, best achieved with frequent monitoring of plasma aPTT. Subtherapeutic dosing within the first 24 hours of a documented DVT resulted in a significantly greater frequency of venous thromboembolus recurrence when compared to those patients who reached a supratherapeutic threshold within 24 hours (82).

The weight-based method was developed by Raschke et al. (83) who found that a weight-based titration of UH resulted in a significant decrease in the time required to reach therapeutic levels as compared to a standard dosing scheme of heparin. These clinicians found that 97% of patients dosed using the weight-based nomogram achieve therapeutic levels within 24 hours of initiation as opposed to 77% in the standard dosing group (Tables 145.2 and 145.3).

Typically, the Raschke method of anticoagulation in the acute phase of venous thromboembolism is initiated with an intravenous loading dose of 80 units/kg, followed by 18 units/kg/hr. Subsequent doses should be adjusted using a standard nomogram to rapidly reach and maintain an aPTT that corresponds to therapeutic heparin levels of 1.5 to 2.5 times the

TABLE 145.2 Weight-Based Heparin Dosing Nomogram

aPTT[a], s[b]	Dose Change (U/kg/hr)	Additional Action	Next aPTT (hrs)
<35 (<1.2 × mean normal)	+4	Rebolus with 80 IU/kg	6
35–45 (1.2–1.5 × mean normal)	+2	Rebolus with 40 IU/kg	6
46–70[a] (1.5–2.3 × mean normal)	0	0	6[c]
71–90 (2.3–3.0 × mean normal)	−2	0	6
>90 (> × mean normal)	−3	Stop infusion 1 hrs	6

aPTT, activated prothrombin time.
Initial dosing: Loading 80 IU/kg; maintenance infusion: 18 IU/kg/hr (aPTT in 6 hrs)
[a]Therapeutic range in seconds should correspond to a plasma heparin level of 0.2–0.4 IU/mL by protamine sulfate or 0.3–0.6 IU/mL by amidolytic assay. When aPTT is checked at 6 hrs or longer, steady-state kinetics can be assumed.
[b]Heparin, 25,000 IU in 250 mL D_5W. Infuse at rate dictated by body weight.
[c]During the first 24 hrs, repeat aPTT every 6 hrs. Thereafter, monitor aPTT once every morning unless it is outside the therapeutic range.
From Hyers TM, Agnelli G, Hull RD, et al. Antithrombotic therapy for venous thromboembolic disease. *Chest.* 2001;119(Suppl):179S.

TABLE 145.3 Guidelines for Anticoagulation Using Unfractionated Heparin

Indication	Guidelines
VTE suspected	• Obtain baseline aPTT, PT, CBC • Check for contraindication to heparin therapy • Order imaging study, consider giving heparin 5,000 IU IV
VTE confirmed	• Rebolus with heparin 80 IU/kg IV and start maintenance infusion at 18 U/kg (see Table 145.2) • Check aPTT at 6 hrs to keep aPTT in a range that corresponds to a therapeutic blood heparin level (see text and Table 145.2) • Check a platelet count between days 3 and 5 • Start warfarin therapy on day 1 at 5 mg and adjust subsequent daily dose according to INR • Stop heparin therapy after at least 4–5 of combined therapy when INR is >2.0 • Anticoagulate with warfarin for at least 3 mo at an INR of 2.5; range: 2.0–3.0 (see Table 145.6)

aPTT, activated prothrombin time; PT, prothrombin time; CBC, complete blood count; IV, intravenously; INR, international normalized ratio.
For subcutaneous treatment with unfractionated heparin, give 250 IU/kg subcutaneously every 12 hrs to obtain a therapeutic aPTT at 6–8 hrs.
From Hyers TM, Agnelli G, Hull RD, et al. Antithrombotic therapy for venous thromboembolic disease. *Chest.* 2001;119(Suppl):180S.

baseline (83–88). Alternatively, therapeutic heparin anticoagulation is determined by achieving a plasma anti–factor Xa level of 0.35 to 0.7 units/mL (89,90). This therapeutic range is recommended based on animal studies (91), prospective studies and analysis of patients with established DVT (90), studies on the prevention of mural thrombus formation following MI (91) and prevention of recurrent ischemia following coronary thrombolysis (93). Heparin anticoagulation should be continued for up to 5 days so that adequate anticoagulation is achieved. During this time, the aPTT should be monitored every 6 hours until the therapeutic range is achieved, and once daily thereafter. Preferably on day 1, the patient may be transitioned to long-term warfarin (5 mg), a vitamin K–antagonist agent that may be administered orally if the patient can tolerate enteral intake. The anticoagulation effect of warfarin is monitored by the international normalized ratio (INR) to achieve a therapeutic range of two to three times the normal level for a first thrombotic episode. Warfarin is considered to be at therapeutic level if the INR of 2 to 3 is maintained for 2 consecutive days. If the patient is unstable and unable to tolerate oral anticoagulation, intravenous heparin may need to be continued. It is important to keep in mind that warfarin interacts with many commonly used drugs in the ICU, and its metabolism may be affected by hepatic and renal impairment. This may lead to erratic variation in the anticoagulant effect of warfarin, exposing the patient to increased risks of bleeding and thrombotic complications (7). The minimum recommended duration of warfarin therapy is 3 months (66,94) based upon the clinical scenario and patient risk factors, with follow-up evaluation to determine if longer therapy is necessary. Further studies have demonstrated that longer treatment may be beneficial (95–97) in higher-risk patients. In accordance with the American College of Chest Physicians Conference on Antithrombotic and

Thrombolytic Therapy, it is now recommended that warfarin therapy be continued following a first unprovoked proximal or second unprovoked DVT or those with active cancer. For those with recurrent events or who have permanent or long-term risk factors, the panel recommends indefinite therapy (94).

Acute Coronary Syndromes. The ACC/AHA updated guidelines for the management of patients with acute myocardial infarction (AMI) (98) evaluated multiple trials comparing the use of LMWH with UH in non–ST elevation ACS (99–101). The studies cited demonstrate, as a whole, a benefit of LMWH over UH when it came to a lower event rate and relative risk reduction (102). These guidelines suggest considering LMWH, as opposed to UH due to its greater inhibition of factor Xa, the ability to administer the drug subcutaneously, and its high bioavailability. In those patients with impaired renal function (CrCl <30 mL/min) it may be necessary to consider a reduction in dose to one-half recommended and/or frequency of administration to only once daily. It should be noted that a sub study of the Enoxaparin and Thrombolysis Reperfusion for AMI-TIMI 25 trial demonstrated that for every 30 mL/min decrease in CrCl, the risk of major and minor bleeding increased by 50% (103,104). Until conclusive results are available regarding optimal dosing, it may be safer to use UFH in patients with impaired renal function presenting with ACS. However, other benefits of the drug are cited as well, such as the potential to prevent thrombin generation and inhibit thrombin, the lack of need to monitor coagulation, and the lower incidence of heparin-associated thrombocytopenia (105).

Monitoring UH

The most widely used test for evaluating the adequacy of heparin anticoagulation is the aPTT, a global coagulation test that is not always a reliable indicator of plasma heparin levels and/or the antithrombotic activity of heparin. The aPTT can be impacted by various acute phase reactant plasma proteins, including factor VIII. Additionally, the aPTT can be influenced by the coagulation timer and reagents used to perform the test (103). If a hospital is unable to measure plasma heparin levels directly, it is recommended that each laboratory standardize the therapeutic range of the aPTT to correspond to plasma levels of 0.3 to 0.7 IU/mL anti–factor Xa activity by an amidolytic assay.

Complications of Anticoagulation Therapy

Heparin Resistance

Patients are considered heparin resistant if their daily requirement of heparin exceeds 35,000 units/24 hr; unfortunately, multiple studies demonstrate that at least 25% of patients with venous thromboemboli are heparin resistant. Heparin resistance may be associated with antithrombin deficiency, increased heparin clearance, increases in heparin-binding proteins, and increases in factor VIII, fibrinogen, and platelet factor 4. Aprotinin and nitroglycerin have been reported to cause drug-induced resistance, but the association with nitroglycerin remains controversial (106). Factor VIII and fibrinogen are elevated in response to acute illness or pregnancy. Elevation of factor VIII alters the response of the aPTT to heparin without decreasing the antithrombotic effect, as the anticoagulant effect measured by the plasma aPTT and the antithrombotic effect is measured by anti–factor Xa activity become dissociated.

For those patients considered heparin resistant, the dose of heparin should be adjusted to maintain the anti–factor Xa heparin levels between 0.35 and 0.7 mIU/mL. In a randomized, controlled study by Levine and Hirsch (107), evaluating 131 patients with venous thromboembolism and manifesting heparin resistance, monitoring the aPTT was compared to anti–factor Xa activity; while there were no difference in clinical outcomes, it was found that the patient group monitored with anti–factor Xa heparin levels required significantly less heparin with no differences in bleeding.

Hemorrhagic Complications

The incidence of major hemorrhagic complications—defined as intracranial or retroperitoneal hemorrhage, hemorrhage requiring a transfusion, or hemorrhage directly related to death—from therapeutic anticoagulation is less than 5% (105). The risk increases with age, total dose of heparin/24 hr. patient premorbid condition, concomitant use of aspirin, GPIIb/IIIa antagonists, or thrombolytic therapy. Intravenous (IV) heparin infusion appears to produce less marked bleeding complications than when the agent is administered (107) subcutaneously. This may be due to a lower total dose of heparin via the IV, as compared to the subcutaneous, route (106).

The anticoagulant effect of UH can be neutralized rapidly by intravenous protamine. Protamine is a cationic protein derived from fish sperm that strongly binds to the anionic heparin compound in a ratio of approximately 100 units of UH/mg of protamine. When heparin has been infused, only the heparin given over the prior 2 hours should be included in the calculation. If the heparin infusion was discontinued for more than 30 minutes but less than 2 hours, use one-half of the calculated protamine dose. If the infusion was discontinued for longer than 2 hours, use one-quarter of the calculated protamine dose. One should avoid giving 50 mg of protamine at one time and, if given by infusion, it should not exceed 5 mg per minute to reduce the incidence of adverse reactions. Heparin neutralization can be confirmed by a fall in the aPTT.

The risks of severe adverse reactions to protamine, such as hypotension and bradycardia, are reduced with a slow administration of the drug over more than 3 minutes. Some clinicians will begin the protamine infusion following a 3- to 5-mg test dose administered over 1 minute (107,108). Allergic reactions including anaphylaxis are associated with a previous exposure to protamine-containing insulin—for example, NPH-insulin (108)—fish hypersensitivity (109), and vasectomy. Patients at risk for developing antiprotamine antibodies can be pretreated with corticosteroid and antihistamine medications.

Heparin-Associated (Induced) Thrombocytopenia

Heparin-induced thrombocytopenia (HIT) is an antibody-mediated adverse reaction to the administration of heparin and/or LMWH and may lead to both arterial and venous thrombosis. The diagnosis is made both on clinical and serologic findings. HIT antibody formation, accompanied by an otherwise unexplained fall in platelet count by more than 50% from baseline and/or skin lesions at injection sites are the manifestations of HIT (110).

The incidence of HIT is less than 1% when heparin is given for less than 7 days; thereafter, when given to patients with an extended need for anticoagulation (such as ICU patients), the incidence may rise as high as 10% to 20% for the mild form (type 1) of HIT and to more than 5% for type 2, the more severe manifestation. A precipitous fall in platelet count from baseline is usually seen with the type 1 syndrome, and 50% to 75% of these patients may go on to develop the more ominous type 2 syndrome, which manifests with either the development of arterial, or more commonly, venous thrombotic complications.

Patients who develop HIT generate large amounts of thrombin. In vivo, platelet activation results from binding of the heparin PF4-IgG immune complexes to platelet factor IIa receptors. These increased levels of thrombin are demonstrated by elevated levels of thrombin–antithrombin complexes, which serve as an in vivo marker of thrombin generation, much higher than that seen in control patients with DVT (111). The diagnosis can be confirmed with platelet function testing or the identification in the blood of the antibody to heparin-platelet factor 4 complex using an enzyme-linked immunosorbent assay (ELISA) (111) (see Fig. 145.5).

Once the determination of HIT is made, it is not adequate simply to stop anticoagulation therapy with heparin or LMWH. Multiple studies document that patients continue to be at risk of thrombosis if no anticoagulation is given (112,113). Currently, alternative antithrombotic agents are being used and have been approved in many countries for the treatment of HIT. Three of the agents are direct thrombin inhibitors: argatroban, hirudin (lepirudin), and bivalirudin, and the other agent is a heparinoid, danaparoid (Table 145.4).

Argatroban is a small (MW 526) synthetic molecule derived from L-arginine that reversibly binds to thrombin. It is approved for prophylaxis and treatment of patients with HIT in both the United States and Canada. It reportedly has been associated with a lower thrombotic event rate in one prospective study. The half-life is less than 1 hour, and the drug is excreted normally, even in those with moderate renal failure. In the event of hepatic dysfunction, the dose of argatroban must be reduced. The anticoagulant effect is monitored by the aPTT.

TABLE 145.4 Alternatives to Heparin for the Treatment of Heparin-Induced Thrombocytopenia

Agent (Direct Thrombin Inhibitors)	Clearance	Therapeutic Dose	Therapeutic Dose	Adverse Effects
Lepirudin (Refludan, Berlex)[a]	Renal	IV, 0.4 mg/kg of body weight (up to 110 kg); IV bolus[b] followed by 0.15 mg/kg/hr (up to 110 kg) (maximal initial infusion, 16.5 mg/hr)	Measure aPTT 2 hrs after therapy started and after each dose adjustment[c]; therapeutic range, 1.5–2.5 times the baseline value (optimal aPTT, <65 s); check baseline PT before switching therapy to warfarin[d]	Bleeding with therapeutic dose in 17.6% of patients; antilepirudin antibodies develop in 30% of patients
Argatroban (Novastan, GlaxoSmithKline)[a]	Hepatic	2 μg/kg/min continuous infusion (maximal infusion, 10 μg/kg/min)	Measure aPTT 2 hrs after therapy started and after each dose adjustment; therapeutic range, 1.5–2.5 times the baseline value (optimal aPTT; <65 s); check baseline PT before switching therapy to warfarin[e]	Bleeding with therapeutic dose in 17.6% of patients; antilepirudin antibodies develop in 30% of patients
Bivalirudin (Angiomax, The Medicines Company)[f]	Enzymatic (80%) and renal (20%)	2 μg/kg/min continuous infusion (maximal infusion, 10 μg/kg/min)	Measure aPTT 2 hrs after therapy started and after each dose adjustment therapeutic range, 1.5–2.5 times the baseline value (optimal aPTT, <65 s): check baseline PT before switching therapy to warfarin	Bleeding with therapeutic dose in 17.6% of patients; antilepirudin antibodies develop in 30% of patients
Anti-factor Xa therapy Danaparoid (Orgaran, Diosynth)[g]	Renal	IV, 2,250 U bolus followed by 400 U/hr for 4 hrs, then 150–200 U/hr	Nor required, but if needed, maintain anti–factor Xa level, 0.5–0.8 U/mL	Bleeding with therapeutic dose in 8.1% of patients; cross-reactivity with PF4–heparin antibodies develop in 3.2% of patients

aPTT, activated partial thromboplastin time; PT, prothrombin time; hr, hour; s, second.

Except where indicated, the guidelines for dosing and monitoring are from the manufacturers of the drugs. Guidelines for therapeutic dosing are for intravenous (IV) infusion, except for bivalirudin, which is used in patients undergoing percutaneous coronary intervention (PCI). The guidelines of the American College of Chest Physicians recommend overlap use of direct thrombin inhibitor therapy and warfarin therapy for more than 5 days, whereas the Hemostasis and Thrombosis Task Force of the British Committee for Standards in Hemotology recommend overlap use of direct thrombin inhibitor therapy and warfarin therapy until the international normalized ratio (INR) is at a therapeutic level for at least 48 hrs.

[a]These drugs have been approved in the United States for the treatment of heparin-induced thrombocytopenia.

[b]Bolus therapy is not advised in older patients or patients with renal insufficiency.

[c]This value is the maximal aPTT recommended by Lubenow et al.

[d]Therapeutic lepirudin may prolong the baseline PT slightly, but it generally does not interfere with conversion from lepirudin to warfarin therapy. If the PT is prolonged by more than a few seconds, further evaluation should be undertaken before initiating warfarin.

[e]Combined anticoagulant therapy with argatroban and warfarin produces an INR response that is significantly greater than that obtained with warfarin alone. To change therapy from argatroban to warfarin for outpatient anticoagulant therapy, the INR should be monitored daily, and when the INR is greater than 4, the argatroban infusion should be withheld and the INR rechecked to determine whether it is therapeutic. An alternative strategy would be to use a chromogenic factor X assay to monitor warfarin therapy while the patient is also receiving argatroban.

[f]This drug has been approved in the United States for the treatment of patients undergoing percutaneous coronary intervention (PCI) who have heparin-induced thrombocytopenia or a history of heparin-induced thrombocytopenia.

[g]This drug is not available in the United States.

From Arepally GM, Ortel TL. Clinical practice. Heparin-induced thrombocytopenia. *N Engl J Med.* 2006;355:809–817.

Lepirudin is a recombinant polypeptide originally derived from the medicinal leech (see below). It inhibits thrombin directly and is approved only for the treatment of HIT. The anticoagulant effect of lepirudin is monitored by the aPTT. It is renally excreted, and the risk for accumulation and bleeding is high in patients with renal failure; the half-life of lepirudin is 1.3 hours.

Danaparoid is a mixture of heparan sulfate, dermatan sulfate, and chondroitin sulfate; the drug reduces thrombin generation in vivo by the inhibition of factor Xa. Although no longer available in the United States, it is used for the treatment of HIT elsewhere. It is important to consider that cross-reactivity between heparin and danaparoid may occur in up to 30% of cases; in this case, a direct thrombin inhibitor should be used for treatment.

A third direct thrombin inhibitor, *bivalirudin,* is not approved for the treatment of HIT but has been successfully used and reported off-label for this use (113). An early transition from intravenous heparin or LMWH anticoagulation to warfarin (or an equivalent anticoagulant) has been standard therapy for most patients with acute venous and arterial thromboembolism. This approach may also help prevent HIT by limiting a patient's total dose-time exposure to heparin medications. One complication to be considered is that early transition has been associated with further thrombotic complications of venous limb gangrene and warfarin-induced skin necrosis (112,113).

Warfarin and other equivalent vitamin K antagonists counter thrombin generation by slowly decreasing the plasma levels of the vitamin K factors (II, VII, IX, X) while concurrently decreasing the natural anticoagulant factors C and S. During the transition to oral vitamin K antagonist therapy in patients with HIT, thrombin is still being generated (warfarin having failed to control this). Due to their shorter half-lives, factors VII and protein C are reduced faster than the prothrombotic factors II, IX, and X (Table 145.5). This results in a supratherapeutic INR secondary to factor VII depletion and a *transient hypercoagulable state* due to the decrease in protein C without a concurrent decrease in the prothrombotic levels of factors II and X. Throughout this process, there is still increased thrombin generation due to the HIT, and venous limb gangrene and/or warfarin-induced skin necrosis may develop as a result (110,113).

In these patients, it has been recommended to use the direct thrombin inhibitors available—argatroban, lepirudin, and bivalirudin or danaparoid—once HIT has been established and discontinue the use of heparin or LMWH. Anticoagulation needs to be ensured, and with use of these alternatives, there should be no interruption in anticoagulation therapy. Oral therapy with warfarin or an equivalent vitamin K–antagonist agent should be avoided until the patient's platelet count has recovered to near-normal levels (>150,000 platelets/μL). Thereafter, one may begin administering warfarin at modest doses (2.5 to 5.0 mg orally [PO]), titrating to and maintaining the target INR; warfarin should not be used as the initial treatment for HIT (112,113,116).

TABLE 145.5 Half-Lives of the Vitamin K–Dependent Procoagulant and Natural Anticoagulant Factors

Factor	Half-Life (hrs)
VII	5–6
IX	24
X	30–50
II	96
Protein C	8–10
Protein S	42–60

Low-Molecular-Weight Heparin

LMWH is prepared from UH by controlled depolymerization of the parent drug into short segments. The molecular weight of LMWH ranges from 1,000 to 10,000, and about 20% of the LMWH chains contain pentasaccharide sequences that are needed for antithrombin binding.

Mechanism of Action

LMWH chains bind to antithrombin and brings about conformational changes that lead to inhibition of factor Xa. The ratio of inhibition of thrombin to factor Xa varies from 1:2 to 1:4 for different preparations of LMWH (117). LMWH is being increasingly used for the treatment of venous thromboembolic disease in non-ICU patients. It can be administered as a subcutaneous injection once or twice daily and intravenously when a rapid anticoagulant effect is needed. It is as safe and effective as intravenous and subcutaneous UH (76).

The shorter chains of LMWH bind less avidly to endothelial cells, macrophages, and heparin-binding proteins and have better bioavailability (118). They tend to accumulate in vivo, leading to longer half-life, and have more predictable renal clearance and a greater ability to inactivate factor Xa compared to inactivation of thrombin and, consequently, have a negligible effect on the aPTT. The clearance of LMWH is dose independent and is accomplished almost exclusively by the kidneys; hence the drug can accumulate in renal insufficiency. LMWH has proved to be cost effective because of the reduced need for monitoring, and there are several advantages of LMWH over the UH (Table 145.6).

The disadvantages of LMWH, which may be more pertinent to the ICU, include the absence of an established dose for obese patients and impaired clearance in patients with renal failure. These can be overcome by monitoring anti–factor-Xa levels and adjusting the subsequent doses. Based on the anti–factor-Xa levels, LMWH has a plasma half-life of 4 hours. The therapeutic anti–factor Xa levels with LMWH range from

TABLE 145.6 Advantages of Low-Molecular-Weight Heparin over Unfractionated Heparin

Advantage	Consequence
Better bioavailability and longer half-life	Can be given subcutaneously one or twice after subcutaneous injection daily for both prophylaxis and treatment
Dose-independent clearance	Simplified dosing
Predictable anticoagulant response	Coagulation monitoring is unnecessary in most patients
Lower risk of heparin-induced thrombocytopenia	Safer than heparin for short- or long-term administration
Lower risk of osteoporosis	Safer than heparin for extended administration

From Weitz JI. Anticoagulants and fibrinolytic drugs. In: Hoffman, ed. *Hematology: Basic Principles and Practice.* 4th ed. Orlando, FL: Churchill Livingstone; 2005:2254.

TABLE 145.7 LMWH Dosage Regimens for Patients with Severe Renal Impairment

Indication	Dosage Regimen
Prophylaxis in abdominal surgery	30 mg SC once daily
Prophylaxis in hip or knee replacement surgery	30 mg SC once daily
Prophylaxis in medical patients during acute illness	30 mg SC once daily
Prophylaxis of ischemic complications of unstable angina and non–Q wave myocardial infarction when concurrently administered with aspirin	1 mg/kg SC once daily
Inpatient treatment of acute deep vein thrombosis with or without pulmonary embolism when administered in conjunction with warfarin sodium	1 mg/kg SC once daily
Outpatient treatment of acute deep vein thrombosis without pulmonary embolism when administered in conjunction with warfarin sodium	1 mg/kg SC once daily

SC, subcutaneously.

0.5 to 1.2 units/mL when measured 3 to 4 hours after drug administration. There is no rapid and complete antagonist to the anticoagulant effect of LMWH, which may complicate and hinder ICU and surgical procedures (Table 145.7) (7).

Dosing

The most commonly prescribed LMWHs are enoxaparin, dalteparin, and newer agents like tinzaparin. Enoxaparin is primarily metabolized in the liver by desulfation and/or depolymerization to lower–molecular-weight species with much reduced biologic potency. Renal clearance of active fragments represents about 10% of the administered dose, and total renal excretion of active and nonactive fragments represents about 40% of the dose.

Prophylaxis of DVT following Abdominal Surgery in Patients at Risk for Thromboembolic Complications. Abdominal surgery patients at risk include those who are older than 40 years, obese, undergoing surgery with general anesthesia lasting longer than 30 minutes, or who have additional risk factors such as malignancy or a history of DVT or PE (119). The recommended dose of enoxaparin for this indication is 40 mg subcutaneously (SC) daily, beginning 2 hours preoperatively.

Treatment of DVT with or without PE. In patients with acute DVT with PE, or patients with acute DVT without PE, but who are not candidates for outpatient treatment, the recommended dose of enoxaparin is 1 mg/kg every 12 hours administered SC (119).

Unstable Angina and Non–Q Wave Myocardial Infarction. In patients with unstable angina or non–Q wave MI, the recommended dose of enoxaparin is 1 mg/kg administered SC every 12 hours in conjunction with oral aspirin therapy (100 to 325 mg daily) (111). Based on the currently available data on the efficacy and safety of LMWHs in the treatment of non–ST segment MI and unstable angina, enoxaparin is the only LMWH to have consistently demonstrated both short- and long-term improvements in major ischemic outcomes compared with UH (100,102,120).

Hip or Knee Replacement Surgery. In patients undergoing hip or knee replacement surgery, the recommended dose of enoxaparin is 30 mg every 12 hours, administered by SC injection. Provided that hemostasis has been established, the initial dose should be given 12 to 24 hours after surgery. For hip replacement surgery, a dose of 40 mg once a day SC, given initially 12 (±3) hours prior to surgery, may be considered. Following the initial phase of thromboprophylaxis in hip replacement surgery patients, continued prophylaxis with enoxaparin 40 mg once a day administered by SC injection for 3 weeks is recommended; the usual duration of administration is 7 to 10 days.

Restricted Mobility. In medical patients at risk for thromboembolic complications due to severely restricted mobility during acute illness, the recommended dose of enoxaparin is 40 mg once a day administered by SC injection (119).

Mechanical Prosthetic Heart Valves. The use of enoxaparin has not been adequately studied for thromboprophylaxis or for long-term use in patients with mechanical prosthetic heart valves. Isolated cases of prosthetic heart valve thrombosis have been reported in patients with mechanical prosthetic heart valves who have received enoxaparin for thromboprophylaxis. Some of these patients were pregnant women in whom thrombosis led to maternal and fetal deaths. Insufficient data, issues related to the underlying disease state, and the possibility of inadequate anticoagulation complicates evaluation of these cases. Pregnant women with mechanical prosthetic heart valves may be at higher risk for thromboembolism (119).

Like enoxaparin, dalteparin consists of small heparin molecules ranging from 2,000 to 9,000 d. It is administered subcutaneously and has better availability and a longer half-life than UFH. It has a similar mechanism of action as enoxaparin, selectively inhibiting factor Xa. The inhibitory activity is 2.7:1 compared to 1:1 for UH. The inhibition of factor Xa prevents the formation of fibrin clots. The elimination of the drug occurs via the renal route and is dose independent, with a plasma half-life of 3 to 5 hours. Dalteparin does not significantly affect the platelet activity, prothrombin time (PT), or aPTT and has been shown to be superior to warfarin in preventing DVT following total hip replacement surgery (120). The FRISC trial (Low–Molecular-Weight Heparin [Fragmin] during Instability in Coronary Artery Disease) showed that dalteparin decreased the risk of death or AMI by 36% as compared to aspirin alone (121).

In the FRIC trial (Fragmin in Unstable Coronary Artery Disease), dalteparin was found to be as effective as intravenous heparin in preventing death or AMI in the acute phase following unstable angina or non–Q wave MI (119).

Tinzaparin is a relatively new drug with a similar mechanism of action and pharmacokinetic profile as enoxaparin and dalteparin. It was approved for the treatment of symptomatic DVT in 2000.

Complications

Bleeding. The major complication of the LMWHs is bleeding and is as frequent as with UH. It is, of course, more common in patients receiving antiplatelet or antifibrinolytic therapy in addition to LMWH. Recent surgery, coagulopathy, or trauma also increases the risk of bleeding (99). Protamine sulfate can be used as an antidote, although it incompletely neutralizes the anticoagulant activity by binding only to the longer chains of LMWH. The longer chains are responsible for the antithrombin activity, but the short chains, which inhibit factor Xa activity, will not bind to protamine sulfate, resulting in the latter's ability to only partially reverse the effect of LMWH (122).

Thrombocytopenia. LMWH binds less avidly to platelets, causes less release of PF4, and has a reduced affinity for PF4; it is thus less likely to trigger the formation of antibodies, resulting in a lower incidence of HIT as compared to UH. Unfortunately, antibodies already formed in established HIT cases can exhibit cross-reactivity with LMWH and lead to thrombosis and other complications of this disorder (123,124); for this reason LMWHs should not be used as a substitute for heparin in HIT patients.

Warfarin (Coumadin)

Warfarin, an antagonist of vitamin K, prevents the vitamin K–mediated posttranslational modification of clotting factors II, VII, IX, and X, as well as the naturally occurring endogenous anticoagulant proteins C and S. These factors are biologically inactive without the carboxylation of selected glutamic acid residues, a process requiring reduced vitamin K as a cofactor.

Warfarin is well absorbed in the gut and transported in plasma bound to albumin. Therapeutic doses of warfarin reduce the production of functional vitamin K–dependent clotting factors by 30% to 50%; a concomitant reduction in the carboxylation of secreted clotting factors yields a 10% to 40% decrease in the biologic activity of the clotting factors. As a result, the coagulation system becomes functionally deficient (125).

The PT is the primary assay used in monitoring warfarin therapy. Changes in the PT noted in the first few days of warfarin therapy are primarily due to the reduction in factors VII and IX, with the shortest half-lives, 6 and 24 hours respectively. Commercially available tissue thromboplastins differ in their sensitivity to the warfarin effect; hence, PTs performed with different thromboplastins are not always directly comparable, and for this reason, the INR has been adopted using thromboplastins with international sensitivity index values near 1.0 (125).

Warfarin is used in patients with lower extremity DVT to prevent extension and to reduce the risk of PE. Patients with PE are treated with warfarin to prevent further thromboemboli. Warfarin is used in patients with atrial fibrillation and artificial heart valves to reduce the risk of embolic strokes. It is also helpful in preventing blood clot formation in certain orthopedic surgeries such as knee or hip replacements and in preventing thrombotic stenosis of coronary artery stents (Table 145.8).

The most common complication of warfarin therapy is bleeding, occurring in 6% to 39% of patients annually (126,127); the incidence of bleeding is related to the intensity of anticoagulation. As the need for intense anticoagulation has evolved and been reduced over the last 20 years, the incidence of bleeding has decreased significantly. Moderate bleeding (manifested by elevated INR) can be treated by adjusting down the warfarin dose. If severe bleeding is encountered, this can be adequately treated with fresh-frozen plasma.

TABLE 145.8 Therapeutic Goals and Duration of Warfarin Anticoagulation

Indication	INR	Duration
Prophylaxis of venous thrombosis for high-risk surgery	2–3	Clinical judgment
Treatment of venous thrombosis		
First episode	2–3	3–6 mo[a]
High risk of recurrent thrombosis	2–3	Lifelong
Thrombosis associated with antiphospholipid antibody	3–4	Lifelong
Treatment of pulmonary embolism		
First episode	2–3	3–6 mo
High risk of recurrent embolism	2–3	Lifelong
Prevention of systemic embolism		
Tissue heart valves	2–3	3 mo
Acute myocardial infarction (to prevent systemic embolism)[b]	2–3	Clinical judgment
Valvular heart disease (after thrombotic event or dilated left)	2–3	Lifelong
Atrial fibrillation		
Chronic or intermittent	2–3	Lifelong
Cardioversion	2–3	3 weeks before and 4 weeks after atrial fibrillation if normal sinus rhythm is maintained
Prosthetic heart valves		
Aortic position		
Mechanical	2.5–3.5[c]	Lifelong
Bioprosthetic	2–3	Clinical judgment (3 mo optional)
Mitral position		
Mechanical	2.5–3.5[c]	Lifelong
Bioprosthetic	2–3	3 mo

INR, international normalized ratio.
[a]All recommendations are subject to modification by individual characteristics. First event with reversible or time limited risk factors (surgery, trauma, immobilization, estrogen use). Hyers TM, Agnelli G, Hull RD, et al. Antithrombotic therapy for venous thromboembolic disease. *Chest.* 2001;119(Suppl):176s–193s.
[b]If oral anticoagulant therapy is elected to prevent recurrent myocardial infarction, an INR of 2.5–3.5 is recommended.
[c]Depending on the type of prosthetic valve and valve position (mitral), some patients may benefit from INR in upper therapeutic range.
From Horton JD, Bushwick BM. Warfarin therapy: evolving strategies in anticoagulation. *Am Fam Physician.* 1999;59(3):635–646.

Alternative Therapies

Thrombin Inhibitors

Heparin, and subsequently LMWH, in addition to warfarin have been used effectively for the treatment of both venous and arterial thromboemboli, but these drugs have drawbacks. The biophysical limitations of heparin include the inability of the heparin/antithrombin complex to inhibit factor Xa within the prothrombinase complex and thrombin bound to fibrin, clotting enzymes that are important triggers of thrombin growth (128).

Thrombin, a trypsinlike serine protease, is the enzyme that converts fibrinogen to fibrin; it may be inhibited either directly or indirectly. Indirect thrombin inhibitors act by catalyzing the reaction of antithrombin and/or heparin cofactor II. Thrombin has great substrate specificity secondary to its surface binding sites (e.g., exosite 1). Direct thrombin inhibitors directly bind thrombin at the exosite 1 site or the other active site of thrombin, thereby blocking this procoagulant from reacting further. Direct thrombin inhibitors do not bind PF4, and their anticoagulant activity is unaffected by the large quantities of PF4 released in the surrounding region of platelet-rich thrombi. Additionally, direct thrombin inhibitors inactivate fibrin-bound thrombin as well as fluid-phase thrombin (128,129).

Three parenteral direct thrombin inhibitors have been approved for limited use in the United States and Canada. Hirudin and argatroban are approved for treatment of patients diagnosed with heparin-associated thrombocytopenia. Bivalirudin has been approved as an alternative therapy for heparin-sensitive patients undergoing PCIs.

Hirudin

This agent is a 65 amino acid polypeptide originally isolated from the salivary glands of the medicinal leech; it is now available in recombinant DNA technology (130). The recombinant form exhibits an approximate 20-fold reduced affinity for thrombin as compared to the native form of the drug (131). Hirudin directly inhibits thrombin in a bivalent manner in that the globular amino-terminal domain interacts with the active site of thrombin. The anionic carboxy-terminal tail binds to exosite 1 on thrombin, the substrate recognition site (131). The hirudin/thrombin complex is essentially irreversible. This may create a problem if significant bleeding should occur, as there is no specific antidote. Recombinant hirudins—for example, desirudin and lepirudin—have a leucine substituted for an isoleucine at the N-terminal end of the molecule. Lepirudin (Refludan) has been approved in North America for the treatment of HIT subtypes 1 and 2 (132).

The plasma half-life of hirudin is approximately 60 minutes following intravenous injection and 120 minutes following subcutaneous administration (133). It is cleared via the kidneys and should be used with caution, if at all, in patients with renal insufficiency. The anticoagulant activity can be measured using the aPTT. Dose adjustment must be made to maintain the aPTT within a therapeutic range ratio of 1.5 to 2.0 time normal, measured approximately 4 hours after drug initiation. The correlation between plasma hirudin levels and the aPTT is nonlinear, and therefore the ecarin clotting time is the more preferable means of monitoring anticoagulation. Dose adjustments need to be made in those with renal impairment. Antibodies to lepirudin develop in approximately 30% of patients following their first exposure; this number may rise to 70% following repeat exposure. Serious anaphylactic reactions have occurred following initial and subsequent exposures to lepirudin, resulting in shock and death. Therefore, patients should not be treated with this agent more than one time. Rarely, in the hirudin-treated patient, there may develop non neutraliing hirudin antibodies that prolong its anticoagulant effect because of delayed hirudin–antibody complex clearance (131). Thus, continued close monitoring of the aPTT is needed during the course of therapy, even when the initial anticoagulant effects appear stable, to avoid the risk of bleeding.

Hirudin has been successfully used, and is licensed for, the treatment of arterial or venous thrombosis complicating heparin-induced thrombocytopenia. It has also been used in patients with HIT undergoing cardiopulmonary bypass. Hirudin has been shown to be superior to heparin or LMWHs for thromboprophylaxis in patients undergoing elective hip arthroplasty, and it does not increase the risk of bleeding in this high-risk setting. Hirudin has been used extensively in patients with ACSs and for venous thromboprophylaxis. However, because of its narrow therapeutic index and high risk of bleeding, it must be used with extreme caution and is not currently approved for this use (128).

Desirudin

Desirudin is a recombinant form of hirudin for subcutaneous administration; it is a direct thrombin inhibitor indicated for the prevention of DVT that puts the patient at risk for PE. It directly inhibits free and fibrin-bound thrombin (133–135), and has demonstrated improved efficacy and comparable bleeding outcomes to both UFH and enoxaparin for the prevention of thromboembolism in patients undergoing elective total hip replacement (136–138). The benefit of using a direct thrombin inhibitor over either LMWH or UFH has the advantage of minimizing the potential of developing HIT (139,140,141). The typical dose in patients with normal renal function is 15 mg subcutaneously every 12 hours following an initial dose; it is given 30 minutes prior to hip surgery or in the postoperative period. The half-life is approximately 2 hours (133,140,141).

Bivalirudin

This is a 20 amino acid synthetic polypeptide analog of hirudin; the amino-terminal D-Phe-Pro-Arg-Pro sequence, which binds to the active site of thrombin, is connected via four Gly residues to a carboxyl-terminal (142,143) dodecapeptide that interacts with exosite 1 on thrombin (139,140). Bivalirudin differs from hirudin in that, once bound to thrombin, the Arg-Pro bond on the amino-terminal extension of bivalirudin is cleaved, converting bivalirudin into a lower-affinity thrombin inhibitor, therefore producing only transient inhibition of the active site (143) of thrombin and thereby allowing recovery of thrombin activity (140). The shorter half-life of bivalirudin, 25 minutes after intravenous injection, and the fact that only about 20% is renally excreted (144), may make bivalirudin a safer alternative to hirudin. In patients with a high risk of developing HIT, bivalirudin is typically administered as a weight-adjusted (1 mg/kg) bolus dose given prior to PCIs and followed by a 4-hour infusion (0.2 to 0.5 mg/kg/hr); the dose is adjusted according to renal function. Robson et al. demonstrated that the plasma clearance of bivalirudin in patients with moderate or severe renal impairment is reduced by approximately 20% as compared to that in patients with normal or mild renal function, and suggests that bivalirudin infusion should be reduced by 20% in patients with moderate-to-severe renal impairment (144). The anticoagulant effect is monitored by the activated clotting time (ACT), and an additional bolus dose is given if the ACT is less than 350 seconds.

Argatroban

This is a synthetic L-arginine derivative competitive inhibitor of thrombin. Argatroban binds noncovalently to the active site of thrombin to form a reversible complex (145). The plasma half-life of this agent is 45 minutes. It is monitored using the aPTT, and the dose is adjusted to maintain a therapeutic aPTT ratio of 1.5 to 3.0. It is metabolized in the liver and needs to be used with caution in patients with hepatic dysfunction (143).

Argatroban is considered the drug of choice for patients with severe renal impairment. Therapy with this agent can prolong plasma INR more than the other direct thrombin inhibitors and may complicate overlap therapy with vitamin K antagonists. Argatroban has been approved for use in patients with documented HIT and for anticoagulation in HIT patients undergoing PCI (132).

Melagatran/Ximelagatran

Melagatran is a dipeptide mimetic of the region of fibrinopeptide A that interacts with the active site of thrombin. This drug has poor oral bioavailability and must be given via the subcutaneous route. Ximelagatran is an uncharged lipophilic prodrug exhibiting about 20% bioavailability after oral administration. Once absorbed, ximelagatran is rapidly transformed to melagatran, which has a half-life of approximately 4 to 5 hours. The primary route of excretion for melagatran is the kidneys, where approximately 80% is eliminated. Dose adjustments may be needed in the elderly and in those patients with renal impairment. There appears to be no adverse food or drug interaction to influence the absorption of ximelagatran, and it therefore produces a predictable anticoagulant effect. The need for routine monitoring of this drug is usually unnecessary. Ximelagatran is under evaluation for thromboprophylaxis in orthopedic patients (146) and for the treatment of venous thromboembolism and atrial fibrillation (147).

Dabigatran

Dabigatran etexilate is an orally administered prodrug metabolized in the liver to dabigatran. This is the only orally administered, reversible direct thrombin inhibitor approved for prevention of stroke and systemic embolism in people with nonvalvular atrial fibrillation. It should not be used in patients with prosthetic heart valves or during pregnancy.

The RE-LY trial (Randomised evaluation of long-term anticoagulation therapy) compared two doses of dabigatran, 110 and 150 mg administered twice daily with warfarin for noninferiority in prevention of stroke or systemic embolus in patients with a history of atrial fibrillation. When dabigatran was compared to patients receiving warfarin and who were titrated to a therapeutic target INR of 2 to 3, both doses of the dabigatran significantly decreased the annual rate of stroke or systemic embolus, the primary outcomes, by 1.69% per year in the warfarin group, as compared with 1.53% per year in the group that received 110 mg of dabigatran (relative risk with dabigatran, 0.91; 95% confidence interval [CI], 0.74 to 1.11; $p < 0.001$ for noninferiority) and 1.11% per year in the group that received 150 mg of dabigatran (relative risk, 0.66; 95% CI, 0.53 to 0.82; $p < 0.001$ for superiority). The rate of major bleeding was 3.36% per year in the warfarin group, as compared with 2.71% per year in the group receiving 110 mg of dabigatran ($p = 0.003$) and 3.11% per year in the group receiving 150 mg of dabigatran ($p = 0.31$) (149).

Dabigatran is typically given at a fixed dose without monitoring. The maximum anticoagulant effect is achieved within 2 to 3 hours following administration. In patients with normal renal function, when administered for prevention of venous thromboembolism in surgical patients, a dose of dabigatran, 150 mg given twice daily is indicated following 5 to 10 days of parenteral anticoagulant therapy. When patients with atrial fibrillation are being treated for stroke prevention the suggested dose in patients is 150 mg taken orally twice daily (149).

Even though dabigatran has been associated with less severe bleeding than warfarin (149), life-threatening hemorrhage can occur especially during emergency surgical procedures. It has been reported that a monoclonal antibody fragment, idarucizumab, binds dabigatran with an affinity which is 350 times that observed with thrombin, neutralizing its activity (150,151). An interim analysis was reported in 2015 from the Reversal Effects of Idarucizumab on Active Dabigatran (RE-VERSE AD) study evaluating the safety and capacity of 5 g of intravenous idarucizumab to reverse the anticoagulant effects of dabigatran in patients who had serious bleeding or requiring an urgent intervention. This analysis demonstrated that idarucizumab was able to completely reverse anticoagulant activity in 88% to 98% of patients within minutes (152).

Factor Xa Inhibitors

Drugs that block factor Xa are considered as either indirect or direct inhibitors. Indirect factor Xa inhibitors act by binding to and activating antithrombin, which then inhibits free factor Xa. Direct factor Xa inhibitors actually bind to and inhibit factor Xa without requiring antithrombin to be present.

Indirect Factor Xa Inhibitors

Fondaparinux and *idraparinux* are two relatively new parenteral indirect factor Xa inhibitors. They are synthetic analogs of the antithrombin-binding pentasaccharide sequence found in heparin and LMWH. However, these drugs are modified to increase their affinity for antithrombin as compared to both heparin and LMWH. The chain length of these molecules is too short to bridge thrombin to antithrombin; therefore, these agents act by catalyzing factor Xa inhibition by antithrombin. Their properties are quite different from those of LMWH (Table 145.9).

There are potential benefits of fondaparinux over LMWH. It is synthetically produced, has a longer half-life, and does not bind to plasma proteins other than antithrombin. Additionally,

TABLE 145.9 Properties of Low-Molecular-Weight Heparin, Fondaparinux, and Idraparinux

Property	LMWH	Fondaparinux	Idraparinux
Source	Porcine mucosal heparin	Chemical synthesis	Chemical synthesis
Molecular weight (daltons)	Mean 5,000	1,728	1,727
SC bioavailability	~90%	100%	100%
Target(s)	Multiple: FXa > FIIa > FIXa, FXIa, FXIIa	FXa only	FXa only
Binding to proteins other than target	Yes	No	No
Anti-Xa:anti-IIa	2–5:1	Anti-Xa only	Anti-Xa only
TFPI release from endothelium	Yes	No	No
Clearance	Renal primarily	Renal	Renal
Half-life (SC route)	3–4 hrs	17–21 hrs	80–130 hrs
Effects of protamine	Partial neutralization	No effect	No effect
Potential for HIT	Low	Very low	Very low

LMWH, low-molecular-weight heparin; SC, subcutaneous; FXa, factor Xa; FIIa, factor IIa; FIXa, factor IXa; FXIa, factor XIa; FXIIa, factor XIIa; TFPI, tissue factor pathway inhibitor; HIT, heparin-induced thrombocytopenia.

From Weitz JI, Middledorp S, Geerts W, Heit JA. Thrombophilia and new anticoagulant drugs. *Hematology Am Soc Hematol Educ Program.* 2004;1:424–438.

it does not bind to PF4 to form the heparin/PF4 complexes that serve as the antigenic target for the antibodies that cause heparin-induced thrombocytopenia, and may be safer to use in these patients (153,154). Fondaparinux has been extensively studied and has been found to be effective as an antithrombotic agent for the prevention and treatment of both venous and arterial disorders. It is currently approved as thromboprophylaxis following orthopedic procedures, as initial treatment for venous thromboembolism, and is being investigated as an antithrombotic agent in cardiac disease.

Idraparinux is a chemically modified analog of fondaparinux that binds to antithrombin with such a high affinity that its half-life approximates that of antithrombin (155). This drug requires subcutaneous dosing only once a week, has a long half-life and lacks an antidote. In one study, bleeding occurred in healthy volunteers, but the anticoagulant effect reversed by recombinant factor VIIa (132). The Amadeus study demonstrated that clinically relevant bleeding was evident when compared to vitamin K antagonist *medication and* did not appear to reduce the risk of stroke. Further development of this medication has been suspended (156).

Direct Factor Xa Inhibitors

Several oral acting synthetic direct factor Xa inhibitors are currently available; none are available for parenteral use. These drugs inhibit both free and activated platelet-bound factor Xa trapped within a thrombus as part of the prothrombinase complex.

Rivaroxaban is an orally active oxazolidinone derivative that reversibly inhibits factor Xa. It achieves 80% bioavailability after a single oral dose, with peak plasma levels in 2 to 3 hours and a half-life of 7 to 17 hours. It is approved for stroke prevention in atrial fibrillation and venous thromboembolism prophylaxis following orthopedic surgery; the medication should be used with extreme caution in patients with severe hepatic or renal impairment. Rivaroxaban interacts with dual inhibitors of the cytochrome P450–3A4 and P-glycoprotein, and should not be administered with these medications (e.g., azole antifungals and ritinovair). It is administered initially 6 to 10 hours postoperatively and continued for 2 weeks following knee replacement surgery and 5 weeks following hip replacement. When administered for prevention of stroke and systemic embolus in patients with atrial fibrillation, 20 mg of rivaroxaban should be given once daily for those with a creatinine clearance greater than 50 mL/min. Routine coagulation monitoring is not required because blood levels of the drug are relatively predictable for a certain dose (157,158).

The efficacy of rivaroxaban was demonstrated in the ROCKET–AF trial which was a noninferiority trial comparing rivaroxaban 20 mg by mouth, once daily with warfarin for stroke prevention in over 14,000 patients with atrial fibrillation. The rivaroxaban group demonstrated benefit in the primary endpoints of stroke and systemic embolization (2.1%/yr vs. 2.4%/yr, $p < 0.001$). The overall rates of bleeding for both medications were comparable (158).

Apixaban has an identical mechanism of action and indications to rivaroxaban. It is administered orally in a dose of 5 mg twice daily. This is adjusted to 2.5 mg twice daily for patients greater than 80 years, less than 60 kg, and with renal insufficiency (creatinine >1.5 mg/dL). Similarly to rivaroxaban, it has a high oral bioavailability and short onset to peak action of 3 hours; the plasma half-life is approximately 12 hours and thus a twice daily dosing schedule is required. A dose reduction or avoidance should be considered in patients taking dual inhibitors of the cytochrome P-3A4 and P-glycoprotein (159).

The efficacy of apixaban was demonstrated in the apixaban for reduction in stroke and other thromboembolic events in atrial fibrillation (the ARISTOTLE Trial), a noninferiority trial comparing apixaban, 5 mg orally administered twice daily with warfarin (target range INR = 2–3) for the prevention of stroke and systemic embolization in atrial fibrillation in 18,206 patients followed for 12 months. Apixaban was associated with significantly lower rate of stroke and systemic embolization than warfarin (1.27% vs. 1.60%, $p < 0.001$). Apixaban was also associated with a significant reduction in major bleeding (2.13% vs. 3.09%, $p < 0.001$) (160).

Thrombolytic Therapy

Thrombolytic agents act as plasminogen-activating agents, catalyzing the conversion of endogenous plasminogen to plasmin. These agents will dissolve both fibrin deposits and pathologic thrombi at sites of vascular injury and, thus, may be associated with significant hemorrhage.

In the treatment of pulmonary embolus, thrombolytic therapy followed by heparin administration has been shown to be more efficacious in thromboembolus dissolution than heparin alone in the acute (first 24 hours) setting (161,162). These agents lead to a more rapid resolution of lung scan abnormalities and hemodynamic improvements, but the benefit over the longer term is questionable. Recent guidelines do not recommend thrombolysis for the treatment of DVT unless limb ischemia and limb loss is imminent (162).

Although beyond the scope of this review, thrombolytic therapy has become a standard treatment for patients presenting with acute ST-segment elevation MI and new-onset left bundle branch block. Various clinical trials have demonstrated the importance and benefit of early and full reperfusion in improving clinical outcomes following an acute MI (163–166). Thrombolytic therapy is also indicated in the treatment of ischemic stroke (167), cerebral vein and sinus thrombosis (168), thrombosed mechanical valves, and thrombosed arteriovenous shunts and catheters. These agents have evolved from the non–fibrin-selective first-generation agents to the more fibrin-selective third-generation agents. As there are still limitations with the currently available agents, work continues to achieve an ideal drug.

First-generation thrombolytic agents are not fibrin specific and convert circulating plasminogen to plasmin. There is constant equilibrium between circulating plasminogen and plasminogen that is in the thrombus. There is eventual depletion of plasminogen, reducing clot lysis. Additionally, the first-generation agents are associated with increased risk of allergic reaction and have comparatively short half-lives.

Streptokinase is a single-chain polypeptide, with a molecular weight of 47 to 50.2 kd, produced by group C β-hemolytic streptococci (169). It works by binding with circulating plasminogen to form an activator complex that converts plasminogen to plasmin by proteolytic cleavage, forming a streptokinase–plasmin complex (170). This 1:1 complex has increased catalytic activity compared with plasmin. The streptokinase–plasmin complex–mediated degradation of fibrin leads to stimulation of locally bound streptokinase–plasmin and streptokinase–plasminogen complexes, which results in an acceleration in plasminogen activation and clot dissolution. In addition, streptokinase can increase levels of activated protein C, enhancing clot lysis. The half-life of the streptokinase–plasminogen complex is approximately 23 minutes, with a lytic effect ranging from 82 to 184 minutes. There are no metabolites of streptokinase; it is eliminated by the liver (171,172).

Adverse reactions include allergic reactions—rarely anaphylaxis—and bleeding. Hypotension not related to bleeding or anaphylaxis may also be seen during streptokinase infusion in 1% to 10% of patients. For PE, the FDA recommends that streptokinase be given as a 1 million IU dose infusion over 24 hours. For acute MI, the adult dose is 1.5 million IU in 50 mL 5% dextrose in water given intravenously over 5 minutes.

Anistreplase has a longer half-life compared to streptokinase so can be used as a bolus. It is antigenic as streptokinase so repeat administration within 1 year is avoided. The lack of any compelling advantages (other than bolus administration) and cost higher than streptokinase has reduced anistreplase to an infrequently prescribed drug for acute myocardial infarction.

Urokinase is a two-chain serine protease containing 41 amino acid residues, isolated from human urine and fetal kidney cell cultures as a single-chain precursor, with a molecular weight of 54 kd. In plasma, the single-chain precursor is converted to the active two-chain urokinase plasminogen activator through limited hydrolysis by plasmin and kallikrein. The two-chain active form increases the efficacy of plasmin activation, which enhances further conversion of the single-chain precursor to the two-chain urokinase plasminogen activator form. Urokinase has a 15- to 20-minute half-life and is metabolized in the liver (173,174). Because it has a shorter half-life than streptokinase, urokinase produces a less sustained fibrinolysis. It has the same potential disadvantages—significant bleeding—as do all thrombolytics. Human-derived urokinase is no longer available in North America and has been replaced by a recombinant product.

For PE, the FDA-approved regimen of urokinase is the administration of a 4,400 IU/kg body weight loading dose, followed by an infusion of 4,400 IU/kg for 12 to 24 hours. Urokinase for acute MI is less well studied than other agents, but the most commonly used regimen is 1 to 2 million U given as an intravenous load, over 15 to 30 minutes depending on side effect profile (rigors, febrile episode).

Second-generation thrombolytics are fibrin selective and were developed with the intention to limit or avoid systemic thrombolysis. The present agents may cause a mild-to-moderate depletion in levels of circulation fibrinogen and plasminogen.

Tissue-type plasminogen activator (Alteplase), a glycoprotein of 527 amino acids, was the first recombinant tissue-type plasminogen activator (rtPA) and is identical to the native form of the drug. Native tissue plasminogen activator (tPA) is naturally synthesized and made available by vascular endothelial cells. It is the enzyme that is responsible for most of the body's natural physiologic responses to clear and reduce excessive thrombus propagation. Tissue plasminogen activator binds fibrin with a greater affinity than streptokinase, converting plasminogen to plasmin once bound to a fibrin clot surface—hence the term "clot selective." Fibrin provides the platform for which tPA and fibrin may interact to enhance the catalytic efficiency of the plasminogen activation of tPA. Alteplase (rtPA) is rapidly cleared from plasma, primarily by the liver, having an initial half-life of less than 5 minutes. Heparin is usually administered with alteplase due to the very short half-life of this agent and to avoid reocclusion. This drug is not antigenic and is almost never associated with allergic reactions. Alteplase is the lytic agent most commonly used for the acute treatment of myocardial ischemia (174), pulmonary embolism, and acute ischemic stroke. There are two different forms of tissue-type plasminogen activator based on the number of chains: the two-chain alteplase (recombinant) and the recombinant one-chain form.

For acute MI, this drug may be given as an accelerated infusion (over 1.5 hours) or a long infusion (>3 hours). It must be given in a 1 mg/mL concentration and be reconstituted with sterile water. The accelerated infusion of rtPA is 15 mg intravenously, followed by 0.75 mg/kg, up to 50 mg, intravenously over 60 minutes with a maximum total dose of 100 mg. This is the most common regimen used for acute MI. Alternatively, the greater than 3-hour infusion begins as a 10-mg intravenous loading dose over 2 minutes, followed by a 50-mg infusion over the first hour, and by a 20-mg/kg infusion over the next 2 hours.

Alteplase is the only drug that has been studied and approved by the FDA for use in acute ischemic stroke with a well-established time of symptom onset of less than 3 hours. Once diagnosed, and within the defined time period, it is recommended that two peripheral intravenous lines—one for rtPA infusion and one for complications that may occur from therapy—be initiated. The recommended dose of alteplase for acute ischemic stroke is 0.9 mg/kg, to a maximum of 90 mg, infused over 60 minutes; 10% of the total dose is to be administered as an initial intravenous bolus over 1 minute (175).

The FDA-approved regimen for thrombolysis of PE is 100 mg of rtPA given as a continuous infusion over 2 hours: an initial 15-mg intravenous loading dose is followed by 85 mg over 2 hours. Heparin has been shown to improve the clinical course in hemodynamically stable patients with acute submassive PE when receiving rtPA. Given the short half-life of the drug, if the patient can tolerate it, it would seem beneficial to administer alteplase with heparin (176).

Third-generation thrombolytics are based on modifications of the tPA structure. These modifications may give the agents longer half-lives, increased resistance to plasma protease inhibitors, and/or cause more selective binding to fibrin.

Reteplase (rtPA) is a synthetic, nonglycosylated deletion-mutant form of tPA containing 355 of the 527 amino acids of native tPA; the drug is produced in *Escherichia coli* via recombinant technology. Reteplase binds fibrin five times less avidly than native tissue plasminogen activator, thus allowing the drug to diffuse through the clot rather than just binding to the surface as is the mechanism of tissue plasminogen activator. In high concentrations, reteplase does not compete with plasminogen for fibrin-binding sites, but rather it allows plasminogen at the clot to be converted into plasmin. These reasons may explain why reteplase results in faster clot resolution in contrast to alteplase.

Reteplase is more rapidly cleared from plasma and has a somewhat extended half-life—11 to 19 minutes—than does alteplase. Reteplase undergoes primarily renal and some hepatic clearance; the agent is not antigenic and is rarely associated with allergic reactions. It must not be given with heparin due to physical incompatibility (176).

In the setting of acute MI, the FDA has approved the adult dose of reteplase to be two intravenous loads of 10 U each. Each loading dose is to be given over 2 minutes, with the second loading dose given 30 minutes following the first (176). Although approved by the FDA only for use in the setting of acute MI, reteplase has achieved wide off-label use for acute

TABLE 145.10 Characteristics of U.S. Food and Drug Administration–Approved Thrombolytic Agents

	Streptokinase	Amistreplace	Alteplase	Reteplase	Tenecteplase
Molecular weight (daltons)	47,000	131,000	70,000	39,000	70,000
Half-life (min)	23	100	<5	13–16	20–24
Dose/time	1.5 MU × 30–60 min	30 mg × 5 min	100 mg × 90 min	10 + 10 U × 30 min	0.5 mg/kg × 5–10 s
Bolus administration	No	Yes	No	Yes	Yes
Metabolism	Hepatic	Hepatic	Hepatic	—	—
Allergic reactions	1–4%		<0.2%	No	<1%
Hypotension	Yes	Yes	No	No	No
Early heparin[a]	?Yes	?Yes	Yes	Yes	Yes
Fibrin selective	No	No	Yes	Yes	Yes
Systemic fibrinogen	Marked	Marked	Mild	Moderate	—
Fibrinogen breakdown	4+		1–2+	Unknown	4–15
Plasminogen binding	Indirect	Indirect	Direct	Direct	Direct
TIMI 3 flow (%)	32	43	54	60	66
≈90-min patency (%)	50	65	75	80	75
Intracerebral hemorrhage (%)	0.5	0.6	0.8	0.9	
Mortality rates (%)	7.3	10.5	7.2	7.5	

[a]The need for concomitant heparin has been formally tested with only streptokinase and alteplase may be of little benefit and can increase risk of bleeding.
?, may or may not be effective.
From Khan IJ, Gowda RM. Clinical perspectives and therapeutics of thrombolysis. *Int J Cardiol.* 2003;91:117.

DVT and PE. The dosing schedule is the same as that approved for treatment of acute MI.

Tenecteplase was approved as a fibrinolytic agent by the FDA in 2000. It is a genetically engineered mutation of tPA with a similar mechanism of action to alteplase. It is produced by recombinant technology using Chinese hamster ovary cells as a 527 amino acid glycoprotein, with several modifications in the amino acid sequence. As a result, tenecteplase has a decreased plasma clearance, a 15- to 19-minute half-life, a reduced sensitivity to plasminogen activator inhibitor (165), and greater fibrin specificity, which may lead to a reduction in hemorrhagic complications (177). Tenecteplase is administered as a 30- to 50-mg intravenous bolus over 5 seconds; the dose is calculated as follows: 0.5 mg/kg (166). The drug is currently under investigation for use in ischemic stroke.

Thrombolytic agents differ in their ability to cause clot lysis, as well as fibrin selectivity, and their ability to activate thrombosis and platelet aggregation. The clinical effectiveness of the same agent can be altered by dose, route of administration, and concomitant use of adjunctive agents. All thrombolytic agents are administered via the intravenous route in dosing regimens designed to achieve greater than 90% activation of the fibrinolytic system (178) (Table 145.10).

Key Points

- The coagulation system depends on normal vascular endothelium to maintain antithrombotic activity and promote laminar fluid blood flow. When vascular injury occurs, it can immediately respond through thrombin generation and fibrin production at the site of vascular damage.
- Venous thrombi typically form under conditions of low flow and are mainly composed of fibrin and red blood cells. Arterial thrombi typically form under conditions of high flow and are predominantly composed of platelet aggregates held together by fibrin strands.
- The coagulation cascade is regulated by the TF pathway inhibitor, the protein C pathway, and the fibrinolytic degradation of fibrin.
- UH has been used in multiple clinical scenarios including prevention of venous thromboembolism, treatment of DVT and pulmonary embolism, and ACSs. Until recently, it has been the most widely used antithrombotic agent, although it has several disadvantages.
- The most efficient and safe method for initiating intravenous heparin therapy is using weight-adjusted nomograms.
- A single dose of aspirin is sufficient to inhibit platelet function for the life span of the platelets (30).
- Clopidogrel is more effective than aspirin in reducing atherosclerotic events, including MI, stroke, and peripheral vascular disease (45).
- The incidence of bleeding is higher among patients taking antiplatelet agents, requiring urgent surgical procedures (47).
- In the event of bleeding, the antiplatelet agent must be stopped, and platelet transfusion will be required to normalize platelet function.
- LMWH inhibits predominantly factor Xa to produce its anticoagulant effect. It can be administered as a subcutaneous injection once or twice a day.
- LMWH has proved to be cost effective as compared to UH because of reduced need for monitoring.
- LMWH tends to accumulate in patients with renal failure.
- There is no rapid and complete antagonist to the anticoagulant effects of LMWH, which may complicate ICU and surgical procedures (7).
- Direct thrombin inhibitors directly bind thrombin, thereby blocking its procoagulant effect. This class of drugs may be advantageous over indirect thrombin inhibitors such as heparin because they do not bind plasma proteins and produce a more predictable response.

- Drugs that block factor Xa are considered either indirect or direct inhibitors. Indirect agents act by binding to and activating antithrombin, which inhibits free factor Xa. Direct factor Xa inhibitors bind to and inhibit free factor and inactivate factor Xa bound to platelets.
- Thrombolytic agents act as plasminogen-activating agents, catalyzing the conversion of endogenous plasminogen to plasmin. These agents will dissolve both fibrin deposits and pathologic thrombi at sites of vascular injury and thus may be associated with significant hemorrhage.

References

1. Weitz JI, Hirsh J. New anticoagulant drugs. *Chest.* 2001;119(1 Suppl): 95S–107S.
2. Turpie AG. State of the art: a journey through the world of antithrombotic therapy. *Semin Thromb Hemost.* 2002;28(Suppl 3):3–11.
3. Puggioni A, Kalra M, Gloviczki P. Practical aspects of the postthrombotic syndrome. *Dis Mon.* 2005;51(2–3):166–175.
4. Hirsch DR, Ingenito EP, Goldhaber SZ. Prevalence of deep venous thrombosis among patients in medical intensive care. *JAMA.* 1995;274(4): 335–337.
5. Cade JF. High risk of the critically ill for venous thromboembolism. *Crit Care Med.* 1982;10(7):448–450.
6. Cook D, Attia J, Weaver B, et al. Venous thromboembolic disease: an observational study in medical-surgical intensive care unit patients. *J Crit Care.* 2000;15(4):127–132.
7. Williams MT, Aravindan N, Wallace MJ, et al. Venous thromboembolism in the intensive care unit. *Crit Care Clin.* 2003;19(2):185–207.
8. Schafer AI, Levine MN, Konkle BA, Kearon C. Thrombotic disorders: diagnosis and treatment. *Hematology Am Soc Hematol Educ Program.* 2003:520–539.
9. Hirsh J, Hoak J. Management of deep vein thrombosis and pulmonary embolism: a statement for healthcare professionals. Council on Thrombosis (in consultation with the Council on Cardiovascular Radiology), American Heart Association. *Circulation.* 1996;93(12):2212–2245.
10. Lopez JA, Kearon C, Lee AY. Deep venous thrombosis. *Hematol Am Soc Hematol Educ Progr.* 2004:439–456.
11. Cumming AM, Shiach CR. The investigation and management of inherited thrombophilia. *Clin Lab Haematol.* 1999;21(2):77–92.
12. Broze GJ Jr. Tissue factor pathway inhibitor. *Thromb Haemost.* 1995;74(1): 90–93.
13. Drake TA, Morrissey JH, Edgington TS. Selective cellular expression of tissue factor in human tissues: implications for disorders of hemostasis and thrombosis. *Am J Pathol.* 1989;134(5):1087–1097.
14. Fleck RA, Rao LV, Rapaport SI, Varki N. Localization of human tissue factor antigen by immunostaining with monospecific, polyclonal anti-human tissue factor antibody. *Thromb Res.* 1990;59(2):421–437.
15. Fuster V, Badimon L, Badimon JJ, Chesebro JH. The pathogenesis of coronary artery disease and the acute coronary syndromes (2). *N Engl J Med.* 1992;326(5):310–318.
16. Eisenberg PR, Ghigliotti G. Platelet-dependent and procoagulant mechanisms in arterial thrombosis. *Int J Cardiol.* 1999;68(Suppl 1):S3–S10.
17. Ruggeri ZM. The role of von Willebrand factor and fibrinogen in the initiation of platelet adhesion to thrombogenic surfaces. *Thromb Haemost.* 1995;74:460–463.
18. Sakariassen KS, Fressinaud E, Girma JP, et al. Role of platelet membrane glycoproteins and von Willebrand factor in adhesion of platelets to subendothelium and collagen. *Ann N Y Acad Sci.* 1987;516:52–65.
19. Furie B, Furie BC. Molecular and cellular biology of blood coagulation. *N Engl J Med.* 1992;326(12):800–806.
20. Gailani D, Broze GJ Jr. Factor XI activation by thrombin and factor XIa. *Semin Thromb Hemost.* 1993;19(4):396–404.
21. Esmon CT, Ding W, Yasuhiro K, et al. The protein C pathway: new insights. *Thromb Haemost.* 1997;78(1):70–74.
22. Hirsh J. Heparin. *N Engl J Med.* 1991;324(22):1565–1574.
23. de Agostini AI, Watkins SC, Slayter HS, et al. Localization of anticoagulantly active heparan sulfate proteoglycans in vascular endothelium: antithrombin binding on cultured endothelial cells and perfused rat aorta. *J Cell Biol.* 1990;111(3):1293–1304.
24. Collen D. The plasminogen (fibrinolytic) system. *Thromb Haemost.* 1999; 82(2):259–270.
25. Brown MD, Rowe BH, Reeves MJ, et al. The accuracy of the enzyme-linked immunosorbent assay D-dimer test in the diagnosis of pulmonary embolism: a meta-analysis. *Ann Emerg Med.* 2002;40(2):133–144.
26. Perrier A, Desmarais S, Miron MJ, et al. Non-invasive diagnosis of venous thromboembolism in outpatients. *Lancet.* 1999;353(9148):190–195.
27. Ohlmann P, Faure A, Morel O, et al. Diagnostic and prognostic value of circulating D-Dimers in patients with acute aortic dissection. *Crit Care Med.* 2006;34(5):1358–1364.
28. Shorr AF, Thomas SJ, Alkins SA, et al. D-dimer correlates with proinflammatory cytokine levels and outcomes in critically ill patients. *Chest.* 2002;121(4):1262–1268.
29. Randomised trial of intravenous streptokinase, oral aspirin, both, or neither among 17,187 cases of suspected acute myocardial infarction: ISIS-2. ISIS-2 (Second International Study of Infarct Survival) Collaborative Group. *Lancet.* 1988;2(8607):349–360.
30. Antithrombotic Trialists' Collaboration. Collaborative meta-analysis of randomised trials of antiplatelet therapy for prevention of death, myocardial infarction, and stroke in high risk patients. *BMJ.* 2002;324(7329):71–86.
31. CURRENT-OASIS 7 Investigators, Mehta SR, Bassand JP, et al. Dose comparisons of clopidogrel and aspirin in acute coronary syndromes. *N Engl J Med.* 2010;363(10):930–42.
32. Gullov AL, Koefoed BG, Petersen P, et al. Fixed minidose warfarin and aspirin alone and in combination vs adjusted-dose warfarin for stroke prevention in atrial fibrillation: Second Copenhagen Atrial Fibrillation, Aspirin, and Anticoagulation Study. *Arch Intern Med.* 1998;158(14):1513–1521.
33. Singer DE, Hughes RA, Gress DR, et al. The effect of aspirin on the risk of stroke in patients with nonrheumatic atrial fibrillation: The BAATAF Study. *Am Heart J.* 1992;124(6):1567–1573.
34. Grotemeyer KH, Scharafinski HW, Husstedt IW. Two-year follow-up of aspirin responder and aspirin non responder: a pilot-study including 180 post-stroke patients. *Thromb Res.* 1993;71(5):397–403.
35. Eikelboom JW, Hankey GJ. Aspirin resistance: a new independent predictor of vascular events? *J Am Coll Cardiol.* 2003;41(6):966–968.
36. Gum PA, Kottke-Marchant K, Poggio ED, et al. Profile and prevalence of aspirin resistance in patients with cardiovascular disease. *Am J Cardiol.* 2001;88(3):230–235.
37. Bhatt DL, Topol EJ. Scientific and therapeutic advances in antiplatelet therapy. *Nat Rev Drug Discov.* 2003;2(1):15–28.
38. Cambria-Kiely JA, Gandhi PJ. Aspirin resistance and genetic polymorphisms. *J Thromb Thrombolysis.* 2002;14(1):51–58.
39. Ferraris VA, Ferraris SP, Joseph O, et al. Aspirin and postoperative bleeding after coronary artery bypass grafting. *Ann Surg.* 2002;235(6):820–827.
40. Clagett GP, Anderson FA Jr, Levine MN, et al. Prevention of venous thromboembolism. *Chest.* 1992;102(4 Suppl):391S–407S.
41. Storey RF, Newby LJ, Heptinstall S. Effects of P2Y(1) and P2Y(12) receptor antagonists on platelet aggregation induced by different agonists in human whole blood. *Platelets.* 2001;12(7):443–447.
42. Wijeyeratne YD, Heptinstall S. Anti-platelet therapy: ADP receptor antagonists. *Br J Clin Pharmacol.* 2011;72(4):647–657.
43. Helft G, Osende JI, Worthley SG, et al. Acute antithrombotic effect of a front-loaded regimen of clopidogrel in patients with atherosclerosis on aspirin. *Arterioscler Thromb Vasc Biol.* 2000;20(10):2316–2321.
44. Curtin R. *Clopidogrel and Ticlopidine. Platelets,* Amsterdam, The Netherlands: Academic Press; 2002:787–801.
45. CAPRIE Steering Committee. A randomised, blinded, trial of clopidogrel versus aspirin in patients at risk of ischaemic events (CAPRIE). CAPRIE Steering Committee. *Lancet.* 1996;348(9038):1329–1339.
46. Yusuf S, Zhao F, Mehta SR, et al.; Clopidogrel in Unstable Angina to Prevent Recurrent Events Trial Investigators. Effects of clopidogrel in addition to aspirin in patients with acute coronary syndromes without ST-segment elevation. *N Engl J Med.* 2001;345(7):494–502.
47. Genoni M, Tavakoli R, Hofer C, et al. Clopidogrel before urgent coronary artery bypass graft. *J Thorac Cardiovasc Surg.* 2003;126(1):288–289.
48. Wiviott SD, Braunwald E, McCabe CH, et al.; TRITON-TIMI 38 Investigators. Prasugrel versus clopidogrel in patients with acute coronary syndromes. *N Engl J Med.* 2007;357(20):2001–2015.
49. Price MJ, Walder JS, Baker BA, et al. Recovery of platelet function after discontinuation of prasugrel or clopidogrel maintenance dosing in aspirin-treated patients with stable coronary disease: the recovery trial. *J Am Coll Cardiol.* 2012;59(25):2338–2343.
50. Ferreiro JL, Angiolillo DJ. New directions in antiplatelet therapy. *Circ Cardiovasc Interv.* 2012;5(3):433–445.
51. Gurbel PA, Bliden KP, Butler K, et al. Randomized double-blind assessment of the ONSET and OFFSET of the antiplatelet effects of ticagre-

lor versus clopidogrel in patients with stable coronary artery disease: the ONSET/OFFSET study. *Circulation.* 2009;120(25):2577–2585.

52. Wallentin L, Becker RC, Budaj A, et al. Ticagrelor versus clopidogrel in patients with acute coronary syndromes. *N Engl J Med.* 2009;361(11): 1045–1057.
53. Angiolillo DJ, Schneider DJ, Bhatt DL, et al. Pharmacodynamic effects of cangrelor and clopidogrel: the platelet function substudy from the cangrelor versus standard therapy to achieve optimal management of platelet inhibition (CHAMPION) trials. *J Thromb Thrombolysis.* 2012;34(1):44–55.
54. Bhatt DL, Stone GW, Mahaffey KW, et al.; CHAMPION PHOENIX Investigators. Effect of platelet inhibition with cangrelor during PCI on ischemic events. *N Engl J Med.* 2013;368(14):1303–1313.
55. Scirica BM, Bonaca MP, Braunwald E, et al.; TRA 2°P-TIMI 50 Steering Committee Investigators. Vorapaxar for secondary prevention of thrombotic events for patients with previous myocardial infarction: a prespecified subgroup analysis of the TRA 2 degrees P-TIMI 50 trial. *Lancet.* 2013; 380(9850):1317–1324.
56. EPILOG Investigators. Platelet glycoprotein IIb/IIIa receptor blockade and low-dose heparin during percutaneous coronary revascularization. *N Engl J Med.* 1997;336(24):1689–1696.
57. EPISTENT Investigators. Randomised placebo-controlled and balloon-angioplasty-controlled trial to assess safety of coronary stenting with use of platelet glycoprotein-IIb/IIIa blockade. *Lancet.* 1998;352(9122):87–92.
58. Use of a monoclonal antibody directed against the platelet glycoprotein IIb/IIIa receptor in high-risk coronary angioplasty. The EPIC Investigation. *N Engl J Med.* 1994;330(14):956–961.
59. Sane DC, Damaraju LV, Topol EJ, et al. Occurrence and clinical significance of pseudothrombocytopenia during abciximab therapy. *J Am Coll Cardiol.* 2000;36(1):75–83.
60. Reiter RA, Mayr F, Blazicek H, et al. Desmopressin antagonizes the in vitro platelet dysfunction induced by GPIIb/IIIa inhibitors and aspirin. *Blood.* 2003;102(13):4594–4599.
61. Ronner E, Boersma E, Akkerhuis KM, et al. Patients with acute coronary syndromes without persistent ST elevation undergoing percutaneous coronary intervention benefit most from early intervention with protection by a glycoprotein IIb/IIIa receptor blocker. *Eur Heart J.* 2002;23(3): 239–246.
62. A comparison of aspirin plus tirofiban with aspirin plus heparin for unstable angina. Platelet Receptor Inhibition in Ischemic Syndrome Management (PRISM) Study Investigators. *N Engl J Med.* 1998;338(21):1498–1505.
63. Sacco RL, Sivenius J, Diener HC. Efficacy of aspirin plus extended-release dipyridamole in preventing recurrent stroke in high-risk populations. *Arch Neurol.* 2005;62(3):403–408.
64. Beguin S, Lindhout T, Hemker HC. The mode of action of heparin in plasma. *Thromb Haemost.* 1988;60(3):457–462.
65. Ofosu FA, Hirsh J, Esmon CT, et al. Unfractionated heparin inhibits thrombin-catalysed amplification reactions of coagulation more efficiently than those catalysed by factor Xa. *Biochem J.* 1989;257(1):143–150.
66. Hyers TM, Agnelli G, Hull RD, et al. Antithrombotic therapy for venous thromboembolic disease. *Chest.* 2001;119(1 Suppl):176S–193S.
67. Collins R, Scrimgeour A, Yusuf S, Peto R. Reduction in fatal pulmonary embolism and venous thrombosis by perioperative administration of subcutaneous heparin. Overview of results of randomized trials in general, orthopedic, and urologic surgery. *N Engl J Med.* 1988;318(18):1162–1173.
68. Noble S, Peters DH, Goa KL. Enoxaparin. A reappraisal of its pharmacology and clinical applications in the prevention and treatment of thromboembolic disease. *Drugs.* 1995;49(3):388–410.
69. Samama MM, Cohen AT, Darmon JY, et al. A comparison of enoxaparin with placebo for the prevention of venous thromboembolism in acutely ill medical patients. Prophylaxis in Medical Patients with Enoxaparin Study Group. *N Engl J Med.* 1999;341(11):793–800.
70. Jacobs DG, Piotrowski JJ, Hoppensteadt DA, et al. Hemodynamic and fibrinolytic consequences of intermittent pneumatic compression: preliminary results. *J Trauma.* 1996;40(5):710–716; discussion 716–717.
71. Barritt DW, Jordan SC. Anticoagulant drugs in the treatment of pulmonary embolism: a controlled trial. *Lancet.* 1960;1(7138):1309–1312.
72. Kernohan RJ, Todd C. Heparin therapy in thromboembolic disease. *Lancet.* 1966;1(7438):621–623.
73. Alpert JS, Smith R, Carlson J, et al. Mortality in patients treated for pulmonary embolism. *JAMA.* 1976;236(13):1477–1480.
74. Kanis JA. Heparin in the treatment of pulmonary thromboembolism. *Thromb Diath Haemorrh.* 1974;32(2–3):519–527.
75. Levine M, Gent M, Hirsh J, et al. A comparison of low-molecular-weight heparin administered primarily at home with unfractionated heparin administered in the hospital for proximal deep-vein thrombosis. *N Engl J Med.* 1996;334(11):677–681.
76. Koopman MM, Prandoni P, Piovella F, et al. Treatment of venous thrombosis with intravenous unfractionated heparin administered in the hospital as compared with subcutaneous low-molecular-weight heparin administered at home. The Tasman Study Group. *N Engl J Med.* 1996;334(11):682–687.
77. Low-molecular-weight heparin in the treatment of patients with venous thromboembolism. The Columbus Investigators. *N Engl J Med.* 1997;337 (10):657–662.
78. Doyle DJ, Turpie AG, Hirsh J, et al. Adjusted subcutaneous heparin or continuous intravenous heparin in patients with acute deep vein thrombosis: a randomized trial. *Ann Intern Med.* 1987;107(4):441–445.
79. Pini M, Pattachini C, Quintavalla R, et al. Subcutaneous vs intravenous heparin in the treatment of deep venous thrombosis: a randomized clinical trial. *Thromb Haemost.* 1990;64(2):222–226.
80. Andersson G, Fagrell B, Holmgren K, et al. Subcutaneous administration of heparin: a randomised comparison with intravenous administration of heparin to patients with deep-vein thrombosis. *Thromb Res.* 1982;27(6): 631–639.
81. Kearon C, Ginsberg JS, Julian JA, et al.; Fixed-Dose Heparin (FIDO) Investigators. Comparison of fixed-dose weight-adjusted unfractionated heparin and low-molecular-weight heparin for acute treatment of venous thromboembolism. *JAMA.* 2006;296(8):935–942.
82. Hull RD, Raskob GE, Brant RF, et al. Relation between the time to achieve the lower limit of the APTT therapeutic range and recurrent venous thromboembolism during heparin treatment for deep vein thrombosis. *Arch Intern Med.* 1997;157(22):2562–2568.
83. Raschke RA, Reilly BM, Guidry JR, et al. The weight-based heparin dosing nomogram compared with a “standard care” nomogram: a randomized controlled trial. *Ann Intern Med.* 1993;119(9):874–881.
84. Hull RD, Pineo GF. Heparin and low-molecular-weight heparin therapy for venous thromboembolism: will unfractionated heparin survive? *Semin Thromb Hemost.* 2004;30Suppl 1:11–23.
85. Anand SS, Bates S, Ginsberg JS, et al. Recurrent venous thrombosis and heparin therapy: an evaluation of the importance of early activated partial thromboplastin times. *Arch Intern Med.* 1999;159(17):2029–2032.
86. Cruickshank MK, Levine MN, Hirsh J, et al. A standard heparin nomogram for the management of heparin therapy. *Arch Intern Med.* 1991;151(2):333–337.
87. Hollingsworth JA, Rowe BH, Brisebois FJ, et al. The successful application of a heparin nomogram in a community hospital. *Arch Intern Med.* 1995;155(19):2095–2100.
88. Brown G, Dodek P. An evaluation of empiric vs. nomogram-based dosing of heparin in an intensive care unit. *Crit Care Med.* 1997;25(9):1534–1538.
89. Basu D, Gallus A, Hirsh J, Cade J. A prospective study of the value of monitoring heparin treatment with the activated partial thromboplastin time. *N Engl J Med.* 1972;287(7):324–327.
90. Hull RD, Raskob GE, Hirsh J, et al. Continuous intravenous heparin compared with intermittent subcutaneous heparin in the initial treatment of proximal-vein thrombosis. *N Engl J Med.* 1986;315(18):1109–1114.
91. Chiu HM, Hirsh J, Yung WL, et al. Relationship between the anticoagulant and antithrombotic effects of heparin in experimental venous thrombosis. *Blood.* 1977;49(2):171–184.
92. Turpie AG, Robinson JG, Doyle DJ, et al. Comparison of high-dose with low-dose subcutaneous heparin to prevent left ventricular mural thrombosis in patients with acute transmural anterior myocardial infarction. *N Engl J Med.* 1989;320(6):352–357.
93. Kaplan K, Davison R, Parker M, et al. Role of heparin after intravenous thrombolytic therapy for acute myocardial infarction. *Am J Cardiol.* 1987;59(4):241–244.
94. Kearon C, Akl EA, Comerota AJ, et al.; American College of Chest Physicians. Antithrombotic therapy for VTE disease antithrombotic therapy and prevention of thrombosis, 9th ed: American College of Chest Physicians evidence-based clinical practice guidelines. *Chest.* 2012;141(2 Suppl):e419S–e494S.
95. Kearon C, Gent M, Hirsh J, et al. A comparison of three months of anticoagulation with extended anticoagulation for a first episode of idiopathic venous thromboembolism. *N Engl J Med.* 1999;340(12):901–907.
96. Schulman S, Rhedin AS, Lindmarker P, et al. A comparison of six weeks with six months of oral anticoagulant therapy after a first episode of venous thromboembolism: duration of Anticoagulation Trial Study Group. *N Engl J Med.* 1995;332(25):1661–1665.
97. Agnelli G, Prandoni P, Santamaria MG, et al. Three months versus one year of oral anticoagulant therapy for idiopathic deep venous thrombosis. Warfarin Optimal Duration Italian Trial Investigators. *N Engl J Med.* 2001;345(3):165–169.
98. Amsterdam EA, Wenger NK, Brindis RG, et al. 2014 AHA/ACC Guideline for the Management of Patients with Non-ST-Elevation Acute Coronary Syndromes: a report of the American College of Cardiology/American

Heart Association Task Force on Practice Guidelines. *J Am Coll Cardiol.* 2014;64(24):e139–e228.

99. Klein W, Buchwald A, Hillis SE, et al. Comparison of low-molecular-weight heparin with unfractionated heparin acutely and with placebo for 6 weeks in the management of unstable coronary artery disease. Fragmin in unstable coronary artery disease study (FRIC). *Circulation.* 1997;96(1):61–68.
100. Cohen M, Demers C, Gurfinkel EP, et al. A comparison of low-molecular-weight heparin with unfractionated heparin for unstable coronary artery disease. Efficacy and Safety of Subcutaneous Enoxaparin in Non-Q-Wave Coronary Events Study Group. *N Engl J Med.* 1997;337(7):447–452.
101. Antman EM, McCabe CH, Gurfinkel EP, et al. Enoxaparin prevents death and cardiac ischemic events in unstable angina/non-Q-wave myocardial infarction: results of the thrombolysis in myocardial infarction (TIMI) 11B trial. *Circulation.* 1999;100(15):1593–1601.
102. Mahaffey KW, Ferguson JJ. Exploring the role of enoxaparin in the management of high-risk patients with non-ST-elevation acute coronary syndromes: the SYNERGY trial. *Am Heart J.* 2005;149(4 Suppl):S81–S90.
103. Brill-Edwards P, Ginsberg JS, Johnston M, Hirsh J. Establishing a therapeutic range for heparin therapy. *Ann Intern Med.* 1993;119(2):104–109.
104. Fernandez JS, Sadaniantz BT, Sadaniantz A. Review of antithrombotic agents used for acute coronary syndromes in renal patients. *Am J Kidney Dis.* 2003;42:446–455.
105. Fox KA, Antman EM, Montalescot G, et al. The impact of renal dysfunction on outcomes in the ExTRACT-TIMI 25 trial. *J Am Coll Cardiol.* 2007;49:2249–2255.
106. Raschke R. Heparin-nitroglcerin interaction. *Am Heart J.* 1991;121:1849–1850.
107. Levine MN, Hirsh J, Gent M, et al. A randomized trial comparing activated thromboplastin time with heparin assay in patients with acute venous thromboembolism requiring large daily doses of heparin. *Arch Intern Med.* 1994;154(1):49–56.
108. Levine MN, Raskob G, Beyth RJ, et al. Hemorrhagic complications of anticoagulant treatment: the Seventh ACCP Conference on Antithrombotic and Thrombolytic Therapy. *Chest.* 2004;126(3 Suppl):287S–310S.
109. Glazier RL, Crowell EB. Randomized prospective trial of continuous vs intermittent heparin therapy. *JAMA.* 1976;236(12):1365–1367.
110. Horrow JC. Protamine: a review of its toxicity. *Anesth Analg.* 1985;64(3):348–361.
111. Stewart WJ, McSweeney SM, Kellett MA, et al. Increased risk of severe protamine reactions in NPH insulin-dependent diabetics undergoing cardiac catheterization. *Circulation.* 1984;70(5):788–792.
112. Caplan SN, Berkman EM. Letter: Protamine sulfate and fish allergy. *N Engl J Med.* 1976;295(3):146.
113. Warkentin TE, Sikov WM, Lillicrap DP. Multicentric warfarin-induced skin necrosis complicating heparin-induced thrombocytopenia. *Am J Hematol.* 1999;62(1):44–48.
114. Griffiths E, Dzik WH. Assays for heparin-induced thrombocytopenia. *Transfus Med.* 1997;7(1):1–11.
115. Bartholomew JR. Transition to an oral anticoagulant in patients with heparin-induced thrombocytopenia. *Chest.* 2005;127(2 Suppl):27S–34S.
116. Warkentin TE, Elavathil LJ, Hayward CP, et al. The pathogenesis of venous limb gangrene associated with heparin-induced thrombocytopenia. *Ann Intern Med.* 1997;127(9):804–812.
117. Majerus P, Brose GJ, Miletich JP, et al. *Anticoagulant, Thrombolytic, and Antiplatelet Drugs.* 9th ed. New York, NY: McGraw-Hill; 1996.
118. Srinivasan AF, Rice L, Bartholomew JR, et al. Warfarin-induced skin necrosis and venous limb gangrene in the setting of heparin-induced thrombocytopenia. *Arch Intern Med.* 2004;164(1):66–70.
119. Weitz JI. Low-molecular-weight heparins. *N Engl J Med.* 1997;337(10):688–698.
120. Cosmi B, Fredenburgh JC, Rischke J, et al. Effect of nonspecific binding to plasma proteins on the antithrombin activities of unfractionated heparin, low-molecular-weight heparin, and dermatan sulfate. *Circulation.* 1997;95(1):118–124.
121. MD Consult website. http://home.mdconsult.com/das/drug/view. Accessed December 8, 2016.
122. Francis CW, Pellegrini VD Jr, Totterman S, et al. Prevention of deep-vein thrombosis after total hip arthroplasty: comparison of warfarin and dalteparin. *J Bone Joint Surg Am.* 1997;79(9):1365–1372.
123. Low-molecular-weight heparin during instability in coronary artery disease, Fragmin during Instability in Coronary Artery Disease (FRISC) study group. *Lancet.* 1996;347(9001):561–568.
124. Levine MN, Raskob G, Landefeld S, Kearon C. Hemorrhagic complications of anticoagulant treatment. *Chest.* 2001;119(1 Suppl):108S-121S.
125. Holst J, Lindblad B, Bergqvist D, et al. Protamine neutralization of intravenous and subcutaneous low-molecular-weight heparin (tinzaparin, Logiparin): an experimental investigation in healthy volunteers. *Blood Coagul Fibrinolysis.* 1994;5(5):795–803.
126. Warkentin TE, Levine MN, Hirsh J, et al. Heparin-induced thrombocytopenia in patients treated with low-molecular-weight heparin or unfractionated heparin. *N Engl J Med.* 1995;332(20):1330–1335.
127. Newman PM, Swanson RL, Chong BH. Heparin-induced thrombocytopenia: IgG binding to PF4-heparin complexes in the fluid phase and cross-reactivity with low molecular weight heparin and heparinoid. *Thromb Haemost.* 1998;80(2):292–297.
128. Hirsh J, Dalen JE, Deykin D, et al. Oral anticoagulants: mechanism of action, clinical effectiveness, and optimal therapeutic range. *Chest.* 1995;108(4 Suppl):231S–246S.
129. Routledge PA, Chapman PH, Davies DM, Rawlins MD. Pharmacokinetics and pharmacodynamics of warfarin at steady state. *Br J Clin Pharmacol.* 1979;8(3):243–247.
130. Levine MN, Raskob G, Landefeld S, Hirsh J. Hemorrhagic complications of anticoagulant treatment. *Chest.* 1995;108(4 Suppl):276S–290S.
131. Weitz JI, Crowther M. Direct thrombin inhibitors. *Thromb Res.* 2002;106(3):V275–V284.
132. Linkins LA, Weitz JI. New anticoagulants. *Semin Thromb Hemost.* 2003;29(6):619–631.
133. Wallis RB. Hirudins: from leeches to man. *Semin Thromb Hemost.* 1996;22(2):185–196.
134. Hofsteenge J, Stone SR, Donella-Deana A, Pinna LA. The effect of substituting phosphotyrosine for sulphotyrosine on the activity of hirudin. *Eur J Biochem.* 1990;188(1):55–59.
135. Weitz JI, Middeldorp S, Geerts W, Heit JA. Thrombophilia and new anticoagulant drugs. *Hematol Am Soc Hematol Educ Progr.* 2004:424–438.
136. Eriksson BI, Ekman S, Lindbratt S, et al. Prevention of thromboembolism with use of recombinant hirudin: results of a double-blind, multicenter trial comparing the efficacy of desirudin (Revasc) with that of unfractionated heparin in patients having a total hip replacement. *J Bone Joint Surg Am.* 1997;79(3):326–333.
137. Maraganore JM, Bourdon P, Jablonski J, et al. Design and characterization of hirulogs: a novel class of bivalent peptide inhibitors of thrombin. *Biochemistry.* 1990;29(30):7095–7101.
138. Eriksson BI, Wille-Jorgensen P, Kalebo P, et al. A comparison of recombinant hirudin with a low-molecular-weight heparin to prevent thromboembolic complications after total hip replacement. *N Engl J Med.* 1997;337(19):1329–1335.
139. Jove M, Maslanka M, Minkowitz HS, Jaffer AK. Safety of desirudin in thrombosis prevention after total knee arthroplasty: the DESIR-ABLE study. *Am J Ther.* 2014;21(6):496–499.
140. Lefevre G, Duval M, Gauron S, et al. Effect of renal impairment on the pharmacokinetics and pharmacodynamics of desirudin. *Clin Pharmacol Ther.* 1997;62(1):50–59.
141. Graetz TJ, Tellor BR, Smith JR, Avidan MS. Desirudin: a review of the pharmacology and clinical application for the prevention of deep vein thrombosis. *Expert Rev Cardiovasc Ther.* 2011;9(9):1101–1109.
142. Skrzypczak-Jankun E, Carperos VE, Ravichandran KG, et al. Structure of the hirugen and hirulog 1 complexes of alpha-thrombin. *J Mol Biol.* 1991;221(4):1379–1393.
143. Witting JI, Bourdon P, Brezniak DV, et al. Thrombin-specific inhibition by and slow cleavage of hirulog-1. *Biochem J.* 1992;283(Pt 3):737–743.
144. Robson R, White H, Aylward P, Frampton C. Bivalirudin pharmacokinetics and pharmacodynamics: effect of renal function, dose, and gender. *Clin Pharmacol Ther.* 2002;71(6):433–439.
145. Hursting MJ, Alford KL, Becker JC, et al. Novastan (brand of argatroban): a small-molecule, direct thrombin inhibitor. *Semin Thromb Hemost.* 1997;23(6):503–516.
146. Francis CW, Berkowitz SD, Comp PC, et al. Comparison of ximelagatran with warfarin for the prevention of venous thromboembolism after total knee replacement. *N Engl J Med.* 2003 30;349(18):1703–1712.
147. O'Brien CL, Gage BF. Costs and effectiveness of ximelagatran for stroke prophylaxis in chronic atrial fibrillation. *JAMA.* 2005;293(6):699–706.
148. Cohen A, Davidson, BL, Gallus, AS, et al. Fondaparinux for the prevention of VTE in acutely ill medical patients. *Blood.* 2003;102:15a.
149. Connolly SJ, Ezekowitz MD, Yusuf S, et al. Dabigatran versus warfarin in patients with atrial fibrillation. *N Engl J Med.* 2009;361(12):1139–1151.
150. Stangier J, Rathgen K, Stahle H, Mazur D. Influence of renal impairment on the pharmacokinetics and pharmacodynamics of oral dabigatran etexilate: an open-label, parallel-group, single-centre study. *Clin Pharmacokinet.* 2010;49(4):259–268.

151. Van Ryan J, Stangier J, Haertter S, et al. A novel, reversible, oral direct thrombin inhibitor: interpretation of coagulation assays and reversal of anticoagulant activity. *Thromb Haemost.* 2010;103: 1116–1127.
152. Pollack CV, Reilly PA, Eikelboom J, et al. Idarucizumab for Dabigatran reversal. *N Engl J Med.* 2015;373:511–520.
153. Herbert JM, Herault JP, Bernat A, et al. Biochemical and pharmacological properties of SANORG 34006, a potent and long-acting synthetic pentasaccharide. *Blood.* 1998;91(11):4197–4205.
154. Bijsterveld NR, Vink R, van Aken BE, et al. Recombinant factor VIIa reverses the anticoagulant effect of the long-acting pentasaccharide idraparinux in healthy volunteers. *Br J Haematol.* 2004;124(5):653–658.
155. Levine M, Hirsh J, Weitz J, et al. A randomized trial of a single bolus dosage regimen of recombinant tissue plasminogen activator in patients with acute pulmonary embolism. *Chest.* 1990;98(6):1473–1479.
156. Lane DA, Kamphuisen PW, et al. Bleeding risk in patients with atrial fibrillation: the AMADAEUS study. *Chest.* 2011;140:146–155.
157. EINSTEIN Investigators, Bauersachs R, Berkowitz SD, et al. Oral rivaroxaban for symptomatic venous thromboembolism. *N Engl J Med.* 2010;363(26):2499–2510.
158. Patel MR, Mahaffey KW, Garg J, et al. Rivaroxaban versus warfarin in nonvalvular atrial fibrillation. *N Engl J Med.* 2011;365(10):883–891.
159. Raghavan N, Frost CE, Yu Z, et al. Apixaban metabolism and pharmacokinetics after oral administration to humans. *Drug Metab Dispos.* 2009;37(1):74–81.
160. Lopes RD, Alexander JH, Al-Khatib SM, et al. Apixaban for Reduction In STroke and Other ThromboemboLic Events in atrial fibrillation (ARISTOTLE) trial: design and rationale. *Am Heart J.* 2010;159(3):331–339.
161. Dalla-Volta S, Palla A, Santolicandro A, et al. PAIMS 2: alteplase combined with heparin versus heparin in the treatment of acute pulmonary embolism. Plasminogen Activator Italian Multicenter Study 2. *J Am Coll Cardiol.* 1992;20(3):520–526.
162. Garcia D, Ageno W, Libby E. Update on the diagnosis and management of pulmonary embolism. *Br J Haematol.* 2005;131(3):301–312.
163. ISIS-3: a randomised comparison of streptokinase vs tissue plasminogen activator vs anistreplase and of aspirin plus heparin vs aspirin alone among 41,299 cases of suspected acute myocardial infarction. ISIS-3 (Third International Study of Infarct Survival) Collaborative Group. *Lancet.* 1992;339(8796):753–770.
164. An international randomized trial comparing four thrombolytic strategies for acute myocardial infarction. The GUSTO investigators. *N Engl J Med.* 1993;329(10):673–682.
165. A comparison of reteplase with alteplase for acute myocardial infarction. The Global Use of Strategies to Open Occluded Coronary Arteries (GUSTO III) Investigators. *N Engl J Med.* 1997;337(16):1118–1123.
166. Assessment of the Safety and Efficacy of a New Thrombolytic (ASSENT-2) Investigators. Van De Werf F, Adgey J, et al. Single-bolus tenecteplase compared with front-loaded alteplase in acute myocardial infarction: the ASSENT-2 double-blind randomised trial. *Lancet.* 1999;354(9180):716–722.
167. Clark WM, Wissman S, Albers GW, et al. Recombinant tissue-type plasminogen activator (Alteplase) for ischemic stroke 3 to 5 hours after symptom onset. The ATLANTIS Study: a randomized controlled trial. Alteplase Thrombolysis for Acute Noninterventional Therapy in Ischemic Stroke. *JAMA.* 1999;282(21):2019–2026.
168. Stam J. Thrombosis of the cerebral veins and sinuses. *N Engl J Med.* 2005;352(17):1791–1798.
169. Jackson KW, Tang J. Complete amino acid sequence of streptokinase and its homology with serine proteases. *Biochemistry.* 1982;21(26): 6620–6625.
170. Reddy KN, Markus G. Mechanism of activation of human plasminogen by streptokinase. Presence of active center in streptokinase-plasminogen complex. *J Biol Chem.* 1972;247(6):1683–1691.
171. Mentzer RL, Budzynski AZ, Sherry S. High-dose, brief-duration intravenous infusion of streptokinase in acute myocardial infarction: description of effects in the circulation. *Am J Cardiol.* 1986;57(15):1220–1226.
172. Col JJ, Col-De Beys CM, Renkin JP, et al. Pharmacokinetics, thrombolytic efficacy and hemorrhagic risk of different streptokinase regimens in heparin-treated acute myocardial infarction. *Am J Cardiol.* 1989;63(17):1185–1192.
173. Collen D, De Cock F, Lijnen HR. Biological and thrombolytic properties of proenzyme and active forms of human urokinase. II. Turnover of natural and recombinant urokinase in rabbits and squirrel monkeys. *Thromb Haemost.* 1984;52(1):24–26.
174. Kohler M, Sen S, Miyashita C, et al. Half-life of single-chain urokinase-type plasminogen activator (scu-PA) and two-chain urokinase-type plasminogen activator (tcu-PA) in patients with acute myocardial infarction. *Thromb Res.* 1991;62(1–2):75–81.
175. Konstantinides S, Geibel A, Heusel G, et al. Heparin plus alteplase compared with heparin alone in patients with submassive pulmonary embolism. *N Engl J Med.* 2002;347(15):1143–1150.
176. Verstraete M. Third-generation thrombolytic drugs. *Am J Med.* 2000;109 (1):52–58.
177. Bozeman WP, Kleiner DM, Ferguson KL. Empiric tenecteplase is associated with increased return of spontaneous circulation and short term survival in cardiac arrest patients unresponsive to standard interventions. *Resuscitation.* 2006;69(3):399–406.
178. Khan IA, Gowda RM. Clinical perspectives and therapeutics of thrombolysis. *Int J Cardiol.* 2003;91(2–3):115–127.

CHAPTER

146

Hematologic Conditions

JAN S. MOREB and GAURAV TRIKHA

INTRODUCTION

Hematopoiesis is a polyclonal process responsible for the production and maintenance of blood and immune cells, thereby producing billions of new blood cells each day. Large numbers of blood and immune cells can be traced to a pool of hematopoietic stem cells (HSCs) from which these clones have originated (1). It is also known that these HSCs can mobilize out of the bone marrow into circulating blood and can undergo programmed cell death, called *apoptosis*—a process by which cells that are detrimental or unneeded self-destruct, all for the purpose of maintaining homeostasis. The most primitive stem cell, in the bone marrow, is responsible for the production of all peripheral blood cell lineages, while maintaining sufficient numbers of pluripotent stem cells to sustain hematopoiesis throughout adult life. These cells are characterized by the surface expression of CD34 molecule and by lack of markers of differentiation.

The HSC population supports a tremendous production of blood cells over an animal's life span; for example, adult humans produce their body weight of red cells, white cells, and platelets every 7 years, whereas the mouse produces 60% of its body weight over a 2-year life span. Using DNA labeling data, investigators in the field have tried to characterize the HSC kinetics in the mouse. Based on such data, MacKey (2) was able to calculate that in the course of producing a mature, circulating blood cell, the original single HSC will undergo between 17 and 19.5 divisions, providing a net output between approximately 170,000 and 720,000 blood cells.

A wide array of environmental factors, both humoral and cellular, regulate the quantity and behavior of HSCs, including cytokines and chemokines, extracellular matrix components, as well as hematopoietic and nonhematopoietic cells such as natural killer (NK) cells, T cells, macrophages, fibroblasts, osteoblasts, adipocytes and, perhaps, even neurons. In addition to this wide array of microenvironmental factors, several intrinsic genetic events are critical to hematopoiesis and are currently the subject of intense research (3). This complex interplay determines whether HSCs, progenitors, and mature blood cells remain quiescent, proliferate, differentiate, self-renew, or undergo apoptosis (4–6).

Production of a specific type of differentiated blood cell from a stem cell is thought to occur randomly. Cytokines promote proliferation and survival of certain types of cells but do not affect which cell type is produced from a stem cell. Cytokines are made and secreted mainly by helper T lymphocytes and macrophages, but also by other stroma cells such as fibroblasts and endothelial cells. A few of these cytokines have been synthesized and are FDA approved for clinical use (7).

PATHOPHYSIOLOGY

In the event of stress, such as bleeding or infection, several processes occur. Stored pools of cells in the marrow or adherent to the endothelium are quickly released into the circulation to localize to the site of injury; additionally, fewer progenitors and mature cells undergo apoptosis. Furthermore, quiescent progenitors and HSCs are stimulated by various growth factors to proliferate and differentiate into mature white cells, red blood cells (RBCs), and platelets. Finally, when the bleeding, infection, or other underlying stress ceases, the kinetics of hematopoiesis return to baseline levels. This process repeats itself innumerable times during the life span of an individual, and is seen in an exaggerated form following chemotherapy or bone marrow transplantation.

Cytokines are very important in critical care medicine, especially those proinflammatory cytokines released by monocytes/macrophages in response to infectious and noninfectious inflammation. The release of these cytokines results in whole body inflammation such as that seen in the systemic inflammatory response syndrome (SIRS). These patients also undergo an anti-inflammatory phase, which includes the release of cytokines with opposing—anti-inflammatory—biologic effects or naturally occurring cytokine antagonists, such as interleukin-1 receptor antagonist and tumor necrosis factor-α (TNF-α) soluble receptors p55 and p75 (8,9). Clinical studies to intervene in the inflammatory response using these and other anticytokine therapy have been more than a little disappointing, but efforts continue with several FDA-approved cytokines antagonists. On the other hand, many studies have shown that plasma concentrations of certain cytokines correlate with severity and outcome of sepsis (10–12). New fundamental understanding of the inflammatory signaling that regulates hematopoiesis in health and disease will facilitate the development of new interventions (13).

Many acquired and inherited abnormalities that interfere with the normal mechanisms of hematopoiesis result in known diseases of decreased, or increased, production of one or more of the blood cell lineages; any one of these can be encountered in patients hospitalized in the ICU. The pathophysiology, diagnosis and treatment of these diseases will be the main subject of this chapter.

DECREASED BLOOD COUNTS

Anemias

Diagnosis and Transfusions Guidelines

Anemia—hemoglobin concentration less than 12 g/dL—is present in 95% of patients in the intensive care unit, with

TABLE 146.1 Anemia Classification

Anemias Secondary to Marrow Underproduction
- **Decreased erythropoietin production**
  - Renal disease
  - Endocrine deficiency
  - Starvation
- **Inadequate response to erythropoietin**
  - Iron deficiency
  - B_{12} deficiency
  - Folic acid deficiency
  - Anemia of chronic disease
  - Marrow infiltration
  - Sideroblastic anemia
  - Myelodysplastic syndrome
- **Marrow failure**
  - Congenital dyserythropoietic anemia
  - Aplastic anemia
  - Pure red cell aplasia
  - Toxic marrow damage

Anemias Secondary to Increased Destruction
- **Acquired**
  - Immune-mediated hemolytic anemia
  - Paroxysmal nocturnal hemoglobinuria
  - Hemolytic anemia due to red cell fragmentation (TTP, DIC)
  - Hemolytic anemia due to chemical or physical agents
  - Infections
  - Acquired hemoglobinopathies (methemoglobinemia)
- **Hereditary**
  - Congenital hemoglobinopathies (sickle cell disease)
  - Enzyme deficiency (G6PD, pyruvate kinase)
  - Red cell membrane defects (spherocytosis, elliptocytosis)

TTP, thrombotic thrombocytopenic purpura; DIC, disseminated intravascular coagulopathy.

about one-third of those having, upon admission, a concentration of less than 10 g/dL. In the assessment, particular attention should be paid to the time of onset, patient's ethnic origin, concurrent illness, procedures patient has undergone, drugs patient is receiving, and history of transfusions. One practical approach is to classify anemia into two major categories: anemia resulting from underproduction versus anemia due to increased destruction of RBCs (Table 146.1). These considerations will affect the type of laboratory tests and the need for transfusions.

Every effort should be exerted to obtain diagnostic tests prior to any transfusions. These should include a complete blood count, including hematocrit, hemoglobin, mean corpuscular volume (MCV) and hemoglobin (MCH), reticulocyte count, and a stained blood smear. In addition, serum bilirubin and lactic acid dehydrogenase are useful to determine the presence of hemolysis. If immune hemolysis is suspected, direct Coombs test should be ordered (indirect Coombs test is done routinely with any cross-match request sent to the blood bank); or if hemoglobinopathy is suspected, hemoglobin electrophoresis should be obtained before transfusion.

The physician in the ICU may be faced with the immediate decision of whether the patient requires transfusion with packed red blood cells (PRBC). For years, many physicians firmly believed that hemoglobin of 10 g/dL or hematocrit of 30% was desirable in anemic patients, especially those undergoing surgical procedures or with critical illness (14). This approach—of using fixed transfusion triggers—has been recognized as the main reason for high transfusion rates in ICU patients and is finally being replaced by a more physiologic approach in which the patient's intravascular volume and tissue oxygen needs are considered. A restrictive transfusion policy, in which hemoglobin concentration is maintained between 7 and 9 g/dL, has proved to be effective and yields decreased death rates in comparison to the liberal strategy (14–17). More recent studies and a meta-analysis, as discussed below (18–20), concluded that there is no difference in outcomes of patients receiving restrictive versus liberal PRBC transfusion approaches. Indeed, in young traumatized patients, the hemoglobin is sometimes allowed to drift to as low as 5 g/dL, as long as there are no signs of oxygen delivery deficit, such as elevated lactate levels, an unacceptable heart rate, or other symptoms. These patients are most often started on recombinant erythropoietin and have iron stores repleted, if necessary, to keep from undergoing transfusion.

There are few specific questions regarding transfusions that pertain to specific conditions encountered in the ICU, which the American Association of Blood Banks (AABB) recent guidelines (based on the TRICC, TRIBPICU, and FOCUS trials) has addressed (21):

- When to transfuse hospitalized hemodynamically stable patient? Consider transfusion when Hgb 7 g/dL or less for adult and pediatric patients in the ICU and 8 g/dL or less for postoperative surgical patients (based on studies done in surgical patients).
- When to transfuse hospitalized hemodynamically stable patient with pre-existing cardiovascular disease? Based on the FOCUS trial, transfuse for Hgb 8 g/dL or less, or if symptoms are present.
- When to transfuse in hospitalized hemodynamically stable patient with acute coronary syndrome? No definite recommendation was given because of lack of randomized trials.
- Should symptoms rather than Hgb levels guide transfusions in hospitalized hemodynamically stable patient? Again without significant evidence, it was recommended to consider both.

Recently published randomized studies address two other important questions, one regarding transfusions in patients with gastrointestinal bleeding (18) and another in patients with septic shock (19). Both studies support the use of 7 g/dL threshold in these situations. Finally, a meta-analysis of 31 trials comparing the benefit and harms of restrictive versus liberal transfusion strategies showed that liberal transfusion strategies have not been shown to convey any benefit to patients and, overall, there was no differences in mortality, morbidity, or myocardial infarction incidence (20). A key principle is that one should not give blood unless one can show benefit from its administration. Obviously, different transfusion approaches will be addressed under the specific types of anemia discussed in this chapter.

Anemia in Critical Illness

Anemia with a hemoglobin 8.5 g/dL or less is the most frequent type of anemia encountered in the ICU. As a result, over 50% of these patients receive RBC transfusions during their ICU stay, as do over 85% of patients with an ICU length of stay longer than 7 days. This trend was confirmed by two historic studies: the CRIT study in the United States (22) and the ABC trial in Europe (23). Both studies also showed that the number of RBC transfusions a patient received was independently associated with longer ICU stay and increase in mortality. These and other similar epidemiologic studies have revealed some similarities. First, the vast majority of critically ill patients have anemia on admission to the ICU. Second, the most common indication for RBC transfusion in the ICU was treatment of the anemia. Third, the transfusion trigger in all these studies was hemoglobin of about 8.5 g/dL. Finally, RBC transfusions were increased in patients with prolonged ICU length of stay and increased age.

Pathophysiology

Possible mechanisms involved in anemia of acute critically ill patients include a blunted erythropoietin (EPO) response to anemia, with blood concentrations being inappropriately low in these patients; suppression of erythropoiesis by proinflammatory cytokines; possible blood loss from frequent phlebotomies; and blood loss from gastrointestinal bleeding as a result of gastric tubes, stress-induced mucosal ulcerations, acute renal failure, and frequent coagulation problems in ICU patients. This anemia shares characteristics with anemia of chronic inflammation such as high ferritin concentrations and low-to-normal transferrin saturation with functional iron deficiency.

Until recently, we understood little about the pathogenesis of anemia of chronic inflammation. It now appears that the inflammatory cytokine interleukin-6 (IL-6) induces the production of hepcidin, an iron-regulatory hormone that may be responsible for the hypoferremia and suppressed erythropoiesis (24). This discovery has led to multiple studies focused on the role of hepcidin in the anemia of the critically ill patient, and exploring potential therapeutic applications.

Treatment

The approach to treatment of this type of anemia should include measures to reduce blood loss, a restrictive blood transfusion policy, and possibly the use of recombinant human EPO (rh-EPO). Multiple studies have shown that the subcutaneous administration of rh-EPO at 40,000 units weekly, starting between days 3 and 7 of the ICU stay, resulted in a significant reduction in RBC transfusions and a higher hemoglobin level (25,26). Because iron is locked up in the phagocytic system and hardly available, the administration of intravenous iron, together with rh-EPO, may result in an enhanced rh-EPO effect. As only about 10% of oral iron is bioavailable, this route may not be appropriate in ICU patients. Additionally, several intravenous formulations are available including iron dextran, iron gluconate, and iron sucrose. Typically, intravenous iron is administered at small doses over several sessions up to a total cumulative dose of 1,000 mg.

Autoimmune Hemolytic Anemia

Pathophysiology and Diagnosis

When a patient is critically ill from autoimmune hemolytic anemia (AIHA), the presenting signs and symptoms are those of normovolemic anemia, unless massive hemolysis is associated with hypotension, significant hemoglobinuria, and acute renal failure. Variable levels of jaundice may also be present in the nonmassive AIHA. Initial laboratory data may show an elevated reticulocyte index of more than 2, decreased haptoglobin, hemoglobinuria, and an elevated indirect bilirubinemia and lactate dehydrogenase (LDH); the blood smear shows increased numbers of diffusely basophilic red cells, reflecting the increased reticulocytes, and variable numbers of microspherocytes and fragmented cells, indicative of the hemolysis (Fig. 146.1). A positive result on direct antiglobulin (Coombs) test, indicating that immunoglobulin or complement is on the surface of the circulating red cells, identifies the immune etiology of the hemolysis. This information may first become available when the blood bank attempts to cross-match the patient's blood for transfusion.

It is important to determine, by history and appropriate laboratory studies, whether the hemolysis could be related to a drug the patient is taking and whether it is caused by warm-reacting (usually IgG) or cold-reacting (usually IgM) antibodies. In some instances, the drug must be present for hemolysis to occur (e.g., quinidine, penicillin); in others, hemolysis occurs even in the absence of the drug (e.g., methyldopa). Underlying diseases that may be associated with AIHA include infections, such as infectious mononucleosis and pneumonia caused by *Mycoplasma pneumonia;* collagen vascular diseases, especially systemic lupus erythematosus; and lymphoproliferative disorders such as chronic lymphocytic leukemia. In other instances,

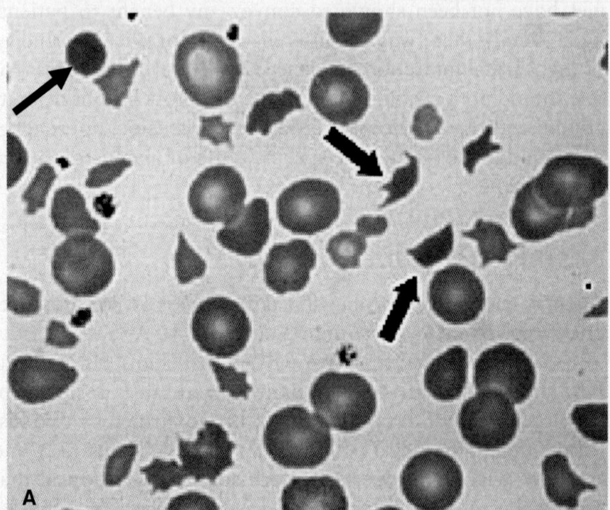

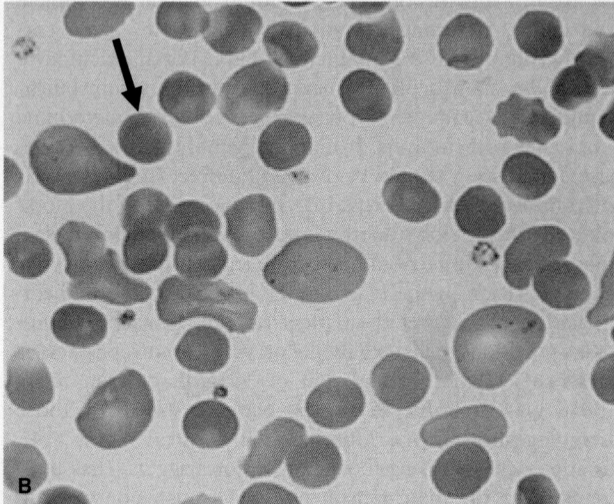

FIGURE 146.1 Microspherocytes (*thin arrows*) and schistocytes (fragmented cells, *thick arrows*) **(A)**, spherocytes with increased reticulocytes (the large cells) **(B)** are usually seen in the peripheral blood smear of a patient with hemolytic anemia.

the AIHA may be associated with idiopathic thrombocytopenic purpura (ITP) as part of Evans syndrome.

Treatment

The mainstay of treatment of AIHA caused by warm-reacting antibodies is the administration of corticosteroids, usually given in dosages equivalent to 60 to 80 mg/day of prednisone. In patients who do not respond to steroids, splenectomy, high-dose intravenous gamma globulin, rituximab chimeric anti-CD20 antibody, alemtuzumab humanized anti-CD52 antibody, or other immunosuppressive drugs may be useful.

Steroids are usually ineffective in AIHA caused by cold-reactive antibodies (cold agglutinin disease), but responses have been observed using larger doses. Patients with cold agglutinins may have symptoms related to impaired blood flow in acral parts where the blood temperature is low enough to permit agglutination of RBCs by antibodies. Warming usually prevents or alleviates such symptoms; however, in a small percentage of cases, plasmapheresis to reduce the concentration of the offending IgM antibodies may be required. In drug-induced immune hemolysis, discontinuing the drug is usually the only treatment needed.

In a patient with AIHA with a critical degree of anemia, transfusion must be considered (27). It may be impossible to find compatible RBCs by the usual cross-matching procedures, and transfused cells may be subject to rapid antibody-mediated destruction. On the other hand, the patient must not be allowed to die because of undue caution regarding the transfusion of incompatible red cells. The key to optimal care in this critical situation is close communication between the intensivist and the blood bank physician. When an AIHA patient is transfused, the patient must be observed closely for signs of accelerated hemolysis, such as visible hemoglobin in the plasma or urine.

Certain special considerations pertain to transfusion of patients with cold-reacting antibodies. Administered blood should be warmed to body temperature. Transfusion of plasma, which contains complement, should be avoided because hemolysis is complement mediated and may be limited by depletion of complement in vivo. In massive hemolysis, therapeutic efforts should be directed at maintenance of blood pressure, renal blood flow, and urinary output; intravenous fluids and diuretics such as furosemide should be used to maintain a urine flow of 100 mL/hr.

Hemolytic Anemia from G6PD Deficiency

Pathophysiology

RBC glucose-6-phosphate dehydrogenase (G6PD) deficiency is inherited as an X-linked recessive disorder, affecting various population groups around the world. In the United States, African Americans are the group most often affected, with a gene frequency of about 11%. They have the G6PD A variant of the enzyme and a mild-to-moderate deficiency. A recent study by the US army found that 2.5% of males and 1.6% of females were deficient. The highest rates of G6PD deficiency were in African American males (12.2%) and females (4.1%), along with Asian males (4.3%) (28). Among drugs producing hemolysis are some sulfonamides, nitrofurantoins, and antimalarials, such as primaquine. Illnesses most likely to trigger hemolysis are acute infections. Infectious hepatitis, in particular, has been associated with severe hemolytic episodes in G6PD-deficient patients.

Diagnosis and Treatment

Hemolysis in the G6PD-deficient patient may be sudden and massive, usually becoming apparent 1 to 3 days after the inciting stress, such as administration of an oxidant drug. Hemoglobinemia and hemoglobinuria may occur; the blood smear shows polychromatophilia within a few days, reflecting the developing reticulocytosis. Early in the course of the hemolytic episode, Heinz bodies may be identified in red cells by special staining methods. These precipitates of oxidatively denatured hemoglobin provide a useful diagnostic clue and should be sought if G6PD deficiency is suspected as a cause of acute hemolysis. However, the absence of Heinz bodies does not exclude this diagnosis. The red cell enzyme deficiency may be readily detected by laboratory assay when the patient is in a stable state but may be more difficult to demonstrate during a hemolytic episode. This is because the enzyme deficiency is greatest in the oldest red cells. These cells are the first destroyed in a hemolytic episode and, as they are replaced by newly produced young cells, the overall red cell enzyme level may rise to the normal range. This replacement of susceptible erythrocytes by more resistant cells also tends to ameliorate the hemolysis with time.

If the diagnosis is suspected, any potentially offending drugs should be stopped. Otherwise, supportive care is usually all that is necessary. Although the deficiency is an X-linked trait, female heterozygotes may have hemolytic episodes.

Hemolytic Anemia from Red Cell Injury in the Circulation

Pathophysiology

Fragmentation and destruction of red cells in the circulation may result from increased shear stresses caused by turbulent blood flow. The two major categories of disease in which this kind of hemolysis occurs are malfunctioning intravascular prosthetic devices (e.g., heart valves, vascular grafts, and shunts) and disorders affecting blood vessels that result in microangiopathic hemolytic disease, such as disseminated intravascular coagulopathy (DIC) or thrombotic microangiopathy (TMA).

TMA encompasses the spectrum of thrombotic thrombocytopenic purpura (TTP) and hemolytic uremic syndrome (HUS). These forms of hemolytic disease are rarely of sufficient severity to require critical care. However, they can be seen in critically ill patients admitted to the ICU, and have been associated with various initiating factors such as severe infections, drug intake, malignancies, connective tissue diseases, and pregnancy (29). Characteristically, the blood smear shows red cell fragmentation producing micropoikilocytes (schistocytes, similar to that shown in Fig. 146.1). Typically, the TMA patients will also have thrombocytopenia (TP), fever, and possibly neurologic and renal involvement. TTP must be considered in the presence of TP and microangiopathic hemolytic anemia (29). ADAMTS13 assays help to confirm the diagnosis and monitor the course of the disease.

Treatment

The diagnosis of TMA/TTP should be treated as a medical emergency. The treatment of TMA with plasma administration, either infusion or plasmapheresis, is the only effective therapy that has dramatically improved the prognosis of these patients, and should be initiated within 4 to 8 hours to prevent early deaths from TTP.

Specific treatment is directed at the underlying disorder. Supportive measures may be required for the effects of hemolysis itself and to minimize any adverse renal consequences of hypotension and hemoglobinuria. These may include blood transfusion and hydration to ensure good urine flow. Occasionally, a badly malfunctioning prosthesis, such as an artificial heart valve, may require replacement, but this is more often necessary to correct a life-threatening hemodynamic abnormality than to alleviate severe hemolysis.

Sickle Cell Anemia

Pathophysiology and Clinical Symptoms

Sickle cell hemoglobin (hemoglobin S) is the result of a single nucleotide mutation in the sixth codon of the β-globin gene ($β^s$). Heterozygous inheritance of hemoglobin S does not usually cause disease or symptoms but is detectable as sickle cell trait (30). Homozygous inheritance or compound heterozygous inheritance with another β-globin gene results in disease. The discussion here is directed primarily toward homozygous sickle cell disease (SCD) which includes those genotypes associated with chronic hemolytic anemia and vaso-occlusive pain: homozygous SCD (hemoglobin SS), hemoglobin SC disease (hemoglobin SC), sickle-$β^0$ thalassemia (hemoglobin S$β^0$), and sickle-$β^+$ thalassemia (hemoglobin S$β^+$), and other less common hemoglobin mutants. The clinical manifestations are related to the degree of intracellular polymerization of deoxyhemoglobin S (Table 146.2), and it is different among the various genotypes.

The clinical symptoms of SCD affect multiple organs and may vary widely among patients. Chief among the clinical features are episodes of severe pain—namely, crises—in the chest, back, abdomen, or extremities. The acute chest syndrome (ACS), sometimes fatal complication, affects over 40% of all patients with SCD and can lead to acute and chronic respiratory insufficiency, including pulmonary hypertension. Its cardinal features are fever, pleuritic chest pain, referred abdominal pain, cough, lung infiltrates, and hypoxia. Other complications of SCD include recurrent strokes in young adults; parvovirus B19-induced aplastic crisis; hyperbilirubinemia from cholestatic syndrome or cholecystitis; liver disease; splenic infarctions; autosplenectomy with increased risk of fulminant septicemia caused by encapsulated organisms such as *Streptococcus pneumoniae* and *Haemophilus influenzae;* hematuria; priapism; bone infarctions with the risk of avascular necrosis; osteomyelitis and other musculoskeletal manifestations; leg ulcers; and spontaneous abortions (32). Despite the fact that some of these complications are fatal, many patients with SCD survive into their fifth and sixth decades in industrialized countries.

Treatment

The reasons for ICU admission may result from SCD-related or SCD-unrelated causes. ACS is the most frequent cause for ICU admission; it can be a life-threatening condition when it precipitates acute respiratory syndrome (ARDS) and multiorgan failure. Expanding on prior small studies, Cecchini et al. (33) showed that SC patients still face death in ICU with 7% mortality in 138 consecutive ICU admissions. About 20% of 119 SC patients required vital support including mechanical ventilation, vasopressors, and hemodialysis. This complicated outcome correlated to more rapid deterioration in the 48 hours prior to ICU transfer, rapidly declining hemoglobin, and progressive renal injury. Expert consensus holds that early recognition of deterioration and timely transfusion can abort an impending catastrophe (34). However, one should always remember the double-edged sword of transfusions. Because there is no clear evidence that transfusion therapy shortens a simple painful crisis, and because the crisis is unpredictable and self-limited, transfusion is not a treatment for the uncomplicated painful crisis. Urgent transfusions are needed when there is a severe sudden drop in hemoglobin, especially in children in whom splenic sequestration or aplastic crises present in this manner, and in severe ACS with hypoxia. Exchange transfusion is the most rapid method to reduce the hemoglobin S concentration to less than 30% in urgent situations that arise from complications of SCD, including stroke and cholestatic syndrome with signs of liver failure.

TABLE 146.2 Clinical and Hematologic Findings in the Common Variants of Sickle Cell Disease after the Age of 5 Years[a]

		Hemoglobin Electrophoresis				Hematologic Values[b]			
Disease group	Clinical severity	S (%)	F (%)	A_2 (%)	A (%)	Hb g/dL	Retic (%)	MCV (fL)	RBC morphology
SS	Usually marked	>90	<10	<3.5	0	6–11	5–20	>80	Sickle cells, NRBCs, normochromia, anisocytosis, poikilocytosis, target cells, Howell–Jolly bodies
S$β^0$ Thal	Marked to moderate	>80	<20	>3.5	0	6–10	5–20	<80	Sickle cells, NRBCs, hypochromia, microcytosis, anisocytosis, poikilocytosis, target cells
S$β^+$ Thal	Mild to moderate	>60	<20	>3.5	10–30	9–12	5–10	<75	No sickle cells, hypochromia, microcytosis, anisocytosis, poikilocytosis, target cells
SC	Mild to moderate	50	<5	50% Hb C	0	10–15	5–10	75–95	"Fat" sickle cells, anisocytosis, poikilocytosis, target cells
S HPFH	Asymptomatic	<70	>30	<2.5	0	12–14	1–2	<80	No sickle cells, anisocytosis, poikilocytosis, rare target cells

MCV, mean corpuscular volume; NRBCs, nucleated red blood cells.
[a]For findings in younger children, see Brown AK et al. (31).
[b]Hematologic values are approximate. There is tremendous variability between disease groups and between individual patients of the same group, particularly regarding clinical severity.
Adapted from NIH Publication No. 96-2117.

The goals of the SCD treatment are either to relieve symptoms of the complications or to prevent complications by using some of the new treatments targeting disease mechanisms. The treatment of the painful crisis is supportive. Dehydration, acidosis, infection, and hypoxemia all promote red cell sickling and should be prevented or corrected. Summary points regarding the treatment of SCD patients include:

- Sufficient analgesics should be used to relieve pain without worrying about addiction or side effects of opiates; patients can be given oral analgesics to take at home.
- Oxygen is often administered in sickle cell crisis, although its benefits are uncertain.
- Antibiotics that cover major pulmonary pathogens should be administered in patients with ACS.
- Chronic red cell transfusions have been shown to prevent strokes in patients with SCD.
- For patients undergoing general anesthesia, preoperative transfusion to a hematocrit above 30% reduced postoperative complications.
- Preventive treatments should include early vaccinations against *S. pneumoniae* and *H. influenzae;* prophylactic penicillin in children until the age of 5 years.
- Folic acid (1 mg daily) to all patients to prevent megaloblastic erythropoiesis.
- Hydroxyurea treatment should be reserved for patients with SCD who have severe complications.

Aplastic Crisis in Hemolytic Anemia

Pathophysiology

Sudden intensification of anemia in hemolytic disease resulting from a precipitous reduction in the rate of red cell production is known as *aplastic crisis.* It may occur in the course of any hemolytic disease but has been most commonly reported in congenital hemolytic disorders such as hereditary spherocytosis and sickle cell anemia. It is most common in children but also occurs in adults. Patients characteristically have fever, anorexia, nausea, and vomiting; abdominal pain and headache are common. Their anemia is usually severe and may be life-threatening; mild leukopenia and TP are often present. The episode is self-limited, and recovery usually begins by 2 weeks. In the recovery phase, there is a return of vigorous erythropoiesis and often an outpouring of nucleated red cells and reticulocytes into the blood, frequently accompanied by leukocytosis and immature white blood cells. There is convincing evidence that parvovirus B19 is the cause of most aplastic crises (35).

Diagnosis and Treatment

Prompt recognition of this syndrome is important because of the suddenness and severity of the anemia. A low reticulocyte count in a patient with hemolytic disease is usually the main clue to the diagnosis. Treatment is via transfusion with RBCs. The volume given should be sufficient to alleviate signs or symptoms of inadequate tissue oxygenation; that amount need not be exceeded, as episodes are self-limited, and the patient's hematocrit will return rapidly to its baseline level.

Leukopenias

The term *leukopenia* refers to a total white blood cell (WBC) count of less than 4,000 cells/μL, whereas granulocytopenia or neutropenia refers to a circulating granulocyte count below 1,500 cells/μL. WBC and granulocyte levels are lower in some ethnic groups, for example, Africans, African Americans, and Yemenite Jews, without any clinical significance. The clinical importance of granulocytopenia relates to the associated increased risk of bacterial infection. If the absolute neutrophil count is less than or equal to 500 cells/μL, bacterial infection becomes the rule. Agranulocytosis implies severe neutropenia or a complete absence of granulocytes. The pathophysiology of three patient groups is discussed below as most pertinent to critical care situations.

Primary Bone Marrow Diseases and Cytotoxic Treatment

This is the largest and most frequent entity that causes neutropenia. Bone marrow diseases such as leukemias, myelodysplastic syndrome, and marrow fibrosis frequently present with neutropenia. Chemotherapy-induced neutropenia is a common complication of the treatment of cancer. The risk of life-threatening infections increases with the increased severity of neutropenia and its duration, increasing patient age, and the coexistence of other severe illnesses. Many of these patients, whether inpatient or outpatient, end up in the ICU due to a rapid onset of septic shock. In current practice, the occurrence of neutropenic fever is an indication for hospitalization and prompt institution of intravenous wide-spectrum antibiotics. Before starting antibiotics, cultures of blood,* sputum, and urine should be obtained in all patients, and other sites should be cultured as indicated in individual patients. All patients should have chest radiographs taken as well. The common effects of bacterial infections—purulent sputum in pneumonia, pyuria in urinary tract infection, or abscess formation—are usually absent because of lack of granulocytes.

Bone Marrow Aplasia

Neutropenia is part of the pancytopenia commonly present in aplastic anemia. Some cases of aplastic anemia seem to have an autoimmune basis; in others, a drug or chemical exposure may be suspected as a cause; no tests are available to prove an association in individual cases. Benzene and its derivatives are potentially toxic to the bone marrow, and many other chemicals, such as dichlorodiphenyltrichloroethane (DDT) and other insecticides, are suspect. Toluene exposure in glue sniffers may be associated with aplastic anemia. Many medications have been linked with aplastic anemia, which occurs as an idiosyncratic reaction in a small percentage of patients exposed to a given drug. Drugs for which an etiologic role seems likely include chloramphenicol, phenylbutazone, indomethacin, diphenylhydantoin, sulfonamides, and gold preparations. In at least half the cases of aplastic anemia, no cause is found or suspected.

Immune and Drug-related Granulocytopenia

Neutropenia in adults often occurs as an isolated finding or in association with autoimmune disease such as rheumatoid arthritis, systemic lupus erythematosus, and other similar conditions. The evaluation should include peripheral blood smear to seek

*When blood cultures are drawn, there should never be any less than two full sets—four bottles—drawn. This routine is needed to prevent the possibility of a contaminated specimen being overtreated, or worse, undertreated.

out large granular lymphocytes (LGL); measurement of antinuclear antibodies, rheumatoid factor, and other autoantibodies; and possibly a bone marrow examination. Patients with chronic neutropenia, either idiopathic or autoimmune, usually do not require treatment. Patients with an absolute neutrophil count less than 500 cells/μL are prone to develop recurrent fevers and infections. In addition to antibiotics, G-CSF administration may improve the neutrophil count during the infection. Patients with LGL syndrome may not respond well to G-CSF, and may require immunosuppressive therapy, such as methotrexate or cyclosporine, alone or with G-CSF. Chronic neutropenia in association with rheumatoid arthritis, or Felty syndrome, is usually seen in severe cases with elevated rheumatoid factor. These patients who have recurrent fevers and infection require treatment similar to patients with LGL syndrome; splenectomy should be considered in refractory cases.

Drug-induced agranulocytosis is a serious medical problem and occurs in 1% to 3% of patients treated with certain medications. The characteristic clinical syndrome includes high fever, chills, and severe sore throat (agranulocytic angina) caused by bacterial infection. Oral and pharyngeal ulcers, necrotizing tonsillitis, pharyngeal abscesses, and bacteremia may occur. The blood will demonstrate a virtual absence of granulocytes. The bone marrow may show absence of all granulocyte precursors or only the mature cells. The picture may superficially resemble acute leukemia, or a state of maturation arrest; the disease mechanism is often unclear. In some cases, it is an antibody against the drug acting as a hapten in association with endogenous antigen on neutrophil surface. Other drugs may impair production of neutrophils by direct toxic mechanism.

Serial blood counts are now recommended for patients on some drugs such as phenothiazines, clozapine, sulfasalazine, and antithyroid drugs because of the relatively high frequency of drug-induced neutropenia. Otherwise, management should include prompt withdrawal of all potentially offending drugs and the use of broad-spectrum antibiotics. Bone marrow examination is not usually indicated. The time to recovery may be proportional to the severity but is usually within about a week after withdrawal of the offending drug.

Prophylactic Antibiotics and Treatment Approaches

Many antibiotic regimens have been tested, and guidelines for a rational approach to therapy have been formulated (36). The choice of an antibiotic regimen should take into account any findings in the individual patient that suggest a specific site of infection and any knowledge of patterns of infection in a given institution. If cultures are positive, the antibiotic treatment should be adjusted accordingly. If cultures are negative, as is frequently the case, empirical therapy should be continued if the patient remains neutropenic and until counts recover. If, on the other hand, fever continues and the patient's general condition deteriorates with persistent neutropenia, it is appropriate in selected patients to prescribe empirical treatment with an antifungal agent, such as amphotericin B, because of the frequency of fungal infections in patients with prolonged neutropenia. Patients should be screened by obtaining a CT scan of sinuses, chest, abdomen, and pelvis for possible foci of invasive fungal infections. The galactomannan antigen test for aspergillus should be done routinely on blood and sputum (usually bronchoalveolar lavage) of immunosuppressed patients with neutropenia. If patients have central venous catheter, fungal and bacterial blood cultures should be obtained[†], and removal of catheters should be considered if blood cultures are positive for fungal infection or certain bacterial infections that are difficult to eradicate.

Various regimens of prophylactic antibiotics have been investigated for their efficacy in preventing infection in the neutropenic patient. The results have been too variable to justify blanket recommendations (37,38). The routine therapeutic use of colony-stimulating factors—such as G-CSF and GM-CSF—in febrile neutropenia to stimulate the proliferation and maturation of neutrophil progenitor cells was not recommended by the American Society of Clinical Oncology (ASCO). However, these factors should be considered in such patients at high risk for infection-related complications or who have prognostic factors that are predictive of poor clinical outcomes. High-risk features include expected prolonged (>10 days) and profound (<0.1 × 10^3 cells/μL) neutropenia, age older than 65 years, uncontrolled primary disease, pneumonia, hypotension, multiorgan dysfunction, invasive fungal infection, or being hospitalized at the time of the development of the fever. On the other hand, colony-stimulating factors are recommended for primary and secondary prophylaxes used to prevent chemotherapy-induced neutropenia (39).

ICU physicians should be aware of respiratory status deterioration or the development of ARDS during neutropenia recovery with or without the use of G-CSF (40,41). This could be related to the release of inflammatory cytokines by resident alveolar neutrophils and macrophages. Mortality can be as high as 62% in these patients, and therefore, immediate evaluation by bronchoscopy to rule out infection and early use of high-dose steroids could be critical for their survival.

The principles of treating infectious complications resulting from neutropenia in aplastic states are the same as those outlined earlier for neutropenia in malignant diseases. The treatment of aplastic anemia includes allogeneic bone marrow transplantation in suitable patients, immunosuppressive therapy including antithymocyte globulin, and other supportive care measures such as antibiotic prophylaxis and colony-stimulating factors.

Thrombocytopenias

TP is a common laboratory abnormality in ICU patients that has been associated with adverse outcomes. The incidence of TP—defined as a platelet count (PC) below 150 × 10^3 cells/μL—has been reported to be 23% to 41.3%, with mortality rates up to 54% (42). The incidence of more severe TP—less than 50 × 10^3 cells/μL—is lower, about 10% to 17%, but is associated with greater mortality (42,43). Two more recent studies showed hospital and ICU mortality were independently associated with moderate and severe TP (44,45). The relationship between the time course of platelet counts and mortality in 1,449 critically ill patients was examined in a prospective multicenter observational study in 40 ICUs from Europe, the United States, and Australia (42). There was a documented increase in mortality in patients who had TP on

†The CDC recommends against the routine culturing of CVLs. However, in the neutropenic patient with difficult IV access, cultures could be obtained from the CVL as long as the preparation of the hub is acceptable.

TABLE 146.3 Potential Causes of Thrombocytopenia

- Sepsis, infections
- Disseminated intravascular coagulopathy
- Perioperative and postresuscitation hemodilution
- Immune thrombocytopenias
- Drug-induced thrombocytopenias
- Liver disease/hypersplenism
- Massive transfusion
- Primary marrow disorder
- Antiphospholipid antibody syndrome/lupus anticoagulant
- Intravascular devices

day 4 of admission to the ICU and even higher mortality in those patients with documented TP by day 14 (42).

Pathophysiology

Systematic evaluation of TP is essential to the identification and management of the causes (43). There are numerous potential causes of TP in the ICU (Table 146.3). Although sepsis is the most common cause, accounting for more than 48% of TP cases in the ICU, more than 25% of ICU patients have more than one cause (46). Drug-induced thrombocytopenia (DIT) presents a diagnostic challenge inasmuch as many medications can cause TP, and critically ill patients often receive multiple drugs. One such drug is heparin, the most common cause of DIT due to immune mechanisms (47).

Diagnosis

A thorough history could elucidate the following: chronicity (familial thrombocytopenia), temporal relationship to a medication or travel history (tick-borne infection), past medical history of autoimmune disorders, infections, or malignancies; pregnancy status in premenopausal woman; recent medications and vaccinations (MMR); recent organ transplantation; ingestion of alcohol and quinine-containing beverages; viral hepatitis (hepatitis C) and other liver conditions associated with splenomegaly. Physical examination should focus on finding the cause and severity of the process. A hepatosplenomegaly could be the etiology of TP, and bleeding in joints with muscle as opposed to mucocutaneous bleeding suggests coagulopathy alongside TP and potentially a more severe process.

Given the multiple causes of the TP, a clinical context is essential prior to ensuing diagnostic workup. Any change in PC over time—duration, speed of decrease or rise, etc.—should be considered to be associated with the prognosis. The following should be the rough guide to initiate a thorough workup (45,48):

- More than 30% decrease in PC
- Rapid decline in PC over 24 to 48 hours
- Failure to rebound after 5 to 7 days
- Decline in PC after initial recovery
- PC less than 100,000 cells/μL

Peripheral smear in the initial workup and in a specific clinical context can lead to the appropriate diagnosis (48):

- Platelet clumping is a common but a benign cause of TP and does not require any further diagnostics
- If the transfusion of blood products is associated with an abrupt PC fall within hours, TP can be caused by bacterial contamination or passive alloimmunization.
- Schistocytes in the context of TP and hemolytic anemia suggest potentially catastrophic conditions TTP/HUS and should obligate emergent workup.
- Blasts, nucleated RBCs and Pelger–Huet anomaly of neutrophils suggest underlying bone marrow process necessitating bone marrow aspirate (BMA) and biopsy.
- Macrospherocytes, RBC clumping or agglutination suggest autoimmune process.
- Lymphocytosis, atypical lymphocytes, neutrophilia, toxic granulation suggest underlying infection.
- Isolated TP requires astute clinical acumen and workup should be based on the clinical context with the differential diagnosis including the different entities mentioned in this section.

BMA is often not indicated in the initial workup and the information gathered often does not change the management. However in the context of severe sepsis if hemophagocytosis is suspected, BMA can be life-saving.

HIT, even though it is a rare cause of TP in ICU settings, should be suspected in the context of thrombosis and TP. The presence of anti-PF4/heparin antibodies alone cannot confirm the diagnosis given that the seroprevalence is high in ICU patients, being 10.8% on admission and increasing to 29.4% on day 7 (45,49). Therefore patients suspecting of having HIT after an initial antibody test need a confirmation with functional assays (e.g., serotonin release assay [SRA]). Given the low prevalence of HIT in ICU in comparison to incidence of TP, calculating 4Ts score is helpful and only patients scoring 4 or more should have heparin stopped and be tested further for HIT (Table 146.4) (50). A meta-analysis of 12 studies

TABLE 146.4 The 4Ts Scoring System for Heparin-Induced Thrombocytopenia

4Ts Category	2 Points	1 Point	0 Points
Thrombocytopenia	Platelet count fall >50% and platelet nadir 20K or more	Platelet count fall 30–50% or platelet nadir 10–19K	Platelet count fall <30% or platelet nadir 10K
Timing of platelet count fall	Clear onset days 5–10 or platelet fall ≤1 day (prior heparin exposure within 30 days)	Consistent with days 5–10 fall, but not clear (e.g., missing platelet counts); onset after day 10; or fall ≤1 day (prior heparin exposure 30–100 days ago)	Platelet count 4 days or less without recent exposure
Thrombosis or other sequelae	New thrombosis (confirmed); skin necrosis; acute systemic reaction after intravenous unfractionated heparin bolus	Progressive or recurrent thrombosis; non-necrotizing (erythematous) skin lesions; suspected thrombosis (not proven)	None
Other causes of thrombocytopenia	None apparent	Possible	Definite

The 4Ts score is the sum of the values for each of the four categories. Scores of 1–3, 4–5, and 6–8 are considered to correspond to a low, intermediate, and high probability of HIT, respectively.

applying 4Ts score reported a negative predictive value (NPV) of 99.8% (51). However, the addition of rapid particle gel immunoassay for PF4-H/PaGIA to the 4Ts score was better able to exclude HIT in patients with low or intermediate 4Ts score (52). This is on condition that the results of the immunoassay are available within 24 hrs.

Treatment

Multiple studies have shown TP to be associated with mortality, whether increasing PCs lead to decrease in mortality is yet to be established (44). Considering this, we suggest that the management of TP in the ICU is challenging and should address platelet transfusion, anticoagulation, and etiology-specific treatments (i.e., addressing the underlying cause). When TP is caused by destruction or sequestration of the patient's own platelets, transfused platelets are subject to the same fate. Thus, platelet transfusions most often are of little benefit, and are reserved for the treatment of severe bleeding. Transfusion of one random donor platelet unit per 10 kg of recipient weight, or single-donor unit from apheresis, is usually used to achieve that goal, which can be confirmed by a repeat PC within an hour posttransfusion. The effectiveness of platelet transfusions is diminished in febrile, infected patients who may require larger and more frequent transfusions.

Platelet prophylaxis, as compared with a therapeutic transfusion strategy, has shown interval reduction in bleeding in hospitalized patients with therapy-induced hypo proliferative thrombocytopenia. Per the AABB 2015 guidelines, patients with less than 10,000 platelets/μL should be transfused (53). This recommendation is based on two trials in which prophylactic platelet transfusions to achieve counts greater than 10,000 cells/μL had reduction in severe bleeding (54,55). The evidence for platelet transfusion in the setting of instrumentation–placement of central venous catheter (CVC) and lumbar puncture (LP), is weak. Based on several observational studies, a CVC placement obligates a PC of greater than 20,000 cells/μL and for an LP, a PC of greater than 50,000 cells/μL is desired (53).

For patients undergoing invasive surgery, the recommendations are now based on the locations and type of surgery. Per AABB 2015 guidelines, nonbleeding patients can undergo major nonneuraxial surgery with PC more than 50,000 cells/μL; patients undergoing neuraxial surgery have a threshold set at a PC of greater than 100,000 cells/μL.

In patients with sepsis, there is not much evidence for the threshold for transfusion, but given the underlying consumption potentially causing acute drop in PC, maintaining higher PC could be considered (45). In the setting of severe hemorrhage, patients should be considered for transfusion if PC is less than 30,000 cells/μL (48). Following the transfusion, depending on the context, a posttransfusion PC could be checked within 1 hour; this would be helpful in conditions where transfusion refractoriness is suspected (splenomegaly, sepsis, fever, medications, active bleeding, and alloimmunization).

Chemoprophylaxis, using unfractionated heparin (UFH) or low–molecular-weight heparin (LMWH), is usually prescribed routinely in all adult patients admitted to the ICU, except when the PC is less than 30,000 cells/μL or when there is a major risk of hemorrhage (48). In a retrospective multivariate analysis, LMWH was found to have a lower risk of bleeding in all patients with TP, and therefore should be the preferred agent unless contraindicated (44).

Thrombocytopenia with Infection

Mild and transient TP occurs with many systemic infections; the mechanism for this may be a combination of suppressed bone marrow production, increased destruction, and increased splenic sequestration. In bacteremia, platelets may be consumed because of DIC, whereas in viral infection, platelet production may be suppressed. TP is commonly associated with human immunodeficiency virus (HIV) infection, mainly due to decreased production, although sometimes an autoimmune mechanism is also involved. TTP or TMA may be associated with HIV as well as other infections, such as streptococcal and *Escherichia coli* (56–58). Treating the underlying infection in most cases is usually adequate to correct the TP.

Drug-Induced Thrombocytopenia

DIT presents a diagnostic challenge because many medications can cause TP, and patients in ICU are often on multiple medications (59). The most commonly reported drugs with probable or definite relation to TP were quinidine, quinine, rifampin, and trimethoprim-sulfamethoxazole. Many other drugs can cause TP, including heparin, which is discussed in detail below, intravenous antibiotics, anticonvulsants, diuretics, and the platelet GP IIb/IIIa antagonists used in acute coronary syndrome. The underlying mechanism of DIT is usually immune, and at least three different types of antibodies appear to play a role: hapten-dependent antibodies, drug-induced platelet-reactive autoantibodies, and drug-dependent antibodies. Targets for drug-dependent antibodies are glycoproteins (GP) on the cell membrane of platelets, such as GP Ib/IX and GPIIb/IIIa. The diagnosis of DIT is usually supported by recovery to a normal PC within 5 to 7 days.

Treatment of DIT may only require withdrawal of the offending drug. Prednisone may be given if the diagnosis of idiopathic autoimmune thrombocytopenia (ITP) cannot be ruled out. Patients with severe TP caused by GP IIb/IIIa antagonists may require platelet transfusions because they are typically also receiving heparin and aspirin for their acute coronary syndrome. Although platelet serology tests are available, the results may not be available in a time frame that allows such information to be used in the decision-making process for drug-induced immune thrombocytopenia.

Heparin-Induced Thrombocytopenia

Heparin-induced thrombocytopenia (HIT) is an anticoagulant-induced prothrombotic disorder caused by platelet activation of heparin-dependent antibodies of the immunoglobulin G class. The diagnosis of HIT should be considered when the PC falls to less than 150×10^3 cells/μL, or more than 50% decrease of the PC from baseline, between days 5 and 14 from start of heparin therapy; a high index of suspicion on the physician's part is key in making the diagnosis. The TP is usually moderate and resolves within a few days of discontinuing heparin. HIT without thrombosis is called *isolated HIT,* whereas *HIT thrombotic syndrome* (HITTS) denotes HIT complicated with thrombosis. The mortality rate associated with HIT ranges between 10% and 20%.

HIT is an immune-mediated hypersensitivity reaction to platelet factor 4 (PF4)/heparin complex. PF4 is a heparin-binding protein found naturally in platelet α granules, which undergoes conformational changes once bound to heparin. Anti-PF4/heparin antibodies are produced by many patients taking heparin, but only a few will develop TP. Anti-PF4/heparin antibodies are transient and usually become undetectable within a median of 50 to 85 days. If heparin is readministered to a patient with high levels of HIT antibodies, abrupt TP can occur. However, this likely will be more than 100 days after the last exposure to heparin. It is important to note that seroconversion can be found by ELISA (enzyme-linked immunosorbent assay) in up to 15% of patients on heparin; however, this does not constitute a diagnosis of HIT. In general, surgical patients, individuals exposed to higher doses of heparin for a longer time, and patients receiving UFH, as opposed to LMWH, are more likely to develop HIT.

The frequency of HIT in ICU patients was examined in two major studies (56,57). The results suggested that only a small minority of ICU patients with TP receiving UFH have HIT, and that the PF4/heparin-reactive antibodies are more likely to be detected by ELISA assay than SRA, suggesting a possible *over* diagnosis—due to a high false-positive rate by ELISA—of HIT. The Complications After Thrombocytopenia Caused by Heparin (CATCH) registry is a recent attempt to achieve better understanding of the prevalence, consequences, and temporal relationship of HIT and TP among patients treated with anticoagulants. The thrombotic sequelae of HIT carry significant morbidity and may even be lethal. Some of the morbid events include deep venous thrombosis (DVT), pulmonary embolism, skin necrosis, limb ischemia, thrombotic stroke, and myocardial infarction. Venous thrombosis is the most common manifestation, with lower limb DVT predominating.

All strategies should be used to prevent HIT in ICU patients. Heparin locks for central venous catheters and hemodialysis catheters are commonly used in the ICU setting and may need to be reconsidered. Hemodialysis without heparin has been shown to be safe and effective. However, once the diagnosis of HIT is recognized, heparin should promptly be substituted with a direct thrombin inhibitor, such as argatroban or lepirudin, or the heparinoid danaparoid—which is not available in the United States—to reduce the risk of life-threatening thromboembolic events. Because warfarin can temporarily reduce the synthesis of protein C and S, causing a hypercoagulable state, it should never be used alone in the initial treatment of HIT, and its use should be postponed until substantial platelet recovery has occurred. Consultation with a hematologist in these situations should be considered in all critically ill patients. The argatroban dose is 2 μg/kg/min in continuous infusion and dilution of 1 mg/mL. Dose adjustment is needed for hepatic impairment (use 25% of the dose), with the aim of a 1.5 to 3 times prolongation of activated prothrombin time (aPTT) in comparison to baseline. On the other hand, lepirudin treatment consists of a bolus 0.4 mg/kg (maximum of 44 mg), given over 10 to 15 seconds and followed by continuous infusion at 0.15 mg/kg/hr, with the goal of a 1.5 to 3 times prolongation of aPTT over baseline. The dose should be modified if creatinine is more than 1.5 mg/dL or clearance is less than 60 mL/min. If given with warfarin, discontinue lepirudin when an international normalized ratio (INR) of 2.0 is obtained.

IDIOPATHIC THROMBOCYTOPENIC PURPURA

Pathophysiology and Diagnosis

ITP, also known as immune thrombocytopenic purpura, is a common cause of TP in both adults and children. Although it is usually in the differential diagnosis of TP, the diagnosis of ITP can usually be made only after exclusion of other causes. When the history, physical examination, and blood count with peripheral smear are consistent with ITP and do not suggest other causes of TP, few diagnostic tests are necessary. Bone marrow examination may be important to rule out other primary marrow diseases such as myelodysplastic syndrome or lymphoproliferative disorders. In ITP, the marrow will show an increased number of megakaryocytes with immature forms and normal erythroid and myeloid lineages. A test for HIV is important in patients with risk factors for infection with this agent. Tests for platelet antibodies are not helpful because of lack of limited specificity and sensitivity. Thrombocytopenic purpura also may occur as one of the autoimmune complications of collagen vascular diseases such as systemic lupus erythematosus, or lymphoproliferative diseases such as chronic lymphocytic leukemia, and may even be the presenting manifestation of these disorders. ITP is categorized as acute, chronic, and refractory.

Treatment

Many forms of treatment have demonstrated effectiveness in ITP. Because of the numerous therapeutic options, individualization of therapy is possible. Platelet transfusions are used only in the case of severe, life-threatening hemorrhage. Initial therapy is usually with corticosteroids in a dosage equivalent to 1 mg/kg/day of prednisone. If the PC does not rise substantially within 2 to 3 weeks, splenectomy is usually the next step. Splenectomy produces prolonged remissions in two-thirds of cases, with additional partial remission in 15% of patients. Splenectomy also may be necessary in patients who have responded to steroids but cannot be weaned from the drug without the recurrence of thrombocytopenia. The 10% to 20% of patients who fail to respond to splenectomy may benefit from treatment with vincristine or immunosuppressive agents such as cyclophosphamide. The anabolic steroid, danazol, when given for periods of several months, also has been effective in some cases of ITP. Large doses of intravenous gamma globulin also may increase the PC in ITP, perhaps through blockage of reticuloendothelial sites of platelet destruction. The high cost of this therapy and the short duration of responses—usually 2 to 3 weeks—limit its use to certain specific circumstances such as active bleeding or prior to surgery. Anti-D therapy is effective only in Rh(D)+ patients and is not effective in splenectomized patients. Rituximab, a chimeric anti-CD20 monoclonal antibody, has been shown to be effective in chronic ITP. The overall goal in treating chronic/refractory ITP is to maintain a safe PC, defined as greater than about 10,000 to 20,000 cells/μL, and minimal therapy to minimize the morbidity and mortality associated with treatment.

When ITP occurs during pregnancy, there is an additional concern that the IgG autoantibody may cross the placenta and produce TP in the fetus and newborn. The lowest PC is usually seen several days after birth. The current practice is to use standard obstetric management of pregnancy and delivery. ITP should be differentiated from gestational TP that occurs in about 5% of normal women with uncomplicated pregnancies. The most important clue to differentiating the two is a history of previous TP when the woman was not pregnant. Additionally, more severe TP occurring before the third trimester is more likely to be ITP.

THROMBOTIC THROMBOCYTOPENIC PURPURA

Pathophysiology and Diagnosis

TTP and its closely related disorders—HUS, TMA, and peripartum HELLP (hemolysis, elevated liver enzymes, and low platelets) syndrome—may be catastrophic and rapidly fatal. This disease entity was discussed in the first section of this chapter in regard to microangiopathic hemolytic anemia. TTP was defined by a pentad of abnormalities: TP from increased platelet destruction; microangiopathic hemolytic anemia caused by mechanical damage to red cells as a result of the vascular lesions; neurologic abnormalities; renal abnormalities; and fever. With the advent of curative plasma exchange in the 1970s, the urgency to establish a diagnosis and start treatment has resulted in using limited diagnostic criteria. Now only TP and microangiopathic hemolytic anemia are sufficient to begin plasmapheresis.

The clinical presentation is variable, but the TP and hemolytic anemia are often severe. A wide variety of fluctuating neurologic abnormalities may be present, including seizures, altered consciousness, delirium, and paresis. Renal abnormalities may include uremia, hematuria, and proteinuria. The reasons for fever are unclear. The typical presentation for young children is to have a prodrome of bloody diarrhea caused by the Shiga toxin-producing enterohemorrhagic strain of *E. coli.* The laboratory findings in TTP are basically those related above: TP, hemolytic anemia with red cell fragmentation, and renal dysfunction. Elevation of serum lactic acid dehydrogenase from intravascular hemolysis, and perhaps also damage to other tissues, is an index of activity of the disease; coagulation tests are usually normal.

The basic pathogenic mechanism behind these syndromes is likely related to the vascular endothelial cells. A role for ultralarge von Willebrand factor (vWF) multimers has been identified and is linked to endothelial damage and the occurrence of disseminated platelet thrombi. Recently, a specific metalloprotease (ADAMTS13) that rapidly cleaves these multimers has been identified (60,61). Deficiency of this metalloprotease activity appears to be associated with many, but not all, TTP cases (62).

Treatment

Plasma exchange has dramatically changed TTP-HUS prognosis and outcome. Plasma infusion is less effective in adults, but it may be adequate in congenital TTP caused by ADAMTS13 deficiency. The duration of plasma exchange is unpredictable. Long durations, up to several months, may be required in patients with repeated relapses. The efficacy of additional treatments such as prednisone, platelet aggregation inhibitors, and splenectomy is unknown (see http://moon.ouhsc.edu/jgeorge).

Alcoholism-Associated Thrombocytopenia

Platelet counts less than 100,000 cells/μL are present in over one-fourth of critically ill alcoholic patients. There are many possible causes for TP in such patients, including hypersplenism and folic acid deficiency. However, it is important to recognize that reversible severe TP may occur as a direct effect of alcohol ingestion in some patients. Studies of the mechanism have demonstrated elements of both decreased effective platelet production and shortened platelet survival; abnormalities of platelet function have been noted as well. Recovery begins 2 to 3 days after cessation of alcohol ingestion, and maximum PC is reached in 1 to 3 weeks. There is often an overshoot to abnormally high platelet counts, which then return to baseline levels. Therapy consists of having the patient discontinue alcohol ingestion and providing appropriate supportive measures.

Thrombocytopenia Associated with Bone Marrow Disorders

Severe TP from impaired platelet production is a frequent concomitant of bone marrow disorders, such as aplastic anemia, leukemia, or other malignancies metastatic to the bone marrow, as well as cytotoxic chemotherapy of such disorders. Treatment is directed at the underlying disease.

INCREASED BLOOD COUNTS

Erythrocytosis

Erythrocytosis, defined as an abnormally increased red cell mass, may require critical care due to complications of blood hyperviscosity or because of hemorrhagic or thromboembolic complications that may threaten these patients. The initial clue to the presence of erythrocytosis is usually a high value for hematocrit or hemoglobin concentration. Such values may be present without true erythrocytosis—that is, in the presence of a normal red cell mass—if the plasma volume is contracted. This circumstance is usually apparent, although it is often advisable to quantify the red cell mass (RCM) by direct measurement using radioisotopic red cell labels. The RCM is usually increased when the hematocrit is above 60% in a man or 57% in a woman.

Pathophysiology

True erythrocytosis results from one of two general mechanisms:

- Polycythemia vera (PV) is a clonal abnormality of bone marrow stem cells resulting in autonomous overproduction of red cells and often of granulocytes and platelets;
- Secondary erythrocytosis results from excess erythropoietin production in response to hypoxemia, abnormalities of oxygen release from hemoglobin, or autonomous hormone production (e.g., by renal or other tumors).

When the RCM is expanded and the hematocrit increased, blood viscosity is increased, and diminished blood flow, stasis, thrombosis, and tissue hypoxia may ensue. On the other hand, hemorrhagic tendency is also increased, particularly in PV, where elevated platelet counts and abnormalities of platelet function may also be present.

Diagnosis

Criteria for the diagnosis of PV have been modified multiple times since the first criteria were published by Modan and Lilienfeld (63) in 1965; modified diagnostic criteria are shown in Table 146.5 (64). The detection by PCR of Janus kinase 2 (JAK2) tyrosine kinase in up to 97% of patients with PV increases the sensitivity and specificity of early diagnosis. The JAK2 V617F point mutation makes hematopoietic progenitors hypersensitive to the different growth factors, resulting in proliferation of all lineages (65). Risks in uncontrolled PV are primarily hyperviscosity and thromboembolic or hemorrhagic events. Symptoms resulting from decreased cerebral flow, such as headache, dizziness, and changes in vision are the most common manifestations of hyperviscosity. Hemorrhage or thrombosis can affect almost any body part; peptic ulcer disease with bleeding is common and thromboses may be arterial or venous. Fatigue, plethora, pruritus–particularly with hot bath, excessive sweating, paresthesias (erythromelalgia), fullness in the left upper abdomen (splenomegaly), and shortness of breath are also some manifestations of PV. Surgery poses an enormous risk in the patient with uncontrolled PV because of a high incidence of thrombotic or hemorrhagic complications.

The diagnosis of secondary erythrocytosis is made in a patient with an increased RCM in whom the criteria for PV are not met. These patients could either have physiologically appropriate increased RCM (e.g., secondary to tissue hypoxemia) or inappropriate increased RCM (e.g., secondary to increased erythropoietin production). Additional studies are needed to differentiate the diverse causes of polycythemia.

Treatment

Patients with uncontrolled PV may present as medical emergencies requiring ICU care and urgent therapy. The mainstay of such therapy is phlebotomy to reduce hematocrit to less than 45%. This may be done as rapidly as 1 unit of blood every other day in young adults. Electrolyte solutions or plasma expanders should be administered with phlebotomy, as necessary, to avoid circulatory instability from sudden changes in blood volume. Elderly patients may tolerate phlebotomy less well, so that removal of volumes of 200 to 300 mL at less frequent intervals may be necessary. Because of the clinical observations of increased thrombosis with aggressive phlebotomy, the simultaneous use of cytotoxic chemotherapy is recommended as part of the initial therapy of patients older than 60 years of age, as well as in younger patients with thrombotic risk factors or a history of thrombosis. Hydroxyurea is often used for this purpose in an initial dose of 15 to 30 mg/kg/day. Emergency plateletpheresis may also be considered in such emergencies to lower an elevated platelet count. The FDA approved a new drug in December 2014, Jakafi (ruxolitinib, a JAK2 inhibitor), to be used in PV patients who have an inadequate response to or intolerance to hydroxyurea.

Other treatment options include low-dose aspirin (81 mg/day), interferon-α, and anagrelide; these may be used together with phlebotomy as needed. In general, patients with PV should avoid practices and habits that augment hypercoagulability such as smoking, use of oral contraceptives, or hormone replacement therapy. Aggressive antithrombotic prophylaxis should be given postoperatively in addition to maintaining normal hematocrit and platelet counts.

Indications for phlebotomy in secondary erythrocytosis are less clear than in PV. The best current advice is to individualize therapy so as to maximize the patient's exercise tolerance and overall sense of well-being.

TABLE 146.5 Proposed Modified Criteria for the Diagnosis of Polycythemia Vera

Symptom categories	
A1	Raised red cell mass (>25% above mean normal predicted value, or a hematocrit value >60% in males or >56% in females)
A2	Absence of causes of secondary erythrocytosis
A3	Palpable splenomegaly
A4	Clonality marker (i.e., acquired abnormal marrow karyotype)
B1	Thrombocytosis (platelet count >400 × 10³ cells/μL)
B2	Neutrophil leukocytosis (neutrophil count >10 × 10³ cells/μL, or >12.5 × 10³ cells/μL in smokers)
B3	Splenomegaly demonstrated on isotope or ultrasound scanning
B4	Characteristic erythroid burst-forming unit growth or reduced serum erythropoietin
Diagnostic scoring	
A1 + A2 + A3 or A4 establishes polycythemia vera.	
A1 + A2 + two of B establishes polycythemia vera.	

Adapted from Pearson TC, Messinezy M, Westwood N, et al. A polycythemia vera updated: diagnosis, pathobiology, and treatment. *Hematology Am Soc Hematol Educ Program*. 2000;51–68.

Thrombocytosis

With the availability of a PC as part of a routine blood count, an elevated platelet count, or thrombocytosis, has become an important clinical problem in hospitalized patients. Unlike TP, the literature dealing with thrombocytosis in ICU patients is very scant, however the presence of thrombocytosis predicts a favorable outcome in ICU patients, whereas a blunted rise in PC may be associated with worse outcome.

Pathophysiology and Diagnosis

Thrombocytosis in hospitalized patients is classified into primary (clonal) and secondary (reactive) forms. Primary thrombocytosis refers to a persistent elevation of PC due to clonal thrombopoiesis, as it occurs in myeloproliferative disorders including essential thrombocythemia (ET), PV, myelodysplastic syndrome, chronic myelogenous leukemia, and primary myelofibrosis (PMF). The discovery of JAK2 V617F and MPL exon 10 mutations allows for the positive identification of ET in more than 50% of patients, although differentiation from PV and PMF is still needed. Secondary thrombocytosis is due to various conditions, some of them short-lived, such as acute bleeding, infection, trauma or other tissue injury, and surgery; other causes, such as malignancy, postsplenectomy, chronic infection, iron deficiency, or chronic inflammatory disease may persist for a longer time. Multiple studies have been conducted on adult and pediatric hospitalized patients (66–70) with an elevated PC (>500 × 10³ cells/μL), and the main conclusions suggest that whereas most patients have secondary thrombocytosis, a higher PC and increased thromboembolic complications are significantly associated with primary thrombocytosis. In one study, even when using greater than or equal to $1,000 \times 10^3$ cells/μL as the basis for defining extreme thrombocytosis, 82% of 231 patients analyzed were found to have an elevated PC due to reactive (secondary) thrombocytosis (71). In this study, the risk of bleeding and/or thrombosis was 56% in primary thrombocytosis, but only 4% in the secondary type. Unless additional risk factors are present, secondary thrombocytosis is not associated with an increased risk of thromboembolic events.

Treatment

Treatment for primary thrombocytosis, such as ET, is based on risks for thrombosis or bleeding in the presence of vasomotor symptoms. Patients at increased risk (age >60 years, history of thromboembolism, PC >1,500,000 cells/μL) should receive platelet-lowering agents such as hydroxyurea, anagrelide, or interferon-α (IFN-α). Low-dose aspirin can be used for the relief of vasomotor symptoms, but if there is no relief, platelet-lowering agents should be added. Hydroxyurea is the recommended drug in patients 60 years of age or older, whereas IFN-α is the cytoreductive agent of choice for childbearing women. The aim should be to lower the PC to less than 400,000 cells/μL. Arterial or venous thrombosis should be treated with heparin and, possibly, thrombolysis in some arterial events; plateletpheresis may be indicated in both types of events. Low-dose aspirin may be useful in arterial thrombosis. In hemorrhage, it is appropriate to stop antiplatelet agents and transfuse platelets if the bleeding is persistent. Some patients with uncontrolled thrombocytosis (>1,500,000 cells/μL) were found to have an acquired defect of von Willebrand factor, which contributes to the risk of bleeding. Thus, DDAVP, cryoprecipitate, or factor VIII concentrate may be indicated to treat hemorrhage in these patients.

LEUKOCYTOSIS

Pathophysiology

As in thrombocytosis, leukocytosis can be due to primary bone marrow disorders or secondary disorders in response to acute infection or inflammation. Secondary leukocytosis is physiologic and transient, resolving after treating the underlying cause. *Leukemoid reaction* refers to a persistent leukocytosis of more than 50,000 cells/μL, with shift to the left. The major causes for such a reaction include severe infections, severe hemorrhage, acute hemolysis, hypersensitivity, and a malignancy-induced paraneoplastic syndrome.

Diagnosis

Leukocytosis due to a primary bone marrow disorder with uncontrolled clonal growth of immature cells can result in an emergency situation known as the hyperleukocytosis syndrome. This occurs in leukemic states when the WBC count is high. Signs and symptoms are most commonly related to the central nervous system, eyes, and lungs. They include stupor, altered mentation, dizziness, visual blurring, retinal abnormalities, dyspnea, tachypnea, and hypoxia. Intracranial and pulmonary infarction or hemorrhage and sudden death may occur. Priapism and peripheral vascular insufficiency have also been linked with the syndrome. Although the pathogenesis is incompletely understood, autopsies have shown white cell aggregates, microthrombi, and microvascular invasion (leukostatic tumors). The syndrome occurs more commonly in acute (AML) and chronic myelogenous leukemia (CML) than in acute lymphoblastic leukemia, and occurs rarely, if ever, in chronic lymphocytic leukemia. The level of the WBC count at which the syndrome appears is variable, depending perhaps on the maturity and size of the white blood cells present and the degree of coexisting anemia. A white count exceeding 100,000 cells/μL in acute myelogenous leukemia or the accelerated phase of CML is usually an alarming sign and an indication for prompt treatment.

Treatment

If there are signs or symptoms attributable to the hyperleukocytosis syndrome, then leukopheresis is indicated to rapidly and safely decrease the white count. At the same time, chemotherapy should be initiated, and treatment with allopurinol and intravenous hydration with urine alkalinization should be started in anticipation of the hyperuricemia. Hydroxyurea (6 g by mouth) is frequently used initially to produce rapid leukemic cell kill.

OTHER HEMATOLOGIC DISORDERS

Plasma Cell Dyscrasias

The presenting symptoms for these malignant disorders may include severe infection, spinal cord compression, or hyperviscosity syndrome that can lead to admission to the ICU. Total serum protein will be abnormally high on routine chemistry blood test. Subsequent evaluation will reveal an IgM monoclonal gammopathy in Waldenstrom macroglobulinemia or IgG/IgA in multiple myeloma. Hyperviscosity syndrome is rare and less frequent when IgG or IgA, respectively, are the abnormal proteins. The most common manifestations of the hyperviscosity syndrome are neurologic and include headache, visual disturbances, hearing loss, vertigo, altered consciousness—ranging from stupor to coma—paresis, seizures, and peripheral neuropathy. A bleeding tendency may exist because of the associated TP or interference by the abnormal protein with the function of platelets or plasma coagulation factors. The most rapidly effective form of therapy for hyperviscosity from serum protein abnormalities is plasmapheresis. At the same time, hydration and specific therapy for the underlying disease should be started.

STEM CELL TRANSPLANTATION

Patients after stem cell transplantation (SCT)—mainly allogeneic—constitute a large proportion of those with hematologic disorders who are admitted to the ICU. These patients are usually admitted with respiratory distress requiring mechanical ventilation, multiorgan failure, or septic shock, and have the highest mortality among cancer patients admitted to the ICU (72,73). Because of the generally poor outcome, especially for patients requiring mechanical ventilation, the utility of such support has been questioned (74,75). It is generally accepted that patients admitted to the ICU during the engraftment period should be fully supported because of better outcome (76). These patients may have the *engraftment syndrome,* which can result in cytokine-induced capillary leak syndrome with multiorgan failure or alveolar hemorrhage; early high-dose steroids can dramatically reverse the downhill course. These patients should also undergo bronchoscopy to rule out infection while receiving the steroid therapy. Early intervention and transfer to ICU in septic shock will result in improved outcome. After autologous SCT, patients usually have better survival in the ICU than after allogeneic SCT, even those requiring mechanical ventilation.

Admission to the surgical ICU is less frequent for patients after SCT, but some of the most frequent reasons include intestinal perforation and intracranial bleeding. This topic is dealt with in more detail elsewhere in this textbook.

Key Points

- Benign and malignant hematologic disorders are frequently encountered in patients admitted to the intensive care units. Some of these disorders develop while patients are in the ICU for other reasons, such as anemia, HIT, TTP, and other drug-induced cytopenias.
- Other disorders are the primary reason for admission to the ICU and include neutropenic fever and septic shock, respiratory distress, serious life-threatening bleeding, and other disease-specific and chemotherapy-related complications.
- Familiarity with these problems and the early involvement of the hematology service in the evaluation and treatment of these specific entities are essential for better outcome and improved survival.
- The approach to patients with suspected (4Ts score 4 or more) or confirmed HIT includes the following:
  - Discontinuation of all heparin.
  - Administration of alternative nonheparin anticoagulation, such as argatroban or lepirudin.
  - Testing for anti-PF4/heparin antibodies, followed, if positive, by an SRA.
  - Avoiding prophylactic platelet transfusions.
  - Allowing platelet recovery before starting warfarin.
  - Assessing for lower extremity DVT.
- Patients with previous HIT:
  - Those who are antibody-negative and require cardiac surgery should receive UFH in preference to other anticoagulants, which are less validated for this purpose.
  - Preoperative and postoperative anticoagulation should be handled with an anticoagulant other than UFH or LMWH.
  - Patients with recent or active HIT should have surgery delayed until antibody is negative, if possible; otherwise, an alternative anticoagulant should be used (77).

References

1. Till JL, McCulloch EA, Siminovitch L. A stochastic model of stem cell proliferation, based on the growth of spleen colony-forming cells. *Proc Natl Acad Sci U S A.* 1964;51:29–36.
2. MacKey MC. Cell kinetic status of haematopoietic stem cells. *Cell Prolif.* 2001;34:71–83.
3. Smith C. Hematopoietic stem cells and hematopoiesis. *Cancer Control.* 2003; 10:9–16.
4. Domen J, Weissman IL. Self-renewal, differentiation or death: regulation and manipulation of hematopoietic stem cell fate. *Mol Med Today.* 1999; 5:201–208.
5. Domen J, Cheshier SH, Weissman IL. The role of apoptosis in the regulation of hematopoietic stem cells: overexpression of Bcl-2 increases both their number and repopulation potential. *J Exp Med.* 2000;191:253–264.
6. Orkin SH, Zon LI. Hematopoiesis and stem cells: plasticity versus developmental heterogeneity. *Nat Immunol.* 2002;3:323–328.
7. Baldo BA. Side effects of cytokines approved for therapy. *Drug Saf.* 2014; 37:921–943.
8. Arend WP, Malyak M, Bigler CF, et al. The biological role of naturally-occurring cytokine inhibitors. *Br J Rheumatol.* 1991;30(Suppl 2):49–52.
9. Moldawer LL. Interleukin-1, TNF alpha and their naturally occurring antagonists in sepsis. *Blood Purif.* 1993;11:128–133.
10. Blackwell TS, Christman JW. Sepsis and cytokines: current status. *Br J Anaesth.* 1996;77:110–117.
11. Kox WJ, Volk T, Kox SN, Volk HD. Immunomodulatory therapies in sepsis. *Intensive Care Med.* 2000;26(Suppl 1):S124–S128.
12. Osuchowski MF, Welch K, Siddiqui J, Remick DG. Circulating cytokine/inhibitor profiles reshape the understanding of the SIRS/CARS continuum in sepsis and predict mortality. *J Immunol.* 2006;177:1967–1974.
13. Zhao JL, Baltimore D. Regualtion of stress-induced hematopoiesis. *Curr Opin Hematol.* 2015;22:286–292.
14. Fakhry SM, Fata P. How low is too low? Cardiac risks with anemia. *Crit Care.* 2004;8(Suppl 2):S11–S14.
15. Napolitano LM. Scope of the problem: epidemiology of anemia and use of blood transfusions in critical care. *Crit Care.* 2004;8(Suppl 2):S1–S8.
16. van de Wiel A. Anemia in critically ill patients. *Eur J Int Med.* 2004;15:481–486.
17. Hébert PC, Wells G, Blajchman MA, et al. A multicenter, randomized, controlled clinical trial of transfusion requirements in critical care. Transfusion Requirements in Critical Care Investigators, Canadian Critical Care Trials Group. *N Engl J Med.* 1999;340:409–417.
18. Villanueva C, Colomo A, Bosch A, et al. Transfusion strategies for acute upper gastrointestinal bleeding. *N Engl J Med.* 2013;368:11–21.
19. Holst LB, Haase N, Wetterslev J, et al. Lower versus higher hemoglobin threshold for transfusion in septic shock. *N Engl J Med.* 2014;371:1381–1391.
20. Holst LB, Petersen MW, Haase N, et al. Restrictive versus liberal transfusion strategy for red blood cell transfusion: systematic review of randomised trials with meta-analysis and trial sequential analysis. *BMJ.* 2015;350:h1354.
21. Carson JL, Grossman BJ, Kleinman S, et al.; Clinical Transfusion Medicine Committee of the AABB. Red blood cell transfusion: a clinical practice guideline from the AABB. *Ann Intern Med.* 2012;157:49–58.
22. Corwin HL, Gettinger A, Pearl RG, et al. The CRIT study: anemia and blood transfusion in the critically ill–current clinical practice in the United States. *Crit Care Med.* 2004;32:39–52.
23. Vincent JL, Baron JF, Reinhart K, et al. Anemia and blood transfusion in critically ill patients. *JAMA.* 2002;288:1499–1507.
24. Andrews NC. Anemia of inflammation: the cytokine-hepcidin link. *J Clin Invest.* 2004;113:1251–1253.
25. Corwin HL, Gettinger A, Pearl RG, et al.; EPO Critical Care Trials Group. Efficacy of recombinant human erythropoietin in critically ill patients: a randomized controlled trial. *JAMA.* 2002;288:2827–2835.
26. Silver M, Corwin MJ, Bazan A, et al. Efficacy of recombinant human erythropoietin in critically ill patients admitted to a long-term acute care facility: a randomized, double-blind, placebo-controlled trial. *Crit Care Med.* 2006;34:2310–2316.
27. Reardon JE, Marquea MB. Laboratory evaluation and transfusion support of patients with autoimmune hemolytic anemia. *Am J Clin Pathol.* 2006;125(Suppl 1):S71–S77.
28. Chinevere TD, Murray CK, Grant E Jr, et al. Prevalence of glucose-6-phosphate dehydrogenase deficiency in U.S. Army personnel. *Mil Med.* 2006;171:905–907.
29. Scully M, Hunt BJ, Benjamin S, et al. Guidelines on the diagnosis and management of thrombotic thrombocytopenic purpura and other thrombotic microangiopathies. *Br J Haematol.* 2012;158:323–335.
30. Sears DA. Sickle cell trait. In: Embury SH, Hebbel RP, Mohandas N, et al., eds. *Sickle Cell Disease: Basic Principles and Clinical Practice.* New York: Raven Press; 1994:381.
31. Brown AK, Sleeper LA, Miller ST, et al. Reference values and hematological changes from birth to five years in patients with sickle cell disease. *Arch Pediatr Adolesc Med.* 1994;48:796–804.
32. Steinberg MH. Management of sickle cell anemia. *N Engl J Med.* 1999;340: 1021–1030.

33. Cecchini J, Lionnet F, Djibré M, et al. Outcomes of adult patients with sickle cell disease admitted to the ICU: a case series. *Crit Care Med.* 2014;42:1629–1639.
34. Rice L, Teruya M. Sickle cell patients face death in the ICU. *Crit Care Med.* 2014;42:1730–1731.
35. Lefrere JJ, Courouce AM, Bertrand Y, et al. Human parvovirus and aplastic crisis in chronic hemolytic anemias: a study of 24 observations. *Am J Hematol.* 1986;23:271–275.
36. Hughes WT, Armstrong D, Bodey GP, et al. 2002 guidelines for the use of antimicrobial agents in neutropenic patients with cancer. *Clin Infect Dis.* 2002;34:730–751.
37. van de Wetering MD, de Witte MA, Kremer LC, et al. Efficacy of oral prophylactic antibiotics in neutropenic afebrile oncology patients: a systematic review of randomised controlled trials. *Eur J Cancer.* 2005;41:1372–1382.
38. Gafter-Gvili A, Fraser A, Paul M, Leibovici L. Meta-analysis: antibiotic prophylaxis reduces mortality in neutropenic patients. *Ann Intern Med.* 2005;142:979–995.
39. Smith TJ, Bohlke K, Lyman GH, et al. Recommendations for the use of WBC growth factors: American Society of Clinical Oncology clinical practice guideline update. *J Clin Oncol.* 2015;33(28):3199–3212.
40. Azoulay E, Darmon M, Delclaux C, et al. Deterioration of previous acute lung injury during neutropenia recovery. *Crit Care Med.* 2002;30:781–786.
41. Karlin L, Darmon M, Thiery G, et al. Respiratory status deterioration during G-CSF-induced neutropenia recovery. *Bone Marrow Transplant.* 2005;36:245–250.
42. Akca S, Haji-Michael P, de Mendonca A, et al. Time course of platelet counts in critically ill patients. *Crit Care Med.* 2002;30:753–756.
43. Williamson DR, Albert M, Heels-Ansdell D, et al. Thrombocytopenia in critically ill patients receiving thromboprophylaxis: frequency, risk factors, and outcomes. *Chest.* 2013;144:1207–1215.
44. Williamson DR, Lesur O, Tétrault JP, et al. Thrombocytopenia in the critically ill: prevalence, incidence, risk factors, and clinical outcomes. *Can J Anaesth.* 2013;60:641–651.
45. Thiele T, Selleng K, Selleng S, et al. Thrombocytopenia in the intensive care unit-diagnostic approach and management. *Semin Hematol.* 2013;50: 239–250.
46. Vanderschueren S, De Weerdt A, Malbrain M, et al. Thrombocytopenia and prognosis in intensive care. *Crit Care Med.* 2000;28:1871–1876.
47. Napolitano LM, Warkentin TE, Almahameed A, Nasraway SA. Heparin-induced thrombocytopenia in the critical care setting: diagnosis and Management. *Crit Care Med.* 2006;34:2898–2911.
48. Van der Linden T, Souweine B, Dupic L, et al. Management of thrombocytopenia in the ICU (pregnancy excluded). *Ann Intensive Care.* 2012;2:42.
49. Levine RL, Hergenroeder GW, Francis JL, et al. Heparin-platelet factor 4 antibodies in intensive care patients: an observational seroprevalence study. *J Thromb Thrombolysis.* 2010;30:142–148.
50. Warkentin TE. Management of heparin-induced thrombocytopenia: a critical comparison of lepirudin and argatroban. *Thromb Res.* 2003;110:73–82.
51. Cuker A, Gimotty PA, Crowther MA, Warkentin TE. Predictive value of the 4Ts scoring system for heparin-induced thrombocytopenia: a systematic review and meta-analysis. *Blood.* 2012;120:4160–4167.
52. Linkins LA, Bates SM, Lee AY, et al. Combination of 4Ts score and PF4/H-PaGIA for diagnosis and management of heparin-induced thrombocytopenia: prospective cohort study. *Blood.* 2015;126:597–603.
53. Kaufman RM, Djulbegovic B, Gernsheimer T, et al. Clinical guidelines platelet transfusion: a clinical practice guideline. *Ann Intern Med.* 2015;162:20.
54. Wandt H, Schaefer-Eckart K, Wendelin K, et al.; Study Alliance Leukemia. Therapeutic platelet transfusion versus routine prophylactic transfusion in patients with haematological malignancies: an open-label, multicentre, randomised study. *Lancet.* 2012;380:1309–1316.
55. Stanworth SJ, Estcourt LJ, Powter G, et al.; TOPPS Investigators. A no-prophylaxis platelet-transfusion strategy for hematologic cancers. *N Engl J Med.* 2013;368:1771–1780.
56. Coppo P, Adrie C, Azoulay E, et al. Infectious diseases as a trigger in thrombotic microangiopathies in intensive care unit (ICU) patients? *Intensive Care Med.* 2003;29:564–569.
57. Drews RE, Weinberger SE. Thrombocytopenic disorders in critically ill patients. *Am J Respir Crit Care Med.* 2000;162(2 Pt 1):347–351.
58. Morrin MJ, Jones FG, McConville J, et al. Thrombotic thrombocytopenic purpura secondary to Streptococcus. *Transfus Apher Sci.* 2006;34:153–155.
59. Drews RE. Critical issues in hematology: anemia, thrombocytopenia, coagulopathy, and blood product transfusions in critically ill patients. *Clin Chest Med.* 2003;24:607–622.
60. Tsai HM. Physiologic cleavage of von Willebrand factor by a plasma protease is dependent on its conformation and requires calcium ion. *Blood.* 1996;87:4235–4244.
61. Furlan M, Robles R, Galbusera M, et al. von Willebrand factor-cleaving protease in thrombotic thrombocytopenic purpura and the hemolytic-uremic syndrome. *N Engl J Med.* 1998;339:1578–1584.
62. Dlott JS, Danielson CF, Blue-Hnidy DE, McCarthy LJ. Drug-induced thrombotic thrombocytopenic purpura/hemolytic uremic syndrome: a concise review. *Ther Apher Dial.* 2004;8:102–111.
63. Modan B, Lilienfeld AM. Polycythemia vera and leukemia—the role of radiation treatment. a study of 1222 patients. *Medicine (Baltimore).* 1965;44: 305–344.
64. Pearson TC, Messinezy M, Westwood N, et al. A polycythemia vera updated: diagnosis, pathobiology, and treatment. *Hematology Am Soc Hematol Educ Program.* 2000;51–68.
65. Bellucci S, Michiels JJ. The role of JAK2 V617F mutation, spontaneous erythropoiesis and megakaryocytopoiesis, hypersensitive platelets, activated leukocytes, and endothelial cells in the etiology of thrombotic manifestations in polycythemia vera and essential thrombocythemia. *Semin Thromb Hemost.* 2006;32(4 Pt 2):381–398.
66. Santhosh-Kumar CR, Yohannan MD, Higgy KE, al-Mashhadani SA. Thrombocytosis in adults: analysis of 777 patients. *J Intern Med.* 1991;229: 493–495.
67. Griesshammer M, Bangerter M, Sauer T, et al. Aetiology and clinical significance of thrombocytosis: analysis of 732 patients with an elevated platelet count. *J Intern Med.* 1999;245:295–300.
68. Chen HL, Chiou SS, Sheen JM, et al. Thrombocytosis in children at one medical center of southern Taiwan. *Acta Paediatr Taiwan.* 1999;40:309–313.
69. Gurung AM, Carr B, Smith I. Thrombocytosis in intensive care. *Br J Anaesth.* 2001;87:926–928.
70. Valade N, Decailliot F, Rebufat Y, et al. Thrombocytosis after trauma: incidence, aetiology, and clinical significance. *Br J Anaesth.* 2005;94:18–23.
71. Buss DH, Cashell AW, O'Connor ML, et al. Occurrence, etiology, and clinical significance of extreme thrombocytosis: a study of 280 cases. *Am J Med.* 1994;96:247–253.
72. Staudinger T, Stoiser B, Mullner M, et al. Outcome and prognostic factors in critically ill cancer patients admitted to the intensive care unit. *Crit Care Med.* 2000;28:1322–1328.
73. Benz R, Schanz U, Maggiorini M, et al. Risk factors for ICU admission and ICU survival after allogeneic hematopoietic SCT. *Bone Marrow Transplant.* 2014;49:62–65.
74. Naeem N, Reed MD, Creger RJ, et al. Transfer of the hematopoietic stem cell transplant patient to the intensive care unit: does it really matter? *Bone Marrow Transplant.* 2006;37:119–133.
75. Kew AK, Couban S, Patrick W, et al. Outcome of hematopoietic stem cell transplant recipients admitted to the intensive care unit. *Biol Blood Marrow Transplant.* 2006;12:301–305.
76. Pene F, Aubron C, Azoulay E, et al. Outcome of critically ill allogeneic hematopoietic stem-cell transplantation recipients: a reappraisal of indications for organ failure supports. *J Clin Oncol.* 2006;24:643–649.
77. Keeling D, Davidson S, Watson H. Haemostasis and thrombosis task force of the British committee for standards in haematology: The management of heparin-induced thrombocytopenia. *Br J Haematol.* 2006;133:259–269.

CHAPTER

147

Oncologic Emergencies

ADAM KLOTZ and JEFFREY GROEGER

INTRODUCTION

Cancer is the second leading cause of death in the United States, surpassed only by heart disease (1). New chemotherapeutic regimens, advances in hematopoietic stem cell transplantation (2), and the expansion of molecular targeted therapies (3,4) offer hope but may lead to complications rarely seen in the nononcologic patient. It is beyond the scope of this chapter to discuss all aspects of cancer that warrant admission to an intensive care unit. Topics such as infection in the immunocompromised host, shock, coagulation abnormalities, and multisystem organ failure are discussed elsewhere in this book. Herein, we focus on clinical conditions that arise either as a direct result of a neoplasm or antineoplastic therapies.

HYPERCALCEMIA

Hypercalcemia is the most common of the paraneoplastic syndromes, developing in 10% to 30% of all patients with malignancy at some time during their disease course (5–7). Breast cancer, lung cancer, and multiple myeloma represent the most common malignancies associated with hypercalcemia (5). The presence of hypercalcemia in a patient with cancer portends a poor prognosis, particularly when elevated parathyroid hormone–related protein (PTHrP) levels are detected (8–10).

Pathophysiology

Hypercalcemia of malignancy results from increased bone resorption and subsequent release of calcium from bone into the extracellular fluid (11). *Humoral hypercalcemia* of malignancy is the most common cause of cancer-induced hypercalcemia, seen in 80% of cases (7,12). The mechanism is mediated by PTHrP, which is secreted into the systemic circulation by malignant tumors (12–15). *Local osteolytic hypercalcemia* accounts for about 20% of cases of malignant hypercalcemia, and occurs when tumor cells present in bone metastases secrete cytokines which induce osteoclastic bone resorption. These agents stimulate local macrophages within the tumor to differentiate into osteoclasts. Local osteolytic hypercalcemia occurs frequently in breast cancer, non–small cell lung cancer (NSCLC), and multiple myeloma (9).

Symptoms of hypercalcemia correlate with the absolute concentration and the rapidity in rise of the serum calcium (Table 147.1) (16,17). Neurologic symptoms may be mild at lower serum calcium levels or when hypercalcemia develops slowly. Drowsiness or fatigue may progress to weakness, lethargy, stupor, and eventually coma in hypercalcemic crisis or in acutely rising hypercalcemia (11). Psychotic behavior, visual and speech abnormalities, hypotonia, and occasionally localizing signs on neurologic examination may be exhibited; these resolve with normalization of serum calcium (18,19). In older patients, neurologic dysfunction may be more pronounced even at lower concentrations of serum calcium (5).

Gastrointestinal (GI) symptoms are secondary to smooth muscle hypotonicity and include anorexia, nausea, vomiting, constipation, and abdominal pain (11). Infrequently, hypercalcemia may present as peptic ulcer disease (16) and pancreatitis (20).

Renal manifestations result from impaired water-concentrating ability as antidiuretic hormone secretion is inhibited by hypercalcemia. Dehydration decreases the glomerular filtration rate and further reduces renal excretion of excess serum calcium. To expand the extracellular volume, compensatory proximal tubular resorption of sodium and calcium occurs, leading to a paradoxical increase in serum calcium (21). Frank renal failure may ensue, particularly in the patient with multiple myeloma (11). In contrast to primary hyperparathyroidism, hypercalcemia of malignancy is rarely associated with nephrolithiasis and nephrocalcinosis (11,22).

Cardiovascular manifestations of hypercalcemia stem from increased myocardial contractility and irritability (11). Electrocardiographic changes include a PR-interval prolongation, QRS-complex widening, QT-interval shortening, and T-wave changes (16). At increasing serum calcium levels, patients may experience bradydysrhythmias and bundle branch block, with progression to AV nodal block and cardiac arrest at serum concentrations above 18 mg/dL (11).

Patients with hypercalcemia, may experience bone pain or pathologic fractures secondary to osteolytic metastases or humorally mediated bone resorption (11).

Diagnosis

Calcium is present in the extracellular fluid in three fractions: 50% is the ionized free fraction, 40% is protein bound (primarily to albumin and not renally filtered), and 10% is complexed to anions (13,23). Hypercalcemia is diagnosed by measuring the ionized calcium level, as this is the biologically active level that correlates with the signs and symptoms of hypercalcemia. Except in the presence of hypoalbuminemia, the ionized calcium level can be inferred from the total plasma calcium. In cancer patients with hypoalbuminemia, the following correction must be performed: for each 1 g/dL decrease in serum albumin, there is a 0.8 mg/dL decrease in serum calcium. This method of calculation is inaccurate in the presence of calcium-binding immunoglobulins, as seen in multiple myeloma.

Once the diagnosis of hypercalcemia is confirmed by obtaining corrected calcium levels, measurement of the intact PTH level can elucidate the mechanism. The intact PTH level is suppressed in hypercalcemia of malignancy and elevated in primary hyperparathyroidism. A low serum chloride (<100 mEq/L) suggests hypercalcemia of malignancy, whereas elevation of serum chloride is caused by hyperchloremic acidosis

TABLE 147.1 Clinical Manifestations in Hypercalcemia

NEUROLOGIC
Drowsiness, weakness, lethargy
Stupor, coma
Psychosis
Visual and speech impairment
Focal neurologic deficits
GASTROINTESTINAL
Anorexia
Nausea, vomiting
Constipation
Abdominal pain
Peptic ulcer disease
Pancreatitis
RENAL
Nephrogenic diabetes insipidus
Acute renal failure
CARDIAC
PR interval prolongation
QRS complex widening
QT interval shortening
T-wave changes
Bradyarrhythmias
Bundle branch block
AV nodal block
Cardiac arrest
BONE
Pain
Pathologic fractures

resulting from PTH-induced renal bicarbonate loss seen in hyperparathyroidism (22).

Treatment

The only effective long-term means of reversing malignancy-associated hypercalcemia is reduction in tumor burden (Table 147.2). Antihypercalcemic therapy is a temporizing measure that does not affect survival (5). The aggressiveness of the therapeutic approach depends on the potential for palliation and cure. When all antitumor strategies have failed, or in patients who do not wish to pursue further treatment of their cancer, an ethical, humane, and appropriate approach may involve withholding antihypercalcemic treatment (5,9).

Stewart (5) has classified hypercalcemia based on serum calcium levels into mild hypercalcemia (10.5 to 11.9 mg/dL), moderate hypercalcemia (12.0 to 13.9 mg/dL), and severe hypercalcemia (14.0 mg/dL or greater). In addition to the magnitude of hypercalcemia, the severity of symptoms and the underlying cause are important factors in formulating an appropriate treatment strategy. In general, severe hypercalcemia requires emergent, aggressive treatment in the presence or absence of symptoms, whereas interventions in mild-to-moderate hypercalcemia are contingent on the severity of the symptoms. Prior to initiating therapy, the clinician should assess the patient for correctable factors that may contribute to hypercalcemia such as calcium-containing intravenous fluids, parenteral nutrition, and oral calcium supplements. In addition, thiazide diuretics, vitamins A and D, calcitriol, lithium, and estrogens or antiestrogens should be held (11). Immobilization is a well-established cause of hypercalcemia, and weight-bearing ambulation is recommended whenever possible (24). Finally, hypercalcemia is more difficult to treat in the setting of hypophosphatemia; oral or nasogastric phosphate supplementation should be administered to keep the calcium-phosphate product between 30 and 40. Intravenous phosphorous replacement may precipitate hypocalcemia, seizures, and acute renal failure, and is reserved for patients in whom oral or nasogastric administration cannot be performed (5).

Fluids and Diuretics

The initial intervention in the treatment of hypercalcemia is the administration of isotonic saline at a rate of 200 to 500 mL/hr based on the degree of hypovolemia and renal and cardiovascular dysfunction to maintain urine output of 150 to 200 mL/hr (5). Once the fluid deficit is replaced, the infusion rate should be decreased to 100 to 200 mL/hr in patients without cardiac or renal impairment (20). The patient must be carefully monitored to prevent fluid overload. Saline hydration reduces serum calcium level by increasing the glomerular filtration rate and increasing calcium delivery to the proximal tubule where urinary calcium excretion is augmented by the calciuric effects of saline (5).

Loop diuretics inhibit calcium reabsorption at the loop of Henle, increasing calciuresis. These agents should be used

TABLE 147.2 Treatment of Hypercalcemia of Malignancy

DEFINITIVE TREATMENT	
Antitumor therapy to reduce tumor burden	
INITIAL TREATMENT	
Removal of exogenous calcium sources: Intravenous fluids parenteral nutrition, oral calcium supplements, thiazide diuretics, vitamins A and D, calcitriol, lithium, estrogens, antiestrogens	
Weight-bearing ambulation	
Phosphate repletion	
Fluids and diuresis	
Saline hydration	
Loop diuretics	Judicious use in euvolemic or hypervolemic patients; now less favorable because of hypokalemia, hypomagnesemia, volume depletion
PHARMACOLOGIC TREATMENT	
Bisphosphonate therapy	
Principal agents in hypercalcemic treatment	
Zoledronate	15-minute infusion
Pamidronate	2-hour infusion
	Bisphosphonate adverse effects: Acute and chronic renal failure, fever arthralgias, ocular inflammation, electrolyte imbalance, osteonecrosis of the jaw
Other agents	
Calcitonin	Useful in congestive heart failure or renal failure
Glucocorticoids	Used in lymphomas with elevated levels of 1,25-vitamin D
Denosumab	For bisphosphonate-refractory hypercalcemia or renal insufficiency
DIALYSIS	
For patients with renal failure or congestive heart failure	

judiciously and only after euvolemia is achieved in hypovolemic patients or in patients who present with volume overload (5,9,18). Because of ensuing complications such as hypokalemia, hypomagnesemia, and volume depletion, and because of the availability of bisphosphonates, loop diuretics are used less favorably in clinical practice (24).

Bisphosphonate Therapy

Bisphosphonates inhibit osteoclastic bone resorption and are the principal agents used in the management of hypercalcemia of malignancy (25,26). When compared to saline and diuretics alone, and other antiresorptive agents including calcitonin, bisphosphonates are superior in treating hypercalcemia of malignancy (5). Because only 1% to 2% of oral bisphosphonates are absorbed, these drugs are administered intravenously (7). Pamidronate and zoledronate are the most commonly used bisphosphonates for the treatment of hypercalcemia of malignancy. Patients respond to bisphosphonate therapy within 2 to 4 days, with a nadir in serum calcium occurring within 4 to 7 days; normocalcemia may persist for 2 to 4 weeks (5,16). Zoledronate is 850 times more potent than pamidronate and is considered first-line therapy (9,27). In a pooled analysis of two randomized controlled trials comparing a single 4-mg dose of zoledronic acid to a 90-mg dose of pamidronate, serum calcium concentrations normalized within 10 days in 88% versus 70% of patients, respectively, and the duration of response was 32 days versus 18 days, respectively, within the two groups (27). Both zoledronate and pamidronate have been associated with acute and chronic renal failure, with more adverse events reported with zoledronate. Dose reduction of zoledronate is recommended in patients with a creatinine clearance between 30 and 60 mL/min. Other complications of bisphosphonates include acute systemic inflammatory reactions such as fever and arthralgias, ocular inflammation, electrolyte imbalances, and osteonecrosis of the jaw (28).

Other Agents

Calcitonin is a well-tolerated synthetic polypeptide analog of salmon calcitonin, which reduces serum calcium levels by inhibiting bone resorption. When administered subcutaneously or intramuscularly, it produces a rapid but transient decrease in serum calcium levels within 12 to 24 hours (5,9). This agent is useful in patients with congestive heart failure (CHF) or renal failure where saline, diuresis, and bisphosphonates may be contraindicated. Tachyphylaxis may occur with continued use (7). Glucocorticoids are effective in decreasing serum calcium in hypercalcemia of malignancy associated with some lymphomas, particularly Hodgkin lymphoma (HL). These agents have limited utility in the acute setting because a reduction in serum calcium may not be observed for 1 to 2 weeks (11).

Denosumab is a human monoclonal antibody that inhibits osteoclast formation by preventing human receptor activator of nuclear factor kappa-β ligand (RANKL) from binding with its receptor. It is metabolized and excreted by the liver and considered safe to give to patients with renal insufficiency although optimal dosing is uncertain. In patients with multiple myeloma, hypercalcemia, and severe renal impairment (serum creatinine 2.5 to 5.7 mg/dL), denosumab improved serum calcium and was associated with improved in renal function (29). In patients with breast cancer metastatic to bone, denosumab proved superior to zoledronic acid in preventing skeletal-related events such as pathologic fractures (30). It has also proved efficacious in patients with persistent hypercalcemia despite bisphosphonate therapy (31,32).

Dialysis may be necessary for patients with severe malignancy-associated hypercalcemia and concomitant renal insufficiency or heart failure, who will not tolerate the therapies outlined above (5,16).

Controversies

As noted above, the use of loop diuretics has fallen out of favor in the routine management of hypercalcemia. These agents may be necessary, however, to prevent fluid overload in selected individuals with renal insufficiency or heart failure.

ACUTE TUMOR LYSIS SYNDROME

Acute tumor lysis syndrome (ATLS) occurs as a consequence of the rapid and massive destruction of tumor cells resulting in the release of intracellular metabolites into the circulation in quantities sufficient to exceed renal excretory capacity (33,34). The four biochemical disturbances generated by this process that characterize the syndrome are life threatening (35):

- Hyperkalemia
- Hyperphosphatemia
- Hypocalcemia
- Hyperuricemia

These metabolic abnormalities have widespread adverse effects on the cardiac, musculoskeletal, nervous, and renal systems.

ATLS is most frequently observed after the administration of cytotoxic chemotherapy in patients with high-grade hematologic malignancies—classically, Burkitt lymphoma and acute lymphocytic leukemia (ALL) (7,36,37). The incidence of clinically significant ATLS in non-Hodgkin lymphoma (NHL) and ALL has been reported as 6% (38) and 5.2% (7), respectively. Metabolic derangements in these patients may develop within a few hours to a few days after initiating chemotherapy (7,39–41). Other malignancies in which ATLS has been described include chronic leukemia, low-grade lymphoma, and, rarely, solid tumors such as metastatic breast carcinoma, lung carcinoma, seminoma, thymoma, medulloblastoma, ovarian carcinoma, rhabdomyosarcoma, melanoma, vulvar carcinoma, and Merkel cell carcinoma (34). The syndrome can also occur after radiation therapy, immunotherapy with rituximab, and endocrine therapy (7,34,36). Spontaneous tumor lysis syndrome (STLS) is a rare entity that develops primarily in Burkitt lymphoma and leukemia in the absence of any treatment. Prompt recognition of ATLS is essential because it is associated with poor outcomes and high mortality rates (41). Predisposing factors for developing ATLS include large tumor burdens (36), bulky lymphadenopathy (7), extensive bone marrow involvement (37), rapid tumor cell proliferation, leukocytosis (more than 50×10^3 cells/μL) (34), lactate dehydrogenase (LDH) more than 1,500 IU/L (37), and high tumor chemosensitivity (7,35). Pretreatment hyperuricemia, renal dysfunction, and hypovolemia, as well as treatment with nephrotoxic agents, also confer an increased risk of ATLS (34).

Pathophysiology

Rapid dissolution of cells with aggressive cytotoxic therapy results in an increase in plasma uric acid, potassium, and phosphorus levels. Hyperphosphatemia then leads to secondary hypocalcemia; hyperkalemia occurs 6 to 72 hours after the administration of chemotherapy (39). Associated manifestations include lethargy, nausea, vomiting, diarrhea, muscle weakness, paresthesias, and electrocardiographic abnormalities such as peaked T waves, PR-interval prolongation, and QRS-complex widening. Ventricular arrhythmias may lead to sudden death (7,34). Hyperphosphatemia is seen 24 to 48 hours following chemotherapy (39). Malignant cells may contain up to four times more phosphorous than non-neoplastic cells and, as plasma phosphorous increases with cell lysis, the normal renal mechanism that excretes excess phosphate and prevents distal tubular reabsorption becomes overwhelmed, leading to hyperphosphatemia (42). Acute hyperphosphatemia manifests as secondary hypocalcemia with a range of signs and symptoms including anorexia, vomiting, confusion, neuromuscular irritability, tetany, carpopedal spasm, seizures, dysrhythmias, and cardiac arrest (7,34). Secondary hypocalcemia occurs in association with hyperphosphatemia when the calcium phosphate product exceeds 60. Calcium phosphate then precipitates into tissues, including the renal interstitium and tubules, resulting in nephrocalcinosis (35). However, hypocalcemia may persist even after correction of hyperphosphatemia when an inappropriately low plasma calcitriol level is present (43). Hypocalcemia itself causes a rise in serum parathyroid hormone, which, in turn, increases phosphate resorption in the proximal tubule, leading to nephrocalcinosis and acute renal failure (ARF) (7).

Hyperuricemia occurs 48 to 72 hours after chemotherapy (39). Patients may exhibit nonspecific symptoms such as nausea, vomiting, anorexia, and lethargy. ARF with associated oliguria, edema, hypertension, and altered sensorium will be seen in untreated patients (36). Uric acid is generated from purine metabolism in the liver. Adenosine and guanosine nucleotides are degraded to hypoxanthine and xanthine, respectively, and xanthine oxidase converts these products to uric acid (7). Rapidly proliferating neoplastic cells have high turnover rates with accelerated purine catabolism from DNA and RNA degradation (44), and these cells contain large amounts of purine nucleotides; consequently, with cytotoxic therapy, there is a rapid rise in plasma uric acid (36). Uric acid is excreted by the kidneys through the processes of glomerular filtration, partial proximal tubular reabsorption, and distal tubular secretion (35). The clearance of uric acid is independently proportional to intravascular volume status (34) and the urinary flow rate (35), and may be significantly reduced in the presence of dehydration or tubular obstruction from acute nephrocalcinosis or uric acid nephropathy. Uric acid nephropathy develops when uric acid crystals deposit in the renal tubules and collecting ducts under acidic conditions. The urinary pKa of uric acid is 5.4, and the luminal pH of the distal tubules and collecting ducts is 5.0, resulting in the poor solubility of uric acid in acidic urine (7). This poor solubility, coupled with the marked hyperuricosuria present in ATLS, leads to uric acid precipitation, intraluminal obstruction, oliguria, and ARF (7,45). ARF in ATLS may also be caused by renal calculi from phosphate and uric acid precipitation (34), as well as ischemic acute tubular necrosis caused by renal hypoperfusion (36). Drug toxicity, sepsis, and tumor-associated obstructive uropathy or renal parenchymal infiltration may exacerbate ATLS-induced ARF (42).

Diagnosis and Classification

Hande and Garrow (38) first classified ATLS into laboratory TLS and clinical TLS. Cairo and Bishop (42) have modified and further developed this classification system into the Cairo–Bishop definition, which uses laboratory and clinical data in conjunction with a grading scale to assess the severity of ATLS. Laboratory TLS (LTLS) is defined as two or more of the following metabolic abnormalities occurring 3 days before or 7 days after chemotherapy: uric acid 8 mg/dL or greater, potassium 6 mEq/dL or greater, phosphorous 6.5 mg/dL or greater, or a 25% increase in baseline levels of these metabolites, and calcium up to 7 mg/dL, or a 25% decrease from baseline level. Clinical tumor lysis syndrome is defined as LTLS in addition to one or more of the following findings: serum creatinine at least 1.5 times the upper limit of normal, cardiac dysrhythmia/sudden death, or seizure. The grading of ATLS from 0 through 5 is determined by the presence or absence of LTLS, the degree of serum creatinine elevation, and the presence and severity of the cardiac arrhythmia and seizure (42).

Prevention and Treatment

Early recognition of patients at high risk for ATLS is an essential component of the management strategy so that appropriate prophylactic interventions can be instituted.

Fluids and Alkalinization

Except in patients at risk for CHF, aggressive intravenous hydration with isotonic or hypotonic saline (46) is the single most important intervention for both prevention and treatment of ATLS. Cytotoxic therapy should be delayed whenever possible to administer appropriate hydration (7,46). Intravenous hydration should commence 2 days before and for 2 to 3 days after chemotherapy (34,36) at a rate of 2,000 to 3,000 mL/m^2/day (7,9,38,46,47), or two to four times the daily fluid maintenance requirement to achieve a urine output of greater than or equal to 80 to 100 mL/m^2/hr (30,38,46). Aggressive administration of intravenous fluid increases the intravascular volume, renal blood flow, glomerular filtration rate, and urinary flow rate, resulting in correction of electrolyte derangements by dilution of the extracellular fluid and prevention of phosphate and uric acid precipitation by increasing urinary excretion of these metabolites (48). Volume expansion alone may be insufficient to maintain adequate urine output, necessitating the administration of diuretics. Once euvolemia is achieved, and no signs of acute obstructive uropathy are present, a dose of furosemide (0.5 to 1 mg/kg or 2 to 4 mg/kg for severe oliguria or anuria, respectively) may induce or improve urine output (34). The effectiveness of furosemide is diminished in the setting of uric acid precipitation in the renal tubules; in this circumstance, mannitol, at a dose of 0.5 mg/kg, may be administered.

Alkalinization of the urine to a pH of 7.0 has fallen out of favor (7,9,46). This practice is based on the biochemical properties of uric acid, that is, uric acid is 13 times more soluble at pH 7.0 than at pH 5.0 (35), maximal solubility of uric acid is attained at pH 7.5, and urine alkalinization (pH ≥6.5) enhances renal excretion of uric acid (42). What limits this approach is that calcium phosphate precipitation increases with systemic alkalinization, exacerbating nephrocalcinosis (7,34). Additionally, hypoxanthine and xanthine solubility are substantially reduced, leading to xanthine nephropathy with concurrent allopurinol therapy (9,34,40). At this time, use of sodium bicarbonate can only be recommended in patients with metabolic acidosis and high levels of uric acid. It should be discontinued when serum phosphate levels begin to rise (47).

Management of Hyperuricemia

Allopurinol reduces the risk of ATLS when administered 2 to 3 days prior to chemotherapy by inhibiting the production of uric acid (9). Allopurinol is both a synthetic structural analog of the purine base, hypoxanthine, and a competitive inhibitor of xanthine oxidase (36), and, therefore, in the presence of allopurinol, xanthine oxidase cannot catalyze the conversion of hypoxanthine to xanthine and xanthine to uric acid (34). Allopurinol is administered orally at 300 to 800 mg daily (10 mg/kg/day or up to 400 mg/m^2/day) in one to three divided doses, and should be titrated to uric acid level. Intravenous allopurinol can be administered in doses of 200 to 400 mg/m^2/day, to a maximum of 600 mg/day, in patients unable to tolerate oral medications (7,49). Dose adjustment of allopurinol is required for reduced creatinine clearance (7,49). There are several limitations with allopurinol therapy:

- A reduction in serum uric acid level is not seen before 48 to 72 hours after initiating allopurinol because the drug inhibits the synthesis of uric acid but does not affect the pretreatment uric acid concentration (7).
- Inhibition of xanthine oxidase by allopurinol leads to increased plasma levels of xanthine and hypoxanthine, which may precipitate in the renal tubules (36).
- Three percent of patients develop hypersensitivity reactions, including Stevens–Johnson syndrome.
- Allopurinol interacts with many drugs, including chemotherapeutic agents such as cyclosporine and azathioprine (45).

Another agent that lowers uric acid concentration is urate oxidase (48). Urate oxidase converts uric acid to allantoin, which is five to ten times more soluble in urine than uric acid. Rasburicase, a recombinant urate oxidase, normalizes uric acid levels within 4 hours of administration in children and adults at doses of 0.15 to 0.20 mg/kg (7,45). This dose may be repeated daily for a total of 5 days, and chemotherapy should be initiated 4 to 24 hours after the first dose. In addition to being more effective than allopurinol in reducing pretreatment and posttreatment uric acid levels, rasburicase does not generate increased xanthine and hypoxanthine levels, thereby minimizing the risk of uric acid nephropathy that may be seen with allopurinol use (7,34,45). Of note, rasburicase is contraindicated in patients with glucose-6-phosphate dehydrogenase (G6PD) deficiency; additionally, bronchospasm and anaphylaxis may rarely occur with rasburicase therapy (50). There is insufficient evidence that rasburicase reduces the incidence of dialysis in ATLS, and because a 5-day course of therapy is considerably more expensive than a 5-day course of oral allopurinol (7,42), cost-effectiveness must be considered in formulating a treatment plan.

Correction of Electrolyte Abnormalities

Because of the potential for life-threatening dysrhythmias, prompt recognition of electrolyte derangements is imperative. Laboratory monitoring should be performed every 4 to 6 hours in the first 24 hours of chemotherapy in patients at high risk for ATLS, and then every 6 to 8 hours thereafter. A baseline electrocardiogram (ECG) should be obtained to assess for cardiac effects related to electrolyte abnormalities. Hyperkalemia is treated with calcium gluconate to stabilize the cardiac membrane and with intravenous insulin/dextrose and inhaled beta$_2$ agonists to facilitate intracellular shift of potassium. Although sodium bicarbonate may also shift potassium intracellularly by improving the metabolic acidosis, its use may result in inappropriate volume expansion. Potassium-binding resins such as sodium polystyrene sulfate increase potassium elimination in the GI tract and have a delayed hypokalemic effect. Diuretics can be administered to reduce serum potassium in patients without renal failure. When ARF occurs, dialysis may be required to emergently reduce serum potassium. Asymptomatic hypocalcemia should be left untreated to preclude calcium phosphate precipitation; however, symptomatic hypocalcemia is managed with intravenous calcium gluconate. Treatment of hyperphosphatemia with oral phosphate binders such as aluminum hydroxide or aluminum carbonate will usually concurrently correct the hypocalcemia (7,34).

Dialysis

Dialysis is indicated in patients with marked elevations in serum uric acid, phosphate, and potassium that do not respond to aggressive treatment, and in patients with ARF with volume overload, severe uremia, or acidosis (33,36,42,46). Hemodialysis is used in ATLS because it is superior to peritoneal dialysis in the clearance of both uric acid and phosphorous (34,42).

Controversies

- Administration of urine alkalinizing agent such as sodium bicarbonate or acetazolamide can only be recommended in patients with metabolic acidosis and high levels of uric acid. It should be discontinued when serum phosphate levels begin to rise (47).
- The preferred regimen for lowering serum uric oxide remains unclear. Although rasburicase is a more effective hypouricemic agent than allopurinol, it is unknown if its use results in improved clinical outcomes such as reduced AKI and mortality.

SUPERIOR VENA CAVA SYNDROME

Superior vena cava syndrome (SVCS) describes the set of signs and symptoms associated with obstruction of the superior vena cava (SVC), which may be caused by extrinsic compression, vascular invasion, or intraluminal thrombosis of the vein (51–53). The SVC is a thin-walled, compliant, low-pressure middle mediastinal vessel, rendering it easily vulnerable to disease processes in the adjacent right lung, the paratracheal and perihilar lymph nodes, the mainstem bronchi, the esophagus, and the thoracic spinal cord (53,54).

First described by Hunter (55) in 1757 in a patient with an aortic aneurysm secondary to syphilis, SVCS was—prior to the widespread use of antibiotics—primarily a complication of infectious diseases, as seen in syphilitic aortitis, histoplasmosis-induced fibrosing mediastinitis, and tuberculous mediastinitis (56,57). Currently, malignancy is the most common cause of SVCS accounting for approximately 60% to 85% of cases (57,58,59). Benign etiologies of SVCS account for the remaining 15% to 40% and appear to be increasing due to the increasing use of intravascular devices, such as central venous catheters and pacemaker wires (71%) (57). Other nonmalignant causes of SVCS include fibrosing mediastinitis from prior irradiation or histoplasmosis, aortic dissection, and complications of surgery, such as aortic dissection repair (57,58,60,61). Bronchogenic carcinoma accounts for 85% to 90% of the malignancies in which SVCS presents (61–64). Overall, SVCS develops in 2% to 10% of lung malignancies (46,51,55,58,60), and the risk of SVCS is higher in small cell lung cancer, with an incidence of 6.6% to 12% (65) because it involves the central mediastinal structures. In addition, because of the anatomic location of the SVC, right-sided lung cancers cause SVCS four times as often as left-sided lung cancers (63). Other neoplasms causing SVCS include malignant lymphomas; although HL more often involves the mediastinum, it rarely causes SVCS (61,64). Primary germ cell cancers, thymoma, mesothelioma (66), and metastatic disease (primarily breast carcinoma) constitute a small proportion of SVCS cases (57,61,66).

Pathophysiology

The severity of signs and symptoms depends on the extent, location, and rapidity of onset of the SVC occlusion (62). In general, obstruction within or below the azygos vein results in more pronounced symptoms. Normally, azygos venous capacity increases from 11% to 35% to augment drainage of the head and neck (52), but impedance of flow from obstruction precludes this auxiliary function (52,61,66). With slowly developing SVCS, collateral vessels in the chest wall and upper extremities are recruited as a diversion for the existing SVC engorgement; hence, SVCS in this population is of insidious onset, as in fibrosing mediastinitis (62). The most commonly reported symptom in SVCS is dyspnea followed by head and facial swelling (53,57). Other cardiopulmonary symptoms include cough, orthopnea, and chest pain. Associated signs are neck and arm vein distention, plethora or cyanosis of the head and neck (53), venous collateralization in the arms and upper chest wall (61), and chronic pleural effusions (61,62). More extensive airway or vascular obstruction is predicted when positional maneuvers such as lying supine or leaning forward exacerbate respiratory or cardiac symptoms; for example, respiratory insufficiency in the supine position worsens as the weight of the mediastinal structures impinges on the tracheobronchial tree. In the substantially compromised patient with SVCS, cardiopulmonary arrest may ensue simply with the administration of sedatives and general anesthesia (61). Other head and neck signs and symptoms range from conjunctival and periorbital edema, nasal congestion, dysphagia, and hoarseness due to laryngeal nerve compression (67) to proptosis, glossal edema, stridor secondary to laryngeal edema, and tracheal obstruction (61,62). Patients with central nervous system (CNS) manifestations may exhibit mild headaches, dizziness, and lethargy with progression to syncope in rapidly developing or complete SVC obstruction, seizures, or coma from cerebral edema and increased intracranial pressure (52,61). Bleeding complications such as epistaxis, hemoptysis, and GI hemorrhage from esophageal varices in long-standing SVC may occur (61).

Diagnosis

Once the clinical diagnosis of SVC syndrome is suspected, confirmation can be obtained using radiologic techniques. Chest radiography reveals widening of the superior mediastinum in approximately 60% of patients (60,61,63) and pleural effusions, most frequently right-sided, in up to 25% of patients (53,61). A normal chest radiograph, however, does not exclude the diagnosis. Contrast-enhanced helical computed tomography (CT) accurately delineates the site, extent, and cause of the occlusion (63,66), as well as any associated thrombus and collateral vessel development (66). The radiologic diagnosis of SVCS is made by demonstrating both decreased or absent venous opacification below the level of obstruction and prominent collateral vessel opacification (63). MRI is an alternative imaging method in patients with iodinated contrast allergy or without adequate venous access for contrast administration, but offers no distinct advantage over CT (52,61,68). Venography is most useful when planning bypass or stenting procedures (52,66). Although venography is superior to CT in identifying the site and extent of obstruction and in mapping the collateral circulation, it does not elucidate the underlying cause of the SVCS (68), unless SVC thrombosis alone is the causative factor (58,63,66).

Treatment

The primary goals of treatment are symptom relief and eradication or palliation of the underlying malignancy. Initial symptomatic management involves bed rest, head elevation to reduce venous pressure, and supplemental oxygen administration. Diuretics and sodium restriction may decrease edema, but reports are anecdotal. Use of glucocorticoids to minimize inflammatory responses to tumor or radiotherapy (XRT) is controversial (64), but steroids are a mainstay of treatment in NHL (61,63). Urgency of treatment is guided by the severity of symptoms (58,69–72). The American College of Chest Physicians (ACCP) and the National Comprehensive Cancer Network (NCCN) recommend expedited stent placement or radiotherapy for patients with symptomatic SVCS (73,74). Patients with evidence of cerebral or laryngeal edema or those with hemodynamic compromise require an emergent intervention.

Endovascular Stenting

If conservative measures are ineffectual in controlling symptoms, a percutaneously placed endovascular stent can be inserted with or without balloon angioplasty (63,75–77). Prior series note relief of symptoms immediately after stent placement in over 90% of patients with few complications (78,79). Recurrence of SVCS occurs in up to 40% of patients after primary stenting (average 13%) and is usually successfully treated with a second interventional procedure. Complications of stent placement occur in up to 7% of patients and include infection, bleeding, pulmonary embolus, stent migration, and SVC perforation (79–81).

Thrombolysis

With the increased use of intravascular devices, thrombus now accounts for a larger proportion of the benign causes of SVCS (57). When SVC syndrome is attributable to thrombosis of a central venous catheter, and catheter preservation is desired, thrombolytic therapy given within 5 days of symptom onset is associated with an 88% success rate versus 25% after 5 days (63,82). Patients with extensive thrombosis in the context of SVCS may benefit from catheter-directed thrombolysis (83).

Radiotherapy and Chemotherapy

The treatment modality selected should be individualized to the type of malignancy, stage, and performance status of each patient (66). Primary management of radiosensitive tumors such as NSCLC involves XRT. NSCLC associated with SVCS carries a poor prognosis, with 1-year survival, in one series, of 17% (84). The treatment of choice in NSCLC is XRT and, when possible, stent insertion (73). Within 72 hours of XRT, patients have relief of symptoms, and within 2 weeks, 70% to 90% of patients are symptom free (63). In a large systematic review, 60% of the NSCLC patients had relief of SVCS after chemotherapy and/or radiotherapy, and SVCS recurred in 19% (66).

Chemotherapy prolongs survival and improves quality of life in patients with small cell lung cancer (SCLC), and addition of thoracic irradiation may reduce the recurrence risk of SVCS. In the aforementioned systematic review, SVCS was relieved in 77% of patients receiving chemotherapy and/or radiation, with relapse in 17% of patients (66). Lymphoma and germ cell tumors are usually treated with chemotherapy based on the histologic type, grade, and stage of the disease. In HL, chemotherapy followed by XRT to areas of bulky disease may be indicated (63). In NHL, XRT alone may be used in early-stage disease, and chemotherapy is the treatment for higher-stage tumors. Whether to irradiate areas of bulky disease in NHL after chemotherapeutic remission is less clear; however, with residual tumor or progression of disease after chemotherapy, radiotherapy is administered (63).

Surgery

Surgical bypass of the obstruction with vein grafts or prosthetic grafts may be appropriate in patients with benign causes of SVCS. In patients with malignancy, surgical intervention, when no further treatment options are possible, at best, is a palliative measure with poor long-term survival (62,63,84).

Controversies

The need for long-term anticoagulation following SVC stent placement remains unclear. Given the poor prognosis of many of these patients, there is little data to guide choice of anticoagulant and duration of therapy. Most practitioners favor a short course (4 to 12 weeks) of dual antiplatelet therapy. Anticoagulation with low–molecular-weight heparin is indicated when SVC occurs in the presence of an upper extremity DVT.

ACUTE AIRWAY OBSTRUCTION

Oropharyngeal and Tracheal Obstruction

Sudden upper airway obstruction (UAO) of the larynx, pharynx, or extrathoracic trachea is uncommon with cancers of the head and neck. Tumors of the larynx, pharynx, base of tongue, and thyroid are primarily slow growing and, as they progressively enlarge, obvious signs and symptoms of airway compromise are usually evident prior to the development of acute obstruction (85); tracheal masses, which take years to be discovered, first become symptomatic when the airway lumen is narrowed by 75% (86). Mechanisms of UAO include direct tracheal invasion as well as extrinsic tracheal compression (87).

In the head and neck, direct tracheal invasion is seen with locally advanced oropharyngeal tumors, laryngeal neoplasms associated with bulky or supraglottic lesions, and rarely, thyroid cancer and primary tracheal tumors (85). In thyroid cancer, tracheal invasion develops in 1% to 6.5% of patients, and UAO is the most common cause of death in this group (88). Direct tumor extension into the trachea from adjacent structures by malignancies of the lung, esophagus, and mediastinum occurs more frequently than metastatic disease spread (89).

Tracheal impingement in lung cancer occurs when there is tracheal ingrowth of the primary tumor originating in a mainstem bronchus or from enlarging paratracheal or subcarinal lymph nodes. Bilateral vocal cord paralysis with recurrent laryngeal nerve paralysis may also be associated with lung malignancies (85,90). Extrathoracic malignancies may metastasize to mediastinal and endobronchial lymph nodes, causing airway obstruction. Renal cell carcinoma, sarcomas, breast cancer, and colon cancer are most commonly involved (91). Melanoma may arise as a primary tracheal tumor but more often is a metastatic lesion (89).

Tracheal compression, which is usually attributable to benign disease, is a secondary mechanism of UAO in neoplastic disease and is often the initial presentation of mediastinal tumors and extensive lymphoma (92).

Pathophysiology

Patients may present with dysphagia, hoarseness, intractable cough, hemoptysis, dyspnea, or stridor (85). Important goals during physical examination are to determine whether impending airway obstruction is present and to localize the site of the lesion. Once stridor is apparent, the airway caliber has narrowed to approximately 6 mm and, without intervention, complete UAO is imminent. Inspiratory stridor implies an extrathoracic lesion at the level of the glottis or above, whereas expiratory stridor suggests an intrathoracic lesion. Biphasic stridor may be indicative of a subglottic or tracheal mass. Voice alteration, such as muffling and hoarseness, accompanies subglottic lesions and unilateral vocal cord paralysis, respectively (52).

Diagnosis

A chest radiograph may identify an obstructive neck mass and consequent tracheal deviation. Flexible oropharyngeal or nasopharyngeal endoscopy can be performed to assess the airway. Once the airway is stabilized, high-resolution CT of the head and neck provides comprehensive evaluation of the sites of narrowing and the size and extent of the tumor in relation to adjacent structures. Spirometry demonstrates a plateau in the inspiratory limb of the flow–volume loop if there is a fixed obstructive lesion in the extrathoracic trachea (93).

Treatment

Initial management includes head elevation and administration of cool humidified oxygen. Case reports have demonstrated that inhalation of a helium–oxygen mixture, consequent to its lower density compared to oxygen supplementation alone, reduces the work of breathing (61,94,95). Airway obstruction in patients with bulky oropharyngeal, laryngeal, or thyroid carcinomas will require emergent or elective tracheostomy. Endotracheal intubation is not recommended for patients with bulky, friable, laryngeal, and/or pharyngeal disease, as it may exacerbate existing airway edema and hemorrhage (86). For intraluminal tracheal lesions, bronchoscopy with interventions such as laser therapy (96,97), brachytherapy, photodynamic therapy, or stenting may be performed to rapidly alleviate symptoms (97). Stents are also useful in palliating symptomatic extrinsic compression (98). Endotracheal intubation or stenting may be used to maintain the airway when there is extrinsic compression from lymphoma (98) or other highly radiosensitive or chemosensitive tumors with anticipation of rapid reduction of tumor mass. Surgical resection is indicated for primary airway tumors (99) and for lung cancers without mediastinal lymph node involvement. In lung and thyroid cancers that directly invade the trachea, surgery may be curative (89); metastatic disease to the trachea requires palliative treatment.

Intrathoracic Obstruction

Pathophysiology

Intrathoracic airway obstruction may be present with intrinsic primary endobronchial tumors such as bronchogenic carcinoma and carcinoid, with metastatic tumors or their associated lymphadenopathy—lung, renal, breast, thyroid, and colon cancers, and sarcoma or melanoma—or with bulky disease causing airway compression. Symptoms often progress slowly over time, and patients may complain of dyspnea, wheezing, or chest discomfort, leading to the misdiagnosis of asthma or bronchitis prior to the development of fulminant airway obstruction (100); postobstructive pneumonia may be a finding on initial presentation. With impending obstruction, patients may exhibit hypertension, tachycardia, tachypnea, and significant pulsus paradoxus. Poor air movement, use of accessory muscles, and mental status changes are indicators of severe obstruction. Progressive symptoms may result in negative pressure pulmonary edema and anoxic brain injury (93). Chest examination may reveal a prolonged expiratory time and wheezing.

Diagnosis

Respiratory symptoms are unilateral with lesions below the carina (100), and the chest radiograph reveals asymmetric lung fields, particularly on end-expiration. Stable patients should have a flow–volume loop performed. An intrathoracic, mobile tracheal lesion above the carina will demonstrate airway compression during the expiratory phase, producing flattening of the expiratory limb of the flow–volume loop, whereas a plateau in both inspiratory and expiratory limbs will be observed with fixed obstructive lesions (93). Chest CT defines tumor extent and location, but rigid bronchoscopy is usually necessary to evaluate the airway in impending obstruction and those in whom significant bleeding is likely. When airway obstruction is severe, flexible bronchoscopy is hazardous because this technique does not permit ventilatory support, and, additionally, the bronchoscope may obstruct the already narrowed airway lumen (100).

Treatment

Treatment proceeds with the general measures of oxygen or helium/oxygen supplementation and, possibly, steroids. If endotracheal intubation is required, the clinician must recognize the potential for hemodynamic compromise associated with asymmetric obstruction and significant increases in airway pressure distal to the obstruction (93). Bronchoscopy with various interventions, including debridement, dilation, endotracheal stent placement, laser ablation, photodynamic therapy, and placement of brachytherapy catheters may relieve symptoms (100); external beam radiotherapy may also play a role. In lung cancer, tracheal and carinal resection is indicated in patients without mediastinal lymph node involvement for a potential cure (61).

SPINAL CORD COMPRESSION

Malignant spinal cord compression (MSCC) is a profoundly debilitating, but usually nonfatal, manifestation of metastatic cancer, occurring in 5% to 10% of cancer patients (102–105). The term, *MSCC*, refers to epidural, intramedullary, and leptomeningeal disease; however, the focus of this section is on epidural spinal cord compression (ESCC) because the literature primarily discusses this population (103). Although any malignancy capable of metastatic spread may give rise to MSCC, prostate, breast, and lung cancers are most commonly involved, with each accounting for 15% to 20% of cases (101,104) or, in combination, 60% of cases (103,105). The cumulative incidence of MSCC is specific to tumor type, with the highest rates occurring in multiple myeloma (8%), prostate cancer (7%), and nasopharyngeal cancer (6.5%) (105). Other tumors include NHL and renal cell carcinoma, with each representing 5% to 10% of cases (106), and GI cancers, sarcoma, melanoma, thyroid cancer (92,93), and unknown primary carcinoma (105,106). Enlarging meningiomas, nerve sheath tumors, and leptomeningeal metastases may also compress the spinal cord. Nonmalignant causes of MSCC in the cancer patient are epidural abscesses in the presence of immune compromise and hematoma with bleeding diatheses (107).

MSCC has a proclivity for the thoracic spine (102,106,108–110) and is estimated to occur in this location in approximately 60% to 66% of cases (107,109). Twenty percent of cases involve the lumbar spine (102,107); MSCC in the cervical spine is uncommon, seen in 7% to 10% of cases (109,110). Prostate and colorectal carcinomas favor the lumbosacral spine (107); MSCC is the initial manifestation of malignancy in 20% of patients.

Pathophysiology

The mechanisms by which MSCC occurs include vertebral body invasion by tumor with possible vertebral collapse causing encroachment on the anterior spinal cord (85%); direct extension into the intervertebral space by paraspinal lymphoma, sarcoma, or lung cancer, seen in 10% to 15% of cases; and epidural or intramedullary space invasion, seen in less than 5% of cases (102). The mechanism of injury to the spinal cord is mediated by white matter vasogenic edema and axonal swelling that result from cord compression. Venous hypertension, decreased spinal cord blood flow, and cord infarction ensue, resulting in ischemic hypoxic neuronal injury.

Pain, which may be characterized as localized, radicular, or referred, is the primary presenting symptom in MSCC, occurring in 83% to 95% (106,108,111) of patients for a median of 8 weeks prior to diagnosis (106,108). Focal bony pain is typically localized, dull or aching, and constant. Direct tenderness of the involved vertebral body may be evident with periosteal destruction (112). With time, radicular pain occurs in the dermatome of the affected nerve root and is severe, deep, and lancinating. Radicular symptoms occur most often in the lumbosacral spine and may be unilateral or bilateral, the latter more frequent with thoracic spine involvement (107,113). Referred pain does not radiate, but appears in a region distal to the area of pathology; for example, sacroiliac pain may result from L1 compression (113). The pain of MSCC is typified by worsening with recumbency secondary to distention of the epidural venous plexus (106,107); coughing, sneezing, or Valsalva maneuvers will also exacerbate the pain (102). Straight-leg raising identifies a lumbosacral radiculopathy, and neck flexion reproduces symptoms of thoracic radiculopathy (107,111,113).

Motor weakness is present in 60% to 85% of patients on diagnosis of MSCC. Although only one-third of patients complain of lower extremity weakness on initial presentation (107), two-thirds are not ambulatory at the time of diagnosis (106,107). Motor deficits at the level of the conus medullaris or above generally have a symmetric distribution. Paresis is usually seen in the extensors of the upper extremities or the flexors of the lower extremities, depending on the location of the lesion in the spine. Upper motor neuron signs such as spasticity, hyperreflexia, and Babinski responses, may be present. Cervical lesions may lead to quadriplegia and respiratory collapse (112).

Sensory deficits, reported as varying degrees of paresthesias, are less common than motor deficits but can still be found in 40% to 90% of patients. The level of hyperesthesia on examination occurs one to five levels below the actual anatomic level of cord compression (106). The sensation of an electric shock radiating through the spine and extremities with neck flexion, termed the *Lhermitte sign,* is seen infrequently with cervical or thoracic neoplasms. Perineal paresthesias may occur with cauda equina lesions. Gait ataxia may follow sensory loss impairment, but in the absence of sensory findings, impairment of the spinocerebellar tract should be considered.

Bowel and bladder dysfunction reflects autonomic dysfunction and is a late manifestation of MSCC (113). Patients report urinary hesitancy and frequency, and both incontinence of urine, from poor sphincter tone or overflow of urine, and urinary retention may ensue. At the time of diagnosis, 50% of patients are incontinent or catheter-dependent (114); patients may also exhibit erectile dysfunction and impotence. Constipation and incontinence of stool with diminished sphincter tone may be present (113).

Diagnosis

The imaging study of choice in evaluating MSCC is magnetic resonance imaging (MRI); this noninvasive test provides high resolution of the soft tissues, including bony metastases and intramedullary pathology. One study found that MRI had a sensitivity, specificity, and overall accuracy of 93%, 97%, and 95%, respectively, in detecting MSCC in patients with known malignancies, excluding primary CNS tumors (114). When the entire spine is imaged beyond the area of clinically determined cord compression, multiple epidural metastases (MEMs) are found in 30% of patients. Because the presence of MEMs may alter treatment strategy, several studies have purported using whole-spine MRI in all patients undergoing imaging (104,109,114,115). Myelography, with or without CT myelogram, is a more invasive tool than MRI and is used in imaging MSCC when MRI is contraindicated. CT alone does not adequately define the soft tissues and spinal cord, and plain radiographs and radionuclide testing have low sensitivity and specificity for demonstrating MSCC. Plain films detect vertebral metastases at the site of known cord compression only 80% of the time, and many metastases are missed because the ability to visualize these lesions requires that 30% to 40% of the bone be eroded (116).

Delay in diagnosis may be attributed to the patient's failure to identify symptoms and diagnostic delays by the generalist and hospital practitioner, leading to potentially avoidable deterioration in motor or bladder function (117).

Treatment

The goals of therapy are pain control and preservation of neurologic function. Treatment options include narcotics, corticosteroids, radiation, and surgery. Pretreatment neurologic function is the most important predictor of posttreatment outcome (118,119).

Corticosteroids

In a randomized trial that established the efficacy of corticosteroids in cord compression, patients were assigned to XRT with or without dexamethasone. At the conclusion of the study, 81% of those receiving corticosteroids and XRT versus 63% of those receiving XRT alone remained ambulatory. At 6 months, the percentages were 59% and 33% in the two groups, respectively (120). There are less well-established data regarding the use of high-dose dexamethasone regimens because, although higher doses (100-mg vs. 10-mg boluses) may have greater clinical efficacy in improving posttreatment ambulation, they are associated with a higher proportion of adverse effects. Typical regimens include a 10-mg bolus, followed by 16 mg divided four times daily, tapered over 2 weeks. High-dose regimens (100-mg bolus, then 96 mg divided four times daily, tapered over 2 weeks) (103) may be reserved for patients with paresis or paraplegia. In ambulatory patients who are asymptomatic and undergoing XRT, corticosteroids may be withheld (103,104,121).

Surgery and Radiation

Definitive management of MSCC includes decompressive surgery and/or radiotherapy. Individuals with mechanical instability of the spine and a favorable overall prognosis should proceed directly to surgery (122). Vertebroplasty or kyphoplasty is an option for patients who are not suitable candidates for spine surgery. The same is true of individuals with stable spine lesions that are not radiosensitive. Patients with mechanically stable MSCC should proceed with radiotherapy. This may be administered via external beam radiation therapy (EBRT) or stereotactic radiosurgery (SRS). Occasionally, embolization of vascular tumors may be performed preoperatively.

Controversies

The role of high-dose steroids remains unclear. As noted above, only one of three studies demonstrated improved motor function at higher doses of dexamethasone (with an increased incidence of side effects). Current practice favors the use of high-dose steroids only for patients with severe myelopathy upon presentation.

CARDIAC TAMPONADE

Primary neoplasms of the myocardium and pericardium are uncommon, but metastatic disease to the pericardial space is frequently seen (123). Primary pericardial tumors, of which mesothelioma represents the largest proportion, are 40 times less common than metastatic disease. Secondary malignancies include, most frequently, lung, breast, ovarian carcinomas, and melanoma, lymphoma, and leukemia (124). Malignancy is a primary cause of pericardial effusion in the United States (125), and pericardial tamponade resulting from malignant pericardial effusion (MPCE) represents at least 50% of reported cases of pericardial fluid collection requiring intervention (126,127). Autopsy series have reported, with varying estimates, that MPCE is seen in 2% to 22% of cancer patients (125,126,128), and that these effusions are clinically quiescent, remaining unrecognized (52). In some patients, MPCE may be the initial presentation of cancer, but in any patient, it signifies a dismal prognosis, with most patients dying within 1 year (129). Pericardial effusions in some cancer patients may be attributable to comorbid conditions rather than to malignant disease, and other causes must be considered, such as radiation-induced pericarditis, infection, uremia, myocardial infarction, CHF, and pneumonia (124).

Pathophysiology

The pericardium is a fibroserous sac, composed of two layers that surround the heart. The outer layer is the fibrous pericardium, which attaches to the diaphragm and securely anchors the heart within the thoracic cavity. The serous pericardium is a single layer of mesothelial cells and its underlying connective tissue, which lines the fibrous pericardium. During embryonic development, the heart invaginates the walls of the serous pericardium, creating a potential space between an inner serous layer that is adherent to the heart (visceral pericardium) and an outer serous layer that lines the fibrous pericardium (parietal pericardium). The pericardial space is formed between the two serous layers, and it normally contains 15 to 50 mL of fluid for lubrication. The fluid is drained from the right pleural space into the right lymphatic duct, and from the parietal pericardium into the thoracic duct (130,131); any interruption in this flow will result in accumulation of fluid and pericardial effusion. The mechanisms by which malignant disease generates MPCEs include direct invasion of the pericardium or myocardium, and disruption of lymphatic flow from lymph node metastases or from prior radiotherapy to the chest or mediastinum (126,128). The tumors that invade the pericardium directly or hematogenously are most often lung cancer, followed by lymphoma and breast cancer (52,126).

With either of the aforementioned mechanisms, pericardial fluid accumulates and inhibits passive diastolic filling of the normally low-pressure right heart structures, producing jugular and abdominal venous hypertension (126). As the pericardial effusion expands, the heart is further compressed, leading to reduced diastolic compliance, decreased diastolic filling, and, ultimately, decreased stroke volume, cardiac output, and blood pressure. Right atrial and right ventricular collapse ensues, resulting in frank tamponade, which, untreated, will lead to shock (133). *Pericardial reserve volume,* defined as the volume that will just distend the pericardium, is approximately 10 to 20 mL. As the pericardial effusion enlarges, capacity for stretch is exceeded. Therefore, when fluid accumulates rapidly, the pericardium cannot stretch rapidly enough to accommodate the added volume, and the heart becomes compressed (131). Under these circumstances, acute tamponade may occur with as little as 50 mL of fluid (132). When effusions develop chronically, the pericardium is able to compensate by stretching slowly over time—the phenomenon of stretch relaxation (131–133). In cancer patients, the MPCE develops slowly, and as much as 2 L of pericardial fluid may be present before critical symptoms occur (132).

Patients may be asymptomatic with small pericardial effusions (9,124) and, in general, symptoms correlate with the compressive effect of the effusion on surrounding structures, including the lung, trachea, and esophagus. Symptoms include dyspnea, cough, chest pain, hoarseness, hiccups, and dysphagia (131). The most commonly reported physical sign is distension of the jugular veins. The classic finding of the Beck triad of hypotension, increased jugular venous pressure, and quiet heart sounds may be present, in addition to the Kussmaul sign, which is paradoxical jugular venous distention and increased jugular venous pressure on inspiration. Sinus tachycardia, hepatomegaly, and peripheral edema may all be apparent. On cardiac examination, dullness beyond the apical impulse and râles can be detected, and in patients with inflammatory effusions, a pericardial rub is often heard. A narrow pulse pressure is frequently noted, and pulsus paradoxus, a decrease in systolic blood pressure greater than 10 mmHg, is observed in 77% of patients with acute tamponade; patients may report a feeling of uneasiness (132). When low-output shock results from failure of compensatory mechanisms to maintain cardiac output, the patient exhibits cold, clammy skin, cyanosis, oliguria, and altered mental status (133).

Diagnosis

Chest radiograph reveals a water bottle–shaped heart with widening of the cardiac silhouette and, occasionally, pericardial calcifications (132); pleural effusions will be present in one-third of cases (126). The ECG may demonstrate a low-voltage QRS or nonspecific ST-T wave changes (9). Electrical alternans in the P wave and QRS complex is a rare finding, noted in 0% to 10% of patients (131), in which every other QRS complex has a lower-voltage and/or reversed polarity (132). The echocardiogram precisely localizes the pericardial fluid, discerns the quality of the effusion (homogeneous vs. heterogeneous), determines whether loculations or bulky tumor are present, assesses right and left ventricular function, and ascertains whether right atrial and right ventricular diastolic collapse are present. On echocardiography, the heart may be seen to swing in a pendular fashion within the pericardial fluid. Right heart catheterization is the definitive standard for further defining the pericardial effusion. Classically, there will be equalization of diastolic pressures across all cardiac chambers (126).

Treatment

There are no randomized control trials to guide the management of malignant pericardial effusions. Treatment strategy should be individualized to each patient based on age, comorbid conditions, malignancy type, and overall prognosis (125). Although temporizing measures such as volume repletion and inotropic support may provide some benefit, definitive treatment requires removal of fluid from the pericardial space. The initial emergent intervention in malignant cardiac tamponade is to drain the effusion, usually with echocardiographic guidance (124). Fluid should be sent for chemical analysis, microbiology, and cytology; the effusion is removed successfully in 97% of patients (134). In the absence of tamponade, systemic chemotherapy is administered as baseline treatment (124), thereby precluding recurrences in 67% of cases (134). Systemic chemotherapy is effective in controlling malignant effusions when the tumors are chemosensitive, as in lymphoma, leukemia, and breast cancer. Notably, XRT is highly effective (93%) in controlling malignant pericardial effusions in patients with lymphoma and leukemia, although radiation myocarditis or pericarditis is, in itself, a complication of radiotherapy (134). Pericardiocentesis should be performed in MPCE, especially when these are large, for symptomatic relief and to establish a cause. Because fluid reaccumulates within 48 hours of the initial pericardiocentesis (135), intrapericardial sclerosing or cytostatic agents, selected according to tumor type, should be administered to prevent recurrence. The mechanism of action of sclerosing agents is to effect symphysis of the visceral and parietal pericardia (124). A surgical approach to MPCE management is subxiphoid pericardiotomy to create a pericardial window. An advantage of this technique is that it is performed using local anesthesia and has a low recurrence rate. Additionally, tissue can be obtained for pathologic review. However, there is a small risk of myocardial laceration, pneumothorax, and mortality with this procedure. One study showed a 12% recurrence at 1 year and a 4% reoperation rate for subxiphoid pericardiotomy (125). Pleuropericardiotomy and pericardiectomy, which require general anesthesia, have higher morbidity and mortality rates, and are rarely used in MPCE management (124). Percutaneous balloon pericardiotomy is a treatment option for patients with large recurrent neoplastic pericardial effusions. Requiring only local anesthesia, it facilitates passage of pericardial fluid into the left pleural or peritoneal spaces, which have greater resorptive capacity. The major side effect is asymptomatic pleural effusion in most patients (52,136). Percutaneous balloon pericardiotomy appears to be a safe and effective technique in patients with large MPCEs and recurrent tamponade (90 to 97%) (136,137). Reaccumulation rates with this method are 0% to 6%. Reaccumulation rates for other therapies that are administered after initial pericardiocentesis is performed are radiotherapy, 33%; systemic chemotherapy, 30%; sclerotherapy with tetracycline, 15% to 30%; and mechanical therapies, including indwelling pericardial catheter placement, balloon pericardiotomy, and thoracotomy with pericardiostomy, 0% to 15% (52).

Even if there is no reaccumulation of fluid, cardiac function may remain impaired in the presence of epicardial infiltration by tumor. Diastolic dysfunction occurs because of the constrictive effect of a diseased epicardium surrounding the heart. Effusive-constrictive pericarditis results in a combination of tamponade and cardiac restriction. This entity must be considered in the differential diagnosis when a patient develops hemodynamic collapse a few days after pericardiocentesis. Pericardiectomy may be useful in alleviating the constrictive component; irrespective of this procedure, mortality is extremely high (52,138–140).

NEUTROPENIC ENTEROCOLITIS

Neutropenic enterocolitis (NE) is also known as necrotizing enteropathy, ileocecal syndrome, or typhlitis (141), from the Greek derivation of the word "typhlon," or cecum (142). The disorder is a life-threatening inflammatory syndrome in the immunocompromised patient that involves the terminal ileum, ascending colon, and cecum (143). Because the disease affects both the small and large bowel, the term, *neutropenic enterocolitis,* is most commonly used (144). The cardinal features that define the syndrome are fever, abdominal pain, and bowel wall thickening in a patient with neutropenia (143,145), where *neutropenia* is defined as a neutrophil count of either less than 500 neutrophils/μL, or less than 1,000 neutrophils/μL with an expected precipitous decline to below 500 neutrophils/μL (146,147). In its natural history, the disease may progress to bowel ulceration, necrosis, and perforation, and ultimately, sepsis and death (148).

NE occurs primarily in patients following aggressive cytotoxic therapy for acute leukemia (143,149) and other hematologic malignancies such as lymphoma (143,145,150), chronic leukemia (143), multiple myeloma (143–145), and rarely in solid tumors, such as colon, breast, testicular, lung (141,151), and pancreatic cancer (151). In leukemia, administration of drugs toxic to the bowel mucosa, such as cytosine arabinoside (152), which cause changes ranging from cellular atypia to frank ulceration, increases the risk of NE (151). Other agents include cytarabine, cisplatin, paclitaxel, fluorouracil, vincristine, doxorubicin, 5-fluorouracil, thioguanine, and mercaptopurine (152,153). Patients receiving immunosuppressive therapy for bone marrow (154) or renal transplantation (155) are also at risk.

The incidence of NE in adults varies widely in the literature, ranging from 0.8% to 26%. The increased use of cytotoxic chemotherapies that lead to GI tract mucosal inflammation is believed to result in an increased incidence of NEC (142,156,157). Early case reports described mortality rates ranging from 50% to 100% (158). Although no large recent case series have been published, early recognition and timely interventions described below have significantly reduced mortality from NE (159).

Pathophysiology

NE has a predilection for the terminal ileum, cecum, and appendix (160). One factor that may explain this predisposition is the overall decreased blood supply to the colon (145). Also, inherent to the cecum is decreased vascularity and increased distensibility compared to other colonic segments (151,161), and progressive distention in the cecum may cause increasing intraluminal pressure and exacerbation of submucosal edema (151). The pathogenesis of NE is multifactorial and remains unclear (141,145). Drug-induced cytotoxic mucosal injury (141,142,151) initiates the process by limiting cellular proliferation and generating glandular epithelial atypia and necrosis (cytosine arabinoside), and by producing myenteric plexus degeneration (vincristine) (151). Subsequently, mucosal barrier integrity is breached because cells cannot rapidly regenerate to repair the damaged surface (151). Once mucosal damage develops, bacterial translocation occurs, resulting in microbial infection and sepsis (141,151). Marked neutropenia impairs host defense and promotes further microbial invasion; bowel flora becomes altered (145). Blood cultures are often positive for *Clostridium septicum, C. difficile, Escherichia coli, Pseudomonas, Klebsiella, Enterobacter,* and *Staphylococcus* (144,151). Candidiasis, primarily *Candida albicans,* which colonizes mucosal surfaces, is the most common fungal infection in neutropenic patients and is associated with a high morbidity and mortality (162). These microbial infections lead to inflammation and edema. With sustained profound neutropenia, bacterial invasion is unconstrained, resulting in transmural necrosis, hemorrhage, ulceration, and perforation (144,145,151,163). In addition to drug-induced mucosal injury, infiltration of mucosa with leukemic and lymphoproliferative cells and mucosal ischemia from sepsis-related hypotension may also participate in initiating and perpetuating mucosal injury (151,160).

Diagnosis

The onset of NE is 7 to 10 days after treatment when neutropenia is evident. The clinical presentation includes fever, occurring in 90% of all hospitalized neutropenic patients at any time (163), nausea and vomiting, abdominal pain, and watery or bloody diarrhea. Physical examination may reveal stomatitis with diffuse mucositis, abdominal tenderness, abdominal distention, and peritoneal signs suggestive of bowel perforation (151,152,164). In 60% to 80% of patients, right lower quadrant (RLQ) tenderness is elicited. Palpation of a mass in the RLQ usually indicates a thickened, dilated, fluid-filled cecum (151).

On laboratory analysis, in addition to neutropenia, thrombocytopenia may be seen. Blood cultures are positive in 50% to 82% of cases for bowel organisms as described above (144). Stool studies may be notable for absence of *C. difficile* toxin A because *C. difficile* is not the primary pathogen in NE (143,161).

Plain radiographs of the abdomen are usually normal or nonspecific. Findings may include a decrease in RLQ gas with dilated small bowel loops and air–fluid levels consistent with a distal bowel obstruction. Free intraperitoneal air after perforation, pneumatosis coli, or localized or diffuse "thumbprinting" characteristic of mucosal edema may be exhibited (141,151). Sonography assists in confirming the diagnosis of NE and in excluding other differential diagnoses by detecting bowel wall thickening. Additionally, ultrasound is useful in following the clinical course of the disease (145,165). Sonographic manifestations of NE include a rounded mass with dense central echoes and a wider hyperechoic periphery (141), pseudopolypoid changes of the cecal mucosa, and pericolic fluid collections (151). CT is a more accurate modality for assessing cecal wall thickening and evaluating the extent of the colitis (141,145). It also has utility in differentiating NE from appendicitis, appendiceal abscess, or pseudomembranous colitis (167). CT findings include diffuse submucosal thickening and edema of the terminal ileum and ascending colon, mural hemorrhage, pericolic fluid collections, abscess formation, pneumatosis coli, and intraperitoneal free air (145). The false-negative rates in identifying NE for CT, ultrasound, and plain radiographs are 15%, 23%, and 48%, respectively (149).

Barium enema is unsafe because it may result in bowel perforation in the presence of severely damaged, necrotic bowel (142,167). Endoscopic evaluation is generally avoided because it involves a high risk of perforation in addition to hemorrhagic and infectious complications, and it may precipitate fulminant mural necrosis (141). Colonoscopy has been performed in a small number of patients and shows irregular nodular mucosa, ulcerations, hemorrhagic friability, and a masslike lesion resembling carcinoma (142).

Management

Prospective trials or case-control studies evaluating therapeutic interventions in NE are lacking (143). Conservative management of NE is indicated for patients without overt perforation, peritonitis, or bleeding; this includes bowel rest, intravenous fluid and blood product resuscitation, broad-spectrum antibiotics, granulocyte colony-stimulating factor (G-CSF), and nasogastric decompression. Medications that inhibit bowel motility, such as antidiarrheal and narcotic agents should be avoided because they perpetuate ileus and promote bacterial overgrowth (152). Patients with chemotherapy-induced NE may suffer from repeated episodes with future treatment; therefore, further chemotherapy should be withheld until NE has completely resolved. Bowel decontamination may be helpful before subsequent chemotherapy (142). Empiric antibiotic therapy with a carbapenem, piperacillin–tazobactam, or cefepime plus metronidazole should be initiated immediately (143,151,168). Empiric antifungal therapy with voriconazole or amphotericin B therapy should be considered in profoundly neutropenic patients whose fevers persist beyond 3 days of appropriately dosed broad-spectrum antibiotics (146).

G-CSF increases cell division in myeloid precursor cells, decreases bone marrow transit time, and modulates activity and function of developing and mature neutrophils (163). As clinical improvement in NE patients is usually seen after normalization of the neutrophil count, G-CSF is often given as part of initial management of this condition; it should be noted that there are no data to support its use. Furthermore, there is a theoretical risk that bowel inflammation during immune recovery may lead to further inflammation and perforation (142).

There are no standard recommendations, but rather, general guidelines in the literature regarding surgical intervention in NE. Most patients are unlikely to be surgical candidates. Early reports recommended aggressive and early surgical resection of involved bowel, anticipating that in the natural history of NE, bowel perforation is inevitable (143). Subsequent series demonstrate successful nonsurgical management (143,169,170). More recent publications support surgery with laparotomy alone for patients with perforation and ileus (143). Some advocate that patients who fail to improve or develop bowel perforation and peritonitis after 2 or 3 days of conservative therapy warrant consideration for surgery (161,171). Several authors recommend surgery for severe complications such as abscess, necrotic bowel, and obstruction (145). In general, definitive indications for surgery include intraperitoneal free air/perforation, generalized peritonitis, and persistent bleeding in spite of correction of coagulopathy (141,151). Important considerations that must influence the decision to surgically intervene are the patient's prognosis and comorbidities (151). If surgery is warranted, the procedure of choice is colectomy with ileostomy and mucous fistula; a primary anastomosis is used in very few patients (172). Of note, the extent of mucosal necrosis may be underestimated by the appearance of the serosa. A surgeon must ensure complete resection of edematous bowel, even in the absence of necrosis and inflammation, to preclude a fatal outcome (151).

Controversies

The management of NE is not based on prospective studies of medical versus surgical intervention. Treatment is usually individualized and based on past experience. Although it appears reasonable to treat patients with early NE conservatively, there are no data to support superior outcomes with this approach.

TOXICITY OF CHEMOTHERAPY

Most antineoplastic agents exert their therapeutic actions by targeting rapidly proliferating malignant cells. Because these agents interrupt fundamental cellular processes such as DNA, RNA, and protein synthesis, they are not completely specific to malignant cells and will also act on normal tissues, causing multiple toxicities. Rapidly regenerating cells, such as the hematopoietic lineage, GI mucosa, spermatogonia, and hair follicles may suffer transient toxicity compared to cells that have limited regenerative capacity, including those of the myocardium, and nerves (173–175). This section focuses on the major life-threatening toxicities that occur with commonly used chemotherapeutic agents. Molecularly targeted therapies and immunotherapy often have organ-specific adverse effects, which will be discussed below.

Pulmonary Toxicities

Pulmonary toxicity, both acute and chronic, is seen increasingly with numerous antineoplastic agents (176). Chemotherapy-induced lung disease describes lung injury with multiple etiologic agents and varying pathophysiologic mechanisms. These major mechanisms include direct lung toxicity, immunologic response, and increased capillary permeability. The corresponding clinical presentations are interstitial pneumonitis/fibrosis, hypersensitivity syndrome, and capillary leak syndrome, respectively, and each may eventuate in fulminant respiratory failure. Symptoms can appear immediately or months after termination of therapy (177).

Antitumor Antibiotics

Bleomycin

Bleomycin is an antitumor antibiotic used in the treatment of lymphoma, germ cell tumors, cervical carcinoma, and head and neck squamous cell carcinoma. The absence of bleomycin hydrolase in the skin and lungs prevents deactivation of the drug, accounting for its selective toxicity. Bleomycin interstitial pneumonitis is the most ominous toxicity, associated with a 3% mortality rate (178) and occurring in up to 10% of patients receiving bleomycin-containing regimens, either during treatment or up to 6 months after discontinuation (179). Toxicity is mediated by the mechanism of direct lung injury via generation of cytokines and free radicals, the sequelae of which are endothelial damage, inflammatory cell infiltration, fibroblast activation, and fibrosis (177,179). There is conflicting evidence in the literature as to whether perioperative oxygen supplementation exceeding a concentration of 24% fractional inspired oxygen causes synergistic toxicity with bleomycin through the production of free radicals (180,181); older patients and those with renal insufficiency are more susceptible. Drug withdrawal, steroids, and avoidance of supplemental oxygen may be helpful (182).

Mitomycin C

This is an antibiotic used in treating solid tumors, primarily breast and lung carcinomas. The mechanism of injury is alkylation of endothelial cell DNA, precluding cell division. This agent is associated with the development of an interstitial pneumonitis/fibrosis (184,185), usually 3 to 12 months after therapy (182,184), with a 3% to 14% incidence. Mortality is as high as 14% to 50% (183–185). Risk factors include oxygen exposure, prior irradiation, and other cytotoxic drug administration, such as bleomycin, cisplatin, the vinca alkaloids, cyclophosphamide, and doxorubicin. Drug withdrawal, steroids, and avoidance of supplemental oxygen may be helpful (182).

Alkylating Agents

Carmustine

Carmustine (BCNU) is a nitrosourea used in the management of CNS tumors and in induction therapy for bone marrow transplantation (BMT). Its cytotoxicity is mediated by alkylation of guanine in DNA (180). Carmustine causes dose-dependent pulmonary fibrosis and carries the highest incidence of fibrosis among the nitrosoureas. The mortality rate ranges from 24% to as high as 90% in some reports (182,185). Sixty percent of patients will respond dramatically to steroids (182).

Microtubule-Targeting Agents

Taxanes

Paclitaxel inhibits microtubule disassembly (186), and has activity against solid tumors such as non–small cell lung carcinoma, breast carcinoma, and ovarian carcinoma (177); it is prepared in Cremophor, a castor oil-based solution (177,186). A type I hypersensitivity reaction, characterized by urticaria, bronchospasm, angioedema, and hypotension, occurs within 2 to 10 minutes of infusion of paclitaxel (186,187) with a 3% to 10% incidence (182), and is attributable to the Cremophor vehicle rather than paclitaxel itself (177). Premedication with steroids and H_1 and H_2 blockers can curtail this reaction (186).

Antimetabolites

Cytosine Arabinoside

Ara-C is a substituted nucleoside antimetabolite that disrupts DNA replication and is used in the therapy of leukemia and NHL. One of its toxicities is the abrupt onset of endothelial inflammation and capillary leak syndrome (177), causing noncardiogenic pulmonary edema, acute dyspnea, and a diffuse interstitial and alveolar pattern. Management is supportive and includes oxygen, diuretics, and mechanical ventilation when needed (182).

Gemcitabine

This pyrimidine analog, structurally similar to ara-C (187), has activity against a variety of solid tumors and lymphoma. The reported incidence of lung toxicity is less than 1.4% (188). The proposed mechanism of injury involves pulmonary endothelial cell damage resulting in capillary leak syndrome (177,187). The symptoms of gemcitabine pulmonary toxicity range from mild dyspnea to fatal ARDS. Increasing age, pulmonary neoplasm, and prior radiotherapy may be contributing risk factors (177,189). Patients respond rapidly to corticosteroids (177), but fatalities do occur (177,185,187,189,190).

Differentiation Agents

All-trans-Retinoic Acid

ATRA is a differentiation agent used for the treatment of acute promyelocytic leukemia (APL). It is associated with retinoic acid syndrome, developing in 20% to 50% of APL patients receiving ATRA (191) a median of 7 days (range 0 to 35 days) after induction therapy (192). The clinical presentation includes fluid retention, weight gain, fever, and musculoskeletal pain, with progression to respiratory distress, pulmonary infiltrates, pleural (191) and pericardial effusions (182), renal insufficiency, skin infiltrates, hypotension, and death (191). Corticosteroids are highly effective when the syndrome commences but have limited utility once pulmonary symptoms are apparent. The putative mechanism of the pulmonary toxicity of ATRA is a capillary leak syndrome (182). Treatment is supportive.

Cardiac Toxicities

Antitumor Antibiotics

Anthracyclines. These are red-pigmented antibiotics (rhodomycins), which include doxorubicin, daunorubicin, idarubicin, and epirubicin (175). They are active against a broad spectrum of tumors, such as breast and esophageal carcinomas, HL and NHL, osteosarcomas, Kaposi sarcoma, and soft-tissue sarcomas. Acute cardiotoxicities include nonspecific ST-T wave changes (193), supraventricular tachycardia (SVT), ventricular dysrhythmias, myopericarditis, cardiomyopathy, and sudden death. The cardiomyopathy is dose dependent, and is classified as subacute and late. Subacute cardiomyopathy presents within 8 months of therapy, with a peak onset of 3 months, whereas late cardiomyopathy is observed after 5 or more years. A continual decline in left ventricular function results in CHF (175). Reduced cardiotoxicity has been observed with liposomal doxorubicin (194). Dexrazoxane, an iron chelator with cardioprotective properties, has been demonstrated to substantially reduce toxicity (195,196). Toxic effects may be compounded by other therapies, including trastuzumab, cyclophosphamide, dactinomycin, mithramycin, mitomycin, etoposide, melphalan vincristine, bleomycin, dacarbazine (175), and taxanes (197,198). In a recent study of patients with anthracycline-induced decrease in left ventricular ejection fraction (LVEF), treatment with enalapril and carvedilol resulted in normalization of LVEF in 42% of patients (199). Patients with CHF resulting from anthracycline-induced cardiomyopathy respond to standard treatment including ACE inhibitors, beta blockers, and loop diuretics (200).

Mitoxantrone. This agent has structural similarity to the anthracyclines, and is used in managing metastatic breast cancer, acute myeloid leukemia, and NHL (198). The mechanism of cardiac injury, like that of the anthracyclines, may involve iron chelation complexes (201); dysrhythmias and dose-dependent heart failure are toxicities. The incidence of a moderate-to-severe decrease in LVEF and of CHF is 13% and 2.6%, respectively, with a cumulative dose of less than or equal to 140 mg/m^2. Doses below 110 mg/m^2 decrease the incidence of heart failure, whereas incidence increases with doses greater than 160 mg/m^2 (175). Again, standard therapy with ACE inhibitors, beta blockers, and diuretics are indicated for CHF.

Mitomycin C. In addition to its lung toxicity, mitomycin is cardiotoxic, resulting in an increased incidence of cardiac failure with cumulative doses exceeding 30 mg/m^2 (175,202). Additive cardiotoxicity occurs when mitomycin is used in conjunction with anthracyclines (202); superoxide free radicals may mediate this toxicity (193).

Alkylating Agents

Cyclophosphamide. This agent is a nitrogen mustard alkylating agent effective in treating a variety of solid and liquid tumors. Acute cardiotoxicity may develop with doses of 120 to 170 mg/kg given over 1 to 7 days. ECG may reveal decreased QRS amplitude, nonspecific T-wave abnormalities, poor R-wave progression, supraventricular and ventricular tachydysrhythmias, and second-degree atrioventricular block (201). Acute fulminant CHF may occur in up to 28% of patients treated with high-dose cyclophosphamide (175), but CHF is usually short lived and reversible (201). The drug is metabolized to its active form in the liver by the cytochrome P-450, and more rapid metabolism amplifies the risk of CHF (203). Another cyclophosphamide-related cardiotoxicity is hemorrhagic myocarditis, putatively mediated by endothelial capillary injury, which results in pericardial effusion, tamponade, and death. Most effusions are treatable with corticosteroids and analgesics.

Ifosfamide. This is an alkylating agent, with similar properties to cyclophosphamide, used to treat lymphoma, leukemia, and testicular and bladder tumors. Dysrhythmias and transient, reversible, dose-dependent CHF—as with cyclophosphamide—may be seen (201,204).

Cisplatin. This agent cross-links interstrand DNA. It is used in treating cancers of the testes, bladder, ovaries, and other tumors. Bradycardia, SVT (175), acute ischemia (205), myocardial infarction, and ischemic cardiomyopathy may be observed (175). Acute chest pain and palpitations may be associated with cisplatin infusion. Hypomagnesemia and hypokalemia generated by cisplatin-induced tubular defects (175) may exacerbate arrhythmias (193). Venous thrombosis and pulmonary embolism have also been recognized (206).

Antimetabolites

5-Fluorouracil and Capecitabine. 5-Fluorouracil (5-FU) is a synthetic pyrimidine antimetabolite used in regimens for managing multiple solid tumors including GI, breast, ovarian, and head and neck malignancies. Myocardial ischemia, possibly triggered by coronary vasospasm, is a well-known cardiac toxicity that occurs with increased frequency in combination with cisplatin. In one study, silent ischemic ECG changes were identified during 24 hours of observation in up to 68% of patients receiving a continuous 5-FU infusion (207). Other cardiac manifestations include chest pain, angina, atrial and ventricular dysrhythmias, myocardial infarction, persistent ventricular dysfunction, sudden death, and cardiogenic shock (175) requiring inotropic support (175). Pre-existing cardiac morbidity significantly increases the risk of cardiotoxicity compared to no prior cardiac disease (15.1% vs. 1.5%). The oral equivalent of infused 5-FU is capecitabine, which exhibits a similar cardiotoxicity profile to 5-FU (208). Given the potential for severe cardiotoxicity, infusions should be terminated when chest pain occurs. If chest pain persists despite discontinuation of drug, administration of nitrates or calcium channel blockers results in resolution of symptoms in 70% to 90% of patients (209).

Differentiation Agents

All-trans-Retinoic Acid. Pericardial effusions, cardiac tamponade, myocardial ischemia (175), fatal infarction, and thrombosis (193), in addition to pulmonary toxicity, may occur with the retinoic acid syndrome as described above (175). (See also Pulmonary Toxicities.)

Arsenic Trioxide. Arsenic trioxide is a differentiation agent effective in treating relapsed acute promyelocytic leukemia. Like all-*trans*-retinoic acid, it may also cause the retinoic acid syndrome. Prolongation of the QT interval is another complication seen in up to 63% of patients, leading to torsades de pointes (175) and sudden death. The degree of QT prolongation is higher in the presence of hypokalemia; therefore, careful monitoring of electrolytes and maintaining levels in the high normal range is prudent (210).

Monoclonal Antibodies

Trastuzumab. There is an increased risk of cardiotoxicity associated with trastuzumab, which is highest in patients receiving concurrent anthracycline plus cyclophosphamide (27%) (211). The mechanism of cardiac toxicity of trastuzumab is not well understood, but cardiac erbB2 is essential for myocyte function, and trastuzumab targets both HER2 and erbB2 receptors (211). Early following initial treatment, there may be an asymptomatic decline in LVEF with late progression to dilated cardiomyopathy. Risk factors for cardiovascular toxicity include older age, cumulative doxorubicin dosage 400 mg/m^2 or greater (213), and concurrent anthracycline and trastuzumab administration, rather than temporally separated dosing (212). Pertuzumab and ado-trastuzumab emtansine, other monoclonal antibodies that target HER2, are also associated with a decline in LVEF, although not as severe as trastuzumab. Trastuzumab-related cardiomyopathy is reversible with discontinuation of drug (212).

Rituximab. The CD20 antigen, present on normal and malignant B cells, is the target of the chimeric murine/human monoclonal antibody rituximab, which is used to treat leukemias and lymphomas, as well as benign diseases. Cardiac toxicity involves dysrhythmias and angina in less than 1% of infusions (175). Most adverse effects with rituximab are infusion related, usually occurring within 2 hours of the first infusion (213). Acute infusion-related deaths have been reported in 0.04% to 0.07% of cases. The clinical presentation in these patients includes hypoxia, pulmonary infiltrates, adult respiratory distress syndrome, myocardial infarction, ventricular fibrillation, and cardiogenic shock (213). Hypersensitivity reactions, including hypotension, angioedema, hypoxia, or bronchospasm, may occur in up to 10% of cases. Management is supportive, using intravenous fluids, antihistamines, acetaminophen, bronchodilators, and vasopressors (193).

Bevacizumab. This agent is associated with CHF, hypertension, and arterial thromboembolism. With bevacizumab monotherapy, 2% of patients developed moderate to life-threatening (grades 2 to 4) left ventricular dysfunction (see also Pulmonary Toxicities) (213). CHF developed in 14% of patients concurrently receiving anthracyclines, and in 4% of patients who had previously received anthracyclines or left chest wall irradiation (214). Clinical trials have also documented hypertension in 5% of patients, with reports of hypertensive crisis, hypertensive encephalopathy, and subarachnoid hemorrhage (193). The risk of fatal arterial thrombotic events is doubled to 5% in patients receiving intravenous 5-FU and bevacizumab (214,215).

Small Molecule Kinase Inhibitors

The drugs sunitinib, sorafenib, dasatanib, and lapatinib belong to the family of small molecule tyrosine kinase inhibitors (TKI). These agents interfere with VEGF, FLT, and PDGF-mediated pathways and have activity across a wide spectrum of malignancies.

Sunitinib

Hypertension induced by this agent is noted in 3% to 8% of individuals (216). Grade 3 or higher hypertension occurred in 7.3% of patients during phase I trials. In the phase II clinical trials of sunitinib for renal cell carcinoma 8.9% of patients developed a reduction in LVEF, and 3% developed NYHA stage 3 or 4 heart failure (216). Sunitinib-induced hypertension is usually reversible with discontinuation of drug (217); antihypertensive therapy is often necessary although no particular class has proved most efficacious in this setting.

Sorafenib

This agent is associated with an increased risk of myocardial ischemia and infarction of approximately 3% (218). In phase II studies with sorafenib 12% of patients developed grade 1 or 2 hypertension and 13.8% developed grade 3 hypertension (217). Antihypertensive therapy is often necessary with no particular class of medication favored.

Imatinib

This drug is used in the treatment of CML and ALL, and is associated with an incidence of symptomatic CHF of approximately 1% (219). Most patients will respond to diuresis and medical management.

Dasatanib

This is another TKI used in the treatment of CML and ALL and is associated with QT prolongation and CHF (<2%). No deaths have been attributed to cardiac adverse effects from dasatanib (220). Initial management includes reversal of other proximate causes of QT prolongation such as electrolyte derangements and discontinuation of medications affecting the QT interval.

Lapatinib

This agent, used in the treatment of herceptin refractory breast cancer that over-expresses HER2, is associated with an incidence of symptomatic heart failure in 1.3% patients treated longer than 6 months (221). Of note, many of these have already been exposed to anthracycline and herceptin-based therapy. Drug discontinuation and standard medical therapy for heart failure may be indicated.

Gastrointestinal Toxicities

Bevacizumab

Bevacizumab is associated with both bowel perforation in 0.2% to 3.2% of recipients, and grades 3 to 4 GI hemorrhage in 3.8% of patients (222). Perforation may occur at the site of a primary tumor, prior resection, prior radiation, or even in patients without evidence of peritoneal metastases. Although surgical exploration with repair or diversion is indicated in most patients with a perforated viscus, this decision must be made within the larger context of a patient's overall prognosis and desire for aggressive interventions. When possible, surgery should be avoided for at least 28 days following bevacizumab.

Immunomodulatory Agents

The successful use of immunomodulatory antibodies in the treatment of melanoma and other malignancies heralds a new front in the treatment of cancer. The anti–cytotoxic T-lymphocyte–associated antigen 4 (CTLA-4) antibodies ipilimumab and tremelimumab (currently under development) as well as the anti–programmed cell death-1 receptor antibodies nivolumab and pembrolizumab carry a unique set immune-related toxicities affecting the skin, GI tract, liver, and endocrine system. These adverse events are triggered by a release of natural immunologic inhibition and are often successfully managed with a course of immunosuppressive therapy such as corticosteroids, tumor necrosis factor-alpha antagonists, or mycophenolate mofetil. The approach to treatment of these adverse events is based upon clinical experience, as there no prospective trials to guide therapy.

Diarrhea/Colitis

Diarrhea is a common side effect in patients undergoing treatment with checkpoint blocking antibodies and typically presents 6 weeks after initiation of therapy. It is more frequently seen in patients receiving anti–CTLA-4 immunotherapy than anti–PD-1 therapy (223,224). It is important to exclude other etiologies such as infection with bacterial or viral pathogens. Diarrhea was reported in approximately 30% of patients treated with ipilimumab for melanoma (223). Severe diarrhea—an increase of 7 or more stools above baseline—occurred in less than 10% of cases and significant colitis was reported in approximately 5% of patients (224).

Patients with mild symptoms (less than four stools per day over baseline) can be managed symptomatically with an American Dietetic Association colitis diet, antimotility agents, and oral budesonide. For patients with more than four to six stools per day above baseline, CT scan or, if unrevealing, colonoscopy may establish the diagnosis of colitis. If present, mild colitis is treated with IV corticosteroids (1 mg/kg prednisone). For patients with an increase of seven or more stools above baseline, high-dose corticosteroids (2 mg/kg prednisone) should be initiated. If the patient does not improve, infliximab at a dose of 5 mg/kg once every 2 weeks should be given, a regimen based upon treatment of inflammatory bowel disease (225,226). Mycophenolate may be necessary for colitis does not improve with infliximab.

Hepatotoxicity

Therapy with anti–CTLA-4 and PD-1 antibodies is associated with elevations in serum levels of the hepatic enzymes aspartate aminotransferase (AST) and alanine aminotransferase (ALT) (227,228). This occurs less than 10% of the time and is usually asymptomatic. Some patients have an associated fever. Hepatotoxicity most commonly occurs 8 to 12 weeks after initiation of treatment (229). CT scan may show mild hepatomegaly, periportal edema, or periportal lymphadenopathy (232). Liver biopsy, although not necessary to make the diagnosis, shows severe panlobular hepatitis with prominent perivenular infiltrate with endothelialitis (230).

Once elevated transaminases are identified, other causes of hepatotoxicity must be excluded. If no other etiology is identified, treatment with 1 to 2 mg/kg prednisone should be initiated as soon as possible. Elevated transaminases may persist for several weeks and may require prolonged or repeated corticosteroid tapers. Mycophenolate mofetil (500 mg every 12 hours) and antithymocyte globulin therapy may be used for patients with elevations in transaminases that do not improve with steroids (231).

Adrenal insufficiency is a rare but critical endocrinopathy associated with checkpoint blockade therapy, seen in less than 2% of cases (232). Patients present with hypotension, dehydration, and electrolyte derangements, which must be differentiated from other acute causes of hemodynamic instability. Emergent therapy includes intravenous corticosteroids (hydrocortisone 100 mg or dexamethasone 4 mg), aggressive management of fluid status, and correction of electrolyte abnormalities.

Key Points

Hypercalcemia

- The severity of symptoms correlates with both the degree of hypercalcemia and the rate at which the calcium is rising.
- Initial therapy consists of normal saline hydration to maintain a urine output of 150 to 200 mL/hr. Calcitonin and bisphosphonates are indicated for patients with severe hypercalcemia. Denosumab is indicated for patients with bisphosphonate-refractory hypercalcemia or renal insufficiency.

Tumor Lysis Syndrome

- Cornerstones of therapy include aggressive hydration with maintenance urine output of 80 to 100 mL/m^2/hr or greater, frequent monitoring and correction of electrolyte derangements, and administration of a hypouricemic agent such as rasburicase or allopurinol.

SVCS

- CT scan with IV contrast can often establish the diagnosis, define the level of blockage, document collateral circulation, and identify the underlying cause.
- The relative ease and availability of endovascular stenting has obviated the need for emergent RT prior to histologic diagnosis in most cases.

Malignant Spinal Cord Compression

- Pretreatment neurologic function is the most important predictor of posttreatment outcome.
- The choice of definitive therapy must take into account the patient's overall prognosis; Surgery is recommended for patients with unstable spine lesions or radiation resistant tumors.

Malignant Pericardial Effusion

- The diagnosis is suspected based on physical examination, ECG, chest x-ray, and echocardiography.
- Percutaneous and surgical approaches are both effective and lead to prompt improvement in hemodynamic compromise. When technically feasible, percutaneous drainage is preferred in most patients.

Neutropenic Enterocolitis

- Patients with uncomplicated NE should receive empiric broad-spectrum antibiotics, bowel rest, NG decompression, transfusional support, and hydration. Surgery is reserved for patients with overt perforation or uncontrolled bleeding.

References

1. Alteri R, Bertaut T, Brooks D, et al. *Cancer Facts & Figures 2015*. Atlanta, GA: American Cancer Society; 2015:1–52.
2. Copelan EA. Hematopoietic stem-cell transplantation. *N Engl J Med.* 2006;354:1813–1826.
3. Hojjat-Farsangi M. Novel and emerging target-based cancer agents and methods. *Tumour Biol.* 2015;36(2):543–546.
4. Widakowich C, de Castro G Jr, de Azambuja E, et al. Review: side effects of approved molecular targeted therapies in solid cancers. *Oncologist.* 2007;12(12):1443–1455.
5. Stewart AF. Hypercalcemia associated with cancer. *N Engl J Med.* 2005;352:373–379.
6. Rosol TJ, Capen CC. Mechanisms of cancer-induced hypercalcemia. *Lab Invest.* 1992;67:680–702.
7. Fojo AT. Oncologic emergencies: metabolic emergencies. In: DeVita VT, Hellman S, Rosenberg SA, eds. *Cancer: Principles and Practice of Oncology.* 9th ed. Philadelphia, PA: Lippincott Williams & Wilkins; 2011:2142–2152.
8. Pecherstorfer M, Schilling T, Blind E, et al. Parathyroid hormone-related protein and life expectancy in hypercalcemic patients. *J Clin Endocrinol Metab.* 1994;78:1268–1270.
9. Halfdanarson TR, Hogan WJ, Moynihan TJ. Oncological emergencies: diagnosis and treatment. *Mayo Clin Proc.* 2006;81(6):835–848.
10. Ralston SH, Gallagher SJ, Patel U, et al. Cancer-associated hypercalcemia: morbidity and mortality: clinical experience in 126 treated patients. *Ann Intern Med.* 1990;112:499–504.
11. Lumachi F, Brunello A, Roma A, Basso U. Cancer-induced hypercalcemia. *Anticancer Res.* 2009 29(5):1551–1555.
12. Dunbar ME, Wysolmerski JJ, Broadus AE. Parathyroid hormone-related protein: from hypercalcemia of malignancy to developmental regulatory molecule. *Am J Med Sci.* 1996;312(6):287–294.
13. Rizzoli R, Ferrari SL, Pizurki L, et al. Actions of parathyroid hormone and parathyroid hormone-related protein. *J Endocrinol Invest.* 1992;15(9 Suppl 6):51–56.
14. Walls J, Ratcliffe WA, Howell A, Bundred NJ. Parathyroid hormone and parathyroid hormone-related protein in the investigation of hypercalcaemia in two hospital populations. *Clin Endocrinol (Oxf).* 1994;41(4):407–413.
15. Bringhurst F, Demay M, Krane S, et al. Bone and mineral metabolism in health and disease. In: Kasper D, Braunwald E, Fauci A, et al. *Harrison's Internal Medicine.* 17th ed. New York, NY: McGraw-Hill; 2008:2365–2377.
16. Bushinsky DA, Monk RD. Calcium. *Lancet.* 1998;352:306–311.
17. Bilezekian JP, Silverberg SJ. Asymptomatic primary hyperparathyroidism. *N Engl J Med.* 2004:350:1746–1751.
18. Germano T. The parathyroid gland and calcium-related emergencies. *Top Emerg Med.* 2001;23(4):51–56.
19. Cogan MG, Covey GM, Arieff AL, et al. Central nervous system manifestations of hyperparathyroidism. *Am J Med.* 1978;65:963–970.
20. Ward JB, Petersen OH, Jenkins SA, Sutton R. Is an elevated concentration of acinar cytosolic free ionised calcium the trigger for acute pancreatitis? *Lancet.* 1995;346(8981):1016–1019.
21. Berenson JR. Treatment of hypercalcemia with bisphosphonates. *Semin Oncol.* 2002:29(6 Suppl 21):12–18.
22. al Zaharani A, Levine ML. Primary hyperparathyroidism. *Lancet.* 1997;349:1233–1238.
23. Wang S, McDonnell EH, Sedor FA, Toffaletti JG. pH effects on measurements of ionized calcium and ionized magnesium in the blood. *Arch Pathol Lab Med.* 2002;126:947–950.
24. Body JJ. Hypercalcemia of malignancy. *Semin Nephrol.* 2004;24:48–54.
25. Gurney H, Grill V, Martin TJ. Parathyroid hormone-related protein and response to pamidronate in tumour induced hypercalcemia. *Lancet.* 1993;341:1611–1613.
26. Berenson JR, Lipton A. Bisphosphonates in the treatment of malignant bone disease. *Annu Rev Med.* 1999;50:237–248.
27. Major P, Lortholary A, Hon J, et al. Zoledronic acid is superior to pamidronate in the treatment of hypercalcemia of malignancy: a pooled analysis of two randomized, controlled clinical trials. *J Clin Oncol.* 2001;19:558–567.
28. Tanveyanon T, Stiff PJ. Management of the adverse effects associated with intravenous bisphosphonates. *Ann Oncol.* 2006;17(6):897–907.
29. Cicci JD, Buie L, Bates J, van Deventer H. Denosumab for the management of hypercalcemia of malignancy in patients with multiple myeloma and renal dysfunction. *Clin Lymphoma Myeloma Leuk.* 2014;14:e207–e211.
30. Adhikaree J, Newby Y, Sundar S. Denosumab should be the treatment of choice for bisphosphonate refractory hypercalcemia of malignancy. *BMJ Case Rep.* 2014: pii. bcr2013202861.
31. Stopeck AT, Lipton A, Body JJ, et al. Denosumab compared with zoledronic acid for the treatment of bone metastases in patients with advanced breast cancer: a randomized, double-blind study. *J Clin Oncol.* 2010;28(35)5132–5139.
32. Karuppiah D, Thanabalasingham G, Shine B, et al. Refractory hypercalcemia secondary to parathyroid carcinoma: response to high-dose denosumab. *Eur J Endocrinol.* 2014;171:K1–K5.
33. Silverman P, Distelhorst CW. Metabolic emergencies in clinical oncology. *Semin Oncol.* 1989;16(6):504–515.
34. Rampello E, Fricia T, Malaguarnera M. The management of tumor lysis syndrome. *Nat Clin Pract Oncol.* 2006;3(8):438–447.
35. Chasty RC, Liu-Yin JA. Acute tumor lysis syndrome. *Br J Hosp Med.* 1993;49(70):488–492.
36. Davidson MD, Thakkar S, Hix JK, et al. Pathophysiology, clinical consequences, and treatment of tumor lysis syndrome. *Am J Med.* 2004;116:546–554.
37. Cohen LF, Balow JE, Magrath IT, et al. Acute tumor lysis syndrome: a review of 37 patients with Burkitt's lymphoma. *Am J Med.* 1980;68:486–491.
38. Hande KR, Garrow GC. Acute tumor lysis syndrome in patients with high-grade non-Hodgkin's lymphoma. *Am J Med.* 1993;94:133–139.
39. Flombaum CD. Metabolic emergencies in the cancer patient. *Semin Oncol.* 2000;27:322–334.
40. Jasek AM, Day HJ. Acute spontaneous tumor lysis syndrome. *Am J Hematol.* 1994;47:129–131.
41. Hsu H, Chan Y, Huang C. Acute spontaneous tumor lysis presenting with hyperuricemic acute renal failure: clinical features and therapeutic approach. *J Nephrol.* 2004;17:50–56.
42. Cairo MS, Bishop M. Tumour lysis syndrome: new therapeutic strategies and classification. *Br J Haematol.* 2004;127:3–11.
43. Dunlay RW, Camp MA, Allon M, et al. Calcitriol in prolonged hypocalcemia due to the tumor lysis syndrome. *Ann Intern Med.* 1989;110:162–164.
44. Altman A. Acute tumor lysis syndrome. *Semin Oncol.* 2001;28 (Suppl 5):3–8.

45. Navolanic PM, Pui C-H, Larson RA, et al. Elitek-rasburicase: an effective means to prevent and treat hyperuricemia associated with tumor lysis syndrome, a Meeting Report, Dallas, Texas, January 2002. *Leukemia.* 2003;17(3):499–514.
46. Howard SC, Jones DP, Pui CH. The tumor lysis syndrome. *N Engl J Med.* 2011;364:1844–1854.
47. Coiffier B, Altman A, Pui CH, et al. Guidelines for the management of pediatric and adult tumor lysis syndrome: an evidence-based review. *J Clin Oncol.* 2008;26:2767–2778.
48. Yeldani AV, Yeldani V, Kumar S, et al. Molecular evolution of the urate oxidase-encoding gene in hominoid primates: nonsense mutations. *Gene.* 1991;109:281–284.
49. Ueng S. Rasburicase (Elitek): a novel agent for tumor lysis syndrome. *Proc (Bayl Univ Med Cent).* 2005;18(3):275–279.
50. Bertrand Y, Mechinaud F, Brethon B, et al. SFCE (SociétéFrançaise de Lutte contre les Cancers et Leucémies de l'Enfant et de l'Adolescent) recommendations for the management of tumor lysis syndrome (TLS) with rasburicase: an observational survey. *J Pediatr Hematol Oncol.* 2008;30(4):267–271.
51. Abner A. Approach to the patient who presents with superior vena cava obstruction. *Chest.* 1993;103(4 Suppl):394S–397S.
52. Lamont EB, Hoffman PC. Chapter 72. Oncologic emergencies. In: Hall JB, Schmidt GA, Wood LH, eds. *Principles of Critical Care.* 3rd ed. New York, NY: McGraw-Hill; 2005:1099–1110.
53. Yahalom J. Oncologic emergencies: superior vena cava syndrome. In: DeVita VT, Hellman S, Rosenberg SA, eds. *Cancer: Principles and Practice of Oncology.* 7th ed. Vol 2. Philadelphia, PA: Lippincott Williams & Wilkins; 2005:2274–2280.
54. Duwe BV, Sterman DH, Musani AI. Tumors of the mediastinum. *Chest.* 2005;128(4):2893–2909.
55. Hunter W. The history of an aneurysm of the aorta with some remarks on aneurysms in general. *Med Observ Inq.* 1757;1:323.
56. Schechter MM. The superior vena cava syndrome. *Am J Med Sci.* 1954;227:46–56.
57. Rice TW, Rodriguez RM, Light RW. The superior vena cava syndrome: clinical characteristics and evolving etiology. *Medicine (Baltimore).* 2006; 85(1):37–42.
58. Yu JB, Wilson LD, Detterbeck FC. Superior vena cava syndrome: a proposed classification system and algorithm for management. *J Thorac Oncol.* 2008;3(8):811–814.
59. Wilson LD, Detterbeck FC, Yahalom J. Superior vena cava syndrome with malignant causes. *N Engl J Med.* 2007;356:1862–1869.
60. Parish JM, Marschke RF Jr,Dines DE, Lee RE. Etiologic considerations in superior vena cava syndrome. *Mayo Clin Proc.* 1981;56(7):407–413.
61. Gucalp R, Dutcher J. Oncologic emergencies. In: Kasper D, Braunwald E, Fauci A, et al., eds. *Harrison's Internal Medicine.* 18th ed. New York, NY: McGraw-Hill; 2012:2266–2278.
62. Lochridge SK, Knibbe WP, Doty DB. Obstruction of the superior vena cava. *Surgery.* 1979;85:14–24.
63. Ostler PJ, Clarke DP, Watkinson AF, et al. Superior vena cava obstruction: a modern management strategy. *Clin Oncol.* 1997;9:83–89.
64. Theodore PR, Jablons D. In: Doherty GM, Way LW, eds. *Current Surgical Diagnosis and Treatment.* 12th ed. New York, NY: McGraw-Hill, 2006:325–389.
65. Ahmann FR. A reassessment of the clinical implications of the superior vena cava syndrome. *J Clin Oncol.* 1984;2:961–969.
66. Rowell NP, Gleeson FV. Steroids, radiotherapy, chemotherapy and stents for superior vena caval obstruction in carcinoma of the bronchus: a systematic review. *Clin Oncol (R Coll Radiol).* 2002;14(5):338–351.
67. Crausman RS, De Palo VA, Sid RL. Diseases of the mediastinum. In: Hanley ME, Welsh CH, eds. *Current Diagnosis and Treatment in Pulmonary Medicine.* New York, NY: McGraw-Hill; 2003:241–250.
68. Qanadli SD, El Hajjam M, Bruckert F, et al. Helical CT phlebography of the superior vena cava: diagnosis and evaluation of venous obstruction. *AJR Am J Roentgenol.* 1999;172(5):1327–1333.
69. Schraufnagel DE, Hill R, Leech JA, Pare JA. Superior vena caval obstruction: is it a medical emergency? *Am J Med.* 1981;70(6):1169–1174.
70. Gauden SJ. Superior vena cava syndrome induced by bronchogenic carcinoma: is this an oncological emergency? *Australas Radiol.* 1993;37(4):363–366.
71. Yellin A, Rosen A, Reichert N, Lieberman Y. Superior vena cava syndrome: the myth—the facts. *Am Rev Respir Dis.* 1990;141(5):1114–1990.
72. Escalante CP. Causes and management of superior vena cava syndrome. *Oncology (Williston Park).* 1993;7:61–68; discussion 71–72, 75–77.
73. Kvale PA, Selecky PA, Prakash UB, American College of Chest Physicians. Palliative care in lung cancer: ACCP evidence-based clinical practice guidelines (2nd edition). *Chest.* 2007;132(3 Suppl):368S-403S.
74. *Nation Comprehensive Cancer Network (NCCN) clinical practice guidelines in oncology.* Available at http://www.nccn.org/professionals/physician_gls/f_guidelines.asp. Accessed April 10, 2015.
75. Urruticoechea A, Mesia R, Dominguez J, et al. Treatment of malignant superior vena cava syndrome by endovascular stent insertion: experience on 52 patients with lung cancer. *Lung Cancer.* 2004;43(2):209–214.
76. Courtheoux P, Alkofer B, Al Refaï M, et al. Stent placement in superior vena cava syndrome. *Ann Thorac Surg.* 2003;75(1):158–161.
77. Chatziioannou A, Alexopoulos T, Mourikis D, et al. Stent therapy for malignant superior vena cava syndrome: should be first line therapy or simple adjunct to radiotherapy. *Eur J Radiol.* 2003;47(3):247–250.
78. Uberoi R. Quality assurance guidelines for superior vena cava stenting in malignant disease. *Cardiovasc Intervent Radiol.* 2006;29(3):319–322.
79. Nagata T, Makutani S, Uchida H, et al. Follow-up results of 71 patients undergoing metallic stent placement for the treatment of a malignant obstruction of the superior vena cava. *Cardiovasc Intervent Radiol.* 2007;30:959–967.
80. Martin M, Baumgartner I, Kolb M, et al. Fatal pericardial tamponade after Wallstent implementation for malignant superior vena cava syndrome. *J Endovasc Ther.* 2002;9:680–684.
81. Smith SL, Manhire AR, Clark DM. Delayed spontaneous superior vena cava perforation associated with a SVC wallstent. *Cardiovasc Intervent Radiol.* 2001;24:286–287.
82. Gray BH, Olin JW, Graor RA, et al. Safety and efficacy of thrombolytic therapy for superior vena cava syndrome. *Chest.* 1991;99(1):54–59.
83. Kee ST, Kinoshita L, Razavi MK, et al. Superior vena cava syndrome: treatment with catheter-directed thrombolysis and endovascular stent placement. *Radiology.* 1998:206(1):187–193.
84. Porte H, Metois D, Finzi L, et al. Superior vena cava syndrome of malignant origin. Which surgical procedure for which diagnosis? *Eur J Cardiothorac Surg.* 2000;17(4):384–388.
85. Strong EW. Head and neck emergencies. *Curr Probl Cancer.* 1979;4:36–41.
86. McCarthy MJ, Rosado-de-Christenson ML. Tumors of the trachea. *J Thorac Imag.* 1995 Summer;10:180–198.
87. Noppen M, Poppe K, D'Haese J, et al. Interventional bronchoscopy for treatment of tracheal obstruction secondary to benign or malignant thyroid disease. *Chest.* 2004;125:723–730.
88. Muehrcke DD. Surgical treatment of thyroid cancer invading the airway. *Surg Rounds.* 1994;669.
89. Chen A, Otto KJ. Diagnosis and management of tracheal neoplasms. In: Cummings CW, Flint PW, Haughey BH, et al., eds. *Otolaryngology: Head & Neck Surgery.* 5th ed. Philadelphia, PA: Elsevier Mosby; 2010:1636–1642.
90. Balkissoon RC, Baroody FM, Togias A. Disorders of the upper airways. In: Mason RJ, Murray JF, Broaddus VC, et al., eds. *Textbook of Respiratory Medicine.* 5th ed. Philadelphia, PA: Elsevier Saunders, 2010:1047–1065.
91. Wood DE. Management of malignant tracheobronchial obstruction. *Surg Clin North Am.* 2002;82:621–642.
92. Yu K. Airway management and tracheostomy. In: Lalwani AK, ed. *Current Diagnosis & Treatment in Otolaryngology–Head & Neck Surgery.* 3rd ed. New York, NY: McGraw-Hill, 2012:541–548.
93. Gehlbach B, Kress JK. Upper airway obstruction. In: Hall JB, Schmidt GA, Wood LDH, eds. *Principles of Critical Care.* 3rd ed. New York, NY: McGraw-Hill; 2005:455–464.
94. Boorstein JM, Boorstein SM, Humphries GN, Johnston CC. Using helium-oxygen mixtures in the emergency management of acute upper airway obstruction. *Ann Emerg Med.* 1989;18(6):688–690.
95. Jaber S, Carlucci A, Boussarsar M, et al. Helium-oxygen in the postextubation period decreases inspiratory effort. *Am J Respir Crit Care Med.* 2001;164:633–637.
96. Lund ME, Garland R, Ernst A. Airway stenting: applications and practice management considerations. *Chest.* 2007;131:579–587.
97. Wood DE, Liu Y, Vallières E, et al. Airway stenting for malignant and benign tracheobronchial stenosis. *Ann Thorac Surg.* 2003;76:167–172; discussion 173–174.
98. Fan AC, Baron TH, Utz JP. Combined tracheal and esophageal stenting for palliation of tracheoesophageal symptoms from mediastinal lymphoma. *Mayo Clin Proc.* 2002;77(12):1347–1350.
99. Regnard JF, Fourquier P, Levasseur P. Results and prognostic factors in resections of primary tracheal tumors: a multicenter retrospective study. *J Thorac Cardiovasc Surg.* 1996;111(4):808–813; discussion 813–814.
100. Ernst A, Feller-Kopman D, Becker HD, Mehta AC. Central airway obstruction. *Am J Respir Crit Care Med.* 2004;169:1278–1297.
101. Helweg-Larsen S, Sorensen PS, Kreiner S. Prognostic factors in metastatic spinal cord compression: a prospective study using multivariate analysis of variables influencing survival and gait function in 153 patients. *Int J Radiat Oncol Biol Phys.* 2000;46:1163–1169.

102. Klimo P Jr,Schmidt MH. Surgical management of spinal metastases. *Oncologist.* 2004;9(2):188–196.
103. Loblaw DA, Laperriere NJ. Emergency treatment of malignant extradural spinal cord compression: an evidence-based guideline. *J Clin Oncol.* 1998;16:1613–1624.
104. Loblaw DA, Perry J, Chambers A, Laperriere NJ. Systematic review of the diagnosis and management of malignant extradural spinal cord compression: the Cancer Care Ontario practice guidelines initiative's Neuro-Oncology Disease Site Group. *J Clin Oncol.* 2005;23(9):2028–2037.
105. Loblaw DA, Laperriere NJ, Mackillop WJ. A population-based study of malignant spinal cord compression in Ontario. *Clin Oncol (R Coll Radiol).* 2003;15:211–217.
106. Prasad D, Schiff D. Malignant spinal-cord compression. *Lancet Oncol.* 2005;6(1):15–24.
107. Becker KP, Baehring JM. Spinal cord compression. In: DeVita VT, Hellman S, Rosenberg SA, eds. *Cancer: Principles and Practice of Oncology.* 9th ed. Philadelphia, PA: Lippincott Williams & Wilkins; 2011:2136–2152.
108. Helweg-Larsen S, Sorensen PS. Symptoms and signs in metastatic spinal cord compression: a study of progression from first symptom until diagnosis in 153 patients. *Eur J Cancer.* 1994;30A(3):396–398.
109. Schiff D, O'Neill BP, Wang CH, O'Fallon JR. Neuroimaging and treatment implications of patients with multiple epidural spinal metastases. *Cancer.* 1998;83:1593–1601.
110. Schiff D, O'Neill BP, Suman VJ. Spinal epidural metastasis as the initial manifestation of malignancy: clinical features and diagnostic approach. *Neurology.* 1997;49(2):452–456.
111. Bach F, Larsen BH, Rohde K, et al. Metastatic spinal cord compression. Occurrence, symptoms, clinical presentations and prognosis in 398 patients with spinal cord compression. *Acta Neurochir (Wien).* 1990;107(1–2):37–43.
112. Willson JK, Masaryk TJ. Neurologic emergencies in the cancer patient. *Semin Oncol.* 1989;16:490–503.
113. Portenoy RK, Lipton RB, Foley KM. Back pain in the cancer patient: an algorithm for evaluation and management. *Neurology.* 1987;37:134–138.
114. Li KC, Poon PY. Sensitivity and specificity of MRI in detecting malignant spinal cord compression and in distinguishing malignant from benign compression fractures of vertebrae. *Magn Reson Imaging.* 1988;6:547–556.
115. Cook AM, Lau TN, Tomlinson MJ, et al. Magnetic resonance imaging of the whole spine in suspected malignant spinal cord compression: impact on management. *Clin Oncol (R Coll Radiol).* 1998;10(1):39–43.
116. Ecker RD, Endo T, Wetjen NM, Krauss WE. Diagnosis and treatment of vertebral column metastases. *Mayo Clin Proc.* 2005;80(9):1177–1186.
117. Husband DJ. Malignant spinal cord compression: prospective study of delays in referral and treatment. *BMJ.* 1998;317(7150):18–21.
118. Maranzano E, Latini P. Effectiveness of radiation therapy without surgery in metastatic spinal cord compression: final results from a prospective trial. *Int J Radiat Oncol Biol Phys.* 1995;32(4):959–967.
119. Kim RY, Spencer SA, Meredith RF, et al. Extradural spinal cord compression: analysis of factors determining functional prognosis- prospective study. *Radiology.* 1990;176(1);279–282.
120. Sorensen S, Helweg-Larsen S, Mouridsen H, et al. Effect of high-dose dexamethasone in carcinomatous metastatic spinal cord compression treated with radiotherapy: a randomised trial. *Eur J Cancer.* 1994;30A(1):22–27.
121. Maranzano E, Latini P, Beneventi S, et al. Radiotherapy without steroids in selected metastatic spinal cord compression patients: a phase II trial. *Am J Clin Oncol.* 1996;19:179–183.
122. Patchell RA, Tibbs PA, Regine WF, et al. Direct decompressive surgical resection in the treatment of spinal cord compression caused by metastatic cancer: a randomised trial. *Lancet.* 2005;366(9486):643–648.
123. Pierri MK. Heart disease. In: Groeger JS, ed. *Critical Care of the Cancer Patient.* St. Louis, MO: Mosby-Year Book; 1991:64.
124. Maisch B, Seferovi PM, Ristic AD, et al.; Task Force on the Diagnosis and Management of Pricardial Diseases of the European Society of Cardiology. Guidelines on the diagnosis and management of pericardial diseases executive summary: the task force on the diagnosis and management of pericardial diseases of the European Society of Cardiology. *Eur Heart J.* 2004;25:587–610.
125. Campbell PT, Van Trigt P, Wall TC, et al. Subxiphoid pericardiotomy in the diagnosis and management of large pericardial effusions associated with malignancy. *Chest.* 1992;101:938–943.
126. Decamp MM Jr,Mentzer SJ, Swanson SJ, Sugarbaker DJ. Malignant effusive disease of the pleura and pericardium. *Chest.* 1997;112(4 Suppl):291S–295S.
127. Kwong KF, Nguyen DM. Malignant effusions of the pleural and pericardium. In: DeVita VT, Hellman S, Rosenberg SA, eds. *Cancer: Principles and Practice of Oncology.* 9th ed. Philadelphia, PA: Lippincott Williams & Wilkins; 2011:2205–2219.
128. Cullinane CA, Paz IB, Smith D, et al. Prognostic factors in the surgical management of pericardial effusion in the patient with concurrent malignancy. *Chest.* 2004;125:1328–1334.
129. Garcia-Riego A, Cuinas C, Vilanova JJ. Malignant pericardial effusion. *Acta Cytol.* 2001;45:561–566.
130. Spodick DH. Macrophysiology, microphysiology, and anatomy of the pericardium: a synopsis. *Am Heart J.* 1992;124:1046–1051.
131. Stouffer GA, Sheahan RG, Lenihan DJ, et al. Diagnosis and management of chronic pericardial effusions. *Am J Med Sci.* 2001;322:79–87.
132. Fiedler M, Nelson LA. Cardiac tamponade. *Int Anesthesiol Clin.* 2005 Fall;43(4):33–43.
133. Spodick DH. Acute cardiac tamponade. *N Engl J Med.* 2003;349:684–690.
134. Vaitkus PT, Herrmann HC, LeWinter MM. Treatment of malignant pericardial effusion. *JAMA.* 1994;272:59–64.
135. Tsang TS, Seward JB, Barnes ME, et al. Outcomes of primary and secondary treatment of pericardial effusion in patients with malignancy. *Mayo Clin Proc.* 2000;75(3):248–253.
136. Galli M, Politi A, Pedretti F, et al. Percutaneous balloon pericardiotomy for malignant pericardial tamponade. *Chest.* 1995;108:1499–1501.
137. Ziskind AA, Pearce AC, Lemmon CC, et al. Percutaneous balloon pericardiotomy for the treatment of cardiac tamponade and large pericardial effusions: description of technique and report of the first 50 cases. *J Am Coll Cardiol.* 1993;21:1–5.
138. Sagristà-Sauleda J, Angel J, Sànchez A, et al. Effusive-constrictive pericarditis. *N Engl J Med.* 2004;350:469–475.
139. Wang HJ, Hsu K, Chiang FT, et al. Technical and prognostic outcomes of double- balloon pericardiotomy for large malignancy-related pericardial effusions. *Chest.* 2002;122:893–899.
140. Gornik HL, Gerhard-Herman M, Beckman J. Abnormal cytology predicts poor prognosis in cancer patients with pericardial effusion. *J Clin Oncol.* 2005;23(22):5211–5216.
141. O'Connor K, Dijkstra B, Kelly L, et al. Successful conservative management of neutropenic enterocolitis: a report of two cases and review of the literature. *ANZ J Surg.* 2003;73(6):463–465.
142. Nesher L, Rolston KV. Neutropenic enterocolitis, a growing concern in the era of widespread use of aggressive chemotherapy. *Clin Infect Dis.* 2013;56(5):711–717.
143. Gorschlüter M, Mey U, Strehl J, et al. Neutropenic enterocolitis in adults: systematic analysis of evidence quality. *Eur J Haematol.* 2005;75(1):1–13.
144. Bibbo C, Barbieri RA, Deitch EA, Brolin RE. Neutropenic enterocolitis in a trauma patient during antibiotic therapy for osteomyelitis. *J Trauma.* 2000;49:760–763.
145. Hsu T, Huang HH, Yen DH. ED presentation of neutropenic enterocolitis in adult patients with acute leukemia. *Am J of Emerg Med.* 2004;22(4):276–279.
146. Hughes WT, Armstrong D, Bodey GP, et al. 2002 guidelines for the use of antimicrobial agents in neutropenic patients with cancer. *Clin Infect Dis.* 2002;34:730–751.
147. Gea-Banacloche JC, Segal BH. Infections in the cancer patient. In: DeVita VT, Hellman S, Rosenberg SA, eds. *Cancer: Principles and Practice of Oncology.* 9th ed. Vol 2. Philadelphia, PA: Lippincott Williams & Wilkins; 2011:2262–2299.
148. Wagner ML, Rosenberg HS, Fernbach DJ, Singleton EB. Typhlitis: a complication of leukemia in childhood. *Am J Roentgenol Radium Ther Nucl Med.* 1970;109:341–350.
149. Sloas MM, Flynn PM, Kaste SC, Patrick CC. Typhlitis in children with cancer: a 30-year experience. *Clin Infect Dis.* 1993;17:484–490.
150. Amromin GD, Solomon RD. Necrotizing enteropathy: a complication of treated leukemia or lymphoma patients. *JAMA.* 1962;182:23–29.
151. Williams N, Scott AD. Neutropenic colitis: a continuing surgical challenge. *Br J Surg.* 1997;84(9):1200–1205.
152. Cappell MS. Colonic toxicity of administered drugs and chemicals. *Am J Gastroenterol.* 2004;99(6):1175–1190.
153. Daniele B, Rossi GB, Losito S, et al. Ischemic colitis associated with paclitaxel. *J Clin Gastroenterol.* 2001;33(2):159–160.
154. Mehta J, Nagler A, Or R, et al. Neutropenic enterocolitis and intestinal perforation associated with carboplatin-containing conditioning regimen for autologous bone marrow transplantation. *Acta Oncol.* 1992;31:591.
155. Frankel AH, Barker F, Williams G, et al. Neutropenic enterocolitis in a renal transplant patient. *Transplantation.* 1991;52:913–914.
156. Ibrahim NK, Sahin AA, Dubrow RA, et al. Colitis associated with docetaxel-based chemotherapy in patients with metastatic breast cancer. *Lancet.* 2000;355:281–283.
157. Pestalozzi BC, Sotos GA, Choyke PL, et al. Typhlitis resulting from treatment with Taxol and doxorubicin in patients with metastatic breast cancer. *Cancer.* 1993;71:1797–1800.

158. Shamberger RC, Weinstein HJ, Delorey MJ, Levey RH. The medical and surgical management of typhlitis in children with acute nonlymphocytic (myelogenous) leukemia. *Cancer.* 1986;57:603–609.
159. Moran H, Yaniv I, Ashkenazi S, et al. Risk factors for typhlitis in pediatric patients with cancer. *J Pediatr Hematol Oncol.* 2009;31(9):630–634.
160. Mourra N, Nion-Larmurier I, Parc R, Flejou JF. Neutropenic enterocolitis in acute myeloblastic leukaemia. *Histopathology.* 2005;46(3):353–355.
161. Kouroussis C, Samonis G, Androulakis N, et al. Successful conservative treatment of neutropenic enterocolitis complicating taxane-based chemotherapy: a report of five cases. *Am J Clin Oncol.* 2000;23(3):309–313.
162. Guiot HF, Fibbe WE, van't Wout JW, et al. Risk factors for fungal infection in patients with malignant hematologic disorders: implications for empirical therapy and prophylaxis. *Clin Infect Dis.* 1994;18:525–532.
163. Lord BI, Bronchud MH, Owens S, et al. The kinetics of human granulopoiesis following treatment with granulocyte colony-stimulating factor in vivo. *Proc Natl Acad Sci U S A.* 1989;86:9499–9503.
164. Katz JA, Wagner ML, Gresik MV, et al. Typhlitis: an 18-year experience and postmortem review. *Cancer.* 1990;65:1041–1047.
165. Cartoni C, Dragoni F, Micozzi A, et al. Neutropenic enterocolitis in patients with acute leukemia: prognostic significance of bowel wall thickening detected by ultrasonography. *J Clin Oncol.* 2001;19:756–761.
166. de Brito D, Barton E, Spears KL, et al. Acute right lower quadrant pain in a patient with leukemia. *Ann Emerg Med.* 1998;32:98–101.
167. Kaste SC, Flynn PM, Furman WL. Acute lymphoblastic leukemia presenting with typhlitis. *Med Pediatr Oncol.* 1997;28(3):209–212.
168. Solomkin JS, Mazuski JE, Baron EJ, et al.; Infectious Diseases Society of America. Guidelines for the selection of anti-infective agents for complicated intra-abdominal infections. *Clin Infect Dis.* 2003;37(8):997–1005.
169. Gandy W, Greenberg BR. Successful medical management of neutropenic enterocolitis. *Cancer.* 1983;51:1551–1555.
170. O'Brien S, Kantarjian HM, Anaissie E, et al. Successful medical management of neutropenic enterocolitis in adults with acute leukemia. *South Med J.* 1987;80:1233–1235.
171. Wade DS, Nava HR, Douglass HO. Neutropenic enterocolitis. Clinical diagnosis and treatment. *Cancer.* 1992;69:17–23.
172. Moir CR, Scudamore CH, Benny WB. Typhlitis: selective surgical management. *Am J Surg.* 1986;151:563–566.
173. Small EJ. Chemotherapy of urologic tumors. In: Tanagho EA, McAninch JW, eds. *Smith's General Urology.* 17th ed. New York, NY: McGraw-Hill; 2008:302–307.
174. Tew K, Reed E, Chu E, et al. Pharmacology of cancer therapeutics: drug development. In: DeVita VT, Hellman S, Rosenberg SA, eds. *Cancer: Principles and Practice of Oncology.* 9th ed. Philadelphia, PA: Lippincott Williams & Wilkins, 2011:360–521.
175. Floyd JD, Nguyen DT, Lobins RL, et al. Cardiotoxicity of cancer therapy. *J Clin Oncol.* 2005;23:7685–7696.
176. White DA, Orenstein M, Godwin TA, Stover DE. Chemotherapy-associated pulmonary toxic reactions during the treatment of breast cancer. *Arch Intern Med.* 1984;144:953–956.
177. Vander Els NJ, Stover DE. Chemotherapy-induced lung disease. *Clin Pulm Med.* 2004;11(2):84–91.
178. Simpson AB, Paul J, Graham J, Kaye SB. Fatal bleomycin pulmonary toxicity in the west of Scotland 1991–95: a review of patients with germ cell tumours. *Br J Cancer.* 1998;78(8):1061–1066.
179. Sleijffer S. Bleomycin-induced pneumonitis. *Chest.* 2001;120:617–624.
180. Donat SM, Levy DA. Bleomycin associated pulmonary toxicity: is perioperative oxygen restriction necessary? *J Urol.* 1998;60(4):1347–1352.
181. Goldiner PL, Schweizer O. The hazards of anesthesia and surgery in bleomycin-treated patients. *Semin Oncol.* 1979;6:121–124.
182. Abid SH, Malhotra V, Perry MC. Radiation-induced and chemotherapy-induced pulmonary injury. *Curr Opin Oncol.* 2001;13(4):242–248.
183. Rivera MP, Kris MG, Gralla RV, White DA. Syndrome of acute dyspnea related to combined mitomycin plus vinca alkaloid chemotherapy. *Am J Clin Oncol.* 1995;18:245–250.
184. Castro M, Veeder MH, Mailliard JA. A prospective study of pulmonary function in patients receiving mitomycin. *Chest.* 1996;109:939–944.
185. Stover DE, Kaner RJ. Adverse effects of treatment: pulmonary toxicity. In: DeVita VT, Hellman S, Rosenberg SA, eds. *Cancer: Principles and Practice of Oncology.* 7th ed. Vol 2. Philadelphia, PA: Lippincott Williams & Wilkins; 2005:2536–2545.
186. Rowinsky EK, Donehower RC. Paclitaxel (Taxol). *N Engl J Med.* 1995; 332:1004–1014.
187. Dimopoulou I, Bamias A, Lyberopoulos P, Dimopoulos MA. Pulmonary toxicity from novel antineoplastic agents. *Ann Oncol.* 2006;17(3):372–379.
188. Aapro MS, Martin C, Hatty S. Gemcitabine: a safety review. *Anticancer Drugs.* 1998;9:191–201.
189. Gupta N, Ahmed I, Steinberg H, et al. Gemcitabine-induced pulmonary toxicity: case report and review of the literature. *Am J Clin Oncol.* 2002;25(1):96–100.
190. Pavlakis N, Bell DR, Millward MJ, Levi JA. Fatal pulmonary toxicity resulting from treatment with gemcitabine. *Cancer.* 1997;80:286–291.
191. Camacho LH, Soignet SL, Chanel S, et al. Leukocytosis and the retinoic acid syndrome in patients with acute promyelocytic leukemia treated with arsenic trioxide. *J Clin Oncol.* 2000;18:2620–2625.
192. De Botton S, Dombret H, Sanz M. Incidence, clinical features, and outcome of all trans- retinoic acid syndrome in 413 cases of newly diagnosed acute promyelocytic leukemia. The European APL group. *Blood.* 1998;92(8):2712–2718.
193. Yeh ET, Tong AT, Lenihan DJ, et al. Cardiovascular complications of cancer therapy: diagnosis, pathogenesis, and management. *Circulation.* 2004;109(25):3122–3131.
194. Batist G, Ramakrishnan G, Rao CS, et al. Reduced cardiotoxicity and preserved antitumor efficacy of liposome-encapsulated doxorubicin and cyclophosphamide compared with conventional doxorubicin and cyclophosphamide in a randomized, multicenter trial of metastatic breast cancer. *J Clin Oncol.* 2001;19:1444–1454.
195. Singal PK, Iliskovic N. Doxorubicin-induced cardiomyopathy. *N Engl J Med.* 1998;339:900–905.
196. Swaim S, Whaley FS, Gerber M, et al. Cardioprotection with dexrazoxane for doxorubicin-containing therapy in advanced breast cancer. *J Clin Oncol.* 1997;15:1318–1332.
197. Gehl J, Boesgaard M, Paaske T, et al. Combined doxorubicin and paclitaxel in advanced breast cancer: effective and cardiotoxic. *Ann Oncol.* 1996;7(7):687–693.
198. Malhotra V, Dorr VJ, Lyss AP, et al. Neoadjuvant and adjuvant chemotherapy with doxorubicin and docetaxel in locally advanced breast cancer. *Clin Breast Cancer.* 2004;5(5):377.
199. Cardinale D, Colombo A, Lamantia G, et al. Anthracycline-induced cardiomyopathy: clinical relevance and response to pharmacologic therapy. *J Am Coll Cardiol.* 2010;55(3):213–220.
200. Volkova M, Russell R 3rd. Anthracycline cardiotoxicity: prevalence, pathogenesis and treatment. *Curr Cardiol Rev.* 2011;7(4):214–220.
201. Shenkenberg TD, Von Hoff DD. Mitoxantrone: a new anticancer drug with significant clinical activity. *Ann Intern Med.* 1986;105:67–81.
202. Yahalom J, Portlock CS. Cardiac Toxicity. In: DeVita VT, Hellman S, Rosenberg SA, eds. *Cancer: Principles and Practice of Oncology.* 9th ed. Vol 2. Philadelphia, PA: Lippincott Williams & Wilkins; 2011:2360–2367.
203. Verweij J, Funke-Kupper AJ, Teule GJ, Pinedo HM. A prospective study on the dose dependency of cardiotoxicity induced by mitomycin C. *Med Oncol Tumor Pharmacother.* 1988;5:159–163.
204. Ayash LJ, Wright JE, Tretyakov O, et al. Cyclophosphamide pharmacokinetics: correlation with cardiac toxicity and tumor response. *J Clin Oncol.* 1992;10(6):995–1000.
205. Quezado ZM, Wilson WH, Cunnion RE, et al. High-dose ifosfamide is associated with severe, reversible cardiac dysfunction. *Ann Intern Med.* 1993;118(1):31–36.
206. Talcott JA, Herman TS. Acute ischemic vascular events and cisplatin. *Ann Intern Med.* 1987;107:121–122.
207. Rezkalla S, Kloner RA, Ensley J, et al. Continuous ambulatory ECG monitoring during fluorouracil therapy: a prospective clinical study. *J Clin Oncol.* 1989;7:509–514.
208. Van Cutse ME, Hoff PM, Blum JL, et al. Incidence of cardiotoxicity with the oral fluoropyrimidine capecitabine is typical of that reported with 5-fluorouracil. *Ann Oncol.* 2002;13:484–485.
209. Sorrentino MF, Kim J, Foderaro AE, Truesdell AG. 5-fluorouracil induced cardiotoxicity: review of the literature. *Cardiol J.* 2012;19(5):453–458.
210. Barbey J, Pezzullo JC, Soignet SL. Effect of arsenic trioxide on QT interval in patients with advanced malignancies. *J Clin Oncol.* 2003;21:3609–3615.
211. Seidman A, Hudis C, Pierri MK, et al. Cardiac dysfunction in the trastuzumab clinical trials experience. *J Clin Oncol.* 2002;20:1215–1221.
212. Keefe DL. Trastuzumab-associated cardiotoxicity. *Cancer.* 2002;95(7): 1592–1600.
213. Cersosimo RJ. Monoclonal antibodies in the treatment of cancer, part 1. *Am J Health Syst Pharm.* 2003;60(15):1531–1548.
214. Choueiri TK, Mayer EL, Je Y, et al. Congestive heart failure risk in patients with breast cancer treated with bevacizumab. *J Clin Oncol.* 2011;29(6):632–638.
215. Ranpura V, Hapani S, Chuang J, Wu S. Risk of cardiac ischemia and arterial thromboembolic events with the angiogenesis inhibitor bevacizumab in cancer patients: a meta-analysis of randomized controlled trials. *Acta Oncol.* 2010;49(3):287–297.

216. Khakoo AY, Kassiotis CM, Tannir N, et al. Heart failure associated with sunitinib malate: a multitargeted receptor tyrosine kinase inhibitor. *Cancer.* 2008;112(11):2500–2508.
217. Chintalgattu V, Patel SS, Khakoo AY. Cardiovascular effects of tyrosine kinase inhibitors used for gastrointestinal stromal tumors. *Hematol Oncol Clin North Am.* 2009;23(1):97–107, viii–ix.
218. Escudier B, Eisen T, Stadler WM, et al. Sorafenib in advanced clear-cell renal-cell carcinoma. *N Engl J Med.* 2007;356(2):125–134.
219. Kerkelä R, Grazette L, Yacobi R, et al. Cardiotoxicity of the cancer therapeutic agent imatinib mesylate. *Nat Med.* 2006;12(8):908–916.
220. Strevel EL, Ing DJ, Siu LL. Molecularly targeted oncology therapeutics and prolongation of the QT interval. *J Clin Oncol.* 2007;25(22):3362–3371.
221. Blackwell KL, Burstein HJ, Storniolo AM, et al. Randomized study of Lapatinib alone or in combination with trastuzumab in women with ErbB2-positive, trastuzumab-refractory metastatic breast cancer. *J Clin Oncol.* 2010;28(7):1124–1130.
222. Hang XF, Xu WS, Wang JX, et al. Risk of high-grade bleeding in patients with cancer treated with bevacizumab: a meta-analysis of randomized controlled trials. *Eur J Clin Pharmacol.* 2011;67(6):613–623.
223. Weber JS, Dummer R, de Pril V, et al. Patterns of onset and resolution of immune-related adverse events of special interest with ipilimumab: detailed safety analysis from a phase 3 trial in patients with advanced melanoma. *Cancer.* 2013;119(9):1675–1682.
224. Wolchok JD, Neyns B, Linette G, et al. Ipilimumab monotherapy in patients with pretreated advanced melanoma: a randomised, double-blind, multicentre, phase 2, dose-ranging study. *Lancet Oncol.* 2010;11(2):155–164.
225. Pagès C, Gornet JM, Monsel G, et al. Ipilimumab-induced acute severe colitis treated by infliximab. *Melanoma Res.* 2013;23(3):227–230.
226. Minor DR, Chin K, Kashani-Sabet M. Infliximab in the treatment of anti-CTLA4 antibody (ipilimumab) induced immune-related colitis. *Cancer Biother Radiopharm.* 2009;24(3):321–325.
227. Bernardo SG, Moskalenko M, Pan M, et al. Elevated rates of transaminitis during ipilimumab therapy for metastatic melanoma. *Melanoma Res.* 2013;23(1):47–54.
228. Ribas A, Kefford R, Marshall MA, et al. Phase III randomized clinical trial comparing tremelimumab with standard-of-care chemotherapy in patients with advanced melanoma. *J Clin Oncol.* 2013;31(5):616–622.
229. Weber JS, Kähler KC, Hauschild A. Management of immune-related adverse events and kinetics of response with ipilimumab. *J Clin Oncol.* 2012;30(21):2691–2697.
230. Kim KW, Ramaiya NH, Krajewski KM, et al. Ipilimumab associated hepatitis: imaging and clinicopathologic findings. *Invest New Drugs.* 2013;31(4):1071–1077.
231. Chmiel KD, Suan D, Liddle C, et al. Resolution of severe ipilimumab-induced hepatitis after antithymocyte globulin therapy. *J Clin Oncol.* 2011;29(9):e237–e240.
232. Corsello SM, Barnabei A, Marchetti P, et al. Endocrine side effects induced by immune checkpoint inhibitor. *J Clin Endocrinol Metab.* 2013;98(4):1361–1375.

SECTION 18 PHARMACOLOGY, NUTRITION, TOXICOLOGY, AND THE ENVIRONMENT

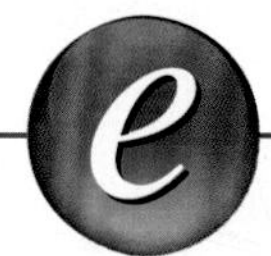

This chapter can be accessed in the accompanying eBook (see inside front cover for access instructions).

CHAPTER
148

Pharmacologic Principles

ANGELA A. SLAMPAK-CINDRIC

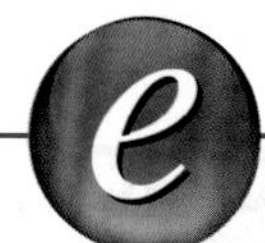

This chapter can be accessed in the accompanying eBook (see inside front cover for access instructions).

CHAPTER
149

Sedation and Neuromuscular Blockade

MICHAEL J. MURRAY

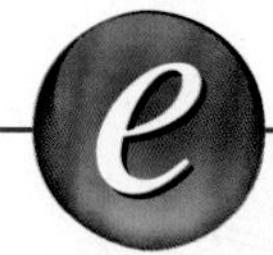

This chapter can be accessed in the accompanying eBook (see inside front cover for access instructions).

CHAPTER
150

Nutritional Issues and Practical Aspects of Nutritional Support

PATRICIA MARIE BYERS

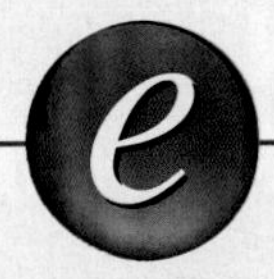

This chapter can be accessed in the accompanying eBook (see inside front cover for access instructions).

CHAPTER
151
Toxicology

KAROLINA PAZIANA and ANDREW STOLBACH

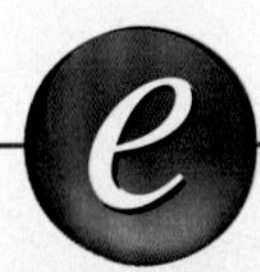

This chapter can be accessed in the accompanying eBook (see inside front cover for access instructions).

CHAPTER
152
Substance Abuse and Withdrawal: Alcohol, Cocaine, Opioids, and Other Drugs

ADITYA UPPALAPATI and JANICE L. ZIMMERMAN

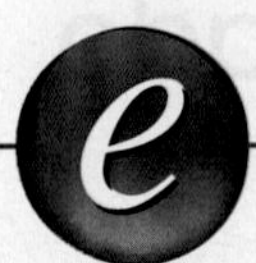

This chapter can be accessed in the accompanying eBook (see inside front cover for access instructions).

CHAPTER
153
Envenomation

CRAIG S. KITCHENS – Snakes Native to the United States, STEVEN A. SEIFERT – Snakes Non-Native to the United States, CLAUDIA L. BARTHOLD – Spiders and Scorpions, and JENNIFER A. OAKES – Marine Envenomation

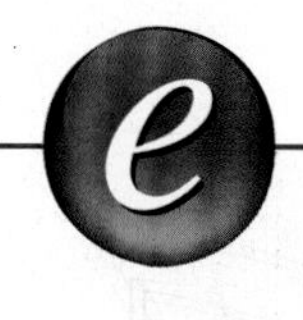

This chapter can be accessed in the accompanying eBook (see inside front cover for access instructions).

CHAPTER
154

Molecular and Metabolic Perspectives on Genetics in the ICU

ANDREAS G. ZORI, BRYCE A. HEESE, ROBERTO T. ZORI, and PETR STAROSTIK

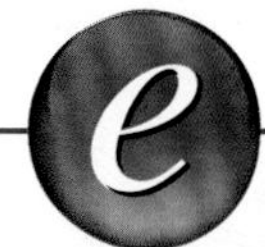

This chapter can be accessed in the accompanying eBook (see inside front cover for access instructions).

CHAPTER
155

Mass Casualty Incidents: Organizational and Triage Management Issues

JAMES A. GEILING and FREDERICK M. BURKLE JR.

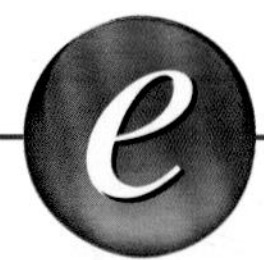

This chapter can be accessed in the accompanying eBook (see inside front cover for access instructions).

CHAPTER
156

Bioterrorism and High-Consequence Biologic Threats

EDGAR JIMENEZ, ALFREDO VAZQUEZ-SANDOVAL, and F. ELIZABETH POALILLO

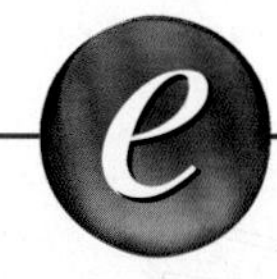

This chapter can be accessed in the accompanying eBook (see inside front cover for access instructions).

CHAPTER
157

Disaster Response

DONALD R. SESSIONS, KATHERINE KEMBERLING, and W. CRAIG FUGATE

JOSEPH VARON AND SANTIAGO HERRERO

APPENDIX A

Prefixes and Conversions

TABLE A.1 Metric Prefixes

Multiple	Prefix	Abbreviation
10^{12}	tera-	T
10^{9}	giga-	G
10^{6}	mega-	M
10^{3}	kilo-	k
10	deca-	da
10^{-1}	deci-	d
10^{-2}	centi-	c
10^{-3}	milli-	m
10^{-6}	micro-	μ
10^{-9}	nano-	n
10^{-12}	pico-	p
10^{-15}	femto-	f
10^{-16}	atto-	a

TABLE A.2 Fahrenheit and Celsius Temperature Conversions

Celsius scale (°C): Degree of Celsius (or centigrade) equals 1/100th of the difference in temperature of melting ice and boiling water at the atmospheric pressure of 760 mmHg.

Fahrenheit scale (°F): The interval between freezing and boiling is divided into 180°.

°C = (5/9°F) − 32

°F = (9/5°C) + 32

°C	°F	°C	°F
45	113.0	32	89.6
44	111.2	31	87.8
43	109.4	30	86.0
42	107.6	29	84.2
41	105.8	28	82.4
40	104.0	27	80.6
39	102.2	26	78.8
38	100.4	25	77.0
37	98.6	24	75.2
36	96.8	23	73.4
35	95.0	22	71.6
34	93.2	21	69.8
33	91.4	20	68.0

APPENDIX

B

Dubois Body Surface Area Nomogram

Body surface area (in m^2) = [(Height in cm)$^{0.725}$ × (Weight in kg)$^{0.4259}$] × 0.007184

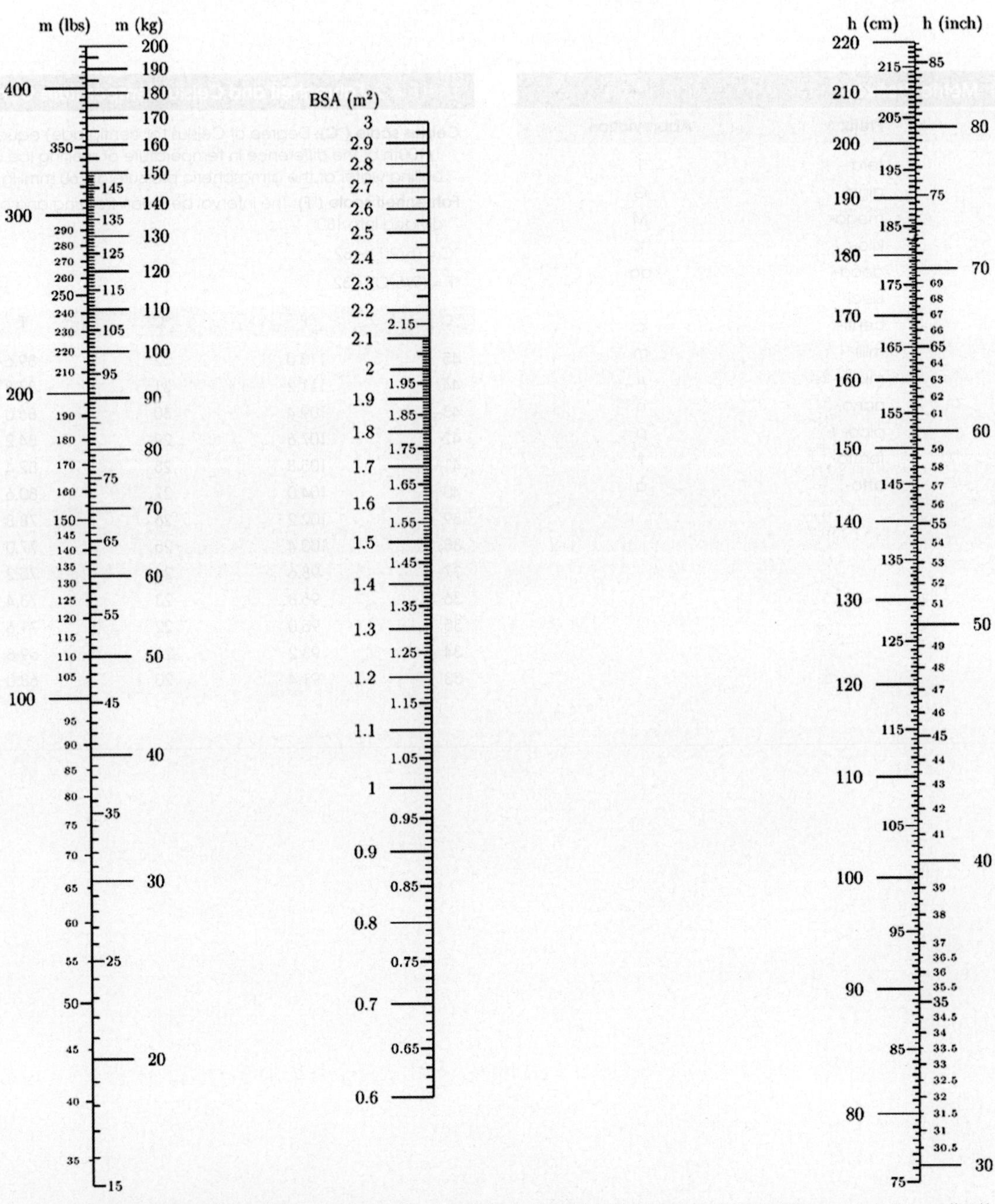

FIGURE B.1 Nomogram for determination of body surface area in adults. A straight edge is placed so that it connects the patient's height (*left column*) with his or her weight (*right column*) crossing the center column at the point indicating the body surface area. (From Carey CC, et al. *The Washington Manual of Medical Therapeutics*. Philadelphia, PA: Lippincott Williams & Wilkins, 1998:562.)

APPENDIX C

Fluids and Electrolytes

TABLE C.1 Intravenous Fluids

Solution			Na^+	Cl^-	K^+	Ca	Mg	Acetate	Gluconate	Albumin	Lactate	Dextrose
Units	**mOsm/L**	**pH**	**mmol/L**			**mg/dL**				**g/L**		
5% dextrose (D_5 W)	250–253	5	—	—	—	—	—	—	—	—	—	50
0.45% NaCl (½ NS)	155	5–5.6	77	77	—	—	—	—	—	—	—	—
0.9% NaCl (NS)	308	5.7	154	154	—	—	—	—	—	—	—	—
0.45% NaCl + D_5 W (D_5 ½ NS)	406	4–4.4	77	77	—	—	—	—	—	—	—	50
0.9% NaCl + D_5 W (D_5NS)	561	4–4.4	154	154	—	—	—	—	—	—	—	50
Ringer solution	309	6	147	156	4	4–4.5	—	—	—	—	—	—
Lactated Ringer solution (LR)	275	6.7	130	109	4	3	—	—	—	—	28	—
5% dextrose + lactated Ringer (D_5LR)	525–530	4.7–5	130	109	4	3	—	—	—	—	28	50
Plasma protein fractions 5%	294	6.7–7.3	130–160	90	0–5	—	0–3	0–27	0–23	0–12.5	—	—
3% NaCl	1,026	5.8	513	513	—	—	—	—	—	—	—	—
5% NaCl	1,710	5–6	855	855	—	—	—	—	—	—	—	—
Mannitol 5%	275	6										
Mannitol 1.0%	550	6										
Mannitol 15%	825	6										
Mannitol 20%	7.100	6										
Mannitol 25%	1,375	6										
Fresh frozen plasma	31.0–33.0		7.68	76	3.2	3.2	8.2	—	—	—	—	—
Dextran-40 in NS	310	5–5.5	154	154	—	—	—	—	—	—	—	—
Dextran-70 in D_5 W	287	3.5–7										50
5% albumin	300	6.9	145	145						50		
25% albumin		6.9	145	145						250		
Hydroxyethyl starch 6% (Hetastarch)	310	5.5	1.54	154								

Na^+, sodium; Cl^-, chloride; K^+, potassium; Ca, calcium; Mg, magnesium; D_5 W, 5% dextrose in water; NaCl, sodium chloride; NS, normal saline.

TABLE C.2 Electrolyte Composition of Various Body Fluids

Fluid (mmol/L)	Na^+	K^+	Cl^-	HCO_3^-	Volume (L/d)
Saliva	30	20	35	15	1–1.5
Gastric fluid (pH <4)	60	10	90	—	2.5
Gastric fluid (pH >4)	100	10	100	—	2
Bile	145	5	110	40	1.5
Duodenum	140	5	80	50	—
Pancreas	140	5	75	90	0.7–1.0
Ileum	130	10	110	30	3.5
Cecum	80	20	50	20	—
Colon	60	30	40	20	—
Sweat	50	5	55	—	0–3
New ileostomy	130	20	110	30	0.5–2.0
Adapted ileostomy	50	5	30	25	0.4
Colostomy	50	10	40	20	0.3

Osmolality

CALCULATED SERUM OSMOLALITY

$$= 2[Na^+] + \frac{[glucose]}{18}$$

$$+ \frac{[BUN]}{2.8} + \frac{[mannitol]}{18} + \frac{[EtOH]}{4.6} + \frac{[ethylene\ glycol]}{6.2}$$

$$+ \frac{[methanol]}{3.2}$$

[Normal: 275–290 mmol/kg]
Osmolar gap = measured serum osmolality – calculated serum osmolality
[Normal: 0–5 mOsm/kg]

SODIUM (NA^+)

Pseudohyponatremia with hyperglycemia:
Each 100-mg/dL increase in serum glucose (above 100 mg/dL) decreases Na^+ by 1.6 mmol/L.

Free water deficit in hypernatremia

$$= (0.6)(\text{body weight in kg})\left(\frac{[Na^+]}{140} - 1\right)$$

Free water excess in hyponatremia

$$= (0.6)(\text{body weight in kg})\left(1 - \frac{[Na^+]}{140}\right)$$

POTASSIUM (K^+)

Potassium concentration ($[K^+]$) increases 0.6 mmol/L for each 0.1-unit decrease in pH.

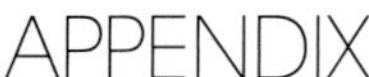

APPENDIX D

Acid–Base Balance

TABLE D.1 Anticipated Changes in Simple Disturbances

Primary Disorder	Primary	Secondary	Compensation	Limit	Net Effect
Metabolic acidosis	↓ (HCO_3)	↓ $PaCO_2$	Δ $PaCO_2$ = 1.0–1.4 × Δ (HCO_3)	10 mmHg	↑ (H^+)(↓ pH)
Metabolic alkalosis	↑ (HCO_3)	↑ $PaCO_2$	Δ $PaCO_2$ = 0.5–1.0 × Δ (HCO_3)	55 mmHg No hypoxia	↓ (H^+)(↑ pH)
Respiratory acidosis	↑ $PaCO_2$	↑ (HCO_3)	Acute: Δ (H^+) = 0.75 $\Delta PaCO_2$ Δ (HCO_3) = 1 mmol/L ↑ /10 mmHg ↑ $PaCO_2$ Δ (HCO_3) = 0.1 × $\Delta PaCO_2$	30 mmol/L HCO_3	↑ (H^+)(↓ pH)
			Chronic: Δ (HCO_3) = 0.35 × $PaCO_2$ Δ (HCO_3) = mmol/L ↑ /10 mmHg ↑ $PaCO_2$	45 mmol/L HCO_3	
Respiratory alkalosis	↓ $PaCO_2$	↓ (HCO_3)	Acute: Δ (HCO_3) = 0.2 × $\Delta PaCO_2$ Δ (HCO_3) = 1 mmol/L ↓ /10 mmHg ↓ $PaCO_2$ Δ (H^+) = 0.75 $\Delta PaCO_2$	18 mmol/L	↓ (H^+)(↑ pH)
			Chronic: Δ (HCO_3) = 0.5 × $\Delta PaCO_2$ Δ (HCO_3) = 2–5 mmol/L ↓ /10 mmHg ↓ $PaCO_2$	12–15 mmol/L	

Causes of Simple Acid–Base Disturbances

METABOLIC ACIDOSIS

- Increased anion gap (usually decreased chloride)
  - Acidosis
    - Alcoholic ketoacidosis
    - Diabetic ketoacidosis
    - Starvation ketoacidosis
    - Ethylene glycol ingestion
    - Paraldehyde
    - Methanol ingestion
    - Lactic acidosis
    - Uremic acidosis
    - Hyperosmolar nonketotic coma
  - Nonacidosis
    - Hypokalemia
    - Hypocalcemia
    - Hypomagnesemia
    - Hyperalbuminemia
    - Nitrate usage
    - Penicillin/carbenicillin
    - Pseudohypernatremia
    - Pseudohypochloremia
    - False decrease in serum HCO_3^-
- Normal anion gap (usually increased chloride)
  - Acidosis
    - Carbonic anhydrase inhibitors
    - Ureterosigmoidostomy
    - Ileostomy
    - Diarrhea
    - Pancreatic fistula
    - Parenteral nutrition
    - Ingestion of NH_4Cl
    - Ingestion of HCl or other acid
    - Renal tubular acidosis
    - Dilutional acidosis
    - Following respiratory alkalosis
    - Cholestyramine
    - Normal saline infusions
  - Nonacidosis
    - Hyperkalemia
    - Hypocalcemia
    - Hypomagnesemia
    - Hypoalbuminemia
    - IgG
    - Lithium
    - Pseudohyponatremia
    - Pseudohyperchloremia
    - False increase in serum HCO_3^-

METABOLIC ALKALOSIS

- Loss of H^+
  - Gastrointestinal loss
    - Vomiting, nasogastric suction
    - Antacids
    - Chloride-depleting diarrhea
  - Renal loss
    - Diuretics
    - Excess mineralocorticoid
    - Postchronic hypercapnia
    - Decreased chloride intake
    - High-dose penicillins
    - Hypercalcemia
  - Intracellular H^+ shift
    - Hypokalemia
    - Refeeding
- HCO_3^- retention
  - Massive transfusions
  - $NaHCO_3$ therapy
  - Milk-alkali syndrome
- Volume contraction
  - Diuretics
  - Gastrointestinal losses in patients with achlorhydria
  - Sweat losses in cystic fibrosis

RESPIRATORY ACIDOSIS

- CNS depression
- Chronic obstructive lung disease
- Severe asthma
- Pneumothorax
- Abdominal distention
- Pulmonary edema
- Mechanical hypoventilation
- Idiopathic hypoventilation
- Neuromuscular disease

RESPIRATORY ALKALOSIS

- Salicylate toxicity
- Hepatic failure
- Psychogenic hyperventilation
- Pulmonary edema
- Asthma
- Systemic inflammatory response syndrome
- Restrictive lung disease
- Primary CNS disease
- Mechanical hyperventilation
- Hypoxemia

APPENDIX

E

Formulas

Cerebral/Neurologic Formulas

Intracranial pressure (ICP)
[Normal: <20 cm H_2O, <15 mmHg]

Cerebral perfusion pressure (CPP) = MAP – ICP

[Normal: 70–100 mmHg]

Cerebral vascular resistance (CVR)
[Normal: 1.5–2.1 mmHg/100 g/min/mL]

Cerebral blood flow (CBF) = CPP/CVR

[Normal: 75 mL/100 g gray matter/min]
[Normal: 45 mL/100 g white matter/min]

Jugular bulb saturation ($S_{jv}O_2$)
[Normal: 55–70%]

Cerebral metabolic rate ($CMRO_2$) = $(CBF)(CaO_2 - C_{jv}O_2)$

[Normal: 3–3.5 mL/100 g/min]

$$\text{Cerebral oxygen extraction} = \frac{CMO_2}{(CBF)(CaO_2)} = \frac{CaO_2 - C_{jv}O_2}{CaO_2}$$

Hemodynamic Formulas

Pulse pressure = systolic BP – diastolic BP

$$\text{Mean arterial pressure (MAP)} = \frac{SBP + 2(DBP)}{3}$$

[Normal: 70–105 mmHg]

Central venous pressure (CVP)
[Normal: 0–8 mmHg]

Pulse pressure variation = PPV = (PPmax – PPmin)/PPmean
(Over a respiratory cycle or other period of time; Normal: ≤10%)

Stroke volume variation = SVV = (SVmax – SVmin)/SVmean
(Over a respiratory cycle or other period of time; Normal: ≤10%)

Mean pulmonary artery pressure ($\overline{PA}$)
[Normal: 10–20 mmHg]

Pulmonary artery occlusion pressure (PAOP)
[Normal: 4–12 mmHg]

Cardiac output (CO) = Stroke volume (SV) × Heart rate (HR)
[Normal: 4–8 L/min]

$$\text{Cardiac index (CI)} = \frac{CO}{BSA}$$

[Normal: 2.5–4.0 L/min/m^2]

$$\text{Pulmonary vascular resistance (PVR)} = \frac{(\overline{PA} - PAOP)80}{CO}$$

[Normal: 150–250 dyne/s/cm^{-5}]

$$\text{Pulmonary vascular resistance index (PVRI)} = \frac{(\overline{PA} - PAOP)80}{CI}$$

[Normal: 100–240 dyne/s/cm^{-5}/m^2]

$$\text{Systemic vascular resistance (SVR)} = \frac{(MAP - CVP)80}{CO}$$

[Normal: 800–1,200 dyne/s/cm^{-5}]

$$\text{Systemic vascular resistance index (SVRI)} = \frac{(MAP - CVP)80}{CI}$$

[1,300–2,900 dyne/s/cm^{-5}/m^2]

$$\text{Stroke volume index (SVI)} = \frac{CI}{HR}$$

[Normal: 40 ± 7 mL/beat/m^2]

Right ventricular stroke work index (RVSWI)

$$= SVI(\overline{PA} - CVP)(0.0136)$$

[Normal: 6–10 gm·meter/m^2 per beat]

Left ventricular stroke work index (LVSWI)

$$= SVI(MAP - PAOP)(0.0136)$$

[Normal: 43–56 gm·meter/m^2 per beat]

Arterial O_2 content (CaO_2) = O_2 combined with hemoglobin + O_2 dissolved in the plasma

[1 g Hb binds 1.36 mL O_2]

$$= (1.36)(Hb)(SaO_2) + 0.0031(PaO_2)$$

[Normal: 20 mL O_2/dL]

Mixed venous O_2 saturation ($S\bar{v}O_2$)
[Normal: 75%]

$$\text{Mixed venous } O_2 \text{ content } (C\bar{v}O_2) = (1.36)(Hb)(S\bar{v}O_2) + 0.0031(PvO_2)$$

[Normal: 15 mL O_2/dL]

$$O_2 \text{ delivery } (\dot{D}O_2) = CO \times CaO_2 \times 10$$

[Normal: 600–1,000 mL O_2/min]

$$\text{Oxygen delivery indexed } (DO_2I) = CI \times CaO_2 \times 10$$

[Normal: 500–600 mL/min/m^2]

$$O_2 \text{ consumption } (\dot{V}O_2) = CI(CaO_2 - C\bar{v}O_2)$$

[Normal: 110–150 mL/min/m^2]

$$O_2 \text{ extraction ratio} = \frac{(CaO_2 - C\bar{v}O_2)}{CaO_2}$$

[Normal: 25%]

Respiratory Formulas

OXYGENATION

Fraction of inspired O_2 (FIO_2)
[Range: 0.21–1.0]

Respiratory quotient (R) = VCO_2 expired/VO_2 inspired

[Normal: 0.8]

Barometric pressure (PB)
[760 mmHg at sea level]

Partial pressure of H_2O (PH_2O)
[47 mmHg at 37°C]

Partial pressure of inspired O_2 (PIO_2) = FIO_2 (PB – PH_2O)

[150 mmHg at sea level breathing room air (FIO_2 = 0.21)]

Partial pressure of alveolar O_2 (PAO_2) (alveolar gas equation)

$$PAO_2 = FIO_2\ (PB - PH_2O) - \frac{PaCO_2}{R}$$
$$= (FIO_2 \times 713) - (PaCO_2/0.8) \text{ (at sea level)}$$
$$= 150 - (PaCO_2/0.8) \text{ (at sea level on room air)}$$

[Range: 100 mmHg on room air; 673 mmHg on 100% O_2]

Partial pressure of arterial O_2 (PaO_2)
[Normal: 70–100 mmHg on room air]

Increased: hyperventilation, increased FIO_2, contaminated sample

Decreased: hypoventilation, decreased FIO_2, $\dot{V}/\dot{Q}$mismatch, intrapulmonary or anatomic R → L shunt, diffusion abnormalities

Alveolar–arterial O_2 gradient ($P(A - a)O_2$) = $PAO_2 - PaO_2$

[Normal: 3–16 mmHg on room air; 25–65 mmHg on 100% O_2]

VENTILATION

Partial pressure of arterial CO_2 ($PaCO_2$)
[Normal: 46 mmHg]

Partial pressure of alveolar (expired) CO_2 ($PetCO_2$)

Dead-space ventilation (VD): Portion of VT that does not participate in gas exchange

VD = anatomic dead space + physiologic dead space

[Normal: 150 mL]

Engelhoff modification of the Bohr formula for dead space

$$\frac{VD}{VT} = \frac{PaCO_2 - PetCO_2}{PaCO_2}$$

Minute ventilation (VE) = respiratory rate × VT

Pulmonary capillary blood O_2 content (CcO_2)

$$= 1.36\ (Hb)(SaO_2)(FIO_2) + 0.003(PBH_2O - PaCO_2)(FIO_2)$$

$$\text{Shunt fraction } (\dot{Q}s/\dot{Q}t) = \frac{CcO_2 - CaO_2}{CcO_2 - CvO_2}$$

LUNG VOLUMES

Tidal volume (VT): Volume inspired/expired with each breath
[Normal: 500 mL; 6–7 mL/kg lean body weight]

Inspiratory reserve volume (IRV): Maximal inspired volume end-tidal inspiration
[Normal: 25% of vital capacity (VC)]

Inspiratory capacity (IC): Maximal volume inspired from resting expiratory level

$$IC = IRV + VT$$

[Normal: 1–2.4 L]

Expiratory reserve volume (ERV): Maximal expired volume from end-tidal inspiration
[Normal: 25% of vital capacity (VC)]

Residual volume (RV): Volume remaining in lungs after maximal expiration
[Normal: 1–2.4 L]

Functional residual capacity (FRC): Volume remaining in lungs at end-tidal expiration

$$FRC = ERV + RV$$

[Normal: 1.8–3.4 L]

Vital capacity (VC): Maximal volume expelled by forceful effort after maximal inspiration

$$VC = IRV + ERV + VT$$

[Normal: 3–5 L; 50–60 mL/kg lean body weight in females; 70 mL/kg lean body weight in males]

Total lung capacity (TLC): Volume in lungs at end of maximal inspiration

$$TLC = VC + RV$$

[Normal: 4–6 L]

Lung Mechanics

Plateau pressure (P_{plat})

Peak inspiratory pressure (PIP)

Esophageal pressure (P_{esoph})

Transpulmonary pressure = $P_{tp} = P_{plat} - P_{esoph}$
[Normal: For recruitment P_{tp} = 25 cm H_2O; to set PEEP $P_{tp-end\text{-}exp}$ = 0 – 5 cm H_2O; to set Vt or P_{insp} $P_{tp-end\text{-}insp}$ = <15 cm H_2O]

Positive end-expiratory pressure (PEEP)

Compliance = change in volume/change in pressure

$$\text{Static compliance (Cst)} = \frac{VT}{Pplat - PEEP}$$

[Normal: 70–160 mL/cm H_2O (paralyzed/anesthetized and supine)]

$$\text{Dynamic compliance (Cdyn)} = \frac{VT}{PIP - PEEP}$$

[Normal: 50–80 mL/cm H_2O (paralyzed/anesthetized and supine)]

Renal Formulas

$$\text{Creatinine clearance } (Cl_{Creat}) = \frac{(U_{Creat})(\text{urine volume})}{P_{Creat}}$$

Fractional excretion of sodium ($FeNa^+$)

$$= \frac{\text{urine } [Na^+]}{\text{plasma } [Na^+]} \times \frac{\text{plasma [creatinine]}}{\text{urine [creatinine]}} \times 100$$

Free water clearance

$$= \text{urine vol} - \frac{\text{urine osmolality}}{\text{plasma osmolality}} \times \text{urine vol}$$

Toxicology Formulas

Serum methanol concentration [MeOH] in mg/dL
$= 3.2\ (Osm_s - (2 \times [Na^+]) - ([BUN]/2.8) - ([glucose]/18) - ([ETOH]/4.6) - 10)$

Ethylene glycol concentration
$= 6.2\ (Osm_s - (2 \times [Na^+]) - ([BUN]/2.8) - ([glucose]/18) - ([EtOH]/4.6) - 10)$

TABLE E.1 Daily Renal Excretion of Cations and Anions in Normals

Electrolyte	Urinary Excretion (mmol/d)
CATIONS	
Na	127 ± 6
K	49 ± 2
Ca	4 ± 1
Mg	11 ± 1
NH_4	28 ± 2
Total	**219 ± 3**
ANIONS	
Cl	135 ± 5
SO_4	34 ± 1
PO_4	20 ± 1
Organic anions	29 ± 1
Total	**221 ± 6**

Na, sodium; K, potassium; Ca, calcium; Mg, magnesium; NH_4, ammonia; Cl, chloride; SO_4, sulfate; PO_4, phosphate.

TABLE E.2 Use of Urine Electrolytes

Diagnostic Problem	Urinary Value	Primary Diagnostic Possibilities
Volume depletion	Na = 0–10 mmol/L	Extrarenal sodium loss
	Na >10 mmol/L	Renal salt wasting or adrenal insufficiency
Acute oliguria	Na = 0–10 mmol/L	Prerenal azotemia
	Na >30 mmol/L	Acute tubular necrosis
Hyponatremia	Na = 0–10 mmol/L	Severe volume depletion, edematous
	Na >dietary intake	Inappropriate antidiuretic hormone secretion; adrenal insufficiency
Hypokalemia	K = 0–10 mmol/L	Extrarenal K loss
	K >10 mmol/L	Renal K loss
Metabolic alkalosis	Cl = 0–10 mmol/L	Cl-responsive alkalosis
	Cl = dietary intake	Cl-resistant alkalosis

Na, sodium; K, potassium; Cl, chloride.

Infectious Diseases Formulas

ANTIBIOTIC KINETICS

The *volume of distribution* (V_D) of an antimicrobial is calculated as:

$$V_D = \frac{A}{C_p}$$

where A = total amount of antibiotic in the body and C_p = antibiotic plasma concentration.

Repetitive dosing of antibiotics depends on the principle of *minimal plasma concentrations* (C_{min}):

$$C_{min} = \frac{D}{(V_D)(2^n - 1)}$$

where D = dose and n = dosing interval expressed in half-lives.

The *plasma concentration at steady state* (C_{ss}) of an antimicrobial can be estimated utilizing the following formula:

$$C_{ss} = \frac{\text{Dose per half-life}}{(0.693)(V_D)}$$

ANTIBIOTIC ADJUSTMENTS

Renal dysfunction in critically ill patients is common. In those patients receiving aminoglycosides, dosage modification is required according to the *aminoglycoside clearance:*

$$\text{Aminoglycoside clearance} = (C_{cr})(0.6) + 10$$

where C_{cr} = creatinine clearance in mL/minute.

In order to estimate the creatinine clearance, the Cockcrof and Gault formula is utilized:

$$C_{cr}\ (\text{mL/min}) = \frac{(140 - \text{age}) \times \text{weight}}{\text{Cr} \times 72}$$

where Cr = serum creatinine in mg/dL. Another modification to this formula is the *Spyker and Guerrant method:*

$$C_{cr}\ (\text{mL/min}) = \frac{(140 - \text{age}) \times (1.03 - 0.053 \times \text{Cr})}{\text{Cr}}$$

TABLE E.3 Interpretation of Urine Electrolytes

Electrolyte	Normal Response	Patient Response	Potential Pitfalls
Na^+	Reflects diet and ECF volume; <10 mmol if ECF volume contracted	>20 mmol in ECF volume contraction suggests renal tubular damage	Diuretic use No reabsorbed anions Recent vomiting, drugs
Cl^-	Reflects diet and ECF volume; <10 mmol if ECF volume contracted	>20 mmol with ECF volume contraction suggests renal damage	Diuretic Diarrhea
K^+	Reflects diet, plasma (K), aldosterone action	If hypokalemia and urine (K): >20 mM or rate of K excretion >30 mmol/d then K excretion too high	K-sparing diuretics Low urine (Na) Water diuresis
pH	Depends on acid–base status Useful for bicarbonaturia	Useful once low NH_4^+ excretion confirmed to define cause of low NH_4^+	Unreliable for urine NH_4^+ Urinary tract infection
HCO_3^-	Depends on diet and acid–base status; >10 mM indicates HCO_3^- load 0 in acidemia	High urine HCO_3^- with chronic metabolic alkalosis indicates vomiting or HCO_3^- input High urine HCO_3 with acidemia in pRTA	Urinary tract infection Carbonic anhydrase inhibitors
(Na^+, K^+, Cl^-)	Depends on diet and acid–base status	Na + K > Cl = low urine NH_4^+ Cl > Na + K = high urine NH_4^+	Ketonuria Drug anions Alkaline urine

Na^+, sodium; Cl, chloride; K^+, potassium; HCO_3^-, carbonate; NH_4, ammonia; ECF, extracellular fluid; pRTA, partial renal tubular acidosis.
From Halperin ML, Goldstein MB. *Fluid, Electrolyte and Acid-Base Emergencies.* Philadelphia, PA: WB Saunders; 1988.

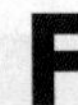

APPENDIX

F

Pharmacology

Drug Formulas

$$\text{Drug clearance} = V_d \times K_{el}$$

$$\text{Drug half-life } (T_{1/2}) = 0.693/K_{el}$$

$$\text{Drug elimination constant } (K_{el}) = \frac{\ln([\text{peak}]/[\text{trough}])}{{}^{t}\text{peak} - {}^{t}\text{trough}}$$

$$\text{Drug loading dose} = V_d \times [\text{target peak}]$$

$$\text{Drug dosing interval} = (-1/K_{el}) \times \ln([\text{desired trough}]/[\text{desired peak}]) + \text{infusion time (h)}$$

Dosage Adjustments in Renal Failure

TABLE F.1 Drug Dosage Adjustments in Renal Failure

	Dose Adjustment	GFR (mL/min)			Removed By	
		>50	10–50	<10	Hemodialysis	Peritoneal Dialysis
Aminoglycosides						
Gentamicin	D	60–90	30–70	20–30	Yes	Yes
	I	8–12	12	24		
Tobramycin	D	60–90	30–70	20–30	Yes	Yes
	I	8–12	12	24		
Antifungals						
Amphotericin B	I	24	24	24–36	No	No
Flucytosine	I	6	12–24	24–48	Yes	Yes
Antituberculous						
Ethambutol	I	24	24–36	48	Yes	Yes
Isoniazid	D	100	100	66–75	Yes	Yes
Rifampin	I	None	None	None	No	No
Antivirals						
Acyclovir	I	8	24	48	Yes	—
Amantadine	I	12–24	48–72	168	No	No
Cephalosporins						
Cefamandole	I	6	6–8	8	Yes	—
Cefazolin	I	6	12	24–48	Yes	—
Cefotaxime	I	6–8	8–12	12–24	Yes	—
Cefoxitin	I	8	8–12	24–48	Yes	—
Cephalothin	I	6	6	8–12	Yes	Yes
Chloramphenicol	D	None	None	None	Yes	No
Clindamycin	D	None	None	None	No	No
Erythromycin	D	None	None	None	No	No
Metronidazole	I	8	8–12	12–24	Yes	No
Nitrofurantoin	D	100	Avoid	Avoid	Yes	—
Penicillins						
Amoxicillin	I	6	6–12	12–16	Yes	No
Ampicillin	I	6	6–12	12–16	Yes	No
Carbenicillin	I	8–12	12–24	24–48	Yes	Yes
Dicloxacillin	D	None	None	None	No	—
Nafcillin	D	None	None	None	No	—
PCN G	I	6–8	8–12	12–16	Yes	No
Piperacillin	I	4–6	6–8	8	Yes	—
Ticarcillin	I	8–12	12–24	24–28	Yes	Yes
Sulfas/trimethoprim						
Sulfamethoxazole	I	12	18	24	Yes	No

TABLE F.1 Drug Dosage Adjustments in Renal Failure (*Continued*)

	Dose Adjustment	GFR (mL/min)			Removed By	
		>50	10–50	<10	Hemodialysis	Peritoneal Dialysis
Trimethoprim	I	12	18	24	Yes	No
Tetracyclines						
Doxycycline	I	12	12–18	18–24	No	No
Minocycline	D	None	None	None	No	No
Vancomycin	I	24–72	72–240	240	No	No
Antihypertensives						
Atenolol	D	None	50	25	Yes	—
Captopril	D	None	None	50	Yes	—
Clonidine	D	None	None	50–75	No	—
Hydralazine	D	8	8	12–24	No	No
Methyldopa	I	6	9–18	12–24	Yes	Yes
Metoprolol	D	None	None	None	Yes	—
Minoxidil	D	None	None	None	Yes	
Nadolol	D	None	50	25	Yes	—
Nitroprusside	D	None	None	None	Yes	—
Prazosin	D	None	None	None	No	No
Propranolol	D	None	None	None	No	—
Antidysrhythmics						
Disopyramide	I	None	12–24	24–40	Yes	—
Lidocaine	D	None	None	None	No	—
Procainamide	I	4	6–12	8–24	Yes	—
Quinidine	I	None	None	None	Yes	Yes
Calcium blockers						
Diltiazem	D	None	None	None	—	—
Nifedipine	D	None	None	None	—	—
Verapamil	D	None	None	None	No	—
Digoxin	D	100	25–75	10–25	No	No
	I	24	36	48		
H_2 blockers						
Cimetidine	D	800/d	600/d	400/d	No	No
Ranitidine	D	None	150/d	150/d	No	—
Nizatidine	D	None	150/d	150 qod	—	—
Famotidine	D	None	None	20/d or (40 qod)	—	—

GFR, glomerular filtration rate; PCN G, penicillin G; D, dosage reduction method of dosage adjustment; I, interval extension method of dosage adjustment; qod, every other day; H_2, histamine.
From Bennett WM, Aronoff GR, Golper TA, et al. *Drug Prescribing in Renal Failure*. Philadelphia: American College of Physicians; 1987.

Drugs Commonly Used in the Intensive Care Unit (In Alphabetical Order), Excluding Antibiotics

ADENOSINE

a. Action: Slows atrioventricular (AV) nodal conduction; produces short-term (seconds) high-degree AV blockade
b. Indications: Antiarrhythmic; useful for diagnosing supraventricular tachycardias and effective for terminating reentrant AV tachyarrhythmias
c. Loading dose: 6- or 12-mg intravenous (IV) bolus followed with a rapid saline flush
d. Dose interval/infusion: Wait 1–2 min between doses; no continuous infusion
e. Comments: Give through central venous catheter; contraindicated in heart block; sick sinus syndrome (except if pacemaker present), ventricular arrhythmias

AMINOPHYLLINE

a. Action: Bronchodilator, improves diaphragm contractility; positive inotrope and chronotrope; natriuretic and diuretic
b. Indications: Bronchoconstriction
c. Loading dose: 5–6 mg/kg lean body weight over 20 min (if patient already taking aminophylline/theophylline then check level, begin infusion, and then adjust dose based on baseline value)
d. Dose interval/infusion: 0.2–0.8 mg/kg/min (use increased dosage with smokers; decreased dosage with the elderly, patients with heart or liver disease)
e. Comments: Produces increased irritability, agitation, tachycardia, arrhythmias, nausea, and vomiting

AMRINONE/MILRINONE

a. Action: Inhibit cellular phosphodiesterase, producing extracellular to intracellular calcium shift; increased contractility but with arterial and venous dilatation
b. Indications: Positive inotrope

c. Loading dose: Amrinone 0.75–3.0 mg/kg over 2–3 min; milrinone 50 μg/kg over 10 min
d. Dose interval/infusion: Amrinone 5–10 μg/kg/min continuous infusion; milrinone 0.375–0.75 μg/kg/min
e. Comments: Synergistic with dobutamine (because of receptor downregulation in congestive heart failure); hepatic metabolism; renal excretion; rapid onset of action; dose-related thrombocytopenia with prolonged use of amrinone

ATRACURIUM

a. Action: Nondepolarizing neuromuscular blocker; minimal dose-dependent histamine (H_2) release; no vagal activity
b. Indications: Intermediate-acting neuromuscular blockade
c. Loading dose: 0.4–0.5 mg/kg intubating dose
d. Dose interval/infusion: 4–12 μg/kg/min continuous infusion
e. Comments: Titrate to effect in intensive care unit (ICU) patients (monitor with train-of-four testing); onset within 3–5 min; 25–35 min duration; 40–60 min recovery; no dose adjustment in hepatorenal dysfunction

BUMETANIDE

a. Action: Acts at loop of Henle to prevent chloride and sodium uptake; diuretic
b. Indications: Decreased urine output, mobilize edema fluid, pulmonary edema, treat hypercalcemia
c. Loading dose: 0.5–1.0 mg over 1–2 min
d. Dose interval/infusion: Repeat dose every 2–3 h; up to 10 mg/d
e. Comments: Observe for secondary electrolyte disturbances (hyponatremia, hypokalemia)

CALCIUM CHLORIDE/GLUCONATE

a. Action: Required for wide variety of cellular functions
b. Indications: Ionized hypocalcemia; vasopressor; hypermagnesemia/hyperkalemia (stabilizes cell membrane); calcium channel blocker overdose
c. Loading dose: 90 mg Ca IV bolus (chloride: 1 g = 272 mg [13.6 mmol] Ca) (gluconate: 1 g = 90 mg [4.65 mmol] Ca)
d. Dose interval/infusion: 0.5–2.0 mg/h adjust to ionized calcium value
e. Comments: Monitor for hypercalcemia, hypophosphatemia, and decreased sensorium

CLONIDINE

a. Action: Central α_2-receptor agonist
b. Indications: Hypertension; withdrawal syndromes (opiates, nicotine); modulate sympathetic hyperactivity of closed head injury
c. Loading dose: 0.1 mg transdermal weekly (may require 2–3 d for response); for hypertensive urgencies use 0.2–0.3 mg orally every 20 min until target blood pressure is reached (maximum 0.9 mg)
d. Dose interval/infusion: Usually twice daily when taken orally, no intravenous formulation
e. Comments: Usual maximum dose 2.4 mg/d; rebound hypertension with acute withdrawal

DIAZEPAM

a. Action: Benzodiazepine
b. Indications: Sedation, anxiety, agitation; ethanol withdrawal; seizures
c. Loading dose: 5 mg
d. Dose interval/infusion: Begin at 5 mg/h and titrate to effect
e. Comments: Central nervous system (CNS) depression

DILTIAZEM

a. Action: Calcium channel blockade; negative inotrope and peripheral vasodilator; depresses sinoatrial (SA) and AV node
b. Indications: Hypertension, angina; rate control in atrial fibrillation/flutter
c. Loading dose: 0.25 mg/kg IV over 2 min
d. Dose interval/infusion: 5–15 mg/h
e. Comments: Maximum dose 360 mg/d

DEXMEDETOMIDINE

a. Action: Central α_2-receptor agonist
b. Indications: Short-acting sedative
c. Loading dose: 0.1 mg transdermal weekly (may require 2–3 d for response); for hypertensive urgencies use 0.2–0.3 mg orally every 20 min until target blood pressure is reached (maximum 0.9 mg)
d. Dose interval/infusion: Usually twice daily when taken orally, no intravenous formulation
e. Comments: Usual maximum dose 2.4 mg/d; rebound hypertension with acute withdrawal

dDAVP

a. Action: Synthetic vasopressin; decreased excretion of free water; increases factor VIII levels
b. Indications: Central (neurogenic) diabetes insipidus (DI); bleeding in patients with decreased factor VIII levels
c. Loading dose: 2–4 μg IV or subcutaneously (SQ) for DI; 0.3 μg/kg IV over 15–30 min for bleeding
d. Dose interval/infusion: Twice daily
e. Comments: Dose for central DI by following urine output/osmolarity and serum sodium/osmolarity

DOBUTAMINE

a. Action: Positive inotrope, peripheral vasodilator, increases automaticity of SA node and enhances conduction through AV node and ventricles
b. Indications: Low cardiac output states, especially with increased systemic vascular resistance
c. Loading dose: 2.5–20.0 μg/kg/min
d. Dose interval/infusion: Titrate to effect
e. Comments: No dopaminergic effects on renal vessels; tachycardia may be a problem; contraindicated in idiopathic hypertrophic subaortic stenosis; tolerance may develop

DOPAMINE

a. Action: Dose-dependent vasopressor acting at multiple receptor sites
b. Indications: Bradycardia and refractory hypotension after cardiac insult while patient is waiting to place a pacemaker; not demonstrate that increases renal blood flow and subsequently urine output

c. Loading dose: None
d. Dose interval/infusion: Dopaminergic 0.5–2.0 μg/kg/min; β plus dopaminergic 2–10 μg/kg/min; α, β, and dopaminergic at >10 μg/kg/min
e. Comments: Tachycardia may be significant; necrosis at injection site with extravasation (treat with phentolamine)

EPINEPHRINE

a. Action: α- and β-receptor agonist; vasopressor, positive inotrope and chronotrope; bronchodilatation; increased glycogenolysis
b. Indications: Bronchoconstriction; allergic reactions; advanced cardiac life support; refractory hypotension
c. Loading dose: 1-mg bolus IV
d. Dose interval/infusion: 0.01–0.3 μg/kg/min titrated to effect
e. Comments: Increased myocardial oxygen consumption with arrhythmias and ischemia; hypertension; hyperglycemia; poor renal perfusion

ESMOLOL

a. Action: Short-acting β-blockade ($\beta_1 > \beta_2$)
b. Indications: Supraventricular tachyarrhythmias; hypertension
c. Loading dose: 0.5–1.0 mg/kg over 1 min
d. Dose interval/infusion: 10–300 μg/kg/min
e. Comments: Hypotension; bradycardia; bronchospasm; may prolong neuromuscular blockade effects of succinylcholine; contraindicated in bradycardia, heart block, cardiogenic shock

FENTANYL

a. Action: Potent opiate receptor ligand; produces decreases in heart rate, blood pressure, and cardiac index; respiratory depressant; may produce skeletal muscle rigidity
b. Indications: Opioid analgesia
c. Loading dose: 1–3 μg/kg, depending on additional anesthetic agents used
d. Dose interval/infusion: 0.01–0.3 μg/kg/h
e. Comments: Approximately 100 times as potent as morphine; no histamine release

FLUMAZENIL

a. Action: Benzodiazepine antagonist; acts centrally at benzodiazepine receptors
b. Indications: Complete or partial reversal of sedative effects of benzodiazepines; reversal effects occur within 1 min of intravenous dose
c. Loading dose: 0.2 mg IV over 15–30 s
d. Dose interval/infusion: Can repeat 0.2 mg every 60 s up to total dose of 1 mg; may use up to 3 mg in suspected benzodiazepine overdose; no continuous infusion
e. Comments: Effective reversal of benzodiazepine effects lasts 20 min, so repeated dosing with flumazenil may be necessary; liver metabolism

FUROSEMIDE

a. Action: Inhibits chloride and sodium reabsorption in ascending loop of Henle, producing a diuretic effect
b. Indications: Decreased urine output, acute oliguric renal failure, mobilize edema fluid, pulmonary edema, hypercalcemia
c. Loading dose: 10–200 mg, depending on the clinical situation
d. Dose interval/infusion: Begin at 5 mg/h and titrate to effect
e. Comments: Hepatic metabolism, renal excretion; up to 6 g/d has been given by continuous infusion; observe for electrolyte disturbances (hyponatremia, hypomagnesemia, hypokalemia)

GLUCAGON

a. Action: Increases glycogenolysis and gluconeogenesis producing hyperglycemia; increases lipolysis; positive inotrope; decreases gastrointestinal (GI) motility and secretions
b. Indications: Hypoglycemia; β-blocker and calcium channel blocker overdoses; hypotension
c. Loading dose: 0.5–1.0 mg SQ/IV/intramuscularly (IM)
d. Dose interval/infusion: Repeat loading dose every 15 min; 1–20 mg/h as continuous infusion
e. Comments: Hyperglycemia; tachycardia; hypokalemia

HALOPERIDOL

a. Action: Dopaminergic blockade acting as an antipsychotic
b. Indications: Agitation; acute psychosis, Delirium (hyperactive)
c. Loading dose: 0.5–5.0 mg IV/IM
d. Dose interval/infusion: Can be given hourly; 1–20 mg/h as continuous infusion
e. Comments: Decrease dose in hepatic dysfunction; observe closely for dystonic reactions and sedative effects; α-blockade

HEPARIN

a. Action: Anticoagulant acting through antithrombin III complexes
b. Indications: Deep venous thrombosis (acute and prophylaxis); pulmonary embolism; acute myocardial infarction; hemodialysis; catheter patency
c. Loading dose: Wide variety, depending on clinical situation
d. Dose interval/infusion: Adjusted to desired anticoagulant effect, usually based on following serial activated partial thromboplastin time (aPTT)
e. Comments: Side effects include hemorrhage, thrombocytopenia, fever

H_2 BLOCKERS (CIMETIDINE, FAMOTIDINE, RANITIDINE)

a. Action: H_2 receptor competitive antagonist decreasing gastric acid secretion
b. Indications: Prophylaxis for stress ulcer GI bleeding, acute/chronic peptic ulcer disease, acid hypersecretory diseases, reflux disease
c. Loading dose for stress ulcer prophylaxis: Cimetidine 300 mg IV every 6 h; famotidine 20 mg IV every 12 h; ranitidine 50 mg IV every 8 h

d. Dose interval/infusion: Total daily dose divided into continuous infusion, may be placed in parenteral nutritional formulas
e. Comments: Adjust dose based on creatinine clearance

ISOPROTERENOL
a. Action: Nonspecific β-agonist; positive inotrope and chronotrope; bronchodilator
b. Indications: Bronchoconstriction; symptomatic bradycardia; β-blocker overdose
c. Loading dose: 0.02–0.06 mg IV
d. Dose interval/infusion: 2–20 μg/min
e. Comments: Tachycardia; arrhythmias (torsade de pointes); myocardial ischemia; anxiety

LABETALOL
a. Action: α_1- and nonspecific β-blocker
b. Indications: Hypertension
c. Loading dose: 0.1, 0.2, 0.4, 0.8, 1.6 mg/kg IV. Start at lowest dose and advance to the next highest dose every 10 min until BP control is achieved. May repeat hourly; when repeating start with the dose one step below that which allowed control of BP.
d. Dose interval/infusion: Boluses can be repeated every 10 min; continuous infusion of 1–10 mg/min titrated to effect
e. Comments: Observe for bronchospasm, bradycardia

LEVOSIMENDAN
a. Action: Calcium sensitization for positive inotrope effect and activation of adenosine triphosphate (ATP)-dependent potassium channels for vasodilation and cardioprotective effect
b. Indication: Decompensated low-output heart failure (cardiac index <2.5 L/min/m^2 or pulmonary capillary wedge pressure [PCWP] >16 mmHg or left ventricular ejection fraction [LVEF] <0.4)
c. Dose infusion/interval: Infusion 0.05–0.2 μg/kg/min for 24 h
d. Comments: Most common adverse reaction is headache and hypotension (both 5%); caution in renal, hepatic impairment, severe hypotension, severe tachycardia, history of torsades de pointes; correct hypovolemia

LIDOCAINE
a. Action: Antidysrhythmic and local anesthetic
b. Indications: Local anesthesia; ventricular arrhythmias; prophylaxis in acute myocardial infarction
c. Loading dose: 1.0–1.5 mg/kg bolus IV (maximum load, 3 mg/kg)
d. Dose interval/infusion: Bolus repeated in 20 min; 1–4 mg/min continuous infusion
e. Comments: Observe for metabolic acidosis, altered mental status (including seizures), and myocardial depression; hepatic metabolism; methemoglobinemia

LORAZEPAM
a. Action: Benzodiazepine
b. Indications: Agitation; seizures; supplemental sedation with neuromuscular blockade
c. Loading dose: 0.5–2-mg bolus IV (In an older person start with lower dose)
d. Dose interval/infusion: Begin at 1 mg/h and titrate to effect
e. Comments: CNS depression

MAGNESIUM
a. Action: Coenzyme; muscular contractility; nerve conduction; membrane stabilization; antiseizure; inhibits uterine contractility
b. Indications: Hypomagnesemia; arrhythmias; preeclampsia and eclampsia
c. Loading dose: 1–4 g IV over 15 min (infuse over 4 h for treatment of asymptomatic hypomagnesemia)
d. Dose interval/infusion: Subsequent dosing based on desired clinical effect and serum levels
e. Comments: Observe for hypotension and heart block; respiratory and CNS depressant (primarily in patients with renal dysfunction)

MIDAZOLAM
a. Action: Short-acting benzodiazepine
b. Indications: Sedation, anxiety, agitation; ETOH withdrawal; seizures
c. Loading dose: 0.5–4 mg (in older person start at low dose)
d. Dose interval/infusion: 1–20 mg/h titrated to effect
e. Comments: CNS depression; active metabolites; respiratory depression when used in combination with narcotics; three to four times the potency of diazepam

MIVACURIUM
a. Action: Nondepolarizing neuromuscular blocker; minimal to moderate H_2 release; minimal tachycardia
b. Indications: Short-acting neuromuscular blockade
c. Loading dose: 0.1–0.25 mg/kg intubating dose
d. Dose interval/infusion: 5–15 μg/kg/min continuous infusion; onset in 2–4 min; 13–40 min duration of action; 6–14 min recovery
e. Comments: Titrate to effect in ICU patients (monitor with train-of-four testing)

MORPHINE
a. Action: Opioid analgesia; venodilation
b. Indications: Analgesia, sedation; pulmonary edema
c. Loading dose: 1–5 mg IV
d. Dose interval/infusion: Rebolus every 2–3 h; 1–10 mg/h continuous infusion titrated to effect
e. Comments: CNS disturbances; hypotension (especially if intravascular volume depletion is present); respiratory depression; histamine release

NICARDIPINE
a. Action: Noncardiosuppressive calcium channel antagonist
b. Indications: Postoperative hypertension, prevention of vasospasm from subarachnoid hemorrhage; angina
c. Loading dose: 5 mg/h and increase by 2.5 mg/h every 15 min
d. Dose interval/infusion: 1–15 mg/h; 20–40 mg orally three times daily
e. Comments: Hypotension; reflex tachycardia

NIFEDIPINE

a. Action: Calcium channel blocker; minimal myocardial depression with slowing of conduction; smooth muscle relaxation
b. Indications: Angina, hypertension
c. Loading dose: 10–20 mg orally or sublingually
d. Dose interval/infusion: Hourly as needed, no intravenous preparation; maximum dose 180 mg/d
e. Comments: Hypotension and reflex tachycardia

NIMODIPINE

a. Action: Calcium channel antagonist; minimal cardiovascular effect
b. Indications: Prevention of vasospasm due to subarachnoid hemorrhage
c. Loading dose: None, no IV formulation available
d. Dose interval/infusion: 60 mg orally or sublingually every 4 h for 21 d
e. Comments: Hypotension may occur

NITROGLYCERIN

a. Action: Smooth muscle relaxation through nitric oxide pathway; pulmonary vasculature and venous vasodilator; decreased preload; improved coronary blood flow
b. Indications: Myocardial ischemia; hypertension; congestive heart failure; esophageal spasm
c. Loading dose: None necessary in intravenous dosing
d. Dose interval/infusion: 10–400 μg/min titrated to effect
e. Comments: Liver metabolism; renal excretion; tolerance; rare methemoglobinemia; increased cerebral blood flow (CBF); hypotension

NITROPRUSSIDE

a. Action: Arterial and venous vasodilatation through nitric oxide pathway; coronary vasodilatation; increased CBF and volume with subsequent increased intracranial pressure
b. Indications: Hypertension; acute left ventricular failure
c. Loading dose: Not indicated
d. Dose interval/infusion: 0.5–10 μg/kg/min and titrate to effect
e. Comments: Coronary steal (angina) possible with coronary vasodilatation; metabolic acidosis; follow thiocyanate levels if toxicity suspected (toxicity: Amyl nitrate and sodium nitrite converts hemoglobin to methemoglobin; methemoglobin binds cyanide; sodium thiosulfate converts cyanide to thiocyanate)

NOREPINEPHRINE

a. Action: α- and β_1-agonists; arterial and venous vasoconstriction; minimal chronotropic effect
b. Indications: Hypotension
c. Loading dose: Not indicated
d. Dose interval/infusion: 0.01–0.1 μg/kg/min titrated to effect
e. Comments: Decreased renal perfusion; peripheral vasoconstriction; arrhythmias; tissue necrosis with extravasation

OCTREOTIDE

a. Action: Mimics effects of somatostatin; increases GI motility while decreasing GI and pancreatic secretions; decreases splanchnic blood flow
b. Indications: Gut neuroendocrine tumors, diarrhea, excess GI/pancreatic secretions; variceal hemorrhage
c. Loading dose: 250-μg bolus
d. Dose interval/infusion: 25–100 μg three times daily or 50–250 μg/h infusion
e. Comments: Total dose, 50–1,500 μg/d; both hypoglycemia and hyperglycemia

PANCURONIUM

a. Action: Nondepolarizing neuromuscular blocker; no histamine release, modest to marked vagal block with tachycardia
b. Indications: Long-acting neuromuscular blockade
c. Loading dose: 0.1-mg/kg intubating dose
d. Dose interval/infusion: 1–2 μg/kg/min continuous infusion
e. Comments: Titrate to effect in ICU patient (monitor with train-of-four testing); onset within 2–4 min and duration of action of 60–100 min; recovery within 120–180 min; primarily renal excretion

PHENTOLAMINE

a. Action: α-blocker; vasodilatation
b. Indications: Hypertension; pheochromocytoma
c. Loading dose: 5 mg IV/IM to effect
d. Dose interval/infusion: No continuous infusion
e. Comments: Monitor for hypotension

PHENYLEPHRINE

a. Action: α-agonist; arterial and venous vasoconstriction; vasopressor with reflex decrease in heart rate
b. Indications: Hypotension
c. Loading dose: Not indicated
d. Dose interval/infusion: 0.1–1 μg/kg/min titrated to effect
e. Comments: Hypertension, bradycardia, myocardial ischemia, decreased renal perfusion

PROCAINAMIDE

a. Action: Antiarrhythmic; vasodilatation
b. Indications: Supraventricular and ventricular arrhythmias; recurrent atrial fibrillation/flutter
c. Loading dose: 50 mg/min to effect or total dose of 17 mg/kg
d. Dose interval/infusion: 2–6 mg/min continuous infusion
e. Comments: Observe for conduction disturbances (including torsade) and myocardial depression

PROPOFOL

a. Action: Alkylphenol
b. Indications: Short-acting sedative
c. Loading dose: 1.5–3 mg/kg
d. Dose interval/infusion: Titrate to effect; usual dose is 10–50 μg/kg/min
e. Comments: No analgesic properties; very short duration of action (2–3 min); reduce dosage in the elderly; monitor triglyceride values

PROPRANOLOL

a. Action: Nonspecific β-blockade; decreased heart rate and contractility; antiarrhythmic
b. Indications: Supraventricular tachyarrhythmias, angina, hypertension, acute myocardial infarct
c. Loading dose: 0.5–1.0 mg bolus IV
d. Dose interval/infusion: Repeat bolus every 5 min to effect
e. Comments: Bradycardia, hypotension, bronchospasm

PROTAMINE

a. Action: Heparin antagonist (complexes with heparin)
b. Indications: Reverse the effects of heparin
c. Loading dose: 1 mg/90 IU bovine heparin; 1 mg/115 IU porcine heparin over 1–3 min
d. Dose interval/infusion: Titrate to aPTT
e. Comments: Maximum dose of 50 mg in any 10-min period; observe for bleeding after large dosages; hypotension

REMIFENTANIL

a. Action: Potent opiate receptor ligand; produces decreases in heart rate and blood pressure; respiratory depressant; may produce skeletal muscle rigidity and vocal cord closure
b. Indications: Opioid analgesia
c. Loading dose: If needed, bolus 0.1–0.2 μg/kg
d. Dose interval/infusion: Usually ranges between 0.05 and 0.25 μg/kg/min, higher doses have been used
e. Comments: About twice as potent as fentanyl; rapid onset of action with short duration—about 6.5 min to wake up after turning off infusion

ROCURONIUM

a. Action: Nondepolarizing neuromuscular blocker; minimal H_2 release; minimal to moderate vagal blockade
b. Indications: Intermediate-acting neuromuscular blockade
c. Loading dose: 0.4–1.2 mg/kg intubating dose
d. Dose interval/infusion: 10–12 μg/kg/min continuous infusion
e. Comments: Titrate to effect in ICU patients (monitor with train-of-four testing); 1–3 min onset of action; 22–67 min duration of action; recovery in 10–20 min

SUCCINYLCHOLINE

a. Action: Depolarizing neuromuscular blocker; no H_2 release, some vagal stimulation
b. Indications: Rapid onset of paralysis; short-acting neuromuscular blockade
c. Loading dose: 0.25–1.5 mg/kg (ED_{95} is 0.25 mg/kg)
d. Dose interval/infusion: Continuous infusion of 7.1–142 μg/kg/min
e. Comments: Onset in 0.5–5 min with duration of action of 2–3 min and recovery within 10 min; hyperkalemia; prolonged blockade in patients with atypical pseudocholinesterase; increased intracranial pressure (ICP)

SUFENTANIL

a. Action: Potent opiate receptor ligand; produces decreases in heart rate, blood pressure, and cardiac index; respiratory depressant; may increase ICP in patients with compromised intracranial compliance; may produce skeletal muscle rigidity
b. Indications: Opioid analgesia
c. Loading dose: 1–30 μg/kg, depending on other anesthetic agents used
d. Dose interval/infusion: As needed, no infusion
e. Comments: Five to ten times as potent as fentanyl with a shorter duration of action; muscle rigidity

THIOPENTAL

a. Action: Barbiturate with hypnotic and anesthetic properties
b. Indications: General anesthesia, seizures, increased ICP
c. Loading dose: 3–5 mg/kg for induction of anesthesia; 75–125 mg for treatment of seizures
d. Dose interval/infusion: Additional doses as clinically indicated; no continuous infusion
e. Comments: Observe clinically and use blood levels as necessary; respiratory depression

THROMBOLYTICS (STREPTOKINASE, UROKINASE, TISSUE PLASMINOGEN ACTIVATOR)

a. Action: Plasminogen activators; plasmin produced; plasmin degrades fibrinogen and fibrin, dissolving preexisting thrombi
b. Indications: Pulmonary embolism, acute myocardial infarction, venous thrombosis, graft thrombosis, catheter occlusion
c. Loading dose: Varies, depending on agent used and clinical condition
d. Dose interval/infusion: Variable
e. Comments: Bleeding (about 5% of patients); absolute contraindications include active hemorrhage, recent (2 mo) neurologic injury/surgery/tumor

VASOPRESSIN

a. Action: Decreases hepatic blood flow and portal pressure; increased clotting; decreased free water excretion; increases gut motility
b. Indications: Central (neurogenic) DI; bleeding esophageal varices, septic shock, and cardiopulmonary resuscitation
c. Loading dose: Central DI—aqueous vasopressin 5–10 IU IM/SQ
d. Dose interval/infusion: Sepsis–0.02–0.04 Units/min IV; Central DI—two to four times daily dosing (follow polyuria and serum sodium); GI bleeding—aqueous vasopressin 0.2–1.0 U/min IV
e. Comments: CNS disturbances, hypertension, angina, hyponatremia; metabolic acidosis

VECURONIUM

a. Action: Nondepolarizing neuromuscular blocker; no H_2 release; no vagal activity or tachycardia
b. Indications: Intermediate-acting neuromuscular blockade

c. Loading dose: 0.08 mg/kg intubating dose
d. Dose interval/infusion: 1–2 μg/kg/min continuous infusion
e. Comments: Titrate to effect in ICU patients (monitor with train-of-four testing); onset within 2.5–4.5 min; 35–45 min duration; recovery within 45–60 min; renal and hepatic excretion

VERAPAMIL

a. Action: Antiarrhythmic; calcium channel blockade
b. Indications: Treatment of angina, hypertension, hypertrophic cardiomyopathy, and supraventricular tachyarrhythmias (SVTs) (slows ventricular response in atrial fibrillation or flutter and may convert SVT to sinus rhythm)
c. Loading dose: 0.075–0.15 mg/kg (5–10 mg) IV over 2–3 min; may repeat bolus in 10 min
d. Dose interval/infusion: Continuous infusion of 5 mg/h titrated to effect
e. Comments: May produce hypotension: Bradycardia and AV block in patients treated with concomitant β-blockers

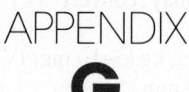

APPENDIX G

Dermatomes and Rule of Nines

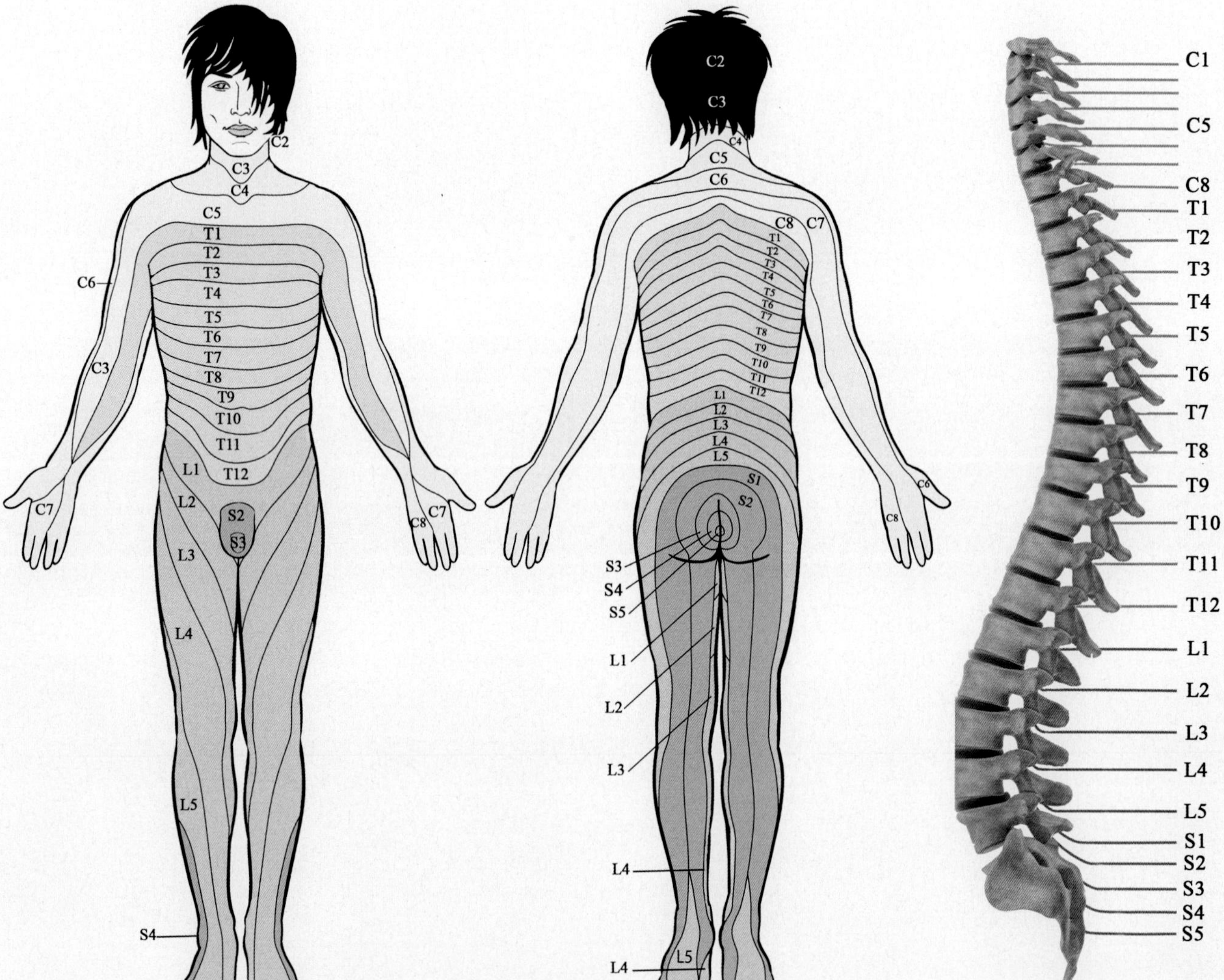

FIGURE G.1 Spinal nerves transmit impulses to specific areas, or dermatomes.

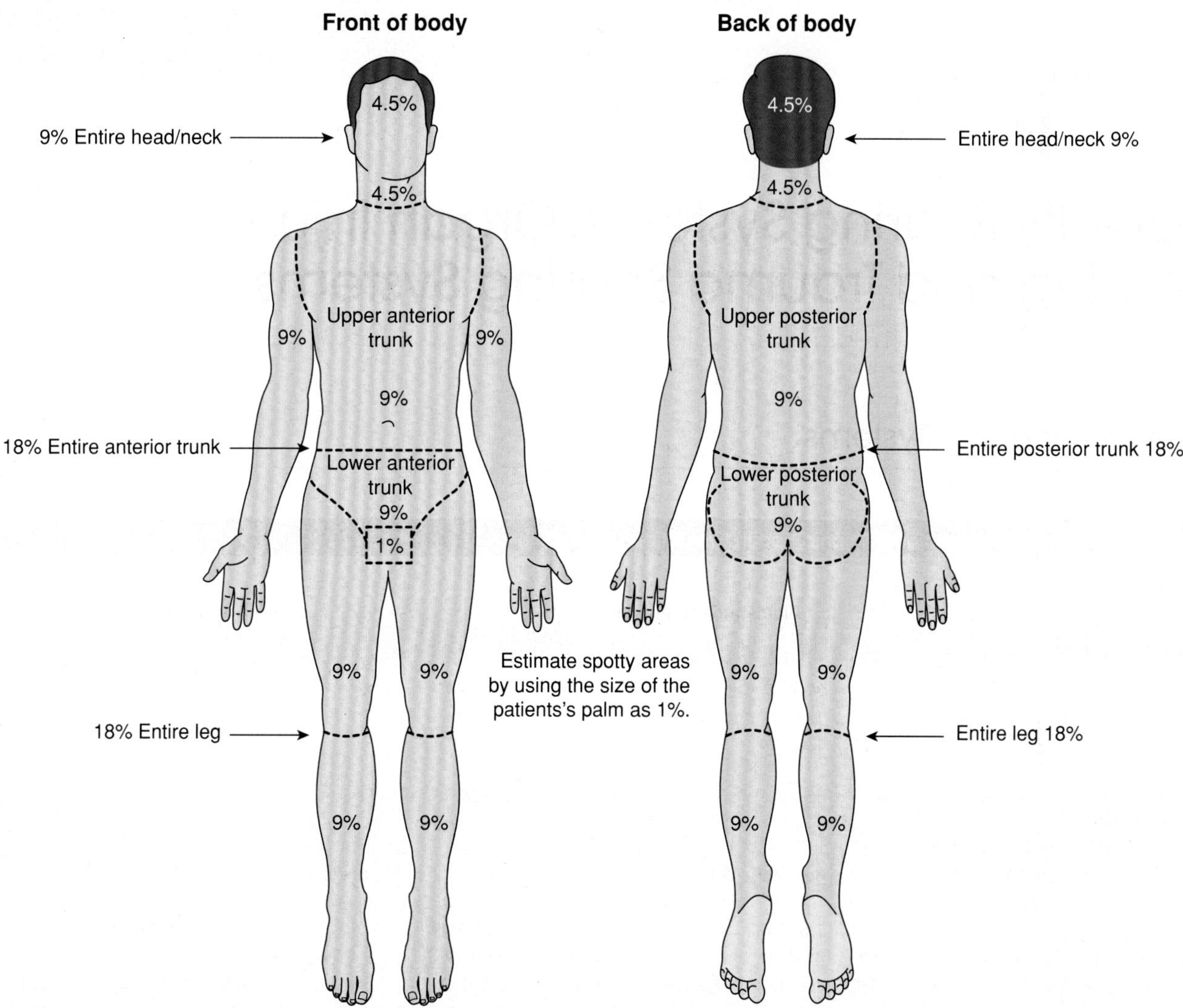

FIGURE G.2 To estimate the extent of burn, the *rule of nines* for body surface area is commonly used. In children: arms 9% each; legs 9% each; head 13%; trunk 18% anterior, 18% posterior; genitalia 1%.

APPENDIX

H

Severity Scoring Systems, Organ Injury Scaling and Trauma Scoring Systems

Severity Scoring Systems

TABLE H.1 Acute Physiologic and Chronic Health Evaluation (APACHE II)

A: Acute Physiologic Score (APS; 12 Variables)

	High Abnormal Range					Low Abnormal Range			
Physiologic Variable	+4	+3	+2	+1	0	+1	+2	+3	+4
Temperature rectal (°C)	≥41	39–40.9		38.5–38.9	36–38.4	34–35.9	32–33.9	30–31.9	≤29.0
Mean arterial pressure (mmHg)	≥160	130–159	110–129		70–109		50–69		≤49
Heart rate—ventricular response	≥180	140–179	110–139		70–109		55–69	40–54	≤39
Respiratory rate—nonventilated or ventilated	≥50	35–49		25–34	12–24	10–11	6–9		≤5
Oxygen: A-a DO_2 or PaO_2 (mmHg)									
a. FiO_2 ≥0.5 record A-a DO_2	≥500	350–499	200–349		≤200	PO_2 61–70		PO_2 55–60	PO_2 <55
b. FiO_2 <0.5 record only PaO_2					PO_2 >70				
Arterial pH	≥7.7	7.6–7.69		7.5–7.59	7.33–7.49		7.25–7.32	7.15–7.24	<7.15
Serum HCO_3—only if no ABGs	≥52	41–51.9		32–40.9	23–31.9		18–21.9	15–17.9	<15
Serum sodium (mmoL/L)	≥180	160–179	155–159	150–154	130–149		120–129	111–119	≤110
Serum potassium (mmoL/L)	≥7	6–6.9		5.5–5.9	3.5–5.4	3–3.4	2.5–2.9		≤2.5
Serum creatinine (μmoL/L)	≥350	200–340	150–190		60–140		<60		
Hematocrit (%)	≥60		50–50.9	46–49.9	30–45.9		20–29.9		≤20
White blood cell count (×1,000 mm^3)	≥40		20–39.9	15–19.9	3–14.9		1–2.9		<1
Glasgow coma score (GCS) Score = 15 – actual GCS									

B: Age points		C: Chronic health points			Apache II score
Age (years)	**Points**	**History**	**Points for elective surgery**	**Points for emergency surgery**	**Sum of A + B + C**
≤44	0	**Liver:** Biopsy-proven cirrhosis and documented portal hypertension or prior episodes of hepatic failure	2	5	**A: APS**
45–54	2	**Cardiovascular:** NYHA Class IV	2	5	**B: Age points score**
55–64	3	**Respiratory:** e.g., severe COPD, hypercapnia, home O_2, pulmonary hypertension	2	5	
65–74	5	**Immunocompromised**	2	5	**C: Chronic health points score**
≥75	6	**Renal:** Chronic dialysis	2	5	**Total:**

ABG, arterial blood gas; NYHA, New York Heart Association; COPD, chronic obstructive pulmonary disease.
From Knaus WA, et al. APACHE II: a severity of disease classification system. *Crit Care Med.* 1985;13:818–829.

TABLE H.2 Simplified Acute Physiology (SAPS II) Score

Variable	26	13	12	11	9	7	6	5	4	3	2	0	1	2	3	4	6	7	8	9	10	12	15	16	17	18
Age in years												<40						40–59				60–69	70–74	75–79		≥80
Heart rate (beat/min)			<40								40–69	70–119				120–159		≥160								
Systolic blood pressure (mmHg)		<70						70–99				100–199		≥200												
Body temperature (°C)												<39°C			≥39°C											
PaO_2/FiO_2 (mmHg) only if VENT or CPAP				<100	100–199	≥200																				
Urinary output (L/d)				<0.500					0.500–0.999			≥1.000														
Blood urea (mmol/L) (g/L)												<10.0 <0.60					10.0–29.9 0.60–1.79				≥30.0 ≥1.80					
WBC count (10^3/mL)			<1.0									1.0–19.9		≥20.0												
Serum K^+ (mEq/L)										<3.0		3.0–4.9		≥5.0												
Serum Na^+ (mEq/L)								<125				125–144	≥145													
Serum HCO_3 (mEq/L)							<15			15–19		≥20														
Bilirubin (if jaundice µmol/L) (mg/L)												<68.4 <40.0				68.4–102.4 40.0–59.9				≥102.5 ≥60.0						
Glasgow coma score (points)	<6	6–8				9–10		11–13				14–15														
Chronic diseases																				Met. cancer	Hem. mal				AIDS	
Type of admission												Elective surgery			Medical		Surgery emergency									

VENT, ventilator; CPAP, continuous positive airway pressure; WBC, white blood cell; Met. cancer, metastatic carcinoma; Met, metastatic; Hem. mal, hematologic malignancy; AIDS, acquired immunodeficiency syndrome.
The SAPS II score registers the worst value of selected variables, within the first 24 hours after admission.
From Le Gall JR, Lemeshow S, Saulnier F, et al. A new simplified acute physiology score (SAPS II) based on a European/North American multicenter study. *JAMA.* 1993;270:2957–2963.

TABLE H.3 Sequential Organ Failure Assessment (SOFA) Score

Organ System		Score 0	Score 1	Score 2	Score 3	Score 4
Respiration	Lowest PaO_2/FiO_2 (mmHg) or (Kpa) Respiratory support (yes/no)	>400 >53.33	≤400 40–53.33	≤300 26.67–40	≤200 13.33–26.67 and yes	≤100 ≤13.33 and yes
Coagulation	Lowest platelet ($10^3/mm^3$)	>150	≤150	≤100	≤50	≤20
Hepatic	Highest bilirubin (mg/dL) or (µmol/L)	<1.2 <20	1.2–1.9 20–32	2.0–5.9 33–101	6.0–11.9 102–204	≥12 >204
Circulatory	Lowest mean arterial pressure (mmHg)	>70	<70			
	Highest dopamine dose (µg/kg/min)			≤5	>5	>15
	Highest epinephrine dose (µg/kg/min)				≤0.1	>0.1
	Highest norepinephrine dose (µg/kg/min)				≤0.1	>0.1
	Dobutamine (yes/no)			Any dose		
Neurologic	(GCS, see Table H.6)	15	13–14	10–12	6–9	<6
Renal	Highest creatinine level (mg/dL)	<1.2	1.2–1.9	2.0–3.4	3.0–4.9	≥5.0
	or (µmol/L)	<110	110–170	171–299	300–440	>440
	Total urine output (mL/24 h)				<500	<200

GCS, Glasgow Coma Score.
SOFA total (Σ 6 items). The SOFA score assesses the function of 6 different organ systems: respiratory (partial arterial oxygen pressure (PaO_2)/fraction of inspired oxygen (FiO_2)), cardiovascular (blood pressure, vasoactive drugs), renal (creatine and diuresis), hepatic (bilirubin), neurologic (Glasgow Coma Score), and hematologic (platelet count).
From Vincent JL, Moreno R, Takala J, et al. The SOFA (Sepsis-related Organ Failure Assessment) score to describe organ dysfunction/failure. On behalf of the Working Group on sepsis-related problems of the European Society of Intensive Care Medicine. *Intensive Care Med.* 1996;22:707–710.

TABLE H.4 Multiple Organ Dysfunction Score (MODS)

Variables	0	1	2	3	4
PaO_2/FiO_2	<300	226–300	151–225	76–150	≤75
Creatinine serum	≤100	101–200	201–350	351–500	≥500
Bilirubin	≤20	21–60	61–120	121–240	>240
Heart rate	≤10	10.1–15	15.1–20	20.1–30	>30
Platelet count	>120	81–120	51–80	21–50	≤20
Glasgow Coma Score	15	13–14	10–12	7–9	≤6

From Marshall JC, Cook DJ, Christou NV, et al. Multiple organ dysfunction score: a reliable descriptor of a complex clinical outcome. *Crit Care Med.* 1995;23:1638–1652.

Injury/Trauma Scoring Systems

TABLE H.5 Abbreviated Injury Score (AIS)

Score	Injury[a]
1	Minor
2	Moderate
3	Serious
4	Severe
5	Critical
6	Unsurvivable

[a]Injuries are ranked on a scale of 1–6, with 1 being minor, 5 severe, and 6 an unsurvivable injury. This represents the "threat to life" associated with an injury and is not meant to represent a comprehensive measure of severity.

From Copes WS, Sacco WJ, Champion HR, Bain LW. Progress in characterising anatomic injury. In: *Proceedings of the 33rd Annual Meeting of the Association for the Advancement of Automotive Medicine.* Baltimore, MD; 1993;205–218.

TABLE H.6 Glasgow Coma Score (GCS)[a]

	Score[b]
Best Eye Response (E)	
No eye opening	1
Eye opening to pain	2
Eye opening to verbal command	3
Eyes open spontaneously	4
Best verbal response (V)	
No verbal response	1
Incomprehensible sounds	2
Inappropriate words	3
Confused	4
Orientated	5
Best motor response (M)	
No motor response	1
Extension to pain	2
Flexion to pain	3
Withdrawal from pain	4
Localizing pain	5
Obeys commands	6

[a]Note that the phrase "GCS of 11" is essentially meaningless, and it is important to break the figure down into its components, such as E3V3M5 = GCS 11.

[b]A coma score of 13 or higher correlates with a mild brain injury, 9–12 is a moderate injury, and 8 or less a severe brain injury.

From Teasdale G, Jennett B. Assessment of coma and impaired consciousness. *Lancet.* 1974;2:81–83.

TABLE H.7 Revised Trauma Score (RTS)[a]

Glasgow Coma Score (GCS)[b]	Systolic Blood Pressure (SBP)	Respiratory Rate (RR)	Coded Value
13–15	>89	10–29	4
9–12	76–89	>29	3
6–8	50–75	6–9	2
4–5	1–49	1–5	1
3	0	0	0

[a]The coded form of the RTS is calculated as follows: RTS = 0.9368 GCS + 0.7326 SBP + 0.2908 RR. Values for the RTS are in the range 0–7.8408. The RTS is heavily weighted toward the GCS to compensate for major head injury without multisystem injury or major physiologic changes. A threshold of RTS <4 has been proposed to identify those patients who should be treated in a trauma center, although this value may be somewhat low.

From Champion HR, Sacco JW, Copes WS. A revision of the trauma score. *J Trauma.* 1989;29:623–629.

TABLE H.8 Injury Severity Score (ISS)[a]

Region	Injury Description	Abbreviated Injury Score (AIS[b])	Square Top Three
Head and neck	Cerebral contusion	3	9
Face	No injury	0	
Chest	Flail chest	4	16
Abdomen	Minor contusion of liver	2	
	Complex rupture of spleen	5	25
Extremity	Fractured femur	3	
External	No injury	0	
Injury severity score	50		

[a]The ISS takes values from 0 to 75. If an injury is assigned an AIS[b] of 6 (unsurvivable injury), the ISS is automatically assigned to 75. The ISS is virtually the only anatomic scoring system in use and correlates linearly with mortality, morbidity, hospital stay, and other measures of severity.

From Baker SP, O'Neill B, Haddon W, et al. The injury severity score: a method for describing patients with multiple injuries and evaluating emergency care. *J Trauma.* 1974;14:187–196.

APPENDIX I

Analgesia–Sedation Scores and Tools

TABLE I.1 Ramsay Scale

Level	Characteristics
1	Patient awake, anxious, agitated, or restless
2	Patient awake, cooperative, orientated, and tranquil
3	Patient drowsy, with response to commands
4	Patient asleep, brisk response to glabella tap or loud auditory
5	Patient asleep, sluggish response to stimulus
6	Patient has no response to firm nailbed pressure or other noxious stimuli

From Ramsay MAE, Savege TM, Simpson BRJ, et al. Controlled sedation with alphaxolone/alphadolone. *BMJ.* 1974;ii:656–659.

TABLE I.2 Richmond Agitation–Sedation Scale (RASS)

Score	Term	Description
+4	Combative	Overtly combative or violent; immediate danger to staff
+3	Very agitated	Pulls on or removes tube(s) or catheter(s) or has aggressive behavior toward staff
+2	Agitated	Frequent nonpurposeful movement or patient–ventilator dyssynchrony
+1	Restless	Anxious or apprehensive but movements not aggressive or vigorous
0	Alert and calm	
−1	Drowsy	Not fully alert, but has sustained (>10 s) awakening, with eye contact, to voice
−2	Light sedation	Briefly (<10 s) awakens with eye contact to voice
−3	Moderate sedation	Any movement (but no eye contact) to voice
−4	Deep sedation	No response to voice, but any movement to physical stimulation
−5	Unarousable	No response to voice or physical stimulation

From Sessler CN, Gosnell MS, Grap MJ, et al. The Richmond agitation-sedation scale: validity and reliability in adult intensive care unit patients. *Am J Respir Crit Care Med.* 2002;166:1338–1344.

TABLE I.3 Behavioral Pain Scale (BPS)

Indicator	Description	Score
Facial expression	Relaxed	1
	Partially tightened (e.g., brow lowering)	2
	Fully tightened (e.g., eyelid closing)	3
	Grimacing	4
Upper limb movements	No movement	1
	Partially bent	2
	Fully bent with finger flexion	3
	Permanent retracted	4
Compliance with mechanical ventilation	Tolerating movement	1
	Coughing but tolerating ventilation for the most time	2
	Fighting ventilator	3
	Unable to control ventilation	4
Total, range		3–12

Aissaoui Y, Zeggawagh AA, Zekraoui A, et al. Validation of a behavioral pain scale in critically ill, sedated, and mechanically ventilated patients. *Anesth Analg.* 2006;101(5):1470–1478.

TABLE I.4 Critical Care Pain Observation Tool (CPOT)

Indicator	Description	Observation	Score
Facial expression	No muscular tension observed	Relaxed, neutral	0
	Presence of frowning, brow lowering, orbit tightening and levator contraction	Tense	1
	All of the above facial movements plus eyelid tightly	Grimacing	2
Body movements	Does not move at all (does not necessarily mean absence of pain)	Absence of movements	0
	Slow, cautious movements, touching or rubbing the pain site, seeking attention through movements	Protection	1
	Pulling tube, attempting to sit up, moving limbs/thrashing, not following commands, striking at staff, trying to climb out of bed	Restlessness	2
Muscle tension Evaluation by passive flexion and extension of upper extremities	No resistance to passive movements	Relaxed	0
	Resistance to passive movements	Tense, rigid	1
	Strong resistance to passive movements, inability to complete them	Restlessness	2
Compliance with ventilator (intubated patients)	Alarms not activated, easy ventilation	Tolerating ventilator or movement	0
	Alert stop spontaneously	Coughing but tolerating	1
	Asynchrony: Blocking ventilation, alarms frequently activated	Fighting ventilator	2
Or			
Vocalization (extubated patients)	Talking in normal tone or no sound	Talking in normal tone or no sound	0
	Sighing, moaning	Sighing, moaning	1
	Crying out, sobbing	Crying out, sobbing	2
Total, range			0–8

Gélinas C, Fillion L, Puntillo KA, Viens C, Fortier M. Validation of the critical-care pain observation tool in adult patients. *Am J Crit Care.* 2006:15(4):420–427.

APPENDIX J

Antibiotics

TABLE J.1 Aminopenicillins

Drug	Drug class	Usual dose in adults	Actions, interactions, and others	Spectrum of activity, indications, and active against most strains of	Route, reduce dose, and contraindications
Ampicillin	Aminopenicillin	IV: 2.0 g IV q4 h PO: 500 mg q6 h	Allopurinol (increased frequency of rash) Warfarin (increased INR)	*Streptococcus pneumoniae; Staphylococcus aureus* (penicillinase and nonpenicillinase producing); *Haemophilus influenzae*, and group A β-hemolytic *Streptococci* Bacterial meningitis caused by *Escherichia coli*, group B *Streptococci*, and other gram-negative bacteria (*Listeria monocytogenes, Neisseria meningitidis*) Endocarditis caused by susceptible gram-positive organisms including *Streptococcus* sp., penicillin G–susceptible *Staphylococci*, and *Enterococci*. Endocarditis due to enterococcal strains usually respond to intravenous therapy Gram-negative sepsis caused by *E. coli, Proteus mirabilis*, and *Salmonella* sp. Gastrointestinal infections caused by *Salmonella typhosa* (typhoid fever), other *Salmonella* sp., and *Shigella* sp. Urinary tract infections caused by *E. coli* and *Proteus mirabilis*	• Primary mode of elimination: Renal • Reduce dose in moderate to severe renal impairment
Amoxicillin	Aminopenicillin	IV: 500 mg–1 g tds (higher doses: 2 g 4 hourly in endocarditis PO: 1 g q8 h	Bactericide Some gram-negative activity	• *Streptococcus pneumoniae* • *Haemophilus influenzae* (except COPD patients) • β-Hemolytic *Streptococci* • *Streptococcus pyogenes* do not produce β-lactamase • *Enterococcus faecalis*	• Primary mode of elimination: Renal • Reasonable oral absorption (oral preparation) • Reduce dose in moderate to severe renal impairment
Amoxicillin/ clavulanate	Aminopenicillin/β-lactam inhibitor combination	PO: 500/125 mg q8 h or 875/125 mg q12 h for severe infections or respiratory tract infections		**Aerobic gram-positive micro-organisms** *Streptococcus pneumoniae* (including isolates with penicillin MICs ≤2 μg/mL) **Aerobic gram-negative micro-organisms** *Haemophilus influenzae* (including β-lactamase—producing isolates) *Moraxella catarrhalis* (including β-lactamase—producing isolates) The following in vitro data are available, but their clinical significance is unknown. **Aerobic gram-positive micro-organisms** *Staphylococcus aureus* (including β-lactamase—producing isolates) NOTE: *Staphylococci* that are resistant to methicillin/oxacillin must be considered resistant to amoxicillin/clavulanic acid *S. pyogenes*	• Primary mode of elimination: Renal • Reduce dose in moderate to severe renal impairment • 875/125 mg formulation should not be used in patients with CrCl <30 mL/min

TABLE J.1 Aminopenicillins (*Continued*)

Drug	Drug class	Usual dose in adults	Actions, interactions, and others	Spectrum of activity, indications, and active against most strains of	Route, reduce dose, and contraindications
Ampicillin/ sulbactam	Aminopenicillin/β-lactam inhibitor combination	IV: 1.5–3.0 g q6 h Remember: Na^+ content = 4.2 mEq/g Total dose of sulbactam should not exceed 4 g/d	Bactericide Broad-spectrum antibiotic and a β-lactamase inhibitor For mild or moderate infection, 1.5 g IV q6 h Pseudoresistance with *E. coli/Klebsiella* (in vitro)	**Gram-negative bacteria** *Haemophilus influenzae* (β-lactamase and non–β-lactamase producing); *Moraxella* (Branhamella) *catarrhalis* (β-lactamase and non–β-lactamase producing); *Escherichia coli* (β-lactamase and non–β-lactamase producing); *Klebsiella* spp. (all known strains are β-lactamase producing); *Proteus mirabilis* (β-lactamase and non–β-lactamase producing); *Proteus vulgaris; Providencia rettgeri; Providencia stuartii; Morganella morganii; Neisseria gonorrhoeae* (β-lactamase and non–β-lactamase producing). **Anaerobes** *Clostridium* sp.; *Peptococcus* sp.; *Peptostreptococcus* sp.; *Bacteroides* sp., including *B. fragilis*	• Primary mode of elimination: Renal and hepatic • Ampicillin and sulbactam for injection may be administered by either the IV or the IM routes • In patients with impairment of renal function, the elimination kinetics of ampicillin and sulbactam are similarly affected

INR, international normalized ratio; COPD, chronic obstructive pulmonary disease; MIC, minimum inhibitory concentration; CrCl, creatinine clearance.
Data from Cunha BA. *Antibiotic Essentials.* 12th ed. Burlington, MA: Jones & Bartlett Learning, 2013. Available at http://www.drugs.com. Revised January 2015.

TABLE J.2 Antipseudomonal Penicillins

Drug	Drug class	Usual dose in adults	Actions, interactions, and others	Spectrum of activity, indications, and active against most strains of	Route, reduce dose, and contraindications
Piperacillin	Antipseudomonal penicillin	IV: 34 g q48 h	Drug interaction with aminoglycosides in renal failure	Prophylaxis: Piperacillin is indicated for prophylactic use in surgery including intra-abdominal (gastrointestinal and biliary) procedures, vaginal hysterectomy, abdominal hysterectomy, and cesarean section. Piperacillin should only be used to treat or prevent infections that are proven or strongly suspected to be caused by susceptible bacteria. **Indications and use** Intra-abdominal infections including hepatobiliary and surgical infections caused by *E. coli*, *Pseudomonas aeruginosa*, *Enterococci*, *Clostridium* spp., anaerobic cocci, or *Bacteroides* spp., including *B. fragilis*. Urinary tract infections caused by *E. coli*, *Klebsiella* spp., *P. aeruginosa*, *Proteus* spp. including *P. mirabilis*, or *Enterococci* Gynecologic infections including endometritis, pelvic inflammatory disease, pelvic cellulitis caused by *Bacteroides* spp. including *B. fragilis*, anaerobic cocci, *Neisseria gonorrhoeae*, or *Enterococci (E. faecalis)* Septicemia including bacteremia caused by *E. coli*, *Klebsiella* spp., *Enterobacter* spp., *Serratia* spp., *P. mirabilis*, *S. pneumoniae*, *Enterococci*, *P. aeruginosa*, *Bacteroides* spp., or anaerobic cocci. Lower respiratory tract infections caused by *E. coli*, *Klebsiella* spp., *Enterobacter* spp., *P. aeruginosa*, *Serratia* spp., *H. influenzae*, *Bacteroides* spp., or anaerobic cocci. Skin and skin structure infections caused by *E. coli*, *Klebsiella* spp., *Serratia* spp., *Acinetobacter* spp., *Enterobacter* spp., *P. aeruginosa*, *Morganella morganii*, *Providencia rettgeri*, *Proteus vulgaris*, *P. mirabilis*, *Bacteroides* spp. including *B. fragilis*, anaerobic cocci, or *Enterococci* Bone and joint infections caused by *P. aeruginosa*, *Enterococci*, *Bacteroides* spp., or anaerobic cocci	• Primary mode of elimination: Renal • Reduce dose in moderate to severe renal impairment
Piperacillin/ tazobactam	Antipseudomonal penicillin	IV: 4.5 g q8 h Pneumonia nosocomial, use 4.5 g (IV) q6 h	Drug interaction with aminoglycosides and vecuronium	Indicated for nosocomial pneumonia (moderate to severe) caused by piperacillin-resistant, β-lactamase–producing strains of *Staphylococcus aureus* and by piperacillin/tazobactam-susceptible *Acinetobacter baumannii*, *Haemophilus influenzae*, *Klebsiella pneumoniae*, and *Pseudomonas aeruginosa* (nosocomial pneumonia caused by *P. aeruginosa* should be treated in combination with an aminoglycoside) Community-acquired pneumonia (moderate severity only) caused by piperacillin-resistant, β-lactamase–producing strains of *H. influenzae* Appendicitis (complicated by rupture or abscess) and peritonitis caused by piperacillin-resistant, β-lactamase–producing strains of *Escherichia coli* or the following members of the *Bacteroides fragilis* group: *B. fragilis*, *B. ovatus*, *B. thetaiotaomicron*, or *B. vulgatus* Uncomplicated and complicated skin and skin structure infections, including cellulitis, cutaneous abscesses, and ischemic/diabetic foot infections caused by piperacillin-resistant, β-lactamase–producing strains of *S. aureus* Infections caused by piperacillin-susceptible organisms for which piperacillin has been shown to be effective are also amenable to piperacillin tazobactam content. Postpartum endometritis or pelvic inflammatory disease caused by piperacillin-resistant, β-lactamase–producing strains of *E. coli*	• Mode of elimination: 20% in bile, 80% unchanged in urine • Reduce dose in moderate to severe renal impairment

TABLE J.2 Antipseudomonal Penicillins (*Continued*)

Drug	Drug class	Usual dose in adults	Actions, interactions, and others	Spectrum of activity, indications, and active against most strains of	Route, reduce dose, and contraindications
Ticarcillin disodium	Antipseudomonal penicillin	IV: 3 g q6 h	Drug interaction with aminoglycosides in renal failure	Ticarcillin is a semisynthetic antibiotic with a broad spectrum of bactericidal activity against many gram-positive and gram-negative aerobic and anaerobic bacteria. Ticarcillin is, however, susceptible to degradation by β-lactamases, and therefore, the spectrum of activity does not normally include organisms that produce these enzymes.	• Primary mode of elimination: Renal • Reduce dose in moderate to severe renal impairment
Ticarcillin/ clavulanate	Ticarcillin disodium (Antipseudomonal penicillin) + β-lactamase inhibitor clavulanate potassium (the potassium salt of clavulanic acid), for intravenous administration	IV: 3.1 g q4–6 h (3.1 g vial containing 3-g ticarcillin and 100-mg clavulanic acid) Moderate infections 200 mg/kg/d in divided doses every 6 h Severe infections 300 mg/kg/d in divided doses every 4 h For patients weighing <60 kg, the recommended dosage is 200–300 mg/kg/d, based on ticarcillin content, given in divided doses every 4–6 hours.	Drug interaction with aminoglycosides in renal failure	Ticarcillin is a semisynthetic antibiotic with a broad spectrum of bactericidal activity against many gram-positive and gram-negative aerobic and anaerobic bacteria. Ticarcillin is, however, susceptible to degradation by β-lactamases, and therefore, the spectrum of activity does not normally include organisms that produce these enzymes. **Gram-positive aerobes** *Staphylococcus aureus; Staphylococcus epidermidis* **Gram-negative aerobes** *Citrobacter* sp.; *Enterobacter* sp., including *E. cloacae; Escherichia coli; Haemophilus influenzae; Klebsiella* sp. including *K. pneumoniae; Pseudomonas* sp. including *P. aeruginosa; Serratia marcescens* **Anaerobic bacteria** *Bacteroides fragilis* group; *Prevotella* (formerly *Bacteroides*) *melaninogenicus* **Gram-positive aerobes** *Staphylococcus saprophyticus; Streptococcus agalactiae* (group B); *Streptococcus bovis; Streptococcus pneumoniae* (penicillin-susceptible strains only); *Streptococcus pyogenes; Viridans group streptococci* **Gram-negative aerobes** *Acinetobacter baumannii; Acinetobacter calcoaceticus; Acinetobacter haemolyticus; Acinetobacter lwoffi; Moraxella catarrhalis; Morganella morganii; Neisseria gonorrhoeae; Pasteurella multocida; Proteus mirabilis; Proteus penneri; Proteus vulgaris; Providencia rettgeri; Providencia stuartii; Stenotrophomonas maltophilia* **Anaerobic bacteria** *Clostridium* sp. including *C. perfringens, C. difficile, C. sporogenes, C. ramosum,* and *C. bifermentans; Eubacterium* sp.; *Fusobacterium* sp. including *F. nucleatum* and *F. necrophorum; Peptostreptococcus* sp.; *Veillonella* sp.	• Primary mode of elimination: Renal • Reduce dose in moderate to severe renal impairment

Data from Cunha BA. *Antibiotic Essentials.* 12th ed. Burlington, MA: Jones & Bartlett Learning, 2013. Available at http://www.drugs.com. Revised January 2015.

TABLE J.3 Carbapenems

Drug	Drug class	Usual dose in adults	Actions, interactions, and others	Spectrum of activity, indications, and active against most strains of	Route, reduce dose, and contraindications
			Not a substrate/inhibitor of cytochrome P450 enzymes	**Aerobic and facultative gram-positive micro-organisms** *Staphylococcus aureus* (methicillin-susceptible isolates only); *Streptococcus agalactiae; Streptococcus pneumoniae* (penicillin susceptible isolates only); *Streptococcus pyogenes* Note: Methicillin-resistant *Staphylococci* and *Enterococcus* spp. are resistant to ertapenem. **Aerobic and facultative gram-positive micro-organisms**	
Ertapenem	Carbapenem	IV/IM: 1 g q24 h	Probenecid (decrease clearance of ertapenem)	*Escherichia coli; Haemophilus influenzae* (β-lactamase negative isolates only); *Klebsiella pneumoniae; Moraxella catarrhalis; Proteus mirabilis* **Anaerobic micro-organisms** *Bacteroides fragilis; Bacteroides distasonis; Bacteroides ovatus; Bacteroides thetaiotaomicron; Bacteroides uniformis; Clostridium clostridiiforme; Eubacterium lentum; Peptostreptococcus* sp.; *Porphyromonas asaccharolytica; Prevotella bivia*	Primary mode of elimination: Renal Reduce dose in moderate to severe renal impairment.
Imipenem/ cilastatin	Carbapenem	IV: 1,000 mg q6 h (4 g) only in severe life-threatening infections (mainly in some Pseudomonas species) no more than 50 mg/kg/24 h IV: 250 mg q6 h in mild infections IV: 500 mg q8 h (1.5 g) or q6 h (2.0 g) in moderate infections Total dose of sodium 37.5 mg (1.6 mEq) by 500-mg imipenem	The bactericidal activity of imipenem results from the inhibition of cell wall synthesis	**Conditions:** Bacterial septicemia. Lower respiratory tract infections. Urinary tract infections (complicated and uncomplicated). Nosocomial pneumonia, peritonitis, sepsis. Gynecologic infections. Bone and joint infections. Skin and skin structure infections. Endocarditis. Polymicrobic infections. **Gram-positive aerobes** *Enterococcus faecalis* (formerly *S. faecalis*) (NOTE: Imipenem is inactive in vitro against *Enterococcus faecium* (formerly *S. faecium*)); *Staphylococcus aureus* including penicillinase-producing strains; *Staphylococcus epidermidis* including penicillinase-producing strains; *Streptococcus agalactiae* (group B streptococci); *Streptococcus pneumoniae; Streptococcus pyogenes* **Gram-negative aerobes** *Acinetobacter* spp.; *Citrobacter* spp.; *Enterobacter* spp.; *Escherichia coli; Gardnerella vaginalis; Haemophilus influenzae; Haemophilus parainfluenzae* *Klebsiella* spp.; *Morganella morganii; Proteus vulgaris; Providencia rettgeri; Pseudomonas aeruginosa* (NOTE: Imipenem is inactive in vitro against *Xanthomonas (Pseudomonas) maltophilia* and some strains of *P. cepacia*); *Serratia* spp., including *S. marcescens* **Gram-positive anaerobes** *Bifidobacterium* spp.; *Clostridium* spp.; *Eubacterium* spp.; *Peptococcus* spp.; *Peptostreptococcus* spp.; *Propionibacterium* spp. **Gram-negative anaerobes** *Bacteroides* spp., *including B. fragilis; Fusobacterium* spp. **Gram-positive aerobes** *Bacillus* spp.; *Listeria monocytogenes; Nocardia spp.; Staphylococcus saprophyticus;* group C *streptococci;* group G *streptococci; Viridans group streptococci*	Central nervous system adverse experiences such as confusional states, myoclonic activity, and seizures have been reported during treatment with imipenem. Reduce dose in moderate to severe renal impairment. For patients on hemodialysis, imipenem is recommended only when the benefit outweighs the potential risk of seizures.

TABLE J.3 Carbapenems (*Continued*)

Drug	Drug class	Usual dose in adults	Actions, interactions, and others	Spectrum of activity, indications, and active against most strains of	Route, reduce dose, and contraindications
				Gram-negative aerobes *Aeromonas hydrophila; Alcaligenes* spp.; *Capnocytophaga* spp.; *Haemophilus ducreyi; Neisseria gonorrhoeae* including penicillinase-producing strains *Pasteurella* spp.; *Providencia stuartii.* **Gram-negative anaerobes** *Prevotella bivia; Prevotella disiens; Prevotella melaninogenica; Veillonella* spp. In vitro tests show imipenem to act synergistically with aminoglycoside antibiotics against some isolates of *Pseudomonas aeruginosa.*	
Meropenem	Carbapenem	IV: 500 mg q8 h	Pneumonia, urinary tract infection, gynecologic infections, skin and skin structure infections	Meropenem is a broad-spectrum carbapenem antibiotic. It is active against gram-positive and gram-negative bacteria. Meropenem has significant stability to hydrolysis by β-lactamases of most categories, both penicillinases and cephalosporinases produced by gram-positive and gram-negative bacteria. Meropenem should not be used to treat methicillin-resistant *Staphylococcus aureus* (MRSA). In vitro tests show meropenem to act synergistically with aminoglycoside antibiotics against some isolates of *Pseudomonas aeruginosa.*	Reduce dose in moderate to severe renal impairment.
		IV: 1 g q8 h	Nosocomial pneumonia, peritonitis, neutropenic patients, sepsis		
		IV: 2 g q8 h	Meningitis and cystic fibrosis		

Data from Cunha BA. *Antibiotic Essentials.* 12th ed. Burlington, MA: Jones & Bartlett Learning, 2013. Available at http://www.drugs.com. Revised January 2015.

TABLE J.4 Monobactams

Drug	Drug class	Usual dose in adults	Actions, interactions, and others	Spectrum of activity, indications, and active against most strains of	Route, reduce dose, and contraindications
Aztreonam	Monobactam It was originally isolated from *Chromobacterium violaceum.*	IV: 1–2 g q8 h IV: 2 g q6 h	• Synthetic bactericidal antibiotic • Synthetic bactericidal antibiotic • Meningeal dose	Aerobic gram-negative micro-organisms: *Citrobacter* spp., including *C. freundii; Enterobacter* spp., including *E. cloacae; Escherichia coli; Haemophilus influenzae* (including ampicillin-resistant and other penicillinase-producing strains); *Klebsiella, Proteus,* and *Serratia* species.	Reduce dose in moderate to severe renal impairment.

Data from Cunha BA. *Antibiotic Essentials.* 12th ed. Burlington, MA: Jones & Bartlett Learning, 2013. Available at http://www.drugs.com. Revised January 2015.

TABLE J.5 Cephalosporins (Parenteral)

Drug	Drug class	Usual dose in adults	Actions, interactions, and others	Spectrum of activity, indications, and active against most strains of	Route, reduce dose, and contraindications
Cefazolin	First-generation cephalosporin	IV: 1 g q8 h Remember: Na^+ content = 46 mg per g cefazolin	In vitro tests demonstrate that the bactericidal action of cephalosporins results from inhibition of cell wall synthesis **Drug interactions:** None	*Staphylococcus aureus* (including penicillinase-producing strains); *Staphylococcus epidermidis;* Methicillin-resistant staphylococci are uniformly resistant to cefazolin. Group A β-hemolytic *Streptococci* and other strains of streptococci (many strains of enterococci are resistant) *Streptococcus pneumoniae; Escherichia coli; Proteus mirabilis; Klebsiella* sp.; *Enterobacter aerogenes; Haemophilus influenzae*	Reduce dose in moderate to severe renal impairment.
Cefuroxime	Second-generation IV/oral cephalosporin	IV: 1.5 g q8 h PO: 500 mg q12 h Remember: Na^+ content = 2.4 mEq/g	Cefuroxime has in vitro activity against a wide range of gram-positive and gram-negative organisms, and it is highly stable in the presence of β-lactamases of certain gram-negative bacteria. The bactericidal action of cefuroxime results from inhibition of cell wall synthesis.	**Aerobes, gram-positive** *Staphylococcus aureus; Staphylococcus epidermidis; Streptococcus pneumoniae; Streptococcus pyogenes* (and other streptococci) NOTE: Most strains of enterococci (e.g., *Enterococcus faecalis* (formerly *Streptococcus faecalis*)), are resistant to cefuroxime. Methicillin-resistant staphylococci and *Listeria monocytogenes* are resistant to cefuroxime. **Aerobes, gram-negative** *Citrobacter* spp.; *Enterobacter* spp.; *Escherichia coli; Haemophilus influenzae* (including ampicillin-resistant strains); *Haemophilus parainfluenzae; Klebsiella* spp. (including *Klebsiella pneumoniae*); *Moraxella* (*Branhamella*) *catarrhalis* (including ampicillin- and cephalothin-resistant strains); *Morganella morganii* (formerly *Proteus morganii*); *Neisseria gonorrhoeae* (including penicillinase- and non–penicillinase-producing strains); *Neisseria meningitidis; Proteus mirabilis; Providencia rettgeri* (formerly *Proteus rettgeri*); *Salmonella* spp.; *Shigella* spp.	Reduce dose in moderate to severe renal impairment. Do not use for meningitis prophylaxis.
Cefotaxime	Third-generation cephalosporin	IV: 2 g q6 h	Administer by IV injection or infusion or by deep IM injection.	**Lower respiratory tract infections,** including pneumonia, caused by *Streptococcus pneumoniae* (formerly *Diplococcus pneumoniae*), *Streptococcus pyogenes*[a] (group A streptococci) and other streptococci (excluding enterococci, e.g., *Enterococcus faecalis*), *Staphylococcus aureus* (penicillinase and nonpenicillinase producing), *Escherichia coli, Klebsiella* sp., *Haemophilus influenzae* (including ampicillin-resistant strains), *Haemophilus parainfluenzae, Proteus mirabilis, Serratia marcescens,*[a] *Enterobacter* sp., indole-positive *Proteus* and *Pseudomonas* sp. (including *P. aeruginosa*). **Genitourinary infections** Urinary tract infections caused by *Enterococcus* sp., *Staphylococcus epidermidis, Staphylococcus aureus*[a] (penicillinase and nonpenicillinase producing), *Citrobacter* sp., *Enterobacter* sp., *Escherichia coli, Klebsiella* sp., *Proteus mirabilis, Proteus vulgaris,*[a] *Providencia stuartii, Morganella morganii,*[a] *Providencia rettgeri,*[a] *Serratia marcescens*, and *Pseudomonas* sp. (including *P. aeruginosa*). Also, uncomplicated gonorrhea (cervical/urethral and rectal) caused by *Neisseria gonorrhoeae,* including penicillinase-producing strains. **Gynecologic infections,** including pelvic inflammatory disease, endometritis, and pelvic cellulitis caused by *Staphylococcus epidermidis, Streptococcus* sp., *Enterococcus* sp., *Enterobacter* species,[a] *Klebsiella* sp.,[a] *Escherichia coli, Proteus mirabilis, Bacteroides* sp. (including *Bacteroides fragilis*[a]), *Clostridium* sp., and anaerobic cocci (including *Peptostreptococcus* sp. and *Peptococcus* sp.) and *Fusobacterium* sp. (including *F. nucleatum*[a])	Reduce dose in moderate to severe renal impairment.

(Continued)

TABLE J.5 Cephalosporins (Parenteral) (*Continued*)

Drug	Drug class	Usual dose in adults	Actions, interactions, and others	Spectrum of activity, indications, and active against most strains of	Route, reduce dose, and contraindications
				Bacteremia/septicemia caused by *Escherichia coli, Klebsiella* sp., *Serratia marcescens, Staphylococcus aureus,* and *Streptococcus* sp. (including *S. pneumoniae*) **Skin and skin structure infections** caused by *Staphylococcus aureus* (penicillinase and nonpenicillinase producing), *Staphylococcus epidermidis, Streptococcus pyogenes* (group A streptococci) and other streptococci, *Enterococcus* sp., *Acinetobacter* species,[a] *Escherichia coli, Citrobacter* species (including *C. freundii*[a]), *Enterobacter* sp., *Klebsiella* sp., *Proteus mirabilis, Proteus vulgaris,*[a] *Morganella morganii, Providencia rettgeri,*[a] *Pseudomonas* sp., *Serratia marcescens, Bacteroides* sp., and anaerobic cocci (including *Peptostreptococcus*[a] sp. and *Peptococcus* sp.) **Intra-abdominal infections** including peritonitis caused by *Streptococcus* sp.,[a] *Escherichia coli, Klebsiella* sp., *Bacteroides* sp., and anaerobic cocci (including *Peptostreptococcus*[a] sp. and *Peptococcus*[a] sp.) *Proteus mirabilis,*[a] and *Clostridium* species[a] **Bone and/or joint infections** caused by *Staphylococcus aureus* (penicillinase- and non–penicillinase-producing strains), *Streptococcus* sp. (including *S. pyogenes*[a]), *Pseudomonas* sp. (including *P. aeruginosa*[a]), and *Proteus mirabilis*[a] **Central nervous system infections** (e.g., meningitis and ventriculitis), caused by *Neisseria meningitidis, Haemophilus influenzae, Streptococcus pneumoniae, Klebsiella pneumoniae,*[a] and *Escherichia coli*[a]	
Ceftazidime	Third-generation cephalosporin	IV: 2 g q8 h	Ceftazidime is bactericidal in action, exerting its effect by inhibition of enzymes responsible for cell wall synthesis.	**Lower respiratory tract infections, including pneumonia, caused by** *Pseudomonas aeruginosa* and other *Pseudomonas* spp.; *Haemophilus influenzae,* including ampicillin-resistant strains; *Klebsiella* spp.; *Enterobacter* spp.; *Proteus mirabilis; Escherichia coli; Serratia* spp.; *Citrobacter* spp.; *Streptococcus pneumoniae;* and *Staphylococcus aureus* (methicillin-susceptible strains). **Skin and skin structure infections caused by** *Pseudomonas aeruginosa; Klebsiella* spp.; *Escherichia coli; Proteus* spp., including *Proteus mirabilis* and indole-positive *Proteus; Enterobacter* spp.; *Serratia* spp.; *Staphylococcus aureus* (methicillin-susceptible strains); and *Streptococcus pyogenes* (group A β-hemolytic streptococci). **Urinary tract infections, both complicated and uncomplicated, caused by** *Pseudomonas aeruginosa; Enterobacter* spp.; *Proteus* spp., including *Proteus mirabilis* and indole-positive *Proteus; Klebsiella* spp.; *and Escherichia coli* **Bacterial septicemia caused by** *Pseudomonas aeruginosa, Klebsiella* spp., *Haemophilus influenzae, Escherichia coli, Serratia* spp., *Streptococcus pneumoniae,* and *Staphylococcus aureus* (methicillin-susceptible strains) **Bone and joint infections caused by** *Pseudomonas aeruginosa, Klebsiella* spp., *Enterobacter* spp., and *Staphylococcus aureus* (methicillin-susceptible strains)	Reduce dose in moderate to severe renal impairment.

TABLE J.5 Cephalosporins (Parenteral) (*Continued*)

Drug	Drug class	Usual dose in adults	Actions, interactions, and others	Spectrum of activity, indications, and active against most strains of	Route, reduce dose, and contraindications
				Gynecologic infections, including endometritis, pelvic cellulitis, and other infections of the female genital tract caused by *Escherichia coli* **Intra-abdominal infections, including peritonitis caused by** *Escherichia coli, Klebsiella* spp., and *Staphylococcus aureus* (methicillin-susceptible strains) and polymicrobial infections caused by aerobic and anaerobic organisms and *Bacteroides* spp. (many strains of *Bacteroides fragilis* are resistant) **Central nervous system infections, including meningitis, caused by** *Haemophilus influenzae* and *Neisseria meningitidis.* Ceftazidime has also been used successfully in a limited number of cases of meningitis due to *Pseudomonas aeruginosa* and *Streptococcus pneumoniae.*	
Cefepime	Fourth-generation cephalosporin	IV: 1–2 g q12 h For proven serious systemic *P. aeruginosa* infections, febrile neutropenia, or cystic fibrosis: 2 g (IV) q8 h (max dose) Meningeal dose: 2 g (IV) q8 h (max dose)	Local intolerances to IV or IM administration of cefepime were not statistically different from those of ceftazidime administration	*In vitro*, activity against gram-**positive organisms** including *Streptococcus agalactiae, Streptococcus pneumoniae, Streptococcus pyogenes*, and penicillin-susceptible *Staphylococcus aureus* **The broad range of gram-negative organisms sensitive to include** family Enterobacteriaceae, *Klebsiella pneumoniae, Haemophilus influenza, Neisseria meningitidis, Neisseria gonorrhoeae*, and *Pseudomonas aeruginosa*	Reduce dose in moderate to severe renal impairment

[a]Usual dose, assumes normal renal/hepatic function.
Data from Cunha BA. *Antibiotic Essentials.* 12th ed. Burlington, MA: Jones & Bartlett Learning, 2013. Available at http://www.drugs.com. Revised January 2015.

TABLE J.6 Glycopeptides

Drug	Drug class	Usual dose in adults	Actions, interactions, and others	Spectrum of activity, indications, and active against most strains of	Route, reduce dose, and contraindications
Vancomycin	Glycopeptide	The initial dose should be no <15 mg/kg, even in patients with mild to moderate renal insufficiency IV: 1 g q12 h	The bactericidal action of vancomycin results primarily from inhibition of cell wall biosynthesis. In addition, vancomycin alters bacterial cell membrane permeability and RNA synthesis. Concomitant administration of vancomycin and anesthetic agents has been associated with erythema and histaminelike flushing and anaphylactoid reactions.	Indicated for the treatment of serious or severe infections caused by susceptible strains of methicillin-resistant (β-lactam–resistant) staphylococci. It is indicated for penicillin-allergic patients; for patients who cannot receive or who have failed to respond to other drugs, including the penicillins or cephalosporins; and for infections caused by vancomycin-susceptible organisms that are resistant to other antimicrobial drugs. Also indicated for initial therapy when methicillin-resistant staphylococci are suspected, but after susceptibility data are available, therapy should be adjusted accordingly. Effective in the treatment of *Staphylococcal endocarditis*. Its effectiveness has been documented in other infections due to staphylococci, including septicemia, bone infections, lower respiratory tract infections, and skin and skin structure infections. Effective alone or in combination with an aminoglycoside for endocarditis caused by *S. viridans* or *S. bovis*. For endocarditis caused by *enterococci* (e.g., *E. faecalis*), vancomycin hydrochloride has been reported to be effective only in combination with an aminoglycoside. Effective for the treatment of *diphtheroid* endocarditis Has been used successfully in combination with rifampin, an aminoglycoside, or both, in early-onset prosthetic valve endocarditis caused by *S. epidermidis* or *diphtheroids* The parenteral form of vancomycin may be administered orally for the treatment of antibiotic-associated pseudomembranous colitis produced by *C. difficile* and for staphylococcal enterocolitis	Dosage adjustment must be made in patients with impaired renal function. Vancomycin dosage schedules should be adjusted in elderly patients Dosage table for vancomycin (Adapted from Moellering et al.)[b] Creatine Clearance/Dose mL/min—mg/24 h 100—1,545 90—1,390 80—1,235 70—1,080 60—925 50—770 40—620 30—465 20—310 10—155

Data from Cunha BA. *Antibiotic Essentials.* 12th ed. Burlington, MA: Jones & Bartlett Learning, 2013. Available at http://www.drugs.com. Revised January 2015.

TABLE J.7 Chloramphenicol, Clindamycin, Erythromycin Group, Ketolides

Drug	Drug class	Usual dose in adults	Actions, interactions, and others	Spectrum of activity, indications, and active against most strains of	Route, reduce dose, and contraindications
Chloramphenicol	Chloramphenicol sodium succinate	Chloramphenicol sodium succinate is intended for intravenous use only. It has been demonstrated to be ineffective when given intramuscularly. 0.25–1 g IV q6 h (max of 4 g/d) Administration of 50 mg/kg/d in divided doses will produce blood levels of the magnitude to which the majority of susceptible micro-organisms will respond.	The most serious adverse effect of chloramphenicol is bone marrow depression. Serious and fatal blood dyscrasias (aplastic anemia, hypoplastic anemia, thrombocytopenia, and granulocytopenia) are known to occur after the administration of chloramphenicol.	Chloramphenicol must be used only in those serious infections for which less potentially dangerous drugs are ineffective or contraindicated: 1. Acute infections caused by *Salmonella typhi* 2. Serious infections caused by susceptible strains: • *Salmonella* sp. • *H. influenzae*, especially meningeal infections • Rickettsia • Lymphogranuloma-psittacosis group • Various gram-negative bacteria causing bacteremia, meningitis, or other serious gram-negative infections • Other susceptible organisms that have been demonstrated to be resistant to all other appropriate antimicrobial agents 3. Cystic fibrosis regimens	Total urinary excretion of chloramphenicol in these studies ranged from a low of 68% to a high of 99% over a 3-day period. From 8% to 12% of the antibiotic excreted is in the form of free chloramphenicol
Clindamycin	Clindamycin phosphate	IV or IM: 600–900 mg q8 h PO: 0.15–0.45 g q6 h	Pseudomembranous colitis has been reported with nearly all antibacterial agents, including clindamycin, and may range in severity from mild to life threatening.	**Aerobic gram-positive cocci,** including: *Staphylococcus aureus* (penicillinase and non–penicillinase-producing strains); *Staphylococcus epidermidis* (penicillinase- and non–penicillinase-producing strains); *Streptococci* (except *Enterococcus faecalis*); *Pneumococci* **Anaerobic gram-negative bacilli,** including *Bacteroides* sp. (including *Bacteroides fragilis* group and *Bacteroides melaninogenicus* group) and *Fusobacterium* species **Anaerobic gram-positive non-spore-forming bacilli,** including *Propionibacterium, Eubacterium*, and *Actinomyces* sp. **Anaerobic and microaerophilic gram-positive cocci,** including *Peptococcus* sp., *Peptostreptococcus* sp., *Microaerophilic streptococci*, and *Clostridia*	The elimination half-life of clindamycin is increased slightly in patients with markedly reduced renal or hepatic function. Hemodialysis and peritoneal dialysis are not effective in removing clindamycin from the serum.

(Continued)

TABLE J.7 Chloramphenicol, Clindamycin, Erythromycin Group, Ketolides (*Continued*)

Drug	Drug class	Usual dose in adults	Actions, interactions, and others	Spectrum of activity, indications, and active against most strains of	Route, reduce dose, and contraindications
Clarithromycin	Semi-synthetic macrolide antibiotic	PO: 0.5 g q12 h	**Drug Interactions:** Patients who are receiving single doses of clarithromycin and theophylline or carbamazepine may be associated with an increase of serum theophylline and carbamazepine concentrations.	**Aerobic gram-positive micro-organisms** *Staphylococcus aureus; Streptococcus pneumoniae; Streptococcus pyogenes* **Aerobic gram-negative micro-organisms** *Haemophilus influenzae; Haemophilus parainfluenzae; Moraxella catarrhalis* **Other micro-organisms** *Mycoplasma pneumoniae; Chlamydia pneumoniae* **Mycobacteria** *Mycobacterium avium* complex consisting of *Mycobacterium avium* and *Mycobacterium intracellulare* β-Lactamase production should have no effect on clarithromycin activity. Most strains of methicillin-resistant and oxacillin-resistant staphylococci are resistant to clarithromycin. **Helicobacter** *Helicobacter pylori*	Contraindications: Any of the following drugs: cisapride, pimozide, astemizole, terfenadine, and ergotamine or dihydroergotamine. If clarithromycin is coadministered with cisapride, pimozide, astemizole, or terfenadine resulting in cardiac arrhythmias (QT prolongation, ventricular tachycardia, ventricular fibrillation, and torsades de pointes), this is most likely due to inhibition of metabolism of these drugs.
Linezolid	Oxazolidinone	PO or IV: 600 mg q12 h all indications except 400 mg q12 h for uncomplicated skin infections	**Reversible myelosuppression** including anemia, leukopenia, pancytopenia, and thrombocytopenia has been reported in patients. In cases where the outcome is known, when linezolid was discontinued, the affected hematologic parameters have risen toward pretreatment levels. **Lactic acidosis** has been reported with the use of linezolid. Spontaneous reports of **serotonin syndrome** associated with the coadministration of linezolid and serotonergic agents, including antidepressants **Peripheral and optic neuropathy** have been reported in patients treated with Linezolid	**Aerobic and facultative gram-positive micro-organisms** *Enterococcus faecium* (vancomycin-resistant strains only); *Staphylococcus aureus* (including methicillin-resistant strains); *Streptococcus agalactiae; Streptococcus pneumoniae* (including multidrug-resistant isolates); *Streptococcus pyogenes* **Aerobic and facultative gram-positive micro-organisms** *Enterococcus faecalis* (including vancomycin-resistant strains); *Enterococcus faecium* (vancomycin-susceptible strains); *Staphylococcus epidermidis* (including methicillin-resistant strains); *Staphylococcus haemolyticus; Viridans group streptococci* **Aerobic and facultative gram-negative micro-organisms** *Pasteurella multocida*	Linezolid is primarily metabolized by oxidation of the morpholine ring, which results in two inactive ring-opened carboxylic acid metabolites: The aminoethoxyacetic acid metabolite (A) and the hydroxyethyl glycine metabolite (B). Nonrenal clearance accounts for approximately 65% of the total clearance of linezolid. Under steady-state conditions, approximately 30% of the dose appears in the urine as linezolid, 40% as metabolite B, and 10% as metabolite A.

Data from Cunha BA. *Antibiotic Essentials.* 12th ed. Burlington, MA: Jones & Bartlett Learning, 2013. Available at http://www.drugs.com. Revised January 2015.

TABLE J.8 Tetracyclines

Drug	Drug class	Usual dose in adults	Actions, interactions, and others	Spectrum of activity, indications, and active against most strains of	Route, reduce dose, and contraindications
Doxycycline	Derived from oxytetracycline	PO: 0.1 g q12 h IV: 0.1 g q12 h	The tetracyclines are primarily bacteriostatic and are thought to exert their antimicrobial effect by the inhibition of protein synthesis.	Wide range of gram-positive and gram-negative micro-organisms **Aerobic gram-positive micro-organisms** *Bacillus anthracis; Listeria monocytogenes; Staphylococcus aureus* **Aerobic gram-negative micro-organisms** *Bartonella bacilliformis; Brucella* sp.; *Calymmatobacterium granulomatis; Campylobacter fetus; Francisella tularensis; Haemophilus ducreyi; Haemophilus influenzae; Neisseria gonorrhoeae; Vibrio cholerae; Yersinia pestis.* **Anaerobic micro-organisms** *Actinomyces israelii; Fusobacterium fusiforme; Clostridium* sp. **Other micro-organisms** *Borrelia recurrentis; Chlamydia psittaci; Chlamydia trachomatis; Mycoplasma pneumoniae; Rickettsiae; Treponema pallidum; Treponema pertenue*	Can be used in patients with renal failure Hemodialysis does not alter serum half-life.
Oxytetracycline	Tetracycline	PO: 0.25–0.5 g q6 h IV: 0.5–1.0 g q12 h	Primarily bacteriostatic	Wide range of gram-positive and gram-negative micro-organisms, similar to other tetracyclines	Contraindicated in pregnancy, hepatotoxicity in mother, transplacental to fetus. Intravenous dosage over 2.0 g/d may be associated with fatal hepatotoxicity

Data from Cunha BA. *Antibiotic Essentials.* 12th ed. Burlington, MA: Jones & Bartlett Learning, 2013. Available at http://www.drugs.com. Revised January 2015.

TABLE J.9 Fluoroquinolones

Drug	Drug class	Usual dose in adults	Actions, interactions, and others	Spectrum of activity, indications, and active against most strains of	Route, reduce dose, and contraindications
Ciprofloxacin	Fluoroquinolone	IV: 400 mg q8–12 h (infusion over a period of 60 min) PO: 500–750 mg q12 h	Inhibition of bacterial topoisomerase IV and DNA gyrase (both of which are type II topoisomerases), enzymes required for DNA replication, transcription, repair, and recombination **Drug interactions** with theophylline, caffeine, warfarin phenytoin, sulfonylurea glyburide, metronidazole, probenecid, piperacillin sodium, and cyclosporine	**Aerobic gram-positive micro-organisms** *Enterococcus faecalis* (many strains are only moderately susceptible); *Staphylococcus aureus* (methicillin-susceptible strains only); *Staphylococcus epidermidis* (methicillin-susceptible strains only); *Staphylococcus saprophyticus; Staphylococcus pneumoniae* (penicillin-susceptible strains); *Staphylococcus pyogenes* **Aerobic gram-negative micro-organism** *Citrobacter (diversus, freundii); Enterobacter cloacae; Escherichia coli; Haemophilus (influenzae, parainfluenzae); Klebsiella pneumoniae; Moraxella catarrhalis; Morganella morganii; Proteus (mirabilis, vulgaris), Providencia (rettgeri, stuartii); Pseudomonas aeruginosa; Serratia marcescens.* Also ciprofloxacin has been shown to be active against *Bacillus anthracis* both in vitro and by use of serum levels as a surrogate marker.	Contraindications: Concomitant administration with tizanidine Patients with impaired renal function: Creatinine clearance (mL/min): • >30 (see usual dose) • 5–29 (200–400 mg q18–24 h)
Levofloxacin	Fluoroquinolone	250–750 mg qd PO or IV	Inhibition of bacterial topoisomerase IV and DNA gyrase (both of which are type II topoisomerases), enzymes required for DNA replication, transcription, repair, and recombination **Drug interactions** with theophylline, caffeine, warfarin, phenytoin, sulfonylurea glyburide, metronidazole, probenecid, piperacillin sodium, and cyclosporine	**Acute bacterial sinusitis** due to *Streptococcus pneumoniae, Haemophilus influenzae*, or *Moraxella catarrhalis* **Acute bacterial exacerbation of chronic bronchitis** due to *Staphylococcus aureus, Streptococcus pneumoniae, Haemophilus influenzae, Haemophilus parainfluenzae*, or *Moraxella catarrhalis.* **Nosocomial pneumonia** due to methicillin-susceptible *Staphylococcus aureus, Pseudomonas aeruginosa, Serratia marcescens, Escherichia coli, Klebsiella pneumoniae, Haemophilus influenzae*, or *Streptococcus pneumoniae.* Adjunctive therapy should be used as clinically indicated. Where *Pseudomonas aeruginosa* is a documented or presumptive pathogen, combination therapy with an antipseudomonal β-lactam is recommended. **Community-acquired pneumonia** due to *Staphylococcus aureus, Streptococcus pneumoniae* (including multidrug-resistant strains (MDRSP)),[a] *Haemophilus influenzae, Haemophilus parainfluenzae, Klebsiella pneumoniae, Moraxella catarrhalis, Chlamydia pneumoniae, Legionella pneumophila*, or *Mycoplasma pneumoniae*	Clearance of levofloxacin is substantially reduced and plasma elimination half-life is substantially prolonged in patients with impaired renal function (creatinine clearance <50 mL/min), requiring dosage adjustment in such patients to avoid accumulation. Neither hemodialysis nor continuous ambulatory peritoneal dialysis (CAPD) is effective in removal of levofloxacin from the body, indicating that supplemental doses of levofloxacin are not required following hemodialysis or CAPD. Adverse reactions: Opiate screen false positives; photosensitivity; QTc interval prolongation and tendinopathy

TABLE J.9 Fluoroquinolones (*Continued*)

Drug	Drug class	Usual dose in adults	Actions, interactions, and others	Spectrum of activity, indications, and active against most strains of	Route, reduce dose, and contraindications
				Complicated skin and skin structure infections due to methicillin-susceptible *Staphylococcus aureus, Enterococcus faecalis, Streptococcus pyogenes*, or *Porteus mirabilis.* **Uncomplicated skin and skin structure infections** (mild to moderate) including abscesses, cellulites, furuncles, impetigo, pyoderma, and wound infections, due to *Staphylococcus aureus* or *Streptococcus pyogenes* **Chronic bacterial prostatitis** due to *Escherichia coli, Enterococcus faecalis*, or *Staphylococcus epidermidis* **Complicated urinary tract infections** (mild to moderate) due to *Enterococcus faecalis, Enterobacter cloacae, Escherichia coli, Klebsiella pneumoniae, Proteus mirabilis*, or *Pseudomonas aeruginosa* **Acute pyelonephritis** (mild to moderate) caused by *Escherichia coli* **Uncomplicated urinary tract infections** (mild to moderate) due to *Escherichia coli, Klebsiella pneumoniae*, or *Staphylococcus saprophyticus*	
Moxifloxacin	Fluoroquinolone	400 mg PO or IV qd	The bactericidal action of moxifloxacin results from the interference with topoisomerase II and IV	Community-acquired pneumonia (CAP), including CAP caused by multidrug-resistant *Streptococcus pneumoniae*[b] Complicated skin and skin structure infections, including diabetic foot infections Complicated intra-abdominal infections, including polymicrobial infections such as abscesses	Similar to other fluoroquinolones

[a]MDRSP (multidrug-resistant *Streptococcus pneumoniae*) are strains resistant to two or more of the following antibiotics: penicillin (minimum inhibitory concentration (MIC) = 2 μg/mL), second-generation cephalosporins (e.g., cefuroxime, macrolides, tetracyclines, and trimethoprim/sulfamethoxazole).

[b]Multidrug-resistant *S. pneumoniae* includes isolates previously known as PRSP (penicillin-resistant *S. pneumoniae*), and are strains resistant to two or more of the following antibiotics: Penicillin (MIC ≥2 mg/mL), second-generation cephalosporins (e.g., cefuroxime), macrolides, tetracyclines, and trimethoprim/sulfamethoxazole.

Data from Cunha BA. *Antibiotic Essentials.* 12th ed. Burlington, MA: Jones & Bartlett Learning, 2013. Available at http://www.drugs.com. Revised January 2015.

TABLE J.10 Polymyxins

Drug	Drug class	Usual dose in adults	Actions, interactions, and others	Spectrum of activity, indications, and active against most strains of	Route, reduce dose, and contraindications
Polymyxin B	Phospholipid cell membrane-altering antibiotic	0.75–1.25 mg/kg (IV) q12 h (1 mg = 10,000 units)	Colistin is polycationic and has both hydrophilic and lipophilic moieties. These interact with the bacterial cytoplasmic membrane, changing its permeability. This effect is bactericidal. The main toxicities described with intravenous treatment are nephrotoxicity and neurotoxicity. At a dose of 160 mg colistimethate IV q8 h, very little nephrotoxicity is seen.	Colistin is effective against gram-negative bacilli, except *Proteus* and *Burkholderia cepacia*, and is used as a polypeptide antibiotic. Multidrug-resistant *Acinetobacter baumanii*, even in *Acinetobacter* meningitis with intrathecal polymyxin E *Mycobacterium aurum* is susceptible to the antibiotic colistin (polymyxin E), which has an MIC of 5 μg/mL and an apparent bactericidal effect at concentrations >50 μg/mL.	Usage in pregnancy: The safety of this drug in human pregnancy has not been established.
Polymyxin E	Colistin (polymyxin E) is a polymyxin antibiotic produced by certain strains of *Bacillus polymyxa* var. colistinus. Two forms of colistin available commercially: colistin sulfate and colistimethate sodium (colistin methanesulfonate sodium, colistin sulfomethate sodium)	Colomycin 1,000,000 units is 80-mg colistimethate Coly-mycin M 150 mg "colistin base" is 360-mg colistimethate, or 4,500,000 units	Polymyxins bind to the cell membrane and alter its structure making it more permeable. The resulting water uptake leads to cell death. They are cationic, basic proteins that act like detergents. Interactions: Amphotericin B, amikacin, gentamicin, tobramycin, vancomycin. Adverse effects: Renal failure (tubular necrosis). Neurotoxicity associated with very prolonged or high serum levels; neuromuscular blockade with renal failure and or neuromuscular disorders	Bactericidal for gram-negative; little to no effect on gram-positive since cell wall is too thick to permit access to membrane	Colistin sulfate and colistimethate sodium are eliminated from the body by different routes.

Data from Cunha BA. *Antibiotic Essentials.* 12th ed. Burlington, MA: Jones & Bartlett Learning, 2013. Available at http://www.drugs.com. Revised January 2015.

TABLE J.11 Aminoglycosides

Drug	Drug class	Usual dose in adults	Actions, interactions, and others	Spectrum of activity, indications, and active against most strains of	Route, reduce dose, and contraindications
Gentamicin	Aminoglycoside antibiotic, derived from *Micromonospora purpurea*, an actinomycete	Intravenous use only for gentamicin sulfate in 0.9% sodium chloride. Gentamicin sulfate IV: 3 mg/kg/d q8 h In patients with life-threatening infections: 5 mg/kg/d q24 h (preferred over q8 h dosing)	Bactericidal antibiotic that acts by inhibiting normal protein synthesis in susceptible micro-organisms **Drug interactions:** Amphotericin B, cephalothin, cyclosporine, enflurane, methoxyflurane, polymyxin B, radiographic contrast, vancomycin (increase nephrotoxicity), cisplatinum, etc. (see specifications of the product)	*Escherichia coli; Proteus* sp. (indole-positive and indole-negative); *Pseudomonas aeruginosa;* species of *Klebsiella-Enterobacter-Serratia* group; *Citrobacter* sp.; and *Staphylococcus* sp. (including penicillin and methicillin-resistant strains) Gentamicin is also active in vitro against species of *Salmonella* and *Shigella.*	To adjust the doses for patients with renal impairment Adverse reactions: Nephrotoxicity: Adverse renal effects have been reported. They occur more frequently in patients with a history of renal impairment and in patients treated for longer periods or with larger dosages than recommended. Others such as neurotoxicity (serious adverse effects on both vestibular and auditory branches of the eighth nerve), peripheral neuropathy, or encephalopathy, including numbness, skin tingling, muscle twitching, convulsions, and a myasthenia gravis-like syndrome, have been reported (see specifications of the product).
Amikacin	Semi-synthetic aminoglycoside antibiotic, derived from kanamycin	Amikacin sulfate IV: 15 mg/kg or 1 g q24 h (preferred to q12 h dosing)	**Drug interactions:** Amphotericin B, cephalothin, cyclosporine, enflurane, methoxyflurane, polymyxin B, radiographic contrast, vancomycin (increase nephrotoxicity), cisplatinum, etc. (see specifications of the product)	**Gram negative** Amikacin is active in vitro against *Pseudomonas* sp., *Escherichia coli, Proteus* sp. (indole-positive and indole-negative), *Providencia* sp., *Klebsiella-Enterobacter-Serratia* sp., *Acinetobacter* (formerly Mima-Herellea) sp., and *Citrobacter freundii* When strains of the above organisms are found to be resistant to other aminoglycosides, including gentamicin, tobramycin, and kanamycin, many are susceptible to amikacin in vitro. **Gram positive** Amikacin is active in vitro against penicillinase and non–penicillinase-producing *Staphylococcus* sp. including methicillin-resistant strains. However, aminoglycosides in general have a low order of activity against other gram-positive organisms.	See gentamicin sulfate.
Tobramycin	Aminoglycoside antibiotic, derived from the actinomycete *Streptomyces tenebrarius*	Tobramycin sulfate: IV: 5 mg/kg q24 h or 240 mg q24 h (preferred over q8 h dosing). The dosage should be reduced to 3 mg/kg/d as soon as clinically indicated.	Tobramycin acts by inhibiting synthesis of protein in bacterial cells. **Drug interactions:** Amphotericin B, cephalothin, cyclosporine, enflurane, methoxyflurane, polymyxin B, radiographic contrast, vancomycin (increase nephrotoxicity), cisplatinum, etc. (see specifications of the product)	**Gram-positive aerobes** *Staphylococcus aureus* **Gram-negative aerobes** *Citrobacter* sp., *Enterobacter* sp., *Escherichia coli, Klebsiella* sp., *Morganella morganii, Pseudomonas aeruginosa, Proteus mirabilis, Proteus vulgaris, Providencia* sp., *Serratia* sp. Aminoglycosides have a low order of activity against most gram-positive organisms, including *Streptococcus pyogenes, Streptococcus pneumoniae*, and *Enterococci*	See gentamicin sulfate.

Data from Cunha BA. *Antibiotic Essentials.* 12th ed. Burlington, MA: Jones & Bartlett Learning, 2013. Available at http://www.drugs.com. Revised January 2015.

TABLE J.12 Miscellaneous

Drug	Drug class	Usual dose in adults	Actions, interactions, and others	Spectrum of activity, indications, and active against most strains of	Route, reduce dose, and contraindications
Metronidazole	Nitroimidazole antiparasitic/ antibiotic	IV: 1 g q/24 h PO: 500 mg q12 h	Metronidazole is a synthetic antibacterial compound. **Drug interactions:** Warfarin and other oral coumarin anticoagulants, phenytoin or phenobarbital, cimetidine, and disulfiram	**Anaerobic gram-negative bacilli,** including *Bacteroides* sp., including the *Bacteroides fragilis* group (*B. fragilis, B. distasonis, B. ovatus, B. thetaiotaomicron, B. vulgatus*); *Fusobacterium* sp. **Anaerobic gram-positive bacilli,** including *Clostridium* sp. and susceptible strains of *Eubacterium* **Anaerobic gram-positive cocci,** including *Peptococcus* sp.; *Peptostreptococcus* sp.	Primary mode of elimination: Hepatic
Trimethoprim (TMP)/ sulfamethoxazole (SMX) or cotrimoxazole	Synthetic folate antagonist/ sulfonamide	IV or PO: 2.5–5 mg/kg q6 h	Sulfamethoxazole is bacteriostatic and trimethoprim is bactericidal **Drug interactions:** Warfarin (monitoring carefully); phenytoin (folate deficiencies when is used concomitantly); thiazides increased incidence of thrombocytopenia with purpura in elderly patients; cyclosporine (nephrotoxicity reversible); digoxin; indomethacin; pyrimethamine; tricyclic antidepressants; amantadine; methotrexate; and oral hypoglycemic agents	Primary agent in the treatment of *Pneumocystis carinii pneumonia* (PCP), an opportunistic infection in patients with HIV/AIDS, and as secondary prophylaxis of PCP in patients who have already had at least one episode of PCP. Also is indicated for the treatment of chronic bronchitis, enterocolitis caused by strains of *Shigella* (*flexneri and sonnei*), acute otitis media in children, traveler's diarrhea caused by enterotoxigenic *Escherichia coli* and *Shigella* sp., and bacterial urinary tract infections	SMX-TMP is metabolized in the liver. Urinary concentrations of both active drugs are decreased in patients with impaired renal function. Only small amounts of trimethoprim are excreted in feces via biliary elimination. Trimethoprim and active sulfamethoxazole are moderately removed by hemodialysis.

Data from Cunha BA. *Antibiotic Essentials*. 12th ed. Burlington, MA: Jones & Bartlett Learning, 2013. Available at http://www.drugs.com. Revised January 2015.

TABLE J.13 Antifungals

Drug	Drug class	Usual dose in adults	Actions, interactions, and others	Spectrum of activity, indications, and active against most strains of	Route, reduce dose, and contraindications
Amphotericin B	Antifungal Polyene macrolide antibiotic produced by soil bacteria *Streptomyces nodosus*	IV: 0.5–0.8 mg/kg q24 h	Amphotericin B is the gold standard for the treatment of serious and invasive systemic mycosis as well as for kala azar. **Drug interactions:** Avoid concomitant administration of nephrotoxic drugs and bone marrow suppressants.	Amphotericin B has useful activity against candidiasis, cryptococcosis, histoplasmosis, blastomycosis, paracoccidioidomycosis, coccidioidomycosis, aspergillosis, extracutaneous sporotrichosis, zygomycosis (mucormycosis), penicilliosis (*Penicilliosis marneffei*) pseudallescheriasis, hyalohyphomycosis (including infection due to *Acremonium, Fusarium, Penicillium*, etc.) and phaeohyphomycosis (including infection due to *Alternaria, Bipolaris, Cladosporium, Cladophialophora, Curvularia, Exophiala, Exserohilum, Fonsecaea, Phialophora, Wangiella*, etc.). Empirical antifungal therapy is useful to granulocytopenic patients with persistent or recurrent fever.[a]	Primary mode of elimination: Metabolized The most common cause for withdrawal of or failure to continue amphotericin B therapy is its severe renal toxicity in nearly half of all the patients. The second problem, which is a major one, is the nephrotoxicity of amphotericin B.
Liposomal amphotericin B	Antifungal Polyene macrolide antibiotic True liposomal preparation of amphotericin B in which lipid complex of liposomes is constituted of lecithin and cholesterol	IV: 3–6 mg/kg q24 h	Is the most effective and affordable drug for treatment of both systemic mycosis and kala azar. **Drug interactions:** As with conventional amphotericin B, avoid concomitant administration of nephrotoxic drugs and bone marrow suppressants, only and in patients with hypokalemia.	Amphotericin B shows a high order of in vitro activity against many species of fungi *viz. Histoplasma capsulatum, Cryptococcus immitis, Candida* sp., *Blastomyces dermatitidis, Rhodotorula, Cryptococcus neoformans, Sporothrix schenckii, Mucor* sp., *Aspergillus fumigatus, Malassezia furfur, Trichosporon beigelii, Saccharomyces cerevisiae, Scedosporium* sp., *Paecilomyces* sp., *Penicillium* sp., *Fusarium* sp., *Bipolaris* sp., *Exophiala* sp., *Cladophialophora* sp., *Absidia* sp., *Apophysomyces* sp., *Cunninghamella* sp., *Rhizomucor* sp., *Rhizopus* sp., *and Saksenaea* sp. These fungi are inhibited by concentrations of amphotericin B ranging from 0.03 to 1 μg/mL in vitro. Amphotericin B also has activity against species of *Leishmania* and is found to be effective in the treatment of Kala-Azar.	Primary mode of elimination: Metabolized

(*Continued*)

TABLE J.13 Antifungals (*Continued*)

Drug	Drug class	Usual dose in adults	Actions, interactions, and others	Spectrum of activity, indications, and active against most strains of	Route, reduce dose, and contraindications
Fluconazole	Triazole antifungal agent	IV or PO: 400 mg for 1 dose, then 200 mg q24 h For candidemia, IV or PO: 400 mg q24 h after loading dose of 800 mg Meningeal dose, IV or PO: 400 mg q24 h	Fluconazole is a highly selective inhibitor of fungal cytochrome P450 sterol C-14 α-demethylation. **Drug interactions:** Oral contraceptives, cimetidine, antacid, hydrochlorothiazide, rifampin, warfarin, phenytoin, cyclosporine, zidovudine, theophylline, terfenadine, oral hypoglycemic agents, tolbutamide, glipizide, glyburide, rifabutin, tacrolimus, cisapride, midazolam, azithromycin (not significant)	**Prophylaxis:** Fluconazole is indicated to decrease the incidence of candidiasis in patients undergoing bone marrow transplantation who receive cytotoxic chemotherapy and/or radiation therapy. Fluconazole exhibits in vitro activity against *Cryptococcus neoformans* and *Candida* spp. Fungistatic activity has also been demonstrated in normal and immunocompromised animal models for systemic and intracranial fungal infections due to *Cryptococcus neoformans* and for systemic infections due to *Candida albicans.* **Fluconazole is indicated for the treatment of:** 1. Vaginal candidiasis (vaginal yeast infections due to *Candida*) 2. Oropharyngeal and esophageal candidiasis. In open noncomparative studies of relatively small numbers of patients, fluconazole was also effective for the treatment of *Candida* urinary tract infections, peritonitis, and systemic *Candida* infections including candidemia, disseminated candidiasis, and pneumonia. 3. Cryptococcal meningitis	Primary mode of elimination: Renal Contraindications: Terfenadine and cisapride Fluconazole has been associated with rare cases of serious hepatic toxicity.
Voriconazole	Triazole antifungal agent	IV: Loading dose of 6 mg/kg (IV) q12 h × 1 day, then maintenance dose of 4 mg/kg (IV) q12 h. It is possible to switch to weight-based PO maintenance IV dose. PO: If weight ≥40 kg: Loading dose of 400 mg (PO) q12 h × 1 day, then maintenance dose of 200 mg (PO) q12 h. If response is inadequate, increase dose to 300 mg (PO) q12 h. If weight <40 kg: Loading dose of 200 mg (PO) × 1 day, then maintenance dose of 100 mg (PO) q12 h. If response is inadequate, increase dose to 150 mg (PO) q12 h. In patients with chronic and/or non–life-threatening infections, loading dose may be given PO.	**Mode of action** of voriconazole is the inhibition of fungal cytochrome P450–mediated 14 α-lanosterol demethylation, an essential step in fungal ergosterol biosynthesis. **Drug interactions:** Benzodiazepines, vinca alkaloids, carbamazepine, ergo alkaloids, rifampin, rifabutin, sirolimus, long-acting barbiturates (see contraindications), cyclosporine, omeprazole, tacrolimus, phenytoin, warfarin, statins, dihydropyridine, calcium channel blockers (low arterial pressure), sulfonylureas (hypoglycemia). Potential hepatotoxicity risk.	**Invasive aspergillosis** Indicated for the primary treatment of acute invasive aspergillosis (*Aspergillus* spp.). Also with *Fusarium* spp. and *Scedosporium* spp. **Other disease-causing agents** Voriconazole was shown to be effective against both *Scedosporium apiospermum* and *Fusarium* spp. For *Scedosporium apiospermum,* a successful response to Vfend was reported in 15 of 24 subjects (63%). In those with *Fusarium* spp., 9 of 21 (43%) were successfully treated with voriconazole.	Primary mode of elimination: Hepatic Contraindications: Long-acting barbiturates

TABLE J.13 Antifungals (*Continued*)

Drug	Drug class	Usual dose in adults	Actions, interactions, and others	Spectrum of activity, indications, and active against most strains of	Route, reduce dose, and contraindications
Itraconazole	Antifungal agent	IV or PO: 200 mg q24 h 200-mg capsule/solution (PO) q24 h. Begin itraconazole for acute/severe infections with a loading regimen of 200 mg (IV) q12 h × 2 days (4 doses), then give 200 mg (IV or PO) q24 h maintenance dose. Each IV dose should be infused over 60 min.	**Drug interactions:** Coadministration of cisapride, pimozide, quinidine, *dofetilide*, or levacetylmethadol (levomethadyl) with itraconazole.	Itraconazole exhibits in vitro activity against *Blastomyces dermatitidis, Histoplasma capsulatum, Histoplasma duboisii, Aspergillus flavus, Aspergillus fumigatus, Candida albicans*, and *Cryptococcus neoformans*. Itraconazole also exhibits varying in vitro activity against *Sporothrix schenckii, Trichophyton* species, *Candida krusei*, and other *Candida* species. Fungistatic activity has been demonstrated against disseminated fungal infections caused by *Blastomyces dermatitidis, Histoplasma duboisii, Aspergillus fumigatus, Coccidioides immitis, Cryptococcus neoformans, Paracoccidioides brasiliensis, Sporothrix schenckii, Trichophyton rubrum*, and *Trichophyton mentagrophytes*.	Primary mode of elimination: Hepatic; metabolized predominantly by the cytochrome P450 3A4 isoenzyme system (CYP3A4) Patients with impaired hepatic function should be carefully monitored when taking itraconazole. If signs or symptoms of congestive heart failure appear during administration of itraconazole, monitor carefully and consider other treatment alternatives. **Contraindications:** Cisapride, oral midazolam, pimozide, quinidine, dofetilide, triazolam, and levacetylmethadol (levomethadyl) are contraindicated with itraconazole.
Caspofungin	Echinocandin antifungal	70 mg (IV) × 1 dose, then 50 mg (IV) q24 h. In patients >80 kg, give 70 mg/d rather than 50 mg/d. Patients with moderate liver insufficiency should receive a dose of 35 mg/d	Caspofungin is not an inhibitor and is a poor substrate for cytochrome P450 enzymes. **Drug interactions:** Cyclosporine, tacrolimus, carbamazepine, rifampin, dexamethasone, efavirenz, nelfinavir, nevirapine, phenytoin	Caspofungin is active against all species of *Candida*. It is extremely active against all species except *Candida parapsilosis, Candida guilliermondii*, and *Candida lusitaniae*, against which it is moderately active. Caspofungin is also very active against all *Aspergillus* sp. It does not kill *Aspergillus* completely in test tubes. There is a very limited amount of activity against *Coccidioides immitis, Blastomyces dermatitidis, Scedosporium* sp., *Paecilomyces variotii*, and *Histoplasma capsulata* but it is likely that the activity is not sufficient for clinical use.	Primary mode of elimination: Hepatic
Anidulafungin	Semisynthetic product of echinocandin B	200 mg (IV) x 1 dose, then 100 mg IV q24 h. No dosage adjustments are required for renal or hepatic insufficiency Administer IV infusions at a rate ≤1.1 mg/min (1.4 mL/min) Treatment should be given for ≥14 days and then for ≥7 days following resolution of symptoms.	Anidulafungin is not an inhibitor and is a poor substrate for cytochrome P450 enzymes. **Drug interactions:** Cyclosporine	Anidulafungin is recommended in the treatment of candidemia in *nonneutropenic* patients or for empiric treatment of suspected invasive candidiasis (intra-abdominal abscess and peritonitis). Anidulafungin b is active against all species of *Candida*. It is extremely active and usually rapidly fungicidal against all species except *Candida parapsilosis, Candida guilliermondii* and *Candida famata* against which it is moderately active. Anidulafungin is also active against all *Aspergillus* spp., but is not fungicidal. Anidulafungin has limited activity against *Coccidioides* spp., *Blastomyces dermatitidis, Scedosporium* spp., *Paecilomyces varioti* and *Histoplasma* spp., which is not sufficient for clinical use	Hepatic metabolism of anidulafungin has not been observed. Anidulafungin is not a clinically relevant substrate, inducer, or inhibitor of cytochrome P450 isoenzymes. The commonest **side effects** (all <1 in 40 patients) were flushing or a hot flush, pruritus, rash and/or urticaria. Raised liver enzymes occur in about 1 in 40 patients. Other side effects appear to be rare. **Contraindications:** Hypersensitivity to the active substance. Hypersensitivity to other medicinal products of the echinocandin class

[a]Walsh TJ, Lee J, Lecciones J. Empiric therapy with amphotericin B in febrile granulocytopenic patients. *Rev Infect Dis.* 1991;13:496–503.
Data from Cunha BA. *Antibiotic Essentials.* 12th ed. Burlington, MA: Jones & Bartlett Learning, 2013. Available at http://www.drugs.com. Revised January 2015.

Index

Note: Page number followed by "f" and "t" indicates figure and table only. Page number from e-only chapter has alpha "e" before page number.

E

F

M

T